RED BOOK®

PHARMACY'S FUNDAMENTAL REFERENCE™

2010 Edition

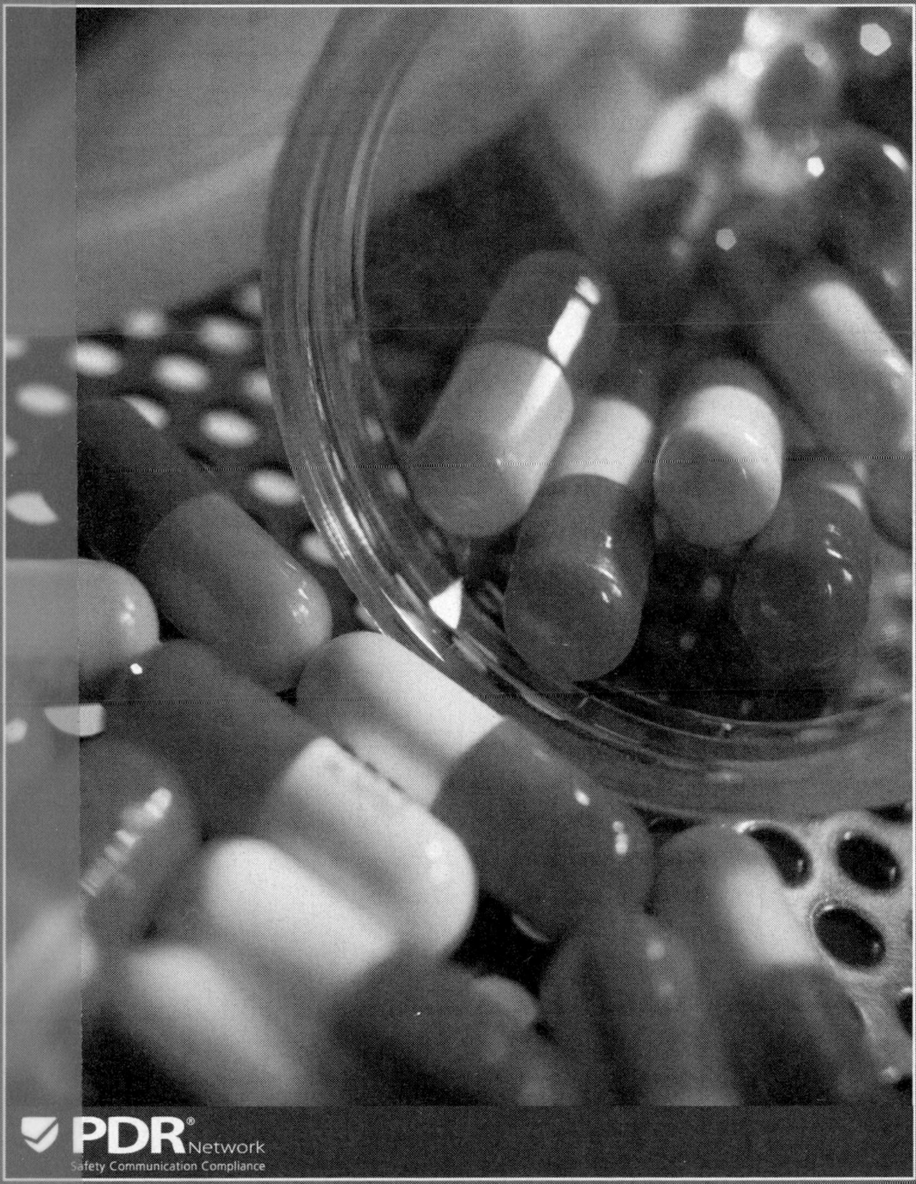

Prices and product information, plus so much more:

- Emergency Contacts, Poison Antidotes
- Clinical Reference Guide
- Practice Management Resources
- Pharmacy and Healthcare Directories
- Reimbursement Information
- Manufacturer/Wholesaler Directories
- Full-Color Drug Identification Section
- Guide to Medicinal Herbs

PDR® Network
Safety Communication Compliance

2010 RED BOOK®

PHARMACY'S FUNDAMENTAL REFERENCE™

114th YEAR OF PUBLICATION

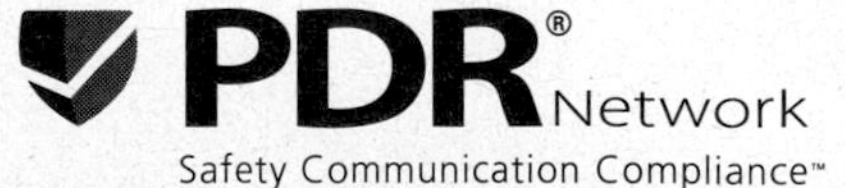

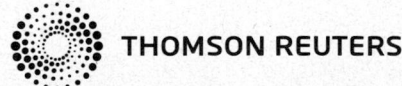

ISBN: 978-1-56363-751-3

FOREWORD

Dear Reader:

We are pleased to present the 2010 print edition of the *Red Book*® online database, published by PDR Network, LLC and licensed from Thomson Reuters (Healthcare) Inc. ("Thomson Reuters"). For more than a century, this unique reference has provided pharmacists, buyers, and other pharmaceutical industry decision makers with important clinical and practical information about today's drug products. It's a resource that you'll turn to again and again.

Red Book continues to be a fast and economical way to find key information. Inside this latest edition you'll find updated listings of more than 160,000 prescription and over-the-counter drugs, medical devices, and accessories. Of course, *Red Book* is more than just a pricing guide. In addition to Average Wholesale Price and Direct Price, each drug listing also contains a wealth of information: supplier name, trademarked and generic names, National Drug Code (NDC) numbers, route of administration, strength and quantity, and Orange Book Code (OBC), if applicable.

AWP POLICY
Please refer to this AWP Policy as you review the pricing information contained in the publication.

The Average Wholesale Price (AWP) as published by Thomson Reuters (Healthcare) Inc. is in most cases the manufacturer's[1] suggested AWP and does not necessarily reflect the *actual* AWP charged by a wholesaler. Thomson Reuters bases the AWP data it publishes on the following:

- AWP is reported by the manufacturer, **or**
- AWP is calculated based on a markup specified by the manufacturer. This markup is typically based on the Wholesale Acquisition Cost (WAC) or Direct Price (DP), as provided by the manufacturer, but may be based on other pricing data provided by the manufacturer.

When the manufacturer does not provide an AWP or markup formula from which AWP can be calculated, the AWP will be calculated by applying a standard 20% markup over the manufacturer-supplied WAC. If a WAC is not provided, the standard markup will be applied to the DP.

Please note that Thomson Reuters does not perform any independent analysis to determine or calculate the *actual* AWP paid by providers[2] to wholesalers. Thomson Reuters also does not independently investigate the *actual* WAC paid by wholesalers to manufacturers or DP paid by providers to manufacturers. Thomson Reuters relies on the manufacturers to report the values for these categories as described above.

Thomson Reuters provides a list of the manufacturers that do not provide the AWP or a markup formula. The list of these manufacturers and products is available at *http://www.micromedex.com/products/redbook/awp/*. Additionally, an ASCII text file with this same information is available to download. For more information on this file and instructions on downloading, please contact *Red Book* Technical Support at *http://www.micromedex.com/support/request/*.

If you'd like to order additional copies of *Red Book*, please call Customer Service at 800-678-5689. We hope you find this edition helpful and welcome your comments and suggestions.

Christine Côté, MD
Chief Medical Officer
PDR Network, LLC

[1] The term "manufacturer" includes manufacturers, repackagers, and private labelers.
[2] The term "provider" includes retailers, hospitals, physicians, and others buying either from the wholesaler or directly from the manufacturer for distribution to a patient.

CONTENTS

2010 RED BOOK

PDR Network, LLC
Red Book
Five Paragon Drive
Montvale, NJ 07645-1725

Main Number: (201) 358-7200
Customer Service: (800) 222-3045
Red Book Electronic Sales:
Phone: +1 (877) 843-6796
Speak the product name, then select option 7
Advertising Sales: (201) 358-7290

To order additional copies of the ***2010 Red Book***, call (800) 678-5689 or fax (802) 864-7626.

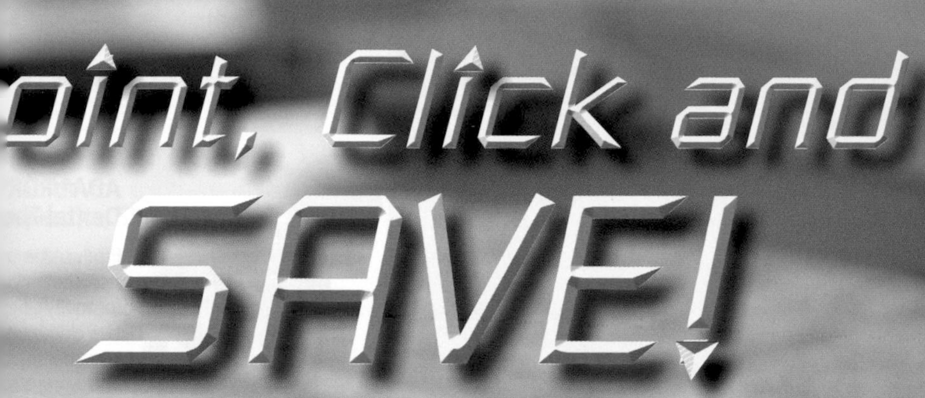

oint, Click and
SAVE!

U.S. Department of Health and Human Services

Form Approved: OMB No. 0910-0291, Expires: 12/31/2011
See OMB statement on reverse.

MEDWATCH

The FDA Safety Information and Adverse Event Reporting Program

For VOLUNTARY reporting of adverse events, product problems and product use errors

Page 1 of____

FDA USE ONLY

Triage unit sequence #

A. PATIENT INFORMATION

1. **Patient Identifier** — In confidence
2. **Age at Time of Event or Date of Birth:**
3. **Sex** — ☐ Female ☐ Male
4. **Weight** — ____ lb or ____ kg

B. ADVERSE EVENT, PRODUCT PROBLEM OR ERROR

Check all that apply:

1. ☐ **Adverse Event** ☐ **Product Problem** *(e.g., defects/malfunctions)*
☐ **Product Use Error** ☐ **Problem with Different Manufacturer of Same Medicine**

2. **Outcomes Attributed to Adverse Event** *(Check all that apply)*
☐ Death: ________ *(mm/dd/yyyy)*
☐ Disability or Permanent Damage
☐ Life-threatening
☐ Congenital Anomaly/Birth Defect
☐ Hospitalization - initial or prolonged
☐ Other Serious (Important Medical Events)
☐ Required Intervention to Prevent Permanent Impairment/Damage (Devices)

3. **Date of Event** *(mm/dd/yyyy)*
4. **Date of this Report** *(mm/dd/yyyy)*
5. **Describe Event, Problem or Product Use Error**
6. **Relevant Tests/Laboratory Data, Including Dates**
7. **Other Relevant History, Including Preexisting Medical Conditions** *(e.g., allergies, race, pregnancy, smoking and alcohol use, liver/kidney problems, etc.)*

C. PRODUCT AVAILABILITY

Product Available for Evaluation? *(Do not send product to FDA)*

☐ Yes ☐ No ☐ Returned to Manufacturer on: ________ *(mm/dd/yyyy)*

D. SUSPECT PRODUCT(S)

1. **Name, Strength, Manufacturer** *(from product label)*
#1 Name:
Strength:
Manufacturer:
#2 Name:
Strength:
Manufacturer:

2. **Dose or Amount** | **Frequency** | **Route**
#1
#2

3. **Dates of Use** *(If unknown, give duration) from/to (or best estimate)*
#1
#2

4. **Diagnosis or Reason for Use** *(Indication)*
#1
#2

5. **Event Abated After Use Stopped or Dose Reduced?**
#1 ☐ Yes ☐ No ☐ Doesn't Apply
#2 ☐ Yes ☐ No ☐ Doesn't Apply

6. **Lot #**
#1
#2

7. **Expiration Date**
#1
#2

8. **Event Reappeared After Reintroduction?**
#1 ☐ Yes ☐ No ☐ Doesn't Apply
#2 ☐ Yes ☐ No ☐ Doesn't Apply

9. **NDC # or Unique ID**

E. SUSPECT MEDICAL DEVICE

1. **Brand Name**
2. **Common Device Name**
3. **Manufacturer Name, City and State**
4. **Model #** | **Lot #**
Catalog # | **Expiration Date** *(mm/dd/yyyy)*
Serial # | **Other #**
5. **Operator of Device**
☐ Health Professional
☐ Lay User/Patient
☐ Other:
6. **If Implanted, Give Date** *(mm/dd/yyyy)*
7. **If Explanted, Give Date** *(mm/dd/yyyy)*
8. **Is this a Single-use Device that was Reprocessed and Reused on a Patient?**
☐ Yes ☐ No
9. **If Yes to Item No. 8, Enter Name and Address of Reprocessor**

F. OTHER (CONCOMITANT) MEDICAL PRODUCTS

Product names and therapy dates *(exclude treatment of event)*

G. REPORTER *(See confidentiality section on back)*

1. **Name and Address**
Name:
Address:
City: State: ZIP:
Phone # **E-mail**
2. **Health Professional?** ☐ Yes ☐ No
3. **Occupation**
4. **Also Reported to:**
☐ Manufacturer
☐ User Facility
☐ Distributor/Importer
5. **If you do NOT want your identity disclosed to the manufacturer, place an "X" in this box:** ☐

PLEASE TYPE OR USE BLACK INK

FORM FDA 3500 (1/09) Submission of a report does not constitute an admission that medical personnel or the product caused or contributed to the event.

ADVICE ABOUT VOLUNTARY REPORTING

Detailed instructions available at: http://www.fda.gov/medwatch/report/consumer/instruct.htm

Report adverse events, product problems or product use errors with:

- Medications *(drugs or biologics)*
- Medical devices *(including in-vitro diagnostics)*
- Combination products *(medication & medical devices)*
- Human cells, tissues, and cellular and tissue-based products
- Special nutritional products *(dietary supplements, medical foods, infant formulas)*
- Cosmetics

Report product problems - quality, performance or safety concerns such as:

- Suspected counterfeit product
- Suspected contamination
- Questionable stability
- Defective components
- Poor packaging or labeling
- Therapeutic failures (product didn't work)

Report SERIOUS adverse events. An event is serious when the patient outcome is:

- Death
- Life-threatening
- Hospitalization - initial or prolonged
- Disability or permanent damage
- Congenital anomaly/birth defect
- Required intervention to prevent permanent impairment or damage (devices)
- Other serious (important medical events)

Report even if:

- You're not certain the product caused the event
- You don't have all the details

How to report:

- Just fill in the sections that apply to your report
- Use section D for all products except medical devices
- Attach additional pages if needed
- Use a separate form for each patient
- Report either to FDA or the manufacturer *(or both)*

Other methods of reporting:

- 1-800-FDA-0178 - To FAX report
- 1-800-FDA-1088 - To report by phone
- www.fda.gov/medwatch/report.htm - To report online

If your report involves a serious adverse event with a device and it occurred in a facility outside a doctor's office, that facility may be legally required to report to FDA and/or the manufacturer. Please notify the person in that facility who would handle such reporting.

If your report involves a serious adverse event with a vaccine, call 1-800-822-7967 to report.

Confidentiality: The patient's identity is held in strict confidence by FDA and protected to the fullest extent of the law. FDA will not disclose the reporter's identity in response to a request from the public, pursuant to the Freedom of Information Act. The reporter's identity, including the identity of a self-reporter, may be shared with the manufacturer unless requested otherwise.

The public reporting burden for this collection of information has been estimated to average 36 minutes per response, including the time for reviewing instructions, searching existing data sources, gathering and maintaining the data needed, and completing and reviewing the collection of information. Send comments regarding this burden estimate or any other aspect of this collection of information, including suggestions for reducing this burden to:

Department of Health and Human Services
Food and Drug Administration
Office of Chief Information Officer (HFA-710)
5600 Fishers Lane
Rockville, MD 20857

Please DO NOT RETURN this form to this address.

OMB statement:
"An agency may not conduct or sponsor, and a person is not required to respond to, a collection of information unless it displays a currently valid OMB control number."

U.S. DEPARTMENT OF HEALTH AND HUMAN SERVICES
Food and Drug Administration

MEDI-CATION ERRORS REPORTING PROGRAM

ISMP Medication Errors Reporting Program

ISMP is a federally certified Patient Safety Organization and an FDA MedWatch partner

Reporters should not provide any individually identifiable health information, including names of practitioners, names of patients, names of healthcare facilities, or dates of birth (age is acceptable).

Date and time of event:

Please describe the error. Include description/sequence of events, type of staff involved, and work environment (e.g., code situation, change of shift, no 24-hr. pharmacy, floor stock). If more space is needed, please attach a separate page.

Did the error reach the patient? ☐ Yes ☐ No

Was the incorrect medication, dose, or dosage form administered to or taken by the patient? ☐ Yes ☐ No

Circle the appropriate Error Outcome Category (select one—see back for details): A B C D E F G H I

Describe the direct result of the error on the patient (e.g., death, type of harm, additional patient monitoring).

Indicate the possible error cause(s) and contributing factor(s) (e.g., abbreviation, similar names, distractions).

Indicate the location of the error (e.g., hospital, community pharmacy, clinic, nursing home, patient's home).

What type of staff or healthcare practitioner made the initial error?

Indicate if other practitioner(s) were also involved in the error (type of staff perpetuating error).

What type of staff or healthcare practitioner discovered the error or recognized the potential for error?

How was the error (or potential for error) discovered/intercepted?

If available, provide patient age, gender, diagnosis. Do not provide any patient identifiers.

Please complete the following for the product(s) involved. (If more space is needed for additional products, please attach a separate page.)

	Product #1	Product #2
Brand/Product Name (If Applicable)		
Generic Name		
Manufacturer		
Labeler		
Dosage Form		
Strength/Concentration		
Type and Size of Container		

Reports are most useful when relevant materials such as product label, copy of prescription/order, etc., can be reviewed.

Can these materials be provided? ☐ Yes ☐ No Please specify:

Suggest any recommendations to prevent recurrence of this error, or describe policies or procedures you instituted or plan to institute to prevent future similar errors.

Name and Title/Profession — Telephone Number ( ) — Fax Number ( )

Facility/Address and Zip — E-mail

Address/Zip (where correspondence should be sent)

Please check the box that applies: ☐ Consumer ☐ Licensed Healthcare Practitioner ☐ Student/Technician

Copies of reports, without any identifying information, will be sent to third parties such as the manufacturer/labeler and to the Food and Drug Administration (FDA). You have the option of including your name on these copies.

ISMP may release my identity to these third parties as follows (check boxes that apply):

☐ FDA ☐ The manufacturer and/or labeler as listed above ☐ Anonymous to all third parties

Signature — Date

Return to: **ISMP**, 200 Lakeside Dr., Ste. 200, Horsham, PA 19044 Fax: 215-914-1492
Submit via the web at: www.ismp.org/merp Phone: 800-Fail-Saf(e) (800-324-5723)

Date Received by ISMP	File Access Number

NCC MERP Index for Categorizing Medication Errors

Category A: Circumstances or events that have the capacity to cause error

Category B: An error occurred but the error did not reach the patient (An "error of omission" *does* reach the patient)

Category C: An error occurred that reached the patient but did not cause patient harm

Category D: An error occurred that reached the patient and required monitoring to confirm that it resulted in no harm to the patient and/or required intervention to preclude harm

Category E: An error occurred that may have contributed to or resulted in temporary harm to the patient and required intervention

Category F: An error occurred that may have contributed to or resulted in temporary harm to the patient and required initial or prolonged hospitalization

Category G: An error occurred that may have contributed to or resulted in permanent patient harm

Category H: An error occurred that required intervention necessary to sustain life

Category I: An error occurred that may have contributed to or resulted in the patient's death

No Error | Error, No Harm | Error, Harm | Error, Death

NCC MERP Index for Categorizing Medication Errors Algorithm

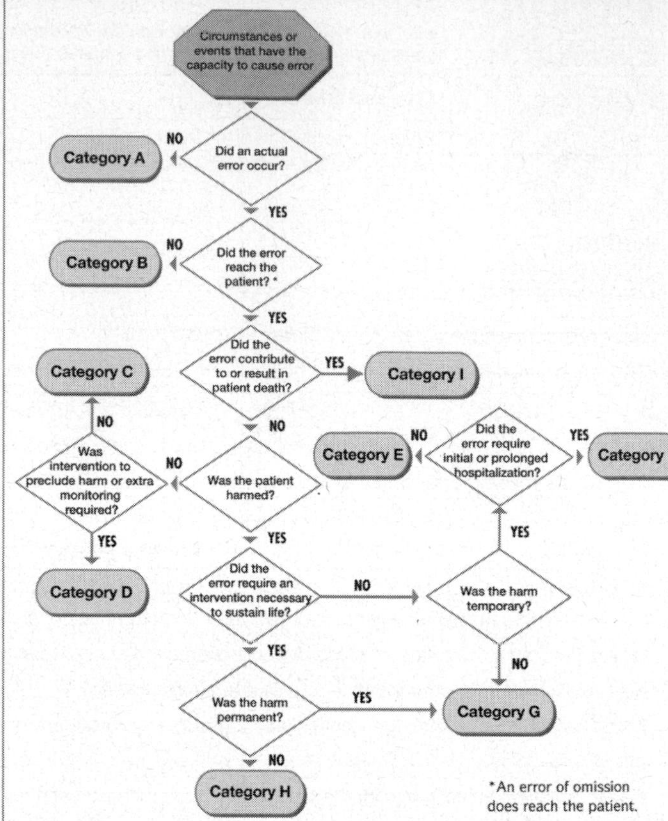

Full-size copies are available: INDEX—www.nccmerp.org/010612_color_index.pdf; ALGORITHM—www.nccmerp.org/010612_color_algo.pdf

Definitions from ISMP and NCC MERP

Hazardous Condition (ISMP)
A condition or situation that could lead to or cause an error (i.e., Category A).

Near Miss (ISMP)
A medication error that was detected and corrected before it reached the patient (i.e., Category B).

Harm (NCC MERP)
Impairment of the physical, emotional, or psychological function or structure of the body and/or pain resulting therefrom.

Monitoring (NCC MERP)
To observe or record relevant physiological or psychological signs.

Intervention (NCC MERP)
May include change in therapy or active medical/surgical treatment.

Intervention Necessary to Sustain Life (NCC MERP)
Includes cardiovascular and respiratory support (e.g., CPR, defibrillation, intubation, etc.).

Submit a Report to the ISMP Medication Errors Reporting Program (MERP)

Mail:
ISMP
200 Lakeside Drive
Suite 200
Horsham, PA 19044

Internet:
www.ismp.org/merp

Email:
merp@ismp.org

Phone:
800-Fail-Saf(e) (800-324-5723)

Fax:
215-914-1492

About ISMP

The Institute for Safe Medication Practices (ISMP) is the nation's only nonprofit, charitable organization devoted entirely to medication error prevention. ISMP provides independent recommendations for the safe use of medications to healthcare professionals, government agencies, accrediting organizations, the pharmaceutical industry and consumers. Its effective error prevention strategies, recognized and respected worldwide, are based on information gained through analysis of reports to a voluntary national program as well as onsite visits to individual healthcare organizations. ISMP is a federally certified patient safety organization (PSO), providing legal protection and confidentiality for patient safety data and error reports it receives. For more information or to make a donation to support ISMP's lifesaving work, visit www.ismp.org.

A federally certified Patient Safety Organization

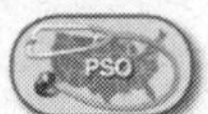

WEBSITE: www.vaers.hhs.gov E-MAIL: info@vaers.org FAX: 1-877-721-0366

VAERS

VACCINE ADVERSE EVENT REPORTING SYSTEM

24 Hour Toll-Free Information 1-800-822-7967
P.O. Box 1100, Rockville, MD 20849-1100
PATIENT IDENTITY KEPT CONFIDENTIAL

For CDC/FDA Use Only
VAERS Number ______
Date Received ______

Patient Name: ______
Last First M.I.
Address ______
City State Zip
Telephone no. (____) ______

Vaccine administered by (Name): ______
Responsible Physician ______
Facility Name/Address ______
City State Zip
Telephone no. (____) ______

Form completed by (Name): ______
Relation to Patient ☐ Vaccine Provider ☐ Patient/Parent ☐ Manufacturer ☐ Other
Address *(if different from patient or provider)* ______
City State Zip
Telephone no. (____) ______

1. State
2. County where administered
3. Date of birth __/__/__ mm dd yy
4. Patient age
5. Sex ☐ M ☐ F
6. Date form completed __/__/__ mm dd yy

7. Describe adverse events(s) (symptoms, signs, time course) and treatment, if any

8. Check all appropriate:
☐ Patient died (date __/__/__ mm dd yy)
☐ Life threatening illness
☐ Required emergency room/doctor visit
☐ Required hospitalization (______days)
☐ Resulted in prolongation of hospitalization
☐ Resulted in permanent disability
☐ None of the above

9. Patient recovered ☐ YES ☐ NO ☐ UNKNOWN

10. Date of vaccination __/__/__ mm dd yy Time ______ AM PM

11. Adverse event onset __/__/__ mm dd yy Time ______ AM PM

12. Relevant diagnostic tests/laboratory data

13. Enter all vaccines given on date listed in no. 10

	Vaccine (type)	Manufacturer	Lot number	Route/Site	No. Previous Doses
a.					
b.					
c.					
d.					

14. Any other vaccinations within 4 weeks prior to the date listed in no. 10

	Vaccine (type)	Manufacturer	Lot number	Route/Site	No. Previous doses	Date given
a.						
b.						

15. Vaccinated at:
☐ Private doctor's office/hospital
☐ Public health clinic/hospital
☐ Military clinic/hospital
☐ Other/unknown

16. Vaccine purchased with:
☐ Private funds
☐ Public funds
☐ Military funds
☐ Other/unknown

17. Other medications

18. Illness at time of vaccination (specify)

19. Pre-existing physician-diagnosed allergies, birth defects, medical conditions (specify)

20. Have you reported this adverse event previously? ☐ No ☐ To health department ☐ To doctor ☐ To manufacturer

Only for children 5 and under

22. Birth weight ______ lb. ______ oz.

23. No. of brothers and sisters

21. Adverse event following prior vaccination (check all applicable, specify)

	Adverse Event	Onset Age	Type Vaccine	Dose no. in series
☐ In patient				
☐ In brother or sister				

Only for reports submitted by manufacturer/immunization project

24. Mfr./imm. proj. report no.

25. Date received by mfr./imm.proj.

26. 15 day report? ☐ Yes ☐ No

27. Report type ☐ Initial ☐ Follow-Up

Health care providers and manufacturers are required by law (42 USC 300aa-25) to report reactions to vaccines listed in the Table of Reportable Events Following Immunization. Reports for reactions to other vaccines are voluntary except when required as a condition of immunization grant awards.

Form VAERS-1(FDA)

TABLE OF REPORTABLE EVENTS FOLLOWING VACCINATION

Vaccine/Toxoid	Event	Interval from Vaccination
Tetanus in any combination; DTaP, DTP, DTP-HiB, DT, Td, TT, Tdap	A. Anaphylaxis or anaphylactic shock B. Brachial neuritis C. Any acute complications or sequela (including death) of above events D. Events described in manufacturer's package insert as contraindications to additional doses of vaccine	7 days 28 days Not applicable See package insert
Pertussis in any combination; DTaP, DTP, DTP-HiB, P, Tdap	A. Anaphylaxis or anaphylactic shock B. Encephalopathy (or encephalitis) C. Any acute complications or sequela (including death) of above events D. Events described in manufacturer's package insert as contraindications to additional doses of vaccine	7 days 7 days Not applicable See package insert
Measles, mumps and rubella in any combination; MMR, MR, M, MMRV, R	A. Anaphylaxis or anaphylactic shock B. Encephalopathy (or encephalitis) C. Any acute complications or sequela (including death) of above events D. Events described in manufacturer's package insert as contraindications to additional doses of vaccine	7 days 15 days Not applicable See package insert
Rubella in any combination; MMR, MMRV, MR, R	A. Chronic arthritis B. Any acute complications or sequela (including death) of above event C. Events described in manufacturer's package insert as contraindications to additional doses of vaccine	42 days Not applicable See package insert
Measles in any combination; MMR, MMRV, MR, M	A. Thrombocytopenic purpura B. Vaccine-strain measles viral infection in an immunodeficient recipient C. Any acute complications or sequela (including death) of above events D. Events described in manufacturer's package insert as contraindications to additional doses of vaccine	7-30 days 6 months Not applicable See package insert
Oral Polio (OPV)	A. Paralytic polio – in a non-immunodeficient recipient – in an immunodeficient recipient – in a vaccine associated community case B. Vaccine-strain polio viral infection – in a non-immunodeficient recipient – in an immunodeficient recipient – in a vaccine associated community case C. Any sequela (including death) of above events D. Events described in manufacturer's package insert as contraindications to additional doses of vaccine	 30 days 6 months Not applicable 30 days 6 months Not applicable Not applicable See package insert
Inactivated Polio (IPV)	A. Anaphylaxis or anaphylactic shock B. Any sequela (including death) of the above event C. Events described in manufacturer's package insert as contraindications to additional doses of vaccine	7 days Not applicable See package insert
Hepatitis B	A. Anaphylaxis or anaphylactic shock B. Any acute complications or sequela (including death) of the above event C. Events described in manufacturer's package insert as contraindications to additional doses of vaccine	7 days Not applicable See package insert
Hemophilus influenzae type b (conjugate)	A. Events described in manufacturer's package insert as contraindications to additional doses of vaccine	See package insert
Varicella	A. Events described in manufacturer's package insert as contraindications to additional doses of vaccine	See package insert
Rotavirus	A. Intussusception B. Any acute complications or sequela (including death) of the above event C. Events described in manufacturer's package insert as contraindications to additional doses of vaccine	30 days Not applicable See package insert
Pneumococcal conjugate	A. Events described in manufacturer's package insert as contraindications to additional doses of vaccine	See package insert
Hepatitis A	A. Events described in manufacturer's package insert as contraindications to additional doses of vaccine	See package insert
Influenza	A. Events described in manufacturer's package insert as contraindications to additional doses of vaccine	See package insert

Effective date: July 01, 2005. The Reportable Events Table (RET) reflects what is reportable by law (42 USC 300aa-25) to the Vaccine Adverse Event Reporting System (VAERS) including conditions found in the manufacturers package insert. In addition, individuals are encouraged to report **any** clinically significant or unexpected events (even if you are not certain the vaccine caused the event) for **any** vaccine, whether or not it is listed on the RET. Manufacturers are also required by regulation (21CFR 600.80) to report to the VAERS program all adverse events made known to them for any vaccine.

POISON ANTIDOTE CHART

WARNING: While every effort has been made to ensure the accuracy of this chart, it is not intended to serve as the sole source of information on antidotes. Guidelines may need to be adjusted based on factors such as anticipated usage in the hospital's local area, the nearest alternate sources of antidotes, and distance to tertiary care institutions. Contact your nearest regional poison control center (1-800-222-1222) for treatment information regarding any exposure, including indications for use of antidote therapy. Directions in this chart assume that all basic life support and decontamination measures have been initiated as needed.

Antidote	Poison/Drug/Toxin	Suggested Minimum Stock Quantity	Comments
N-Acetylcysteine (Acetadote®, Mucomyst®)	Acetaminophen Carbon tetrachloride Other hepatotoxins	Oral product: 600 mL in 10 mL or 30 mL vials of 20% solution IV product: One carton of four 30 mL vials of 20% solution	Acetaminophen is the most common drug involved in intentional and unintentional poisonings. 600 mL (120 g) of the oral product provides enough antidote to treat an adult for an entire 3-day course of therapy, or enough to treat three adults for 24 h. Several vials may be stocked in the ED to provide a loading dose and the remaining vials in the pharmacy for the q 4 h maintenance doses. The IV product dose of 120 mL (24 g) will treat one adult patient for an entire 20-hour IV protocol.
Amyl nitrite, sodium nitrite, and sodium thiosulfate (Cyanide antidote kit)	Acetonitrile Acrylonitrile Bromates (thiosulfate only) Chlorates (thiosulfate only) Cyanide (e.g., HCN, KCN and NaCN) Cyanogen chloride Cyanogenic glycoside natural sources (e.g., apricot pits and peach pits) Hydrogen sulfide (nitrites only) Laetrile Mustard agents (thiosulfate only) Nitroprusside (thiosulfate only) Smoke inhalation (combustion of synthetic materials)	One to two kits Each kit contains: Twelve 0.3 mL amyl nitrite ampules Two vials 3% sodium nitrite, 10 mL each Two vials 25% sodium thiosulfate, 50 mL each	Stock one kit in the ED. Consider also stocking one kit in the pharmacy. Note: This kit has a short shelf life of 24 months. Note: Stocking this kit may be unnecessary if an adequate supply of hydroxocobalamin is available.
Antivenin, *Crotalidae* Polyvalent (equine origin)	Pit viper envenomation (e.g., rattlesnakes, cottonmouths, copperheads, and timber rattlers)	None	As of March 31, 2007, this product is no longer available from the manufacturer. See Antivenin, *Crotalidae* Polyvalent Immune Fab–Ovine below.
Antivenin, *Crotalidae* Polyvalent Immune Fab–Ovine (CroFab®)	Pit viper envenomation (e.g., rattlesnakes, cottonmouths, copperheads, and timber rattlers)	Four to six vials	Advised in geographic areas with endemic populations of copperhead, water moccasin, eastern massasauga, or timber rattlesnake. In low-risk areas, know nearest alternate source of antivenin. This product may have a lower risk of hypersensitivity reaction than previously marketed equine product. Average dose in pre-marketing trials was 12 vials, but more may be needed. Stock in pharmacy. Store in refrigerator. Equine unavailable after March 31, 2007.
Antivenin, *Latrodectus mactans* (Black widow spider)	Black widow spider envenomation	Zero to one vial	Serious *Latrodectus* envenomations are rare. This product is only used for severe envenomations. Antivenin must be given in a critical care setting since it is an equine-derived product. Know the nearest source of antidote. Note: Product must be refrigerated at all times.
Atropine sulfate	Alpha$_2$ agonists (e.g., clonidine, guanabenz, and guanfacine) Alzheimer's drugs (e.g., donepezil, galantamine, rivastigmine, tacrine) Antimyesthenic agents (e.g., pyridostigmine) Bradyarrhythmia-producing agents (e.g., beta blockers, calcium channel blockers, and digitalis glycosides) Cholinergic agonists (e.g., bethanechol) Muscarine-containing mushrooms (e.g., Clitocybe and Inocybe) Nerve agents (e.g., sarin, soman, tabun, and VX) Organophosphate and carbamate insecticides	Total 100 mg to 150 mg Available in various formulations: 0.4 mg/mL (1 mL, 0.4 mg ampules) 0.4 mg/mL (20 mL, 8 mg vials) 0.1 mg/mL (10 mL, 1 mg ampules) Atropine sulfate military-style auto-injectors: (Atropen®) 2 mg/0.7 mL, 1 mg/0.7 mL, 0.5 mg/0.7 mL, 0.25 mg/0.3 mL Atropine sulfate 2.1 mg/0.7 mL with pralidoxime chloride 600 mg/2 mL (DuoDote®)	The product should be immediately available in the ED. Some may also be stored in the pharmacy or other hospital sites, but should be easily mobilized if a severely poisoned patient needs treatment. Note: Product is necessary for adequate preparedness for a weapon of mass destruction (WMD) incident; the suggested amount may not be sufficient for mass-casualty events. Auto-injectors are available from Bound Tree Medical, Inc. Drug stocked in chempack container is intended only for use in mass-casualty events.

This chart is adapted from material furnished by the Illinois Poison Center, a program of the Metropolitan Chicago Healthcare Council (MCHC).

Antidote	Poison/Drug/Toxin	Suggested Minimum Stock Quantity	Comments
Calcium disodium EDTA (Versenate®)	Lead Zinc salts (e.g., zinc chloride)	One 5-mL ampule (200 mg/mL)	Stock in pharmacy. One vial provides one day of therapy for a child. More may be needed in lead-endemic areas. Important note: Edetate disodium (Endrate®) is not the same as calcium disodium EDTA, and is used primarily as an IV chelator for emergent treatment of hypercalcemia, etc.
Calcium chloride and Calcium gluconate	Beta blockers Calcium channel blockers Fluoride salts (e.g., NaF) Hydrofluoric acid (HF) Hyperkalemia (not digoxin-induced) Hypermagnesemia	10% calcium chloride: fifteen 10-mL vials 10% calcium gluconate: five 10-mL vials	Stock in ED. More may be stocked in pharmacy. Many ampules of calcium chloride may be necessary in life-threatening calcium channel blocker or hydrofluoric acid poisoning.
Deferoxamine mesylate (Desferal®)	Iron	Twelve 500-mg vials	Stock in pharmacy. Note: Per package insert, the maximum daily dose is 6 g (12 vials). However, this dose may be exceeded in serious poisonings.
Digoxin immune Fab (Digibind®, DigiFab®)	Cardiac glycoside-containing plants (e.g., foxglove and oleander) Digitoxin Digoxin	Ten vials	Stock in ED or pharmacy. This amount (ten vials) may be given to a digoxin-poisoned patient in whom the digoxin level is unknown. This amount would effectively neutralize a steady-state digoxin level of 14.2 ng/mL in a 70-kg patient. More may be necessary in severe intoxications. Know nearest source of additional supply.
Dimercaprol (BAL in oil)	Arsenic Copper Gold Lead Lewisite Mercury	Two 3-mL ampules (100 mg/mL)	Stock in pharmacy. This amount provides two doses of 3 to 5 mg/kg/dose given q 4 h to treat one seriously poisoned adult or provides enough to treat a 15-kg child for 24 h.
Ethanol	Ethylene glycol Methanol	10% alcohol in D_5W was discontinued in 2004; 5% alcohol in D_5W was discontinued in 2007. However, 10% alcohol can be prepared from dehydrated alcohol and D_5W. 180 mL of 100% ethanol or equivalents. Consult regional poison control center.	Stock in pharmacy. This amount provides enough to treat two adults with a loading dose followed by a maintenance infusion for 4 hours each. More alcohol or fomepizole will be needed during dialysis or prolonged treatment. 95% or 40% alcohol diluted in juice may be given po if IV alcohol is unavailable. Note: Ethanol is unnecessary if fomepizole is stocked. See also fomepizole in this chart.
Flumazenil (Romazicon®)	Benzodiazepines Zaleplon Zolpidem	Total 1 mg: two 5 mL vials (0.1 mg/mL)	Suggested minimum is for ED stocking. Due to risk of seizures, use with extreme caution, if at all, in poisoned patients. More may be stocked in the pharmacy for use in reversal of conscious sedation.
Folic acid and Folinic acid (Leucovorin)	Formaldehyde/Formic Acid Methanol Methotrexate, trimetrexate Pyrimethamine Trimethoprim	Folic acid: three 50-mg vials Folinic acid: one 50-mg vial	Stock in pharmacy. For methanol-poisoned patients with an acidosis, give 50 mg folinic acid initially, then 50 mg of folic acid q 4 h for six doses.
Fomepizole (Antizol®)	Ethylene glycol Methanol	Two 1.5-g vials Note: Available in a kit of four 1.5-g vials	Stock in pharmacy. Know where nearest alternate supply is located. One vial will provide at least one initial adult dose. Hospitals with critical care and hemodialysis capabilities should consider stocking one kit of four vials (enough to treat one patient for up to several days). Note: Product has a 2-year shelf life; however, the manufacturer offers a credit for unused, expired product. Ethanol is unnecessary if adequate supply of fomepizole is stocked.
Glucagon	Beta blockers Calcium channel blockers Hypoglycemia Hypoglycemic agents	Fifty 1-mg vials	Stock 20 mg in ED and remainder in pharmacy. The total amount (50 mg) provides approximately 5 to 10 hours of high-dose therapy in life-threatening beta blocker or calcium channel blocker poisoning. A protocol using high doses of insulin/dextrose also may be considered. Consult regional poison center for guidelines.

Antidote	Poison/Drug/Toxin	Suggested Minimum Stock Quantity	Comments
Hydroxocobalamin (Cyanokit®)	Acetonitrile Acrylonitrile Cyanide (e.g., HCN, KCN and NaCN) Cyanogen chloride Cyanogenic glycoside natural sources (e.g., apricot pits and peach pits) Laetrile Nitroprusside Smoke inhalation (combustion of synthetic materials)	Two to four kits Each kit contains two 2.5-g vials Note: Diluent is not included in the kit.	Seriously poisoned cyanide patients may require 5-10 g (one or two kits). Stock two kits in ED. Consider also stocking two kits in the pharmacy. The product has a shelf-life of 30 months post-manufacture. Due to its favorable safety profile, this product may be used in a pre-hospital setting.
Hyperbaric oxygen (HBO)	Carbon monoxide Carbon tetrachloride Cyanide Hydrogen sulfide Methemoglobinemia	Post the location and phone number of nearest HBO chamber in the ED.	Consult IPC to determine if HBO treatment is indicated.
Methylene blue	Methemoglobin-inducing agents including: Aniline dyes Dapsone Dinitrophenol Local anesthetics (e.g., benzocaine) Metoclopramide Monomethylhydrazine-containing mushrooms (e.g., Gyromitra) Naphthalene Nitrates and nitrites Nitrobenzene Phenazopyridine	Three 10-mL ampules (10 mg/mL)	Stock in pharmacy. This amount provides three doses of 1 to 2 mg/kg (0.1 to 0.2 mL/kg) for an adult patient.
Nalmefene (Revex®) and Naloxone (Narcan®)	ACE inhibitors Alpha$_2$ agonists (e.g., clonidine, guanabenz, and guanfacine) Coma of unknown cause Imidazoline decongestants (e.g., oxymetazoline and tetrahydrozoline) Loperamide Opioids (e.g., codeine, dextromethorphan, diphenoxylate, fentanyl, heroin, meperidine, morphine, and propoxyphene)	Nalmefene: none required Naloxone: total 40 mg, any combination of 0.4 mg, 1 mg, and 2 mg ampules	Stock 20 mg naloxone in the ED and 20 mg elsewhere in the institution. Note: Nalmefene has a longer duration of action but it offers no therapeutic advantage over a naloxone infusion.
D-Penicillamine (Cuprimine®)	Arsenic Copper Lead Mercury	None required as an antidote. Available in bottles of 100 capsules (125 mg or 250 mg/capsule)	D-Penicillamine is no longer considered the drug of choice for heavy-metal poisonings. It may be stocked in the pharmacy for other indications such as Wilson's disease or rheumatoid arthritis.
Physostigmine salicylate (Antilirium®)	Anticholinergic alkaloid-containing plants (e.g., deadly nightshade and jimson weed) Antihistamines Atropine and other anticholinergic agents Intrathecal baclofen	Two 2-mL ampules (1 mg/mL)	Stock in ED or pharmacy. Usual adult dose is 1 to 2 mg slow IV push. Note: Duration of effect is 30 to 60 min.
Phytonadione (Vitamin K$_1$) (AquaMEPHYTON®, Mephyton®)	Indandione derivatives Long-acting anticoagulant rodenticides (e.g., brodifacoum and bromadiolone) Warfarin	Two 0.5-mL ampules (2 mg/mL) and ten 1-mL ampules (10 mg/mL) 5-mg tablets available in packages of 10, 14, 20, 30, and 100	Stock in pharmacy.
Pralidoxime chloride (2-PAM) (Protopam®)	Antimyesthenic agents (e.g., pyridostigmine) Nerve agents (e.g., sarin, soman, tabun, and VX) Organophosphate insecticides Tacrine	Six 1-g vials Pralidoxime chloride military-style auto-injectors: 600 mg/2 mL	Stock in ED or pharmacy. Note: Serious intoxications may require 500 mg/h (12 g/day). Product is necessary for adequate preparedness for a weapon of mass destruction (WMD) incident; the suggested amount may not be sufficient for mass-casualty events. Auto-injectors are available from Bound Tree Medical, Inc. Drug stocked in chempack container is intended only for use in mass-casualty events.
Protamine sulfate	Enoxaparin Heparin	Variable, consider recommendation of hospital P&T Committee Available as 5-mL ampules (10 mg/mL) and 25-mL vials (250 mg/25 mL)	Stock in pharmacy.
Pyridoxine hydrochloride (Vitamin B$_6$)	Acrylamide Ethylene glycol Hydrazine Isoniazid (INH) Monomethylhydrazine-containing mushrooms (e.g., Gyromitra)	100 1-mL vials (100 mg/mL vials)	Stock in ED or pharmacy. Usual dose is 1 g pyridoxine HCl for each gram of INH ingested. If amount ingested is unknown, give 5 g of pyridoxine. Repeat dose if seizures are uncontrolled. Know nearest source of additional supply. For ethylene glycol, a dose of 100 mg/day enhances the clearance of toxic metabolite.

Antidote	Poison/Drug/Toxin	Suggested Minimum Stock Quantity	Comments
Sodium bicarbonate	Chlorine gas Hyperkalemia Serum alkalinization: Agents producing a quinidine-like effect as noted by widened QRS complex on EKG (e.g., amantadine, carbamazepine, chloroquine, cocaine, diphenhydramine, flecainide, propafenone, propoxyphene, tricyclic antidepressants, quinidine, and related agents) Urine alkalinization: Weakly acidic agents (e.g., chlorophenoxy herbicides, chlorpropamide, phenobarbital, and salicylates)	Twenty 50-mEq vials	Stock 10 vials in the ED and 10 vials elsewhere in the hospital.
Succimer (Chemet®)	Arsenic Lead Lewisite Mercury	One bottle of 100 capsules (100 mg/capsule)	Stock in pharmacy. FDA-approved only for pediatric lead poisoning; however, it has shown efficacy for other heavy-metal poisonings.

POISON CONTROL CENTERS

The American Association of Poison Control Centers (AAPCC) uses a single, nationwide emergency number to automatically link callers with their regional poison center. This toll-free number, **800-222-1222**, also works for **teletype lines (TTY)** for the hearing-impaired and **telecommunication devices (TTD)** for individuals who are deaf. However, a few local poison centers and the ASPCA/Animal Poison Control Center are not part of this nationwide system and continue to use separate numbers.

Most of the centers listed below are accredited by the AAPCC. **Certified centers are marked by an asterisk after the name.**

Each has to meet certain criteria. It must, for example, serve a large geographic area; it must be open 24 hours a day and provide direct-dial or toll-free access; it must be supervised by a medical director; and it must have registered pharmacists or nurses available to answer questions from the public.

Within each state, centers are listed alphabetically by city. Some state poison centers also list their original emergency numbers (including TTY/TDD) that only work within that state. For these listings, callers may use either the state number or the nationwide 800 number.

ALABAMA

BIRMINGHAM

Regional Poison Control Center (*)
Children's Hospital of Alabama

1600 7th Ave. South
Birmingham, AL 35233
Business: 205-939-6334
Emergency: 800-222-1222
www.chsys.org

TUSCALOOSA

Alabama Poison Center (*)

2503 Phoenix Dr.
Tuscaloosa, AL 35405
Business: 800-462-0609
Emergency: 800-222-1222
800-462-0800 (AL)
www.alapoisoncenter.org

ALASKA

JUNEAU

Alaska Poison Control System
Section of Injury Prevention and EMS

410 Willoughby Ave., Room 103
Box 110616
Juneau, AK 99811-0616
Business: 907-465-3027
Emergency: 800-222-1222
www.chems.alaska.gov

(PORTLAND, OR)

Oregon Poison Center (*)
Oregon Health and Science University

3181 SW Sam Jackson Park Rd.
CB550
Portland, OR 97239
Business: 503-494-8600
Emergency: 800-222-1222
www.oregonpoison.com

ARIZONA

PHOENIX

Banner Poison Control Center (*)
Banner Good Samaritan Medical Center

1111 E. McDowell
Phoenix, AZ 85006
Business: 602-495-4884
Emergency: 800-222-1222
www.bannerpoisoncontrol.com

TUCSON

Arizona Poison and Drug Information Center (*)
Arizona Health Sciences Center

1295 N. Martin Ave., Room B308
Tucson, AZ 85721
Business: 520-626-7899
Emergency: 800-222-1222
www.pharmacy.arizona.edu/outreach/poison

ARKANSAS

LITTLE ROCK

Arkansas Poison and Drug Information Center (*)
College of Pharmacy - UAMS

4301 West Markham St.
Mail Slot 522-2
Little Rock, AR 72205
Business: 501-686-6161
Emergency: 800-222-1222
800-376-4766 (AR)
TDD/TTY: 800-641-3805

ASPCA/ ANIMAL POISON CONTROL CENTER

1717 South Philo Rd.
Suite 36
Urbana, IL 61802
Business: 217-337-5030
Emergency: 888-426-4435
800-548-2423
www.aspca.org/apcc

CALIFORNIA

FRESNO/MADERA

California Poison Control System-Fresno/Madera Div. (*)
Children's Hospital Central California

9300 Valley Children's Place, MB 15
Madera, CA 93638-8762
Business: 559-622-2300
Emergency: 800-222-1222
800-876-4766 (CA)
TDD/TTY: 800-972-3323
www.calpoison.org

SACRAMENTO

California Poison Control System-Sacramento Div. (*)
UC Davis Medical Center

2315 Stockton Blvd.
Sacramento, CA 95817
Business: 916-227-1400
Emergency: 800-222-1222
800-876-4766 (CA)
TDD/TTY: 800-972-3323
www.calpoison.org

SAN DIEGO

California Poison Control System-San Diego Div. (*)
UC San Diego Medical Center

200 West Arbor Dr.
San Diego, CA 92103-8925
Business: 858-715-6300
Emergency: 800-222-1222
800-876-4766 (CA)
TDD/TTY: 800-972-3323
www.calpoison.org

SAN FRANCISCO

California Poison Control System-San Francisco Div. (*)
University of California San Francisco

Box 1369
San Francisco, CA 94143-1369
Business: 415-502-6000
Emergency: 800-222-1222
800-876-4766 (CA)
TDD/TTY: 800-972-3323
www.calpoison.org

COLORADO

DENVER

Rocky Mountain Poison and Drug Center (*)

777 Bannock St., Mail Code 0180
Denver, CO 80204
Business: 303-739-1100
Emergency: 800-222-1222
TDD/TTY: 303-739-1127 (CO)
www.RMPDC.org

CONNECTICUT

FARMINGTON

Connecticut Poison Control Center (*)
University of Connecticut Health Center

263 Farmington Ave.
Farmington, CT 06030-5365
Business: 860-679-4540
Emergency: 800-222-1222
TDD/TTY: 866-218-5372
http://poisoncontrol.uchc.edu

DELAWARE

(PHILADELPHIA, PA)

The Poison Control Center (*)
Children's Hospital of Philadelphia

34th St. & Civic Center Blvd.
Philadelphia, PA 19104-4399
Business: 215-590-2003
Emergency: 800-222-1222
TDD/TTY: 215-590-8789
www.poisoncontrol.chop.edu

DISTRICT OF COLUMBIA

WASHINGTON, DC

National Capital Poison Center (*)

3201 New Mexico Ave., NW
Suite 310
Washington, DC 20016
Business: 202-362-3867
Emergency: 800-222-1222
www.poison.org

FLORIDA

JACKSONVILLE

Florida Poison Information Center-Jacksonville (*)

655 West 8th St.
Box C23
Jacksonville, FL 32209
Business: 904-244-4465
Emergency: 800-222-1222
http://fpicjax.org

MIAMI

Florida Poison Information Center (*)
University of Miami, Dept. of Pediatrics

P.O. Box 016960 (R-131)
Miami, FL 33101
Business: 305-585-5250
Emergency: 800-222-1222
www.med.miami.edu/poisoncontrol

TAMPA

Florida Poison Information Center (*)
Tampa General Hospital

P.O. Box 1289
Tampa, FL 33601-1289
Business: 813-844-7044
Emergency: 800-222-1222
www.poisoncentertampa.org

GEORGIA

ATLANTA

Georgia Poison Center (*)
Hughes Spalding Children's Hospital, Grady Health System

80 Jesse Hill Jr. Dr., SE
P.O. Box 26066
Atlanta, GA 30303-3050
Business: 404-616-9237
Emergency: 800-222-1222
(Atlanta) 404-616-9000
TDD: 404-616-9287
www.georgiapoisoncenter.org

HAWAII

(DENVER, CO)

Rocky Mountain Poison and Drug Center (*)

777 Bannock St., Mail Code 0180
Denver, CO 80204
Business: 303-739-1100
Emergency: 800-222-1222
TDD/TTY: 303-739-1127 (CO)
www.RMPDC.org

IDAHO

(DENVER, CO)

Rocky Mountain Poison and Drug Center (*)

777 Bannock St., Mail Code 0180
Denver, CO 80204
Business: 303-739-1100
Emergency: 800-222-1222
TDD/TTY: 303-739-1127 (CO)
www.RMPDC.org

ILLINOIS

CHICAGO

Illinois Poison Center (*)

222 South Riverside Plaza
Suite 1900
Chicago, IL 60606
Business: 312-906-6136
Emergency: 800-222-1222
TDD/TTY: 312-906-6185
www.mchc.org/ipc

INDIANA

INDIANAPOLIS

Indiana Poison Control Center (*)
Methodist Hospital, Clarian Health Partners

I-65 at 21st St.
P.O. Box 1367
Indianapolis, IN 46206-1367
Business: 317-962-2335
Emergency: 800-222-1222
800-382-9097
317-962-2323
(Indianapolis)
www.clarian.org/poisoncontrol

IOWA

SIOUX CITY

Iowa Statewide Poison Control Center (*)
Iowa Health System and the University of Iowa Hospitals and Clinics

401 Douglas St., Suite 402
Sioux City, IA 51101
Business: 712-279-3710
Emergency: 800-222-1222
712-277-2222 (IA)
www.iowapoison.org

KANSAS

KANSAS CITY

University of Kansas Poison Control Hospital Center

3901 Rainbow Blvd.
Delp - Room 4043
Kansas City, KS 66160-7231
Business: 913-588-6638
Emergency: 800-222-1222
800-332-6633 (KS)
www.kumed.com/poison

KENTUCKY

LOUISVILLE

Kentucky Regional Poison Center (*)
Medical Towers South

234 E Gray St, Suite 847
Louisville, KY 40202
Business: 502-629-7264
Emergency: 800-222-1222
www.krpc.com

LOUISIANA

SHREVEPORT

Louisiana Poison Center (*)
LSUHSC - Shreveport
Dept. of Emergency Medicine
Section of Clinical Toxology

1455 Wilkinson St
Shreveport, LA 71130
Business: 318-813-3314
Emergency: 800-222-1222

MAINE

PORTLAND

Northern New England Poison Center (*)

22 Bramhall St.
Portland, ME 04102
Business: 207-662-7042
Emergency: 800-222-1222
800-442-6035
207-871-2879
(ME)
TDD/TTY: 207-662-2879 (ME)
www.nnepc.org

MARYLAND

BALTIMORE

Maryland Poison Center (*)
University of Maryland at Baltimore School of Pharmacy
220 Arch St.
Office Level 01
Baltimore, MD 21201
Business: 410-706-7604
Emergency: 800-222-1222
TDD: 410-528-7530
www.mdpoison.com

(WASHINGTON, DC)

National Capital Poison Center (*)
3201 New Mexico Ave., NW
Suite 310
Washington, DC 20016
Business: 202-362-3867
Emergency: 800-222-1222
www.poison.org

MASSACHUSETTS

BOSTON

Regional Center for Poison Control and Prevention (*) (Serving Massachusetts and Rhode Island)
300 Longwood Ave.
Boston, MA 02115
Business: 617-355-6609
Emergency: 800-222-1222
TDD/TTY: 888-244-5313
www.maripoisoncenter.com

MICHIGAN

DETROIT

Regional Poison Control Center (*)
Children's Hospital of Michigan
4160 John R. Harper Professional Office Bldg.
Suite 616
Detroit, MI 48201
Business: 313-745-5335
Emergency: 800-222-1222
www.mitoxic.org/pcc

MINNESOTA

MINNEAPOLIS

Hennepin Regional Poison Center (*)
Hennepin County Medical Center
701 Park Ave.
Mail Code RL
Minneapolis, MN 55415
Business: 612-873-3144
Emergency: 800-222-1222
www.mnpoison.org

MISSISSIPPI

JACKSON

Mississippi Regional Poison Control Center
University of Mississippi Medical Center
2500 North State St.
Jackson, MS 39216
Business: 601-984-1680
Emergency: 800-222-1222
http://poisoncontrol.umc.edu

MISSOURI

ST. LOUIS

Missouri Regional Poison Center (*)
7980 Clayton Rd. Suite 200
St. Louis, MO 63117
Business: 314-772-8300
Emergency: 800-222-1222
www.cardinalglennon.com

MONTANA

(DENVER, CO)

Rocky Mountain Poison and Drug Center (*)
777 Bannock St., Mail Code 0180
Denver, CO 80204
Business: 303-739-1100
Emergency: 800-222-1222
TDD/TTY: 303-739-1127 (CO)
www.RMPDC.org

NEBRASKA

OMAHA

Nebraska Regional Poison Center (*)
8401 W. Dodge Rd., Suite 115
Omaha, NE 68114
Business: 402-390-5555
Emergency: 800-222-1222
www.nebraskapoison.com

NEVADA

(DENVER, CO)

Rocky Mountain Poison and Drug Center (*)
777 Bannock St., Mail Code 0180
Denver, CO 80204
Business: 303-739-1100
Emergency: 800-222-1222
TDD/TTY: 303-739-1127 (CO)
www.RMPDC.org

NEW HAMPSHIRE

(PORTLAND, ME)

Northern New England Poison Center
Maine Medical Center
22 Bramhall St.
Portland, ME 04102
Business: 207-662-0111
Emergency: 800-222-1222
www.nnepc.org

NEW JERSEY

NEWARK

New Jersey Poison Information and Education System (*)
UMDNJ
140 Bergen St. PO Box 1709
Newark, NJ 07101
Business: 973-972-9280
Emergency: 800-222-1222
TDD/TTY: 973-926-8008
www.njpies.org

NEW MEXICO

ALBUQUERQUE

New Mexico Poison and Drug Information Center (*)
MSC09/5080
1 University of New Mexico
Albuquerque, NM 87131-0001
Business: 505-272-4261
Emergency: 800-222-1222
http://hsc.unm.edu/pharmacy/poison

NEW YORK

MINEOLA

Long Island Regional Poison and Drug Information Center (*)
Winthrop University Hospital
259 First St.
Mineola, NY 11501
Business: 516-663-4574
Emergency: 800-222-1222
www.lirpdic.org

NEW YORK CITY

New York City Poison Control Center (*)
NYC Bureau of Public Health
455 First Ave., Room 123, Box 81
New York, NY 10016
Business: 212-447-8152
Emergency: 800-222-1222
(English) 212-340-4494
212-POISONS
(212-764-7667)
Emergency: 212-venenos
(Spanish) (212-836-3667)
TDD: 212-689-9014
www.nyc.gov/html/doh/html/poison/poison.shtml

ROCHESTER

The Ruth A. Lawrence Regional Poison and Drug Information Center (*)
University of Rochester Medical Center
601 Elmwood Ave.
Box 321
Rochester, NY 14642
Business: 585-273-4155
Emergency: 800-222-1222
TTY: 585-273-3854
www.fingerlakespoison.org

SYRACUSE

Upstate New York Poison Center (*)
SUNY Upstate Medical University
750 East Adams St.
Syracuse, NY 13210
Business: 315-464-7078
Emergency: 800-222-1222
TTY: 315-464-5424
www.upstatepoison.org

NORTH CAROLINA

CHARLOTTE

Carolinas Poison Center (*)
Carolinas Medical Center
PO Box 32861
Charlotte, NC 28232-2861
Business: 704-512-3795
Emergency: 800-222-1222
www.ncpoisoncenter.org

NORTH DAKOTA

(MINNEAPOLIS, MN)

Hennepin Regional Poison Center (*)
Hennepin County Medical Center
701 Park Ave., Mail Code RL
Minneapolis, MN 55415
Business: 612-873-3144
Emergency: 800-222-1222
www.mnpoison.org

OHIO

CINCINNATI

Cincinnati Drug and Poison Information Center (*)
3333 Burnet Ave., MLC 9004
Cincinnati, OH 45229
Business: 513-636-5063
Emergency: 800-222-1222
www.cincinnatichildrens.org/dpic

CLEVELAND

Northern Ohio Poison Center
Rainbow Babies and Children's Hospital
11100 Euclid Ave.
B261 MP 6007
Cleveland, OH 44106-6010
Business: 216-844-1573
Emergency: 800-222-1222
www.uhhospitals.org/rainbowchildren/tabid/195/Default.aspx

COLUMBUS

Central Ohio Poison Center (*)
700 Children's Dr.
Columbus, OH 43205
Business: 614-355-0435
Emergency: 800-222-1222
TTY: 866-688-0088
www.bepoisonsmart.com

OKLAHOMA

OKLAHOMA CITY

Oklahoma Poison Control Center (*)
OU Health Sciences Center
940 Northeast 13th St.
Room 3N3510
Oklahoma City, OK 73104
Business: 405-271-5062
Emergency: 800-222-1222
www.oklahomapoison.org

OREGON

PORTLAND

Oregon Poison Center (*)
Oregon Health and Science University
3181 S.W. Sam Jackson Park Rd.
CB550
Portland, OR 97239
Business: 503-494-8600
Emergency: 800-222-1222
www.ohsu.edu/poison

PENNSYLVANIA

PHILADELPHIA

The Poison Control Center (*)
Children's Hospital of Philadelphia
34th Street & Civic Center Blvd.
Philadelphia, PA 19104
Business: 215-590-2003
Emergency: 800-222-1222
215-386-2100 (PA)
TDD/TTY: 215-590-8789
www.poisoncontrol.chop.edu

PITTSBURGH

Pittsburgh Poison Center (*)
University of Pittsburgh
200 Lothrop Street
Pittsburgh, PA 15213
Business: 412-390-3300
Emergency: 800-222-1222
412-681-6669
www.upmc.com/services/poison-center

RHODE ISLAND

(BOSTON, MA)

Regional Center for Poison Control and Prevention (*) (Serving Massachusetts and Rhode Island)
300 Longwood Ave.
Boston, MA 02115
Business: 617-355-6609
Emergency: 800-222-1222
TDD/TTY: 888-244-5313
www.maripoisoncenter.com

SOUTH CAROLINA

COLUMBIA

Palmetto Poison Center (*)
South Carolina College of Pharmacy
University of South Carolina
Columbia, SC 29208
Business: 803-777-7909
Emergency: 800-222-1222
http://poison.sc.edu

SOUTH DAKOTA

(MINNEAPOLIS, MN)

Hennepin Regional Poison Center (*)
Hennepin County Medical Center
701 Park Ave., Mail Code RL
Minneapolis, MN 55415
Business: 612-873-3144
Emergency: 800-222-1222
www.mnpoison.org

TENNESSEE

NASHVILLE

Tennessee Poison Center (*)
1161 21st Ave. South
501 Oxford House
Nashville, TN 37232-4632
Business: 615-936-0760
Emergency: 800-222-1222
www.tnpoisoncenter.org

TEXAS

AMARILLO

Texas Panhandle Poison Center (*)
1501 S. Coulter Dr.
Amarillo, TX 79106
Business: 806-354-1630
Emergency: 800-222-1222
www.poisoncontrol.org

DALLAS

North Texas Poison Center (*)
Texas Poison Center Network
Parkland Memorial Hospital
5201 Harry Hines Blvd.
Dallas, TX 75235
Business: 214-589-0911
Emergency: 800-222-1222
www.poisoncontrol.org

EL PASO

West Texas Regional Poison Center (*)
At University Medical Center of El Paso

4815 Alameda Ave.
El Paso, TX 79905
Business 915-534-3800
Emergency: 800-222-1222
www.poisoncontrol.org

GALVESTON

Southeast Texas Poison Center (*)
The University of Texas Medical Branch

3.112 Trauma Center
Galveston, TX 77555-1175
Business: 409-772-3332
Emergency: 800-222-1222
www.utmb.edu/setpc

SAN ANTONIO

South Texas Poison Center (*)
The University of Texas Health Science Center–San Antonio Dept. of Surgery

7703 Floyd Curl Dr., MSC 7849
San Antonio, TX 78229-3900
Business: 210-567-5762
Emergency: 800-222-1222
www.texaspoison.com

TEMPLE

Central Texas Poison Center (*)
Scott & White Memorial Hospital

2401 South 31st St.
Temple, TX 76508
Business: 254-724-7405
Emergency: 800-222-1222
http://www.sw.org/web/patientsAndVisitors/iwcontent/public/poison/en_us/html/poison.jsp

UTAH

SALT LAKE CITY

Utah Poison Control Center (*)
University of Utah

585 Komas Dr. Suite #200
Salt Lake City, UT 84108-1234
Business: 801-587-0600
Emergency: 800-222-1222
http://uuhsc.utah.edu/poison

VERMONT

(PORTLAND, ME)

Northern New England Poison Center (*)
Maine Medical Center

22 Bramhall St.
Portland, ME 04102
Business: 207-662-0111
Emergency: 800-222-1222
www.nnepc.org

VIRGINIA

CHARLOTTESVILLE

Blue Ridge Poison Center (*)
Jefferson Park Place

1222 Jefferson Park Ave.
Charlottesville, VA 22908-0774
Business: 434-924-0347
Emergency: 800-222-1222
www.healthsystem.virginia.edu/brpc

RICHMOND

Virginia Poison Center (*)
Medical College of Virginia Hospitals
Virginia Commonwealth University Health System

P.O. Box 980522
Richmond, VA 23298-0522
Business: 804-828-4780
Emergency: 800-222-1222
www.poison.vcu.edu

WASHINGTON

SEATTLE

Washington Poison Center (*)

155 NE 100th St.
Seattle, WA 98125-8007
Business: 206-517-2350
Emergency: 800-222-1222
www.wapc.org

WEST VIRGINIA

CHARLESTON

West Virginia Poison Center (*)
WVU Charleston Division

3110 MacCorkle Ave. SE
Charleston, WV 25314
Business: 304-347-1212
Emergency: 800-222-1222
www.wvpoisoncenter.org

WISCONSIN

MILWAUKEE

Wisconsin Poison Center

Mail Station 660
P.O. Box 1997
Milwaukee, WI 53201-1997
Business: 414-266-6973
Emergency: 800-222-1222
www.wisconsinpoison.org

WYOMING

(OMAHA, NE)

Nebraska Regional Poison Center (*)

8401 W. Dodge St., Suite 115
Omaha, NE 68114
Business: 402-390-5555
Emergency: 800-222-1222
www.nebraskapoison.com

BE CRUSHED

articles, though. (Patients should,
ny medication unless it is specif-

-inclusive. Generic and alternate
ablets intended for sublingual or
this list) should also be adminis-
n.

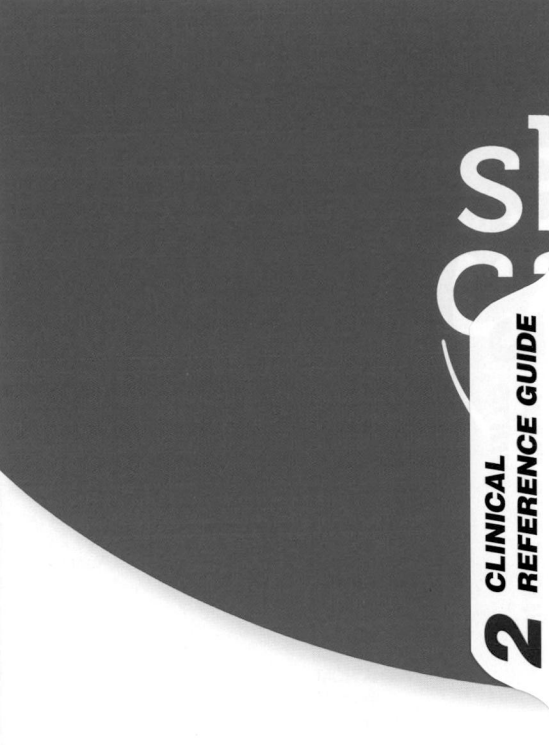

Manufacturer	Form
Schering Plough	sr
Schering Plough	sr
Schering Plough	sr
Schering	sr
Schering	sr
Schering	sr
Breckenridge	sr
McNeil Pediatrics	sr
GlaxoSmithKline	sr
Schering Plough	ec
GlaxoSmithKline	sr
Pfizer	sr
Cypress	sr
Brighton	sr
Solvay	ec
Solvay	ec
Solvay	ec
Eli Lilly	ec
Plainview	ec
Laser	sr
Laser	sr
Kenwood Therapeutics	sr
Cornerstone	sr
Poly	sr
Poly	sr
Abbott	ec
Abbott	sr
Abbott	ec
International Ethical	sr
Pfizer	sr
GlaxoSmithKline	sr
Dexo	sr
Midlothian	sr
Mason Vitamins	sr
Duramed	sr
Watson	sr
Pfizer	sr
Pfizer	sr
UCB	sr
Andrx	sr
Apotex	sr
Schering Plough	sr
Ortho-McNeil	sr
PBM	sr
Warner Chilcott	ec
Midlothian	sr
Prasco	sr
A.G. Marin	sr
Palm	sr
Boehringer Ingelheim	ec
Capellon	sr
Kowa	sr
Kowa	sr
Kowa	sr
Physicians Total Care	sr
Victory	sr
GlaxoSmithKline	sr
Breckenridge	sr
Athlon	sr
Athlon	sr
Hawthorn	sr
Rosedale	ec
Roche	ec
GlaxoSmithKline	ec
GlaxoSmithKline	ec
GlaxoSmithKline	ec
Prime Marketing	ec
Edwards	sr

Drug	Manufacturer	Form
Effexor-XR	Wyeth	sr
Embeda	Alpharma	sr
Enablex	Novartis	sr
Entercote	Global Source	ec
Entex LA	Andrx	sr
Entex PSE	Andrx	sr
Entocort EC	Prometheus	ec
Equetro	Shire U.S.	sr
ERYC	Warner Chilcott	sr
Ery-Tab	Abbott	ec
Eskalith-CR	GlaxoSmithKline	sr
Extendryl G	Auriga	sr
Extendryl Jr	Auriga	sr
Extendryl SR	Auriga	sr
Extress-30	Key	sr
Exetuss-DM	Larken	sr
Extress-60	Key	sr
Feen-A-Mint	Schering Plough	ec
Femilax	G & W	ec
Fero-Folic-500	Abbott	sr
Fero-Grad-500	Abbott	sr
Ferro-Sequels	Inverness Medical	sr
Ferrous Fumarate DS	Vita-Rx	sr
Fetrin	Lunsco	sr
Flagyl ER	Pharmacia	sr
Fleet Bisacodyl	Fleet, C.B.	ec
Focalin XR	Novartis	sr
Folitab 500	Rising	sr
Fortamet	First Horizon	sr
Fumatinic	Laser	sr
Genacote	Teva	ec
GFN 600/Phenylephrine 20	Cypress	sr
GFN 600/PSE 60/DM 30	Cypress	sr
GFN 1200/DM 60	Cypress	sr
GFN 1200/ Phenylephrine 40	Cypress	sr
Gilphex TR	Gil	sr
Giltuss TR	Gil	sr
Glucophage XR	Bristol-Myers Squibb	sr
Glucotrol XL	Pfizer	sr
Glumetza	Depomed	sr
Guaifenex DM	Ethex	sr
Guaifenex GP	Ethex	sr
Guaifenex PSE 60	Ethex	sr
Guaifenex PSE 80	Ethex	sr
Guaifenex PSE 85	Ethex	sr
Guaifenex PSE 120	Ethex	sr
Halfprin	Kramer	ec
Hemax	Pronova	sr
Histacol LA	Breckenridge	sr
Humavent LA	Dexo	sr
Humibid	Adams	sr
Humibid DM	Cornerstone	sr
Humibid LA	Cornerstone	sr
Iberet-500	Abbott	sr
Iberet-Folic-500	Abbott	sr
Icar-C Plus SR	Hawthorn	sr
Imdur	AstraZeneca	sr
Inderal LA	Wyeth	sr
Indocin SR	Forte Pharma	sr
Innopran XL	GlaxoSmithKline	sr
Intuniv	Shire	sr
Invega	Janssen	sr
Isochron	Forest	sr
Isopro	Rugby	sr
Isoptin SR	Ranbaxy	sr
Kadian	Alpharma	sr
Kapidex	Takeda	sr
Kaon-Cl 10	Savage	sr
Keppra XR	UCB	sr
Klor-Con 8	Upsher-Smith	sr
Klor-Con 10	Upsher-Smith	sr
Klor-Con M10	Upsher-Smith	sr
Klor-Con M15	Upsher-Smith	sr
Klor-Con M20	Upsher-Smith	sr
K-Tab	Abbott	sr
K-Tan	Prasco	sr
Lamictal XR	GlaxoSmithKline	sr
Lescol XL	Novartis	sr
Levall G	Auriga	sr
Levbid	Alaven	sr
Levsinex	Alaven	sr
Lialda	Shire	ec
Lipram 4500	Global	ec
Lipram-PN10	Global	ec
Lipram-PN16	Global	ec
Lipram-PN20	Global	ec
Liquibid-D	Capellon	sr
Liquibid-D 1200	Capellon	sr
Liquibid-PD	Capellon	sr
Lithobid	JDS Pharmaceuticals	sr
Lodrane-12 Hour	ECR	sr
Lodrane-12D	ECR	sr
Lodrane 24	ECR	sr
Lodrane 24D	ECR	sr
Lohist-12	Larken	sr
Lohist-12D	Larken	sr
Luvox CR	Jazz Pharmaceuticals	sr
Mag Delay	Major	ec
Mag64	Rising	ec
Mag-SR Plus Calcium	Cypress	sr
Mag-Tab SR	Niche	sr
Maxifed	MCR American	sr
Maxifed DM	MCR American	sr
Maxifed DMX	MCR American	sr
Maxifed-G	MCR American	sr
Maxiphen DM	MCR American	sr
Medent DM	SJ	sr
Medent PE	SJ	sr
Mega-C	Merit	sr
Menopause Trio	Mason Vitamins	sr
Mestinon Timespan	Valeant	sr
Metadate CD	UCB	sr
Metadate ER	UCB	sr
Methylin ER	Mallinckrodt	sr
Micro-K	Ther-Rx	sr
Micro-K 10	Ther-Rx	sr
Mild-C	Carlson, J.R.	sr
Montephen	Monte Sano	sr
Moxatag	Middlebrook	sr
MS Contin	Purdue	sr
Mucinex	Adams	sr
Mucinex D	Adams	sr
Mucinex DM	Adams	sr
Multiret Folic-500	Actavis	sr
Mydocs	Centurion	sr
Myfortic	Novartis	ec
Nalex-A	Blansett	sr
Naprelan	Victory	sr
Nasatab LA	ECR	sr
New Ami-Tex LA	Actavis	sr
Nexium	AstraZeneca	ec
Niaspan	Abbott	sr
Nicomide	Sirius	sr
Nifediac CC	Teva	sr
Nifedical XL	Teva	sr
Nitro-Time	Time-Cap	sr
Nohist	Larken	sr
Nohist-Plus	Larken	sr
Nohist-Plus Jr	Larken	sr
Norel SR	U.S. Pharmaceutical	sr
Norpace CR	Pfizer	sr
Obstetrix EC	Seyer Pharmatec	ec
Omnihist LA	Dexo	sr
Opana ER	Endo	sr
Oramorph SR	Xanodyne	sr
Oracea	Collagenex	sr
Oxycontin	Purdue	sr
Palcaps 10	Breckenridge	ec
Palcaps 20	Breckenridge	ec
Pancrease MT 10	McNeil Consumer	ec
Pancrease MT 16	McNeil Consumer	ec
Pancrease MT 20	McNeil Consumer	ec
Pancrecarb MS-4	Digestive Care	ec
Pancrecarb MS-8	Digestive Care	ec
Pancrecarb MS-16	Digestive Care	ec
Pangestyme CN-10	Ethex	ec
Pangestyme CN-20	Ethex	ec
Pangestyme EC	Ethex	ec
Pangestyme MT16	Ethex	ec
Pangestyme UL12	Ethex	ec
Pangestyme UL18	Ethex	ec

Enteric-coated = ec **Slow-release = sr**

Drug	Manufacturer	Form
Pangestyme UL20	Ethex	ec
Panocaps	Breckenridge	ec
Panocaps MT 16	Breckenridge	ec
Panocaps MT 20	Breckenridge	ec
Para-Time SR	Time-Cap	sr
Paser	Jacobus	sr
Pavacot	Truxton	sr
Paxil CR	GlaxoSmithKline	sr
PCE Dispertab	Abbott	sr
PCM LA	Cypress	sr
Pendex	Cypress	sr
Pentasa	Shire U.S.	sr
Pentoxil	Upsher-Smith	sr
Phenabid	Gil	sr
Phenabid DM	Gil	sr
Phenavent D	Ethex	sr
Phendiet-105	Truxton	sr
Phenytek	Mylan Bertek	sr
Phlemex-PE	Cypress	sr
Plendil	AstraZeneca	sr
Poly Hist Forte	Poly	sr
Poly-Vent	Poly	sr
Poly-Vent Jr	Poly	sr
Prehist D	Marnel	sr
Prevacid	Tap	ec
Prilosec	AstraZeneca	ec
Prilosec OTC	Procter & Gamble	sr
Pristiq	Wyeth	sr
Procardia XL	Pfizer	sr
Prolex PD	Blansett	sr
Prolex-D	Blansett	sr
Pronestyl-SR	Bristol-Myers Squibb	sr
Proquin XR	Depomed	sr
Protid	Lunsco	sr
Protonix	Wyeth	ec
Prozac Weekly	Eli Lilly	ec
Pseudocot-C	Truxton	sr
Pseudocot-G	Truxton	sr
Pseudovent DM	Ethex	sr
Ralix	Cypress	sr
Ranexa	CV Therapeutics	sr
Razadyne ER	Ortho-McNeil	sr
Reliable Gentle Laxative	Ivax	ec
Requip XL	GlaxoSmithKline	sr
Rescon-Jr	Capellon	sr
Rescon-MX	Capellon	sr
Respa-AR	Respa	sr
Respa-BR	Respa	sr
Respahist-II	Respa	sr
Respaire-60 SR	Laser	sr
Respaire-120 SR	Laser	sr
Rhinacon A	Breckenridge	sr
Risperdal Consta	Janssen	sr
Ritalin LA	Novartis	sr
Ritalin-SR	Novartis	sr
Rodex Forte	Legere	sr
Ru-Tuss	Carwin	sr
Rythmol SR	GlaxoSmithKline	sr
Ryzolt	Purdue	sr
SAM-e	Pharmavite	ec
Sanctura XR	Allergan	sr
Scopohist-PE	Larken	sr
Seroquel XR	AstraZeneca	sr
Simcor	Abbott	sr
Sinemet CR	Bristol-Myers Squibb	sr
Sinutuss DM	Dexo	sr
Sinuvent PE	Dexo	sr
Slo-Niacin	Upsher-Smith	sr
Slow Fe	Novartis Consumer	sr
Slow Fe With Folic Acid	Novartis Consumer	sr
Slow-Mag	Purdue	ec
Solodyn	Medicis	sr
St. Joseph Pain Reliever	McNeil Consumer	ec
Stahist	Magna	sr
Stavzor	Noven	sr
Sudafed 12 Hour	Johnson & Johnson	sr
Sudafed 24 Hour	Johnson & Johnson	sr
Sudahist	Larken	sr
Sudatrate	Larken	sr
Sudex Tab	Atley	sr
Sular	Sciele	sr

Drug	Manufacturer	Form
Sulfazine EC	Qualitest	ec
Symax Duotab	Capellon	sr
Symax-SR	Capellon	sr
Tarka	Abbott	sr
Taztia XT	Andrx	sr
Tegretol-XR	Novartis	sr
Theo-24	UCB	sr
Theochron	Forest	sr
Theo-Time	Major	sr
Tiazac	Forest	sr
Toprol XL	AstraZeneca	sr
Totalday	National Vitamin	sr
Touro Allergy	Dartmouth	sr
Touro CC	Dartmouth	sr
Touro CC-LD	Dartmouth	sr
Touro DM	Dartmouth	sr
Touro HC	Dartmouth	sr
Touro LA	Dartmouth	sr
Touro LA-LD	Dartmouth	sr
Toviaz	Pfizer	sr
Tranxene-SD	Ovation	sr
Trental	sanofi-aventis	sr
Treximet	GlaxoSmithKline	ec
Trilipix	Abbott	ec
Trituss-ER	Everett	sr
Tussafed-LA	Everett	sr
Tussall-ER	Everett	sr
Tussi-Bid	Capellon	sr
Tussicaps	Mallinckrodt	sr
Tusso-DM	Everett	sr
Tusso-HC	Everett	sr
Tylenol Arthritis	McNeil Consumer	sr
Ultrabrom	Dexo	sr
Ultrabrom PD	Dexo	sr
Ultracaps MT 20	Breckenridge	ec
Ultram ER	Ortho-McNeil	sr
Ultrase	Axcan Scandipharm	ec
Ultrase MT12	Axcan Scandipharm	ec
Ultrase MT18	Axcan Scandipharm	ec
Ultrase MT20	Axcan Scandipharm	ec
Uniphyl	Purdue	sr
Urocit-K 5	Mission	sr
Urocit-K 10	Mission	sr
Uroxatral	sanofi-aventis	sr
Utira	Hawthorn	sr
Veracolate	Numark	ec
Verelan	UCB	sr
Verelan PM	UCB	sr
Videx EC	Bristol-Myers Squibb	ec
Vivitrol	Cephalon	sr
Voltaren	Novartis	ec
Voltaren-XR	Novartis	sr
Vospire	Dava	sr
Vospire ER	Dava	sr
Votrient	GlaxoSmithKline	ec
We Mist LA	WE Pharmaceuticals	sr
We Mist II LA	WE Pharmaceuticals	sr
Wellbid-D	Prasco	sr
Wellbid-D 1200	Prasco	sr
Wellbutrin SR	GlaxoSmithKline	sr
Wellbutrin XL	GlaxoSmithKline	sr
Wobenzym N	Marlyn	ec
Woman's Wellbeing Menopause Relief	Consumer Choice	sr
Xanax XR	Pfizer	sr
Xedec II	Cypress	sr
Xpect-AT	Hawthorn	sr
Xpect-HC	Hawthorn	sr
Xpect PE	Hawthorn	sr
Zenpep	Eurand	ec
Zmax	Pfizer	sr
Zorprin	Par	sr
Zotex-12D	Vertical	sr
Zyban	GlaxoSmithKline	sr
Zyflo CR	Critical Therapeutics	sr
Zyrtec-D	McNeil Consumer	sr

Enteric-coated = ec **Slow-release = sr**

SUGAR-FREE PRODUCTS

The following is a selection of products by therapeutic category that contain no sugar. When recommending these products to diabetic patients, keep in mind that many may contain sorbitol, alcohol, or other sources of carbohydrates. This list is not all-inclusive and generics and alternate brands may be available. Check product labeling for a current listing of inactive ingredients.

Analgesics

Product	Manufacturer
Addaprin Tablets	Dover
Aminofen Tablets	Dover
Aminofen Max Tablets	Dover
Aspirtab Tablets	Dover
Back Pain-Off Tablets ‡	Medique
Buffasal Tablets	Dover
Dyspel Tablets	Dover
I-Prin Tablets ‡	Medique
Medi-Seltzer Effervescent Tablets	Medique
Methadose Sugar Free Oral Concentrate	Mallinckrodt
Ms.-Aid Tablets ‡	Medique
Children's Silapap Liquid	Silarx

Antacids/Antiflatulants

Product	Manufacturer
Alcalak Chewable Tablets*† ‡ §	Medique
Dimacid Chewable Tablets	Otis Clapp & Son
Diotame Chewable Tablets*† ‡ §	Medique
Neutralin Tablets	Dover
Pepto-Bismol Caplets † ‡	Procter & Gamble
Tums E-X Sugar Free Tablets* §	GlaxoSmithKline Consumer

Anti-asthmatic/Respiratory Agents

Product	Manufacturer
Jay-Phyl Syrup	JayMac

Antidiarrheals

Product	Manufacturer
Diarrest Tablets	Dover
Imogen Liquid	Pharm Generic

Blood Modifiers/Iron Preparations

Product	Manufacturer
I.L.X. B-12 Elixir	Kenwood
Nephro-Fer Tablets ‡	Rugby

Corticosteroid

Product	Manufacturer
Pediapred Solution* §	UCB

Cough/Cold/Allergy Preparations

Product	Manufacturer
Alacol DM Syrup	Ballay
Alacol Solution	Ballay
Anaplex DMX Syrup	ECR
Andehist DM NR Syrup	Cypress
Andehist NR Syrup	Cypress
Aquatab C Tablets	Deston
Aridex Solution	Gentex
Baltussin Solution	Ballay
Children's Benadryl-D Allergy & Sinus Liquid*† §	Johnson & Johnson
Bromhist-DM Solution	Cypress
Bromhist Pediatric Solution	Cypress
Bromphenex DM Solution*† §	Breckenridge
Bromplex DM Solution*† §	Prasco
Broncotron Liquid	Seyer Pharmatec
Broncotron-D Suspension	Seyer Pharmatec
B-Tuss Liquid	Blansett
Carbaphen 12 Ped Suspension	Gil
Carbaphen 12 Suspension	Gil
Carbatuss-12 Suspension	GM
Carbatuss-CL Solution	GM
Carbetaplex Liquid* §	Breckenridge
Carbofed DM Liquid	Hi-Tech
Carbofed DM Syrup	Hi-Tech
Cardec DM Syrup	Qualitest
Cardec Solution	Qualitest
Cetafen Cough & Cold Tablets ‡	Hart Health and Safety
Cetafen Cold Tablets ‡	Hart Health and Safety
Cheratussin DAC Liquid	Qualitest
Chlordex GP Syrup	Cypress
Codal-DM Syrup	Cypress
Coldcough PD Syrup* §	Breckenridge
Coldcough Syrup* §	Breckenridge
Coldonyl Tablets	Dover
Corfen DM Solution	Cypress
Crantex Syrup	Breckenridge
Dacex-DM Solution	Cypress
Dallergy Drops*† §	Laser
De-Chlor DM Solution	Cypress
De-Chlor DR Solution	Cypress
De-Chlor HD Solution	Cypress
Despec Liquid	International Ethical
Despec-SF Liquid	International Ethical
Diabetic Tussin	Health Care Products
Diabetic Tussin Allergy Relief Tablets	Health Care Products
Diabetic Tussin Cold & Flu Gelcaplets †	Health Care Products
Diabetic Tussin DM Liquid §	Health Care Products
Diabetic Tussin EX Liquid §	Health Care Products
Diabetic Tussin Solution§	Health Care Products
Diphen Capsules ‡	Medique
Donatussin Drops*† §	Laser
Double Tussin DM Liquid	Reese
Duratuss DM Elixir*† ‡ §	Victory
Dytan-CS Tablets	Hawthorn
Emagrin Forte Tablets	Otis Clapp & Son
Emagrin Tablets	Otis Clapp & Son
Endacof-PD Solution † §	Larken Laboratories
Ganidin NR Liquid	Cypress
Gani-Tuss NR Liquid	Cypress
Gani-Tuss-DM NR Liquid	Cypress
Genebronco-D Liquid	Pharm Generic
Genecof-HC Liquid	Pharm Generic
Genecof-XP Liquid	Pharm Generic
Genedel Syrup	Pharm Generic
Genedotuss-DM Liquid	Pharm Generic
Genelan Liquid	Pharm Generic
Genetuss-2 Liquid	Pharm Generic

* Contains sorbitol.

† May contain other sugar alcohols (eg, glycerol, isomalt, maltitol, mannitol, xylitol).

‡ May contain other sources of carbohydrates (eg, cellulose, lactose, maltodextrin, polydextrose, starch).

§ May contain natural or artificial flavors.

Genexpect DM Liquid	Pharm Generic
Genexpect SF Liquid	Pharm Generic
Gilphex TR Tablets	Gil
Giltuss Liquid§	Gil
Giltuss Ped-C Solution§	Gil
Giltuss Pediatric Liquid§	Gil
Giltuss TR Tablets	Gil
Guiadex DM Liquid*† §	Breckenridge
Halotussin AC Liquid	Axiom
Halotussin DAC Solution	Axiom
Lodrane D Suspension	ECR
Lohist-PD Solution*† §	Larken
Marcof Expectorant Syrup	Marnel
Metanx Tablets‡	Pamlab
Nalex DH Liquid	Blansett
Nalex A Liquid	Blansett
Neo DM Drops*† §	Laser
Neo DM Syrup*† §	Laser
Neotuss-D Liquid † §	A.G. Marin
Neotuss S/F Liquid † §	A.G. Marin
Niferex Elixir* ‡ §	Ther-Rx
Norel DM Liquid*† §	U.S. Pharmaceutical
Nycoff Tablets	Dover
Organidin NR Liquid † §	Meda
Organidin NR Tablets ‡	Meda
Phanasin Syrup	Pharmakon
Phanasin Diabetic Choice Syrup	Pharmakon
Phanatuss Syrup	Pharmakon
Phanatuss DM Diabetic Choice Syrup	Pharmakon
Phanatuss-HC Diabetic Choice Solution	Pharmakon
Phena-HC Solution	GM
Phenabid Tablets	Gil
Phenabid DM Tablets	Gil
Phena-S 12 Suspension	GM
Phena-S Liquid	GM
Poly Hist DM	Poly
Poly Hist PD Solution	Poly
Prolex DM Liquid	Blansett
Quintex Syrup	Qualitest
Rescon-DM Liquid* §	Capellon
Rondec DM*†	Sciele
Ru-Tuss DM Syrup*† §	Carwin
Safetussin Liquid	Kramer
Scot-Tussin Diabetes CF Liquid	Scot-Tussin
Scot-Tussin DM Cough Chasers Lozenge	Scot-Tussin
Scot-Tussin DM Maximum Strength	Scot-Tussin
Scot-Tussin Diabetes CF	Scot-Tussin
Scot-Tussin Expectorant Solution	Scot-Tussin
Scot-Tussin Senior Solution	Scot-Tussin
Siladryl Allergy Solution* §	Silarx
Sildec Syrup*† §	Silarx
Sildec DM Syrup*† §	Silarx
Sildec PE-DM Syrup*† §	Silarx
Sildec-PE Syrup*† §	Silarx
Siltussin DAS Liquid*† §	Silarx
Siltussin DM DAS Cough Formula Syrup*† §	Silarx
Siltussin SA Liquid*† §	Silarx
Statuss Green Liquid* §	Magna
Children's Sudafed PE Cough & Cold Liquid*† §	Pfizer
Children's Sudafed Nasal Decongestant Liquid*† §	Pfizer
Sudanyl Tablets	Dover
Sudatuss-SF Liquid	Pharm Generic Developers
Supress DX Pediatric Drops † §	Kramer-Novis
Suttar-SF Syrup	Gil
Tanacof XR Suspension*† ‡ §	Larken
Tusdec-DM Solution*† §	Cypress
Tusnel Solution	Llorens
Tussall Solution* §	Everett
Tussi-Pres Liquid † §	Kramer-Novis
Vazol Solution	Wraser
Z-Tuss DM Syrup † §	Magna
Ztuss Expectorant Solution* §	Magna

Fluoride Preparations

Fluor-A-Day Tablets*† §	Pharmascience
Fluor-A-Day Liquid	Pharmascience
Lozi-Flur Lozenge* §	Dreir
Sensodyne with Fluoride Cool Gel*† ‡ §	GlaxoSmithKline Consumer
Sensodyne Tartar Control with Whitening † ‡ §	GlaxoSmithKline Consumer
Sensodyne w/Fluoride Toothpaste Original Flavor*† ‡ §	GlaxoSmithKline Consumer

Laxatives

Benefiber Powder	Novartis
Citrucel Powder ‡ §	GlaxoSmithKline Consumer
Colace Liquid 1% Solution	Purdue Products
Fiber Choice Tablets* ‡ §	GlaxoSmithKline Consumer
Fibro-XL Capsules	Key
Genfiber Powder	Teva
Konsyl Easy Mix Formula Powder ‡	Konsyl
Konsyl Orange Powder ‡ §	Konsyl
Konsyl Powder ‡	Konsyl
Metamucil Smooth Texture Powder ‡	Procter & Gamble
Reguloid Powder Regular Flavor ‡	Rugby
Reguloid Powder Orange Flavor ‡ §	Rugby

Mouth/Throat Preparations

Cepacol Dual Relief Sore Throat Spray † §	Combe
Cepacol Maximum Strength Spray*† §	Combe
Cepacol Sore Throat + Coating Relief Lozenge † §	Combe
Cepacol Sore Throat Lozenges † §	Combe
Cheracol Sore Throat Spray †	Lee
Chloraseptic Spray*† §	Prestige
Diabetic Tussin Cough Drops † §	Health Care Products
Fisherman's Friend Sugar Free Mint Lozenges*	Mentholatum
Fresh N Free Liquid	Geritrex
Larynex Lozenges	Dover
Listerine Pocketpaks Film ‡ §	Johnson & Johnson
Luden's Sugar Free & Wild Cherry Throat Drops † §	Johnson Johnson
Medikoff Sugar Free Drops †	Medique
N'ice Lozenges* §	Heritage/Insight
Oragesic Solution* §	Parnell
Oragel Dry Mouth Moisturizing Gel*† ‡ §	Del
Orajel Dry Mouth Moisturizing Spray † ‡ §	Del
Sepasoothe Lozenges* ‡ §	Medique
Thorets Maximum Strength Lozenges	Otis Clapp & Son
Triaminic Sore Throat Spray*† §	Novartis

Vitamins/Minerals/Supplements

Action Tabs Made for Men ‡	Action Labs
Adaptoside R+R For Stress Liquid	HVS
Adaptoside R+R For Acute Stress Liquid	HVS
Alamag Tablets*† ‡ §	Medique
Alcalak Tablets*† ‡	Medique
Apetigen Elixir*†	Kramer-Novis
Apptrim Capsules	Physician Therapeutics

Product	Manufacturer
Apptrim-D Capsules	Physician Therapeutics
Bevitamel Tablets	Westlake
Biosode Liquid	HVS
Biotect Plus Caplet	Gil
Bugs Bunny Complete	Bayer
C&M Caps-375 Capsules	Key
Cal-Cee Tablets	Key
Calcet Plus Tablets	Mission Pharmacal
Calcimin-300 Tablets	Key
Cal-Mint Chewable Tablets*† ‡	Freeda Vitamins
Cerefolin NAC Tablets	Pamlab
Chromacaps ‡	Key
Delta D3 Tablets ‡	Freeda Vitamins
Detoxosode Liquids	HVS
Dexfol Tablets ‡	Rising
DHEA Capsules	ADH Health Products
Diatx ZN Tablets ‡	Pamlab
Dimacid Tablets	Otis Clapp & Son
Diucaps Capsules	Legere
DL-Phen-500 Capsules	Key
Enterex Diabetic Liquid ‡	Victus
Evening Primose Oil Capsules †	National Vitamin
Ex-L Tablets Tablets ‡	Key
Extress Tablets	Key
Eyetamins Tablets ‡	Rexall Consumer
Fem-Cal Citrate Tablets ‡	Freeda Vitamins
Fem-Cal Tablets ‡	Freeda Vitamins
Fem-Cal Plus Tablets	Freeda Vitamins
Ferrocite Plus Tablets ‡	Breckenridge
Folacin-800 Tablets ‡	Key
Folbee Plus Tablets ‡	Breckenridge
Folbee Tablets ‡	Breckenridge
Folplex 2.2 Tablets ‡	Breckenridge
Foltx Tablets ‡	Pamlab
Gabadone Capsules	Physician Therapeutics
Gram-O-Leci Tablets*† ‡	Freeda Vitamins
Herbal Slim Complex Products Capsules	ADH Health
Hypertensa Capsules ‡	Physician Therapeutics
Lynae Calcium/Vitamin C Chewable Tablets	Boscogen
Lynae Chondroitin/ Glucosamine Capsules	Boscogen
Lynae Ginse-Cool Chewable Tablets	Boscogen
Mag-Ox 400 Tablets	Blaine
Mag-SR Tablets ‡	Cypress
Mag-SR Plus Calcium Tablets ‡	Cypress
Magimin Tablets ‡	Key
Maginex Tablets ‡	Logan
Magnacaps Capsules ‡	Key
Mangimin Tablets ‡	Key
Medi-Lyte Tablets ‡	Medique
Metanx Tablets ‡	Pamlab
Multi-Delyn with Iron Liquid †	Silarx
Natelle C Tablets	Azur
Natelle Tablets	Azur
Nephro-Fer Tablets ‡	Rugby
New Life Hair Tablets ‡	Rexall Consumer
Niferex Elixir* ‡ §	Ther-Rx
Nutrisure OTC Tablets	Westlake
Nutrivit Solution*† §	Llorens
Ob Complete Tablets	Vertical
O-Cal Fa Tablets ‡	Pharmics
Os-Cal 500 + D Tablets ‡	GlaxoSmithKline Consumer
Powervites Tablets ‡	Green Turtle Bay Vitamin
Prostaplex Herbal Complex Capsules	ADH Health Products
Protect Plus Liquid	Gil
Protect Plus Liquid NR Softgels	Gil
Pulmona Capsules	Physician Therapeutics
Quintabs-M Tablets ‡	Freeda Vitamins
Replace Capsules ‡	Key
Replace w/o Iron Capsules ‡	Key
Resource Arginaid Powder ‡	Novartis Nutrition
Ribo-100 T.D. Capsules	Key
Samolinic Softgels †	Key
Sea Omega 30 Softgels †	Rugby
Sea Omega 50 Softgels †	Rugby
Sentra AM Capsules	Physician Therapeutics
Sentra PM Capsules	Physician Therapeutics
Soy Care for Menopause Capsules	Inverness Medical
Span C Tablets ‡	Freeda Vitamins
Strovite Forte Syrup	Everett
Sunnie Tablets	Green Turtle Bay Vitamin
Sunvite Tablets † ‡	Rexall Naturalist
Super Dec B100 Tablets ‡	Freeda Vitamins
Super Quints B-50 Tablets ‡	Freeda Vitamins
Supervite Liquid	Seyer Pharmatec
Suplevit Liquid	Gil
Theramine Capsules	Physician Therapeutics
Triamin Tablets	Key
Triamino Tablets* ‡	Freeda Vitamins
Ultramino Powder	Freeda Vitamins
Uro-Mag Capsules ‡	Blaine
Vitafol Tablets † ‡	Everett
Vitamin C/Rose Hips Tablets	ADH Health Products
Vitrim Jr Chewable Tablets † ‡ §	Mason Vitamins
Xtramins Tablets	Key
Yohimbe Power Max 1500 for Women Tablets ‡	Action Labs
Ze Plus Softgel	Everett

Miscellaneous

Product	Manufacturer
Acidoll Capsules	Key
Alka-Gest Tablets	Key
Bicitra Solution † §	Ortho-McNeil
Cafergot Tablets ‡	Sandoz
Cytra-2 Solution* §	Cypress
Cytra-K Solution* §	Cypress
Cytra-K Crystals	Cypress
Melatin Tablets ‡	Mason Vitamins
Namenda Solution*† §	Forest
Polycitra-K Crystals	Ortho-McNeil
Prosed/DS Tablets ‡	Ferring
Questran Light Powder ‡ §	Par
Soltamox Solution*† ‡	Cytogen

* Contains sorbitol.

† May contain other sugar alcohols (eg, glycerol, isomalt, maltitol, mannitol, xylitol).

‡ May contain other sources of carbohydrates (eg, cellulose, lactose, maltodextrin, polydextrose, starch).

§ May contain natural or artificial flavors.

ALCOHOL-FREE PRODUCTS

The following is a selection of alcohol-free products grouped by therapeutic category. This list is not comprehensive. Generic and alternate brands may exist. Always check product labeling for definitive information on specific ingredients.

Analgesics

Product	Manufacturer
Advil Children's Suspension	Wyeth Consumer
APAP Elixir	Bio-Pharm
Motrin Children's Suspension	McNeil Consumer
Motrin Infants' Suspension	McNeil Consumer
Silapap Infant's Drops	Silarx
Tylenol Children's Suspension	McNeil Consumer
Tylenol Extra Strength Solution	McNeil Consumer
Tylenol Infant's Suspension	McNeil Consumer

Antiasthmatic Agent

Product	Manufacturer
Dy-G Liquid	Cypress

Anticonvulsant

Product	Manufacturer
Zarontin Syrup	Pfizer

Antiviral Agent

Product	Manufacturer
Epivir Oral Solution	GlaxoSmithKline

Cough/Cold/Allergy Preparations

Product	Manufacturer
Accuhist PDX Drops Solution	Pediamed
Accuhist PDX Syrup	Pediamed
Alacol Solution	Ballay
Alacol DM Syrup	Ballay
Allanhist PDX Syrup	Allan
Andehist DM NR Syrup	Cypress
Andehist NR Syrup	Cypress
Aridex Solution	Gentex
Aridex-D Solution	Gentex
Baltussin Solution	Ballay
Banophen Elixir	Major
Benadryl Allergy Solution	Pfizer Consumer
Benadryl-D Allergy & Sinus Children's Solution	Johnson & Johnson Consumer
Bromaline Syrup	Rugby
Bromaline DM Elixir	Rugby
Bromhist PDX Solution	Cypress
Bromhist Pediatric Solution	Cypress
Bromhist-DM Pediatric Syrup	Cypress
Bromhist-DM Solution	Cypress
Bromhist-NR Solution	Cypress
Bromhist-PDX Syrup	Cypress
Bromphenex DM Solution	Breckenridge
Bromphenex HD Solution	Breckenridge
Bromplex DM Solution	Prasco
Bromplex HD Solution	Prasco
Bromtuss DM Solution	Breckenridge
Broncotron Liquid	Seyer Pharmatec
Broncotron-D Suspension	Seyer Pharmatec
B-Tuss Liquid	Blansett
Carbaphen 12 Ped Suspension	Gil
Carbaphen 12 Suspension	Gil
Carbatuss Liquid	GM
Carbatuss-12 Suspension	GM
Carbatuss-CL Solution	GM
Carbetaplex Solution	Breckenridge
Carbetaplex TS Suspension	Breckenridge
Carbofed DM Syrup	Hi-Tech Pharmacal
Cardec DM Solution	Qualitest
Children's Dimetapp Cold & Allergy Solution	Wyeth Consumer
Children's Dimetapp Long Acting Cough Plus Cold Solution	Wyeth Consumer
Children's Dimetapp Nighttime Flu Syrup	Wyeth Consumer
Children's Dimetapp DM Cold & Cough Solution	Wyeth Consumer
Children's Mucinex Cold Solution	Adams
Children's Mucinex Cough Syrup	Adams
Children's Mucinex Syrup	Adams
Chlordex GP Syrup	Cypress
Chlor-Mes D Solution	Cypress
Codal-DM Syrup	Cypress
Complete Allergy Elixir	Cardinal Health
Corfen DM Solution	Cypress
Coughtuss Solution	Breckenridge
Crantex HC Syrup	Breckenridge
Crantex Syrup	Breckenridge
Creomulsion Cough Syrup	Summit Industries
Creomulsion for Children Syrup	Summit Industries
Dacex-DM Solution	Cypress
Dallergy Solution	Laser
De-Chlor DM Solution	Cypress
De-Chlor DR Solution	Cypress
Dehistine Syrup	Cypress
Despec Liquid	International Ethical
Dex PC Syrup	Boca Pharmacal
Diabetic Tussin Allergy Relief Liquid	Health Care Products
Diabetic Tussin Cough Lozenges	Health Care Products
Diabetic Tussin Night Time Formula Solution	Health Care Products
Diabetic Tussin Solution	Health Care Products
Diabetic Tussin DM Solution	Health Care Products
Diabetic Tussin DM Maximum Strength Liquid	Health Care Products
Diabetic Tussin EX Liquid	Health Care Products
Dimetapp Decongestant Pediatric Drops	Wyeth Consumer
Donatussin Solution	Laser
Donatussin DC Syrup	Laser
Donatussin DM Solution	Laser
Donatussin DM Suspension	Laser
Donatussin DM Syrup	Laser
Double-Tussin DM Liquid	Reese
Duratuss AC12 Suspension	Victory
Duratuss DM Solution	Victory
Duratuss DM12 Suspension	Victory
Dynatuss EX Syrup	Breckenridge
Dynatuss HC Solution	Breckenridge
Father John's Medicine Plus Drops	Oakhurst
Ganidin NR Liquid	Cypress
Gani-Tuss NR Liquid	Cypress
Gani-Tuss-DM NR Liquid	Cypress
Genebronco-D Liquid	PGD
Genecof-HC Liquid	PGD
Genecof-XP Liquid	PGD
Genecof-XP Syrup	PGD
Genedel Syrup	PGD
Genedotuss-DM Liquid	PGD
Genepatuss Liquid	PGD
Genetuss-2 Liquid	PGD
Genexpect-DM Liquid	PGD
Genexpect-PE Liquid	PGD
Genexpect-SF Liquid	PGD
Giltuss Liquid	Gil
Giltuss Pediatric Liquid	Gil
Giltuss Ped-C Solution	Gil
H-C Tussive Syrup	Vintage
Histacol DM Pediatric Syrup	Breckenridge
Histinex HC Syrup	Ethex
Histinex PV Syrup	Ethex
Hydramine Elixir	Teva
Hydro-Tussin HC Syrup	Ethex
Hydro-Tussin HD Liquid	Ethex
Hydro-Tussin XP Syrup	Ethex
Jaycof Expectorant Syrup	Pharmakon
Jaycof-HC Liquid	Pharmakon
Jaycof-XP Syrup	Pharmakon
Lodrane D Suspension	ECR
Lohist D Syrup	Larken
Lohist DM Syrup	Larken
Marcof Expectorant Syrup	Marnel
M-Clear Jr Solution	McNeil, R.A.
M-Clear Solution	McNeil, R.A.
Medi-Brom Elixir	Medicine Shoppe
Mintuss G Syrup	Breckenridge
Mintuss MR Syrup	Breckenridge
Mintuss MS Syrup	Breckenridge
Mintuss NX Solution	Breckenridge
Motrin Cold Children's Suspension	McNeil Consumer
Myhist-DM Solution	Larken
Myhist-PD Solution	Larken
Nalex DH Liquid	Blansett Pharmacal
Nalex-A Liquid	Blansett Pharmacal
Nasop Suspension	Hawthorn
Neotuss S/F Liquid	A.G. Marin
Neotuss-D Liquid	A.G. Marin
Norel DM Liquid	U.S. Pharmaceutical
Organidin NR Liquid	Meda
PediaCare Cough + Cold Children's Liquid	Johnson & Johnson Consumer
PediaCare Decongestant & Cough Liquid	Johnson & Johnson Consumer
PediaCare Long-Acting Cough Solution	Johnson & Johnson Consumer
PediaCare Multi-Symptom Cold Liquid	Johnson & Johnson Consumer
PediaCare Nightrest Liquid	Johnson & Johnson Consumer
Pediahist DM Syrup	Boca Pharmacal
Pedia-Relief Liquid	Major
Phanasin Diabetic Choice Syrup	Pharmakon
Phanasin Syrup	Pharmakon
Phanatuss Syrup	Pharmakon
Phanatuss DM Diabetic Choice Syrup	Pharmakon

Product	Manufacturer
Phanatuss-HC Diabetic Choice Solution	Pharmakon
Phena-HC Solution	GM
Phena-S Liquid	GM
Phena-S 12 Suspension	GM
Poly Hist DM Solution	Poly
Poly Hist HC Solution	Poly
Poly Hist PD Solution	Poly
Poly-Tussin Solution	Poly
Poly-Tussin AC	Poly
Poly-Tussin DHC	Poly
Poly-Tussin DM Syrup	Poly
Poly-Tussin HD Syrup	Poly
Poly-Tussin XP Solution	Poly
Pro-Clear Solution	Pro-Pharma
Prolex DM Liquid	Blansett Pharmacal
Pro-Red Solution	Pro-Pharma
Q-Tussin Liquid	Qualitest
Q-Tussin PE Liquid	Qualitest
Rescon-DM Liquid	Capellon
Rescon-GG Liquid	Capellon
Rindal HD Liquid	Breckenridge
Rindal HD Plus Solution	Breckenridge
Robitussin Chest Congestion Syrup	Wyeth Consumer
Robitussin Cough & Allergy Solution	Wyeth Consumer
Robitussin Cough & Cold CF Syrup	Wyeth Consumer
Robitussin Cough, Cold & Flu Nighttime Solution	Wyeth Consumer
Robitussin Cough & Congestion Liquid	Wyeth Consumer
Robitussin Cough DM Syrup	Wyeth Consumer
Robitussin Head & Chest Congestion PE Syrup	Wyeth Consumer
Robitussin Pediatric Cough & Cold CF Solution	Wyeth Consumer
Robitussin Pediatric Cough & Cold Long-Acting Solution	Wyeth Consumer
Robitussin Pediatric Night Relief Liquid	Wyeth Consumer
Rondec Solution	Sciele
Rondec DM Drops	Sciele
Rondec DM Solution	Sciele
Ru-Tuss DM Solution	Carwin
Scot-Tussin Diabetes CF Liquid	Scot-Tussin
Scot-Tussin DM Solution	Scot-Tussin
Scot-Tussin Expectorant Solution	Scot-Tussin
Scot-Tussin Original Solution	Scot-Tussin
Scot-Tussin Senior Solution	Scot-Tussin
Siladryl Allergy Solution	Silarx
Sildec Syrup	Silarx
Sildec-DM Syrup	Silarx
Sildec-PE Solution	Silarx
Sildec PE-DM Solution	Silarx
Siltussin DAS Liquid	Silarx
Siltussin DM DAS Cough Formula Syrup	Silarx
Siltussin SA Syrup	Silarx
Simply Cough Liquid	McNeil Consumer
Sudafed Children's Cold & Cough Solution	Johnson & Johnson
Sudafed Children's Solution	Johnson & Johnson
Sudatuss DM Syrup	PGD
Sudatuss-2 Liquid	PGD
Sudatuss-SF Liquid	PGD
Triant-HC Solution	Hawthorn
TriTuss Solution	Everett
Tusdec-DM Solution	Cypress
Tusnel Pediatric Solution	Llorens
Tusnel Solution	Llorens
Tussafed-EX Syrup	Everett
Tussafed-EX Pediatric Drops	Everett
Tussafed-HC Syrup	Everett
Tussafed-HCG Solution	Everett
Tussall Solution	Everett
Tussinate Syrup	Pediamed
Tussi-Organidin DM NR Solution	Victory
Tussi-Organidin DM-S NR Solution	Victory
Tussi-Organidin NR Solution	Victory
Tussi-Organidin-S NR Solution	Victory
Tussi-Pres Liquid	Kramer-Novis
Tussi-Pres Pediatric Solution	Kramer-Novis
Tylenol Cold Children's Suspension	McNeil Consumer
Tylenol Cold Infants' Drops	McNeil Consumer
Tylenol Cold Plus Cough Children's Suspension	McNeil Consumer
Tylenol Cold Plus Cough Infants' Suspension	McNeil Consumer
Tylenol Flu Children's Suspension	McNeil Consumer
Tylenol Flu Night Time Max Strength Liquid	McNeil Consumer
Tylenol Sinus Children's Suspension	McNeil Consumer
Vazol Solution	Wraser Pharm
Vicks 44E Pediatric Liquid	Procter & Gamble
Vicks 44M Pediatric Liquid	Procter & Gamble
Vicks Dayquil Multi-Symptom Liquid	Procter & Gamble
Vicks Nyquil Children's Liquid	Procter & Gamble
V-Tann Suspension	Breckenridge
Welltuss EXP Solution	Prasco
Z-Cof 12 DM Suspension	Zyber
Z-Cof 8 DM Suspension	Zyber
Z-Cof DM Solution	Zyber
Z-Cof DMX Solution	Zyber
Z-Cof HC Solution	Zyber
Z-Cof HCX Solution	Zyber
Z-Tuss DM Syrup	Magna

Ear/Nose/Throat Products

Product	Manufacturer
4-Way Saline Moisturizing Mist Spray	Bristol-Myers
Ayr Baby Saline Spray	Ascher
Bucalcide Spray	Seyer Pharmatec
Bucalsep Solution	Gil
Bucalsep Spray	Gil
Cheracol Sore Throat Spray	Lee
Fresh N Free Solution	Geritrex
Gly-Oxide Solution	GlaxoSmithKline
Larynex Lozenges	Dover
Listermint Solution	Johnson & Johnson Consumer
Nasal Moist Gel	Blairex
Orajel Baby Day & Night Gel	Del
Orajel Baby Nighttime Teething Pain Medicine Gel	Del
OraMagic Plus Powder	MPM Medical
OraMagicRx Powder	MPM Medical
Orasept Mouthwash/ Gargle Liquid	Pharmakon
Tanac Liquid	Del
Throto-Ceptic Spray	S.S.S.
Triaminic Sore Throat Spray	Novartis Consumer
Vicks Sinex Spray	P&G Company
Vicks Sinex 12 Hour Spray	P&G Company
Zilactin Baby Extra Strength Gel	Zila

Gastrointestinal Agents

Product	Manufacturer
Axid Solution	Braintree
Colidrops Pediatric Drops	A.G. Marin
Colace Solution	Purdue
Gas Relief Solution	Perrigo
Imogen Liquid	PGD
Kaodene NN Suspension	Pfeiffer
Kaopectate Advanced Formula Suspension	Pharmacia Consumer
Liqui-Doss Liquid	Ferndale
Mylicon Infants' Drops	Johnson & Johnson/Merck

Topical Products

Product	Manufacturer
Aloe Vesta 2-N-1 Antifungal Ointment	Convatec
Dermatone Lips N Face Protector Ointment	Dermatone
Dermatone Moisturizing Sunblock Cream	Dermatone
Dermatone Skin Protector Cream	Dermatone
Fleet Pain Relief Pads	Fleet
Fresh & Pure Douche Solution	Unico
Handclens Solution	Woodward
Joint-Ritis Maximum Strength Ointment	Naturopathic
Neutrogena Acne Wash Liquid	Neutrogena
Neutrogena Antiseptic Solution	Neutrogena
Neutrogena Clear Pore Gel	Neutrogena
Neutrogena T/Derm Liquid	Neutrogena
Neutrogena Toner Solution	Neutrogena
Podiclens Spray	Woodward
Sea Breeze Foaming Face Wash Gel	Clairol
Sportz Bloc Cream	Med-Derm
Therasoft Anti-Acne Cream	SFC
Therasoft Skin Protectant Cream	SFC
Tiger Balm Arthritis Rub Lotion	Prince of Peace

Vitamins/Minerals/Supplements

Product	Manufacturer
Adaptosode For Stress Liquid	HVS
Adaptosode R+R For Acute Stress Liquid	HVS
Apetigen Elixir	Kramer-Novis
Biosode Liquid	HVS
Detoxosode Products Liquid	HVS
Genesupp-500 Liquid	PGD
Genetect Plus Liquid	PGD
Multi-Delyn Liquid	Silarx
Multi-Delyn w/Iron Liquid	Silarx
Nutrivit Solution	Llorens
Poly-Vi-Sol Drops	Mead Johnson
Poly-Vi-Sol w/Iron Drops	Mead Johnson
Protect Plus Liquid	Gil
Strovite Forte Syrup	Everett
Supervite Liquid	Seyer Pharmatec
Suplevit Liquid	Gil
Tri-Vi-Sol w/Iron Drops	Mead Johnson
Vitafol Syrup	Everett

Miscellaneous

Product	Manufacturer
Cytra-2 Solution	Cypress
Cytra-K Solution	Cypress
Fluorinse Solution	Oral B
Namenda Solution	Forest
Primsol Solution	FSC

SULFITE-CONTAINING PRODUCTS

The following is a selection of products that contain sulfites, a common allergic trigger. Please remember, however, that the list is not comprehensive. Always check product labeling for definitive information on specific ingredients.

Product	Generic Name
Alphaquin HP	Hydroquinone
Amikacin Sulfate Injection	Amikacin sulfate
Amikin Injectable	Amikacin sulfate
Apokyn	Apomorphine hydrochloride
Aramine Injection	Metaraminol
Betagan Liquifilm	Levobunolol
Betagan Ophthalmic Solution, USP	Levobunolol hydrochloride
Campral (residual traces)	Acamprosate calcium
Corlopam Injection	Fenoldopam mesylate
Cortisporin Otic Solution	Hydrocortisone/neomycin sulfate/polymyxin B
Dilaudid Ampules, Dilaudid Tablets, Dilaudid Non-Sterile Powder	Hydromorphone
Dilaudid-HP Injection, Dilaudid-HP Lyophilized Powder 250 mg	Hydromorphone
Dilaudid Oral Liquid; Dilaudid Tablets - 2 mg, 4 mg, 8 mg	Hydromorphone
Dobutamine Injection	Dobutamine Injection
Dopamine HCl Injection	Dopamine HCl
Eldopaque Forte 4%	Hydroquinone
Eldoquin Forte 4%	Hydroquinone
EpiPen Auto-Injector	Epinephrine
EpiPen Jr. Auto-Injector	Epinephrine
EpiQuin Micro	Hydroquinone
Gentamicin Sulfate Injection	Gentamicin sulfate
Innohep Injection	Tinzaparin sodium
Ketoconazole Cream	Ketoconazole
Klaron Lotion 10%	Sodium sulfacetamide
Levophed Injection	Norepinephrine
Lustra	Hydroquinone
Lustra-AF	Hydroquinone
Marcaine Hydrochloride/ Epinephrine 1:200,000	Bupivacaine/epinephrine bitartrate
Melpaque HP	Hydroquinone
Melquin HP	Hydroquinone
Morphine Sulfate Injection	Morphine sulfate
Nizoral A-D	Ketoconazole
Norflex Injection	Orphenadrine
Novocain Hydrochloride for Spinal Anesthesia	Procaine
Nubain Ampules/ Multiple-Dose Vials	Nalbuphine
Nuquin HP	Hydroquinone
Orphenadrine Citrate Injection	Orphenadrine citrate
Perphenazine Tablets	Perphenazine
Phenergan Injection	Promethazine hydrochloride
Pred Forte Ophthalmic Solution	Prednisolone acetate
Pred Mild Ophthalmic Solution	Prednisolone acetate
Propofol Injectable Emulsion	Propofol
Rowasa Enema	Mesalamine
Sensorcaine with Epinephrine Injection	Bupivacaine/epinephrine bitartrate
Sensorcaine-MPF with Epinephrine Injection	Bupivacaine/epinephrine bitartrate
SMZ-TMP Concentrate	Trimethoprim/sulfamethoxazole
Solaquin Forte 4% Cream; 4% Gel	Hydroquinone
Soma Compound with Codeine	Carisoprodol/aspirin/codeine
Streptomycin Sulfate Injection	Streptomycin sulfate
Sulfamylon Cream	Mafenide acetate
Sumycin Suspension	Tetracycline hydrochloride
Talacen	Pentazocine hydrochloride/ acetaminophen
Tobramycin Sulfate Injection	Tobramycin sulfate
Torecan Injection	Triethylperazine maleate
Tri-Luma	Fluocinolone acetonide/ hydroquinone/tretinoin
Twinject Injection	Epinephrine
Tylenol with Codeine Tablets	Acetaminophen/codeine
Tylox Capsules	Acetaminophen/oxycodone
Vibramycin Syrup	Doxycycline calcium
Xibrom Ophthalmic	Bromfenac
Xylocaine with Epinephrine Injection	Lidocaine/epinephrine

DRUGS THAT MAY CAUSE PHOTOSENSITIVITY

The drugs in this table are known to cause photosensitivity in some individuals. Effects can range from itching, scaling, rash, and swelling to skin cancer, premature skin aging, skin and eye burns, cataracts, reduced immunity, blood vessel damage, and allergic reactions.

The list is not all-inclusive, and shows only representative brands of each generic. When in doubt, always check specific product labeling. Individuals should be advised to wear protective clothing and to apply sunscreens while taking the medications listed below.

Generic	Brand
Acamprosate calcium	Campral
Acetazolamide	Diamox
Acitretin	Soriatane
Acyclovir	Zovirax
Alendronate	Fosamax
Alendronate/cholecalciferol	Fosamax Plus D
Almotriptan malate	Axert
Amiloride HCl/HCTZ	
Aminolevulinic acid HCl	Levulan Kerastick
Amiodarone HCl	Cordarone, Pacerone
Amitriptyline HCl	
Amitryptyline HCl/ chlordiazepoxide	Limbitrol, Limbitrol DS
Amitryptyline HCl/ perphenazine	
Amlodipine/HCTZ/ valsartan	Exforge HCT
Amphetamine aspartate/ amphetamine sulfate/ dextroamphetamine saccharate/ dextroamphetamine sulfate	Adderall XR
Anagrelide HCl	Agrylin
Atenolol/chlorthalidone	Tenoretic
Atorvastatin	Lipitor
Atorvastatin/Amlodipine	Caduet
Atovaquone/proguanil HCl	Malarone
Azithromycin	Zithromax, Zmax
Benazepril HCl	Lotensin
Benazepril HCl/HCTZ	Lotensin HCT
Bendoflumethizaide/nadolol	Corzide
Benzoyl proxide/erythromycin	Benzamycin Pak
Bexarotene	Targretin
Bismuth subcitrate potassium/metronidazole/ tetracycline HCl	Pylera
Bismuth subsalicylate/ metronidazole/ tetracycline HCl	Helidac Therapy
Brompheniramine maleate/ carbetapentane citrate/ phenylephrine HCl	Vazotan Tannate
Brompheniramine maleate/ dextromethorphan HBr/ phenylephrine HCl	Alacol DM
Brompheniramine maleate/ phenylephrine HCl	Vazobid Tannate
Bupropion HBr	Aplenzin
Bupropion HCl	Budeprion SR, Budeprion XL, Buproban, Wellbutrin SR, Zyban
Candesartan Cilexetil/HCTZ	Atacand HCT
Capecitabine	Xeloda
Captopril	Capoten
Captopril/HCTZ	Capozide
Carbamazepine	Carbatrol, Epitol, Equetro, Tegretol, Tegretol-XR
Carbinoxamine maleate	Palgic
Carvedilol	Coreg
Carvedilol phosphate	Coreg CR
Celecoxib	Celebrex
Cetirizine HCl/ pseudoephedrine HCl	Zyrtec-D 12 Hour
Cevimeline HCl	Evoxac
Chloroquine Phosphate	Aralen
Chlorothiazide	Diuril
Chlorpheniramine maleate/ dextromethorphan HBr/ pseudoephedrine HCl	Atuss DS
Chlorpheniramine maleate/ pseudoephedrine HCl	Sudal-12
Chlorpheniramine tannate/ dextromethorphan tannate/ pseudoephedrine tannate	Dicel DM
Chlorpromazine HCl	
Chlorpropamide	Diabinese
Chlorthalidone	Thalitone
Chlorthalidone/clonidine HCl	Clorpres
Cidofovir	Vistide
Ciprofloxacin HCl	Cipro, Cipro XR, Proquin XR
Citalopram HBr	Celexa
Clemastine Fumarate	
Clindamycin phosphate	Clindagel
Clomipramine HCl	Anafranil
Clozapine	Clozaril, FazaClo
Codeine phosphate/ phenylephrine HCl/ promethazine HCl	Promethazine VC with Codeine
Codeine phosphate/ promethazine HCl	Promethazine with Codeine
Cyclobenzaprine HCl	Flexeril
Cyproheptadine HCl	
Dacarbazine	DTIC-Dome
Demeclocycline HCl	Declomycin
Desipramine HCl	Norpramin
Dextromethorphan HBR/ Promethazine HCl	Dextromethorphan HBR/ Promethazine HCl
Diclofenac potassium	Cataflam, Zipsor
Diclofenac sodium	
Diclofenac sodium/ misoprostol	Arthrotec
Diflunisal	
Diltiazem HCl	Cardizem LA, Tiazac
Diphenhydramine HCl	Benadryl
Divalproex sodium	Depakote, Depakote ER
Doxepin HCl	Sinequan
Doxorubicin HCl	
Doxycycline	Oracea
Doxycycline hyclate	Doryx, Periostat
Duloxetine HCl	Cymbalta Delayed-Release
Enalapril maleate	
Enalapril maleate/felodipine	
Enalapril maleate/HCTZ	
Enalaprilat	Enalaprilat
Epirubicin HCl	Ellence
Eprosartan mesylate/HCTZ	Teveten HCT
Erythromycin ethylsuccinate/ sulfisoxazole acetyl	
Escitalopram oxalate	Lexapro
Esomeprazole magnesium	Nexium
Esomeprazole sodium	Nexium I.V.
Estazolam	
Estradiol	Elestrin
Estradiol cypionate	Depo- Estradiol
Ethinyl Estradiol/ Norelgestromin	Ortho Evra
Ethionamide	Trecator
Etodolac, Etodolac ER	
Ezetimibe/simvastatin	Vytorin
Feboxostat	Uloric
Felbamate	Felbatol
Fenofibrate	Antara, Lipofen, Lofibra, Tricor, Triglide
Floxuridine	Sterile FUDR for Intra-Arterial Infusion
Flucytosine	Ancobon
Fluorouracil	Efudex
Fluoxetine HCl	Prozac, Sarafem
Fluoxetine/Olanzapine	Symbyax
Fluphenazine HCl	
Flurbiprofen	Ansaid
Flutamide	Eulexin
Fluvoxamine maleate	
Fosinopril sodium	Monopril
Fosinopril sodium/HCTZ	
Fosphenytoin	Cerebyx
Furosemide	Lasix
Gabapentin	Neurontin
Gemfibrozil	Lopid
Gemifloxacin mesylate	Factive
Gentamicin sulfate	
Glatiramer acetate	Copaxone
Glimepiride/pioglitazone HCl	Duetact
Glimeperide	Amaryl
Glimeperide/ rosiglitazone maleate	Avandaryl
Glipizide	Glucotrol
Glyburide	DiaBeta, Glynase PresTab, Micronase
Griseofulvin	Grifulvin V
Haloperidol decanoate	Haldol Decanoate
Haloperidol lactate	Haldol
Hexachlorophene	pHisoHex Detergent Cleanser
HCTZ	
HCTZ/aliskiren hemifumarate	Tekturna HCT
HCTZ/bisoprolol fumarate	Ziac
HCTZ/irbesartan	Avalide
HCTZ/lisinopril	Prinzide, Zestoretic
HCTZ/losartan potassium	Hyzaar
HCTZ/methyldopa	
HCTZ/metoprolol succinate	Dutoprol
HCTZ/metoprolol tartrate	Lopressor HCT

Generic	Brand
HCTZ/moexipril HCl	Uniretic
HCTZ/propranolol HCl	Inderide
HCTZ/quinapril HCl	Accuretic
HCTZ/spironolactone	Aldactazide
HCTZ/telmisartan	Micardis HCT
HCTZ/triamterene	Dyazide, Maxzide
HCTZ/valsartan	Diovan HCT
Hydroxychloroquine sulfate	Plaquenil
Ibuprofen	Motrin
Imatinib mesylate	Gleevec
Imipramine HCl	Tofranil
Imipramine pamoate	Tofranil-PM
Indapamide	Indapamide
Interferon alfa-2b	Intron A
Interferon alfa-n3	Alferon-N
Interferon beta-1a	Avonex
Inferferon beta-1b	Betaseron
Isocarboxazid	Marplan
Isoniazid/ pyrazinamide/rifampin	Rifater
Isotretinoin	Accutane, Amnesteem, Claravis, Sotret
Itraconazole	Sporanox
Ketoprofen	Ketoprofen
Ketorolac tromethamine	Toradol
Lamotrigine	Lamictal, Lamictal XR
Lansoprazole/naproxen	Prevacid NapraPAC 500
Leuprolide acetate	Lupron, Lupron Depot
Levofloxacin	Levaquin
Lisinopril	Prinivil, Zestril
Losartan potassium	Cozaar
Lovastatin	Altoprev, Mevacor
Maprotiline HCl, USP	
Mefenamic acid	Ponstel
Mesalamine	Pentasa
Methotrexate	
Methyclothiazide	
Methyl aminolevulinate HCl	Metvixia
Metolazone	Zaroxolyn
Metoprolol succinate	Toprol-XL
Metoprolol tartrate	Lopressor
Minocycline HCl	Dynacin, Minocin, Solodyn
Mirtazapine	Remeron, RemeronSolTab
Moexipril HCl	Univasc
Moxifloxacin HCl	Avelox
Nabilone	Cesamet
Nabumetone	
Naproxen	EC-Naprosyn, Naprosyn
Naproxen sodium	Anaprox, Anaprox DS, Naprelan
Naratriptan HCl	Amerge
Nefazodone HCl	Nefazodone HCl
Nifedipine	Adalat CC, Nifediac CC, Nifedical XL, Procardia, Procardia XL
Nilotinib HCl monohydrate	Tasigna
Nisoldipine	Sular
Norfloxacin	Noroxin
Nortriptyline HCl	Pamelor
Ofloxacin	Floxin
Olanzapine	Zyprexa, Zyprexa ZYDIS
Olsalazine sodium	Dipentum
Omeprazole magnesium	Prilosec
Omeprazole/ sodium bicarbonate	Zegerid
Oxaprozin	Daypro, Daypro Alta
Oxcarbazepine	Trileptal
Paclitaxel	Abraxane
Panitumumab	Vectibix
Pantoprazole sodium	Protonix
Paroxetine HCl	Paxil, Paxil CR
Paroxetine mesylate	Pexeva
Pentosan polysulfate sodium	Elmiron
Perphenazine	Perphenazine
Phenylephrine HCl/ promethazine HCl	Promethazine VC
Pilocarpine HCl	Salagen
Pimozide	Orap
Poly-L-lactic acid	Sculptra
Porfimer sodium	Photofrin
Pramipexole DiHCl	Mirapex
Pravastatin sodium	Pravachol
Pregabalin	Lyrica
Prochlorperazine	Compro Suppositories
Promethazine HCl	Phenadoz, Phenergan, Promethegan
Protriptyline HCl	Vivactil
Pyrazinamide	
Quetiapine fumarate	Seroquel
Quinapril HCl	Accupril
Quinidine gluconate	
Quinidine sulfate	
Quinine sulfate	Qualaquin
Ramipril	Altace
Rasagiline mesylate	Azilect
Riluzole	Rilutek
Ritonavir	Norvir
Rizatriptan benzoate	Maxalt, Maxalt-MLT
Ropinirole HCl	Requip
Saquinavir mesylate	Invirase
Selegiline	Emsam Transdermal System
Selegiline HCl	Eldepryl
Sertraline HCl	Zoloft
Sibutramine HCl	Meridia
Sildenafil citrate	Viagra
Simvastatin	Zocor
Sotalol HCl	Betapace, Betapace AF, Sorine
Sulfamethoxazole/ trimethoprim	Bactrim, Bactrim DS, Septra, Septra DS, Sulfatrim
Sulfasalazine	Azulfidine, Azulfidine EN-tabs
Sulindac	Clinoril
Sumatriptan	Imitrex Nasal Spray
Sumatriptan succinate	Imitrex
Tacrolimus	Prograf, Protopic
Tetracycline HCl	Sumycin
Thalidomide	Thalomid
Thioridazine HCl	Thioridazine HCl
Thiothixene	Navane
Tiagabine HCl	Gabitril
Tigecycline	Tygacil
Tipranavir	Aptivus Oral Solution
Tolazamide	
Tolbutamide	
Topiramate	Topamax
Tretinoin	Avita, Retin-A
Triamcinolone acetonide	Azmacort Inhalation Aerosol
Triamterene	Dyrenium
Trifluoperazine HCl	Trifluoperazine HCl
Trimipramine maleate	Surmontil
Valacyclovir HCl	Valtrex Caplets
Valproate sodium	Depacon
Valproic acid	Depakene, Stavzor
Vardenafil HCl	Levitra
Varenicline	Chantix
Venlafaxine HCl	Effexor, Effexor XR
Verteporfin	Visudyne
Vibramycin calcium	Vibramycin Calcium
Vibramycin hyclate	Vibra-Tabs
Vibramycin monohydrate	Vibramycin Monohydrate
Voriconazole	VFEND
Zaleplon	Sonata
Ziprasidone HCl	Geodon
Zolmitriptan	Zomig, Zomig-ZMT
Zolpidem tartrate	Ambien, Ambien CR, Edluar, Zolpimist

LACTOSE- AND GALACTOSE-FREE DRUGS

The following is a selection of lactose- and galactose-free products. This list is not comprehensive. Generic and alternate brands may exist. Always check product labeling for definitive information on specific ingredients.

Trade Name (OTC)	Form
Advil	Tablets, Caplets, Gel Caplets, Liquigels
Advil PM	Liquigels
Advil Cold and Sinus	Caplets
Aleve	Caplets, Gelcaps, Tablets, Gel Tablets
Aleve Smooth Gels	Gel Tablets
Align	Capsules
Alka-Mints	Tablets
Alka-Seltzer	Effervescent Tablets
Alka-Seltzer Plus Cold	Effervescent Tablets
Ascriptin	Tablets
Axid AR	Tablets
Benadryl	Liquid, Tablets
Benadryl Allergy & Cold	Caplets
Caltrate 600 PLUS	Tablets
Claritin-D 24	Tablets
Claritin-D Reditabs	Tablets
Colace	Capsules
Dramamine Chewable	Tablets
Elecare	Powder
Enfamil Poly-Vi-Sol	Drops
Enfamil Poly-Vi-Sol with Iron	Drops
Enfamil Tri-Vi-Sol	Drops
Enfamil Tri-Vi-Sol with Iron	Drops
Ensure	Liquid, Powder, Pudding
Ensure Fiber	Liquid
Ensure High Calcium	Liquid
Ensure High Protein	Liquid
Ensure Plus	Liquid
Excedrin Extra-Strength	Caplets
Ex-Lax Maximum Strength	Tablets
Ex-Lax Regular Strength	Tablets
Ex-Lax Regular Strength Chocolate	Chewable
Fergon Iron	Tablets
Gaviscon Regular Strength	Tablets
Imodium A-D	Liquid, Tablets
Imodium A-D EZ Chews	Tablets
Imodium Multi Symptom Relief Chewable	Tablets, Caplets
Jevity	Liquid
Kaopectate Cherry	Liquid
Kaopectate Peppermint	Liquid
Kaopectate Peppermint Extra Strength	Liquid
Kaopectate Stool Softener	Softgel
Kaopectate Vanilla	Liquid
Konsyl	Powder
Lactaid	Tablets
Lactaid Fast Act	Caplets, Chewables
MCT Oil	Oil
Medi-Lyte	Tablets
Metamucil	Powder, Wafers
Metamucil Heart and Digestive Health	Capsules
Metamucil Strong Bones	Capsules
Motrin Children's	Suspension
Motrin Children's Cold	Suspension
Motrin IB	Tablets
Motrin Infant's	Drops
Motrin Junior Strength	Caplets, Tablets
Mylanta Children's	Tablets
Mylanta Gas	Tablets
Mylanta Gas Maximum Strength	Softgels
Mylanta Maximum Strength	Liquid
Mylanta Regular Strength	Liquid
Mylanta Supreme	Liquid
Mylanta Ultimate Strength	Liquid, Tablets
Mylicon Infants'	Drops
Nepro	Liquid
Ocuvite Vitamin and Mineral Supplement	Tablets
One-A-Day Cholesterol Plus	Tablets
One-A-Day Energy	Tablets
One-A-Day Essential	Tablets
One-A-Day Maximum	Tablets
One-A-Day Men's	Tablets
One-A-Day Men's Health Formula	Tablets
One-A-Day Men's 50+ Advantage	Tablets
One-A-Day Weightsmart Advanced	Tablets
One-A-Day Women's	Tablets
One-A-Day Women's 50+ Advantage	Tablets
One-A-Day Women's Active Mind & Body	Tablets
One-A-Day Women's Prenatal	Tablets
Pepto-Bismol	Suspension, Tablets
Pepto-Bismol Max. Strength	Suspension
Percy Medicine	Liquid
Polycose	Liquid, Powder
Portagen	Powder
Prilosec OTC	Tablets
Promote	Liquid
Promote with Fiber	Liquid
Pulmocare	Liquid
RCF	Liquid
Simply Sleep	Caplets
St. Joseph Adult Low Strength Aspirin	Tablets
Sucrets Maximum Strength	Lozenges
Sudafed	Tablets
Sudafed Children's	Liquid
Sudafed OM Sinus Congestion Spray	Liquid
Sudafed PE Cold and Cough	Caplets
Sudafed PE Maximum Strength Sinus & Allergy	Tablets
Sudafed PE Nighttime Cold	Caplets
Sudafed PE Non-Drying Sinus	Caplets
Sudafed PE Severe Cold Formula	Caplets
Sudafed PE Sinus Headache	Caplets
Sudafed Sinus	Tablets
Titralac	Tablets
Titralac Plus	Tablets
Tums	Tablets
Tums E-X 750	Tablets
Tums E-X Sugar Free	Tablets
Tums Kids	Tablets
Tums Quik Pak	Powder
Tums Smoothies	Tablets
Tums Ultra 1000	Tablets
Tylenol	Drops, Liquid, Tablets
Tylenol Children's Plus Cold	Liquid
Tylenol Children's Plus Cold & Allergy	Liquid
Tylenol Children's Plus Cough & Runny Nose	Liquid
Tylenol Children's Plus Cough & Sore Throat	Liquid
Tylenol Children's Plus Flu	Liquid
Tylenol Children's Plus Multi-Symptom Cold	Liquid
Tylenol Meltaways Jr.	Tablets
Unisom SleepTabs	Gels, Melts, Tablets
Zantac 75	Tablets
Zantac 150 Cool Mint	Tablets
Zantac Maximum Strength 150	Tablets

Trade Name (Rx)	Form
Actigall	Capsules
Advicor	Tablets
Aldactazide	Tablets
Aldactone	Tablets
Allegra Oral	Suspension
Allegra	Solution, Tablets
Allegra-D 12 Hr, 24 Hr	Tablets
Allernase	Liquid
Altace	Capsules
Amicar	Solution, Tablets
Amnesteem	Capsules
Antivert	Tablets
Aplenzin	Tablets
Apriso	Capsule
Aromasin	Tablets
Augmentin Chewable	Tablets
Augmentin ES 600	Powder
Augmentin XR	Tablets
Augmentin	Suspension, Tablets
Axid	Capsules, Solution
Bactrim	Tablets
Biaxin Granules	Suspension
Calan SR	Tablets
Cambia	Solution
Carafate	Suspension, Tablets
Cardene	Capsules
Cardizem CD	Capsules
Ceftin	Suspension, Tablets
Cefzil	Suspension, Tablets
Cipro XR	Tablets
Cipro	Suspension, Tablets
Citranatal RX	Tablets
Clinoril	Tablets
Coartim	Tablets
Combivir	Tablets
Comtan	Tablets
Covera-HS	Tablets
Creon	Capsules
Cytotec	Tablets
Daypro	Tablets
Demerol	Tablets
Depakene	Capsules
Depakote Sprinkle	Capsules
Depakote	Tablets
Detrol LA	Tablets
Detrol	Tablets
DiaBeta	Tablets
Diabinese	Tablets
Diovan HCT	Tablets
Diovan	Tablets
E.E.S.	Suspension, Tablets
Edluar	Tablets
Embeda	Capsules

Entereg	Capsules
Epivir	Tablets, Solution
Epivir-HBV	Tablets
Ery-Tab	Tablets
Esgic-Plus	Capsules, Tablets
Exelon	Capsules
Exforge HCT	Tablets
Fibricor (fenofibric acid)	Tablets
Fioricet with Codeine	Capsules
Fioricet	Tablets
Flomax	Capsules
Gleevec	Tablets
Glucotrol XL	Tablets
Glucovance	Tablets
Glyset	Tablets
GoLYTELY	Powder
Granisol	Liquid
Grifulvin V	Suspension, Tablets
Inderal LA	Capsules
Isoptin SR	Tablets
Kaletra	Solution, Tablets
Kapidex	Capsules
Keppra	Solution, Tablets
K-Lor	Powder
K-Phos Neutral	Tablets
K-Phos Original Formula	Tablets
K-Tab	Tablets
Lamisil	Tablets
Lescol XL	Tablets
Lescol	Capsules
Levaquin	Solution, Tablets
Levothroid	Tablets
Levoxyl	Tablets
Lexapro	Suspension, Tablets
Librium	Capsules
Lomotil	Solution, Tablets
Lopid	Tablets
Lysteda	Tablets
Malarone Pediatric	Tablets
Malarone	Tablets
Maxzide	Tablets
Methylin ER	Tablets
Micardis	Tablets
Micro-K	Capsules
Micronase	Tablets
Minipress	Capsules
Minocin	Capsules
Moxatag	Tablets
Niaspan	Tablets
Niferex-150	Capsules, Elixir
Niferex-150-Forte	Capsules
Norpramin	Tablets
Norvasc	Tablets
Omnicef	Capsules, Suspension
Onsolis	Buccal film
Pamelor	Capsules, Suspension
Pamine Forte	Tablets
Pancrease MT	Capsules
Patanase	Liquid
Paxil	Suspension, Tablets
Pepcid	Suspension, Tablets
Percocet	Tablets
Percodan	Tablets
Plaquenil	Tablets
Pletal	Tablets
PrandiMet	tablets
Prandin	Tablets
Precare	Tablets
Precose	Tablets
Prevacid	Capsules, Suspension
Prinivil	Tablets
Pristiq	Tablets
ProAmatine	Tablets
Procardia XL	Tablets
Procardia	Capsules
Promacta	Tablets
Prometrium	Capsules
Protonix	Suspension, Tablets
Prozac	Capsules, Solution
Qualaquin	Tablets
Questran Light	Powder
Questran	Powder
Rapaflo	Capsules
Remeron SolTab	Tablets
Rifadin	Capsules
Robaxin	Tablets
Ryzolt	Tablets
Sabril	Solution, Tablets
Saphris	Tablets
Sarafem	Pulvules, Tablets
Savella	Tablets
Sectral	Capsules
Sinemet CR	Tablets
Sinemet	Tablets
Soma	Tablets
Stalevo	Tablets
Stavzor	Capsules
Sucraid	Solution
Symmetrel	Syrup, Tablets
Tamiflu	Capsules, Suspension
Tegretol/Tegretol-XR	Suspension, Tablets
Tenoretic	Tablets
Tenormin	Tablets
Tessalon	Capsules
Tiazac	Capsules
Ticlid	Tablets
Tikosyn	Capsules
Tofranil-PM	Capsules
Toprol-XL	Tablets
Treanda	Powder
Trental	Tablets
Treximet	Tablets
Trileptal	Suspension, Tablets
Trilipix	Capsules
Trizivir	Tablets
Twynsta	Tablets
Tyvaso	Liquid
Ultrase MT	Capsules
Ultrase	Capsules
Uniphyl	Tablets
Urex	Tablets
Valcyte	Tablets
Valtrex	Caplets
Valturna	Tablets
Vibramycin Hyclate	Capsules, Suspension
Vicodin ES	Tablets
Vicodin HP	Tablets
Vicodin	Tablets
Vicoprofen	Tablets
Videx EC	Capsules, Delayed Release
Vimpat	Capsules
Visicol	Tablets
Vistaril	Capsules, Suspension
Votrient	Tablets
Welchol	Tablets
Wellbutrin SR	Tablets
Wellbutrin XL	Tablets
Wellbutrin	Tablets
Xenical	Capsules
Zantac	Efferdose Tablets, Syrup, Tablets
Zarontin	Capsules, Solution
Zebeta	Tablets
Zenpep	Capsules
Zestril	Tablets
Ziac	Tablets
Ziagen	Solution, Tablets
Zipsor	Capsules
Zofran	Solution, Tablets (disintegrating)
Zoloft	Oral Concentrate, Tablets
Zolpimist	Solution
Zonegran	Capsules
Zyban	Tablets
Zyvox	Suspension, Tablets

VITAMIN COMPARISON TABLE

For easy comparison, the grid below lists the contents of an assortment of widely available vitamin/mineral supplements. It includes entries for all vitamins and minerals—except sodium—assigned a Recommended Dietary Allowance (Daily Value) by the U.S. Food and Drug Administration.

The grid is divided into two parts: the first covers general multivitamin/mineral supplements for adults; the second focuses on supplements sold especially for children.

Many of the brands in the grid include other ingredients that have nutritional importance but lack an official Recommended Dietary Allowance from the government. The presence of additional ingredients is noted in the last column of the grid.

The amounts listed are drawn from the manufacturer's package labeling, primarily as published in the *PDR® for Nutritional Supplements, 2nd Edition*. For easy comparison, the figures have been converted as necessary from the unit of measure used by the manufacturer to the measurement most frequently employed in the industry. **Amounts listed are those found in the total daily dose.** Check package labeling for other usage information provided by the manufacturer.

To conserve space, units of measure are not shown in the grid; see the following key for the measurement used for a particular ingredient.

Ingredient	Measure
Vitamin A (retinol, beta-carotene)	International Units
Vitamin B1 (thiamin)	Milligrams
Vitamin B2 (riboflavin)	Milligrams
Vitamin B3 (niacin)	Milligrams
Vitamin B5 (pantothenic acid)	Milligrams
Vitamin B6 (pyridoxine)	Milligrams
Vitamin B9 (folic acid)	Micrograms
Vitamin B12 (cobalamin)	Micrograms
Vitamin C (ascorbic acid)	Milligrams
Vitamin D	International Units
Vitamin E	International Units
Biotin	Micrograms
Calcium	Milligrams
Copper	Milligrams
Iodine	Micrograms
Iron	Milligrams
Magnesium	Milligrams
Phosphorus	Milligrams
Potassium	Milligrams
Zinc	Milligrams

ADULTS

BRAND	A	B1	B2	B3	B5	B6	B9	B12	C	D	E	BIOTIN	CALCIUM	COPPER	IODINE	IRON	MAGNESIUM	PHOSPHORUS	POTASSIUM	ZINC	OTHER
ACES (Carlson)	5,000	—	—	—	—	—	—	—	500	—	200	—	—	—	—	—	—	—	—	—	y
Adult Chewable Multivitamin (Puritan's Pride)	5,000	15	15	—	20	15	400	15	150	400	100	20	10	0.05	100	5	0.145	—	—	0.325	y
Advanced Prenatal *per 3 tabs*	2,700	3	3.4	—	10	3	800	12	120	400	45	300	125	2	75	30	125	—	25	25	y
Centamin Liquid *per 15 ml*	1,300	1.5	1.7	20	10	2	—	6	60	400	30	300	—	—	150	9	—	—	—	3	
Centrum	3,500	1.5	1.7	20	10	2	400	6	60	400	30	30	200	0.5	150	18	50	20	80	11	y
Centrum Cardio	1,750	0.75	0.85	10	5	2.5	200	100	30	200	15	15	54	0.35	75	3	20	40	32	3.75	y
Centrum Chewable	3,500	1.5	1.7	20	10	2	400	6	60	400	30	45	108	2	150	18	40	50	—	15	y
Centrum Performance	3,500	4.5	5.1	40	12	6	400	18	120	400	60	50	100	0.9	150	18	40	48	80	11	y
Centrum Silver	2,500	1.5	1.7	20	10	3	400	25	60	500	50	30	220	0.5	150	—	50	20	80	11	y
Daily Multi (Sundown)	2,500	1.5	1.7	20	10	2	400	6	60	400	30	30	155	2	150	18	100	105	80	15	y
Duet by Stuartnatal	3,000	1.8	4	20	—	25	1,000	12	120	400	30	—	200	2	—	29	25	—	—	25	y
Duet Chewable by Stuartnatal	3,000	1.8	4	—	—	25	—	12	120	400	30	—	100	2	—	29	25	—	—	25	y
Folgard Rx 2.2	—	—	—	—	—	25	2,200	1,000	—	—	—	—	—	—	—	—	—	—	—	—	
Formula 100 (Puritan's Pride)	10,000	100	100	100	100	100	400	100	250	400	150	100	100	0.5	150	18	50	—	10	15	y
Geritol Complete	6,100	1.5	1.7	20	13	2	380	6.7	57	400	30	44	148	1.8	120	16	86	118	36	13.5	y
Goldline Prenatal S	4,000	1.84	1.7	—	—	2.6	800	4	100	400	11	—	200	—	—	27	—	—	—	25	y
Green Source *per 3 tabs*	5,000	25	25	25	30	25	400	250	500	800	100	300	237	0.5	150	15	125	—	50	15	y
Hair, Skin & Nails Formula (Nature's Bounty) *per 3 tabs*	5,000	5	5	25	15	5	200	8	120	100	15	3,000	707	—	112.5	3	100	150	—	7.5	y
Hep-Forte	1,200	1	1	10	2	0.5	60	1	10	—	10	3.3	—	—	—	—	—	—	—	2	y

BRAND	A	B1	B2	B3	B5	B6	B9	B12	C	D	E	BIOTIN	CALCIUM	COPPER	IODINE	IRON	MAGNESIUM	PHOSPHORUS	POTASSIUM	ZINC	OTHER
Mega Vita Gel Iron Free *per 2 softgels*	10,000	50	50	50	50	50	400	50	300	400	300	50	200	2	150	—	50	50	30	15	y
Mini-Multi (Carlson Laboratories)	5,000	1.5	1.7	20	10	2	400	6	120	400	60	30	20	2	75	—	40	—	—	15	
Mini-Prenatal (Freeda Vitamins)	2,000	2	3	20	10	3	800	10	100	400	15	100	200	2	—	27	60	—	—	15	
Multi-Day Plus Minerals (Nature's Bounty)	5,000	1.5	1.7	20	10	2	400	6	60	400	30	30	162	2	150	18	100	109	80	15	
Myadec	5,000	1.7	2	20	10	3	400	6	60	400	30	30	162	2	150	18	100	125	40	15	y
Ocuvite	1,000	—	—	—	—	—	—	—	200	—	60	—	—	2	—	—	—	—	—	40	
One A Day Active	5,000	4.5	5.1	40	10	6	400	18	120	400	60	40	110	2	150	9	40	48	200	15	y
One A Day Men's 50+ Advantage	2,500	4.5	3.4	20	15	6	400	25	120	400	33	30	120	2	150	—	100	—	40	22.5	y
One A Day Men's	3,500	1.2	1.7	16	5	3	400	18	90	400	45	30	210	2	—	—	120	—	100	15	y
One A Day Women's	2,500	1.5	1.7	10	5	2	400	6	60	800	30	30	450	2	—	18	50	—	—	15	y
One A Day Women's 50+ Advantage	2,500	4.5	3.4	20	15	6	400	25	60	800	33	30	405	2	150	—	50	—	—	22.5	y
One A Day Women's Prenatal	4,000	1.7	2	20	10	2.5	800	8	60	400	30	300	300	2	150	28	50	—	—	15	y
Optisource Chewable	1,875	0.375	0.425	5	2.5	0.5	200	125	15	100	125	75	250	0.5	37.5	7.5	100	50	—	7.5	y
PreCare Chewable	—	—	2	—	—	2	1,000	—	50	6mcg	3.5	—	250	2	—	40	50	—	—	15	y
PreCare Conceive	—	3	3.4	20	—	50	1,000	12	60	—	30	—	200	2	—	30	100	—	—	15	y
PremesisRx Tablets	—	—	—	—	—	75	1,000	12	—	—	—	—	200	—	—	—	—	—	—	—	
Prenatal Vitamins (Nature's Bounty)	4,000	1.8	1.7	20	—	2.6	800	8	120	400	30	—	200	—	—	28	—	—	—	25	
Prenatal Vitamin (Puritan's Pride)	4,000	1.84	1.7	18	—	2.6	800	4	100	400	11	—	200	—	—	27	—	—	—	25	
Puritan's Pride Complete One	10,000	25	25	50	50	50	400	50	250	400	30	50	54	2	150	10	100	23	1	15	y
Strovite Advance	3,000	20	5	25	15	25	1,000	50	300	400	100	100	—	1.5	—	—	50	—	—	25	y
Stuart Prenatal	4,000	1.8	1.7	20	—	2.6	800	8	120	400	30	—	200	—	—	28	—	—	—	25	
Viactiv Chews	2,500	1.5	1.7	15	10	2	400	6	60	400	33	30	200	—	—	—	—	—	—	—	

CHILDREN

BRAND	A	B1	B2	B3	B5	B6	B9	B12	C	D	E	BIOTIN	CALCIUM	COPPER	IODINE	IRON	MAGNESIUM	PHOSPHORUS	POTASSIUM	ZINC	OTHER
Carlson for Kids Chewable	5,000	1.5	1.7	5	10	2	400	6	120	400	60	150	50	1	75	9	25	22	2.5	7.5	y
Centrum Kids	3,500	1.5	1.7	20	10	2	400	6	60	400	30	45	108	2	150	18	40	50	—	15	y
Flintstones	3,000	1.5	1.7	15	10	2	400	6	60	400	30	40	100	2	150	18	20	100	—	12	y
GNC Kid's Chewable *per 2 tabs*	5,000	5	5	20	15	5	400	10	90	400	30	100	30	0.2	100	12	15	15	—	3	y
One A Day Kids Bugs Bunny	3,000	1.5	1.7	15	10	2	400	6	60	400	30	40	100	2	150	18	20	100	—	12	y
One A Day Kids Scooby-Doo Complete	3,000	1.5	1.7	15	10	2	400	6	60	400	30	40	100	2	150	18	20	100	—	12	y
One A Day Kids Scooby-Doo Plus Calcium	2,500	1.05	1.2	13.5	—	1.05	300	4.5	60	400	15	—	200	—	—	—	—	—	—	—	y

*USP units.

USE-IN-PREGNANCY RATINGS

The U.S. Food and Drug Administration's Use-in-Pregnancy rating system weighs the degree to which available information has ruled out risk to the fetus against the drug's potential benefit to the patient. Below is a listing of drugs (by generic name) for which ratings are available.

CONTRAINDICATED IN PREGNANCY

Studies in animals or humans, or investigational or post-marketing reports, have demonstrated fetal risk, which clearly outweighs any possible benefit to the patient.

Acetohydroxamic Acid
Acitretin
Ambrisentan
Amlodipine Besylate/Atorvastatin Calcium
Atorvastatin Calcium
Bexarotene
Bicalutamide
Bosentan
Cetrorelix Acetate
Clomiphene Citrate
Degarelix Acteate
Desogestrel/Ethinyl Estradiol
Diclofenac Sodium/Misoprostol
Dihydroergotamine Mesylate
Dronedarone
Dutasteride
Estazolam
Estradiol
Estradiol Acetate
Estradiol Valerate
Estradiol/Levonorgestrel
Estradiol/Norethindrone Acetate
Estrogens, Conjugated
Estrogens, Conjugated, Synthetic A
Estrogens, Conjugated/Medroxyprogesterone Acetate
Estrogens, Esterified
Estrogens, Esterified/Methyltestosterone
Estropipate
Ethinyl Estradiol/Drospirenone
Ethinyl Estradiol/Ethynodiol Diacetate
Ethinyl Estradiol/Etonogestrel
Ethinyl Estradiol/Ferrous Fumarate/Norethindrone Acetate
Ethinyl Estradiol/Levonorgestrel
Ethinyl Estradiol/Norelgestromin
Ethinyl Estradiol/Norethindrone Acetate
Ethinyl Estradiol/Norgestimate
Ethinyl Estradiol/Norgestrel
Ezetimibe/Simvastatin
Finasteride
Fluorouracil
Flurazepam Hydrochloride
Fluvastatin Sodium
Follitropin Alfa
Follitropin Beta
Ganirelix Acetate
Goserelin Acetate
Histrelin Acetate
Iodine I 131 Tositumomab/Tositumomab
Isotretinoin
Leflunomide
Leuprolide Acetate
Levonorgestrel
Lovastatin
Lovastatin/Niacin
Medroxyprogesterone Acetate
Megestrol Acetate
Mequinol/Tretinoin
Mestranol/Norethindrone
Methotrexate Sodium
Methyltestosterone
Miglustat
Misoprostol
Nafarelin Acetate
Niacin/Simvastatin
Norethindrone
Norethindrone Acetate
Oxandrolone
Oxymetholone
Pitavastatin Calcium
Pravastatin Sodium
Raloxifene Hydrochloride
Ribavirin
Rosuvastatin Calcium
Simvastatin
Tazarotene
Testosterone
Testosterone Enanthate
Thalidomide
Tositumomab
Triptorelin Pamoate
Warfarin Sodium

D

POSITIVE EVIDENCE OF RISK

Investigational or postmarketing data show risk to the fetus. Nevertheless, potential benefits may outweigh the potential risk.

Aliskiren*
Aliskiren/Hydrochlorothiazide
Aliskiren/Valsartan
Alitretinoin
Alprazolam
Altretamine
Amiodarone Hydrochloride
Amlodipine Besylate/Benazepril Hydrochloride
Amlodipine Besylate/Olmesartan Medoxomil*
Amlodipine Besylate/Valsartan
Amlodipine Besykate/Valsartan/HCTZ
Amlodipine/Telmisartan
Anastrozole
Arsenic Trioxide
Aspirin/Dipyridamole
Atenolol
Azacitidine
Azathioprine
Azathioprine Sodium
Benazepril Hydrochloride
Benazepril Hydrochloride/Hydrochlorothiazide
Bendamustine Hydrochloride
Bortezomib
Busulfan
Candesartan Cilexetil*
Candesartan Cilexetil/Hydrochlorothiazide*
Capecitabine
Captopril*
Carbamazepine
Carboplatin
Carmustine (BiCNU)
Chlorambucil
Cladribine
Clofarabine
Clonazepam
Cytarabine Liposome
Dactinomycin
Dasatinib
Daunorubicin Citrate Liposome
Daunorubicin Hydrochloride
Demeclocycline Hydrochloride
Dexrazoxane
Diazepam
Divalproex Sodium
Docetaxel
Doxorubicin Hydrochloride
Doxorubicin Hydrochloride Liposome
Doxycycline
Doxycycline Calcium
Doxycycline Hyclate
Doxycycline Monohydrate
Efavirenz
Enalapril Maleate*
Enalapril Maleate/Hydrochlorothiazide*
Epirubicin Hydrochloride
Eprosartan Mesylate
Erlotinib
Everolimus
Exemestane
Floxuridine
Fludarabine Phosphate
Flutamide
Fosinopril Sodium*
Fosinopril Sodium/Hydrochlorothiazide*
Fosphenytoin Sodium
Fulvestrant
Gemcitabine Hydrochloride
Gemtuzumab Ozogamicin
Goserelin Acetate
Idarubicin Hydrochloride
Ifosfamide
Imatinib Mesylate
Irbesartan*
Irbesartan/Hydrochlorothiazide*
Irinotecan Hydrochloride
Ixabepilone
Letrozole
Lisinopril*
Lisinopril/Hydrochlorothiazide*
Lithium Carbonate
Losartan Potassium*
Losartan Potassium/Hydrochlorothiazide*
Mechlorethamine Hydrochloride
Melphalan Hydrochloride
Mephobarbital
Mercaptopurine
Methimazole
Midazolam Hydrochloride
Minocycline Hydrochloride
Mitoxantrone Hydrochloride
Moexipril Hydrochloride*
Moexipril Hydrochloride/Hydrochlorothiazide
Mycophenolate Mofetil
Mycophenolic Acid
Nelarabine
Neomycin Sulfate/Polymyxin B Sulfate
Nicotine
Nilotinib
Nilotinib Hydrochloride Monohydrate
Olmesartan Medoxomil
Oxaliplatin
Pamidronate Disodium
Paroxetine Hydrochloride
Paroxetine Mesylate
Pazopanib HCl
Pemetrexed
Penicillamine
Pentobarbital Sodium
Pentostatin
Perindopril Erbumine
Phenytoin
Procarbazine Hydrochloride
Quinapril Hydrochloride*
Quinapril Hydrochloride/Hydrochlorothiazide*
Ramipril*
Romidepsin
Sorafenib
Streptomycin Sulfate
Sunitinib
Tamoxifen Citrate
Telmisartan*
Telmisartan/Hydrochlorothiazide*
Temozolomide
Temsirolimus
Thioguanine
Tigecycline
Tobramycin
Topotecan Hydrochloride
Toremifene Citrate
Trandolapril*
Trandolapril/Verapamil Hydrochloride*
Tretinoin
Valproate Sodium
Valproic Acid
Valsartan
Valsartan/Hydrochlorothiazide
Vinorelbine Tartrate
Voriconazole
Zoledronic Acid

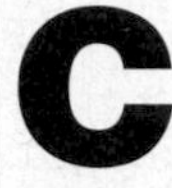

RISK CANNOT BE RULED OUT

Human studies are lacking, and animal studies are either positive for risk or are lacking as well. However, potential benefits may outweigh the potential risk.

Abacavir Sulfate
Abacavir Sulfate/Lamivudine
Abacavir Sulfate/Lamivudine/Zidovudine
Abciximab
Acamprosate Calcium
Acetaminophen
Acetaminophen/Butalbital/Caffeine
Acetaminophen/Caffeine/Chlorpheniramine Maleate/Hydrocodone Bitartrate/Phenylephrine Hydrochloride
Acetazolamide
Acetazolamide Sodium
Acyclovir
Adapalene
Adefovir Dipivoxil
Adenosine
Albendazole
Albumin (Human)
Albuterol Sulfate
Albuterol Sulfate/Ipratropium Bromide
Alclometasone Dipropionate
Aldesleukin
Alemtuzumab
Alendronate Sodium
Alendronate Sodium/Cholecalciferol
Aliskiren*
Allopurinol Sodium
Almotriptan Malate
Alpha1-Proteinase Inhibitor (Human)
Alprostadil
Alteplase
Amantadine Hydrochloride
Amifostine
Aminocaproic Acid
Aminohippurate Sodium
Aminolevulinic Acid Hydrochloride
Amlodipine Besylate

* Category C or D depending on the trimester the drug is given.

Amlodipine Besylate/ Olmesartan Medoxomil*
Amoxicillin/Clarithromycin/ Lansoprazole
Amphetamine Aspartate/ Amphetamine Sulfate/ Dextroamphetamine Saccharate/ Dextroamphetamine Sulfate
Anagrelide Hydrochloride
Anthralin
Antihemophilic Factor (Human)
Antihemophilic Factor (Recombinant)
Anti-Inhibitor Coagulant Complex
Anti-Thymocyte Globulin
Apomorphine Hydrochloride
Aripiprazole
Armodafinil
Arnica Montana/Herbals, Multiple/Sulfur
Artemther/Lumefantrine
Asenapine Maleate
Asparaginase
Atomoxetine Hydrochloride
Atovaquone
Atovaquone/Proguanil Hydrochloride
Atropine Sulfate/Hyoscyamine Sulfate/Scopolamine Hydrobromide
Azelastine Hydrochloride
Bacitracin Zinc/Neomycin Sulfate/Polymyxin B Sulfate
Baclofen
BCG, Live (Intravesical)
Becaplermin
Beclomethasone Dipropionate
Beclomethasone Dipropionate Monohydrate
Bendroflumethiazide
Benzocaine
Benzonatate
Benzoyl Peroxide
Benzoyl Peroxide/Clindamycin
Benzoyl Peroxide/Erythromycin
Bepotastine Besilate
Besifloxacin HCl
Betamethasone Dipropionate
Betamethasone Dipropionate/Clotrimazole
Betamethasone Valerate
Betaxolol Hydrochloride
Bethanechol Chloride
Bevacizumab
Bimatoprost
Bisacodyl/Polyethylene Glycol/ Potassium Chloride/Sodium Bicarbonate/Sodium Chloride
Bisoprolol Fumarate
Bisoprolol Fumarate/ Hydrochlorothiazide
Black Widow Spider Antivenin (Equine)
Botulinum Toxin Type A
Botulinum Toxin Type B
Brimonidine Tartrate/ Timolol Maleate
Brinzolamide
Brompheniramine Maleate/ Dextromethorphan Hydrobromide/Phenylephrine Hydrochloride
Budesonide

Bupivacaine Hydrochloride
Bupivacaine Hydrochloride/ Epinephrine Bitartrate
Buprenorphine Hydrochloride
Buprenorphine Hydrochloride/ Naloxone Hydrochloride
Bupropion Hydrobromide
Bupropion Hydrochloride
Butalbital/Acetaminophen
Butenafine Hydrochloride
Butoconazole Nitrate
Butorphanol Tartrate
Caffeine Citrate
Calcipotriene
Calcitonin-Salmon
Calcitriol
Calcium Acetate
Canakinumab
Candesartan Cilexetil*
Candesartan Cilexetil/ Hydrochlorothiazide*
Capreomycin Sulfate
Captopril*
Carbetapentane Tannate/ Chlorpheniramine Tannate
Carbidopa/Entacapone/ Levodopa
Carbidopa/Levodopa
Carbinoxamine Maleate/ Dextromethorphan Hydrobromide/ Pseudoephedrine Hydrochloride
Carteolol Hydrochloride
Carvedilol
Caspofungin Acetate
Celecoxib
Cetirizine Hydrochloride
Cetuximab
Cevimeline Hydrochloride
Chloramphenicol
Chloroprocaine Hydrochloride
Chlorothiazide
Chlorothiazide Sodium
Chlorpheniramine Maleate/ Pseudoephedrine Hydrochloride
Chlorpheniramine Polistirex/Hydrocodone Polistirex
Chlorpheniramine Tannate/ Phenylephrine Tannate
Chlorpropamide
Chlorthalidone/Clonidine Hydrochloride
Choline Magnesium Trisalicylate
Ciclesonide
Cidofovir
Cilostazol
Cinacalcet Hydrochloride
Ciprofloxacin Hydrochloride
Ciprofloxacin Hydrochloride/ Hydrocortisone
Ciprofloxacin/Dexamethasone
Citalopram Hydrobromide
Clarithromycin
Clobetasol Propionate
Clonidine
Clonidine Hydrochloride
Codeine Phosphate/ Acetaminophen
Colistimethate Sodium
Colistin Sulfate/Hydrocortisone Acetate/Neomycin Sulfate/ Thonzonium Bromide

Corticorelin Ovine Triflutate
Cyanocobalamin
Cycloserine
Cyclosporine
Cytomegalovirus Immune Globulin
Dacarbazine
Daclizumab
Dantrolene Sodium
Dapsone
Darbepoetin Alfa
Darifenacin
Deferoxamine Mesylate
Delavirdine Mesylate
Denileukin Diftitox
Desloratadine
Desloratadine/ Pseudoephedrine Sulfate
Desoximetasone
Desvenlafaxine
Dexamethasone
Dexamethasone Sodium Phosphate
Dexmethylphenidate Hydrochloride
Dexrazoxane
Dextroamphetamine Sulfate
Diazoxide
Diclofenac Epolamine
Diclofenac Potassium
Diclofenac Sodium
Diflorasone Diacetate
Diflunisal
Digoxin
Digoxin Immune Fab (Ovine)
Diltiazem Hydrochloride
Dimethyl Sulfoxide
Dinoprostone
Diphtheria & Tetanus Toxoids and Acellular Pertussis Vaccine Adsorbed
Diphtheria & Tetanus Toxoids and Acellular Pertussis Vaccine Adsorbed/ Hepatitis B Vaccine, Recombinant/Poliovirus Vaccine Inactivated
Dofetilide
Donepezil Hydrochloride
Dorzolamide Hydrochloride
Dorzolamide Hydrochloride/ Timolol Maleate
Doxazosin Mesylate
Dronabinol
Drotrecogin Alfa (Activated)
Duloxetine Hydrochloride
Echothiophate Iodide
Econazole Nitrate
Eflornithine Hydrochloride
Eletriptan Hydrobromide
Enalapril Maleate*
Enalapril Maleate/ Hydrochlorothiazide*
Entacapone
Entecavir
Epinastine Hydrochloride
Epinephrine
Epoetin Alfa
Eprosartan Mesylate
Erythromycin Ethylsuccinate/ Sulfisoxazole Acetyl
Escitalopram Oxalate
Eszopiclone
Ethionamide
Ethotoin

Etidronate Disodium
Exenatide
Ezetimibe
Factor IX Complex
Febuxostat
Felodipine
Fenofibrate
Fentanyl
Fentanyl Citrate
Fentanyl Hydrochloride
Ferumoxytol
Fexofenadine Hydrochloride
Fexofenadine Hydrochloride/ Pseudoephedrine Hydrochloride
Filgrastim
Flecainide Acetate
Fluconazole
Flucytosine
Fludrocortisone Acetate
Flumazenil
Flunisolide
Fluocinolone Acetonide
Fluocinolone Acetonide/ Hydroquinone/Tretinoin
Fluocinonide
Fluorometholone
Fluorometholone/ Sulfacetamide Sodium
Fluoxetine Hydrochloride
Fluoxetine Hydrochloride/ Olanzapine
Flurandrenolide
Flurbiprofen Sodium
Fluticasone Furoate
Fluticasone Propionate
Fluticasone Propionate HFA
Fluticasone Propionate/ Salmeterol Xinafoate
Fluvoxamine Maleate
Formoterol Fumarate
Fosamprenavir Calcium
Foscarnet Sodium*
Fosinopril Sodium*
Fosinopril Sodium/ Hydrochlorothiazide*
Frovatriptan Succinate
Furosemide
Gabapentin
Gallium Nitrate
Ganciclovir
Ganciclovir Sodium
Gemfibrozil
Gemifloxacin Mesylate
Gentamicin Sulfate
Gentamicin Sulfate/ Prednisolone Acetate
Glimepiride
Glimepiride/Rosiglitazone Maleate
Glipizide
Glipizide/Metformin Hydrochloride
Globulin, Immune (Human)
Globulin, Immune (Human)/ Rho (D) Immune Globulin (Human)
Glyburide
Gramicidin/Neomycin Sulfate/ Polymyxin B Sulfate
Guaifenesin/Hydrocodone Bitartrate
Haemophilus B Conjugate Vaccine

Haemophilus B Conjugate Vaccine/Hepatitis B Vaccine, Recombinant
Halobetasol Propionate
Haloperidol Decanoate
Hemin
Heparin Sodium
Hepatitis A Vaccine, Inactivated
Hepatitis A Vaccine, Inactivated/Hepatitis B Vaccine, Recombinant
Hepatitis B Immune Globulin (Human)
Hepatitis B Vaccine, Recombinant
Homatropine Methylbromide/ Hydrocodone Bitartrate
Homeopathic Formulations
Hyaluronidase Recombinant Human
Hydralazine Hydrochloride/ Isosorbide Dinitrate
Hydrochlorothiazide
Hydrocodone Bitartrate
Hydrocodone Bitartrate/ Acetaminophen
Hydrocodone Bitartrate/ Ibuprofen
Hydrocortisone
Hydrocortisone Acetate
Hydrocortisone Acetate/ Neomycin Sulfate/ Polymyxin B Sulfate
Hydrocortisone Butyrate
Hydrocortisone Probutate
Hydrocortisone/Neomycin Sulfate/Polymyxin B Sulfate
Hydromorphone Hydrochloride
Hydroquinone
Hyoscyamine Sulfate
Ibandronate Sodium
Ibutilide Fumarate
Iloperidone
Iloprost
Imiglucerase
Imipenem/Cilastatin
Imiquimod
Immune Globulin Intravenous (Human)
Indinavir Sulfate
Indocyanine Green
Influenza Virus Vaccine
Insulin Aspart Protamine, Human/Insulin Aspart, Human
Insulin Glargine
Insulin Glulisine
Interferon Alfa-2B, Recombinant
Interferon Alfacon-1
Interferon Alfa-N3 (Human Leukocyte Derived)
Interferon Beta-1A
Interferon Beta-1B
Interferon Gamma-1B
Iodoquinol/Hydrocortisone
Irbesartan*
Irbesartan/Hydrochlorothiazide*
Iron Dextran
Isoniazid/Pyrazinamide/ Rifampin
Isosorbide Mononitrate
Isradipine
Itraconazole
Ivermectin

* Category C or D depending on the trimester the drug is given.

Ketoconazole
Ketorolac Tromethamine
Ketotifen Fumarate
Labetalol Hydrochloride
Lamivudine
Lamivudine/Zidovudine
Lamotrigine
Lanreotide Acetate
Lanthanum Carbonate
Latanoprost
Levalbuterol Hydrochloride
Levalbuterol Tartrate
Levamisole Hydrochloride
Levetiracetam
Levobunolol Hydrochloride
Levofloxacin
Linezolid
Lisdexamfetamine
Lisinopril*
Lisinopril/Hydrochlorothiazide*
Lopinavir/Ritonavir
Losartan Potassium*
Losartan Potassium/ Hydrochlorothiazide*
Loteprednol Etabonate
Lubiprostone
Mafenide Acetate
Magnesium Salicylate Tetrahydrate
Measles Virus Vaccine, Live
Measles, Mumps & Rubella Virus Vaccine, Live
Mebendazole
Mecasermin [rDNA Origin]
Mefenamic Acid
Mefloquine Hydrochloride
Meloxicam
Meningoccal Polysaccharide Diphtheria Toxoid Conjugate Vaccine
Meningococcal Polysaccharide Vaccine
Meperidine Hydrochloride
Mepivacaine Hydrochloride
Metaproterenol Sulfate
Metaraminol Bitartrate
Metformin Hydrochloride/ Pioglitazone Hydrochloride
Metformin Hydrochloride/ Repaglinide
Metformin Hydrochloride/ Rosiglitazone Maleate
Methamphetamine Hydrochloride
Methazolamide
Methenamine Mandelate/ Sodium Acid Phosphate
Methocarbamol
Methoxsalen
Methoxy Polyethylene Glycol/ Epoetin Beta
Methscopolamine Nitrate/ Pseudoephedrine Hydrochloride
Methyldopa/Hydrochlorothiazide
Methylphenidate Hydrochloride
Metipranolol
Metoprolol Succinate
Metoprolol Tartrate
Metoprolol Tartrate/ Hydrochlorothiazide
Metyrosine
Mexiletine Hydrochloride
Micafungin Sodium
Midodrine Hydrochloride
Milnacipran HCl
Modafinil
Moexipril Hydrochloride*
Moexipril Hydrochloride/ Hydrochlorothiazide*
Mometasone Furoate
Mometasone Furoate Monohydrate
Morphine Sulfate
Morphine Sulfate, Liposomal
Morphine sulfate/Naltrexone HCl
Moxifloxacin Hydrochloride
Mumps Virus Vaccine, Live
Muromonab-CD3
Nabumetone
Nadolol
Nadolol/Bendroflumethiazide
Naloxone Hydrochloride/ Pentazocine Hydrochloride
Naltrexone Hydrochloride
Naphazoline Hydrochloride
Naproxen Sodium
Naratriptan Hydrochloride
Natamycin
Nateglinide
Nebivolol
Nefazodone Hydrochloride
Neomycin Sulfate/Polymyxin B Sulfate/Prednisolone Acetate
Nesiritide
Nevirapine
Niacin
Nicardipine Hydrochloride
Nifedipine
Nilutamide
Nimodipine
Nisoldipine
Nitroglycerin
Norfloxacin
Ofatumumab
Ofloxacin
Olanzapine
Olmesartan Medoxomil/ Hydrochlorothiazide
Olopatadine Hydrochloride
Olsalazine Sodium
Omega-3-Acid Ethyl Esters
Omeprazole
Oprelvekin
Orphenadrine Citrate
Oseltamivir Phosphate
Oxcarbazepine
Oxycodone Hydrochloride/ Acetaminophen
Oxycodone Hydrochloride/ Ibuprofen
Oxymorphone Hydrochloride
Palifermin
Paliperidone
Palivizumab
Pancrelipase
Paricalcitol
Peg-3350/Potassium Chloride/ Sodium Bicarbonate/ Sodium Chloride
Pegademase Bovine
Pegaspargase
Pegfilgrastim
Peginterferon Alfa-2A
Peginterferon Alfa-2B
Pemirolast Potassium
Pentazocine Hydrochloride/ Acetaminophen
Pentoxifylline
Phenoxybenzamine Hydrochloride
Phentermine Hydrochloride
Pilocarpine Hydrochloride
Pimecrolimus
Pimozide
Pioglitazone Hydrochloride
Pirbuterol Acetate
Piroxicam
Plasma Fractions, Human/ Rabies Immune Globulin (Human)
Plasma Protein Fraction (Human)
Pneumococcal Vaccine, Diphtheria Conjugate
Pneumococcal Vaccine, Polyvalent
Podofilox
Polyethylene Glycol
Polyethylene Glycol/ Potassium Chloride/Sodium Bicarbonate/Sodium Chloride
Polyethylene Glycol/Potassium Chloride/Sodium Bicarbonate/Sodium Chloride/Sodium Sulfate
Polymyxin B Sulfate/ Trimethoprim Sulfate
Porfimer Sodium
Potassium Acid Phosphate
Potassium Chloride
Potassium Citrate
Pralidoxime Chloride
Pramipexole Dihydrochloride
Pramlintide Acetate
Pramoxine Hydrochloride/ Hydrocortisone Acetate
Prazosin Hydrochloride
Prednisolone Acetate
Prednisolone Acetate/ Sulfacetamide Sodium
Prednisolone Sodium
Phosphate
Pregabalin
Promethazine Hydrochloride
Propafenone Hydrochloride
Proparacaine Hydrochloride
Propranolol Hydrochloride
Pseudoephedrine Hydrochloride
Pyrimethamine
Quetiapine Fumarate
Quinapril Hydrochloride*
Quinidine Sulfate
Rabies Vaccine
Raltegravir Potassium
Ramelteon
Ramipril*
Ranolazine
Rasburicase
Remifentanil Hydrochloride
Repaglinide
Reteplase
Rho (D) Immune Globulin (Human)
Rifampin
Rifapentine
Rifaximin
Riluzole
Rimantadine Hydrochloride
Risedronate Sodium
Risedronate Sodium/ Calcium Carbonate
Risperidone
Rituximab
Rizatriptan Benzoate
Rocuronium Bromide
Romiplostim
Ropinirole Hydrochloride
Rosiglitazone Maleate
Rubella Virus Vaccine, Live
Sacrosidase
Salmeterol Xinafoate
Sapropterin Dihydrochloride
Sargramostim
Scopolamine
Selegiline Hydrochloride
Selenium Sulfide
Sertaconazole Nitrate
Sertraline Hydrochloride
Sevelamer Carbonate
Sevelamer Hydrochloride
Sibutramine Hydrochloride Monohydrate
Sirolimus
Sodium Benzoate/ Sodium Phenylacelate
Sodium Phenylbutyrate
Sodium Polysterene Sulfonate
Sodium Sulfacetamide/Sulfur
Solifenacin Succinate
Somatropin
Somatropin (rDNA Origin)
Stavudine
Streptokinase
Succimer
Sulfacetamide Sodium
Sulfamethoxazole/Trimethoprim
Sulfanilamide
Sumatriptan
Sumatriptan Succinate
Tacrine Hydrochloride
Tacrolimus
Tapendalol HCl
Televancin HCl
Telithromycin
Telmisartan*
Telmisartan/ Hydrochlorothiazide*
Tenecteplase
Terazosin Hydrochloride
Teriparatide
Tetanus & Diphtheria Toxoids Adsorbed
Tetanus Immune Globulin (Human)
Theophylline
Theophylline Anhydrous
Thiabendazole
Thrombin
Thyrotropin Alfa
Tiagabine Hydrochloride
Tiludronate Disodium
Timolol Maleate
Tinidazole
Tiotropium Bromide
Tipranavir
Tizanidine Hydrochloride
Tobramycin/Dexamethasone
Tobramycin/Loteprednol Etabonate
Tolcapone
Tolterodine Tartrate
Tolvaptan
Topiramate
Tramadol Hydrochloride
Tramadol Hydrochloride/ Acetaminophen
Trandolapril*
Trandolapril/Verapamil Hydrochloride*
Travoprost
Tretinoin
Triamcinolone Acetonide
Triamterene
Triamterene/Hydrochlorothiazide
Trientine Hydrochloride
Triethanolamine Polypeptide Oleate-Condensate
Trifluridine
Trimethoprim Hydrochloride
Trimipramine Maleate
Tropicamide/ Hydroxyamphetamine Hydrobromide
Trospium Chloride
Tuberculin Purified Protein Derivative, Diluted
Typhoid Vaccine Live Oral Ty21a
Urea
Valganciclovir Hydrochloride
Varenicline Tartrate
Varicella Virus Vaccine, Live
Venlafaxine Hydrochloride
Verapamil Hydrochloride
Verteporfin
Vigabatrin
Vitamin K1
Yellow Fever Vaccine
Zaleplon
Zanamivir
Zidovudine
Ziprasidone Mesylate
Zolmitriptan
Zolpidem Tartrate
Zonisamide

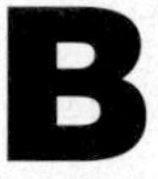

NO EVIDENCE OF RISK IN HUMANS

Either animal findings show risk while human findings do not, or, if no adequate human studies have been done, animal findings are negative.

Acarbose
Acrivastine
Acyclovir
Acyclovir Sodium
Adalimumab
Agalsidase Beta
Alefacept
Alfuzosin Hydrochloride
Alosetron Hydrochloride
Alvimopan
Amiloride Hydrochloride
Amiloride Hydrochloride/ Hydrochlorothiazide
Amoxicillin
Amoxicillin/Clavulanate Potassium
Amphotericin B
Amphotericin B Lipid Complex
Amphotericin B, Liposomal
Amphotericin B/Cholesteryl Sulfate Complex
Ampicillin Sodium/ Sulbactam Sodium
Anakinra

* Category C or D depending on the trimester the drug is given.

Antithrombin III
Aprepitant
Aprotinin
Argatroban
Arginine Hydrochloride
Atazanavir Sulfate
Azelaic Acid
Azithromycin
Azithromycin Dihydrate
Aztreonam
Balsalazide Disodium
Basiliximab
Bivalirudin
Brimonidine Tartrate
Bromocriptine Besylate
Budesonide
Cabergoline
Cefaclor
Cefazolin Sodium
Cefdinir
Cefditoren Pivoxil
Cefepime Hydrochloride
Cefixime
Cefotetan Disodium
Cefoxitin Sodium
Cefpodoxime Proxetil
Cefprozil
Ceftazidime Sodium
Ceftibuten Dihydrate
Ceftriaxone Sodium
Cefuroxime
Cefuroxime Axetil
Cephalexin
Cetirizine Hydrochloride
Certolizumab Pegol
Ciclopirox
Ciclopirox Olamine
Cimetidine Hydrochloride
Cisatracurium Besylate
Clindamycin Hydrochloride/ Clindamycin Phosphate
Clindamycin Palmitate Hydrochloride
Clindamycin Phosphate
Clopidogrel Bisulfate
Clotrimazole
Clozapine
Colesevelam Hydrochloride
Cromolyn Sodium
Cyclobenzaprine Hydrochloride
Cyproheptadine Hydrochloride
Dalfopristin/Quinupristin
Dalteparin Sodium
Dapiprazole Hydrochloride
Daptomycin
Desflurane
Desmopressin Acetate
Dexlansoprazole
Dicyclomine Hydrochloride
Didanosine
Diphenhydramine Hydrochloride
Dipivefrin Hydrochloride
Dipyridamole
Dolasetron Mesylate
Doripenem
Dornase Alfa
Doxapram Hydrochloride
Doxepin Hydrochloride
Doxercalciferol
Edetate Calcium Disodium
Emtricitabine
Emtricitabine/Tenofovir Disoproxil Fumarate
Enfuvirtide
Enoxaparin Sodium
Eplerenone
Epoprostenol Sodium
Ertapenem
Erythromycin
Erythromycin Ethylsuccinate
Erythromycin Stearate
Esomeprazole Magnesium
Esomeprazole Sodium
Etanercept
Ethacrynate Sodium
Ethacrynic Acid
Etravirine
Famciclovir
Famotidine
Fenoldopam Mesylate
Fondaparinux Sodium
Galantamine Hydrobromide
Glatiramer Acetate
Glucagon
Glyburide/Metformin Hydrochloride
Guanfacine HCl
Granisetron Hydrochloride
Hydrochlorothiazide
Ibuprofen
Indapamide
Infliximab
Insulin Aspart
Insulin Lispro Protamine, Human/Insulin Lispro, Human
Insulin Lispro, Recombinant
Ipratropium Bromide
Iron Sucrose
Isosorbide Mononitrate
Lactulose
Lansoprazole
Lansoprazole/Naproxen
Laronidase
Lepirudin
Levocarnitine
Levocetirizine Dihydrochloride
Lidocaine Hydrochloride
Lidocaine/Prilocaine
Lindane
Loperamide Hydrochloride
Loratadine
Malathion
Maraviroc
Meclizine Hydrochloride
Memantine Hydrochloride
Meropenem
Mesalamine
Metformin Hydrochloride
Metformin Hydrochloride/ Sitagliptin
Methohexital Sodium
Methyldopa
Methylnaltrexone Bromide
Metolazone
Metronidazole
Miglitol
Montelukast Sodium
Mupirocin
Mupirocin Calcium
Naftifine Hydrochloride
Nalbuphine Hydrochloride
Naloxone Hydrochloride
Naproxen Sodium
Nedocromil Sodium
Nelfinavir Mesylate
Nitazoxanide
Nitrofurantoin Macrocrystals
Nitrofurantoin Macrocrystals/ Nitrofurantoin Monohydrate
Nizatidine
Octreotide Acetate
Omalizumab
Ondansetron Hydrochloride
Orlistat
Oxiconazole Nitrate
Oxybutynin
Oxybutynin Chloride
Oxycodone Hydrochloride
Palonosetron Hydrochloride
Pancrelipase
Pantoprazole Sodium
Pegvisomant
Penciclovir
Penicillin G Benzathine
Penicillin G Benzathine/ Penicillin G Procaine
Penicillin G Potassium
Pentosan Polysulfate Sodium
Permethrin
Piperacillin Sodium
Piperacillin Sodium/ Tazobactam Sodium
Prasugrel HCl
Praziquantel
Progesterone
Propofol
Pseudoephedrine Hydrochloride
Psyllium Preparations
Rabeprazole Sodium
Ranitidine Hydrochloride
Retapamulin
Rifabutin
Ritonavir
Rivastigmine Tartrate
Ropivacaine Hydrochloride
Saquinavir Mesylate
Saxagliptin
Sevoflurane
Sildenafil Citrate
Silver Sulfadiazine
Sitagliptin Phosphate
Sodium Ferric Gluconate
Somatropin
Sotalol Hydrochloride
Sucralfate
Sulfasalazine
Tadalafil
Tamsulosin Hydrochloride
Tenofovir Disoproxil Fumarate
Teprostinil
Terbinafine Hydrochloride
Ticarcillin Disodium/ Clavulanate Potassium
Ticlopidine Hydrochloride
Tirofiban Hydrochloride
Torsemide
Tranexamic Acid
Trastuzumab
Treprostinil Sodium
Urokinase
Ursodiol
Ustekinumab
Valacyclovir Hydrochloride
Vancomycin Hydrochloride
Vardenafil Hydrochloride
Zafirlukast

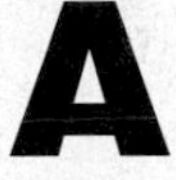

CONTROLLED STUDIES SHOW NO RISK

Adequate, well-controlled studies in pregnant women have failed to demonstrate risk to the fetus.

Liothyronine Sodium
Liotrix
Nystatin

* Category C or D depending on the trimester the drug is given.

DRUGS EXCRETED IN BREAST MILK

The following list is not comprehensive; generic forms and alternate brands of some products may be available. When recommending drugs to pregnant or nursing patients, always check product labeling for specific precautions.

Accolate
Accuretic
Aciphex
Actiq
Activella
Actonel
Actonel with Calcium
ActoPlus Met
Adalat
Adderall
Advicor
Aggrenox
Aldactazide
Aldactone
Alesse
Alfenta
Allegra-D
Aloprim
Altace
Ambien
Amerge
Anafranil
Anaprox
Androderm
Aplenzin
Apresoline
Aralen
Arthrotec
Asacol
Ativan
Augmentin
Avalide
Avandamet
Axid
Azactam
Azasan
Azathioprine
Azulfidine
Bactrim
Baraclude
Benadryl
Bentyl
Betapace
Bexxar
Bicillin
Boniva
Brethine
Brevicon
Brontex
Byetta
Caduet
Cafergot
Calan
Campral
Capoten
Capozide
Captopril
Carbatrol
Cardizem
Cataflam
Catapres
Ceclor
Cefotan
Ceftin
Celebrex
Celexa
Cerebyx
Ceredase
Cipro
Ciprodex
Claforan
Clarinex
Claritin
Claritin-D
Cleocin
Climara
Clozaril
Codeine
Combigan
CombiPatch
Combivir
Combunox
Compazine
Cordarone
Corgard
Cortisporin
Corzide
Cosopt
Coumadin
Covera-HS
Cozaar
Crestor
Crinone
Cyclessa
Cymbalta
Cytomel
Cytotec
Dapsone
Daraprim
Darvon
Darvon-N
Deconsal II
Demerol
Demulen
Depacon
Depakene
Depakote
DepoDur
Depo-Provera
Desogen
Desoxyn
Desyrel
Dexedrine
DextroStat
D.H.E. 45
Diabinese
Diastat
Diflucan
Digitek
Dilacor
Dilantin
Dilaudid
Diovan
Diprivan
Diuril
Dolobid
Dolophine
Doral
Doryx
Droxia
Duraclon
Duragesic
Duramorph
Duratuss
Duricef
Dyazide
Dyrenium
E.E.S.
EC-Naprosyn
Ecotrin
Effexor
Elavil
EMLA
Enduron
Epzicom
Equetro
ERYC
EryPed
Ery-Tab
Erythrocin
Erythromycin
Esgic-plus
Eskalith
Estrogel
Estrostep
Evista
Factive
FazaClo
Felbatol
Feldene
femhrt
Fiorinal
Flagyl
Floxin
Foradil
Fortamet
Fortaz
Fosamax
Furosemide
Gabitril
Galzin
Garamycin
Glucophage
Glucovance
Glumetza
Glyset
Halcion
Haldol
Helidac
Hycamtin
Hydrocortone
Ifex
Imitrex
Imuran
Inderal
Indocin
INFeD
Inspra
Invanz
Invega
Isoptin
Janumet
Kadian
Kaletra
Keflex
Keppra
Kerlone
Ketek
Klonopin
Kronofed-A
Lamictal
Lamisil
Lamprene
Lanoxicaps
Lanoxin
Lariam
Lescol
Letairis
Levbid
Levitra
Levlen
Levlite
Levora
Levothroid
Levoxyl
Levsin
Levsinex
Lexapro
Lexiva
Lialda
Lindane
Lioresal
Lithium
Lithobid
Lo/Ovral
Loestrin
Lomotil
Lopressor
Lortab
Lotensin
Lotrel
Luminal
Luvox
Lyrica
Macrobid
Macrodantin
Marinol
Maxipime
Maxzide
Menostar
Metaglip
Methergine
Methotrexate
MetroCream/Gel/Lotion
Micronor
Microzide
Migranal
Minocin
Mirapex
Mircette
M-M-R II
Mobic
Modicon
Monodox
Monopril
Morphine
MS Contin
Myambutol
Mycamine
Mysoline
Namenda
Naprelan
Naprosyn
Nascobal
Necon
Nembutal
Neoral
Neurontin
Niaspan
Nicotrol
Niravam
Nizoral
Norco
Nor-QD
Nordette
Norinyl
Noritate
Normodyne
Norpace
Norpramin
Novantrone
Nubain
Nucofed
Nydrazid
Oramorph
Ortho-Cept
Ortho-Cyclen
Ortho-Novum
Ortho Tri-Cyclen
Orudis
Ovcon
Oxistat
OxyContin
OxyIR
Pacerone
Pamelor
Pancrease
Paxil
PCE
Pediapred
Pediazole
Pediotic
Pentasa
Pepcid
Periostat
Persantine
Pfizerpen
Phenergan
Phenobarbital
Phenytek
Phrenilin
Plan B
Ponstel
Prandimet
Pravachol
Premphase
Prempro
Prevacid
Prevacid NapraPAC
PREVPAC
Prinzide
Pristiq
Prograf
Prometrium
Pronestyl
Propofol
Prosed/DS
Protonix
Provera
Prozac
Pseudoephedrine
Pulmicort
Pyrazinamide
Quinidex
Quinine
Reglan
Relpax
Renese
Requip
Reserpine
Restoril
Retrovir
Rifadin
Rifamate
Rifater
Risperdal
Rocaltrol
Rocephin
Roxanol
Rozerem
Sanctura
Sanctura XR
Sandimmune
Sarafem
Seconal
Sectral
Semprex-D
Septra
Seroquel
Seroquel XR
Soma
Sonata
Soriatane
Spiriva
Sprycel
Stadol
Stavzor
Streptomycin
Stromectol
Symbyax
Synthroid
Tagamet
Tambocor
Tapazole
Tarka
Tasigna
Tavist
Tazicef
Tegretol
Tenoretic
Tenormin
Thalitone
Theo-24
Theo-Dur
Thorazine
Tiazac
Timoptic
Tindamax
Tobi
Tofranil
Toprol-XL
Toradol
Trandate
Tranxene
Trental
Tricor
Triglide
Trileptal
Tri-Levlen
Tri-Norinyl
Triostat
Triphasil
Trisenox
Trivora
Trizivir
Truvada
Tygacil
Tylenol
Tylenol with Codeine
Ultane
Ultram
Unasyn
Uniphyl
Uniretic
Unithroid
Valium
Valtrex
Vancocin
Vantin
Vaseretic
Vasotec
Ventavis
Verelan
Vermox
Vibramycin
Vibra-Tabs
Vicodin
Vigamox
Viramune
Voltaren
Vytorin
Vyvanse
Wellbutrin
Xanax
Xolair
Zantac
Zarontin
Zaroxolyn
Zegerid
Zemplar
Zestoretic
Zetia
Ziac
Zinacef
Zithromax
Zoloft
Zomig
Zonalon
Zonegran
Zosyn
Zovia
Zovirax
Zyban
Zydone
Zyloprim
Zyprexa
Zyrtec

TABLES FOR PHARMACY CALCULATIONS

WEIGHTS AND MEASURES

Metric Measure

Weight

1 kilogram (kg)	=	1,000 g
1 gram (g)	=	1,000 mg
1 milligram (mg)	=	0.001 g
1 microgram (mcg)	=	0.001 mg
1 gamma	=	1 mcg

Liquid

1 liter (L)	=	1,000 mL
1 milliliter (mL)	=	1 cc (cubic centimeter)

Apothecary (Ap)

Weight

1 scruple	=	20 grains (gr)
1 drachm	=	3 scruples
	=	60 gr
1 ounce (oz)	=	8 drachms
	=	24 scruples
	=	480 gr
1 pound (lb)	=	12 oz
	=	96 drachms
	=	288 scruples
	=	5,760 gr

U.S. Fluid Measure

1 fluidrachm	=	60 minim (min)
1 fluidounce	=	8 fld drachm
	=	480 min
1 pint (pt)	=	16 fl oz
	=	7,680 min
1 quart (qt)	=	2 pt
	=	32 fl oz
1 gallon (gal)	=	4 qts
	=	128 fl oz

Avoirdupois (Av)

Weight

1 ounce	=	437.5 gr
1 pound	=	16 oz

Conversion Factors

1 gram	=	15.4 gr
1 grain	=	64.8 mg
1 ounce (Av)	=	28.35 g
	=	437.5 gr
1 ounce (Ap)	=	31.1 g
	=	480 gr
1 pound (Av)	=	453.6 g
1 kilogram	=	2.68 pounds Ap
	=	2.20 lbs Av
1 fluidounce	=	29.57 mL
1 fluidrachm	=	3.697 mL
1 minim	=	0.06 mL

Converting °F to °C

For °F to °C, the formula is: °C=$\frac{5}{9}$ (°F- 32)
For °C to °F, the formula is: °F=($\frac{9}{5}$ × °C) + 32

Common Measures

1 teaspoonful	=	5 mL
	=	$\frac{1}{6}$ fl oz
1 tablespoonful	=	15 mL
	=	$\frac{1}{2}$ fl oz
1 wineglassful	=	60 mL
	=	2 fl oz
1 teacupful	=	120 mL
	=	4 fl oz

TABLE OF SATURATED SOLUTIONS

This table shows the quantity of the substance and milliliters (mL) of water for 100 mL of a saturated solution at about 25° C.

Substance	Gram	mL Water
Alum	13.00	92.0
Ammonium Carbonate	22.00	88.0
Ammonium Chloride	28.30	79.3
Ammonium Nitrate	90.20	41.8
Ammonium Sulfate	53.10	71.7
Borax	5.90	98.0
Boric Acid	5.10	97.0
Calcium Lactate	5.00	96.0
Chloral Hydrate	120.00	31.0
Citric Acid	88.60	42.7
Copper Sulfate	22.30	98.7
Dextrose	59.00	60.0
Ferric Chloride	125.00	29.0
Ferrous Sulfate	52.80	72.7
Lactose	17.00	90.0
Lead Acetate	55.00	79.0
Lithium Chloride	59.50	70.2
Lithium Sulfate	33.00	88.5
Magnesium Sulfate	72.00	58.5
Manganese Chloride	90.00	54.0
Mercuric Chloride	6.96	98.5
Methylene Blue	4.30	97.0
Oxalic Acid	10.30	94.2
Potassium Bromide	56.00	82.0
Potassium Carbonate	82.20	73.5
Potassium Chloride	8.41	96.6
Potassium Citrate	92.00	56.5
Potassium Iodide	103.20	69.1
Potassium Nitrate	33.40	86.0
Potassium Permanganate	7.43	97.3
Resorcinol	67.20	47.2
Rochelle Salt	51.90	78.8
Silver Nitrate	164.00	65.5
Sodium Acetate	65.00	53.0
Sodium Benzoate	41.50	73.9
Sodium Bicarbonate	8.80	97.6
Sodium Bromide	73.00	78.0
Sodium Carbonate	27.50	96.0
Sodium Chloride	31.50	88.1
Sodium Citrate	55.50	72.5
Sodium Iodide	124.30	67.7
Sodium Nitrate	62.30	73.8
Sodium Salicylate	67.00	58.0
Sodium Sulfate	33.30	87.0
Sodium Thiocyanate	87.00	51.0
Sodium Thiosulfate	93.00	46.0
Tartaric Acid	76.90	54.7
Urea	62.00	53.5
Zinc Sulfate	93.00	56.0

DOSE EQUIVALENTS

These approximate dose equivalents have been adopted by U.S.P. XXII, N.F. XVII. They are approved by the Food and Drug Administration. When converting specific quantities or a prescription that requires compounding, or when converting a pharmaceutical formula from one system of weights or measures to the other, the following must be used.

Weight

Metric	Apothecary
030 g	1 ounce
015 g	4 drachms
010 g	$2\frac{1}{2}$ drachms
07.5 g	2 drachms
006 g	90 grains
005 g	75 grains
004 g	60 grains (1 drachm)
003 g	45 grains
002 g	30 grains ($\frac{1}{2}$ drachm)
01.5 g	22 grains
001 g	15 grains
750 mg	12 grains
600 mg	10 grains
500 mg	$7\frac{1}{2}$ grains
400 mg	6 grains
300 mg	5 grains
250 mg	4 grains
200 mg	3 grains
150 mg	$2\frac{1}{2}$ grains
125 mg	2 grains
100 mg	$1\frac{1}{2}$ grains
75 mg	$1\frac{1}{4}$ grains
60 mg	1 grain
50 mg	$\frac{3}{4}$ grain
40 mg	$\frac{2}{3}$ grain
30 mg	$\frac{1}{2}$ grain
25 mg	$\frac{3}{8}$ grain
20 mg	$\frac{1}{3}$ grain
15 mg	$\frac{1}{4}$ grain
12 mg	$\frac{1}{5}$ grain
10 mg	$\frac{1}{6}$ grain
08 mg	$\frac{1}{8}$ grain
06 mg	$\frac{1}{10}$ grain
05 mg	$\frac{1}{12}$ grain
04 mg	$\frac{1}{15}$ grain
03 mg	$\frac{1}{20}$ grain
02 mg	$\frac{1}{30}$ grain
1.5 mg	$\frac{1}{40}$ grain
1.2 mg	$\frac{1}{50}$ grain
01 mg	$\frac{1}{60}$ grain

Liquid Measure

Metric	Apothecary
1000 mL	1 quart
0750 mL	$1\frac{1}{2}$ pints
0500 mL	1 pint
0250 mL	8 fluidounces
0200 mL	7 fluidounces
0100 mL	$3\frac{1}{2}$ fluidounces
0050 mL	$1\frac{3}{4}$ fluidounces
0030 mL	1 fluidounce
0015 mL	4 fluidrachms
0010 mL	$2\frac{1}{2}$ fluidrachms
0008 mL	2 fluidrachms
0005 mL	$1\frac{1}{4}$ fluidrachms
0004 mL	1 fluidrachm
0003 mL	45 minims
0002 mL	30 minims
0001 mL	15 minims
0.75 mL	12 minims
00.6 mL	10 minims
00.5 mL	8 minims
00.3 mL	5 minims
0.25 mL	4 minims
00.2 mL	3 minims
00.1 mL	$1\frac{1}{2}$ minims
0.06 mL	1 minim
0.05 mL	$\frac{3}{4}$ minim
0.03 mL	$\frac{1}{2}$ minim

COMMON LABORATORY TEST VALUES

Listed below are generally accepted normal values for a selection of common laboratory assays conducted on serum, plasma, and blood. Remember that norms may vary from laboratory to laboratory in accordance with the methodology and quality control measures employed by the facility. When in doubt, check with the laboratory that performed the analysis.

"SI range" refers to Système International d'Unités, a uniform system of reporting numerical values that permits interchangeability of information among nations and disciplines.

Test	US Range	SI Range
Acid phosphatase	≤2.5 ng/mL	≤2.5 µg/L
Prostatic Total	≤5.8 U/L	<97 nkat/L
Alanine aminotransferase [ALT] (SGPT)	≤48 U/L	≤0.8 µkat/L
Albumin, serum	3.5-5.5 g/dL	35-55 g/L
Alkaline phosphatase	20-125 U/L	0.33-2.08 µkat/L
Ammonia [NH_3+]	10-80 µg/dL	6-47 µmol/L
Amylase, serum	60-180 U/L	0.8-3.2 µkat/L
Antinuclear antibodies (ANA)	Negative at 1:40 dilution	
Aspartate aminotransferase (AST) (SGOT)	≤42 U/L	,0.7 µkat/L
Bilirubin		
Total	0.3-1.0 mg/dL	5.1-17 µmol/L
Direct	0.1-0.3 mg/dL	1.7-5.1 µmol/L
Indirect	0.2-0.7 mg/dL	3.4-12 µmol/L
Blood urea nitrogen/creatinine ratio	10:1-20:1	Average 15:1
Calcium, plasma	9-10.5 mg/dL	2.2-2.6 mmol/L
Calcium, ionized	4.5-5.6 mg/dL	1.1-1.4 mmol/L
Chloride, serum	95-108 mEq/L	95-108 mmol/L
Cholesterol (total plasma)		
Desirable level	<200 mg/dL	<5.20 mmol/L
Moderate risk	200-240 mg/dL	5.2-6.3 mmol/L
High risk	>240 mg/dL	>6.3 mmol/L
Copper	70-140 µg/dL	11-22 µmol/L
Cortisol, serum		
0800 hours	5-25 µg/dL	140-690 nmol/L
1600 hours	3-12 µg/dL	80-330 nmol/L
Creatinine kinase (CK)		
Isoenzymes	CK-MM: 97-100% of total	CK-MM: 0.97-1.00 of total
	CK-MB: <3% of total	CK-MB: <0.03 of total
	CK-BB: 0% of total	CK-BB: 0 of total
Total	Male: ≤235 U/L	Male: ≤3.92 µkat/L
	Female: ≤190 U/L	Female: ≤3.17 µkat/L
Creatinine, serum	<1.5 mg/dL	<133 µmol/L
Creatinine clearance	75-125 mL/min	1.24-2.08 mL/sec
Digoxin		
Therapeutic	0.8-2.0 ng/mL	1.0-2.6 nmol/L
Toxic	>2.5 ng/mL	>3.2 nmol/L
Erythrocyte count (RBC)	4.15-4.90 × 10^6/mm^3	4.15-4.90 × 10^{12}/L
Erythrocyte sedimentation rate (ESR)		
Male	0-20 mm/hr	0-20 mm/hr
Female	0-30 mm/hr	0-30 mm/hr
Ferritin		
Male	15-400 ng/mL	15-400 µg/L
Female	10-200 ng/mL	10-200 µg/L
Folic acid	3-16 ng/mL	7-36 nmol/L

Test	US Range	SI Range
Follicle-stimulating hormone (FSH)		
Female	1.4-9.6 mIU/mL	1.4-9.6 IU/L
Ovulation	2.3-21 mIU/mL	2.3-21 IU/L
Postmenopausal	34-96 mIU/mL	34-96 IU/L
Male	0.9-15 mIU/mL	0.9-15 IU/L
Gamma-glutamyl transferase (GGT)		
Male	≤65 U/L	≤1.08 µkat/L
Female	≤45 U/L	≤0.75 µkat/L
Gases, arterial blood		
pO_2	80-100 mmHg	11-13 kPa
pCO_2	35-45 mmHg	4.7-6 kPa
Glucose, plasma		
Fasting	75-115 mg/dL	4.2-6.4 mmol/L
Postprandial (2 h)	<140 mg/dL	<7.8 mmol/L
Immunoglobulins (Ig)		
IgG	800-1500 mg/dL	8.0-15.0 g/L
IgA	90-325 mg/dL	0.9-3.2 g/L
IgM	45-150 mg/dL	0.45-1.5 g/L
IgD	0-8 mg/dL	0-0.08 g/L
IgE	<0.025 mg/dL	<0.00025 g/L
Iron, serum	50-150 µg/dL	9-27 µmol/L
Iron binding capacity	250-370 µg/dL	45-66 µmol/L
Iron saturation	20-45%	
Lactic acid (plasma, venous)	9-16 mg/dL	1.0-1.8 mmol/L
Lactic dehydrogenase (LDH)	100-190 U/L	1.7-3.2 µkat/L
Lead	<20 µg/dL	1.0 µmol/L
Leukocyte count (WBC)	$4.3\text{-}10.8 \times 10^3$	$4.3\text{-}10.8 \times 10^9$/L
Lipase	0-160 U/L	0-2.66 µkat/L
Lipoproteins (desirable levels)		
Low density (LDL)	<130 mg/dL	<3.36 mmol/L
High density (HDL)	>60 mg/dL	>1.55 mmol/L
Lithium ion (therapeutic)	0.6-1.2 mEq/L	0.6-1.2 mmol/L
Luteinizing hormone		
Female	0.8-26 mIU/mL	0.8-26 IU/L
Ovulation	25-57 mIU/mL	25-57 IU/L
Postmenopausal	40-104 mIU/mL	40-104 IU/L
Male	1.3-13 mIU/mL	1.3-13 IU/L
Osmolality, plasma	285-295 mOsm/kg	285-295 mmol/kg
Phenytoin		
Therapeutic	10-20 mg/L	40-80 µmol/L
Toxic	>30 mg/L	>120 µmol/L
Phosphorus, serum	2.5-4.5 mg/dL	0.8-1.45 mmol/L
Potassium, serum	3.5-5 mEq/L	3.5-5 mmol/L
Prolactin	2-15 ng/mL	2-15 µg/L
Prostate-specific antigen (PSA)	≤4 ng/mL	≤4 µg/L
Protein		
Total	5.5-8.0 g/dL	55-80 g/L
Albumin	3.5-5.5 g/dL	35-55 g/L
Globulin	2.0-3.5 g/dL	20-35 g/L
Reticulocyte count	0.5-2.3% of RBCs	0.005-0.023 of RBCs
Rheumatoid factor	<40 IU/mL	<40 kIU/L
Sodium, serum	136-145 mEq/L	136-145 mmol/L
Theophylline (therapeutic)	10-20 mg/L	55-110 µmol/L

Test	US Range	SI Range
Thyroxine-binding globulin (TBG)	16-34 mg/L	16-34 mg/L
Thyroid-stimulating hormone (TSH)	0.4-5 µU/mL	0.4-5 mU/L
Thyroxine (T_4)		
Free	0.8-1.8 ng/dL	10-23 pmol/L
Total	4.5-12.5 µg/dL	58-161 nmol/L
Transferrin	230-390 µg/dL	2.3-3.9 mg/L
Triglycerides	<160 µg/dL	<1.8 mmol/L
Triiodothyronine (T_3)	70-190 ng/dL	1.1-2.9 nmol/L
T_3 uptake	25-35%	0.25-0.35 (proportion of 1.0)
Urea nitrogen, blood (BUN)	7-30 mg/dL	2.5-10.7 mmol/L
Uric acid		
Male	4.0-8.5 mg/dL	238-506 µmol/L
Female	2.5-7.5 mg/dL	149-446 µmol/L
Vitamin B_{12}	200-600 pg/mL	148-443 pmol/L

Sources:

Beers MH, Porter RS, Jones TV, et al. *Merck Manual of Diagnosis and Therapy*, ed 18. Whitehouse Station, NJ: Merck Research Laboratories; 2006.

Cahill M. *Illustrated Guide to Diagnostic Tests*, ed 2. Springhouse, PA: Springhouse Corporation; 1998.

Fauci AS, Braunwald E, Kasper DL, et al. *Harrison's Principles of Internal Medicine*, ed 17. New York, NY: McGraw Hill; 2008.

Goldman L, Ausiello D. *Cecil Medicine*, ed 23. Philadelphia, PA: Saunders Elsevier; 2008.

Sacher RA, McPherson RA, Campos JM. *Wildmann's Clinical Interpretation of Laboratory Tests*. Philadelphia, PA: FA Davis Company; 2000.

herbs, consult the latest edition of the

culeatus). This herb, native to the
Africa, and western Asia, is used medici-
ry, and for its beneficial effects on circula-
ieve the discomforts of hemorrhoids, such
the leg heaviness, pain, cramping, and
enous insufficiency.

). The root of the South American Cat's
ve immune-stimulating, anti-inflammatory,
is often used to treat cancer; arthritis and
d other viral diseases. It has also been
asthma, menstrual irregularities, and
ects on estradiol and progesterone, Cat's
s a contraceptive.

be used by pregnant or breastfeeding
mmune disorders, multiple sclerosis, or
and children under 2 years of age should
should not be combined with anticoagu-
gents.

xternally, Cayenne is used to relieve the
n, diabetic neuropathy, and rheumatism.
nally to relieve gastrointestinal disorders.

ations should not be used for more than
o-week break between applications. It
kin or near the eyes. When used internal-
not be taken with aspirin or antifungal
avoided by people who have stomach
onic irritable bowel, gastrointestinal dis-
who are undergoing inhalation therapy.

a recutita). Chamomile tea—which has
and muscle-relaxing effects—is used to
h as indigestion and gas. It is also used
ness, and general debility. It is used topi-
and throat, rhinitis, toothache, earache,
used in mouthwashes.

e used by pregnant women.

e). This herb is applied topically as
or bruises and sprains and to promote

adverse effects, Comfrey should not be
indicated in pregnant and breastfeeding
by people with a history of liver or kidney

). Dandelion, commonly used as an addi-
nded as an effective remedy for digestive
nfection, and as an appetite stimulant.

Warning: Although the herb is sometimes used for gallbladder complaints, this should only be done under a doctor's supervision. People with bile duct obstruction or stomach ulcer should not use Dandelion.

Dong Quai *(Angelica sinensis)*. Dong Quai root is used in China as a women's health tonic. It is particularly used as a remedy for fibrocystic breast disease, premenstrual syndrome, painful periods, and menopausal symptoms. Dong Quai is also used in cardiovascular disease to treat high blood pressure and improve poor circulation. It is has also been used for rheumatism, ulcers, anemia, allergies, constipation, as a blood tonic, and to strengthen the uterus and aid patients in supportive functions before pregnancy. In Japan, the herb is used as an analgesic, sedative, and nutrient.

Warning: Dong Quai should not be used by pregnant or breastfeeding women. It is contraindicated in patients with hemorrhagic disease, hypermenorrhea, chronic diarrhea, abdominal bloating, or acute infections including colds and flu. It should not be used by people with bleeding disorders, or by those taking blood thinners. The herb can also cause photosensitivity.

Echinacea *(Echinacea purpurea)*. This species of Echinacea is a well-established immune-system stimulator; it is used to treat flu, fevers, coughs and colds, bronchitis, urinary tract infections, wounds and burns, and inflammation of the mouth and pharynx. It is also used to prevent infection.

Warning: Echinacea should not be used in patients who have autoimmune disorders such as multiple sclerosis, collagen disease, AIDS or HIV infection, leukosis, and tuberculosis. Parenteral administration should not be used in patients with diabetes or those prone to allergies, especially to members of the composite family *(Asteraceae)*. The herb is also contraindicated in pregnant or breastfeeding women. Echinacea should not be used with the following: anticancer agents, drugs used to prevent organ rejection, corticosteroids, immunosuppressants, or drugs metabolized by cytochrome P450 3A4 antibodies.

English Hawthorn *(Crataegus laevigata)*. Hawthorn contains several compounds that are considered beneficial to the heart. It is used for cardiac insufficiency, angina, congestive heart failure, and irregular heartbeat.

Warning: Hawthorn should not be used in children under 12, or in the first trimester of pregnancy. People taking Hawthorn must be carefully monitored by a physician, especially in cases where it is combined with cardiac glycosides, beta-blockers, calcium channel blockers, antiarrhythmics, or antiplatelet agents. Hawthorn should not be taken with cisapride. Overuse can lead to low blood pressure, irregular heartbeat, and excessive sleepiness.

Evening Primrose *(Oenothera biennis)*. The anti-inflammatory compounds in Evening Primrose oil have been extensively studied, but no definitive indication has been accepted. Some herbalists consider the oil useful for treating breast pain, premenstrual syndrome, menopausal symptoms, and cyclic mastalgia. Other common uses include hypertension, rheumatoid arthritis, thrombosis, and autoimmune disease *(*e.g., multiple sclerosis and Raynaud's phenomenon*)*. Capsules containing at least 500 mg of the oil are approved in Germany as a remedy for eczema.

Warning: People with seizure disorder or schizophrenia should not take Evening Primrose oil. It should not be used by people with bleeding disorders or those taking blood thinners.

Feverfew *(Tanacetum parthenium)*. Feverfew is used to treat migraine headaches, allergies, and arthritic and rheumatic diseases. It has also been used to treat tinnitus, vertigo, arthritis, fever, toothache, insect bites, and asthma.

Warning: Feverfew should not be used during pregnancy or breastfeeding. It is also contraindicated in people with bleeding disorders and those using anticoagulants, including aspirin. This herb should not be used in children under 2 years of age.

Flax *(Linum usitatissimum)*. Ground Flax *(*also known as Linseed*)* is used internally to relieve constipation. It is also used externally as a compress to relieve skin inflammation.

Warning: Flax should not be used internally by patients with bowel or esophageal obstruction; or in the presence of gastrointestinal or esophageal inflammation. Flax may delay absorption of other drugs taken simultaneously.

Fo-Ti *(Polygonum multiflorum)*. The Asian herb Fo-Ti is used for constipation, atherosclerosis, fatigue, high cholesterol, and as an immune enhancer.

Warning: Because of its laxative action, the herb may cause diarrhea. Taking the unprocessed root may cause skin rash, and overdosage may cause numbness in the extremities.

Garlic *(Allium sativum)*. Garlic is used as a treatment for hardening of the arteries, high blood pressure, and for reducing cholesterol levels. It may also have antibacterial and antiviral effects. It is used internally as an adjuvant to dietetic measures for elevated lipid levels and the prevention of age-related vascular changes and arteriosclerosis. Recent studies, however, found garlic ineffective for reducing cholesterol.

Warning: Garlic can cause allergic skin and respiratory reactions. It should not be used by people with bleeding disorders, or by those taking blood thinners *(*including aspirin*)* or NSAID therapy. Garlic significantly induces the metabolism of chlorzoxazone and should not be used with this drug. Starting or stopping Garlic intake while taking protease inhibitors should not be done without consulting a physician. Nursing women should also avoid Garlic.

Ginger *(Zingiber officinale)*. Ginger root is a treatment for motion sickness and loss of appetite. It is also indicated for dyspeptic complaints, for nausea and vomiting associated with chemotherapy, and for helping to control nausea and vomiting in postoperative patients.

Warning: Ginger should not be used for morning sickness associated with pregnancy, or by nursing mothers, without physician approval. People who have gallstones or bleeding disorders should not take Ginger. Caution is advised for individuals concomitantly taking ginger and blood thinners or NSAID therapy (including asprin).

Ginkgo *(Gingko biloba)*. Ginkgo may be helpful for treating dementia, Alzheimer's disease, peripheral arterial occlusive disease, vertigo, and tinnitus of vascular origin.

Warning: Ginkgo should not be used by people who have bleeding disorders or who are taking blood thinners or NSAID therapy *(*including aspirin*)*. Patients with a history of seizures should use the herb with caution, since Ginkgo may lower the seizure threshold.

Ginseng *(Panax ginseng)*. The Ginseng root is used for alleviating fatigue and improving concentration and stamina. Ginseng may also have antiviral, antioxidant, and anticancer effects.

Warning: People with cardiovascular disease or diabetes should use the herb cautiously. People who are taking diabetes drugs, diuretics, blood thinners, MAO inhibitors, or NSAIDs *(*including aspirin*)* should not take Ginseng. It should not be used during pregnancy or breastfeeding, or by those with bleeding disorders. Taking large amounts can result in Ginseng abuse syndrome, which is characterized by high blood pressure, insomnia, water retention, skin eruptions, diarrhea, and muscle tension. Concomitant use of Ginseng with conjugated estrogens may result in symptoms of estrogen excess.

Goldenseal *(Hydrastis canadensis)*. Goldenseal contains the compound berberine, which is used for gastritis, gastric ulcer, gallbladder disease, and acute diarrhea. Goldenseal is also used externally as an antiseptic for wounds and *herpes labialis*.

Berberine is also used as an adjunct treatment in various cancers and in neutropenia resulting from radiation and chemotherapy.

Warning: Goldenseal should not be used by pregnant or breastfeeding women, by women with a history of miscarriage, or by individuals with bleeding disorders. It should also not be combined with blood thinners or NSAIDs (including aspirin). In addition, the herb should not be used in people with glucose-6-phosphate-dehydrogenase deficiency. Use of Goldenseal for extended periods can result in digestive disorders, constipation, hallucination or delirium, and decreased vitamin B absorption. Overdosage can result in convulsion, difficulty breathing, and paralysis.

Gotu Kola *(Centella asiatica)*. Gotu Kola is used internally for chronic venous insufficiency and venous hypertension. In animal and lab studies, Gotu Kola was also effective for ulcers and varicose veins. The herb is used externally to treat wounds; if a rash develops, discontinue topical use.

Warning: Gotu Kola should not be used during pregnancy.

Great Burnet *(Sanguisorba officinalis)*. Great Burnet may be used for its astringent, decongestant, and diuretic properties. It is used internally for dysentery, enteritis, hemorrhoids, phlebitis, menopausal symptoms, intestinal bladder problems, and venous disorders. It is also prepared for external use as a plaster for wounds and ulcers.

Green Tea *(Camellia sinensis)*. Green tea, which is rich in catechins and flavonoids, is used to help prevent cancer. The antibacterial effects of Green Tea mouthwash are useful in the prevention of dental cavities. Keep in mind that Green Tea contains caffeine and should be used sparingly by pregnant and breastfeeding women and by those who are caffeine-sensitive. Consuming too much Green Tea may result in hyperacidity, gastric irritation, reduction of appetite, and diarrhea; however, these symptoms can generally be avoided by the addition of milk. Green Tea should be used cautiously by those with weakened cardiovascular systems, renal disease, thyroid hyperfunction, elevated susceptibility to spasm, and psychic disorders such as anxiety. Also be aware that the herb reacts with alkaline medication and may delay resorption.

Horse Chestnut *(Aesculus hippocastanum)*. Both the seed and leaf of Horse Chestnut are used medicinally. The seed is indicated for the symptoms of chronic venous insufficiency, including pain, cramping, swelling, sensations of heaviness, and night cramping. Horse Chestnut leaf is used for venous disorders such as varicose veins, hemorrhoids, and phlebitis.

Warning: People taking blood thinners (including aspirin) should not use Horse Chestnut.

Kava *(Piper methysticum)*. The active compounds in Kava are lactones, which have antispasmodic, muscle-relaxing, and anticonvulsive effects; Kava can also thin the blood. The herb is used for nervousness, insomnia, tension, stress, and agitation.

Warning: The United States Food and Drug Administration advised consumers of the potential risk of severe liver injury associated with Kava. People who have liver problems or are taking drugs that can affect the liver should consult a physician before using Kava. The herb is also contraindicated in patients with depression, in those with neurologic disorders, and in pregnant or nursing women. Overuse of Kava can result in skin rash or weight loss. Kava use for more than three months should be supervised by a physician. The herb should not be combined with the following: alcohol, anti-anxiety or mood-altering drugs (including barbiturates), levodopa, drugs metabolized by P450 (CYP) enzymes, blood thinners, hepatotoxic drugs, and MAO inhibitors.

Licorice *(Glycyrrhiza glabra)*. The sweet root of the Licorice plant has a long history of use in traditional medicine. It contains various compounds with anti-inflammatory and other soothing effects that make it helpful as a treatment for ulcers and digestive disorders such as gastritis. It also acts as an expectorant for cough and bronchitis.

Warning: Licorice is contraindicated in pregnant and breastfeeding women and in people with hepatitis and other liver disorders, kidney disease, diabetes, arrhythmias, high blood pressure, muscle cramping, and low potassium levels. Licorice should not be taken with digoxin, blood thinners, diuretics, or medications that lower blood pressure. It should also not be combined with laxatives, combination contraceptives, MAO inhibitors, potassium supplements, testosterone, or drugs metabolized by P450 (CYP) enzymes.

Ma Huang *(Ephedra sinica)*. Ma Huang contains compounds that alleviate bronchial constriction and is used in folk remedies as a treatment for coughs and bronchitis.

Warning: Because of the severe adverse effects linked to ephedrine alkaloids—including heart attack, stroke, and death—the FDA banned dietary supplements containing ephedra in February 2004. The risks of this herb outweigh any possible benefits, especially for pregnant or breastfeeding women, children and teenagers, and for people with the following: anxiety, depression, high blood pressure, glaucoma, brain tumors, seizure disorders, prostate disorders, stomach ulcers, pheochromocytoma, thyrotoxicosis, cerebral perfusions, adrenal tumors, cardiac arrhythmia, or thyroid disease. Ma Huang should not be combined with caffeine, decongestants, diet medications containing sympathomimetics or caffeine, stimulants, glaucoma medication, MAO inhibitors, anesthetics, or labor-inducing drugs. Overdosage can result in death.

Milk Thistle *(Silybum marianum)*. The compounds in Milk Thistle seed have protective and regenerative effects on the liver. It is used as a treatment for liver and gallbladder disorders such as jaundice, toxic liver damage, cirrhosis of the liver, and gallbladder pain. It is also used for dyspeptic complaints.

Warning: The herb should not be used with antipsychotic drugs, the herb Yohimbe, or male hormones.

Pumpkin Seed *(Cucurbita pepo)*. Pumpkin seed has anti-inflammatory and antioxidant properties. It is used to treat irritable bladder and symptoms of benign prostatic hyperplasia such as obstructed urinary flow. It does not, however, appear to relieve an enlarged prostate.

Warning: INR may increase when Pumpkin Seed is combined with blood thinners, Saw Palmetto, or vitamin E.

Pygeum *(Pygeum africanum)*. Pygeum bark contains compounds that inhibit the inflammation and swelling associated with benign prostatic hyperplasia.

Warning: The herb should not be used by pregnant or breastfeeding women. People with stomach disorders should check with their physician before using Pygeum.

Saw Palmetto *(Serenoa repens)*. The anti-inflammatory and hormone-moderating effects of Saw Palmetto theoretically make it useful for treating symptoms of benign prostatic hyperplasia, but clinical trials are inconclusive. The herb has also been used for treating irritable bladder.

Warning: Saw Palmetto should not be used by pregnant or breastfeeding women. The herb should be avoided by those who have hormone-dependent cancers or a family history of such cancers. People with stomach disorders and those who are taking hormones or hormone-like drugs should check with their physician before using Saw Palmetto.

St. John's Wort *(Hypericum perforatum)*. St. John's Wort is one of the better studied herbs. Various compounds in St. John's Wort have antidepressant, anti-inflammatory, and antibacterial effects. The herb is used internally for depression and anxiety, and externally for wounds, burns, skin inflammation, and blunt injuries.

Warning: St. John's Wort can cause photosensitivity if taken for too long or at high doses. It can also cause gastrointestinal discomfort and headache. Combining St. John's Wort with other antidepressant medications such as MAO inhibitors, selective serotonin reuptake inhibitors (including fluoxetine, paroxetine, sertraline, fluvoxamine, or citalopram), or nefazodone could cause "serotonin syndrome"—a condition characterized by sweating, tremor, confusion, and agitation. The herb should also not be combined with the following: antibiotics that have photosensitizing effects, cyclosporine, indinavir, combination oral contraceptives, reserpine, barbiturates, theophylline, or digoxin. Taking St. John's Wort with drugs that are metabolized by P450 liver enzymes may decrease their effectiveness.

Stinging Nettle *(Urtica dioica)*. Both the flowers and root of the Stinging Nettle plant contain beneficial compounds used in various conditions. The flower is used internally and externally for rheumatism. It is also used internally for urinary tract infections and kidney and bladder stones. The root is used for irritable bladder and to help relieve symptoms of benign prostatic hyperplasia such as obstructed urinary flow, although it does not reduce prostate enlargement.

Warning: Stinging Nettle should not be used by people who suffer from fluid retention due to impaired cardiac or kidney function. The herb should not be used during pregnancy.

Uva-Ursi *(Arctostaphylos uva-ursi)*. Uva-ursi is used in the treatment of urinary tract infections because of its astringent and antibacterial effects.

Warning: The herb should not be used by pregnant or breastfeeding women; it should also not be used in children under 12 years of age, as it could cause liver damage. Uva-ursi should not be combined with diuretics, NSAIDs, or with substances (food or medication) that promote acidity in the urine, since this reduces its antibacterial effect. Individuals with kidney disorders, irritated digestive disorders, and acidic urine should not take Uva-Ursi.

Valerian *(Valeriana officinalis)*. Valerian root contains sedative compounds that are useful in nervousness and insomnia. It is also used for many other unproven uses such as headache, anxiety disorders, premenstrual syndrome, and menopausal symptoms.

Warning: Patients should avoid operating motor vehicles for several hours after taking Valerian. The herb should not be used by pregnant or breastfeeding women. It should also not be used in children less than 14 years old without medical supervision. Valerian extract or bath oils should not be used by people suffering from skin disorders, fever, infectious disease, heart disease, or muscle tension. The herb should be avoided in patients with preexisting liver disease. Valerian should not be combined with the following: alcohol, barbiturates, benzodiazepines, blood thinners, hepatoxic agents, supplemental iron, loperamide, or opioid analgesics.

Vitex *(Vitex agnus-castus)*. Also known as Chaste Tree, Vitex is used as a treatment for premenstrual syndrome and menopausal symptoms, menstrual cycle irregularities, and mastalgia/mastodynia.

Warning: Because of its hormonal effects, Vitex should not be used by pregnant or breastfeeding women. Occasionally, rash can occur. The herb should not be used with drugs that affect dopamine levels.

Wild Yam *(Dioscorea villosa)*. Popular reports have led to the belief that Wild Yam is a "natural" source of the hormone progesterone. While Wild Yam is used as a constituent of artificial progesterone pharmaceutically, the body cannot complete the conversion process by itself. The herb may be useful in treating high cholesterol.

Warning: Because of possible hormonal effects, pregnant and nursing women should not use Wild Yam. The herb should not be taken with estrogen-containing drugs or indomethacin.

Yohimbe *(Pausinystalia yohimbe)*. Yohimbe is prepared pharmaceutically under the brand name Yocon and is used to treat erectile dysfunction. Compounds in Yohimbe stimulate norepinephrine, which improves blood flow to the penis. It is also used for debility and exhaustion. The risks, however, of unregulated ingestion of the herb are thought to outweigh the benefits. Therefore, it is recommended that Yohimbe be taken only under strict medical supervision.

Warning: Yohimbe should not be used by women, especially pregnant or breastfeeding women. Children under 12 years of age should not take the herb. It is also contraindicated in patients with liver or kidney disease, post-traumatic stress disorder, high blood pressure, panic disorder, or Parkinson's disease. The herb should not be combined with the following: alcohol, blood pressure medication, carbamazepine, clomipramine, clonidine, guanabenz, guanadrel, guanethidine, guanfacine, lithium, minoxidil, morphine, naloxone, naltrexone, OTC stimulants, reserpine, sibutramine, or valproic acid. Patients should check with their doctor before taking Yohimbe with any OTC product. It should also not be taken with tyramine-containing foods such as wine and aged cheese.

COMMON HERBAL TERMINOLOGY

In this section, you'll find a brief glossary of the terms that frequently appear in discussions of herbs and herbal remedies. Some are familiar from the current medical literature. Others are now considered archaic, but can still be found in foreign herbal references. The glossary is reproduced from *PDR® for Herbal Medicines,* a compendium of information on more than 700 natural remedies.

abortifacient A drug or chemical that induces abortion.

achene A small 1-seeded fruit which has a pericarp attached to the seed at only one point.

acuminate Pointed, or tapering to a slender point.

adaptogen A preparation that acts to strengthen the body and increase resistance to disease.

alterative Any drug used to favorably alter the course of an ailment and to restore health. To improve the excretion of wastes from the circulatory system.

amarum A bitter herb or herb part.

androgynous In botany, a flower with both a stamen and pistil.

annual A plant that completes its growth cycle in one year.

anthelmintic An agent or drug that is destructive to worms.

anther The part of the stamen that contains pollen.

antiphlogistic An agent that prevents or counteracts inflammation and fever.

antisialagogue An agent that prevents or counteracts the formation or flow of saliva.

autumnalis In botany, referring to producing, gathering, or harvesting in the autumn.

bitter An alcoholic liquid prepared by maceration or distillation of a bitter herb or herb part that is often used to improve appetite or digestion.

blood purification Removal of undesirable agents from the blood.

bracteole A small leaf arising from the floral axis.

brightening agent A substance added to the active constituents.

calculosis The condition or formation of calculi.

calyx The outer set of floral leaves consisting of fused or separate sepals.

campanulate Shaped like a bell.

capitulum A rounded or flattened cluster of sessile flowers.

capsule A closed container that contains seeds or spores.

carminative An aid to relieve gas from the alimentary canal. An agent that acts to relieve colic.

carpel A small pistil or seed vessel comprising the innermost whorl of a flower.

cataplasm A poultice or soft external application.

catarrh An inflammation of the air passages usually involving the nose, throat, or lungs.

catkin A cattail-like inflorescence bearing scaly bracts.

cauline Growing on the upper portion of a stem.

cholagogue An agent that stimulates the flow of bile from the gallbladder to the duodenum.

choleretic An agent that stimulates the production of bile by the liver.

climacteric The syndrome of physical and psychological changes that occurs during the transition to menopause.

comminuted Broken or crushed into small pieces.

cordate Heart-shaped *(a cordate leaf).*

coriaceous Tough, strong, and leather-like.

corolla The inner set of floral leaves that consists of separate or fused leaves.

cortex In botany, the bark of a tree or the rind of a fruit.

cotyledon A seed leaf, or the first set of leaves from the embryo in seed plants.

crenate In reference to leaf structure, having a margin cut into rounded scallops.

cyme An inflorescence where the axes always end in a single flower.

deciduous A tree that sheds its leaves at the end of the growing season.

decoction A liquid substance prepared by boiling plant parts in water or some other liquid for a period of time.

decumbent A plant, stem, or shoot that lays on the ground but terminates with an ascending apex.

dentate Tooth-like projections on the margin of a leaf.

dessertspoon A unit of measure equal to about 2½ fluidrachms.

diaphoretic An agent that causes sweating or excessive perspiration.

dioecious In botany, when a plant has either a stamen or a pistil on each flower.

downy Covered with soft hairs.

dromotropic Affecting nerve fiber conduction.

dropsy An abnormal accumulation of fluid in body tissues or cavities usually related to an underlying disease.

drupe A one-seeded fruit; as in an olive or a peach.

embrocation An external medication applied as a liniment or other liquid form.

emmenagogue A substance that renews or stimulates the menstrual flow.

endosperm The albumin of the seed.

epicalyx An external accessory calyx located outside the true calyx of the flower.

eructation The act of belching.

exocarp The outer wall of a fruit covering.

extraction The portion of a plant that is removed by solvents and used in drug preparations in solid or liquid form.

febrifuge An agent that counteracts fever; an antipyretic.

floret A little flower; one of the small individual flowers that form a cluster or head.

flos Flower.

fluidextract A hydroalcoholic preparation of a botanical drug where 1 mL of the preparation contains 1 gm of the standard botanical.

folium The leaf of a plant.

fructus Fruit.

furuncle A boil or sore caused by bacterial infection of the subcutaneous tissue.

galenic preparation Medications prepared from plants as opposed to refined chemicals.

glabrous Having a smooth surface; without hair or down.

globular Spherical.

hastate Plant leaves with a triangular shape with the base coming together on each side into an acute lobe.

hilum The scar on a seed which indicates its point of attachment.

homeopathic A system of therapy which says that a medicinal substance that can evoke certain symptoms in healthy individuals may be effective in the treatment of illnesses having similar symptoms, if given in very small doses.

imbricate Overlapping flower petals, as in the bud.

indehiscent A fruit or grain that doesn't open spontaneously when ripe.

induration The process of hardening.

inflorescence The mode of disposition of flowers or the act of flowering. The spatial arrangement of flowers along the axis.

infusion The process of steeping or soaking plant matter in a liquid to extract its medicinal properties without boiling.

involucre A ring or rosette of leaves that surround the base of a flower cluster.

labiate A lip-like part of a plant, like a calyx or corolla.

lanceolate Lance-like or spear shaped; often referring to a long, tapering leaf.

lignum Woody tissue.

maceration The softening of a solid preparation by soaking it in a liquid.

meteorism The presence of gas in the intestine or stomach.

monoecious Having stamens and pistils in separate blossoms on the same plant.

mucilage 1. A viscid substance in a plant consisting of a gum dissolved in the juice of the plant. 2. A soothing application made from plant gums.

muscarinic An effect characterized by contraction of smooth muscle, excessive salivation and perspiration, abdominal colic, and excessive bronchial secretion.

nutlet The stone in a drupe.

obstipation Persistent or intractable constipation.

panicle A loose, multiple flower cluster usually formed from numerous branches.

pedicel The stalk that supports a single flower in an inflorescence of flowers arranged upon a common peduncle.

peduncle A stalk that bears a flower or flower cluster.

percolation A liquid containing the soluble portion of a drug that has been filtered or separated from the plant matter.

perennial A plant that grows for three or more years.

perianth The external envelope of a flower which does not include the calyx and corolla if they are distinguishable.

pericarp The wall of the ripened ovary of a flower containing the germ of the fruit.

petal One of the leaves of the corolla.

petiolate The footstalk of a leaf.

pinnate Compound leaves or leaflets that have a feather-like arrangement with leaves arranged on both sides of a common axis.

pinnatisect Cleft pinnately or almost to the midrib.

pistil The seed-bearing organ of flowering plants consisting of the ovary and the stigma; usually with a style.

plaster A viscous substance that is spread on linen or cloth and applied to a part of the body for healing purposes.

poultice A soft, moist mass of plant parts that are wrapped in muslin or gauze and applied warm or hot to the skin.

pubescent In botany, having a fuzzy surface; covered with soft, fine short hairs.

raceme An inflorescence where flowers are borne on stalks at an almost equal distance apart along an elongated axis that continues to grow with flowers opening in succession from below.

radix The root of a plant.

reniform When describing a leaf, kidney or bean-shaped.

resin An amorphous, solid or semi-solid substance produced by plants usually as a result of terpene oxidation.

reticulate Veins, fibers, or lines running like a network across the surface of a leaf.

rhizome An underground stem.

roborant A tonic or substance that gives strength.

runners A plant that spreads or forms by means of runners.

scape A flower stalk or peduncle arising from the surface or from below the ground.

schizocarp A dry fruit that splits at maturity into several one-seeded carpels.

scrofulous Having an ulcerous or diseased appearance on the surface.

secretagogue An agent that promotes secretion.

secretolytic To inhibit or dry secretions.

semen A seed or seed-like fruit.

sepal One of the modified leaves comprising a calyx; usually positioned outside and surrounding the carpels.

serrate Having notched, tooth-like protrusions along the margin of a leaf that points toward the apex.

sessile Attached directly to the base of a main stem or branch without the aid of an intervening stalk.

stamen The organ of the flower that comprises the anther and filament and gives rise to the male gamete.

stipule A stalk.

stomachic An agent that promotes digestion and improves appetite.

subshrub A perennial plant which has woody stems with the exception of the terminal portion of new growth, which drops off annually.

sudorific Causing or inducing sweat.

tendril The portion of a stem, leaf, or stipule that modified into a slender, spiral-shaped, touch-sensitive specialized appendage, which acts as an anchor to aid in climbing.

tepal Any of the modified leaves that combine to make up the perianth.

testa The hard outer coating of a seed; the exocarp.

tincture An alcoholic or hydroalcoholic mixture prepared from plant parts.

tomentose Covered with densely matted hairs.

tonic A medication used to fortify and provide increased vigor.

turiones A shoot or sprout which develops from a bud on a subterranean rootstock.

umbel Numerous flower stalks arising from the same point at the apex of the main stalk and terminating at an equal distance from the joining point.

undulate A wavy formation at the margin of a leaf, or bending in a gradual curve.

villous Having long, soft hairs.

vulnery A preparation applied externally.

wineglassful A measure equal to four fluid ounces.

HERBS THAT REQUIRE SUPERVISION

Although herbal remedies enjoy a benign, "natural" image among consumers, some pose the danger of significant adverse reactions. Indeed, in some instances, overdosage can lead to fatalities. Listed below are herbs that should be used only under direct supervision of a medical expert. Omission from this list does not necessarily imply that an herb presents no possibility of adverse effects. For detailed information on overdosage and side effects of more than 700 botanicals, please consult the latest edition of *PDR® for Herbal Medicines*.

Almond *(Prunus dulcis)*

American Hellebore *(Veratrum viride)*

Belladonna *(Atropa belladonna)*

Birthwort *(Aristolochia clematitis)*

Boxwood *(Buxus sempervirens)*

Digitalis *(Digitalis purpurea)*

Germander *(Teucrium chamaedrys)*

Indian-Hemp *(Apocynum cannabinum)*

Jaborandi *(Pilocarpus microphyllus)*

Lily-of-the-Valley *(Convallaria majalis)*

Ma-Huang *(Ephedra sinica)**

Mandrake *(Mandragora officinarum)*

Mayapple *(Podophyllum peltatum)*

Monkshood *(Aconitum napellus)*

Nutmeg *(Myristica fragrans)*

Poke *(Phytolacca americana)*

Scopolia *(Scopolia carniolica)*

Scotch Broom *(Cytisus scoparius)*

Tonka Beans *(Dipteryx odorata)*

Wahoo *(Euonymus atropurpurea)*

Yohimbe Bark *(Pausinystalia yohimbe)*

*The FDA banned dietary supplements containing ephedra in February 2004.

HERBAL CONTRAINDICATIONS

Listed below is a brief review of the contraindications for the most commonly used herbal remedies. The information is culled from Germany's "Commission E" monographs. Omission of an herb does not necessarily imply that it has no contraindications. For further information on the safe use of more than 700 botanicals, consult the latest edition of *PDR® for Herbal Medicines*.

Herb	*Contraindications*
Adonis	Potassium deficiency, digitalis glycoside therapy
Alfalfa	Systemic lupus erythematosus, gout, pregnancy, internal use
Alkanet	Pregnancy and nursing mothers
Aloe	Intestinal obstruction, acutely inflamed intestinal diseases (eg, Crohn's disease, ulcerative colitis), appendicitis, abdominal pain of unknown origin, ileus, electrolyte abnormalities, pregnancy and nursing mothers, children under 12 years of age
Alpine Cranberry	Pregnancy and nursing mothers, children under 12 years of age
Amargo	Pregnancy and nursing mothers, children under 12 years of age
American Liverwort	Pregnancy
Ammoniac Gum	Pregnancy
Angelica	Pregnancy
Anise	Anise or ethanol allergy, pregnancy
Artichoke	Bile duct blockage, gallstones
Asa Foetida	Pregnancy
Asarum	Pregnancy
Asparagus	Kidney disease, reduced cardiac and/or renal function
Barberry	Pregnancy and nursing mothers
Barley	Pregnancy
Basil	Pregnancy and nursing mothers
Behen	Pregnancy
Beth Root Stock	Pregnancy
Birch	Edema associated with reduced cardiac and/or renal function
Birthwort	Pregnancy
Bittersweet Nightshade	Pregnancy and nursing mothers
Black Cohosh	Pregnancy and nursing mothers
Black Currant	Edema associated with reduced cardiac and/or renal function
Black Mustard	Gastrointestinal ulcer, inflammatory kidney disease, children under 6 years of age
Bladderwrack	Pregnancy and nursing mothers, hyperthyroidism
Blessed Thistle	Pregnancy
Bloodroot	Pregnancy
Blue Cohosh	Pregnancy, heart disease
Bog Bean	Diarrhea, dysentery, colitis
Boldo	Bile duct obstruction, severe liver disease, gallstones (consult a physician before taking)
Borage	Epilepsy, people receiving epileptogenic drugs, schizophrenia, pregnancy and nursing mothers
Brown Kelp	Thyroid illness, hyperthyroidism

Herb	Contraindications
Buckthorn	Intestinal obstruction, inflammatory intestinal disease, appendicitis, abdominal pain of unknown origin, children under 12 years of age, pregnancy and nursing mothers, thyroid hormone preparations
Bugleweed	Hypothyroidism, thyroid enlargement, thyroid hormone preparations, pregnancy and nursing mothers
Bulbous Buttercup	Pregnancy
Cajuput	Gastrointestinal inflammatory disease, biliary duct inflammation, severe liver disease, topical application to facial area of infants and children
California Poppy	Pregnancy
Camphor	Pregnancy
Canadian Golden Rod	Edema resulting from reduced cardiac and/or renal function
Cape Aloe	Pregnancy
Cascara Sagrada	Intestinal and bowel obstruction, acute inflammatory intestinal disease (colitis, Crohn's disease, irritable bowel), fecal impaction, appendicitis, abdominal pain of unknown origin, nausea, vomiting, pregnancy and nursing mothers (consult a physician before taking), children under 12 years of age
Castor Oil	Intestinal obstruction, acute inflammatory intestinal disease, appendicitis, abdominal pain of unknown origin, immunosuppressant therapy, pregnancy and nursing mothers, children under 12 years of age
Cat's Claw	Multiple sclerosis, tuberculosis, autoimmune disease, transplant recipients, children under 2 years of age, pregnancy and nursing mothers
Catnip	Pregnancy
Celandine	Pregnancy
Celery Seed (Fruit)	Pregnancy, kidney infection or disease
Centaury	Stomach or intestinal ulcers
Chamomile (English)	Pregnancy
Chamomile (German)	History of hay fever or asthma, known allergy to species (eg, ragweed), pregnancy
Chaste Tree	Pregnancy or nursing mothers
Chinese Cinnamon	Pregnancy
Chinese Motherwort	Pregnancy
Chinese Rhubarb (Da-Huang)	Intestinal obstruction, acute inflammatory intestinal disease, appendicitis, abdominal pain of unknown origin, pregnancy and nursing mothers (consult a physician before taking)
Chinese Thoroughwax	Pregnancy
Chiretta	Gastric or duodenal ulcers
Chocolate Vine	Pregnancy
Cinnamon	Pregnancy
Cocillana Tree	Pregnancy
Coffee	Pregnancy and nursing mothers
Cola	Pregnancy, stomach or duodenal ulcers
Colt's Foot	Pregnancy and nursing mothers
Comfrey	Pregnancy and nursing mothers, liver or kidney disease

Herb	Contraindications
Common Stonecrop	Inflammatory diseases of the gastrointestinal tract or urinary tract
Congorosa	Pregnancy
Cowslip	Cowslip allergy
Dandelion	Closure of biliary ducts, gallbladder empyema, ileus, biliary ailments
Devil's Claw	Stomach or duodenal ulcers, gallstones
Dyer's Broom	Pregnancy
Echinacea	Autoimmune diseases, multiple sclerosis, leukosis, collagen disease, AIDS, tuberculosis, tendency to allergy, echinacea allergy, diabetes (IV form only), pregnancy
Elecampane	Pregnancy
Elephant Ears	Pregnancy and nursing mothers, children under age 12
English Hawthorn	Pregnancy (first trimester), children under 12 years of age
Ergot	All therapeutic use including peripheral blood flow disorders (eg, Raynaud's), thromboangiitis obliterans, severe arteriosclerotic vascular changes, liver function disorders, severe coronary insufficiency, kidney damage, pregnant and nursing mothers, infectious diseases, sepsis, hypertonia, severe hypotonia
Eucalyptus	Infants and small children (on face or nose), hypersensitivity to eugenol, inflammatory diseases of the gastrointestinal tract or bile ducts, serious liver disease
European Golden Rod	Edema resulting from reduced cardiac and/or renal function
European Mistletoe	Protein hypersensitivity, chronic-progressive infections (eg, tuberculosis, AIDS), hyperthyroidism, inflammatory or febrile disorders, tumors of the CNS, spinal cord tumors, intracranial metastasis affecting intracranial pressure, high fever
Evening Primrose	Schizophrenia (if treated with neuroleptic drugs)
False Unicorn Root	Pregnancy
Fenugreek	Pregnancy
Feverfew	Pregnancy and nursing mothers, children under 2 years of age
Flaxseed	Ileus, stricture of the esophagus and/or gastrointestinal area, acute inflammatory illnesses of the intestine, esophagus, or stomach entrance, thyroid insufficiency, or hypersensitivity to the seed
Frangula	Intestinal obstruction, acute inflammatory intestinal diseases, appendicitis, pregnancy and nursing mothers, children under 12 years of age
Garlic	Nursing mothers, within 10 days of surgery
Germander	The drug is highly toxic and should not be used.
Ginger	Pregnancy or lactation (consult a physician before taking), morning sickness, gallstones (consult a physician before taking), hemorrhage risk
Ginkgo	Known hypersensitivity to ginkgo, risk factors for intracranial hemorrhage, systematic arterial hypertension, diabetes, amyloid senile plaques, seizure risk, during or after surgery
Golden Shower Tree	Ileus, acute inflammatory diseases of the intestine, appendicitis, pregnancy and nursing mothers, children under 12 years of age

Herb	Contraindications
Goldenseal	Pregnancy and nursing mothers, history of miscarriage, glucose-6-phosphate-dehydrogenase deficiency, hypersensitivity to the herb
Goldthread	Pregnancy
Guar Gum	Diseases of the esophagus, stomach, intestine
Guarana	Pregnancy and nursing mothers
Haronga	Acute pancreatitis, severe liver function disorders, gallstone illnesses, obstruction of the biliary ducts, gallbladder empyema, ileus
Hawthorn	Hypersensitivity or history of allergic reaction to crataegus, pregnancy (first trimester), children under 12 years of age
Horehound	Pregnancy
Horsemint	Pregnancy
Horseradish	Stomach or intestinal ulcers, kidney disease, children under 4 years of age
Horsetail	Edema due to reduced cardiac and/or renal function
Hyssop	Pregnancy
Immortelle	Biliary obstruction, gallstones
Indian Squill	First- and second-degree AV-block, hypercalcemia, hypokalemia, hypertrophic cardiomyopathy, carotid sinus syndrome, ventricular tachycardia, thoracic aortic aneurysm, Wolff-Parkinson-White syndrome
Ipecac	Pregnancy
Jaborandi	Pregnancy
Jack-in-the-Pulpit	Pregnancy
Jalap	Pregnancy
Japanese Mint	Occlusion of the biliary ducts, gallbladder inflammation, severe liver damage, gallstones
Jatamansi	Pregnancy
Java Tea	Edema associated with reduced cardiac and/or renal function
Jimson Weed	Glaucoma, suspicion of glaucoma, paralytic ileus, pyloric stenosis, enlarged prostate, tachycardic arrhythmias, acute pulmonary edema
Juniper	Pregnancy and nursing mothers, inflammatory renal disease
Kava	Endogenous depression, neurologic disorders, pregnancy and nursing mothers
Labrador Tea	Pregnancy
Larch	Inhalation may cause acute inflammation of the airway passages
Lemongrass	Pregnancy
Levant Cotton	Pregnancy (except at delivery)
Licorice	Chronic hepatitis, cholestatic diseases of the liver, cirrhosis of the liver, severe renal insufficiency, inflammatory diseases of the gastrointestinal tract or bile ducts, diabetes mellitus, arrhythmias, hypertension, hypertonia, hypokalemia, pregnancy and nursing mothers, tobacco use, hypersensitivity to the herb
Lobelia	Pregnancy and nursing mothers
Lovage	Edema associated with reduced cardiac and/or renal function, inflammation of kidneys or of the urinary drainage passages, pregnancy
Lycium Bark	Pregnancy, common cold, diarrhea
Lycium Berries	Pregnancy

Herb	Contraindications
Ma-Huang (Ephedra)	Numerous contraindications. The FDA banned dietary supplements containing ephedra in Feb. 2004.
Maidenhair	Pregnancy
Malabar Nut	Pregnancy
Male Fern	Anemia, heart disease, liver or kidney diseases, diabetes, pregnancy, children under 4 years of age, the elderly
Manna	Ileus
Mayapple	Pregnancy
Meadowsweet	Childhood febrile illness, salicylate sensitivity
Mexican Scammony Root	Pregnancy
Morning Glory	Pregnancy
Motherwort	Pregnancy
Mountain Grape	Pregnancy
Mugwort	Pregnancy
Myrrh	Pregnancy and nursing mothers
Myrtle	Inflammatory illnesses of the gastrointestinal area or biliary ducts, severe liver disease, faces of infants and small children
Nasturtium	Gastrointestinal ulcer, kidney disease, not for use in infants and small children
Niauli	Inflammatory illnesses of the gastrointestinal area or biliary ducts, severe liver diseases, faces of infants and small children
Northern Prickly Ash	Pregnancy
Nutmeg	Pregnancy
Oak	Large areas of weeping eczema or skin injuries, feverish and infectious illnesses, cardiac insufficiency in stages III and IV (NYHA), hypertonia in stage IV (WHO)
Olive	Gallstones
Orris	Pregnancy
Oswego Tea	Pregnancy
Papaya	Pregnancy
Parsley	Parsley or apiole allergy, pregnancy, kidney inflammation, edema associated with reduced cardiac and/or renal function
Pasque Flower	Pregnancy
Pau d'Arco	Pregnancy and nursing mothers
Pennyroyal	Pregnancy
Peppermint Leaf	Gallstones
Peppermint Oil	Occlusion of the biliary ducts, gallbladder inflammation, severe liver damage, gallstones, infants and small children (on faces, especially nasal areas)
Perilla	Pregnancy
Petasites	Pregnancy and nursing mothers
Pleurisy Root	Pregnancy
Poplar	Hypersensitivity to salicylates, propolis, or balsam of Peru
Poppyseed	Pregnancy and nursing mothers, illnesses connected with reduced respiratory function, pancreatitis, colon ulcers, elevated internal cranial pressure, acute hepatitis porphyria, biliary colic, Addison's disease, hypothyroidism

Herb	Contraindications
Psyllium	Pathological narrowing in the gastrointestinal tract, ileus, severely variable diabetes mellitus
Psyllium Seed	Pathological constriction of the gastrointestinal tract, inflammatory illnesses of the gastrointestinal tract, the threat or presence of ileus, severely variable diabetes mellitus
Quassia	Pregnancy
Quinine	Pregnancy
Rauwolfia	Depression, ulceration, pheochromocytoma, pregnancy and nursing mothers
Red Clover	Pregnancy and nursing mothers, estrogen receptor-positive neoplasias
Rosemary	Pregnancy
Rue	Pregnancy
Safflower	Pregnancy
Saffron	Pregnancy
Sage	Pregnancy and nursing mothers
Sandalwood	Kidney disease
Scopolia	Angle-closure glaucoma, prostatic adenoma with residual urine, tachycardia, mechanical stenosis in the gastrointestinal tract, megacolon
Scotch Broom	High blood pressure, AV block, MAO inhibitor drug therapy, pregnancy
Scotch Pine	Bronchial asthma, whooping cough, children
Seneca Snakeroot	Pregnancy
Senna	Intestinal obstruction, acute inflammatory intestinal diseases, appendicitis, pregnancy and nursing mothers
Shepherd's Purse	Pregnancy
Short Buchu	Pregnancy
Siberian Ginseng	Hypertension, hypersensitivity to the herb or its extracts, diabetes, myocardial infarction
Spikenard	Pregnancy
Spiny Rest Harrow	Edema resulting from reduced cardiac and/or renal function
Spruce	Bronchial asthma, whooping cough, extensive skin injury, acute skin diseases, feverish or infectious diseases, cardiac insufficiency, hypertonia
Squill	Second- or third-degree AV block, hypercalcemia, hypokalemia, hypertrophic cardiomyopathy, carotid sinus syndrome, ventricular tachycardia, thoracic aortic aneurysm, Wolff-Parkinson-White syndrome
St. John's Wort	Hypersensitivity or allergy to the herb or any of its constituents, people with a history of photosensitivity
Stillingia	Nursing mothers
Stinging Nettle	Edema associated with reduced cardiac and/or renal function, pregnancy
Tansy	Pregnancy
Thuja	Pregnancy
Turmeric	Obstructed biliary ducts, gallstones, hyperacidity, gastrointestinal ulcers, pregnancy
Uva Ursi	Kidney disorders, irritated digestive disorders, acidic urine, prolonged unsupervised use, pregnancy, nursing mothers, children under 12 years of age
Vervain	Pregnancy
Watercress	Stomach or intestinal ulcer, inflammatory kidney disease, pregnancy, children under 4 years of age
Wheat	Edema associated with reduced cardiac and/or renal function
White Fir	Bronchial asthma, obstructive bronchial diseases, whooping cough, large skin injuries (consult a physician if taking whole body baths), severe feverish or infectious disease, cardiac insufficiency, hypertonia, acute infection of the respiratory passages
White Mustard	Gastrointestinal ulcer, inflammatory kidney disease, children under 6 years of age
Willow Bark	Hypersensitivity to salicylates, children with flu-like symptoms
Wild Carrot	Pregnancy
Wild Indigo	Pregnancy
Wormwood	History of seizures, stomach or intestinal ulcers, pregnancy and nursing mothers
Yarrow	Yarrow allergy, pregnancy and nursing mothers
Yellow Gentian	Stomach or duodenal ulcer
Yellow Jessamine	Cardiac weakness
Yew	Pregnancy
Yohimbe Bark	Women (especially during pregnancy and breastfeeding), liver and kidney disease, gastric or duodenal ulcers, anxiety disorders, chronic inflammation of the sexual organs or prostate gland, children under 12 years of age, long-term use
Zedoary	Pregnancy

HERB/DRUG INTERACTIONS

Below is a selection of common herbal remedies known to interact with conventional medications. Following the name of each herb is a list of the specific pharmaceutical categories with which it may interact, together with a brief description of each interaction's results. Please remember that this table is not all-inclusive. For further information on any herb of interest, consult the latest edition of *PDR® for Herbal Medicines*, a compendium of information on more than 700 medicinal herbs.

Adonis
(Adonis vernalis)

Calcium, Digoxin, Glucocorticoids (extended therapy), Laxatives, Quinidine, Saluretics May increase the action of Adonis, potentially increasing risk of side effects

Aloe
(Aloe vera)

Antiarrhythmics Aloe-induced hypokalemia may affect cardiac rhythm

Antidiabetic Agents Increased risk of hypoglycemia

Cardiac Glycosides Increases effect of cardiac glycosides

Corticosteroids, Licorice, Thiazide Digoxin Herb may cause hypokalemia, which may increase digoxin toxicity

Diuretics, Loop Diuretics Increased potassium loss

Alpine Cranberry
(Vaccinium vitis-idaea)

Medications and Food That Increase Uric Acid Levels Decreased effect of Alpine Cranberry

Arnica
(Arnica montana)

Anticoagulants, Antiplatelet Agents, Low Molecular Weight Heparins, Thrombolytic Agents Coumarin component in Arnica may increase anticoagulant effect

Astragalus (Huang-Qi)
(Astragalus species)

Anticoagulants, Antiplatelet Agents, Low Molecular Weight Heparins, Thrombolytic Agents Astragalus may potentiate anticoagulant effects

Immunosuppressants Decreased effectiveness of immunosuppressive effect due to immunostimulant effect of Astragalus

Belladonna
(Atropa belladonna)

Amantadine Hydrochloride, Quinidine, Tricyclic Antidepressants Increases anticholinergic effect of herb

Bilberry
(Vaccinium myrtillus)

Anticoagulants, Antiplatelet Agents, Low Molecular Weight Heparins, Thrombolytic Agents Bilberry may potentiate anticoagulant effects with concomitant use

Salicylates, Warfarin Sodium Increases prothrombin time; caution should be observed when used concurrently

Bladderwrack
(Fucus vesiculosus)

Anticoagulants, Antiplatelet Agents, Low Molecular Weight Heparins, Thrombolytic Agents Bladderwrack may potentiate anticoagulant effects with concomitant use

Hypoglycemic Drugs Herb may have an additive hypoglycemic effect when taken with other hypoglycemic drugs

Brewer's Yeast
(Saccharomyces cerevisiae)

MAO Inhibitors Increase in blood pressure

Buckthorn
(Rhamnus catharticus)

Antiarrhythmics Increased effect due to potassium loss with chronic use of herb

Cardiac Glycosides Increased effect due to potassium loss with chronic use of herb

Corticosteroids Increases hypokalemic effects

Digoxin Herb may cause hypokalemia, which may increase digoxin toxicity

Licorice Root Increases hypokalemic effects

Thiazide Diuretics Increases hypokalemic Effects

Other Medications Resorption of other medications could be reduced, due to a laxative effect.

Bugleweed
(Lycopus virginicus)

Diagnostic Procedures Using Radioactive Isotopes Herb interferes with these isotopes

Thyroid Preparations Effect not specified

Cascara Sagrada
(Rhamnus purshiana)

Antiarrhythmics Potentiate arrhythmias with prolonged use of Cascara

Cardiac Glycosides Increased effect due to potassium loss with chronic use of herb

Corticosteroids Increase hypokalemic effect

Digoxin Herb may cause hypokalemia, which may increase digoxin toxicity

Indomethacin Decreases therapeutic effect of Cascara

Iron May result in adverse sequellae with concomitant use

Licorice, Thiazide Diuretics Increased risk of hypokalemic effect

Castor Oil Plant
(Ricinus communis)

Cardioactive Steroids Increased effect due to potassium loss with chronic use of herb

Cayenne
(Capsicum annuum)

Aspirin, Salicylic Acid Compounds Decreased bioavailability of aspirin with concomitant use

Barbiturates Further studies in humans needed for concomitant use

Theophylline Herb may increase absorption, resulting in toxicity; use cautiously and monitor for side effects

Chamomile (German)
(Matricaria recutita)

Alcohol May increase sedative effect

Anticoagulants German Chamomile may increase risk of bleeding with concomitant use

Benzodiazepines May increase sedative effect

Chaste Tree
(Vitex agnus-castus)

Dopamine Agonists May result in increased dopaminergic side effects

Dopamine-2 Antagonists May result in decreased dopaminergic effect of herb

Chinese Rhubarb (Da-Huang)
(Rheum palmatum)

Cardiac Glycosides Increased effect due to potassium loss with chronic use of herb

Digoxin Herb may cause hypokalemia, which may increase digoxin toxicity

Coffee
(Coffea arabica)

Drugs, unspecified Herb can hinder (or decrease) resorption of other drugs

Digitalis
(Digitalis purpurea)

Methylxanthines, Phosphodiesterase Inhibitors, Quinidine, Sympathomimetic Agents Increased risk of cardiac arrhythmias with concomitant use

Echinacea
(Echinacea angustifolia)

Corticosteroids Echinacea may interfere with the anticancer chemotherapeutic effect of corticosteroids

Drugs metabolized by cytochrome P450 (CYP) Inhibits CYP 3A and CYP 1A2; use caution when coadministering the herb withdrugs dependent on CYP enzymes for their elimination

Immunosuppressants The immune-stimulating effect of Echinacea may interfere with drugs that have immunosuppressant effects

Evening Primrose
(Oenothera biennis)

Anticoagulants, Antiplatelet Agents, Low Molecular Weight Heparins, Thrombolytic Agents Evening Primrose oil may potentiate anticoagulant effects with concomitant use

Anticonvulsants Evening Primrose oil may lower seizure threshold and decrease effectiveness of anticonvulsant medications

Phenothiazines Evening Primrose oil may reduce the seizure threshold with concomitant use

Fenugreek
(Trigonella foenum-graecum)

Hypoglycemic Drugs Herb may have an additive hypoglycemic effect when taken with other hypoglycemic drugs

Feverfew
(Tanacetum parthenium)

Anticoagulants, Antiplatelet Agents, Low Molecular Weight Heparins, Thrombolytic Agents Feverfew may potentiate drug effects

Flax
(Linum usitatissimum)

Drugs, unspecified Absorption of other drugs may be delayed when taken simultaneously with Flax

Ginkgo
(Ginkgo biloba)

Anticoagulants, Antiplatelets, Low Molecular Weight Heparins, Thrombolytics, NSAIDs Ginkgo may potentiate drug effects

Anticonvulsants Concomitant use may precipitate seizures in epileptic patients with concomitant use

Buspirone, Fluoxetine, SSRIs Concomitant use resulted in hypomanic episode in a case report

Insulin Ginkgo may alter insulin requirements

MAO Inhibitors Ginkgo may potentiate drug effects

Nicardipine Ginkgo extract may reduce hypotensive effects

Nifedipine Herb may increase mean plasma concentration of nifedipine

Papaverine Herb may increase incidence of adverse effects

Thiazide Diuretics Concomitant use may increase blood pressure

Ginseng
(Panax ginseng)

Estrogen (conjugated) May result in symptoms of estrogen excess or interference

Hypoglycemic Drugs Due to hypoglycemic effects of Ginseng, concomitant use may theoretically increase risk of hypoglycemia

Loop Diuretics Increases diuretic resistance

MAO Inhibitors Combination increases chance for agitation, depression, headache, insomnia, tremors, manic-type symptoms

Nifedipine Herb increases mean plasma concentration of nifedipine

Green Tea
(Camellia sinensis)

Alkaline Drugs Decreased absorption of alkaline drugs due to tannin component in tea

Anticoagulants May interfere with the action of warfarin and other anticoagulants

Guarana
(Paullinia cupana)

Cardiac Glycosides Increased effect due to potassium loss with chronic use of herb

Digoxin Herb may cause hypokalemia, which may increase digoxin toxicity

Hawthorn
(Crataegus oxyacantha)

Antiplatelet Agents May increase risk of bleeding

Digoxin May increase pharmacodynamic effect of digoxin

Henbane
(Hyoscyamus niger)

Amantadine Hydrochloride, Antihistamines, Phenothiazines, Procainamide, Quinidine, Tricyclic Antidepressants Increased anticholinergic action

Horse Chestnut
(Aesculus hippocastanum)

Anticoagulant drugs, unspecified Horse Chestnut has a coumarin component and may interact with warfarin, salicylates, and other drugs with anticoagulant properties

Indian Squill
(Urginea indica)

Methylxanthines, Phosphodiesterase Inhibitors, Quinidine, Sympathomimetic Agents Concomitant use can increase risk of cardiac arrhythmias

Kombe Seed
(Strophanthus hispidus)

Calcium Salts, Glucocorticoids, Laxatives, Quinidine, Saluretics Concomitant use may increase the herb's effects, resulting in adverse events

Licorice
(Glycyrrhiza glabra)

Note: The herb may interact with multiple drugs, including ACE inhibitors, anticoagulants, antiplatelet agents, antidiabetic agents, calcium channel blockers, MAO inhibitors, oral contraceptives, and many others. For a comprehensive list of interactions, consult the fourth edition of *PDR for Herbal Medicines*.

Lily-of-the-Valley
(Convallaria majalis)

Calcium, Digoxin, Glucocorticoids, Laxatives, Quinidine, Saluretics Increases the effect of Lily-of-the-Valley

Ma-Huang
(Ephedra sinica)

Note: Due to the risk of severe side effects, the FDA banned dietary supplements containing ephedra in February 2004.

Milk Thistle
(Silybum marianum)

Butyrophenones, Phenothiazines Silymarin in combination with butyrophenones or phenothiazines causes a decrease in lipid peroxidation

Metronidazole Metronidazole dose may need to be increased with concomitant use.

Phentolamine Mesylate Silymarin antagonizes the effect of phentolamine

Yohimbine Hydrochloride Silymarin antagonizes the effect of yohimbine

Oleander
(Nerium oleander)

Calcium Salts, Glucocorticoids, Laxatives, Quinidine, Saluretics May increase efficacy and side effects when given simultaneously with herb

Papaya
(Carica papaya)

Warfarin Sodium Concomitant use may increase INR levels

Psyllium
(Plantago ovata)

Antidiabetic Agents Mean area-under-the-curve (AUC) for glucose and insulin was reduced when herb was administered with a glucose load

Carbamazepine Reduced bioavailability with concomitant use

Drugs, unspecified Absorption of other drugs may be decreased if taken simultaneously with herb

Insulin Effect unspecified; insulin dose should be decreased

Psyllium Seed
(Plantago afra)

Drugs, unspecified Absorption of other drugs may be delayed or decreased if taken simultaneously with herb

Quinine
(Cinchona pubescens)

Drugs that Cause Thrombocytopenia Herb increases risk of thrombocytopenia

Rauwolfia
(Rauwolfia serpentina)

Alcohol Concurrent use may increase impairment of motor skills

Barbiturates, Neuroleptics Synergistic effect when used concurrently

Digitalis Glycoside Preparations Severe bradycardia when used in combination with digitalis glycosides
Levodopa Decreased effect when used concurrently, along with an increase in extrapyramidal symptoms
Sympathomimetic Agents Concurrent use may increase blood pressure

Saw Palmetto

(Serenoa repens)
Alpha Adrenergic Blockers Concomitant use may result in additive alpha adrenergic blocking effect
Androgens Saw Palmetto antagonizes the effect of androgens
Hormones, Hormone-Like Drugs, or Adrenergic Drugs Herb interferes with therapy due to the possible estrogenic, androgenic, and alpha-adrenergic effects
Warfarin Increased risk of bleeding with concurrent use

Scopolia

(Scopolia carniolica)
Amantadine Hydrochloride, Quinidine, Tricyclic Antidepressants Increased effect when given simultaneously with herb

Scotch Broom

(Cytisus scoparius)
MAO Inhibitors Increased risk of hypertensive crisis when used concomitantly

Senna

(Cassia senna)
Antiarrhythmics Senna-induced hypokalemia may increase risk of arrhythmia
Digitalis Glycoside Preparations Senna-induced hypokalemia may increase toxicity of digitalis preparations
Estrogen Senna decreases estrogen levels when taken with estrogen supplements
Indomethacin Decreased therapeutic effect of Senna
Nifedipine Inhibits activity of Senna via calcium channel blockade

Siberian Ginseng

(Eleutherococcus senticosus)
Antidiabetic agents and insulin May alter the effects of insulin or other medications

Squill

(Urginea maritima)
Arrhythmogenic Substances Increases risk of cardiac arrhythmias
Calcium, Glucocorticoids (extended therapy), Laxatives, Saluretics Increases effectiveness and side effects of herb
Digoxin Squill potentiates the positive inotropic and negative chronopic effects of digoxin
Methylxanthines Increases risk of cardiac arrhythmias
Phosphodiesterase Inhibitors Increases risk of cardiac arrhythmias
Quinidine Increases risk of cardiac arrhythmias; increases effectiveness and side effects of herb

St. John's Wort

(Hypericum perforatum)
Note: The herb may interact with multiple drugs, including antianxiety drugs, anticoagulants, antidepressants, anti-HIV drugs, calcium channel blockers, cardiac glycosides, oral contraceptives, statins, sympathomimetics, and many others. For a comprehensive list of interactions, consult the fourth edition of *PDR for Herbal Medicines.*

Uva-Ursi

(Arctostaphylos uva-ursi)
Iron Uva-Ursi's tannin content may complex with concomitantly administered iron, resulting in nonabsorbable insoluble components, which may result in adverse sequelae on blood components
Loop Diuretics, Thiazide Diuretics The sodium-sparing effect of Uva-Ursi may antagonize the diuretic effect of loop diuretics
Medications and Food That Increase Uric Acid Levels Decreases antibacterial effect of herb
Nonsteroidal Anti-Inflammatory Drugs Uva-Ursi may potentiate the gastrointestinal irritation caused by NSAIDs

Valerian

(Valeriana officinalis)
Alcohol Additive sedation and depressant effects when combined with Valerian
Anticoagulants, Antiplatelet Agents, Low Molecular Weight Heparins, Barbiturates, Benzodiazipines Concurrent use may increase central nervous system depression
Hepatotoxic Agents Concurrent use may result in elevated liver transaminases with or without concomitant hepatic damage
Iron Valerian's tannin content may complex with concomitantly administered iron, resulting in nonabsorbable insoluble components, which may result in adverse sequelae on blood components
Loperamide Concurrent use may result in delirium with symptoms of confusion, agitation, and disorientation
Opioid Analgesics Additive central nervous system depression when combined with Valerian
Thrombolytic Agents Concurrent use may potentiate anticoagulant effects

White Willow

(Salix species)
Alcohol, Barbiturates Enhances toxicity of salicylates
Antiplatelet Drugs, Medications That Prolong PT Time Risk of additive effect with salicylates
Carbonic Anhydrase Inhibitors Potentiates action of salicylates
Nonsteroidal Anti-Inflammatory Drugs Use with caution; salicylate component of herb may decrease serum concentration and clearance of NSAIDs

Wild Yam

(Dioscorea villosa)
Estrogen Concurrent use may result in additive effect
Indomethacin Wild Yam may decrease the anti-inflammatory effect of indomethacin

Wormwood

(Artemisia absinthium)
Iron Wormwood's tannin content may complex with concomitantly administered iron, resulting in nonabsorbable insoluble components, which may result in adverse sequelae on blood components
Phenothiazines, Trazodone Hydrochloride, Tricyclic Antidepressants Wormwood preparations should not be administered with drugs known to lower the seizure threshold

Yohimbe Bark

(Pausinystalia yohimbe)
Antihypertensive agents, unspecified May need to adjust antihypertensive medications due to hypertensive effect of Yohimbe
Carbamazepine, Lithium Herb may exacerbate bipolar disorder by precipitating manic episodes
Clomipramine Increased risk of hypertension with concurrent use
Clonidine Reduced effectiveness with concurrent use
Ethanol Increased intoxication and anxiogenic effects with concurrent use
Guanabenz, Guanadrel, Guanethidine, Guanfacine Herb counteracts the effect of these substances
Minoxidil Yohimbe may counteract antihypertensive effect
Morphine Herb may enhance and/or prolong the effects of morphine
Naloxone Concurrent use may increase cortisol levels as well as symptoms of nervousness, anxiety, tremors, palpitations, hot and cold flashes, and nausea
Naltrexone Yohimbe may increase side effects (anxiety or nervousness), which may decrease compliance with treatment
OTC stimulants Concurrent use may potentiate hypertensive effects

DICTIONARY OF SCIENTIFIC AND COMMON NAMES

In the clinical literature, medicinal herbs are sometimes identified only by their scientific name. To assist you in locating citations relevant to a particular herbal product, this brief dictionary gives you the scientific designation for each of over 500 names found in the vernacular.

Common Name	Scientific Name
Abscess Root	*Polemonium reptans*
Acacia	*Acacia senegal*
Acacia	*Acacia arabica*
Adonis	*Adonis vernalis*
Adrue	*Cyperus articulatus*
African Potato	*Hypoxis rooperi*
Aga	*Amanita muscaria*
Agar	*Gelidium amansii*
Agrimony	*Agrimonia eupatoria*
Alfalfa	*Medicago sativa*
Alisma	*Alisma plantago-aquatica*
Alkanet	*Alkanna tinctoria*
Aloe Vera	*Aloe barbadensis*
Alpine Cranberry	*Vaccinium vitis-idaea*
Alteris	*Aletris farinosa*
Amaranth	*Amaranthus hypochondriacus*
American Adder's Tongue	*Erythronium americanum*
American Bittersweet	*Celastrus scandens*
American Hellebore	*Veratrum viride*
American Liverleaf	*Hepatica nogilis*
American Pawpaw	*Asimina triloba*
American White Pond Lily	*Nymphaea odorata*
Ammoniac Gum	*Dorema ammoniacum*
Angelica	*Angelica archangelica*
Angostura	*Galipea officinalis*
Anise	*Pimpinella anisum*
Apple Tree	*Malus domestica*
Areca Nut	*Areca catechu*
Arenaria Rubra	*Spergularia rubra*
Arjun Tree	*Terminalia arjuna*
Arnica	*Arnica montana*
Arrach	*Chenopodium vulvaria*
Arrowroot	*Maranta arundinacea*
Artichoke	*Cynara scolymus*
Arum	*Arum maculatum*
Asafetida	*Ferula assa-foetida*
Asarum	*Asarum europaeum*
Ash	*Fraxinus excelsior*
Ash	*Sorbus domestica*
Ash	*Sorbus torminalis*
Asiatic Dogwood	*Cornus officinalis*
Asparagus	*Asparagus officinalis*
Bael	*Aegle marmelos*
Balloon-Flower	*Platycodon grandiflorum*
Balmony	*Chelone glabra*
Bamboo	*Arundinaria japonica*
Baneberry	*Actaea spicata*
Barberry	*Berberis vulgaris*
Barley	*Hordeum distichon*
Basil	*Ocimum basilicum*
Bean	*Phaseolus vulgaris*
Bear's Garlic	*Allium ursinum*
Beet	*Beta vulgaris*
Behen	*Moringa oleifera*
Belladonna	*Atropa belladonna*
Bennet's Root	*Geum urbanum*
Benzoin	*Styrax benzoin*
Betel Nut	*Piper betle*
Bethroot	*Trillium erectum*
Bilberry	*Vaccinium myrtillus*
Birch	*Betula species*
Birthwort	*Aristolochia clematitis*
Bishop's Weed	*Ammi visnaga*
Bistort	*Persicaria bistorta*
Bitter Almond	*Prunus dulcis*
Bitter Apple	*Citrullus colocynthis*
Bitter Candytuft	*Iberis amara*
Bitter Milkwort	*Polygala amara*
Bitter Orange	*Citrus aurantium*
Bittersweet Nightshade	*Solanum dulcamara*
Black Alder	*Alnus glutinosa*
Black Bryony	*Tamus communis*
Black Catnip	*Phyllanthus amarus*
Black Cohosh	*Cimicifuga racemosa*
Black Currant	*Ribes nigrum*
Black Hellebore	*Helleborus niger*
Black Horehound	*Ballota nigra*
Black Mulberry	*Morus nigra*
Black Mustard	*Brassica nigra*
Black Nightshade	*Solanum nigrum*
Black Pepper	*Piper nigrum*
Black Root	*Veronica virginica*
Blackberry	*Rubus fruticosus*
Blackhaw	*Viburnum prunifolium*
Bladderwort	*Utricularia vulgaris*
Bladderwrack	*Fucus vesiculosus*
Bloodroot	*Sanguinaria canadensis*
Blue Cohosh	*Caulophyllum thalictroides*
Bog Bean	*Menyanthes trifoliata*
Bog Bilberry	*Vaccinium uliginosum*
Boldo	*Peumus boldus*
Boneset	*Eupatorium perfoliatum*
Borage	*Borago officinalis*
Boxwood	*Buxus sempervirens*
Brewer's Yeast	*Saccharomyces cerevisiae*
British Elecampane	*Inula britannica*
Broad Bean	*Vicia faba*
Brooklime	*Veronica beccabunga*
Broom Corn	*Sorghum vulgare*
Brown Kelp	*Macrocystis pyrifera*
Buckthorn	*Rhamnus catharticus*
Buckwheat	*Fagopyrum esculentum*
Bugle	*Ajuga reptans*
Bugleweed	*Lycopus virginicus*
Bulbous Buttercup	*Ranunculus bulbosus*
Burdock	*Arctium lappa*
Burnet Saxifrage	*Pimpinella major*
Burning Bush	*Dictamnus albus*
Burr Marigold	*Bidens tripartita*
Butcher's Broom	*Ruscus aculeatus*
Buttercup	*Ranunculus acris*
Butternut	*Juglans cinerea*
Cabbage	*Brassica oleracea*
Cajuput	*Melaleuca leucadendra*
Calabar Bean	*Physostigma venenosum*
Calamint	*Calamintha nepeta*
Calamus	*Acorus calamus*
California Poppy	*Eschscholzia californica*
Calotropis	*Calotropis procera*
Camphor Tree	*Cinnamomum camphora*
Canadian Fleabane	*Conyza canadensis*
Canella	*Canella winterana*
Cane-Reed	*Costus speciosa*
Cape Aloe	*Aloe ferox*
Carambola	*Averrhoa carambola*
Caraway	*Carum carvi*
Cardamom	*Elettaria cardamomum*
Carline Thistle	*Carlina acaulis*
Carob	*Ceratonia siliqua*
Carrageen	*Chondrus crispus*
Cascara Sagrada	*Rhamnus purshiana*
Cascarilla	*Croton eluteria*
Cashew	*Anacardium occidentale*
Cassia	*Cassia angustifolia*
Castor Oil Plant	*Ricinus communis*
Catechu	*Acacia catechu*
Catnip	*Nepeta cataria*
Cat's Foot	*Antennaria dioica*
Cayenne	*Capsicum annuum*
Cedar	*Cedrus libani*
Celandine	*Chelidonium majus*
Celery	*Apium graveolens*
Centaury	*Centaurium erythraea*
Chaste Tree	*Vitex agnus-castus*
Chaulmoogra	*Hydnocarpus species*
Cheken	*Eugenia chequen*
Cherry Laurel	*Prunus laurocerasus*
Chickweed	*Stellaria media*
Chicory	*Cichorium intybus*
Chinese Cinnamon	*Cinnamomum aromaticum*
Chinese Motherwort	*Leonurus japonicus*
Chinese Olive	*Canarium species*
Chinese Rhubarb	*Rheum palmatum*
Chinese Thoroughwax	*Bupleurum chinese*
Chiretta	*Swertia chirata*
Chocolate Vine	*Akebia quinata*
Cinnamon	*Cinnamomum verum*
Cinquefoil	*Potentilla erecta*
Cleavers	*Galium aparine*
Clematis	*Clematis recta*
Clove	*Syzygium aromaticum*
Club Moss	*Lycopodium clavatum*
Coca	*Erythroxylum coca*
Cocillana Tree	*Guraea rusbyi*
Cocoa	*Theobroma cacao*
Coconut Palm	*Cocos nucifera*
Coffee	*Coffea arabica*
Cola	*Cola acuminata*
Colchicum	*Colchicum autumnale*

Common Name	Scientific Name
Colombo	Jateorhiza palmata
Coltsfoot	Tussilago farfara
Columbine	Aquilegia vulgaris
Comfrey	Symphytum officinale
Common Stonecrop	Sedum acre
Condurango	Marsdenia condurango
Congorosa	Maytenus ilicifolia
Contrayerva	Dorstenia contrayerva
Coolwort	Tiarella cordifolia
Copaiba Balsam	Copaifera langsdorffi
Coral Root	Corallorhiza odontorhiza
Coriander	Coriandrum sativum
Corn Cockle	Agrostemma githago
Corn Poppy	Papaver rhoeas
Corn Silk	Zea mays
Cornflower	Centaurea cyanus
Corydalis	Corydalis cava
Costus	Saussurea costus
Cotton Tree	Cochlospermum gossypium
Cowhage	Mucuna pruriens
Cowslip	Primula veris
Cranesbill	Geranium maculatum
Croton Seeds	Croton tiglium
Cubeb	Piper cubeba
Cudweed	Gnaphalium uliginosum
Cumin	Cuminum cyminum
Cup Plant	Silphium perfoliatum
Cupmoss	Cladonia pyxidata
Curcuma	Curcuma xanthorrhizia
Cyclamen	Cyclamen europaeum
Cypress	Cupressus sempervirens
Cypress Spurge	Euphorbia cyparissias
Daffodil	Narcissus pseudonarcissus
Damiana	Turnera diffusa
Dandelion	Taraxacum officinale
Date Palm	Phoenix dactylifera
Devil's Claw	Harpagophytum procumbens
Digitalis	Digitalis purpurea
Digitalis Lanata	Digitalis lanata
Dill	Anethum graveolens
Divi-Divi	Caesalpinia bonducella
Dodder	Cuscuta epithymum
Dog Rose	Rosa canina
Dogwood	Cornus florida
Dragon's Blood	Daemonorops draco
Duckweed	Lemna minor
Dusty Miller	Senecio bicolor
Dwarf Elder	Sambucus ebulus
Dyer's Broom	Genista tinctoria
Echinacea Angustifolia	Echinacea angustifolia
Echinacea Pallida	Echinacea pallida
Echinacea Purpurea	Echinacea purpurea
Elecampane	Inula helenium
Elephant-Ears	Bergenia crassifolia
Elm Bark	Ulmus minor
English Adder's Tongue	Ophioglossum vulgatum
English Chamomile	Chamaemelum nobile
English Hawthorn	Crataegus laevigata
English Horsemint	Mentha longifolia
English Ivy	Hedera helix
English Lavender	Lavandula angustifolia
English Plantain	Plantago lanceolata
Ephedra	Ephedra sinica
Ergot	Claviceps purpurea
Eryngo	Eryngium campestre
Eucalyptus	Eucalyptus globulus
European Alder	Sambucus nigra
European Five-Finger Grass	Potentilla reptans
European Golden Rod	Solidago canadensis
European Mistletoe	Viscum album
European Peony	Paeonia officinalis
European Sanicle	Sanicula europaea
European Vervain	Verbena officinalis
European Water Hemlock	Cicuta virosa
Evening Primrose	Oenothera biennis
Eyebright	Euphrasia officinalis
False Schisandra	Kadsura japonica
False Unicorn Root	Veratrum luteum
Fennel	Foeniculum vulgare
Fenugreek	Trigonella foenum-graecum
Fever Bark	Alstonia constricta
Feverfew	Tanacetum parthenium
Field Scabious	Knautia arvensis
Figs	Ficus carica
Figwort	Scrophularia nodosa
Fireweed	Epilobium angustifolium
Fish Berry	Anamirta cocculus
Flax	Linum usitatissimum
Fool's Parsley	Aethusa cynapium
Forget-Me-Not	Myosotis arvensis
Frangula	Rhamnus frangula
Frankincense	Boswellia carteri
French Tarragon	Artemisia dracunculus
Fringetree	Chionanthus virginicus
Frostwort	Helianthemum canadense
Fumitory	Fumaria officinalis
Galbanum	Ferula gummosa
Gambir	Uncaria species
Gamboge	Garcinia hanburyi
Garden Cress	Lepidium sativum
Garlic	Allium sativum
Gentian	Gentiana lutea
German Chamomile	Matricaria recutita
German Ipecac	Cynanchum vincetoxicum
German Sarsaparilla	Carex arenaria
Germander	Teucrium chamaedrys
Giant Milkweed	Calotropis gigantea
Ginger	Zingiber officinale
Ginkgo	Ginkgo biloba
Ginseng	Panax ginseng
Globe Flower	Trollius europaeus
Goa Powder	Andira araroba
Goat's Rue	Galega officinalis
Golden Rod	Solidago virgaurea
Golden Shower Tree	Cassia fistula
Goldenseal	Hydrastis canadensis
Goldthread	Coptis trifolia
Gotu Kola	Centella asiatica
Goutweed	Aegopodium podagraria
Grains-Of-Paradise	Amomum melegueta
Gray Wallflower	Erysimum diffusum
Great Burnet	Sanguisorba officinalis
Greater Bindweed	Calystegia sepium
Green Hellebore	Helleborus viridis
Grindelia	Grindelia species
Ground Ivy	Glechoma hederacea
Ground Pine	Ajuga chamaepitys
Groundsel	Senecio vulgaris
Guaiac	Guaiacum officinale
Guar Gum	Cyamopsis tetragonoloba
Guarana	Paullinia cupana
Haronga	Haronga madagascariensis
Hartstongue	Scolopendrium vulgare
Heal-All	Prunella vulgaris
Heartsease	Viola tricolor
Heather	Calluna vulgaris
Hedge Mustard	Sisymbrium officinale
Hedge-Hyssop	Gratiola officinalis
Hemlock	Conium maculatum
Hemp Agrimony	Eupatorium cannabinum
Hempnettle	Galeopsis segetum
Henbane	Hyoscyamus niger
Herb Paris	Paris quadrifolia
Herb Robert	Geranium robertianum
Hibiscus	Hibiscus sabdariffa
High Mallow	Malva sylvestris
Holly	Ilex aquifolium
Hollyhock	Alcea rosea
Honeysuckle	Lonicera caprifolium
Hops	Humulus lupulus
Horehound	Marrubium vulgare
Horse Chestnut	Aesculus hippocastanum
Horsemint	Monarda punctata
Horseradish	Armoracia rusticana
Horsetail	Equisetum arvense
Hound's Tongue	Cynoglossum officinale
Houseleek	Sempervivum tectorum
Hydrangea	Hydrangea arborescens
Hyssop	Hyssopus officinalis
Iceland Moss	Cetraria islandica
Ignatius Beans	Strychnos ignatii
Immortelle	Helichrysum arenarium
Indian Nettle	Acalypha indica
Indian Physic	Gillenia trifoliata
Indian Squill	Urginea indica
Indian-Hemp	Apocynum cannabinum
Ipecac	Cephaelis ipecacuanha
Iporuru	Alchornea floribunda
Jaborandi	Pilocarpus microphyllus
Jack-in-the-Pulpit	Arisaema atrorubens
Jacob's Ladder	Polemonium caeruleum
Jalap	Ipomoea purga
Jamaica Dogwood	Piscidia piscipula
Jambolan	Syzygium cumini
Japanese Atractylodes	Atractylodes japonica
Japanese Mint	Mentha arvensis piperascens
Jasmine	Jasminum officinale
Jatamansi	Nardostachys jatamansi
Java Tea	Orthosiphon spicatus
Jequirity	Abrus precatorius
Jewel Weed	Impatiens biflora
Jimson Weed	Datura stramonium
Jojoba	Simmondsia chinesis
Jujube	Zyzyphus jujube
Juniper	Juniperus communis
Kamala	Mallotus philippinensis

Common Name	Scientific Name
Kava Kava	*Piper methysticum*
Kelp	*Laminaria hyperborea*
Khat	*Catha edulis*
Knotweed	*Polygonum aviculare*
Kombe Seed	*Strophanthus hispidus*
Kousso	*Hagenia abyssinica*
Labrador Tea	*Ledum latifolium*
Laburnum	*Cytisus laburnum*
Lactucarium	*Lactuca virosa*
Lady Fern	*Athyrium filix-femina*
Lady's Bedstraw	*Galium verum*
Lady's Mantle	*Alchemilla vulgaris*
Larch	*Larix decidua*
Larkspur	*Delphinium consolida*
Laurel	*Laurus nobilis*
Lavender Cotton	*Santolina chamaecyparissias*
Lemon	*Citrus limon*
Lemon Balm	*Melissa officinalis*
Lemon Verbena	*Aloysia triphylla*
Lemongrass	*Cymbopogon citratus*
Lemon-Wood	*Schisandra sphenanthera*
Lesser Celandine	*Ranunculus ficaria*
Lesser Galangal	*Alpinia officinarum*
Levant Cotton	*Gossypium herbaceum*
Licorice	*Glycyrrhiza glabra*
Life Root	*Senecio aureus*
Life Root	*Senecio nemorensis*
Lily-of-the-Valley	*Convallaria majalis*
Lime	*Citrus aurantifolia*
Linden	*Tilia species*
Lobelia	*Lobelia inflata*
Logwood	*Haematoxylon campechianum*
Loosestrife	*Lysimachia vulgaris*
Lotus	*Nelumbo nucifera*
Lovage	*Levisticum officinale*
Luffa	*Luffa aegyptica*
Lungmoss	*Lobaria pulmonaria*
Lungwort	*Pulmonaria officinalis*
Lycium Bark	*Lycium chinense*
Lycium Berries	*Lycium barbarum*
Madder	*Rubia tinctorum*
Magnolia	*Magnolia glauca*
Maidenhair	*Adiantum capillus-veneris*
Malabar Nut	*Justicia adhatoda*
Male Fern	*Dryopteris filix-mas*
Manaca	*Brunfelsia hopeana*
Mandrake	*Mandragora officinarum*
Manna	*Fraxinus ornus*
Marigold	*Calendula officinalis*
Marijuana	*Cannabis sativa*
Marsh Blazing Star	*Liatris spicata*
Marsh Marigold	*Caltha palustris*
Marshmallow	*Althaea officinalis*
Martagon	*Lilium martagon*
Masterwort	*Heracleum sphondylium*
Masterwort	*Peucedanum ostruthium*
Mastic Tree	*Pistacia lentiscus*
Mate	*Ilex paraguariensis*
Matico	*Piper elongatum*
Mayapple	*Podophyllum peltatum*
Meadowsweet	*Filipendula ulmaria*
Mercury Herb	*Mercurialis annua*
Mexican Scammony Root	*Ipomoea orizabensis*
Mezereon	*Daphne mezereum*
Milk Thistle	*Silybum marianum*
Moneywort	*Lysimachia nummularia*
Monkshood	*Aconitum napellus*
Morning Glory	*Ipomoea hederacea*
Motherwort	*Leonurus cardiaca*
Mountain Ash Berry	*Sorbus aucuparia*
Mountain Avens	*Dryas octopetala*
Mountain Flax	*Linum catharticum*
Mountain Laurel	*Kalmia latifolia*
Mouse Ear	*Pilosella officinarum*
Mugwort	*Artemisia vulgaris*
Muira-Puama	*Ptychopetalum olacoides*
Mullein	*Verbascum densiflorum*
Muskmallow	*Abelmoschus moschatus*
Myrrh	*Commiphora molmol*
Myrtle	*Myrtus communis*
Narrow-Leaf Sage	*Salvia lavandulifolia*
Nasturtium	*Tropaeolum majus*
Neem	*Antelaea azadirachta*
Nepalese Cardamom	*Amomum aromaticum*
Nerve Root	*Cypripedium calceolus*
New Jersey Tea	*Ceanothus americanus*
Niauli	*Melaleucea viridiflora*
Night-Blooming Cereus	*Selenicereus grandiflorus*
Noni	*Morinda citrifolia*
Northern Prickly Ash	*Zanthoxylum americanum*
Nutmeg	*Myristica fragrans*
Nux Vomica	*Strychnos nux vomica*
Oak Bark	*Quercus robur*
Oak Gall	*Quercus infectoria*
Oats	*Avena sativa*
Oilseed Rape	*Brassica napus*
Oleander Leaf	*Nerium oleander*
Olive	*Olea europaea*
Onion	*Allium cepa*
Opium Antidote	*Combretum micranthum*
Oregano	*Origanum vulgare*
Oregon Grape	*Mahonia aquifolium*
Oriental Arborvitae	*Thuja orientalis*
Orris	*Iris species*
Oswego Tea	*Monarda didyma*
Ox-Eye Daisy	*Chrysanthemum leucanthemum*
Pagoda Tree	*Sophora japonica*
Papaya	*Carica papaya*
Pareira	*Chondrodendron tomentosum*
Parsley	*Petroselinum crispum*
Parsley Piert	*Aphanes arvensis*
Pasque Flower	*Pulsatilla pratensis*
Passion Flower	*Passiflora incarnata*
Patchouly	*Pogostemon cablin*
Pellitory	*Anacyclus pyrethrum*
Pellitory-Of-The-Wall	*Parietaria officinalis*
Pennyroyal	*Mentha pulegium*
Peppermint	*Mentha piperita*
Perilla	*Perilla fructescens*
Periwinkle	*Vinca minor*
Petasites	*Petasites hybridus*
Peyote	*Lophophora williamsii*
Picrorhiza	*Picrorhiza kurroa*
Pimento	*Pimenta racemosa*
Pineapple	*Ananas comosus*
Pink Root	*Spigelia marilandica*
Pinus Bark	*Tsuga canadensis*
Pipsissewa	*Chimaphila umbellata*
Pitcher Plant	*Sarracenia purpurea*
Pleurisy	*Asclepias tuberosa*
Plumbago	*Plumbago zeylanica*
Poisonous Buttercup	*Ranunculus sceleratus*
Poke	*Phytolacca americana*
Poley	*Teucrium polium*
Pontian Rhododendron	*Rhododendron ponticum*
Poplar Bark	*Populus species*
Potentilla	*Potentilla anserina*
Premorse	*Scabiosa succisa*
Provence	*Rosa centifolia*
Psyllium	*Plantago ovata*
Psyllium Seed	*Plantago afra*
Puff Ball	*Lycoperdon species*
Pumpkin	*Cucurbita pepo*
Purple Gromwell	*Lithospermum erytrorhizon*
Purple Loosestrife	*Lythrum salicaria*
Pyrethrum	*Chrysanthemum cinerariifolium*
Quassia	*Picrasma excelsa*
Quassia	*Quassia amara*
Quebracho	*Aspidosperma quebracho-blanco*
Quillaja	*Quillaja saponaria*
Quince	*Cydonia oblongata*
Quinine	*Cinchona pubescens*
Radish	*Raphanus sativus*
Ragwort	*Senecio jacobaea*
Raspberry	*Rubus idaeus*
Rauwolfia	*Rauwolfia serpentina*
Red Bryony	*Bryonia cretica*
Red Clover	*Trifolium pratense*
Red Currant	*Ribes rubrum*
Red Maple	*Acer rubrum*
Red Sandalwood	*Pterocarpus santalinus*
Red-Rooted Sage	*Salvia miltiorrhiza*
Red-Spur Valerian	*Centranthus ruber*
Reed Herb	*Phragmites communis*
Rehmannia	*Rehmannia glutinosa*
Rhatany	*Krameria triandra*
Rosemary	*Rosmarinus officinalis*
Rosinweed	*Silphium laciniatum*
Rue	*Ruta graveolens*
Rupturewort	*Herniaria glabra*
Rust-Red Rhododendron	*Rhododendron ferrugineum*
Safflower	*Carthamus tinctorius*
Saffron	*Crocus sativus*
Sage	*Salvia officinalis*
Salep	*Orchis species*
Samphire	*Crithum maritimum*
Sandalwood	*Santalum album*
Sandarac	*Tetraclinis articulata*
Sarsaparilla	*Smilax species*
Sassafras	*Sassafras albidum*
Savin Tops	*Juniperus sabina*
Saw Palmetto	*Serenoa repens*
Scarlet Pimpernel	*Anagallis arvensis*
Schisandra	*Schisandra chinensis*
Scopolia	*Scopolia carniolica*
Scotch Broom	*Cytisus scoparius*
Scotch Pine	*Pinus species*
Scotch Thistle	*Onopordum acanthium*
Scullcap	*Scutellaria lateriflora*

Common Name	Scientific Name
Scurvy Grass	*Cochlearia officinalis*
Sea Buckthorn	*Hippophae rhamnoides*
Senburi	*Swertia japonica*
Seneca Snakeroot	*Polygala senega*
Senna	*Cassia senna*
Sesame	*Sesamum orientale*
Shepherd's Purse	*Capsella bursa-pastoris*
Short Buchu	*Barosma betulina*
Siam Benzoin	*Styrax tonkinesis*
Siberian Ginseng	*Eleutherococcus senticosus*
Simaruba	*Simaruba amara*
Skirret	*Sium sisarum*
Skunk Cabbage	*Symplocarpus foetidus*
Slippery Elm	*Ulmus rubra*
Sloe	*Prunus spinosa*
Smartweed	*Persicaria hydropiper*
Sneezewort	*Achillea ptarmica*
Snowdrop	*Galanthus nivalis*
Soapwort	*Saponaria officinalis*
Solomon's Seal	*Polygonatum multiflorum*
Sorrel	*Rumex acetosa*
Southern Bayberry	*Myrica cerifera*
Southern Tsangshu	*Atractylodes*
Soybean	*Glycine soja*
Spanish-Chestnut	*Castanea sativa*
Spearmint	*Mentha spicata*
Speedwell	*Veronica officinalis*
Spikenard	*Aralia racemosa*
Spinach	*Spinacia oleracea*
Spiny Rest Harrow	*Ononis spinosa*
Spurge	*Euphorbia resinifera*
Squill	*Drimia maritima*
St. Benedict Thistle	*Cnicus benedictus*
St. John's Wort	*Hypericum perforatum*
Star Anise	*Illicium verum*
Stavesacre	*Delphinium staphisagria*
Stevia	*Stevia rebaudiana*
Stillingia	*Stillingia sylvatica*
Stinging Nettle	*Urtica dioica*
Stone Root	*Collinsonia canadensis*
Storax	*Liquidambar orientalis*
Strawberry	*Fragaria vesca*
Strophanthus	*Strophanthus Kombe*
Strophanthus Gratus	*Strophanthus gratus*
Sumatra Benzoin	*Styrax paralleloneurum*

Common Name	Scientific Name
Sumbul	*Ferula sumbul*
Summer Savory	*Satureja hortensis*
Sundew	*Drosera rotundifolia*
Sunflower	*Helianthus annuus*
Surinam Cherry	*Eugenia unifloria*
Swamp Milkweed	*Asclepias incarnata*
Sweet Cicely	*Myrrhis odorata*
Sweet Clover	*Melilotus officinalis*
Sweet Gale	*Myrica gale*
Sweet Marjoram	*Origanum majorana*
Sweet Orange	*Citrus sinensis*
Sweet Sumach	*Rhus aromatica*
Sweet Vernal Grass	*Anthoxanthum odoratum*
Sweet Violet	*Viola odorata*
Sweet Woodruff	*Galium odoratum*
Tansy	*Tanacetum vulgare*
Taumelloolch	*Lolium temulentum*
Tea	*Camellia sinensis*
Tea Tree	*Melaleuca alternifolia*
Teazle	*Dipsacus silvestris*
Thuja	*Thuja occidentalis*
Thyme	*Thymus vulgaris*
Tolu Balsam	*Myroxylon balsamum*
Tomato	*Lycopersicon esculentum*
Tonka Beans	*Dipteryx odorata*
Tragacanth	*Astragalus gummifer*
Trailing Arbutus	*Epigae repens*
Traveller's Joy	*Clematis vitalba*
Tree of Heaven	*Ailanthus altissima*
Triticum	*Agropyron repens*
Tropical Almond	*Terminalia chebula*
Tulip Tree	*Liriodendron tulipifera*
Turkey Corn	*Dicentra cucullaria*
Turmeric	*Curcuma domestica*
Usnea	*Usnea species*
Uva-Ursi	*Arctostaphylos uva-ursi*
Uzara	*Xysmalobium undulatum*
Valerian	*Valeriana officinalis*
Virola	*Virola theiodora*
Wafer Ash	*Ptelea trifoliata*
Wahoo	*Euonymus atropurpurea*
Wallflower	*Cheiranthus cheiri*
Walnut	*Juglans regia*
Water Avens	*Geum rivale*
Water Dock	*Rumex aquaticus*

Common Name	Scientific Name
Water Dropwort	*Oenanthe crocata*
Water Fennel	*Oenanthe aquatica*
Water Germander	*Teucrium scordium*
Watercress	*Nasturtium officinale*
Wheat	*Triticum aestivum*
White Bryony	*Bryonia alba*
White Hellebore	*Veratrum album*
White Lily	*Lilium candidium*
White Mustard	*Sinapis alba*
White Nettle	*Lamium album*
White Willow	*Salix species*
Wild Carrot	*Daucus carota*
Wild Cherry	*Prunus serotina*
Wild Daisy	*Bellis perennis*
Wild Indigo	*Baptisia tinctoria*
Wild Mint	*Mentha aquatica*
Wild Radish	*Raphanus raphanistrum*
Wild Thyme	*Thymus serpyllum*
Wild Turnip	*Brassica rapa*
Wild Yam	*Dioscorea villosa*
Winter Cherry	*Physalis alkekengi*
Wintergreen	*Pyrola rotundifolia*
Wintergreen	*Gaultheria procumbens*
Winter's Bark	*Drimys winteri*
Witch Hazel	*Hamamelis virginiana*
Wood Anemone	*Anemone nemorosa*
Wood Betony	*Betonica officinalis*
Wood Sage	*Teucrium scorodonia*
Wood Sorrel	*Oxalis acetosella*
Wormseed	*Artemisia cina*
Wormseed Oil	*Chenopodium ambrosioides*
Wormwood	*Artemisia absinthium*
Wormwood Grass	*Spigelia anthelmia*
Woundwort	*Anthyllis vulneraria*
Woundwort	*Stachys palustris*
Yage	*Banisteriopsis caapi*
Yarrow	*Achillea millefolium*
Yellow Dock	*Rumex crispus*
Yellow Jessamine	*Gelsemium sempervirens*
Yellow Lupin	*Lupinus luteus*
Yellow Toadflax	*Linaria vulgaris*
Yerba Santa	*Eriodictyon californicum*
Yew	*Taxus baccata*
Yohimbe	*Pausinystalia yohimbe*
Yucca	*Yucca filamentosa*
Zedoary	*Curcuma zedoaria*

COMMON HERBAL USES

Claims made for herbs in the popular press often outdistance their actual benefits. Which uses should be taken seriously and which dismissed? Extensive information comes from Germany, where the efficacy of medicinal herbs undergoes official scrutiny by the German Regulatory Authority's "Commission E." This agency has conducted an intensive analysis of the peer-reviewed literature on some 300 common botanicals, weighing the quality of the clinical evidence and identifying the uses for which the herb may be helpful. The results of this effort are summarized in the table below.

Herb	Uses
Adonis *(Adonis vernalis)*	Arrhythmias Anxiety disorders, management of
Agrimony *(Agrimonia eupatoria)*	Diarrhea, symptomatic relief of Skin, inflammatory conditions Stomatitis
Aloe *(A. baradensis, A. capensis)*	Constipation Oral lichen planus
Angelica *(Angelica archangelica)*	Appetite, stimulation of Digestive disorders, symptomatic relief of
Anise *(Pimpinella anisum)*	Appetite, stimulation of Bronchitis, acute Cold, common, symptomatic relief of Cough, symptomatic relief of Digestive disorders, symptomatic relief of Fever associated with common cold Stomatitis
Arnica *(Arnica montana)*	Bronchitis, acute Cold, common, symptomatic relief of Cough, symptomatic relief of Fever associated with common cold Infection, tendency to Rheumatic disorders, unspecified Skin, inflammatory conditions Stomatitis Trauma, blunt
Artichoke *(Cynara scolymus)*	Appetite, stimulation of Liver and gallbladder complaints
Asparagus *(Asparagus officinalis)*	Infections, urinary tract Kidney and bladder stones
Bean Pod *(Phaseolus vulgaris)*	Infections, urinary tract Kidney and bladder stones
Belladonna *(Atropa belladonna)*	Liver and gallbladder complaints
Bilberry *(Vaccinium myrtillus)*	Diarrhea, symptomatic relief of Stomatitis
Bitter Orange *(Citrus aurantium)*	Appetite, stimulation of Digestive disorders, symptomatic relief of
Bittersweet Nightshade *(Solanum dulcamara)*	Acne, unspecified Furunculosis Dermatitis, eczematoid Warts
Black Cohosh *(Cimicifuga racemosa)*	Menopause, climacteric complaints Premenstrual syndrome, management of
Blackberry *(Rubus fruticosus)*	Diarrhea, symptomatic relief of Stomatitis
Blessed Thistle *(Cnicus benedictus)*	Appetite, stimulation of Digestive disorders, symptomatic relief of
Bog Bean *(Menyanthes trifoliata)*	Appetite, stimulation of Digestive disorders, symptomatic relief of
Boldo *(Peumus boldus)*	Digestive disorders, symptomatic relief of
Brewer's Yeast *(Saccharomyces cerevisiae)*	Acne vulgaris Appetite, stimulation of Digestive disorders, symptomatic relief of Eczema Furunculosis
Buckthorn *(Rhamnus catharticus)*	Constipation
Bugleweed *(Lycopus virginicus)*	Anxiety disorders, management of Premenstrual syndrome, management of Sleep, induction of
Butcher's Broom *(Ruscus aculeatus)*	Hemorrhoids, symptomatic relief of Venous conditions
Cajuput *(Melaleuca leucadendra)*	Rheumatic disorders, unspecified Infection, tendency to Pain, muscular, temporary relief of Pain, neurogenic Wound/burn care, adjunctive therapy in
Camphor Tree *(Cinnamomum camphora)*	Anxiety disorders, management of Arrhythmias Bronchitis, acute Cough, symptomatic relief of Hypotension Rheumatic disorders, unspecified
Canadian Golden Rod *(Solidago canadensis)*	Infections, urinary tract Kidney and bladder stones
Caraway *(Carum carvi)*	Digestive disorders, symptomatic relief of
Cardamom *(Elettaria cardamomum)*	Digestive disorders, symptomatic relief of

Herb	Uses
Cascara Sagrada *(Rhamnus purshianus)*	Constipation
Cayenne *(Capsicum annuum)*	Muscle tension Rheumatic disorders, unspecified
Celandine *(Chelidonium majus)*	Liver and gallbladder complaints
Centaury *(Centaurium erythraea)*	Appetite, stimulation of Digestive disorders, symptomatic relief of
Chaste Tree *(Vitex agnus-castus)*	Premenstrual syndrome, management of Menopause, climacteric complaints Mestalgia/mastalgia
Chicory *(Cichorium intybus)*	Appetite, stimulation of Digestive disorders, symptomatic relief of
Chinese Cinnamon *(Cinnamomum aromaticum)*	Appetite, stimulation of Digestive disorders, symptomatic relief of
Chinese Rhubarb *(Rheum palmatum)*	Constipation
Cinnamon *(Cinnamomum verum)*	Appetite, stimulation of Digestive disorders, symptomatic relief of
Cinquefoil *(Potentilla erecta)*	Diarrhea, symptomatic relief of Premenstrual syndrome Stomatitis
Clove *(Syzygium aromaticum)*	Pain, dental Stomatitis
Coffee *(Coffea arabica)*	Diarrhea, symptomatic relief of Stomatitis
Cola *(Cola acuminata)*	Lack of stamina
Colchicum *(Colchicum autumnale)*	Brucellosis (Mediterranean fever) Gout, management of signs and symptoms
Colt's Foot *(Tussilago farfara)*	Bronchitis, acute Cough, symptomatic relief of Stomatitis
Comfrey *(Symphytum officinale)*	Trauma, blunt
Condurango *(Marsdenia condurango)*	Appetite, stimulation of Digestive disorders, symptomatic relief of
Coriander *(Coriandrum sativum)*	Appetite, stimulation of Digestive disorders, symptomatic relief of
Cowslip *(Primula veris)*	Bronchitis, acute Cough, symptomatic relief of
Curcuma *(Curcuma xanthorrhizia)*	Appetite, stimulation of Digestive disorders, symptomatic relief of
Dandelion *(Taraxacum officinale)*	Appetite, stimulation of Digestive disorders, symptomatic relief of Infections, urinary tract Liver and gallbladder complaints
Devil's Claw *(Harpagophytum procumbens)*	Appetite, stimulation of Digestive disorders, symptomatic relief of Rheumatic disorders, unspecified
Dill *(Anethum graveolens)*	Digestive disorders, symptomatic relief of
Echinacea Pallida *(Echinacea pallida)*	Cold, common, symptomatic relief of Fever associated with common cold
Echinacea Purpurea *(Echinacea purpurea)*	Bronchitis, acute Cold, common, symptomatic relief of Cough, symptomatic relief of Fever associated with common cold Infections, tendency to Infections, urinary tract Stomatitis Wound/burn care, adjunctive therapy in
English Hawthorn *(Crataegus laevigata)*	Cardiac output, low
English Ivy *(Hedera helix)*	Bronchitis, acute Cough, symptomatic relief of
English Lavender *(Lavandula angustifolia)*	Anxiety disorders, management of Appetite, stimulation of Circulatory disorders Digestive disorders, symptomatic relief of Sleep, induction of
English Plantain *(Plantago lanceolata)*	Bronchitis, acute Cold, common, symptomatic relief of Cough, symptomatic relief of Fever associated with common cold Skin, inflammatory conditions Stomatitis
Eucalyptus *(Eucalyptus globulus)*	Bronchitis, acute Cough, symptomatic relief of Rheumatic disorders, unspecified
European Elder *(Sambucus nigra)*	Bronchitis, acute Cold, common, symptomatic relief of Cough, symptomatic relief of Fever associated with common cold
European Mistletoe *(Viscum album)*	Rheumatic disorders, unspecified Tumor therapy adjuvant

Herb	Uses
European Sanicle (*Sanicula europaea*)	Bronchitis, acute Cough, symptomatic relief of
Fennel (*Foeniculum vulgare*)	Bronchitis, acute Cough, symptomatic relief of Digestive disorders, symptomatic relief of
Fenugreek (*Trigonella foenum-graecum*)	Appetite, stimulation of Skin, inflammatory conditions
Flax (*Linum usitatissimum*)	Constipation Skin, inflammatory conditions
Frangula (*Rhamnus frangula*)	Constipation
Fumitory (*Fumaria officinalis*)	Liver and gallbladder complaints
Garlic (*Allium sativum*)	Arteriosclerosis Hypercholesterolemia Hyperlipidemia Hypertension
German Chamomile (*Matricaria recutita*)	Bronchitis, acute Cold, common, symptomatic relief of Cough, symptomatic relief of Fever associated with common cold Infection, tendency to Skin, inflammatory conditions Stomatitis Wound/burn care, adjunctive therapy in
Ginger (*Zingiber officinale*)	Appetite, stimulation of Digestive disorders, symptomatic relief of Motion sickness
Ginkgo (*Ginkgo biloba*)	Claudication, intermittent Dementia Organic brain dysfunction, symptomatic relief of Tinnitus Vertigo Vitiligo
Ginseng (*Panax ginseng*)	Lack of stamina
Guaiac (*Guaiacum officinale*)	Rheumatic disorders, unspecified
Gumweed (*Grindelia* species)	Bronchitis, acute Cough, symptomatic relief of
Haronga (*Haronga madagascariensis*)	Digestive disorders, symptomatic relief of Pancreatic insufficiency
Hawthorn (*Crataegus oxyacantha*)	Heart failure, treatment of
Heartsease (*Viola tricolor*)	Skin, inflammatory conditions
Hempnettle (*Galeopsis segetum*)	Bronchitis, acute Cough, symptomatic relief of
Henbane (*Hyoscyamus niger*)	Digestive disorders, symptomatic relief of
High Mallow (*Malva sylvestris*)	Bronchitis, acute Cough, symptomatic relief of Stomatitis
Hops (*Humulus lupulus*)	Anxiety disorders, management of Sleep, induction of
Horehound (*Marrubium vulgare*)	Appetite, stimulation of Digestive disorders, symptomatic relief of
Horse Chestnut (*Aesculus hippocastanum*)	Venous conditions (chronic venous insufficiency)
Horseradish (*Armoracia rusticana*)	Bronchitis, acute Cough, symptomatic relief of Infections, urinary tract
Horsetail (*Equisetum arvense*)	Infections, urinary tract Kidney and bladder stones Wound care, adjunctive therapy in
Iceland Moss (*Cetraria islandica*)	Appetite, stimulation of Bronchitis, acute Cough, symptomatic relief of Digestive disorders, symptomatic relief of Stomatitis
Immortelle (*Helichrysum arenarium*)	Digestive disorders, symptomatic relief of
Jambolan (*Syzygium cumini*)	Diarrhea, symptomatic relief of Skin, inflammatory conditions Stomatitis
Japanese Mint (*Mentha arvensis piperascens*)	Bronchitis, acute Cold, common, symptomatic relief of Cough, symptomatic relief of Fever associated with common cold Liver and gallbladder complaints Pain, unspecified Stomatitis
Java Tea (*Orthosiphon spicatus*)	Infections, urinary tract Kidney and bladder stones
Juniper (*Juniperus communis*)	Digestive disorders, symptomatic relief of
Kava-Kava (*Piper methysticum*)	Anxiety disorders, management of Sleep, induction of
Knotweed (*Polygonum aviculare*)	Bronchitis, acute Cough, symptomatic relief of Stomatitis
Lady's Mantle (*Alchemilla vulgaris*)	Diarrhea, symptomatic relief of

Herb	Uses
Larch *(Larix decidua)*	Blood pressure problems Bronchitis, acute Cold, common, symptomatic relief of Cough, symptomatic relief of Fever associated with common cold Infection, tendency to Rheumatic disorders, unspecified Stomatitis
Lemon Balm *(Melissa officinalis)*	Anxiety disorders, management of Sleep, induction of
Lesser Galangal *(Alpinia officinarum)*	Appetite, stimulation of Digestive disorders, symptomatic relief of
Licorice *(Glycyrrhiza glabra)*	Bronchitis, acute Cough, symptomatic relief of Gastritis
Lily-of-the-Valley *(Convallaria majalis)*	Anxiety disorders, management of Arrhythmias Cardiac output, low
Linden *(Tilia* species*)*	Bronchitis, acute Cough, symptomatic relief of
Lovage *(Levisticum officinale)*	Infections, urinary tract Kidney and bladder stones
Ma-Huang *(Ephedra sinica)*	Bronchitis (acute), cough **Note:** The FDA banned ephedra products in Feb. 2004.
Manna *(Fraxinus ornus)*	Constipation
Marigold *(Calendula officinalis)*	Stomatitis Wound/burn care, adjunctive therapy in
Marshmallow *(Althaea officinalis)*	Bronchitis, acute Cough, symptomatic relief of
MatO *(Ilex paraguariensis)*	Lack of stamina
Mayapple *(Podophyllum peltatum)*	Warts
Meadowsweet *(Filipendula ulmaria)*	Bronchitis, acute Cold, common, symptomatic relief of Cough, symptomatic relief of Fever associated with common cold
Milk Thistle *(Silybum marianum)*	Digestive disorders, symptomatic relief of Liver and gallbladder complaints
Motherwort *(Leonurus cardiaca)*	Anxiety disorders, management of
Mullein *(Verbascum densiflorum)*	Bronchitis, acute Cough, symptomatic relief of
Myrrh *(Commiphora molmol)*	Stomatitis
Nasturtium *(Tropaeolum majus)*	Bronchitis, acute Cough, symptomatic relief of Infections, urinary tract
Niauli *(Melaleucea viridiflora)*	Bronchitis, acute Cough, symptomatic relief of
Oak *(Quercus robur)*	Bronchitis, acute Cough, symptomatic relief of Diarrhea, symptomatic relief of Skin, inflammatory conditions Stomatitis
Oats *(Avena sativa)*	Skin, inflammatory conditions Warts
Onion *(Allium cepa)*	Appetite, stimulation of Arteriosclerosis Bronchitis, acute Cold, common, symptomatic relief of Cough, symptomatic relief of Digestive disorders, symptomatic relief of Fever associated with common cold Hypertension Infection, tendency to Stomatitis
Parsley *(Petroselinum crispum)*	Infections, urinary tract Kidney and bladder stones
Passion Flower *(Passiflora incarnata)*	Anxiety disorders, management of Sleep, induction of
Peppermint *(Mentha piperita)*	Cold, common, symptomatic relief of Cough, symptomatic relief of Digestive disorders, symptomatic relief of Liver and gallbladder complaints Muscle pain (external use) Neuralgia (external use) Stomatitis
Petasites *(Petasites hybridus)*	Kidney and bladder stones
Pimpinella *(Pimpinella major)*	Cough, symptomatic relief of Bronchitis, acute
Pineapple *(Ananas comosus)*	Wound/burn care, adjunctive therapy in
Poplar *(Populus* species*)*	Hemorrhoids, symptomatic relief of Wound/burn care, adjunctive therapy in
Potentilla *(Potentilla anserina)*	Diarrhea, symptomatic relief of Premenstrual syndrome, management of Stomatitis

Herb	Uses
Psyllium *(Plantago ovata)*	Constipation Diarrhea, symptomatic relief of Hemorrhoids Hypercholesterolemia, primary, adjunct to diet
Psyllium Seed *(Plantago afra)*	Cholesterol, lowering of Constipation Diarrhea, symptomatic relief of Hemorrhoids
Pumpkin *(Cucurbita pepo)*	Urinary frequency, symptomatic relief of Prostatic hyperplasia, benign, symptomatic treatment of
Quinine *(Cinchona pubescens)*	Appetite, stimulation of Digestive disorders, symptomatic relief of
Radish *(Raphanus sativus)*	Bronchitis, acute Cough, symptomatic relief of Digestive disorders, symptomatic relief of
Rauwolfia *(Rauwolfia serpentina)*	Anxiety disorders, management of Hypertension Sleep, induction of
Rhatany *(Krameria triandra)*	Stomatitis
Rose *(Rosa centifolia)*	Stomatitis
Rosemary *(Rosmarinus officinalis)*	Appetite, stimulation of Blood pressure problems Digestive disorders, symptomatic relief of Rheumatic disorders, unspecified
Sage *(Salvia officinalis)*	Appetite, stimulation of Hyperhidrosis Stomatitis
Sandalwood *(Santalum album)*	Infections, urinary tract
Saw Palmetto *(Serenoa repens)*	Urinary frequency, symptomatic relief of Prostatic hyperplasia, benign, symptomatic treatment of
Scopolia *(Scopolia carniolica)*	Liver and gallbladder complaints
Scotch Broom *(Cytisus scoparius)*	Hypertension Circulatory disorders
Scotch Pine *(Pinus species)*	Blood pressure problems Bronchitis, acute Cold, common, symptomatic relief of Cough, symptomatic relief of Fever associated with common cold Infection, tendency to Pain, neurogenic Rheumatic disorders, unspecified Stomatitis
Seneca Snakeroot *(Polygala senega)*	Bronchitis, acute Cough, symptomatic relief of
Senna *(Cassia senna)*	Constipation
Shepherd's Purse *(Capsella bursa-pastoris)*	Hemorrhage, nasal Premenstrual syndrome, management of Wound/burn care, adjunctive therapy in
Siberian Ginseng *(Eleutherococcus senticosus)*	Infection, tendency to Lack of stamina
Sloe *(Prunus spinosa)*	Stomatitis
Soapwort *(Saponaria officinalis)*	Bronchitis, acute Cough, symptomatic relief of
Soybean *(Glycine soja)*	Hypercholesterolemia, primary, adjunct to diet
Spiny Rest Harrow *(Ononis spinosa)*	Infections, urinary tract Kidney and bladder stones
Spruce *(Picea* species*)*	Bronchitis, acute Cold, common, symptomatic relief of Cough, symptomatic relief of Fever associated with common cold Infection, tendency to Muscle pain (external use) Neuralgia (external use) Rheumatic disorders, unspecified Stomatitis
Squill *(Drimia maritima)*	Anxiety disorders, management of Arrhythmia Cardiac output, low (NYHA I and II)
St. John's Wort *(Hypericum perforatum)*	Anxiety disorders, management of Depression, relief of symptoms Skin, inflammatory conditions Trauma, blunt Wound/burn care, adjunctive therapy in
Star Anise *(Illicium verum)*	Appetite, stimulation of Bronchitis, acute Cough, symptomatic relief of
Stinging Nettle *(Urtica dioica)*	Infections, urinary tract Kidney and bladder stones Rheumatic disorders, unspecified Prostatic hyperplasia, benign, symptomatic treatment of Urinary frequency, symptomatic relief of Urinary tract infections
Sundew *(Drosera rotundifolia)*	Bronchitis, acute Cough, symptomatic relief of
Sweet Clover *(Melilotus officinalis)*	Hemorrhoids, symptomatic relief of Trauma, blunt Venous conditions

Herb	Uses
Sweet Orange (*Citrus sinensis*)	Appetite, stimulation of Digestive disorders, symptomatic relief of
Thyme (*Thymus vulgaris*)	Bronchitis, acute Cough, symptomatic relief of
Tolu Balsam (*Myroxylon balsamum*)	Bronchitis, acute Cough, symptomatic relief of Hemorrhoids, symptomatic relief of (Peruvian variety) Wound/burn care, adjunctive therapy in (Peruvian variety)
Triticum (*Agropyron repens*)	Infections, urinary tract Kidney and bladder stones
Turmeric (*Curcuma domestica*)	Appetite, stimulation of Digestive disorders, symptomatic relief of
Usnea (*Usnea* species)	Stomatitis
Uva-Ursi (*Arctostaphylos uva-ursi*)	Infections, urinary tract
Uzara (*Xysmalobium undulatum*)	Diarrhea, symptomatic relief of
Valerian (*Valeriana officinalis*)	Anxiety disorders, management of Sleep, induction of
Walnut (*Juglans regia*)	Hyperhidrosis Skin, inflammatory conditions
Watercress (*Nasturtium officinale*)	Bronchitis, acute Cough, symptomatic relief of
White Fir (*Abies alba*)	Neuralgia Rheumatic disorders, unspecified
White Mustard (*Sinapis alba*)	Bronchitis, acute Cold, common, symptomatic relief of Cough, symptomatic relief of Rheumatic disorders, unspecified
White Nettle (*Lamium album*)	Bronchitis, acute Cough, symptomatic relief of Skin, inflammatory conditions Stomatitis
White Willow (*Salix* species)	Pain, unspecified Rheumatic disorders, unspecified
Wild Thyme (*Thymus serpyllum*)	Bronchitis, acute Cough, symptomatic relief of
Witch Hazel (*Hamamelis virginiana*)	Hemorrhoids, symptomatic relief of Skin disorders Skin, inflammatory conditions Stomatitis (leaf only) Venous conditions Wound/burn care, adjunctive therapy in
Wormwood (*Artemisia absinthium*)	Appetite, stimulation of Digestive disorders, symptomatic relief of Liver and gallbladder complaints
Yarrow (*Achillea millefolium*)	Appetite, stimulation of Digestive disorders, symptomatic relief of Liver and gallbladder complaints
Yellow Gentian (*Gentiana lutea*)	Appetite, stimulation of Digestive disorders, symptomatic relief of

4 PRACTICE MANAGEMENT

...CATION PROVIDERS

...tinuing pharmacy education. Some programs
...rds and a list of approved providers, contact
...ceproviders/providers.asp.

...t_ed.html

...k_desc.cfm?LinkID=6

...nuing_education

...m

...tion

...ng_professional_development.asp

...ntinuing-education

...continuing_education

...px

...eOfPharmacy/ContinuingEducation

...y/health_pros_conted.asp

...asp

...on.cfm

...e

...rmacyce/custom/pages/Public/default.aspx

DISEASE MANAGEMENT PROGRAMS

Below is a list of providers for the conditions most commonly chosen for disease management. Many are affiliated with national and governmental groups as well as managed care organizations. Others have close ties to pharmaceutical manufacturers, which some critics say could lead to a conflict of interest. Therefore, it's important for all providers to openly state which groups are sponsoring their programs. And while each provider has its own criteria for developing programs and measuring disease outcomes, the goals should remain the same: to prevent complications, provide continuity of care, and avoid waste of resources.

ALZHEIMER'S DISEASE

SRA International
(formerly Constella Group)
2605 Meridian Pkwy.
Durham, NC 27713
919-544-8500
www.constellagroup.com

University of Pennsylvania
Health System
1 Presidential Blvd.
Suite 421
Philadelphia, PA 19004
(215) 662-4000 (general info)
www.pennhealth.com

AMYOTROPHIC LATERAL SCLEROSIS

Accordant Health Services
4900 Koger Blvd., Suite 100
Greensboro, NC 27407-2710
336-855-5870
www.accordant.com

ASTHMA

American Health Holding, Inc.
100 W. Old Wilson Bridge Rd.
Third Floor
PO Box 6016
Worthington, OH 43085-6016
614-818-3222
888-610-0089
(Disease Management
Nursecare Line)
www.americanhealthholding.com

Caremark
(Adult, Pediatric)
2211 Sanders Rd.
Northbrook, IL 60062
800-426-4488
www.caremark.com

Health Management
Corporation
6800 Paragon Pl., Suite 500
Richmond, VA 23230
800-523-9279
www.choosehmc.com

Lovelace Sandia Health Systems
5400 Gibson Blvd., SE
Albuquerque, NM 87108
505-262-7000
www.lovelace.com

SRA International
(formerly Constella Group)
2605 Meridian Pkwy.
Durham, NC 27713
919-544-8500
www.constellagroup.com

University of Pennsylvania
Health System
(Congestive Heart Failure)
1 Presidential Blvd.
Suite 421
Philadelphia, PA 19004
215-662-4000 (general info)
www.pennhealth.com

CARDIOVASULAR DISEASE

American Health Holding, Inc.
(Coronary Artery Disease,
Congestive Heart Failure,
Hypertension)
100 W. Old Wilson Bridge Rd.
Third Floor
PO Box 6016
Worthington, OH 43085-6016
614-818-3222
www.americanhealthholding.com

Caremark
(Congestive Heart Failure,
Coronary Artery Disease)
2211 Sanders Rd.
Northbrook, IL 60062
800-426-4488
www.caremark.com

Health Management
Corporation
(Congestive Heart Failure,
Coronary Artery Disease)
6800 Paragon Pl., Suite 500
Richmond, VA 23230
800-523-9279
www.choosehmc.com

Lovelace Sandia Health Systems
(Congestive Heart Failure,
Lipid Disorder)
5400 Gibson Blvd., SE
Albuquerque, NM 87108
505-262-7000
www.lovelace.com

SRA International
(formerly Constella Group)
(Stroke)
2605 Meridian Pkwy.
Durham, NC 27713
919-544-8500
www.constellagroup.com

CHRONIC INFLAMMATORY DEMYELINATING POLY-RADICULONEUROPATHY

Accordant Health Services
4900 Koger Blvd., Suite 100
Greensboro, NC 27407-2710
336-855-5870
www.accordant.com

CHRONIC OBSTRUCTIVE PULMONARY DISEASE

American Health Holding, Inc.
100 W. Old Wilson Bridge Rd.
Third Floor
PO Box 6016
Worthington, OH 43085-6016
614-818-3222
www.americanhealthholding.com

Caremark
2211 Sanders Rd.
Northbrook, IL 60062
800-426-4488
www.caremark.com

Health Management
Corporation
6800 Paragon Pl., Suite 500
Richmond, VA 23230
800-523-9279
www.choosehmc.com

SRA International
(formerly Constella Group)
2605 Meridian Pkwy.
Durham, NC 27713
919-544-8500
www.constellagroup.com

CYSTIC FIBROSIS

Accordant Health Services
4900 Koger Blvd., Suite 100
Greensboro, NC 27407-2710
336-855-5870
www.accordant.com

DEPRESSIVE DISORDERS

Caremark
2211 Sanders Rd.
Northbrook, IL 60062
800-426-4488
www.caremark.com

Lovelace Sandia Health Systems
5400 Gibson Blvd., SE
Albuquerque, NM 87108
505-262-7000
www.lovelace.com

DERMATOMYOSITIS

Accordant Health Services
4900 Koger Blvd., Suite 100
Greensboro, NC 27407-2710
336-855-5870
www.accordant.com

DIABETES

American Health Holding, Inc.
100 W. Old Wilson Bridge Rd.
Third Floor
PO Box 6016
Worthington, OH 43085-6016
614-818-3222
www.americanhealthholding.com

Caremark
2211 Sanders Rd.
Northbrook, IL 60062
800-426-4488
www.caremark.com

Health Management
Corporation
6800 Paragon Pl., Suite 500
Richmond, VA 23230
800-523-9279
www.choosehmc.com

Lovelace Sandia Health Systems
5400 Gibson Blvd., SE
Albuquerque, NM 87108
505-262-7000
www.lovelace.com

SRA International
(formerly Constella Group)
2605 Meridian Pkwy.
Durham, NC 27713
919-544-8500
www.constellagroup.com

University of Pennsylvania
Health System
1 Presidential Blvd.
Suite 421
Philadelphia, PA 19004
215-662-4000
www.pennhealth.com

GASTROINTESTINAL DISEASES

Caremark
(Peptic Ulcer Disease)
2211 Sanders Rd.
Northbrook, IL 60062
800-426-4488
www.caremark.com

SRA International
(formerly Constella Group)
(Gastrointestinal Malignancies)
2605 Meridian Pkwy.
Durham, NC 27713
919-544-8500
www.constellagroup.com

GAUCHER DISEASE

Accordant Health Services
4900 Koger Blvd., Suite 100
Greensboro, NC 27407-2710
336-855-5870
www.accordant.com

HEMOPHILIA

Accordant Health Services
4900 Koger Blvd., Suite 100
Greensboro, NC 27407-2710
336-855-5870
www.accordant.com

Caremark
2211 Sanders Rd.
Northbrook, IL 60062
800-426-4488
www.caremark.com

HIV/AIDS

BioScrip
10050 Crosstown Circle
Suite 300
Eden Prairie, MN 55344
800-444-5951
www.bioscrip.com

SRA International
(formerly Constella Group)
2605 Meridian Pkwy.
Durham, NC 27713
919-544-8500
www.constellagroup.com

JOINT DISEASES

Accordant Health Services
(Rheumatoid Arthritis)
4900 Koger Blvd., Suite 100
Greensboro, NC 27407-2710
336-855-5870
www.accordant.com

Caremark
(Osteoarthritis,
Rheumatoid Arthritis)
2211 Sanders Rd.
Northbrook, IL 60062
800-426-4488
www.caremark.com

Lovelace Sandia Health Systems
(Osteoarthritis,
Rheumatoid Arthritis)
5400 Gibson Blvd., SE
Albuquerque, NM 87108
505-262-7000
www.lovelace.com

LOW BACK PAIN

Health Management
Corporation
6800 Paragon Pl., Suite 500
Richmond, VA 23230
800-523-9279
www.choosehmc.com

LUPUS

Accordant Health Services
4900 Koger Blvd., Suite 100
Greensboro, NC 27407-2710
336-855-5870
www.accordant.com

MENTAL HEALTH

SRA International
(formerly Constella Group)
2605 Meridian Pkwy.
Durham, NC 27713
919-544-8500
www.constellagroup.com

MIGRAINE

American Health Holding, Inc.
100 W. Old Wilson Bridge Rd.
Third Floor
PO Box 6016
Worthington, OH 43085-6016
614-818-3222
www.americanhealthholding.com

MULTIPLE SCLEROSIS

Accordant Health Services
4900 Koger Blvd., Suite 100
Greensboro, NC 27407-2710
336-855-5870
www.accordant.com

American Health Holding, Inc.
100 W. Old Wilson Bridge Rd.
Third Floor
PO Box 6016
Worthington, OH 43085-6016
614-818-3222
www.americanhealthholding.com

Caremark
2211 Sanders Rd.
Northbrook, IL 60062
800-426-4488
www.caremark.com

MYASTHENIA GRAVIS

Accordant Health Services
4900 Koger Blvd., Suite 100
Greensboro, NC 27407-2710
336-855-5870
www.accordant.com

ORGAN TRANSPLANT

SRA International
(formerly Constella Group)
2605 Meridian Pkwy.
Durham, NC 27713
919-544-8500
www.constellagroup.com

PAIN

Lovelace Sandia Health Systems
5400 Gibson Blvd., SE
Albuquerque, NM 87108
505-262-7000
www.lovelace.com

SRA International
(formerly Constella Group)
2605 Meridian Pkwy.
Durham, NC 27713
919-544-8500
www.constellagroup.com

PARKINSON'S DISEASE

Accordant Health Services
4900 Koger Blvd., Suite 100
Greensboro, NC 27407-2710
336-855-5870
www.accordant.com

POLYMYOSITIS

Accordant Health Services
4900 Koger Blvd., Suite 100
Greensboro, NC 27407-2710
336-855-5870
www.accordant.com

SCLERODERMA

Accordant Health Services
4900 Koger Blvd., Suite 100
Greensboro, NC 27407-2710
336-855-5870
www.accordant.com

SEIZURE DISORDER

Accordant Health Services
4900 Koger Blvd., Suite 100
Greensboro, NC 27407-2710
336-855-5870
www.accordant.com

SICKLE CELL ANEMIA

Accordant Health Services
4900 Koger Blvd., Suite 100
Greensboro, NC 27407-2710
336-855-5870
www.accordant.com

SLEEP DISORDERS

Lovelace Sandia Health Systems
5400 Gibson Blvd., SE
Albuquerque, NM 87108
505-262-7000
www.lovelace.com

SUBSTANCE ABUSE

Lovelace Sandia Health Systems
5400 Gibson Blvd., SE
Albuquerque, NM 87108
505-262-7000
www.lovelace.com

WOMEN'S HEALTH

Caremark
(Menopause)
2211 Sanders Rd.
Northbrook, IL 60062
800-426-4488
www.caremark.com

Lovelace Sandia Health Systems
(Osteoporosis)
5400 Gibson Blvd., SE
Albuquerque, NM 87108
505-262-7000
www.lovelace.com

SRA International
(formerly Constella Group)
(Osteoporosis)
2605 Meridian Pkwy.
Durham, NC 27713
919-544-8500
www.constellagroup.com

DISEASE MANAGEMENT CREDENTIALING

Disease management is fast becoming a favorite of managed care groups, and many pharmacy organizations now offer training and credentialing in areas where patient monitoring—and, more importantly, patient compliance—make a significant difference, including diabetes, asthma, and hypertension. To qualify for reimbursement, certain third-party payers, including some state Medicaid programs, are requiring pharmacists to complete standardized exams. To find out how to become credentialed, log on to the websites of the sponsoring organizations listed below. Some groups provide training programs. Other groups, including the National Association of Boards of Pharmacy, offer online testing at computerized test centers.

Organization	Website
American Pharmacists Association • diabetes • dyslipidemia • immunization • OTC Advisor™ Pharmacy-Based Self Care Services	**www.aphanet.org**
American Society of Health-System Pharmacists (see website for traineeship programs)	**www.ashp.org**
Board of Pharmaceutical Specialties • nuclear pharmacy • nutrition support pharmacy • oncology pharmacy • pharmacotherapy	**www.bpsweb.org**
Healthcare Quality Certification Board of the National Association for Healthcare Quality (Certified Professional in Healthcare Quality)	**www.cphq.org**
Individual State Pharmacists Associations and Boards of Pharmacy (see website for specific programs)	**www.ncpanet.org**
National Association of Boards of Pharmacy • anticoagulation therapy • asthma • diabetes • dyslipidemia	**www.nabp.net**
National Certification Board for Diabetes Educators	**www.ncbde.org**
National Institute for Pharmacist Care Outcomes (Division of National Community Pharmacists Association) • alternative medicine • arthritis and pain management • cardiovascular care certification program • community aging care • diabetes care certification program • immunization skills certification program • lipid management certification program • men's health care certification program • mental health care certification program • nutrition and weight management certification program • osteoporosis care certification program • respiratory care certification program • therapeutic foot care certification program	**www.ncpanet.org**
National Institute for Standards in Pharmacist Credentialing • diabetes	**www.nispcnet.org**
Pharmacy Technician Certification Board	**www.ptcb.org**

NONTRADITIONAL PHARM.D. PROGRAMS

Getting a Pharm.D. is no longer relegated to the traditional classroom setting. Students can now choose from courses that are given off-site, on weekends and evenings, or by satellite. They can also take advantage of home-study courses delivered via print, video, or the Web. The following tables highlight schools that offer nontraditional pharmacy degrees, outlining their prominent features and comparing first-year tuition and fees. The schools are organized alphabetically by state. All information comes from the American Association of Colleges of Pharmacy, and can be found on the group's website at www.aacp.org.

Table 1. Characteristics of Nontraditional Pharm.D. Programs (includes only colleges and schools for which data were reported)

		As of Fall 2008			Anticipated for 2010–11				
Institution	Location	Total Number of Pharmacists Graduated from Program	Number of Pharmacists Currently Enrolled	Average Calendar Years to Complete Program	Total Credit Hours Required	Didactic Credit Hours Required	Experiential Credit Hours Required	Experiential Component Integrated	Semester or Quarter Hours
Western	CA	20	20	3	131	67	64	•	Sem
Colorado	CO	129	277	3	65	35	30		Sem
Howard	DC	63	13	2	65	35	30	•	Sem
Florida	FL	1377	590	3	63	54	9	•	Sem
Idaho State	ID	238	98	4	55	37	18	•	Sem
Purdue	IN	164	60	6	56	28	28		Sem
Massachusetts–Boston	MA	307	74	3	37	27	10	•	Sem
Shenandoah	VA	394	142	2.5	45	33	12		Sem

Table 2. Didactic Features of Nontraditional Pharm.D. Programs Anticipated for 2010-11

	Delivery Methods						Academic Credit via Other Mechanisms (Max.Credit Hrs.)		
Institution	Off-site Scheduled Live Courses	Weekend/ Evening Courses	Print-based Home Study	Video-based Home Study	Web-based Courses	Other	For Challenge Exams	For Prior Learning	Other
Western						•[a]			• (40)[b]
Colorado					•			• (10)[c]	• (20)[c]
Howard	•	•			•		• (27)		
Florida		•		•	•	•[d]			
Idaho State			•	•	•		• (9)		• (8)[e]
Purdue			•	•	•				
Massachusetts–Boston		•			•	•[f]	• (5)		• (7)[g]
Shenandoah					•				

Notes

a: International students integrated into traditional program

b: Credit given for B.S. degree in Pharmacy prior to enrollment

c: Allow transfer credit if the syllabus and credit hour(s) that were taken match Colorado's course(s). Students can also challenge out of any didactic course if experience/ability is proven and approved via a portfolio process.

d: Clinical training at selected health care facilities

e: Candidates may obtain academic credit via current BCPS certification and shorten the didactic requirements for the degree

f: Off-site experiential; web-based conferencing

g: Transfer credit

Table 3. Experiential Features of Nontraditional Pharm.D. Programs Anticipated for 2010-11

		Rotation Options				Academic Credit Options		
Institution	Location	Completed Part-time	Extended Time Off Between Breaks	Completed at Pharmacist's Practice Site (Max. Credit Hrs.)	Completed in Another State	Challenge Exams (Max. Credit Hrs.)	Prior Learning (Max. Credit Hrs.)	Via Other Mechanisms (Max. Credit Hrs.)
Western	CA				•[a]			
Colorado	CO	•	•	• (10)	•		• (20)	
Howard	DC	•	•	• (10)	•		• (10)	
Florida	FL	•			•			
Idaho State	ID	•	•	• (6)[b]	•		• (6)	
Purdue	IN		•	•	•		• (4)	• (4)[c]
Massachusetts-Boston	MA	•		• (7)	•			• (3)[d]
Shenandoah	VA	•	•	• (12)	•		• (8)	

Notes

a: Must be approved by the College of Pharmacy Office of Experiential Education

b: Candidates can complete one rotation at own practice site upon approval from the program coordinators.

c: Exams

d: Residency training

Table 4. Post-B.S. Pharm.D. Programs Anticipated for 2010-11

	Enrollment Options			Non-Traditional Options Offered to the Following Groups						
Institution	Full-Time	Part-Time	Non-traditional	Alumni	State Practitioners	Geographic Regional Practitioners	U.S. Graduates	Canadian Graduates	Foreign Graduates	Other
Western	•		•				•	•	•	
Colorado			•	•	•	•	•	•		
Howard	•		•	•	•	•	•			•[a]
Florida			•	•	•	•	•	•		
Idaho State	•		•	•	•	•	•	•	•	•[b]
Purdue			•	•	•	•	•			•[c]
Massachusetts–Boston			•	•	•	•	•	•	•	
Mississippi	•	•								
Campbell	•									
Wingate	•									
North Dakota State	•	•								
Toledo	•									
Shenandoah			•	•	•	•	•	•[d]	•[d]	
Virginia Commonwealth	•									
Lebanese American	•									

Notes

a: Foreign pharmacy graduates who are licensed in the United States

b: Must hold a current U.S. or Canadian licensure

c: Graduates of selected schools in the United Arab Emirates region

d: Must reside in the United States and possess a U.S. pharmacy license

HANDHELD Rx SYSTEMS

AdvancePCS
101 Redwood Shores Pkwy., Suite 101
Redwood City, CA 94065
650-381-2155
877-483-1324
www.iscribe.com
Product: iScribe system

Allscripts Healthcare Solutions
222 Merchandise Mart Plaza
Suite 2024
Chicago, Il 60654
800-654-0889
www.allscripts.com
Product: TouchWorks Rx+

Axolotl Corp.
160 W. Santa Clara St., Suite 1000
San Jose, CA 95113
888-296-5685 or 408-920-0800
www.axolotl.com
Product: Elysium

Delphi Medical Systems
4195 E. Thousand Oaks Blvd.
Westlake Village, CA 91362
805-504-2804
www.caretools.com
Product: PocketChart

DrFirst
9420 Key West Ave., Suite 230
Rockville, MD 20850
866-263-6511
www.drfirst.com
Product: Rcopia network

eHealth Solutions
360 W. 31st St., Suite 302
New York, NY 10001
212-268-4242
877-472-3379
www.ehealthsolutions.com
Product: SigmaPoint

ePocrates, Inc.
1100 Park Pl., Suite 300
San Mateo, CA 94403
650-227-1700
www.epocrates.com
Products: ePocrates Rx and ePocrates Rx Pro

HEALTHvision
5030 Riverside Dr., Suite 300
Irving, TX 75039
469-420-2500
www.healthvision.com
Product: e-healthSOURCE

instaCare, Inc.
2660 Townsgate Rd., Suite 300
Westlake Village, CA 91361
805-446-1973
www.instacare.net
Product: MD@Hand

InstantDx, LLC
948 Clopper Rd.
Gaithersburg, MD 20878
301-208-8800
800-576-0526
www.oncalldata.com
Product: OnCallData

MDPad
90 Longwood Ave., Suite 9J
Brookline, MA 02215
617-277-6477
www.mdpad.com
Product: MDPad

med-i-nets.com
20101 S.W. Birch St., Suite 240
Newport Beach, CA 92660
949-955-9546
www.med-i-nets.com
Product: pharm-i-net

MedPlus
4690 Parkway Dr.
Mason, OH 45040
513-229-5500 or 800-444-6235
www.medplus.com
Products: Care360 Physician Portal, ChartMaxx

PD-Rx Pharmaceuticals, Inc.
727 North Ann Arbor St.
Oklahoma City, OK 73127
405-942-3040
800-299-7379
www.pdrx.com
Products: PD-Rx Net, RxWebPad

Rx Networking Technology
1106 West St.
Annapolis, MD 21401
410-626-0089
800-943-7968
www.rxnt.com
Product: RxNT

PDR Network, LLC
5 Paragon Dr.
Montvale, NJ 07645-1725
800-563-6699
www.pdr.net
Product: *mobile*PDR

Zix Corporation
2711 N. Haskell Ave., Suite 2300, LB 36
Dallas, TX 75204-2960
888-771-4049 or 214-370-2000
www.zixcorp.com
Product: PocketScript

DOSING INSTRUCTIONS IN SPANISH

The following list of Spanish numbers and phrases is adapted from "Spanish for the Pharmaceutical Profession," I and II, a set of audiocassettes from Language Unlimited. They are intended to help the pharmacist communicate basic patient instructions to exclusively Spanish-speaking individuals. Numbers are listed first, followed by instructions for the proper administration of various medications, including liquids, tablets and capsules, and those that are externally applied. Phrases are arranged first in English, then Spanish, followed by the pronunciation in parentheses. Capitalized letters and words appearing within the parentheses indicate stressed syllables. Audiocassettes can be ordered from Language Unlimited for $24.99 for one tape, or $45 for both. The cassettes come with a book that provides the audio program verbatim, as well as a grammar guide and glossary. Contact the company at 11109 Emelita St., N. Hollywood, CA 91601; phone: 818-508-6843; fax: 818-761-6784; email: language-unltd@aol.com.

NUMBERS

(0) **Zero**
CERO
(seh-roh)

(1) **One**
UNO
(oo-noh)

(2) **Two**
DOS
(dohs)

(3) **Three**
TRES
(trehs)

(4) **Four**
CUATRO
(koo-ah-troh)

(5) **Five**
CINCO
(seen-koh)

(6) **Six**
SEIS
(seh-ees)

(7) **Seven**
SIETE
(see-eh-tah)

(8) **Eight**
OCHO
(oh-choh)

(9) **Nine**
NUEVE
(noo-eh-veh)

(10) **Ten**
DIEZ
(d-s)

(11) **Eleven**
ONCE
(ohn-seh)

(12) **Twelve**
DOCE
(doh-seh)

(13) **Thirteen**
TRECE
(treh-seh)

(14) **Fourteen**
CATORCE
(ka-tohr-seh)

(15) **Fifteen**
QUINCE
(keen-seh)

(16) **Sixteen**
DIEZ Y SEIS
(d-s e seh-ees)

(17) **Seventeen**
DIEZ Y SIETE
(d-s e see-eh-teh)

(18) **Eighteen**
DIEZ Y OCHO
(d-s e oh-choh)

(19) **Nineteen**
DIEZ Y NUEVE
(d-s e noo-eh-veh)

(20) **Twenty**
VEINTE
(veh-een-teh)

(21) **Twenty-one**
VEINTIUNO
(veh-een-t-oo-noh)

(30) **Thirty**
TREINTA
(treh-een-tah)

(40) **Forty**
CUARENTA
(koo-ah-rehn-tah)

(50) **Fifty**
CINCUENTA
(seen-koo-ehn-tah)

(60) **Sixty**
SESENTA
(seh-sehn-tah)

(70) **Seventy**
SETENTA
(seh-tehn-tah)

(80) **Eighty**
OCHENTA
(oh-chehn-tah)

(90) **Ninety**
NOVENTA
(noh-vehn-tah)

(100) **One hundred**
CIEN
(see-n)

(101) **One hundred and one**
CIENTO UNO
(see-n-toh oo-noh)

(200) **Two hundred**
DOS CIENTOS
(dohs see-n-tohs)

(1,000) **One thousand**
MIL
(meel)

LIQUIDS

Take _____ teaspoonful(s) _____ times a day.
TOME _____ CUCHARADITA(S) _____VECES AL DIA.
(toh-meh…coo-chah-rah-d-tah(s)…veh-sehs ahl Dee-ah)

Take _____ tablespoonful(s) _____ times a day.
TOME _____ CUCHARADA(S) _____ VECES AL DIA.
(toh-meh…coo-chah-rah-dah(s)…veh-sehs ahl Dee-ah)

Take 1/2 teaspoonful _____ times a day.
TOME MEDIA CUCHARADITA _____ VECES AL DIA.
(toh-meh meh-d-ah coo-chah-rah-d-tah…veh-sehs ahl Dee-ah)

Dilute _____ teaspoonful(s) in water and take _____ times daily.
DILUYA _____ CUCHARADITA(S) EN AGUA Y TOME _____ VECES AL DIA.
(d-loo-ya…coo-chah-rah-d-tah(s) n ah-wah e toh-meh…veh-sehs ahl Dee-ah)

Take one dropperful _____ times daily.
LLENE EL GOTERO Y TOME _____ VECES AL DIA.
(yeh-ne el goh-teh-roh e toh-meh…veh-ses-ahl Dee-ah)

Mix _____ drops in a soft drink or juice and take _____ times daily.
MEZCLE _____ GOTAS EN UN REFRESCO O EN JUGO Y TOME _____VECES AL DIA.
(mehs-kleh…goh-tahs n oon reh-fresh-koh oh n hoo-goh e toh-meh…veh-sehs ahl Dee-ah)

Take for _____ days, then discontinue.
TOME POR _____ DIAS, LUEGO PARE DE TOMAR.
(toh-me pohr…D-ahs loo-eh-goh pah-reh deh toh-mahr)

Instill _____ drops in affected eye(s).
ECHESE _____ GOTA(S) EN EL (LOS) OJO(S) AFFECTADO(S).
(EH-cheh-seh…goh-tah(s) n el (lohs) oh-hoh(s) ah-fehk-tah-doh(s)

Left eye.
EL OJO IZQUIERDO.
(el oh-hoh eez-key-ehr-doh)

In each eye.
EN CADA OJO.
(n cah-dah oh-hoh)

Right eye.
EL OJO DERECHO.
(el oh-hoh deh-reh-choh)

Both eyes.
AMBOS OJOS.
(ahm-bohs oh-hohs)

Put _____ drop(s) in each ear/nostril.
PONGASE _____ GOTA(S) EN CADA OIDO/ABERTURA DE LA NARIZ.
(POHN-gah-seh…goh-tah(s) n cah-dah oh E-doh/ah-behr-too-rah deh lah nah-rees)

Shake well before using.
AGITESE BIEN ANTES DE USARSE.
(ah-HE-teh-seh b-n ahn-tehs deh oo-sahr-seh)

Do not refrigerate.
NO REFRIGERE.
(no reh-free-heh-reh)

Shake gently and keep in refrigerator.
AGITESE SUAVEMENTE Y GUARDE EN EL REFRIGERADOR.
(ah-HE-teh-se soo-ah-ve-mehn-teh e goo-ahr-deh n el reh-free-hehr-ah-dohr)

Store in a cool, dry place.
ALMACENE EN UN SITIO FRESCO Y SECO.
(ahl-mah-seh-neh n oon c-t-oh frehs-koh e seh-koh)

Store away from heat and sunlight.
ALMACENE LEJOS DE ALTAS TEMPERATURAS Y FUERA DE LA LUZ DEL SOL.
(ahl-mah-seh-neh leh-hohs deh ahl-tahs tehm-peh-rah-too-rahs e foo-ey-rah deh lah loose dehl sohl)

Do not use after this date.
NO USE DESPUES DE ESTA FECHA.
(noh oo-seh dehs-poo-s deh s-tah feh-chah)

TABLETS AND CAPSULES

Take _____ tablet(s) _____ times a day.
TOME _____ TABLETA(S) _____ VECES AL DIA.
(toh-meh...tah-bleh-ta(s)...veh-sehs ahl D-ah)

Take _____ capsule(s) daily.
TOME _____ CAPSULA(S) DIARIAMENTE.
(toh-meh...cahp-soo-lah(s) d-ahr-e-ah-mehn-teh)

Take 1/2 tablet.
TOME MEDIA TABLETA.
(toh-meh meh-d-ah tah-bleh-tah)

Take 1/4 tablet.
TOME UN CUARTO DE TABLETA.
(toh-meh oon coo-ahr-toh deh tah-bleh-tah)

Take 1 1/2 tablets.
TOME UNA TABLETA Y MEDIA.
(toh-meh oo-nah tah-bleh-tah e meh-d-ah)

Take medication on an empty stomach.
TOME ESTA MEDICINA EN AYUNAS.
(toh-meh s-tah med-d-c-nah n ah-yoo-nahs)

Take a total of _____ capsules daily.
TOME UN TOTAL DE _____ CAPSULAS DIARIAMENTE.
(toh-meh oon toh-tahl deh...cahp-soo-lahs d-ah-ree-ah-mehn-teh)

Take as needed.
TOME SI LA NECESITA.
(toh-meh c lah neh-seh-c-tah)

Chew _____ tablets every day.
MASTIQUE _____ TABLETA(S) CADA DIA.
(Mahs-t-keh...tah-bleh-tah(s) cah-dah D-ah)

Do not chew; swallow whole.
NO LAS MASTIQUE; TRAGUELAS ENTERA
(noh lahs mahs-t-keh; trah-geh-lahs n-teh-rah)

Dissolve _____ tablet(s) in a large glass of cold water and drink.
DISUELVA _____ TABLETA(S) EN UN VASO GRANDE DE AGUA FRIA Y TOMESE.
(d-soo-l-vah...tah-bleh-tah(s) n oon vah-soh grahn-deh ah-wah free-ah e toh-meh-seh)

Dissolve _____ tablet(s) under the tongue.
DISUELVA _____ TABLETA(S) DEBAJO DE LA LENGUA.
(d-soo-l-vah...tah-bleh-tah(s) deh-bah-hoh deh lah lehn-gwah)

Place _____ tablet(s) between gum and cheek.
COLOQUE _____TABLETA(S) ENTRE LA ENCIA Y LA MEJILLA.
(koh-loh-keh...tah-bleh-tah(s) n-treh lah n-C-ah e lah meh-he-ya)

Keep these tablets in original container to prevent loss of potency.
CONSERVE ESTAS TABLETAS EN SU ENVASE ORIGINAL PARA EVITAR QUE PIERDA SU POTENCIA.
(kohn-sehr-veh s-tahs tah-bleh-tas n soon nvah-seh oh-ree-he-nahl pah-rah eh-v-tahr keh p-ehr-dah soo poh-tehn-c-ah)

Close tightly after each use.
CIERRE BIEN DESPUES DE CADA USO.
(c-eh-rreh b-n dehs-poo-s deh cah-dah oo-soh)

This patient requested that a safety cap not be used on this prescription.
ESTE PACIENTE PIDIO QUE LA TAPA DE SEGURIDAD NO SE USARA EN ESTA RECETA.
(s-teh pah-c-n-teh p-d-OH keh lah tah-pah deh seh-goo-ree-dahd noh seh oo-sah-rah n s-tah reh-seh-tah)

EXTERNALS

Apply externally _____ times a day.
APLIQUE EXTERNAMENTE _____ VECES AL DIA.
(ah-plee-keh x-tehr-nah-mehn-teh...veh-sehs ahl D-ah)

Apply to affected area(s).
APLIQUE EN EL(LAS) AREA(S) AFFECTADA(S).
(ah-plee-keh n l (las) ah-reh-ah(s) ah-fehk-tah-dah(s)

Apply to skin sparingly.
APLIQUE UNA PEQUEДA CANTIDAD SOBRE LA PIEL.
(ah-plee-keh oo-nah peh-kehn-yah kahn-t-dahd soh-breh lah p-l)

Apply to skin liberally.
APLIQUE LIBREMENT SOBRE LA PIEL.
(ah-plee-keh lee-brah-mehn-teh soh-breh lah p-l)

Apply a thin film.
APLIQUE UNA CAPA FINA.
(AH-plee-keh oo-nah cah-pah fee-nah)

Apply to wound after each dressing change.
APLIQUE A LA HERIDA DESPUES DE CADA CAMBIO DE VENDAJE.
(ah-plee-keh ah lah eh-ree-dah dehs-poo-ehs deh cah-dah cahm-b-oh deh vehn-dah-heh)

Cut to size and tape on affected area for _____ hours.
CORTELO AL TAMANO NECESARIO Y PEGUELO AL AREA AFECTADA POR _____ HORAS.
(KOHR-teh-loh ahl tah-mahn-yoh neh-seh-sahr-e-oh e peh-geh-loh ahl AH-reh-ah-fehk-tah-dah pohr...oh-rahs)

Add _____ capful(s) to bath water.
AЦADA _____ TAPA(S) LLENA(S) AL AGUA DEL BAЦO.
(ahn-yah-dah...tah-pah(s) yeh-nah(s) ahl ah-wah dehl bahn-yoh)

Cover with plastic wrap as directed.
CUBRA CON ENVOLTURA PLASTICA SEGUN INDICADO.
(koo-brah cohn n-vohl-too-rah PLAHS-t-kah seh-GOON een-d-cah-doh)

Massage into area(s).
APLIQUE CON MASAJE EN EL(LAS) AREA(S).
(AH-plee-keh kohn mah-sah-heh n el (lahs) AH-reh-ah(s)

Rub into affected area(s).
FRICCIONE EN EL(LAS) AREA(S) AFECTADA(S).
(Freek-c-oh-neh n el (las) AH-reh-ah(s) ah-fehk-tah-dah(s)

Shampoo as directed.
LAVESE EL CABELLO SEGUN INDICADO.
(LAH-veh-seh el cah-beh-yoh-seh-GOON een-d-cah-doh)

Spray affected area.
ROCIE EL AREA AFECTADA.
(roh-C-eh el AH-reh-ah-fehk-tah-dah)

Sprinkle powder on affected area.
ROCIE EL POLVO EN EL AREA AFECTADA.
(roh-C-eh el pohl-voh n el AH-reh-ah-fehk-tah-dah)

Use as needed.
USE SI LO NECESITA.
(oo-seh c loh neh-seh-c-tah)

Apply for _____ days, then discontinue.
APLIQUE POR _____ DIAS, LUEGO NO USE MAS.
(ah-plee-keh pohr...D-ahs loo-eh-goh noh oo-seh mahs)

MISCELLANEOUS

Inject ____ units subcutaneously.
INYECTAR _____ UNIDADES DEBAJO DE LA PIEL.
(een-yeck-tahr...oo-nee-dah-dehs deh-bah-hoh deh lah p-l)

Suck one lozenge as needed.
CHUPE UNA PASTILLA CUANDO SE NECESITE.
(shoo-peh oo-nah pahs-t-yah coo-ahn-doh seh neh-seh-c-teh)

Remove wrapping and insert one suppository rectally/vaginally.
QUITE LA ENVOLTURA E INSERTE UN SUPOSITORIO RECTALMENTE/VAGINALMENTE.
(kee-teh lah n-vohl-too-rah eh een-sehr-teh oon soo-poh-c-toh-ree-oh rehk-tahl-mehn-teh/vah-hee-nahl-mehn-teh)

Retain suppository as long as possible.
RETENGA EL SUPOSITORIO EL MAJOR TIEMPO POSIBLE.
(reh-tehn-gah el soo-poh-c-toh-ree el mah-yohr t-m-poh poh-c-bleh)

Moisten suppository with water before inserting.
HUMEDEZCA EL SUPOSITORIO CON AGUA ANTES DE INSERTARLO.
(oo-meh-dehs-cah el soo-pah-c-toh-ree-oh kohn ah-wah ahn-tehs deh een-sehr-tahr-loh)

Insert one applicatorful vaginally after douche.
LLENE EL APLICADOR E INSERTE VAGINALMENTE DESPUES DE UNA DUCHA VAGINAL.
(yeh-neh el ah-plee-cah-dohr eh een-sehr-teh vah-he-nahl-mehn-teh dehs poo-s deh oo-nah doo-chah vah-he-nahl)

Use as mouthwash.
USE PARA ENJUAGARSE LA BOCA.
(oo-seh pah-rah n-hoo-ah-gahr-seh lah boh-kah)

Apply drops to cotton wick.
APLIQUE LAS GOTAS A LA MECHA DE ALGODON.
(ah-plee-keh lahs goh-tahs ah lah meh-chah deh ahl-goh-DOHN)

Do not take at same time as other medicine.
NO TOME ESTE MEDICAMENTO AL MISMO TIEMPO QUE OTRAS MEDICINAS.
(noh toh-meh s-teh meh-d-cah-mehn-toh ahl mees-moh t-m-poh keh oh-trahs meh-d-c nahs)

Do not drink alcoholic beverages while taking this medicine.
NO TOME BEBIDAS ALCOHOLICAS MIENTRAS TOMA ESTA MEDICINA.
(noh toh-meh beh-b-dahs ahl-co-ohl-e-cahs me-n tras toh-mah s-tah meh-d-c-nah)

Do not drive while taking this medication.
NO MANEJE SI TOMA ESTA MEDICINA.
(noh mah-neh-heh c toh-mah s-tah meh-d-c-nah)

Take if _____ does not help.
TOME SI_____ NO LE AYUDA
(toh-me c...noh leh ay-yoo-dah)

Take whenever pain occurs.
TOME CUANDO TENGA DOLOR.
(toh-me coo-ahn-doh tehn-gah dohl-lohr)

NATIONAL PHARMACY ORGANIZATIONS

Academy of Managed Care Pharmacy
100 N. Pitt St.
Suite 400
Alexandria, VA 22314
703-683-8416
800-827-2627
www.amcp.org

Accreditation Council for Pharmacy Education
20 North Clark St.
Suite 2500
Chicago, IL 60602-5109
312-664-3575
www.acpe-accredit.org

American Association of Colleges of Pharmacy
1727 King St.
Alexandria, VA 22314
703-739-2330
www.aacp.org

American Association of Pharmaceutical Scientists
2107 Wilson Blvd.
Suite 700
Arlington, VA 22201
703-243-2800
www.aapspharma-ceutica.com

American College of Apothecaries
Research and Education Resource Center
P.O. Box 341266
Memphis, TN 38184
901-383-8119
www.acainfo.org

American College of Clinical Pharmacy
13000 W. 87th St. Pkwy.
Lenexa, KS 66215
913-492-3311
www.accp.com

American Foundation for Pharmaceutical Education
One Church St.
Suite 202
Rockville, MD 20850
301-738-2160
www.afpenet.org

American Institute of the History of Pharmacy
777 Highland Ave.
Madison, WI 53705-2222
608-262-5378
www.pharmacy.wisc.edu/aihp

American Pharmacists Association
2215 Constitution Ave., NW
Washington, DC 20037
202-628-4410
800-237-2742
www.aphanet.org

American Society for Automation in Pharmacy
492 Norristown Rd.
Suite 160
Blue Bell, PA 19422-2355
610-825-7783
www.asapnet.org

American Society of Consultant Pharmacists
1321 Duke St.
Alexandria, VA
22314-3563
703-739-1300
800-355-2727
www.ascp.com

American Society of Health-System Pharmacists
7272 Wisconsin Ave.
Bethesda, MD 20814
866-279-0681
www.ashp.org

American Society of Pharmacognosy
3149 Dundee Rd.
Suite 260
Northbrook, IL 60062
623-202-3500
www.phcog.org

Board of Pharmaceutical Specialties
2215 Constitution Ave., NW
Washington, DC 20037
202-429-7591
www.bpsweb.org
bps@aphanet.org

Consumer Healthcare Products Association
900 19th St., NW
Suite 700
Washington, DC 20006
202-429-9260
www.chpa-info.org

The Food and Drug Law Institute
1155 15th St., NW
Suite 800
Washington, DC 20005
202-371-1420
800-956-6293
www.fdli.org

Generic Pharmaceutical Association
2300 Clarendon Blvd.
Suite 400
Arlington, VA 22201
703-647-2480
www.gphaonline.org
info@gphonline.org

Healthcare Distribution Management Association
901 North Glebe Rd.
Suite 1000
Arlington, VA 22203
703-787-0000
www.healthcare-distribution.org

International Academy of Compounding Pharmacists
4638 Riverstone Blvd.
Missouri City, TX 77459
281-933-8400
800-927-4227
www.iacprx.org
iacpinfo@iacprx.org

National Association of Boards of Pharmacy
1600 Feehanville Dr.
Mount Prospect, IL 60056
847-391-4406
www.nabp.net

National Association of Chain Drug Stores Inc.
413 North Lee St.
PO Box 1417-D49
Alexandria, VA
22313-1480
703-549-3001
www.nacds.org

National Community Pharmacists Association
100 Daingerfield Rd.
Alexandria, VA 22314
703-683-8200
www.ncpanet.org
info@ncpanet.org

National Council for Prescription Drug Programs
9240 E. Raintree Dr.
Scottsdale, AZ
85260-7518
480-477-1000
www.ncpdp.org

National Council of State Pharmacy Association Executives
2530 Professional Rd.
Richmond, VA 23235
804-285-4431
www.ncspae.org

National Council on Patient Information and Education (NCPIE)
200-A Monroe St.
Suite 212
Rockville, MD 20850
301-340-3940
www.talkaboutrx.org

National Pharmaceutical Council
1894 Preston White Dr.
Reston, VA 20191-5433
703-620-6390
www.npcnow.org

Parenteral Drug Association Inc.
Bethesda Towers
4350 East-West Hwy.
Suite 150
Bethesda, MD 20814
301-656-5900
www.pda.org

Pediatric Pharmacy Advocacy Group, Inc.
7975 Stage Hills Blvd.
Suite 6
Memphis, TN 38133
901-380-3617
www.ppag.org

Pharmaceutical Care Management Association
601 Pennsylvania Ave., NW
Seventh Floor
Washington, DC 20004
202-207-3610
www.pcmanet.org

Pharmaceutical Research and Manufacturers of America
950 F St., NW
Washington, DC 20005
202-835-3400
www.phrma.org
5600 Fishers Lane
Parklawn Building (10-C)
Rockville, MD 20857

Pharmacist Professional Advisory Committee to the U.S. Surgeon General–U.S. Public Health Service
Health Services Div.
Room 1000
320 1st St., NW
Washington, DC 20001
800-800-2676
www.hhs.gov/pharmacy

Pharmacy Technician Certification Board
2215 Constitution Ave., NW
Washington, DC 20037
800-363-8012
www.ptcb.org

U.S. Adopted Names (USAN) Council
American Medical Association
515 N. State St.
8th Floor
Chicago, IL 60610
800-621-8335
www.ama-assn.org/go/usan

The U.S. Pharmacopeia Convention Inc.
12601 Twinbrook Pkwy.
Rockville, MD 20852
800-227-8772
301-881-0666
www.usp.org

STATE PHARMACISTS ASSOCIATIONS

ALABAMA
1211 Carmichael Way
Montgomery, AL 36106
334-271-4222
800-529-7533
www.aparx.org

ALASKA
203 W. 15th Ave., #100
Anchorage, AK 99501
907-563-8880
www.alaskapharmacy.org

ARIZONA
1845 E. Southern Ave.
Tempe, AZ 85282-5831
480-838-3385
www.azpharmacy.org

ARKANSAS
417 S. Victory St.
Little Rock, AR 72201
501-372-5250
www.arpharmacists.org

CALIFORNIA
4030 Lennane Dr.
Suite 300
Sacramento, CA 95834
916-779-1400
800-444-3851
www.cpha.com

COLORADO
6825 E. Tennessee Ave.
Suite 440
Denver, CO 80224
303-756-3069
www.copharm.org

CONNECTICUT
35 Cold Spring Rd.
Suite 121
Rocky Hill, CT 06067
860-563-4619
www.ctpharmacists.org

DELAWARE
Patricia Carroll-Grant
Executive Director
PO Box 454
Smyrna, DE 19977
302-659-3089
800-782-3716
www.dpsrx.org

DISTRICT OF COLUMBIA
908 Caddington Ave.
Silver Spring, MD 20901
301-593-3292

FLORIDA
610 N. Adams St.
Tallahassee, FL 32301
850-222-2400
www.pharmview.com

GEORGIA
50 Lenox Pointe NE
Atlanta, GA 30324
404-231-5074
888-871-5590
www.gpha.org

HAWAII
PO Box 1510
Aiea, HI 96701
808-330-7738
www.hipharm.org

ILLINOIS
204 W. Cook St.
Springfield, IL 62704
217-522-7300
www.ipha.org

INDIANA
729 N. Pennsylvania St.
Indianapolis, IN 46204
317-634-4968
www.indianapharma-cists.org

IOWA
8515 Douglas Ave.
Suite 16
Des Moines, IA 50322
515-270-0713
www.iarx.org

KANSAS
1020 SW Fairlawn Rd.
Topeka, KS 66604
785-228-2327
www.ksrx.org

KENTUCKY
1228 U.S. 127 S
Frankfort, KY 40601
502-227-2303
www.kphanet.org

LOUISIANA
450 Laurel St.
Suite 1400
Baton Rouge, LA 70801
225-346-6883
800-611-8307
www.louisianapharma-cists.com

MAINE
PO Box 174
Turner, ME 04282
207-225-5205
www.mparx.com

MARYLAND
1800 Washington Blvd.
Suite 333
Baltimore, MD 21230
410-727-0746
www.marylandpharma-cist.org

MASSACHUSETTS
500 W. Cummings Park
Suite 3475
Woburn, MA 01801
781-933-1107
www.masspharmacists.org

MICHIGAN
815 N. Washington Ave.
Lansing, MI 48906-5198
517-484-1466
www.michiganpharma-cists.org

MINNESOTA
1935 W. County Rd., B2
Suite 165
Roseville, MN 55113
651-697-1771
800-451-8349
www.mpha.org

MISSISSIPPI
341 Edgewood Terrace Dr.
Jackson, MS 39206
601-981-0416
www.mspharm.org

MISSOURI
211 E. Capitol Ave.
Jefferson City, MO
65101
800-468-4672
573-636-7522
www.morx.com

MONTANA
PO Box 1569
Helena, MT 59624
406-449-3843
www.rxmt.org

NEBRASKA
6221 S. 58th St.
Suite A
Lincoln, NE 68516
402-420-1500
www.npharm.org

NEVADA
PO Box 35668
Las Vegas, NV
89193-5277
702-242-0903
www.nvpharmacist-assoc.com

NEW HAMPSHIRE
26 S. Main St.
Box 188
Concord, NH 03301-4916
www.nhpharmacists.org

NEW JERSEY
760 Alexander Rd.
PO Box 1
Princeton, NJ 08543-0001
609-275-4246
www.njpharma.org

NEW MEXICO
2716 San Pedro NE
Suite C
Albuquerque, NM 87110
505-265-8729
800-464-8729
www.nm-pharmacy.com

NEW YORK
210 Washington Ave. Ext.
Suite 101
Albany, NY 12203
518-869-6595
800-632-8822
www.pssny.org

NORTH CAROLINA
109 Church St.
Chapel Hill, NC 27516
919-967-2237
www.ncpharmacists.org

NORTH DAKOTA
1661 Capitol Way
Bismarck, ND
58501-5600
701-258-4968
www.nodakpharmacy.com

OHIO
2155 Riverside Dr.
Columbus, OH
43221-4052
614-586-1497
www.ohiopharmacists.org

OKLAHOMA
45 NE 52nd St.
PO Box 73154
Oklahoma City, OK
73154
405-528-3338
800-260-7574
www.opha.com

OREGON
147 SE 102nd Ave.
Portland, OR 97216
503-582-9055
www.oregonpharmacy.org

PENNSYLVANIA
508 N. Third St.
Harrisburg, PA
17101-1199
717-234-6151
www.papharmacists.com

RHODE ISLAND
1643 Warwick Ave.
PMB 113
Warwick, RI 02889
401-737-2600
www.ripharmacists.org

SOUTH CAROLINA
1350 Browning Rd.
Columbia, SC
29210-6903
803-354-9977
800-532-4033
www.scrx.org

SOUTH DAKOTA
320 East Capitol
PO Box 518
Pierre, SD 57501-0518
605-224-2338
www.sdpha.org

TENNESSEE
500 Church St.
Suite 650
Nashville, TN 37219
615-256-3023
www.tnpharm.org

TEXAS
12007 Research Blvd.
Suite 201
Austin, TX 78759
512-836-8350
800-505-5463
www.texaspharmacy.org

UTAH
1125 S. Blackhawk Blvd.
Suite B
Mount Pleasant, UT
84647
435-462-5323
www.upha.com

VERMONT
Box 90
Woodstock, VT 05091
877-483-2646
www.vtpharmacists.org

VIRGINIA
2530 Professional Rd.
Richmond, VA 23235
804-285-4145
800-527-8742
www.vapharmacy.org

WASHINGTON
1501 Taylor Ave. SW
Renton, WA 98057
425-228-7171
www.wsparx.org

WEST VIRGINIA
2016 1/2 Kanawha
Blvd. E.
Charleston, WV 25311
304-344-5302
www.pharmacy.org

WISCONSIN
701 Heartland Trail
Madison, WI 53717
608-827-9200
www.pswi.org

WYOMING
PO Box 228
Byron, WY 82412
307-272-3361
www.wpha.net

STATE BOARDS OF PHARMACY

ALABAMA
10 Inverness Center
Suite 110
Birmingham, AL 35242
205-981-2280
www.albop.com

ALASKA
Physical Address:
333 Willoughby Ave.
9th Floor
State Office Bldg.
Juneau, AK 99801
Mailing Address:
PO Box 110806
Juneau, AK 99811-0806
907-465-2534
www.dced.state.ak.us/occ/ppha.htm

ARIZONA
1700 W. Washington
Suite 250
Phoenix, AZ 85007
602-771-2727
www.azpharmacy.gov

ARKANSAS
Executive Director
101 E. Capitol
Suite 218
Little Rock, AR 72201
501-682-0190
www.arkansas.gov/asbp

CALIFORNIA
1625 N. Market Blvd.
Suite N 219
Sacramento, CA 95834
916-574-7900
www.pharmacy.ca.gov

COLORADO
1560 Broadway
Suite 1350
Denver, CO 80202
303-894-7800
www.dora.state.co.us/pharmacy

CONNECTICUT
Dept. of Consumer Protection
Drug Control Division
State Office Building
Room 147
165 Capitol Ave.
Hartford, CT 06106
860-713-6070
www.ct.gov/dcp

DELAWARE
Cannon Bldg.
861 Silver Lake Blvd.
Suite 203
Dover, DE 19904
302-744-4500
www.dpr.delaware.gov

DISTRICT OF COLUMBIA
Dept. of Health
Government of the District of Columbia
825 North Capitol St. NE
Washington, DC 20002
202-442-5955
www.dchealth.dc.gov

FLORIDA
Dept. of Health
Florida Board of Pharmacy
4052 Bald Cypress Way
Bin# C04
Tallahassee, FL
32399-3254
850-245-4292
www.doh.state.fl.us/mqa/pharmacy

GEORGIA
237 Coliseum Dr.
Macon, GA
31217-3858
478-207-2440
www.sos.georgia.gov/plb/pharmacy

HAWAII
PO Box 3469
Honolulu, HI 96801
808-587-3295
www.hawaii.gov/dcca/areas/pvl/boards/pharmacy

IDAHO
3380 Americana Terrace
Suite 320
Boise, ID 83706
208-334-2356
www.accessidaho.org/bop

ILLINOIS
320 W. Washington St.
3rd Floor
Springfield, IL 62786
217-782-3000
www.idfpr.com

INDIANA
402 W. Washington St.
Room W072
Indianapolis, IN 46204
317-234-2067
www.in.gov/pla/

IOWA
400 SW Eighth St.
Suite E
Des Moines, IA
50309-4688
515-281-5944
www.state.ia.us/ibpe

KANSAS
900 SW Jackson St.
Room 560
Topeka, KS
66612-1231
785-296-4056
888-792-6273
www.kansas.gov/pharmacy/

KENTUCKY
Spindletop Admin. Bldg.
Suite 302
2624 Research Park Dr.
Lexington, KY 40511
859-246-2820
www.pharmacy.ky.gov

LOUISIANA
5615 Corporate Blvd., 8E
Baton Rouge, LA
70808-2537
225-925-6496
www.labp.com

MAINE
Maine Board of Pharmacy
35 State House Station
Augusta, ME 04333
207-624-8603
www.maine.gov/professionallicensing

MARYLAND
4201 Patterson Ave.
Baltimore, MD
21215-2299
410-764-4755
800-542-4964 (MD Only)
www.dhmh.state.md.us/pharmacyboard

MASSACHUSETTS
239 Causeway St.
Suite 200
Boston, MA 02114
800-414-0168
www.mass.gov/reg/boards/ph

MICHIGAN
Licensing Division
611 W. Ottawa St.
1st Floor
PO Box 30670
Lansing, MI 48909
517-335-0918
www.michigan.gov/healthlicense

MINNESOTA
2829 University Ave. SE
Suite 530
Minneapolis, MN
55414-3251
651-201-2825
www.phcybrd.state.mn.us

MISSISSIPPI
204 Key Dr.
Suite D
Madison, MS 39110
601-605-5388
www.mbp.state.ms.us

MISSOURI
3605 Missouri Blvd.
Jefferson City, MO
65102
573-751-0091
www.pr.mo.gov/pharmacists.asp

MONTANA
301 South Park
PO Box 200513
Helena, MT
59620-0513
406-841-2371
www.mt.gov/dli/bsd/license/bsd_boards/pha_board/board_page.asp

NEBRASKA
Board of Pharmacy
301 Centennial Mall South
PO Box 94986
Lincoln, NE
68509-4986
402-471-2118
www.hhs.state.ne.us

NEVADA
431 W. Plumb Ln.
Reno, NV 89509
775-850-1440
http://bop.nv.gov

NEW HAMPSHIRE
57 Regional Dr.
Concord, NH 03301
603-271-2350
www.state.nh.us/pharmacy

NEW JERSEY
PO Box 45013
Newark, NJ 07101
973-504-6450
www.njconsumeraffairs.gov/medical/pharmacy.htm

NEW MEXICO
5200 Oakland NE
Suite A
Albuquerque, NM 87113
505-222-9830
www.rld.state.nm.us/Pharmacy

NEW YORK
State Education Bldg.
89 Washington Ave.
2nd Floor
Albany, NY 12234
518-474-3817, ext. 130
www.op.nysed.gov

NORTH CAROLINA
PO Box 4560
Chapel Hill, NC 27517
919-246-1050
www.ncbop.org

NORTH DAKOTA
1906 E. Broadway Ave
Bismarck, ND
58501
701-328-9535
www.nodakpharmacy.com

OHIO
77 S. High St.
Room 1702
Columbus, OH
43215-6126
614-466-4143
www.pharmacy.ohio.gov

OKLAHOMA
4545 Lincoln Blvd.
Suite 112
Oklahoma City, OK
73105
405-521-3815
www.ok.gov/OSBP

OREGON
800 NE Oregon St.
Suite 150
Portland, OR 97232
971-673-0001
www.pharmacy.state.or.us

PENNSYLVANIA
State Board of Pharmacy
PO Box 2649
Harrisburg, PA 17105-2649
717-783-7156
www.dos.state.pa.us/pharm

RHODE ISLAND
Dept. of Health
Three Capitol Hill
Room 205
Providence, RI 02908
401-222-5960
800-942-7434
www.health.ri.gov/hsr/professions/pharmacy.php

SOUTH CAROLINA
Synergy Business Park
Kingstree Bldg.
110 Centerview Dr.
Columbia, SC 29210
803-896-4700
www.llronline.com/POL/pharmacy

SOUTH DAKOTA
4305 S. Louise Ave.
Suite 104
Sioux Falls, SD 57106
605-362-2737
http://doh.sd.gov/boards/pharmacy

TENNESSEE
227 French Landing
Suite 300
Nashville, TN 37243
615-741-2718
http://health.state.tn.us/Boards/Pharmacy/index.shtml

TEXAS
333 Guadalupe
Suite 3-600, Box 21
Austin, TX 78701-3943
512-305-8000
www.tsbp.state.tx.us

UTAH
Utah Dept. of Commerce
PO Box 146741
Salt Lake City, UT 84114-6741
801-530-6179
www.dopl.utah.gov

VERMONT
Office of Professional Regulation
National Life Bldg.
North Floor 2
Montpelier, VT 05620-3402
802-828-2373
www.vtprofessionals.org

VIRGINIA
Perimeter Center
9960 Mayland Dr.
Suite 300
Richmond, VA 23233-1463
804-367-4456
www.dhp.virginia.gov/pharmacy

WASHINGTON
PO Box 47865
Olympia, WA 98504
360-236-4828
https://fortress.wa.gov/doh/hpqa1/HPS4/pharmacy/default.htm

WEST VIRGINIA
General Counsel
232 Capitol St.
Charleston, WV 25301
304-558-0558
www.wvbop.com

WISCONSIN
PO Box 8953
Madison, WI 53708-8935
608-266-2112
www.drl.state.wi.us

WYOMING
1712 Carey Ave.
Suite 200
Cheyenne, WY 82002
307-634-9636
http://pharmacyboard.state.wy.us

STATE DRUG UTILIZATION REVIEW OFFICES

ALABAMA
Alabama Medicaid DUR
501 Dexter Ave.
PO Box 5624
Montgomery, AL 36103
334-353-4596
800-362-1504
www.medicaid.state.al.us

ALASKA
Alaska Medicaid DUR
Div. of Medical Assistance
4501 Business Park Blvd.
Suite 24
Anchorage, AK 99503-7167
907-334-2425
www.hss.state.ak.us/dhcs/pdl/
drugutilizB_pdl.html

ARIZONA
Arizona Medicaid DUR
Pharmacy Program Administration
Office of Medical Management
Arizona Health Care Cost
Containment System
801 E. Jefferson, M/D 8000
Phoenix, AZ 85034
602-417-4000
800-654-8713
www.azahcccs.gov

ARKANSAS
Arkansas Medicaid DUR
Dept. of Human Services –
Pharmacy Program
PO Box 1437, Slot S401
Little Rock, AR 72203
501-683-4124
www.medicaid.state.ar.us

CALIFORNIA
California Medicaid DUR
State Dept. of Health Services
Medi-Cal Policy Div.
1501 Capitol Ave.
PO Box 997413, MS 4604
Sacramento, CA 95899-7413
916-636-1000
www.medi-cal.ca.gov

COLORADO
Colorado Medicaid DUR
1570 Grant St., 3rd Floor
Denver, CO 80203
303-866-2993

CONNECTICUT
Connecticut Medicaid DUR
Medical Operations Unit #4
Dept. of Social Services
25 Sigourney St.
Hartford, CT 06106-5033
860-424-5016
www.ct.gov/dss

DELAWARE
Delaware Division of Medicaid &
Medical Assistance
1901 N. Du Pont Highway
Lewis Bldg.
New Castle, DE 19720
302-255-9500
http://dhss.delaware.gov/
dhss/dmma/drugutilization
reviewboard.html

DISTRICT OF COLUMBIA
District of Columbia Medicaid DUR
Dept. of Health
Medical Assistance Administration
825 North Capitol Street, NE
Suite 500
Washington, DC 20002
202-442-5988
www.dchealth.dc.gov

FLORIDA
Florida Medicaid DUR
Health Care Administration and
Medicaid Pharmacy Services
2727 Mahan Dr.
Suite 2408E
Mail Stop 20
Tallahassee, FL 32308-5407
850-487-2618
www.fdhc.state.fl.us

GEORGIA
Georgia Medicaid DUR
Dept. of Community Health
Div. of Medical Assistance
2 Peachtree St. NW
37th Floor
Atlanta, GA 30803-3159
404-656-4044
www.ghp.georgia.gov
www.dch.state.ga.us

HAWAII
Hawaii Medicaid DUR
Dept. of Human Services
Med-Quest Div.
Medical Standards Branch
PO Box 700190
Kapolei, HI 96709-0190
808-692-8065
PO Box 339
Honolulu, HI 96809
808-587-3521/808-692-7182
www.himed-questffs.org
www.med-quest.us

IDAHO
Idaho DUR
Idaho State University
970 S. 5th St.
Campus Box 8288
Pocatello, ID 83209
208-282-3475
idahodur.isu.edu

ILLINOIS
Illinois Medicaid DUR
Bureau of Pharmacy Services
Prescott Bloom Bldg.
Illinois Dept. of Public Aid
201 S. Grand Ave. East
Springfield, IL 62763
217-782-1200
www.hfs.illinois.gov

INDIANA
Indiana Medicaid DUR
Office of Medicaid and Policy
Planning
Indiana State Govt. Center South
402 W. Washington St.
Room W382
Indianapolis, IN 46204
317-233-4455
www.in.gov/fssa/ompp

IOWA
Iowa Medicaid Enterprise
100 Army Post Rd.
Des Moines, IA 50315
515-725-1287
www.iadur.org

KANSAS
Kansas Medicaid DUR EDS
DHPF
900 SW Jackson Ave., Suite 900
Room 651 South
Topeka, KS 66612-1570
785-296-3981
www.khpa.ks.gov/pharmacy/
pharmacy_dur_program.html

KENTUCKY
Kentucky Medicaid DUR
Dept. for Medicaid Services
275 E. Main St.
Frankfort, KY 40621
502-564-7940
www.chfs.ky.gov/dms

LOUISIANA
Louisiana Medicaid DUR
Dept. of Health and Hospitals
Pharmacy Benifits Management
Bin#24
PO Box 91030
Baton Rouge, LA 70821
225-342-9768
628 N. 4th St., 7th Floor
Baton Rouge, LA 70802-4438
www.dhh.louisiana.gov

MAINE
Office of MaineCare Services
(formerly Bureau of Medical
Services)
442 Civic Center Dr.
11 State House Station
Augusta, ME 04333-0011
207-287-9202
www.maine.gov/dhhs/oms

MARYLAND
Maryland Medicaid DUR
State of Maryland – Dept. of
Health and Mental Hygiene
Maryland Pharmacy Program
201 West Preston St., 4th Floor
Baltimore, MD 21201
410-767-1755
www.dhmh.state.md.us/mma/mpap

MASSACHUSETTS
Massachusetts Office of Medicaid
One Ashburn Place
11th Floor
Boston, MA 02108
617-573-1770
www.mass.gov/masshealth

MICHIGAN
Capitol View Building
201 Townsend St.
Lansing, MI 48913
517-373-3740
www.michigan.gov/mdch
http://michigan.fhsc.com

MINNESOTA
Minnesota Medicaid DUR
Dept. of Human Services
540 Cedar St.
St. Paul, MN 55155-3854
651-431-2000
www.dhs.state.mn.us/provider

MISSISSIPPI
Drug Utilization Review
Sillers Bldg.
550 High St.
Suite 1000
Jackson, MS 39201
601-359-6050
www.medicaid.ms.gov

MISSOURI
The State of Missouri
MO HealthNet Division
615 Howerton Ct.
PO Box 6500
Jefferson City, MO 65102
573-751-3425
www.dss.mo.gov/mhd/index.htm

MONTANA
Montana Medicaid DUR
Medicaid Services Bureau
Pharmacy Program Director
Mountain-Pacific Quality Health
Foundation
1400 Broadway
Helena, MT 59620-2951
406-444-2738
www.dphhs.mt.gov

NEBRASKA
DUR Director
Nebraska Pharmacists
Association
6221 S. 58th St., Suite A
Lincoln, NE 68516
402-420-1500
www.hhs.state.ne.us
www.npharm.org

NEVADA
Nevada Medicaid DUR
1100 E. William St., Suite 101
Carson City, NV 89701
775-684-3676
http://dhcfp.state.nv.us

NEW HAMPSHIRE
NH DHHS Office of
Medicaid Business & Policy
Medicaid Program
129 Pleasant St.
Concord, OH 03301
603-271-5254

NEW JERSEY
Note: The New Jersey DUR
Council was dissolved in 2003.
Please direct queries to the
following:
New Jersey Dept. of Human
Services
Div. of Medical Assistance &
Health Services
Quakerbridge Plaza, Building 7
PO Box 712
Trenton, NJ 08625-0716
609-631-2396
800-356-1561 (NJ)
www.state.nj.us/humanservices

NEW MEXICO
New Mexico Medicaid DUR
Medical Assistance Div.
PO Box 2348
Santa Fe, NM 87504-2348
505-827-3100
888-997-2583
www.state.nm.us/hsd/mad/
Index.html

NEW YORK
New York Medicaid DUR
Office of Health Insurance Programs
New York State Dept. of Health
99 Washington Ave. Suite 720
Albany, NY 12210
518-486-1434
www.health.state.ny.us

NORTH CAROLINA
North Carolina Medicaid DUR
Dept. of Health and Human Services
Div. of Medical Assistance
2501 Mail Service Center
Raleigh, NC 27699-2401
919-855-4307
www.dhhs.state.nc.us/dma

NORTH DAKOTA
North Dakota Medicaid DUR
North Dakota Dept. of Human Services
Medical Services Div.
600 East Blvd. Ave.
Dept. 325
Bismarck, ND 58505
701-328-4023
www.nd.gov/dhs

OHIO
Ohio Medicaid DUR
Ohio Dept. of Job and Family Services
Office of Research Assessment & Accountability
30 E. Broad St.
32nd Fl.
Columbus, OH 43215
http://jfs.ohio.gov.ohp/index.stm
614-466-2100
877-852-0010

OKLAHOMA
Oklahoma Medicaid DUR
Oklahoma Health Care Authority
4545 North Lincoln Blvd.
Suite 124
Oklahoma City, OK 73105
405-522-7300
www.ohca.state.ok.us

OREGON
Oregon Medicaid DUR
Pharmacy Program Manager
Policy, PPS
Human Services Building
500 Summer St., NE, E35
Salem, OR 97301-1077
503-947-5220
www.oregon.gov/DHS/healthplan

PENNSYLVANIA
Pennsylvania Medicaid DUR
Dept. of Public Welfare
Health & Welfare Bldg.
Room 515
PO Box 2675
Harrisburg, PA 17105
717-787-1870

RHODE ISLAND
Rhode Island Medicaid DUR
Dept. of Human Services
600 New London Ave.
Cranston, RI 02920
401-462-6390
www.dhs.state.ri.us

SOUTH CAROLINA
Pharmacy Services
SC State Medicaid DUR Office
Dept. of Health and Human Services
1801 Main Street, 12th Floor
PO Box 8206
Columbia, SC, 29202-8206
803-898-2876
www.dhhs.state.sc.us

SOUTH DAKOTA
South Dakota Medicaid DUR
700 Governor's Dr.
Pierre, SD 57501
605-773-3165
www.state.sd.us/social/medical

TENNESSEE
Tennessee Medicaid DUR
Bureau of TennCare
310 Great Circle Rd.
Nashville, TN 37228
804-217-7397
www.state.tn.us/tenncare

TEXAS
Texas Medicaid DUR
Texas Health and Human Services Commission
Vendor Drug Program
11209 Metric Blvd.
Building H, Suite A
Austin, TX 78758
800-252-8263
www.hhsc.state.tx.us/hcf/vdp/aboutvdp.html

UTAH
Utah Medicaid DUR
Utah State Dept. of Health
Healthcare Financing
PO Box 143106
Salt Lake City, UT 84114-3102
801-538-6155
www.utah.gov

VERMONT
Vermont Medicaid DUR
Office of Vermont Healthcare Access
312 Hurricane Ln.
Suite 201
Williston, VT 05495
802-879-5912

VIRGINIA
Virginia Medicaid DUR
DUR/DSM Program Administrator
Dept. of Medical Assistance Services
600 E. Broad St., Suite 1300
Richmond, VA 23219
804-225-2873
www.dmas.virginia.gov

WASHINGTON
Washington Medicaid DUR
Pharmacy Section
Dept. of SHS
805 Plum St., SE
PO Box 45130
Olympia, WA 98504-5506
360-725-1564
http://maa.dshs.wa.gov

WEST VIRGINIA
West Virginia Medicaid DUR
Bureau for Medical Services
Policy Unit
350 Capitol St., Room 251
Charleston, WV 25301-3707
304-558-1700
www.wvdhhr.org

WISCONSIN
Wisconsin Dept. of Health Services
1 West Wilson St.
Madison, WI 53702
608-266-1865
http://dhs.wisconsin.gov/medicaid/index.htm

WYOMING
Wyoming Medicaid DUR
DUR Manager
Univ. of Wyoming School of Pharmacy
Dept. 3375
Laramie, WY 82071
307-766-6750
http://uwacadweb.uwyo.edu/DUR

FEDERAL GOVERNMENT OFFICES

U.S. Department of
Health and Human Services
Hubert H. Humphrey Bldg.
200 Independence Ave., SW
Washington, DC 20201
202-619-0257
877-696-6775
www.hhs.gov

Centers for Medicare and
Medicaid Services
7500 Security Blvd.
Baltimore, MD 21244-1850
410-786-3000
866-226-1819
www.cms.hhs.gov/default.asp

Food and Drug
Administration
10903 New Hampshire Ave.
W051-2201
Silver Spring, MD 20993-0002
301-827-2410
888-463-6332
www.fda.gov

Drug Enforcement
Administration
Mailstop AXS
8701 Morrissette Dr.
Springfield, VA 22152
202-307-1000
www.dea.gov

STATE MEDICAID-PROGRAM OFFICES

ALABAMA
Alabama Medicaid Agency
501 Dexter Ave.
PO Box 5624
Montgomery, AL 36103-5624
334-242-5050
800-362-1504 (AL)
www.medicaid.state.al.us

ALASKA
Alaska Health and Social Services
4501 Business Park Blvd.
Suite 24
Anchorage, AK 99503
907-334-2425
907-586-4265
www.hss.state.ak.us

ARIZONA
Health Care Cost Containment of Arizona
801 E. Jefferson
Phoenix, AZ 85034
602-417-4726
800-962-6690
TTY: 602-417-4000 (AZ)
www.ahcccs.state.az.us

ARKANSAS
Arkansas Dept. of Human Services
Div. of Medical Services
PO Box 1437, Slot 415
Donaghey Plaza South
Little Rock, AR 72203-1437
501-683-4120
800-482-5431
800-482-8988 (eligibility)
www.medicaid.state.ar.us

CALIFORNIA
California Dept. of Social Services
744 P St.
Sacramento, CA 95814-5512
TTY: 800-541-5555 (CA)

COLORADO
Colorado Dept. of Health Care Policy and Financing
1570 Grant St.
Denver, CO 80203-1714
303-866-2993
800-221-3943
www.chcpf.state.co.us

CONNECTICUT
Connecticut Dept. of Social Services
25 Sigourney St.
Hartford, CT 06106-5033
860-424-5250
800-842-1508
www.dss.state.ct.us

DELAWARE
Delaware Medicaid Office
Health and Social Services of Delaware
1901 N. DuPont Hwy., Levis Bldg.
New Castle, DE 19720
302-255-9500
www.dhss.delaware.gov

DISTRICT OF COLUMBIA
Washington D.C. Dept. of Health
Medical Assistance Administration
825 N. Capitol St., NE
5th Floor
Washington, DC 20002
202-442-5955
888-557-1116
www.dchealth.dc.gov/information/maa_outline.shtm

FLORIDA
Assistant Deputy Secretary for Florida Medicaid Operations
Agency for Health Care Administration
2727 Mahan Dr.
Mail Stop 8
Tallahassee, FL 32308
888-367-6554
www.fdhc.state.fl.us

GEORGIA
Georgia Dept. of Community Health
2 Peachtree St., NW
Atlanta, GA 30303
800-766-4456
www.dch.georgia.gov

HAWAII
Hawaii Dept. of Human Services
Med-Quest Div.
601 Kamokila Blvd., Room 5068
PO Box 700190
Honolulu, HI 96707
808-586-5390
www.med-quest.us

IDAHO
Idaho Dept. of Health and Welfare
Div. of Medicaid
3232 Elder St.
Boise, ID 83705
208-334-5747
www.idahohealth.org

ILLINOIS
Illinois Dept. of Public Aid
201 South Grand Ave., East
Springfield, IL 62763
217-524-7478
TTY: 800-526-5812 (IL)
www.hfs.illinois.gov

INDIANA
Indiana Family and Social Services Administration
402 W. Washington St.
PO Box 7083
Indianapolis, IN 46207-7083
317-234-2407
800-446-1993
www.in.gov/fssa

IOWA
Iowa Dept. of Human Services
Iowa Medicaid Enterprise
1305 E. Walnut St.
Des Moines, IA 50319
515-281-5454
www.dhs.state.ia.us

KANSAS
Pharmacy Program Manager
900 SW Jackson St., Suite 900
Topeka, KS 66612
785-296-3981
www.khpa.ks.gov

KENTUCKY
Cabinet for Health and Family Services of Kentucky
275 E. Main St.
Frankfort, KY 40621
502-564-5492
800-372-2973
www.chfs.ky.gov

LOUISIANA
Louisiana Dept. of Health and Hospitals
628 N. 4th St.
PO Box 629
Baton Rouge, LA 70821-0629
225-342-9500
www.dhh.louisiana.gov

MAINE
Maine Dept. of Human Services
Bureau of Medical Services
221 State St.
Augusta, ME 04333
207-287-3707
www.maine.gov/dhhs

MARYLAND
Maryland Pharmacy Program
DHMH Office
201 W. Preston St., Room 408
Baltimore, MD 21201
410-767-1455
800-492-5231
www.dhr.state.md.us/fia/medicaid.htm

MASSACHUSETTS
Massachusetts Office of Health and Human Services
Div. of Medical Assistance
600 Washington St.
Boston, MA 02111
617-573-1770
617-210-5000

MICHIGAN
Capitol View Building
201 Townsend St.
Lansing, MI 48913
517-373-3740
www.michigan.gov/mdch

MINNESOTA
Minnesota Dept. of Human Services
540 Cedar St.
St. Paul, MN 55155
651-431-2504
800-366-5411
TTY: 651-296-5705 (MN)
www.dhs.state.mn.us

MISSISSIPPI
Mississippi Div. of Medicaid
Sillers Bldg.
550 High St., Suite 1000
Jackson, MS 39201-1399
601-359-6050
www.medicaid.ms.gov

MISSOURI
Missouri Dept. of Social Services
615 Howerton Ct.
PO Box 6500
Jefferson City, MO 65102-1527
573-751-3425
800-735-2966
www.dss.mo.gov

MONTANA
Montana Dept. of Public Health and Human Services
Div. of Child and Adult Health Resources
Cogswell Bldg.
1400 Broadway
PO Box 202951
Helena, MT 59604-8005
406-444-4458
www.dphhs.mt.gov

NEBRASKA
Nebraska Health and Human Services System
PO Box 95026
Lincoln, NE 68509-5044
402-471-9147
www.hhs.state.ne.us

NEVADA
Nevada Dept. of Human Resources
1100 E. William St.
Suite 101
Carson City, NV 89701
775-684-3676
www.dhcfp.state.nv.us

NEW HAMPSHIRE
New Hampshire Dept. of Health and Human Services
129 Pleasant St.
Concord, NH 03301-3857
603-228-4100
800-852-3345
www.dhhs.state.nh.us

NEW JERSEY
New Jersey Dept. of Human Services
Div. of Medical Assistance & Health Services
Quakerbridge Plaza, Building 7
PO Box 712
Trenton, NJ 08625-0716
800-356-1561 (NJ)
www.state.nj.us/humanservices

NEW MEXICO
New Mexico Dept. of Human Services
Medical Assistance Division
PO Box 2348
Sante Fe, NM 87504-2348
505-827-3174
888-997-2583
www.state.nm.us/hsd/mad/Index.html

NEW YORK
New York State Dept. of Health
Office of Medicaid Management
Coming Tower
Empire State Plaza
Albany, NY 12237
518-473-1134
800-541-2831
www.health.state.ny.us/nysdoh
(click on "Medicaid Information?")

NORTH CAROLINA
North Carolina Dept. of Health and Human Services
2501 Mail Service Center
Raleigh, NC 27699-2501
919-855-4300
www.dhhs.state.nc.us/dma

NORTH DAKOTA
North Dakota Dept. of Human Services – Medical Services
600 E. Boulevard Ave.
Bismarck, ND 58505-0250
701-328-2321
800-755-2604 (ND)
www.nd.gov/dhs/services/medicalserv/medicaid

OHIO
Ohio Dept. of Job and Family Services – Ohio Health Plans
50 West Town St.
Columbus, OH 43215
614-466-6420
http://jfs.ohio.gov/ohp

OKLAHOMA
Health Care Authority of Oklahoma
4545 N. Lincoln Blvd.
Suite 124
Oklahoma City, OK 73105
405-522-7325 (claims)
www.ohca.state.ok.us

OREGON
Oregon Dept. of Human Services
500 Summer St., NE
3rd Floor
Salem, OR 97310-1014
503-945-5772
800-527-5772
TTY: 800-375-2863 (OR)
www.oregon.gov/DHS

PENNSYLVANIA
Pennsylvania Dept. of Public Welfare
Office of Medical Assistance Programs
Health and Welfare Building
Room 515
PO Box 2675
Harrisburg, PA 17105
717-787-1870
www.dpw.state.pa.us/omap

RHODE ISLAND
Rhode Island Dept. of Human Services
Louis Pasteur Bldg.
600 New London Ave.
Cranston, RI 02921
401-462-6300
www.dhs.state.ri.us

SOUTH CAROLINA
South Carolina Dept. of Health and Human Services
PO Box 8206
Columbia, SC 29202-8206
803-898-2875
888-549-0820 (eligibility)
www.dhhs.state.sc.us/Default.htm

SOUTH DAKOTA
South Dakota Dept. of Social Services
Office of Medical Eligibility
Richard F. Kneip Building
700 Governors Dr.
Pierre, SD 57501
605-773-4678
www.dss.sd.gov

TENNESSEE
Tenn. Bureau of TennCare
310 Great Circle Rd.
Nashville, TN 37243
800-342-3145
http://state.tn.us/tenncare

TEXAS
Texas Health and Human Services Commission
Brown-Heatly Bldg.
4900 N. Lamar Blvd.
Austin, TX 78751
512-424-6500
www.hhsc.state.tx.us/medicaid

UTAH
Utah Dept. of Health
288 N. 1480 West
PO Box 143102
Salt Lake City, UT 84116
801-538-6155
800-662-9651
http://health.utah.gov/medicaid

VERMONT
Agency of Human Services of Vermont
312 Hurricane Lane, Suite 201
Williston, VT 05495
802-879-5900
800-250-8427 (VT only)
TTY: 802-241-1282 (VT)
www.dpath.state.vt.us

VIRGINIA
Virginia Dept. of Medical Assistance Services
600 E. Broad St.
Suite 1300
Richmond, VA 23219
804-786-8658
800-884-9730 (eligibility verification)
www.dmas.virginia.gov

WASHINGTON
Washington Dept. of Social and Health Services
PO Box 45505
Olympia, WA 98504-5505
800-562-3022
http://fortress.wa.gov/dshs/maa

WEST VIRGINIA
West Virginia Dept. of Health and Human Resources
Bureau for Medical Services
350 Capitol St.
Room 251
Charleston, WV 25301-3709
304-558-5976
http://www.wvdhhr.org/bms

WISCONSIN
Wisconsin Dept. of Health and Family Services
1 W. Wilson St.
PO Box 309
Madison, WI 53701-0309
608-266-2522
800-362-3002
http://dhs.wi.gov/medicaid

WYOMING
Wyoming Dept. of Health
401 Hathaway Bldg.
Cheyenne, WY 82002
307-777-7656
866-571-0944
http://wdh.state.wy.us

PHARMACY BUYING GROUPS

Pharmacy buying groups are particularly important to independent pharmacies and small chain drugstore operations. The volume of prescriptions major chains generate affords them a lot of clout in dealing with managed care organizations and manufacturers. That can put smaller retailers at a competitive disadvantage. By banding together in a pharmacy buying group, however, they can pool their buying power, thereby gaining access to lower prices and other perks usually reserved for higher-volume pharmacies.

American Pharmacy Services Corp.
102 Enterprise Dr.
Frankfort, KY 40601
502-695-8899
www.apscnet.com
States served: AL, FL, GA, IL, IN, KY, MD, MO, OH, PA, TN, TX, VA, WV

Associated Pharmacies, Inc.
211 Lonnie Crawford Blvd.
Scottsboro, AL 35769
800-243-8521
www.apirx.com
States served: 40 states

Association of Northwest Pharmacies
126 3rd Ave. South, Suite 101
Edmonds, WA 98026
425-744-8444
www.anponline.com

EPIC Pharmacies, Inc.
50 Scott Adam Rd., Suite 100
Cockeysville, MD 21030
410-667-7600
800-965-EPIC (3742)
www.epicrx.com
States served: DE, MD, NJ, PA, TN, VA, WV, Washington, DC

Georgia Pharmaceutical Services, Inc.
50 Lenox Pointe, NE
Atlanta, GA 30324
404-231-5074
www.gpha.org
States served: GA

Independent Pharmacy Alliance, Inc.
3 Cedar Brook Dr.
Cranbury, NJ 08512
800-575-2667
www.ipa-rx.org/
States served: CT, NJ, NY, PA

Independent Pharmacy Cooperative
1550 Columbus St.
Sun Prairie, WI 53590
800-755-1531
www.ipcrx.com
States served: All

Keystone Pharmacy Purchasing Alliance, Inc.
2200 Michener St., Suite 10
Philadelphia, PA 19115
215-464-9892
www.kpparx.com
State served: PA

Kunkel Pharmacy
7717 Beechmont Ave.
Cincinnati, OH 45255
513-231-1943
www.kunkelrx.com
States served: IN, KY, OH

National Community Pharmacists Association
100 Dangerfield Rd.
Alexandria, VA 22314
703-683-8200
800-544-7447
www.ncpanet.org

Northeast Pharmacy Service Corp.
1661 Worcester Rd., Suite 405
Framingham, MA 01701
508-875-1866
800-532-3742
www.northeastpharmacy.com
States served: CT, MA, ME, NH, RI

Pace Alliance, Inc.
1429 Oread West, Suite 110A
Lawrence, KS 66049
888-200-0998
www.pacealliance.com
States served: CO, GA, IA, IL, IN, KS, MA, MN, MS, NC, ND, NE, NM, OH, OR, PA, SC, TX

PBA Health
1575 North Universal Ave., Suite 100
Kansas City, MO 64120
816-245-5700
800-333-8097
www.pbahealth.com
States served: All

PDM Healthcare
24700 Center Ridge Rd., Suite 110
Cleveland, OH 44145
440-871-1721
www.pdmhealthcare.com
States served: All

Pharmacy Group of New England
PO Box 1450
Scarborough, ME 04070
207-396-5323
800-639-1609
www.pgnerx.com
States served: AL, CO, CT, FL, IA, IL, KY, LA, MA, ME, MN, NE, NH, NY, OH, PR, RI, TN, TX, VT, WV

Pharmacy Provider Services Corp. (PPSC)
3375-I Capitol Circle NE
Tallahassee, FL 32308
850-656-0100
888-778-9909
www.ppsconline.com
States served: All

Pharmacy Providers of Oklahoma, Inc.
PO Box 18204
Oklahoma City, OK 73154
405-557-5700
877-557-5707
www.ppok.com
States served: All

Pharmacy Services, Inc.
815 North Washington Ave.
Lansing, MI 48906
517-484-1468
800-678-2774
www.pharmacyservicesonline.com
States served: IN, MI, OH (northern)

Southern Pharmacy Cooperative
3055 Lebanon Rd.
Building 11, Suite 2101
Nashville, TN 37214
615-627-3556
States served: AL, AR, KY, LA, MO, MS, TN

Rx Plus Pharmacies
3660 Wadsworth Blvd.
Wheat Ridge, CO 80033
303-463-4875
www.rxplus.com
States served: AK, CO, KS, NE, NM, SD, UT, WA, WY
Claims processing: Outsourced, PCS

United Drugs
7227 North 16th St., Suite 160
Phoenix, AZ 85020-5256
602-678-1179
www.uniteddrugs.com
States served: All

DEA OFFICE DIRECTORY

The DEA has 21 domestic field divisions throughout the United States and in Puerto Rico, each managed by a Special Agent in Charge (SAC). Subordinate to these divisions are resident offices, district offices, and posts of duty, with at least one office located in every state. Overseas, the DEA maintains 80 offices in 58 foreign countries.

Questions about DEA physician registration or the Controlled Substances Act can be directed to: Drug Enforcement Administration, Office of Diversion Control, 2401 Jefferson Davis Hwy., Alexandria, VA 22301; phone: 800-882-9539; or visit their website at www.dea.gov.

ATLANTA DIVISION
404-893-7000
OFFICES
Augusta, GA
Columbus, GA
Macon, GA
Rome, GA
Savannah, GA
Asheville, NC
Charlotte, NC
Greensboro, NC
Raleigh, NC
Wilmington, NC
Beaufort, SC
Charleston, SC
Columbia, SC
Florence, SC
Greenville, SC
Chattanooga, TN
Jackson, TN
Johnson City, TN
Knoxville, TN
Memphis, TN
Nashville, TN

BOSTON DIVISION
617-557-2100
OFFICES
Bridgeport, CT
Hartford, CT
New Haven, CT
Cape Cod, MA
New Bedford, MA
Springfield, MA
Worcester, MA
Portland, ME
Manchester, NH
Portsmouth, NH
Providence, RI
Burlington, VT

CARIBBEAN DIVISION
787-277-4700
OFFICES
Bridgetown, Barbados
Santo-Domingo, D.R.
Port-au-Prince, Haiti
Kingston, Jamaica
Curacao, Neth. Antilles
Fajardo, Puerto Rico
Ponce, Puerto Rico
Paramaribo, Suriname
Port of Spain, Trinidad & Tobago
St. Thomas, V.I.
St. Croix, V.I.

CHICAGO DIVISION
312-353-7875
OFFICES
Rockford, IL
Springfield, IL
Evansville, IN
Ft. Wayne, IN
Indianapolis, IN
Merrillville, IN
Minneapolis/St. Paul, MN
Bismarck, ND
Fargo, ND
Green Bay, WI
Madison, WI
Milwaukee, WI

DALLAS DIVISION
214-366-6900
OFFICES
McAlester, OK
Oklahoma City, OK
Tulsa, OK
Amarillo, TX
Ft. Worth, TX
Lubbock, TX
Tyler, TX

DENVER DIVISION
720-895-4040
OFFICES
Colorado Springs, CO
Durango, CO
Glenwood Springs, CO
Grand Junction, CO
Billings, MT
Salt Lake City, UT
St. George, UT
Casper, WY
Cheyenne, WY

DETROIT DIVISION
313-234-4000
OFFICES
Lexington, KY
London, KY
Louisville, KY
Madisonville, KY
East Lansing, MI
Grand Rapids, MI
Saginaw, MI
Cincinnati, OH
Cleveland, OH
Columbus, OH
Dayton, OH
Toledo, OH
Youngstown, OH

EL PASO DIVISION
915-832-6000
OFFICES
Albuquerque, NM
Las Cruces, NM
Alpine, TX
Midland, TX

HOUSTON DIVISION
713-693-3000
OFFICES
Austin, TX
Beaumont, TX
Brownsville, TX
Corpus Christi, TX
Del Rio, TX
Eagle Pass, TX
Galveston, TX
Laredo, TX
McAllen, TX
San Antonio, TX
Waco, TX

LOS ANGELES DIVISION
213-621-6700
OFFICES
Riverside, CA
Santa Ana, CA
Ventura, CA
Hilo, HI
Honolulu, HI
Maui, HI
Carson City, NV
Las Vegas, NV
Reno, NV

MIAMI DIVISION
954-660-4500
OFFICES
Freeport, Bahamas
Nassau, Bahamas
Ft. Lauderdale, FL
Ft. Myers, FL
Gainesville, FL
Jacksonville, FL
Key Largo, FL
Key West, FL
Orlando, FL
Panama City, FL
Pensacola, FL
Port St. Lucie, FL
Tallahassee, FL
Tampa, FL
W. Palm Beach, FL

NEW JERSEY DIVISION
973-776-1100
OFFICES
Atlantic City, NJ
Camden, NJ
Paterson, NJ

NEW ORLEANS DIVISION
504-840-1100
OFFICES
Birmingham, AL
Huntsville, AL
Mobile, AL
Fayetteville, AR
Ft. Smith, AR
Little Rock, AR
Baton Rouge, LA
Lafayette, LA
Monroe, LA
Shreveport, LA
Gulfport, MS
Jackson, MS
Oxford, MS

NEW YORK DIVISION
212-337-3900
OFFICES
Albany, NY
Buffalo, NY
Long Island, NY
Plattsburgh, NY
Rochester, NY
Syracuse, NY
Westchester Cty., NY

PHILADELPHIA DIVISION
215-861-3474
OFFICES
Dover, DE
Wilmington, DE
Allentown, PA
Harrisburg, PA
Pittsburgh, PA
Scranton, PA

PHOENIX DIVISION
602-664-5600
OFFICES
Flagstaff, AZ
Lake Havasu City, AZ
Nogales, AZ
Sierra Vista, AZ
Tucson, AZ
Yuma, AZ

SAN DIEGO DIVISION

858-616-4100

OFFICES

Carlsbad, CA
Imperial County, CA
San Ysidro, CA

SAN FRANCISCO DIVISION

415-436-7900

OFFICES

Bakersfield, CA
Fresno, CA
Oakland, CA
Sacramento, CA
San Jose, CA
Santa Rosa, CA

SEATTLE DIVISION

206-553-5443

OFFICES

Anchorage, AK
Fairbanks, AK
Boise, ID
Bend, OR
Eugene, OR
Medford, OR
Portland, OR
Salem, OR
Blaine, WA
Spokane, WA
Tacoma, WA
Tri-Cities, WA
Yakima, WA

ST. LOUIS DIVISION

314-538-4600

OFFICES

Cedar Rapids, IA
Des Moines, IA
Sioux City, IA
Carbondale, IL
Fairview Hts., IL
Quad Cities, IL
Garden City, KS
Kansas City, KS
Topeka, KS
Wichita, KS
Cape Giradeau, MO
Springfield, MO
North Platte, NE
Omaha, NE
Rapid City, SD
Sioux Falls, SD

WASHINGTON, DC DIVISION

202-305-8500

OFFICES

Baltimore, MD
Hagerstown, MD
Salisbury, MD
Bristol, VA
Hampton, VA
Norfolk, VA
Richmond, VA
Roanoke, VA
Winchester, VA
Charleston, WV
Clarksburg, WV
Wheeling, WV

DEA REGISTRATION UNIT

The DEA Office of Diversion Control, Registration Unit, has a 24-hour toll-free number: 800-882-9539.

This number is equipped with a voicemail system that may be used to request:

- A listing of the present fee structure
- New applications for registration
- Renewal applications
- Duplicate certificates of registration
- DEA order forms
- Changes of address

Callers may also opt to speak with a registration assistant during normal business hours (8:30 AM to 6:00 PM EST).

Additional information is available on their website at www.deadiversion.usdoj.gov.

STATE CONTROLLED-SUBSTANCES SCHEDULING AUTHORITIES

ALABAMA
Dept. of Public Health
PO Box 303017
Montgomery, AL 36130-3018
334-206-5300
www.adph.org

Alabama Board of Medical Examiners
PO Box 946
848 Washington Ave.
Montgomery, AL 36101
334-242-4116
www.albme.org

ALASKA
Div. of Occupational Licensing
PO Box 110806
Juneau, AK 99811-0806
907-465-2589
www.dced.state.ak.us/occ/ppha.htm

ARIZONA
Board of Pharmacy
1700 W. Washington St.
Suite 250
Phoenix, AZ 85007
602-771-2727
www.pharmacy.state.az.us

ARKANSAS
Div. of Pharmacy Services and Drug Control
Arkansas Dept. of Health
4815 W. Markham Street – Slot 25
Little Rock, AR 72205-3867
Office: 501-661-2325
www.healthyarkansas.com

CALIFORNIA
Board of Pharmacy
1625 N. Market Blvd.
Suite N 219
Sacramento, CA 95834
916-574-7900
www.pharmacy.ca.gov

California Dept. of Justice
Bureau of Narcotic Enforcement
3046 Prospect Park Dr.
Suite 1
Rancho Cordova, CA 95670
916-464-2020
http://ag.ca.gov

COLORADO
Board of Pharmacy
1560 Broadway
Suite 1350
Denver, CO 80202-5146
303-894-7800
www.dora.state.co.us/pharmacy

CONNECTICUT
Dept. of Consumer Protection
Drug Control Division
165 Capitol Ave.
Hartford, CT 06106
860-713-7240
www.ct.gov/dcp

DELAWARE
Board of Pharmacy
Cannon Bldg., Suite 203
861 Silver Lake Blvd.
Dover, DE 19904
302-744-4500
http://dpr.delaware.gov/boards/pharmacy/ index.shtml

DISTRICT OF COLUMBIA
Dept. of Health
Pharmaceutical Control
717 14th St., NW
6th Floor
Washington, DC 20005
202-724-4900
http://doh.dc.gov/doh

FLORIDA
Board of Pharmacy
4052 Bald Cypress Way,
Bin C19
Tallahassee, FL 32399
850-922-9036
www.doh.state.fl.us

GEORGIA
Georgia Drugs and Narcotics Agency
40 Pryor St., SW
Suite 2000
Atlanta, GA 30303
404-656-5100
www.gdna.georgia.gov

HAWAII
Dept. of Public Safety
Bureau of Narcotic Enforcement
3375 Koapaka St.
Suite D100
Honolulu, HI 96819
808-837-8470
http://hawaii.gov/psd

IDAHO
Board of Pharmacy
3380 Americana Terrace
Suite 320
Boise, ID 83706
208-334-2356
www.accessidaho.org/bop

ILLINOIS
Illinois Prescription Monitoring Program
401 N. Fourth St.
Room 133
Springfield, IL 62702
217-524-9074
https://www.ilpmp.org

INDIANA
Board of Pharmacy
Health Professions Bureau
402 W. Washington St.
Room W072
Indianapolis, IN 46204
317-234-2067
www.in.gov/hpb/boards/isbp

IOWA
Governors Office of Drug Control Policy
401 SW 7th St.
Suite N
Des Moines, IA 50309
515-242-6391
www.state.ia.us/government/odcp

KANSAS
Board of Pharmacy
Landon State Office Bldg.
900 SW Jackson St.
Suite 560
Topeka, KS 66612
785-296-4056
www.accesskansas.org/pharmacy

KENTUCKY
Dept. for Public Health
CHR, Drug Enforcement Branch
275 E. Main St. HS2GW-B
Frankfort, KY 40621
502-564-5497
http://chfs.ky.gov

LOUISIANA
Board of Pharmacy
5615 Corporate Blvd.
Suite 8E
Baton Rouge, LA 70808
225-925-6496
www.labp.com

MAINE
Board of Commissioners and Pharmacy
State House Station #35
Augusta, ME 04333
207-624-8620
TTY: 888-577-6690
www.state.me.us/pfr

Dept. of Professions
35 State House Station
Augusta, ME 04333
207-264-8600
www.state.me.us/pfr

MARYLAND
Board of Pharmacy
4201 Patterson Ave.
Baltimore, MD 21215-2299
410-764-4755
www.dhmh.state.md.us/pharmacyboard

MASSACHUSETTS
Drug Control Program
Dept. of Public Health–Div. of Food and Drugs
305 S. St., 2nd floor
Jamaica Plain, MA 02130
617-983-6700
www.mass.gov/dph/dcp

MICHIGAN
Bureau of Health Professions
PO Box 30670
Lansing, MI 48909-8170
517-335-0918
www.michigan.gov/healthlicense

Board of Pharmacy
611 W. Ottawa, 1st Floor
PO Box 30670
Lansing, MI 48909-8170
517-335-0918
www.michigan.gov/cis

MINNESOTA
Board of Pharmacy
2829 University Ave., SE #530
Minneapolis, MN 55414-3251
651-201-2825
www.phcybrd.state.mn.us

MISSISSIPPI
Director of Pharmacy
Dept. of Health
PO Box 1700
Jackson, MS 39205
601-576-7400
www.msdh.state.ms.us

MISSOURI
Bureau of Narcotics and Dangerous Drugs
Dept. of Health and Senior Services
PO Box 570
Jefferson City, MO 65102
573-751-6321
www.dhss.mo.gov/BNDD

MONTANA
Board of Pharmacy
PO Box 200513
Helena, MT 59620-0513
406-841-2371

NEBRASKA
Professional and Occupational Licensing Division
Dept. of Health
PO Box 94986
Lincoln, NE 68509-4986
402-471-2115
www.hhs.state.ne.us/crl/crlindex.htm

Nebraska State Patrol
PO Box 94907
Lincolin, NE 68509
402-471-4545
www.nsp.state.ne.us

NEVADA
Board of Pharmacy
431 W. Plumb Ln.
Reno, NV 89509
775-850-1440
800-364-2081
www.bop.nv.gov

NEW HAMPSHIRE
Compliance Investigation
Board of Pharmacy
57 Regional Dr.
Concord, NH 03301-8518
603-271-2350
www.state.nh.us/pharmacy

NEW JERSEY
Enforcement Bureau, Drug Control Unit
PO Box 45045
124 Halsey St., 3rd Floor
Newark, NJ 07101
973-504-6351
www.state.nj.us/lps/ca/drug/dchome.htm

NEW MEXICO
Board of Pharmacy
5200 Oakland NE
Suite A
Albuquerque, NM 87113
505-222-9830
800-565-9102
www.rld.state.us/pharmacy

NEW YORK
N.Y. Bureau of Controlled Substances
433 River St., Suite 303
Troy, NY 12180
866-811-7957
www.health.state.ny.us/professionals/narcotic

NORTH CAROLINA
Controlled Substances Regulatory Branch
Alcohol and Drug Abuse Services
3008 Mail Service Center
Raleigh, NC 27699
919-733-1765

NORTH DAKOTA
Board of Pharmacy
1906 East Broadway Ave.
Bismarck, ND 58501
701-328-9535
www.nodakpharmacy.com

OHIO
Board of Pharmacy
77 S. High St.
Room 1702
Columbus, OH 43215-6126
614-466-4143
www.pharmacy.ohio.gov

OKLAHOMA
Oklahoma Bureau of Narcotics and Dangerous Drugs Control
440 N.E. 39th St.
Oklahoma City, OK 73105
405-521-2885
800-522-8031
www.ok.gov/obndd

OREGON
Board of Pharmacy
State Office Building #425
800 N.E. Oregon St.
Portland, OR 97232
971-673-0001
www.pharmacy.state.or.us

PENNSYLVANIA
Bureau of Narcotic Investigations and Drug Control
106 Lowther St.
Lemoyne, PA 17043
717-712-1280
www.attorneygeneral.gov

Pennsylvania Dept. of Health
Health & Welfare Bldg.
8th Floor West
625 Foster St.
Harrisburg, PA 17102
877-724-3258
www.dsf.health.state.pa.us/health/site/default.asp

RHODE ISLAND
Compliance and Regulatory Section
Div. of Drug Control
205 Cannon Office Building
3 Capitol Hill, #205
Providence, RI 02908-5097
401-222-2837

SOUTH CAROLINA
Bureau of Drug Control
Dept. of Health and Environmental Control
2600 Bull St.
Columbia, SC 29201
803-896-0636
www.scdhec.net

SOUTH DAKOTA
Dept. of Health
Licensure and Certification
615 E. 4th St.
Pierre, SD 57501-3133
605-773-3356
www.state.sd.us/doh

TENNESSEE
Tennessee Board of Pharmacy
227 French Landing
Suite 300
Nashville, TN 37243
615-253-1299
http://health.state.tn.us/Boards/Pharmacy/index.shtml

TEXAS
Drugs and Medical Devices Division
Texas State Dept. of Health
PO Box 149347
Austin, TX 78714
512-834-6755
www.dshs.state.tx.us/dmd/default.htm

Controlled Substance Programs
Texas Prescription Program
Dept. of Public Safety
PO Box 4087
Austin, TX 78752-0439
512-424-2000

UTAH
Div. of Professional Licensing
PO Box 146741
Salt Lake City, UT 84114-6741
801-530-6628
www.dopl.utah.gov

VIRGINIA
Dept. of Health Professions
Perimeter Ctr.
9960 Mayland Dr.
Suite 300
Richmond, VA 23233
804-367-4456
www.dhp.state.va.us/default.htm

WASHINGTON
Board of Pharmacy
PO Box 47877
Olympia, WA 98504-7863
360-236-4700
www.doh.wa.gov/hsqa/professionals/pharmacy

WEST VIRGINIA
Board of Pharmacy
232 Capitol St.
Charleston, WV 25301
304-558-0558
www.wvbop.com

WISCONSIN
Dept. of Regulation and Licensing
Controlled Substances Board
PO Box 8935
Madison, WI 53708-8935
608-266-2112
http://drl.wi.gov/boards/csb

WYOMING
State Board of Pharmacy
1712 Carey Ave.
Suite 200
Cheyenne, WY 82002
307-634-9636
http://pharmacyboard.state.wy.us

HEALTHCARE WEBSITES

Note: All sites use the Web prefix of http://www.

ACPE-accredit.org
Home of the Accreditation Council for Pharmacy Education (formerly the American Council on Pharmaceutical Education). Independent agency that provides national accreditation for professional pharmacy degrees and continuing education programs.

AHRQ.gov
Site of the Agency for Healthcare Research and Quality; provides clinical guidelines and evidence-based reports for various diseases.

APHAnet.org
Site of the American Pharmacists Association; provides association and pharmacy news, health information, continuing education, and pharmacy training programs.

CDC.gov
Site of the Centers for Disease Control and Prevention; features current public health issues, as well as listings of disease and health topics. The site also links to numerous public health agencies.

ClinicalTrials.gov
Search engine for information on clinical trials and medical research from the National Library of Medicine database. Information can be accessed by trial site, sponsor, treatment, or disease name.

CMS.gov
Site of the Centers for Medicare and Medicaid Services; provides reimbursement information at the federal and state levels. Also features coding instructions and downloadable government forms.

Drugs.com
Searchable database of drugs, medical conditions, drug interactions, and images. Also offers a pill identifier search.

DrugTopics.com
Offers the latest pharmacy and medical news, as well as continuing education and a professional forum for pharmacists.

FDA.gov
Home page of the Food and Drug Administration; offers information on drugs, cosmetics, and food safety.

FDA.gov/cder/index.html
Site of the FDA's Center for Drug Evaluation and Research. Offers drug information and regulatory guidance, with links to Drug Approvals, Orange Book, National Drug Code Directory, MedWatch, and Drug Shortages.

GHX.com
Site of Global Healthcare Exchange, which offers streamlined, Web-based purchasing systems for hospitals, group purchasing organizations, manufacturers, and distributors.

Health.NIH.gov
Provides health reports and studies from the National Institutes of Health database; includes listing of toll-free health hotlines.

Healthsquare.com/drugmain.htm
Contains information on more than 1,000 prescription medications, including side effects and possible food and drug interactions. Data supplied by *The PDR Pocket Guide To Prescription Drugs*®.

Innovatix.com
A group purchasing organization that offers online ordering of pharmaceutical products and medical/surgical supplies.

InteliHealth.com
Sponsored by Aetna U.S. Healthcare; provides health information from Harvard Medical School, as well as listings of health resources and links to medical search engines.

Lib.uiowa.edu/hardin/md
Sponsored by the University of Iowa's Hardin Library for the Health Sciences; provides listing of Web sites by medical specialty.

MayoClinic.com
Offers health and drug information, including a Drug Watch Index that monitors recent approvals and recalls.

Medicare.gov/pdphome.asp
Provides information about Medicare Part D prescription drug coverage, including eligibility and approved drug plans.

MEDLINEplus.gov
Part of the National Library of Medicine database; provides health and drug information, medical dictionaries and encyclopedias, and directories for locating healthcare organizations and providers.

Medscape.com
Provides peer-reviewed, practice-oriented information on diseases, pharmacotherapy, and managed care, and links to medical journals for healthcare professionals and consumers, as well as continuing education courses.

NCPAnet.org
Home of the National Community Pharmacists Association. Represents the political interests of independent pharmacists nationwide at the federal and state levels. Also provides current professional news and continuing education programs.

NLM.NIH.gov
Site of the National Library of Medicine; PubMed and MedlinePlus allow users to search the NLM database, which includes millions of journal citations as well as links to other Web sites and databases.

PDRhealth.com
Consumer site for the *Physicians' Desk Reference*®. Provides practitioners and their patients with drug information on prescription and over-the-counter products as well as herbal and dietary supplements. Also includes links to health information and a leading clinical trial registry.

Pharmacist.com
Features professional resources such as licensing information, monthly updates on drug therapy developments, and online continuing education programs.

PharmScope.com
Reports on current practices and trends affecting managed care pharmacy; resources include formulary kits and drug databases.

PharmWeb.net
Emphasizes international pharmacy news for consumers and healthcare professionals; offers links to pharmacy-related resources and discussion groups.

RxList.com
Offers searchable database of prescription and OTC drug information and interactions.

WebMD.com
Provides news and health information for consumers and healthcare professionals.

STATE AIDS DRUG-ASSISTANCE PROGRAMS

ALABAMA
HIV/AIDS Division
Alabama Dept. of Public Health
RSA Tower, Suite 1400
201 Monroe St., Suite 110
Montgomery, AL 36104-3721
PO Box 303017
Montgomery, AL 36130-3017
334-206-5364

ALASKA
AIDS/STD Program
Dept. of Health and Social Services
Div. of Public Health, Epidemiology
3601 C St., Suite 576
PO Box 240249
Anchorage, AK 99524-0249
907-269-8027

ARIZONA
AIDS Drug Assistance Program
Dept. of Health Services
150 N. 18th Ave., Suite 110
Phoenix, AZ 85007-3233
602-542-1025

ARKANSAS
Arkansas Dept. of Health
4815 W. Markham St., Slot 33
Little Rock, AR 72205-3867
501-661-2000

CALIFORNIA
Dept. of Health Services
611 N. Seventh St.
PO Box 97413
Sacramento, CA 94234-7320
916-449-5900

COLORADO
Ryan White CARE Unit
DCEED-STD-A3
Dept. of Public Health & Environment
4300 Cherry Creek Dr. S.
Denver, CO 80246-1530
303-692-2000

CONNECTICUT
ADAP Coordinator
Dept. of Social Services
25 Sigourney St., 11th Floor
Hartford, CT 06106
860-424-4903

DELAWARE
Delaware Div. of Public Health
Jesse Cooper Building
PO Box 637
Dover, DE 19901
302-744-4700

DISTRICT OF COLUMBIA
Director of Columbia Dept. of Health
HIV/AIDS Administration
64 New York Ave, NE
Suite 5001
Washington, DC 20001
202-671-4900

FLORIDA
HIV/AIDS Program
Florida Dept. of Health
4052 Bald Cypress Way
Mail Bin #A09
Tallahassee, FL 32399-1715
850-245-4300

GEORGIA
Dept. of Human Resources
Div. of Public Health/STD HIV Program
2 Peachtree St., NW
Suite 12-235
Atlanta, GA 30303-3186
404-657-2700

HAWAII
HIV Drug Assistance Program (HDAP)
3627 Kilauea Ave., Suite 306
Honolulu, HI 96816
808-732-0026

IDAHO
STD/AIDS Program
Dept. of Health and Welfare
450 W. State St. 4th Floor
Boise, ID 83720
208-334-6996

ILLINOIS
Illinois Dept. of Public Health
535 W. Jefferson St.
Springfield, IL 62761
217-524-5983

INDIANA
HIV Services
Indiana State Dept. of Health
2 N. Meridian St., Suite 6C
Indianapolis, IN 46204
866-588-4948

IOWA
HIV/AIDS Bureau
Iowa Dept. of Public Health
Lucas State Office Bldg.
321 E. 12th St., 5th Floor
Des Moines, IA 50319-0075
515-242-5316

KANSAS
Bureau of Disease Control & Prevention
1000 SW Jackson
Suite 210
Topeka, KS 66612-1274
785-296-6174

KENTUCKY
KADAP Administrator
Dept. for Public Health
HIV/AIDS Branch
275 E. Main St., HS2C-A
Frankfort, KY 40621-0001
502-564-6539

LOUISIANA
HIV/AIDS Program Office
Dept. of Health and Hospitals
234 Loyola Ave., 5th Floor
New Orleans, LA 70112
504-568-7474

MAINE
Maine Dept. of Human Services
11 State House Station
221 State St.
Augusta, ME 04333
207-287-5551

MARYLAND
The Maryland AIDS Administration
500 N. Calvert St., 5th Floor
Baltimore, MD 21202
410-767-5227

MASSACHUSETTS
HIV/AIDS Bureau
Dept. of Public Health
250 Washington St., 3rd Floor
Boston, MA 02108-4619
617-624-5300

MICHIGAN
Capitol View Building
201 Townsend St.
Lansing, MI 48913
517-373-3740

MINNESOTA
HIV/AIDS Programs
Dept. of Human Services
PO Box 64972
St. Paul, MN 55164-0972
651-431-2414

MISSISSIPPI
Ryan White Programs
Mississippi Dept. of Health
570 E. Woodrow Wilson, Suite 350
PO Box 1700
Jackson, MS 39215-1700
601-576-7723

MISSOURI
ADAP Program Manager
HIV/AIDS Prevention
Missouri Dept. of Health
930 Wildwood Dr.
PO Box 570
Jefferson City, MO 65102-0570
573-751-6439

MONTANA
Ryan White Title II Coordinator
Dept. of Health and Human Services
Cogswell Bldg., C-211
1400 Broadway St.
PO Box 202951
Helena, MT 59620-9910
406-444-3565

NEBRASKA
Ryan White Program Coordinator
Nebraska Dept. of Health
PO Box 95026
Lincoln, NE 68509
402-471-0362

NEVADA
Nevada State Health Division
4150 Technology Way, Suite 300
Carson City, NV 89701-3701
775-684-4200

NEW HAMPSHIRE
Div. of Public Health Services
Office of Health Management
29 Hazen Dr., Suite 210
Concord, NH 03301-6527
603-271-4502

NEW JERSEY
Prevention and Care
Division of AIDS
New Jersey Dept. of Health
50 E. State St.
PO Box 363
Trenton, NJ 08625-0363
609-292-7837

NEW MEXICO
ADAP Administrator
New Mexico Dept. of Health
1190 St. Francis Dr.
Runnels Bldg.
PO Box 26110
Santa Fe, NM 87502-6110
505-827-2389

NEW YORK
Div. of HIV Health Care
AIDS Institute
Dept. of Health
90 Church St., 13th Floor
Albany, NY 12237
800-541-2437

NORTH CAROLINA
HIV/STD Prevention and Care Branch
Div. of Public Health & Human Services
1902 Mail Service Center
225 N. McDowell St., 5th Floor
Raleigh, NC 27699-1902
919-733-7301

NORTH DAKOTA
ADAP Coordinator
Dept. of Health
600 E. Boulevard Ave.
Dept. 301
Bismarck, ND 58505-0200
701-328-2372

OHIO
AIDS Client Resources Supervisor
Dept. of Health
246 N. High St.
Columbus, OH 43215
614-752-2427

Source: The HIV/AIDS Bureau of the U.S. Department of Health and Human Services.

OKLAHOMA
Special Projects Coordinator
HIV/STD Service
Oklahoma State Dept. of Health
1000 NE 10th St.
PO Box 0308
Oklahoma City, OK 73117-1299
800-777-4775

OREGON
HIV Client Services Section
Div. of Health
Dept. of Human Resources
Room 21
800 NE Oregon St.
Portland, OR 97232-2162
971-673-0153

PENNSYLVANIA
Administrator, SPBP
Department of Public Welfare
Cherrywood Building
PO Box 8021
Room 119
Harrisburg, PA 17105-8021
717-772-6057

PUERTO RICO
ADAP Coordinator
Dept. de Salud
RIO Pietres Med
Centro Psiquiatrico Hospital
Pavilion No. 1
PO Box 70184
San Juan, PR 00936-8184
787-274-5500

RHODE ISLAND
Office of AIDS/STD
Rhode Island Dept. of Health
3 Capitol Hill, Room 106
Providence, RI 02908-5097
401-222-7547

SOUTH CAROLINA
ADAP Director
South Carolina Dept. of Health
and Environment Control
Mills/Jarrett Complex
PO Box 101106
State Park, SC 29211-0106
803-898-0829

SOUTH DAKOTA
South Dakota Dept. of Health
Part B ADAP Program
615 E. 4th St.
c/o 500 E. Capitol Ave.
Pierre, SD 57501-3185
605-773-3523

TENNESSEE
Ryan White Services
Tennessee Dept. of Health
Cordell Hall Bldg., 4th Floor
425 Fifth Ave. N.
Nashville, TN 37427-4911
615-532-8520

TEXAS
ADAP Coordinator
HIV/STD Prevention Resources
Texas Dept. of Health,
Medication Program
1100 W. 49th St.
Austin, TX 78756-3199
512-533-3000

UTAH
Bureau of HIV/AIDS
Utah Dept. of Health
288 North, 1460 West
PO Box 142105
Salt Lake City, UT 84114-2105
801-538-6225

VERMONT
Div. of HIV/AIDS
Vermont Dept. of Health Services
108 Cherry St.
PO Box 70
Burlington, VT 05402
802-863-7244

VIRGINIA
Virginia Dept. of Health
PO Box 2448
Richmond, VA 23218-2448
109 Governor St.
Richmond VA, 23219
804-864-7965
800-533-4148

WASHINGTON
ADAP Coordinator
HIV/AIDS Client Services
Dept. of Health
PO Box 47841
Olympia, WA 98504-7841
877-376-9316

WEST VIRGINIA
West Virginia Dept. of Health
and Social Services
350 Capital St., Room 125
Charleston, WV 25301
304-588-2971

WISCONSIN
HIV/AIDS Program
Dept. of Health and
Family Services
1 W. Wilson St., Room 318
PO Box 2659
Madison, WI 53703
608-266-1865
608-267-7371

WYOMING
Title II Coordinator
Wyoming Health Dept.
6101 Yellowstone Rd., Suite 510
Cheyenne, WY 82002
307-777-5932
800-438-1282

PATIENT ASSISTANCE PROGRAMS

The following directory lists some of the manufacturers and states that provide medications free of charge or at a reduced rate for qualified patients. For more information on patient assistance programs, visit RxHope at www.rxhope.com or RxAssist at www.rxassist.org.

Abbott Laboratories
Patient Assistance Program
800-222-6885
Virology Patient Assistance Program
800-222-6885
HUMIRA Medicare Assistance Program
800-4-HUMIRA (800-448-6472)
Ross Medical Nutritionals Patient Assistance Program
800-222-6885
Ross Metabolic Formula and Elecare Patient Assistance Program
800-222-6885

Alabama
ALLKIDS Health Insurance Program
888-373-5437
ALLKIDS Low Fee
888-373-5437
Medicaid 6-18
800-362-1504
Medicaid Under 6
800-362-1504

Alaska
Chronic and Acute Medical Assistance (CAMA)
800-780-9972
Denali KidCare
888-318-8890 or 907-269-6529 (Anchorage area)
Medicaid
800-780-9972 or 907-644-6800

Alcon Labs
Glaucoma Patient Assistance Program
800-222-8103

Allergan, Inc.
Patient Assistance Program
800-553-6783
Botox Reimbursement Hotline and Patient Assistance Program
800-530-6680

Alpharma Pharmaceuticals
Patient Assistance Program
888-206-9743
American Regent Laboratories
Patient Assistance Program
800-282-7712

Amgen Inc.
Enliven
888-4-ENBREL (888-436-2735)
Safety Net Foundation
888-KINERET (888-762-6436)
Safety Net Program
800-272-9376 (choose opion 2)
Encourage Foundation
800-282-7752

Arizona
Family Assistance Administration
800-352-8401
KidsCare
877-764-5437 or
602-417-5437 (Phoenix area)
Pregnant Women's Medicaid
800-352-8401 or
602-417-4000 (Phoenix area)

Arkansas
ARKids First
888-474-8275

Astellas Pharma Inc.
Prograf Patient Assistance Program
800-477-6472
Protopic Patient Assistance Program
866-263-8483

AstraZeneca
Cancer Support Network
866-992-9276
AstraZeneca Foundation
Patient Assistance Program
800-424-3727 (choose option 2)

Aventis Oncology
PACT+ (Providing Access to Cancer Therapy) – Anzemet CINV
800-996-6626
PACT+ – Anzemet PONV
800-996-6626
PACT+ – Nilandron
800-996-6626
PACT+ – Anzemet
800-996-6626
PACT+ – Taxotere
800-996-6626

Axcan Scandipharm, Inc.
Rx Complete Program
866-292-2679
Comprehensive Care Program for CF
866-292-2679

Baxter Healthcare
Factor Plus
888-548-4448 (choose option 2)

Baxter Pharmaceutical Products
Baxter Factor Plus Program
800-548-4448 (choose option 2)

Bayer Healthcare Pharmaceuticals
Patient Assistance Program Information
888-84-BAYER or 888-842-2937 (choose option 7)
Reimbursement Hotline
800-423-7539
The Betaseron Foundation
800-948-5777

Biogen, Inc.
Avonex Patient Services
800-456-2255

Biovail Pharmaceuticals, Inc.
Patient Assistance Program
866-268-7325

Boehringer Ingelheim Pharmaceuticals, Inc.
Boehringer Ingelheim Cares Foundation, Inc.
800-556-8317

Bristol-Myers Squibb Company
Bristol-Myers Squibb – AmeriCares Oncology/Virology Access Program
800-736-0003
Bristol-Myers Squibb Patient Assistance Foundation, Inc.
800-736-0003
Bristol-Myers Squibb Patient Assistance Foundation, Inc. (Abilify)
800-736-0003

California
AIM – Access for Infants and Mothers
800-433-2611
California AIDS Drugs Assistance Program (ADAP)
916-449-5900
Healthy Families
888-747-1222
Medi-Cal (Dept. of Health Services)
800-541-5555 or 916-445-4171

Celgene Corporation
Celgene Customer Care Center
888-423-5436
Innohep Patient Assistance Program
866-742-7646

Cephalon
Gabitril PAP
866-209-7589
Provigil Reimbursement Hotline and PAP
800-675-8415

Chiron
Proleukin Patient Assistance Program
866-385-4729
Tobi Patient Assistance Program
866-598-8624

CLS Behring
Patient Assistance Program
800-676-4266

Colorado
CHP+
800-359-1991

Connecticut
ConnPACE
800-423-5026 or 860-269-2029
Husky Health Plan A
877-284-8759

Daiichi Sankyo Pharma
Sankyo Pharma Open Care Program
866-268-7327 (choose option 1)

Delaware
Delaware Healthy Children Program
800-996-9969
Pharmacy Assistance Program (DPAP) of Delaware
800-996-9969

Dey
Patient Assistance Program
800-755-5560

Digestive Care, Inc.
Digestive Care, Inc. Assistance Program
610-882-5950

Duramed Pharmaceuticals, Inc.
Cenestin Patient Assistance Program
800-425-3122

ECR Pharmaceuticals
Patient Assistance Program
804-527-1950

Eisai Inc.
Aciphex Patient Assistance Program
800-523-5870
Aricept Patient Assistance Program
800-226-2072
Patient Assistance Program
877-873-4724 (choose opion 2)

Elan Pharmaceuticals
Patient Assistance Program
888-638-7605

Eli Lilly and Company
Lilly Cares and Zyprexa PAP
800-545-6962
Lilly Medicare Answers Program
877-RX-LILLY (877-795-4559)

EMD Serono, Inc.
Fertility LifeLines
866-538-7879
MS LifeLines Patient Assistance
877-447-3243
National Organization for Rare Disorders (NORD)
800-999-6673
SeroCare
800-714-2437

Endo Pharmaceuticals, Inc
Endo Patient Assistance Program
866-824-4747

Enzon
Financial Assistance Program for ABELCET
800-345-2252

Ferndale Laboratories, Inc.
Ferndale PAP
800-621-6003, ext. 442

Ferring Pharmaceuticals
Euflexxa Reimbursement Program
866-383-5391
Ferring Pharmaceuticals Prescription Reimbursement Program
888-337-7464

Florida
Department of Elder Affairs
850-414-2000
Kid Care
888-540-5437
Senior Prescription Affordability Program
888-419-3456
SHINE
850-414-2000

Forest Pharmaceuticals
Forest Pharmaceuticals Patient Assistance Program
800-851-0758

Galderma Laboratories, Inc.
Patient Assistance Program
866-730-5074

Genentech, Inc.
Genentech Access to Care Foundation
800-530-3083

Genetics Institute, Inc.
BENEFIX Patient Assistance Program
800-568-9938

Genzyme Corporation
The Charitable Access Program (CAP)
800-745-4447, ext. 16593

Georgia
PeachCare for Kids
877-427-3224

Gilead Sciences, Inc.
Gilead Patient Assistance Program
800-226-2056

GlaxoSmithKline
Bridges to Access
866-728-4368
Commitment to Access
8-ONCOLOGY-1 (866-265-6491)
Medicare Part D
866-518-4357

Glenwood, LLC
Potaba Patient Assistance Program
800-542-0772

Graceway Pharmaceuticals
Patient Assistance Program
800-328-0255

Hawaii
Hawaii AIDS Drug Assistance Program
808-732-0315
Hawaii QUEST for Adults
800-882-4608
Hawaii QUEST for Children
800-882-4608
Hawaii Rx Plus
808-692-7999 (Oahu)
866-878-9769

Hospira
Reimbursement Assistance Program
800-340-8667

Idaho
Idaho CHP – Children's Health Insurance Program
2-1-1 or 800-926-2588 or 866-326-2485
Idaho Medicaid – Adult or Disabled Programs
2-1-1 or 800-926-2588 or 866-326-2485
Idaho Medicaid – Children (between age 6 and 19)
2-1-1 or 800-926-2588 or 866-326-2485
Idaho Medicaid – Children (birth up to age 6)
2-1-1 or 800-926-2588 or 866-326-2485
Idaho Medicaid Families
2-1-1 or 800-926-2588 or 866-326-2485
Idaho Medicaid – Pregnant Women
2-1-1 or 800-926-2588 or 866-326-2485

Illinois
Senior Helpline
800-252-8966 or 217-524-6911
FamilyCare
866-255-5437
Illinois AIDS Drug Assistance Program
217-782-4977
All Kids
866-255-5437

Indiana
Hoosier Healthwise
800-889-9949

Iowa
Hawk-I
800-257-8563
Iowa Priority
866-282-5817

Ivax Pharmaceuticals
Patient Assistance Program
800-507-8334 (choose option 3)

Janssen Pharmaceutica, Inc.
Aciphex Patient Assistance Program
800-523-5870
Janssen Patient Assistance Program
800-652-6227
Risperdal Patient Assistance Program
800-652-6227

Johnson & Johnson
Patient Assistance Program
866-489-5957

Kansas
Healthwave
800-792-4884

Kentucky
KCHIP
877-524-4718

Ligand Pharmaceuticals, Inc.
Ligand Assistance Program
866-613-4724

Louisiana
LA CHIP
877-252-2447

Maine
Maine Rx Plus
866-796-2463
Maine Low Cost Drugs for the Elderly and Disabled Program
866-796-2463
MaineCare
800-321-5557

Maryland
Maryland Children's Health Program
800-456-8900
Maryland Pharmacy Access Hotline
410-767-5800

Massachusetts
Children's Medical Security Plan
800-909-2677
Healthy Start Program
888-488-9161
Massachusetts AIDS Drug Assistance Program
617-624-5762
MassHealth
800-652-6227

McNeil Consumer and Specialty Pharmaceuticals
MCSP Patient Assistance Program
800-652-6227

Mead Johnson Nutritionals
Helping Hands Program for Mead Johnson Nutritionals
812-429-5000

Medicare Drug Coverage
Medicare Prescription Drug Cards
800-MEDICARE (800-633-4227)

Medimmune, Inc.
Ethyll Patient Assistance Program
800-887-2467
Synagis Assistance Program
877-480-8082

MedPointe, Inc.
Felbatol Assistance Program
800-678-4657

Merck & Co., Inc.
ACT (Accessing Coverage Today) for EMEND
866-EMEND-Rx (866-363-6379)
Merck Patient Assistance Program
800-994-2111
Support Program for Crixivan Reimbursement Support and Patient Assistance Services for Crixivan
800-850-3430

Merck/Schering-Plough Pharmaceuticals
Merck/Schering-Plough Assistance Program
800-347-7503

Michigan
Elder Prescription Insurance Plan (EPIC)
866-747-5844
MIChild
888-988-6300
World Medical Relief
313-866-5333

Millennium Pharmaceuticals, Inc.
VELCADE Reimbursement Assistance Program
866-VELCADE (866-835-2233)

Minnesota
GAMC
651-431-2670 (Twin Cities metro area)
800-657-3739 (outside Twin Cities metro area)
TTY: 800-627-3529 or 711
MinnesotaCare
651-297-3862 (Twin Cities metro area)
800-657-3672 (outside Twin Cities metro area)
TTY: 800-627-3529 or 711
Prescription Drug Program
651-431-2670 (Twin Cities metro area)
800-657-3739 (outside Twin Cities metro area)
Senior LinkAge Line: 800-333-2433
TTY: 800-627-3529 or 711

Mission Pharmacal Company
Mission Pharmaceutical Patient Assistance Program
800-292-7364

Mississippi
Mississippi CHIP
877-543-7669
Mississippi Medicaid
877-543-7669

Missouri
MO Healthnet for Kids
888-275-5908

Montana
Montana CHIP
877-543-7669

Nebraska
Kids Connection
877-632-5437

Nevada
Nevada Check Up
877-543-7669

New Hampshire
Healthy Kids
877-464-2447

New Jersey
Medicaid for Families with Children
800-356-1561
Medicaid for Pregnant Women
800-356-1561
Medicaid through General Assistance
800-356-1561
New Jersey AIDS Drugs Distribution Program
877-613-4533
NJFamilyCare
800-701-0710
PAAD
800-792-9745
Senior Gold Prescription Discount Program
800-792-9745

New Mexico
New Mexikids
888-997-2583

New York
Child Health Plus
800-698-4543
EPIC Deductible Plan
800-332-3742

North Carolina
NC Health Choice for Children
800-422-4658

Novartis Pharmaceuticals Corporation
Patient Assistance Foundation
800-277-2254

Novo Nordisk
Novo Nordisk Diabetes Patient Assistance Program
800-727-6500
Novo Nordisk Diabetes Patient Assistance Program (California Residents)
866-310-7549
Novo Nordisk Women's Health Care Patient Assistance Program
866-668-6336

Ohio
Healthy Start
800-324-8680

Oklahoma
Sooner Care
800-987-7767

Oregon
Oregon Health Plan
503-945-5772

Orphan Medical, Inc.
Cystadane Patient Assistance Program
800-999-6673 or 203-744-0100

Ortho Biotech
DOXILine (Alaska)
800-609-1083
DOXILine (Hawaii)
800-609-1083
ORTHOVISCline
866-633-VISC (8472)
ORTHOVISCline (Alaska)
866-633-VISC (8472)
ORTHOVISCline (Hawaii)
866-633-VISC (8472)
PROCRITline (Alaska)
800-553-3851
PROCRITline (Hawaii)
800-553-3851
PROCRITline (Leustatin)
800-553-3851
PROCRITline (PROCRIT)
800-553-3851

Ortho-McNeil
Patient Assistance Program
800-652-6227
Regranex Gel Patient Assistance Program
800-652-6227

Par Pharmaceutical, Inc.
Megace ES Patient Assistance Program
800-589-0841

Pennsylvania
CHIP
800-986-5437
PACE Needs Enhancement Tier (PACENET)
800-225-7223
Pennsylvania Special Pharmaceutical Benefits Program (PSPBP)
800-922-9384
Pharmaceutical Assistance Contract for the Elderly (PACE)
800-225-7223

Pfizer Inc
Connection to Care
866-706-2400
FirstRESOURCE
877-744-5675
Pfizer Bridge Program
800-645-1280

Procter & Gamble Pharmaceuticals
Patient Assistance Program
800-830-9049

Questcor Pharmaceuticals
Acthar Gel Patient Assistance Program
800-247-4963

Rare Disease Therapeutics, Inc.
Orfadin Patient Assistance Program
800-999-6673

Rhode Island
Rhode Island Pharmaceutical Assistance to the Elderly (RIPAE)
401-462-3000

Roche Laboratories, Inc.
CellCept Patient Assistance Program
800-772-5790 (choose option 2)
ONCOLINE Patient Assistance Program
800-443-6676 (choose option 3)
Pegassist Patient Assistance Program
866-247-5084 (choose option 1)
Roche HIV Therapy Assistance Program
800-282-7780

Sanofi-Aventis, Inc.
Patient Assistance Program
800-221-4025

Sanofi-Aventis Pharmaceuticals, Inc.
Patient Assistance Program
800-221-4025
Lovenox Patient Assistance Program
888-632-8607

Sanofi-Pasteur Inc.
Patient Assistance Programs
866-801-5655

Savient Pharmaceuticals
Oxandrin Reimbursement and Patient Assistance Program
866-692-6374, option 2

Schering-Plough
Commitment to Care
800-521-7157
Patient Assistance Program
800-656-9485 (choose option 1)

Sciele Pharma, Inc.
Patient Assistance Program
800-869-4514

Sigma-Tau Pharmaceuticals
Carnitor Drug Assistance (CDA) Program
800-999-6673
Matulane Patient Assistance Program
800-999-6673

Solvay Pharmaceuticals, Inc.
Patient Assistance Program
800-256-8918
Patient Assistance Program (Controlled Products)
800-256-8918

South Dakota
CHIP
800-305-3064 or 605-773-4678

Stiefel Laboratories, Inc.
Stiefel Laboratories Indigent Care Program
888-784-3335
Stiefel Laboratories Patient Assistance Program
888-500-3376

Takeda Pharmaceuticals North America, Inc.
Patient Assistance Program
800-830-9159

Tennessee
TennCare
800-342-3145

Teva Neuroscience, Inc.
Copaxone Patient Assistance Program
800-887-8100

Texas
ADAP
800-255-1090
TexCare Partnership CHIP
800-647-6558

Together Rx Access
Prescription Drug Card
800-444-4106
(discounts of 25%-40%; participating manufacturers include Abbott Laboratories, AstraZeneca, Bristol-Myers Squibb, GlaxoSmithKline, Janssen Pharmaceutica, LifeScan, Novartis, Ortho-McNeil, Pfizer, Sanofi-Aventis, Takeda, and TAP Pharmaceutical)

UCB Pharma, Inc.
UCB Patient Assistance Program
866-395-8366
Ucyclyd Pharma, Inc.
Buphenyl and Urea Cycle Treatment Assistance Program
800-711-0811

Valeant Pharmaceuticals International
Patient Assistance Program
800-511-2120

Vermont
Dr. Dynasaur
800-250-8427
Healthy Vermonters Program
800-250-8427
VHAP and Vscript
800-250-8427

Virginia
Family Access to Medical Insurance Security (FAMIS)
866-873-2647

Washington, DC
DC Healthcare Alliance
866-842-5809
DC Healthy Families
888-557-1116
Medicaid for Children 1-18
202-442-5955
State Child Health Plan
202-442-5955

Watson Laboratories, Inc.
Trelstar Reimbursement Program
866-755-3315
Watson Iron Reimbursement Assistance
800-964-4766

West Virginia
Golden Mountaineer Discount Card
877-987-3646
Low-Income Medicaid & Children
800-642-8589
West Virginia AIDS Drug Assistance Program
304-232-6822
WV CHIP
877-982-2447

Wisconsin
BadgerCare
800-362-3002
Wisconsin AIDS/HIV Drug Assistance Program (ADAP)
800-991-5532 or 608-267-6875

Wyeth Pharmaceuticals
Wyeth Patient Assistance Program
800-568-9938

Wyoming
Medicaid Program
307-772-8401
Wyoming Kid Care
888-996-8786

Xubex Pharmaceutical Services
Patient Assistance Program
866-699-8239

MEDICAID FEDERAL UPPER LIMIT PRICES

The following list provides federal upper limit (FUL) prices for Medicaid reimbursement of multiple-source drugs, effective March 2010. The FUL price list is updated approximately every 6 months. To keep current on pricing information, consult your monthly *Red Book UPDATE*.

In accordance with current policy, federal financial participation will not be provided for any drug on the FUL listing for which the FDA has issued a notice of an opportunity for a hearing as a result of the Drug Efficacy Study and Implementation (DESI) program and the drug has been found to be less than effective or is identical, related or similar (IRS) to the DESI drug. The DESI drug is identified by the Food and Drug Administration or reported by the drug manufacturer for purposes of the Medicaid drug rebate program. For more information on abbreviations and symbols, refer to the Key to Rx Product Listings.

PRODUCT	FUL
ACEBUTOLOL HYDROCHLORIDE	
CAP, PO, 200 mg, 100s ea	46.13
400 mg, 100s ea	67.13
ACETAMINOPHEN/BUTALBITAL/CAFFEINE	
TAB, PO, 500 mg-50 mg-40 mg, 100s ea	68.70
ACETAMINOPHEN/CODEINE PHOSPHATE	
TAB, PO, 300 mg-15 mg, 100s ea	15.00
300 mg-30 mg, 100s ea	21.37
300 mg-60 mg, 100s ea	38.33
ACETAMINOPHEN/HYDROCODONE BITARTRATE	
CAP, PO, 500 mg-5 mg, 100s ea	19.43
ELI, PO, 473 ml	47.96
TAB, PO, 500 mg-2.5 mg, 100s ea	21.90
500 mg-5 mg, 100s ea	47.63
500 mg-7.5 mg, 100s ea	64.26
500 mg-10 mg, 100s ea	51.29
650 mg-7.5 mg, 100s ea	67.08
650 mg-10 mg, 100s ea	18.52
660 mg-10 mg, 100s ea	54.00
750 mg-7.5 mg, 100s ea	15.48
ACETAMINOPHEN/OXYCODONE HYDROCHLORIDE	
CAP, PO, 500 mg-5 mg, 100s ea	32.30
TAB, PO, 325 mg-5 mg, 100s ea	23.40
650 mg-10 mg, 100s ea	141.87
ACETAMINOPHEN/PENTAZOCINE HYDROCHLORIDE	
TAB, PO, 650 mg-25 mg, 100s ea	85.17
ACETAMINOPHEN/PROPOXYPHENE HYDROCHLORIDE	
TAB, PO, 650 mg-65 mg, 100s ea	10.90
ACETAMINOPHEN/PROPOXYPHENE NAPSYLATE	
TAB, PO, 650 mg-100 mg, 100s ea	18.00
ACETYLCYSTEINE	
SOL, IH, 10%, 10 ml	9.78
20%, 30 ml	8.04
ACYCLOVIR	
CAP, PO, 200 mg, 100s ea	14.78
TAB, PO, 400 mg, 100s ea	23.34
800 mg, 100s ea	46.67
ALBUTEROL SULFATE	
SOL, IH, 0.083%, 3 ml	0.35
0.5%, 20 ml	4.67
TAB, PO, 4 mg, 100s ea	14.25
ALCLOMETASONE DIPROPIONATE	
CRE, TP, 0.05%, 45 gm	37.27
OIN, TP, 0.05%, 45 gm	37.27
ALENDRONATE SODIUM	
TAB, PO, 5 mg, 100s ea	42.93
10 mg, 100s ea	42.93
35 mg, 4s ea	61.47
70 mg, 4s ea	61.47
ALLOPURINOL	
TAB, PO, 100 mg, 100s ea	7.85
300 mg, 100s ea	17.39
ALPRAZOLAM	
TAB, PO, 0.25 mg, 100s ea	6.14
0.5 mg, 100s ea	6.98
1 mg, 100s ea	8.85
2 mg, 100s ea	17.45

PRODUCT	FUL
TER, PO, 0.5 mg, 60s ea	116.06
1 mg, 60s ea	144.39
2 mg, 60s ea	191.64
3 mg, 60s ea	287.44
AMANTADINE HYDROCHLORIDE	
SYR, PO, 50 mg/5 ml, 480 ml	31.49
AMILORIDE HYDROCHLORIDE/ HYDROCHLOROTHIAZIDE	
TAB, PO, 5 mg-50 mg, 100s ea	6.75
AMIODARONE HYDROCHLORIDE	
TAB, PO, 200 mg, 60s ea	44.25
AMITRIPTYLINE HYDROCHLORIDE	
TAB, PO, 10 mg, 100s ea	6.08
25 mg, 100s ea	6.53
50 mg, 100s ea	7.58
75 mg, 100s ea	14.25
100 mg, 100s ea	15.68
150 mg, 100s ea	24.30
AMLODIPINE BESYLATE	
TAB, PO, 2.5 mg, 90s ea	11.61
5 mg, 90s ea	11.61
10 mg, 90s ea	16.04
AMOXICILLIN	
CAP, PO, 250 mg, 100s ea	6.53
500 mg, 100s ea	11.93
PDR, PO, 125 mg/5 ml, 150 ml	3.02
250 mg/5 ml, 150 ml	4.49
AMOXICILLIN/CLAVULANATE POTASSIUM	
PDR, PO, 400 mg/5 ml-57 mg/5 ml, 100 ml	53.47
AMPICILLIN	
CAP, PO, 250 mg, 100s ea	17.36
500 mg, 100s ea	29.91
ANAGRELIDE HYDROCHLORIDE	
CAP, PO, 0.5 mg, 100s ea	43.95
1 mg, 100s ea	87.90
ASPIRIN/BUTALBITAL/CAFFEINE	
TAB, PO, 325 mg-50 mg-40 mg, 100s ea	24.00
ASPIRIN/CARISOPRODOL	
TAB, PO, 325 mg-200 mg, 100s ea	27.08
ASPIRIN/CARISOPRODOL/CODEINE PHOSPHATE	
TAB, PO, 325 mg-200 mg-16 mg, 100s ea	183.75
ATENOLOL	
TAB, PO, 25 mg, 100s ea	4.59
50 mg, 100s ea	5.00
100 mg, 100s ea	6.90
ATENOLOL/CHLORTHALIDONE	
TAB, PO, 50 mg-25 mg, 100s ea	11.22
100 mg-25 mg, 100s ea	30.68
ATROPINE SULFATE/DIPHENOXYLATE HYDROCHLORIDE	
TAB, PO, 0.025 mg-2.5 mg, 100s ea	21.38
AZATHIOPRINE	
TAB, PO, 50 mg, 100s ea	65.81

PRODUCT	FUL
AZITHROMYCIN	
TAB, PO, 250 mg, 30s ea	95.63
500 mg, 30s ea	164.55
600 mg, 30s ea	207.24
BACLOFEN	
TAB, PO, 10 mg, 100s ea	5.25
20 mg, 100s ea	8.93
BALSALAZIDE DISODIUM	
CAP, PO, 750 mg, 280s ea	302.29
BENAZEPRIL HYDROCHLORIDE	
TAB, PO, 5 mg, 100s ea	49.05
10 mg, 100s ea	49.05
20 mg, 100s ea	49.05
40 mg, 100s ea	49.05
BENAZEPRIL HYDROCHLORIDE/ HYDROCHLOROTHIAZIDE	
TAB, PO, 5 mg-6.25 mg, 100s ea	49.58
10 mg-12.5 mg, 100s ea	49.58
20 mg-12.5 mg, 100s ea	49.58
20 mg-25 mg, 100s ea	49.58
BENZONATATE	
SGL, PO, 100 mg, 100s ea	43.87
200 mg, 100s ea	24.60
BENZTROPINE MESYLATE	
TAB, PO, 0.5 mg, 100s ea	7.47
1 mg, 100s ea	8.48
2 mg, 100s ea	12.08
BETAMETHASONE DIPROPIONATE	
CRE, TP, 0.05%, 15 gm	3.45
LOT, TP, 0.05%, 60 ml	9.00
BETAMETHASONE DIPROPIONATE/CLOTRIMAZOLE	
CRE, TP, 0.05%-1%, 15 gm	12.35
LOT, TP, 0.05%-1%, 30 gm	54.35
BETAMETHASONE VALERATE	
CRE, TP, 0.1%, 45 gm	5.39
BETHANECHOL CHLORIDE	
TAB, PO, 5 mg, 100s ea	48.89
10 mg, 100s ea	91.71
25 mg, 100s ea	170.79
50 mg, 100s ea	195.65
BICALUTAMIDE	
TAB, PO, 50 mg, 100s ea	348.02
BISOPROLOL FUMARATE	
TAB, PO, 5 mg, 100s ea	106.88
10 mg, 100s ea	106.88
BISOPROLOL FUMARATE/HYDROCHLOROTHIAZIDE	
TAB, PO, 2.5 mg-6.25 mg, 100s ea	102.60
5 mg-6.25 mg, 100s ea	102.60
10 mg-6.25 mg, 100s ea	25.42
BRIMONIDINE TARTRATE	
SOL, OP, 0.2%, 5 ml	22.50
BUMETANIDE	
TAB, PO, 0.5 mg, 100s ea	17.43
1 mg, 100s ea	28.14
2 mg, 100s ea	47.08

PRODUCT	FUL
BUPROPION HYDROCHLORIDE	
T12, PO, 150 mg, 60s ea	109.98
BUSPIRONE HYDROCHLORIDE	
TAB, PO, 5 mg, 100s ea	5.27
10 mg, 100s ea	7.14
15 mg, 100s ea	10.28
CAPTOPRIL	
TAB, PO, 12.5 mg, 100s ea	2.33
25 mg, 100s ea	2.63
50 mg, 100s ea	3.90
100 mg, 100s ea	10.80
CAPTOPRIL/HYDROCHLOROTHIAZIDE	
TAB, PO, 25 mg-15 mg, 100s ea	23.59
25 mg-25 mg, 100s ea	23.60
50 mg-25 mg, 100s ea	37.02
CARBAMAZEPINE	
CTB, PO, 100 mg, 100s ea	20.25
SUS, PO, 100 mg/5 ml, 450 ml	37.67
TAB, PO, 200 mg, 100s ea	8.49
CARBIDOPA/LEVODOPA	
TAB, PO, 10 mg-100 mg, 100s ea	40.43
25 mg-100 mg, 100s ea	46.88
25 mg-250 mg, 100s ea	51.45
CARISOPRODOL	
TAB, PO, 350 mg, 100s ea	8.51
CARTEOLOL HYDROCHLORIDE	
SOL, OP, 1%, 10 ml	36.68
CARVEDILOL	
TAB, PO, 3.125 mg, 100s ea	14.25
6.25 mg, 100s ea	14.25
12.5 mg, 100s ea	14.25
25 mg, 100s ea	14.25
CEFADROXIL	
CAP, PO, 500 mg, 50s ea	39.15
CEFDINIR	
CAP, PO, 300 mg, 60s ea	229.59
PDR, PO, 125 mg/5 ml, 100 ml	62.31
250 mg/5 ml, 100 ml	130.79
CEFPROZIL	
PDR, PO, 125 mg/5 ml, 100 ml	40.80
250 mg/5 ml, 100 ml	73.94
TAB, PO, 250 mg, 100s ea	239.39
500 mg, 100s ea	459.90
CEFUROXIME AXETIL	
TAB, PO, 250 mg, 20s ea	11.03
500 mg, 20s ea	21.33
CEPHALEXIN	
CAP, PO, 250 mg, 100s ea	16.50
500 mg, 100s ea	27.30
CHLORDIAZEPOXIDE HYDROCHLORIDE	
CAP, PO, 5 mg, 100s ea	11.39
10 mg, 100s ea	8.78
25 mg, 100s ea	9.90
CHLORHEXIDINE GLUCONATE	
LIQ, PO, 0.12%, 480 ml	5.23
CHLORPROPAMIDE	
TAB, PO, 100 mg, 100s ea	23.25
250 mg, 100s ea	49.17
CHLORZOXAZONE	
TAB, PO, 500 mg, 100s ea	7.57
CICLOPIROX	
SUS, TP, 0.77%, 30 ml	45.00
CICLOPIROX OLAMINE	
CRE, TP, 0.77%, 30 gm	49.83
CILOSTAZOL	
TAB, PO, 50 mg, 60s ea	32.85
100 mg, 60s ea	32.85

PRODUCT	FUL
CIMETIDINE	
TAB, PO, 200 mg, 100s ea	13.13
300 mg, 100s ea	13.13
400 mg, 100s ea	15.48
800 mg, 100s ea	27.75
CIMETIDINE HYDROCHLORIDE	
SOL, PO, 300 mg/5 ml, 240 ml	27.34
CIPROFLOXACIN HYDROCHLORIDE	
SOL, OP, 0.3%, 5 ml	37.85
TAB, PO, 250 mg, 100s ea	37.50
500 mg, 100s ea	45.00
750 mg, 100s ea	48.00
CITALOPRAM HYDROBROMIDE	
SOL, PO, 10 mg/5 ml, 240 ml	74.98
TAB, PO, 10 mg, 100s ea	16.73
20 mg, 100s ea	17.25
40 mg, 100s ea	17.55
CLARITHROMYCIN	
TAB, PO, 250 mg, 60s ea	142.35
500 mg, 60s ea	51.75
CLINDAMYCIN HYDROCHLORIDE	
CAP, PO, 150 mg, 100s ea	21.53
300 mg, 100s ea	119.75
CLINDAMYCIN PHOSPHATE	
GEL, TP, 1%, 60 gm	45.88
LOT, TP, 1%, 60 ml	47.93
SOL, TP, 1%, 60 ml	12.36
CLOBETASOL PROPIONATE	
CRE, TP, 0.05%, 30 gm	5.48
EMO, TP, 0.05%, 30 gm	13.40
FOA, TP, 100 gm	297.96
0.05%, 100 gm	297.96
GEL, TP, 0.05%, 60 gm	27.84
OIN, TP, 0.05%, 45 gm	8.73
SOL, TP, 0.05%, 50 ml	21.00
CLOMIPHENE CITRATE	
TAB, PO, 50 mg, 30s ea	106.50
CLOMIPRAMINE HYDROCHLORIDE	
CAP, PO, 25 mg, 100s ea	37.50
50 mg, 100s ea	50.36
75 mg, 100s ea	66.23
CLONAZEPAM	
TAB, PO, 0.5 mg, 100s ea	6.00
1 mg, 100s ea	7.80
2 mg, 100s ea	10.80
CLONIDINE HYDROCHLORIDE	
TAB, PO, 0.1 mg, 100s ea	10.50
0.2 mg, 100s ea	14.10
0.3 mg, 100s ea	18.15
CLORAZEPATE DIPOTASSIUM	
TAB, PO, 3.75 mg, 100s ea	13.77
7.5 mg, 100s ea	19.47
15 mg, 100s ea	27.54
CLOTRIMAZOLE	
SOL, TP, 1%, 10 ml	4.73
CODEINE PHOSPHATE/PROMETHAZINE HYDROCHLORIDE	
SYR, PO, 10 mg/5 ml-6.25 mg/5 ml, 480 ml	18.24
CROMOLYN SODIUM	
SOL, OP, 4%, 10 ml	33.75
CYCLOBENZAPRINE HYDROCHLORIDE	
TAB, PO, 5 mg, 100s ea	15.86
10 mg, 100s ea	10.35
DEMECLOCYCLINE HYDROCHLORIDE	
TAB, PO, 150 mg, 100s ea	949.50
300 mg, 48s ea	825.00
DESIPRAMINE HYDROCHLORIDE	
TAB, PO, 150 mg, 50s ea	98.09

PRODUCT	FUL
DESONIDE	
CRE, TP, 0.05%, 60 gm	14.02
KIT, TP, 0.05%, 59 ml	32.10
60 gm	14.02
LOT, TP, 0.05%, 59 ml	32.10
OIN, TP, 0.05%, 60 gm	24.46
DEXAMETHASONE/NEOMYCIN SULFATE/POLYMYXIN B SULFATE	
OIN, OP, 3 gm	3.21
DEXTROAMPHETAMINE SULFATE	
TAB, PO, 10 mg, 100s ea	34.35
DIAZEPAM	
TAB, PO, 2 mg, 100s ea	4.23
5 mg, 100s ea	7.18
10 mg, 100s ea	5.73
DICLOFENAC POTASSIUM	
TAB, PO, 50 mg, 100s ea	47.48
DICLOFENAC SODIUM	
SOL, OP, 0.1%, 5 ml	21.36
TER, PO, 75 mg, 100s ea	58.50
100 mg, 100s ea	236.18
DICYCLOMINE HYDROCHLORIDE	
CAP, PO, 10 mg, 100s ea	8.85
TAB, PO, 20 mg, 100s ea	4.05
DIGOXIN	
TAB, PO, 0.125 mg, 100s ea	21.32
0.25 mg, 100s ea	21.32
DILTIAZEM HYDROCHLORIDE	
TAB, PO, 30 mg, 100s ea	10.19
60 mg, 100s ea	11.14
90 mg, 100s ea	23.12
120 mg, 100s ea	23.31
DIPHENHYDRAMINE HYDROCHLORIDE	
ELI, PO, 12.5 mg/5 ml, 120 ml	1.64
DIPIVEFRIN HYDROCHLORIDE	
SOL, OP, 0.1%, 5 ml	4.35
DIPYRIDAMOLE	
TAB, PO, 25 mg, 100s ea	29.78
50 mg, 100s ea	47.96
75 mg, 100s ea	64.17
DISOPYRAMIDE PHOSPHATE	
CAP, PO, 100 mg, 100s ea	59.79
150 mg, 100s ea	62.88
DIVALPROEX SODIUM	
ECC, PO, 125 mg, 100s ea	82.10
TCP, PO, 125 mg, 100s ea	26.91
250 mg, 100s ea	52.88
500 mg, 100s ea	97.49
DOXAZOSIN MESYLATE	
TAB, PO, 1 mg, 100s ea	59.18
2 mg, 100s ea	59.18
4 mg, 100s ea	62.10
8 mg, 100s ea	65.18
DOXEPIN HYDROCHLORIDE	
CAP, PO, 10 mg, 100s ea	8.91
25 mg, 100s ea	18.22
50 mg, 100s ea	14.47
75 mg, 100s ea	20.52
100 mg, 100s ea	41.74
SOL, PO, 10 mg/ml, 120 ml	13.74
DOXYCYCLINE HYCLATE	
CAP, PO, 50 mg, 50s ea	6.59
100 mg, 50s ea	7.46
TAB, PO, 100 mg, 50s ea	6.44
ENALAPRIL MALEATE	
TAB, PO, 2.5 mg, 100s ea	4.73
5 mg, 100s ea	5.70
10 mg, 100s ea	7.32
20 mg, 100s ea	8.55

PRODUCT	FUL
ERYTHROMYCIN	
GEL, TP, 2%, 30 gm	18.75
ESTAZOLAM	
TAB, PO, 1 mg, 100s ea	59.25
2 mg, 100s ea	64.49
ESTRADIOL	
TAB, PO, 0.5 mg, 100s ea	17.91
1 mg, 100s ea	21.75
2 mg, 100s ea	30.60
ESTROPIPATE	
TAB, PO, 0.75 mg, 100s ea	27.54
1.5 mg, 100s ea	34.50
3 mg, 100s ea	86.22
ETHINYL ESTRADIOL/NORGESTIMATE	
TAB, PO, 35 mcg-0.25 mg, 28s ea	32.58
ETODOLAC	
CAP, PO, 200 mg, 100s ea	58.50
TAB, PO, 400 mg, 100s ea	39.23
500 mg, 100s ea	75.00
FAMOTIDINE	
TAB, PO, 20 mg, 100s ea	15.00
40 mg, 100s ea	30.00
FEXOFENADINE HYDROCHLORIDE	
CAP, PO, 60 mg, 100s ea	115.40
TAB, PO, 30 mg, 100s ea	57.56
60 mg, 100s ea	115.40
180 mg, 100s ea	200.18
FINASTERIDE	
TAB, PO, 5 mg, 100s ea	173.03
FLECAINIDE ACETATE	
TAB, PO, 50 mg, 100s ea	86.10
100 mg, 100s ea	140.70
150 mg, 100s ea	193.28
FLUCONAZOLE	
TAB, PO, 50 mg, 30s ea	15.00
100 mg, 30s ea	26.48
200 mg, 30s ea	42.23
FLUOCINONIDE	
CRE, TP, 0.05%, 60 gm	7.12
EMO, TP, 0.05%, 60 gm	14.72
GEL, TP, 0.05%, 60 gm	29.79
SOL, TP, 0.05%, 60 ml	15.84
FLUOROURACIL	
SOL, TP, 5%, 10 ml	116.90
FLUOXETINE HYDROCHLORIDE	
CAP, PO, 10 mg, 100s ea	13.86
20 mg, 100s ea	14.54
40 mg, 30s ea	34.88
SOL, PO, 20 mg/5 ml, 120 ml	27.00
TAB, PO, 10 mg, 30s ea	18.00
FLUPHENAZINE HYDROCHLORIDE	
TAB, PO, 1 mg, 100s ea	22.73
5 mg, 100s ea	35.46
10 mg, 100s ea	50.99
FLURAZEPAM HYDROCHLORIDE	
CAP, PO, 15 mg, 100s ea	9.75
30 mg, 100s ea	11.48
FLURBIPROFEN	
TAB, PO, 100 mg, 100s ea	24.38
FLURBIPROFEN SODIUM	
SOL, OP, 0.03%, 2 ml	8.14
FLUTICASONE PROPIONATE	
CRE, TP, 0.05%, 30 gm	33.33
OIN, TP, 0.005%, 30 gm	33.33
FLUVOXAMINE MALEATE	
TAB, PO, 25 mg, 100s ea	108.83
50 mg, 100s ea	108.30
100 mg, 100s ea	117.75

PRODUCT	FUL
FOLIC ACID	
TAB, PO, 1 mg, 100s ea	3.78
FOSINOPRIL SODIUM	
TAB, PO, 10 mg, 90s ea	53.82
20 mg, 90s ea	53.82
40 mg, 90s ea	53.82
FOSINOPRIL SODIUM/HYDROCHLOROTHIAZIDE	
TAB, PO, 10 mg-12.5 mg, 100s ea	134.54
20 mg-12.5 mg, 100s ea	134.54
FUROSEMIDE	
SOL, PO, 10 mg/ml, 60 ml	7.80
TAB, PO, 20 mg, 100s ea	5.63
40 mg, 100s ea	5.99
80 mg, 100s ea	10.43
GABAPENTIN	
CAP, PO, 100 mg, 100s ea	8.25
300 mg, 100s ea	12.38
400 mg, 100s ea	15.38
TAB, PO, 600 mg, 100s ea	97.38
800 mg, 100s ea	117.56
GEMFIBROZIL	
TAB, PO, 600 mg, 500s ea	67.50
GENTAMICIN SULFATE	
CRE, TP, 0.1%, 15 gm	3.00
OIN, TP, 0.1%, 15 gm	3.00
SOL, OP, 3 mg/ml, 5 ml	2.85
GLIMEPIRIDE	
TAB, PO, 1 mg, 100s ea	13.41
2 mg, 100s ea	21.74
4 mg, 100s ea	41.00
GLIPIZIDE	
TAB, PO, 5 mg, 100s ea	6.99
10 mg, 100s ea	11.92
GLYBURIDE	
TAB, PO, 1.25 mg, 100s ea	12.44
2.5 mg, 100s ea	18.93
5 mg, 100s ea	28.31
GLYBURIDE/METFORMIN HYDROCHLORIDE	
TAB, PO, 1.25 mg-250 mg, 100s ea	84.05
2.5 mg-500 mg, 100s ea	100.26
5 mg-500 mg, 100s ea	100.26
GRAMICIDIN/NEOMYCIN SULFATE/POLYMYXIN B SULFATE	
SOL, OP, 10 ml	20.25
GUANFACINE HYDROCHLORIDE	
TAB, PO, 1 mg, 100s ea	12.42
2 mg, 100s ea	70.11
HALOBETASOL PROPIONATE	
CRE, TP, 0.05%, 50 gm	24.00
OIN, TP, 0.05%, 50 gm	26.63
HALOPERIDOL LACTATE	
SOL, PO, 2 mg/ml, 120 ml	16.43
HYDRALAZINE HYDROCHLORIDE	
TAB, PO, 10 mg, 100s ea	25.56
25 mg, 100s ea	32.84
50 mg, 100s ea	42.00
100 mg, 100s ea	78.38
HYDROCHLOROTHIAZIDE	
CAP, PO, 12.5 mg, 100s ea	12.00
TAB, PO, 25 mg, 1000s ea	18.00
50 mg, 1000s ea	49.90
HYDROCHLOROTHIAZIDE/LISINOPRIL	
TAB, PO, 12.5 mg-10 mg, 100s ea	20.97
12.5 mg-20 mg, 100s ea	21.99
25 mg-20 mg, 100s ea	22.25

PRODUCT	FUL
HYDROCHLOROTHIAZIDE/MOEXIPRIL HYDROCHLORIDE	
TAB, PO, 12.5 mg-7.5 mg, 100s ea	121.11
12.5 mg-15 mg, 100s ea	121.11
25 mg-15 mg, 100s ea	121.11
HYDROCHLOROTHIAZIDE/PROPRANOLOL HYDROCHLORIDE	
TAB, PO, 25 mg-40 mg, 100s ea	8.77
25 mg-80 mg, 100s ea	13.20
HYDROCHLOROTHIAZIDE/SPIRONOLACTONE	
TAB, PO, 25 mg-25 mg, 100s ea	34.63
HYDROCHLOROTHIAZIDE/TRIAMTERENE	
CAP, PO, 25 mg-37.5 mg, 100s ea	31.77
TAB, PO, 25 mg-37.5 mg, 100s ea	16.83
50 mg-75 mg, 100s ea	4.88
HYDROCORTISONE	
CRE, TP, 0.5%, 30 gm	1.53
1%, 30 gm	1.68
2.5%, 30 gm	4.95
LOT, TP, 1%, 120 ml	6.86
2.5%, 59 ml	44.25
OIN, TP, 1%, 30 gm	1.68
HYDROCORTISONE BUTYRATE	
CRE, TP, 0.1%, 45 gm	50.30
SOL, TP, 0.1%, 20 ml	7.58
HYDROCORTISONE VALERATE	
CRE, TP, 0.2%, 45 gm	29.62
OIN, TP, 0.2%, 45 gm	29.62
HYDROMORPHONE HYDROCHLORIDE	
TAB, PO, 2 mg, 100s ea	21.84
HYDROXYCHLOROQUINE SULFATE	
TAB, PO, 200 mg, 100s ea	22.50
HYDROXYZINE HYDROCHLORIDE	
TAB, PO, 10 mg, 100s ea	48.65
25 mg, 100s ea	71.34
HYDROXYZINE PAMOATE	
CAP, PO, 25 mg, 100s ea	11.50
50 mg, 100s ea	15.72
IBUPROFEN	
TAB, PO, 400 mg, 100s ea	3.45
600 mg, 100s ea	4.17
800 mg, 100s ea	6.38
IMIPRAMINE HYDROCHLORIDE	
TAB, PO, 10 mg, 100s ea	26.43
25 mg, 100s ea	35.51
50 mg, 100s ea	46.04
INDAPAMIDE	
TAB, PO, 1.25 mg, 100s ea	10.35
2.5 mg, 100s ea	11.25
IPRATROPIUM BROMIDE	
SOL, IH, 0.02%, 2.5 ml 25s	6.75
ISONIAZID	
TAB, PO, 100 mg, 100s ea	5.61
300 mg, 100s ea	8.90
ISOSORBIDE DINITRATE	
TAB, PO, 5 mg, 100s ea	4.88
10 mg, 100s ea	5.25
20 mg, 100s ea	5.63
ISOSORBIDE MONONITRATE	
TAB, PO, 10 mg, 100s ea	61.10
20 mg, 100s ea	49.50
TER, PO, 60 mg, 100s ea	60.00
KETOCONAZOLE	
TAB, PO, 200 mg, 100s ea	225.00
KETOROLAC TROMETHAMINE	
TAB, PO, 10 mg, 100s ea	67.73

PRODUCT	FUL
LABETALOL HYDROCHLORIDE	
TAB, PO, 100 mg, 100s ea	21.57
200 mg, 100s ea	35.82
300 mg, 100s ea	53.63
LACTULOSE	
SOL, PO, 10 gm/15 ml, 480 ml	10.61
LAMOTRIGINE	
CTB, PO, 5 mg, 100s ea	66.09
25 mg, 100s ea	69.23
TAB, PO, 25 mg, 100s ea	30.35
100 mg, 100s ea	34.67
150 mg, 60s ea	22.80
200 mg, 60s ea	24.81
LEFLUNOMIDE	
TAB, PO, 10 mg, 30s ea	75.00
20 mg, 30s ea	75.00
LEVETIRACETAM	
SOL, PO, 100 mg/ml, 473 ml	164.98
TAB, PO, 250 mg, 120s ea	51.76
500 mg, 120s ea	63.25
750 mg, 120s ea	85.69
1000 mg, 60s ea	84.43
LEVOBUNOLOL HYDROCHLORIDE	
SOL, OP, 0.25%, 10 ml	12.75
0.5%, 10 ml	14.93
LEVOTHYROXINE SODIUM	
TAB, PO, 0.025 mg, 100s ea	23.18
0.05 mg, 100s ea	26.33
0.075 mg, 100s ea	29.10
0.088 mg, 100s ea	29.55
0.1 mg, 100s ea	29.85
0.112 mg, 100s ea	34.43
0.125 mg, 100s ea	34.95
0.15 mg, 100s ea	36.00
0.175 mg, 100s ea	42.75
0.2 mg, 100s ea	44.18
0.3 mg, 100s ea	60.23
LIDOCAINE HYDROCHLORIDE	
SOL, MM, 2%, 100 ml	5.13
LISINOPRIL	
TAB, PO, 2.5 mg, 100s ea	3.68
5 mg, 100s ea	4.83
10 mg, 100s ea	6.75
20 mg, 100s ea	7.95
30 mg, 100s ea	16.31
40 mg, 100s ea	15.00
LITHIUM CARBONATE	
CAP, PO, 300 mg, 100s ea	13.82
LORAZEPAM	
TAB, PO, 0.5 mg, 100s ea	7.40
1 mg, 100s ea	8.22
2 mg, 100s ea	14.67
LOVASTATIN	
TAB, PO, 10 mg, 60s ea	19.71
20 mg, 60s ea	27.73
40 mg, 60s ea	47.53
MECLIZINE HYDROCHLORIDE	
TAB, PO, 12.5 mg, 100s ea	5.99
MEDROXYPROGESTERONE ACETATE	
TAB, PO, 2.5 mg, 100s ea	20.25
5 mg, 100s ea	30.61
10 mg, 100s ea	37.87
MEGESTROL ACETATE	
TAB, PO, 20 mg, 100s ea	34.89
40 mg, 100s ea	67.55
MELOXICAM	
TAB, PO, 7.5 mg, 100s ea	14.25
15 mg, 100s ea	20.93
MEPERIDINE HYDROCHLORIDE	
TAB, PO, 50 mg, 100s ea	31.88
100 mg, 100s ea	62.93

PRODUCT	FUL
METFORMIN HYDROCHLORIDE	
TAB, PO, 500 mg, 100s ea	7.50
850 mg, 100s ea	14.64
1000 mg, 100s ea	16.58
TER, PO, 500 mg, 100s ea	13.07
750 mg, 100s ea	33.68
METHAZOLAMIDE	
TAB, PO, 25 mg, 100s ea	31.50
50 mg, 100s ea	46.50
METHENAMINE MANDELATE	
TAB, PO, 1 gm, 100s ea	29.23
METHIMAZOLE	
TAB, PO, 5 mg, 100s ea	42.12
15 mg, 100s ea	71.76
METHOCARBAMOL	
TAB, PO, 500 mg, 100s ea	19.43
750 mg, 100s ea	25.20
METHOTREXATE SODIUM	
TAB, PO, 2.5 mg, 100s ea	126.37
METHYLPHENIDATE HYDROCHLORIDE	
TAB, PO, 5 mg, 100s ea	22.53
10 mg, 100s ea	30.06
20 mg, 100s ea	33.09
METHYLPREDNISOLONE	
TAB, PO, 4 mg, 100s ea	43.04
METOCLOPRAMIDE HYDROCHLORIDE	
SOL, PO, 5 mg/5 ml, 480 ml	7.44
TAB, PO, 5 mg, 100s ea	18.42
10 mg, 100s ea	10.95
METOLAZONE	
TAB, PO, 2.5 mg, 100s ea	89.10
5 mg, 100s ea	106.80
10 mg, 100s ea	134.25
METOPROLOL TARTRATE	
TAB, PO, 25 mg, 100s ea	7.20
50 mg, 100s ea	5.00
100 mg, 100s ea	6.90
METRONIDAZOLE	
CRE, TP, 0.75%, 45 gm	73.18
GEL, TP, 0.75%, 45 gm	69.38
LOT, TP, 0.75%, 59 ml	69.00
TAB, PO, 250 mg, 100s ea	8.49
500 mg, 100s ea	21.84
MEXILETINE HYDROCHLORIDE	
CAP, PO, 200 mg, 100s ea	97.12
MIDAZOLAM HYDROCHLORIDE	
SYR, PO, 2 mg/ml, 118 ml	97.50
MIDODRINE HYDROCHLORIDE	
TAB, PO, 2.5 mg, 100s ea	111.72
5 mg, 100s ea	183.83
10 mg, 100s ea	313.38
MINOCYCLINE HYDROCHLORIDE	
CAP, PO, 50 mg, 100s ea	90.00
75 mg, 100s ea	195.75
100 mg, 50s ea	90.00
TAB, PO, 50 mg, 100s ea	300.00
75 mg, 100s ea	444.00
100 mg, 50s ea	262.50
MINOXIDIL	
TAB, PO, 2.5 mg, 100s ea	31.70
10 mg, 100s ea	69.65
MIRTAZAPINE	
ODT, PO, 30 mg, 30s ea	37.95
TAB, PO, 15 mg, 30s ea	36.90
30 mg, 30s ea	37.95
45 mg, 30s ea	38.54
MOMETASONE FUROATE	
CRE, TP, 0.1%, 45 gm	33.00
OIN, TP, 0.1%, 45 gm	42.00

PRODUCT	FUL
MUPIROCIN	
OIN, TP, 2%, 22 gm	41.45
MYCOPHENOLATE MOFETIL	
CAP, PO, 250 mg, 100s ea	52.91
TAB, PO, 500 mg, 100s ea	105.80
NADOLOL	
TAB, PO, 20 mg, 100s ea	46.50
40 mg, 100s ea	42.89
80 mg, 100s ea	80.25
NALTREXONE HYDROCHLORIDE	
TAB, PO, 50 mg, 100s ea	404.00
NAPHAZOLINE HYDROCHLORIDE	
SOL, OP, 0.1%, 15 ml	4.71
NAPROXEN	
TAB, PO, 250 mg, 100s ea	10.32
375 mg, 100s ea	7.61
500 mg, 100s ea	8.24
NIACIN	
TAB, PO, 500 mg, 100s ea	3.90
NICARDIPINE HYDROCHLORIDE	
CAP, PO, 20 mg, 100s ea	33.75
30 mg, 100s ea	40.50
NIZATIDINE	
CAP, PO, 150 mg, 60s ea	109.84
300 mg, 30s ea	109.85
NORTRIPTYLINE HYDROCHLORIDE	
CAP, PO, 10 mg, 100s ea	10.19
25 mg, 100s ea	14.06
50 mg, 100s ea	17.22
75 mg, 100s ea	22.03
NYSTATIN	
CRE, TP, 100000 u/gm, 30 gm	2.97
OIN, TP, 100000 u/gm, 15 gm	1.53
POW, TP, 100000 u/gm, 15 gm	26.22
SUS, PO, 100000 u/ml, 60 ml	12.37
NYSTATIN/TRIAMCINOLONE ACETONIDE	
CRE, TP, 100000 u/gm-0.1%, 30 gm	2.93
OIN, TP, 100000 u/gm-0.1%, 30 gm	2.93
OFLOXACIN	
SOL, OP, 0.3%, 5 ml	17.25
OMEPRAZOLE	
ECC, PO, 10 mg, 100s ea	354.63
20 mg, 100s ea	397.90
40 mg, 100s ea	173.43
ONDANSETRON HYDROCHLORIDE	
TAB, PO, 4 mg, 30s ea	33.00
8 mg, 30s ea	57.00
ORPHENADRINE CITRATE	
TER, PO, 100 mg, 100s ea	104.25
OXAPROZIN	
TAB, PO, 600 mg, 100s ea	67.58
OXAZEPAM	
CAP, PO, 10 mg, 100s ea	53.63
15 mg, 100s ea	57.09
30 mg, 100s ea	123.37
OXCARBAZEPINE	
TAB, PO, 150 mg, 100s ea	90.00
300 mg, 100s ea	171.00
600 mg, 100s ea	342.00
OXYBUTYNIN CHLORIDE	
SYR, PO, 5 mg/5 ml, 473 ml	13.15
TAB, PO, 5 mg, 100s ea	16.50
OXYCODONE HYDROCHLORIDE	
CAP, PO, 5 mg, 100s ea	21.38
SOL, PO, 20 mg/ml, 30 ml	28.50
TAB, PO, 5 mg, 100s ea	23.99
15 mg, 100s ea	66.95
30 mg, 100s ea	130.94

PRODUCT	FUL
PAROXETINE HYDROCHLORIDE	
TAB, PO, 10 mg, 30s ea	10.28
20 mg, 30s ea	10.73
30 mg, 30s ea	12.60
40 mg, 30s ea	14.63
PENICILLIN V POTASSIUM	
TAB, PO, 250 mg, 100s ea	21.12
500 mg, 100s ea	35.90
PENTOXIFYLLINE	
TER, PO, 400 mg, 100s ea	31.47
PHENYTOIN	
SUS, PO, 125 mg/5 ml, 237 ml	36.05
PILOCARPINE HYDROCHLORIDE	
TAB, PO, 7.5 mg, 100s ea	194.25
PIROXICAM	
CAP, PO, 10 mg, 100s ea	8.91
20 mg, 100s ea	11.31
POLYMYXIN B SULFATE/TRIMETHOPRIM SULFATE	
SOL, OP, 10000 u/ml-1 mg/ml, 10 ml	12.36
POTASSIUM CHLORIDE	
TER, PO, 8 meq, 100s ea	10.44
10 meq, 100s ea	25.38
20 meq, 100s ea	46.25
PRAVASTATIN SODIUM	
TAB, PO, 10 mg, 90s ea	22.50
20 mg, 90s ea	26.25
40 mg, 90s ea	32.04
80 mg, 90s ea	51.78
PRAZOSIN HYDROCHLORIDE	
CAP, PO, 5 mg, 250s ea	134.25
PREDNISOLONE	
SYR, PO, 15 mg/5 ml, 480 ml	99.89
PREDNISOLONE ACETATE	
SUS, OP, 1%, 10 ml	16.95
PREDNISOLONE SODIUM PHOSPHATE	
SOL, PO, 15 mg/5 ml, 237 ml	49.51
PREDNISONE	
TAB, PO, 5 mg, 100s ea	2.03
10 mg, 100s ea	6.15
20 mg, 100s ea	8.04
PRIMIDONE	
TAB, PO, 250 mg, 100s ea	80.55
PROBENECID	
TAB, PO, 500 mg, 100s ea	70.59
PROCHLORPERAZINE MALEATE	
TAB, PO, 5 mg, 100s ea	39.86
10 mg, 100s ea	57.66
PROMETHAZINE HYDROCHLORIDE	
SUP, RC, 12.5 mg, 12s ea	11.53
25 mg, 12s ea	12.43
TAB, PO, 12.5 mg, 100s ea	45.00
PROPAFENONE HYDROCHLORIDE	
TAB, PO, 150 mg, 100s ea	110.49
225 mg, 100s ea	156.24
PROPRANOLOL HYDROCHLORIDE	
CER, PO, 60 mg, 100s ea	132.24
80 mg, 100s ea	154.47
120 mg, 100s ea	191.60
160 mg, 100s ea	250.88
TAB, PO, 10 mg, 100s ea	5.85
20 mg, 100s ea	7.05
40 mg, 100s ea	8.48
60 mg, 100s ea	127.92
80 mg, 100s ea	11.40
PSE HCL/TRIPROLIDINE HCL	
TAB, PO, 60 mg-2.5 mg, 100s ea	3.36

PRODUCT	FUL
PYRIDOSTIGMINE BROMIDE	
TAB, PO, 60 mg, 100s ea	58.32
QUINAPRIL HYDROCHLORIDE	
TAB, PO, 5 mg, 90s ea	22.50
10 mg, 90s ea	22.50
20 mg, 90s ea	22.50
40 mg, 90s ea	22.50
RAMIPRIL	
CAP, PO, 1.25 mg, 100s ea	45.90
2.5 mg, 100s ea	48.77
5 mg, 100s ea	51.17
10 mg, 100s ea	59.87
RANITIDINE HYDROCHLORIDE	
SYR, PO, 15 mg/ml, 473 ml	112.48
TAB, PO, 150 mg, 100s ea	6.00
300 mg, 30s ea	3.75
RIBAVIRIN	
CAP, PO, 200 mg, 84s ea	636.42
RIFAMPIN	
CAP, PO, 150 mg, 30s ea	44.34
300 mg, 100s ea	188.60
RIMANTADINE HYDROCHLORIDE	
TAB, PO, 100 mg, 100s ea	151.20
RISPERIDONE	
TAB, PO, 0.25 mg, 60s ea	78.03
0.5 mg, 60s ea	85.64
1 mg, 60s ea	91.04
2 mg, 60s ea	152.15
3 mg, 60s ea	178.70
4 mg, 60s ea	240.01
ROPINIROLE HYDROCHLORIDE	
TAB, PO, 0.25 mg, 100s ea	75.15
0.5 mg, 100s ea	75.15
1 mg, 100s ea	75.15
2 mg, 100s ea	75.15
3 mg, 100s ea	77.96
4 mg, 100s ea	77.96
5 mg, 100s ea	77.96
SELEGILINE HYDROCHLORIDE	
TAB, PO, 5 mg, 60s ea	45.95
SELENIUM SULFIDE	
LOT, TP, 2.5%, 120 ml	9.00
SERTRALINE HYDROCHLORIDE	
TAB, PO, 25 mg, 100s ea	12.83
50 mg, 100s ea	12.83
100 mg, 100s ea	12.83
SILVER SULFADIAZINE	
CRE, TP, 1%, 400 gm	25.12
SIMVASTATIN	
TAB, PO, 5 mg, 90s ea	15.75
10 mg, 90s ea	15.75
20 mg, 90s ea	18.90
40 mg, 90s ea	23.00
80 mg, 90s ea	23.00
SOTALOL HYDROCHLORIDE	
TAB, PO, 80 mg, 100s ea	178.50
120 mg, 100s ea	235.50
160 mg, 100s ea	292.50
240 mg, 100s ea	397.50
SPIRONOLACTONE	
TAB, PO, 25 mg, 100s ea	30.00
STAVUDINE	
CAP, PO, 15 mg, 60s ea	135.33
20 mg, 60s ea	140.74
30 mg, 60s ea	149.47
40 mg, 60s ea	161.25
SUCRALFATE	
TAB, PO, 1 gm, 100s ea	36.90

PRODUCT	FUL
SULFACETAMIDE SODIUM	
SOL, OP, 10%, 15 ml	2.54
SULFAMETHOXAZOLE/TRIMETHOPRIM	
TAB, PO, 400 mg-80 mg, 100s ea	13.25
800 mg-160 mg, 100s ea	37.88
SULFASALAZINE	
TAB, PO, 500 mg, 100s ea	15.65
SULINDAC	
TAB, PO, 150 mg, 100s ea	33.17
200 mg, 100s ea	42.89
TAMOXIFEN CITRATE	
TAB, PO, 10 mg, 60s ea	58.28
20 mg, 30s ea	58.28
TEMAZEPAM	
CAP, PO, 15 mg, 100s ea	13.65
30 mg, 100s ea	17.48
TERAZOSIN HYDROCHLORIDE	
CAP, PO, 1 mg, 100s ea	14.25
2 mg, 100s ea	14.25
5 mg, 100s ea	14.25
10 mg, 100s ea	14.25
TERBINAFINE HYDROCHLORIDE	
TAB, PO, 250 mg, 100s ea	70.50
TERCONAZOLE	
CRE, VG, 0.4%, 45 gm	43.43
0.8%, 20 gm	39.74
TETRACYCLINE HYDROCHLORIDE	
CAP, PO, 500 mg, 100s ea	9.75
THEOPHYLLINE	
TER, PO, 200 mg, 100s ea	21.60
THIOTHIXENE	
CAP, PO, 1 mg, 100s ea	13.88
2 mg, 100s ea	18.60
5 mg, 100s ea	29.63
10 mg, 100s ea	40.65
TICLOPIDINE HYDROCHLORIDE	
TAB, PO, 250 mg, 60s ea	16.39
TIMOLOL MALEATE	
SOL, OP, 0.25%, 10 ml	6.98
0.5%, 15 ml	13.50
TIZANIDINE HYDROCHLORIDE	
TAB, PO, 2 mg, 150s ea	39.00
4 mg, 150s ea	48.00
TOBRAMYCIN	
SOL, OP, 0.3%, 5 ml	3.36
TOPIRAMATE	
TAB, PO, 25 mg, 60s ea	14.52
50 mg, 60s ea	28.89
100 mg, 60s ea	39.56
200 mg, 60s ea	46.31
TORSEMIDE	
TAB, PO, 5 mg, 100s ea	45.00
10 mg, 100s ea	48.00
20 mg, 100s ea	52.50
100 mg, 100s ea	291.75
TRAMADOL HYDROCHLORIDE	
TAB, PO, 50 mg, 100s ea	9.00
TRANDOLAPRIL	
TAB, PO, 1 mg, 100s ea	66.66
2 mg, 100s ea	66.66
4 mg, 100s ea	66.66
TRAZODONE HYDROCHLORIDE	
TAB, PO, 50 mg, 100s ea	7.42
100 mg, 100s ea	11.40
150 mg, 100s ea	31.13

PRODUCT	FUL
TRETINOIN	
CRE, TP, 0.025%, 45 gm	70.62
TRIAMCINOLONE ACETONIDE	
CRE, TP, 0.025%, 80 gm	3.00
0.1%, 80 gm	3.75
0.5%, 15 gm	3.56
OIN, TP, 0.1%, 80 gm	4.02
TRIAZOLAM	
TAB, PO, 0.125 mg, 10s ea	3.01
0.25 mg, 10s ea	3.25
TRIHEXYPHENIDYL HYDROCHLORIDE	
TAB, PO, 2 mg, 100s ea	12.75
5 mg, 100s ea	22.95
TRIMETHOBENZAMIDE HYDROCHLORIDE	
CAP, PO, 300 mg, 100s ea	101.93
TROPICAMIDE	
SOL, OP, 0.5%, 15 ml	9.83
1%, 15 ml	10.50
VALPROIC ACID	
SGL, PO, 250 mg, 100s ea	52.50
SYR, PO, 250 mg/5 ml, 480 ml	28.51
VENLAFAXINE HYDROCHLORIDE	
TAB, PO, 25 mg, 100s ea	116.58
37.5 mg, 100s ea	120.03
50 mg, 100s ea	123.66
75 mg, 100s ea	131.10
100 mg, 100s ea	138.92
VERAPAMIL HYDROCHLORIDE	
TAB, PO, 80 mg, 100s ea	7.73
120 mg, 100s ea	11.48
TER, PO, 120 mg, 100s ea	82.50
180 mg, 100s ea	48.38
240 mg, 100s ea	43.50
WARFARIN SODIUM	
TAB, PO, 1 mg, 100s ea	54.03
2 mg, 100s ea	56.39
2.5 mg, 100s ea	58.16
3 mg, 100s ea	58.43
4 mg, 100s ea	58.56
5 mg, 100s ea	58.97
6 mg, 100s ea	83.64
7.5 mg, 100s ea	86.49
10 mg, 100s ea	89.70
ZALEPLON	
CAP, PO, 5 mg, 100s ea	71.91
10 mg, 100s ea	73.86
ZIDOVUDINE	
TAB, PO, 300 mg, 60s ea	54.66
ZOLPIDEM TARTRATE	
TAB, PO, 5 mg, 100s ea	7.04
10 mg, 100s ea	7.04
ZONISAMIDE	
CAP, PO, 25 mg, 100s ea	19.31
50 mg, 100s ea	21.12
100 mg, 100s ea	49.98

MEDICAID REIMBURSEMENT FOR DRUGS BY STATE

	Medicaid Formula	Dispensing Fee	Co-pay
Alabama	Lower of WAC+9.2% or AWP-10%	$5.40	$0.50-$3.00*
Alaska	AWP-5%	$3.45-$11.46 (based on pharmacy/ Medicaid volume)	$2.00
Arizona	AWP-15%	$2.00 (FFS only)	None
Arkansas	AWP-20% (generic); AWP-14% (brand)	$5.51	$0.50-$3.00*
California	AWP-17%	$7.25; $8.00 (legend: skilled nursing & intermediate-care facilities)	$1.00
Colorado	AWP-45% (generic); AWP-14% (brand); direct price+18%; AWP-12% (approved rural)	$4.00 (retail pharmacy); $1.89 (institutional pharmacy)	$1.00 (generic); $3.00 (brand)
Connecticut	AWP-40% (selected multi-source brand and generic); AWP-14% (brand)	$3.15**	None
Delaware	AWP-14% (traditional: retail independent & retail chain pharmacies); AWP-16% (non-traditional: long-term care & specialty pharmacies)	$3.65	None
District of Columbia	AWP-10%	$4.50	$1.00
Florida	Lower of AWP-16.4%; WAC+4.75%	$3.73 (non 340B billed drugs); $7.50 (340B billed drugs)	2.5% of payment up to $300, capped at 5% total family income (certain beneficiaries)
Georgia	AWP-11%; ASP+6% as determined in Jan. 1st of applicable yr (maximum allowable reimbursement for an injectable drug administered by provider or their designee in outpatient setting)	$4.63 (for profit pharm); $4.33 (not for profit)	$0.50-$3.00
Hawaii	AWP-10.5%	$4.67	None
Idaho	AWP-12%	$4.94; $5.54 (unit dose)	None
Illinois	AWP-25% (generic); AWP-12% (brand)	$4.60 (generic); $3.40 (brand)	$3.00 (brand only)
Indiana	AWP-20% (generic); AWP-16% (brand)	$4.90	$3.00
Iowa	AWP-12%	$4.57	$1.00 (non-preferred brand, no more than $25.00), $2.00 (non-preferred brand, between $25.01 and $50.00), $3.00 (non-preferred brand, $50.01 or more)
Kansas	AWP-27% (generic); AWP-13% (brand)	$3.40	$3.00
Kentucky	AWP-14% (generic); AWP-15% (brand)	$5.00 (generic); $4.50 (brand)	$1.00 (generic or atypical antipsychotic); $2.00 (brand without generic equivalent); $3.00 (non-preferred brand); cap $225 per year per recipient
Louisiana	AWP-13.5% (independent pharmacies); AWP-15% (chains)	$5.77**	$0.50-$3.00*
Maine	AWP-15%; AWP-17%; (on direct supply); AWP-20% (mail-order)	$3.35; $1.00 (mail-order) $4.35 & $5.35 (compounding); $12.50 (insulin syringe)	$3.00 (not to exceed $30 per month) (mail order not subject to co-pay)
Maryland	Lower of AWP-12%, WAC+8%, direct price+8%, or distributor price when available	$3.69 (generic); $2.69 (brand); $4.69 (generic-NH); $3.69 (brand-NH); $7.25 (home IV therapy)	$1.00 (generic and preferred brand); $3.00 (non-preferred brand)
Massachusetts	WAC+5%; (all drugs except 340B billed drugs); actual acquisition cost (340B billed drugs)	$3.00 (all drugs except 340B billed drugs); $10 (340B billed drugs)	$1.00 (multi-source & OTC); $3.00 (all others)
Michigan	AWP-13.5% (independent pharmacies, 1-4 stores); AWP-15.1% (chain, 5+ stores)	$2.75; $3.00 (long-term care)	$1.00 (generic); $3.00 (brand)
Minnesota	AWP-12%	$3.65 (+$0.30 for legend unit dose drugs)	$1.00 (generic); $3.00 (brand)
Mississippi	Lower of AWP-12% or WAC+9% (brand); AWP-25% (generic)	$3.91 (brand); $5.50 (generic)	$3.00 (medically needy only)
Missouri	Lower of AWP-10.43% or WAC+10%	$4.09	$0.50-$2.00*
Montana	AWP-15%	$5.04; $12.50 - $22.50 (compounding)	$1.00
Nebraska	AWP-11%	$3.27-$5.00 (based on service delivery, unit dosage or third-party payors)**	$2.00.
Nevada	AWP-15%	$4.76; $22.40 daily (home IV therapy); $16.80 daily (NH IV therapy)	None
New Hampshire	AWP-16%	$1.75	$1.00 (generic); $2.00 (brand & compound)
New Jersey	AWP-15%	$3.73 up to $3.99 (24-hour emergency service, patient consultation and impact area location)**	None
New Mexico	Lower of AWP-14%; wholesaler average cost as submitted to state; manufacturer price as submitted to state; pharmacy invoice price as obtained through audits	$3.65	None
New York	AWP-16.25% (brand); AWP-25% (generic); AWP-12% (specialized HIV pharmacies)	$4.50 (generic); $3.50 (brand)	$1.00 (generic); $3.00 (brand); $0.50 (OTC)
North Carolina	AWP-10%, ASP+6.7% (physician-administered drugs)	$5.60 (generic); $4.00 (brand)	$1.00 (generic); $3.00 (brand)
North Dakota	Lower of AWP-10%, WAC+12.5%	$5.60 (generic legend); $4.60 (brand legend); 1.5 times allowed amount (EAC, FUL, or MAC) up to a maximum of $4.60 (non-legend drugs prescribed); plus $0.15 per pill (pill splitting)	$3.00 (brand)
Ohio	WAC+7% or AWP-14.4% if WAC cannot be determined	$3.70	$3.00 (non-perferred drugs); $2.00 (preferred brand drugs)
Oklahoma	AWP-12%	$4.15	$1.00-$2.00*
Oregon	AWP-15% (multi-source drugs); AWP-11% (institutional); AWP-68% (mail order); AWP-15% (single-source drugs); AWP-11% (institutional); AWP-21% (mail order)	$3.50 (retail); $3.91 (institutional)	$1.00 (non-preferred generic or generics costing $10.00); No co-pay (preferred generic or brand); $3.00 (all others)
Pennsylvania	Lower of WAC+7%, AWP-14%	$4.00; $5.00 (compounding)	$1.00
Rhode Island	WAC	$3.40 (outpatient), $2.85 (long-term care)	None
South Carolina	AWP-10%	$4.05 (independent pharmacies); $3.15 (institutional)	$3.00
South Dakota	AWP-10.5%	$4.75; $5.55 (unit dose)	$3.00 (brand)

*Variation in co-pay amounts is due to the cost of the prescription. ** CMS-approved state plans or state source if marked. ASP = average sale price; AWP = average wholesale price; DEAC = direct estimated acquisition cost; EAC = estimated acquisition cost; FFS = fee-for-service; FUL = federal upper limit; MAC = maximum allowable cost; NH = nursing home; OTC = over-the-counter; PDL = preferred drug list; RHC = rural health clinic; SMAC = state maximum allowable cost; U&C = usual and customary; WAC = wholesaler's acquisition cost; WEAC = wholesale estimated acquisition cost. **Source:** Centers for Medicare and Medicaid Services, Mar. 2010. For more information, visit www.cms.hhs.gov/home/medicaid.asp.

State	Medicaid Formula	Dispensing Fee	Co-pay
Tennessee	Lower of AWP-16%, MAC or FUL for Pharmacy Benefit Management (PBM) National Network; lower of AWP-13%, MAC or FUL for TennCare Pharmacy Network; special pharmacy rates set separately	$1.50 (PBM National); $2.50 (TennCare Pharmacy Network - brand); $3.00 (generic); $5.00 (brand nursing home); $6.00 (generic nursing home); $25 (compound prescriptions)	$0 (generics and categorically needy); $3.00 (medically needy)
Texas	EAC is WEAC, which is lower of AWP-15% or WAC+12%; DEAC for certain drug products available through direct purchasing	$7.50 plus 2% of cost of drug	None**
Utah	AWP-15%	$3.90 (urban); $4.40 (rural)**	$3.00 **
Vermont	AWP-11.9%	In-state: $4.75; Out-of-state: $3.65	$1.00-$3.00*
Virginia	AWP-10.25%	$3.75; $5.00 (unit-dose drugs)	$1.00
Washington	AWP-16% (single-source drugs & multi-source drugs with 4 or fewer manufacturers/labelers); AWP-50% (multi-source drugs with 5 or more manufacturers/labelers & no MAC or FUL)	$4.24-$5.25 (based on 3-tiered pharmacy volume)	None
West Virginia	AWP-15% (brand), AWP-30% (generic)	$2.50 (brand); $5.30 (generic) $8.25 (340B drugs)	$0.50-$3.00*
Wisconsin	AWP-14%	$3.44 (brand); $3.94 (generic); $0.015 per unit (for repackaging); $9.45-$22.16 (compound drug fee); $9.45-$40.11 (pharmaceutical care dispensing fee)	$0.50 (OTC); $3.00 (brand); $1.00 (generic); cap $12 per pharmacy per recipient per month
Wyoming	AWP-11%	$5.00	$2.00

*Variation in co-pay amounts is due to the cost of the prescription. ** CMS-approved state plans or state source if marked. ASP = average sale price; AWP = average wholesale price; DEAC = direct estimated acquisition cost; EAC = estimated acquisition cost; FFS = fee-for-service; FUL = federal upper limit; MAC = maximum allowable cost; NH = nursing home; OTC = over-the-counter; PDL = preferred drug list; RHC = rural health clinic; SMAC = state maximum allowable cost; U&C = usual and customary; WAC = wholesaler's acquisition cost; WEAC = wholesale estimated acquisition cost. **Source:** Centers for Medicare and Medicaid Services, Mar. 2010. For more information, visit www.cms.hhs.gov/home/medicaid.asp.

PHARMACY BENEFIT MANAGERS

To help pharmacists navigate the growing impact of third-party administrators on their practice, we've compiled a list of pharmacy benefit managers that health insurers often use. Keep in mind that while every effort has been made to verify the following information, the field is rapidly changing, with companies often merging and restructuring. When in doubt, contact the patient's health insurer directly.

ABC Managed Care
800-829-3132
www.amerisourcebergen.com
States served: Nationwide

ACS State Healthcare
214-841-6111
www.acs-inc.com
States served: All

Aetna
860-273-0123
www.aetna.com
States served: All

AmeriScript, Inc.
800-681-6912
www.ameriscript.com
States served: All

BeneScript Services, Inc.
800-345-3189; 800-531-6351
www.benescript.com
States served: All

Blue Cross and Blue Shield of Illinois
312-653-6000
www.bcbsil.com
States served: All

Caremark Research Team
800-552-8159; 615-743-6600
www.caremark.com
States served: All

Catalyst Rx
888-869-4600
www.catalystrx.com
States served: All

Central Fill, Inc.
(A division of Express Scripts)
800-233-7139
www.express-scripts.com
States served: All

CuraScript PBM Services
407-852-4903; 888-773-7386
www.curascript.com
States served: All

EPIC Pharmacy Network, Inc.
804-559-4597; 800-876-EPIC (3742)
www.epicrx.com
States served: CA, DC, DE, MD, NC, NJ, NY, PA, SC, TN, TX, VA, WI, WV

Express Scripts, Inc.
314-770-1666; 800-332-5455
www.express-scripts.com
States served: All

First Health Rx
630-737-7900
www.firsthealth.com
States served: All

First Health Services Corp.
804-965-7400; 800-884-2822
www.fhsc.com
States served: All

GSPO Provider Services (GSPOPS)
800-778-8089
www.gspops.com
States served: All

HealthPlus
800-639-1609
www.pgnerx.com
States served: All

Health Resources Inc.
410-347-1540; 800-727-1444
www.hri-dho.com
States served: All

informedRx
866-533-6977
www.myinformedrx.com
States served: All

MaxorPlus
800-658-6146; 806-324-5400
www.maxor.com
States served: All

Medco Health Solutions, Inc.
Mail Stop E1-MS1
Franklin Lakes, NJ 07417
800-922-1557
www.medco.com/rph
States served: All plus Puerto Rico

NMHCRx Inc.
800-251-3883
www.nmhcrx.com
States served: All

NMHCRx
800-510-8980
www.nmhcrx.com
States served: All plus Puerto Rico

Northwest Pharmacy Services
800-998-2611
www.nwpsrx.com
States served: All

PBM Plus, Inc.
(An Omnicare Company)
513-248-3071; 888-863-1726, ext. 1526
www.pbmplus.com
States served: All

Pequot Pharmaceutical Network
Pharmacy Benefit Management Services
800-219-1226, ext. 66462
www.prxn.com
States served: All

PharmaCare, Inc.
401-334-0069; 800-777-1023
www.pharmacare.com
States served: All

Pharmaceutical Technologies, Inc.
402-964-9030; 888-334-4488
www.pti-nps.com
States served: All

Pharmacy Providers of Oklahoma
877-557-5707; Fax: 405-528-7523
www.ppok.com
States served: All

Pharmacy Provider Services Corp. (PPSC)
850-656-0100; 888-778-9909
www.ppsconline.com
States served: All

Premier Pharmacy Plan
864-591-0025; 800-247-4526
www.smithpremier.com
States served: All

Walgreens Health Initiatives
847-374-2640; 800-926-6779
www.mywhi.com – Pharmacy Benefit Management
www.walgreenshealth.com – All Health Initiatives
States served: All plus Puerto Rico and U.S. Virgin Islands

WellPoint Pharmacy Management
888-809-6084
www.wellpointrx.com
States served: All

NCPDP STANDARD BILLING UNITS

To assist in obtaining the fastest possible reimbursement and avoid over- or under-billing, the National Council for Prescription Drug Programs (NCPDP) has developed industry guidelines for submitting prescription claims. The latest version was released in January 2010. NCPDP standards are available free of charge to NCPDP members. See www.ncpdp.org for membership information. Below is a general description of the standard. For more information, contact the organization at:

NCPDP

9240 E. Raintree Dr.

Scottsdale, AZ 85260-7518

Phone: 480-477-1000

Fax: 480-767-1042

Website: www.ncpdp.org

E-mail: ncpdp@ncpdp.org

Basic Guide to the Billing Unit Standard

Due to the number of processors, fiscal intermediaries, plan administrators, and Medicaid programs, the billing unit standard was created to promote a "common billing unit language" for the submission of prescription claims.

The principal rule of the standard is that there are only three billing units necessary to describe any and all drug products. These billing units are "each", "ml", and "gm". The use of "tablet", "capsule", "kit" and others is not appropriate, since these are dosage forms or package descriptions. Breaking billing units into dosage forms does not add value to the model and violates the goals of the standard. Whether an "each" refers to a tablet, a capsule, a suppository, or a transdermal patch, the price will be the same for each billing unit. Once this definition is in place, the remainder of the standard describes how the various types of pharmaceutical products fit into one of the standard billing units.

Adapted from *NCPDP Basic Guide to Standards*. Reprinted with permission of the National Council for Prescription Drug Programs,

What business problem is this standard trying to overcome?

- Billing unit inconsistencies within the health care delivery industry
- Incorrect reimbursement
- Difficulties defining what constitutes a billing unit

How is/could this standard be used in practical, day-to-day applications?

- Provide a consistent and well-defined billing unit for use in pharmacy transactions
- Provide a method to assign a standard billing unit
- Reduce the time it takes for a pharmacist to accurately bill a prescription and get paid correctly
- Provides a standard billing unit for use in calculation of accurate reimbursement
- Provides a standard size unit of measure for use in DUR

To whom is this standard useful (i.e., target markets)?

- Anyone in the health care delivery industry
- Pharmacies and pharmacists
- Manufacturers
- Payers/processors
- HCFA
- Wholesalers/distributors
- Pricing compendia
- Billing agents
- Software vendors
- EMR
- Physicians

21
3
3N
3N
3N
4U
7
A-
A.
A.
AE
AE
AE
AE
AE
AE
AC
AC

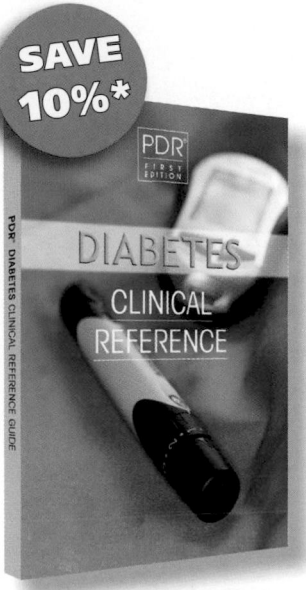

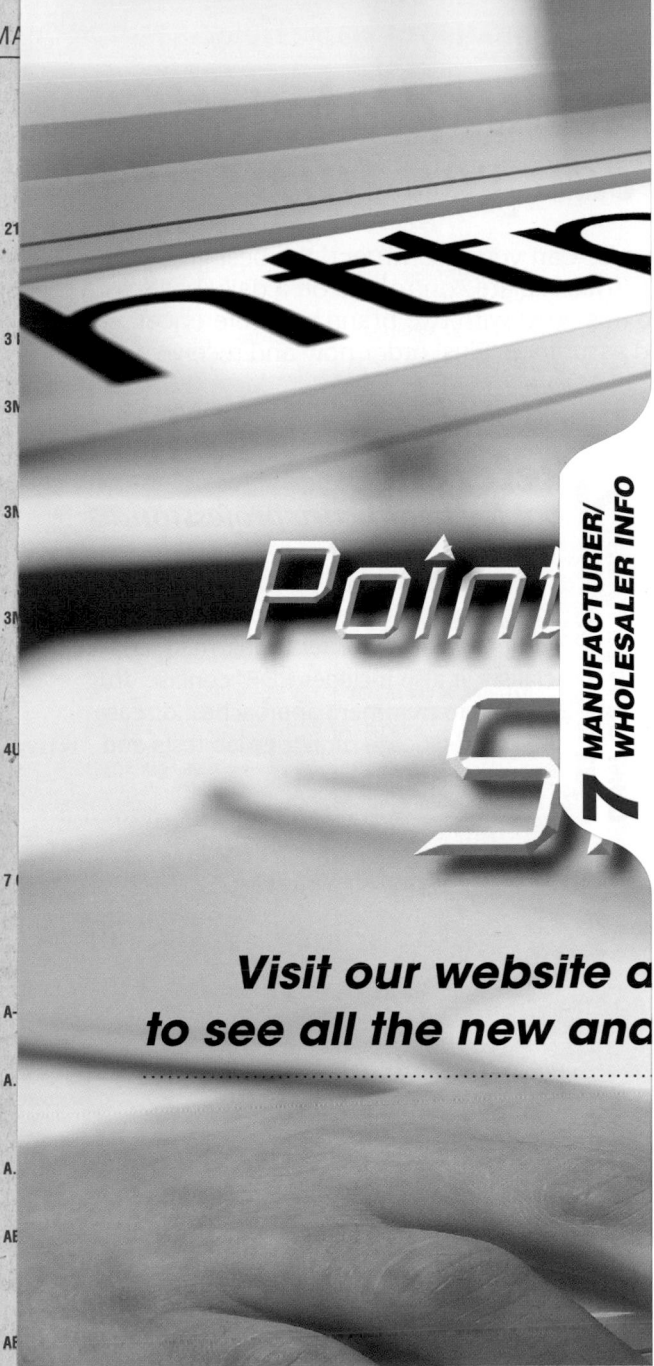

THERAPEUTICS, INC. 303-426-6262
0 CIRCLE POINT ROAD
E 200
TMINSTER, CO 80020

GEN LABORATORIES, INC. 770-475-8973
HEMBREE PARK DRIVE
E 112.
WELL, GA 30076

BIOLOGICS INC. 845-680-2400
NGS HIGHWAY
NGEBURG, NY 10962

E PHARMACEUTICALS, INC. 631-722-5988
WEST LANE
BOX 849
EBOGUE, NY 11931

NATIVA NATURAL 866-630-3001
MILL ROAD
AM, NY 11727

HARMACEUTICALS, INC. 813-968-0522
OX 271150
PA, FL 33688-1150

A PHARMACEUTICALS, INC. 562-906-9000
0 MCCANN DRIVE
TA FE SPRINGS, CA 90670

MCO PHARMACAL PANIES, INC. 847-663-0700
N. MERRIMAC AVENUE
S, IL 60714-3423

EN, INC. 973-796-2412
MPUS DRIVE
FLOOR
SIPPANY, NJ 07054

COMPANY, INC. 800-793-2666
WAY 60 EAST
CRYSTAL, MN 56055

PHARMACEUTICALS, INC. 617-498-3300
HAYDEN AVENUE
NGTON, MA 02421

DRUG & CHEMICAL PANY 973-926-0331
ORDIER STREET
NGTON, NJ 07111

CAN HEALTH PACKAGING 614-492-8177
JOHN GLENN AVENUE,
E A
UMBUS, OH 43217

CAN HYGIENIC LABS., INC. 305-756-4907
NE 79TH STREET
MI, FL 33138

CAN MEDICAL ID 512-826-0688
BEE CAVES ROAD
DING B, SUITE 22
TIN, TX 78746

CAN RED CROSS, OD SERVICES 800-446-8883
rican Red Cross, Plsma Svcs
E. STREET N.W.
HINGTON, DC 20006

CAN REGENT, INC. 631-924-4000
SIDIARY OF
POLD PHARM. INC.
LUITPOLD DRIVE
LEY, NY 11967

DERM LABORATORIES, LTD. 973-279-5100
PENNSYLVANIA AVENUE
RSON, NJ 07503

FIT BRANDS, INC. 860-894-1200
EBETHE DRIVE
E 102
MWELL, CT 06416

SOURCEBERGEN CORP. 610-727-7000
MORRIS DRIVE
TERBROOK, PA 190875594

USA INC. 805-447-1000
n Inc.
AMGEN CENTER DRIVE
USAND OAKS, CA 913201799

L PHARMACEUTICALS LLC 270-629-2596
HIPPOCRATES WAY
GOW, KY 42141

AMPHASTAR PHARMACEUTICALS INC. 800-423-4136
11570 SIXTH ST.
RANCHO CUCAMONGA, CA 91730

AMRITA AROMATHERAPY 641-472-9136
1900 C. WEST STONE AVE
FAIRFIELD, IA 52556

AMSINO MEDICAL USA 619-332-9959
5209 LINBAR DRIVE,
SUITE 640
NASHVILLE, TN 37211

AMYLIN PHARMACEUTICALS, INC. 858-552-2200
9360 TOWNE CENTRE DRIVE
SAN DIEGO, CA 92121

ANCHEN PHARMACEUTICALS, INC. 949-837-6178
9601 JERONIMO
IRVINE, CA 92618

ANDERSEN PHARMACEUTICALS, LLC. 607-334-2877
5851 COUNTY RD 32
P.O. BOX 848
NORWICH, NY 13815

ANI PHARMACEUTICALS, INC. 218-634-3500
210 MAIN STREET WEST
BAUDETTE, MN 56623

ANIMAS CORPORATION 610-644-8990
590 LANCASTER AVENUE
FRAZER, PA 19355

ANSELL HEALTHCARE INC. 732-345-5400
200 SCHULZ DRIVE
RED BANK, NJ 077016745

ANTARES PHARMA, INC. 763-475-7700
13755 1ST AVE NORTH
SUITE 100
MINNEAPOLIS, MN 55441

APACE PACKAGING, LLC 270-434-2722
12954 FOUNTAIN RUN ROAD
P.O.BOX 190
FOUNTAIN RUN, KY 42133

APLICARE, INC. 203-630-0500
550 RESEARCH PARKWAY
MERIDEN, CT 06405

APOTEX CORP. 954-384-8007
2400 N. COMMERCE PARKWAY
#400
WESTON, FL 33326

APOTHECARY PRODUCTS 800-328-2742
11750 12TH AVENUE S.-
BURNSVILLE, MN 553371297

APOTHECARY VISION CARE CO. 305-756-4907
859 NE 79TH STREET
MIAMI, FL 33138

APOTHECUS PHARMACEUTICAL CORP. 516-624-8200
220 TOWNSEND SQUARE
OYSTER BAY, NY 11771

APP (AMERICAN PHARMACEUTICAL PARTNERS, INC.) 888-391-6300
American Bioscience, Inc.
1501 E. WOODFIELD ROAD,
SUITE 300
SCHAUMBURG, IL 60173

APP PHARMACEUTICALS, LLC 847-969-2700
1501 E. WOODFIELD ROAD
SUITE 300 EAST
SCHAUMBURG, IL 60173

APPLIED NUTRITION CORP. 973-734-0023
10 SADDLE ROAD
CEDAR KNOLLS, NJ 07927

APPLIED NUTRITION, INC. 800-883-4851
Linus Pauling Vitamins
5310 BEETHOVEN STREET
LOS ANGELES, CA 90066

AQ PHARMACEUTICALS, INC. 714-903-1000
11555 MONARCH ST.
GARDEN GROVE, CA 92841

AQUA PHARMACEUTICALS, LLC. 610-644-7000
158 WEST GAY STREET
SUITE 310
WEST CHESTER, PA 119380

AR SCIENTIFIC, INC. 877-960-2400
1100 ORTHODOX STREET
PHILADELPHIA, PA 19124

ARBOR PHARMACEUTICALS, INC. 919-792-1700
4505 FALLS OF NEUSE ROAD
SUITE 420
RALEIGH, NC 27609

ARCO PHARMACEUTICALS, INC. 800-645-5412
2100 SMITHTOWN AVE
RONKONKOMA , NY 11717

ARISTOS PHARMACEUTICALS 866-280-5755
1255 CRESCENT GREEN DRIVE
SUITE 250
CARY, NC 27518

ARKRAY 952-646-3200
5198 W 76TH STREET
EDINA, MN 55439

ARMSTRONG PHARMACEUTICALS 800-423-4136
Amphastar Pharmaceuticals Inc.
423 LAGRANGE STREET
WEST ROXBURY, MA 02132

ARZOL CHEMICAL COMPANY 603-352-5242
12 NORWAY AVENUE #2
KEENE, NH 034313740

ASAFI PHARMACEUTICAL 661-294-9509
Home-Aid-Healthcare, Inc.
P.O. BOX 801764
SANTA CLARITA, CA 91380-1764

ASCEND LABORATORIES, LLC 201-476-1977
180 SUMMIT AVENUE
SUITE 200
MONTVALE, NJ 07645

ASCEND THERAPEUTICS INC. 703-471-4744
607 HERNDON PARKWAY
SUITE 210
HERNDON, VA 20170

ASCHER, B. F. & CO., INC. 913-888-1880
15501 WEST 109TH STREET
LENEXA, KS 66219-1308

ASTELLAS PHARMA US, INC. 847-317-8800
THREE PARKWAY NORTH
DEERFIELD, IL 60015

ASTRAZENECA LP 302-886-8800
1800 CONCORD PIKE
P. O. BOX 15437
WILMINGTON, DE 19850-5437

ATHENA FEMININE TECHNOLOGIES, INC. 925-254-6090
21 ORINDA WAY
C246
ORINDA, CA 94563

ATHLON PHARMACEUTICALS, INC. 205-986-1111
P.O. BOX 26708
BIRMINGHAM, AL 35260

ATLEY PHARMACEUTICALS, INC. 804-227-2250
10511 OLD RIDGE ROAD
ASHLAND, VA 23005

ATON PHARMA, INC. 609-671-9010
3150 BRUNSWICK PIKE
SUITE 130
LAWRENCEVILLE, NJ 08648

ATS PHARMACEUTICALS 805-437-7200
5284 ADOLFO ROAD
SUITE 150
CAMARILLO, CA 93012

ATTENDS HEALTHCARE PRODUCTS, INC. 252-752-1100
1029 OLD CREEK ROAD
GREENVILLE, NC 27834

AURIGA PHARMACEUTICALS, LLC. 678-282-1600
5555 TRIANGLE PARKWAY
SUITE 300
NORCROSS, GA 30092

AUROBINDO PHARMA USA, INC. 732-839-9400
2400 ROUTE 130 NORTH
DAYTON, NJ 08810

AURORA HEALTH CARE 414-747-3773
180 WEST GRANGE AVENUE
MILWAUKEE, WI 53207

AUTOMATIC LIQUID PACKAGING, INC. 800-638-9778
2200 LAKE SHORE DRIVE
WOODSTOCK, IL 60098-7498

AUXILIUM PHARMACEUTICALS, INC. 484-321-5900
40 VALLEY STREAM PKWY
MALVERN, PA 19355

AVIDAS PHARMACEUTICALS, LLC 267-895-1755
196 WEST ASHLAND STREET
DOYLESTOWN, PA 18901

AVOCET POLYMER TECHNOLOGIES, INC. 815-609-2170
23560 W MAIN ST., RTE 126
UNIT # 2
PLAINFIELD, NJ 60544

AXCAN PHARMA US, INC. 205-991-8085
22 INVERNESS CENTER PARKWAY
BIRMINGHAM, AL 35242
CORPORATION

AXIOM PHARMACEUTICAL 815-399-2060
695 N. PERRYVILLE ROAD
ROCKFORD, IL 61107

AXOGEN, INC. 386-462-6800
13859 PROGRESS BLVD.
SUITE 100
ALACHUA, FL 32615

AZUR PHARMA, INC. 215-832-3750
1818 MARKET STREET
SUITE 2350
PHILADELPHIA, PA 19103

B

B. BRAUN MEDICAL INC. 610-691-5400
824 12TH AVENUE
BETHLEHEM, PA 18018-3524

B&B PHARMACEUTICALS, INC. 303-755-5110
17200 E OHIO DRIVE
AURORA, CO 80017

BAKER, J.T. 800-582-2537
Mallinckrodt Baker, Inc.
A DIV. OF MALLINCKRODT BAKER, INC.
222 RED SCHOOL LANE
PHILLIPSBURG, NJ 08865

BALLAY PHARMACEUTICALS, INC. 512-847-6458
200 STILLWATER
WIMBERLEY, TX 78676

BASIC ORGANICS, INC. 614-863-3004
885 CLAYCRAFT ROAD
COLUMBUS, OH 43230

BASIC VITAMINS 800-782-2742
P.O. BOX 412
VANDALIA, OH 45377

BAUSCH & LOMB INCORPORATED 800-344-8815
8500 HIDDEN RIVER PARKWAY
PO BOX 450
TAMPA, FL 33637

BAXTER HEALTHCARE BIOSCIENCE DIVISION 800-4232-090
Baxter Healthcare Corp.
ONE BAXTER PARKWAY
BUILDING 3, THIRD FLOOR (DF3 3W)
DEERFIELD, IL 60015

BAXTER HEALTHCARE CORP. 888-229-0001
RTL-10
ROUTE 120 & WILSON ROAD
ROUND LAKE, IL 60073

BAYER CORP., PHARMACEUTICAL/ BIOLOGICAL DIVISION 800-205-0666
400 MORGAN LANE
WEST HAVEN, CT 065164-175

BAYER HEALTHCARE LLC E DIABETES CAR 800-248-2637
430 S. BEIGER STREET
P.O. BOX 2009
MISHAWAKA, IN 46544

BAYER HEALTHCARE PHARMACEUTICALS INC. 888-842-2937
P.O. BOX 1000
MONTVILLE, NJ 07045

BAYER HEALTHCARE, CONSUMER CARE DIVISION 800-348-2240
Bayer Corp., Pharmaceutical/
Biological Division
36 COLUMBIA ROAD
P.O. BOX 1910
MORRISTOWN, NJ 07962-1910

BAYER HEALTHCARE, LLC. 800-248-2637
P.O. BOX 2009
430 SOUTH BEIGER STREET
MISHAWAKA, IN 46544

BAYPHARMA, INC. 218-634-3500
ANI Pharmaceuticals, Inc.
210 MAIN STREET
BAUDETTE, MN 56623

BEACH PHARMACEUTICALS, DIV. OF BEACH PRODUCTS, INC. 800-322-8210
5220 S. MANHATTAN AVENUE
P.O. BOX 13447
TAMPA, FL 33681-3447

BEAUMONT PRODUCTS, INC. 800-451-7096
1560 BIG SHANTY DRIVE
KENNESAW, GA 30144

BECTON DICKINSON CONSUMER PRODUCTS PRODUCTS 201-847-6800
Becton, Dickinson and Company
1 BECTON DRIVE
FRANKLIN LAKES, NJ 07417

BECTON DICKINSON HOSPITAL PRODUCTS PRODUCTS 201-847-6800
Becton, Dickinson and Company
1 BECTON DRIVE
MAIL CODE 364
FRANKLIN LAKES, NJ 07417-1884

BECTON DICKINSON MEDICAL SYSTEMS, IV DIVISION 801-565-2300
Becton, Dickinson and Company
9450 SOUTH STATE STREET
SANDY, UT 84070

BEDFORD LABORATORIES 440-232-3320
Boehringer Ingelheim
Pharmaceuticals, Inc.
300 NORTHFIELD ROAD
BEDFORD, OH 44146

BEIERSDORF, INC. 203-563-5800
187 DANBURY RD.
WILTON, CT 06897

BERNA PRODUCTS 305-443-2900
4216 PONCE DE LEON BLVD.
CORAL GABLES, FL 33146

BESTMED, LLC 303-271-0300
311 CORPORATE CIRCLE
STE E
GOLDEN, CO 80401

BETA DERMACEUTICALS, INC. 210-349-9326
P. O. BOX 691106
SAN ANTONIO, TX 78269-1106

BETHANY PHARMACAL CO., INC. 217-665-3395
P.O. BOX 248
131 W. MAIN STREET
BETHANY, IL 61914

BEUTLICH LP, PHARMACEUTICALS 847-473-1100
1541 SHIELDS DRIVE
WAUKEGAN, IL 60085

BIO-PHARM INC. 215-949-3711
2091 HARTEL STREET
LEVITTOWN, PA 19057

BIO-TECH PHARMACAL, INC. 800-345-1199
P. O. BOX 1992
FAYETTEVILLE, AR 72702

BIOCODEX, INC. PHARMACEUTICAL LABORATORIES 650-243-5320
1250 BAYHILL DRIVE,
SUITE 315
SAN BRUNO, CA 94066

BIOGEN IDEC 617-679-2000
14 CAMBRIDGE CENTER
CAMBRIDGE, MA 02142

BIOMARIN PHARMACEUTICAL INC. 415-506-6700
105 DIGITAL DRIVE
NOVATO, CA 94949

BIOMERICA, INC. 800-854-3002
1533 MONROVIA AVENUE
NEWPORT BEACH, CA 92663

BIONEXUS, LTD. 607-266-9492
30 BROWN ROAD
ITHACA, NY 14850

BIONICHE PHARMA USA LLC 888-258-4199
272 EAST DEERPATH ROAD
SUITE 304
LAKE FOREST, IL 60045

BIONUTRICS HEALTH PRODUCTS, INC. 602-508-0112
2415 E. CAMELBACK RD STE 700
PHOENIX, AZ 85016

BIOPELLE, INC. 866-424-6735
780 WEST EIGHT MILE ROAD
FERNDALE, MI 48220

BIORX LABORATORIES 310-855-0475
369 SOUTH DOHENY DR
#326
BEVERLY HILLS, CA 90211

BIOTEST PHARMACEUTICALS CORPORATION 561-989-5800
5800 PARK OF COMMERCE BLVD., NW
BOCA RATON, FL 33487

BIOTROL INTERNATIONAL 800-822-8550
13705 SHORELINE COURT EAST
EARTH CITY, MO 63045

BIOVITRUM AB 866-276-2078
SE-112 76
STOCKHOLM, SWEDEN 11276

BLAINE LABS 800-307-8818
11037 LOCKPORT PLACE
SANTA FE SPRINGS, CA 90670

BLAINE PHARMACEUTICALS 859-344-9600
1717 DIXIE HIGHWAY
SUITE 700
FORT WRIGHT, KY 41011

BLAIREX LABORATORIES, INC. 812-378-1864
1600 BRIAN DR.
COLUMBUS, IN 47201

BLANSETT PHARMACAL CO., INC. 501-758-8635
P.O. BOX 638
NORTH LITTLE ROCK, AR 72115

BLU PHARMACEUTICALS LLC 270-586-6386
301 ROBEY STREET
FRANKLIN, KY 42134

BOCA PHARMACAL, INC. 954-346-8810
3550 NW 126TH AVENUE
CORAL SPRINGS, FL 33065

BOEHRINGER INGELHEIM CONSUMER HEALTHCARE 888-285-9159
Boehringer Ingelheim
Pharmaceuticals, Inc.
900 RIDGEBURY ROAD
P. O. BOX 368
RIDGEFIELD, CT 06877

BOEHRINGER INGELHEIM PHARMACEUTICALS, INC. 203-798-9988
900 RIDGEBURY ROAD
P. O. BOX 368
RIDGEFIELD, CT 06877-0368

BOIRON USA 610-325-7464
6 CAMPUS BLVD.
NEWTOWN SQUARE, PA 19073

BOSCOGEN, INC. 949-380-4317
11 MORGAN
IRVINE, CA 92618

BOTANICAL LABORATORIES, INC. 360-384-5656
1441 WEST SMITH ROAD
FERNDALE, WA 98248

BOUDREAUX'S BUTT PASTE 800-368-7274
13405 SEYMOUR MYERS BLVD.
SUITE 29
COVINGTON, LA 70433

BRACCO DIAGNOSTICS INC. 800-631-5245
107 COLLEGE ROAD
PRINCETON, NJ 08543

BRAINTREE LABORATORIES, INC. 781-843-2202
60 COLUMBIAN STREET WEST
PO BOX 850929
BRAINTREE, MA 021850929

BRECKENRIDGE PHARMACEUTICAL, INC. 561-443-3314
1141 SOUTH ROGERS CIR
SUITE 3
BOCA RATON, FL 33487

BRIOSCHI, INC. 201-796-4226
19-01 POLLITT DRIVE
FAIR LAWN, NJ 07410

BRISTOL-MYERS SQUIBB & GILEAD SCIENCES, LLC 800-445-3235
333 LAKESIDE DRIVE
FOSTER CITY, CA 94404

BRISTOL-MYERS SQUIBB CONSUMER MEDICINES 609-897-2000
Bristol-Myers Squibb U.S.
Medicines Group
A BRISTOL-MYERS SQUIBB COMPANY
777 SCUDDERS MILL RD
PLAINSBORO, NJ 08536

BRISTOL-MYERS SQUIBB MATURE BRANDS 609-897-2000
Bristol-Myers Squibb U.S.
Medicines Group
BRISTOL-MYERS SQUIBB COMPANY
777 SCUDDERS MILL RD
PLAINSBORO, NJ 08536

BRISTOL-MYERS SQUIBB ONCOLOGY/VIROLOGY 800-426-7644
Bristol-Myers Squibb U.S. Medicines Group
A BRISTOL-MYERS SQUIBB COMPANY
777 SCUDDERS MILL RD
PLAINSBORO, NJ 08536

BRISTOL-MYERS SQUIBB U.S. MEDICINES GROUP 609-897-2000
777 SCUDDERS MILL RD
PLAINSBORO, NJ 08536

BRISTOL-MYERS SQUIBB U.S. PHARMACEUTICALS/INST 800-631-5244
777 SCUDDERS MILL RD
PLAINSBORO, NJ 08536

BRYAN CORPORATION 781-935-0004
4 PLYMPTON STREET
WOBURN, MA 01801

BRYANT RANCH PREPACK 818-764-7225
12623 SHERMAN WAY #A
NORTH HOLLYWOOD, CA 91605

BTA PHARMACEUTICALS, INC. 908-927-1400
700 ROUTE 202-206 NORTH
P.O. BOX 6935
BRIDGEWATER, NJ 08807

C

CADBURY ADAMS USA LLC 973-909-2000
389 INTERPACE PARKWAY
PARSIPPANY, NJ 07054

CADISTA PHARMACEUTICALS, INC. 410-860-8500
207 KILEY DRIVE
SUITE 220
SALISBURY, MD 21801

CALMOSEPTINE, INC. 714-840-3405
16602 BURKE LANE
HUNTINGTON BEACH, CA 92647-4536

CAMBER PHARMACEUTICALS, INC. 732-377-2029
200 CENTENNIAL AVENUE
STE 200
PISCATAWAY, NJ 08854

CAMBROOKE FOODS, LLC 508-782-2300
4 COPELAND DRIVE
AYER, MA 01432

CAN-AM CARE 678-795-3440
Access Product Mktg
3780 MANSELL ROAD, T-50
ALPHARETTA, GA 30022

CAPELLON PHARMACEUTICALS LTD. 817-595-5820
7509 FLAGSTONE STREET
FORT WORTH, TX 76118

CARACO PHARMACEUTICAL LABS., LTD. 313-871-8400
1150 ELIJAH MCCOY DRIVE
DETROIT, MI 48202

CARDINAL HEALTH, INC. 614-757-5000
7000 CARDINAL PLACE
DUBLIN, OH 43016

CARDINAL PHARMACEUTICALS 562-696-1954
12035 E. BURKE ST., STE. 9
SANTA FE SPRINGS, CA 90670

CARE-TECH LABORATORIES, INC. 800-325-9681
DIV. CONSOLIDATED CHEMICAL INC.
3224 SO. KINGSHIGHWAY BLVD
ST. LOUIS, MO 63139-1183

CARLSBAD TECHNOLOGY, INC. 760-431-8284
5923 BALFOUR COURT
CARLSBAD, CA 92008

CARLSON, J. R., LABS., INC. 847-255-1600
15 COLLEGE DRIVE
ARLINGTON HEIGHTS, IL 60004-1985

CARMA LABORATORIES, INC. 414-421-7707
5801 W. AIRWAYS AVENUE
FRANKLIN, WI 53132

CAROLINA MEDICAL PRODUCTS CO. 252-753-7111
P. O. BOX 147
8026 US 264 ALTERNATE
FARMVILLE, NC 27828

CARRINGTON LABORATORIES, INC. 972-518-1300
2001 WALNUT HILL LANE
IRVING, TX 75038

CARWIN ASSOCIATES, INC. 205-369-6857
180 ST. CLAIR SHORES, RD
CROPWELL, AL 35054

CEBERT PHARMACEUTICALS, INC. 205-981-0201
1200 CORPORATE DRIVE,
SUITE 370
BIRMINGHAM, AL 35242

CELGENE CORPORATION 732-271-1001
86 MORRIS AVENUE
SUMMIT, NJ 07901

CENTOCOR ORTHO BIOTECH PRODUCTS, L.P. 610-651-6000
800 RIDGEVIEW DRIVE
HORSHAM, PA 19044

CENTOCOR ORTHO BIOTECH, INC. 610-651-6000
800 RIDGEVIEW DRIVE
HORSHAM, PA 19044

CENTRIX PHARMACEUTICAL INC. 205-991-9878
31 INVERNESS CENTER PARKWAY
SUITE #270
BIRMINGHAM, AL 35242

CENTURION LABS, LLC. 601-720-0111
657 HWY SOUTH
SUITE B
RICHLAND, MS 39218

CENTURY PHARMACEUTICALS, INC. 317-849-4210
10377 HAGUE ROAD
INDIANAPOLIS, IN 46256

CEPHALON, INC. 610-344-0200
41 MOORES ROAD
FRAZER, PA 19355

CEPHAZONE PHARMA, LLC 909-392-8900
250 EAST BONITA AVENUE
POMONA, CA 91767

CERA PRODUCTS, INC. 410-309-1000
9017 MENDEN HALL COURT
COLUMBIA, MD 21045

CETYLITE INDUSTRIES, INC. 856-665-6111
9051 RIVER ROAD
P.O. BOX 90006
PENNSAUKEN, NJ 08110-3293

CHAIN DRUG CONSORTIUM, LLC 412-828-2061
1020 WILLIAM PITT WAY
SUITE 338
PITTSBURG, PA 15238

CHAIN DRUG MARKETING ASSOC., INC. 248-449-9300
43517 W. NINE MILE ROAD
P.O. BOX 995
NOVI, MI 483760995

CHATTEM CONSUMER PRODUCTS 800-366-6833
1715 W. 38TH STREET
CHATTANOOGA, TN 37409

CHIRHOCLIN, INC. 301-476-8333
4000 BLACKBURN LANE
SUITE 270
BURTONSVILLE, MD 20866

CIBA VISION CORPORATION 800-241-5999
Novartis Pharm
11460 JOHNS CREEK PKWY
DULUTH, GA 30097

CITRA ANTICOAGULANTS, INC. 781-848-2174
Cytosol Laboratories, Inc.
55 MESSINA DRIVE
BRAINTREE, MA 02184

CLAIROL, INC. 203-357-5000
1 BALATCHLEY ROAD
STAMFORD, CT 06922

CLARIS LIFESCIENCES, INC. 732-422-9100
1445, US HIGHWAY 130
NORTH BRUNSWICK, NJ 08902

CLINT PHARMACEUTICALS, INC. 800-677-5022
629 SHUTE LANE
OLD HICKORY, TN 37138

COATS ALOE INTERNATIONAL, INC. 210-573-7055
249 HUNTERS DAWN
LA VERNEA, TX 78121

CODADOSE, INC. 678-866-0172
5659 SOUTHFIELD DRIVE
SUITE B
FLOWERT BRANCH, GA 30542

CODY LABORATORIES, INC. 307-587-7099
601 YELLOWSTONE AVE.
CODY, WY 82414

COLGATE ORAL PHARMACEUTICALS 781-821-2880
1 COLGATE WAY
CANTON, MA 02021

COLGATE-PALMOLIVE COMPANY 212-310-2000
300 PARK AVENUE
NEW YORK, NY 10022-7499

COLOPLAST CORP. 612-337-7800
200 SOUTH 6TH STREET
SUITE 900
MINNEAPOLIS, MN 55402

COLORADO BIOLABS, INC. 308-784-2444
404 M STREET
COZAD, NE 69130-0125

COLUMBIA LABORATORIES, INC. 973-994-3999
Columbia Drug Co., Inc.
354 EISENHOWER PARKWAY
PLAZA 1
LIVINGSTON, NJ 07039

COMBE, INC. 914-694-5454
1101 WESTCHESTER AVENUE
WHITE PLAINS, NY 10604

CONCEPTS IN CONFIDENCE 561-369-1700
2500 QUANTUM LAKES DRIVE
SUITE 214
BOYNTON BEACH, FL 33426

CONCORD LABORATORIES, INC. 973-227-6757
140 NEW DUTCH LANE
FAIRFIELD, NJ 07004

CONSOLIDATED MIDLAND CORP. 845-279-6108
20 MAIN STREET
BREWSTER, NY 10509

CONSUMER CHOICE SYSTEMS, INC. 800-479-5232
P.O. BOX 6740
NAPA, CA 94581

CONTINENTAL QUEST CORP. 317-843-2501
220 W. CARMEL DRIVE
CARMEL, IN 46032

CONTRACT PHARMACAL CORPORATION 631-231-4610
135 ADAMS AVENUE
HAUPPAUGE, NY 11788

CONVATEC 908-904-2500
Bristol-Myers Squibb U.S.
Medicines Group
100 HEADQUARTERS PARK
SKILLMAN, NJ 08558

COOK INCORPORATED 800-457-4500
750 DANIELS WAY
P.O. BOX 489
BLOOMINGTON, IN 47404

COOPER SURGICAL, INC. 203-601-5200
95 CORPORATE DRIVE
TRUMBULL, CT 06611

CORE PHARMACEUTICALS, INC. 818-545-1177
434 W. BROADWAY
GLENDALE, CA 91204

COREPHARMA, LLC 732-868-1090
215 WOOD AVENUE
MIDDLESEX, NJ 08846

CORNERSTONE THERAPEUTICS, INC. 919-678-6611
1255 CRESCENT GREEN DRIVE
SUITE 250
CARY, NC 27518

COTHERIX, INC. 650-808-6500
5000 SHORELINE COURT,
SUITE 101
SOUTH SAN FRANCISO, CA 94080

COUNTY LINE PHARMACEUTICALS, LLC 262-439-8109
13890 BISHOP'S DRIVE
SUITE 410
BROOKFIELD, WI 53005

COVIDIEN MALLINCKRODT 314-654-2000
675 MCDONNELL BLVD
HAZELWOOD, MO 63042

COVIDIEN SURGICAL DEVICES 203-845-1000
60 MIDDLETOWN ROAD
NORTH HAVEN, CT 06473

COVIDIEN/KENDALL/ TYCO HEALTHCARE 508-261-8000
15 HAMPSHIRE STREET
MANSFIELD, MA 02048

CREEKWOOD PHARMACEUTICAL, INC. 205-995-7390
31 INVERNESS CENTER PARKWAY
SUITE 270
BIRMINGHAM, AL 35242

CSL BEHRING LLC 610-878-4000
1020 FIRST AVENUE
P O BOX 61501
KING OF PRUSSIA, PA 19406

CSL BIOTHERAPIES, INC. 610-290-7400
1020 FIRST AVENUE
BOX 60446
KING OF PRUSSIA, PA 19406

CUBIST PHARMACEUTICALS, INC. 781-860-8660
65 HAYDEN AVENUE
LEXINGTON, MA 02421

CUMBERLAND PHARMACEUTICALS, INC. 615-255-0068
2525 WEST END AVENUE
SUITE 950
NASHVILLE, TN 37203

CUMBERLAND-SWAN, INC. 800-251-3068
ONE SWAN DRIVE
P. O. BOX 129
SMYRNA, TN 37167-0129

CURA PHARMACEUTICAL COMPANY, INC. 732-982-8300
542 INDUSTRIAL WAY WEST
EATONTOWN, NJ 07742

CUTISPHARMA, INC. 781-935-8141
68 CUMMINGS PARK
WOBURN, MA 01801

CUTIX, INC. 610-246-7518
585 E. SWEDESFORD ROAD
SUITE 200
WAYNE, PA 19087

CVS CORPORATION 401-765-1500
ONE CVS DRIVE
WONSOCKET, RI 02895

CYCLIN PHARMACEUTICALS, INC. 800-558-7046
1289 DEMING WAY
MADISON, WI 53717

CYPRESS PHARMACEUTICAL INC. 601-856-4393
135 INDUSTRIAL BLVD.
MADISON, MS 39110

CYTOSOL OPHTHALMICS, INC. 828-758-2343
PO BOX 1408
1325 WM. WHITE PLACE, NE
LENOIR, NC 28645

D

DAIICHI SANKYO, INC. 973-359-2600
11 PHILLIPS PARKWAY
MONTVALE, NJ 07645-1810

DANCO LABORATORIES, LLC 877-432-7596
PO BOX 4816
NEW YORK, NY 10185

DARTMOUTH PHARMACEUTICALS, INC. 508-295-2200
38 CHURCH AVENUE
WAREHAM, MA 02571

DAVA PHARMACEUTICALS 201-947-7442
400 KELBY ST.
10TH FLOOR PARKER PLAZA
FORT LEE, NJ 07024

DAVOL INC. 401-463-7000
SUB. OF C.R. BARD, INC.
100 SOCKANOSSETT CROSS ROAD
CRANSTON, RI 02920

DAXOR CORPORATION 212-330-8500
350 5TH AVE., STE. 7120
NEW YORK, NY 10118

DECA PHARMACEUTICALS, LLC. 270-842-3002
643 FAIRVIEW AVENUE
BOWLING GREEN, KY 42101

DEEN PRE-FILLED SYRINGES, LLC 615-834-0520
5209 LINBAR DRIVE,
SUITE 630
NASHVILLE, TN 37211

DEL PHARMACEUTICALS, INC. 800-645-4664
Dell Labs., Inc.
SUB. DEL LABORATORIES, INC.
726 RECKSON PLAZA
UNIONDALE, NY 11556

DEL-RAY DERMATOLOGICALS 423-926-4413
Crown Laboratories
P.O. BOX 1425
JOHNSON CITY, TN 37605

DELTA HI-TECH, INC. 801-263-0975
3762 SOUTH 150 EAST
SALT LAKE CITY, UT 84115

DELTA PHARMACEUTICALS INC. 803-407-7733
401 WESTERN LANE SUITE 10-C
IRMO, SC 29063

DENISON PHARMACEUTICALS, INC. 401-723-5500
60 DUNNELL LANE
P. O. BOX 1305
PAWTUCKET, RI 02860

DENT, C. S., & CO. 859-647-0777
Grandpa Brands Company
DIV. OF THE GRANDPA BRANDS
1820 AIRPORT EXCHANGE BLVD.
ERLANGER, KY 41018-3192

DENTSPLY PHARMACEUTICALS 717-767-8500
1301 SMILE WAY
YORK, PA 17404

DEPOMED, INC. 650-462-5900
1360 O'BRIEN DRIVE
MENLO PARK, CA 94025-1436

DEPUY MITEK 508-880-8100
325 PARAMOUNT DRIVE
RAYNHAM, MA 02767

DERMA SCIENCES, INC. 800-825-4325
214 CARNEGIE CENTER
SUITE 100
PRINCETON, NJ 08540

DERMALAB, INC. 847-266-0000
625 CENTRAL AVENUE
HIGHLAND PARK, IL 60035

DERMALOGIX PARTNERS, INC. 207-883-4103
P.O. BOX 1510
SCARBOROUGH, ME 04070

DERMARITE INDUSTRIES LLC. 973-569-9000
3 E. 26TH STREET
PATERSON, NJ 07514

DERMASAVE LABORATORIES, INC. 800-277-7099
3 CHARLES ST., BLDG. 1,
UNIT 4
PLEASANT VALLEY, NY 12569

DERMATONE LABORATORIES, INC. 860-292-1311
334 ELLA GRASSO TURNPIKE
SUITE 121
WINDSOR LOCKS, CT 06096-1150

DERMIK LABORATORIES, INC. 908-981-5000
A DIVISION OF
SANOFI-AVENTIS U.S.,LLC
55 CORP DRIVE.
BRIDGEWATER, NJ 08807

DESTON THERAPEUTICS, LLC 919-314-4730
6320 QUADRANGLE DRIVE
SUITE 100
CHAPEL HILL, NC 27517

DEXCOM, INC. 858-200-0200
6340 SEQUENCE DRIVE
SAN DIEGO, CA 92121

DEXGEN PHARMACEUTICALS, INC. 732-223-8811
P.O. BOX 675
MANASQUAN, NJ 08736

DEXO, LLC 913-339-9688
5370 COLLEGE BLVD
SUITE 115
OVERLAND PARK, KS 66211

DEY, L.P. 707-224-3200
2751 NAPA VALLEY CORP. DRIVE
NAPA, CA 94558

DHS, INC. 770-410-1588
250 HEMBREE PARK DRIVE
SUITE 112 B
ROSWELL, GA 30076

DIABETES TECHNOLOGIES, INC. 229-227-1245
184 BIG STAR DRIVE
PO BOX 1954
THOMASVILLE, GA 31757

DIABETIC SUPPLIES.COM, INC. 877-787-7543
2210 WEST MAIN STREET
107-388
BATTLE GROUND, WA 98604

DIAGNOSTIC DEVICES, INC. 704-285-6400
9300 HARRIS CORNERS PARKWAY
SUITE 450
CHARLOTTE, NC 28269

DICKINSON BRANDS, INC. 860-267-2279
31 EAST HIGH STREET
EAST HAMPTON, CT 06424

DIGESTIVE CARE, INC. 610-882-5950
1120 WIN DRIVE
BETHLEHEM, PA 18017-7058

DIHOMA INC. 843-423-7799
195 DREW ROAD
MULLINS, SC 29574

DIRECT PHARMACEUTICAL, INC. 256-721-2372
7293 WALL TRIANA HIGHWAY
SUITE D
MADISON, AL 35757

DISCUS DENTAL, LLC 310-845-8600
8550 HIGUERA ST.
CULVER CITY, CA 90232

DISETRONIC MEDICAL SYSTEMS, INC. 800-280-7801
Roche Diagnostics
11800 EXIT 5 PARKWAY
SUITE 120
FISHERS, IN 46038

DISPENSING SOLUTIONS, INC. 714-437-0330
3000 WEST WARNER AVE
SANTA ANA, CA 92704

DISTA PRODUCTS COMPANY 317-276-2000
Lilly, Eli & Company
DIV. ELI LILLY & CO.
LILLY CORPORATE CENTER
INDIANAPOLIS, IN 46285

DOAK DERMATOLOGICS 973-514-4240
Bradley Pharmaceuticals, Inc.
210 PARK AVENUE
Florham Park, NJ 07932

DOME INDUSTRIES, INC. 800-432-4352
TEN NEW ENGLAND WAY
WARWICK, RI 02887

DR REDDY'S LABORATORIES, INC. 866-733-3952
3600 ARCO CORPORATE DRIVE
SUITE 310
CHARLOTTE, NC 28273

DSE HEALTHCARE SOLUTIONS, LLC. 732-417-1870
164 NORTHFIELD AVE
P.O. BOX 6321
EDISON, NJ 08837

DUANE READE 212-273-5700
440 9TH AVENUE
NEW YORK, NY 10001

DURAMED PHARMACEUTICALS, INC. 888-482-9522
Teva Pharmaceuticals USA
425 PRIVET ROAD
HORSHAM, PA 19044

DUREX CONSUMER PRODUCTS 770-582-2222
3585 ENGINEERING DRIVE
STE 200
NORCROSS, GA 30092

DUSA PHARMACEUTICALS, INC. 978-657-7500
25 UPTON DRIVE
WILMINGTON, MA 01887

DUTCH OPHTHALMIC, USA 603-778-6929
10 CONTINENTAL DR, BLDG 1
EXETER, NH 03833

DYAX CORP. 617-225-2500
300 TECHNOLOGY SQUARE
CAMBRIDGE, MA 02139

E

E-Z-EM, INC. 800-443-6362
750 SUMMA AVENUE
WESTBURY, NY 11590

E.T. BROWNE DRUG COMPANY 201-894-9020
440 SYLVAN AVENUE
P.O. BOX 1613
ENGLEWOOD CLIFFS, NJ 07632

E5 PHARMA 954-346-8810
3550 NW 126TH AVENUE
CORAL SPRINGS, FL 33065

ECR PHARMACEUTICALS 804-527-1950
3969 DEEP ROCK ROAD
RICHMOND, VA 23233

EDENBRIDGE PHARMACEUTICALS, LLC 201-292-1292
119 CHERRY HILL ROAD
SUITE 310
PARSIPPANY, NJ 07054

EDWARDS PHARMACEUTICALS, INC. 662-837-8182
111 MULBERRY STREET
PO BOX 1110
RIPLEY, MS 38663

EISAI INC. 201-746-1100
100 TICE BLVD
WOODCLIFF LAKE, NJ 07677

EKR THERAPEUTICS, INC. 877-435-2524
7 EAST FREDRICK PLACE
CEDAR KNOLLS, NJ 07927

ELAN PHARMACEUTICALS, INC. 858-457-2553
Elan Corporation
7475 LUSK BLVD
SAN DIEGO, CA 92121

ELECTROLYTE LABORATORIES, INC. 303-757-8767
6803 E. BUCKNELL PLACE
DENVER, CO 80224

ELGE, INC. 281-232-0463
P.O. BOX 944
RICHMOND, TX 77406-0944

ELI RUTLEDGE, INC. 513-891-3400
10999 REED HARTMAN HWY
STE 220 B
CINCINNATI, OH 45242

ELLON TRADITIONAL FLOWER REMEDIES 800-423-2256
302 E WINONA AVE.
WARSAW, IN 46580

ELORAC, INC. 847-362-8200
100 FAIRWAY DRIVE
SUITE 134
VERNON HILLS, IL 60061

EMD SERONO, INC. 781-982-9000
ONE TECHNOLOGY PLACE
ROCKLAND, MA 02370

EMERGENT BIODEFENSE OPERATIONS LANSING INC. 517-327-1500
3500 N. MARTIN LUTER KING JR. BLVD.
LANSING, MI 48906

EMMAUS MEDICAL, INC. 310-214-0065
20725 S. WESTERN AVE.
STE 136
TORRANCE, CA 90501

ENCYTE SYSTEMS, INC. 781-848-2175
Cytosol Laboratories, Inc.
55 MESSINA DRIVE
BRAINTREE, MA 02184

ENDO GENERIC PRODUCTS 610-558-9800
Endo Pharmaceuticals, Inc.
DIV OF ENDO
PHARMACEUTICALS, INC.
100 ENDO BOULEVARD
CHADDS FORD, PA 19317

ENDO LABORATORIES 610-558-9800
Endo Pharmaceuticals, Inc.
DIV OF ENDO
PHARMACEUTICALS, INC.
100 ENDO BOULEVARD
CHADDS FORD, PA 19317

ENDO PHARMACEUTICALS, INC. 610-558-9800
100 ENDO BOULEVARD
CHADDS FORD, PA 19317

ENZON PHARMACEUTICALS, INC. 908-541-8600
685 ROUTE 202/206
BRIDGEWATER, NJ 08807

ESBA LABORATORIES INC. 561-746-0365
1001 JUPITER PARK DRIVE
SUITE 112
JUPITER, FL 33458

ETHEX CORPORATION 314-646-3750
ONE CORPORATE WOODS DRIVE
BRIDGETON, MO 63044

EURAND PHARMACEUTICALS, INC. 267-759-9400
790 TOWNSHIP LINE ROAD
SUITE 250
YARDLEY, PA 19067

EUSA PHARMA, INC. 215-867-4900
ONE SUMMIT SQUARE
1717 LANGHORNE NEWTOWN ROAD
LANGHORNE, PA 19407

EVERETT LABORATORIES, INC. 973-324-0200
29 SPRING STREET
W. ORANGE, NJ 07052-5415

EXCELLIUM PHARMACEUTICALS, INC. 973-276-9600
3G OAK ROAD
FAIRFIELD, NJ 07004

EXCELSIOR MEDICAL CORP 732-776-7525
1933 HECK AVENUE
NEPTUNE, NJ 07753

EXELINT INTERNATIONAL COMPANY 310-649-0707
5840 W. CENTINELA AVE.
LOS ANGELES, CA 90045

EYESUPPLY USA, INC. 813-975-2020
10770 N. 46TH STREET,
SUITE C-700
TAMPA, FL 33617

EYETECH INC. 866-744-6697
11360 JOG ROAD,
SUITE 200
PALM BEACH GARDENS, FL 33418

F

FAICHNEY MEDICAL COMPANY 636-240-9501
433 SCENIC DRIVE
ST. PETERS, MO 63376

FALCON PHARMACEUTICALS, LTD. 800-343-2133
Alcon Laboratories, Inc.
6201 SOUTH FREEWAY
FORT WORTH, TX 76134-2099

FAMILY PHARMACY 800-829-3132
1300 MORRIS DRIVE
GHESTERBROOK, PA 19087

FAULDING LABORATORIES INC. 732-465-3600
Alpharma USPD
ONE NEW ENGLAND AVE
PISCATAWAY, NJ 08854

FEI PRODUCTS LLC 800-322-4966
825 WURLITZER DRIVE
NORTH TONAWANDA, NY 14120

FEMALE HEALTH COMPANY, THE 312-595-9123
515 N. STATE ST.
SUITE 2225
CHICAGO, IL 60610

FERA PHARMACEUTICALS, LLC 516-277-1449
15R BIRCH HILL ROAD
LOCUST VALLEY, NY 11560

FERNDALE LABORATORIES, INC. 800-621-6003
780 W. EIGHT MILE ROAD
FERNDALE, MI 48220

FERRING PHARMACEUTICALS, INC. 973-796-1600
4 GATEHALL DRIVE
3RD FLOOR
PARSIPPANY, GA 07054

FERRIS MFG. CORP. 630-887-9797
16W300 83RD STREET
BURR RIDGE, IL 60527-5848

FLANDERS, INC. 843-571-3363
P. O. BOX 80428
ASHLEY RIVER STATION
CHARLESTON, SC 29416

FLAR MEDICINE OF PUERTO RICO, INC. 787-841-8181
P.O. BOX 981
COTTO LAUREL, PR 00780

FLEET, C. B., CO., INC. 434-528-4000
4615 MURRAY PLACE
P. O. BOX 11349
LYNCHBURG, VA 24506-1349

FLEMING PHARMACEUTICALS 636-343-5306
1733 GILSINN LANE
FENTON, MO 63026

FLEX-POWER INC. 510-529-9955
823 GILMAN STREET
BERKELEY, CA 94710

FLUORITAB CORP. 231-755-9113
1197 LAMBERT DRIVE
MUSKEGON, MI 49441

FOCUS LABORATORIES, INC. 501-753-6006
7645 COUNTS MASSIE RD
NORTH LITTLE ROCK, AR 72113

FORA CARE, INC. 805-498-8188
810 LAWRENCE DR.
SUITE 104
NEWBURY PARK, CA 91320

FORECARE, INC. 877-924-2273
1540 BARCLAY BLVD.
BUFFALO GROVE, IL 60089

FOREST PHARMACEUTICALS, INC. 800-678-1605
SUB. FOREST LABORATORIES, INC.
13600 SHORELINE DRIVE
ST. LOUIS, MO 63045

FORTE PHARMA 877-993-6783
Eon Labs, Inc.
DIVISION OF EON LABS MANUF., INC.
220 LAKE DRIVE
NEWARK, DE 19702

FOUGERA 631-454-6996
60 BAYLIS ROAD P.O. BOX 2006
MELVILLE, NY 11747

FRANK LETTEAU & ASSOC., LTD. 212-268-3400
22 WEST 32ND STREET
10TH FLOOR
NEW YORK, NY 10001

FREEDA VITAMINS, INC. 718-433-4337
47-25 34 TH STREET
SUITE 301
LONG ISLAND CITY, NY 11101

FRESENIUS MEDICAL CARE, NORTH AMERICA 781-699-9000
920 WINTER STREET
WALTHAM, MA 02451

FSC LABORATORIES, INC. 704-941-2500
6000 FAIRVIEW ROAD,
SUITE 600
CHARLOTTE, NC 28210

G

G & W LABORATORIES, INC. 908-753-2000
111 COOLIDGE STREET
SO. PLAINFIELD, NJ 07080

GALDERMA LABORATORIES, L.P. 817-961-5000
14501 N. FREEWAY
FT. WORTH, TX 76177

GALLIPOT, INC. 800-423-6967
2400 PILOT KNOB ROAD
ST. PAUL, MN 55120

GATE PHARMACEUTICALS 215-591-3000
Teva Pharmaceuticals USA
A DIV. OF TEVA
PHARMACEUTICALS USA
650 CATHILL ROAD
SELLERSVILLE, PA 18960

GE HEALTHCARE 609-514-6405
101 CARNEGIE CENTER
PRINCETON, NJ 08540

GEBAUER COMPANY 216-271-5252
4444 E. 153RD STREET
CLEVELAND, OH 44128

GENENTECH, INC. 650-225-1000
1 DNA WAY MS #219
SO. SAN FRANCISCO, CA 94080-4990

GENERAMEDIX INC. 908-504-1300
150 ALLEN ROAD
LIBERTY CORNER, NJ 07938

GENESIS PHARMACEUTICAL INC. 248-548-7846
9 CAMPUS DRIVE
PARSIPPANY, NJ 07054

GENSCO LABORATORIES, INC. 352-726-6284
110 W.HIGHLANDS. BLVD.
INVERNESS, FL 34452

GENTA INCORPORATED 908-286-9800
2 CONNELL DRIVE
BERKELEY HEIGHTS, NJ 07922

GENTEX PHARMA 601-201-7231
276 NISSAN PARKWAY
SUITE B
CANTON, MS 39046

GENZYME CORPORATION 617-252-7500
500 KENDALL STREET
CAMBRIDGE, MA 02142

GERI-CARE PHARMACEUTICALS 718-382-5000
1650 63RD STREET
BROOKLYN, NY 11204

GERITREX CORPORATION 914-668-4003
144 KINGSBRIDGE ROAD EAST
MOUNT VERNON, NY 10550

GIL PHARMACEUTICAL CORPORATION 787-848-9116
P.O. BOX 10489
PONCE, PR 00732-0489

GILEAD SCIENCES, INC. 800-445-3235
333 LAKESIDE DRIVE
FOSTER CITY, CA 94404

GLAXOSMITHKLINE CONSUMER HEALTHCARE 800-456-6670
Glaxo SmithKline Pharmaceuticals
1000 GSK DRIVE
MOON TOWNSHIP, PA 15108

GLAXOSMITHKLINE PHARMACEUTICALS 888-825-5249
3 FRANKLIN PLAZA
P.O. BOX 7929
PHILADELPHIA, PA 19101

GLENMARK PHARMACEUTICALS INC., USA 201-684-8000
750 CORPORATE DRIVE
MAHWAH, NJ 07430

GLENWOOD, LLC 201-569-0050
111 CEDAR LANE
P. O. BOX 5419
ENGLEWOOD, NJ 07631

GLOBAL HEALTH PRODUCTS, INC. 585-235-8815
1099 JAY STREET
SUITE 100E
ROCHESTER, NY 14611

GLOBAL PHARMACEUTICALS 215-933-0323
Impax Laboratories, Inc.
121 NEW BRITAIN BLVD
CHALFONT, PA 18914

GLOBAL SOURCE 954-747-8977
MANAGEMENT & CONSULTING, INC.
5371 N. HIATUS ROAD
SUNRISE, FL 333518718

GM PHARMACEUTICALS, INC. 817-461-8230
P. O. BOX 150312
ARLINGTON, TX 76015

GOLDEN STATE MEDICAL SUPPLY (GSMS) INC. 805-477-9866
5187 CAMINO RUIZ
CAMARILLO, CA 93012

GOLDEN SUNSHINE USA, INC. 714-223-0425
2880 E. IMPERIAL HIGHWAY
BREA, CA 92821

GOOD SAMARITAN LABORATORIES, INC. 215-794-7316
P. O. BOX 2138
DOYLESTOWN, PA 189010649

GORDON LABORATORIES 610-734-2011
6801 LUDLOW STREET
UPPER DARBY, PA 19082

GRACEWAY PHARMACEUTICALS, LLC. 484-321-5600
2 WEST LIBERTY BLVD
SUITE 203
MALVERN, PA 19355

GRANDPA SOAP CO. 859-647-0777
Grandpa Brands Company
DIVISION OF GRANDPA BRANDS CO.
1820 AIRPORT EXCHANGE BLVD.
ERLANGER, KY 410183192

GREEN TURTLE BAY VITAMIN CO., INC., THE 908-277-2240
56 HIGH STREET
P.O. BOX 642
SUMMIT, NJ 07902

GREENSTONE LLC 800-435-7095
100 ROUTE 206 NORTH
PEAPACK, NJ 07977

GRIFOLS USA, INC. 323-225-2221
2410 LILYVALE AVENUE
LOS ANGELES, CA 90032-

GTX, INC. 901-523-9700
175 TOYOTA PLAZA
SUITE 700
MEMPHIS, TN 38103

GUARDIAN LABORATORIES, DIV. UNITED-GUARDIAN, INC. 631-273-0900
230 MARCUS BOULEVARD
P.O. BOX 18050
HAUPPAUGE, NY 11788

H

HALL BIOSCIENCE CORPORATION 678-866-0173
5659 SOUTHFIELD DRIVE
FLOWERY BRANCH, GA 30542

HALLCREST PRODUCTS, INC. 847-998-8580
1820 PICKWICK LANE
GLENVIEW, IL 60025

HALOCARBON LABORATORIES 201-262-8899
P.O. BOX 661
RIVER EDGE, NJ 07661

HARRIS PHARMACEUTICAL, INC. 239-278-4749
9090 PARK ROYAL DRIVE
FT. MYERS, FL 33908

HART HEALTH 800-234-4278
P.O. BOX 94044
SEATTLE, WA 98124-9444

HAWKINS, INC. PHARMACEUTICAL GROUP 612-617-8600
3000 EAST HENNEPIN AVENUE
MINNEAPOLIS, MN 55413

HAWTHORN PHARMACEUTICALS 800-856-4393
Cypress Pharmaceutical Inc.
135 INDUSTRIAL BLVD.
MADISON, MS 39110

HEALTH CARE LABS. INC. 281-659-1591
112 S.COLLEGE AVE,
SUITE 100A
CLEVELAND, TX 77327

HEALTH CARE PRODUCTS 800-899-3116
Hi-Tech Pharmacal Co., Inc.
DIV. OF HI-TECH PHARMACAL,
369 BAYVIEW AVENUE
AMITYVILLE, NY 11701

HEALTH MANAGEMENT RESOURCES 617-357-9876
59 TEMPLE PLACE,
SUITE 704
BOSTON, MA 02111-1346

HEALTH PRODUCTS CORPORATION/HEALTH BRANDS 914-423-2900
1060 NEPPERHAN AVENUE.
YONKERS, NY 10703-1432

HEALTHPOINT 800-441-8227
3909 HULEN
FORT WORTH, TX 76107

HEEL INC. 505-293-3843
11600 COCHITI ROAD SE
ALBUQUERQUE, NM 87123

HEMISPHERX BIOPHARMA, INC. 215-988-0080
ONE PENN CENTER
1617 JFK BLVD
PHILADELPHIA, PA 19103

HERCON LABORATORIES CORPORATION 717-764-1191
P.O. BOX 467
101 SINKING SPRINGS LANE
EMIGSVILLE, PA 17318

HERITAGE BRAND/INSIGHT PHARMACEUTICALS 267-852-0505
550 TOWNSHIP LINE ROAD
SUITE 300
BLUE BELL, PA 19422

HERITAGE PHARMACEUTICALS INC. 732-429-1000
105 FIELDCREST AVE
SUITE 100
EDISON, NJ 08837

HEYLTEX CORPORATION 281-395-7040
1800 S MASON RD.
SUITE 260
KATY, TX 77450

HI-TECH PHARMACAL CO., INC. 631-789-8228
369 BAYVIEW AVENUE
AMITYVILLE, NY 11701-2801

HIGH CHEMICAL COMPANY 800-447-8792
3901A NEBRASKA STREET
LEVITTOWN, PA 19056

HILL DERMACEUTICALS INC. 407-323-1887
2650 SOUTH MELLONVILLE AVENUE
SANFORD, FL 327739311

HILLESTAD PHARMACEUTICALS USA, INC. 715-358-2113
178 U.S. HIGHWAY 51 NORTH
WOODRUFF, WI 54568-9501

HOBART LABORATORIES, INC. 218-751-9505
7736 GRANT CREEK RD NW
BEMIDJI, MN 56601

HOGIL PHARMACEUTICAL CORP. 914-696-7600
TWO MANHATTANVILLE ROAD
PURCHASE, NY 10577-2118

HOLLISTER INCORPORATED 847-680-1000
2000 HOLLISTER DRIVE
LIBERTYVILLE, IL 60048

HOLLISTER-STIER LABORATORIES LLC 509-489-5656
3525 N. REGAL STREET
P.O. BOX 3145
SPOKANE, WA 99220-3145

HOME ACCESS HEALTH 847-781-2500
2401 WEST HASSELL ROAD
SUITE 1510
HOFFMAN ESTATES, IL 60195-5200

HOME DIAGNOSTICS, INC. 954-677-9201
2400 N.W. 55TH COURT
FORT LAUDERDALE, FL 33309

HOMEMED PROVIDER SOLUTIONS 317-522-1637
8875 BASH STREET
INDIANAPOLIS, IN 46256

HOPE PHARMACEUTICALS 480-607-1970
16416 NORTH 92ND STREET
#125
SCOTTSDALE, AZ 85260

HORMEL HEALTHLABS 561-434-6723
1 HORMEL PLACE
AUSTIN, MN 55912

HOSPIRA, INC. 877-946-7747
DEPT 36G, BLDG H-1
275 NORTH FIELD DRIVE
LAKE FOREST, IL 60045

HUB PHARMACEUTICALS, LLC 909-476-8394
9339 CHARLES SMITH AVENUE
BLDG#150
RANCHO CUCAMONGA, CA 91730

HUCKABY PHARMACEUTICALS, INC. 502-241-1570
6316 OLD LAGRANGE ROAD
CRESTWOOD, KY 40014

HUMCO 800-662-3435
7400 ALUMAX DRIVE
TEXARKANA, TX 75501

HVS LABORATORIES, INC. 941-643-4636
3663 ARNOLD AVENUE
NAPLES, FL 34104

HYGENIC PERFORMANCE HEALTH, INC. 800-246-3733
2230 BOYD ROAD
EXPORT, PA 15632

HYLAND'S INC. 310-768-0700
Standard Homeopathic Company
210 W. 131ST STREET
P. O. BOX 61067
LOS ANGELES, CA 90061

I

IKARIA / INO THERAPEUTICS LLC 908-238-6600
6 ROUTE 173
CLINTON, NJ 08809

IMARX THERAPEUTICS, INC. 520-770-1259
1730 EAST RIVER ROAD
SUITE 200
TUCSON, AZ 85719

IMMUNOMEDICS, INC. 973-605-8200
300 AMERICAN ROAD
MORRIS PLAINS, NJ 07950

IMMUNOTEC INC. 450-424-9992
300 JOSEPH-CARRIER
VAUDREUIL-DORION, QC J7V5V5

INJEX-EQUIDYNE SYSTEMS, INC. 714-777-5111
17662 IRVIN BLVD
SUITE 20
TUSTIN, CA 92780

INNOVATIVE HEALTH PRODUCTS, INC. 727-544-8866
695 BRYAN DAIRY ROAD
LARGO, FL 33777

INSIGHT PHARMACEUTICALS 267-852-0505
1170 WHEELER WAY
SUITE 150
LANGHORNE, PA 19047

INSPIRE PHARMACEUTICALS, INC. 919-941-9777
4222 EMPEROR BLVD.
DURHAM, NC 27703

INSTEAD, INC. 858-550-1901
4275 EXECUTIVE SQUARE
SUITE 440
LA JOLLA, CA 92037

INTEGRA LIFESCIENCES CORPORATION 609-275-0500
311 ENTERPRISE DRIVE
PLAINSBORO, NJ 08536

INTENDIS, INC. 866-463-3634
36 COLUMBIA ROAD
PO BOX 1941
MORRISTOWN, NJ 07962

INTERMUNE, INC. 415-466-2200
3280 BAYSHORE BLVD
BRISBANE, CA 94005

INTERNATIONAL ETHICAL LABS. 787-765-3510
AVENUE AMERICO MIRANDA
#1021
REPTO. METROPOLITANO
SAN JUAN, PR 00921

INTERNATIONAL TECHNIDYNE CORP. 732-548-5700
Thoratec
8 OLSEN AVENUE
EDISON, NJ 08820

INVADO PHARMACEUTICALS LLC 914-715-6232
25 RAVENNA DRIVE
POMONA, NY 10970

INVERNESS MEDICAL, INC. 800-899-7353
51 SAWYER RD
WALTHAM, MA 02453

INWOOD LABORATORIES, INC. 631-858-6000
Forest Pharmaceuticals, Inc.
500 COMMACK ROAD
COMMACK, NY 11725-5000

IPI PHARMACEUTICALS 267-725-3222
1800 BYBERRY ROAD
SUITE 1300
HUNTINGDON VALLEY, PA 19006

IROKO PHARMACEUTICALS LLC 367-546-3003
ONE CRESCENT DRIVE
SUITE 400
PHILADELPHIA, PA 19112

ISTA PHARMACEUTICALS 949-788-6000
15295 ALTON PARKWAY
IRVINE, CA 92618

IVAX CORPORATION 800-327-4114
4400 BISCAYNE BLVD
MIAMI, FL 33137

J

JACOBUS PHARMACEUTICAL COMPANY, INC. 609-921-7447
IRL BUILDING
SCHALKS CROSSING ROAD
PLAINSBORO, NJ 08536

JAMOL LABORATORIES, INC. 201-262-6363
13 ACKERMAN AVENUE
EMERSON, NJ 07630

JANSSEN PHARMACEUTICAL PRODUCTS, L.P. 609-526-7736
Johnson & Johnson
1125 TRENTON-HARBOURTON RD
P.O. BOX 200
TITUSVILLE, NJ 08560-0200

JAYMAC PHARMACEUTICALS LLC 337-662-5962
P.O. BOX 510
SUNSET, LA 70584

JAZZ PHARMACEUTICALS, INC. 650-496-3777
3180 PORTER DRIVE
PALO ALTO, CA 94304

JHP PHARMACEUTICALS, LLC 877-547-4547
MORRIS CORPORATE CENTER 2
ONE UPPER POND ROAD
PARSIPPANY, NJ 07054

JOHNSON & JOHNSON CONSUMER PRODUCTS COMPANY 908-874-1000
Johnson & Johnson
199 GRANDVIEW AVENUE
SKILLMAN, NJ 08558

JOHNSON & JOHNSON HEALTHCARE PRODUCTS-DIV. OF MCNEIL-PPC, INC. 908-874-1000
190 GRANDVIEW ROAD
SKILLMAN, NJ 08558

JOHNSON & JOHNSON MEDICAL, INC. 800-423-4018
Johnson & Johnson
2500 EAST ARBROOK BOULEVARD
P.O. BOX 90130
ARLINGTON, TX 76014-3631

JOHNSON & JOHNSON/ MERCK CONSUMER PHARMACEUTICALS CO. 215-273-7000
Johnson & Johnson
7050 CAMP HILL ROAD
FORT WASHINGTON, PA 19034

JOHNSON LABORATORIES
P.O. BOX 2184
EDEN, NC 27289

JSJ PHARMACEUTICALS 264-880-2360
3655 ROUTE 202
STE 116
DOYLESTOWN, PA 18901

K

K-PAX, INC. 415-381-7565
655 REDWOOD HIGHWAY
SUITE 346
MILL VALLEY, CA 94941

KARALEX PHARMA, LLC 201-529-0400
470 CHESTNUT RIDGE ROAD
WOODCLIFF LAKE, NJ 07677

KELTMAN PHARMACEUTICALS, INC. 601-936-7533
1 LAKELAND SQUARE
SUITE A
FLOWOOD, MS 39232

KENDALL HEALTHCARE PRODUCTS COMPANY 508-261-8000
15 HAMPSHIRE STREET
MANSFIELD, MA 02048

KENWOOD THERAPEUTICS 973-514-4240
Bradley Pharmaceuticals, Inc.
210 PARK AVE
FLORHAM PARK, NJ 07932

KEY COMPANY, THE 314-965-6699
1313 W. ESSEX AVE.
P.O. BOX 220370
ST. LOUIS, MO 63122

KIMBERLY-CLARK CORP., HEALTHCARE DIVISION 801-572-6800
12050 LONE PEAK PARKWAY
DRAPER, UT 84020

KING PHARMACEUTICALS, INC. 423-989-8000
501 FIFTH STREET
BRISTOL, TN 37620

KINGSWOOD LABORATORIES, INC. 800-968-7772
10375 HAGUE ROAD
INDIANAPOLIS, IN 46256-3316

KINRAY, INC. 718-767-1234
152-35 10TH AVENUE
WHITESTONE, NY 11357

KIRKMAN LABORATORIES, INC. 503-694-1600
6400 SW ROSEWOOD
LAKE OSWEGO, OR 97035

KLI CORP 317-846-7452
1119 THIRD AVENUE S.W.
CARMEL, IN 46032-2565

KONSYL PHARMACEUTICALS, INC. 410-822-5192
8050 INDUSTRIAL PARK ROAD
EASTON, MD 21601

KOWA PHARMACEUTICALS AMERICA, INC. 334-288-1288
530 INDUSTRIAL PARK BLVD
MONTGOMERY, AL 36124-0969

KRAMER LABORATORIES, INC. 800-824-4894
8778 S.W. 8TH STREET
MIAMI, FL 33174-9990

KRAMER-NOVIS 787-767-2072
Kramer Laboratories, Inc.
P.O. BOX 191775
SAN JUAN, PR 00919-1775

KREMERS URBAN LLC 262-238-9994
Schwarz Pharma
1950 LAKE PARK DRIVE
SMYRNA, GA 30080

KRS GLOBAL BIOTECHNOLOGY, INC. 561-961-4083
791 PARK OF COMMERCE BLVD
SUITE 500
BOCA RATON, FL 33487

KVK-TECH, INC. 215-579-1842
110 TERRY DRIVE
SUITE 200
NEWTOWN, PA 18940

L

L. PERRIGO COMPANY 269-673-8451
515 EASTERN AVE.
ALLEGAN, MI 49010

LAKE CONSUMER PRODUCTS, INC. 262-677-4121
1 PHARMACAL WAY
JACKSON, WI 53037

LANE LABS-USA, INC. 201-236-9090
25 COMMERCE DRIVE
ALLENDALE, NJ 07401

LANNETT COMPANY INC. 215-333-9000
9000 STATE ROAD
PHILADELPHIA, PA 19136

LANSINOH LABORATORIES 703-299-1100
333 NORTH FAIRFAX STREET
SUITE 400
ALEXANDRIA, VA 22314

LANTHEUS MEDICAL IMAGING 800-362-2668
331 TREBLE COVE ROAD
N. BILLERICA, MA 01862

LARKEN LABORATORIES, INC. 601-855-7678
276 NISSAN PKWY
SUITE B
CANTON, MS 39046

LARKSPUR GROUP, INC., THE 203-855-1301
19 CONCORD STREET
S. NORWALK, CT 06854

LASER PHARMACEUTICALS 864-286-8229
6003 PONDERS COURT
GREENVILLE, SC 29615

LCM PHARMACEUTICAL INC. 850-650-0589
1016 AIRPORT ROAD
SUITE 3
DESTIN, FL 32541

LEADING EDGE INNOVATIONS, INC. 805-388-7669
699 MOBIL AVENUE
CAMARILLO, CA 93010

LEC TEC CORPORATION 800-777-2291
10701 RED CIRCLE DRIVE
MINNETONKA, MN 55343

LEE PHARMACEUTICALS 626-442-3141
1434 SANTA ANITA AVENUE
SOUTH EL MONTE, CA 91733

LEGERE PHARMACEUTICALS, INC. 480-991-4033
7326 EAST EVANS ROAD
SCOTTSDALE, AZ 85260

LETCO MEDICAL, INC. 800-350-1297
1316 COMMERCE DRIVE NW
DECATUR, AL 35601

LEX PHARMACEUTICALS MFG. & PACKAGING 305-888-7375
7155 N. W. 77TH TERRACE
MEDLEY, FL 33166

LIBBY LABORATORIES, INC. 510-527-5400
1700 SIXTH STREET
BERKELEY, CA 94710-1806

LIFESCAN, INC. 408-263-9789
Johnson & Johnson
1000 GIBRALTAR DRIVE
MILPITAS, CA 95035-6312

LIL DRUG STORE PRODUCTS 319-294-3772
1201 CONTINENTAL PLACE NE
CEDAR RAPIDS, IA 52402

LILLY, ELI & COMPANY 317-276-2000
LILLY CORPORATE CENTER
INDIANAPOLIS, IN 46285

LINE ONE LABORATORIES, INC. (USA) 818-886-2288
21230 LASSEN STREET
CHATSWORTH, CA 91311

LINUS PAULING VITAMINS 800-841-8448
5310 BEETHOVEN STREET
LOS ANGELES, CA 90066

LIONHEARTED INDUSTRIES 800-464-5655
P.O.BOX 22
LAGUNA BEACH, CA 92652

LIPIVO 303-693-2338
16293 E. PRENTICE PLACE
CENTENNIAL, CO 80015

LLORENS PHARMACEUTICALS INTERNATIONAL DIV. 305-716-0595
6830 NW 77 CT
MIAMI, FL 33166

LOBANA LABORATORIES 800-848-5637
Ulmer Pharmacal
P.O. BOX 408
PARK RAPIDS, MN 56470

LOBOB LABORATORIES 408-432-0580
1440 ATTEBERRY LANE
SAN JOSE, CA 951311410

LOGAN PHARMACEUTICALS 888-644-3478
7672 MONTGOMERY RD.
STE#254
CINCINNATI, OH 45236

LOMA LUX LABORATORIES 918-664-9882
Plymouth Pharmaceuticals, Inc.
5117 S. 110th E. AVE.
TULSA, OK 74146

LORANN OILS 517-882-0215
P. O. BOX 22009
LANSING, MI 48909

LUMISCOPE CO., INC. 732-562-9002
1035 CENTENNIAL AVENUE
PISCATAWAY, NJ 08854

LUNDBECK, INC. 847-282-1000
FOUR PARKWAY NORTH
SUITE 200
DEERFIELD, IL 60015

LUNSCO, INC. 540-980-4358
4657 WURNO ROAD
PULASKI, VA 24301

LUPIN PHARMACEUTICALS, INC. 410-576-2000
HARBOR PLACE TOWER
111 SOUTH CALVERT STREET
BALTIMORE, MD 21202

LUYTIES PHARMACAL CO. 800-325-8080
P.O.BOX 8080
RICHFORD, VT 05476

LWP, INC. 310-783-7450
381 VAN NESS AVENUE
SUITE 1507
TORRANCE, CA 90501

M

M D C ASSOCIATES 847-793-0230
C/O DISTRIBCO, INC.
730 CORPORATE WOODS PARKWAY
VERNON HILLS, IL 60061

MACOVEN PHARMACEUTICALS, LLC 225-644-2494
33219 FOREST WEST DRIVE
MAGNOLIA, TX 77354

MAGNA PHARMACEUTICALS, INC. 502-254-5552
Paradigm Healthcare Solns, Inc.
10801 ELECTRON DRIVE
LOUISVILLE, KY 40299

MAGNO-HUMPHRIES LABORATORIES, INC. 503-684-5464
8800 S.W. COMMERCIAL STREET
TIGARD, OR 97223

MAJESTIC DRUG CO., INC. 845-436-0011
4996 MAIN STREET
P.O. BOX 490
SOUTH FALLSBURG, NY 12779

MAJOR PHARMACEUTICALS 800-875-0123
Apotex Corp.
31778 ENTERPRISE DRIVE
LIVONIA, MI 48150

MALLINCKRODT INC. 314-654-2000
675 MCDONNELL BLVD.
ST. LOUIS, MO 63042

MALLINCKRODT LABORATORY CHEMICALS 800-354-2050
Mallinckrodt Baker, Inc.
222 RED SCHOOL LANE
PHILLIPSBURG, NJ 08865

MANCHESTER PHARMACEUTICALS, INC. 970-685-4119
8236 BENSON COURT
FORT COLLINS, CO 80525

MANN CHEMICAL CORP. 502-585-2001
757 LOGAN STREET
LOUISVILLE, KY 40204-1849

MANNE CO. 800-517-0228
P.O. BOX 825
JOHNS ISLAND, SC 29457

MARATHON PHARMACEUTICALS LLC 866-945-7860
1751 LAKE COOK ROAD
SUITE 400
DEERFIELD, IL 60015

MARLEX PHARMACEUTICALS, INC. 302-328-3355
50 MC CULLOUGH DRIVE
SOUTHGATE CENTER
NEW CASTLE, DE 19720

MARLOP PHARMACEUTICALS, INC. 908-355-8854
230 MARSHALL STREET
ELIZABETH, NJ 07206

MARLYN NUTRACEUTICALS ,INC. 480-991-0200
4404 E. ELWOOD ST.
PHOENIX, AZ 85040

MARNEL PHARMACEUTICALS, INC. 337-232-1396
206 LUKE STREET
LAFAYETTE, LA 70506

MARTEC PHARMACEUTICAL, INC. 816-241-4144
1800 N. TOPPING AVENUE
P. O. BOX 33510
KANSAS CITY, MO 6412-03510

MASON PHARMACEUTICALS, INC. 800-366-2454
4425 JAMBORE
SUITE 250
NEWPORT BEACH, CA 92660

MASON VITAMINS, INC. 800-327-6005
5105 N.W. 159TH STREET
MIAMI LAKES, FL 33014

MAYER LABORATORIES 510-229-5300
1950 ADDISON STREET
SUITE 101
BERKELEY, CA 94704

MAYNE PHARMA (USA) INC. 201-225-5510
MACK CALI CENTRE II
650 FROM RD
PARAMUS, NJ 07652

MAYOR PHARMACEUTICAL LABORATORIES, INC. 602-244-8899
2401 S. 24th STREET
PHOENIX, AZ 85034

MCCOY'S PRODUCTS, INC. 914-472-2737
1075 CENTRAL PARK AVENUE
SCARSDALE, NY 10583

MCGUFF CO. 714-438-0536
2921 W. MACARTHUR BLVD, SUITE
SANTA ANA, CA 92704

MCKEON PRODUCTS, INC. 586-427-7560
25460 GUENTHER
WARREN, MI 48091

MCKESSON DRUG COMPANY 415-983-8300
ONE POST STREET
SAN FRANCISCO, CA 94104-5296

MCKESSON PACKAGING SERVICES 704-784-4301
7101 WEDDINGTON ROAD
CONCORD, NC 28027

MCLEAN, DR. J. H., MEDICINE CO. 516-731-5380
3000 HEMPSTEAD TURNPIKE
LEVITTOWN, NY 11756

MCNEIL CONSUMER HEALTHCARE DIV OF MCNEIL-PPC, INC. 215-213-7000
7050 CAMP HILL ROAD
MAIL STOP 35
FT. WASHINGTON, PA 19034

MCNEIL NUTRITIONALS, LLC 215-273-7000
7050 CAMP HILL ROAD
FORT WASHINGTON, PA 19034

MCNEIL, R.A., CO. 423-493-9170
1150 LATTA STREET
CHATTANOOGA, TN 37406

MCR AMERICAN PHARMACEUTICALS, INC 352-754-8587
16255 AVIATION LOOP
BROOKVILLE, FL 34604

ME PHARMACEUTICALS 765-962-4410
DIV. OF VESCO, INC.
2800 S.E. PKWY., BOX 565
RICHMOND, IN 47374

MEAD JOHNSON & COMPANY 812-429-5000
Bristol-Myers Squibb U.S. Medicines Group
DIV. OF BRISTOL-MYERS SQUIBB
2400 W. LLOYD EXPRESSWAY
EVANSVILLE, IN 47721-0001

MEAD-RAYMOND CORP. 903-509-0663
BOX 130967
TYLER, TX 75713-0967

MED GEN INC. 561-750-1100
7284 W. PALMETTO PARK ROAD
STE. 106
BOCA RATON, FL 33433

MED-DERM PHARMACEUTICALS 423-926-4413
Crown Laboratories
P.O. BOX 1425
JOHNSON CITY, TN 37605

MEDA PHARMACEUTICALS, INC. 732-564-2200
265 DAVIDSON AVENUE
SUITE 300
SOMERSET, NJ 08873

MEDCO LAB INC. 712-255-8770
P. O. BOX 864
SIOUX CITY, IA 51102-0864

MEDEFIL, INC. 630-682-4600
250 WINDY POINT DRIVE
GLENDALE HEIGHTS, IL 60139

MEDICAL ACTION INDUSTRIES 800-645-7042
150 MOTOR PARKWAY
SUITE 205
HAUPPAUGE, NY 11788

MEDICAL NUTRITION USA , INC. 201-569-1188
10 WEST FOREST AVENUE
ENGLEWOOD, NJ 07631

MEDICAL PLASTIC DEVICES 514-694-9835
161 ONEIDA DRIVE
POINT CLAIRE, QC H9R 1A9

MEDICAL PRODUCTS PANAMERICANA INC. 305-545-6524
P. O. BOX 771
CORAL GABLES, FL 33134

MEDICINE SHOPPE, THE 314-993-6000
Cardinal Health, Inc.
1100 NORTH LINDBERGH BLVD
ST. LOUIS, MO 63132

MEDICINES COMPANY, THE 973-956-1616
8 CAMPUS DRIVE
PARSIPPANY, NJ 7054

MEDICIS, THE DERMATOLOGY COMPANY 602-808-8800
Medicis Pharmaceutical Corp.
8125 NORTH DOBSON ROAD
SCOTTSDALE, AZ 85256

MEDICORE 305-556-5085
2337 W. 76TH ST.
HIALEAH, FL 33016

MEDICURE PHARMA 732-584-5231
200 COTTONTAIL LANE
SOMERSET, NJ 08873

MEDIMETRIKS PHARMACEUTICALS, INC. 973-882-7512
363 ROUTE 46 WEST
FAIRFIELD, NJ 07004

MEDIMMUNE ONCOLOGY, INC. 301-398-0000
Medimmune, Inc.
ONE MEDIMUNNE WAY
GAITHERSBURG, MD 20878

MEDIMMUNE, INC. 301-398-0000
ONE MEDIMUNNE WAY
GAITHERSBURG, MD 20878

MEDIQUE PRODUCTS 239-790-1962
17080 ALICO COMMERCE COURT
FT. MYERS, FL 33912

MEDISCA, INC. 866-633-4722
661 ROUTE 3, UNIT C
PLATTSBURGH, NY 12901

MEDITRACK PRODUCTS, LLC. 978-567-9412
433 MAIN STREET
HUDSON, MA 01749

MEDLINE INDUSTRIES, INC. 847-949-3040
ONE MEDLINE PLACE
MUNDELEIN, IL 60060

MEDOP, INC. 727-943-9400
630 BROOKER CREEK BLVD.
SUITE 350
OLDSMAR, FL 34677

MEDSOURCE PHARMACEUTICALS 949-305-2501
26439 RANCHO PARKWAY
SOUTH #155
LAKE FOREST, CA 92630

MEDTECH, INC. 914-524-6810
90 N. BROADWAY
IRVINGTON , NY 10533

MEDTRONIC MINIMED INC. 818-576-4692
Medtronic
18000 DEVONSHIRE STREET
NORTHRIDGE, CA 91325-1219

MEDTRONIC NEUROLOGICAL 763-514-4000
Medtronic
7000 CENTRAL AVE NE
MINNEAPOLIS, MN 55432

MENTHOLATUM CO., THE 716-677-2500
707 STERLING DRIVE
ORCHARD PARK, NY 14127-1587

MENTOR CORP. 805-879-6000
201 MENTOR DRIVE
SANTA BARBARA, CA 93111

MERCK & CO., INC. 800-672-6372
U.S. HUMAN HEALTH
P.O. BOX 1000
NORTH WALES, PA 19454-1099

MERCK/SCHERING-PLOUGH PHARMACEUTICALS 800-672-6372
Merck & Co., Inc.
P.O. BOX 1000
NORTH WALES, PA 19454-2505

MERICON INDUSTRIES, INC. 800-242-6464
8819 N. PIONEER ROAD
PEORIA, IL 61615-1561

MERIT PHARMACEUTICALS 323-227-4831
2611 SAN FERNANDO ROAD
LOS ANGELES, CA 90065

MERLIN TECHNOLOGIES, INC. 805-388-7669
699 MOBIL AVE
CAMARILLO, CA 93010

MERRICK MEDICINE CO., INC. 254-753-3461
P. O. BOX 1489
WACO, TX 76703

MERZ PHARMACEUTICALS 336-856-2003
4215 TUDOR LANE
GREENSBORO, NC 27410

MET-RX USA, INC. 949-930-4400
17861 VON KARMAN AVENUE
IRVINE, CA 92614

METABOLIC PRODUCTS 800-766-7839
508 MAIN STREET
WOBURN, MA 01801-1019

METHAPHARM INC. 954-341-0795
81 SINCLAIR BLVD
BRANTFORD, ON N3S7X6

METTLER ELECTRONICS CORP. 714-533-2221
1333 SOUTH CLAUDINA STREET
ANAHEIM, CA 92805

MICROMEDICS, INC. 651-452-1977
1270 EAGAN INDUSTRIAL ROAD
SUITE 120
EAGAN, MN 55121

MIDDLEBROOK PHARMACEUTICALS, INC. 817-837-1200
7 VILLAGE CIRCLE
SUITE 100
WESTLAKE, TX 76262

MIDLOTHIAN LABORATORIES LLC 334-288-8661
780 INDUSTRIAL PARK BLVD.
UNIT 3
MONTGOMERY, AL 36117

MIDWEST IV 763-780-1500
8400 CORAL SEA STREET
BLAINE, MN 55449

MIKART, INC. 404-351-4510
1750 CHATTAHOOCHEE AVE NW
ATLANTA, GA 30318

MILLENNIUM BIOTECHNOLOGIES, INC. 908-604-2500
665 MARTINSVILLE ROAD
SUITE 219
BASKING RIDGE, NJ 07920

MILLENNIUM PHARMACEUTICALS, INC. 617-679-7000
40 LANDSDOWNE
CAMBRIDGE, MA 02139

MILLER PHARMACAL GROUP INC. 630-871-9557
350 RANDY ROAD UNIT 2
CAROL STREAM, IL 60188

MILUPA NORTH AMERICA INC. 301-217-4160
22513 GATEWAY CENTER DRIVE
CLARKSBURG, MD 20871

MISSION PHARMACAL CO. 210-696-8400
P.O. BOX 786099
SAN ANTONIO, TX 78278-6099

MODERN PRODUCTS, INC. 262-242-2400
6425 W. EXECUTIVE DRIVE
MEQUON, WI 53092

MOLNLYCKE HEALTH CARE, INC. 267-685-2000
826 NEWTOWN-YARDLEY ROAD
SUITE 300
NEWTOWN, PA 18940

MONAGHAN MEDICAL CORPORATION 518-561-7330
5 LATOUR AVENUE
SUITE 1600
PLATTSBURGH, NY 12901

MONARCH PHARMACEUTICALS 423-989-8000
King Pharmaceuticals, Inc.
501 FIFTH STREET
BRISTOL, TN 37620

MONTE SANO PHARMACEUTICALS, INC. 256-382-1196
4801 UNIVERSITY SQUARE
SUITE 31
HUNTSVILLE, AL 35816

MONTICELLO DRUG CO. 800-735-0666
1604 STOCKTON STREET
JACKSONVILLE, FL 32204

MONUMENT PHARMACEUTICAL, INC. 800-880-5882
2228-E PAPERMILL ROAD
WINCHESTER, VA 22601

MORTON GROVE PHARMACEUTICALS, INC. 847-967-5600
6451 WEST MAIN STREET
MORTON GROVE, IL 60053

MORTON PHARMACEUTICALS, INC. 901-386-8840
1625 N. HIGHLAND STREET
MEMPHIS, TN 38108

MPM MEDICAL INC. 972-893-4090
2301 CROWN CT
IRVING, TX 75038

MUTUAL PHARMACEUTICAL COMPANY, INC. 215-288-6500
1100 ORTHODOX STREET
PHILADELPHIA, PA 19124

MYLAN BERTEK PHARMACEUTICALS INC. 919-991-9800
Mylan Pharmaceuticals, Inc.
P.O. BOX 14149
RESEARCH TRIANGLE PK, NC 27709-4149

MYLAN PHARMACEUTICALS, INC. 304-599-2595
781 CHESTNUT RIDGE ROAD
P.O. BOX 4310
MORGANTOWN, WV 26505

N

NATIONAL NUTRITION, INC. 717-569-8561
P.O. BOX 5383
LANCASTER, PA 17606

NATIONAL VITAMIN COMPANY, INC. 559-781-8871
1145 WEST GILA BEND HWY
CASA GRANDE, AZ 85222

NATREN 800-992-3323
3105 WILLOW LANE
WESTLAKE VILLAGE, CA 91361

NATURE'S BOUNTY, INC. 631-567-9500
Arco Pharmaceuticals, Inc.
2100 SMITHTOWN AVE.
RONKONKOMA, NY 11779

NEILMED PHARMACEUTICALS, INC. 707-525-3784
601 AVIATION BLVD.
SANTA ROSA, CA 95403

NEPHRO-TECH, INC. 800-879-4755
P.O. BOX 16106
SHAWNEE, KS 66203

NEPHRON PHARMACEUTICALS CORP. 407-246-1389
4121 34TH STREET
ORLANDO, FL 32811-6458

NEPHRX, LLC 508-583-0943
10 BURKE DRIVE
BROCKTON, MA 02301

NESTLE HEALTHCARE NUTRITION, INC. 952-848-6000
10801 RED CIRCLE DRIVE
MINNETONKA, MD 55343

NESTLE NUTRITION 800-225-2270
Nestle USA
800 BRAND AVE
GLENDALE, CA 91203

NEUE MEDICAL PRODUCTS 310-265-9141
Neue Cosmetic Company, Inc.
904 SILVER SPUR ROAD #465
ROLLING HILLS ESTATE, CA 90274

NEUROVITES 503-228-4119
13595 SE 177TH
DAMASCUS, OR 97089

NEUTROGENA CORPORATION 310-642-1150
Johnson & Johnson
5760 W. 96TH STREET
LOS ANGELES, CA 90045

NEXGEN PHARMA, INC. 949-863-0340
46 CORPRATE PARK
Suite 100
IRVINE, CA 92606

NEXTWAVE PHARMACEUTICALS, INC. 847-996-6200
50 LAKEVIEW PARKWAY
SUITE 134
VERNON HILLS, IL 60061

NEXUS PHARMACEUTICALS, INC. 847-996-3789
175 E. HAWTHORN PARKWAY
SUITE 155
VERNON HILLS, IL 60061

NICHE PHARMACEUTICALS, INC. 817-491-2770
209 N. OAK ST.
P.O. BOX 449
ROANOKE, TX 76262-0449

NITROMED, INC. 781-266-4100
125 SPRING ST.
LEXINGTON, MA 02421

NNODUM CORPORATION 513-861-2329
1761 TENNESSEE AVE
CINCINNATI, OH 45229

NOMAX, INC. 314-961-2500
40 N. ROCK HILL ROAD
ST. LOUIS, MO 63119

NORTECH LABORATORIES 800-935-0425
125 SHERWOOD AVENUE
FARMINGDALE, NY 11735

NORTHSTAR RX LLC 901-255-8001
4971 SOUTHRIDGE BOULEVARD
SUITE 111-115
MEMPHIS, TN 38141

NOSTRUM LABORATORIES, INC. 866-408-6567
1800 N. TOPPING AVENUE
KANSAS CITY, MO 64120

NOVA BIOMEDICAL 781-894-0800
200 PROSPECT STREET
WALTHAM, MA 02454

NOVALAR PHARMACEUTICALS, INC. 858-436-1100
12555 HIGH BLUFF DRIVE
SUITE 300
SAN DIEGO, CA 92130

NOVARTIS CONSUMER HEALTH, INC. 973-503-8000
Novartis Pharm
200 KIMBALL DR.
PARSIPPANY, NJ 07054

NOVARTIS PHARMACEUTICALS CORPORATION 862-778-8300
ONE HEALTH PLAZA
BUILDING 415 ROOM 1014C
EAST HANOVER, NJ 07936

NOVARTIS VACCINES AND DIAGNOSTICS, INC. 215-255-4200
BELL ATLANTIC TOWER
1717 ARCH STREET,
28TH FLOOR
PHILADELPHIA, PA 19103

NOVAVAX, INC. 301-854-3900
8320 GILFORD ROAD,
SUITE C
COLUMBIA, MD 21046

NOVEN THERAPEUTICS, LLC 212-682-4420
CHRYSLER BUILDING
405 LEXINGTON AVENUE,
59TH FLOOR
NEW YORK, NY 10174

NOVO NORDISK, INC. 609-987-5800
100 COLLEGE ROAD WEST
PRINCETON, NJ 08540-7810

NOVOGEN PHARMACEUTICALS 203-327-1188
ONE LANDMARK SQUARE -
2ND FLOOR
STAMFORD, CT 06901

NUAGE LABORATORIES LTD 310-768-0700
Walker Pharmacal Co.
RICHFORD, VT 05476

NUCARE PHARMACEUTICALS, INC. 888-482-9545
622 WEST KATELLA AVENUE
ORANGE, CA 92867

NUMARK LABORATORIES, INC. 732-417-1870
P. O. BOX 6321
EDISON, NJ 08818

NUTRA/BALANCE PRODUCTS 317-356-5478
7155 WADSWORTH WAY
INDIANAPOLIS, IN 46219

NUTRACEUTICS CORPORATION 800-391-0114
3317 NW 10TH TERR. #403-404
FORT LAUDERDALE, FL 33309-5941

NUTRAMAX LABORATORIES INC. 800-925-5187
1506-C QUARRY DRIVE
EDGEWOOD, MD 21040

NUTRICIA NORTH AMERICA 301-795-2300
P.O.BOX 117
GAITHERSBURG
GAITHERSBURG, MD 20884

NUVORA, INC. 408-856-2211
3350 SCOTT BLVD, #502
SANTA CLARA, CA 95054

O

OAKHURST CO. 516-731-5380
Woolfoam Corporation
3000 HEMPSTEAD TURNPIKE
LEVITTOWN, NY 11756

OAKTREE PRODUCTS, INC. 636-530-1664
716 CROWN INDUSTRIAL COURT
SUITE J
CHESTERFIELD, MO 63005

OCEAN BLUE QUALITY PRODUCTS, LLC 561-741-6500
Sancilio & Company, Inc.
3874 FISCAL COURT
SUITE 200
RIVERIA BEACH, FL 33458

OCEANSIDE PHARMACEUTICALS 949-461-6199
ONE ENTERPRISE DRIVE
ALISO VIEJO, CA 92656

OCTAPHARMA USA, INC. 201-604-1130
121 RIVER STREET
SUITE 1201
HOBOKEN, NJ 07030-5891

OCTOGEN PHARMACAL COMPANY, INC. 770-888-8881
2750 CAMBRIDGE HILLS ROAD
CUMMING, GA 30041-8274

OCUSOFT 281-342-3350
CYNACON/OCUSOFT
2317 HIGHWAY 34
SUITE 1E
MANASQUAN, NJ 08736

OHM LABORATORIES, INC. 609-720-1155
Ranbaxy Pharmaceuticals, Inc.
600 COLLEGE ROAD EAST
PRINCETON, NJ 08540

OKAMOTO U.S.A., INC. 203-378-0003
18 KING STREET
STRATFORD, CT 06615

OMNII ORAL PHARMACEUTICALS 800-445-3386
1500 N. FLORIDA MANGO RD.
STE. 1
WEST PALM BEACH, FL 33409-5208

OMNIS HEALTH 877-450-6734
ONE APPLE HILL
SUITE 316
NATICK, MA 01760

OMRON HEALTHCARE, INC. 847-680-6200
1200 LAKESIDE DRIVE
BANNOCKBURN, IL 60015

ONSET THERAPEUTICS, LLC 888-713-8154
400 HIGHLAND CORPORATE DRIVE
CUMBERLAND, RI 02864

ONY, INC. 716-636-9096
1576 SWEET HOME ROAD
AMHERST, NY 14228

OPTICS LABORATORY, INC. 626-350-1926
9480 TELSTAR AVE.
STE. 3
EL MONTE, CA 91731

OPTIMOX CORPORATION 800-722-9040
2720 MONTEREY STREET
SUITE 406
TORRANCE, CA 90503

ORAL B LABORATORIES 800-4467252
DIV. GILLETTE COMPANY
800 BOYLSTON STREET
BOSTON, MA 02199

ORGANON PHARMACEUTICALS 800-222-7579
Merck & Co., Inc.
56 LIVINGSTON AVE
ROSELAND, NJ 07068

ORTEC INTERNATIONAL, INC. 212-740-6999
3960 BROADWAY
2ND FLOOR
NEW YORK, NY 10032

ORTHO DERMATOLOGICS 310-642-1150
5760 WEST 96TH STREET
LOS ANGELES, CA 90045

ORTHO-CLINICAL DIAGNOSTICS, INC. 908-2188000
Johnson & Johnson
1001 U.S. HIGHWAY 202 SOUTH
RARITAN, NJ 08869

ORTHO-MCNEIL NEUROLOGICS 800-523-5961
Ortho-McNeil Pharmaceutical Corporation
1125 TRENTON-HARBOURTON ROAD
TITUSVILLE, NJ 08560

ORTHO-MCNEIL PHARMACEUTICAL CORPORATION 908-218-6000
Johnson & Johnson
1000 U.S. HIGHWAY ROUTE 202
P.O. BOX 300
RARITAN, NJ 08869-0602

OSI PHARMACEUTICALS, INC. 631-962-2000
58 SOUTH SERVICE ROAD
MELVILLE, NY 11747

OTN GENERICS, INC. 650-952-8400
395 OYSTER POINT BLVD.
SUITE 500
SOUTH SAN FRANCISCO, CA 94080

OTSUKA AMERICA PHARMACEUTICALS, INC. 800-562-3974
2440 RESEARCH BOULEVARD
ROCKVILLE, MD 20850

OWEN MUMFORD, INC. 770-977-2226
1755 OAK COMMONS CT
MARIETTA, GA 30062-3165

OWENS & MINOR, INCORPORATED 804-747-9794
4800 COX STREET
GLEN ALLEN, VA 23060-6292

P

PACIFIC PHARMA 800-811-4184
Allergan, Inc.
AN ALLERGAN COMPANY
18600 VON KARMAN AVENUE
IRVINE, CA 92612

PACK PHARMACEUTICALS, LLC 734-743-2701
1110 WEST LAKE COOK ROAD
SUITE 152
BUFFALO GROVE, MI 60089

PADDOCK LABORATORIES, INC. 763-546-4676
3940 QUEBEC AVENUE NORTH
MINNEAPOLIS, MN 55427

PAL MIDWEST LTD. 815-332-9405
P O BOX 624
ROCKFORD, IL 61105

PALM PHARMACEUTICALS LLC 843-3643256
P.O. BOX 13227
CHARLESTON, SC 29422

PALMETTO STATE PHARMACEUTICALS 843-769-7633
2000 SAM RITTENBERG BLVD
SUITE 116
CHARLESTON, SC 29407

PAMLAB, L.L.C. 985-893-4097
4099 HWY 190
COVINGTON, LA 70433

PANATOZ INC. 604-275-8353
#106-12368 VALLEY BOULEVARD
EL MONTE, CA 91732

PAR PHARMACEUTICAL, INC. 201-802-4000
300 TICE BOULEVARD
WOODCLIFF LAKE, NJ 07677

PARENTA PHARMACEUTICALS 267-291-1220
777 TOWNSHIP LINE ROAD
SUITE 180
YARDLEY, PA 19067

PARI RESPIRATORY EQUIPMENT, INC. 978-768-7662
2943 OAKLAKE BLVD
MIDLOTHIAN, VA 23112

PARKER LABORATORIES, INC. 973-276-9500
286 ELDRIDGE ROAD
FAIRFIELD, NJ 07004

PARNELL PHARMACEUTICALS, INC. 415-256-1800
1525 FRANCISCO BLVD.
SUITE 15
SAN RAFAEL, CA 94901

PASCAL CO., INC. 425-827-4694
2929 N. E. NORTHRUP WAY
P. O. BOX 1478
BELLEVUE, WA 98009-1478

PATRIOT PHARMACEUTICALS, LLC. 215-325-7676
200 TOURNAMENT DRIVE
HORSHAM, PA 19044

PATTON MEDICAL DEVICES 512-279-4545
3108 NORTH LAMAR BOULEVARD
AUSTIN, TX 78705

PBM PHARMACEUTICALS, INC. 866-366-6282
THE LINNEY HOUSE
204 NORTH MAIN STREET
GORDONSVILLE, VA 22942

PCA, LLC 317-522-1637
8875 BASH STREET
INDIANAPOLIS, IN 46256

PD-RX PHARMACEUTICALS INC. 405-942-3040
727 NORTH ANN ARBOR AVENUE
OKLAHOMA CITY, OK 73127

PEDINOL PHARMACAL, INC. 631-293-9500
30 BANFI PLAZA NORTH
FARMINGDALE, NY 11735

PENN HERB CO., LTD. 215-632-6100
10601 DECATUR ROAD,
SUITE 2
PHILADELPHIA, PA 19154-3293

PENN LABORATORIES, INC. 800-366-8900
Glaxo SmithKline Pharmaceuticals
3 FRANKLIN PLAZA
P.O. BOX 7929
PHILADELPHIA, PA 19101

PERFECTA PRODUCTS, INC. 800-319-2225
14174 ELLSWORTH ROAD
P.O. BOX 189
BERLIN CENTER, OH 44401

PERRIGO PHARMACEUTICALS COMPANY 269-673-1493
515 EASTERN AVE
ALLEGAN, MI 49010

PERRY MEDICAL PRODUCTS 503-694-1600
Kirkman Laboratories, Inc.
6400 SW ROSEWOOD ST
LAKE OSWEGO, OR 97035

PERSON & COVEY 818-240-1030
616 ALLEN AVENUE
P.O. BOX 25018
GLENDALE, CA 91221-5018

PFEIFFER PHARMACEUTICALS, INC 404-614-0255
71 UNIVERSITY AVENUE, S.W.
P.O. BOX 4447
ATLANTA, GA 30315

PFIZER INC. CONSUMER HEALTH CARE GROUP 973-385-2000
Pfizer U.S. Pharmaceuticals Group
201 TABOR ROAD
MORRIS PLAINS , NJ 07950

PFIZER U.S. PHARMACEUTICALS GROUP 800-533-4535
235 EAST 42ND STREET
NEW YORK, NY 10017-5755

PHARMA PAC (A SERVICE OF H.J. HARKINS CO., INC.) 805-929-1333
513 SANDYDALE DRIVE
NIPOMO, CA 93444

PHARMACEUTICA NORTH AMERICA, INC. 818-291-0547
412 W. BROADWAY
SUITE 200
GLENDALE, CA 91204

PHARMACEUTICAL ASSOCIATES, INC. 864-277-7282
Beach Pharmaceuticals,
Div. Of Beach Products, Inc.
201 DELAWARE ST.
GREENVILLE, SC 29605

PHARMACEUTICAL GENERIC DEVELOPERS, INC. 787-781-6516
P.O. BOX 364761
SAN JUAN, PR 00969-4761

PHARMACEUTICAL INNOVATIONS, INC. 973-242-2900
897 FRELINGHUYSEN AVENUE
NEWARK, NJ 07114

PHARMACEUTICAL SPECIALTIES, INC. 507-288-8500
P. O. BOX 6298
ROCHESTER, MN 55903-6298

PHARMACEUTICS CORPORATION 818-291-0547
P.O. BOX 250580
GLENDALE, CA 91225

PHARMACIA AND UPJOHN COMPANY 212-733-2323
DIVISION OF PFIZER INC.
235 EAST 42ND STREET
NEW YORK, NY 10017

PHARMACIA CONSUMER HEALTHCARE 908-901-8000
Pharmacia Corporation
95 CORPORATE DRIVE
BW 280
BRIDGEWATER, NJ 08807

PHARMADERM 866-337-6457
Altana, Inc.
210 PARK AVENUE
FLORHAM PARK, NJ 07932

PHARMAFORCE, INC. 614-436-2222
960 CRUPPER AVENUE
COLUMBUS, OH 43229

PHARMAKON LABS, INC. 813-886-3216
6050 JET PORT INDUSTRIAL BLVD
TAMPA, FL 33634

PHARMALUCENCE, INC. 781-275-7120
10 DE ANGELO DRIVE
BEDFORD, MA 01730

PHARMASCIENCE LABORATORIES, INC. 800-207-4477
Pharmascience, Inc.
450 OAK TREE AVE
SOUTH PLAINFIELD, NJ 07080

PHARMATON NATURAL HEALTH PRODUCTS 203-798-4628
Boehringer Ingelheim
Pharmaceuticals, Inc.
900 RIDGEBURY ROAD
P.O. BOX 368
RIDGEFIELD, CT 06877

PHARMAVITE CORPORATION 800-423-2405
8510 BALBOA BOULEVARD
NORTHRIDGE, CA 91325

PHARMEDIUM SERVICES, L.L.C. 847-457-2300
2 CONWAY PARKWAY
150 NORTH FIELD DRIVE
LAKE FORREST, IL 60045

PHARMICS, INC. 801-9664138
P.O. BOX 27554
SALT LAKE CITY, UT 84127

PHILIPS CHILDREN'S MEDICAL VENTURES 412-380-8836
191 WYNGATE DRIVE
MONROEVILLE, PA 15146

PHR SYSTEMS, LTD. 719-783-2908
317 COLONY GREEN COURT
WILMINGTON, NC 28412

PHYSICIAN PARTNER 805-375-0800
3607 OLD CONEJO RD.
THOUSAND OAKS, CA 91320

PHYSICIAN THERAPEUTICS, LLC 310-474-9809
2980 BEVERLY GLEN CIRCLE
SUITE 301
LOS ANGELES, CA 90077

PHYSICIANS SCIENCE AND NATURE 714-875-6316
220 NEWPORT CENTER DRIVE
SUITE 11-634
NEWPORT BEACH, CA 92660

PHYSICIANS TOTAL CARE 918-254-2273
12515 E. 55th ST
SUITE 100
TULSA, OK 74146

PHYTO PHARMICA 800-553-2370
825 CHALLENGER DRIVE
GREEN BAY, WI 54311

PIERRE FABRE 973-898-1042

PHARMACEUTICALS, INC.
9 CAMPUS DRIVE
PARSIPPANY, NJ 07054

PINCGOLD, INC. 212-889-8575
36A EAST 36TH STREET,
STE. 200
NEW YORK, NY 10016

PLAINVIEW LLC 732-542-0740
107 MONMOUTH ROAD,
SUITE 202
WEST LONG BRANCH, NJ 07764

POLY PHARMACEUTICALS, INC. 601-776-3497
P. O. BOX 93
QUITMAN, MS 39355

PORTEX, INC. 603-352-3812
10 BOWMAN DRIVE
KEENE, NH 03431

POUND INTERNATIONAL CORPORATION 305-530-8702
1221 BRICKELL AVENUE
SUITE 1060
MIAMI, FL 33131

PRAECIS PHARMACEUTICALS INCORPORATED 781-795-4100
830 WINTER ST.
WALTHAM, MA 02451

PRASCO LABORATORIES 513-618-3333
6125 COMMERCE COURT
MASON, OH 45040

PRECISION DOSE, INC. 815-624-8523
722 PROGRESSIVE LANE
SOUTH BELOIT, IL 61080

PRECISION MILANI FOODS 800-442-5242
11457 OLDE CABIN RD.,
STE.100
ST. LOUIS, MO 63141

PRESS CHEM. & PHARM. LABS. 614-863-2802
P. O. BOX 09103
COLUMBUS, OH 43209

PRESTIGE BRANDS 800-552-7932
90 NORTH BROADWAY
IRVINGTON, NY 10533

PRICARA 908-218-6811
Ortho-McNeil Pharmaceutical Corporation
1000 ROUTE 202
RARITAN, NJ 08876

PRICE CHOPPER 518-379-1865
501 DUANESBURG ROAD
SCHENECTADY, NY 12306

PRIME MARKETING 800-222-5609
1775 JOHN R
TROY, MI 48083

PRIMUS PHARMACEUTICALS, INC. 480-483-1410
4725 N. SCOTTSDALE ROAD
STE#200
SCOTTSDALE, AZ 85251

PRINCE OF PEACE ENTERPRISES, INC. 510-887-1899
3536 ARDEN ROAD
HAYWARD, CA 94545-9906

PRO-PHARMA LLC 660-665-0084
515 N. MAIN
KIRKSVILLE, MO 63501

PROCTER & GAMBLE DISTRIBUTING COMPANY 513-983-1100
8700 MASON MONTGOMERY RD
MAIL BOX #2114
MASON, OH 45040

PROCTER & GAMBLE PHARMACEUTICALS INC. 800-448-4878
8700 MASON MONTGOMERY RD.
MAIL BOX #2114
MASON, OH 45040

PRODIGY DIABETES CARE, LLC 704-285-6400
9300 HARRIS CORNERS PARKWAY
SUITE 450
CHARLOTTE, NC 28269

PROFESSIONAL COMPOUNDING CENTERS OF AMERICA 281-933-6948
9901 S. WILCREST
HOUSTON, TX 77099

PROGRESSIVE HEALTH SUPPLY & SOURCE CORP 732-389-4702
119 AVENUE AT THE COMMON
SUITE 1
SHREWSBURY, NJ 07702

PROGRESSIVE LABORATORIES, INC. 800-527-9512
1701 WEST WALNUT HILL LANE
IRVING, TX 75038

PROMETHEUS LABORATORIES INC. 858-824-0895
9410 CARROLL PARK DRIVE
SAN DIEGO, CA 92121

PROMIUS PHARMA, LLC 908-429-4500
200 SOMERSET CORPORATE BLVD.
7TH FLOOR
BRIDGEWATER, NJ 08807

PRONOVA CORPORATION 305-666-4831
7440 SW 50TH TERRACE
SUITE 105
MIAMI, FL 33155

PROPER NUTRITION INC. 610-939-0414
P.O. BOX 13905
115 LITTLE ROCK ROAD, SUITE A
READING, PA 19612

PROPHARMA, INC. 305-592-9216
Dayton Pharmaceuticals, Inc.
3307 N.W. 74TH AVENUE
MIAMI, FL 33122

PROSTRAKAN, INC. 908-234-1096
1430 US HIGHWAY 206
SUITE 110
BEDMINSTER, NJ 07921

PROSYNTHESIS LABORATORIES INC. 703-430-2221
45975 NOKES BLVD
SUITE 170
STERLING, VA 20166

PROVIDENT PHARMACEUTICAL, INC. 804-2704498
3508 MAYLAND COURT
RICHMOND, VA 23233

PRUGEN, INC. 480-585-0122
8711 E. PINNACLE PEAK RD.
SUITE C-201, PMB 225
SCOTTSDALE, AZ 85255

PRX PHARMACEUTICALS, INC. 201-802-4000
Par Pharmaceutical, Inc.
300 TICE BLVD
WOODCLIFF LAKE, NJ 07677

PRYDE PHARMACEUTICAL CORPORATION 954-941-5080
256 SE 6TH AVE
SUITE 5
DELRAY BEACH, FL 33483

PURDUE PHARMA L.P. 203-588-8000
Purdue
ONE STAMFORD FORUM
STAMFORD, CT 0690-13431

PURDUE PHARMACEUTICAL PRODUCTS L.P. 203-588-8000
Purdue
ONE STAMFORD FORIJM
STAMFORD, CT 0690-13431

PURDUE PRODUCTS L.P. 203-588-8000
Purdue
ONE STAMFORD FORUM
STAMFORD, CT 0690-13431

Q

QOL MEDICAL 866-469-3773
5400 CARILLON POINT
KIRKLAND, WA 98033

QUAKER HOUSE PRODUCTS INC. 800-469-2249
P. O. BOX 21088
HOUSTON, TX 77226

QUALITEST PHARMACEUTICALS 256-859-4011
130 VINTAGE DRIVE
HUNTSVILLE, AL 35811

QUALITY CARE PRODUCTS, LLC 734-847-3847
7560 LEWIS AVENUE
TEMPERANCE, MI 48182

QUEST STAR MEDICAL, INC. 952-941-7345
10180 VIKING DRIVE
EDEN PRAIRIE, MN 55344

QUESTCOR PHARMACEUTICALS, INC. 510-400-0700
3260 WHIPPLE ROAD
UNION CITY, CA 94587

QUIGLEY CORPORATION, THE 215-345-0919
621 SHADY RETREAT ROAD
DOYLESTOWN, PA 18901

QUINNOVA PHARMACEUTICALS, INC. 215-860-6263
411 SOUTH STATE STREET
3RD FLOOR
NEWTOWN, PA 18940

QUINTESSA CORP. 661-940-5600
P.O. BOX 808
LANCASTER, CA 93584

R

R.I.J. PHARMACEUTICAL CORP. 845-692-5799
40 COMMERCIAL AVENUE
MIDDLETOWN, NY 10941

RANBAXY LABORATORIES, INC. 904-470-6000
Ranbaxy Pharmaceuticals, Inc.
9431 FLORIDA MINING BLVD EAST
JACKSONVILLE, FL 32257

RANBAXY PHARMACEUTICALS, INC. 904-296-0019
600 COLLEGE ROAD EAST
PRINCETON, NJ 08540

RANDOB LABORATORIES, LTD. 845-534-2197
P. O. BOX 440
CORNWALL, NY 12518

RARE DISEASE THERAPAUTICS, INC. 615-399-0700
2550 MERIDIAN BLVD
SUITE 150
FRANKLIN, TN 37067

RECKITT BENCKISER PHARMACEUTICALS INC. 804-379-1090
10710 MIDLOTHIAN TNPK
RICHMOND, VA 23235

RECKITT BENCKISER, INC. 973-404-2600
399 INTERPACE PKWY
PARSIPPANY, CO 07054

RECSEI LABORATORIES 805-964-2912
330 S. KELLOGG AVENUE
BUILDING M
GOLETA, CA 93117-9973

REESE PHARMACEUTICAL COMPANY 800-3217-178
10617 FRANK AVE.
P.O. BOX 1957
CLEVELAND, OH 44106

REGENERON PHARMACEUTICALS, INC. 914-345-7690
777 OLD SAW MILL RIVER RD.
TARRYTOWN, NY 10591

REGENT LABS, INC. 954-426-4403
700 W. HILLSBORO BLVD. #2-206
DEERFIELD BEACH, FL 33441

REJUVENESS PHARMACEUTICALS 800-588-7455
480 BROADWAY
SUITE LL10
SARATOGA SPRINGS, NY 12866

RESPA PHARMACEUTICALS, INC. 630-543-3333
P.O. BOX 88222
CAROL STREAM, IL 60188

RESPIRONICS INCORPORATED 973-571-2600
41 CANFIELD ROAD
CEDAR GROVE, NJ 07009

REXALL NATURALIST 800-255-7399
851 BROKEN SOUND PARKWAY, NW
DIV OF REXALL SUNDOWN INC.
BOCA RATON, FL 33487

RHODES PHARMACEUTICALS L.P. 401-262-9400
498 WASHINGTON STREET
COVENTRY, RI 02816

RISING PHARMACEUTICALS 201-961-9000
3 PEARL COURT
SUITES A
ALLENDALE, NJ 07401

RITE AID CORPORATION 717-761-2633
P.O. BOX 3165
HARRISBURG, PA 17105

RIVER'S EDGE PHARMACEUTICALS 770-886-3417
5400 LAUREL SPRINGS PKWY
BUILDING 500, SUITE 504
SUWANEE, GA 30024

RLC LABS, INC. 623-879-8535
2404 W. 12TH ST.
SUITE #4
TEMPE, AZ 85281

ROCHE DIAGNOSTICS 800-428-5074
Roche Laboratories
DIV. OF HOFFMANN-LA ROCHE INC.
9115 HAGUE ROAD
INDIANAPOLIS, IN 46250-0100

ROCHE LABORATORIES 800-526-0625
DIV. OF HOFFMANN-LA ROCHE INC.
340 KINGSLAND STREET
NUTLEY, NJ 071101199

RODLEN LABORATORIES 847-362-8200
Sirius Laboratories, Inc.
100 FAIRWAY DRIVE, STE 134
VERNON HILLS, IL 60061

ROMARK LABORATORIES, L.C. 813-282-8544
3000 BAYPORT DRIVE
SUITE 200
TAMPA, FL 33607

ROSE LABORATORIES 203-245-1210
168 COTTAGE ROAD
MADISON, CT 06443

ROSEDALE THERAPEUTICS 800-247-4896
302 ROSEDALE LANE
BRISTOL, TN 37620

ROSS PRODUCTS DIVISION, NUTRITIONAL PRODUCTS 800-551-5840
Abbott Laboratories, Inc.
DIV. ABBOTT LABORATORIES
625 CLEVELAND AVENUE
COLUMBUS, OH 43215-1724

ROUSES POINT PHARMACEUTICALS, LLC 908-272-7207
11 COMMERCE DR
SUITE 100
CRANFORD, NJ 07016

ROXANE LABORATORIES, INC. 614-276-4000
Boehringer Ingelheim
Pharmaceuticals, Inc.
1809 WILSON ROAD
COLUMBUS, OH 43228

RUGBY LABORATORIES, INC. 678-584-5678
Watson Pharmaceuticals, Inc.
SUBS OF WATSON PHARMACEUTICALS, INC.
1810 PEACHTREE INDUSTRIAL BLVD.
DULUTH, GA 30097

RX VITAMINS, INC. 800-792-2222
200 MYRTLE BOULEVARD
LARCHMONT, NY 10538-2002

RXELITE HOLDINGS, INC. 208-288-5550
172 SO. ACADEMY AVE,
STE 150
EAGLE, ID 83616

S

S.S.S. COMPANY 800-237-3843
Pfeiffer Pharmaceuticals, Inc.
71 UNIVERSITY AVENUE, S.W.
P.O. BOX 4447
ATLANTA, GA 30302

SABEX 847-627-8500
506 CARNEGIE CENTER
SUITE 400
PRINCETON, NJ 08540

SAFECOR HEALTH, LLC 781-933-8780
8 HOVEY STREET
WOBURN, MA 01801

SAGENT PHARMACEUTICALS, INC. 847-908-1600
1901 NORTH ROSELLE ROAD
SUITE 700
SCHAUMBURG, IL 60195

SALIX PHARMACEUTICALS INC. 919-862-1000
1700 PERIMETER PARK DRIVE
MORRISVILLE, NC 27560

SAMSON MEDICAL TECHNOLOGIES, LLC 856-751-5051
2050 SPRINGDALE ROAD
SUITE 400
CHERRY HILL, NJ 08003

SAMSUNG AMERICA, INC. 201-229-5047
105 CHALLENGER ROAD
RIDGEFIELD PARK, NJ 07660

SANCILIO & COMPANY, INC. 561-741-6500
3874 FISCAL COURT
SUITE 200
RIVIERA BEACH, FL 33404

SANDOZ 609-627-8500
Novartis Pharm
506 CARNEGIE CTR.
STE# 400
PRINCETON, NJ 08540

SANKYO PHARMA INC. 973-359-2600
TWO HILTON COURT
PARSIPPANY, NJ 07054

SANOFI PASTEUR INC. 800-822-2463
DISCOVERY DRIVE
SWIFTWATER, PA 18370

SANOFI-AVENTIS U.S. LLC 908-981-5000
55 CORPORATE DRIVE
P.O. BOX 5925
BRIDGEWATER, NJ 08807

SANTARUS, INCORPORATED 858-314-5700
3721 VALLEY CENTRE DRIVE
SUITE 400
SAN DIEGO, CA 92130

SAVAGE LABORATORIES 800-231-0206
60 BAYLIS ROAD
P.O. BOX 2006
MELVILLE, NY 11747

SAVIENT PHARMACEUTICALS INC. 732-418-9300
1 TOWER CENTER BLD.
14TH FLOOR
EAST BRUNSWICK, NJ 08816

SCANDINAVIAN FORMULAS, INC. 215-453-2507
140 E. CHURCH ST.
SELLERSVILLE, PA 18960

SCHERER LABORATORIES, INC. 770-933-1800
Scherer Healthcare, Inc.
2333 WAUKEGAN ROAD
SUITE 300
BANNOCKBURN, IL 60015

SCHERING CORPORATION 800-222-7579
Merck & Co., Inc.
RX BRANDED DIVISON OF
SCHERING-PLOUGH CORPORATION
2000 GALLOPING HILL ROAD
KENILWORTH, NJ 07033

SCHERING PLOUGH HEALTHCARE PRODUCTS INC. 800-842-4090
Merck & Co., Inc.
2000 GALLOPING HILL RD
K-5-1
KENILWORTH, NJ 07033

SCIELE PHARMA, INC. 770-442-9707
5 CONCOURSE PARKWAY
ATLANTA, GA 30328

SCIOS INC. 650-564-5000
1900 CHARLESTON ROAD
P O BOX 7210
MOUNTAIN VIEW, CA 94043

SCIVOLUTIONS, INC. 704-853-0100
2260 RAEFORD COURT
GASTONIA, NC 28052

SCOT-TUSSIN PHARM. CO., INC. 401-942-8555
32 WEST HAMDEN ROAD
P.O. BOX 8217
CRANSTON, RI 02920

SDA LABORATORIES 203-861-0005
280 RAILROAD AVE
GREENWICH, CT 06830

SEA-BAND INTERNATIONAL 401-841-5900
205 SPRING STREET
NEWPORT, RI 02840

SEPRACOR, INC. 508-481-6700
84 WATERFORD DRIVE
MARLBOROUGH, MA 01752

SETON PHARMACEUTICALS, LLC 732-292-2661
2317 HIGHWAY 34
SUITE IE
MANASQUAN, NJ 08736

SEYER PHARMATEC, INC. 787-286-3223
CARRETERA ESTATAL 172
KILOMETRO 2.5
CAGUAS, PR 00725

SFC/SOLVENT FREE CORPORATION 610-916-2949
BOX 278
BLANDON, PA 195109755

SHARPS COMPLIANCE INC. 713-432-0300
9220 KIRBY DRIVE
SUITE 500
HOUSTON, TX 77054

SHIONOGI PHARMA, INC 678-341-1400
5 CONCOURSE PARKWAY
SUITE 1800
ATLANTA, GA 30328

SHIONOGI QUALICAPS, INC. 336-449-3900
6505 FRANZ WARNER PARKWAY
WHITSETT, NC 27377-9215

SHIONOGI USA, INC. 973-966-6900
100 CAMPUS DRIVE
SUITE 105
FLORHAM PARK, NJ 07932

SHIRE HUMAN GENETIC THERAPIES, INC. 866-888-0660
700 MAIN STREET
CAMBRIDGE, MA 02139

SHIRE US INC. 484-595-8800
Shire Pharm. Group plc
725 CHESTERBROOK BOULEVARD
WAYNE, PA 19087

SIEMENS MEDICAL SOLUTIONS DIAGNOSTICS 914-631-8000
511 BENEDICT AVE
TARRYTOWN, NY 10591

SIERRA PRE-FILLED 919-552-9689
455 WEST DEPOT STREET
ANGIER, NC 27501

SIGMA-TAU PHARMACEUTICALS, INC. 301-948-1041
9841 WASHINGTONIAN BLVD.
SUITE 500
GAITHERSBURG, MD 20878

SILARX PHARMACEUTICALS, INC. 845-352-4020
19 WEST STREET
P.O. BOX 449
SPRING VALLEY, NY 10977

SIMILASAN CORPORATION 303-539-4060
1745 SHEA CENTER,
SUITE 380
HIGHLANDS RANCH, CO 80129

SINCLAIR PHARMACAL CO., INC. 631-788-7210
ORIENTAL AVENUE
P. O. DRAWER D
FISHERS ISLAND, NY 06390

SIRION THERAPEUTICS, INC. 866-474-7466
9314 EAST BROADWAY AVENUE
TAMPA, FL 33619

SIRIUS LABORATORIES, INC. 877-533-3872
25 LUPTON DRIVE
WILMINGTON, MA 01887

SJ PHARMACEUTICALS, LLC 877-604-7575
4200 NORTHSIDE PARKWAY NW
BUILDING 12
ATLANTA, GA 30327

SKINMEDICA, INC. 760-448-3600
5909 SEA LION PLACE
SUITE H
CARLSBAD, CA 92008

SLATE PHARMACEUTICALS, INC. 919-682-8800
318 BLACKWELL STREET
SUITE 240
DURHAM, NC 27701

SMC 412-521-1635
143 WAGNER ROAD
EVANS CITY, PA 16033

SMITH & NEPHEW, INC. 800-876-1261
WOUND MANAGEMENT DIVISION
970 LAKE CARILLON DR.
ST. PETERSBURG, FL 33716

SMITH BRISTOL CORPORATION 888-776-6005
P.O. BOX 2040
RANCHO MIRAGE, CA 922701054

SNUVA, INC. 708-731-5100
10323 CANTERBURY STREET
WESTCHESTER, IL 60154

SOLACE NUTRITION 401-352-4831
10 ALICE COURT
PAWCATUCK, CT 06379

SOLCO HEALTHCARE US 714-513-1000
959 SOUTH COAST DRIVE
SUITE 325
COSTA MESA, CA 92626

SOLSTICE NEUROSCIENCES, INC. 267-620-8000
40 GENERAL WARREN BLVD.
SUITE 160
MALERN, PA 19355

SOLVAY PHARMACEUTICALS, INC. 770-578-9000
901 SAWYER ROAD
MARIETTA, GA 30062

SOMBRA COSMETICS INC. 505-888-0288
5951 OFFICE BLVD. NE
ALBUQUERQUE, NM 87109

SOMERSET PHARMACEUTICALS, INC. 800-892-8889
3030 NO. ROCKY POINT DR
SUITE 250
TAMPA, FL 33607

SORE NO MORE 800-842-6622
150 EAST CENTER ST
MOAB, UT 84532

SOURCECF, INC. 256-704-4880
6705 ODYSSEY DR
HUNTSVILLE, AL 35806

SOUTHWEST TECHNOLOGIES, INC. 800-247-9951
1746 LEVEE ROAD
NORTH KANSAS CITY, MO 64116

SOUTHWOOD PHARMACEUTICALS, INC. 800-442-4443
60 EMPIRE DRIVE
LAKE FOREST, CA 92630

SPEAR DERMATOLOGY PRODUCTS, INC. 866-773-2779
1247 SUSSEX TURNPIKE
SUITE 120
RANDOLPH, NJ 07869

SPECIALTY MEDICAL SUPPLIES 954-752-5603
3882 NORTHWEST 124TH AVE
CORAL SPRINGS, FL 33065

SPECTRUM DESIGN MEDICAL, INC. 805-684-7678
6387-B ROSE LANE
CARPINTERIA, CA 93013

SPECTRUM PHARMACEUTICALS 949-788-6700
157 TECHNOLOGY DRIVE
IRVINE, CA 92618

SPECTRUM PHARMACY PRODUCTS 800-791-3210
Spectrum Chem and Lab Prods, Inc.
DIV. OF SPECTRUM CHEMICAL AND LABORATORY PRODS.
14422 SOUTH SAN PEDRO STREET
GARDENA, CA 90248

SPENCO MEDICAL CORPORATION 800-877-3626
P.O. BOX 2501
WACO, TX 76702-2501

ST. MARY'S MPP 520-297-3800
10860 N. MAVINEE DRIVE
ORO VALLEY, AZ 85737

ST. PAUL BRANDS 714-903-1000
11555 MONARCH ST.
GARDEN GROVE, CA 92841

STANDARD HOMEOPATHIC COMPANY 310-768-0700
210 WEST 131 STREET
P. O. BOX 61067
LOS ANGELES, CA 90061-0067

STANMAR LABORATORIES 816-421-8081
DIVISION OF Q.A. LABORATORIES
404 ADMIRAL BOULEVARD
KANSAS CITY, MO 64106

STASON PHARMACEUTICAL, INC. 949-380-0752
11 MORGAN
IRVINE, CA 926182005

STAT RX USA 770-653-3824
2481 HILTON DRIVE
GAINESVILLE, GA 30501

STELLAR HEALTH PRODUCTS, INC. 800-635-8372
71 COLLEGE DRIVE
ORANGE PARK, FL 32065-9024

STIEFEL CONSUMER HEALTHCARE 770-945-0101
Stiefel Laboratories, Inc.
6340 SUGARLOAF PARKWAY
SUITE 400
DULUTH, GA 30097

STIEFEL LABORATORIES, INC. 770-945-0101
6340 SUGARLOAF PARKWAY
SUITE 400
DULUTH, GA 30097

STRATUS PHARMACEUTICALS, INC. 305-254-6793
14377 SOUTHWEST 142ND ST
MIAMI, FL 33186

STRYKER ORTHOPAEDICS 201-831-5684
325 CORPORATE DRIVE
MAHWAH, NJ 07430

STURTEVANT, F. C., CO., THE 914-337-5131
P.O. BOX 607
BRONXVILLE, NY 10708

SUMMERS LABORATORIES, INC. 610-454-1471
103 G.P. CLEMENT DR.
COLLEGEVILLE, PA 19426

SUMMIT INDUSTRIES, INC. 770-590-0600
P. O. BOX 7329
MARIETTA, GA 30065

SUNDOWN, INC. 800-327-0908
851 BROKEN SOUND PARKWAY
BOCA RATON, FL 33487

SUNRISE MEDICAL, INC. 814-443-4881
100 DEVILBISS DRIVE
SOMERSET, PA 15501-2125

SUPERGEN INC. 925-560-0100
4140 DUBLIN BLVD.,
STE. 200
DUBLIN, CA 94568

SUPPOSITORIA LABORATORIES, INC. 800-933-5550
Clay-Park Laboratories, Inc.
SUBSIDIARY OF CLAY-PARK LABS, INC.
1700 BATHGATE AVENUE
BRONX, NY 10457

SWISS BIOCEUTICAL INTERNATIONAL, LTD 775-841-7020
2533 N. CARSON STREET
SUITE 3573
CARSON CITY, NV 89706

SYNOVIS SURGICAL INNOVATIONS 651-796-7300
A DIVISION OF SYNOVIS LIFE TECHNOLOGIES
2575 UNIVERSITY AVENUE
SAINT PAUL, MN 55114

SYNTHON PHARMACEUTICALS LTD. 919-493-6006
9000 DEVELOPMETN DR.
P.O. BOX 110487
RESEARCH TRIANGLE PARK, NC 27709

T

TAKEDA PHARMACEUTICALS AMERICA, INC. 877-872-3700
ONE TAKEDA PARKWAY
DEERFIELD, IL 60015

TALECRIS BIOTHERAPEUTICS, INC. 800-243-4153
79 T.W. ALEXANDER DR
BLDG 4101, SUITE 300
RESEARCH TRIANGLE PARK, NC 27709

TARGET CORPORATION 612-696-5947
1000 NICOLLET MALL, TPS-1153
MINNEAPOLIS, MN 55403

TARMAC PRODUCTS, INC. 305-557-6751
13295 NW 107TH AVENUE
HIALEAH GARDENS, FL 33018

TARO PHARMACEUTICALS U.S.A., INC. 800-544-1449
5 SKYLINE DRIVE
HAWTHORNE, NY 10532

TEC LABORATORIES 541-926-4577
7100 TEC LABS WAY SW
ALBANY, OR 97321

TECHNOLOGICAL INVESTMENTS, LLC/MEDI-FRIDGE 617-510-9395
358 SOUTH 700 EAST B521
SALT LAKE CITY, UT 84102

TEI BIOSCIENCES INC. 617-268-1616
7 ELKINS STREET
BOSTON, MA 02127

TERCICA, INC. 650-624-4900
Ipsen U.S.
2000 SIERRA POINT PARKWAY
SUITE 400
BRISBANE, CA 94005

TERUMO MEDICAL CORPORATION 800-283-7866
2101 COTTONTAIL LANE
SOMERSET, NJ 08873

TEVA NEUROSCIENCE, INC. 888-838-2872
901 E. 104TH ST.
SUITE 900
KANSAS CITY, MO 64131

TEVA PHARMACEUTICALS USA 888-838-2872
1090 HORSHAM RD.
NORTH WALES, PA 19454

TEVA SPECIALTY PHARMACEUTICALS 954-389-1981
425 PRIVET ROAD
HORSHAM, PA 19044

THE CHAO CENTER FOR INDUSTRIAL PHARMACY & CONTRACT MANUFACTURING 765-464-8414
3070 KENT AVENUE
PURDUE RESEARCH PARK
WEST LAFAYETTE, IN 47906

THE COROMEGA COMPANY, INC. 760-599-6088
2525 COMMERCE WAY
VISTA, CA 92081

THE GREAT ATLANTA AND PACIFIC TEA COMPANY 201-571-8334
2 PARAGON DRIVE
MONTVALE, NJ 07645

THE T-LITE COMPANY 800-880-6253
981 HWY 98 EAST
SUITE 3, BOX 404
DESTIN, FL 32541-2525

THE TORRANCE COMPANY 269-327-0722
800 LENOX AVENUE
PORTAGE, MI 49024

THER-RX CORPORATION 314-646-3700
KV Pharmaceutical Co.
1 CORPORATE WOODS DRIVE
BRIDGETON, MO 63044

THERAKOS, INC. 610-280-1000
Johnson & Johnson
437 CREAMERY WAY
EXTON, PA 19341

THREE RIVERS PHARMACEUTICALS, LLC 724-778-6100
119 COMMON WEALTH DRIVE
WARREN DALE, PA 15086

TIBER LABORATORIES 770-886-3417
5400 LAUREL SPRINGS PKWY
BUILDING 500, SUITE 503
SUWANEE, GA 30024

TIBOTEC THERAPEUTICS 908-541-4747
Ortho Biotech Products, LP
440 ROUTE 22 EAST
BRIDGEWATER, NJ 08807

TIME-CAP LABORATORIES, INC. 631-753-9090
7 MICHAEL AVENUE
FARMINGDALE, NY 11735

TISHCON CORPORATION 516-333-3050
30 NEW YORK AVENUE
WESTBURY, NY 11590

TOPIX PHARMACEUTICALS, INC. 631-226-7979
5200 NEW HORIZONS BLVD.
N. AMITYVILLE, NY 11701-1144

TOPOTARGET USA, INC. 973-895-6900
100 ENTERPRISE DRIVE
ROCKAWAY, NJ 07866

TORRENT PHARMA, INC. 269-544-2299
5380 HOLIDAY TERRACE
SUITE 40
KALAMAZOO, MI 49009

TOWER LABORATORIES, LTD. 860-767-2127
8 INDUSTRIAL PARK RD.
CENTERBROOK, CT 06409

TRANSDERMAL TECHNOLOGIES, INC. 800-282-5511
1368 NORTH KILLIAN DRIVE
NORTH PALM BEACH, FL 33403

TRASK INDUSTRIES 732-214-9267
163 FARRELL STREET
SOMERSET, NJ 08873

TRIAD PHARMACEUTICALS 262-538-2900
700 W. NORTH SHORE DR
HARTLAND, WI 53029

TRIAX PHARMACEUTICALS, LLC 908-373-1200
20 COMMERCE DRIVE,
SUITE 232
CRANFORD, NJ 07016

TRIGEN LABORATORIES, INC. 732-721-0070
2400 MAIN STREET EXTENSION
SUITE 6
SAYREVILLE, NJ 08872

TRIMARC LABORATORIES 405-942-3040
PD-Rx Pharmaceuticals Inc.
727 NORTH ANN ARBOR
OKLAHOMA CITY, OK 73127

TRITON CONSUMER PRODUCTS, INC. 847-228-7650
561 WEST GOLF ROAD
ARLINGTON HEIGHTS, IL 60005

TRUXTON CO., INC. 856-933-2333
136 HARDING AVENUE
P.O. BOX 1081
BELLMAWR, NJ 08099

TYCO HEALTHCARE 508-261-8000
15 HAMPSHIRE STREET
MANSFIELD, MA 02048

U

U.S. PHARMACEUTICAL CORP. 770-987-4745
2401-C MELLON COURT
DECATUR, GA 30035

UCB, INC. 770-970-7500
1950 LAKE PARK DRIVE
SMYRNA, GA 30080

UCYCLYD PHARMA 602-808-8800
Medicis Pharmaceutical Corp.
7720 N. DOBSON RD.
SCOTTSDALE, AZ 85256

UDL LABORATORIES, INC. 815-282-1201
Mylan Pharmaceuticals, Inc.
1718 NORTHROCK COURT
ROCKFORD, IL 61103

ULMER PHARMACAL 800-848-5637
P.O. BOX 408
PARK RAPIDS, MN 56470-0408

ULTIMED, INC. 651-291-7909
287 EAST SIXTH STREET
STE 380
ST. PAUL, MN 55101

UNICHEM PHARMACEUTICALS USA, INC. 201-226-0240
201 WEST PASSAIC STREET
SUITE 301A
ROCHELLE PARK, NJ 07662

UNICO, INC. 800-367-4477
1830 2ND AVENUE NORTH
LAKE WORTH, FL 33461

UNIGEN PHARMACEUTICALS, INC. 609-448-5500
55 LAKE DRIVE
EAST WINDSOR, NJ 08520

UNIMED PHARMACEUTICALS, INC. 770-578-9000
Solvay Pharmaceuticals, Inc.
901 SAWYER ROAD
MARIETTA, GA 30062

UNIPATH DIAGNOSTICS CO. 609-430-2740
51 SAWYER ROAD
SUITE 200
WALTHAM, MA 02453

UNITED RESEARCH LABORATORIES, INC. 215-288-6500
Mutual Pharmaceutical Company, Inc.
1100 ORTHODOX STREET
PHILADELPHIA, PA 19124

UNITED THERAPEUTICS CORPORATION 301-608-9292
1110 SPRING STREET
SILVER SPRING, MD 20910

UPSHER-SMITH LABORATORIES, INC. 763-315-2000
6701 EVENSTAD DRIVE NORTH
MAPLE GROVE, MN 55369

UPSTATE PHARMA, LLC 800-477-7877
1950 LAKE PARK DR.
SMYRNA, GA 30080

US DIAGNOSTICS, INC. 866-216-5308
304 PARK AVE. SOUTH
SUITE 218
NEW YORK, NY 10010

US MEDICAL INSTRUMENTS, INC. 619-661-5500
1490 AIR WING ROAD
SAN DIEGO, CA 92154

US WORLDMEDS, LLC 502-714-7800
4010 DUPONT CIRCLE
SUITE L-07
LOUISVILLE, KY 40207

V

VALEANT PHARMACEUTICALS INTERNATIONAL 949-461-6199
ONE ENTERPRISE DRIVE
ALISO VIEJO, CA 92656

VALIDUS PHARMACEUTICALS LLC 973-265-2777
119 CHERRY HILL ROAD
SUITE 310
PARSIPPANY, NJ 07054

VALMED INC. 508-845-3438
221 SPRING STREET
SHREWSBURY, MA 01545

VENTURI, INC. 231-929-7732
PO BOX 6348
TRAVERSE CITY, MI 49696-6348

VENTUS MEDICAL 650-632-4199
1301 SHOREWAY ROAD
SUITE 425
BELMONT, CA 94002

VERSAPHARM INCORPORATED 770-499-8100
1775 WEST OAK PARKWAY,
STE 800
MARIETTA, GA 30062

VERTEX DIAGNOSTICS 888-908-3783
958 CHURCH STREET
BALDWIN, NY 11510

VERTICAL PHARMACEUTICALS, INC. 732-721-0070
2400 MAIN STREET EXTENSION
SUITE 6
SAYREVILLE, NJ 08872

VERUS PHARMACEUTICALS 858-436-1600
12671 HIGH BLUFF DRIVE
SUITE 200
SAN DIEGO, CA 92130

VI-JON, INC. 615-459-8900
ONE SWAN DRIVE
PO BOX 129
SMYRNA, TN 37167

VIBRANTA, INC. 305-691-9906
3123-A N.W. 73RD ST.
MIAMI, FL 33147

VICTORY PHARMA, INC. 858-720-4500
12707 HIGH BLUFF DRIVE
SUITE 200
SAN DIEGO, CA 92130

VICTUS, INC. 305-663-2129
4918 SW 74TH COURT
MIAMI, FL 33155

VINDEX PHARMACEUTICALS, INC. 901-759-4970
P.O. BOX 937
CORDOVA, TN 38088

VINTAGE PHARMACEUTICALS, INC. 256-859-4011
Qualitest Pharmaceuticals
130 VINTAGE DRIVE
HUNTSVILLE, AL 35811

VIROPHARMA, INCORPORATED 610-458-7300
730 STOCKTON DRIVE
EXTON, PA 19341

VISION PHARMA, LLC 732-974-6300
1973 HIGHWAY 34
SUITE E22
WALL, NJ 07719

VISION PHARMACEUTICALS 605-996-3356
1022 N MAIN
P.O. BOX 400
MITCHELL, SD 57301

VISTAKON PHARMACEUTICALS, LLC 800-888-1446
Johnson & Johnson
7500 CENTURION PARKWAY
STE 100
JACKSONVILLE, FL 32256

VISTAPHARM, INC. 205-981-1387
2224 CAHABA VALLEY DRIVE,
SUITE B3
BIRMINGHAM, AL 35242

VITA-RX CORP. 800-241-8276
4625 WARM SPRINGS ROAD
P.O. BOX 8229
COLUMBUS, GA 31908

VITAFLO, LLC 631-547-5984
123 EAST NECK ROAD
HUNTINGTON, NY 11743

VITAL SIGNS, INC. 800-9320760
20 CAMPUS ROAD
TOTOWA, NJ 07512

VITALCARE GROUP INC. 305-620-4007
8935 NW 27 ST
MIAMI, FL 33172

VIVUS, INC. 800-934-5200
1172 CASTRO STREET
MOUNTAIN VIEW, CA 94040

W

WAKUNAGA CONSUMER PRODUCTS 800-527-5200
DIV OF WAKUNAGA PHARMACEUTICAL
23501 MADERO
MISSION VIEJO, CA 92691

WAL-MART 888-922-0400
702 S.W. 8TH STREET
BENTONVILLE, AR 72716

WALGREENS 847-914-2500
CORPORATE OFFICES
200 WILMOT ROAD
DEERFIELD, IL 60015

WALKER PHARMACAL CO. 800-325-8080
P.O.BOX 8080
RICHFORD, VT 05476

WALTMAN PHARMACEUTICALS INC. 601-939-0833
P. O. BOX 12442
JACKSON, MS 39236

WARNER CHILCOTT, INC. 800-521-8813
ROCKAWAY 80 CORPORATE CENTER
100 ENTERPRISE DR,
SUITE 280
ROCKAWAY, NJ 07866

WATSON LABS 973-355-8300
Watson Pharma, Inc.
360 MOUNT KEMBLE AVENUE
MORRISTOWN, NJ 07962

WATSON PHARMA, INC. 973-355-8300
Watson Pharmaceuticals, Inc.
360 MOUNT KEMBLE AVENUE
MORRISTOWN, NJ 07962-1953

WELEDA, INC. 845-268-8572
175 NORTH RT. 9W
P.O.BOX 249
CONGERS, NY 10920

WELLSPRING PHARMACEUTICAL CORP. 941-312-4727
5911 NORTH HONORE AVE
SUITE 211
SARASOTA, FL 34243

WESLEY PHARMACAL CO., INC. 215-953-1680
114 RAILROAD DRIVE
IVYLAND, PA 18974

WEST POINT PHARMA 800-672-6372
Merck & Co., Inc.
P.O. Box 1000
NORTH WALES, PA 19454

WEST-WARD PHARMACEUTICAL CORP. 732-542-1191
465 INDUSTRIAL WAY WEST
EATONTOWN, NJ 07724

WESTERN MEDICAL, LTD. 201-567-4440
64 N. SUMMIT STREET
TENAFLY, NJ 07670

WESTLAKE LABORATORIES, INC. 440-835-1518
24700 CENTER RIDGE ROAD
SUITE 113
CLEVELAND, OH 44145-5606

WG CRITICAL CARE LLC 201-857-8210
120 ROUTE 17 NORTH
PARAMUS, NJ 07652

WILLIAM LABORATORIES, INC. 860-749-1350
5 ANNGINA DRIVE, UNIT B
ENFIELD, CT 06082

WILLIAMS LABORATORY, THE BLACKSTONE CO. 973-772-4004
P. O. BOX 101
ORADELL, NJ 07649

WILSON OPHTHALMIC CORPORATION 405-376-9114
P.O. BOX 496
932 W HIGHWAY 152
MUSTANG, OK 73064

WINTHROP U.S. 908-981-5000
a business of Sanofi-Aventis U.S. LLC
55 CORPORATE DRIVE
BRIDGEWATER, NJ 08807-5925

WOCKHARDT USA 301-869-4945
135 US ROUTE 202/206
BEDMINSTER, NJ 07921

WOODWARD LABORATORIES, INC. 562-598-0800
125 B COLUMBIA
ALISO VIEJO, CA 92656

WORLD GEN LLC. 201-857-8210
120 ROUTE 17 NORTH
PARAMUS, NJ 07652

WOUND CARE INNOVATIONS, LLC 800-205-7719
2589 NORTH STATE ROAD 7
FORT LAUDERDALE, FL 33313

WRASER PHARMACEUTICALS 601-605-0664
PO BOX 1699
MADISON, MS 39130

WRIGHT MEDICAL TECHNOLOGY, INC. 901-867-9971
5677 AIRLINE ROAD
ARLINGTON, TN 38002

WYETH CONSUMER HEALTHCARE 800-322-3129
Wyeth
SUBSIDIARY OF WYETH
5 GIRALDO FARMS
MADISON, NJ 07940-0871

WYETH PHARMACEUTICALS 610-902-1200
Wyeth
SUBSIDIARY OF WYETH
500 ARCOLA ROAD, E5283
COLLEGEVILLE, PA 19426

X

X-GEN PHARMACEUTICALS 607-562-2700
P.O. BOX 445
BIG FLATS, NY 14814

XANODYNE PHARMACEUTICALS, INC. 859-371-6383
ONE RIVERFRONT PLACE
SUITE 900
NEWPORT, KY 41071-4563

XTTRIUM LABORATORIES 773-268-5800
415 W PERSHING ROAD
CHICAGO, IL 60609

Y

YERBA PRIMA 541-488-2228
740 JEFFERSON AVENUE
ASHLAND, OR 975203743

YOUNG, W. F., INC. 413-526-9999
302 BENTON DRIVE
EAST LONGMEADOW, MA 01028

Z

Z M O CO., THE 614-875-0230
4188 ALKIRE ROAD
GROVE CITY, OH 43123

ZANFEL LABORATORIES, INC. 515-267-8099
1370 NW 114TH STREET
SUITE 204
CLIVE, IA 50325

ZARS PHARMA, INC. 801-350-0202
1142 W. 2320 S.
SALT LAKE CITY, UT 84119

ZERXIS PHARMA, L.L.C. 985-893-4097
Pamlab, L.L.C.
4099 HIGHWAY 190
COVINGTON, LA 70433

ZILA CONSUMER PHARMACEUTICALS, INC. 602-266-6700
5227 N. 7TH STREET
PHOENIX, AZ 85014

ZOGENIX, INC. 866-964-3649
12671 HIGH BLUFF DRIVE
SAN DIEGO, CA 92129

ZYBER PHARMACEUTICALS. INC. 225-647-3002
208 W. EASTBANK STREET
GONZALES, LA 70737

ZYDUS PHARMACEUTICALS (USA) INC. 609-2755-125
210 CARNEGIE CENTER
SUITE 103
PRINCETON, NJ 08540

ZYLERA PHARMACEUTICALS, LLC 888-499-5372
510 MEDOWMONT VILLAGE CIRCLE
SUITE 272
CHAPEL HILL, NC 27517

ZYMOGENETICS, INC. 206-442-6600
1201 EASTLAKE AVE. EAST
SEATTLE, WA 98102

PHARMACEUTICAL WHOLESALER DIRECTORY

The following is an alphabetical listing of pharmaceutical wholesalers in the United States and Puerto Rico. The names, addresses, and phone numbers typically represent headquarters locations. Regional office information is available through these main offices.

ALBERS MEDICAL, INC.
4400 Broadway, Suite 106
Kansas City, MO 64111
816-931-0100
www.alberspharmacy.com

ALLIED MED WHOLESALE DRUG CO.
6312 SW Capitol Hwy., Suite 226
Portland, OR 97201
800-272-1544

AMERISOURCE BERGEN CORP.
1300 Morris Dr., Suite 100
Chesterbrook, PA 19087
610-727-7000; 800-829-3132
www.amerisourcebergen.net

ATLANTIC BIOLOGICALS CORP.
(Headquarters/Distribution Center)
20101 NE 16th Place
Miami, FL 33179
305-690-4233; 800-509-7592
www.atlanticbiologicals.com

ATLANTIC HEALTHCARE GROUP, INC.
2401 East Atlantic Blvd.
Suite 410
Pompano Beach, FL 33062
786-207-3400

BELLAMY DRUG CO./KING DRUG CO.OF FLORENCE, INC.
411 Landmark Dr.
Wilmington, NC 28412
800-922-9597
www.pharmacysupplier.com

BELLCO HEALTH
5500 New Horizons Blvd.
N. Amityville, NY 11701
631-789-6900; 800-645-5314
www.bellcoonline.com

J.M. BLANCO, INC.
Diana St. #21
Amelia Industrial Park
Guaynabo, PR 00965
787-793-6262

BORSCHOW DRUG
Centro Internacional de Distribución
Edificio #10 Carr. 869 KM 4.2
Guaynabo, PR 00962
787-625-4100; 800-981-2301
www.borschow.com

BURLINGTON DRUG CO.
91 Catamount Dr.
Milton, VT 05468-1001
802-893-5105; 800-338-8703
www.burlingtondrug.com

CALADON TRADING CO.
4305 Industrial Rd.
Las Vegas, NV 89103

CAPITAL WHOLESALE DRUG CO.
873 Williams Ave.
Columbus, OH 43212
614-297-8221

CARDINAL HEALTH, INC.
7000 Cardinal Place
Dublin, OH 43017
614-757-5000; 800-234-8701
www.cardinal.com

CHAPIN MEDICAL CO.
5100 E. Hunter
Anaheim, CA 92807
800-221-7180

D&K HEALTHCARE RESOURCES, INC.
8235 Forsythe Blvd.
St. Louis, MO 62105

DAKOTA DRUG, INC.
28 N. Main St.
Minot, ND 58703
701-852-2141; 800-437-2018
www.dakdrug.com

DARBY DRUG CO.
300 Jericho Quadrangle
Jericho, NY 11753
800-247-4768
www.darbydental.com

DIK DRUG CO.
160 Tower Dr.
Burr Ridge, IL 60527-5720
630-655-4000
www.dikdrug.com

DMS PHARMACEUTICAL GROUP, INC.
810 Busse Hwy.
Park Ridge, IL 60068
847-518-1100
www.dmspharma.com

DOHMEN DISTRIBUTION
215 N. Winter St., No. 300
Milwaukee, WI 53022
414-299-4900
www.dohmen.com

DROGUERIA BETANCES, INC.
PO Box 368
Caguas, PR 00726
787-746-0951; 800-981-8151
www.drogueriabetances.com

DRUGMAX, INC.
312 Farmington Ave.
Farmington, CT 06032-1968
860-676-1222

EXPERT-MED, INC.
400 Andalusia Ave.
Ormond Beach, FL 32174
386-672-1010; 800-447-5050
www.expert-med.com

FMC DISTRIBUTORS, INC.
De Los Caballeros
3306 Ave. Santiago
Ponce, PR 00611
787-841-8181

GENERICS PUERTO RICO, INC.
Calle Acasia #3
Urb. Monte Rey
Pueblo Viejo
San Juan, PR 00920
787-792-2430

GLOBALRX, INC.
4024 Carrington Lane
Efland, NC 27243
919-304-4278; 800-526-6447
www.globalrx.com

GOODWIN DRUG CO.
1410 Main St.
Wheeling, WV 26003
304-233-0260

H & H WHOLESALE SERVICES, INC.
333 Park St.
Troy, MI 48083
248-616-3030; 800-995-5750

HARVARD DRUG GROUP
31778 Enterprise Dr.
Livonia, MI 48150
734-525-8700; 800-875-0123
www.harvarddrugs.com

FRANK W. KERR CO.
43155 W. Nine Mile Rd.
Novi, MI 48376-8026
248-349-5000
www.fwkerr.com

KING DRUG CO. OF FLORENCE
605 W. Lucas St.
Florence, SC 29501-2823
843-662-0411

KINRAY INC.
152-35 10th Ave.
Whitestone, NY 11357-1123
718-767-1234; 800-854-6729
www.kinray.com

KUEHNE + NAGEL
22 Spencer St.
Naugatuck, CT 06770
203-597-5300; 888-850-USCO
http://usco.kuehne-nagel.com

LETCO COMPANIES, INC.
1316 Commerce Dr. N.W.
Decatur, AL 35601
256-350-1297; 800-239-5288
www.letcoinc.com

LOUISIANA WHOLESALE DRUG CO., INC.
2085 I-49 S. Service Rd.
Sunset, LA 70584
337-662-1040; 800-960-3784

MCKESSON SUPPLY SOLUTIONS
One Post St.
San Francisco, CA 94104
415-983-8300
www.mckesson.com

MCQUEARY BROS. DRUG CO.
4727 E. Kearney St.
PO Box 5955
Springfield, MO 65801
417-869-2577; 800-747-2577
www.McQBros.com

MEDRESOURCE SOLUTIONS, INC.
6855 SW 81st St.
Miami, FL 33143
305-667-7871

METRO MEDICAL SUPPLY WHOLESALE, INC.
200 Cumberland Bend
Nashville, TN 37228
615-329-2002; 800-768-2002
www.metromedical.com

MIAMI-LUKEN, INC.
265 S. Pioneer Blvd.
Springboro, OH 45066
937-743-7775
www.miamiluken.com

MOORE MEDICAL CORP.
PO Box 1500
New Britain, CT 06050-1500
800-234-1464

MORRIS & DICKSON CO., LLC
410 Kay Lane
Shreveport, LA 71115
318-797-7900; 800-388-3833
www.morrisdickson.com

NATIONWIDE MEDICAL/SURGICAL, INC.
14141 Covello St.
Suite 6C
Van Nuys, CA 91405
818-997-8848; 800-997-8846
www.nationwidemedical.net

N.C. MUTUAL WHOLESALE DRUG CO.
816 Ellis Rd.
Durham, NC 27703-9979
919-596-2151; 800-800-8551
www.mutualdrug.com

PREMIUM HEALTH SERVICES, INC.
9121 Red Branch Rd., Suite A
Columbia, MD 21045
410-730-6120; 877-730-4747
www.premiumhealthservices.com

PRESCRIPTION SUPPLY, INC.
2233 Tracy Rd.
Northwood, OH 43619-1326
419-661-6600; 800-777-0761
www.prescriptionsupply.com

PRIORITY PHARMACEUTICALS
4040 Sorrento Valley Rd., Suite B
San Diego, CA 92121
877-577-4674
www.prioritypharm.com

QK HEALTHCARE, INC.
2060 9th Ave.
Ronkonkoma, NY 11779
631-439-2000; 800-676-5554
www.qkrx.com

R & S NORTHEAST
256 Geiger Rd.
Philadelphia, PA 19115
215-673-7770; 800-262-7770
www.rsnortheast.com

R & S SALES, INC.
8407 Austin Tracy Rd.
Fountain Run, KY 42133
800-626-0208

REBEL DISTRIBUTORS, CORP.
3607 Old Conejo Rd.
Thousand Oaks, CA 91320
805-214-0900; 877-Rebel-Rx (877-732-3579)
www.rebelrx.com

ROCHESTER DRUG CO-OPERATIVE INC.
320 Goodman St. N.
Rochester, NY 14607
585-271-7220; 800-333-0538
www.rdcdrug.com

Rx CROSSROADS
4500 Progress Blvd.
Louisville, KY 40218
800-918-3252
www.rxcrossroads.com

HENRY SCHEIN, INC.
135 Duryea Rd.
Melville, NY 11747
631-843-5500; 800-772-4346
www.henryschein.com

H.D. SMITH WHOLESALE DRUG CO.
Corporate Offices
3063 Fiat Ave.
Springfield, IL 62703
217-753-1688; 866-232-1222
www.hdsmith.com

SMITH DRUG CO.
9098 Fairforest Rd.
Spartanburg, SC 29301
864-595-0769; 800-572-1216

SMITH MEDICAL PARTNERS
960 Lively Blvd.
Wood Dale, IL 60191
630-227-9420; 800-292-9653

STONE MEDICAL LLC
1160 S. Rogers Circle #2
Boca Raton, FL 33487
561-998-2402

SUPREME DISTRIBUTORS CO.
5400 Broken Sound Blvd. NW
Suite 100
Boca Raton, FL 33487
800-323-6838

VALLEY WHOLESALE DRUG CO.
1401 W. Fremont St.
Stockton, CA 95203-2697
209-466-0131; 800-247-6255

VALUE DRUG CO.
One Golf View Dr.
Altoona, PA 16601
814-944-9316; 800-252-3786
www.valuedrugco.com

WATSON PHARMACEUTICALS
311 Bonnie Circle
Corona, CA 92880
951-493-5300
www.watsonpharm.com

OBRA PARTICIPATING MANUFACTURERS

Listed below are manufacturers approved by the Centers for Medicare and Medicaid Services as of December 2009 who are participating in the Medicaid Rebate Program established under the Omnibus Budget Reconciliation Act (OBRA). Manufacturers are organized first in alphabetical order, followed by numerical order. The 5-digit labeler codes associated with each manufacturer correspond to the first five digits of the manufacturer's NDC number(s).

ALPHABETICAL INDEX

MANUFACTURER	ID#
(OSI) EYETECH	68782
3M PHARMACEUTICALS	00089
A. AARONS	18754
A. H. ROBINS	00031
AAI PHARMA	66591
ABBOTT LABORATORIES	00074
ABRAXIS BIOSCIENCE	68817
ACCORD HEALTHCARE	16729
ACETO PHARMA	25356
ACORDA THERAPEUTICS	10144
ACTAVIS	00472
ACTAVIS	45963
ACTAVIS ELIZABETH	00228
ACTAVIS KADIAN	46987
ACTAVIS SOUTH ATLANTIC	67767
ACTAVIS TOTOWA	52152
ACTELION PHARMACEUTICALS	66215
ADVANCED VISION RESEARCH	58790
AFFORDABLE PHARMACEUTICALS	10572
AKORN	17478
AKRIMAX PHARMACEUTICALS	24090
ALAVEN PHARMACEUTICAL	68220
ALCON LABORATORIES	00065
ALCON LABORATORIES	00998
ALEXION PHARMACEUTICALS	25682
ALKERMES	65757
ALLAN PHARMACEUTICAL	13279
ALLEGIS PHARMACEUTICALS	28595
ALLERGAN	00023
ALLERGAN	11980
ALLIANT PHARMACEUTICALS	68188
ALLOS THERAPEUTICS	48818
ALPHARMA	63857
ALVOGEN	47781
AMAG PHARMACEUTICALS	59338
AMBI PHARMACEUTICALS	66870
AMERICAN HEALTH PACKAGING	62584
AMERICAN HEALTH PACKAGING	68084
AMERICAN RED CROSS	52769
AMERICAN REGENT LABORATORIES	00517
AMERIDERM LABORATORIES	63921
AMERIFIT PHARMA	61451
AMGEN USA	55513
AMGEN/IMMUNEX	58406
AMNEAL PHARMACEUTICALS	53746
AMNEAL PHARMACEUTICALS	65162
AMYLIN PHARMACEUTICALS	66780
ANCHEN PHARMACEUTICALS	10370
ANIP ACQUISITION COMPANY	62559
APACE KY	15338
APOTEX	60505
APP PHARMACEUTICALS	63323
AR SCIENTIFIC	13310
ARBOR PHARMACEUTICALS	24338
ARISTOS PHARMACEUTICALS	24486

MANUFACTURER	ID#
ASCEND LABORATORIES	67877
ASTELLAS	51248
ASTELLAS PHARMA	00469
ASTRAZENECA LP	00186
ASTRAZENECA LP	00310
ATLEY PHARMACEUTICALS	59702
ATON PHARMA	25010
AURIGA LABORATORIES, CORE PHARMA	64720
AUROBINDO PHARMA	13107
AUROBINDO PHARMA	65862
AUXILIUM PHARMACEUTICALS	66887
AVANIR PHARMACEUTICALS	64597
AVANIR PHARMACEUTICALS	68322
AVENTIS PASTEUR	49281
AVENTIS PHARMACEUTICALS	00066
AVENTIS PHARMACEUTICALS	00068
AVENTIS PHARMACEUTICALS	00075
AVENTIS PHARMACEUTICALS	00088
AXCAN SCANDIPHARM	58914
AYERST LABORATORIES	00046
AZUR PHARMA	18860
B. BRAUN MEDICAL	00264
B. F. ASCHER AND COMPANY	00225
BALLAY PHARMACEUTICALS	63162
BARR LABORATORIES	51285
BARR LABORATORIES	00555
BARRIER THERAPEUTICS	13478
BAUSCH & LOMB	24208
BAUSCH & LOMB	57782
BAXTER HEALTHCARE	00944
BAXTER HEALTHCARE	64193
BAXTER HEALTHCARE	00338
BAXTER HEALTHCARE	00641
BAXTER HEALTHCARE	10019
BAXTER HEALTHCARE	54643
BAXTER HEALTHCARE	60977
BAXTER HEALTHCARE	67108
BAY PHARMA	42769
BAYER ORATION	00026
BEACH PRODUCTS	00486
BEDFORD LABORATORIES	55390
BERGEN BRUNSWIG DRUG COMPANY	24385
BERLEX	50419
BETA DERMACEUTICALS	53062
BIOCOMP PHARMA	44523
BIOGEN IDEC	59627
BIOMARIN PHARMACEUTICALS	68135
BIONICHE PHARMA	67457
BIOTEST PHARMACEUTICALS	59730
BIOVITRUM AB	66658
BLAINE COMPANY	00165
BLANSETT PHARMACAL	51674
BOCA PHARMACAL	64376
BOEHRINGER INGELHEIM PHARMACEUTICALS	00597
BOUDREAUX'S BUTT PASTE	62103

MANUFACTURER	ID#
BRAINTREE LABORATORIES	52268
BRECKENRIDGE PHARMACEUTICAL	51991
BRIGHTON PHARMACEUTICALS	10914
BRISTOL-MYERS SQUIBB	00087
BRISTOL-MYERS SQUIBB & GILEAD	15584
BRISTOL-MYERS SQUIBB COMPANY	19810
BRISTOL-MYERS SQUIBB/SANOFI	63653
BROOKSTONE PHARMACEUTICALS	42192
BTA PHARMACEUTICALS	64455
C B FLEET COMPANY	00132
CADISTA PHARMACEUTICALS	59746
CAMBER PHARMACEUTICALS	31722
CAPELLON PHARMACEUTICALS	64543
CAPITAL PHARMACEUTICAL	29978
CARACO PHARMA	49708
CARACO PHARMACEUTICAL	57664
CARLSBAD TECHNOLOGY	61442
CAROLINA MEDICAL PRODUCTS COMPANY	46287
CARWIN ASSOCIATES	15370
CEBERT PHARMACEUTICALS	64019
CELGENE	59572
CELLTECH PHARMACEUTICALS	53014
CENTRIX PHARMACEUTICAL	11528
CENTURION LABS	23359
CEPHALON	63459
CEPHAZONE PHARMA	68330
CHAIN DRUG CONSORTIUM	68016
CHAIN DRUG MARKETING ASSOCIATION	63868
CHIRON	53905
CIMA LABS	55253
COBALT LABORATORIES	16252
CODADOSE	43378
COLGATE ORAL PHARMACEUTICALS	00126
COLLAGENEX PHARMACEUTICALS	64682
COLOPLAST	11701
CONTRACT PHARMACAL	10267
CONVATEC	43553
CORIA LABORATORIES	13548
CORNERSTONE BIOPHARMA	10122
COTHERIX	10148
COUNTY LINE PHARMACEUTICALS	43199
CRITICAL THERAPEUTICS (CRTX)	68734
CSL BEHRING	00053
CSL BEHRING	44206
CSL BEHRING GMBH	63833
CUBIST PHARMACEUTICALS	67919
CUMBERLAND PHARMACEUTICALS	66220
CURA PHARMACEUTICAL	66860
CV THERAPEUTICS (CVT)	67159
CYPRESS PHARMACEUTICAL	60258
DABUR PHARMA US	10518
DAIICHI SANKYO	63395
DAIICHI SANKYO	65597
DANCO LABORATORIES	64875
DAVA INTERNATIONAL	67253

MANUFACTURER	ID#
DAVA PHARMACEUTICALS	68774
DEPOMED	13913
DERMA SCIENCES	25382
DERMARITE INDUSTRIES	61924
DEY L.P.	49502
DIGESTIVE CARE	59767
DISTA PRODUCTS	00777
DOAK DERMATOLOGICS	10337
DR. REDDY'S LABORATORIES	55111
DUPONT PHARMACEUTICALS	00056
DUPONT PHARMACEUTICALS	00590
DURA PHARMACEUTICALS	51479
DYAX	47783
E FOUGERA	00168
E.R. SQUIBB & SONS	00003
ECR PHARMACEUTICALS	00095
EDENBRIDGE PHARMACEUTICALS	42799
EDWARDS PHARMACEUTICALS	00485
EISAI	62856
EKR THERAPEUTICS	24477
ELAN PHARMACEUTICALS/ATHENA NEURO	59075
ELI LILLY AND COMPANY	00002
EMMAUS MEDICAL	42457
ENDO PHARMACEUTICALS	63481
ENDO PHARMACEUTICALS	60951
ENZON PHARMACEUTICALS	57665
EON LABS	00185
EPIC PHARMA	42806
ESP PHARMA	67286
ESPRIT PHARMA	15456
ETHEX	58177
EURAND PHARMACEUTICALS	42865
EVERETT LABORATORIES	00642
EXCELLIUM PHARMACEUTICAL	64125
FALCON PHARMACEUTICALS	61314
FAMILY PHARMACY	52735
FERA PHARMACEUTICALS	48102
FERNDALE LABORATORIES	00496
FERRING PHARMACEUTICALS	55566
FLEMING AND COMPANY	00256
FLUORITAB	00288
FOCUS LABORATORIES	15821
FOREST LABORATORIES	00456
FRESENIUS MEDICAL CARE	49230
FSC LABORATORIES	13551
G&W LABORATORIES	00713
GALDERMA LABORATORIES	00299
GALLIPOT	51552
GATE PHARMACEUTICALS	57844
GAVIS PHARMACEUTICALS	43386
GEMINI PHARMACEUTICALS	51645
GENENTECH	50242
GENERAMED	52569
GENERAMEDIX	10139
GENETICS INSTITUTE	58394
GENPHARM	15330
GENZYME	58468
GENZYME	64894
GILBERT LABORATORIES	00535
GILEAD SCIENCES	61958
GLADES PHARMACEUTICALS	59366
GLAXOSMITHKLINE	00007
GLAXOSMITHKLINE	00029
GLAXOSMITHKLINE	00135
GLAXOSMITHKLINE	00173
GLAXOSMITHKLINE	10158
GLAXOSMITHKLINE	11530
GLENMARK PHARMACEUTICALS	68462
GLOBAL PHARMACEUTICAL	00115
GM PHARMACEUTICALS	58809
GOLDLINE LABORATORIES	00182

MANUFACTURER	ID#
GRACEWAY PHARMACEUTICALS	13453
GRACEWAY PHARMACEUTICALS	29336
GRIFOLS BIOLOGICALS	61953
GRIFOLS BIOLOGICALS	68516
GTX	11399
GUARDIAN LABS	00327
HARRIS PHARMACEUTICAL	67405
HAWTHORN PHARMACEUTICALS	63717
HEALTH CARE PRODUCTS DIVISION	61787
HEALTHPOINT	00064
HEMISPHERX BIOPHARMA	54746
HERCON LABORATORIES	49730
HERITAGE PHARMACEUTICALS	23155
HILL DERMACEUTICALS	28105
HILLESTAD PHARMACEUTICALS	10542
HI-TECH PHARMACAL	50383
HOFFMANN-LA ROCHE	00004
HOPE PHARMACEUTICALS	60267
HOSPIRA	00409
IDEC PHARMACEUTICALS - BIOGEN IDEC	64406
IMCLONE SYSTEMS	66733
INDEVUS PHARMACEUTICALS	67979
INSPIRE PHARMACEUTICALS	31357
INTEGRITY PHARMACEUTICAL	64731
INTENDIS	10922
INTERMUNE	64116
INTERNATIONAL LABS	54458
INTERNATIONAL MEDICATION SYSTEMS	00548
INWOOD LABORATORIES	00258
IPSEN PHARMECEUTICALS	16887
IROKO PHARMACEUTICALS	42211
ISTA PHARMACEUTICALS	67425
IVAX LABS	59310
IVAX PHARMACEUTICALS	00172
IVAX RESEARCH	00575
JACOBUS PHARMACEUTICALS	49938
JAYMAC PHARMACEUTICALS	64661
JAZZ PHARMACEUTICALS	68727
JHP PHARMACEUTICALS	42023
JOHNSON & JOHNSON	10147
JOHNSON & JOHNSON	57894
JOHNSON & JOHNSON	59676
JOHNSON & JOHNSON	65847
JOHNSON & JOHNSON	68669
JONES PHARMA	52604
JSJ PHARMACEUTICALS	68712
KARALEX PHARMA	42043
KENWOOD THERAPEUTICS	00482
KING PHARMACEUTICALS	60793
KIRKMAN LABORATORIES	58223
KONSYL PHARMACEUTICALS	00224
KOS PHARMACEUTICALS	60598
KOWA PHARMACEUTICALS AMERICA	66869
KREMERS URBAN	62175
KVK-TECH	10702
L. PERRIGO COMPANY	00113
LANNETT COMPANY	00527
LARKEN LABORATORIES	68047
LASER PHARMACEUTICALS	00277
LASER PHARMACEUTICALS	16477
LE VISTA	42212
LEADER	37205
LEDERLE LABORATORIES	00005
LEDERLE PIPERACILLIN	00206
LEGACY PHARMACEUTICAL PACKAGING	68645
LEK PHARMACEUTICALS	66685
LEV PHARMACEUTICALS	42227
LLORENS PHARMACEUTICALS	54859
LNK INTERNATIONAL	50844
LTC PRODUCTS	61598
LUNDBECK	67386

MANUFACTURER	ID#
LUNSCO	10892
LUPIN PHARMACEUTICALS	27437
LUPIN PHARMACEUTICALS	68180
MACOVEN PHARMACEUTICALS	44183
MAGNA PHARMACEUTICALS	58407
MAJOR PHARMACEUTICALS	00904
MALLINCKRODT	00406
MALLINCKRODT	23635
MANCHESTER PHARMACEUTICALS	45043
MARATHON PHARMAEUTICALS	42998
MARLOP PHARMACEUTICALS	12939
MARNEL PHARMACEUTICAL	00682
MAYNE PHARMA (USA)	61703
MCKESSON	49348
MCKESSON , RX PAK DIVISION	65084
MCKESSON PACKAGING SERVICE	63739
MCR-AMERICAN PHARMACEUTICALS	58605
MEAD JOHNSON AND COMPANY	00015
MEDA PHARMACEUTICALS	00037
MEDECOR PHARMA	67112
MEDICINE SHOPPE INTERNATIONAL	49614
MEDICIS DERMATOLOGICS	99207
MEDICURE	25208
MEDIMETRIKS PHARMACEUTICALS	43538
MEDIMMUNE	60574
MEDIMMUNE ONCOLOGY	58178
MEDISCA	38779
MEDLINE INDUSTRIES	53329
MEDTRONIC	58281
MERCK & CO	00006
MERCK/SCHERING-PLOUGH JV	66582
MERZ PHARMACEUTICALS	00259
MGI PHARMA	58063
MICROBIX BIOSYSTEMS	24430
MIDDLEBROOK PHARMACEUTICALS	11042
MIDLAND HEALTHCARE	15686
MIDLOTHIAN LABORATORIES	68308
MIKART	46672
MILLENNIUM PHARMACEUTICALS	63020
MISEMER PHARMACEUTICAL	00276
MISSION PHARMACAL COMPANY	00178
MONARCH PHARMACEUTICALS	61570
MORTON GROVE PHARMACEUTICALS	60432
MPM MEDICAL	66977
MULTI-PAK PACKAGING	66789
MUTUAL PHARMACEUTICAL COMPANY	53489
MYLAN BERTEK PHARMACEUTICALS	62794
MYLAN PHARMACEUTICALS	00378
NEPHRON PHARMACEUTICALS	00487
NEPHRO-TECH	59528
NEXTWAVE PHARMACEUTICALS	24478
NITROMED	12948
NNODUM PHARMACEUTICAL	63044
NOMAX	51801
NORTHSTAR RX	68820
NORTHSTAR RX	16714
NOSTRUM LABORATORIES	29033
NOVARTIS	00028
NOVARTIS	00078
NOVARTIS	00083
NOVARTIS	58768
NOVARTIS CONSUMER HEALTH	00067
NOVAVAX	66500
NOVAVAX (FORMERLY FIELDING)	00421
NOVEN THERAPEUTICS	68968
NOVO NORDISK	00169
NOVO NORDISK	59060
OCEANSIDE PHARMACEUTICALS	68682
OCTAPHARMA A.B.	68209
OCTAPHARMA PHARMAZEUTIKA GM	67467
ODYSSEY PHARMACEUTICAL	65473

MANUFACTURER	ID#
OHM PHARMACEUTICALS	51660
ONSET THERAPEUTICS	16781
OPTICS LABORATORY	64108
ORGANON	00052
ORPHAN MEDICAL	62161
ORTHO-MCNEIL JANSSEN	00062
ORTHO-MCNEIL JANSSEN	50458
ORTHO-MCNEIL-JANSSEN	00045
ORTHO-MCNEIL-JANSSEN	17314
OSCIENT PHARMACEUTICALS	67707
OTN GENERICS	15210
OTSUKA AMERICA	59148
PACIFIC PHARMA	60758
PACK PHARMACEUTICALS	16571
PADDOCK LABORATORIES	00574
PALADIN LABS (USA)	46129
PAMLAB	00525
PAR PHARMACEUTICAL	49884
PARENTA PHARMACEUTICALS	66758
PARKEDALE PHARMACEUTICALS	64029
PBM PHARMACEUTICALS	66213
PEDINOL PHARMACAL	00884
PERRIGO PHARMACEUTICALS	00414
PERRIGO PHARMACEUTICALS	10768
PERRIGO PHARMACEUTICALS	45802
PERSON & COVEY	00096
PFIZER	00009
PFIZER	00013
PFIZER	00025
PFIZER	00049
PFIZER	00069
PFIZER	00071
PFIZER	59762
PFIZER	63010
PHARBEST PHARMACEUTICALS	16103
PHARMACEUTICAL ASSOCIATES	00121
PHARMADERM	00462
PHARMAFORCE	40042
PHARMASCIENCE LABORATORIES	51817
PHARMELLE	66663
PHARMICS	00813
PHARMION	67211
PIERRE FABRE MEDICAMENT	64370
PLIVA	50111
PLYMOUTH PHARMACEUTICALS	61480
POLY PHARMACEUTICAL	50991
PRASCO LABORATORIES	66993
PRECISION DOSE	68094
PRIME MARKETING	62107
PRIMUS PHARMACEUTICALS	68040
PROBACTIVE BIOTECH	23110
PROCTER & GAMBLE	37000
PROCTER & GAMBLE PHARMACEUTICALS	00149
PROMETHEUS LABORATORIES	65483
PROMIUS PHARMA	67857
PRO-PHARMA	66594
PROSTRAKAN	42747
PRUGEN	42546
PURDUE GMP CENTER	13845
PURDUE PHARMA	59011
PURDUE PHARMACEUTICAL PRODUCTS	67781
PURDUE PRODUCTS	67618
QOL MEDICAL	67871
QUALITEST PHARMACEUTICALS	00603
QUESTCOR PHARMACEUTICALS	63004
R.A. MCNEIL COMPANY	12830
RANBAXY LABORATORIES	10631
RANBAXY PHARMACEUTICALS	63304
RARE DISEASE THERAPEUTICS	66607
RARE DISEASE THERAPEUTICS	66621
RECKITT BENCKISER	12496

MANUFACTURER	ID#
RECKITT BENCKISER	63824
RED RIVER PHARMA MANUFACTURING	12593
REGENERON PHARMACEUTICALS	61755
RELIANT PHARMACEUTICALS	65726
RESPA PHARMACEUTICALS	60575
RHODES PHARMACEUTICALS	42858
RISING PHARMACEUTICALS	64980
RIVER'S EDGE PHARMACEUTICALS	68032
ROMARK LABORATORIES	67546
ROSEMONT PHARMACEUTICALS	13632
ROUSES POINT PHARMACEUTICALS	43478
ROXANE LABORATORIES	00054
RX ELITE HOLDINGS	66794
SAGE PHARMACEUTICALS	59243
SAGENT PHARMACEUTICALS	25021
SALIX PHARMACEUTICALS	65649
SANCILIO & COMPANY	44946
SANDOZ	00781
SANOFI-AVENTIS	00024
SANOFI-AVENTIS	00039
SANOFI-SYNTHELABO	00955
SAVAGE LABORATORIES	00281
SAVIENT PHARMACEUTICALS	54396
SCHERING	00085
SCHERING HEALTHCARE PRODUCTS	11523
SCHWARZ PHARMA	00091
SCHWARZ PHARMA	00131
SCIELE PHARMA	59630
SDA LABORATORIES	66424
SELECT BRAND DISTRIBUTORS	15127
SEPRACOR	63402
SERONO	44087
SETON PHARMACEUTICALS	13925
SEVEN OAKS PHARMACEUTICAL	63801
SHERWOOD MEDICAL	08880
SHIONOGI USA	45809
SHIRE US	54092
SHIRE US	59417
SICOR PHARMACEUTICALS	00703
SIGMA-TAU PHARMACEUTICALS	54482
SILARX PHARMACEUTICALS	54838
SIRION THERAPEUTICS	42826
SJ PHARMACEUTICALS	24839
SKIN MEDICA	67402
SLATE PHARMACEUTICALS	43773
SMITH & NEPHEW	50484
SOLCO HEALTHCARE US	43547
SOLSTICE NEUROSCIENCES	10454
SOLVAY PHARMACEUTICALS	00032
SOMERSET PHARMACEUTICALS	39506
SPEAR DERMATOLOGY PRODUCTS	66530
SPECTRUM PHARMACEUTICALS	68152
STAT-TRADE	68850
STEWART-JACKSON PHARMACAL	45985
STIEFEL LABORATORIES	00145
STIEFEL LABORATORIES	63032
STONEBRIDGE PHARMA	14168
STRATUS PHARMACEUTICALS	58980
SUMMIT PHARMACEUTICALS	17433
SUN PHARMA GLOBAL	41616
SUN PHARMA GLOBAL FZE	47335
SUN PHARMACEUTICAL INDUSTRIES	14508
SUN PHARMACEUTICAL INDUSTRIES	62756
SYNTHON PHARMACEUTICALS	63672
TAKEDA PHARMACEUTICALS AMERICA	64764
TALECRIS BIOTHERAPEUTICS	13533
TAP PHARMACEUTICALS	00300
TARGACEPT	17205
TARO PHARMACEUTICALS USA	51672
TAYLOR PHARMACEUTICALS	11098
TEC LABORATORIES	51879

MANUFACTURER	ID#
TERCICA	15054
TEVA NEUROSCIENCE	68546
TEVA PHARMACEUTICALS USA	00093
THAMES PHARMACEUTICALS	49158
THE MEDICINES COMPANY	65293
THER-RX	64011
THREE RIVERS PHARMACEUTICALS	66435
TIBER LABORATORIES	23589
TIME-CAP LABS	49483
TOPIX PHARMACEUTICALS	58211
TORRENT PHARMA	13668
TOWER LABORATORIES	50201
TRIGEN LABORATORIES	13811
TRI-MED LABORATORIES	55654
U.S. PHARMACEUTICAL	52747
UAD LABORATORIES	00785
UCB PHARMA	50474
UCYCLYD PHARMA	62592
UDL LABORATORIES	51079
UNICHEM PHARMACEUTICALS	29300
UNIMED PHARMACEUTICALS	00051
UNITED RESEARCH LABORATORIES	00677
UNITED THERAPEUTICS	66302
UPSHER-SMITH LABORATORIES	00245
UPSHER-SMITH LABORATORIES	00832
UPSTATE PHARMA	65580
VALEANT PHARMACEUTICALS	00187
VALEANT PHARMACEUTICALS	65234
VALEANT PHARMACEUTICALS	66490
VALEANT/DOW/DESCARTES ACQUISITION	59987
VALIDUS PHARMACEUTICALS	30698
VANDA PHARMACEUTICALS	43068
VANGARD LABS	00615
VATRING PHARMACEUTICALS	65199
VERSAPHARM	61748
VERTICAL PHARMACEUTICALS	68025
VERUS	13436
VICTORY PHARMA	68453
VIROPHARMA	66593
VISION PHARMA	68013
VISTA PHARMACEUTICALS	61971
VISTAPHARM	66689
VIVUS	62541
WARNER CHILCOTT LABORATORIES	00430
WARRICK PHARMACEUTICALS	59930
WATSON PHARMA	00536
WATSON PHARMA	00591
WATSON PHARMA	52544
WATSON PHARMA	54391
WATSON PHARMA	55515
WATSON PHARMA	62037
WEEKS & LEO	11383
WEST-WARD PHARMACEUTICAL	00143
WESTWOOD-SQUIBB	00072
WG CRITICAL CARE	44567
WOCKHARDT AMERICAS	64679
WORLD GEN	66814
WRASER PHARMACEUTICALS	66992
WYETH CONSUMER HEALTHCARE	00573
WYETH LABORATORIES	00008
XANODYNE PHARMACEUTICAL	66479
X-GEN PHARMACEUTICALS	39822
XTTRIUM LABORATORIES	00116
ZARS PHARMA	43469
ZERXIS PHARMA	18011
ZYBER PHARMACEUTICALS	65224
ZYDUS PHARMACEUTICALS	68382

NUMERICAL INDEX

ID#	MANUFACTURER
00002	ELI LILLY AND COMPANY
00003	E.R. SQUIBB & SONS
00004	HOFFMANN-LA ROCHE
00005	LEDERLE LABORATORIES
00006	MERCK & CO
00007	GLAXOSMITHKLINE
00008	WYETH LABORATORIES
00009	PFIZER
00013	PFIZER
00015	MEAD JOHNSON AND COMPANY
00023	ALLERGAN
00024	SANOFI-AVENTIS
00025	PFIZER
00026	BAYER
00028	NOVARTIS
00029	GLAXOSMITHKLINE
00031	A. H. ROBINS
00032	SOLVAY PHARMACEUTICALS
00037	MEDA PHARMACEUTICALS
00039	SANOFI-AVENTIS
00045	ORTHO-MCNEIL-JANSSEN
00046	AYERST LABORATORIES
00049	PFIZER
00051	UNIMED PHARMACEUTICALS
00052	ORGANON
00053	CSL BEHRING
00054	ROXANE LABORATORIES
00056	DUPONT PHARMACEUTICALS
00062	ORTHO-MCNEIL JANSSEN
00064	HEALTHPOINT
00065	ALCON LABORATORIES
00066	AVENTIS PHARMACEUTICALS
00067	NOVARTIS CONSUMER HEALTH
00068	AVENTIS PHARMACEUTICALS
00069	PFIZER
00071	PFIZER
00072	WESTWOOD-SQUIBB
00074	ABBOTT LABORATORIES
00075	AVENTIS PHARMACEUTICALS
00078	NOVARTIS
00083	NOVARTIS
00085	SCHERING
00087	BRISTOL-MYERS SQUIBB
00088	AVENTIS PHARMACEUTICALS
00089	3M PHARMACEUTICALS
00091	SCHWARZ PHARMA
00093	TEVA PHARMACEUTICALS USA
00095	ECR PHARMACEUTICALS
00096	PERSON & COVEY
00113	L. PERRIGO COMPANY
00115	GLOBAL PHARMACEUTICAL
00116	XTTRIUM LABORATORIES
00121	PHARMACEUTICAL ASSOCIATES
00126	COLGATE ORAL PHARMACEUTICALS
00131	SCHWARZ PHARMA
00132	C B FLEET COMPANY
00135	GLAXOSMITHKLINE
00143	WEST-WARD PHARMACEUTICAL
00145	STIEFEL LABORATORIES
00149	PROCTER & GAMBLE PHARMACEUTICALS
00165	BLAINE COMPANY
00168	E FOUGERA
00169	NOVO NORDISK
00172	IVAX PHARMACEUTICALS
00173	GLAXOSMITHKLINE
00178	MISSION PHARMACAL COMPANY
00182	GOLDLINE LABORATORIES
00185	EON LABS
00186	ASTRAZENECA LP
00187	VALEANT PHARMACEUTICALS
00206	LEDERLE PIPERACILLIN
00224	KONSYL PHARMACEUTICALS
00225	B. F. ASCHER AND COMPANY
00228	ACTAVIS ELIZABETH
00245	UPSHER-SMITH LABORATORIES
00256	FLEMING AND COMPANY
00258	INWOOD LABORATORIES
00259	MERZ PHARMACEUTICALS
00264	B. BRAUN MEDICAL
00276	MISEMER PHARMACEUTICAL
00277	LASER PHARMACEUTICALS
00281	SAVAGE LABORATORIES
00288	FLUORITAB
00299	GALDERMA LABORATORIES
00300	TAP PHARMACEUTICALS
00310	ASTRAZENECA LP
00327	GUARDIAN LABS
00338	BAXTER HEALTHCARE
00378	MYLAN PHARMACEUTICALS
00406	MALLINCKRODT
00409	HOSPIRA
00414	PERRIGO PHARMACEUTICALS
00421	NOVAVAX (FORMERLY FIELDING)
00430	WARNER CHILCOTT LABORATORIES
00456	FOREST LABORATORIES
00462	PHARMADERM
00469	ASTELLAS PHARMA
00472	ACTAVIS
00482	KENWOOD THERAPEUTICS
00485	EDWARDS PHARMACEUTICALS
00486	BEACH PRODUCTS
00487	NEPHRON PHARMACEUTICALS
00496	FERNDALE LABORATORIES
00517	AMERICAN REGENT LABORATORIES
00525	PAMLAB
00527	LANNETT COMPANY
00535	GILBERT LABORATORIES
00536	WATSON PHARMA
00548	INTERNATIONAL MEDICATION SYSTEMS
00555	BARR LABORATORIES
00573	WYETH CONSUMER HEALTHCARE
00574	PADDOCK LABORATORIES
00575	IVAX RESEARCH
00590	DUPONT PHARMACEUTICALS
00591	WATSON PHARMA
00597	BOEHRINGER INGELHEIM
00603	QUALITEST PHARMACEUTICALS
00615	VANGARD LABS
00641	BAXTER HEALTHCARE
00642	EVERETT LABORATORIES
00677	UNITED RESEARCH LABORATORIES
00682	MARNEL PHARMACEUTICAL
00703	SICOR PHARMACEUTICALS
00713	G&W LABORATORIES
00777	DISTA PRODUCTS
00781	SANDOZ
00785	UAD LABORATORIES
00813	PHARMICS
00832	UPSHER-SMITH LABORATORIES
00884	PEDINOL PHARMACAL
00904	MAJOR PHARMACEUTICALS
00944	BAXTER HEALTHCARE
00955	SANOFI-SYNTHELABO
00998	ALCON LABORATORIES
08880	SHERWOOD MEDICAL
10019	BAXTER HEALTHCARE
10122	CORNERSTONE BIOPHARMA
10139	GENERAMEDIX
10144	ACORDA THERAPEUTICS
10147	JOHNSON & JOHNSON
10148	COTHERIX
10158	GLAXOSMITHKLINE
10267	CONTRACT PHARMACAL
10337	DOAK DERMATOLOGICS
10370	ANCHEN PHARMACEUTICALS
10454	SOLSTICE NEUROSCIENCES
10518	DABUR PHARMA US
10542	HILLESTAD PHARMACEUTICALS
10572	AFFORDABLE PHARMACEUTICALS
10631	RANBAXY LABORATORIES
10702	KVK-TECH
10768	PERRIGO PHARMACEUTICALS
10892	LUNSCO
10914	BRIGHTON PHARMACEUTICALS
10922	INTENDIS
11042	MIDDLEBROOK PHARMACEUTICALS
11098	TAYLOR PHARMACEUTICALS
11383	WEEKS & LEO
11399	GTX
11523	SCHERING HEALTHCARE PRODUCTS
11528	CENTRIX PHARMACEUTICAL
11530	GLAXOSMITHKLINE
11701	COLOPLAST
11980	ALLERGAN
12496	RECKITT BENCKISER
12593	RED RIVER PHARMA MANUFACTURING
12830	R.A. MCNEIL COMPANY
12939	MARLOP PHARMACEUTICALS
12948	NITROMED
13107	AUROBINDO PHARMA
13279	ALLAN PHARMACEUTICAL
13310	AR SCIENTIFIC
13436	VERUS
13453	GRACEWAY PHARMACEUTICALS
13478	BARRIER THERAPEUTICS
13533	TALECRIS BIOTHERAPEUTICS
13548	CORIA LABORATORIES
13551	FSC LABORATORIES
13632	ROSEMONT PHARMACEUTICALS
13668	TORRENT PHARMA
13811	TRIGEN LABORATORIES
13845	PURDUE GMP CENTER
13913	DEPOMED
13925	SETON PHARMACEUTICALS
14168	STONEBRIDGE PHARMA
14508	SUN PHARMACEUTICAL INDUSTRIES
15054	TERCICA
15127	SELECT BRAND DISTRIBUTORS
15210	OTN GENERICS
15330	GENPHARM
15338	APACE KY
15370	CARWIN ASSOCIATES
15456	ESPRIT PHARMA
15584	BRISTOL-MYERS SQUIBB & GILEAD
15686	MIDLAND HEALTHCARE

ID#	MANUFACTURER
15821	FOCUS LABORATORIES
16103	PHARBEST PHARMACEUTICALS
16252	COBALT LABORATORIES
16477	LASER PHARMACEUTICALS
16571	PACK PHARMACEUTICALS
16714	NORTHSTAR RX
16729	ACCORD HEALTHCARE
16781	ONSET THERAPEUTICS
16887	IPSEN PHARMECEUTICALS
17205	TARGACEPT
17314	ORTHO-MCNEIL-JANSSEN
17433	SUMMIT PHARMACEUTICALS
17478	AKORN
18011	ZERXIS PHARMA
18754	A. AARONS
18860	AZUR PHARMA
19810	BRISTOL-MYERS SQUIBB COMPANY
23110	PROBACTIVE BIOTECH
23155	HERITAGE PHARMACEUTICALS
23359	CENTURION LABS
23589	TIBER LABORATORIES
23635	MALLINCKRODT
24090	AKRIMAX PHARMACEUTICALS
24208	BAUSCH & LOMB
24338	ARBOR PHARMACEUTICALS
24385	BERGEN BRUNSWIG DRUG COMPANY
24430	MICROBIX BIOSYSTEMS
24477	EKR THERAPEUTICS
24478	NEXTWAVE PHARMACEUTICALS
24486	ARISTOS PHARMACEUTICALS
24839	SJ PHARMACEUTICALS
25010	ATON PHARMA
25021	SAGENT PHARMACEUTICALS
25208	MEDICURE
25356	ACETO PHARMA
25382	DERMA SCIENCES
25682	ALEXION PHARMACEUTICALS
27437	LUPIN PHARMACEUTICALS
28105	HILL DERMACEUTICALS
28595	ALLEGIS PHARMACEUTICALS
29033	NOSTRUM LABORATORIES
29300	UNICHEM PHARMACEUTICALS
29336	GRACEWAY PHARMACEUTICALS
29978	CAPITAL PHARMACEUTICAL
30698	VALIDUS PHARMACEUTICALS
31357	INSPIRE PHARMACEUTICALS
31722	CAMBER PHARMACEUTICALS
37000	PROCTER & GAMBLE
37205	LEADER
38779	MEDISCA
39506	SOMERSET PHARMACEUTICALS
39822	X-GEN PHARMACEUTICALS
40042	PHARMAFORCE
41616	SUN PHARMA GLOBAL
42023	JHP PHARMACEUTICALS
42043	KARALEX PHARMA
42192	BROOKSTONE PHARMACEUTICALS
42211	IROKO PHARMACEUTICALS
42212	LE VISTA
42227	LEV PHARMACEUTICALS
42457	EMMAUS MEDICAL
42546	PRUGEN
42747	PROSTRAKAN
42769	BAY PHARMA
42799	EDENBRIDGE PHARMACEUTICALS
42806	EPIC PHARMA
42826	SIRION THERAPEUTICS
42858	RHODES PHARMACEUTICALS
42865	EURAND PHARMACEUTICALS
42998	MARATHON PHARMAEUTICALS
43068	VANDA PHARMACEUTICALS

ID#	MANUFACTURER
43199	COUNTY LINE PHARMACEUTICALS
43378	CODADOSE
43386	GAVIS PHARMACEUTICALS
43469	ZARS PHARMA
43478	ROUSES POINT PHARMACEUTICALS
43538	MEDIMETRIKS PHARMACEUTICALS
43547	SOLCO HEALTHCARE US
43553	CONVATEC
43773	SLATE PHARMACEUTICALS
44087	SERONO
44183	MACOVEN PHARMACEUTICALS
44206	CSL BEHRING
44523	BIOCOMP PHARMA
44567	WG CRITICAL CARE
44946	SANCILIO & COMPANY
45043	MANCHESTER PHARMACEUTICALS
45802	PERRIGO PHARMACEUTICALS
45809	SHIONOGI USA
45963	ACTAVIS
45985	STEWART-JACKSON PHARMACAL
46129	PALADIN LABS (USA)
46287	CAROLINA MEDICAL PRODUCTS COMPANY
46672	MIKART
46987	ACTAVIS KADIAN
47335	SUN PHARMA GLOBAL FZE
47781	ALVOGEN
47783	DYAX
48102	FERA PHARMACEUTICALS
48818	ALLOS THERAPEUTICS
49158	THAMES PHARMACEUTICALS
49230	FRESENIUS MEDICAL CARE
49281	AVENTIS PASTEUR
49348	MCKESSON
49483	TIME-CAP LABS
49502	DEY L.P.
49614	MEDICINE SHOPPE INTERNATIONAL
49708	CARACO PHARMA
49730	HERCON LABORATORIES
49884	PAR PHARMACEUTICAL
49938	JACOBUS PHARMACEUTICALS
50111	PLIVA
50201	TOWER LABORATORIES
50242	GENENTECH
50383	HI-TECH PHARMACAL
50419	BERLEX
50458	ORTHO-MCNEIL JANSSEN
50474	UCB PHARMA
50484	SMITH & NEPHEW
50844	LNK INTERNATIONAL
50991	POLY PHARMACEUTICAL
51079	UDL LABORATORIES
51248	ASTELLAS
51285	BARR LABORATORIES
51479	DURA PHARMACEUTICALS
51552	GALLIPOT
51645	GEMINI PHARMACEUTICALS
51660	OHM PHARMACEUTICALS
51672	TARO PHARMACEUTICALS USA
51674	BLANSETT PHARMACAL
51801	NOMAX
51817	PHARMASCIENCE LABORATORIES
51879	TEC LABORATORIES
51991	BRECKENRIDGE PHARMACEUTICAL
52152	ACTAVIS TOTOWA
52268	BRAINTREE LABORATORIES
52544	WATSON PHARMA
52569	GENERAMED
52604	JONES PHARMA
52735	FAMILY PHARMACY
52747	U.S. PHARMACEUTICAL
52769	AMERICAN RED CROSS

ID#	MANUFACTURER
53014	CELLTECH PHARMACEUTICALS
53062	BETA DERMACEUTICALS
53329	MEDLINE INDUSTRIES
53489	MUTUAL PHARMACEUTICAL COMPANY
53746	AMNEAL PHARMACEUTICALS
53905	CHIRON
54092	SHIRE US
54391	WATSON PHARMA
54396	SAVIENT PHARMACEUTICALS
54458	INTERNATIONAL LABS
54482	SIGMA-TAU PHARMACEUTICALS
54643	BAXTER HEALTHCARE
54746	HEMISPHERX BIOPHARMA
54838	SILARX PHARMACEUTICALS
54859	LLORENS PHARMACEUTICALS
55111	DR. REDDY'S LABORATORIES
55253	CIMA LABS
55390	BEDFORD LABORATORIES
55513	AMGEN USA
55515	WATSON PHARMA
55566	FERRING PHARMACEUTICALS
55654	TRI-MED LABORATORIES
57664	CARACO PHARMACEUTICAL
57665	ENZON PHARMACEUTICALS
57782	BAUSCH & LOMB
57844	GATE PHARMACEUTICALS
57894	JOHNSON & JOHNSON
58063	MGI PHARMA
58177	ETHEX
58178	MEDIMMUNE ONCOLOGY
58211	TOPIX PHARMACEUTICALS
58223	KIRKMAN LABORATORIES
58281	MEDTRONIC
58394	GENETICS INSTITUTE
58406	AMGEN/IMMUNEX
58407	MAGNA PHARMACEUTICALS
58468	GENZYME
58605	MCR-AMERICAN PHARMACEUTICALS
58768	NOVARTIS
58790	ADVANCED VISION RESEARCH
58809	GM PHARMACEUTICALS
58914	AXCAN SCANDIPHARM
58980	STRATUS PHARMACEUTICALS
59011	PURDUE PHARMA
59060	NOVO NORDISK
59075	ELAN PHARMACEUTICALS/ATHENA NEURO
59148	OTSUKA AMERICA
59243	SAGE PHARMACEUTICALS
59310	IVAX LABS
59338	AMAG PHARMACEUTICALS
59366	GLADES PHARMACEUTICALS
59417	SHIRE US
59528	NEPHRO-TECH
59572	CELGENE
59627	BIOGEN IDEC
59630	SCIELE PHARMA
59676	JOHNSON & JOHNSON
59702	ATLEY PHARMACEUTICALS
59730	BIOTEST PHARMACEUTICALS
59746	CADISTA PHARMACEUTICALS
59762	PFIZER
59767	DIGESTIVE CARE
59930	WARRICK PHARMACEUTICALS
59987	VALEANT/DOW/DESCARTES ACQUISITION
60258	CYPRESS PHARMACEUTICAL
60267	HOPE PHARMACEUTICALS
60432	MORTON GROVE PHARMACEUTICALS
60505	APOTEX
60574	MEDIMMUNE
60575	RESPA PHARMACEUTICALS
60598	KOS PHARMACEUTICALS

ID#	MANUFACTURER
60758	PACIFIC PHARMA
60793	KING PHARMACEUTICALS
60951	ENDO PHARMACEUTICALS
60977	BAXTER HEALTHCARE
61314	FALCON PHARMACEUTICALS
61442	CARLSBAD TECHNOLOGY
61451	AMERIFIT PHARMA
61480	PLYMOUTH PHARMACEUTICALS
61570	MONARCH PHARMACEUTICALS
61598	LTC PRODUCTS
61703	MAYNE PHARMA (USA)
61748	VERSAPHARM
61755	REGENERON PHARMACEUTICALS
61787	HEALTH CARE PRODUCTS DIVISION
61924	DERMARITE INDUSTRIES
61953	GRIFOLS BIOLOGICALS
61958	GILEAD SCIENCES
61971	VISTA PHARMACEUTICALS
62037	WATSON PHARMA
62103	BOUDREAUX'S BUTT PASTE
62107	PRIME MARKETING
62161	ORPHAN MEDICAL
62175	KREMERS URBAN
62541	VIVUS
62559	ANIP ACQUISITION COMPANY
62584	AMERICAN HEALTH PACKAGING
62592	UCYCLYD PHARMA
62756	SUN PHARMACEUTICAL INDUSTRIES
62794	MYLAN BERTEK PHARMACEUTICALS
62856	EISAI
63004	QUESTCOR PHARMACEUTICALS
63010	PFIZER
63020	MILLENNIUM PHARMACEUTICALS
63032	STIEFEL LABORATORIES
63044	NNODUM PHARMACEUTICAL
63162	BALLAY PHARMACEUTICALS
63304	RANBAXY PHARMACEUTICALS
63323	APP PHARMACEUTICALS
63395	DAIICHI SANKYO
63402	SEPRACOR
63459	CEPHALON
63481	ENDO PHARMACEUTICALS
63653	BRISTOL-MYERS SQUIBB/SANOFI
63672	SYNTHON PHARMACEUTICALS
63717	HAWTHORN PHARMACEUTICALS
63739	MCKESSON PACKAGING SERVICE
63801	SEVEN OAKS PHARMACEUTICAL
63824	RECKITT BENCKISER
63833	CSL BEHRING GMBH
63857	ALPHARMA
63868	CHAIN DRUG MARKETING ASSOCIATION
63921	AMERIDERM LABORATORIES
64011	THER-RX
64019	CEBERT PHARMACEUTICALS
64029	PARKEDALE PHARMACEUTICALS
64108	OPTICS LABORATORY
64116	INTERMUNE
64125	EXCELLIUM PHARMACEUTICAL
64193	BAXTER HEALTHCARE
64370	PIERRE FABRE MEDICAMENT

ID#	MANUFACTURER
64376	BOCA PHARMACAL
64406	IDEC PHARMACEUTICALS - BIOGEN IDEC
64455	BTA PHARMACEUTICALS
64543	CAPELLON PHARMACEUTICALS
64597	AVANIR PHARMACEUTICALS
64661	JAYMAC PHARMACEUTICALS
64679	WOCKHARDT AMERICAS
64682	COLLAGENEX PHARMACEUTICALS
64720	AURIGA LABORATORIES, CORE PHARMA
64731	INTEGRITY PHARMACEUTICAL
64764	TAKEDA PHARMACEUTICALS AMERICA
64875	DANCO LABORATORIES
64894	GENZYME
64980	RISING PHARMACEUTICALS
65084	MCKESSON , RX PAK DIVISION
65162	AMNEAL PHARMACEUTICALS
65199	VATRING PHARMACEUTICALS
65224	ZYBER PHARMACEUTICALS
65234	VALEANT PHARMACEUTICALS
65293	THE MEDICINES COMPANY
65473	ODYSSEY PHARMACEUTICAL
65483	PROMETHEUS LABORATORIES
65580	UPSTATE PHARMA
65597	DAIICHI SANKYO
65649	SALIX PHARMACEUTICALS
65726	RELIANT PHARMACEUTICALS
65757	ALKERMES
65847	JOHNSON & JOHNSON
65862	AUROBINDO PHARMA
66213	PBM PHARMACEUTICALS
66215	ACTELION PHARMACEUTICALS
66220	CUMBERLAND PHARMACEUTICALS
66302	UNITED THERAPEUTICS
66424	SDA LABORATORIES
66435	THREE RIVERS PHARMACEUTICALS
66479	XANODYNE PHARMACEUTICAL
66490	VALEANT PHARMACEUTICALS
66500	NOVAVAX
66530	SPEAR DERMATOLOGY PRODUCTS
66582	MERCK/SCHERING-PLOUGH JV
66591	AAI PHARMA
66593	VIROPHARMA
66594	PRO-PHARMA
66607	RARE DISEASE THERAPEUTICS
66621	RARE DISEASE THERAPEUTICS
66658	BIOVITRUM AB
66663	PHARMELLE
66685	LEK PHARMACEUTICALS
66689	VISTAPHARM
66733	IMCLONE SYSTEMS
66758	PARENTA PHARMACEUTICALS
66780	AMYLIN PHARMACEUTICALS
66789	MULTI-PAK PACKAGING
66794	RX ELITE HOLDINGS
66814	WORLD GEN
66860	CURA PHARMACEUTICAL
66869	KOWA PHARMACEUTICALS AMERICA
66870	AMBI PHARMACEUTICALS
66887	AUXILIUM PHARMACEUTICALS
66977	MPM MEDICAL

ID#	MANUFACTURER
66992	WRASER PHARMACEUTICALS
66993	PRASCO LABORATORIES
67108	BAXTER HEALTHCARE
67112	MEDECOR PHARMA
67159	CV THERAPEUTICS (CVT)
67211	PHARMION
67253	DAVA INTERNATIONAL
67286	ESP PHARMA
67386	LUNDBECK
67402	SKIN MEDICA
67405	HARRIS PHARMACEUTICAL
67425	ISTA PHARMACEUTICALS
67457	BIONICHE PHARMA
67467	OCTAPHARMA PHARMAZEUTIKA GM
67546	ROMARK LABORATORIES
67618	PURDUE PRODUCTS
67707	OSCIENT PHARMACEUTICALS
67767	ACTAVIS SOUTH ATLANTIC
67781	PURDUE PHARMACEUTICAL PRODUCTS
67857	PROMIUS PHARMA
67871	QOL MEDICAL
67877	ASCEND LABORATORIES
67919	CUBIST PHARMACEUTICALS
67979	INDEVUS PHARMACEUTICALS
68013	VISION PHARMA
68016	CHAIN DRUG CONSORTIUM
68025	VERTICAL PHARMACEUTICALS
68032	RIVER'S EDGE PHARMACEUTICALS
68040	PRIMUS PHARMACEUTICALS
68047	LARKEN LABORATORIES
68084	AMERICAN HEALTH PACKAGING
68094	PRECISION DOSE
68135	BIOMARIN PHARMACEUTICALS
68152	SPECTRUM PHARMACEUTICALS
68180	LUPIN PHARMACEUTICALS
68188	ALLIANT PHARMACEUTICALS
68209	OCTAPHARMA A.B.
68220	ALAVEN PHARMACEUTICAL
68308	MIDLOTHIAN LABORATORIES
68322	AVANIR PHARMACEUTICALS
68330	CEPHAZONE PHARMA
68382	ZYDUS PHARMACEUTICALS
68453	VICTORY PHARMA
68462	GLENMARK PHARMACEUTICALS
68516	GRIFOLS BIOLOGICALS
68546	TEVA NEUROSCIENCE
68645	LEGACY PHARMACEUTICAL PACKAGING
68669	JOHNSON & JOHNSON
68682	OCEANSIDE PHARMACEUTICALS
68712	JSJ PHARMACEUTICALS
68727	JAZZ PHARMACEUTICALS
68734	CRITICAL THERAPEUTICS (CRTX)
68774	DAVA PHARMACEUTICALS
68782	(OSI) EYETECH
68817	ABRAXIS BIOSCIENCE
68820	NORTHSTAR RX
68850	STAT-TRADE
68968	NOVEN THERAPEUTICS
99207	MEDICIS DERMATOLOGICS

When exces

MUCINE

12 hours of co

That's

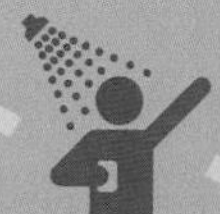

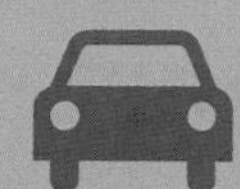

8 PRODUCT IDENTIFICATION

• Dels
OTC
relie

• Give
elim

EX

Mucine

Sinus pres
congest

12-hour symptom rel

Recommend
extended-rel

Please visit our Web site a

Use as directed.
MUCINEX products are indicate

For more information, c
or visit www.delsym.co

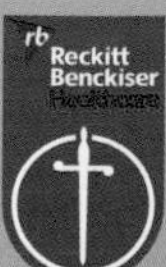

Use as directed.
Do not use in children under 4 yea

Refe
Ora
http

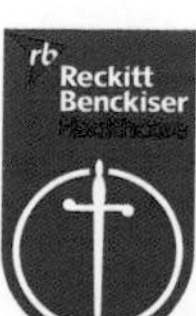

*Combination produ
†Per dose.

References: 1. Data on
Parsippany, NJ. **2.** Electr
Drug Administration W
scripts/cder/ob. Accesse

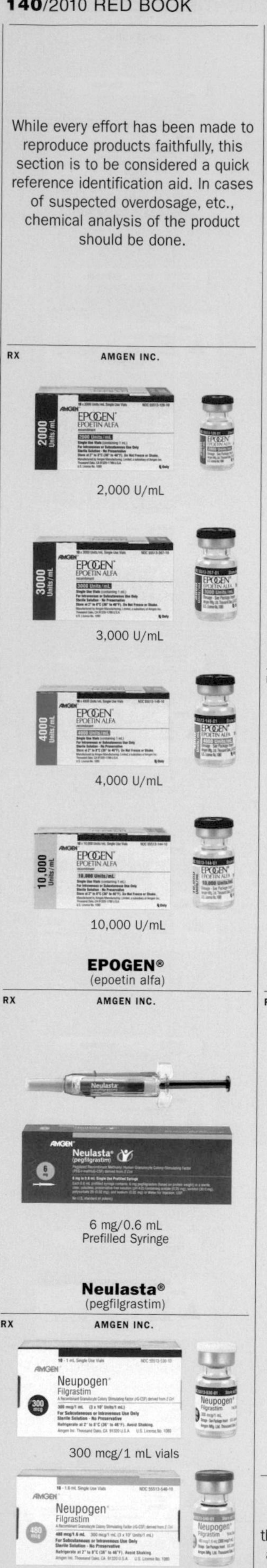

While every effort has been made to reproduce products faithfully, this section is to be considered a quick reference identification aid. In cases of suspected overdosage, etc., chemical analysis of the product should be done.

RX AMGEN INC.

2,000 U/mL

3,000 U/mL

4,000 U/mL

10,000 U/mL

EPOGEN®
(epoetin alfa)

RX AMGEN INC.

6 mg/0.6 mL
Prefilled Syringe

Neulasta®
(pegfilgrastim)

RX AMGEN INC.

300 mcg/1 mL vials

480 mcg/1.6 mL vials

Neupogen®
(filgrastim)

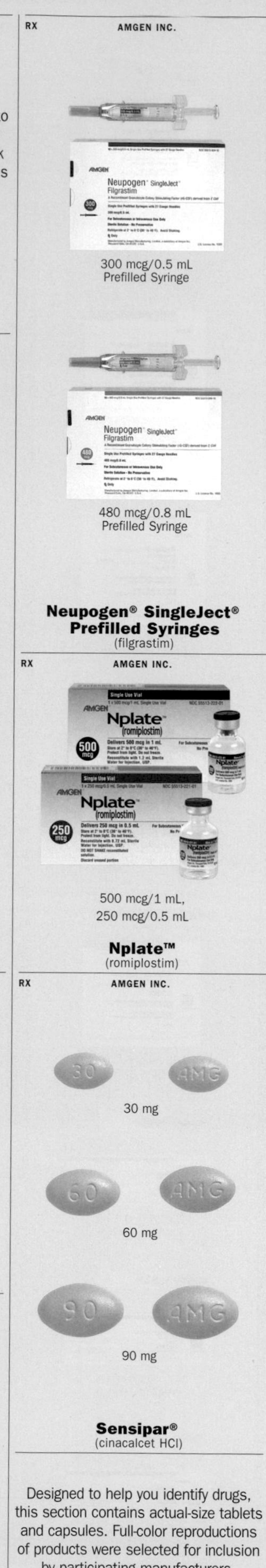

RX AMGEN INC.

300 mcg/0.5 mL
Prefilled Syringe

480 mcg/0.8 mL
Prefilled Syringe

Neupogen® SingleJect® Prefilled Syringes
(filgrastim)

RX AMGEN INC.

500 mcg/1 mL,
250 mcg/0.5 mL

Nplate™
(romiplostim)

RX AMGEN INC.

30 mg

60 mg

90 mg

Sensipar®
(cinacalcet HCl)

Designed to help you identify drugs, this section contains actual-size tablets and capsules. Full-color reproductions of products were selected for inclusion by participating manufacturers.

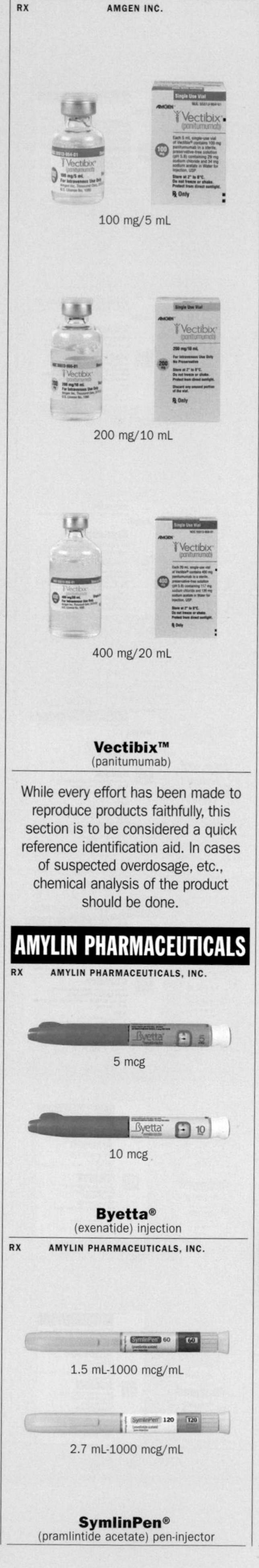

RX AMGEN INC.

100 mg/5 mL

200 mg/10 mL

400 mg/20 mL

Vectibix™
(panitumumab)

While every effort has been made to reproduce products faithfully, this section is to be considered a quick reference identification aid. In cases of suspected overdosage, etc., chemical analysis of the product should be done.

AMYLIN PHARMACEUTICALS

RX AMYLIN PHARMACEUTICALS, INC.

5 mcg

10 mcg

Byetta®
(exenatide) injection

RX AMYLIN PHARMACEUTICALS, INC.

1.5 mL-1000 mcg/mL

2.7 mL-1000 mcg/mL

SymlinPen®
(pramlintide acetate) pen-injector

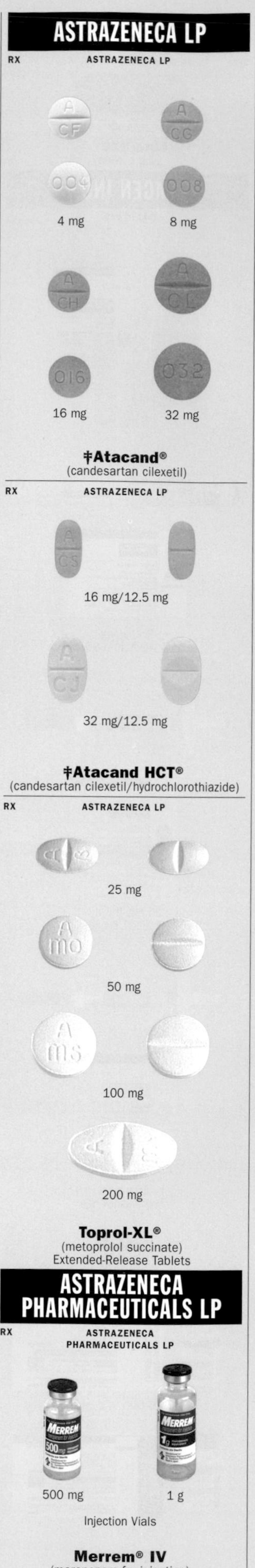

ASTRAZENECA LP

RX ASTRAZENECA LP

4 mg 8 mg

16 mg 32 mg

‡Atacand®
(candesartan cilexetil)

RX ASTRAZENECA LP

16 mg/12.5 mg

32 mg/12.5 mg

‡Atacand HCT®
(candesartan cilexetil/hydrochlorothiazide)

RX ASTRAZENECA LP

25 mg

50 mg

100 mg

200 mg

Toprol-XL®
(metoprolol succinate)
Extended-Release Tablets

ASTRAZENECA PHARMACEUTICALS LP

RX ASTRAZENECA PHARMACEUTICALS LP

500 mg 1 g

Injection Vials

Merrem® IV
(meropenem for injection)

‡ Registered trademark of the AstraZeneca group of companies.

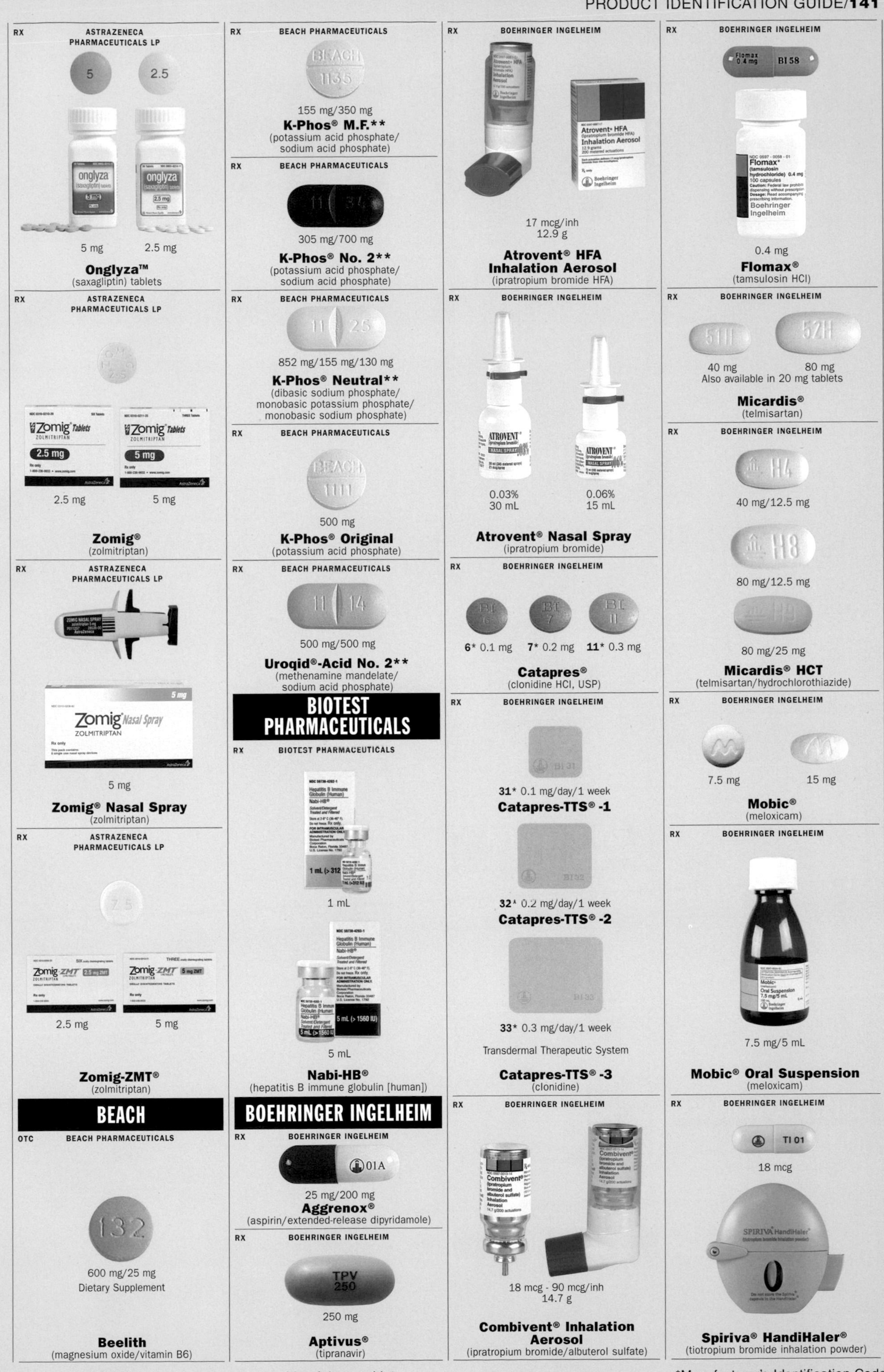

RX ASTRAZENECA PHARMACEUTICALS LP

5 mg 2.5 mg

Onglyza™
(saxagliptin) tablets

RX ASTRAZENECA PHARMACEUTICALS LP

2.5 mg 5 mg

Zomig®
(zolmitriptan)

RX ASTRAZENECA PHARMACEUTICALS LP

5 mg

Zomig® Nasal Spray
(zolmitriptan)

RX ASTRAZENECA PHARMACEUTICALS LP

2.5 mg 5 mg

Zomig-ZMT®
(zolmitriptan)

BEACH

OTC BEACH PHARMACEUTICALS

600 mg/25 mg
Dietary Supplement

Beelith
(magnesium oxide/vitamin B6)

RX BEACH PHARMACEUTICALS

155 mg/350 mg

K-Phos® M.F.**
(potassium acid phosphate/sodium acid phosphate)

RX BEACH PHARMACEUTICALS

305 mg/700 mg

K-Phos® No. 2**
(potassium acid phosphate/sodium acid phosphate)

RX BEACH PHARMACEUTICALS

852 mg/155 mg/130 mg

K-Phos® Neutral**
(dibasic sodium phosphate/monobasic potassium phosphate/monobasic sodium phosphate)

RX BEACH PHARMACEUTICALS

500 mg

K-Phos® Original
(potassium acid phosphate)

RX BEACH PHARMACEUTICALS

500 mg/500 mg

Uroqid®-Acid No. 2**
(methenamine mandelate/sodium acid phosphate)

BIOTEST PHARMACEUTICALS

RX BIOTEST PHARMACEUTICALS

1 mL

5 mL

Nabi-HB®
(hepatitis B immune globulin [human])

BOEHRINGER INGELHEIM

RX BOEHRINGER INGELHEIM

25 mg/200 mg

Aggrenox®
(aspirin/extended-release dipyridamole)

RX BOEHRINGER INGELHEIM

250 mg

Aptivus®
(tipranavir)

RX BOEHRINGER INGELHEIM

17 mcg/inh
12.9 g

Atrovent® HFA Inhalation Aerosol
(ipratropium bromide HFA)

RX BOEHRINGER INGELHEIM

0.03% 30 mL
0.06% 15 mL

Atrovent® Nasal Spray
(ipratropium bromide)

RX BOEHRINGER INGELHEIM

6* 0.1 mg **7*** 0.2 mg **11*** 0.3 mg

Catapres®
(clonidine HCl, USP)

RX BOEHRINGER INGELHEIM

31* 0.1 mg/day/1 week

Catapres-TTS® -1

32* 0.2 mg/day/1 week

Catapres-TTS® -2

33* 0.3 mg/day/1 week

Transdermal Therapeutic System

Catapres-TTS® -3
(clonidine)

RX BOEHRINGER INGELHEIM

18 mcg - 90 mcg/inh
14.7 g

Combivent® Inhalation Aerosol
(ipratropium bromide/albuterol sulfate)

RX BOEHRINGER INGELHEIM

0.4 mg

Flomax®
(tamsulosin HCl)

RX BOEHRINGER INGELHEIM

40 mg 80 mg
Also available in 20 mg tablets

Micardis®
(telmisartan)

RX BOEHRINGER INGELHEIM

40 mg/12.5 mg

80 mg/12.5 mg

80 mg/25 mg

Micardis® HCT
(telmisartan/hydrochlorothiazide)

RX BOEHRINGER INGELHEIM

7.5 mg 15 mg

Mobic®
(meloxicam)

RX BOEHRINGER INGELHEIM

7.5 mg/5 mL

Mobic® Oral Suspension
(meloxicam)

RX BOEHRINGER INGELHEIM

18 mcg

Spiriva® HandiHaler®
(tiotropium bromide inhalation powder)

**The name BEACH appears on the reverse side of these tablets.

*Manufacturer's Identification Code

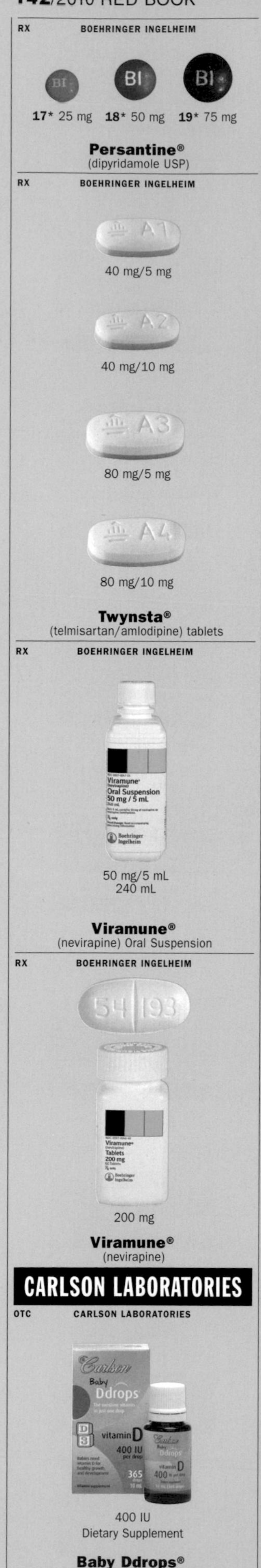

RX BOEHRINGER INGELHEIM

17* 25 mg 18* 50 mg 19* 75 mg

Persantine®
(dipyridamole USP)

RX BOEHRINGER INGELHEIM

40 mg/5 mg

40 mg/10 mg

80 mg/5 mg

80 mg/10 mg

Twynsta®
(telmisartan/amlodipine) tablets

RX BOEHRINGER INGELHEIM

50 mg/5 mL
240 mL

Viramune®
(nevirapine) Oral Suspension

RX BOEHRINGER INGELHEIM

200 mg

Viramune®
(nevirapine)

CARLSON LABORATORIES

OTC CARLSON LABORATORIES

400 IU
Dietary Supplement

Baby Ddrops®

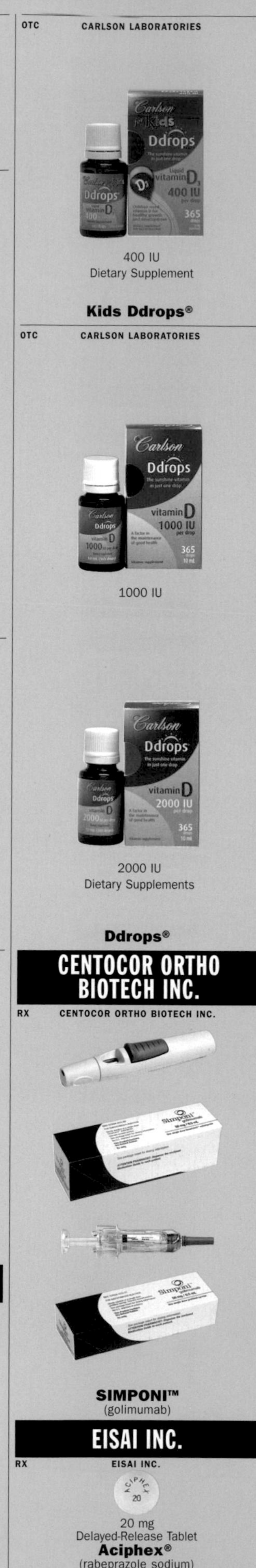

OTC CARLSON LABORATORIES

400 IU
Dietary Supplement

Kids Ddrops®

OTC CARLSON LABORATORIES

1000 IU

2000 IU
Dietary Supplements

Ddrops®

CENTOCOR ORTHO BIOTECH INC.

RX CENTOCOR ORTHO BIOTECH INC.

SIMPONI™
(golimumab)

EISAI INC.

RX EISAI INC.

20 mg
Delayed-Release Tablet

Aciphex®
(rabeprazole sodium)

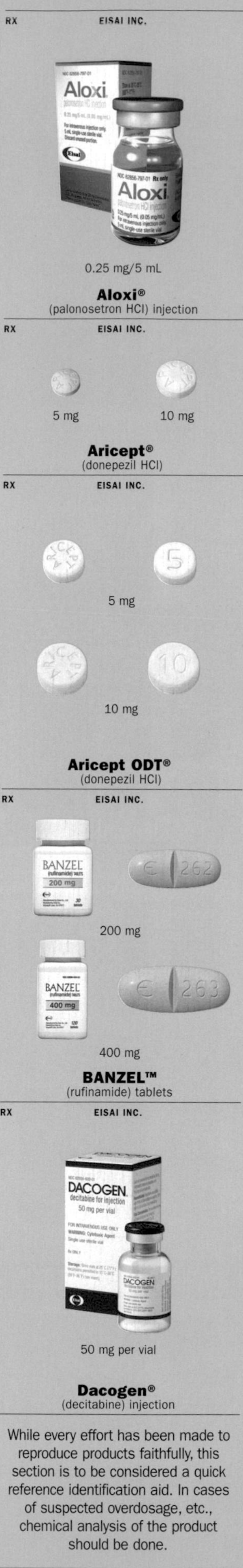

RX EISAI INC.

0.25 mg/5 mL

Aloxi®
(palonosetron HCl) injection

RX EISAI INC.

5 mg 10 mg

Aricept®
(donepezil HCl)

RX EISAI INC.

5 mg

10 mg

Aricept ODT®
(donepezil HCl)

RX EISAI INC.

200 mg

400 mg

BANZEL™
(rufinamide) tablets

RX EISAI INC.

50 mg per vial

Dacogen®
(decitabine) injection

While every effort has been made to reproduce products faithfully, this section is to be considered a quick reference identification aid. In cases of suspected overdosage, etc., chemical analysis of the product should be done.

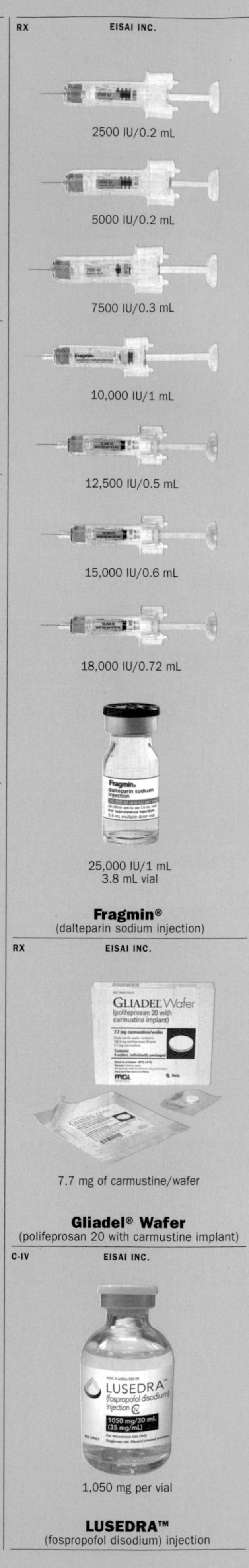

RX EISAI INC.

2500 IU/0.2 mL

5000 IU/0.2 mL

7500 IU/0.3 mL

10,000 IU/1 mL

12,500 IU/0.5 mL

15,000 IU/0.6 mL

18,000 IU/0.72 mL

25,000 IU/1 mL
3.8 mL vial

Fragmin®
(dalteparin sodium injection)

RX EISAI INC.

7.7 mg of carmustine/wafer

Gliadel® Wafer
(polifeprosan 20 with carmustine implant)

C-IV EISAI INC.

1,050 mg per vial

LUSEDRA™
(fospropofol disodium) injection

*Manufacturer's Identification Code

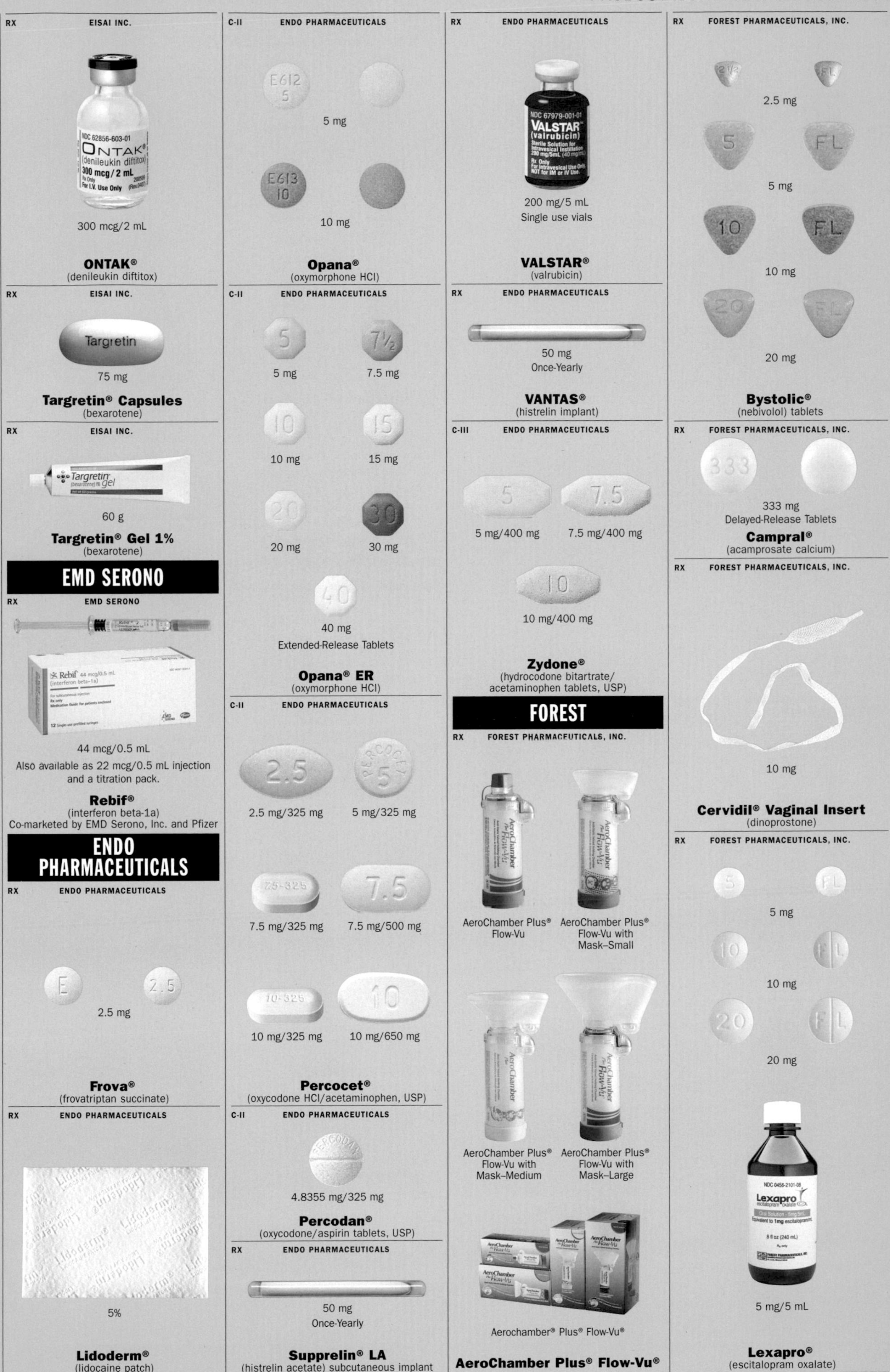
RX EISAI INC.
NDC 62856-603-01
ONTAK
(denileukin diftitox)
300 mcg / 2 mL
For I.V. Use Only
300 mcg/2 mL
ONTAK®
(denileukin diftitox)
RX EISAI INC.
Targretin
75 mg
Targretin® Capsules
(bexarotene)
RX EISAI INC.
Targretin gel
60 g
Targretin® Gel 1%
(bexarotene)
EMD SERONO
RX EMD SERONO
Rebif 44 mcg/0.5 mL
(interferon beta-1a)
44 mcg/0.5 mL
Also available as 22 mcg/0.5 mL injection and a titration pack.
Rebif®
(interferon beta-1a)
Co-marketed by EMD Serono, Inc. and Pfizer
ENDO PHARMACEUTICALS
RX ENDO PHARMACEUTICALS
E
2.5
2.5 mg
Frova®
(frovatriptan succinate)
RX ENDO PHARMACEUTICALS
Lidoderm
5%
Lidoderm®
(lidocaine patch)
C-II ENDO PHARMACEUTICALS
E612 5
5 mg
E613 10
10 mg
Opana®
(oxymorphone HCl)
C-II ENDO PHARMACEUTICALS
5
7½
5 mg
7.5 mg
10
15
10 mg
15 mg
20
30
20 mg
30 mg
40
40 mg
Extended-Release Tablets
Opana® ER
(oxymorphone HCl)
C-II ENDO PHARMACEUTICALS
2.5
PERCOCET 5
2.5 mg/325 mg
5 mg/325 mg
7.5
7.5 mg/325 mg
7.5 mg/500 mg
10
10 mg/325 mg
10 mg/650 mg
Percocet®
(oxycodone HCl/acetaminophen, USP)
C-II ENDO PHARMACEUTICALS
PERCODAN
4.8355 mg/325 mg
Percodan®
(oxycodone/aspirin tablets, USP)
RX ENDO PHARMACEUTICALS
50 mg
Once-Yearly
Supprelin® LA
(histrelin acetate) subcutaneous implant
RX ENDO PHARMACEUTICALS
NDC 67979-001-01
VALSTAR
(valrubicin)
Sterile Solution for Intravesical Instillation
200 mg/5 mL
Single use vials
VALSTAR®
(valrubicin)
RX ENDO PHARMACEUTICALS
50 mg
Once-Yearly
VANTAS®
(histrelin implant)
C-III ENDO PHARMACEUTICALS
5
7.5
5 mg/400 mg
7.5 mg/400 mg
10
10 mg/400 mg
Zydone®
(hydrocodone bitartrate/acetaminophen tablets, USP)
FOREST
RX FOREST PHARMACEUTICALS, INC.
AeroChamber Plus Flow-Vu
AeroChamber Plus® Flow-Vu
AeroChamber Plus® Flow-Vu with Mask–Small
AeroChamber Plus® Flow-Vu with Mask–Medium
AeroChamber Plus® Flow-Vu with Mask–Large
Aerochamber® Plus® Flow-Vu®
AeroChamber Plus® Flow-Vu®
RX FOREST PHARMACEUTICALS, INC.
2½
FL
2.5 mg
5
FL
5 mg
10
FL
10 mg
20
FL
20 mg
Bystolic®
(nebivolol) tablets
RX FOREST PHARMACEUTICALS, INC.
333
333 mg
Delayed-Release Tablets
Campral®
(acamprosate calcium)
RX FOREST PHARMACEUTICALS, INC.
10 mg
Cervidil® Vaginal Insert
(dinoprostone)
RX FOREST PHARMACEUTICALS, INC.
5
FL
5 mg
10
FL
10 mg
20
FL
20 mg
NDC 0456-2101-08
Lexapro
escitalopram oxalate
8 fl oz (240 mL)
5 mg/5 mL
Lexapro®
(escitalopram oxalate)

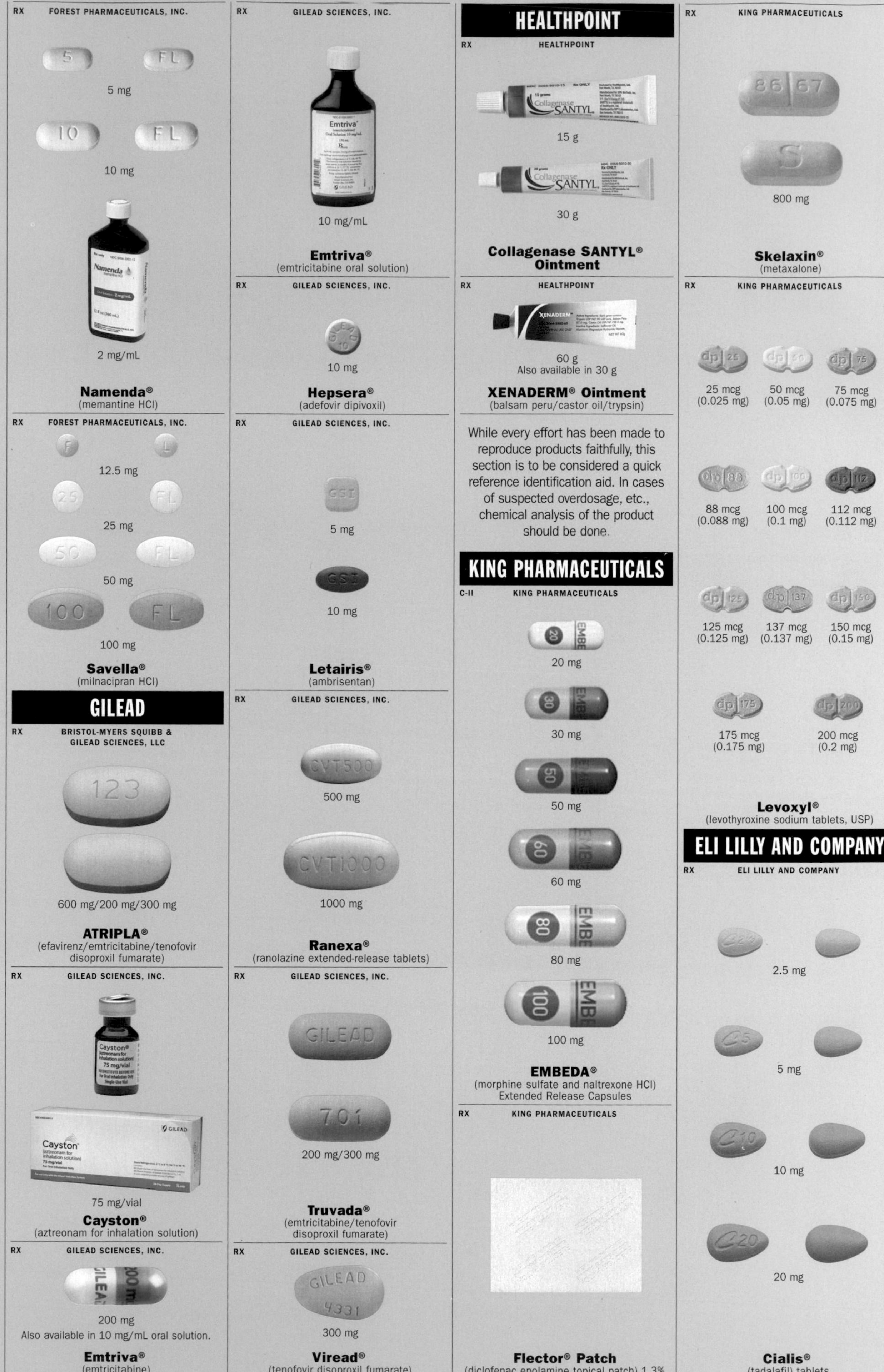

RX FOREST PHARMACEUTICALS, INC.
5 mg
10 mg
2 mg/mL
Namenda®
(memantine HCl)
RX FOREST PHARMACEUTICALS, INC.
12.5 mg
25 mg
50 mg
100 mg
Savella®
(milnacipran HCl)
GILEAD
RX BRISTOL-MYERS SQUIBB & GILEAD SCIENCES, LLC
600 mg/200 mg/300 mg
ATRIPLA®
(efavirenz/emtricitabine/tenofovir disoproxil fumarate)
RX GILEAD SCIENCES, INC.
75 mg/vial
Cayston®
(aztreonam for inhalation solution)
RX GILEAD SCIENCES, INC.
200 mg
Also available in 10 mg/mL oral solution.
Emtriva®
(emtricitabine)
RX GILEAD SCIENCES, INC.
10 mg/mL
Emtriva®
(emtricitabine oral solution)
RX GILEAD SCIENCES, INC.
10 mg
Hepsera®
(adefovir dipivoxil)
RX GILEAD SCIENCES, INC.
5 mg
10 mg
Letairis®
(ambrisentan)
RX GILEAD SCIENCES, INC.
500 mg
1000 mg
Ranexa®
(ranolazine extended-release tablets)
RX GILEAD SCIENCES, INC.
200 mg/300 mg
Truvada®
(emtricitabine/tenofovir disoproxil fumarate)
RX GILEAD SCIENCES, INC.
300 mg
Viread®
(tenofovir disoproxil fumarate)
HEALTHPOINT
RX HEALTHPOINT
15 g
30 g
Collagenase SANTYL® Ointment
RX HEALTHPOINT
60 g
Also available in 30 g
XENADERM® Ointment
(balsam peru/castor oil/trypsin)
While every effort has been made to reproduce products faithfully, this section is to be considered a quick reference identification aid. In cases of suspected overdosage, etc., chemical analysis of the product should be done.
KING PHARMACEUTICALS
C-II KING PHARMACEUTICALS
20 mg
30 mg
50 mg
60 mg
80 mg
100 mg
EMBEDA®
(morphine sulfate and naltrexone HCl) Extended Release Capsules
RX KING PHARMACEUTICALS
Flector® Patch
(diclofenac epolamine topical patch) 1.3%
RX KING PHARMACEUTICALS
800 mg
Skelaxin®
(metaxalone)
RX KING PHARMACEUTICALS
25 mcg (0.025 mg)
50 mcg (0.05 mg)
75 mcg (0.075 mg)
88 mcg (0.088 mg)
100 mcg (0.1 mg)
112 mcg (0.112 mg)
125 mcg (0.125 mg)
137 mcg (0.137 mg)
150 mcg (0.15 mg)
175 mcg (0.175 mg)
200 mcg (0.2 mg)
Levoxyl®
(levothyroxine sodium tablets, USP)
ELI LILLY AND COMPANY
RX ELI LILLY AND COMPANY
2.5 mg
5 mg
10 mg
20 mg
Cialis®
(tadalafil) tablets

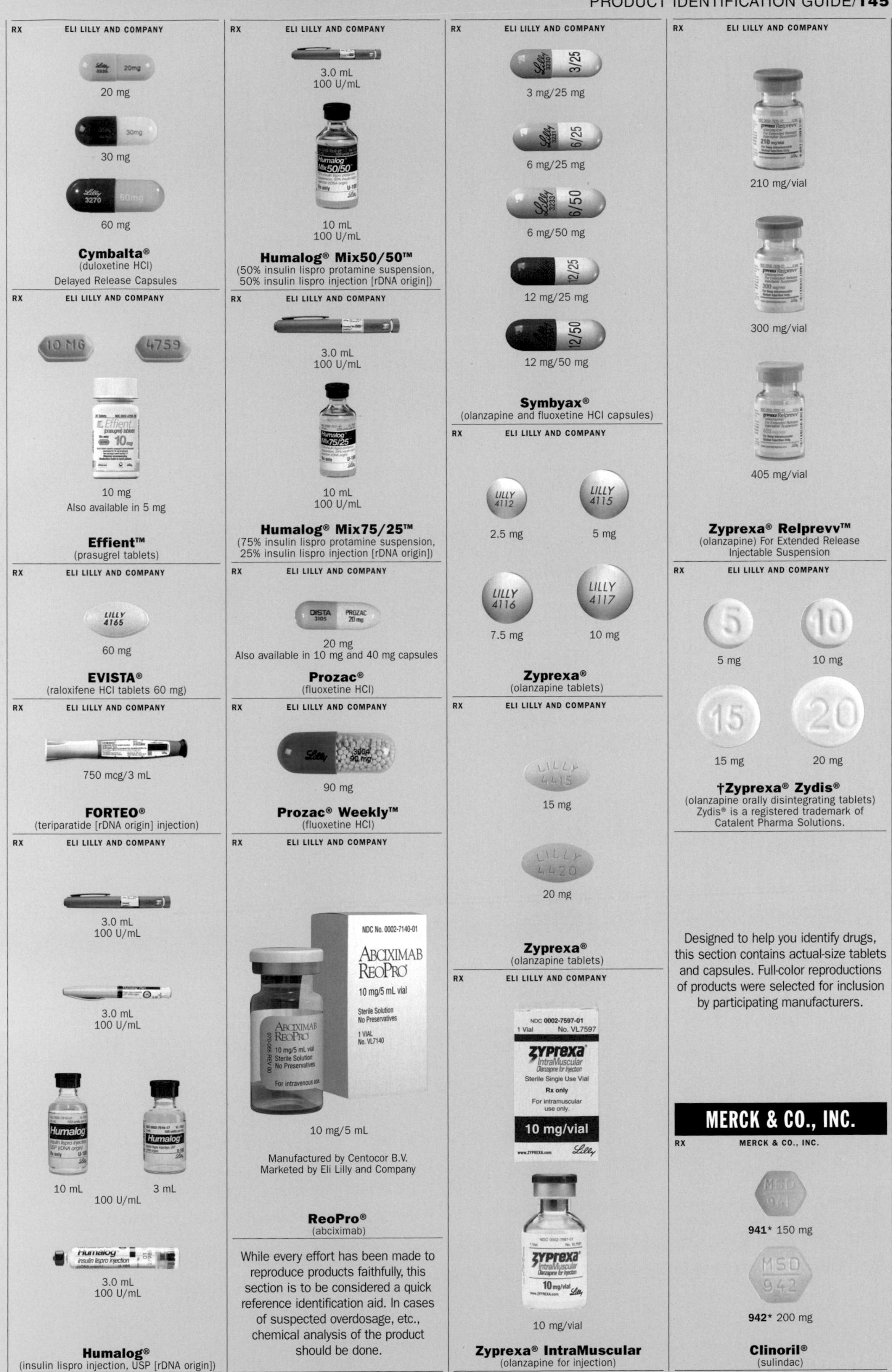

RX ELI LILLY AND COMPANY

20 mg

30 mg

60 mg

Cymbalta®
(duloxetine HCl)
Delayed Release Capsules

RX ELI LILLY AND COMPANY

10 mg
Also available in 5 mg

Effient™
(prasugrel tablets)

RX ELI LILLY AND COMPANY

60 mg

EVISTA®
(raloxifene HCl tablets 60 mg)

RX ELI LILLY AND COMPANY

750 mcg/3 mL

FORTEO®
(teriparatide [rDNA origin] injection)

RX ELI LILLY AND COMPANY

3.0 mL
100 U/mL

3.0 mL
100 U/mL

10 mL 3 mL
100 U/mL

3.0 mL
100 U/mL

Humalog®
(insulin lispro injection, USP [rDNA origin])

RX ELI LILLY AND COMPANY

3.0 mL
100 U/mL

10 mL
100 U/mL

Humalog® Mix50/50™
(50% insulin lispro protamine suspension, 50% insulin lispro injection [rDNA origin])

RX ELI LILLY AND COMPANY

3.0 mL
100 U/mL

10 mL
100 U/mL

Humalog® Mix75/25™
(75% insulin lispro protamine suspension, 25% insulin lispro injection [rDNA origin])

RX ELI LILLY AND COMPANY

20 mg
Also available in 10 mg and 40 mg capsules

Prozac®
(fluoxetine HCl)

RX ELI LILLY AND COMPANY

90 mg

Prozac® Weekly™
(fluoxetine HCl)

RX ELI LILLY AND COMPANY

10 mg/5 mL

Manufactured by Centocor B.V.
Marketed by Eli Lilly and Company

ReoPro®
(abciximab)

While every effort has been made to reproduce products faithfully, this section is to be considered a quick reference identification aid. In cases of suspected overdosage, etc., chemical analysis of the product should be done.

RX ELI LILLY AND COMPANY

3 mg/25 mg

6 mg/25 mg

6 mg/50 mg

12 mg/25 mg

12 mg/50 mg

Symbyax®
(olanzapine and fluoxetine HCl capsules)

RX ELI LILLY AND COMPANY

2.5 mg 5 mg

7.5 mg 10 mg

Zyprexa®
(olanzapine tablets)

RX ELI LILLY AND COMPANY

15 mg

20 mg

Zyprexa®
(olanzapine tablets)

RX ELI LILLY AND COMPANY

10 mg/vial

Zyprexa® IntraMuscular
(olanzapine for injection)

RX ELI LILLY AND COMPANY

210 mg/vial

300 mg/vial

405 mg/vial

Zyprexa® Relprevv™
(olanzapine) For Extended Release Injectable Suspension

RX ELI LILLY AND COMPANY

5 mg 10 mg

15 mg 20 mg

†Zyprexa® Zydis®
(olanzapine orally disintegrating tablets)
Zydis® is a registered trademark of Catalent Pharma Solutions.

Designed to help you identify drugs, this section contains actual-size tablets and capsules. Full-color reproductions of products were selected for inclusion by participating manufacturers.

MERCK & CO., INC.

RX MERCK & CO., INC.

941* 150 mg

942* 200 mg

Clinoril®
(sulindac)

*Manufacturer's Identification Code

† Additional dosage forms and sizes available.

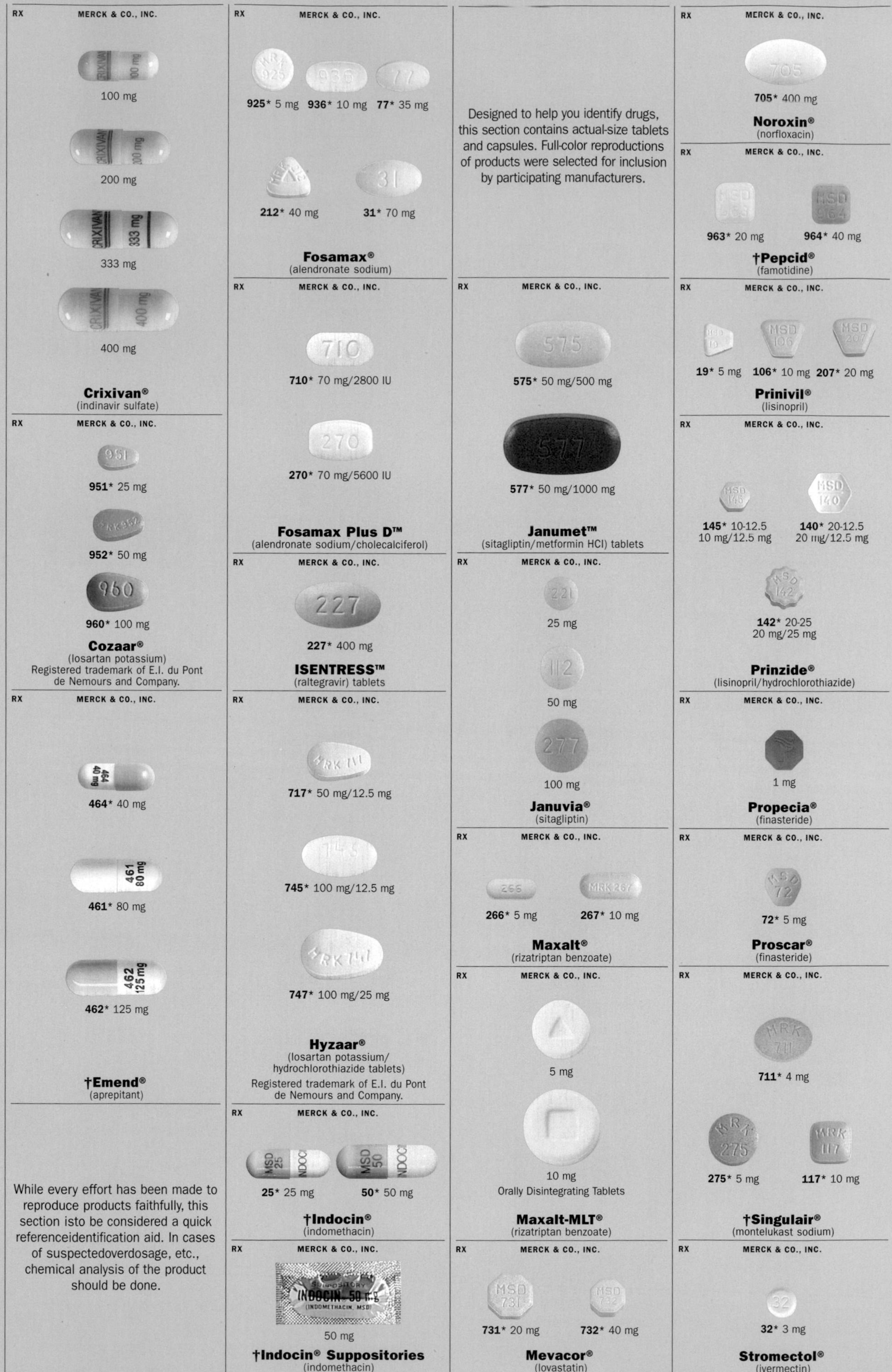

RX MERCK & CO., INC.

100 mg

200 mg

333 mg

400 mg

Crixivan®
(indinavir sulfate)

RX MERCK & CO., INC.

951* 25 mg

952* 50 mg

960* 100 mg

Cozaar®
(losartan potassium)
Registered trademark of E.I. du Pont de Nemours and Company.

RX MERCK & CO., INC.

464* 40 mg

461* 80 mg

462* 125 mg

†Emend®
(aprepitant)

While every effort has been made to reproduce products faithfully, this section isto be considered a quick referenceidentification aid. In cases of suspectedoverdosage, etc., chemical analysis of the product should be done.

RX MERCK & CO., INC.

925* 5 mg **936*** 10 mg **77*** 35 mg

212* 40 mg **31*** 70 mg

Fosamax®
(alendronate sodium)

RX MERCK & CO., INC.

710* 70 mg/2800 IU

270* 70 mg/5600 IU

Fosamax Plus D™
(alendronate sodium/cholecalciferol)

RX MERCK & CO., INC.

227* 400 mg

ISENTRESS™
(raltegravir) tablets

RX MERCK & CO., INC.

717* 50 mg/12.5 mg

745* 100 mg/12.5 mg

747* 100 mg/25 mg

Hyzaar®
(losartan potassium/ hydrochlorothiazide tablets)
Registered trademark of E.I. du Pont de Nemours and Company.

RX MERCK & CO., INC.

25* 25 mg **50*** 50 mg

†Indocin®
(indomethacin)

RX MERCK & CO., INC.

50 mg

†Indocin® Suppositories
(indomethacin)

Designed to help you identify drugs, this section contains actual-size tablets and capsules. Full-color reproductions of products were selected for inclusion by participating manufacturers.

RX MERCK & CO., INC.

575* 50 mg/500 mg

577* 50 mg/1000 mg

Janumet™
(sitagliptin/metformin HCl) tablets

RX MERCK & CO., INC.

25 mg

50 mg

100 mg

Januvia®
(sitagliptin)

RX MERCK & CO., INC.

266* 5 mg **267*** 10 mg

Maxalt®
(rizatriptan benzoate)

RX MERCK & CO., INC.

5 mg

10 mg
Orally Disintegrating Tablets

Maxalt-MLT®
(rizatriptan benzoate)

RX MERCK & CO., INC.

731* 20 mg **732*** 40 mg

Mevacor®
(lovastatin)

RX MERCK & CO., INC.

705* 400 mg

Noroxin®
(norfloxacin)

RX MERCK & CO., INC.

963* 20 mg **964*** 40 mg

†Pepcid®
(famotidine)

RX MERCK & CO., INC.

19* 5 mg **106*** 10 mg **207*** 20 mg

Prinivil®
(lisinopril)

RX MERCK & CO., INC.

145* 10-12.5
10 mg/12.5 mg

140* 20-12.5
20 mg/12.5 mg

142* 20-25
20 mg/25 mg

Prinzide®
(lisinopril/hydrochlorothiazide)

RX MERCK & CO., INC.

1 mg

Propecia®
(finasteride)

RX MERCK & CO., INC.

72* 5 mg

Proscar®
(finasteride)

RX MERCK & CO., INC.

711* 4 mg

275* 5 mg **117*** 10 mg

†Singulair®
(montelukast sodium)

RX MERCK & CO., INC.

32* 3 mg

Stromectol®
(ivermectin)

*Manufacturer's Identification Code

† Additional dosage forms and sizes available.

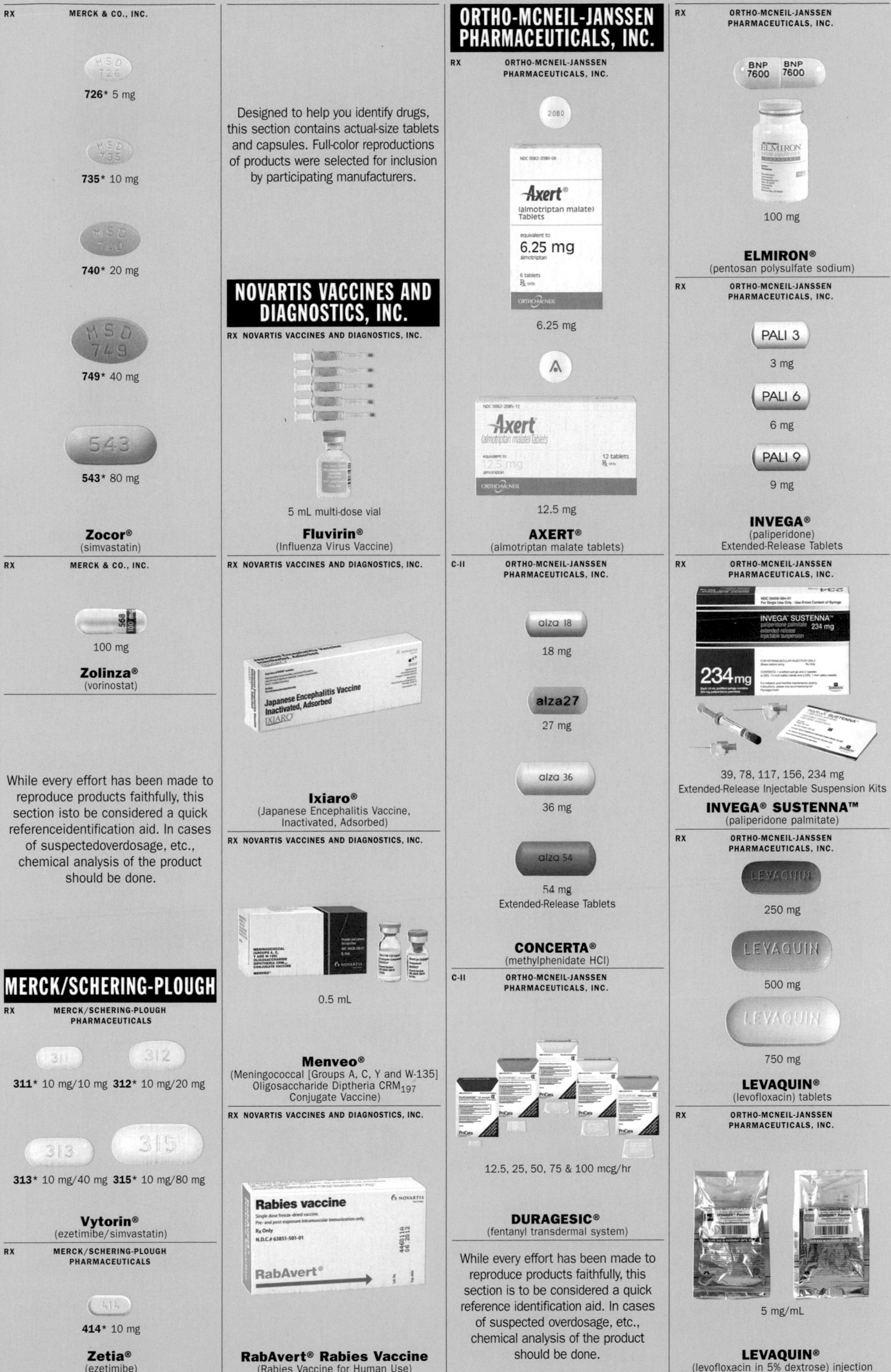

RX MERCK & CO., INC.

726* 5 mg

735* 10 mg

740* 20 mg

749* 40 mg

543* 80 mg

Zocor®
(simvastatin)

RX MERCK & CO., INC.

100 mg

Zolinza®
(vorinostat)

While every effort has been made to reproduce products faithfully, this section isto be considered a quick referenceidentification aid. In cases of suspectedoverdosage, etc., chemical analysis of the product should be done.

MERCK/SCHERING-PLOUGH

RX MERCK/SCHERING-PLOUGH PHARMACEUTICALS

311* 10 mg/10 mg 312* 10 mg/20 mg

313* 10 mg/40 mg 315* 10 mg/80 mg

Vytorin®
(ezetimibe/simvastatin)

RX MERCK/SCHERING-PLOUGH PHARMACEUTICALS

414* 10 mg

Zetia®
(ezetimibe)

Designed to help you identify drugs, this section contains actual-size tablets and capsules. Full-color reproductions of products were selected for inclusion by participating manufacturers.

NOVARTIS VACCINES AND DIAGNOSTICS, INC.

RX NOVARTIS VACCINES AND DIAGNOSTICS, INC.

5 mL multi-dose vial

Fluvirin®
(Influenza Virus Vaccine)

RX NOVARTIS VACCINES AND DIAGNOSTICS, INC.

Ixiaro®
(Japanese Encephalitis Vaccine, Inactivated, Adsorbed)

RX NOVARTIS VACCINES AND DIAGNOSTICS, INC.

0.5 mL

Menveo®
(Meningococcal [Groups A, C, Y and W-135] Oligosaccharide Diptheria CRM_{197} Conjugate Vaccine)

RX NOVARTIS VACCINES AND DIAGNOSTICS, INC.

RabAvert® Rabies Vaccine
(Rabies Vaccine for Human Use)

ORTHO-MCNEIL-JANSSEN PHARMACEUTICALS, INC.

RX ORTHO-MCNEIL-JANSSEN PHARMACEUTICALS, INC.

6.25 mg

12.5 mg

AXERT®
(almotriptan malate tablets)

C-II ORTHO-MCNEIL-JANSSEN PHARMACEUTICALS, INC.

18 mg

27 mg

36 mg

54 mg
Extended-Release Tablets

CONCERTA®
(methylphenidate HCl)

C-II ORTHO-MCNEIL-JANSSEN PHARMACEUTICALS, INC.

12.5, 25, 50, 75 & 100 mcg/hr

DURAGESIC®
(fentanyl transdermal system)

While every effort has been made to reproduce products faithfully, this section is to be considered a quick reference identification aid. In cases of suspected overdosage, etc., chemical analysis of the product should be done.

RX ORTHO-MCNEIL-JANSSEN PHARMACEUTICALS, INC.

100 mg

ELMIRON®
(pentosan polysulfate sodium)

RX ORTHO-MCNEIL-JANSSEN PHARMACEUTICALS, INC.

3 mg

6 mg

9 mg

INVEGA®
(paliperidone)
Extended-Release Tablets

RX ORTHO-MCNEIL-JANSSEN PHARMACEUTICALS, INC.

39, 78, 117, 156, 234 mg
Extended-Release Injectable Suspension Kits

INVEGA® SUSTENNA™
(paliperidone palmitate)

RX ORTHO-MCNEIL-JANSSEN PHARMACEUTICALS, INC.

250 mg

500 mg

750 mg

LEVAQUIN®
(levofloxacin) tablets

RX ORTHO-MCNEIL-JANSSEN PHARMACEUTICALS, INC.

5 mg/mL

LEVAQUIN®
(levofloxacin in 5% dextrose) injection

*Manufacturer's Identification Code

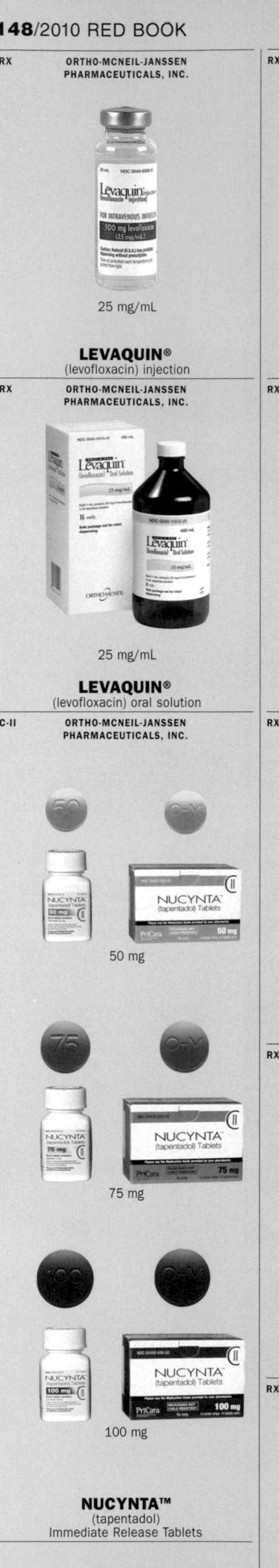

RX ORTHO-MCNEIL-JANSSEN PHARMACEUTICALS, INC.

25 mg/mL

LEVAQUIN®
(levofloxacin) injection

RX ORTHO-MCNEIL-JANSSEN PHARMACEUTICALS, INC.

25 mg/mL

LEVAQUIN®
(levofloxacin) oral solution

C-II ORTHO-MCNEIL-JANSSEN PHARMACEUTICALS, INC.

50 mg

75 mg

100 mg

NUCYNTA™
(tapentadol)
Immediate Release Tablets

Designed to help you identify drugs, this section contains actual-size tablets and capsules. Full-color reproductions of products were selected for inclusion by participating manufacturers.

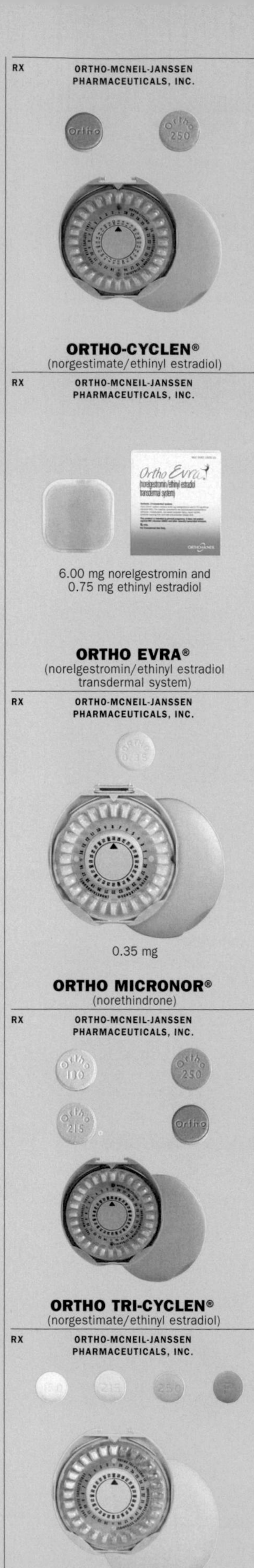

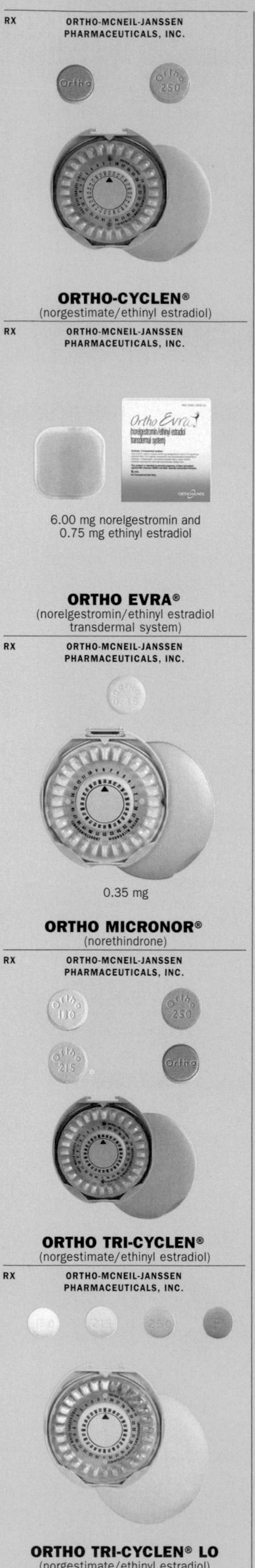

RX ORTHO-MCNEIL-JANSSEN PHARMACEUTICALS, INC.

ORTHO-CYCLEN®
(norgestimate/ethinyl estradiol)

RX ORTHO-MCNEIL-JANSSEN PHARMACEUTICALS, INC.

6.00 mg norelgestromin and 0.75 mg ethinyl estradiol

ORTHO EVRA®
(norelgestromin/ethinyl estradiol transdermal system)

RX ORTHO-MCNEIL-JANSSEN PHARMACEUTICALS, INC.

0.35 mg

ORTHO MICRONOR®
(norethindrone)

RX ORTHO-MCNEIL-JANSSEN PHARMACEUTICALS, INC.

ORTHO TRI-CYCLEN®
(norgestimate/ethinyl estradiol)

RX ORTHO-MCNEIL-JANSSEN PHARMACEUTICALS, INC.

ORTHO TRI-CYCLEN® LO
(norgestimate/ethinyl estradiol)

While every effort has been made to reproduce products faithfully, this section isto be considered a quick referenceidentification aid. In cases of suspectedoverdosage, etc., chemical analysis of the product should be done.

RX ORTHO-MCNEIL-JANSSEN PHARMACEUTICALS, INC.

4 mg 8 mg 12 mg

Razadyne®
(galantamine HBr tablets)

RX ORTHO-MCNEIL-JANSSEN PHARMACEUTICALS, INC.

4 mg/mL

Razadyne®
(galantamine HBr oral solution)

RX ORTHO-MCNEIL-JANSSEN PHARMACEUTICALS, INC.

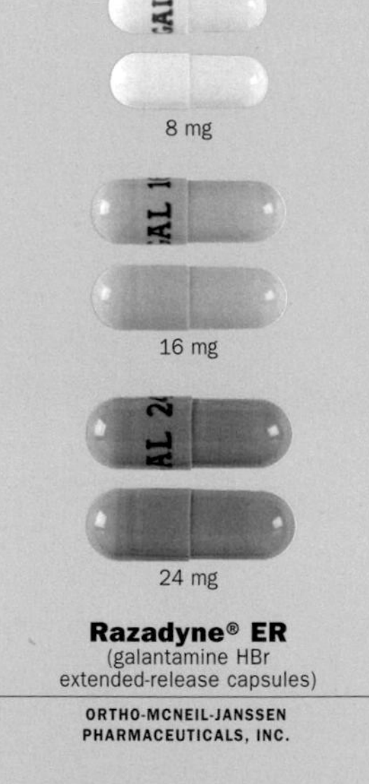

8 mg

16 mg

24 mg

Razadyne® ER
(galantamine HBr extended-release capsules)

RX ORTHO-MCNEIL-JANSSEN PHARMACEUTICALS, INC.

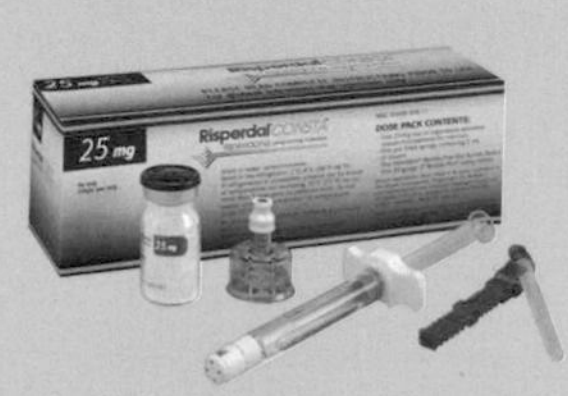

Available in 12.5, 25, 37.5, & 50 mg Dose Pack Long-Acting Injection

RISPERDAL® CONSTA®
(risperidone)

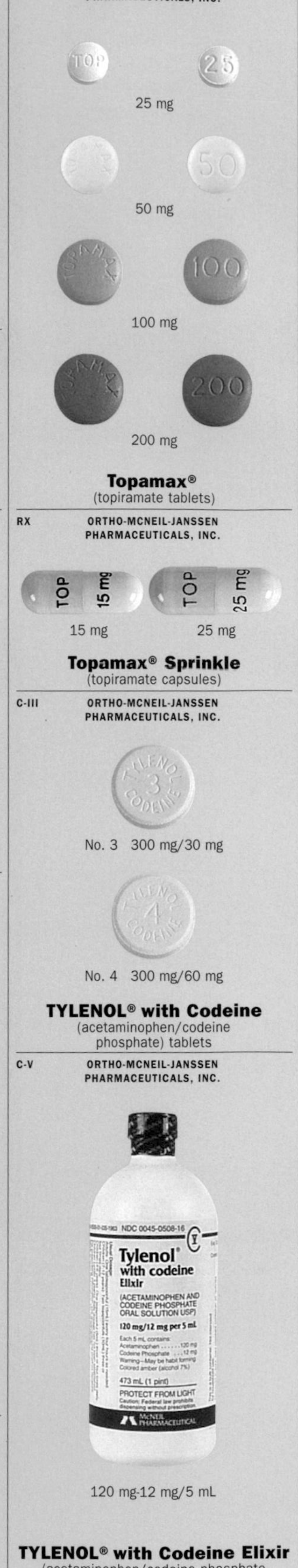

RX ORTHO-MCNEIL-JANSSEN PHARMACEUTICALS, INC.

25 mg

50 mg

100 mg

200 mg

Topamax®
(topiramate tablets)

RX ORTHO-MCNEIL-JANSSEN PHARMACEUTICALS, INC.

15 mg 25 mg

Topamax® Sprinkle
(topiramate capsules)

C-III ORTHO-MCNEIL-JANSSEN PHARMACEUTICALS, INC.

No. 3 300 mg/30 mg

No. 4 300 mg/60 mg

TYLENOL® with Codeine
(acetaminophen/codeine phosphate) tablets

C-V ORTHO-MCNEIL-JANSSEN PHARMACEUTICALS, INC.

120 mg-12 mg/5 mL

TYLENOL® with Codeine Elixir
(acetaminophen/codeine phosphate oral solution) USP

While every effort has been made to reproduce products faithfully, this section is to be considered a quick reference identification aid. In cases of suspected overdosage, etc., chemical analysis of the product should be done.

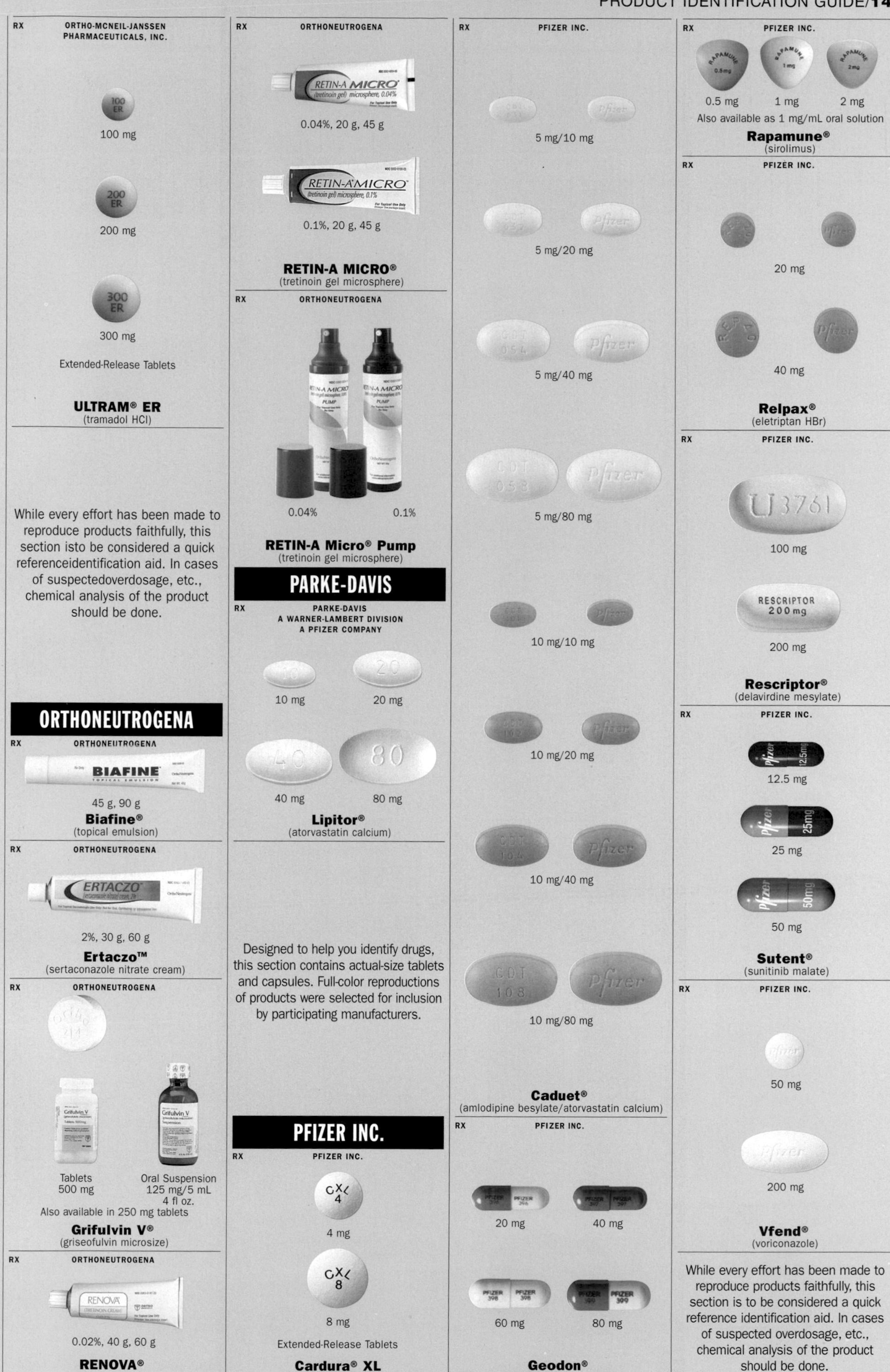

RX ORTHO-MCNEIL-JANSSEN PHARMACEUTICALS, INC.

100 mg

200 mg

300 mg

Extended-Release Tablets

ULTRAM® ER
(tramadol HCl)

While every effort has been made to reproduce products faithfully, this section isto be considered a quick referenceidentification aid. In cases of suspectedoverdosage, etc., chemical analysis of the product should be done.

ORTHONEUTROGENA

RX ORTHONEUTROGENA

45 g, 90 g

Biafine®
(topical emulsion)

RX ORTHONEUTROGENA

2%, 30 g, 60 g

Ertaczo™
(sertaconazole nitrate cream)

RX ORTHONEUTROGENA

Tablets 500 mg

Oral Suspension 125 mg/5 mL 4 fl oz.

Also available in 250 mg tablets

Grifulvin V®
(griseofulvin microsize)

RX ORTHONEUTROGENA

0.02%, 40 g, 60 g

RENOVA®
(tretinoin cream)

RX ORTHONEUTROGENA

0.04%, 20 g, 45 g

0.1%, 20 g, 45 g

RETIN-A MICRO®
(tretinoin gel microsphere)

RX ORTHONEUTROGENA

0.04% 0.1%

RETIN-A Micro® Pump
(tretinoin gel microsphere)

PARKE-DAVIS

RX PARKE-DAVIS
A WARNER-LAMBERT DIVISION
A PFIZER COMPANY

10 mg 20 mg

40 mg 80 mg

Lipitor®
(atorvastatin calcium)

Designed to help you identify drugs, this section contains actual-size tablets and capsules. Full-color reproductions of products were selected for inclusion by participating manufacturers.

PFIZER INC.

RX PFIZER INC.

4 mg

8 mg

Extended-Release Tablets

Cardura® XL
(doxazosin mesylate)

RX PFIZER INC.

5 mg/10 mg

5 mg/20 mg

5 mg/40 mg

5 mg/80 mg

10 mg/10 mg

10 mg/20 mg

10 mg/40 mg

10 mg/80 mg

Caduet®
(amlodipine besylate/atorvastatin calcium)

RX PFIZER INC.

20 mg 40 mg

60 mg 80 mg

Geodon®
(ziprasidone HCl)

RX PFIZER INC.

0.5 mg 1 mg 2 mg

Also available as 1 mg/mL oral solution

Rapamune®
(sirolimus)

RX PFIZER INC.

20 mg

40 mg

Relpax®
(eletriptan HBr)

RX PFIZER INC.

100 mg

200 mg

Rescriptor®
(delavirdine mesylate)

RX PFIZER INC.

12.5 mg

25 mg

50 mg

Sutent®
(sunitinib malate)

RX PFIZER INC.

50 mg

200 mg

Vfend®
(voriconazole)

While every effort has been made to reproduce products faithfully, this section is to be considered a quick reference identification aid. In cases of suspected overdosage, etc., chemical analysis of the product should be done.

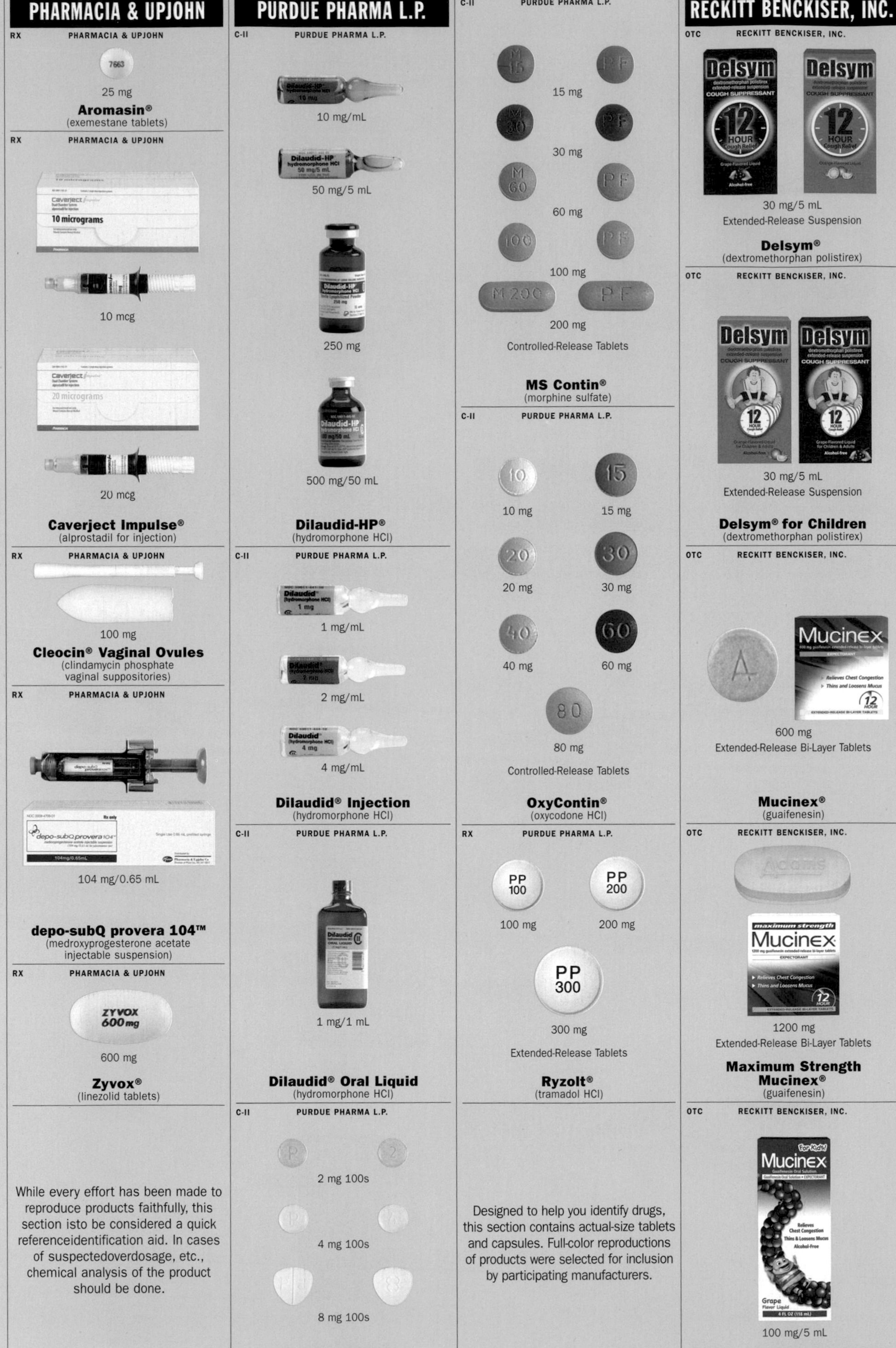

PHARMACIA & UPJOHN

RX PHARMACIA & UPJOHN

25 mg

Aromasin®
(exemestane tablets)

RX PHARMACIA & UPJOHN

10 mcg

20 mcg

Caverject Impulse®
(alprostadil for injection)

RX PHARMACIA & UPJOHN

100 mg

Cleocin® Vaginal Ovules
(clindamycin phosphate vaginal suppositories)

RX PHARMACIA & UPJOHN

104 mg/0.65 mL

depo-subQ provera 104™
(medroxyprogesterone acetate injectable suspension)

RX PHARMACIA & UPJOHN

600 mg

Zyvox®
(linezolid tablets)

While every effort has been made to reproduce products faithfully, this section isto be considered a quick referenceidentification aid. In cases of suspectedoverdosage, etc., chemical analysis of the product should be done.

PURDUE PHARMA L.P.

C-II PURDUE PHARMA L.P.

10 mg/mL

50 mg/5 mL

250 mg

500 mg/50 mL

Dilaudid-HP®
(hydromorphone HCl)

C-II PURDUE PHARMA L.P.

1 mg/mL

2 mg/mL

4 mg/mL

Dilaudid® Injection
(hydromorphone HCl)

C-II PURDUE PHARMA L.P.

1 mg/1 mL

Dilaudid® Oral Liquid
(hydromorphone HCl)

C-II PURDUE PHARMA L.P.

2 mg 100s

4 mg 100s

8 mg 100s

Dilaudid® Tablets
(hydromorphone HCl)

C-II PURDUE PHARMA L.P.

15 mg

30 mg

60 mg

100 mg

200 mg

Controlled-Release Tablets

MS Contin®
(morphine sulfate)

C-II PURDUE PHARMA L.P.

10 mg 15 mg

20 mg 30 mg

40 mg 60 mg

80 mg

Controlled-Release Tablets

OxyContin®
(oxycodone HCl)

RX PURDUE PHARMA L.P.

100 mg 200 mg

300 mg

Extended-Release Tablets

Ryzolt®
(tramadol HCl)

Designed to help you identify drugs, this section contains actual-size tablets and capsules. Full-color reproductions of products were selected for inclusion by participating manufacturers.

RECKITT BENCKISER, INC.

OTC RECKITT BENCKISER, INC.

30 mg/5 mL
Extended-Release Suspension

Delsym®
(dextromethorphan polistirex)

OTC RECKITT BENCKISER, INC.

30 mg/5 mL
Extended-Release Suspension

Delsym® for Children
(dextromethorphan polistirex)

OTC RECKITT BENCKISER, INC.

600 mg
Extended-Release Bi-Layer Tablets

Mucinex®
(guaifenesin)

OTC RECKITT BENCKISER, INC.

1200 mg
Extended-Release Bi-Layer Tablets

Maximum Strength Mucinex®
(guaifenesin)

OTC RECKITT BENCKISER, INC.

100 mg/5 mL

Mucinex® Liquid for Children
(guaifenesin)

OTC RECKITT BENCKISER, INC.

100 mg - 2.5 mg/5 mL

Mucinex® Cold Liquid for Children
(guaifenesin/phenylephrine HCl)

OTC RECKITT BENCKISER, INC.

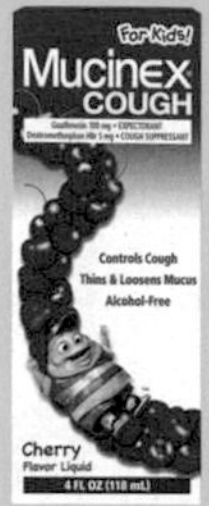

100 mg - 5 mg/5 mL

Mucinex® Cough Liquid for Children
(guaifenesin/dextromethorphan HBr)

OTC RECKITT BENCKISER, INC.

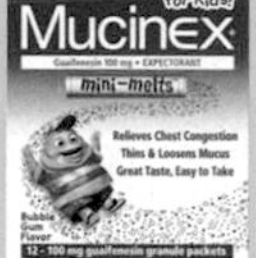

50 mg 100 mg

Mucinex® Mini-Melts™ for Children
(guaifenesin)

OTC RECKITT BENCKISER, INC.

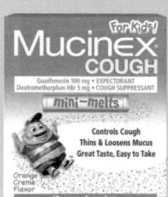

100 mg/5 mg

Mucinex® Cough Mini-Melts™ for Children
(guaifenesin/dextromethorphan HBr)

OTC RECKITT BENCKISER, INC.

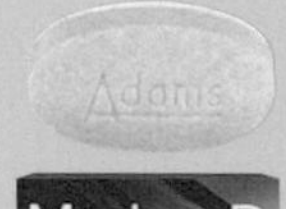

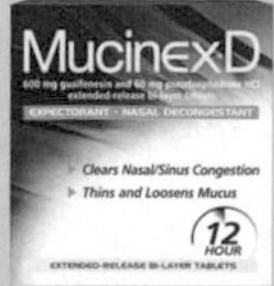

600 mg/60 mg
Extended-Release Bi-Layer Tablets

Mucinex® D
(guaifenesin/pseudoephedrine HCl)

OTC RECKITT BENCKISER, INC.

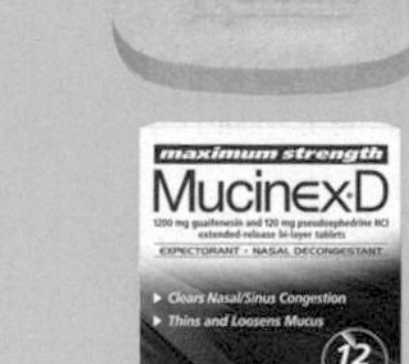

1200 mg/120 mg
Extended-Release Bi-Layer Tablets

Maximum Strength Mucinex® D
(guaifenesin/pseudoephedrine HCl)

OTC RECKITT BENCKISER, INC.

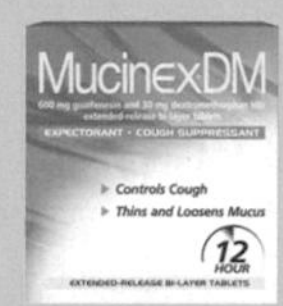

600 mg/30 mg
Extended-Release Bi-Layer Tablets

Mucinex® DM
(guaifenesin/dextromethorphan HBr)

OTC RECKITT BENCKISER, INC.

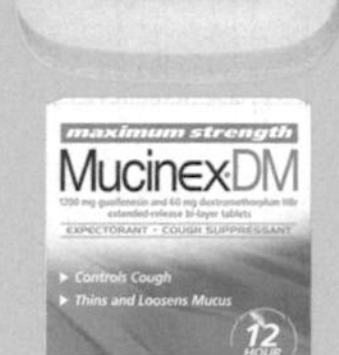

1200 mg/60 mg
Extended-Release Bi-Layer Tablets

Maximum Strength Mucinex® DM
(guaifenesin/dextromethorphan HBr)

While every effort has been made to reproduce products faithfully, this section is to be considered a quick reference identification aid. In cases of suspected overdosage, etc., chemical analysis of the product should be done.

RLC LABS, INC.

RX RLC LABS, INC.

16.25 mg (1/4 gr.) 32.5 mg (1/2 gr.)

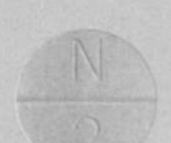

65 mg (1 gr.) 130 mg (2 gr.)

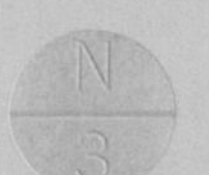

195 mg (3 gr.)

Nature-Throid™
(Thyroid USP) tablets

RX RLC LABS, INC.

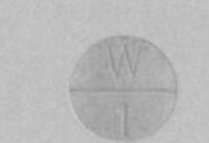

32.5 mg (1/2 gr.) 65 mg (1 gr.)

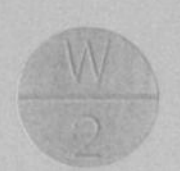

130 mg (2 gr.)

Westhroid™
(Thyroid USP) tablets

SALIX PHARMACEUTICALS

RX SALIX PHARMACEUTICALS, INC.

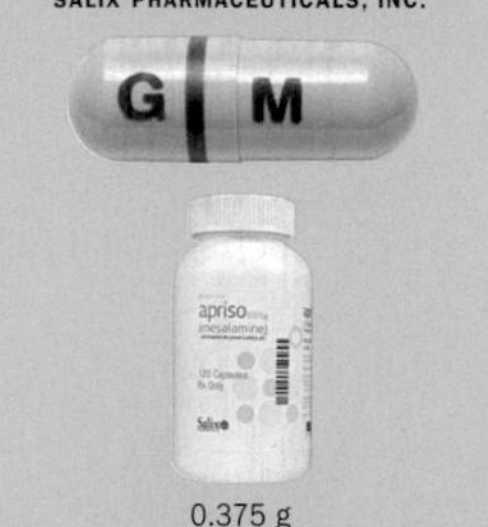

0.375 g
Extended-Release Capsules

Apriso™
(mesalamine)

RX SALIX PHARMACEUTICALS, INC.

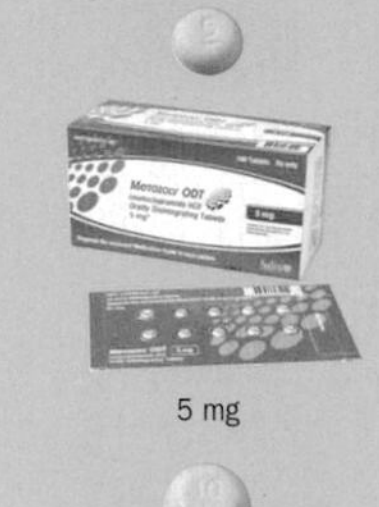

5 mg

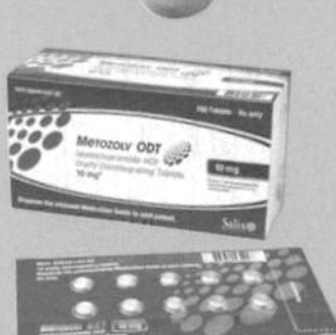

10 mg
Orally Disintegrating Tablets

Metozolv® ODT
(metoclopramide HCl)

RX SALIX PHARMACEUTICALS, INC.

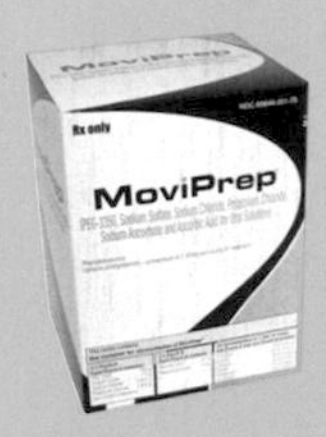

MoviPrep®
(PEG-3350, sodium sulfate, sodium chloride, potassium chloride, sodium ascorbate and ascorbic acid for oral solution)

RX SALIX PHARMACEUTICALS, INC.

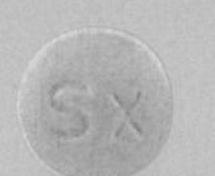

200 mg

Xifaxan®
(rifaximin)

RX SALIX PHARMACEUTICALS, INC.

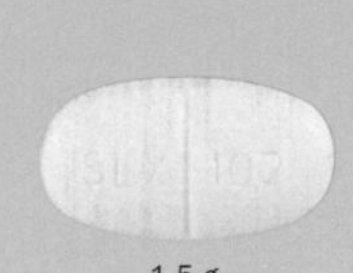

1.5 g

OsmoPrep®
(sodium phosphate monobasic monohydrate, USP, and sodium phosphate dibasic anhydrous, USP)

SEARLE

RX G.D. SEARLE & CO.

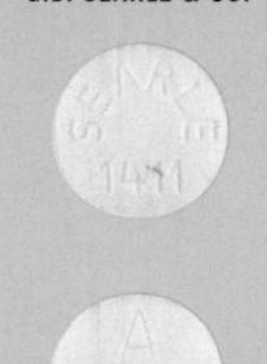

50 mg and 75 mg/200 mcg

Arthrotec®
(diclofenac sodium/misoprostol)

RX G.D. SEARLE & CO.

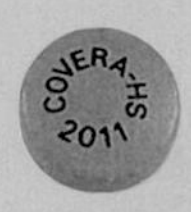

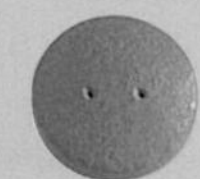

2011* 180 mg

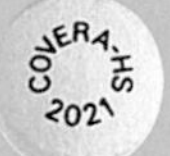

2021* 240 mg
Extended-Release Tablets

Covera-HS®
(verapamil HCl)

TIBOTEC THERAPEUTICS

RX TIBOTEC THERAPEUTICS, DIVISION OF CENTOCOR ORTHO BIOTECH PRODUCTS, L.P.

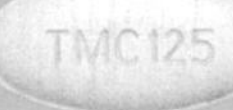

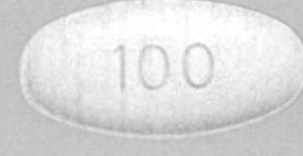

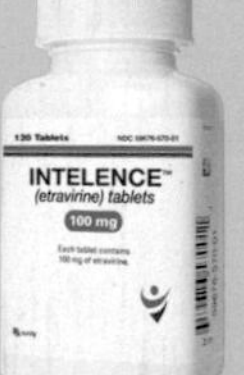

100 mg

Intelence™
(etravirine)

*Manufacturer's Identification Code

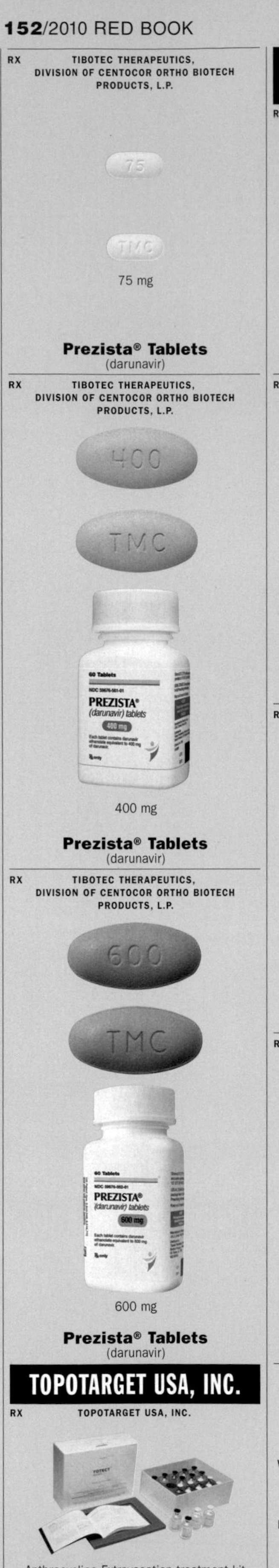

RX TIBOTEC THERAPEUTICS, DIVISION OF CENTOCOR ORTHO BIOTECH PRODUCTS, L.P.

75 mg

Prezista® Tablets
(darunavir)

RX TIBOTEC THERAPEUTICS, DIVISION OF CENTOCOR ORTHO BIOTECH PRODUCTS, L.P.

400 mg

Prezista® Tablets
(darunavir)

RX TIBOTEC THERAPEUTICS, DIVISION OF CENTOCOR ORTHO BIOTECH PRODUCTS, L.P.

600 mg

Prezista® Tablets
(darunavir)

TOPOTARGET USA, INC.

RX TOPOTARGET USA, INC.

Anthracycline Extravasation treatment kit for single patient use. 5,000 mg Totect® is packaged in a carton consisting of 10 vials of dexrazoxane for injection and 10 vials of diluent.

Totect® Kit
(dexrazoxane) for injection, for intravenous infusion only

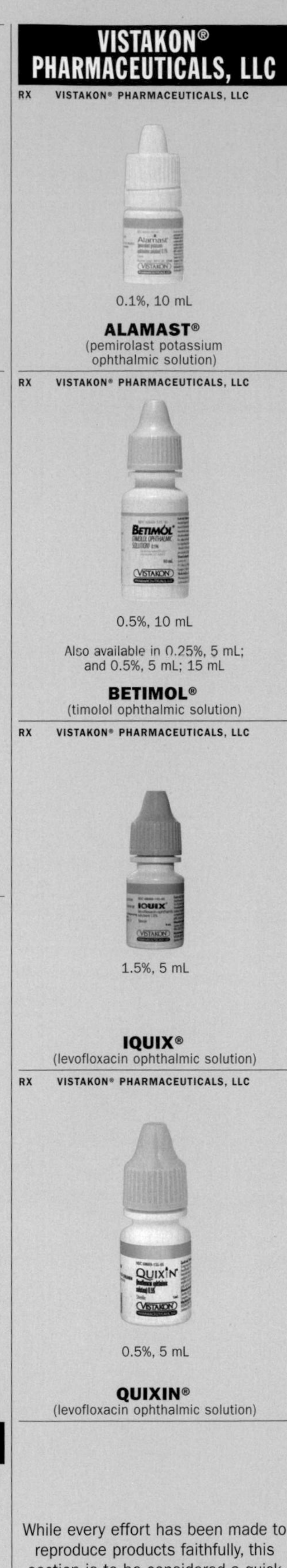

VISTAKON® PHARMACEUTICALS, LLC

RX VISTAKON® PHARMACEUTICALS, LLC

0.1%, 10 mL

ALAMAST®
(pemirolast potassium ophthalmic solution)

RX VISTAKON® PHARMACEUTICALS, LLC

0.5%, 10 mL

Also available in 0.25%, 5 mL; and 0.5%, 5 mL; 15 mL

BETIMOL®
(timolol ophthalmic solution)

RX VISTAKON® PHARMACEUTICALS, LLC

1.5%, 5 mL

IQUIX®
(levofloxacin ophthalmic solution)

RX VISTAKON® PHARMACEUTICALS, LLC

0.5%, 5 mL

QUIXIN®
(levofloxacin ophthalmic solution)

While every effort has been made to reproduce products faithfully, this section is to be considered a quick reference identification aid. In cases of suspected overdosage, etc., chemical analysis of the product should be done.

WYETH PHARMACEUTICALS

RX WYETH PHARMACEUTICALS

837* 37.5 mg

833* 75 mg

836* 150 mg

Extended-Release Capsules

‡Effexor XR®
(venlafaxine HCl)

RX WYETH PHARMACEUTICALS

Lybrel®
(90 mcg levonorgestrel and 20 mcg ethinyl estradiol)

RX WYETH PHARMACEUTICALS

20 mg 40 mg

Protonix®
(pantoprazole sodium)

*Manufacturer's Identification Code

‡ The appearance of these capsules is a trademark of Wyeth Pharmaceuticals.

9 Rx PRODUCTS

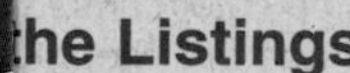

the Listings

ntry features the product or generic name.
mit price information is provided for all appli-
duct categories. The FUL symbol can be
owing the generic product name. A complete
er Limit prices appears in Section 6, "Drug
nation."

ted alphabetically within generic listings.
cts feature the REPACK symbol next to their
listings, generic cross-references appear in
wing line.

ion indicates the form of the drug; e.g., CAP
AB indicates tablets, etc. For a key to
s, refer to the table on the following page.

, descriptive information, strength, quantity,
(where applicable) appear next, followed by
DC) number. The Average Wholesale Price
P), and the Orange Book Code (OBC) com-
h product. For more information on Orange
e next page.

ss	NDC (National Drug Code)		DP (Direct Price)	
....	00839-7713-06	9.79	7.25	AB
....	00839-7713-16	93.96	69.60	AB
....	00839-7714-06	23.69	17.55	AB
Quantity		AWP (Average Wholesale Price)		OBC (Orange Book Code)

Red Book are based on data *reported* by
blisher has not performed any independent
ices paid by wholesalers and providers in the
ual prices paid by wholesalers and providers
prices contained in this publication and all
ange without notice. Further, while care has
piling all of the information contained herein,
warrant its accuracy. For further explanation,
"AWP Policy" in the *Red Book* Foreword.
plemented by subscribing to the monthly *Red*
Price™, *Red Book* for Windows™, *Red Book*
taining prices published in catalogs or other
minated by manufacturers or distributors.

RATION ABBREVIATIONS

(ROA) refers to the intake or application
he following abbreviations are used to

	MR	Multiple routes
	NA	Not applicable
	NS	Nasal
osal	**OP**	Ophthalmic
	OT	Otic
	PL	Intrapleural
	PO	Oral
ar	**PT**	Intraperitoneal
	RC	Rectal
	SC	Subcutaneous
	SG	Subgingival
	SL	Sublingual
	TD	Transdermal
	TP	Topical
	UR	Intraurethral
nbrane	**VG**	Vaginal

ORANGE BOOK CODES

The Orange Book Codes supply the FDA's therapeutic equivalence rating for applicable multisource categories. Codes beginning with "A" signify that the product is deemed therapeutically equivalent to the reference product for the category. Codes beginning with "B" indicate that bioequivalence has not been confirmed. In certain instances, a number is added to the end of the **AB** code to make it a three-character code (i.e., **AB1**, **AB2**, **AB3**, **etc.**). Three-character codes are assigned only in situations where more than one reference drug of the same strength has been designated under the same heading. "EE" is assigned by *Red Book* to products that have been evaluated by the FDA but for which an equivalence rating is not available.

Products appearing in the Orange Book have historically been limited to those manufacturers holding the original approved New Drug Application (NDA) or Abbreviated New Drug Application (ANDA). However, in recognition of the fact that generic products are available from a widespread number of sources, *Red Book* publications and database services extend Orange Book ratings to distributors and generic labelers other than the holder of the NDA or ANDA. All ratings applied to such labelers have been directly supplied to *Red Book* through written certification attesting to the accuracy of the codes supplied.

AA..........No bioequivalence problems in conventional dosage forms
AB..........Meets bioequivalence requirements
AB1........Meets bioequivalence requirements to AB1 rated reference drug
AB2........Meets bioequivalence requirements to AB2 rated reference drug
AB3........Meets bioequivalence requirements to AB3 rated reference drug
AN..........Solution or powder for aerosolization
AO..........Injectable oil solution
AP..........Injectable aqueous solution
AT..........Topical product
BC..........Controlled-release tablet, capsule, or injectable
BD..........Documented bioequivalence problem
BN..........Product in aerosol-nebulizer delivery system
BP..........Potential bioequivalence problem
BR..........Suppository or enema for systemic use
BS..........Testing standards are insufficient for determination
BT..........Topical product with bioequivalence issues
BX..........Insufficient data to confirm therapeutic equivalence
EE..........This entry has been evaluated by the FDA, but a rating is not available for this labeler's product

OTHER DESCRIPTIVE ABBREVIATIONS

The following abbreviations are used to provide additional descriptive information about products:

A.F..............Alcohol-free
AMP...........Ampule
D.F..............Dye-free
EXT. STR......Extra strength
F.C..............Film coated
F.F..............Fragrance-free
FR...............French
INSTIT. USE .Institutional use
MAX. STR. ..Maximum strength
M.D.V..........Multi-dose vial
N.F..............National Formulary
P.B..............Piggyback
P.C.............Plastic container
P.F..............Preservative-free
R.N.P. ....Reversed number package
S.D.............Single dose
S.D.V..........Single-dose vial
S.F. ....Sugar-free
SRN...........Syringe
TAX INCL ..Federal excise tax included
U.D. ....Unit dose
U.S.P..........U.S. Pharmacopeia

STANDARD DOSAGE FORM DESCRIPTIONS

The following three-character abbreviations are used to indicate the form in which a product is available:

ACC Accesory
AER Aerosol liquid
ARO Aerosol powder
BAN Bandage
BAR Bar
BEA Beads
C12 Capsule, extended release, 12-hr.
C24 Capsule, extended release, 24-hr.
CAK Cake
CAP Capsule
CER Capsule, extended release
CHI Chip
CRE Cream
CRY Crystal
CTB Tablet, chewable
DAP Patch, device assisted
DEV Device
DRE Dressing
DSK Disk
ECC Capsule, delayed release
ECT Tablet, enteric-coated
ELI Elixir
EMO Emollient cream
EMU Emulsion
FIL Film
FLA Flake
FOA Foam
GAS Gas
GEF Powder, effervescent
GEL Gel/jelly
GER Granules, extended release
GFS Gel-forming solution
GRA Granules
GUM Gum
ICR Insert, extended release
IMP Implant
INJ Injection
KIT Kit
LEA Leaf
LIQ Liquid
LOT Lotion
LOZ Lozenge/troche
LUM Lump
NMA Enema
ODT Tablet, disintegrating
OEM Emollient ointment
OIL Oil
OIN Ointment
PAD Pad
PAS Paste
PDR Powder for suspension
PDS Powder for solution
PEL Pellet
PI1 Powder for suspension, 1-month
PI3 Powder for suspension, 3-month
PI4 Powder for suspension, 4-month
PI6 Powder for suspension, 6-month
PKT Packet
POD Pod
POW Powder
PRO Prophylactic
PUD Pudding
SER Suspension, extended release
SGL Capsule, liquid-filled
SHA Shampoo
SHE Sheet
SOA Soap
SOL Solution
SPE Suppository, extended release
SPG Sponge
SPR Spray
STI Stick
SUP Suppository
SUS Suspension
SWA Swab
SYR Syrup
T12 Tablet, extended release, 12-hr.
T24 Tablet, extended release, 24-hr.
TAB Tablet
TAM Tampon
TAP Tape
TBS Tablet for suspension
TCP Tablet, coated particles
TDM Patch, extended release
TDR Tablet disintegrating, delayed
TEF Tablet, effervescent
TER Tablet, extended release
TES Test
TIN Tincture
TSN Tablet for solution
WAF Wafer
WAX Wax

ABBREVIATED INGREDIENT DESCRIPTIONS

Generic names are listed according to the following guidelines:

- Single-ingredient generic names will be spelled out in full (e.g., ACETAMINOPHEN)
- Multi-ingredient products (two or more) are listed in the alphabetical order of their ingredients using the following standard abbreviations:

ACE ....ACETATE
ALK ....ALKALOIDS
APAP .................................ACETAMINOPHEN
ASA ....ASPIRIN
BELL ....BELLADONNA
BENZO ....BENZOCAINE
BICARB ....BICARBONATE
BIT ....BITARTRATE
BPM .................................BROMPHENIRAMINE
CA ....CALCIUM
CAFF ....CAFFEINE
CIT ....CITRATE
CL ....CHLORIDE
CPM .................................CHLORPHENIRAMINE
CR ....CHROMIUM
CU ....COPPER
DM .................................DEXTROMETHORPHAN
DSS ....DOCUSATE SODIUM
EPH ....EPHEDRINE
EPI ....EPINEPHRINE
FE ....IRON
FUM ....FUMARATE
GG ....GUAIFENESIN
HC .................................HYDROCORTISONE
HCL .................................HYDROCHLORIDE
HCTZ .................................HYDROCHLOROTHIAZIDE
HEP ....HEPATITIS
HYDROBROM .................................HYDROBROMIDE
HYDROCOD ....HYDROCODONE
IF ....INTRINSIC FACTOR
K ....POTASSIUM
GUAI .................................GUAIACOLSULFONATE
KI ....POTASSIUM IODIDE
LACT ....LACTATE
MAL ....MALEATE
MG ....MAGNESIUM
MN ....MANGANESE
NA ....SODIUM
PB .................................PHENOBARBITAL
PEG .................................POLYETHYLENE GLYCOL
PENTOBARB .................................PENTOBARBITAL
PHENYLEPH .................................PHENYLEPHRINE
PHOS ....PHOSPHATE
PPA .................................PHENYLPROPANOLAMINE
PSE .................................PSEUDOEPHEDRINE
PYRIL ....PYRILAMINE
SCOP ....SCOPOLAMINE
SE ....SELENIUM
SULF ....SULFATE
TAN ....TANNATE
TART ....TARTRATE
THEOPH .................................THEOPHYLLINE
VAC ....VACCINE
VIT ....VITAMIN
ZN ....ZINC

LOOK-ALIKE, SOUND-ALIKE DRUG NAMES

The following list is adapted from the April 2004 *USP Quality Review* newsletter. It includes reports submitted to two medication error reporting programs—MEDMARX® and the USP-ISMP Medication Errors Reporting (MER) Program—from their inception through December 31, 2002. Similarity of drug names involves confusion between look-alike and/or sound-alike brand names, generic names, and brand to generic names. This confusion is compounded by illegible handwriting, lack of knowledge of drug names, newly available products, similar packaging or labeling, and incorrect selection of a similar name from a computerized product list.

It's important to remember that these names may not sound alike as you read them or look alike in print, but when handwritten or communicated verbally, these names have caused or could cause confusion. For more information, contact USP at 800-23-ERROR (800-233-7767) or uspcaps@usp.org, or visit their website at www.usp.org/hqi/patientSafety.

Note: USP has transferred its reporting program MEDMARX to Quantros (www.quantros.com) and the MER program to the Institute for Safe Medication Practices (www.ismp.org).

Accolate	Accupril
Accolate	Accutane
Accupril	Aciphex
Accupril	Accolate
Accupril	Accutane
Accupril	Altace
Accupril	Aricept
Accupril	Monopril
Accutane	Accolate
Accutane	Accupril
Acebutolol	Albuterol
Acetaminophen and Codeine	Acetaminophen and Hydrocodone
Acetaminophen and Codeine	Acetaminophen and Oxycodone
Acetaminophen and Hydrocodone	Acetaminophen and Codeine
Acetaminophen and Oxycodone	Acetaminophen and Codeine
Acetazolamide	Acetohexamide
Acetazolamide	Acetylcysteine
Acetazolamide	Acyclovir
Acetohexamide	Acetazolamide
Acetylcysteine	Acetazolamide
Aciphex	Accupril
Aciphex	Adipex-P
Aciphex	Aricept
Aciphex	Vioxx
Activase	Retavase
Actonel	Actos
Actos	Actonel
Acular	Ocular Lubricants
Acyclovir	Acetazolamide
Acyclovir	Famciclovir
Adalat CC	Aldomet
Adalat CC	Allegra
Adderall	Inderal
Adenosine	Adenosine Phosphate
Adenosine Phosphate	Adenosine
Adipex-P	Aciphex
Adriamycin	Aredia
Adriamycin	Idamycin
Advair	Advicor
Advicor	Advair
Aggrastat	Aggrenox
Aggrastat	Argatroban
Aggrenox	Aggrastat
Akarpine	Atropine
Albuterol	Acebutolol
Aldara	Alora
Aldesleukin	Oprelvekin
Aldomet	Adalat CC
Alkeran	Leukeran
Allegra	Adalat CC
Allegra	Allegra-D
Allegra	Asacol
Allegra	Viagra
Allegra-D	Allegra
Allegra-D	Allerx-D
Allerx-D	Allegra-D
Allopurinol	Apresoline
Alora	Aldara
Alprazolam	Clonazepam
Alprazolam	Diazepam
Alprazolam	Lorazepam
Altace	Accupril
Altace	Amaryl, Amerge
Altace	Artane
Altace	Norvasc
Alupent	Atrovent
Amantadine	Amiodarone
Amantadine	Ranitidine, Rimantadine
Amaryl	Altace, Amerge
Amaryl	Avandia
Amaryl	Reminyl
Amaryl	Symmetrel
Ambien	Amen
Ambien	Ativan
Ambien	Coumadin
Amen	Ambien
Amerge	Altace, Amaryl
Amicar	Amikin
Amikacin	Anakinra
Amikin	Amicar
Amiloride	Amlodipine
Aminophylline	Amitriptyline
Amiodarone	Trazodone
Amiodarone	Amantadine
Amiodarone	Amlodipine
Amiodarone	Amrinone (Former nomenclature for Inamrinone)
Amitriptyline	Aminophylline
Amitriptyline	Imipramine
Amitriptyline	Nortriptyline
Amlodipine	Amiloride
Amlodipine	Amiodarone
Amlodipine	Felodipine
Amoxicillin	Amoxil
Amoxicillin	Ampicillin
Amoxicillin	Atarax
Amoxicillin	Augmentin
Amoxil	Amoxicillin
Amphotericin B, Lipid Complex	Amphotericin B, Liposomal
Amphotericin B, Liposomal	Amphotericin B, Lipid Complex
Ampicillin	Amoxicillin
Ampicillin	Augmentin
Ampicillin	Oxacillin
Amrinone (Former nomenclature for Inamrinone)	Amiodarone
Anaflex	Zanaflex
Anakinra	Amikacin
Anaprox	Avapro
Anaspaz	Antispas
Anbesol	Anusol
Ansaid	Asacol
Antacid	Atacand
Antispas	Anaspaz
Anusol	Anbesol
Anusol	Anusol-HC
Anusol-HC	Anusol
Anzemet	Aricept
Apresoline	Allopurinol
Apresoline	Priscoline
Aredia	Adriamycin
Argatroban	Aggrastat
Argatroban	Orgaran
Aricept	Accupril
Aricept	Aciphex
Aricept	Anzemet
Artane	Altace
Asacol	Allegra
Asacol	Ansaid
Asacol	Os-Cal
Asparaginase	Pegaspargase
Atacand	Antacid
Atacand	Avandia
Atarax	Amoxicillin
Atarax	Ativan
Atenolol	Metoprolol
Atgam	Ratgam (Synonym for Thymoglobulin)
Ativan	Ambien
Ativan	Atarax
Atorvastatin	Pravastatin
Atropine	Akarpine
Atrovent	Alupent
Atrovent	Azmacort
Atrovent	Flovent
Atrovent	Natru-Vent
Atrovent	Serevent
Attenuvax	Meruvax
Augmentin	Amoxicillin
Augmentin	Ampicillin
Avandia	Amaryl
Avandia	Atacand
Avandia	Avelox
Avandia	Coumadin
Avandia	Prandin
Avapro	Anaprox
Avapro	Avelox
Avelox	Avandia
Avelox	Avapro
Avelox	Cerebyx
Avinza	Invanz
Avonex	Lovenox
Azithromycin	Erythromycin
Azithromycin	Vancomycin
Azithromycin	Aztreonam
Azmacort	Atrovent
Azmacort	Nasacort
Aztreonam	Azithromycin
Bactrim	Biaxin
Bactrim DS	Bancap HC
Bancap HC	Bactrim DS
Baycol	Bellergal
Beclovent	Beconase
Beconase	Beclovent
Beconase	Beconase AQ
Beconase AQ	Beconase
Bellergal	Baycol
Benadryl	Benazepril
Benadryl	Bentyl
Benadryl	Benylin
Benazepril	Benadryl
Benazepril	Benzonatate
Benazepril	Donepezil
Benazepril	Lisinopril
Bentyl	Benadryl
Bentyl	Bumex
Bentyl	Proventil
Benylin	Benadryl
Benylin	Ventolin
Benzonatate	Benazepril
Benzonatate	Benztropine
Benztropine	Benzonatate
Bepridil	Prepidil
Betagan	Betoptic
Betapace	Betapace AF
Betapace AF	Betapace
Betoptic	Betagan
Betoptic	Betoptic S
Betoptic S	Betoptic

Biaxin	Bactrim
Bisacodyl	Bisoprolol
Bisacodyl	Visicol
Bisoprolol	Bisacodyl
Bisoprolol	Fosinopril
Boost bar	Buspar
Brevibloc	Brevital
Brevital	Brevibloc
Bumex	Bentyl
Bumex	Buprenex
Bumex	Nimbex
Bumex	Permax
Bupivacaine	Ropivacaine
Buprenex	Bumex
Bupropion	Buspirone
Buspar	Boost bar
Buspirone	Bupropion
Butalbital, Acetaminophen, and Caffeine	Butalbital, Aspirin, and Caffeine
Butalbital, Aspirin, and Caffeine	Butalbital, Acetaminophen, and Caffeine
Cafergot	Carafate
Calan	Calan SR
Calan	Colace
Calan SR	Calan
Calan SR	Cardizem CD
Calan SR	Cardizem SR
Calciferol	Calcitriol
Calcitriol	Calciferol
Calcium Acetate	Calcium Carbonate
Calcium Carbonate	Calcium Acetate
Calcium Carbonate	Calcium Gluconate
Calcium Chloride	Calcium Gluconate
Calcium Gluconate	Calcium Carbonate
Calcium Gluconate	Calcium Chloride
Capoten	Catapres
Captopril	Carvedilol
Carafate	Cafergot
Carbatrol (Carbamezapine in U.S.)	Carbrital (Pentobarbitone Sodium in Australia)
Carbidopa	Levodopa and Carbidopa
Carboplatin	Cisplatin
Carbrital (Pentobarbitone Sodium in Australia)	Carbatrol (Carbamezapine in U.S.)
Cardene	Cardizem
Cardene	Cardura
Cardene	Codeine
Cardene SR	Cardizem SR
Cardiem	Cardizem
Cardizem	Cardene
Cardizem	Cardiem
Cardizem	Cardizem SR
Cardizem	Clonidine
Cardizem CD	Calan SR
Cardizem CD	Cardizem SR
Cardizem SR	Calan SR
Cardizem SR	Cardene SR
Cardizem SR	Cardizem
Cardizem SR	Cardizem CD
Cardura	Cardene
Cardura	Cordarone
Cardura	Coumadin
Cardura	K-Dur
Cardura	Ridaura
Carteolol	Carvedilol
Cartia (Aspirin in New Zealand)	Cartia XT (Diltiazem in U.S.)
Cartia XT	Diltia XT
Cartia XT	Procardia XL
Cartia XT (Diltiazem in U.S.)	Cartia (Aspirin in New Zealand)
Carvedilol	Captopril
Carvedilol	Carteolol
Cataflam	Catapres
Catapres	Capoten
Catapres	Cataflam
Ceclor	Ceclor CD
Ceclor CD	Ceclor
Cefaclor	Cephalexin
Cefazolin	Cefepime
Cefazolin	Cefotaxime
Cefazolin	Cefotetan
Cefazolin	Cefoxitin
Cefazolin	Cefprozil
Cefazolin	Ceftazidime
Cefazolin	Ceftizoxime
Cefazolin	Ceftriaxone
Cefazolin	Cefuroxime
Cefazolin	Cephalexin
Cefepime	Cefazolin
Cefepime	Cefotetan
Cefepime	Cefotan
Cefixime	Cefpodoxime
Cefobid	Celecoxib
Cefobid	Levbid
Cefol	Cefzil
Cefotan	Ceftin
Cefotan	Claforan
Cefotan	Cefepime
Cefotan	Ceftriaxone
Cefotaxime	Cefazolin
Cefotaxime	Cefotetan
Cefotaxime	Cefoxitin
Cefotaxime	Ceftazidime
Cefotaxime	Ceftizoxime
Cefotaxime	Ceftriaxone
Cefotaxime	Cefuroxime
Cefotetan	Cefazolin
Cefotetan	Cefepime
Cefotetan	Cefotaxime
Cefotetan	Cefoxitin
Cefotetan	Ceftazidime
Cefotetan	Ceftizoxime
Cefotetan	Ceftriaxone
Cefoxitin	Cefazolin
Cefoxitin	Cefotaxime
Cefoxitin	Cefotetan
Cefoxitin	Ceftriaxone
Cefoxitin	Cefuroxime
Cefpodoxime	Cefixime
Cefprozil	Cefazolin
Cefprozil	Cefuroxime
Ceftazidime	Cefazolin
Ceftazidime	Cefotaxime
Ceftazidime	Cefotetan
Ceftazidime	Ceftizoxime
Ceftazidime	Ceftriaxone
Ceftazidime	Cefuroxime
Ceftin	Cefotan
Ceftin	Cefzil
Ceftin	Cipro
Ceftin	Rocephin
Ceftizoxime	Cefazolin
Ceftizoxime	Cefotaxime
Ceftizoxime	Cefotetan
Ceftizoxime	Ceftazidime
Ceftizoxime	Cefuroxime
Ceftriaxone	Cefazolin
Ceftriaxone	Cefotaxime
Ceftriaxone	Cefotetan
Ceftriaxone	Cefoxitin
Ceftriaxone	Ceftazidime
Ceftriaxone	Cefuroxime
Ceftriaxone	Cefotan
Cefuroxime	Cefazolin
Cefuroxime	Cefotaxime
Cefuroxime	Cefprozil
Cefuroxime	Ceftazidime
Cefuroxime	Ceftizoxime
Cefuroxime	Ceftriaxone
Cefuroxime	Cephalexin
Cefuroxime	Deferoxamine
Cefuroxime	Cefoxitin
Cefzil	Cefol
Cefzil	Ceftin
Cefzil	Kefzol
Celebrex	Celexa, Cerebyx
Celebrex	Celexa, Cerebra
Celecoxib	Cefobid
Celexa	Zyprexa
Celexa	Celebrex, Cerebra
Celexa	Cerebyx, Celebrex
Cephalexin	Cefaclor
Cephalexin	Cefazolin
Cephalexin	Cefuroxime
Cephalexin	Ciprofloxacin
Cerebra	Celebrex, Celexa
Cerebyx	Avelox
Cerebyx	Celebrex, Celexa
Cetirizine	Cyclobenzaprine
Chlordiazepoxide	Chlorpromazine
Chlorhexidine	Chlorpromazine
Chlorpromazine	Chlordiazepoxide
Chlorpromazine	Chlorhexidine
Chlorpromazine	Chlorpropamide
Chlorpromazine	Chlorthalidone
Chlorpromazine	Prochlorperazine
Chlorpromazine	Thioridazine
Chlorpropamide	Chlorpromazine
Chlorthalidone	Chlorpromazine
Cipro	Ceftin
Ciprofloxacin	Cephalexin
Ciprofloxacin	Levofloxacin
Ciprofloxacin	Ofloxacin
Cisplatin	Carboplatin
Citracal	Citrucel
Citrucel	Hydrocil
Citrucel	Citracal
Claforan	Cefotan
Claritin	Claritin-D
Claritin-D	Claritin
Clinoril	Clozaril
Clinoril	Oruvail
Clomiphene	Clomipramine
Clomipramine	Clomiphene
Clomipramine	Desipramine
Clonapam (Clonazepam in Canada)	Corlopam (Fenoldopam in U.S.)
Clonazepam	Alprazolam
Clonazepam	Clonidine, Klonopin
Clonazepam	Clorazepate
Clonazepam	Diazepam
Clonazepam	Lorazepam
Clonidine	Colchicine
Clonidine	Cardizem
Clonidine	Klonopin, Clonazepam
Clorazepate	Clonazepam
Clozaril	Clinoril
Clozaril	Colazal
Codeine	Cardene
Codeine	Iodine
Codeine	Lodine
Codiclear DH	Codimal DH
Codimal DH	Codiclear DH
Cognex	Corgard
Colace	Calan
Colace	Peri-Colace
Colace (Docusate Sodium)	Colace (Glycerin suppository)
Colace (Glycerin suppository)	Colace (Docusate Sodium)
Colazal	Clozaril
Colchicine	Clonidine
Combivir	Epivir
Cordarone	Cardura
Cordarone	Coumadin
Corgard	Cognex
Corgard	Cozaar
Corlopam (Fenoldopam in U.S.)	Clonapam (Clonazepam in Canada)
Cortane	Cortane-B
Cortane-B	Cortane
Cortef	Lortab
Cortisone	Hydrocortisone
Cortisporin (Ophthalmic)	Cortisporin (Otic)
Cortisporin (Otic)	Cortisporin (Ophthalmic)
Cosopt	Trusopt
Coumadin	Avandia
Coumadin	Cardura
Coumadin	Cordarone
Coumadin	Ambien
Covera	Provera
Cozaar	Corgard
Cozaar	Hyzaar
Cozaar	Zocor
Cyclobenzaprine	Cetirizine
Cyclobenzaprine	Cyproheptadine
Cyclophosphamide	Cyclosporine
Cycloserine	Cyclosporine
Cyclosporine	Cyclophosphamide
Cyclosporine	Cycloserine
Cyproheptadine	Cyclobenzaprine
Cytarabine	Cytosar, Cytoxan
CytoGam	Gamimune N
Cytosar	Cytovene
Cytosar	Cytoxan, Cytarabine
Cytosar-U	Neosar
Cytotec	Cytoxan
Cytovene	Cytosar
Cytoxan	Cytosar, Cytarabine
Cytoxan	Cytotec
Danazol	Dantrium
Danocrine	Dantrium

Dantrium	Danazol
Dantrium	Danocrine
Darvocet	Percocet
Darvocet-N	Darvon
Darvocet-N	Darvon-N
Darvon	Darvocet-N
Darvon	Diovan
Darvon-N	Darvocet-N
Datril	Detrol
Daunorubicin	Doxorubicin
Deferoxamine	Cefuroxime
Demadex	Demerol
Demeclocycline	Dicyclomine
Demerol	Demadex
Demerol	Desyrel
Demerol	Dilaudid
Denavir	Indinavir
Depakene	Depakote
Depakote	Depakene
Depakote	Senokot
Depakote (Delayed Release)	Depakote ER (Extended Release)
Depakote ER (Extended Release)	Depakote (Delayed Release)
Depo-Estradiol	Depo-Testadiol
Depo-Medrol	Depo-Provera
Depo-Provera	Depo-Medrol
Depo-Testadiol	Depo-Estradiol
Deseril (Methysergide Maleate in Australia)	Desyrel (Trazodone in U.S.)
Desferal	DexFerrum
Desipramine	Imipramine
Desipramine	Clomipramine
Desipramine	Nortriptyline
Desyrel	Demerol
Desyrel (Trazodone in U.S.)	Deseril (Methysergide Maleate in Australia)
Detrol	Datril
Detrol	Dextrostat
DexFerrum	Desferal
Dextroamphetamine	Dextroamphetamine and Amphetamine
Dextroamphetamine and Amphetamine	Dextroamphetamine
Dextrostat	Detrol
DiaBeta	Zebeta
Diamox	Dobutrex
Diastix	Keto-Diastix
Diatex (Diazepam in Mexico)	Diatx (Multivitamin in U.S.)
Diatx (Multivitamin in U.S.)	Diatex (Diazepam in Mexico)
Diazepam	Alprazolam
Diazepam	Clonazepam
Diazepam	Ditropan
Diazepam	Ditropan XL
Diazepam	Lorazepam
Diazepam	Midazolam
Dicloxacillin	Doxycycline
Dicyclomine	Demeclocycline
Dicyclomine	Diphenhydramine
Dicyclomine	Doxycycline
Diflucan	Dilantin
Diflucan	Diprivan
Digoxin	Doxepin
Dilantin	Diflucan
Dilaudid	Demerol
Diltia XT	Cartia XT
Dimetapp	Donnatal
Diovan	Darvon
Diovan	Zyban
Diphenhydramine	Dicyclomine
Diphenhydramine	Dipyridamole
Diphtheria and Tetanus Toxoid	Tetanus Toxoid
Diprivan	Diflucan
Diprivan	Ditropan
Dipyridamole	Diphenhydramine
Ditropan	Diazepam
Ditropan	Diprivan
Ditropan XL	Diazepam
Dobutamine	Dopamine
Dobutrex	Diamox
Dobutrex	Dopamine
Docetaxel	Paclitaxel
Docusate Calcium	Docusate Sodium
Docusate Sodium	Docusate Calcium
Dolobid	Slo-bid
Donepezil	Benazepril
Donepezil	Doxazosin
Donnatal	Dimetapp
Donnatal	Donnatal Extentabs
Donnatal Extentabs	Donnatal
Dopamine	Dobutrex
Dopamine	Dobutamine
Doxazosin	Terazosin
Doxazosin	Donepezil
Doxepin	Digoxin
Doxepin	Doxycycline
Doxorubicin	Daunorubicin
Doxorubicin	Doxorubicin Liposomal
Doxorubicin	Idarubicin
Doxorubicin Liposomal	Doxorubicin
Doxycycline	Dicloxacillin
Doxycycline	Dicyclomine
Doxycycline	Doxepin
Duratuss	Duratuss-G
Duratuss-G	Duratuss
Dynabac	DynaCirc
Dynacin	DynaCirc
DynaCirc	Dynabac
DynaCirc	Dynacin
Edecrin	Eulexin
Efavirenz	Nelfinavir
Effexor	Effexor XR
Effexor XR	Effexor
Efudex	Eurax
Elavil	Enbrel
Elavil	Oruvail
Elavil	Plavix
Eldepryl	Enalapril
Eldopaque Forte	Eldoquin Forte
Eldoquin Forte	Eldopaque Forte
Elidel	Eligard
Eligard	Elidel
Elmiron	Imuran
Enalapril	Eldepryl
Enalapril	Lisinopril
Enbrel	Elavil
Enoxacin	Enoxaparin
Enoxaparin	Enoxacin
Entex LA	Eulexin
Entuss	Entuss-D
Entuss-D	Entuss
Ephedrine	Epinephrine
Epinephrine	Ephedrine
Epinephrine	Neo-Synephrine
Epinephrine	Norepinephrine
Epivir	Combivir
Epogen	Neupogen
Equagesic	EquiGesic
EquiGesic	Equagesic
Erex	Urex
Erythrocin	Ethmozine
Erythromycin	Azithromycin
Eskalith	Estratest
Esmolol	Osmitrol
Esomeprazole	Omeprazole
Estrace	Evista
Estraderm	Testoderm
Estradiol	Ethinyl Estradiol
Estradiol	Risperdal
Estramustine	Exemestane
Estratab	Estratest
Estratest	Eskalith
Estratest	Estratab
Estratest	Estratest HS
Estratest HS	Estratest
Ethinyl Estradiol	Estradiol
Ethinyl Estradiol and Levonorgestrel	Ethinyl Estradiol and Norgestrel
Ethinyl Estradiol and Norgestrel	Ethinyl Estradiol and Levonorgestrel
Ethmozine	Erythrocin
Etidronate	Etomidate
Etomidate	Etidronate
Eulexin	Edecrin
Eulexin	Entex LA
Eurax	Efudex
Evista	Estrace
Evista	E-Vista (Monograph in Nursing Drug References)
E-Vista (Monograph in Nursing Drug References)	Evista
Exemestane	Estramustine
Famciclovir	Acyclovir
Famotidine	Fluoxetine
Famotidine	Furosemide
Felodipine	Amlodipine
Felodipine	Nifedipine
Felodipine	Ranitidine
Fentanyl Citrate	Sufentanil Citrate
Fer-In-Sol	Poly-Vi-Sol
Fioricet	Fiorinal
Fioricet	Florinef
Fiorinal	Fioricet
Fleet Enema	Fleet Phospho-Soda
Fleet Phospho-Soda	Fleet Enema
Flomax	Flonase
Flomax	Flovent
Flomax	Fosamax
Flomax	Volmax
Flonase	Flomax
Flonase	Flovent
Florinef	Fioricet
Florinef	Fluoride
Flovent	Atrovent
Flovent	Flomax
Flovent	Flonase
Flucytosine	Fluorouracil
Fludara	FUDR
Fludarabine	Flumadine
Flumadine	Fludarabine
Fluocinolone	Fluocinonide
Fluocinonide	Fluocinolone
Fluocinonide	Fluorouracil
Fluoride	Florinef
Fluorouracil	Flucytosine
Fluorouracil	Fluocinonide
Fluoxetine	Fluphenazine
Fluoxetine	Fluvoxamine
Fluoxetine	Famotidine
Fluoxetine	Fluvastatin
Fluoxetine	Furosemide
Fluoxetine	Paroxetine
Fluphenazine	Fluoxetine
Fluphenazine	Perphenazine
Fluphenazine	Trifluoperazine
Flurazepam	Temazepam
Fluvastatin	Fluoxetine
Fluvoxamine	Fluoxetine
FML Forte	FML S.O.P.
FML S.O.P.	FML Forte
Folic Acid	Folinic Acid
Folinic Acid	Folic Acid
Foltex PFS	FOLTX
FOLTX	Foltex PFS
Foradil	Toradol
Fortovase	Invirase
Fosamax	Flomax
Fosinopril	Bisoprolol
Fosinopril	Furosemide
Fosinopril	Lisinopril
Fosinopril	Minoxidil
Fosphenytoin	Phenytoin
FUDR	Fludara
Furosemide	Famotidine
Furosemide	Fluoxetine
Furosemide	Fosinopril
Furosemide	Torsemide
Gamimune N	CytoGam
Gemzar	Zinecard
Gengraf	Prograf
Gentamicin	Tobramycin
Gentamicin	Vancomycin
Glipizide	Glyburide
Glucophage	Glucophage XR
Glucophage	Glucotrol
Glucophage	Glutofac
Glucophage	Glucophage XR, Glucotrol
Glucophage XR	Glucotrol XL
Glucophage XR	Glucophage
Glucophage XR	Glucotrol, Glucophage
Glucotrol	Glucophage, Glucophage XR
Glucotrol	Glucophage
Glucotrol	Glucotrol XL
Glucotrol	Glyburide
Glucotrol XL	Glucophage XR
Glucotrol XL	Glucotrol
Glutofac	Glucophage
Glyburide	Glipizide
Glyburide	Glucotrol
Glycerin	Nitroglycerin
Granulex	Regranex
Guaifenesin	Guanfacine

Guanfacine	Guaifenesin
Halcion	Haldol
Haldol	Halcion
Haldol	Haldol Decanoate
Haldol	Inderal
Haldol	Stadol
Haldol Decanoate	Haldol
Haloperidol	Halotestin
Halotestin	Haloperidol
Hemoccult	Seracult
Heparin	Levaquin
Heparin	Hespan
Herceptin	Perceptin
Hespan	Heparin
Humalog	Humalog Mix
Humalog Mix	Humalog
Humalog, Insulin Human	Humulin, Insulin Human
Humulin 70/30	Humulin N
Humulin 70/30	Humulin R
Humulin L	Humulin N
Humulin L (Lente)	Humulin U (Ultralente)
Humulin N	Humulin 70/30
Humulin N	Humulin R
Humulin N	Humulin U
Humulin N	Novolin N
Humulin N	Humulin L
Humulin R	Humulin 70/30
Humulin R	Humulin N
Humulin R	Humulin U
Humulin R	Novolin R
Humulin U	Humulin N
Humulin U	Humulin R
Humulin U (Ultralente)	Humulin L (Lente)
Humulin, Insulin Human	Humalog, Insulin Human
Hydralazine	Hydrochlorothiazide
Hydralazine	Hydrocortisone
Hydralazine	Hydroxyzine
Hydrochlorothiazide	Hydralazine
Hydrochlorothiazide	Hydroxychloroquine
Hydrocil	Citrucel
Hydrocodone	Hydrocortisone
Hydrocodone and Acetaminophen	Oxycodone and Acetaminophen
Hydrocodone and Acetaminophen	Hydromorphone
Hydrocortisone	Cortisone
Hydrocortisone	Hydralazine
Hydrocortisone	Hydrocodone
Hydromorphone	Hydrocodone and Acetaminophen
Hydromorphone	Morphine
Hydroxychloroquine	Hydrochlorothiazide
Hydroxyurea	Hydroxyzine
Hydroxyzine	Hydralazine
Hydroxyzine	Hydroxyurea
Hypergel	MPM GelPad Hydrogel Saturated Dressing
Hyzaar	Cozaar
Idamycin	Adriamycin
Idarubicin	Doxorubicin
IMDUR	Imuran
IMDUR	Inderal LA
IMDUR	K-Dur
Imipenem	Meropenem
Imipenem	Omnipen
Imipramine	Amitriptyline
Imipramine	Desipramine
Imodium	Indocin
Imovax	Imovax I.D.
Imovax I.D.	Imovax
Imuran	Elmiron
Imuran	IMDUR
Imuran	Tenormin
Inapsine	Lanoxin
Inderal	Adderall
Inderal	Haldol
Inderal	Isordil
Inderal	Toradol
Inderal LA	IMDUR
Indinavir	Denavir
Indocin	Imodium
Infliximab	Rituximab
Insulin	Integrilin
Insulin Human	Lispro, Insulin Human
Insulin Human	Isophane, Insulin Human
Integrilin	Insulin
Invanz	Avinza
Invirase	Fortovase
Iodine	Codeine
Iodine	Lodine
Ismo	Isordil
Isophane, Insulin Human	Insulin Human
Isopto Carpine	Propine
Isordil	Inderal
Isordil	Ismo
Isosorbide Dinitrate	Isosorbide Mononitrate
Isosorbide Mononitrate	Isosorbide Dinitrate
Kaletra	Keppra
Kaopectate	Kayexalate
Kayexalate	Kaopectate
Kayexalate	Potassium Acetate
K-Dur	Cardura
K-Dur	IMDUR
K-Dur	K-Lor
Keflex	Kefzol
Keflex	Norflex
Kefurox	Kefzol
Kefzol	Cefzil
Kefzol	Keflex
Kefzol	Kefurox
Kenalog	Ketalar
Keppra	Kaletra
Ketalar	Kenalog
Keto-Diastix	Diastix
Ketorolac	Ketotifen
Ketotifen	Ketorolac
Klonopin	Clonidine, Clonazepam
K-Lor	K-Dur
K-Lor	K-Lyte
K-Lyte	K-Lor
K-Lyte	K-Lyte Cl
K-Lyte Cl	K-Lyte
Kogenate	Kogenate-2
Kogenate-2	Kogenate
K-Phos Neutral	Neutra-Phos-K
Labetolol	Lamictal
Lacrilube	Surgilube
Lamicel	Lamisil
Lamictal	Labetolol
Lamictal	Lamisil
Lamictal	Lomotil
Lamictal	Ludiomil
Lamisil	Lamicel
Lamisil	Lamictal
Lamisil	Lomotil
Lamivudine	Lamotrigine
Lamivudine	Zidovudine
Lamotrigine	Lamivudine
Lanoxin	Levothyroxine
Lanoxin	Inapsine
Lanoxin	Lasix, Lomotil
Lanoxin	Levoxyl
Lanoxin	Levsin
Lanoxin	Lonox
Lanoxin	Lovenox
Lanoxin	Xanax
Lantus, Insulin Human	Lente, Insulin Human
Lasix	Lomotil, Lanoxin
Lasix	Luvox
L-Dopa	Levodopa, Methyldopa
Lente, Insulin Human	Lispro, Insulin Human
Lente, Insulin Human	Lantus, Insulin Human
Leucovorin	Leukine, Leukeran
Leucovorin	Levothyroxine
Leukeran	Alkeran
Leukeran	Leucovorin, Leukine
Leukine	Leukeran, Leucovorin
Levaquin	Heparin
Levaquin	Lovenox
Levaquin	Tequin
Levbid	Cefobid
Levbid	Lithobid
Levbid	Lopid
Levbid	Lorabid
Levlen	Tri-Levlen
Levobunolol	Levocabastine
Levocabastine	Levobunolol
Levocarnitine	Levofloxacin
Levodopa	L-Dopa, Methyldopa
Levodopa and Carbidopa	Carbidopa
Levofloxacin	Ciprofloxacin
Levofloxacin	Levocarnitine
Levothyroxine	Lanoxin
Levothyroxine	Leucovorin
Levothyroxine	Liothyronine
Levoxyl	Lanoxin
Levoxyl	Luvox
Levsin	Lanoxin
Lexapro	Loxapine
Librax	Librium
Librium	Librax
Lioresal	Lotensin
Liothyronine	Levothyroxine
Lipitor	Zocor
Lisinopril	Benazepril
Lisinopril	Enalapril
Lisinopril	Fosinopril
Lisinopril	Quinapril
Lisinopril	Risperdal
Lispro, Insulin Human	Insulin Human
Lispro, Insulin Human	Lente, Insulin Human
Lithobid	Levbid
Lithobid	Lithostat
Lithostat	Lithobid
Lodine	Codeine
Lodine	Iodine
Lomotil	Lamictal
Lomotil	Lamisil
Lomotil	Lanoxin, Lasix
Loniten	Lotensin
Lonox	Lanoxin
Loperamide	Lorazepam
Lopid	Levbid
Lopid	Lorabid, Slo-bid
Lorabid	Levbid
Lorabid	Lortab
Lorabid	Slo-bid, Lopid
Loratadine	Losartan
Lorazepam	Alprazolam
Lorazepam	Clonazepam
Lorazepam	Diazepam
Lorazepam	Loperamide
Lorazepam	Midazolam
Lorazepam	Temazepam
Lorcet	Lortab
Lortab	Cortef
Lortab	Lorabid
Lortab	Lorcet
Lortab	Luride
Losartan	Loratadine
Losartan	Valsartan
Lotensin	Lioresal
Lotensin	Loniten
Lotensin	Lovastatin
Lotrimin	Lotrisone
Lotrisone	Lotrimin
Lotronex	Lovenox
Lotronex	Protonix
Lovastatin	Lotensin
Lovenox	Avonex
Lovenox	Lanoxin
Lovenox	Levaquin
Lovenox	Lotronex
Lovenox	Luvox
Loxapine	Lexapro
Loxitane	Soriatane
Ludiomil	Lamictal
Luride	Lortab
Luvox	Lasix
Luvox	Levoxyl
Luvox	Lovenox
Magnesium Citrate	Magnesium Sulfate
Magnesium Sulfate	Magnesium Citrate
Maxipime (Cefepime Hydrochloride in U.S.)	Moxapen (Amoxacillin Trihydrate in Thailand)
Meclofenamate	Mycophenolate
Medigesic	Medi-Gesic
Medi-Gesic	Medigesic
Medroxyprogesterone	Methylprednisolone
Medroxyprogesterone	Metolazone
Mefloquine	Meloxicam
Megace	Reglan
Mellaril	Melphalan
Meloxicam	Mefloquine
Melphalan	Mellaril
Melphalan	Myleran
Meperidine	Methadone
Meperidine	Morphine

Mepron (Atovaquone in U.S.)	Mepron (Meprobamate in Australia)
Meropenem	Imipenem
Meruvax	Attenuvax
Mesalamine	Sulfasalazine
Metadate CD	Metadate ER
Metadate ER	Metadate CD
Metaxalone	Metolazone
Metformin	Metronidazole
Methadone	Meperidine
Methadone	Methylphenidate
Methazolamide	Methimazole
Methazolamide	Metronidazole
Methimazole	Methazolamide
Methohexital	Methotrexate
Methotrexate	Methohexital
Methotrexate	Metolazone
Methyldopa	L-Dopa, Levodopa
Methylphenidate	Methadone
Methylprednisolone	Medroxyprogesterone
Methylprednisolone	Prednisone
Metoclopramide	Metolazone
Metoclopramide	Metoprolol
Metoclopramide	Metronidazole
Metolazone	Medroxyprogesterone
Metolazone	Metaxalone
Metolazone	Methotrexate
Metolazone	Metoclopramide
Metolazone	Metoprolol
Metoprolol	Atenolol
Metoprolol	Metoclopramide
Metoprolol	Metolazone
Metoprolol	Metronidazole
Metoprolol	Misoprostol
Metoprolol Succinate	Metoprolol Tartrate
Metoprolol Tartrate	Metoprolol Succinate
MetroGel	MetroGel-Vaginal
MetroGel-Vaginal	MetroGel
Metronidazole	Metformin
Metronidazole	Methazolamide
Metronidazole	Metoclopramide
Metronidazole	Metoprolol
Metronidazole	Miconazole
Miacalcin	Micatin
Micatin	Miacalcin
Miconazole	Metronidazole
Micro-K	Micronase
Micronase	Micro-K
Micronase	Microzide
Microzide	Micronase
Midazolam	Diazepam
Midazolam	Lorazepam
Midodrin	Midrin
Midodrine	Molindone
Midrin	Midodrin
Mifepristone	Misoprostol
Minoxidil	Fosinopril
Minoxidil	Monopril
MiraLax	Mirapex
Mirapex	MiraLax
Misoprostol	Metoprolol
Misoprostol	Mifepristone
Mitomycin	Mitoxantrone
Mitoxantrone	Mitomycin
Moban	Mobic
Mobic	Moban
Molindone	Midodrine
Monoket	Monopril
Monopril	Accupril
Monopril	Minoxidil
Monopril	Monoket
Morphine	Hydromorphone
Morphine	Meperidine
Moxapen (Amoxacillin Trihydrate in Hydrochloride Thailand)	Maxipime (Cefepime in U.S.)
MPM GelPad Hydrogel Saturated Dressing	Hypergel
MS Contin	OxyContin
Murocel	Murocoll-2
Murocoll-2	Murocel
Mycelex	Mycolog
Mycolog	Mycelex
Mycophenolate	Meclofenamate
Mylanta	Mylicon
Myleran	Melphalan
Mylicon	Mylanta
Naprelan	Naprosyn
Naprosyn	Naprelan
Naprosyn	Niaspan
Narcan	Norcuron
Narcan	Nubain
Nasacort	Azmacort
Nasalcrom	Nasalide
Nasalide	Nasalcrom
Nasarel	Nizoral
Natru-Vent	Atrovent
Navane	Norvasc
Nebcin	Nubain
Nefazodone	Nelfinavir
Nelfinavir	Efavirenz
Nelfinavir	Nefazodone
Nelfinavir	Nevirapine
Neoral	Neurontin
Neoral	Nizoral
Neosar	Cytosar-U
Neo-Synephrine	Epinephrine
Neo-Synephrine	Neo-Synephrine 12-Hour
Neo-Synephrine 12-Hour	Neo-Synephrine
Neo-Synephrine	Norepinephrine
Nephrox	Niferex
Neumega	Neupogen
Neupogen	Epogen
Neupogen	Neumega
Neurontin	Neoral
Neurontin	Noroxin
Neutra-Phos	Neutra-Phos-K
Neutra-Phos-K	K-Phos Neutral
Neutra-Phos-K	Neutra-Phos
Nevirapine	Nelfinavir
Niacin	Niaspan
Niaspan	Naprosyn
Niaspan	Niacin
Nicardipine	Nifedipine, Nimodipine
Nicoderm	Nitroderm
NicoDerm CQ	Nitro-Dur
Nifedipine	Felodipine
Nifedipine	Nicardipine, Nimodipine
Niferex	Nephrox
Nimbex	Bumex
Nimbex	Revex
Nimodipine	Nicardipine, Nifedipine
Nitro-Bid	Nitro-Dur
Nitroderm	Nicoderm
Nitro-Dur	NicoDerm CQ
Nitro-Dur	Nitro-Bid
Nitro-Dur	NitroQuick
Nitroglycerin	Glycerin
NitroQuick	Nitro-Dur
Nizatidine	Tizanidine
Nizoral	Nasarel
Nizoral	Neoral
Nolvadex	Norvasc
Norcuron	Narcan
Norepinephrine	Epinephrine
Norepinephrine	Neo-Synephrine
Norepinephrine	Phenylephrine
Norflex	Keflex
Norflex	Noroxin, Norfloxacin
Norflex	Norvasc
Norfloxacin	Norflex, Noroxin
Noroxin	Neurontin
Noroxin	Norflex, Norfloxacin
Norpramin	Nortriptyline
Nortriptyline	Amitriptyline
Nortriptyline	Desipramine
Nortriptyline	Norpramin
Norvasc	Altace
Norvasc	Navane
Norvasc	Nolvadex
Norvasc	Norflex
Norvasc	Vasotec
Norvir	Retrovir
Novolin 70/30	Novolin N
Novolin L	Novolin N
Novolin N	Humulin N
Novolin N	Novolin 70/30
Novolin N	Novolin L
Novolin N	Novolin R
Novolin R	Humulin R
Novolin R	Novolin N
Nubain	Narcan
Nubain	Nebcin
Nutropin	Nutropin AQ
Nutropin AQ	Nutropin
Ocufen	Ocuflox
Ocufen	Ocupress
Ocuflox	Ocufen
Ocular Lubricants	Acular
Ocumycin	Ocu-Mycin
Ocu-Mycin	Ocumycin
Ocupress	Ocufen
Ofloxacin	Ciprofloxacin
Olanzapine	Oxcarbazepine
Omeprazole	Esomeprazole
Omnipen	Imipenem
Opium Tincture, Deodorized	Opium, Camphorated
Opium, Camphorated	Opium Tincture, Deodorized
Oprelvekin	Aldesleukin
Orgaran	Argatroban
Ortho Tri-Cyclen	Ortho-Cyclen
Ortho Tri-Cyclen	Tri-Levlen
Ortho-Cept	Ortho-Cyclen
Ortho-Cept	Ortho-Est
Ortho-Cyclen	Ortho-Cept
Ortho-Cyclen	Ortho Tri-Cyclen
Ortho-Est	Ortho-Cept
Oruvail	Clinoril
Oruvail	Elavil
Os-Cal	Asacol
Osmitrol	Esmolol
Oxacillin	Ampicillin
Oxazepam	Oxycodone
Oxazepam	Temazepam
Oxcarbazepine	Olanzapine
Oxybutynin	OxyContin
Oxycodone	Oxazepam
Oxycodone	OxyContin
Oxycodone and Acetaminophen	Hydrocodone and Acetaminophen
Oxycodone and Acetaminophen	Oxycodone and Aspirin
Oxycodone and Aspirin	Oxycodone and Acetaminophen
OxyContin	MS Contin
OxyContin	Oxybutynin
OxyContin	Oxycodone
Paclitaxel	Docetaxel
Paclitaxel	Paroxetine
Paclitaxel	Paxil
Pamelor	Panlor SS
Panlor SS	Pamelor
Papaverine	Propafenone
Parafon Forte DSC	Profen Forte
Paraplatin	Platinol
Parlodel	Pindolol
Parlodel	Provera
Paroxetine	Fluoxetine
Paroxetine	Paclitaxel
Paroxetine	Pyridoxine
Paxil	Paclitaxel
Paxil	Plavix
Paxil	Taxol
Pediapred	Pediazole
Pediapred	Risperdal
Pediazole	Pediapred
Pegaspargase	Asparaginase
Penicillamine	Penicillin
Penicillin	Penicillamine
Penicillin G Potassium	Penicillin G Procaine
Penicillin G Procaine	Penicillin G Potassium
Pentobarbital	Phenobarbital
Pepcid	Prevacid
Perative	Periactin
Perceptin	Herceptin
Percocet	Darvocet
Percocet	Percodan
Percocet	Procet
Percodan	Percocet
Percodan	Peri-Colace
Percodan	Vicodin
Periactin	Perative
Peri-Colace	Colace
Peri-Colace	Percodan
Peri-Colace	Procardia
Permax	Bumex
Permethrin	Pyrethrins, Piperonyl Butoxide
Perphenazine	Fluphenazine
Phenazopyridine	Promethazine
Phenobarbital	Pentobarbital
Phenylephrine	Norepinephrine
Phenylephrine	Phenytoin
Phenytoin	Fosphenytoin

Phenytoin	Phenylephrine
Physostigmine	Pyridostigmine
Pilocar	Polocaine
Pilocarpine	Proparacaine
Pindolol	Parlodel
Pindolol	Plendil
Pioglitazone	Rosiglitazone
Pitocin	Pitressin
Pitressin	Pitocin
Platinol	Paraplatin
Plavix	Elavil
Plavix	Paxil
Plendil	Pindolol
Plendil	Pletal
Plendil	Prilosec
Plendil	Prinivil
Pletal	Plendil
Pneumococcal Vaccine, 23-Valent (Polyvalent)	Pneumococcal Vaccine, 7-Valent
Pneumococcal Vaccine, 7-Valent	Pneumococcal Vaccine, 23-Valent (Polyvalent)
Polocaine	Pilocar
Poly-Vi-Sol	Fer-In-Sol
Potassium	Prednisone
Potassium Acetate	Kayexalate
Potassium Acetate	Potassium Chloride
Potassium Bicarbonate and Potassium Chloride	Potassium Bicarbonate and Potassium Citrate
Potassium Bicarbonate and Potassium Citrate	Potassium Bicarbonate and Potassium Chloride
Potassium Chloride	Potassium Acetate
Potassium Chloride	Potassium Citrate
Potassium Chloride	Sodium Chloride
Potassium Citrate	Potassium Chloride
Potassium Phosphates	Sodium Phosphates
Prandin	Avandia
Pravachol	Prevacid
Pravachol	Prinivil
Pravachol	Propranolol
Pravastatin	Atorvastatin
Prazosin	Terazosin
Precare	Precose
Precose	Precare
Prednisolone	Prednisone
Prednisone	Methylprednisolone
Prednisone	Potassium
Prednisone	Prednisolone
Prednisone	Prilosec
Prednisone	Primidone
Prednisone	Pseudoephedrine
Premarin	Prempro
Premarin	Prevacid
Premarin	Primaxin
Premarin	Provera
Premphase	Prempro
Premphase	Vancenase
Prempro	Premarin
Prempro	Premphase
Prepidil	Bepridil
Prevacid	Prinivil
Prevacid	Pepcid
Prevacid	Pravachol
Prevacid	Premarin
Prevacid	Prilosec
Preven	Preveon
Preveon	Preven
Prilosec	Plendil
Prilosec	Prednisone
Prilosec	Prevacid
Prilosec	Prinivil
Prilosec	Prozac
Primacor	Primaxin
Primatene	ProAmantine
Primaxin	Premarin
Primaxin	Primacor
Primidone	Prednisone
Prinivil	Plendil
Prinivil	Pravachol
Prinivil	Prevacid
Prinivil	Prilosec
Prinivil	Prinzide
Prinivil	Proventil
Prinzide	Prinivil
Priscoline	Apresoline
ProAmantine	Primatene
Probenecid	Procanbid
Procainamide	Prochlorperazine
Procan SR	Proscar
Procanbid	Probenecid
Procardia	Peri-Colace
Procardia	Provera
Procardia XL	Cartia XT
Procet	Percocet
Prochlorperazine	Chlorpromazine
Prochlorperazine	Procainamide
Prochlorperazine	Promethazine
Proctocort	Proctocream HC
Proctocream HC	Proctocort
Profen	Profen II, Profen LA
Profen Forte	Parafon Forte DSC
Profen II	Profen, Profen LA
Profen LA	Profen, Profen II
Prograf	Gengraf
Promethazine	Phenazopyridine
Promethazine	Prochlorperazine
Promethazine VC	Promethazine w/ Codeine
Promethazine VC w/ Codeine	Promethazine w/ Codeine
Promethazine w/ Codeine	Promethazine VC w/ Codeine
Promethazine w/ Codeine	Promethazine VC
Propafenone	Papaverine
Proparacaine	Pilocarpine
Propine	Isopto Carpine
Propranolol	Pravachol
Propranolol	Propulsid
Propulsid	Propranolol
Propylthiouracil	Purinethol
Proscar	Procan SR
Proscar	ProSom
Proscar	ProSom, Prozac
Proscar	Provera
ProSom	Proscar
ProSom	Prozac, Proscar
Protonix	Lotronex
Proventil	Bentyl
Proventil	Prinivil
Provera	Covera
Provera	Parlodel
Provera	Premarin
Provera	Procardia
Provera	Proscar
Prozac	Prilosec
Prozac	Proscar, ProSom
Pseudoephedrine	Prednisone
Pulmicort	Pulmozyme
Pulmozyme	Pulmicort
Purinethol	Propylthiouracil
Pyrazinamide	Pyridostigmine
Pyrethrins, Piperonyl Butoxide	Permethrin
Pyridium	Pyridoxine
Pyridostigmine	Physostigmine
Pyridostigmine	Pyrazinamide
Pyridostigmine	Pyridoxine
Pyridoxine	Paroxetine
Pyridoxine	Pyridium
Pyridoxine	Pyridostigmine
Pyridoxine	Pyrimethamine
Pyrimethamine	Pyridoxine
Quibron	Quibron-T, Quibron-T/SR
Quibron-T	Quibron, Quibron-T/SR
Quibron-T/SR	Quibron, Quibron-T
Quinacrine	Quinidine
Quinapril	Lisinopril
Quinidine	Quinacrine
Quinidine	Quinine
Quinine	Quinidine
Raloxifene	Ropinirole
Ramipril	Rifampin
Ranitidine	Amantadine, Rimantadine
Ranitidine	Felodipine
Ratgam (Synonym for Thymoglobulin)	Atgam
ReFresh (breath drops)	Refresh (lubricant eye drops)
Refresh (lubricant eye drops)	ReFresh (breath drops)
Reglan	Megace
Reglan	Renagel
Reglan	Robitussin
Reglan	Zofran
Regranex	Granulex
Relafen	Rezulin
Remegel	Renagel
Remeron	Restoril
Remeron	Zemuron
Reminyl	Amaryl
Reminyl	Robinul
Renagel	Reglan
Renagel	Remegel
Reno-60	Renografin-60
Renografin-60	Reno-60
Reopro	Rheomacrodex
Repaglinide	Rosiglitazone
Requip	Risperdal
Reserpine	Risperdal, Risperidone
Restoril	Remeron
Restoril	Risperdal
Restoril	Vistaril
Retavase	Activase
Retrovir	Norvir
Retrovir	Ritonavir
Revex	Nimbex
Revex	ReVia
ReVia	Revex
Rezulin	Relafen
Rheomacrodex	Reopro
Ridaura	Cardura
Rifabutin	Rifampin
Rifadin	Rifater
Rifampin	Ramipril
Rifampin	Rifabutin
Rifater	Rifadin
Rimantadine	Amantadine, Ranitidine
Risedronate	Risperidone
Risperdal	Estradiol
Risperdal	Lisinopril
Risperdal	Pediapred
Risperdal	Requip
Risperdal	Reserpine, Risperidone
Risperdal	Restoril
Risperidone	Reserpine, Risperdal
Risperidone	Risedronate
Risperidone	Ropinirole
Ritalin	Ritalin SR
Ritalin SR	Ritalin
Ritonavir	Retrovir
Rituximab	Infliximab
Robinul	Reminyl
Robitussin	Reglan
Robitussin	Robitussin DM
Robitussin AC	Robitussin DAC
Robitussin AC	Robitussin DM
Robitussin DAC	Robitussin AC
Robitussin DM	Robitussin
Robitussin DM	Robitussin AC
Robitussin DM	Rondec DM
Rocephin	Ceftin
Rondec DM	Robitussin DM
Ropinirole	Raloxifene
Ropinirole	Risperidone
Ropivacaine	Bupivacaine
Rosiglitazone	Pioglitazone
Rosiglitazone	Repaglinide
Roxanol	Roxicet
Roxanol	Roxicodone
Roxanol	Roxicodone Intensol
Roxicet	Roxanol
Roxicet	Roxicodone
Roxicodone	Roxanol
Roxicodone	Roxicet
Roxicodone	Roxicodone Intensol
Roxicodone Intensol	Roxanol
Roxicodone Intensol	Roxicodone
Rynatan	Rynatuss
Rynatuss	Rynatan
Salagen	Selegiline
Salbutamol (Albuterol in other countries)	Salmeterol
Salmeterol	Salbutamol (Albuterol in other countries)
Salsalate	Sulfasalazine
Sarafem	Serophene
Selegiline	Salagen
Selegiline	Serentil, Sertraline, Serzone
Selegiline	Sertraline
Senna	Soma
Senokot	Depakote

Senokot	Sinemet
Seracult	Hemoccult
Serentil	Selegiline, Sertraline, Serzone
Serentil	Seroquel
Serentil	Serzone
Serentil	Sinequan
Serevent	Atrovent
Serevent	Serevent Diskus
Serevent Diskus	Serevent
Serophene	Sarafem
Seroquel	Serentil
Seroquel	Serzone, Sinequan
Seroquel	Symmetrel
Seroquel	Sertraline
Sertraline	Selegiline, Serentil, Serzone
Sertraline	Seroquel
Serzone	Seroquel, Sinequan
Serzone	Sertraline, Selegiline, Serentil
Sinemet	Senokot
Sinemet	Sinemet CR
Sinemet CR	Sinemet
Sinequan	Serentil
Sinequan	Seroquel, Serzone
Sinequan	Singulair
Singulair	Sinequan
Slo-bid	Dolobid
Slo-bid	Lopid, Lorabid
Slow Fe	Slow-K
Slow-K	Slow Fe
Sodium Bicarbonate	Sodium Chloride
Sodium Chloride	Potassium Chloride
Sodium Chloride	Sodium Bicarbonate
Sodium Phosphates	Potassium Phosphates
Solu-Cortef	Solu-Medrol
Solu-Medrol	Depo-Medrol
Solu-Medrol	Solu-Cortef
Soma	Senna
Soma	Soma Compound
Soma Compound	Soma
Soriatane	Loxitane
Sotalol	Subdue
Stadol	Haldol
Stadol	Toradol
Subdue	Sotalol
Sufentanil Citrate	Fentanyl Citrate
Sulfadiazine	Sulfasalazine
Sulfasalazine	Mesalamine
Sulfasalazine	Salsalate
Sulfasalazine	Sulfadiazine
Sulfasalazine	Sulfisoxazole
Sulfisoxazole	Sulfasalazine
Sumatriptan	Zolmitriptan
Suprax	Surfak
Surfak	Suprax
Surgilube	Lacrilube
Symmetrel	Amaryl
Symmetrel	Seroquel
Symmetrel	Synthroid
Synagis	Synvisc
Synthroid	Symmetrel
Synvisc	Synagis
Tambocor	Temodar
Tamiflu	Tamoxifen
Tamiflu	Theraflu
Tamoxifen	Tamiflu
Tamoxifen	Tamsulosin
Tamsulosin	Tamoxifen
Taxol	Paxil
Taxol	Taxotere
Taxotere	Taxol
Tegretol	Toradol
Tegretol	Trental
Tegretol	Trileptal
Tegretol-XR	Toprol-XL
Temazepam	Flurazepam
Temazepam	Lorazepam
Temazepam	Oxazepam
Temodar	Tambocor
Tenormin	Imuran
Tenormin	Thiamine
Tenormin	Trovan
Tequin	Levaquin
Tequin	Ticlid
Terazosin	Prazosin
Terazosin	Doxazosin
Testoderm	Estraderm
Tetanus Toxoid	Diphtheria and Tetanus Toxoid
Tetracycline	Tetradecyl Sulfate
Tetradecyl Sulfate	Tetracycline
Thalitone	Thalomid
Thalomid	Thalitone
Theraflu	Tamiflu
Thiamine	Tenormin
Thioridazine	Chlorpromazine
Thorazine	Thioridazine
Thioridazine	Thorazine
Tiagabine	Tizanidine
Tiazac	Tigan
Tiazac	Ziac
Ticlid	Tequin
Tigan	Tiazac
Timoptic	Timoptic-XE
Timoptic-XE	Timoptic
Tizanidine	Nizatidine
Tizanidine	Tiagabine
TNKase	t-PA (Synonym for Alteplase, recombinant)
Tobradex	Tobrex
Tobramycin	Gentamicin
Tobrex	Tobradex
Tolazamide	Tolbutamide
Tolbutamide	Tolazamide
Tolcapone	Tolterodine
Tolterodine	Tolcapone
Topamax	Toprol-XL
Topiramate	Torsemide
Toprol-XL	Tegretol-XR
Toprol-XL	Topamax
Toradol	Foradil
Toradol	Inderal
Toradol	Stadol
Toradol	Tegretol
Toradol	Torecan
Toradol	Tramadol
Torecan	Toradol
Torsemide	Furosemide
Torsemide	Topiramate
t-PA (Synonym for Alteplase, recombinant)	TNKase
Tramadol	Toradol
Tramadol	Trandolapril
Tramadol	Trazodone
Tramadol	Voltaren
Trandate	Trental
Trandate	Tridrate
Trandolapril	Tramadol
Trazodone	Amiodarone
Trazodone	Tramadol
Trental	Tegretol
Trental	Trandate
Triad (Butalbital/ Acetaminophen/ Caffeine)	Triad (topical)
Triad (topical)	Triad (Butalbital/ Acetaminophen/ Caffeine)
Triamterene	Trimethoprim
Tridrate	Trandate
Trifluoperazine	Fluphenazine
Trifluoperazine	Trihexyphenidyl
Trihexyphenidyl	Trifluoperazine
Trileptal	Tegretol
Tri-Levlen	Levlen
Tri-Levlen	Ortho Tri-Cyclen
Trimethoprim	Triamterene
Tri-Nasal	Triphasil
Tri-Norinyl	Triphasil
Triphasil	Tri-Nasal
Triphasil	Tri-Norinyl
Trovan	Tenormin
Trusopt	Cosopt
Tylenol	Tylenol w/ Codeine
Tylenol Children's	Tylenol w/ Codeine
Tylenol w/ Codeine	Tylenol
Tylenol w/ Codeine	Tylenol Children's
Ultane	Ultram
Ultracef (Cefadroxil in other countries)	Ultracet (Acetaminophen/ Tramadol Hydrochloride in U.S.)
Ultracet (Acetaminophen/ Tramadol Hydrochloride in U.S.)	Ultracef (Cefadroxil in other countries)
Ultram	Ultane
Ultram	Voltaren
Unasyn	Zosyn
Uniretic	Univasc
Univasc	Uniretic
Univasc	Urispas
Urex	Erex
Uridon	Vicodin
Urised	Urocit-K
Urispas	Univasc
Urispas	Uro-Mag
Urocit-K	Urised
Uro-Mag	Urispas
Valacyclovir	Valgancyclovir
Valcyte	Valtrex
Valgancyclovir	Valacyclovir
Valium	Versed
Valium	Vicodin
Valsartan	Losartan
Valtrex	Valcyte
Vancenase	Premphase
Vancenase	Vanceril
Vancenase AQ	Vanceril DS
Vanceril	Vancenase
Vanceril DS	Vancenase AQ
Vancomycin	Azithromycin
Vancomycin	Gentamicin
Vancomycin	Vecuronium
Vancomycin	Vibramycin
Vantin	Ventolin
Vasocon	Vasocon A
Vasocon A	Vasocon
Vasotec	Norvasc
Vecuronium	Vancomycin
Ventolin	Benylin
Ventolin	Vantin
Vepesid	Versed
Verapamil	Verelan
Verelan	Verapamil
Verelan	Virilon
Versed	Valium
Versed	Vepesid
Versed	Vistaril
Vexol	VoSol
Viagra	Allegra
Vibramycin	Vancomycin
Vicodin	Percodan
Vicodin	Uridon
Vicodin	Valium
Vicodin	Vicodin ES
Vicodin	Vioxx
Vicodin ES	Vicodin
Vinblastine	Vincristine
Vincristine	Vinblastine
Vioxx	Aciphex
Vioxx	Vicodin
Vioxx	Zyvox
Viracept	Viramune
Viramune	Viracept
Virilon	Verelan
Visicol	Bisacodyl
Vistaril	Restoril
Vistaril	Versed
Vistaril	Zestril
Vitamin C	Vitamin E
Vitamin D	Vitamin E
Vitamin E	Vitamin C
Vitamin E	Vitamin D
Volmax	Flomax
Voltaren	Tramadol
Voltaren	Ultram
VoSol	Vexol
Wellbutrin	Wellbutrin SR
Wellbutrin SR	Wellbutrin
Xalatan	Xalcom (Latanoprost/ Timolol in other countries)
Xalcom (Latanoprost/ Timolol in other countries)	Xalatan
Xanax	Lanoxin
Xanax	Zanaflex
Xanax	Zantac
Xanax	Zantac, Zyrtec
Xigris	Zydis (Dosage Form Trademark)
Yocon	Zocor
Zagam	Zyban
Zaleplon	Zolpidem
Zanaflex	Anaflex

Zanaflex	Xanax
Zantac	Xanax
Zantac	Xanax, Zyrtec
Zantac	Zofran
Zaroxolyn	Zyprexa
Zebeta	DiaBeta
Zemuron	Remeron
Zerit	Zestril
Zestril	Vistaril
Zestril	Zerit
Zestril	Zocor
Zestril	Zyrtec
Ziac	Tiazac
Ziac	Zocor
Zidovudine	Lamivudine
Zidovudine	Zidovudine and Lamivudine
Zidovudine	Ziprasidone
Zidovudine and Lamivudine	Zidovudine
Zinacef	Zithromax
Zinecard	Gemzar
Ziprasidone	Zidovudine
Zithromax	Zinacef
Zocor	Cozaar
Zocor	Lipitor
Zocor	Yocon
Zocor	Zestril
Zocor	Ziac
Zocor	Zoloft
Zofran	Reglan
Zofran	Zantac
Zofran	Zosyn
Zolmitriptan	Sumatriptan
Zoloft	Zocor
Zoloft	Zyloprim
Zolpidem	Zaleplon
Zonalon	Zone A Forte
Zone A Forte	Zonalon
Zosyn	Unasyn
Zosyn	Zofran
Zovirax	Zyvox
Zyban	Zagam
Zydis (Dosage Form Trademark)	Xigris
Zyloprim	Zoloft
Zyprexa	Celexa
Zyprexa	Zaroxolyn
Zyprexa	Zyprexa Zydis
Zyprexa	Zyrtec
Zyprexa Zydis	Zyprexa
Zyrtec	Xanax, Zantac
Zyrtec	Zestril
Zyrtec	Zyprexa
Zyvox	Vioxx
Zyvox	Zovirax

NEW Rx DRUG AND BIOLOGIC APPROVALS IN 2009

Drug	Indication	Company
Actoplus Met XR (Metformin HCl/Pioglitazone HCl)	Adjunct to diet and exercise to improve glycemic control in adults with type 2 diabetes mellitus who are already treated with pioglitazone and metformin or who have inadequate glycemic control on pioglitazone alone or metformin alone	Takeda
Afinitor (Everolimus)	Advanced renal cell carcinoma after failure of treatment with sunitinib or sorafenib	Novartis
Arzerra (Ofatumumab)	Chronic lymphocytic leukemia (CLL) refractory to fludarabine and alemtuzumab	GlaxoSmithKline
Bepreve (Bepotastine besilate)	Itching associated with allergic conjunctivitis	Ista
Besivance (Besifloxacin HCl)	Bacterial conjunctivitis caused by susceptible isolates of the following bacteria: *CDC coryneform group G, Corynebacterium pseudodiphtheriticum, Corynebacterium striatum, Haemophilus influenzae, Moraxella lacunata, Staphylococcus aureus, Staphylococcus epidermidis, Staphylococcus hominis, Staphylococcus lugdunensis, Streptococcus mitis group, Streptococcus oralis, Streptococcus pneumoniae, Streptococcus salivarius*	Bausch & Lomb
Caldolor (Ibuprofen)	Management of mild to moderate pain; management of moderate to severe pain as an adjunct to opioid analgesics; reduction of fever	Cumberland
Cambia (Diclofenac potassium)	Migraine attacks with or without aura in adults 18 years of age or older	Kowa
Cetraxal (Ciprofloxacin HCl)	Acute otitis externa due to susceptible isolates of *Pseudomonas aeruginosa* or *Staphylococcus aureus*	Wraser
Coartem (Artemether/Lumefantrine)	Acute, uncomplicated malaria infections due to *Plasmodium falciparum* in patients of 5 kg bodyweight and above	Novartis
Colcrys (Colchine)	Familial Mediterranean fever in adults and children 4 years or older	Mutual Pharma, AR Holding Co
Cycloset (Bromocriptine mesylate)	An adjunct to diet and exercise to improve glycemic control in adults with type 2 diabetes mellitus	Veroscience
Dysport (abobotulinumtoxinA)	Treatment of adults with cervical dystonia to reduce the severity of abnormal head position and neck pain in both toxin-naïve and previously treated patients; temporary improvement in the appearance of moderate to severe glabellar lines associated with procerus and corrugator muscle activity in adult patients < 65 years of age	Ipsen Biopharm
Edular (Zolpidem tartrate)	Insomnia characterized by difficulties with sleep initiation	Meda

Source: FDA's Center for Drug Evaluation and Research. List includes only new molecular entities and new combinations.

Effient (Prasugrel HCl)	Reduction of thrombotic cardiovascular events (including stent thrombosis) in patients with acute coronary syndrome who are to be managed with PCI as follows: patients with unstable angina or non-ST-elevation myocardial infarction (NSTEMI); patients with ST-elevation myocardial infarction (STEMI) when managed with either primary or delayed PCI	Eli Lilly
Embeda (Morphine sulfate/ Naltrexone HCl)	Moderate to severe pain when a continuous, around-the-clock opioid analgesic is needed for an extended period of time	King
Exforge HCT (Hydrochlorothiazide/Valsartan)	Hypertension	Novartis
Extavia (Interferon Beta-1B)	Relapsing fonns of multiple sclerosis to reduce the frequency of clinical exacerbations	Novartis
Fanapt (Iloperidone)	Schizophrenia in adults	Vanda
Feraheme (Ferumoxytol)	Iron deficiency anemia in adult patients with chronic kidney disease (CKD)	Amag
Folotyn (Pralatrexate)	Relapsed or refractory peripheral T-cell lymphoma (PTCL)	Allos
Gelnique (Oxybutynin chloride)	Overactive bladder with symptoms of urge urinary incontinence, urgency, and frequency	Watson
Ilaris (Canakinumab)	Cryopyrin-associated periodic syndromes (CAPS), in adults and children 4 years of age and older including familial cold autoinflammatory syndrome (FCAS) and Muckle-Wells syndrome (MWS)	Novartis
Intuniv (Guafacine HCl)	Attention deficit hyperactivity disorder (ADHD)	Shire
Invega Sustenna (Paliperidone palmitate)	Acute and maintenance treatment of schizophrenia in adults	Johnson & Johnson
Istodax (Romidepsin)	Cutaneous T-cell lymphoma (CTCL) in patients who have received at least one prior systemic therapy	Gloucester
Jenloga (Clonidine HCl)	Hypertension	Sciele Pharma
Kalbitor (Ecallantide)	Acute attacks of hereditar angioedema (HAE) in patients 6 years of age and older	Dyax
Kapidex (Dexlansoprazole)	Healing of all grades of erosive esophagitis (EE); maintaining healing of EE; treating heartburn associated with non-erosive gastroesophageal reflux disease (GERD)	Takeda
Lamictal XR (Lamotrigine)	Adjunctive therapy for partial onset seizures with or without secondary generalization in patients ≥13 years of age	SmithKline Beecham
Livalo (Pitavastatin calcium)	Adjunctive therapy to diet to reduce elevated total cholesterol (TC), low-density lipoprotein cholesterol (LDL-C), apolipoprotein B (Apo B), triglycerides (TG), and to increase high-density lipoprotein cholesterol (HDL-C)	Kowa
Lysteda (Tranexamic acid)	Cyclic heavy menstrual bleeding	Xanodyne

Metozolv ODT (Metoclopramide HCl)	Symptomatic gastroesophageal reflux: short-term (4-12 weeks) therapy for adults with symptomatic, documented gastroesophageal reflux who fail to respond to conventional therapy; diabetic gastroparesis (diabetic gastric stasis): the relief of symptoms in adults associated with acute and recurrent diabetic gastroparesis (gastric stasis)	Salix
Multaq (Dronedarone HCl)	Reduction in the risk of cardiovascular hospitalization in patients with paroxysmal or persistent atrial fibrillation (AF) or atrial flutter (AFL), with a recent episode of AF/AFL and associated cardiovascular risk factors (i.e., age >70, hypertension, diabetes, prior cerebrovascular accident, left atrial diameter ≥50 mm or left ventricular ejection fraction [LVEF] <40%), who are in sinus rhythm or who will be cardioverted	Sanofi Aventis
Onglyza (Saxagliptin HCl)	Adjunct to diet and exercise to improve glycemic control in adults with type 2 diabetes mellitus	Bristol-Myers Squibb
Onsolis (Fentanyl citrate)	Breakthrough pain in patients with cancer, 18 years of age and older, who are already receiving and who are tolerant to opioid therapy for their underlying persistent cancer pain	Meda
Ozurdex (Dexamethasone)	Macular edema following branch retinal vein occlusion (BRVO) or central retinal vein occlusion (CRVO)	Allergan
Pennsaid (Diclofenac sodium)	Signs and symptoms of osteoarthritis of the knee(s)	Nuvo
Plan B One Step (Levonorgestrel)	Prevention of pregnancy following unprotected intercourse or a known or suspected contraceptive failure	Duramed
Renvela Suspension (Sevelamer carbonate)	Control of serum phosphorus in patients with chronic kidney disease on dialysis	Genzyme
Sabril (Vigabatrin)	Refractory complex partial seizures in adults, used as adjunctive therapy in patients who have responded inadequately to several alternative treatments	Lundbeck
Samsca (Tolvaptan)	Clinically significant hypervolemic and euvolemic hyponatremia [serum sodium <125 mEq/L or less marked hyponatremia that is symptomatic and has resisted correction with fluid restriction], including patients with heart failure, cirrhosis, and syndrome of inappropriate antidiuretic hormone (SIADH)	Otsuka America
Saphris (Asenapine maleate)	Acute treatment of schizophrenia in adults; acute treatment of manic or mixed episodes associated with bipolar I disorder in adults	Organon
Savella (Minalcipran HCl)	Fibromyalgia	Cypress Bioscience
Simponi (Golimumab)	Moderately to severely active rheumatoid arthritis (RA) in adults, in combination with methotrexate; active psoriatic arthritis (PsA) in adults, alone or in combination with methotrexate; active ankylosing spondylitis in adults (AS)	Centocor Ortho Biotech
Stelara (Ustekinumab)	Adult patients (18 years or older) with moderate to severe plaque psoriasis who are candidates for phototherapy or systemic therapy	Centocor Ortho Biotech
Sumavel Dosepro (Sumatriptan succinate)	Migraine attacks, with or without aura; cluster headache episodes	Zogenix

Tobradex ST (Dexamethasone/Tobramycin)	Steroid-responsive inflammatory ocular conditions for which a corticosteroid is indicated and where superficial bacterial ocular infection or a risk of bacterial ocular infection exists	Alcon
Twynsta (Amlodipine besylate/ Temisartan)	Hypertension alone or with other antihypertensive agents; initial therapy in patients likely to need multiple antihypertensive agents to achieve their blood pressure goals	Boehringer
Tyvaso (Treprostinil sodium)	Pulmonary arterial hypertension (WHO Group I) in patients with NYHA Class III symptoms, to increase walk distance	United Therapies
Ulesfia (Benzyl alcolhol)	Head lice infestation in patients 6 months of age and older	Sciele Pharma
Uloric (Febuxostat)	Chronic management of hyperuricemia in patients with gout	Takeda
Valturna (Aliskiren hemifumarate/ Valsartan)	Hypertension in patients not adequately controlled with monotherapy; may be substituted for titrated components; as initial therapy in patients likely to need multiple drugs to achieve their blood pressure goals	Novartis
Vectical (Calcitrol)	Mild to moderate plaque psoriasis in adults 18 years and older	Galderma Labs
Vibativ (Telavancin HCl)	Complicated skin and skin structure infections (cSSSI) caused by susceptible gram-positive bacteria	Theravance
Votrient (Pazopanib HCl)	Advanced renal cell carcinoma	GlaxoSmithKline
Zipsor (Diclofenac potassium)	Mild to moderate acute pain	Xanodyne
Zirgan (Ganciclovir)	Acute herpetic keratitis (dendritic ulcers)	Sirion Therapeutics
Zyprexa Relprevv (Olanzapine pamoate)	Schizophrenia	Eli Lilly

GENERICS APPROVED FOR THE FIRST TIME IN 2009

Generic Name	Company
Alprazolam ODT 0.25mg, 0.5mg, 1mg, 2mg	Kali Laboratories
Apraclonidine oph. solution, 0.5%	Akorn
ASA/Dipyridamole 25mg/200mg ER caplets	Barr Laboratories
Azelastine HCl 0.1% nasal spray	Apotex
Azelastine HCl oph. soln. 0.05%	Apotex
Benzoyl peroxide 5%/ Clindamycin 1% gel	Dow Pharmaceutical Sciences
Benztropine mesylate injection 1mg/mL	Nexus Pharmaceuticals
Betamethasone acetate/ Betamethasone sodium phosphate injectable suspension, 3mg/mL and 6mg/mL	Pharmaforce
Bicalutamide tablets 50mg	Accord Healthcare, Kudco Ireland, Mylan Pharmaceuticals, Sandoz, Sun Pharma Global, Synthon Pharmaceuticals, Teva Pharmaceutcials, Zydus Pharmaceuticals
Buprenorphine HCl 2mg, 8mg	Roxane Laboratories
Carbamazepine ER 100mg, 200mg, 400mg tablets	Taro Pharmaceuticals
Chenodiol 250mg tablets	Nexgen Pharma
Chlorothiazide sodium injection 500mg/vial	APP Pharmaceuticals
Clonidine HCl 0.1mg/mL, 0.5mg/mL	Pharmaforce
Clonidine transdermal system 0.1mg, 0.2mg, 0.3mg/day	Aveva Drug Delivery Systems
Cosyntropin for Inj 0.25mg/vial	Generamedix
Cromolyn sodium oral solution 100mg/5mL	Genera Pharmaceuticals
Divalproex sodium DR capsules 125mg	Dr. Reddy's Laboratories
Divalproex sodium ER 250mg, 500mg tablets	Mylan Pharmaceuticals
Donepezil HCl ODT 5mg,10mg	Mutual Pharmaceutical
Drospirenone/EE 3mg/0.02mg	Barr Laboratories
Fentanyl citrate transmucosal lozenge 20mcg, 400mcg, 600mcg, 800mcg, 1200mcg, 1600mcg	Barr Laboratories, Mallinckrodt

Generic Name	Company
Galantamine oral solution 4mg/mL	Roxane Laboratories
Ketorolac 0.4% oph. soln.	Apotex, Alcon, Akorn
Ketoroloc 0.5% oph. soln.	Alcon, Akorn, Sun Pharma Global
Lansoprazole 15mg, 30mg DR capsules	Teva Pharmaceuticals, Matrix Laboratories
Levalbuterol solution 0.25%	Dey LP
Levetiracetam oral solution (100mg/5mL)	Actavis Mid Atlantic, Aurobindo Pharma, Roxane Laboratories, Tolmar
Levonorgestrel 0.75mg tablets	Watson Laboratories
Liothyronine 5mcg, 25mcg, 50mcg	Coastal Pharmaceuticals
Lorazepam 2mg/mL oral concentrate	Paddock Laboratories
Malathion lotion USP, 0.5%	Synerx Pharma
Melphalan HCl for injection 50mg/vial	Synerx Pharma
Minocycline HCl ER 45mg, 90mg, 135mg tablets	Impax Laboratories
Mivacurium chloride injection 2mg/mL	Ebewe Parenta Pharmaceuticals
Nateglinide 60mg,120mg tablets	Par Pharmaceutical, Dr. Reddy's Laboratories, Teva Pharmaceuticals
Nicardipine HCl injection 2.5/mL	Generamedix, Navinta, Pharmaforce, Sun Pharma Global, Wockhardt
Nizatidine 15mg/mL oral solution	Amneal Pharmaceuticals
Norethindrone acetate/fumarate EE 1mg/0.02mg with 75mg ferrous fumarate	Barr Laboratories, Watson Laboratories
Norethindrone/EE 1mg/0.005mg	Barr Laboratories
Norgestimate/EE 0.180mg/0.025mg, 0.215mg/0.025mg, 0.250mg/0.025mg	Barr Laboratories
Omeprazole DR capsules 20mg	Dr. Reddy's Laboratories
Oxaliplatin for injection, packaged in 50mg and 100mg single-use vials	Hospira Worldwide, Sun Pharma Global, Fresenius Kabi Oncology
Oxcarbazepine oral suspension 300mg/5mL	Ranbaxy Laboratories

Source: Food and Drug Administration's Office of Generic Drugs.

Generic Name	Company
PEG 3350 OTC powder	Kremers Urban Development, Mylan Pharmaceuticals, Novel Laboratories, Perrigo R&D
Perindopril erbumine 2mg, 4mg, 8mg tablets	Aurobindo Pharma, Ivax Pharmaceuticals, Roxane Laboratories
Piperacillin/Tazobactam for injection	Orchid Healthcare
Risperidone ODT 0.25mg, 0.5mg, 2mg, 3mg, 4mg	Dr. Reddy's Laboratories, Kali Laboratories
Risperidone oral solution 1mg/mL	Teva Pharmaceuticals
Sumatriptan succinate injections, 4mg, 6mg	Bedford Laboratories, Sandoz Canada, Teva Parenteral Medicines
Sumatriptan succinate tablets 25mg, 50mg, 100mg	Ranbaxy Laboratories, Teva Pharmaceuticals
Tacrolimus 0.5mg, 1mg, 5mg	Sandoz
Temazepam 7.5mg capsules	Mutual Pharmaceutical
Topiramate 25mg, 50mg, 100mg, 200mg tablets	Apotex, Aurobindo Pharma, Barr Laboratories, Cipla Limited, Cobalt Laboratories, Glenmark Generics, Invagen Pharmaceuticals, Mylan Pharmaceuticals, Par Pharmaceutical, Ranbaxy Laboratories, Roxane Laboratories, Sun Pharmaceutical, Teva Pharmaceuticals, Torrent Pharmaceuticals, Zydus Pharmaceuticals
Topiramate sprinkle capsules 15mg, 25mg	Barr Laboratories, Cobalt Laboratories
Tramadol HCl ER 100mg, 200mg tablets	Par Pharmaceutical
Triamcinolone acetonide 10mg/mL, 40mg/mL	Sandoz Canada
Triamcinolone acetonide nasal spray	Barr Laboratories

PROD/MFR	NDC	AWP	DP	OBC
(Atley) *See SUDAL-12*				
(Auriga) *See ZINX KIDS SNEEZE*				
(Braintree) *See HALFLYTELY & BISACODYL TABLETS BOWEL PREP*				
(Braintree) *See HALFLYTELY AND BISACODYL TABLET BOWEL PREP KIT*				
(Doak) *See ROSULA CLK*				
(Sanofi) *See PENTACEL*				
1,1,1,3,3-PENTAFLUOROPROPANE/NORFLURANE				
(Gebauer) *See GEBAUER'S PAIN EASE*				
(Gebauer) *See SPRAY AND STRETCH*				
14C UREA				
(Kimberly-Clark Hc) *See PYTEST*				
2-MERCAPTOETHANOL				
(PCCA) *See MERCAPTOETHANOL*				
2,6-DICHLOROINDOPHENOL SODIUM				
(PCCA) *See DICHLOROINDOPHENOL SODIUM*				
3-(CYCLOHEXYLAMINO)-1-PROPANESULFONIC ACID				
(Baker, J.T.) *See CAPS*				
3,3'-DIINDOLYLMETHANE				
(PCCA) *See DIINDOLYLMETHANE (3,3)*				
3,4-DIAMINOPYRIDINE				
(PCCA) *See DIAMINOPYRIDINE*				
3,5-DIIODO-L-THYRONINE				
(PCCA) *See DIIODO-L-THYRONINE (3,5)*				
7-OXODEHYDROEPIANDROSTERONE				
(Spectrum Pharmacy) *See DEHYDROEPIANDRO-STEARONE, 7-KETO*				
A-AMYLASE (Gallipot)				
alpha amylase				
POW, NA (BACTERIAL)				
100 gm	**51552-0748-05**	151.69	108.35	
A-C-D MODIFIED BRACCO (Bracco Diag)				
citric acid/dextrose/sodium citrate				
SOL, IV (VIAL)				
10 ml 10s	**00270-0013-20**	451.25	361.00	
A-HYDROCORT (Hospira)				
hydrocortisone sodium succinate				
PDS, IJ (SINGLE-DOSE)				
100 mg, 10s ea	**00409-4856-05**	24.60	21.50	**AP**
A-METHAPRED (Hospira)				
methylprednisolone sodium succinate				
PDS, IJ (SDV)				
40 mg, 10s ea	**00409-3217-05**	23.64	20.70	**AP**
10s ea	**00409-5684-23**	21.00	18.40	**AP**
(UNIVIAL,LATEX-FREE)				
40 mg, 10s ea	**00409-5684-01**	23.40	20.50	**AP**
(SDV)				
125 mg, 10s ea	**00409-3218-05**	36.84	32.20	**AP**
(SINGLE-DOSE)				
125 mg, 10s ea	**00409-5685-23**	33.96	29.70	**AP**
(UNIVIAL,LATEX-FREE)				
125 mg, 10s ea	**00409-5685-02**	41.52	36.30	**AP**
A/B OTIC (Altura)				
REPACK				
antipyrine/benzocaine				
SOL, OT, 54 mg/ml-14 mg/ml,				
15 ml	**63874-0719-15**	7.06		
(Stat Rx)				
REPACK				
SOL, OT, 54 mg/ml-14 mg/ml,				
15 ml	**16590-0001-15**	10.00		
AABP (Acella)				
acetic acid/antipyrine/benzocaine/policosanol				
SOL, OT (1X15ML)				
15 ml	**42192-0701-15**	170.18		
ABACAVIR SULFATE				
(Glaxo) *See ZIAGEN*				
ABACAVIR SULFATE/LAMIVUDINE				
(Glaxo) *See EPZICOM*				
ABACAVIR SULFATE/LAMIVUDINE/ZIDOVUDINE				
(Glaxo) *See TRIZIVIR*				
ABARELIX/SODIUM CHLORIDE				
(Praecis Pharma Inc) *See PLENAXIS*				
ABATACEPT				
(Bristol-Myers) *See ORENCIA*				
ABBOCATH-T (Abbott Hosp)				
catheter				
DEV, NA (14G, 5-1/2" SUBCLAVIAN)				
60s ea	**00074-4535-84**	435.34	366.60	
(16G, 5-1/2" SUBCLAVIAN)				
60s ea	**00074-4535-76**	120.96	120.60	
(14 GAUGE, 2")				
100s ea	**00074-4535-14**	147.60	148.00	
(16GX1-1/4")				
100s ea	**00074-4535-06**	147.60	148.00	
(16GX2")				
100s ea	**00074-4535-16**	147.60	148.00	
(18GX1-1/4")				
100s ea	**00074-4535-08**	147.60	148.00	
(18GX2")				
100s ea	**00074-4535-18**	147.60	148.00	
(20 GAUGE, 1-1/4")				
100s ea	**00074-4535-20**	147.60	148.00	
(20 GAUGE, 2")				
100s ea	**00074-4535-02**	414.00	414.00	
(22 GAUGE, 1-1/4")				
100s ea	**00074-4535-22**	154.80	154.00	
(22 GAUGE, 1")				
100s ea	**00074-4535-32**	154.80	154.00	
(24 GAUGE, 3/4")				
100s ea	**00074-4535-24**	240.00	240.00	
(26 GAUGE, 3/4")				
120s ea	**00074-4535-26**	475.20	475.20	
(W/SYRINGE, 16 GAUGE, 2")				
120s ea	**00074-4536-16**	194.40	194.40	
(W/SYRINGE, 18 GAUGE, 2")				
120s ea	**00074-4536-18**	194.40	194.40	
(W/SYRINGE, 18G, 1-1/4")				
120s ea	**00074-4536-08**	194.40	194.40	
(W/SYRINGE, 20G, 1-1/4")				
120s ea	**00074-4536-20**	194.40	194.40	
(W/SYRINGE, 22G, 1-1/4")				
120s ea	**00074-4536-22**	201.60	202.80	
ABCIXIMAB				
(Lilly) *See REOPRO*				
ABELCET (Enzon Pharma, Inc.)				
amphotericin b lipid complex				
SUS, IV (W/FILTER NEEDLE)				
5 mg/ml, 20 ml	**57665-0101-41**	240.00		
ABILIFY (Bristol-Myers)				
aripiprazole				
SOL, IM (SDV)				
9.75 mg/1.3 ml,				
1.3 ml	**59148-0016-65**	16.04		
PO (ORANGE CREAM)				
1 mg/ml, 150 ml	**59148-0013-15**	565.69		
TAB, PO, 2 mg, 30s ea	**59148-0006-13**	514.04		
5 mg, 30s ea	**59148-0007-13**	514.04		
100s ea UD	**59148-0007-35**	1713.41		
10 mg, 30s ea	**59148-0008-13**	514.04		
100s ea UD	**59148-0008-35**	1713.41		
15 mg, 30s ea	**59148-0009-13**	514.04		
100s ea UD	**59148-0009-35**	1713.41		
20 mg, 30s ea	**59148-0010-13**	726.94		
100s ea	**59148-0010-35**	2423.12		
30 mg, 30s ea	**59148-0011-13**	726.94		
100s ea UD	**59148-0011-35**	2423.12		
(Nucare Pharm)				
REPACK				
TAB, PO, 5 mg, 15s ea	**68071-0792-15**	277.00		
10 mg, 15s ea	**68071-0793-15**	277.00		
15 mg, 15s ea	**68071-0794-15**	277.00		
(PD-Rx Pharm)				
REPACK				
TAB, PO, 10 mg, 30s ea	**55289-0251-30**	720.77		
30 mg, 30s ea	**55289-0566-30**	1019.27		
(Pharma Pac)				
REPACK				
TAB, PO, 5 mg, 30s ea	**52959-0604-30**	679.90		
10 mg, 30s ea	**52959-0605-30**	569.90		
(Phys Total Care)				
REPACK				
TAB, PO, 10 mg, 30s ea	**54868-5202-00**	435.71		
(Physician Partner)				
REPACK				
TAB, PO, 5 mg, 15s ea	**21695-0002-15**	514.84		
30s ea	**21695-0002-30**	969.88		
10 mg, 15s ea	**21695-0003-15**	514.84		
30s ea	**21695-0003-30**	969.88		
45s ea	**21695-0003-45**	1444.80		
15 mg, 15s ea	**21695-0004-15**	514.84		
20 mg, 30s ea	**21695-0005-30**	1371.58		
(Quality Care Prod)				
REPACK				
TAB, PO, 5 mg, 30s ea	**49999-0816-30**	829.56		
90s ea	**49999-0816-90**	2272.68		
10 mg, 30s ea	**49999-0598-30**	829.56		
15 mg, 30s ea	**49999-0817-30**	829.56		
20 mg, 30s ea	**49999-0818-30**	1171.11		
30 mg, 30s ea	**35356-0171-30**	1171.11		
(Southwood)				
REPACK				
TAB, PO, 5 mg, 30s ea	**58016-0054-30**	457.50		
60s ea	**58016-0054-60**	915.00		
90s ea	**58016-0054-90**	1372.50		
100s ea	**58016-0054-00**	1525.00		
(Stat Rx)				
REPACK				
TAB, PO, 2 mg, 30s ea	**16590-0323-30**	550.35		
5 mg, 30s ea	**16590-0745-30**	563.81		
60s ea	**16590-0745-60**	1124.36		
20 mg, 30s ea	**16590-0573-30**	698.89		
ABILIFY DISCMELT (Bristol-Myers)				
aripiprazole				
ODT, PO (CREME DE VANILLA)				
10 mg, 30s ea	**59148-0640-23**	611.83		
15 mg, 30s ea	**59148-0641-23**	611.83		
ABLAVAR (Lantheus)				
gadofosveset trisodium				
SOL, IJ (10X10ML,SINGLE USE)				
244 mg/ml,				
10 ml 10s	**11994-0012-01**	1458.96	1215.80	
(10X15ML,SINGLE USE)				
244 mg/ml,				
15 ml 10s	**11994-0012-02**	2188.44	1823.70	
ABOBOTULINUMTOXINA				
(Tercica) *See DYSPORT*				
ABRAXANE (Abraxis)				
paclitaxel protein-bound				
PDR, IV, 100 mg, ea	**68817-0134-50**	1119.60		
ABSINTHIUM OIL (PCCA)				
wormwood oil				
OIL, NA (AMERICAN)				
1 gm	**51927-2131-00**	2.16		
ACACIA (Baker, J.T.)				
POW, NA (N.F., F.C.C.)				
500 gm	**10106-0430-01**	44.35		
2000 gm	**10106-0430-05**	180.44		
(Letco)				
POW, NA (U.S.P./N.F.)				
100 gm	**62991-1332-01**	30.00		
500 gm	**62991-1332-02**	57.00		
(Lorann Oil)				
POW, NA (N.F.)				
30 gm	**23535-0600-35**	2.00		
120 gm	**23535-0600-38**	4.25		
480 gm	**23535-0600-31**	8.00		
(Medisca)				
POW, NA (N.F.)				
500 gm	**38779-0060-08**	64.35		
(NF,SPRAY DRIED)				
2500 gm	**38779-0060-01**	270.00		
(PCCA) *See ACACIA SYRUP*				
(PCCA)				
POW, NA (NF SPRAYDRIED GUMARABIC)				
1 gm	**51927-3140-00**	0.30		
(Spectrum Pharmacy)				
POW, NA (MILLED,N.F.)				
500 gm	**49452-3443-01**	97.30		
(N.F., SPRAY DRIED)				
500 gm	**49452-3440-01**	97.30		
(MILLED,N.F.)				
2500 gm	**49452-3443-02**	399.00		
(N.F., SPRAY DRIED)				
2500 gm	**49452-3440-02**	399.00		
ACACIA SYRUP (PCCA)				
acacia				
SYR, NA, 1 gm	**51927-3321-00**	0.16		
ACAMPROSATE CALCIUM				
(Forest Pharm) *See CAMPRAL*				
ACANYA (Valeant Pharm Intl)				
benzoyl peroxide/clindamycin phosphate				
GEL, TP (1X50GM)				
2.5%-1.2%, 50 gm	**59987-0101-25**	192.50		
ACAPELLA (Adamis)				
spacer, inhalation				
DEV, NA (LATEX-FREE)				
ea	**38739-0277-00**	54.00		
ACARBOSE				
(Bayer Corp.) *See PRECOSE*				
(Roxane)				
TAB, PO, 25 mg, 100s ea	**00054-0140-25**	90.95		**AB**
50 mg, 100s ea	**00054-0141-25**	97.93		**AB**

PROD/MFR	NDC	AWP	DP	OBC
(10X10)				
50 mg, 100s ea UD	00054-0141-20	102.88		AB
100 mg, 100s ea	00054-0142-25	117.28		AB
(Watson Labs)				
TAB, PO, 25 mg, 100s ea	16252-0523-01	55.80		AB
50 mg, 100s ea	16252-0524-01	61.20		AB
100 mg, 100s ea	16252-0525-01	72.60		AB
(A-S Medication)				
REPACK				
TAB, PO, 50 mg, 42s ea	54569-6061-00	40.67		AB
(Phys Total Care)				
REPACK				
TAB, PO, 25 mg, 90s ea	54868-5945-00	139.09		AB
ACCOLATE (AstraZeneca)				
zafirlukast				
TAB, PO, 10 mg, 60s ea	00310-0401-60	119.30		
20 mg, 60s ea	00310-0402-60	119.30		
(AQ)				
REPACK				
TAB, PO, 10 mg, 60s ea	66105-0501-06	123.36		
20 mg, 60s ea	66105-0502-06	123.36		
(Phys Total Care)				
REPACK				
TAB, PO, 20 mg, 6s ea	54868-4172-00	12.10		
30s ea	54868-4172-01	53.03		
60s ea	54868-4172-02	103.56		
ACCU-CHECK CMPAC TEST STRP/DRUMS				
(Phys Total Care)				
glucose, blood test				
DEV, NA, 51s ea	54868-3243-00	63.13		
102s ea	54868-3243-01	121.21		
ACCUNEB (Dey, L.P.)				
albuterol sulfate				
SOL, IH (PF)				
0.021%,				
3 ml 25s UD	49502-0692-03	51.10		
0.042%,				
3 ml 25s UD	49502-0693-03	51.10		
ACCUPRIL (Pfizer)				
quinapril hydrochloride				
TAB, PO (FILM-COATED)				
5 mg, 90s ea	00071-0527-23	174.56	145.47	
(10X10,FILM-COATED)				
5 mg, 100s ea UD	00071-0527-40	193.96	161.63	
(FILM-COATED)				
10 mg, 90s ea	00071-0530-23	174.56	145.47	
(10X10,FILM-COATED)				
10 mg, 100s ea UD	00071-0530-40	193.96	161.63	
(FILM-COATED)				
20 mg, 90s ea	00071-0532-23	174.56	145.47	
(10X10,FILM-COATED)				
20 mg, 100s ea UD	00071-0532-40	193.96	161.63	
(FILM-COATED)				
40 mg, 90s ea	00071-0535-23	174.56	145.47	
(AQ)				
REPACK				
TAB, PO, 5 mg, 90s ea	66105-0524-09	178.18		
10 mg, 90s ea	66105-0101-09	178.18		
20 mg, 90s ea	66105-0102-09	178.18		
40 mg, 90s ea	66105-0103-09	178.18		
(Bryant Ranch)				
REPACK				
TAB, PO, 10 mg, 30s ea	63629-1240-01	42.92		
40 mg, 30s ea	63629-1242-01	42.92		
(PD-Rx Pharm)				
REPACK				
TAB, PO (FILM-COATED)				
5 mg, 30s ea	55289-0552-30	82.37		
10 mg, 30s ea	55289-0553-30	82.37		
(REDI-SCRIPT,FILM-COATED)				
10 mg, 30s ea	58864-0859-30	82.37		
(FILM-COATED)				
20 mg, 30s ea	55289-0554-30	82.37		
(REDI-SCRIPT,FILM-COATED)				
20 mg, 30s ea	58864-0869-30	82.37		
(FILM-COATED)				
40 mg, 30s ea	55289-0555-30	82.37		
(REDI-SCRIPT,FILM-COATED)				
40 mg, 30s ea	58864-0863-30	82.37		
(Phys Total Care)				
REPACK				
TAB, PO, 5 mg, 30s ea	54868-3307-01	43.78		
60s ea	54868-3307-00	85.68		
10 mg, 30s ea	54868-2665-01	51.99		
90s ea	54868-2665-00	143.24		
20 mg, 30s ea	54868-2666-01	68.11		
50s ea	54868-2666-02	112.21		
(FILM-COATED)				
20 mg, 60s ea	54868-2666-04	134.26		
90s ea	54868-2666-03	200.41		
40 mg, 30s ea	54868-3445-00	51.99		
90s ea	54868-3445-01	151.59		
(Vibranta)				
REPACK				
TAB, PO (FILM-COATED)				
5 mg, 30s ea	57866-4423-01	37.72		
10 mg, 30s ea	57866-4420-01	37.72		
20 mg, 30s ea	57866-4421-01	37.72		
40 mg, 30s ea	57866-4424-01	37.72		
ACCURETIC (Pfizer)				
hydrochlorothiazide/quinapril hydrochloride				
TAB, PO (FILM-COATED)				
12.5 mg-10 mg,				
90s ea	00071-0222-23	172.90	144.08	
12.5 mg-20 mg,				
90s ea	00071-0220-23	172.90	144.08	
25 mg-20 mg,				
90s ea	00071-0223-23	172.90	144.08	
ACCUTANE (Phys Total Care)				
REPACK				
isotretinoin				
SGL, PO (RX PAK, 10X10)				
40 mg, 100s ea	54868-0955-00	1655.93		
ACCUZYME (Healthpoint)				
papain/urea				
SPR, TP (DEBRIDING)				
830000 u/gm-10%,				
30 ml	00064-1001-33	54.55		
(Dispensing Solutions)				
REPACK				
OIN, TP, 30 gm	55045-3730-03	55.00		
ACE AEROSOL CLOUD ENHANCER (Dey, L.P.)				
spacer, inhalation				
DEV, NA, ea	49502-0203-01	18.00		
ACEBUTOLOL (Southwood)				
REPACK				
acebutolol hydrochloride				
CAP, PO, 200 mg, 30s ea	58016-0300-30	30.22		
60s ea	58016-0300-60	60.44		
90s ea	58016-0300-90	90.66		
100s ea	58016-0300-00	100.73		
ACEBUTOLOL HCL (Mylan)				
acebutolol hydrochloride				
CAP, PO, 200 mg, 100s ea	00378-1200-01	100.73		AB
400 mg, 100s ea	00378-1400-01	133.97		AB
(PCCA)				
POW, NA (U.S.P.)				
1 gm	51927-2906-00	7.08		
(Phys Total Care)				
REPACK				
CAP, PO, 200 mg, 30s ea	54868-5520-00	28.95		
ACEBUTOLOL HYDROCHLORIDE				
FUL				
CAP, PO, 200 mg, 100s ea		46.13		
400 mg, 100s ea		67.13		
(Amneal)				
CAP, PO (HARD GELATIN)				
200 mg, 100s ea	65162-0669-10	100.73		AB
400 mg, 100s ea	65162-0670-10	133.97		AB
(Mylan) *See ACEBUTOLOL HCL*				
(PCCA) *See ACEBUTOLOL HCL*				
(Promius) *See SECTRAL*				
ACEFYLLINE				
(PCCA) *See THEOPHYLLINE ACETIC ACID*				
ACEON (Solvay)				
perindopril erbumine				
TAB, PO, 2 mg, 100s ea	00032-1101-01	217.18		
4 mg, 100s ea	00032-1102-01	253.24		
8 mg, 100s ea	00032-1103-01	307.58		
(Phys Total Care)				
REPACK				
TAB, PO, 4 mg, 10s ea	54868-4552-01	33.43		
30s ea	54868-4552-00	95.06		
8 mg, 10s ea	54868-4555-01	29.59		
30s ea	54868-4555-00	85.00		
ACEPROMAZINE MALEATE (Medisca)				
POW, NA (USP,1X25GM)				
25 gm	38779-0172-04	165.00		
(U.S.P.)				
100 gm	38779-0172-05	450.00		
(USP,1X500GM)				
500 gm	38779-0172-08	1725.00		
(USP,1X1000GM)				
1000 gm	38779-0172-09	3150.00		
(PCCA)				
POW, NA (U.S.P.)				
1 gm	51927-3574-00	34.80		
ACESULFAME POTASSIUM (PCCA)				
POW, NA, 1 gm	51927-3159-00	2.40		
(Spectrum Pharmacy)				
POW, NA (1X25GM)				
25 gm	49452-3449-01	103.25		
(1X100GM)				
100 gm	49452-3449-02	304.15		
(1X1000GM)				
1000 gm	49452-3449-03	2086.00		
ACET W/ HYDROCODONE (PD-Rx Pharm)				
REPACK				
acetaminophen/hydrocodone bitartrate				
TAB, PO, 500 mg-10 mg,				
60s ea, C-III	55289-0965-60	51.55		
ACETADOTE (Cumberland Pharma)				
acetylcysteine				
SOL, IV (PF)				
200 mg/ml,				
30 ml 4s	66220-0107-30	755.28		
ACETAMIDE (Baker, J.T.)				
acetic acid amide				
CRY, NA (REAGENT)				
500 gm	10106-0006-01	112.48		
ACETAMIN W/ CODEINE (Core)				
REPACK				
acetaminophen/codeine phosphate				
TAB, PO, 300 mg-60 mg,				
30s ea, C-III	33358-0002-30	46.27		
60s ea, C-III	33358-0002-60	64.56		
100s ea, C-III	33358-0002-00	120.34		
ACETAMIN W/CODEINE (Core)				
acetaminophen/codeine phosphate				
TAB, PO, 300 mg-30 mg,				
15s ea, C-III	33358-0001-15	16.37		
20s ea, C-III	33358-0001-20	21.45		
30s ea, C-III	33358-0001-30	31.71		
40s ea, C-III	33358-0001-40	40.64		
50s ea, C-III	33358-0001-50	56.89		
60s ea, C-III	33358-0001-60	60.12		
90s ea, C-III	33358-0001-90	95.99		
100s ea, C-III	33358-0001-00	103.33		
120s ea, C-III	33358-0001-01	123.79		
ACETAMIN/BUTAL/CAFF/COD (Stat Rx)				
REPACK				
apap/butalbital/caff/codeine phos				
CAP, PO				
325 mg-50 mg-40 mg-30 mg,				
20s ea, C-III	16590-0470-20	38.00		
30s ea, C-III	16590-0470-30	57.00		
60s ea, C-III	16590-0470-60	114.00		
90s ea, C-III	16590-0470-90	171.00		
ACETAMINOPHEN (Gallipot)				
POW, NA (U.S.P.)				
28.35 gm	51552-0086-02	5.60		
113.4 gm	51552-0086-04	12.04		
454 gm	51552-0086-06	30.66		
1000 gm	51552-0086-07	54.60		
2270 gm	51552-0086-09	90.65		
(Hawkins)				
POW, NA (U.S.P.)				
1000 gm	63370-0003-50	115.00		
2500 gm	63370-0003-53	259.00		
(Letco)				
POW, NA (U.S.P./N.F.)				
500 gm	62991-1002-02	45.00		
2500 gm	62991-1002-03	150.00		
(Mallinckrodt Lab)				
POW, NA (U.S.P.)				
125 gm	00406-5543-01	11.87		
500 gm	00406-5543-03	26.86		
(Medisca)				
POW, NA (U.S.P.)				
100 gm	38779-0409-05	24.75		
500 gm	38779-0409-08	62.85		
1000 gm	38779-0409-09	105.00		
2500 gm	38779-0409-01	195.00		
(PCCA)				
GRA, NA (U.S.P.)				
1 gm	51927-1191-00	0.21		
POW, NA, 1 gm	51927-2633-00	0.27		

PROD/MFR	NDC	AWP	DP	OBC
(Spectrum Pharmacy)				
GRA, NA (U.S.P.)				
125 gm	**49452-0009-01**	49.70		
500 gm	**49452-0009-02**	96.95		
2500 gm	**49452-0009-03**	283.15		
POW, NA, 125 gm	**49452-0010-01**	47.25		
500 gm	**49452-0010-02**	92.05		
2500 gm	**49452-0010-03**	267.40		
(Bryant Ranch)				
REPACK				
TAB, PO, 325 mg, 20s ea	**63629-1518-01**	8.99		
30s ea	**63629-1518-03**	10.99		
100s ea	**63629-1518-02**	15.99		
(Core)				
REPACK				
TAB, PO, 325 mg, 20s ea	**33358-0006-20**	9.21		
30s ea	**33358-0006-30**	11.26		
60s ea	**33358-0006-60**	14.34		
500 mg, 15s ea	**33358-0007-15**	6.52		
20s ea	**33358-0007-20**	9.20		
30s ea	**33358-0007-30**	14.33		
40s ea	**33358-0007-40**	17.37		
45s ea	**33358-0007-45**	17.41		
100s ea	**33358-0007-00**	43.44		
120s ea	**33358-0007-01**	47.14		
(DHS, Inc.)				
REPACK				
TAB, PO, 325 mg, 30s ea	**55887-0167-30**	3.41		
60s ea	**55887-0167-60**	6.82		
(Keltman Pharma., Inc.)				
REPACK				
TAB, PO, 500 mg, 30s ea	**68387-0214-30**	6.85		
ACETAMINOPHEN & HYDROCODONE (PD-Rx Pharm)				
REPACK				
acetaminophen/hydrocodone bitartrate				
TAB, PO, 325 mg-10 mg,				
20s ea, C-III	**55289-0737-20**	42.20		
(USP MAY BE HABIT FORMNG)				
325 mg-10 mg,				
30s ea, C-III	**55289-0737-30**	55.00		
90s ea, C-III	**55289-0737-90**	111.50		
120s ea, C-III	**55289-0737-98**	115.00		
ACETAMINOPHEN AND CODEINE PHOSPHATE (Southwood)				
REPACK				
acetaminophen/codeine phosphate				
TAB, PO, 300 mg-30 mg,				
30s ea, C-III	**58016-0271-30**	25.80		AA
60s ea, C-III	**58016-0271-60**	51.60		AA
90s ea, C-III	**58016-0271-90**	77.40		AA
100s ea, C-III	**58016-0271-00**	86.00		AA
120s ea, C-III	**58016-0271-02**	103.20		AA
ACETAMINOPHEN AND CODEINE PHOSPHATE #3 (CorePharma)				
acetaminophen/codeine phosphate				
TAB, PO (USP)				
300 mg-30 mg,				
100s ea, C-III	**64720-0304-10**	36.14		
500s ea, C-III	**64720-0304-50**	148.56		
1000s ea, C-III	**64720-0304-11**	288.34		
(4u)				
REPACK				
TAB, PO, 300 mg-30 mg,				
30s ea, C-III	**42549-0501-30**	24.36		
(Medsource)				
REPACK				
TAB, PO, 300 mg-30 mg,				
30s ea, C-III	**45865-0439-30**	16.50		
60s ea, C-III	**45865-0439-60**	33.00		
90s ea, C-III	**45865-0439-90**	49.50		
100s ea, C-III	**45865-0439-49**	26.95		
120s ea, C-III	**45865-0439-51**	28.05		
(PD-Rx Pharm)				
REPACK				
TAB, PO (USP)				
300 mg-30 mg,				
25s ea, C-III	**55289-0005-25**	31.96		
ACETAMINOPHEN AND CODEINE PHOSPHATE #4 (CorePharma)				
acetaminophen/codeine phosphate				
TAB, PO (USP)				
300 mg-60 mg,				
100s ea, C-III	**64720-0305-10**	63.87		AA
500s ea, C-III	**64720-0305-50**	275.95		AA
1000s ea, C-III	**64720-0305-11**	535.31		AA
(Dispensing Solutions)				
REPACK				
TAB, PO, 300 mg-60 mg,				
60s ea, C-III	**66336-0632-60**	60.00		AA
90s ea, C-III	**66336-0632-90**	90.00		AA
(Southwood)				
REPACK				
TAB, PO, 300 mg-60 mg,				
30s ea, C-III	**58016-0272-30**	36.00		AA
60s ea, C-III	**58016-0272-60**	72.00		AA
90s ea, C-III	**58016-0272-90**	108.00		AA
100s ea, C-III	**58016-0272-00**	120.00		AA
120s ea, C-III	**58016-0272-02**	144.00		AA
ACETAMINOPHEN ER (Dispensing Solutions)				
REPACK				
acetaminophen				
TER, PO, 650 mg, 50s ea	**55045-3374-05**	14.00		
100s ea	**55045-3374-01**	28.00		
ACETAMINOPHEN W/ CODEINE (DHS, Inc.)				
REPACK				
acetaminophen/codeine phosphate				
TAB, PO, 300 mg-60 mg,				
30s ea, C-III	**55887-0309-30**	34.00		
40s ea, C-III	**55887-0309-40**	45.33		
60s ea, C-III	**55887-0309-60**	67.99		
(HomeMed)				
REPACK				
TAB, PO, 300 mg-60 mg,				
90s ea, C-III	**51655-0816-26**	85.99		
ACETAMINOPHEN WITH CODEINE (IPI)				
REPACK				
acetaminophen/codeine phosphate				
TAB, PO, 300 mg-30 mg,				
60s ea, C-III	**18837-0193-60**	37.29		
90s ea, C-III	**18837-0193-90**	25.59		
120s ea, C-III	**18837-0193-98**	74.58		
ACETAMINOPHEN-HYDROCODONE (A-S Medication)				
REPACK				
acetaminophen/hydrocodone bitartrate				
TAB, PO, 325 mg-10 mg,				
6s ea, C-III	**54569-5240-06**	4.20		
ACETAMINOPHEN, CAFFEINE, AND DIHYDROCODEINE (Boca Pharmacal)				
acetaminophen/caffeine/dihydrocodeine bitartrate				
TAB, PO, 712.8 mg-60 mg-32 mg,				
30s ea, C-III	**64376-0611-31**	46.40		AA
100s ea, C-III	**64376-0611-01**	146.95		AA
(Phys Total Care)				
REPACK				
TAB, PO, 712.8 mg-60 mg-32 mg,				
30s ea, C-III	**54868-5900-00**	111.83		AA
(Quality Care Prod)				
REPACK				
TAB, PO, 712.8 mg-60 mg-32 mg,				
30s ea, C-III	**35356-0328-30**	86.40		AA
(Stat Rx)				
REPACK				
TAB, PO, 712.8 mg-60 mg-32 mg,				
30s ea, C-III	**16590-0555-30**	96.75		AA
60s ea, C-III	**16590-0555-60**	190.00		AA
90s ea, C-III	**16590-0555-90**	280.00		AA
100s ea, C-III	**16590-0555-71**	311.10		AA
ACETAMINOPHEN/ASPIRIN/CAFFEINE/SALICYLAMIDE				
(Wraser Pharm) *See LEVACET*				
ACETAMINOPHEN/BUTALBITAL				
(Athlon Pharm) *See BUTEX FORTE*				
(Atley) *See CEPHADYN*				
(ECR) *See BUPAP*				
(Everett) *See REPAN CF*				
(Intl Ethical) *See TENCON*				
(Marnel) *See MARTEN-TAB*				
(MCR American) *See PROMACET*				
(Merz) *See SEDAPAP*				
(Qualitest)				
TAB, PO, 325 mg-50 mg,				
100s ea	**00603-2540-21**	37.79		AB
(Valeant Pharm Intl) *See PHRENILIN*				
(Valeant Pharm Intl) *See PHRENILIN FORTE*				
(DHS, Inc.)				
REPACK				
TAB, PO, 325 mg-50 mg,				
60s ea	**55887-0566-60**	51.04		AB
(IPI)				
REPACK				
TAB, PO, 325 mg-50 mg,				
60s ea	**18837-0333-60**	48.55		AB
90s ea	**18837-0333-90**	72.83		AB
(Nucare Pharm)				
REPACK				
TAB, PO, 325 mg-50 mg,				
30s ea	**68071-0421-30**	31.39		AB
60s ea	**68071-0421-60**	53.41		AB
90s ea	**68071-0421-90**	82.49		AB
ACETAMINOPHEN/BUTALBITAL/CAFFEINE				
FUL				
TAB, PO, 500 mg-50 mg-40 mg,				
100s ea		68.70		
(Alphagen) *See GEONE*				
(Athlon Pharm) *See DOLGIC LQ*				
(Axiom Pharmaceutical) *See APAP/BUTALBITAL/CAFFEINE*				
(Blansett) *See ANOLOR 300*				
(Everett) *See REPAN*				
(Forest Pharm) *See ESGIC*				
(Forest Pharm) *See ESGIC-PLUS*				
(Lunsco) *See PACAPS*				
(Major) *See APAP/BUTALBITAL/CAFFEINE*				
(Marnel) *See MARGESIC*				
(Mikart) *See APAP/BUTALBITAL/CAFFEINE*				
(Poly) *See ALAGESIC*				
(Poly) *See ALAGESIC LQ*				
(Qualitest) *See APAP/BUTALBITAL/CAFFEINE*				
(Rising) *See BUTALBITAL, ACETAMINOPHEN AND CAFFEINE*				
(Rising) *See BUTALBITAL/ACETAMINOPHEN/CAFFEINE*				
(Teva) *See APAP/BUTALBITAL/CAFFEINE*				
(Truxton) *See NONBAC*				
(Victory Pharma, Inc.) *See DOLGIC PLUS*				
(Victory Pharma, Inc.) *See ZEBUTAL*				
(Watson) *See FIORICET*				
(Watson Labs) *See BUTALBITAL/ACETAMINOPHEN/CAFFEINE*				
(West-Ward) *See APAP/BUTALBITAL/CAFFEINE*				
(Palmetto)				
REPACK				
CAP, PO, 325 mg-50 mg-40 mg,				
30s ea	**23490-5179-03**	23.60		
TAB, PO, 325 mg-50 mg-40 mg,				
20s ea	**23490-5180-00**	16.12		
30s ea	**23490-5180-01**	24.18		
45s ea	**23490-5180-03**	36.27		
60s ea	**23490-5180-02**	48.36		
500s ea	**23490-9070-00**	875.00		
500 mg-50 mg-40 mg,				
30s ea	**23490-7867-03**	72.00		
60s ea	**23490-7867-06**	144.00		
120s ea	**23490-5181-08**	144.00		
120s ea	**23490-7867-00**	288.00		
ACETAMINOPHEN/BUTALBITAL/CAFFEINE/CODEINE (Breckenridge Pharm)				
apap/butalbital/caff/codeine phos				
CAP, PO				
325 mg-50 mg-40 mg-30 mg,				
100s ea, C-III	**51991-0073-01**	149.95		AB
(Qualitest)				
CAP, PO				
325 mg-50 mg-40 mg-30 mg,				
100s ea, C-III	**00603-2553-21**	149.00		EE
(Teva)				
CAP, PO				
325 mg-50 mg-40 mg-30 mg,				
100s ea, C-III	**00182-2693-01**	209.82		AB
(Watson Labs)				
CAP, PO				
325 mg-50 mg-40 mg-30 mg,				
100s ea, C-III	**00591-3220-01**	149.00		AB
(Phys Total Care)				
REPACK				
CAP, PO				
325 mg-50 mg-40 mg-30 mg,				
10s ea, C-III	**54868-5162-01**	21.12		AB
90s ea, C-III	**54868-5162-02**	101.27		AB

PROD/MFR	NDC	AWP	DP	OBC
(Physician Partner)				
REPACK				
CAP, PO				
325 mg-50 mg-40 mg-30 mg,				
28s ea, C-III	21695-0258-28	41.99		AB
30s ea, C-III	21695-0258-30	53.40		AB
60s ea, C-III	21695-0258-60	106.80		AB
ACETAMINOPHEN/CAFFEINE/DIHYDROCODEINE BITARTRATE				
(Boca Pharmacal) *See ACETAMINOPHEN, CAFFEINE, AND DIHYDROCODEINE*				
(Pamlab) *See PANLOR SS*				
(Pamlab) *See ZERLOR*				
(Wraser Pharm) *See TREZIX*				
ACETAMINOPHEN/CAFFEINE/ISOMETHEPTENE MUCATE				
(Azur Pharma, Inc.) *See MIGRATEN*				
(Wraser Pharm) *See PRODRIN*				
ACETAMINOPHEN/CAFFEINE/MAGNESIUM SALICYLATE				
(Hart Health) *See BACKPRIN*				
ACETAMINOPHEN/CAFFEINE/PHENYLTOLOXAMINE CITRATE				
(Poly) *See FLEXTRA*				
ACETAMINOPHEN/COD #4 (Dispensing Solutions)				
REPACK				
acetaminophen/codeine phosphate				
TAB, PO, 300 mg-60 mg,				
30s ea, C-III	66336-0632-30	30.00		
ACETAMINOPHEN/CODEINE (Actavis Mid Atlantic)				
acetaminophen/codeine phosphate				
SOL, PO, 120 mg/5 ml-12 mg/5 ml,				
118 ml, C-V	00472-1419-04	5.74		AA
473 ml, C-V	00472-1419-16	18.55		AA
(Covidien)				
TAB, PO, 300 mg-15 mg,				
100s ea, C-III	00406-0483-01	51.41		AA
300 mg-30 mg,				
100s ea, C-III	00406-0484-01	61.40		AA
(10X10)				
300 mg-30 mg,				
100s ea UD, C-III	00406-0484-62	36.12		AA
1000s ea, C-III	00406-0484-10	483.31		AA
300 mg-60 mg,				
100s ea, C-III	00406-0485-01	108.55		AA
500s ea, C-III	00406-0485-05	468.35		AA
(Hi-Tech)				
SOL, PO (CHERRY)				
120 mg/5 ml-12 mg/5 ml,				
473 ml, C-V	50383-0079-16	18.00		AA
(Mallinckrodt Lab)				
TAB, PO, 300 mg-30 mg,				
20s ea, C-III	00406-0484-20	12.27		AA
30s ea, C-III	00406-0484-03	18.43		AA
50s ea, C-III	00406-0484-50	30.70		AA
(Mikart)				
ELI, PO, 120 mg/5 ml-12 mg/5 ml,				
480 ml, C-V	46672-0561-16	12.50		AA
(Morton Grove)				
ELI, PO (CHERRY)				
120 mg/5 ml-12 mg/5 ml,				
118 ml, C-V	60432-0245-04	7.30		AA
473 ml, C-V	60432-0245-16	19.55		AA
(Pharm Assoc Inc)				
SOL, PO, 120 mg/5 ml-12 mg/5 ml,				
5 ml 100s UD, C-V	00121-0504-05	71.80		AA
10 ml 100s UD, C-V	00121-0504-10	80.76		AA
12.5 ml 100s UD, C-V	00121-0504-12	85.00		AA
15 ml 100s UD, C-V	00121-0504-15	89.00		AA
118 ml, C-V	00121-0504-04	6.75		AA
473 ml, C-V	00121-0504-16	19.85		AA
(Qualitest)				
ELI, PO, 120 mg/5 ml-12 mg/5 ml,				
473 ml, C-V	00603-1020-58	19.85		AA
TAB, PO, 300 mg-15 mg,				
100s ea, C-III	00603-2337-21	30.44		AA
300 mg-30 mg,				
30s ea, C-III	00603-2338-16	10.84		AA
50s ea, C-III	00603-2338-19	18.07		AA
60s ea, C-III	00603-2338-20	21.68		AA
90s ea, C-III	00603-2338-02	32.53		AA
100s ea, C-III	00603-2338-21	36.14		AA
120s ea, C-III	00603-2338-22	43.37		AA
180s ea, C-III	00603-2338-04	53.87		AA
1000s ea, C-III	00603-2338-32	284.34		AA
300 mg-60 mg,				
100s ea, C-III	00603-2339-21	63.88		AA
500s ea, C-III	00603-2339-28	275.92		AA
(Ranbaxy Pharm)				
TAB, PO, 300 mg-30 mg,				
100s ea, C-III	63304-0562-01	36.14		EE
1000s ea, C-III	63304-0562-10	284.35		EE
300 mg-60 mg,				
100s ea, C-III	63304-0561-01	63.88		EE
500s ea, C-III	63304-0561-05	275.93		EE
(Teva)				
TAB, PO, 300 mg-15 mg,				
100s ea, C-III	00093-0050-01	30.44		AA
100s ea, C-III	00555-0305-02	33.26		AA
300 mg-30 mg,				
100s ea, C-III	00093-0150-01	36.14		AA
100s ea, C-III	00555-0303-02	36.14		AA
1000s ea, C-III	00093-0150-10	284.35		AA
1000s ea, C-III	00555-0303-05	284.35		AA
300 mg-60 mg,				
100s ea, C-III	00093-0350-01	63.87		AA
100s ea, C-III	00555-0304-02	63.87		AA
500s ea, C-III	00093-0350-05	275.93		AA
500s ea, C-III	00555-0304-04	275.93		AA
1000s ea, C-III	00093-0350-10	535.31		AA
(UDL)				
TAB, PO (EMERGI-SCRIPT, 15X6)				
300 mg-30 mg,				
90s ea, C-III	51079-0161-99	60.00		AA
(10X10)				
300 mg-30 mg,				
100s ea UD, C-III	51079-0161-20	32.35		AA
(R.N.P., 5X20)				
300 mg-30 mg,				
100s ea UD, C-III	51079-0161-21	33.97		AA
(A-S Medication)				
REPACK				
ELI, PO, 120 mg/5 ml-12 mg/5 ml,				
120 ml, C-V	54569-1001-00	6.86		EE
TAB, PO, 300 mg-15 mg,				
12s ea, C-III	54569-0311-00	3.73		EE
30s ea, C-III	54569-0311-02	9.33		EE
300 mg-30 mg,				
4s ea, C-III	54569-2523-04	1.78		AA
6s ea, C-III	54569-0025-06	2.67		AA
10s ea, C-III	54569-0025-00	4.46		AA
12s ea, C-III	54569-0025-01	5.35		AA
15s ea, C-III	54569-0025-02	6.68		AA
16s ea, C-III	54569-2523-01	7.13		AA
20s ea, C-III	54569-0025-03	8.91		AA
24s ea, C-III	54569-0025-09	10.69		AA
30s ea, C-III	54569-0025-04	13.37		AA
60s ea, C-III	54569-2523-06	26.74		AA
90s ea, C-III	54569-2523-07	40.10		AA
100s ea, C-III	54569-0025-07	44.56		AA
300 mg-60 mg,				
30s ea, C-III	54569-0302-01	19.16		EE
60s ea, C-III	54569-0302-08	38.33		EE
90s ea, C-III	54569-0302-02	57.49		EE
(Aidarex)				
REPACK				
TAB, PO, 300 mg-30 mg,				
7s ea, C-III	33261-0001-07	5.11		AA
12s ea, C-III	33261-0001-12	8.82		AA
14s ea, C-III	33261-0001-14	10.29		AA
18s ea, C-III	33261-0001-18	13.23		AA
20s ea, C-III	33261-0001-20	14.70		AA
21s ea, C-III	33261-0001-21	15.44		AA
24s ea, C-III	33261-0001-24	17.64		AA
25s ea, C-III	33261-0001-25	18.38		AA
28s ea, C-III	33261-0001-28	20.58		AA
30s ea, C-III	33261-0001-30	22.05		AA
40s ea, C-III	33261-0001-40	29.40		AA
42s ea, C-III	33261-0001-42	30.87		AA
48s ea, C-III	33261-0001-48	35.28		AA
50s ea, C-III	33261-0001-50	36.75		AA
60s ea, C-III	33261-0001-60	44.10		AA
64s ea, C-III	33261-0001-64	47.04		AA
72s ea, C-III	33261-0001-72	52.92		AA
84s ea, C-III	33261-0001-84	61.74		AA
90s ea, C-III	33261-0001-90	66.15		AA
120s ea, C-III	33261-0001-02	88.20		AA
120s ea, C-III	33261-0124-02	229.20		EE
140s ea, C-III	33261-0001-03	102.90		AA
180s ea, C-III	33261-0001-04	132.30		AA
300 mg-60 mg,				
56s ea, C-III	33261-0002-56	110.88		AA
90s ea, C-III	33261-0002-90	178.20		AA
120s ea, C-III	33261-0002-02	237.60		AA
(Altura)				
REPACK				
ELI, PO, 120 mg/5 ml-12 mg/5 ml,				
90 ml, C-V	63874-0266-90	6.55		EE
120 ml, C-V	63874-0266-12	12.18		EE
3840 ml, C-V	63874-0266-38	109.61		EE
SOL, PO (1X480ML)				
120 mg/5 ml-12 mg/5 ml,				
480 ml, C-V	63874-0266-48	48.72		AA
TAB, PO, 300 mg-15 mg,				
12s ea, C-III	63874-0259-12	4.63		AA
15s ea, C-III	63874-0259-15	5.40		AA
20s ea, C-III	63874-0259-20	5.73		AA
24s ea, C-III	63874-0259-24	6.04		AA
30s ea, C-III	63874-0259-30	16.20		AA
60s ea, C-III	63874-0259-60	32.40		AA
100s ea, C-III	63874-0259-01	27.98		AA
120s ea, C-III	63874-0259-04	62.80		AA
300 mg-30 mg,				
6s ea, C-III	63874-0202-06	4.50		AA
8s ea, C-III	63874-0202-08	6.00		AA
10s ea, C-III	63874-0202-10	7.50		AA
12s ea, C-III	63874-0202-12	9.00		AA
14s ea, C-III	63874-0202-14	10.50		AA
15s ea, C-III	63874-0202-15	11.25		AA
16s ea, C-III	63874-0202-16	12.00		AA
18s ea, C-III	63874-0202-18	13.50		AA
20s ea, C-III	63874-0202-20	15.00		AA
24s ea, C-III	63874-0202-24	18.00		AA
25s ea, C-III	63874-0202-25	18.75		AA
28s ea, C-III	63874-0202-28	21.00		AA
30s ea, C-III	63874-0202-30	28.73		AA
40s ea, C-III	63874-0202-40	30.00		AA
42s ea, C-III	63874-0202-42	31.50		AA
50s ea, C-III	63874-0202-50	37.50		AA
60s ea, C-III	63874-0202-60	45.00		AA
90s ea, C-III	63874-0202-90	67.50		AA
100s ea, C-III	63874-0202-01	75.00		AA
120s ea, C-III	63874-0202-04	90.00		AA
500s ea, C-III	63874-0202-05	322.00		AA
1000s ea, C-III	63874-0202-02	204.15		AA
300 mg-60 mg,				
5s ea, C-III	63874-0267-05	5.19		EE
8s ea, C-III	63874-0267-08	8.31		AA
10s ea, C-III	63874-0267-10	10.39		AA
12s ea, C-III	63874-0267-12	12.46		AA
15s ea, C-III	63874-0267-15	15.58		AA
20s ea, C-III	63874-0267-20	20.77		AA
28s ea, C-III	63874-0267-28	29.08		EE
30s ea, C-III	63874-0267-30	31.16		AA
40s ea, C-III	63874-0267-40	41.55		EE
50s ea, C-III	63874-0267-50	51.93		EE
60s ea, C-III	63874-0267-60	62.32		AA
90s ea, C-III	63874-0267-90	93.48		EE
100s ea, C-III	63874-0267-01	103.87		AA
120s ea, C-III	63874-0267-04	124.64		EE
500s ea, C-III	63874-0267-03	355.00		EE
1000s ea, C-III	63874-0267-02	545.50		AA
(American Health)				
REPACK				
TAB, PO, 300 mg-30 mg,				
100s ea UD, C-III	68084-0372-01	16.75		AA
300 mg-60 mg,				
100s ea UD, C-III	68084-0373-01	21.25		AA
(Bryant Ranch)				
REPACK				
TAB, PO, 300 mg-30 mg,				
6s ea, C-III	63629-1494-01	7.78		AA
84s ea, C-III	63629-1494-04	12.45		AA
100s ea, C-III	63629-1494-07	103.73		AA
300 mg-60 mg,				
40s ea, C-III	63629-3031-05	55.23		AA
(DHS, Inc.)				
REPACK				
SOL, PO, 120 mg/5 ml-12 mg/5 ml,				
120 ml, C-V	55887-0756-04	16.00		AA
TAB, PO, 300 mg-30 mg,				
10s ea, C-III	55887-0951-10	8.00		AA
15s ea, C-III	55887-0951-15	12.95		AA
16s ea, C-III	55887-0951-16	13.50		AA
20s ea, C-III	55887-0951-20	16.00		AA
30s ea, C-III	55887-0951-30	24.00		AA
40s ea, C-III	55887-0951-40	32.00		AA
60s ea, C-III	55887-0951-60	48.00		AA
90s ea, C-III	55887-0951-90	60.00		AA
(Dispensing Solutions)				
REPACK				
ELI, PO (CHERRY)				
120 mg/5 ml-12 mg/5 ml,				
118 ml, C-V	55045-1616-02	13.65		AA

PROD/MFR	NDC	AWP	DP	OBC
TAB, PO, 300 mg-15 mg,				
15s ea, C-III	55045-1580-05	6.50		AA
20s ea, C-III	55045-1580-07	8.60		AA
30s ea, C-III	55045-1580-08	12.90		AA
50s ea, C-III	55045-1580-06	21.50		AA
300 mg-30 mg,				
6s ea, C-III	55045-1112-02	4.50		AA
10s ea, C-III	66336-0059-10	8.63		AA
12s ea, C-III	55045-1112-04	9.00		EE
12s ea, C-III	66336-0059-12	10.36		EE
15s ea, C-III	55045-1112-05	11.25		EE
15s ea, C-III	66336-0059-15	12.95		AA
16s ea, C-III	66336-0059-16	13.50		EE
20s ea, C-III	55045-1112-07	15.00		EE
20s ea, C-III	66336-0059-20	16.00		EE
24s ea, C-III	55045-1112-06	18.00		EE
25s ea, C-III	55045-3094-05	18.75		AA
30s ea, C-III	55045-1112-08	22.50		EE
30s ea, C-III	66336-0059-30	24.00		EE
40s ea, C-III	55045-1112-09	30.00		AA
40s ea, C-III	66336-0059-40	32.00		AA
45s ea, C-III	55045-3094-04	33.75		AA
50s ea, C-III	55045-1112-03	37.50		AA
60s ea, C-III	55045-2853-06	45.00		EE
60s ea, C-III	66336-0059-60	48.00		EE
(USP)				
300 mg-30 mg,				
90s ea, C-III	55045-2853-09	67.50		AA
100s ea, C-III	55045-1112-01	75.00		
120s ea, C-III	55045-3094-01	90.00		
135s ea, C-III	55045-3094-03	101.25		AA
200s ea, C-III	55045-3094-02	150.00		EE
300 mg-60 mg,				
10s ea, C-III	55045-1897-02	10.00		AA
12s ea, C-III	55045-1897-03	12.00		AA
20s ea, C-III	55045-1897-07	20.05		AA
30s ea, C-III	55045-1897-08	30.00		AA
40s ea, C-III	55045-1897-04	40.00		AA
50s ea, C-III	55045-3357-05	50.00		AA
60s ea, C-III	55045-1897-06	60.00		AA
90s ea, C-III	55045-1897-09	90.00		AA
100s ea, C-III	55045-1897-01	100.25		AA
120s ea, C-III	55045-1897-05	120.00		AA
200s ea, C-III	55045-1897-00	200.00		AA
(GSMS) REPACK				
TAB, PO (UNIT OF USE)				
300 mg-30 mg,				
30s ea, C-III	60429-0500-30	17.85	5.95	AA
60s ea, C-III	60429-0500-60	25.20	8.40	AA
90s ea, C-III	60429-0500-90	36.60	12.20	AA
(HomeMed) REPACK				
TAB, PO, 300 mg-30 mg,				
10s ea, C-III	51655-0802-53	6.35		
15s ea, C-III	51655-0802-54	12.99		
20s ea, C-III	51655-0802-52	17.89		
30s ea, C-III	51655-0802-24	29.99		
40s ea, C-III	51655-0802-51	6.27		
50s ea, C-III	51655-0802-77	11.95		
60s ea, C-III	51655-0802-25	57.89		
90s ea, C-III	51655-0802-26	20.71		
120s ea, C-III	51655-0802-82	27.27		
300 mg-60 mg,				
15s ea, C-III	51655-0816-54	5.26		
30s ea, C-III	51655-0816-24	8.78		
(IPI) REPACK				
TAB, PO, 300 mg-30 mg,				
40s ea, C-III	18837-0193-40	24.86		EE
300 mg-60 mg,				
60s ea, C-III	18837-0192-60	33.11		AA
(Keltman Pharma., Inc.) REPACK				
TAB, PO (USP)				
300 mg-30 mg,				
15s ea, C-III	68387-0250-15	10.00		AA
30s ea, C-III	68387-0250-30	20.00		
(USP)				
300 mg-30 mg,				
60s ea, C-III	68387-0250-60	40.00		AA
90s ea, C-III	68387-0250-90	60.00		AA
300 mg-60 mg,				
60s ea, C-III	68387-0252-60	63.82		
(McKesson Packaging) REPACK				
TAB, PO, 300 mg-30 mg,				
100s ea UD, C-III	63739-0004-10	35.54		AA
(Medsource) REPACK				
TAB, PO, 300 mg-60 mg,				
30s ea, C-III	45865-0466-30	19.50		AA
60s ea, C-III	45865-0466-60	39.00		AA
90s ea, C-III	45865-0466-90	58.50		AA
100s ea, C-III	45865-0466-49	31.85		AA
120s ea, C-III	45865-0466-51	33.15		AA
(Nucare Pharm) REPACK				
ELI, PO, 120 mg/5 ml-12 mg/5 ml,				
120 ml, C-V	66267-0997-04	13.95		EE
TAB, PO, 300 mg-15 mg,				
30s ea, C-III	66267-0221-30	19.66		AA
300 mg-30 mg,				
6s ea, C-III	66267-0001-06	4.70		EE
10s ea, C-III	66267-0001-10	6.29		EE
12s ea, C-III	66267-0001-12	8.49		EE
15s ea, C-III	66267-0001-15	12.65		AA
20s ea, C-III	66267-0001-20	12.12		EE
24s ea, C-III	66267-0001-24	14.59		EE
30s ea, C-III	66267-0001-30	32.99		EE
40s ea, C-III	66267-0001-40	27.35		AA
60s ea, C-III	66267-0001-60	41.02		AA
90s ea, C-III	66267-0001-90	61.53		AA
120s ea, C-III	66267-0001-91	69.64		AA
300 mg-60 mg,				
20s ea, C-III	66267-0002-20	23.48		EE
30s ea, C-III	66267-0002-30	29.99		EE
40s ea, C-III	66267-0002-40	41.14		AA
60s ea, C-III	66267-0002-60	61.71		AA
(Palmetto) REPACK				
SOL, PO, 120 mg/5 ml-12 mg/5 ml,				
120 ml, C-V	23490-7969-01	14.82		
(PD-Rx Pharm) REPACK				
TAB, PO, 300 mg-30 mg,				
4s ea, C-III	43063-0014-04	15.96		EE
6s ea, C-III	43063-0014-06	17.68		EE
6s ea, C-III	55289-0005-06	17.69		AA
10s ea, C-III	55289-0005-10	20.58		AA
12s ea, C-III	55289-0005-12	22.04		AA
12s ea, C-III	55289-0005-90	78.52		AA
15s ea, C-III	55289-0005-15	24.22		AA
(REDI-SCRIPT)				
300 mg-30 mg,				
15s ea, C-III	58864-0004-15	24.24		AA
20s ea, C-III	55289-0005-20	27.82		AA
20s ea, C-III	58864-0004-20	27.84		AA
24s ea, C-III	55289-0005-24	30.76		AA
30s ea, C-III	55289-0005-30	35.07		AA
30s ea, C-III	58864-0004-30	35.08		AA
60s ea, C-III	55289-0005-60	56.80		AA
300 mg-60 mg,				
20s ea, C-III	55289-0916-20	56.00		AA
30s ea, C-III	55289-0916-30	84.00		AA
90s ea, C-III	55289-0916-90	112.00		AA
(Pharma Pac) REPACK				
ELI, PO, 120 mg/5 ml-12 mg/5 ml,				
90 ml, C-V	52959-0141-04	14.25		EE
120 ml, C-V	52959-0141-03	18.53		EE
TAB, PO, 300 mg-15 mg,				
15s ea, C-III	52959-0208-15	5.68		EE
30s ea, C-III	52959-0208-30	10.36		EE
300 mg-30 mg,				
4s ea, C-III	52959-0003-04	2.93		EE
6s ea, C-III	52959-0003-06	4.40		EE
10s ea, C-III	52959-0003-10	7.32		EE
12s ea, C-III	52959-0003-12	8.78		EE
15s ea, C-III	52959-0003-15	10.95		EE
16s ea, C-III	52959-0003-16	11.76		EE
20s ea, C-III	52959-0003-20	14.59		EE
24s ea, C-III	52959-0003-24	17.49		EE
25s ea, C-III	52959-0003-25	18.22		EE
28s ea, C-III	52959-0003-28	20.37		EE
30s ea, C-III	52959-0003-30	21.82		EE
40s ea, C-III	52959-0003-40	29.07		EE
42s ea, C-III	52959-0003-42	30.52		EE
45s ea, C-III	52959-0003-45	32.67		EE
50s ea, C-III	52959-0003-50	36.29		EE
60s ea, C-III	52959-0003-60	43.52		EE
84s ea, C-III	52959-0003-84	60.90		EE
90s ea, C-III	52959-0003-90	65.20		EE
100s ea, C-III	52959-0003-00	72.40		EE
120s ea, C-III	52959-0003-02	86.76		EE
300 mg-60 mg,				
20s ea, C-III	52959-0446-20	22.50		EE
24s ea, C-III	52959-0446-24	26.52		EE
30s ea, C-III	52959-0446-30	30.50		EE
50s ea, C-III	52959-0446-50	50.49		EE
60s ea, C-III	52959-0446-60	60.00		EE
90s ea, C-III	52959-0446-90	89.09		EE
100s ea, C-III	52959-0446-00	96.75		EE
120s ea, C-III	52959-0446-02	121.08		EE
(Phys Total Care) REPACK				
ELI, PO, 120 mg/5 ml-12 mg/5 ml,				
120 ml, C-V	54868-0378-01	12.93		EE
480 ml, C-V	54868-0378-02	29.04		EE
TAB, PO, 300 mg-15 mg,				
40s ea, C-III	54868-2130-01	20.19		EE
300 mg-30 mg,				
10s ea, C-III	54868-0072-09	7.41		EE
15s ea, C-III	54868-0072-02	9.18		EE
20s ea, C-III	54868-0072-03	10.74		EE
30s ea, C-III	54868-0072-01	14.73		EE
40s ea, C-III	54868-0072-05	16.98		EE
50s ea, C-III	54868-0072-04	20.10		EE
60s ea, C-III	54868-0072-07	23.22		EE
100s ea, C-III	54868-0072-08	35.70		EE
300 mg-60 mg,				
30s ea, C-III	54868-0860-01	21.21		EE
40s ea, C-III	54868-0860-02	26.28		EE
90s ea, C-III	54868-0860-03	50.91		AA
100s ea, C-III	54868-0860-00	56.73		AA
(Physician Partner) REPACK				
TAB, PO, 300 mg-30 mg,				
12s ea, C-III	21695-0242-12	15.23		AA
15s ea, C-III	21695-0242-15	19.04		AA
18s ea, C-III	21695-0242-18	22.85		
20s ea, C-III	21695-0242-20	25.38		
28s ea, C-III	21695-0242-28	21.29		AA
30s ea, C-III	21695-0242-30	31.67		
40s ea, C-III	21695-0242-40	42.23		AA
60s ea, C-III	21695-0242-60	43.34		
90s ea, C-III	21695-0242-90	65.02		
300 mg-60 mg,				
28s ea, C-III	21695-0243-28	30.86		
30s ea, C-III	21695-0243-30	33.06		
60s ea, C-III	21695-0243-60	66.12		AA
(Quality Care Prod) REPACK				
ELI, PO (CHERRY)				
120 mg/5 ml-12 mg/5 ml,				
120 ml, C-V	49999-0323-04	22.72		AA
TAB, PO, 300 mg-30 mg,				
6s ea, C-III	49999-0060-06	4.32		AA
10s ea, C-III	49999-0060-10	7.18		EE
12s ea, C-III	49999-0060-12	8.61		EE
15s ea, C-III	49999-0060-15	10.77		EE
20s ea, C-III	49999-0060-20	18.25		EE
24s ea, C-III	49999-0060-24	17.28		AA
30s ea, C-III	49999-0060-30	33.70		EE
50s ea, C-III	49999-0060-50	36.22		EE
60s ea, C-III	49999-0060-60	67.40		EE
90s ea, C-III	49999-0060-90	64.62		EE
100s ea, C-III	49999-0060-00	112.33		AA
120s ea, C-III	49999-0060-01	112.00		AA
300 mg-60 mg,				
30s ea, C-III	49999-0026-30	36.72		EE
40s ea, C-III	49999-0026-40	49.87		EE
60s ea, C-III	49999-0026-60	73.44		EE
90s ea, C-III	49999-0026-90	110.16		AA
120s ea, C-III	49999-0026-01	146.88		AA
(Southwood) REPACK				
TAB, PO, 300 mg-15 mg,				
12s ea, C-III	58016-0269-12	6.28		EE
15s ea, C-III	58016-0269-15	7.85		EE
20s ea, C-III	58016-0269-20	10.47		EE
24s ea, C-III	58016-0269-24	12.56		EE
30s ea, C-III	58016-0269-30	15.70		EE
100s ea, C-III	58016-0269-00	26.65		EE
300 mg-30 mg,				
6s ea, C-III	58016-0271-06	3.53		EE
8s ea, C-III	58016-0271-08	4.70		EE
10s ea, C-III	58016-0271-10	5.88		EE
12s ea, C-III	58016-0271-12	7.06		EE
14s ea, C-III	58016-0271-14	8.23		EE
15s ea, C-III	58016-0271-15	8.82		EE
16s ea, C-III	58016-0271-16	9.41		EE
18s ea, C-III	58016-0271-18	10.58		EE
20s ea, C-III	58016-0271-20	11.76		EE
24s ea, C-III	58016-0271-24	14.11		EE
25s ea, C-III	58016-0271-25	14.70		EE
28s ea, C-III	58016-0271-28	16.46		EE
40s ea, C-III	58016-0271-40	23.52		EE
42s ea, C-III	58016-0271-42	24.70		EE
45s ea, C-III	58016-0271-45	26.46		AA
50s ea, C-III	58016-0271-50	29.40		EE

PROD/MFR	NDC	AWP	DP	OBC
56s ea, C-III	58016-0271-56	32.93		EE
84s ea, C-III	58016-0271-84	49.39		EE
(USP)				
300 mg-30 mg,				
240s ea, C-III	58016-0271-04	141.12		AA
300 mg-60 mg,				
8s ea, C-III	58016-0272-08	8.31		EE
10s ea, C-III	58016-0272-10	10.39		EE
12s ea, C-III	58016-0272-12	12.47		EE
15s ea, C-III	58016-0272-15	15.59		EE
20s ea, C-III	58016-0272-20	20.78		EE
28s ea, C-III	58016-0272-28	29.09		EE
40s ea, C-III	58016-0272-40	41.56		EE
50s ea, C-III	58016-0272-50	51.95		EE
56s ea, C-III	58016-0272-56	58.18		EE
84s ea, C-III	58016-0272-84	87.28		EE

(St. Mary's MPP)
REPACK
TAB, PO, 300 mg-30 mg,

PROD/MFR	NDC	AWP	DP	OBC
15s ea, C-III	60760-0022-15	10.69		AA
30s ea, C-III	60760-0022-30	15.39		AA

(Stat Rx)
REPACK
TAB, PO, 300 mg-30 mg,

PROD/MFR	NDC	AWP	DP	OBC
20s ea, C-III	16590-0023-20	12.33		EE
84s ea, C-III	16590-0023-62	52.81		EE
180s ea, C-III	16590-0023-82	113.16		EE
300 mg-60 mg,				
28s ea, C-III	16590-0472-28	28.00		AA
56s ea, C-III	16590-0472-56	56.00		AA

ACETAMINOPHEN/CODEINE #3 (Palmetto)
REPACK
acetaminophen/codeine phosphate
TAB, PO, 300 mg-30 mg,

PROD/MFR	NDC	AWP	DP	OBC
30s ea, C-III	23490-0010-03	32.99		
60s ea, C-III	23490-0010-06	65.40		
90s ea, C-III	23490-0010-09	98.10		

ACETAMINOPHEN/CODEINE PHOSPHATE
FUL
TAB, PO, 300 mg-15 mg,

PROD/MFR	NDC	AWP	DP	OBC
100s ea		15.00		
300 mg-30 mg,				
100s ea		21.37		
300 mg-60 mg,				
100s ea		38.33		

(Actavis Mid Atlantic) *See ACETAMINOPHEN/CODEINE*
(Athlon Pharm) *See VOPAC*
(CorePharma) *See ACETAMINOPHEN AND CODEINE PHOSPHATE #3*
(CorePharma) *See ACETAMINOPHEN AND CODEINE PHOSPHATE #4*
(Covidien) *See ACETAMINOPHEN/CODEINE*
(Hi-Tech) *See ACETAMINOPHEN/CODEINE*
(Mallinckrodt Lab) *See ACETAMINOPHEN/CODEINE*
(Mikart) *See ACETAMINOPHEN/CODEINE*
(Morton Grove) *See ACETAMINOPHEN/CODEINE*
(Ortho-McNeil Pharm) *See TYLENOL W/CODEINE #3*
(Ortho-McNeil Pharm) *See TYLENOL W/CODEINE #4*
(Pharm Assoc Inc) *See ACETAMINOPHEN/CODEINE*
(Poly) *See COCET*
(PriCara) *See TYLENOL WITH CODEINE NO. 4*
(Qualitest) *See ACETAMINOPHEN/CODEINE*
(Ranbaxy Pharm) *See ACETAMINOPHEN/CODEINE*
(Teva) *See ACETAMINOPHEN/CODEINE*
(UDL) *See ACETAMINOPHEN/CODEINE*
(Valeant Pharm Intl) *See CAPITAL W/CODEINE*

(Aidarex)
REPACK
TAB, PO, 300 mg-60 mg,

PROD/MFR	NDC	AWP	DP	OBC
8s ea, C-III	33261-0002-08	15.84		
10s ea, C-III	33261-0002-10	19.90		
12s ea, C-III	33261-0002-12	23.76		
14s ea, C-III	33261-0002-14	27.72		
20s ea, C-III	33261-0002-20	39.60		
21s ea, C-III	33261-0002-21	41.58		
28s ea, C-III	33261-0002-28	55.44		
30s ea, C-III	33261-0002-30	59.40		
40s ea, C-III	33261-0002-40	76.00		
42s ea, C-III	33261-0002-42	83.16		
48s ea, C-III	33261-0002-48	95.04		
60s ea, C-III	33261-0002-60	118.80		

(Palmetto)
REPACK
TAB, PO, 300 mg-30 mg,

PROD/MFR	NDC	AWP	DP	OBC
6s ea, C-III	23490-5004-01	9.82		
10s ea, C-III	23490-5004-02	11.69		
12s ea, C-III	23490-5004-03	14.03		
15s ea, C-III	23490-5004-04	17.54		
16s ea, C-III	23490-5004-05	18.71		
20s ea, C-III	23490-5004-06	23.39		
28s ea, C-III	23490-5004-00	32.74		
30s ea, C-III	23490-5004-07	35.08		
60s ea, C-III	23490-5004-08	70.16		
120s ea, C-III	23490-5004-09	140.32		
300 mg-60 mg,				
20s ea, C-III	23490-5005-00	20.78		
30s ea, C-III	23490-5005-01	31.17		
60s ea, C-III	23490-5005-03	62.34		
90s ea, C-III	23490-5005-02	93.51		

(Physician Partner)
REPACK
SOL, PO (1X120ML)
120 mg/5 ml-12 mg/5 ml,

PROD/MFR	NDC	AWP	DP	OBC
120 ml, C-V	21695-0547-04	13.50		

ACETAMINOPHEN/DICHLORALPHENAZONE/ISOMETHEPTENE (American Health)
REPACK
apap/dichloralphenazone/isometheptene mucate
CAP, PO (10X10)
325 mg-100 mg-65 mg,

PROD/MFR	NDC	AWP	DP	OBC
100s ea UD, C-IV	62584-0139-01	83.70		

ACETAMINOPHEN/HYDROCODONE (A-S Medication)
REPACK
acetaminophen/hydrocodone bitartrate
TAB, PO, 325 mg-5 mg,

PROD/MFR	NDC	AWP	DP	OBC
30s ea, C-III	54569-5523-03	16.27		

ACETAMINOPHEN/HYDROCODONE BITARTRATE
FUL
CAP, PO, 500 mg-5 mg,

PROD/MFR	NDC	AWP	DP	OBC
100s ea		19.43		
ELI, PO, 473 ml		47.96		
TAB, PO, 500 mg-2.5 mg,				
100s ea		21.90		
500 mg-5 mg,				
100s ea		47.63		
500 mg-7.5 mg,				
100s ea		64.26		
500 mg-10 mg,				
100s ea		51.29		
650 mg-7.5 mg,				
100s ea		67.08		
650 mg-10 mg,				
100s ea		18.52		
660 mg-10 mg,				
100s ea		54.00		
750 mg-7.5 mg,				
100s ea		15.48		

(A. G. Marin) *See DOLOREX FORTE*
(Abbott Pharm) *See VICODIN*
(Abbott Pharm) *See VICODIN ES*
(Abbott Pharm) *See VICODIN HP*
(Amneal) *See HYDROCODONE BITARTRATE AND ACETAMINOPHEN*
(Caraco) *See HYDROCODONE BITARTRATE AND ACETAMINOPHEN*
(Covidien) *See APAP/HYDROCODONE BITARTRATE*
(Cypress Pharm) *See APAP/HYDROCODONE BITARTRATE*
(Edwards) *See HYDROGESIC*
(Endo Labs) *See ZYDONE*
(Ethex) *See APAP/HYDROCODONE BITARTRATE*
(Forest Pharm) *See LORCET 10/650*
(Forest Pharm) *See LORCET PLUS*
(Hawthorn Pharm) *See ZAMICET*
(MAGNA Pharm) *See STAGESIC*
(Major) *See APAP/HYDROCODONE BITARTRATE*
(Marnel) *See MARGESIC-H*
(Pharm Assoc Inc) *See HYDROCODONE BITARTRATE AND ACETAMINOPHEN*
(Qualitest) *See APAP/HYDROCODONE BITARTRATE*
(Qualitest) *See APAP/HYDROCODONE BITARTRATE HS*
(Qualitest) *See HYDROCODONE BITARTRATE AND ACETAMINOPHEN*
(Ranbaxy Pharm) *See HYDROCODONE BITARTRATE/APAP*
(St. Mary's MPP) *See APAP/HYDROCODONE BITARTRATE*
(UCB) *See CO-GESIC*
(UCB) *See LORTAB*
(UCB) *See LORTAB 10/500*
(UCB) *See LORTAB 5/500*
(UCB) *See LORTAB 7.5/500*
(UDL) *See HYDROCODONE BITARTRATE AND ACETAMINOPHEN*
(Victory Pharma, Inc.) *See XODOL*
(Victory Pharma, Inc.) *See XODOL 5/300*
(Victory Pharma, Inc.) *See XODOL 7.5/300*
(Vintage) *See APAP/HYDROCODONE BITARTRATE*
(Watson) *See APAP/HYDROCODONE BITARTRATE*
(Watson) *See MAXIDONE*
(Watson) *See NORCO*
(Watson Labs) *See APAP/HYDROCODONE BITARTRATE*
(Xanodyne Pharma) *See HYCET*

(Palmetto)
REPACK
TAB, PO, 325 mg-5 mg,

PROD/MFR	NDC	AWP	DP	OBC
30s ea, C-III	23490-7487-03	18.00		
40s ea, C-III	23490-7487-01	25.88		
90s ea, C-III	23490-7487-09	58.23		
100s ea, C-III	23490-7487-00	60.00		
120s ea, C-III	23490-7487-02	48.00		
500 mg-2.5 mg,				
20s ea, C-III	23490-7849-00	11.00		
30s ea, C-III	23490-7849-03	16.50		
40s ea, C-III	23490-7849-04	22.00		
60s ea, C-III	23490-7849-06	33.00		
90s ea, C-III	23490-7849-09	49.50		
500 mg-5 mg,				
25s ea, C-III	23490-7842-03	37.03		
45s ea, C-III	23490-7842-01	66.60		
90s ea, C-III	23490-7842-00	52.88		
100s ea, C-III	23490-7842-02	145.93		
120s ea, C-III	23490-7842-04	150.96		
180s ea, C-III	23490-7842-05	213.12		
500 mg-10 mg,				
6s ea, C-III	23490-6966-01	8.65		
20s ea, C-III	23490-6966-04	20.60		
30s ea, C-III	23490-6966-02	31.00		
60s ea, C-III	23490-6966-03	62.00		
90s ea, C-III	23490-6966-05	93.00		
100s ea, C-III	23490-6966-07	87.55		
120s ea, C-III	23490-6966-06	98.88		
650 mg-7.5 mg,				
100s ea, C-III	23490-5689-01	106.67		
650 mg-10 mg,				
6s ea, C-III	23490-5694-01	11.17		
15s ea, C-III	23490-5694-06	20.00		
30s ea, C-III	23490-5694-05	39.99		
60s ea, C-III	23490-5694-02	79.98		
90s ea, C-III	23490-5694-04	119.97		
100s ea, C-III	23490-5694-03	133.30		
120s ea, C-III	23490-5694-07	120.00		
750 mg-7.5 mg,				
12s ea, C-III	23490-5692-01	12.00		
15s ea, C-III	23490-5692-02	15.00		
16s ea, C-III	23490-5692-03	16.00		
20s ea, C-III	23490-5692-04	20.00		
25s ea, C-III	23490-7945-01	22.71		
30s ea, C-III	23490-5692-05	30.00		
40s ea, C-III	23490-5692-00	40.00		
60s ea, C-III	23490-5692-06	60.00		
90s ea, C-III	23490-5692-07	90.00		
100s ea, C-III	23490-5692-08	100.00		
120s ea, C-III	23490-5692-09	102.00		

ACETAMINOPHEN/OXYCODONE HYDROCHLORIDE
FUL
CAP, PO, 500 mg-5 mg,

PROD/MFR	NDC	AWP	DP	OBC
100s ea		32.30		
TAB, PO, 325 mg-5 mg,				
100s ea		23.40		
650 mg-10 mg,				
100s ea		141.87		

(Amneal) *See OXYCODONE AND ACETAMINOPHEN*
(Atley) *See PRIMALEV*
(Covidien) *See APAP/OXYCODONE*
(Endo Generics) *See ENDOCET*
(Endo Labs) *See PERCOCET*
(Endo Pharm) *See PERCOCET*

PROD/MFR NDC AWP DP OBC

(Mylan) *See OXYCODONE AND ACETAMINOPHEN*
(Ortho-McNeil Pharm) *See TYLOX*
(Qualitest) *See APAP/OXYCODONE*
(Roxane) *See APAP/OXYCODONE*
(Roxane) *See ROXICET*
(Teva) *See APAP/OXYCODONE*
(Victory Pharma, Inc.) *See MAGNACET*
(Vintage) *See APAP/OXYCODONE*
(Watson Labs) *See APAP/OXYCODONE*
(Watson Labs) *See OXYCODONE AND ACETAMINOPHEN*
(Wraser Pharm) *See XOLOX*

(Palmetto)
REPACK
CAP, PO, 500 mg-5 mg,
30s ea, C-II **23490-7910-03** 49.50
90s ea, C-II **23490-7910-09** 148.50
TAB, PO, 325 mg-5 mg,
6s ea, C-II **23490-6053-00** 9.48
10s ea, C-II **23490-6053-01** 15.81
15s ea, C-II **23490-6053-02** 23.71
20s ea, C-II **23490-6053-03** 31.61
30s ea, C-II **23490-6053-04** 47.42
40s ea, C-II **23490-6053-08** 63.23
60s ea, C-II **23490-6053-05** 94.84
90s ea, C-II **23490-6053-09** 142.26
100s ea, C-II **23490-6053-06** 158.07
120s ea, C-II **23490-6053-07** 189.68
325 mg-7.5 mg,
30s ea, C-II **23490-7826-03** 114.53
60s ea, C-II **23490-7826-06** 229.06
90s ea, C-II **23490-7826-09** 381.00
120s ea, C-II **23490-7826-07** 458.17
325 mg-10 mg,
30s ea, C-II **23490-7592-01** 105.20
40s ea, C-II **23490-7592-04** 144.00
60s ea, C-II **23490-7592-02** 210.40
90s ea, C-II **23490-7592-09** 324.00
100s ea, C-II **23490-7592-03** 350.67
120s ea, C-II **23490-7592-07** 432.00
500 mg-7.5 mg,
30s ea, C-II **23490-7909-03** 66.00

ACETAMINOPHEN/PENTAZOCINE HCL **(Watson Labs)**
acetaminophen/pentazocine hydrochloride
TAB, PO (CAPLET)
650 mg-25 mg,
100s ea, C-IV ...... **00591-0396-01** 109.02 AB

(Stat Rx)
REPACK
TAB, PO (CAPLET)
650 mg-25 mg,
30s ea, C-IV........ **16590-0582-30** 42.67 AB
60s ea, C-IV........ **16590-0582-60** 76.00 AB
90s ea, C-IV........ **16590-0582-90** 114.00 AB

ACETAMINOPHEN/PENTAZOCINE HYDROCHLORIDE
FUL
TAB, PO, 650 mg-25 mg,
100s ea 85.17

(Sanofi-Aventis) *See TALACEN*
(Watson Labs) *See ACETAMINOPHEN/PENTAZOCINE HCL*

ACETAMINOPHEN/PHENYLTOLOXAMINE
(Llorens Pharma Int) *See DOLOGESIC*

ACETAMINOPHEN/PHENYLTOLOXAMINE CITRATE
(A. G. Marin) *See DOLOREX*
(A. G. Marin) *See NOVAGESIC*
(Acella) *See BP POLY-650*
(Breckenridge Pharm) *See HYFLEX-DS*
(Capellon) *See ZGESIC*
(Carwin) *See RHINOFLEX*
(Carwin) *See RHINOFLEX-650*
(Intl Ethical) *See RELAGESIC*
(Laser Pharma) *See LAGESIC*
(MAGNA Pharm) *See STAFLEX*
(PGD, Inc.) *See GENECAR*
(Poly) *See FLEXTRA-650*
(Poly) *See FLEXTRA-DS*
(Vertical) *See ACUFLEX*
(Vision) *See VISTRA 650*

ACETAMINOPHEN/PROPOXYPHENE HCL
(A-S Medication)
REPACK
acetaminophen/propoxyphene hydrochloride
TAB, PO, 650 mg-65 mg,
20s ea, C-IV........ **54569-2588-00** 6.08 EE
30s ea, C-IV........ **54569-2588-01** 9.12 EE

(Pharma Pac)
REPACK
TAB, PO, 650 mg-65 mg,
20s ea, C-IV........ **52959-0165-20** 11.66 EE

ACETAMINOPHEN/PROPOXYPHENE HYDROCHLORIDE
FUL
TAB, PO, 650 mg-65 mg,
100s ea 10.90

(Mylan) *See APAP/PROPOXYPHENE*
(Qualitest) *See APAP/PROPOXYPHENE HCL*
(UDL) *See APAP/PROPOXYPHENE*

ACETAMINOPHEN/PROPOXYPHENE NAPSYLATE
FUL
TAB, PO, 650 mg-100 mg,
100s ea 18.00

(Aristos) *See PROPOXYPHENE NAPSYLATE AND ACETAMINOPHEN*
(Cornerstone) *See BALACET 325*
(Covidien) *See APAP/PROPOXYPHENE NAPSYLATE*
(Mylan) *See APAP/PROPOXYPHENE NAPSYLATE*
(Qualitest) *See APAP/PROPOXYPHENE NAPSYLATE*
(Qualitest) *See PROPOXYPHENE NAPSYLATE AND ACETAMINOPHEN*
(Teva) *See APAP/PROPOXYPHENE NAPSYLATE*
(Teva) *See PROPOXYPHENE NAPSYLATE AND ACETAMINOPHEN*
(UDL) *See APAP/PROPOXYPHENE NAPSYLATE*
(Xanodyne Pharma) *See DARVOCET A500*
(Xanodyne Pharma) *See DARVOCET-N 100*
(Xanodyne Pharma) *See DARVOCET-N 50*

(Palmetto)
REPACK
TAB, PO, 650 mg-100 mg,
10s ea, C-IV........ **23490-6197-01** 11.00
12s ea, C-IV........ **23490-6197-02** 13.20
15s ea, C-IV........ **23490-6197-03** 16.50
16s ea, C-IV........ **23490-6197-04** 17.60
20s ea, C-IV........ **23490-6197-05** 22.00
25s ea, C-IV........ **23490-7930-07** 31.02
30s ea, C-IV........ **23490-6197-06** 33.00
40s ea, C-IV........ **23490-7930-04** 40.80
50s ea, C-IV........ **23490-6197-07** 55.00
60s ea, C-IV........ **23490-6197-08** 66.00
100s ea, C-IV **23490-7930-08** 110.00
120s ea, C-IV **23490-6197-09** 99.00

ACETAMINOPHEN/SALICYLAMIDE
(A. G. Marin) *See FRENADOL*

ACETAMINOPHEN/TRAMADOL **(A-S Medication)**
REPACK
acetaminophen/tramadol hydrochloride
TAB, PO, 325 mg-37.5 mg,
60s ea............ **54569-5680-02** 61.49
120s ea........... **54569-5680-03** 122.98

ACETAMINOPHEN/TRAMADOL HYDROCHLORIDE
(Amneal) *See TRAMADOL HYDROCHLORIDE AND ACETAMINOPHEN*
(Caraco) *See TRAMADOL HYDROCHLORIDE/ ACETAMINOPHEN*
(Mylan) *See TRAMADOL HYDROCHLORIDE AND ACETAMINOPHEN*
(Ortho-McNeil Pharm) *See ULTRACET*
(Par) *See TRAMADOL HYDROCHLORIDE AND ACETAMINOPHEN*
(PriCara) *See ULTRACET*
(Teva) *See APAP/TRAMADOL HYDROCHLORIDE*
(Teva) *See TRAMADOL HYDROCHLORIDE/ ACETAMINOPHEN*

(Palmetto)
REPACK
TAB, PO, 325 mg-37.5 mg,
6s ea............. **23490-7586-01** 10.50
30s ea............ **23490-7586-02** 37.50
60s ea............ **23490-7586-03** 75.00
90s ea............ **23490-7586-04** 112.50
120s ea........... **23490-7586-05** 127.50
180s ea........... **23490-7586-06** 191.25

ACETANILIDE **(PCCA)**
POW, NA (REAGENT)
1 gm **51927-2788-00** 0.60

ACETASOL **(Southwood)**
REPACK
acetic acid
SOL, OT, 2%, 15 ml .... **58016-6082-01** 31.00 AT

ACETASOL HC **(Actavis Mid Atlantic)**
acetic acid/hydrocortisone
SOL, OT, 2%-1%, 10 ml ... **00472-0882-82** 226.29 AT

(Altura)
REPACK
SOL, OT, 2%-1%, 10 ml ... **63874-0756-10** 40.64

(Nucare Pharm)
REPACK
SOL, OT, 2%-1%, 10 ml ... **66267-0996-10** 38.70 AT

(Pharma Pac)
REPACK
SOL, OT, 2%-1%, 10 ml ... **52959-0319-01** 35.30 AT

(Phys Total Care)
REPACK
SOL, OT, 2%-1%, 10 ml ... **54868-0799-01** 59.73 AT

ACETAZOLAMIDE **(Consolidated Midland)**
TAB, PO, 250 mg, 100s ea . **00223-0039-01** 8.95 AB
1000s ea .... **00223-0039-02** 85.00 AB

(Gallipot)
CRY, NA (U.S.P.)
5 gm **51552-0855-02** 19.88 14.20
25 gm **51552-0855-04** 48.65 34.75
100 gm **51552-0855-05** 132.30 94.50

(Lannett)
TAB, PO, 250 mg, 100s ea . **00527-1050-01** 39.24 AB

(Letco)
POW, NA (U.S.P.)
1000 gm............ **62991-2517-01** 900.00
5000 gm............ **62991-2517-02** 2700.00

(Medisca)
POW, NA (U.S.P.)
25 gm **38779-0410-04** 111.00
100 gm............. **38779-0410-05** 297.00
1000 gm............ **38779-0410-09** 2085.00

(PCCA)
POW, NA (U.S.P.)
1 gm **51927-2276-00** 8.28

(Spectrum Pharmacy)
POW, NA (U.S.P.)
25 gm **49452-0018-02** 195.30
100 gm............. **49452-0018-03** 497.00

(Taro)
TAB, PO, 125 mg, 100s ea . **51672-4022-01** 37.18 AB
250 mg, 100s ea ..... **51672-4023-01** 54.15 AB

(Teva)
CER, PO (HARD GELATIN)
500 mg, 100s ea...... **00555-0513-02** 429.35 AB

(Teva) *See DIAMOX SEQUELS*
(X-Gen) *See NOVAPLUS ACETAZOLAMIDE*

(X-Gen)
PDS, IV (USP,1X500MG,LYOPHILIZED)
500 mg, 500 ml ...... **39822-0190-01** 51.75 AP

(Zydus Pharm.)
CER, PO, 500 mg, 100s ea. **68382-0261-01** 428.90 AB

(A-S Medication)
REPACK
TAB, PO, 125 mg, 12s ea .. **54569-4387-01** 4.06 EE
250 mg, 12s ea ...... **54569-1697-00** 5.23 EE

(Dispensing Solutions)
REPACK
TAB, PO, 125 mg, 12s ea .. **55045-1703-04** 5.55 AB

(Palmetto)
REPACK
TAB, PO, 125 mg, 120s ea . **23490-5007-07** 55.20

(PD-Rx Pharm)
REPACK
TAB, PO (USP)
125 mg, 12s ea ...... **55289-0720-12** 10.08 AB
250 mg, 24s ea ...... **55289-0221-24** 10.03 AB

(Phys Total Care)
REPACK
TAB, PO, 125 mg, 15s ea .. **54868-2819-00** 7.89

PROD/MFR	NDC	AWP	DP	OBC
250 mg, 12s ea	54868-1195-02	15.30		EE
(USP)				
250 mg, 15s ea	54868-1195-00	18.00		EE
20s ea	54868-1195-03	30.27		AB
60s ea	54868-1195-04	78.80		AB
100s ea	54868-1195-01	92.94		EE
(Quality Care Prod)				
REPACK				
TAB, PO, 250 mg, 12s ea	49999-0892-12	11.36		
(Vibranta)				
REPACK				
TAB, PO, 250 mg, 12s ea	57866-3002-02	39.36		
ACETAZOLAMIDE SODIUM (Bedford)				
PDS, IV (S.D.V.,PF)				
500 mg, ea	55390-0460-01	54.00		AP
ACETIC ACID				
(Amend) *See ACETIC ACID 36%*				
(Amend) *See ACETIC ACID GLACIAL*				
(B. Braun)				
SOL, IL (PIC CONTAINER)				
0.25%, 500 ml	00264-2304-10	2.64		AT
1000 ml	00264-2304-00	2.50		AT
(Baker, J.T.) *See ACETIC ACID GLACIAL*				
(Baxter)				
SOL, IL, 0.25%,				
1000 ml 12s	00338-0656-04	248.40		AT
(Gallipot) *See ACETIC ACID 3%*				
(Gallipot) *See ACETIC ACID 36%*				
(Gallipot) *See ACETIC ACID 5%*				
(Gallipot) *See ACETIC ACID 50%*				
(Gallipot) *See ACETIC ACID GLACIAL*				
(Hi-Tech)				
SOL, OT (1X15ML,USP)				
2%, 15 ml	50383-0889-15	40.00		
(Hospira)				
SOL, IL (AQUALITE, 24X250ML,PF)				
0.25%, 250 ml 24s	00409-6143-22	135.94	119.04	AT
(AQUALITE,PF,LATEX-FREE)				
0.25%, 1000 ml 12s	00409-6143-09	34.56	30.24	AT
(Mallinckrodt Lab) *See ACETIC ACID 36%*				
(Mallinckrodt Lab) *See ACETIC ACID GLACIAL*				
(Medisca) *See ACETIC ACID GLACIAL*				
(Morton Grove)				
SOL, OT, 2%, 15 ml	60432-0741-15	40.00		AT
(PCCA) *See GLACIAL ACETIC ACID*				
(Qualitest)				
SOL, OT, 2%, 15 ml	00603-7038-41	39.99		AT
(Spectrum Pharmacy) *See ACETIC ACID 3%*				
(Spectrum Pharmacy) *See ACETIC ACID 36%*				
(Spectrum Pharmacy) *See ACETIC ACID 5%*				
(Spectrum Pharmacy) *See ACETIC ACID GLACIAL*				
(A-S Medication)				
REPACK				
SOL, OT, 2%, 15 ml	54569-2311-00	40.00		EE
(Dispensing Solutions)				
REPACK				
SOL, OT, 2%, 15 ml	55045-1243-00	40.00		AT
ACETIC ACID 3% (Gallipot)				
acetic acid				
SOL, NA, 473 ml	51552-0051-06	17.50		
3785 ml	51552-0051-08	55.72		
(Spectrum Pharmacy)				
SOL, NA, 500 ml	49452-0042-01	77.00		
4000 ml	49452-0042-02	205.45		
ACETIC ACID 36% (Amend)				
acetic acid				
SOL, NA (N.F.)				
500 ml	17317-0210-01	28.00		
(Gallipot)				
SOL, NA (U.S.P.,N.F.)				
473 ml	51552-0211-06	21.70		
(Mallinckrodt Lab)				
LIQ, NA (N.F.)				
500 ml	00406-2488-14	19.62		
2500 ml	00406-2488-44	43.71		
(Spectrum Pharmacy)				
LIQ, NA (N.F.)				
500 ml	49452-0040-01	232.75		
2500 ml	49452-0040-02	927.50		
ACETIC ACID 5% (Gallipot)				
acetic acid				
SOL, NA, 473 ml	51552-0055-06	17.50		
3785 ml	51552-0055-08	55.72		
(Spectrum Pharmacy)				
SOL, NA, 500 ml	49452-0047-01	85.05		
4000 ml	49452-0047-02	215.60		
ACETIC ACID 50% (Gallipot)				
acetic acid				
SOL, NA, 473 ml	51552-0386-06	24.71		
3785 ml	51552-0386-08	62.86		
ACETIC ACID AMIDE				
(Baker, J.T.) *See ACETAMIDE*				
ACETIC ACID GLACIAL (Amend)				
acetic acid				
SOL, NA (A.C.S.)				
500 ml	17317-0211-01	14.00		
(U.S.P.)				
500 ml	17317-2435-01	14.00		
(A.C.S.)				
2500 ml	17317-0211-05	23.80		
(U.S.P.)				
3840 ml	17317-2435-06	31.50		
20352 ml	17317-2435-08	138.60		
(Baker, J.T.)				
SOL, NA (U.S.P., F.C.C.)				
500 ml	10106-9522-02	18.52		
2500 ml	10106-9522-03	32.21		
(Gallipot)				
LIQ, NA (U.S.P.,N.F.)				
473 ml	51552-0209-06	34.65		
(Mallinckrodt Lab)				
LIQ, NA, 500 ml	00406-2504-03	14.68		
(Medisca)				
LIQ, NA (U.S.P.)				
500 ml	38779-0582-08	40.50		
(USP,1X2500ML)				
2500 ml	38779-0582-01	76.50		
(Spectrum Pharmacy)				
LIQ, NA (U.S.P.)				
500 ml	49452-0030-01	73.85		
2500 ml	49452-0030-02	152.95		
4000 ml	49452-0030-03	214.55		
ACETIC ACID GLACIAL/OXYQUINOLINE SULFATE				
(Blansett) *See RELAGARD*				
(Pharmics) *See FEM PH*				
ACETIC ACID/ALUMINUM ACETATE				
(Bausch & Lomb Inc.)				
SOL, OT, 2%-0.79%, 60 ml	24208-0615-77	72.00		AT
(Major) *See BOROFAIR*				
(Dispensing Solutions)				
REPACK				
SOL, OT, 2%-0.79%, 60 ml	55045-3190-06	10.00		
ACETIC ACID/ANTIPYRINE/BENZOCAINE/ POLICOSANOL				
(Acella) *See AABP*				
(Deston Therapeutics, LLC) *See AURALGAN*				
(PruGen) *See PR OTIC SOLUTION*				
ACETIC ACID/HC (Taro)				
acetic acid/hydrocortisone				
SOL, OT, 2%-1%, 10 ml	51672-3007-01	26.79		AT
(Dispensing Solutions)				
REPACK				
SOL, OT, 2%-1%, 10 ml	55045-1263-02	26.75		AT
(Southwood)				
REPACK				
SOL, OT, 2%-1%, 10 ml	58016-6081-01	38.70		EE
ACETIC ACID/HYDROCORTISONE				
(Actavis) *See HYDROCORTISONE AND ACETIC ACID*				
(Actavis Mid Atlantic) *See ACETASOL HC*				
(ECR) *See VOSOL HC*				
(Hi-Tech) *See HYDROCORTISONE AND ACETIC ACID*				
(Taro) *See ACETIC ACID/HC*				
(Truxton) *See OTICOT HC*				
ACETIC ACID/OXYQUINOLINE SULFATE/ RICINOLEIC ACID				
(Hope) *See ACID JELLY*				
ACETIC ANHYDRIDE (Baker, J.T.)				
SOL, NA (A.C.S., REAGENT)				
500 ml	10106-0018-01	41.66		
4000 ml	10106-0018-03	173.97		
ACETOHYDROXAMIC ACID				
(Mission) *See LITHOSTAT*				
(PCCA)				
POW, NA, 1 gm	51927-3352-00	87.60		
ACETONE (Baker, J.T.)				
LIQ, NA (N.F., F.C.C.)				
500 ml	10106-9008-01	7.98		
(Mallinckrodt Lab)				
LIQ, NA (N.F.)				
500 ml	00406-2432-04	10.66		
4000 ml	00406-2432-08	49.17		
(Medisca)				
LIQ, NA (1X500ML)				
500 ml	38779-0913-08	37.50		
(A.C.S., REAGENT)				
500 ml	38779-0954-08	37.50		
(PCCA)				
LIQ, NA (NF)				
1 ml	15927-1888-00	0.09		
(Spectrum Pharmacy)				
LIQ, NA (U.S.P., NF, EP, BP)				
500 ml	49452-0050-01	70.35		
1000 ml	49452-0050-03	114.10		
(N.F.)				
4000 ml	49452-0050-02	189.00		
ACETONE/FUCHSIN/RESORCINOL				
(Amend) *See RESORCINOL*				
(Gallipot) *See RESORCINOL*				
ACETONITRILE				
(Baker, J.T.) *See ACETONITRILE LOW WATER*				
(Baker, J.T.)				
LIQ, NA (A.C.S., REAGENT)				
500 ml	10106-9011-01	47.23		
(HPLC)				
1000 ml	10106-9017-02	62.73		
(ULTRA RESI-ANALYZED)				
1000 ml	10106-9255-02	40.17		
(A.C.S., REAGENT)				
4000 ml	10106-9011-03	191.84		
(HPLC)				
4000 ml	10106-9017-03	165.47		
(ULTRA RESI-ANALYZED)				
4000 ml	10106-9255-03	116.49		
(A.C.S., REAGENT)				
20000 ml	10106-9011-07	319.25		
ACETONITRILE LOW WATER (Baker, J.T.)				
acetonitrile				
LIQ, NA (BIO-ANALYZED)				
4000 ml	10106-9018-03	187.41		
ACETOPHENONE (Baker, J.T.)				
LIQ, NA, 500 ml	10106-9012-01	60.20		
ACETYL-D-GLUCOSAMINE (Letco)				
n-acetyl glucosamine				
POW, NA (U.S.P.)				
100 gm	62991-1169-02	135.00		
500 gm	62991-1169-03	360.00		
(Medisca)				
POW, NA, 5 gm	38779-0956-03	46.50		
25 gm	38779-0956-04	67.50		
(1X100GM)				
100 gm	38779-0956-05	225.00		
(1X500GM)				
500 gm	38779-0956-08	675.00		
(1X1000GM)				
1000 gm	38779-0956-09	1095.00		
(PCCA)				
POW, NA (N)				
1 gm	51927-2573-00	9.00		
ACETYL-DL-PENICILLAMINE (PCCA)				
n-acetyl-penicillamine				
POW, NA (1X1GM)				
1 gm	51927-2018-00	81.00		
ACETYL-L-CARNITINE HCL (Gallipot)				
levocarnitine hydrochloride				
POW, NA, 1000 gm	51552-0994-07	651.00	465.00	
(Medisca)				
POW, NA, 25 gm	38779-0958-04	129.00		
100 gm	38779-0958-05	420.00		
(1X500GM)				
500 gm	38779-0958-08	1635.00		
(PCCA)				
POW, NA (N)				
1 gm	51927-2611-00	5.88		

PROD/MFR	NDC	AWP	DP	OBC
(Spectrum Pharmacy)				
POW, NA (1X25GM)				
25 gm	**49452-0057-02**	199.15		
(1X100GM)				
100 gm	**49452-0057-03**	658.00		
(1X500GM)				
500 gm	**49452-0057-04**	2443.00		
ACETYLCHOLINE CHLORIDE				
(Novartis Pharm) *See MIOCHOL-E*				
(PCCA)				
POW, NA, 1 gm	**51927-2326-00**	7.08		
(Spectrum Pharmacy)				
POW, NA (CRYSTALLINE)				
25 gm	**49452-0070-01**	305.20		
100 gm	**49452-0070-02**	539.00		
ACETYLCYSTEINE				
FUL				
SOL, IH, 10%, 10 ml		9.78		
20%, 30 ml		8.04		
(Amer Regent)				
SOL, IH (PF)				
10%, 4 ml 25s	**00517-7504-25**	132.50		AN
10 ml 3s	**00517-7510-03**	39.30		AN
20%, 4 ml 25s	**00517-7604-25**	163.75		AN
10 ml 3s	**00517-7610-03**	45.90		AN
30 ml 3s	**00517-7630-03**	37.50		AN
(Cumberland Pharma) *See ACETADOTE*				
(Gallipot)				
POW, NA (U.S.P.,N.F.)				
25 gm	**51552-0201-04**	21.70		
100 gm	**51552-0201-05**	61.39		
1000 gm	**51552-0201-07**	343.00		
(Hawkins)				
POW, NA (U.S.P.)				
25 gm	**63370-0005-25**	28.00		
100 gm	**63370-0005-35**	96.00		
500 gm	**63370-0005-45**	240.00		
1000 gm	**63370-0005-50**	460.00		
5000 gm	**63370-0005-55**	2200.00		
25000 gm	**63370-0005-62**	10800.00		
(Hospira)				
SOL, IH, 10%, 30 ml 3s	**00409-3307-03**	19.48	17.04	AN
(3X30ML)				
20%, 30 ml 3s	**00409-3308-03**	18.36	16.08	AN
30 ml 10s	**61703-0204-31**	71.88	62.90	AN
(Letco)				
POW, NA (U.S.P.)				
100 gm	**62991-1003-02**	60.00		
500 gm	**62991-1003-03**	150.00		
1000 gm	**62991-1003-04**	240.00		
(Mayne Pharma)				
SOL, IH, 10%, 30 ml 10s	**61703-0203-31**	51.84	45.36	AN
(Medisca)				
POW, NA (U.S.P.)				
25 gm	**38779-0495-04**	45.00		
100 gm	**38779-0495-05**	111.00		
500 gm	**38779-0495-08**	447.00		
1000 gm	**38779-0495-09**	795.00		
(PCCA)				
POW, NA (U.S.P.)				
1 gm	**51927-1601-00**	2.28		
(Roxane)				
SOL, IH, 10%, 10 ml 3s	**00054-3027-02**	19.56		AN
30 ml 3s	**00054-3025-02**	34.94		AN
20%, 10 ml 3s	**00054-3028-02**	24.45		AN
30 ml 3s	**00054-3026-02**	39.13		AN
(Spectrum Pharmacy) *See N-ACETYL-L-CYSTEINE*				
(Phys Total Care)				
REPACK				
SOL, IH, 20%, 30 ml	**54868-5670-00**	84.40		
(3X30ML)				
20%, 30 ml 3s	**54868-5670-01**	250.19		
ACETYLCYSTEINE/L-METHYLFOLATE/ METHYLCOBALAMIN				
(Pamlab) *See CEREFOLIN NAC*				
ACETYLMANDELIC ACID				
(PCCA) *See ALPHA-ACETYLMANDELIC ACID*				
ACETYLSALICYLIC ACID (Medisca)				
aspirin				
POW, NA (USP,1X100GM)				
100 gm	**38779-0955-05**	39.00		
(U.S.P.)				
500 gm	**38779-0955-08**	55.50		
2500 gm	**38779-0955-01**	195.00		
12000 gm	**38779-0955-07**	597.00		

PROD/MFR	NDC	AWP	DP	OBC
(USP,1X12000GM)				
12000 gm	**38779-0955-06**	597.00		
ACID BRILLIANT GREEN BS				
(PCCA) *See LISSAMINE GREEN B*				
ACID JELLY (Hope)				
acetic acid/oxyquinoline sulfate/ricinoleic acid				
GEL, VG (W/APPLICATOR)				
0.92%-0.025%-0.7%,				
85 gm	**60267-0125-85**	36.00		
ACID RED 52 (PCCA)				
color additive				
POW, NA, 1 gm	**51927-2668-00**	8.76		
(Spectrum Pharmacy)				
POW, NA (1X25GM)				
25 gm	**49452-0109-02**	295.05		
ACIDOPHILUS LACTOBACILLUS (Letco)				
lactobacillus acidophilus				
POW, NA, 500 gm	**62991-2001-01**	108.00		
1000 gm	**62991-2001-02**	177.00		
2500 gm	**62991-2001-03**	375.00		
5000 gm	**62991-2001-04**	600.00		
(Medisca)				
POW, NA (1X1000GM)				
1000 gm	**38779-2427-09**	465.00		
(PCCA)				
POW, NA, 1 gm	**51927-3055-00**	0.28		
(DDS-1)				
10 billion u/gm,				
1 gm	**51927-3522-00**	57.00		
(Spectrum Pharmacy)				
POW, NA (1X100GM)				
1 billion u/gm,				
100 gm	**49452-0107-01**	98.00		
(1X500GM)				
1 billion u/gm,				
500 gm	**49452-0107-02**	226.10		
(1X2500GM)				
1 billion u/gm,				
2500 gm	**49452-0107-03**	616.00		
(1X100GM)				
2 billion u/gm,				
100 gm	**49452-0108-01**	144.90		
(1X500GM)				
2 billion u/gm,				
500 gm	**49452-0108-02**	360.50		
(1X2500GM)				
2 billion u/gm,				
2500 gm	**49452-0108-03**	1015.00		
ACIDOPHILUS LACTOBACILLUS PLANTARUM (PCCA)				
lactobacillus combination				
POW, NA (1X1GM)				
1 gm	**51927-3523-00**	0.57		
ACIDULATED PHOSPHATE FLUORIDE				
(Omnii Intl) *See ORTHOWASH*				
ACIPHEX (Eisai)				
rabeprazole sodium				
ECT, PO, 20 mg, 30s ea	**62856-0243-30**	215.62		
90s ea	**62856-0243-90**	646.87		
(10X10 BLISTER PACK)				
20 mg, 100s ea UD	**62856-0243-41**	718.74		
(A-S Medication)				
REPACK				
ECT, PO, 20 mg, 30s ea	**54569-4980-00**	266.94		
(Core)				
REPACK				
ECT, PO, 20 mg, 30s ea	**33358-0008-30**	154.35		
60s ea	**33358-0008-60**	297.58		
(Dispensing Solutions)				
REPACK				
ECT, PO, 20 mg, 30s ea	**55045-3495-01**	269.63		
(Keltman Pharma., Inc.)				
REPACK				
ECT, PO, 20 mg, 15s ea	**68387-0371-15**	82.00		
30s ea	**68387-0371-30**	164.00		
(Phys Total Care)				
REPACK				
ECT, PO, 20 mg, 30s ea	**54868-4185-00**	245.69		
60s ea	**54868-4185-02**	488.78		
90s ea	**54868-4185-01**	707.68		
(Quality Care Prod)				
REPACK				
ECT, PO, 20 mg, 30s ea	**49999-0447-30**	348.80		
90s ea	**49999-0447-90**	643.50		
(Southwood)				
REPACK				
ECT, PO, 20 mg, 30s ea	**58016-0597-30**	179.41		

PROD/MFR	NDC	AWP	DP	OBC
60s ea	**58016-0597-60**	358.82		
90s ea	**58016-0597-90**	538.23		
100s ea	**58016-0597-00**	598.03		
(Stat Rx)				
REPACK				
ECT, PO, 20 mg, 30s ea	**16590-0467-30**	240.59		
60s ea	**16590-0467-60**	365.00		
90s ea	**16590-0467-90**	547.50		
100s ea	**16590-0467-71**	608.34		
ACITRETIN				
(Stiefel Labs) *See SORIATANE*				
ACLARO (JSJ Pharma)				
hydroquinone				
EMU, TP (AIRLESS PUMP)				
4%, 50.28 ml	**68712-0003-01**	100.68		
ACLOVATE (PharmaDerm)				
alclometasone dipropionate				
CRE, TP (1X15GM)				
0.05%, 15 gm	**00462-0263-15**	52.44		
(1X60GM)				
0.05%, 60 gm	**00462-0263-60**	123.35		
OIN, TP (1X15GM)				
0.05%, 15 gm	**00462-0264-15**	52.44		AB
60 gm	**00173-0402-06**	104.69		
60 gm	**00462-0264-60**	135.67		AB
(Phys Total Care)				
REPACK				
CRE, TP, 0.05%, 15 gm	**54868-0975-01**	18.79		
OIN, TP, 0.05%, 15 gm	**54868-3336-00**	18.79		
ACONITE (PCCA)				
aconitum napellus				
TIN, NA, 1 ml	**51927-3388-00**	0.34		
ACONITE EXTRACT (PCCA)				
SOL, NA, 1 ml	**51927-1982-00**	1.50		
ACONITUM NAPELLUS				
(PCCA) *See ACONITE*				
ACRIFLAVINE				
(Amend) *See ACRIFLAVINF NEUTRAL*				
(Gallipot) *See ACRIFLAVINE NEUTRAL*				
(Medisca)				
POW, NA (NEUTRAL)				
25 gm	**38779-0962-04**	73.50		
50 gm	**38779-0962-02**	150.00		
100 gm	**38779-0962-05**	211.50		
(PCCA) *See ACRIFLAVINE NEUTRAL*				
(Spectrum Pharmacy)				
POW, NA (NEUTRAL)				
25 gm	**49452-0120-01**	133.00		
100 gm	**49452-0120-02**	378.00		
ACRIFLAVINE HYDROCHLORIDE (Amend)				
POW, NA (C.P.)				
25 gm	**17317-0807-02**	19.30		
(Gallipot)				
POW, NA, 25 gm	**51552-0749-04**	33.95	24.25	
(Spectrum Pharmacy)				
POW, NA, 25 gm	**49452-0110-01**	143.15		
100 gm	**49452-0110-02**	399.00		
ACRIFLAVINE NEUTRAL (Amend)				
acriflavine				
POW, NA (C.P.)				
25 gm	**17317-0008-02**	19.30		
(Gallipot)				
POW, NA, 25 gm	**51552-1077-04**	38.50	27.50	
(PCCA)				
POW, NA, 1 gm	**51927-1394-00**	3.72		
ACRIVASTINE/PSEUDOEPHEDRINE HYDROCHLORIDE				
(UCB) *See SEMPREX-D*				
ACRYLAMIDE (Baker, J.T.)				
acrylic acid amide				
POW, NA (ULTRAPURE, BIOREAGENT)				
100 gm	**10106-4081-00**	33.94		
500 gm	**10106-4081-01**	111.19		
2500 gm	**10106-4081-05**	442.44		
12000 gm	**10106-4081-07**	1597.79		
ACRYLATES COPOLYMER				
(PCCA) *See EUDRAGIT S-100*				
ACRYLIC ACID AMIDE				
(Baker, J.T.) *See ACRYLAMIDE*				
ACTEMRA (Genentech)				
tocilizumab				
SOL, IV (1X4ML,PF)				
20 mg/ml, 4 ml	**50242-0135-01**	318.72		

PROD/MFR	NDC	AWP	DP	OBC
(1X10ML,PF)				
20 mg/ml, 10 ml	50242-0136-01	796.80		
(1X20ML,PF)				
20 mg/ml, 20 ml	50242-0137-01	1593.60		
ACTHIB (Sanofi)				
haemophilus b conjugate vaccine				
PDS, IM (SDV W/DIL,TAX INCL,PF)				
10 mcg, 5s ea	49281-0545-05	140.89	118.03	
ACTHREL (Ferring)				
corticorelin ovine triflutate				
PDS, IV (S.D.V.)				
0.1 mg, ea	55566-0302-01	599.10		
ACTICIN (Mylan)				
permethrin				
CRE, TP, 5%, 60 gm	00378-6131-06	29.15		
ACTIGALL (Watson)				
ursodiol				
CAP, PO, 300 mg, 100s ea	52544-0930-01	549.95		AB
ACTIMMUNE (Intermune)				
interferon gamma-1b				
SOL, SC (VIAL)				
2 million iu/0.5 ml,				
0.5 ml 12s	64116-0011-12	4132.80		
ACTIQ (Cephalon)				
fentanyl citrate				
LOZ, MM (BERRY)				
0.2 mg,				
30s ea, C-II	63459-0502-30	1116.00		
0.4 mg,				
30s ea, C-II	63459-0504-30	1412.40		
0.6 mg,				
30s ea, C-II	63459-0506-30	1730.40		
0.8 mg,				
30s ea, C-II	63459-0508-30	2049.60		
1.2 mg,				
30s ea, C-II	63459-0512-30	2664.00		
1.6 mg,				
30s ea, C-II	63459-0516-30	3286.80		
(Quality Care Prod)				
REPACK				
LOZ, MM (BERRY)				
0.2 mg,				
30s ea, C-II	35356-0456-30	1531.40		
0.4 mg,				
30s ea, C-II	35356-0457-30	1938.64		
0.6 mg,				
30s ea, C-II	35356-0458-30	2374.66		
0.8 mg,				
30s ea, C-II	35356-0459-30	2812.85		
1.2 mg,				
30s ea, C-II	35356-0460-30	3654.48		
1.6 mg,				
30s ea, C-II	35356-0461-30	4508.60		
ACTIVASE (Genentech)				
alteplase, recombinant				
PDS, IV (W/DILUENT)				
50 mg, ea	50242-0044-13	2389.85		
100 mg, ea	50242-0085-27	4779.71		
ACTIVATED CHARCOAL				
(Amend) *See CHARCOAL WOOD*				
(Amend) *See DARCO G-60*				
(Amend) *See LAMP BLACK POWDER*				
(Amend) *See NORIT A*				
(Baker, J.T.) *See CHARCOAL ACTIVATED*				
(Gallipot) *See CHARCOAL*				
(Mallinckrodt Lab) *See CHARCOAL ACTIVATED*				
(Medisca) *See CHARCOAL ACTIVATED*				
(Spectrum Pharmacy) *See CHARCOAL ACTIVATED*				
ACTIVE CATH SELF-ADHERING (Mentor)				
catheter				
DEV, NA (MALE, 23 MM)				
30s ea	81317-0081-30	61.80		
(MALE, 28 MM)				
30s ea	81317-0083-30	61.80		
(MALE, 31 MM)				
30s ea	81317-0083-35	61.80		
(MALE, 35 MM)				
30s ea	81317-0085-30	61.80		
(MALE, 23 MM)				
100s ea	81317-0081-00	180.00		
(MALE, 28 MM)				
100s ea	81317-0083-00	180.00		
(MALE, 31 MM)				
100s ea	81317-0083-05	180.00		
(MALE, 35 MM)				
100s ea	81317-0085-00	180.00		
ACTIVELLA (Novo Nordisk)				
estradiol/norethindrone acetate				
TAB, PO (DIALPACK,FILM-COATED)				
0.5 mg-0.1 mg,				
28s ea UD	00169-5175-10	72.91		EE
(5X28,DIALPACK)				
0.5 mg-0.1 mg,				
140s ea UD	00169-5175-11	364.56		EE
(DIALPACK,FILM-COATED)				
1 mg-0.5 mg,				
28s ea	00169-5174-02	80.14	20.87	
(5X28 DIALPACK)				
1 mg-0.5 mg,				
140s ea	00169-5174-01	400.68	119.37	
(Phys Total Care)				
REPACK				
TAB, PO (1X28 DIALPACK)				
1 mg-0.5 mg,				
28s ea	54868-4830-00	53.66		
ACTONEL (P & G Pharm)				
risedronate sodium				
TAB, PO (FILM-COATED)				
5 mg, 30s ea	00149-0471-01	117.46	97.88	
2000s ea	00149-0471-03	7830.40	6525.33	
30 mg, 30s ea	00149-0470-01	822.17	685.14	
(DOSEPACK,FILM-COATED)				
35 mg, 4s ea	00149-0472-01	109.62	91.35	
(FILM-COATED)				
35 mg, 12s ea	00149-0472-04	328.86	274.05	
(DOSE PACK,FILM-COATED)				
150 mg, ea	00149-0478-01	118.75	98.96	EE
3s ea	00149-0478-03	356.26	296.88	EE
(A-S Medication)				
REPACK				
TAB, PO (FILM-COATED)				
35 mg, 4s ea	54569-5462-00	142.51		
(AQ)				
REPACK				
TAB, PO, 5 mg, 30s ea	66105-0157-03	117.98		
30 mg, 30s ea	66105-0158-03	795.79		
(DHS, Inc.)				
REPACK				
TAB, PO, 35 mg, 4s ea	55887-0685-04	119.98		
(Palmetto)				
REPACK				
TAB, PO, 35 mg, 4s ea	23490-9245-00	95.73		
(Phys Total Care)				
REPACK				
TAB, PO, 5 mg, 30s ea	54868-4386-00	111.85		
35 mg, 4s ea	54868-4671-00	128.84		
(FILM-COATED)				
150 mg, ea	54868-6069-00	142.54		EE
(Quality Care Prod)				
REPACK				
TAB, PO (FILM-COATED)				
35 mg, 4s ea	49999-0448-04	162.30		
(Stat Rx)				
REPACK				
TAB, PO (FILM-COATED)				
35 mg, 4s ea	16590-0721-04	119.22		
ACTONEL WITH CALCIUM (P & G Pharm)				
calcium carbonate/risedronate sodium				
TAB, PO (FILM-COATED)				
1250 mg-35 mg,				
28s ea	00149-0475-01	109.62	91.35	
(Phys Total Care)				
REPACK				
TAB, PO, 1250 mg-35 mg,				
28s ea	54868-5518-00	117.17		
ACTOPLUS MET (Takeda)				
metformin hydrochloride/pioglitazone hydrochloride				
TAB, PO (FILM-COATED)				
500 mg-15 mg,				
60s ea	64764-0155-60	241.38		EE
180s ea	64764-0155-18	724.15		EE
850 mg-15 mg,				
60s ea	64764-0158-60	241.38		
180s ea	64764-0158-18	724.15		
(Phys Total Care)				
REPACK				
TAB, PO, 500 mg-15 mg,				
60s ea	54868-5500-01	288.35		
90s ea	54868-5500-00	431.22		
(FILM-COATED)				
850 mg-15 mg,				
30s ea	54868-5553-02	145.48		
60s ea	54868-5553-00	287.69		
(FILM-COATED)				
850 mg-15 mg,				
90s ea	54868-5553-01	431.22		
(Quality Care Prod)				
REPACK				
TAB, PO (FILM-COATED)				
850 mg-15 mg,				
60s ea	35356-0130-60	341.86		
ACTOS (Takeda)				
pioglitazone hydrochloride				
TAB, PO, 15 mg, 30s ea	64764-0151-04	158.84		
90s ea	64764-0151-05	476.52		
500s ea	64764-0151-06	2647.49		
30 mg, 30s ea	64764-0301-14	242.76		
90s ea	64764-0301-15	728.28		
500s ea	64764-0301-16	4046.00		
45 mg, 30s ea	64764-0451-24	263.32		
90s ea	64764-0451-25	790.01		
500s ea	64764-0451-26	4388.96		
(A-S Medication)				
REPACK				
TAB, PO, 15 mg, 30s ea	54569-4880-00	206.02		
30 mg, 30s ea	54569-4881-00	315.59		
45 mg, 30s ea	54569-4882-00	342.32		
(Advanced Pharm Serv, Inc.)				
REPACK				
TAB, PO, 15 mg, 10s ea	13411-0101-01	57.83		
15s ea	13411-0101-05	86.75		
30s ea	13411-0101-03	173.51		
60s ea	13411-0101-06	347.02		
90s ea	13411-0101-09	520.50		
30 mg, 10s ea	13411-0102-01	88.38		
15s ea	13411-0102-15	132.58		
30s ea	13411-0102-03	265.16		
60s ea	13411-0102-06	530.33		
90s ea	13411-0102-09	795.50		
45 mg, 10s ea	13411-0103-01	95.87		
15s ea	13411-0103-15	143.81		
30s ea	13411-0103-03	287.62		
60s ea	13411-0103-06	572.25		
90s ea	13411-0103-09	862.93		
(AQ)				
REPACK				
TAB, PO, 15 mg, 10s ea	66105-0156-01	74.80		
15s ea	66105-0156-15	112.20		
30s ea	66105-0156-03	224.40		
60s ea	66105-0156-06	448.80		
90s ea	66105-0156-09	673.20		
30 mg, 10s ea	66105-0154-01	109.40		
15s ea	66105-0154-15	164.10		
30s ea	66105-0154-03	328.20		
60s ea	66105-0154-06	656.40		
90s ea	66105-0154-09	984.60		
45 mg, 10s ea	66105-0732-01	95.87		
15s ea	66105-0732-15	143.81		
30s ea	66105-0732-03	287.62		
60s ea	66105-0732-06	572.25		
90s ea	66105-0732-09	862.93		
(DHS, Inc.)				
REPACK				
TAB, PO, 45 mg, 30s ea	55887-0975-30	299.98		
(Nucare Pharm)				
REPACK				
TAB, PO, 15 mg, 15s ea	68071-0405-15	132.00		
30 mg, 15s ea	68071-0406-15	157.00		
45 mg, 15s ea	68071-0407-15	173.00		
(PD-Rx Pharm)				
REPACK				
TAB, PO (REDI-SCRIPT)				
15 mg, 14s ea	58864-0670-14	105.00		
30s ea	58864-0670-30	225.00		
30 mg, 15s ea	55289-0862-15	163.94		
(REDI-SCRIPT)				
30 mg, 15s ea	58864-0745-15	163.94		
30s ea	55289-0862-30	360.81		
30s ea	58864-0745-30	343.95		
45 mg, 30s ea	55289-0540-30	391.40		
(Phys Total Care)				
REPACK				
TAB, PO, 15 mg, 30s ea	54868-4343-00	189.99		
90s ea	54868-4343-01	548.51		
30 mg, 30s ea	54868-4354-00	289.32		
90s ea	54868-4354-01	836.24		
45 mg, 30s ea	54868-4391-00	313.67		
90s ea	54868-4391-01	906.92		
(Physician Partner)				
REPACK				
TAB, PO, 15 mg, 15s ea	21695-0147-15	152.01		
30 mg, 15s ea	21695-0148-15	243.37		

PROD/MFR	NDC	AWP	DP	OBC
(Quality Care Prod)				
REPACK				
TAB, PO, 15 mg, 30s ea	49999-0449-30	170.40		
30 mg, 30s ea	49999-0450-30	328.10		
45 mg, 30s ea	49999-0451-30	379.35		
90s ea	49999-0451-90	1138.50		
ACUFLEX (Vertical)				
acetaminophen/phenyltoloxamine citrate				
TAB, PO (CAPLET)				
635 mg-55 mg,				
100s ea	68025-0004-10	159.37		
ACULAR (Allergan Inc)				
ketorolac tromethamine				
SOL, OP, 0.5%, 5 ml	00023-2181-05	122.32		
10 ml	00023-2181-10	244.61		
(A-S Medication)				
REPACK				
SOL, OP, 0.5%, 3 ml	54569-4573-00	51.00		
5 ml	54569-4083-00	154.38		
(DHS, Inc.)				
REPACK				
SOL, OP (DROPS)				
0.5%, 5 ml	55887-0195-05	84.98		
(Dispensing Solutions)				
REPACK				
SOL, OP, 0.5%, 3 ml	55045-2168-03	62.00		
5 ml	55045-2168-05	110.00		
(Pharma Pac)				
REPACK				
SOL, OP, 0.5%, 5 ml	52959-0114-05	145.50		
(Phys Total Care)				
REPACK				
SOL, OP, 0.5%, 3 ml	54868-3950-00	65.21		
5 ml	54868-3950-02	139.78		
10 ml	54868-3950-01	202.56		
(Physician Partner)				
REPACK				
SOL, OP, 0.5%, 5 ml	21695-0463-05	229.08		
(Quality Care Prod)				
REPACK				
SOL, OP (1X3ML)				
0.5%, 3 ml	49999-0695-03	87.24		
5 ml	49999-0695-05	80.22		
(Southwood)				
REPACK				
SOL, OP, 0.5%, 3 ml	58016-4598-01	40.11		
5 ml	58016-6461-01	93.40		
10 ml	58016-6461-02	99.80		
(Stat Rx)				
REPACK				
SOL, OP, 0.5%, 3 ml	16590-0002-03	67.21		
5 ml	16590-0002-05	140.52		
10 ml	16590-0002-10	256.00		
ACULAR LS (Allergan Inc)				
ketorolac tromethamine				
SOL, OP, 0.4%, 5 ml	00023-9277-05	122.32		
(Phys Total Care)				
REPACK				
SOL, OP, 0.4%, 5 ml	54868-4913-00	91.77		
ACULAR PF (Dispensing Solutions)				
REPACK				
ketorolac tromethamine				
SOL, OP (12X0.4ML)				
0.5%, 0.4 ml 12s	55045-2745-01	71.00		
(Phys Total Care)				
REPACK				
SOL, OP (SINGLE USE VIALS)				
0.5%, 12s ea	54868-4704-00	53.33		
ACUNOL (Loma Lux)				
homeopathic				
TAB, PO, 1 x-1 x-1 x-1 x-1 x,				
90s ea	61480-0137-05	90.00		
ACUVAIL (Allergan Inc)				
ketorolac tromethamine				
SOL, OP (30X0.4ML,SINGLE-USE,PF)				
0.45%, 0.4 ml 30s	00023-3507-30	124.97		EE
ACYCLOVIR				
FUL				
CAP, PO, 200 mg, 100s ea		14.78		
TAB, PO, 400 mg, 100s ea		23.34		
800 mg, 100s ea		46.67		
(Actavis Mid Atlantic)				
SUS, PO, 200 mg/5 ml,				
473 ml	00472-0082-16	137.77		AB
(Apotex Corp.)				
CAP, PO (USP)				
200 mg, 100s ea	60505-0042-06	97.70		AB
TAB, PO, 400 mg, 100s ea	60505-5306-01	216.91		AB
1000s ea	60505-5306-08	2169.10		AB
(USP)				
800 mg, 100s ea	60505-5307-01	421.60		AB
500s ea	60505-5307-05	2108.00		AB
(Boscogen)				
CAP, PO, 200 mg, 100s ea	62033-0204-10	45.00		AB
400s ea	62033-0204-14	105.60		AB
(BTA) *See ZOVIRAX*				
(Carlsbad Tech)				
CAP, PO (USP)				
200 mg, 100s ea	61442-0111-01	97.20		AB
TAB, PO, 400 mg, 100s ea	61442-0112-01	188.60		AB
800 mg, 100s ea	61442-0113-01	366.65		AB
(Dava Pharma)				
CAP, PO, 200 mg, 100s ea	67253-0100-10	111.65		AB
1000s ea	67253-0100-11	1004.85		AB
TAB, PO, 400 mg, 100s ea	67253-0101-10	216.70		AB
1000s ea	67253-0101-11	1950.30		AB
800 mg, 100s ea	67253-0102-10	421.42		AB
500s ea	67253-0102-50	2001.75		AB
(Gallipot)				
POW, NA (U.S.P.)				
1 gm	51552-0671-01	7.00	5.00	
5 gm	51552-0671-02	16.80	12.00	
10 gm	51552-0671-03	38.50	27.50	
25 gm	51552-0671-04	56.00	40.00	
100 gm	51552-0671-05	210.00	150.00	
500 gm	51552-0671-06	1164.24	831.60	
(Glaxo) *See ZOVIRAX*				
(Hawkins)				
POW, NA (U.S.P.)				
25 gm	63370-0007-25	160.00		
100 gm	63370-0007-35	600.00		
1000 gm	63370-0007-50	5400.00		
(Hi-Tech)				
SUS, PO (BANANA)				
200 mg/5 ml,				
473 ml	50383-0810-16	137.70		AB
(Letco)				
POW, NA (U.S.P.)				
25 gm	62991-1004-01	120.00		
100 gm	62991-1004-02	405.00		
(Major)				
CAP, PO (10X10,USP)				
200 mg, 100s ea UD	00904-5789-61	152.90		AB
TAB, PO, 400 mg,				
100s ea UD	00904-5790-61	172.44		AB
800 mg, 100s ea UD	00904-5799-61	412.66		AB
(Medisca)				
POW, NA (U.S.P.)				
10 gm	38779-0173-01	70.50		
25 gm	38779-0173-04	135.00		
100 gm	38779-0173-05	465.00		
500 gm	38779-0173-08	1785.00		
(Mylan)				
TAB, PO, 400 mg, 100s ea	00378-0253-01	217.00		AB
800 mg, 100s ea	00378-0302-01	421.70		AB
(PCCA)				
POW, NA (U.S.P.)				
1 gm	51927-2994-00	7.20		
(Ranbaxy Pharm)				
CAP, PO, 200 mg, 100s ea	63304-0652-01	111.95		AB
500s ea	63304-0652-05	531.76		AB
TAB, PO, 400 mg, 100s ea	63304-0504-01	216.97		AB
800 mg, 100s ea	63304-0505-01	421.67		AB
(Spectrum Pharmacy)				
POW, NA (U.S.P.)				
25 gm	49452-0001-03	220.85		
100 gm	49452-0001-04	714.00		
(Stason Pharm)				
CAP, PO, 200 mg, 100s ea	60763-2041-00	97.70		AB
400s ea	60763-2041-04	550.70		AB
(Teva)				
CAP, PO, 200 mg, 100s ea	00093-8940-01	97.20		AB
(USP,HARD GELATIN)				
200 mg, 100s ea UD	00093-8940-93	111.88		AB
500s ea	00093-8940-05	461.70		AB
TAB, PO, 400 mg,				
100s ea UD	00093-8943-93	216.91		AB
(COMPRESSED)				
400 mg, 100s ea	00093-8943-01	216.91		AB
500s ea	00093-8943-05	947.30		AB
800 mg, 100s ea UD	00093-8947-93	421.60		AB
(COMPRESSED)				
800 mg, 100s ea	00093-8947-01	421.60		AB
500s ea	00093-8947-05	1751.09		AB
(UDL)				
CAP, PO (10X10)				
200 mg, 100s ea UD	51079-0876-20	99.15		AB
TAB, PO, 400 mg,				
100s ea UD	51079-0877-20	194.40		AB
800 mg, 100s ea UD	51079-0878-20	355.10		AB
(A-S Medication)				
REPACK				
CAP, PO, 200 mg, 21s ea	54569-4482-06	21.98		AB
25s ea	54569-4482-00	26.16		EE
40s ea	54569-4482-04	41.43		AB
50s ea	54569-4482-01	51.79		AB
TAB, PO, 400 mg, 14s ea	54569-4765-01	30.34		EE
15s ea	54569-4765-04	32.51		EE
25s ea	54569-4765-02	54.18		EE
45s ea	54569-4765-05	65.02		EE
45s ea	54569-4765-09	97.52		EE
50s ea	54569-4765-03	108.36		EE
60s ea	54569-4765-06	130.03		EE
800 mg, 35s ea	54569-4724-00	147.50		EE
(Advanced Pharm Serv, Inc.)				
REPACK				
TAB, PO, 400 mg, 10s ea	13411-0182-01	31.90		
30s ea	13411-0182-03	95.70		
60s ea	13411-0182-06	191.40		
90s ea	13411-0182-09	287.10		
100s ea	13411-0182-10	300.98		
800 mg, 10s ea	13411-0183-01	44.80		
30s ea	13411-0183-03	134.40		
60s ea	13411-0183-06	268.80		
90s ea	13411-0183-09	403.20		
100s ea	13411-0183-10	484.63		
(Altura)				
REPACK				
CAP, PO, 200 mg, 10s ea	63874-0404-10	16.07		EE
14s ea	63874-0404-14	21.65		EE
15s ea	63874-0404-15	23.19		EE
20s ea	63874-0404-20	30.87		EE
24s ea	63874-0404-24	33.80		EE
25s ea	63874-0404-25	40.16		EE
30s ea	63874-0404-30	47.15		EE
35s ea	63874-0404-35	55.00		EE
40s ea	63874-0404-40	55.13		EE
50s ea	63874-0404-50	65.30		EE
60s ea	63874-0404-60	74.00		EE
70s ea	63874-0404-70	86.33		AB
100s ea	63874-0404-01	102.51		EE
TAB, PO, 400 mg, 15s ea	63874-0500-15	30.15		EE
20s ea	63874-0500-20	40.20		EE
21s ea	63874-0500-21	42.21		EE
25s ea	63874-0500-25	50.25		EE
30s ea	63874-0500-30	60.30		EE
40s ea	63874-0500-40	80.40		EE
60s ea	63874-0500-60	120.60		EE
100s ea	63874-0500-01	201.00		EE
800 mg, 10s ea	63874-0405-10	40.13		
20s ea	63874-0405-20	80.27		
25s ea	63874-0405-25	100.34		
30s ea	63874-0405-30	120.41		
35s ea	63874-0405-35	140.47		
100s ea	63874-0405-01	401.37		
(Bryant Ranch)				
REPACK				
CAP, PO, 200 mg, 25s ea	63629-1676-02	37.22		
30s ea	63629-1676-01	44.67		
35s ea	63629-1676-03	52.11		
TAB, PO, 400 mg, 15s ea	63629-1677-05	31.25		EE
20s ea	63629-1677-01	53.05		
28s ea	63629-1677-02	74.27		
30s ea	63629-1677-03	79.57		
800 mg, 25s ea	63629-1678-01	147.58		
30s ea	63629-1678-03	177.10		
35s ea	63629-1678-02	206.62		
(Core)				
REPACK				
CAP, PO, 200 mg, 25s ea	33358-0009-25	38.15		
TAB, PO, 400 mg, 15s ea	33358-0010-15	56.75		
28s ea	33358-0010-28	76.13		
30s ea	33358-0010-30	81.56		
60s ea	33358-0010-60	103.70		
800 mg, 25s ea	33358-0011-25	151.27		
30s ea	33358-0011-30	181.53		
35s ea	33358-0011-35	211.79		
(DHS, Inc.)				
REPACK				
CAP, PO, 200 mg, 30s ea	55887-0977-30	29.16		

PROD/MFR	NDC	AWP	DP	OBC
40s ea	**55887-0977-40**	39.95		
TAB, PO, 400 mg, 15s ea	**55887-0246-15**	29.29		
25s ea	**55887-0246-25**	46.67		AB
30s ea	**55887-0246-30**	56.00		EE
40s ea	**55887-0246-40**	70.00		
50s ea	**55887-0246-50**	91.06		EE
60s ea	**55887-0246-60**	81.57		
800 mg, 25s ea	**55887-0853-25**	100.24		EE
30s ea	**55887-0853-30**	120.30		EE
35s ea	**55887-0853-35**	140.33		
50s ea	**55887-0853-50**	200.00		
60s ea	**55887-0853-60**	240.60		EE
90s ea	**55887-0853-90**	360.90		EE
(Dispensing Solutions)				
REPACK				
CAP, PO, 200 mg, 15s ea	**55045-2565-05**	16.80		
25s ea	**55045-2565-02**	28.00		AB
30s ea	**55045-2565-08**	33.60		
30s ea	**66336-0642-30**	34.99		
40s ea	**66336-0642-40**	46.66		AB
50s ea	**55045-2565-04**	56.00		
50s ea	**66336-0642-50**	58.32		
100s ea	**55045-2565-00**	112.00		
TAB, PO, 400 mg, 15s ea	**55045-2571-04**	42.15		AB
15s ea	**66336-0735-15**	39.60		AB
25s ea	**55045-2571-02**	70.25		
25s ea	**66336-0735-25**	65.64		AB
30s ea	**55045-2571-08**	84.30		
40s ea	**66336-0735-40**	104.70		AB
50s ea	**55045-2571-05**	140.50		
60s ea	**55045-2571-06**	168.60		
100s ea	**55045-2571-00**	281.00		
800 mg, 15s ea	**55045-2648-02**	60.00		AB
25s ea	**55045-2648-03**	100.00		
(COMPRESSED)				
800 mg, 30s ea	**66336-0862-30**	151.71		AB
50s ea	**55045-2648-05**	200.00		
50s ea	**66336-0862-50**	252.85		
60s ea	**55045-2648-06**	240.00		
100s ea	**55045-2648-00**	400.00		
(GSMS)				
REPACK				
CAP, PO (UNIT OF USE)				
200 mg, 50s ea	**60429-0711-50**	53.71	6.25	AB
TAB, PO, 800 mg, 50s ea	**60429-0713-50**	175.15	31.18	AB
(HomeMed)				
REPACK				
CAP, PO, 200 mg, 15s ea	**51655-0296-54**	23.19		
25s ea	**51655-0296-76**	40.89		
40s ea	**51655-0296-51**	55.13		
TAB, PO, 400 mg, 15s ea	**51655-0300-54**	32.89		
25s ea	**51655-0300-76**	62.79		
40s ea	**51655-0300-51**	65.09		
(McKesson Packaging)				
REPACK				
CAP, PO, 200 mg,				
100s ea UD	**63739-0314-10**	115.43		
TAB, PO, 400 mg,				
100s ea UD	**63739-0315-10**	223.75		
800 mg, 100s ea UD	**63739-0316-10**	435.25		
(Nucare Pharm)				
REPACK				
CAP, PO, 200 mg, 25s ea	**66267-0006-25**	18.56		EE
40s ea	**66267-0006-40**	25.56		EE
50s ea	**66267-0006-50**	31.95		EE
TAB, PO, 400 mg, 15s ea	**66267-0007-15**	31.36		EE
21s ea	**66267-0007-21**	40.89		AB
25s ea	**66267-0007-25**	48.56		EE
30s ea	**66267-0007-30**	56.99		EE
800 mg, 30s ea	**66267-0399-30**	120.45		
35s ea	**66267-0399-35**	140.53		AB
(Palmetto)				
REPACK				
CAP, PO, 200 mg, 25s ea	**23490-5012-01**	44.40		
30s ea	**23490-5012-02**	53.28		
40s ea	**23490-5012-03**	71.04		
100s ea	**23490-5012-04**	177.60		
SUS, PO, 200 mg/5 ml,				
120 ml	**23490-5011-01**	52.54		
TAB, PO, 400 mg, 15s ea	**23490-5013-01**	28.50		
25s ea	**23490-5013-02**	47.49		
30s ea	**23490-5013-04**	56.99		
40s ea	**23490-5013-03**	75.99		
800 mg, 25s ea	**23490-5015-01**	100.41		
30s ea	**23490-5015-02**	120.49		
(PD-Rx Pharm)				
REPACK				
CAP, PO, 200 mg, 10s ea	**55289-0273-10**	20.49		AB
25s ea	**55289-0273-25**	32.22		AB
30s ea	**55289-0273-30**	34.40		AB

PROD/MFR	NDC	AWP	DP	OBC
35s ea	**55289-0273-35**	39.78		AB
35s ea	**58864-0876-35**	39.76		AB
50s ea	**55289-0273-50**	51.11		AB
TAB, PO, 400 mg, 5s ea	**55289-0462-05**	22.84		AB
12s ea	**55289-0462-12**	26.76		AB
15s ea	**55289-0462-15**	28.48		AB
21s ea	**55289-0462-21**	31.88		AB
25s ea	**55289-0462-25**	34.16		AB
30s ea	**55289-0462-30**	37.00		AB
(REDI-SCRIPT)				
400 mg, 30s ea	**58864-0602-30**	32.00		AB
(USP)				
400 mg, 35s ea	**55289-0462-35**	39.80		AB
60s ea	**55289-0462-60**	50.68		AB
100s ea	**43063-0001-01**	216.91		AB
(REDI-SCRIPT)				
400 mg, 100s ea	**58864-0602-01**	75.56		AB
800 mg, 10s ea	**55289-0629-10**	28.20		AB
20s ea	**55289-0629-20**	36.36		AB
(REDI-SCRIPT)				
800 mg, 25s ea	**58864-0191-25**	56.00		AB
30s ea	**55289-0629-30**	44.56		AB
35s ea	**55289-0629-35**	48.68		AB
(REDI-SCRIPT)				
800 mg, 35s ea	**58864-0191-35**	45.07		AB
(USP)				
800 mg, 40s ea	**55289-0629-40**	52.72		AB
50s ea	**55289-0629-50**	61.00		EE
(Pharma Pac)				
REPACK				
CAP, PO, 200 mg, 25s ea	**52959-0517-25**	17.48		AB
30s ea	**52959-0517-30**	20.10		AB
35s ea	**52959-0517-35**	21.00		AB
TAB, PO, 400 mg, 10s ea	**52959-0544-10**	20.99		AB
12s ea	**52959-0544-12**	24.63		AB
15s ea	**52959-0544-15**	30.15		AB
21s ea	**52959-0544-21**	40.90		AB
25s ea	**52959-0544-25**	48.14		AB
30s ea	**52959-0544-30**	56.98		AB
40s ea	**52959-0544-40**	74.14		AB
50s ea	**52959-0544-50**	90.46		AB
100s ea	**52959-0544-01**	217.00		AB
800 mg, 30s ea	**52959-0678-30**	145.20		
40s ea	**52959-0678-40**	157.26		AB
50s ea	**52959-0678-50**	182.36		AB
(Phys Total Care)				
REPACK				
CAP, PO, 200 mg, 25s ea	**54868-3996-00**	9.03		EE
30s ea	**54868-3996-02**	10.23		EE
40s ea	**54868-3996-01**	12.66		EE
50s ea	**54868-3996-03**	15.06		EE
60s ea	**54868-3996-05**	17.49		EE
100s ea	**54868-3996-04**	27.15		AB
TAB, PO, 400 mg, 10s ea	**54868-3997-03**	5.88		EE
20s ea	**54868-3997-02**	8.76		EE
30s ea	**54868-3997-00**	11.64		EE
40s ea	**54868-3997-04**	14.55		EE
60s ea	**54868-3997-05**	20.31		EE
100s ea	**54868-3997-01**	30.36		EE
800 mg, 15s ea	**54868-3998-02**	12.18		EE
20s ea	**54868-3998-03**	15.24		EE
30s ea	**54868-3998-00**	21.36		EE
35s ea	**54868-3998-06**	24.39		EE
40s ea	**54868-3998-04**	27.45		EE
50s ea	**54868-3998-01**	33.57		EE
60s ea	**54868-3998-08**	39.69		EE
100s ea	**54868-3998-05**	62.64		EE
500s ea	**54868-3998-07**	222.33		EE
(Physician Partner)				
REPACK				
CAP, PO, 200 mg, 25s ea	**21695-0009-25**	48.85		AB
TAB, PO, 400 mg, 20s ea	**21695-0010-20**	86.78		
25s ea	**21695-0010-25**	108.48		AB
30s ea	**21695-0010-30**	130.18		
60s ea	**21695-0010-60**	260.36		
800 mg, 25s ea	**21695-0011-25**	248.04		AB
30s ea	**21695-0011-30**	252.85		AB
35s ea	**21695-0011-35**	397.65		AB
40s ea	**21695-0011-40**	387.14		AB
(Quality Care Prod)				
REPACK				
CAP, PO, 200 mg, 10s ea	**49999-0385-10**	31.20		AB
15s ea	**49999-0385-15**	46.80		AB
25s ea	**49999-0385-25**	78.00		AB
40s ea	**49999-0385-40**	53.74		AB
TAB, PO, 400 mg, 21s ea	**49999-0086-21**	51.37		AB
25s ea	**49999-0086-25**	61.16		EE
30s ea	**49999-0086-30**	65.01		AB
90s ea	**49999-0086-90**	195.03		AB
100s ea	**49999-0086-00**	216.71		EE
800 mg, 35s ea	**49999-0231-35**	158.64		AB

PROD/MFR	NDC	AWP	DP	OBC
(Southwood)				
REPACK				
CAP, PO, 200 mg, 15s ea	**58016-0111-15**	26.64		
20s ea	**58016-0111-20**	35.52		
25s ea	**58016-0111-25**	44.40		
30s ea	**58016-0111-30**	53.28		
60s ea	**58016-0111-60**	106.57		
90s ea	**58016-0111-90**	159.85		
100s ea	**58016-0111-00**	177.61		
TAB, PO, 400 mg, 20s ea	**58016-0112-20**	36.01		AB
30s ea	**58016-0112-30**	54.01		AB
60s ea	**58016-0112-60**	108.02		EE
90s ea	**58016-0112-90**	162.04		AB
100s ea	**58016-0112-00**	180.04		AB
800 mg, 20s ea	**58016-0627-20**	80.27		EE
30s ea	**58016-0627-30**	120.41		EE
60s ea	**58016-0627-60**	240.82		EE
90s ea	**58016-0627-90**	361.23		EE
100s ea	**58016-0627-00**	401.37		EE
(St. Mary's MPP)				
REPACK				
CAP, PO (USP)				
200 mg, 25s ea	**60760-0652-25**	36.78		AB
(Stat Rx)				
REPACK				
TAB, PO, 400 mg, 20s ea	**16590-0370-20**	54.25		
30s ea	**16590-0370-30**	81.38		
40s ea	**16590-0370-40**	100.08		
800 mg, 30s ea	**16590-0003-30**	120.00		
35s ea	**16590-0003-35**	140.00		AB
50s ea	**16590-0003-50**	231.94		AB
60s ea	**16590-0003-60**	240.00		
(Vibranta)				
REPACK				
CAP, PO, 200 mg, 25s ea	**57866-6950-02**	18.60		EE
50s ea	**57866-6950-03**	82.12		EE
ACYCLOVIR SODIUM (APP)				
PDS, IV (VIAL,PF)				
500 mg, ea	**63323-0105-10**	56.51		AP
SOL, IV (S.D.V.,PF)				
50 mg/ml, 10 ml	**63323-0325-10**	22.82		AP
20 ml	**63323-0325-20**	42.59		AP
(Bedford)				
PDS, IV (PF)				
500 mg, 10s ea	**55390-0612-10**	96.00		AP
1000 mg, 10s ea	**55390-0613-20**	192.00		AP
ACZONE (Allergan Inc)				
dapsone				
GEL, TP (1X30GM)				
5%, 30 gm	**00023-3670-30**	165.50		
(1X60GM)				
5%, 60 gm	**00023-3670-60**	313.87		
ADACEL (Sanofi)				
tdap vaccine				
SUS, IM, 0.5 ml 5s	**49281-0400-15**	222.31	187.13	
(S.D.V.,TAX INCL)				
0.5 ml 10s	**49281-0400-10**	444.60	374.25	
ADAGEN (Enzon Pharma, Inc.)				
pegademase bovine				
SOL, IM (VIAL)				
250 u/ml, 1.5 ml	**57665-0001-01**	4375.00		
ADALAT CC (Schering)				
nifedipine				
TER, PO, 30 mg, 100s ea	**00085-1701-02**	161.36		AB1
100s ea UD	**00085-1701-03**	169.42		AB1
1000s ea	**00085-1701-01**	1613.51		AB1
(FILM-COATED)				
60 mg, 100s ea	**00085-1716-02**	287.44		AB1
100s ea UD	**00085-1716-03**	301.79		AB1
1000s ea	**00085-1716-01**	2874.22		AB1
90 mg, 100s ea	**00085-1722-01**	336.86		BC
100s ea UD	**00085-1722-02**	353.75		BC
(PD-Rx Pharm)				
REPACK				
TER, PO, 30 mg, 14s ea	**58864-0669-14**	46.28		AB1
60 mg, 30s ea	**55289-0543-30**	114.42		AB1
90 mg, 30s ea	**55289-0545-30**	133.13		BC
(Phys Total Care)				
REPACK				
TER, PO, 30 mg, 10s ea	**54868-2868-05**	19.88		AB1
30s ea	**54868-2868-01**	56.32		AB1
60s ea	**54868-2868-00**	110.79		AB1
100s ea	**54868-2868-02**	172.68		AB1
60 mg, 30s ea	**54868-2869-03**	98.87		AB1
60s ea	**54868-2869-00**	185.10		AB1
100s ea	**54868-2869-01**	307.25		AB1
90 mg, 30s ea	**54868-2870-00**	115.56		BC

PROD/MFR	NDC	AWP	DP	OBC
ADALIMUMAB				
(Abbott Pharm) *See HUMIRA*				
ADAPALENE				
(Galderma) *See DIFFERIN*				
ADAPALENE/BENZOYL PEROXIDE				
(Galderma) *See EPIDUO*				
ADAPTER, SYRINGE				
(APP) *See UNIVERSAL SYRINGE TIP ADAPTER*				
ADCIRCA (Lilly)				
tadalafil				
TAB, PO (FILM-COATED)				
20 mg, 60s ea	66302-0467-60	1176.48	980.40	
ADDERALL (Teva)				
amphetamine salt combination				
TAB, PO (DYE-FREE)				
5 mg,				
100s ea, C-II	00555-0762-02	360.50		
7.5 mg,				
100s ea, C-II	00555-0763-02	360.50		
10 mg,				
100s ea, C-II	00555-0764-02	360.50		
12.5 mg,				
100s ea, C-II	00555-0765-02	360.50		
15 mg,				
100s ea, C-II	00555-0766-02	360.50		
20 mg,				
100s ea, C-II	00555-0767-02	360.50		
30 mg,				
100s ea, C-II	00555-0768-02	360.50		
(Bryant Ranch)				
REPACK				
TAB, PO, 10 mg,				
30s ea, C-II	63629-3768-01	104.70		
20 mg,				
30s ea, C-II	63629-3769-01	104.70		
(Palmetto)				
REPACK				
TAB, PO, 20 mg,				
30s ea, C-II	23490-7911-03	46.50		
60s ea, C-II	23490-7911-06	93.00		
90s ea, C-II	23490-7911-09	139.50		
(Phys Total Care)				
REPACK				
TAB, PO, 5 mg,				
100s ea, C-II	54868-3976-00	203.41		AB
10 mg,				
10s ea, C-II	54868-3674-02	35.09		AB
30s ea, C-II	54868-3674-01	99.00		AB
100s ea, C-II	54868-3674-00	304.98		AB
20 mg,				
20s ea, C-II	54868-4410-01	58.35		AB
60s ea, C-II	54868-4410-00	168.53		AB
30 mg,				
10s ea, C-II	54868-5470-00	29.68		
30s ea, C-II	54868-5470-01	82.77		
(Stat Rx)				
REPACK				
TAB, PO, 10 mg,				
30s ea, C-II	16590-0739-30	116.49		
20 mg,				
30s ea, C-II	16590-0738-30	116.49		
ADDERALL XR (Shire US Inc.)				
amphetamine salt combination				
CER, PO, 5 mg,				
100s ea, C-II	54092-0381-01	719.42	599.52	EE
10 mg,				
100s ea, C-II	54092-0383-01	719.42	599.52	EE
15 mg,				
100s ea, C-II	54092-0385-01	719.42	599.52	EE
20 mg,				
100s ea, C-II	54092-0387-01	719.42	599.52	EE
25 mg,				
100s ea, C-II	54092-0389-01	719.42	599.52	EE
30 mg,				
100s ea, C-II	54092-0391-01	719.42	599.52	
(Phys Total Care)				
REPACK				
CER, PO, 5 mg,				
10s ea, C-II	54868-5007-01	85.89		EE
30s ea, C-II	54868-5007-00	236.18		EE
60s ea, C-II	54868-5007-02	453.45		EE
10 mg,				
10s ea, C-II	54868-4760-03	85.89		
20s ea, C-II	54868-4760-01	158.76		
30s ea, C-II	54868-4760-02	236.18		
60s ea, C-II	54868-4760-00	468.44		
15 mg,				
10s ea, C-II	54868-5140-01	85.89		EE
30s ea, C-II	54868-5140-00	236.18		EE
20 mg,				
10s ea, C-II	54868-4640-01	85.89		
30s ea, C-II	54868-4640-00	236.18		
60s ea, C-II	54868-4640-02	453.45		
25 mg,				
10s ea, C-II	54868-5368-01	85.89		EE
30s ea, C-II	54868-5368-00	236.18		EE
30 mg,				
10s ea, C-II	54868-5142-01	85.89		
30s ea, C-II	54868-5142-00	236.18		
60s ea, C-II	54868-5142-02	453.45		
(Quality Care Prod)				
REPACK				
CER, PO, 10 mg,				
30s ea, C-II	35356-0147-30	173.69		
90s ea, C-II	35356-0147-90	513.06		
15 mg,				
30s ea, C-II	35356-0148-30	173.69		EE
90s ea, C-II	35356-0148-90	513.06		EE
20 mg,				
30s ea, C-II	35356-0149-30	173.69		
90s ea, C-II	35356-0149-90	513.06		
30 mg,				
30s ea, C-II	35356-0150-30	173.69		
90s ea, C-II	35356-0150-90	513.06		
ADEFOVIR DIPIVOXIL				
(Gilead Sciences) *See HEPSERA*				
ADENOCARD (Astellas)				
adenosine				
SOL, IV (ANSYR,LUER LOK)				
3 mg/ml, 2 ml	00469-8234-12	43.24		
4 ml	00469-8234-14	82.01		
ADENOSCAN (Astellas)				
adenosine				
SOL, IV (S.D.V.,PF)				
3 mg/ml, 20 ml	00469-0871-20	201.72		
30 ml	00469-0871-30	302.58		
(Phys Total Care)				
REPACK				
SOL, IV, 3 mg/ml, 20 ml	54868-5825-01	195.92		
30 ml	54868-5825-00	293.25		
ADENOSINE (APP)				
SOL, IV (PF)				
3 mg/ml, 2 ml 10s	63323-0651-02	136.90		
4 ml 10s	63323-0651-04	273.80		
(Astellas) *See ADENOCARD*				
(Astellas) *See ADENOSCAN*				
(Baxter)				
SOL, IV (SDV,PF)				
3 mg/ml, 2 ml	10019-0063-02	15.30		
(SINGLE DOSE,PF)				
3 mg/ml, 2 ml	10019-0063-34	37.33		
(PF)				
3 mg/ml, 2 ml 10s	10019-0063-03	153.00		
(SINGLE-DOSE SYRINGES,PF)				
3 mg/ml, 2 ml 10s	10019-0063-08	373.32		
(Bedford)				
SOL, IV (S.D.V.)				
3 mg/ml, 2 ml 10s	55390-0067-10	109.20		AP
4 ml	55390-0068-01	17.04		AP
(PCCA)				
POW, NA (9B-RIBOFURANOSYLADENINE)				
1 gm	51927-2116-00	16.80		
(TRIHYDRATE)				
1 gm	51927-2132-00	12.00		
(Sagent)				
SOL, IV (10X2ML,USP,PRF SYRINGE)				
3 mg/ml, 2 ml 10s	25021-0301-72	388.00		AP
(10X2ML,USP,SDV,PF)				
3 mg/ml, 2 ml 10s	25021-0301-02	75.00		AP
(10X4ML,USP,PRF SYRINGE)				
3 mg/ml, 4 ml 10s	25021-0301-76	739.00		AP
(Spectrum Pharmacy)				
POW, NA (USP,1X5GM)				
5 gm	49452-0131-01	129.50		
(USP,1X25GM)				
25 gm	49452-0131-02	243.95		
(USP,1X100GM)				
100 gm	49452-0131-03	549.50		
(Teva)				
SOL, IV (INNER VIAL)				
3 mg/ml, 2 ml	00703-8771-01	16.20		
2 ml 10s	00703-8771-03	162.00		
(USP,10X2ML)				
3 mg/ml, 2 ml 10s	00703-8781-23	255.30		
4 ml	00703-8773-01	32.40		
(Wockhardt USA)				
SOL, IV (1X2ML,SINGLE DOSE,USP)				
3 mg/ml, 2 ml	64679-0630-01	26.59		AP
(10X2ML,SINGLE DOSE,USP)				
3 mg/ml, 2 ml 10s	64679-0630-07	265.94		AP
(1X4ML,SINGLE DOSE,USP)				
3 mg/ml, 4 ml	64679-0630-02	50.45		AP
(10X4ML,SINGLE DOSE,USP)				
3 mg/ml, 4 ml 10s	64679-0630-08	504.51		AP
(A-S Medication)				
REPACK				
SOL, IV, 3 mg/ml, 2 ml	54569-5610-00	32.73		
(Phys Total Care)				
REPACK				
SOL, IV, 3 mg/ml, 2 ml 10s	54868-5551-00	367.98		
ADENOSINE PHOSPHATE				
(Legere) *See MY-O-DEN*				
(Medisca) *See ADENOSINE-5-MONOPHOSPHATE*				
(PCCA) *See ADENOSINE-5-MONOPHOSPHATE*				
ADENOSINE TRIPHOSPHATE				
(Medisca) *See ADENOSINE-5-TRIPHOSPHATE DISODIUM SALT*				
ADENOSINE-5-MONOPHOSPHATE (Medisca)				
adenosine phosphate				
POW, NA, 100 gm	38779-0556-05	10.50		
(PCCA)				
POW, NA, 1 gm	51927-2027-00	6.84		
ADENOSINE-5-TRIPHOSPHATE DISODIUM SALT (Medisca)				
adenosine triphosphate				
POW, NA (1X5GM)				
5 gm	38779-0964-03	39.00		
(1X25GM)				
25 gm	38779-0964-04	178.50		
(1X100GM)				
100 gm	38779-0964-05	520.50		
ADIPEX-P (Gate)				
phentermine hydrochloride				
CAP, PO, 37.5 mg,				
100s ea, C-IV	57844-0019-01	218.81		AA
TAB, PO, 37.5 mg,				
100s ea, C-IV	57844-0009-01	214.97		AA
(A-S Medication)				
REPACK				
TAB, PO, 37.5 mg,				
30s ea, C-IV	54569-1718-00	64.49		AA
(PD-Rx Pharm)				
REPACK				
TAB, PO, 37.5 mg,				
30s ea, C-IV	55289-0379-30	86.93		AA
(Phys Total Care)				
REPACK				
TAB, PO, 37.5 mg,				
10s ea, C-IV	54868-0479-00	29.13		AA
30s ea, C-IV	54868-0479-01	80.84		AA
(Southwood)				
REPACK				
TAB, PO, 37.5 mg,				
30s ea, C-IV	58016-0043-30	61.42		AA
60s ea, C-IV	58016-0043-60	122.84		AA
90s ea, C-IV	58016-0043-90	184.26		AA
100s ea, C-IV	58016-0043-00	204.73		AA
ADIPIC ACID (Spectrum Pharmacy)				
POW, NA (F.C.C.)				
500 gm	49452-0150-01	193.20		
3000 gm	49452-0150-02	360.50		
ADOXA (Doak)				
doxycycline				
CAP, PO (USP)				
150 mg, 60s ea	10337-0815-06	1059.84		
TAB, PO, 50 mg, 100s ea	10337-0800-01	929.00		
75 mg, 100s ea	10337-0801-01	1277.12		
500s ea	10337-0801-50	3669.91		
(PAK 1/100MG,FILM-COATED)				
100 mg, 31s ea	10337-0802-03	306.20		
(FILM-COATED)				
100 mg, 50s ea	10337-0802-05	692.95		
(PAK 2/100MG,FILM-COATED)				
100 mg, 60s ea	10337-0802-06	592.63		
(FILM-COATED)				
100 mg, 250s ea	10337-0802-25	3377.04		
ADOXA CK (Doak)				
doxycycline				
KIT, MR, 150 mg, ea	10337-0819-01	645.95		

PROD/MFR	NDC	AWP	DP	OBC
ADOXA PAK 1/150 (Doak)				
doxycycline				
TAB, PO (DOSE PACK,FILM-COATED)				
150 mg, 30s ea	10337-0814-03	597.90		
ADOXA PAK 1/75 (Doak)				
doxycycline				
TAB, PO (FILM-COATED)				
75 mg, 31s ea	10337-0801-03	392.78		
ADOXA TT (Doak)				
doxycycline				
KIT, MR (FILM-COATED)				
150 mg, ea	10337-0818-01	403.40		
ADRENACLICK (Shionogi)				
epinephrine				
SOL, IJ (0.15MG AUTO-INJECTOR)				
1 mg/ml, ea	59630-0803-01	73.09		
(0.3MG AUTO-INJECTOR)				
1 mg/ml, ea	59630-0804-01	73.09		
(0.15MG AUTO-INJECTOR)				
1 mg/ml, 2s ea	59630-0803-02	146.17		
(0.3MG AUTO-INJECTOR)				
1 mg/ml, 2s ea	59630-0804-02	146.17		
ADRENALIN (JHP)				
epinephrine hydrochloride				
SOL, IJ (1X30ML,MDV)				
1 mg/ml, 30 ml	42023-0101-01	24.80		
NS (1X30ML)				
1:1000, 30 ml	42023-0103-01	24.80		
(Phys Total Care) REPACK				
SOL, IJ (AMP)				
1 mg/ml, 1 ml 10s	54868-1363-00	24.73		
ADRENALIN CHLORIDE (JHP)				
epinephrine				
SOL, IJ (25X1ML,SDV)				
1 mg/ml, 1 ml 25s	42023-0122-25	50.40		
(Dispensing Solutions) REPACK				
epinephrine hydrochloride				
SOL, IJ, 1 mg/ml, 30 ml	55045-3696-03	26.00		
ADRENOCHROME SEMICARBAZONE REAGENT (PCCA)				
carbazochrome				
POW, NA (1X1GM)				
1 gm	51927-2857-00	75.00		
ADREVIEW (GE)				
iobenguane i 123				
SOL, IV, 2 mci/ml, 5 ml	17156-0235-01	2200.00	2200.00	
ADRIAMYCIN (Bedford)				
doxorubicin hydrochloride				
PDS, IV (S.D.V.,PF)				
10 mg, 10s ea	55390-0231-10	132.00		AP
20 mg, 10s ea	55390-0232-10	264.00		AP
50 mg, ea	55390-0233-01	64.80		AP
SOL, IV (S.D.V.)				
2 mg/ml, 5 ml 10s	55390-0235-10	132.00		AP
(S.D.V.,PF)				
2 mg/ml, 10 ml 10s	55390-0236-10	264.00		AP
(S.D.V.)				
2 mg/ml, 25 ml	55390-0237-01	64.80		AP
(M.D.V.)				
2 mg/ml, 100 ml	55390-0238-01	264.00		AP
ADRUCIL (Teva)				
fluorouracil				
SOL, IV (S.D.V.)				
50 mg/ml, 10 ml 10s	00703-3015-13	69.38		AP
(PHARMACY BULK PACKAGE)				
50 mg/ml, 50 ml 5s	00703-3018-12	121.25		AP
100 ml 5s	00703-3019-12	208.12		AP
ADVAIR DISKUS (Dispensing Solutions) REPACK				
fluticasone propionate/salmeterol xinafoate				
DSK, IH, 60s ea	55045-3686-01	210.00		
(Palmetto) REPACK				
DSK, IH, 60s ea	23490-7541-01	200.00		
60s ea	23490-7542-01	250.00		
(Southwood) REPACK				
DSK, IH, 60s ea	58016-4812-01	146.22		
ADVAIR DISKUS 100/50 (Glaxo)				
fluticasone propionate/salmeterol xinafoate				
DSK, IH, 14s ea	00173-0695-04	92.40		
60s ea	00173-0695-00	193.07		
(A-S Medication) REPACK				
DSK, IH, 60s ea	54569-5241-00	239.04		
(Dispensing Solutions) REPACK				
DSK, IH, 60s ea	55045-3388-01	168.00		
(Phys Total Care) REPACK				
DSK, IH, 60s ea	54868-4518-00	230.50		
(Quality Care Prod) REPACK				
DSK, IH, 60s ea	49999-0984-60	260.60		
ADVAIR DISKUS 250/50 (Glaxo)				
fluticasone propionate/salmeterol xinafoate				
DSK, IH, 14s ea	00173-0696-04	92.40		
60s ea	00173-0696-00	239.88		
(A-S Medication) REPACK				
DSK, IH, 60s ea	54569-5242-00	297.00		
(Phys Total Care) REPACK				
DSK, IH, 60s ea	54868-4517-00	285.93		
(Physician Partner) REPACK				
DSK, IH, 60s ea	21695-0196-01	475.96		
(Quality Care Prod) REPACK				
DSK, IH, 60s ea	49999-0819-60	310.40		
(Southwood) REPACK				
DSK, IH, 28s ea	58016-4601-01	217.57		
28s ea	58016-4604-01	163.41		
ADVAIR DISKUS 500/50 (Glaxo)				
fluticasone propionate/salmeterol xinafoate				
DSK, IH, 14s ea	00173-0697-04	150.61		
60s ea	00173-0697-00	315.52		
(A-S Medication) REPACK				
DSK, IH, 60s ea	54569-5243-00	390.64		
(Phys Total Care) REPACK				
DSK, IH, 60s ea	54868-4516-00	375.45		
(Physician Partner) REPACK				
DSK, IH, 60s ea	21695-0197-01	626.02		
(Quality Care Prod) REPACK				
DSK, IH, 60s ea	49999-0985-60	450.45		
(Southwood) REPACK				
DSK, IH, 60s ea	58016-4813-01	300.49		
ADVAIR HFA (Glaxo)				
fluticasone propionate/salmeterol xinafoate				
AER, IH (ADVAIR HFA 45/21)				
8 gm	00173-0715-22	129.38		
12 gm	00173-0715-20	193.07		
(ADVAIR HFA 115/21)				
8 gm	00173-0716-22	129.38		
12 gm	00173-0716-20	239.88		
(ADVAIR HFA 230/21)				
8 gm	00173-0717-22	191.89		
12 gm	00173-0717-20	315.52		
(Palmetto) REPACK				
AER, IH, 12 gm	23490-7540-01	250.00		
ADVATE (Baxter Bioscience)				
antihemophilic factor (recomb) plasma/albumin-free				
PDS, IV (2400-3600,PF)				
1 iu, ea	00944-2946-10	1.68		
(AP 250IU/VIAL,W/DILUENT)				
1 iu, ea	00944-2941-10	1.68		
(AP 500IU/VIAL,W/DILUENT)				
1 iu, ea	00944-2942-10	1.68		
(AP1000IU/VIAL,W/DILUENT)				
1 iu, ea	00944-2943-10	1.68		
(AP1500IU/VIAL,W/DILUENT)				
1 iu, ea	00944-2944-10	1.68		
(AP2000IU/VIAL,W/DILUENT)				
1 iu, ea	00944-2945-10	1.68		
ADVICOR (Abbott Pharm)				
lovastatin/niacin				
TER, PO, 20 mg-500 mg,				
90s ea	00074-3005-90	326.33	286.25	
20 mg-750 mg,				
90s ea	00074-3072-90	350.02	307.03	
20 mg-1000 mg,				
90s ea	00074-3007-90	375.23	329.15	
(COATED)				
40 mg-1000 mg,				
90s ea	00074-3010-90	434.42	381.07	
(Phys Total Care) REPACK				
TER, PO, 20 mg-500 mg,				
30s ea	54868-4807-01	149.35		
60s ea	54868-4807-00	279.79		
20 mg-750 mg,				
30s ea	54868-4999-01	94.50		
60s ea	54868-4999-00	176.83		
90s ea	54868-4807-02	417.73		
20 mg-1000 mg,				
30s ea	54868-5087-00	145.93		
40 mg-1000 mg,				
30s ea	54868-5653-00	187.11		
AERO OTIC HC (Adamis)				
chloroxylenol/hc/pramoxine hcl				
SOL, OT, 10 ml	38739-3767-01	14.27		
AEROBID (Forest Pharm)				
flunisolide				
ARO, IH, 0.25 mg/actuation,				
7 gm	00456-0672-99	98.03		
(Dispensing Solutions) REPACK				
ARO, IH, 0.25 mg/actuation,				
7 gm	55045-1868-03	107.00		
(Phys Total Care) REPACK				
ARO, IH, 0.25 mg/actuation,				
7 gm	54868-1883-01	95.84		
AEROBID M (Dispensing Solutions) REPACK				
flunisolide				
ARO, IH, 0.25 mg/actuation,				
7 gm	55045-2520-07	107.00		
AEROBID-M (Forest Pharm)				
flunisolide				
ARO, IH (MENTHOL)				
0.25 mg/actuation,				
7 gm	00456-0670-99	98.03		
(Phys Total Care) REPACK				
ARO, IH (MENTHOL)				
0.25 mg/actuation,				
7 gm	54868-5294-00	243.63		
AEROCHAMBER (Forest Pharm)				
spacer, inhalation				
DEV, NA, ea	00456-3154-67	39.62		
(W/MASK, LARGE)				
ea	00456-0746-13	53.42		
(W/MASK,SMALL)				
ea	00456-0744-13	53.42		
(W/MASK)				
ea	00456-0745-13	53.42		
(A-S Medication) REPACK				
DEV, NA, ea	54569-2294-00	41.28		
(W/MASK, SMALL)				
ea	54569-4344-00	55.65		
(Phys Total Care) REPACK				
DEV, NA (VHC W/FLOW SIGNAL)				
ea	54868-4519-00	49.18		
AEROCHAMBER Z-STAT PLUS (Monaghan Medical)				
spacer, inhalation				
DEV, NA (VHC W/FLOWSIGNAL)				
ea	04351-0797-10	9.50		
(VHC W/MASK,LARGE)				
ea	04351-0807-10	17.50		
(VHC W/MASK,MEDIUM)				
ea	04351-0787-10	16.00		
(VHC W/MASK,SMALL)				
ea	04351-0887-10	16.00		
AEROECLIPSE NEBULIZER (Monaghan Medical)				
nebulizer, direct patient interface				
DEV, NA (BREATH ACTIVATED)				
ea	04351-0440-50	5.40		
AEROHIST (Adamis)				
chlorpheniramine maleate/methscopolamine nitrate				
TER, PO (CAPLET)				
8 mg-2.5 mg,				
100s ea	38739-0082-51	135.99		

PROD/MFR	NDC	AWP	DP	OBC
AEROHIST PLUS (Adamis)				
cpm/methscopolamine nitrate/phenyleph hcl				
TER, PO (CAPLET)				
8 mg-2.5 mg-20 mg,				
100s ea	38739-2376-01	68.25		
AEROKID (Adamis)				
cpm/methscopolamine nitrate/phenyleph hcl				
SYR, PO (BLUE RASPBERRY)				
118 ml	38739-0110-02	138.60		
473 ml	38739-0110-03	138.60		
AEROPEP PLUS (Monaghan Medical)				
spacer, inhalation				
DEV, NA (VHC,PEP COMBO)				
ea	04351-0475-00	11.00		
10s ea	04351-0475-10	110.00		
AEROSIL 200 (Amend)				
silicon dioxide				
POW, NA, 4540 gm	17317-1187-06	129.50		
AEROTRACH PLUS (Monaghan Medical)				
spacer, inhalation				
DEV, NA (VHC)				
ea	04351-0525-10	9.00		
AEROVENT CHC (Monaghan Medical)				
device, inhalation				
DEV, NA, ea	04351-0859-50	4.50		
(W/ ADAPTERS)				
50s ea	04351-0859-55	240.00		
AFEDITAB CR (Watson Labs)				
nifedipine				
TER, PO (FILM-COATED)				
30 mg, 100s ea	00591-3193-01	103.81		AB1
500s ea	00591-3193-05	493.10		AB1
60 mg, 100s ea	00591-3194-01	195.11		AB
500s ea	00591-3194-05	926.76		AB
(PD-Rx Pharm) REPACK				
TER, PO (REDI-SCRIPT,USP)				
30 mg, 100s ea	58864-0966-01	103.96		
AFINITOR (Novartis Pharm)				
everolimus				
TAB, PO (INNER PACK)				
5 mg, ea	00078-0566-61	234.76		
28s ea	00078-0566-51	6573.07		
(INNER PACK)				
10 mg, ea	00078-0567-61	247.58		
28s ea	00078-0567-51	6932.26		
AFLAXEN (Intl Ethical)				
naproxen sodium				
TAB, PO, 550 mg,				
100s ea UD	11584-0465-01	95.77		EE
AFLURIA (CSL Biotherapies)				
influenza virus vaccine				
SUS, IM (10X0.5ML,2009-2010,PF)				
45 mcg/0.5 ml,				
0.5 ml 10s	33332-0009-01	172.50	145.00	
(1X5ML,2009-2010,MDV)				
45 mcg/0.5 ml,				
5 ml	33332-0109-10	130.50	110.00	
AFRICAN PYGEUM BARK (PCCA) *See PYGEUM BARK*				
AGALSIDASE BETA (Genzyme) *See FABRAZYME*				
AGAR (Medisca)				
POW, NA (N.F.)				
100 gm	38779-0965-05	31.50		
500 gm	38779-0965-08	87.00		
(PCCA)				
POW, NA (NF)				
1 gm	51927-1421-00	0.42		
(Spectrum Pharmacy)				
GRA, NA (U.S.P./N.F.)				
500 gm	49452-0170-02	281.05		
2500 gm	49452-0170-03	1130.50		
POW, NA, 500 gm	49452-0180-02	255.50		
AGGRASTAT (Medicure)				
tirofiban hydrochloride				
SOL, IV (1X100ML)				
0.05 mg/ml, 100 ml	25208-0002-01	287.55		
(1X250ML)				
0.05 mg/ml, 250 ml	25208-0002-02	602.10		
AGGRENOX (Boehr Ingelheim Phar)				
aspirin/dipyridamole				
CER, PO, 25 mg-200 mg,				
60s ea	00597-0001-60	194.95		
(Phys Total Care) REPACK				
CER, PO, 25 mg-200 mg,				
60s ea	54868-5143-00	232.74		
(Physician Partner) REPACK				
CER, PO, 25 mg-200 mg,				
60s ea	21695-0656-60	372.62		
(Quality Care Prod) REPACK				
CER, PO, 25 mg-200 mg,				
60s ea	49999-0919-60	256.76		
AGRIFLU (Novartis)				
influenza virus vaccine				
SUS, IM (PF,LATEX-FREE)				
45 mcg/0.5 ml,				
0.5 ml 10s	46028-0108-01	92.50	92.50	
AGRYLIN (Shire US Inc.)				
anagrelide hydrochloride				
CAP, PO, 0.5 mg, 100s ea	54092-0063-01	675.44	562.87	
AH-CHEW (Dexo)				
cpm/methscopolamine nitrate/phenyleph hcl				
CTB, PO, 2 mg-1.25 mg-10 mg,				
100s ea	59196-0003-01	57.60		
AH-CHEW D (Dexo)				
phenylephrine hydrochloride				
CTB, PO (BUBBLEGUM)				
10 mg, 100s ea	59196-0007-01	57.60		
AHF HUMAN/VON WILLEBRAND FACTOR (CSL) *See HUMATE-P*				
(Grifols USA, Inc.) *See ALPHANATE*				
(Octapharma USA) *See WILATE*				
AHF VIII (RECOMBINANT) SUCROSE FORMULATED (CSL) *See HELIXATE FS*				
AHIST (MAGNA Pharm)				
chlorpheniramine tannate				
TAB, PO, 12 mg, 100s ea	58407-0012-01	110.40	78.86	
AIMSCO (Delta Hi-Tech)				
insulin syringe/needle				
DEV, NA (28G,0.5CC,1/2")				
100s ea	51709-0005-02	17.55		
(28G,1CC,1/2")				
100s ea	51709-0005-03	17.55		
(29G,0.5CC,1/2",10/10'S)				
100s ea	51709-0005-28	21.05		
(29G,1CC,1/2",10/10'S)				
100s ea	51709-0005-29	21.05		
AIMSCO ULTRA-THIN II (Delta Hi-Tech)				
insulin syringe/needle				
DEV, NA ((3/10CC,29GX1/2")				
100s ea	51709-0007-24	22.10		
((3/10CC,30GX5/16")				
100s ea	51709-0007-22	24.20		
(30G,1CC,5/16")				
100s ea	51709-0006-20	23.10		
(30G,5CC,5/16")				
100s ea	51709-0006-18	23.10		
AK-CIDE (Phys Total Care) REPACK				
prednisolone acetate/sulfacetamide sodium				
OIN, OP, 0.5%-10%, 4 gm	54868-3696-00	8.47		AT
AK-CON (Akorn)				
naphazoline hydrochloride				
SOL, OP, 0.1%, 15 ml	17478-0216-12	7.13		AT
(Altura) REPACK				
SOL, OP, 0.1%, 15 ml	63874-0198-15	19.89		AT
(Phys Total Care) REPACK				
SOL, OP, 0.1%, 15 ml	54868-2109-00	10.56		AT
AK-DILATE (Akorn)				
phenylephrine hydrochloride				
SOL, OP, 2.5%, 2 ml	17478-0200-20	4.10		
15 ml	17478-0200-12	6.70		
10%, 5 ml	17478-0205-10	6.70		
AK-FLUOR (Akorn)				
fluorescein sodium				
SOL, IV (S.D.V.)				
10%, 5 ml	17478-0253-10	7.80		
25%, 2 ml	17478-0250-20	7.80		
AK-PENTOLATE (Akorn)				
cyclopentolate hydrochloride				
SOL, OP, 1%, 2 ml	17478-0100-20	5.35		AT
15 ml	17478-0100-12	10.61		AT
(Physician Partner) REPACK				
SOL, OP (1X15ML)				
1%, 15 ml	21695-0883-15	21.22		AT
AK-POLY-BAC (Akorn)				
bacitracin zinc/polymyxin b sulfate				
OIN, OP (PF)				
500 u/gm-10000 u/gm,				
3.5 gm	17478-0238-35	25.70		AT
(Pharma Pac) REPACK				
OIN, OP (PF)				
500 u/gm-10000 u/gm,				
3.5 gm	52959-0618-05	34.97		AT
AK-TROL (Phys Total Care) REPACK				
dexamethasone/neomycin sulfate/polymyxin b sulfate				
OIN, OP, 3.5 gm	54868-2943-00	10.22		EE
AKINETON (Phys Total Care)				
biperiden hydrochloride				
TAB, PO, 2 mg, 100s ea	54868-2432-00	37.07		
AKNE-MYCIN (Valeant Pharm Intl)				
erythromycin				
OIN, TP, 2%, 25 gm	13548-0030-25	103.12		
AKTEN (Akorn)				
lidocaine hydrochloride				
GEL, OP (1X5ML,PF)				
3.5%, 5 ml	17478-0792-10	37.49		
AKTOB (Akorn)				
tobramycin				
SOL, OP, 0.3%, 5 ml	17478-0290-10	14.25		AT
AKURZA (Auriga)				
salicylic acid				
CRE, TP, 6%, 340 gm	14629-0501-12	125.00		
LOT, TP, 6%, 355 ml	14629-0502-12	125.00		
ALA-CORT (Del-Ray)				
hydrocortisone				
CRE, TP, 1%, 30 gm	00316-0126-01	12.46		AT
90 gm	00316-0126-03	19.96		AT
ALA-HIST (Poly)				
bpm/diphenhydramine hcl				
TER, PO, 6 mg-25 mg,				
100s ea	50991-0527-01	95.94	79.95	
ALA-HIST AC (Poly)				
codeine phosphate/phenylephrine hydrochloride				
SOL, PO (1X473ML,TUTTI FRUTTI)				
10 mg/5 ml-7.5 mg/5 ml,				
473 ml, C-V	50991-0901-16	86.46	69.17	
ALA-HIST D (Poly)				
bpm/diphenhydramine hcl/phenyleph hcl				
TER, PO, 6 mg-25 mg-20 mg,				
100s ea	50991-0513-01	95.94	79.95	
ALA-QUIN (Del-Ray)				
clioquinol/hydrocortisone				
CRE, TP, 3%-0.5%, 30 gm	00316-0123-01	29.46		
ALA-SCALP HP (Del-Ray)				
hydrocortisone				
LOT, TP, 2%, 30 ml	00316-0140-01	31.18		
ALACOL (Ballay Pharm., Inc)				
bpm/phenyleph hcl				
SOL, PO (W/DROPPER,2X30ML,AF,SF)				
0.4 mg/ml-1 mg/ml,				
30 ml 2s	63162-0517-60	31.59	27.47	
(AF,SF,BLACK RASPBERRY)				
2 mg/5 ml-5 mg/5 ml,				
473 ml	63162-0515-16	77.30	67.22	
ALACOL DM (Ballay Pharm., Inc)				
bpm/dm/phenyleph hcl				
SOL, PO (W/DROPPER,2X30ML,AF,SF)				
30 ml 2s	63162-0516-60	32.92	28.62	
SYR, PO (AF,SF,BLACK RASPBERRY)				
473 ml	63162-0507-16	85.64	74.47	
ALAGESIC (Poly)				
acetaminophen/butalbital/caffeine				
CAP, PO, 325 mg-50 mg-40 mg,				
100s ea	50991-0302-01	56.24	46.85	EE
ALAGESIC LQ (Poly)				
acetaminophen/butalbital/caffeine				
SOL, PO (1X473ML)				
473 ml	50991-0514-16	124.99	99.99	
ALAHIST DHC (Poly)				
dihydrocodeine bitartrate/phenyleph hcl				
SOL, PO (1X473ML,MANGO CANDY)				
3 mg/5 ml-7.5 mg/5 ml,				
473 ml, C-V	50991-0325-16	86.46	69.17	

PROD/MFR	NDC	AWP	DP	OBC
ALAHIST DM (Poly)				
bpm/dm/phenyleph hcl				
SOL, PO (1X473ML,AF,SF,DYE-FREE)				
473 ml	**50991-0814-16**	74.35	59.48	
ALAHIST LQ (Poly)				
diphenhydramine hcl/phenyleph hcl				
SOL, PO (1X473ML,AF,SF)				
25 mg/5 ml-7.5 mg/5 ml, 473 ml	**50991-0607-16**	74.35	59.48	
ALAMAST (Vistakon)				
pemirolast potassium				
SOL, OP, 0.1%, 10 ml	**68669-0711-10**	113.88		
ALANINE				
(Amend) *See DL-ALANINE*				
(Amend) *See L-ALANINE*				
(PCCA)				
POW, NA, 1 gm	**51927-3060-00**	24.00		
(BETA) 1 gm	**51927-2499-00**	0.36		
(FCC) 1 gm	**51927-3357-00**	1.68		
(USP) 1 gm	**51927-2579-00**	1.26		
(Spectrum Pharmacy) *See D-ALANINE*				
(Spectrum Pharmacy) *See DL-ALANINE*				
(Spectrum Pharmacy) *See L-ALANINE*				
ALBA PROTOPET (Amend)				
petrolatum				
POW, NA (U.S.P.)				
454 gm	**17317-1048-01**	4.90		
3178 gm	**17317-1048-06**	21.00		
16344 gm	**17317-1048-08**	88.20		
ALBA-DERM (Pharmaceutica North)				
cream base				
CRE, NA (1X1GM)				
1 gm	**45861-0002-00**	2.15		
ALBENDAZOLE				
(Glaxo) *See ALBENZA*				
(Medisca)				
POW, NA (U.S.P.)				
100 gm	**38779-0772-05**	147.00		
500 gm	**38779-0772-08**	199.50		
1000 gm	**38779-0772-09**	435.00		
(PCCA)				
POW, NA (USP)				
1 gm	**51927-1763-00**	5.52		
(Spectrum Pharmacy)				
POW, NA (U.S.P.)				
25 gm	**49452-0003-02**	144.90		
100 gm	**49452-0003-03**	395.50		
1000 gm	**49452-0003-05**	679.00		
ALBENZA (Glaxo)				
albendazole				
TAB, PO, 200 mg, 112s ea	**00007-5500-40**	176.93		
(Southwood) REPACK				
TAB, PO, 200 mg, 30s ea	**00490-0055-30**	47.39		
60s ea	**00490-0055-60**	94.78		
90s ea	**00490-0055-90**	142.18		
100s ea	**00490-0055-00**	157.97		
112s ea	**00490-0055-92**	176.93		
ALBUMARC (Amer Red Cross-Blood)				
albumin human				
SOL, IV, 5%, 250 ml	**52769-0450-25**	98.50		
500 ml	**52769-0450-50**	197.00		
25%, 50 ml	**52769-0451-05**	98.50		
100 ml	**52769-0451-10**	197.00		
ALBUMIN (Octapharma USA)				
albumin human				
SOL, IV (SINGLE USE,PF)				
5%, 100 ml	**67467-0623-01**	30.00		
250 ml	**67467-0623-02**	75.00		
(25GM,SINGLE USE,PF) 5%, 500 ml	**67467-0623-03**	150.00		
(12.5GM,SINGLE USE,PF) 25%, 50 ml	**67467-0643-01**	64.50		
(25GM/,SINGLE USE,PF) 25%, 100 ml	**67467-0643-02**	129.00		
ALBUMIN BOVINE				
(Spectrum Pharmacy) *See ALBUMIN BOVINE FRACTION V*				
ALBUMIN BOVINE FRACTION V (Spectrum Pharmacy)				
albumin bovine				
POW, NA (LYOPHILIZED)				
10 gm	**49452-0223-01**	212.80		
100 gm	**49452-0223-02**	847.00		
ALBUMIN HUMAN				
(Alpine Biologics) *See ALBUMIN-ALPINE*				
(Amer Red Cross-Blood) *See ALBUMARC*				
(Amer Red Cross-Blood)				
SOL, IV (PF)				
5%, 250 ml	**52769-0250-25**	98.50		
500 ml	**52769-0250-50**	197.00		
25%, 50 ml	**52769-0251-05**	98.50		
100 ml	**52769-0251-10**	197.00		
(Baxter Bioscience) *See BUMINATE*				
(Baxter Bioscience) *See FLEXBUMIN*				
(CSL) *See ALBUMINAR-25*				
(CSL) *See ALBUMINAR-5*				
(CSL) *See ALBURX*				
(Grifols USA, Inc.) *See ALBUTEIN*				
(Octapharma USA) *See ALBUMIN*				
(Talecris) *See PLASBUMIN-25*				
(Talecris) *See PLASBUMIN-5*				
ALBUMIN-ALPINE (Alpine Biologics)				
albumin human				
SOL, IV (W/ADMIN. SET/SAFETY NDL)				
5%, 250 ml	**63546-0310-25**	99.00		
500 ml	**63546-0310-50**	198.00		
25%, 50 ml	**63546-0251-05**	99.00		
100 ml	**63546-0251-10**	198.00		
ALBUMIN, IODINATED I-131				
(Daxor Corp) *See VOLUMEX*				
ALBUMINAR-25 (CSL)				
albumin human				
SOL, IV, 25%, 50 ml	**00053-7680-32**	112.50		
(W/OUT IV SETS) 25%, 100 ml	**00053-7680-33**	225.00		
ALBUMINAR-5 (CSL)				
albumin human				
SOL, IV, 5%, 250 ml	**00053-7670-31**	112.50		
500 ml	**00053-7670-32**	225.00		
ALBURX (CSL)				
albumin human				
SOL, IV, 5%, 250 ml	**44206-0310-25**	58.00		
500 ml	**44206-0310-50**	116.00		
25%, 50 ml	**44206-0251-05**	58.00		
100 ml	**44206-0251-10**	116.00		
ALBUTEIN (Grifols USA, Inc.)				
albumin human				
SOL, IV (1X250ML,SINGLE-DOSE)				
5%, 250 ml	**68516-5214-01**	108.00	90.00	
(1X500ML,SINGLE-DOSE) 5%, 500 ml	**68516-5214-02**	216.00	180.00	
25%, 50 ml	**61953-0002-01**	108.00	90.00	
(1X50ML,SINGLE-DOSE) 25%, 50 ml	**68516-5216-01**	108.00	90.00	
100 ml	**61953-0002-02**	216.00	180.00	
(1X100ML,SINGLE-DOSE) 25%, 100 ml	**68516-5216-02**	216.00	180.00	
ALBUTEROL (PCCA)				
POW, NA (U.S.P.)				
1 gm	**51927-2859-00**	10.32		
(Spectrum Pharmacy)				
POW, NA (U.S.P.)				
5 gm	**49452-0225-03**	164.15		
25 gm	**49452-0225-01**	497.00		
(Altura) REPACK				
ARO, IH, 0.09 mg/actuation, 17 gm	**63874-0749-17**	31.71		EE
(Bryant Ranch) REPACK				
albuterol sulfate				
SYR, PO, 2 mg/5 ml,				
120 ml	**63629-1828-01**	13.86		
240 ml	**63629-1828-02**	27.72		
TAB, PO, 4 mg, 20s ea	**63629-2611-01**	10.79		
30s ea	**63629-2611-02**	20.99		
30s ea	**63629-2736-01**	18.83		
ALBUTEROL (DHS, Inc.) REPACK				
ARO, IH, 0.09 mg/actuation, 17 gm	**55887-0812-18**	29.82		BN
(DHS, Inc.)				
albuterol sulfate				
SOL, IH, 0.5%, 20 ml	**55887-0382-20**	19.96		
ALBUTEROL (Dispensing Solutions) REPACK				
ARO, IH, 0.09 mg/actuation, 17 gm	**55045-2390-05**	32.00		AB
(HomeMed) REPACK				
albuterol sulfate				
TAB, PO, 2 mg, 30s ea	**51655-0563-24**	8.10		
90s ea	**51655-0563-26**	24.30		
ALBUTEROL (Nucare Pharm) REPACK				
ARO, IH, 0.09 mg/actuation, 17 gm	**66267-0995-17**	25.95		EE
(Palmetto) REPACK				
ARO, IH, 0.09 mg/actuation,				
8.5 gm	**23490-7022-01**	36.72		
17 gm	**23490-5019-01**	39.99		
(Pharma Pac) REPACK				
albuterol sulfate				
TAB, PO, 4 mg, 20s ea	**52959-0906-20**	11.10		
ALBUTEROL (Phys Total Care) REPACK				
ARO, IH, 0.09 mg/actuation, 17 gm	**54868-3709-00**	58.44		EE
(Phys Total Care)				
albuterol sulfate				
SOL, IH (30X3ML)				
0.042%, 3 ml 30s	**54868-5709-00**	137.46		
ALBUTEROL (Southwood) REPACK				
ARO, IH, 0.09 mg/actuation, 17 gm	**58016-6569-01**	35.70		EE
(Stat Rx) REPACK				
ARO, IH, 0.09 mg/actuation, 17 gm	**16590-0004-17**	39.85		
(Vibranta) REPACK				
ARO, IH, 0.09 mg/actuation, 17 gm	**57866-0051-01**	29.95		
ALBUTEROL HFA (Phys Total Care) REPACK				
albuterol sulfate				
ARO, IH, 0.09 mg/actuation, 8.5 gm	**54868-5646-00**	99.97		
ALBUTEROL INHALER (Physician Partner) REPACK				
albuterol				
ARO, IH, 0.09 mg/actuation, 17 gm	**21695-0198-01**	42.82		
ALBUTEROL SULFATE FUL				
SOL, IH, 0.083%, 3 ml		0.35		
0.5%, 20 ml		4.67		
TAB, PO, 4 mg, 100s ea		14.25		
(Actavis Mid Atlantic)				
SYR, PO (BERRY)				
2 mg/5 ml, 120 ml	**00472-0825-04**	11.07		AA
473 ml	**00472-0825-16**	40.15		AA
(Bausch & Lomb Inc.)				
SOL, IH (STERILE)				
0.5%, 20 ml	**24208-0347-20**	17.00		AN
(Dava Pharma)				
TER, PO (COATED)				
4 mg, 100s ea	**68774-0400-01**	140.23		
8 mg, 100s ea	**68774-0401-01**	262.94		
(Dava Pharma) *See VOSPIRE*				
(Dey, L.P.) *See ACCUNEB*				
(Dey, L.P.)				
SOL, IH (VIAL)				
0.083%, 3 ml 25s UD	**49502-0697-24**	30.25		AN
(SINGLE-PAK) 0.083%, 3 ml 30s UD	**49502-0697-30**	36.90		AN
(VIAL) 0.083%, 3 ml 30s UD	**49502-0697-29**	36.30		AN
3 ml 60s UD	**49502-0697-61**	72.60		AN
(Gallipot)				
POW, NA (U.S.P.,N.F.)				
5 gm	**51552-0044-02**	11.20		

PROD/MFR	NDC	AWP	DP	OBC
(U.S.P.)				
25 gm	51552-0044-04	32.20		
(U.S.P.,N.F.)				
100 gm	51552-0044-05	98.00		
500 gm	51552-0044-06	392.00	280.00	
1000 gm	51552-0044-07	595.00		
(Glaxo) *See NOVAPLUS VENTOLIN HFA*				
(Glaxo) *See RELION VENTOLIN HFA*				
(Glaxo) *See VENTOLIN HFA*				
(Hawkins)				
POW, NA (U.S.P.)				
25 gm	63370-0010-25	76.80		
100 gm	63370-0010-35	254.40		
500 gm	63370-0010-45	1056.00		
1000 gm	63370-0010-50	1992.00		
(Hi-Tech)				
SOL, IH, 0.5%, 20 ml	50383-0741-20	16.50		AN
SYR, PO, 2 mg/5 ml, 473 ml	50383-0740-16	39.60		AA
(Letco)				
POW, NA (U.S.P.)				
25 gm	62991-1006-01	48.00		
100 gm	62991-1006-02	159.00		
500 gm	62991-1006-03	660.00		
(U.S.P., MICRONIZED)				
1000 gm	62991-1006-04	1245.00		
(Major)				
SOL, IH, 0.5%, 20 ml	00904-7658-55	16.80		AN
(Medisca)				
POW, NA (USP,1X10GM)				
10 gm	38779-0185-01	37.50		
(U.S.P.)				
25 gm	38779-0185-04	76.50		
100 gm	38779-0185-05	217.50		
500 gm	38779-0185-08	660.00		
1000 gm	38779-0185-09	1245.00		
(Mutual)				
TAB, PO, 2 mg, 100s ea	53489-0176-01	31.14		AB
500s ea	53489-0176-05	154.18		AB
4 mg, 100s ea	53489-0177-01	45.76		AB
500s ea	53489-0177-05	224.20		AB
(Mylan)				
SOL, IH (5X5)				
0.083%, 3 ml 25s UD	00378-6990-52	33.28		AN
(1X30)				
0.083%, 3 ml 30s UD	00378-6990-93	46.98		AN
(6X5)				
0.083%, 3 ml 30s UD	00378-6990-58	39.93		AN
(12X5)				
0.083%, 3 ml 60s UD	00378-6990-91	79.86		AN
(25X3ML,PF)				
0.63 mg/3 ml, 3 ml 25s UD	00378-6991-52	41.50		
1.25 mg/3 ml, 3 ml 25s UD	00378-6992-52	41.50		
TAB, PO, 2 mg, 100s ea	00378-0255-01	31.14		AB
500s ea	00378-0255-05	154.18		AB
4 mg, 100s ea	00378-0572-01	45.76		AB
500s ea	00378-0572-05	224.20		AB
TER, PO (FILM-COATED)				
4 mg, 100s ea	00378-4122-01	121.95		AB
8 mg, 100s ea	00378-4124-01	228.65		AB
(Nephron)				
SOL, IH (LDPE VIAL)				
0.042%, 3 ml 25s UD	00487-9904-25	41.50		AN
(PF)				
0.042%, 3 ml 30s UD	00487-9904-01	49.80		AN
(ROBOT READY,LDPE VIAL)				
0.042%, 3 ml 30s UD	00487-9904-02	53.55		AN
(PF)				
0.083%, 3 ml 25s UD	00487-9501-25	20.00		AN
3 ml 30s UD	00487-9501-01	24.00		AN
3 ml 30s UD	00487-9501-03	24.00		AN
(ROBOT READY,PF)				
0.083%, 3 ml 30s UD	00487-9501-02	24.00		AN
(PF)				
0.083%, 3 ml 60s UD	00487-9501-60	48.00		AN
(UNIT OF USE,PF)				
0.5%, 30s ea	00487-9901-30	27.00		AN
(UNIT OF USE,ROBOT READY)				
0.5%, 30s ea	00487-9901-02	30.00		AN
(PCCA)				
POW, NA (U.S.P.)				
1 gm	51927-1573-00	6.90		
(Prasco Labs)				
SYR, PO (1X473ML,STRAWBERRY)				
2 mg/5 ml, 473 ml	66993-0230-57	30.79		
(Qualitest)				
SYR, PO (STRAWBERRY)				
2 mg/5 ml, 473 ml	00603-1008-58	30.79		AA
(Schering) *See PROVENTIL*				
(Schering) *See PROVENTIL HFA*				
(Spectrum Pharmacy)				
POW, NA (U.S.P.)				
25 gm	49452-0227-02	133.00		
100 gm	49452-0227-03	329.35		
(Teva) *See PROAIR HFA*				
(Teva)				
SYR, PO, 2 mg/5 ml, 473 ml	00093-0661-16	30.79		AA
(UDL)				
TAB, PO (10X10)				
2 mg, 100s ea UD	51079-0657-20	32.07		AB
4 mg, 100s ea UD	51079-0658-20	47.13		AB
(Watson Labs)				
SOL, IH (25X3ML,PF)				
0.021%, 3 ml 25s UD	00591-3467-53	39.84		AN
0.042%, 3 ml 25s UD	00591-3468-53	39.84		AN
(25X3ML,LDPE)				
0.083%, 3 ml 25s UD	16252-0097-22	4.50		
(30X3ML,LDPE)				
0.083%, 3 ml 30s UD	16252-0097-33	5.40		
(60X3ML,LDPE)				
0.083%, 3 ml 60s UD	16252-0097-66	10.80		
(A-S Medication) REPACK				
SOL, IH, 0.083%, 3 ml 25s UD	54569-3899-00	30.25		EE
0.5%, 20 ml	54569-3900-00	17.00		EE
SYR, PO, 2 mg/5 ml, 120 ml 4s	54569-3700-02	34.42		AA
TAB, PO, 2 mg, 30s ea	54569-3409-00	9.34		EE
4 mg, 60s ea	54569-2874-01	27.46		EE
(Altura) REPACK				
SOL, IH, 0.5%, 20 ml	63874-0708-20	14.21		EE
SYR, PO, 2 mg/5 ml, 90 ml	63874-0709-90	14.21		EE
100 ml	63874-0709-01	16.28		EE
120 ml	63874-0709-12	19.20		EE
240 ml	63874-0709-24	28.40		EE
480 ml	63874-0709-48	28.40		EE
TAB, PO, 2 mg, 12s ea	63874-0377-12	4.56		EE
15s ea	63874-0377-15	13.77		EE
20s ea	63874-0377-20	18.36		EE
24s ea	63874-0377-24	22.03		EE
100s ea	63874-0377-01	37.98		EE
4 mg, 12s ea	63874-0485-12	6.79		EE
15s ea	63874-0485-15	8.49		EE
20s ea	63874-0485-20	11.33		EE
24s ea	63874-0485-24	13.59		EE
30s ea	63874-0485-30	16.98		EE
60s ea	63874-0485-60	32.34		EE
100s ea	63874-0485-01	56.65		EE
500s ea	63874-0485-05	208.82		EE
(B&B Pharm, Inc) REPACK				
POW, NA (U.S.P.)				
25 gm	63275-9999-04	81.00		
100 gm	63275-9999-05	310.00		
(Bryant Ranch) REPACK				
TAB, PO (USP)				
2 mg, 20s ea	63629-2638-01	8.72		
30s ea	63629-2638-02	13.08		
(Dispensing Solutions) REPACK				
SOL, IH (3MLX25)				
0.083%, 3 ml 25s	55045-2043-07	31.00		
0.5%, 20 ml	55045-2470-02	17.00		
TAB, PO, 2 mg, 30s ea	66336-0054-30	11.81		AB
4 mg, 30s ea	66336-0285-30	15.10		AB
(Nucare Pharm) REPACK				
TAB, PO, 2 mg, 30s ea	66267-0010-30	10.86		EE
(Palmetto) REPACK				
SOL, IH (24X3ML)				
0.083%, 3 ml 24s	23490-5020-01	25.00		
(25X3ML)				
0.083%, 3 ml 25s	23490-5020-02	27.00		
(30X3ML)				
0.083%, 3 ml 30s	23490-5020-03	30.00		
(1X20ML)				
0.5%, 20 ml	23490-5021-02	17.00		
SYR, PO, 2 mg/5 ml, 120 ml	23490-5023-00	18.29		
180 ml	23490-5023-01	27.00		
480 ml	23490-5023-02	42.43		
TAB, PO, 2 mg, 30s ea	23490-5022-01	10.87		
90s ea	23490-5022-02	32.61		
4 mg, 20s ea	23490-5025-01	10.78		
(PD-Rx Pharm) REPACK				
TAB, PO, 2 mg, 20s ea	55289-0363-20	10.22		AB
24s ea	55289-0363-24	10.93		AB
30s ea	55289-0363-30	12.00		AB
4 mg, 30s ea	55289-0045-30	13.33		AB
(Pharma Pac) REPACK				
SOL, IH, 0.5%, 20 ml	52959-0741-20	22.64		AN
SYR, PO, 2 mg/5 ml, 120 ml	52959-0153-03	19.97		EE
180 ml	52959-0153-06	29.20		EE
480 ml	52959-0153-09	33.10		EE
TAB, PO, 2 mg, 20s ea	52959-0425-20	8.95		EE
30s ea	52959-0425-30	13.50		EE
(Phys Total Care) REPACK				
SOL, IH, 0.083%, 3 ml 60s UD	54868-2472-00	34.56		AN
0.5%, 3 ml 25s	54868-2472-01	13.17		EE
20 ml	54868-3407-00	14.55		EE
SYR, PO, 2 mg/5 ml, 480 ml	54868-2887-00	24.93		EE
TAB, PO, 2 mg, 30s ea	54868-1073-03	13.50		EE
50s ea	54868-1073-06	19.50		EE
60s ea	54868-1073-04	22.55		EE
100s ea	54868-1073-02	33.00		EE
4 mg, 30s ea	54868-1074-03	15.45		EE
60s ea	54868-1074-07	27.92		EE
100s ea	54868-1074-05	43.05		EE
(Physician Partner) REPACK				
SOL, IH (3MLX25)				
0.083%, 3 ml 25s	21695-0332-25	60.50		
0.5%, 20 ml	21695-0245-20	33.00		
SYR, PO (1X16ML)				
2 mg/5 ml, 16 ml	21695-0350-16	79.20		AA
(Quality Care Prod) REPACK				
SOL, IH, 0.083%, 3 ml 25s UD	49999-0344-25	42.34		AN
0.5%, 17 gm	49999-0171-17	34.50		
SYR, PO (BERRY)				
2 mg/5 ml, 473 ml	49999-0338-16	48.18		AA
TAB, PO, 2 mg, 20s ea	49999-0901-20	13.29		
(Southwood) REPACK				
SOL, IH, 0.5%, 20 ml	58016-6404-01	15.53		EE
TAB, PO, 2 mg, 12s ea	58016-0473-12	4.34		EE
15s ea	58016-0473-15	5.42		EE
20s ea	58016-0473-20	7.23		EE
24s ea	58016-0473-24	8.68		EE
30s ea	58016-0473-30	10.85		EE
90s ea	58016-0473-90	32.55		EE
100s ea	58016-0473-00	36.17		EE
4 mg, 12s ea	58016-0603-12	6.47		EE
15s ea	58016-0603-15	8.09		EE
20s ea	58016-0603-20	10.79		EE
24s ea	58016-0603-24	12.94		EE
30s ea	58016-0603-30	16.17		EE
100s ea	58016-0603-00	53.95		EE
ALBUTEROL SULFATE HFA (Dispensing Solutions) REPACK				
albuterol sulfate				
ARO, IH, 0.09 mg/actuation, 8.5 gm	55045-3494-01	41.00		

ALBUTEROL SULFATE/IPRATROPIUM BROMIDE

(Boehr Ingelheim Phar) *See COMBIVENT*

(Dey, L.P.) *See DUONEB*

(Mylan) *See IPRATROPIUM BROMIDE AND ALBUTEROL SULFATE*

(Nephron) *See IPRATROPIUM BROMIDE AND ALBUTEROL SULFATE*

PROD/MFR	NDC	AWP	DP	OBC
(Sandoz) *See IPRATROPIUM BROMIDE AND ALBUTEROL SULFATE*				
(Teva) *See IPRATROPIUM BROMIDE AND ALBUTEROL SULFATE*				
(Watson Labs) *See IPRATROPIUM BROMIDE AND ALBUTEROL SULFATE*				
(Watson Labs) *See IPRATROPIUM BROMIDE/ALBUTEROL SULFATE*				
ALCAINE **(Alcon Ophthalmic)**				
proparacaine hydrochloride				
SOL, OP, 0.5%, 15 ml	**00998-0016-15**	32.88		AT
(A-S Medication)				
REPACK				
SOL, OP, 0.5%, 15 ml	**54569-4368-00**	32.63		AT
(Dispensing Solutions)				
REPACK				
SOL, OP, 0.5%, 15 ml	**55045-3687-01**	32.00		
(Quality Care Prod)				
REPACK				
SOL, OP, 0.5%, 15 ml	**49999-0353-15**	57.34		AT
(Southwood)				
REPACK				
SOL, OP, 0.5%, 15 ml	**58016-5564-01**	25.81		AT
ALCLOMETASONE DIPROPIONATE				
FUL				
CRE, TP, 0.05%, 45 gm		37.27		
OIN, TP, 0.05%, 45 gm		37.27		
(Fougera)				
CRE, TP, 0.05%, 15 gm	**00168-0263-15**	20.29		AB
45 gm	**00168-0263-45**	42.32		AB
60 gm	**00168-0263-60**	53.60		AB
OIN, TP, 0.05%, 15 gm	**00168-0264-15**	19.08		AB
45 gm	**00168-0264-45**	39.70		AB
60 gm	**00168-0264-60**	50.32		AB
(PharmaDerm) *See ACLOVATE*				
(Taro)				
CRE, TP, 0.05%, 15 gm	**51672-1306-01**	19.05		AB
45 gm	**51672-1306-06**	39.72		AB
60 gm	**51672-1306-03**	50.30		AB
OIN, TP, 0.05%, 15 gm	**51672-1316-01**	19.05		
45 gm	**51672-1316-06**	39.72		
60 gm	**51672-1316-03**	50.30		
(Phys Total Care)				
REPACK				
CRE, TP, 0.05%, 15 gm	**54868-2861-00**	54.99		
ALCOHOL ABSOLUTE **(Abbott Hosp)**				
ethanol				
SOL, IV (AMP,LATEX-FREE)				
99.5%, 1 ml 25s	**00074-3772-04**	614.40	537.50	
(Consolidated Midland)				
SOL, IV (AMPULE)				
98%, 1 ml 10s	**00223-7115-01**	150.00		
5 ml 10s	**00223-7115-05**	250.00		
(Mallinckrodt Lab)				
SOL, NA (A.C.S., REAGENT)				
4000 ml	**00406-7019-10**	42.81		
ALCOHOL BENZYL **(Amend)**				
benzyl alcohol				
LIQ, NA (N.F.)				
500 ml	**17317-0056-01**	19.60		
3840 ml	**17317-0056-06**	84.00		
(Baker, J.T.)				
LIQ, NA (REAGENT)				
500 ml	**10106-9050-01**	59.95		
(N.F.)				
4000 ml	**10106-9040-03**	160.19		
(Gallipot)				
SOL, NA (U.S.P.,N.F.)				
473 ml	**51552-0242-06**	24.85		
3785 ml	**51552-0242-08**	151.20		
(Letco)				
LIQ, NA (N.F.)				
500 ml	**62991-1318-01**	49.50		
(Mallinckrodt Lab)				
LIQ, NA, 500 ml	**00406-1816-04**	29.55		
(Spectrum Pharmacy)				
LIQ, NA (N.F.)				
500 ml	**49452-1020-01**	102.20		
4000 ml	**49452-1020-02**	437.50		
ALCOHOL BUTYL **(Spectrum Pharmacy)**				
butyl alcohol				
LIQ, NA (N.F.)				
500 ml	**49452-1315-01**	102.55		
1000 ml	**49452-1315-02**	148.40		
4000 ml	**49452-1315-03**	360.50		

PROD/MFR	NDC	AWP	DP	OBC
ALCOHOL CETOSTEARYL **(Spectrum Pharmacy)**				
cetostearyl alcohol				
OIN, NA (N.F.)				
500 gm	**49452-1878-01**	191.80		
2500 gm	**49452-1878-02**	577.50		
ALCOHOL CETYL **(Amend)**				
cetyl alcohol				
FLA, NA (N.F.)				
500 gm	**17317-0011-01**	9.80		
2270 gm	**17317-0011-05**	35.00		
11350 gm	**17317-0011-08**	150.00		
(Gallipot)				
POW, NA (U.S.P.,N.F.)				
100 gm	**51552-0227-05**	10.64		
454 gm	**51552-0227-06**	13.16		
2270 gm	**51552-0227-08**	43.33		
(Hawkins)				
POW, NA (N.F.)				
1000 gm	**63370-0046-50**	60.00		
2500 gm	**63370-0046-53**	120.00		
(Letco)				
POW, NA (N.F.)				
500 gm	**62991-1181-01**	30.00		
(Medisca)				
POW, NA (N.F.)				
500 gm	**38779-0618-08**	27.00		
1000 gm	**38779-0618-09**	46.50		
(Spectrum Pharmacy)				
LIQ, NA (N.F.)				
500 gm	**49452-1880-01**	64.75		
2500 gm	**49452-1880-02**	183.75		
ALCOHOL D-PANTHENOL **(Amend)**				
dexpanthenol				
LIQ, NA (U.S.P.)				
100 ml	**17317-2408-03**	23.10		
1000 ml	**17317-2408-06**	82.60		
ALCOHOL DEHYDRATED **(Amer Regent)**				
ethanol				
SOL, IV (AMP,PF)				
99.5%, 1 ml 10s	**00517-8571-10**	81.25		
5 ml 10s	**00517-8575-10**	462.50		
ALCOHOL DENATURED **(Spectrum Pharmacy)**				
ethanol				
SOL, NA (REAGENT, A.C.S.)				
500 ml	**49452-0235-01**	130.55		
1000 ml	**49452-0235-02**	163.45		
4000 ml	**49452-0235-03**	254.80		
ALCOHOL DENATURED ANHYDROUS **(Spectrum Pharmacy)**				
ethanol				
SOL, NA, 500 ml	**49452-0230-01**	84.70		
1000 ml	**49452-0230-04**	114.10		
4000 ml	**49452-0230-02**	223.65		
ALCOHOL ETHYL 200% ANHYDROUS **(Gallipot)**				
ethanol				
SOL, NA (1X100ML,USP)				
100 ml	**51552-0256-05**	14.00	10.00	
(1X473ML,USP)				
473 ml	**51552-0256-06**	45.50	32.50	
(1X1000ML,USP)				
1000 ml	**51552-0256-07**	76.44	54.60	
(1X4000ML,USP)				
4000 ml	**51552-0256-08**	216.72	154.80	
ALCOHOL ETHYL 95% **(Letco)**				
ethanol				
SOL, NA, 500 ml	**62991-1663-01**	93.00		
3840 ml	**62991-1663-02**	237.00		
ALCOHOL ETHYL ANHYDROUS 190 PROOF **(Spectrum Pharmacy)**				
ethanol				
SOL, NA (U.S.P.)				
100 ml	**49452-2840-06**	76.65		
500 ml	**49452-2840-01**	156.80		
1000 ml	**49452-2840-02**	284.90		
4000 ml	**49452-2840-04**	693.00		
ALCOHOL ETHYL ANHYDROUS 200 PROOF **(Spectrum Pharmacy)**				
ethanol				
SOL, NA (U.S.P.)				
100 ml	**49452-2850-06**	76.65		
500 ml	**49452-2850-01**	156.80		
1000 ml	**49452-2850-02**	284.90		
4000 ml	**49452-2850-04**	693.00		
ALCOHOL ISOBUTYL **(Baker, J.T.)**				
isobutyl alcohol				
LIQ, NA (A.C.S., REAGENT)				
500 ml	**10106-9044-01**	25.80		
4000 ml	**10106-9044-03**	102.85		

PROD/MFR	NDC	AWP	DP	OBC
ALCOHOL ISOPROPYL **(Baker, J.T.)**				
isopropyl alcohol				
LIQ, NA (U.S.P.)				
500 ml	**10106-9080-01**	11.75		
4000 ml	**10106-9080-03**	61.16		
(Mallinckrodt Lab)				
LIQ, NA (U.S.P.)				
500 ml	**00406-3031-04**	10.34		
4000 ml	**00406-3031-08**	45.77		
ALCOHOL ISOPROPYL 50% **(Gallipot)**				
isopropyl alcohol				
LIQ, NA, 473 ml	**51552-0466-06**	2.10		
ALCOHOL ISOPROPYL 70% **(Gallipot)**				
isopropyl alcohol				
LIQ, NA, 3785 ml	**51552-0404-08**	14.91		
(Humco)				
LIQ, NA (U.S.P.)				
120 ml	**00395-5701-94**	0.46		
480 ml	**00395-5701-16**	1.02		
(Spectrum Pharmacy)				
LIQ, NA (U.S.P.)				
500 ml	**49452-3810-01**	52.85		
1000 ml	**49452-3810-06**	63.00		
4000 ml	**49452-3810-02**	192.50		
ALCOHOL ISOPROPYL 91% **(Gallipot)**				
isopropyl alcohol				
LIQ, NA, 3785 ml	**51552-0420-08**	17.99		
ALCOHOL ISOPROPYL 99% **(Spectrum Pharmacy)**				
isopropyl alcohol				
LIQ, NA (U.S.P.)				
500 ml	**49452-3820-01**	58.10		
1000 ml	**49452-3820-04**	72.80		
4000 ml	**49452-3820-02**	194.25		
ALCOHOL METHYL **(Amend)**				
methyl alcohol				
LIQ, NA (N.F.)				
480 ml	**17317-0362-01**	5.60		
(A.C.S., REAGENT)				
500 ml	**17317-1331-01**	7.00		
3840 ml	**17317-1331-06**	18.20		
(N.F.)				
3840 ml	**17317-0362-06**	16.80		
19200 ml	**17317-0362-08**	49.00		
(A.C.S., REAGENT)				
19200 ml	**17317-1331-08**	52.50		
(Mallinckrodt Lab)				
LIQ, NA (N.F.)				
500 ml	**00406-8814-04**	7.96		
4000 ml	**00406-8814-06**	30.34		
ALCOHOL METHYL ANHYDROUS **(Mallinckrodt Lab)**				
methyl alcohol				
LIQ, NA (A.C.S.)				
500 ml	**00406-3016-04**	7.11		
4000 ml	**00406-3016-07**	29.07		
ALCOHOL PHENETHYL **(Spectrum Pharmacy)**				
phenylethyl alcohol				
LIQ, NA (U.S.P.)				
100 gm	**49452-5168-01**	95.20		
1000 gm	**49452-5168-02**	218.40		
ALCOHOL POLYVINYL **(Spectrum Pharmacy)**				
polyvinyl alcohol				
POW, NA (U.S.P.)				
250 gm	**49452-5665-01**	630.00		
1000 gm	**49452-5665-02**	2607.50		
ALCOHOL STEARYL **(Amend)**				
stearyl alcohol				
FLA, NA (N.F.)				
454 gm	**17317-0542-01**	8.40		
2270 gm	**17317-0542-05**	35.00		
11350 gm	**17317-0542-08**	113.75		
(Gallipot)				
FLA, NA, 454 gm	**51552-0417-06**	15.40		
(Letco)				
POW, NA (N.F.)				
500 gm	**62991-1212-01**	31.50		
2500 gm	**62991-1212-02**	90.00		
(Medisca)				
POW, NA (N.F.)				
100 gm	**38779-1630-05**	34.50		
500 gm	**38779-1630-08**	76.50		
1000 gm	**38779-1630-09**	135.00		
(NF)				
5000 gm	**38779-1630-03**	555.00		
(Spectrum Pharmacy)				
POW, NA (N.F.)				
500 gm	**49452-7300-01**	63.00		
2500 gm	**49452-7300-02**	221.90		
12000 gm	**49452-7300-03**	717.50		

PROD/MFR	NDC	AWP	DP	OBC
ALCORTIN A (Primus Pharma)				
aloe/hydrocortisone acetate/iodoquinol				
GEL, TP (24X2GM)				
1%-2%-1%, 2 gm 24s	**68040-0705-13**	118.15		
ALDACTAZIDE (Pfizer)				
hydrochlorothiazide/spironolactone				
TAB, PO (FILM COATED)				
25 mg-25 mg,				
100s ea	**00025-1011-31**	103.92	86.60	**AB**
50 mg-50 mg,				
100s ea	**00025-1021-31**	191.68	159.73	
ALDACTONE (Pfizer)				
spironolactone				
TAB, PO, 25 mg, 100s ea	**00025-1001-31**	101.24	84.37	**AB**
500s ea	**00025-1001-51**	506.21	421.84	**AB**
50 mg, 100s ea	**00025-1041-31**	177.83	148.19	**AB**
100 mg, 100s ea	**00025-1031-31**	298.12	248.43	**AB**
(Phys Total Care)				
REPACK				
TAB, PO, 50 mg, 30s ea	**54868-3087-00**	34.81		**AB**
ALDARA (Graceway)				
imiquimod				
CRE, TP, 5%, 24s ea	**29336-0610-24**	681.14		
(A-S Medication)				
REPACK				
CRE, TP (CREAM)				
5%, 12s ea	**54569-4894-00**	268.38		
24s ea	**54569-6103-00**	619.95		
(Phys Total Care)				
REPACK				
CRE, TP, 5%, 24s ea	**54868-4554-01**	683.08		
(Quality Care Prod)				
REPACK				
CRE, TP, 5%, 12s ea	**35356-0010-12**	322.06		
ALDESLEUKIN				
(Prometheus Labs) *See PROLEUKIN*				
ALDEX AN (Zyber)				
doxylamine succinate				
CTB, PO (ORANGE)				
5 mg, 100s ea	**65224-0542-01**	249.20		
ALDEX D (Zyber)				
phenylephrine hydrochloride/pyrilamine maleate				
SUS, PO (GRAPE)				
5 mg/5 ml-16 mg/5 ml,				
473 ml	**65224-0550-16**	291.74		
ALDEX DM (Zyber)				
dm/phenyleph hcl/pyril mal				
SUS, PO (GRAPE)				
473 ml	**65224-0555-16**	294.55		
ALDEX-CT (Zyber)				
diphenhydramine hcl/phenyleph hcl				
CTB, PO (STRAWBERRY)				
12.5 mg-5 mg,				
100s ea	**65224-0545-01**	294.55		
ALDOSTERONE (PCCA)				
POW, NA (1X0.001GM)				
0.001 gm	**51927-2092-00**	99.00		
ALDURAZYME (Genzyme)				
laronidase				
SOL, IV (PF)				
0.58 mg/ml, 5 ml	**58468-0070-01**	840.00	700.00	
ALEFACEPT				
(Astellas) *See AMEVIVE*				
ALEMTUZUMAB				
(Genzyme) *See CAMPATH*				
ALENDRONATE SOD (Phys Total Care)				
REPACK				
alendronate sodium				
TAB, PO, 10 mg, 30s ea	**54868-5862-00**	154.91		
35 mg, 4s ea	**54868-5860-00**	77.31		
70 mg, 4s ea	**54868-5861-00**	77.31		
ALENDRONATE SODIUM				
FUL				
TAB, PO, 5 mg, 100s ea		42.93		
10 mg, 100s ea		42.93		
35 mg, 4s ea		61.47		
70 mg, 4s ea		61.47		
(Apotex Corp.)				
TAB, PO (USP)				
5 mg, 30s ea	**60505-2592-03**	87.80		**AB**
100s ea	**60505-2592-01**	292.68		**AB**
10 mg, 30s ea	**60505-2593-03**	87.80		**AB**
100s ea	**60505-2593-01**	292.68		**AB**
35 mg, 4s ea	**60505-2594-04**	81.95		**AB**
70 mg, 4s ea	**60505-2596-04**	81.95		**AB**
20s ea UD	**60505-2596-02**	409.76		**AB**
1000s ea	**60505-2596-08**	19873.36		**AB**
(Aurobindo Pharma)				
TAB, PO (USP)				
10 mg, 30s ea	**65862-0327-30**	87.80		**AB**
(USP,1X4)				
35 mg, 4s ea	**65862-0328-04**	81.95		**AB**
70 mg, 4s ea	**65862-0329-04**	81.95		**AB**
(Caraco)				
TAB, PO (USP)				
5 mg, 30s ea	**41616-0635-83**	87.80		**AB**
100s ea	**41616-0635-88**	292.50		**AB**
10 mg, 30s ea	**41616-0636-83**	87.80		**AB**
100s ea	**41616-0636-88**	292.50		**AB**
35 mg, 4s ea	**41616-0637-68**	81.93		**AB**
70 mg, 4s ea	**41616-0638-68**	81.93		**AB**
(Dr Reddy's)				
TAB, PO (USP)				
5 mg, 30s ea	**55111-0589-30**	87.80		**AB**
100s ea	**55111-0589-01**	292.68		**AB**
10 mg, 30s ea	**55111-0588-30**	87.80		**AB**
100s ea	**55111-0588-01**	292.68		**AB**
35 mg, 4s ea	**55111-0590-48**	81.95		**AB**
70 mg, 4s ea	**55111-0592-48**	81.95		**AB**
(Merck) *See FOSAMAX*				
(Mylan)				
TAB, PO (USP)				
5 mg, 100s ea	**00378-3566-01**	292.25		**AB**
10 mg, 100s ea	**00378-3567-01**	292.25		**AB**
(USP,12X4)				
35 mg, 48s ea UD	**00378-3568-22**	982.20		**AB**
70 mg, 48s ea UD	**00378-3569-22**	982.20		**AB**
(Northstar)				
TAB, PO (USP)				
10 mg, 30s ea	**16714-0631-01**	87.80		**AB**
100s ea	**16714-0631-02**	242.59		**AB**
35 mg, 4s ea	**16714-0632-01**	81.95		**AB**
20s ea	**16714-0632-02**	409.76		**AB**
70 mg, 4s ea	**16714-0633-01**	81.94		**AB**
20s ea	**16714-0633-02**	409.51		**AB**
(Teva)				
TAB, PO (USP)				
5 mg, 30s ea	**00093-5140-56**	87.80		**AB**
100s ea	**00093-5140-01**	292.68		**AB**
10 mg, 30s ea	**00093-5141-56**	87.80		**AB**
100s ea	**00093-5141-01**	292.68		**AB**
35 mg, 4s ea	**00093-5172-44**	81.95		**AB**
(2X10,USP)				
35 mg, 20s ea UD	**00093-5172-20**	409.76		**AB**
(USP,2X10)				
35 mg, 20s ea	**00555-0719-51**	409.75		**AB**
(USP)				
40 mg, 30s ea	**00093-5142-56**	197.96		**AB**
70 mg, 4s ea	**00093-5171-44**	81.95		**AB**
(2X10,USP)				
70 mg, 20s ea UD	**00093-5171-20**	409.76		**AB**
(UDL)				
TAB, PO (2X10,USP)				
10 mg, 20s ea UD	**51079-0941-05**	58.45		**AB**
70 mg, 20s ea UD	**51079-0942-05**	409.25		**AB**
(Watson Labs)				
TAB, PO (USP)				
35 mg, 4s ea	**00591-3171-04**	9.00		**AB**
4s ea	**16252-0599-44**	9.00		
12s ea	**16252-0599-02**	27.00		
70 mg, 4s ea	**00591-3173-04**	9.00		**AB**
4s ea	**16252-0601-44**	9.60		
12s ea	**16252-0601-02**	28.80		
(A-S Medication)				
REPACK				
TAB, PO, 35 mg, 4s ea	**54569-6047-00**	81.96		**EE**
70 mg, 4s ea	**54569-6050-00**	81.96		**EE**
(American Health)				
REPACK				
TAB, PO (USP,2X10)				
70 mg, 20s ea	**68084-0322-64**	409.72		
(Dispensing Solutions)				
REPACK				
TAB, PO, 35 mg, 4s ea	**55045-3908-01**	88.81		**EE**
70 mg, 4s ea	**68258-3014-01**	88.81		
(GSMS)				
REPACK				
TAB, PO, 70 mg, 4s ea UD	**60429-0773-04**	7.02	2.34	**AB**
12s ea UD	**60429-0773-12**	21.42	7.14	**AB**
(Nucare Pharm)				
REPACK				
TAB, PO, 5 mg, 30s ea	**68071-0791-30**	97.56		**AB**
10 mg, 30s ea	**68071-0790-30**	97.56		**AB**
(Physician Partner)				
REPACK				
TAB, PO, 35 mg, 4s ea	**21695-0901-04**	163.92		**AB**
70 mg, 4s ea	**21695-0902-04**	163.92		**AB**
(Stat Rx)				
REPACK				
TAB, PO, 70 mg, 4s ea	**16590-0718-04**	90.25		**AB**
20s ea	**16590-0718-20**	425.00		**AB**
30s ea	**16590-0718-30**	172.50		**AB**
ALENDRONATE SODIUM/CHOLECALCIFEROL				
(Merck) *See FOSAMAX PLUS D*				
ALESSE 28 (Phys Total Care)				
REPACK				
ethinyl estradiol/levonorgestrel				
TAB, PO (MINIPACK DISPENSER)				
0.02 mg-0.1 mg,				
28s ea	**54868-3951-00**	47.83		**AB1**
ALESSE-28 (Palmetto)				
REPACK				
ethinyl estradiol/levonorgestrel				
TAB, PO, 0.02 mg-0.1 mg,				
28s ea	**23490-7654-01**	43.90		
ALEVE (Dispensing Solutions)				
REPACK				
naproxen sodium				
TAB, PO, 220 mg, 24s ea	**55045-2149-02**	6.00		
100s ea	**55045-2149-01**	25.00		
ALFADEX				
(PCCA) *See CASHEW NUT OIL*				
(PCCA) *See CYCLODEXTRIN*				
ALFENTA (Akorn)				
alfentanil hydrochloride				
SOL, IJ (AMP,PF)				
0.5 mg/ml,				
2 ml 10s, C-II	**11098-0060-02**	105.22		**AP**
5 ml 10s, C-II	**11098-0060-05**	188.60		**AP**
10 ml 5s, C-II	**11098-0060-10**	152.27		**AP**
ALFENTANIL (Hospira)				
alfentanil hydrochloride				
SOL, IJ (10X2ML,NONPYROGENIC,SDA)				
0.5 mg/ml,				
2 ml 10s, C-II	**00409-2266-02**	51.60	45.20	**AP**
(10X5ML,PF)				
0.5 mg/ml,				
5 ml 10s, C-II	**00409-2266-05**	96.72	84.60	**AP**
ALFENTANIL HYDROCHLORIDE				
(Akorn) *See ALFENTA*				
(Hospira) *See ALFENTANIL*				
(Hospira) *See NOVAPLUS ALFENTANIL*				
ALFERON N (Hemispherx)				
interferon alfa-n3				
SOL, IJ (M.D.V.)				
5 million iu/ml,				
1 ml	**54746-0001-01**	430.08		
ALFUZOSIN HYDROCHLORIDE				
(Sanofi-Aventis) *See UROXATRAL*				
ALGINIC ACID (Gallipot)				
POW, NA (U.S.P.)				
125 gm	**51552-0856-09**	27.30	19.50	
(PCCA)				
POW, NA (NF)				
1 gm	**51927-2768-00**	2.40		
(Spectrum Pharmacy)				
POW, NA (N.F.)				
125 gm	**49452-0250-04**	113.05		
500 gm	**49452-0250-01**	339.15		
2500 gm	**49452-0250-02**	1228.50		
ALGLUCERASE				
(Genzyme) *See CEREDASE*				
ALGLUCOSIDASE ALFA				
(Genzyme) *See MYOZYME*				
ALICLEN (Prasco Labs)				
salicylic acid				
SHA, TP (1X177ML)				
6%, 177 ml	**66993-0887-71**	69.40		
ALIMTA (Lilly)				
pemetrexed				
PDS, IV (SINGLE-USE)				
100 mg, ea	**00002-7640-01**	606.72	505.60	
500 mg, ea	**00002-7623-01**	3033.60	2528.00	
ALINIA (Romark)				
nitazoxanide				
PDR, PO (STRAWBERRY)				
100 mg/5 ml, 60 ml	**67546-0212-21**	91.50		

PROD/MFR	NDC	AWP	DP	OBC
TAB, PO (FILM-COATED)				
500 mg, 30s ea	67546-0111-12	706.80		
60s ea	67546-0111-11	1365.60		
ALISKIREN				
(Novartis Pharm) *See TEKTURNA*				
ALISKIREN/HYDROCHLOROTHIAZIDE				
(Novartis Pharm) *See TEKTURNA HCT*				
ALISKIREN/VALSARTAN				
(Novartis Pharm) *See VALTURNA*				
ALITRETINOIN				
(Eisai) *See PANRETIN*				
ALKERAN (Celgene Corp)				
melphalan				
TAB, PO (FILM-COATED)				
2 mg, 50s ea	59572-0302-50	283.96		
(Glaxo)				
melphalan hydrochloride				
PDS, IV, 50 mg, ea	00173-0130-93	1971.72		
(Glaxo)				
melphalan				
TAB, PO (FILM-COATED)				
2 mg, 50s ea	00173-0045-35	283.96		
(Phys Total Care)				
REPACK				
TAB, PO (FILM-COATED)				
2 mg, 4s ea	54868-4339-00	28.03		
24s ea	54868-4339-02	150.08		
28s ea	54868-4339-03	184.95		
32s ea	54868-4339-04	199.48		
50s ea	54868-4339-01	310.01		
ALKERAN IV (Celgene Corp)				
melphalan hydrochloride				
PDS, IV, 50 mg, ea	59572-0301-01	1971.72		
ALKYL BENZOATE (PCCA)				
c12-15 alkyl benzoate				
SOL, NA, 1 ml	51927-2433-00	0.31		
ALLANDERM-T (IPI)				
REPACK				
castor oil/peru balsam/trypsin				
OIN, TP, 30 gm	18837-0308-30	69.50		
ALLANFIL (Allan Pharmaceutical)				
chlorophyllin copper complex/papain/urea				
SPR, TP, 0.5%-10%, 33 ml	13279-0103-33	78.95		
ALLANFIL 405 OINTMENT (Allan Pharmaceutical)				
chlorophyllin copper complex, sodium/papain/urea				
OIN, TP (U.S.P.)				
0.5%-405900 u/gm-10%,				
30 gm	13279-0101-30	78.32		
(IPI)				
REPACK				
OIN, TP, 0.5%-405900 u/gm-10%,				
30 gm	18837-0309-30	98.88		
ALLANHIST PDX (Allan Pharmaceutical)				
bpm/dm/gg/phenyleph hcl				
SYR, PO (AF,GRAPE)				
473 ml	13279-0300-16	48.60		
ALLANTOIN (Amend)				
POW, NA (T.G.A.)				
125 gm	17317-0683-04	9.80		
454 gm	17317-0683-01	30.80		
2270 gm	17317-0683-05	133.00		
11350 gm	17317-0683-08	420.00		
(Gallipot)				
POW, NA, 100 gm	51552-0179-05	16.10		
(Medisca)				
POW, NA, 100 gm	38779-0492-05	64.50		
(PCCA)				
POW, NA, 1 gm	51927-1258-00	1.20		
(Spectrum Pharmacy)				
POW, NA, 100 gm	49452-0260-01	89.95		
500 gm	49452-0260-02	252.35		
2500 gm	49452-0260-03	913.50		
ALLANVAN-S (Allan Pharmaceutical)				
phenylephrine tannate/pyrilamine tannate				
SUS, PO (GRAPE)				
12.5 mg/5 ml-30 mg/5 ml,				
473 ml	13279-0306-16	139.50		
ALLANZYME (Allan Pharmaceutical)				
papain/urea				
SPR, TP, 650000 u/gm-10%,				
33 ml	13279-0102-33	49.00		

PROD/MFR	NDC	AWP	DP	OBC
ALLANZYME 650 OINTMENT (Allan Pharmaceutical)				
papain/urea				
OIN, TP, 650000 u/gm-10%,				
30 gm	13279-0100-30	48.56		
ALLEGRA (Sanofi-Aventis)				
fexofenadine hydrochloride				
SUS, PO, 30 mg/5 ml,				
300 ml	00088-1097-20	70.99		
TAB, PO (FILM-COATED)				
60 mg, 100s ea	00088-1107-47	163.37		
500s ea	00088-1107-55	816.85		
180 mg, 100s ea	00088-1109-47	283.39		
500s ea	00088-1109-55	1416.95		
(A-S Medication)				
REPACK				
TAB, PO, 60 mg, ea	54569-5378-03	1.70		
10s ea	54569-5378-01	17.02		
30s ea	54569-5378-02	51.05		
60s ea	54569-5378-00	102.11		
180 mg, 30s ea	54569-4938-00	88.56		
(DHS, Inc.)				
REPACK				
CAP, PO, 60 mg, 14s ea	55887-0869-14	33.01		
TAB, PO, 60 mg, 60s ea	55887-0720-60	184.28		
(Direct Pharmaceutical, Inc.)				
REPACK				
TAB, PO, 60 mg,				
30s ea UD	67801-0336-03	58.81		
30s ea	67801-0436-03	58.81		
(Dispensing Solutions)				
REPACK				
TAB, PO (FILM-COATED)				
60 mg, 10s ea	55045-3048-02	19.70		
14s ea	55045-3048-07	27.58		
30s ea	55045-3048-08	59.10		
100s ea	55045-3048-01	197.00		
180 mg, 30s ea	66336-0261-30	123.73		
(HomeMed)				
REPACK				
CAP, PO, 60 mg, 14s ea	51655-0781-84	33.01		
TAB, PO, 180 mg, 10s ea	51655-0782-53	33.91		
20s ea	51655-0782-52	68.08		
(Nucare Pharm)				
REPACK				
TAB, PO (FILM-COATED)				
60 mg, 20s ea	66267-0536-20	50.58		
(PD-Rx Pharm)				
REPACK				
TAB, PO (FILM-COATED)				
60 mg, 6s ea	55289-0628-06	12.62		
14s ea	55289-0628-14	30.43		
28s ea	55289-0628-28	58.93		
60s ea	55289-0628-60	126.26		
(REDI-SCRIPT,FILM-COATED)				
60 mg, 60s ea	58864-0514-60	123.59		
(FILM-COATED)				
180 mg, 20s ea	55289-0732-20	73.01		
30s ea	55289-0732-30	110.28		
(REDI-SCRIPT,FILM-COATED)				
180 mg, 30s ea	58864-0747-30	105.07		
(Pharma Pac)				
REPACK				
TAB, PO, 60 mg, 30s ea	52959-0698-30	53.90		
100s ea	52959-0698-00	179.20		
(Phys Total Care)				
REPACK				
TAB, PO, 60 mg, 10s ea	54868-4632-01	21.64		
30s ea	54868-4632-00	61.15		
60s ea	54868-4632-02	120.44		
180 mg, 10s ea	54868-4259-01	37.48		
(FILM-COATED)				
180 mg, 15s ea	54868-4259-03	55.24		
30s ea	54868-4259-00	108.52		
(FILM-COATED)				
180 mg, 60s ea	54868-4259-04	203.24		
100s ea	54868-4259-02	336.78		
(Quality Care Prod)				
REPACK				
CAP, PO, 60 mg, 14s ea	49999-0196-14	30.10		
TAB, PO (FILM-COATED)				
60 mg, 8s ea	49999-0196-08	17.20		
20s ea	49999-0196-20	42.99		
30s ea	49999-0196-30	64.50		
60s ea	49999-0196-60	129.00		
90s ea	49999-0196-90	193.50		
180 mg, 30s ea	49999-0452-30	164.98		
60s ea	49999-0452-60	327.65		
90s ea	49999-0452-90	490.33		

PROD/MFR	NDC	AWP	DP	OBC
(Southwood)				
REPACK				
CAP, PO, 60 mg, 10s ea	58016-0131-10	10.77		
12s ea	58016-0131-12	12.92		
15s ea	58016-0131-15	16.15		
20s ea	58016-0131-20	21.53		
30s ea	58016-0131-30	32.30		
60s ea	58016-0131-60	64.60		
100s ea	58016-0131-00	107.67		
TAB, PO (FILM-COATED)				
60 mg, 10s ea	58016-0692-10	16.34		
12s ea	58016-0692-12	19.60		
15s ea	58016-0692-15	24.51		
20s ea	58016-0692-20	32.67		
25s ea	58016-0692-25	40.84		
30s ea	58016-0692-30	49.01		
40s ea	58016-0692-40	65.35		
50s ea	58016-0692-50	81.69		
60s ea	58016-0692-60	98.02		
70s ea	58016-0692-70	114.36		
80s ea	58016-0692-80	130.70		
90s ea	58016-0692-90	147.03		
100s ea	58016-0692-00	163.37		
120s ea	58016-0692-02	196.04		
180 mg, 30s ea	58016-0026-30	85.02		
60s ea	58016-0026-60	170.03		
90s ea	58016-0026-90	255.05		
100s ea	58016-0026-00	283.39		
ALLEGRA D 12 HOUR (Quality Care Prod)				
REPACK				
fexofenadine hcl/pse hcl				
TER, PO, 60 mg-120 mg,				
100s ea	49999-0195-00	346.02		
ALLEGRA ODT (Sanofi-Aventis)				
fexofenadine hydrochloride				
ODT, PO (10X6)				
30 mg, 60s ea	00088-1113-30	119.08		
ALLEGRA-D (A-S Medication)				
REPACK				
fexofenadine hcl/pse hcl				
TER, PO (FILM-COATED)				
60 mg-120 mg,				
30s ea	54569-4658-01	97.06		
60s ea	54569-4658-00	194.12		
(Bryant Ranch)				
REPACK				
TER,,PO, 60 mg-120 mg,				
30s ea	63629-1249-01	47.93		
(PD-Rx Pharm)				
REPACK				
TER, PO, 60 mg-120 mg,				
30s ea	55289-0783-30	96.17		
(Pharma Pac)				
REPACK				
TER, PO, 60 mg-120 mg,				
14s ea	52959-0918-14	43.10		
(Phys Total Care)				
REPACK				
TER, PO, 60 mg-120 mg,				
10s ea	54868-4258-03	33.81		
20s ea	54868-4258-02	65.00		
30s ea	54868-4258-00	96.19		
60s ea	54868-4258-01	179.37		
(Quality Care Prod)				
REPACK				
TER, PO (FILM-COATED)				
60 mg-120 mg,				
30s ea	49999-0195-30	92.25		
(Vibranta)				
REPACK				
TER, PO, 60 mg-120 mg,				
30s ea	57866-1250-01	56.93		
ALLEGRA-D 12 HOUR (Sanofi-Aventis)				
fexofenadine hcl/pse hcl				
TER, PO (FILM-COATED)				
60 mg-120 mg,				
100s ea	00088-1090-47	248.87		
500s ea	00088-1090-55	1244.40		
(A-S Medication)				
REPACK				
TER, PO (FILM-COATED)				
60 mg-120 mg,				
14s ea	54569-4658-02	36.29		
(PD-Rx Pharm)				
REPACK				
TER, PO (FILM-COATED)				
60 mg-120 mg,				
60s ea	55289-0783-60	221.94		

PROD/MFR	NDC	AWP	DP	OBC
(REDI-SCRIPT,FILM-COATED)				
60 mg-120 mg,				
60s ea	58864-0855-60	172.35		
(Quality Care Prod)				
REPACK				
TER, PO (FILM-COATED)				
60 mg-120 mg,				
8s ea	49999-0195-08	29.93		
14s ea	49999-0195-14	52.38		
20s ea	49999-0195-20	74.83		
60s ea	49999-0195-60	224.49		
(Southwood)				
REPACK				
TER, PO (FILM-COATED)				
60 mg-120 mg,				
30s ea	00490-0076-30	62.84		
60s ea	00490-0076-60	125.68		
90s ea	00490-0076-90	188.52		
100s ea	00490-0076-00	209.47		
ALLEGRA-D 24HOUR (Sanofi-Aventis)				
fexofenadine hcl/pse hcl				
T24, PO (FILM-COATED)				
180 mg-240 mg,				
100s ea	00088-1095-47	497.76		
(Phys Total Care)				
REPACK				
T24, PO (FILM-COATED)				
180 mg-240 mg,				
10s ea	54868-5419-00	59.85		
30s ea	54868-5419-01	164.78		
(Stat Rx)				
REPACK				
T24, PO (FILM-COATED)				
180 mg-240 mg,				
28s ea	16590-0852-28	149.58		
ALLEGRA-D 24HR (Phys Total Care)				
REPACK				
fexofenadine hcl/pse hcl				
T24, PO, 180 mg-240 mg,				
60s ea	54868-5419-02	326.95		
ALLERGY DN II (Breckenridge Pharm)				
chlorpheniramine maleate/methscopolamine nitrate				
TAB, PO, 20s ea	51991-0534-20	69.10		
ALLERGY DN PE (Breckenridge Pharm)				
cpm/methscopolamine nitrate/phenyleph hcl				
TAB, PO, 20s ea	51991-0558-20	69.10		
ALLERX (Phys Total Care)				
REPACK				
cpm/methscopolamine nitrate/pse hcl				
TER, PO (DOSE PACK)				
20s ea	54868-5198-00	62.75		
ALLERX DOSE PACK (Cornerstone)				
cpm/methscopolamine nitrate/pse hcl/phenyleph hcl				
KIT, PO (AM/PM DOSE PACK 10)				
20s ea	10122-0650-20	182.19	145.75	
(AM/PM DOSE PACK 30)				
60s ea	10122-0650-60	546.56	437.25	
ALLERX DOSE PACK DF (Cornerstone)				
chlorpheniramine maleate/methscopolamine nitrate				
TAB, PO (10AM,10PM)				
20s ea	10122-0704-20	165.63	132.50	
ALLERX DOSE PACK DF 30 (Cornerstone)				
chlorpheniramine maleate/methscopolamine nitrate				
TAB, PO, 60s ea	10122-0704-60	496.88	397.50	
ALLERX DOSEPACK PE (Cornerstone)				
cpm/methscopolamine nitrate/phenyleph hcl				
TAB, PO (10AM,10PM)				
20s ea	10122-0705-20	165.63	132.50	
(30AM,30PM)				
60s ea	10122-0705-60	496.88	397.50	
ALLERX-D (Cornerstone)				
methscopolamine nitrate/pse hcl				
TER, PO, 2.5 mg-120 mg,				
60s ea	10122-0702-60	178.86	143.09	
ALLFEN CD (MCR American)				
codeine phosphate/guaifenesin				
TAB, PO, 10 mg-400 mg,				
100s ea, C-III	58605-0404-01	105.96		
ALLFEN CDX (MCR American)				
codeine phosphate/guaifenesin				
TAB, PO, 20 mg-400 mg,				
100s ea, C-III	58605-0405-01	110.80		
ALLOPURINOL				
FUL				
TAB, PO, 100 mg, 100s ea		7.85		
300 mg, 100s ea		17.39		
(Apotex Corp.)				
TAB, PO (USP)				
100 mg, 100s ea	60505-2516-02	24.25		AB
1000s ea	60505-2516-03	242.50		AB
300 mg, 100s ea	60505-2517-02	59.25		AB
1000s ea	60505-2517-03	592.50		AB
(Ascend)				
TAB, PO (USP)				
100 mg, 100s ea	67877-0122-01	24.63		AB
1000s ea	67877-0122-10	244.25		AB
300 mg, 100s ea	67877-0123-01	67.43		AB
500s ea	67877-0123-05	331.58		AB
1000s ea	67877-0123-10	661.48		AB
(Caraco)				
TAB, PO (USP)				
100 mg, 100s ea	57664-0434-88	21.95		AB
500s ea	57664-0434-13	109.75		AB
1000s ea	57664-0434-18	219.50		AB
300 mg, 100s ea	57664-0436-88	59.25		AB
500s ea	57664-0436-13	296.25		AB
1000s ea	57664-0436-18	592.50		AB
(Consolidated Midland)				
TAB, PO, 100 mg, 100s ea	00223-0114-01	9.75		EE
500s ea	00223-0114-05	39.00		EE
1000s ea	00223-0114-02	75.00		EE
300 mg, 100s ea	00223-0115-01	21.00		EE
500s ea	00223-0115-05	95.00		EE
1000s ea	00223-0115-02	190.00		EE
(Dr Reddy's)				
TAB, PO (USP)				
100 mg, 100s ea	55111-0729-01	24.25		AB
1000s ea	55111-0729-10	242.50		AB
300 mg, 100s ea	55111-0730-01	59.25		AB
500s ea	55111-0730-05	296.25		AB
1000s ea	55111-0730-10	592.50		AB
(Major)				
TAB, PO (10X10)				
100 mg, 100s ea UD	00904-2613-61	26.87		AB
300 mg, 100s ea UD	00904-2614-61	73.53		AB
(Medisca)				
POW, NA (U.S.P.)				
5 gm	38779-0186-03	31.50		
25 gm	38779-0186-04	117.00		
(Mutual)				
TAB, PO, 100 mg, 100s ea	53489-0156-01	24.25		AB
500s ea	53489-0156-05	115.19		AB
1000s ea	53489-0156-10	218.86		AB
300 mg, 100s ea	53489-0157-01	59.25		AB
500s ea	53489-0157-05	288.99		AB
1000s ea	53489-0157-10	577.95		AB
(Mylan)				
TAB, PO, 100 mg, 100s ea	00378-0137-01	21.72		AB
1000s ea	00378-0137-10	212.78		AB
300 mg, 100s ea	00378-0181-01	59.04		AB
500s ea	00378-0181-05	288.86		AB
(Northstar)				
TAB, PO (USP)				
100 mg, 30s ea	16714-0041-01	6.52		AB
100s ea	16714-0041-04	21.72		AB
1000s ea	16714-0041-06	212.78		AB
(USP)				
300 mg, 30s ea	16714-0042-01	17.71		AB
100s ea	16714-0042-04	59.04		AB
500s ea	16714-0042-05	288.86		AB
(PCCA)				
POW, NA (U.S.P.)				
1 gm	51927-1915-00	6.60		
(Prometheus Labs) *See ZYLOPRIM*				
(Qualitest)				
TAB, PO, 100 mg, 100s ea	00603-2115-21	24.42		AB
1000s ea	00603-2115-32	249.95		AB
300 mg, 100s ea	00603-2116-21	66.89		AB
500s ea	00603-2116-28	330.92		AB
1000s ea	00603-2116-32	651.49		AB
(Spectrum Pharmacy)				
POW, NA (U.S.P.)				
5 gm	49452-0008-01	79.45		
25 gm	49452-0008-02	215.95		
(USP,1X500GM)				
500 gm	49452-0008-03	1501.50		
(UDL)				
TAB, PO (ROBOT READY 25X1)				
100 mg, 25s ea UD	51079-0205-19	5.59		AB
(10X10)				
100 mg, 100s ea UD	51079-0205-20	22.37		AB
(ROBOT READY 25X1)				
300 mg, 25s ea UD	51079-0206-19	15.20		AB
(10X10)				
300 mg, 100s ea UD	51079-0206-20	60.81		AB
(Watson Labs)				
TAB, PO, 100 mg, 100s ea	00591-5543-01	24.24		AB
1000s ea	00591-5543-10	249.95		AB
300 mg, 100s ea	00591-5544-01	64.50		AB
500s ea	00591-5544-05	330.93		AB
(A-S Medication)				
REPACK				
TAB, PO, 100 mg, 30s ea	54569-0233-03	7.27		EE
300 mg, 30s ea	54569-0235-01	19.35		EE
100s ea	54569-0235-00	64.50		EE
(Altura)				
REPACK				
TAB, PO, 100 mg, 30s ea	63874-0754-30	6.13		EE
300 mg, 10s ea	63874-0755-10	6.06		AB
12s ea	63874-0755-12	7.28		EE
14s ea	63874-0755-14	8.49		AB
20s ea	63874-0755-20	11.18		EE
30s ea	63874-0755-30	16.78		EE
40s ea	63874-0755-40	24.27		AB
100s ea	63874-0755-01	56.47		EE
500s ea	63874-0755-50	303.33		AB
(American Health)				
REPACK				
TAB, PO (10X10)				
100 mg, 100s ea UD	62584-0988-01	26.30		AB
(15X30)				
100 mg, 450s ea	62584-0988-85	166.05		AB
(10X10)				
300 mg, 100s ea UD	62584-0713-01	70.49		AB
(Bryant Ranch)				
REPACK				
TAB, PO, 100 mg, 30s ea	63629-1675-02	7.26		
60s ea	63629-1675-03	14.52		
100s ea	63629-1675-01	24.20		
300 mg, 30s ea	63629-1781-01	14.40		
60s ea	63629-1781-02	28.80		
(Core)				
REPACK				
TAB, PO, 100 mg, 100s ea	33358-0012-00	24.81		
300 mg, 60s ea	33358-0013-60	29.52		
(DHS, Inc.)				
REPACK				
TAB, PO, 100 mg, 30s ea	55887-0337-30	11.00		AB
90s ea	55887-0337-90	31.08		AB
100s ea	55887-0337-01	36.67		
300 mg, 30s ea	55887-0370-30	16.17		AB
90s ea	55887-0370-90	37.00		AB
100s ea	55887-0370-01	41.00		
(Dispensing Solutions)				
REPACK				
TAB, PO, 100 mg, 30s ea	55045-1948-08	7.50		AB
300 mg, 30s ea	55045-1340-08	15.75		AB
60s ea	55045-1340-06	31.80		AB
(GSMS)				
REPACK				
TAB, PO (UNIT OF USE)				
300 mg, 30s ea	60429-0014-30	13.20	4.40	AB
90s ea	60429-0014-90	34.50	11.50	AB
(HomeMed)				
REPACK				
TAB, PO, 300 mg, 30s ea	51655-0038-24	15.40		
(Palmetto)				
REPACK				
TAB, PO, 300 mg, 30s ea	23490-5031-03	22.66		
90s ea	23490-5031-01	67.98		
(PD-Rx Pharm)				
REPACK				
TAB, PO (USP)				
100 mg, 20s ea	43063-0079-20	9.88		AB
300 mg, 3s ea	55289-0010-03	10.50		AB
30s ea	55289-0010-30	14.98		AB
90s ea	55289-0010-90	24.96		AB
100s ea	55289-0010-01	26.62		AB
(Pharma Pac)				
REPACK				
TAB, PO, 100 mg, 30s ea	52959-0473-30	10.38		AB
100s ea	52959-0311-00	56.29		AB
100s ea	52959-0473-00	34.50		AB
300 mg, 30s ea	52959-0311-30	18.28		AB
60s ea	52959-0311-60	17.93		
(Phys Total Care)				
REPACK				
TAB, PO, 100 mg, 30s ea	54868-0075-00	8.04		EE
60s ea	54868-0075-03	13.11		EE
90s ea	54868-0075-05	18.15		AB
100s ea	54868-0075-04	19.86		EE
300 mg, 30s ea	54868-0076-06	11.76		EE

PROD/MFR	NDC	AWP	DP	OBC
50s ea	54868-0076-05	17.58		EE
60s ea	54868-0076-02	20.49		EE
90s ea	54868-0076-07	30.75		EE
100s ea	54868-0076-03	32.16		EE
500s ea	54868-0076-00	147.36		EE
(Physician Partner)				
REPACK				
TAB, PO, 100 mg, 90s ea	21695-0836-90	102.71		AB
300 mg, 30s ea	21695-0246-30	38.70		AB
(Quality Care Prod)				
REPACK				
TAB, PO, 100 mg, 30s ea	49999-0374-30	12.46		AB
300 mg, 30s ea	49999-0245-30	21.24		EE
300s ea	49999-0245-03	212.40		EE
(Southwood)				
REPACK				
TAB, PO, 100 mg, 12s ea	58016-0941-12	2.33		EE
20s ea	58016-0941-20	3.89		EE
30s ea	58016-0941-30	5.84		EE
100s ea	58016-0941-00	19.45		EE
300 mg, 12s ea	58016-0942-12	6.93		EE
20s ea	58016-0942-20	10.65		EE
30s ea	58016-0942-30	15.98		EE
100s ea	58016-0942-00	53.27		EE
(Vibranta)				
REPACK				
TAB, PO, 100 mg, 30s ea	57866-3027-01	8.50		AB
300 mg, 30s ea	57866-3028-01	26.18		AB
ALLOPURINOL SODIUM (Bedford)				
PDS, IV (S.D.V.,PF)				
500 mg, ea	55390-0106-01	485.95		AP
(Bioniche Pharma) *See ALOPRIM*				
ALLRES G (Allegis)				
carbetapentane citrate/guaifenesin				
SUS, PO (1X473ML,GRAPE)				
7.5 mg/5 ml-200 mg/5 ml,				
473 ml	28595-0602-16	146.79		
ALLRES PD (Allegis)				
carbetapentane cit/pse hcl				
SUS, PO (GRAPE BUBBLEGUM)				
7.5 mg/5 ml-30 mg/5 ml,				
473 ml	28595-0601-16	146.79		
ALMOND FLAVOR BITTER (PCCA)				
almond oil				
OIL, NA (BITTER ALMOND)				
1 ml	51927-2172-00	0.90		
ALMOND OIL				
(Gallipot) *See ALMOND OIL BITTER*				
(Gallipot) *See ALMOND OIL SWEET*				
(Letco) *See ALMOND OIL SWEET*				
(Medisca)				
OIL, NA (1X100ML,SWEET NATURAL)				
100 ml	38779-0975-05	31.50		
(NF 24,SWEET NATURAL)				
100 ml	38779-2490-05	31.50		
(1X500ML,NF SWEETNATURAL)				
500 ml	38779-0975-08	61.50		
(NF 24,SWEET NATURAL)				
500 ml	38779-2490-08	61.50		
(1X1000ML,SWEET NATURAL)				
1000 ml	38779-0975-09	108.00		
(NF 24,SWEET NATURAL)				
1000 ml	38779-2490-09	108.00		
(1X4000ML, SWEET NATURAL)				
4000 ml	38779-0975-01	255.00		
(NF 24,SWEET NATURAL)				
4000 ml	38779-2490-01	255.00		
(PCCA) *See ALMOND FLAVOR BITTER*				
(PCCA) *See ALMOND OIL SWEET*				
(Spectrum Pharmacy) *See ALMOND OIL SWEET*				
ALMOND OIL BITTER (Gallipot)				
almond oil				
OIL, NA, 118.28 ml	51552-0625-04	11.97		
ALMOND OIL SWEET (Gallipot)				
almond oil				
OIL, NA (N.F.)				
118.28 ml	51552-0128-04	9.10		
473 ml	51552-0128-06	29.19		
3785 ml	51552-0128-08	83.30		
(Letco)				
OIL, NA, 500 ml	62991-1331-01	45.00		
3840 ml	62991-1331-02	177.00		
(PCCA)				
OIL, NA (BASE G; NF)				
1 ml	51927-9027-00	0.14		

PROD/MFR	NDC	AWP	DP	OBC
(Spectrum Pharmacy)				
OIL, NA (N.F.)				
100 ml	49452-0270-04	67.90		
(U.S.P./N.F.)				
500 ml	49452-0270-01	104.30		
4000 ml	49452-0270-02	406.00		
(NF)				
20000 ml	49452-0270-03	1428.00		
ALMOTRIPTAN MALATE				
(Ortho-McNeil Pharm) *See AXERT*				
ALOCRIL (Allergan Inc)				
nedocromil sodium				
SOL, OP, 2%, 5 ml	00023-8842-05	96.70		
ALODOX (Ocusoft)				
doxycycline hyclate				
TAB, PO (CONVENIENCE KIT)				
20 mg, ea	54799-0534-66	94.80		
ALOE				
(Spectrum Pharmacy) *See ALOE CAPE*				
ALOE CAPE (Spectrum Pharmacy)				
aloe				
LUM, NA (U.S.P., N.F.)				
100 gm	49452-0285-03	160.30		
500 gm	49452-0285-01	451.50		
ALOE VERA				
(Gallipot) *See ALOE VERA EXTRACT 200:1*				
(Letco)				
POW, NA (FREEZE-DRIED)				
25 gm	62991-2532-01	60.00		
100 gm	62991-2532-02	165.00		
(Medisca)				
POW, NA (1X5GM,FREEZE DRIED)				
5 gm	38779-0977-03	31.50		
(1X25GM,FREEZE DRIED)				
25 gm	38779-0977-04	70.50		
(1X100GM,FREEZE DRIED)				
100 gm	38779-0977-05	225.00		
(MPM Medical Inc.) *See ORAMAGICRX*				
ALOE VERA (PCCA)				
aloe vera oil				
OIL, NA, 1 ml	51927-2634-00	0.16		
ALOE VERA (PCCA)				
POW, NA, 1 gm	51927-1806-00	6.00		
(Spectrum Pharmacy) *See ALOE VERA EXTRACT 200:1*				
ALOE VERA EXTRACT 200:1 (Gallipot)				
aloe vera				
POW, NA (NATURAL)				
5 gm	51552-0571-02	14.00		
(Spectrum Pharmacy)				
POW, NA (1X25GM)				
25 gm	49452-0287-01	116.90		
(1X100GM)				
100 gm	49452-0287-02	345.80		
(1X500GM)				
500 gm	49452-0287-03	955.50		
ALOE VERA OIL (Medisca)				
OIL, NA (1X100ML)				
100 ml	38779-0976-05	28.50		
(1X500ML)				
500 ml	38779-0976-08	75.00		
(PCCA) *See ALOE VERA*				
ALOE/COLLAGEN/LIDOCAINE HYDROCHLORIDE				
(MPM Medical Inc.) *See REGENECARE WOUND*				
ALOE/HC ACE/PRAMOXINE HCL				
(Primus Pharma) *See NOVACORT*				
ALOE/HYDROCORTISONE ACETATE/IODOQUINOL				
(Primus Pharma) *See ALCORTIN A*				
ALOE/IODOQUINOL				
(Primus Pharma) *See ALOQUIN*				
ALOIN (PCCA)				
POW, NA, 1 gm	51927-3264-00	1.17		
ALOMIDE (Alcon Ophthalmic)				
lodoxamide tromethamine				
SOL, OP, 0.1%, 10 ml	00065-0345-10	100.56		
ALOPRIM (Bioniche Pharma)				
allopurinol sodium				
PDS, IV (SINGLE USE VIAL)				
500 mg, ea	67457-0187-50	637.81		AP
ALOQUIN (Primus Pharma)				
aloe/iodoquinol				
GEL, TP (1X60GM)				
1%-1.25%, 60 gm	68040-0706-16	175.00		

PROD/MFR	NDC	AWP	DP	OBC
ALORA (Watson)				
estradiol				
TDM, TD, 0.025 mg/24 hr,				
8s ea	52544-0884-08	50.10		BX
0.05 mg/24 hr,				
8s ea	52544-0471-08	54.86		BX
0.075 mg/24 hr,				
8s ea	52544-0472-08	56.03		BX
0.1 mg/24 hr,				
8s ea	52544-0473-08	57.25		BX
ALOSETRON HYDROCHLORIDE				
(Prometheus Labs) *See LOTRONEX*				
ALOXI (Eisai)				
palonosetron hydrochloride				
SOL, IV (SINGLE-USE)				
0.05 mg/ml,				
1.5 ml 5s	62856-0798-01	264.00		EE
5 ml	62856-0797-01	418.80		EE
ALPHA AMYLASE				
(Gallipot) *See A-AMYLASE*				
(PCCA)				
POW, NA (FCC)				
1 gm	51927-1071-00	6.00		
ALPHA KETOGLUTARIC ACID (Medisca)				
POW, NA, 25 gm	38779-0978-04	37.50		
100 gm	38779-0978-05	135.00		
(1X1000GM)				
1000 gm	38779-0978-09	585.00		
(PCCA) *See KETOGLUTARIC ACID*				
ALPHA-1 PROTEINASE INHIBITOR HUMAN				
(Baxter Bioscience) *See ARALAST*				
(Baxter Bioscience) *See ARALAST NP*				
(CSL) *See ZEMAIRA*				
(Talecris) *See PROLASTIN*				
(Talecris) *See PROLASTIN-C*				
ALPHA-ACETYLMANDELIC ACID (PCCA)				
acetylmandelic acid				
CRY, NA (1X1GM)				
1 gm	51927-1187-00	17.25		
ALPHAGAN P (Allergan Inc)				
brimonidine tartrate				
SOL, OP, 0.1%, 5 ml	00023-9321-05	69.24		
10 ml	00023-9321-10	138.43		
15 ml	00023-9321-15	207.67		
0.15%, 5 ml	00023-9177-05	73.25		
10 ml	00023-9177-10	146.46		
15 ml	00023-9177-15	219.71		
(Phys Total Care)				
REPACK				
SOL, OP, 0.15%, 5 ml	54868-4690-02	93.77		
10 ml	54868-4690-00	175.34		
15 ml	54868-4690-01	262.05		
(Southwood)				
REPACK				
SOL, OP, 0.15%, 10 ml	58016-4566-01	116.27		
ALPHANATE (Grifols USA, Inc.)				
ahf human/von willebrand factor				
PDS, IV (SINGLE DOSE,1000IU/10ML)				
1 iu-1 iu, ea	68516-4603-02	1.32	1.10	
(SINGLE DOSE,1500IU/10ML)				
1 iu-1 iu, ea	68516-4604-02	1.32	1.10	
(SINGLE DOSE,250IU/5ML)				
1 iu-1 iu, ea	68516-4601-01	1.32	1.10	
(SINGLE DOSE,500IU/5ML)				
1 iu-1 iu, ea	68516-4602-01	1.32	1.10	
ALPHANINE SD (Grifols USA, Inc.)				
factor ix human, purified				
PDS, IV (1000IU FIX/10ML SDV)				
1 iu, ea	68516-3600-05	1.42	1.18	
(1500IU FIX/10ML SDV)				
1 iu, ea	68516-3600-06	1.42	1.18	
(500IU FIX/10ML SDV)				
1 iu, ea	68516-3600-04	1.42	1.18	
ALPHAQUIN HP (Stratus)				
hydroquinone				
CRE, TP (SUNSCREEN/GLYCOLIC ACID)				
4%, 28.4 gm	58980-0580-10	44,00		
(SUNSCREEN)				
4%, 56.8 gm	58980-0580-20	70.75		
ALPRAZOLAM				
FUL				
TAB, PO, 0.25 mg,				
100s ea		6.14		
0.5 mg, 100s ea		6.98		
1 mg, 100s ea		8.85		

PROD/MFR	NDC	AWP	DP	OBC
2 mg, 100s ea		17.45		
TER, PO, 0.5 mg, 60s ea		116.06		
1 mg, 60s ea		144.39		
2 mg, 60s ea		191.64		
3 mg, 60s ea		287.44		
(Actavis)				
TAB, PO, 0.25 mg,				
100s ea, C-IV	**00228-2027-10**	69.50		AB
500s ea, C-IV	**00228-2027-50**	347.45		AB
1000s ea, C-IV	**00228-2027-96**	649.10		AB
0.5 mg,				
100s ea, C-IV	**00228-2029-10**	93.25		AB
500s ea, C-IV	**00228-2029-50**	466.25		AB
1000s ea, C-IV	**00228-2029-96**	808.75		AB
1 mg, 100s ea, C-IV	**00228-2031-10**	115.50		AB
500s ea, C-IV	**00228-2031-50**	570.00		AB
1000s ea, C-IV	**00228-2031-96**	1079.00		AB
2 mg, 100s ea, C-IV	**00228-2039-10**	196.45		AB
500s ea, C-IV	**00228-2039-50**	920.30		AB
TER, PO, 0.5 mg,				
60s ea, C-IV	**00228-3083-06**	135.40		AB
1 mg, 60s ea, C-IV	**00228-3084-06**	168.46		AB
2 mg, 60s ea, C-IV	**00228-3087-06**	223.58		AB
3 mg, 60s ea, C-IV	**00228-3086-06**	335.36		AB
(Amneal)				
TER, PO, 0.5 mg,				
60s ea, C-IV	**65162-0809-06**	128.95		AB
1 mg, 60s ea, C-IV	**65162-0810-06**	160.44		AB
2 mg, 60s ea, C-IV	**65162-0812-06**	212.93		AB
3 mg, 60s ea, C-IV	**65162-0813-06**	319.38		AB
(Azur Pharma, Inc.) *See NIRAVAM*				
(Dava Pharma)				
TAB, PO (USP)				
0.25 mg,				
100s ea, C-IV	**67253-0900-10**	69.50		AB
500s ea, C-IV	**67253-0900-50**	347.50		AB
1000s ea, C-IV	**67253-0900-11**	660.25		AB
0.5 mg,				
100s ea, C-IV	**67253-0901-10**	93.50		AB
500s ea, C-IV	**67253-0901-50**	467.50		AB
1000s ea, C-IV	**67253-0901-11**	688.25		AB
1 mg, 100s ea, C-IV	**67253-0902-10**	115.50		AB
500s ea, C-IV	**67253-0902-50**	577.50		AB
1000s ea, C-IV	**67253-0902-11**	1097.25		AB
2 mg, 100s ea, C-IV	**67253-0903-10**	196.45		AB
500s ea, C-IV	**67253-0903-50**	982.55		AB
(Gallipot)				
POW, NA (U.S.P.,N.F.)				
0.025 gm, C-IV	**51552-0537-04**	70.00		
0.1 gm, C-IV	**51552-0537-05**	210.00	150.00	
(Greenstone) *See ALPRAZOLAM XR*				
(Greenstone)				
TAB, PO (UNIT OF USE)				
0.25 mg,				
100s ea, C-IV	**59762-3719-01**	61.67		AB
500s ea, C-IV	**59762-3719-03**	302.11		AB
1000s ea, C-IV	**59762-3719-04**	534.07		AB
(UNIT OF USE)				
0.5 mg,				
100s ea, C-IV	**59762-3720-01**	74.29		AB
500s ea, C-IV	**59762-3720-03**	380.47		AB
1000s ea, C-IV	**59762-3720-04**	665.31		AB
(UNIT OF USE)				
1 mg,				
100s ea, C-IV	**59762-3721-01**	98.42		AB
500s ea, C-IV	**59762-3721-03**	481.81		AB
1000s ea, C-IV	**59762-3721-04**	887.64		AB
(UNIT OF USE)				
2 mg,				
100s ea, C-IV	**59762-3722-01**	169.36		AB
500s ea, C-IV	**59762-3722-03**	771.23		AB
(Major)				
TAB, PO (10X10,USP)				
1 mg,				
100s ea UD, C-IV	**00904-5860-61**	89.75		AB
(10X10)				
2 mg,				
100s ea UD, C-IV	**00904-5861-61**	385.97		AB
TER, PO, 0.5 mg,				
100s ea UD, C-IV	**00904-5862-61**	156.92		AB
1 mg,				
100s ea UD, C-IV	**00904-5863-61**	156.92		AB
2 mg,				
100s ea UD, C-IV	**00904-5864-61**	385.97		AB
3 mg,				
100s ea UD, C-IV	**00904-5865-61**	355.35		AB
(Medisca)				
POW, NA (U.S.P.)				
0.025 gm, C-IV	**38779-1993-04**	133.95		
0.1 gm, C-IV	**38779-1993-09**	450.00		
(Mylan)				
TAB, PO, 0.25 mg,				
100s ea, C-IV	**00378-4001-01**	69.50		AB
500s ea, C-IV	**00378-4001-05**	347.50		AB
0.5 mg,				
100s ea, C-IV	**00378-4003-01**	95.85		AB
500s ea, C-IV	**00378-4003-05**	494.60		AB
1 mg, 100s ea, C-IV	**00378-4005-01**	115.55		AB
500s ea, C-IV	**00378-4005-05**	577.75		AB
2 mg, 100s ea, C-IV	**00378-4007-01**	196.45		AB
TER, PO, 0.5 mg,				
60s ea, C-IV	**00378-5021-91**	128.95		AB
1 mg, 60s ea, C-IV	**00378-5022-91**	160.40		AB
2 mg, 60s ea, C-IV	**00378-5023-91**	212.90		AB
3 mg, 60s ea, C-IV	**00378-5024-91**	319.35		AB
(Par)				
ODT, PO (10X10)				
0.25 mg,				
100s ea UD, C-IV	**49884-0110-74**	151.73		
0.5 mg,				
100s ea UD, C-IV	**49884-0111-74**	189.04		
(10X10)				
1 mg,				
100s ea UD, C-IV	**49884-0213-74**	252.22		
2 mg,				
100s ea UD, C-IV	**49884-0214-74**	428.86		
(Pfizer) *See XANAX*				
(Pfizer) *See XANAX XR*				
(Qualitest)				
TAB, PO (USP)				
0.25 mg,				
100s ea, C-IV	**00603-2127-21**	69.50		AB
500s ea, C-IV	**00603-2127-28**	347.45		AB
1000s ea, C-IV	**00603-2127-32**	649.10		AB
0.5 mg,				
100s ea, C-IV	**00603-2128-21**	95.80		AB
500s ea, C-IV	**00603-2128-28**	494.59		AB
1000s ea, C-IV	**00603-2128-32**	939.72		AB
1 mg, 100s ea, C-IV	**00603-2129-21**	115.55		AB
500s ea, C-IV	**00603-2129-28**	577.70		AB
1000s ea, C-IV	**00603-2129-32**	1097.20		AB
(USP)				
2 mg,				
100s ea, C-IV	**00603-2130-21**	196.45		AB
500s ea, C-IV	**00603-2130-28**	957.75		AB
TER, PO, 0.5 mg,				
60s ea, C-IV	**00603-2131-20**	135.40		AB
1 mg, 60s ea, C-IV	**00603-2132-20**	168.45		AB
2 mg, 60s ea, C-IV	**00603-2133-20**	223.57		AB
3 mg, 60s ea, C-IV	**00603-2134-20**	335.35		AB
(Rising)				
TER, PO, 0.5 mg,				
60s ea, C-IV	**64980-0140-06**	128.95		AB
1 mg, 60s ea, C-IV	**64980-0141-06**	160.44		AB
2 mg, 60s ea, C-IV	**64980-0142-06**	212.93		AB
3 mg, 60s ea, C-IV	**64980-0143-06**	319.38		AB
(Roxane) *See ALPRAZOLAM INTENSOL*				
(Sandoz)				
TAB, PO, 0.25 mg,				
100s ea, C-IV	**00781-1061-01**	69.52		AB
500s ea, C-IV	**00781-1061-05**	338.91		AB
1000s ea, C-IV	**00781-1061-10**	660.44		AB
0.5 mg,				
100s ea, C-IV	**00781-1077-01**	86.61		AB
500s ea, C-IV	**00781-1077-05**	422.22		AB
1000s ea, C-IV	**00781-1077-10**	822.80		AB
1 mg, 100s ea, C-IV	**00781-1079-01**	115.56		AB
500s ea, C-IV	**00781-1079-05**	563.36		AB
1000s ea, C-IV	**00781-1079-10**	1097.82		AB
2 mg, 100s ea, C-IV	**00781-1089-01**	196.47		AB
500s ea, C-IV	**00781-1089-05**	957.79		AB
TER, PO, 0.5 mg,				
60s ea, C-IV	**00185-0195-60**	128.95		AB
1 mg, 60s ea, C-IV	**00185-0196-60**	160.44		AB
2 mg, 60s ea, C-IV	**00185-0197-60**	212.93		AB
3 mg, 60s ea, C-IV	**00185-0198-60**	319.38		AB
(Spectrum Pharmacy)				
POW, NA (U.S.P.)				
0.025 gm, C-IV	**49452-0295-01**	221.65		
0.1 gm, C-IV	**49452-0295-02**	735.00		
(Teva)				
TER, PO, 0.5 mg,				
60s ea, C-IV	**00093-5450-06**	135.55		AB
1 mg, 60s ea, C-IV	**00093-5451-06**	168.65		AB
2 mg, 60s ea, C-IV	**00093-5452-06**	223.83		AB
3 mg, 60s ea, C-IV	**00093-5453-06**	335.74		AB
(UDL)				
TAB, PO (10X10)				
0.25 mg,				
100s ea UD, C-IV	**51079-0788-20**	63.54		AB
(R.N.P., 5X20)				
0.25 mg,				
100s ea UD, C-IV	**51079-0788-21**	73.82		AB
(10X10)				
0.5 mg,				
100s ea UD, C-IV	**51079-0789-20**	75.97		AB
(R.N.P., 5X20)				
0.5 mg,				
100s ea UD, C-IV	**51079-0789-21**	86.02		AB
(10X10)				
1 mg,				
100s ea UD, C-IV	**51079-0790-20**	101.35		AB
(A-S Medication)				
REPACK				
TAB, PO, 0.25 mg,				
4s ea, C-IV	**54569-3755-05**	2.72		AB
14s ea, C-IV	**54569-3755-02**	9.51		AB
30s ea, C-IV	**54569-3755-00**	20.38		AB
60s ea, C-IV	**54569-3755-01**	40.76		AB
90s ea, C-IV	**54569-3755-04**	61.15		AB
0.5 mg, 20s ea, C-IV	**54569-3756-01**	17.74		AB
30s ea, C-IV	**54569-3756-00**	26.61		AB
45s ea, C-IV	**54569-3756-04**	39.92		AB
60s ea, C-IV	**54569-3756-02**	53.22		AB
90s ea, C-IV	**54569-3756-03**	79.83		AB
1 mg, 30s ea, C-IV	**54569-4619-01**	33.63		EE
45s ea, C-IV	**54569-4619-06**	50.45		EE
60s ea, C-IV	**54569-4619-02**	67.27		EE
90s ea, C-IV	**54569-4619-00**	100.90		EE
100s ea, C-IV	**54569-4619-03**	112.11		EE
2 mg, 40s ea, C-IV	**54569-4900-02**	76.42		EE
60s ea, C-IV	**54569-4900-00**	114.62		EE
90s ea, C-IV	**54569-4900-01**	171.94		EE
(Aidarex)				
REPACK				
TAB, PO, 0.5 mg,				
7s ea, C-IV	**33261-0004-07**	9.94		AB
14s ea, C-IV	**33261-0004-14**	19.88		AB
20s ea, C-IV	**33261-0004-20**	28.40		AB
21s ea, C-IV	**33261-0004-21**	29.82		AB
28s ea, C-IV	**33261-0004-28**	39.76		AB
30s ea, C-IV	**33261-0004-30**	42.60		AB
40s ea, C-IV	**33261-0004-40**	56.80		AB
60s ea, C-IV	**33261-0004-60**	85.20		AB
90s ea, C-IV	**33261-0004-90**	127.80		AB
120s ea, C-IV	**33261-0004-02**	170.40		AB
2 mg, 30s ea, C-IV	**33261-0500-30**	111.00		AB
60s ea, C-IV	**33261-0500-60**	222.00		AB
90s ea, C-IV	**33261-0500-90**	338.00		AB
120s ea, C-IV	**33261-0500-02**	444.00		AB
(Altura)				
REPACK				
TAB, PO, 0.25 mg,				
10s ea, C-IV	**63874-0251-10**	5.91		AB
12s ea, C-IV	**63874-0251-12**	7.08		EE
14s ea, C-IV	**63874-0251-14**	8.26		EE
15s ea, C-IV	**63874-0251-15**	8.85		EE
20s ea, C-IV	**63874-0251-20**	11.80		EE
30s ea, C-IV	**63874-0251-30**	17.70		EE
60s ea, C-IV	**63874-0251-60**	35.40		EE
90s ea, C-IV	**63874-0251-90**	75.26		AB
100s ea, C-IV	**63874-0251-01**	59.00		EE
150s ea, C-IV	**63874-0251-72**	120.32		EE
200s ea, C-IV	**63874-0251-74**	160.42		EE
300s ea, C-IV	**63874-0251-77**	240.63		EE
1000s ea, C-IV	**63874-0251-02**	296.41		EE
0.5 mg, 6s ea, C-IV	**63874-0252-06**	5.25		EE
9s ea, C-IV	**63874-0252-09**	7.88		EE
10s ea, C-IV	**63874-0252-10**	8.75		EE
12s ea, C-IV	**63874-0252-12**	10.50		EE
14s ea, C-IV	**63874-0252-14**	12.25		EE
15s ea, C-IV	**63874-0252-15**	13.13		EE
18s ea, C-IV	**63874-0252-18**	15.75		EE
20s ea, C-IV	**63874-0252-20**	17.50		EE
24s ea, C-IV	**63874-0252-24**	21.00		EE
30s ea, C-IV	**63874-0252-30**	26.25		EE
50s ea, C-IV	**63874-0252-50**	43.75		EE
60s ea, C-IV	**63874-0252-60**	52.50		EE
90s ea, C-IV	**63874-0252-90**	78.75		EE
100s ea, C-IV	**63874-0252-01**	87.50		EE
120s ea, C-IV	**63874-0252-04**	105.00		EE
150s ea, C-IV	**63874-0252-72**	131.25		EE
200s ea, C-IV	**63874-0252-74**	175.00		EE
300s ea, C-IV	**63874-0252-77**	262.50		EE
1000s ea, C-IV	**63874-0252-02**	726.75		EE
1 mg, 10s ea, C-IV	**63874-0253-10**	11.80		EE
12s ea, C-IV	**63874-0253-12**	14.16		EE
14s ea, C-IV	**63874-0253-14**	16.52		EE

PROD/MFR	NDC	AWP	DP	OBC
15s ea, C-IV	**63874-0253-15**	17.70		EE
18s ea, C-IV	**63874-0253-18**	21.24		EE
20s ea, C-IV	**63874-0253-20**	23.60		EE
21s ea, C-IV	**63874-0253-21**	24.78		EE
24s ea, C-IV	**63874-0253-24**	28.32		EE
25s ea, C-IV	**63874-0253-25**	29.50		EE
28s ea, C-IV	**63874-0253-28**	33.04		EE
30s ea, C-IV	**63874-0253-30**	35.04		EE
40s ea, C-IV	**63874-0253-40**	47.20		EE
50s ea, C-IV	**63874-0253-50**	66.67		AB
60s ea, C-IV	**63874-0253-60**	70.80		EE
90s ea, C-IV	**63874-0253-90**	106.20		AB
100s ea, C-IV	**63874-0253-01**	118.00		EE
120s ea, C-IV	**63874-0253-04**	160.01		EE
150s ea, C-IV	**63874-0253-72**	200.01		EE
200s ea, C-IV	**63874-0253-74**	266.68		EE
300s ea, C-IV	**63874-0253-77**	400.02		EE
500s ea, C-IV	**63874-0253-03**	666.70		AB
2 mg, 14s ea, C-IV	**63874-1016-04**	27.72		
15s ea, C-IV	**63874-1016-05**	29.70		
20s ea, C-IV	**63874-1016-02**	39.60		
28s ea, C-IV	**63874-1016-08**	55.44		
30s ea, C-IV	**63874-1016-03**	59.40		
60s ea, C-IV	**63874-1016-06**	118.80		
90s ea, C-IV	**63874-1016-09**	178.20		AB
100s ea, C-IV	**63874-1016-01**	198.00		
(American Health)				
REPACK				
TAB, PO (10X10)				
0.25 mg,				
100s ea UD, C-IV	**68084-0018-01**	65.15		AB
(15X30)				
0.25 mg,				
450s ea, C-IV	**68084-0018-85**	305.02		AB
(10X10)				
0.5 mg,				
100s ea UD, C-IV	**68084-0019-01**	79.57		AB
(15X30)				
0.5 mg,				
450s ea, C-IV	**68084-0019-85**	380.00		AB
(10X10)				
1 mg,				
100s ea UD, C-IV	**68084-0020-01**	103.95		AB
(15X30)				
1 mg,				
450s ea, C-IV	**68084-0020-85**	507.02		AB
(B&B Pharm, Inc)				
REPACK				
POW, NA, 1 gm, C-IV	**63275-9961-01**	210.00		
5 gm, C-IV	**63275-9961-02**	1000.00		
25 gm, C-IV	**63275-9961-04**	4900.00		
(Bryant Ranch)				
REPACK				
TAB, PO, 0.25 mg,				
20s ea, C-IV	**63629-2955-04**	28.95		
30s ea, C-IV	**63629-2955-01**	34.45		
60s ea, C-IV	**63629-2955-03**	62.03		
90s ea, C-IV	**63629-2955-06**	109.23		AB
100s ea, C-IV	**63629-2955-02**	101.32		
0.5 mg, 15s ea, C-IV	**63629-1541-01**	17.28		
20s ea, C-IV	**63629-1541-03**	23.04		
30s ea, C-IV	**63629-1541-02**	34.56		
60s ea, C-IV	**63629-1541-06**	69.12		
90s ea, C-IV	**63629-1541-05**	103.67		
100s ea, C-IV	**63629-1541-04**	115.19		
1 mg, 10s ea, C-IV	**63629-2942-01**	16.96		
20s ea, C-IV	**63629-2942-02**	33.92		
30s ea, C-IV	**63629-2942-03**	50.88		
60s ea, C-IV	**63629-2942-04**	70.00		
(USP)				
1 mg, 90s ea, C-IV	**63629-2942-05**	152.64		AB
2 mg, 30s ea, C-IV	**63629-3308-01**	106.90		
60s ea, C-IV	**63629-3308-02**	212.03		
90s ea, C-IV	**63629-3308-03**	319.56		
(Core)				
REPACK				
TAB, PO, 0.25 mg,				
30s ea, C-IV	**33358-0014-30**	35.31		
60s ea, C-IV	**33358-0014-60**	63.58		
0.5 mg, 20s ea, C-IV	**33358-0015-20**	23.62		
30s ea, C-IV	**33358-0015-30**	35.42		
40s ea, C-IV	**33358-0015-40**	49.28		
60s ea, C-IV	**33358-0015-60**	70.85		
90s ea, C-IV	**33358-0015-90**	106.26		
1 mg, 10s ea, C-IV	**33358-0016-10**	17.38		
20s ea, C-IV	**33358-0016-20**	34.77		
30s ea, C-IV	**33358-0016-30**	52.15		
40s ea, C-IV	**33358-0016-40**	67.64		
60s ea, C-IV	**33358-0016-60**	71.75		
100s ea, C-IV	**33358-0016-00**	103.99		
2 mg, 40s ea, C-IV	**33358-0017-40**	79.25		
60s ea, C-IV	**33358-0017-60**	118.53		
90s ea, C-IV	**33358-0017-90**	177.43		

PROD/MFR	NDC	AWP	DP	OBC
(DHS, Inc.)				
REPACK				
TAB, PO, 0.25 mg,				
20s ea, C-IV	**55887-0280-20**	16.00		
30s ea, C-IV	**55887-0280-30**	24.00		
60s ea, C-IV	**55887-0280-60**	48.00		
90s ea, C-IV	**55887-0280-90**	72.00		
0.5 mg, 20s ea, C-IV	**55887-0648-20**	21.09		AB
21s ea, C-IV	**55887-0648-21**	22.11		
30s ea, C-IV	**55887-0648-30**	32.02		AB
60s ea, C-IV	**55887-0648-60**	59.66		AB
90s ea, C-IV	**55887-0648-90**	87.49		AB
1 mg, 5s ea, C-IV	**55887-0245-05**	6.79		
30s ea, C-IV	**55887-0245-30**	40.79		AB
60s ea, C-IV	**55887-0245-60**	81.58		AB
90s ea, C-IV	**55887-0245-90**	99.00		AB
2 mg, 30s ea, C-IV	**55887-0182-30**	65.00		AB
60s ea, C-IV	**55887-0182-60**	130.00		AB
90s ea, C-IV	**55887-0182-90**	195.00		
(Dispensing Solutions)				
REPACK				
TAB, PO, 0.25 mg,				
6s ea, C-IV	**55045-2102-06**	3.66		AB
15s ea, C-IV	**55045-2102-05**	9.15		AB
20s ea, C-IV	**66336-0876-20**	17.28		
30s ea, C-IV	**55045-2102-08**	18.30		AB
30s ea, C-IV	**55045-3756-08**	18.30		
30s ea, C-IV	**66336-0876-30**	25.62		AB
45s ea, C-IV	**55045-2102-09**	27.45		AB
60s ea, C-IV	**55045-2102-07**	36.60		AB
60s ea, C-IV	**66336-0876-60**	50.64		AB
90s ea, C-IV	**55045-2102-01**	54.90		AB
100s ea, C-IV	**55045-2102-00**	61.00		AB
112s ea, C-IV	**55045-2102-03**	68.32		AB
120s ea, C-IV	**55045-2102-02**	73.20		AB
0.5 mg, 10s ea, C-IV	**55045-2110-02**	7.70		
20s ea, C-IV	**55045-2110-07**	15.40		
30s ea, C-IV	**55045-2110-08**	23.10		AB
30s ea, C-IV	**66336-0861-30**	27.86		AB
60s ea, C-IV	**55045-2110-06**	46.35		AB
60s ea, C-IV	**66336-0861-60**	55.73		AB
90s ea, C-IV	**55045-2110-09**	69.30		AB
90s ea, C-IV	**66336-0861-90**	83.60		AB
100s ea, C-IV	**55045-2110-01**	77.00		AB
112s ea, C-IV	**55045-2110-03**	86.24		AB
120s ea, C-IV	**55045-2110-00**	92.40		
1 mg, 10s ea, C-IV	**55045-2278-00**	11.60		
30s ea, C-IV	**55045-2278-08**	34.85		AB
30s ea, C-IV	**66336-0932-30**	40.79		
40s ea, C-IV	**55045-2278-04**	46.40		AB
60s ea, C-IV	**55045-2278-06**	69.60		AB
60s ea, C-IV	**66336-0932-60**	81.58		
90s ea, C-IV	**55045-2278-09**	104.40		AB
90s ea, C-IV	**66336-0932-90**	122.37		AB
100s ea, C-IV	**55045-2278-01**	116.00		AB
120s ea, C-IV	**55045-2278-02**	139.20		
2 mg, 30s ea, C-IV	**55045-2568-03**	66.60		AB
30s ea, C-IV	**66336-0403-30**	70.72		
40s ea, C-IV	**55045-2568-04**	88.80		AB
60s ea, C-IV	**66336-0403-60**	130.00		AB
90s ea, C-IV	**66336-0403-90**	195.00		
100s ea, C-IV	**55045-2568-01**	222.00		
(GSMS)				
REPACK				
TAB, PO (UNIT OF USE)				
0.25 mg,				
30s ea, C-IV	**60429-0502-30**	8.55	2.85	EE
60s ea, C-IV	**60429-0502-60**	14.55	4.85	EE
90s ea, C-IV	**60429-0502-90**	20.55	6.85	EE
0.5 mg, 60s ea, C-IV	**60429-0503-60**	8.10	2.70	EE
90s ea, C-IV	**60429-0503-90**	10.95	3.65	EE
(HomeMed)				
REPACK				
TAB, PO, 0.25 mg,				
30s ea, C-IV	**51655-0861-24**	15.60		
60s ea, C-IV	**51655-0861-25**	61.99		
90s ea, C-IV	**51655-0861-26**	24.40		
0.5 mg, 30s ea, C-IV	**51655-0860-24**	38.99		
60s ea, C-IV	**51655-0860-25**	69.99		
90s ea, C-IV	**51655-0860-26**	63.10		
120s ea, C-IV	**51655-0860-82**	83.80		
1 mg, 30s ea, C-IV	**51655-0863-24**	50.89		
60s ea, C-IV	**51655-0863-25**	52.80		
90s ea, C-IV	**51655-0863-26**	78.70		
120s ea, C-IV	**51655-0863-82**	104.60		
(IPI)				
REPACK				
TAB, PO, 0.5 mg,				
60s ea, C-IV	**18837-0001-60**	50.67		AB
90s ea, C-IV	**18837-0001-90**	76.00		AB
1 mg, 30s ea, C-IV	**18837-0002-30**	33.80		AB
60s ea, C-IV	**18837-0002-60**	67.60		AB

PROD/MFR	NDC	AWP	DP	OBC
90s ea, C-IV	**18837-0002-90**	101.40		AB
120s ea, C-IV	**18837-0002-98**	135.21		AB
2 mg, 60s ea, C-IV	**18837-0003-60**	143.67		AB
90s ea, C-IV	**18837-0003-90**	215.50		AB
120s ea, C-IV	**18837-0003-98**	229.87		AB
(Keltman Pharma., Inc.)				
REPACK				
TAB, PO, 0.25 mg,				
30s ea, C-IV	**68387-0465-30**	18.00		AB
45s ea, C-IV	**68387-0465-45**	27.00		
90s ea, C-IV	**68387-0465-90**	79.20		
0.5 mg, 30s ea, C-IV	**68387-0460-30**	30.00		AB
60s ea, C-IV	**68387-0460-60**	76.80		AB
60s ea, C-IV	**68387-0465-60**	52.84		AB
90s ea, C-IV	**68387-0460-90**	90.00		
180s ea, C-IV	**68387-0460-18**	160.20		
1 mg, 30s ea, C-IV	**68387-0466-30**	43.10		AB
45s ea, C-IV	**68387-0466-45**	64.65		
60s ea, C-IV	**68387-0466-60**	86.20		
90s ea, C-IV	**68387-0466-90**	129.30		
(McKesson Packaging)				
REPACK				
TAB, PO, 0.25 mg,				
100s ea UD, C-IV	**63739-0010-10**	85.00		AB
0.5 mg,				
100s ea UD, C-IV	**63739-0011-10**	105.00		AB
1 mg,				
100s ea UD, C-IV	**63739-0012-10**	141.25		AB
(Medsource)				
REPACK				
TAB, PO, 0.25 mg,				
30s ea, C-IV	**45865-0484-30**	19.47		AB
60s ea, C-IV	**45865-0484-60**	39.00		AB
0.5 mg, 30s ea, C-IV	**45865-0424-30**	27.90		AB
60s ea, C-IV	**45865-0424-60**	55.80		AB
TER, PO, 0.5 mg,				
30s ea, C-IV	**45865-0481-30**	67.80		AB
60s ea, C-IV	**45865-0481-60**	135.60		AB
(Nucare Pharm)				
REPACK				
TAB, PO, 0.25 mg,				
30s ea, C-IV	**66267-0219-30**	25.98		AB
60s ea, C-IV	**66267-0219-60**	41.60		AB
90s ea, C-IV	**66267-0219-90**	83.88		AB
0.5 mg, 30s ea, C-IV	**66267-0013-30**	32.45		AB
60s ea, C-IV	**66267-0013-60**	61.00		AB
90s ea, C-IV	**66267-0013-90**	86.45		AB
1 mg, 30s ea, C-IV	**66267-0014-30**	49.78		AB
60s ea, C-IV	**66267-0014-60**	92.93		AB
90s ea, C-IV	**66267-0014-90**	137.30		AB
120s ea, C-IV	**66267-0014-91**	180.61		AB
2 mg, 120s ea, C-IV	**66267-0564-91**	295.96		AB
(Palmetto)				
REPACK				
TAB, PO, 0.25 mg,				
10s ea, C-IV	**23490-5032-07**	11.93		
20s ea, C-IV	**23490-5032-01**	23.85		
30s ea, C-IV	**23490-5032-02**	35.78		
60s ea, C-IV	**23490-5032-04**	71.56		
90s ea, C-IV	**23490-5032-05**	107.34		
100s ea, C-IV	**23490-5032-06**	119.27		
0.5 mg, 6s ea, C-IV	**23490-5033-01**	9.24		
10s ea, C-IV	**23490-5033-05**	11.00		
30s ea, C-IV	**23490-5033-02**	33.00		
60s ea, C-IV	**23490-5033-03**	66.00		
90s ea, C-IV	**23490-5033-04**	99.00		
1 mg, 30s ea, C-IV	**23490-5034-01**	45.00		
60s ea, C-IV	**23490-5034-02**	90.00		
90s ea, C-IV	**23490-5034-04**	135.00		
100s ea, C-IV	**23490-5034-03**	150.00		
2 mg, 30s ea, C-IV	**23490-5035-03**	82.05		
60s ea, C-IV	**23490-5035-06**	164.10		
90s ea, C-IV	**23490-5035-09**	246.15		
100s ea, C-IV	**23490-5035-08**	273.50		
(PD-Rx Pharm)				
REPACK				
TAB, PO, 0.25 mg,				
5s ea, C-IV	**55289-0962-05**	25.28		AB
6s ea, C-IV	**43063-0088-06**	26.32		AB
20s ea, C-IV	**55289-0962-20**	33.32		AB
30s ea, C-IV	**55289-0962-30**	35.78		AB
60s ea, C-IV	**55289-0962-60**	48.14		AB
90s ea, C-IV	**55289-0962-90**	60.48		AB
120s ea, C-IV	**55289-0962-98**	72.96		AB
(USP)				
0.5 mg,				
6s ea, C-IV	**43063-0061-06**	25.48		AB
15s ea, C-IV	**55289-0945-15**	32.98		AB
30s ea, C-IV	**55289-0945-30**	39.67		AB
60s ea, C-IV	**55289-0945-60**	56.00		AB
90s ea, C-IV	**55289-0945-90**	72.33		AB

PROD/MFR	NDC	AWP	DP	OBC
120s ea, C-IV	55289-0945-98	97.07		AB
1 mg, 30s ea, C-IV	55289-0920-30	48.37		AB
40s ea, C-IV	55289-0920-40	49.07		AB
60s ea, C-IV	55289-0920-60	56.00		AB
90s ea, C-IV	55289-0920-90	72.33		AB
120s ea, C-IV	55289-0920-98	88.67		AB
2 mg, 30s ea, C-IV	55289-0523-30	53.67		AB
40s ea, C-IV	55289-0523-40	74.34		AB
60s ea, C-IV	55289-0523-60	84.00		AB

(Pharma Pac)

REPACK

TAB, PO, 0.25 mg,

PROD/MFR	NDC	AWP	DP	OBC
10s ea, C-IV	52959-0321-10	10.19		EE
14s ea, C-IV	52959-0321-14	14.16		EE
20s ea, C-IV	52959-0321-20	20.39		EE
30s ea, C-IV	52959-0321-30	30.58		EE
60s ea, C-IV	52959-0321-60	66.54		AB
90s ea, C-IV	52959-0321-90	91.73		EE
100s ea, C-IV	52959-0321-00	101.89		EE
120s ea, C-IV	52959-0321-02	122.16		EE
0.5 mg, 15s ea, C-IV	52959-0457-15	17.00		EE
20s ea, C-IV	52959-0457-20	22.66		EE
24s ea, C-IV	52959-0457-24	27.18		AB
30s ea, C-IV	52959-0457-30	33.98		EE
45s ea, C-IV	52959-0457-45	50.96		EE
60s ea, C-IV	52959-0457-60	67.92		EE
90s ea, C-IV	52959-0457-90	101.74		EE
100s ea, C-IV	52959-0457-00	112.99		EE
120s ea, C-IV	52959-0457-02	119.99		EE
1 mg, 6s ea, C-IV	52959-0524-06	10.18		AB
10s ea, C-IV	52959-0524-10	16.97		AB
30s ea, C-IV	52959-0524-30	50.89		AB
60s ea, C-IV	52959-0524-60	101.76		AB
90s ea, C-IV	52959-0524-90	152.62		AB
100s ea, C-IV	52959-0524-00	169.58		AB
120s ea, C-IV	52959-0524-02	202.80		AB
2 mg, 10s ea, C-IV	52959-0864-10	22.74		AB
30s ea, C-IV	52959-0864-30	68.20		
40s ea, C-IV	52959-0864-40	90.92		
60s ea, C-IV	52959-0864-60	135.48		
90s ea, C-IV	52959-0864-90	203.17		
100s ea, C-IV	52959-0864-00	225.60		
TER, PO, 1 mg,				
30s ea, C-IV	52959-0965-30	79.81		AB
60s ea, C-IV	52959-0965-60	155.50		AB

(Phys Total Care)

REPACK

TAB, PO, 0.25 mg,

PROD/MFR	NDC	AWP	DP	OBC
10s ea, C-IV	54868-2929-07	6.06		EE
15s ea, C-IV	54868-2929-00	6.87		EE
20s ea, C-IV	54868-2929-05	6.15		EE
30s ea, C-IV	54868-2929-02	9.21		EE
50s ea, C-IV	54868-2929-01	12.36		EE
60s ea, C-IV	54868-2929-06	12.45		EE
90s ea, C-IV	54868-2929-08	18.66		EE
100s ea, C-IV	54868-2929-03	20.25		EE
0.5 mg, 10s ea, C-IV	54868-2930-00	6.24		AB
20s ea, C-IV	54868-2930-07	8.16		FF
25s ea, C-IV	54868-2930-06	9.06		EE
30s ea, C-IV	54868-2930-03	9.96		EE
50s ea, C-IV	54868-2930-02	13.62		EE
60s ea, C-IV	54868-2930-04	15.45		EE
90s ea, C-IV	54868-2930-05	20.91		EE
100s ea, C-IV	54868-2930-01	21.99		EE
120s ea, C-IV	54868-2930-09	25.94		EE
1 mg, 20s ea, C-IV	54868-3005-04	8.07		EE
30s ea, C-IV	54868-3005-02	9.84		EE
45s ea, C-IV	54868-3005-05	12.51		AB
60s ea, C-IV	54868-3005-03	15.45		EE
(USP)				
1 mg, 90s ea, C-IV	54868-3005-07	19.03		EE
100s ea, C-IV	54868-3005-01	20.82		EE
500s ea, C-IV	54868-3005-06	72.72		AB
2 mg, 30s ea, C-IV	54868-4663-02	17.46		AB
40s ea, C-IV	54868-4663-00	21.30		AB
60s ea, C-IV	54868-4663-05	24.27		AB
90s ea, C-IV	54868-4663-01	40.38		AB
100s ea, C-IV	54868-4663-06	40.45		AB
120s ea, C-IV	54868-4663-04	55.46		
500s ea, C-IV	54868-4663-03	162.36		AB

(Physician Partner)

REPACK

TAB, PO, 0.25 mg,

PROD/MFR	NDC	AWP	DP	OBC
30s ea, C-IV	21695-0247-30	40.67		
60s ea, C-IV	21695-0247-60	81.34		
0.5 mg, 15s ea, C-IV	21695-0248-15	25.98		AB
30s ea, C-IV	21695-0248-30	51.96		
60s ea, C-IV	21695-0248-60	103.93		
100s ea, C-IV	21695-0248-00	173.22		AB
1 mg, 30s ea, C-IV	21695-0249-30	65.87		
45s ea, C-IV	21695-0249-45	116.24		AB
60s ea, C-IV	21695-0249-60	131.74		
90s ea, C-IV	21695-0249-90	202.81		
2 mg, 30s ea, C-IV	21695-0250-30	114.93		
60s ea, C-IV	21695-0250-60	229.86		

(Quality Care Prod)

REPACK

TAB, PO, 0.25 mg,

PROD/MFR	NDC	AWP	DP	OBC
10s ea, C-IV	49999-0039-10	7.00		AB
15s ea, C-IV	49999-0039-15	10.50		AB
30s ea, C-IV	49999-0039-30	21.06		EE
60s ea, C-IV	49999-0039-60	42.00		EE
90s ea, C-IV	49999-0039-90	63.18		AB
0.5 mg, 2s ea, C-IV	49999-0032-02	2.10		EE
4s ea, C-IV	49999-0032-04	4.20		EE
15s ea, C-IV	49999-0032-15	15.75		AB
30s ea, C-IV	49999-0032-30	31.50		EE
60s ea, C-IV	49999-0032-60	63.00		EE
90s ea, C-IV	49999-0032-90	94.50		EE
100s ea, C-IV	49999-0032-00	105.00		AB
1 mg, 2s ea, C-IV	49999-0252-02	2.80		EE
4s ea, C-IV	49999-0252-04	5.60		EE
10s ea, C-IV	49999-0252-10	13.98		AB
30s ea, C-IV	49999-0252-30	41.94		AB
60s ea, C-IV	49999-0252-60	83.88		AB
90s ea, C-IV	49999-0252-90	125.82		EE
100s ea, C-IV	49999-0252-00	139.80		AB
2 mg, 60s ea, C-IV	49999-0253-60	142.92		AB
90s ea, C-IV	49999-0253-90	214.38		AB
100s ea, C-IV	49999-0253-00	272.04		AB

(Southwood)

REPACK

TAB, PO, 0.25 mg,

PROD/MFR	NDC	AWP	DP	OBC
12s ea, C-IV	58016-0198-12	9.63		EE
15s ea, C-IV	58016-0198-15	12.03		EE
20s ea, C-IV	58016-0198-20	16.04		EE
30s ea, C-IV	58016-0198-30	27.90		AB
60s ea, C-IV	58016-0198-60	55.80		AB
90s ea, C-IV	58016-0198-90	83.70		AB
100s ea, C-IV	58016-0198-00	93.00		AB
120s ea, C-IV	58016-0198-02	96.25		EE
150s ea, C-IV	58016-0198-03	120.32		EE
200s ea, C-IV	58016-0198-89	160.42		EE
300s ea, C-IV	58016-0198-73	240.63		EE
0.5 mg, 6s ea, C-IV	58016-0197-06	6.00		EE
9s ea, C-IV	58016-0197-09	8.99		EE
10s ea, C-IV	58016-0197-10	9.99		EE
12s ea, C-IV	58016-0197-12	11.99		EE
14s ea, C-IV	58016-0197-14	13.99		EE
15s ea, C-IV	58016-0197-15	14.99		EE
18s ea, C-IV	58016-0197-18	17.99		EE
20s ea, C-IV	58016-0197-20	19.99		EE
24s ea, C-IV	58016-0197-24	23.98		EE
30s ea, C-IV	58016-0197-30	34.50		AB
50s ea, C-IV	58016-0197-50	49.97		EE
60s ea, C-IV	58016-0197-60	69.00		AB
90s ea, C-IV	58016-0197-90	103.50		AB
100s ea, C-IV	58016-0197-00	115.00		AB
120s ea, C-IV	58016-0197-02	119.92		EE
150s ea, C-IV	58016-0197-03	149.90		EE
200s ea, C-IV	58016-0197-89	199.86		EE
300s ea, C-IV	58016-0197-73	299.79		EE
1 mg, 10s ea, C-IV	58016-0840-10	13.33		EE
12s ea, C-IV	58016-0840-12	16.00		EE
14s ea, C-IV	58016-0840-14	18.67		EE
15s ea, C-IV	58016-0840-15	20.00		EE
18s ea, C-IV	58016-0840-18	24.00		EE
20s ea, C-IV	58016-0840-20	26.67		EE
21s ea, C-IV	58016-0840-21	28.00		EE
24s ea, C-IV	58016-0840-24	32.00		EE
25s ea, C-IV	58016-0840-25	33.34		EE
28s ea, C-IV	58016-0840-28	37.34		EE
30s ea, C-IV	58016-0840-30	46.20		AB
40s ea, C-IV	58016-0840-40	53.34		EE
60s ea, C-IV	58016-0840-60	92.40		AB
90s ea, C-IV	58016-0840-90	138.60		AB
100s ea, C-IV	58016-0840-00	154.00		AB
120s ea, C-IV	58016-0840-02	160.01		EE
150s ea, C-IV	58016-0840-03	200.01		EE
200s ea, C-IV	58016-0840-89	266.68		EE
300s ea, C-IV	58016-0840-73	400.02		EE
2 mg, 10s ea, C-IV	58016-0379-10	22.67		EE
12s ea, C-IV	58016-0379-12	27.20		EE
14s ea, C-IV	58016-0379-14	31.74		EE
15s ea, C-IV	58016-0379-15	34.01		EE
20s ea, C-IV	58016-0379-20	45.34		EE
21s ea, C-IV	58016-0379-21	47.61		EE
24s ea, C-IV	58016-0379-24	54.41		EE
25s ea, C-IV	58016-0379-25	56.68		EE
28s ea, C-IV	58016-0379-28	63.48		EE
30s ea, C-IV	58016-0379-30	78.00		AB
40s ea, C-IV	58016-0379-40	90.68		EE
60s ea, C-IV	58016-0379-60	156.00		AB
90s ea, C-IV	58016-0379-90	234.00		AB
100s ea, C-IV	58016-0379-00	260.00		AB
120s ea, C-IV	58016-0379-02	272.04		EE
150s ea, C-IV	58016-0379-03	340.05		EE
200s ea, C-IV	58016-0379-89	453.40		EE
300s ea, C-IV	58016-0379-73	680.10		EE

(Stat Rx)

REPACK

TAB, PO, 0.25 mg,

PROD/MFR	NDC	AWP	DP	OBC
14s ea, C-IV	16590-0447-14	8.84		
20s ea, C-IV	16590-0447-20	14.50		
30s ea, C-IV	16590-0447-30	25.47		AB
60s ea, C-IV	16590-0447-60	43.50		
90s ea, C-IV	16590-0447-90	65.25		
100s ea, C-IV	16590-0447-71	72.50		AB
0.5 mg, 20s ea, C-IV	16590-0005-20	19.70		
30s ea, C-IV	16590-0005-30	29.50		
60s ea, C-IV	16590-0005-60	59.00		
90s ea, C-IV	16590-0005-90	88.50		
120s ea, C-IV	16590-0005-72	118.00		
1 mg, 15s ea, C-IV	16590-0006-15	20.58		AB
28s ea, C-IV	16590-0006-28	40.04		AB
30s ea, C-IV	16590-0006-30	41.17		AB
60s ea, C-IV	16590-0006-60	83.82		AB
90s ea, C-IV	16590-0006-90	123.51		AB
120s ea, C-IV	16590-0006-72	167.64		AB
2 mg, 30s ea, C-IV	16590-0576-30	19.00		AB
60s ea, C-IV	16590-0576-60	37.75		AB
90s ea, C-IV	16590-0576-90	56.00		AB
120s ea, C-IV	16590-0576-72	70.00		AB
TER, PO, 1 mg,				
30s ea, C-IV	16590-0571-30	54.75		AB
60s ea, C-IV	16590-0571-60	90.00		AB
90s ea, C-IV	16590-0571-90	104.00		AB
120s ea, C-IV	16590-0571-72	140.00		AB
2 mg, 30s ea, C-IV	16590-0588-30	100.00		AB
60s ea, C-IV	16590-0588-60	190.00		AB
90s ea, C-IV	16590-0588-90	275.00		AB
120s ea, C-IV	16590-0588-72	290.00		AB

ALPRAZOLAM INTENSOL (Roxane)

alprazolam

SOL, PO (W/DROPPER)

PROD/MFR	NDC	AWP	DP	OBC
1 mg/ml,				
30 ml, C-IV	00054-3068-44	67.03		

ALPRAZOLAM XR (Greenstone)

alprazolam

TER, PO, 0.5 mg,

PROD/MFR	NDC	AWP	DP	OBC
60s ea, C-IV	59762-0057-01	128.95		
1 mg, 60s ea, C-IV	59762-0059-01	160.44		
2 mg, 60s ea, C-IV	59762-0066-01	212.93		
3 mg, 60s ea, C-IV	59762-0068-01	319.38		

(Phys Total Care)

REPACK

TER, PO, 0.5 mg,

PROD/MFR	NDC	AWP	DP	OBC
20s ea, C-IV	54868-5515-00	68.58		

(Quality Care Prod)

REPACK

TER, PO, 1 mg,

PROD/MFR	NDC	AWP	DP	OBC
60s ea, C-IV	35356-0503-60	158.60		
2 mg, 60s ea, C-IV	35356-0504-60	210.33		
3 mg, 60s ea, C-IV	35356-0505-60	234.40		

ALPROSTADIL

(B&B Pharm, Inc) *See PROSTAGLANDIN E1*

(Bedford) *See ALPROSTADIL NOVAPLUS*

(Bedford)

SOL, IV (S.D.V.,USP)

PROD/MFR	NDC	AWP	DP	OBC
0.5 mg/ml, 1 ml	55390-0506-10	62.40		AP

(Gallipot) *See PROSTAGLANDIN E1*

(Hawkins)

POW, NA (U.S.P.)

PROD/MFR	NDC	AWP	DP	OBC
0.01 gm	63370-0210-04	360.00		
0.1 gm	63370-0210-06	1932.00		
1 gm	63370-0210-10	6720.00		

(Letco)

POW, NA (U.S.P.)

PROD/MFR	NDC	AWP	DP	OBC
0.05 gm	62991-1128-08	375.00		
0.1 gm	62991-1128-07	600.00		
0.5 gm	62991-1128-06	1950.00		
1 gm	62991-1128-02	3600.00		

PROD/MFR | NDC | AWP | DP | OBC

(Medisca)
POW, NA (U.S.P.)
0.01 gm **38779-0944-07** 267.00
0.1 gm **38779-0944-09** 1563.00
(USP,1X1GM)
1 gm **38779-0944-06** 4950.00

(PCCA)
POW, NA (U.S.P.)
0.001 gm **51927-2196-00** 75.00

(Pfizer) *See CAVERJECT*

(Pfizer) *See CAVERJECT IMPULSE*

(Pfizer) *See PROSTIN VR PEDIATRIC*

(Spectrum Pharmacy)
POW, NA (U.S.P.)
0.025 gm **49452-0073-04** 903.00
0.1 gm **49452-0073-03** 1603.00

(Teva)
SOL, IV (S.D.V.)
0.5 mg/ml, 1 ml 5s ... **00703-1501-02** 330.00 **AP**

(UCB) *See EDEX*

(Vivus) *See MUSE*

ALPROSTADIL NOVAPLUS (Bedford)
alprostadil
SOL, IV (S.D.V.,USP)
0.5 mg/ml, 1 ml ...... **55390-0503-10** 37.20 **AP**

ALREX (Bausch & Lomb Inc.)
loteprednol etabonate
SUS, OP, 0.2%, 5 ml **24208-0353-05** 82.36
10 ml............ **24208-0353-10** 164.70

(Phys Total Care)
REPACK
SUS, OP, 0.2%, 10 ml **54868-4277-00** 112.10

(Stat Rx)
REPACK
SUS, OP, 0.2%, 1 ml **16590-0007-01** 58.00
5 ml............ **16590-0007-05** 116.00

ALTABAX (Glaxo)
retapamulin
OIN, TP, 1%, 5 gm **00007-5180-05** 41.14
15 gm **00007-5180-22** 89.48
(1X30GM)
1%, 30 gm.......... **00007-5180-25** 178.97

(Phys Total Care)
REPACK
OIN, TP, 1%, 15 gm **54868-6096-00** 114.12

(Physician Partner)
REPACK
OIN, TP (1X10GM)
1%, 10 gm.......... **21695-0644-10** 152.48

ALTACAINE (Altaire)
tetracaine hydrochloride
SOL, OP (STERILE)
0.5%, 15 ml **59390-0181-13** 8.39
30 ml............ **59390-0181-18** 12.00

ALTACE (King Pharm)
ramipril
TAB, PO, 1.25 mg,
100s ea............ **60793-0500-01** 163.21 **EE**
2.5 mg, 100s ea...... **60793-0501-01** 192.65 **EE**
5 mg, 100s ea........ **60793-0502-01** 202.12 **EE**
10 mg, 100s ea **60793-0503-01** 236.51

(Monarch)
CAP, PO, 1.25 mg,
100s ea............ **61570-0110-01** 211.20
2.5 mg, 100s ea...... **61570-0111-01** 249.29
100s ea UD **61570-0111-56** 235.18
500s ea............ **61570-0111-05** 963.18
5 mg, 100s ea........ **61570-0112-01** 261.55
100s ea UD **61570-0112-56** 246.74
10 mg, 100s ea **61570-0120-01** 306.06

(A-S Medication)
REPACK
CAP, PO, 5 mg, 30s ea **54569-3714-00** 77.11
10 mg, 30s ea........ **54569-5936-00** 112.60

(Bryant Ranch)
REPACK
CAP, PO, 5 mg, 30s ea **63629-1254-01** 70.72
10 mg, 30s ea........ **63629-1253-01** 97.14

PROD/MFR | NDC | AWP | DP | OBC

(PD-Rx Pharm)
REPACK
CAP, PO (REDI-SCRIPT)
5 mg, 30s ea......... **58864-0674-30** 83.10
10 mg, 30s ea........ **55289-0867-30** 106.01
30s ea............ **58864-0847-30** 97.24

(Phys Total Care)
REPACK
CAP, PO, 1.25 mg, 10s ea.. **54868-5747-00** 27.69
30s ea............ **54868-5747-01** 61.10
2.5 mg, 10s ea **54868-2644-02** 25.18
30s ea............ **54868-2644-01** 71.78
100s ea............ **54868-2644-00** 221.33
5 mg, 10s ea **54868-2645-02** 26.32
30s ea............ **54868-2645-01** 75.22
60s ea............ **54868-2645-03** 140.41
100s ea............ **54868-2645-00** 232.14
10 mg, 10s ea........ **54868-3846-02** 30.48
30s ea............ **54868-3846-00** 87.70
60s ea............ **54868-3846-03** 163.98
100s ea............ **54868-3846-01** 271.43

(Quality Care Prod)
REPACK
CAP, PO, 5 mg, 30s ea **49999-0934-30** 109.40
10 mg, 30s ea........ **49999-0871-30** 152.36
90s ea............ **49999-0871-90** 455.01

ALTAFRIN (Altaire)
phenylephrine hydrochloride
SOL, OP (STERILE)
2.5%, 5 ml.......... **59390-0193-05** 4.10
15 ml............ **59390-0193-13** 6.70
10%, 5 ml **59390-0194-05** 6.70

ALTEPLASE, RECOMBINANT
(Genentech) *See ACTIVASE*

(Genentech) *See CATHFLO ACTIVASE*

ALTOPREV (Shionogi)
lovastatin
TER, PO, 20 mg, 30s ea ... **59630-0628-30** 198.36
40 mg, 30s ea........ **59630-0629-30** 209.06
60 mg, 30s ea........ **59630-0630-30** 230.51

(Phys Total Care)
REPACK
TER, PO, 40 mg, 30s ea ... **54868-5513-00** 126.03
60 mg, 30s ea........ **54868-5358-00** 196.08

ALTRETAMINE
(Eisai) *See HEXALEN*

ALUM (Gallipot)
POW, NA (U.S.P.,N.F.)
56.7 gm **51552-0218-03** 2.24
113.4 gm............ **51552-0218-04** 3.01
454 gm............ **51552-0218-06** 10.50

(Humco) *See ALUM AMMONIUM*

ALUM AMMONIUM (Amend)
alum, ammonium
POW, NA (U.S.P./F.C.C.)
454 gm............ **17317-0018-01** 9.80
2270 gm............ **17317-0018-05** 39.20
11350 gm **17317-0018-08** 122.50

(Humco)
alum
POW, NA (U.S.P.)
360 gm............ **00395-0049-12** 5.41

(Lorann Oil)
alum, ammonium
POW, NA (U.S.P.)
120 gm............ **23535-0600-58** 2.50
480 gm............ **23535-0600-51** 7.95

ALUM POTASSIUM (Amend)
alum, potassium
POW, NA (U.S.P.)
500 gm............ **17317-0021-01** 9.80
2270 gm............ **17317-0021-05** 29.40
11350 gm **17317-0021-08** 105.00

ALUM, AMMONIUM
(Amend) *See ALUM AMMONIUM*

(Lorann Oil) *See ALUM AMMONIUM*

(Mallinckrodt Lab) *See ALUMINUM AMMONIUM SULFATE*

(Spectrum Pharmacy) *See ALUMINUM AMMONIUM SULFATE*

PROD/MFR | NDC | AWP | DP | OBC

ALUM, POTASSIUM
(Amend) *See ALUM POTASSIUM*

(Baker, J.T.) *See ALUMINUM POTASSIUM SULFATE*

(Gallipot) *See ALUMINUM POTASSIUM SULFATE*

(Mallinckrodt Lab) *See ALUMINUM POTASSIUM SULFATE*

(Medisca) *See POTASSIUM ALUM DODECAHYDRATE*

(PCCA) *See ALUMINUM POTASSIUM SULFATE*

(Spectrum Pharmacy) *See ALUMINUM POTASSIUM SULFATE*

ALUMINUM (Baker, J.T.)
POW, NA (PURIFIED, 325 MESH)
500 gm............ **10106-0446-01** 60.82

(Mallinckrodt Lab)
POW, NA (PURIFIED)
500 gm............ **00406-3116-03** 49.49

(PCCA)
POW, NA, 1 gm.......... **51927-2844-00** 1.05

ALUMINUM ACETATE
(Amend) *See ALUMINUM ACETATE BASIC*

(Baker, J.T.) *See ALUMINUM ACETATE BASIC*

(Gallipot) *See ALUMINUM ACETATE BASIC*

(Mallinckrodt Lab) *See ALUMINUM ACETATE BASIC*

(PCCA) *See ALUMINUM ACETATE, BASIC*

ALUMINUM ACETATE BASIC (Amend)
aluminum acetate
POW, NA (PURIFIED)
454 gm............ **17317-0017-01** 28.00
2270 gm............ **17317-0017-05** 98.00

(Baker, J.T.)
POW, NA (C.P.)
500 gm............ **10106-0491-01** 114.33

(Gallipot)
POW, NA, 113.4 gm....... **51552-0246-04** 20.16
454 gm............ **51552-0246-06** 38.08

(Mallinckrodt Lab)
POW, NA, 125 gm......... **00406-6957-01** 25.14
500 gm............ **00406-6957-03** 56.81

ALUMINUM ACETATE, BASIC (PCCA)
aluminum acetate
POW, NA, 1 gm.......... **51927-3387-00** 1.32

ALUMINUM ACETATE/ACETIC ACID (Palmetto)
REPACK
acetic acid/aluminum acetate
SOL, OT (1X60ML,DROPS)
2%-0.79%, 60 ml **23490-7382-06** 19.75

ALUMINUM AMMONIUM SULFATE (Mallinckrodt Lab)
alum, ammonium
CRY, NA, 500 gm **00406-3212-12** 48.21

(Spectrum Pharmacy)
POW, NA (FCC,1X500GM)
500 gm............ **49452-0325-01** 66.50
(U.S.P.)
500 gm............ **49452-0012-01** 67.55
(FCC,1X2500GM)
2500 gm............ **49452-0325-02** 184.80
(U.S.P.)
2500 gm............ **49452-0012-02** 184.80
(FCC,1X12000GM)
12000 gm **49452-0325-03** 640.50
(U.S.P.)
12000 gm **49452-0012-03** 616.00

ALUMINUM CHLORIDE (Amend)
POW, NA (U.S.P.)
500 gm............ **17317-0019-01** 19.60
2270 gm............ **17317-0019-05** 77.00
11350 gm **17317-0019-08** 262.50

(Baker, J.T.) *See ALUMINUM CHLORIDE ANHYDROUS*

(Baker, J.T.) *See ALUMINUM CHLORIDE HEXAHYDRATE*

(Gallipot)
CRY, NA (U.S.P.,N.F.)
100 gm............ **51552-0185-05** 17.50
454 gm............ **51552-0185-06** 42.00

(Mallinckrodt Lab)
CRY, NA (U.S.P.)
500 gm............ **00406-3132-12** 19.89

(Medisca) *See ALUMINUM CHLORIDE ANHYDROUS*

PROD/MFR	NDC	AWP	DP	OBC
(PCCA)				
CRY, NA (USP; HEXAHYDRATE)				
1 gm	**51927-1286-00**	0.35		
(Person & Covey) *See DRYSOL*				
(Person & Covey) *See XERAC AC*				
(Spectrum Pharmacy) *See ALUMINUM CHLORIDE HEXAHYDRATE*				
(Stratus) *See HYPERCARE*				
ALUMINUM CHLORIDE ANHYDROUS (Baker, J.T.)				
aluminum chloride				
POW, NA (REAGENT)				
125 gm	**10106-0504-04**	64.53		
500 gm	**10106-0504-01**	100.22		
(Medisca)				
POW, NA (U.S.P.)				
100 gm	**38779-0685-05**	22.50		
500 gm	**38779-0685-08**	55.50		
1000 gm	**38779-0685-09**	87.00		
ALUMINUM CHLORIDE HEXAHYDRATE (Baker, J.T.)				
aluminum chloride				
CRY, NA (U.S.P.)				
500 gm	**10106-0500-01**	20.42		
(Spectrum Pharmacy)				
POW, NA (U.S.P.)				
100 gm	**49452-0330-06**	138.25		
500 gm	**49452-0330-01**	259.88		
2500 gm	**49452-0330-02**	857.50		
ALUMINUM CHLOROHYDRATE (Gallipot)				
POW, NA, 25 gm	**51552-0245-04**	7.00		
100 gm	**51552-0245-05**	17.50		
454 gm	**51552-0245-06**	32.55		
(PCCA)				
POW, NA (USP; ANHYDROUS)				
1 gm	**51927-1092-00**	0.60		
(Spectrum Pharmacy)				
POW, NA (U.S.P.)				
500 gm	**49452-0335-01**	163.10		
2500 gm	**49452-0335-02**	395.50		
ALUMINUM HYDROXIDE (Baker, J.T.)				
POW, NA (U.S.P., DRIED GEL)				
500 gm	**10106-0526-01**	32.14		
(Medisca) *See ALUMINUM HYDROXIDE GEL*				
(PCCA)				
POW, NA (USP; DRIED)				
1 gm	**51927-1091-00**	0.54		
(Spectrum Pharmacy) *See ALUMINUM HYDROXIDE GEL*				
ALUMINUM HYDROXIDE GEL (Medisca)				
aluminum hydroxide				
POW, NA (DRIED,U.S.P.)				
500 gm	**38779-1255-08**	61.50		
1000 gm	**38779-1255-09**	108.00		
(Spectrum Pharmacy)				
POW, NA (U.S.P.)				
500 gm	**49452-0350-01**	131.95		
2500 gm	**49452-0350-02**	378.00		
ALUMINUM MONOSTEARATE (PCCA)				
POW, NA (NF)				
1 gm	**51927-3472-00**	7.20		
(Spectrum Pharmacy)				
POW, NA (N.F.)				
500 gm	**49452-0360-01**	1064.00		
ALUMINUM NITRATE				
(Baker, J.T.) *See ALUMINUM NITRATE 9-HYDRATE*				
ALUMINUM NITRATE 9-HYDRATE (Baker, J.T.)				
aluminum nitrate				
CRY, NA (A.C.S., REAGENT)				
500 gm	**10106-0528-01**	74.88		
2500 gm	**10106-0528-05**	253.79		
ALUMINUM OXIDE				
(Baker, J.T.) *See ALUMINUM OXIDE ACID*				
(Baker, J.T.) *See ALUMINUM OXIDE BASIC*				
(Baker, J.T.) *See ALUMINUM OXIDE NEUTRAL*				
(Baker, J.T.)				
POW, NA (REAGENT)				
500 gm	**10106-0536-01**	36.26		
2500 gm	**10106-0536-05**	130.96		
ALUMINUM OXIDE ACID (Baker, J.T.)				
aluminum oxide				
POW, NA (REAGENT)				
500 gm	**10106-0538-01**	89.97		
2500 gm	**10106-0538-05**	302.56		
ALUMINUM OXIDE BASIC (Baker, J.T.)				
aluminum oxide				
POW, NA (REAGENT)				
500 gm	**10106-0539-01**	105.11		
2500 gm	**10106-0539-05**	349.58		
ALUMINUM OXIDE NEUTRAL (Baker, J.T.)				
aluminum oxide				
POW, NA (REAGENT)				
500 gm	**10106-0540-01**	99.40		
2500 gm	**10106-0540-05**	397.01		
ALUMINUM POTASSIUM SULFATE (Baker, J.T.)				
alum, potassium				
CRY, NA (A.C.S.,12-H2O,REAGENT)				
500 gm	**10106-0546-01**	90.64		
2500 gm	**10106-0546-05**	376.52		
(Gallipot)				
GRA, NA (U.S.P.,GRANULAR)				
454 gm	**51552-0714-06**	20.16	14.40	
2268 gm	**51552-0714-09**	62.93	44.95	
(Mallinckrodt Lab)				
POW, NA (U.S.P.)				
2500 gm	**00406-3076-12**	68.50		
(PCCA)				
POW, NA (U.S.P, 0.12 H2O)				
1 gm	**51927-1692-00**	0.11		
(Spectrum Pharmacy)				
GRA, NA (U.S.P.)				
500 gm	**49452-0370-01**	84.35		
2500 gm	**49452-0370-02**	268.10		
ALUMINUM SULFATE (Amend)				
POW, NA (U.S.P.)				
454 gm	**17317-0023-01**	14.00		
2270 gm	**17317-0023-05**	56.00		
11350 gm	**17317-0023-08**	210.00		
(Baker, J.T.) *See ALUMINUM SULFATE 18-HYDRATE*				
(Medisca)				
POW, NA (U.S.P.)				
500 gm	**38779-0983-08**	31.50		
(PCCA)				
POW, NA (USP; HYDRATE)				
1 gm	**51927-1646-00**	0.33		
(Spectrum Pharmacy)				
POW, NA (U.S.P.,E.P.,B.P.)				
500 gm	**49452-0380-01**	103.95		
2500 gm	**49452-0380-02**	371.00		
ALUMINUM SULFATE 18-HYDRATE (Baker, J.T.)				
aluminum sulfate				
CRY, NA (A.C.S., REAGENT)				
500 gm	**10106-0564-01**	121.08		
2500 gm	**10106-0564-05**	505.47		
ALUPENT (HomeMed)				
REPACK				
metaproterenol sulfate				
TAB, PO, 10 mg, 25s ea	**51655-0177-76**	4.35		AB
(Pharma Pac)				
REPACK				
ARO, IH, 0.65 mg/actuation, 14 gm	**52959-0155-00**	41.50		
SOL, IH (VIAL) 0.6%, 2.5 ml 25s	**52959-0158-06**	54.23		AN
(Phys Total Care)				
REPACK				
ARO, IH, 0.65 mg/actuation, 14 gm	**54868-1043-01**	51.39		
SOL, IH (VIAL) 0.6%, 2.5 ml 25s UD	**54868-3179-00**	57.78		AN
(Southwood)				
REPACK				
ARO, IH, 0.65 mg/actuation, 14 gm	**58016-6537-01**	35.16		
ALVESCO (Sepracor)				
ciclesonide				
AER, IH, 80 mcg/actuation, 6.1 gm	**63402-0711-01**	156.00		EE
160 mcg/actuation, 6.1 gm	**63402-0712-01**	156.00		
(Phys Total Care)				
REPACK				
AER, IH (1X6.1GM) 80 mcg/actuation, 6.1 gm	**54868-5989-00**	186.62		EE
160 mcg/actuation, 6.1 gm	**54868-5990-00**	186.62		
ALVIMOPAN				
(Glaxo) *See ENTEREG*				
AMANTADINE (Dispensing Solutions)				
REPACK				
amantadine hydrochloride				
SGL, PO, 100 mg, 10s ea	**55045-1297-03**	10.00		
12s ea	**55045-1297-04**	12.00		
20s ea	**55045-1297-07**	20.00		
50s ea	**55045-1297-05**	50.00		
AMANTADINE HCL (Hi-Tech)				
amantadine hydrochloride				
SYR, PO, 50 mg/5 ml, 473 ml	**50383-0807-16**	64.00		AA
(Letco)				
POW, NA, 100 gm	**62991-2559-01**	135.00		
1000 gm	**62991-2559-02**	720.00		
(Medisca)				
POW, NA (U.S.P.)				
25 gm	**38779-0411-04**	87.00		
100 gm	**38779-0411-05**	297.00		
(Mikart)				
SYR, PO, 50 mg/5 ml, 480 ml	**46672-0606-16**	62.50		AA
(Morton Grove)				
SYR, PO (RASPBERRY) 50 mg/5 ml, 473 ml	**60432-0093-16**	70.70		AA
(PCCA)				
POW, NA (U.S.P.)				
1 gm	**51927-1754-00**	3.60		
(Pharm Assoc Inc)				
SYR, PO (AF,SF,DYE-FREE) 50 mg/5 ml, 10 ml 100s UD	**00121-0646-10**	247.47		AA
473 ml	**00121-0646-16**	72.75		AA
(Sandoz)				
CAP, PO, 100 mg, 100s ea	**00781-2048-01**	74.63		AB
500s ea	**00781-2048-05**	363.79		AB
(Silarx)				
SYR, PO (U.S.P.,RASPBERRY) 50 mg/5 ml, 480 ml	**54838-0509-80**	72.75		AA
(Spectrum Pharmacy)				
POW, NA (U.S.P./N.F.)				
25 gm	**49452-0395-01**	144.55		
100 gm	**49452-0395-02**	472.50		
(UDL)				
SGL, PO (10X10) 100 mg, 100s ea UD	**51079-0481-20**	74.63		AB
(Upsher-Smith)				
SGL, PO, 100 mg, 100s ea	**00832-1015-00**	61.23		AB
500s ea	**00832-1015-50**	311.04		AB
TAB, PO, 100 mg, 100s ea	**00832-0111-00**	120.03		AB
500s ea	**00832-0111-50**	570.15		AB
(A-S Medication)				
REPACK				
CAP, PO, 100 mg, 10s ea	**54569-0084-03**	7.02		AB
14s ea	**54569-0084-02**	9.82		AB
SYR, PO (RASPBERRY) 50 mg/5 ml, 480 ml	**54569-5635-00**	71.75		AA
(Altura)				
REPACK				
SGL, PO, 100 mg, 10s ea	**63874-0529-10**	9.98		EE
14s ea	**63874-0529-14**	12.45		EE
20s ea	**63874-0529-20**	17.79		EE
30s ea	**63874-0529-30**	21.71		EE
100s ea	**63874-0529-01**	88.96		EE
(DHS, Inc.)				
REPACK				
SGL, PO, 100 mg, 10s ea	**55887-0767-10**	14.50		AB
30s ea	**55887-0767-30**	35.00		AB
(Dispensing Solutions)				
REPACK				
SGL, PO, 100 mg, 14s ea	**55045-1297-02**	14.00		AB
14s ea	**66336-0079-14**	15.55		
(HomeMed)				
REPACK				
SGL, PO, 100 mg, 10s ea	**51655-0499-53**	9.98		
20s ea	**51655-0499-52**	17.79		

PROD/MFR	NDC	AWP	DP	OBC
PD-Rx Pharm)				
REPACK				
CAP, PO, 100 mg, 10s ea	58864-0795-10	13.34		AB
TAB, PO, 100 mg, 10s ea	55289-0012-10	17.94		AB
14s ea	55289-0012-14	21.10		AB
20s ea	55289-0012-20	25.84		AB
(Pharma Pac)				
REPACK				
SGL, PO, 100 mg, 10s ea	52959-0007-10	9.73		EE
14s ea	52959-0007-14	12.96		EE
15s ea	52959-0007-15	13.88		EE
20s ea	52959-0007-20	18.01		EE
30s ea	52959-0007-30	26.70		EE
60s ea	52959-0007-60	53.39		EE
(Phys Total Care)				
REPACK				
SGL, PO, 100 mg, 10s ea	54868-0800-01	13.38		EE
15s ea	54868-0800-07	18.36		EE
20s ea	54868-0800-02	23.76		EE
30s ea	54868-0800-03	34.14		EE
60s ea	54868-0800-00	65.31		AB
100s ea	54868-0800-04	105.45		EE
SYR, PO (RASPBERRY)				
50 mg/5 ml, 473 ml	54868-3216-00	55.74		AA
(Quality Care Prod)				
REPACK				
SGL, PO, 100 mg, 14s ea	49999-0324-14	14.23		EE
20s ea	49999-0324-20	20.33		AB
AMANTADINE HYDROCHLORIDE				
FUL				
SYR, PO, 50 mg/5 ml,				
480 ml		31.49		
(Carolina)				
SOL, PO, 50 mg/5 ml,				
473 ml	46287-0015-01	22.40	16.25	AA
(Hi-Tech) *See AMANTADINE HCL*				
(Lannett)				
SGL, PO (USP,SOFTGEL)				
100 mg, 100s ea	00527-1704-01	89.56		AB
(SOFTGEL)				
100 mg, 500s ea	00527-1704-05	684.18		AB
(Letco) *See AMANTADINE HCL*				
(Medisca) *See AMANTADINE HCL*				
(Mikart) *See AMANTADINE HCL*				
(Morton Grove) *See AMANTADINE HCL*				
(PCCA) *See AMANTADINE HCL*				
(Pharm Assoc Inc) *See AMANTADINE HCL*				
(Qualitest)				
SYR, PO, 50 mg/5 ml,				
473 ml	00603-1011-58	59.95		AA
(Sandoz) *See AMANTADINE HCL*				
(Silarx) *See AMANTADINE HCL*				
(Spectrum Pharmacy) *See AMANTADINE HCL*				
(UDL) *See AMANTADINE HCL*				
(Upsher-Smith) *See AMANTADINE HCL*				
(Nucare Pharm)				
REPACK				
SGL, PO, 100 mg, 14s ea	66267-0015-14	11.96		AB
20s ea	66267-0015-20	17.65		AB
(Palmetto)				
REPACK				
SGL, PO, 100 mg, 6s ea	23490-5037-01	6.72		
14s ea	23490-5037-02	11.20		
(Physician Partner)				
REPACK				
SGL, PO (SOFTGEL)				
100 mg, 10s ea	21695-0564-10	13.90		AB
(Southwood)				
REPACK				
SGL, PO, 100 mg, 10s ea	58016-0153-10	6.22		AB
14s ea	58016-0153-14	8.71		AB
15s ea	58016-0153-15	9.33		AB
20s ea	58016-0153-20	12.44		AB
30s ea	58016-0153-30	18.66		AB
100s ea	58016-0153-00	62.19		AB
120s ea	58016-0153-02	74.63		AB
(Stat Rx)				
REPACK				
SGL, PO, 100 mg, 10s ea	16590-0008-10	10.00		
14s ea	16590-0008-14	14.00		
20s ea	16590-0008-20	20.00		
30s ea	16590-0008-30	30.00		
AMARANTH (Spectrum Pharmacy)				
POW, NA (1X25GM)				
25 gm	49452-0390-01	81.55		
(1X100GM)				
100 gm	49452-0390-02	211.40		
AMARYL (Sanofi-Aventis)				
glimepiride				
TAB, PO, 1 mg, 100s ea	00039-0221-10	60.29		
2 mg, 100s ea	00039-0222-10	97.72		
4 mg, 100s ea	00039-0223-10	184.28		
(Phys Total Care)				
REPACK				
TAB, PO, 1 mg, 10s ea	54868-4412-02	7.10		
30s ea	54868-4412-00	17.56		
100s ea	54868-4412-01	53.56		
2 mg, 20s ea	54868-4205-02	18.84		
30s ea	54868-4205-00	27.31		
60s ea	54868-4205-01	52.75		
4 mg, 10s ea	54868-4026-01	17.74		
30s ea	54868-4206-00	49.47		
60s ea	54868-4206-04	97.06		
100s ea	54868-4206-03	151.09		
AMBENONIUM CHLORIDE				
(Sanofi-Aventis) *See MYTELASE CHLORIDE*				
AMBI 40PSE/400GFN (MCR American)				
guaifenesin/pseudoephedrine hydrochloride				
TAB, PO, 400 mg-40 mg,				
100s ea	66870-0408-01	56.25		
AMBI 40PSE/400GFN/20DM (MCR American)				
dm/gg/pse hcl				
TAB, PO, 20 mg-400 mg-40 mg,				
100s ea	66870-0409-01	57.50		
AMBI 60PSE/400GFN (MCR American)				
guaifenesin/pseudoephedrine hydrochloride				
TAB, PO, 400 mg-60 mg,				
100s ea	66870-0406-01	56.25		
AMBI 60PSE/400GFN/20DM (MCR American)				
dm/gg/pse hcl				
TAB, PO, 20 mg-400 mg-60 mg,				
100s ea	66870-0407-01	58.75		
AMBIEN (Sanofi-Aventis)				
zolpidem tartrate				
TAB, PO (FILM-COATED)				
5 mg,				
100s ea, C-IV	00024-5401-31	586.16		
10 mg,				
100s ea, C-IV	00024-5421-31	586.16		
(FILM-COATED)				
10 mg,				
500s ea, C-IV	00024-5421-50	2930.81		
(A-S Medication)				
REPACK				
TAB, PO (FILM-COATED)				
5 mg, 6s ea, C-IV	54569-3827-03	45.72		
20s ea, C-IV	54569-3827-00	102.79		
10 mg, 2s ea, C-IV	54569-3828-08	12.21		
10s ea, C-IV	54569-3828-01	76.20		
30s ea, C-IV	54569-3828-03	228.60		
(Altura)				
REPACK				
TAB, PO (FILM-COATED)				
5 mg, 6s ea, C-IV	63874-0924-06	77.16		
8s ea, C-IV	63874-0924-08	102.88		
10s ea, C-IV	63874-0924-10	128.60		
20s ea, C-IV	63874-0924-20	257.20		
30s ea, C-IV	63874-0924-30	385.80		
40s ea, C-IV	63874-0924-40	514.40		
60s ea, C-IV	63874-0924-60	771.60		
90s ea, C-IV	63874-0924-90	1157.40		
100s ea, C-IV	63874-0924-01	1286.00		
10 mg, 4s ea, C-IV	63874-0280-04	51.44		
6s ea, C-IV	63874-0280-06	77.16		
10s ea, C-IV	63874-0280-10	128.60		
15s ea, C-IV	63874-0280-15	192.90		
20s ea, C-IV	63874-0280-20	257.20		
30s ea, C-IV	63874-0280-30	385.80		
40s ea, C-IV	63874-0280-40	514.40		
60s ea, C-IV	63874-0280-60	771.60		
90s ea, C-IV	63874-0280-90	1157.00		
100s ea, C-IV	63874-0280-01	1286.00		
(Bryant Ranch)				
REPACK				
TAB, PO, 10 mg,				
20s ea, C-IV	63629-1256-02	140.24		
30s ea, C-IV	63629-1256-01	211.86		
(DHS, Inc.)				
REPACK				
TAB, PO (FILM-COATED)				
5 mg, 20s ea, C-IV	55887-0514-20	85.00		
10 mg,				
20s ea, C-IV	55887-0806-20	79.00		
(Dispensing Solutions)				
REPACK				
TAB, PO (FILM-COATED)				
5 mg, 20s ea, C-IV	55045-2812-07	108.40		
30s ea, C-IV	55045-2812-08	162.60		
60s ea, C-IV	55045-2812-06	325.20		
10 mg, 6s ea, C-IV	55045-2271-06	32.52		
10s ea, C-IV	55045-2271-01	54.20		
15s ea, C-IV	55045-2271-02	81.30		
20s ea, C-IV	55045-2271-07	108.40		
30s ea, C-IV	55045-2271-08	162.60		
60s ea, C-IV	55045-2271-09	325.20		
100s ea, C-IV	55045-2271-00	542.00		
AMBIEN (Keltman Pharma., Inc.)				
REPACK				
zolpidem tartrate				
TAB, PO, 10 mg,				
15s ea, C-IV	68387-0485-15	87.97		
(FILM-COATED)				
10 mg,				
30s ea, C-IV	68387-0485-30	175.95		
(Nucare Pharm)				
REPACK				
TAB, PO, 5 mg,				
10s ea, C-IV	66267-0017-10	47.44		
30s ea, C-IV	66267-0017-30	125.35		
10 mg,				
10s ea, C-IV	66267-0016-10	54.99		
20s ea, C-IV	66267-0016-20	109.80		
28s ea, C-IV	66267-0016-28	153.72		
30s ea, C-IV	66267-0016-30	164.70		
60s ea, C-IV	66267-0016-60	329.40		
(PD-Rx Pharm)				
REPACK				
TAB, PO (FILM-COATED)				
5 mg, 6s ea, C-IV	55289-0729-06	57.15		
6s ea, C-IV	58864-0891-06	57.15		
12s ea, C-IV	55289-0729-12	109.19		
30s ea, C-IV	55289-0729-30	261.36		
10 mg, 6s ea, C-IV	55289-0792-06	57.15		
10s ea, C-IV	55289-0792-10	73.70		
(FILM-COATED)				
10 mg,				
12s ea, C-IV	55289-0792-12	88.45		
(REDI-SCRIPT,FILM-COATED)				
10 mg,				
15s ea, C-IV	58864-0700-15	81.45		
20s ea, C-IV	55289-0792-20	147.40		
30s ea, C-IV	55289-0792-30	221.12		
(Phys Total Care)				
REPACK				
TAB, PO, 5 mg,				
3s ea, C-IV	54868-2642-03	20.40		
10s ea, C-IV	54868-2642-02	62.18		
20s ea, C-IV	54868-2642-04	121.23		
30s ea, C-IV	54868-2642-01	171.59		
60s ea, C-IV	54868-2642-00	340.04		
10 mg, 5s ea, C-IV	54868-2643-00	36.97		
10s ea, C-IV	54868-2643-02	70.67		
15s ea, C-IV	54868-2643-04	104.37		
20s ea, C-IV	54868-2643-06	138.07		
30s ea, C-IV	54868-2643-01	194.24		
60s ea, C-IV	54868-2643-07	385.21		
90s ea, C-IV	54868-2643-08	557.70		
100s ea, C-IV	54868-2643-05	619.31		
(Physician Partner)				
REPACK				
TAB, PO, 5 mg,				
15s ea, C-IV	21695-0211-15	181.38		
30s ea, C-IV	21695-0211-30	308.35		
10 mg,				
15s ea, C-IV	21695-0212-15	181.38		
30s ea, C-IV	21695-0212-30	308.35		
45s ea, C-IV	21695-0212-45	544.15		
(Quality Care Prod)				
REPACK				
TAB, PO (FILM-COATED)				
5 mg, 15s ea, C-IV	49999-0453-15	116.10		
30s ea, C-IV	49999-0453-30	232.21		
10 mg,				
10s ea, C-IV	49999-0037-10	77.40		
15s ea, C-IV	49999-0037-15	116.10		
20s ea, C-IV	49999-0037-20	154.80		
30s ea, C-IV	49999-0037-30	232.21		

PROD/MFR	NDC	AWP	DP	OBC
60s ea, C-IV	49999-0037-60	464.42		
90s ea, C-IV	49999-0037-90	696.60		
100s ea, C-IV	49999-0037-00	774.00		
TER, PO, 12.5 mg,				
100s ea, C-IV	49999-0763-00	216.60		
(Southwood)				
REPACK				
TAB, PO, 5 mg,				
10s ea, C-IV	58016-0342-10	53.78		
20s ea, C-IV	58016-0342-20	107.55		
30s ea, C-IV	58016-0342-30	161.33		
40s ea, C-IV	58016-0342-40	215.11		
60s ea, C-IV	58016-0342-60	322.66		
90s ea, C-IV	58016-0342-90	483.99		
100s ea, C-IV	58016-0342-00	537.77		
10 mg,				
10s ea, C-IV	58016-0341-10	53.78		
20s ea, C-IV	58016-0341-20	107.55		
30s ea, C-IV	58016-0341-30	161.33		
40s ea, C-IV	58016-0341-40	215.11		
60s ea, C-IV	58016-0341-60	322.66		
90s ea, C-IV	58016-0341-90	483.99		
100s ea, C-IV	58016-0341-00	537.77		
(Stat Rx)				
REPACK				
TAB, PO, 5 mg,				
20s ea, C-IV	16590-0009-20	88.00		
30s ea, C-IV	16590-0009-30	132.00		
60s ea, C-IV	16590-0009-60	264.00		
90s ea, C-IV	16590-0009-90	396.00		
(FILM-COATED)				
10 mg,				
20s ea, C-IV	16590-0010-20	138.76		
28s ea, C-IV	16590-0010-28	192.97		
30s ea, C-IV	16590-0010-30	206.52		
56s ea, C-IV	16590-0010-56	382.69		
60s ea, C-IV	16590-0010-60	293.00		
90s ea, C-IV	16590-0010-90	474.00		
AMBIEN CR (Sanofi-Aventis)				
zolpidem tartrate				
TER, PO (3X10)				
6.25 mg,				
30s ea UD, C-IV	00024-5501-10	185.66		
(TWO LAYER FILM-COATED)				
6.25 mg,				
100s ea, C-IV	00024-5501-31	619.06		
(3X10,FILM-COATED)				
12.5 mg,				
30s ea UD, C-IV	00024-5521-10	185.66		
(FILM-COATED)				
12.5 mg,				
100s ea, C-IV	00024-5521-31	619.06		
500s ea, C-IV	00024-5521-50	3095.24		
(A-S Medication)				
REPACK				
TER, PO (FILM-COATED)				
12.5 mg,				
20s ea, C-IV	54569-5760-01	117.35		
30s ea, C-IV	54569-5760-00	176.03		
(Aidarex)				
REPACK				
TER, PO (FILM-COATED)				
12.5 mg,				
7s ea, C-IV	33261-0652-07	43.16		
14s ea, C-IV	33261-0652-14	86.33		
30s ea, C-IV	33261-0652-30	185.00		
60s ea, C-IV	33261-0652-60	370.00		
(Bryant Ranch)				
REPACK				
TER, PO, 12.5 mg,				
30s ea, C-IV	63629-3141-01	126.60		
(Dispensing Solutions)				
REPACK				
TER, PO, 6.25 mg,				
30s ea, C-IV	55045-3438-08	195.00		
12.5 mg,				
30s ea, C-IV	55045-3633-01	195.00		
100s ea, C-IV	55045-3633-02	650.00		
(IPI)				
REPACK				
TER, PO, 12.5 mg,				
90s ea, C-IV	18837-0005-90	516.47		
(Keltman Pharma., Inc.)				
REPACK				
TER, PO, 12.5 mg,				
15s ea, C-IV	68387-0486-15	74.48		
30s ea, C-IV	68387-0486-30	148.96		
(Nucare Pharm)				
REPACK				
TER, PO (FILM-COATED)				
12.5 mg,				
30s ea, C-IV	68071-0361-30	235.45		
(Palmetto)				
REPACK				
TER, PO, 12.5 mg,				
30s ea, C-IV	23490-0060-03	115.83		
(PD-Rx Pharm)				
REPACK				
TER, PO (TWO LAYER FILM-COATED)				
6.25 mg,				
30s ea, C-IV	55289-0572-30	274.61		
(FILM-COATED)				
12.5 mg,				
30s ea, C-IV	55289-0205-30	274.61		
(Pharma Pac)				
REPACK				
TER, PO, 12.5 mg,				
30s ea, C-IV	52959-0870-30	153.21		
(Phys Total Care)				
REPACK				
TER, PO (TWO LAYER FILM-COATED)				
6.25 mg,				
10s ea, C-IV	54868-5461-00	73.21		
15s ea, C-IV	54868-5461-02	108.52		
(TWO LAYER FILM-COATED)				
6.25 mg,				
30s ea, C-IV	54868-5461-01	203.30		
60s ea, C-IV	54868-5461-03	322.16		
(FILM-COATED)				
12.5 mg,				
10s ea, C-IV	54868-5426-00	80.86		
15s ea, C-IV	54868-5426-02	119.00		
(FILM-COATED)				
12.5 mg,				
30s ea, C-IV	54868-5426-01	223.11		
60s ea, C-IV	54868-5426-03	442.29		
(FILM-COATED)				
12.5 mg,				
90s ea, C-IV	54868-5426-04	641.51		
(Physician Partner)				
REPACK				
TER, PO, 6.25 mg,				
30s ea, C-IV	21695-0319-30	371 44		
12.5 mg,				
15s ea, C-IV	21695-0213-15	218.49		
30s ea, C-IV	21695-0213-30	371.44		
(Quality Care Prod)				
REPACK				
TER, PO (TWO LAYER FILM-COATED)				
6.25 mg,				
30s ea, C-IV	49999-0764-30	280.86		
60s ea, C-IV	49999-0764-60	481.72		
(FILM-COATED)				
12.5 mg,				
30s ea, C-IV	49999-0763-30	280.86		
(Southwood)				
REPACK				
TER, PO (FILM-COATED)				
12.5 mg,				
30s ea, C-IV	58016-0863-30	153.76		
60s ea, C-IV	58016-0863-60	307.52		
90s ea, C-IV	58016-0863-90	461.29		
100s ea, C-IV	58016-0863-00	512.54		
(St. Mary's MPP)				
REPACK				
TER, PO (FILM-COATED)				
12.5 mg,				
30s ea, C-IV	60760-0551-30	284.58		
(Stat Rx)				
REPACK				
TER, PO (TWO LAYER FILM-COATED)				
6.25 mg,				
15s ea, C-IV	16590-0562-15	110.59		
25s ea, C-IV	16590-0562-25	182.14		
28s ea, C-IV	16590-0562-28	203.61		
30s ea, C-IV	16590-0562-30	217.92		
60s ea, C-IV	16590-0562-60	310.00		
90s ea, C-IV	16590-0562-90	459.50		
12.5 mg,				
6s ea, C-IV	16590-0436-06	67.00		
10s ea, C-IV	16590-0436-10	101.00		
20s ea, C-IV	16590-0436-20	111.16		
(FILM-COATED)				
12.5 mg,				
25s ea, C-IV	16590-0436-25	182.14		
28s ea, C-IV	16590-0436-28	286.00		
30s ea, C-IV	16590-0436-30	217.92		
60s ea, C-IV	16590-0436-60	303.50		
90s ea, C-IV	16590-0436-90	390.00		
AMBIENPAK (Bryant Ranch)				
REPACK				
zolpidem tartrate				
TAB, PO (FILM-COATED)				
10 mg,				
10s ea, C-IV	63629-1256-05	70.12		
15s ea, C-IV	63629-1256-03	105.18		
90s ea, C-IV	63629-1256-04	631.08		
AMBIFED CD (MCR American)				
codeine phos/gg/pse hcl				
TAB, PO, 10 mg-400 mg-30 mg,				
100s ea, C-III	58605-0420-01	105.84		
AMBIFED CDX (MCR American)				
codeine phos/gg/pse hcl				
TAB, PO, 20 mg-400 mg-30 mg,				
100s ea, C-III	58605-0421-01	110.01		
AMBIFED-G CD (MCR American)				
codeine phos/gg/pse hcl				
TAB, PO, 10 mg-400 mg-20 mg,				
100s ea, C-III	58605-0418-01	106.10		
AMBIFED-G CDX (MCR American)				
codeine phos/gg/pse hcl				
TAB, PO, 20 mg-400 mg-20 mg,				
100s ea, C-III	58605-0419-01	111.11		
AMBISOME (Astellas)				
amphotericin b liposome				
PDS, IV, 50 mg, ea	00469-3051-30	188.40		
AMBRISENTAN				
(Gilead Sciences) *See LETAIRIS*				
AMCINONIDE (Fougera)				
CRE, TP, 0.1%, 15 gm	00168-0278-15	18.42		AB
30 gm	00168-0278-30	27.46		AB
60 gm	00168-0278-60	46.12		AB
LOT, TP, 0.1%, 60 ml	00168-0280-60	42.18		AB
OIN, TP, 0.1%, 60 gm	00168-0279-60	46.12		AB
(Taro)				
CRE, TP, 0.1%, 15 gm	51672-4054-01	18.52		
30 gm	51672-4054-02	27.61		
60 gm	51672-4054-03	46.38		
AMDRY-D (Prasco Labs)				
methscopolamine nitrate/pse hcl				
TER, PO, 2.5 mg-120 mg,				
60s ea	66993-0120-60	55.51		
AMERGE (Glaxo)				
naratriptan hydrochloride				
TAB, PO (BLISTER PACK)				
1 mg, 9s ea	00173-0561-00	294.90		
2.5 mg, 9s ea	00173-0562-00	294.90		
AMERICAINE (Pharma Pac)				
REPACK				
benzocaine				
SOL, OT, 20%, 15 ml	52959-0038-15	25.00		
(Phys Total Care)				
REPACK				
SOL, OT, 20%, 15 ml	54868-1609-02	24.81		
AMERINET CHOICE AMPICILLIN AND SULBACTAM (Baxter)				
ampicillin sodium/sulbactam sodium				
PDS, IJ (PRIVATE LABEL)				
1 gm-0.5 gm, ea	10019-0634-31	4.74		AP
(10X10MLVIALS)				
1 gm-0.5 gm,				
10s ea	10019-0634-01	47.40		AP
(PRIVATE LABEL)				
2 gm-1 gm, ea	10019-0633-33	8.06		AP
10s ea	10019-0633-02	80.64		AP
(PHARMACYBULKPACKAGE,USP)				
10 gm-5 gm, ea	10019-0635-15	43.15		AP
AMERINET CHOICE BACITRACIN (Pfizer)				
bacitracin				
PDS, IM (PRIVATE LABEL)				
50000 u, ea	00009-0233-44	13.31	11.09	EE
AMERINET CHOICE CARBOPLATIN (Hospira)				
carboplatin				
SOL, IV (MDV,1X5ML,PRIVATE LABEL)				
10 mg/ml, 5 ml	61703-0339-61	7.54	6.59	AP
(MDV,1X15ML)				
10 mg/ml, 15 ml	61703-0339-62	17.80	15.57	AP
(MDV,1X45ML)				
10 mg/ml, 45 ml	61703-0339-63	50.08	43.82	AP

PROD/MFR	NDC	AWP	DP	OBC
AMERINET CHOICE CEFTRIAXONE (Hospira)				
ceftriaxone sodium				
PDS, IJ (USP, SINGLE USE)				
1 gm, 10s ea	00409-7332-61	28.08	24.60	AP
2 gm, 10s ea	00409-7335-61	45.12	39.50	AP
AMERINET CHOICE CIPROFLOXACIN (Hospira)				
ciprofloxacin				
SOL, IV (24X100ML,SINGLEDOSE,USP)				
200 mg/100 ml, 100 ml 24s	00409-4777-61	53.57	46.80	AP
(24X200ML,SINGLEDOSE,USP) 400 mg/200 ml, 200 ml 24s	00409-4777-62	70.56	61.68	AP
AMERINET CHOICE CORVERT (Pfizer)				
ibutilide fumarate				
SOL, IV (1X10ML,SDV,FLIPTOPVIAL)				
0.1 mg/ml, 10 ml	00009-3794-44	542.72	452.27	
AMERINET CHOICE DILTIAZEM HYDROCHLORIDE (Bedford)				
diltiazem hydrochloride				
SOL, IV (10X5ML,SINGLE USE)				
5 mg/ml, 5 ml 10s	55390-0374-05	13.20		AP
(10X10ML,SINGLE USE) 5 mg/ml, 10 ml 10s	55390-0374-10	21.60		AP
(10X25ML,SINGLE USE) 5 mg/ml, 25 ml 10s	55390-0374-30	43.20		AP
(Hospira)				
SOL, IV (10X10ML,PRIVATE LABEL)				
5 mg/ml, 10 ml 10s	00409-1171-62	16.08	14.10	AP
AMERINET CHOICE FLUCONAZOLE (Hospira)				
fluconazole				
SOL, IV (100MLX6,LATEX-FREE)				
200 mg/100 ml, 100 ml 6s	00409-4688-27	56.09	49.08	AP
(6X200ML,LATEX-FREE) 200 mg/100 ml, 200 ml 6s	00074-4688-33	207.36	181.44	AP
200 ml 6s	00409-4688-33	63.79	55.80	AP
AMERINET CHOICE IRINOTECAN HYDROCHLORIDE (Hospira)				
irinotecan hydrochloride				
SOL, IV (1X2ML,PRIVATE LABEL)				
20 mg/ml, 2 ml	61703-0349-61	25.68	22.47	AP
(1X5ML,PRIVATE LABEL) 20 mg/ml, 5 ml	61703-0349-62	36.37	31.83	AP
AMERINET CHOICE METOCLOPRAMIDE (Hospira)				
metoclopramide hydrochloride				
SOL, IJ (USP,25X2ML,SDV,PF)				
5 mg/ml, 2 ml 25s	00409-3414-61	10.80	9.50	AP
AMERINET CHOICE METOPROLOL TARTRATE (Bedford)				
metoprolol tartrate				
SOL, IV (USP,10X5ML,SDV)				
1 mg/ml, 5 ml 10s	55390-0373-10	15.60		AP
AMERINET CHOICE NALBUPHINE HYDROCHLORIDE (Hospira)				
nalbuphine hydrochloride				
SOL, IJ (10X1ML,PRIVATE LABEL)				
10 mg/ml, 1 ml 10s	00409-1463-61	13.56	11.90	AP
20 mg/ml, 1 ml 10s	00409-1465-61	27.12	23.70	AP
AMERINET CHOICE OCTREOTIDE ACETATE (Bedford)				
octreotide acetate				
SOL, IJ (10X1ML,SINGLE DOSE)				
100 mcg/ml, 1 ml 10s	55390-0375-10	42.00		AP
(1X5ML,MULTIPLE DOSE) 200 mcg/ml, 5 ml	55390-0377-01	42.00		AP
(10X1ML,SINGLE DOSE) 500 mcg/ml, 1 ml 10s	55390-0376-10	198.00		AP
AMERINET CHOICE ONDANSETRON (Hospira)				
ondansetron hydrochloride				
SOL, IJ (5X2ML,SDV,USP)				
2 mg/ml, 2 ml 5s	00409-4755-61	3.84	3.35	AP
(10X2ML,SDV,USP) 2 mg/ml, 2 ml 10s	00409-4755-62	7.68	6.70	AP
(25X2ML,SDV,USP) 2 mg/ml, 2 ml 25s	00409-4755-63	19.20	16.75	AP
AMERINET CHOICE PFIZERPEN (Pfizer)				
penicillin g potassium				
PDS, IJ (PRIVATE LABEL)				
5000000 u, 10s ea	00049-0520-44	79.86	66.55	AP
IV, 20 million u, ea	00049-0530-44	23.41	19.51	AP
AMERINET CHOICE PROPOFOL (Hospira)				
propofol				
EMU, IV (5X20ML,SDV,PF)				
10 mg/ml, 20 ml 5s	00409-4699-61	8.64	7.55	AB

PROD/MFR	NDC	AWP	DP	OBC
(20X50ML,SDV,PF) 10 mg/ml, 50 ml 20s	00409-4699-62	89.04	78.00	AB
(10X100ML,SDV,PF) 10 mg/ml, 100 ml 10s	00409-4699-63	89.28	78.10	AB
AMERINET CHOICE SEVOFLURANE (Baxter)				
sevoflurane				
LIQ, IH (PRIVATE LABEL)				
250 ml 6s	10019-0653-64	1332.00		
AMERINET CHOICE SUCCINYLCHOLINE CHLORIDE (Hospira)				
succinylcholine chloride				
SOL, IJ (USP,25X10ML,MD FLIPTOP)				
20 mg/ml, 10 ml 25s	00409-6629-61	52.20	45.75	
AMERINET CHOICE SUPRANE (Baxter)				
desflurane				
LIQ, IH (PRIVATE LABEL)				
240 ml 6s	10019-0646-24	1088.28		
AMERINET CHOICE VANCOMYCIN HYDROCHLORIDE (Hospira)				
vancomycin hydrochloride				
PDS, IV (SDV,FLIPTOP,USP)				
1 gm, 10s ea	00409-6533-61	61.32	53.70	AP
AMERINET CHOICE VINORELBINE TARTRATE (Pierre Fabre)				
vinorelbine tartrate				
SOL, IV (1X1ML,PRIVATE LABEL)				
10 mg/ml, 1 ml	64370-0210-01	28.80		
(1X5ML,PRIVATE LABEL) 10 mg/ml, 5 ml	64370-0250-01	144.00		
AMERINET CLAFORAN (Hospira)				
cefotaxime sodium				
PDS, IJ (PRIVATE LABEL)				
1 gm, 50s ea	00039-0023-61	197.40	172.50	
AMEVIVE (Astellas)				
alefacept				
PDS, IM (W/DILUENT PACK,PF)				
15 mg, ea	00469-0021-04	1092.00		EE
4s ea	00469-0021-03	4368.00		EE
AMIBID DM (Quality Care Prod) REPACK				
dextromethorphan hydrobromide/guaifenesin				
TER, PO, 30 mg-600 mg, 30s ea	49999-0888-30	7.58		
AMICAR (Xanodyne Pharma)				
aminocaproic acid				
SYR, PO (RASPBERRY)				
1.25 gm/5 ml, 473 ml	66479-0023-56	794.66		AA
TAB, PO, 500 mg, 100s ea	66479-0021-82	333.53		AB
1000 mg, 100s ea	66479-0022-82	716.74		
(Phys Total Care) REPACK				
TAB, PO, 500 mg, 10s ea	54868-0180-02	39.96		
30s ea	54868-0180-01	115.97		
50s ea	54868-0180-00	191.98		
AMIDATE (Hospira)				
etomidate				
SOL, IV (5X10ML)				
2 mg/ml, 10 ml 5s	00409-8062-01	82.62	72.30	AP
(10X10ML,LATEX-FREE) 2 mg/ml, 10 ml 10s	00409-6695-01	147.60	129.20	AP
(5X20ML) 2 mg/ml, 20 ml 5s	00409-8061-01	94.80	82.95	AP
(FTV,10X20ML,LATEX-FREE) 2 mg/ml, 20 ml 10s	00409-6695-02	168.36	147.30	AP
(LATEX-FREE) 2 mg/ml, 20 ml 10s	00074-8060-19	243.84	213.40	AP
(LIFESHIELD,LATEX-FREE) 2 mg/ml, 20 ml 10s	00409-8060-29	304.56	266.50	AP
AMIDRINE (DHS, Inc.) REPACK				
apap/dichloralphenazone/isometheptene mucate				
CAP, PO, 325 mg-100 mg-65 mg, 30s ea, C-IV	55887-0776-30	21.49		
AMIFOSTINE (Bedford)				
PDS, IV (3X10ML, SINGLE USE VIAL)				
500 mg, 3s ea	55390-0308-03	1800.00		
(Caraco)				
PDS, IV (USP)				
500 mg, ea	62756-0581-40	564.95		AP
3s ea	62756-0581-42	1694.75		AP
(Medimmune Oncology) *See ETHYOL*				

PROD/MFR	NDC	AWP	DP	OBC
AMIKACIN SULFATE				
(Bedford) *See AMIKACIN SULFATE NOVAPLUS*				
(Bedford) *See AMIKACIN SULFATE PEDIATRIC*				
(Bedford) *See AMIKACIN SULFATE PEDIATRIC NOVAPLUS*				
(Bedford)				
SOL, IJ (S.D.V.,PF)				
250 mg/ml, 2 ml 10s	55390-0226-02	78.00		AP
(PF) 250 mg/ml, 4 ml 10s	55390-0226-04	156.00		AP
(Hawkins)				
POW, NA (U.S.P.)				
5 gm	63370-0016-15	160.00		
25 gm	63370-0016-25	660.00		
100 gm	63370-0016-35	1200.00		
1000 gm	63370-0016-50	6800.00		
(Hospira)				
SOL, IJ (VIAL,FLIPTOP,LATEX-FREE)				
50 mg/ml, 2 ml 10s	00409-1955-01	36.00	31.50	AP
(10X2ML) 250 mg/ml, 2 ml 10s	00409-1956-01	50.52	44.20	AP
(10X4ML) 250 mg/ml, 4 ml 10s	00409-1957-01	83.52	73.10	AP
(Medisca)				
POW, NA (1X5GM,USP)				
5 gm	38779-2488-03	127.50		
(U.S.P.) 5 gm	38779-0295-03	127.50		
(1X25GM,USP) 25 gm	38779-2488-04	525.00		
(U.S.P.) 25 gm	38779-0295-04	525.00		
(1X100GM,USP) 100 gm	38779-2488-05	1425.00		
(U.S.P.) 100 gm	38779-0295-05	1425.00		
(1X1000GM,USP) 1000 gm	38779-2488-09	2685.00		
(USP,1X1000GM) 1000 gm	38779-0295-09	2685.00		
(PCCA)				
POW, NA (U.S.P.)				
1 gm	51927-2704-00	34.20		
(Sandoz) *See AMIKIN*				
(Sandoz) *See AMIKIN PEDIATRIC*				
(Spectrum Pharmacy)				
POW, NA, 5 gm	49452-0013-01	220.85		
(USP,1X25GM) 25 gm	49452-0013-02	892.50		
1000 gm	49452-0013-04	3825.50		
(Teva)				
SOL, IJ (S.D.V.)				
250 mg/ml, 2 ml 10s	00703-9032-03	44.40		AP
(VIAL) 250 mg/ml, 4 ml 10s	00703-9040-03	87.60		AP
AMIKACIN SULFATE NOVAPLUS (Bedford)				
amikacin sulfate				
SOL, IJ (S.D.V.,PF)				
250 mg/ml, 2 ml 10s	55390-0224-02	39.60		AP
(PF) 250 mg/ml, 4 ml 10s	55390-0224-04	93.60		AP
AMIKACIN SULFATE PEDIATRIC (Bedford)				
amikacin sulfate				
SOL, IJ (S.D.V.,PF)				
50 mg/ml, 2 ml 10s	55390-0225-02	78.00		AP
AMIKACIN SULFATE PEDIATRIC NOVAPLUS (Bedford)				
amikacin sulfate				
SOL, IJ (S.D.V.,PF)				
50 mg/ml, 2 ml 10s	55390-0223-02	43.20		AP
AMIKIN (Sandoz)				
amikacin sulfate				
SOL, IJ (VIAL)				
250 mg/ml, 4 ml	00015-3023-20	67.71		AP
AMIKIN PEDIATRIC (Sandoz)				
amikacin sulfate				
SOL, IJ (VIAL)				
50 mg/ml, 2 ml	00015-3015-20	33.04		AP

PROD/MFR	NDC	AWP	DP	OBC

AMILORIDE HCL (Par)
amiloride hydrochloride
TAB, PO, 5 mg, 100s ea . . . **49884-0117-01** 128.97 **AB**
1000s ea . . . . **49884-0117-10** 1289.70 **AB**

(PCCA)
POW, NA (USP; DIHYDRATE)
1 gm **51927-1993-00** 13.20

(Spectrum Pharmacy)
POW, NA (U.S.P./N.F.)
5 gm **49452-0397-02** 214.20
25 gm **49452-0397-03** 693.00

(Phys Total Care)
REPACK
TAB, PO, 5 mg, 10s ea **54868-5214-03** 21.33
20s ea . . . . **54868-5214-01** 38.19 **AB**
30s ea **54868-5214-02** 55.02
60s ea . . . . **54868-5214-00** 105.54 **AB**

AMILORIDE HCL/HCTZ (West Point)
amiloride hydrochloride/hydrochlorothiazide
TAB, PO, 5 mg-50 mg,
100s ea. . . . . **59591-0162-68** 32.75 **AB**

(Dispensing Solutions)
REPACK
TAB, PO, 5 mg-50 mg,
28s ea . . . . **55045-2392-09** 12.32 **AB**

AMILORIDE HYDROCHLORIDE
(Paddock) *See MIDAMOR*

(Paddock)
TAB, PO (USP,COMPRESSED)
5 mg, 100s ea. **00574-0292-01** 128.97

(Par) *See AMILORIDE HCL*

(PCCA) *See AMILORIDE HCL*

(Rising)
TAB, PO (USP,COMPRESSED)
5 mg, 100s ea. . . . . **64980-0151-01** 127.95 **AB**

(Spectrum Pharmacy) *See AMILORIDE HCL*

AMILORIDE HYDROCHLORIDE/ HYDROCHLOROTHIAZIDE
FUL
TAB, PO, 5 mg-50 mg,
100s ea 6.75

(Mylan) *See AMILORIDE/HCTZ*

(Teva) *See AMILORIDE/HCTZ*

(West Point) *See AMILORIDE HCL/HCTZ*

AMILORIDE/HCTZ (Mylan)
amiloride hydrochloride/hydrochlorothiazide
TAB, PO, 5 mg-50 mg,
100s ea. . . . . **00378-0577-01** 42.45 **AB**
500s ea. . . . . **00378-0577-05** 207.83 **AB**

(Teva)
TAB, PO, 5 mg-50 mg,
100s ea. . . . . **00555-0483-02** 32.86 **AB**
1000s ea . . . . **00555-0483-05** 330.16 **AB**

(A-S Medication)
REPACK
TAB, PO, 5 mg-50 mg,
28s ea . . . . **54569-3869-00** 11.89 **EE**

(Phys Total Care)
REPACK
TAB, PO, 5 mg-50 mg,
30s ea . . . . **54868-0667-01** 10.17 **EE**
90s ea . . . . **54868-0667-02** 21.49 **AB**
100s ea . . . . **54868-0667-00** 23.37 **EE**

AMILORIDE/HYDROCHLOROTHIAZIDE (DHS, Inc.)
REPACK
amiloride hydrochloride/hydrochlorothiazide
TAB, PO, 5 mg-50 mg,
30s ea **55887-0199-30** 12.73

AMINACRINE HYDROCHLORIDE
(PCCA) *See AMINOACRIDINE HYDROCHLORIDE MONO-HYDRATE*

(Spectrum Pharmacy) *See 9-AMINOACRIDINE HYDROCHLORIDE*

AMINO ACETIC ACID (Amend)
glycine
POW, NA (U.S.P.)
454 gm **17317-0189-01** 15.40
2270 gm **17317-0189-05** 58.80
11350 gm **17317-0189-08** 245.00

AMINO ACIDS
(B. Braun) *See FREAMINE HBC*

(B. Braun) *See FREAMINE III*

(B. Braun) *See HEPATAMINE*

(B. Braun) *See NEPHRAMINE*

(B. Braun) *See TROPHAMINE*

(Baxter) *See CLINISOL*

(Baxter) *See HEPATASOL*

(Baxter) *See PREMASOL*

(Baxter) *See PROSOL*

(Baxter) *See RENAMIN*

(Baxter) *See TRAVASOL*

(Hospira) *See AMINOSYN*

(Hospira) *See AMINOSYN (PH6)*

(Hospira) *See AMINOSYN HBC*

(Hospira) *See AMINOSYN II*

(Hospira) *See AMINOSYN-HBC*

(Hospira) *See AMINOSYN-HF*

(Hospira) *See AMINOSYN-PF*

(Hospira) *See AMINOSYN-RF*

(Hospira) *See NOVAMINE*

(Nestle) *See BRANCHAMIN*

(Physician Thera, LLC) *See APPTRIM-D*

(Spectrum Pharmacy) *See BRANCHED CHAIN AMINO ACIDS*

AMINO ACIDS AND ELECTROLYTES
(B. Braun) *See FREAMINE III W/ELECTROLYTES*

(B. Braun) *See PROCALAMINE*

AMINO ACIDS AND NUTRICEUTICALS
(Physician Thera, LLC) *See APPTRIM*

(Physician Thera, LLC) *See APPTRIM LIFESTYLES POST-BARIATRIC SURGERY PROGRAM*

(Physician Thera, LLC) *See APPTRIM LIFESTYLES PRE-BARIATRIC SURGERY PROGRAM*

(Physician Thera, LLC) *See APPTRIM WEIGHT MANAGEMENT PROGRAM*

(Physician Thera, LLC) *See GABADONE*

(Physician Thera, LLC) *See HYPERTENSA*

(Physician Thera, LLC) *See PULMONA*

(Physician Thera, LLC) *See SENTRA AM*

(Physician Thera, LLC) *See SENTRA PM*

(Physician Thera, LLC) *See THERAMINE*

(Physician Thera, LLC) *See VIRILEX*

AMINO ACIDS, DEXTROSE, AND ELECTROLYTES
(Baxter) *See CLINIMIX E 2.75/10*

(Baxter) *See CLINIMIX E 2.75/5*

(Baxter) *See CLINIMIX E 4.25/10*

(Baxter) *See CLINIMIX E 4.25/25*

(Baxter) *See CLINIMIX E 4.25/5*

(Baxter) *See CLINIMIX E 5/15*

(Baxter) *See CLINIMIX E 5/20*

(Baxter) *See CLINIMIX E 5/25*

AMINO ACIDS, MULTIVITAMIN, AND MINERALS
(VITAFLO, LLC) *See MMA/PA GEL*

AMINO ACIDS/CA CL/DEXTROSE/ K CL/K PHOS/MG CL/NA CL
(Hospira) *See AMINOSYN II 4.25%*

(Hospira) *See AMINOSYN II WITH ELECTROLYTES*

AMINO ACIDS/DEXTROSE
(Baxter) *See CLINIMIX*

(Hospira) *See AMINOSYN II W/ ELECTROLYTES*

(Hospira) *See AMINOSYN II W/DEXTROSE*

(Hospira) *See NUTRIMIX*

AMINO ACIDS/DEXTROSE/ K CL/MG CL/NA CL/NA PHOS
(Hospira) *See AMINOSYN II M W/DEXTROSE*

(Hospira) *See NUTRIMIX W/ELECTROLYTES*

AMINO ACIDS/K ACE/MG ACE/NA CL/ PHOSPHORIC ACID
(Hospira) *See AMINOSYN M W/ELECTROLYTES*

AMINO ACIDS/K CL/MG CL/NA CL/NA PHOS
(Hospira) *See AMINOSYN II WITH ELECTROLYTES*

(Hospira) *See AMINOSYN W/ELECTROLYTES*

(Hospira) *See AMINOSYN WITH ELECTROLYTES*

AMINO-CERV (Phys Total Care)
REPACK
cystine/inositol/methionine/sodium propionate/urea
CRE, VG, 78 gm **54868-0482-00** 22.30

AMINOACETIC ACID (Spectrum Pharmacy)
glycine
POW, NA (F.C.C.)
100 gm **49452-3378-01** 67.90
(U.S.P.)
100 gm **49452-0400-04** 65.80
(F.C.C.)
500 gm **49452-3378-02** 116.55
(U.S.P.)
500 gm **49452-0400-01** 114.45
(F.C.C.)
2500 gm **49452-3378-03** 335.65
(U.S.P.)
2500 gm **49452-0400-02** 332.85

9-AMINOACRIDINE HYDROCHLORIDE (Spectrum Pharmacy)
aminacrine hydrochloride
CRY, NA, 5 gm **49452-0404-01** 150.50
25 gm **49452-0404-02** 357.00

AMINOACRIDINE HYDROCHLORIDE MONOHYDRATE (PCCA)
aminacrine hydrochloride
CRY, NA (1X1GM)
1 gm **51927-1538-00** 12.00

AMINOBENZOATE POTASSIUM (Cypress Pharm)
PDR, PO (50X2GM)
2 gm/packet,
2 gm 50s **60258-0841-50** 87.20

(Glenwood) *See POTABA*

(Hope)
CAP, PO (U.S.P.)
0.5 gm, 250s ea **60267-0953-25** 118.00

AMINOBENZOIC ACID
(Gallipot) *See PARA-AMINOBENZOIC ACID*

(Medisca) *See PARA-AMINOBENZOIC ACID*

(PCCA) *See PARA-AMINOBENZOIC ACID*

(Spectrum Pharmacy) *See PARA-AMINOBENZOIC ACID*

AMINOBUTYRIC ACID (PCCA)
gamma aminobutyric acid
POW, NA (1X1GM)
1 gm **51927-2325-00** 1.50
(DL-2)
1 gm **51927-3134-00** 9.36

4-AMINOBUTYRIC ACID (Spectrum Pharmacy)
gamma aminobutyric acid
CRY, NA (1X100GM,REAGENT)
100 gm **49452-0412-02** 156.10
(1X500GM,REAGENT)
500 gm **49452-0412-03** 507.50

AMINOCAPROIC ACID (Amer Regent)
SOL, IV (M.D.V.)
250 mg/ml,
20 ml 25s . . . . **00517-9120-25** 67.20 **AP**

(Consolidated Midland)
SOL, IV (VIAL)
250 mg/ml, 20 ml . . . . **00223-7126-20** 17.50 **EE**

(Hospira)
SOL, IV (VIAL,FLIPTOP)
250 mg/ml,
20 ml 25s . . . . **00409-4346-73** 27.90 24.50 **AP**

(Medisca)
POW, NA (U.S.P.)
25 gm **38779-0989-04** 31.50
100 gm **38779-0989-05** 96.00
500 gm **38779-0989-08** 405.00
1000 gm **38779-0989-09** 675.00

(PCCA)
POW, NA (USP (6))
1 gm **51927-1776-00** 1.92

(Spectrum Pharmacy)
POW, NA (U.S.P.)
25 gm **49452-0409-01** 72.45
100 gm **49452-0409-02** 159.60
500 gm **49452-0409-03** 626.50
2500 gm **49452-0409-04** 1407.00

(VersaPharm)
SOL, PO (RASPBERRY)
1.25 gm/5 ml,
237 ml . . . . **61748-0044-08** 312.88 **AA**
473 ml . . . . **61748-0044-16** 650.79 **AA**

PROD/MFR	NDC	AWP	DP	OBC
TAB, PO, 500 mg, 100s ea	61748-0045-01	262.63		AB
10(2X5))				
500 mg, 100s ea UD	61748-0045-11	262.63		AB
(Xanodyne Pharma) *See AMICAR*				
AMINOGUANIDINE BICARBONATE (PCCA)				
POW, NA (HYDROGEN CARBONATE)				
1 gm	51927-2822-00	1.38		
AMINOHIPPURATE SODIUM (Merck)				
SOL, IV (AMP)				
20%, 10 ml	00006-3395-11	6.65		
AMINOLEVULINIC ACID				
(Dusa Pharmaceuticals) *See LEVULAN KERASTICK*				
AMINOLEVULINIC ACID HYDROCHLORIDE (Medisca)				
POW, NA (1X1GM)				
1 gm	38779-2362-06	195.00		
(1X5GM)				
5 gm	38779-2362-03	837.00		
(1X500MG)				
500 ml	38779-2362-00	112.50		
AMINOMETHANE HYDROCHLORIDE (PCCA)				
methylamine hydrochloride				
POW, NA (1X1GM)				
1 gm	51927-1478-00	1.05		
AMINOPHYLLINE				
(Amend) *See AMINOPHYLLINE ANHYDROUS*				
(Amer Regent)				
SOL, IV (S.D.V.,PF)				
25 mg/ml,				
10 ml 25s	00517-3810-25	19.69		AP
20 ml 25s	00517-3820-25	22.19		AP
(Consolidated Midland)				
SOL, IV, 25 mg/ml,				
10 ml 25s	00223-7130-10	30.00		EE
(VIAL)				
25 mg/ml,				
10 ml 25s	00223-7128-10	27.50		EE
10 ml 100s	00223-7130-00	110.00		EE
(VIAL)				
25 mg/ml,				
10 ml 100s	00223-7128-02	70.00		EE
(S.D.V.)				
25 mg/ml,				
20 ml 25s	00223-7136-20	40.00		EE
TAB, PO, 100 mg, 100s ea	00223-0100-01	3.25		EE
1000s ea	00223-0100-02	21.50		EE
200 mg, 100s ea	00223-0102-01	4.50		EE
1000s ea	00223-0102-02	29.50		EE
(Gallipot) *See AMINOPHYLLINE ANHYDROUS*				
(Hospira)				
SOL, IV (10X10ML,ABBOJECT)				
25 mg/ml,				
10 ml 10s	00074-4909-18	38.24	32.20	AP
(AMP,LATEX-FREE)				
25 mg/ml,				
10 ml 25s	00409-7385-01	19.80	17.25	AP
(VIAL,FLIPTOP,25X10ML)				
25 mg/ml,				
10 ml 25s	00409-5921-01	17.10	15.00	AP
(AMP,LATEX-FREE)				
25 mg/ml,				
20 ml 25s	00409-7386-01	48.30	42.25	AP
(VIAL, FLIPTOP,ABBOJECT)				
25 mg/ml,				
20 ml 25s	00409-5922-01	27.00	23.75	AP
(Letco) *See AMINOPHYLLINE ANHYDROUS*				
(Medisca) *See AMINOPHYLLINE DIHYDRATE*				
(PCCA)				
POW, NA (U.S.P.; ANHYDROUS)				
1 gm	51927-1444-00	1.02		
(Spectrum Pharmacy) *See AMINOPHYLLINE ANHYDROUS*				
(West-Ward)				
TAB, PO, 100 mg, 100s ea	00143-1020-01	7.85		AB
1000s ea	00143-1020-10	30.22		AB
200 mg, 100s ea	00143-1025-01	8.45		AB
1000s ea	00143-1025-10	48.45		AB
(Phys Total Care)				
REPACK				
SOL, IV (S.D.V.)				
25 mg/ml,				
10 ml 25s	54868-0004-00	75.67		EE
(Quality Care Prod)				
REPACK				
TAB, PO, 200 mg, 100s ea	49999-0550-00	13.05		AB
AMINOPHYLLINE ANHYDROUS (Amend)				
aminophylline				
POW, NA (U.S.P.)				
125 gm	17317-0022-04	19.60		
454 gm	17317-0022-01	42.00		
2270 gm	17317-0022-05	196.00		
(Gallipot)				
POW, NA (U.S.P.)				
100 gm	51552-0313-05	16.59		
454 gm	51552-0313-06	52.92		
(Letco)				
POW, NA (U.S.P.)				
100 gm	62991-2003-02	31.50		
500 gm	62991-2003-03	117.00		
(Spectrum Pharmacy)				
POW, NA (U.S.P.)				
100 gm	49452-0430-01	67.90		
500 gm	49452-0430-02	203.70		
(USP,1X2500GM)				
2500 gm	49452-0430-03	854.00		
AMINOPHYLLINE DIHYDRATE (Medisca)				
aminophylline				
POW, NA (U.S.P.)				
25 gm	38779-0571-04	24.00		
100 gm	38779-0571-05	34.50		
500 gm	38779-0571-08	108.00		
AMINOPYRIDINE (PCCA)				
POW, NA (4)				
1 gm	51927-2423-00	7.20		
(Spectrum Pharmacy) *See 4-AMINOPYRIDINE*				
4-AMINOPYRIDINE (Spectrum Pharmacy)				
aminopyridine				
POW, NA (REAGENT)				
25 gm	49452-0452-01	183.75		
100 gm	49452-0452-02	570.50		
AMINOSALICYLIC (PCCA)				
aminosalicylic acid				
POW, NA (USP; (5))				
1 gm	51927-1078-00	1.80		
AMINOSALICYLIC ACID				
(Gallipot) *See 5-AMINOSALICYLIC ACID*				
5-AMINOSALICYLIC ACID (Gallipot)				
aminosalicylic acid				
POW, NA (USP)				
25 gm	51552-0302-04	14.28	10.20	
100 gm	51552-0302-05	34.65		
500 gm	51552-0302-06	147.00		
AMINOSALICYLIC ACID				
(Hawkins) *See MESALAMINE*				
(Jacobus) *See PASER*				
(Medisca) *See 5-AMINOSALICYLIC ACID*				
5-AMINOSALICYLIC ACID (Medisca)				
aminosalicylic acid				
POW, NA, 25 gm	38779-0012-04	42.00		
100 gm	38779-0012-05	72.00		
500 gm	38779-0012-08	264.00		
1000 gm	38779-0012-09	468.00		
AMINOSALICYLIC ACID				
(PCCA) *See AMINOSALICYLIC*				
(PCCA)				
POW, NA (4)				
1 gm	51927-1608-00	1.17		
AMINOSYN (Hospira)				
amino acids				
SOL, IV, 3.5%,				
1000 ml 6s	00074-2989-05	124.76	105.06	
1000 ml 6s	00074-4154-05	124.76	105.06	
(6X1000ML,LATEX-FREE)				
3.5%, 1000 ml 6s	00409-4159-05	73.66	64.44	
5%, 500 ml 12s	00074-2990-03	111.01	93.48	
(LATEX-FREE,SULFITE-FREE)				
5%, 500 ml 12s	00409-4181-03	149.62	130.92	EE
(1000MLX6,LATEX-FREE)				
5%, 1000 ml 6s	00409-4181-05	163.80	143.34	EE
(500MLX12,LATEX-FREE)				
7%, 500 ml 12s	00409-4184-03	155.23	135.84	EE
8.5%, 500 ml 12s	00074-5855-03	121.84	102.60	
(500MLX12,SINGLE DOSE)				
8.5%, 500 ml 12s	00409-4187-03	130.61	114.24	EE
(LATEX-FREE,SULFITE-FREE)				
8.5%, 1000 ml 6s	00074-4187-05	146.02	127.74	
10%, 500 ml 12s	00074-2991-03	136.52	114.96	
(12X500ML,LATEX-FREE)				
10%, 500 ml 12s	00409-4191-03	204.19	178.68	
(LATEX-FREE,SULFITE-FREE)				
10%, 500 ml 12s	00049-4191-03	167.62	146.64	
(6X1000ML,LATEX-FREE)				
10%, 1000 ml 6s	00409-4191-05	153.65	134.46	
AMINOSYN (PH6) (Hospira)				
amino acids				
SOL, IV (6X1000ML,LATEX-FREE)				
10%, 1000 ml 6s	00409-4192-05	153.50	134.34	
AMINOSYN HBC (Hospira)				
amino acids				
SOL, IV (HIGH BRANCHED CHAIN)				
7%, 1000 ml 6s	00074-4168-05	822.96	720.06	
AMINOSYN II (Hospira)				
amino acids				
SOL, IV (LATEX-FREE,SULFITE-FREE)				
7%, 500 ml 12s	00409-4160-03	150.05	131.28	
(12X500ML,LATEX-FREE)				
8.5%, 500 ml 12s	00409-4162-03	145.01	126.84	EE
(6X1000ML,LATEX-FREE)				
8.5%, 1000 ml 6s	00409-4162-05	127.51	111.60	
(LATEX-FREE,SULFITE-FREE)				
10%, 500 ml 12s	00409-4164-03	163.30	142.92	
1000 ml 6s	00409-4164-05	139.32	121.92	
(BULK PACKAGE,LATEX-FREE)				
10%, 2000 ml 6s	00409-7121-07	232.56	203.52	
(BULK PACKAGE,6X2000ML)				
15%, 2000 ml 6s	00409-7122-07	411.77	360.30	
AMINOSYN II 4.25% (Hospira)				
amino acids/ca cl/dextrose/k cl/k phos/mg cl/na cl				
SOL, IV (IN 20% DEXTROSE W/CA)				
1000 ml 6s	00409-7753-29	210.60	184.26	
AMINOSYN II M W/DEXTROSE (Hospira)				
amino acids/dextrose/k cl/mg cl/na cl/na phos				
SOL, IV (DUAL CHAMBER,LATEX-FREE)				
1000 ml 6s	00409-7740-29	176.40	154.38	
AMINOSYN II W/ ELECTROLYTES (Hospira)				
amino acids/dextrose				
SOL, IV (NUTRIMIX DUAL CHAMBER)				
3.5%-25%,				
1000 ml 6s	00409-7756-29	206.28	180.48	EE
AMINOSYN II W/DEXTROSE (Hospira)				
amino acids/dextrose				
SOL, IV (DUAL CHAMBER,6X1000ML)				
3.5%-5%,				
1000 ml 6s	00409-7701-29	172.44	150.90	
4.25%-10%,				
1000 ml 6s	00409-7751-29	178.34	156.06	
(DUAL CHAMBER,LATEX-FREE)				
4.25%-20%,				
1000 ml 6s	00409-7752-29	190.08	166.32	
(DUAL CHAMBER,6X1000ML)				
4.25%-25%,				
1000 ml 6s	00409-7702-29	169.63	148.44	
AMINOSYN II WITH ELECTROLYTES (Hospira)				
amino acids/ca cl/dextrose/k cl/k phos/mg cl/na cl				
SOL, IV (NUTRIMIX,LATEX-FREE)				
1000 ml 6s	00409-7757-29	180.50	157.92	EE
(Hospira)				
amino acids/k cl/mg cl/na cl/na phos				
(12X500ML,SINGLE DOSE)				
500 ml 12s	00409-4171-03	133.92	117.24	EE
AMINOSYN M W/ELECTROLYTES (Hospira)				
amino acids/k ace/mg ace/na cl/phosphoric acid				
SOL, IV (6X1000ML,LATEX-FREE)				
1000 ml 6s	00409-4196-05	72.29	63.24	
AMINOSYN W/ELECTROLYTES (Hospira)				
amino acids/k cl/mg cl/na cl/na phos				
SOL, IV (12X500ML,W/DEHP)				
500 ml 12s	00409-4200-03	170.35	149.04	
(6X1000ML,LATEX-FREE)				
1000 ml 6s	00409-4203-05	128.81	112.68	EE
AMINOSYN WITH ELECTROLYTES (Hospira)				
amino acids/k cl/mg cl/na cl/na phos				
SOL, IV (12X500ML,LATEX-FREE)				
500 ml 12s	00409-4203-03	153.79	134.52	EE
AMINOSYN-HBC (Hospira)				
amino acids				
SOL, IV (12X500ML,SD,LATEX-FREE)				
7%, 500 ml 12s	00409-4168-03	904.75	791.64	EE
AMINOSYN-HF (Hospira)				
amino acids				
SOL, IV (12X500ML,LATEX-FREE)				
8%, 500 ml 12s	00409-4167-03	915.98	801.48	
AMINOSYN-PF (Hospira)				
amino acids				
SOL, IV, 7%, 250 ml 12s	00074-1616-02	530.53	446.76	
(12X500ML,LATEX-FREE)				
7%, 500 ml 12s	00409-4178-03	531.50	465.12	
(PED, FORMULA, 6X1000ML)				
10%, 1000 ml 6s	00409-4179-05	549.00	480.36	EE

PROD/MFR	NDC	AWP	DP	OBC
AMINOSYN-RF (Hospira)				
amino acids				
SOL, IV (12X500ML,SINGLE-DOSE)				
5.2%, 500 ml 12s	**00409-4166-03**	331.63	290.16	
AMIODARONE (DHS, Inc.)				
REPACK				
amiodarone hydrochloride				
TAB, PO, 200 mg, 30s ea	**55887-0798-30**	47.96		
100s ea	**55887-0798-01**	127.56		
(Dispensing Solutions)				
REPACK				
TAB, PO, 200 mg, 60s ea	**55045-2864-06**	198.00		
100s ea	**55045-2864-00**	330.00		
(Phys Total Care)				
REPACK				
SOL, IV (SDV,10X3ML)				
50 mg/ml, 3 ml 10s	**54868-5722-00**	81.48		
(Quality Care Prod)				
REPACK				
TAB, PO, 200 mg, 10s ea	**35356-0001-10**	39.60		
(Southwood)				
REPACK				
TAB, PO, 200 mg, 30s ea	**58016-0304-30**	59.45		
60s ea	**58016-0304-60**	118.89		
90s ea	**58016-0304-90**	178.34		
100s ea	**58016-0304-00**	198.15		
AMIODARONE HCL (Apotex Corp.)				
amiodarone hydrochloride				
SOL, IV (SDS,10X3ML)				
50 mg/ml, 3 ml 10s	**60505-0722-01**	112.50		AP
(SDV)				
50 mg/ml, 3 ml 10s	**60505-0722-00**	112.50		AP
(Baxter)				
SOL, IV, 50 mg/ml, 9 ml	**10019-0133-19**	7.20		
9 ml 10s	**10019-0133-04**	72.00		
(SDV,1X18ML)				
50 mg/ml, 18 ml	**10019-0133-02**	9.00		
(SINGLE DOSE, INNER PACK)				
50 mg/ml, 18 ml	**10019-0133-89**	9.00		
(Bedford)				
SOL, IV (S.D.V.,PF)				
50 mg/ml, 3 ml 10s	**55390-0057-10**	24.00		AP
(M.D.V.)				
50 mg/ml, 9 ml	**55390-0105-01**	7.20		AP
(18ML MULTIPLE USE VIAL)				
50 mg/ml, 18 ml	**55390-0057-01**	14.40		AP
(Bioniche Pharma)				
SOL, IV, 50 mg/ml,				
3 ml 10s	**67457-0153-03**	16.69		
(Hospira)				
SOL, IV, 50 mg/ml,				
3 ml 10s	**00074-4348-35**	23.28	20.40	AP
3 ml 10s	**61703-0241-03**	25.20	22.05	AP
(Par)				
TAB, PO, 200 mg, 250s ea	**49884-0458-04**	826.07		AB
(Sandoz)				
TAB, PO, 200 mg, 60s ea	**00185-0144-60**	202.91		AB
60s ea	**00781-1203-60**	197.93		AB
90s ea	**00185-0144-09**	290.96		AB
90s ea	**00781-1203-92**	290.96		AB
500s ea	**00185-0144-05**	1691.01		AB
(Taro)				
TAB, PO, 200 mg, 60s ea	**51672-4025-04**	198.16		AB
400 mg, 30s ea	**51672-4057-06**	169.69		AB
100s ea UD	**51672-4057-00**	632.02		AB
(Teva)				
SOL, IV, 50 mg/ml, 9 ml	**00703-1335-01**	5.10		AP
(1X18ML,SINGLE-USE)				
50 mg/ml, 18 ml	**00703-1336-01**	10.20		AP
TAB, PO, 200 mg, 60s ea	**00093-9133-06**	198.15		AB
60s ea	**00555-0917-09**	200.66		AB
250s ea	**00093-9133-52**	825.00		AB
500s ea	**00555-0917-04**	1601.71		AB
(UDL)				
TAB, PO (10X10)				
200 mg, 100s ea UD	**51079-0906-20**	329.00		AB
(A-S Medication)				
REPACK				
TAB, PO, 200 mg, 30s ea	**54569-5140-01**	99.67		AB
400 mg, 30s ea	**54569-6129-00**	169.69		AB
(Phys Total Care)				
REPACK				
TAB, PO, 200 mg, 30s ea	**54868-4618-01**	27.12		AB
60s ea	**54868-4618-00**	49.74		AB
90s ea	**54868-4618-03**	76.86		AB
100s ea	**54868-4618-02**	62.97		AB
(Quality Care Prod)				
REPACK				
TAB, PO, 200 mg, 90s ea	**35356-0001-90**	49.60		AB
AMIODARONE HYDROCHLORIDE				
FUL				
TAB, PO, 200 mg, 60s ea		44.25		
(Apotex Corp.) *See AMIODARONE HCL*				
(APP)				
SOL, IV (S.D.V.)				
50 mg/ml, 3 ml 25s	**63323-0616-03**	154.69		AP
9 ml 10s	**63323-0616-09**	179.50		AP
(Baxter) *See AMIODARONE HCL*				
(Bedford) *See AMIODARONE HCL*				
(Bedford) *See AMIODARONE HYDROCHLORIDE NOVAPLUS*				
(Bioniche Pharma) *See AMIODARONE HCL*				
(Bioniche Pharma)				
SOL, IV (10X9ML)				
50 mg/ml, 9 ml 10s	**67457-0153-09**	52.31		AP
18 ml	**67457-0153-18**	9.81		AP
(Hospira) *See AMIODARONE HCL*				
(Hospira) *See NOVAPLUS AMIODARONE HYDROCHLORIDE*				
(Hospira)				
SOL, IV (3MLX10,SINGLE-DOSE)				
50 mg/ml, 3 ml 10s	**00409-4348-35**	21.60	18.90	AP
(Par) *See AMIODARONE HCL*				
(PCCA)				
POW, NA, 1 gm	**51927-3760-00**	288.60		
(Sagent)				
SOL, IV (10X3ML,PRF SYRINGE)				
50 mg/ml, 3 ml 10s	**25021-0302-73**	112.50		AP
(Sandoz) *See AMIODARONE HCL*				
(Taro) *See AMIODARONE HCL*				
(Teva) *See AMIODARONE HCL*				
(Teva)				
SOL, IV (10X3ML,SINGLE USE)				
50 mg/ml, 3 ml 10s	**00703-1332-03**	27.60		AP
(UDL) *See AMIODARONE HCL*				
(UDL)				
TAB, PO (ROBOT READY,25X1)				
200 mg, 25s ea	**51079-0906-19**	82.25		AB
(Upsher-Smith) *See PACERONE*				
(West-Ward)				
SOL, IV (10X3ML)				
50 mg/ml, 3 ml 10s	**00143-9875-10**	25.00		AP
(Wyeth) *See CORDARONE*				
(Zydus Pharm.)				
TAB, PO, 200 mg, 60s ea	**68382-0227-14**	199.33		AB
500s ea	**68382-0227-05**	1615.35		AB
(American Health)				
REPACK				
TAB, PO, 200 mg,				
100s ea UD	**68084-0371-01**	60.63		AB
(McKesson Packaging)				
REPACK				
TAB, PO, 200 mg,				
100s ea UD	**63739-0387-10**	338.00		
AMIODARONE HYDROCHLORIDE NOVAPLUS				
(Bedford)				
amiodarone hydrochloride				
SOL, IV (S.D.V.,PRIVATE LABEL)				
50 mg/ml, 3 ml 10s	**55390-0097-10**	14.40		AP
AMITHIOZONE				
(PCCA) *See THIACETAZONE*				
AMITIZA (Takeda)				
lubiprostone				
SGL, PO (SOFT GELATIN)				
8 mcg, 60s ea	**64764-0080-60**	251.35		
(SOFT GELATIN CAPSULE)				
24 mcg, 60s ea	**64764-0240-60**	251.35		
(Phys Total Care)				
REPACK				
SGL, PO (SOFT GELATIN CAPSULE)				
24 mcg, 60s ea	**54868-5971-00**	272.10		
(Quality Care Prod)				
REPACK				
SGL, PO (SOFT GELATIN CAPSULE)				
24 mcg, 60s ea	**35356-0500-60**	388.50		
(Stat Rx)				
REPACK				
SGL, PO (SOFT GELATIN)				
8 mcg, 30s ea	**16590-0622-30**	128.84		
60s ea	**16590-0622-60**	280.28		
90s ea	**16590-0622-90**	334.90		
(SOFT GELATIN CAPSULE)				
24 mcg, 28s ea	**16590-0471-28**	138.84		
30s ea	**16590-0471-30**	148.53		
60s ea	**16590-0471-60**	293.80		
(SOFTGEL)				
24 mcg, 90s ea	**16590-0471-90**	381.00		
AMITRAZ (PCCA)				
POW, NA, 1 gm	**51927-3540-00**	12.15		
AMITRIPTYLINE (Core)				
REPACK				
amitriptyline hydrochloride				
TAB, PO, 10 mg, 15s ea	**33358-0022-15**	11.60		
30s ea	**33358-0022-30**	20.49		
60s ea	**33358-0022-60**	46.08		
25 mg, 20s ea	**33358-0023-20**	20.46		
30s ea	**33358-0023-30**	27.61		
60s ea	**33358-0023-60**	53.97		
100s ea	**33358-0023-00**	92.05		
50 mg, 30s ea	**33358-0024-30**	31.80		
60s ea	**33358-0024-60**	71.74		
100s ea	**33358-0024-00**	105.99		
(DHS, Inc.)				
REPACK				
TAB, PO, 10 mg, 14s ea	**55887-0572-14**	6.30		
50s ea	**55887-0572-50**	20.85		
25 mg, 40s ea	**55887-0570-40**	14.44		
180s ea	**55887-0570-92**	114.00		
(Dispensing Solutions)				
REPACK				
TAB, PO, 10 mg, 60s ea	**55045-1682-09**	28.80		
90s ea	**55045-1682-06**	43.20		
120s ea	**55045-1682-01**	57.60		
25 mg, 90s ea	**55045-1463-06**	63.00		
120s ea	**55045-1463-02**	84.00		
50 mg, 60s ea	**66336-0673-60**	63.60		
120s ea	**55045-1741-00**	126.00		
135s ea	**55045-1741-02**	141.75		
75 mg, 30s ea	**55045-2153-08**	33.00		
100s ea	**55045-2153-01**	110.00		
100 mg, 15s ea	**55045-1592-05**	19.80		
30s ea	**55045-1592-08**	39.60		
90s ea	**55045-1592-09**	118.80		
100s ea	**55045-1592-00**	132.00		
120s ea	**55045-1592-01**	158.40		
(Keltman Pharma., Inc.)				
REPACK				
TAB, PO, 75 mg, 30s ea	**68387-0338-30**	27.89		
100 mg, 30s ea	**68387-0339-30**	41.38		
(Nucare Pharm)				
REPACK				
TAB, PO, 10 mg, 30s ea	**66267-0018-30**	22.48		
60s ea	**66267-0018-60**	44.96		
(Palmetto)				
REPACK				
TAB, PO, 10 mg, 10s ea	**23490-5047-00**	7.49		
14s ea	**23490-5047-04**	11.20		
30s ea	**23490-0065-03**	19.41		
30s ea	**23490-5047-01**	22.48		
60s ea	**23490-5047-02**	44.96		
90s ea	**23490-5047-03**	67.44		
25 mg, 12s ea	**23490-5050-00**	8.40		
30s ea	**23490-5050-01**	21.00		
40s ea	**23490-5050-05**	28.00		
60s ea	**23490-0067-06**	20.25		
60s ea	**23490-5050-06**	42.00		
90s ea	**23490-5050-08**	63.00		
100s ea	**23490-5050-04**	70.00		
180s ea	**23490-5050-09**	126.00		
(Southwood)				
REPACK				
TAB, PO, 75 mg, 30s ea	**58016-0808-30**	26.88		
60s ea	**58016-0808-60**	53.76		
90s ea	**58016-0808-90**	80.64		
100s ea	**58016-0808-00**	89.60		
(Stat Rx)				
REPACK				
TAB, PO, 10 mg, 30s ea	**16590-0011-30**	19.50		
60s ea	**16590-0011-60**	39.00		
25 mg, 30s ea	**16590-0012-30**	25.00		
60s ea	**16590-0012-60**	50.00		
90s ea	**16590-0012-90**	75.00		
50 mg, 30s ea	**16590-0013-30**	30.00		
60s ea	**16590-0013-60**	60.00		

PROD/MFR	NDC	AWP	DP	OBC
90s ea	**16590-0013-90**	80.00		
100 mg, 30s ea	**16590-0437-30**	38.50		
60s ea	**16590-0437-60**	77.00		
90s ea	**16590-0437-90**	110.25		
120s ea	**16590-0437-72**	135.00		
(Vibranta)				
REPACK				
TAB, PO, 75 mg, 30s ea	**57866-3906-01**	67.49		
150 mg, 30s ea	**57866-3907-01**	99.99		
AMITRIPTYLINE HCL (Consolidated Midland)				
amitriptyline hydrochloride				
TAB, PO, 10 mg, 100s ea	**00223-0195-01**	2.25		EE
1000s ea	**00223-0195-02**	17.50		EE
25 mg, 100s ea	**00223-0196-01**	2.75		EE
100s ea	**00223-0196-02**	19.00		EE
50 mg, 100s ea	**00223-0197-01**	3.25		EE
1000s ea	**00223-0197-02**	25.00		EE
75 mg, 100s ea	**00223-0198-01**	3.75		EE
100s ea UD	**00223-0199-01**	7.25		EE
1000s ea	**00223-0198-02**	29.00		EE
100 mg, 100s ea	**00223-0201-01**	6.00		EE
150 mg, 100s ea	**00223-0200-01**	7.75		EE
(Gallipot)				
POW, NA (1X5GM)				
5 gm	**51552-0464-02**	11.55	8.25	
25 gm	**51552-0464-04**	42.00		
(1X100GM)				
100 gm	**51552-0464-05**	100.10	71.50	
(1X500GM)				
500 gm	**51552-0464-06**	406.00	290.00	
(Hawkins)				
POW, NA (U.S.P.)				
5 gm	**63370-0018-15**	36.00		
25 gm	**63370-0018-25**	96.00		
100 gm	**63370-0018-35**	312.00		
(Letco)				
POW, NA (U.S.P.)				
5 gm	**62991-2004-01**	22.50		
25 gm	**62991-2004-02**	57.00		
100 gm	**62991-2004-03**	180.00		
(Major)				
TAB, PO (10X10)				
25 mg, 100s ea UD	**00904-0201-61**	48.67		AB
50 mg, 100s ea UD	**00904-0202-61**	70.56		AB
(Medisca)				
POW, NA (U.S.P.)				
5 gm	**38779-0189-03**	36.00		
25 gm	**38779-0189-04**	99.00		
100 gm	**38779-0189-05**	300.00		
(USP,1X500GM)				
500 gm	**38779-0189-08**	975.00		
(USP,1X1000GM)				
1000 gm	**38779-0189-09**	1770.00		
(Mutual)				
TAB, PO, 10 mg, 100s ea	**53489-0104-01**	18.08		AB
25 mg, 100s ea	**53489-0105-01**	36.11		AB
50 mg, 100s ea	**53489-0106-01**	64.14		AB
100 mg, 100s ea	**53489-0108-01**	111.11		AB
150 mg, 100s ea	**53489-0109-01**	116.16		AB
(Mylan)				
TAB, PO, 10 mg, 100s ea	**00378-2610-01**	18.05		AB
1000s ea	**00378-2610-10**	176.55		AB
25 mg, 100s ea	**00378-2625-01**	36.10		AB
1000s ea	**00378-2625-10**	338.75		AB
50 mg, 100s ea	**00378-2650-01**	64.15		AB
1000s ea	**00378-2650-10**	602.00		AB
75 mg, 30s ea	**00378-2675-93**	26.43		AB
100s ea	**00378-2675-01**	88.10		AB
100 mg, 30s ea	**00378-2685-93**	33.33		AB
100s ea	**00378-2685-01**	111.10		AB
150 mg, 30s ea	**00378-2695-93**	34.85		AB
100s ea	**00378-2695-01**	116.15		AB
(PCCA)				
POW, NA (U.S.P.)				
1 gm	**51927-1603-00**	9.60		
(Qualitest)				
TAB, PO (FILM COATED)				
10 mg, 100s ea	**00603-2212-21**	17.50		AB
1000s ea	**00603-2212-32**	177.45		AB
25 mg, 100s ea	**00603-2213-21**	36.10		AB
1000s ea	**00603-2213-32**	338.75		AB
50 mg, 100s ea	**00603-2214-21**	64.15		AB
1000s ea	**00603-2214-32**	602.00		AB
75 mg, 100s ea	**00603-2215-21**	88.13		AB
100 mg, 100s ea	**00603-2216-21**	111.10		AB
150 mg, 100s ea	**00603-2217-21**	116.16		AB
(Sandoz)				
TAB, PO, 10 mg, 100s ea	**00781-1486-01**	18.08		AB
1000s ea	**00781-1486-10**	177.45		AB
25 mg, 100s ea	**00781-1487-01**	36.11		AB
1000s ea	**00781-1487-10**	338.75		AB
50 mg, 100s ea	**00781-1488-01**	64.14		AB
1000s ea	**00781-1488-10**	602.00		AB
75 mg, 100s ea	**00781-1489-01**	88.13		AB
100 mg, 100s ea	**00781-1490-01**	111.11		AB
150 mg, 100s ea	**00781-1491-01**	116.16		AB
(Spectrum Pharmacy)				
CRY, NA (U.S.P.)				
5 gm	**49452-0460-01**	67.90		
25 gm	**49452-0460-02**	157.50		
100 gm	**49452-0460-03**	448.00		
(UDL)				
TAB, PO (USP)				
10 mg, 30s ea	**51079-0131-63**	32.46		AB
(10X10)				
10 mg, 100s ea UD	**51079-0131-20**	18.03		AB
(ROBOT READY 25X1)				
25 mg, 25s ea UD	**51079-0107-19**	9.14		AB
(10X10)				
25 mg, 100s ea UD	**51079-0107-20**	36.57		AB
50 mg, 100s ea UD	**51079-0133-20**	64.89		AB
75 mg, 100s ea UD	**51079-0147-20**	89.61		AB
100 mg, 100s ea UD	**51079-0563-20**	111.24		AB
(Vita-Rx)				
TAB, PO, 10 mg, 100s ea	**49727-0159-02**	2.86		EE
1000s ea	**49727-0159-05**	17.21		EE
25 mg, 100s ea	**49727-0162-02**	3.08		EE
1000s ea	**49727-0162-05**	19.89		EE
50 mg, 100s ea	**49727-0163-02**	4.51		EE
1000s ea	**49727-0163-05**	32.29		EE
75 mg, 100s ea	**49727-0164-02**	7.66		EE
100 mg, 1000s ea	**49727-0165-02**	9.63		EE
150 mg, 100s ea	**49727-0166-02**	14.93		EE
(4u)				
REPACK				
TAB, PO, 10 mg, 30s ea	**10544-0413-30**	28.68		AB
30s ea	**42549-0613-30**	28.68		AB
25 mg, 30s ea	**42549-0329-30**	25.98		AB
30s ea	**42549-0529-30**	32.46		AB
75 mg, 30s ea	**10544-0405-30**	38.86		AB
30s ea	**42549-0605-30**	38.86		AB
60s ea	**42549-0605-60**	58.18		AB
(A-S Medication)				
REPACK				
TAB, PO, 10 mg, 14s ea	**54569-0172-04**	2.53		EE
30s ea	**54569-0172-00**	5.42		EE
90s ea	**54569-0172-06**	16.27		EE
100s ea	**54569-0172-01**	18.08		EE
25 mg, 15s ea	**54569-0175-02**	5.42		EE
30s ea	**54569-0175-00**	10.83		EE
60s ea	**54569-0175-04**	21.67		EE
90s ea	**54569-0175-08**	32.50		EE
100s ea	**54569-0175-01**	36.11		EE
50 mg, 30s ea	**54569-1519-01**	19.25		AB
60s ea	**54569-1519-02**	38.49		AB
100 mg, 30s ea	**54569-2146-01**	33.33		EE
60s ea	**54569-2146-02**	66.67		EE
(Aidarex)				
REPACK				
TAB, PO, 10 mg, 30s ea	**33261-0459-30**	21.95		AB
60s ea	**33261-0459-60**	43.90		AB
90s ea	**33261-0459-90**	65.85		AB
120s ea	**33261-0459-02**	87.80		AB
25 mg, 14s ea	**33261-0007-14**	11.76		AB
20s ea	**33261-0007-20**	16.84		AB
21s ea	**33261-0007-21**	17.64		AB
28s ea	**33261-0007-28**	23.52		AB
30s ea	**33261-0007-30**	25.20		AB
60s ea	**33261-0007-60**	50.40		AB
90s ea	**33261-0007-90**	75.60		AB
(Altura)				
REPACK				
TAB, PO, 10 mg, 10s ea	**63874-0311-10**	1.85		EE
12s ea	**63874-0311-12**	2.28		EE
15s ea	**63874-0311-15**	2.85		EE
20s ea	**63874-0311-20**	3.80		EE
24s ea	**63874-0311-24**	4.56		EE
30s ea	**63874-0311-30**	5.70		EE
(FILM COATED)				
10 mg, 40s ea	**63874-0311-40**	7.60		AB
50s ea	**63874-0311-50**	9.50		EE
60s ea	**63874-0311-60**	11.40		EE
(FILM COATED)				
10 mg, 90s ea	**63874-0311-90**	18.57		AB
100s ea	**63874-0311-01**	18.59		EE
120s ea	**63874-0311-04**	22.30		EE
(FILM COATED)				
10 mg, 150s ea	**63874-0311-72**	30.95		AB
200s ea	**63874-0311-74**	41.26		AB
300s ea	**63874-0311-77**	61.89		AB
1000s ea	**63874-0311-02**	216.00		AB
25 mg, 14s ea	**63874-0430-14**	9.99		AB
15s ea	**63874-0430-15**	10.70		EE
20s ea	**63874-0430-20**	14.27		EE
25s ea	**63874-0430-25**	17.83		EE
(FILM COATED)				
25 mg, 28s ea	**63874-0430-28**	19.97		AB
30s ea	**63874-0430-30**	21.40		EE
40s ea	**63874-0430-40**	28.53		EE
50s ea	**63874-0430-50**	35.67		EE
60s ea	**63874-0430-60**	42.80		EE
(FILM COATED)				
25 mg, 90s ea	**63874-0430-90**	64.20		AB
100s ea	**63874-0430-01**	71.33		EE
(FILM COATED)				
25 mg, 120s ea	**63874-0430-04**	85.60		AB
1000s ea	**63874-0430-02**	741.00		AB
50 mg, 14s ea	**63874-0359-14**	16.45		EE
15s ea	**63874-0359-15**	17.62		EE
20s ea	**63874-0359-20**	23.49		EE
28s ea	**63874-0359-28**	32.61		EE
30s ea	**63874-0359-30**	35.24		EE
40s ea	**63874-0359-40**	46.99		EE
50s ea	**63874-0359-50**	58.73		EE
60s ea	**63874-0359-60**	70.48		EE
90s ea	**63874-0359-90**	105.72		EE
100s ea	**63874-0359-01**	117.47		EE
120s ea	**63874-0359-04**	140.96		AB
1000s ea	**63874-0359-02**	703.33		EE
75 mg, 30s ea	**63874-0296-30**	22.01		EE
(FILM COATED)				
75 mg, 100s ea	**63874-0296-01**	24.00		EE
(Bryant Ranch)				
REPACK				
TAB, PO, 10 mg, 90s ea	**63629-1370-04**	59.24		AB
(DHS, Inc.)				
REPACK				
TAB, PO, 10 mg, 30s ea	**55887-0572-30**	13.50		AB
60s ea	**55887-0572-60**	25.00		AB
90s ea	**55887-0572-90**	37.00		AB
(FILM COATED)				
25 mg, 30s ea	**55887-0570-30**	20.63		AB
60s ea	**55887-0570-60**	38.00		AB
90s ea	**55887-0570-90**	57.00		AB
50 mg, 30s ea	**55887-0552-30**	29.75		AB
90s ea	**55887-0552-90**	71.00		AB
(FILM COATED)				
75 mg, 60s ea	**55887-0398-60**	42.00		AB
(Dispensing Solutions)				
REPACK				
TAB, PO (FILM COATED)				
10 mg, 14s ea	**55045-1682-05**	6.75		AB
30s ea	**66336-0354-30**	9.82		
(FILM COATED)				
10 mg, 30s ea	**55045-1682-08**	14.40		AB
45s ea	**55045-1682-03**	21.60		AB
50s ea	**55045-1682-04**	24.00		AB
60s ea	**66336-0354-60**	19.65		
100s ea	**55045-1682-00**	48.00		
(FILM COATED)				
10 mg, 135s ea	**55045-1682-02**	64.80		AB
25 mg, 10s ea	**55045-1463-01**	7.00		AB
14s ea	**55045-1463-04**	9.80		
(FILM COATED)				
25 mg, 20s ea	**55045-1463-07**	14.00		AB
30s ea	**66336-0027-30**	12.61		EE
(FILM COATED)				
25 mg, 30s ea	**55045-1463-08**	21.00		AB
45s ea	**55045-1463-03**	31.50		AB
60s ea	**55045-1463-09**	42.00		
60s ea	**66336-0027-60**	25.22		
(FILM COATED)				
25 mg, 90s ea	**66336-0027-90**	37.83		AB
100s ea	**55045-1463-00**	70.00		AB
50 mg, 15s ea	**55045-1741-05**	15.75		
30s ea	**55045-1741-08**	31.50		
30s ea	**66336-0673-30**	31.80		
45s ea	**55045-1741-03**	47.25		AB
60s ea	**55045-1741-09**	63.00		
90s ea	**55045-1741-06**	94.50		
100s ea	**55045-1741-01**	105.00		
135s ea	**55045-1742-02**	141.75		AB
100 mg, 30s ea	**66336-0224-30**	39.25		AB
60s ea	**55045-1592-06**	79.00		AB
(GSMS)				
REPACK				
TAB, PO (UNIT OF USE)				
25 mg, 30s ea	**60429-0016-30**	8.40	2.10	AB
60s ea	**60429-0016-60**	14.00	3.50	AB

PROD/MFR	NDC	AWP	DP	OBC
90s ea	60429-0016-90	19.60	4.90	AB
120s ea	60429-0016-12	25.40	6.25	AB
180s ea	60429-0016-18	37.00	9.25	AB
50 mg, 30s ea	60429-0017-30	9.00	2.25	AB
(HomeMed)				
REPACK				
TAB, PO, 10 mg, 30s ea	51655-0633-24	6.10		
25 mg, 30s ea	51655-0121-24	23.99		
60s ea	51655-0121-25	21.20		
50 mg, 30s ea	51655-0082-24	34.99		
75 mg, 30s ea	51655-0062-24	9.40		
(IPI)				
REPACK				
TAB, PO, 25 mg, 30s ea	18837-0008-30	10.16		AB
60s ea	18837-0008-60	20.33		AB
50 mg, 30s ea	18837-0009-30	18.06		AB
100 mg, 90s ea	18837-0364-90	100.00		AB
(Keltman Pharma., Inc.)				
REPACK				
TAB, PO, 10 mg, 30s ea	68387-0336-30	8.32		AB
90s ea	68387-0336-90	18.84		AB
25 mg, 24s ea	68387-0335-24	17.25		AB
30s ea	68387-0335-30	21.56		AB
60s ea	68387-0335-60	43.12		AB
90s ea	68387-0335-90	64.68		AB
50 mg, 24s ea	68387-0337-24	20.66		AB
(LWP)				
REPACK				
TAB, PO (FILM COATED)				
25 mg, 30s ea	64038-0009-30	18.08		AB
100s ea	64038-0009-01	46.10		AB
50 mg, 30s ea	64038-0010-30	38.46		AB
100s ea	64038-0010-01	69.15		AB
(Nucare Pharm)				
REPACK				
TAB, PO, 10 mg, 90s ea	66267-0018-90	63.54		AB
25 mg, 14s ea	66267-0019-14	9.79		EE
(FILM COATED)				
25 mg, 30s ea	66267-0019-30	25.95		AB
60s ea	66267-0019-60	46.71		AB
90s ea	66267-0019-90	70.05		AB
120s ea	66267-0019-91	89.42		AB
(FILM COATED)				
50 mg, 30s ea	66267-0020-30	34.99		AB
60s ea	66267-0020-60	69.99		AB
90s ea	66267-0020-90	104.98		AB
100 mg, 90s ea	66267-0560-90	131.24		AB
(PD-Rx Pharm)				
REPACK				
TAB, PO (FILM COATED)				
10 mg, 12s ea	55289-0124-12	7.28		AB
30s ea	55289-0124-30	20.84		AB
(REDI-SCRIPT)				
10 mg, 30s ea	58864-0024-30	20.84		AB
25 mg, 12s ea	55289-0730-12	15.60		AB
(REDI-SCRIPT)				
25 mg, 15s ea	58864-0022-15	16.18		
25s ea	55289-0730-25	17.02		AB
30s ea	55289-0730-30	17.24		AB
((REDI-SCRIPT),USP)				
25 mg, 30s ea	58864-0022-30	17.24		AB
60s ea	55289-0730-60	21.16		AB
(FILM COATED)				
25 mg, 90s ea	55289-0730-90	23.76		AB
100s ea	55289-0730-01	26.31		AB
50 mg, 30s ea	55289-0016-30	17.73		AB
30s ea	58864-0023-30	17.72		AB
60s ea	55289-0016-60	22.09		AB
100 mg, 30s ea	58864-0757-30	23.51		AB
(USP,FILM COATED)				
100 mg, 60s ea	43063-0193-60	32.08		AB
(Pharma Pac)				
REPACK				
TAB, PO, 10 mg, 15s ea	52959-0008-15	11.41		EE
20s ea	52959-0008-20	15.18		EE
30s ea	52959-0008-30	22.70		EE
40s ea	52959-0008-40	30.25		EE
60s ea	52959-0008-60	45.34		EE
90s ea	52959-0008-90	67.48		EE
120s ea	52959-0008-02	89.82		EE
25 mg, 5s ea	52959-0348-05	3.58		AB
10s ea	52959-0348-10	7.05		EE
12s ea	52959-0348-12	8.35		EE
14s ea	52959-0348-14	9.75		EE
15s ea	52959-0348-15	10.65		EE
20s ea	52959-0348-20	14.20		EE
30s ea	52959-0348-30	21.30		EE
50s ea	52959-0348-50	35.50		EE
60s ea	52959-0348-60	42.60		EE
90s ea	52959-0348-90	63.90		EE
100s ea	52959-0348-00	71.26		EE
50 mg, 10s ea	52959-0514-10	11.99		EE
21s ea	52959-0514-21	25.01		AB
30s ea	52959-0514-30	35.53		EE
60s ea	52959-0514-60	70.99		EE
90s ea	52959-0514-90	106.15		EE
100s ea	52959-0514-01	117.67		EE
150s ea	52959-0514-00	175.18		EE
75 mg, 30s ea	52959-0284-30	7.08		AB
100s ea	52959-0284-00	23.00		EE
100 mg, 14s ea	52959-0542-14	25.48		EE
15s ea	52959-0542-15	27.15		EE
21s ea	52959-0542-21	29.75		AB
28s ea	52959-0542-28	38.56		EE
30s ea	52959-0542-30	41.29		EE
40s ea	52959-0542-40	55.02		EE
(Phys Total Care)				
REPACK				
TAB, PO, 10 mg, 20s ea	54868-0064-03	6.15		EE
30s ea	54868-0064-07	6.99		EE
50s ea	54868-0064-04	8.64		EE
60s ea	54868-0064-02	9.45		EE
90s ea	54868-0064-06	12.52		AB
100s ea	54868-0064-05	12.75		EE
25 mg, 15s ea	54868-0065-09	5.88		EE
20s ea	54868-0065-04	6.36		EE
30s ea	54868-0065-02	7.26		EE
50s ea	54868-0065-05	9.12		EE
60s ea	54868-0065-03	10.05		EE
100s ea	54868-0065-08	13.74		EE
1000s ea	54868-0065-00	83.19		EE
50 mg, 30s ea	54868-0066-05	6.63		EE
50s ea	54868-0066-03	9.06		EE
60s ea	54868-0066-02	10.26		EE
100s ea	54868-0066-06	15.09		EE
1000s ea	54868-0066-00	95.64		EE
75 mg, 30s ea	54868-2357-02	8.49		EE
60s ea	54868-2357-03	13.98		EE
100s ea	54868-2357-00	21.33		EE
100 mg, 30s ea	54868-2433-02	10.20		EE
100s ea	54868-2433-00	22.02		EE
(USP)				
150 mg, 30s ea	54868-2434-02	19.86		EE
100s ea	54868-2434-00	55.68		EE
(Physician Partner)				
REPACK				
TAB, PO, 10 mg, 90s ea	21695-0446-90	32.55		AB
25 mg, 90s ea	21695-0251-90	65.00		AB
(Quality Care Prod)				
REPACK				
TAB, PO (FILM COATED)				
10 mg, 30s ea	49999-0205-30	11.78		AB
60s ea	49999-0205-60	13.38		AB
25 mg, 15s ea	49999-0063-15	12.59		AB
30s ea	49999-0063-30	25.18		EE
50s ea	49999-0063-50	69.87		AB
60s ea	49999-0063-60	50.36		EE
90s ea	49999-0063-90	75.60		EE
100s ea	49999-0063-00	83.94		EE
50 mg, 30s ea	49999-0228-30	41.92		AB
60s ea	49999-0228-60	83.84		AB
90s ea	49999-0228-90	125.76		EE
100s ea	49999-0228-00	139.73		AB
75 mg, 60s ea	49999-0909-60	67.20		AB
100 mg, 60s ea	49999-0318-60	96.12		AB
100s ea	49999-0318-00	160.20		AB
(Southwood)				
REPACK				
TAB, PO, 10 mg, 10s ea	58016-0813-10	2.06		EE
12s ea	58016-0813-12	2.48		AB
15s ea	58016-0813-15	3.09		AB
20s ea	58016-0813-20	4.13		AB
24s ea	58016-0813-24	4.95		AB
30s ea	58016-0813-30	6.19		AB
50s ea	58016-0813-50	10.32		AB
60s ea	58016-0813-60	12.38		AB
90s ea	58016-0813-90	18.57		AB
100s ea	58016-0813-00	20.63		AB
120s ea	58016-0813-02	24.76		AB
150s ea	58016-0813-03	30.95		AB
180s ea	58016-0813-99	37.13		
200s ea	58016-0813-89	41.26		AB
300s ea	58016-0813-73	61.89		AB
25 mg, 15s ea	58016-0814-15	10.49		EE
20s ea	58016-0814-20	13.99		EE
25s ea	58016-0814-25	17.49		EE
30s ea	58016-0814-30	20.98		EE
40s ea	58016-0814-40	27.98		EE
45s ea	58016-0814-45	31.34		EE
50s ea	58016-0814-50	34.97		EE
60s ea	58016-0814-60	41.97		EE
90s ea	58016-0814-90	62.96		EE
100s ea	58016-0814-00	69.95		EE
120s ea	58016-0814-02	83.94		EE
180s ea	58016-0814-99	125.91		
(FILM COATED)				
25 mg, 200s ea	58016-0814-89	139.30		AB
50 mg, 15s ea	58016-0815-15	17.47		EE
20s ea	58016-0815-20	23.29		EE
21s ea	58016-0815-21	24.45		EE
28s ea	58016-0815-28	32.61		EE
30s ea	58016-0815-30	34.94		EE
60s ea	58016-0815-60	69.87		EE
90s ea	58016-0815-90	104.80		EE
100s ea	58016-0815-00	116.45		EE
180s ea	58016-0815-99	209.61		
100 mg, 14s ea	58016-0858-14	18.69		EE
21s ea	58016-0858-21	28.04		EE
28s ea	58016-0858-28	37.38		EE
30s ea	58016-0858-30	40.05		EE
40s ea	58016-0858-40	53.40		EE
50s ea	58016-0858-50	66.75		EE
60s ea	58016-0858-60	80.10		EE
100s ea	58016-0858-00	133.50		EE
180s ea	58016-0858-99	240.30		AB
150 mg, 30s ea	58016-0710-30	62.00		EE
60s ea	58016-0710-60	124.00		EE
90s ea	58016-0710-90	186.00		EE
100s ea	58016-0710-00	206.67		EE
180s ea	58016-0710-99	372.00		
(St. Mary's MPP)				
REPACK				
TAB, PO (FILM COATED)				
10 mg, 15s ea	60760-0212-15	8.93		AB
30s ea	60760-0212-30	11.83		AB
25 mg, 30s ea	60760-0367-30	17.18		AB
60s ea	60760-0367-60	28.36		AB
(FILM COATED)				
50 mg, 30s ea	60760-0214-30	27.17		AB
(Stat Rx)				
REPACK				
TAB, PO, 10 mg, 56s ea	16590-0011-56	38.04		AB
90s ea	16590-0011-90	59.55		AB
(FILM COATED)				
25 mg, 15s ea	16590-0012-15	13.00		AB
56s ea	16590-0012-56	43.35		AB
120s ea	16590-0012-72	93.67		AB
180s ea	16590-0012-82	140.50		AB
50 mg, 28s ea	16590-0013-28	21.00		AB
75 mg, 30s ea	16590-0541-30	24.00		AB
60s ea	16590-0541-60	35.00		AB
90s ea	16590-0541-90	44.00		AB
120s ea	16590-0541-72	54.00		AB
(FILM COATED)				
150 mg, 30s ea	16590-0565-30	34.80		AB
60s ea	16590-0565-60	61.75		AB
90s ea	16590-0565-90	90.00		AB
120s ea	16590-0565-72	115.00		AB
(Vibranta)				
REPACK				
TAB, PO, 25 mg, 30s ea	57866-3072-01	25.18		AB
60s ea	57866-3072-02	50.36		AB
50 mg, 30s ea	57866-3073-01	34.99		AB
60s ea	57866-3073-02	83.84		AB
90s ea	57866-3073-03	69.25		AB

AMITRIPTYLINE HYDROCHLORIDE

FUL

TAB, PO, 10 mg, 100s ea	6.08
25 mg, 100s ea	6.53
50 mg, 100s ea	7.58
75 mg, 100s ea	14.25
100 mg, 100s ea	15.68
150 mg, 100s ea	24.30

(Consolidated Midland) *See AMITRIPTYLINE HCL*
(Gallipot) *See AMITRIPTYLINE HCL*
(Hawkins) *See AMITRIPTYLINE HCL*
(Letco) *See AMITRIPTYLINE HCL*
(Major) *See AMITRIPTYLINE HCL*
(Medisca) *See AMITRIPTYLINE HCL*
(Mutual) *See AMITRIPTYLINE HCL*
(Mylan) *See AMITRIPTYLINE HCL*
(PCCA) *See AMITRIPTYLINE HCL*
(Qualitest) *See AMITRIPTYLINE HCL*
(Sandoz) *See AMITRIPTYLINE HCL*
(Spectrum Pharmacy) *See AMITRIPTYLINE HCL*
(UDL) *See AMITRIPTYLINE HCL*

PROD/MFR	NDC	AWP	DP	OBC
(UDL)				
TAB, PO (USP,FILM-COATED)				
25 mg, 30s ea	51079-0107-63	65.82		AB
50 mg, 30s ea	51079-0133-63	116.82		AB
(Vita-Rx) *See AMITRIPTYLINE HCL*				
(4u)				
REPACK				
TAB, PO, 25 mg, 30s ea	10544-0329-30	32.46		
(Altura)				
REPACK				
TAB, PO (FILM COATED)				
100 mg, 30s ea	63874-1158-03	40.05		
(B&B Pharm, Inc)				
REPACK				
POW, NA (1X5GM, USP)				
5 gm	63275-9936-02	18.00		
(1X25GM, USP)				
25 gm	63275-9936-04	51.00		
(1X100GM, USP)				
100 gm	63275-9936-05	156.00		
(1X500GM, USP)				
500 gm	63275-9936-08	750.00		
(Bryant Ranch)				
REPACK				
TAB, PO, 10 mg, 15s ea	63629-1370-02	11.32		
30s ea	63629-1370-01	19.99		
25 mg, 20s ea	63629-1369-01	19.96		
30s ea	63629-1369-02	26.94		
50s ea	63629-1369-05	47.65		
60s ea	63629-1369-04	52.65		
100s ea	63629-1369-03	89.80		
50 mg, 30s ea	63629-1368-02	31.02		
60s ea	63629-1368-03	69.99		
100s ea	63629-1368-01	103.40		
(IPI)				
REPACK				
TAB, PO, 10 mg, 30s ea	18837-0006-30	19.00		
90s ea	18837-0006-90	57.76		
25 mg, 90s ea	18837-0008-90	63.68		
50 mg, 60s ea	18837-0009-60	36.12		
150 mg, 30s ea	18837-0007-30	34.85		
(Keltman Pharma., Inc.)				
REPACK				
TAB, PO, 25 mg, 15s ea	68387-0335-15	10.78		
50 mg, 30s ea	68387-0337-30	37.24		
(Palmetto)				
REPACK				
TAB, PO, 50 mg, 30s ea	23490-5051-01	39.60		
60s ea	23490-5051-02	79.20		
90s ea	23490-5051-03	104.97		
75 mg, 30s ea	23490-5052-03	36.00		
(Physician Partner)				
REPACK				
TAB, PO, 10 mg, 30s ea	21695-0446-30	10.85		
25 mg, 30s ea	21695-0251-30	21.67		
60s ea	21695-0251-60	43.33		
50 mg, 30s ea	21695-0252-30	36.12		
60s ea	21695-0252-60	72.24		
100 mg, 30s ea	21695-0253-30	66.67		
60s ea	21695-0253-60	133.34		
(Quality Care Prod)				
REPACK				
TAB, PO, 10 mg, 100s ea	49999-0205-00	40.00		
75 mg, 30s ea	49999-0909-30	33.60		
100s ea	49999-0909-00	25.31		
100 mg, 30s ea	49999-0318-30	48.06		
(St. Mary's MPP)				
REPACK				
TAB, PO (USP)				
75 mg, 30s ea	60760-0221-30	35.08		
(Vibranta)				
REPACK				
TAB, PO, 10 mg, 30s ea	57866-3071-01	11.78		
25 mg, 90s ea	57866-3072-03	75.60		
AMITRIPTYLINE HYDROCHLORIDE/CHLOR-DIAZEPOXIDE				
(Mylan) *See AMITRIPTYLINE/CHLORDIAZEPOXIDE*				
(Par) *See CHLORDIAZEPOXIDE AND AMITRIPTYLINE HYDROCHLORIDE*				
AMITRIPTYLINE HYDROCHLORIDE/PERPHENAZINE				
(Mylan) *See AMITRIPTYLINE/PERPHENAZINE*				
AMITRIPTYLINE/CHLORDIAZEPOXIDE (Mylan)				
amitriptyline hydrochloride/chlordiazepoxide				
TAB, PO, 12.5 mg-5 mg,				
100s ea, C-IV	00378-0211-01	83.95		AB
500s ea, C-IV	00378-0211-05	419.75		AB
25 mg-10 mg,				
100s ea, C-IV	00378-0277-01	118.45		AB
500s ea, C-IV	00378-0277-05	592.25		AB
(Phys Total Care)				
REPACK				
TAB, PO, 12.5 mg-5 mg,				
30s ea, C-IV	54868-2206-00	63.39		EE
100s ea, C-IV	54868-2206-01	152.25		EE
25 mg-10 mg,				
10s ea, C-IV	54868-1534-00	30.30		EE
30s ea, C-IV	54868-1534-01	83.43		EE
(Stat Rx)				
REPACK				
TAB, PO, 25 mg-10 mg,				
30s ea, C-IV	16590-0800-30	47.00		AB
AMITRIPTYLINE/PERPHENAZINE (Mylan)				
amitriptyline hydrochloride/perphenazine				
TAB, PO, 10 mg-2 mg,				
100s ea	00378-0330-01	26.20		AB
500s ea	00378-0330-05	128.10		AB
10 mg-4 mg,				
100s ea	00378-0042-01	29.90		AB
25 mg-2 mg,				
100s ea	00378-0442-01	30.40		AB
500s ea	00378-0442-05	148.60		AB
25 mg-4 mg,				
100s ea	00378-0574-01	32.90		AB
500s ea	00378-0574-05	159.30		AB
50 mg-4 mg,				
100s ea	00378-0073-01	74.25		AB
(Phys Total Care)				
REPACK				
TAB, PO, 50 mg-4 mg,				
100s ea	54868-3927-00	54.48		EE
(Quality Care Prod)				
REPACK				
TAB, PO, 25 mg-2 mg,				
30s ea	49999-0551-30	10.20		AB
AMLEXANOX				
(Discus Dental) *See APHTHASOL*				
AMLODIPINE (Quality Care Prod)				
REPACK				
amlodipine besylate				
TAB, PO, 10 mg, 10s ea	49999-0248-10	28.40		
(Southwood)				
REPACK				
TAB, PO, 5 mg, 30s ea	00490-0126-30	51.89		
60s ea	00490-0126-60	103.79		
90s ea	00490-0126-90	155.68		
100s ea	00490-0126-00	172.98		
(Vibranta)				
REPACK				
TAB, PO, 5 mg, 30s ea	57866-7076-01	60.52		
10 mg, 30s ea	57866-0284-01	66.95		
AMLODIPINE BESYLATE				
FUL				
TAB, PO, 2.5 mg, 90s ea		11.61		
5 mg, 90s ea		11.61		
10 mg, 90s ea		16.04		
(Actavis)				
TAB, PO, 2.5 mg, 90s ea	52152-0507-08	167.36		AB
5 mg, 90s ea	52152-0508-08	167.36		AB
10 mg, 90s ea	52152-0509-08	229.68		AB
(Amneal)				
TAB, PO, 2.5 mg, 90s ea	65162-0006-09	155.00		AB
500s ea	65162-0006-50	947.15		AB
5 mg, 90s ea	65162-0007-09	155.00		AB
500s ea	65162-0007-50	951.17		AB
10 mg, 90s ea	65162-0008-09	213.59		AB
500s ea	65162-0008-50	1305.32		AB
(Apotex Corp.)				
TAB, PO, 2.5 mg, 90s ea	60505-0193-03	155.86		AB
1000s ea	60505-0193-02	1731.78		AB
5 mg, 90s ea	60505-0194-02	155.86		AB
1000s ea	60505-0194-03	1731.78		AB
10 mg, 90s ea	60505-0195-02	213.88		AB
1000s ea	60505-0195-03	2376.47		AB
(Aurobindo Pharma)				
TAB, PO, 2.5 mg, 90s ea	65862-0101-90	155.68		AB
500s ea	65862-0101-05	864.70		AB
1000s ea	65862-0101-99	1731.77		AB
5 mg, 90s ea	65862-0102-90	155.68		AB
500s ea	65862-0102-05	864.70		AB
1000s ea	65862-0102-99	1731.77		AB
10 mg, 90s ea	65862-0103-90	213.65		AB
500s ea	65862-0103-05	1186.65		AB
1000s ea	65862-0103-99	2376.46		AB
(Breckenridge Pharm)				
TAB, PO, 2.5 mg, 90s ea	51991-0666-90	175.36		AB
5 mg, 90s ea	51991-0667-90	175.36		AB
10 mg, 90s ea	51991-0668-90	240.65		AB
(Camber)				
TAB, PO, 2.5 mg, 90s ea	31722-0237-90	156.50		AB
1000s ea	31722-0237-10	1730.00		AB
5 mg, 90s ea	31722-0238-90	156.50		AB
1000s ea	31722-0238-10	1730.00		AB
10 mg, 90s ea	31722-0239-90	214.75		AB
1000s ea	31722-0239-10	2375.00		AB
(Caraco)				
TAB, PO, 2.5 mg, 90s ea	57664-0568-99	155.65		AB
500s ea	57664-0568-13	864.70		AB
5 mg, 90s ea	57664-0569-99	155.65		AB
500s ea	57664-0569-13	864.70		AB
10 mg, 90s ea	57664-0570-99	213.60		AB
500s ea	57664-0570-13	1186.65		AB
1000s ea	57664-0570-18	2373.30		AB
(Dr Reddy's)				
TAB, PO, 2.5 mg, 90s ea	55111-0269-90	155.65		AB
5 mg, 90s ea	55111-0270-90	155.65		AB
500s ea	55111-0270-05	864.70		AB
10 mg, 90s ea	55111-0271-90	213.60		AB
500s ea	55111-0271-05	1186.65		AB
(Glenmark Pharmaceuticals)				
TAB, PO, 2.5 mg, 1000s ea	68462-0210-10	1673.60		AB
5 mg, 1000s ea	68462-0211-10	1673.60		AB
10 mg, 1000s ea	68462-0212-10	2296.80		AB
(Greenstone)				
TAB, PO, 2.5 mg, 90s ea	59762-1520-01	155.69		AB
300s ea	59762-1520-02	518.97		AB
5 mg, 90s ea	59762-1530-01	155.69		AB
100s ea UD	59762-1530-05	172.98		AB
300s ea	59762-1530-02	518.95		AB
1000s ea	59762-1530-03	1729.89		AB
2500s ea	59762-1530-04	4324.72		AB
10 mg, 90s ea	59762-1540-01	213.65		AB
100s ea UD	59762-1540-04	237.38		AB
300s ea	59762-1540-02	712.17		AB
1000s ea	59762-1540-03	2373.89		AB
(Lupin Pharma, Inc.)				
TAB, PO, 2.5 mg, 90s ea	68180-0750-09	155.86		AB
5 mg, 90s ea	68180-0751-09	155.86		AB
1000s ea	68180-0751-03	1731.78		AB
10 mg, 90s ea	68180-0752-09	213.88		AB
1000s ea	68180-0752-03	2376.47		AB
(Major)				
TAB, PO (10X10)				
2.5 mg, 100s ea UD	00904-5991-61	159.29		AB
(10X10,CAPLET)				
5 mg, 100s ea UD	00904-5992-61	164.29		AB
(10X10)				
10 mg, 100s ea UD	00904-5993-61	225.50		AB
(Marlex)				
TAB, PO, 2.5 mg, 90s ea	10135-0524-90	8.40		AB
300s ea	10135-0524-03	32.40		AB
500s ea	10135-0524-05	79.00		AB
1000s ea	10135-0524-10	93.31		AB
5 mg, 90s ea	10135-0525-90	8.40		AB
300s ea	10135-0525-03	30.07		AB
500s ea	10135-0525-05	44.91		AB
1000s ea	10135-0525-10	93.31		AB
10 mg, 90s ea	10135-0526-90	9.91		AB
100s ea	10135-0526-01	13.05		AB
300s ea	10135-0526-03	36.07		AB
500s ea	10135-0526-05	54.43		AB
1000s ea	10135-0526-10	132.19		AB
(Medisca)				
POW, NA (1X25GM)				
25 gm	38779-2335-04	244.80		
(1X100GM)				
100 gm	38779-2335-05	825.00		
(1X500GM)				
500 gm	38779-2335-08	3300.00		
(1X1000GM)				
1000 gm	38779-2335-09	5700.00		
(Mylan)				
TAB, PO, 2.5 mg, 90s ea	00378-5208-77	155.65		AB
500s ea	00378-5208-05	864.70		AB
5 mg, 90s ea	00378-5209-77	155.65		AB
500s ea	00378-5209-05	864.70		AB
10 mg, 90s ea	00378-5210-77	213.60		AB
500s ea	00378-5210-05	1186.65		AB
(PCCA)				
POW, NA (1X1GM)				
1 gm	51927-4216-00	5.25		
(Pfizer) *See NORVASC*				

PROD/MFR	NDC	AWP	DP	OBC
(Roxane)				
TAB, PO, 2.5 mg, 90s ea	00054-0100-22	155.65		AB
5 mg, 90s ea	00054-0101-22	155.65		AB
(10X10)				
5 mg, 100s ea UD	00054-0101-20	172.94		AB
300s ea	00054-0101-28	518.95		AB
10 mg, 90s ea	00054-0102-22	213.60		AB
(10X10)				
10 mg, 100s ea UD	00054-0102-20	237.33		AB
300s ea	00054-0102-28	712.00		AB
(Solco)				
TAB, PO, 2.5 mg, 90s ea	43547-0230-09	155.66		AB
1000s ea	43547-0230-11	1729.57		AB
5 mg, 90s ea	43547-0231-09	155.66		AB
1000s ea	43547-0231-11	1729.57		AB
10 mg, 90s ea	43547-0232-09	213.59		AB
1000s ea	43547-0232-11	2373.22		AB
(Synthon)				
TAB, PO, 2.5 mg, 90s ea	63672-0044-03	155.75		AB
5 mg, 90s ea	63672-0045-03	155.75		AB
10 mg, 90s ea	63672-0046-03	213.72		AB
(Teva)				
TAB, PO, 2.5 mg, 90s ea	00093-0083-98	155.86		AB
5 mg, 90s ea	00093-7167-98	155.86		AB
300s ea	00093-7167-55	519.53		AB
10 mg, 90s ea	00093-7168-98	213.89		AB
(Torrent)				
TAB, PO, 2.5 mg, 300s ea	13668-0022-03	518.82		AB
500s ea	13668-0022-05	864.70		AB
5 mg, 300s ea	13668-0023-03	518.82		AB
500s ea	13668-0023-05	864.70		AB
10 mg, 500s ea	13668-0024-05	1260.00		AB
1000s ea	13668-0024-10	2376.00		AB
(UDL)				
TAB, PO (10X10)				
2.5 mg, 100s ea UD	51079-0450-20	172.94		AB
(ROBOT READY,25X1)				
5 mg, 25s ea UD	51079-0451-19	43.24		AB
(10X10)				
5 mg, 100s ea UD	51079-0451-20	172.94		AB
(10X30 PUNCH CARDS)				
5 mg, 300s ea UD	51079-0451-56	518.82		AB
(ROBOT READY,25X1)				
10 mg, 25s ea UD	51079-0452-19	59.33		AB
(10X10)				
10 mg, 100s ea UD	51079-0452-20	237.33		AB
(10X30 PUNCH CARDS)				
10 mg, 300s ea UD	51079-0452-56	711.99		AB
(Upsher-Smith)				
TAB, PO, 2.5 mg, 90s ea	00832-0042-09	155.65		AB
1000s ea	00832-0042-10	1556.50		AB
5 mg, 90s ea	00832-0043-09	155.65		AB
1000s ea	00832-0043-10	1556.50		AB
10 mg, 90s ea	00832-0044-09	213.60		AB
1000s ea	00832-0044-10	2136.00		AB
(Watson Labs)				
TAB, PO, 2.5 mg, 90s ea	16252-0544-90	6.00		AB
5 mg, 90s ea	16252-0545-90	6.60		AB
500s ea	16252-0545-50	36.60		AB
10 mg, 90s ea	16252-0546-90	8.40		AB
500s ea	16252-0546-50	46.68		AB
(Wockhardt USA)				
TAB, PO, 2.5 mg, 90s ea	64679-0421-01	155.65		AB
(CAPLET)				
5 mg, 90s ea	64679-0422-01	155.65		AB
1000s ea	64679-0422-02	1731.75		AB
10 mg, 90s ea	64679-0423-01	213.60		AB
1000s ea	64679-0423-02	2373.89		AB
(Zydus Pharm.)				
TAB, PO, 2.5 mg, 90s ea	68382-0121-16	155.86		AB
500s ea	68382-0121-05	864.70		AB
5 mg, 90s ea	68382-0122-16	155.86		AB
500s ea	68382-0122-05	864.70		AB
10 mg, 90s ea	68382-0123-16	213.88		AB
500s ea	68382-0123-05	1186.65		AB
(A-S Medication) REPACK				
TAB, PO, 5 mg, 30s ea	54569-5901-00	51.90		AB
90s ea	54569-5901-01	155.69		AB
10 mg, 30s ea	54569-5902-00	71.22		AB
90s ea	54569-5902-01	213.65		AB
(Aidarex) REPACK				
TAB, PO, 5 mg, 30s ea	33261-0437-30	68.70		AB
60s ea	33261-0437-60	137.40		AB
90s ea	33261-0437-90	206.10		AB
120s ea	33261-0437-02	274.80		AB
10 mg, 30s ea	33261-0535-30	84.90		AB
60s ea	33261-0535-60	169.80		AB
90s ea	33261-0535-90	254.70		AB
120s ea	33261-0535-02	339.60		AB
(American Health) REPACK				
TAB, PO (10X10)				
2.5 mg, 100s ea UD	68084-0237-01	39.59		
5 mg, 100s ea UD	68084-0238-01	39.59		
10 mg, 100s ea UD	68084-0239-01	56.91		
(DHS, Inc.) REPACK				
TAB, PO, 5 mg, 30s ea	55887-0136-30	51.89		
90s ea	55887-0136-90	225.00		
10 mg, 30s ea	55887-0135-30	75.51		
90s ea	55887-0135-90	155.00		
(Dispensing Solutions) REPACK				
TAB, PO, 2.5 mg, 90s ea	55045-3795-09	157.50		
5 mg, 30s ea	66336-0809-30	56.45		
90s ea	55045-3794-09	157.50		
10 mg, 30s ea	66336-0894-30	74.76		AB
90s ea	55045-3796-09	216.00		
90s ea	66336-0894-90	224.28		AB
(Nucare Pharm) REPACK				
TAB, PO, 5 mg, 30s ea	68071-0728-30	55.78		AB
90s ea	68071-1348-00	167.34		AB
10 mg, 30s ea	68071-0707-30	58.78		AB
90s ea	68071-1349-00	177.04		AB
(Palmetto) REPACK				
TAB, PO, 5 mg, 30s ea	23490-5057-03	63.00		
90s ea	23490-5057-09	175.00		AB
10 mg, 30s ea	23490-5056-01	75.51		
(PD-Rx Pharm) REPACK				
TAB, PO, 2.5 mg, 30s ea	55289-0448-30	54.90		AB
5 mg, 90s ea	55289-0270-90	64.85		AB
10 mg, 30s ea	55289-0299-30	58.15		AB
90s ea	55289-0299-90	74.45		AB
(Pharma Pac) REPACK				
TAB, PO, 2.5 mg, 90s ea	52959-0910-90	156.83		
5 mg, 90s ea	52959-0911-90	156.59		
10 mg, 90s ea	52959-0209-90	255.59		
(Phys Total Care) REPACK				
TAB, PO, 2.5 mg, 30s ea	54868-5764-00	117.06		
90s ea	54868-5764-01	31.16		AB
5 mg, 30s ea	54868-5761-00	19.11		
60s ea	54868-5761-02	11.51		AB
90s ea	54868-5761-01	48.36		
10 mg, 30s ea	54868-5762-00	18.50		
60s ea	54868-5762-02	17.35		AB
90s ea	54868-5762-01	46.50		
(Physician Partner) REPACK				
TAB, PO, 2.5 mg, 60s ea	21695-0541-60	207.82		
5 mg, 30s ea	21695-0542-30	103.91		
90s ea	21695-0542-90	311.73		AB
10 mg, 30s ea	21695-0543-30	142.59		
90s ea	21695-0543-90	427.77		AB
(Quality Care Prod) REPACK				
TAB, PO, 5 mg, 10s ea	35356-0059-10	20.80		
(Stat Rx) REPACK				
TAB, PO, 5 mg, 30s ea	16590-0295-30	51.89		
10 mg, 60s ea	16590-0460-60	142.41		AB

AMLODIPINE BESYLATE AND BENAZEPRIL HYDROCHLORIDE (Lupin Pharma, Inc.)
amlodipine besylate/benazepril hydrochloride

PROD/MFR	NDC	AWP	DP	OBC
CAP, PO, 2.5 mg-10 mg,				
100s ea	68180-0755-01	265.45		
5 mg-10 mg,				
100s ea	68180-0756-01	270.71		
5 mg-20 mg,				
100s ea	68180-0757-01	285.87		
10 mg-20 mg,				
100s ea	68180-0758-01	332.10		
(Sandoz)				
CAP, PO, 2.5 mg-10 mg,				
100s ea	00781-2271-01	265.45		AB
5 mg-10 mg,				
100s ea	00781-2272-01	270.71		AB
1000s ea	00781-2272-10	2707.10		
5 mg-20 mg,				
100s ea	00781-2273-01	285.87		AB
1000s ea	00781-2273-10	2858.70		
10 mg-20 mg,				
100s ea	00781-2274-01	332.10		AB
1000s ea	00781-2274-10	3321.00		
(Teva)				
CAP, PO (HARD GELATIN CAPSULE)				
2.5 mg-10 mg,				
100s ea	00093-7370-01	265.45		AB
5 mg-10 mg,				
100s ea	00093-7371-01	270.71		AB
5 mg-20 mg,				
100s ea	00093-7372-01	285.87		AB
10 mg-20 mg,				
100s ea	00093-7373-01	332.10		AB
(PD-Rx Pharm) REPACK				
CAP, PO, 2.5 mg-10 mg,				
14s ea	43063-0171-14	160.00		AB
(Phys Total Care) REPACK				
CAP, PO, 5 mg-20 mg,				
90s ea	54868-5782-04	475.83		AB
(HARD GELATIN CAPSULE)				
10 mg-20 mg,				
90s ea	54868-5781-03	561.18		AB

AMLODIPINE BESYLATE/ATORVASTATIN CALCIUM
(Pfizer) *See CADUET*

AMLODIPINE BESYLATE/ BENAZEPRIL HYDROCHLORIDE
(Lupin Pharma, Inc.) *See AMLODIPINE BESYLATE AND BENAZEPRIL HYDROCHLORIDE*

(Novartis Pharm) *See LOTREL*

(Sandoz) *See AMLODIPINE BESYLATE AND BENAZEPRIL HYDROCHLORIDE*

(Teva) *See AMLODIPINE BESYLATE AND BENAZEPRIL HYDROCHLORIDE*

PROD/MFR	NDC	AWP	DP	OBC
(A-S Medication) REPACK				
CAP, PO, 5 mg-10 mg,				
30s ea	54569-5937-00	81.21		
5 mg-20 mg, 30s ea	54569-5938-00	85.76		

AMLODIPINE BESYLATE/HYDROCHLOROTHIAZIDE/VALSARTAN
(Novartis Pharm) *See EXFORGE HCT*

AMLODIPINE BESYLATE/OLMESARTAN MEDOXOMIL
(Daiichi Sankyo) *See AZOR*

AMLODIPINE BESYLATE/TELMISARTAN
(Boehr Ingelheim Phar) *See TWYNSTA*

AMLODIPINE BESYLATE/VALSARTAN
(Novartis Pharm) *See EXFORGE*

AMLODIPINE/BENAZEPRIL (Phys Total Care) REPACK
amlodipine besylate/benazepril hydrochloride

PROD/MFR	NDC	AWP	DP	OBC
CAP, PO, 5 mg-10 mg,				
10s ea	54868-5792-01	79.37		
30s ea	54868-5792-00	202.27		
90s ea	54868-5792-02	491.13		
5 mg-20 mg, 10s ea	54868-5782-03	83.64		
30s ea	54868-5782-00	217.56		
60s ea	54868-5782-01	408.28		
100s ea	54868-5782-02	664.43		
10 mg-20 mg,				
10s ea	54868-5781-02	88.85		
30s ea	54868-5781-00	256.05		
60s ea	54868-5781-01	509.10		

AMMONIA
(Amend) *See AMMONIA 27%*

PROD/MFR	NDC	AWP	DP	OBC
(Baker, J.T.)				
SOL, NA (STRONG, N.F., F.C.C.)				
500 ml	10106-9726-02	33.02		
2500 ml	10106-9726-05	21.93		

(Mallinckrodt Lab) *See AMMONIA 27%*

AMMONIA 27% (Amend)
ammonia

PROD/MFR	NDC	AWP	DP	OBC
SOL, NA (N.F., STRONG)				
500 ml	17317-0216-01	12.60		
35000 ml	17317-0216-06	24.50		
(Mallinckrodt Lab)				
SOL, NA (N.F.)				
500 ml	00406-3248-14	25.52		
2500 ml	00406-3248-44	34.08		

AMMONIATED GLYCYRRHIZIN
(PCCA) *See AMMONIUM GLYCYRRHIZINATE*

(Spectrum Pharmacy) *See MAGNASWEET 135*

PROD/MFR	NDC	AWP	DP	OBC
AMMONIATED MERCURY				
(Amend) *See MERCURY AMMONIATED*				
(Baker, J.T.) *See MERCURY AMMONIATED*				
(Gallipot) *See MERCURY AMMONIATED*				
(Medisca) *See MERCURY*				
(Spectrum Pharmacy) *See MERCURY AMMONIATED*				
AMMONIUM ACETATE (Baker, J.T.)				
CRY, NA (A.C.S., REAGENT)				
500 gm	**10106-0596-01**	76.43		
2000 gm	**10106-0596-05**	177.21		
(PCCA)				
POW, NA, 1 gm	**51927-3368-00**	0.69		
(Spectrum Pharmacy)				
CRY, NA (1X500GM,REAGENT,ACS)				
500 gm	**49452-0473-02**	243.60		
AMMONIUM BICARBONATE (Amend)				
POW, NA (PURIFIED)				
454 gm	**17317-1868-01**	11.20		
2270 gm	**17317-1868-05**	29.40		
(Baker, J.T.)				
POW, NA (REAGENT)				
500 gm	**10106-3003-01**	23.74		
2500 gm	**10106-3003-05**	69.78		
(Gallipot)				
GRA, NA (F.C.C.)				
113.4 gm	**51552-0338-04**	6.93		
454 gm	**51552-0338-06**	27.65		
(PCCA)				
POW, NA (FCC)				
1 gm	**51927-2288-00**	0.15		
(Spectrum Pharmacy)				
POW, NA (F.C.C.)				
500 gm	**49452-0480-01**	73.15		
AMMONIUM BROMIDE (Amend)				
POW, NA (PURIFIED)				
2270 gm	**17317-0025-01**	21.00		
2270 gm	**17317-0025-05**	84.00		
(Mallinckrodt Lab)				
GRA, NA, 500 gm	**00406-0424-03**	40.91		
(PCCA)				
POW, NA (PURIFIED)				
1 gm	**51927-1675-00**	0.36		
(Spectrum Pharmacy)				
GRA, NA (REAGENT)				
500 gm	**49452-0490-02**	208.25		
AMMONIUM CARBONATE (Amend)				
CHI, NA (N.F.)				
125 gm	**17317-0027-04**	7.00		
454 gm	**17317-0027-01**	14.00		
2270 gm	**17317-0027-05**	49.00		
11350 gm	**17317-0027-08**	161.25		
POW, NA, 125 gm	**17317-0207-04**	9.80		
454 gm	**17317-0207-01**	18.20		
2270 gm	**17317-0207-05**	51.80		
11350 gm	**17317-0207-08**	175.00		
(Baker, J.T.)				
CHI, NA (N.F., F.C.C.)				
125 gm	**10106-0647-04**	16.57		
500 gm	**10106-0647-01**	27.45		
POW, NA, 500 gm	**10106-0650-01**	29.50		
(Gallipot)				
CHI, NA (PURIFIED)				
113.4 gm	**51552-0226-04**	11.20		
454 gm	**51552-0226-06**	34.65		
POW, NA (F.C.C.)				
113.4 gm	**51552-0270-04**	8.75		
454 gm	**51552-0270-06**	22.75		
(N.F.)				
454 gm	**51552-0572-06**	22.75		
(Lorann Oil)				
POW, NA (N.F.)				
30 gm	**23535-0600-75**	2.00		
120 gm	**23535-0600-78**	5.00		
480 gm	**23535-0600-71**	9.00		
(Mallinckrodt Lab)				
CHI, NA (N.F.)				
125 gm	**00406-3330-02**	12.10		
(Medisca)				
POW, NA (N.F.)				
500 gm	**38779-0638-08**	58.50		
(PCCA)				
POW, NA (N.F.;CHIPS)				
1 gm	**51927-1522-00**	0.36		
(NF)				
1 gm	**51927-2979-00**	0.13		
(Spectrum Pharmacy)				
POW, NA (F.C.C.)				
500 gm	**49452-0510-01**	115.85		
(N.F.)				
500 gm	**49452-0014-01**	96.25		
(F.C.C.)				
2500 gm	**49452-0510-02**	374.50		
(N.F.)				
2500 gm	**49452-0014-02**	312.90		
AMMONIUM CERIC NITRATE				
(Baker, J.T.) *See CERIC AMMONIUM NITRATE*				
AMMONIUM CHLORIDE (Amend)				
GRA, NA (A.C.S., REAGENT)				
500 gm	**17317-1470-01**	17.50		
(U.S.P.)				
500 gm	**17317-0028-01**	12.60		
2270 gm	**17317-0028-05**	42.00		
(A.C.S., REAGENT)				
2500 gm	**17317-1470-05**	56.00		
10442 gm	**17317-1470-08**	140.00		
(U.S.P.)				
11350 gm	**17317-0028-08**	113.75		
(Baker, J.T.)				
GRA, NA (U.S.P., F.C.C., A.C.S.)				
500 gm	**10106-0666-01**	41.25		
(A.C.S., REAGENT)				
1000 gm	**10106-0660-19**	65.55		
(Gallipot)				
GRA, NA (U.S.P.,N.F.)				
113.4 gm	**51552-0514-04**	8.61		
(U.S.P./N.F.)				
454 gm	**51552-0514-06**	15.05		
(Hospira)				
SOL, IV (VIAL,FLIPTOP)				
5 meq/ml,				
20 ml 25s	**00409-6043-01**	110.40	96.50	
(Mallinckrodt Lab)				
GRA, NA (U.S.P.)				
500 gm	**00406-3364-12**	28.73		
(Medisca)				
POW, NA (U.S.P.)				
500 gm	**38779-0595-08**	31.50		
1000 gm	**38779-0595-09**	55.50		
(PCCA)				
GRA, NA (U.S.P.)				
1 gm	**51927-1189-00**	0.10		
(Spectrum Pharmacy)				
GRA, NA (U.S.P.)				
500 gm	**49452-0520-01**	76.30		
2500 gm	**49452-0520-02**	220.15		
AMMONIUM CITRATE				
(Baker, J.T.) *See AMMONIUM CITRATE DIBASIC*				
AMMONIUM CITRATE DIBASIC (Baker, J.T.)				
ammonium citrate				
CRY, NA (A.C.S., REAGENT)				
500 gm	**10106-0682-01**	88.01		
2500 gm	**10106-0682-05**	344.54		
AMMONIUM DICHROMATE (Amend)				
POW, NA (PURIFIED)				
125 gm	**17317-0217-04**	9.80		
500 gm	**17317-0217-01**	18.20		
2270 gm	**17317-0217-05**	84.00		
11350 gm	**17317-0217-08**	140.00		
(Baker, J.T.)				
CRY, NA (A.C.S., REAGENT)				
125 gm	**10106-0688-04**	46.61		
500 gm	**10106-0688-01**	71.38		
2500 gm	**10106-0688-05**	283.66		
(Mallinckrodt Lab)				
CRY, NA (PURIFIED)				
500 gm	**00406-3284-12**	70.70		
2500 gm	**00406-3284-05**	208.73		
(PCCA)				
POW, NA (PURIFIED)				
1 gm	**51927-1630-00**	0.45		
(Spectrum Pharmacy)				
CRY, NA (1X500GM,PURIFIED)				
500 gm	**49452-0530-02**	167.30		
(1X2500GM,PURIFIED)				
2500 gm	**49452-0530-03**	665.00		
AMMONIUM FERRIC SULFATE				
(Baker, J.T.) *See FERRIC AMMONIUM SULFATE 12-HYDRATE*				
AMMONIUM FLUORIDE (Baker, J.T.)				
CRY, NA (A.C.S., REAGENT)				
125 gm	**10106-0698-04**	76.94		
500 gm	**10106-0698-01**	130.71		
2500 gm	**10106-0698-05**	327.08		
12000 gm	**10106-0698-07**	1429.95		
AMMONIUM GLYCYRRHIZINATE (PCCA)				
ammoniated glycyrrhizin				
POW, NA (PENTAHYDRATE)				
1 gm	**51927-3543-00**	0.66		
AMMONIUM HYDROXIDE				
(Baker, J.T.) *See AMMONIUM HYDROXIDE 28-30%*				
(PCCA)				
LIQ, NA (NF)				
1 ml	**51927-1318-00**	0.16		
AMMONIUM HYDROXIDE 28-30% (Baker, J.T.)				
ammonium hydroxide				
SOL, NA (A.C.S., REAGENT)				
500 ml	**10106-9721-00**	19.36		
500 ml	**10106-9721-01**	15.45		
500 ml	**10106-9721-02**	27.04		
2500 ml	**10106-9721-03**	23.33		
2500 ml	**10106-9721-04**	25.85		
2500 ml	**10106-9721-05**	40.84		
AMMONIUM IODIDE (Baker, J.T.)				
CRY, NA (A.C.S., REAGENT)				
125 gm	**10106-0708-04**	75.19		
500 gm	**10106-0708-01**	227.37		
(Spectrum Pharmacy)				
GRA, NA (1X25GM,REAGENT,ACS)				
25 gm	**49452-0560-01**	119.35		
(1X125GM,REAGENT,ACS)				
125 gm	**49452-0560-02**	235.55		
(1X500GM,REAGENT,ACS)				
500 gm	**49452-0560-03**	644.00		
AMMONIUM LACTATE (Paddock)				
CRE, TP (2X140GM TUBES)				
12%, 140 gm 2s	**00574-2121-28**	38.30		AB
385 gm	**00574-2121-38**	50.10		AB
(Paddock) *See LAC-LOTION*				
(PCCA) *See AMMONIUM LACTATE 70%*				
(Perrigo)				
CRE, TP (FRAGRANCE-FREE)				
12%, 140 gm	**45802-0513-77**	13.95		
(2X140 GM)				
12%, 280 gm	**45802-0493-83**	38.30		AB
(PUMP BOTTLE)				
12%, 385 gm	**45802-0493-26**	50.10		AB
LOT, TP, 12%, 225 gm	**45802-0419-54**	33.05		AB
400 gm	**45802-0419-26**	56.65		AB
(Ranbaxy Labs) *See LAC-HYDRIN*				
(Spectrum Pharmacy) *See AMMONIUM LACTATE 70%*				
(Taro)				
CRE, TP, 12%, 140 gm 2s	**51672-1301-04**	37.90		AB
(PUMP)				
12%, 385 gm	**51672-1301-00**	48.93		AB
LOT, TP, 12%, 225 gm	**51672-1300-05**	35.87		
400 gm	**51672-1300-09**	56.00		
(Phys Total Care)				
REPACK				
CRE, TP (FRAGRANCE-FREE)				
12%, 140 gm	**54868-5107-00**	27.93		
AMMONIUM LACTATE 70% (PCCA)				
ammonium lactate				
SOL, NA (W/V)				
1 ml	**51927-1767-00**	0.17		
(Spectrum Pharmacy)				
SOL, NA (1X500ML)				
500 ml	**49452-0565-01**	108.50		
(1X2500ML)				
2500 ml	**49452-0565-02**	364.00		
AMMONIUM LACTATE/HALOBETASOL PROPIONATE				
(Ranbaxy Labs) *See ULTRAVATE PAC*				
AMMONIUM LAURYL SULFATE (PCCA)				
SOL, NA, 28%, 1 ml	**51927-2437-00**	0.18		
AMMONIUM MOLYBDATE				
(Amend) *See MOLYBDIC ACID 85%*				
(Amend)				
POW, NA (A.C.S., REAGENT)				
500 gm	**17317-1435-01**	49.00		
2500 gm	**17317-1435-05**	189.00		
(Amer Regent)				
SOL, IV (S.D.V.)				
25 mcg/ml,				
10 ml 25s	**00517-6610-25**	157.19		
(Baker, J.T.) *See AMMONIUM MOLYBDATE TETRAHYDRATE*				

PROD/MFR	NDC	AWP	DP	OBC
(Baker, J.T.) *See MOLYBDIC ACID 85%*				
(PCCA)				
POW, NA (ACS; TETRAHYDRATE)				
1 gm	**51927-1984-00**	1.80		
(Spectrum Pharmacy) *See AMMONIUM MOLYBDATE TETRAHYDRATE*				
AMMONIUM MOLYBDATE TETRAHYDRATE (Baker, J.T.)				
ammonium molybdate				
CRY, NA (A.C.S., REAGENT)				
500 gm	**10106-0716-01**	137.30		
2500 gm	**10106-0716-05**	550.28		
(Spectrum Pharmacy)				
CRY, NA (U.S.P.)				
100 gm	**49452-0015-01**	179.20		
500 gm	**49452-0015-02**	693.00		
AMMONIUM MOLYBDENUM SULFIDE				
(PCCA) *See AMMONIUM TETRATHIOMOLYBDATE*				
(Spectrum Pharmacy) *See AMMONIUM TETRATHIOMOLYBDATE*				
AMMONIUM NITRATE (Amend)				
POW, NA (PURIFIED)				
454 gm	**17317-0218-01**	10.50		
2270 gm	**17317-0218-05**	39.20		
11350 gm	**17317-0218-08**	105.00		
(Baker, J.T.)				
POW, NA (A.C.S., REAGENT)				
500 gm	**10106-0729-01**	43.52		
2500 gm	**10106-0729-05**	134.57		
(PCCA)				
POW, NA (ACS 98% MIN.)				
1 gm	**51927-3528-00**	0.59		
AMMONIUM OXALATE				
(Baker, J.T.) *See AMMONIUM OXALATE MONOHYDRATE*				
AMMONIUM OXALATE MONOHYDRATE (Baker, J.T.)				
ammonium oxalate				
CRY, NA (A.C.S., REAGENT)				
125 gm	**10106-0746-04**	64.58		
500 gm	**10106-0746-01**	116.29		
2500 gm	**10106-0746-05**	399.18		
AMMONIUM PEROXYDISULFATE				
(Baker, J.T.) *See AMMONIUM PERSULFATE*				
AMMONIUM PERSULFATE (Baker, J.T.)				
ammonium peroxydisulfate				
CRY, NA (A.C.S., REAGENT)				
500 gm	**10106-0762-01**	48.05		
2500 gm	**10106-0762-05**	177.37		
AMMONIUM PHOSPHATE				
(Amend) *See AMMONIUM PHOSPHATE DIBASIC*				
(Amend) *See AMMONIUM PHOSPHATE MONOBASIC*				
(Baker, J.T.) *See AMMONIUM PHOSPHATE DIBASIC*				
(Baker, J.T.) *See AMMONIUM PHOSPHATE MONOBASIC*				
(Spectrum Pharmacy) *See AMMONIUM PHOSPHATE DIBASIC*				
AMMONIUM PHOSPHATE DIBASIC (Amend)				
ammonium phosphate				
POW, NA (F.C.C.)				
454 gm	**17317-0684-01**	8.10		
2270 gm	**17317-0684-05**	35.00		
11350 gm	**17317-0684-08**	140.00		
(Baker, J.T.)				
CRY, NA (A.C.S., REAGENT)				
500 gm	**10106-0784-01**	67.36		
2500 gm	**10106-0784-05**	251.17		
(Spectrum Pharmacy)				
GRA, NA (N.F.)				
500 gm	**49452-0585-01**	173.95		
2500 gm	**49452-0585-02**	535.50		
12000 gm	**49452-0585-03**	1379.00		
AMMONIUM PHOSPHATE MONOBASIC (Amend)				
ammonium phosphate				
GRA, NA (F.C.C.)				
454 gm	**17317-0810-01**	8.10		
2270 gm	**17317-0810-05**	35.00		
11350 gm	**17317-0810-08**	140.00		
(Baker, J.T.)				
CRY, NA (A.C.S., REAGENT)				
500 gm	**10106-0776-01**	51.09		
2500 gm	**10106-0776-05**	182.26		
AMMONIUM SULFATE (Amend)				
GRA, NA (F.C.C.)				
454 gm	**17317-0219-01**	7.00		
(REAGENT)				
500 gm	**17317-1669-05**	14.00		
(F.C.C.)				
2270 gm	**17317-0219-05**	29.40		
(REAGENT)				
2500 gm	**17317-1669-01**	35.00		
(F.C.C.)				
11350 gm	**17317-0219-08**	140.00		
(REAGENT)				
12000 gm	**17317-1669-08**	100.80		
(Baker, J.T.)				
GRA, NA (F.C.C.)				
2500 gm	**10106-0800-05**	65.56		
(Gallipot)				
GRA, NA (F.C.C.)				
454 gm	**51552-0237-06**	27.30		
2270 gm	**51552-0237-09**	38.50		
(PCCA)				
GRA, NA (FCC,GRANULAR)				
1 gm	**51927-1936-00**	0.09		
(Spectrum Pharmacy)				
GRA, NA (F.C.C.)				
500 gm	**49452-0600-01**	74.20		
2500 gm	**49452-0600-02**	184.45		
12000 gm	**49452-0600-03**	511.00		
AMMONIUM TARTRATE (Baker, J.T.)				
CRY, NA (REAGENT)				
500 gm	**10106-0810-01**	96.00		
2500 gm	**10106-0810-05**	510.73		
AMMONIUM TETRATHIOMOLYBDATE (PCCA)				
ammonium molybdenum sulfide				
POW, NA (1X1GM)				
1 gm	**51927-3291-00**	135.00		
(Spectrum Pharmacy)				
POW, NA (1X1GM)				
1 gm	**49452-0610-01**	228.55		
(1X10GM)				
10 gm	**49452-0610-02**	1001.00		
AMMONIUM THIOCYANATE (Baker, J.T.)				
CRY, NA (A.C.S., REAGENT)				
500 gm	**10106-0818-01**	98.52		
2500 gm	**10106-0818-05**	334.34		
AMMONUL (Ucyclyd)				
sodium benzoate/sodium phenylacetate				
SOL, IV (S.D.V.)				
10%-10%, 50 ml	**62592-0720-50**	2666.80		
AMNESTEEM (Mylan Bertek)				
isotretinoin				
SGL, PO, 10 mg, 30s ea	**00378-6611-93**	244.60		
100s ea	**62794-0611-88**	731.43		
20 mg, 30s ea	**00378-6612-93**	290.05		
100s ea	**62794-0612-88**	867.46		
40 mg, 30s ea	**00378-6614-93**	336.95		
(Phys Total Care)				
REPACK				
SGL, PO, 20 mg, 30s ea	**54868-5041-00**	784.90		
40 mg, 30s ea	**54868-5043-00**	870.40		
AMNIOCENTESIS TRAY (Portex)				
lidocaine hydrochloride				
KIT, IJ, 1%, 10s ea	**00074-4379-20**	391.64	329.80	
AMNISCREEN (Teva)				
device				
DEV, NA, ea	**51285-0786-03**	46.88		
AMOBARBITAL SODIUM				
(Marathon) *See AMYTAL SODIUM*				
AMOCLAN (West-Ward)				
amoxicillin/clavulanate potassium				
PDR, PO (FRUITY)				
200 mg/5 ml-28.5 mg/5 ml,				
50 ml	**00143-9981-50**	19.85		
75 ml	**00143-9981-75**	26.45		
100 ml	**00143-9981-01**	38.85		
400 mg/5 ml-57 mg/5 ml,				
50 ml	**00143-9982-50**	37.75		
75 ml	**00143-9982-75**	50.30		
100 ml	**00143-9982-01**	74.05		
AMODIAQUINE HCL (PCCA)				
amodiaquine hydrochloride				
POW, NA (U.S.P.; DIHYDRATE)				
1 gm	**51927-3162-00**	1.35		
AMODIAQUINE HYDROCHLORIDE				
(PCCA) *See AMODIAQUINE HCL*				
AMOX/CLAV POT (Phys Total Care)				
REPACK				
amoxicillin/clavulanate potassium				
CTB, PO, 400 mg-57 mg,				
20s ea	**54868-0286-00**	100.06		
(Physician Partner)				
REPACK				
TAB, PO, 875 mg-125 mg,				
20s ea	**21695-0215-20**	202.06		
28s ea	**21695-0215-28**	274.40		
AMOXAPINE (Watson Labs)				
TAB, PO, 25 mg, 100s ea	**00591-5713-01**	61.51		AB
(AF,SF)				
50 mg, 100s ea	**00591-5714-01**	99.89		AB
100 mg, 100s ea	**00591-5715-01**	166.95		AB
150 mg, 30s ea	**00591-5716-30**	78.99		AB
AMOXI/CLAVULANATE (Bryant Ranch)				
REPACK				
amoxicillin/clavulanate potassium				
TAB, PO, 500 mg-125 mg,				
20s ea	**63629-2895-01**	105.97		
AMOXICILLIN				
FUL				
CAP, PO, 250 mg, 100s ea		6.53		
500 mg, 100s ea		11.93		
PDR, PO, 125 mg/5 ml,				
150 ml		3.02		
250 mg/5 ml,				
150 ml		4.49		
(Aurobindo Pharma)				
CAP, PO (USP,HARD GELATIN)				
250 mg, 100s ea	**65862-0016-01**	25.00		AB
500s ea	**65862-0016-05**	118.00		AB
500 mg, 100s ea	**65862-0017-01**	44.00		AB
500s ea	**65862-0017-05**	190.50		AB
PDR, PO (1X50ML,BUBBLE-GUM)				
200 mg/5 ml, 50 ml	**65862-0070-50**	4.59		AB
(1X75ML,BUBBLE-GUM)				
200 mg/5 ml, 75 ml	**65862-0070-75**	6.84		AB
(1X100ML,BUBBLE-GUM)				
200 mg/5 ml,				
100 ml	**65862-0070-01**	9.14		AB
(1X50ML,BUBBLE-GUM)				
400 mg/5 ml, 50 ml	**65862-0071-50**	4.85		AB
(1X75ML,BUBBLE-GUM)				
400 mg/5 ml, 75 ml	**65862-0071-75**	7.30		AB
(1X100ML,BUBBLE-GUM)				
400 mg/5 ml,				
100 ml	**65862-0071-01**	9.81		AB
TAB, PO (FILM-COATED)				
500 mg, 100s ea	**65862-0014-01**	49.80		AB
875 mg, 100s ea	**65862-0015-01**	87.00		AB
(Dava Pharma)				
CAP, PO, 250 mg, 100s ea	**67253-0140-10**	24.94		AB
500s ea	**67253-0140-50**	118.92		AB
500 mg, 100s ea	**67253-0141-10**	58.75		AB
500s ea	**67253-0141-50**	196.82		AB
PDR, PO (BUBBLE GUM)				
125 mg/5 ml,				
150 ml	**67253-0142-15**	4.69		AB
(BUBBLEGUM)				
250 mg/5 ml, 80 ml	**67253-0143-08**	5.42		AB
(BUBBLE GUM)				
250 mg/5 ml,				
100 ml	**67253-0143-10**	6.09		AB
150 ml	**67253-0143-15**	7.08		AB
TAB, PO (USP,FILM-COATED)				
875 mg, 100s ea	**67253-0145-10**	87.25		AB
(Greenstone)				
CAP, PO (USP,HARD GELATIN)				
250 mg, 100s ea	**59762-1020-01**	24.89		
500s ea	**59762-1020-03**	118.53		
500 mg, 100s ea	**59762-1021-07**	43.41		
500s ea	**59762-1021-01**	190.31		
PDR, PO (1X50ML, USP,BUBBLE-GUM)				
200 mg/5 ml, 50 ml	**59762-1022-02**	4.59		
(1X75ML, USP,BUBBLE-GUM)				
200 mg/5 ml, 75 ml	**59762-1022-04**	6.84		
(1X100ML, USP,BUBBLE-GUM)				
200 mg/5 ml,				
100 ml	**59762-1022-07**	9.14		
(1X50ML, USP,BUBBLE-GUM)				
400 mg/5 ml, 50 ml	**59762-1023-04**	4.90		
(1X75ML, USP,BUBBLE-GUM)				
400 mg/5 ml, 75 ml	**59762-1023-05**	7.33		
(1X100ML, USP,BUBBLE-GUM)				
400 mg/5 ml,				
100 ml	**59762-1023-06**	9.81		
TAB, PO (USP,FILM-COATED)				
875 mg, 20s ea	**59762-1050-02**	18.25		
100s ea	**59762-1050-05**	87.00		
(Intl Ethical) *See MOXILIN*				
(MiddleBrook) *See MOXATAG*				

PROD/MFR	NDC	AWP	DP	OBC
(Par)				
PDR, PO (BUBBLE GUM)				
400 mg/5 ml, 50 ml	**49884-0073-27**	4.89		
75 ml	**49884-0073-28**	7.30		
100 ml	**49884-0073-47**	9.80		
TAB, PO (FILM-COATED)				
875 mg, 100s ea	**49884-0041-01**	87.25		
(Ranbaxy Pharm)				
CAP, PO, 250 mg, 100s ea	**63304-0654-01**	24.97		AB
500s ea	**63304-0654-05**	118.95		AB
500 mg, 100s ea	**63304-0655-01**	43.41		AB
500s ea	**63304-0655-05**	191.82		AB
CTB, PO (BERRY)				
200 mg, 20s ea	**63304-0760-20**	8.93		AB
(STRAWBERRY)				
250 mg, 100s ea	**63304-0515-01**	45.00		AB
250s ea	**63304-0515-04**	109.86		AB
(BERRY)				
400 mg, 20s ea	**63304-0761-20**	10.91		AB
100s ea	**63304-0761-01**	54.56		AB
PDR, PO (FRUITY)				
200 mg/5 ml, 50 ml	**63304-0969-03**	4.59		AB
75 ml	**63304-0969-01**	6.84		AB
100 ml	**63304-0969-04**	9.14		AB
400 mg/5 ml, 50 ml	**63304-0970-03**	4.90		AB
75 ml	**63304-0970-01**	7.33		AB
100 ml	**63304-0970-04**	9.81		AB
TAB, PO, 500 mg, 20s ea	**63304-0762-20**	11.70		AB
875 mg, 20s ea	**63304-0763-20**	18.25		AB
100s ea	**63304-0763-01**	87.16		AB
500s ea	**63304-0763-05**	419.25		AB
(Sandoz)				
CAP, PO (USP)				
250 mg, 30s ea	**00781-2020-31**	7.47		AB
100s ea	**00781-2020-01**	24.89		AB
(12X30COUNT)				
250 mg, 360s ea	**00781-2020-76**	89.60		AB
500s ea	**00781-2020-05**	118.53		AB
500 mg, 30s ea	**00781-2613-31**	13.02		AB
100s ea	**00781-2613-01**	43.41		AB
360s ea	**00781-2613-76**	156.28		AB
500s ea	**00781-2613-05**	190.31		AB
PDR, PO (RASPBERRY-STRAWBERRY)				
125 mg/5 ml, 80 ml	**00781-6039-58**	3.10		
100 ml	**00781-6039-46**	3.56		
150 ml	**00781-6039-55**	4.11		
(1X50ML,USP,FRUITY)				
200 mg/5 ml, 50 ml	**00781-6156-52**	4.59		AB
(1X75ML,USP,FRUITY)				
200 mg/5 ml, 75 ml	**00781-6156-57**	6.84		AB
(1X100ML,USP,FRUITY)				
200 mg/5 ml,				
100 ml	**00781-6156-46**	9.14		AB
(RASPBERRY-STRAWBERRY)				
250 mg/5 ml, 80 ml	**00781-6041-58**	5.31		
100 ml	**00781-6041-46**	6.09		
150 ml	**00781-6041-55**	7.06		
(1X50ML,USP,FRUITY)				
400 mg/5 ml, 50 ml	**00781-6157-52**	4.90		AB
(1X75ML,USP,FRUITY)				
400 mg/5 ml, 75 ml	**00781-6157-57**	7.33		AB
(1X100ML,USP,FRUITY)				
400 mg/5 ml,				
100 ml	**00781-6157-46**	9.81		AB
TAB, PO (USP,FILM-COATED)				
500 mg, 20s ea	**00781-5060-20**	10.55		AB
100s ea	**00781-5060-01**	49.85		AB
875 mg, 20s ea	**00781-5061-20**	18.30		AB
100s ea	**00781-5061-01**	87.25		AB
(Sandoz) *See TRIMOX*				
(Spectrum Pharmacy) *See AMOXICILLIN TRIHYDRATE*				
(Teva)				
CAP, PO, 250 mg, 100s ea	**00093-3107-01**	25.00		AB
(10X10,USP)				
250 mg, 100s ea UD	**00093-3107-93**	26.29		AB
500s ea	**00093-3107-05**	118.95		AB
500 mg, 50s ea	**00093-3109-53**	23.35		AB
(10X10,USP)				
500 mg, 100s ea UD	**00093-3109-93**	49.09		AB
500s ea	**00093-3109-05**	184.50		AB
CTB, PO (CHERRY)				
125 mg, 100s ea	**00093-2267-01**	22.50		AB
250 mg, 100s ea	**00093-2268-01**	45.00		AB
500s ea	**00093-2268-05**	218.25		AB
PDR, PO, 125 mg/5 ml,				
80 ml	**00093-4150-79**	3.12		AB
100 ml	**00093-4150-73**	3.59		AB
150 ml	**00093-4150-80**	4.71		AB
(FRUIT GUM)				
200 mg/5 ml, 50 ml	**00093-4160-76**	4.59		AB
75 ml	**00093-4160-78**	6.84		AB
100 ml	**00093-4160-73**	9.14		AB
250 mg/5 ml, 80 ml	**00093-4155-79**	5.35		AB
100 ml	**00093-4155-73**	6.13		AB
150 ml	**00093-4155-80**	7.11		AB
(FRUIT GUM)				
400 mg/5 ml, 50 ml	**00093-4161-76**	4.90		AB
75 ml	**00093-4161-78**	7.33		AB
100 ml	**00093-4161-73**	9.81		AB
TAB, PO, 500 mg, 100s ea	**00093-2263-01**	49.81		AB
875 mg, 100s ea	**00093-2264-01**	87.21		AB
(Truxton) *See AMOXICOT*				
(West-Ward)				
CAP, PO (USP)				
250 mg, 500s ea	**00143-9938-05**	118.90		AB
500 mg, 500s ea	**00143-9939-05**	195.50		AB
PDR, PO (1X80ML,FRUITY)				
125 mg/5 ml, 80 ml	**00143-9888-80**	3.10		AB
(1X100ML,FRUITY)				
125 mg/5 ml,				
100 ml	**00143-9888-01**	3.56		AB
(1X150ML,FRUITY)				
125 mg/5 ml,				
150 ml	**00143-9888-15**	4.11		AB
(1X50ML,FRUITY)				
200 mg/5 ml, 50 ml	**00143-9886-50**	4.59		AB
(1X75ML,FRUITY)				
200 mg/5 ml, 75 ml	**00143-9886-75**	6.84		AB
(1X100ML,FRUITY)				
200 mg/5 ml,				
100 ml	**00143-9886-01**	9.14		AB
(1X80ML,FRUITY)				
250 mg/5 ml, 80 ml	**00143-9889-80**	5.31		AB
(1X100ML,FRUITY)				
250 mg/5 ml,				
100 ml	**00143-9889-01**	6.09		AB
(1X150ML,FRUITY)				
250 mg/5 ml,				
150 ml	**00143-9889-15**	7.06		AB
(1X50ML,FRUITY)				
400 mg/5 ml, 50 ml	**00143-9887-50**	4.90		AB
(1X75ML,FRUITY)				
400 mg/5 ml, 75 ml	**00143-9887-75**	7.33		AB
(1X100ML,FRUITY)				
400 mg/5 ml,				
100 ml	**00143-9887-01**	9.81		AB
TAB, PO (FILM COATED)				
875 mg, 20s ea	**00143-9951-20**	18.30		
100s ea	**00143-9951-01**	87.20		
(A-S Medication) REPACK				
CAP, PO, 250 mg, 9s ea	**54569-1746-09**	2.25		EE
15s ea	**54569-1746-05**	3.75		EE
21s ea	**54569-1746-01**	5.24		EE
30s ea	**54569-1746-00**	7.49		EE
(HARD GELATIN)				
500 mg, 4s ea	**54569-3335-05**	1.85		AB
9s ea	**54569-1861-08**	4.16		AB
14s ea	**54569-5727-00**	6.47		AB
15s ea	**54569-1861-05**	6.93		AB
20s ea	**54569-3335-06**	9.24		AB
21s ea	**54569-1861-02**	9.70		AB
30s ea	**54569-1861-00**	13.86		AB
40s ea	**54569-1861-01**	18.48		AB
42s ea	**54569-1861-09**	19.41		AB
56s ea	**54569-3335-04**	25.88		AB
100s ea	**54569-3335-07**	46.21		AB
CTB, PO, 250 mg, 21s ea	**54569-3689-01**	9.45		EE
30s ea	**54569-3689-00**	13.50		EE
40s ea	**54569-3689-05**	18.00		EE
(BERRY)				
400 mg, 20s ea	**54569-5622-00**	10.91		AB
PDR, PO, 125 mg/5 ml,				
100 ml	**54569-2928-00**	3.59		EE
150 ml	**54569-2930-00**	4.71		EE
250 mg/5 ml, 80 ml	**54569-2954-00**	5.35		EE
100 ml	**54569-2929-00**	6.13		EE
150 ml	**54569-2931-00**	7.11		EE
(1X75ML)				
400 mg/5 ml, 75 ml	**54569-6037-00**	7.33		
(FRUITY)				
400 mg/5 ml,				
100 ml	**54569-5553-00**	9.81		AB
TAB, PO, 500 mg, 4s ea	**54569-5182-00**	11.70		EE
875 mg, 20s ea	**54569-5193-00**	17.43		AB
(Aidarex) REPACK				
CAP, PO, 250 mg, 7s ea	**33261-0144-07**	3.50		AB
12s ea	**33261-0144-12**	6.00		AB
14s ea	**33261-0144-14**	7.00		AB
20s ea	**33261-0144-20**	10.00		AB
30s ea	**33261-0144-30**	15.00		AB
40s ea	**33261-0144-40**	20.00		AB
60s ea	**33261-0144-60**	30.00		AB
90s ea	**33261-0144-90**	45.00		AB
500 mg, 10s ea	**33261-0137-10**	8.46		
12s ea	**33261-0137-12**	10.15		
14s ea	**33261-0137-14**	11.90		
20s ea	**33261-0137-20**	17.00		
21s ea	**33261-0137-21**	17.85		
28s ea	**33261-0137-28**	23.80		
30s ea	**33261-0137-30**	25.50		
40s ea	**33261-0137-40**	34.00		
60s ea	**33261-0137-60**	51.00		
84s ea	**33261-0137-84**	71.40		
(Altura) REPACK				
CAP, PO, 250 mg, 5s ea	**63874-0101-05**	2.90		EE
9s ea	**63874-0101-09**	1.98		EE
15s ea	**63874-0101-15**	3.31		EE
18s ea	**63874-0101-18**	6.28		EE
20s ea	**63874-0101-20**	7.97		EE
21s ea	**63874-0101-21**	8.40		EE
24s ea	**63874-0101-24**	9.60		EE
28s ea	**63874-0101-28**	11.15		EE
30s ea	**63874-0101-30**	17.42		EE
40s ea	**63874-0101-40**	23.23		EE
45s ea	**63874-0101-45**	26.13		EE
50s ea	**63874-0101-50**	29.03		EE
100s ea	**63874-0101-01**	58.06		EE
500s ea	**63874-0101-03**	118.92		EE
500 mg, 9s ea	**63874-0102-09**	5.54		EE
12s ea	**63874-0102-12**	7.39		EE
14s ea	**63874-0102-14**	8.63		EE
15s ea	**63874-0102-15**	9.24		EE
18s ea	**63874-0102-18**	11.07		EE
20s ea	**63874-0102-20**	12.32		EE
21s ea	**63874-0102-21**	14.31		EE
24s ea	**63874-0102-24**	14.79		EE
28s ea	**63874-0102-28**	18.02		EE
30s ea	**63874-0102-30**	19.45		EE
40s ea	**63874-0102-40**	25.95		EE
45s ea	**63874-0102-45**	27.55		EE
100s ea	**63874-0102-01**	61.62		EE
CTB, PO, 125 mg, 20s ea	**63874-0239-20**	10.91		EE
30s ea	**63874-0239-30**	13.34		EE
PDR, PO, 125 mg/5 ml,				
80 ml	**63874-0143-80**	6.06		EE
100 ml	**63874-0143-10**	7.41		EE
150 ml	**63874-0143-15**	8.34		EE
250 mg/5 ml, 100 ml	**63874-0144-10**	6.83		EE
150 ml	**63874-0144-15**	9.15		EE
(American Health) REPACK				
CAP, PO (10X10)				
250 mg, 100s ea UD	**62584-0237-01**	26.29		AB
500 mg, 100s ea UD	**62584-0238-01**	49.09		AB
(Bryant Ranch) REPACK				
CAP, PO, 250 mg, 21s ea	**63629-1257-02**	6.99		
30s ea	**63629-1257-01**	9.99		
45s ea	**63629-1257-03**	14.99		
500 mg, 4s ea	**63629-1236-08**	9.99		AB
15s ea	**63629-1236-02**	15.86		AB
16s ea	**63629-1236-03**	15.86		AB
20s ea	**63629-1236-04**	16.68		AB
21s ea	**63629-1236-06**	16.68		AB
24s ea	**63629-1236-00**	17.58		AB
30s ea	**63629-1236-05**	29.73		AB
40s ea	**63629-1236-07**	44.59		AB
45s ea	**63629-1236-01**	44.59		AB
60s ea	**63629-1236-09**	54.32		AB
CTB, PO, 250 mg, 20s ea	**63629-1759-02**	12.30		
30s ea	**63629-1759-01**	18.46		
45s ea	**63629-1759-03**	27.68		
64s ea	**63629-1759-04**	39.37		
84s ea	**63629-1759-05**	51.68		
TAB, PO, 875 mg, 20s ea	**63629-2871-01**	23.48		
(Core) REPACK				
CAP, PO, 250 mg, 10s ea	**33358-0025-10**	6.08		
20s ea	**33358-0025-20**	7.64		
30s ea	**33358-0025-30**	10.24		
500 mg, 10s ea	**33358-0028-10**	8.77		
16s ea	**33358-0028-16**	16.22		
20s ea	**33358-0028-20**	18.99		
21s ea	**33358-0028-21**	22.11		
30s ea	**33358-0028-30**	29.24		
40s ea	**33358-0028-40**	40.02		
45s ea	**33358-0028-45**	45.92		
60s ea	**33358-0028-60**	60.72		
100s ea	**33358-0028-00**	71.76		
CTB, PO, 250 mg, 30s ea	**33358-0026-30**	18.92		
45s ea	**33358-0026-45**	28.37		

PROD/MFR	NDC	AWP	DP	OBC
64s ea	33358-0026-64	40.35		
84s ea	33358-0026-84	52.97		
TAB, PO, 875 mg, 20s ea	33358-0029-20	24.07		
(DHS, Inc.)				
REPACK				
CAP, PO, 250 mg, 20s ea	55887-0993-20	7.24		AB
21s ea	55887-0993-21	7.60		AB
30s ea	55887-0993-30	10.85		AB
40s ea	55887-0993-40	14.00		AB
500 mg, 8s ea	55887-0982-08	4.89		AB
10s ea	55887-0982-10	6.15		AB
12s ea	55887-0982-12	7.35		AB
14s ea	55887-0982-14	8.55		AB
15s ea	55887-0982-15	9.15		AB
20s ea	55887-0982-20	12.22		AB
21s ea	55887-0982-21	12.81		AB
28s ea	55887-0982-28	17.08		AB
30s ea	55887-0982-30	18.30		AB
36s ea	55887-0982-36	21.95		AB
40s ea	55887-0982-40	24.40		AB
42s ea	55887-0982-42	26.66		AB
45s ea	55887-0982-45	28.50		AB
50s ea	55887-0982-50	31.00		AB
60s ea	55887-0982-60	36.60		AB
500s ea	55887-0982-05	199.00		AB
CTB, PO (STRAWBERRY)				
250 mg, 21s ea	55887-0622-21	13.00		AB
30s ea	55887-0622-30	19.00		AB
100s ea	55887-0622-01	61.90		
PDR, PO, 125 mg/5 ml,				
150 ml	55887-0814-14	9.25		AB
250 mg/5 ml, 100 ml	55887-0823-01	7.91		
(BUBBLEGUM)				
250 mg/5 ml,				
150 ml	55887-0823-14	9.09		AB
400 mg/5 ml, 100 ml	55887-0867-01	13.60		
TAB, PO, 875 mg, 14s ea	55887-0659-14	37.05		AB
20s ea	55887-0659-20	50.96		AB
(Dispensing Solutions)				
REPACK				
CAP, PO, 250 mg, 4s ea	55045-1122-04	1.76		
9s ea	55045-1122-03	3.96		AB
15s ea	55045-1122-05	6.60		AB
20s ea	55045-1122-07	8.80		
21s ea	55045-1122-00	9.24		AB
21s ea	66336-0655-21	8.37		EE
30s ea	55045-1122-08	13.20		AB
30s ea	55045-3918-01	13.20		AB
30s ea	66336-0655-30	9.59		EE
40s ea	66336-0655-40	12.79		AB
42s ea	55045-1122-09	18.48		
56s ea	55045-1122-02	24.64		
60s ea	55045-3260-06	26.40		AB
90s ea	55045-3260-09	39.60		AB
100s ea	55045-1122-01	44.00		AB
120s ea	55045-3260-01	52.80		
500 mg, 4s ea	55045-1226-01	2.80		AB
8s ea	66336-0634-08	4.77		AB
9s ea	55045-1226-02	6.30		AB
14s ea	55045-3194-04	9.80		AB
15s ea	55045-1226-05	10.50		AB
15s ea	66336-0634-15	8.76		AB
21s ea	55045-1226-09	14.70		AB
21s ea	66336-0634-21	12.26		AB
25s ea	55045-3194-03	17.50		
30s ea	55045-1226-08	21.00		AB
30s ea	55045-3919-01	21.00		AB
30s ea	66336-0634-30	17.52		EE
40s ea	55045-1226-03	28.00		AB
40s ea	66336-0634-40	23.36		AB
45s ea	55045-1226-04	31.50		
50s ea	55045-1226-06	35.00		
60s ea	55045-3194-06	42.00		AB
60s ea	55045-3921-01	42.00		AB
60s ea	66336-0634-60	42.00		AB
90s ea	55045-3194-09	63.00		AB
100s ea	55045-1226-00	70.00		AB
120s ea	55045-3194-01	84.00		
CTB, PO (CHERRY)				
125 mg, 30s ea	55045-2672-08	14.10		AB
60s ea	55045-2672-09	28.20		AB
90s ea	55045-2672-06	42.30		AB
100s ea	55045-2672-01	47.00		AB
120s ea	55045-2672-02	56.40		AB
(STRAWBERRY)				
250 mg, 15s ea	55045-2004-05	7.35		AB
30s ea	66336-0113-30	22.76		AB
(STRAWBERRY)				
250 mg, 30s ea	55045-2004-08	14.70		AB
30s ea	55045-3920-01	14.70		AB
40s ea	55045-2004-04	19.60		AB
60s ea	55045-2004-06	29.40		

PROD/MFR	NDC	AWP	DP	OBC
(STRAWBERRY)				
250 mg, 100s ea	55045-2004-00	49.00		AB
(BERRY)				
400 mg, 20s ea	55045-2993-02	15.00		AB
20s ea	66336-0648-20	18.50		AB
40s ea	66336-0648-40	36.97		AB
PDR, PO, 125 mg/5 ml,				
150 ml	55045-1199-03	12.46		AB
(BUBBLEGUM)				
250 mg/5 ml, 80 ml	55045-1200-00	7.95		AB
100 ml	55045-1189-01	8.05		AB
(FRUITY)				
250 mg/5 ml,				
150 ml	55045-1200-03	12.46		AB
(RASPBERRY-STRAWBERRY)				
250 mg/5 ml,				
150 ml	55045-3934-01	8.75		
400 mg/5 ml, 100 ml	55045-2992-02	10.25		
TAB, PO, 500 mg, 30s ea	66336-0293-30	20.48		
875 mg, 20s ea	55045-3016-07	20.00		
20s ea	66336-0074-20	21.52		
(GSMS)				
REPACK				
CAP, PO (UNIT OF USE)				
250 mg, 30s ea	60429-0021-30	23.00	5.75	AB
500 mg, 30s ea	60429-0022-30	31.60	7.90	AB
(HomeMed)				
REPACK				
CAP, PO, 250 mg, 6s ea	51655-0075-87	11.20		
21s ea	51655-0075-28	15.89		
30s ea	51655-0075-24	18.99		
40s ea	51655-0075-51	9.24		
500 mg, 30s ea	51655-0157-24	24.99		
40s ea	51655-0157-51	29.49		
42s ea	51655-0157-49	30.96		
CTB, PO, 250 mg, 30s ea	51655-0917-24	25.99		
(IPI)				
REPACK				
CAP, PO, 500 mg, 30s ea	18837-0268-30	18.99		
(IPI)				
amoxicillin/clavulanate potassium				
TAB, PO, 875 mg-125 mg,				
20s ea	18837-0216-20	122.50		
30s ea	18837-0216-30	183.75		
AMOXICILLIN (Keltman Pharma., Inc.)				
REPACK				
CAP, PO, 500 mg, 30s ea	68387-0430-30	19.68		
40s ea	68387-0430-40	26.24		
(Nucare Pharm)				
REPACK				
CAP, PO, 250 mg, 21s ea	66267-0021-21	7.89		EE
30s ea	66267-0021-30	10.89		EE
500 mg, 4s ea	66267-0023-04	4.35		AB
8s ea	66267-0023-08	7.97		AB
9s ea	66267-0023-09	8.97		AB
15s ea	66267-0023-15	14.94		AB
20s ea	66267-0023-20	16.60		AB
21s ea	66267-0023-21	17.43		AB
30s ea	66267-0023-30	24.89		AB
40s ea	66267-0023-40	33.20		AB
60s ea	66267-0023-60	49.78		AB
CTB, PO, 250 mg, 30s ea	66267-0022-30	22.69		EE
PDR, PO, 250 mg/5 ml,				
100 ml	66267-0994-00	7.89		EE
150 ml	66267-0993-15	9.89		EE
TAB, PO, 875 mg, 20s ea	66267-1309-02	24.79		AB
(Palmetto)				
REPACK				
CAP, PO, 250 mg, 6s ea	23490-5066-01	5.29		
21s ea	23490-5066-02	13.23		
30s ea	23490-5066-03	18.90		
500 mg, 6s ea	23490-5070-01	7.53		
8s ea	23490-5070-02	6.97		
15s ea	23490-5070-03	10.01		
20s ea	23490-5070-07	13.34		
21s ea	23490-0076-02	58.35		
21s ea	23490-5070-04	14.01		
30s ea	23490-0076-03	83.36		
30s ea	23490-5070-05	20.01		
40s ea	23490-5070-06	26.68		
CTB, PO, 250 mg, 30s ea	23490-5067-01	28.00		
400 mg, 30s ea	23490-5071-03	52.50		
PDR, PO, 125 mg/5 ml,				
150 ml	23490-5065-01	9.25		
200 mg/5 ml, 100 ml	23490-7311-01	10.10		
250 mg/5 ml, 100 ml	23490-5068-01	8.99		
150 ml	23490-5068-02	11.99		
400 mg/5 ml, 100 ml	23490-7312-01	16.99		
TAB, PO, 500 mg, 30s ea	23490-7220-03	19.99		
875 mg, 20s ea	23490-7950-02	34.48		
30s ea	23490-7950-00	51.72		

PROD/MFR	NDC	AWP	DP	OBC
(PD-Rx Pharm)				
REPACK				
CAP, PO, 250 mg, 4s ea	43063-0015-04	11.97		AB
6s ea	43063-0015-06	12.93		AB
6s ea	55289-0019-06	19.59		AB
15s ea	43063-0015-15	14.31		AB
15s ea	55289-0019-15	21.96		AB
21s ea	43063-0015-21	15.21		AB
21s ea	55289-0019-21	23.55		AB
24s ea	43063-0015-24	15.66		AB
24s ea	55289-0019-24	24.33		AB
30s ea	43063-0015-30	16.59		AB
30s ea	55289-0019-30	25.92		AB
(REDI-SCRIPT)				
250 mg, 30s ea	58864-0028-30	15.99		AB
40s ea	43063-0015-40	18.12		AB
40s ea	55289-0019-40	28.56		AB
60s ea	43063-0015-60	21.18		AB
60s ea	55289-0019-60	33.84		AB
500 mg, 4s ea	55289-0020-04	16.47		AB
6s ea	43063-0017-06	13.50		AB
6s ea	55289-0020-06	20.04		AB
9s ea	43063-0017-09	14.25		AB
9s ea	55289-0020-09	21.60		AB
14s ea	43063-0017-14	15.51		AB
14s ea	55289-0020-14	23.58		AB
15s ea	43063-0017-15	15.78		AB
15s ea	55289-0020-15	24.00		AB
21s ea	43063-0017-21	17.28		AB
21s ea	55289-0020-21	26.37		EE
24s ea	43063-0017-24	18.03		AB
24s ea	55289-0020-24	27.57		AB
28s ea	43063-0017-28	19.02		AB
28s ea	55289-0020-28	29.16		AB
30s ea	43063-0017-30	19.53		AB
30s ea	55289-0020-30	29.97		AB
(REDI-SCRIPT)				
500 mg, 30s ea	58864-0029-30	20.01		AB
40s ea	43063-0017-40	22.05		AB
40s ea	55289-0020-40	33.96		EE
(REDI-SCRIPT)				
500 mg, 40s ea	58864-0029-40	23.34		AB
42s ea	43063-0017-42	22.56		AB
42s ea	55289-0020-42	34.77		AB
50s ea	43063-0017-50	24.57		AB
50s ea	55289-0020-50	37.95		AB
56s ea	43063-0017-56	26.07		AB
56s ea	55289-0020-56	40.35		AB
60s ea	43063-0017-60	27.06		AB
60s ea	55289-0020-60	41.94		AB
63s ea	43063-0017-63	27.81		AB
63s ea	55289-0020-63	43.14		AB
CTB, PO (STRAWBERRY)				
250 mg, 6s ea	55289-0182-06	19.35		AB
9s ea	55289-0182-09	21.51		AB
14s ea	55289-0182-14	25.14		AB
(REDI-SCRIPT,STRAWBERRY)				
250 mg, 30s ea	58864-0675-30	27.99		AB
(STRAWBERRY)				
250 mg, 30s ea	55289-0182-30	36.75		AB
(REDI-SCRIPT,STRAWBERRY)				
250 mg, 40s ea	58864-0675-40	56.25		AB
(USP,STRAWBERRY)				
250 mg, 40s ea	55289-0182-40	43.98		AB
(BERRY)				
400 mg, 20s ea	55289-0727-20	37.37		AB
(USP,BERRY)				
400 mg, 30s ea	55289-0727-30	45.18		AB
TAB, PO, 875 mg, 20s ea	55289-0707-20	56.97		AB
28s ea	55289-0707-28	60.81		AB
(Pharma Pac)				
REPACK				
CAP, PO, 250 mg, 20s ea	52959-0011-20	8.05		EE
21s ea	52959-0011-21	8.37		EE
24s ea	52959-0011-24	9.36		EE
30s ea	52959-0011-30	11.55		EE
40s ea	52959-0011-40	15.20		EE
60s ea	52959-0011-60	22.79		EE
500 mg, 4s ea	52959-0020-04	6.01		EE
5s ea	52959-0020-05	7.01		EE
6s ea	52959-0020-06	7.85		EE
18s ea	52959-0020-18	17.88		EE
20s ea	52959-0020-20	17.85		EE
21s ea	52959-0020-21	18.64		EE
24s ea	52959-0020-24	20.70		EE
28s ea	52959-0020-28	23.62		EE
30s ea	52959-0020-30	24.80		EE
40s ea	52959-0020-40	29.07		EE
42s ea	52959-0020-42	29.54		EE
60s ea	52959-0020-60	37.55		EE
100s ea	52959-0020-00	62.54		EE
CTB, PO, 250 mg, 19s ea	52959-0246-19	16.53		EE
21s ea	52959-0246-21	17.01		EE

PROD/MFR	NDC	AWP	DP	OBC
30s ea	52959-0246-30	22.77		EE
PDR, PO, 125 mg/5 ml,				
80 ml	52959-0181-80	6.12		AB
100 ml	52959-0181-00	5.36		AB
150 ml	52959-0181-01	8.01		AB
200 mg/5 ml, 100 ml	52959-0843-01	9.80		
250 mg/5 ml, 100 ml	52959-0613-02	8.99		AB
150 ml	52959-0613-03	9.15		AB
400 mg/5 ml, 100 ml	52959-0296-05	9.95		
TAB, PO, 875 mg, 20s ea	52959-0661-20	29.39		AB
30s ea	52959-0661-30	36.37		AB
(Phys Total Care) REPACK				
CAP, PO, 250 mg, 15s ea	54868-3107-09	5.85		EE
20s ea	54868-3107-07	6.78		EE
21s ea	54868-3107-06	6.96		EE
30s ea	54868-3107-01	8.67		EE
40s ea	54868-3107-03	10.56		EE
500s ea	54868-3107-02	79.74		EE
500 mg, 9s ea	54868-3109-06	10.86		EE
15s ea	54868-3109-08	14.10		EE
20s ea	54868-3109-07	16.80		EE
21s ea	54868-3109-03	17.34		EE
30s ea	54868-3109-01	22.20		EE
40s ea	54868-3109-09	27.60		EE
50s ea	54868-3109-04	33.00		EE
100s ea	54868-3109-02	60.00		EE
500s ea	54868-3109-00	210.97		EE
CTB, PO (STRAWBERRY)				
250 mg, 20s ea	54868-3105-02	14.76		AB
30s ea	54868-3105-00	19.86		EE
40s ea	54868-3105-03	24.99		EE
100s ea	54868-3105-01	54.24		EE
(BERRY)				
400 mg, 20s ea	54868-4614-00	30.69		AB
30s ea	54868-4614-01	46.05		AB
40s ea	54868-4614-02	59.88		AB
PDR, PO, 125 mg/5 ml,				
80 ml	54868-4150-00	9.81		AB
100 ml	54868-4150-02	7.96		EE
150 ml	54868-4150-01	9.12		EE
200 mg/5 ml, 100 ml	54868-4468-00	22.20		
250 mg/5 ml, 80 ml	54868-4155-00	17.94		EE
100 ml	54868-4155-02	18.76		EE
150 ml	54868-4155-01	16.20		EE
300 ml	54868-4155-04	22.39		AB
(FRUITY)				
400 mg/5 ml,				
75s ea	54868-5101-02	17.61		AB
50 ml	54868-5101-01	15.24		
(FRUITY)				
400 mg/5 ml,				
100 ml	54868-5101-00	23.76		AB
TAB, PO, 875 mg, 14s ea	54868-4543-01	21.75		AB
20s ea	54868-4543-00	28.26		AB
30s ea	54868-4543-02	43.14		AB
(Physician Partner) REPACK				
CAP, PO, 250 mg, 21s ea	21695-0314-21	19.99		
30s ea	21695-0314-30	24.27		
500 mg, 8s ea	21695-0315-08	16.29		
9s ea	21695-0315-09	18.32		AB
21s ea	21695-0315-21	21.45		
30s ea	21695-0315-30	26.05		
40s ea	21695-0315-40	40.86		AB
42s ea	21695-0315-42	42.90		AB
CTB, PO, 250 mg, 30s ea	21695-0418-30	27.00		
PDR, PO (1X80ML)				
125 mg/5 ml, 80 ml	21695-0384-80	15.18		AB
150 ml	21695-0384-15	19.42		
250 mg/5 ml, 80 ml	21695-0385-80	10.70		
(1X100ML)				
250 mg/5 ml,				
100 ml	21695-0385-00	12.18		AB
150 ml	21695-0385-15	24.22		
400 mg/5 ml, 100 ml	21695-0294-00	29.81		
(Quality Care Prod) REPACK				
CAP, PO, 250 mg, 4s ea	49999-0016-04	5.57		EE
21s ea	49999-0016-21	8.37		EE
30s ea	49999-0016-30	11.96		EE
40s ea	49999-0016-40	15.93		EE
500 mg, 6s ea	49999-0015-06	5.88		EE
8s ea	49999-0015-08	5.67		EE
12s ea	49999-0015-12	8.44		EE
14s ea	49999-0015-14	13.72		EE
15s ea	49999-0015-15	10.56		EE
20s ea	49999-0015-20	14.09		EE
21s ea	49999-0015-21	14.78		EE
28s ea	49999-0015-28	19.71		EE
30s ea	49999-0015-30	21.13		EE
40s ea	49999-0015-40	28.18		EE
42s ea	49999-0015-42	29.82		AB
45s ea	49999-0015-45	31.78		EE
100s ea	49999-0015-00	70.45		AB
CTB, PO, 250 mg, 30s ea	49999-0033-30	17.42		EE
(STRAWBERRY)				
250 mg, 100s ea	49999-0033-00	58.07		AB
(BERRY)				
400 mg, 20s ea	49999-0745-20	44.80		AB
PDR, PO, 125 mg/5 ml,				
80 ml	49999-0191-80	6.42		EE
100 ml	49999-0191-00	6.48		
150 ml	49999-0191-50	9.72		
250 mg/5 ml, 80 ml	49999-0168-80	6.42		AB
100 ml	49999-0168-00	8.20		AB
150 ml	49999-0168-50	10.98		AB
(BUBBLE GUM)				
400 mg/5 ml,				
100 ml	49999-0983-00	29.70		
TAB, PO, 500 mg, 30s ea	49999-0651-30	20.16		AB
875 mg, 20s ea	49999-0766-20	62.71		
28s ea	49999-0766-28	87.79		
(Southwood) REPACK				
CAP, PO, 250 mg, 9s ea	58016-0103-09	1.89		EE
12s ea	58016-0103-12	2.52		EE
15s ea	58016-0103-15	3.15		EE
18s ea	58016-0103-18	5.98		EE
20s ea	58016-0103-20	6.65		EE
21s ea	58016-0103-21	6.98		EE
24s ea	58016-0103-24	7.98		EE
30s ea	58016-0103-30	9.97		EE
40s ea	58016-0103-40	13.27		EE
100s ea	58016-0103-00	33.24		EE
500 mg, 9s ea	58016-0104-09	5.28		EE
12s ea	58016-0104-12	7.04		EE
14s ea	58016-0104-14	8.22		EE
15s ea	58016-0104-15	8.80		EE
18s ea	58016-0104-18	10.56		EE
20s ea	58016-0104-20	11.74		EE
21s ea	58016-0104-21	12.32		EE
24s ea	58016-0104-24	14.09		EE
28s ea	58016-0104-28	16.43		EE
30s ea	58016-0104-30	17.61		EE
40s ea	58016-0104-40	23.48		EE
100s ea	58016-0104-00	58.69		EE
CTB, PO, 250 mg, 60s ea	58016-0105-60	22.41		AB
90s ea	58016-0105-90	33.62		AB
100s ea	58016-0105-00	37.35		AB
PDR, PO (80ML)				
125 mg/5 ml, 80 ml	58016-1004-01	2.71		AB
100 ml	58016-1003-01	3.88		AB
250 mg/5 ml, 80 ml	58016-1007-01	5.35		EE
150 ml	58016-1006-01	7.11		AB
150 ml	58016-1006-05	7.11		EE
TAB, PO, 875 mg, 9s ea	58016-0643-09	7.85		AB
12s ea	58016-0643-12	10.47		AB
15s ea	58016-0643-15	13.09		AB
18s ea	58016-0643-18	15.71		AB
20s ea	58016-0643-20	17.45		AB
21s ea	58016-0643-21	18.32		AB
24s ea	58016-0643-24	20.94		AB
30s ea	58016-0643-30	26.18		AB
40s ea	58016-0643-40	34.90		AB
50s ea	58016-0643-50	43.63		AB
60s ea	58016-0643-60	52.35		AB
90s ea	58016-0643-90	78.53		AB
100s ea	58016-0643-00	87.25		AB
120s ea	58016-0643-02	104.70		AB
180s ea	58016-0643-99	157.05		AB
200s ea	58016-0643-89	174.50		AB
240s ea	58016-0643-04	209.40		AB
(Stat Rx) REPACK				
CAP, PO, 250 mg, 30s ea	16590-0014-30	18.00		
100s ea	16590-0014-71	60.00		AB
500 mg, 4s ea	16590-0016-04	3.37		AB
15s ea	16590-0016-15	12.00		
20s ea	16590-0016-20	12.66		AB
28s ea	16590-0016-28	17.72		AB
30s ea	16590-0016-30	24.00		
40s ea	16590-0016-40	32.00		
CTB, PO (CHERRY)				
125 mg, 30s ea	16590-0647-33	25.95		AB
250 mg, 20s ea	16590-0424-20	26.55		
30s ea	16590-0424-30	24.00		
40s ea	16590-0424-40	32.00		
PDR, PO, 125 mg/5 ml,				
150 ml	16590-0018-33	10.00		
(1X100ML)				
250 mg/5 ml,				
100 ml	16590-0015-32	10.69		AB
150 ml	16590-0015-33	13.00		AB
400 mg/5 ml, 100 ml	16590-0401-32	14.95		
TAB, PO, 875 mg, 15s ea	16590-0017-15	41.00		AB
20s ea	16590-0017-20	54.67		
28s ea	16590-0017-28	76.54		AB
30s ea	16590-0017-30	82.50		
(Vibranta) REPACK				
CAP, PO, 250 mg, 21s ea	57866-7218-02	7.00		EE
30s ea	57866-7218-01	8.51		EE
500 mg, 21s ea	57866-0106-02	11.00		EE
30s ea	57866-0106-01	11.62		EE
AMOXICILLIN AND CLAVULANATE POTASSIUM				
(Apotex Corp.)				
amoxicillin/clavulanate potassium				
TAB, PO (FILM COATED)				
250 mg-125 mg,				
30s ea	60505-2539-03	123.50		AB
500 mg-125 mg,				
20s ea	60505-2540-02	75.69		AB
875 mg-125 mg,				
20s ea	60505-2541-02	101.03		AB
(Ranbaxy Pharm)				
PDR, PO (USP,STRAWBERRY)				
600 mg/5 ml-42.9 mg/5 ml,				
75 ml	63304-0768-01	46.85		AB
125 ml	63304-0768-07	75.01		AB
200 ml	63304-0768-02	117.80		AB
(Sandoz)				
PDR, PO (USP)				
600 mg/5 ml-42.9 mg/5 ml,				
75 ml	00781-6139-57	51.83		AB
125 ml	00781-6139-54	83.03		AB
200 ml	00781-6139-48	130.37		AB
TAB, PO (FILM-COATED)				
250 mg-125 mg,				
30s ea	00781-1874-31	148.08		AB
(Wockhardt USA)				
PDR, PO (1X75ML,USP,ORANGE)				
250 mg/5 ml-62.5 mg/5 ml,				
75 ml	60432-0065-75	64.73		EE
(1X100ML,USP,ORANGE)				
250 mg/5 ml-62.5 mg/5 ml,				
100 ml	60432-0065-00	86.43		EE
(1X150ML,USP,ORANGE)				
250 mg/5 ml-62.5 mg/5 ml,				
150 ml	60432-0065-47	127.00		EE
(DHS, Inc.) REPACK				
PDR, PO (1X75ML,STRAWBERRY)				
600 mg/5 ml-42.9 mg/5 ml,				
75 ml	55887-0032-75	50.00		AB
(Physician Partner) REPACK				
PDR, PO (1X125ML,STRAWBERRY)				
600 mg/5 ml-42.9 mg/5 ml,				
125 ml	21695-0401-12	150.02		AB
AMOXICILLIN TRIHYDRATE (Spectrum Pharmacy)				
amoxicillin				
POW, NA (U.S.P.)				
25 gm	49452-0016-01	294.00		
100 gm	49452-0016-02	927.50		
AMOXICILLIN/CLARITHROMYCIN/LANSOPRAZOLE (Takeda) *See PREVPAC*				
AMOXICILLIN/CLAV (DHS, Inc.) REPACK				
amoxicillin/clavulanate potassium				
PDR, PO, 400 mg/5 ml-57 mg/5 ml,				
100 ml	55887-0714-01	130.00		
TAB, PO, 250 mg-125 mg,				
14s ea	55887-0862-14	167.96		
AMOXICILLIN/CLAV ACID (Southwood) REPACK				
amoxicillin/clavulanate potassium				
CTB, PO, 200 mg-28.5 mg,				
20s ea	58016-4869-01	37.20		
TAB, PO, 875 mg-125 mg,				
20s ea	58016-4990-01	101.03		
AMOXICILLIN/CLAV POT (Physician Partner) REPACK				
amoxicillin/clavulanate potassium				
TAB, PO (FILM-COATED)				
500 mg-125 mg,				
20s ea	21695-0214-20	151.38		
(Southwood) REPACK				
PDR, PO				
200 mg/5 ml-28.5 mg/5 ml,				
100 ml	58016-4842-01	12.83		

PROD/MFR	NDC	AWP	DP	OBC
AMOXICILLIN/CLAV.POT. (Stat Rx)				
REPACK				
amoxicillin/clavulanate potassium				
TAB, PO, 500 mg-125 mg,				
20s ea	**16590-0019-20**	91.00		
AMOXICILLIN/CLAVU/POTASSIUM (Vibranta)				
REPACK				
amoxicillin/clavulanate potassium				
TAB, PO, 875 mg-125 mg,				
20s ea	**57866-3129-01**	169.27		
AMOXICILLIN/CLAVULANATE (Bryant Ranch)				
REPACK				
amoxicillin/clavulanate potassium				
TAB, PO, 875 mg-125 mg,				
10s ea	**63629-1248-03**	53.65		
14s ea	**63629-1248-02**	77.32		
20s ea	**63629-1248-01**	140.28		
AMOXICILLIN/CLAVULANATE ACID (Palmetto)				
REPACK				
amoxicillin/clavulanate potassium				
TAB, PO, 500 mg-125 mg,				
3s ea	**23490-5074-01**	22.95		
20s ea	**23490-0081-00**	84.60		
20s ea	**23490-5074-02**	90.00		
21s ea	**23490-0081-02**	89.05		
30s ea	**23490-0081-03**	126.90		
30s ea	**23490-5074-03**	135.00		
AMOXICILLIN/CLAVULANATE POT (Aidarex)				
REPACK				
amoxicillin/clavulanate potassium				
TAB, PO (FILM-COATED)				
500 mg-125 mg,				
20s ea	**33261-0112-01**	89.27		
875 mg-125 mg,				
20s ea	**33261-0111-01**	175.00		
AMOXICILLIN/CLAVULANATE POTASSIUM				
FUL				
PDR, PO, 400 mg/5 ml-57 mg/5 ml,				
100 ml		53.47		
(Apotex Corp.) *See AMOXICILLIN AND CLAVULANATE POTASSIUM*				
(Glaxo) *See AUGMENTIN*				
(Glaxo) *See AUGMENTIN ES-600*				
(Glaxo) *See AUGMENTIN XR*				
(Par)				
PDR, PO (ORANGE)				
400 mg/5 ml-57 mg/5 ml,				
50 ml	**49884-0168-27**	35.19		
75 ml	**49884-0168-28**	46.85		
100 ml	**49884-0168-47**	68.95		
(STRAWBERRY CREAM)				
600 mg/5 ml-42.9 mg/5 ml,				
75 ml	**49884-0201-28**	38.16		
125 ml	**49884-0201-49**	61.12		
200 ml	**49884-0201-70**	95.98		
TAB, PO (FILM-COATED)				
500 mg-125 mg,				
20s ea	**49884-0298-07**	75.70		
875 mg-125 mg,				
20s ea	**49884-0299-07**	101.05		
100s ea UD	**49884-0299-12**	529.39		
(Ranbaxy Pharm) *See AMOXICILLIN AND CLAVULANATE POTASSIUM*				
(Ranbaxy Pharm)				
CTB, PO, 200 mg-28.5 mg,				
20s ea	**63304-0753-20**	37.20	27.15	**AB**
400 mg-57 mg, 20s ea	**63304-0754-20**	70.88	51.75	**AB**
PDR, PO (STRAWBERRY)				
200 mg/5 ml-28.5 mg/5 ml,				
50 ml	**63304-0977-03**	18.45		**AB**
75 ml	**63304-0977-01**	24.63		**AB**
100 ml	**63304-0977-04**	36.17		**AB**
400 mg/5 ml-57 mg/5 ml,				
50 ml	**63304-0979-03**	35.15		**AB**
75 ml	**63304-0979-01**	46.82		**AB**
100 ml	**63304-0979-04**	68.93		**AB**
TAB, PO (USP)				
500 mg-125 mg,				
20s ea	**63304-0713-20**	75.69		**AB**
875 mg-125 mg,				
20s ea	**63304-0509-20**	101.03		**AB**
100s ea	**63304-0509-01**	501.00		**AB**
(Sandoz) *See AMOXICILLIN AND CLAVULANATE POTASSIUM*				
(Sandoz)				
CTB, PO (BANANA-CHERRY)				
200 mg-28.5 mg,				
20s ea	**00781-1619-66**	36.17		**AB**
400 mg-57 mg, 20s ea	**00781-1643-66**	68.93		**AB**
PDR, PO (CARAMEL-ORANG-RASPBERRY)				
200 mg/5 ml-28.5 mg/5 ml,				
50 ml	**66685-1011-00**	18.45		**AB**
75 ml	**66685-1011-01**	24.63		**AB**
100 ml	**66685-1011-02**	36.17		**AB**
(ORANGE)				
200 mg/5 ml-28.5 mg/5 ml,				
100 ml	**00781-6102-46**	36.17		**AB**
(CARAMEL-ORANG-RASPBERRY)				
400 mg/5 ml-57 mg/5 ml,				
50 ml	**66685-1012-00**	35.15		**AB**
75 ml	**66685-1012-01**	46.82		**AB**
100 ml	**66685-1012-02**	68.93		**AB**
(ORANGE)				
400 mg/5 ml-57 mg/5 ml,				
100 ml	**00781-6104-46**	68.93		**AB**
TAB, PO, 500 mg-125 mg,				
20s ea	**00781-1831-20**	75.69		**AB**
20s ea	**66685-1002-00**	75.69		**AB**
100s ea	**66685-1002-02**	367.10		**AB**
875 mg-125 mg,				
20s ea	**00781-1852-20**	101.03		**AB**
20s ea	**66685-1001-00**	101.03		**AB**
100s ea	**66685-1001-01**	490.00		**AB**
(Teva)				
CTB, PO (BANANA-CHERRY)				
200 mg-28.5 mg,				
20s ea	**00093-2270-34**	36.21		**AB**
400 mg-57 mg, 20s ea	**00093-2272-34**	69.00		**AB**
PDR, PO (ORANGE-RASPBERRY)				
200 mg/5 ml-28.5 mg/5 ml,				
100 ml	**00093-2277-73**	36.17		**AB**
400 mg/5 ml-57 mg/5 ml,				
100 ml	**00093-2279-73**	68.95		**AB**
(ORANGE)				
600 mg/5 ml-42.9 mg/5 ml,				
75 ml	**00093-8675-78**	38.38		**AB**
75 ml	**00172-7407-22**	38.16		
125 ml	**00093-8675-75**	61.46		**AB**
125 ml	**00172-7407-14**	61.12		
200 ml	**00093-8675-74**	96.52		**AB**
200 ml	**00172-7407-26**	95.98		
TAB, PO, 500 mg-125 mg,				
20s ea	**00093-2274-34**	75.69		**AB**
875 mg-125 mg,				
20s ea	**00093-2275-34**	101.03		**AB**
(West-Ward) *See AMOCLAN*				
(Wockhardt USA) *See AMOXICILLIN AND CLAVULANATE POTASSIUM*				
(4u)				
REPACK				
TAB, PO, 500 mg-125 mg,				
20s ea	**42549-0531-20**	95.24		**AB**
875 mg-125 mg,				
20s ea	**42549-0570-20**	158.40		**AB**
(A-S Medication)				
REPACK				
CTB, PO, 400 mg-57 mg,				
20s ea	**54569-5638-00**	69.94		**AB**
PDR, PO (STRAWBERRY)				
200 mg/5 ml-28.5 mg/5 ml,				
100 ml	**54569-5488-00**	36.71		**AB**
400 mg/5 ml-57 mg/5 ml,				
50 ml	**54569-5689-00**	35.81		**AB**
75 ml	**54569-5690-00**	47.70		**AB**
(CARAMEL-ORANG-RASPBERRY)				
400 mg/5 ml-57 mg/5 ml,				
100 ml	**54569-5487-00**	69.79		**AB**
(STRAWBERRY CREAM)				
600 mg/5 ml-42.9 mg/5 ml,				
75 ml	**54569-6043-00**	41.94		
125 ml	**54569-5831-00**	68.35		
TAB, PO, 500 mg-125 mg,				
20s ea	**54569-5470-00**	75.69		**AB**
(USP)				
500 mg-125 mg,				
21s ea	**54569-5470-01**	79.47		**AB**
875 mg-125 mg,				
10s ea	**54569-5471-01**	50.52		**AB**
20s ea	**54569-5471-00**	101.03		**AB**
28s ea	**54569-5471-03**	141.44		**AB**
(Altura)				
REPACK				
TAB, PO, 500 mg-125 mg,				
20s ea	**63874-1226-02**	70.07		**AB**
875 mg-125 mg,				
20s ea	**63874-1112-02**	203.99		
(American Health)				
REPACK				
TAB, PO (10X10,USP)				
500 mg-125 mg,				
100s ea UD	**68084-0235-01**	356.82		**AB**
875 mg-125 mg,				
100s ea UD	**68084-0236-01**	502.38		**AB**
(Core)				
REPACK				
TAB, PO, 500 mg-125 mg,				
20s ea	**33358-0030-20**	108.62		
875 mg-125 mg,				
20s ea	**33358-0031-20**	143.79		
(DHS, Inc.)				
REPACK				
CTB, PO, 400 mg-57 mg,				
20s ea	**55887-0216-20**	70.88		
TAB, PO, 500 mg-125 mg,				
14s ea	**55887-0637-14**	62.50		
20s ea	**55887-0637-20**	88.99		**AB**
30s ea	**55887-0637-30**	133.00		**AB**
875 mg-125 mg,				
20s ea	**55887-0629-20**	102.32		**AB**
(Dispensing Solutions)				
REPACK				
PDR, PO				
200 mg/5 ml-28.5 mg/5 ml,				
50 ml	**55045-3355-01**	21.00		
(STRAWBERRY)				
200 mg/5 ml-28.5 mg/5 ml,				
100 ml	**55045-3355-00**	36.17		**AB**
400 mg/5 ml-57 mg/5 ml,				
50 ml	**55045-2965-01**	38.00		**AB**
100 ml	**55045-2965-00**	75.00		**AB**
TAB, PO, 500 mg-125 mg,				
4s ea	**55045-2953-04**	16.56		**AB**
7s ea	**55045-2953-07**	29.00		**AB**
15s ea	**55045-2953-05**	62.10		**AB**
20s ea	**55045-2953-02**	113.24		**AB**
21s ea	**55045-2953-06**	86.94		
30s ea	**55045-2953-08**	124.20		**AB**
875 mg-125 mg,				
14s ea	**55045-2966-03**	77.00		**AB**
20s ea	**55045-2966-07**	110.00		**AB**
30s ea	**55045-2966-08**	165.00		**AB**
(HomeMed)				
REPACK				
TAB, PO, 875 mg-125 mg,				
2s ea	**51655-0110-31**	11.88		
(Keltman Pharma., Inc.)				
REPACK				
TAB, PO, 500 mg-125 mg,				
15s ea	**68387-0580-15**	94.00		
875 mg-125 mg,				
30s ea	**68387-0585-30**	179.25		**AB**
(Nucare Pharm)				
REPACK				
TAB, PO, 500 mg-125 mg,				
3s ea	**66267-0857-03**	13.35		
4s ea	**66267-0857-04**	17.81		
6s ea	**68071-0063-06**	26.70		**AB**
20s ea	**66267-1001-01**	89.05		
30s ea	**68071-0063-30**	125.13		**AB**
875 mg-125 mg, 3s ea	**66267-0712-03**	17.83		
3s ea	**66267-0859-03**	17.83		
4s ea	**66267-0859-04**	23.77		
10s ea	**66267-0712-10**	59.44		
14s ea	**66267-0712-14**	83.25		**AB**
20s ea	**66267-1002-01**	118.88		
21s ea	**66267-0712-21**	124.82		**AB**
30s ea	**66267-0712-30**	192.47		**AB**
(Palmetto)				
REPACK				
CTB, PO, 200 mg-28.5 mg,				
20s ea	**23490-6977-01**	37.20		
PDR, PO (1X50ML)				
200 mg/5 ml-28.5 mg/5 ml,				
50 ml	**23490-6979-00**	18.31		
100 ml	**23490-6979-01**	36.62		
400 mg/5 ml-57 mg/5 ml,				
50 ml	**23490-7961-03**	41.01		
75 ml	**23490-7961-02**	61.52		
100 ml	**23490-7961-01**	82.03		
600 mg/5 ml-42.9.mg/5 ml,				
75 ml	**23490-7585-03**	40.52		
125 ml	**23490-7585-01**	61.23		
200 ml	**23490-7585-02**	110.62		

PROD/MFR	NDC	AWP	DP	OBC
TAB, PO, 250 mg-125 mg,				
14s ea	23490-5075-01	63.00		
875 mg-125 mg, 4s ea	23490-6940-01	38.40		
14s ea	23490-6940-00	84.00		
20s ea	23490-6940-02	120.00		
30s ea	23490-6940-03	180.00		
(PD-Rx Pharm)				
REPACK				
TAB, PO (USP)				
500 mg-125 mg,				
21s ea	55289-0845-21	95.40		AB
(REDI-SCRIPT,USP)				
500 mg-125 mg,				
30s ea	58864-0777-30	109.78		AB
(USP)				
500 mg-125 mg,				
30s ea	55289-0845-30	109.77		AB
875 mg-125 mg, 3s ea	43063-0077-03	13.24		AB
(USP)				
875 mg-125 mg,				
4s ea	43063-0077-04	15.50		AB
6s ea	43063-0077-06	19.98		AB
14s ea	55289-0767-14	46.66		
20s ea	55289-0767-20	66.66		
(USP)				
875 mg-125 mg,				
20s ea	58864-0767-20	155.00		
21s ea	55289-0767-21	70.00		AB
30s ea	55289-0767-30	109.78		AB
(Pharma Pac)				
REPACK				
TAB, PO, 500 mg-125 mg,				
4s ea	52959-0702-04	22.95		AB
9s ea	52959-0702-09	51.58		AB
12s ea	52959-0702-12	68.70		AB
14s ea	52959-0702-14	80.15		AB
15s ea	52959-0702-15	85.90		AB
20s ea	52959-0702-20	114.52		AB
21s ea	52959-0702-21	120.09		AB
30s ea	52959-0702-30	171.45		AB
40s ea	52959-0702-40	228.70		AB
875 mg-125 mg,				
10s ea	52959-0707-10	57.45		AB
14s ea	52959-0707-14	80.42		AB
15s ea	52959-0707-15	86.17		AB
20s ea	52959-0707-20	114.88		AB
30s ea	52959-0707-30	172.29		
60s ea	52959-0707-60	344.49		
(Phys Total Care)				
REPACK				
PDR, PO (CARAMEL-ORANG-RASPBERRY)				
200 mg/5 ml-28.5 mg/5 ml,				
100 ml	54868-4990-00	72.24		AB
(1X200ML)				
600 mg/5 ml-42.9 mg/5 ml,				
200 ml	54868-5165-01	110.22		
TAB, PO (USP)				
500 mg-125 mg,				
15s ea	54868-4743-02	63.84		
20s ea	54868-4743-00	63.54		AB
30s ea	54868-4743-01	96.06		
875 mg-125 mg,				
10s ea	54868-4951-00	55.65		AB
14s ea	54868-4951-02	79.77		
20s ea	54868-4951-01	82.05		AB
28s ea	54868-4951-04	110.65		AB
30s ea	54868-4951-03	82.48		AB
(Physician Partner)				
REPACK				
PDR, PO (1X100ML,STRAWBERRY)				
400 mg/5 ml-57 mg/5 ml,				
100 ml	21695-0546-00	137.86		AB
(Quality Care Prod)				
REPACK				
PDR, PO (CARAMEL-ORANG-RASPBERRY)				
200 mg/5 ml-28.5 mg/5 ml,				
100 ml	49999-0356-00	64.11		AB
TAB, PO, 500 mg-125 mg,				
20s ea	49999-0246-20	159.60		AB
(USP)				
875 mg-125 mg,				
14s ea	49999-0177-14	52.30		AB
20s ea	49999-0177-20	210.76		AB
(Southwood)				
REPACK				
TAB, PO, 500 mg-125 mg,				
20s ea	58016-1002-01	82.42		AB
875 mg-125 mg,				
20s ea	58016-1000-01	110.01		AB

PROD/MFR	NDC	AWP	DP	OBC
(Stat Rx)				
REPACK				
TAB, PO (USP)				
500 mg-125 mg,				
30s ea	16590-0019-30	136.50		AB
875 mg-125 mg,				
10s ea	16590-0020-10	61.25		AB
14s ea	16590-0020-14	85.75		AB
20s ea	16590-0020-20	122.51		AB
28s ea	16590-0020-28	171.51		AB
30s ea	16590-0020-30	183.76		AB
AMOXICOT (Truxton)				
amoxicillin				
CAP, PO, 250 mg, 100s ea	00463-5019-01	14.40		EE
500 mg, 50s ea	00463-5020-55	15.00		EE
PDR, PO, 125 mg/5 ml,				
100 ml	00463-5015-01	3.00		EE
150 ml	00463-5015-15	3.90		EE
250 mg/5 ml,				
100 ml	00463-5016-01	4.80		EE
150 ml	00463-5016-15	6.00		EE
AMOXIL (Altura)				
REPACK				
amoxicillin				
CAP, PO, 500 mg, 4s ea	63874-0102-04	2.35		AB
5s ea	63874-0102-05	3.07		AB
10s ea	63874-0102-10	6.15		AB
50s ea	63874-0102-50	30.61		AB
500s ea	63874-0102-03	196.83		AB
(Dispensing Solutions)				
REPACK				
CAP, PO, 500 mg, 24s ea	55045-2067-07	18.00		AB
PDR, PO, 250 mg/5 ml,				
150 ml	55045-1843-03	9.50		
(BUBBLEGUM,BUBBLEGUM)				
250 mg/5 ml,				
150 ml	55045-1848-03	9.50		AB
(BUBBLEGUM)				
400 mg/5 ml,				
100 ml	55045-2756-00	16.20		
(PD-Rx Pharm)				
REPACK				
CAP, PO (REDI-SCRIPT)				
250 mg, 40s ea	58864-0663-40	10.93		AB
(Pharma Pac)				
REPACK				
CTB, PO, 250 mg, 40s ea	52959-0246-40	30.35		AB
PDR, PO, 125 mg/5 ml,				
80 ml	52959-0614-02	7.82		AB
100 ml	52959-0614-03	8.72		AB
150 ml	52959-0614-01	9.55		AB
(Phys Total Care)				
REPACK				
CAP, PO, 250 mg, 30s ea	54868-0193-01	3.49		AB
500 mg, 20s ea	54868-0348-02	21.66		AB
30s ea	54868-0348-01	31.55		AB
CTB, PO (BANANA-CHERRY MINT)				
400 mg, 20s ea	54868-4470-00	15.66		AB
PDR, PO, 125 mg/5 ml,				
100 ml	54868-0195-02	2.39		AB
150 ml	54868-0195-01	3.75		AB
(BUBBLEGUM)				
200 mg/5 ml,				
100 ml	54868-4472-00	13.00		
250 mg/5 ml,				
100 ml	54868-0196-02	4.15		AB
150 ml	54868-0196-01	5.93		AB
(BUBBLEGUM)				
400 mg/5 ml, 75 ml	54868-4473-01	10.80		
100 ml	54868-4473-00	16.65		
(Southwood)				
REPACK				
CAP, PO, 500 mg, 21s ea	58016-0356-21	2.94		
30s ea	58016-0356-30	4.20		
60s ea	58016-0356-60	8.40		
90s ea	58016-0356-90	12.60		
100s ea	58016-0356-00	14.00		
CTB, PO, 250 mg, 20s ea	58016-0105-20	7.47		AB
30s ea	58016-0105-30	11.21		AB
AMOXIL PEDIATRIC (Phys Total Care)				
REPACK				
amoxicillin				
PDR, PO (BUBBLEGUM,DROPS)				
50 mg/ml, 15 ml	54868-3016-00	2.83		AB
30 ml	54868-3016-01	3.43		AB
AMPHADASE (Amphastar)				
hyaluronidase				
SOL, SC, 150 u/ml,				
10s ea	00548-9090-10	300.00	200.00	
25s ea	00548-9090-00	750.00		

PROD/MFR	NDC	AWP	DP	OBC
AMPHETAMINE SALT COMBINATION				
(CorePharma) *See DEXTROAMP SAC/AMP ASPART/DEXTROAMP SULF/AMP SULF*				
(CorePharma) *See DEXTROAMPH SACC/AMPH ASP/DEXTROAM SULF/AMPHET SULF*				
(Global Pharm) *See MIXED AMPHETAMINE SALTS*				
(Ranbaxy Pharm) *See AMPHETAMINE SALT COMBO*				
(Sandoz) *See AMPHETAMINE SALT COMBO*				
(Shire US Inc.) *See ADDERALL XR*				
(Teva) *See ADDERALL*				
(Teva) *See AMPHETAMINE SALT COMBO*				
(Teva) *See MIXED AMPHETAMINE SALT*				
AMPHETAMINE SALT COMBO (Ranbaxy Pharm)				
amphetamine salt combination				
TAB, PO, 5 mg,				
100s ea, C-II	63304-0908-01	137.16		AB
10 mg,				
100s ea, C-II	63304-0909-01	137.16		AB
20 mg,				
100s ea, C-II	63304-0910-01	137.16		AB
30 mg,				
100s ea, C-II	63304-0911-01	137.16		AB
(Sandoz)				
TAB, PO, 5 mg,				
100s ea, C-II	00185-0084-01	137.16		AB
10 mg,				
100s ea, C-II	00185-0111-01	137.16		AB
20 mg,				
100s ea, C-II	00185-0401-01	137.16		AB
30 mg,				
100s ea, C-II	00185-0404-01	137.16		AB
(Teva)				
TAB, PO, 5 mg,				
100s ea, C-II	00555-0971-02	137.16		AB
7.5 mg,				
100s ea, C-II	00555-0775-02	142.85		AB
10 mg,				
100s ea, C-II	00555-0972-02	137.16		AB
12.5 mg,				
100s ea, C-II	00555-0776-02	142.85		AB
15 mg,				
100s ea, C-II	00555-0777-02	142.85		AB
20 mg,				
100s ea, C-II	00555-0973-02	137.16		AB
30 mg,				
100s ea, C-II	00555-0974-02	137.16		AB
(Bryant Ranch)				
REPACK				
TAB, PO, 10 mg,				
60s ea, C-II	63629-3730-01	86.32		AB
(Phys Total Care)				
REPACK				
TAB, PO, 5 mg,				
20s ea, C-II	54868-4631-01	34.32		AB
30s ea, C-II	54868-4631-02	48.48		AB
60s ea, C-II	54868-4631-03	90.96		AB
100s ea, C-II	54868-4631-00	114.27		AB
10 mg,				
10s ea, C-II	54868-4728-00	17.16		AB
30s ea, C-II	54868-4728-01	33.95		AB
60s ea, C-II	54868-4728-02	61.91		AB
90s ea, C-II	54868-4728-03	89.85		
100s ea, C-II	54868-4728-04	94.00		AB
15 mg,				
90s ea, C-II	54868-5387-00	106.32		AB
20 mg,				
20s ea, C-II	54868-5103-03	22.98		AB
30s ea, C-II	54868-5103-00	31.47		AB
60s ea, C-II	54868-5103-01	56.94		AB
90s ea, C-II	54868-5103-02	82.44		AB
30 mg,				
10s ea, C-II	54868-4863-01	17.17		AB
30s ea, C-II	54868-4863-00	39.51		AB
60s ea, C-II	54868-4863-02	73.02		
AMPHETAMINE SALTS (Palmetto)				
REPACK				
amphetamine salt combination				
TAB, PO, 5 mg,				
30s ea, C-II	23490-7973-03	127.50		
10 mg,				
30s ea, C-II	23490-7974-03	112.50		
20 mg,				
60s ea, C-II	23490-7975-06	225.00		
AMPHOTEC (Three Rivers Pharm)				
amphotericin b cholesteryl sulfate complex				
PDS, IV (SDV)				
50 mg, ea	66435-0301-51	93.33	70.00	
100 mg, ea	66435-0302-01	160.00	120.00	

PROD/MFR	NDC	AWP	DP	OBC
AMPHOTERICIN B (Abbott Hosp)				
PDS, IV (S.D.V.)				
50 mg, ea	00703-9785-01	11.64	9.80	AP
(Gallipot)				
POW, NA, 0.1 gm	51552-0304-03	3.15		
0.5 gm	51552-0304-09	12.60		
1 gm	51552-0304-01	12.50		
5 gm	51552-0304-02	38.50		
(1X25GM)				
25 gm	51552-0304-04	112.00	80.00	
(1X100GM)				
100 gm	51552-0304-05	392.00	280.00	
(1X500GM)				
500 gm	51552-0304-06	1862.00	1330.00	
(U.S.P.)				
1000 gm	51552-0304-07	4200.00		
(Hawkins)				
POW, NA (U.S.P.,ORAL)				
1 gm	63370-0020-10	48.00		
5 gm	63370-0020-15	158.40		
25 gm	63370-0020-25	384.00		
100 gm	63370-0020-35	1368.00		
1000 gm	63370-0020-50	8880.00		
(Letco)				
POW, NA (U.S.P., ORAL GRADE)				
5 gm	62991-1173-02	90.00		
25 gm	62991-1173-04	240.00		
(USP)				
100 gm	62991-1173-05	885,00		
(Medisca)				
POW, NA (U.S.P.)				
1 gm	38779-0191-06	43.50		
5 gm	38779-0191-03	147.00		
25 gm	38779-0191-04	594.00		
100 gm	38779-0191-05	1365.00		
500 gm	38779-0191-08	5805.00		
1000 gm	38779-0191-09	9870.00		
(PCCA)				
POW, NA (U.S.P.; ORAL GRADE)				
1 gm	51927-1726-00	69.00		
(Spectrum Pharmacy)				
POW, NA (U.S.P.)				
1 gm	49452-0023-01	84.00		
5 gm	49452-0023-02	227.85		
25 gm	49452-0023-03	868.00		
(X-Gen) *See NOVAPLUS AMPHOTERICIN B*				
(X-Gen)				
PDS, IV (STERILE)				
50 mg, ea	39822-1055-05	24.50		AP
(Phys Total Care)				
REPACK				
PDS, IV, 50 mg, ea	54868-5752-00	50.31		
AMPHOTERICIN B CHOLESTERYL SULFATE COMPLEX				
(Three Rivers Pharm) *See AMPHOTEC*				
AMPHOTERICIN B LIPID COMPLEX				
(Enzon Pharma, Inc.) *See ABELCET*				
AMPHOTERICIN B LIPOSOME				
(Astellas) *See AMBISOME*				
AMPICILLIN				
FUL				
CAP, PO, 250 mg, 100s ea		17.36		
500 mg, 100s ea		29.91		
(Cura Pharm)				
ampicillin sodium				
PDS, IJ (USP)				
1 gm, 10s ea	66860-0011-02	90.00		AP
2 gm, 10s ea	66860-0012-02	175.00		AP
(USP,PHARMACY BULK PKG)				
10 gm, 10s ea	66860-0013-02	950.00		AP
(USP)				
500 mg, 10s ea	66860-0015-02	50.00		AP
AMPICILLIN (Dava Pharma)				
CAP, PO, 250 mg, 100s ea	67253-0180-10	42.22		AB
500s ea	67253-0180-50	205.86		
500 mg, 100s ea	67253-0181-10	71.78		AB
500s ea	67253-0181-50	349.96		AB
PDR, PO (BUBBLEGUM)				
125 mg/5 ml,				
100 ml	67253-0182-10	9.54		AB
200 ml	67253-0182-20	16.56		AB
250 mg/5 ml, 100 ml	67253-0183-10	14.08		AB
200 ml	67253-0183-20	28.16		AB
(Sandoz)				
CAP, PO, 250 mg, 100s ea	00781-2144-01	23.46		AB
500s ea	00781-2144-05	114.37		AB
500 mg, 100s ea	00781-2145-01	39.88		AB

PROD/MFR	NDC	AWP	DP	OBC
500s ea	00781-2145-05	194.42		AB
(WG)				
ampicillin sodium				
PDS, IJ (USP)				
1 gm, 10s ea	44567-0102-10	83.37		AP
2 gm, 10s ea	44567-0103-10	161.30		AP
(PHARMACY BULK)				
10 gm, 10s ea	44567-0104-10	1013.87		AP
(USP)				
500 mg, 10s ea	44567-0101-10	47.60		AP
AMPICILLIN (A-S Medication)				
REPACK				
CAP, PO, 250 mg, 28s ea	54569-1719-02	6.41		AB
40s ea	54569-1719-00	9.15		AB
500 mg, 28s ea	54569-2411-01	15.63		AB
(Altura)				
REPACK				
CAP, PO, 250 mg, 8s ea	63874-0113-08	1.56		EE
9s ea	63874-0113-09	1.75		EE
10s ea	63874-0113-01	29.95		EE
10s ea	63874-0113-10	1.95		EE
12s ea	63874-0113-12	2.34		EE
14s ea	63874-0113-14	2.73		EE
15s ea	63874-0113-15	2.92		EE
20s ea	63874-0113-20	3.90		EE
21s ea	63874-0113-21	6.29		EE
24s ea	63874-0113-24	7.19		EE
28s ea	63874-0113-28	8.39		EE
30s ea	63874-0113-30	8.99		EE
40s ea	63874-0113-40	11.98		EE
50s ea	63874-0113-50	14.97		EE
500s ea	63874-0113-03	149.76		EE
500 mg, 7s ea	63874-0114-07	2.44		EE
10s ea	63874-0114-10	3.48		EE
20s ea	63874-0114-20	6.95		EE
21s ea	63874-0114-21	7.99		EE
24s ea	63874-0114-24	8.35		EE
25s ea	63874-0114-25	8.69		EE
28s ea	63874-0114-28	11.75		EE
30s ea	63874-0114-30	11.58		EE
40s ea	63874-0114-40	13.91		EE
100s ea	63874-0114-01	34.78		EE
500s ea	63874-0114-50	164.15		EE
PDR, PO, 125 mg/5 ml,				
100 ml	63874-0145-10	7.49		EE
200 ml	63874-0145-20	9.69		EE
250 mg/5 ml, 100 ml	63874-0146-10	10.87		EE
150 ml	63874-0146-15	8.09		EE
200 ml	63874-0146-20	12.59		EE
(Bryant Ranch)				
REPACK				
CAP, PO, 250 mg, 21s ea	63629-2609-01	6.39		
30s ea	63629-2609-02	9.13		
40s ea	63629-2609-03	12.17		
500 mg, 20s ea	63629-2610-01	10.34		
30s ea	63629-2610-02	15.51		
40s ea	63629-2610-03	20.69		
(Core)				
REPACK				
CAP, PO, 250 mg, 20s ea	33358-0032-20	6.55		
28s ea	33358-0032-28	8.19		
30s ea	33358-0032-30	9.36		
40s ea	33358-0032-40	12.47		
500 mg, 20s ea	33358-0033-20	10.60		
30s ea	33358-0033-30	15.90		
40s ea	33358-0033-40	21.21		
(DHS, Inc.)				
REPACK				
CAP, PO, 500 mg, 21s ea	55887-0463-21	15.91		AB
28s ea	55887-0463-28	19.09		AB
40s ea	55887-0463-40	15.95		AB
60s ea	55887-0463-60	23.93		
PDR, PO, 125 mg/5 ml,				
100 ml	55887-0691-01	37.00		
(Dispensing Solutions)				
REPACK				
CAP, PO, 500 mg, 28s ea	55045-1204-09	11.75		AB
40s ea	55045-1204-03	16.80		AB
(HomeMed)				
REPACK				
CAP, PO, 250 mg, 28s ea	51655-0104-29	14.89		
40s ea	51655-0104-51	7.21		
500 mg, 28s ea	51655-0258-29	22.65		EE
(Nucare Pharm)				
REPACK				
CAP, PO, 250 mg, 28s ea	66267-0024-28	7.99		AB

PROD/MFR	NDC	AWP	DP	OBC
30s ea	66267-0024-30	8.40		AB
40s ea	66267-0024-40	9.86		AB
500 mg, 28s ea	66267-0025-28	10.96		AB
30s ea	66267-0025-30	11.25		AB
40s ea	66267-0025-40	13.89		AB
(Palmetto)				
REPACK				
CAP, PO, 250 mg, 4s ea	23490-5079-01	4.98		
500 mg, 30s ea	23490-5081-01	22.16		
(PD-Rx Pharm)				
REPACK				
CAP, PO, 250 mg, 10s ea	55289-0023-10	7.00		AB
20s ea	55289-0023-20	9.00		AB
28s ea	55289-0023-28	10.60		AB
30s ea	55289-0023-30	11.00		AB
40s ea	55289-0023-40	13.00		AB
100s ea	55289-0023-01	24.08		AB
500 mg, 4s ea	55289-0024-04	6.27		AB
7s ea	55289-0024-07	7.22		AB
10s ea	55289-0024-10	8.17		AB
20s ea	55289-0024-20	11.33		AB
28s ea	55289-0024-28	13.87		AB
30s ea	55289-0024-30	14.50		AB
40s ea	55289-0024-40	17.67		AB
(Pharma Pac)				
REPACK				
CAP, PO, 500 mg, 20s ea	52959-0389-20	9.05		EE
28s ea	52959-0389-28	10.80		EE
30s ea	52959-0389-30	11.30		EE
40s ea	52959-0389-40	13.50		EE
(Phys Total Care)				
REPACK				
CAP, PO, 250 mg, 30s ea	54868-3111-03	17.22		EE
40s ea	54868-3111-01	21.48		EE
100s ea	54868-3111-05	46.92		EE
500s ea	54868-3111-00	104.42		EE
500 mg, 20s ea	54868-3113-07	25.14		EE
21s ea	54868-3113-09	26.16		EE
30s ea	54868-3113-05	35.46		EE
40s ea	54868-3113-03	45.75		EE
60s ea	54868-3113-08	66.39		EE
100s ea	54868-3113-00	81.87		EE
PDR, PO, 125 mg/5 ml,				
100 ml	54868-4129-01	6.07		EE
200 ml	54868-4129-02	10.15		EE
250 mg/5 ml, 200 ml	54868-4131-01	39.36		EE
(Quality Care Prod)				
REPACK				
CAP, PO, 250 mg, 28s ea	49999-0001-28	6.23		AB
40s ea	49999-0001-40	8.90		EE
500 mg, 20s ea	49999-0117-20	15.20		EE
(Southwood)				
REPACK				
CAP, PO, 250 mg, 8s ea	58016-0148-08	1.49		EE
9s ea	58016-0148-09	1.67		EE
10s ea	58016-0148-10	1.86		EE
12s ea	58016-0148-12	2.23		EE
14s ea	58016-0148-14	2.60		EE
15s ea	58016-0148-15	2.78		EE
20s ea	58016-0148-20	3.71		EE
24s ea	58016-0148-24	4.45		EE
28s ea	58016-0148-28	5.20		EE
30s ea	58016-0148-30	5.57		EE
40s ea	58016-0148-40	7.42		EE
50s ea	58016-0148-50	9.28		EE
100s ea	58016-0148-00	18.56		EE
500 mg, 7s ea	58016-0149-07	2.32		EE
10s ea	58016-0149-10	3.31		EE
20s ea	58016-0149-20	6.62		EE
21s ea	58016-0149-21	6.96		EE
24s ea	58016-0149-24	7.95		EE
25s ea	58016-0149-25	8.28		EE
28s ea	58016-0149-28	9.27		EE
30s ea	58016-0149-30	9.94		EE
40s ea	58016-0149-40	13.25		EE
100s ea	58016-0149-00	33.12		EE
PDR, PO, 125 mg/5 ml,				
100 ml	58016-1031-01	3.90		EE
200 ml	58016-1032-01	7.00		EE
250 mg/5 ml, 100 ml	58016-1033-01	6.71		EE
150 ml	58016-1062-01	7.70		EE
200 ml	58016-1034-01	9.10		EE
AMPICILLIN AND SULBACTAM (APP)				
ampicillin sodium/sulbactam sodium				
PDS, IJ (USP,W/LATEX)				
1 gm-0.5 gm,				
10s ea	63323-0368-20	81.40		
2 gm-1 gm, 10s ea	63323-0369-20	153.50		

PROD/MFR | NDC | AWP | DP | OBC

IV (USP,PHARMACY BULK PKG)
10 gm-5 gm, ea 63323-0370-62 77.31

(GeneraMedix)
PDS, IJ, 1 gm-0.5 gm, ea .. 10139-0070-12 7.50 AP
(USP)
1 gm-0.5 gm,
10s ea .... 10139-0070-11 75.00 AP
2 gm-1 gm, ea .... 10139-0071-18 13.80 AP
(USP)
2 gm-1 gm, 10s ea ... 10139-0071-10 138.00 AP

(Hospira)
PDS, IJ (USP)
1 gm-0.5 gm,
10s ea .... 00409-2988-01 42.96 37.60 AP
2 gm-1 gm, 10s ea ... 00409-2998-03 84.36 73.80 AP
IV (SDV,ADD-VANTAGE)
1 gm-0.5 gm,
10s ea .... 00409-2689-01 74.64 65.30 AP
2 gm-1 gm, 10s ea ... 00409-2987-03 120.00 105.00 AP
10 gm-5 gm, ea ...... 00409-2687-15 45.59 39.89 AP

(Sandoz)
PDS, IJ (USP)
1 gm-0.5 gm,
10s ea .... 00781-3032-95 81.41 AP
2 gm-1 gm, 10s ea ... 00781-3033-95 153.67 AP
IV, 10 gm-5 gm, ea ..... 00781-3034-46 76.85 AP

AMPICILLIN SODIUM (APP)
PDS, IJ (VIAL)
1 gm, ea 63323-0389-10 7.38
2 gm, ea 63323-0399-23 14.14
250 mg, ea 63323-0387-10 3.13
500 mg, 10s ea 63323-0388-10 48.80

(Cura Pharm) *See AMPICILLIN*

(Sandoz) *See NOVAPLUS AMPICILLIN*

(Sandoz)
PDS, IJ (ADD-VANTAGE)
1 gm, ea .... 00015-7404-18 10.36 AP
ea .... 00781-3412-15 14.90 AP
(ADD-VANTAGE,USP)
1 gm, 10s ea .... 00781-3412-92 148.99 AP
(ADD-VANTAGE)
1 gm, 10s ea .... 00015-7404-89 103.62 AP
(U.S.P.)
1 gm, 10s ea .... 00781-3404-95 86.35 AP
(ADD-VANTAGE,USP)
2 gm, ea .... 00781-3413-15 28.90 AP
(ADD-VANTAGE)
2 gm, ea .... 00015-7405-18 20.11 AP
(VIAL,PIGGYBACK)
2 gm, ea .... 00015-7405-20 16.75 AP
(ADD-VANTAGE,ADD-VANTAGE)
2 gm, 10s ea .... 00015-7405-89 201.03 AP
10s ea .... 00781-3413-92 289.01 AP
(U.S.P.)
2 gm, 10s ea .... 00781-3408-95 167.53 AP
10 gm, 10s ea .... 00781-3409-95 1077.73 AP
125 mg, 10s ea ...... 00781-3400-95 52.20 AP
250 mg, ea .... 00781-3402-78 4.19 AP
(VIAL)
250 mg, ea .... 00015-7402-20 4.19 AP
(U.S.P.)
250 mg, 10s ea ...... 00781-3402-95 41.86 AP
(VIAL)
500 mg, ea .... 00015-7403-20 4.41 AP
(U.S.P.)
500 mg, 10s ea ...... 00781-3407-95 44.06 AP

(WG) *See AMPICILLIN*

(Phys Total Care)
REPACK
PDS, IJ, 1 gm, 10s ea ..... 54868-3481-00 61.27 EE
(VIAL)
500 mg, 10s ea ...... 54868-4047-00 101.45 EE

AMPICILLIN SODIUM/SULBACTAM SODIUM
(APP) *See AMPICILLIN AND SULBACTAM*

(Baxter) *See AMERINET CHOICE AMPICILLIN AND SULBACTAM*

(Baxter) *See AMPICILLIN/SULBACTAM*

(Baxter) *See NOVAPLUS AMPICILLIN AND SULBACTAM*

(GeneraMedix) *See AMPICILLIN AND SULBACTAM*

(Hospira) *See AMPICILLIN AND SULBACTAM*

(Hospira) *See NOVAPLUS AMPICILLIN AND SULBACTAM*

(Pfizer) *See UNASYN*

(Sandoz) *See AMPICILLIN AND SULBACTAM*

AMPICILLIN/SULBACTAM (Baxter)
ampicillin sodium/sulbactam sodium
PDS, IJ, 1 gm-0.5 gm, ea .. 10019-0631-31 4.74 AP
10s ea .... 10019-0631-01 47.40 AP
2 gm-1 gm, ea .... 10019-0630-33 8.06 AP
(VIAL)
2 gm-1 gm, 10s ea ... 10019-0630-02 80.64 AP
IV (BULK PACKAGE)
10 gm-5 gm, ea ...... 10019-0632-03 43.15 AP
(PHARMACYBULKPACKAGE,USP)
10 gm-5 gm, ea ...... 10019-0632-15 43.15 AP

AMPYRA (Acorda Therapeutics)
dalfampridine
TER, PO (FILM-COATED)
10 mg, 60s ea 10144-0427-60 1267.39

AMRIX (Cephalon)
cyclobenzaprine hydrochloride
CER, PO, 15 mg, 60s ea ... 63459-0700-60 612.00
30 mg, 60s ea 63459-0701-60 612.00

(A-S Medication)
REPACK
CER, PO, 15 mg, 5s ea 54569-6064-01 50.63
10s ea 54569-6064-00 101.25

(Phys Total Care)
REPACK
CER, PO, 15 mg, 30s ea ... 54868-6022-00 347.79

(Physician Partner)
REPACK
CER, PO, 15 mg, 14s ea ... 21695-0723-14 336.00
28s ea 21695-0723-28 672.00
60s ea 21695-0723-60 1224.00

(Quality Care Prod)
REPACK
CER, PO, 15 mg, 10s ea ... 35356-0262-10 251.16
30s ea 35356-0262-30 496.24
60s ea 35356-0262-60 992.48
90s ea 35356-0262-90 1488.72
30 mg, 30s ea 35356-0263-30 496.24
120s ea 35356-0263-01 1675.60

(Stat Rx)
REPACK
CER, PO, 15 mg, 10s ea ... 16590-0596-10 121.15
15s ea 16590-0596-15 180.10
28s ea 16590-0596-28 333.38
30s ea 16590-0596-30 356.96
60s ea 16590-0596-60 545.00
90s ea 16590-0596-90 815.00

AMVISC PLUS (Bausch & Lomb Inc.)
hyaluronate sodium
SOL, IO, 16 mg/ml,
0.8 ml 61772-0600-81 162.50

AMYL ACETATE (Amend)
LIQ, NA (PURIFIED)
500 ml 17317-1414-01 10.50
3840 ml 17317-1414-06 49.00
19200 ml 17317-1414-08 196.00

(Baker, J.T.)
LIQ, NA (PURIFIED)
500 ml 10106-9094-01 40.58
4000 ml 10106-9094-03 170.41

(PCCA)
LIQ, NA (PURIFIED)
1 ml 51927-1581-00 0.16

AMYL NITRITE (Alexander, James)
SOL, IH, 12s ea 46414-2222-01 4.55

(Consolidated Midland)
SOL, IH (AMP)
12s ea 00223-7002-12 6.60

(X-Gen)
SOL, IH (CRUSHABLE AMP)
12s ea 39822-9950-02 7.50

AMYL NITRITE/SODIUM NITRITE/ SODIUM THIOSULFATE
(Akorn) *See CYANIDE ANTIDOTE*

AMYLASE/LIPASE/PROTEASE
(Axcan) *See ULTRASE*

(Axcan) *See ULTRASE MT12*

(Axcan) *See ULTRASE MT18*

(Axcan) *See ULTRASE MT20*

(Axcan) *See VIOKASE*

(Axcan) *See VIOKASE 16*

(Breckenridge Pharm) *See PALCAPS 10*

(Breckenridge Pharm) *See PALCAPS 20*

(Breckenridge Pharm) *See PANOCAPS*

(Breckenridge Pharm) *See PANOCAPS MT 16*

(Breckenridge Pharm) *See PANOCAPS MT 20*

(Breckenridge Pharm) *See PANOKASE*

(Breckenridge Pharm) *See PANOKASE 16*

(Breckenridge Pharm) *See ULTRACAPS MT 20*

(Contract Pharmacal) *See PANCRELIPASE 8000*

(Contract Pharmacal) *See PANCRELIPASE MT 16*

(Cypress Pharm) *See DYGASE*

(Cypress Pharm) *See LAPASE*

(Digestive Care Inc) *See PANCRECARB MS-16*

(Digestive Care Inc) *See PANCRECARB MS-4*

(Digestive Care Inc) *See PANCRECARB MS-8*

(Eurand) *See ZENPEP*

(Global Pharm) *See LIPRAM 4500*

(Global Pharm) *See LIPRAM-PN10*

(Global Pharm) *See LIPRAM-PN16*

(Global Pharm) *See LIPRAM-PN20*

(Ortho-McNeil Pharm) *See PANCREASE MT 10*

(Ortho-McNeil Pharm) *See PANCREASE MT 16*

(Ortho-McNeil Pharm) *See PANCREASE MT 20*

(Ortho-McNeil Pharm) *See PANCREASE MT 4*

(Solvay) *See CREON*

(Solvay) *See CREON 10*

(Solvay) *See CREON 20*

(Solvay) *See CREON 5*

(X-Gen) *See PANCRELIPASE*

AMYTAL SODIUM (Marathon)
amobarbital sodium
PDS, IJ, 0.5 gm,
ea, C-II 42998-0303-01 122.24

ANABAR (Lunsco)
apap/phenyltoloxamine cit/salicylamide
TAB, PO (CAPLET)
300 mg-20 mg-200 mg,
100s ea 10892-0153-10 47.88

ANACAINE (Gordon)
benzocaine
OIN, TP, 10%, 30 gm 10481-1002-01 13.45

ANADROL-50 (Alaven)
oxymetholone
TAB, PO, 50 mg,
100s ea, C-III 68220-0055-10 2850.80

ANAEMODORON (Weleda)
homeopathic substance
LIQ, PO, 50 ml 55946-0060-15 12.00

ANAFRANIL (Covidien)
clomipramine hydrochloride
CAP, PO (USP)
25 mg, 30s ea 00406-9906-03 397.28
50 mg, 30s ea 00406-9907-03 397.28
75 mg, 30s ea 00406-9908-03 397.28

(Phys Total Care)
REPACK
CAP, PO, 50 mg, 30s ea ... 54868-1447-00 157.11 AB

ANAGRELIDE HCL (Mylan)
anagrelide hydrochloride
CAP, PO, 0.5 mg, 100s ea .. 00378-6868-01 585.70 AB
1 mg, 100s ea .... 00378-6869-01 1171.35 AB

(Sandoz)
CAP, PO, 0.5 mg, 100s ea .. 00185-0155-01 586.33 AB
1 mg, 100s ea .... 00185-0156-01 1172.64 AB

(Phys Total Care)
REPACK
CAP, PO, 0.5 mg, 30s ea ... 54868-5443-02 52.05
60s ea 54868-5443-00 99.60
100s ea 54868-5443-01 124.20

ANAGRELIDE HYDROCHLORIDE
FUL
CAP, PO, 0.5 mg, 100s ea 43.95
1 mg, 100s ea 87.90

(Mylan) *See ANAGRELIDE HCL*

(Sandoz) *See ANAGRELIDE HCL*

(Shire US Inc.) *See AGRYLIN*

PROD/MFR	NDC	AWP	DP	OBC
(Teva)				
CAP, PO, 0.5 mg, 100s ea	**00172-5241-60**	586.27		AB
1 mg, 100s ea	**00172-5240-60**	1172.51		AB
(Phys Total Care)				
REPACK				
CAP, PO, 1 mg, 10s ea	**54868-5385-01**	26.52		AB
30s ea	**54868-5385-00**	70.53		AB
ANAKINRA				
(Amgen USA Inc.) *See KINERET*				
(Biovitrum) *See KINERET*				
ANALPRAM E (Ferndale)				
hydrocortisone acetate/pramoxine hydrochloride				
KIT, MR, ea	**00496-0751-64**	204.00		
ea	**00496-0752-04**	90.00		
ANALPRAM HC (Ferndale)				
hydrocortisone acetate/pramoxine hydrochloride				
CRE, TP (SINGLES,12X4GM)				
1%-1%, 4 gm 12s	**00496-0778-65**	113.69		
(12X4GM,PARABEN-FREE)				
2.5%-1%, 4 gm 12s	**00496-0799-65**	113.69		
(30X4GM,PARABEN-FREE)				
2.5%-1%, 4 gm 30s	**00496-0799-64**	226.03		
(1X30GM,PARABEN-FREE)				
2.5%-1%, 30 gm	**00496-0799-04**	92.70		
ANALPRAM-HC (Ferndale)				
hydrocortisone acetate/pramoxine hydrochloride				
CRE, TP (30X4GM)				
1%-1%, 4 gm 30s	**00496-0778-64**	226.03		
30 gm	**00496-0778-04**	92.70		
LOT, TP, 2.5%-1%, 59 ml	**00496-0829-04**	109.61		
(Pharma Pac)				
REPACK				
CRE, TP, 1%-1%, 30 gm	**52959-0500-01**	29.95		
ANAMANTLE HC (Kenwood)				
hydrocortisone acetate/lidocaine hydrochloride				
CRE, RC (SINGLEUSE UNITS W/APP)				
0.5%-3%, 7 gm 14s	**00482-4800-14**	246.41		
KIT, MR, 0.5%-3%, ea	**00482-4800-20**	351.90		
2.5%-3%, ea	**00482-4804-20**	351.90		
ANAMANTLE HC FORTE (Kenwood)				
hydrocortisone acetate/lidocaine hydrochloride				
KIT, MR, 1%-3%, 20s ea	**00482-4802-20**	351.90		
ANAPLEX DM (ECR)				
bpm/dm/pse hcl				
SYR, PO (AF,SF,DYE-FREE,FRUIT)				
480 ml	**00095-0131-16**	30.00		
(Phys Total Care)				
REPACK				
SYR, PO (AF,SF,DYE-FREE,FRUIT)				
473 ml	**54868-5335-00**	53.93		
ANAPLEX DMX (ECR)				
brompheniramine tan/dm tan/pse tan				
SUS, PO (AF,SF,GRAPE)				
480 ml	**00095-0132-16**	57.60		
(Phys Total Care)				
REPACK				
SUS, PO (AF,SF,GRAPE)				
473 ml	**54868-5441-00**	107.14		
ANAPROX (Roche Labs)				
naproxen sodium				
TAB, PO, 275 mg, 100s ea	**00004-6202-01**	233.16		AB
(PD-Rx Pharm)				
REPACK				
TAB, PO, 275 mg, 10s ea	**55289-0837-10**	30.14		AB
20s ea	**55289-0837-20**	60.27		AB
(Phys Total Care)				
REPACK				
TAB, PO, 275 mg, 30s ea	**54868-1872-01**	31.55		AB
ANAPROX DS (Roche Labs)				
naproxen sodium				
TAB, PO (CAPLET)				
550 mg, 100s ea	**00004-6203-01**	363.04		AB
500s ea	**00004-6203-14**	1096.99		AB
(PD-Rx Pharm)				
REPACK				
TAB, PO, 550 mg, 6s ea	**55289-0332-06**	30.88		AB
15s ea	**55289-0332-15**	52.15		AB
20s ea	**55289-0332-20**	57.00		AB
30s ea	**55289-0332-30**	83.00		AB
(Phys Total Care)				
REPACK				
TAB, PO, 550 mg, 15s ea	**54868-0197-02**	36.30		AB
20s ea	**54868-0197-03**	47.78		AB
30s ea	**54868-0197-04**	70.71		AB
ANASPAZ (Ascher)				
hyoscyamine sulfate				
TAB, PO, 0.125 mg,				
100s ea	**00225-0295-15**	25.80	21.50	
500s ea	**00225-0295-20**	124.80	104.00	
(Phys Total Care)				
REPACK				
TAB, PO, 0.125 mg,				
10s ea	**54868-3451-00**	3.64		
ANASTROZOLE				
(AstraZeneca) *See ARIMIDEX*				
(Medisca)				
POW, NA (1X1GM)				
1 gm	**38779-2274-06**	1300.50		
(1X5GM)				
5 gm	**38779-2274-03**	5463.00		
(1X25GM)				
25 gm	**38779-2274-04**	21420.00		
ANCOBON (Valeant Pharm Intl)				
flucytosine				
CAP, PO, 250 mg, 100s ea	**00187-3554-10**	2358.25		
500 mg, 100s ea	**00187-3555-10**	4563.25		
ANDEHIST DM NR (Cypress Pharm)				
bpm/dm/pse hcl				
SYR, PO (AF,SF,GRAPE)				
473 ml	**60258-0444-16**	99.99		
ANDEHIST NR (Cypress Pharm)				
bpm/pse hcl				
SYR, PO (AF,SF,RASPBERRY)				
4 mg/5 ml-45 mg/5 ml,				
473 ml	**60258-0434-16**	58.30		
ANDRODERM (Watson)				
testosterone				
TDM, TD, 2.5 mg/24 hr,				
60s ea, C-III	**52544-0469-60**	301.93		
5 mg/24 hr,				
30s ea, C-III	**52544-0470-30**	301.93		BX
(Phys Total Care)				
REPACK				
TDM, TD, 2.5 mg/24 hr,				
60s ea, C-III	**54868-3704-00**	266.93		
5 mg/24 hr,				
30s ea, C-III	**54868-6032-00**	334.20		BX
ANDROGEL (Unimed Pharm)				
testosterone				
GEL, TP (PACKET)				
1%,				
2.5 gm 30s UD,				
C-III	**00051-8425-30**	290.88		
5 gm 30s UD, C-III	**00051-8450-30**	298.94		
(2X75GM PUMPS)				
1%,				
75 gm 2s UD,				
C-III	**00051-8488-88**	298.94		
(A-S Medication)				
REPACK				
GEL, TP, 1%,				
5 gm 30s, C-III	**54569-5339-00**	374.84		
(Phys Total Care)				
REPACK				
GEL, TP (PACKET)				
1%,				
2.5 gm 30s UD,				
C-III	**54868-4792-00**	347.60		
5 gm 30s, C-III	**54868-4810-00**	355.83		
150 gm, C-III	**54868-5814-00**	357.14		
(Physician Partner)				
REPACK				
GEL, TP, 1%,				
30s ea UD, C-III	**21695-0112-30**	576.60		
(Quality Care Prod)				
REPACK				
GEL, TP (1X5GM)				
1%, 5 gm, C-III	**35356-0376-05**	35.74		
(Stat Rx)				
REPACK				
GEL, TP (1X30GM)				
1%, 30 gm, C-III	**16590-0719-30**	348.80		
ANDROID (Valeant Pharm Intl)				
methyltestosterone				
CAP, PO, 10 mg,				
100s ea, C-III	**00187-0902-01**	1182.01		AB
ANDROSTENEDIOL (PCCA)				
POW, NA, 1 gm	**51927-3376-00**	10.20		
ANDROSTENEDIONE (PCCA)				
POW, NA, 1 gm	**51927-1595-00**	36.00		
ANDROSTERONE				
(PCCA) *See ANDROSTERONE (CIS)*				
ANDROSTERONE (CIS) (PCCA)				
androsterone				
POW, NA (1X1GM)				
1 gm	**51927-2183-00**	255.00		
ANDROXY (Upsher-Smith)				
fluoxymesterone				
TAB, PO, 10 mg,				
100s ea, C-III	**00832-0086-00**	356.69		
ANECTINE (Sandoz)				
succinylcholine chloride				
SOL, IV (MDV,10MLX10VIALS)				
20 mg/ml,				
10 ml 10s	**00781-3009-95**	29.00		AP
ANESTACAINE (Clint)				
lidocaine hydrochloride				
SOL, EP (VIAL)				
1%, 50 ml	**55553-0055-50**	4.20		EE
IJ, 2%, 50 ml	**55553-0056-50**	4.20		EE
ANETHOLE (PCCA)				
SOL, NA (NF,SYNTHETIC)				
1 ml	**51927-2893-00**	1.35		
ANEXSIA (Dispensing Solutions)				
REPACK				
acetaminophen/hydrocodone bitartrate				
TAB, PO, 650 mg-7.5 mg,				
15s ea, C-III	**55045-1590-05**	18.75		AA
20s ea, C-III	**55045-1590-08**	25.00		AA
ANEXTUSS (Cypress Pharm)				
dm/gg/phenyleph hcl				
TER, PO, 60 mg-600 mg-40 mg,				
100s ea	**60258-0241-01**	81.65		
ANGELIQ (Bayer)				
drospirenone/estradiol				
TAB, PO (3X28,FILM-COATED)				
0.5 mg-1 mg,				
84s ea	**50419-0483-03**	215.82		
ANGIO SET IV (Becton Dickinson)				
catheter, central venous, peripheral insertion				
DEV, NA (20GX1", W/PRN)				
ea	**08290-3862-20**	2.50		
(22GX3/4", W/PRN)				
ea	**08290-3862-22**	2.50		
ANGIOMAX (Medicines Company)				
bivalirudin				
PDS, IV (VIAL,GLASS)				
250 mg, 10s ea	**65293-0001-01**	7800.00		
ANGIOSCEIN (Eyesupply USA)				
fluorescein sodium				
SOL, IV (S.D.V.)				
10%, 5 ml	**59414-0010-05**	3.90		
25%, 2 ml	**59414-0025-02**	3.90		
ANIDULAFUNGIN				
(Pfizer) *See ERAXIS*				
ANILINE (Baker, J.T.)				
LIQ, NA (A.C.S., REAGENT)				
500 ml	**10106-9110-01**	54.64		
4000 ml	**10106-9110-03**	230.67		
ANIMAS INFUSION (Animas Corp.)				
kit, administration, intravenous				
DEV, NA (23" COMFORT, STD 5/5)				
5s ea	**65781-0212-05**	112.23	87.00	
(43" COMFORT, STD 5/5)				
5s ea	**65781-0213-05**	112.23	87.00	
(23" COMFORT)				
10s ea	**65781-0210-10**	132.23	102.50	
(43" COMFORT)				
10s ea	**65781-0211-10**	132.00	102.50	
(24" MICRO,STRAIGHT 6MM)				
12s ea	**65781-0232-12**	174.15	135.00	
(24" STRAIGHT ULT.,9MM)				
12s ea	**65781-0230-12**	174.15	135.00	
(42" MICRO,STRAIGHT 6MM)				
12s ea	**65781-0233-12**	174.15	135.00	
(42" STRAIGHT ULT.,9MM)				
12s ea	**65781-0231-12**	174.15	135.00	
(23"CONTACT, 10MM)				
15s ea	**65781-0221-15**	121.26	94.00	
(23"CONTACT, 8MM)				
15s ea	**65781-0222-15**	121.26	94.00	
(43"CONTACT, 10MM)				
15s ea	**65781-0220-15**	121.26	94.00	

PROD/MFR NDC AWP DP OBC

(23" BASIC W/BUTTERFLY)
25s ea..............65781-0240-25 161.25 125.00
(23" BASIC,W/O BUTTERFLY)
25s ea..............65781-0242-25 154.80 120.00
(43" BASIC W/BUTTERFLY)
25s ea..............65781-0241-25 161.25 125.00
(43"BASIC, W/O BUTTERFLY)
25s ea..............65781-0243-25 154.80 120.00

ANIMAS INSULIN PUMP R1000 (Animas Corp.)
infusion pump, parenteral
DEV, NA (ENGLISH/FRENCH)
ea..................65781-0111-01 6500.00 5050.00
(ENGLISH/GERMAN)
ea..................65781-0112-01 6500.00 5050.00
(ENGLISH/SPANISH)
ea..................65781-0110-01 6500.00 5050.00

ANIMI-3 (PBM Pharmaceuticals)
folic acid/omega-3 fatty acids/vit b12/vit b6
CAP, PO, 60s ea 66213-0540-60 82.13

ANISE
(Lorann Oil) *See ANISE OIL NATURAL*

ANISE EXTRACT
(PCCA) *See ANISE EXTRACT FLAVOR*

ANISE EXTRACT FLAVOR (PCCA)
anise extract
SOL, NA, 1 ml............51927-1465-00 0.30

ANISE OIL (Medisca)
OIL, NA (1X14ML,NATURAL)
14 ml...............38779-0894-03 12.00
(1X25ML,NATURAL)
25 ml...............38779-0894-04 16.50
(1X100ML,NATURAL)
100 ml..............38779-0894-05 31.50
(1X500ML,NATURAL)
500 ml..............38779-0894-08 76.50

(PCCA)
OIL, NA (FCC)
1 ml................51927-1580-00 0.62

(Spectrum Pharmacy)
OIL, NA (F.C.C.)
100 ml..............49452-0645-01 74.20
500 ml..............49452-0645-02 203.70

ANISE OIL NATURAL (Lorann Oil)
anise
OIL, NA (U.S.P.)
3.75 ml.............23535-0100-01 0.57
7.5 ml..............23535-0100-02 1.14
30 ml...............23535-0100-05 3.75
120 ml..............23535-0100-08 11.75
480 ml..............23535-0100-10 40.00
1920 ml.............23535-0100-15 145.00
3840 ml.............23535-0100-11 265.00

ANISE PYRITE (Weleda)
homeopathic substance
TAB, PO (3X)
100s ea.............55946-0070-30 6.60

ANOLOR 300 (Blansett)
acetaminophen/butalbital/caffeine
CAP, PO, 325 mg-50 mg-40 mg,.
100s ea.............51674-0009-01 39.95 AB

ANSAID (PD-Rx Pharm)
REPACK
flurbiprofen
TAB, PO, 100 mg, 14s ea ..55289-0647-14 67.83 AB
20s ea..............55289-0647-20 83.27 AB
30s ea..............55289-0647-30 124.91 AB

(Phys Total Care)
REPACK
TAB, PO, 100 mg, 12s ea ..54868-1113-01 36.94 AB
60s ea..............54868-1113-03 177.43 AB
100s ea.............54868-1113-02 278.20 AB

ANTABUSE (Teva)
disulfiram
TAB, PO, 250 mg, 100s ea .65473-0706-01 154.49
(USP)
250 mg, 100s ea 51285-0523-02 397.07
500 mg, 100s ea .....65473-0707-01 247.10 EE
(USP)
500 mg, 100s ea 51285-0524-02 635.30

(Phys Total Care)
REPACK
TAB, PO, 250 mg, 10s ea ..54868-5034-02 43.30
30s ea..............54868-5034-01 126.15
100s ea.............54868-5034-00 379.87

PROD/MFR NDC AWP DP OBC

ANTACID COMBINATION
(Cutispharma) *See FIRST-MOUTHWASH BLM*

ANTARA (Lupin Pharma, Inc.)
fenofibrate, micronized
CAP, PO, 43 mg, 30s ea ...67707-0043-30 48.79
130 mg, 30s ea 27437-0110-06 143.64
100s ea.............67707-0130-99 478.80

(Phys Total Care)
REPACK
CAP, PO, 130 mg, 30s ea ..54868-5498-00 121.43

ANTHRALIN (Amend)
POW, NA (U.S.P.)
25 gm...............17317-0208-02 67.20
100 gm..............17317-0208-04 210.00

(Elorac) *See ZITHRANOL-RR*

(Gallipot)
POW, NA (1X10GM,BP)
10 gm...............51552-1010-03 41.93 29.95
(U.S.P.,N.F.)
10 gm...............51552-0253-03 41.44
(1X25GM,BP)
25 gm...............51552-1010-04 91.00 65.00
(U.S.P.,N.F.)
25 gm...............51552-0253-04 93.24
(1X100GM,BP)
100 gm..............51552-1010-05 299.60 214.00
(U.S.P.,N.F.)
100 gm..............51552-0253-05 299.60

(Medisca)
POW, NA (U.S.P.)
25 gm...............38779-0003-04 181.50
100 gm..............38779-0003-05 616.50

(PCCA)
POW, NA (BP)
1 gm................51927-3444-00 10.20

(Spectrum Pharmacy)
POW, NA (U.S.P.)
10 gm...............49452-0660-01 192.85
25 gm...............49452-0660-02 378.00
100 gm..............49452-0660-03 1162.00

(Summers) *See DRITHO-SCALP*

(Summers) *See DRITHOCREME*

ANTHRAX VACCINE ADSORBED
(Emergent) *See BIOTHRAX*

ANTI-INHIBITOR COAGULANT COMPLEX
(Baxter Bioscience) *See FEIBA-VH IMMUNO*

ANTIBACTERIAL/ANALGESIC COMBINATION
(Azur Pharma, Inc.) *See URELLE*

ANTIBACTERIAL/ANTI-INFLAMMATORY COMBINATION
(JHP) *See COLY-MYCIN S*

(JHP) *See CORTISPORIN-TC*

ANTIBIOTIC EAR (A-S Medication)
REPACK
hc/neomycin sulf/polymyxin b sulf
SOL, OT, 1%-0.35%-10000 u/ml,
10 ml...............54569-3341-00 30.80 EE

(Phys Total Care)
REPACK
SOL, OT, 1%-0.35%-10000 u/ml,
10 ml...............54868-0708-01 62.49 EE
SUS, OT, 1%-0.35%-10000 u/ml,
10 ml...............54868-0736-01 63.99 EE

ANTIBIOTIC OTIC (Quality Care Prod)
REPACK
hc/neomycin sulf/polymyxin b sulf
SOL, OT, 1%-0.35%-10000 u/ml,
10 ml...............49999-0254-10 60.48 AT
10 ml...............49999-0744-10 60.48 AT

ANTIBIOTIC-CORT EAR (A-S Medication)
REPACK
hc/neomycin sulf/polymyxin b sulf
SUS, OT, 1%-0.35%-10000 u/ml,
10 ml...............54569-3259-00 30.80 EE

ANTICOAGULANT CPD (Hospira)
citric acid/dextrose/na cit/na phos
SOL, IV (12X500ML)
500 ml..............00409-1967-03 305.28 267.12

ANTIDIARRHEAL COMBINATION
(Hall) *See CESINEX*

(Hall) *See CESINEX 100*

PROD/MFR NDC AWP DP OBC

(Hall) *See CESINEX 125*

(Hall) *See CESINEX 150*

(Hall) *See CESINEX 20*

(Hall) *See CESINEX 25*

(Hall) *See CESINEX 30*

(Hall) *See CESINEX 35*

(Hall) *See CESINEX 40*

(Hall) *See CESINEX 50*

(Hall) *See CESINEX 60*

(Hall) *See CESINEX 80*

ANTIFLEX (Clint)
orphenadrine citrate
SOL, IJ (AMP)
30 mg/ml, 10 ml .....55553-0129-10 19.75 EE

ANTIHEMOPHILIC FACTOR (RECOMB) PLASMA/ALBUMIN-FREE
(Baxter Bioscience) *See ADVATE*

(Wyeth) *See XYNTHA*

ANTIHEMOPHILIC FACTOR VIII (RECOMBINANT)
(Baxter Bioscience) *See RECOMBINATE*

(Bayer) *See KOGENATE FS*

(Bayer) *See KOGENATE FS WITH BIO-SET*

(Bayer Corp.) *See KOGENATE FS*

(Bayer Corp.) *See KOGENATE FS WITH BIO-SET*

(CSL) *See HELIXATE FS*

(Wyeth) *See REFACTO*

ANTIHEMOPHILIC FACTOR VIII HUMAN
(Talecris) *See KOATE-DVI*

ANTIHEMOPHILIC FACTOR VIII:C HUMAN
(Amer Red Cross-Blood) *See MONARC-M*

(Baxter Bioscience) *See HEMOFIL M*

(Baxter Bioscience) *See MONARC-M*

(CSL) *See MONOCLATE-P*

ANTIMONY (Baker, J.T.)
LUM, NA (REAGENT)
125 gm..............10106-0848-04 59.38
500 gm..............10106-0848-01 117.47

ANTIMONY POTASSIUM TARTRATE (Amend)
POW, NA (U.S.P.)
125 gm..............17317-0031-04 14.00
454 gm..............17317-0031-01 35.00
2270 gm.............17317-0031-05 105.00

(Baker, J.T.)
POW, NA (U.S.P., TRIHYDRATE)
125 gm..............10106-0864-04 41.12
500 gm..............10106-0864-01 111.01

(Gallipot)
POW, NA (U.S.P.)
113.4 gm............51552-0868-04 29.40 21.00

(PCCA)
POW, NA (U.S.P.;TRIHYDRATE)
1 gm................51927-2500-00 0.87

(Spectrum Pharmacy)
POW, NA (U.S.P.)
125 gm..............49452-0670-04 142.45
500 gm..............49452-0670-01 285.25
2500 gm.............49452-0670-02 892.50

ANTIMONY TRICHLORIDE (Baker, J.T.)
CRY, NA (A.C.S., REAGENT)
125 gm..............10106-0878-04 126.23
500 gm..............10106-0878-01 266.00

(PCCA) *See ANTIMONY TRICHLORIDE CRYSTALS*

(Spectrum Pharmacy)
CRY, NA (1X25GM,REAGENT,ACS)
25 gm...............49452-0673-01 185.85
(1X100GM,REAGENT,ACS)
100 gm..............49452-0673-02 327.25
(1X500GM,REAGENT,ACS)
500 gm..............49452-0673-03 983.50

ANTIMONY TRICHLORIDE CRYSTALS (PCCA)
antimony trichloride
CRY, NA (ACS REAGENT)
1 gm................51927-1426-00 2.04

ANTIMONY TRIOXIDE (Baker, J.T.)
POW, NA (REAGENT)
125 gm..............10106-0886-04 53.35
500 gm..............10106-0886-01 69.11
2500 gm.............10106-0886-05 282.79

PROD/MFR NDC AWP DP OBC

ANTIMONY TRISULFIDE (PCCA)
POW, NA (TECHNICAL)
1 gm 51927-1957-00 1.32

ANTIPYRINE (Amend)
CRY, NA (U.S.P.)
125 gm 17317-0032-04 13.30
500 gm 17317-0032-01 35.00
2270 gm 17317-0032-05 140.00
11350 gm 17317-0032-08 499.00

(PCCA)
CRY, NA (U.S.P.)
1 gm 51927-1292-00 1.20

ANTIPYRINE AND BENZOCAINE (Boca Pharmacal)
antipyrine/benzocaine
SOL, OT, 54 mg/ml-14 mg/ml,
15 ml 64376-0438-15 12.91

(County Line)
SOL, OT (1X15ML,USP)
54 mg/ml-14 mg/ml,
15 ml 43199-0016-15 12.90

ANTIPYRINE W/ BENZOCAINE (DHS, Inc.)
REPACK
antipyrine/benzocaine
SOL, OT, 54 mg/ml-14 mg/ml,
15 ml 55887-0699-15 7.02

ANTIPYRINE/BENZOCAINE (Bausch & Lomb Inc.)
SOL, OT, 54 mg/ml-14 mg/ml,
10 ml 24208-0561-62 11.95

(Boca Pharmacal) *See ANTIPYRINE AND BENZOCAINE*

(County Line) *See ANTIPYRINE AND BENZOCAINE*

(Major) *See AURODEX*

(Taro) *See RX-OTIC DROPS*

(Altura)
REPACK
SOL, OT, 54 mg/ml-14 mg/ml,
10 ml 63874-0719-10 5.30

(Dispensing Solutions)
REPACK
SOL, OT, 54 mg/ml-14 mg/ml,
15 ml 55045-1186-05 19.26

(Palmetto)
REPACK
SOL, OT, 54 mg/ml-14 mg/ml,
15 ml 23490-5088-01 11.01

(Phys Total Care)
REPACK
SOL, OT, 54 mg/ml-14 mg/ml,
10 ml 54868-2034-00 15.66
15 ml 54868-2034-01 6.81

(Physician Partner)
REPACK
SOL, OT, 54 mg/ml-14 mg/ml,
15 ml 21695-0216-15 25.82

(Quality Care Prod)
REPACK
SOL, OT, 54 mg/ml-14 mg/ml,
15 ml 49999-0204-05 39.60

(Southwood)
REPACK
SOL, OT, 54 mg/ml-14 mg/ml,
10 ml 58016-6482-01 3.37
15 ml 58016-6003-01 6.51

ANTIPYRINE/BENZOCAINE/GLYCERIN
(SDA) *See AUROGUARD*

ANTIPYRINE/BENZOCAINE/GLYCERIN/ZINC ACETATE
(Arbor) *See NEOTIC*

ANTISPASMODIC (Bryant Ranch)
REPACK
atropine sulf/hyoscyamine sulf/pb/scop hydrobrom
ELI, PO, 480 ml 63629-1356-02 61.31

(Phys Total Care)
REPACK
ELI, PO, 120 ml 54868-2087-01 11.04
480 ml 54868-2087-00 16.50

(Quality Care Prod)
REPACK
ELI, PO (LIME-ORANGE)
120 ml 49999-0746-04 4.52

ANTITHROMBIN III HUMAN
(Talecris) *See THROMBATE III*

ANTITHROMBIN, RECOMBINANT
(Lundbeck) *See ATRYN*

ANTITHYMOCYTE GLOBULIN EQUINE
(Pfizer) *See ATGAM*

ANTITHYMOCYTE GLOBULIN RABBIT
(Genzyme) *See THYMOGLOBULIN*

ANTIVENIN (Wyeth)
antivenin (micrurus fulvius)
KIT, IV, ea 00008-0407-03 1867.72 1556.43

ANTIVENIN (CROTALIDAE) POLYVALENT IMMUNE FAB
(Savage) *See CROFAB*

ANTIVENIN (LATRODECTUS MACTANS)
(Merck) *See ANTIVENIN-SPIDER*

ANTIVENIN (MICRURUS FULVIUS)
(Wyeth) *See ANTIVENIN*

ANTIVENIN-SPIDER (Merck)
antivenin (latrodectus mactans)
PDS, IJ (BLACK WIDOW)
6000 u, ea 00006-4084-00 33.25

ANTIVERT (Pfizer)
meclizine hydrochloride
TAB, PO, 12.5 mg,
100s ea .... 00049-2100-66 67.62 56.35 AA

ANTIVERT/25 (Pfizer)
meclizine hydrochloride
TAB, PO, 25 mg, 100s ea .. 00049-2110-66 106.93 89.11 AA

(Phys Total Care)
REPACK
TAB, PO, 25 mg, 30s ea ... 54868-0882-02 29.44 AA

ANTIVERT/50 (Pfizer)
meclizine hydrochloride
TAB, PO, 50 mg, 100s ea .. 00049-2140-66 203.20 169.33 AA

(Quality Care Prod)
REPACK
TAB, PO, 50 mg, 60s ea ... 35356-0520-60 234.33 AA

ANTIZOL (Jazz)
fomepizole
SOL, IV (4X1.5ML,PF)
1 gm/ml, 1.5 ml 4s ... 68727-0200-02 7399.20
(PF)
1 gm/ml, 1.5 ml 4s ... 62161-0003-34 6066.00 4814.00

ANU-MED HC (Major)
hydrocortisone acetate
SUP, RC, 25 mg, 12s ea ... 00904-0160-12 7.29

(Pharma Pac)
REPACK
SUP, RC, 25 mg, 12s ea ... 52959-0250-03 9.15

ANUCORT HC (Physician Partner)
REPACK
hydrocortisone acetate
SUP, RC, 25 mg, 12s ea ... 21695-0200-12 21.72

ANUCORT-HC (G&W)
hydrocortisone acetate
SUP, RC, 25 mg, 12s ea ... 00713-0503-12 10.86
24s ea 00713-0503-24 21.26
100s ea 00713-0503-01 96.84

(DHS, Inc.)
REPACK
SUP, RC, 25 mg, 12s ea ... 55887-0253-12 18.00

(Quality Care Prod)
REPACK
SUP, RC, 25 mg, 12s ea ... 49999-0717-12 14.38

ANUSOL-HC (Salix Pharm)
hydrocortisone
CRE, RC, 2.5%, 30 gm .... 65649-0401-30 89.95 AT

(Salix Pharm)
hydrocortisone acetate
SUP, RC, 25 mg, 12s ea ... 65649-0411-12 100.12
24s ea 65649-0411-24 175.37

(Southwood)
REPACK
hydrocortisone
CRE, RC (W/APPLICATOR)
2.5%, 30 gm .... 58016-3004-01 30.13 AT

ANZEMET (Sanofi-Aventis)
dolasetron mesylate
SOL, IV (S.D.V.)
20 mg/ml,
0.625 ml 6s 00088-1208-06 112.46
5 ml 00088-1206-32 46.80
(M.D.V.)
20 mg/ml, 25 ml 00088-1209-26 234.00

TAB, PO, 50 mg, 5s ea 00088-1202-05 287.60
10s ea UD 00088-1202-43 575.27
100 mg, 5s ea 00088-1203-05 381.20
10s ea UD 00088-1203-43 762.41

(Phys Total Care)
REPACK
TAB, PO, 100 mg, ea 54868-4138-01 94.09
5s ea 54868-4138-00 422.68

APAP (Stat Rx)
REPACK
acetaminophen
TAB, PO, 500 mg, 20s ea .. 16590-0021-20 5.00
40s ea 16590-0021-40 10.00
50s ea 16590-0021-50 12.50

APAP AND CODEINE (Southwood)
REPACK
acetaminophen/codeine phosphate
SOL, PO, 120 mg/5 ml-12 mg/5 ml,
120 ml, C-V 58016-5598-01 5.74

APAP W/ CODEINE (Bryant Ranch)
REPACK
acetaminophen/codeine phosphate
TAB, PO, 300 mg-15 mg,
12s ea, C-III 63629-2945-01 4.54
300 mg-30 mg,
15s ea, C-III 63629-1494-05 15.56
20s ea, C-III 63629-1494-02 20.75
30s ea, C-III 63629-1494-03 31.12
50s ea, C-III 63629-1494-00 56.23
60s ea, C-III 63629-1494-08 62.24
90s ea, C-III 63629-1494-09 93.35
120s ea, C-III 63629-1494-06 119.99
300 mg-60 mg,
30s ea, C-III 63629-3031-01 45.14
60s ea, C-III 63629-3031-03 62.99
90s ea, C-III 63629-3031-04 145.28
120s ea, C-III 63629-3031-02 179.57

APAP/ASA/CAFF/CODEINE PHOS/SALICYLAMIDE
(Pfeiffer) *See RID-A-PAIN W/CODEINE*

APAP/BUTALBITAL/CAFF/CODEINE PHOS
(Breckenridge Pharm) *See ACETAMINOPHEN/BUTALBITAL/CAFFEINE/CODEINE*

(Qualitest) *See ACETAMINOPHEN/BUTALBITAL/CAFFEINE/CODEINE*

(Teva) *See ACETAMINOPHEN/BUTALBITAL/CAFFEINE/CODEINE*

(Watson) *See FIORICET WITH CODEINE*

(Watson Labs) *See ACETAMINOPHEN/BUTALBITAL/CAFFEINE/CODEINE*

(West-Ward) *See BUTALBITAL, ACETAMINOPHEN AND CAFFEINE W/ CODEINE*

APAP/BUTALBITAL/CAFFEINE (Axiom Pharmaceutical)
acetaminophen/butalbital/caffeine
TAB, PO, 325 mg-50 mg-40 mg,
100s ea 67870-0111-01 44.10
500s ea 67870-0111-05 165.10

(Major)
TAB, PO, 325 mg-50 mg-40 mg,
100s ea .... 00904-3280-60 63.35 AB
500s ea .... 00904-3280-40 247.52 AB

(Mikart)
TAB, PO, 325 mg-50 mg-40 mg,
100s ea .... 46672-0053-10 59.25 AB
500s ea .... 46672-0053-50 247.52 AB

(Qualitest)
CAP, PO, 325 mg-50 mg-40 mg,
100s ea .... 00603-2546-21 41.99 AB
TAB, PO, 325 mg-50 mg-40 mg,
100s ea .... 00603-2544-21 64.15 AB
500s ea .... 00603-2544-28 305.05 AB
1000s ea .... 00603-2544-32 591.80 AB
500 mg-50 mg-40 mg,
100s ea .... 00603-2545-21 119.99 EE
500s ea .... 00603-2545-28 565.31 EE

(Teva)
TAB, PO, 325 mg-50 mg-40 mg,
100s ea .... 00093-0854-01 43.95 AB

(West-Ward)
TAB, PO, 325 mg-50 mg-40 mg,
100s ea .... 00143-1787-01 64.15 AB
500s ea .... 00143-1787-05 305.05 AB
500 mg-50 mg-40 mg,
100s ea .... 00143-1115-01 120.00 AB
500s ea .... 00143-1115-05 565.31 AB

PROD/MFR	NDC	AWP	DP	OBC
(4u)				
REPACK				
TAB, PO, 325 mg-50 mg-40 mg,				
30s ea	10544-0353-30	29.68		AB
30s ea	42549-0553-30	29.68		AB
(A-S Medication)				
REPACK				
TAB, PO, 325 mg-50 mg-40 mg,				
30s ea	54569-2538-00	20.11		AB
60s ea	54569-2538-05	40.21		AB
100s ea	54569-2538-03	67.02		AB
500 mg-50 mg-40 mg,				
30s ea	54569-4935-00	36.00		EE
(Aidarex)				
REPACK				
TAB, PO, 325 mg-50 mg-40 mg,				
10s ea	33261-0008-10	10.70		AB
14s ea	33261-0008-14	14.98		AB
20s ea	33261-0008-20	21.40		AB
21s ea	33261-0008-21	22.47		AB
28s ea	33261-0008-28	29.96		AB
30s ea	33261-0008-30	32.00		AB
56s ea	33261-0008-56	59.92		AB
60s ea	33261-0008-60	64.20		AB
90s ea	33261-0008-90	96.30		AB
100s ea	33261-0008-00	107.00		AB
120s ea	33261-0008-02	128.40		AB
180s ea	33261-0008-03	192.60		AB
(Altura)				
REPACK				
TAB, PO, 325 mg-50 mg-40 mg,				
10s ea	63874-0448-10	4.78		AB
20s ea	63874-0448-20	9.55		AB
30s ea	63874-0448-30	14.33		AB
50s ea	63874-0448-50	23.88		AB
60s ea	63874-0448-60	28.66		AB
90s ea	63874-0448-90	42.98		AB
100s ea	63874-0448-01	47.76		AB
500s ea	63874-0448-03	238.80		AB
1000s ea	63874-0448-02	477.60		AB
(American Health)				
REPACK				
TAB, PO, 325 mg-50 mg-40 mg,				
100s ea UD	68084-0396-01	22.50		AB
(Bryant Ranch)				
REPACK				
TAB, PO, 325 mg-50 mg-40 mg,				
50s ea	63629-1774-05	108.79		AB
(DHS, Inc.)				
REPACK				
TAB, PO, 325 mg-50 mg-40 mg,				
6s ea	55887-0988-06	7.00		
20s ea	55887-0988-20	11.28		AB
30s ea	55887-0988-30	16.92		AB
40s ea	55887-0988-40	22.56		
60s ea	55887-0988-60	30.05		AB
90s ea	55887-0988-90	45.07		AB
120s ea	55887-0988-82	76.98		AB
500s ea	55887-0988-05	199.00		
(Dispensing Solutions)				
REPACK				
TAB, PO, 325 mg-50 mg-40 mg,				
12s ea	55045-1582-04	8.28		AB
20s ea	55045-1582-07	13.80		AB
30s ea	55045-1582-08	20.70		
30s ea	66336-0703-30	19.01		
45s ea	55045-1582-02	31.05		AB
50s ea	55045-1582-05	34.50		AB
60s ea	55045-1582-09	41.40		AB
60s ea	66336-0703-60	38.01		
90s ea	55045-1582-03	62.10		AB
100s ea	55045-1582-00	69.00		AB
120s ea	55045-1582-01	82.80		AB
120s ea	66336-0703-94	76.98		AB
135s ea	55045-3313-03	93.15		
(Keltman Pharma., Inc.)				
REPACK				
TAB, PO, 325 mg-50 mg-40 mg,				
60s ea	68387-0520-60	68.55		AB
120s ea	68387-0520-12	137.10		AB
(Nucare Pharm)				
REPACK				
TAB, PO, 325 mg-50 mg-40 mg,				
12s ea	66267-0039-12	7.65		AB
30s ea	66267-0039-30	17.67		EE
60s ea	66267-0039-60	53.41		
90s ea	66267-0039-90	82.49		
(PD-Rx Pharm)				
REPACK				
TAB, PO, 325 mg-50 mg-40 mg,				
10s ea	55289-0879-10	10.67		AB
15s ea	55289-0879-15	15.98		AB
20s ea	55289-0879-20	16.33		AB
30s ea	55289-0879-30	22.00		AB
(REDI-SCRIPT)				
325 mg-50 mg-40 mg,				
30s ea	58864-0857-30	22.01		AB
60s ea	55289-0879-60	39.20		AB
500 mg-50 mg-40 mg,				
12s ea	55289-0439-12	16.37		AB
(Pharma Pac)				
REPACK				
TAB, PO, 325 mg-50 mg-40 mg,				
12s ea	52959-0370-12	8.24		EE
20s ea	52959-0370-20	12.24		EE
25s ea	52959-0370-25	14.88		EE
30s ea	52959-0370-30	17.67		EE
50s ea	52959-0370-50	26.95		EE
60s ea	52959-0370-60	31.38		EE
90s ea	52959-0370-90	42.82		AB
100s ea	52959-0370-00	48.77		EE
500 mg-50 mg-40 mg,				
30s ea	52959-0913-30	27.38		AB
120s ea	52959-0913-02	102.82		AB
(Phys Total Care)				
REPACK				
TAB, PO, 325 mg-50 mg-40 mg,				
15s ea	54868-1036-00	6.90		EE
30s ea	54868-1036-01	21.00		EE
40s ea	54868-1036-05	13.43		EE
50s ea	54868-1036-03	16.95		EE
60s ea	54868-1036-04	18.66		AB
100s ea	54868-1036-02	29.07		EE
180s ea	54868-1036-06	51.53		AB
500 mg-50 mg-40 mg,				
30s ea	54868-5943-01	20.15		AB
60s ea	54868-5943-00	42.44		AB
(Physician Partner)				
REPACK				
TAB, PO, 325 mg-50 mg-40 mg,				
60s ea	21695-0209-60	76.80		AB
120s ea	21695-0209-72	153.60		AB
500 mg-50 mg-40 mg,				
8s ea	21695-0257-08	9.76		AB
(Quality Care Prod)				
REPACK				
TAB, PO, 325 mg-50 mg-40 mg,				
20s ea	49999-0151-20	11.46		EE
30s ea	49999-0151-30	17.19		EE
60s ea	49999-0151-60	34.38		EE
(Southwood)				
REPACK				
TAB, PO, 325 mg-50 mg-40 mg,				
10s ea	58016-0995-10	4.78		EE
12s ea	58016-0995-12	5.73		EE
14s ea	58016-0995-14	6.69		EE
15s ea	58016-0995-15	7.16		EE
20s ea	58016-0995-20	9.55		EE
21s ea	58016-0995-21	10.03		EE
24s ea	58016-0995-24	11.46		EE
28s ea	58016-0995-28	13.37		EE
30s ea	58016-0995-30	14.33		EE
40s ea	58016-0995-40	19.10		EE
45s ea	58016-0995-45	21.49		EE
50s ea	58016-0995-50	23.88		EE
60s ea	58016-0995-60	28.66		EE
75s ea	58016-0995-75	35.82		EE
100s ea	58016-0995-00	47.76		EE
(Stat Rx)				
REPACK				
TAB, PO, 325 mg-50 mg-40 mg,				
20s ea	16590-0022-20	21.75		
30s ea	16590-0022-30	32.62		
60s ea	16590-0022-60	65.25		
90s ea	16590-0022-90	90.50		
120s ea	16590-0022-72	120.00		
500 mg-50 mg-40 mg,				
30s ea	16590-0581-30	35.00		EE
60s ea	16590-0581-60	68.00		EE
90s ea	16590-0581-90	102.00		EE
120s ea	16590-0581-72	134.00		EE
APAP/CAFF/MAGNESIUM SAL/ PHENYLTOLOXAMINE CIT				
(Breckenridge Pharm) *See COMBIFLEX ES*				
(Cypress Pharm) *See CAFGESIC FORTE*				
(Poly) *See DURABAC FORTE*				
APAP/CAFF/PHENYLTOLOXAMINE CIT/SALICYLAMIDE				
(Breckenridge Pharm) *See COMBIFLEX*				
(Cypress Pharm) *See CAFGESIC*				
(Poly) *See DURABAC*				
APAP/CODEINE (4u)				
REPACK				
acetaminophen/codeine phosphate				
TAB, PO, 300 mg-30 mg,				
30s ea, C-III	10544-0301-30	24.36		
(DHS, Inc.)				
REPACK				
TAB, PO, 300 mg-15 mg,				
30s ea, C-III	55887-0287-30	12.00		
60s ea, C-III	55887-0287-60	24.00		
90s ea, C-III	55887-0287-90	36.00		
(Stat Rx)				
REPACK				
SOL, PO, 120 mg/5 ml-12 mg/5 ml,				
120 ml, C-V	16590-0361-04	12.00		
TAB, PO, 300 mg-30 mg,				
15s ea, C-III	16590-0023-15	13.00		
30s ea, C-III	16590-0023-30	18.50		
40s ea, C-III	16590-0023-40	24.86		
60s ea, C-III	16590-0023-60	49.20		
90s ea, C-III	16590-0023-90	56.58		
120s ea, C-III	16590-0023-72	75.44		
300 mg-60 mg,				
30s ea, C-III	16590-0472-30	30.00		
60s ea, C-III	16590-0472-60	60.00		
90s ea, C-III	16590-0472-90	90.00		
120s ea, C-III	16590-0472-72	120.00		
APAP/CODEINE PHOS/GG/PHENYLEPH HCL				
(MCR American) *See PHENFLU CD*				
(MCR American) *See PHENFLU CDX*				
APAP/CODEINE PHOS/GG/PSE HCL				
(MCR American) *See MAXIFLU CD*				
(MCR American) *See MAXIFLU CDX*				
APAP/CPM/CODEINE PHOS				
(MCR American) *See COTABFLU*				
APAP/CPM/PHENYLEPH HCL				
(Lunsco) *See PROTID*				
APAP/CPM/PHENYLEPH HCL/ PHENYLTOLOXAMINE CIT				
(Breckenridge Pharm) *See TRITAL SR*				
(U.S. Pharm) *See NOREL SR*				
APAP/DICHLORAL/ISOMETHEPTENE (Amneal)				
apap/dichloralphenazone/isometheptene mucate				
CAP, PO (GELATIN CAPSULE)				
325 mg-100 mg-65 mg,				
100s ea, C-IV	53746-0141-01	53.05		
(Aidarex)				
REPACK				
CAP, PO (GELATIN CAPSULE)				
325 mg-100 mg-65 mg,				
7s ea, C-IV	33261-0406-07	5.25		
14s ea, C-IV	33261-0406-14	10.50		
20s ea, C-IV	33261-0406-20	15.00		
21s ea, C-IV	33261-0406-21	15.75		
28s ea, C-IV	33261-0406-28	21.00		
30s ea, C-IV	33261-0406-30	22.50		
60s ea, C-IV	33261-0406-60	45.00		
90s ea, C-IV	33261-0406-90	67.50		
(Altura)				
REPACK				
CAP, PO, 325 mg-100 mg-65 mg,				
20s ea, C-IV	63874-0504-20	11.12		
28s ea, C-IV	63874-0504-28	15.56		
30s ea, C-IV	63874-0504-30	16.68		
40s ea, C-IV	63874-0504-40	22.24		
60s ea, C-IV	63874-0504-60	23.31		
75s ea, C-IV	63874-0504-75	29.13		
90s ea, C-IV	63874-0504-90	50.04		
100s ea, C-IV	63874-0504-01	38.85		
120s ea, C-IV	63874-0504-04	66.72		
(Dispensing Solutions)				
REPACK				
CAP, PO (GELATIN CAPSULE)				
325 mg-100 mg-65 mg,				
30s ea, C-IV	66336-0625-30	22.50		
90s ea, C-IV	66336-0625-90	60.07		

PROD/MFR	NDC	AWP	DP	OBC
(Nucare Pharm)				
REPACK				
CAP, PO (GELATIN CAPSULE)				
325 mg-100 mg-65 mg,				
20s ea, C-IV	**66267-0354-20**	26.42		
30s ea, C-IV	**66267-0354-30**	39.60		
(PD-Rx Pharm)				
REPACK				
CAP, PO (GELATIN CAPSULE)				
325 mg-100 mg-65 mg,				
30s ea, C-IV	**55289-0842-30**	9.12		
(Pharma Pac)				
REPACK				
CAP, PO, 325 mg-100 mg-65 mg,				
20s ea, C-IV	**52959-0447-20**	12.57		
24s ea, C-IV	**52959-0447-24**	23.17		
30s ea, C-IV	**52959-0447-30**	28.81		
50s ea, C-IV	**52959-0447-50**	28.89		
60s ea, C-IV	**52959-0447-60**	42.61		
100s ea, C-IV	**52959-0447-00**	42.17		
(Phys Total Care)				
REPACK				
CAP, PO, 325 mg-100 mg-65 mg,				
10s ea, C-IV	**54868-1514-07**	22.45		
15s ea, C-IV	**54868-1514-05**	32.12		
30s ea, C-IV	**54868-1514-03**	61.26		
50s ea, C-IV	**54868-1514-04**	76.41		
60s ea, C-IV	**54868-1514-01**	90.48		
90s ea, C-IV	**54868-1514-06**	132.75		
100s ea, C-IV	**54868-1514-00**	146.82		
(Physician Partner)				
REPACK				
CAP, PO (GELATIN CAPSULE)				
325 mg-100 mg-65 mg,				
30s ea, C-IV	**21695-0275-30**	36.83		
(Southwood)				
REPACK				
CAP, PO, 325 mg-100 mg-65 mg,				
12s ea, C-IV	**58016-0288-12**	4.66		
14s ea, C-IV	**58016-0288-14**	5.44		
15s ea, C-IV	**58016-0288-15**	5.83		
18s ea, C-IV	**58016-0288-18**	6.99		
20s ea, C-IV	**58016-0288-20**	7.77		
21s ea, C-IV	**58016-0288-21**	8.16		
24s ea, C-IV	**58016-0288-24**	9.32		
25s ea, C-IV	**58016-0288-25**	9.71		
28s ea, C-IV	**58016-0288-28**	10.88		
30s ea, C-IV	**58016-0288-30**	14.62		
50s ea, C-IV	**58016-0288-50**	21.25		
60s ea, C-IV	**58016-0288-60**	23.31		
90s ea, C-IV	**58016-0288-90**	34.97		
100s ea, C-IV	**58016-0288-00**	38.85		
(Stat Rx)				
REPACK				
CAP, PO (GELATIN CAPSULE)				
325 mg-100 mg-65 mg,				
30s ea, C-IV	**16590-0318-30**	30.50		
60s ea, C-IV	**16590-0318-60**	61.00		
APAP/DICHLORALPHENAZONE/ ISOMETHEPTENE MUCATE				
(Amneal) *See APAP/DICHLORAL/ISOMETHEPTENE*				
(Breckenridge Pharm) *See MIGRAZONE*				
(Caraco) *See MIDRIN*				
(Excellium) *See EPIDRIN*				
(Palmetto)				
REPACK				
CAP, PO, 325 mg-100 mg-65 mg,				
20s ea, C-IV	**23490-5765-01**	26.40		
30s ea, C-IV	**23490-5765-03**	39.60		
APAP/DM/DIPHENHYDRAMINE HCL/PHENYLEPH HCL				
(Respa Pharm) *See RESPA C&C IR*				
APAP/DM/GG/PSE HCL				
(Breckenridge Pharm) *See FLUTABS*				
(Kowa) *See DURAFLU*				
APAP/HYDROCODONE (Dispensing Solutions)				
REPACK				
acetaminophen/hydrocodone bitartrate				
TAB, PO, 325 mg-5 mg,				
10s ea, C-III	**55045-3098-01**	7.20		
30s ea, C-III	**55045-3098-08**	21.60		
60s ea, C-III	**55045-3098-06**	43.20		
325 mg-7.5 mg,				
40s ea, C-III	**55045-3057-04**	30.80		
50s ea, C-III	**55045-3057-05**	38.50		
60s ea, C-III	**55045-3057-06**	46.20		
90s ea, C-III	**55045-3057-09**	69.30		
100s ea, C-III	**55045-3057-01**	77.00		
(Keltman Pharma., Inc.)				
REPACK				
TAB, PO, 500 mg-7.5 mg,				
15s ea, C-III	**68387-0230-15**	18.45		
750 mg-7.5 mg,				
120s ea, C-III	**68387-0400-12**	96.00		
APAP/HYDROCODONE BITARTRATE (Covidien)				
acetaminophen/hydrocodone bitartrate				
CAP, PO, 500 mg-5 mg,				
100s ea, C-III	**00406-4357-01**	22.61		AA
ELI, PO, 473 ml, C-III	**00406-0375-16**	58.12		AA
TAB, PO, 325 mg-5 mg,				
100s ea, C-III	**00406-0365-01**	54.20		
(10X10)				
325 mg-5 mg,				
100s ea UD, C-III	**00406-0365-62**	54.20		
325 mg-7.5 mg,				
100s ea, C-III	**00406-0366-01**	61.83		
(10X10)				
325 mg-7.5 mg,				
100s ea UD, C-III	**00406-0366-62**	61.83		
325 mg-10 mg,				
100s ea, C-III	**00406-0367-01**	70.25		AA
(10X10)				
325 mg-10 mg,				
100s ea UD, C-III	**00406-0367-62**	110.00		AA
500s ea, C-III	**00406-0367-05**	338.95		AA
5000s ea, C-III	**00406-0367-91**	3400.00		AA
500 mg-5 mg,				
100s ea, C-III	**00406-0357-01**	31.75		AA
(10X10)				
500 mg-5 mg,				
100s ea UD, C-III	**00406-0357-62**	43.75		AA
500s ea, C-III	**00406-0357-05**	98.43		AA
(BULK)				
500 mg-5 mg,				
5000s ea, C-III	**00406-0357-91**	1000.00		AA
500 mg-7.5 mg,				
100s ea, C-III	**00406-0358-01**	42.84		AA
(10X10)				
500 mg-7.5 mg,				
100s ea UD, C-III	**00406-0358-62**	50.50		AA
500s ea, C-III	**00406-0358-05**	172.80		AA
(BULK)				
500 mg-7.5 mg,				
5000s ea, C-III	**00406-0358-91**	1750.00		AA
500 mg-10 mg,				
100s ea, C-III	**00406-0363-01**	53.27		AA
(10X10)				
500 mg-10 mg,				
100s ea UD, C-III	**00406-0363-62**	53.75		AA
500s ea, C-III	**00406-0363-05**	253.03		AA
5000s ea, C-III	**00406-0363-91**	2550.00		AA
650 mg-7.5 mg,				
100s ea, C-III	**00406-0359-01**	44.72		AA
500s ea, C-III	**00406-0359-05**	178.88		AA
650 mg-10 mg,				
100s ea, C-III	**00406-0361-01**	53.20		AA
(10X10)				
650 mg-10 mg,				
100s ea UD, C-III	**00406-0361-62**	115.55		AA
500s ea, C-III	**00406-0361-05**	244.72		AA
5000s ea, C-III	**00406-0361-91**	2450.00		AA
660 mg-10 mg,				
100s ea, C-III	**00406-0362-01**	61.17		AA
750 mg-7.5 mg,				
100s ea, C-III	**00406-0360-01**	39.50		AA
500s ea, C-III	**00406-0360-05**	177.75		AA
5000s ea, C-III	**00406-0360-91**	1800.00		AA
750 mg-10 mg,				
100s ea, C-III	**00406-0364-01**	111.55		
(Cypress Pharm)				
ELI, PO (FRUIT)				
473 ml, C-III	**60258-0720-16**	56.79		AA
(Ethex)				
ELI, PO (FRUIT)				
473 ml, C-III	**58177-0909-07**	61.85		AA
(Major)				
TAB, PO (10X10,CAPLET)				
500 mg-5 mg,				
100s ea UD, C-III	**00904-3440-61**	51.46		AA
(10X10)				
750 mg-7.5 mg,				
100s ea UD, C-III	**00904-7632-61**	51.25		AA
(Qualitest)				
ELI, PO, 473 ml, C-III	**00603-1295-58**	58.12		AA
TAB, PO, 325 mg-10 mg,				
100s ea, C-III	**00603-3887-21**	69.90		AA
500s ea, C-III	**00603-3887-28**	337.28		AA
1000s ea, C-III	**00603-3887-32**	667.81		AA
(CAPLET)				
500 mg-5 mg,				
30s ea, C-III	**00603-3881-16**	13.50		AA
50s ea, C-III	**00603-3881-19**	22.50		AA
60s ea, C-III	**00603-3881-20**	26.99		AA
90s ea, C-III	**00603-3881-02**	40.49		AA
100s ea, C-III	**00603-3881-21**	44.99		AA
(CAPLET)				
500 mg-5 mg,				
120s ea, C-III	**00603-3881-22**	53.99		AA
180s ea, C-III	**00603-3881-04**	79.29		AA
500s ea, C-III	**00603-3881-28**	209.26		AA
(CAPLET)				
500 mg-5 mg,				
1000s ea, C-III	**00603-3881-32**	414.34		AA
500 mg-7.5 mg,				
30s ea, C-III	**00603-3882-16**	17.69		AA
60s ea, C-III	**00603-3882-20**	35.39		AA
90s ea, C-III	**00603-3882-02**	53.08		AA
100s ea, C-III	**00603-3882-21**	57.21		AA
120s ea, C-III	**00603-3882-22**	63.71		AA
500s ea, C-III	**00603-3882-28**	257.46		AA
(CAPLET)				
500 mg-7.5 mg,				
1000s ea, C-III	**00603-3882-32**	489.17		AA
500 mg-10 mg,				
30s ea, C-III	**00603-3888-16**	16.47		AA
60s ea, C-III	**00603-3888-20**	32.95		AA
90s ea, C-III	**00603-3888-02**	49.42		AA
100s ea, C-III	**00603-3888-21**	53.27		AA
120s ea, C-III	**00603-3888-22**	62.60		AA
180s ea, C-III	**00603-3888-04**	93.91		AA
500s ea, C-III	**00603-3888-28**	253.03		AA
1000s ea, C-III	**00603-3888-32**	480.76		AA
(CAPLET)				
650 mg-7.5 mg,				
100s ea, C-III	**00603-3884-21**	69.51		AA
500s ea, C-III	**00603-3884-28**	292.51		AA
650 mg-10 mg,				
30s ea, C-III	**00603-3885-16**	30.24		AA
60s ea, C-III	**00603-3885-20**	60.47		AA
90s ea, C-III	**00603-3885-02**	90.70		AA
100s ea, C-III	**00603-3885-21**	97.76		AA
120s ea, C-III	**00603-3885-22**	112.47		AA
180s ea, C-III	**00603-3885-04**	168.71		AA
500s ea, C-III	**00603-3885-28**	454.57		AA
1000s ea, C-III	**00603-3885-32**	890.95		AA
660 mg-10 mg,				
100s ea, C-III	**00603-3886-21**	61.17		AA
500s ea, C-III	**00603-3886-28**	296.67		AA
(CAPLET)				
750 mg-7.5 mg,				
100s ea, C-III	**00603-3883-21**	43.78		AA
500s ea, C-III	**00603-3883-28**	204.54		AA
1000s ea, C-III	**00603-3883-32**	400.89		AA
(St. Mary's MPP)				
TAB, PO (CAPLET)				
500 mg-10 mg,				
30s ea, C-III	**60760-0540-30**	22.70		AA
(Vintage)				
TAB, PO, 325 mg-10 mg,				
100s ea, C-III	**00254-3601-28**	69.90		AA
(CAPLET)				
500 mg-7.5 mg,				
500s ea, C-III	**00254-3594-35**	257.46		AA
(Watson)				
TAB, PO, 660 mg-10 mg,				
100s ea, C-III	**62037-0567-01**	26.93		AA
(Watson Labs)				
TAB, PO (CAPLET)				
325 mg-5 mg,				
100s ea, C-III	**00591-3202-01**	36.01		AA
325 mg-7.5 mg,				
100s ea, C-III	**00591-3203-01**	40.68		AA
325 mg-10 mg,				
100s ea, C-III	**00591-0853-01**	38.41		AA
500s ea, C-III	**00591-0853-05**	199.50		AA
500 mg-2.5 mg,				
100s ea, C-III	**00591-0388-01**	33.35		AA
500 mg-5 mg,				
100s ea, C-III	**00591-0349-01**	5.51		AA
500s ea, C-III	**00591-0349-05**	29.05		AA
500 mg-7.5 mg,				
100s ea, C-III	**00591-0385-01**	7.69		AA
500s ea, C-III	**00591-0385-05**	32.66		AA

PROD/MFR	NDC	AWP	DP	OBC
(CAPLET)				
500 mg-10 mg,				
100s ea, C-III	00591-0540-01	22.72		AA
500s ea, C-III	00591-0540-05	94.06		AA
650 mg-7.5 mg,				
100s ea, C-III	00591-0502-01	7.13		AA
500s ea, C-III	00591-0502-05	31.69		AA
650 mg-10 mg,				
100s ea, C-III	00591-0503-01	9.30		AA
500s ea, C-III	00591-0503-05	38.89		AA
750 mg-7.5 mg,				
100s ea, C-III	00591-0387-01	9.92		AA
500s ea, C-III	00591-0387-05	32.96		AA
750 mg-10 mg,				
100s ea, C-III	00591-3228-01	111.55		AA
(4u)				
REPACK				
TAB, PO (CAPLET)				
325 mg-5 mg,				
30s ea, C-III	10544-0356-30	48.86		AA
30s ea, C-III	42549-0556-30	48.86		AA
60s ea, C-III	10544-0356-60	86.26		AA
60s ea, C-III	42549-0556-60	86.26		AA
90s ea, C-III	10544-0356-90	118.32		AA
90s ea, C-III	42549-0556-90	118.32		AA
325 mg-7.5 mg,				
28s ea, C-III	10544-0357-28	47.08		AA
28s ea, C-III	42549-0557-28	49.56		AA
30s ea, C-III	10544-0357-30	48.28		AA
30s ea, C-III	42549-0557-30	50.54		AA
40s ea, C-III	42549-0557-40	98.86		AA
56s ea, C-III	10544-0357-56	72.28		AA
56s ea, C-III	42549-0557-56	74.69		AA
60s ea, C-III	10544-0357-60	73.82		AA
60s ea, C-III	42549-0557-60	75.90		AA
90s ea, C-III	10544-0357-90	92.16		AA
90s ea, C-III	42549-0557-90	95.48		AA
112s ea, C-III	10544-0357-02	114.82		AA
112s ea, C-III	42549-0557-02	117.80		AA
325 mg-10 mg,				
28s ea, C-III	10544-0314-28	58.12		AA
28s ea, C-III	42549-0514-28	58.12		AA
30s ea, C-III	10544-0314-30	57.26		AA
30s ea, C-III	42549-0514-30	59.96		AA
40s ea, C-III	42549-0514-40	65.46		AA
60s ea, C-III	42549-0514-60	76.26		AA
90s ea, C-III	42549-0514-90	106.88		AA
112s ea, C-III	10544-0314-02	128.92		AA
112s ea, C-III	42549-0514-02	128.92		AA
120s ea, C-III	42549-0514-12	138.24		AA
140s ea, C-III	10544-0314-04	156.82		AA
140s ea, C-III	42549-0514-04	156.82		AA
500 mg-5 mg,				
28s ea, C-III	42549-0609-28	46.88		AA
30s ea, C-III	42549-0609-30	48.22		AA
40s ea, C-III	42549-0609-40	58.08		AA
60s ea, C-III	42549-0609-60	86.26		AA
84s ea, C-III	42549-0609-84	122.24		AA
90s ea, C-III	42549-0609-90	128.78		AA
112s ea, C-III	42549-0609-02	154.76		AA
140s ea, C-III	42549-0609-04	204.58		AA
(A-S Medication)				
REPACK				
TAB, PO, 325 mg-5 mg,				
10s ea, C-III	54569-5523-01	5.42		AA
20s ea, C-III	54569-5523-00	10.84		AA
(CAPLET)				
325 mg-5 mg,				
60s ea, C-III	54569-5523-02	32.53		AA
500 mg-5 mg,				
4s ea, C-III	54569-3322-05	2.52		AA
6s ea, C-III	54569-0303-07	3.78		AA
10s ea, C-III	54569-0303-06	6.29		AA
12s ea, C-III	54569-0303-09	7.55		AA
14s ea, C-III	54569-5962-01	8.39		AA
15s ea, C-III	54569-0303-00	9.44		AA
16s ea, C-III	54569-3322-01	10.07		AA
20s ea, C-III	54569-0303-01	12.59		AA
24s ea, C-III	54569-0303-08	15.11		AA
30s ea, C-III	54569-0303-02	18.88		AA
40s ea, C-III	54569-0303-03	25.18		AA
50s ea, C-III	54569-0303-05	31.25		AA
60s ea, C-III	54569-3322-07	37.50		AA
90s ea, C-III	54569-3322-08	56.25		AA
100s ea, C-III	54569-0303-04	62.50		AA
120s ea, C-III	54569-5962-00	75.00		AA
180s ea, C-III	54569-3322-09	107.86		AA
500 mg-7.5 mg,				
15s ea, C-III	54569-3911-06	8.58		EE
20s ea, C-III	54569-3911-01	11.44		EE
30s ea, C-III	54569-3911-05	17.16		EE
40s ea, C-III	54569-5945-00	22.88		EE
50s ea, C-III	54569-3911-00	28.61		EE
60s ea, C-III	54569-3911-04	34.33		EE
150s ea, C-III	54569-5963-00	85.82		EE
500 mg-10 mg,				
30s ea, C-III	54569-5481-02	15.98		AA
40s ea, C-III	54569-5481-05	21.31		
60s ea, C-III	54569-5481-00	31.96		AA
90s ea, C-III	54569-5481-07	47.94		
100s ea, C-III	54569-5481-01	53.27		
120s ea, C-III	54569-5481-03	63.92		AA
150s ea, C-III	54569-5481-06	79.91		
(CAPLET)				
650 mg-10 mg,				
10s ea, C-III	54569-4272-07	9.78		AA
15s ea, C-III	54569-5964-01	14.66		AA
20s ea, C-III	54569-4272-01	19.55		EE
30s ea, C-III	54569-4272-04	29.33		EE
40s ea, C-III	54569-4272-05	39.10		EE
45s ea, C-III	54569-4272-08	43.99		EE
60s ea, C-III	54569-4272-00	58.66		EE
90s ea, C-III	54569-4272-02	87.98		EE
100s ea, C-III	54569-4272-03	97.76		EE
120s ea, C-III	54569-4272-06	117.31		EE
150s ea, C-III	54569-5964-00	146.64		EE
750 mg-7.5 mg,				
6s ea, C-III	54569-3909-03	2.63		EE
10s ea, C-III	54569-3909-04	4.38		EE
15s ea, C-III	54569-3909-01	6.57		EE
20s ea, C-III	54569-3909-00	8.76		EE
30s ea, C-III	54569-3909-02	13.13		EE
60s ea, C-III	54569-3909-05	26.27		EE
90s ea, C-III	54569-5517-01	39.40		EE
(CAPLET)				
750 mg-7.5 mg,				
120s ea, C-III	54569-5517-00	52.54		AA
150s ea, C-III	54569-5965-00	65.67		EE
(Aidarex)				
REPACK				
TAB, PO (CAPLET)				
325 mg-5 mg,				
7s ea, C-III	33261-0053-07	5.60		AA
14s ea, C-III	33261-0053-14	11.20		AA
20s ea, C-III	33261-0053-20	16.00		AA
21s ea, C-III	33261-0053-21	16.80		AA
28s ea, C-III	33261-0053-28	22.40		AA
30s ea, C-III	33261-0053-30	24.00		AA
60s ea, C-III	33261-0053-60	48.00		AA
90s ea, C-III	33261-0053-90	72.00		AA
120s ea, C-III	33261-0053-02	96.00		AA
325 mg-7.5 mg,				
7s ea, C-III	33261-0055-07	6.58		AA
14s ea, C-III	33261-0055-14	13.16		AA
20s ea, C-III	33261-0055-20	18.80		AA
21s ea, C-III	33261-0055-21	19.74		AA
28s ea, C-III	33261-0055-28	26.32		AA
30s ea, C-III	33261-0055-30	28.20		AA
60s ea, C-III	33261-0055-60	56.40		AA
90s ea, C-III	33261-0055-90	84.60		AA
100s ea, C-III	33261-0055-00	94.00		AA
120s ea, C-III	33261-0055-02	117.60		AA
180s ea, C-III	33261-0055-03	176.40		AA
325 mg-10 mg,				
56s ea, C-III	33261-0058-56	81.20		AA
500 mg-5 mg,				
36s ea, C-III	33261-0054-36	43.92		AA
500 mg-7.5 mg,				
7s ea, C-III	33261-0056-07	6.86		AA
10s ea, C-III	33261-0056-10	9.80		AA
14s ea, C-III	33261-0056-14	13.72		AA
20s ea, C-III	33261-0056-20	19.60		AA
21s ea, C-III	33261-0056-21	20.58		AA
25s ea, C-III	33261-0056-25	24.50		AA
28s ea, C-III	33261-0056-28	27.44		AA
30s ea, C-III	33261-0056-30	29.40		AA
36s ea, C-III	33261-0056-36	35.28		AA
40s ea, C-III	33261-0056-40	39.20		AA
50s ea, C-III	33261-0056-50	49.00		AA
60s ea, C-III	33261-0056-60	58.80		AA
90s ea, C-III	33261-0056-90	88.20		AA
120s ea, C-III	33261-0056-02	117.60		AA
(CAPLET)				
500 mg-10 mg,				
7s ea, C-III	33261-0218-07	9.87		AA
14s ea, C-III	33261-0218-14	19.74		AA
20s ea, C-III	33261-0218-20	28.20		AA
21s ea, C-III	33261-0218-21	29.61		AA
25s ea, C-III	33261-0218-25	35.25		AA
28s ea, C-III	33261-0218-28	39.48		AA
30s ea, C-III	33261-0218-30	42.30		AA
36s ea, C-III	33261-0218-36	50.76		AA
40s ea, C-III	33261-0218-40	56.40		AA
50s ea, C-III	33261-0218-50	70.50		AA
60s ea, C-III	33261-0218-60	84.60		AA
90s ea, C-III	33261-0218-90	126.90		AA
100s ea, C-III	33261-0218-00	141.00		AA
120s ea, C-III	33261-0218-02	169.20		AA
180s ea, C-III	33261-0218-03	253.80		AA
650 mg-7.5 mg,				
14s ea, C-III	33261-0379-14	23.80		AA
20s ea, C-III	33261-0379-20	34.00		AA
28s ea, C-III	33261-0379-28	47.60		AA
30s ea, C-III	33261-0379-30	51.00		AA
60s ea, C-III	33261-0379-60	102.00		AA
90s ea, C-III	33261-0379-90	153.00		AA
120s ea, C-III	33261-0379-02	204.00		AA
180s ea, C-III	33261-0379-03	306.00		AA
650 mg-10 mg,				
24s ea, C-III	33261-0059-24	40.80		AA
25s ea, C-III	33261-0059-25	42.50		AA
36s ea, C-III	33261-0059-36	61.20		AA
50s ea, C-III	33261-0059-50	85.00		AA
180s ea, C-III	33261-0059-03	306.00		AA
750 mg-7.5 mg,				
7s ea, C-III	33261-0057-07	7.84		AA
14s ea, C-III	33261-0057-14	15.68		AA
20s ea, C-III	33261-0057-20	22.40		AA
21s ea, C-III	33261-0057-21	23.52		AA
28s ea, C-III	33261-0057-28	31.36		AA
30s ea, C-III	33261-0057-30	33.60		AA
40s ea, C-III	33261-0057-40	44.80		AA
56s ea, C-III	33261-0057-56	62.72		AA
60s ea, C-III	33261-0057-60	67.20		AA
90s ea, C-III	33261-0057-90	100.80		AA
120s ea, C-III	33261-0057-02	134.40		AA
180s ea, C-III	33261-0057-03	201.60		AA
(Altura)				
REPACK				
TAB, PO (CAPLET)				
325 mg-5 mg,				
45s ea, C-III	63874-1092-05	29.70		AA
90s ea, C-III	63874-1092-09	59.40		AA
325 mg-10 mg,				
10s ea, C-III	63874-0834-10	8.30		AA
15s ea, C-III	63874-0834-15	12.45		AA
20s ea, C-III	63874-0834-20	16.60		AA
24s ea, C-III	63874-0834-24	19.92		AA
28s ea, C-III	63874-0834-28	23.24		AA
30s ea, C-III	63874-0834-30	24.90		AA
40s ea, C-III	63874-0834-40	33.20		AA
42s ea, C-III	63874-0834-42	34.86		AA
50s ea, C-III	63874-0834-50	41.50		AA
56s ea, C-III	63874-0834-56	46.48		AA
60s ea, C-III	63874-0834-60	49.80		AA
84s ea, C-III	63874-0834-84	69.72		AA
90s ea, C-III	63874-0834-90	74.70		AA
99s ea, C-III	63874-0834-99	86.24		AA
100s ea, C-III	63874-0834-01	83.00		AA
112s ea, C-III	63874-0834-71	92.96		AA
120s ea, C-III	63874-0834-04	99.60		AA
126s ea, C-III	63874-0834-79	104.58		AA
150s ea, C-III	63874-0834-72	124.50		AA
168s ea, C-III	63874-0834-73	139.44		AA
180s ea, C-III	63874-0834-88	139.44		AA
200s ea, C-III	63874-0834-74	166.00		AA
224s ea, C-III	63874-0834-76	185.92		AA
252s ea, C-III	63874-0834-83	209.16		AA
300s ea, C-III	63874-0834-77	249.00		AA
500 mg-5 mg,				
5s ea, C-III	63874-0203-05	3.10		AA
6s ea, C-III	63874-0203-06	3.72		AA
9s ea, C-III	63874-0203-09	5.58		AA
10s ea, C-III	63874-0203-10	6.20		AA
12s ea, C-III	63874-0203-12	7.44		EE
14s ea, C-III	63874-0203-14	8.68		AA
15s ea, C-III	63874-0203-15	9.30		EE
16s ea, C-III	63874-0203-16	9.92		AA
18s ea, C-III	63874-0203-18	11.16		AA
20s ea, C-III	63874-0203-20	12.40		EE
24s ea, C-III	63874-0203-24	14.88		EE
25s ea, C-III	63874-0203-25	15.50		AA
27s ea, C-III	63874-0203-27	16.74		AA
28s ea, C-III	63874-0203-28	17.36		AA
30s ea, C-III	63874-0203-30	18.60		EE
35s ea, C-III	63874-0203-35	21.70		AA
36s ea, C-III	63874-0203-36	22.32		AA
40s ea, C-III	63874-0203-40	24.80		AA
42s ea, C-III	63874-0203-42	26.04		AA
45s ea, C-III	63874-0203-45	25.58		AA
50s ea, C-III	63874-0203-50	31.00		EE
56s ea, C-III	63874-0203-56	34.72		AA
60s ea, C-III	63874-0203-60	37.20		AA

PROD/MFR	NDC	AWP	DP	OBC
80s ea, C-III	63874-0203-80	45.48		AA
84s ea, C-III	63874-0203-84	52.08		AA
90s ea, C-III	63874-0203-90	55.80		AA
96s ea, C-III	63874-0203-96	59.52		AA
100s ea, C-III	63874-0203-01	62.00		EE
112s ea, C-III	63874-0203-71	69.44		AA
120s ea, C-III	63874-0203-04	74.40		AA
126s ea, C-III	63874-0203-79	78.12		AA
150s ea, C-III	63874-0203-72	93.00		AA
168s ea, C-III	63874-0203-73	104.16		AA
180s ea, C-III	63874-0203-88	111.60		AA
200s ea, C-III	63874-0203-74	124.00		AA
224s ea, C-III	63874-0203-76	138.88		AA
300s ea, C-III	63874-0203-77	186.00		AA
500s ea, C-III	63874-0203-03	574.00		AA
500 mg-7.5 mg,				
12s ea, C-III	63874-0295-12	10.08		AA
15s ea, C-III	63874-0295-15	12.60		AA
20s ea, C-III	63874-0295-20	16.80		AA
25s ea, C-III	63874-0295-25	21.00		AA
30s ea, C-III	63874-0295-30	25.20		AA
35s ea, C-III	63874-0295-35	29.40		AA
40s ea, C-III	63874-0295-40	33.60		AA
42s ea, C-III	63874-0295-42	35.28		AA
50s ea, C-III	63874-0295-50	42.00		AA
56s ea, C-III	63874-0295-56	47.04		AA
60s ea, C-III	63874-0295-60	50.40		AA
84s ea, C-III	63874-0295-84	70.56		AA
90s ea, C-III	63874-0295-90	75.60		AA
100s ea, C-III	63874-0295-01	84.00		AA
112s ea, C-III	63874-0295-71	94.08		AA
120s ea, C-III	63874-0295-04	100.80		AA
150s ea, C-III	63874-0295-72	126.00		AA
168s ea, C-III	63874-0295-73	141.12		AA
180s ea, C-III	63874-0295-88	141.12		AA
200s ea, C-III	63874-0295-74	168.00		AA
224s ea, C-III	63874-0295-76	188.16		AA
300s ea, C-III	63874-0295-77	252.00		AA
(CAPLET)				
500 mg-10 mg,				
10s ea, C-III	63874-0293-10	8.60		AA
14s ea, C-III	63874-0293-14	12.04		AA
15s ea, C-III	63874-0293-15	12.90		AA
18s ea, C-III	63874-0293-08	15.48		AA
20s ea, C-III	63874-0293-20	17.20		AA
21s ea, C-III	63874-0293-21	18.06		AA
28s ea, C-III	63874-0293-28	24.08		AA
30s ea, C-III	63874-0293-30	25.80		AA
40s ea, C-III	63874-0293-40	34.40		AA
42s ea, C-III	63874-0293-42	36.12		AA
50s ea, C-III	63874-0293-50	43.00		AA
56s ea, C-III	63874-0293-56	48.16		AA
60s ea, C-III	63874-0293-60	51.60		AA
84s ea, C-III	63874-0293-84	72.24		AA
90s ea, C-III	63874-0293-90	77.40		AA
100s ea, C-III	63874-0293-01	86.00		AA
112s ea, C-III	63874-0293-71	96.32		AA
120s ea, C-III	63874-0293-04	103.20		AA
150s ea, C-III	63874-0293-72	129.00		AA
168s ea, C-III	63874-0293-73	144.48		AA
180s ea, C-III	63874-0293-18	154.80		AA
180s ea, C-III	63874-0293-88	144.48		AA
200s ea, C-III	63874-0293-74	172.00		AA
224s ea, C-III	63874-0293-76	192.64		AA
300s ea, C-III	63874-0293-77	258.00		AA
650 mg-7.5 mg,				
20s ea, C-III	63874-1074-02	18.80		AA
30s ea, C-III	63874-1074-03	28.20		AA
60s ea, C-III	63874-1074-06	56.40		AA
90s ea, C-III	63874-1074-09	84.60		AA
100s ea, C-III	63874-1074-00	94.00		AA
120s ea, C-III	63874-1074-04	112.80		AA
180s ea, C-III	63874-1074-08	112.80		AA
650 mg-10 mg,				
6s ea, C-III	63874-0861-06	7.38		AA
10s ea, C-III	63874-0861-10	12.30		AA
12s ea, C-III	63874-0861-12	14.76		AA
15s ea, C-III	63874-0861-15	18.45		AA
20s ea, C-III	63874-0861-20	24.60		AA
25s ea, C-III	63874-0861-25	30.75		AA
30s ea, C-III	63874-0861-30	36.90		AA
35s ea, C-III	63874-0861-35	43.05		AA
40s ea, C-III	63874-0861-40	49.20		AA
42s ea, C-III	63874-0861-42	51.66		AA
50s ea, C-III	63874-0861-50	61.50		AA
56s ea, C-III	63874-0861-56	68.88		AA
60s ea, C-III	63874-0861-60	73.80		AA
84s ea, C-III	63874-0861-84	103.32		AA
90s ea, C-III	63874-0861-90	110.70		AA
100s ea, C-III	63874-0861-01	123.00		AA
112s ea, C-III	63874-0861-71	137.76		AA
115s ea, C-III	63874-0861-78	141.45		AA
120s ea, C-III	63874-0861-04	147.60		AA
126s ea, C-III	63874-0861-79	154.98		AA
150s ea, C-III	63874-0861-72	184.50		AA
168s ea, C-III	63874-0861-73	206.64		AA
180s ea, C-III	63874-0861-88	206.64		AA
200s ea, C-III	63874-0861-74	246.00		AA
224s ea, C-III	63874-0861-76	275.52		AA
252s ea, C-III	63874-0861-83	309.96		AA
300s ea, C-III	63874-0861-77	369.00		AA
750 mg-7.5 mg,				
5s ea, C-III	63874-0230-05	3.33		AA
10s ea, C-III	63874-0230-10	6.60		AA
12s ea, C-III	63874-0230-12	7.92		AA
14s ea, C-III	63874-0230-14	9.24		AA
15s ea, C-III	63874-0230-15	9.90		AA
16s ea, C-III	63874-0230-16	10.56		AA
20s ea, C-III	63874-0230-20	13.20		AA
24s ea, C-III	63874-0230-24	15.84		AA
25s ea, C-III	63874-0230-25	16.50		AA
28s ea, C-III	63874-0230-28	18.48		AA
30s ea, C-III	63874-0230-30	19.80		AA
35s ea, C-III	63874-0230-35	23.10		AA
40s ea, C-III	63874-0230-40	26.40		AA
42s ea, C-III	63874-0230-42	27.72		AA
45s ea, C-III	63874-0230-45	29.70		AA
50s ea, C-III	63874-0230-50	33.00		AA
56s ea, C-III	63874-0230-56	36.96		AA
60s ea, C-III	63874-0230-60	39.60		AA
70s ea, C-III	63874-0230-70	46.20		AA
75s ea, C-III	63874-0230-75	49.50		AA
84s ea, C-III	63874-0230-84	55.44		AA
90s ea, C-III	63874-0230-90	59.40		AA
100s ea, C-III	63874-0230-01	66.00		AA
112s ea, C-III	63874-0230-71	73.92		AA
120s ea, C-III	63874-0230-04	79.20		AA
150s ea, C-III	63874-0230-72	99.00		AA
168s ea, C-III	63874-0230-73	110.88		AA
180s ea, C-III	63874-0230-88	118.80		AA
200s ea, C-III	63874-0230-74	132.00		AA
224s ea, C-III	63874-0230-76	147.84		AA
300s ea, C-III	63874-0230-77	198.00		AA
500s ea, C-III	63874-0230-03	400.25		AA
(American Health)				
REPACK				
TAB, PO, 500 mg-5 mg,				
100s ea UD, C-III	62584-0738-01	15.00		AA
(10X10)				
750 mg-7.5 mg,				
100s ea UD, C-III	68084-0144-01	17.50		AA
(Bryant Ranch)				
REPACK				
TAB, PO (CAPLET)				
325 mg-7.5 mg,				
40s ea, C-III	63629-3342-05	33.99		AA
500 mg-5 mg,				
6s ea, C-III	63629-1532-00	8.23		AA
500 mg-10 mg,				
20s ea, C-III	63629-3092-09	20.83		AA
84s ea, C-III	63629-3092-06	87.50		AA
(DHS, Inc.)				
REPACK				
TAB, PO (CAPLET)				
325 mg-7.5 mg,				
30s ea, C-III	55887-0444-30	28.00		AA
60s ea, C-III	55887-0444-60	55.00		AA
90s ea, C-III	55887-0444-90	68.00		AA
325 mg-10 mg,				
30s ea, C-III	55887-0443-30	38.00		AA
60s ea, C-III	55887-0443-60	62.00		AA
90s ea, C-III	55887-0443-90	82.00		AA
120s ea, C-III	55887-0443-82	108.00		AA
500 mg-5 mg,				
6s ea, C-III	55887-0952-06	6.00		AA
10s ea, C-III	55887-0952-10	10.00		AA
12s ea, C-III	55887-0952-12	12.00		EE
13s ea, C-III	55887-0952-13	17.40		AA
15s ea, C-III	55887-0952-15	15.00		AA
20s ea, C-III	55887-0952-20	20.00		EE
25s ea, C-III	55887-0952-25	25.00		AA
30s ea, C-III	55887-0952-30	30.00		EE
40s ea, C-III	55887-0952-40	33.00		AA
45s ea, C-III	55887-0952-45	36.00		AA
50s ea, C-III	55887-0952-50	39.00		AA
60s ea, C-III	55887-0952-60	42.00		AA
90s ea, C-III	55887-0952-90	120.45		AA
120s ea, C-III	55887-0952-82	82.00		AA
500 mg-7.5 mg,				
20s ea, C-III	55887-0447-20	19.00		AA
30s ea, C-III	55887-0447-30	27.00		AA
60s ea, C-III	55887-0447-60	46.00		AA
90s ea, C-III	55887-0447-90	65.61		AA
120s ea, C-III	55887-0447-82	91.59		AA
(CAPLET)				
500 mg-10 mg,				
20s ea, C-III	55887-0538-20	21.00		AA
30s ea, C-III	55887-0538-30	31.00		AA
60s ea, C-III	55887-0538-60	53.95		AA
90s ea, C-III	55887-0538-90	72.55		AA
120s ea, C-III	55887-0538-82	105.75		AA
650 mg-7.5 mg,				
15s ea, C-III	55887-0680-15	15.26		AA
20s ea, C-III	55887-0680-20	21.00		AA
30s ea, C-III	55887-0680-30	32.00		AA
40s ea, C-III	55887-0680-40	40.70		AA
45s ea, C-III	55887-0680-45	44.00		AA
60s ea, C-III	55887-0680-60	61.04		AA
650 mg-10 mg,				
10s ea, C-III	55887-0679-10	14.22		AA
15s ea, C-III	55887-0679-15	19.00		
20s ea, C-III	55887-0679-20	24.00		AA
(CAPLET)				
650 mg-10 mg,				
21s ea, C-III	55887-0679-21	25.19		AA
30s ea, C-III	55887-0679-30	35.99		AA
32s ea, C-III	55887-0679-32	38.39		
40s ea, C-III	55887-0679-40	47.98		AA
50s ea, C-III	55887-0679-50	60.00		
60s ea, C-III	55887-0679-60	71.68		AA
90s ea, C-III	55887-0679-90	107.61		AA
(CAPLET)				
650 mg-10 mg,				
150s ea, C-III	55887-0679-86	134.52		AA
180s ea, C-III	55887-0679-92	161.42		AA
750 mg-7.5 mg,				
10s ea, C-III	55887-0623-10	10.00		AA
14s ea, C-III	55887-0623-14	13.50		AA
20s ea, C-III	55887-0623-20	18.00		AA
30s ea, C-III	55887-0623-30	27.00		AA
60s ea, C-III	55887-0623-60	40.01		AA
90s ea, C-III	55887-0623-90	53.89		AA
120s ea, C-III	55887-0623-82	66.99		AA
(Dispensing Solutions)				
REPACK				
TAB, PO (CAPLET)				
325 mg-5 mg,				
30s ea, C-III	66336-0670-30	27.50		AA
40s ea, C-III	55045-3098-04	28.80		AA
60s ea, C-III	66336-0670-60	55.00		AA
100s ea, C-III	55045-3098-00	72.00		
325 mg-7.5 mg,				
30s ea, C-III	55045-3057-08	23.15		
30s ea, C-III	66336-0115-30	28.00		AA
60s ea, C-III	66336-0116 60	55.00		AA
90s ea, C-III	66336-0115-90	68.00		AA
120s ea, C-III	55045-3057-02	92.40		
325 mg-10 mg,				
20s ea, C-III	55045-2849-07	17.20		AA
20s ea, C-III	55045-2921-07	16.50		AA
21s ea, C-III	66336-0444-21	21.70		AA
30s ea, C-III	55045-2921-08	24.90		AA
30s ea, C-III	66336-0444-30	31.00		AA
45s ea, C-III	55045-2921-03	37.35		AA
50s ea, C-III	55045-2921-05	41.50		AA
60s ea, C-III	55045-2921-09	49.80		AA
60s ea, C-III	55045-3753-06	49.80		
60s ea, C-III	66336-0444-60	62.00		AA
90s ea, C-III	55045-2921-06	74.70		AA
90s ea, C-III	66336-0444-90	93.00		AA
100s ea, C-III	55045-2921-01	83.00		AA
120s ea, C-III	55045-2921-02	99.60		
120s ea, C-III	66336-0444-94	124.00		AA
126s ea, C-III	55045-3713-01	104.58		
135s ea, C-III	55045-3304-03	112.05		AA
160s ea, C-III	55045-2921-04	132.80		AA
180s ea, C-III	66336-0444-62	186.00		AA
200s ea, C-III	55045-2921-00	166.00		AA
240s ea, C-III	55045-3304-04	199.20		AA
252s ea, C-III	55045-3713-02	209.16		
500 mg-2.5 mg,				
20s ea, C-III	55045-2935-07	10.80		AA
500 mg-5 mg,				
6s ea, C-III	55045-1213-02	3.30		AA
10s ea, C-III	55045-3331-01	5.50		AA
10s ea, C-III	66336-0442-10	6.80		AA

PROD/MFR	NDC	AWP	DP	OBC
12s ea, C-III	55045-1213-04	6.60		AA
12s ea, C-III	66336-0442-12	8.17		AA
15s ea, C-III	55045-1213-05	8.25		AA
15s ea, C-III	66336-0442-15	8.81		AA
16s ea, C-III	66336-0442-16	12.42		AA
20s ea, C-III	55045-1213-07	11.00		AA
20s ea, C-III	66336-0442-20	13.62		AA
24s ea, C-III	55045-1213-06	13.20		AA
24s ea, C-III	66336-0442-24	16.34		AA
30s ea, C-III	55045-1213-08	16.40		AA
30s ea, C-III	66336-0442-30	22.45		AA
35s ea, C-III	55045-3125-05	19.25		AA
40s ea, C-III	55045-1213-03	21.98		AA
45s ea, C-III	55045-3125-04	24.55		AA
50s ea, C-III	55045-3125-02	27.50		AA
60s ea, C-III	55045-1213-09	32.99		AA
60s ea, C-III	66336-0442-60	40.85		AA
90s ea, C-III	55045-3125-09	49.50		AA
90s ea, C-III	66336-0442-90	61.26		AA
100s ea, C-III	55045-1213-01	55.90		AA
120s ea, C-III	55045-1213-00	65.95		AA
(CAPLET)				
500 mg-5 mg,				
120s ea, C-III	66336-0442-94	81.68		AA
135s ea, C-III	55045-3125-03	74.25		AA
180s ea, C-III	55045-3125-00	99.00		AA
500 mg-7.5 mg,				
6s ea, C-III	55045-3010-02	5.04		AA
10s ea, C-III	55045-3330-01	8.40		AA
14s ea, C-III	55045-3010-03	11.76		AA
15s ea, C-III	66336-0012-15	13.19		EE
20s ea, C-III	55045-3010-07	16.85		AA
20s ea, C-III	66336-0012-20	17.59		EE
30s ea, C-III	55045-3010-08	25.50		AA
30s ea, C-III	66336-0012-30	26.39		EE
40s ea, C-III	55045-3010-04	33.50		AA
50s ea, C-III	55045-3330-05	42.00		AA
60s ea, C-III	55045-3010-06	50.40		AA
60s ea, C-III	66336-0012-60	52.78		AA
90s ea, C-III	55045-3010-09	75.60		AA
90s ea, C-III	66336-0012-90	79.16		AA
100s ea, C-III	55045-3010-00	84.00		AA
120s ea, C-III	55045-3010-01	100.80		AA
500 mg-10 mg,				
ea, C-III	66336-0408-30	28.67		AA
(CAPLET)				
500 mg-10 mg,				
15s ea, C-III	66336-0408-15	16.78		AA
24s ea, C-III	55045-2849-02	20.64		AA
(CAPLET)				
500 mg-10 mg,				
28s ea, C-III	66336-0408-28	26.76		AA
30s ea, C-III	55045-2849-08	25.75		AA
(CAPLET)				
500 mg-10 mg,				
32s ea, C-III	66336-0408-32	30.58		AA
40s ea, C-III	55045-2849-04	34.25		AA
50s ea, C-III	55045-2849-05	43.00		AA
60s ea, C-III	66336-0408-60	57.34		AA
(CAPLET)				
500 mg-10 mg,				
60s ea, C-III	55045-2849-06	51.65		AA
90s ea, C-III	55045-2849-09	77.40		AA
90s ea, C-III	66336-0408-90	86.01		AA
100s ea, C-III	55045-2849-00	86.00		AA
120s ea, C-III	55045-2849-01	103.20		AA
(CAPLET)				
500 mg-10 mg,				
120s ea, C-III	66336-0408-94	114.68		AA
150s ea, C-III	66336-0408-97	143.35		AA
650 mg-7.5 mg,				
20s ea, C-III	55045-2539-07	18.85		AA
30s ea, C-III	55045-2539-08	28.20		AA
(CAPLET)				
650 mg-7.5 mg,				
40s ea, C-III	55045-2539-04	37.60		AA
60s ea, C-III	55045-2539-06	56.40		AA
90s ea, C-III	55045-2539-09	84.60		AA
100s ea, C-III	55045-2539-01	94.00		AA
APAP/HYDROCODONE BITARTRATE				
(Dispensing Solutions)				
REPACK				
acetaminophen/hydrocodone bitartrate				
TAB, PO (CAPLET)				
650 mg-7.5 mg,				
120s ea, C-III	55045-2539-00	112.80		AA
650 mg-10 mg,				
15s ea, C-III	66336-0406-15	17.74		AA
(CAPLET)				
650 mg-10 mg,				
20s ea, C-III	55045-2386-07	24.60		AA
21s ea, C-III	66336-0406-21	24.83		AA
(CAPLET)				
650 mg-10 mg,				
30s ea, C-III	55045-2386-08	36.90		AA
30s ea, C-III	55045-2623-08	36.90		AA
40s ea, C-III	55045-2386-09	49.20		
(CAPLET)				
650 mg-10 mg,				
50s ea, C-III	55045-2386-06	61.50		AA
60s ea, C-III	55045-3752-06	73.80		
60s ea, C-III	66336-0406-60	70.94		AA
(CAPLET)				
650 mg-10 mg,				
60s ea, C-III	55045-2623-06	73.80		AA
84s ea, C-III	55045-2386-04	103.32		AA
90s ea, C-III	55045-2623-09	110.70		AA
90s ea, C-III	66336-0406-90	107.61		AA
100s ea, C-III	55045-2623-00	123.00		AA
120s ea, C-III	66336-0406-94	120.00		AA
(CAPLET)				
650 mg-10 mg,				
120s ea, C-III	55045-2386-01	147.60		AA
120s ea, C-III	55045-2623-01	147.60		AA
126s ea, C-III	55045-3714-01	154.98		
660 mg-10 mg,				
30s ea, C-III	55045-3265-08	29.75		AA
90s ea, C-III	55045-3265-09	89.10		AA
750 mg-7.5 mg,				
12s ea, C-III	55045-1980-04	7.20		AA
12s ea, C-III	66336-0106-12	9.41		AA
15s ea, C-III	55045-1980-02	9.00		AA
15s ea, C-III	66336-0106-15	11.76		AA
20s ea, C-III	55045-1980-07	12.00		AA
20s ea, C-III	66336-0106-20	15.69		AA
30s ea, C-III	55045-1980-05	18.00		AA
30s ea, C-III	66336-0106-30	23.53		AA
40s ea, C-III	55045-1980-06	24.10		AA
45s ea, C-III	55045-3151-04	27.10		AA
50s ea, C-III	55045-1980-03	30.10		AA
60s ea, C-III	55045-1980-09	36.00		AA
60s ea, C-III	66336-0106-60	47.06		AA
84s ea, C-III	55045-3151-01	50.00		AA
90s ea, C-III	55045-1980-08	54.00		AA
90s ea, C-III	66336-0106-90	70.59		AA
100s ea, C-III	55045-1980-00	60.00		AA
120s ea, C-III	55045-3151-02	72.00		AA
135s ea, C-III	55045-3151-03	81.00		AA
(CAPLET)				
750 mg-7.5 mg,				
180s ea, C-III	55045-3151-08	108.00		AA
(GSMS)				
REPACK				
TAB, PO, 500 mg-5 mg,				
10s ea, C-III	60429-0509-10	4.35	1.45	EE
25s ea, C-III	60429-0509-25	6.90	2.30	EE
(HomeMed)				
REPACK				
TAB, PO, 500 mg-5 mg,				
90s ea, C-III	51655-0812-26	24.74		
120s ea, C-III	51655-0812-82	32.66		
(IPI)				
REPACK				
TAB, PO (CAPLET)				
325 mg-5 mg,				
60s ea, C-III	18837-0067-60	40.67		AA
120s ea, C-III	18837-0067-98	81.30		
325 mg-7.5 mg,				
60s ea, C-III	18837-0068-60	62.66		
500 mg-7.5 mg,				
30s ea, C-III	18837-0065-30	10.37		AA
(CAPLET)				
500 mg-7.5 mg,				
40s ea, C-III	18837-0065-40	29.29		AA
50s ea, C-III	18837-0065-50	38.50		AA
650 mg-7.5 mg,				
30s ea, C-III	18837-0062-30	21.94		AA
750 mg-7.5 mg,				
120s ea, C-III	18837-0069-98	42.66		AA
(Keltman Pharma., Inc.)				
REPACK				
TAB, PO (CAPLET)				
325 mg-5 mg,				
40s ea, C-III	68387-0236-40	39.25		AA
90s ea, C-III	68387-0236-90	88.31		AA
325 mg-7.5 mg,				
40s ea, C-III	68387-0237-40	42.35		AA
90s ea, C-III	68387-0237-90	95.28		AA
120s ea, C-III	68387-0237-12	127.05		AA
325 mg-10 mg,				
40s ea, C-III	68387-0235-40	45.64		AA
90s ea, C-III	68387-0235-90	102.69		AA
120s ea, C-III	68387-0235-12	136.92		AA
500 mg-5 mg,				
30s ea, C-III	68387-0300-30	21.25		AA
60s ea, C-III	68387-0300-60	42.50		AA
90s ea, C-III	68387-0300-90	63.75		AA
120s ea, C-III	68387-0300-12	85.00		AA
500 mg-7.5 mg,				
10s ea, C-III	68387-0230-10	12.30		AA
30s ea, C-III	68387-0230-30	36.90		AA
36s ea, C-III	68387-0230-36	44.28		AA
40s ea, C-III	68387-0230-40	52.40		AA
42s ea, C-III	68387-0230-42	51.66		AA
50s ea, C-III	68387-0230-50	61.50		AA
60s ea, C-III	68387-0230-60	73.80		AA
90s ea, C-III	68387-0230-90	110.70		AA
100s ea, C-III	68387-0230-01	123.00		AA
120s ea, C-III	68387-0230-12	147.60		AA
150s ea, C-III	68387-0230-51	187.50		AA
(CAPLET)				
500 mg-10 mg,				
30s ea, C-III	68387-0220-30	36.90		AA
50s ea, C-III	68387-0220-50	65.50		AA
60s ea, C-III	68387-0220-60	78.60		AA
(CAPLET)				
500 mg-10 mg,				
90s ea, C-III	68387-0220-90	117.90		AA
100s ea, C-III	68387-0220-01	131.00		AA
(CAPLET)				
500 mg-10 mg,				
150s ea, C-III	68387-0220-51	196.50		AA
650 mg-10 mg,				
30s ea, C-III	68387-0200-30	36.78		AA
60s ea, C-III	68387-0200-60	73.56		AA
90s ea, C-III	68387-0200-90	110.34		AA
100s ea, C-III	68387-0200-12	147.12		AA
750 mg-7.5 mg,				
30s ea, C-III	68387-0400-30	24.00		AA
36s ea, C-III	68387-0400-36	28.80		AA
42s ea, C-III	68387-0400-42	33.60		AA
50s ea, C-III	68387-0400-50	30.13		AA
60s ea, C-III	68387-0400-60	48.00		AA
90s ea, C-III	68387-0400-90	72.00		AA
100s ea, C-III	68387-0400-01	80.00		AA
(McKesson Packaging)				
REPACK				
TAB, PO, 500 mg-5 mg,				
100s ea UD, C-III	63739-0130-10	52.31		AA
(BLISTER PACK)				
500 mg-5 mg,				
750s ea UD, C-III	63739-0130-01	392.36		AA
(PUNCH CARD 25X30)				
500 mg-5 mg,				
750s ea, C-III	63739-0130-03	392.36		AA
500 mg-7.5 mg,				
100s ea UD, C-III	63739-0141-10	46.58		EE
750 mg-7.5 mg,				
100s ea UD, C-III	63739-0131-10	48.92		EE
(Medsource)				
REPACK				
TAB, PO (CAPLET)				
325 mg-7.5 mg,				
30s ea, C-III	45865-0419-30	28.50		AA
60s ea, C-III	45865-0419-60	57.00		AA
84s ea, C-III	45865-0419-84	79.80		AA
90s ea, C-III	45865-0419-90	85.50		AA
100s ea, C-III	45865-0419-00	95.00		AA
100s ea, C-III	45865-0419-49	95.00		AA
120s ea, C-III	45865-0419-01	114.00		AA
120s ea, C-III	45865-0419-51	114.00		AA
126s ea, C-III	45865-0419-52	119.70		AA
150s ea, C-III	45865-0419-02	142.50		AA
252s ea, C-III	45865-0419-59	239.40		AA
300s ea, C-III	45865-0419-05	285.00		AA
325 mg-10 mg,				
30s ea, C-III	45865-0411-30	28.50		AA
60s ea, C-III	45865-0411-60	57.00		AA
84s ea, C-III	45865-0411-84	79.80		AA
90s ea, C-III	45865-0411-90	85.50		AA
100s ea, C-III	45865-0411-00	95.00		AA
100s ea, C-III	45865-0411-49	95.00		AA
120s ea, C-III	45865-0411-01	114.00		AA
126s ea, C-III	45865-0411-52	119.70		AA
150s ea, C-III	45865-0411-02	142.50		AA
252s ea, C-III	45865-0411-59	239.40		AA
300s ea, C-III	45865-0411-05	285.00		AA
500 mg-5 mg,				
30s ea, C-III	45865-0407-30	22.50		AA
60s ea, C-III	45865-0407-60	45.00		AA
90s ea, C-III	45865-0407-90	67.50		AA
100s ea, C-III	45865-0407-00	75.00		AA
120s ea, C-III	45865-0407-01	90.00		AA
150s ea, C-III	45865-0407-02	112.50		AA
300s ea, C-III	45865-0407-05	225.00		AA

PROD/MFR	NDC	AWP	DP	OBC
650 mg-7.5 mg,				
100s ea, C-III	45865-0412-00	75.00		AA
120s ea, C-III	45865-0412-01	90.00		AA
150s ea, C-III	45865-0412-02	112.50		AA
300s ea, C-III	45865-0412-05	225.00		AA
750 mg-7.5 mg,				
30s ea, C-III	45865-0410-30	25.50		AA
60s ea, C-III	45865-0410-60	51.24		AA
90s ea, C-III	45865-0410-90	76.86		AA
100s ea, C-III	45865-0410-00	85.40		AA
120s ea, C-III	45865-0410-01	102.48		AA
150s ea, C-III	45865-0410-02	128.10		AA
300s ea, C-III	45865-0410-05	256.20		AA
(Nucare Pharm)				
REPACK				
TAB, PO, 325 mg-5 mg,				
30s ea, C-III	68071-0296-30	22.35		
40s ea, C-III	68071-0296-40	29.70		
60s ea, C-III	68071-0296-60	44.74		
90s ea, C-III	68071-0296-90	66.83		
120s ea, C-III	68071-0296-91	89.43		
325 mg-7.5 mg,				
30s ea, C-III	68071-0301-30	25.51		
40s ea, C-III	68071-0301-40	34.01		
60s ea, C-III	68071-0301-60	68.93		
90s ea, C-III	68071-0301-90	76.55		
325 mg-10 mg,				
20s ea, C-III	66267-0319-20	38.78		EE
30s ea, C-III	66267-0319-30	58.16		AA
40s ea, C-III	66267-0319-40	77.55		AA
60s ea, C-III	66267-0319-60	116.35		EE
90s ea, C-III	66267-0319-90	176.96		AA
100s ea, C-III	68071-1361-00	193.95		AA
120s ea, C-III	66267-0319-91	235.95		AA
140s ea, C-III	66267-0319-88	275.28		EE
180s ea, C-III	66267-0319-92	353.93		AA
500 mg-5 mg,				
4s ea, C-III	66267-0109-04	8.99		EE
6s ea, C-III	66267-0109-06	10.97		EE
12s ea, C-III	66267-0109-12	20.67		EE
15s ea, C-III	66267-0109-15	28.91		AA
20s ea, C-III	66267-0109-20	33.29		EE
24s ea, C-III	66267-0109-24	36.45		EE
30s ea, C-III	66267-0109-30	43.78		EE
40s ea, C-III	66267-0109-40	58.37		AA
45s ea, C-III	66267-0109-45	72.23		AA
50s ea, C-III	66267-0109-50	80.25		AA
60s ea, C-III	66267-0109-60	91.93		AA
90s ea, C-III	66267-0109-90	137.90		AA
100s ea, C-III	68071-1360-00	145.00		AA
120s ea, C-III	66267-0109-91	175.12		AA
500 mg-7.5 mg,				
12s ea, C-III	66267-0110-12	11.05		EE
15s ea, C-III	66267-0110-15	21.09		AA
20s ea, C-III	66267-0110-20	17.89		EE
30s ea, C-III	66267-0110-30	28.26		AA
40s ea, C-III	66267-0110-40	33.33		EE
50s ea, C-III	66267-0110-50	42.35		AA
60s ea, C-III	66267-0110-60	46.75		AA
90s ea, C-III	66267-0110-90	72.17		AA
120s ea, C-III	66267-0110-91	90.85		AA
140s ea, C-III	66267-0110-88	85.12		EE
150s ea, C-III	66267-0110-81	113.56		AA
180s ea, C-III	66267-0110-92	109.80		EE
500 mg-10 mg,				
30s ea, C-III	66267-0108-30	44.86		EE
60s ea, C-III	66267-0108-60	76.49		EE
90s ea, C-III	66267-0108-90	68.36		EE
120s ea, C-III	66267-0108-91	128.52		AA
140s ea, C-III	66267-0108-88	103.69		EE
180s ea, C-III	66267-0108-92	136.39		EE
650 mg-7.5 mg,				
30s ea, C-III	66267-0405-30	24.13		AA
60s ea, C-III	66267-0405-60	48.27		AA
650 mg-10 mg,				
15s ea, C-III	66267-0297-15	18.76		AA
30s ea, C-III	66267-0297-30	36.89		EE
40s ea, C-III	66267-0297-40	49.18		AA
50s ea, C-III	66267-0297-50	62.50		AA
60s ea, C-III	66267-0297-60	73.78		EE
90s ea, C-III	66267-0297-90	110.66		AA
120s ea, C-III	66267-0297-91	179.40		AA
750 mg-7.5 mg,				
15s ea, C-III	66267-0111-15	11.40		AA
20s ea, C-III	66267-0111-20	15.20		AA
30s ea, C-III	66267-0111-30	22.89		AA
40s ea, C-III	66267-0111-40	33.60		AA
60s ea, C-III	66267-0111-60	45.60		AA
90s ea, C-III	66267-0111-90	75.60		AA
120s ea, C-III	66267-0111-91	100.80		AA
(Palmetto)				
REPACK				
ELI, PO (1X120ML,FRUIT)				
120 ml, C-III	23490-7085-00	166.00		AA
(PD-Rx Pharm)				
REPACK				
TAB, PO, 325 mg-7.5 mg,				
20s ea, C-III	55289-0802-20	51.50		AA
(CAPLET)				
325 mg-7.5 mg,				
60s ea, C-III	55289-0802-60	75.90		AA
90s ea, C-III	55289-0802-90	113.80		AA
325 mg-10 mg,				
6s ea, C-III	55289-0737-06	24.65		AA
60s ea, C-III	55289-0737-60	93.35		AA
100s ea, C-III	55289-0737-01	122.25		AA
500 mg-5 mg,				
6s ea, C-III	55289-0137-06	18.65		AA
10s ea, C-III	55289-0137-10	20.00		AA
(REDI-SCRIPT)				
500 mg-5 mg,				
10s ea, C-III	58864-0271-10	20.00		AA
12s ea, C-III	55289-0137-12	20.65		AA
15s ea, C-III	55289-0137-15	21.65		AA
16s ea, C-III	58864-0271-16	21.98		AA
20s ea, C-III	55289-0137-20	23.35		AA
(REDI-SCRIPT)				
500 mg-5 mg,				
20s ea, C-III	58864-0271-20	23.35		AA
24s ea, C-III	55289-0137-24	24.65		AA
25s ea, C-III	55289-0137-25	25.00		AA
(REDI-SCRIPT)				
500 mg-5 mg,				
25s ea, C-III	58864-0271-25	25.00		AA
30s ea, C-III	55289-0137-30	26.65		AA
30s ea, C-III	58864-0271-30	26.65		AA
40s ea, C-III	55289-0137-40	30.00		AA
60s ea, C-III	55289-0137-60	36.65		AA
90s ea, C-III	55289-0137-90	46.65		AA
120s ea, C-III	55289-0137-98	56.65		AA
500 mg-7.5 mg,				
10s ea, C-III	55289-0268-10	21.10		AA
(REDI-SCRIPT)				
500 mg-7.5 mg,				
15s ea, C-III	58864-0699-15	23.35		AA
16s ea, C-III	58864-0699-16	23.80		AA
20s ea, C-III	55289-0268-20	25.55		AA
(REDI-SCRIPT)				
500 mg-7.5 mg,				
20s ea, C-III	58864-0699-20	25.55		AA
30s ea, C-III	55289-0268-30	30.00		
45s ea, C-III	55289-0268-45	37.50		AA
60s ea, C-III	55289-0268-60	43.35		AA
90s ea, C-III	55289-0268-90	56.65		AA
500 mg-10 mg,				
40s ea, C-III	55289-0965-40	48.25		AA
(CAPLET)				
500 mg-10 mg,				
100s ea, C-III	55289-0965-01	90.40		AA
120s ea, C-III	55289-0965-98	103.00		AA
650 mg-7.5 mg,				
15s ea, C-III	55289-0534-15	25.85		AA
90s ea, C-III	55289-0534-90	71.65		EE
650 mg-10 mg,				
20s ea, C-III	55289-0311-20	24.45		AA
60s ea, C-III	55289-0311-60	40.00		AA
90s ea, C-III	55289-0311-90	56.65		AA
750 mg-7.5 mg,				
6s ea, C-III	55289-0360-06	19.35		AA
12s ea, C-III	55289-0360-12	22.00		AA
15s ea, C-III	55289-0360-15	22.90		AA
16s ea, C-III	55289-0360-16	23.80		AA
20s ea, C-III	55289-0360-20	25.55		AA
24s ea, C-III	55289-0360-24	27.35		AA
30s ea, C-III	55289-0360-30	30.00		AA
60s ea, C-III	55289-0360-60	43.35		AA
90s ea, C-III	55289-0360-90	56.65		AA
100s ea, C-III	55289-0360-01	63.65		AA
(Pharma Pac)				
REPACK				
TAB, PO, 325 mg-5 mg,				
15s ea, C-III	52959-0737-15	9.76		
20s ea, C-III	52959-0737-20	12.99		
25s ea, C-III	52959-0737-25	14.32		
30s ea, C-III	52959-0737-30	19.18		
40s ea, C-III	52959-0737-40	25.21		
45s ea, C-III	52959-0737-45	28.37		
50s ea, C-III	52959-0737-50	30.98		
60s ea, C-III	52959-0737-60	34.19		
90s ea, C-III	52959-0737-90	49.51		
120s ea, C-III	52959-0737-02	65.98		
325 mg-7.5 mg,				
30s ea, C-III	52959-0735-30	38.73		
60s ea, C-III	52959-0735-60	77.25		
90s ea, C-III	52959-0735-90	115.02		
100s ea, C-III	52959-0735-00	127.60		
120s ea, C-III	52959-0735-12	152.88		
(CAPLET)				
325 mg-7.5 mg,				
126s ea, C-III	52959-0735-03	160.39		AA
325 mg-10 mg,				
10s ea, C-III	52959-0324-10	10.39		AA
15s ea, C-III	52959-0324-15	15.58		AA
20s ea, C-III	52959-0324-20	20.77		AA
24s ea, C-III	52959-0324-24	24.92		EE
25s ea, C-III	52959-0324-25	25.95		AA
30s ea, C-III	52959-0324-30	31.14		AA
40s ea, C-III	52959-0324-40	41.52		AA
50s ea, C-III	52959-0324-50	51.89		EE
60s ea, C-III	52959-0324-60	62.26		AA
90s ea, C-III	52959-0324-90	93.35		AA
100s ea, C-III	52959-0324-00	117.08		AA
120s ea, C-III	52959-0324-02	124.42		AA
126s ea, C-III	52959-0324-06	130.57		AA
150s ea, C-III	52959-0324-05	155.40		AA
180s ea, C-III	52959-0324-08	186.56		AA
240s ea, C-III	52959-0324-03	248.40		AA
252s ea, C-III	52959-0324-01	260.69		AA
500 mg-5 mg,				
4s ea, C-III	52959-0312-04	2.88		EE
6s ea, C-III	52959-0312-06	4.32		EE
8s ea, C-III	52959-0312-08	5.75		EE
10s ea, C-III	52959-0312-10	7.19		EE
12s ea, C-III	52959-0312-12	8.62		EE
14s ea, C-III	52959-0312-14	10.06		EE
15s ea, C-III	52959-0312-15	10.77		EE
16s ea, C-III	52959-0312-16	11.49		EE
20s ea, C-III	52959-0312-20	14.35		EE
24s ea, C-III	52959-0312-24	17.22		EE
25s ea, C-III	52959-0312-25	17.93		EE
28s ea, C-III	52959-0312-28	20.08		EE
30s ea, C-III	52959-0312-30	21.50		EE
35s ea, C-III	52959-0312-35	25.08		EE
40s ea, C-III	52959-0312-40	28.66		EE
45s ea, C-III	52959-0312-45	32.22		EE
50s ea, C-III	52959-0312-50	35.79		EE
58s ea, C-III	52959-0312-58	41.49		EE
60s ea, C-III	52959-0312-60	42.91		EE
84s ea, C-III	52959-0312-84	60.03		EE
90s ea, C-III	52959-0312-90	64.30		EE
100s ea, C-III	52959-0312-00	71.39		EE
120s ea, C-III	52959-0312-02	85.62		EE
180s ea, C-III	52959-0312-88	128.36		AA
500 mg-7.5 mg,				
10s ea, C-III	52959-0380-10	8.96		EE
12s ea, C-III	52959-0380-12	10.74		EE
14s ea, C-III	52959-0380-14	12.53		EE
15s ea, C-III	52959-0380-15	13.43		EE
16s ea, C-III	52959-0380-16	14.32		AA
20s ea, C-III	52959-0380-20	17.89		EE
24s ea, C-III	52959-0380-24	21.47		EE
28s ea, C-III	52959-0380-28	25.04		EE
30s ea, C-III	52959-0380-30	26.82		EE
35s ea, C-III	52959-0380-35	31.29		EE
40s ea, C-III	52959-0380-40	35.74		EE
42s ea, C-III	52959-0380-42	37.54		EE
45s ea, C-III	52959-0380-45	40.20		EE
60s ea, C-III	52959-0380-60	53.59		EE
75s ea, C-III	52959-0380-75	66.98		EE
84s ea, C-III	52959-0380-84	75.01		EE
90s ea, C-III	52959-0380-90	80.37		EE
100s ea, C-III	52959-0380-00	89.25		EE
120s ea, C-III	52959-0380-02	107.08		EE
180s ea, C-III	52959-0380-08	160.55		EE
(CAPLET)				
500 mg-10 mg,				
10s ea, C-III	52959-0521-10	10.50		AA
14s ea, C-III	52959-0521-14	12.53		AA
15s ea, C-III	52959-0521-15	13.43		AA
16s ea, C-III	52959-0521-16	14.32		AA
20s ea, C-III	52959-0521-20	17.90		AA
24s ea, C-III	52959-0521-24	20.44		AA
24s ea, C-III	52959-0521-28	23.59		AA
30s ea, C-III	52959-0521-30	25.80		AA
40s ea, C-III	52959-0521-40	33.70		AA
42s ea, C-III	52959-0521-42	35.38		AA
50s ea, C-III	52959-0521-50	41.00		AA
60s ea, C-III	52959-0521-60	47.76		AA
80s ea, C-III	52959-0521-80	63.64		AA
84s ea, C-III	52959-0521-84	66.82		AA
90s ea, C-III	52959-0521-90	71.56		AA
100s ea, C-III	52959-0521-00	79.50		AA
120s ea, C-III	52959-0521-02	95.37		AA
126s ea, C-III	52959-0521-03	100.06		AA
180s ea, C-III	52959-0521-18	142.83		AA

PROD/MFR	NDC	AWP	DP	OBC
650 mg-7.5 mg,				
20s ea, C-III	52959-0372-20	15.90		EE
30s ea, C-III	52959-0372-30	23.50		EE
40s ea, C-III	52959-0372-40	30.50		EE
50s ea, C-III	52959-0372-50	37.50		EE
60s ea, C-III	52959-0372-60	44.50		EE
90s ea, C-III	52959-0372-90	62.57		EE
100s ea, C-III	52959-0372-00	69.50		EE
120s ea, C-III	52959-0372-02	83.37		EE
650 mg-10 mg,				
4s ea, C-III	52959-0371-04	6.48		EE
12s ea, C-III	52959-0371-12	19.32		EE
15s ea, C-III	52959-0371-15	24.00		EE
20s ea, C-III	52959-0371-20	31.80		EE
24s ea, C-III	52959-0371-24	34.82		AA
30s ea, C-III	52959-0371-30	42.00		EE
35s ea, C-III	52959-0371-35	40.24		EE
40s ea, C-III	52959-0371-40	55.60		EE
50s ea, C-III	52959-0371-50	69.25		EE
60s ea, C-III	52959-0371-60	82.80		EE
75s ea, C-III	52959-0371-75	103.31		EE
90s ea, C-III	52959-0371-90	124.20		EE
100s ea, C-III	52959-0371-00	137.00		EE
120s ea, C-III	52959-0371-02	164.40		EE
180s ea, C-III	52959-0371-18	246.60		EE
660 mg-10 mg,				
20s ea, C-III	52959-0071-20	9.20		AA
120s ea, C-III	52959-0071-02	75.75		AA
750 mg-7.5 mg,				
10s ea, C-III	52959-0415-10	7.20		EE
12s ea, C-III	52959-0415-12	8.69		EE
15s ea, C-III	52959-0415-15	10.80		AA
20s ea, C-III	52959-0415-20	14.39		EE
24s ea, C-III	52959-0415-24	17.26		EE
30s ea, C-III	52959-0415-30	21.59		EE
35s ea, C-III	52959-0415-35	25.19		EE
40s ea, C-III	52959-0415-40	28.78		EE
45s ea, C-III	52959-0415-45	32.38		EE
50s ea, C-III	52959-0415-50	35.98		EE
56s ea, C-III	52959-0415-56	40.28		EE
60s ea, C-III	52959-0415-60	43.17		EE
70s ea, C-III	52959-0415-70	50.37		EE
90s ea, C-III	52959-0415-90	64.76		EE
100s ea, C-III	52959-0415-01	71.95		EE
120s ea, C-III	52959-0415-02	86.34		EE
(Phys Total Care)				
REPACK				
TAB, PO (CAPLET)				
325 mg-5 mg,				
120s ea, C-III	54868-5146-05	101.59		AA
325 mg-7.5 mg,				
150s ea, C-III	54868-5167-08	122.21		AA
325 mg-10 mg,				
150s ea, C-III	54868-4974-08	92.03		AA
180s ea, C-III	54868-4974-09	134.94		AA
500 mg-5 mg,				
120s ea, C-III	54868-0071-06	27.54		AA
(CAPLET)				
500 mg-10 mg,				
10s ea, C-III	54868-4237-09	13.38		AA
150s ea, C-III	54868-4237-08	94.27		AA
650 mg-7.5 mg,				
30s ea, C-III	54868-3585-04	15.72		AA
660 mg-10 mg,				
60s ea, C-III	54868-5059-04	44.29		AA
90s ea, C-III	54868-5059-07	57.72		AA
120s ea, C-III	54868-5059-05	74.95		AA
150s ea, C-III	54868-5059-06	92.19		AA
(Physician Partner)				
REPACK				
ELI, PO, 480 ml, C-III	21695-0816-16	116.24		AA
TAB, PO (CAPLET)				
325 mg-5 mg,				
30s ea, C-III	21695-0268-30	32.53		AA
325 mg-7.5 mg,				
30s ea, C-III	21695-0386-30	37.12		AA
325 mg-10 mg,				
28s ea, C-III	21695-0272-28	40.25		AA
500 mg-2.5 mg,				
8s ea, C-III	21695-0579-08	6.28		AA
16s ea, C-III	21695-0579-16	12.56		AA
28s ea, C-III	21695-0579-28	21.98		AA
30s ea, C-III	21695-0579-30	23.55		AA
500 mg-5 mg,				
8s ea, C-III	21695-0269-08	8.75		AA
10s ea, C-III	21695-0269-10	10.93		AA
12s ea, C-III	21695-0269-12	13.12		AA
16s ea, C-III	21695-0269-16	17.49		AA
40s ea, C-III	21695-0269-40	43.75		AA
45s ea, C-III	21695-0269-45	49.22		AA
500 mg-7.5 mg,				
8s ea, C-III	21695-0270-08	9.69		AA
12s ea, C-III	21695-0270-12	14.54		AA
45s ea, C-III	21695-0270-45	54.52		AA
72s ea, C-III	21695-0270-72	145.37		AA
90s ea, C-III	21695-0270-90	92.67		AA
(CAPLET)				
500 mg-10 mg,				
8s ea, C-III	21695-0273-08	9.53		AA
12s ea, C-III	21695-0273-12	14.29		AA
45s ea, C-III	21695-0273-45	53.58		AA
72s ea, C-III	21695-0273-72	142.90		AA
(Quality Care Prod)				
REPACK				
TAB, PO (CAPLET)				
325 mg-5 mg,				
50s ea, C-III	49999-0608-50	110.91		AA
325 mg-7.5 mg,				
30s ea, C-III	49999-0609-30	44.40		AA
60s ea, C-III	49999-0609-60	88.80		AA
90s ea, C-III	49999-0609-90	132.20		AA
120s ea, C-III	49999-0609-01	177.60		AA
325 mg-10 mg,				
20s ea, C-III	49999-0169-20	38.18		AA
30s ea, C-III	49999-0169-30	57.27		AA
50s ea, C-III	49999-0169-50	95.50		AA
60s ea, C-III	49999-0169-60	114.54		AA
100s ea, C-III	49999-0169-00	190.90		AA
120s ea, C-III	49999-0169-01	229.08		AA
180s ea, C-III	49999-0169-18	343.62		AA
500 mg-5 mg,				
6s ea, C-III	49999-0017-06	6.66		EE
10s ea, C-III	49999-0017-10	11.10		EE
12s ea, C-III	49999-0017-12	13.32		EE
15s ea, C-III	49999-0017-15	16.65		EE
20s ea, C-III	49999-0017-20	22.20		EE
30s ea, C-III	49999-0017-30	32.80		EE
40s ea, C-III	49999-0017-40	44.40		EE
(CAPLET)				
500 mg-5 mg,				
45s ea, C-III	49999-0017-45	49.95		AA
50s ea, C-III	49999-0017-50	55.50		AA
60s ea, C-III	49999-0017-60	66.60		EE
90s ea, C-III	49999-0017-90	99.87		AA
100s ea, C-III	49999-0017-00	111.00		EE
120s ea, C-III	49999-0017-01	133.16		AA
180s ea, C-III	49999-0017-18	199.80		AA
500 mg-7.5 mg,				
ea, C-III	49999-0053-10	8.08		EE
ea, C-III	49999-0053-30	24.23		EE
5s ea, C-III	49999-0053-05	3.69		AA
15s ea, C-III	49999-0053-15	11.07		AA
20s ea, C-III	49999-0053-20	14.74		EE
40s ea, C-III	49999-0053-40	34.44		EE
50s ea, C-III	49999-0053-50	36.84		AA
60s ea, C-III	49999-0053-60	48.47		EE
90s ea, C-III	49999-0053-90	72.90		AA
100s ea, C-III	49999-0053-00	73.66		AA
120s ea, C-III	49999-0053-01	97.20		AA
500 mg-10 mg,				
15s ea, C-III	49999-0327-15	22.50		AA
30s ea, C-III	49999-0327-30	27.96		AA
60s ea, C-III	49999-0327-60	55.92		AA
90s ea, C-III	49999-0327-90	134.83		AA
100s ea, C-III	49999-0327-00	93.20		AA
120s ea, C-III	49999-0327-01	111.84		AA
650 mg-7.5 mg,				
20s ea, C-III	49999-0054-20	29.02		EE
30s ea, C-III	49999-0054-30	43.53		AA
650 mg-10 mg,				
10s ea, C-III	49999-0277-10	15.94		AA
15s ea, C-III	49999-0277-05	24.00		AA
20s ea, C-III	49999-0277-20	31.87		
30s ea, C-III	49999-0277-30	47.81		AA
60s ea, C-III	49999-0277-60	95.62		AA
90s ea, C-III	49999-0277-90	143.43		AA
100s ea, C-III	49999-0277-00	159.37		AA
120s ea, C-III	49999-0277-01	191.24		AA
180s ea, C-III	49999-0277-18	286.87		AA
750 mg-7.5 mg,				
2s ea, C-III	49999-0052-02	3.30		AA
5s ea, C-III	49999-0052-05	4.38		AA
15s ea, C-III	49999-0052-15	9.56		EE
20s ea, C-III	49999-0052-20	14.34		EE
30s ea, C-III	49999-0052-30	24.29		EE
40s ea, C-III	49999-0052-40	28.68		EE
60s ea, C-III	49999-0052-60	48.58		EE
90s ea, C-III	49999-0052-90	72.90		EE
100s ea, C-III	49999-0052-00	71.70		EE
120s ea, C-III	49999-0052-01	97.16		EE
(Southwood)				
REPACK				
TAB, PO, 325 mg-5 mg,				
10s ea, C-III	58016-0949-10	5.42		
12s ea, C-III	58016-0949-12	6.50		
15s ea, C-III	58016-0949-15	8.13		
20s ea, C-III	58016-0949-20	10.84		
25s ea, C-III	58016-0949-25	13.55		
30s ea, C-III	58016-0949-30	16.26		
40s ea, C-III	58016-0949-40	21.68		
50s ea, C-III	58016-0949-50	27.10		
60s ea, C-III	58016-0949-60	32.52		
70s ea, C-III	58016-0949-70	37.94		
80s ea, C-III	58016-0949-80	43.36		
90s ea, C-III	58016-0949-90	48.78		
100s ea, C-III	58016-0949-00	54.20		
120s ea, C-III	58016-0949-02	65.04		
325 mg-7.5 mg,				
30s ea, C-III	58016-0928-30	18.56		
60s ea, C-III	58016-0928-60	37.12		
90s ea, C-III	58016-0928-90	55.67		
100s ea, C-III	58016-0928-00	61.86		
120s ea, C-III	58016-0928-02	74.23		
325 mg-10 mg,				
20s ea, C-III	58016-0495-20	15.69		EE
28s ea, C-III	58016-0495-28	21.97		EE
30s ea, C-III	58016-0495-30	29.10		AA
40s ea, C-III	58016-0495-40	31.39		EE
50s ea, C-III	58016-0495-50	39.24		EE
56s ea, C-III	58016-0495-56	43.94		EE
60s ea, C-III	58016-0495-60	58.20		AA
80s ea, C-III	58016-0495-80	30.80		EE
84s ea, C-III	58016-0495-84	65.91		EE
90s ea, C-III	58016-0495-90	87.30		AA
99s ea, C-III	58016-0495-99	141.24		EE
100s ea, C-III	58016-0495-00	97.00		AA
112s ea, C-III	58016-0495-92	87.89		AA
120s ea, C-III	58016-0495-02	116.40		AA
150s ea, C-III	58016-0495-03	117.71		AA
160s ea, C-III	58016-0495-71	125.55		EE
168s ea, C-III	58016-0495-93	131.83		AA
200s ea, C-III	58016-0495-89	156.94		AA
224s ea, C-III	58016-0495-91	175.77		AA
240s ea, C-III	58016-0495-04	188.33		EE
300s ea, C-III	58016-0495-73	235.41		AA
500 mg-2.5 mg,				
30s ea, C-III	58016-0436-30	2.22		AA
60s ea, C-III	58016-0436-60	4.43		AA
90s ea, C-III	58016-0436-90	6.65		AA
100s ea, C-III	58016-0436-00	7.39		AA
120s ea, C-III	58016-0436-02	8.87		AA
150s ea, C-III	58016-0436-03	11.09		AA
500 mg-5 mg,				
6s ea, C-III	58016-0276-06	3.41		EE
9s ea, C-III	58016-0276-09	5.12		EE
10s ea, C-III	58016-0276-10	5.69		EE
12s ea, C-III	58016-0276-12	6.82		EE
14s ea, C-III	58016-0276-14	7.96		EE
15s ea, C-III	58016-0276-15	8.53		EE
16s ea, C-III	58016-0276-16	9.10		EE
18s ea, C-III	58016-0276-18	10.23		EE
20s ea, C-III	58016-0276-20	11.37		EE
24s ea, C-III	58016-0276-24	13.64		EE
25s ea, C-III	58016-0276-25	14.21		EE
27s ea, C-III	58016-0276-27	15.35		EE
28s ea, C-III	58016-0276-28	15.92		EE
(CAPLET)				
500 mg-5 mg,				
30s ea, C-III	58016-0276-30	23.40		AA
36s ea, C-III	58016-0276-36	20.47		EE
40s ea, C-III	58016-0276-40	22.74		EE
42s ea, C-III	58016-0276-42	23.88		EE
45s ea, C-III	58016-0276-45	25.58		EE
50s ea, C-III	58016-0276-50	28.43		EE
56s ea, C-III	58016-0276-56	31.84		EE
(CAPLET)				
500 mg-5 mg,				
60s ea, C-III	58016-0276-60	46.80		AA
80s ea, C-III	58016-0276-80	45.48		AA
84s ea, C-III	58016-0276-84	47.75		EE
(CAPLET)				
500 mg-5 mg,				
90s ea, C-III	58016-0276-90	70.20		AA
100s ea, C-III	58016-0276-00	78.00		AA
112s ea, C-III	58016-0276-92	63.67		AA
(CAPLET)				
500 mg-5 mg,				
120s ea, C-III	58016-0276-02	93.60		AA
135s ea, C-III	58016-0276-67	76.74		AA
150s ea, C-III	58016-0276-03	85.28		AA
160s ea, C-III	58016-0276-71	90.96		AA
180s ea, C-III	58016-0276-99	102.00		AA
200s ea, C-III	58016-0276-89	113.70		AA
300s ea, C-III	58016-0276-73	170.55		AA
500 mg-7.5 mg,				
10s ea, C-III	58016-0195-10	7.49		EE
12s ea, C-III	58016-0195-12	8.99		EE
15s ea, C-III	58016-0195-15	11.23		EE
20s ea, C-III	58016-0195-20	14.98		EE

PROD/MFR	NDC	AWP	DP	OBC
25s ea, C-III	58016-0195-25	18.72		EE
30s ea, C-III	58016-0195-30	27.60		AA
50s ea, C-III	58016-0195-50	37.45		EE
60s ea, C-III	58016-0195-60	55.20		AA
90s ea, C-III	58016-0195-90	82.80		AA
100s ea, C-III	58016-0195-00	92.00		AA
120s ea, C-III	58016-0195-02	110.40		AA
150s ea, C-III	58016-0195-03	112.34		AA
200s ea, C-III	58016-0195-89	149.78		AA
300s ea, C-III	58016-0195-73	224.67		AA
500 mg-10 mg,				
10s ea, C-III	58016-0229-10	7.85		EE
14s ea, C-III	58016-0229-14	10.99		EE
20s ea, C-III	58016-0229-20	15.70		EE
21s ea, C-III	58016-0229-21	16.49		EE
28s ea, C-III	58016-0229-28	21.98		EE
30s ea, C-III	58016-0229-30	23.55		EE
40s ea, C-III	58016-0229-40	31.40		EE
50s ea, C-III	58016-0229-50	39.26		EE
(CAPLET)				
500 mg-10 mg,				
56s ea, C-III	58016-0229-56	43.97		AA
60s ea, C-III	58016-0229-60	47.11		EE
80s ea, C-III	58016-0229-80	62.81		EE
(CAPLET)				
500 mg-10 mg,				
84s ea, C-III	58016-0229-84	65.95		AA
90s ea, C-III	58016-0229-90	70.66		EE
100s ea, C-III	58016-0229-00	78.51		EE
(CAPLET)				
500 mg-10 mg,				
112s ea, C-III	58016-0229-92	87.93		AA
120s ea, C-III	58016-0229-02	94.21		EE
(CAPLET)				
500 mg-10 mg,				
150s ea, C-III	58016-0229-03	117.77		AA
168s ea, C-III	58016-0229-93	131.90		AA
180s ea, C-III	58016-0229-99	141.32		EE
(CAPLET)				
500 mg-10 mg,				
200s ea, C-III	58016-0229-89	157.02		AA
224s ea, C-III	58016-0229-91	175.86		AA
240s ea, C-III	58016-0229-04	188.42		EE
(CAPLET)				
500 mg-10 mg,				
300s ea, C-III	58016-0229-73	235.53		AA
650 mg-7.5 mg,				
6s ea, C-III	58016-0239-06	3.63		EE
10s ea, C-III	58016-0239-10	6.05		EE
12s ea, C-III	58016-0239-12	7.26		EE
15s ea, C-III	58016-0239-15	9.08		EE
20s ea, C-III	58016-0239-20	12.10		EE
25s ea, C-III	58016-0239-25	15.13		EE
30s ea, C-III	58016-0239-30	18.15		EE
40s ea, C-III	58016-0239-40	24.20		AA
60s ea, C-III	58016-0239-60	36.30		AA
90s ea, C-III	58016-0239-90	54.45		AA
100s ea, C-III	58016-0239-00	60.50		AA
120s ea, C-III	58016-0239-02	72.60		AA
150s ea, C-III	58016-0239-03	90.75		AA
200s ea, C-III	58016-0239-89	121.00		AA
300s ea, C-III	58016-0239-73	181.50		AA
650 mg-10 mg,				
6s ea, C-III	58016-0232-06	7.26		EE
10s ea, C-III	58016-0232-10	12.10		EE
12s ea, C-III	58016-0232-12	14.51		EE
15s ea, C-III	58016-0232-15	18.14		EE
20s ea, C-III	58016-0232-20	24.19		EE
25s ea, C-III	58016-0232-25	30.24		EE
30s ea, C-III	58016-0232-30	40.50		AA
40s ea, C-III	58016-0232-40	48.38		EE
50s ea, C-III	58016-0232-50	60.48		EE
60s ea, C-III	58016-0232-60	81.00		AA
90s ea, C-III	58016-0232-90	121.50		AA
100s ea, C-III	58016-0232-00	135.00		AA
120s ea, C-III	58016-0232-02	162.00		AA
126s ea, C-III	58016-0232-97	152.40		EE
150s ea, C-III	58016-0232-03	181.43		AA
200s ea, C-III	58016-0232-89	241.90		AA
300s ea, C-III	58016-0232-73	362.85		AA
660 mg-10 mg,				
10s ea, C-III	58016-0950-10	6.12		AA
20s ea, C-III	58016-0950-20	12.23		AA
30s ea, C-III	58016-0950-30	18.35		AA
40s ea, C-III	58016-0950-40	24.47		AA
50s ea, C-III	58016-0950-50	30.59		AA
60s ea, C-III	58016-0950-60	36.70		AA
90s ea, C-III	58016-0950-90	55.05		AA
100s ea, C-III	58016-0950-00	61.17		AA
120s ea, C-III	58016-0950-02	73.40		AA
750 mg-7.5 mg,				
12s ea, C-III	58016-0758-12	7.26		EE
14s ea, C-III	58016-0758-14	8.47		EE
15s ea, C-III	58016-0758-15	9.08		EE
16s ea, C-III	58016-0758-16	9.68		EE
20s ea, C-III	58016-0758-20	12.10		EE
25s ea, C-III	58016-0758-25	15.13		EE
28s ea, C-III	58016-0758-28	16.94		EE
30s ea, C-III	58016-0758-30	22.80		AA
35s ea, C-III	58016-0758-35	21.18		EE
40s ea, C-III	58016-0758-40	24.20		EE
42s ea, C-III	58016-0758-42	25.41		EE
45s ea, C-III	58016-0758-45	27.23		EE
50s ea, C-III	58016-0758-50	30.25		EE
56s ea, C-III	58016-0758-56	33.88		EE
60s ea, C-III	58016-0758-60	45.60		AA
70s ea, C-III	58016-0758-70	42.35		EE
75s ea, C-III	58016-0758-75	45.38		EE
84s ea, C-III	58016-0758-84	50.82		EE
90s ea, C-III	58016-0758-90	68.40		AA
100s ea, C-III	58016-0758-00	76.00		AA
120s ea, C-III	58016-0758-02	91.20		AA
150s ea, C-III	58016-0758-03	90.75		AA
180s ea, C-III	58016-0758-99	108.90		AA
200s ea, C-III	58016-0758-89	121.00		AA
240s ea, C-III	58016-0758-04	145.20		AA
300s ea, C-III	58016-0758-73	181.50		AA
(St. Mary's MPP)				
REPACK				
TAB, PO (CAPLET)				
325 mg-7.5 mg,				
30s ea, C-III	60760-0032-30	26.42		AA
60s ea, C-III	60760-0032-60	46.83		AA
90s ea, C-III	60760-0032-90	67.25		AA
325 mg-10 mg,				
30s ea, C-III	60760-0388-30	28.26		AA
60s ea, C-III	60760-0388-60	50.52		AA
90s ea, C-III	60760-0388-90	72.78		AA
120s ea, C-III	60760-0388-92	95.04		AA
180s ea, C-III	60760-0388-98	139.48		AA
500 mg-5 mg,				
15s ea, C-III	60760-0349-15	13.67		AA
30s ea, C-III	60760-0349-30	21.34		AA
60s ea, C-III	60760-0349-60	36.68		AA
90s ea, C-III	60760-0349-90	52.02		AA
500 mg-7.5 mg,				
15s ea, C-III	60760-0594-15	14.50		EE
30s ea, C-III	60760-0594-30	22.99		EE
60s ea, C-III	60760-0594-60	39.98		AA
90s ea, C-III	60760-0594-90	56.98		AA
(Stat Rx)				
REPACK				
TAB, PO, 325 mg-7.5 mg,				
28s ea, C-III	16590-0114-28	29.62		
40s ea, C-III	16590-0114-40	32.00		
56s ea, C-III	16590-0114-56	59.25		
240s ea, C-III	16590-0114-84	216.00		
325 mg-10 mg,				
20s ea, C-III	16590-0118-20	35.50		AA
28s ea, C-III	16590-0118-28	50.43		AA
40s ea, C-III	16590-0118-40	72.05		AA
56s ea, C-III	16590-0118-56	100.87		AA
84s ea, C-III	16590-0118-62	151.32		AA
112s ea, C-III	16590-0118-73	175.44		AA
150s ea, C-III	16590-0118-83	396.31		AA
180s ea, C-III	16590-0118-82	142.50		AA
500 mg-5 mg,				
15s ea, C-III	16590-0113-15	46.66		AA
45s ea, C-III	16590-0113-45	61.65		AA
56s ea, C-III	16590-0113-56	81.57		AA
75s ea, C-III	16590-0113-75	102.75		AA
84s ea, C-III	16590-0113-62	122.36		AA
100s ea, C-III	16590-0113-71	145.67		AA
112s ea, C-III	16590-0113-73	163.15		AA
240s ea, C-III	16590-0113-84	349.60		AA
500 mg-7.5 mg,				
15s ea, C-III	16590-0115-15	19.17		AA
20s ea, C-III	16590-0115-20	25.55		AA
28s ea, C-III	16590-0115-28	35.78		AA
30s ea, C-III	16590-0115-30	38.33		AA
40s ea, C-III	16590-0115-40	51.11		AA
45s ea, C-III	16590-0115-45	57.60		AA
50s ea, C-III	16590-0115-50	63.89		AA
56s ea, C-III	16590-0115-56	71.55		AA
60s ea, C-III	16590-0115-60	76.66		AA
75s ea, C-III	16590-0115-75	96.00		AA
84s ea, C-III	16590-0115-62	107.33		AA
90s ea, C-III	16590-0115-90	114.99		AA
100s ea, C-III	16590-0115-71	175.78		AA
112s ea, C-III	16590-0115-73	75.85		AA
120s ea, C-III	16590-0115-72	210.94		AA
150s ea, C-III	16590-0115-83	191.66		AA
180s ea, C-III	16590-0115-82	154.14		AA
240s ea, C-III	16590-0115-84	173.68		AA
500 mg-10 mg,				
40s ea, C-III	16590-0119-40	54.93		AA
56s ea, C-III	16590-0119-56	58.24		AA
75s ea, C-III	16590-0119-75	89.25		AA
84s ea, C-III	16590-0119-62	86.00		AA
112s ea, C-III	16590-0119-73	113.36		AA
150s ea, C-III	16590-0119-83	156.00		AA
180s ea, C-III	16590-0119-82	196.50		AA
240s ea, C-III	16590-0119-84	249.60		AA
650 mg-10 mg,				
50s ea, C-III	16590-0120-50	60.00		AA
660 mg-10 mg,				
30s ea, C-III	16590-0875-30	35.25		AA
60s ea, C-III	16590-0875-60	42.70		AA
90s ea, C-III	16590-0875-90	64.29		AA
120s ea, C-III	16590-0875-72	84.30		AA
750 mg-7.5 mg,				
60s ea, C-III	16590-0117-60	48.11		AA
APAP/HYDROCODONE BITARTRATE HS (Qualitest)				
acetaminophen/hydrocodone bitartrate				
TAB, PO, 500 mg-2.5 mg,				
100s ea, C-III	00603-3880-21	30.30		AA
APAP/OXYCODONE (Covidien)				
acetaminophen/oxycodone hydrochloride				
CAP, PO, 500 mg-5 mg,				
100s ea, C-II	00406-0532-01	40.25		AA
500s ea, C-II	00406-0532-05	181.13		AA
TAB, PO, 325 mg-5 mg,				
100s ea, C-II	00406-0512-01	31.05		AA
100s ea UD, C-II	00406-0512-62	32.91		AA
500s ea, C-II	00406-0512-05	108.55		AA
5000s ea, C-II	00406-0512-91	1100.00		AA
(CAPLET)				
325 mg-7.5 mg,				
100s ea, C-II	00406-0522-01	135.77		AA
(USP,CAPLET)				
325 mg-7.5 mg,				
100s ea UD, C-II	00406-0522-62	135.77		AA
(CAPLET)				
325 mg-10 mg,				
100s ea, C-II	00406-0523-01	177.54		
100s ea UD, C-II	00406-0523-62	177.54		
500 mg-7.5 mg,				
100s ea, C-II	00406-0582-01	106.05		AA
650 mg-10 mg,				
100s ea, C-II	00406-0562-01	145.65		
(Qualitest)				
CAP, PO, 500 mg-5 mg,				
100s ea, C-II	00603-4997-21	58.98		AA
TAB, PO, 325 mg-5 mg,				
100s ea, C-II	00603-4998-21	51.23		AA
500s ea, C-II	00603-4998-28	230.98		AA
(Roxane)				
CAP, PO (HARD GEL)				
500 mg-5 mg,				
100s ea, C-II	00054-2795-25	57.72		
(Teva)				
CAP, PO, 500 mg-5 mg,				
100s ea, C-II	00555-0658-02	49.50		AA
(Vintage)				
CAP, PO, 500 mg-5 mg,				
100s ea, C-II	00254-4832-28	41.67		AA
(Watson Labs)				
TAB, PO, 325 mg-5 mg,				
100s ea, C-II	00591-0749-01	5.94		AA
500s ea, C-II	00591-0749-05	28.36		AA
325 mg-7.5 mg,				
100s ea, C-II	00591-0933-01	79.64		AA
325 mg-10 mg,				
100s ea, C-II	00591-0932-01	93.12		AA
500 mg-7.5 mg,				
100s ea, C-II	00591-0824-01	82.72		AA
650 mg-10 mg,				
100s ea, C-II	00591-0825-01	82.19		AA
(4u)				
REPACK				
TAB, PO, 325 mg-5 mg,				
30s ea, C-II	10544-0382-30	66.94		AA
60s ea, C-II	10544-0382-60	120.22		AA
(CAPLET)				
325 mg-7.5 mg,				
28s ea, C-II	10544-0383-28	118.86		AA
30s ea, C-II	42549-0615-30	123.46		AA
(CAPLET)				
325 mg-7.5 mg,				
30s ea, C-II	10544-0383-30	123.46		AA
30s ea, C-II	42549-0625-30	123.46		AA
40s ea, C-II	42549-0615-40	146.68		AA
60s ea, C-II	42549-0615-60	216.72		AA
(CAPLET)				
325 mg-7.5 mg,				
60s ea, C-II	10544-0383-60	216.72		AA

PROD/MFR	NDC	AWP	DP	OBC
60s ea, C-II	42549-0625-60	216.72		AA
84s ea, C-II	10544-0383-84	358.34		AA
90s ea, C-II	42549-0615-90	364.44		AA
120s ea, C-II	42549-0615-12	398.26		AA
(CAPLET)				
325 mg-7.5 mg,				
168s ea, C-II	10544-0383-08	462.22		AA
325 mg-10 mg,				
28s ea, C-II	10544-0384-28	101.76		
84s ea, C-II	10544-0384-84	278.14		
112s ea, C-II	10544-0384-02	326.86		
650 mg-10 mg,				
168s ea, C-II	10544-0385-08	462.92		AA
(Altura)				
REPACK				
TAB, PO, 325 mg-5 mg,				
10s ea, C-II	63874-1227-01	11.91		AA
30s ea, C-II	63874-1227-03	35.74		AA
60s ea, C-II	63874-1227-06	71.47		AA
90s ea, C-II	63874-1227-09	107.21		AA
120s ea, C-II	63874-1227-00	142.94		AA
(CAPLET)				
325 mg-10 mg,				
30s ea, C-II	63874-1233-03	91.11		
60s ea, C-II	63874-1233-06	182.24		
90s ea, C-II	63874-1233-09	273.35		
120s ea, C-II	63874-1233-00	306.89		
(American Health)				
REPACK				
TAB, PO, 325 mg-7.5 mg,				
100s ea UD, C-II	68084-0379-01	100.00		AA
325 mg-10 mg,				
100s ea UD, C-II	68084-0378-01	81.70		AA
(Core)				
REPACK				
TAB, PO, 325 mg-5 mg,				
90s ea, C-II	33358-0279-90	61.98		AA
(DHS, Inc.)				
REPACK				
TAB, PO (CAPLET)				
325 mg-10 mg,				
60s ea, C-II	55887-0129-60	143.31		
(Dispensing Solutions)				
REPACK				
TAB, PO, 325 mg-5 mg,				
10s ea, C-II	66336-0145-10	14.52		AA
15s ea, C-II	66336-0145-15	21.85		AA
30s ea, C-II	66336-0145-30	43.72		AA
325 mg-7.5 mg,				
60s ea, C-II	66336-0177-60	93.89		AA
90s ea, C-II	66336-0177-90	140.93		AA
120s ea, C-II	66336-0177-94	187.78		AA
(Nucare Pharm)				
REPACK				
TAB, PO, 325 mg-5 mg,				
10s ea, C-II	68071-0158-10	15.39		AA
12s ea, C-II	68071-0158-12	18.69		AA
20s ea, C-II	68071-0158-20	30.83		AA
30s ea, C-II	68071-0158-30	46.23		AA
40s ea, C-II	68071-0158-40	103.79		AA
60s ea, C-II	68071-0158-60	155.69		AA
90s ea, C-II	68071-0158-90	234.02		AA
120s ea, C-II	68071-0158-91	312.39		AA
(CAPLET)				
325 mg-10 mg,				
10s ea, C-II	68071-0344-10	45.99		
20s ea, C-II	68071-0344-20	77.39		
30s ea, C-II	68071-0344-30	116.89		
40s ea, C-II	68071-0344-40	154.79		
90s ea, C-II	68071-0344-90	347.49		
(Phys Total Care)				
REPACK				
CAP, PO, 500 mg-5 mg,				
20s ea, C-II	54868-2771-00	23.94		EE
30s ea, C-II	54868-2771-04	21.36		AA
60s ea, C-II	54868-2771-01	56.82		EE
90s ea, C-II	54868-2771-05	49.08		AA
120s ea, C-II	54868-2771-03	82.93		EE
TAB, PO, 325 mg-5 mg,				
10s ea, C-II	54868-1700-02	10.20		EE
20s ea, C-II	54868-1700-04	14.40		EE
30s ea, C-II	54868-1700-01	18.60		EE
40s ea, C-II	54868-1700-06	22.83		EE
60s ea, C-II	54868-1700-08	31.23		AA
90s ea, C-II	54868-1700-09	43.84		AA
100s ea, C-II	54868-1700-07	49.29		AA
120s ea, C-II	54868-1700-00	39.85		AA
325 mg-7.5 mg,				
10s ea, C-II	54868-5076-00	44.28		AA
(CAPLET)				
325 mg-7.5 mg,				
10s ea, C-II	54868-5338-01	16.68		AA
20s ea, C-II	54868-5076-01	82.53		AA
30s ea, C-II	54868-5076-02	93.81		AA
(CAPLET)				
325 mg-7.5 mg,				
30s ea, C-II	54868-5338-00	59.73		AA
60s ea, C-II	54868-5338-02	88.17		AA
150s ea, C-II	54868-5338-07	207.11		AA
325 mg-10 mg,				
10s ea, C-II	54868-5024-04	26.55		AA
20s ea, C-II	54868-5024-02	47.10		AA
30s ea, C-II	54868-5024-03	67.65		AA
40s ea, C-II	54868-5024-06	121.32		
60s ea, C-II	54868-5024-00	100.29		AA
(USP)				
325 mg-10 mg,				
90s ea, C-II	54868-5024-07	207.01		
100s ea, C-II	54868-5024-01	163.17		AA
120s ea, C-II	54868-5024-05	174.30		
500 mg-7.5 mg,				
40s ea, C-II	54868-5076-04	123.06		
60s ea, C-II	54868-5076-05	108.85		
90s ea, C-II	54868-5076-06	115.71		AA
100s ea, C-II	54868-5076-03	298.65		AA
650 mg-10 mg,				
10s ea, C-II	54868-5004-01	25.77		AA
20s ea, C-II	54868-5004-02	45.57		AA
30s ea, C-II	54868-5004-03	65.34		AA
40s ea, C-II	54868-5004-04	85.14		AA
60s ea, C-II	54868-5004-00	96.76		AA
90s ea, C-II	54868-5004-05	142.14		AA
100s ea, C-II	54868-5004-07	158.77		AA
120s ea, C-II	54868-5004-06	194.49		AA
(Quality Care Prod)				
REPACK				
CAP, PO, 500 mg-5 mg,				
30s ea, C-II	35356-0343-30	129.00		AA
TAB, PO, 325 mg-5 mg,				
15s ea, C-II	49999-0852-15	49.05		AA
40s ea, C-II	49999-0852-40	130.93		AA
325 mg-10 mg,				
15s ea, C-II	49999-0854-15	49.80		AA
500 mg-7.5 mg,				
120s ea, C-II	35356-0063-01	664.00		AA
650 mg-10 mg,				
90s ea, C-II	49999-0855-90	270.25		AA
(St. Mary's MPP)				
REPACK				
TAB, PO (USP)				
325 mg-7.5 mg,				
60s ea, C-II	60760-0933-60	95.71		AA
(Stat Rx)				
REPACK				
CAP, PO, 500 mg-5 mg,				
30s ea, C-II	16590-0723-30	17.83		
40s ea, C-II	16590-0723-40	23.77		
60s ea, C-II	16590-0723-60	44.50		
90s ea, C-II	16590-0723-90	66.75		
120s ea, C-II	16590-0723-72	71.30		
TAB, PO, 325 mg-5 mg,				
15s ea, C-II	16590-0614-15	18.00		AA
30s ea, C-II	16590-0614-30	36.00		AA
45s ea, C-II	16590-0614-45	54.00		AA
60s ea, C-II	16590-0614-60	61.00		AA
75s ea, C-II	16590-0614-75	90.00		AA
84s ea, C-II	16590-0614-62	95.57		AA
90s ea, C-II	16590-0614-90	89.00		AA
100s ea, C-II	16590-0614-71	98.75		AA
120s ea, C-II	16590-0614-72	118.00		AA
180s ea, C-II	16590-0614-82	183.00		AA
325 mg-7.5 mg,				
30s ea, C-II	16590-0655-30	64.20		AA
30s ea, C-II	16590-0655-40	85.60		AA
45s ea, C-II	16590-0655-45	96.30		AA
60s ea, C-II	16590-0655-60	128.40		AA
75s ea, C-II	16590-0655-75	160.50		AA
84s ea, C-II	16590-0655-62	181.76		AA
90s ea, C-II	16590-0655-90	194.75		AA
100s ea, C-II	16590-0655-71	214.00		AA
120s ea, C-II	16590-0655-72	256.80		AA
325 mg-10 mg,				
20s ea, C-II	16590-0612-20	40.00		AA
30s ea, C-II	16590-0612-30	67.85		AA
40s ea, C-II	16590-0612-40	90.47		AA
45s ea, C-II	16590-0612-45	101.70		AA
56s ea, C-II	16590-0612-56	72.85		AA
60s ea, C-II	16590-0612-60	135.70		AA
75s ea, C-II	16590-0612-75	169.50		AA
84s ea, C-II	16590-0612-62	325.32		AA
90s ea, C-II	16590-0612-90	192.00		AA
100s ea, C-II	16590-0612-71	387.28		AA
112s ea, C-II	16590-0612-73	228.00		AA
120s ea, C-II	16590-0612-72	120.20		AA
150s ea, C-II	16590-0612-83	150.50		AA
180s ea, C-II	16590-0612-82	180.25		AA
650 mg-10 mg,				
30s ea, C-II	16590-0613-30	64.00		AA
60s ea, C-II	16590-0613-60	116.00		AA
90s ea, C-II	16590-0613-90	172.00		AA
120s ea, C-II	16590-0613-72	226.25		AA
APAP/PENTAZOCINE HCL (Dispensing Solutions)				
REPACK				
acetaminophen/pentazocine hydrochloride				
TAB, PO, 650 mg-25 mg,				
30s ea, C-IV	55045-3037-08	32.50		AB
(Southwood)				
REPACK				
TAB, PO (CAPLET)				
650 mg-25 mg,				
20s ea, C-IV	58016-0461-20	21.80		AB
30s ea, C-IV	58016-0461-30	32.70		AB
60s ea, C-IV	58016-0461-60	65.40		AB
90s ea, C-IV	58016-0461-90	98.10		AB
100s ea, C-IV	58016-0461-00	109.00		AB
APAP/PHENYLTOLOXAMINE CIT/SALICYLAMIDE				
(Cypress Pharm) *See BY-ACHE*				
(Edwards) *See ED-FLEX*				
(Larken Labs, Inc.) *See BE-FLEX PLUS*				
(Lunsco) *See ANABAR*				
(PGD, Inc.) *See ASP 300/200/20*				
APAP/PROPOXYPHENE (Mylan)				
acetaminophen/propoxyphene hydrochloride				
TAB, PO (CAPLET)				
650 mg-65 mg,				
100s ea, C-IV	00378-0130-01	30.40		AA
500s ea, C-IV	00378-0130-05	144.40		AA
(UDL)				
TAB, PO (10X10)				
650 mg-65 mg,				
100s ea UD, C-IV	51079-0741-20	34.78		AA
(Dispensing Solutions)				
REPACK				
TAB, PO, 650 mg-65 mg,				
90s ea, C-IV	55045-1380-09	46.80		AA
(PD-Rx Pharm)				
REPACK				
TAB, PO, 650 mg-65 mg,				
30s ea, C-IV	55289-0321-30	70.40		AA
(Pharma Pac)				
REPACK				
TAB, PO, 650 mg-65 mg,				
30s ea, C-IV	52959-0165-30	17.46		AA
(Phys Total Care)				
REPACK				
TAB, PO, 650 mg-65 mg,				
10s ea, C-IV	54868-3646-01	9.63		EE
100s ea, C-IV	54868-3646-00	42.33		EE
(Southwood)				
REPACK				
TAB, PO, 650 mg-65 mg,				
10s ea, C-IV	58016-0279-10	3.80		EE
12s ea, C-IV	58016-0279-12	4.56		EE
15s ea, C-IV	58016-0279-15	5.70		EE
20s ea, C-IV	58016-0279-20	7.59		EE
25s ea, C-IV	58016-0279-25	9.49		EE
30s ea, C-IV	58016-0279-30	11.39		EE
40s ea, C-IV	58016-0279-40	15.19		EE
50s ea, C-IV	58016-0279-50	18.98		EE
60s ea, C-IV	58016-0279-60	22.78		EE
70s ea, C-IV	58016-0279-70	26.58		EE
80s ea, C-IV	58016-0279-80	30.37		EE
90s ea, C-IV	58016-0279-90	34.17		EE
100s ea, C-IV	58016-0279-00	37.97		EE
120s ea, C-IV	58016-0279-02	45.56		EE
APAP/PROPOXYPHENE HCL (Qualitest)				
acetaminophen/propoxyphene hydrochloride				
TAB, PO, 650 mg-65 mg,				
100s ea, C-IV	00603-5462-21	30.40		AA
500s ea, C-IV	00603-5462-28	144.40		AA
(A-S Medication)				
REPACK				
TAB, PO, 650 mg-65 mg,				
10s ea, C-IV	54569-2588-05	3.04		AA

PROD/MFR	NDC	AWP	DP	OBC
APAP/PROPOXYPHENE NAPSYLATE (Covidien)				
acetaminophen/propoxyphene napsylate				
TAB, PO (PINK)				
650 mg-100 mg,				
30s ea, C-IV	**00406-1772-03**	24.08		AB
60s ea, C-IV	**00406-1772-60**	45.75		AB
90s ea, C-IV	**00406-1772-90**	65.19		AB
120s ea, C-IV	**00406-1772-12**	76.24		AB
5000s ea, C-IV	**00406-1772-91**	2850.00		AB
(WHITE)				
650 mg-100 mg,				
5000s ea, C-IV	**00406-1721-91**	2850.00		AB
(Mylan)				
TAB, PO (PINK)				
650 mg-100 mg,				
100s ea, C-IV	**00378-0155-01**	60.25		AB
500s ea, C-IV	**00378-0155-05**	286.10		AB
(Qualitest)				
TAB, PO, 325 mg-50 mg,				
100s ea, C-IV	**00603-5465-21**	93.05		EE
(PINK)				
650 mg-100 mg,				
30s ea, C-IV	**00603-5468-16**	20.01		AB
60s ea, C-IV	**00603-5468-20**	40.01		AB
90s ea, C-IV	**00603-5468-02**	60.02		AB
100s ea, C-IV	**00603-5466-21**	66.69		AB
(PINK)				
650 mg-100 mg,				
100s ea, C-IV	**00603-5468-21**	66.69		AB
(WHITE)				
650 mg-100 mg,				
100s ea, C-IV	**00603-5467-21**	66.69		AB
(PINK)				
650 mg-100 mg,				
120s ea, C-IV	**00603-5468-22**	80.03		AB
180s ea, C-IV	**00603-5468-04**	120.04		AB
500s ea, C-IV	**00603-5466-28**	285.99		AB
(PINK)				
650 mg-100 mg,				
500s ea, C-IV	**00603-5468-28**	285.99		AB
(WHITE)				
650 mg-100 mg,				
500s ea, C-IV	**00603-5467-28**	285.99		AB
1000s ea, C-IV	**00603-5466-32**	554.82		AB
(PINK)				
650 mg-100 mg,				
1000s ea, C-IV	**00603-5468-32**	554.82		AB
(WHITE)				
650 mg-100 mg,				
1000s ea, C-IV	**00603-5467-32**	554.82		AB
(Teva)				
TAB, PO, 650 mg-100 mg,				
100s ea, C-IV	**00093-0490-01**	54.50		AB
(R.N.S.,5X20)				
650 mg-100 mg,				
100s ea UD, C-IV	**00182-0317-89**	51.95		AB
500s ea, C-IV	**00093-0490-05**	267.30		AB
500s ea, C-IV	**00093-0890-05**	267.30		AB
(CAPLET)				
650 mg-100 mg,				
500s ea, C-IV	**00172-4980-70**	286.00		AB
1000s ea, C-IV	**00172-4980-80**	459.50		AB
(UDL)				
TAB, PO (EMRGI-SCRPT,15X6)				
650 mg-100 mg,				
90s ea, C-IV	**51079-0322-99**	60.00		AB
(10X10,FILM-COATED)				
650 mg-100 mg,				
100s ea UD, C-IV	**51079-0322-20**	56.14		AB
(R.N.P., 5X20)				
650 mg-100 mg,				
100s ea UD, C-IV	**51079-0322-21**	56.14		AB
(10X30,FILM-COATED)				
650 mg-100 mg,				
300s ea UD, C-IV	**51079-0322-56**	168.42		AB
(4u)				
REPACK				
TAB, PO, 650 mg-100 mg,				
30s ea, C-IV	**10544-0364-30**	39.24		AB
30s ea, C-IV	**42549-0502-30**	39.24		AB
30s ea, C-IV	**42549-0564-30**	39.24		AB
40s ea, C-IV	**42549-0502-40**	49.56		AB
60s ea, C-IV	**10544-0364-60**	68.86		AB
60s ea, C-IV	**42549-0502-60**	68.86		AB
60s ea, C-IV	**42549-0564-60**	68.86		AB
84s ea, C-IV	**42549-0564-84**	88.28		AB
112s ea, C-IV	**42549-0502-02**	115.36		AB
112s ea, C-IV	**42549-0564-02**	115.36		AB
120s ea, C-IV	**42549-0502-12**	118.12		AB
(A-S Medication)				
REPACK				
TAB, PO, 650 mg-100 mg,				
6s ea, C-IV	**54569-0015-08**	4.00		EE
10s ea, C-IV	**54569-3292-00**	6.67		EE
12s ea, C-IV	**54569-0015-05**	8.00		EE
15s ea, C-IV	**54569-0015-00**	10.00		EE
16s ea, C-IV	**54569-0015-06**	10.67		EE
20s ea, C-IV	**54569-0015-03**	13.34		EE
30s ea, C-IV	**54569-0015-01**	20.01		EE
50s ea, C-IV	**54569-0015-04**	33.35		EE
60s ea, C-IV	**54569-0015-09**	40.01		EE
90s ea, C-IV	**54569-3292-01**	60.02		EE
100s ea, C-IV	**54569-0015-02**	66.69		EE
120s ea, C-IV	**54569-3292-06**	80.03		EE
180s ea, C-IV	**54569-3292-04**	120.04		EE
(Altura)				
REPACK				
TAB, PO, 650 mg-100 mg,				
5s ea, C-IV	**63874-0201-05**	465.00		AB
8s ea, C-IV	**63874-0201-08**	7.44		AB
10s ea, C-IV	**63874-0201-10**	9.30		AB
12s ea, C-IV	**63874-0201-12**	11.16		AB
14s ea, C-IV	**63874-0201-14**	13.02		AB
15s ea, C-IV	**63874-0201-15**	13.95		AB
16s ea, C-IV	**63874-0201-16**	14.88		AB
18s ea, C-IV	**63874-0201-18**	16.74		AB
20s ea, C-IV	**63874-0201-20**	18.60		AB
20s ea, C-IV	**63874-0212-20**	18.71		EE
21s ea, C-IV	**63874-0201-21**	19.53		AB
24s ea, C-IV	**63874-0201-24**	22.32		AB
25s ea, C-IV	**63874-0201-25**	23.25		AB
28s ea, C-IV	**63874-0201-28**	26.04		AB
30s ea, C-IV	**63874-0201-30**	27.90		AB
30s ea, C-IV	**63874-0212-30**	27.28		EE
35s ea, C-IV	**63874-0201-35**	32.55		AB
36s ea, C-IV	**63874-0201-36**	33.48		AB
40s ea, C-IV	**63874-0201-40**	37.20		AB
42s ea, C-IV	**63874-0201-42**	39.06		AB
45s ea, C-IV	**63874-0201-45**	41.85		AB
48s ea, C-IV	**63874-0201-48**	44.64		AB
50s ea, C-IV	**63874-0201-50**	46.50		AB
56s ea, C-IV	**63874-0201-56**	52.08		AB
60s ea, C-IV	**63874-0201-60**	55.80		AB
80s ea, C-IV	**63874-0201-80**	74.40		AB
84s ea, C-IV	**63874-0201-84**	78.12		AB
90s ea, C-IV	**63874-0201-90**	83.70		AB
100s ea, C-IV	**63874-0201-01**	93.00		AB
112s ea, C-IV	**63874-0201-71**	104.16		AB
120s ea, C-IV	**63874-0201-04**	111.60		AB
150s ea, C-IV	**63874-0201-72**	139.50		AB
200s ea, C-IV	**63874-0201-74**	186.00		AB
300s ea, C-IV	**63874-0201-77**	279.00		AB
500s ea, C-IV	**63874-0201-03**	472.17		AB
(American Health)				
REPACK				
TAB, PO, 650 mg-100 mg,				
100s ea UD, C-IV	**68084-0393-01**	17.75		AB
(Dispensing Solutions)				
REPACK				
TAB, PO, 650 mg-100 mg,				
6s ea, C-IV	**55045-1127-01**	4.92		
10s ea, C-IV	**66336-0628-10**	11.29		AB
12s ea, C-IV	**55045-1127-04**	9.84		AB
12s ea, C-IV	**55045-2999-04**	9.84		AB
12s ea, C-IV	**66336-0628-12**	13.57		AB
15s ea, C-IV	**55045-1127-05**	12.30		
15s ea, C-IV	**55045-2999-05**	12.30		AB
15s ea, C-IV	**66336-0628-15**	16.97		AB
16s ea, C-IV	**66336-0628-16**	18.10		AB
20s ea, C-IV	**55045-1127-07**	16.40		AB
20s ea, C-IV	**55045-2999-07**	16.40		AB
20s ea, C-IV	**66336-0628-20**	22.61		AB
30s ea, C-IV	**55045-1127-08**	24.60		AB
30s ea, C-IV	**55045-2999-08**	24.60		AB
30s ea, C-IV	**66336-0628-30**	33.89		AB
36s ea, C-IV	**55045-3095-05**	29.52		
36s ea, C-IV	**55045-3377-05**	29.52		AB
40s ea, C-IV	**55045-1127-03**	32.80		AB
40s ea, C-IV	**55045-2999-03**	32.80		AB
45s ea, C-IV	**55045-3095-04**	36.90		AB
45s ea, C-IV	**55045-3377-04**	36.90		AB
50s ea, C-IV	**55045-1127-09**	41.00		AB
50s ea, C-IV	**55045-2999-09**	41.00		AB
60s ea, C-IV	**55045-1127-00**	49.20		AB
60s ea, C-IV	**55045-2999-00**	49.20		AB
60s ea, C-IV	**66336-0628-60**	47.15		AB
84s ea, C-IV	**55045-3095-02**	68.88		AB
90s ea, C-IV	**55045-3095-09**	73.80		
90s ea, C-IV	**55045-3377-09**	73.80		AB
100s ea, C-IV	**55045-1127-02**	82.00		AB
100s ea, C-IV	**55045-2999-02**	82.00		AB
120s ea, C-IV	**55045-3095-01**	98.40		AB
120s ea, C-IV	**55045-3377-01**	98.40		AB
135s ea, C-IV	**55045-3095-03**	110.70		AB
135s ea, C-IV	**55045-3377-05**	110.70		AB
160s ea, C-IV	**55045-3095-00**	131.20		AB
160s ea, C-IV	**55045-3377-00**	131.20		AB
180s ea, C-IV	**55045-3095-08**	147.60		
(GSMS)				
REPACK				
TAB, PO (UNIT OF USE)				
650 mg-100 mg,				
30s ea, C-IV	**60429-0518-30**	14.43	4.81	AB
60s ea, C-IV	**60429-0518-60**	25.92	8.64	AB
(IPI)				
REPACK				
TAB, PO, 650 mg-100 mg,				
90s ea, C-IV	**18837-0128-90**	49.93		AB
(Keltman Pharma., Inc.)				
REPACK				
TAB, PO (USP)				
650 mg-100 mg,				
10s ea, C-IV	**68387-0100-10**	12.50		AB
(McKesson Packaging)				
REPACK				
TAB, PO, 650 mg-100 mg,				
100s ea UD, C-IV	**63739-0215-10**	37.68		AB
(BLISTER PACK)				
650 mg-100 mg,				
750s ea UD, C-IV	**63739-0215-01**	282.60		AB
(PUNCH CARD 25X30)				
650 mg-100 mg,				
750s ea, C-IV	**63739-0215-03**	282.60		AB
(Medsource)				
REPACK				
TAB, PO, 650 mg-100 mg,				
30s ea, C-IV	**45865-0414-30**	16.35		AB
60s ea, C-IV	**45865-0414-60**	32.70		AB
84s ea, C-IV	**45865-0414-84**	45.78		AB
90s ea, C-IV	**45865-0414-90**	49.05		AB
100s ea, C-IV	**45865-0414-49**	54.50		AB
120s ea, C-IV	**45865-0414-51**	65.40		AB
150s ea, C-IV	**45865-0414-53**	81.75		AB
200s ea, C-IV	**45865-0414-62**	109.00		AB
(Nucare Pharm)				
REPACK				
TAB, PO, 650 mg-100 mg,				
6s ea, C-IV	**66267-0178-06**	6.20		AB
12s ea, C-IV	**66267-0178-12**	12.40		AB
15s ea, C-IV	**66267-0178-15**	15.50		AB
20s ea, C-IV	**66267-0178-20**	20.66		AB
30s ea, C-IV	**66267-0178-30**	30.99		AB
40s ea, C-IV	**66267-0178-40**	41.32		AB
50s ea, C-IV	**66267-0178-50**	51.65		AB
60s ea, C-IV	**66267-0178-60**	61.98		AB
90s ea, C-IV	**66267-0178-90**	92.97		AB
100s ea, C-IV	**68071-1363-00**	103.30		AB
120s ea, C-IV	**66267-0178-91**	111.60		AB
(PD-Rx Pharm)				
REPACK				
TAB, PO, 650 mg-100 mg,				
4s ea, C-IV	**43063-0023-04**	15.57		AB
4s ea, C-IV	**55289-0231-04**	42.00		AB
6s ea, C-IV	**43063-0023-06**	14.10		AB
6s ea, C-IV	**55289-0231-06**	43.60		AB
8s ea, C-IV	**55289-0231-08**	45.11		AB
10s ea, C-IV	**55289-0231-10**	46.70		AB
12s ea, C-IV	**55289-0231-12**	48.22		AB
15s ea, C-IV	**55289-0231-15**	50.60		AB
16s ea, C-IV	**55289-0231-16**	51.33		AB
20s ea, C-IV	**55289-0231-20**	54.40		AB
(REDI-SCRIPT)				
650 mg-100 mg,				
20s ea, C-IV	**58864-0428-20**	54.40		AB
30s ea, C-IV	**55289-0231-30**	62.22		AB
(REDI-SCRIPT)				
650 mg-100 mg,				
30s ea, C-IV	**58864-0428-30**	62.20		AB
40s ea, C-IV	**55289-0231-40**	70.00		AB
50s ea, C-IV	**55289-0231-50**	77.78		AB
60s ea, C-IV	**55289-0231-60**	80.00		AB
90s ea, C-IV	**55289-0231-90**	108.89		AB
(Pharma Pac)				
REPACK				
TAB, PO, 650 mg-100 mg,				
10s ea, C-IV	**52959-0335-10**	16.02		EE
12s ea, C-IV	**52959-0335-12**	19.22		EE
14s ea, C-IV	**52959-0335-14**	22.42		EE
15s ea, C-IV	**52959-0335-15**	24.00		EE
20s ea, C-IV	**52959-0335-20**	31.85		EE
21s ea, C-IV	**52959-0335-21**	33.43		EE

PROD/MFR	NDC	AWP	DP	OBC
24s ea, C-IV	**52959-0335-24**	38.20		EE
25s ea, C-IV	**52959-0335-25**	39.80		EE
28s ea, C-IV	**52959-0335-28**	44.54		EE
30s ea, C-IV	**52959-0335-30**	47.70		EE
35s ea, C-IV	**52959-0335-35**	55.63		AB
36s ea, C-IV	**52959-0335-36**	56.08		EE
40s ea, C-IV	**52959-0335-40**	63.48		EE
42s ea, C-IV	**52959-0335-42**	66.66		EE
45s ea, C-IV	**52959-0335-45**	71.40		EE
50s ea, C-IV	**52959-0335-50**	79.29		EE
60s ea, C-IV	**52959-0335-60**	95.07		EE
80s ea, C-IV	**52959-0335-80**	126.70		EE
84s ea, C-IV	**52959-0335-84**	132.99		EE
90s ea, C-IV	**52959-0335-90**	142.38		EE
100s ea, C-IV	**52959-0335-00**	158.15		EE
120s ea, C-IV	**52959-0335-02**	189.66		EE
(Phys Total Care)				
REPACK				
TAB, PO, 650 mg-100 mg,				
15s ea, C-IV	**54868-0073-03**	8.28		EE
20s ea, C-IV	**54868-0073-04**	9.66		EE
30s ea, C-IV	**54868-0073-01**	12.06		EE
40s ea, C-IV	**54868-0073-07**	14.61		EE
50s ea, C-IV	**54868-0073-05**	17.13		EE
100s ea, C-IV	**54868-0073-09**	29.76		EE
180s ea, C-IV	**54868-0073-08**	49.95		EE
(Physician Partner)				
REPACK				
TAB, PO, 650 mg-100 mg,				
8s ea, C-IV	**21695-0280-08**	10.06		AB
16s ea, C-IV	**21695-0280-16**	20.12		AB
(Quality Care Prod)				
REPACK				
TAB, PO, 650 mg-100 mg,				
15s ea, C-IV	**49999-0025-15**	9.97		AB
20s ea, C-IV	**49999-0025-20**	20.75		AB
30s ea, C-IV	**49999-0025-30**	29.49		AB
60s ea, C-IV	**49999-0025-60**	57.55		AB
(Southwood)				
REPACK				
TAB, PO, 650 mg-100 mg,				
8s ea, C-IV	**58016-0212-08**	6.06		EE
10s ea, C-IV	**58016-0212-10**	7.58		EE
12s ea, C-IV	**58016-0212-12**	9.09		EE
14s ea, C-IV	**58016-0212-14**	10.61		EE
15s ea, C-IV	**58016-0212-15**	11.36		EE
16s ea, C-IV	**58016-0212-16**	12.12		EE
18s ea, C-IV	**58016-0212-18**	13.64		EE
20s ea, C-IV	**58016-0212-20**	15.15		EE
21s ea, C-IV	**58016-0212-21**	15.91		EE
24s ea, C-IV	**58016-0212-24**	18.18		EE
28s ea, C-IV	**58016-0212-28**	21.21		EE
30s ea, C-IV	**58016-0212-30**	47.00		AB
36s ea, C-IV	**58016-0212-36**	27.27		EE
40s ea, C-IV	**58016-0212-40**	30.30		EE
42s ea, C-IV	**58016-0212-42**	31.82		EE
45s ea, C-IV	**58016-0212-45**	34.09		EE
50s ea, C-IV	**58016-0212-50**	37.88		EE
56s ea, C-IV	**58016-0212-56**	42.42		EE
60s ea, C-IV	**58016-0212-60**	94.00		AB
80s ea, C-IV	**58016-0212-80**	60.60		EE
84s ea, C-IV	**58016-0212-84**	63.63		EE
90s ea, C-IV	**58016-0212-90**	141.00		AB
100s ea, C-IV	**58016-0212-00**	156.67		AB
112s ea, C-IV	**58016-0212-92**	84.84		EE
120s ea, C-IV	**58016-0212-02**	188.00		AB
150s ea, C-IV	**58016-0212-03**	113.63		EE
180s ea, C-IV	**58016-0212-99**	181.80		EE
200s ea, C-IV	**58016-0212-89**	151.50		EE
300s ea, C-IV	**58016-0212-73**	227.25		EE
(St. Mary's MPP)				
REPACK				
TAB, PO, 650 mg-100 mg,				
15s ea, C-IV	**60760-0890-15**	14.82		AB
30s ea, C-IV	**60760-0890-30**	24.88		AB
60s ea, C-IV	**60760-0890-60**	43.77		AB
90s ea, C-IV	**60760-0890-90**	62.64		AB
(Stat Rx)				
REPACK				
TAB, PO, 325 mg-50 mg,				
60s ea, C-IV	**16590-0377-60**	51.17		EE
90s ea, C-IV	**16590-0377-90**	75.97		EE
650 mg-100 mg,				
20s ea, C-IV	**16590-0197-20**	20.00		AB
28s ea, C-IV	**16590-0197-28**	25.26		AB
50s ea, C-IV	**16590-0197-50**	33.33		AB
56s ea, C-IV	**16590-0197-56**	50.51		AB
84s ea, C-IV	**16590-0197-62**	63.24		AB
112s ea, C-IV	**16590-0197-73**	84.31		AB
APAP/TRAMADOL (Keltman Pharma., Inc.)				
REPACK				
acetaminophen/tramadol hydrochloride				
TAB, PO, 325 mg-37.5 mg,				
90s ea	**68387-0497-90**	119.70		
120s ea	**68387-0497-12**	159.60		
APAP/TRAMADOL HCL (Keltman Pharma., Inc.)				
acetaminophen/tramadol hydrochloride				
TAB, PO, 325 mg-37.5 mg,				
30s ea	**68387-0497-30**	40.00		
60s ea	**68387-0497-60**	79.80		
(PD-Rx Pharm)				
REPACK				
TAB, PO, 325 mg-37.5 mg,				
20s ea	**55289-0895-20**	52.93		
30s ea	**55289-0895-30**	57.69		
(Pharma Pac)				
REPACK				
TAB, PO (FILM-COATED)				
325 mg-37.5 mg,				
20s ea	**52959-0814-20**	25.18		AB
30s ea	**52959-0814-30**	37.74		AB
60s ea	**52959-0814-60**	75.36		AB
90s ea	**52959-0814-90**	112.95		AB
(Phys Total Care)				
REPACK				
TAB, PO (FILM-COATED)				
325 mg-37.5 mg,				
30s ea	**54868-5291-00**	50.85		AB
40s ea	**54868-5291-01**	63.90		AB
60s ea	**54868-5291-03**	72.87		AB
90s ea	**54868-5291-02**	107.79		AB
(Southwood)				
REPACK				
TAB, PO (FILM-COATED)				
325 mg-37.5 mg,				
30s ea	**58016-0617-30**	30.60		AB
60s ea	**58016-0617-60**	61.20		AB
90s ea	**58016-0617-90**	91.80		AB
100s ea	**58016-0617-00**	102.00		AB
120s ea	**58016-0617-02**	122.40		AB
APAP/TRAMADOL HYDROCHLORIDE (Teva)				
acetaminophen/tramadol hydrochloride				
TAB, PO (10X10,FILM-COATED)				
325 mg-37.5 mg,				
100s ea UD	**00172-6359-10**	112.73		
(FILM-COATED)				
325 mg-37.5 mg,				
100s ea	**00172-6359-60**	102.49		
(A-S Medication)				
REPACK				
TAB, PO (FILM-COATED)				
325 mg-37.5 mg,				
20s ea	**54569-5680-00**	20.50		
30s ea	**54569-5680-01**	30.74		
(Dispensing Solutions)				
REPACK				
TAB, PO (FILM-COATED)				
325 mg-37.5 mg,				
20s ea	**55045-3350-07**	20.40		
25s ea	**55045-3350-02**	25.50		
30s ea	**55045-3350-08**	30.60		
60s ea	**55045-3350-06**	61.20		
90s ea	**55045-3350-09**	91.80		
100s ea	**55045-3350-00**	102.00		
180s ea	**55045-3350-01**	183.60		
(Pharma Pac)				
REPACK				
TAB, PO, 325 mg-37.5 mg,				
40s ea	**52959-0814-40**	50.28		
(Physician Partner)				
REPACK				
TAB, PO (FILM-COATED)				
325 mg-37.5 mg,				
20s ea	**21695-0236-20**	49.01		
(Quality Care Prod)				
REPACK				
TAB, PO (FILM-COATED)				
325 mg-37.5 mg,				
20s ea	**49999-0693-20**	49.36		
30s ea	**49999-0693-30**	68.40		
40s ea	**49999-0693-40**	98.72		
(Stat Rx)				
REPACK				
TAB, PO (FILM-COATED)				
325 mg-37.5 mg,				
15s ea	**16590-0230-15**	31.05		
50s ea	**16590-0230-50**	124.87		
180s ea	**16590-0230-82**	234.30		
APEXICON (PharmaDerm)				
diflorasone diacetate				
OIN, TP, 0.05%, 30 gm	**00462-0394-30**	117.00		
60 gm	**00462-0394-60**	234.01		
APEXICON E (PharmaDerm)				
diflorasone diacetate				
CRE, TP, 0.05%, 30 gm	**00462-0395-30**	120.60		
60 gm	**00462-0395-60**	241.09		
APHTHASOL (Discus Dental)				
amlexanox				
PAS, MM (1X3GM)				
5%, 3 gm	**64854-0029-01**	18.40		
APIDRA (Sanofi-Aventis)				
insulin glulisine				
SOL, IJ (5X3ML,OPTICLIK PEN)				
100 u/ml, 3 ml 5s	**00088-2500-52**	199.49		
10 ml	**00088-2500-33**	107.36		
APIDRA SOLOSTAR (Sanofi-Aventis)				
insulin glulisine				
SOL, IJ (5X3ML)				
100 u/ml, 3 ml 5s	**00088-2502-05**	207.42		EE
APLENZIN (Sanofi-Aventis)				
bupropion hydrobromide				
TER, PO, 174 mg, 30s ea	**00024-5810-30**	167.40		
348 mg, 30s ea	**00024-5811-30**	220.68		EE
522 mg, 30s ea	**00024-5812-30**	502.20		EE
APLIGRAF (Novartis Pharm)				
graftskin				
SHE, TP (75MM DIAM DISK)				
ea	**09978-0001-99**	1362.50		
APLISOL (JHP)				
tuberculin				
SOL, ID (1X1ML)				
5 tu/0.1 ml, 1 ml	**42023-0104-01**	38.86		
(1X5ML)				
5 tu/0.1 ml, 5 ml	**42023-0104-05**	138.86		
(Phys Total Care)				
REPACK				
SOL, ID (10 TEST VIAL)				
5 tu/0.1 ml, 1 ml	**54868-2696-00**	43.09		
(VIAL, 50 TEST)				
5 tu/0.1 ml, 5 ml	**54868-2328-01**	103.92		
APOKYN (Tercica)				
apomorphine hydrochloride				
SOL, SC (1X3ML)				
10 mg/ml, 3 ml	**15054-0211-01**	157.44		
(5X3ML)				
10 mg/ml, 3 ml 5s	**15054-0211-05**	787.20		
APOMORPHINE HCL (Gallipot)				
apomorphine hydrochloride				
POW, NA (1X1GM)				
1 gm	**51552-0652-01**	168.00	120.00	
(1X5GM)				
5 gm	**51552-0652-02**	693.00	495.00	
(U.S.P.)				
25 gm	**51552-0652-04**	3003.00		
(Hawkins)				
POW, NA (U.S.P.)				
0.1 gm	**63370-0022-06**	70.00		
0.5 gm	**63370-0022-09**	248.00		
5 gm	**63370-0022-15**	1920.00		
(Letco)				
POW, NA (U.S.P.)				
0.25 gm	**62991-1513-01**	105.00		
1 gm	**62991-1513-02**	270.00		
5 gm	**62991-1513-03**	1125.00		
(Medisca)				
POW, NA (U.S.P.)				
0.5 gm	**38779-1764-00**	229.50		
1 gm	**38779-1764-06**	414.00		
5 gm	**38779-1764-03**	1759.50		
(PCCA)				
POW, NA (U.S.P., HEMIHYDRATE)				
1 gm	**51927-2303-00**	960.00		

APOMORPHINE HYDROCHLORIDE

(Gallipot) *See APOMORPHINE HCL*

(Hawkins) *See APOMORPHINE HCL*

(Letco) *See APOMORPHINE HCL*

(Medisca) *See APOMORPHINE HCL*

(PCCA) *See APOMORPHINE HCL*

(Spectrum Pharmacy) *See APOMORPHINE HYDROCHLORIDE, HEMIHYDRATE*

(Tercica) *See APOKYN*

PROD/MFR	NDC	AWP	DP	OBC
APOMORPHINE HYDROCHLORIDE, HEMIHYDRATE				
(Spectrum Pharmacy)				
apomorphine hydrochloride				
POW, NA (1X5GM)				
5 gm	49452-0700-04	3650.50		
(1X100MG) 100 ml	49452-0700-01	223.30		
(1X500MG) 500 ml	49452-0700-02	696.50		
APPLE (Medisca)				
flavoring aid				
SOL, NA (1X50ML,APPLE) 50 ml	38779-1999-02	22.50		
(1X100ML,APPLE) 100 ml	38779-1999-05	34.50		
(1X500ML,APPLE) 500 ml	38779-1999-08	87.00		
(1X4000ML,APPLE) 4000 ml	38779-1999-01	585.00		
APPLE FLAVOR (Gallipot)				
flavoring aid				
POW, NA (ARTIFICIAL,APPLE) 454 gm	51552-0885-06	44.87	32.05	
(PCCA)				
POW, NA, 1 gm	51927-3411-00	0.20		
SOL, NA (ARTIFICIAL) 1 ml	51927-2171-00	0.90		
(Spectrum Pharmacy)				
POW, NA (1X500GM) 500 gm	49452-0691-03	140.35		
(1X2500GM) 2500 gm	49452-0691-04	413.00		
APPLE FLAVORING (Gallipot)				
flavoring aid				
SOL, NA (ARTIFICIAL,APPLE) 473 ml	51552-0772-06	35.00	25.00	
APPLE POWDER (Medisca)				
flavoring aid				
POW, NA (1X500GM,APPLE) 500 gm	38779-2000-08	78.00		
(1X2500GM,APPLE) 2500 gm	38779-2000-01	276.00		
APPLE POWDER FLAVOR (PCCA)				
flavoring aid				
POW, NA (WATER MISCIBLE) 1 gm	51927-2896-00	0.17		
APPLE-ADE FLAVOR (PCCA)				
flavoring aid				
SOL, NA (LIQUID,WATER MISCIBLE) 1 ml	51927-3009-00	0.38		
APPTRIM (Physician Thera, LLC)				
amino acids and nutriceuticals				
CAP, PO (PF,SF,STARCH-FREE) 40 mg-101 mg, 120s ea	68405-1001-01	190.08		
(Altura) REPACK				
CAP, PO, 40 mg-101 mg, 120s ea	63874-1177-04	148.50		
(Dispensing Solutions) REPACK				
CAP, PO (PF,SF,STARCH-FREE) 40 mg-101 mg, 120s ea	55045-3393-02	148.50		
APPTRIM LIFESTYLES POST-BARIATRIC SURGERY PROGRAM (Physician Thera, LLC)				
amino acids and nutriceuticals				
CAP, PO, 120s ea	68405-1015-01	318.72		
APPTRIM LIFESTYLES PRE-BARIATRIC SURGERY PROGRAM (Physician Thera, LLC)				
amino acids and nutriceuticals				
CAP, PO, 120s ea	68405-1014-01	318.72		
APPTRIM WEIGHT MANAGEMENT PROGRAM (Physician Thera, LLC)				
amino acids and nutriceuticals				
CAP, PO, 120s ea	68405-1013-01	318.72		
APPTRIM-D (Physician Thera, LLC)				
amino acids				
CAP, PO (PF,SF,DYE-FREE) 120s ea	68405-1009-01	190.08		
(Altura) REPACK				
CAP, PO, 120s ea	63874-1178-04	148.50		

PROD/MFR	NDC	AWP	DP	OBC
(Dispensing Solutions) REPACK				
CAP, PO (PF,SF,DYE-FREE) 120s ea	55045-3394-02	148.50		
APRACLONIDINE (Akorn)				
apraclonidine hydrochloride				
SOL, OP (1X5ML,USP) 0.5%, 5 ml	17478-0716-10	90.54		AT
(1X10ML,USP) 0.5%, 10 ml	17478-0716-11	179.82		AT
(Falcon Ophthalmics)				
SOL, OP (1X5ML) 0.5%, 5 ml	61314-0665-05	77.10		AT
(1X10ML) 0.5%, 10 ml	61314-0665-10	152.88		AT
APRACLONIDINE HYDROCHLORIDE				
(Akorn) *See APRACLONIDINE*				
(Alcon Ophthalmic) *See IOPIDINE*				
(Falcon Ophthalmics) *See APRACLONIDINE*				
APREPITANT				
(Merck) *See EMEND*				
APRESOLINE (Phys Total Care) REPACK				
hydralazine hydrochloride				
TAB, PO, 50 mg, 100s ea	54868-3369-00	64.83		AA
APRI (Teva)				
desogestrel/ethinyl estradiol				
TAB, PO (6X28) 0.15 mg-0.03 mg, 168s ea	00555-9043-58	183.10		AB
(Phys Total Care) REPACK				
TAB, PO, 0.15 mg-0.03 mg, 28s ea	54868-4754-00	61.47		AB
APRICOT FLAVOR (PCCA)				
flavoring aid				
POW, NA, 1 gm	51927-3297-00	0.54		
SOL, NA (ARTIFICIAL,APRICOT) 1 ml	51927-2170-00	0.90		
APRISO (Salix Pharm)				
mesalamine				
CER, PO (HARD GELATIN CAPSULE) 0.375 gm, 120s ea	65649-0103-02	237.60		
APROTININ				
(Bayer Corp.) *See TRASYLOL*				
APROTININ/CALCIUM CHLORIDE/FIBRINOGEN/THROMBIN				
(Baxter Bioscience) *See ARTISS*				
(Baxter Bioscience) *See TISSEEL*				
APTIVUS (Boehr Ingelheim Phar)				
tipranavir				
SGL, PO, 250 mg, 120s ea	00597-0003-02	1187.27		
SOL, PO (1X95ML,W/5MLSYRINGE) 100 mg/ml, 95 ml	00597-0002-01	395.75		
AQUACOT (Truxton)				
trichlormethiazide				
TAB, PO, 4 mg, 1000s ea	00463-6248-10	24.00		EE
AQUAFRESH SENSITIVE (Glaxo)				
potassium nitrate/sodium fluoride				
PAS, DE, 5%-0.15%, 121.9 gm	53100-0324-25	2.28		
AQUAMEPHYTON (Phys Total Care) REPACK				
phytonadione				
SOL, IJ (VIAL) 10 mg/ml, 5 ml	54868-3806-00	24.94		BP
AQUAPHOR (Amend)				
ointment base				
OIN, NA, 454 gm	17317-1347-01	29.40		
2270 gm	17317-1347-05	119.00		
AQUASATE-P (Quintess Corp)				
ointment base				
OIN, NA (FRAGRANCE-FREE) 400 gm	53982-0302-12	14.98		
AQUASOL A (Hospira)				
vitamin a palmitate				
SOL, IM (SDV) 50000 u/ml, 2 ml 10s	61703-0418-07	340.68	298.10	
AQUORAL (Auriga)				
saliva substitutes				
SPR, MM, 40 ml	08546-0001-40	87.50		

PROD/MFR	NDC	AWP	DP	OBC
ARALAST (Baxter Bioscience)				
alpha-1 proteinase inhibitor human				
PDS, IV (1000MG VIAL,PF) 1 mg, ea	00944-2801-02	0.50		
(500MG VIAL,PF) 1 mg, ea	00944-2801-01	0.50		
ARALAST NP (Baxter Bioscience)				
alpha-1 proteinase inhibitor human				
PDS, IV (SDV,APPROX 500MG,PF) 1 mg, ea	00944-2802-01	0.52		
(SDV,APRROX 1000MG,PF) 1 mg, ea	00944-2802-02	0.52		
ARALEN PHOSPHATE (Sanofi-Aventis)				
chloroquine phosphate				
TAB, PO, 500 mg, 25s ea	00024-0084-01	194.39		AA
(Phys Total Care) REPACK				
TAB, PO, 500 mg, 25s ea	54868-3953-00	128.73		AA
ARAMINE (Phys Total Care)				
metaraminol bitartrate				
SOL, IJ, 10 mg/ml, 10 ml	54868-3692-00	14.34		AP
ARANELLE (Teva)				
ethinyl estradiol/norethindrone				
TAB, PO (BLISTER PACK,3 X 28) 84s ea	00555-9066-67	118.05		AB
ARANESP (Amgen USA Inc.)				
darbepoetin alfa				
SOL, IJ (PF) 0.025 mg/ml, 1 ml	55513-0002-01	156.36		
(S.D.V.,ALBUMIN SOL,PF) 0.025 mg/ml, 1 ml	55513-0010-01	148.20		
(4X1ML,PF) 0.025 mg/ml, 1 ml 4s	55513-0002-04	625.44		
(S.D.V.,ALBUMIN SOL,PF) 0.025 mg/ml, 1 ml 4s	55513-0010-04	592.80		
(PF) 0.04 mg/ml, 1 ml	55513-0003-01	250.20		
(S.D.V.,ALBUMIN SOL,PF) 0.04 mg/ml, 1 ml	55513-0011-01	237.12		
(1MLX4,PF) 0.04 mg/ml, 1 ml 4s	55513-0003-04	1000.80		
(S.D.V.,ALBUMIN SOL,PF) 0.04 mg/ml, 1 ml 4s	55513-0011-04	948.48		
(PF) 0.025 mg/0.42 ml, 0.42 ml	55513-0057-01	156.36		
(SINGLEJECT,PF) 0.025 mg/0.42 ml, 0.42 ml	55513-0058-01	148.20		
(PF) 0.025 mg/0.42 ml, 0.42 ml 4s	55513-0057-04	625.44		
(SINGLEJECT,PF) 0.025 mg/0.42 ml, 0.42 ml 4s	55513-0058-04	592.80		
(PF) 0.06 mg/ml, 1 ml	55513-0004-01	375.30		
(S.D.V.,ALBUMIN SOL,PF) 0.06 mg/ml, 1 ml	55513-0012-01	355.68		
(1MLX4,PF) 0.06 mg/ml, 1 ml 4s	55513-0004-04	1501.20		
(S.D.V.,ALBUMIN SOL,PF) 0.06 mg/ml, 1 ml 4s	55513-0012-04	1422.72		
(PF) 0.04 mg/0.4 ml, 0.4 ml	55513-0021-01	250.20		
(SINGLEJECT,PF) 0.04 mg/0.4 ml, 0.4 ml	55513-0037-01	237.12		
(PF) 0.04 mg/0.4 ml, 0.4 ml 4s	55513-0021-04	1000.80		
(SINGLEJECT,PF) 0.04 mg/0.4 ml, 0.4 ml 4s	55513-0037-04	948.48		
(PF) 0.1 mg/ml, 1 ml	55513-0005-01	625.44		
(S.D.V.,ALBUMIN SOL,PF) 0.1 mg/ml, 1 ml	55513-0013-01	592.80		
(1MLX4,PF) 0.1 mg/ml, 1 ml 4s	55513-0005-04	2501.76		
(S.D.V.,ALBUMIN SOL,PF) 0.1 mg/ml, 1 ml 4s	55513-0013-04	2371.20		

PROD/MFR	NDC	AWP	DP	OBC
(PF,PREFILLED SYRINGE)				
0.06 mg/0.3 ml,				
0.3 ml	**55513-0039-01**	355.68		
(PF)				
0.06 mg/0.3 ml,				
0.3 ml	**55513-0023-01**	375.30		
(PF,PREFILLED SYRINGE)				
0.06 mg/0.3 ml,				
0.3 ml 4s	**55513-0039-04**	1422.72		
(PF)				
0.06 mg/0.3 ml,				
0.3 ml 4s	**55513-0023-04**	1501.20		
(PF,PREFILLED SYRINGE)				
0.1 mg/0.5 ml,				
0.5 ml	**55513-0041-01**	592.80		
(PF)				
0.1 mg/0.5 ml,				
0.5 ml	**55513-0025-01**	625.44		
(PF,PREFILLED SYRINGE)				
0.1 mg/0.5 ml,				
0.5 ml 4s	**55513-0041-04**	2371.20		
(PF)				
0.1 mg/0.5 ml,				
0.5 ml 4s	**55513-0025-04**	2501.76		
0.15 mg/0.75 ml,				
0.75 ml	**55513-0053-01**	938.16		
(S.D.V.,ALBUMIN SOL,PF)				
0.15 mg/0.75 ml,				
0.75 ml	**55513-0054-01**	889.20		
(1MLX4,PF)				
0.15 mg/0.75 ml,				
0.75 ml 4s	**55513-0053-04**	3752.64		
(SDV,ALBUMIN SOLN,PF)				
0.15 mg/0.75 ml,				
0.75 ml 4s	**55513-0054-04**	3556.80		
(PF)				
0.2 mg/ml, 1 ml	**55513-0006-01**	1250.88		
(S.D.V.,ALBUMIN SOL,PF)				
0.2 mg/ml, 1 ml	**55513-0014-01**	1185.60		
1 ml 4s	**55513-0014-04**	4533.12		
(PF)				
0.3 mg/ml, 1 ml	**55513-0110-01**	1876.32		
(S.D.V.,ALBUMIN SOL,PF)				
0.3 mg/ml, 1 ml	**55513-0015-01**	1778.40		
(PF,PFS)				
0.15 mg/0.3 ml,				
0.3 ml	**55513-0043-01**	889.20		
(PF)				
0.15 mg/0.3 ml,				
0.3 ml	**55513-0027-01**	938.16		
(0.3MLX4,PF)				
0.15 mg/0.3 ml,				
0.3 ml 4s	**55513-0027-04**	3752.64		
(PF,PFS)				
0.15 mg/0.3 ml,				
0.3 ml 4s	**55513-0043-04**	3556.80		
(PF,PREFILLED SYRINGE)				
0.2 mg/0.4 ml,				
0.4 ml	**55513-0044-01**	1185.60		
(PF)				
0.2 mg/0.4 ml,				
0.4 ml	**55513-0028-01**	1250.88		
(PF,PREFILLED SYRINGE)				
0.3 mg/0.6 ml,				
0.6 ml	**55513-0046-01**	1778.40		
(PF)				
0.3 mg/0.6 ml,				
0.6 ml	**55513-0111-01**	1876.32		
(SINGLEJECT,G27,1/2",PF)				
0.5 mg/ml, 1 ml	**55513-0032-01**	3127.20		
(SINGLEJECT,PF)				
0.5 mg/ml, 1 ml	**55513-0048-01**	2964.00		
(Phys Total Care)				
REPACK				
SOL, IJ, 0.2 mg/0.4 ml,				
0.4 ml	**54868-5428-00**	1331.54		
(1X0.6ML, PREFILLED,PF)				
0.3 mg/0.6 ml,				
0.6 ml	**54868-5429-00**	1996.32		
(1X1ML, PREFILLED,PF)				
0.5 mg/ml, 1 ml	**54868-5867-00**	3325.88		
ARAVA (Sanofi-Aventis)				
leflunomide				
TAB, PO (FILM-COATED)				
10 mg, 30s ea	**00088-2160-30**	674.39		
20 mg, 30s ea	**00088-2161-30**	674.39		
(AQ)				
REPACK				
TAB, PO, 10 mg, 30s ea	**66105-0565-03**	541.38		
20 mg, 30s ea	**66105-0566-03**	541.38		

PROD/MFR	NDC	AWP	DP	OBC
(Bryant Ranch)				
REPACK				
TAB, PO, 20 mg, 30s ea	**63629-1263-01**	652.95		
(Phys Total Care)				
REPACK				
TAB, PO (FILM-COATED)				
10 mg, 30s ea	**54868-4902-00**	430.03		
ARCALYST (Regeneron)				
rilonacept				
PDS, SC (PF)				
220 mg, 4s ea	**61755-0001-01**	24000.00		
ARCITUMOMAB				
(Immunomedics, Inc.) *See CEA-SCAN*				
AREDIA (Novartis Pharm)				
pamidronate disodium				
PDS, IV, 30 mg, 4s ea	**00078-0463-91**	1119.44		AP
90 mg, ea	**00078-0464-61**	839.59		AP
ARFORMOTEROL TARTRATE				
(Sepracor) *See BROVANA*				
ARGATROBAN				
(Glaxo) *See NOVAPLUS ARGATROBAN*				
(Glaxo)				
SOL, IV (SDV)				
100 mg/ml, 2.5 ml	**00007-4407-01**	1486.98		
ARGININE (Medisca)				
POW, NA (U.S.P.,L-ARGININE)				
100 gm	**38779-0502-05**	43.50		
500 gm	**38779-0502-08**	211.50		
1000 gm	**38779-0502-09**	367.50		
(PCCA)				
POW, NA (U.S.P.)				
1 gm	**51927-3096-00**	0.51		
(Spectrum Pharmacy) *See ARGININE HYDROCHLORIDE*				
(Spectrum Pharmacy) *See L-ARGININE*				
ARGININE HCL (PCCA)				
arginine hydrochloride				
POW, NA (USP)				
1 gm	**51927-2056-00**	0.51		
ARGININE HCL/FOLIC ACID/VIT B12/VIT B6				
(SJ) *See CARDIOTEK RX*				
ARGININE HYDROCHLORIDE				
(Amend) *See L-ARGININE MONOHYDROCHLORIDE*				
(PCCA) *See ARGININE HCL*				
(Pfizer) *See R-GENE 10*				
ARGININE HYDROCHLORIDE (Spectrum Pharmacy)				
arginine				
POW, NA (U.S.P.)				
100 gm	**49452-0715-01**	68.60		
1000 gm	**49452-0715-02**	504.00		
ARICEPT (Eisai)				
donepezil hydrochloride				
TAB, PO, 5 mg, 30s ea	**62856-0245-30**	240.82		
90s ea	**62856-0245-90**	722.51		
(10 X 10)				
5 mg, 100s ea UD	**62856-0245-41**	802.78		
1000s ea	**62856-0245-11**	8027.64		
(FILM-COATED)				
10 mg, 30s ea	**62856-0246-30**	240.82		
90s ea	**62856-0246-90**	722.51		
(10 X 10,FILM-COATED)				
10 mg, 100s ea UD	**62856-0246-41**	802.78		
(FILM-COATED)				
10 mg, 1000s ea	**62856-0246-11**	8027.64		
(AQ)				
REPACK				
TAB, PO, 5 mg, 10s ea	**66105-0739-01**	99.46		
15s ea	**66105-0739-15**	149.19		
30s ea	**66105-0739-03**	298.38		
60s ea	**66105-0739-06**	596.76		
90s ea	**66105-0739-09**	895.13		
10 mg, 10s ea	**66105-0737-01**	99.46		
15s ea	**66105-0737-15**	149.19		
30s ea	**66105-0737-03**	298.38		
60s ea	**66105-0737-06**	596.76		
90s ea	**66105-0737-09**	895.13		
(Bryant Ranch)				
REPACK				
TAB, PO, 10 mg, 30s ea	**63629-3632-01**	184.38		
(PD-Rx Pharm)				
REPACK				
TAB, PO, 5 mg, 30s ea	**58864-0886-30**	351.02		
(FILM-COATED)				
10 mg, 21s ea	**55289-0151-21**	247.97		
30s ea	**55289-0151-30**	351.02		
(REDI-SCRIPT,FILM-COATED)				
10 mg, 30s ea	**58864-0895-30**	247.43		

PROD/MFR	NDC	AWP	DP	OBC
(Phys Total Care)				
REPACK				
TAB, PO, 5 mg, 30s ea	**54868-3952-00**	287.03		
90s ea	**54868-3952-01**	829.58		
(FILM-COATED)				
10 mg, 30s ea	**54868-4245-00**	287.03		
90s ea	**54868-4245-01**	829.58		
(Quality Care Prod)				
REPACK				
TAB, PO, 5 mg, 30s ea	**49999-0753-30**	295.57		
(FILM-COATED)				
10 mg, 30s ea	**49999-0754-30**	295.57		
90s ea	**49999-0754-90**	886.71		
ARICEPT ODT (Eisai)				
donepezil hydrochloride				
ODT, PO (10X3)				
5 mg, 30s ea UD	**62856-0831-30**	240.82		
10 mg, 30s ea UD	**62856-0832-30**	240.82		
ARIDEX (Gentex Pharma)				
carbetapentane cit/carbinoxamine mal/phenyleph hcl				
SOL, PO (W/DROPPER,AF,SF)				
4 mg/ml-1 mg/ml-2 mg/ml,				
30 ml	**15014-0902-30**	27.09		
ARIDEX-D (Gentex Pharma)				
carbinoxamine maleate/phenylephrine hydrochloride				
SOL, PO (W/DROPPER,AF,SF)				
1 mg/ml-2 mg/ml,				
30 ml	**15014-0901-30**	32.24		
ARIMIDEX (AstraZeneca)				
anastrozole				
TAB, PO (FILM-COATED)				
1 mg, 30s ea	**00310-0201-30**	449.86		
(A-S Medication)				
REPACK				
TAB, PO (FILM-COATED)				
1 mg, 30s ea	**54569-5731-00**	508.53		
(Phys Total Care)				
REPACK				
TAB, PO (FILM-COATED)				
1 mg, 30s ea	**54868-5000-00**	517.30		
(Quality Care Prod)				
REPACK				
TAB, PO (FILM-COATED)				
1 mg, 30s ea	**35356-0270-30**	637.77		
ARIPIPRAZOLE				
(Bristol-Myers) *See ABILIFY*				
(Bristol-Myers) *See ABILIFY DISCMELT*				
ARISTOSPAN (Sabex)				
triamcinolone hexacetonide				
SUS, IJ (VIAL)				
5 mg/ml, 5 ml	**54643-1054-00**	16.18		
20 mg/ml, 1 ml	**54643-1055-00**	12.96		
5 ml	**54643-1056-00**	32.50		
(Sandoz)				
SUS, IJ, 5 mg/ml, 5 ml	**00781-3084-75**	17.72		
20 mg/ml, 1 ml	**00781-3085-71**	14.19		
(Phys Total Care)				
REPACK				
SUS, IJ (M.D.V.)				
20 mg/ml, 1 ml	**54868-3344-00**	12.53		
(Southwood)				
REPACK				
SUS, IJ, 20 mg/ml, 5 ml	**58016-4855-01**	32.50		
ARISTOWAX 143 (Amend)				
paraffin wax				
WAX, NA, 24970 gm	**17317-1080-00**	96.25		
ARISTOWAX 165 (Amend)				
paraffin wax				
WAX, NA, 24970 gm	**17317-1081-00**	77.00		
ARIXTRA (Glaxo)				
fondaparinux sodium				
SOL, SC (PREFL,27GX1/2",PF)				
2.5 mg/0.5 ml,				
0.5 ml 2s	**00007-3230-02**	121.44		
(SRN,PREFL,27GX1/2",PF)				
2.5 mg/0.5 ml,				
0.5 ml 10s	**00007-3230-11**	578.33		
0.5 ml 10s	**66203-2300-01**	435.00		
(PREFL,27GX1/2",PF)				
5 mg/0.4 ml,				
0.4 ml 2s	**00007-3232-02**	285.82		
0.4 ml 10s	**00007-3232-11**	1360.97		
7.5 mg/0.6 ml,				
0.6 ml 2s	**00007-3234-02**	285.82		
0.6 ml 10s	**00007-3234-11**	1360.97		

PROD/MFR	NDC	AWP	DP	OBC
10 mg/0.8 ml,				
0.8 ml 2s	00007-3236-02	285.82		
0.8 ml 10s	00007-3236-11	1360.97		
(Phys Total Care)				
REPACK				
SOL, SC, 7.5 mg/0.6 ml,				
0.6 ml	54868-5501-01	134.78		
0.6 ml 2s	54868-5501-02	245.70		
0.6 ml 10s	54868-5501-00	1329.48		
5 mg/0.4 ml, 10 ml	54868-5652-00	1180.51		
(Quality Care Prod)				
REPACK				
SOL, SC (10X0.5ML)				
2.5 mg/0.5 ml,				
0.5 ml 10s	35356-0078-10	1322.17		
(2X0.4ML)				
5 mg/0.4 ml,				
0.4 ml 2s	35356-0079-02	653.42		
(10X0.4ML)				
5 mg/0.4 ml,				
0.4 ml 10s	35356-0079-10	3207.62		
(2X0.6ML)				
7.5 mg/0.6 ml,				
0.6 ml 2s	35356-0080-02	653.42		
(10X0.6ML)				
7.5 mg/0.6 ml,				
0.6 ml 10s	35356-0080-10	3207.62		
(2X0.8ML)				
10 mg/0.8 ml,				
0.8 ml 2s	35356-0081-02	653.42		
(10X0.8ML)				
10 mg/0.8 ml,				
0.8 ml 10s	35356-0081-10	3207.62		
ARLACEL 165 (PCCA)				
glyceryl monostearate/peg-100 stearate				
POW, NA, 1 gm	51927-1803-00	0.08		
ARLACEL 186 (Amend)				
diglycerides/monoglycerides				
LIQ, NA, 480 ml	17317-0947-01	15.00		
3840 ml	17317-0947-06	60.00		
ARLACEL 20 (Amend)				
sorbitan monolaurate				
LIQ, NA (N.F.)				
480 ml	17317-0941-01	15.00		
3840 ml	17317-0941-06	60.00		
ARLACEL 40 (Amend)				
sorbitan monopalmitate				
LIQ, NA (N.F.)				
480 gm	17317-0942-01	15.00		
4800 gm	17317-0942-02	60.00		
24000 gm	17317-0942-03	215.00		
ARLACEL 60 (Amend)				
sorbitan monostearate				
LIQ, NA (N.F.)				
480 gm	17317-0943-01	15.00		
4800 gm	17317-0943-02	60.00		
24000 gm	17317-0943-03	201.00		
ARLACEL 80 (Amend)				
sorbitan monooleate				
LIQ, NA (N.F.)				
480 ml	17317-0944-01	15.00		
3840 ml	17317-0944-06	60.00		
21600 ml	17317-0944-09	182.25		
ARLACEL 83 (Amend)				
sorbitan sesquioleate				
LIQ, NA, 480 ml	17317-0945-01	15.00		
3840 ml	17317-0945-06	60.00		
21600 ml	17317-0945-02	183.60		
(PCCA)				
LIQ, NA (SORBITAN SESQUIOLEATE)				
1 ml	51927-1666-00	0.16		
ARLACEL C (Amend)				
sorbitan sesquioleate				
LIQ, NA, 480 ml	17317-0940-01	15.00		
3840 ml	17317-0940-06	60.00		
ARLAMOL E (Amend)				
polyoxy propylene (15) stearyl ether				
SOL, NA, 454 gm	17317-0948-01	15.00		
3840 ml	17317-0948-06	60.00		
20640 gm	17317-0948-08	200.81		
ARLASOLVE 200 (Amend)				
polyoxyethylene (20) isohexadecyl ether				
SOL, NA, 454 gm	17317-0949-01	15.00		
454 gm	17317-0949-08	192.40		
3632 gm	17317-0949-06	60.00		

PROD/MFR	NDC	AWP	DP	OBC
ARLATONE G (Amend)				
polyoxyethylene fatty glyceride				
LIQ, NA, 480 ml	17317-0951-01	15.00		
3840 ml	17317-0951-06	60.00		
21600 ml	17317-0951-07	202.05		
ARLATONE T (Amend)				
polyoxyethylene (40) sorbitol septaoleate				
LIQ, NA, 480 ml	17317-0952-01	15.00		
3840 ml	17317-0952-06	60.00		
21600 ml	17317-0952-03	207.00		
ARLEX (Amend)				
sorbitol				
LIQ, NA, 480 ml	17317-0953-01	15.00		
3840 ml	17317-0953-06	60.00		
28800 ml	17317-0953-08	240.00		
ARMODAFINIL				
(Cephalon) *See NUVIGIL*				
ARMOUR THYROID (Forest Pharm)				
thyroid				
TAB, PO, 15 mg, 100s ea	00456-0457-01	12.34		
30 mg, 100s ea	00456-0458-01	14.48		
(10X10)				
30 mg, 100s ea UD	00456-0458-63	25.38		
60 mg, 100s ea	00456-0459-01	16.08		
(10X10)				
60 mg, 100s ea UD	00456-0459-63	27.00		
90 mg, 100s ea	00456-0460-01	25.38		
120 mg, 100s ea	00456-0461-01	29.74		
(10X10)				
120 mg, 100s ea UD	00456-0461-63	33.68		
180 mg, 100s ea	00456-0462-01	47.18		
240 mg, 100s ea	00456-0463-01	70.73		
300 mg, 100s ea	00456-0464-01	87.67		
(A-S Medication)				
REPACK				
TAB, PO, 30 mg, 30s ea	54569-0917-01	4.53		
100s ea	54569-0917-00	15.09		
60 mg, 30s ea	54569-0918-01	5.03		
100s ea	54569-0918-00	16.75		
90 mg, 100s ea	54569-4471-00	26.44		
120 mg, 30s ea	54569-0919-02	9.29		
100s ea	54569-0919-00	30.98		
(Dispensing Solutions)				
REPACK				
TAB, PO, 30 mg, 30s ea	55045-2930-08	9.00		
100s ea	55045-2930-00	30.00		
60 mg, 30s ea	55045-1620-08	10.50		
100s ea	55045-1620-00	35.00		
(Phys Total Care)				
REPACK				
TAB, PO, 15 mg, 30s ea	54868-4979-00	7.71		
100s ea	54868-4979-01	16.14		
30 mg, 30s ea	54868-4982-00	6.81		
90s ea	54868-4982-01	16.70		
100s ea	54868-4982-02	17.73		
60 mg, 30s ea	54868-1253-01	7.35		
60s ea	54868-1253-02	12.81		
100s ea	54868-1253-00	20.11		
90 mg, 30s ea	54868-5159-01	11.51		
90s ea	54868-5159-00	30.60		
120 mg, 100s ea	54868-1746-00	35.00		
(Quality Care Prod)				
REPACK				
TAB, PO, 15 mg, 60s ea	49999-0289-60	22.68		
60 mg, 30s ea	49999-0702-30	4.95		
90 mg, 100s ea	49999-0281-00	89.92		
ARNICA FLOWER				
(PCCA) *See ARNICA FLOWER TINCTURE*				
ARNICA FLOWER TINCTURE (PCCA)				
arnica flower				
TIN, NA (1X1ML)				
1 ml	51927-2228-00	0.50		
AROMASIN (Pfizer)				
exemestane				
TAB, PO, 25 mg, 30s ea	00009-7663-04	404.90	337.42	
(Bryant Ranch)				
REPACK				
TAB, PO, 25 mg, 30s ea	63629-1262-01	265.31		
(Phys Total Care)				
REPACK				
TAB, PO, 25 mg, 30s ea	54868-5261-00	465.80		
(Quality Care Prod)				
REPACK				
TAB, PO, 25 mg, 30s ea	49999-0986-30	357.90		
AROMATIC ELIXIR (Gallipot)				
ELI, NA, 473 ml	51552-0428-06	16.73		

PROD/MFR	NDC	AWP	DP	OBC
ARRANON (Glaxo)				
nelarabine				
SOL, IV (LATEX-FREE)				
5 mg/ml, 50 ml	00007-4401-01	615.94		
(6X50ML,LATEX-FREE)				
5 mg/ml, 50 ml 6s	00007-4401-06	3695.60		
ARSENIC TRIOXIDE (Baker, J.T.)				
POW, NA (A.C.S., REAGENT)				
125 gm	10106-0061-04	105.21		
(REAGENT)				
125 gm	10106-0062-04	70.50		
(A.C.S., REAGENT)				
500 gm	10106-0061-01	267.29		
(REAGENT)				
500 gm	10106-0062-01	192.51		
(Cephalon) *See TRISENOX*				
(PCCA)				
POW, NA (TECHNICAL)				
1 gm	51927-1441-00	1.95		
(Spectrum Pharmacy)				
POW, NA (A.C.S.,REAGENT)				
25 gm	49452-0735-04	208.25		
125 gm	49452-0735-01	647.50		
500 gm	49452-0735-02	2327.50		
ARTEMETHER/LUMEFANTRINE				
(Novartis Pharm) *See COARTEM*				
ARTHRICREAM W/ ALOE (Physician Partner)				
REPACK				
trolamine salicylate				
CRE, TP, 10%, 85 gm	21695-0310-03	17.80		
ARTHROTEC (Pfizer)				
diclofenac sodium/misoprostol				
ECT, PO, 50 mg-0.2 mg,				
60s ea	00025-1411-60	170.64	142.20	
90s ea	00025-1411-90	255.95	213.29	
100s ea UD	00025-1411-34	298.66	248.88	
75 mg-0.2 mg,				
60s ea	00025-1421-60	170.64	142.20	
100s ea UD	00025-1421-34	298.66	248.88	
(A-S Medication)				
REPACK				
ECT, PO, 50 mg-0.2 mg,				
60s ea	54569-6097-00	211.28		
75 mg-0.2 mg,				
60s ea	54569-4579-00	211.28		
(AQ)				
REPACK				
ECT, PO, 50 mg-0.2 mg,				
60s ea	66105-0130-06	174.29		
(ENTERIC COATED)				
75 mg-0.2 mg,				
60s ea	66105-0131-06	174.29		
(DHS, Inc.)				
REPACK				
ECT, PO, 75 mg-0.2 mg,				
30s ea	66887-0643-30	89.50		
(Dispensing Solutions)				
REPACK				
ECT, PO, 50 mg-0.2 mg,				
30s ea	55045-2548-08	75.90		
60s ea	55045-2548-06	151.80		
75 mg-0.2 mg,				
14s ea	55045-3047-01	35.42		
60s ea	55045-3047-09	151.80		
(Nucare Pharm)				
REPACK				
ECT, PO, 75 mg-0.2 mg,				
30s ea	68071-0695-30	122.46		
60s ea	68071-1310-00	244.92		
(Palmetto)				
REPACK				
ECT, PO, 75 mg-0.2 mg,				
60s ea	23490-9246-06	140.38		
(PD-Rx Pharm)				
REPACK				
ECT, PO, 50 mg-0.2 mg,				
15s ea	55289-0406-15	60.39		
30s ea	55289-0406-30	120.77		
(Pharma Pac)				
REPACK				
ECT, PO, 50 mg-0.2 mg,				
20s ea	52959-0531-20	58.90		
30s ea	52959-0531-30	87.60		
42s ea	52959-0531-42	122.64		
60s ea	52959-0531-60	175.20		
90s ea	52959-0531-90	262.80		

PROD/MFR	NDC	AWP	DP	OBC
75 mg-0.2 mg,				
14s ea	52959-0525-14	46.95		
20s ea	52959-0525-20	66.95		
30s ea	52959-0525-30	100.10		
60s ea	52959-0525-60	199.70		
(Phys Total Care)				
REPACK				
ECT, PO, 50 mg-0.2 mg,				
30s ea	54868-4164-01	104.46		
60s ea	54868-4164-00	146.73		
75 mg-0.2 mg,				
30s ea	54868-4165-01	109.56		
60s ea	54868-4165-00	203.97		
(Physician Partner)				
REPACK				
ECT, PO, 75 mg-0.2 mg,				
60s ea	21695-0425-60	341.28		
(Quality Care Prod)				
REPACK				
ECT, PO, 50 mg-0.2 mg,				
60s ea	35356-0467-60	264.00		
75 mg-0.2 mg,				
60s ea	49999-0987-60	264.00		
(Southwood)				
REPACK				
ECT, PO, 50 mg-0.2 mg,				
30s ea	58016-0577-30	77.39		
60s ea	58016-0577-60	154.78		
90s ea	58016-0577-90	232.17		
100s ea	58016-0577-00	257.97		
120s ea	58016-0577-02	309.56		
150s ea	58016-0577-03	386.95		
200s ea	58016-0577-89	515.93		
300s ea	58016-0577-73	773.90		
75 mg-0.2 mg,				
30s ea	58016-0498-30	81.27		
60s ea	58016-0498-60	162.53		
90s ea	58016-0498-90	243.80		
100s ea	58016-0498-00	270.89		
(Stat Rx)				
REPACK				
ECT, PO, 50 mg-0.2 mg,				
60s ea	16590-0564-60	189.35		
75 mg-0.2 mg,				
30s ea	16590-0024-30	95.38		
56s ea	16590-0024-56	176.81		
60s ea	16590-0024-60	191.11		
ARTHROTEC 75 (Altura)				
REPACK				
diclofenac sodium/misoprostol				
ECT, PO (FILM COATED)				
75 mg-0.2 mg,				
14s ea	63874-0944-14	32.63		
15s ea	63874-0944-15	34.96		
20s ea	63874-0944-20	46.61		
30s ea	63874-0944-30	69.92		
60s ea	63874-0944-60	139.83		
100s ea	63874-0944-01	233.05		
ARTISS (Baxter Bioscience)				
aprotinin/calcium chloride/fibrinogen/thrombin				
KIT, TP (10ML TOTAL VOLUME)				
ea	00944-4351-10	899.05		
(4ML TOTAL VOLUME)				
ea	00944-4351-08	400.67		
SOL, TP (1X2ML)				
2 ml	00944-8503-02	230.20		
(1X4ML)				
4 ml	00944-8503-04	391.99		
(1X10ML)				
10 ml	00944-8503-10	877.38		
ARZERRA (Glaxo)				
ofatumumab				
SOL, IV (SINGLE-USE W/2 FILTERS)				
20 mg/ml, 5 ml 3s	00173-0808-02	1584.00		
5 ml 10s	00173-0808-05	5280.00		
ASA/OXYCODONE HCL/OXYCODONE TEREPHTHALATE				
(Watson Labs) *See ASPIRIN/OXYCODONE*				
ASACOL (P & G Pharm)				
mesalamine				
ECT, PO, 400 mg, 180s ea	00149-0752-15	332.82	277.35	
(PD-Rx Pharm)				
REPACK				
ECT, PO, 400 mg, 30s ea	55289-0833-30	87.00		
(Phys Total Care)				
REPACK				
ECT, PO, 400 mg, 40s ea	54868-2515-02	63.35		
60s ea	54868-2515-00	111.33		
90s ea	54868-2515-05	156.90		
100s ea	54868-2515-01	183.59		

PROD/MFR	NDC	AWP	DP	OBC
120s ea	54868-2515-04	208.55		
180s ea	54868-2515-03	311.84		
(Quality Care Prod)				
REPACK				
ECT, PO, 400 mg, 180s ea	49999-0969-18	516.28		
ASACOL HD (P & G Pharm)				
mesalamine				
TCP, PO, 800 mg, 180s ea	00149-0783-01	665.64	554.70	
ASAFETIDA				
(PCCA) *See ASAFETIDA GUM*				
ASAFETIDA GUM (PCCA)				
asafetida				
POW, NA, 1 gm	51927-1967-00	0.92		
ASCOMP W/CODEINE (Breckenridge Pharm)				
aspirin/butalbital/caffeine/codeine phosphate				
CAP, PO				
325 mg-50 mg-40 mg-30 mg,				
100s ea, C-III	51991-0074-01	139.95		AB
500s ea, C-III	51991-0074-05	664.75		AB
ASCOR L 500 (McGuff)				
ascorbic acid				
SOL, IJ (SDV,PF)				
500 mg/ml,				
50 ml 25s	67157-0101-50	11.95		
ASCOR L NC (McGuff)				
ascorbic acid				
SOL, IJ (NON-CORN SOURCE,PF)				
500 mg/ml,				
50 ml 25s	67157-0103-50	16.95		
ASCORBIC ACID (Amer Regent)				
SOL, IJ (S.D.V.,PF)				
500 mg/ml, 50 ml	00517-5050-01	12.50		
(Baker, J.T.)				
GRA, NA (USP, FCC, 20-80 MESH)				
125 gm	10106-0938-05	38.33		
500 gm	10106-0938-07	25.71		
1000 gm	10106-0938-08	71.82		
POW, NA (USP, FCC, 2-200 MESH)				
500 gm	10106-0936-07	42.52		
(USP, FCC, 200-325 MESH)				
500 gm	10106-0937-07	39.34		
(USP, FCC, 2-200 MESH)				
1000 gm	10106-0936-08	63.33		
(USP, FCC, 200-325 MESH)				
1000 gm	10106-0937-08	160.28		
(Bioniche Pharma)				
SOL, IJ (PF)				
500 mg/ml, 50 ml	67457-0118-50	17.38		
(Consolidated Midland)				
SOL, IJ (AMP)				
250 mg/ml,				
2 ml 25s	00223-8875-02	60.00		
30 ml	00223-8873-30	6.00		
(VIAL)				
250 mg/ml, 30 ml	00223-7185-30	6.00		
(AMP)				
500 mg/ml, 50 ml	00223-7186-50	7.50		
(Gallipot)				
GRA, NA (U.S.P.,N.F.)				
118.28 gm	51552-0164-04	14.00		
454 gm	51552-0164-06	23.03		
(U.S.P.)				
1000 gm	51552-0164-07	55.16		
POW, NA (U.S.P.,N.F.)				
113.4 gm	51552-0163-04	14.00		
454 gm	51552-0163-06	23.03		
(Hospira) *See CENOLATE*				
(Letco)				
POW, NA (U.S.P./N.F.)				
100 gm	62991-1011-01	27.00		
500 gm	62991-1011-02	57.00		
(U.S.P.)				
1000 gm	62991-1011-03	75.00		
5000 gm	62991-1011-04	270.00		
(Lorann Oil)				
POW, NA (F.C.C.)				
30 gm	23535-0601-55	1.75		
120 gm	23535-0601-58	4.95		
454 gm	23535-0601-51	16.00		
(Mallinckrodt Lab)				
POW, NA (U.S.P.)				
100 gm	00406-1852-57	26.24		
(U.S.P.,FINE)				
500 gm	00406-8829-03	58.78		
(U.S.P.)				
500 gm	00406-1852-10	86.57		

PROD/MFR	NDC	AWP	DP	OBC
(McGuff) *See ASCOR L 500*				
(McGuff) *See ASCOR L NC*				
(Medisca)				
POW, NA (U.S.P.)				
100 gm	38779-0634-05	88.50		
500 gm	38779-0634-08	148.50		
1000 gm	38779-0634-09	262.50		
5000 gm	38779-0634-03	645.00		
(Merit) *See MEGA-C/A PLUS*				
(Merit) *See ORTHO/CS*				
(Neurovites) *See VITAMIN C*				
(PCCA)				
GRA, NA (USP)				
1 gm	51927-1173-00	0.57		
POW, NA (U.S.P.,FINE)				
1 gm	51927-1483-00	1.44		
(USP)				
1 gm	51927-3204-00	0.30		
(Spectrum Pharmacy)				
GRA, NA (U.S.P.)				
100 gm	49452-0740-06	93.10		
500 gm	49452-0740-01	144.90		
1000 gm	49452-0740-02	219.45		
5000 gm	49452-0740-03	840.00		
POW, NA (1X25GM,USP)				
25 gm	49452-0739-01	86.45		
(1X100GM,USP)				
100 gm	49452-0739-02	163.10		
(U.S.P.)				
100 gm	49452-0750-06	93.10		
(1X500GM,USP)				
500 gm	49452-0739-03	264.25		
(U.S.P.)				
500 gm	49452-0750-02	144.90		
(1X1000GM,USP)				
1000 gm	49452-0739-04	423.50		
(U.S.P.)				
1000 gm	49452-0750-03	219.45		
(1X5000GM,USP)				
5000 gm	49452-0739-05	1596.00		
(U.S.P.)				
5000 gm	49452-0750-04	840.00		
ASCORBIC ACID/CYANOCOBALAMIN/ FERROUS FUMARATE				
(Laser Pharma) *See FUMATINIC*				
(Lunsco) *See FETRIN*				
ASCORBIC ACID/CYANOCOBALAMIN/FOLIC ACID/IRON				
(Hawthorn Pharm) *See ICAR-C PLUS SR*				
(River's Edge) *See RE KAR C PLUS SR*				
ASCORBIC ACID/FERROUS SULFATE/FOLIC ACID				
(Contract Pharmacal) *See FOLI-IRON & C*				
(Rising) *See FOLITAB 500*				
ASCORBIC ACID/IRON/SUCCINIC ACID				
(Ther-RX) *See NIFEREX-150*				
ASCORBIC ACID/SODIUM FLUORIDE/VITAMIN A /VITAMIN D				
(Hi-Tech) *See TRI-VITAMIN W/FLUORIDE*				
(Perry Med) *See FLOR-DAC TRI-VITAMIN*				
(Qualitest) *See TRI-VIT W/FLUORIDE*				
(Qualitest) *See TRI-VIT WITH FLUORIDE*				
(Silarx) *See TRI-VITAMIN WITH 0.25MG FLUORIDE*				
(Vintage) *See TRIPLE VITAMIN W/FLUORIDE*				
ASCORBIC ACID/VITAMIN B COMPLEX				
(Consolidated Midland) *See VITAMIN B COMPLEX W/VITAMIN C*				
(Intl Ethical) *See NEUROFORTE-SIX*				
ASCORBYL PALMITATE (Letco)				
POW, NA (NF, FCC)				
25 gm	62991-1560-01	30.00		
100 gm	62991-1560-02	66.75		
(Medisca)				
POW, NA (1X25GM)				
25 gm	38779-0908-04	31.50		
(1X100GM)				
100 gm	38779-0908-05	67.50		
(1X500GM)				
500 gm	38779-0908-08	297.00		
(PCCA)				
POW, NA (FCC)				
1 gm	51927-2728-00	1.80		

PROD/MFR	NDC	AWP	DP	OBC
(Spectrum Pharmacy)				
POW, NA (N.F.)				
25 gm	**49452-0754-03**	84.00		
125 gm	**49452-0754-01**	208.60		
500 gm	**49452-0754-02**	535.50		
ASENAPINE				
(Schering) *See SAPHRIS*				
ASMANEX TWIST (Phys Total Care)				
REPACK				
mometasone furoate				
POW, IH, 0.22 mg/actuation,				
0.24 gm	**54868-5547-00**	177.81		
(1X0.24GM)				
0.22 mg/actuation,				
0.24 gm	**54868-5547-01**	151.62		
ASMANEX TWISTHALER (Schering)				
mometasone furoate				
POW, IH (120-INHALATION)				
0.22 mg/actuation,				
0.24 gm	**00085-1341-01**	221.41		
(30-INHALATION)				
0.22 mg/actuation,				
0.24 gm	**00085-1341-03**	131.47		
(60-INHALATION)				
0.22 mg/actuation,				
0.24 gm	**00085-1341-02**	154.49		
(30-INHALATION UNITS)				
110 mcg/actuation,				
0.135 gm	**00085-1461-02**	121.76		EE
(Phys Total Care)				
REPACK				
POW, IH (1X0.24GM)				
0.22 mg/actuation,				
0.24 gm	**54868-5547-02**	112.56		
(Quality Care Prod)				
REPACK				
POW, IH (14-INHALATION)				
0.22 mg/actuation,				
0.24 gm	**35356-0099-14**	154.53		
ASP 300/200/20 (PGD, Inc.)				
apap/phenyltoloxamine cit/salicylamide				
CAP, PO, 300 mg-20 mg-200 mg,				
60s ea	**65615-0200-60**	12.03		
ASPARAGINASE				
(Lundbeck) *See ELSPAR*				
ASPARAGINE (PCCA)				
asparagine monohydrate				
POW, NA (FCC,MONOHYDRATE)				
1 gm	**51927-2717-00**	1.05		
ASPARAGINE MONOHYDRATE				
(PCCA) *See ASPARAGINE*				
(Spectrum Pharmacy) *See L-ASPARAGINE MONOHYDRATE*				
ASPARTAME				
(Gallipot) *See NUTRASWEET ASPARTAME APM*				
(Letco)				
POW, NA (U.S.P.,N.F.)				
100 gm	**62991-1175-02**	75.00		
500 gm	**62991-1175-03**	225.00		
1000 gm	**62991-1175-04**	345.00		
(Medisca)				
POW, NA (N.F.)				
10 gm	**38779-0061-01**	27.00		
100 gm	**38779-0061-05**	165.00		
(NF,1X500GM)				
500 gm	**38779-0061-08**	292.50		
(NF,1X1000GM)				
1000 gm	**38779-0061-09**	526.50		
(PCCA)				
POW, NA (NF)				
1 gm	**51927-1134-00**	1.67		
(Spectrum Pharmacy)				
POW, NA (N.F.)				
25 gm	**49452-0762-01**	67.90		
125 gm	**49452-0762-02**	191.80		
500 gm	**49452-0762-03**	434.00		
ASPARTIC ACID (PCCA)				
POW, NA (FCC)				
1 gm	**51927-2887-00**	0.63		
(Spectrum Pharmacy) *See L-ASPARTIC ACID*				
ASPARTIC ACID MAGNESIUM SALT (PCCA)				
magnesium aspartate				
POW, NA (L,DIHYDRATE)				
1 gm	**51927-2191-00**	0.75		

PROD/MFR	NDC	AWP	DP	OBC
ASPARTIC ACID SODIUM				
(PCCA) *See ASPARTIC ACID SODIUM SALT*				
(Spectrum Pharmacy) *See L-ASPARTIC ACID SODIUM SALT*				
ASPARTIC ACID SODIUM SALT (PCCA)				
aspartic acid sodium				
POW, NA, 1 gm	**51927-2864-00**	2.07		
ASPIRIN (Baker, J.T.)				
POW, NA (U.S.P.)				
500 gm	**10106-0033-01**	36.07		
(Gallipot)				
POW, NA (U.S.P.,N.F.)				
454 gm	**51552-0175-06**	22.96		
2270 gm	**51552-0175-09**	85.40		
(Hawkins)				
POW, NA (U.S.P.)				
100 gm	**63370-0024-35**	24.00		
500 gm	**63370-0024-45**	64.00		
2500 gm	**63370-0024-53**	196.00		
(Medisca) *See ACETYLSALICYLIC ACID*				
(Par) *See ZORPRIN*				
(PCCA)				
POW, NA (U.S.P.)				
1 gm	**51927-1157-00**	0.21		
(Rosedale) *See EASPRIN*				
(Spectrum Pharmacy)				
POW, NA (U.S.P.)				
500 gm	**49452-0760-01**	88.20		
2500 gm	**49452-0760-02**	269.15		
12000 gm	**49452-0760-03**	983.50		
(Bryant Ranch)				
REPACK				
TAB, PO, 325 mg, 30s ea	**63629-1881-02**	2.50		
100s ea	**63629-1881-01**	6.70		
(Dispensing Solutions)				
REPACK				
ECT, PO, 325 mg, 15s ea	**55045-1222-05**	1.50		
30s ea	**55045-1222-08**	3.00		
100s ea	**55045-1222-01**	10.00		
650 mg, 100s ea	**55045-2790-01**	11.00		
ASPIRIN/BUTALBITAL/CAFFEINE				
FUL				
TAB, PO, 325 mg-50 mg-40 mg,				
100s ea		24.00		
(Actavis)				
TAB, PO, 325 mg-50 mg-40 mg,				
100s ea, C-III	**00228-2023-10**	70.25		AB
(Lannett)				
CAP, PO, 325 mg-50 mg-40 mg,				
100s ea, C-III	**00527-1552-01**	89.00		AB
(Major)				
TAB, PO, 325 mg-50 mg-40 mg,				
100s ea, C-III	**00904-3092-60**	64.20		AB
(Qualitest) *See BUTALBITAL COMPOUND*				
(Watson) *See FIORINAL*				
(Watson Labs)				
CAP, PO, 325 mg-50 mg-40 mg,				
100s ea, C-III	**00591-3219-01**	89.00		AB
(West-Ward)				
TAB, PO, 325 mg-50 mg-40 mg,				
100s ea, C-III	**00143-1785-01**	70.25		AB
1000s ea, C-III	**00143-1785-10**	662.50		AB
(A-S Medication)				
REPACK				
TAB, PO, 325 mg-50 mg-40 mg,				
30s ea, C-III	**54569-0339-04**	24.71		EE
(Aidarex)				
REPACK				
CAP, PO, 325 mg-50 mg-40 mg,				
7s ea, C-III	**33261-0177-07**	9.63		AB
14s ea, C-III	**33261-0177-14**	19.25		AB
20s ea, C-III	**33261-0177-20**	27.51		AB
21s ea, C-III	**33261-0177-21**	28.89		AB
28s ea, C-III	**33261-0177-28**	38.51		AB
30s ea, C-III	**33261-0177-30**	41.27		AB
60s ea, C-III	**33261-0177-60**	82.54		AB
90s ea, C-III	**33261-0177-90**	123.80		AB
120s ea, C-III	**33261-0177-02**	165.06		AB
(Palmetto)				
REPACK				
CAP, PO, 325 mg-50 mg-40 mg,				
30s ea, C-III	**23490-5182-01**	49.99		

PROD/MFR	NDC	AWP	DP	OBC
ASPIRIN/BUTALBITAL/CAFFEINE (Palmetto)				
TAB, PO, 325 mg-50 mg-40 mg,				
10s ea, C-III	**23490-5183-01**	16.66		
20s ea, C-III	**23490-5183-02**	33.32		
30s ea, C-III	**23490-5183-03**	49.99		
60s ea, C-III	**23490-5183-06**	99.98		
90s ea, C-III	**23490-5183-09**	149.97		
ASPIRIN/BUTALBITAL/CAFFEINE (PD-Rx Pharm)				
REPACK				
TAB, PO, 325 mg-50 mg-40 mg,				
15s ea, C-III	**55289-0040-15**	21.88		AB
20s ea, C-III	**55289-0040-20**	27.52		AB
30s ea, C-III	**55289-0040-30**	38.77		AB
(Pharma Pac)				
REPACK				
CAP, PO, 325 mg-50 mg-40 mg,				
30s ea, C-III	**52959-0767-30**	32.10		
60s ea, C-III	**52959-0767-60**	64.35		
TAB, PO, 325 mg-50 mg-40 mg,				
20s ea, C-III	**52959-0399-20**	21.46		EE
30s ea, C-III	**52959-0399-30**	32.10		EE
50s ea, C-III	**52959-0399-50**	53.61		AB
60s ea, C-III	**52959-0399-60**	64.35		EE
90s ea, C-III	**52959-0399-90**	96.25		EE
100s ea, C-III	**52959-0399-00**	107.00		EE
(Physician Partner)				
REPACK				
TAB, PO, 325 mg-50 mg-40 mg,				
60s ea, C-III	**21695-0354-60**	84.30		AB
(Quality Care Prod)				
REPACK				
TAB, PO, 325 mg-50 mg-40 mg,				
20s ea, C-III	**49999-0115-20**	48.78		EE
30s ea, C-III	**49999-0115-30**	73.17		AB
60s ea, C-III	**49999-0115-60**	146.34		AB
(Southwood)				
REPACK				
TAB, PO, 325 mg-50 mg-40 mg,				
10s ea, C-III	**58016-0233-10**	4.78		EE
12s ea, C-III	**58016-0233-12**	5.73		EE
14s ea, C-III	**58016-0233-14**	6.69		EE
15s ea, C-III	**58016-0233-15**	7.16		EE
20s ea, C-III	**58016-0233-20**	9.55		EE
21s ea, C-III	**58016-0233-21**	10.03		EE
24s ea, C-III	**58016-0233-24**	11.46		EE
25s ea, C-III	**58016-0233-25**	11.94		EE
28s ea, C-III	**58016-0233-28**	13.37		EE
30s ea, C-III	**58016-0233-30**	14.33		EE
40s ea, C-III	**58016-0233-40**	19.10		EE
50s ea, C-III	**58016-0233-50**	23.25		EE
60s ea, C-III	**58016-0233-60**	28.66		EE
90s ea, C-III	**58016-0233-90**	41.85		EE
100s ea, C-III	**58016-0233-00**	46.50		EE
120s ea, C-III	**58016-0233-02**	57.32		AB
ASPIRIN/BUTALBITAL/CAFFEINE/CODEINE (Lannett)				
aspirin/butalbital/caffeine/codeine phosphate				
CAP, PO				
325 mg-50 mg-40 mg-30 mg,				
100s ea, C-III	**00527-1312-01**	138.00		AB
(Major)				
CAP, PO				
325 mg-50 mg-40 mg-30 mg,				
100s ea, C-III	**00904-5140-60**	157.37		AB
(Watson Labs)				
CAP, PO (USP)				
325 mg-50 mg-40 mg-30 mg,				
100s ea, C-III	**00591-3546-01**	126.41		AB
(Altura)				
REPACK				
CAP, PO				
325 mg-50 mg-40 mg-30 mg,				
20s ea, C-III	**63874-0219-20**	28.20		EE
25s ea, C-III	**63874-0219-25**	35.25		EE
30s ea, C-III	**63874-0219-30**	42.30		EE
100s ea, C-III	**63874-0219-01**	141.00		EE
(Dispensing Solutions)				
REPACK				
CAP, PO				
325 mg-50 mg-40 mg-30 mg,				
30s ea, C-III	**55045-2352-08**	42.00		AB
30s ea, C-III	**66336-0314-30**	44.15		AB
(Pharma Pac)				
REPACK				
CAP, PO				
325 mg-50 mg-40 mg-30 mg,				
30s ea, C-III	**52959-0865-30**	84.30		
100s ea, C-III	**52959-0865-00**	142.50		

PROD/MFR	NDC	AWP	DP	OBC

ASPIRIN/BUTALBITAL/CAFFEINE/ CODEINE PHOSPHATE
(Breckenridge Pharm) *See ASCOMP W/CODEINE*
(Lannett) *See ASPIRIN/BUTALBITAL/CAFFEINE/CODEINE*
(Major) *See ASPIRIN/BUTALBITAL/CAFFEINE/CODEINE*
(Watson) *See FIORINAL W/CODEINE*
(Watson Labs) *See ASPIRIN/BUTALBITAL/CAFFEINE/CODEINE*
(Watson Labs) *See BUTALBITAL,ASPIRIN,CAFFEINE, AND CODEINE PHOSPHATE*

(Palmetto)
REPACK
CAP, PO
325 mg-50 mg-40 mg-30 mg,
30s ea, C-III 23490-6825-03 45.00

ASPIRIN/CAFFEINE/DIHYDROCODEINE BITARTRATE
(Caraco) *See SYNALGOS-DC*

ASPIRIN/CAFFEINE/ORPHENADRINE (Mylan)
aspirin/caffeine/orphenadrine citrate
TAB, PO, 385 mg-30 mg-25 mg,
100s ea .... 00378-3354-01 79.50 AB

(Sandoz)
TAB, PO, 385 mg-30 mg-25 mg,
100s ea .... 00185-0713-01 180.94 AB
500s ea .... 00185-0713-05 904.72 AB
770 mg-60 mg-50 mg,
100s ea .... 00185-0714-01 261.89 AB

(Dispensing Solutions)
REPACK
TAB, PO (CAPLET)
770 mg-60 mg-50 mg,
30s ea .... 55045-2777-08 33.00 AB

(Pharma Pac)
REPACK
TAB, PO, 385 mg-30 mg-25 mg,
60s ea .... 52959-0673-60 48.60 EE

(Physician Partner)
REPACK
TAB, PO, 770 mg-60 mg-50 mg,
30s ea .... 21695-0726-30 157.13 AB
(MULTILAYER)
770 mg-60 mg-50 mg,
45s ea .... 21695-0726-45 231.27 AB

ASPIRIN/CAFFEINE/ORPHENADRINE CITRATE
(Mylan) *See ASPIRIN/CAFFEINE/ORPHENADRINE*
(Sandoz) *See ASPIRIN/CAFFEINE/ORPHENADRINE*

ASPIRIN/CARISOPRODOL
FUL
TAB, PO, 325 mg-200 mg,
100s ea 27.08

(Consolidated Midland) *See CARISOPRODOL COMPOUND*

(Sandoz)
TAB, PO, 325 mg-200 mg,
100s ea .... 00185-0724-01 239.20 AB
500s ea .... 00185-0724-05 1160.13 AB

(PD-Rx Pharm)
REPACK
TAB, PO, 325 mg-200 mg,
28s ea .... 55289-0695-28 192.25 AB
40s ea .... 55289-0695-40 239.00 AB

(Pharma Pac)
REPACK
TAB, PO, 325 mg-200 mg,
14s ea .... 52959-0454-14 21.28 EE
60s ea .... 52959-0454-60 90.60 EE
120s ea .... 52959-0454-02 181.20 EE

ASPIRIN/CARISOPRODOL/CODEINE (Sandoz)
aspirin/carisoprodol/codeine phosphate
TAB, PO, 325 mg-200 mg-16 mg,
100s ea, C-III ...... 00185-0749-01 277.50 AB

ASPIRIN/CARISOPRODOL/CODEINE PHOSPHATE
FUL
TAB, PO, 325 mg-200 mg-16 mg,
100s ea 183.75

(Sandoz) *See ASPIRIN/CARISOPRODOL/CODEINE*

ASPIRIN/CODEINE (Altura)
REPACK
aspirin/codeine phosphate
TAB, PO, 325 mg-30 mg,
12s ea, C-III 63874-0217-12 4.41
15s ea, C-III 63874-0217-15 5.51
20s ea, C-III 63874-0217-20 7.49
24s ea, C-III 63874-0217-24 14.38
30s ea, C-III 63874-0217-30 37.71
100s ea, C-III 63874-0217-01 36.75
325 mg-60 mg,
12s ea, C-III 63874-0218-12 10.29
15s ea, C-III 63874-0218-15 12.87
20s ea, C-III 63874-0218-20 17.16
30s ea, C-III 63874-0218-30 25.74
100s ea, C-III 63874-0218-01 85.79

(HomeMed)
REPACK
TAB, PO, 325 mg-30 mg,
15s ea, C-III 51655-0817-54 4.69
30s ea, C-III 51655-0817-24 4.55
325 mg-60 mg,
15s ea, C-III 51655-0818-54 6.15
30s ea, C-III 51655-0818-24 7.07

(PD-Rx Pharm)
REPACK
TAB, PO, 325 mg-30 mg,
15s ea, C-III 55289-0331-15 8.07

(Phys Total Care)
REPACK
TAB, PO, 325 mg-60 mg,
15s ea, C-III 54868-0386-00 19.68

ASPIRIN/DIPYRIDAMOLE
(Boehr Ingelheim Phar) *See AGGRENOX*

ASPIRIN/HYDROCODONE BITARTRATE
(Mason Pharm) *See DAMASON-P*

ASPIRIN/MEPROBAMATE
(Caraco) *See EQUAGESIC*

ASPIRIN/METHOCARBAMOL (PD-Rx Pharm)
REPACK
TAB, PO, 325 mg-400 mg,
30s ea .... 55289-0496-30 28.96 AB

ASPIRIN/OXYCODONE (Watson Labs)
asa/oxycodone hcl/oxycodone terephthalate
TAB, PO, 325 mg-4.5 mg-0.38 mg,
100s ea, C-II .... 00591-0820-01 113.74 AA

(Phys Total Care)
REPACK
TAB, PO, 325 mg-4.5 mg-0.38 mg,
20s ea, C-II .... 54868-2094-00 77.46 EE
30s ea, C-II .... 54868-2094-01 112.44 EE

ASPIRIN/OXYCODONE HYDROCHLORIDE
(Endo Pharm) *See ENDODAN*
(Endo Pharm) *See PERCODAN*

ASSESS PEAK FLOW METER ZONE SYSTEM (Respironics)
meter, peak flow, spirometry
DEV, NA (ASTHMA MGMNT,FULL RANGE)
ea 83730-0718-00 20.60
(ASTHMA MGMNT,LOW RANGE)
ea 83730-0719-00 22.74

ASTELIN READY-SPRAY (Meda)
azelastine hydrochloride
SPR, NS, 137 mcg/actuation,
30 ml 00037-0241-30 111.36

(A-S Medication)
REPACK
SPR, NS, 137 mcg/actuation,
30 ml 54569-5625-00 144.77

(Pharma Pac)
REPACK
SPR, NS, 137 mcg/actuation,
30 ml 52959-0813-03 77.35

(Phys Total Care)
REPACK
SPR, NS, 137 mcg/actuation,
30 ml 54868-5072-00 141.54

ASTEPRO (Meda)
azelastine hydrochloride
SPR, NS, 205.5 mcg/actuation,
30 ml 00037-0243-30 107.13 85.70

ASTHMA PACK II PEAK FLOW METER (Respironics)
meter, peak flow, spirometry
DEV, NA (W/OPTICHAMBER)
ea 83730-0722-00 38.00

ASTHMA PACK III PEAK FLOW METER (Respironics)
meter, peak flow, spirometry
DEV, NA (W/OPTICHAMBER)
ea 83730-0724-00 38.00

ASTHMA PACK PEAK FLOW METER (Respironics)
meter, peak flow, spirometry
DEV, NA (W/OPTIHALER)
ea 83730-0720-00 35.00

ASTRAGALUS ROOT (PCCA)
POW, NA, 1 gm 51927-3481-00 0.60

ASTRAMORPH/PF (APP)
morphine sulfate
SOL, IJ (SINGLE USE,10X2ML,PF)
0.5 mg/ml,
2 ml 10s, C-II ...... 63323-0291-80 98.40 AP
(5X10ML,SINGLEUSEONLY,PF)
0.5 mg/ml,
10 ml 5s, C-II ...... 63323-0291-97 36.18 AP
(S.D.V.,E-Z O CLOSURE,PF)
0.5 mg/ml,
10 ml 5s, C-II ...... 00186-1152-12 63.48 AP
(10X2ML,SINGLE USE,PF)
1 mg/ml,
2 ml 10s, C-II ...... 63323-0292-80 108.84 AP
(5X10ML,SDV,PF)
1 mg/ml,
10 ml 5s, C-II ...... 63323-0292-10 64.44 AP
(5X10ML,SINGLE USE,PF)
1 mg/ml,
10 ml 5s, C-II ...... 63323-0292-97 57.66 AP

ASTRINGYN (Cooper Surgical)
ferric subsulfate
GEL, TP (MODIFIED MONSEL'S)
8 gm 12s 59365-6065-01 141.40 11.00

ATACAND (AstraZeneca)
candesartan cilexetil
TAB, PO (UNIT OF USE)
4 mg, 30s ea .... 00186-0004-31 73.06 EE
8 mg, 30s ea .... 00186-0008-31 73.06 EE
16 mg, 30s ea .... 00186-0016-31 73.06 EE
(NON FILM-COATED)
16 mg, 90s ea .... 00186-0016-54 219.35 EE
100s ea UD .... 00186-0016-28 243.71 EE
(UNIT OF USE)
32 mg, 30s ea 00186-0032-31 98.93
(NON FILM-COATED)
32 mg, 90s ea 00186-0032-54 296.71
100s ea UD 00186-0032-28 329.68

(A-S Medication)
REPACK
TAB, PO (NON FILM-COATED)
16 mg, 30s ea .... 54569-4714-00 72.48 EE

(AQ)
REPACK
TAB, PO, 32 mg, 32s ea ... 66105-0559-03 103.14

(Phys Total Care)
REPACK
TAB, PO, 4 mg, 30s ea 54868-5591-00 64.68
8 mg, 30s ea 54868-5489-00 71.16
16 mg, 30s ea 54868-4413-00 89.24
32 mg, 30s ea 54868-4612-00 114.43

(Quality Care Prod)
REPACK
TAB, PO (NON FILM-COATED)
8 mg, 30s ea .... 35356-0427-30 106.48 EE
16 mg, 30s ea 49999-0305-30 95.98
(NON FILM-COATED)
32 mg, 30s ea 49999-0988-30 121.40

ATACAND HCT (AstraZeneca)
candesartan cilexetil/hydrochlorothiazide
TAB, PO (NON FILM-COATED)
16 mg-12.5 mg,
90s ea .... 00186-0162-54 296.71 EE
100s ea UD .... 00186-0162-28 EE
32 mg-12.5 mg,
90s ea 00186-0322-54 302.62
100s ea UD 00186-0322-28 336.25
(NON-FILM COATED)
32 mg-25 mg,
90s ea 00186-0324-54 327.56

(A-S Medication)
REPACK
TAB, PO (NON FILM-COATED)
32 mg-12.5 mg,
30s ea 54569-5801-00 124.89

(Phys Total Care)
REPACK
TAB, PO, 16 mg-12.5 mg,
30s ea 54868-4729-00 87.73
32 mg-12.5 mg,
30s ea 54868-4869-00 129.05

ATAZANAVIR SULFATE
(Bristol-Myers) *See REYATAZ*

ATENOLOL
FUL
TAB, PO, 25 mg, 100s ea 4.59
50 mg, 100s ea 5.00
100 mg, 100s ea 6.90

PROD/MFR	NDC	AWP	DP	OBC
(AstraZeneca) *See TENORMIN*				
(Aurobindo Pharma)				
TAB, PO (USP)				
25 mg, 100s ea	**65862-0168-01**	81.77		AB
1000s ea	**65862-0168-99**	817.70		AB
50 mg, 100s ea	**65862-0169-01**	83.42		AB
1000s ea	**65862-0169-99**	834.20		AB
100 mg, 100s ea	**65862-0170-01**	125.15		AB
1000s ea	**65862-0170-99**	1251.50		AB
(Dava Pharma)				
TAB, PO, 25 mg, 100s ea	**67253-0420-10**	81.73		
1000s ea	**67253-0420-11**	810.45		
50 mg, 100s ea	**67253-0421-10**	84.65		AB
1000s ea	**67253-0421-11**	804.95		AB
100 mg, 100s ea	**67253-0422-10**	121.75		AB
1000s ea	**67253-0422-11**	1180.97		AB
(Gallipot)				
POW, NA (1X25GM,USP)				
25 gm	**51552-0914-04**	57.40	41.00	
(1X100GM,USP)				
100 gm	**51552-0914-05**	249.20	178.00	
(Major)				
TAB, PO, 25 mg, 100s ea	**00904-5392-60**	69.50		AB
(10X10,USP)				
25 mg, 100s ea UD	**00904-5392-61**	72.03		AB
(Medisca)				
POW, NA (USP,1X5GM)				
5 gm	**38779-0262-03**	31.50		
(U.S.P.)				
25 gm	**38779-0262-04**	126.00		
100 gm	**38779-0262-05**	432.00		
(Mutual)				
TAB, PO, 25 mg, 100s ea	**53489-0536-01**	81.77		AB
1000s ea	**53489-0536-10**	776.74		AB
50 mg, 100s ea	**53489-0529-01**	83.41		AB
1000s ea	**53489-0529-10**	792.48		AB
100 mg, 100s ea	**53489-0530-01**	125.14		AB
1000s ea	**53489-0530-10**	1188.93		AB
(Mylan)				
TAB, PO, 25 mg, 100s ea	**00378-0218-01**	81.75		EE
1000s ea	**00378-0218-10**	817.50		EE
50 mg, 100s ea	**00378-0231-01**	84.70		AB
1000s ea	**00378-0231-10**	805.00		AB
100 mg, 30s ea	**00378-0757-93**	36.54		AB
100s ea	**00378-0757-01**	121.80		AB
1000s ea	**00378-0757-10**	1218.00		AB
(Northstar)				
TAB, PO (USP)				
25 mg, 100s ea	**16714-0031-04**	81.75		AB
1000s ea	**16714-0031-06**	799.10		AB
50 mg, 100s ea	**16714-0032-04**	83.42		AB
1000s ea	**16714-0032-06**	798.72		AB
100 mg, 100s ea	**16714-0033-04**	125.15		AB
1000s ea	**16714-0033-06**	1189.93		AB
(PCCA)				
POW, NA (U.S.P.,FINE POWDER)				
1 gm	**51927-2467-00**	5.52		
(Ranbaxy Pharm)				
TAB, PO (USP)				
25 mg, 100s ea	**63304-0621-01**	81.75		AB
1000s ea	**63304-0621-10**	817.50		AB
50 mg, 100s ea	**63304-0622-01**	84.65		AB
1000s ea	**63304-0622-10**	846.45		AB
100 mg, 100s ea	**63304-0623-01**	125.15		AB
1000s ea	**63304-0623-10**	1251.50		AB
(Sandoz)				
TAB, PO, 25 mg, 100s ea	**00781-1078-01**	81.76		AB
1000s ea	**00781-1078-10**	776.72		AB
50 mg, 100s ea	**00781-1506-01**	83.42		AB
1000s ea	**00781-1506-10**	792.49		AB
100 mg, 100s ea	**00781-1507-01**	125.15		AB
1000s ea	**00781-1507-10**	1188.93		AB
(Spectrum Pharmacy)				
POW, NA (U.S.P.)				
5 gm	**49452-0020-02**	132.65		
25 gm	**49452-0020-03**	194.60		
100 gm	**49452-0020-04**	668.50		
(Teva)				
TAB, PO, 25 mg, 100s ea	**00093-0787-01**	81.77		AB
100s ea UD	**00182-8235-89**	80.01		AB
1000s ea	**00093-0787-10**	776.82		AB
50 mg, 100s ea	**00093-0752-01**	83.42		AB
100s ea UD	**00182-8236-89**	89.12		AB
1000s ea	**00093-0752-10**	792.49		AB
100 mg, 100s ea	**00093-0753-01**	125.15		AB
(USP)				
100 mg, 500s ea	**00093-0753-05**	610.11		AB
(UDL)				
TAB, PO (ROBOT READY 25X1)				
25 mg, 25s ea UD	**51079-0759-19**	20.00		AB
(1X30)				
25 mg, 30s ea	**51079-0759-63**	24.53		AB
(10X10)				
25 mg, 100s ea UD	**51079-0759-20**	80.03		AB
(ROBOT READY 25X1)				
50 mg, 25s ea UD	**51079-0684-19**	24.34		AB
(1X30)				
50 mg, 30s ea	**51079-0684-63**	24.15		AB
(10X10)				
50 mg, 100s ea UD	**51079-0684-20**	89.15		AB
100 mg, 100s ea UD	**51079-0685-20**	149.25		AB
(Zydus Pharm.)				
TAB, PO, 25 mg, 100s ea	**68382-0022-01**	81.77		AB
1000s ea	**68382-0022-10**	799.10		AB
50 mg, 100s ea	**68382-0023-01**	84.60		AB
1000s ea	**68382-0023-10**	804.95		AB
100 mg, 100s ea	**68382-0024-01**	125.14		AB
1000s ea	**68382-0024-10**	1190.60		AB
(A-S Medication)				
REPACK				
TAB, PO, 25 mg, 30s ea	**54569-3885-00**	24.53		EE
100s ea	**54569-3885-02**	81.76		EE
200s ea	**54569-3885-04**	163.52		EE
50 mg, 30s ea	**54569-3432-01**	25.16		AB
60s ea	**54569-3432-04**	50.32		AB
100s ea	**54569-3432-00**	83.86		AB
200s ea	**54569-3432-07**	167.72		AB
100 mg, 30s ea	**54569-3654-00**	37.55		AB
60s ea	**54569-3654-03**	75.09		AB
200s ea	**54569-3654-04**	250.30		AB
(Advanced Pharm Serv, Inc.)				
REPACK				
TAB, PO, 50 mg, 10s ea	**13411-0169-01**	44.60		
30s ea	**13411-0169-03**	133.80		
60s ea	**13411-0169-06**	267.60		
90s ea	**13411-0169-09**	401.40		
100s ea	**13411-0169-10**	95.93		
100 mg, 10s ea	**13411-0176-01**	22.30		
30s ea	**13411-0176-03**	66.90		
60s ea	**13411-0176-06**	133.80		
90s ea	**13411-0176-09**	200.70		
100s ea	**13411-0176-10**	143.92		
(Aidarex)				
REPACK				
TAB, PO, 25 mg, 7s ea	**33261-0220-07**	11.83		AB
14s ea	**33261-0220-14**	23.66		AB
20s ea	**33261-0220-20**	33.80		AB
21s ea	**33261-0220-21**	35.49		AB
28s ea	**33261-0220-28**	47.32		AB
30s ea	**33261-0220-30**	50.70		AB
40s ea	**33261-0220-40**	67.60		AB
60s ea	**33261-0220-60**	101.40		AB
90s ea	**33261-0220-90**	152.10		AB
120s ea	**33261-0220-02**	202.80		AB
(Altura)				
REPACK				
TAB, PO, 25 mg, 10s ea	**63874-0468-10**	7.02		
14s ea	**63874-0468-14**	9.83		
15s ea	**63874-0468-15**	10.53		
20s ea	**63874-0468-20**	14.05		
30s ea	**63874-0468-30**	21.07		
60s ea	**63874-0468-60**	42.14		
90s ea	**63874-0468-90**	63.20		
100s ea	**63874-0468-01**	70.23		
50 mg, 15s ea	**63874-0332-15**	14.09		EE
30s ea	**63874-0332-30**	28.14		EE
60s ea	**63874-0332-60**	56.36		EE
100s ea	**63874-0332-01**	93.98		EE
100 mg, 7s ea	**63874-0388-07**	11.03		EE
10s ea	**63874-0388-10**	15.75		EE
12s ea	**63874-0388-12**	18.90		EE
15s ea	**63874-0388-15**	23.63		EE
20s ea	**63874-0388-20**	31.50		EE
30s ea	**63874-0388-30**	47.25		EE
100s ea	**63874-0388-01**	157.50		EE
(American Health)				
REPACK				
TAB, PO (10X10)				
50 mg, 100s ea UD	**62584-0467-01**	113.02		AB
(15X30)				
50 mg, 450s ea	**62584-0467-85**	356.62		AB
(10X10)				
100 mg, 100s ea UD	**62584-0715-01**	223.90		AB
(Bryant Ranch)				
REPACK				
TAB, PO, 25 mg, 30s ea	**63629-1785-01**	32.62		
60s ea	**63629-1785-03**	65.25		
100s ea	**63629-1785-02**	108.74		
50 mg, 30s ea	**63629-1740-01**	42.81		
60s ea	**63629-1740-03**	67.62		
100s ea	**63629-1740-02**	139.69		
100 mg, 30s ea	**63629-2626-02**	49.60		
100s ea	**63629-2626-01**	165.34		
(Core)				
REPACK				
TAB, PO, 25 mg, 30s ea	**33358-0037-30**	33.44		
60s ea	**33358-0037-60**	66.88		
100s ea	**33358-0037-00**	111.46		
50 mg, 30s ea	**33358-0038-30**	43.88		
60s ea	**33358-0038-60**	69.31		
100s ea	**33358-0038-00**	143.18		
100 mg, 30s ea	**33358-0039-30**	50.84		
100s ea	**33358-0039-00**	169.47		
(DHS, Inc.)				
REPACK				
TAB, PO, 25 mg, 30s ea	**55887-0599-30**	22.66		EE
60s ea	**55887-0599-60**	44.00		EE
90s ea	**55887-0599-90**	63.49		EE
50 mg, 30s ea	**55887-0838-30**	31.01		AB
60s ea	**55887-0838-60**	60.83		AB
90s ea	**55887-0838-90**	89.05		AB
100s ea	**55887-0838-01**	99.00		
100 mg, 30s ea	**55887-0998-30**	51.81		AB
60s ea	**55887-0998-60**	102.62		AB
90s ea	**55887-0998-90**	154.43		AB
(Dispensing Solutions)				
REPACK				
TAB, PO, 25 mg, 30s ea	**55045-2498-08**	21.00		AB
30s ea	**66336-0587-30**	24.58		EE
60s ea	**66336-0587-60**	49.16		EE
90s ea	**66336-0587-90**	73.74		
100s ea	**55045-2498-01**	70.00		AB
100s ea	**66336-0587-00**	81.93		
50 mg, 30s ea	**55045-1860-08**	32.00		AB
30s ea	**66336-0719-30**	31.01		EE
60s ea	**55045-1860-06**	64.20		AB
60s ea	**66336-0719-60**	60.83		
90s ea	**55045-1860-09**	96.30		AB
90s ea	**66336-0719-90**	89.05		AB
100s ea	**55045-1860-01**	107.00		AB
120s ea	**55045-1860-02**	128.40		AB
100 mg, 30s ea	**55045-2269-08**	44.35		AB
30s ea	**66336-0914-30**	41.30		
60s ea	**53489-2269-06**	88.80		AB
60s ea	**66336-0914-60**	82.60		
90s ea	**55045-2269-09**	133.20		AB
90s ea	**66336-0914-90**	123.89		AB
100s ea	**55045-2269-01**	148.00		AB
120s ea	**55045-2269-02**	177.60		AB
(GSMS)				
REPACK				
TAB, PO (UNIT OF USE)				
25 mg, 90s ea	**60429-0211-90**	15.00	10.00	AB
50 mg, 30s ea	**60429-0025-30**	7.05	2.35	AB
90s ea	**60429-0025-90**	10.05	3.35	AB
100 mg, 30s ea	**60429-0026-30**	15.30	5.10	AB
(HomeMed)				
REPACK				
TAB, PO, 25 mg, 30s ea	**51655-0926-24**	28.89		
50 mg, 30s ea	**51655-0530-24**	39.99		
60s ea	**51655-0530-25**	59.99		
100 mg, 30s ea	**51655-0532-24**	66.99		EE
(Keltman Pharma., Inc.)				
REPACK				
TAB, PO, 50 mg, 30s ea	**68387-0538-30**	39.87		
100 mg, 30s ea	**68387-0539-30**	52.65		
(McKesson Packaging)				
REPACK				
TAB, PO (USP)				
25 mg, 100s ea UD	**63739-0027-10**	83.76		AB
50 mg, 100s ea UD	**63739-0028-10**	99.06		AB
(Nucare Pharm)				
REPACK				
TAB, PO, 25 mg, 60s ea	**66267-0030-60**	49.79		AB
50 mg, 30s ea	**66267-0031-30**	27.99		AB
(Palmetto)				
REPACK				
TAB, PO, 25 mg, 30s ea	**23490-5097-01**	38.12		
60s ea	**23490-5097-02**	76.24		
100s ea	**23490-5097-03**	127.07		
50 mg, 30s ea	**23490-0139-03**	36.95		
30s ea	**23490-5098-01**	39.00		
60s ea	**23490-0139-06**	73.89		
60s ea	**23490-5098-02**	78.00		
100 mg, 30s ea	**23490-5096-01**	49.50		
60s ea	**23490-5096-02**	99.00		
90s ea	**23490-5096-03**	148.50		

PROD/MFR	NDC	AWP	DP	OBC
(PD-Rx Pharm)				
REPACK				
TAB, PO, 25 mg, 30s ea	55289-0227-30	20.00		AB
(REDI-SCRIPT)				
25 mg, 30s ea	58864-0749-30	20.00		AB
90s ea	55289-0227-90	34.75		EE
(REDI-SCRIPT)				
25 mg, 90s ea	58864-0749-90	34.75		EE
50 mg, 3s ea	55289-0228-03	13.65		AB
(USP)				
50 mg, 6s ea	55289-0228-06	14.35		AB
14s ea	55289-0228-14	16.35		AB
30s ea	55289-0228-30	20.90		AB
(REDI-SCRIPT)				
50 mg, 30s ea	58864-0065-30	20.90		AB
60s ea	55289-0228-60	28.05		AB
(USP)				
50 mg, 90s ea	55289-0228-90	44.10		AB
100s ea	55289-0228-01	46.45		AB
(REDI-SCRIPT)				
50 mg, 100s ea	58864-0065-01	46.45		AB
100 mg, 30s ea	55289-0653-30	29.45		AB
(REDI-SCRIPT)				
100 mg, 30s ea	58864-0717-30	29.45		AB
90s ea	55289-0653-90	58.95		AB
(Pharma Pac)				
REPACK				
TAB, PO, 25 mg, 30s ea	52959-0463-30	21.40		EE
60s ea	52959-0463-60	42.78		EE
100s ea	52959-0463-01	71.25		EE
50 mg, 20s ea	52959-0253-20	20.80		AB
30s ea	52959-0253-30	28.50		EE
40s ea	52959-0253-40	34.70		EE
100s ea	52959-0253-00	71.90		EE
100 mg, 60s ea	52959-0258-60	94.26		AB
(Phys Total Care)				
REPACK				
TAB, PO, 25 mg, 15s ea	54868-2349-04	6.48		AB
30s ea	54868-2349-02	7.08		EE
60s ea	54868-2349-03	12.39		EE
90s ea	54868-2349-05	16.35		EE
100s ea	54868-2349-01	16.14		EE
50 mg, 30s ea	54868-1871-01	8.58		EE
60s ea	54868-1871-00	12.66		EE
90s ea	54868-1871-04	16.74		EE
100s ea	54868-1871-02	18.12		EE
100 mg, 30s ea	54868-1971-03	10.95		EE
60s ea	54868-1971-00	18.90		EE
90s ea	54868-1971-04	23.40		AB
100s ea	54868-1971-01	29.49		EE
(Physician Partner)				
REPACK				
TAB, PO, 25 mg, 30s ea	21695-0322-30	40.40		
90s ea	21695-0322-90	121.20		AB
50 mg, 30s ea	21695-0323-30	47.55		
60s ea	21695-0323-60	95.10		AB
90s ea	21695-0323-90	142.65		AB
100 mg, 30s ea	21695-0324-30	71.33		
(Quality Care Prod)				
REPACK				
TAB, PO, 25 mg, 10s ea	49999-0454-10	8.43		
30s ea	49999-0454-30	25.28		AB
60s ea	49999-0454-60	50.56		AB
90s ea	49999-0454-90	75.84		AB
100s ea	49999-0454-00	84.30		
50 mg, 30s ea	49999-0104-30	32.16		EE
60s ea	49999-0104-60	65.34		EE
90s ea	49999-0104-90	96.48		AB
100s ea	49999-0104-00	107.40		EE
100 mg, 30s ea	49999-0178-30	56.70		
100s ea	49999-0178-00	157.50		AB
(Southwood)				
REPACK				
TAB, PO, 25 mg, 15s ea	58016-0582-15	7.02		EE
20s ea	58016-0582-20	14.05		EE
30s ea	58016-0582-30	21.07		EE
60s ea	58016-0582-60	42.14		EE
100s ea	58016-0582-00	70.23		EE
50 mg, 15s ea	58016-0333-15	13.42		EE
30s ea	58016-0333-30	26.80		EE
60s ea	58016-0333-60	53.70		EE
100s ea	58016-0333-00	89.50		EE
100 mg, 12s ea	58016-0771-12	18.90		EE
15s ea	58016-0771-15	23.63		EE
20s ea	58016-0771-20	31.50		EE
30s ea	58016-0771-30	47.25		EE
60s ea	58016-0771-60	94.50		EE
100s ea	58016-0771-00	157.50		EE

PROD/MFR	NDC	AWP	DP	OBC
(Stat Rx)				
REPACK				
TAB, PO, 100 mg, 28s ea	16590-0851-28	35.00		AB
(Vibranta)				
REPACK				
TAB, PO, 25 mg, 30s ea	57866-3332-01	22.55		EE
50 mg, 30s ea	57866-3330-01	55.75		EE
90s ea	57866-3330-03	66.56		EE
100 mg, 30s ea	57866-3331-01	84.25		EE
60s ea	57866-3331-02	93.12		EE
ATENOLOL/CHLORTHALIDONE				
FUL				
TAB, PO, 50 mg-25 mg, 100s ea		11.22		
100 mg-25 mg, 100s ea		30.68		
(AstraZeneca) *See TENORETIC 100*				
(AstraZeneca) *See TENORETIC 50*				
(Major)				
TAB, PO, 50 mg-25 mg, 100s ea	00904-7881-60	96.93		AB
(Mutual)				
TAB, PO, 50 mg-25 mg, 100s ea	53489-0531-01	97.15		AB
100 mg-25 mg, 100s ea	53489-0532-01	136.49		AB
(Mylan)				
TAB, PO, 50 mg-25 mg, 100s ea	00378-2063-01	97.21		AB
100 mg-25 mg, 30s ea	00378-2064-93	40.97		AB
100s ea	00378-2064-01	136.55		AB
(Watson Labs)				
TAB, PO, 50 mg-25 mg, 100s ea	00591-5782-01	12.83		AB
100 mg-25 mg, 100s ea	00591-5783-01	24.54		AB
(Altura)				
REPACK				
TAB, PO, 100 mg-25 mg, 12s ea	63874-0676-12	18.21		EE
15s ea	63874-0676-15	22.76		EE
20s ea	63874-0676-20	30.35		EE
100s ea	63874-0676-01	151.73		EE
(Bryant Ranch)				
REPACK				
TAB, PO, 50 mg-25 mg, 10s ea	63629-2909-03	8.90		
30s ea	63629-2909-01	26.70		
60s ea	63629-2909-02	53.40		
90s ea	63629-2909-04	80.10		
(DHS, Inc.)				
REPACK				
TAB, PO, 50 mg-25 mg, 30s ea	55887-0585-30	26.87		AB
60s ea	55887-0585-60	52.74		AB
90s ea	55887-0585-90	80.61		AB
120s ea	55887-0585-82	107.48		AB
100 mg-25 mg, 30s ea	55887-0613-30	29.09		AB
60s ea	55887-0613-60	57.18		AB
120s ea	55887-0613-82	112.08		AB
(Dispensing Solutions)				
REPACK				
TAB, PO, 50 mg-25 mg, 30s ea	55045-2755-08	29.10		AB
90s ea	66336-0811-90	87.44		AB
(PD-Rx Pharm)				
REPACK				
TAB, PO, 50 mg-25 mg, 30s ea	55289-0993-30	23.85		AB
60s ea	55289-0993-60	32.16		AB
90s ea	55289-0993-90	40.47		AB
100 mg-25 mg, 30s ea	55289-0988-30	19.20		AB
(Phys Total Care)				
REPACK				
TAB, PO, 50 mg-25 mg, 30s ea	54868-2683-01	10.50		EE
90s ea	54868-2683-02	25.47		AB
100s ea	54868-2683-00	27.96		EE
100 mg-25 mg, 30s ea	54868-3064-00	15.20		AB
90s ea	54868-3064-01	41.10		AB

PROD/MFR	NDC	AWP	DP	OBC
(Physician Partner)				
REPACK				
TAB, PO, 50 mg-25 mg, 30s ea	21695-0743-30	55.50		AB
(Quality Care Prod)				
REPACK				
TAB, PO, 50 mg-25 mg, 30s ea	49999-0512-30	32.60		AB
(Southwood)				
REPACK				
TAB, PO, 50 mg-25 mg, 30s ea	58016-0526-30	42.11		
60s ea	58016-0526-60	84.22		
90s ea	58016-0526-90	126.32		
100s ea	58016-0526-00	140.36		
120s ea	58016-0526-02	168.43		
100 mg-25 mg, 30s ea	58016-0331-30	38.13		AB
60s ea	58016-0331-60	76.27		AB
90s ea	58016-0331-90	114.40		AB
100s ea	58016-0331-00	127.11		AB
ATGAM (Pfizer)				
antithymocyte globulin equine				
SOL, IV (AMP,5X5ML)				
50 mg/ml, 5 ml 5s	00009-7224-02	3216.04	2680.03	
ATIVAN (Baxter)				
lorazepam				
SOL, IJ (SDV)				
2 mg/ml, 1 ml, C-IV	60977-0112-81	2.08		AP
(S.D.V.)				
2 mg/ml, 1 ml 25s, C-IV	60977-0112-01	51.90	133.96	AP
(1X10ML,MULTIPLE-DOSE)				
2 mg/ml, 10 ml, C-IV	60997-0116-01	19.26		AP
(10X10ML,MULTIPLE-DOSE)				
2 mg/ml, 10 ml 10s, C-IV	60997-0116-02	192.60		AP
4 mg/ml, 1 ml, C-IV	60977-0113-81	2.88		AP
(S.D.V.)				
4 mg/ml, 1 ml 25s, C-IV	60977-0113-01	72.00	163.88	AP
(MDV)				
4 mg/ml, 10 ml, C-IV	60977-0113-71	19.32		AP
(M.D.V.)				
4 mg/ml, 10 ml 10s, C-IV	60977-0113-02	193.20	596.56	AP
(BTA)				
TAB, PO, 0.5 mg, 100s ea, C-IV	64455-0063-01	219.90	183.25	AB
1 mg, 100s ea, C-IV	64455-0064-01	293.77	244.81	AB
1000s ea, C-IV	64455-0064-10	2877.07	2397.56	AB
2 mg, 100s ea, C-IV	64455-0065-01	468.16	390.13	AB
(A-S Medication)				
REPACK				
TAB, PO, 1 mg, 3s ea, C-IV	54569-0927-01	8.74		AB
(Nucare Pharm)				
REPACK				
TAB, PO, 1 mg, 100s ea, C-IV	66267-1295-00	292.39		AB
(Phys Total Care)				
REPACK				
SOL, IJ, 2 mg/ml, 10 ml, C-IV	54868-2407-01	97.04		AP
TAB, PO, 0.5 mg, 30s ea, C-IV	54868-2144-00	41.51		AB
1 mg, 20s ea, C-IV	54868-1339-05	37.58		AB
30s ea, C-IV	54868-1339-02	55.10		AB
60s ea, C-IV	54868-1339-01	107.71		AB
90s ea, C-IV	54868-1339-00	151.55		AB
(Stat Rx)				
REPACK				
TAB, PO, 1 mg, 120s ea, C-IV	16590-0813-72	391.34		AB
ATMOS 300 (Amend)				
diglycerides/monoglycerides				
LIQ, NA, 480 ml	17317-0955-01	21.00		
3840 ml	17317-0955-06	84.00		
ATMUL 84 (Amend)				
glyceryl monostearate				
SOL, NA, 22700 gm	17317-0957-03	217.50		

PROD/MFR	NDC	AWP	DP	OBC
ATOMOXETINE HYDROCHLORIDE				
(Lilly) *See STRATTERA*				
ATOPICLAIR (Graceway)				
cream, multi ingredient				
CRE, TP (1X56GM,NON-STEROIDAL)				
100 gm	**29336-0100-11**	117.73		
ATORVASTATIN CALCIUM				
(Pfizer) *See LIPITOR*				
ATOVAQUONE				
(Glaxo) *See MEPRON*				
ATOVAQUONE/PROGUANIL HYDROCHLORIDE				
(Glaxo) *See MALARONE*				
(Glaxo) *See MALARONE PEDIATRIC*				
ATRACURIUM BESYLATE				
(Bedford) *See ATRACURIUM BESYLATE NOVAPLUS*				
(Bedford)				
SOL, IV (S.D.V.)				
10 mg/ml, 5 ml 10s	**55390-0102-05**	96.00		**AP**
(M.D.V.)				
10 mg/ml, 10 ml 10s	**55390-0103-10**	156.00		**AP**
(Hospira)				
SOL, IV (S.D.V.)				
10 mg/ml, 5 ml 10s	**61703-0312-53**	47.76	41.80	**AP**
(M.D.V.)				
10 mg/ml, 10 ml 10s	**61703-0313-32**	98.76	86.40	**AP**
ATRACURIUM BESYLATE NOVAPLUS (Bedford)				
atracurium besylate				
SOL, IV (S.D.V.,PRIVATE LABEL)				
10 mg/ml, 5 ml 10s	**55390-0180-05**	52.80		**AP**
(M.D.V.,PRIVATE LABEL)				
10 mg/ml, 10 ml 10s	**55390-0179-10**	84.00		**AP**
ATRALIN (Valeant Pharm Intl)				
tretinoin				
GEL, TP (1X45GM)				
0.05%, 45 gm	**13548-0070-45**	189.00		
ATRIPLA (Bristol-Myers Squibb)				
efavirenz/emtricitabine/tenofovir disoproxil fum				
TAB, PO (FILM-COATED)				
600 mg-200 mg-300 mg, 30s ea	**15584-0101-01**	1755.50		
(A-S Medication)				
REPACK				
TAB, PO (FILM-COATED)				
600 mg-200 mg-300 mg, 30s ea	**54569-5805-00**	2235.97		
(Phys Total Care)				
REPACK				
TAB, PO (FILM-COATED)				
600 mg-200 mg-300 mg, 30s ea	**54868-5643-00**	1718.94		
(Quality Care Prod)				
REPACK				
TAB, PO (FILM-COATED)				
600 mg-200 mg-300 mg, 6s ea	**35356-0064-06**	714.20		
30s ea	**35356-0064-30**	3306.60		
ATROHIST PEDIATRIC (Phys Total Care)				
REPACK				
cpm tan/phenyleph tan/pyril tan				
SUS, PO, 120 ml	**54868-3385-00**	38.01		
ATROPINE (Gallipot)				
POW, NA (1X5GM)				
5 gm	**51552-0999-02**	34.65	24.75	
(1X25GM)				
25 gm	**51552-0999-04**	111.72	79.80	
(Spectrum Pharmacy)				
CRY, NA (U.S.P.)				
5 gm	**49452-0770-01**	148.75		
25 gm	**49452-0770-02**	455.00		
100 gm	**49452-0770-03**	1533.00		
ATROPINE CARE (Akorn)				
atropine sulfate				
SOL, OP, 1%, 2 ml	**17478-0214-20**	4.05		
ATROPINE SULF/HYOSCYAMINE SULF/PB/SCOP HYDROBROM				
(Excellium) *See BELLADONNA ALKALOIDS/ PHENOBARBITAL*				
(PBM Pharmaceuticals) *See DONNATAL*				
(PBM Pharmaceuticals) *See DONNATAL EXTENTABS*				
(River's Edge) *See RE-PB HYOS*				
(Vintage) *See BELLADONNA ALKALOIDS/ PHENOBARBITAL*				
(West-Ward) *See BELLADONNA ALKALOIDS/ PHENOBARBITAL*				
ATROPINE SULF/HYOSCYAMINE SULF/ SCOP HYDROBROM				
(Llorens Pharma Int) *See COLYTROL*				
ATROPINE SULFATE				
(Akorn) *See ATROPINE CARE*				
(Alcon Ophthalmic) *See ISOPTO ATROPINE*				
(Alcon Surgical)				
SOL, OP, 1%, 2 ml 12s	**00065-0702-12**	69.12		
(Altaire)				
SOL, OP (STERILE)				
1%, 5 ml	**59390-0191-05**	7.72		
15 ml	**59390-0191-13**	13.40		
(Amend)				
POW, NA (U.S.P.)				
5 gm	**17317-0036-07**	11.20		
125 gm	**17317-0036-02**	44.80		
125 gm	**17317-0036-05**	189.00		
(Amer Regent)				
SOL, IJ (AMP,PF)				
0.4 mg/ml, 0.5 ml 25s	**00517-0805-25**	31.25		
(S.D.V.,PF)				
0.4 mg/ml, 1 ml 25s	**00517-0401-25**	25.00		
(AMP,PF)				
1 mg/ml, 1 ml 25s	**00517-0101-25**	31.25		
(S.D.V.,PF)				
1 mg/ml, 1 ml 25s	**00517-1010-25**	37.50		
(Amphastar)				
SOL, IJ (SRN,PREFILLED,LUER-JET)				
0.1 mg/ml, 10 ml 10s	**00548-3339-00**	53.20		
(MIN-I-JET,21GX1 1/2")				
0.1 mg/ml, 10 ml 25s	**00548-1039-00**	171.90		
(SRN,PREFILLED,STICKGARD)				
0.1 mg/ml, 10 ml 25s	**00548-2039-00**	181.88		
(Bausch & Lomb Inc.)				
OIN, OP, 1%, 3.5 gm	**24208-0825-55**	15.31		
SOL, OP, 1%, 5 ml	**24208-0750-60**	16.82		
15 ml	**24208-0750-06**	37.85		
(Baxter)				
SOL, IJ (SDV,1X1ML,USP)				
0.4 mg/ml, 1 ml	**10019-0250-39**	0.82		
(S.D.V.)				
0.4 mg/ml, 1 ml 25s	**10019-0250-12**	20.40		
(MDV,1X20ML,USP)				
0.4 mg/ml, 20 ml	**10019-0250-37**	18.00		
(M.D.V.)				
0.4 mg/ml, 20 ml 10s	**10019-0250-20**	180.00		
(SDV,1X1ML,USP)				
1 mg/ml, 1 ml	**10019-0251-39**	1.93		
(S.D.V.)				
1 mg/ml, 1 ml 25s	**10019-0251-12**	48.30		
(Consolidated Midland)				
OIN, OP, 1%, 3.5 gm	**00223-4105-03**	2.75		
SOL, IJ (AMP)				
0.4 mg/ml, 1 ml 25s	**00223-7193-25**	15.00		
(VIAL)				
0.4 mg/ml, 1 ml 25s	**00223-7191-25**	16.25		
1 ml 100s	**00223-7192-00**	45.75		
1 mg/ml, 1 ml 25s	**00223-7206-01**	16.25		
OP, 1%, 15 ml	**00223-6101-15**	3.00		
(Falcon Ophthalmics)				
SOL, OP, 1%, 5 ml	**61314-0303-01**	15.60		
15 ml	**61314-0303-02**	33.60		
(Gallipot) *See ATROPINE SULFATE MONOHYDRATE*				
(Hope) *See SAL-TROPINE*				
(Hospira)				
SOL, IJ (ANSYR PLASTIC SYRINGE)				
0.05 mg/ml, 5 ml 10s	**00409-9630-05**	70.68	61.80	
(10X5ML)				
0.1 mg/ml, 5 ml 10s	**00409-9629-05**	29.16	25.50	
(LIFESHIELD,LATEX-FREE)				
0.1 mg/ml, 5 ml 10s	**00409-4910-34**	42.72	37.40	
(ANSYR,10X10ML)				
0.1 mg/ml, 10 ml 10s	**00409-1630-10**	24.96	21.80	
(LIFESHIELD, 21GX1-1/2)				
0.1 mg/ml, 10 ml 10s	**00074-4911-34**	38.16	33.40	
(LIFESHIELD,21GX1-1/2)				
0.1 mg/ml, 10 ml 10s	**00409-4911-34**	42.12	36.90	
(Medisca)				
POW, NA (U.S.P.,MICRONIZED)				
10 gm	**38779-0014-01**	73.50		
25 gm	**38779-0014-04**	108.00		
100 gm	**38779-0014-05**	382.50		
(PCCA)				
POW, NA (U.S.P.)				
1 gm	**51927-1001-00**	8.40		
(Spectrum Pharmacy) *See ATROPINE SULFATE MONOHYDRATE*				
(A-S Medication)				
REPACK				
SOL, IJ, 1 mg/ml, 1 ml	**54569-5607-00**	1.98		
OP, 1%, 5 ml	**54569-2784-00**	4.55		
(Dispensing Solutions)				
REPACK				
SOL, OP, 1%, 5 ml	**55045-3611-01**	7.00		
(Palmetto)				
REPACK				
SOL, OP, 1%, 10 ml	**23490-5102-01**	6.50		
(Phys Total Care)				
REPACK				
SOL, IJ (SRN, 21GX1-1/2")				
0.1 mg/ml, 10 ml	**54868-0006-00**	91.44		
(M.D.V.)				
0.4 mg/ml, 20 ml	**54868-0740-00**	10.05		
20 ml 10s	**54868-0740-01**	73.62		
(S.D.V.)				
1 mg/ml, 1 ml 25s	**54868-3893-00**	47.31		
OP, 1%, 5 ml	**54868-1178-00**	13.20		
ATROPINE SULFATE MONOHYDRATE (Gallipot)				
atropine sulfate				
POW, NA (U.S.P.,N.F.)				
5 gm	**51552-0156-02**	17.92		
25 gm	**51552-0156-04**	56.00		
(Spectrum Pharmacy)				
POW, NA (U.S.P.)				
5 gm	**49452-0780-01**	72.45		
25 gm	**49452-0780-02**	200.55		
125 gm	**49452-0780-03**	616.00		
ATROPINE SULFATE/DIFENOXIN HYDROCHLORIDE				
(Valeant Pharm Intl) *See MOTOFEN*				
ATROPINE SULFATE/DIPHENOXYLATE HCL (Lannett)				
atropine sulfate/diphenoxylate hydrochloride				
TAB, PO, 0.025 mg-2.5 mg,				
100s ea, C-V	**00527-1170-01**	48.00		**AA**
1000s ea, C-V	**00527-1170-10**	445.00		**AA**
(Mylan)				
TAB, PO, 0.025 mg-2.5 mg,				
100s ea, C-V	**00378-0415-01**	48.00		**AA**
1000s ea, C-V	**00378-0415-10**	445.00		**AA**
(Roxane)				
SOL, PO (CHERRY)				
60 ml, C-V	**00054-3194-46**	8.42		**AA**
(Sandoz)				
TAB, PO, 0.025 mg-2.5 mg,				
100s ea, C-V	**00185-0024-01**	45.95		**AA**
500s ea, C-V	**00185-0024-05**	218.26		**AA**
1000s ea, C-V	**00185-0024-10**	413.55		**AA**
(UDL)				
TAB, PO (10X10)				
0.025 mg-2.5 mg, 100s ea UD, C-V	**51079-0067-20**	47.80		**AA**
(A-S Medication)				
REPACK				
TAB, PO, 0.025 mg-2.5 mg,				
15s ea, C-V	**54569-0222-00**	7.20		**EE**
20s ea, C-V	**54569-0222-01**	9.60		**EE**
30s ea, C-V	**54569-0222-02**	14.40		**EE**

PROD/MFR	NDC	AWP	DP	OBC
(Altura)				
REPACK				
SOL, PO (1X60ML,CHERRY)				
60 ml, C-V	63874-0277-60	9.80		AA
(1X120ML,CHERRY)				
120 ml, C-V	63874-0277-12	19.60		AA
TAB, PO, 0.025 mg-2.5 mg,				
10s ea, C-V	63874-0261-10	17.27		AA
12s ea, C-V	63874-0261-12	20.72		AA
14s ea, C-V	63874-0261-14	5.95		AA
15s ea, C-V	63874-0261-15	6.37		AA
20s ea, C-V	63874-0261-20	34.53		AA
21s ea, C-V	63874-0261-21	8.93		AA
24s ea, C-V	63874-0261-24	41.44		AA
28s ea, C-V	63874-0261-28	11.90		AA
30s ea, C-V	63874-0261-30	51.80		AA
40s ea, C-V	63874-0261-40	69.06		AA
60s ea, C-V	63874-0261-60	25.50		AA
100s ea, C-V	63874-0261-01	172.65		AA
(DHS, Inc.)				
REPACK				
TAB, PO, 0.025 mg-2.5 mg,				
20s ea, C-V	55887-0841-20	13.30		AA
30s ea, C-V	55887-0841-30	15.50		AA
(Dispensing Solutions)				
REPACK				
TAB, PO, 0.025 mg-2.5 mg,				
15s ea, C-V	55045-1130-05	7.20		AA
15s ea, C-V	66336-0437-15	33.53		AA
20s ea, C-V	55045-1130-07	9.60		AA
20s ea, C-V	66336-0437-20	44.71		AA
30s ea, C-V	55045-1130-08	14.40		AA
(Palmetto)				
REPACK				
TAB, PO, 0.025 mg-2.5 mg,				
10s ea, C-V	23490-5461-05	10.00		AA
30s ea, C-V	23490-5461-04	38.00		AA
(PD-Rx Pharm)				
REPACK				
TAB, PO, 0.025 mg-2.5 mg,				
4s ea, C-V	43063-0089-04	16.76		AA
6s ea, C-V	43063-0089-06	17.12		AA
10s ea, C-V	55289-0102-10	17.94		AA
15s ea, C-V	55289-0102-15	20.25		AA
20s ea, C-V	55289-0102-20	22.55		AA
30s ea, C-V	55289-0102-30	27.16		AA
30s ea, C-V	58864-0166-30	27.16		AA
(Pharma Pac)				
REPACK				
SOL, PO (1X60ML,CHERRY)				
60 ml, C-V	52959-0949-60	21.58		AA
TAB, PO, 0.025 mg-2.5 mg,				
10s ea, C-V	52959-0157-10	18.71		EE
12s ea, C-V	52959-0157-12	22.46		EE
15s ea, C-V	52959-0157-15	27.18		EE
20s ea, C-V	52959-0157-20	33.53		EE
30s ea, C-V	52959-0157-30	46.92		EE
50s ea, C-V	52959-0157-50	72.50		EE
100s ea, C-V	52959-0157-00	121.31		EE
(Phys Total Care)				
REPACK				
TAB, PO, 0.025 mg-2.5 mg,				
10s ea, C-V	54868-0032-00	6.30		EE
15s ea, C-V	54868-0032-04	7.20		EE
20s ea, C-V	54868-0032-03	8.10		EE
30s ea, C-V	54868-0032-06	9.90		EE
40s ea, C-V	54868-0032-07	11.70		EE
100s ea, C-V	54868-0032-09	21.00		EE
1000s ea, C-V	54868-0032-01	143.01		EE
(Quality Care Prod)				
REPACK				
TAB, PO, 0.025 mg-2.5 mg,				
10s ea, C-V	49999-0207-10	18.72		AA
100s ea, C-V	49999-0207-00	187.20		AA
(Southwood)				
REPACK				
TAB, PO, 0.025 mg-2.5 mg,				
10s ea, C-V	58016-0713-10	4.25		EE
12s ea, C-V	58016-0713-12	5.10		EE
14s ea, C-V	58016-0713-14	5.95		EE
15s ea, C-V	58016-0713-15	6.37		EE
20s ea, C-V	58016-0713-20	8.79		EE
21s ea, C-V	58016-0713-21	8.93		EE
24s ea, C-V	58016-0713-24	10.20		EE
28s ea, C-V	58016-0713-28	11.90		EE
30s ea, C-V	58016-0713-30	12.75		EE
40s ea, C-V	58016-0713-40	17.00		EE
60s ea, C-V	58016-0713-60	25.50		EE
100s ea, C-V	58016-0713-00	42.50		EE

ATROPINE SULFATE/DIPHENOXYLATE HYDROCHLORIDE

PROD/MFR	NDC	AWP	DP	OBC
FUL				
TAB, PO, 0.025 mg-2.5 mg,				
100s ea		21.38		

(Lannett) *See ATROPINE SULFATE/DIPHENOXYLATE HCL*

(Mylan) *See ATROPINE SULFATE/DIPHENOXYLATE HCL*

(Pfizer) *See LOMOTIL*

(Roxane) *See ATROPINE SULFATE/DIPHENOXYLATE HCL*

(Sandoz) *See ATROPINE SULFATE/DIPHENOXYLATE HCL*

(Sandoz) *See LONOX*

(Truxton) *See LOMOCOT*

(UDL) *See ATROPINE SULFATE/DIPHENOXYLATE HCL*

(Vita-Rx) *See VI-ATRO*

PROD/MFR	NDC	AWP	DP	OBC
(Dispensing Solutions)				
REPACK				
TAB, PO, 0.025 mg-2.5 mg,				
10s ea, C-V	55045-1130-06	4.80		
(Palmetto)				
REPACK				
TAB, PO, 0.025 mg-2.5 mg,				
12s ea, C-V	23490-5461-02	15.20		
15s ea, C-V	23490-5461-01	18.99		
20s ea, C-V	23490-5461-03	25.33		

ATROPINE SULFATE/EDROPHONIUM CHLORIDE

(Bioniche Pharma) *See ENLON-PLUS*

ATROVENT (Boehr Ingelheim Phar)
ipratropium bromide

PROD/MFR	NDC	AWP	DP	OBC
SPR, NS, 0.03%, 30 ml	00597-0081-30	93.22		
0.06%, 15 ml	00597-0086-76	79.90		
(Phys Total Care)				
REPACK				
SPR, NS, 0.03%, 30 ml	54868-5565-00	85.97		
0.06%, 15 ml	54868-4284-00	93.00		

ATROVENT HFA (Boehr Ingelheim Phar)
ipratropium bromide

PROD/MFR	NDC	AWP	DP	OBC
SOL, IH, 0.017 mg/actuation,				
12.9 gm	00597-0087-17	142.72		
(A-S Medication)				
REPACK				
SOL, IH (ACTIVATION INHALER)				
0.017 mg/actuation,				
12.9 gm	54569-5757-00	165.66		
(Phys Total Care)				
REPACK				
SOL, IH, 0.017 mg/actuation,				
12.9 gm	54868-5511-00	161.68		

ATRYN (Lundbeck)
antithrombin, recombinant

PROD/MFR	NDC	AWP	DP	OBC
PDS, IV (1750IU/VIAL)				
1 iu, ea	67386-0521-51	2.34		

ATTAPULGITE (PCCA)

PROD/MFR	NDC	AWP	DP	OBC
POW, NA (COLLOIDAL ACTIVATED USP)				
1 gm	51927-2405-00	0.15		
(Spectrum Pharmacy)				
POW, NA (1X500GM,USP)				
500 gm	49452-0781-02	158.55		

ATTENUVAX (Merck)
measles virus vaccine, live

PROD/MFR	NDC	AWP	DP	OBC
PDS, SC (SDV W/DILUENT,TAX INCL)				
1000 tcid50,				
10s ea	00006-4589-00	204.79		

ATUSS DS (Atley)
cpm/dm/pse hcl

PROD/MFR	NDC	AWP	DP	OBC
SUS, PO (GRAPE BUBBLEGUM)				
473 ml	59702-0800-16	299.28		

AUGMENTED BETAMETHASONE DIPROPIONATE
(Dispensing Solutions)

PROD/MFR	NDC	AWP	DP	OBC
REPACK				
betamethasone dipropionate, augmented				
OIN, TP, 0.05%, 45 gm	55045-3008-02	62.00		

AUGMENTIN (Glaxo)
amoxicillin/clavulanate potassium

PROD/MFR	NDC	AWP	DP	OBC
PDR, PO, 75 ml	00029-6085-39	39.66		
(BANANA)				
100 ml	00029-6085-23	52.84		
150 ml	00029-6085-22	77.68		
(ORANGE)				
250 mg/5 ml-62.5 mg/5 ml,				
75 ml	00029-6090-39	75.53		
100 ml	00029-6090-23	100.84		
150 ml	00029-6090-22	148.18		
TAB, PO, 250 mg-125 mg,				
30s ea	00029-6075-27	121.42		
500 mg-125 mg,				
20s ea	00029-6080-12	119.11		AB
875 mg-125 mg,				
20s ea	00029-6086-12	158.99		
(A-S Medication)				
REPACK				
PDR, PO, 150 ml	54569-0137-00	77.06		
(ORANGE)				
250 mg/5 ml-62.5 mg/5 ml,				
150 ml	54569-0117-00	147.00		
TAB, PO, 250 mg-125 mg,				
30s ea	54569-0142-01	129.59		
500 mg-125 mg,				
14s ea UD	54569-1959-04	88.99		AB
21s ea UD	54569-1959-01	133.49		AB
30s ea UD	54569-1959-06	190.70		AB
875 mg-125 mg,				
10s ea UD	54569-4458-00	84.85		
14s ea UD	54569-4458-02	118.79		
20s ea	54569-4325-00	206.69		
(Altura)				
REPACK				
CTB, PO, 125 mg-31.25 mg,				
12s ea	63874-0116-12	11.55		
15s ea	63874-0116-15	16.16		
20s ea	63874-0116-20	22.86		
21s ea	63874-0116-21	25.19		
30s ea	63874-0116-30	38.04		
250 mg-62.5 mg,				
10s ea	63874-0117-10	24.94		
12s ea	63874-0117-12	29.92		
14s ea	63874-0117-14	34.92		
15s ea	63874-0117-15	37.41		
20s ea	63874-0117-20	49.88		
30s ea	63874-0117-30	79.13		
PDR, PO, 75 ml	63874-0148-75	14.70		
100 ml	63874-0148-10	21.84		
150 ml	63874-0148-15	32.24		
250 mg/5 ml-62.5 mg/5 ml,				
75 ml	63874-0147-75	27.98		
100 ml	63874-0147-10	43.37		
150 ml	63874-0147-15	63.44		
TAB, PO, 250 mg-125 mg,				
21s ea	63874-0103-21	65.02		
30s ea	63874-0103-30	82.97		
100s ea	63874-0103-01	255.48		
500 mg-125 mg,				
8s ea	63874-0115-08	28.81		
10s ea	63874-0115-10	32.29		
12s ea	63874-0115-12	35.21		
14s ea	63874-0115-14	43.31		
15s ea	63874-0115-15	46.15		
20s ea	63874-0115-20	69.68		
21s ea	63874-0115-21	72.80		
30s ea	63874-0115-30	107.12		
100s ea	63874-0115-01	332.32		
875 mg-125 mg,				
10s ea	63874-0249-10	59.82		
20s ea	63874-0249-20	112.26		
30s ea	63874-0249-30	179.46		
(DHS, Inc.)				
REPACK				
PDR, PO (ORANGE)				
250 mg/5 ml-62.5 mg/5 ml,				
150 ml	55887-0817-22	109.50		
(Dispensing Solutions)				
REPACK				
CTB, PO (LEMON-LIME)				
250 mg-62.5 mg,				
30s ea	55045-1373-08	97.50		
PDR, PO (ORANGE)				
250 mg/5 ml-62.5 mg/5 ml,				
150 ml	55045-1345-03	84.50		
TAB, PO, 500 mg-125 mg,				
20s ea	55045-1258-07	85.88		AB
875 mg-125 mg,				
20s ea	55045-2446-07	129.00		
(Nucare Pharm)				
REPACK				
TAB, PO, 500 mg-125 mg,				
15s ea	66267-0444-15	81.99		AB
20s ea	66267-0992-20	109.32		AB
875 mg-125 mg,				
20s ea	66267-0991-20	117.49		AB

PROD/MFR	NDC	AWP	DP	OBC
(PD-Rx Pharm)				
REPACK				
CTB, PO, 125 mg-31.25 mg,				
15s ea	**55289-0240-15**	63.35		
TAB, PO, 250 mg-125 mg,				
9s ea	**55289-0242-09**	59.46		
15s ea	**55289-0242-15**	94.10		
21s ea	**55289-0242-21**	128.81		
500 mg-125 mg,				
15s ea	**55289-0296-15**	134.93		AB
30s ea	**55289-0296-30**	262.37		AB
(REDI-SCRIPT)				
500 mg-125 mg,				
30s ea	**58864-0740-30**	194.24		AB
875 mg-125 mg,				
10s ea	**55289-0512-10**	120.90		
14s ea	**55289-0512-14**	166.26		
(REDI-SCRIPT)				
875 mg-125 mg,				
20s ea	**58864-0697-20**	198.55		
28s ea	**55289-0512-28**	325.02		
(Pharma Pac)				
REPACK				
CTB, PO (LEMON-LIME)				
125 mg-31.25 mg,				
30s ea	**52959-0470-30**	35.03		
250 mg-62.5 mg,				
30s ea	**52959-0022-30**	75.96		
PDR, PO				
250 mg/5 ml-62.5 mg/5 ml,				
75 ml	**52959-0616-01**	33.54		
100 ml	**52959-0616-02**	45.25		
150 ml	**52959-0616-00**	64.84		
(ORANGE-RASPBERRY)				
400 mg/5 ml-57 mg/5 ml,				
100 ml	**52959-0617-00**	70.25		
TAB, PO, 250 mg-125 mg,				
9s ea	**52959-0343-09**	28.90		
15s ea	**52959-0343-15**	44.75		
21s ea	**52959-0343-21**	58.15		
30s ea	**52959-0343-30**	94.50		
500 mg-125 mg,				
4s ea	**52959-0021-01**	32.52		
14s ea	**52959-0021-14**	75.88		
15s ea	**52959-0021-15**	81.25		
20s ea	**52959-0021-20**	102.10		
21s ea	**52959-0021-21**	105.21		
30s ea	**52959-0021-30**	149.10		
875 mg-125 mg,				
10s ea	**52959-0478-10**	77.87		
14s ea	**52959-0478-14**	95.38		
15s ea	**52959-0478-15**	104.43		
20s ea	**52959-0478-20**	117.97		
(Phys Total Care)				
REPACK				
CTB, PO, 250 mg-62.5 mg,				
10s ea	**54868-0387-00**	52.69		
20s ea	**54868-0387-02**	103.42		
30s ea	**54868-0387-01**	153.50		
(LEMON-LIME)				
250 mg-62.5 mg,				
30s ea	**54868-1709-01**	100.91		
(BANANA-CHERRY)				
400 mg-57 mg,				
20s ea	**54868-4471-00**	114.94		AB
PDR, PO, 75 ml	**54868-0199-03**	30.36		
(BANANA)				
100 ml	**54868-0199-00**	43.18		
(1X150ML)				
150 ml	**54868-0199-02**	90.27		
(ORANGE-RASPBERRY)				
200 mg/5 ml-28.5 mg/5 ml,				
100 ml	**54868-4208-00**	57.00		
(ORANGE)				
250 mg/5 ml-62.5 mg/5 ml,				
100 ml	**54868-0200-00**	81.30		
(1X150ML)				
250 mg/5 ml-62.5 mg/5 ml,				
150 ml	**54868-0200-01**	161.06		
(ORANGE-RASPBERRY)				
400 mg/5 ml-57 mg/5 ml,				
100 ml	**54868-4080-00**	103.26		
TAB, PO, 500 mg-125 mg,				
10s ea	**54868-0388-00**	64.30		AB
15s ea	**54868-0388-02**	90.31		AB
20s ea	**54868-0388-01**	119.79		AB
30s ea	**54868-0388-04**	178.13		AB
875 mg-125 mg,				
10s ea	**54868-3903-00**	80.57		
15s ea	**54868-3903-02**	126.86		
20s ea	**54868-3903-01**	159.26		
30s ea	**54868-3903-03**	237.96		
(Quality Care Prod)				
REPACK				
PDR, PO (ORANGE)				
250 mg/5 ml-62.5 mg/5 ml,				
150 ml	**49999-0365-50**	107.16		
TAB, PO, 500 mg-125 mg,				
20s ea	**49999-0213-20**	204.54		AB
875 mg-125 mg,				
14s ea	**35356-0188-14**	232.03		
20s ea	**35356-0188-20**	313.43		
28s ea	**35356-0463-28**	76.07		
(Southwood)				
REPACK				
CTB, PO (LEMON-LIME)				
250 mg-62.5 mg,				
30s ea	**58016-0106-30**	134.40		
PDR, PO, 75 ml	**58016-1009-03**	14.00		
(ORANGE)				
250 mg/5 ml-62.5 mg/5 ml,				
150 ml	**58016-1011-01**	134.40		
TAB, PO, 500 mg-125 mg,				
20s ea	**58016-0107-20**	119.11		AB
20s ea	**58016-4808-01**	95.70		
875 mg-125 mg,				
20s ea	**58016-0512-20**	162.91		
AUGMENTIN ES-600 (Glaxo)				
amoxicillin/clavulanate potassium				
PDR, PO (STRAWBERRY CREAM)				
600 mg/5 ml-42.9 mg/5 ml,				
75 ml	**00029-6094-40**	55.28		AB
(A-S Medication)				
REPACK				
PDR, PO (ORANGE-RASPBERRY)				
600 mg/5 ml-42.9 mg/5 ml,				
125 ml	**54569-5522-00**	92.25		
(Phys Total Care)				
REPACK				
PDR, PO				
600 mg/5 ml-42.9 mg/5 ml,				
125 ml	**54868-4680-01**	94.08		
AUGMENTIN XR (Glaxo)				
amoxicillin/clavulanate potassium				
TER, PO (SCORED, 7 DAY XR PACK)				
1000 mg-62.5 mg,				
28s ea	**00029-6096-48**	115.86		
(SCORED,10 DAY XR PACK)				
1000 mg-62.5 mg,				
40s ea	**00029-6096-60**	165.50		
(Pharma Pac)				
REPACK				
TER, PO (FILM-COATED)				
1000 mg-62.5 mg,				
28s ea	**52959-0793-28**	90.95		
40s ea	**52959-0793-40**	129.91		
(Phys Total Care)				
REPACK				
TER, PO (FILM-COATED)				
1000 mg-62.5 mg,				
20s ea	**54868-4735-00**	100.74		
28s ea	**54868-4735-02**	128.83		
40s ea	**54868-4735-01**	187.89		
(Quality Care Prod)				
REPACK				
TER, PO, 1000 mg-62.5 mg,				
40s ea	**35356-0037-40**	180.00		
(Stat Rx)				
REPACK				
TER, PO, 1000 mg-62.5 mg,				
40s ea	**16590-0369-40**	143.25		
AURALGAN (Deston Therapeutics, LLC)				
acetic acid/antipyrine/benzocaine/policosanol				
SOL, OT, 14 ml	**16881-0300-15**	191.21		
(Quality Care Prod)				
REPACK				
SOL, OT (1X14ML,DROPS)				
14 ml	**35356-0189-14**	296.40		
AURANOFIN				
(Prometheus Labs) *See RIDAURA*				
AURODEX (Major)				
antipyrine/benzocaine				
SOL, OT (1X10ML)				
54 mg/ml-14 mg/ml,				
10 ml	**00904-0793-10**	11.37		
(Pharma Pac)				
REPACK				
SOL, OT, 54 mg/ml-14 mg/ml,				
15 ml	**52959-0135-03**	18.80		
AUROGUARD (SDA)				
antipyrine/benzocaine/glycerin				
SOL, OT, 54 mg/ml-14 mg/ml,				
15 ml	**66424-0520-35**	2.75	2.00	
(Physician Partner)				
REPACK				
SOL, OT, 54 mg/ml-14 mg/ml,				
14.79 ml	**21695-0199-01**	7.90		
AURORA HEALTH CARE LANCETS (Medicore)				
lancet				
DEV, NA, 100s ea	**32671-0201-44**	7.00	3.00	
200s ea	**32671-0202-44**	12.00	4.50	
AUROTO (Nucare Pharm)				
REPACK				
antipyrine/benzocaine				
SOL, OT, 54 mg/ml-14 mg/ml,				
15 ml	**66267-0990-15**	21.90		
(Quality Care Prod)				
REPACK				
SOL, OT, 54 mg/ml-14 mg/ml,				
15 ml	**49999-0329-15**	8.84		
AURUM (Weleda)				
homeopathic substance				
LIQ, PO (12X)				
50 ml	**55946-0133-15**	9.00		
AURUMHEEL (Heel/BHI)				
homeopathic substance				
LIQ, PO (DROPS)				
50 ml	**50114-1015-04**	5.95	5.95	
AVAGE (Allergan Inc)				
tazarotene				
CRE, TP, 0.1%, 30 gm	**00023-9236-30**	167.68		
AVAILNEX (Hall)				
carbocysteine				
CTB, PO, 750 mg, 60s ea	**44411-0103-60**	40.63		
AVALIDE (Bristol-Myers)				
hydrochlorothiazide/irbesartan				
TAB, PO, 12.5 mg-150 mg,				
30s ea	**00087-2775-31**	98.00		
90s ea	**00087-2775-32**	293.92		
12.5 mg-300 mg,				
30s ea	**00087-2776-31**	106.74		
90s ea	**00087-2776-32**	320.27		
(FILM-COATED)				
25 mg-300 mg,				
30s ea	**00087-2788-31**	117.20		
90s ea	**00087-2788-32**	351.58		
(Phys Total Care)				
REPACK				
TAB, PO, 12.5 mg-150 mg,				
30s ea	**54868-4494-00**	111.53		
12.5 mg-300 mg,				
30s ea	**54868-4526-00**	125.96		
90s ea	**54868-4526-01**	353.29		
25 mg-300 mg,				
30s ea	**54868-5465-00**	138.11		
(Quality Care Prod)				
REPACK				
TAB, PO, 12.5 mg-150 mg,				
30s ea	**35356-0374-30**	169.46		
150s ea	**35356-0374-15**	759.82		
12.5 mg-300 mg,				
30s ea	**35356-0406-30**	184.28		
(FILM-COATED)				
25 mg-300 mg,				
30s ea	**35356-0407-30**	203.55		
AVANCE NERVE GRAFT (AxoGen)				
implant insertion device				
DEV, NA (1-2MM X 15MM)				
ea	**08624-1111-15**	1450.00	1450.00	
ea	**08624-1112-15**	1450.00	1450.00	
(1-2MM X 30MM)				
ea	**08624-1111-30**	1750.00	1750.00	
ea	**08624-1112-30**	1750.00	1750.00	
(1-2MM X 50MM)				
ea	**08624-1111-50**	2149.26	2150.00	
ea	**08624-1112-50**	2150.00	2150.00	
(1-2MM X 70MM)				
ea	**08624-1111-70**	2550.00	2550.00	
ea	**08624-1112-70**	2550.00	2550.00	

PROD/MFR	NDC	AWP	DP	OBC
(2-3MM X 15MM)				
ea	08624-2111-15	1450.00	1450.00	
ea	08624-2112-15	1450.00	1450.00	
(2-3MM X 30MM)				
ea	08624-2111-30	1750.00	1750.00	
ea	08624-2112-30	1750.00	1750.00	
(2-3MM X 50MM)				
ea	08624-2111-50	2150.00	2150.00	
ea	08624-2112-50	2150.00	2150.00	
(2-3MM X 70MM)				
ea	08624-2111-70	2550.00	2550.00	
ea	08624-2112-70	2550.00	2550.00	
(3-4MM X 15MM)				
ea	08624-3111-15	1450.00	1450.00	
ea	08624-3112-15	1450.00	1450.00	
(3-4MM X 30MM)				
ea	08624-3111-30	1750.00	1750.00	
ea	08624-3112-30	1750.00	1750.00	
(3-4MM X 50MM)				
ea	08624-3111-50	2150.00	2150.00	
ea	08624-3112-50	2150.00	2150.00	
(3-4MM X 70MM)				
ea	08624-3111-70	2550.00	2550.00	
ea	08624-3112-70	2550.00	2550.00	
(4-5MM X 15MM)				
ea	08624-4111-15	1450.00	1450.00	
ea	08624-4112-15	1450.00	1450.00	
(4-5MM X 30MM)				
ea	08624-4111-30	1750.00	1750.00	
ea	08624-4112-30	1750.00	1750.00	
(4-5MM X 50MM)				
ea	08624-4111-50	2150.00	2150.00	
ea	08624-4112-50	2150.00	2150.00	
(4-5MM X 70MM)				
ea	08624-4111-70	2550.00	2550.00	
ea	08624-4112-70	2550.00	2550.00	
AVANDAMET (Glaxo)				
metformin hydrochloride/rosiglitazone maleate				
TAB, PO (FILM COATED)				
500 mg-2 mg, 60s ea	00007-3167-18	165.31		
(FILM-COATED)				
500 mg-4 mg, 60s ea	00007-3168-18	280.07		
(FILM COATED)				
1000 mg-2 mg, 60s ea	00007-3163-18	165.31		
1000 mg-4 mg, 60s ea	00007-3164-18	280.07		
(Phys Total Care)				
REPACK				
TAB, PO (FILM COATED)				
500 mg-2 mg, 20s ea	54868-4965-01	59.97		
30s ea	54868-4965-02	88.97		
60s ea	54868-4965-00	166.32		
500 mg-4 mg, 30s ea	54868-5157-01	133.56		
(FILM-COATED)				
500 mg-4 mg, 60s ea	54868-5157-00	249.99		
(FILM COATED)				
1000 mg-2 mg, 60s ea	54868-5376-00	141.06		
1000 mg-4 mg, 30s ea	54868-5262-00	141.18		
60s ea	54868-5262-01	279.74		
AVANDARYL (Glaxo)				
glimepiride/rosiglitazone maleate				
TAB, PO, 1 mg-4 mg, 30s ea	00007-3151-13	156.64		
2 mg-4 mg, 30s ea	00007-3152-13	156.64		
2 mg-8 mg, 30s ea	00007-3148-13	269.45		
4 mg-4 mg, 30s ea	00007-3153-13	156.64		
4 mg-8 mg, 30s ea	00007-3149-13	269.45		
(Phys Total Care)				
REPACK				
TAB, PO, 4 mg-4 mg, 60s ea	54868-5739-00	280.10		
AVANDIA (Glaxo)				
rosiglitazone maleate				
TAB, PO (FILM-COATED)				
2 mg, 60s ea	00029-3158-18	189.25		
(FILM-COATED TILTAB)				
4 mg, 30s ea	00029-3159-13	140.45		
90s ea	00029-3159-00	421.31		
(FILM-COATED, TILTAB)				
8 mg, 30s ea	00029-3160-13	255.17		
90s ea	00029-3160-59	765.42		
(A-S Medication)				
REPACK				
TAB, PO, 4 mg, 30s ea	54569-4802-00	113.72		
(FILM-COATED, TILTAB)				
8 mg, 30s ea	54569-4803-00	298.10		
(Advanced Pharm Serv, Inc.)				
REPACK				
TAB, PO (FILM-COATED TILTAB)				
4 mg, 30s ea	13411-0104-03	144.60		
(FILM-COATED, TILTAB)				
8 mg, 30s ea	13411-0105-03	262.74		
(Altura)				
REPACK				
TAB, PO (FILM COATED)				
4 mg, 10s ea	63874-0510-10	28.85		
30s ea	63874-0510-30	89.85		
90s ea	63874-0510-90	249.30		
100s ea	63874-0510-01	288.53		
(AQ)				
REPACK				
TAB, PO, 2 mg, 10s ea	66105-0145-01	47.02		
15s ea	66105-0145-15	70.54		
30s ea	66105-0145-03	141.08		
60s ea	66105-0145-06	282.17		
90s ea	66105-0145-09	423.25		
4 mg, 10s ea	66105-0159-01	48.20		
15s ea	66105-0159-15	72.30		
30s ea	66105-0159-03	114.60		
60s ea	66105-0159-06	289.20		
90s ea	66105-0159-09	433.80		
8 mg, 30s ea	66105-0146-03	262.74		
(DHS, Inc.)				
REPACK				
TAB, PO, 4 mg, 30s ea	55887-0646-30	156.75		
60s ea	55887-0646-60	313.50		
90s ea	55887-0646-90	470.25		
(PD-Rx Pharm)				
REPACK				
TAB, PO (REDI-SCRIPT)				
4 mg, 30s ea	58864-0687-30	163.10		
60s ea	58864-0687-60	258.07		
8 mg, 30s ea	55289-0938-30	296.34		
(Phys Total Care)				
REPACK				
TAB, PO (FILM-COATED)				
2 mg, 30s ea	54868-5249-00	109.20		
60s ea	54868-5249-01	203.29		
4 mg, 30s ea	54868-4198-00	140.93		
60s ea	54868-4198-01	281.20		
8 mg, 30s ea	54868-4221-00	227.24		
(Quality Care Prod)				
REPACK				
TAB, PO (FILM-COATED)				
2 mg, 60s ea	35356-0271-60	297.02		
(FILM-COATED TILTAB)				
4 mg, 30s ea	49999-0304-30	210.42		
8 mg, 30s ea	49999-0935-30	302.45		
(Southwood)				
REPACK				
TAB, PO (FILM-COATED)				
2 mg, 30s ea	58016-0082-30	79.47		
60s ea	58016-0082-60	158.94		
90s ea	58016-0082-90	238.41		
100s ea	58016-0082-00	264.90		
(FILM-COATED, TILTAB)				
8 mg, 30s ea	58016-0081-30	214.31		
60s ea	58016-0081-60	428.62		
90s ea	58016-0081-90	642.93		
100s ea	58016-0081-00	714.37		
AVAPRO (Bristol-Myers)				
irbesartan				
TAB, PO (UNIT OF USE)				
75 mg, 30s ea	00087-2771-31	76.97		
90s ea	00087-2771-32	230.89		
150 mg, 30s ea	00087-2772-31	81.00		
90s ea	00087-2772-32	243.06		
(10X10,BLISTER PACK)				
150 mg, 100s ea UD	00087-2772-35	270.06		
(UNIT OF USE)				
150 mg, 500s ea	00087-2772-15	1350.26		
300 mg, 30s ea	00087-2773-31	97.39		
90s ea	00087-2773-32	292.14		
500s ea	00087-2773-15	1622.95		
(A-S Medication)				
REPACK				
TAB, PO, 75 mg, 30s ea	54569-5867-00	63.05		
150 mg, 30s ea	54569-4572-00	75.26		
(Advanced Pharm Serv, Inc.)				
REPACK				
TAB, PO, 150 mg, 10s ea	13411-0106-01	39.45		
15s ea	13411-0106-15	59.18		
30s ea	13411-0106-03	118.36		
60s ea	13411-0106-06	236.72		
90s ea	13411-0106-09	355.08		
300 mg, 10s ea	13411-0107-01	44.36		
15s ea	13411-0107-15	66.54		
30s ea	13411-0107-03	133.09		
60s ea	13411-0107-06	266.17		
90s ea	13411-0107-09	399.26		
(Altura)				
REPACK				
TAB, PO, 150 mg, 10s ea	63874-0647-10	16.63		
14s ea	63874-0647-14	23.28		
30s ea	63874-0647-30	47.89		
(AQ)				
REPACK				
TAB, PO, 150 mg, 10s ea	66105-0503-01	39.45		
15s ea	66105-0503-15	59.18		
30s ea	66105-0503-03	118.36		
60s ea	66105-0503-06	236.72		
90s ea	66105-0503-09	355.08		
300 mg, 10s ea	66105-0504-01	44.36		
15s ea	66105-0504-15	66.54		
30s ea	66105-0504-03	133.09		
60s ea	66105-0504-06	266.17		
90s ea	66105-0504-09	399.26		
(DHS, Inc.)				
REPACK				
TAB, PO, 75 mg, 30s ea	55887-0962-30	74.98		
150 mg, 30s ea	55887-0956-30	77.25		
300 mg, 30s ea	55887-0963-30	93.75		
(PD-Rx Pharm)				
REPACK				
TAB, PO, 150 mg, 15s ea	58864-0726-15	55.82		
(REDI-SCRIPT)				
150 mg, 30s ea	58864-0726-30	111.60		
300 mg, 15s ea	58864-0771-15	78.86		
(Phys Total Care)				
REPACK				
TAB, PO, 150 mg, 30s ea	54868-4199-00	96.06		
60s ea	54868-4199-02	180.37		
90s ea	54868-4199-01	268.59		
300 mg, 30s ea	54868-4414-00	115.10		
(Quality Care Prod)				
REPACK				
TAB, PO, 150 mg, 30s ea	35356-0428-30	124.59		
300 mg, 30s ea	35356-0131-30	132.90		
AVAR CLEANSER (Tiber)				
sulfacetamide sodium/sulfur				
SOA, TP (1X226.8GM)				
10%-5%, 226.8 gm	23589-0025-08	118.75		
AVAR GEL (Tiber)				
sulfacetamide sodium/sulfur				
GEL, TP (1X45GM)				
10%-5%, 45 gm	23589-0026-45	100.00		
AVAR-E (Tiber)				
sulfacetamide sodium/sulfur				
CRE, TP (1X45GM)				
10%-5%, 45 gm	23589-0027-45	100.00		
AVAR-E GREEN (Tiber)				
sulfacetamide sodium/sulfur				
CRE, TP (1X45GM)				
10%-5%, 45 gm	23589-0028-45	100.00		
AVASTIN (Genentech)				
bevacizumab				
SOL, IV (PF)				
25 mg/ml, 4 ml	50242-0060-01	669.90		
16 ml	50242-0061-01	2679.60		
AVC (Azur Pharma, Inc.)				
sulfanilamide				
CRE, VG (W/APPLICATOR)				
15%, 120 gm	66663-0103-04	106.70		EE
(Phys Total Care)				
REPACK				
CRE, VG, 15%, 120 gm	54868-0389-01	39.51		AT
AVELOX (Schering)				
moxifloxacin hydrochloride				
TAB, PO (FILM-COATED)				
400 mg, 5s ea	00085-1733-03	81.77		
30s ea	00085-1733-01	490.63		
50s ea UD	00085-1733-02	817.82		

PROD/MFR	NDC	AWP	DP	OBC
(A-S Medication)				
REPACK				
TAB, PO, 400 mg, 5s ea	**54569-4922-00**	66.87		
(BRONCHITIS COURSE)				
400 mg, 5s ea	**54569-5149-00**	106.30		
(FILM-COATED)				
400 mg, 10s ea	**54569-4922-01**	212.61		
(Advanced Pharm Serv, Inc.)				
REPACK				
TAB, PO, 400 mg, 10s ea	**13411-0108-01**	159.47		
15s ea	**13411-0108-15**	239.21		
20s ea	**13411-0108-02**	318.95		
(FILM-COATED)				
400 mg, 30s ea	**13411-0108-03**	478.43		
60s ea	**13411-0108-06**	956.86		
(AQ)				
REPACK				
TAB, PO, 400 mg, 10s ea	**66105-0537-01**	193.30		
15s ea	**66105-0537-15**	289.95		
30s ea	**66105-0537-03**	579.90		
60s ea	**66105-0537-06**	1159.80		
90s ea	**66105-0537-09**	1739.70		
(Dispensing Solutions)				
REPACK				
TAB, PO (FILM-COATED)				
400 mg, 5s ea	**55045-2843-05**	72.50		
7s ea	**55045-2843-07**	101.50		
10s ea	**55045-2843-01**	145.00		
(FILM-COATED)				
400 mg, 10s ea	**66336-0040-10**	188.07		
(PD-Rx Pharm)				
REPACK				
TAB, PO (REDI-SCRIPT,FILM-COATED)				
400 mg, 5s ea	**58864-0621-05**	120.92		
(FILM-COATED)				
400 mg, 10s ea	**55289-0077-10**	241.83		
(REDI-SCRIPT,FILM-COATED)				
400 mg, 10s ea	**58864-0621-10**	241.83		
(FILM-COATED)				
400 mg, 30s ea	**58864-0621-30**	729.23		
(Pharma Pac)				
REPACK				
TAB, PO (FILM-COATED)				
400 mg, 5s ea	**52959-0004-05**	99.90		
(Phys Total Care)				
REPACK				
TAB, PO (FILM-COATED)				
400 mg, 2s ea	**54868-4367-05**	40.43		
5s ea	**54868-4367-00**	105.11		
7s ea	**54868-4367-03**	138.13		
10s ea	**54868-4367-01**	196.21		
(FILM-COATED)				
400 mg, 14s ea	**54868-4367-04**	273.65		
30s ea	**54868-4367-02**	564.66		
(Quality Care Prod)				
REPACK				
TAB, PO (FILM-COATED)				
400 mg, 5s ea	**49999-0455-05**	131.65		
10s ea	**49999-0455-10**	182.00		
30s ea	**49999-0455-30**	743.30		
(Southwood)				
REPACK				
TAB, PO (FILM-COATED)				
400 mg, 30s ea	**00490-0085-30**	417.54		
60s ea	**00490-0085-60**	835.08		
90s ea	**00490-0085-90**	1252.62		
100s ea	**00490-0085-00**	1391.80		
(Stat Rx)				
REPACK				
TAB, PO (FILM-COATED)				
400 mg, 5s ea	**16590-0881-05**	95.95		
AVELOX I.V. (Schering)				
moxifloxacin hydrochloride				
SOL, IV (FLEXIBAG,PF)				
400 mg/250 ml,				
250 ml 12s	**00085-1737-01**	504.00		
AVIANE (Teva)				
ethinyl estradiol/levonorgestrel				
TAB, PO (6X28)				
0.02 mg-0.1 mg,				
168s ea	**00555-9045-58**	210.96	DP	AB1
(Phys Total Care)				
REPACK				
TAB, PO, 0.02 mg-0.1 mg,				
28s ea	**54868-5356-00**	27.38		AB1

PROD/MFR	NDC	AWP	DP	OBC
AVIDOXY (Avidas)				
doxycycline				
TAB, PO (FILM COATED,CAPLET)				
100 mg, 50s ea	**43684-0200-20**	576.00		
AVIDOXY DK (Avidas)				
doxycycline/octinoxate/salicylic acid/zinc oxide				
KIT, MR, 100 mg-5.5%-2%-8%,				
ea	**43684-0200-21**	576.00		
AVINZA (King Pharm)				
morphine sulfate				
C24, PO, 30 mg,				
100s ea, C-II	**60793-0605-01**	436.68		BX
45 mg,				
100s ea, C-II	**60793-0603-01**	647.46		
60 mg,				
100s ea, C-II	**60793-0606-01**	847.97		BX
75 mg,				
100s ea, C-II	**60793-0604-01**	1079.10		
90 mg,				
100s ea, C-II	**60793-0607-01**	1274.99		
120 mg,				
100s ea, C-II	**60793-0608-01**	1504.36		
(Bryant Ranch)				
REPACK				
C24, PO, 30 mg,				
30s ea, C-II	**63629-3766-01**	115.21		BX
60s ea, C-II	**63629-3766-02**	232.33		BX
60 mg,				
30s ea, C-II	**63629-3764-01**	220.32		BX
60s ea, C-II	**63629-3764-02**	438.95		BX
90s ea, C-II	**63629-3764-03**	672.85		BX
(Phys Total Care)				
REPACK				
C24, PO, 30 mg,				
10s ea, C-II	**54868-4941-01**	54.13		
30s ea, C-II	**54868-4941-00**	154.56		
60s ea, C-II	**54868-4941-02**	288.46		
60 mg,				
10s ea, C-II	**54868-4942-01**	84.95		
30s ea, C-II	**54868-4942-00**	234.97		
90 mg,				
10s ea, C-II	**54868-4943-01**	116.42		
30s ea, C-II	**54868-4943-00**	325.28		
120 mg,				
10s ea, C-II	**54868-4944-01**	135.68		
30s ea, C-II	**54868-4944-00**	379.85		
(Quality Care Prod)				
REPACK				
C24, PO, 30 mg,				
30s ea, C-II	**35356-0238-30**	263.47		BX
100s ea, C-II	**35356-0238-00**	600.06		BX
45 mg,				
30s ea, C-II	**35356-0548-30**	306.60		
60 mg,				
30s ea, C-II	**35356-0118-30**	349.60		BX
100s ea, C-II	**35356-0118-00**	1158.42		BX
90 mg,				
30s ea, C-II	**35356-0333-30**	664.28		
100s ea, C-II	**35356-0333-00**	1755.91		
120 mg,				
100s ea, C-II	**35356-0339-00**	2048.25		
(Stat Rx)				
REPACK				
C24, PO, 30 mg,				
30s ea, C-II	**16590-0594-30**	154.68		BX
60s ea, C-II	**16590-0594-60**	306.12		BX
90s ea, C-II	**16590-0594-90**	457.55		BX
60 mg,				
30s ea, C-II	**16590-0593-30**	297.31		BX
60s ea, C-II	**16590-0593-60**	591.36		BX
90s ea, C-II	**16590-0593-90**	885.41		BX
75 mg,				
30s ea, C-II	**16590-0842-30**	316.72		
60s ea, C-II	**16590-0842-60**	633.45		
90s ea, C-II	**16590-0842-90**	945.50		
90 mg,				
30s ea, C-II	**16590-0597-30**	445.39		
60s ea, C-II	**16590-0597-60**	658.00		
90s ea, C-II	**16590-0597-90**	1329.66		
120 mg,				
30s ea, C-II	**16590-0473-30**	524.92		
60s ea, C-II	**16590-0473-60**	694.00		
90s ea, C-II	**16590-0473-90**	1026.00		
100s ea, C-II	**16590-0842-71**	1145.79		
120s ea, C-II	**16590-0473-72**	2089.95		
AVITA (Mylan)				
tretinoin				
CRE, TP, 0.025%, 20 gm	**00378-6141-44**	58.05		AB
45 gm	**00378-6141-45**	130.58		AB

PROD/MFR	NDC	AWP	DP	OBC
GEL, TP, 0.025%, 20 gm	**00378-6140-44**	58.05		BT
45 gm	**00378-6140-45**	130.58		BT
AVITENE MICROFIBRILLAR COLLAGEN HEMOSTAT (Davol)				
collagen hemostat				
POW, NA (FLOUR,5GM)				
2s ea	**03031-0105-90**	1042.44	868.70	
(FLOUR,0.5GM)				
6s ea	**03031-0100-10**	428.04	356.70	
(FLOUR,1GM)				
6s ea	**03031-0100-20**	859.02	715.85	
AVITENE ULTRAFOAM COLLAGEN (Davol)				
collagen hemostat				
SHE, NA (SPONGE,100 SQ.CM)				
6s ea	**03031-0500-40**	284.04	236.70	
(SPONGE,100/THIN)				
6s ea	**03031-0500-50**	283.50	236.25	
(SPONGE,50 SQ.CM)				
6s ea	**03031-0500-30**	189.96	158.30	
(SPONGE,12.5 SQ.CM)				
12s ea	**03031-0500-20**	117.18	97.65	
AVOCADO OIL (Amend)				
OIL, NA (REFINED)				
500 ml	**17317-1290-01**	19.60		
3840 ml	**17317-1290-06**	126.00		
19200 ml	**17317-1290-08**	462.00		
(PCCA)				
OIL, NA (REFINED)				
1 ml	**51927-2829-00**	0.43		
AVODART (Glaxo)				
dutasteride				
SGL, PO (SOFT GELATIN CAPSULE)				
0.5 mg, 30s ea	**00173-0712-15**	121.96		
(SOFT GELATIN)				
0.5 mg, 30s ea	**00173-0712-25**	121.96		
(SOFT GELATIN CAPSULE)				
0.5 mg, 90s ea	**00173-0712-04**	365.83		
(AQ)				
REPACK				
SGL, PO (SOFT GELATIN CAPSULE)				
0.5 mg, 30s ea	**66105-0987-03**	198.43		
(Phys Total Care)				
REPACK				
SGL, PO, 0.5 mg, 30s ea	**54868-5114-00**	139.45		
(SOFT GELATIN CAPSULE)				
0.5 mg, 90s ea	**54868-5114-01**	414.42		
(Quality Care Prod)				
REPACK				
SGL, PO (SOFT GELATIN CAPSULE)				
0.5 mg, 30s ea	**35356-0210-30**	208.87		
(Southwood)				
REPACK				
SGL, PO (SOFT GELATIN)				
0.5 mg, 30s ea	**58016-0846-30**	108.55		
60s ea	**58016-0846-60**	217.10		
90s ea	**58016-0846-90**	325.65		
100s ea	**58016-0846-00**	361.83		
AVONEX (Biogen Idec)				
interferon beta-1a				
KIT, IM (S.D.V.)				
33 mcg, 4s ea	**59627-0001-03**	2964.00		
MR (ALBUMIN-FREE)				
30 mcg/0.5 ml,				
4s ea	**59627-0002-05**	2964.00		
AXERT (Ortho-McNeil Pharm)				
almotriptan malate				
TAB, PO (BLISTER PACK)				
6.25 mg, 6s ea	**00062-2080-06**	144.28	120.23	
(BLISTER PACK,2X6)				
12.5 mg, 12s ea	**00062-2085-12**	288.60	240.50	
(Phys Total Care)				
REPACK				
TAB, PO, 12.5 mg, 6s ea	**54868-5527-00**	138.01		
12s ea	**54868-5527-01**	318.42		
AXID (Braintree)				
nizatidine				
SOL, PO (AF,BUBBLE GUM)				
15 mg/ml, 480 ml	**52268-0147-62**	386.71		
(Glaxo)				
CAP, PO (PULVULES)				
150 mg, 60s ea	**65726-0144-15**	192.76		

PROD/MFR	NDC	AWP	DP	OBC
(Phys Total Care)				
REPACK				
SOL, PO, 15 mg/ml,				
480 ml	54868-5710-00	353.68		
AXID PULVULES (PD-Rx Pharm)				
REPACK				
nizatidine				
CAP, PO, 150 mg, 20s ea	55289-0637-20	105.90		
(Pharma Pac)				
REPACK				
CAP, PO, 150 mg, 30s ea	52959-0366-30	75.10		
50s ea	52959-0366-50	114.80		
60s ea	52959-0366-60	120.15		
(Phys Total Care)				
REPACK				
CAP, PO, 150 mg, 30s ea	54868-1130-00	113.80		
60s ea	54868-1130-01	213.29		
120s ea	54868-1130-02	424.71		
300 mg, 30s ea	54868-1131-01	221.28		
AXOGUARD NERVE CONNECTOR (AxoGen)				
implant insertion device				
DEV, NA (1.5MM X 10MM,SINGLE USE)				
ea	08624-0114-10	600.00	600.00	
(2MM X 10MM,SINGLE USE)				
ea	08624-0214-10	600.00	600.00	
(3MM X 10MM,SINGLE USE)				
ea	08624-0314-10	600.00	600.00	
(4MM X 10MM,SINGLE USE)				
ea	08624-0414-10	600.00	600.00	
(5MM X 10MM,SINGLE USE)				
ea	08624-0514-10	600.00	600.00	
(6MM X 10MM,SINGLE USE)				
ea	08624-0614-10	600.00	600.00	
(7MM X 10MM,SINGLE USE)				
ea	08624-0714-10	600.00	600.00	
AXOGUARD NERVE PROTECTOR (AxoGen)				
implant insertion device				
DEV, NA (10MM X 20MM,SINGLE USE)				
ea	08624-1013-20	1200.00	1200.00	
(10MM X 40MM,SINGLE USE)				
ea	08624-1013-40	1377.50	1450.00	
(2MM X 20MM,SINGLE USE)				
ea	08624-0213-20	1200.00	1200.00	
(3.5MM X 20MM,SINGLE USE)				
ea	08624-0313-20	1200.00	1200.00	
(3.5MM X 40MM,SINGLE USE)				
ea	08624-0313-40	1450.00	1450.00	
(5MM X 20MM,SINGLE USE)				
ea	08624-0513-20	1200.00	1200.00	
(5MM X 40MM,SINGLE USE)				
ea	08624-0513-40	1450.00	1450.00	
(7MM X 20MM,SINGLE USE)				
ea	08624-0713-20	1200.00	1200.00	
(7MM X 40MM,SINGLE USE)				
ea	08624-0713-40	1341.25	1450.00	
AXONA (Accera)				
medical food				
PDS, PO (30X40GM)				
40 gm 30s	42907-0040-30	86.40		
AYGESTIN (Teva)				
norethindrone acetate				
TAB, PO, 5 mg, 50s ea	51285-0424-10	153.27	67.42	AB
AZACITIDINE				
(Celgene Corp) *See VIDAZA*				
AZACTAM (Elan Pharmaceuticals)				
aztreonam				
PDS, IJ (S.D.V.)				
1 gm, 10s ea	51479-0041-15	407.72		
2 gm, 10s ea	51479-0042-15	813.94		
SOL, IV (GALAXY P.C.,24X50ML)				
1 gm/50 ml,				
50 ml 24s	51479-0048-01	958.20		
2 gm/50 ml,				
50 ml 24s	51479-0049-01	1919.04		
AZASAN (Salix Pharm)				
azathioprine				
TAB, PO, 75 mg, 100s ea	65649-0231-41	377.00		
100 mg, 100s ea	65649-0241-41	504.44		
AZASITE (Inspire)				
azithromycin				
SOL, OP (2.5ML FILL IN 5ML)				
1%, 2.5 ml	31357-0040-25	85.69		
AZATADINE MALEATE (PCCA)				
POW, NA (U.S.P.)				
1 gm	51927-2306-00	672.00		

PROD/MFR	NDC	AWP	DP	OBC
AZATHIOPRINE				
FUL				
TAB, PO, 50 mg, 100s ea		65.81		
(Gallipot)				
POW, NA (1X5GM)				
5 gm	51552-0779-02	87.50	62.50	
(1X25GM)				
25 gm	51552-0779-04	210.00	150.00	
(1X100GM)				
100 gm	51552-0779-05	700.00	500.00	
(Hawkins)				
POW, NA (U.S.P.)				
1 gm	63370-0025-10	32.00		
5 gm	63370-0025-15	136.00		
25 gm	63370-0025-25	600.00		
100 gm	63370-0025-35	2000.00		
(Medisca)				
POW, NA (1X1GM)				
1 gm	38779-2313-06	34.50		
(U.S.P.)				
1 gm	38779-0312-06	34.50		
(1X5GM)				
5 gm	38779-2313-03	138.00		
(U.S.P.)				
5 gm	38779-0312-03	138.00		
(1X25GM)				
25 gm	38779-2313-04	585.00		
(U.S.P.)				
25 gm	38779-0312-04	585.00		
(Mylan)				
TAB, PO, 50 mg, 100s ea	00378-1005-01	131.93		AB
(PCCA)				
POW, NA (USP)				
1 gm	51927-2258-00	33.00		
(Prometheus Labs) *See IMURAN*				
(Roxane)				
TAB, PO, 50 mg, 100s ea	00054-4084-25	131.08		AB
(10X10)				
50 mg, 100s ea UD	00054-8084-25	144.18		AB
(Salix Pharm) *See AZASAN*				
(Sandoz)				
TAB, PO, 50 mg, 100s ea	00781-5075-01	130.93		
(Spectrum Pharmacy)				
POW, NA (U.S.P.)				
1 gm	49452-0783-01	77.00		
5 gm	49452-0783-02	239.40		
25 gm	49452-0783-03	966.00		
(Zydus Pharm.)				
TAB, PO (USP)				
50 mg, 100s ea	68382-0003-01	131.08		AB
500s ea	68382-0003-05	655.40		AB
(American Health)				
REPACK				
TAB, PO, 50 mg,				
100s ea UD	68084-0229-01	84.50		
(Dispensing Solutions)				
REPACK				
TAB, PO, 50 mg, 100s ea	55045-3471-01	131.00		
(Palmetto)				
REPACK				
TAB, PO, 50 mg, 90s ea	23490-5110-09	135.00		
(Phys Total Care)				
REPACK				
TAB, PO, 50 mg, 30s ea	54868-5310-00	27.90		AB
(USP)				
50 mg, 60s ea	54868-5310-03	51.30		
90s ea	54868-5310-04	74.70		
100s ea	54868-5310-02	82.50		AB
120s ea	54868-5310-01	76.08		AB
(Physician Partner)				
REPACK				
TAB, PO, 50 mg, 75s ea	21695-0484-75	231.31		AB
(Vibranta)				
REPACK				
TAB, PO, 50 mg, 30s ea	57866-9021-01	59.25		
AZATHIOPRINE SODIUM (Bedford)				
PDS, IV (PF)				
100 mg, ea	55390-0600-20	132.00		AP
AZELAIC ACID				
(Allergan Inc) *See AZELEX*				
(Gallipot) *See AZELAIC ACID*				

PROD/MFR	NDC	AWP	DP	OBC
(Gallipot)				
FLA, NA, 100 gm	51552-0112-05	43.40		
AZELAIC ACID (Gallipot)				
500 gm	51552-0112-06	182.00		
AZELAIC ACID				
(Intendis, Inc.) *See FINACEA*				
(Intendis, Inc.) *See FINACEA PLUS*				
(Medisca)				
FLA, NA, 100 gm	38779-0628-05	93.00		
500 gm	38779-0628-08	166.50		
1000 gm	38779-0628-09	330.00		
(PCCA)				
FLA, NA, 1 gm	51927-1179-00	1.05		
(Spectrum Pharmacy)				
CRY, NA, 25 gm	49452-0021-01	97.30		
100 gm	49452-0021-02	177.45		
1000 gm	49452-0021-03	535.50		
AZELASTINE HYDROCHLORIDE (Apotex Corp.)				
SOL, OP (1X6ML)				
0.05%, 6 ml	60505-0578-04	104.07		AT
(Meda) *See ASTELIN READY-SPRAY*				
(Meda) *See ASTEPRO*				
(Meda) *See OPTIVAR*				
AZELEX (Allergan Inc)				
azelaic acid				
CRE, TP, 20%, 30 gm	00023-8694-30	156.34		
50 gm	00023-8694-50	229.90		
(Quality Care Prod)				
REPACK				
CRE, TP (1X30GM)				
20%, 30 gm	35356-0217-30	187.73		
(1X50GM)				
20%, 50 gm	35356-0218-50	309.49		
AZILECT (Teva Neuroscience)				
rasagiline				
TAB, PO, 0.5 mg, 30s ea	68546-0142-56	356.20		
1 mg, 30s ea	68546-0229-56	356.20		
AZITHROMYCIN				
FUL				
TAB, PO, 250 mg, 30s ea		95.63		
500 mg, 30s ea		164.55		
600 mg, 30s ea		207.24		
(APP) *See NOVAPLUS AZITHROMYCIN*				
(APP)				
PDS, IV (10X10ML,LATEX-FREE)				
500 mg, 10s ea	63323-0398-10	299.50		
(Baxter)				
PDS, IV, 500 mg, ea	10019-0648-71	8.75		AP
(LYOPHILIZED)				
500 mg, 10s ea	10019-0648-02	87.48		
(Greenstone)				
PDR, PO, 1 gm/packet,				
3s ea	59762-3051-02	72.45		
10s ea	59762-3051-01	241.50		
(CHERRY)				
100 mg/5 ml, 15 ml	59762-3110-01	32.93		
200 mg/5 ml, 15 ml	59762-3120-01	32.93		
22.5 ml	59762-3130-01	32.93		
30 ml	59762-3140-01	32.93		
TAB, PO (3BLISTER CARDSX6TABS)				
250 mg, 18s ea	59762-3060-01	139.95		
(FILM-COATED)				
250 mg, 30s ea	59762-3060-02	233.25		
50s ea UD	59762-3060-03	388.77		
(3 TAB BLISTER CARDSX3)				
500 mg, 9s ea	59762-3070-01	139.97		
(FILM-COATED)				
500 mg, 30s ea	59762-3070-02	466.50		
600 mg, 30s ea	59762-3080-01	559.83		
(Hospira)				
PDS, IV (SINGLE USE,LYOPHILIZED)				
500 mg, 10s ea	00409-0144-11	134.40	117.60	AP
(Inspire) *See AZASITE*				
(Letco) *See AZITHROMYCIN DIHYDRATE*				
(Major)				
TAB, PO (10X3,FILM-COATED)				
250 mg, 30s ea UD	00904-6010-04	221.67		AB
(10X3,FILM COATED)				
500 mg, 30s ea UD	00904-6011-04	582.21		AB
(Medisca)				
POW, NA (1X25GM,DIHYDRATE,USP)				
25 gm	38779-2246-04	267.00		

PROD/MFR	NDC	AWP	DP	OBC
(1X100GM,DIHYDRATE,USP)				
100 gm	38779-2246-05	705.00		
(1X500GM,DIHYDRATE,USP)				
500 gm	38779-2246-08	1912.50		
(1X1000GM,DIHYDRATE,USP)				
1000 gm	38779-2246-09	3366.00		
(Mylan)				
TAB, PO (3X6,FILM-COATED)				
250 mg, 18s ea UD	00378-1533-83	140.10		AB
(3X3,FILM-COATED)				
500 mg, 9s ea UD	00378-1534-59	140.10		AB
(FILM-COATED)				
600 mg, 30s ea	00378-1535-93	560.46		AB
(Pfizer) *See ZITHROMAX*				
(Pfizer) *See ZITHROMAX TRI-PAK*				
(Pfizer) *See ZITHROMAX Z-PAK*				
(Pfizer) *See ZMAX*				
(Sagent)				
PDS, IV (PF,LATEX-FREE)				
500 mg, 10s ea	25021-0112-10	206.25		AP
(Sandoz)				
PDR, PO (USP,CHERRY)				
100 mg/5 ml, 15 ml	00185-7203-70	34.88		AB
200 mg/5 ml, 15 ml	00185-7206-70	34.88		AB
22.5 ml	00185-7209-69	34.88		AB
30 ml	00185-7212-68	34.88		AB
TAB, PO (3X6,UNIT OF USE)				
250 mg, 3s ea	00781-1496-68	140.10		AB
(FILM-COATED)				
250 mg, 30s ea	00781-1496-31	233.51		AB
50s ea UD	00781-1496-69	389.21		AB
(3X3,UNIT OF USE)				
500 mg, 3s ea	00781-1941-33	140.10		AB
(FILM-COATED)				
500 mg, 30s ea	00781-1941-31	467.02		AB
600 mg, 30s ea	00781-1497-31	560.46		AB
(Teva)				
PDR, PO (1X15ML USP,CHERRY)				
100 mg/5 ml, 15 ml	00093-7148-23	35.02		AB
(USP,CHERRY)				
100 mg/5 ml, 15 ml	50111-0793-20	34.88		AB
(1X15ML, USP,CHERRY)				
200 mg/5 ml, 15 ml	00093-7149-23	35.02		AB
(USP,CHERRY)				
200 mg/5 ml, 15 ml	50111-0791-20	34.88		AB
(1X22.5ML, USP,CHERRY)				
200 mg/5 ml, 22.5 ml	00093-7149-94	35.02		AB
(USP,CHERRY)				
200 mg/5 ml, 22.5 ml	50111-0767-28	34.88		AB
(1X30ML, USP,CHERRY)				
200 mg/5 ml, 30 ml	00093-7149-31	35.02		AB
(USP,CHERRY)				
200 mg/5 ml, 30 ml	50111-0792-22	34.88		AB
PDS, IV (PHARMACY BULK PKG)				
2.5 gm, ea	00703-9089-01	102.02		
(USP)				
500 mg, 10s ea	50111-0794-78	206.25		AP
TAB, PO (FILM-COATED)				
250 mg, 6s ea	00093-7146-18	46.70		AB
(3X6,FILM-COATED)				
250 mg, 18s ea	00093-7146-09	140.10		AB
(6X3,FILM-COATED)				
250 mg, 18s ea	50111-0787-66	139.99		AB
(FILM-COATED)				
250 mg, 30s ea	00093-7146-56	233.33		AB
500 mg, 3s ea	00093-7169-33	46.70		AB
(3X3,FILM-COATED)				
500 mg, 9s ea	00093-7169-90	140.10		AB
9s ea	50111-0788-67	139.99		AB
(FILM-COATED)				
500 mg, 30s ea	00093-7169-56	467.02		AB
30s ea	50111-0788-10	466.66		AB
600 mg, 30s ea	00093-7147-56	560.46		AB
30s ea	50111-0789-10	560.02		AB
(UDL)				
TAB, PO (10X10,FILM-COATED)				
250 mg, 100s ea UD	51079-0591-20	777.60		AB
(Wockhardt USA)				
TAB, PO (FILM-COATED)				
250 mg, 6s ea	64679-0961-04	46.62		AB
(3X6,FILM-COATED)				
250 mg, 18s ea	64679-0961-05	139.87		AB
(FILM-COATED)				
250 mg, 30s ea	64679-0961-01	233.15		AB
(FILM COATED)				
500 mg, 3s ea	64679-0964-03	46.62		AB
(3X3,FILM COATED)				
500 mg, 9s ea	64679-0964-05	139.87		AB
(FILM COATED)				
500 mg, 30s ea	64679-0964-01	466.28		AB
600 mg, 30s ea	64679-0962-01	559.80		AB
(A-S Medication)				
REPACK				
PDR, PO, 1 gm/packet, ea	54569-5806-00	24.15		
(CHERRY)				
100 mg/5 ml, 15 ml	54569-5807-00	34.43		
200 mg/5 ml, 15 ml	54569-5808-00	34.43		
22.5 ml	54569-5809-00	34.43		
30 ml	54569-5810-00	34.43		
TAB, PO (FILM-COATED)				
250 mg, 4s ea	54569-5754-00	31.10		
6s ea	54569-5755-00	46.68		
500 mg, 3s ea	54569-5756-00	46.68		
600 mg, 8s ea	54569-5804-00	149.40		
(Aidarex)				
REPACK				
TAB, PO (FILM-COATED)				
250 mg, 6s ea	33261-0139-06	63.00		AB
500 mg, 6s ea	33261-0402-06	127.26		AB
7s ea	33261-0402-07	148.47		AB
10s ea	33261-0402-10	212.10		AB
12s ea	33261-0402-12	254.52		AB
14s ea	33261-0402-14	296.94		AB
20s ea	33261-0402-20	424.20		AB
28s ea	33261-0402-28	593.88		AB
30s ea	33261-0402-30	636.30		AB
(Altura)				
REPACK				
TAB, PO (3X6,FILM-COATED)				
250 mg, 18s ea	63874-1197-06	72.67		AB
(American Health)				
REPACK				
TAB, PO (10X10,FILM-COATED)				
250 mg, 100s ea UD	68084-0278-01	716.91		AB
(3X10,FILM COATED)				
500 mg, 30s ea UD	68084-0279-21	612.86		AB
(AQ)				
REPACK				
TAB, PO, 250 mg, 10s ea	66105-0670-01	87.61		
18s ea	66105-0670-18	156.07		
30s ea	66105-0670-03	258.86		
50s ea	66105-0670-05	430.06		
60s ea	66105-0670-06	515.72		
500 mg, 9s ea	66105-0653-19	139.95		
10s ea	66105-0653-01	155.50		
30s ea	66105-0653-03	513.15		
50s ea	66105-0653-05	777.50		
60s ea	66105-0653-06	933.00		
(Core)				
REPACK				
TAB, PO, 250 mg, 6s ea	33358-0040-06	62.41		
500 mg, 10s ea	33358-0041-10	160.28		
(DHS, Inc.)				
REPACK				
PDR, PO (1X15ML,CHERRY)				
100 mg/5 ml, 15 ml	55887-0033-15	34.00		AB
200 mg/5 ml, 30 ml	55887-0311-30	138.00		
TAB, PO, 250 mg, 6s ea	55887-0785-06	49.00		
(Dispensing Solutions)				
REPACK				
PDR, PO, 100 mg/5 ml, 15 ml	55045-3725-01	35.00		
200 mg/5 ml, 15 ml	55045-3727-01	35.00		
22.5 ml	55045-3726-02	35.00		
30 ml	55045-3698-03	35.00		
TAB, PO, 250 mg, 6s ea	55045-3442-06	47.10		
500 mg, 3s ea	55045-3693-01	47.10		
(FILM COATED)				
500 mg, 3s ea	68258-3012-01	55.94		AB
5s ea	66336-0400-05	91.50		
(IPI)				
REPACK				
TAB, PO (FILM-COATED)				
250 mg, 6s ea	18837-0338-06	46.66		AB
(Keltman Pharma., Inc.)				
REPACK				
TAB, PO, 250 mg, 6s ea	68387-0565-06	84.59		
(Nucare Pharm)				
REPACK				
TAB, PO (FILM-COATED)				
250 mg, 6s ea	68071-1323-06	46.70		AB
(Palmetto)				
REPACK				
PDR, PO (1X15ML)				
100 mg/5 ml, 15 ml	23490-6904-01	95.92		
TAB, PO, 250 mg, 4s ea	23490-7760-01	31.60		
6s ea	23490-7760-02	47.40		
500 mg, 3s ea	23490-7758-01	82.50		
(PD-Rx Pharm)				
REPACK				
TAB, PO (FILM-COATED)				
250 mg, 2s ea	43063-0090-02	41.19		AB
4s ea	55289-0964-04	106.47		
14s ea	55289-0964-14	196.63		
500 mg, 2s ea	55289-0274-02	70.47		
(FILM-COATED)				
500 mg, 3s ea	55289-0274-03	70.47		AB
(Pharma Pac)				
REPACK				
PDR, PO (1X30ML,CHERRY)				
200 mg/5 ml, 30 ml	52959-0932-30	39.81		AB
TAB, PO, 250 mg, 6s ea	52959-0838-06	49.70		
(FILM-COATED)				
500 mg, 3s ea	52959-0927-03	78.52		AB
(Phys Total Care)				
REPACK				
PDR, PO, 1 gm/packet, 3s ea	54868-5938-00	180.56		
100 mg/5 ml, 15 ml	54868-5647-00	63.12		
200 mg/5 ml, 15 ml	54868-5648-02	68.22		
23 ml	54868-5648-01	68.22		
30 ml	54868-5648-00	68.22		
TAB, PO, 250 mg, 6s ea	54868-5478-00	61.02		
(PAK)				
250 mg, 6s ea	54868-5471-00	55.20		
10s ea	54868-5478-02	98.70		
30s ea	54868-5478-01	269.88		
(TRI-PACK)				
500 mg, 3s ea	54868-3648-00	55.20		
6s ea	54868-5487-00	126.15		
60s ea	54868-5487-01	1116.24		
(Physician Partner)				
REPACK				
PDR, PO (1X15ML,CHERRY)				
100 mg/5 ml, 15 ml	21695-0548-15	65.86		AB
200 mg/5 ml, 15 ml	21695-0549-15	65.86		AB
(1X30ML,CHERRY)				
200 mg/5 ml, 30 ml	21695-0549-30	69.76		AB
TAB, PO, 250 mg, 6s ea	21695-0012-06	93.40		
(FILM-COATED)				
500 mg, 3s ea	21695-0013-03	93.40		AB
(Quality Care Prod)				
REPACK				
PDR, PO (1X1GM)				
1 gm/packet, 1 gm	35356-0487-01	126.64		
100 mg/5 ml, 15 ml	35356-0044-15	40.00		
(1X15ML,CHERRY)				
200 mg/5 ml, 15 ml	35356-0199-15	79.00		AB
(CHERRY)				
200 mg/5 ml, 30 ml	35356-0199-30	312.00		AB
TAB, PO, 250 mg, 6s ea	49999-0786-06	90.08		
500 mg, 3s ea	35356-0017-03	167.97		
(Southwood)				
REPACK				
TAB, PO, 250 mg, 6s ea	58016-4814-01	46.67		
30s ea	58016-0086-30	70.00		
60s ea	58016-0086-60	140.00		
90s ea	58016-0086-90	210.00		
100s ea	58016-0086-00	233.33		
(Stat Rx)				
REPACK				
TAB, PO (FILM-COATED)				
500 mg, 3s ea	16590-0383-03	49.25		AB
(Vibranta)				
REPACK				
TAB, PO, 250 mg, 6s ea	57866-4356-01	90.08		
500 mg, 3s ea	57866-3136-01	89.90		
AZITHROMYCIN DIHYDRATE (Letco)				
azithromycin				
POW, NA (1X100GM,USP)				
100 gm	62991-2577-02	465.00		
(1X500GM,USP)				
500 gm	62991-2577-03	1800.00		
(1X1000GM,USP)				
1000 gm	62991-2577-01	2550.00		

PROD/MFR	NDC	AWP	DP	OBC
(B&B Pharm, Inc)				
REPACK				
POW, NA (1X5GM, USP)				
5 gm	63275-9965-02	195.00		
(1X10GM, USP)				
10 gm	63275-9965-03	351.00		
(1X25GM, USP)				
25 gm	63275-9965-04	780.00		
(1X100GM, USP)				
100 gm	63275-9965-05	2730.00		
(Palmetto)				
REPACK				
PDR, PO, 200 mg/5 ml,				
15 ml	23490-6905-00	43.82		
22.5 ml	23490-6905-01	43.82		
30 ml	23490-6905-02	43.82		
(PD-Rx Pharm)				
REPACK				
TAB, PO, 250 mg, 6s ea	58864-0791-06	126.29		
AZMACORT (Altura)				
REPACK				
triamcinolone acetonide				
ARO, IH, 100 mcg/actuation,				
20 gm	63874-0714-20	100.05		
(Palmetto)				
REPACK				
ARO, IH (1X20GM)				
100 mcg/actuation,				
20 gm	23490-9405-00	175.00		
(Pharma Pac)				
REPACK				
ARO, IH, 100 mcg/actuation,				
20 gm	52959-0286-03	63.12		
(Stat Rx)				
REPACK				
ARO, IH, 100 mcg/actuation,				
20 gm	16590-0025-20	169.78		
AZOPT (Alcon Ophthalmic)				
brinzolamide				
SUS, OP (DROP-TAINER)				
1%, 10 ml	00065-0275-10	104.64		
15 ml	00065-0275-15	156.84		
(Phys Total Care)				
REPACK				
SUS, OP, 1%, 5 ml	54868-4281-01	38.24		
15 ml	54868-4281-00	115.07		
AZOR (Daiichi Sankyo)				
amlodipine besylate/olmesartan medoxomil				
TAB, PO, 5 mg-20 mg,				
30s ea	65597-0110-30	101.88		
90s ea	65597-0110-90	305.64		
(10X10)				
5 mg-20 mg,				
100s ea UD	65597-0110-10	294.00		
5 mg-40 mg, 30s ea	65597-0112-30	128.88		
90s ea	65597-0112-90	386.64		
(10X10)				
5 mg-40 mg,				
100s ea UD	65597-0112-10	369.60		
10 mg-20 mg,				
30s ea	65597-0111-30	101.88		
90s ea	65597-0111-90	305.64		
(10X10)				
10 mg-20 mg,				
100s ea UD	65597-0111-10	332.40		
10 mg-40 mg,				
30s ea	65597-0113-30	128.88		
90s ea	65597-0113-90	386.64		
(10X10)				
10 mg-40 mg,				
100s ea UD	65597-0113-10	421.20		
(Phys Total Care)				
REPACK				
TAB, PO, 5 mg-20 mg,				
30s ea	54868-6036-00	112.52		
AZTREONAM (APP)				
PDS, IJ (SDV,USP,SODIUM-FREE)				
1 gm, 10s ea	63323-0401-20	395.40		
2 gm, 10s ea	63323-0402-20	803.40		
(Elan Pharmaceuticals) *See AZACTAM*				
(Gilead Sciences) *See CAYSTON*				
AZULFIDINE (Pfizer)				
sulfasalazine				
TAB, PO, 500 mg, 100s ea	00013-0101-01	57.76	48.13	AB
300s ea	00013-0101-20	173.29	144.41	AB
(Phys Total Care)				
REPACK				
TAB, PO, 500 mg, 100s ea	54868-1123-01	51.51		AB
AZULFIDINE ENTABS (Pfizer)				
sulfasalazine				
ECT, PO (CAPLET)				
500 mg, 100s ea	00013-0102-01	69.22	57.68	AB
300s ea	00013-0102-20	207.62	173.02	AB
AZURETTE (Watson)				
desogestrel/ethinyl estradiol				
TAB, PO (6X28)				
168s ea	52544-0940-28	310.84		
B-COMPLEX (Merit)				
dexpanthenol/niacinamide/vit b1/vit b2/vit b6				
SOL, IJ, 30 ml	30727-0300-80	50.90	25.45	
B-COMPLEX PLUS (A-S Medication)				
REPACK				
multivitamin and minerals				
TAB, PO, 100s ea	54569-2739-00	37.77		
B-D ALLERGIST TRAY (BD Dickinson Hosp Prod)				
syringe, allergy				
DEV, NA (26GX1/2,1CC,INTRADERMAL)				
25s ea	82903-0055-38	2.48		
(26GX1/2,1CC,REG. BEVEL)				
25s ea	82903-0055-37	2.48		
(26GX3/8,1CC,INTRADERMAL)				
25s ea	82903-0055-39	2.48		
(27GX1/2,1/2CC,REG BEVEL)				
25s ea	82903-0055-35	2.48		
(27GX1/2,1CC,REG. BEVEL)				
25s ea	82903-0055-40	2.48		
(27GX3/8,1/2CC)				
25s ea	82903-0055-36	2.48		
(27GX3/8,1CC,INTRADERMAL)				
25s ea	82903-0055-41	2.48		
(27GX3/8,1CC,REG. BEVEL)				
25s ea	82903-0055-42	2.48		
B-D ALLERGY SYRINGE (BD Dickinson Hosp Prod)				
syringe, allergy				
DEV, NA (28GX1/2, 1CC)				
100s ea	08290-3055-00	19.58		
B-D BLUNT FILL NEEDLE (BD Dickinson Hosp Prod)				
needle and/or syringe supplies				
DEV, NA (18GX11/2" W/FILTER)				
100s ea	08290-3052-11	35.51		
(18GX11/2",18GX11/2")				
100s ea	08290-3051-80	20.15		
B-D BULK NEEDLES REGULAR BEVEL				
(BD Dickinson Hosp Prod)				
needle, hypodermic				
DEV, NA (18GX1-1/2, NON-STERILE)				
5000s ea	08290-3030-05	300.00		
(19GX1-1/2, NON-STERILE)				
5000s ea	08290-3030-06	300.00		
(20GX1-1/2, NON-STERILE)				
5000s ea	08290-3030-07	300.00		
(21GX1-1/2, NON-STERILE)				
5000s ea	08290-3030-08	300.00		
(22GX1-1/2, NON-STERILE)				
5000s ea	08290-3030-09	300.00		
(23GX1, NON-STERILE)				
5000s ea	08290-3030-11	300.00		
(25GX1, NON-STERILE)				
5000s ea	08290-3030-12	300.00		
(25GX5/8, NON-STERILE)				
5000s ea	08290-3030-10	300.00		
B-D BULK NEEDLES SHORT BEVEL				
(BD Dickinson Hosp Prod)				
needle, hypodermic				
DEV, NA (18GX1-1/2, NON-STERILE)				
5000s ea	08290-3030-13	300.00		
(22GX1-1/2, NON-STERILE)				
5000s ea	08290-3030-15	300.00		
B-D BULK SYRINGES CATHETER TIP				
(BD Dickinson Hosp Prod)				
syringe and needle				
DEV, NA (2 OZ., NON-STERILE)				
125s ea	08290-3010-37	122.40		
B-D BULK SYRINGES LUER-LOK TIP				
(BD Dickinson Hosp Prod)				
syringe and needle				
DEV, NA (60CC, NON-STERILE)				
125s ea	08290-3010-35	122.40		
(30CC, NON-STERILE)				
225s ea	08290-3010-33	137.25		
(20CC, NON-STERILE)				
325s ea	08290-3010-31	165.75		
(10CC, NON-STERILE)				
850s ea	08290-3010-29	148.58		
(5CC, NON-STERILE)				
1400s ea	08290-3010-27	196.85		
B-D BULK SYRINGES SLIP TIP				
(BD Dickinson Hosp Prod)				
syringe and needle				
DEV, NA (60CC, NON-STERILE)				
125s ea	08290-3010-36	122.40		
(30CC, NON-STERILE)				
225s ea	08290-3010-34	137.25		
(20CC, NON-STERILE)				
325s ea	08290-3010-32	165.75		
(10CC, NON-STERILE)				
850s ea	08290-3010-30	148.58		
(5CC, NON-STERILE)				
1400s ea	08290-3010-28	196.85		
(1CC, NON-STERILE)				
3000s ea	08290-3010-25	246.90		
B-D CORNWALL FLUID DISPENSING				
(BD Dickinson Hosp Prod)				
syringe and needle				
DEV, NA (10CC)				
10s ea	08290-3052-24	101.40		
B-D FILTER NEEDLES (BD Dickinson Hosp Prod)				
needle				
DEV, NA (18GX1-1/2, THIN WALL)				
100s ea	08290-3052-01	32.87		
(19GX1-1/2, THIN WALL)				
100s ea	08290-3052-00	29.25		
B-D INSULIN LO-DOSE BLISTER PACKAGE				
(BD Dickinson Hosp Prod)				
insulin syringe/needle				
DEV, NA (28GX1/2,1/2CC,U100)				
100s ea	08290-3294-61	25.12		
B-D INSULIN SYRINGE BLISTER PACKAGE				
(BD Dickinson Hosp Prod)				
insulin syringe/needle				
DEV, NA (28GX1/2,1CC,U100)				
100s ea	08290-3294-20	25.12		
100s ea	08290-3294-24	25.12		
B-D INSULIN SYRINGE SELF-CONTAINED				
(BD Dickinson Hosp Prod)				
insulin syringe/needle				
DEV, NA (27GX5/8,1CC,U100)				
100s ea	08290-3294-12	25.12		
B-D INSULIN W/DETACHABLE NEEDLE				
(BD Dickinson Hosp Prod)				
insulin syringe/needle				
DEV, NA (25GX1,1CC,U100)				
100s ea	08290-3296-22	28.41		
(25GX5/8,1CC,U100)				
100s ea	08290-3296-51	28.41		
(26GX1/2,1CC,U100)				
100s ea	08290-3296-52	28.41		
B-D INTEGRA SYRINGE (BD Dickinson Hosp Prod)				
needle and/or syringe supplies				
DEV, NA (23GX1"3CCDETACHABLE NDL)				
100s ea	08290-3052-71	54.63		
(25GX5/8",3CC)				
100s ea	08290-3052-69	54.63		
B-D LAB SYRINGE ECCENTRIC TIP				
(BD Dickinson Hosp Prod)				
syringe and needle				
DEV, NA (10CC, NON-STERILE)				
100s ea	08290-3054-62	15.65		
B-D LO-DOSE MICRO-FINE IV				
(BD Dickinson Hosp Prod)				
insulin syringe/needle				
DEV, NA (28G,1/2ML,1/2",U100)				
100s ea	08290-3294-65	25.12		
B-D NEEDLES (BD Dickinson Hosp Prod)				
needle, hypodermic				
DEV, NA (26GX3/8,INTRADERMAL BVL)				
100s ea	08290-3051-10	8.13		
(27GX1/2)				
100s ea	08290-3051-09	8.13		
B-D NEEDLES REGULAR BEVEL				
(BD Dickinson Hosp Prod)				
needle, hypodermic				
DEV, NA (18G,FILL,1-1/2)				
100s ea	08290-3051-85	8.78		
(18GX1-1/2)				
100s ea	08290-3051-96	8.05		
(18GX1)				
100s ea	08290-3051-95	8.05		

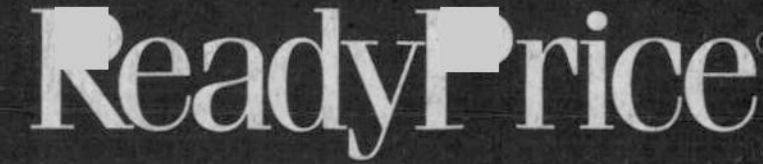

PROD/MFR	NDC	AWP	DP	OBC
(19GX1-1/2, THIN WAL)				
100s ea	08290-3051-87	8.05		
(19GX1, THIN WALL)				
100s ea	08290-3051-86	8.05		
(20GX1-1/2)				
100s ea	08290-3051-76	8.05		
(20GX1)				
100s ea	08290-3051-75	8.05		
(21G, I.V., 1-1/2)				
100s ea	08290-3051-90	8.87		
(21G, I.V.1, THIN WALL)				
100s ea	08290-3051-77	8.78		
(21GX1-1/2)				
100s ea	08290-3051-67	8.13		
(21GX1)				
100s ea	08290-3051-65	8.13		
(22GX1-1/2)				
100s ea	08290-3051-56	8.13		
(22GX1)				
100s ea	08290-3051-55	8.13		
(23G, IM, 1, THIN WALL)				
100s ea	08290-3051-93	8.87		
(23G,IM,1-1/2,THIN WALL)				
100s ea	08290-3051-94	8.87		
(23GX1)				
100s ea	08290-3051-45	8.13		
(23GX3/4)				
100s ea	08290-3051-43	8.13		
(25GX1-1/2)				
100s ea	08290-3051-27	8.13		
(25GX1)				
100s ea	08290-3051-25	8.13		
(25GX5/8)				
100s ea	08290-3051-22	8.13		
(26GX1/2)				
100s ea	08290-3051-11	8.13		
B-D NEEDLES SHORT BEVEL (BD Dickinson Hosp Prod)				
needle, hypodermic				
DEV, NA (18GX1-1/2)				
100s ea	08290-3051-99	8.05		
(19GX1-1/2, THIN WALL)				
100s ea	08290-3051-89	8.05		
(19GX1, THIN WALL)				
100s ea	08290-3051-88	8.05		
(20GX1-1/2)				
100s ea	08290-3051-79	8.05		
(20GX1)				
100s ea	08290-3051-78	8.05		
(22GX1-1/2)				
100s ea	08290-3051-59	8.13		
B-D NOKOR ADMIX NEEDLES				
(BD Dickinson Hosp Prod)				
needle				
DEV, NA (16GX1, THIN WALL)				
100s ea	08290-3052-16	19.09		
(18GX1-1/2, THIN WALL)				
100s ea	08290-3052-15	13.03		
B-D NOKOR VENTED NEEDLE				
(BD Dickinson Hosp Prod)				
needle				
DEV, NA (16GX1, THIN WALL)				
100s ea	08290-3052-13	39.50		
(18GX1, THIN WALL)				
100s ea	08290-3052-14	33.80		
B-D SAFETY GLIDE (BD Consumer)				
syringe and needle				
DEV, NA (26GX3/8",1CC,TRAY)				
25s ea	08290-3059-51	9.67		
(23GX1,3CC)				
50s ea	08290-3059-05	21.94		
(BD Consumer)				
insulin syringe/needle				
(29GX1/2",1/2CC)				
100s ea	08290-3059-32	47.35		
(29GX1/2",1CC)				
100s ea	08290-3059-30	47.35		
(29GX1/2",3/10CC)				
100s ea	08290-3059-35	47.35		
B-D SAFETY GLIDE TB (BD Consumer)				
syringe and needle				
DEV, NA (27GX1/2,1CC)				
100s ea	08290-3059-45	47.35		
(29GX1/2",0.5CC)				
100s ea	08290-5932-01	40.00		
B-D SAFETY-LOK W/ATTACHED NEEDLE				
(BD Dickinson Hosp Prod)				
syringe and needle				
DEV, NA (25GX5/8,1CC,TUBERCULIN)				
100s ea	08290-3055-54	38.41		

PROD/MFR	NDC	AWP	DP	OBC
(BD Dickinson Hosp Prod)				
insulin syringe/needle				
(29GX1/2, 1CC)				
100s ea	08290-3294-64	35.22		
B-D SPECIALTY USE NEEDLES				
(BD Dickinson Hosp Prod)				
needle, hypodermic				
DEV, NA (16GX1-1/2)				
100s ea	08290-3051-98	20.79		
(16GX1)				
100s ea	08290-3051-97	20.79		
(21GX2)				
100s ea	08290-3051-29	20.99		
(23GX1-1/4)				
100s ea	08290-3051-20	9.16		
(25GX7/8)				
100s ea	08290-3051-24	9.16		
(27GX1-1/4)				
100s ea	08290-3051-36	11.76		
(30GX1)				
100s ea	08290-3051-28	26.57		
(30GX1/2)				
100s ea	08290-3051-06	26.57		
B-D SYRINGE CONVENIENCE PAK TRAY				
(BD Dickinson Hosp Prod)				
syringe and needle				
DEV, NA (20CC, LUER-LOK TIP)				
10s ea	82903-0056-17	5.30		
(30CC, LUER-LOK TIP)				
10s ea	82903-0056-18	7.30		
(10CC, LUER-LOK TIP)				
20s ea	82903-0096-05	3.63		
(60CC, LUER-LOK TIP)				
20s ea	82903-0096-80	18.40		
(1ML,STERILE ,SLIP TIP)				
25s ea	82903-0097-01	3.65		
(3ML,STERILE,LUER-LOKTIP)				
25s ea	82903-0097-02	2.63		
(5ML,STERILE,LUER-LOKTIP)				
25s ea	82903-0097-03	5.03		
B-D SYRINGE ECCENTRIC TIP				
(BD Dickinson Hosp Prod)				
insulin syringe/needle				
DEV, NA (10CC)				
100s ea	08290-3054-82	18.45		
B-D SYRINGE LUER-LOK (BD Consumer)				
insulin syringe/needle				
DEV, NA (1CC)				
100s ea	08290-3096-28	49.80		
B-D SYRINGE LUER-LOK TIP (BD Dickinson Hosp Prod)				
syringe and needle				
DEV, NA (10CC)				
25s ea	08290-3096-95	31.50		
(20CC)				
40s ea	08290-3096-61	20.16		
(30CC)				
40s ea	08290-3096-50	23.80		
(10CC)				
100s ea	08290-3096-04	18.16		
(3CC)				
100s ea	08290-3095-85	8.92		
(5CC)				
100s ea	08290-3096-03	16.81		
B-D SYRINGE SLIP TIP (BD Dickinson Hosp Prod)				
syringe and needle				
DEV, NA (20CC)				
40s ea	08290-3016-25	20.00		
(10CC)				
100s ea	08290-3016-04	18.16		
(3CC)				
100s ea	08290-3095-86	8.92		
(5CC)				
100s ea	08290-3016-03	16.81		
B-D SYRINGE W/BLUNT FILL NEEDLE				
(BD Dickinson Hosp Prod)				
needle and/or syringe supplies				
DEV, NA (18GX11/2,3ML,LUER-LOK)				
100s ea	08290-3050-60	20.25		
(18GX11/2",10ML,LUER-LOK)				
100s ea	08290-3050-64	42.00		
(18GX11/2",5ML,LUER-LOK)				
100s ea	08290-3050-62	39.50		
B-D SYRINGE/NEEDLE COMBO LUER-LOK				
(BD Dickinson Hosp Prod)				
insulin syringe/needle				
DEV, NA (18GX1-1/2, 3CC)				
100s ea	08290-3095-80	13.15		
(20GX1-1/2, 10CC)				
100s ea	08290-3096-45	27.27		

PROD/MFR	NDC	AWP	DP	OBC
(20GX1-1/2, 3CC)				
100s ea	08290-3095-79	13.15		
(20GX1-1/2, 5CC)				
100s ea	08290-3096-35	25.59		
(20GX1, 10CC)				
100s ea	08290-3096-44	27.27		
(20GX1, 3CC)				
100s ea	08290-3095-78	13.15		
100s ea	08290-3096-37	55.55		
(20GX1, 5CC)				
100s ea	08290-3096-34	25.59		
(21G I.V.1,3CC,THIN WALL)				
100s ea	08290-3095-98	13.15		
(21G, I.V., 1-1/2,10CC)				
100s ea	08290-3096-39	27.27		
(21G, I.V.1-1/2, 3CC)				
100s ea	08290-3095-99	13.15		
(21GX1-1/2, 10CC)				
100s ea	08290-3096-43	27.27		
(21GX1-1/2, 3CC)				
100s ea	08290-3095-77	13.15		
(21GX1-1/2, 5CC)				
100s ea	08290-3096-33	25.59		
(21GX1, 10CC)				
100s ea	08290-3096-42	27.27		
(21GX1, 3CC)				
100s ea	08290-3095-75	13.15		
(21GX1, 5CC)				
100s ea	08290-3096-32	25.59		
(22GX1-1/2, 3CC)				
100s ea	08290-3095-74	13.15		
(22GX1-1/2, 5CC)				
100s ea	08290-3096-31	25.59		
(22GX1-1/4, 3CC)				
100s ea	08290-3095-73	13.15		
(22GX1, 3CC)				
100s ea	08290-3095-72	13.15		
(22GX1, 5CC)				
100s ea	08290-3096-30	25.59		
(22GX1,10CC)				
100s ea	08290-3096-40	27.27		
(22GX3/4, 3CC)				
100s ea	08290-3095-69	13.15		
(23G, IM, 1-1/2, 3CC)				
100s ea	08290-3095-89	13.15		
(23G,IM,1,3CC,THIN WALL)				
100s ea	08290-3095-88	13.15		
(23GX1, 3CC)				
100s ea	08290-3095-71	13.15		
(25GX1-1/2, 3CC)				
100s ea	08290-3095-82	13.15		
(25GX1, 3CC)				
100s ea	08290-3095-81	13.15		
(25GX5/8, 3CC)				
100s ea	08290-3095-70	13.15		
(26G,SUB-Q 5/8,THIN WALL)				
100s ea	08290-3095-87	13.15		
B-D TUBERCULIN COMBINATION SLIP TIP				
(BD Dickinson Hosp Prod)				
insulin syringe/needle				
DEV, NA (26GXSUB-Q 5/8,1CC)				
100s ea	08290-3095-97	17.80		
B-D TUBERCULIN SYRINGE (BD Dickinson Hosp Prod)				
insulin syringe/needle				
DEV, NA (1CC, SLIP TIP)				
100s ea	08290-3096-02	12.10		
(27GX1/2,1/2CC,REG BEVEL)				
100s ea	08290-3056-20	19.40		
B-D TUBERCULIN W/DETACHABLE NEEDLE				
(BD Dickinson Hosp Prod)				
insulin syringe/needle				
DEV, NA (21GX1, 1CC, SLIP TIP)				
100s ea	08290-3096-24	17.51		
(25GX5/8,1CC,SLIP TIP)				
100s ea	08290-3096-26	17.51		
(26GX3/8,1CC,SLIP TIP)				
100s ea	08290-3096-25	17.51		
(27GX1/2,1CC,SLIP TIP)				
100s ea	08290-3096-23	17.51		
B-PLEX (Contract Pharmacal)				
vitamin b complex and vitamin c				
TAB, PO, 100s ea	10267-1025-01	10.20		
1000s ea	10267-1025-05	46.30		
B-PLEX PLUS (Contract Pharmacal)				
multivitamin and minerals				
TAB, PO, 100s ea	10267-1027-01	18.30		
500s ea	10267-1027-05	85.10		

PROD/MFR	NDC	AWP	DP	OBC
B-TUSS (Blansett)				
cpm/hydrocod bit/phenyleph hcl				
LIQ, PO (AF,SF,CANDY APPLE)				
480 ml, C-III	51674-0645-07	53.26		
B/CA/FOLIC ACID/MG/VIT B12/VIT B6/VIT D				
(Upsher-Smith) *See FOLGARD OS*				
BAC (IPI)				
REPACK				
acetaminophen/butalbital/caffeine				
TAB, PO, 325 mg-50 mg-40 mg,				
60s ea	18837-0017-60	48.55		
BACI-RX (X-Gen)				
bacitracin				
POW, NA (U.S.P.,5 MMU,MICRONIZED)				
ea	39822-0200-05	355.15		AA
BACIIM (X-Gen)				
bacitracin				
PDS, IM (STERILE)				
50000 u, 10s ea	39822-0277-02	198.00		AP
BACILLUS OF CALMETTE AND GUERIN VACCINE, LIVE				
(Organon) *See BCG VACCINE*				
(Organon) *See TICE BCG*				
(Sanofi) *See THERACYS*				
BACITRACIN (APP)				
PDS, IM (LATEX-FREE)				
50000 u, ea	63323-0329-30	24.95		AP
(Consolidated Midland)				
OIN, OP, 500 u/gm, 3.5 gm	00223-4107-03	1.95		EE
(Fera)				
OIN, OP, 500 u/gm, 3.5 gm	00168-0026-38	57.46		AT
(1X3.5GM,USP)				
500 u/gm, 3.5 gm	48102-0007-35	57.46		AT
(Medisca)				
POW, NA (U.S.P.,MICRONIZED)				
10 gm	38779-0015-01	150.45		EE
25 gm	38779-0015-04	402.90		EE
100 gm	38779-0015-05	1134.75		EE
(Pfizer) *See AMERINET CHOICE BACITRACIN*				
(Pfizer)				
PDS, IM, 50000 u, ea	00009-0233-01	13.31	11.09	AP
(Spectrum Pharmacy)				
POW, NA (MICRNZD, U.S.P./5MU)				
ea	49452-0800-01	2247.00		EE
(U.S.P. STERILE)				
1 gm	49452-0801-01	190.75		EE
(X-Gen) *See BACI-RX*				
(X-Gen) *See BACIIM*				
(X-Gen) *See NOVAPLUS BACIIM*				
(Altura)				
REPACK				
OIN, OP, 500 u/gm, 3.5 gm	63874-0033-04	9.05		EE
3.5 gm	63874-0149-04	9.81		EE
(Dispensing Solutions)				
REPACK				
OIN, OP, 500 u/gm, 3.5 gm	55045-1700-09	7.00		AT
PDS, IM, 50000 u, ea	55045-3773-05	18.00		
(Nucare Pharm)				
REPACK				
OIN, OP, 500 u/gm, 3.5 gm	66267-0987-35	14.62		EE
BACITRACIN (Palmetto)				
REPACK				
OIN, OP (1X3.5GM)				
500 u/gm, 3.5 gm	23490-7651-00	13.54		
BACITRACIN (Pharma Pac)				
REPACK				
OIN, OP, 500 u/gm, 3.5 gm	52959-0228-03	11.96		EE
(Phys Total Care)				
REPACK				
OIN, OP, 500 u/gm, 3.5 gm	54868-0649-01	9.45		EE
(Physician Partner)				
REPACK				
OIN, TP, 500 u/gm, 14 gm	21695-0347-15	12.96		
(Southwood)				
REPACK				
OIN, OP, 500 u/gm, 3.5 gm	58016-6004-01	10.40		EE
BACITRACIN METHYLENE DISALICYLATE				
(PCCA) *See BACITRACIN METHYLENE DISALICYLATE-FEED GRADE*				
BACITRACIN METHYLENE DISALICYLATE-FEED GRADE (PCCA)				
bacitracin methylene disalicylate				
GRA, NA (1X1GM)				
1 gm	51927-2292-00	0.06		
BACITRACIN MICRONIZED (PCCA)				
bacitracin, micronized				
POW, NA (USP,NONSTERILE)				
1 gm	51927-1669-00	16.80		
BACITRACIN ZINC (Medisca)				
POW, NA (USP,68 U/MG,MICRONIZED)				
5 gm	38779-1763-03	67.50		
10 gm	38779-1763-01	111.00		
(USP,73U/MG,1X10GM)				
10 gm	38779-2264-01	375.00		
(USP,68 U/MG,MICRONIZED)				
25 gm	38779-1763-04	243.00		
BACITRACIN ZINC & POLYMYXIN B SULFATE (Dispensing Solutions)				
REPACK				
bacitracin zinc/polymyxin b sulfate				
OIN, OP, 500 u/gm-10000 u/gm,				
3.5 gm	55045-1388-09	25.00		
BACITRACIN ZINC MICRONIZED (PCCA)				
bacitracin zinc, micronized				
POW, NA (USP; NONSTERILE)				
1 gm	51927-1176-00	37.20		
BACITRACIN ZINC, MICRONIZED				
(PCCA) *See BACITRACIN ZINC MICRONIZED*				
BACITRACIN ZINC/NEOMYCIN/ POLYMYXIN B SULFATE				
(Bausch & Lomb Inc.) *See BACITRACIN/NEOMYCIN/POLYMYXIN*				
(Consolidated Midland) *See BACITRACIN-NEO-POLY*				
(Truxton) *See TRIPLE ANTIBIOTIC*				
(Palmetto)				
REPACK				
OIN, OP, 3.5 gm	23490-5974-01	17.63		
15 gm	23490-5974-04	25.00		
BACITRACIN ZINC/POLYMYXIN B SULFATE				
(Akorn) *See AK-POLY-BAC*				
(Bausch & Lomb Inc.)				
OIN, OP, 500 u/gm-10000 u/gm,				
3.5 gm	24208-0555-55	28.65		AT
(Ocusoft) *See POLYCIN-B*				
(A-S Medication)				
REPACK				
OIN, OP, 500 u/gm-10000 u/gm,				
3.5 gm	54569-3570-00	25.77		AT
(Dispensing Solutions)				
REPACK				
OIN, TP, 500 u/gm-10000 u/gm,				
15 gm	55045-2199-05	5.99		
30 gm	55045-2199-08	8.99		
(Nucare Pharm)				
REPACK				
OIN, OP, 500 u/gm-10000 u/gm,				
3.5 gm	66267-0925-35	21.22		EE
(Phys Total Care)				
REPACK				
OIN, OP, 500 u/gm-10000 u/gm,				
4 gm	54868-1199-00	22.62		EE
(Physician Partner)				
REPACK				
OIN, OP (PF)				
500 u/gm-10000 u/gm,				
3.5 gm	21695-0156-35	51.40		
(Quality Care Prod)				
REPACK				
OIN, OP, 500 u/gm-10000 u/gm,				
3.5 gm	49999-0406-35	30.92		AT
(Southwood)				
REPACK				
OIN, OP, 500 u/gm-10000 u/gm,				
3.5 gm	58016-5556-01	28.00		EE
BACITRACIN ZN/HC/NEOMYCIN SULF/ POLYMYXIN B SULF				
(Bausch & Lomb Inc.) *See BACITRACIN/HC/NEOMYCIN/POLYMYXIN*				
(Consolidated Midland) *See HC W/BACITRACIN-NEOMYCIN-POLYMYXIN*				
(Monarch) *See CORTISPORIN*				
(Truxton) *See TRIPLE ANTIBIOTIC W/HYDROCORTISONE*				
BACITRACIN ZN/NEOMYCIN/POLYMYXIN B SULFATE (Pharma Pac)				
REPACK				
bacitracin zinc/neomycin/polymyxin b sulfate				
OIN, OP, 3.5 gm	52959-0239-00	15.99		EE
3.5 gm	52959-0239-03	15.99		EE
(Phys Total Care)				
REPACK				
OIN, OP, 3.5 gm	54868-2971-01	7.36		EE
BACITRACIN-NEO-POLY (Consolidated Midland)				
bacitracin zinc/neomycin/polymyxin b sulfate				
OIN, OP, 3.5 gm	00223-4109-03	2.75		EE
BACITRACIN, MICRONIZED				
(PCCA) *See BACITRACIN MICRONIZED*				
BACITRACIN/HC/NEOMYCIN/POLYMYXIN (Bausch & Lomb Inc.)				
bacitracin zn/hc/neomycin sulf/polymyxin b sulf				
OIN, OP, 3.5 gm	24208-0785-55	50.04		AT
(A-S Medication)				
REPACK				
OIN, OP, 3.5 gm	54569-5389-00	27.41		AT
(Altura)				
REPACK				
OIN, OP, 3.5 gm	63874-0140-04	17.33		
(Dispensing Solutions)				
REPACK				
OIN, OP, 3.5 gm	55045-1184-09	16.00		AT
(Pharma Pac)				
REPACK				
OIN, OP, 3.5 gm	52959-0238-03	8.77		EE
(Physician Partner)				
REPACK				
OIN, OP (1X3.5GM)				
3.5 gm	21695-0736-35	32.66		AT
(Quality Care Prod)				
REPACK				
OIN, OP, 3.5 gm	49999-0653-35	37.20		AT
(Southwood)				
REPACK				
OIN, OP, 3.5 gm	58016-6015-01	31.00		EE
BACITRACIN/NEOMYCIN/POLYMYXIN (Bausch & Lomb Inc.)				
bacitracin zinc/neomycin/polymyxin b sulfate				
OIN, OP, 3.5 gm	24208-0780-55	43.81		AT
(A-S Medication)				
REPACK				
OIN, OP, 3.5 gm	54569-2391-00	33.70		AT
(DHS, Inc.)				
REPACK				
OIN, OP, 3.5 gm	55887-0740-35	37.02		AT
(Dispensing Solutions)				
REPACK				
OIN, OP, 3.5 gm	55045-1183-09	27.55		AT
BACKPRIN (Hart Health)				
acetaminophen/caffeine/magnesium salicylate				
TAB, PO (50X2,SF)				
250 mg-50 mg-290 mg,				
100s ea UD	50332-0120-04	9.86		
(125X2,SF)				
250 mg-50 mg-290 mg,				
250s ea UD	50332-0120-07	22.77		
BACLOFEN				
FUL				
TAB, PO, 10 mg, 100s ea		5.25		
20 mg, 100s ea		8.93		
(Caraco)				
TAB, PO (USP)				
10 mg, 100s ea	57664-0291-88	59.60		AB
500s ea	57664-0291-13	298.00		AB
1000s ea	57664-0291-18	596.00		AB
20 mg, 100s ea	57664-0292-88	109.60		AB
500s ea	57664-0292-13	548.00		AB
1000s ea	57664-0292-18	1096.00		AB
(Gallipot)				
POW, NA (1X5GM)				
5 gm	51552-0613-02	32.20	23.00	
(1X25GM)				
25 gm	51552-0613-04	126.00	90.00	
(1X100GM)				
100 gm	51552-0613-05	448.00	320.00	

PROD/MFR	NDC	AWP	DP	OBC
(Hawkins)				
POW, NA (U.S.P.)				
5 gm	**63370-0026-15**	110.40		
25 gm	**63370-0026-25**	432.00		
100 gm	**63370-0026-35**	1584.00		
500 gm	**63370-0026-45**	6240.00		
(Lannett)				
TAB, PO (USP)				
10 mg, 100s ea	**00527-1330-01**	4.20		AB
500s ea	**00527-1330-05**	38.40		AB
1000s ea	**00527-1330-10**	72.00		AB
20 mg, 100s ea (USP)	**00527-1337-01**	7.14		AB
20 mg, 500s ea	**00527-1337-05**	72.00		AB
(Letco)				
POW, NA (U.S.P.)				
5 gm	**62991-1013-01**	60.00		
25 gm	**62991-1013-02**	240.00		
100 gm (U.S.P.)	**62991-1013-03**	855.00		
500 gm	**62991-1013-04**	3900.00		
(Major)				
TAB, PO (10X10)				
10 mg, 100s ea UD	**00904-3365-61**	43.27		AB
20 mg, 100s ea UD	**00904-5222-61**	108.52		AB
(Medisca)				
POW, NA (U.S.P.)				
5 gm	**38779-0388-03**	70.50		
25 gm	**38779-0388-04**	276.00		
100 gm (USP,1X500GM)	**38779-0388-05**	897.00		
500 gm (U.S.P.)	**38779-0388-08**	3525.00		
1000 gm	**38779-0388-09**	5475.00		
(Medtronic Neurologic) *See LIORESAL INTRATHECAL REFILL KIT*				
(Medtronic Neurologic) *See LIORESAL INTRATHECAL SCREENING KIT*				
(Mylan)				
TAB, PO (USP)				
10 mg, 100s ea	**00378-6010-01**	59.65		AB
500s ea	**00378-6010-05**	284.23		AB
20 mg, 100s ea	**00378-6020-01**	106.99		AB
500s ea	**00378-6020-05**	509.81		AB
(Northstar)				
TAB, PO (USP)				
10 mg, 100s ea	**16714-0071-04**	59.65		AB
1000s ea	**16714-0071-06**	558.60		AB
20 mg, 100s ea	**16714-0072-04**	109.60		AB
500s ea	**16714-0072-05**	520.70		AB
(PCCA)				
POW, NA (U.S.P.)				
1 gm	**51927-2007-00**	19.80		
(Qualitest)				
TAB, PO, 10 mg, 100s ea	**00603-2406-21**	59.64		AB
500s ea	**00603-2406-28**	289.80		AB
1000s ea	**00603-2406-32**	550.62		AB
20 mg, 100s ea	**00603-2407-21**	106.98		AB
500s ea	**00603-2407-28**	520.69		AB
1000s ea	**00603-2407-32**	989.31		AB
(Spectrum Pharmacy)				
CRY, NA (U.S.P.)				
5 gm	**49452-0807-02**	106.05		
25 gm	**49452-0807-03**	448.00		
100 gm	**49452-0807-04**	1375.50		
(Teva)				
TAB, PO, 10 mg, 100s ea	**00172-4096-60**	61.01		AB
1000s ea	**00172-4096-80**	558.60		AB
20 mg, 100s ea	**00172-4097-60**	109.62		AB
1000s ea	**00172-4097-80**	1041.39		AB
(UDL)				
TAB, PO (10X10)				
10 mg, 100s ea UD	**51079-0668-20**	54.91		AB
20 mg, 100s ea UD	**51079-0669-20**	98.66		AB
(Upsher-Smith)				
TAB, PO, 10 mg, 90s ea	**00832-1024-09**	49.42		AB
100s ea	**00832-1024-00**	54.91		AB
500s ea	**00832-1024-50**	251.37		AB
1000s ea	**00832-1024-10**	502.74		AB
20 mg, 90s ea	**00832-1025-09**	88.79		AB
100s ea	**00832-1025-00**	98.66		AB
500s ea	**00832-1025-50**	491.45		AB
1000s ea	**00832-1025-10**	539.88		AB
(Watson Labs)				
TAB, PO, 10 mg, 100s ea	**00591-5730-01**	7.98		AB
500s ea	**00591-5730-05**	37.91		AB
20 mg, 100s ea	**00591-5731-01**	11.40		AB
500s ea	**00591-5731-05**	54.16		AB

PROD/MFR	NDC	AWP	DP	OBC
(A-S Medication)				
REPACK				
TAB, PO, 10 mg, 30s ea	**54569-4330-01**	17.39		AB
60s ea	**54569-4330-00**	34.78		EE
90s ea	**54569-4330-03**	52.16		AB
20 mg, 30s ea	**54569-4171-02**	32.28		AB
60s ea	**54569-4171-01**	64.55		AB
(Aidarex)				
REPACK				
TAB, PO, 10 mg, 7s ea	**33261-0010-07**	5.81		AB
14s ea	**33261-0010-14**	11.62		AB
20s ea	**33261-0010-20**	16.60		AB
21s ea	**33261-0010-21**	17.43		AB
28s ea	**33261-0010-28**	23.52		AB
30s ea	**33261-0010-30**	24.90		AB
60s ea	**33261-0010-60**	49.80		AB
90s ea	**33261-0010-90**	74.70		AB
20 mg, 7s ea	**33261-0011-07**	9.45		AB
10s ea	**33261-0011-10**	13.50		AB
14s ea	**33261-0011-14**	18.90		AB
20s ea	**33261-0011-20**	27.00		AB
28s ea	**33261-0011-28**	37.80		AB
30s ea	**33261-0011-30**	40.50		AB
60s ea	**33261-0011-60**	81.20		AB
90s ea	**33261-0011-90**	121.50		AB
(Altura)				
REPACK				
TAB, PO, 10 mg, 10s ea	**63874-0620-10**	6.49		AB
20s ea	**63874-0620-20**	12.98		EE
30s ea	**63874-0620-30**	19.47		EE
40s ea	**63874-0620-40**	25.96		AB
60s ea	**63874-0620-60**	38.94		AB
90s ea	**63874-0620-90**	58.41		AB
100s ea	**63874-0620-01**	64.90		EE
120s ea	**63874-0620-04**	77.88		AB
20 mg, 20s ea	**63874-1025-02**	23.80		AB
30s ea	**63874-1025-03**	35.70		AB
40s ea	**63874-1025-04**	47.60		AB
60s ea	**63874-1025-06**	71.40		AB
90s ea	**63874-1025-09**	107.10		AB
100s ea	**63874-1025-00**	119.00		AB
120s ea	**63874-1025-01**	142.80		AB
(American Health)				
REPACK				
TAB, PO (10X10)				
10 mg, 100s ea UD (15X30)	**68084-0038-01**	43.87		AB
10 mg, 450s ea (10X10)	**68084-0038-85**	260.82		AB
20 mg, 100s ea UD (15X30)	**68084-0039-01**	85.98		AB
20 mg, 450s ea	**68084-0039-85**	468.63		AB
(B&B Pharm, Inc)				
REPACK				
POW, NA (U.S.P.)				
5 gm	**63275-9992-02**	68.00		
25 gm	**63275-9992-04**	285.00		
100 gm (USP,1X500GM)	**63275-9992-05**	972.00		
500 gm	**63275-9992-08**	3000.00		
(Bryant Ranch)				
REPACK				
TAB, PO, 10 mg, 30s ea	**63629-1286-01**	24.65		
50s ea	**63629-1286-06**	42.11		
60s ea	**63629-1286-03**	44.95		AB
120s ea	**63629-1286-02**	98.01		
20 mg, 28s ea	**63629-3193-05**	35.98		AB
30s ea	**63629-3193-06**	35.98		AB
45s ea	**63629-3193-04**	55.22		AB
60s ea	**63629-3193-03**	69.89		AB
90s ea	**63629-3193-01**	102.68		
100s ea	**63629-3193-02**	112.54		AB
(Core)				
REPACK				
TAB, PO, 10 mg, 30s ea	**33358-0042-30**	25.27		
60s ea	**33358-0042-60**	51.38		
120s ea	**33358-0042-01**	100.46		
20 mg, 30s ea	**33358-0043-30**	40.87		
60s ea	**33358-0043-60**	71.21		
90s ea	**33358-0043-90**	105.25		
(DHS, Inc.)				
REPACK				
TAB, PO, 10 mg, 30s ea	**55887-0420-30**	21.00		AB
20 mg, 30s ea	**55887-0526-30**	32.25		AB
60s ea	**55887-0526-60**	64.50		AB
90s ea	**55887-0526-90**	96.75		AB

PROD/MFR	NDC	AWP	DP	OBC
(Dispensing Solutions)				
REPACK				
TAB, PO, 10 mg, 30s ea	**55045-3122-08**	18.95		AB
30s ea	**66336-0834-30**	20.37		AB
60s ea	**55045-3122-06**	37.85		AB
90s ea	**55045-3122-09**	56.70		AB
90s ea	**66336-0834-90**	61.11		AB
100s ea	**55045-3122-00**	63.00		AB
120s ea	**55045-3122-02**	75.60		AB
20 mg, 30s ea	**55045-3074-08**	33.60		AB
60s ea	**55045-3074-06**	67.20		AB
90s ea	**66336-0486-90**	107.46		AB
(IPI)				
REPACK				
TAB, PO, 10 mg, 30s ea	**18837-0018-30**	17.39		
60s ea	**18837-0018-60**	43.47		
90s ea	**18837-0018-90**	52.16		AB
20 mg, 60s ea	**18837-0019-60**	58.97		AB
90s ea	**18837-0019-90**	110.58		
120s ea	**18837-0019-98**	117.95		AB
(Keltman Pharma., Inc.)				
REPACK				
TAB, PO, 10 mg, 30s ea	**68387-0110-30**	20.03		AB
60s ea	**68387-0110-60**	40.06		AB
90s ea	**68387-0110-90**	60.09		AB
20 mg, 90s ea	**68387-0111-90**	111.80		AB
(McKesson Packaging)				
REPACK				
TAB, PO (USP)				
10 mg, 100s ea UD (BLISTER PACK)	**63739-0031-10**	72.45		AB
10 mg, 750s ea UD (PUNCH CARD 25X30)	**63739-0031-01**	543.38		AB
10 mg, 750s ea (USP)	**63739-0031-03**	543.38		AB
20 mg, 100s ea UD (BLISTER PACK)	**63739-0032-10**	130.17		AB
20 mg, 750s ea UD	**63739-0032-01**	976.31		AB
(Medsource)				
REPACK				
TAB, PO, 10 mg, 30s ea	**45865-0452-30**	21.90		AB
60s ea	**45865-0452-60**	43.80		AB
90s ea	**45865-0452-90**	65.70		AB
100s ea	**45865-0452-00**	73.00		AB
120s ea	**45865-0452-01**	87.60		AB
150s ea	**45865-0452-02**	109.50		AB
300s ea	**45865-0452-05**	219.00		AB
20 mg, 30s ea	**45865-0355-30**	39.00		AB
60s ea	**45865-0355-60**	78.00		AB
90s ea	**45865-0355-90**	117.00		AB
100s ea	**45865-0355-00**	130.00		AB
120s ea	**45865-0355-01**	156.00		AB
150s ea	**45865-0355-02**	195.00		AB
300s ea	**45865-0355-05**	390.00		AB
(Nucare Pharm)				
REPACK				
TAB, PO, 10 mg, 30s ea	**66267-0617-30**	25.25		AB
60s ea	**66267-0617-60**	47.82		AB
90s ea	**66267-0617-90**	71.73		AB
20 mg, 60s ea	**66267-0872-60**	81.09		AB
90s ea	**66267-0872-90**	116.11		AB
120s ea	**66267-0872-91**	164.02		AB
(Palmetto)				
REPACK				
TAB, PO, 10 mg, 30s ea	**23490-5114-01**	23.36		
60s ea	**23490-5114-06**	46.72		
90s ea	**23490-5114-02**	70.08		
120s ea	**23490-5114-07**	93.44		
180s ea	**23490-5114-08**	140.17		
270s ea	**23490-5114-03**	210.25		
20 mg, 30s ea	**23490-5115-02**	35.70		
60s ea	**23490-5115-01**	71.40		
90s ea	**23490-5115-09**	107.10		
120s ea	**23490-5115-07**	142.80		
(PD-Rx Pharm)				
REPACK				
TAB, PO, 10 mg, 30s ea (USP)	**55289-0757-30**	29.50		AB
10 mg, 60s ea	**55289-0757-60**	44.75		AB
90s ea	**55289-0757-90**	60.00		
20 mg, 30s ea	**43063-0085-30**	40.75		AB
(Pharma Pac)				
REPACK				
TAB, PO, 10 mg, 10s ea	**52959-0733-10**	7.98		AB
12s ea	**52959-0733-12**	9.15		AB
20s ea	**52959-0733-20**	13.00		AB

PROD/MFR	NDC	AWP	DP	OBC
30s ea	52959-0733-30	18.98		AB
40s ea	52959-0733-40	25.00		AB
60s ea	52959-0733-60	36.78		AB
90s ea	52959-0733-90	55.15		AB
100s ea	52959-0733-00	60.20		AB
120s ea	52959-0733-02	72.25		
180s ea	52959-0733-18	108.29		AB
20 mg, 10s ea	52959-0677-10	12.87		
30s ea	52959-0677-30	38.55		
45s ea	52959-0677-45	57.60		
60s ea	52959-0677-60	74.42		
90s ea	52959-0677-90	111.60		
120s ea	52959-0677-02	148.77		
(Phys Total Care)				
REPACK				
TAB, PO, 10 mg, 30s ea	54868-3405-00	10.50		EE
60s ea	54868-3405-02	17.97		AB
90s ea	54868-3405-03	25.47		AB
100s ea	54868-3405-04	107.55		EE
100s ea	54868-3405-05	26.03		AB
(USP)				
20 mg, 30s ea	54868-3006-04	16.20		AB
60s ea	54868-3006-01	53.28		AB
90s ea	54868-3006-03	38.69		AB
100s ea	54868-3006-02	44.49		
180s ea	54868-3006-05	67.14		AB
(Physician Partner)				
REPACK				
TAB, PO, 10 mg, 30s ea	21695-0014-30	36.61		AB
42s ea	21695-0014-42	54.10		AB
60s ea	21695-0014-60	69.55		
90s ea	21695-0014-90	104.33		
120s ea	21695-0014-72	139.10		
20 mg, 60s ea	21695-0015-60	124.97		
90s ea	21695-0015-90	187.45		
(Quality Care Prod)				
REPACK				
TAB, PO, 10 mg, 30s ea	49999-0607-30	23.36		AB
45s ea	49999-0607-45	35.04		AB
60s ea	49999-0607-60	46.72		
90s ea	49999-0607-90	70.08		
100s ea	49999-0607-00	77.87		
120s ea	49999-0607-01	93.60		
20 mg, 60s ea	49999-0691-60	68.73		
90s ea	49999-0691-90	103.50		
(Southwood)				
REPACK				
TAB, PO, 10 mg, 10s ea	58016-0486-10	6.49		EE
20s ea	58016-0486-20	12.98		EE
30s ea	58016-0486-30	19.47		EE
40s ea	58016-0486-40	25.96		EE
60s ea	58016-0486-60	38.94		EE
90s ea	58016-0486-90	58.40		EE
100s ea	58016-0486-00	64.90		EE
120s ea	58016-0486-02	77.88		AB
180s ea	58016-0486-99	116.82		EE
224s ea	58016-0486-91	145.38		AB
240s ea	58016-0486-04	155.76		AB
270s ea	58016-0486-79	175.23		EE
450s ea	58016-0486-59	292.00		EE
20 mg, 10s ea	58016-0477-10	11.90		EE
20s ea	58016-0477-20	23.80		EE
30s ea	58016-0477-30	39.90		AB
40s ea	58016-0477-40	47.60		EE
60s ea	58016-0477-60	79.80		AB
90s ea	58016-0477-90	119.70		AB
100s ea	58016-0477-00	133.00		AB
120s ea	58016-0477-02	159.60		AB
360s ea	58016-0477-98	427.86		EE
(St. Mary's MPP)				
REPACK				
TAB, PO, 10 mg, 60s ea	60760-0409-60	42.87		AB
90s ea	60760-0409-90	63.38		AB
(Stat Rx)				
REPACK				
TAB, PO, 10 mg, 28s ea	16590-0026-28	21.56		AB
30s ea	16590-0026-30	22.95		AB
60s ea	16590-0026-60	43.47		AB
90s ea	16590-0026-90	63.00		
100s ea	16590-0026-71	70.00		
112s ea	16590-0026-73	78.40		AB
120s ea	16590-0026-72	84.00		
180s ea	16590-0026-82	126.00		AB
240s ea	16590-0026-84	168.00		AB
270s ea	16590-0026-86	189.00		AB
20 mg, 30s ea	16590-0027-30	32.00		
60s ea	16590-0027-60	64.00		
84s ea	16590-0027-62	102.90		AB
90s ea	16590-0027-90	96.00		
112s ea	16590-0027-73	145.82		AB
120s ea	16590-0027-72	147.00		AB
270s ea	16590-0027-86	533.27		AB
(Vibranta)				
REPACK				
TAB, PO, 10 mg, 30s ea	57866-9022-01	23.36		EE
90s ea	57866-9022-02	70.08		EE
20 mg, 30s ea	57866-9023-01	25.15		EE
BACMIN (Marnel)				
multivitamin, minerals, iron, and nutriceuticals				
TAB, PO (CAPLET)				
100s ea	00682-3001-01	36.40		
BACON FLAVOR (Gallipot)				
flavoring aid				
LIQ, NA (NATURAL)				
59.14 ml	51552-0662-09	10.22		
(Medisca)				
SOL, NA (NATURAL,1X25ML,BACON)				
25 ml	38779-2420-04	25.50		
(NATURAL,1X100ML,BACON)				
100 ml	38779-2420-05	46.50		
(NATURAL,1X500ML,BACON)				
500 ml	38779-2420-08	108.00		
BACTRIM (AR Scientific)				
sulfamethoxazole/trimethoprim				
TAB, PO (U.S.P.)				
400 mg-80 mg,				
100s ea	13310-0145-01	160.06		AB
(Quality Care Prod)				
REPACK				
TAB, PO, 400 mg-80 mg,				
20s ea	49999-0232-20	52.20		
BACTRIM DS (AR Scientific)				
sulfamethoxazole/trimethoprim				
TAB, PO (U.S.P.)				
800 mg-160 mg,				
100s ea	13310-0146-01	288.84		AB
(Phys Total Care)				
REPACK				
TAB, PO, 800 mg-160 mg,				
10s ea	54868-0337-03	28.57		AB
20s ea	54868-0337-00	55.18		AB
30s ea	54868-0337-01	88.83		AB
(Quality Care Prod)				
REPACK				
TAB, PO, 800 mg-160 mg,				
10s ea	49999-0649-10	52.20		AB
20s ea	49999-0649-20	68.40		AB
30s ea	49999-0649-30	72.71		AB
60s ea	49999-0649-60	144.43		AB
90s ea	49999-0649-90	216.65		AB
BACTROBAN (Glaxo)				
mupirocin calcium				
CRE, TP, 2%, 15 gm	00029-1527-22	51.06		
30 gm	00029-1527-25	86.53		
OIN, NS (10X1GM)				
2%, 1 gm 10s	00029-1526-11	95.51		
(Glaxo)				
mupirocin				
OIN, TP, 2%, 22 gm	00029-1525-44	74.05		
(A-S Medication)				
REPACK				
mupirocin calcium				
CRE, TP, 2%, 15 gm	54569-4664-00	53.19		
30 gm	54569-5552-00	90.14		
(A-S Medication)				
mupirocin				
OIN, TP, 2%, 22 gm	54569-4960-00	77.14		
(DHS, Inc.)				
REPACK				
mupirocin calcium				
CRE, TP, 2%, 15 gm	55887-0709-15	49.00		
(Dispensing Solutions)				
REPACK				
CRE, TP, 2%, 15 gm	55045-2677-05	44.00		
(Dispensing Solutions)				
mupirocin				
OIN, TP, 2%, 22 gm	55045-1561-07	58.00		
(Nucare Pharm)				
REPACK				
mupirocin calcium				
CRE, TP, 2%, 15 gm	66267-0986-15	36.06		
22 gm	66267-0986-22	52.88		
(Pharma Pac)				
REPACK				
CRE, TP, 2%, 15 gm	52959-0723-15	39.75		
30 gm	52959-0723-30	49.55		
(Pharma Pac)				
mupirocin				
OIN, TP, 2%, 22 gm	52959-0166-22	51.59		
(Phys Total Care)				
REPACK				
mupirocin calcium				
CRE, TP, 2%, 15 gm	54868-4642-01	65.97		
30 gm	54868-4642-00	93.18		
OIN, NS, 2%, 1 gm 10s	54868-4325-00	121.67		
(Phys Total Care)				
mupirocin				
OIN, TP, 2%, 22 gm	54868-0202-00	65.82		
(Quality Care Prod)				
REPACK				
mupirocin calcium				
CRE, TP, 2%, 15 gm	49999-0521-15	107.68		
30 gm	49999-0521-30	67.79		
OIN, NS (10X1GM)				
2%, 1 gm 10s	35356-0468-01	366.00		
(Quality Care Prod)				
mupirocin				
OIN, TP, 2%, 22 gm	49999-0278-22	54.40		
(Southwood)				
REPACK				
mupirocin calcium				
CRE, TP, 2%, 30 gm	58016-5645-01	58.28		
OIN, NS, 2%, 1 gm 10s	58016-4568-01	64.33		
(Southwood)				
mupirocin				
OIN, TP, 2%, 15 gm	58016-3154-01	34.38		
22 gm	58016-5571-01	41.43		
(Stat Rx)				
REPACK				
mupirocin calcium				
CRE, TP, 2%, 15 gm	16590-0028-15	37.00		
30 gm	16590-0028-30	72.00		
BAG, URINARY COLLECTION				
(Covidien) *See PRECISION DRAINAGE BAG*				
BAL IN OIL (Akorn)				
dimercaprol				
OIL, IM (AMP)				
10%, 3 ml 10s	11098-0526-03	988.69		
BALACALL DM (Centurion)				
bpm/dm/phenyleph hcl				
SOL, PO (1X473ML,AF,SF,DYE-FREE)				
473 ml	23359-0005-16	63.77		
BALACET 325 (Cornerstone)				
acetaminophen/propoxyphene napsylate				
TAB, PO (FILM-COATED)				
325 mg-100 mg,				
100s ea, C-IV	10122-0301-10	326.05	260.84	
(Dispensing Solutions)				
REPACK				
TAB, PO (FILM-COATED)				
325 mg-100 mg,				
100s ea, C-IV	55045-3419-00	156.00		
BALANCED SALT (Akorn)				
ca cl/k cl/na cl				
SOL, IR (BLISTER PACK,PF)				
0.48%-0.075%-0.64%,				
18 ml	17478-0920-19	6.46		
BALANCED SALT SOLUTION				
(Alcon Surgical) *See BSS PLUS*				
(Allergan Medical) *See OCUSURG*				
BALANCED SALT SOLUTION (Baxter)				
ca cl/k cl/mg cl/na ace/na cit/na cl				
SOL, IR (OPHTHALMIC)				
1000 ml 6s	00338-0058-03	212.82		
(Cytosol Ophth)				
SOL, IR (NOT FOR INTRAVENOUS USE)				
18 ml 30s	61534-8100-08	112.50		
200 ml 12s	61534-8100-02	43.70		
250 ml 12s	61534-8100-03	48.00		
500 ml 6s	61534-8100-01	34.50		
500 ml 12s	61534-8100-05	69.00		
(Hospira)				
SOL, IR (12X500ML)				
500 ml 12s	00409-3911-03	237.46	207.72	

PROD/MFR NDC AWP DP OBC

(HUB Pharma)
SOL, IR (SINGLE DOSE,PF)
500 ml **17238-0950-50** 110.50
500 ml **17238-0975-50** 110.50

BALSALAZIDE DISODIUM
FUL
CAP, PO, 750 mg, 280s ea 302.29

(Apotex Corp.)
CAP, PO (HARD GELATIN)
750 mg, 280s ea ..... **60505-2575-07** 447.77 **AB**

(Mylan)
CAP, PO (HARD GELATIN)
750 mg, 280s ea ..... **00378-6750-82** 357.27 **AB**

(Roxane)
CAP, PO (HARD GELATIN)
750 mg, 280s ea ..... **00054-0079-28** 399.83 **AB**

(Salix Pharm) *See COLAZAL*

(Watson Labs)
CAP, PO (HARD GELATIN)
750 mg, 280s ea **00591-3570-35** 241.82

BALSAM CANADA
(Medisca) *See CANADA BALSAM*

(PCCA) *See CANADA BALSAM*

(Spectrum Pharmacy) *See CANADIAN BALSAM*

BALSAM PERU (Lorann Oil)
peru balsam
OIL, NA (N.F.)
30 ml............ **23535-0717-05** 2.20
120 ml **23535-0717-08** 6.50
480 ml **23535-0717-01** 22.00
3840 ml **23535-0717-11** 150.00

BALSAM TOLU (Amend)
tolu balsam
POW, NA (U.S.P.)
454 gm............ **17317-0037-01** 70.00

BALTUSSIN (Ballay Pharm., Inc)
cpm/dihydrocodeine bitartrate/phenyleph hcl
SOL, PO (AF,SF,GRAPE)
473 ml, C-V.......... **63162-0513-16** 101.06 88.40

BALZIVA (Teva)
ethinyl estradiol/norethindrone
TAB, PO (6X28)
35 mcg-0.4 mg,
168s ea........... **00555-9034-58** 269.01 **AB**

BANALG (Stat Rx)
REPACK
camphor/menthol/methyl salicylate
LOT, TP, 2%-1%-4.9%,
60 ml............ **16590-0029-02** 16.00

BANANA (Medisca)
flavoring aid
SOL, NA (1X500ML,ARTIFICIAL)
500 ml **38779-2253-08** 37.50

BANANA ARTIFICIAL FLAVOR (Spectrum Pharmacy)
flavoring aid
LIQ, NA (1X100ML)
100 ml **49452-0809-01** 53.20
(1X500ML)
500 ml **49452-0809-02** 118.30

BANANA CREAM (Medisca)
flavoring aid
SOL, NA (1X25ML,BANANA CREAM)
25 ml............ **38779-1016-04** 21.00
(1X100ML,BANANA CREAM)
100 ml **38779-1016-05** 34.50
(1X500ML,BANANA CREAM)
500 ml **38779-1016-08** 81.00

(Spectrum Pharmacy)
LIQ, NA (NATURAL&ARTIFICIAL,CONC)
100 ml **49452-0811-02** 59.50
500 ml **49452-0811-03** 142.45

BANANA CREME FLAVOR (PCCA)
flavoring aid
SOL, NA (ARTIFICIAL)
1 ml............ **51927-2169-00** 0.90

BANANA DAIQUIRI (Medisca)
flavoring aid
SOL, NA (1X100ML,BANANA DAIQUIRI)
100 ml **38779-1017-05** 31.50
(1X500ML,BANANA DAIQUIRI)
500 ml **38779-1017-08** 58.50

PROD/MFR NDC AWP DP OBC

BANANA FLAVOR (Gallipot)
flavoring aid
LIQ, NA (ARTIFICIAL)
59.14 ml............ **51552-0168-03** 6.02

(PCCA)
SOL, NA (CONCENTRATE,BANANA)
1 ml............ **51927-2039-00** 0.23

BANARIL (Clint)
diphenhydramine hydrochloride
SOL, IJ (VIAL)
50 mg/ml, 10 ml ..... **55553-0827-10** 9.75 **EE**

BANDAGE
(Carrington) *See DIAB F.D.G.*

(Carrington) *See DIAB GEL*

(Carrington) *See RADIAFDG*

(Carrington) *See RADIAGEL*

(Carrington) *See SALICEPT*

BANZEL (Eisai)
rufinamide
TAB, PO (FILM-COATED)
200 mg, 30s ea **62856-0582-30** 99.00
400 mg, 120s ea **62856-0583-52** 792.00

BAR-TEST (Glenwood)
barium sulfate
TAB, PO, 650 mg, 100s ea . **00516-0130-01** 170.90

BARACLUDE (Bristol-Myers)
entecavir
SOL, PO (ORANGE)
0.05 mg/ml, 210 ml... **00003-1614-12** 595.74
TAB, PO (FILM-COATED)
0.5 mg, 30s ea **00003-1611-12** 851.08
90s ea........... **00003-1611-13** 2553.20
1 mg, 30s ea......... **00003-1612-12** 851.08

BARBITAL SODIUM (PCCA)
POW, NA, 1 gm, C-IV...... **51927-1009-00** 1.80

BARIUM ACETATE (Baker, J.T.)
CRY, NA (A.C.S., REAGENT)
125 gm............ **10106-0942-04** 30.44
500 gm............ **10106-0942-01** 58.09
2500 gm............ **10106-0942-05** 227.53

BARIUM CARBONATE (Baker, J.T.)
POW, NA (A.C.S., REAGENT)
500 gm............ **10106-0950-01** 129.47
2500 gm............ **10106-0950-05** 454.23
12000 gm **10106-0950-07** 1183.62

BARIUM CHLORIDE
(Baker, J.T.) *See BARIUM CHLORIDE ANHYDROUS*

(Baker, J.T.) *See BARIUM CHLORIDE DIHYDRATE*

(PCCA) *See BARIUM CHLORIDE DIHYDRATE*

(Spectrum Pharmacy) *See BARIUM CHLORIDE DIHYDRATE*

BARIUM CHLORIDE ANHYDROUS (Baker, J.T.)
barium chloride
POW, NA (PURIFIED)
500 gm............ **10106-0980-01** 60.51
2500 gm............ **10106-0980-05** 229.90

BARIUM CHLORIDE DIHYDRATE (Baker, J.T.)
barium chloride
CRY, NA (REAGENT, A.C.S.)
125 gm............ **10106-0970-04** 35.95
500 gm............ **10106-0970-01** 65.04
2500 gm............ **10106-0970-05** 265.74

(PCCA)
POW, NA (A.C.S., REAGENT)
1 gm **51927-1850-00** 0.30

(Spectrum Pharmacy)
CRY, NA (REAGENT, A.C.S.)
500 gm............ **49452-0830-01** 142.80
2500 gm............ **49452-0830-02** 584.50

BARIUM DIOXIDE (Baker, J.T.)
POW, NA (REAGENT)
125 gm............ **10106-0992-04** 53.61
500 gm............ **10106-0992-01** 107.33

BARIUM HYDROXIDE
(Baker, J.T.) *See BARIUM HYDROXIDE 8-HYDRATE*

BARIUM HYDROXIDE 8-HYDRATE (Baker, J.T.)
barium hydroxide
CRY, NA (A.C.S., REAGENT)
125 gm............ **10106-1006-04** 47.07
500 gm............ **10106-1006-01** 85.59
2500 gm............ **10106-1006-05** 152.03

PROD/MFR NDC AWP DP OBC

BARIUM NITRATE (Baker, J.T.)
CRY, NA (A.C.S., REAGENT)
125 gm............ **10106-1018-04** 31.83
500 gm............ **10106-1018-01** 59.95
2500 gm............ **10106-1018-05** 161.71

BARIUM SULFATE (Amend)
POW, NA (U.S.P.)
454 gm............ **17317-0039-01** 14.80
2270 gm............ **17317-0039-05** 49.00
11350 gm **17317-0039-08** 157.50

(Baker, J.T.)
POW, NA (REAGENT)
500 gm............ **10106-1030-01** 145.64
(U.S.P.)
500 gm............ **10106-1040-01** 59.35
(REAGENT)
2500 gm............ **10106-1030-05** 587.98

(E-Z-EM) *See CAT-PAK*

(E-Z-EM) *See E-Z-DISK*

(E-Z-EM) *See READI-CAT*

(E-Z-EM) *See READI-CAT 2*

(Gallipot)
POW, NA (U.S.P.,N.F.)
454 gm............ **51552-0154-06** 22.40

(Glenwood) *See BAR-TEST*

(Humco)
POW, NA (U.S.P.)
454 gm............ **00395-0200-01** 21.22

(Mallinckrodt Lab)
POW, NA (U.S.P.)
500 gm............ **00406-8821-04** 49.35

(PCCA)
POW, NA (USP)
1 gm **51927-1146-00** 0.36

(Spectrum Pharmacy)
POW, NA (USP,1X100GM)
100 gm............ **49452-0840-01** 80.85
(USP,1X500GM)
500 gm............ **49452-0840-02** 152.60
(USP,1X2500GM)
2500 gm............ **49452-0840-03** 315.70

BASE E (PCCA)
peg-150
POW, NA (1X1GM)
1 gm............ **51927-1016-00** 0.07

BASE L (PCCA)
peg-8 distearate
WAX, NA (1X1GM)
1 gm **51927-1058-00** 0.11

BASE, ALCOHOL GEL (Spectrum Pharmacy)
ethanol
GEL, NA (1X500GM)
500 gm............ **49452-0237-01** 148.75
(1X2500GM)
2500 gm............ **49452-0237-02** 532.00

BASE, COA (Spectrum Pharmacy)
cream base
CRE, NA, 500 gm **49452-0836-01** 104.30

BASE, CREAM-HEAVY WITH LIPOSOME (Spectrum Pharmacy)
cream base
CRE, NA (1X453.6GM)
453.6 gm **49452-0833-01** 284.90
(1X2268GM)
2268 gm............ **49452-0833-02** 1263.50

BASE, HORMONE (Spectrum Pharmacy)
cream base
CRE, NA (1X453.6GM)
453.6 gm **49452-0835-01** 220.15
(1X2268GM)
2268 gm............ **49452-0835-02** 896.00

BASE, HORMONE CREAM-BOTANICAL (Spectrum Pharmacy)
cream base
CRE, NA (1X453.6GM)
453.6 gm **49452-0826-01** 239.75
(1X2268GM)
2268 gm............ **49452-0826-02** 976.50

PROD/MFR | NDC | AWP | DP | OBC

BASE, HORMONE CREAM-HEAVY (Spectrum Pharmacy)
cream base
CRE, NA (1X453.6GM)
453.6 gm 49452-0829-01 220.15
(1X2268GM)
2268 gm 49452-0829-02 896.00

BASE, LIPOSOME (Spectrum Pharmacy)
cream base
CRE, NA (1X453.6GM)
453.6 gm 49452-0834-01 284.90
(1X2268GM)
2268 gm 49452-0834-02 1263.50

BASE, OINTMENT (Spectrum Pharmacy)
ointment base
OIN, NA (HYDRATED,HYDROPHILIC)
453.6 gm 49452-0849-01 108.50

BASE, PCCA FIXED OIL SUSPENSION VEHICLE (PCCA)
liquid base
OIL, NA, 1 ml 51927-4316-00 0.25

BASE, PCCA MBK (PCCA)
suppository base
WAX, NA, 1 gm 51927-1056-00 0.13

BASE, PEG (Spectrum Pharmacy)
ointment base
OIN, NA (1X453.6GM)
453.6 gm 49452-0851-01 109.90

BASE, PLURONIC (Spectrum Pharmacy)
gel base
GEL, NA (1X500ML,20%)
500 ml 49452-0858-01 95.90
(1X500ML,30%)
500 ml 49452-0859-01 150.50
(1X4000ML,20%)
4000 ml 49452-0858-02 647.50
(1X4000ML,30%)
4000 ml 49452-0859-02 612.50

BASE, SUPPOSIBASE (Spectrum Pharmacy)
suppository base
WAX, NA (1X500GM)
500 gm 49452-0838-01 101.85
(1X2500GM)
2500 gm 49452-0838-02 423.50

BASE, WATER (Spectrum Pharmacy)
gel base
GEL, NA (1X500GM)
500 gm 49452-0841-01 127.40

BASIC FUCHSIN (Medisca)
color additive
POW, NA (1X5GM,USP,MAGENTA)
5 gm 38779-0826-03 25.50
(1X25GM,USP,MAGENTA)
25 gm 38779-0826-04 70.50

(Spectrum Pharmacy)
fuchsin, basic
CRY, NA (C.I. 42500)
25 gm 49452-0832-01 165.90
100 gm 49452-0832-02 483.00

BASIC FUCHSIN HYDROCHLORIDE (PCCA)
fuchsin, basic
POW, NA, 1 gm 51927-1319-00 11.40

(Spectrum Pharmacy)
CRY, NA (1X25GM)
25 gm 49452-0850-01 330.75

BASILIXIMAB
(Novartis Pharm) *See SIMULECT*

BAY LEAF OIL (PCCA)
bay oil
OIL, NA, 1 ml 51927-2371-00 1.60

BAY OIL (Lorann Oil)
OIL, NA, 9.9 ml 23535-0151-03 3.90

(PCCA) *See BAY LEAF OIL*

(Spectrum Pharmacy)
OIL, NA (F.C.C.)
25 ml 49452-0875-03 131.60
100 ml 49452-0875-01 275.80
500 ml 49452-0875-02 756.00

BAYCADRON ELIXIR (Wockhardt USA)
dexamethasone
ELI, PO (NO DROPPER,RASPBERRY)
0.5 mg/5 ml,
237 ml 64679-0810-08 79.10

BAYHEP B (Phys Total Care)
REPACK
hepatitis b immune globulin
SOL, IM (S.D.V.,200 IU/ML)
1 ml 54868-2289-01 184.18

BCG VACCINE (Organon)
bacillus of calmette and guerin vaccine, live
PDS, ID (VIAL)
ea 00052-0603-02 169.10

BD INSULIN SYRINGE (BD Consumer)
insulin syringe/needle
DEV, NA (1CC,U100,SLIP TIP)
100s ea 08290-3296-50 18.45

BD LANCET (BD Consumer)
lancet device
DEV, NA, ea 08290-3257-75 10.40
(33 GAUGE)
100s ea 08290-3220-57 8.81

BD MICRO-FINE (BD Consumer)
insulin syringe/needle
DEV, NA (27GX5/8",1CC)
10s ea 08290-8412-01 2.47
10s ea 82908-0412-03 2.47
(28GX1/2",1/2CC,9X10)
90s ea 08290-3282-82 23.76
(28GX1/2",1CC,9X10)
90s ea 08290-3282-81 23.76
(28GX1/2",3/10CC,9X10)
90s ea 08290-3282-83 23.76
(27GX5/8",1CC)
500s ea 08290-3284-12 123.25

BD MICRO-FINE IV (BD Consumer)
insulin syringe/needle
DEV, NA (28GX1/2",1CC)
10s ea 08290-8410-02 2.73
(28GX1/2",3/10CC)
10s ea 08290-8430-02 2.73
(28GX1/2",1/2CC)
100s ea 08290-3284-65 27.30
(28GX1/2",1CC)
100s ea 08290-3284-10 27.30
(28GX1/2",3/10CC)
100s ea 08290-3284-30 27.30

BD POSIFLUSH SF (BD Dickinson Hosp Prod)
sodium chloride
SOL, IV (SALINE FLUSH SYRINGEUSP)
0.9%, 10 ml 30s 08290-0950-10 36.60

BD ULTRA-FINE (BD Consumer)
insulin syringe/needle
DEV, NA (30GX1/2",1/2CC)
10s ea 08290-8466-01 2.73
(30GX1/2",1CC)
10s ea 08290-8411-01 2.73
(30GX1/2",3/10CC)
10s ea 08290-8431-01 2.73
(30GX1/2",1/2CC,9X10)
90s ea 08290-3282-79 23.76
(30GX1/2",1CC,9X10)
90s ea 08290-3282-78 23.76
(30GX1/2",3/10CC,9X10)
90s ea 08290-3282-80 23.76
(30GX1/2",1/2CC,100X5)
100s ea 08290-3284-66 27.30
(30GX1/2",1CC,100X5)
100s ea 08290-3284-11 27.30
(30GX1/2",3/10CC,100X5)
100s ea 08290-3284-31 27.30

BD ULTRA-FINE PEN (BD Consumer)
insulin syringe/needle
DEV, NA (29GX1/2")
100s ea 08290-3282-03 32.56

BE-FLEX PLUS (Larken Labs, Inc.)
apap/phenyltoloxamine cit/salicylamide
CAP, PO, 300 mg-20 mg-200 mg,
100s ea 68047-0116-01 38.55

BEBULIN VH (Baxter Bioscience)
factor ix complex human
PDS, IV (VAPOR HEATED)
1 iu, ea 64193-0244-02 1.07

BECAPLERMIN
(Ortho-McNeil Pharm) *See REGRANEX*

BECLOMETHASONE DIPROPIONATE (Gallipot)
POW, NA (1X250MG,USP)
0.25 gm 51552-0883-09 26.95 19.25
(1X1GM,USP)
1 gm 51552-0883-01 69.30 49.50
(1X5GM,USP)
5 gm 51552-0883-02 277.20 198.00

(Medisca)
POW, NA (U.S.P.,MICRONIZED)
1 gm 38779-0364-06 105.00
5 gm 38779-0364-03 435.00
10 gm 38779-0364-01 796.50

(PCCA)
POW, NA (U.S.P. (ANHYDROUS))
1 gm 51927-1641-00 126.00

(Spectrum Pharmacy)
POW, NA (U.S.P.,MICRONIZED)
0.25 gm 49452-0802-01 73.15
1 gm 49452-0802-02 160.65
5 gm 49452-0802-03 717.50

(Teva) *See QVAR*

BECLOMETHASONE DIPROPIONATE MONOHYDRATE
(Glaxo) *See BECONASE AQ*

BECLOVENT (Phys Total Care)
REPACK
beclomethasone dipropionate
ARO, IH, 0.042 mg/actuation,
16.8 gm 54868-1269-01 57.43 BN

(Southwood)
REPACK
ARO, IH, 0.042 mg/actuation,
16.8 gm 58016-6207-01 38.13 BN

BECONASE (Phys Total Care)
REPACK
beclomethasone dipropionate
ARO, NS, 0.042 mg/actuation,
16.8 gm 54868-1243-01 66.64 BN

(Southwood)
REPACK
ARO, NS, 0.042 mg/actuation,
16.8 gm 58016-6092-01 37.44 BN

BECONASE AQ (Glaxo)
beclomethasone dipropionate monohydrate
SPR, NS, 0.042 mg/actuation,
25 gm 00173-0388-79 148.74 BN

(A-S Medication)
REPACK
SPR, NS, 0.042 mg/actuation,
25 gm 54569-1729-01 124.51 BN

(Altura)
REPACK
SPR, NS, 0.042 mg/actuation,
25 gm 63874-0721-25 38.98 BN

(Palmetto)
REPACK
SPR, NS (1X25GM)
0.042 mg/actuation,
25 gm 23490-9406-00 175.00 BN

(Phys Total Care)
REPACK
SPR, NS, 0.042 mg/actuation,
25 gm 54868-0175-01 178.02 BN

(Southwood)
REPACK
SPR, NS, 0.042 mg/actuation,
25 gm 58016-6451-01 148.74 BN

(Stat Rx)
REPACK
SPR, NS, 0.042 mg/actuation,
15 gm 16590-0030-25 173.38 BN

BEE PROPOLIS EXTRACT (Gallipot)
propolis extract
POW, NA, 100 gm 51552-0816-05 25.90 18.50

BEE VENOM
(Alk-Abello) *See HONEY BEE TREATMENT*
(Hollister-Stier) *See HONEY BEE VENOM PROTEIN*
(Hollister-Stier) *See VENOMIL*

BEEF (Medisca)
flavoring aid
POW, NA (1X25GM)
25 gm 38779-1942-04 22.50
(1X100GM)
100 gm 38779-1942-05 43.50

PROD/MFR NDC AWP DP OBC

BEEF (Medisca)
flavoring aid
POW, NA (1X500GM)
500 gm.............38779-1942-08 105.00

BEEF FLAVOR (Gallipot)
flavoring aid
LIQ, NA (NATURAL)
59.14 ml.............51552-0634-09 10.22

(PCCA)
LIQ, NA (OIL SOLUBLE)
1 ml.................51927-2897-00 0.38
(WATER MISCIBLE)
1 ml.................51927-2898-00 0.45

BEEF-ADE FLAVOR (PCCA)
flavoring aid
POW, NA (DRY,BEEF-ADE)
1 gm.................51927-3450-00 0.12

BEESWAX WHITE (Humco)
yellow wax
WAX, NA (N.F.)
30 gm...............00395-0207-91 25.44

(Spectrum Pharmacy)
WAX, NA (N.F.)
500 gm..............49452-8140-01 101.50

BEESWAX YELLOW (Spectrum Pharmacy)
yellow wax
WAX, NA (N.F.)
500 gm..............49452-8150-01 103.95

BELL ALK/CPM/PSE HCL
(Carwin) *See RU-TUSS*

BELLADONNA (Amend)
belladonna alkaloids
TIN, NA (U.S.P.)
120 ml..............17317-0044-04 11.20
500 ml..............17317-0044-01 29.40

BELLADONNA
(Medisca) *See BELLADONNA TINCTURE*

BELLADONNA (PCCA)
belladonna alkaloids
TIN, NA (U.S.P.)
1 ml.................51927-1823-00 0.22

BELLADONNA (Spectrum Pharmacy)
TIN, NA (U.S.P.)
500 ml..............49452-0136-02 198.98

BELLADONNA ALK W/ PHENOBARBITAL (HomeMed)
REPACK
atropine sulf/hyoscyamine sulf/pb/scop hydrobrom
TAB, PO, 30s ea..........51655-0119-24 10.99

BELLADONNA ALK/PHEN (Core)
REPACK
atropine sulf/hyoscyamine sulf/pb/scop hydrobrom
TAB, PO, 30s ea..........33358-0045-30 3.54

BELLADONNA ALK/PHEN I (Core)
atropine sulf/hyoscyamine sulf/pb/scop hydrobrom
ELI, PO, 120 ml..........33358-0046-04 55.84

BELLADONNA ALKALOIDS
(Amend) *See BELLADONNA*
(Gallipot) *See BELLADONNA LEAF*
(PCCA) *See BELLADONNA*
(PCCA) *See BELLADONNA LEAF*
(Spectrum Pharmacy) *See BELLADONNA LEAF*

BELLADONNA ALKALOIDS AND ANALGESICS
(A. G. Marin) *See URETRON D/S*
(Azur Pharma, Inc.) *See PYRELLE HB*
(Breckenridge Pharm) *See PHENAZOPYRIDINE PLUS*
(Contract Pharmacal) *See PHENAZOPYRIDINE PLUS*
(Cypress Pharm) *See UTICAP*
(Cypress Pharm) *See UTRONA-C*
(Edwards) *See UROGESIC-BLUE*
(Ferring) *See PROSED/DS*
(Hawthorn Pharm) *See UTIRA*
(Hawthorn Pharm) *See UTIRA-C*
(Marnel) *See URIMAR-T*
(SJ) *See UTA*
(Truxton) *See CYSTEMMS-V*

BELLADONNA ALKALOIDS/OPIUM ALKALOIDS
(Paddock) *See BELLADONNA/OPIUM*

BELLADONNA ALKALOIDS/PHENOBARBITAL
(Excellium)
atropine sulf/hyoscyamine sulf/pb/scop hydrobrom
TAB, PO, 1000s ea........64125-0128-10 82.07

(Vintage)
ELI, PO, 480 ml..........00254-9035-58 14.75
TAB, PO, 100s ea.........00254-2320-28 5.80

(West-Ward)
TAB, PO (W/ALKALOIDS)
1000s ea..........00143-1140-10 60.00
5000s ea..........00143-1140-51 260.00

(A-S Medication)
REPACK
TAB, PO, 20s ea..........54569-0427-04 1.73
30s ea..............54569-0427-01 2.59

(Altura)
REPACK
ELI, PO, 120 ml..........63874-0724-12 8.67
TAB, PO, 20s ea..........63874-0309-20 4.36
30s ea..............63874-0309-30 6.98
40s ea..............63874-0309-40 9.31
42s ea..............63874-0309-42 9.77
50s ea..............63874-0309-50 11.63

(Apace)
REPACK
TAB, PO, 60s ea..........15338-0600-60 1.51

(Dispensing Solutions)
REPACK
ELI, PO (LIME-ORANGE)
118 ml..............55045-1324-09 5.75
TAB, PO, 20s ea..........66336-0042-20 5.84
30s ea..............55045-1234-08 6.10
60s ea..............55045-1234-09 12.00

(PD-Rx Pharm)
REPACK
TAB, PO, 14s ea..........55289-0035-14 7.32
20s ea..............55289-0035-20 7.73
(REDI-SCRIPT)
20s ea..............58864-0734-20 5.99
28s ea..............55289-0035-28 8.27
28s ea..............55289-0053-28 6.27
30s ea..............55289-0035-30 8.40
60s ea..............55289-0035-60 10.43
100s ea.............66289-0035-01 16.94

(Pharma Pac)
REPACK
ELI, PO, 90 ml...........52959-0274-30 7.42
120 ml..............52959-0274-03 9.90
180 ml..............52959-0274-06 14.85
TAB, PO, 6s ea...........52959-0023-06 4.70
20s ea..............52959-0023-20 4.87
30s ea..............52959-0023-30 5.25
50s ea..............52959-0023-50 6.01
60s ea..............52959-0023-60 8.85

(Phys Total Care)
REPACK
TAB, PO, 30s ea..........54868-0031-04 12.92
50s ea..............54868-0031-01 17.54
60s ea..............54868-0031-02 19.85
100s ea.............54868-0031-00 27.58

(Physician Partner)
REPACK
TAB, PO, 30s ea..........21695-0890-30 15.18

(Quality Care Prod)
REPACK
TAB, PO, 16s ea..........49999-0076-16 5.61
20s ea..............49999-0076-20 7.48
30s ea..............49999-0076-30 8.38
90s ea..............49999-0076-90 15.94

(Southwood)
REPACK
TAB, PO, 20s ea..........58016-0709-20 4.98
30s ea..............58016-0709-30 7.47
40s ea..............58016-0709-40 9.96
42s ea..............58016-0709-42 10.45
50s ea..............58016-0709-50 12.45
100s ea.............58016-0709-00 24.89
120s ea.............58016-0709-02 29.87
150s ea.............58016-0709-03 37.34
200s ea.............58016-0709-89 49.78
300s ea.............58016-0709-73 74.67

(Stat Rx)
REPACK
TAB, PO, 30s ea..........16590-0290-30 3.61

BELLADONNA ALKALOIDS/SIMETHICONE
(Kramer-Novis) *See SIMETYL*

BELLADONNA LEAF (Gallipot)
belladonna alkaloids
POW, NA (U.S.P.)
113.4 gm............51552-0655-04 38.50

(PCCA)
POW, NA (U.S.P.)
1 gm................51927-1120-00 1.68

(Spectrum Pharmacy)
POW, NA (U.S.P. EXTRACT)
125 gm..............49452-0135-01 167.30
500 gm..............49452-0135-02 535.50

BELLADONNA TINCTURE (Medisca)
belladonna
TIN, NA (USP,1X500ML)
500 ml..............38779-1022-08 94.50

BELLADONNA WITH PHENOBARBITAL (Bryant Ranch)
REPACK
atropine sulf/hyoscyamine sulf/pb/scop hydrobrom
TAB, PO, 20s ea..........63629-1719-02 2.30
30s ea..............63629-1719-01 3.45
60s ea..............63629-1719-03 6.89

BELLADONNA/OPIUM (Paddock)
belladonna alkaloids/opium alkaloids
SUP, RC, 16.2 mg-30 mg,
12s ea UD, C-II.....00574-7045-12 123.45
16.2 mg-60 mg,
12s ea UD, C-II.....00574-7040-12 150.15

BELLADONNA/PHENOBARBITAL (DHS, Inc.)
REPACK
atropine sulf/hyoscyamine sulf/pb/scop hydrobrom
TAB, PO, 30s ea..........55887-0066-30 3.90

BENACTYZINE HYDROCHLORIDE (PCCA)
POW, NA, 1 gm...........51927-2023-00 32.40

BENADRYL (Pfizer)
diphenhydramine hydrochloride
SOL, IJ (SRN, STERI-DOSE)
50 mg/ml, 1 ml 10s...00071-4259-45 18.64 14.91 AP

(Dispensing Solutions)
REPACK
SOL, IJ, 50 mg/ml, 10 ml...55045-3298-01 13.00

(Phys Total Care)
REPACK
SOL, IJ (AMP)
50 mg/ml, 1 ml 10s...54868-0554-00 21.00 AP
(VIAL)
50 mg/ml, 10 ml......54868-0007-00 12.67 AP
25 ml...............54868-3053-00 30.35 AP

BENALG (Physician Partner)
REPACK
menthol/methyl salicylate
LOT, TP (HOSPITAL STRENGTH)
3%-14%, 60 ml......21695-0440-02 17.36

BENAZEPRIL (Bryant Ranch)
REPACK
benazepril hydrochloride
TAB, PO, 10 mg, 30s ea...63629-2672-01 29.70
60s ea..............63629-2672-02 59.40
40 mg, 30s ea........63629-2923-01 45.00

(Core)
REPACK
TAB, PO, 10 mg, 30s ea...33358-0048-30 30.44
20 mg, 30s ea........33358-0049-30 45.20

(DHS, Inc.)
REPACK
TAB, PO, 20 mg, 30s ea...55887-0322-30 20.12
40 mg, 30s ea........55887-0223-30 33.00

(Pharma Pac)
REPACK
TAB, PO, 20 mg, 30s ea...52959-0831-30 48.01
40 mg, 30s ea........52959-0835-30 36.23
60s ea..............52959-0835-60 72.40

(Physician Partner)
REPACK
TAB, PO, 10 mg, 30s ea...21695-0326-30 58.75
20 mg, 30s ea........21695-0327-30 58.75

BENAZEPRIL HCL/HYDROCHLOROTHIAZIDE (Mylan)
benazepril hydrochloride/hydrochlorothiazide
TAB, PO, 5 mg-6.25 mg,
100s ea.............00378-4725-01 105.00
10 mg-12.5 mg,
100s ea.............00378-4735-01 105.00
20 mg-12.5 mg,
100s ea.............00378-4745-01 105.00
20 mg-25 mg,
100s ea.............00378-4775-01 105.00

PROD/MFR	NDC	AWP	DP	OBC
(Sandoz)				
TAB, PO, 5 mg-6.25 mg, 100s ea	**00781-5131-01**	105.11		
(FILM-COATED) 5 mg-6.25 mg, 100s ea	**00185-0124-01**	100.91		
10 mg-12.5 mg, 100s ea	**00781-5132-01**	105.11		
(FILM-COATED) 10 mg-12.5 mg, 100s ea	**00185-0204-01**	100.91		
20 mg-12.5 mg, 100s ea	**00781-5133-01**	105.11		
(FILM-COATED) 20 mg-12.5 mg, 100s ea	**00185-0211-01**	100.91		
20 mg-25 mg, 100s ea	**00781-5134-01**	105.11		
(FILM-COATED) 20 mg-25 mg, 100s ea	**00185-0277-01**	100.91		
(A-S Medication)				
REPACK				
TAB, PO (FILM-COATED) 20 mg-25 mg, 30s ea	**54569-5685-00**	31.21		
(Dispensing Solutions)				
REPACK				
TAB, PO, 20 mg-12.5 mg, 100s ea	**55045-3170-00**	105.00		
(Phys Total Care)				
REPACK				
TAB, PO (FILM-COATED) 10 mg-12.5 mg, 30s ea	**54868-5256-00**	22.14		
20 mg-12.5 mg, 30s ea	**54868-3906-00**	21.36		
100s ea	**54868-3906-01**	62.76		
20 mg-25 mg, 30s ea	**54868-5296-00**	25.95		
BENAZEPRIL HCT (Pharma Pac)				
REPACK				
benazepril hydrochloride/hydrochlorothiazide				
TAB, PO, 20 mg-25 mg, 30s ea	**52959-0907-30**	45.20		
BENAZEPRIL HYDROCHLORIDE				
FUL				
TAB, PO, 5 mg, 100s ea		49.05		
10 mg, 100s ea		49.05		
20 mg, 100s ea		49.05		
40 mg, 100s ea		49.05		
(Amneal)				
TAB, PO, 5 mg, 100s ea	**65162-0751-10**	105.11		
500s ea	**65162-0751-50**	525.56		
10 mg, 100s ea	**65162-0752-10**	105.11		
500s ea	**65162-0752-50**	525.56		
20 mg, 100s ea	**65162-0753-10**	105.11		
500s ea	**65162-0753-50**	525.56		
40 mg, 100s ea	**65162-0754-10**	105.11		
500s ea	**65162-0754-50**	525.56		
(Apotex Corp.)				
TAB, PO (FILM COATED) 5 mg, 100s ea	**60505-0265-01**	105.11		**AB**
10 mg, 100s ea	**60505-0266-01**	105.11		**AB**
500s ea	**60505-0266-05**	525.56		**AB**
20 mg, 100s ea	**60505-0267-01**	105.11		**AB**
500s ea	**60505-0267-05**	525.56		**AB**
40 mg, 100s ea	**60505-0268-01**	105.11		**AB**
500s ea	**60505-0268-05**	525.56		**AB**
(Aurobindo Pharma)				
TAB, PO (USP,FILM-COATED) 10 mg, 100s ea	**65862-0116-01**	105.11		**AB**
20 mg, 100s ea	**65862-0117-01**	105.11		**AB**
40 mg, 100s ea	**65862-0118-01**	105.11		**AB**
(Ethex)				
TAB, PO, 5 mg, 100s ea	**58177-0341-04**	104.99		
10 mg, 100s ea	**58177-0342-04**	104.99		
500s ea	**58177-0342-08**	498.70		
20 mg, 100s ea	**58177-0343-04**	104.99		
500s ea	**58177-0343-08**	498.70		
40 mg, 100s ea	**58177-0344-04**	104.99		
500s ea	**58177-0344-08**	498.70		
(Mylan)				
TAB, PO, 5 mg, 100s ea	**00378-0441-01**	105.00		
10 mg, 100s ea	**00378-0443-01**	105.00		
20 mg, 100s ea	**00378-0444-01**	105.00		
40 mg, 100s ea	**00378-0447-01**	105.00		
(Novartis Pharm) *See LOTENSIN*				
(Sandoz)				
TAB, PO, 5 mg, 100s ea	**00781-1891-01**	105.11		
(FILM-COATED) 5 mg, 100s ea	**00185-0505-01**	100.91		
500s ea	**00185-0505-05**	489.55		
10 mg, 100s ea	**00185-0053-01**	100.91		
100s ea	**00781-1892-01**	105.11		
500s ea	**00185-0053-05**	489.55		
20 mg, 100s ea	**00781-1893-01**	105.11		
(FILM-COATED) 20 mg, 100s ea	**00185-0820-01**	100.91		
500s ea	**00185-0820-05**	489.55		
40 mg, 100s ea	**00781-1894-01**	105.11		
(FILM-COATED) 40 mg, 100s ea	**00185-0048-01**	100.91		
500s ea	**00185-0048-05**	489.55		
(Teva)				
TAB, PO (FILM-COATED) 5 mg, 100s ea	**00093-5124-01**	105.11		
(10X10,FILM-COATED) 10 mg, 100s ea UD	**00172-5351-10**	106.53		
(FILM-COATED) 10 mg, 100s ea	**00093-5125-01**	105.11		
500s ea	**00093-5125-05**	525.56		
500s ea	**00172-5351-70**	496.50		
(10X10,FILM-COATED) 20 mg, 100s ea UD	**00172-5352-10**	106.53		
(FILM-COATED) 20 mg, 100s ea	**00093-5126-01**	105.11		
500s ea	**00093-5126-05**	525.56		
500s ea	**00172-5352-70**	496.50		
(10X10,FILM-COATED) 40 mg, 100s ea UD	**00172-5353-10**	106.53		
(FILM-COATED) 40 mg, 100s ea	**00093-5127-01**	105.11		
500s ea	**00172-5353-70**	496.50		
(UDL)				
TAB, PO (10X10) 10 mg, 100s ea UD	**51079-0145-20**	95.20		**AB**
20 mg, 100s ea UD	**51079-0146-20**	95.20		**AB**
(A-S Medication)				
REPACK				
TAB, PO (FILM-COATED) 10 mg, 30s ea	**54569-5668-00**	31.38		
60s ea	**54569-5668-01**	62.77		
20 mg, 30s ea	**54569-5669-00**	31.50		
40 mg, 30s ea	**54569-5670-00**	31.50		
(Altura)				
REPACK				
TAB, PO, 10 mg, 10s ea	**63874-1149-00**	11.49		
20 mg, 30s ea	**63874-1123-03**	114.99		
100s ea	**63874-1123-01**	114.99		
(Bryant Ranch)				
REPACK				
TAB, PO, 20 mg, 30s ea	**63629-1728-01**	44.10		
60s ea	**63629-1728-02**	88.20		
100s ea	**63629-1728-03**	147.00		
(Dispensing Solutions)				
REPACK				
TAB, PO, 5 mg, 30s ea	**66336-0232-30**	17.69		
10 mg, 30s ea	**66336-0773-30**	17.69		
(FILM-COATED) 10 mg, 100s ea	**55045-3164-00**	104.00		
20 mg, 30s ea	**66336-0691-30**	17.69		
40 mg, 30s ea	**66336-0124-30**	36.38		
(Nucare Pharm)				
REPACK				
TAB, PO, 20 mg, 30s ea	**68071-0146-30**	39.69		
(Palmetto)				
REPACK				
TAB, PO, 5 mg, 30s ea	**23490-5121-01**	40.36		
10 mg, 30s ea	**23490-5118-01**	40.36		
20 mg, 30s ea	**23490-5119-01**	40.36		
40 mg, 30s ea	**23490-5120-03**	40.36		
90s ea	**23490-5120-09**	121.08		
(PD-Rx Pharm)				
REPACK				
TAB, PO (FILM-COATED) 5 mg, 30s ea	**55289-0963-30**	8.37		
(FILM COATED) 20 mg, 30s ea	**43063-0131-30**	41.00		**AB**
40 mg, 30s ea	**43063-0132-30**	42.35		**AB**
(Pharma Pac)				
REPACK				
TAB, PO, 10 mg, 30s ea	**52959-0841-30**	36.28		
60s ea	**52959-0841-60**	72.57		
(Phys Total Care)				
REPACK				
TAB, PO (FILM-COATED) 5 mg, 30s ea	**54868-5392-00**	18.90		
10 mg, 30s ea	**54868-5001-00**	13.05		
100s ea	**54868-5001-01**	31.53		
20 mg, 30s ea	**54868-5079-00**	12.12		
(FILM-COATED) 20 mg, 100s ea	**54868-5079-01**	31.86		
40 mg, 30s ea	**54868-5204-00**	18.33		
60s ea	**54868-5204-02**	25.27		
90s ea	**54868-5204-01**	45.99		
100s ea	**54868-5204-03**	39.12		
(Physician Partner)				
REPACK				
TAB, PO (FILM-COATED) 10 mg, 60s ea	**21695-0326-60**	117.50		
20 mg, 60s ea	**21695-0327-60**	117.50		
90s ea	**21695-0327-90**	176.25		
40 mg, 30s ea	**21695-0877-30**	60.55		
90s ea	**21695-0877-90**	181.65		
(Quality Care Prod)				
REPACK				
TAB, PO, 20 mg, 30s ea	**49999-0759-30**	47.25		
(FILM-COATED) 40 mg, 30s ea	**35356-0432-30**	36.20		
(Stat Rx)				
REPACK				
TAB, PO, 10 mg, 30s ea	**16590-0280-30**	34.60		
20 mg, 30s ea	**16590-0259-30**	34.60		
BENAZEPRIL HYDROCHLORIDE/HCTZ (Bryant Ranch)				
REPACK				
benazepril hydrochloride/hydrochlorothiazide				
TAB, PO, 10 mg-12.5 mg, 30s ea	**63629-1809-01**	31.53		
(Core)				
REPACK				
TAB, PO, 10 mg-12.5 mg, 30s ea	**33358-0047-30**	32.32		
20 mg-25 mg, 30s ea	**33358-0050-30**	45.25		
BENAZEPRIL HYDROCHLORIDE/HYDROCHLOROTHIAZIDE				
FUL				
TAB, PO, 5 mg-6.25 mg, 100s ea		49.58		
10 mg-12.5 mg, 100s ea		49.58		
20 mg-12.5 mg, 100s ea		49.58		
20 mg-25 mg, 100s ea		49.58		
(Mylan) *See BENAZEPRIL HCL/HYDROCHLOROTHIAZIDE*				
(Novartis Pharm) *See LOTENSIN HCT*				
(Sandoz) *See BENAZEPRIL HCL/HYDROCHLOROTHIAZIDE*				
BENAZEPRIL/HCTZ (Bryant Ranch)				
REPACK				
benazepril hydrochloride/hydrochlorothiazide				
TAB, PO, 20 mg-25 mg, 30s ea	**63629-2735-01**	44.15		
(DHS, Inc.)				
REPACK				
TAB, PO, 20 mg-12.5 mg, 30s ea	**55887-0175-30**	31.50		
(Southwood)				
REPACK				
TAB, PO, 20 mg-12.5 mg, 30s ea	**58016-0065-30**	31.50		
60s ea	**58016-0065-60**	63.00		
90s ea	**58016-0065-90**	94.50		
100s ea	**58016-0065-00**	105.00		

PROD/MFR	NDC	AWP	DP	OBC
BENAZEPRIL/HYDROCHLOROTHIAZIDE (Bryant Ranch)				
REPACK				
benazepril hydrochloride/hydrochlorothiazide				
TAB, PO, 20 mg-12.5 mg,				
30s ea	**63629-2680-01**	50.45		
90s ea	**63629-2680-02**	149.35		
BENDAMUSTINE HYDROCHLORIDE				
(Cephalon) *See TREANDA*				
BENDROFLUMETHIAZIDE (PCCA)				
POW, NA (U.S.P. BENDROFLUAZIDE)				
1 gm	**51927-1969-00**	41.40		
BENDROFLUMETHIAZIDE/NADOLOL				
(Global Pharm) *See NADOLOL AND BENDROFLUMETHIAZIDE*				
(King Pharm) *See CORZIDE 40/5*				
(King Pharm) *See CORZIDE 80/5*				
(Mylan) *See NADOLOL AND BENDROFLUMETHIAZIDE*				
BENEFIX (Wyeth)				
coagulation factor ix recombinant				
PDS, IV (1000IU,PF)				
1 iu, ea	**58394-0001-06**	1.12	0.93	
(2000IU,PF)				
1 iu, ea	**58394-0008-02**	1.12	0.93	
(250IU,PF)				
1 iu, ea	**58394-0003-06**	1.12	0.93	
(500IU,PF)				
1 iu, ea	**58394-0002-06**	1.12	0.93	
(S.D.V.,W/DILUENT,1000IU)				
1 iu, ea	**58394-0001-01**	1.00	0.83	
(S.D.V.,W/DILUENT,250 IU)				
1 iu, ea	**58394-0003-01**	1.00	0.83	
(S.D.V.,W/DILUENT,500 IU)				
1 iu, ea	**58394-0002-01**	1.00	0.83	
BENICAR (Daiichi Sankyo)				
olmesartan medoxomil				
TAB, PO (FILM-COATED)				
5 mg, 30s ea	**65597-0101-30**	66.60		
20 mg, 30s ea	**65597-0103-30**	76.32		
90s ea	**65597-0103-90**	228.96		
(BLISTER CARD,10X10)				
20 mg, 100s ea UD	**65597-0103-10**	254.40		
(FILM-COATED)				
40 mg, 30s ea	**65597-0104-30**	102.24		
90s ea	**65597-0104-90**	306.72		
(BLISTER CARD,10X10)				
40 mg, 100s ea UD	**65597-0104-10**	340.80		
(A-S Medication)				
REPACK				
TAB, PO (FILM-COATED)				
20 mg, 30s ea	**54569-5606-00**	71.63		
(Dispensing Solutions)				
REPACK				
TAB, PO (FILM-COATED)				
40 mg, 90s ea	**55045-3356-00**	165.60		
(Palmetto)				
REPACK				
TAB, PO, 20 mg, 30s ea	**23490-9409-03**	90.00		
90s ea	**23490-9409-09**	270.00		
40 mg, 30s ea	**23490-9410-03**	90.00		
90s ea	**23490-9410-09**	270.00		
(PD-Rx Pharm)				
REPACK				
TAB, PO (FILM-COATED)				
40 mg, 30s ea	**55289-0436-30**	118.53		
(Phys Total Care)				
REPACK				
TAB, PO (FILM-COATED)				
20 mg, 30s ea	**54868-4986-00**	80.28		
90s ea	**54868-4986-02**	225.71		
(FILM-COATED)				
20 mg, 100s ea	**54868-4986-01**	251.23		
40 mg, 30s ea	**54868-4885-00**	110.70		
90s ea	**54868-4885-01**	310.72		
(Quality Care Prod)				
REPACK				
TAB, PO (FILM-COATED)				
5 mg, 20s ea	**35356-0287-20**	465.85		
30s ea	**35356-0287-30**	112.90		
20 mg, 30s ea	**49999-0815-30**	121.65		
90s ea	**49999-0815-90**	356.70		
(FILM-COATED)				
40 mg, 30s ea	**35356-0216-30**	145.29		
90s ea	**35356-0216-90**	783.48		

PROD/MFR	NDC	AWP	DP	OBC
(Southwood)				
REPACK				
TAB, PO (FILM-COATED)				
20 mg, 30s ea	**58016-0066-30**	63.00		
60s ea	**58016-0066-60**	126.00		
90s ea	**58016-0066-90**	189.00		
100s ea	**58016-0066-00**	210.00		
40 mg, 30s ea	**58016-0053-30**	73.08		
60s ea	**58016-0053-60**	146.16		
90s ea	**58016-0053-90**	219.24		
100s ea	**58016-0053-00**	243.60		
BENICAR HCT (Daiichi Sankyo)				
hydrochlorothiazide/olmesartan medoxomil				
TAB, PO (FILM-COATED)				
12.5 mg-20 mg,				
30s ea	**65597-0105-30**	81.72		
90s ea	**65597-0105-90**	245.16		
12.5 mg-40 mg,				
30s ea	**65597-0106-30**	103.32		
90s ea	**65597-0106-90**	309.96		
25 mg-40 mg,				
30s ea	**65597-0107-30**	108.36		
90s ea	**65597-0107-90**	325.08		
(A-S Medication)				
REPACK				
TAB, PO (FILM-COATED)				
12.5 mg-40 mg,				
30s ea	**54569-5998-00**	92.63		
25 mg-40 mg,				
30s ea	**54569-5903-00**	104.63		
(PD-Rx Pharm)				
REPACK				
TAB, PO (FILM-COATED)				
25 mg-40 mg,				
30s ea	**55289-0443-30**	149.28		
(Phys Total Care)				
REPACK				
TAB, PO (FILM-COATED)				
12.5 mg-20 mg,				
30s ea	**54868-5170-00**	104.40		
90s ea	**54868-5170-01**	292.85		
(FILM-COATED)				
12.5 mg-40 mg,				
30s ea	**54868-5075-00**	117.47		
90s ea	**54868-5075-01**	329.24		
25 mg-40 mg,				
30s ea	**54868-5078-00**	132.37		
90s ea	**54868-5078-01**	371.46		
(Quality Care Prod)				
REPACK				
TAB, PO (FILM-COATED)				
12.5 mg-20 mg,				
30s ea	**35356-0256-30**	152.44		
90s ea	**35356-0256-90**	444.98		
12.5 mg-40 mg,				
30s ea	**35356-0257-30**	172.75		
90s ea	**35356-0257-90**	503.55		
25 mg-40 mg,				
30s ea	**35356-0258-30**	182.97		
90s ea	**35356-0258-90**	533.82		
BENOL (Amend)				
mineral oil				
OIL, NA (N.F.)				
19200 ml	**17317-1065-08**	84.00		
BENOXINATE HCL (PCCA)				
benoxinate hydrochloride				
POW, NA (U.S.P.)				
1 gm	**51927-2256-00**	196.80		
BENOXINATE HYDROCHLORIDE				
(PCCA) *See BENOXINATE HCL*				
BENOXINATE HYDROCHLORIDE/ FLUORESCEIN SODIUM				
(Akorn) *See FLURESS*				
(Altaire) *See BENOXINATE/FLUORESCEIN*				
(Bausch & Lomb Inc.) *See BENOXINATE/FLUORESCEIN*				
(HUB Pharma) *See FLUORESCEIN SODIUM AND BENOXINATE HYDROCHLORIDE*				
(Ocusoft) *See FLUROX*				
BENOXINATE HYDROCHLORIDE/ FLUOREXON DISODIUM				
(Altaire) *See FLURA-SAFE*				
BENOXINATE/FLUORESCEIN (Altaire)				
benoxinate hydrochloride/fluorescein sodium				
SOL, OP (W/STERILE DROPPER)				
0.4%-0.25%, 5 ml	**59390-0206-05**	11.81		

PROD/MFR	NDC	AWP	DP	OBC
(Bausch & Lomb Inc.)				
SOL, OP, 0.4%-0.25%,				
5 ml	**24208-0732-05**	11.81		
BENSAL HP (7 Oaks Pharma.)				
benzoic acid/salicylic acid				
OIN, TP (1X4GM)				
60 mg/gm-30 mg/gm,				
4 gm	**63801-0107-12**	48.69		
15 gm	**63801-0107-09**	159.34		
30 gm	**63801-0107-01**	273.63		
BENTONITE (Amend)				
POW, NA (N.F.)				
500 gm	**17317-0046-01**	9.80		
2270 gm	**17317-0046-05**	29.40		
11350 gm	**17317-0046-08**	113.75		
(Gallipot) *See BENTONITE GRAY*				
(Gallipot) *See BENTONITE WHITE*				
(PCCA)				
POW, NA (N.F.)				
1 gm	**51927-1195-00**	0.09		
(Spectrum Pharmacy) *See BENTONITE MAGMA*				
(Spectrum Pharmacy)				
POW, NA (N.F.)				
500 gm	**49452-0920-01**	72.10		
2500 gm	**49452-0920-02**	205.10		
BENTONITE GRAY (Gallipot)				
bentonite				
POW, NA (U.S.P.,N.F.)				
454 gm	**51552-0091-06**	9.52		
BENTONITE MAGMA (Spectrum Pharmacy)				
bentonite				
LIQ, NA (N.F.)				
500 ml	**49452-0910-01**	160.65		
BENTONITE WHITE (Gallipot)				
bentonite				
POW, NA (U.S.P.,N.F.)				
113.4 gm	**51552-0135-04**	5.95		
454 gm	**51552-0135-06**	13.93		
BENTYL (Axcan)				
dicyclomine hydrochloride				
CAP, PO, 10 mg, 100s ea	**58914-0012-10**	47.88		AB
SOL, IM (AMP)				
10 mg/ml, 2 ml 5s	**58914-0080-52**	122.78		AP
SYR, PO, 10 mg/5 ml,				
480 ml	**58914-0015-16**	53.18		AA
TAB, PO, 20 mg, 100s ea	**58914-0013-10**	68.32		AB
(Pharma Pac)				
REPACK				
TAB, PO, 20 mg, 30s ea	**52959-0390-30**	15.01		AB
(Phys Total Care)				
REPACK				
TAB, PO, 20 mg, 30s ea	**54868-0392-01**	19.41		AB
BENZAC AC (Galderma)				
benzoyl peroxide				
GEL, TP, 5%, 60 gm	**00299-3625-60**	93.13		
10%, 60 gm	**00299-3630-60**	93.13		
(Phys Total Care)				
REPACK				
GEL, TP, 2.5%, 90 gm	**54868-2392-01**	24.32		
LIQ, TP, 5%, 90 ml	**54868-2393-01**	27.35		
240 ml	**54868-2691-01**	27.35		
10%, 60 ml	**54868-2394-01**	21.57		
90 ml	**54868-2394-02**	28.65		
240 ml	**54868-2689-01**	30.03		
BENZAC AC 5 (DHS, Inc.)				
REPACK				
benzoyl peroxide				
GEL, TP, 5%, 60 gm	**55887-0317-60**	19.48		
BENZAC AC WASH (Galderma)				
benzoyl peroxide				
LIQ, TP, 5%, 226 ml	**00299-3640-08**	137.50		
10%, 240 ml	**00299-3645-08**	137.50		
(Phys Total Care)				
REPACK				
LIQ, TP, 2.5%, 240 ml	**54868-2690-01**	24.25		
BENZAC W (Phys Total Care)				
benzoyl peroxide				
GEL, TP, 5%, 60 gm	**54868-2396-00**	24.50		
10%, 60 gm	**54868-2397-01**	21.42		
BENZAC W WASH (Galderma)				
benzoyl peroxide				
LIQ, TP, 5%, 226 ml	**00299-3670-08**	137.50		
10%, 240 ml	**00299-3672-08**	137.50		

PROD/MFR	NDC	AWP	DP	OBC
BENZACLIN (Dermik)				
benzoyl peroxide/clindamycin phosphate				
GEL, TP, 5%-1%, 25 gm (1X35GM)	00066-0494-25	106.16		
5%-1%, 35 gm (1X50GM)	00066-0494-35	148.68		
5%-1%, 50 gm (W/PUMP)	00066-0495-55	181.16		
5%-1%, 50 gm	00066-0494-55	181.16		
(A-S Medication) REPACK				
GEL, TP, 5%-1%, 25 gm	54569-5259-00	90.21		
(Phys Total Care) REPACK				
GEL, TP (1X25GM)				
5%-1%, 25 gm	54868-4650-01	118.54		
50 gm (1X50GM+20AMPULES)	54868-4650-00	206.09		
5%-1%, 50 gm	54868-6062-00	216.41		
(Quality Care Prod) REPACK				
GEL, TP (1X50GM,PUMP KIT)				
5%-1%, 50 gm	35356-0220-50	321.10		
BENZACOT (Truxton)				
trimethobenzamide hydrochloride				
SOL, IM (VIAL)				
100 mg/ml, 20 ml	00463-1108-20	14.40		EE
BENZALDEHYDE (Amend)				
LIQ, NA (N.F.)				
500 ml	17317-0047-01	21.00		
(Baker, J.T.)				
LIQ, NA (REAGENT)				
500 ml	10106-9144-01	39.71		
(Gallipot)				
LIQ, NA (U.S.P.)				
100 ml	51552-0241-05	8.75		
473 ml	51552-0241-06	34.65		
(PCCA)				
LIQ, NA (NF)				
1 ml	51927-1198-00	0.38		
(Spectrum Pharmacy)				
LIQ, NA (N.F.)				
500 ml	49452-0930-01	100.45		
4000 ml	49452-0930-02	367.50		
BENZALKONIUM CHLORIDE				
(Amend) *See BENZALKONIUM CHLORIDE 17%*				
(Amend) *See BENZALKONIUM CHLORIDE 50%*				
(Gallipot) *See BENZALKONIUM CHLORIDE 17%*				
(Gallipot) *See BENZALKONIUM CHLORIDE 50%*				
(Letco) *See BENZALKONIUM CHLORIDE 17%*				
(Letco)				
SOL, NA, 17%, 500 ml	62991-2011-02	66.00		
(Medisca)				
SOL, NA (1X100ML)				
100 ml (1X500ML)	38779-0264-05	31.50		
500 ml (1X1000ML)	38779-0264-08	72.00		
1000 ml	38779-0264-09	84.00		
(PCCA)				
POW, NA (NF)				
1 gm	51927-3219-00	1.95		
SOL, NA, 1 ml	51927-1568-00	0.32		
(Spectrum Pharmacy) *See BENZALKONIUM CHLORIDE 17%*				
(Spectrum Pharmacy) *See BENZALKONIUM CHLORIDE 50%*				
BENZALKONIUM CHLORIDE 17% (Amend)				
benzalkonium chloride				
SOL, NA (N.F.)				
500 ml	17317-1860-01	11.20		
3840 ml	17317-1860-06	44.80		
20000 ml	17317-1860-08	210.00		
(Gallipot)				
SOL, NA (N.F.)				
473 ml	51552-0648-06	13.16		
3785 ml	51552-0648-08	75.32		
(Letco)				
SOL, NA, 120 ml	62991-2011-01	38.85		
(Spectrum Pharmacy)				
SOL, NA, 500 ml	49452-0940-01	134.40		
4000 ml	49452-0940-02	700.00		
BENZALKONIUM CHLORIDE 50% (Amend)				
benzalkonium chloride				
SOL, NA (N.F.)				
500 ml	17317-0048-01	16.80		
3840 ml	17317-0048-06	70.00		
20000 ml	17317-0048-08	245.00		
(Gallipot)				
SOL, NA (U.S.P.,N.F.)				
118.28 ml	51552-0153-04	12.11		
473 ml	51552-0153-06	24.71		
3785 ml	51552-0153-08	114.80		
(Spectrum Pharmacy)				
SOL, NA (N.F.)				
500 ml	49452-0950-01	121.45		
4000 ml	49452-0950-02	423.50		
BENZALKONIUM CL/CHLOROXYLENOL/ HC/PRAMOXINE HCL				
(A. G. Marin) *See OTOMAX HC*				
(Everett) *See CORTIC-ND*				
(Marnel) *See OTOMAR-HC*				
BENZAMYCIN (Dermik)				
benzoyl peroxide/erythromycin				
GEL, TP, 5%-3%, 46.6 gm	00066-0510-46	227.53		
(Pharma Pac) REPACK				
GEL, TP, 5%-3%, 23.3 gm	52959-0259-01	30.57		
(Phys Total Care) REPACK				
GEL, TP, 5%-3%, 24 gm	54868-2246-00	56.95		
46.6 gm	54868-2246-01	139.09		
BENZAMYCIN PAK (Dermik)				
benzoyl peroxide/erythromycin				
GEL, TP (GEL)				
5%-3%, 60s ea	00066-0577-60	142.09		
(A-S Medication) REPACK				
GEL, TP (GEL)				
5%-3%, 60s ea	54569-5478-00	135.79		
(Dispensing Solutions) REPACK				
GEL, TP, 5%-3%, 60s ea	55045-3694-06	115.00		
BENZASHAVE (Doak)				
benzoyl peroxide				
CRE, TP (MEDICATED SHAVE CREAM)				
5%, 113.4 gm	10337-0805-41	83.29		
10%, 113.4 gm	10337-0806-41	90.83		
BENZEFOAM (Onset)				
benzoyl peroxide				
FOA, TP (1X60GM)				
5.3%, 60 gm	16781-0194-60	173.12	173.12	
BENZENE				
(PCCA) *See BENZENE ACS CERTIFIED*				
BENZENE ACS CERTIFIED (PCCA)				
benzene				
SOL, NA (1X1ML)				
1 ml	51927-1579-00	0.24		
BENZETHONIUM CHLORIDE				
(Amend) *See HYAMINE 1622*				
(Amend)				
POW, NA (U.S.P.)				
454 gm	17317-0728-01	70.00		
2270 gm	17317-0728-05	315.00		
(PCCA)				
POW, NA (U.S.P.)				
1 gm	51927-2978-00	1.05		
(Spectrum Pharmacy)				
POW, NA (U.S.P.)				
125 gm	49452-0960-01	189.70		
500 gm	49452-0960-02	427.00		
BENZIQ (Graceway)				
benzoyl peroxide				
GEL, TP, 5.25%, 50 gm	29336-0240-50	83.18		
BENZIQ LS (Graceway)				
benzoyl peroxide				
GEL, TP, 2.75%, 50 gm	13453-0225-50	84.54		
BENZIQ WASH (Graceway)				
benzoyl peroxide				
SOL, TP (1X175GM)				
5.25%, 175 gm	29336-0210-18	80.09		
BENZO/CETYLPYRIDINIUM CL/MENTHOL/ZN CL				
(Gil Pharmaceutical) *See BUCALSEP*				
(Seyer Pharmatec) *See BUCALCIDE*				
BENZOCAINE				
(Athlon Pharm) *See OMEDIA*				
(Baker, J.T.)				
POW, NA (FINE, U.S.P.)				
500 gm	10106-1080-01	47.35		
(Gallipot)				
POW, NA (U.S.P.,N.F.)				
28.35 gm	51552-0130-02	10.57		
113.4 gm	51552-0130-04	16.80		
454 gm	51552-0130-06	49.21		
(Gordon) *See ANACAINE*				
(Hawkins)				
POW, NA (U.S.P.)				
25 gm	63370-0031-25	33.60		
100 gm	63370-0031-35	57.60		
500 gm	63370-0031-45	148.80		
(Letco)				
POW, NA (U.S.P./N.F.)				
100 gm (U.S.P.)	62991-1021-02	33.00		
500 gm	62991-1021-04	75.00		
(Medisca)				
POW, NA (U.S.P.)				
25 gm	38779-0063-04	25.50		
100 gm	38779-0063-05	37.50		
500 gm	38779-0063-08	128.10		
1000 gm	38779-0063-09	225.00		
(PCCA)				
POW, NA, 1 gm	51927-1194-00	0.96		
(Spectrum Pharmacy)				
POW, NA (U.S.P.)				
125 gm	49452-0970-01	64.40		
500 gm	49452-0970-02	182.70		
2500 gm	49452-0970-03	759.50		
BENZOCAINE/BUTAMBEN/TETRACAINE				
(Cetylite) *See CETACAINE*				
(Onset) *See EXACTACAIN*				
BENZOCAINE/BUTAMBEN/TETRACAINE HYDROCHLORIDE				
(Healthpoint) *See EXACTACAIN*				
BENZOCAINE/CHLOROXYLENOL/ HYDROCORTISONE ACETATE				
(Vertical) *See TRIOXIN*				
BENZOCAINE/ TRIMETHOBENZAMIDE HYDROCHLORIDE				
(Consolidated Midland) *See TRIMETHOBENZAMIDE HCL*				
(Intl Ethical) *See NAVOGAN*				
BENZOIC ACID (Amend)				
CRY, NA (U.S.P.)				
125 gm	17317-0050-04	7.00		
500 gm	17317-0050-01	18.20		
2270 gm	17317-0050-05	56.00		
11350 gm	17317-0050-08	175.00		
(Baker, J.T.)				
CRY, NA (U.S.P., F.C.C.)				
500 gm	10106-0080-01	51.10		
(Gallipot)				
CRY, NA (U.S.P.,N.F.)				
454 gm	51552-0225-06	23.24		
(Mallinckrodt Lab)				
CRY, NA (U.S.P.)				
500 gm	00406-0108-03	74.05		
(Medisca)				
CRY, NA (U.S.P.)				
100 gm	38779-0615-05	28.50		
500 gm (USP,1X2500GM)	38779-0615-08	52.50		
2500 gm	38779-0615-01	153.00		
(PCCA)				
POW, NA (USP)				
1 gm	51927-1114-00	0.32		
(Spectrum Pharmacy)				
CRY, NA (U.S.P.,E.P.,B.P.,J.P.)				
500 gm (U.S.P.E.P.,B.P.,J.P.)	49452-0980-01	100.10		
2500 gm	49452-0980-02	304.15		
BENZOIC ACID/SALICYLIC ACID				
(7 Oaks Pharma.) *See BENSAL HP*				
BENZOIN (Amend)				
TIN, NA (N.F.)				
120 ml	17317-0052-04	3.50		
500 ml	17317-0052-01	10.50		
4000 ml	17317-0052-06	58.80		

PROD/MFR	NDC	AWP	DP	OBC
(Gallipot)				
TIN, NA (N.F.)				
15 ml	51552-0177-01	3.01		
60 ml	51552-0177-03	4.76		
118.28 ml	51552-0177-04	7.28		
473 ml	51552-0177-06	16.59		
(Medisca) *See BENZOIN TINCTURE*				
(PCCA) *See BENZOIN GUM*				
(PCCA)				
TIN, NA (NF,ALCOHOL 75-83%)				
1 ml	51927-1420-00	0.12		
(Spectrum Pharmacy)				
TIN, NA, 500 ml	49452-1000-01	88.90		
4000 ml	49452-1000-02	388.50		
BENZOIN COMPOUND (Amend)				
TIN, NA (U.S.P.)				
120 ml	17317-0054-04	3.50		
500 ml	17317-0054-01	10.50		
4000 ml	17317-0054-06	58.80		
(Gallipot)				
TIN, NA (U.S.P.,N.F.)				
118.28 ml	51552-0228-04	5.81		
473 ml	51552-0228-06	16.59		
3785 ml	51552-0228-08	74.41		
(PCCA) *See COMPOUND BENZOIN*				
(Spectrum Pharmacy)				
TIN, NA (U.S.P.)				
500 ml	49452-0990-01	192.50		
4000 ml	49452-0990-02	857.50		
BENZOIN COMPOUND/PODOPHYLLUM				
(Paddock) *See PODOCON-25*				
BENZOIN GUM (PCCA)				
benzoin				
POW, NA (1X1GM)				
1 gm	51927-2054-00	3.00		
BENZOIN TINCTURE (Medisca)				
benzoin				
TIN, NA (ALCOHOL 75-83%,1X500ML)				
500 ml	38779-1027-08	52.50		
BENZONATATE				
FUL				
SGL, PO, 100 mg, 100s ea		43.87		
200 mg, 100s ea		24.60		
(Amneal)				
SGL, PO (USP,SOFT GELATIN)				
100 mg, 100s ea	65162-0536-10	101.33		AA
500s ea	65162-0536-50	504.44		AA
200 mg, 100s ea	65162-0537-10	197.73		AA
(Ascend)				
SGL, PO (USP,SOFT GELATIN)				
100 mg, 100s ea	67877-0105-01	102.10		
200 mg, 100s ea	67877-0106-01	199.75		
(Caraco)				
SGL, PO (USP,SOFTGEL)				
100 mg, 100s ea	57664-0133-88	95.48		AA
200 mg, 100s ea	57664-0134-88	197.73		AA
(Ethex)				
SGL, PO (USP,10X10,SOFT GELATIN)				
100 mg, 100s ea UD	58177-0091-11	129.27		
(USP,SOFT GELATIN)				
100 mg, 100s ea	58177-0091-04	101.33		
500s ea	58177-0091-08	504.44		
200 mg, 100s ea	58177-0092-04	197.73		
(Forest Pharm) *See TESSALON PERLES*				
(Inwood)				
SGL, PO, 100 mg, 100s ea	00258-3654-01	95.48		AA
(Major)				
SGL, PO (USP,SOFT GELATIN)				
100 mg, 100s ea	00904-5904-60	76.45		
500s ea	00904-5904-40	614.14		
200 mg, 100s ea	00904-5905-60	76.40		
(Provident)				
SGL, PO (USP)				
100 mg, 100s ea	20091-0536-01	98.41		
500s ea	20091-0536-05	478.99		
200 mg, 100s ea	20091-0537-01	196.82		
(Teva)				
SGL, PO, 100 mg, 100s ea	00182-1080-01	77.19		AA
(SOFTGEL)				
100 mg, 100s ea	50111-0851-01	101.33		AA
500s ea	50111-0851-02	504.44		AA
(USP,SOFTGEL)				
200 mg, 100s ea	00555-1883-02	197.72		

PROD/MFR	NDC	AWP	DP	OBC
(Zydus Pharm.)				
SGL, PO (USP,SOFT GELATIN)				
100 mg, 100s ea	68382-0247-01	101.33		AA
200 mg, 100s ea	68382-0248-01	197.73		AA
(A-S Medication)				
REPACK				
SGL, PO, 100 mg, 20s ea	54569-4091-00	20.27		EE
24s ea	54569-4091-01	24.32		EE
30s ea	54569-4091-02	30.40		EE
(SOFTGEL)				
200 mg, 30s ea	54569-5590-00	59.32		
(Altura)				
REPACK				
SGL, PO, 100 mg, 12s ea	63874-0530-12	9.89		EE
15s ea	63874-0530-15	12.29		EE
20s ea	63874-0530-20	16.38		EE
30s ea	63874-0530-30	24.57		EE
100s ea	63874-0530-01	82.43		EE
(American Health)				
REPACK				
SGL, PO (USP,10X10,SOFT GELATIN)				
100 mg, 100s ea UD	68084-0214-01	72.90		AA
(Bryant Ranch)				
REPACK				
SGL, PO, 100 mg, 20s ea	63629-2655-02	28.37		
30s ea	63629-2655-01	42.56		
(DHS, Inc.)				
REPACK				
SGL, PO (SOFTGEL)				
100 mg, 20s ea	55887-0816-20	21.00		AA
30s ea	55887-0816-30	31.50		AA
(Dispensing Solutions)				
REPACK				
SGL, PO, 100 mg, 15s ea	55045-2025-01	16.05		AA
15s ea	66336-0101-15	17.79		
(SOFT GELATIN)				
100 mg, 20s ea	66336-0101-20	23.72		
(SOFTGEL)				
100 mg, 20s ea	55045-2025-07	21.40		AA
30s ea	55045-3931-01	32.10		
30s ea	66336-0101-30	35.51		
(SOFTGEL)				
100 mg, 30s ea	55045-2025-08	32.10		AA
(HomeMed)				
REPACK				
SGL, PO, 100 mg, 9s ea	51655-0769-05	11.40		EE
(SOFTGEL)				
100 mg, 9s ea	51655-0769-85	11.40		
30s ea	51655-0769-24	24.19		EE
(Nucare Pharm)				
REPACK				
SGL, PO (SOFT GELATIN)				
100 mg, 15s ea	66267-0033-15	15.85		
20s ea	66267-0033-20	21.14		
21s ea	66267-0033-21	22.19		
30s ea	66267-0033-30	31.70		
(Palmetto)				
REPACK				
SGL, PO, 100 mg, 6s ea	23490-5124-01	13.52		
15s ea	23490-5124-02	24.18		
20s ea	23490-5124-03	32.24		
30s ea	23490-5124-04	48.36		
(PD-Rx Pharm)				
REPACK				
SGL, PO (USP,SOFT GELATIN)				
100 mg, 6s ea	43063-0111-06	14.04		AA
(USP)				
100 mg, 10s ea	55289-0175-10	8.21		AA
12s ea	55289-0175-12	16.80		EE
20s ea	55289-0175-20	35.25		EE
21s ea	55289-0175-21	38.77		EE
30s ea	55289-0175-30	39.07		EE
(REDI-SCRIPT)				
100 mg, 30s ea	58864-0676-30	39.06		EE
(USP,SOFTGEL)				
200 mg, 21s ea	55289-0996-21	45.09		
30s ea	58864-0854-30	59.50		
(USP)				
200 mg, 30s ea	55289-0996-30	56.82		
(Pharma Pac)				
REPACK				
SGL, PO, 100 mg, 10s ea	52959-0411-10	13.90		EE
15s ea	52959-0411-15	18.55		EE
20s ea	52959-0411-20	21.48		EE
30s ea	52959-0411-30	30.66		EE
(Phys Total Care)				
REPACK				
SGL, PO, 100 mg, 15s ea	54868-3457-03	18.63		AA

PROD/MFR	NDC	AWP	DP	OBC
20s ea	54868-3457-00	23.82		EE
30s ea	54868-3457-01	34.26		EE
60s ea	54868-3457-02	65.49		EE
(SOFTGEL)				
100 mg, 60s ea	64868-3457-02	119.25		AA
200 mg, 20s ea	54868-4482-00	47.25		
(SOFTGEL)				
200 mg, 30s ea	54868-4482-01	69.39		
(SOFT GELATIN)				
200 mg, 90s ea	54868-4482-02	68.14		
(Physician Partner)				
REPACK				
SGL, PO, 100 mg, 10s ea	21695-0191-10	23.84		
20s ea	21695-0191-20	47.68		
(SOFTGEL)				
100 mg, 30s ea	21695-0191-30	60.80		AA
200 mg, 15s ea	21695-0760-15	59.32		
20s ea	21695-0760-20	79.09		
30s ea	21695-0760-30	118.09		
(Quality Care Prod)				
REPACK				
SGL, PO (SOFTGEL)				
100 mg, 20s ea	49999-0297-20	38.64		AA
30s ea	49999-0297-30	57.96		
50s ea	49999-0297-50	96.60		AA
(SOFTGEL)				
200 mg, 15s ea	49999-0552-15	49.90		
30s ea	49999-0552-30	59.76		
(Southwood)				
REPACK				
SGL, PO, 200 mg, 30s ea	58016-0098-30	78.10		
60s ea	58016-0098-60	156.20		
90s ea	58016-0098-90	234.30		
100s ea	58016-0098-00	260.33		
(Stat Rx)				
REPACK				
SGL, PO, 100 mg, 15s ea	16590-0031-15	24.00		
20s ea	16590-0031-20	32.00		
30s ea	16590-0031-30	48.00		
(SOFT GELATIN)				
200 mg, 30s ea	16590-0638-30	35.25		
(Vibranta)				
REPACK				
SGL, PO, 100 mg, 20s ea	57866-5995-01	23.64		
21s ea	57866-5995-05	24.77		
30s ea	57866-5995-03	48.36		
BENZOYL CHLORIDE				
(Baker, J.T.) *See BENZYL CHLORIDE*				
(Baker, J.T.)				
LIQ, NA (A.C.S., REAGENT)				
500 ml	10106-1066-01	91.26		
BENZOYL PEROXIDE				
(Acella) *See BPO 4% CREAMY WASH COMPLETE PACK*				
(Acella) *See BPO 4% GEL*				
(Acella) *See BPO 8% CREAMY WASH COMPLETE PACK*				
(Acella) *See BPO 8% GEL*				
(Actavis Mid Atlantic)				
PAD, TP, 3%, 30s ea	00472-0463-30	138.25		
60s ea	00472-0463-60	193.82		
6%, 30s ea	00472-0464-30	138.25		
60s ea	00472-0464-60	193.82		
9%, 30s ea	00472-0465-30	138.25		
60s ea	00472-0465-60	193.82		
SOA, TP (1X170.3GM)				
3%, 170.3 gm	00472-0469-06	54.37		
(1X340.2GM)				
3%, 340.2 gm	00472-0469-12	97.37		
(1X170.3GM)				
6%, 170.3 gm	00472-0470-06	56.01		
(1X340.2GM)				
6%, 340.2 gm	00472-0470-12	100.63		
(1X170.3GM)				
9%, 170.3 gm	00472-0471-06	58.08		
(1X340.2GM)				
9%, 340.2 gm	00472-0471-12	104.28		
(ATS) *See BREZE*				
(Consolidated Midland)				
GEL, TP, 5%, 45 gm	00223-4254-45	2.25		
10%, 45 gm	00223-4256-45	2.50		
LOT, TP, 5%, 30 ml	00223-4252-30	2.25		
10%, 30 ml	00223-4253-30	2.50		
(Doak) *See BENZASHAVE*				
(Doak) *See ZODERM*				
(Doak) *See ZODERM HYDRATING WASH*				
(Ferndale) *See CLINAC BPO*				

PROD/MFR NDC AWP DP OBC

(Fougera) *See BENZOYL PEROXIDE WASH*

(Fougera)
PAD, TP, 4.5%, 30s ea..... **18754-0752-10** 95.43
(SINGLE-USE)
6.5%, 30s ea......... **00168-0477-01** 75.18
8.5%, 30s ea......... **00168-0478-01** 75.25

(Galderma) *See BENZAC AC*

(Galderma) *See BENZAC AC WASH*

(Galderma) *See BENZAC W WASH*

(Gallipot) *See BENZOYL PEROXIDE HYDROUS*

(Glaxo) *See BREVOXYL-8*

(Graceway) *See BENZIQ*

(Graceway) *See BENZIQ LS*

(Graceway) *See BENZIQ WASH*

(Harris)
SOA, TP (1X148GM)
5%, 148 gm **67405-0425-05** 12.02
(1X237GM)
5%, 237 gm **67405-0425-08** 22.66
(1X148GM)
10%, 148 gm **67405-0430-05** 12.86
(1X237GM)
10%, 237 gm **67405-0430-08** 24.73

(Hawthorn Pharm) *See ZACLIR 4%*

(Hawthorn Pharm) *See ZACLIR 8%*

(Intendis, Inc.) *See NEOBENZ MICRO*

(Intendis, Inc.) *See NEOBENZ MICRO CREAM PLUS PACK*

(Intendis, Inc.) *See NEOBENZ MICRO SD*

(Intendis, Inc.) *See NEOBENZ MICRO WASH PLUS PACK*

(Medicis) *See TRIAZ*

(Medicis) *See TRIAZ CLEANSER*

(Medicis) *See TRIAZ FOAMING CLOTHS*

(Medimetriks) *See PACNEX*

(Onset) *See BENZEFOAM*

(PCCA) *See BENZOYL PEROXIDE 70%*

(Perrigo) *See BENZOYL PEROXIDE GEL*

(Perrigo) *See BENZOYL PEROXIDE WASH*

(Perrigo)
GEL, TP, 5%, 60 gm....... **45802-0995-96** 19.79
(1X60GM)
5%, 60 gm........... **45802-0910-96** 20.25
(1X90GM)
5%, 90 gm........... **45802-0910-01** 23.91
(1X60GM)
10%, 60 gm **45802-0921-96** 20.66
SOL, TP (1X227GM)
2.5%, 227 gm......... **45802-0907-34** 27.37

(Prasco Labs) *See LAVOCLEN-4*

(Prasco Labs) *See LAVOCLEN-4 ACNE WASH*

(Prasco Labs) *See LAVOCLEN-4 CREAMY WASH*

(Prasco Labs) *See LAVOCLEN-8*

(Prasco Labs) *See LAVOCLEN-8 ACNE WASH*

(Prasco Labs) *See LAVOCLEN-8 CREAMY WASH*

(Prasco Labs) *See OSCION*

(Prasco Labs) *See OSCION CLEANSER*

(PruGen) *See PR BENZOYL PEROXIDE*

(Ranbaxy Labs) *See DESQUAM-X 10*

(Ranbaxy Labs) *See DESQUAM-X 5*

(Seton) *See SE BPO WASH*

(Spectrum Pharmacy) *See BENZOYL PEROXIDE HYDROUS*

(Stiefel Labs) *See BREVOXYL-4*

(TriMarc Labs) *See BENZOYL PEROXIDE 10 GEL*

(TriMarc Labs) *See BENZOYL PEROXIDE 5 GEL*

(A-S Medication)
REPACK
GEL, TP, 2.5%, 60 gm..... **54569-5356-00** 19.79

(Altura)
REPACK
GEL, TP, 5%, 60 gm....... **63874-0827-60** 16.05

(Palmetto)
REPACK
GEL, TP, 5%, 60 gm....... **23490-5131-01** 33.22
10%, 60 gm **23490-5126-01** 34.89

(Phys Total Care)
REPACK
PAD, TP, 9%, 60s ea **54868-5940-00** 389.56
SOA, TP, 6%, 340.2 gm.... **54868-5939-00** 202.68
SOL, TP (CLEANSER)
8.5%, 400 ml **54868-5552-00** 190.23

BENZOYL PEROXIDE 10 GEL **(TriMarc Labs)**
benzoyl peroxide
GEL, TP, 10%, 60 gm...... **68752-0698-60** 15.50

(Pharma Pac)
REPACK
GEL, TP (1X60GM)
10%, 60 gm **52959-0959-02** 13.09

BENZOYL PEROXIDE 10 WASH **(PD-Rx Pharm)**
REPACK
benzoyl peroxide
SOA, TP, 10%, 227 gm **68752-0410-08** 30.60

BENZOYL PEROXIDE 5 GEL **(TriMarc Labs)**
benzoyl peroxide
GEL, TP (AQUEOUS BASE)
5%, 60 gm........... **68752-0692-60** 14.95

BENZOYL PEROXIDE 5 WASH **(PD-Rx Pharm)**
REPACK
benzoyl peroxide
SOA, TP, 5%, 227 gm **68752-0405-08** 27.90

BENZOYL PEROXIDE 70% **(PCCA)**
benzoyl peroxide
POW, NA (USP)
1 gm **51927-3085-00** 0.75

BENZOYL PEROXIDE AQUEOUS **(Phys Total Care)**
REPACK
benzoyl peroxide
GEL, TP, 10%, 60 gm...... **54868-2057-00** 70.05

BENZOYL PEROXIDE CLEANSER **(Fougera)**
benzoyl peroxide/urea
SOA, TP (1X400ML)
4.5%-10%, 400 ml ... **00168-0473-40** 61.45
6.5%-10%, 400 ml ... **00168-0474-40** 61.45
8.5%-10%, 400 ml ... **00168-0475-40** 63.53

BENZOYL PEROXIDE CREAMY WASH **(Phys Total Care)**
REPACK
benzoyl peroxide
SOA, TP, 4%, 170.1 gm.... **54868-5881-00** 58.54
(1X170.1GM)
8%, 170.1 gm........ **54868-5235-00** 60.85

BENZOYL PEROXIDE GEL **(Perrigo)**
benzoyl peroxide
GEL, TP (1X60GM,AQUEOUS BASE)
2.5%, 60 gm......... **45802-0905-96** 19.79

BENZOYL PEROXIDE HYDROUS **(Gallipot)**
benzoyl peroxide
POW, NA (U.S.P.,N.F.)
25 gm............... **51552-0521-04** 16.73
(U.S.P.)
113.4 gm **51552-0521-09** 31.78
(U.S.P.,N.F.)
454 gm.............. **51552-0521-06** 61.04

(Spectrum Pharmacy)
POW, NA (U.S.P.)
125 gm.............. **49452-1010-01** 126.35
500 gm.............. **49452-1010-02** 176.40

BENZOYL PEROXIDE WASH **(Fougera)**
benzoyl peroxide
SOL, TP (1X473ML)
5.75%, 473 ml **00168-0758-51** 103.26

(Perrigo)
LIQ, TP (1X227GM)
5%, 227 gm **45802-0913-34** 30.86
SOA, TP (1X113GM)
5%, 113 gm **45802-0913-26** 18.65
(1X142GM)
5%, 142 gm **45802-0913-01** 15.76
10%, 142 gm **45802-0918-01** 16.87
(1X227GM)
10%, 227 gm **45802-0918-34** 33.74

(Phys Total Care)
REPACK
LIQ, TP, 5%, 113 ml....... **54868-4450-01** 54.39
140 ml **54868-4450-00** 89.76

(Quality Care Prod)
REPACK
LIQ, TP, 10%, 240 ml **49999-0508-08** 42.81

BENZOYL PEROXIDE/CLINDAMYCIN PHOSPHATE
(Dermik) *See BENZACLIN*

(Mylan) *See CLINDAMYCIN/BENZOYL PEROXIDE*

(Stiefel Labs) *See DUAC CS*

(Valeant Pharm Intl) *See ACANYA*

BENZOYL PEROXIDE/ERYTHROMYCIN
(Dermik) *See BENZAMYCIN*

(Dermik) *See BENZAMYCIN PAK*

(Perrigo)
GEL, TP, 5%-3%, 23.3 gm . **45802-0083-02** 68.60
46.6 gm **45802-0083-86** 128.00

(Sandoz)
GEL, TP, 5%-3%, 23.3 gm . **00781-7054-49** 58.35
46.6 gm **00781-7054-59** 111.64

(Phys Total Care)
REPACK
GEL, TP (1X23.6GM)
5%-3%, 23.6 gm **54868-5617-00** 91.55

BENZOYL PEROXIDE/HYALURONATE SODIUM
(Hawthorn Pharm) *See ZACARE 4%*

(Hawthorn Pharm) *See ZACARE 8%*

BENZOYL PEROXIDE/HYDROCORTISONE
(Summers) *See VANOXIDE HC*

(Summers) *See VANOXIDE-HC*

BENZOYL PEROXIDE/SALICYLIC ACID
(Quinnova) *See CLEANSE & TREAT*

BENZOYL PEROXIDE/SULFUR
(Breckenridge Pharm) *See BPS GEL*

(Wraser Pharm) *See NUOX*

BENZOYL PEROXIDE/UREA
(Breckenridge Pharm) *See PERODERM*

(Breckenridge Pharm) *See PERODERM CLEANSER*

(Doak) *See ZODERM*

(Fougera) *See BENZOYL PEROXIDE CLEANSER*

BENZPHETAMINE HYDROCHLORIDE **(Boca Pharmacal)**
TAB, PO, 50 mg,
30s ea, C-III .... **64376-0650-31** 41.39 AA
90s ea, C-III .... **64376-0650-90** 124.17 AA
100s ea, C-III ...... **64376-0650-01** 131.07 AA
500s ea, C-III ...... **64376-0650-05** 655.33 AA

(CorePharma)
TAB, PO (FILM-COATED)
50 mg,
30s ea, C-III .... **64720-0194-03** 41.39 AA
100s ea, C-III ...... **64720-0194-10** 131.07 AA
500s ea, C-III ...... **64720-0194-50** 655.33 AA

(Global Pharm)
TAB, PO, 50 mg,
90s ea, C-III .... **00115-1205-10** 137.90 AA
100s ea, C-III ...... **00115-1205-01** 153.23 AA
500s ea, C-III ...... **00115-1205-02** 766.11 AA

(Paddock)
TAB, PO (FILM-COATED)
50 mg,
30s ea, C-III .... **00574-0116-30** 40.87 AA
100s ea, C-III ...... **00574-0116-01** 130.19 AA
500s ea, C-III ...... **00574-0116-05** 650.95 AA

(Pfizer) *See DIDREX*

(A-S Medication)
REPACK
TAB, PO, 50 mg,
30s ea, C-III .... **54569-5912-00** 40.60 AA
60s ea, C-III .... **54569-5912-01** 81.20 AA
90s ea, C-III .... **54569-5912-02** 121.80 AA
(FILM-COATED)
50 mg,
90s ea, C-III .... **54569-6078-00** 121.79 AA

(Dispensing Solutions)
REPACK
TAB, PO, 50 mg,
14s ea, C-III .... **66336-0992-14** 19.19 AA
30s ea, C-III .... **66336-0992-30** 41.13 AA
60s ea, C-III .... **66336-0992-60** 82.26 AA

PROD/MFR	NDC	AWP	DP	OBC
(Palmetto)				
REPACK				
TAB, PO, 50 mg,				
21s ea, C-III	**23490-5133-01**	30.13		
30s ea, C-III	**23490-5133-03**	46.04		
100s ea, C-III	**23490-5133-02**	138.19		
(PD-Rx Pharm)				
REPACK				
TAB, PO, 50 mg,				
14s ea, C-III	**55289-0158-14**	43.05		AA
60s ea, C-III	**55289-0158-60**	142.47		AA
90s ea, C-III	**55289-0158-90**	167.40		AA
BENZTROPINE (Southwood)				
REPACK				
benztropine mesylate				
TAB, PO, 1 mg, 30s ea	**58016-0018-30**	6.50		
60s ea	**58016-0018-60**	12.99		
90s ea	**58016-0018-90**	19.49		
100s ea	**58016-0018-00**	21.65		
BENZTROPINE MESYLATE				
FUL				
TAB, PO, 0.5 mg, 100s ea		7.47		
1 mg, 100s ea		8.48		
2 mg, 100s ea		12.08		
(Gallipot)				
POW, NA (1X1GM,USP)				
1 gm	**51552-0952-01**	24.50	17.50	
(Lundbeck) *See COGENTIN*				
(Major)				
TAB, PO, 0.5 mg, 100s ea (10X10)	**00904-1055-60**	18.75		AA
0.5 mg, 100s ea UD	**00904-1055-61**	20.83		AA
1 mg, 100s ea (10X10)	**00904-1056-60**	21.74		AA
1 mg, 100s ea UD	**00904-1056-61**	23.93		AA
1000s ea	**00904-1056-80**	213.84		AA
2 mg, 100s ea (10X10)	**00904-1057-60**	27.03		AA
2 mg, 100s ea UD	**00904-1057-61**	30.03		AA
1000s ea	**00904-1057-80**	269.87		AA
(Medisca)				
POW, NA (U.S.P.)				
1 gm	**38779-0194-06**	32.85		
5 gm	**38779-0194-03**	129.30		
25 gm	**38779-0194-04**	597.00		
(Nexus)				
SOL, IJ (5X2ML,USP,SDV)				
1 mg/ml, 2 ml 5s	**14789-0300-02**	343.75	275.00	AP
(PCCA)				
POW, NA (USP,1X1GM)				
1 gm	**51927-2421-00**	186.00		
(Qualitest)				
TAB, PO (USP)				
0.5 mg, 100s ea	**00603-2433-21**	18.94		AA
1000s ea	**00603-2433-32**	185.65		AA
1 mg, 100s ea	**00603-2434-21**	21.64		AA
1000s ea	**00603-2434-32**	216.00		AA
2 mg, 100s ea	**00603-2435-21**	27.31		AA
1000s ea	**00603-2435-32**	272.60		AA
(Rising)				
TAB, PO, 0.5 mg, 100s ea (USP,COMPRESSED)	**64980-0111-01**	18.94		AA
0.5 mg, 1000s ea	**64980-0111-10**	180.00		AA
1 mg, 100s ea	**64980-0112-01**	21.65		AA
1000s ea	**64980-0112-10**	216.00		AA
2 mg, 100s ea	**64980-0113-01**	27.31		AA
1000s ea	**64980-0113-10**	272.60		AA
(Spectrum Pharmacy)				
CRY, NA (U.S.P.)				
1 gm	**49452-1016-01**	88.55		
5 gm	**49452-1016-02**	285.60		
25 gm	**49452-1016-03**	1165.50		
(Teva)				
TAB, PO, 0.5 mg, 100s ea	**50111-0393-01**	18.94		
1 mg, 100s ea	**50111-0394-01**	19.26		
1000s ea	**50111-0394-03**	183.00		
2 mg, 100s ea	**50111-0395-01**	24.29		
1000s ea	**50111-0395-03**	230.87		
(UDL)				
TAB, PO (10X10,USP)				
0.5 mg, 100s ea UD (1X25)	**51079-0404-20**	26.07		AA
1 mg, 25s ea UD (10X10)	**51079-0406-19**	8.11		AA
1 mg, 100s ea UD (10X10,USP)	**51079-0406-20**	25.74		AA
2 mg, 100s ea UD	**51079-0407-20**	32.03		AA
(Upsher-Smith)				
TAB, PO, 0.5 mg, 100s ea	**00832-1080-00**	18.42		AA
1000s ea	**00832-1080-10**	184.26		AA
1 mg, 100s ea	**00832-1081-00**	19.48		AA
1000s ea	**00832-1081-10**	185.06		AA
2 mg, 100s ea	**00832-1082-00**	24.71		AA
1000s ea	**00832-1082-10**	234.75		AA
(West-Ward)				
SOL, IJ (5X2ML,USP)				
1 mg/ml, 2 ml 5s	**00143-9729-05**	375.00		AP
(Altura)				
REPACK				
TAB, PO, 2 mg, 12s ea	**63874-0565-12**	3.20		EE
15s ea	**63874-0565-15**	4.01		EE
20s ea	**63874-0565-20**	5.34		EE
30s ea	**63874-0565-30**	8.02		EE
100s ea	**63874-0565-01**	26.72		EE
(American Health)				
REPACK				
TAB, PO, 0.5 mg,				
100s ea UD	**68084-0381-01**	12.50		AA
(Dispensing Solutions)				
REPACK				
TAB, PO, 1 mg, 30s ea	**55045-3279-08**	9.00		AA
(HomeMed)				
REPACK				
TAB, PO, 1 mg, 30s ea	**51655-0233-24**	5.24		EE
60s ea	**51655-0233-25**	7.60		EE
2 mg, 30s ea	**51655-0234-24**	4.02		EE
(McKesson Packaging)				
REPACK				
TAB, PO, 1 mg, 100s ea UD (BLISTER PACK)	**63739-0034-10**	26.85		AA
1 mg, 750s ea UD	**63739-0034-01**	201.38		AA
2 mg, 100s ea UD	**63739-0035-10**	27.89		AA
(Palmetto)				
REPACK				
TAB, PO, 2 mg, 30s ea	**23490-5136-01**	13.99		
(PD-Rx Pharm)				
REPACK				
TAB, PO (REDI-SCRIPT)				
1 mg, 6s ea	**58864-0055-06**	13.90		AA
2 mg, 30s ea	**58864-0056-30**	26.00		AA
(Phys Total Care)				
REPACK				
TAB, PO, 1 mg, 30s ea	**54868-2301-02**	11.94		EE
1000s ea	**54868-2301-00**	72.12		EE
2 mg, 30s ea	**54868-2292-02**	5.92		EE
1000s ea	**54868-2292-00**	89.19		EE
(Physician Partner)				
REPACK				
TAB, PO, 2 mg, 30s ea	**21695-0286-30**	16.39		AA
(Vibranta)				
REPACK				
TAB, PO, 1 mg, 30s ea	**57866-3371-01**	6.20		AA
60s ea	**57866-3371-02**	10.94		AA
90s ea	**57866-3371-03**	15.86		AA
120s ea	**57866-3371-04**	20.71		AA
2 mg, 30s ea	**57866-3372-01**	7.79		AA
60s ea	**57866-3372-02**	14.48		AA
90s ea	**57866-3372-03**	21.17		AA
120s ea	**57866-3372-04**	27.86		AA
BENZYL ALCOHOL				
(Amend) *See ALCOHOL BENZYL*				
(Baker, J.T.) *See ALCOHOL BENZYL*				
(Gallipot) *See ALCOHOL BENZYL*				
(Letco) *See ALCOHOL BENZYL*				
(Letco)				
SOL, NA (NF)				
3840 ml	**62991-1318-02**	150.00		
(Mallinckrodt Lab) *See ALCOHOL BENZYL*				
(Medisca)				
SOL, NA (1X500ML)				
500 ml (1X4000ML)	**38779-1029-08**	58.50		
4000 ml	**38779-1029-01**	271.50		
(PCCA)				
SOL, NA (NF)				
1 ml	**51927-1391-00**	0.15		
(Shionogi) *See ULESFIA*				
(Spectrum Pharmacy) *See ALCOHOL BENZYL*				
BENZYL BENZOATE (Letco)				
SOL, NA (U.S.P.)				
99%, 480 ml	**62991-1645-01**	40.50		
(Medisca)				
LIQ, NA (U.S.P)				
500 ml (USP,1X1000ML)	**38779-1030-08**	46.50		
1000 ml (U.S.P.)	**38779-1030-09**	70.50		
4000 ml	**38779-1030-01**	226.50		
(PCCA)				
LIQ, NA (U.S.P.)				
1 ml	**51927-1422-00**	0.25		
(Spectrum Pharmacy)				
LIQ, NA (U.S.P.)				
500 ml	**49452-1025-01**	73.50		
4000 ml	**49452-1025-02**	360.50		
BENZYL CHLORIDE (Baker, J.T.)				
benzoyl chloride				
LIQ, NA (STABILIZED, REAGENT)				
500 ml	**10106-1076-01**	121.90		
4-BENZYLOXYPHENOL (Spectrum Pharmacy)				
monobenzone				
POW, NA, 5 gm	**49452-1037-03**	98.70		
50 gm	**49452-1037-01**	329.35		
250 gm	**49452-1037-02**	1151.50		
BENZYLPENICILLOYL POLYLYSINE				
(Alk-Abello) *See PRE-PEN*				
BEPOTASTINE BESILATE				
(ISTA Pharm.) *See BEPREVE*				
BEPREVE (ISTA Pharm.)				
bepotastine besilate				
SOL, OP, 15 mg/ml, 10 ml	**67425-0007-75**	112.50	90.00	
BERACTANT				
(Abbott Pharm) *See SURVANTA*				
BERBERINE HCL (PCCA)				
berberine hydrochloride				
POW, NA (HYDRATE)				
1 gm	**51927-2574-00**	8.70		
BERBERINE HYDROCHLORIDE				
(PCCA) *See BERBERINE HCL*				
BERGAMOT OIL (Amend)				
OIL, NA (IMITATION)				
30 ml (TRUE)	**17317-0229-02**	4.20		
30 ml (IMITATION)	**17317-0230-02**	10.50		
120 ml (TRUE)	**17317-0229-04**	11.20		
120 ml (IMITATION)	**17317-0230-04**	28.00		
500 ml (TRUE)	**17317-0229-01**	29.40		
500 ml	**17317-0230-01**	84.00		
(Lorann Oil)				
OIL, NA, 9.9 ml	**23535-0151-06**	8.50		
(PCCA)				
OIL, NA (FRAGRANCE)				
1 ml	**51927-2458-00**	0.38		
(Spectrum Pharmacy)				
OIL, NA (1X25ML,NATURAL)				
25 ml (1X100ML,NATURAL)	**49452-1050-01**	72.75		
100 ml (1X500ML,NATURAL)	**49452-1050-02**	194.95		
500 ml	**49452-1050-03**	770.00		
BERINERT (CSL)				
c1 esterase inhibitor, human				
PDS, IV (500U VIAL, 10ML DILUENT)				
500 u, ea	**63833-0825-02**	2070.00		
BESIFLOXACIN HYDROCHLORIDE				
(Bausch & Lomb Inc.) *See BESIVANCE*				
BESIVANCE (Bausch & Lomb Inc.)				
besifloxacin hydrochloride				
SUS, OP, 0.6%, 5 ml	**24208-0446-05**	83.18		
BETA AMYLASE (PCCA)				
POW, NA, 1 gm	**51927-3477-00**	9.60		
BETA CAROTENE (Medisca)				
POW, NA (U.S.P.)				
5 gm	**38779-0414-03**	61.50		
25 gm	**38779-0414-04**	184.50		
(PCCA)				
BEA, NA (WS,167 IU/MG,BEADLETS)				
10%, 1 gm	**51927-2356-00**	1.38		
BETA GLUCAN (PCCA)				
POW, NA (NQ)				
1 gm	**51927-2949-00**	60.00		

PROD/MFR	NDC	AWP	DP	OBC
BETA NAPHTHOL (Amend)				
naphthol				
SOL, NA (PURIFIED)				
454 gm	17317-0058-01	14.00		
2270 gm	17317-0058-05	56.00		
BETA SITOSTEROL (PCCA)				
POW, NA (40% GRANULAR)				
1 gm	51927-3516-00	0.84		
BETA-NICOTINAMIDE ADENINE DINUCLEOTIDE				
(Spectrum Pharmacy)				
nadide				
POW, NA (1X0.25GM)				
0.25 gm	49452-1082-01	177.80		
(1X1GM)				
1 gm	49452-1082-02	437.50		
1 gm	49452-4851-02	133.35		
(1X5GM)				
5 gm	49452-1082-03	1620.50		
5 gm	49452-4851-03	539.00		
(1X25GM)				
25 gm	49452-4851-04	1557.50		
BETA-VAL (Teva)				
betamethasone valerate				
CRE, TP, 0.1%, 15 gm	00093-0673-15	4.85		AB
45 gm	00093-0673-95	8.03		AB
LOT, TP, 0.1%, 60 ml	00093-0671-39	11.45		AB
BETADEX				
(PCCA) *See CYCLODEXTRIN*				
BETADINE (Alcon Surgical)				
povidone iodine				
SOL, OP (STERILE)				
5%, 30 ml 24s	00065-0411-30	293.76		
BETAGAN (Allergan Inc)				
levobunolol hydrochloride				
SOL, OP (B.I.D. C CAP)				
0.25%, 5 ml	00023-4526-05	24.58		AT
0.5%, 2 ml	11980-0252-02	12.65		AT
5 ml	00023-4385-05	30.48		AT
10 ml	00023-4385-10	63.38		AT
15 ml	00023-4385-15	92.38		AT
(Phys Total Care)				
REPACK				
SOL, OP, 0.5%, 5 ml	54868-0629-01	26.55		AT
(B.I.D. C CAP)				
0.5%, 5 ml	54868-2624-01	29.33		AT
15 ml	54868-2624-00	105.40		AT
BETAHISTINE DIHYDROCHLORIDE (PCCA)				
betahistine hydrochloride				
POW, NA, 1 gm	51927-1882-00	75.00		
(Spectrum Pharmacy)				
POW, NA (1X5GM)				
5 gm	49452-1065-01	147.00		
(1X25GM)				
25 gm	49452-1065-02	528.50		
(1X100GM)				
100 gm	49452-1065-03	1445.50		
BETAHISTINE HYDROCHLORIDE				
(PCCA) *See BETAHISTINE DIHYDROCHLORIDE*				
(Spectrum Pharmacy) *See BETAHISTINE DIHYDROCHLORIDE*				
BETAINE				
(Medisca) *See BETAINE ANHYDROUS*				
(PCCA) *See BETAINE MONOHYDRATE*				
(PCCA)				
POW, NA (BASE; ANHYDROUS)				
1 gm	51927-2548-00	1.17		
(Rare Disease) *See CYSTADANE*				
(Spectrum Pharmacy) *See BETAINE ANHYDROUS*				
BETAINE ANHYDROUS (Medisca)				
betaine				
POW, NA, 100 gm	38779-1040-05	46.50		
500 gm	38779-1040-08	112.50		
(Spectrum Pharmacy)				
POW, NA, 100 gm	49452-0803-01	85.75		
500 gm	49452-0803-02	186.20		
BETAINE HYDROCHLORIDE (Amend)				
POW, NA (U.S.P.)				
454 gm	17317-0845-01	21.00		
2270 gm	17317-0845-05	84.00		
11350 gm	17317-0845-08	280.00		
(PCCA)				
POW, NA (USP)				
1 gm	51927-1557-00	0.53		
(Spectrum Pharmacy)				
POW, NA (U.S.P.)				
100 gm	49452-1055-01	81.55		
1000 gm	49452-1055-02	324.45		
BETAINE MONOHYDRATE (PCCA)				
betaine				
POW, NA, 1 gm	51927-3594-00	1.65		
BETAMETHASONE				
(Schering) *See CELESTONE*				
(Spectrum Pharmacy)				
POW, NA (U.S.P.)				
0.025 gm	49452-1070-04	128.45		
0.1 gm	49452-1070-05	413.00		
0.5 gm	49452-1070-06	1120.00		
BETAMETHASONE ACE/BETAMETHASONE NA PHOS				
(PharmaForce) *See BETAMETHASONE SODIUM PHOSPHATE-BETAMETHASONE ACE*				
(Schering) *See CELESTONE SOLUSPAN*				
BETAMETHASONE ACETATE MICRONIZED (Gallipot)				
betamethasone acetate, micronized				
POW, NA (U.S.P.)				
1 gm	51552-0628-01	55.44		
(Hawkins)				
POW, NA (U.S.P.)				
1 gm	63370-0032-10	168.00		
5 gm	63370-0032-15	696.00		
25 gm	63370-0032-25	2496.00		
100 gm	63370-0032-35	8640.00		
(Letco)				
POW, NA (U.S.P., 24)				
25 gm	62991-2501-02	870.00		
100 gm	62991-2501-01	3378.00		
(Medisca)				
POW, NA (U.S.P.)				
1 gm	38779-0126-06	108.00		
5 gm	38779-0126-03	462.00		
10 gm	38779-0126-01	765.00		
25 gm	38779-0126-04	1635.00		
(PCCA)				
POW, NA (U.S.P.)				
1 gm	51927-1954-00	129.00		
(Spectrum Pharmacy)				
POW, NA (U.S.P.)				
1 gm	49452-1072-02	183.05		
5 gm	49452-1072-03	686.00		
(USP)				
100 gm	49452-1072-01	5810.00		
BETAMETHASONE ACETATE, MICRONIZED				
(Gallipot) *See BETAMETHASONE ACETATE MICRONIZED*				
(Hawkins) *See BETAMETHASONE ACETATE MICRONIZED*				
(Letco) *See BETAMETHASONE ACETATE MICRONIZED*				
(Medisca) *See BETAMETHASONE ACETATE MICRONIZED*				
(PCCA) *See BETAMETHASONE ACETATE MICRONIZED*				
(Spectrum Pharmacy) *See BETAMETHASONE ACETATE MICRONIZED*				
BETAMETHASONE DIP. (Stat Rx)				
REPACK				
betamethasone dipropionate				
CRE, TP, 0.05%, 15 gm	16590-0032-15	20.00		
BETAMETHASONE DIP./CLOTRIMAZOLE (Stat Rx)				
betamethasone dipropionate/clotrimazole				
CRE, TP, 0.05%-1%, 15 gm	16590-0033-15	32.00		
BETAMETHASONE DIPROPIONATE				
FUL				
CRE, TP, 0.05%, 15 gm		3.45		
LOT, TP, 0.05%, 60 ml		9.00		
(Actavis Mid Atlantic)				
CRE, TP, 0.05%, 15 gm	00472-0380-15	7.80		AB
45 gm	00472-0380-45	18.17		AB
OIN, TP, 0.05%, 15 gm	00472-0381-15	7.80		AB
45 gm	00472-0381-45	18.17		AB
(Actavis Mid Atlantic)				
betamethasone dipropionate, augmented				
(AUGMENTED)				
0.05%, 50 gm	00472-0382-50	84.87		AB
BETAMETHASONE DIPROPIONATE (Consolidated Midland)				
CRE, TP, 0.05%, 15 gm	00223-4260-15	4.25		EE
45 gm	00223-4260-45	7.50		EE
60 gm	00223-4260-60	17.50		EE
OIN, TP, 0.05%, 15 gm	00223-4261-15	3.75		EE
45 gm	00223-4261-45	7.50		EE
(Fougera)				
CRE, TP, 0.05%, 15 gm	00168-0055-15	7.80		AB
45 gm	00168-0055-46	18.17		AB
(Fougera)				
betamethasone dipropionate, augmented				
LOT, TP (USP)				
0.05%, 30 ml	00168-0267-30	57.23		AB
BETAMETHASONE DIPROPIONATE (Fougera)				
60 ml	00168-0057-60	30.49		AB
(Fougera)				
betamethasone dipropionate, augmented				
(USP)				
0.05%, 60 ml	00168-0267-60	112.77		AB
BETAMETHASONE DIPROPIONATE (Fougera)				
OIN, TP, 0.05%, 15 gm	00168-0056-15	9.40		AB
45 gm	00168-0056-46	25.46		AB
(Gallipot)				
CRE, NA, 1 gm	51552-0022-01	27.79		
5 gm	51552-0022-02	111.16		
10 gm	51552-0022-03	210.00		
(Letco)				
POW, NA (U.S.P.,MICRONIZED)				
5 gm	62991-1023-02	225.00		
10 gm	62991-1023-03	390.00		
(Medisca)				
POW, NA (U.S.P.,MICRONIZED)				
1 gm	*38779-0017-06	58.50		
5 gm	38779-0017-03	240.00		
10 gm	38779-0017-01	399.00		
25 gm	38779-0017-04	1005.00		
(PCCA)				
POW, NA (U.S.P.,MICRONIZED)				
1 gm	51927-1454-00	78.00		
(Perrigo)				
LOT, TP, 0.05%, 60 ml	45802-0021-46	11.85		AB
(Sandoz)				
CRE, TP, 0.05%, 15 gm	00781-7074-27	38.16		AB
50 gm	00781-7074-50	85.34		AB
(Spectrum Pharmacy)				
POW, NA (U.S.P.)				
1 gm	49452-1075-01	101.15		
5 gm	49452-1075-02	367.50		
(U.S.P.,MICRONIZED)				
25 gm	49452-1075-03	1375.50		
(Taro)				
CRE, TP, 0.05%, 15 gm	51672-1274-01	7.65		AB
45 gm	51672-1274-06	17.58		AB
(Taro)				
betamethasone dipropionate, augmented				
LOT, TP (USP,1X30ML)				
0.05%, 30 ml	51672-1340-03	57.17		AB
(USP,1X60ML)				
0.05%, 60 ml	51672-1340-04	112.66		AB
BETAMETHASONE DIPROPIONATE (Teva)				
LOT, TP, 0.05%, 60 ml	00093-0302-39	38.85		AB
(A-S Medication)				
REPACK				
CRE, TP, 0.05%, 15 gm	54569-1113-00	7.65		EE
45 gm	54569-2556-00	15.92		EE
LOT, TP, 0.05%, 60 ml	54569-1556-00	26.50		EE
OIN, TP, 0.05%, 15 gm	54569-1114-00	9.40		EE
45 gm	54569-2613-00	25.46		EE
(Altura)				
REPACK				
CRE, TP, 0.05%, 15 gm	63874-0825-15	20.90		EE
45 gm	63874-0825-45	22.31		EE
LOT, TP, 0.05%, 60 ml	63874-0781-60	20.07		EE
(Dispensing Solutions)				
REPACK				
CRE, TP, 0.05%, 15 gm	55045-2071-05	11.99		AB
45 gm	55045-1673-08	18.00		
OIN, TP (1X15GM)				
0.05%, 15 gm	55045-1978-05	11.99		AB
(1X45GM)				
0.05%, 45 gm	55045-1978-08	18.00		AB
(Nucare Pharm)				
REPACK				
OIN, TP, 0.05%, 15 gm	66267-1296-01	19.47		AB
(Palmetto)				
REPACK				
CRE, TP, 0.05%, 15 gm	23490-5139-01	18.00		
45 gm	23490-5139-02	21.19		
OIN, TP, 0.05%, 15 gm	23490-5141-02	10.00		

PROD/MFR	NDC	AWP	DP	OBC
(Pharma Pac) REPACK				
CRE, TP, 0.05%, 15 gm	52959-0721-15	20.50		AB
OIN, TP, 0.05%, 15 gm	52959-0262-15	10.70		EE
45 gm	52959-0262-00	10.65		EE
(Phys Total Care) REPACK				
CRE, TP, 0.05%, 15 gm	54868-0973-01	5.88		EE
45 gm	54868-0973-02	10.26		EE
OIN, TP, 0.05%, 45 gm	54868-3280-00	27.53		EE
(Physician Partner) REPACK				
CRE, TP, 0.05%, 15 gm	21695-0521-15	15.30		AB
(Quality Care Prod) REPACK				
CRE, TP, 0.05%, 15 gm	49999-0222-15	28.05		AB
45 gm	49999-0222-45	56.10		AB
(Southwood) REPACK				
CRE, TP, 0.05%, 15 gm	58016-6338-01	19.90		EE
OIN, TP (1X45GM) 0.05%, 45 gm	58016-5594-01	59.70		AB
BETAMETHASONE DIPROPIONATE AUGMENTED (Actavis Mid Atlantic) betamethasone dipropionate, augmented				
OIN, TP, 0.05%, 15 gm	00472-0382-15	56.57		AB
45 gm	00472-0382-45	113.87		AB
(Fougera)				
CRE, TP, 0.05%, 15 gm	00168-0265-15	36.43		AB
50 gm	00168-0265-50	81.65		AB
(Perrigo)				
CRE, TP (AUGMENTED) 0.05%, 15 gm	45802-0376-35	38.10		
50 gm	45802-0376-32	85.25		
(Taro)				
CRE, TP, 0.05%, 15 gm	51672-1310-01	37.95		
50 gm	51672-1310-03	84.87		
GEL, TP, 0.05%, 15 gm	51672-1309-01	37.95		AB
50 gm	51672-1309-03	84.87		AB
OIN, TP (AUGMENTED) 0.05%, 15 gm	51672-1317-01	30.00		AB
50 gm	51672-1317-03	73.00		AB
(Dispensing Solutions) REPACK				
CRE, TP (1X50GM) 0.05%, 50 gm	55045-3254-05	75.00		AB
OIN, TP, 0.05%, 15 gm	55045-3008-01	31.50		AB
(1X50GM) 0.05%, 50 gm	55045-3008-05	65.00		AB
(Pharma Pac) REPACK				
OIN, TP (1X50GM) 0.05%, 50 gm	52959-0962-01	83.20		AB
(Quality Care Prod) REPACK				
CRE, TP (1X15GM) 0.05%, 15 gm	35356-0496-15	28.05		
GEL, TP, 0.05%, 15 gm	49999-0757-15	49.32		
BETAMETHASONE DIPROPIONATE, AUGMENTED				
(Actavis Mid Atlantic) *See BETAMETHASONE DIPROPIONATE*				
(Actavis Mid Atlantic) *See BETAMETHASONE DIPROPIONATE AUGMENTED*				
(Fougera) *See BETAMETHASONE DIPROPIONATE*				
(Fougera) *See BETAMETHASONE DIPROPIONATE AUGMENTED*				
(Perrigo) *See BETAMETHASONE DIPROPIONATE AUGMENTED*				
(Schering) *See DIPROLENE*				
(Schering) *See DIPROLENE AF*				
(Taro) *See BETAMETHASONE DIPROPIONATE*				
(Taro) *See BETAMETHASONE DIPROPIONATE AUGMENTED*				
BETAMETHASONE DIPROPIONATE/CALCIPOTRIENE				
(Warner Chilcott) *See TACLONEX*				
(Warner Chilcott) *See TACLONEX SCALP*				
BETAMETHASONE DIPROPIONATE/CLOTRIMAZOLE FUL				
CRE, TP, 0.05%-1%, 15 gm		12.35		
LOT, TP, 0.05%-1%, 30 gm		54.35		
(Actavis Mid Atlantic)				
CRE, TP, 0.05%-1%, 15 gm	00472-0379-15	23.55		AB
45 gm	00472-0379-45	50.70		AB
(Fougera) *See BETAMETHASONE/CLOTRIMAZOLE*				
(Schering) *See LOTRISONE*				
(Taro) *See BETAMETHASONE/CLOTRIMAZOLE*				
(Keltman Pharma., Inc.) REPACK				
CRE, TP (1X15GM) 0.05%-1%, 15 gm	68387-0626-01	27.85		
(Palmetto) REPACK				
CRE, TP, 0.05%-1%, 15 gm	23490-7619-00	24.50		
45 gm	23490-7619-01	50.00		
BETAMETHASONE SODIUM PHOSPHATE (Consolidated Midland)				
SOL, IJ (VIAL) 3 mg/ml, 5 ml	00223-7265-05	4.25		EE
(Gallipot)				
POW, NA (U.S.P.) 1 gm	51552-0064-01	42.00		
5 gm	51552-0064-02	147.00		
(Hawkins)				
POW, NA (U.S.P.) 0.1 gm	63370-0028-06	38.40		
1 gm	63370-0028-10	115.20		
5 gm	63370-0028-15	417.60		
25 gm	63370-0028-25	1776.00		
100 gm	63370-0028-35	6000.00		
(Letco)				
POW, NA (U.S.P.) 1 gm	62991-1024-01	60.00		
5 gm	62991-1024-02	247.50		
(U.S.P., 25) 10 gm	62991-1024-04	450.00		
100 gm	62991-1024-05	2100.00		
(Medisca)				
POW, NA (U.S.P.) 1 gm	38779-0195-06	82.50		
5 gm	38779-0195-03	297.00		
10 gm	38779-0195-01	555.00		
(USP,1X100GM) 100 gm	38779-0195-05	3750.00		
(PCCA)				
POW, NA (U.S.P.) 1 gm	51927-1951-00	102.00		
(Spectrum Pharmacy)				
POW, NA (U.S.P.) 1 gm	49452-1077-01	144.90		
5 gm	49452-1077-02	497.00		
25 gm	49452-1077-04	1704.50		
(1X100GM,USP) 100 gm	49452-1077-06	4609.50		
BETAMETHASONE SODIUM PHOSPHATE-BETAMETHASONE ACE (PharmaForce) betamethasone ace/betamethasone na phos				
SUS, IJ (MULTI-DOSE) 3 mg/ml-3 mg/ml, 5 ml	40042-0048-05	35.85		AB
BETAMETHASONE VAL. (Stat Rx) REPACK betamethasone valerate				
CRE, TP, 0.1%, 15 gm	16590-0034-15	17.05		
30 gm	16590-0034-45	21.50		
BETAMETHASONE VALERATE FUL				
CRE, TP, 0.1%, 45 gm		5.39		
(Actavis Mid Atlantic)				
CRE, TP, 0.1%, 15 gm	00472-0370-15	4.95		AB
45 gm	00472-0370-45	8.05		AB
OIN, TP, 0.1%, 15 gm	00472-0371-15	4.95		AB
45 gm	00472-0371-45	8.05		AB
(Consolidated Midland)				
CRE, TP, 0.1%, 15 gm	00223-4258-15	2.75		EE
45 gm	00223-4258-45	5.75		EE
LOT, TP, 0.1%, 60 ml	00223-6432-60	12.50		EE
OIN, TP, 0.1%, 15 gm	00223-4259-15	4.00		EE
45 gm	00223-4259-45	7.95		EE
(Fougera)				
CRE, TP, 0.1%, 15 gm	00168-0040-15	6.06		AB
45 gm	00168-0040-46	8.96		AB
LOT, TP, 0.1%, 60 ml	00168-0041-60	13.13		AB
OIN, TP, 0.1%, 15 gm	00168-0033-15	6.31		AB
45 gm	00168-0033-46	9.78		AB
(Gallipot)				
CRE, NA (U.S.P.) 1 gm	51552-0023-01	59.50		
5 gm	51552-0023-02	110.60		
10 gm	51552-0023-03	229.60		
(Medisca)				
POW, NA (U.S.P.,MICRONIZED) 1 gm	38779-0004-06	70.50		
5 gm	38779-0004-03	262.50		
10 gm	38779-0004-01	469.50		
(PCCA)				
POW, NA (U.S.P. : MICRONIZED) 1 gm	51927-1160-00	78.00		
(Spectrum Pharmacy)				
POW, NA (U.S.P.,MICRONIZED) 1 gm	49452-1080-01	115.15		
5 gm	49452-1080-02	395.50		
(Stiefel Labs) *See LUXIQ*				
(Taro)				
CRE, TP, 0.1%, 15 gm	51672-1269-01	4.95		AB
45 gm	51672-1269-06	8.01		AB
(Teva) *See BETA-VAL*				
(A-S Medication) REPACK				
CRE, TP, 0.1%, 15 gm	54569-1115-00	6.06		EE
45 gm	54569-1873-01	8.96		EE
LOT, TP, 0.1%, 60 ml	54569-1874-01	13.13		EE
OIN, TP, 0.1%, 15 gm	54569-0793-00	6.31		EE
(Altura) REPACK				
CRE, TP, 0.1%, 15 gm	63874-0842-15	17.07		EE
45 gm	63874-0842-45	15.36		EE
OIN, TP, 0.1%, 15 gm	63874-0925-15	6.02		EE
(DHS, Inc.) REPACK				
CRE, TP, 0.1%, 45 gm	55887-0879-45	17.88		AB
(Dispensing Solutions) REPACK				
CRE, TP, 0.1%, 15 gm	55045-1815-05	15.45		AB
(1X45GM) 0.1%, 45 gm	55045-1815-08	28.15		AB
LOT, TP (1X60ML) 0.1%, 60 ml	55045-2472-02	28.00		AB
OIN, TP (1X15GM) 0.1%, 15 gm	55045-3019-05	6.25		AB
(1X45GM) 0.1%, 45 gm	55045-3019-04	9.75		AB
(Nucare Pharm) REPACK				
CRE, TP, 0.1%, 15 gm	66267-0984-15	9.89		EE
(Palmetto) REPACK				
CRE, TP, 0.1%, 15 gm	23490-5142-01	17.19		
(1X45GM) 0.1%, 45 gm	23490-5142-02	24.64		
LOT, TP, 0.1%, 60 ml	23490-5143-06	37.55		
(Pharma Pac) REPACK				
CRE, TP, 0.1%, 15 gm	52959-0263-00	10.03		EE
45 gm	52959-0263-01	15.41		EE
LOT, TP, 0.1%, 60 ml	52959-0243-03	14.55		EE
(Phys Total Care) REPACK				
CRE, TP, 0.1%, 15 gm	54868-0520-01	5.16		EE
45 gm	54868-0520-00	9.21		EE
LOT, TP, 0.1%, 60 ml	54868-5002-00	13.62		AB
OIN, TP, 0.1%, 15 gm	54868-2994-01	5.16		EE
45 gm	54868-2994-02	6.75		EE
(Physician Partner) REPACK				
CRE, TP (1X15GM) 0.1%, 15 gm	21695-0583-15	14.90		AB
OIN, TP (1X45GM) 0.1%, 45 gm	21695-0586-45	49.56		AB
(Quality Care Prod) REPACK				
CRE, TP, 0.1%, 15 gm	49999-0218-15	19.52		
(Southwood) REPACK				
CRE, TP, 0.1%, 15 gm	58016-3097-01	16.26		EE
45 gm	58016-3109-01	18.65		EE
OIN, TP, 0.1%, 15 gm	58016-3099-01	7.75		EE
BETAMETHASONE/CLOTRIMAZOLE (Fougera) betamethasone dipropionate/clotrimazole				
CRE, TP, 0.05%-1%, 15 gm	00168-0258-15	23.57		AB
45 gm	00168-0258-46	50.75		AB
LOT, TP, 0.05%-1%, 30 ml	00168-0370-30	55.80		

PROD/MFR	NDC	AWP	DP	OBC
(Taro)				
CRE, TP, 0.05%-1%, 15 gm	**51672-4048-01**	22.87		**AB**
45 gm	**51672-4048-06**	49.27		**AB**
LOT, TP, 0.05%-1%, 30 ml	**51672-1308-03**	55.74		
(A-S Medication) REPACK				
CRE, TP, 0.05%-1%, 15 gm	**54569-5266-00**	23.55		**EE**
(DHS, Inc.) REPACK				
CRE, TP, 0.05%-1%, 15 gm	**55887-0692-15**	26.92		**AB**
45 gm	**55887-0692-45**	50.05		**AB**
(Dispensing Solutions) REPACK				
CRE, TP, 0.05%-1%, 15 gm	**55045-2883-05**	23.99		**AB**
(Pharma Pac) REPACK				
CRE, TP, 0.05%-1%, 15 gm	**52959-0633-15**	25.25		**AB**
45 gm	**52959-0633-45**	14.32		**AB**
(Phys Total Care) REPACK				
CRE, TP, 0.05%-1%, 15 gm	**54868-4546-01**	18.99		**AB**
45 gm	**54868-4546-00**	28.23		**AB**
LOT, TP, 0.05%-1%, 30 ml	**54868-5232-00**	71.04		
(Physician Partner) REPACK				
CRE, TP (15GMX45) 0.05%-1%, 15 gm 45s	**21695-0333-45**	98.54		**AB**
(Quality Care Prod) REPACK				
CRE, TP (1X45GM) 0.05%-1%, 45 gm	**35356-0120-45**	58.60		**AB**
(Southwood) REPACK				
CRE, TP, 0.05%-1%, 15 gm	**58016-5612-01**	23.95		**EE**
BETANAPHTHOL				
(Spectrum Pharmacy) *See 2-NAPHTHOL*				
BETAPACE (Bayer) sotalol hydrochloride				
TAB, PO, 80 mg, 100s ea	**50419-0105-10**	408.96		**AB**
120 mg, 100s ea	**50419-0109-10**	545.70		**AB**
160 mg, 100s ea	**50419-0106-10**	682.14		**AB**
(CAPLET) 240 mg, 100s ea	**50419-0107-10**	886.74		**AB**
BETAPACE AF (Bayer) sotalol hydrochloride				
TAB, PO (CAPLET) 80 mg, 60s ea	**50419-0115-06**	224.16		
120 mg, 60s ea	**50419-0119-06**	299.10		
160 mg, 60s ea	**50419-0116-06**	374.10		
(Phys Total Care) REPACK				
TAB, PO (CAPLET) 80 mg, 30s ea	**54868-4423-00**	108.81		
60s ea	**54868-4423-01**	203.88		
BETASERON (Bayer) interferon beta-1b/sodium chloride				
KIT, MR (15 BLISTER UNITS,PF) 0.3 mg-0.54%, 15s ea	**50419-0523-25**	2951.46		
(Bayer) interferon beta-1b				
PDS, SC (BLISTER UNITS,W/DILUENT) 0.3 mg, 14s ea	**50419-0523-35**	2951.46		
BETAXOLOL (KVK) betaxolol hydrochloride				
TAB, PO (USP,FILM-COATED) 10 mg, 100s ea	**10702-0013-01**	124.25		**AB**
20 mg, 100s ea	**10702-0014-01**	186.10		**AB**
(GSMS) REPACK				
TAB, PO (FILM-COATED) 10 mg, 100s ea	**60429-0753-01**	281.55	93.85	**AB**
20 mg, 100s ea	**60429-0754-01**	368.55	122.85	**AB**
BETAXOLOL HCL (Falcon Ophthalmics) betaxolol hydrochloride				
SOL, OP, 0.5%, 5 ml	**61314-0245-01**	31.31		**AT**
10 ml	**61314-0245-03**	58.24		**AT**
15 ml	**61314-0245-02**	86.93		**AT**
(Phys Total Care) REPACK				
TAB, PO (FILM-COATED) 10 mg, 10s ea	**54868-4932-01**	39.15		**AB**
30s ea	**54868-4932-00**	108.48		**AB**
BETAXOLOL HYDROCHLORIDE				
(Alcon Ophthalmic) *See BETOPTIC S*				
(Falcon Ophthalmics) *See BETAXOLOL HCL*				
(KVK) *See BETAXOLOL*				
(Sanofi-Aventis) *See KERLONE*				
BETHANECHOL (Southwood) REPACK bethanechol chloride				
TAB, PO, 25 mg, 30s ea	**58016-0358-30**	53.52		
60s ea	**58016-0358-60**	107.05		
90s ea	**58016-0358-90**	160.57		
100s ea	**58016-0358-00**	178.41		
BETHANECHOL CHLORIDE FUL				
TAB, PO, 5 mg, 100s ea		48.89		
10 mg, 100s ea		91.71		
25 mg, 100s ea		170.79		
50 mg, 100s ea		195.65		
(Actavis)				
TAB, PO, 5 mg, 100s ea	**52152-0268-02**	71.32		**AA**
10 mg, 100s ea	**52152-0269-02**	133.83		**AA**
25 mg, 100s ea	**52152-0270-02**	178.41		**AA**
(Amneal)				
TAB, PO (USP) 5 mg, 100s ea	**65162-0571-10**	71.32		**AA**
10 mg, 100s ea	**65162-0572-10**	133.83		**AA**
25 mg, 100s ea	**65162-0573-10**	178.41		**AA**
50 mg, 100s ea	**65162-0574-10**	285.46		**AA**
(Caraco)				
TAB, PO (USP,UNCOATED) 5 mg, 100s ea	**57664-0137-88**	71.34		**AA**
10 mg, 100s ea	**57664-0104-88**	133.85		**AA**
25 mg, 100s ea	**57664-0138-88**	178.45		**AA**
50 mg, 100s ea	**57664-0106-88**	285.50		**AA**
(Gallipot)				
POW, NA (1X5GM,USP) 5 gm	**51552-0879-02**	30.80	22.00	
(1X25GM,USP) 25 gm	**51552-0879-04**	118.30	84.50	
(Global Pharm)				
TAB, PO (USP) 5 mg, 100s ea	**00115-9511-01**	71.32		**AA**
10 mg, 100s ea	**00115-9522-01**	133.83		**AA**
25 mg, 100s ea	**00115-9533-01**	178.41		**AA**
50 mg, 100s ea	**00115-9544-01**	285.46		**AA**
(Lannett)				
TAB, PO (USP) 5 mg, 100s ea	**00527-1332-01**	85.58		**AA**
10 mg, 100s ea	**00527-1340-01**	160.60		**AA**
25 mg, 100s ea	**00527-1356-01**	214.49		**AA**
50 mg, 100s ea	**00527-1329-01**	342.55		**AA**
(Letco)				
POW, NA (U.S.P.) 5 gm	**62991-1530-02**	46.50		
25 gm	**62991-1530-03**	150.00		
(Major)				
TAB, PO (USP) 10 mg, 100s ea	**00904-6029-60**	138.21		**AA**
25 mg, 100s ea	**00904-6030-60**	183.50		**AA**
50 mg, 100s ea	**00904-6031-60**	195.17		**AA**
(Marlex)				
TAB, PO (USP) 5 mg, 100s ea	**10135-0515-01**	71.32		**AA**
10 mg, 100s ea	**10135-0516-01**	133.83		**AA**
25 mg, 100s ea	**10135-0517-01**	178.41		**AA**
500s ea	**10135-0517-05**	1100.00		**AA**
50 mg, 100s ea	**10135-0518-01**	285.46		**AA**
(Medisca)				
POW, NA (U.S.P.) 1 gm	**38779-0393-06**	25.50		
5 gm	**38779-0393-03**	49.50		
25 gm	**38779-0393-04**	268.50		
100 gm	**38779-0393-05**	717.00		
(PCCA)				
POW, NA (U.S.P.) 1 gm	**51927-2097-00**	54.00		
(Spectrum Pharmacy)				
CRY, NA (U.S.P.) 5 gm	**49452-1083-02**	108.50		
25 gm	**49452-1083-03**	476.00		
(Teva)				
TAB, PO, 5 mg, 100s ea	**50111-0323-01**	71.32		**AA**
10 mg, 100s ea	**50111-0324-01**	133.83		**AA**
25 mg, 100s ea	**50111-0325-01**	178.41		**AA**
50 mg, 100s ea	**50111-0326-01**	285.46		**AA**
(Teva) *See URECHOLINE*				
(Upsher-Smith)				
TAB, PO, 5 mg, 100s ea	**00832-0510-00**	72.07		**AA**
10 mg, ea (10X10)	**00832-0511-89**	1.60		**AA**
10 mg, 10s ea UD	**00832-0511-01**	160.18		**AA**
100s ea	**00832-0511-00**	133.83		**AA**
25 mg, ea (10X10)	**00832-0512-89**	2.14		**AA**
25 mg, 10s ea UD	**00832-0512-01**	213.56		**AA**
100s ea	**00832-0512-00**	178.41		**AA**
500s ea	**00832-0512-50**	889.93		**AA**
50 mg, ea (10X10)	**00832-0513-89**	3.42		**AA**
50 mg, 10s ea UD	**00832-0513-01**	341.70		**AA**
100s ea	**00832-0513-00**	285.46		**AA**
(Wockhardt USA)				
TAB, PO, 5 mg, 100s ea (USP)	**64679-0965-01**	71.32		**AA**
10 mg, 100s ea	**64679-0966-01**	133.83		**AA**
25 mg, 100s ea	**64679-0967-01**	178.41		**AA**
50 mg, 100s ea	**64679-0968-01**	285.46		**AA**
(American Health) REPACK				
TAB, PO (10X10) 10 mg, 100s ea UD	**68084-0166-01**	149.38		**AA**
25 mg, 100s ea UD	**68084-0010-01**	178.41		**AA**
(10X10) 25 mg, 100s ea UD	**68084-0110-01**	178.41		**AA**
(Phys Total Care) REPACK				
TAB, PO, 10 mg, 40s ea	**54868-1624-00**	113.13		**AA**
25 mg, 20s ea	**54868-1625-02**	42.99		**AA**
30s ea	**54868-1625-05**	55.11		
100s ea	**54868-1625-04**	133.50		
120s ea	**54868-1625-03**	181.14		
50 mg, 60s ea	**54868-1625-01**	92.82		**AA**
60s ea	**54868-5154-00**	193.50		**AA**
(USP) 50 mg, 90s ea	**54868-5154-01**	288.00		
(Stat Rx) REPACK				
TAB, PO, 10 mg, 30s ea	**16590-0812-30**	40.15		**AA**
BETIMOL (Vistakon) timolol				
SOL, OP, 0.25%, 5 ml	**68669-0522-05**	45.96		
0.5%, 5 ml	**68669-0525-05**	50.76		
10 ml	**68669-0525-10**	97.56		
15 ml	**68669-0525-15**	146.52		
BETOPTIC S (Alcon Ophthalmic) betaxolol hydrochloride				
SUS, OP, 0.25%, 10 ml	**00065-0246-10**	125.28		
15 ml	**00065-0246-15**	187.92		
(Phys Total Care) REPACK				
SUS, OP, 0.25%, 5 ml	**54868-1639-02**	48.26		
10 ml	**54868-1639-01**	89.60		
15 ml	**54868-1639-03**	135.64		
BEVACIZUMAB				
(Genentech) *See AVASTIN*				
BEXAROTENE				
(Eisai) *See TARGRETIN*				
BEXXAR (Glaxo) iodine i 131 tositumomab				
SOL, IV (DOSIMETRIC,PF) 20 ml	**00007-3261-01**	3615.30		
(THERAPEUTIC STEP,PF) 20 ml	**00007-3262-01**	34873.19		
(Glaxo) tositumomab				
(DOSIMETRIC STEP,PF) 14 mg/ml, 34.7 ml	**00007-3260-31**	3414.46		
(THERAPEUTIC STEP,PF) 14 mg/ml, 34.7 ml	**00007-3260-36**	3414.46		
BHA (Amend) butylated hydroxyanisole				
POW, NA (N.F., F.C.C.) 454 gm	**17317-0815-01**	35.00		
2270 gm	**17317-0815-05**	140.00		
(Spectrum Pharmacy)				
FLA, NA (N.F.) 125 gm	**49452-1095-01**	97.30		
500 gm	**49452-1095-02**	247.80		
2500 gm	**49452-1095-03**	955.50		
BHRTBASE (Gallipot) paste base				
PAS, NA, 454 gm	**51552-1021-06**	56.70	40.50	

PROD/MFR	NDC	AWP	DP	OBC
BHT (Amend)				
butylated hydroxytoluene				
GRA, NA (N.F., F.C.C.)				
454 gm	**17317-0816-01**	19.60		
2270 gm	**17317-0816-05**	84.00		
(Gallipot)				
GRA, NA (F.C.C.)				
100 gm	**51552-0098-05**	11.76		
POW, NA, 500 gm	**51552-0098-06**	55.30		
(Spectrum Pharmacy)				
GRA, NA (N.F.)				
125 gm	**49452-1105-01**	53.20		
500 gm	**49452-1105-02**	161.35		
BI SUBCITRATE K/METRONIDAZOLE/ TETRACYCLINE HCL				
(Axcan) *See PYLERA*				
BI SUBSALICYLATE/METRONIDAZOLE/ TETRACYCLINE HCL				
(Prometheus Labs) *See HELIDAC THERAPY*				
BIAFINE (Ortho)				
cream, multi ingredient				
CRE, TP, 45 gm	**00062-0205-02**	33.64	28.03	
90 gm	**00062-0205-03**	53.82	44.85	
BIAXIN (Abbott Pharm)				
clarithromycin				
PDR, PO (FRUIT)				
125 mg/5 ml, 50 ml	**00074-3163-50**	28.44	24.95	
100 ml	**00074-3163-13**	52.57	46.12	
250 mg/5 ml, 50 ml	**00074-3188-50**	54.12	47.47	
100 ml	**00074-3188-13**	100.24	87.93	
(A-S Medication) REPACK				
PDR, PO (FRUIT)				
125 mg/5 ml, 100 ml	**54569-3896-00**	53.18		
250 mg/5 ml, 100 ml	**54569-3897-00**	96.64		
(AQ) REPACK				
TAB, PO, 250 mg, 10s ea	**66105-0743-01**	83.40		
15s ea	**66105-0743-15**	125.10		
30s ea	**66105-0743-03**	250.20		
60s ea	**66105-0743-06**	500.40		
90s ea	**66105-0743-09**	750.60		
500 mg, 10s ea	**66105-0744-01**	85.80		
15s ea	**66105-0744-15**	128.70		
30s ea	**66105-0744-03**	257.40		
60s ea	**66105-0744-06**	514.80		
90s ea	**66105-0744-09**	772.20		
(Phys Total Care) REPACK				
PDR, PO (FRUIT)				
125 mg/5 ml, 100 ml	**54868-4919-00**	47.89		
250 mg/5 ml, 100 ml	**54868-3384-00**	115.34		
(Stat Rx) REPACK				
TAB, PO, 500 mg, 14s ea	**16590-0035-14**	79.50		
21s ea	**16590-0035-21**	119.25		
30s ea	**16590-0035-30**	170.36		
BIAXIN FILMTAB (Abbott Pharm)				
clarithromycin				
TAB, PO, 250 mg, 60s ea	**00074-3368-60**	364.90	320.08	
(10X10,ABBO-PAC)				
250 mg, 100s ea UD	**00074-3368-11**	642.42	535.35	
500 mg, 60s ea	**00074-2586-60**	364.90	320.08	
(10X10,ABBO-PAC)				
500 mg, 100s ea UD	**00074-2586-11**	642.42	535.35	
(A-S Medication) REPACK				
TAB, PO, 500 mg, 2s ea	**54569-3439-04**	12.39		
14s ea	**54569-3439-01**	90.96		
20s ea	**54569-3439-00**	129.94		
28s ea	**54569-3439-03**	173.42		
(DHS, Inc.) REPACK				
TAB, PO, 500 mg, 30s ea	**55887-0813-30**	186.19		
(Dispensing Solutions) REPACK				
TAB, PO, 500 mg, 20s ea	**55045-1865-07**	105.00		
(PD-Rx Pharm) REPACK				
TAB, PO, 500 mg, 10s ea	**55289-0021-10**	86.80		
14s ea	**55289-0021-14**	121.02		
20s ea	**55289-0021-20**	168.60		
(REDI-SCRIPT)				
500 mg, 20s ea	**58864-0067-20**	168.60		
28s ea	**55289-0021-28**	209.55		
(Pharma Pac) REPACK				
TAB, PO, 250 mg, 10s ea	**52959-0442-10**	48.70		
14s ea	**52959-0442-14**	67.20		
20s ea	**52959-0442-20**	94.45		
500 mg, 10s ea	**52959-0230-10**	53.71		
20s ea	**52959-0230-20**	102.32		
(Phys Total Care) REPACK				
TAB, PO, 250 mg, 20s ea	**54868-3820-00**	97.54		
500 mg, 5s ea	**54868-2338-00**	29.18		
10s ea	**54868-2338-06**	57.13		
15s ea	**54868-2338-07**	80.43		
20s ea	**54868-2338-01**	119.39		
60s ea	**54868-2338-03**	353.78		
(Quality Care Prod) REPACK				
TAB, PO, 500 mg, 20s ea	**49999-0407-20**	78.12		
(Southwood) REPACK				
TAB, PO, 500 mg, 10s ea	**58016-0550-10**	59.46		
12s ea	**58016-0550-12**	71.35		
14s ea	**58016-0550-14**	83.24		
15s ea	**58016-0550-15**	89.19		
20s ea	**58016-0550-20**	118.92		
30s ea	**58016-0550-30**	178.37		
40s ea	**58016-0550-40**	237.83		
100s ea	**58016-0550-00**	594.58		
BIAXIN XL (Abbott Pharm)				
clarithromycin				
TER, PO (4X14,FILM-COATED)				
500 mg, 56s ea	**00074-3165-41**	361.30	316.93	
(FILM-COATED)				
500 mg, 60s ea	**00074-3165-60**	390.37	342.43	
(ABBO-PAC,10X2X5)				
500 mg, 100s ea UD	**00074-3165-11**	687.23	572.69	
(A-S Medication) REPACK				
TER, PO (FILM-COATED)				
500 mg, 14s ea	**54569-4953-00**	91.35		
(Bryant Ranch) REPACK				
TER, PO, 500 mg, 14s ea	**63629-1284-01**	73.25		
(Core) REPACK				
TER, PO, 500 mg, 14s ea	**33358-0087-14**	75.08		
(DHS, Inc.) REPACK				
TER, PO (FILM-COATED)				
500 mg, 30s ea	**55887-0372-30**	175.00		
60s ea	**55887-0372-60**	335.25		
(Dispensing Solutions) REPACK				
TER, PO, 500 mg, 14s ea	**55045-3452-01**	89.88		
(Phys Total Care) REPACK				
TER, PO, 500 mg, 14s ea	**54868-4191-01**	96.89		
20s ea	**54868-4191-00**	130.74		
BICALUTAMIDE FUL				
TAB, PO, 50 mg, 100s ea		348.02		
(Accord)				
TAB, PO (FILM COATED)				
50 mg, 30s ea	**16729-0023-10**	550.61		AB
100s ea	**16729-0023-01**	1835.44		AB
(Actavis)				
TAB, PO (FILM-COATED)				
50 mg, 30s ea	**52152-0526-30**	556.18		AB
100s ea	**52152-0526-02**	1853.93		AB
(Apotex Corp.)				
TAB, PO (FILM COATED)				
50 mg, 30s ea	**60505-2642-03**	556.79		AB
100s ea	**60505-2642-01**	1856.04		AB
(AstraZeneca) *See CASODEX*				
(Caraco)				
TAB, PO (FILM-COATED)				
50 mg, 30s ea	**41616-0485-83**	556.00		AB
100s ea	**41616-0485-88**	1853.00		AB
(Dava Pharma)				
TAB, PO (USP,FILM-COATED)				
50 mg, 30s ea	**67253-0191-03**	550.60		AB
100s ea	**67253-0191-10**	1835.43		AB
(Kremers Urban)				
TAB, PO (FILM-COATED)				
50 mg, 30s ea	**62175-0132-32**	550.61		AB
(Major)				
TAB, PO (FILM-COATED)				
50 mg, 30s ea	**00904-6019-46**	493.95		
100s ea	**00904-6019-60**	1651.89		
(Mylan)				
TAB, PO (FILM COATED)				
50 mg, 30s ea	**00378-7017-93**	556.11		AB
500s ea	**00378-7017-05**	9268.56		AB
(Northstar)				
TAB, PO (USP,FILM-COATED)				
50 mg, 30s ea	**16714-0571-01**	556.11		
100s ea	**16714-0571-02**	1856.04		
(Sandoz)				
TAB, PO (3X10,FILM-COATED)				
50 mg, 30s ea UD	**00781-5409-64**	556.79		AB
(FILM-COATED)				
50 mg, 30s ea	**00781-5409-31**	556.79		AB
100s ea	**00781-5409-01**	1856.06		AB
(Teva)				
TAB, PO (USP,FILM COATED)				
50 mg, 30s ea	**00093-0220-56**	556.79		AB
100s ea	**00093-0220-01**	1856.06		AB
(UDL)				
TAB, PO (3X10,FILM COATED)				
50 mg, 30s ea UD	**51079-0692-03**	556.18		AB
(Zydus Pharm.)				
TAB, PO (FILM-COATED)				
50 mg, 30s ea	**68382-0224-06**	556.17		AB
100s ea	**68382-0224-01**	1853.90		AB
500s ea	**68382-0224-05**	9269.50		AB
1000s ea	**68382-0224-10**	18539.00		AB
(American Health) REPACK				
TAB, PO (3X10,FILM-COATED)				
50 mg, 30s ea UD	**68084-0374-21**	50.00		AB
BICILLIN C-R (King Pharm)				
penicillin g benzathine/penicillin g procaine				
SUS, IM (2MLX10,21GX1",PEDIA)				
2 ml 10s	**60793-0601-10**	459.18		
(2MLX10,21GX1&1/2")				
2 ml 10s	**60793-0600-10**	459.18		
(A-S Medication) REPACK				
SUS, IM (10X2ML)				
2 ml 10s	**54569-5957-00**	405.51		
(Phys Total Care) REPACK				
SUS, IM (10X2ML)				
2 ml 10s	**54868-5932-00**	474.02		
BICILLIN C-R 900/300 (King Pharm)				
penicillin g benzathine/penicillin g procaine				
SUS, IM (2MLX10,21GX1",PEDIA)				
2 ml 10s	**60793-0602-10**	477.97		
(A-S Medication) REPACK				
SUS, IM (10X2ML)				
2 ml 10s	**54569-5958-00**	422.09		
BICILLIN CR 900/300 (Dispensing Solutions) REPACK				
penicillin g benzathine/penicillin g procaine				
SUS, IM (10X2ML)				
2 ml 10s	**55045-3684-02**	400.00		
BICILLIN L-A (King Pharm)				
penicillin g benzathine				
SUS, IM (10X1ML)				
600000 u/ml,				
1 ml 10s	**60793-0700-10**	332.60		BC
2 ml 10s	**60793-0701-10**	576.05		BC
4 ml 10s	**60793-0702-10**	1180.40		BC
(A-S Medication) REPACK				
SUS, IM (10X1ML)				
600000 u/ml,				
1 ml 10s	**54569-5876-00**	293.73		BC
(1200M U)				
600000 u/ml, 2 ml	**54569-5877-01**	50.87		BC
(10X2ML,1200M U)				
600000 u/ml,				
2 ml 10s	**54569-5877-00**	508.70		BC
(Phys Total Care) REPACK				
SUS, IM (M.D.V.)				
300000 u/ml, 10 ml	**54868-3349-00**	37.98		

PROD/MFR NDC AWP DP OBC

(10X1ML)
600000 u/ml,
1 ml 10s.......... 54868-5933-00 355.12 BC
(TUBEX)
600000 u/ml, 2 ml.... 54868-0753-00 60.33 BC
2 ml 10s.......... 54868-0753-01 559.13 BC
(10X4ML)
600000 u/ml,
4 ml 10s.......... 54868-2466-00 1016.19 BC

BICNU (B/M Squibb Onc/Vir)
carmustine
PDS, IV (W/DILUENT)
100 mg, ea 00015-3012-60 205.69

BIDEX-A (SJ)
dextromethorphan hydrobromide/guaifenesin
TER, PO (DYE-FREE)
25 mg-600 mg,
100s ea........... 24839-0223-01 100.79

BIDHIST (Cypress Pharm)
brompheniramine maleate
TER, PO (CAPLET)
6 mg, 100s ea........ 60258-0471-01 38.66

BIDIL (Nitromed)
hydralazine hydrochloride/isosorbide dinitrate
TAB, PO (FILM-COATED)
37.5 mg-20 mg,
180s ea........... 12948-0001-12 405.00

BIFIDOBACTERIUM BIFIDUM
(PCCA) *See BIFIDOBACTERIUM BIFIDUS*

BIFIDOBACTERIUM BIFIDUS (PCCA)
bifidobacterium bifidum
POW, NA, 1 gm.......... 51927-3504-00 1.35

BILBERRY EXTRACT/EVENING PRIMROSE OIL/FLAXSEED OIL
(Ocusoft) *See TEARS AGAIN HYDRATE*

BILE SALTS (PCCA)
POW, NA, 1 gm.......... 51927-3132-00 7.08

BILTRICIDE (Schering)
praziquantel
TAB, PO, 600 mg, 6s ea ... 00085-1747-01 85.93

BIMATOPROST
(Allergan Inc) *See LATISSE*
(Allergan Inc) *See LUMIGAN*

BIO GLO (HUB Pharma)
fluorescein sodium
TES, OP, 1 mg, 100s ea.... 17238-0900-11 14.06
300s ea........... 17238-0900-30 36.25

BIO-CEF (Intl Ethical)
cephalexin
CAP, PO, 500 mg, 100s ea . 11584-1034-05 162.02 EE
PDR, PO, 125 mg/5 ml,
100 ml .... 11584-1035-01 10.49 EE
250 mg/5 ml,
100 ml .... 11584-1036-02 20.34 EE

BIO-STATIN (Bio-Tech Pharm)
nystatin
CAP, PO, 1 million u,
100s ea.......... 53191-0192-01 35.00
500000 u, 100s ea.... 53191-0009-01 24.00
POW, NA, ea............ 53191-0103-03 48.00 EE

BIOFLAVONOID
(PCCA) *See BIOFLAVONOIDS CITRUS*

BIOFLAVONOID/CALCIUM/MAGNESIUM/VITAMIN D
(PGD, Inc.) *See GENETICAL*

BIOFLAVONOIDS CITRUS (PCCA)
bioflavonoid
POW, NA (GRANULAR POWDER)
1 gm 51927-2221-00 0.09

BIOFREEZE (Dispensing Solutions)
REPACK
camphor/menthol
GEL, TP, 0.2%-3.5%,
90 gm 55045-9800-02 17.95

BIONECT (JSJ Pharma)
hyaluronate sodium
CRE, TP, 0.2%, 25 gm..... 68712-0007-02 54.00
GEL, TP, 0.2%, 30 gm..... 68712-0008-02 63.00
(2X30GM)
0.2%, 30 gm 2s...... 68712-0008-03 114.00
SPR, TP, 0.2%, 20 ml 68712-0009-01 54.00

(Physician Partner)
REPACK
CRE, TP (1X25GM)
0.2%, 25 gm........ 21695-0451-25 137.82
GEL, TP (1X30GM)
0.2%, 30 gm........ 21695-0452-25 137.82

BIOTECT PLUS (Gil Pharmaceutical)
multivitamin, minerals, and nutriceuticals
SGL, PO (SF,SOFTGEL)
60s ea.............. 58552-0308-60 7.94

BIOTHRAX (Emergent)
anthrax vaccine adsorbed
SUS, IM (M.D.V.)
5 ml................ 64678-0211-05 1331.19

BIOTIN
(Amend) *See D-BIOTIN*
(Gallipot) *See D-BIOTIN*

(Medisca)
POW, NA (VITAMIN H,USP,1X1GM)
1 gm 38779-2004-06 55.50
(VITAMIN H,USP,1X5GM)
5 gm 38779-2004-03 208.50
(VITAMIN H,USP,1X25GM)
25 gm 38779-2004-04 918.00

(PCCA)
POW, NA (USP; VITAMIN H)
1 gm 51927-1323-00 75.00

(Spectrum Pharmacy)
POW, NA (F.C.C.)
1 gm 49452-1120-02 117.60
(U.S.P.)
1 gm 49452-1115-02 105.35
(F.C.C.)
5 gm 49452-1120-03 323.05
(U.S.P.)
5 gm 49452-1115-03 392.00
(F.C.C.)
25 gm 49452-1120-04 1491.00
(U.S.P.)
25 gm 49452-1115-04 1596.00

BIOTIN/CU/DSS/FE/FOLIC ACID/ VIT B12/VIT C/VIT E
(Pronova) *See HEMAX*

BIOTUSS (Gil Pharmaceutical)
dm/gg/phenyleph hcl
SOL, PO (AF,SF,GRAPE)
473 ml 58552-0113-16 9.95

BIOTUSS PEDIATRIC (Gil Pharmaceutical)
dm/gg/phenyleph hcl
SOL, PO (AF,SF,GRAPE)
60 ml............... 58552-0119-02 5.99

BIOTUSSIN AC (Bio-Pharm)
codeine phosphate/guaifenesin
SYR, PO, 10 mg/5 ml-100 mg/5 ml,
120 ml, C-V........ 59741-0113-04 3.75
480 ml, C-V........ 59741-0113-16 12.25

BIOTUSSIN DAC (Bio-Pharm)
codeine phos/gg/pse hcl
LIQ, PO, 120 ml, C-V...... 59741-0115-04 5.25
480 ml, C-V......... 59741-0115-16 19.40

BIOVUE LONG-TERM PICC PROCEDURE (J&J Medical)
catheter, central venous, peripheral insertion
DEV, NA (4FR/18G,SING LUMEN,60CM)
ea.................. 56091-0979-10 71.50

BIOVUE MIDLINE PROCEDURE (J&J Medical)
catheter, central venous
DEV, NA (3FR/20G,SING LUMEN,20CM)
ea.................. 56091-0979-25 71.50
(4FR/18G,DUAL LUMEN,20CM)
ea.................. 56091-0979-19 88.40
(4FR/18G,SING LUMEN,20CM)
ea.................. 56091-0979-22 71.50

BIOVUE MIDLINE STARTER (J&J Medical)
catheter, central venous
DEV, NA (3FR/20G,SING LUMEN,20CM)
ea.................. 56091-0979-24 52.00
(4FR/18G,DUAL LUMEN,20CM)
ea.................. 56091-0979-18 71.50
(4FR/18G,SING LUMEN,20CM)
ea.................. 56091-0979-21 52.00

BIOVUE PICC PROCEDURE (J&J Medical)
catheter, central venous, peripheral insertion
DEV, NA (2FR/24G,SING LUMEN,30CM)
ea.................. 56091-0979-16 71.50
(3FR/20G,SING LUMEN,60CM)
ea.................. 56091-0979-13 71.50
(4FR/18G,DUAL LUMEN,60CM)
ea.................. 56091-0979-07 88.40
(5FR/16G,DUAL LUMEN,60CM)
ea.................. 56091-0979-01 88.40

BIOVUE PICC STARTER (J&J Medical)
catheter, central venous, peripheral insertion
DEV, NA (2FR/24G,SING LUMEN,30CM)
ea.................. 56091-0979-15 52.00
(3FR/20G,SING LUMEN,60CM)
ea.................. 56091-0979-12 52.00
(4FR/18G,DUAL LUMEN,60CM)
ea.................. 56091-0979-06 71.50
(4FR/18G,SING LUMEN,60CM)
ea.................. 56091-0979-09 52.00
(5FR/16G,DUAL LUMEN,60CM)
ea.................. 56091-0979-00 71.50

BIOVUE PROCEDURE TRAY (J&J Medical)
vascular catheter supplies
DEV, NA (CENTRAL CATH/OCRILON II)
ea.................. 56091-0979-94 19.50

BISACODYL (Medisca)
POW, NA (U,S.P.)
25 gm 38779-0113-04 76.50
100 gm 38779-0113-05 261.00
500 gm 38779-0113-08 1224.00

(PCCA)
POW, NA (U.S.P.)
1 gm 51927-2553-00 5.40

(Spectrum Pharmacy)
CRY, NA (U.S.P.)
5 gm 49452-1123-01 154.00
25 gm 49452-1123-02 395.50
100 gm 49452-1123-03 1211.00

(Bryant Ranch)
REPACK
ECT, PO, 5 mg, 30s ea..... 63629-3049-01 12.99

(Pharma Pac)
REPACK
ECT, PO, 5 mg, 30s ea..... 52959-0674-30 8.26
60s ea............ 52959-0674-60 15.18
100s ea........... 52959-0674-00 21.00

BISMUTH (Baker, J.T.)
POW, NA (REAGENT)
500 gm 10106-1084-01 242.93

BISMUTH CHLORIDE
(Baker, J.T.) *See BISMUTH TRICHLORIDE*

BISMUTH CITRATE (Amend)
POW, NA, 125 gm......... 17317-0059-04 21.35
500 gm 17317-0059-01 84.00
2270 gm............ 17317-0059-05 315.00

(Gallipot)
POW, NA, 113 gm......... 51552-0271-04 38.71
(U.S.P. VIII)
454 gm 51552-0271-06 111.72

(Medisca)
POW, NA, 25 gm.......... 38779-0717-04 25.50 9.90
100 gm 38779-0717-05 64.50
500 gm 38779-0717-08 211.50
(1X1000GM)
1000 gm............ 38779-0717-09 399.00

(PCCA)
POW, NA, 1 gm 51927-2008-00 1.44

(Spectrum Pharmacy)
POW, NA, 25 gm.......... 49452-0804-01 72.45
125 gm 49452-0804-02 144.20
500 gm 49452-0804-03 455.00

BISMUTH NITRATE
(Baker, J.T.) *See BISMUTH NITRATE PENTAHYDRATE*

BISMUTH NITRATE PENTAHYDRATE (Baker, J.T.)
bismuth nitrate
CRY, NA (A.C.S., REAGENT)
125 gm 10106-1092-04 85.08
500 gm 10106-1092-01 170.36

BISMUTH SALICYLATE (Medisca)
bismuth subsalicylate
POW, NA (U.S.P.)
100 gm 38779-0881-05 55.50
500 gm 38779-0881-08 187.50

(PCCA)
POW, NA (U.S.P.)
1 gm 51927-3102-00 1.17

BISMUTH SUBCARBONATE (Amend)
POW, NA (PURIFIED)
125 gm 17317-0061-04 19.60
500 gm 17317-0061-01 58.80
2500 gm............ 17317-0061-05 210.00
11350 gm 17317-0061-08 875.00

PROD/MFR	NDC	AWP	DP	OBC
(Baker, J.T.)				
POW, NA (REAGENT)				
125 gm	**10106-1116-04**	101.61		
(Gallipot)				
POW, NA (PURIFIED)				
120 gm	**51552-0455-04**	26.46		
2270 gm	**51552-0455-09**	404.88		
(Mallinckrodt Lab)				
POW, NA (PURIFIED)				
125 gm	**00406-0292-02**	22.30		
500 gm	**00406-0292-12**	65.87		
(Medisca)				
POW, NA, 25 gm	**38779-0659-04**	22.50		
100 gm	**38779-0659-05**	55.50		
500 gm	**38779-0659-08**	207.00		
(PCCA)				
POW, NA (USP)				
1 gm	**51927-1119-00**	1.44		
BISMUTH SUBGALLATE (Amend)				
POW, NA (PURIFIED)				
125 gm	**17317-0062-04**	25.20		
500 gm	**17317-0062-01**	78.40		
2500 gm	**17317-0062-05**	280.00		
(Baker, J.T.)				
POW, NA (PURIFIED)				
125 gm	**10106-1131-04**	35.05		
500 gm	**10106-1131-01**	113.52		
(Gallipot)				
POW, NA (PURIFIED)				
100 gm	**51552-0202-05**	33.53		
454 gm	**51552-0202-06**	95.90		
(Mallinckrodt Lab)				
POW, NA, 125 gm	**00406-0304-02**	33.49		
500 gm	**00406-0304-12**	110.97		
(Medisca)				
POW, NA, 25 gm	**38779-1046-04**	28.50		
100 gm	**38779-1046-05**	64.50		
(USP,1X500GM)				
500 gm	**38779-1046-08**	217.50		
(PCCA)				
POW, NA (USP)				
1 gm	**51927-1262-00**	1.68		
(Spectrum Pharmacy)				
POW, NA (U.S.P.)				
125 gm	**49452-1155-01**	109.90		
500 gm	**49452-1155-02**	320.60		
2500 gm	**49452-1155-03**	1347.50		
BISMUTH SUBNITRATE (Amend)				
POW, NA (U.S.P.)				
125 gm	**17317-0063-04**	16.80		
454 gm	**17317-0063-01**	52.50		
2270 gm	**17317-0063-05**	231.00		
(Baker, J.T.)				
POW, NA (U.S.P.)				
125 gm	**10106-1140-04**	55.18		
500 gm	**10106-1140-01**	94.85		
(Gallipot)				
POW, NA (U.S.P.,N.F.)				
25 gm	**51552-0162-04**	15.40		
113.4 gm	**51552-0162-09**	23.80		
454 gm	**51552-0162-06**	78.40		
(Mallinckrodt Lab)				
POW, NA (U.S.P.)				
125 gm	**00406-0308-02**	51.37		
500 gm	**00406-0308-04**	148.97		
(Medisca)				
POW, NA (U.S.P.)				
25 gm	**38779-1047-04**	34.50		
100 gm	**38779-1047-05**	76.50		
500 gm	**38779-1047-08**	208.50		
(PCCA)				
POW, NA (USP)				
1 gm	**51927-1145-00**	1.68		
(Spectrum Pharmacy)				
POW, NA (U.S.P.)				
125 gm	**49452-1180-01**	117.60		
500 gm	**49452-1180-02**	323.05		
2500 gm	**49452-1180-03**	1491.00		
BISMUTH SUBSALICYLATE (Amend)				
POW, NA (PURIFIED)				
454 gm	**17317-0064-01**	56.00		
2270 gm	**17317-0064-05**	245.00		
11350 gm	**17317-0064-08**	875.00		
(Medisca) *See BISMUTH SALICYLATE*				
(PCCA) *See BISMUTH SALICYLATE*				
(Palmetto)				
REPACK				
CTB, PO, 262 mg, 30s ea	**23490-7252-01**	7.50		
BISMUTH TRIBROMOPHENATE (PCCA)				
POW, NA, 1 gm	**51927-1399-00**	4.80		
BISMUTH TRICHLORIDE (Baker, J.T.)				
bismuth chloride				
POW, NA (REAGENT)				
500 gm	**10106-1150-01**	259.05		
BISOPROLOL (Vibranta)				
REPACK				
bisoprolol fumarate				
TAB, PO, 5 mg, 30s ea	**57866-7068-01**	74.25		
90s ea	**57866-7068-02**	215.10		
10 mg, 30s ea	**57866-4655-01**	74.25		
90s ea	**57866-4655-02**	215.10		
BISOPROLOL FM (Quality Care Prod)				
REPACK				
bisoprolol fumarate				
TAB, PO, 5 mg, 100s ea	**49999-0866-00**	146.36		
BISOPROLOL FUMARATE				
FUL				
TAB, PO, 5 mg, 100s ea		106.88		
10 mg, 100s ea		106.88		
(Aurobindo Pharma)				
TAB, PO (USP,FILM-COATED)				
5 mg, 30s ea	**65862-0086-30**	36.59		AB
100s ea	**65862-0086-01**	121.97		AB
10 mg, 30s ea	**65862-0087-30**	36.59		AB
100s ea	**65862-0087-01**	121.97		AB
(Greenstone)				
TAB, PO (USP,FILM COATED)				
5 mg, 30s ea	**59762-1258-01**	36.59		
100s ea	**59762-1258-02**	121.97		
10 mg, 30s ea	**59762-1261-01**	36.59		
100s ea	**59762-1261-02**	121.97		
(Mylan)				
TAB, PO (FILM-COATED)				
5 mg, 30s ea	**00378-0523-93**	67.60		AB
100s ea	**00378-0523-01**	225.30		AB
10 mg, 30s ea	**00378-0524-93**	67.60		AB
100s ea	**00378-0524-01**	225.30		AB
(Sandoz)				
TAB, PO, 5 mg, 30s ea	**00185-0771-30**	36.59		AB
100s ea	**00185-0771-01**	121.97		AB
10 mg, 30s ea	**00185-0774-30**	36.59		AB
100s ea	**00185-0774-01**	121.97		AB
(Teva)				
TAB, PO (FILM-COATED)				
5 mg, 30s ea	**00093-5270-56**	36.59		
10 mg, 30s ea	**00093-5271-56**	36.59		
(Teva) *See ZEBETA*				
(Unichem)				
TAB, PO (USP,FILM COATED)				
5 mg, 30s ea	**29300-0126-13**	36.59		AB
100s ea	**29300-0126-01**	121.97		AB
10 mg, 30s ea	**29300-0127-13**	36.59		AB
100s ea	**29300-0127-01**	121.97		AB
(Phys Total Care)				
REPACK				
TAB, PO, 5 mg, 30s ea	**54868-5095-00**	72.15		AB
(FILM-COATED)				
5 mg, 60s ea	**54868-5095-01**	119.36		
90s ea	**54868-5095-03**	176.04		
100s ea	**54868-5095-02**	223.46		AB
BISOPROLOL FUMARATE AND HYDROCHLOROTHIAZIDE (Phys Total Care)				
bisoprolol fumarate/hydrochlorothiazide				
TAB, PO (USP)				
2.5 mg-6.25 mg,				
30s ea	**54868-4577-00**	9.42		
60s ea	**54868-4577-02**	15.84		
BISOPROLOL FUMARATE/HYDROCHLOROTHIAZIDE				
FUL				
TAB, PO, 2.5 mg-6.25 mg,				
100s ea		102.60		
5 mg-6.25 mg,				
100s ea		102.60		
10 mg-6.25 mg,				
100s ea		25.42		
(Mylan) *See BISOPROLOL/HCTZ*				
(Sandoz) *See BISOPROLOL/HCTZ*				
(Teva) *See ZIAC*				
(Palmetto)				
REPACK				
TAB, PO, 5 mg-6.25 mg,				
30s ea	**23490-6504-03**	43.50		
60s ea	**23490-6504-06**	87.00		
90s ea	**23490-6504-09**	130.50		
BISOPROLOL FUMARATE/HYDROCHLOROTHIAZIDE				
(Palmetto)				
10 mg-6.25 mg,				
30s ea	**23490-6503-03**	34.25		
BISOPROLOL/HCTZ (Mylan)				
bisoprolol fumarate/hydrochlorothiazide				
TAB, PO, 2.5 mg-6.25 mg,				
100s ea	**00378-0501-01**	114.00		AB
1000s ea	**00378-0501-10**	1140.00		AB
5 mg-6.25 mg,				
100s ea	**00378-0503-01**	114.00		AB
1000s ea	**00378-0503-10**	1140.00		AB
10 mg-6.25 mg,				
100s ea	**00378-0505-01**	114.00		AB
500s ea	**00378-0505-05**	570.00		AB
(Sandoz)				
TAB, PO, 2.5 mg-6.25 mg,				
30s ea	**00185-0701-30**	34.24		AB
100s ea	**00185-0701-01**	114.15		AB
500s ea	**00185-0701-05**	570.75		AB
5 mg-6.25 mg,				
30s ea	**00185-0704-30**	34.24		AB
100s ea	**00185-0704-01**	114.15		AB
500s ea	**00185-0704-05**	570.75		AB
10 mg-6.25 mg,				
30s ea	**00185-0707-30**	34.24		AB
100s ea	**00185-0707-01**	114.15		AB
500s ea	**00185-0707-05**	570.75		AB
(A-S Medication)				
REPACK				
TAB, PO, 2.5 mg-6.25 mg,				
30s ea	**54569-5417-00**	34.22		AB
200s ea	**54569-5417-01**	228.16		AB
5 mg-6.25 mg,				
30s ea	**54569-5404-00**	34.25		EE
200s ea	**54569-5404-01**	228.30		EE
10 mg-6.25 mg,				
30s ea	**54569-5419-00**	34.25		EE
200s ca	**54569-5419-01**	228.30		EE
(DHS, Inc.)				
REPACK				
TAB, PO, 2.5 mg-6.25 mg,				
30s ea	**55887-0267-30**	21.00		AB
10 mg-6.25 mg,				
30s ea	**55887-0625-30**	24.99		AB
60s ea	**55887-0625-60**	40.83		AB
90s ea	**55887-0625-90**	61.05		AB
(Dispensing Solutions)				
REPACK				
TAB, PO, 5 mg-6.25 mg,				
30s ea	**55045-2990-08**	34.00		AB
10 mg-6.25 mg,				
30s ea	**55045-3006-08**	34.20		AB
90s ea	**66336-0612-90**	102.60		AB
(Palmetto)				
REPACK				
TAB, PO, 2.5 mg-6.25 mg,				
30s ea	**23490-7861-03**	34.50		
(PD-Rx Pharm)				
REPACK				
TAB, PO, 2.5 mg-6.25 mg,				
90s ea	**43063-0135-90**	40.60		AB
5 mg-6.25 mg,				
30s ea	**55289-0630-30**	26.92		AB
30s ea	**58864-0784-30**	20.80		AB
90s ea	**55289-0630-90**	42.20		AB
10 mg-6.25 mg,				
90s ea	**43063-0134-90**	44.28		AB
(Pharma Pac)				
REPACK				
TAB, PO, 5 mg-6.25 mg,				
10s ea	**52959-0337-10**	11.69		AB
30s ea	**52959-0337-30**	35.07		AB
10 mg-6.25 mg,				
30s ea	**52959-0241-30**	35.08		AB
(Phys Total Care)				
REPACK				
TAB, PO, 2.5 mg-6.25 mg,				
90s ea	**54868-4577-03**	25.27		AB
100s ea	**54868-4577-01**	22.92		AB
5 mg-6.25 mg,				
30s ea	**54868-4576-00**	9.93		EE

PROD/MFR	NDC	AWP	DP	OBC
(USP)				
5 mg-6.25 mg,				
60s ea	**54868-4576-02**	16.86		EE
90s ea	**54868-4576-03**	25.19		AB
100s ea	**54868-4576-01**	24.57		AB
10 mg-6.25 mg,				
30s ea	**54868-4578-00**	15.84		
60s ea	**54868-4578-02**	17.68		AB
90s ea	**54868-4578-03**	25.77		AB
100s ea	**54868-4578-01**	40.86		AB
(Physician Partner)				
REPACK				
TAB, PO (FILM COATED)				
5 mg-6.25 mg,				
30s ea	**21695-0808-30**	68.10		AB
10 mg-6.25 mg,				
30s ea	**21695-0809-30**	68.40		AB
(Southwood)				
REPACK				
TAB, PO, 2.5 mg-6.25 mg,				
30s ea	**00490-0053-30**	34.05		
60s ea	**00490-0053-60**	68.10		
90s ea	**00490-0053-90**	102.15		
100s ea	**00490-0053-00**	113.50		
5 mg-6.25 mg,				
30s ea	**58016-0286-30**	27.92		AB
60s ea	**58016-0286-60**	55.84		AB
90s ea	**58016-0286-90**	83.76		AB
100s ea	**58016-0286-00**	93.07		AB
120s ea	**58016-0286-02**	111.68		AB
BITREX (Spectrum Pharmacy)				
denatonium benzoate				
POW, NA (N.F.)				
1 gm	**49452-2445-01**	88.55		
5 gm	**49452-2445-02**	277.90		
25 gm	**49452-2445-03**	906.50		
BITTER MELON (PCCA)				
POW, NA, 1 gm	**51927-3460-00**	0.19		
BITTER STOP FLAVOR (PCCA)				
flavoring aid				
SOL, NA (THE MASKED SUPPRESSOR)				
1 ml	**51927-3519-00**	1.50		
BITTERNESS MASKING AGENT				
(Gallipot) *See NATURAL BITTERNESS MASKING*				
(Spectrum Pharmacy) *See BITTERNESS SUPPRESSOR FLAVOR*				
BITTERNESS SUPPRESSOR FLAVOR (Spectrum Pharmacy)				
bitterness masking agent				
SOL, NA (1X100ML)				
100 ml	**49452-1203-01**	82.25		
(1X500ML)				
500 ml	**49452-1203-02**	321.65		
BIVALIRUDIN				
(Medicines Company) *See ANGIOMAX*				
BLACK COHOSH ROOT (PCCA)				
POW, NA, 1 gm	**51927-2991-00**	0.26		
BLACK FOOD COLOR (PCCA)				
color additive				
POW, NA, 1 gm	**51927-1734-00**	4.95		
BLACK WALNUT FLAVOR (PCCA)				
flavoring aid				
SOL, NA, 1 ml	**51927-2167-00**	1.20		
BLACKBERRY (Medisca)				
flavoring aid				
SOL, NA (1X25ML,BLACKBERRY)				
25 ml	**38779-1051-04**	24.00		
(1X100ML,BLACKBERRY)				
100 ml	**38779-1051-05**	34.50		
BLACKBERRY FLAVOR (PCCA)				
flavoring aid				
SOL, NA (ARTIFICIAL)				
1 ml	**51927-2168-00**	0.90		
BLANDOL (Amend)				
mineral oil				
OIL, NA (N.F.)				
480 ml	**17317-1066-01**	4.90		
3840 ml	**17317-1066-06**	21.00		
19200 ml	**17317-1066-08**	70.00		
BLANEX-A (Blansett)				
cpm/phenyleph hcl/phenyltoloxamine cit				
TER, PO, 4 mg-20 mg-40 mg,				
100s ea	**51674-0058-01**	59.12		
BLEOMYCIN (APP)				
bleomycin sulfate				
PDS, IJ (USP,LYOPHILIZED)				
15 u, ea	**63323-0136-10**	41.40		AP
30 u, ea	**63323-0137-20**	91.54		AP
BLEOMYCIN SULFATE				
(APP) *See BLEOMYCIN*				
(Bedford)				
PDS, IJ (S.D.V.,USP)				
15 u, ea	**55390-0005-01**	49.20		AP
30 u, ea	**55390-0006-01**	98.40		AP
(Hospira)				
PDS, IJ, 15 u, ea	**61703-0332-18**	35.80	31.32	AP
30 u, ea	**61703-0323-22**	84.62	74.05	AP
(Teva)				
PDS, IJ (S.D.V.)				
15 u, ea	**00703-3154-01**	85.00		AP
30 u, ea	**00703-3155-01**	120.00		EE
BLEPH-10 (Allergan Inc)				
sulfacetamide sodium				
SOL, OP, 10%, 5 ml	**11980-0011-05**	19.43		AT
(Dispensing Solutions)				
REPACK				
SOL, OP, 10%, 5 ml	**55045-1955-05**	20.00		AT
(Pharma Pac)				
REPACK				
SOL, OP, 10%, 5 ml	**52959-0272-00**	22.99		AT
15 ml	**52959-0272-01**	24.00		AT
BLEPHAMIDE (Allergan Inc)				
prednisolone acetate/sulfacetamide sodium				
SUS, OP, 0.2%-10%, 5 ml	**11980-0022-05**	64.38		
10 ml	**11980-0022-10**	95.47		
(A-S Medication)				
REPACK				
SUS, OP, 0.2%-10%, 5 ml	**54569-0860-00**	62.01		
(Dispensing Solutions)				
REPACK				
SUS, OP, 0.2%-10%, 5 ml	**55045-1873-05**	56.00		
(Nucare Pharm)				
REPACK				
SUS, OP, 0.2%-10%, 5 ml	**66267-0983-05**	34.38		
(Pharma Pac)				
REPACK				
SUS, OP, 0.2%-10%, 5 ml	**52959-0068-01**	79.97		
10 ml	**52959-0068-00**	93.24		
(Phys Total Care)				
REPACK				
SUS, OP, 0.2%-10%, 5 ml	**54868-0634-01**	50.13		
10 ml	**54868-0634-02**	72.25		
(Quality Care Prod)				
REPACK				
SUS, OP, 0.2%-10%, 5 ml	**49999-0408-05**	28.74		
(Southwood)				
REPACK				
SUS, OP, 0.2%-10%, 5 ml	**58016-6234-01**	55.63		
10 ml	**58016-6238-01**	82.50		
BLEPHAMIDE S.O.P. (Allergan Inc)				
prednisolone acetate/sulfacetamide sodium				
OIN, OP, 0.2%-10%,				
3.5 gm	**00023-0313-04**	62.98		
(A-S Medication)				
REPACK				
OIN, OP, 0.2%-10%,				
3.5 gm	**54569-0861-00**	75.69		
(Dispensing Solutions)				
REPACK				
OIN, OP, 0.2%-10%,				
3.5 gm	**55045-2117-09**	55.00		
(Pharma Pac)				
REPACK				
OIN, OP, 0.2%-10%,				
3.5 gm	**52959-0276-03**	64.66		
(Phys Total Care)				
REPACK				
OIN, OP, 0.2%-10%,				
3.5 gm	**54868-1157-00**	44.09		EE
(Southwood)				
REPACK				
OIN, OP, 0.2%-10%,				
3.5 gm	**58016-6428-00**	22.98		
3.5 gm	**58016-6428-01**	54.42		
BLOOD ADMINISTRATION W/CAIR CLAMP (Abbott Hosp)				
kit, administration, blood				
DEV, NA (105", OL)				
48s ea	**00074-3039-48**	702.81	591.84	
BLOOD COLLECTION (Abbott Hosp)				
kit, blood collection, phlebotomy				
DEV, NA (36", 17GX1-7/8" IV NDL)				
48s ea	**00074-4736-48**	147.46	245.76	
BLOOD SECONDARY (Abbott Hosp)				
kit, administration, blood				
DEV, NA (26", SLIDE CLAMP)				
48s ea	**00074-4602-58**	264.96	442.08	
BLOODROOT (PCCA)				
POW, NA (SANGUINARIA CANADENSIS)				
1 gm	**51927-3020-00**	0.88		
BLUE FOOD COLOR (PCCA)				
color additive				
POW, NA, 1 gm	**51927-1276-00**	4.95		
SOL, NA (LIQUID)				
1 ml	**51927-1006-00**	3.86		
BLUEBERRY (Medisca)				
flavoring aid				
SOL, NA (1X25ML,BLUEBERRY)				
25 ml	**38779-1052-04**	19.50		
(1X100ML,BLUEBERRY)				
100 ml	**38779-1052-05**	25.50		
(1X500ML,BLUEBERRY)				
500 ml	**38779-1052-08**	76.50		
BLUEBERRY FLAVOR (PCCA)				
flavoring aid				
POW, NA (ARTIFICIAL)				
1 gm	**51927-3274-00**	0.60		
SOL, NA, 1 ml	**51927-2164-00**	0.90		
BOLDENONE UNDECYLENATE (Medisca)				
OIL, NA, 25 gm, C-III	**38779-2221-04**	2250.00		
1000 gm, C-III	**38779-2221-09**	12825.00		
BONIVA (Roche Labs)				
ibandronate sodium				
SOL, IV, 1 mg/ml, ea	**00004-0188-09**	504.06		
TAB, PO (FILM-COATED)				
2.5 mg, 30s ea	**00004-0185-23**	124.67		
150 mg, 3s ea	**00004-0186-82**	373.97		
(DHS, Inc.)				
REPACK				
TAB, PO, 150 mg, 3s ea	**55887-0641-03**	260.32		
(Phys Total Care)				
REPACK				
SOL, IV (PFS)				
1 mg/ml, ea	**54868-5823-00**	536.87		
TAB, PO (FILM-COATED)				
150 mg, ea	**54868-5322-01**	150.76		
3s ea	**54868-5322-00**	423.56		
(Quality Care Prod)				
REPACK				
TAB, PO (FILM-COATED)				
150 mg, 3s ea	**35356-0423-03**	492.00		
BONTRIL (Dispensing Solutions)				
REPACK				
phendimetrazine tartrate				
CER, PO, 105 mg,				
7s ea, C-III	**66336-0779-07**	19.83		
14s ea, C-III	**66336-0779-14**	33.24		
28s ea, C-III	**66336-0779-28**	56.52		
BONTRIL PDM (Valeant Pharm Intl)				
phendimetrazine tartrate				
TAB, PO, 35 mg,				
100s ea, C-III	**00187-0497-01**	67.36		AA
1000s ea, C-III	**00187-0497-02**	485.10		AA
BONTRIL SLOW-RELEASE (Valeant Pharm Intl)				
phendimetrazine tartrate				
CER, PO, 105 mg,				
100s ea, C-III	**00187-0498-01**	147.31		BC
1000s ea, C-III	**00187-0498-02**	1060.70		BC
(A-S Medication)				
REPACK				
CER, PO, 105 mg,				
ea, C-III	**54569-1798-09**	143.03		BC
14s ea, C-III	**54569-1798-02**	20.02		BC
28s ea, C-III	**54569-1798-06**	40.05		BC
30s ea, C-III	**54569-1798-03**	42.91		BC
(Dispensing Solutions)				
REPACK				
CER, PO, 105 mg,				
30s ea, C-III	**55045-1745-08**	22.80		BC
60s ea, C-III	**55045-1745-06**	45.60		BC

PROD/MFR	NDC	AWP	DP	OBC
(PD-Rx Pharm)				
REPACK				
CER, PO, 105 mg,				
30s ea, C-III	55289-0537-30	60.23		BC
(Pharma Pac)				
REPACK				
CER, PO, 105 mg,				
28s ea, C-III	52959-0628-28	21.89		BC
BOOSTRIX (Glaxo)				
tdap vaccine				
SUS, IM (S.D.V.,TAX INCL)				
0.5 ml 5s	58160-0842-46	223.05		
0.5 ml 10s	58160-0842-11	446.10		
BORAX (Gallipot)				
sodium borate				
GRA, NA (TECHNICAL)				
113.4 gm	51552-0281-04	4.90		
454 gm	51552-0281-06	14.35		
BORIC ACID (Amend)				
GRA, NA (N.F.)				
500 gm	17317-0687-01	9.80		
2270 gm	17317-0687-05	35.00		
11350 gm	17317-0687-08	122.50		
POW, NA (A.C.S., REAGENT)				
500 gm	17317-1512-01	21.00		
(N.F.)				
500 gm	17317-0069-01	9.80		
2270 gm	17317-0069-05	35.00		
(A.C.S., REAGENT)				
2500 gm	17317-1512-05	70.00		
(N.F.)				
11350 gm	17317-0069-08	122.50		
(A.C.S., REAGENT)				
12000 gm	17317-1512-08	176.40		
(Baker, J.T.)				
GRA, NA (N.F.)				
500 gm	10106-0091-01	32.75		
2500 gm	10106-0091-05	125.47		
POW, NA (N.F., IMPALPABLE)				
500 gm	10106-0090-01	33.53		
(Gallipot)				
GRA, NA (N.F.)				
56.7 gm	51552-0046-03	4.90		
113.4 gm	51552-0046-04	6.65		
226.8 gm	51552-0046-05	7.28		
454 gm	51552-0046-06	12.18		
(TECHNICAL)				
2270 gm	51552-0298-02	41.30		
11350 gm	51552-0298-03	83.44		
POW, NA (N.F.)				
56.7 gm	51552-0343-03	2.87		
113.4 gm	51552-0343-04	3.57		
454 gm	51552-0343-06	8.33		
(Humco)				
POW, NA (N.F.)				
120 gm	00395-0303-94	1.68		
360 gm	00395-0303-12	3.94		
(Mallinckrodt Lab)				
POW, NA (N.F.)				
500 gm	00406-2536-04	44.13		
(Medisca)				
GRA, NA (N.F.)				
500 gm	38779-0706-08	25.50		
999 gm	38779-0706-09	49.50		
2500 gm	38779-0706-01	93.00		
POW, NA, 500 gm	38779-0064-08	28.50		
999 gm	38779-0064-09	51.00		
(1X2500GM)				
2500 gm	38779-0064-01	108.00		
(Neurovites)				
POW, NA, 0.5 gm 100s	93595-2021-01	22.50		
(PCCA)				
CRY, NA (ACS)				
1 gm	51927-2476-00	0.17		
GRA, NA (NF,GRANULAR)				
1 gm	51927-1004-00	0.07		
POW, NA (NF)				
1 gm	51927-2010-00	0.08		
(Spectrum Pharmacy)				
CRY, NA (N.F.)				
500 gm	49452-1210-01	64.75		
2500 gm	49452-1210-02	181.65		
12000 gm	49452-1210-03	665.00		
GRA, NA, 500 gm	49452-1220-02	64.75		
2500 gm	49452-1220-03	181.65		
12000 gm	49452-1220-04	665.00		
POW, NA, 500 gm	49452-1230-01	64.75		
2500 gm	49452-1230-02	181.65		
12000 gm	49452-1230-03	665.00		
(Palmetto)				
REPACK				
GRA, NA, 120 gm	23490-7791-04	7.50		
BORIC ANHYDRIDE (Baker, J.T.)				
POW, NA (PURIFIED)				
500 gm	10106-1176-01	58.81		
2500 gm	10106-1176-05	209.81		
BOROFAIR (Major)				
acetic acid/aluminum acetate				
SOL, OT, 2%-0.79%, 60 ml	00904-3524-03	72.00		AT
BORON (PCCA)				
POW, NA, 1 gm	51927-1217-00	10.80		
BORON CITRATE (PCCA)				
POW, NA (5%)				
5%, 1 gm	51927-3343-00	0.57		
BORTEZOMIB				
(Millennium Pharm) *See VELCADE*				
BOSENTAN				
(Actelion Pharm) *See TRACLEER*				
BOSWELLIA SERRATA EXTRACT (PCCA)				
POW, NA (1X1GM)				
1 gm	51927-3064-00	1.29		
BOTOX (Allergan Inc)				
onabotulinumtoxina				
PDS, IJ (SINGLE USE)				
200 u, ea	00023-3921-02	1260.00		
IM, 100 u, ea	00023-1145-01	630.00		
(Phys Total Care)				
REPACK				
PDS, IM, 100 u, ea	54868-4123-00	624.46		
BOTOX COSMETIC (Allergan Inc)				
onabotulinumtoxina				
PDS, IM, 100 u, ea	00023-9232-01	630.00		
BOVINE CARTILAGE (PCCA)				
POW, NA, 1 gm	51927-2941-00	0.75		
BP 10-1 (Acella)				
sulfacetamide sodium/sulfur				
SOA, TP (1X170.1GM)				
10%-1%, 170.1 gm	42192-0104-06	75.64		
BP 8 COUGH (Acella)				
dm/gg/pse hcl				
SUS, PO (AF,GRAPE)				
473 ml	42192-0507-16	246.06		
BP CLEANSING WASH (Acella)				
sulfacetamide sodium/sulfur				
SOA, TP (1X473ML)				
10%-4%, 473 ml	42192-0103-16	144.18		
BP FOLINATAL PLUS B (Acella)				
calcium/cyanocobalamin/folic acid/pyridoxine				
TAB, PO (FILM-COATED)				
200 mg-12 mcg-1 mg-75 mg,				
30s ea	42192-0324-30	34.75		
BP MULTINATAL PLUS (Acella)				
prenatal vitamins				
CTB, PO, 30s ea	42192-0318-30	34.75		
BP POLY-650 (Acella)				
acetaminophen/phenyltoloxamine citrate				
TAB, PO, 650 mg-60 mg,				
100s ea	42192-0304-01	57.57		
BP VIT 3 (Acella)				
nutriceutical				
CAP, PO, 60s ea	42192-0301-60	65.17		
BP-50% UREA EMULSION (Acella)				
urea				
EMU, TP (1X300GM)				
50%, 300 gm	42192-0101-10	181.56		
BPM 6MG (Boca Pharmacal)				
brompheniramine maleate				
TER, PO, 6 mg, 30s ea	64376-0543-31	11.97		
100s ea	64376-0543-01	38.70		
BPM PE (Boca Pharmacal)				
bpm/phenyleph hcl				
SOL, PO (AF,SF,DYE-FREE)				
4 mg/5 ml-7.5 mg/5 ml,				
118 ml	64376-0432-40	14.50		
474 ml	64376-0432-16	55.08		
BPM PSEUDO 6/45MG (Boca Pharmacal)				
bpm/pse hcl				
TER, PO, 6 mg-45 mg,				
30s ea	64376-0544-31	11.97		
100s ea	64376-0544-01	38.70		
BPM/CARBETAPENTANE CIT/PHENYLEPH HCL				
(Capellon) *See TREXBROM*				
(Gentex Pharma) *See SERADEX*				
(Macoven) *See V-COF*				
(Wraser Pharm) *See VAZOTAN*				
BPM/CODEINE PHOS/PHENYLEPH HCL				
(McNeil,R.A.) *See M-END PE*				
(MCR American) *See BROVEX PB C*				
(MCR American) *See BROVEX PB CX*				
(Poly) *See POLY-TUSSIN AC*				
BPM/CODEINE PHOS/PSE HCL				
(McNeil,R.A.) *See M-END WC*				
BPM/DIHYDROCODEINE BITARTRATE/ PHENYLEPH HCL				
(Larken Labs, Inc.) *See ENDACOF-DH*				
(Poly) *See POLY-TUSSIN DHC*				
BPM/DIHYDROCODEINE BITARTRATE/PSE HCL				
(JayMac Pharma) *See J-COF DHC*				
BPM/DIPHENHYDRAMINE HCL				
(Poly) *See ALA-HIST*				
BPM/DIPHENHYDRAMINE HCL/PHENYLEPH HCL				
(Poly) *See ALA-HIST D*				
BPM/DM/GG				
(Llorens Pharma Int) *See TUSNEL*				
BPM/DM/GG/PHENYLEPH HCL				
(Allan Pharmaceutical) *See ALLANHIST PDX*				
(Cypress Pharm) *See BROMHIST-PDX*				
BPM/DM/GG/PSE HCL				
(Boca Pharmacal) *See PEDIAHIST DM*				
(Breckenridge Pharm) *See HISTACOL DM PEDIATRIC*				
(Cypress Pharm) *See BROMHIST-DM PEDIATRIC*				
BPM/DM/PHENYLEPH HCL				
(Auriga) *See DURAVENT DPB*				
(Ballay Pharm., Inc) *See ALACOL DM*				
(Breckenridge Pharm) *See BROMTUSS DM*				
(Breckenridge Pharm) *See PHENYLEPHRINE COMPLEX*				
(Centurion) *See BALACALL DM*				
(Cypress Pharm) *See TUSDEC-DM*				
(Larken Labs, Inc.) *See LOHIST-DM*				
(MCR American) *See BROVEX PEB DM*				
(Poly) *See ALAHIST DM*				
BPM/DM/PSE HCL				
(Boca Pharmacal) *See PBM ALLERGY*				
(Boca Pharmacal) *See PEDIAHIST DM*				
(Boca Pharmacal) *See PSE BROM DM*				
(Breckenridge Pharm) *See BROMDEX D*				
(Cypress Pharm) *See ANDEHIST DM NR*				
(Cypress Pharm) *See BROMHIST PDX*				
(Cypress Pharm) *See BROMHIST-DM*				
(Cypress Pharm) *See RESPERAL-DM*				
(ECR) *See ANAPLEX DM*				
(Larken Labs, Inc.) *See ENDACOF-PD*				
(Laser Pharma) *See DALLERGY DM*				
(Laser Pharma) *See NEO DM*				
(MCR American) *See BROVEX PSB DM*				
(Morton Grove) *See BROMFED DM COUGH*				
(Morton Grove) *See MYPHETANE DX COUGH*				
(PGD, Inc.) *See GENEBROM DM*				
(Prasco Labs) *See BROMPLEX DM*				
(Silarx) *See SILDEC-DM*				
BPM/DM/PSE HYDROCHLORIDE (Pharma Pac)				
REPACK				
bpm/dm/pse hcl				
SYR, PO, 90 ml	52959-0716-03	27.99		
120 ml	52959-0716-04	37.32		
BPM/HYDROCOD BIT/PSE HCL				
(Breckenridge Pharm) *See BROMCOMP HC*				

PROD/MFR | NDC | AWP | DP | OBC

(Breckenridge Pharm) See *BROMPHENEX HD*
(JayMac Pharma) See *J-TAN D HC*

BPM/PHENYLEPH HCL
(Ballay Pharm., Inc) See *ALACOL*
(Boca Pharmacal) See *BPM PE*
(JayMac Pharma) See *J-TAN D SR*
(Macoven) See *V-HIST*
(MCR American) See *BROVEX PEB*
(Respa Pharm) See *RESPAHIST-II*
(Vertical) See *ZOTEX-PE*
(Wraser Pharm) See *VAZOBID*
(Wraser Pharm) See *VAZOL-D*
(Wraser Pharm) See *VAZOTAB*

BPM/PSE HCL
(Boca Pharmacal) See *BPM PSEUDO 6/45MG*
(Boca Pharmacal) See *PSE-BPM*
(Cypress Pharm) See *ANDEHIST NR*
(Cypress Pharm) See *BROMHIST PEDIATRIC*
(Cypress Pharm) See *BROMHIST-NR*
(Dexo) See *ULTRABROM*
(Dexo) See *ULTRABROM PD*
(ECR) See *LODRANE 12D*
(ECR) See *LODRANE 24D*
(JayMac Pharma) See *J-TAN D PD*
(Larken Labs, Inc.) See *LOHIST-12D*
(Larken Labs, Inc.) See *LOHIST-PD*
(MCR American) See *BROVEX PSB*
(Silarx) See *SILDEC*
(Tiber) See *HISTEX SR*

BPO 4% CREAMY WASH COMPLETE PACK (Acella)
benzoyl peroxide
KIT, MR, 212.1 gm........42192-0110-03 81.17

BPO 4% GEL (Acella)
benzoyl peroxide
GEL, TP (1X42.5GM)
4%, 42.5 gm........42192-0105-15 79.46

BPO 8% CREAMY WASH COMPLETE PACK (Acella)
benzoyl peroxide
KIT, MR, 212.1 gm........42192-0111-03 84.19

BPO 8% GEL (Acella)
benzoyl peroxide
GEL, TP (1X42.5GM)
8%, 42.5 gm........42192-0106-15 82.24

BPS GEL (Breckenridge Pharm)
benzoyl peroxide/sulfur
GEL, TP (1X43GM)
6%-3%, 43 gm.......51991-0634-83 37.92

BRANCHAMIN (Nestle)
amino acids
SOL, IV, 4%, 500 ml 18s ..00338-0477-03 1684.80

BRANCHED CHAIN AMINO ACIDS (Spectrum Pharmacy)
amino acids
POW, NA (1X100GM)
100 gm.............49452-1243-01 185.15
(1X500GM)
500 gm.............49452-1243-02 623.00

BRAVELLE (Ferring)
urofollitropin
PDS, IJ (S.D.V. W/DILUENT)
75 iu, 5s ea..........55566-8505-02 427.86 BX
(SDV W/Q-CAP)
75 iu, 5s ea..........55566-8505-06 469.27 BX

BRETHINE (Phys Total Care)
REPACK
terbutaline sulfate
TAB, PO, 2.5 mg, 30s ea...54868-2849-02 20.01 AB
100s ea...........54868-2849-01 61.73 AB
5 mg, 30s ea........54868-1240-00 25.63 AB
100s ea...........54868-1240-01 84.20 AB
200s ea...........54868-1240-02 106.53 AB

BREVIBLOC (Baxter)
esmolol hydrochloride
SOL, IV (SDV,1X10ML,ISOTONIC,PF)
10 mg/ml, 10 ml 10019-0115-39 22.07
(S.D.V., ISOTONIC)
10 mg/ml,
10 ml 100s 10019-0115-01 551.70
(PREMIX,DUAL PORT)
10 mg/ml,
250 ml 10s 10019-0055-61 1535.04
(DOUBLESTRENGTH,PREMIX)
20 mg/ml,
100 ml 10s 10019-0075-87 1535.04

BREVICON (Watson)
ethinyl estradiol/norethindrone
TAB, PO (WALLETTE, 3X28)
35 mcg-0.5 mg,
84s ea.............52544-0254-28 151.24 AB

BREVITAL SODIUM (JHP)
methohexital sodium
PDS, IJ (MDV,USP,FREEZE-DRIED)
2.5 gm, ea, C-IV......42023-0106-01 221.20
(MDV,FREEZE-DRIED PLUG)
500 mg, ea, C-IV 42023-0105-01 51.52
(Phys Total Care)
REPACK
PDS, IV (VIAL)
2.5 gm,
25s ea, C-IV........54868-3727-00 1372.76
5 gm, ea, C-IV........54868-4194-00 137.96
(M.D.V.)
500 mg,
50s ea, C-IV........54868-3694-00 63.00

BREVOXYL-4 (Stiefel Labs)
benzoyl peroxide
GEL, TP, 4%, 42.5 gm.....00145-2374-06 85.70
(Phys Total Care)
REPACK
LOT, TP, 4%, 297 gm......54868-5206-00 79.01

BREVOXYL-8 (Glaxo)
benzoyl peroxide
GEL, TP, 8%, 42.5 gm.....00145-2384-06 93.14
(Phys Total Care)
REPACK
GEL, TP, 8%, 90 gm.......54868-5352-00 100.31

BREZE (ATS)
benzoyl peroxide
PAD, TP, 4.75%, 31s ea 14629-0521-01 111.25
7.75%, 31s ea........14629-0522-01 111.25

BRIJ 30 (Amend)
laureth-4
LIQ, NA, 480 ml 17317-0962-01 15.00
3840 ml 17317-0962-06 60.00
20880 ml 17317-0962-07 193.58
(Spectrum Pharmacy)
polyoxyethylene lauryl ether
POW, NA, 500 gm..........49452-1250-02 103.60

BRIJ 35 (Amend)
laureth-23
SOL, NA, 480 ml..........17317-0964-01 15.00
3840 ml 17317-0964-06 60.00
19200 ml 17317-0964-08 176.40
(Gallipot)
POW, NA, 454 gm.........51552-0614-06 26.81
(PCCA)
POW, NA, 1 gm...........51927-2301-00 0.12
(Spectrum Pharmacy)
polyoxyethylene (2) oleyl ether
POW, NA (1X500GM)
500 gm..............49452-1260-02 122.85
(1X2500GM)
2500 gm............49452-1260-03 423.50

BRIJ 35 SP (Amend)
laureth-23
SOL, NA, 480 ml..........17317-0965-01 15.00
3840 ml 17317-0965-06 60.00
19200 ml 17317-0965-08 176.40

BRIJ 52 (Amend)
ceteth-2
SOL, NA, 480 ml..........17317-0966-01 15.00
3360 ml 17317-0966-06 60.00
16800 ml 17317-0966-08 175.35

BRIJ 56 (Amend)
ceteth-10
SOL, NA, 480 ml..........17317-0967-01 15.00
19200 ml 17317-0967-08 183.60

BRIJ 58 (Amend)
polyoxyethylene (200) cetyl ether
SOL, NA, 480 ml..........17317-0968-01 15.00
3840 ml 17317-0968-06 60.00
19200 ml 17317-0968-08 176.00
(Spectrum Pharmacy)
ceteth-20
POW, NA (1X500GM)
500 gm..............49452-1270-02 185.15
(1X2500GM)
2500 gm............49452-1270-03 472.50

BRIJ 700 (Gallipot)
peg-100 stearate
POW, NA, 454 gm.........51552-0615-06 22.33

BRIJ 78 (Spectrum Pharmacy)
steareth-20
POW, NA (1X500GM)
500 gm..............49452-1280-02 185.15
(1X2500GM)
2500 gm............49452-1280-03 472.50

BRIJ 93 (Gallipot)
polyoxyethylene (2) oleyl ether
SOL, NA, 473 ml..........51552-1007-06 38.50 27.50
(PCCA)
SOL, NA, 1 ml 51927-2143-00 0.38

BRIJ 98 (Spectrum Pharmacy)
polyoxyethylene (20) oleyl ether
POW, NA, 500 gm.........49452-1290-01 191.10
2500 gm............49452-1290-02 493.50

BRILLIANT GREEN (Medisca)
color additive
CRY, NA (1X5GM)
5 gm 38779-1056-03 25.50
25 gm 38779-1056-04 52.50
(PCCA)
POW, NA, 1 gm...........51927-1583-00 8.40
(Spectrum Pharmacy)
POW, NA, 25 gm..........49452-1300-01 108.50
(1X100GM)
100 gm.............49452-1300-02 297.50
SOL, NA, 100 ml..........49452-1303-01 103.60
500 ml 49452-1303-02 215.60

BRILLIANT GREEN/GENTIAN VIOLET/ PROFLAVINE SULFATE
(William Labs) See *TRIPLE DYE*

BRIMONIDINE TARTRATE
FUL
SOL, OP, 0.2%, 5 ml.......................... 22.50
(Akorn)
SOL, OP, 0.2%, 5 ml ......17478-0715-10 32.65 AT
10 ml.............17478-0715-11 65.24 AT
15 ml.............17478-0715-12 97.92 AT
(Allergan Inc) See *ALPHAGAN P*
(Bausch & Lomb Inc.)
SOL, OP, 0.2%, 5 ml ......24208-0411-05 18.13 AT
10 ml.............24208-0411-10 34.06 AT
15 ml.............24208-0411-15 54.69 AT
(Falcon Ophthalmics)
SOL, OP (1X5ML)
0.15%, 5 ml ....61314-0144-05 51.30 AT
(1X10ML)
0.15%, 10 ml ....61314-0144-10 102.60 AT
(1X15ML)
0.15%, 15 ml ....61314-0144-15 153.90 AT
0.2%, 5 ml...........61314-0143-05 32.65
10 ml..............61314-0143-10 65.24
15 ml..............61314-0143-15 97.92
(Pacific Pharma) See *BRIMONIDINE TARTRATE*

BRIMONIDINE TARTRATE (Pacific Pharma)
brimonidine tartrate
SOL, OP, 0.2%, 5 ml 60758-0866-05 32.25
10 ml.............60758-0866-10 64.50
15 ml.............60758-0866-15 96.75

BRIMONIDINE TARTRATE (Teva)
SOL, OP (USP)
0.2%, 5 ml...........00172-4997-16 32.60 AT
10 ml.............00172-4997-17 65.20 AT
15 ml.............00172-4997-24 97.90 AT
(Phys Total Care)
REPACK
SOL, OP, 0.15%, 10 ml ....54868-6094-00 298.15 AT
(Stat Rx)
REPACK
SOL, OP (1X10ML)
0.2%, 10 ml ....16590-0883-10 65.12 AT

BRIMONIDINE TARTRATE/TIMOLOL MALEATE
(Allergan Inc) See *COMBIGAN*

BRINZOLAMIDE
(Alcon Ophthalmic) See *AZOPT*

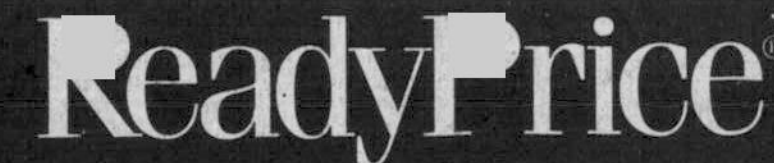

PROD/MFR | NDC | AWP | DP | OBC

BROM/PSEUD/DM (Phys Total Care)
REPACK
bpm/dm/pse hcl
SYR, PO, 473 ml.......... 54868-5496-00 82.98

BROMATAN PLUS (Cypress Pharm)
dm tan/dexchlorpheniramine tan/pse tan
SUS, PO (ORANGE-PINEAPPLE)
473 ml 60258-0410-16 134.12

BROMAX (Poly)
brompheniramine maleate
TER, PO, 11 mg, 100s ea .. 50991-0911-01 112.49

BROMAXEFED DM RF (DHS, Inc.)
REPACK
bpm/dm/pse hcl
SYR, PO (AF,SF,GRAPE)
120 ml 55887-0364-04 25.01

(Quality Care Prod)
REPACK
SYR, PO (AF,SF,GRAPE)
120 ml 49999-0330-04 18.40

BROMAXEFED RF (Quality Care Prod)
bpm/pse hcl
SYR, PO (AF,SF,CHERRY)
4 mg/5 ml-45 mg/5 ml,
120 ml 49999-0553-04 18.40

BROMCOMP HC (Breckenridge Pharm)
bpm/hydrocod bit/pse hcl
SOL, PO (AF,SF,BUBBLE GUM)
473 ml, C-III 51991-0441-16 56.74

BROMDEX D (Breckenridge Pharm)
bpm/dm/pse hcl
SOL, PO (1X473ML,AF,SF)
473 ml 51991-0637-16 44.28

BROMELAIN (Gallipot)
bromelains
POW, NA (600 GDU)
25 gm 51552-1074-04 29.33 20.95

(Spectrum Pharmacy)
POW, NA, 25 gm.......... 49452-1306-01 129.15
100 gm.............. 49452-1306-02 378.00
500 gm.............. 49452-1306-03 1144.50

BROMELAIN 1200 (Gallipot)
bromelains
POW, NA, 1000 gm 51552-1058-07 553.00 395.00

(PCCA)
POW, NA (GDU/GM)
1 gm 51927-3267-00 3.00

BROMELAINS
(Gallipot) *See BROMELAIN*
(Gallipot) *See BROMELAIN 1200*
(PCCA) *See BROMELAIN 1200*
(Spectrum Pharmacy) *See BROMELAIN*

BROMFED (Phys Total Care)
REPACK
bpm/pse hcl
CER, PO, 12 mg-120 mg,
20s ea............ 54868-1211-01 33.05

BROMFED DM COUGH (Morton Grove)
bpm/dm/pse hcl
SYR, PO (1X473ML,BUTTERSCOTCH)
473 ml .... 60432-0837-16 99.93 AA

BROMFENAC
(ISTA Pharm.) *See XIBROM*

BROMFENEX (Quality Care Prod)
REPACK
bpm/pse hcl
CER, PO, 12 mg-120 mg,
60s ea............ 49999-0734-60 36.50

BROMFENEX PD (Quality Care Prod)
bpm/pse hcl
CER, PO, 6 mg-60 mg,
60s ea............ 49999-0735-60 33.37

BROMHEXINE HCL (Spectrum Pharmacy)
bromhexine hydrochloride
POW, NA (B.P.)
1 gm 49452-1305-01 131.60
5 gm 49452-1305-02 423.50
25 gm.............. 49452-1305-03 1680.00

BROMHEXINE HYDROCHLORIDE (Medisca)
CRY, NA (B.P.)
1 gm 38779-0320-06 93.00
5 gm 38779-0320-03 306.00

(PCCA)
POW, NA, 1 gm 51927-1793-00 96.00

(Spectrum Pharmacy) *See BROMHEXINE HCL*

BROMHIST PDX (Cypress Pharm)
bpm/dm/pse hcl
SOL, PO (AF,SF,GRAPE,DROPS)
30 ml............... 60258-0428-30 35.62

BROMHIST PEDIATRIC (Cypress Pharm)
bpm/pse hcl
SOL, PO (AF,SF,DYE-FREE,CHERRY)
1 mg/ml-15 mg/ml,
30 ml............ 60258-0433-30 21.51

BROMHIST-DM (Cypress Pharm)
bpm/dm/pse hcl
SOL, PO (AF,SF,DYE-FREE,GRAPE)
1 mg/ml-4 mg/ml-15 mg/ml,
30 ml............ 60258-0447-30 21.51

BROMHIST-DM PEDIATRIC (Cypress Pharm)
bpm/dm/gg/pse hcl
SYR, PO (AF,DYE-FREE,GRAPE)
473 ml 60258-0446-16 35.97

BROMHIST-NR (Cypress Pharm)
bpm/pse hcl
SOL, PO (AF,SF,CHERRY,DROPS)
1 mg/ml-12.5 mg/ml,
30 ml............ 60258-0427-30 31.25

BROMHIST-PDX (Cypress Pharm)
bpm/dm/gg/phenyleph hcl
SYR, PO (AF,GRAPE)
473 ml 60258-0429-16 54.09

BROMINE (Baker, J.T.)
SOL, NA (A.C.S., REAGENT)
30 ml............... 10106-9760-04 95.07
150 ml 10106-9760-01 121.08
300 ml 10106-9760-06 242.10

BROMOCRIPTINE (Phys Total Care)
REPACK
bromocriptine mesylate
TAB, PO, 2.5 mg, 10s ea... 54868-5667-02 59.97
30s ea............ 54868-5667-00 136.95
60s ea............ 54868-5667-03 272.37
100s ea........... 54868-5667-01 402.06

BROMOCRIPTINE MESYLATE (Gallipot)
POW, NA (1X5GM,USP)
5 gm 51552-1040-02 959.00 685.00

(Medisca)
POW, NA (U.S.P.)
1 gm 38779-0196-06 475.50
5 gm 38779-0196-03 1882.50
10 gm 38779-0196-01 3336.00

(Mylan)
CAP, PO, 5 mg, 30s ea .... 00378-7096-93 158.70 AB
100s ea........... 00378-7096-01 501.20 AB
TAB, PO, 2.5 mg, 30s ea... 00378-2042-93 65.70 AB
100s ea........... 00378-2042-01 218.25 AB

(Novartis Pharm) *See PARLODEL*

(Paddock)
TAB, PO (USP)
2.5 mg, 30s ea .... 00574-0106-03 65.66 AB
100s ea........... 00574-0106-01 218.29 AB

(PCCA)
POW, NA (U.S.P.)
1 gm 51927-2274-00 465.00

(Sandoz)
CAP, PO (USP)
5 mg, 30s ea......... 00781-2119-31 171.44
100s ea........... 00781-2119-01 541.39
TAB, PO, 2.5 mg, 30s ea... 66685-5905-03 70.18 AB
(USP)
2.5 mg, 30s ea .... 00781-5325-31 65.66 AB
100s ea........... 00781-5325-01 218.29 AB
100s ea........... 66685-5905-00 233.31 AB

(Spectrum Pharmacy)
POW, NA (U.S.P.)
1 gm 49452-1308-01 868.00

(Zydus Pharm.)
CAP, PO (USP,HARD GELATIN)
5 mg, 30s ea......... 68382-0110-06 171.40 AB
100s ea........... 68382-0110-01 541.35 AB

BROMOFORM (Baker, J.T.)
LIQ, NA (PURIFIED)
230 ml 10106-9158-04 215.48
500 ml 10106-9158-01 374.20

BROMPHENEX HD (Breckenridge Pharm)
bpm/hydrocod bit/pse hcl
SOL, PO (AF,SF,DYE-FREE)
473 ml, C-III 51991-0148-16 36.31

BROMPHENIRAMINE MALEATE
(Boca Pharmacal) *See BPM 6MG*
(Cypress Pharm) *See BIDHIST*
(ECR) *See LODRANE 24*
(Gallipot)
POW, NA (1X5GM,USP)
5 gm 51552-0894-02 15.26 10.90
(1X25GM,USP)
25 gm.............. 51552-0894-04 36.19 25.85
(1X100GM,USP)
100 gm............. 51552-0894-05 125.30 89.50
(JayMac Pharma) *See J-TAN PD*
(Larken Labs, Inc.) *See LOHIST-12*
(PCCA)
POW, NA (U.S.P.)
1 gm 51927-1950-00 6.00
(Poly) *See BROMAX*
(Respa Pharm) *See RESPA-BR*
(Spectrum Pharmacy)
POW, NA (U.S.P.)
5 gm 49452-1309-04 89.60
25 gm.............. 49452-1309-01 212.10
100 gm............. 49452-1309-05 665.00
(Wraser Pharm) *See VAZOL*

BROMPHENIRAMINE MALEATE/ CODEINE PHOSPHATE
(Larken Labs, Inc.) *See ENDACOF-AC*
(MCR American) *See BROVEX CB*
(MCR American) *See BROVEX CBX*

BROMPHENIRAMINE TAN/DM TAN/PHENYLEPH TAN
(Laser Pharma) *See NEO DM*

BROMPHENIRAMINE TAN/DM TAN/PSE TAN
(ECR) *See ANAPLEX DMX*

BROMPHENIRAMINE TAN/ HYDROCODONE TANNATE/PSE TAN
(Athlon Pharm) *See SYMTAN A*

BROMPHENIRAMINE TANNATE
(JayMac Pharma) *See J-TAN*

BROMPHENIRAMINE TANNATE/ PHENYLEPHRINE TANNATE
(Centurion) *See C-TAN D*
(Centurion) *See C-TAN D PLUS*
(JayMac Pharma) *See J-TAN D*
(MCR American) *See BROVEX ADT*

BROMPHENIRAMINE TANNATE/ PSEUDOEPHEDRINE TANNATE
(ECR) *See LODRANE D*
(MCR American) *See BROVEX PD*

BROMPHENIRAMINE/PSEUDOEPHEDRINE/ DEXTROMETHORPHAN (Dispensing Solutions)
REPACK
bpm/dm/pse hcl
SOL, PO, 118 ml......... 55045-2957-02 25.00

BROMPLEX DM (Prasco Labs)
bpm/dm/pse hcl
SOL, PO (AF,SF,DYE-FREE,FRUIT)
480 ml 66993-0220-57 38.88

BROMTUSS DM (Breckenridge Pharm)
bpm/dm/phenyleph hcl
SOL, PO (AF,SF,DYE-FREE)
473 ml 51991-0443-16 43.25

BRONCHO SALINE 0.9% AEROSAL (Southwood)
REPACK
sodium chloride
SOL, IH, 0.9%, 240 ml 58016-4838-01 7.33

BRONCOMAR (Marlop)
gg/pse hcl/theoph
ELI, PO, 480 ml.......... 12939-0132-16 48.29

BRONCOTRON-D (Seyer Pharmatec)
dm/gg/pse hcl
SUS, PO (AF,SF,DYE-FREE,CHERRY)
118 ml 11026-2680-04 11.40

PROD/MFR NDC AWP DP OBC

BRONTEX (Kenwood)
codeine phosphate/guaifenesin
LIQ, PO, 2.5 mg/5 ml-75 mg/5 ml,
473 ml, C-V **00482-0441-16** 162.30
TAB, PO, 10 mg-300 mg,
100s ea, C-III **00482-0440-01** 408.08

BROVANA (Sepracor)
arformoterol tartrate
SOL, IH, 15 mcg/2 ml,
2 ml 30s UD **63402-0911-30** 204.48
(60X2ML)
15 mcg/2 ml,
2 ml 60s UD **63402-0911-64** 408.96

BROVEX ADT (MCR American)
brompheniramine tannate/phenylephrine tannate
SUS, PO (1X473ML,BUBBLE GUM)
12 mg/5 ml-10 mg/5 ml,
473 ml **58605-0274-01** 115.80

BROVEX CB (MCR American)
brompheniramine maleate/codeine phosphate
TAB, PO, 4 mg-10 mg,
100s ea, C-III **42819-0105-01** 113.39

BROVEX CBX (MCR American)
brompheniramine maleate/codeine phosphate
TAB, PO, 4 mg-20 mg,
100s ea, C-III **42819-0106-01** 113.85

BROVEX PB C (MCR American)
bpm/codeine phos/phenyleph hcl
TAB, PO, 4 mg-10 mg-10 mg,
100s ea, C-III **42819-0103-01** 112.03

BROVEX PB CX (MCR American)
bpm/codeine phos/phenyleph hcl
TAB, PO, 4 mg-20 mg-10 mg,
100s ea, C-III **42819-0104-01** 115.23

BROVEX PD (MCR American)
brompheniramine tannate/pseudoephedrine tannate
SUS, PO (1X473ML,COTTON CANDY)
6 mg/5 ml-30 mg/5 ml,
473 ml **58605-0277-01** 111.45

BROVEX PEB (MCR American)
bpm/phenyleph hcl
SOL, PO (1X473ML,BUBBLE GUM)
4 mg/5 ml-10 mg/5 ml,
473 ml **58605-0152-01** 108.09

BROVEX PEB DM (MCR American)
bpm/dm/phenyleph hcl
SOL, PO (1X473ML,AF,BUBBLE GUM)
473 ml **58605-0153-01** 109.74

BROVEX PSB (MCR American)
bpm/pse hcl
SOL, PO (1X473ML,COTTON CANDY)
4 mg/5 ml-20 mg/5 ml,
473 ml **58605-0150-01** 102.34

BROVEX PSB DM (MCR American)
bpm/dm/pse hcl
SOL, PO (1X473ML,AF,COTTON CANDY)
473 ml **58605-0151-01** 104.71

BROWN FOOD COLOR (PCCA)
color additive
POW, NA, 1 gm **51927-1737-00** 4.95

BRYOPHYLLUM (ARGENTO CULTUM) (Weleda)
homeopathic substance
LIQ, PO (2X)
50 ml **55946-0144-15** 9.00

BSS (Alcon Surgical)
ca cl/k cl/na cl
SOL, IR (OPHTHALMIC)
0.48%-0.075%-0.64%,
15 ml 36s **00065-0795-15** 272.16
30 ml 20s **00065-0795-30** 223.68
250 ml 6s **00065-0795-25** 132.55
500 ml 6s **00065-0795-50** 158.62

BSS & BSS PLUS (Alcon Surgical)
tubing, irrigation
DEV, NA (IRRIGATION SOL ADMIN)
50s ea **00065-0826-50** 420.00

BSS PLUS (Alcon Surgical)
balanced salt solution
SOL, IR (6X250ML)
250 ml 6s .... **00065-0800-25** 298.66 AT
(OPHTHALMIC)
500 ml 6s .... **00065-0800-50** 437.47 AT

BUBBLE GUM (Medisca)
flavoring aid
SOL, NA (1X25ML,ARTIFICIAL)
25 ml **38779-1058-04** 22.50
(1X25ML,CONCENTRATE)
25 ml **38779-1059-04** 19.50
(1X100ML,ARTIFICIAL)
100 ml **38779-1058-05** 37.50
(1X100ML,CONCENTRATE)
100 ml **38779-1059-05** 34.50
(1X500ML,ARTIFICIAL)
500 ml **38779-1058-08** 82.50
(1X500ML,CONCENTRATE)
500 ml **38779-1059-08** 58.50
(1X1000ML,CONCENTRATE)
1000 ml **38779-1059-09** 105.00

BUBBLE GUM ARTIFICIAL FLAVOR (Spectrum Pharmacy)
flavoring aid
LIQ, NA (1X100ML,CONCENTRATE)
100 ml **49452-1287-02** 53.20
(1X500ML,CONCENTRATE)
500 ml **49452-1287-03** 118.30

BUBBLE GUM FLAVOR (PCCA)
flavoring aid
SOL, NA (ANHYDROUS; ARTIFICIAL)
1 ml **51927-2242-00** 0.90
(CONCENTRATE)
1 ml **51927-1820-00** 0.30
1 ml **51927-1898-00** 0.23
1 ml **51927-2233-00** 0.23

BUBBLE GUM SYRUP (Gallipot)
flavoring aid
SYR, NA (PH BUFFERED,SWEETENED)
473 ml **51552-0830-06** 13.09 9.35

BUCALCIDE (Seyer Pharmatec)
benzo/cetylpyridinium cl/menthol/zn cl
SPR, MM (AF)
60 ml **11026-2704-02** 13.20

BUCALSEP (Gil Pharmaceutical)
benzo/cetylpyridinium cl/menthol/zn cl
SOL, TP (AF,PEPPERMINT)
30 ml **58552-0103-01** 11.96
SPR, TP, 30 ml **58552-0104-01** 13.26

BUDEPRION SR (Teva)
bupropion hydrochloride
T12, PO (FILM-COATED)
100 mg, 100s ea **00093-5501-01** 168.90
150 mg, 100s ea **00093-5502-01** 181.04

(Nucare Pharm)
REPACK
T12, PO (FILM-COATED)
150 mg, 30s ea **68071-0122-30** 74.67
60s ea **68071-0122-60** 142.54

(Physician Partner)
REPACK
T12, PO (FILM-COATED)
150 mg, 30s ea **21695-0577-30** 108.62

BUDEPRION XL (Teva)
bupropion hydrochloride
T24, PO (FILM-COATED)
300 mg, 30s ea **00093-5351-56** 143.14 AB3
500s ea **00093-5351-05** 2385.67 AB3
TER, PO, 150 mg, 30s ea .. **00093-5350-56** 143.24
500s ea **00093-5350-05** 2387.33

(IPI)
REPACK
TER, PO, 150 mg, 30s ea .. **18837-0354-30** 143.24

(Phys Total Care)
REPACK
TER, PO, 150 mg, 30s ea .. **54868-5927-00** 335.97

(Physician Partner)
REPACK
T24, PO (FILM-COATED)
300 mg, 30s ea **21695-0578-30** 286.28

(Quality Care Prod)
REPACK
T24, PO (FILM-COATED)
300 mg, 30s ea **35356-0087-30** 191.60 AB3

(Stat Rx)
REPACK
T24, PO (FILM-COATED)
300 mg, 30s ea **16590-0601-30** 146.25 AB3
60s ea **16590-0601-60** 242.50 AB3
90s ea **16590-0601-90** 345.75 AB3
TER, PO, 150 mg, 30s ea .. **16590-0589-30** 199.23
60s ea **16590-0589-60** 295.98
90s ea **16590-0589-90** 443.26

BUDESONIDE
(AstraZeneca) *See PULMICORT FLEXHALER*
(AstraZeneca) *See PULMICORT RESPULES*
(AstraZeneca) *See RHINOCORT AQUA*

(Gallipot)
POW, NA (MICRONIZED)
1 gm **51552-0668-01** 161.00

(Medisca)
POW, NA (MICRONIZED)
0.5 gm **38779-0198-00** 220.50
1 gm **38779-0198-06** 367.50
5 gm **38779-0198-03** 1347.00
25 gm **38779-0198-04** 2985.00
(MICRONIZED,MICRONIZED)
100 gm **38779-0198-05** 9450.00

(Prometheus Labs) *See ENTOCORT EC*

(Spectrum Pharmacy)
POW, NA (EP,MICRONIZED)
0.5 gm **49452-1291-01** 318.85
1 gm **49452-1291-02** 528.50
5 gm **49452-1291-03** 1834.00
(1X25GM,MICRONIZED)
25 gm **49452-1291-04** 4994.50

(Teva)
SUS, IH (30X2ML,MICRONIZED)
0.25 mg/2 ml,
2 ml 30s UD .... **00093-6815-73** 185.22 AN
0.5 mg/2 ml,
2 ml 30s UD .... **00093-6816-73** 218.16 AN

(Phys Total Care)
REPACK
SUS, IH (30X2ML,MICRONIZED)
0.25 mg/2 ml,
2 ml 30s .... **54868-3423-00** 493.93 AN
0.5 mg/2 ml,
2 ml 30s UD .... **54868-3550-00** 498.10 AN

BUDESONIDE MICRONIZED (Hawkins)
budesonide, micronized
POW, NA, 0.5 gm **63370-0035-09** 576.00
1 gm **63370-0035-10** 912.00
5 gm **63370-0035-15** 4080.00
25 gm **63370-0035-25** 16800.00

(Letco)
POW, NA (EP)
0.5 gm **62991-1179-02** 145.50
1 gm **62991-1179-01** 267.00
5 gm **62991-1179-03** 1170.00
25 gm **62991-1179-05** 4800.00

(PCCA)
POW, NA, 1 gm **51927-2834-00** 900.00

BUDESONIDE, MICRONIZED
(Hawkins) *See BUDESONIDE MICRONIZED*
(Letco) *See BUDESONIDE MICRONIZED*
(PCCA) *See BUDESONIDE MICRONIZED*

BUDESONIDE/FORMOTEROL FUMARATE
(AstraZeneca) *See SYMBICORT*

BUFFER PH5 (Gallipot)
buffer solution
SOL, NA, 473 ml **51552-0551-06** 28.00

BUFFER SOLUTION
(Gallipot) *See BUFFER PH5*

BUMETANIDE
FUL
TAB, PO, 0.5 mg, 100s ea 17.43
1 mg, 100s ea 28.14
2 mg, 100s ea 47.08

(Baxter)
SOL, IJ (SDV,1X2ML,USP)
0.25 mg/ml, 2 ml ..... **10019-0506-39** 1.66 AP
(S.D.V.,LATEX-FREE)
0.25 mg/ml,
2 ml 10s .... **10019-0506-02** 16.56 AP
(SDV,1X4ML,USP)
0.25 mg/ml, 4 ml ..... **10019-0506-37** 1.32 AP
(S.D.V.,LATEX-FREE)
0.25 mg/ml,
4 ml 10s .... **10019-0506-45** 13.20 AP
(MDV,1X10ML,USP)
0.25 mg/ml, 10 ml .... **10019-0506-36** 1.93 AP
(M.D.V.,LATEX-FREE)
0.25 mg/ml,
10 ml 10s .... **10019-0506-10** 19.32 AP

(Bedford)
SOL, IJ, 0.25 mg/ml,
2 ml 10s .... **55390-0500-02** 16.20 AP
4 ml 10s .... **55390-0500-05** 16.80 AP

PROD/MFR	NDC	AWP	DP	OBC
(M.D.V.)				
0.25 mg/ml,				
10 ml 10s	55390-0500-10	60.00		AP
(Hospira) *See NOVAPLUS BUMETANIDE*				
(Hospira)				
SOL, IJ (10X4ML)				
0.25 mg/ml,				
4 ml 10s	**00074-1412-04**	10.32	9.00	**AP**
(SD,FLIPTOP,USP,10X4ML)				
0.25 mg/ml,				
4 ml 10s	**00409-1412-04**	10.32	9.00	**AP**
(10X10ML, M.D.V.)				
0.25 mg/ml,				
10 ml 10s	**00074-1412-10**	19.32	16.90	**AP**
(MDV,USP,10X10ML)				
0.25 mg/ml,				
10 ml 10s	**00409-1412-10**	19.32	16.90	**AP**
(Mylan)				
TAB, PO, 0.5 mg, 100s ea	**00378-0245-01**	30.20		**AB**
1 mg, 100s ea	**00378-0370-01**	44.52		**AB**
2 mg, 100s ea	**00378-0417-01**	75.18		**AB**
(Roche Labs) *See BUMEX*				
(Sandoz)				
TAB, PO, 0.5 mg, 100s ea	**00185-0128-01**	55.58		**AB**
500s ea	**00185-0128-05**	274.95		**AB**
1 mg, 100s ea	**00185-0129-01**	79.89		**AB**
500s ea	**00185-0129-05**	366.19		**AB**
2 mg, 100s ea	**00185-0130-01**	133.61		**AB**
500s ea	**00185-0130-05**	663.88		**AB**
(Teva)				
TAB, PO (USP)				
0.5 mg, 100s ea	**00093-4232-01**	36.95		
1 mg, 100s ea	**00093-4233-01**	49.95		
1000s ea	**00093-4233-10**	499.50		
2 mg, 100s ea	**00093-4234-01**	85.69		
1000s ea	**00093-4234-10**	856.90		
(UDL)				
TAB, PO (10X10)				
0.5 mg, 100s ea UD	**51079-0891-20**	29.00		**AB**
(ROBOT READY 25X1)				
1 mg, 25s ea UD	**51079-0892-19**	8.83		**AB**
(10X10)				
1 mg, 100s ea UD	**51079-0892-20**	40.85		**AB**
2 mg, 100s ea UD	**51079-0893-20**	68.90		**AB**
(Dispensing Solutions)				
REPACK				
TAB, PO, 1 mg, 100s ea	**55045-3554-01**	45.00		
2 mg, 30s ea	**55045-2699-08**	10.50		**AB**
BUMETANIDE (Palmetto)				
REPACK				
TAB, PO, 0.5 mg, 30s ea	**23490-9361-03**	45.85		
1 mg, 30s ea	**23490-9362-03**	65.91		
BUMETANIDE (Phys Total Care)				
REPACK				
TAB, PO, 0.5 mg, 30s ea	**54868-3765-00**	11.96		**EE**
1 mg, 30s ea	**54868-3764-00**	19.71		**EE**
60s ea	**54868-3764-01**	42.69		**AB**
2 mg, 15s ea	**54868-4352-02**	15.06		**AB**
20s ea	**54868-4352-03**	18.57		**AB**
30s ea	**54868-4352-00**	25.59		**EE**
60s ea	**54868-4352-04**	46.71		**AB**
90s ea	**54868-4352-05**	67.80		**EE**
120s ea	**54868-4352-01**	88.92		**AB**
(Vibranta)				
REPACK				
TAB, PO, 2 mg, 30s ea	**57866-6069-01**	23.40		
BUMEX (Roche Labs)				
bumetanide				
TAB, PO, 0.5 mg, 100s ea	**00004-0125-01**	69.58		**AB**
5000s ea	**00004-0125-11**	2884.34		**AB**
1 mg, 100s ea	**00004-0121-01**	97.70		**AB**
500s ea	**00004-0121-14**	452.39		**AB**
5000s ea	**00004-0121-11**	4062.06		**AB**
2 mg, 100s ea	**00004-0162-01**	165.17		**AB**
5000s ea	**00004-0162-11**	7048.39		**AB**
(Phys Total Care)				
REPACK				
TAB, PO, 1 mg, 30s ea	**54868-1293-01**	26.38		**AB**
300s ea	**54868-1293-00**	233.29		**AB**
BUMINATE (Baxter Bioscience)				
albumin human				
SOL, IV, 5%, 250 ml	**00944-0491-01**	111.10		
500 ml	**00944-0491-02**	222.19		
25%, 20 ml	**00944-0490-01**	44.44		
50 ml	**00944-0490-02**	109.60		
100 ml	**00944-0490-03**	219.19		

PROD/MFR	NDC	AWP	DP	OBC
BUPAP (ECR)				
acetaminophen/butalbital				
TAB, PO, 650 mg-50 mg,				
100s ea	**00095-0240-01**	47.19		
BUPHENYL (Ucyclyd)				
sodium phenylbutyrate				
POW, PO (WITH MEASURER)				
3 gm/tsp, 250 gm	**62592-0188-64**	3857.38		
TAB, PO, 500 mg, 250s ea	**62592-0496-03**	1928.69		
BUPIV/FENTANYL CITR/SOD CL (PharMEDium Services)				
bupivacaine hcl/fentanyl citrate/na cl				
SOL, EP (INTRAVIA)				
0.0375%-0.005 mg/ml-0.9%,				
50 ml, C-II	**61553-0133-41**	29.23	24.36	
250 ml, C-II	**61553-0127-02**	37.19	30.99	
(IPUMP BAG)				
250 ml, C-II	**61553-0126-02**	53.12	44.27	
(INTRAVIA)				
100 ml, C-II	**61553-0135-48**	31.70	26.42	
250 ml, C-II	**61553-0136-02**	38.68	32.23	
(IPUMP BAG)				
250 ml, C-II	**61553-0137-02**	54.63	45.52	
(INTRAVIA)				
0.1%-0.2 mg/100 ml-0.9%,				
100 ml, C-II	**61553-0123-48**	31.37	26.14	
(IPUMP BAG)				
0.1%-0.2 mg/100 ml-0.9%,				
100 ml, C-II	**61553-0122-48**	45.32	37.77	
(INTRAVIA)				
0.1%-0.4 mg/100 ml-0.9%,				
250 ml, C-II	**61553-0128-02**	39.17	32.64	
0.1%-0.5 mg/100 ml-0.9%,				
250 ml, C-II	**61553-0138-02**	42.02	35.02	
(IPUMP BAG)				
0.1%-0.5 mg/100 ml-0.9%,				
250 ml, C-II	**61553-0141-02**	57.93	48.28	
(INTRAVIA)				
0.1%-1 mg/100 ml-0.9%,				
250 ml, C-II	**61553-0142-02**	49.49	41.24	
100 ml, C-II	**61553-0124-48**	31.55	26.30	
(IPUMP BAG)				
100 ml, C-II	**61553-0125-48**	45.47	37.89	
(INTRAVIA)				
250 ml, C-II	**61553-0139-02**	42.02	35.02	
(IPUMP BAG)				
250 ml, C-II	**61553-0140-02**	57.93	48.28	
(INTRAVIA)				
0.25%-2 mg/100 ml-0.9%,				
250 ml, C-II	**61553-0145-02**	72.22	60.18	
BUPIV/HYDROMORPH/SOD CL (PharMEDium Services)				
bupivacaine hcl/hydromorphone hcl/na cl				
SOL, EP (INTRAVIA)				
0.06%-2 mg/100 ml-0.9%,				
200 ml, C-II	**61553-0157-37**	73.24	61.03	
(IPUMP BAG)				
0.06%-2 mg/100 ml-0.9%,				
200 ml, C-II	**61553-0620-37**	88.86	74.05	
0.125%-2 mg/100 ml-0.9%,				
100 ml, C-II	**61553-0622-48**	70.96	59.13	
(INTRAVIA)				
0.125%-2 mg/100 ml-0.9%,				
200 ml, C-II	**61553-0158-37**	78.03	65.03	
(IPUMP BAG)				
0.125%-2 mg/100 ml-0.9%,				
200 ml, C-II	**61553-0621-37**	92.14	76.78	
BUPIVACAINE HCL (Hawkins)				
bupivacaine hydrochloride				
POW, NA (U.S.P.)				
5 gm	**63370-0040-15**	100.80		
25 gm	**63370-0040-25**	456.00		
100 gm	**63370-0040-35**	1728.00		
(Hospira)				
SOL, IJ (USP,25X2ML,LATEX-FREE)				
0.25%, 10 ml 25s	**00409-1159-01**	42.90	37.50	**AP**
(AMP,STERILE,USP,5X20ML)				
0.25%, 20 ml 5s	**00409-4272-01**	16.14	14.10	**AP**
(AMP,5X30ML,LATEX-FREE)				
0.25%, 30 ml 5s	**00409-1158-01**	15.96	13.95	**AP**
(25X30ML,LATEX-FREE)				
0.25%, 30 ml 25s	**00409-1159-02**	37.80	33.00	**AP**
(W/MALE ADAPTER)				
0.25%, 50 ml 10s	**00074-5749-22**	146.23	127.95	**AP**
(AMP,25X50ML,LATEX-FREE)				
0.25%, 50 ml 25s	**00409-1158-02**	88.80	77.75	**AP**
(VIAL,FLIPTOP,LATEX-FREE)				
0.25%, 50 ml 25s	**00409-1160-01**	72.60	63.50	**AP**
(25X10ML)				
0.5%, 10 ml 25s	**00409-1162-01**	57.60	50.50	**AP**
(VIAL,LATEX-FREE)				
0.5%, 10 ml 25s	**00074-1162-01**	55.80	48.75	**AP**

PROD/MFR	NDC	AWP	DP	OBC
(AMP,LATEX-FREE)				
0.5%, 30 ml 5s	**00409-1161-01**	16.08	14.05	**AP**
(VIAL,LATEX-FREE)				
0.5%, 30 ml 25s	**00409-1162-02**	44.10	38.50	**AP**
(VIAL,FLIPTOP,LATEX-FREE)				
0.5%, 50 ml 25s	**00409-1163-01**	74.40	65.00	**AP**
(VIAL,LATEX-FREE)				
0.75%, 10 ml 25s	**00409-1165-01**	51.30	45.00	**AP**
(AMP,STERILE,USP,5X20ML)				
0.75%, 20 ml 5s	**00409-4274-01**	18.30	16.00	**AP**
(TTV,LATEX-FREE)				
0.75%, 30 ml 25s	**00409-1165-02**	83.70	73.25	**AP**
(Medisca)				
POW, NA (U.S.P.)				
5 gm	**38779-0524-03**	90.00		
25 gm	**38779-0524-04**	405.00		
100 gm	**38779-0524-05**	1167.00		
1000 gm	**38779-0524-09**	5508.00		
(PCCA)				
POW, NA (U.S.P.; MONOHYDRATE)				
1 gm	**51927-2358-00**	27.00		
(B&B Pharm, Inc)				
REPACK				
POW, NA (U.S.P.)				
5 gm	**63275-9993-02**	68.00		
25 gm	**63275-9993-04**	310.00		
100 gm	**63275-9993-05**	1015.00		
BUPIVACAINE HCL MONOHYDRATE (Gallipot)				
bupivacaine hydrochloride				
POW, NA (U.S.P.)				
5 gm	**51552-0456-02**	32.55		
25 gm	**51552-0456-04**	146.30		
(Letco)				
POW, NA (U.S.P.)				
5 gm	**62991-2014-01**	60.00		
25 gm	**62991-2014-02**	255.00		
(Spectrum Pharmacy)				
CRY, NA (U.S.P.)				
1 gm	**49452-1313-01**	64.75		
5 gm	**49452-1313-02**	130.55		
25 gm	**49452-1313-03**	574.00		
(USP)				
100 gm	**49452-1313-04**	1554.00		
BUPIVACAINE HCL W/EPINEPHRINE (Hospira)				
bupivacaine hydrochloride/epinephrine				
SOL, IJ (10X10ML)				
0.25%-1:200000,				
10 ml 10s	**00409-9042-01**	18.96	16.60	
(10X30ML)				
0.25%-1:200000,				
30 ml 10s	**00409-9042-02**	29.40	25.70	
(VIAL, FLIPTOP)				
0.25%-1:200000,				
50 ml 25s	**00409-9043-01**	165.30	144.75	
(VIAL, TEARTOP)				
0.5%-1:200000,				
10 ml 10s	**00409-9045-01**	21.24	18.60	
(VIAL,TEARTOP)				
0.5%-1:200000,				
30 ml 10s	**00409-9045-02**	25.08	21.90	
(25X50ML)				
0.5%-1:200000,				
50 ml 25s	**00409-9046-01**	151.20	132.25	

BUPIVACAINE HCL/DEXTROSE/EPI HCL/LIDO HCL
(Portex) *See SPINAL-22 ANESTHESIA TRAY*
(Portex) *See SPINAL-25 ANESTHESIA TRAY*
(Portex) *See SPINAL-26 ANESTHESIA TRAY*

BUPIVACAINE HCL/FENTANYL CITRATE/NA CL
(PharMEDium Services) *See BUPIV/FENTANYL CITR/SOD CL*

BUPIVACAINE HCL/HYDROMORPHONE HCL/NA CL
(PharMEDium Services) *See BUPIV/HYDROMORPH/SOD CL*

BUPIVACAINE HYDROCHLORIDE
(APP) *See SENSORCAINE*
(APP) *See SENSORCAINE-MPF*
(Gallipot) *See BUPIVACAINE HCL MONOHYDRATE*
(Hawkins) *See BUPIVACAINE HCL*
(Hospira) *See BUPIVACAINE HCL*
(Hospira) *See BUPIVACAINE SPINAL AMPUL*
(Hospira) *See MARCAINE HCL*
(Hospira) *See MARCAINE SPINAL*

PROD/MFR	NDC	AWP	DP	OBC
(Hospira)				
SOL, IJ (SINGLE-DOSE,5X20ML,PF)				
0.5%, 20 ml 5s	00409-4273-01	16.08	14.05	AP
(5X30ML,USP)				
0.75%, 30 ml 5s	00409-1164-01	16.26	14.25	AP
(Letco) *See BUPIVACAINE HCL MONOHYDRATE*				
(Letco)				
POW, NA, 1000 gm	62991-2014-03	7500.00		
(Medisca) *See BUPIVACAINE HCL*				
(PCCA) *See BUPIVACAINE HCL*				
(Spectrum Pharmacy) *See BUPIVACAINE HCL MONOHYDRATE*				
BUPIVACAINE HYDROCHLORIDE WITH EPINEPHRINE (Hospira)				
bupivacaine hydrochloride/epinephrine				
SOL, IJ (DENTAL USE,50X1.8ML)				
0.5%-1:200000,				
1.8 ml 50s	00409-7600-01	33.60	29.50	EE
BUPIVACAINE HYDROCHLORIDE/EPINEPHRINE				
(APP) *See SENSORCAINE-MPF WITH EPINEPHRINE*				
(Hospira) *See BUPIVACAINE HCL W/EPINEPHRINE*				
(Hospira) *See BUPIVACAINE HYDROCHLORIDE WITH EPINEPHRINE*				
BUPIVACAINE HYDROCHLORIDE/EPINEPHRINE BITARTRATE				
(Abbott Hosp) *See MARCAINE HCL/EPINEPHRINE*				
(APP) *See SENSORCAINE WITH EPINEPHRINE*				
(APP) *See SENSORCAINE-MPF WITH EPINEPHRINE*				
(Hospira) *See MARCAINE HCL/EPINEPHRINE*				
(Hospira) *See MARCAINE W/ EPINEPHRINE*				
(Hospira) *See MARCAINE WITH EPINEPHRINE*				
BUPIVACAINE HYDROCHLORIDE/SODIUM CHLORIDE				
(PharMEDium Services) *See BUPIVACAINE/SODIUM CHLORIDE*				
BUPIVACAINE SPINAL AMPUL (Hospira)				
bupivacaine hydrochloride				
SOL, IJ (AMP,LATEX-FREE)				
0.25%, 2 ml 10s	00409-3613-01	23.04	20.20	AP
BUPIVACAINE/SODIUM CHLORIDE (PharMEDium Services)				
bupivacaine hydrochloride/sodium chloride				
SOL, IV (INTRAVIA)				
0.0625%-0.9%,				
100 ml	61553-0189-48	24.76	20.63	
(IPUMP BAG)				
0.0625%-0.9%,				
100 ml	61553-0190-48	37.72	31.43	
(INTRAVIA)				
0.125%-0.9%,				
100 ml	61553-0191-48	26.72	22.27	
(IPUMP BAG)				
0.125%-0.9%,				
100 ml	61553-0194-48	40.67	33.89	
(INTRAVIA)				
0.125%-0.9%,				
250 ml	61553-0192-02	31.03	25.86	
0.25%-0.9%, 50 ml	61553-0193-41	26.72	22.27	
BUPRENEX (Reckitt Benckiser)				
buprenorphine hydrochloride				
SOL, IJ (AMP)				
0.3 mg/ml,				
1 ml 5s, C-III	12496-0757-01	34.80		AP
BUPRENORPHINE HYDROCHLORIDE (Bedford)				
SOL, IJ (S.D.V.)				
0.3 mg/ml,				
1 ml 10s, C-III	55390-0100-10	33.60		AP
(Hawkins)				
POW, NA (USP)				
0.1 gm, C-III	63370-0905-06	480.00		
0.5 gm, C-III	63370-0905-09	1920.00		
1 gm, C-III	63370-0905-10	3072.00		
5 gm, C-III	63370-0905-15	12000.00		
(Hospira)				
SOL, IJ (10X1ML,CARPUJECT)				
0.3 mg/ml,				
1 ml 10s, C-III	00409-2012-32	44.64	39.10	AP
(Letco)				
POW, NA, 0.1 gm, C-III	62991-1583-01	255.00		
0.5 gm, C-III	62991-1583-02	1221.00		
1 gm, C-III	62991-1583-03	1800.00		

PROD/MFR	NDC	AWP	DP	OBC
(Medisca)				
POW, NA (U.S.P.)				
0.1 gm, C-III	38779-0888-09	267.00		
0.5 gm, C-III	38779-0888-00	1125.00		
1 gm, C-III	38779-0888-06	1875.00		
(PCCA)				
POW, NA (U.S.P.;CIII)				
1 gm, C-III	51927-1012-00	4650.00		
(PharmaForce)				
SOL, IJ (5X1ML)				
0.3 mg/ml,				
1 ml 5s, C-III	40042-0010-01	15.44		AP
(Reckitt Benckiser) *See BUPRENEX*				
(Reckitt Benckiser) *See SUBUTEX*				
(Roxane)				
TAB, SL, 2 mg,				
30s ea, C-III	00054-0176-13	124.20		AB
8 mg, 30s ea, C-III	00054-0177-13	232.20		AB
(Spectrum Pharmacy)				
POW, NA (U.S.P.)				
0.1 gm, C-III	49452-8253-01	469.00		
0.5 gm, C-III	49452-8253-02	1732.50		
1 gm, C-III	49452-8253-03	2681.00		
5 gm, C-III	49452-8253-04	9737.00		
(Quality Care Prod)				
REPACK				
TAB, SL, 2 mg,				
30s ea, C-III	35356-0555-30	114.77		AB
8 mg, 30s ea, C-III	35356-0556-30	212.03		AB
BUPRENORPHINE HYDROCHLORIDE/NALOXONE HYDROCHLORIDE				
(Reckitt Benckiser) *See SUBOXONE*				
BUPROBAN (Teva)				
bupropion hydrochloride				
TER, PO (FILM-COATED)				
150 mg, 100s ea	00093-5703-01	181.04		
BUPROPION (Bryant Ranch)				
REPACK				
bupropion hydrochloride				
TAB, PO, 75 mg, 30s ea	63629-3449-01	59.99		
60s ea	63629-3449-02	119.95		
(DHS, Inc.)				
REPACK				
TAB, PO, 100 mg, 20s ea	55887-0151-20	19.23		
30s ea	55887-0151-30	28.84		
60s ea	55887-0151-60	57.69		
90s ea	55887-0151-90	86.54		
100s ea	55887-0151-01	96.16		
120s ea	55887-0151-82	115.39		
(IPI)				
REPACK				
TAB, PO, 100 mg, 30s ea	18837-0298-30	36.06		
(Keltman Pharma., Inc.)				
REPACK				
TAB, PO, 100 mg, 30s ea	68387-0353-30	54.65		
(Quality Care Prod)				
REPACK				
T24, PO, 300 mg, 60s ea	35356-0087-60	382.60		
90s ea	35356-0087-90	865.81		
BUPROPION ER (Stat Rx)				
REPACK				
bupropion hydrochloride				
TER, PO, 100 mg, 60s ea	16590-0036-60	140.00		
BUPROPION HCL (Global Pharm)				
bupropion hydrochloride				
TER, PO (FILM-COATED)				
200 mg, 60s ea	00115-5445-13	226.12		AB1
(Mylan)				
TAB, PO, 75 mg, 100s ea	00378-0433-01	72.05		AB
100 mg, 100s ea	00378-0435-01	96.15		AB
(PCCA)				
POW, NA, 1 gm	51927-3358-00	8.28		
(Sandoz)				
TAB, PO, 75 mg, 100s ea	00781-1053-01	72.00		AB
100 mg, 100s ea	00781-1064-01	96.06		AB
TER, PO (FILM-COATED)				
100 mg, 60s ea	00185-0410-60	101.34		AB1
100s ea	00185-0410-01	168.90		AB1
500s ea	00185-0410-05	844.50		AB1
150 mg, 60s ea	00185-0415-60	116.23		AB1
100s ea	00185-0415-01	193.72		AB1
500s ea	00185-0415-05	968.55		AB1
200 mg, 60s ea	00185-1111-60	229.98		AB1

PROD/MFR	NDC	AWP	DP	OBC
(Teva)				
TAB, PO (FILM-COATED)				
75 mg, 100s ea	00093-0280-01	72.08		AB
500s ea	00093-0280-05	360.40		AB
100 mg, 100s ea	00093-0290-01	96.16		AB
500s ea	00093-0290-05	480.80		AB
(UDL)				
TAB, PO (10X10)				
75 mg, 100s ea UD	51079-0943-20	73.00		AB
100 mg, 100s ea UD	51079-0944-20	97.00		AB
(A-S Medication)				
REPACK				
TAB, PO, 100 mg, 90s ea	54569-5391-03	86.54		EE
TER, PO, 100 mg, 60s ea	54569-5568-00	101.29		
(FILM-COATED)				
150 mg, 60s ea	54569-5569-00	135.59		AB1
(Aidarex)				
REPACK				
TAB, PO, 75 mg, 7s ea	33261-0012-07	13.23		AB
12s ea	33261-0012-12	22.68		AB
14s ea	33261-0012-14	26.46		AB
20s ea	33261-0012-20	37.80		AB
21s ea	33261-0012-21	59.69		AB
28s ea	33261-0012-28	52.92		AB
30s ea	33261-0012-30	56.70		AB
60s ea	33261-0012-60	113.40		AB
90s ea	33261-0012-90	170.10		AB
120s ea	33261-0012-02	226.80		AB
100 mg, 7s ea	33261-0013-07	23.45		AB
14s ea	33261-0013-14	46.90		AB
21s ea	33261-0013-21	70.35		AB
28s ea	33261-0013-28	93.80		AB
30s ea	33261-0013-30	100.50		AB
40s ea	33261-0013-40	134.00		AB
60s ea	33261-0013-60	201.00		AB
90s ea	33261-0013-90	301.50		AB
(Altura)				
REPACK				
TAB, PO (FILM COATED)				
75 mg, 20s ea	63874-0567-20	21.95		EE
28s ea	63874-0567-28	30.73		EE
30s ea	63874-0567-30	32.93		EE
(FILM COATED)				
75 mg, 40s ea	63874-0567-40	32.50		EE
50s ea	63874-0567-50	40.63		EE
60s ea	63874-0567-60	65.86		EE
(FILM COATED)				
75 mg, 70s ea	63874-0567-70	56.88		EE
80s ea	63874-0567-80	65.00		EE
90s ea	63874-0567-90	98.79		EE
100s ea	63874-0567-01	109.77		EE
120s ea	63874-0567-04	131.72		EE
150s ea	63874-0567-72	121.88		EE
200s ea	63874-0567-74	162.50		EE
300s ea	63874-0567-77	243.75		EE
100 mg, 10s ea	63874-0616-10	12.65		EE
12s ea	63874-0616-12	16.97		EE
15s ea	63874-0616-15	21.21		EE
20s ea	63874-0616-20	25.31		EE
25s ea	63874-0616-25	35.35		EE
28s ea	63874-0616-28	35.43		EE
30s ea	63874-0616-30	37.96		EE
40s ea	63874-0616-40	56.57		EE
50s ea	63874-0616-50	70.71		EE
60s ea	63874-0616-60	84.85		EE
70s ea	63874-0616-70	98.99		EE
80s ea	63874-0616-80	113.13		EE
90s ea	63874-0616-90	113.88		EE
100s ea	63874-0616-01	126.53		EE
120s ea	63874-0616-04	169.70		EE
150s ea	63874-0616-72	212.13		EE
200s ea	63874-0616-74	282.83		EE
300s ea	63874-0616-77	424.25		EE
(DHS, Inc.)				
REPACK				
T12, PO, 150 mg, 30s ea	55887-0496-30	55.98		
90s ea	55887-0496-90	128.23		
TAB, PO (FILM-COATED)				
75 mg, 30s ea	55887-0650-30	25.23		AB
60s ea	55887-0650-60	49.00		AB
90s ea	55887-0650-90	68.00		AB
TER, PO, 100 mg, 60s ea	55887-0409-60	140.88		AB1
(Dispensing Solutions)				
REPACK				
TAB, PO (FILM-COATED)				
75 mg, 30s ea	55045-3276-08	21.60		AB
60s ea	55045-3276-06	43.20		AB
90s ea	55045-3276-09	64.80		AB
100s ea	55045-3276-01	72.00		AB
120s ea	55045-3276-02	86.40		AB
100 mg, 30s ea	55045-3195-08	28.80		AB

PROD/MFR	NDC	AWP	DP	OBC
60s ea	55045-3195-06	57.60		AB
90s ea	55045-3195-09	86.40		AB
100s ea	55045-3195-01	96.00		AB
120s ea	55045-3195-02	115.20		AB
TER, PO, 150 mg, 60s ea	55045-3197-06	116.00		AB1
(GSMS)				
REPACK				
TAB, PO, 75 mg, 100s ea	60429-0946-01	25.95	8.65	AB
100 mg, 100s ea	60429-0947-01	25.95	8.65	AB
(Keltman Pharma., Inc.)				
REPACK				
TAB, PO, 75 mg, 60s ea	68387-0350-60	91.30		AB
100 mg, 60s ea	68387-0353-60	109.30		AB
(Nucare Pharm)				
REPACK				
TAB, PO (FILM-COATED)				
100 mg, 30s ea	66267-0614-30	36.99		AB
60s ea	66267-0614-60	69.60		AB
(PD-Rx Pharm)				
REPACK				
T12, PO (REDI-SCRIPT)				
150 mg, 30s ea	58864-0840-30	139.79		
TAB, PO, 75 mg, 30s ea	58864-0794-30	13.85		AB
100 mg, 30s ea	55289-0733-30	45.00		AB
(USP)				
100 mg, 60s ea	55289-0733-60	67.50		AB
90s ea	58864-0808-90	162.45		AB
TER, PO, 100 mg, 30s ea	58864-0808-30	45.00		
(REDI-SCRIPT,FILM-COATED)				
150 mg, 60s ea	58864-0840-60	116.00		AB1
(FILM-COATED)				
200 mg, 60s ea	43063-0183-60	284.22		
(Pharma Pac)				
REPACK				
T12, PO, 100 mg, 60s ea	52959-0805-60	114.90		
TAB, PO (FILM-COATED)				
100 mg, 30s ea	52959-0655-30	47.31		AB
40s ea	52959-0655-40	63.04		AB
(Phys Total Care)				
REPACK				
T12, PO, 150 mg, 90s ea	54868-4892-03	176.74		
180s ea	54868-4892-02	328.50		
TAB, PO, 75 mg, 60s ea	54868-4134-00	50.19		AB
100 mg, 30s ea	54868-4550-02	27.90		AB
60s ea	54868-4550-00	52.83		
100s ea	54868-4550-01	84.54		AB
TER, PO (FILM-COATED)				
100 mg, 60s ea	54868-5377-00	150.60		AB1
150 mg, 30s ea	54868-4892-01	83.10		AB1
60s ea	54868-4892-00	161.70		AB1
(Quality Care Prod)				
REPACK				
TER, PO (FILM-COATED)				
100 mg, 60s ea	49999-0349-60	56.60		AB1
150 mg, 30s ea	49999-0381-30	105.62		AB1
(Southwood)				
REPACK				
T12, PO, 150 mg, 30s ea	58016-0881-30	79.91		
60s ea	58016-0881-60	159.82		
90s ea	58016-0881-90	239.73		
100s ea	58016-0881-00	266.37		
120s ea	58016-0881-02	319.64		
150s ea	58016-0881-03	399.55		
TAB, PO, 75 mg, 20s ea	58016-0722-20	16.25		AB
30s ea	58016-0722-30	24.38		AB
40s ea	58016-0722-40	32.50		AB
50s ea	58016-0722-50	40.63		AB
60s ea	58016-0722-60	48.75		EE
70s ea	58016-0722-70	56.88		AB
80s ea	58016-0722-80	65.00		AB
90s ea	58016-0722-90	73.13		AB
100s ea	58016-0722-00	81.25		AB
120s ea	58016-0722-02	97.50		AB
150s ea	58016-0722-03	121.88		AB
200s ea	58016-0722-89	162.50		AB
300s ea	58016-0722-73	243.75		AB
(FILM-COATED)				
100 mg, 10s ea	58016-0584-10	14.14		AB
12s ea	58016-0584-12	16.97		AB
15s ea	58016-0584-15	21.21		AB
20s ea	58016-0584-20	28.28		AB
25s ea	58016-0584-25	35.35		AB
30s ea	58016-0584-30	42.43		AB
40s ea	58016-0584-40	56.57		AB
50s ea	58016-0584-50	70.71		AB
60s ea	58016-0584-60	84.85		AB
70s ea	58016-0584-70	98.99		AB
80s ea	58016-0584-80	113.13		AB
90s ea	58016-0584-90	127.28		AB
100s ea	58016-0584-00	141.42		AB

PROD/MFR	NDC	AWP	DP	OBC
120s ea	58016-0584-02	169.70		AB
150s ea	58016-0584-03	212.13		AB
200s ea	58016-0584-89	282.83		AB
300s ea	58016-0584-73	424.25		AB
TER, PO, 100 mg, 30s ea	58016-0240-30	51.88		
60s ea	58016-0240-60	103.75		
90s ea	58016-0240-90	155.63		
100s ea	58016-0240-00	172.92		
120s ea	58016-0240-02	207.50		
150s ea	58016-0240-03	259.38		
(St. Mary's MPP)				
REPACK				
T12, PO, 150 mg, 60s ea	60760-0839-60	176.15		

BUPROPION HCL XL (Global Pharm)
bupropion hydrochloride

PROD/MFR	NDC	AWP	DP	OBC
T24, PO (FILM-COATED)				
150 mg, 30s ea	00115-6811-08	156.42		AB2
90s ea	00115-6811-10	469.29		AB2
500s ea	00115-6811-02	2607.04		AB2

BUPROPION HYDROBROMIDE
(Sanofi-Aventis) *See APLENZIN*

BUPROPION HYDROCHLORIDE

PROD/MFR	NDC	AWP	DP	OBC
FUL				
T12, PO, 150 mg, 60s ea		109.98		
(Actavis) *See BUPROPION HYDROCHLORIDE XL*				
(Actavis)				
T12, PO (USP,FILM-COATED)				
150 mg, 60s ea	67767-0117-60	174.45		AB2
60s ea	67767-0133-60	174.45		AB1
250s ea	67767-0133-25	726.88		AB1
500s ea	67767-0133-05	1453.75		AB1
(Anchen) *See BUPROPION HYDROCHLORIDE XL*				
(Anchen)				
T24, PO (USP)				
150 mg, 30s ea	10370-0101-03	143.20		AB3
500s ea	10370-0101-50	2386.67		AB3
1000s ea	10370-0101-00	4773.33		AB3
(Apotex Corp.)				
TAB, PO (FILM-COATED)				
75 mg, 90s ea	60505-0158-09	64.89		AB
(USP,FILM-COATED)				
75 mg, 100s ea	60505-0158-01	72.05		AB
(FILM-COATED)				
75 mg, 500s ea	60505-0158-05	360.25		AB
100 mg, 90s ea	60505-0157-09	86.54		AB
(USP,FILM-COATED)				
100 mg, 100s ea	60505-0157-01	96.15		AB
(FILM-COATED)				
100 mg, 500s ea	60505-0157-05	480.75		AB
(BTA) *See WELLBUTRIN XL*				
(Glaxo) *See WELLBUTRIN*				
(Glaxo) *See WELLBUTRIN SR*				
(Glaxo) *See ZYBAN*				
(Global Pharm) *See BUPROPION HCL*				
(Global Pharm) *See BUPROPION HCL XL*				
(Major)				
TAB, PO (10X10,USP,FILM-COATED)				
75 mg, 100s ea UD	00904-5914-61	65.70		AB
100 mg, 100s ea UD	00904-5913-61	87.30		AB
(Mylan) *See BUPROPION HCL*				
(PCCA) *See BUPROPION HCL*				
(Sandoz) *See BUPROPION HCL*				
(Sandoz) *See BUPROPION HYDROCHLORIDE SR*				
(Sandoz)				
TAB, PO (FILM-COATED)				
75 mg, 1000s ea	00781-1053-10	720.00		AB
100 mg, 1000s ea	00781-1064-10	960.60		AB
(Spectrum Pharmacy)				
POW, NA (1X25GM)				
25 gm	49452-8255-05	392.00		
(1X100GM)				
100 gm	49452-8255-06	1354.50		
(Teva) *See BUDEPRION SR*				
(Teva) *See BUDEPRION XL*				
(Teva) *See BUPROBAN*				
(Teva) *See BUPROPION HCL*				
(Teva)				
TAB, PO (10X10,FILM-COATED)				
75 mg, 100s ea UD	00093-0280-93	73.00		AB
100 mg, 100s ea UD	00093-0290-93	97.00		AB
(UDL) *See BUPROPION HCL*				

PROD/MFR	NDC	AWP	DP	OBC
(UDL)				
TAB, PO (USP,10X30,FILM-COATED)				
75 mg, 300s ea UD	51079-0943-56	219.00		AB
(Watson) *See BUPROPION HYDROCHLORIDE SR*				
(Watson Labs) *See BUPROPION HYDROCHLORIDE SR*				
(Watson Labs) *See BUPROPION HYDROCHLORIDE XL*				
(Bryant Ranch)				
REPACK				
TAB, PO (FILM-COATED)				
100 mg, 60s ea	63629-3233-01	111.65		AB
TER, PO, 150 mg, 60s ea	63629-2873-01	152.07		
(Core)				
REPACK				
TER, PO, 100 mg, 30s ea	33358-0052-30	37.91		
60s ea	33358-0053-60	71.34		
(Dispensing Solutions)				
REPACK				
TAB, PO, 75 mg, 30s ea	55045-3770-08	21.60		
(GSMS)				
REPACK				
TAB, PO (USP,FILM-COATED)				
75 mg, 100s ea	60429-0746-01	25.95	8.65	AB
100 mg, 100s ea	60429-0747-01	30.30	10.10	AB
(IPI)				
REPACK				
T12, PO (FILM-COATED)				
150 mg, 30s ea	18837-0246-30	109.03		AB1
60s ea	18837-0246-60	218.06		AB1
(Keltman Pharma., Inc.)				
REPACK				
TAB, PO, 75 mg, 30s ea	68387-0350-30	45.65		
(McKesson Packaging)				
REPACK				
TAB, PO, 75 mg,				
100s ea UD	63739-0317-10	90.10		
100 mg, 100s ea UD	63739-0318-10	120.20		
(Medsource)				
REPACK				
TAB, PO (FILM-COATED)				
100 mg, 30s ea	45865-0375-30	28.50		AB
60s ea	45865-0375-60	57.00		AB
90s ea	45865-0375-90	85.50		AB
100s ea	45865-0375-00	95.00		AB
(Palmetto)				
REPACK				
TAB, PO, 75 mg, 30s ea	23490-5173-03	25.50		
100 mg, 30s ea	23490-5172-03	43.50		
60s ea	23490-5172-06	87.00		
(Pharma Pac)				
REPACK				
T24, PO, 300 mg, 30s ea	52959-0869-30	147.15		
TAB, PO, 75 mg, 60s ea	52959-0898-60	49.54		
100 mg, 60s ea	52959-0655-60	94.50		
90s ea	52959-0655-90	129.90		
(FILM-COATED)				
100 mg, 100s ea	52959-0665-00	157.28		AB
120s ea	52959-0655-02	188.76		
(Phys Total Care)				
REPACK				
TAB, PO, 100 mg, 90s ea	54868-4550-03	77.73		
(Physician Partner)				
REPACK				
T24, PO, 300 mg, 30s ea	21695-0641-30	286.28		
TAB, PO, 75 mg, 60s ea	21695-0017-60	86.46		
100s ea	21695-0017-00	144.10		
100 mg, 30s ea	21695-0018-30	57.69		
60s ea	21695-0018-60	115.38		
90s ea	21695-0018-90	173.07		
100s ea	21695-0018-00	192.30		
TER, PO, 100 mg, 60s ea	21695-0295-60	202.68		
150 mg, 30s ea	21695-0019-30	116.23		
60s ea	21695-0019-60	232.46		
(Quality Care Prod)				
REPACK				
TAB, PO, 75 mg, 30s ea	49999-0918-30	25.95		
100 mg, 30s ea	49999-0349-30	28.30		
90s ea	49999-0349-90	84.90		
100s ea	49999-0349-00	94.33		
(Stat Rx)				
REPACK				
TAB, PO, 75 mg, 30s ea	16590-0037-30	32.25		
60s ea	16590-0037-60	66.50		
(FILM-COATED)				
75 mg, 120s ea	16590-0037-72	203.61		AB
100 mg, 30s ea	16590-0468-30	53.75		

PROD/MFR	NDC	AWP	DP	OBC
(FILM-COATED)				
100 mg, 30s ea	16590-0036-30	111.80		AB
60s ea	16590-0468-60	107.50		
90s ea	16590-0468-90	161.25		
(FILM-COATED)				
100 mg, 90s ea	16590-0036-90	210.00		AB
120s ea	16590-0468-72	215.00		
TER, PO, 150 mg, 30s ea	16590-0038-30	56.00		
60s ea	16590-0038-60	112.00		
BUPROPION HYDROCHLORIDE ER (A-S Medication)				
REPACK				
bupropion hydrochloride				
T24, PO, 300 mg, 30s ea	54569-5969-00	143.04		
BUPROPION HYDROCHLORIDE SR (Sandoz)				
bupropion hydrochloride				
T12, PO (FILM COATED)				
150 mg, 60s ea	00781-1529-60	120.36		AB1
(Watson)				
TER, PO (USP,FILM-COATED)				
100 mg, 60s ea	00591-3540-60	92.56		AB1
(FILM-COATED)				
200 mg, 60s ea	00591-3542-60	206.96		AB1
(Watson Labs)				
T12, PO (FILM-COATED)				
150 mg, 60s ea	00591-3541-60	87.98		AB1
60s ea	00591-3543-60	99.19		AB2
(USP,STARTER PACK)				
150 mg, 60s ea	00591-3543-76	99.19		AB2
(FILM-COATED)				
150 mg, 250s ea	00591-3541-25	366.60		AB1
(Aidarex)				
REPACK				
T12, PO (FILM COATED)				
150 mg, 30s ea	33261-0449-30	105.00		
60s ea	33261-0449-60	210.00		
90s ea	33261-0449-90	315.00		
120s ea	33261-0449-02	420.00		
(Dispensing Solutions)				
REPACK				
T12, PO (FILM COATED)				
150 mg, 60s ea	66336-0897-60	122.52		
90s ea	66336-0897-90	182.86		
(Physician Partner)				
REPACK				
T12, PO, 200 mg, 60s ea	21695-0020-60	431.18		
(Stat Rx)				
REPACK				
T12, PO (FILM COATED)				
150 mg, 90s ea	16590-0038-90	204.15		
BUPROPION HYDROCHLORIDE XL (Actavis)				
bupropion hydrochloride				
T24, PO (USP)				
150 mg, 30s ea	67767-0141-30	156.60		AB3
90s ea	67767-0141-90	469.80		AB3
300 mg, 30s ea	67767-0142-30	188.88		AB3
90s ea	67767-0142-90	566.64		AB3
(Anchen)				
T24, PO (USP)				
300 mg, 30s ea	10370-0102-03	143.04		AB3
500s ea	10370-0102-50	2384.05		AB3
1000s ea	10370-0102-00	4768.10		AB3
(Watson Labs)				
T24, PO (FILM-COATED)				
150 mg, 30s ea	00591-3331-30	90.30		AB3
90s ea	00591-3331-19	270.90		AB3
500s ea	00591-3331-05	1505.00		AB3
300 mg, 30s ea	00591-3332-30	120.12		AB3
500s ea	00591-3332-05	2002.00		AB3
(Aidarex)				
REPACK				
T24, PO (FILM-COATED)				
300 mg, 30s ea	33261-0627-30	215.00		AB3
60s ea	33261-0627-60	430.00		AB3
90s ea	33261-0627-90	645.00		AB3
120s ea	33261-0627-02	860.00		AB3
(American Health)				
REPACK				
T24, PO (10X10)				
150 mg, 100s ea UD	68084-0251-01	465.80		AB3
(3X10)				
300 mg, 30s ea UD	68084-0252-21	143.04		AB3
(Phys Total Care)				
REPACK				
T24, PO (FILM-COATED)				
150 mg, 90s ea	54868-5927-01	295.40		AB3
300 mg, 90s ea	54868-5736-01	300.99		AB3
(Southwood)				
REPACK				
T24, PO (FILM-COATED)				
300 mg, 30s ea	00490-0163-30	177.49		AB3
60s ea	00490-0163-60	354.98		AB3
90s ea	00490-0163-90	532.47		AB3
100s ea	00490-0163-00	591.63		AB3
(Stat Rx)				
REPACK				
T24, PO, 300 mg, 30s ea	16590-0474-30	135.25		
60s ea	16590-0474-60	270.50		
90s ea	16590-0474-90	390.00		
120s ea	16590-0474-72	525.50		
BUPROPION SR (Bryant Ranch)				
REPACK				
bupropion hydrochloride				
T12, PO, 100 mg, 60s ea	63629-3196-01	165.32		
(Core)				
REPACK				
T12, PO, 100 mg, 60s ea	33358-0363-60	169.45		
150 mg, 30s ea	33358-0364-30	90.25		
60s ea	33358-0364-60	155.87		
90s ea	33358-0364-90	199.00		
(Palmetto)				
REPACK				
T12, PO, 150 mg, 30s ea	23490-7689-03	63.50		
60s ea	23490-7689-06	147.00		
(Pharma Pac)				
REPACK				
T12, PO, 150 mg, 30s ea	52959-0806-30	61.59		
60s ea	52959-0806-60	123.15		
(Phys Total Care)				
REPACK				
TER, PO, 100 mg, 30s ea	54868-5377-01	78.30		
(Quality Care Prod)				
REPACK				
T12, PO, 150 mg, 30s ea	49999-0965-30	69.90		
60s ea	49999-0965-60	192.40		
(Southwood)				
REPACK				
T12, PO, 150 mg, 30s ea	58016-0024-30	58.05		
60s ea	58016-0024-60	116.10		
90s ea	58016-0024-90	174.15		
100s ea	58016-0024-00	193.50		
BUPROPION XL (Core)				
REPACK				
bupropion hydrochloride				
T12, PO, 100 mg, 60s ea	33358-0362-60	107.11		
T24, PO, 300 mg, 30s ea	33358-0365-30	161.08		
(Nucare Pharm)				
REPACK				
T24, PO, 300 mg, 30s ea	68071-1311-00	189.88		
(Phys Total Care)				
REPACK				
T24, PO, 300 mg, 30s ea	54868-5736-00	405.60		
BUSPAR (Bristol-Myers)				
buspirone hydrochloride				
TAB, PO, 5 mg, 100s ea	00087-0818-41	117.65		AB
(Pharma Pac)				
REPACK				
TAB, PO, 5 mg, 30s ea	52959-0654-30	48.75		AB
(Phys Total Care)				
REPACK				
TAB, PO, 5 mg, 60s ea	54868-1098-02	60.29		AB
10 mg, 30s ea	54868-1099-00	59.50		AB
60s ea	54868-1099-02	117.13		AB
100s ea	54868-1099-03	182.66		AB
BUSPAR DIVIDOSE (Phys Total Care)				
buspirone hydrochloride				
TAB, PO, 15 mg, 30s ea	54868-4212-00	87.97		AB
60s ea	54868-4212-01	163.89		AB
BUSPIRONE (Bryant Ranch)				
REPACK				
buspirone hydrochloride				
TAB, PO, 5 mg, 45s ea	63629-3197-02	37.23		
90s ea	63629-3197-01	72.32		
10 mg, 30s ea	63629-3047-01	59.45		
60s ea	63629-3047-02	75.05		
(Core)				
REPACK				
TAB, PO, 5 mg, 30s ea	33358-0054-30	32.34		
90s ea	33358-0054-90	74.13		
10 mg, 30s ea	33358-0055-10	60.94		
60s ea	33358-0055-60	76.93		
15 mg, 30s ea	33358-0056-30	89.74		
30 mg, 30s ea	33358-0057-30	138.94		
60s ea	33358-0057-60	223.83		
(DHS, Inc.)				
REPACK				
TAB, PO, 5 mg, 20s ea	55887-0176-20	18.13		
28s ea	55887-0176-28	25.38		
30s ea	55887-0176-30	27.20		
60s ea	55887-0176-60	54.41		
90s ea	55887-0176-90	81.62		
(Keltman Pharma., Inc.)				
REPACK				
TAB, PO, 5 mg, 30s ea	68387-0355-30	25.86		
(Pharma Pac)				
REPACK				
TAB, PO, 10 mg, 30s ea	52959-0676-30	41.45		
60s ea	52959-0676-60	82.80		
30 mg, 60s ea	52959-0834-60	218.37		
(Quality Care Prod)				
REPACK				
TAB, PO, 10 mg, 30s ea	49999-0812-30	46.50		
100s ea	49999-0812-00	155.71		
BUSPIRONE HCL (Ethex)				
buspirone hydrochloride				
TAB, PO, 5 mg, 100s ea	58177-0264-04	81.55		AB
500s ea	58177-0264-08	396.47		AB
10 mg, 100s ea	58177-0265-04	142.21		AB
500s ea	58177-0265-08	691.30		AB
15 mg, 100s ea	58177-0309-04	212.49		AB
500s ea	58177-0309-08	1047.19		AB
(Medisca)				
POW, NA (USP,1X5GM)				
5 gm	38779-0199-03	68.25		
(U.S.P.)				
10 gm	38779-0199-01	118.50		
25 gm	38779-0199-04	285.00		
100 gm	38779-0199-05	975.00		
(Mylan)				
TAB, PO, 5 mg, 100s ea	00378-1140-01	77.10		AB
500s ea	00378-1140-05	374.00		AB
10 mg, 100s ea	00378-1150-01	134.50		AB
500s ea	00378-1150-05	652.30		AB
15 mg, 60s ea	00378-1165-91	121.15		AB
180s ea	00378-1165-80	358.30		AB
30 mg, 60s ea	00378-1175-91	218.10		AB
(Par)				
TAB, PO, 7.5 mg, 100s ea	49884-0725-01	158.03		AB
500s ea	49884-0725-05	790.15		AB
(PCCA)				
POW, NA (U.S.P.)				
1 gm	51927-3399-00	21.60		
(Teva)				
TAB, PO, 5 mg, 100s ea	00093-0053-01	77.12		AB
10 mg, 100s ea	00093-0054-01	134.50		AB
15 mg, 100s ea	00093-1003-01	201.92		AB
500s ea	00093-1003-05	995.28		AB
30 mg, 60s ea	00093-5200-06	218.10		
500s ea	00093-5200-05	1817.50		
(UDL)				
TAB, PO (10X10)				
5 mg, 100s ea UD	51079-0985-20	77.12		AB
10 mg, 100s ea UD	51079-0986-20	134.50		AB
15 mg, 100s ea UD	51079-0960-20	201.90		AB
30 mg, 100s ea UD	51079-0994-20	363.50		AB
(Watson Labs)				
TAB, PO, 5 mg, 100s ea	00591-0657-01	14.70		AB
500s ea	00591-0657-05	69.83		AB
1000s ea	00591-0657-10	132.67		AB
10 mg, 100s ea	00591-0658-01	17.34		AB
500s ea	00591-0658-05	82.37		AB
1000s ea	00591-0658-10	156.49		AB
15 mg, 60s ea	00591-0718-60	18.68		AB
180s ea	00591-0718-18	56.05		AB
500s ea	00591-0718-05	155.70		AB
(A-S Medication)				
REPACK				
TAB, PO, 10 mg, 45s ea	54569-5253-04	62.56		AB
60s ea	54569-5253-05	83.41		AB
90s ea	54569-5253-01	125.12		AB

PROD/MFR	NDC	AWP	DP	OBC
(Aidarex)				
REPACK				
TAB, PO, 5 mg, 7s ea	33261-0388-07	7.35		AB
10s ea	33261-0388-10	10.50		AB
14s ea	33261-0388-14	14.70		AB
20s ea	33261-0388-20	21.00		AB
21s ea	33261-0388-21	22.05		AB
28s ea	33261-0388-28	29.40		AB
30s ea	33261-0388-30	31.50		AB
60s ea	33261-0388-60	63.00		AB
90s ea	33261-0388-90	94.50		AB
100s ea	33261-0388-00	105.00		AB
120s ea	33261-0388-02	126.00		AB
180s ea	33261-0388-03	113.40		AB
(Altura)				
REPACK				
TAB, PO, 5 mg, 20s ea	63874-0688-20	22.97		EE
90s ea	63874-0688-90	103.37		EE
15 mg, 10s ea	63874-0954-10	21.15		AB
15s ea	63874-0954-15	31.72		AB
20s ea	63874-0954-20	42.29		AB
30s ea	63874-0954-30	63.44		AB
60s ea	63874-0954-60	126.87		AB
100s ea	63874-0954-01	211.45		AB
(DHS, Inc.)				
REPACK				
TAB, PO, 10 mg, 30s ea	55887-0576-30	35.00		EE
15 mg, 30s ea	55887-0533-30	49.67		AB
60s ea	55887-0533-60	80.00		AB
90s ea	55887-0533-90	102.00		AB
(Dispensing Solutions)				
REPACK				
TAB, PO, 5 mg, 20s ea	55045-3277-07	16.40		AB
30s ea	55045-3277-08	24.60		AB
60s ea	55045-3277-06	49.20		AB
90s ea	55045-3277-09	73.80		AB
100s ea	55045-3277-01	82.00		AB
120s ea	55045-3277-02	98.40		AB
10 mg, 30s ea	55045-2879-08	37.20		AB
60s ea	55045-2879-06	74.40		AB
90s ea	55045-2879-09	111.60		AB
100s ea	55045-2879-01	124.00		AB
120s ea	55045-2879-02	148.80		AB
(Keltman Pharma., Inc.)				
REPACK				
TAB, PO, 5 mg, 60s ea	68387-0355-60	51.72		AB
(Nucare Pharm)				
REPACK				
TAB, PO, 10 mg, 20s ea	66267-0528-20	39.99		AB
60s ea	66267-0528-60	74.50		AB
(PD-Rx Pharm)				
REPACK				
TAB, PO, 10 mg, 30s ea (USP)	58864-0782-30	37.87		
10 mg, 45s ea	43063-0186-45	12.60		AB
60s ea	43063-0186-60	13.80		AB
(Pharma Pac)				
REPACK				
TAB, PO, 15 mg, 45s ea	52959-0713-45	106.07		AB
60s ea	52959-0713-60	141.41		AB
(Phys Total Care)				
REPACK				
TAB, PO, 5 mg, 60s ea	54868-4565-00	18.06		
10 mg, 30s ea	54868-4568-01	10.71		AB
60s ea	54868-4568-00	15.42		AB
100s ea	54868-4568-02	22.23		AB
120s ea	54868-4568-05	30.87		AB
15 mg, 30s ea	54868-4647-01	18.21		AB
60s ea	54868-4647-00	31.92		AB
90s ea	54868-4647-03	33.58		AB
100s ea	54868-4647-02	124.75		AB
(Physician Partner)				
REPACK				
TAB, PO, 5 mg, 60s ea	21695-0256-60	92.56		AB
(Southwood)				
REPACK				
TAB, PO, 5 mg, 20s ea	58016-0720-20	17.76		EE
28s ea	58016-0720-28	24.86		EE
30s ea	58016-0720-30	26.64		EE
60s ea	58016-0720-60	53.28		EE
100s ea	58016-0720-00	88.80		EE
10 mg, 20s ea	58016-0586-20	25.00		EE
28s ea	58016-0586-28	35.00		EE
30s ea	58016-0586-30	37.50		EE
60s ea	58016-0586-60	75.00		EE
100s ea	58016-0586-00	125.00		EE
(Stat Rx)				
REPACK				
TAB, PO, 7.5 mg, 60s ea	16590-0727-60	98.50		AB
10 mg, 30s ea	16590-0600-30	47.91		AB
45s ea	16590-0600-45	71.87		AB
90s ea	16590-0600-90	143.73		AB
15 mg, 30s ea	16590-0579-30	75.00		AB
60s ea	16590-0579-60	150.00		AB
90s ea	16590-0579-90	205.00		AB
120s ea	16590-0579-72	270.25		AB
(Vibranta)				
REPACK				
TAB, PO, 15 mg, 30s ea	57866-0919-01	61.67		AB
60s ea	57866-0919-02	122.25		AB
90s ea	57866-0919-03	182.82		AB
BUSPIRONE HYDROCHLORIDE				
FUL				
TAB, PO, 5 mg, 100s ea		5.27		
10 mg, 100s ea		7.14		
15 mg, 100s ea		10.28		
(Bristol-Myers) *See BUSPAR*				
(Ethex) *See BUSPIRONE HCL*				
(Major)				
TAB, PO (10X10)				
15 mg, 100s ea UD	00904-6061-61	191.80		
(Medisca) *See BUSPIRONE HCL*				
(Mylan) *See BUSPIRONE HCL*				
(Par) *See BUSPIRONE HCL*				
(PCCA) *See BUSPIRONE HCL*				
(PRX) *See VANSPAR*				
(Teva) *See BUSPIRONE HCL*				
(Teva)				
TAB, PO, 5 mg, 100s ea UD	00172-5663-10	78.05		AB
100s ea	00172-5663-60	81.15		AB
500s ea	00172-5663-70	394.65		AB
10 mg, 100s ea (10X10)	00172-5664-60	141.55		AB
10 mg, 100s ea UD	00172-5664-10	136.25		AB
500s ea	00172-5664-70	688.15		AB
15 mg, 100s ea	00172-5665-60	211.45		AB
500s ea	00172-5665-70	1042.30		AB
(UDL) *See BUSPIRONE HCL*				
(Watson Labs) *See BUSPIRONE HCL*				
(Altura)				
REPACK				
TAB, PO, 15 mg, 90s ea	63874-0954-90	190.30		
(American Health)				
REPACK				
TAB, PO (10X10,USP)				
5 mg, 100s ea UD	68084-0028-01	76.88		
10 mg, 100s ea UD	68084-0029-01	127.55		
15 mg, 100s ea UD	68084-0030-01	211.50		
(Bryant Ranch)				
REPACK				
TAB, PO, 15 mg, 30s ea	63629-1747-01	87.55		
(Dispensing Solutions)				
REPACK				
TAB, PO, 10 mg, 30s ea	66336-0052-30	40.35		AB
(IPI)				
REPACK				
TAB, PO, 15 mg, 30s ea	18837-0341-30	62.54		AB
(McKesson Packaging)				
REPACK				
TAB, PO, 5 mg, 100s ea UD	63739-0319-10	91.58		
(Nucare Pharm)				
REPACK				
TAB, PO, 10 mg, 45s ea	66267-0528-45	79.06		AB
90s ea	66267-0528-90	150.94		AB
15 mg, 30s ea	66267-0875-30	85.99		AB
(Palmetto)				
REPACK				
TAB, PO, 10 mg, 30s ea	23490-5174-01	42.71		
90s ea	23490-5174-09	128.13		
(PD-Rx Pharm)				
REPACK				
TAB, PO (USP)				
15 mg, 15s ea	58864-0963-15	7.99		
(Pharma Pac)				
REPACK				
TAB, PO, 15 mg, 30s ea	52959-0713-30	70.73		
90s ea	52959-0713-90	212.09		
100s ea	52959-0713-00	235.63		
(Phys Total Care)				
REPACK				
TAB, PO, 10 mg, 90s ea	54868-4568-03	21.66		
(Physician Partner)				
REPACK				
TAB, PO, 10 mg, 14s ea	21695-0217-14	42.98		
30s ea	21695-0217-30	78.28		
60s ea	21695-0217-60	156.56		
90s ea	21695-0217-90	234.84		
15 mg, 60s ea	21695-0172-60	253.84		
100s ea	21695-0172-00	424.98		
30 mg, 30s ea	21695-0195-30	218.10		
60s ea	21695-0195-60	436.20		
(Quality Care Prod)				
REPACK				
TAB, PO, 10 mg, 60s ea	49999-0812-60	98.36		AB
BUSULFAN				
(Glaxo) *See MYLERAN*				
(Otsuka) *See BUSULFEX*				
BUSULFEX (Otsuka)				
busulfan				
SOL, IV (8X10ML)				
6 mg/ml, 10 ml 8s	59148-0070-91	9206.40		
BUT/APAP/CAFF/COD (Bryant Ranch)				
REPACK				
apap/butalbital/caff/codeine phos				
CAP, PO				
325 mg-50 mg-40 mg-30 mg, 20s ea, C-III	63629-3152-01	55.32		
BUT/ASP/CAFF W/CODEINE (Bryant Ranch)				
aspirin/butalbital/caffeine/codeine phosphate				
CAP, PO				
325 mg-50 mg-40 mg-30 mg, 20s ea, C-III	63629-2952-02	38.64		
30s ea, C-III	63629-2952-01	57.96		
90s ea, C-III	63629-2952-03	147.27		
BUTABARBITAL SODIUM				
(Meda) *See BUTISOL SODIUM*				
BUTAL/APAP/CAFF/COD (Pharma Pac)				
REPACK				
apap/butalbital/caff/codeine phos				
CAP, PO				
325 mg-50 mg-40 mg-30 mg, 60s ea, C-III	52959-0912-60	163.77		
BUTALB/APAP (Core)				
REPACK				
acetaminophen/butalbital				
TAB, PO, 325 mg-50 mg, 30s ea	33358-0058-30	29.08		
(Phys Total Care)				
REPACK				
TAB, PO, 325 mg-50 mg, 100s ea	54868-5766-00	77.55		
BUTALB/APAP/CAFF (Core)				
REPACK				
acetaminophen/butalbital/caffeine				
TAB, PO, 325 mg-50 mg-40 mg, 20s ea	33358-0059-20	40.45		
30s ea	33358-0059-30	55.54		
60s ea	33358-0059-60	112.11		
500 mg-50 mg-40 mg, 30s ea	33358-0060-30	42.59		
BUTALB/APAP/CAFFEINE (Physician Partner)				
REPACK				
acetaminophen/butalbital/caffeine				
TAB, PO, 500 mg-50 mg-40 mg, 28s ea	21695-0257-28	34.17		
30s ea	21695-0257-30	36.61		
60s ea	21695-0257-60	73.22		
BUTALBITAL (Medisca)				
POW, NA (U.S.P.)				
25 gm, C-III	38779-0922-04	120.00		
100 gm, C-III	38779-0922-05	375.00		
500 gm, C-III	38779-0922-08	1350.00		
(PCCA)				
POW, NA (U.S.P.)				
1 gm, C-III	51927-2446-00	8.28		
BUTALBITAL COMPOUND (Qualitest)				
aspirin/butalbital/caffeine				
CAP, PO, 325 mg-50 mg-40 mg, 100s ea, C-III	00603-2550-21	89.00		AB
TAB, PO, 325 mg-50 mg-40 mg, 100s ea, C-III	00603-2548-21	103.60		AB

PROD/MFR NDC AWP DP OBC

(Bryant Ranch)
REPACK
TAB, PO, 325 mg-50 mg-40 mg,
20s ea, C-III 63629-2951-02 18.55
30s ea, C-III 63629-2951-01 27.83
90s ea, C-III 63629-2951-03 72.00

(Dispensing Solutions)
REPACK
TAB, PO, 325 mg-50 mg-40 mg,
20s ea, C-III 55045-1208-07 16.00
30s ea, C-III 55045-1208-08 24.00
60s ea, C-III 55045-1208-06 48.00
84s ea, C-III 55045-1208-03 67.20
90s ea, C-III 55045-1208-09 72.00
100s ea, C-III 55045-1208-00 80.00
120s ea, C-III 55045-1208-02 96.00

(HomeMed)
REPACK
TAB, PO, 325 mg-50 mg-40 mg,
20s ea, C-III .... 51655-0588-52 26.79 EE
30s ea, C-III .... 51655-0588-24 40.19 EE
60s ea, C-III .... 51655-0588-25 80.37 EE

(Phys Total Care)
REPACK
TAB, PO, 325 mg-50 mg-40 mg,
20s ea, C-III .... 54868-1075-03 14.76 EE
30s ea, C-III .... 54868-1075-02 19.14 EE
50s ea, C-III .... 54868-1075-01 22.77 EE
100s ea, C-III ...... 54868-1075-00 38.04 EE

BUTALBITAL COMPOUND W/CODEINE (Nucare Pharm)
REPACK
aspirin/butalbital/caffeine/codeine phosphate
CAP, PO
325 mg-50 mg-40 mg-30 mg,
15s ea, C-III .... 66267-0038-15 19.47 EE

(Phys Total Care)
REPACK
CAP, PO
325 mg-50 mg-40 mg-30 mg,
20s ea, C-III .... 54868-1037-01 81.66 EE
30s ea, C-III .... 54868-1037-03 92.76 EE
50s ea, C-III .... 54868-1037-00 195.12 EE
60s ea, C-III .... 54868-1037-05 179.55 EE
120s ea, C-III ...... 54868-1037-04 333.81 EE
500s ea, C-III ...... 54868-1037-06 1327.77 EE

BUTALBITAL, ACETAMINOPHEN AND CAFFEINE (Rising)
acetaminophen/butalbital/caffeine
TAB, PO (USP)
500 mg-50 mg-40 mg,
100s ea............ 64980-0155-01 119.00 AB
500s ea............ 64980-0155-05 564.00 AB

BUTALBITAL, ACETAMINOPHEN AND CAFFEINE W/ CODEINE (West-Ward)
apap/butalbital/caff/codeine phos
CAP, PO
325 mg-50 mg-40 mg-30 mg,
100s ea, C-III ...... 00143-3000-01 149.00 AB

BUTALBITAL, ASPIRIN, CAFFEINE & CODEINE (Dispensing Solutions)
REPACK
aspirin/butalbital/caffeine/codeine phosphate
CAP, PO
325 mg-50 mg-40 mg-30 mg,
90s ea, C-III 55045-2352-09 126.00
120s ea, C-III 55045-2352-02 168.00

BUTALBITAL,ASPIRIN,CAFFEINE, AND CODEINE PHOSPHATE (Watson Labs)
aspirin/butalbital/caffeine/codeine phosphate
CAP, PO (USP)
325 mg-50 mg-40 mg-30 mg,
500s ea, C-III ...... 00591-3546-05 665.77 AB

BUTALBITAL/ACET/CAFFEINE (Physician Partner)
REPACK
acetaminophen/butalbital/caffeine
TAB, PO (FILM-COATED)
325 mg-50 mg-40 mg,
20s ea............ 21695-0209-20 30.11
30s ea............ 21695-0209-30 38.40

BUTALBITAL/ACETAMINOPHEN (Southwood)
REPACK
acetaminophen/butalbital
TAB, PO, 325 mg-50 mg,
30s ea............ 58016-0002-30 11.34
60s ea............ 58016-0002-60 22.67
90s ea............ 58016-0002-90 34.01
100s ea........... 58016-0002-00 37.79

PROD/MFR NDC AWP DP OBC

BUTALBITAL/ACETAMINOPHEN/CAFFEINE (Rising)
acetaminophen/butalbital/caffeine
TAB, PO (USP)
325 mg-50 mg-40 mg,
100s ea............ 64980-0154-01 62.00 AB
500s ea............ 64980-0154-05 294.50 AB

(Watson Labs)
TAB, PO (USP)
325 mg-50 mg-40 mg,
100s ea............ 00591-3369-01 11.66 AB
500s ea............ 00591-3369-05 53.33 AB

BUTALBITAL/APAP W/CAFFEINE (Bryant Ranch)
REPACK
acetaminophen/butalbital/caffeine
TAB, PO, 325 mg-50 mg-40 mg,
20s ea............ 63629-1774-01 39.46
30s ea............ 63629-1774-02 54.19
60s ea............ 63629-1774-03 109.38

BUTALBITAL/APAP/CAFF/COD (Phys Total Care)
REPACK
apap/butalbital/caff/codeine phos
CAP, PO
325 mg-50 mg-40 mg-30 mg,
100s ea, C-III 54868-5162-00 115.99

(Southwood)
REPACK
CAP, PO
325 mg-50 mg-40 mg-30 mg,
30s ea, C-III 58016-0493-30 67.15
60s ea, C-III 58016-0493-60 134.29
90s ea, C-III 58016-0493-90 201.45
100s ea, C-III 58016-0493-00 223.82
120s ea, C-III 58016-0493-02 268.60

BUTALBITAL/APAP/CAFFEINE (DHS, Inc.)
REPACK
acetaminophen/butalbital/caffeine
TAB, PO, 500 mg-50 mg-40 mg,
15s ea............ 55887-0149-15 18.00
30s ea............ 55887-0149-30 36.00
60s ea............ 55887-0149-60 54.00
90s ea............ 55887-0149-90 81.00

(Keltman Pharma., Inc.)
REPACK
TAB, PO, 325 mg-50 mg-40 mg,
20s ea............ 68387-0520-20 25.78
30s ea............ 68387-0520-30 34.28

BUTALBITAL/APAP/CAFFEINE/CODEINE (Dispensing Solutions)
REPACK
apap/butalbital/caff/codeine phos
CAP, PO
325 mg-50 mg-40 mg-30 mg,
60s ea, C-III 55045-3702-06 89.40
100s ea, C-III 55045-3702-01 149.00

BUTALBITAL/ASA/CAFF/COD (Southwood)
REPACK
aspirin/butalbital/caffeine/codeine phosphate
CAP, PO
325 mg-50 mg-40 mg-30 mg,
30s ea, C-III 58016-0322-30 55.00
60s ea, C-III 58016-0322-60 110.00
90s ea, C-III 58016-0322-90 165.00
100s ea, C-III 58016-0322-00 183.33
120s ea, C-III 58016-0322-02 220.00

BUTALBITAL/ASA/CAFFEINE (Dispensing Solutions)
REPACK
aspirin/butalbital/caffeine
TAB, PO, 325 mg-50 mg-40 mg,
30s ea, C-III 66336-0619-30 39.94

BUTALBITAL/ASP/CAFFEINE (Altura)
REPACK
aspirin/butalbital/caffeine
CAP, PO, 325 mg-50 mg-40 mg,
10s ea, C-III 63874-0268-10 8.90
12s ea, C-III 63874-0268-12 10.68
14s ea, C-III 63874-0268-14 12.46
15s ea, C-III 63874-0268-15 13.35
20s ea, C-III 63874-0268-20 17.80
21s ea, C-III 63874-0268-21 18.69
24s ea, C-III 63874-0268-24 21.36
25s ea, C-III 63874-0268-25 22.25
28s ea, C-III 63874-0268-28 24.92
30s ea, C-III 63874-0268-30 26.70
40s ea, C-III 63874-0268-40 35.60
50s ea, C-III 63874-0268-50 44.50
60s ea, C-III 63874-0268-60 53.40
100s ea, C-III 63874-0268-01 89.00
1000s ea, C-III 63874-0268-02 890.00

PROD/MFR NDC AWP DP OBC

1-BUTANOL (Baker, J.T.)
butyl alcohol
LIQ, NA (A.C.S., REAGENT)
500 ml 10106-9054-01 30.85
(PHOTREX)
500 ml 10106-9189-01 53.30
(A.C.S., REAGENT)
4000 ml 10106-9054-03 120.30
20000 ml 10106-9054-07 241.02

BUTENAFINE HYDROCHLORIDE
(Mylan) *See MENTAX*

BUTEX FORTE (Athlon Pharm)
acetaminophen/butalbital
CAP, PO, 650 mg-50 mg,
100s ea............ 62022-0070-01 33.99 AB

BUTISOL SODIUM (Meda)
butabarbital sodium
ELI, PO, 30 mg/5 ml,
473 ml, C-III 00037-0110-16 266.34
TAB, PO, 30 mg,
100s ea, C-III ...... 00037-0113-60 188.88 AA
50 mg,
100s ea, C-III 00037-0114-60 245.71

BUTOCONAZOLE NITRATE
(Ther-RX) *See GYNAZOLE-1*

BUTORPHANOL (Southwood)
REPACK
butorphanol tartrate
SPR, NS, 10 mg/ml,
2.5 ml, C-IV 58016-4833-01 79.26

BUTORPHANOL TARTRATE (Abbott Hosp)
SOL, IJ (CARPUJECT)
2 mg/ml,
1 ml 10s, C-IV ..... 00074-2302-01 93.58 78.80 AP

(Apotex Corp.)
SOL, IJ (VIAL)
1 mg/ml,
1 ml, C-IV .... 60505-0658-00 67.50 AP
2 mg/ml, 1 ml, C-IV .. 60505-0659-00 72.50 AP
(M.D.V.)
2 mg/ml,
10 ml, C-IV .... 60505-0660-00 65.00 AP
SPR, NS, 10 mg/ml,
2.5 ml, C-IV .... 60505-0813-01 79.26 AB

(Bedford) *See BUTORPHANOL TARTRATE NOVAPLUS*

(Bedford)
SOL, IJ (S.D.V.)
1 mg/ml,
1 ml 10s, C-IV ..... 55390-0183-01 26.40 AP
2 mg/ml,
1 ml 10s, C-IV ..... 55390-0184-01 36.00 AP
2 ml 10s, C-IV ..... 55390-0184-02 72.00 AP
(M.D.V.)
2 mg/ml,
10 ml, C-IV .... 55390-0185-10 43.20 AP

(Hospira) *See BUTORPHANOL TARTRATE NOVATION*

(Hospira) *See NOVAPLUS BUTORPHANOL TARTRATE*

(Hospira)
SOL, IJ (10X1ML)
1 mg/ml,
1 ml 10s, C-IV ..... 00409-1623-01 15.00 13.10 AP
(CARPUJECT)
1 mg/ml,
1 ml 10s, C-IV ..... 00074-2301-01 87.28 73.50 AP
(S.D.V.)
1 mg/ml,
1 ml 10s, C-IV ..... 61703-0317-45 29.88 26.15 AP
(10X1ML)
2 mg/ml,
1 ml 10s, C-IV ..... 00409-1626-01 16.20 14.20 AP
(S.D.V.)
2 mg/ml,
1 ml 10s, C-IV ..... 61703-0318-45 54.96 48.10 AP
(10X2ML)
2 mg/ml,
2 ml 10s, C-IV ..... 00409-1626-02 45.84 40.10 AP

(Mylan)
SPR, NS, 10 mg/ml,
2.5 ml, C-IV .... 00378-9639-43 75.25 AB

(PCCA)
POW, NA (U.S.P.; CIV)
1 gm, C-IV 51927-2986-00 3600.00

(Roxane)
SPR, NS, 10 mg/ml,
2.5 ml, C-IV .... 00054-3090-36 79.26 AB

(Sandoz) *See STADOL*

PROD/MFR	NDC	AWP	DP	OBC
(Spectrum Pharmacy)				
POW, NA (U.S.P.)				
0.1 gm, C-IV	49452-1317-01	465.50		
1 gm, C-IV	49452-1317-02	2481.50		
(A-S Medication)				
REPACK				
SPR, NS, 10 mg/ml,				
2.5 ml, C-IV	54569-5988-00	77.92		
(Dispensing Solutions)				
REPACK				
SOL, IJ, 2 mg/ml,				
1 ml, C-IV	55045-2968-02	8.50		
(10X1ML)				
2 mg/ml,				
1 ml 10s, C-IV	55045-2968-01	85.00		
(Palmetto)				
REPACK				
SOL, IJ, 2 mg/ml,				
10 ml, C-IV	23490-5186-02	80.00		
(Phys Total Care)				
REPACK				
SPR, NS, 10 mg/ml,				
2.5 ml, C-IV	54868-4583-00	95.07		AB
(Southwood)				
REPACK				
SOL, IJ (10X1ML)				
2 mg/ml,				
1 ml 10s, C-IV	58016-4868-01	72.50		
BUTORPHANOL TARTRATE NOVAPLUS (Bedford)				
butorphanol tartrate				
SOL, IJ (S.D.V.,USP)				
1 mg/ml,				
1 ml 10s, C-IV	55390-0341-10	21.60		AP
2 mg/ml,				
1 ml 10s, C-IV	55390-0342-10	21.60		AP
BUTORPHANOL TARTRATE NOVATION (Hospira)				
butorphanol tartrate				
SOL, IJ (10X2ML)				
2 mg/ml,				
2 ml 10s, C-IV	00409-1626-51	43.68	38.20	AP
BUTTER (Medisca)				
flavoring aid				
SOL, NA (1X25ML,BUTTER)				
25 ml	38779-1061-04	25.50		
(1X100ML,BUTTER)				
100 ml	38779-1061-05	37.50		
BUTTER FLAVOR (PCCA)				
flavoring aid				
SOL, NA (ARTIFICIAL)				
1 ml	51927-2166-00	1.20		
BUTTER RUM FLAVOR (PCCA)				
flavoring aid				
SOL, NA, 1 ml	51927-2165-00	0.90		
BUTTERFLY INFUSION (Abbott Hosp)				
kit, catheterization, intravenous, winged				
DEV, NA (19GX7/8", 12" TUBING)				
120s ea	00074-4590-01	74.88	124.80	
(21GX3/4", 12" TUBING)				
120s ea	00074-4492-01	72.00	120.00	
(21GX3/4", 3-1/2" TUBING)				
120s ea	00074-4821-01	83.52	139.20	
(23GX3/4", 12" TUBING)				
120s ea	00074-4565-01	76.32	127.20	
(23GX3/4", 3-1/2" TUBING)				
120s ea	00074-4867-01	83.52	139.20	
BUTTERFLY INFUSION PEDIATRIC (Abbott Hosp)				
kit, catheterization, intravenous, winged				
DEV, NA (25GX3/4", 12" TUBING)				
120s ea	00074-4506-01	79.20	132.00	
(25GX3/8", 3-1/2" TUBING)				
120s ea	00074-4573-01	74.88	124.80	
(25GX3/8", 8" TUBING)				
120s ea	00074-5588-01	74.88	124.80	
(27GX3/8", 8" TUBING)				
120s ea	00074-4995-01	106.56	177.60	
BUTTERFLY INT INFUSION (Abbott Hosp)				
kit, catheterization, intravenous, winged				
DEV, NA (19GX7/8", 3-1/2" TUBING)				
100s ea	00074-4550-02	88.80	148.00	
(21GX3/4", 3-1/2" TUBING)				
100s ea	00074-4721-02	82.80	138.00	
(23GX3/4", 3-1/2" TUBING)				
100s ea	00074-4871-02	82.80	138.00	
(25GX3/4", 3-1/2" TUBING)				
100s ea	00074-5827-02	88.80	148.00	
BUTTERSCOTCH (Medisca)				
flavoring aid				
SOL, NA (1X100ML,CONCENTRATE)				
100 ml	38779-1063-05	36.00		
(1X500ML,CONCENTRATE)				
500 ml	38779-1063-08	58.50		
BUTTERSCOTCH FLAVOR (PCCA)				
flavoring aid				
SOL, NA, 1 ml	51927-3072-00	0.30		
(Spectrum Pharmacy)				
LIQ, NA (1X100ML)				
100 ml	49452-1289-01	76.65		
(1X500ML)				
500 ml	49452-1289-02	146.65		
BUTYL ACETATE (PCCA)				
LIQ, NA (N)				
1 ml	51927-2412-00	0.28		
BUTYL ALCOHOL				
(Baker, J.T.) *See 1-BUTANOL*				
(Baker, J.T.) *See TERT-BUTYL ALCOHOL*				
(PCCA)				
LIQ, NA (A.C.S.)				
1 gm	51927-1846-00	0.17		
(Spectrum Pharmacy) *See ALCOHOL BUTYL*				
BUTYLATED HYDROXYANISOLE				
(Amend) *See BHA*				
(PCCA)				
POW, NA, 1 gm	51927-1587-00	0.48		
(Spectrum Pharmacy) *See BHA*				
BUTYLATED HYDROXYTOLUENCE (Medisca)				
butylated hydroxytoluene				
POW, NA (N.F.)				
100 gm	38779-0065-05	37.50		
500 gm	38779-0065-08	114.00		
BUTYLATED HYDROXYTOLUENE				
(Amend) *See BHT*				
(Gallipot) *See BHT*				
(Letco)				
POW, NA (NF)				
100 gm	62991-1316-01	30.00		
500 gm	62991-1316-02	90.00		
(Medisca) *See BUTYLATED HYDROXYTOLUENCE*				
(PCCA)				
POW, NA (N.F.,BHT)				
1 gm	51927-1463-00	0.33		
(Spectrum Pharmacy) *See BHT*				
BUTYLENE GLYCOL (PCCA)				
LIQ, NA, 1 ml	51927-3007-00	0.21		
BUTYLPARABEN (Amend)				
POW, NA (N.F.)				
125 gm	17317-0071-04	8.40		
454 gm	17317-0071-01	22.40		
2270 gm	17317-0071-05	91.00		
11350 gm	17317-0071-08	350.00		
(Baker, J.T.)				
POW, NA (N.F.)				
500 gm	10106-0104-01	61.53		
(Gallipot)				
POW, NA (U.S.P.,N.F.)				
454 gm	51552-0161-06	32.20		
(PCCA)				
POW, NA (NF)				
1 gm	51927-1253-00	0.48		
(Spectrum Pharmacy)				
POW, NA (N.F.)				
125 gm	49452-1310-01	97.30		
500 gm	49452-1310-02	202.30		
BUTYRIC ACID (Baker, J.T.)				
LIQ, NA (PURIFIED)				
500 ml	10106-0098-01	30.44		
(PCCA)				
LIQ, NA (REAGENT)				
1 gm	51927-2271-00	0.14		
BY-ACHE (Cypress Pharm)				
apap/phenyltoloxamine cit/salicylamide				
CAP, PO, 300 mg-20 mg-200 mg,				
100s ea	60258-0055-01	40.25		
BYETTA (Amylin)				
exenatide				
SOL, SC (5MCG PER DOSEX60 DOSE)				
250 mcg/ml, 1.2 ml	66780-0210-07	265.93		
(10MCG PER DOSEX60 DOSE)				
250 mcg/ml, 2.4 ml	66780-0210-08	288.96		
(Phys Total Care)				
REPACK				
SOL, SC, 250 mcg/ml, ea	54868-5384-00	275.66		
2s ea	54868-5384-01	344.02		
BYSTOLIC (Forest Pharm)				
nebivolol hydrochloride				
TAB, PO, 2.5 mg, 30s ea	00456-1402-30	59.53		
100s ea	00456-1402-01	198.46		
(10X10)				
2.5 mg, 100s ea UD	00456-1402-63	202.24		
5 mg, 30s ea	00456-1405-30	59.53		
100s ea	00456-1405-01	198.46		
(10X10)				
5 mg, 100s ea UD	00456-1405-63	202.24		
10 mg, 30s ea	00456-1410-30	59.53		
100s ea	00456-1410-01	198.46		
(10X10)				
10 mg, 100s ea UD	00456-1410-63	202.24		
20 mg, 30s ea	00456-1420-30	60.48		EE
100s ea	00456-1420-01	201.60		EE
(A-S Medication)				
REPACK				
TAB, PO, 5 mg, 30s ea	54569-6119-00	59.06		
(Phys Total Care)				
REPACK				
TAB, PO, 5 mg, 30s ea	54868-5944-00	73.02		
90s ea	54868-5944-01	203.96		
10 mg, 90s ea	54868-6018-00	203.96		
C-PHEN (Boca Pharmacal)				
cpm/phenyleph hcl				
SOL, PO (AF,SF)				
4 mg/5 ml-12.5 mg/5 ml,				
118 ml	64376-0729-40	16.51		
473 ml	64376-0729-16	61.18		
(AF,SF,DROPS)				
1 mg/ml-3.5 mg/ml,				
30 ml	64376-0728-30	33.48		
(Phys Total Care)				
REPACK				
SOL, PO (AF,SF,DROPS)				
1 mg/ml-3.5 mg/ml,				
30 ml	54868-6011-00	35.28		
C-PHEN DM (Boca Pharmacal)				
cpm/dm/phenyleph hcl				
SOL, PO (AF,SF,GRAPE)				
118 ml	64376-0727-40	29.06		
473 ml	64376-0727-16	105.73		
(W/DROPPER,AF,SF,DROPS)				
30 ml	64376-0726-30	46.09		
(A-S Medication)				
REPACK				
SOL, PO (AF,SF,DROPS)				
30 ml	54569-5802-00	46.05		
(Keltman Pharma., Inc.)				
REPACK				
SOL, PO, 120 ml	68387-0630-01	36.75		
(Palmetto)				
REPACK				
SOL, PO (DROPS)				
30 ml	23490-7848-00	11.36		
(Physician Partner)				
REPACK				
SOL, PO (1X120ML,DROPS)				
120 ml	21695-0626-04	58.12		
C-TAN D (Centurion)				
brompheniramine tannate/phenylephrine tannate				
SUS, PO (1X473ML,AF,SF,RASPBERRY)				
4 mg/5 ml-5 mg/5 ml,				
473 ml	23359-0006-16	101.77		
C-TAN D PLUS (Centurion)				
brompheniramine tannate/phenylephrine tannate				
SUS, PO (AF,SF,RASPBERRY)				
5 mg/5 ml-5 mg/5 ml,				
473 ml	23359-0007-16	109.77		
C-TANNA 12 (Prasco Labs)				
carbetapentane tannate/chlorpheniramine tannate				
SUS, PO (STRAWBERRY-BLK CURRANT)				
30 mg/5 ml-4 mg/5 ml,				
473 ml	66993-0550-57	138.11		

PROD/MFR NDC AWP DP OBC

C1 ESTERASE INHIBITOR, HUMAN
(CSL) *See BERINERT*
(ViroPharma, Inc.) *See CINRYZE*

C12-15 ALKYL BENZOATE
(PCCA) *See ALKYL BENZOATE*

CA ACE/K ACE/K CL/MG ACE/NA ACE/ NA GLUCONATE
(Amer Regent) *See NUTRILYTE*
(APP) *See LYPHOLYTE*

CA CL/DEXTROSE/HETASTARCH/K CL/ MG CL/NA CL/NA LACT
(Hospira) *See HEXTEND*

CA CL/DEXTROSE/K CL/NA CL
(B. Braun) *See DEXTROSE 5%/RINGERS*
(Baxter) *See DEXTROSE 5% IN RINGERS*
(Hospira) *See DEXTROSE 5% IN RINGERS*

CA CL/DEXTROSE/K CL/NA CL/NA LACT
(B. Braun) *See DEXTROSE 5%/LACTATED RINGERS*
(Baxter) *See LACTATED RINGER'S AND DEXTROSE*
(Baxter) *See LACTATED RINGER'S/DEXTROSE 5%*
(Baxter) *See POTASSIUM CHLORIDE SOLUTION*
(Hospira) *See DEX/LACT. RINGERS/POTASSIUM CHL*
(Hospira) *See DEXTROSE 5% IN RINGERS*
(Hospira) *See DEXTROSE/LACTATED RINGERS/POTASSIUM CHLORIDE*

CA CL/DEXTROSE/MG CL/NA CL/NA LACT
(Baxter) *See DIANEAL LOW CALCIUM PERITONEAL DIALYSIS W/DEXTROSE*
(Baxter) *See DIANEAL PD-2 PERITONEAL DIALYSIS SOLN W/DEXTROSE*

CA CL/ICODEXTRIN/MG CL/NA CL/NA LACT
(Baxter) *See EXTRANEAL*

CA CL/K CL/MG CL/NA ACE/NA CIT/NA CL
(Baxter) *See BALANCED SALT SOLUTION*
(Cytosol Ophth) *See BALANCED SALT SOLUTION*
(Hospira) *See BALANCED SALT SOLUTION*
(HUB Pharma) *See BALANCED SALT SOLUTION*

CA CL/K CL/MG CL/NA ACE/NA CL
(Amer Regent) *See NUTRILYTE II*
(APP) *See LYPHOLYTE-II*
(Hospira) *See TPN ELECTROLYTES*
(Hospira) *See TPN ELECTROLYTES II*
(Hospira) *See TPN ELECTROLYTES II MULTIPLE ELECTROLYTE ADDITIVE*

CA CL/K CL/MG CL/NA CL
(Baxter) *See CARDIOPLEGIC SOLUTION*
(Hospira) *See PLEGISOL*

CA CL/K CL/NA CL
(Akorn) *See BALANCED SALT*
(Alcon Surgical) *See BSS*
(Allergan Medical) *See OCULAR*
(B. Braun) *See RINGER'S INJECTION*
(B. Braun) *See RINGER'S IRRIGATION*
(Baxter) *See RINGER'S INJECTION*
(Baxter) *See RINGER'S IRRIGATION*
(Hospira) *See RINGER'S INJECTION*
(Hospira) *See RINGER'S IRRIGATION*

CA CL/K CL/NA CL/NA LACT
(B. Braun) *See LACTATED RINGER'S*
(Baxter) *See LACTATED RINGER'S*
(Baxter) *See LACTATED RINGER'S IRRIGATION*
(Hospira) *See LACTATED RINGER'S*

CA/CHOLECALCIFEROL/FE/FOLIC ACID/VIT B6/VIT C
(Mission) *See CITRANATAL B-CALM*

CABERGOLINE (Greenstone)
TAB, PO, 0.5 mg, 8s ea.... **59762-0100-01** 276.62
(Par)
TAB, PO, 0.5 mg, 8s ea.... **49884-0673-14** 276.91 AB
(Teva)
TAB, PO, 0.5 mg, 8s ea.... **00093-5420-88** 293.27 AB
(Watson Labs)
TAB, PO, 0.5 mg, 8s ea.... **16252-0536-08** 156.00 AB

(American Health)
REPACK
TAB, PO (3X10)
0.5 mg, 30s ea UD.... **68084-0245-21** 1038.41 AB

CABOSIL M-5 (Amend)
silicon dioxide
POW, NA, 4540 gm **17317-1199-00** 119.00

CACODYLIC ACID (Spectrum Pharmacy)
CRY, NA, 25 gm........... **49452-1319-02** 262.50
100 gm............... **49452-1319-03** 714.00

CADEXOMER IODINE
(Smith & Nephew) *See IODOFLEX*
(Smith & Nephew) *See IODOSORB*

CADMIUM ACETATE
(Baker, J.T.) *See CADMIUM ACETATE DIHYDRATE*

CADMIUM ACETATE DIHYDRATE (Baker, J.T.)
cadmium acetate
CRY, NA (REAGENT)
125 gm.............. **10106-1190-04** 128.03
500 gm.............. **10106-1190-01** 229.38

CADMIUM CHLORIDE
(Baker, J.T.) *See CADMIUM CHLORIDE 2.5-HYDRATE*
(Baker, J.T.) *See CADMIUM CHLORIDE ANHYDROUS*

CADMIUM CHLORIDE 2.5-HYDRATE (Baker, J.T.)
cadmium chloride
CRY, NA (A.C.S., REAGENT)
125 gm.............. **10106-1208-04** 79.57
500 gm.............. **10106-1208-01** 152.23

CADMIUM CHLORIDE ANHYDROUS (Baker, J.T.)
cadmium chloride
POW, NA (A.C.S., REAGENT)
125 gm.............. **10106-1212-04** 79.05
500 gm.............. **10106-1212-01** 219.85

CADMIUM IODIDE (Baker, J.T.)
CRY, NA (REAGENT)
125 gm.............. **10106-1218-04** 85.75

CADMIUM NITRATE
(Baker, J.T.) *See CADMIUM NITRATE TETRAHYDRATE*

CADMIUM NITRATE TETRAHYDRATE (Baker, J.T.)
cadmium nitrate
POW, NA (REAGENT)
125 gm.............. **10106-1226-04** 108.51
500 gm.............. **10106-1226-01** 264.86

CADMIUM OXIDE (Baker, J.T.)
POW, NA (REAGENT)
125 gm.............. **10106-1234-04** 103.62
500 gm.............. **10106-1234-01** 232.16

CADMIUM SULFATE
(Baker, J.T.) *See CADMIUM SULFATE ANHYDROUS*
(Baker, J.T.) *See CADMIUM SULFATE HYDRATE*

CADMIUM SULFATE ANHYDROUS (Baker, J.T.)
cadmium sulfate
POW, NA (REAGENT)
500 gm.............. **10106-1240-01** 552.44

CADMIUM SULFATE HYDRATE (Baker, J.T.)
cadmium sulfate
CRY, NA (A.C.S., REAGENT)
125 gm.............. **10106-1243-04** 85.90
500 gm.............. **10106-1243-01** 245.45

CADUET (Pfizer)
amlodipine besylate/atorvastatin calcium
TAB, PO (FILM-COATED)
2.5 mg-10 mg,
30s ea........... **00069-2960-30** 134.84 112.37
2.5 mg-20 mg,
30s ea........... **00069-2970-30** 184.49 153.74
2.5 mg-40 mg,
30s ea........... **00069-2980-30** 184.49 153.74
5 mg-10 mg, 30s ea.. **00069-2150-30** 134.84 112.37
5 mg-20 mg, 30s ea.. **00069-2170-30** 184.49 153.74
5 mg-40 mg, 30s ea.. **00069-2190-30** 184.49 153.74
5 mg-80 mg, 30s ea.. **00069-2260-30** 184.49 153.74
10 mg-10 mg,
30s ea........... **00069-2160-30** 134.84 112.37
10 mg-20 mg,
30s ea........... **00069-2180-30** 184.49 153.74
10 mg-40 mg,
30s ea........... **00069-2250-30** 184.49 153.74
10 mg-80 mg,
30s ea........... **00069-2270-30** 184.49 153.74

(A-S Medication)
REPACK
TAB, PO (FILM-COATED)
5 mg-10 mg, 30s ea.. **54569-5704-00** 131.28
10 mg-10 mg,
30s ea........... **54569-5881-00** 131.28
10 mg-20 mg,
30s ea........... **54569-5951-00** 224.15
10 mg-40 mg,
30s ea........... **54569-6099-00** 224.15

(Phys Total Care)
REPACK
TAB, PO, 2.5 mg-40 mg,
30s ea........... **54868-5699-00** 225.26
(FILM-COATED)
5 mg-10 mg, 30s ea.. **54868-3287-00** 151.14
90s ea........... **54868-3287-01** 435.72
5 mg-20 mg, 30s ea.. **54868-1207-00** 206.06
90s ea........... **54868-1207-01** 595.15
5 mg-40 mg, 30s ea.. **54868-5179-00** 188.85
5 mg-80 mg, 30s ea.. **54868-5420-00** 195.69
10 mg-10 mg,
30s ea........... **54868-5567-00** 151.14
(FILM-COATED)
10 mg-20 mg,
30s ea........... **54868-5209-00** 206.06
90s ea........... **54868-5209-01** 595.15
10 mg-40 mg,
30s ea........... **54868-5200-00** 206.06
90s ea........... **54868-5200-01** 595.15
10 mg-80 mg,
30s ea........... **54868-5523-00** 206.06
(FILM-COATED)
10 mg-80 mg,
90s ea........... **54868-5523-01** 595.15

(Quality Care Prod)
REPACK
TAB, PO, 5 mg-10 mg,
30s ea........... **49999-0989-30** 142.80

CAFCIT (Bedford)
caffeine citrate
SOL, IV (SINGLE USE,1X3ML,PF)
20 mg/ml, 3 ml....... **55390-0357-03** 49.21
PO (10X3ML,SINGLE USE,PF)
20 mg/ml, 3 ml 10s... **55390-0358-03** 492.12

CAFERGOT (Sandoz)
caffeine/ergotamine tartrate
TAB, PO (FILM COATED)
100 mg-1 mg,
100s ea........... **00781-5405-01** 189.48 AA
(SUGAR-COATED)
100 mg-1 mg,
100s ea........... **00781-5995-01** 158.03 AA

(Altura)
REPACK
TAB, PO, 100 mg-1 mg,
30s ea........... **63874-1072-03** 40.50

(PD-Rx Pharm)
REPACK
TAB, PO (USP,SUGAR-COATED)
100 mg-1 mg,
12s ea........... **55289-0960-12** 27.20 AA

CAFF/IBUPROFEN/VIT B1/VIT B12/VIT B2/VIT B6
(GM Pharm) *See IC400*
(GM Pharm) *See IC800*

CAFFEINE
(Amend) *See CAFFEINE ANHYDROUS*
(Gallipot) *See CAFFEINE ANHYDROUS*
(Letco) *See CAFFEINE ANHYDROUS*
(Medisca) *See CAFFEINE ANHYDROUS*
(PCCA) *See CAFFEINE ANHYDROUS*
(Spectrum Pharmacy) *See CAFFEINE ANHYDROUS*

CAFFEINE ANHYDROUS (Amend)
caffeine
POW, NA (U.S.P.)
125 gm.............. **17317-0072-04** 9.80
454 gm.............. **17317-0072-01** 22.40
2270 gm............. **17317-0072-05** 98.00
11350 gm **17317-0072-08** 350.00

(Gallipot)
POW, NA (U.S.P.,N.F.)
100 gm.............. **51552-0200-05** 11.20
454 gm.............. **51552-0200-06** 30.10

(Letco)
POW, NA (U.S.P.)
500 gm.............. **62991-2015-02** 60.00

PROD/MFR	NDC	AWP	DP	OBC
(Medisca)				
POW, NA (U.S.P.)				
100 gm	**38779-0419-05**	25.50		
500 gm	**38779-0419-08**	67.50		
(PCCA)				
POW, NA (USP)				
1 gm	**51927-1158-00**	0.30		
(Spectrum Pharmacy)				
POW, NA (U.S.P.)				
125 gm	**49452-1320-01**	49.00		
500 gm	**49452-1320-02**	104.30		
2500 gm	**49452-1320-03**	462.00		
CAFFEINE CITRATE				
(Amend) *See CAFFEINE CITRATED*				
(Amer Regent)				
SOL, IV (USP,10X3ML,SINGLE-DOSE)				
20 mg/ml, 3 ml 10s	**00517-0020-10**	400.00		
(APP)				
SOL, IV (USP,SDV,PF)				
20 mg/ml, 3 ml	**63323-0407-03**	48.44		**AP**
PO (5X3ML,SDV,USP,PF)				
20 mg/ml, 3 ml 5s	**63323-0406-03**	242.20		
(Baker, J.T.) *See CAFFEINE CITRATED*				
(Bedford) *See CAFCIT*				
(Gallipot)				
POW, NA (PURIFIED)				
100 gm	**51552-0178-05**	14.00		
454 gm	**51552-0178-06**	44.10		
(Letco) *See CAFFEINE CITRATED*				
(Mallinckrodt Lab) *See CAFFEINE CITRATED*				
(Medisca)				
POW, NA (PURIFIED)				
100 gm	**38779-1073-05**	40.50		
500 gm	**38779-1073-08**	142.50		
(Paddock) *See NOVAPLUS CAFFEINE CITRATE*				
(Paddock)				
SOL, IV (USP,PF)				
20 mg/ml, 3 ml	**00574-0823-01**	45.62		
PO (USP,10X3ML,PF)				
20 mg/ml, 3 ml 10s	**00574-0152-10**	456.25		
(PCCA)				
POW, NA (PURIFIED)				
1 gm	**51927-1202-00**	0.60		
CAFFEINE CITRATED (Amend)				
caffeine citrate				
POW, NA (PURIFIED)				
125 gm	**17317-0073-04**	14.00		
454 gm	**17317-0073-01**	35.00		
2270 gm	**17317-0073-05**	154.00		
11350 gm	**17317-0073-08**	525.00		
(Baker, J.T.)				
POW, NA (PURIFIED)				
125 gm	**10106-1649-04**	42.90		
500 gm	**10106-1649-01**	131.79		
(Letco)				
POW, NA (PURIFIED)				
500 gm	**62991-1509-02**	147.00		
(Mallinckrodt Lab)				
POW, NA (PURIFIED)				
125 gm	**00406-0646-02**	21.69		
CAFFEINE/ERGOTAMINE TARTRATE				
(Cypress Pharm) *See ERGOTAMINE TARTRATE AND CAFFEINE*				
(G&W) *See MIGERGOT*				
(Sandoz) *See CAFERGOT*				
(West-Ward)				
TAB, PO (U.S.P.,FILM-COATED)				
100 mg-1 mg,				
100s ea	**00143-2120-01**	113.80		**AA**
CAFFEINE/SODIUM BENZOATE (Amend)				
POW, NA (PURIFIED)				
454 gm	**17317-0074-01**	42.00		
2270 gm	**17317-0074-05**	140.00		
(Amer Regent)				
SOL, IJ (S.D.V.)				
125 mg/ml-125 mg/ml,				
2 ml 10s	**00517-2502-10**	81.25		
(Consolidated Midland)				
SOL, IJ (AMP)				
125 mg/ml-125 mg/ml,				
2 ml 10s	**00223-7273-10**	160.00		
2 ml 25s	**00223-7273-25**	375.00		
CAFGESIC (Cypress Pharm)				
apap/caff/phenyltoloxamine cit/salicylamide				
CAP, PO, 100s ea	**60258-0053-01**	60.58		
CAFGESIC FORTE (Cypress Pharm)				
apap/caff/magnesium sal/phenyltoloxamine cit				
TAB, PO, 100s ea	**60258-0058-01**	89.59		
CAJEPUT (PCCA)				
cajeput oil				
OIL, NA, 1 ml	**51927-1300-00**	0.62		
CAJEPUT OIL (Amend)				
OIL, NA, 30 ml	**17317-0233-02**	4.20		
120 ml	**17317-0233-04**	14.00		
500 ml	**17317-0233-01**	49.00		
(PCCA) *See CAJEPUT*				
CAL GLUCEPTATE HEMIHEPTAHYDRATE				
(Spectrum Pharmacy)				
calcium gluceptate				
POW, NA (U.S.P.)				
25 gm	**49452-1445-01**	273.70		
100 gm	**49452-1445-02**	693.00		
CAL-NATE (Ethex)				
prenatal vitamins				
TAB, PO (FILM COATED)				
100s ea	**58177-0439-04**	35.56		
CALAFOL RX (Alaven)				
multivitamin and minerals				
TAB, PO (SF,DYE-FREE)				
90s ea	**68220-0099-90**	57.57		
CALAMINE (Amend)				
POW, NA (U.S.P.)				
120 gm	**17317-0075-04**	4.20		
500 gm	**17317-0075-01**	14.00		
2270 gm	**17317-0075-05**	42.00		
11350 gm	**17317-0075-08**	148.75		
(Baker, J.T.)				
POW, NA (U.S.P.)				
500 gm	**10106-1260-01**	21.24		
(Gallipot)				
POW, NA (U.S.P.)				
113.4 gm	**51552-0223-04**	6.37		
454 gm	**51552-0223-06**	14.00		
(Medisca)				
POW, NA (1X500GM,USP)				
500 gm	**38779-0066-08**	40.50		
(1X1000GM,USP)				
1000 gm	**38779-0066-09**	64.50		
(PCCA)				
POW, NA (USP)				
1 gm	**51927-1022-00**	0.11		
(Spectrum Pharmacy)				
POW, NA (U.S.P.)				
500 gm	**49452-1350-01**	78.75		
2500 gm	**49452-1350-02**	324.80		
CALAN (Pfizer)				
verapamil hydrochloride				
TAB, PO, 80 mg, 100s ea	**00025-1851-31**	113.41	94.51	**AB**
500s ea	**00025-1851-51**	399.54	332.95	**AB**
120 mg, 100s ea	**00025-1861-31**	153.38	127.82	**AB**
(Phys Total Care)				
REPACK				
TAB, PO, 120 mg, 30s ea	**54868-0933-00**	41.41		**AB**
CALAN SR (Pfizer)				
verapamil hydrochloride				
TER, PO (CAPLET)				
120 mg, 100s ea	**00025-1901-31**	213.28	177.73	**AB**
180 mg, 100s ea	**00025-1911-31**	270.34	225.28	**AB**
240 mg, 100s ea	**00025-1891-31**	309.24	257.70	**AB**
100s ea UD	**00025-1891-34**	324.72	270.60	**AB**
500s ea	**00025-1891-51**	1546.20	1288.50	**AB**
(Phys Total Care)				
REPACK				
TER, PO (CAPLET)				
120 mg, 30s ea	**54868-2147-02**	41.74		**AB**
180 mg, 100s ea	**54868-1550-03**	203.50		**AB**
CALCIFOL (Everett)				
multivitamin and minerals				
WAF, PO, 30s ea	**00642-0066-30**	34.23		
CALCIFOLIC-D (Everett)				
multivitamin and minerals				
WAF, PO (GLUTEN-FREE)				
60s ea	**00642-0068-60**	48.98		
CALCIJEX (Abbott Pharm)				
calcitriol				
SOL, IV (AMP,LOW-ALUMINUM)				
1 mcg/ml,				
1 ml 100s	**00074-8110-31**	1454.69	1225.00	**AP**
CALCIPOTRIENE (Fougera)				
SOL, TP (1X60ML)				
0.005%, 60 ml	**00168-0400-60**	207.04		**AT**
(Hi-Tech)				
SOL, TP (1X60ML,SCALP)				
0.005%, 60 ml	**50383-0732-02**	220.08		**EE**
(Sandoz)				
SOL, TP (1X60ML)				
0.005%, 60 ml	**00781-7092-61**	181.28		**AT**
(Warner Chilcott) *See DOVONEX*				
CALCITONIN (SALMON)				
(Apotex Corp.) *See CALCITONIN-SALMON*				
(Novartis Pharm) *See MIACALCIN*				
(Par) *See CALCITONIN-SALMON*				
(Sandoz) *See CALCITONIN-SALMON*				
(Upsher-Smith) *See FORTICAL*				
CALCITONIN-SALMON (Apotex Corp.)				
calcitonin (salmon)				
SPR, NS (1X3.7ML)				
200 iu/actuation,				
3.7 ml	**60505-0823-06**	118.54		**AB**
(Par)				
SPR, NS (1X3.8ML,30DOSES,USP)				
200 iu/actuation,				
3.8 ml	**49884-0161-11**	118.54		**EE**
(Sandoz)				
SPR, NS (1X3.7ML)				
200 iu/actuation,				
3.7 ml	**00781-6320-79**	118.54		
CALCITRIOL				
(Abbott Pharm) *See CALCIJEX*				
(Amer Regent)				
SOL, IV (1MLX25)				
1 mcg/ml, 1 ml 25s	**00517-0132-25**	156.25		
(APP)				
SOL, IV, 1 mcg/ml,				
1 ml 50s	**63323-0731-01**	765.50		**AP**
(Galderma) *See VECTICAL*				
(Mayne Pharma)				
SOL, IV, 1 mcg/ml, 1 ml 5s	**61703-0234-29**	76.40		**AP**
(Nephrx)				
SOL, IV, 1 mcg/ml, 1 ml	**68830-0319-80**	14.20		
(PCCA) *See CALCITRIOL IN ALMOND OIL*				
(Ranbaxy Pharm)				
SGL, PO (SOFTGEL)				
0.25 mcg, 30s ea	**63304-0239-30**	47.71		
100s ea	**63304-0239-01**	156.47		
0.5 mcg, 100s ea	**63304-0240-01**	250.41		
SOL, PO, 1 mcg/ml, 15 ml	**63304-0241-59**	179.00		
(Roxane)				
SGL, PO, 0.25 mcg, 30s ea	**00054-0007-13**	38.39		**AB**
100s ea	**00054-0007-25**	120.95		**AB**
SOL, PO (W/GRADUATED DISPENSERS)				
1 mcg/ml, 15 ml	**00054-3120-41**	179.00		**AA**
(Teva)				
SGL, PO, 0.25 mcg,				
100s ea	**00093-0657-01**	120.95		**AB**
0.5 mcg, 100s ea	**00093-0658-01**	193.38		**AB**
SOL, IV (25X1ML)				
1 mcg/ml, 1 ml 25s	**00703-7311-04**	128.40		**AP**
(Validus) *See ROCALTROL*				
(Phys Total Care)				
REPACK				
SGL, PO, 0.25 mcg, 30s ea	**54868-4584-00**	118.32		
CALCITRIOL IN ALMOND OIL (PCCA)				
calcitriol				
SOL, NA (NF)				
1 mcg/ml, 1 ml	**51927-3422-00**	13.80		
CALCIUM ACETATE (Amend)				
POW, NA (F.C.C.)				
454 gm	**17317-1095-01**	14.00		
2270 gm	**17317-1905-05**	49.00		
11350 gm	**17317-1905-08**	140.00		
(Baker, J.T.) *See CALCIUM ACETATE MONOHYDRATE*				
(Fresenius) *See PHOSLO*				
(Hawthorn Pharm) *See ELIPHOS*				

PROD/MFR	NDC	AWP	DP	OBC
(Medisca)				
POW, NA (1X100GM,USP)				
100 gm	**38779-1075-05**	22.50		
(1X500GM,USP)				
500 gm	**38779-1075-08**	46.50		
(PCCA)				
POW, NA (USP)				
1 gm	**51927-1828-00**	0.36		
(Roxane)				
CAP, PO, 667 mg, 200s ea	**00054-0088-26**	157.92		**AB**
(Sandoz)				
CAP, PO (GELCAP)				
667 mg, 200s ea	**00781-2672-02**	157.92		
(Spectrum Pharmacy)				
POW, NA (1X500GM)				
500 gm	**49452-1355-02**	109.90		
(U.S.P.)				
2500 gm	**49452-1355-03**	337.75		
CALCIUM ACETATE MONOHYDRATE (Baker, J.T.)				
calcium acetate				
POW, NA (A.C.S., REAGENT)				
500 gm	**10106-1266-01**	135.96		
CALCIUM ALGINATE (PCCA)				
POW, NA, 1 gm	**51927-2361-00**	9.60		
CALCIUM ASCORBATE (Medisca)				
POW, NA (1X100GM,USP)				
100 gm	**38779-1077-05**	22.50		
(1X500GM,USP)				
500 gm	**38779-1077-08**	64.50		
(1X1000GM,USP)				
1000 gm	**38779-1077-09**	120.00		
(1X5000GM,USP)				
5000 gm	**38779-1077-03**	520.50		
(PCCA) *See CALCIUM ASCORBATE DIHYDRATE*				
(Spectrum Pharmacy) *See CALCIUM ASCORBATE DIHYDRATE*				
CALCIUM ASCORBATE DIHYDRATE (PCCA)				
calcium ascorbate				
POW, NA (USP)				
1 gm	**51927-1635-00**	0.30		
(Spectrum Pharmacy)				
POW, NA (F.C.C.)				
100 gm	**49452-1365-01**	67.90		
(U.S.P.)				
100 gm	**49452-1366-01**	67.90		
(F.C.C.)				
500 gm	**49452-1365-02**	183.75		
(U.S.P.)				
500 gm	**49452-1366-02**	183.75		
(F.C.C.)				
2500 gm	**49452-1365-03**	665.00		
(U.S.P.)				
2500 gm	**49452-1366-03**	665.00		
CALCIUM BROMIDE (PCCA)				
POW, NA (REAGENT)				
1 gm	**51927-2562-00**	0.96		
CALCIUM CARBIMIDE				
(PCCA) *See CALCIUM CYANAMIDE*				
CALCIUM CARBONATE				
(Amend) *See CALCIUM CARBONATE HEAVY*				
(Amend) *See CALCIUM CARBONATE LIGHT*				
(Baker, J.T.) *See CALCIUM CARBONATE LIGHT*				
(Baker, J.T.)				
POW, NA (A.C.S., REAGENT)				
500 gm	**10106-1288-01**	138.28		
(Gallipot) *See CALCIUM CARBONATE HEAVY*				
(Gallipot) *See CALCIUM CARBONATE LIGHT*				
(Gallipot) *See WHITING GROUND CACO3*				
(Mallinckrodt Lab)				
POW, NA (U.S.P.)				
500 gm	**00406-4052-12**	15.09		
(Medisca)				
POW, NA (U.S.P.)				
500 gm	**38779-0549-08**	28.50		
2500 gm	**38779-0549-01**	82.50		
(PCCA) *See CALCIUM CARBONATE HEAVY*				
(PCCA) *See CORAL CALCIUM*				
(PCCA) *See OYSTER SHELL CALCIUM*				
(Spectrum Pharmacy) *See CALCIUM CARBONATE HEAVY*				
(Spectrum Pharmacy) *See CALCIUM CARBONATE LIGHT*				

PROD/MFR	NDC	AWP	DP	OBC
CALCIUM CARBONATE HEAVY (Amend)				
calcium carbonate				
POW, NA (U.S.P.)				
500 gm	**17317-0078-01**	9.80		
2270 gm	**17317-0078-05**	35.00		
11350 gm	**17317-0078-08**	87.50		
(Gallipot)				
POW, NA (U.S.P.,PRECIPITATED)				
454 gm	**51552-0018-06**	11.90		
2270 gm	**51552-0018-08**	43.05		
(PCCA)				
POW, NA (USP PRECIPITATED LIGHT)				
1 gm	**51927-1944-00**	0.07		
(USP, PRECIPITATED)				
1 gm	**51927-1044-00**	0.08		
(Spectrum Pharmacy)				
POW, NA (U.S.P.)				
500 gm	**49452-1370-01**	53.90		
2500 gm	**49452-1370-02**	128.10		
12000 gm	**49452-1370-03**	455.00		
CALCIUM CARBONATE LIGHT (Amend)				
calcium carbonate				
POW, NA (U.S.P.)				
500 gm	**17317-0077-01**	9.80		
2270 gm	**17317-0077-05**	35.00		
11350 gm	**17317-0077-08**	87.50		
(Baker, J.T.)				
POW, NA (U.S.P./ F.C.C.)				
500 gm	**10106-1301-01**	15.01		
(U.S.P./F.C.C.)				
2500 gm	**10106-1301-05**	378.55		
(Gallipot)				
POW, NA (U.S.P.,N.F.)				
454 gm	**51552-0231-06**	11.90		
(U.S.P.)				
11350 gm	**51552-0231-09**	154.00		
(Spectrum Pharmacy)				
POW, NA (U.S.P.)				
500 gm	**49452-1380-01**	53.90		
2500 gm	**49452-1380-02**	128.10		
12000 gm	**49452-1380-03**	455.00		
CALCIUM CARBONATE/FOLIC ACID/ MAGNESIUM CARBONATE				
(Nephro-Tech) *See MAGNEBIND 400 RX*				
CALCIUM CARBONATE/RISEDRONATE SODIUM				
(P & G Pharm) *See ACTONEL WITH CALCIUM*				
CALCIUM CHLORIDE (Abbott Hosp)				
SOL, IV (18GX3 1/2",LATEX-FREE)				
100 mg/ml,				
10 ml 10s	**00074-4908-18**	39.19	33.00	
(Amend) *See CALCIUM CHLORIDE ANHYDROUS*				
(Amend) *See CALCIUM CHLORIDE DIHYDRATE*				
(Amer Regent)				
SOL, IV (S.D.V.;PF)				
100 mg/ml,				
10 ml 25s	**00517-2710-25**	46.88		
(Amphastar)				
SOL, IV (SRN,PREFILLED,LUER-JET)				
100 mg/ml,				
10 ml 10s	**00548-3304-00**	39.90		
(MIN-I-JET,21GX1 1/2")				
100 mg/ml,				
10 ml 25s	**00548-1004-00**	131.01		
(SRN,PREFILLED,STICKGARD)				
100 mg/ml,				
10 ml 25s	**00548-2004-00**	140.98		
(Baker, J.T.) *See CALCIUM CHLORIDE DIHYDRATE*				
(Consolidated Midland) *See CALCIUM CHLORIDE SOLUTION*				
(Gallipot) *See CALCIUM CHLORIDE DIHYDRATE*				
(Hospira)				
SOL, IV (ANYSR,LATEX-FREE)				
100 mg/ml,				
10 ml 10s	**00409-1631-10**	22.56	19.70	
(SRN,LATEX-FREE)				
100 mg/ml,				
10 ml 10s	**00074-4928-34**	39.24	34.30	
10 ml 10s	**00409-4928-34**	40.80	35.70	
(Mallinckrodt Lab) *See CALCIUM CHLORIDE DIHYDRATE*				
(Medisca)				
GRA, NA (DIHYDRATE,1X500GM,USP)				
500 gm	**38779-1079-08**	46.50		
(DIHYDRATE,1X1000GM,USP)				
1000 gm	**38779-1079-09**	76.50		

PROD/MFR	NDC	AWP	DP	OBC
(PCCA) *See CALCIUM CHLORIDE ANHYDROUS*				
(PCCA) *See CALCIUM CHLORIDE DIHYDRATE*				
(Spectrum Pharmacy) *See CALCIUM CHLORIDE ANHYDROUS*				
(Spectrum Pharmacy) *See CALCIUM CHLORIDE DIHYDRATE*				
(Spectrum Pharmacy)				
GRA, NA (BIOTECH)				
500 gm	**49452-1402-01**	171.50	50.90	
2500 gm	**49452-1402-02**	518.00	175.05	
12000 gm	**49452-1402-03**	1340.50		
(Phys Total Care)				
REPACK				
SOL, IV (SDV,25X10ML)				
100 mg/ml,				
10 ml 25s	**54868-0741-00**	63.57		
CALCIUM CHLORIDE ANHYDROUS (Amend)				
calcium chloride				
POW, NA (F.C.C.)				
500 gm	**17317-1511-01**	11.20		
2270 gm	**17317-1511-05**	49.00		
11350 gm	**17317-1511-08**	122.50		
(PCCA)				
POW, NA (F.C.C.)				
1 gm	**51927-2856-00**	0.12		
(Spectrum Pharmacy)				
GRA, NA (F.C.C.)				
500 gm	**49452-1400-01**	77.70		
2500 gm	**49452-1400-02**	236.25		
(PEL F.C.C.)				
2500 gm	**49452-1401-02**	345.10		
PEL, NA (F.C.C.)				
500 gm	**49452-1401-01**	113.40		
CALCIUM CHLORIDE DIHYDRATE (Amend)				
calcium chloride				
POW, NA (F.C.C., U.S.P.)				
500 gm	**17317-0079-01**	11.90		
2270 gm	**17317-0079-05**	42.00		
11350 gm	**17317-0079-08**	140.00		
(Baker, J.T.)				
GRA, NA (U.S.P./F.C.C.)				
500 gm	**10106-1336-01**	13.66		
2500 gm	**10106-1336-05**	125.33		
(Gallipot)				
POW, NA (U.S.P.)				
454 gm	**51552-0325-06**	16.80		
(Mallinckrodt Lab)				
POW, NA (U.S.P.)				
500 gm	**00406-4616-04**	36.89		
2500 gm	**00406-4616-06**	103.24		
(PCCA)				
POW, NA (USP)				
1 gm	**51927-1205-00**	0.12		
(Spectrum Pharmacy)				
GRA, NA (U.S.P.,E.P.,B.P.,J.P.)				
500 gm	**49452-1410-01**	79.80		
2500 gm	**49452-1410-02**	237.65		
12000 gm	**49452-1410-03**	941.50		
CALCIUM CHLORIDE SOLUTION				
(Consolidated Midland)				
calcium chloride				
SOL, IV (AMP)				
100 mg/ml,				
10 ml 25s	**00223-7277-10**	37.50		
CALCIUM CITRATE				
(Amend) *See CALCIUM CITRATE TETRAHYDRATE*				
(Gallipot)				
POW, NA (U.S.P., N.F.)				
1000 gm	**51552-0819-07**	43.05	30.75	
(Medisca)				
POW, NA (1X100GM,USP)				
100 gm	**38779-1080-05**	22.50		
(1X500GM,USP)				
500 gm	**38779-1080-08**	49.50		
(1X1000GM,USP)				
1000 gm	**38779-1080-09**	82.50		
(PCCA) *See CALCIUM CITRATE TETRAHYDRATE*				
(Spectrum Pharmacy) *See CALCIUM CITRATE TETRAHYDRATE*				
CALCIUM CITRATE TETRAHYDRATE (Amend)				
calcium citrate				
POW, NA (F.C.C.)				
500 gm	**17317-0729-01**	14.00		

PROD/MFR | NDC | AWP | DP | OBC

2270 gm............17317-0729-05 56.00
11350 gm...........17317-0729-08 245.00

(PCCA)
POW, NA (USP)
1 gm...............51927-1346-00 0.36

(Spectrum Pharmacy)
GRA, NA (F.C.C.)
500 gm.............49452-1433-01 117.25
2500 gm............49452-1433-02 371.00
12000 gm...........49452-1433-03 1501.50
POW, NA, 500 gm.......49452-1430-01 110.25
(U.S.P.)
500 gm.............49452-1425-01 110.25
(F.C.C.)
2500 gm............49452-1430-02 357.00
(U.S.P.)
2500 gm............49452-1425-02 357.00
(FCC)
12000 gm...........49452-1430-03 1494.50
(U.S.P.)
12000 gm...........49452-1425-03 1494.50

CALCIUM CYANAMIDE (PCCA)
calcium carbimide
POW, NA (1X1GM)
1 gm...............51927-3206-00 0.47

CALCIUM D-PANTOTHENATE (Amend)
calcium pantothenate
POW, NA (U.S.P.)
25 gm..............17317-0084-02 4.20
100 gm.............17317-0084-03 10.50
500 gm.............17317-0084-05 42.00
1000 gm............17317-0084-06 70.00

CALCIUM DISODIUM VERSENATE (Graceway)
edetate calcium disodium
SOL, IJ, 200 mg/ml,
2.5 ml 10s.........29336-0510-10 1140.00
(10X2.5ML)
200 mg/ml,
2.5 ml 10s.........29336-0400-10 1140.00

CALCIUM FLUORIDE (Baker, J.T.)
POW, NA (REAGENT)
500 gm.............10106-1354-01 97.34
2500 gm............10106-1354-05 296.28

(PCCA)
POW, NA, 1 gm..........51927-2033-00 0.72

CALCIUM GLUBIONATE (PCCA)
POW, NA (ORAL GRADE; MONOHYDRATE)
1 gm...............51927-3398-00 0.78

CALCIUM GLUCEPTATE
(Spectrum Pharmacy) *See CAL GLUCEPTATE HEMIHEPTAHYDRATE*

CALCIUM GLUCONATE
(Amend) *See CALCIUM GLUCONATE ANHYDROUS*
(Amend) *See CALCIUM GLUCONATE MONOHYDRATE*

(Amer Regent)
SOL, IV (S.D.V.,PF)
100 mg/ml,
10 ml 25s..........00517-3910-25 22.19
50 ml 25s..........00517-3950-25 81.88
(VIAL,PF)
100 mg/ml,
100 ml 25s.........00517-3900-25 93.75

(APP)
SOL, IV (S.D.V.)
100 mg/ml, 10 ml.....63323-0311-10 1.52
50 ml..............63323-0311-50 4.52
(MAXIVIAL,BULK PACK)
100 mg/ml, 100 ml....63323-0311-61 9.24
200 ml.............63323-0311-63 14.63

(Baker, J.T.) *See CALCIUM GLUCONATE ANHYDROUS*

(Consolidated Midland)
SOL, IV (VIAL)
100 mg/ml,
10 ml 25s..........00223-7280-10 26.80
10 ml 100s.........00223-7280-00 105.00

(Gallipot) *See CALCIUM GLUCONATE ANHYDROUS*

(Mallinckrodt Lab)
POW, NA (U.S.P.)
500 gm.............00406-6924-04 46.20

(PCCA) *See CALCIUM GLUCONATE ANHYDROUS*
(Spectrum Pharmacy) *See CALCIUM GLUCONATE ANHYDROUS*
(Spectrum Pharmacy) *See CALCIUM GLUCONATE MONOHYDRATE*

CALCIUM GLUCONATE ANHYDROUS (Amend)
calcium gluconate
GRA, NA (U.S.P.)
500 gm.............17317-2322-01 11.90
2270 gm............17317-2322-05 42.00
11350 gm...........17317-2322-08 122.50

(Baker, J.T.)
POW, NA (U.S.P., F.C.C.)
500 gm.............10106-1272-01 23.97

(Gallipot)
POW, NA (U.S.P./N.F.)
454 gm.............51552-0515-06 16.66

(PCCA)
POW, NA (USP)
1 gm...............51927-1117-00 0.36

(Spectrum Pharmacy)
POW, NA (U.S.P.)
500 gm.............49452-1461-01 99.75
2500 gm............49452-1461-02 367.50
12000 gm...........49452-1461-03 1225.00

CALCIUM GLUCONATE MONOHYDRATE (Amend)
calcium gluconate
GRA, NA (U.S.P.)
500 gm.............17317-1812-01 11.90
2270 gm............17317-1812-05 42.00
11350 gm...........17317-1812-08 175.00

(Spectrum Pharmacy)
POW, NA (U.S.P.)
500 gm.............49452-1465-01 99.75
2500 gm............49452-1465-02 367.50
2500 gm............49452-1465-03 1225.00

CALCIUM GLUCONATE-SODIUM CHLORIDE (PharMEDium Services)
calcium gluconate/sodium chloride
SOL, IV (24X50ML, INTRAVIA BAG)
1 gm-0.9%,
50 ml 24s..........61553-0050-41 396.00 330.00
(INTRAVIA BAG,PF)
2 gm-0.9%,
50 ml 24s..........61553-0057-41 460.80 384.00
(24X100ML, INTRAVIA BAG)
2 gm-0.9%,
100 ml 24s.........61553-0051-48 432.00 360.00

CALCIUM GLUCONATE/SODIUM CHLORIDE
(PharMEDium Services) *See CALCIUM GLUCONATE-SODIUM CHLORIDE*

CALCIUM GLYCEROPHOSPHATE (Amend)
POW, NA (N.F., F.C.C.)
500 gm.............17317-0080-01 35.00
2270 gm............17317-0080-05 133.00
11350 gm...........17317-0080-08 525.00

(PCCA)
POW, NA (FCC)
1 gm...............51927-1631-00 0.48

(Spectrum Pharmacy)
POW, NA (F.C.C.)
125 gm.............49452-1470-01 72.45
500 gm.............49452-1470-02 237.65
2500 gm............49452-1470-03 910.00

CALCIUM GLYCEROPHOSPHATE/CALCIUM LACTATE
(Glenwood) *See CALPHOSAN*

CALCIUM HYDROXIDE
(Amend) *See LIME*
(Amend) *See LIME SOLUTION, SULFURATED*

(Amend)
POW, NA (U.S.P.)
500 gm.............17317-2699-01 9.80
(U.S.P., F.C.C.)
2500 gm............17317-2699-05 28.00
11350 gm...........17317-2699-08 96.60

(Baker, J.T.)
POW, NA (U.S.P.)
500 gm.............10106-1374-01 32.70
2500 gm............10106-1374-05 111.17

(Gallipot)
POW, NA (F.C.C.)
454 gm.............51552-0421-06 16.17
(U.S.P.,N.F.)
454 gm.............51552-0167-06 16.17

(Medisca)
POW, NA (1X100GM,USP)
100 gm.............38779-0067-05 25.50
(U.S.P.)
500 gm.............38779-0067-08 31.50
1000 gm............38779-0067-09 55.50

(PCCA)
POW, NA (U.S.P.)
1 gm...............51927-1206-00 0.27

(Spectrum Pharmacy)
POW, NA (U.S.P.,E.P.,B.P.,J.P.)
500 gm.............49452-1480-01 72.10
2500 gm............49452-1480-02 186.90
12000 gm...........49452-1480-03 574.00

CALCIUM HYDROXYAPATITE (PCCA)
durapatite
POW, NA, 1 gm..........51927-2876-00 0.33

CALCIUM HYPOCHLORITE (Baker, J.T.)
POW, NA (PURIFIED)
500 gm.............10106-1378-01 32.39
2500 gm............10106-1378-05 92.49

(Spectrum Pharmacy)
GRA, NA (1X500GM)
500 gm.............49452-1485-02 102.90

CALCIUM IODATE (PCCA)
POW, NA (FCC; MONOHYDRATE)
1 gm...............51927-2448-00 1.66

(Spectrum Pharmacy) *See CALCIUM IODATE MONOHYDRATE*

CALCIUM IODATE MONOHYDRATE (Spectrum Pharmacy)
calcium iodate
POW, NA (F.C.C.)
125 gm.............49452-1487-01 176.40
500 gm.............49452-1487-02 518.00

CALCIUM IODIDE
(Amend) *See CALCIUM IODIDE HEXAHYDRATE*

CALCIUM IODIDE HEXAHYDRATE (Amend)
calcium iodide
LUM, NA (PURIFIED)
500 gm.............17317-0688-01 84.00

CALCIUM LACTATE
(Amend) *See CALCIUM LACTATE PENTAHYDRATE*
(Baker, J.T.) *See CALCIUM LACTATE PENTAHYDRATE*
(Gallipot) *See CALCIUM LACTATE MONOHYDRATE*
(Gallipot) *See CALCIUM LACTATE PENTAHYDRATE*

(Mallinckrodt Lab)
POW, NA (U.S.P.)
500 gm.............00406-4208-12 24.72

(Medisca) *See CALCIUM LACTATE PENTAHYDRATE*

(PCCA)
POW, NA ((U.S.P.) PENTAHYDRATE)
1 gm...............51927-1582-00 0.42

(Spectrum Pharmacy) *See CALCIUM LACTATE MONOHYDRATE*
(Spectrum Pharmacy) *See CALCIUM LACTATE PENTAHYDRATE*
(Spectrum Pharmacy) *See CALCIUM LACTATE TRIHYDRATE*

CALCIUM LACTATE MONOHYDRATE (Gallipot)
calcium lactate
POW, NA (U.S.P.,N.F.)
454 gm.............51552-0081-06 33.25

(Spectrum Pharmacy)
POW, NA (U.S.P.)
500 gm.............49452-1500-01 170.45
2500 gm............49452-1500-02 532.00

CALCIUM LACTATE PENTAHYDRATE (Amend)
calcium lactate
POW, NA (U.S.P.)
500 gm.............17317-0083-01 14.00
2270 gm............17317-0083-05 49.00
11350 gm...........17317-0083-08 175.00

(Baker, J.T.)
POW, NA (U.S.P./F.C.C.)
500 gm.............10106-1390-01 35.25

(Gallipot)
POW, NA (U.S.P.)
454 gm.............51552-0295-06 19.60
2270 gm............51552-0295-09 60.55

(Medisca)
POW, NA (USP,1X100GM)
100 gm.............38779-0797-05 31.50

(Spectrum Pharmacy)
POW, NA (U.S.P.)
500 gm.............49452-1520-01 94.15
2500 gm............49452-1520-02 316.40

PROD/MFR | NDC | AWP | DP | OBC

CALCIUM LACTATE TRIHYDRATE (Spectrum Pharmacy)
calcium lactate
POW, NA (U.S.P.)
500 gm............ 49452-1510-01 162.75
2500 gm............ 49452-1510-02 493.50

CALCIUM LEVULINATE (PCCA)
POW, NA (U.S.P.; DIHYDRATE)
1 gm............ 51927-2679-00 3.00

CALCIUM MALATE (PCCA)
POW, NA (1X1GM)
1 gm............ 51927-3587-00 0.12

CALCIUM NITRATE
(Baker, J.T.) *See CALCIUM NITRATE TETRAHYDRATE*

(PCCA)
POW, NA (TETRAHYDRATE)
1 gm............ 51927-1790-00 0.39

CALCIUM NITRATE TETRAHYDRATE (Baker, J.T.)
calcium nitrate
GRA, NA (A.C.S., REAGENT)
500 gm............ 10106-1395-01 49.54
2500 gm............ 10106-1395-05 195.13
12000 gm............ 10106-1395-07 500.63

CALCIUM OXIDE (Baker, J.T.)
POW, NA (REAGENT)
500 gm............ 10106-1410-01 36.87
2500 gm............ 10106-1410-05 125.61

(PCCA)
POW, NA (USP; LIME)
1 gm............ 51927-1964-00 0.18

(Spectrum Pharmacy)
POW, NA (U.S.P.)
500 gm............ 49452-1530-01 130.55
2500 gm............ 49452-1530-02 455.00

CALCIUM OXIDE/SODIUM HYDROXIDE
(Baker, J.T.) *See SODA LIME INDICATING TYPE*

CALCIUM PANTOTHENATE
(Amend) *See CALCIUM D-PANTOTHENATE*

(Baker, J.T.)
POW, NA (U.S.P.)
25 gm............ 10106-1443-03 18.34

(Gallipot) *See D-CALCIUM PANTOTHENATE*

(Medisca)
POW, NA (U.S.P.)
100 gm............ 38779-0876-05 37.50
500 gm............ 38779-0876-08 126.00

(PCCA)
POW, NA (USP)
1 gm............ 51927-1920-00 0.40

(Spectrum Pharmacy)
POW, NA (U.S.P.)
100 gm............ 49452-1540-01 64.75
500 gm............ 49452-1540-02 203.00

CALCIUM PEROXIDE (Spectrum Pharmacy)
POW, NA, 25 gm............ 49452-1546-01 241.50
125 gm............ 49452-1546-02 497.00
500 gm............ 49452-1546-03 1470.00

CALCIUM PHOSPHATE
(Amend) *See CALCIUM PHOSPHATE DIBASIC ANHYDROUS*

(Amend) *See CALCIUM PHOSPHATE DIBASIC DIHYDRATE*

(Amend) *See CALCIUM PHOSPHATE MONOBASIC*

(Amend) *See CALCIUM PHOSPHATE TRIBASIC*

(Baker, J.T.) *See CALCIUM PHOSPHATE DIBASIC ANHYDROUS*

(Baker, J.T.) *See CALCIUM PHOSPHATE MONOBASIC*

(Baker, J.T.) *See CALCIUM PHOSPHATE TRIBASIC*

(Gallipot) *See CALCIUM PHOSPHATE DIBASIC ANHYDROUS*

(Gallipot) *See CALCIUM PHOSPHATE DIBASIC DIHYDRATE*

(Gallipot) *See CALCIUM PHOSPHATE TRIBASIC*

(PCCA) *See CALCIUM PHOSPHATE DIBASIC ANHY-DROUS*

(PCCA) *See CALCIUM PHOSPHATE MONOBASIC*

(PCCA) *See CALCIUM PHOSPHATE TRIBASIC*

(Spectrum Pharmacy) *See CALCIUM PHOSPHATE DIBASIC*

(Spectrum Pharmacy) *See CALCIUM PHOSPHATE DIBASIC ANHYDROUS*

(Spectrum Pharmacy) *See CALCIUM PHOSPHATE MONOBASIC*

PROD/MFR | NDC | AWP | DP | OBC

(Spectrum Pharmacy) *See CALCIUM PHOSPHATE TRIBASIC*

CALCIUM PHOSPHATE DIBASIC (Spectrum Pharmacy)
calcium phosphate
POW, NA (DIHYDRATE, U.S.P.)
500 gm............ 49452-1570-01 76.30
2500 gm............ 49452-1570-02 218.75

CALCIUM PHOSPHATE DIBASIC ANHYDROUS (Amend)
calcium phosphate
POW, NA (U.S.P./F.C.C)
500 gm............ 17317-0234-01 9.80
(U.S.P./F.C.C.)
2270 gm............ 17317-0234-05 35.00
11350 gm............ 17317-0234-08 113.75

(Baker, J.T.)
POW, NA (REAGENT)
2500 gm............ 10106-1430-05 157.54
12000 gm............ 10106-1430-07 762.97

(Gallipot)
GRA, NA (U.S.P.,F.C.C.)
454 gm............ 51552-0474-06 15.40

(PCCA)
POW, NA (USP)
1 gm............ 51927-1249-00 0.10

(Spectrum Pharmacy)
POW, NA (U.S.P.)
500 gm............ 49452-1552-01 84.35
2500 gm............ 49452-1552-02 248.50

CALCIUM PHOSPHATE DIBASIC DIHYDRATE (Amend)
calcium phosphate
POW, NA (U.S.P./F.C.C., UNMILLED)
500 gm............ 17317-0817-01 9.80
2270 gm............ 17317-0817-05 35.00
11350 gm............ 17317-0817-08 113.75

(Gallipot)
POW, NA (U.S.P.,N.F.)
454 gm............ 51552-0530-06 27.30

CALCIUM PHOSPHATE MONOBASIC (Amend)
calcium phosphate
POW, NA (MONOHYDRATE, F.C.C.)
500 gm............ 17317-0766-01 9.80
2270 gm............ 17317-0766-05 35.00
11350 gm............ 17317-0766-08 87.50

(Baker, J.T.)
CRY, NA (MONOHYDRATE, REAGENT)
500 gm............ 10106-1426-01 89.46
2500 gm............ 10106-1426-05 327.75

(PCCA)
POW, NA (MONOHYDRATE, F.C.C.)
1 gm............ 51927-1937-00 0.27

(Spectrum Pharmacy)
POW, NA (MONOHYDRATE, F.C.C.)
500 gm............ 49452-1550-02 110.25
2500 gm............ 49452-1550-03 350.00

CALCIUM PHOSPHATE TRIBASIC (Amend)
calcium phosphate
POW, NA (N.F., F.C.C.)
500 gm............ 17317-0235-01 14.00
2270 gm............ 17317-0235-05 56.00
11350 gm............ 17317-0235-08 122.50

(Baker, J.T.)
POW, NA (REAGENT)
500 gm............ 10106-1436-01 210.27

(Gallipot)
POW, NA (U.S.P.)
454 gm............ 51552-0594-06 16.10

(PCCA)
POW, NA (NF)
1 gm............ 51927-1250-00 0.11

(Spectrum Pharmacy)
POW, NA (N.F.)
500 gm............ 49452-1580-01 84.35
2500 gm............ 49452-1580-02 326.90

CALCIUM PHOSPHATE, DIBASIC/SELENOMETHIONINE
(Spectrum Pharmacy) *See L-SELENOME-THIONINE BLEND*

CALCIUM POLYCARBOPHIL (PCCA)
POW, NA, 1 gm............ 51927-3535-00 1.80

CALCIUM PROPIONATE (Amend)
POW, NA (F.C.C.)
454 gm............ 17317-1206-01 11.20
2270 gm............ 17317-1206-05 35.00
11350 gm............ 17317-1206-08 140.00

(PCCA)
POW, NA (F.C.C.)
1 gm............ 51927-1095-00 0.39

PROD/MFR | NDC | AWP | DP | OBC

(Spectrum Pharmacy)
POW, NA (F.C.C.)
500 gm............ 49452-1590-01 69.65
2500 gm............ 49452-1590-02 253.40
12000 gm............ 49452-1590-03 829.50

CALCIUM PYRUVATE (PCCA)
POW, NA (1X1GM)
1 gm............ 51927-3052-00 1.20

CALCIUM SACCHARATE (PCCA)
POW, NA (USP; TETRAHYDRATE)
1 gm............ 51927-2860-00 5.88

CALCIUM SACCHARIN (Amend)
saccharin calcium
POW, NA (U.S.P. , F.C.C.)
500 gm............ 17317-0765-01 21.00
(U.S.P./F.C.C.)
2270 gm............ 17317-0765-05 77.00
11350 gm............ 17317-0765-08 350.00

CALCIUM STEARATE (Amend)
POW, NA (N.F.)
500 gm............ 17317-0086-01 9.80
2270 gm............ 17317-0086-05 35.00

(PCCA)
POW, NA (NF)
1 gm............ 51927-2782-00 0.11

(Spectrum Pharmacy)
POW, NA (N.F.)
500 gm............ 49452-1610-01 89.25
2500 gm............ 49452-1610-02 276.85

CALCIUM SULFATE
(Amend) *See CALCIUM SULFATE ANHYDROUS*

(Amend) *See CALCIUM SULFATE DIHYDRATE*

(Baker, J.T.) *See CALCIUM SULFATE ANHYDROUS*

(Baker, J.T.) *See CALCIUM SULFATE DIHYDRATE*

(Baker, J.T.) *See CALCIUM SULFATE HEMIHYDRATE*

(Medisca)
POW, NA (DIHYDRATE,1X500GM)
500 gm............ 38779-1820-08 30.00
(DIHYDRATE,1X2500GM)
2500 gm............ 38779-1820-01 96.00

(PCCA)
POW, NA (HEMIHYDRATE)
1 gm............ 51927-2654-00 0.09
(NF; ANHYDROUS)
1 gm............ 51927-3092-00 0.11

(Spectrum Pharmacy) *See CALCIUM SULFATE ANHYDROUS*

(Spectrum Pharmacy) *See CALCIUM SULFATE DIHYDRATE*

CALCIUM SULFATE ANHYDROUS (Amend)
calcium sulfate
POW, NA (N.F., F.C.C.)
454 gm............ 17317-1210-01 9.80
2270 gm............ 17317-1210-05 29.40
11350 gm............ 17317-1210-08 87.50

(Baker, J.T.)
POW, NA (REAGENT)
500 gm............ 10106-1458-01 164.49

(Spectrum Pharmacy)
POW, NA (F.C.C.)
500 gm............ 49452-1620-01 78.75
2500 gm............ 49452-1620-02 207.20

CALCIUM SULFATE DIHYDRATE (Amend)
calcium sulfate
POW, NA (N.F.)
500 gm............ 17317-0087-01 9.80
2270 gm............ 17317-0087-05 29.40
11350 gm............ 17317-0087-08 87.50

(Baker, J.T.)
POW, NA (A.C.S., REAGENT)
500 gm............ 10106-1452-01 104.24
1000 gm............ 10106-1452-05 187.51

(Spectrum Pharmacy)
POW, NA (N.F.)
500 gm............ 49452-1630-01 78.75
2500 gm............ 49452-1630-02 207.20

CALCIUM SULFATE HEMIHYDRATE (Baker, J.T.)
calcium sulfate
POW, NA (REAGENT)
500 gm............ 10106-1463-01 35.90

CALCIUM SULFATE, DRIED
(Gallipot) *See PLASTER OF PARIS*

(Humco) *See PLASTER OF PARIS*

CALCIUM SULFIDE
(Medisca) *See SULFURATED LIME*

PROD/MFR | NDC | AWP | DP | OBC

(PCCA) *See SULFURATED LIME*

CALCIUM THIOGLYCOLATE
(PCCA) *See CALCIUM THIOGLYCOLATE TRIHYDRATE*

CALCIUM THIOGLYCOLATE TRIHYDRATE (PCCA)
calcium thioglycolate
POW, NA (1X1GM)
1 gm 51927-2090-00 6.60

CALCIUM UNDECYLENATE (PCCA)
POW, NA, 1 gm 51927-1939-00 1.08

CALCIUM-FOLIC ACID PLUS D CHEWABLE WAFER
(Acella)
multivitamin and minerals
WAF, PO (CHOCOLATE)
60s ea 42192-0706-60 37.07

CALCIUM/CYANOCOBALAMIN/FOLIC ACID/PYRIDOXINE
(Acella) *See BP FOLINATAL PLUS B*
(Breckenridge Pharm) *See FOLBECAL*
(Midlothian Labs) *See PREVITE RX*
(Ther-RX) *See PREMESIS RX*

CALCON II (Weleda)
homeopathic substance
POW, PO, 30 gm 55946-0148-40 9.00

CALCON-AM (Weleda)
homeopathic substance
POW, PO, 30 gm 55946-0145-40 9.00

CALDOLOR (Cumberland Pharma)
ibuprofen
SOL, IV, 100 mg/ml,
4 ml 25s 66220-0247-04 230.00
8 ml 25s 66220-0287-08 328.13

CALFACTANT
(ONY) *See INFASURF*

CALOMEL (Amend)
mercurous chloride
POW, NA (PURIFIED, MILD)
30 gm 17317-0088-02 21.00
125 gm 17317-0088-04 35.00
454 gm 17317-0088-01 105.00
(Medisca)
POW, NA (1X25GM)
25 gm 38779-1094-04 55.50
(1X100GM)
100 gm 38779-1094-05 30.00

CALOMEL MILD (Baker, J.T.)
mercurous chloride
POW, NA (PURIFIED)
125 gm 10106-1363-04 66.33

CALOMIST (Fleming)
cyanocobalamin
SPR, NS (1X10.7ML),
25 mcg/0.1 ml,
10.7 ml 00256-0203-01 123.71

CALPHOSAN (Glenwood)
calcium glycerophosphate/calcium lactate
SOL, IJ (M.D.V.)
50 mg/10 ml-50 mg/10 ml,
60 ml 00516-0060-60 92.42

CALTRATE 600+D (Phys Total Care)
REPACK
calcium carbonate/vitamin d
TAB, PO, 600 mg-200 iu,
120s ea 54868-5786-00 13.35

CAMILA (Teva)
norethindrone
TAB, PO, 0.35 mg,
168s ea 00555-0715-58 221.49 AB1
(Phys Total Care)
REPACK
TAB, PO, 0.35 mg, 28s ea .. 54868-4814-00 84.42 AB1

CAMPATH (Genzyme)
alemtuzumab
SOL, IV (CLEAR GLASS VIAL,PF)
30 mg/ml, 1 ml 3s 50419-0357-03 6126.55 5105.46

CAMPHENE (PCCA)
POW, NA, 1 gm 51927-3466-00 7.50

CAMPHOR
(Amend) *See CAMPHOR SQUARES*
(Amend)
POW, NA (U.S.P., SYNTHETIC)
500 gm 17317-0090-01 11.20
2270 gm 17317-0090-05 43.40
11350 gm 17317-0090-08 161.25
(Gallipot)
CRY, NA (SYNTHETIC,U.S.P.)
113.4 gm 51552-0396-04 10.01
454 gm 51552-0396-06 20.58
(Humco) *See CAMPHOR GUM*
(Letco)
CRY, NA (SYNTHETIC)
500 gm 62991-1224-02 49.50
2500 gm 62991-1224-01 150.00
(Medisca)
CRY, NA (U.S.P., SYNTHETIC)
500 gm 38779-0386-08 50.70
(PCCA)
POW, NA (SYNTHETIC)
1 gm 51927-1200-00 0.30
(Spectrum Pharmacy)
CAK, NA (SYNTHETIC, 1 OZ. CUBES)
500 gm 49452-1650-01 199.15
CRY, NA (SYNTHETIC, U.S.P.)
500 gm 49452-1640-01 91.00
2500 gm 49452-1640-02 247.80
12000 gm 49452-1640-03 941.50

CAMPHOR GUM (Humco)
camphor
CAK, NA (U.S.P., SYNTHETIC)
30 gm 00395-0455-91 19.50

CAMPHOR OIL (Medisca)
OIL, NA (1X25ML,LIGHT,NATURAL)
25 ml 38779-1095-04 19.50
(1X100ML,LIGHT,NATURAL)
100 ml 38779-1095-05 43.50
(1X500ML,LIGHT,NATURAL)
500 ml 38779-1095-08 120.00
(1X1000ML,LIGHT,NATURAL)
1000 ml 38779-1095-09 303.00

CAMPHOR SQUARES (Amend)
camphor
LUM, NA (SYNTHETIC)
454 gm 17317-0932-01 21.00

CAMPRAL (Forest Pharm)
acamprosate calcium
ECT, PO (10X10)
333 mg, 100s ea UD .. 00456-3330-63 97.79
180s ea 00456-3330-01 170.14
(DOSE PAK)
333 mg, 100s ea 00456-3330-60 170.14
(Dispensing Solutions)
REPACK
ECT, PO, 333 mg, 180s ea . 55045-3296-01 127.80
(Phys Total Care)
REPACK
ECT, PO (DOSE PAK)
333 mg, 180s ea 54868-5293-00 152.73

CAMPTOSAR (Pfizer)
irinotecan hydrochloride
SOL, IV (S.D.V.)
20 mg/ml, 2 ml 00009-7529-02 294.55 245.46
5 ml 00009-7529-01 736.38 613.65

CANADA BALSAM (Medisca)
balsam canada
SOL, NA (1X25ML)
25 ml 38779-1096-04 22.50
(1X100ML)
100 ml 38779-1096-05 46.50
(1X500ML)
500 ml 38779-1096-08 267.00
(PCCA)
POW, NA, 1 gm 51927-2295-00 1.00

CANADIAN BALSAM (Spectrum Pharmacy)
balsam canada
POW, NA (1X100GM,NEUTRAL)
100 gm 49452-1660-02 156.10
(1X500GM,NEUTRAL)
500 gm 49452-1660-03 605.50

CANAKINUMAB
(Novartis Pharm) *See ILARIS*

CANASA (Axcan)
mesalamine
SUP, RC, 1000 mg, 30s ea . 58914-0501-56 424.34
(USP,PAC)
1000 mg, 42s ea 58914-0501-42 594.08
1080s ea 58914-0501-1814991.26

CANCIDAS (Merck)
caspofungin acetate
PDS, IV (VIAL)
50 mg, ea 00006-3822-10 405.25
70 mg, ea 00006-3823-10 421.06

CANDESARTAN CILEXETIL
(AstraZeneca) *See ATACAND*

CANDESARTAN CILEXETIL/HYDROCHLOROTHIAZIDE
(AstraZeneca) *See ATACAND HCT*

CANDIN (Phys Total Care)
REPACK
candida albicans antigen
INJ, ID (SKIN TEST)
1 ml 54868-5559-00 138.34

CANNULA, INJECTION
(Patton) *See I-PORT*

CANTHARIDIN (Gallipot)
POW, NA (BP 1949)
0.0525 gm 51552-0306-02 34.30
0.075 gm 51552-0306-03 47.60
0.5 gm 51552-0306-04 161.00
1 gm 51552-0306-01 264.60
(Letco)
POW, NA, 0.1 gm 62991-1652-01 90.00
0.5 gm 62991-1652-02 300.00
1 gm 62991-1652-03 510.00
(Medisca)
POW, NA (B.P.)
ea 38779-0389-09 117.00
0.5 gm 38779-0389-00 382.50
1 gm 38779-0389-06 588.00
5 gm 38779-0389-03 2479.50
(PCCA)
POW, NA, 1 gm 51927-2638-00 1110.00
(Spectrum Pharmacy)
POW, NA (BP 49)
0.1 gm 49452-1674-02 193.55
0.5 gm 49452-1674-03 647.50
1 gm 49452-1674-06 868.00

CANTIL (Sanofi-Aventis)
mepenzolate bromide
TAB, PO, 25 mg, 100s ea .. 00068-0037-01 154.20

CAPASTAT SULFATE (Akorn)
capreomycin
PDS, IJ (USP)
1 gm, ea 17478-0080-50 175.00

CAPECITABINE
(Roche Labs) *See XELODA*

CAPEX (Galderma)
fluocinolone acetonide
SHA, TP, 0.01%, 120 ml ... 00299-5500-04 217.50

CAPHOSOL (EUSA)
saliva substitutes
SOL, MM (30 DOSES)
15 ml 60s 84898-0000-01 221.38
(120 DOSES)
15 ml 240s 84898-0000-04 839.04

CAPITAL W/CODEINE (Valeant Pharm Intl)
acetaminophen/codeine phosphate
SUS, PO, 120 mg/5 ml-12 mg/5 ml,
473 ml, C-V .... 00187-0003-01 383.69 AA

CAPOTEN (HomeMed)
REPACK
captopril
TAB, PO, 12.5 mg, 30s ea . 51655-0975-24 19.75 AB
(PD-Rx Pharm)
REPACK
TAB, PO, 25 mg, 30s ea ... 55289-0506-30 64.75 AB
(Phys Total Care)
REPACK
TAB, PO, 12.5 mg, 30s ea . 54868-1775-01 46.91 AB
90s ea .... 54868-1775-04 136.98 AB
50 mg, 60s ea .... 54868-1415-01 168.84 AB

CAPOZIDE 25/15 (Phys Total Care)
captopril/hydrochlorothiazide
TAB, PO, 25 mg-15 mg,
30s ea .... 54868-3769-00 52.75 AB

CAPOZIDE 50/25 (Phys Total Care)
captopril/hydrochlorothiazide
TAB, PO, 50 mg-25 mg,
30s ea .... 54868-3891-00 64.92 AB

CAPREOMYCIN
(Akorn) *See CAPASTAT SULFATE*

CAPRYLIC ACID (PCCA)
octanoic acid
SOL, NA (REAGENT)
1 gm 51927-1397-00 0.54

PROD/MFR	NDC	AWP	DP	OBC
CAPRYLIC TRIGLYCERIDES (PCCA)				
caprylic/capric/myristic/stearic triglyceride				
POW, NA (CAPRIC)				
1 gm	51927-2604-00	0.27		
CAPRYLIC/CAPRIC/MYRISTIC/STEARIC TRIGLYCERIDE (PCCA) *See CAPRYLIC TRIGLYCERIDES*				
CAPS (Baker, J.T.)				
3-(cyclohexylamino)-1-propanesulfonic acid				
POW, NA (ULTRAPURE BIOREAGENT)				
25 gm	10106-4118-00	11.54		
100 gm	10106-4118-01	33.17		
1000 gm	10106-4118-04	232.01		
CAPSAICIN (Gallipot)				
POW, NA (SYNTHETIC)				
1 gm	51552-0129-01	53.90		
5 gm	51552-0129-02	235.20		
(Letco)				
POW, NA (NATURAL)				
95%, 1 gm	62991-2017-01	90.00		
5 gm	62991-2017-02	270.00		
(Medisca) *See CAPSAICIN 2%*				
(Medisca) *See CAPSAICIN 95%*				
(PCCA)				
POW, NA (USP; SYNTHETIC)				
1 gm	51927-1807-00	267.00		
(Spectrum Pharmacy) *See CAPSAICIN SYNTHETIC*				
(Spectrum Pharmacy)				
POW, NA (U.S.P.,NATURAL, KOSHER)				
1 gm	49452-1321-01	292.60		
(Dispensing Solutions)				
REPACK				
CRE, TP, 0.025%, 60 gm	55045-2655-06	15.99		
0.075%, 60 gm	55045-2654-06	26.75		
CAPSAICIN 2% (Medisca)				
capsaicin				
POW, NA (DECOLORIZED)				
454 gm	38779-0664-08	123.00		
CAPSAICIN 95% (Medisca)				
capsaicin				
POW, NA (NATURAL,1X1GM)				
1 gm	38779-0837-06	85.50		
(NATURAL,1X5GM)				
5 gm	38779-0837-03	357.00		
(NATURAL,1X100GM)				
100 gm	38779-0837-05	5355.00		
CAPSAICIN SYNTHETIC (Spectrum Pharmacy)				
capsaicin				
POW, NA (CRYSTALLINE)				
1 gm	49452-1675-01	291.90		
5 gm	49452-1675-02	1102.50		
25 gm	49452-1675-04	2835.00		
CAPSICUM (Amend)				
TIN, NA (N.F.)				
120 ml	17317-0091-04	9.80		
500 ml	17317-0091-01	29.40		
(Medisca)				
TIN, NA, 100 ml	38779-1098-05	34.50		
(PCCA) *See CAPSICUM TINCTURE*				
(Spectrum Pharmacy) *See CAPSICUM OLEORESIN*				
CAPSICUM FRUTESCENS RESIN (PCCA) *See CAPSICUM OLEORESIN*				
CAPSICUM OLEORESIN (PCCA)				
capsicum frutescens resin				
SOL, NA (USP)				
1 gm	51927-3091-00	1.80		
(Spectrum Pharmacy)				
capsicum				
POW, NA (U.S.P.)				
25 gm	49452-4883-01	149.10		
100 gm	49452-4883-02	423.50		
CAPSICUM TINCTURE (PCCA)				
capsicum				
TIN, NA, 1 ml	51927-1843-00	0.75		
CAPSULE 0 BLUE (Gallipot)				
capsules, empty gelatin				
DEV, NA, 100s ea	51552-0387-01	4.13		
1000s ea	51552-0387-02	29.75		
CAPSULE 0 BLUE/BLUE (Medisca)				
capsules, empty gelatin				
DEV, NA (OPAQUE,CONI-SNAP)				
1000s ea	38779-1782-09	30.00		
5000s ea	38779-1782-02	147.00		
10000s ea	38779-1782-01	285.00		
CAPSULE 0 CLEAR (Gallipot)				
capsules, empty gelatin				
DEV, NA, 100s ea	51552-0405-01	4.13		
1000s ea	51552-0405-02	21.70		
CAPSULE 0 CLEAR/CLEAR (Letco)				
capsules, empty gelatin				
DEV, NA, 1000s ea	62991-1389-01	45.00		
5000s ea	62991-1389-02	180.00		
10000s ea	62991-1389-03	300.00		
(Medisca)				
DEV, NA (CONI-SNAP)				
1000s ea	38779-1105-09	30.00		
5000s ea	38779-1105-02	147.00		
10000s ea	38779-1105-01	285.00		
CAPSULE 0 CLEAR/WHITE (Letco)				
capsules, empty gelatin				
DEV, NA, 1000s ea	62991-1386-01	45.00		
1000s ea	62991-1390-01	45.00		
5000s ea	62991-1386-02	180.00		
5000s ea	62991-1390-02	180.00		
10000s ea	62991-1386-03	300.00		
10000s ea	62991-1390-03	300.00		
CAPSULE 0 DARK BLUE/DARK BLUE (Medisca)				
capsules, empty gelatin				
DEV, NA (CONI-SNAP)				
1000s ea	38779-1958-09	30.00		
5000s ea	38779-1958-02	147.00		
CAPSULE 0 LACTOSE BLUE (Gallipot)				
capsules, empty gelatin				
DEV, NA, 100s ea	51552-0484-01	13.86		
CAPSULE 0 LACTOSE WHITE (Gallipot)				
capsules, empty gelatin				
DEV, NA, 100s ea	51552-0485-01	13.86		
CAPSULE 0 ORANGE/ORANGE (Medisca)				
capsules, empty gelatin				
DEV, NA (OPAQUE,POSILOK)				
1000s ea	38779-2008-09	30.00		
5000s ea	38779-2008-02	147.00		
CAPSULE 0 PINK/PINK (Medisca)				
capsules, empty gelatin				
DEV, NA (OPAQUE,CONI-SNAP)				
1000s ea	38779-2009-09	30.00		
5000s ea	38779-2009-02	147.00		
10000s ea	38779-2009-01	285.00		
CAPSULE 0 RED (Gallipot)				
capsules, empty gelatin				
DEV, NA, 100s ea	51552-0333-01	3.43		
1000s ea	51552-0333-02	29.33		
CAPSULE 0 RED/BLACK (Gallipot)				
capsules, empty gelatin				
DEV, NA, 100s ea	51552-0490-01	3.43		
1000s ea	51552-0490-02	29.33		
CAPSULE 0 WHITE (Gallipot)				
capsules, empty gelatin				
DEV, NA, 100s ea	51552-0340-01	4.13		
100s ea	51552-0372-01	5.53		
1000s ea	51552-0340-02	21.70		
1000s ea	51552-0372-02	41.30		
CAPSULE 0 WHITE/WHITE (Letco)				
capsules, empty gelatin				
DEV, NA, 1000s ea	62991-1391-01	45.00		
5000s ea	62991-1391-02	180.00		
10000s ea	62991-1391-03	300.00		
(Medisca)				
DEV, NA (OPAQUE,CONI-SNAP)				
1000s ea	38779-1107-09	30.00		
5000s ea	38779-1107-02	147.00		
10000s ea	38779-1107-01	285.00		
CAPSULE 00 BLUE (Gallipot)				
capsules, empty gelatin				
DEV, NA, 100s ea	51552-0371-01	5.53		
1000s ea	51552-0371-02	43.75		
CAPSULE 00 BLUE/BLUE (Medisca)				
capsules, empty gelatin				
DEV, NA (OPAQUE,CONI-SNAP)				
1000s ea	38779-1883-09	30.00		
5000s ea	38779-1883-02	147.00		
10000s ea	38779-1883-01	285.00		
CAPSULE 00 CLEAR (Gallipot)				
capsules, empty gelatin				
DEV, NA, 100s ea	51552-0382-01	5.53		
1000s ea	51552-0382-02	41.30		
CAPSULE 00 CLEAR/CLEAR (Letco)				
capsules, empty gelatin				
DEV, NA, 1000s ea	62991-1385-01	75.00		
5000s ea	62991-1385-02	300.00		
10000s ea	62991-1385-03	510.00		
(Medisca)				
DEV, NA (CONI-SNAP)				
1000s ea	38779-1108-09	90.00		
5000s ea	38779-1108-02	399.00		
10000s ea	38779-1108-01	750.00		
CAPSULE 00 WHITE/CLEAR (Letco)				
capsules, empty gelatin				
DEV, NA, 1000s ea	62991-1387-01	75.00		
5000s ea	62991-1387-02	300.00		
10000s ea	62991-1387-03	510.00		
CAPSULE 00 WHITE/WHITE (Letco)				
capsules, empty gelatin				
DEV, NA, 1000s ea	62991-1388-01	75.00		
5000s ea	62991-1388-02	300.00		
10000s ea	62991-1388-03	510.00		
(Medisca)				
DEV, NA (OPAQUE,CONI-SNAP)				
1000s ea	38779-1109-09	90.00		
5000s ea	38779-1109-02	399.00		
10000s ea	38779-1109-01	750.00		
CAPSULE 000 CLEAR (Gallipot)				
capsules, empty gelatin				
DEV, NA, 100s ea	51552-0395-01	7.56		
1000s ea	51552-0395-02	68.53		
CAPSULE 000 CLEAR/CLEAR (Medisca)				
capsules, empty gelatin				
DEV, NA (CONI-SNAP)				
1000s ea	38779-1110-09	147.00		
5000s ea	38779-1110-02	888.00		
10000s ea	38779-1110-01	1623.00		
CAPSULE 1 BLUE (Gallipot)				
capsules, empty gelatin				
DEV, NA, 100s ea	51552-0330-01	3.92		
1000s ea	51552-0330-02	26.95		
CAPSULE 1 BLUE/BLUE (Medisca)				
capsules, empty gelatin				
DEV, NA (OPAQUE,CONI-SNAP)				
1000s ea	38779-1889-09	30.00		
5000s ea	38779-1889-02	147.00		
10000s ea	38779-1889-01	285.00		
CAPSULE 1 BLUE/WHITE (Gallipot)				
capsules, empty gelatin				
DEV, NA, 100s ea	51552-0379-01	3.92		
1000s ea	51552-0379-02	26.95		
CAPSULE 1 BROWN/LIGHT TAN (Medisca)				
capsules, empty gelatin				
DEV, NA (OPAQUE,CONI-SNAP)				
1000s ea	38779-1892-09	30.00		
5000s ea	38779-1892-02	147.00		
10000s ea	38779-1892-01	285.00		
CAPSULE 1 CLEAR (Gallipot)				
capsules, empty gelatin				
DEV, NA, 100s ea	51552-0353-01	3.92		
1000s ea	51552-0353-02	21.35		
CAPSULE 1 CLEAR/CLEAR (Letco)				
capsules, empty gelatin				
DEV, NA, 1000s ea	62991-1392-01	45.00		
5000s ea	62991-1392-02	180.00		
10000s ea	62991-1392-03	300.00		
(Medisca)				
DEV, NA (CONI-SNAP)				
1000s ea	38779-1111-09	30.00		
5000s ea	38779-1111-02	147.00		
10000s ea	38779-1111-01	285.00		
CAPSULE 1 CLEAR/WHITE (Letco)				
capsules, empty gelatin				
DEV, NA, 1000s ea	62991-1393-01	45.00		
5000s ea	62991-1393-02	180.00		
10000s ea	62991-1393-03	300.00		
CAPSULE 1 GRAY/PINK (Gallipot)				
capsules, empty gelatin				
DEV, NA, 100s ea	51552-0391-01	3.92		
1000s ea	51552-0391-02	26.95		
CAPSULE 1 GREEN (Gallipot)				
capsules, empty gelatin				
DEV, NA, 100s ea	51552-0360-01	3.22		
1000s ea	51552-0360-02	26.95		
CAPSULE 1 LIGHT BLUE/DARK BLUE (Gallipot)				
capsules, empty gelatin				
DEV, NA, 100s ea	51552-0336-01	3.22		
CAPSULE 1 LIGHT BLUE/POWDER BLUE (Gallipot)				
capsules, empty gelatin				
DEV, NA, 100s ea	51552-0429-01	3.92		
1000s ea	51552-0429-02	26.95		
CAPSULE 1 ORANGE/ORANGE (Medisca)				
capsules, empty gelatin				
DEV, NA (OPAQUE,CONI-SNAP)				
1000s ea	38779-1113-09	30.00		
5000s ea	38779-1113-02	147.00		
10000s ea	38779-1113-01	285.00		

PROD/MFR	NDC	AWP	DP	OBC
CAPSULE 1 ORANGE/YELLOW (Gallipot)				
capsules, empty gelatin				
DEV, NA, 100s ea	51552-0432-01	3.22		
1000s ea	51552-0432-02	26.95		
CAPSULE 1 PINK/BLUE (Medisca)				
capsules, empty gelatin				
DEV, NA (CONI-SNAP)				
1000s ea	38779-1114-09	30.00		
5000s ea	38779-1114-02	147.00		
10000s ea	38779-1114-01	285.00		
CAPSULE 1 PINK/PINK (Medisca)				
capsules, empty gelatin				
DEV, NA (OPAQUE,CONI-SNAP)				
1000s ea	38779-2018-09	30.00		
5000s ea	38779-2018-02	147.00		
10000s ea	38779-2018-01	285.00		
CAPSULE 1 PINK/WHITE (Gallipot)				
capsules, empty gelatin				
DEV, NA, 100s ea	51552-0459-01	3.92		
1000s ea	51552-0459-02	26.95		
CAPSULE 1 PURPLE/PURPLE (Medisca)				
capsules, empty gelatin				
DEV, NA (OPAQUE,CONI-SNAP)				
1000s ea	38779-2019-09	30.00		
5000s ea	38779-2019-02	147.00		
10000s ea	38779-2019-01	285.00		
CAPSULE 1 RED (Gallipot)				
capsules, empty gelatin				
DEV, NA, 100s ea	51552-0362-01	3.92		
1000s ea	51552-0362-02	26.95		
CAPSULE 1 RED/BLUE (Medisca)				
capsules, empty gelatin				
DEV, NA (OPAQUE,CONI-SNAP)				
1000s ea	38779-1891-09	30.00		
5000s ea	38779-1891-02	147.00		
10000s ea	38779-1891-01	285.00		
CAPSULE 1 RED/WHITE (Gallipot)				
capsules, empty gelatin				
DEV, NA, 100s ea	51552-0390-01	3.92		
1000s ea	51552-0390-02	26.95		
CAPSULE 1 RUBY RED (Gallipot)				
capsules, empty gelatin				
DEV, NA, 100s ea	51552-0460-01	3.22		
1000s ea	51552-0460-02	26.95		
CAPSULE 1 TURQUOISE/VIOLET (Gallipot)				
capsules, empty gelatin				
DEV, NA, 100s ea	51552-0407-01	3.22		
1000s ea	51552-0407-02	26.95		
CAPSULE 1 WHITE (Gallipot)				
capsules, empty gelatin				
DEV, NA, 100s ea	51552-0331-01	3.92		
1000s ea	51552-0331-02	21.35		
50000s ea	51552-0331-09	1078.00		
CAPSULE 1 WHITE/CLEAR (Letco)				
capsules, empty gelatin				
DEV, NA, 1000s ea	62991-1394-01	45.00		
5000s ea	62991-1394-02	180.00		
10000s ea	62991-1394-03	300.00		
(Medisca)				
DEV, NA (CONI-SNAP)				
1000s ea	38779-1895-09	30.00		
5000s ea	38779-1895-02	147.00		
10000s ea	38779-1895-01	285.00		
CAPSULE 1 WHITE/GREEN (Medisca)				
capsules, empty gelatin				
DEV, NA (OPAQUE,CONI-SNAP)				
1000s ea	38779-1890-09	30.00		
5000s ea	38779-1890-02	147.00		
10000s ea	38779-1890-01	285.00		
CAPSULE 1 WHITE/ORANGE (Gallipot)				
capsules, empty gelatin				
DEV, NA, 100s ea	51552-0431-01	3.22		
1000s ea	51552-0431-02	26.95		
CAPSULE 1 WHITE/WHITE (Letco)				
capsules, empty gelatin				
DEV, NA, 1000s ea	62991-1395-01	45.00		
5000s ea	62991-1395-02	180.00		
10000s ea	62991-1395-03	300.00		
(Medisca)				
DEV, NA (OPAQUE,CONI-SNAP)				
1000s ea	38779-1112-09	30.00		
5000s ea	38779-1112-02	147.00		
10000s ea	38779-1112-01	285.00		
CAPSULE 1 YELLOW/GREEN (Gallipot)				
capsules, empty gelatin				
DEV, NA, 100s ea	51552-0334-01	3.92		
1000s ea	51552-0334-02	26.95		
(Medisca)				
DEV, NA (CONI-SNAP)				
1000s ea	38779-1115-01	30.00		
5000s ea	38779-1115-02	147.00		
10000s ea	38779-1115-03	285.00		
CAPSULE 13 CLEAR/CLEAR (Letco)				
capsules, empty gelatin				
DEV, NA, 50s ea	62991-1402-01	45.00		
CAPSULE 2 BLUE/BLUE (Medisca)				
capsules, empty gelatin				
DEV, NA (OPAQUE,CONI-SNAP)				
1000s ea	38779-2287-09	46.50		
5000s ea	38779-2287-02	199.50		
10000s ea	38779-2287-01	367.50		
CAPSULE 2 CLEAR (Gallipot)				
capsules, empty gelatin				
DEV, NA, 100s ea	51552-0332-01	3.85		
1000s ea	51552-0332-02	21.35		
CAPSULE 2 CLEAR/CLEAR (Medisca)				
capsules, empty gelatin				
DEV, NA (CONI-SNAP)				
1000s ea	38779-1880-09	30.00		
5000s ea	38779-1880-02	147.00		
10000s ea	38779-1880-01	285.00		
CAPSULE 2 GREEN (Gallipot)				
capsules, empty gelatin				
DEV, NA, 100s ea	51552-0570-01	3.85		
1000s ea	51552-0570-02	26.60		
CAPSULE 2 POWDER BLUE (Gallipot)				
capsules, empty gelatin				
DEV, NA, 100s ea	51552-0581-01	3.15		
1000s ea	51552-0581-02	24.15		
CAPSULE 2 WHITE (Gallipot)				
capsules, empty gelatin				
DEV, NA, 100s ea	51552-0351-01	3.85		
1000s ea	51552-0351-02	21.35		
CAPSULE 2 WHITE/WHITE (Medisca)				
capsules, empty gelatin				
DEV, NA (CONI-SNAP)				
1000s ea	38779-1116-09	30.00		
5000s ea	38779-1116-02	147.00		
10000s ea	38779-1116-01	285.00		
CAPSULE 3 BLUE OPAQUE (Gallipot)				
capsules, empty gelatin				
DEV, NA, 100s ea	51552-0370-01	3.85		
1000s ea	51552-0370-02	26.60		
CAPSULE 3 BLUE/GREEN (Medisca)				
capsules, empty gelatin				
DEV, NA (CONI-SNAP)				
1000s ea	38779-1117-01	30.00		
(OPAQUE,CONI-SNAP)				
1000s ea	38779-1118-09	30.00		
(CONI-SNAP)				
5000s ea	38779-1117-02	147.00		
(OPAQUE,CONI-SNAP)				
5000s ea	38779-1118-02	147.00		
(CONI-SNAP)				
10000s ea	38779-1117-03	285.00		
(OPAQUE,CONI-SNAP)				
10000s ea	38779-1118-01	285.00		
CAPSULE 3 BROWN/LIGHT BLUE (Medisca)				
capsules, empty gelatin				
DEV, NA (OPAQUE,CONI-SNAP)				
1000s ea	38779-2346-09	30.00		
5000s ea	38779-2346-02	199.50		
10000s ea	38779-2346-01	285.00		
CAPSULE 3 CLEAR (Gallipot)				
capsules, empty gelatin				
DEV, NA, 100s ea	51552-0374-01	3.85		
CAPSULE 3 CLEAR/CLEAR (Letco)				
capsules, empty gelatin				
DEV, NA, 1000s ea	62991-1396-01	45.00		
5000s ea	62991-1396-02	180.00		
10000s ea	62991-1396-03	300.00		
(Medisca)				
DEV, NA (CONI-SNAP)				
1000s ea	38779-1121-09	30.00		
(VEGETABLE,CONI-SNAP)				
1000s ea	38779-2414-09	34.50		
(CONI-SNAP)				
5000s ea	38779-1121-02	147.00		
(VEGETABLE,CONI-SNAP)				
5000s ea	38779-2414-02	157.50		
(CONI-SNAP)				
10000s ea	38779-1121-01	285.00		
(VEGETABLE,CONI-SNAP)				
10000s ea	38779-2414-01	291.00		
CAPSULE 3 CLEAR/WHITE (Letco)				
capsules, empty gelatin				
DEV, NA, 1000s ea	62991-1397-01	45.00		
5000s ea	62991-1397-02	180.00		
10000s ea	62991-1397-03	300.00		
CAPSULE 3 DARK RED/DARK RED (Medisca)				
capsules, empty gelatin				
DEV, NA (CONI-SNAP)				
1000s ea	38779-1893-01	30.00		
5000s ea	38779-1893-02	147.00		
10000s ea	38779-1893-03	285.00		
CAPSULE 3 GREEN OPAQUE (Gallipot)				
capsules, empty gelatin				
DEV, NA, 100s ea	51552-0437-01	3.85		
1000s ea	51552-0437-02	26.60		
CAPSULE 3 GREEN TRANSLUCENT (Gallipot)				
capsules, empty gelatin				
DEV, NA, 100s ea	51552-0335-01	2.80		
1000s ea	51552-0335-02	21.35		
CAPSULE 3 GREEN/GREEN (Medisca)				
capsules, empty gelatin				
DEV, NA (OPAQUE,CONI-SNAP)				
1000s ea	38779-1793-09	30.00		
5000s ea	38779-1793-02	147.00		
10000s ea	38779-1793-01	285.00		
CAPSULE 3 MAROON/BLUE (Medisca)				
capsules, empty gelatin				
DEV, NA (OPAQUE,CONI-SNAP)				
1000s ea	38779-1119-09	30.00		
5000s ea	38779-1119-02	147.00		
10000s ea	38779-1119-01	285.00		
CAPSULE 3 ORANGE/ORANGE (Medisca)				
capsules, empty gelatin				
DEV, NA (OPAQUE,CONI-SNAP)				
1000s ea	38779-2020-09	30.00		
5000s ea	38779-2020-02	147.00		
10000s ea	38779-2020-01	285.00		
CAPSULE 3 PINK/PINK (Medisca)				
capsules, empty gelatin				
DEV, NA (OPAQUE,CONI-SNAP)				
1000s ea	38779-1894-09	30.00		
5000s ea	38779-1894-02	147.00		
10000s ea	38779-1894-01	285.00		
CAPSULE 3 RED/RED (Medisca)				
capsules, empty gelatin				
DEV, NA (OPAQUE,CONI-SNAP)				
1000s ea	38779-2021-03	30.00		
5000s ea	38779-2021-02	147.00		
10000s ea	38779-2021-01	285.00		
CAPSULE 3 SWEDISH ORANGE/SWEDISH ORANGE (Medisca)				
capsules, empty gelatin				
DEV, NA (OPAQUE,CONI-SNAP)				
1000s ea	38779-2332-09	30.00		
5000s ea	38779-2332-02	147.00		
10000s ea	38779-2332-01	285.00		
CAPSULE 3 WHITE (Gallipot)				
capsules, empty gelatin				
DEV, NA, 100s ea	51552-0565-01	3.85		
1000s ea	51552-0565-02	21.35		
CAPSULE 3 WHITE/CLEAR (Letco)				
capsules, empty gelatin				
DEV, NA, 1000s ea	62991-1398-01	45.00		
5000s ea	62991-1398-02	180.00		
10000s ea	62991-1398-03	300.00		
(Medisca)				
DEV, NA (CONI-SNAP)				
1000s ea	38779-1896-09	30.00		
5000s ea	38779-1896-02	147.00		
10000s ea	38779-1896-01	285.00		
CAPSULE 3 WHITE/WHITE (Letco)				
capsules, empty gelatin				
DEV, NA, 1000s ea	62991-1399-01	45.00		
5000s ea	62991-1399-02	180.00		
10000s ea	62991-1399-03	300.00		
(Medisca)				
DEV, NA (OPAQUE,CONI-SNAP)				
1000s ea	38779-1122-09	30.00		
5000s ea	38779-1122-02	147.00		
10000s ea	38779-1122-01	285.00		
50000s ea	38779-1122-03	1453.50		

PROD/MFR NDC AWP DP OBC

CAPSULE 3 YELLOW/GRAY (Medisca)
capsules, empty gelatin
DEV, NA (CONI-SNAP)
1000s ea **38779-1124-09** 30.00
5000s ea **38779-1124-02** 147.00
10000s ea **38779-1124-01** 285.00

CAPSULE 4 BLACK/GREEN (Medisca)
capsules, empty gelatin
DEV, NA (OPAQUE,CONI-SNAP)
1000s ea **38779-1126-09** 30.00
5000s ea **38779-1126-02** 147.00
10000s ea **38779-1126-01** 285.00

CAPSULE 4 BLUE/WHITE (Gallipot)
capsules, empty gelatin
DEV, NA, 100s ea **51552-0562-01** 3.50
1000s ea **51552-0562-02** 25.20

CAPSULE 4 CANARY YELLOW (Gallipot)
capsules, empty gelatin
DEV, NA, 100s ea **51552-0415-01** 2.73
1000s ea **51552-0415-02** 19.95

CAPSULE 4 CLEAR (Gallipot)
capsules, empty gelatin
DEV, NA, 100s ea **51552-0375-01** 3.50
1000s ea **51552-0375-02** 21.35

CAPSULE 4 CLEAR/CLEAR (Letco)
capsules, empty gelatin
DEV, NA, 1000s ea **62991-1400-01** 45.00
5000s ea **62991-1400-02** 180.00
10000s ea **62991-1400-03** 300.00

(Medisca)
DEV, NA (CONI-SNAP)
1000s ea **38779-1125-09** 30.00
5000s ea **38779-1125-02** 147.00
10000s ea **38779-1125-01** 285.00

CAPSULE 4 RED/WHITE (Gallipot)
capsules, empty gelatin
DEV, NA, 100s ea **51552-0640-01** 3.50
1000s ea **51552-0561-02** 25.20

CAPSULE 4 WHITE (Gallipot)
capsules, empty gelatin
DEV, NA, 100s ea **51552-0392-01** 3.50
1000s ea **51552-0392-02** 21.35

CAPSULE 4 WHITE/WHITE (Medisca)
capsules, empty gelatin
DEV, NA (OPAQUE,CONI-SNAP)
1000s ea **38779-2022-09** 30.00
5000s ea **38779-2022-02** 147.00
10000s ea **38779-2022-01** 285.00

CAPSULE 5 CLEAR (Gallipot)
capsules, empty gelatin
DEV, NA, 100s ea **51552-0573-01** 5.32
1000s ea **51552-0573-02** 43.75

CAPSULE 5 WHITE (Gallipot)
capsules, empty gelatin
DEV, NA, 100s ea **51552-0574-01** 5.32
1000s ea **51552-0574-02** 43.75

CAPSULE 7 CLEAR/CLEAR (Letco)
capsules, empty gelatin
DEV, NA, 50s ea **62991-1401-01** 57.00
100s ea.............. **62991-1401-02** 90.00

CAPSULE EMPTY GELATIN (PCCA)
capsules, empty gelatin
DEV, NA (#4, LOCKING)
1 gm **51927-3617-00** 0.01

CAPSULE VEGETABLE 0 CLEAR (Medisca)
capsules, empty gelatin
DEV, NA, 1000s ea **38779-1127-09** 84.00
5000s ea **38779-1127-02** 285.00

CAPSULE VEGETABLE 1 CLEAR (Medisca)
capsules, empty gelatin
DEV, NA, 1000s ea **38779-2235-09** 84.00
5000s ea **38779-2235-02** 285.00

CAPSULES EMPTY GELATIN (Shionogi Qualicaps)
capsules, empty gelatin
DEV, NA (SIZE 0 CLEAR/CLEAR)
100s ea.............. **95306-0001-01** 3.85
(SIZE 00 CLEAR/CLEAR)
100s ea.............. **95306-0001-81** 6.80
(SIZE 1 CLEAR/CLEAR)
100s ea.............. **95306-0001-11** 3.70
(SIZE 2 CLEAR/CLEAR)
100s ea.............. **95306-0001-21** 3.50
(SIZE 3 CLEAR/CLEAR)
100s ea.............. **95306-0001-31** 3.30
(SIZE 4 CLEAR/CLEAR)
100s ea.............. **95306-0001-41** 3.20
(SIZE 0 CLEAR/CLEAR)
1000s ea **95306-0002-01** 32.00
(SIZE 00 CLEAR/CLEAR)
1000s ea **95306-0002-81** 56.50

CAPSULES, EMPTY GELATIN
(Gallipot) *See CAPSULE 0 BLUE*
(Gallipot) *See CAPSULE 0 CLEAR*
(Gallipot) *See CAPSULE 0 LACTOSE BLUE*
(Gallipot) *See CAPSULE 0 LACTOSE WHITE*
(Gallipot) *See CAPSULE 0 RED*
(Gallipot) *See CAPSULE 0 RED/BLACK*
(Gallipot) *See CAPSULE 0 WHITE*
(Gallipot) *See CAPSULE 00 BLUE*
(Gallipot) *See CAPSULE 00 CLEAR*
(Gallipot) *See CAPSULE 000 CLEAR*
(Gallipot) *See CAPSULE 1 BLUE*
(Gallipot) *See CAPSULE 1 BLUE/WHITE*
(Gallipot) *See CAPSULE 1 CLEAR*
(Gallipot) *See CAPSULE 1 GRAY/PINK*
(Gallipot) *See CAPSULE 1 GREEN*
(Gallipot) *See CAPSULE 1 LIGHT BLUE/DARK BLUE*
(Gallipot) *See CAPSULE 1 LIGHT BLUE/POWDER BLUE*
(Gallipot) *See CAPSULE 1 ORANGE/YELLOW*
(Gallipot) *See CAPSULE 1 PINK/WHITE*
(Gallipot) *See CAPSULE 1 RED*
(Gallipot) *See CAPSULE 1 RED/WHITE*
(Gallipot) *See CAPSULE 1 RUBY RED*
(Gallipot) *See CAPSULE 1 TURQUOISE/VIOLET*
(Gallipot) *See CAPSULE 1 WHITE*
(Gallipot) *See CAPSULE 1 WHITE/ORANGE*
(Gallipot) *See CAPSULE 1 YELLOW/GREEN*
(Gallipot) *See CAPSULE 2 CLEAR*
(Gallipot) *See CAPSULE 2 GREEN*
(Gallipot) *See CAPSULE 2 POWDER BLUE*
(Gallipot) *See CAPSULE 2 WHITE*
(Gallipot) *See CAPSULE 3 BLUE OPAQUE*
(Gallipot) *See CAPSULE 3 CLEAR*
(Gallipot) *See CAPSULE 3 GREEN OPAQUE*
(Gallipot) *See CAPSULE 3 GREEN TRANSLUCENT*
(Gallipot) *See CAPSULE 3 WHITE*
(Gallipot) *See CAPSULE 4 BLUE/WHITE*
(Gallipot) *See CAPSULE 4 CANARY YELLOW*
(Gallipot) *See CAPSULE 4 CLEAR*
(Gallipot) *See CAPSULE 4 RED/WHITE*
(Gallipot) *See CAPSULE 4 WHITE*
(Gallipot) *See CAPSULE 5 CLEAR*
(Gallipot) *See CAPSULE 5 WHITE*
(Letco) *See CAPSULE 0 CLEAR/CLEAR*
(Letco) *See CAPSULE 0 CLEAR/WHITE*
(Letco) *See CAPSULE 0 WHITE/WHITE*
(Letco) *See CAPSULE 00 CLEAR/CLEAR*
(Letco) *See CAPSULE 00 WHITE/CLEAR*
(Letco) *See CAPSULE 00 WHITE/WHITE*
(Letco) *See CAPSULE 1 CLEAR/CLEAR*
(Letco) *See CAPSULE 1 CLEAR/WHITE*
(Letco) *See CAPSULE 1 WHITE/CLEAR*
(Letco) *See CAPSULE 1 WHITE/WHITE*
(Letco) *See CAPSULE 13 CLEAR/CLEAR*
(Letco) *See CAPSULE 3 CLEAR/CLEAR*
(Letco) *See CAPSULE 3 CLEAR/WHITE*
(Letco) *See CAPSULE 3 WHITE/CLEAR*
(Letco) *See CAPSULE 3 WHITE/WHITE*
(Letco) *See CAPSULE 4 CLEAR/CLEAR*
(Letco) *See CAPSULE 7 CLEAR/CLEAR*
(Medisca) *See CAPSULE 0 BLUE/BLUE*
(Medisca) *See CAPSULE 0 CLEAR/CLEAR*
(Medisca) *See CAPSULE 0 DARK BLUE/DARK BLUE*
(Medisca) *See CAPSULE 0 ORANGE/ORANGE*
(Medisca) *See CAPSULE 0 PINK/PINK*
(Medisca) *See CAPSULE 0 WHITE/WHITE*
(Medisca) *See CAPSULE 00 BLUE/BLUE*
(Medisca) *See CAPSULE 00 CLEAR/CLEAR*
(Medisca) *See CAPSULE 00 WHITE/WHITE*
(Medisca) *See CAPSULE 000 CLEAR/CLEAR*
(Medisca) *See CAPSULE 1 BLUE/BLUE*
(Medisca) *See CAPSULE 1 BROWN/LIGHT TAN*
(Medisca) *See CAPSULE 1 CLEAR/CLEAR*
(Medisca) *See CAPSULE 1 ORANGE/ORANGE*
(Medisca) *See CAPSULE 1 PINK/BLUE*
(Medisca) *See CAPSULE 1 PINK/PINK*
(Medisca) *See CAPSULE 1 PURPLE/PURPLE*
(Medisca) *See CAPSULE 1 RED/BLUE*
(Medisca) *See CAPSULE 1 WHITE/CLEAR*
(Medisca) *See CAPSULE 1 WHITE/GREEN*
(Medisca) *See CAPSULE 1 WHITE/WHITE*
(Medisca) *See CAPSULE 1 YELLOW/GREEN*
(Medisca) *See CAPSULE 2 BLUE/BLUE*
(Medisca) *See CAPSULE 2 CLEAR/CLEAR*
(Medisca) *See CAPSULE 2 WHITE/WHITE*
(Medisca) *See CAPSULE 3 BLUE/GREEN*
(Medisca) *See CAPSULE 3 BROWN/LIGHT BLUE*
(Medisca) *See CAPSULE 3 CLEAR/CLEAR*
(Medisca) *See CAPSULE 3 DARK RED/DARK RED*
(Medisca) *See CAPSULE 3 GREEN/GREEN*
(Medisca) *See CAPSULE 3 MAROON/BLUE*
(Medisca) *See CAPSULE 3 ORANGE/ORANGE*
(Medisca) *See CAPSULE 3 PINK/PINK*
(Medisca) *See CAPSULE 3 RED/RED*
(Medisca) *See CAPSULE 3 SWEDISH ORANGE/SWEDISH ORANGE*
(Medisca) *See CAPSULE 3 WHITE/CLEAR*
(Medisca) *See CAPSULE 3 WHITE/WHITE*
(Medisca) *See CAPSULE 3 YELLOW/GRAY*
(Medisca) *See CAPSULE 4 BLACK/GREEN*
(Medisca) *See CAPSULE 4 CLEAR/CLEAR*
(Medisca) *See CAPSULE 4 WHITE/WHITE*
(Medisca) *See CAPSULE VEGETABLE 0 CLEAR*
(Medisca) *See CAPSULE VEGETABLE 1 CLEAR*
(PCCA) *See CAPSULE EMPTY GELATIN*
(Shionogi Qualicaps) *See CAPSULES EMPTY GELATIN*

CAPTOPRIL
FUL
TAB, PO, 12.5 mg,
100s ea 2.33
25 mg, 100s ea.................... 2.63
50 mg, 100s ea.................... 3.90
100 mg, 100s ea................... 10.80

(Apotex Corp.)
TAB, PO, 12.5 mg, 100s ea **60505-0003-06** 70.67 **AB**
(USP)
12.5 mg, 1000s ea.... **60505-0003-09** 706.70 **AB**
25 mg, 100s ea ...... **60505-0004-06** 75.71 **AB**
(USP)
25 mg, 1000s ea ..... **60505-0004-09** 757.10 **AB**
50 mg, 100s ea ...... **60505-0005-06** 131.46 **AB**
(USP)
50 mg, 1000s ea ..... **60505-0005-09** 1314.60 **AB**
100 mg, 100s ea ..... **60505-0006-06** 172.62 **AB**
(USP)
100 mg, 1000s ea .... **60505-0006-09** 1726.20 **AB**

(Boscogen)
TAB, PO, 25 mg, 100s ea .. **62033-0101-20** 65.00 **AB**

(Gallipot)
POW, NA (1X5GM,USP)
5 gm **51552-1072-02** 63.70 45.50

(Major)
TAB, PO, 12.5 mg,
100s ea UD .... **00904-5045-61** 69.95 **AB**
25 mg, 100s ea UD ... **00904-5046-61** 79.95 **AB**
50 mg, 100s ea UD ... **00904-5047-61** 129.95 **AB**

PROD/MFR	NDC	AWP	DP	OBC
(Medisca)				
POW, NA (U.S.P.)				
1 gm	**38779-0488-06**	37.50		
5 gm	**38779-0488-03**	108.00		
25 gm	**38779-0488-04**	472.50		
(Mylan)				
TAB, PO, 12.5 mg, 100s ea.	**00378-3007-01**	70.67		AB
1000s ea	**00378-3007-10**	693.00		AB
25 mg, 100s ea	**00378-3012-01**	75.71		AB
1000s ea	**00378-3012-10**	749.49		AB
50 mg, 100s ea	**00378-3017-01**	131.46		AB
1000s ea	**00378-3017-10**	1284.78		AB
100 mg, 100s ea	**00378-3022-01**	172.62		AB
(PCCA)				
POW, NA (U.S.P.)				
1 gm	**51927-2907-00**	23.40		
(Sandoz)				
TAB, PO, 12.5 mg, 100s ea.	**00781-1828-01**	77.18		AB
1000s ea	**00781-1828-10**	733.21		AB
50 mg, 100s ea	**00781-1838-01**	143.08		AB
100s ea.	**59772-7047-01**	143.08		AB
1000s ea	**00781-1838-10**	1359.26		AB
1000s ea	**59772-7047-03**	1359.26		AB
100 mg, 100s ea	**00781-1839-01**	190.54		AB
100s ea.	**59772-7048-01**	190.54		AB
(Spectrum Pharmacy)				
POW, NA (U.S.P.)				
1 gm	**49452-1681-01**	79.45		
5 gm	**49452-1681-02**	165.55		
25 gm	**49452-1681-03**	658.00		
100 gm	**49452-1681-04**	2026.50		
(Stason Pharm)				
TAB, PO, 12.5 mg, 100s ea.	**60763-1011-00**	77.50		AB
1000s ea	**60763-1011-02**	760.00		AB
25 mg, 100s ea	**60763-1012-00**	65.00		AB
1000s ea	**60763-1012-02**	790.50		AB
50 mg, 100s ea	**60763-1013-00**	100.50		AB
(Teva)				
TAB, PO, 12.5 mg, 100s ea.	**00093-8132-01**	60.38		AB
25 mg, 100s ea	**00093-8133-01**	65.27		AB
100s ea UD	**00182-2623-89**	77.95		AB
1000s ea	**00093-8133-10**	646.05		AB
50 mg, 100s ea	**00093-8134-01**	111.93		AB
100 mg, 100s ea	**00093-8135-01**	149.98		AB
(UDL)				
TAB, PO (10X10)				
12.5 mg,				
100s ea UD	**51079-0863-20**	72.79		AB
25 mg, 100s ea UD	**51079-0864-20**	77.98		AB
(West-Ward)				
TAB, PO, 12.5 mg, 100s ea.	**00143-1171-01**	63.00		AB
1000s ea	**00143-1171-10**	575.45		AB
25 mg, 100s ea	**00143-1172-01**	68.25		AB
1000s ea	**00143-1172-10**	625.50		AB
50 mg, 100s ea	**00143-1173-01**	116.50		AB
1000s ea	**00143-1173-10**	1075.00		AB
100 mg, 100s ea	**00143-1174-01**	148.00		AB
(Wockhardt USA)				
TAB, PO, 12.5 mg, 100s ea.	**64679-0902-01**	77.18		AB
1000s ea	**64679-0902-02**	733.21		AB
25 mg, 100s ea	**64679-0903-01**	83.44		AB
1000s ea	**64679-0903-02**	792.68		AB
50 mg, 100s ea	**64679-0904-01**	143.08		AB
1000s ea	**64679-0904-02**	1359.26		AB
100 mg, 100s ea	**64679-0905-01**	190.54		AB
(A-S Medication) REPACK				
TAB, PO, 12.5 mg, 60s ea.	**54569-4593-01**	41.91		EE
100s ea.	**54569-4593-00**	69.85		EE
25 mg, 30s ea.	**54569-4246-05**	22.59		EE
60s ea.	**54569-4246-03**	45.18		EE
90s ea.	**54569-4246-04**	67.77		EE
100s ea.	**54569-4246-00**	75.30		EE
50 mg, 60s ea.	**54569-4247-02**	78.91		EE
100s ea.	**54569-4247-00**	131.51		EE
(Advanced Pharm Serv, Inc.) REPACK				
TAB, PO, 50 mg, 20s ea	**13411-0184-02**	26.00		
30s ea.	**13411-0184-03**	42.92		
60s ea.	**13411-0184-06**	85.84		
90s ea.	**13411-0184-09**	128.77		
100s ea.	**13411-0184-10**	143.08		
(Altura) REPACK				
TAB, PO, 25 mg, 5s ea	**63874-0347-05**	5.58		EE
100s ea.	**63874-0347-01**	91.41		EE
(Bryant Ranch) REPACK				
TAB, PO, 12.5 mg, 30s ea.	**63629-2896-01**	9.32		
25 mg, 30s ea.	**63629-1338-02**	26.27		
90s ea.	**63629-1338-03**	78.81		
100s ea.	**63629-1338-01**	87.57		
50 mg, 30s ea.	**63629-2541-02**	31.67		
60s ea.	**63629-2541-01**	59.99		
100 mg, 30s ea	**63629-1706-01**	62.16		
60s ea.	**63629-1706-02**	124.32		
100s ea.	**63629-1706-03**	207.20		
(DHS, Inc.) REPACK				
TAB, PO, 12.5 mg, 30s ea.	**55887-0987-30**	18.99		
25 mg, 30s ea.	**55887-0430-30**	16.96		
50 mg, 30s ea.	**55887-0582-30**	27.08		AB
(Dispensing Solutions) REPACK				
TAB, PO, 25 mg, 30s ea	**55045-2376-08**	20.40		AB
30s ea.	**66336-0946-30**	25.17		AB
60s ea.	**55045-2376-09**	40.80		AB
60s ea.	**66336-0946-60**	49.88		AB
90s ea.	**66336-0946-90**	74.82		AB
100s ea.	**55045-2376-00**	68.00		AB
50 mg, 60s ea.	**55045-2424-06**	72.60		AB
60s ea.	**66336-0750-60**	84.43		AB
90s ea.	**66336-0750-90**	126.37		AB
100s ea.	**55045-2424-00**	121.15		AB
100 mg, 60s ea	**66336-0794-60**	64.20		AB
(GSMS) REPACK				
TAB, PO (UNIT OF USE)				
12.5 mg, 90s ea.	**60429-0029-90**	6.75	2.25	AB
25 mg, 60s ea.	**60429-0030-60**	5.70	1.90	AB
90s ea.	**60429-0030-90**	15.00	2.45	AB
120s ea.	**60429-0030-12**	9.00	3.00	AB
270s ea.	**60429-0030-27**	17.10	5.70	AB
50 mg, 30s ea.	**60429-0031-30**	5.70	1.90	AB
60s ea.	**60429-0031-60**	8.85	2.95	AB
90s ea.	**60429-0031-90**	11.70	3.90	AB
120s ea.	**60429-0031-12**	14.40	4.80	AB
270s ea.	**60429-0031-27**	30.60	10.20	AB
(Palmetto) REPACK				
TAB, PO, 12.5 mg, 60s ea.	**23490-5192-01**	42.36		
25 mg, 30s ea.	**23490-5193-01**	33.73		
60s ea.	**23490-5193-02**	67.46		
90s ea.	**23490-5193-03**	101.19		
50 mg, 30s ea.	**23490-5194-00**	45.44		
60s ea.	**23490-5194-01**	90.88		
90s ea.	**23490-5194-02**	136.32		
100 mg, 60s ea	**23490-5191-01**	116.75		
(PD-Rx Pharm) REPACK				
TAB, PO (USP)				
12.5 mg, 30s ea.	**43063-0146-30**	28.32		AB
(REDI-SCRIPT)				
25 mg, 28s ea.	**58864-0066-28**	32.87		AB
30s ea.	**55289-0344-30**	33.73		AB
90s ea.	**55289-0344-90**	61.07		AB
50 mg, 30s ea.	**55289-0212-30**	42.07		AB
90s ea.	**55289-0212-90**	86.07		AB
(Phys Total Care) REPACK				
TAB, PO, 12.5 mg, 15s ea.	**54868-3723-04**	6.39		AB
30s ea.	**54868-3723-01**	8.31		EE
60s ea.	**54868-3723-02**	12.12		EE
90s ea.	**54868-3723-03**	15.93		AB
100s ea.	**54868-3723-05**	15.69		EE
25 mg, 30s ea.	**54868-3724-01**	4.98		EE
60s ea.	**54868-3724-04**	6.93		AB
90s ea.	**54868-3724-02**	8.91		EE
100s ea.	**54868-3724-03**	9.54		EE
50 mg, 30s ea.	**54868-3725-02**	6.12		EE
60s ea.	**54868-3725-04**	10.87		EE
90s ea.	**54868-3725-03**	12.36		EE
100s ea.	**54868-3725-01**	11.88		EE
100 mg, 20s ea	**54868-5196-01**	10.50		AB
45s ea.	**54868-5196-02**	17.97		
60s ea.	**54868-5196-00**	22.47		AB
(Physician Partner) REPACK				
TAB, PO, 25 mg, 30s ea	**21695-0477-30**	40.95		AB
50 mg, 30s ea.	**21695-0478-30**	69.60		AB
(Quality Care Prod) REPACK				
TAB, PO, 25 mg, 10s ea	**49999-0105-10**	9.08		EE
30s ea.	**49999-0105-30**	27.25		EE
60s ea.	**49999-0105-60**	54.50		AB
100s ea.	**49999-0105-00**	90.83		AB
50 mg, 30s ea.	**49999-0511-30**	44.87		
60s ea.	**49999-0511-60**	89.74		AB
(Vibranta) REPACK				
TAB, PO, 25 mg, 30s ea	**57866-6106-02**	23.81		AB
60s ea.	**57866-6106-01**	74.19		AB
90s ea.	**57866-6106-04**	69.23		AB
120s ea.	**57866-6106-03**	91.94		AB
50 mg, 30s ea.	**57866-6103-01**	40.55		AB
60s ea.	**57866-6103-02**	80.00		AB
90s ea.	**57866-6103-03**	119.45		AB
120s ea.	**57866-6103-04**	158.90		AB
CAPTOPRIL/HCTZ (Mylan)				
captopril/hydrochlorothiazide				
TAB, PO, 25 mg-15 mg,				
100s ea.	**00378-0081-01**	79.59		AB
25 mg-25 mg,				
100s ea.	**00378-0083-01**	79.59		AB
50 mg-15 mg,				
100s ea.	**00378-0084-01**	136.61		AB
50 mg-25 mg,				
100s ea.	**00378-0086-01**	136.61		AB
(Teva)				
TAB, PO, 25 mg-15 mg,				
100s ea.	**00093-0176-01**	71.78		AB
25 mg-25 mg,				
100s ea.	**00093-0177-01**	71.78		AB
50 mg-15 mg,				
100s ea.	**00093-0181-01**	123.28		AB
50 mg-25 mg,				
100s ea.	**00093-0182-01**	123.28		AB
(Phys Total Care) REPACK				
TAB, PO, 25 mg-25 mg,				
30s ea.	**54868-5787-00**	12.35		
50 mg-25 mg,				
30s ea.	**54868-4062-00**	23.19		AB
100s ea.	**54868-4062-01**	65.31		
CAPTOPRIL/HYDROCHLOROTHIAZIDE FUL				
TAB, PO, 25 mg-15 mg,				
100s ea		23.59		
25 mg-25 mg,				
100s ea		23.60		
50 mg-25 mg,				
100s ea		37.02		
(Mylan) *See CAPTOPRIL/HCTZ*				
(Sandoz)				
TAB, PO, 25 mg-15 mg,				
100s ea.	**59772-5160-05**	79.25		AB
25 mg-25 mg, 100s ea.	**59772-5161-05**	79.25		AB
50 mg-15 mg, 100s ea.	**59772-5162-05**	135.00		AB
(Teva) *See CAPTOPRIL/HCTZ*				
CARAC (Dermik)				
fluorouracil				
CRE, TP, 0.5%, 30 gm	**00066-7150-30**	177.05		
(Phys Total Care) REPACK				
CRE, TP, 0.5%, 30 gm	**54868-5450-00**	147.20		
CARAFATE (Axcan)				
sucralfate				
SUS, PO, 1 gm/10 ml,				
420 ml	**58914-0170-14**	75.47		
TAB, PO, 1 gm, 100s ea	**58914-0171-10**	150.62		AB
(Pharma Pac) REPACK				
TAB, PO, 1 gm, 30s ea	**52959-0052-30**	33.90		AB
(Phys Total Care) REPACK				
SUS, PO, 1 gm/10 ml,				
414 ml	**54868-3735-00**	96.56		
TAB, PO, 1 gm, 60s ea	**54868-0312-05**	68.78		AB
(Quality Care Prod) REPACK				
TAB, PO, 1 gm, 60s ea	**35356-0534-60**	158.15		AB
CARAMEL				
(Amend) *See CARAMEL COLOR*				
(Medisca)				
LIQ, NA (1X25ML)				
25 ml.	**38779-1129-04**	22.50		
(1X100ML)				
100 ml	**38779-1129-05**	34.50		
(1X500ML)				
500 ml	**38779-1129-08**	87.00		

PROD/MFR	NDC	AWP	DP	OBC
(PCCA)				
LIQ, NA (NF)				
1 ml	51927-1527-00	0.23		
(Spectrum Pharmacy)				
LIQ, NA (N.F.)				
500 ml	49452-1690-01	70.70		
4000 ml	49452-1690-02	304.85		
CARAMEL COLOR (Amend)				
caramel				
LIQ, NA (FOOD GRADE)				
500 ml	17317-0237-01	7.00		
3840 ml	17317-0237-06	29.40		
CARAMEL FLAVOR (PCCA)				
flavoring aid				
SOL, NA (ARTIFICIAL)				
1 ml	51927-2163-00	0.90		
CARAMIPHEN EDISYLATE (PCCA)				
POW, NA, 1 gm	51927-2238-00	1.05		
CARAWAY (Amend)				
caraway oil				
OIL, NA (N.F.)				
30 ml	17317-0239-02	7.00		
120 ml	17317-0239-04	14.00		
(Medisca)				
OIL, NA (1X14ML,NATURAL)				
14 ml	38779-0895-03	37.50		
(1X25ML, NATURAL)				
25 ml	38779-0895-04	28.50		
(1X100ML,NATURAL)				
100 ml	38779-0895-05	70.50		
(1X500ML,NATURAL)				
500 ml	38779-0895-08	264.00		
CARAWAY OIL				
(Amend) *See CARAWAY*				
(Medisca) *See CARAWAY*				
(PCCA)				
OIL, NA, 1 gm	51927-1881-00	1.56		
(Spectrum Pharmacy)				
OIL, NA (F.C.C.)				
100 ml	49452-1702-02	128.80		
500 ml	49452-1702-03	462.00		
CARBA-XP (GM Pharm)				
carbetapentane citrate/guaifenesin				
LIQ, PO (AF,DYE-FREE,RASPBERRY)				
20 mg/5 ml-100 mg/5 ml,				
473 ml	58809-0303-01	74.00	59.20	
CARBACHOL				
(Alcon Ophthalmic) *See ISOPTO CARBACHOL*				
(Alcon Surgical) *See MIOSTAT*				
(PCCA) *See CARBACHOL 99%*				
CARBACHOL 99% (PCCA)				
carbachol				
POW, NA, 1 gm	51927-1703-00	28.80		
CARBAMAZEPINE				
FUL				
CTB, PO, 100 mg, 100s ea		20.25		
SUS, PO, 100 mg/5 ml,				
450 ml		37.67		
TAB, PO, 200 mg, 100s ea		8.49		
(Apotex Corp.)				
TAB, PO, 200 mg, 100s ea	60505-0183-00	40.65		AB
500s ea	60505-0183-05	203.25		AB
1000s ea	60505-0183-01	406.50		AB
(Gallipot)				
POW, NA (U.S.P.)				
25 gm	51552-0653-04	26.60		
100 gm	51552-0653-05	91.00		
(Hawkins)				
POW, NA (U.S.P.)				
100 gm	63370-0041-35	112.00		
500 gm	63370-0041-45	480.00		
(Letco)				
POW, NA (U.S.P.)				
25 gm	62991-1027-01	48.00		
100 gm	62991-1027-02	135.00		
(Major)				
CTB, PO (USP,STRAWBERRY VANILLA)				
100 mg, 100s ea UD	00904-3854-61	28.65		AB
TAB, PO, 200 mg,				
100s ea UD	00904-3855-61	45.35		AB
(Medisca)				
POW, NA (U.S.P.)				
25 gm	38779-0114-04	55.50		
100 gm	38779-0114-05	175.50		
500 gm	38779-0114-08	810.00		
1000 gm	38779-0114-09	1410.00		
(Morton Grove)				
SUS, PO (CITRUS-VANILLA)				
100 mg/5 ml,				
450 ml	60432-0129-16	31.11		AB
(Novartis Pharm) *See TEGRETOL*				
(Novartis Pharm) *See TEGRETOL-XR*				
(PCCA)				
POW, NA (USP)				
1 gm	51927-2176-00	2.28		
(Precision Dose)				
SUS, PO (1X5ML,USP,ORANGE)				
100 mg/5 ml,				
5 ml UD	68094-0301-59	0.73		
(USP,ORANGE)				
100 mg/5 ml,				
5 ml 30s UD	68094-0301-62	21.95		
(1X10ML,USP)				
100 mg/5 ml,				
10 ml UD	68094-0214-59	1.05		
(USP,CITRUS-VANILLA)				
100 mg/5 ml,				
10 ml 30s UD	68094-0214-62	31.60		
(Sandoz)				
TER, PO (COATED)				
200 mg, 100s ea	00781-5087-01	93.64		
400 mg, 100s ea	00781-5088-01	187.12		
(Shire US Inc.) *See CARBATROL*				
(Spectrum Pharmacy)				
POW, NA (U.S.P.)				
25 gm	49452-1705-01	86.45		
100 gm	49452-1705-02	265.65		
1000 gm	49452-1705-03	1925.00		
(Taro)				
CTB, PO, 100 mg, 100s ea	51672-4041-01	23.11		AB
500s ea	51672-4041-02	114.00		AB
SUS, PO (ORANGE)				
100 mg/5 ml,				
450 ml	51672-4047-09	62.55		AB
TAB, PO, 200 mg, 100s ea	51672-4005-01	30.25		AB
500s ea	51672-4005-02	146.71		AB
1000s ea	51672-4005-03	287.38		AB
TER, PO, 200 mg, 100s ea	51672-4124-01	98.83		AB
400 mg, 100s ea	51672-4125-01	197.50		AB
(Teva)				
CTB, PO, 100 mg, 100s ea	00093-0778-01	23.11		AB
(10X10)				
100 mg, 100s ea UD	00182-1331-89	30.15		AB
(Teva) *See EPITOL*				
(Teva)				
TAB, PO, 200 mg, 100s ea	00093-0109-01	30.17		AB
(10X10)				
200 mg, 100s ea UD	00093-1233-93	45.98		AB
1000s ea	00093-0109-10	301.70		AB
(Torrent)				
CTB, PO (BERRY,VANILLA)				
100 mg, 100s ea	57664-0342-88	23.10		AB
(USP,STRAWBERRY/VANILLA)				
100 mg, 100s ea	13668-0271-01	23.10		AB
(BERRY,VANILLA)				
100 mg, 500s ea	57664-0342-13	144.00		AB
(USP,STRAWBERRY/VANILLA)				
100 mg, 500s ea	13668-0271-05	144.00		AB
TAB, PO (U.S.P.)				
200 mg, 100s ea	57664-0533-88	44.50		AB
(USP)				
200 mg, 100s ea	13668-0268-01	44.50		AB
(U.S.P.)				
200 mg, 500s ea	57664-0533-13	222.00		AB
(USP)				
200 mg, 500s ea	13668-0268-05	222.00		AB
(U.S.P.)				
200 mg, 1000s ea	57664-0533-18	440.00		AB
(USP)				
200 mg, 1000s ea	13668-0268-10	440.00		AB
(UDL)				
CTB, PO (10X10)				
100 mg, 100s ea UD	51079-0870-20	29.48		AB
TAB, PO (ROBOT READY 25X1)				
200 mg, 25s ea UD	51079-0385-19	8.93		AB
(10X10)				
200 mg, 100s ea UD	51079-0385-20	35.70		AB
(Validus) *See EQUETRO*				
(VistaPharm, Inc.)				
SUS, PO (ORANGE)				
100 mg/5 ml,				
10 ml 50s UD	66689-0323-50	83.40		AB
(A-S Medication)				
REPACK				
CTB, PO, 100 mg, 60s ea	54569-2795-01	13.87		EE
TAB, PO, 200 mg, 12s ea	54569-2655-05	3.93		AB
28s ea	54569-2655-03	9.16		AB
60s ea	54569-2655-01	19.63		AB
100s ea	54569-2655-00	32.71		AB
(Altura)				
REPACK				
TAB, PO, 200 mg, 10s ea	63874-0492-10	3.65		AB
20s ea	63874-0492-20	7.30		AB
30s ea	63874-0492-30	10.95		AB
40s ea	63874-0492-40	14.60		AB
45s ea	63874-0492-45	16.43		AB
60s ea	63874-0492-60	21.90		AB
90s ea	63874-0492-90	32.85		AB
100s ea	63874-0492-01	67.84		AB
120s ea	63874-0492-04	43.80		AB
1000s ea	63874-0492-02	678.40		AB
(American Health)				
REPACK				
CTB, PO (10X10)				
100 mg, 100s ea UD	62584-0639-01	29.82		AB
(DHS, Inc.)				
REPACK				
TAB, PO, 200 mg, 30s ea	55887-0345-30	13.35		
60s ea	55887-0345-60	26.70		
90s ea	55887-0345-90	40.05		
(Dispensing Solutions)				
REPACK				
CTB, PO, 100 mg, 100s ea	55045-3027-01	26.00		
TAB, PO, 200 mg, 30s ea	55045-2088-08	13.50		AB
30s ea	66336-0731-30	10.00		
(GSMS)				
REPACK				
TAB, PO, 200 mg, 100s ea	60429-0032-01	12.45	4.15	AB
100s ea	60429-0932-01	12.45	4.15	AB
1000s ea	60429-0032-10	100.35	33.45	AB
1000s ea	60429-0932-10	100.35	33.45	AB
(HomeMed)				
REPACK				
TAB, PO, 200 mg, 12s ea	51655-0953-27	4.38		
(IPI)				
REPACK				
TAB, PO, 200 mg, 90s ea	18837-0313-90	25.86		
(McKesson Packaging)				
REPACK				
TAB, PO, 200 mg,				
100s ea UD	63739-0045-10	36.89		AB
(BLISTER PACK)				
200 mg, 750s ea UD	63739-0045-01	276.68		AB
(PUNCH CARD 25X30)				
200 mg, 750s ea	63739-0045-03	276.68		AB
(Nucare Pharm)				
REPACK				
TAB, PO, 200 mg, 90s ea	66267-0278-90	44.36		AB
120s ea	66267-0278-91	62.82		AB
(Palmetto)				
REPACK				
TAB, PO, 200 mg, 30s ea	23490-5200-01	13.50		
(PD-Rx Pharm)				
REPACK				
TAB, PO (REDI-SCRIPT,USP)				
200 mg, 30s ea	58864-0843-30	11.12		AB
(Phys Total Care)				
REPACK				
CTB, PO, 100 mg, 30s ea	54868-2462-03	12.75		AB
60s ea	54868-2462-02	20.97		AB
100s ea	54868-2462-01	30.45		EE
TAB, PO, 200 mg, 30s ea	54868-0147-04	10.59		EE
60s ea	54868-0147-05	18.60		EE
90s ea	54868-0147-06	24.15		AB
100s ea	54868-0147-01	45.53		EE
100s ea	54868-0147-02	26.07		EE
1000s ea	54868-0147-00	200.22		EE
TER, PO, 400 mg, 30s ea	54868-6074-00	147.53		AB
(Quality Care Prod)				
REPACK				
CTB, PO, 100 mg, 60s ea	49999-0782-60	20.80		
120s ea	49999-0782-01	41.60		
TAB, PO, 200 mg, 60s ea	49999-0616-60	26.28		
100s ea	49999-0616-00	43.80		
120s ea	49999-0616-01	52.56		

PROD/MFR	NDC	AWP	DP	OBC
(Southwood) REPACK				
CTB, PO, 100 mg, 10s ea	**58016-0501-10**	2.31		
15s ea	**58016-0501-15**	3.47		
20s ea	**58016-0501-20**	4.62		
30s ea	**58016-0501-30**	6.93		
40s ea	**58016-0501-40**	9.24		
60s ea	**58016-0501-60**	13.87		
90s ea	**58016-0501-90**	20.80		
100s ea	**58016-0501-00**	23.11		
TAB, PO, 200 mg, 30s ea	**58016-0968-30**	10.95		EE
60s ea	**58016-0968-60**	21.90		EE
90s ea	**58016-0968-90**	32.85		EE
100s ea	**58016-0968-00**	36.50		EE
120s ea	**58016-0968-02**	43.80		EE
(Stat Rx) REPACK				
TAB, PO, 200 mg, 30s ea	**16590-0475-30**	14.50		
60s ea	**16590-0475-60**	29.00		
90s ea	**16590-0475-90**	43.50		
120s ea	**16590-0475-72**	58.00		
(Vibranta) REPACK				
TAB, PO, 200 mg, 30s ea	**57866-3415-01**	26.88		
60s ea	**57866-3415-02**	16.10		
90s ea	**57866-3415-03**	23.60		
120s ea	**57866-3415-04**	36.50		
CARBAMIDE PEROXIDE (PCCA)				
POW, NA, 1 gm	**51927-1476-00**	1.05		
(Spectrum Pharmacy)				
POW, NA (U.S.P.)				
100 gm	**49452-8077-01**	152.95		
500 gm	**49452-8077-02**	514.50		
CARBAPHEN 12 (Gil Pharmaceutical)				
cpm tan/carbetapentane tan/phenyleph tan				
SUS, PO (AF,SF,BLUEBERRY BANNA)				
473 ml	**58552-0117-16**	178.53		
CARBAPHEN 12 PED (Gil Pharmaceutical)				
cpm tan/carbetapentane tan/phenyleph tan				
SUS, PO (AF,SF,BANANA-BLUEBERRY)				
60 ml	**58552-0118-02**	39.93		
CARBATAB-12 (GM Pharm)				
carbetapentane cit/gg/phenyleph hcl				
T12, PO, 60 mg-600 mg-15 mg,				
100s ea	**58809-0615-01**	55.12	42.78	
CARBATROL (Shire US Inc.)				
carbamazepine				
CER, PO, 100 mg, 120s ea	**54092-0171-12**	220.91	184.09	
200 mg, 120s ea	**54092-0172-12**	220.91	184.09	
300 mg, 120s ea	**54092-0173-12**	220.91	184.09	
(Phys Total Care) REPACK				
CER, PO, 300 mg, 120s ea	**54868-5432-00**	244.09		
CARBATUSS (GM Pharm)				
carbetapentane cit/gg/phenyleph hcl				
LIQ, PO (AF,SPEARMINT)				
473 ml	**58809-0536-01**	39.95	31.96	
CARBATUSS-12 (GM Pharm)				
cough/cold combination				
SUS, PO, (AF,SF,TROPICAL FRUIT)				
473 ml	**58809-0818-01**	89.25	69.80	
CARBATUSS-CL (GM Pharm)				
carbetapentane cit/k guai/phenyleph hcl				
SOL, PO (AF,SF,DYE-FREE)				
473 ml	**58809-0707-01**	74.00	59.20	
CARBAXEFED DM RF (Phys Total Care) REPACK				
carbinoxamine mal/dm/pse hcl				
LIQ, PO (AF,SF,GRAPE,DROPS)				
1 mg/ml-4 mg/ml-15 mg/ml,				
30 ml	**54868-4727-00**	15.69		
CARBAXEFED RF (Quality Care Prod) REPACK				
carbinoxamine mal/pse hcl				
SOL, PO (AF,SF,CHERRY)				
1 mg/ml-15 mg/ml,				
30 ml	**49999-0554-30**	11.74		
CARBAZOCHROME (Medisca)				
POW, NA (1X1GM)				
1 gm	**38779-1953-06**	189.00		
(1X10GM)				
10 gm	**38779-1953-01**	1515.00		
(PCCA) *See ADRENOCHROME SEMICARBAZONE REAGENT*				
CARBETAPENTANE CIT/CARBINOXAMINE				

PROD/MFR	NDC	AWP	DP	OBC
MAL/PHENYLEPH HCL				
(Gentex Pharma) *See ARIDEX*				
CARBETAPENTANE CIT/GG/PHENYLEPH HCL				
(Auriga) *See EXTENDRYL GCP*				
(Auriga) *See LEVALL*				
(Boca Pharmacal) *See PHENCARB GG*				
(Breckenridge Pharm) *See CARBETAPLEX*				
(Gentex Pharma) *See GENTEX 30*				
(Gentex Pharma) *See GENTEX-LQ*				
(GM Pharm) *See CARBATAB-12*				
(GM Pharm) *See CARBATUSS*				
CARBETAPENTANE CIT/GG/PSE HCL				
(Hawthorn Pharm) *See EXALL-D*				
CARBETAPENTANE CIT/K GUAI/PHENYLEPH HCL				
(GM Pharm) *See CARBATUSS-CL*				
CARBETAPENTANE CIT/PSE HCL				
(Accentia) *See RESPI-TANN PD*				
(Allegis) *See ALLRES PD*				
(Hawthorn Pharm) *See CORZALL*				
CARBETAPENTANE CIT/PSE HCL/PYRIL MAL				
(Hawthorn Pharm) *See CORZALL PLUS*				
(Vertical) *See ZOTEX-D*				
CARBETAPENTANE CITRATE (PCCA)				
POW, NA, 1 gm	**51927-1965-00**	9.60		
CARBETAPENTANE CITRATE/GUAIFENESIN				
(Allegis) *See ALLRES G*				
(Athlon Pharm) *See DYNEX VR*				
(Capellon) *See CERTUSS*				
(Centurion) *See EXPECTUSS*				
(Cypress Pharm) *See PULMARI-GP*				
(Everett) *See TUSSO-ZMR*				
(Everett) *See TUSSO-ZR*				
(GM Pharm) *See CARBA-XP*				
(Hawthorn Pharm) *See EXALL*				
(Hawthorn Pharm) *See XPECT-AT*				
(Vindex Pharma Inc) *See ORATUSS*				
CARBETAPENTANE TAN/PHENYLEPH TAN/ PYRIL TAN				
(Meda) *See TUSSI-12D*				
(Meda) *See TUSSI-12D S*				
CARBETAPENTANE TAN/PHENYLEPH TAN/ ZINCUM ACETICUM				
(Auriga) *See ZINX COLD*				
CARBETAPENTANE TANNATE				
(Hawthorn Pharm) *See SOLOTUSS*				
CARBETAPENTANE TANNATE/ CHLORPHENIRAMINE TANNATE				
(Breckenridge Pharm) *See TRIONATE*				
(Breckenridge Pharm) *See TRIONATE NF*				
(Cypress Pharm) *See TANNIC-12*				
(Meda) *See TUSSI-12*				
(Meda) *See TUSSI-12 S*				
(Prasco Labs) *See C-TANNA 12*				
CARBETAPENTANE TANNATE/ DIPHENHYDRAMINE TANNATE				
(Hawthorn Pharm) *See DYTAN-AT*				
CARBETAPENTANE TANNATE/ PHENYLEPHRINE TANNATE				
(Athlon Pharm) *See DYNEX 12*				
(Auriga) *See LEVALL-12*				
(Breckenridge Pharm) *See CARBETAPLEX TS*				
CARBETAPENTANE TANNATE/ PSEUDOEPHEDRINE TANNATE				
(Accentia) *See RESPI-TANN*				
(Breckenridge Pharm) *See PSEUDACARB*				
CARBETAPENTANE TANNATE/PYRILAMINE TANNATE				
(Athlon Pharm) *See PYRLEX CB*				
CARBETAPLEX (Breckenridge Pharm)				
carbetapentane cit/gg/phenyleph hcl				
SOL, PO (AF,SF,DYE-FREE)				
473 ml	**51991-0083-16**	48.72		

PROD/MFR	NDC	AWP	DP	OBC
CARBETAPLEX TS (Breckenridge Pharm)				
carbetapentane tannate/phenylephrine tannate				
SUS, PO (AF,SF,STRAWBERRY)				
30 mg/5 ml-30 mg/5 ml,				
118 ml	**51991-0482-04**	30.93		
CARBIDOPA				
(Bristol-Myers) *See LODOSYN*				
(Hawkins)				
POW, NA (U.S.P.,MONOHYDRATE)				
5 gm	**63370-0039-15**	116.00		
25 gm	**63370-0039-25**	480.00		
100 gm	**63370-0039-35**	1600.00		
(Medisca)				
POW, NA (U.S.P.)				
5 gm	**38779-0202-03**	135.00		
25 gm	**38779-0202-04**	537.00		
100 gm	**38779-0202-05**	1575.00		
(PCCA)				
POW, NA (U.S.P.)				
1 gm	**51927-2480-00**	30.60		
(Spectrum Pharmacy)				
CRY, NA (U.S.P)				
5 gm	**49452-1692-02**	201.60		
(U.S.P.)				
25 gm	**49452-1692-03**	808.50		
CARBIDOPA AND LEVODOPA (Actavis)				
carbidopa/levodopa				
TAB, PO, 25 mg-250 mg,				
500s ea	**00228-2540-50**	539.01		AB
(Apotex Corp.)				
TAB, PO (USP)				
10 mg-100 mg,				
100s ea	**60505-0128-01**	77.23		AB
1000s ea	**60505-0128-02**	733.69		AB
25 mg-100 mg,				
100s ea	**60505-0129-01**	87.20		AB
1000s ea	**60505-0129-02**	828.40		AB
25 mg-250 mg,				
100s ea	**60505-0130-01**	111.13		AB
1000s ea	**60505-0130-02**	1055.74		AB
(Caraco)				
ODT, PO (TUTTI FRUTTI,UNCOATED)				
10 mg-100 mg,				
100s ea	**62756-0186-88**	122.00		AB
25 mg-100 mg,				
100s ea	**62756-0187-88**	138.00		AB
25 mg-250 mg,				
100s ea	**62756-0188-88**	174.76		AB
TAB, PO (USP)				
10 mg-100 mg,				
100s ea	**62756-0517-88**	70.88		AB
500s ea	**62756-0517-13**	343.74		AB
25 mg-100 mg,				
100s ea	**62756-0518-88**	80.02		AB
500s ea	**62756-0518-13**	388.10		AB
1000s ea	**62756-0518-18**	760.20		AB
25 mg-250 mg,				
100s ea	**62756-0519-88**	94.95		AB
500s ea	**62756-0519-13**	509.85		AB
TER, PO (COMPRESSED TABLET)				
25 mg-100 mg,				
100s ea	**62756-0461-88**	93.90		AB
50 mg-200 mg,				
100s ea	**62756-0457-88**	180.50		AB
(Major)				
TER, PO (10X10)				
25 mg-100 mg,				
100s ea UD	**00904-5749-61**	91.05		AB
50 mg-200 mg,				
100s ea UD	**00904-5750-61**	156.95		AB
(Mylan)				
TAB, PO (USP)				
10 mg-100 mg,				
100s ea	**00378-0078-01**	77.23		AB
25 mg-100 mg,				
100s ea	**00378-0085-01**	87.20		AB
25 mg-250 mg,				
100s ea	**00378-1133-01**	111.13		AB
(UDL)				
TAB, PO (USP,10X10)				
25 mg-100 mg,				
100s ea UD	**51079-0884-20**	79.80		AB
(American Health) REPACK				
TER, PO (10X10,COMPRESSED TABLET)				
25 mg-100 mg,				
100s ea UD	**68084-0281-01**	83.50		AB

PROD/MFR	NDC	AWP	DP	OBC
50 mg-200 mg,				
100s ea UD	68084-0282-01	158.22		AB
(Phys Total Care)				
REPACK				
TER, PO, 25 mg-100 mg,				
20s ea	54868-5659-01	39.21		
60s ea	54868-5659-00	84.09		
CARBIDOPA/ENTACAPONE/LEVODOPA				
(Novartis Pharm) *See STALEVO 100*				
(Novartis Pharm) *See STALEVO 125*				
(Novartis Pharm) *See STALEVO 150*				
(Novartis Pharm) *See STALEVO 200*				
(Novartis Pharm) *See STALEVO 50*				
(Novartis Pharm) *See STALEVO 75*				
CARBIDOPA/LEVODOPA				
FUL				
TAB, PO, 10 mg-100 mg,				
100s ea		40.43		
25 mg-100 mg,				
100s ea		46.88		
25 mg-250 mg,				
100s ea		51.45		
(Actavis) *See CARBIDOPA AND LEVODOPA*				
(Actavis)				
TAB, PO, 10 mg-100 mg,				
100s ea	00228-2538-10	77.23		AB
500s ea	00228-2538-50	374.63		AB
25 mg-100 mg,				
100s ea	00228-2539-10	87.20		AB
500s ea	00228-2539-50	422.97		AB
1000s ea	00228-2539-96	828.56		AB
25 mg-250 mg,				
100s ea	00228-2540-10	111.13		AB
1000s ea	00228-2540-96	1055.88		AB
(Apotex Corp.) *See CARBIDOPA AND LEVODOPA*				
(Apotex Corp.)				
TER, PO, 25 mg-100 mg,				
100s ea	60505-0131-01	94.00		AB
1000s ea	60505-0131-00	939.95		AB
50 mg-200 mg,				
100s ea	60505-0132-01	180.85		AB
1000s ea	60505-0132-00	1808.53		AB
(Azur Pharma, Inc.) *See PARCOPA*				
(Bristol-Myers) *See SINEMET 10-100*				
(Bristol-Myers) *See SINEMET 25-100*				
(Bristol-Myers) *See SINEMET 25-250*				
(Bristol-Myers) *See SINEMET CR*				
(Caraco) *See CARBIDOPA AND LEVODOPA*				
(Endo Generics)				
TAB, PO, 25 mg-100 mg,				
500s ea	60951-0605-85	400.10		AB
25 mg-250 mg,				
100s ea	60951-0607-68	101.97		AB
500s ea	60951-0607-85	509.85		AB
(Global Pharm)				
TER, PO, 25 mg-100 mg,				
100s ea	00115-3922-01	93.92		AB
500s ea	00115-3922-02	469.60		AB
50 mg-200 mg,				
100s ea	00115-3911-01	180.64		AB
500s ea	00115-3911-02	903.20		AB
(Major) *See CARBIDOPA AND LEVODOPA*				
(Major)				
TAB, PO (10X10)				
10 mg-100 mg,				
100s ea UD	00904-7718-61	121.30		AB
25 mg-100 mg,				
100s ea UD	00904-7719-61	145.41		AB
25 mg-250 mg,				
100s ea UD	00904-7720-61	107.30		AB
(Mylan) *See CARBIDOPA AND LEVODOPA*				
(Mylan)				
ODT, PO, 10 mg-100 mg,				
100s ea	00378-5051-01	121.48		
25 mg-100 mg,				
100s ea	00378-5052-01	137.18		
25 mg-250 mg,				
100s ea	00378-5053-01	174.76		
TER, PO, 25 mg-100 mg,				
100s ea	00378-0088-01	94.00		AB
50 mg-200 mg,				
100s ea	00378-0094-01	180.85		AB
(Teva)				
TAB, PO, 10 mg-100 mg,				
100s ea	00093-0292-01	70.88		AB
500s ea	00093-0292-05	343.74		AB
25 mg-100 mg,				
100s ea	00093-0293-01	80.02		AB
(10X10)				
25 mg-100 mg,				
100s ea UD	00182-1949-89	132.85		AB
500s ea	00093-0293-05	388.10		AB
1000s ea	00093-0293-10	760.20		AB
25 mg-250 mg,				
100s ea	00093-0294-01	101.97		AB
500s ea	00093-0294-05	494.55		AB
1000s ea	00093-0294-10	968.72		AB
(UDL) *See CARBIDOPA AND LEVODOPA*				
(UDL)				
TAB, PO (10X10)				
10 mg-100 mg,				
100s ea UD	51079-0755-20	72.10		AB
(ROBOT READY 25X1)				
25 mg-100 mg,				
25s ea UD	51079-0756-19	19.95		AB
(10X10)				
25 mg-100 mg,				
100s ea UD	51079-0756-20	79.80		AB
25 mg-250 mg,				
100s ea UD	51079-0783-20	98.20		AB
TER, PO, 25 mg-100 mg,				
100s ea UD	51079-0978-20	93.10		AB
50 mg-200 mg,				
100s ea UD	51079-0923-20	174.15		AB
(American Health)				
REPACK				
TAB, PO (10X10)				
10 mg-100 mg,				
100s ea UD	68084-0092-01	53.78		AB
25 mg-100 mg,				
100s ea UD	68084-0093-01	82.00		AB
25 mg-250 mg,				
100s ea UD	68084-0094-01	94.66		AB
(McKesson Packaging)				
REPACK				
TAB, PO, 10 mg-100 mg,				
100s ea UD	63739-0046-10	114.58		AB
(USP)				
25 mg-100 mg,				
100s ea UD	63739-0047-10	126.70		AB
(BLISTER PACK)				
25 mg-100 mg,				
750s ea UD	63739-0047-01	950.25		AB
(PUNCH CARD 25X30)				
25 mg-100 mg,				
750s ea	63739-0047-03	950.25		AB
25 mg-250 mg,				
100s ea UD	63739-0048-10	161.45		AB
(Phys Total Care)				
REPACK				
TAB, PO (USP)				
10 mg-100 mg,				
90s ea	54868-2866-00	74.70		EE
100s ea	54868-2866-01	128.21		EE
25 mg-100 mg, 30s ea	54868-1334-01	26.31		EE
(USP)				
25 mg-100 mg,				
50s ea	54868-1334-05	40.86		EE
60s ea	54868-1334-04	48.12		EE
90s ea	54868-1334-06	69.92		EE
100s ea	54868-1334-02	75.69		EE
25 mg-250 mg, 30s ea	54868-2834-00	30.35		EE
(Quality Care Prod)				
REPACK				
TAB, PO, 25 mg-100 mg,				
30s ea	35356-0355-30	22.30		AB
(Southwood)				
REPACK				
TAB, PO, 25 mg-100 mg,				
20s ea	58016-0958-20	25.34		AB
30s ea	58016-0958-30	38.01		AB
40s ea	58016-0958-40	50.68		AB
56s ea	58016-0958-56	70.95		AB
90s ea	58016-0958-90	114.03		AB
100s ea	58016-0958-00	126.70		AB
(Vibranta)				
REPACK				
TAB, PO, 10 mg-100 mg,				
30s ea	57866-6736-01	37.73		
25 mg-100 mg, 30s ea	57866-6735-01	41.18		
25 mg-250 mg, 30s ea	57866-6737-01	38.08		
TER, PO, 25 mg-100 mg,				
30s ea	57866-6739-01	46.25		AB
50 mg-200 mg, 30s ea	57866-6738-01	95.92		AB
CARBIMAZOLE (PCCA)				
POW, NA, 1 gm	51927-2828-00	96.00		
CARBINOXAMINE COMPOUND (Dispensing Solutions)				
REPACK				
carbinoxamine mal/dm/pse hcl				
SYR, PO, 118 ml	55045-1248-02	25.00		
CARBINOXAMINE MAL/DM/PHENYLEPH HCL				
(Hawthorn Pharm) *See XIRAHISTDM PEDIATRIC DROPS*				
CARBINOXAMINE MAL/DM/PSE HYDROCHLORIDE				
(Palmetto)				
REPACK				
carbinoxamine mal/dm/pse hcl				
LIQ, PO				
1 mg/ml-4 mg/ml-15 mg/ml,				
30 ml	23490-7584-01	42.47		
CARBINOXAMINE MALEATE ()				
SOL, PO (1X118ML)				
4 mg/5 ml, 118 ml	64376-0612-40	17.92		AA
(1X473ML)				
4 mg/5 ml, 473 ml	64376-0612-16	68.09		AA
(Boca Pharmacal)				
TAB, PO, 4 mg, 100s ea	64376-0605-01	68.09		AA
(Pamlab) *See PALGIC*				
(PCCA)				
POW, NA (USP)				
1 gm	51927-3431-00	7.80		
(Zerxis)				
SOL, PO, 4 mg/5 ml,				
473 ml	18011-0675-16	73.94		
CARBINOXAMINE MALEATE/ PHENYLEPHRINE HYDROCHLORIDE				
(Gentex Pharma) *See ARIDEX-D*				
(Hawthorn Pharm) *See XIRAHIST PEDIATRIC DROPS*				
CARBINOXAMINE PSE (Phys Total Care)				
REPACK				
carbinoxamine mal/pse hcl				
SYR, PO, 2 mg/5 ml-25 mg/5 ml,				
473 ml	54868-5017-00	84.24		
CARBINOXAMINE/DM/PSEUDOEPH (Dispensing Solutions)				
REPACK				
carbinoxamine mal/dm/pse hcl				
LIQ, PO (AF,SF,DROPS)				
2 mg/ml-4 mg/ml-25 mg/ml,				
30 ml	55045-1288-07	39.85		
CARBINOXAMINE/PSEUDOEPHEDRINE/ DEXTROMETHORPHAN (Dispensing Solutions)				
carbinoxamine mal/dm/pse hcl				
SOL, PO (DROPS)				
1 mg/ml-4 mg/ml-15 mg/ml,				
30 ml	55045-2982-07	39.85		
CARBOCAINE (Hospira)				
mepivacaine hydrochloride				
SOL, IJ, 1%, 30 ml	00409-1036-30	5.48	4.80	AP
(MDV)				
1%, 50 ml	00409-1038-50	16.84	14.73	AP
(PF)				
1.5%, 30 ml	00409-1041-30	5.80	5.07	AP
(SDV,USP,PF)				
2%, 20 ml	00409-1067-20	8.40	7.35	AP
(M.D.V.,USP)				
2%, 50 ml	00409-2047-50	19.80	17.33	AP
CARBOCAINE HCL (Hospira)				
mepivacaine hydrochloride				
SOL, IJ (S.D.V.)				
2%, 20 ml	00074-1067-20	8.40	7.35	AP
(M.D.V.)				
2%, 50 ml	00074-2047-50	19.80	17.33	AP
CARBOCYSTEINE				
(Hall) *See AVAILNEX*				
(PCCA) *See S-CARBOXYMETHYL-L-CYSTEINE*				
CARBOFED DM (Palmetto)				
REPACK				
bpm/dm/pse hcl				
SYR, PO, 120 ml	23490-0249-05	36.47		
(Quality Care Prod)				
REPACK				
carbinoxamine mal/dm/pse hcl				
SOL, PO (DROPS)				
1 mg/ml-4 mg/ml-15 mg/ml,				
30 ml	49999-0814-30	31.80		

PROD/MFR	NDC	AWP	DP	OBC
CARBOGEL (Gallipot)				
gel base				
GEL, NA (BUFFERED)				
100 gm	50552-0724-05	8.26	5.90	
CARBOHOL (Gallipot)				
gel base				
GEL, NA, 100 gm	51552-0727-05	8.26	5.90	
CARBOMER				
(Amend) *See CARBOPOL 934*				
(Amend) *See CARBOPOL 934 P*				
(Amend) *See CARBOPOL 941*				
(Gallipot) *See CARBOPOL 934*				
(Gallipot) *See CARBOPOL 940 RESIN*				
(Letco) *See CARBOPOL 940*				
(Medisca) *See CARBOMER 934P*				
(PCCA) *See CARBOMER 934P*				
(PCCA) *See CARBOMER 940*				
(Spectrum Pharmacy) *See CARBOMER 1342*				
(Spectrum Pharmacy) *See CARBOMER 934*				
(Spectrum Pharmacy) *See CARBOMER 934P*				
(Spectrum Pharmacy) *See CARBOMER 940*				
(Spectrum Pharmacy) *See CARBOMER 941*				
CARBOMER 1342 (Spectrum Pharmacy)				
carbomer				
POW, NA (N.F.)				
500 gm	49452-1709-02	216.65		
2500 gm	49452-1709-03	672.00		
CARBOMER 934 (Spectrum Pharmacy)				
carbomer				
POW, NA (N.F.)				
500 gm	49452-1704-02	199.50		
2500 gm	49452-1704-03	672.00		
CARBOMER 934P (Medisca)				
carbomer				
POW, NA (N.F.)				
25 gm	38779-0563-04	28.50		
100 gm	38779-0563-05	58.50		
500 gm	38779-0563-08	126.00		
(PCCA)				
POW, NA (N.F.)				
1 gm	51927-2273-00	1.20		
(Spectrum Pharmacy)				
POW, NA (N.F.)				
100 gm	49452-1706-01	101.50		
500 gm	49452-1706-02	213.50		
2500 gm	49452-1706-03	973.00		
CARBOMER 940 (PCCA)				
carbomer				
POW, NA (NF)				
1 gm	51927-3094-00	1.44		
(Spectrum Pharmacy)				
POW, NA (N.F.)				
100 gm	49452-1707-01	86.80		
500 gm	49452-1707-02	189.70		
2500 gm	49452-1707-03	714.00		
CARBOMER 941 (Spectrum Pharmacy)				
carbomer				
POW, NA (N.F.)				
500 gm	49452-1708-02	222.60		
2500 gm	49452-1708-03	773.50		
CARBON ACID WASHED (Baker, J.T.)				
graphite				
POW, NA (REAGENT, 60 MESH)				
500 gm	10106-3370-07	69.53		
3000 gm	10106-3370-09	243.13		
CARBON DISULFIDE (Baker, J.T.)				
LIQ, NA (A.C.S., REAGENT)				
500 ml	10106-9172-01	54.49		
CARBON TETRACHLORIDE (Baker, J.T.)				
SOL, NA (A.C.S., REAGENT)				
500 ml	10106-1512-01	85.90		
(PCCA)				
SOL, NA (REAGENT ACS)				
1 ml	51927-1777-00	1.09		
CARBOPLATIN (APP)				
PDS, IV, 150 mg, ea	63323-0167-21	268.75		
SOL, IV (1X10ML,MDV,PF)				
10 mg/ml, 10 ml	63323-0172-05	12.12		
(1X20ML,MDV,PF)				
10 mg/ml, 20 ml	63323-0172-15	32.40		
(MDV,LATEX-FREE)				
10 mg/ml, 45 ml	63323-0172-45	805.88		AP
(600MG/60ML,LATEX-FREE)				
10 mg/ml, 60 ml	63323-0172-60	562.50		AP
(Bedford) *See CARBOPLATIN AMERINET CHOICE*				
(Bedford)				
PDS, IV (S.D.V.,USP)				
50 mg, ea	55390-0150-01	12.00		AP
150 mg, ea	55390-0151-01	36.00		AP
450 mg, ea	55390-0152-01	108.00		AP
SOL, IV (M.D.V.,PF)				
10 mg/ml, 5 ml	55390-0153-01	12.00		AP
15 ml	55390-0154-01	36.00		AP
45 ml	55390-0155-01	108.00		AP
(MDV,PF)				
10 mg/ml, 60 ml	55390-0156-01	120.00		AP
(GeneraMedix)				
SOL, IV (MDV,YELLOWSEAL,1X5ML)				
10 mg/ml, 5 ml	10139-0060-05	13.20		AP
(MDV,PURPLESEAL,1X15ML)				
10 mg/ml, 15 ml	10139-0060-15	38.36		AP
(MDV,BLUESEAL,1X45ML)				
10 mg/ml, 45 ml	10139-0060-45	108.00		AP
(Hospira) *See AMERINET CHOICE CARBOPLATIN*				
(Hospira) *See NOVAPLUS CARBOPLATIN*				
(Hospira)				
SOL, IV, 10 mg/ml, 5 ml	00409-1129-10	19.25	16.84	AP
(MDV)				
10 mg/ml, 5 ml	61703-0339-18	11.70	10.24	
15 ml	00409-1129-11	41.06	35.93	AP
(MDV)				
10 mg/ml, 15 ml	61703-0339-22	28.80	25.20	
45 ml	00409-1129-12	119.53	104.59	AP
(MDV)				
10 mg/ml, 45 ml	61703-0339-50	67.08	58.70	
60 ml	61703-0339-56	80.17	70.15	
(OTN)				
SOL, IV (MDV)				
10 mg/ml, 5 ml	15210-0061-12	20.00		AP
15 ml	15210-0063-12	59.38		AP
45 ml	15210-0066-12	177.50		AP
60 ml	15210-0067-12	236.25		AP
(Parenta Pharma)				
SOL, IV (1X5ML,MDV,USP)				
10 mg/ml, 5 ml	66758-0047-01	15.00		AP
(1X15ML,MDV,USP)				
10 mg/ml, 15 ml	66758-0047-02	45.00		AP
(1X45ML,MDV,USP)				
10 mg/ml, 45 ml	66758-0047-03	135.00		AP
(Teva)				
PDS, IV, 50 mg, ea	00703-3264-01	20.00		
(VIAL)				
150 mg, ea	00703-3266-01	59.38		
450 mg, ea	00703-3268-01	177.50		
ea	00703-3268-71	177.50		
SOL, IV (1X5ML)				
10 mg/ml, 5 ml	00703-4244-01	20.00		
(M.D.V.)				
10 mg/ml, 5 ml	00703-3244-11	20.00		
(1X15ML)				
10 mg/ml, 15 ml	00703-4246-01	48.00		
(M.D.V.)				
10 mg/ml, 15 ml	00703-3246-11	59.38		
45 ml	00703-4248-01	108.00		AP
(M.D.V.)				
10 mg/ml, 45 ml	00703-3248-11	177.50		
(AQUEOUS SOLUTION)				
10 mg/ml, 60 ml	00703-3249-11	114.00		AP
CARBOPLATIN AMERINET CHOICE (Bedford)				
carboplatin				
SOL, IV (M.D.V.,PF)				
10 mg/ml, 5 ml	55390-0220-01	24.00		AP
15 ml	55390-0221-01	72.00		AP
45 ml	55390-0222-01	216.00		AP
CARBOPOL 934 (Amend)				
carbomer				
POW, NA, 454 gm	17317-0867-01	28.00		
2270 gm	17317-0867-05	112.00		
11350 gm	17317-0867-08	420.00		
(Gallipot)				
POW, NA, 500 gm	51552-0776-06	48.30	34.50	
CARBOPOL 934 P (Amend)				
carbomer				
POW, NA (N.F.)				
454 gm	17317-0870-01	37.80		
2270 gm	17317-0870-05	154.00		
11350 gm	17317-0870-08	630.00		
CARBOPOL 940 (Letco)				
carbomer				
POW, NA, 25 gm	62991-1345-01	27.00		
100 gm	62991-1345-02	37.50		
500 gm	62991-1345-03	75.00		
CARBOPOL 940 RESIN (Gallipot)				
carbomer				
POW, NA, 113.4 gm	51552-0107-04	22.40		
454 gm	51552-0107-06	55.30		
CARBOPOL 941 (Amend)				
carbomer				
POW, NA, 454 gm	17317-0868-01	21.00		
2270 gm	17317-0868-05	84.00		
11350 gm	17317-0868-08	350.00		
CARBOPROST TROMETHAMINE				
(Pfizer) *See HEMABATE*				
CARBOXYMETHYLCELLULOSE SODIUM (Gallipot)				
POW, NA (LOW VISCOSITY)				
100 gm	51552-0510-05	11.90		
(MEDIUM VISCOSITY,U.S.P.)				
100 gm	51552-0099-05	11.90		
(N.A.,U.S.P.,HIGH VISC.)				
100 gm	51552-0476-05	11.90		
(128MP)				
113.4 gm	51552-0436-04	11.83		
(MEDIUM VISCOSITY,U.S.P.)				
454 gm	51552-0099-06	32.48		
(Letco)				
POW, NA (U.S.P.)				
100 gm	62991-1029-01	30.00		
(USP)				
500 gm	62991-1029-02	105.00		
(USP, 1X2500GM)				
2500 gm	62991-1029-03	435.00		
(Medisca)				
POW, NA (U.S.P.)				
100 gm	38779-1130-05	28.50		
500 gm	38779-1130-08	72.00		
(USP,400-800 CPS)				
2500 gm	38779-1130-01	285.00		
(PCCA)				
POW, NA (BASE H)				
1 gm	51927-1077-00	0.36		
(USP)				
1 gm	51927-1235-00	0.36		
1 gm	51927-1800-00	0.36		
(Spectrum Pharmacy)				
POW, NA (HIGH VISCOSITY,U.S.P.)				
125 gm	49452-1750-03	63.70		
(LOW VISCOSITY,U.S.P.)				
125 gm	49452-1730-03	63.70		
(MEDIUM VISCOSITY,USP)				
125 gm	49452-1740-00	63.70		
(HIGH VISCOSITY,U.S.P.)				
500 gm	49452-1750-01	106.05		
(LOW VISCOSITY,U.S.P.)				
500 gm	49452-1730-01	106.05		
(MEDIUM VISCOSITY,USP)				
500 gm	49452-1740-01	106.05		
(HIGH VISCOSITY,U.S.P.)				
2500 gm	49452-1750-02	416.50		
(LOW VISCOSITY,U.S.P.)				
2500 gm	49452-1730-02	416.50		
(MEDIUM VISCOSITY,U.S.P.)				
2500 gm	49452-1740-03	416.50		
CARBOXYMETHYLCELLULOSE/ HYALURONATE SODIUM				
(Genzyme) *See SEPRAFILM*				
CARDAMOM OIL (Lorann Oil)				
OIL, NA, 9.9 ml	23535-0151-09	7.50		
(PCCA)				
OIL, NA, 1 ml	51927-2910-00	3.50		
(Spectrum Pharmacy)				
OIL, NA (F.C.C.)				
5 ml	49452-1755-01	99.75		
25 ml	49452-1755-02	250.25		
125 ml	49452-1755-03	735.00		
CARDEC DM (DHS, Inc.)				
REPACK				
cpm/dm/phenyleph hcl				
SOL, PO (AF,SF,GRAPE,DROPS)				
30 ml	55887-0030-30	33.00		

PROD/MFR	NDC	AWP	DP	OBC
(Pharma Pac)				
REPACK				
carbinoxamine mal/dm/pse hcl				
LIQ, PO (DROPS)				
2 mg/ml-4 mg/ml-25 mg/ml,				
30 ml	**52959-0125-30**	9.95		
SYR, PO, 120 ml	**52959-0073-04**	8.50		
(Phys Total Care)				
REPACK				
SYR, PO, 120 ml	**54868-1979-00**	12.54		
473 ml	**54868-1979-01**	67.83		
CARDEC-DM (DHS, Inc.)				
REPACK				
carbinoxamine mal/dm/pse hcl				
SYR, PO, 120 ml	**55887-0605-04**	29.95		
CARDENE (EKR)				
nicardipine hydrochloride/sodium chloride				
SOL, IV (10X200ML,PREMIXED)				
0.2 mg/ml-8.3 mg/ml,				
200 ml 10s	**24477-0323-02**	2693.04		
(EKR)				
nicardipine hydrochloride				
(10X10ML)				
2.5 mg/ml,				
10 ml 10s	**24477-0030-25**	2810.40		
(EKR)				
dextrose/nicardipine hydrochloride				
(10X200ML,PREMIXED)				
50 mg/ml-0.2 mg/ml,				
200 ml 10s	**24477-0324-02**	2693.04		
CARDENE I.V. (EKR)				
nicardipine hydrochloride				
SOL, IV (10X200ML,SINGLE-USE)				
0.1 mg/ml,				
200 ml 10s	**24477-0311-02**	1346.52		
200 ml 10s	**24477-0312-02**	1346.52		**EE**
CARDENE SR (EKR)				
nicardipine hydrochloride				
CER, PO (HARD GELATIN)				
30 mg, 60s ea	**67286-0814-04**	109.78		
200s ea	**67286-0814-03**	365.57		
45 mg, 60s ea	**67286-0813-04**	174.29		
200s ea	**67286-0813-03**	580.67		
60 mg, 60s ea	**67286-0815-04**	208.61		
(Phys Total Care)				
REPACK				
CER, PO, 30 mg, 50s ea	**54868-3817-00**	43.29		
CARDIODORON (Weleda)				
homeopathic substance				
LIQ, PO, 50 ml	**55946-0170-15**	9.00		
CARDIODORON/MAGNESIA PHOSPHORICA 6X (Weleda)				
homeopathic substance				
LIQ, PO, 50 ml	**55946-0180-15**	9.00		
CARDIOGEN-82 GENERATOR (Bracco Diag)				
rubidium chloride rb 82				
KIT, IV, ea	**00270-0150-00**	36868.75	29495.00	
CARDIOGEN-82 INFUSION SYSTEM (Bracco Diag)				
laboratory tests and/or supplies				
DEV, NA, ea	**00270-0153-70**	90000.00	72000.00	
CARDIOGEN-82 WASTE BOTTLE (Bracco Diag)				
laboratory tests and/or supplies				
DEV, NA, ea	**00270-0152-00**	25.12	20.10	
CARDIOLITE (Lantheus)				
technetium tc 99m sestamibi				
KIT, IV (SRN,PREFILLED)				
ea	**11994-0001-00**	128.10		
CARDIOPLEGIC SOLUTION (Baxter)				
ca cl/k cl/mg cl/na cl				
SOL, IR (P.C.)				
1000 ml	**00338-0341-04**	58.00	48.33	**AT**
CARDIOTEK RX (SJ)				
arginine hcl/folic acid/vit b12/vit b6				
TAB, PO (SF,LACTOSE-FREE)				
500 mg-0.5 mg-2 mg-50 mg,				
30s ea	**45985-0651-30**	19.93		
CARDIOTEK-RX (SJ)				
multivitamin and nutriceuticals				
TAB, PO (SF,GLUTEN-FREE)				
30s ea	**24839-0333-30**	27.00		
CARDIZEM (BTA)				
diltiazem hydrochloride				
TAB, PO, 30 mg, 100s ea	**64455-0771-47**	120.82	100.68	**AB**
500s ea	**64455-0771-55**	593.80	494.83	**AB**
60 mg, 100s ea	**64455-0772-47**	189.59	157.99	**AB**
90 mg, 100s ea	**64455-0791-47**	266.60	222.17	**AB**
(CAPLET)				
120 mg, 100s ea	**64455-0792-47**	348.98	290.82	**AB**

PROD/MFR	NDC	AWP	DP	OBC
(Phys Total Care)				
REPACK				
TAB, PO, 60 mg, 100s ea	**54868-0671-00**	92.92		**AB**
CARDIZEM CD (BTA)				
diltiazem hydrochloride				
C24, PO, 120 mg, 30s ea	**64455-0795-30**	96.96	80.80	**AB3**
90s ea	**64455-0795-42**	284.70	237.25	**AB3**
100s ea UD	**64455-0795-49**	315.55	262.96	**AB3**
180 mg, 30s ea	**64455-0796-30**	119.98	99.98	**AB3**
90s ea	**64455-0796-42**	343.57	286.31	**AB3**
100s ea UD	**64455-0796-49**	379.57	316.31	**AB3**
5000s ea	**64455-0796-50**	19099.66	15916.38	**AB3**
240 mg, 30s ea	**64455-0797-30**	162.64	135.53	**AB3**
90s ea	**64455-0797-42**	487.38	406.15	**AB3**
100s ea UD	**64455-0797-49**	539.59	449.66	**AB3**
300 mg, 30s ea	**64455-0798-30**	213.05	177.54	**AB3**
90s ea	**64455-0798-42**	631.66	526.38	**AB3**
360 mg, 90s ea	**64455-0799-42**	687.12	572.60	
(Altura)				
REPACK				
C24, PO, 240 mg, 30s ea	**63874-1139-03**	82.49		**AB3**
(Phys Total Care)				
REPACK				
C24, PO, 180 mg, 30s ea	**54868-2148-03**	61.59		**AB3**
240 mg, 30s ea	**54868-2149-02**	179.76		**AB3**
60s ea	**54868-2149-00**	337.80		**AB3**
300 mg, 30s ea	**54868-2150-01**	109.23		**AB3**
(Quality Care Prod)				
REPACK				
C24, PO, 120 mg, 30s ea	**35356-0510-30**	178.20		**AB3**
CARDIZEM LA (Abbott Pharm)				
diltiazem hydrochloride				
TER, PO, 120 mg, 30s ea	**00074-3045-30**	89.41	78.43	**AB3**
90s ea	**00074-3045-90**	267.82	234.93	**AB3**
180 mg, 30s ea	**00074-3061-30**	94.46	82.86	**AB3**
90s ea	**00074-3061-90**	283.38	248.58	**AB3**
240 mg, 30s ea	**00074-3062-30**	105.89	92.88	**AB3**
90s ea	**00074-3062-90**	317.59	278.59	**AB3**
300 mg, 30s ea	**00074-3063-30**	137.74	120.82	**EE**
90s ea	**00074-3063-90**	413.16	362.42	**EE**
360 mg, 30s ea	**00074-3064-30**	148.08	129.89	**EE**
90s ea	**00074-3064-90**	444.52	389.93	**EE**
420 mg, 30s ea	**00074-3069-30**	160.49	140.78	
90s ea	**00074-3069-90**	482.35	423.12	
(Phys Total Care)				
REPACK				
TER, PO, 120 mg, 90s ea	**54868-4808-00**	131.88		
240 mg, 30s ea	**54868-5301-00**	62.54		
CARDIZEM SR (Phys Total Care)				
diltiazem hydrochloride				
C12, PO, 120 mg, 30s ea	**54868-1005-00**	54.85		**AB1**
CARDURA (Pfizer)				
doxazosin mesylate				
TAB, PO, 1 mg, 100s ea	**00049-2750-66**	168.55	140.46	**AB**
2 mg, 100s ea	**00049-2760-66**	168.55	140.46	**AB**
4 mg, 100s ea	**00049-2770-66**	176.89	147.41	**AB**
8 mg, 100s ea	**00049-2780-66**	185.75	154.79	**AB**
(PD-Rx Pharm)				
REPACK				
TAB, PO (REDI-SCRIPT)				
4 mg, 30s ea	**58864-0860-30**	57.22		**AB**
8 mg, 30s ea	**55289-0584-30**	59.80		**AB**
(REDI-SCRIPT)				
8 mg, 30s ea	**58864-0856-30**	59.81		**AB**
(Phys Total Care)				
REPACK				
TAB, PO, 1 mg, 30s ea	**54868-1768-01**	50.26		**AB**
100s ea	**54868-1768-02**	163.15		**AB**
2 mg, 30s ea	**54868-2151-01**	45.74		**AB**
60s ea	**54868-2151-00**	89.60		**AB**
100s ea	**54868-2151-02**	147.45		**AB**
4 mg, 30s ea	**54868-2640-01**	47.91		**AB**
8 mg, 10s ea	**54868-3419-01**	17.99		**AB**
30s ea	**54868-3419-00**	50.12		**AB**
CARDURA XL (Pfizer)				
doxazosin mesylate				
TER, PO, 4 mg, 30s ea	**00049-2710-30**	58.13	48.44	**EE**
8 mg, 30s ea	**00049-2720-30**	61.06	50.88	
CARIMUNE NF (CSL)				
immune globulin				
PDS, IV (PF,NANOFILTERED)				
3 gm, ea	**44206-0416-03**	303.00		
6 gm, ea	**44206-0417-06**	606.00		
12 gm, ea	**44206-0418-12**	1212.00		
CARISOPRODOL				
FUL				
TAB, PO, 350 mg, 100s ea		8.51		

PROD/MFR	NDC	AWP	DP	OBC
(Aurobindo Pharma)				
TAB, PO (USP)				
350 mg, 100s ea	**65862-0158-01**	83.95		**AA**
(Caraco)				
TAB, PO (USP)				
350 mg, 100s ea	**62756-0446-02**	59.60		**AA**
500s ea	**62756-0446-05**	286.30		**AA**
1000s ea	**62756-0446-04**	566.30		**AA**
(Consolidated Midland)				
TAB, PO, 350 mg, 100s ea	**00223-0657-01**	8.75		**EE**
500s ea	**00223-0657-05**	40.00		**EE**
1000s ea	**00223-0657-02**	77.50		**EE**
(CorePharma)				
TAB, PO (USP)				
350 mg, 100s ea	**64720-0103-10**	60.23		**AA**
500s ea	**64720-0103-50**	318.20		**AA**
1000s ea	**64720-0103-11**	579.00		**AA**
(Gallipot)				
POW, NA (U.S.P.)				
25 gm	**51552-1052-04**	31.50	22.50	
(GM Pharm)				
TAB, PO, 350 mg, 500s ea	**58809-0424-05**	1590.00		**AA**
(Letco)				
POW, NA (USP)				
25 gm	**62991-2173-01**	67.50		
100 gm	**62991-2173-02**	126.00		
(Major)				
TAB, PO, 350 mg, 100s ea	**00904-0355-60**	59.63		**AA**
(Meda) *See SOMA*				
(Medisca)				
POW, NA (U.S.P.)				
100 gm	**38779-0499-05**	114.75		
500 gm	**38779-0499-08**	501.00		
(USP,1X1000GM)				
1000 gm	**38779-0499-09**	994.50		
(Mutual)				
TAB, PO, 350 mg, 100s ea	**53489-0110-01**	60.23		**AA**
(PCCA)				
POW, NA (U.S.P.)				
1 gm	**51927-3169-00**	1.77		
(Qualitest)				
TAB, PO, 350 mg, 100s ea	**00603-2582-21**	59.61		**AA**
500s ea	**00603-2582-28**	286.36		**AA**
1000s ea	**00603-2582-32**	566.30		**AA**
(Sandoz)				
TAB, PO, 350 mg, 100s ea	**00781-5005-01**	59.62		**AA**
500s ea	**00781-5005-05**	286.38		**AA**
(Spectrum Pharmacy)				
POW, NA (U.S.P.)				
25 gm	**49452-1761-01**	96.25		
100 gm	**49452-1761-02**	183.75		
500 gm	**49452-1761-03**	724.50		
(UDL)				
TAB, PO (10X10)				
350 mg, 100s ea UD	**51079-0055-20**	60.03		**AA**
(Watson Labs)				
TAB, PO, 350 mg, 100s ea	**00591-5513-01**	9.59		**AA**
500s ea	**00591-5513-05**	46.02		**AA**
1000s ea	**00591-5513-10**	91.09		**AA**
(West-Ward)				
TAB, PO, 350 mg, 100s ea	**00143-1176-01**	59.75		**AA**
500s ea	**00143-1176-05**	289.10		**AA**
1000s ea	**00143-1176-10**	524.65		**AA**
(4u)				
REPACK				
TAB, PO, 350 mg, 28s ea	**10544-0303-28**	108.26		**AA**
28s ea	**42549-0503-28**	108.26		**AA**
30s ea	**10544-0303-30**	112.26		
30s ea	**42549-0303-30**	112.26		**AA**
30s ea	**42549-0503-30**	112.26		**AA**
40s ea	**10544-0303-40**	136.82		
40s ea	**42549-0503-40**	136.82		**AA**
60s ea	**10544-0303-60**	188.24		
60s ea	**42549-0503-60**	188.24		**AA**
90s ea	**10544-0303-90**	246.56		
90s ea	**42549-0303-90**	246.56		**AA**
90s ea	**42549-0503-90**	246.56		**AA**
(A-S Medication)				
REPACK				
TAB, PO, 350 mg, 7s ea	**54569-3403-01**	5.57		**AA**
12s ea	**54569-3403-04**	9.55		**AA**
14s ea	**54569-1709-07**	11.14		**AA**
20s ea	**54569-1709-03**	15.92		**AA**
28s ea	**54569-3403-00**	22.29		**AA**
30s ea	**54569-1709-00**	23.88		**AA**

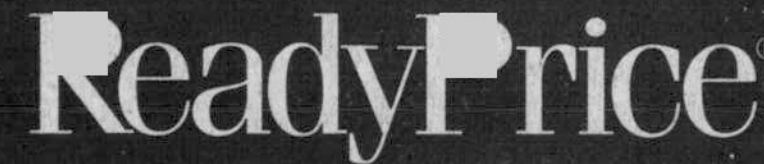

PROD/MFR	NDC	AWP	DP	OBC
40s ea	54569-1709-02	31.84		AA
45s ea	54569-3403-09	35.82		AA
50s ea	54569-1709-01	39.80		AA
60s ea	54569-1709-08	47.75		AA
90s ea	54569-3403-05	71.63		AA
100s ea	54569-1709-04	79.59		AA
120s ea	54569-1709-09	98.17		EE
(Aidarex)				
REPACK				
TAB, PO, 350 mg, 7s ea	33261-0016-07	30.94		
12s ea	33261-0016-12	53.04		
14s ea	33261-0016-14	61.88		
20s ea	33261-0016-20	88.40		
21s ea	33261-0016-21	92.82		
24s ea	33261-0016-24	106.08		
25s ea	33261-0016-25	110.50		AA
28s ea	33261-0016-28	123.76		
30s ea	33261-0016-30	132.30		
36s ea	33261-0016-36	159.12		AA
40s ea	33261-0016-40	176.80		
50s ea	33261-0016-50	221.00		AA
60s ea	33261-0016-60	265.20		
90s ea	33261-0016-90	397.80		
100s ea	33261-0016-00	442.00		
120s ea	33261-0016-02	530.40		
180s ea	33261-0016-03	795.60		
(Altura)				
REPACK				
TAB, PO, 350 mg, 7s ea	63874-0330-07	19.47		EE
10s ea	63874-0330-10	27.80		EE
12s ea	63874-0330-12	33.36		EE
14s ea	63874-0330-14	38.93		EE
15s ea	63874-0330-15	41.71		EE
16s ea	63874-0330-16	44.49		EE
18s ea	63874-0330-18	50.06		EE
20s ea	63874-0330-20	55.64		EE
21s ea	63874-0330-21	58.40		EE
24s ea	63874-0330-24	66.75		EE
25s ea	63874-0330-25	69.54		EE
28s ea	63874-0330-28	77.90		EE
30s ea	63874-0330-30	83.45		EE
40s ea	63874-0330-40	111.28		EE
42s ea	63874-0330-42	116.83		EE
45s ea	63874-0330-45	125.19		EE
50s ea	63874-0330-50	139.05		EE
56s ea	63874-0330-56	155.75		EE
60s ea	63874-0330-60	166.92		EE
75s ea	63874-0330-75	208.65		EE
80s ea	63874-0330-80	222.56		EE
84s ea	63874-0330-84	233.68		EE
90s ea	63874-0330-90	250.38		EE
100s ea	63874-0330-01	278.18		EE
112s ea	63874-0330-11	311.51		EE
120s ea	63874-0330-04	333.83		EE
150s ea	63874-0330-72	417.30		EE
200s ea	63874-0330-74	556.40		EE
300s ea	63874-0330-77	834.60		EE
500s ea	63874-0330-03	2191.00		EE
1000s ea	63874-0330-02	4382.00		EE
(American Health)				
REPACK				
TAB, PO, 350 mg, 100s ea UD	68084-0380-01	18.75		AA
(Bryant Ranch)				
REPACK				
TAB, PO, 350 mg, 14s ea	63629-1308-01	57.49		
15s ea	63629-1308-06	62.32		
20s ea	63629-1308-04	82.42		
28s ea	63629-1308-02	115.99		
30s ea	63629-1308-05	123.63		
50s ea	63629-1308-00	202.65		
60s ea	63629-1308-03	232.99		
90s ea	63629-1308-07	395.56		
100s ea	63629-1308-08	379.99		
120s ea	63629-1308-09	526.99		
(Core)				
REPACK				
TAB, PO, 350 mg, 15s ea	33358-0064-15	63.88		
20s ea	33358-0064-20	84.48		
30s ea	33358-0064-30	126.72		
50s ea	33358-0064-50	203.68		
60s ea	33358-0064-60	251.39		
90s ea	33358-0064-90	405.45		
100s ea	33358-0064-00	389.49		
120s ea	33358-0064-01	540.16		
(DHS, Inc.)				
REPACK				
TAB, PO, 350 mg, 10s ea	55887-0990-10	27.83		AA
20s ea	55887-0990-20	56.00		AA
25s ea	55887-0990-25	55.66		AA
30s ea	55887-0990-30	83.49		AA
40s ea	55887-0990-40	110.00		AA
(USP)				
350 mg, 60s ea	55887-0990-60	150.00		AA
90s ea	55887-0990-90	199.00		AA
120s ea	55887-0990-82	260.00		AA
(Dispensing Solutions)				
REPACK				
TAB, PO, 350 mg, 10s ea	55045-1433-01	29.50		
15s ea	55045-1433-05	44.25		AA
15s ea	66336-0635-15	40.00		AA
20s ea	55045-1433-07	59.00		
20s ea	66336-0635-20	53.33		EE
30s ea	55045-1433-08	88.50		AA
30s ea	55045-3767-08	88.50		
30s ea	66336-0635-30	80.00		EE
40s ea	55045-1433-09	118.00		AA
45s ea	55045-1433-02	132.75		AA
50s ea	55045-1433-03	147.50		AA
56s ea	55045-3123-06	165.20		AA
60s ea	55045-1433-04	177.00		AA
60s ea	66336-0635-60	160.00		EE
84s ea	55045-3716-04	247.80		
90s ea	55045-3123-09	265.50		AA
90s ea	55045-3546-01	265.50		
90s ea	66336-0635-90	240.00		EE
100s ea	55045-1433-00	295.00		
112s ea	55045-3123-02	330.40		AA
120s ea	55045-1433-06	354.00		
120s ea	66336-0635-94	320.00		EE
135s ea	55045-3123-03	398.25		AA
180s ea	55045-3123-04	531.00		AA
(GSMS)				
REPACK				
TAB, PO (UNIT OF USE)				
350 mg, 90s ea	60429-0035-90	120.80	30.20	AA
120s ea	60429-0035-12	160.40	40.10	AA
(HomeMed)				
REPACK				
TAB, PO, 350 mg, 20s ea	51655-0376-52	12.46		EE
30s ea	51655-0376-24	30.56		EE
(IPI)				
REPACK				
TAB, PO, 350 mg, 21s ea	18837-0022-21	68.50		AA
30s ea	18837-0022-30	74.49		
40s ea	18837-0022-40	99.32		
60s ea	18837-0022-60	138.98		
90s ea	18837-0022-90	177.57		
120s ea	18837-0022-98	62.96		AA
(Keltman Pharma., Inc.)				
REPACK				
TAB, PO, 350 mg, 15s ea	68387-0600-15	41.96		AA
30s ea	68387-0600-30	83.91		AA
45s ea	68387-0600-45	125.87		AA
60s ea	68387-0600-60	167.82		AA
90s ea	68387-0600-90	251.73		AA
120s ea	68387-0600-12	335.64		AA
(LWP)				
REPACK				
TAB, PO, 350 mg, 30s ea	64038-0022-30	22.93		AA
60s ea	64038-0022-60	43.85		AA
100s ea	64038-0022-01	64.75		AA
(McKesson Packaging)				
REPACK				
TAB, PO (USP)				
350 mg, 100s ea UD	63739-0049-10	70.79		AA
(Medsource)				
REPACK				
TAB, PO, 350 mg, 30s ea	45865-0408-30	75.00		AA
60s ea	45865-0408-60	150.00		AA
90s ea	45865-0408-90	225.00		AA
100s ea	45865-0408-00	250.00		AA
120s ea	45865-0408-01	300.00		AA
150s ea	45865-0408-02	375.00		AA
300s ea	45865-0408-05	750.00		AA
(Nucare Pharm)				
REPACK				
TAB, PO, 350 mg, 12s ea	66267-0043-12	46.32		AA
15s ea	66267-0043-15	72.42		EE
20s ea	66267-0043-20	94.92		EE
30s ea	66267-0043-30	115.80		AA
40s ea	66267-0043-40	154.39		AA
45s ea	66267-0043-45	125.09		EE
60s ea	66267-0043-60	231.60		AA
90s ea	66267-0043-90	406.92		AA
120s ea	66267-0043-91	463.20		AA
(Palmetto)				
REPACK				
TAB, PO, 350 mg, 4s ea	23490-5212-01	48.64		
10s ea	23490-5212-07	27.80		
15s ea	23490-5212-02	41.70		
20s ea	23490-5212-03	55.60		
24s ea	23490-5212-00	66.72		
25s ea	23490-7917-08	69.50		
28s ea	23490-5212-08	77.84		
30s ea	23490-0252-03	137.60		
30s ea	23490-5212-04	83.40		
40s ea	23490-7917-04	111.20		
45s ea	23490-5212-09	125.10		
50s ea	23490-7917-05	139.00		
60s ea	23490-0252-06	275.20		
60s ea	23490-5212-05	166.80		
90s ea	23490-0252-09	412.79		
90s ea	23490-5212-06	250.20		
100s ea	23490-7917-00	278.00		
120s ea	23490-7917-07	333.60		
(PD-Rx Pharm)				
REPACK				
TAB, PO, 350 mg, 10s ea	55289-0049-10	137.00		AA
14s ea	55289-0049-14	142.00		AA
15s ea	55289-0049-15	143.00		AA
20s ea	55289-0049-20	148.75		AA
21s ea	55289-0049-21	150.00		AA
24s ea	55289-0049-24	153.75		AA
30s ea	55289-0049-30	161.25		AA
30s ea	58864-0778-30	133.25		AA
40s ea	55289-0049-40	173.00		AA
60s ea	55289-0049-60	197.00		AA
90s ea	55289-0049-90	233.00		AA
100s ea	55289-0049-01	245.00		AA
120s ea	55289-0049-98	268.75		AA
(Pharma Pac)				
REPACK				
TAB, PO, 350 mg, 6s ea	52959-0026-06	30.65		AA
10s ea	52959-0026-10	51.08		EE
12s ea	52959-0026-12	61.29		AA
14s ea	52959-0026-14	71.50		EE
15s ea	52959-0026-15	76.60		EE
20s ea	52959-0026-20	102.12		EE
21s ea	52959-0026-21	107.22		EE
24s ea	52959-0026-24	122.50		EE
25s ea	52959-0026-25	127.60		EE
28s ea	52959-0026-28	142.90		EE
30s ea	52959-0026-30	138.29		EE
32s ea	52959-0026-32	147.44		EE
40s ea	52959-0026-40	184.30		EE
45s ea	52959-0026-45	207.31		EE
50s ea	52959-0026-50	230.33		EE
52s ea	52959-0026-52	239.53		EE
56s ea	52959-0026-56	257.95		EE
60s ea	52959-0026-60	276.30		EE
80s ea	52959-0026-80	368.65		AA
90s ea	52959-0026-90	414.36		EE
100s ea	52959-0026-00	460.35		EE
120s ea	52959-0026-03	552.33		EE
(Phys Total Care)				
REPACK				
TAB, PO, 350 mg, 10s ea	54868-0816-07	6.57		EE
20s ea	54868-0816-02	8.64		EE
30s ea	54868-0816-03	10.71		EE
(USP)				
350 mg, 40s ea	54868-0816-09	12.79		EE
50s ea	54868-0816-05	14.85		EE
60s ea	54868-0816-04	16.92		EE
90s ea	54868-0816-08	23.16		AA
100s ea	54868-0816-06	25.23		EE
(Physician Partner)				
REPACK				
TAB, PO, 350 mg, 15s ea	21695-0021-15	77.46		
20s ea	21695-0021-20	103.28		
21s ea	21695-0021-21	108.45		
30s ea	21695-0021-30	131.69		
42s ea	21695-0021-42	216.86		AA
45s ea	21695-0021-45	232.39		
60s ea	21695-0021-60	263.38		
90s ea	21695-0021-90	395.07		
120s ea	21695-0021-72	526.65		
(Quality Care Prod)				
REPACK				
TAB, PO, 350 mg, 6s ea	49999-0064-06	20.04		AA
7s ea	49999-0064-07	23.34		EE
10s ea	49999-0064-10	33.38		AA
14s ea	49999-0064-14	46.74		EE
15s ea	49999-0064-15	50.08		EE
20s ea	49999-0064-20	66.76		EE
30s ea	49999-0064-30	131.69		EE

PROD/MFR	NDC	AWP	DP	OBC
40s ea	49999-0064-40	157.19		EE
50s ea	49999-0064-50	166.92		EE
60s ea	49999-0064-60	262.89		EE
90s ea	49999-0064-90	395.07		AA
100s ea	49999-0064-00	333.84		EE
120s ea	49999-0064-01	523.98		EE
180s ea	49999-0064-18	600.84		EE

(Southwood)
REPACK

PROD/MFR	NDC	AWP	DP	OBC
TAB, PO, 350 mg, 7s ea	58016-0261-07	19.47		EE
7s ea	58016-0488-07	19.47		AA
10s ea	58016-0261-10	27.82		EE
10s ea	58016-0488-10	27.82		AA
12s ea	58016-0261-12	33.38		EE
12s ea	58016-0488-12	33.38		AA
14s ea	58016-0261-14	38.95		EE
14s ea	58016-0488-14	38.95		AA
15s ea	58016-0261-15	41.73		EE
15s ea	58016-0488-15	41.73		AA
16s ea	58016-0261-16	44.51		EE
16s ea	58016-0488-16	44.51		AA
18s ea	58016-0261-18	50.08		EE
18s ea	58016-0488-18	50.08		AA
20s ea	58016-0261-20	55.64		EE
20s ea	58016-0488-20	55.64		AA
21s ea	58016-0261-21	58.42		EE
21s ea	58016-0488-21	58.42		AA
24s ea	58016-0261-24	66.77		EE
24s ea	58016-0488-24	66.77		AA
25s ea	58016-0261-25	69.55		EE
25s ea	58016-0488-25	69.55		AA
28s ea	58016-0261-28	77.90		EE
28s ea	58016-0488-28	77.90		AA
30s ea	58016-0261-30	109.50		AA
30s ea	58016-0488-30	109.50		AA
40s ea	58016-0261-40	111.28		EE
40s ea	58016-0488-40	111.28		AA
42s ea	58016-0261-42	116.84		EE
42s ea	58016-0488-42	116.84		AA
45s ea	58016-0261-45	125.19		EE
45s ea	58016-0488-45	125.19		AA
50s ea	58016-0261-50	139.10		EE
50s ea	58016-0488-50	139.10		AA
56s ea	58016-0261-56	155.79		EE
56s ea	58016-0488-56	155.79		AA
60s ea	58016-0261-60	219.00		AA
60s ea	58016-0488-60	219.00		AA
62s ea	58016-0261-62	172.48		EE
62s ea	58016-0488-62	172.48		AA
80s ea	58016-0261-80	222.56		AA
80s ea	58016-0488-80	222.56		AA
90s ea	58016-0261-90	328.50		AA
90s ea	58016-0488-90	328.50		AA
100s ea	58016-0261-00	365.00		AA
100s ea	58016-0488-00	365.00		AA
112s ea	58016-0261-92	311.58		EE
112s ea	58016-0488-92	311.58		AA
120s ea	58016-0261-02	438.00		AA
120s ea	58016-0488-02	438.00		AA
150s ea	58016-0261-03	417.30		AA
150s ea	58016-0488-03	417.30		AA
160s ea	58016-0261-71	445.12		AA
180s ea	58016-0261-99	500.76		AA
180s ea	58016-0488-99	500.76		AA
200s ea	58016-0261-89	556.40		AA
200s ea	58016-0488-89	556.40		AA
240s ea	58016-0261-04	667.68		AA
240s ea	58016-0488-04	667.68		AA
300s ea	58016-0261-73	834.60		AA
300s ea	58016-0488-73	834.60		AA

(St. Mary's MPP)
REPACK

PROD/MFR	NDC	AWP	DP	OBC
TAB, PO, 350 mg, 20s ea	60760-0110-20	69.67		AA
30s ea	60760-0110-30	101.51		AA
40s ea	60760-0110-40	133.34		AA
60s ea	60760-0110-60	197.01		AA
90s ea	60760-0110-90	292.52		AA
120s ea	60760-0110-92	388.02		AA

(Stat Rx)
REPACK

PROD/MFR	NDC	AWP	DP	OBC
TAB, PO, 350 mg, 20s ea	16590-0039-20	49.66		AA
28s ea	16590-0039-28	69.44		AA
30s ea	16590-0039-30	74.49		AA
40s ea	16590-0039-40	177.91		AA
45s ea	16590-0039-45	111.74		AA
56s ea	16590-0039-56	139.05		AA
60s ea	16590-0039-60			AA
84s ea	16590-0039-62	208.57		AA
90s ea	16590-0039-90	241.68		AA
120s ea	16590-0039-72	245.00		AA
180s ea	16590-0039-82	446.94		AA

(Vibranta)
REPACK

PROD/MFR	NDC	AWP	DP	OBC
TAB, PO, 350 mg, 7s ea	57866-3435-02	21.00		AA
14s ea	57866-3435-04	26.00		AA
20s ea	57866-3435-03	64.16		AA
30s ea	57866-3435-01	142.50		AA
60s ea	57866-3435-05	262.89		AA
90s ea	57866-3435-06	395.07		
120s ea	57866-3435-08	523.98		

CARISOPRODOL COMPOUND (Consolidated Midland)
aspirin/carisoprodol

PROD/MFR	NDC	AWP	DP	OBC
TAB, PO, 325 mg-200 mg,				
100s ea	00223-0658-01	32.50		EE
500s ea	00223-0658-05	150.00		EE
1000s ea	00223-0658-03	275.00		EE

(Phys Total Care)
REPACK

PROD/MFR	NDC	AWP	DP	OBC
TAB, PO, 325 mg-200 mg,				
30s ea	54868-1826-01	22.71		EE

CARISOPRODOL/ASPIRIN (Physician Partner)
REPACK
aspirin/carisoprodol

PROD/MFR	NDC	AWP	DP	OBC
TAB, PO (FILM-COATED)				
325 mg-200 mg,				
30s ea	21695-0570-30	120.00		

CARISOPRODOL/ASPIRIN/CODEINE (Pharma Pac)
REPACK
aspirin/carisoprodol/codeine phosphate

PROD/MFR	NDC	AWP	DP	OBC
TAB, PO, 325 mg-200 mg-16 mg,				
60s ea, C-III	52959-0868-60	138.30		
90s ea, C-III	52959-0868-90	207.63		
100s ea, C-III	52959-0868-00	230.06		

(Southwood)
REPACK

PROD/MFR	NDC	AWP	DP	OBC
TAB, PO, 325 mg-200 mg-16 mg,				
20s ea, C-III	58016-0199-20	45.00		
30s ea, C-III	58016-0199-30	67.50		
40s ea, C-III	58016-0199-40	90.00		
60s ea, C-III	58016-0199-60	135.00		
90s ea, C-III	58016-0199-90	202.50		
100s ea, C-III	58016-0199-00	225.00		
120s ea, C-III	58016-0199-02	270.00		
150s ea, C-III	58016-0199-03	337.50		
180s ea, C-III	58016-0199-99	405.00		
200s ea, C-III	58016-0199-89	450.00		

CARMINE
(Amend) *See CARMINE #40*
(Medisca) *See CARMINE #40*
(PCCA) *See CARMINE NO.40*
(Spectrum Pharmacy)

PROD/MFR	NDC	AWP	DP	OBC
POW, NA (1X10GM)				
10 gm	49452-1760-01	140.70		
(1X25GM)				
25 gm	49452-1760-02	282.80		

CARMINE #40 (Amend)
carmine

PROD/MFR	NDC	AWP	DP	OBC
POW, NA, 30 gm	17317-0095-02	44.80		

(Medisca)

PROD/MFR	NDC	AWP	DP	OBC
POW, NA, 10 gm	38779-1132-01	91.50		
25 gm	38779-1132-04	195.00		

CARMINE NO.40 (PCCA)
carmine

PROD/MFR	NDC	AWP	DP	OBC
POW, NA, 1 gm	51927-1254-00	9.60		

CARMOL 40 (Doak)
urea

PROD/MFR	NDC	AWP	DP	OBC
CRE, TP, 40%, 28.35 gm	10337-0652-52	102.66		
85 gm	10337-0652-19	159.54		
198.6 gm	10337-0652-49	290.78		
GEL, TP (W/APPLICATOR BRUSH)				
40%, 15 ml	10337-0657-15	282.10		
LOT, TP, 40%, 236.6 ml	10337-0656-51	285.84		

CARMOL HC (Doak)
hydrocortisone acetate/urea

PROD/MFR	NDC	AWP	DP	OBC
CRE, TP, 1%-10%, 85 gm	10337-0550-19	205.10		AT

CARMOL SCALP TREATMENT (Doak)
sulfacetamide sodium/urea

PROD/MFR	NDC	AWP	DP	OBC
KIT, TP (KIT WITH BRUSH)				
10%-10%, ea	10337-0655-01	151.25		

(Doak)
sulfacetamide sodium

PROD/MFR	NDC	AWP	DP	OBC
LOT, TP, 10%, 85 gm	10337-0653-19	131.64		

CARMUSTINE
(B/M Squibb Onc/Vir) *See BICNU*
(Eisai) *See GLIADEL*

CARNATION LIGHT (Amend)
mineral oil

PROD/MFR	NDC	AWP	DP	OBC
OIL, NA, 480 ml	17317-1067-01	4.90		
3840 ml	17317-1067-06	21.00		
19200 ml	17317-1067-08	70.00		

CARNAUBA WAX
(Amend) *See CARNAUBA WAX LIGHT*
(PCCA)

PROD/MFR	NDC	AWP	DP	OBC
POW, NA (NF;YELLOW FLAKES)				
1 gm	51927-1825-00	0.17		

CARNAUBA WAX LIGHT (Amend)
carnauba wax

PROD/MFR	NDC	AWP	DP	OBC
FLA, NA (YELLOW #1)				
454 gm	17317-0753-01	14.70		
2270 gm	17317-0753-05	50.40		
11350 gm	17317-0753-08	227.50		
POW, NA (YELLOW #120)				
454 gm	17317-1220-01	14.70		
2270 gm	17317-1220-05	50.40		
11350 gm	17317-1220-08	227.50		

CARNITINE (Medisca)
levocarnitine

PROD/MFR	NDC	AWP	DP	OBC
POW, NA, 25 gm	38779-0306-04	49.50		
100 gm	38779-0306-05	157.50		
500 gm	38779-0306-08	673.50		

CARNITOR (Sigma-Tau)
levocarnitine

PROD/MFR	NDC	AWP	DP	OBC
SOL, IV (S.D.V.)				
200 mg/ml, 5 ml 5s	54482-0147-01	192.00		AP
PO, 100 mg/ml,				
118 ml	54482-0145-08	34.55		AA
TAB, PO, 330 mg,				
90s ea UD	54482-0144-07	86.96		

CARNITOR SF (Sigma-Tau)
levocarnitine

PROD/MFR	NDC	AWP	DP	OBC
SOL, PO (SF)				
100 mg/ml, 118 ml	54482-0148-01	34.55	34.55	AA

CARNOSINE
(Letco) *See L-CARNOSINE*
(PCCA)

PROD/MFR	NDC	AWP	DP	OBC
POW, NA (L-CARNOSINE)				
1 gm	51927-2795-00	13.80		

CARRAGEENAN (Medisca)

PROD/MFR	NDC	AWP	DP	OBC
POW, NA (1X25GM,IRISH MOSS)				
25 gm	38779-1133-04	111.00		
(1X100GM,IRISH MOSS)				
100 gm	38779-1133-05	297.00		
(1X500GM,IRISH MOSS)				
500 gm	38779-1133-08	1300.50		

(PCCA) *See IRISH MOSS*
(Spectrum Pharmacy)

PROD/MFR	NDC	AWP	DP	OBC
POW, NA (1X500GM)				
500 gm	49452-1782-04	122.15		

CARTEOLOL HCL (Apotex Corp.)
carteolol hydrochloride

PROD/MFR	NDC	AWP	DP	OBC
SOL, OP, 1%, 5 ml	60505-1001-01	21.28		AT
10 ml	60505-1001-02	40.10		AT
15 ml	60505-1001-03	55.59		AT

(Bausch & Lomb Inc.)

PROD/MFR	NDC	AWP	DP	OBC
SOL, OP, 1%, 5 ml	24208-0367-05	19.64		AT
10 ml	24208-0367-10	37.07		AT
15 ml	24208-0367-15	55.60		AT

(Falcon Ophthalmics)

PROD/MFR	NDC	AWP	DP	OBC
SOL, OP, 1%, 5 ml	61314-0238-05	21.28		AT
10 ml	61314-0238-10	40.10		AT
15 ml	61314-0238-15	57.25		AT

CARTEOLOL HYDROCHLORIDE
FUL

PROD/MFR	NDC	AWP	DP	OBC
SOL, OP, 1%, 10 ml		36.68		

(Apotex Corp.) *See CARTEOLOL HCL*
(Bausch & Lomb Inc.) *See CARTEOLOL HCL*
(Falcon Ophthalmics) *See CARTEOLOL HCL*

CARTIA XT (Watson)
diltiazem hydrochloride

PROD/MFR	NDC	AWP	DP	OBC
C24, PO, 120 mg, 90s ea	62037-0597-90	83.66		AB3
500s ea	62037-0597-05	464.80		AB3
180 mg, 90s ea	62037-0598-90	100.99		AB3
500s ea	62037-0598-05	561.07		AB3
240 mg, 90s ea	62037-0599-90	143.27		AB3
500s ea	62037-0599-05	795.94		AB3
300 mg, 90s ea	62037-0600-90	185.68		AB3
500s ea	62037-0600-05	1031.53		AB3

(Phys Total Care)
REPACK

PROD/MFR	NDC	AWP	DP	OBC
C24, PO, 180 mg, 30s ea	54868-5150-00	49.95		AB3
240 mg, 30s ea	54868-5316-00	70.35		AB3

PROD/MFR	NDC	AWP	DP	OBC
CARTICEL (Genzyme)				
chondrocytes, autologous cultured				
IMP, IP (APPR 12 MIL CELLS/0.4ML)				
ea	**63861-1025-01**	30654.00	25545.00	
CARVEDILOL				
FUL				
TAB, PO, 3.125 mg, 100s ea		14.25		
6.25 mg, 100s ea		14.25		
12.5 mg, 100s ea		14.25		
25 mg, 100s ea		14.25		
(Actavis)				
TAB, PO (FILM-COATED)				
3.125 mg, 100s ea	**00228-2175-11**	213.45		**AB**
6.25 mg, 100s ea	**00228-2176-11**	213.45		**AB**
12.5 mg, 100s ea	**00228-2177-11**	213.45		**AB**
25 mg, 100s ea	**00228-2178-11**	213.45		**AB**
(Apotex Corp.)				
TAB, PO (FILM-COATED)				
3.125 mg, 100s ea	**60505-2606-01**	213.66		**AB**
1000s ea	**60505-2606-08**	2136.60		**AB**
6.25 mg, 100s ea	**60505-2607-01**	213.60		**AB**
1000s ea	**60505-2607-08**	2136.60		**AB**
12.5 mg, 100s ea	**60505-2608-01**	213.66		**AB**
1000s ea	**60505-2608-08**	2136.60		**AB**
25 mg, 100s ea	**60505-2609-01**	213.66		**AB**
1000s ea	**60505-2609-08**	2136.60		**AB**
(Aurobindo Pharma)				
TAB, PO (FILM-COATED)				
3.125 mg, 100s ea	**65862-0142-01**	194.87		**AB**
6.25 mg, 100s ea	**65862-0143-01**	194.87		**AB**
12.5 mg, 100s ea	**65862-0144-01**	194.87		**AB**
25 mg, 100s ea	**65862-0145-01**	194.87		**AB**
(Caraco)				
TAB, PO (FILM-COATED)				
3.125 mg, 100s ea	**57664-0242-88**	211.31		**AB**
500s ea	**57664-0242-13**	1056.56		**AB**
1000s ea	**57664-0242-18**	2113.13		**AB**
6.25 mg, 100s ea	**57664-0244-88**	211.31		**AB**
500s ea	**57664-0244-13**	1056.56		**AB**
1000s ea	**57664-0244-18**	2113.13		**AB**
12.5 mg, 100s ea	**57664-0245-88**	211.31		**AB**
500s ea	**57664-0245-13**	1056.56		**AB**
1000s ea	**57664-0245-18**	2113.13		**AB**
25 mg, 100s ea	**57664-0247-88**	211.31		**AB**
500s ea	**57664-0247-13**	1056.56		**AB**
1000s ea	**57664-0247-18**	2113.13		**AB**
(Dr Reddy's)				
TAB, PO (FILM-COATED)				
3.125 mg, 100s ea	**55111-0252-01**	213.45		**AB**
500s ea	**55111-0252-05**	1067.25		**AB**
6.25 mg, 100s ea	**55111-0253-01**	213.45		**AB**
500s ea	**55111-0253-05**	1067.25		**AB**
12.5 mg, 100s ea	**55111-0254-01**	213.45		**AB**
500s ea	**55111-0254-05**	1067.25		**AB**
25 mg, 100s ea	**55111-0255-01**	213.45		**AB**
500s ea	**55111-0255-05**	1067.25		**AB**
(Glaxo) *See COREG*				
(Glenmark Pharmaceuticals)				
TAB, PO (FILM COATED)				
3.125 mg, 100s ea	**68462-0162-01**	210.13		**AB**
500s ea	**68462-0162-05**	1050.50		**AB**
6.25 mg, 100s ea	**68462-0163-01**	210.13		**AB**
500s ea	**68462-0163-05**	1050.50		**AB**
12.5 mg, 100s ea	**68462-0164-01**	210.13		**AB**
500s ea	**68462-0164-05**	1050.50		**AB**
25 mg, 100s ea	**68462-0165-01**	210.13		**AB**
500s ea	**68462-0165-05**	1050.50		**AB**
(Major)				
TAB, PO (10X10,FILM-COATED)				
3.125 mg, 100s ea UD	**00904-5870-61**	202.73		**AB**
6.25 mg, 100s ea UD	**00904-5871-61**	202.73		**AB**
12.5 mg, 100s ea UD	**00904-5872-61**	202.73		**AB**
25 mg, 100s ea UD	**00904-5873-61**	202.73		**AB**
(Mylan)				
TAB, PO (FILM-COATED)				
3.125 mg, 100s ea	**00378-3631-01**	213.40		**AB**
500s ea	**00378-3631-05**	1067.00		**AB**
6.25 mg, 100s ea	**00378-3632-01**	213.40		**AB**
500s ea	**00378-3632-05**	1067.00		**AB**
12.5 mg, 100s ea	**00378-3633-01**	213.40		**AB**
500s ea	**00378-3633-05**	1067.00		**AB**
25 mg, 100s ea	**00378-3634-01**	213.40		**AB**
500s ea	**00378-3634-05**	1067.00		**AB**
(Sandoz)				
TAB, PO (FILM-COATED)				
3.125 mg, 100s ea	**00781-5221-01**	213.69		**AB**
6.25 mg, 100s ea	**00781-5222-01**	213.69		**AB**
12.5 mg, 100s ea	**00781-5223-01**	213.69		**AB**
25 mg, 100s ea	**00781-5224-01**	213.69		**AB**
(Teva)				
TAB, PO (FILM-COATED)				
3.125 mg, 100s ea	**00093-0051-01**	213.69		**AB**
500s ea	**00093-0051-05**	1041.74		**AB**
6.25 mg, 100s ea	**00093-0135-01**	213.69		**AB**
500s ea	**00093-0135-05**	1041.74		**AB**
12.5 mg, 100s ea	**00093-7295-01**	213.69		**AB**
500s ea	**00093-7295-05**	1041.74		**AB**
25 mg, 100s ea	**00093-7296-01**	213.69		**AB**
500s ea	**00093-7296-05**	1041.74		**AB**
(UDL)				
TAB, PO (FILM-COATED)				
3.125 mg, 25s ea UD	**51079-0771-19**	53.35		**AB**
(10X10,FILM-COATED)				
3.125 mg, 100s ea UD	**51079-0771-20**	213.40		**AB**
(ROBOT READY 25X1)				
6.25 mg, 25s ea UD	**51079-0930-19**	53.35		**AB**
(10X10,FILM-COATED)				
6.25 mg, 100s ea UD	**51079-0930-20**	213.40		**AB**
(ROBOT READY 25X1)				
12.5 mg, 25s ea UD	**51079-0931-19**	53.35		**AB**
(10X10,FILM-COATED)				
12.5 mg, 100s ea UD	**51079-0931-20**	213.40		**AB**
(FILM-COATED)				
25 mg, 100s ea UD	**51079-0932-20**	213.40		**AB**
(Zydus Pharm.)				
TAB, PO (FILM-COATED)				
3.125 mg, 100s ea	**68382-0092-01**	213.69		**EE**
500s ea	**68382-0092-05**	1068.44		**EE**
6.25 mg, 100s ea	**68382-0093-01**	213.69		**EE**
500s ea	**68382-0093-05**	1068.44		**EE**
12.5 mg, 100s ea	**68382-0094-01**	213.69		**EE**
500s ea	**68382-0094-05**	1068.44		**EE**
25 mg, 100s ea	**68382-0095-01**	213.69		**EE**
500s ea	**68382-0095-05**	1068.44		**EE**
(A-S Medication)				
REPACK				
TAB, PO, 3.125 mg, 60s ea	**54569-5974-00**	128.21		
6.25 mg, 60s ea	**54569-5975-00**	128.21		
12.5 mg, 60s ea	**54569-5976-00**	128.21		
25 mg, 60s ea	**54569-5977-00**	128.41		
(American Health)				
REPACK				
TAB, PO (10X10,FILM-COATED)				
3.125 mg, 100s ea UD	**68084-0261-01**	194.93		**EE**
6.25 mg, 100s ea UD	**68084-0262-01**	194.93		**EE**
12.5 mg, 100s ea UD	**68084-0263-01**	194.93		**EE**
25 mg, 100s ea UD	**68084-0264-01**	194.93		**EE**
(Dispensing Solutions)				
REPACK				
TAB, PO (FILM-COATED)				
3.125 mg, 30s ea	**55045-3867-08**	63.90		**AB**
100s ea	**55045-3867-01**	213.00		**AB**
6.25 mg, 30s ea	**66336-0808-30**	63.17		
(FILM-COATED)				
6.25 mg, 30s ea	**55045-3868-08**	63.90		**AB**
60s ea	**66336-0808-60**	126.34		**AB**
100s ea	**55045-3868-01**	213.00		**AB**
12.5 mg, 30s ea	**66336-0772-30**	63.17		
(FILM-COATED)				
12.5 mg, 30s ea	**55045-3869-08**	63.90		**AB**
100s ea	**55045-3869-01**	213.00		**AB**
25 mg, 30s ea	**66336-0837-30**	63.17		
(FILM-COATED)				
25 mg, 30s ea	**55045-3870-08**	63.90		**AB**
100s ea	**55045-3870-01**	213.00		**AB**
(Palmetto)				
REPACK				
TAB, PO, 3.125 mg, 30s ea	**23490-9369-03**	176.29		
60s ea	**23490-9369-06**	352.59		
6.25 mg, 30s ea	**23490-9370-03**	176.29		
60s ea	**23490-9370-06**	352.59		
12.5 mg, 30s ea	**23490-9371-03**	176.29		
60s ea	**23490-9371-06**	352.59		
25 mg, 30s ea	**23490-9372-03**	176.90		
60s ea	**23490-9372-06**	352.59		
(PD-Rx Pharm)				
REPACK				
TAB, PO (FILM-COATED)				
3.125 mg, 180s ea	**43063-0126-93**	178.00		**AB**
6.25 mg, 180s ea	**43063-0127-93**	178.00		**AB**
12.5 mg, 180s ea	**43063-0125-93**	178.00		**AB**
25 mg, 180s ea	**43063-0129-93**	178.00		**AB**
(Phys Total Care)				
REPACK				
TAB, PO, 3.125 mg, 30s ea	**54868-1980-00**	11.63		
60s ea	**54868-1980-01**	18.76		
6.25 mg, 30s ea	**54868-3062-00**	11.63		
60s ea	**54868-3062-01**	18.90		
(FILM-COATED)				
6.25 mg, 90s ea	**54868-3062-02**	24.85		**EE**
12.5 mg, 30s ea	**54868-5773-01**	11.40		**AB**
60s ea	**54868-5773-00**	18.35		
(FILM-COATED)				
12.5 mg, 90s ea	**54868-5773-02**	20.21		**AB**
180s ea	**54868-5773-03**	40.98		**AB**
25 mg, 30s ea	**54868-5817-01**	11.66		**AB**
60s ea	**54868-5817-00**	18.76		
(Physician Partner)				
REPACK				
TAB, PO, 3.125 mg, 60s ea	**21695-0645-60**	256.39		
6.25 mg, 60s ea	**21695-0646-60**	256.39		
(FILM-COATED)				
12.5 mg, 60s ea	**21695-0647-60**	256.39		**AB**
25 mg, 60s ea	**21695-0648-60**	256.39		**AB**
(Quality Care Prod)				
REPACK				
TAB, PO (FILM-COATED)				
3.125 mg, 30s ea	**35356-0513-30**	63.90		**EE**
6.25 mg, 30s ea	**35356-0512-30**	63.90		**EE**
25 mg, 100s ea	**35356-0526-00**	62.30		**EE**
(Stat Rx)				
REPACK				
TAB, PO (FILM-COATED)				
25 mg, 30s ea	**16590-0533-30**	35.50		**AB**
60s ea	**16590-0533-60**	56.00		**AB**
90s ea	**16590-0533-90**	77.00		**AB**
120s ea	**16590-0533-72**	85.00		**AB**
(Vibranta)				
REPACK				
TAB, PO (FILM-COATED)				
6.25 mg, 60s ea	**57866-2607-02**	10.91		**AB**
12.5 mg, 60s ea	**57866-2608-02**	10.91		**AB**
25 mg, 60s ea	**57866-7067-01**	65.00		
180s ea	**57866-7067-02**	84.84		
CARVEDILOL PHOSPHATE				
(Glaxo) *See COREG CR*				
CASCARA SAGRADA				
(Medisca) *See CASCARA SAGRADA FLUIDEXTRACT*				
(PCCA) *See CASCARA SAGRADA EXTRACT*				
CASCARA SAGRADA EXTRACT (PCCA)				
cascara sagrada				
POW, NA (1:3)				
1 gm	**51927-3318-00**	0.54		
CASCARA SAGRADA FLUIDEXTRACT (Medisca)				
cascara sagrada				
LIQ, NA (1X100ML;USP)				
100 ml	**38779-1134-05**	38.00		
(1X500ML,USP)				
500 ml	**38779-1134-08**	105.00		
CASEIN				
(PCCA) *See SOYABEAN CASEIN DIGEST MEDIUM*				
CASHEW NUT OIL (PCCA)				
alfadex				
POW, NA, 1 gm	**51927-3113-00**	0.75		
CASODEX (AstraZeneca)				
bicalutamide				
TAB, PO (FILM-COATED)				
50 mg, 30s ea	**00310-0705-30**	593.92		
100s ea	**00310-0705-10**	1979.80		
(A-S Medication)				
REPACK				
TAB, PO (FILM-COATED)				
50 mg, 30s ea	**54569-5859-00**	772.10		
(Phys Total Care)				
REPACK				
TAB, PO, 50 mg, 30s ea	**54868-4503-00**	682.33		
CASPOFUNGIN ACETATE				
(Merck) *See CANCIDAS*				
CASTILE SOAP (PCCA)				
POW, NA, 1 gm	**51927-2801-00**	0.20		
CASTOR (Medisca)				
castor oil				
OIL, NA (1X500ML,USP)				
500 ml	**38779-0910-08**	31.50		
(1X4000ML,USP)				
4000 ml	**38779-0910-01**	160.50		

PROD/MFR	NDC	AWP	DP	OBC
CASTOR OIL				
(Amend) *See CASTOR OIL ODORLESS*				
(Gallipot)				
OIL, NA (U.S.P.)				
59.14 ml	**51552-0414-03**	2.52		
118.28 ml	**51552-0414-04**	3.71		
473 ml	**51552-0414-06**	12.88		
3785 ml	**51552-0414-08**	74.97		
18925 ml	**51552-0414-09**	209.72		
(Letco)				
OIL, NA, 500 ml	**62991-1225-01**	36.00		
3840 ml	**62991-1225-02**	150.00		
(Lorann Oil)				
OIL, NA (U.S.P.)				
120 ml	**23535-0902-08**	2.00		
480 ml	**23535-0902-01**	5.00		
3840 ml	**23535-0902-11**	20.00		
(Medisca) *See CASTOR*				
(PCCA) *See CASTOR OIL, SULFATED*				
(PCCA)				
OIL, NA (USP)				
1 ml	**51927-2866-00**	0.12		
(PCCA) *See PEG-40 CASTOR*				
(Spectrum Pharmacy) *See CASTOR OIL SULFONATED*				
(Spectrum Pharmacy)				
OIL, NA (U.S.P.)				
500 ml	**49452-1830-01**	98.35		
4000 ml	**49452-1830-02**	283.85		
20000 ml	**49452-1830-03**	938.00		
CASTOR OIL ODORLESS (Amend)				
castor oil				
OIL, NA (TASTELESS, U.S.P.)				
500 ml	**17317-0100-01**	4.20		
3840 ml	**17317-0100-06**	35.00		
19200 ml	**17317-0100-08**	126.00		
CASTOR OIL SULFONATED (Spectrum Pharmacy)				
castor oil				
OIL, NA, 500 ml	**49452-1840-01**	98.35		
4000 ml	**49452-1840-02**	381.50		
20000 ml	**49452-1840-03**	1120.00		
CASTOR OIL, SULFATED (PCCA)				
castor oil				
OIL, NA (TURKEY RED OIL,1X1ML)				
1 ml	**51927-2504-00**	0.12		
CASTOR OIL/PERU BALSAM/TRYPSIN				
(Breckenridge Pharm) *See TRYPSIN COMPLEX*				
(Delta Pharm) *See TBC*				
(Healthpoint) *See XENADERM*				
(Onset) *See OPTASE*				
(Prasco Labs) *See REVINA*				
(UDL) *See GRANULEX*				
CAT HAIR EXTRACT				
(Alk-Abello) *See SQ CAT HAIR*				
CAT-PAK (E-Z-EM)				
barium sulfate				
SUS, NA (1X400ML)				
1.3%, 400 ml	**32909-0410-01**	82.30	68.58	
CAT'S CLAW (PCCA)				
POW, NA (1X1GM)				
1 gm	**51927-2992-00**	0.23		
CAT'S CLAW EXTRACT (Gallipot)				
POW, NA (3% EXTRACT)				
1000 gm	**51552-0996-07**	126.00	90.00	
CATAFLAM (Novartis Pharm)				
diclofenac potassium				
TAB, PO, 50 mg, 100s ea	**00078-0436-05**	439.74		AB
(Pharma Pac)				
REPACK				
TAB, PO, 50 mg, 20s ea	**52959-0344-20**	47.43		AB
21s ea	**52959-0344-21**	49.80		AB
30s ea	**52959-0344-30**	63.80		AB
(Phys Total Care)				
REPACK				
TAB, PO, 50 mg, 20s ea	**54868-3199-02**	63.30		AB
25s ea	**54868-3199-00**	80.36		AB
30s ea	**54868-3199-01**	96.06		AB
CATAPRES (Boehr Ingelheim Phar)				
clonidine hydrochloride				
TAB, PO, 0.1 mg, 100s ea	**00597-0006-01**	152.00		AB
0.2 mg, 100s ea	**00597-0007-01**	232.55		AB
0.3 mg, 100s ea	**00597-0011-01**	291.82		AB

PROD/MFR	NDC	AWP	DP	OBC
(Phys Total Care)				
REPACK				
TAB, PO, 0.1 mg, 30s ea	**54868-0535-00**	36.33		AB
0.2 mg, 30s ea	**54868-0931-00**	41.08		AB
CATAPRES TTS-3 (Stat Rx)				
REPACK				
clonidine				
TDM, TD, 0.3 mg/24 hr,				
30s ea	**16590-0476-30**	140.50		
CATAPRES-TTS-1 (Boehr Ingelheim Phar)				
clonidine				
TDM, TD, 0.1 mg/24 hr,				
4s ea	**00597-0031-34**	135.20		EE
(Phys Total Care)				
REPACK				
TDM, TD, 0.1 mg/24 hr,				
4s ea	**54868-0537-01**	124.12		
(Physician Partner)				
REPACK				
TDM, TD, 0.1 mg/24 hr,				
4s ea	**21695-0567-04**	194.16		EE
(Stat Rx)				
REPACK				
TDM, TD, 0.1 mg/24 hr,				
4s ea	**16590-0477-04**	68.00		
12s ea	**16590-0477-12**	136.00		
CATAPRES-TTS-2 (Boehr Ingelheim Phar)				
clonidine				
TDM, TD (ADHESIVECOVERS,7(CM)2)				
0.2 mg/24 hr,				
4s ea	**00597-0032-34**	227.64		EE
(Pharma Pac)				
REPACK				
TDM, TD, 0.2 mg/24 hr,				
12s ea	**52959-0679-12**	225.25		
(Phys Total Care)				
REPACK				
TDM, TD, 0.2 mg/24 hr,				
4s ea	**54868-0532-01**	73.06		
CATAPRES-TTS-3 (Boehr Ingelheim Phar)				
clonidine				
TDM, TD, 0.3 mg/24 hr,				
4s ea	**00597-0033-34**	315.79		
(Phys Total Care)				
REPACK				
TDM, TD, 0.3 mg/24 hr,				
4s ea	**54868-0533-00**	341.80		
CATECHIN				
(PCCA) *See CATECHIN (+)*				
CATECHIN (+) (PCCA)				
catechin				
POW, NA (1X1GM)				
1 gm	**51927-3584-00**	375.00		
CATHETER				
(Abbott Hosp) *See ABBOCATH-T*				
(Abbott Hosp) *See CLEAR-CATH*				
(Abbott Hosp) *See INPERSOL ADMINISTRATION SET*				
(Arkray) *See INSUFLON*				
(Coloplast) *See CONVEEN INTERMITTENT CATHETER*				
(Coloplast) *See CONVEEN SECURITY + CATHETER & LINER*				
(Coloplast) *See CONVEEN SECURITY + SELF SEALING*				
(Coloplast) *See CONVEEN SELF SEALING URISHEATH*				
(Coloplast) *See CONVEEN ULTRA SECURE SELF-SEALING*				
(Coloplast) *See CONVEEN URISHEATH/URILINER*				
(J&J Medical) *See CATHLON CLEAR IV CATHETER/FEP*				
(J&J Medical) *See CATHLON IV CATHETER/FEP*				
(J&J Medical) *See CATHLON STRIPED IV CATHETER/FEP*				
(J&J Medical) *See JELCO IV CATHETER/FEP*				
(J&J Medical) *See JELCO STRIPED IV CATHETER/FEP*				
(J&J Medical) *See JELCO WINGED IV CATHETER/FEP*				
(J&J Medical) *See OPTIVA IV CATHETER/OCR*				
(J&J Medical) *See PROTECTIV IV CATHETER/ SAFETY SYSTEM*				

PROD/MFR	NDC	AWP	DP	OBC
(J&J Medical) *See PROTECTIV PLUS IV CATH SAFETY SYST*				
(Medtronic Minimed) *See SILHOUETTE CATHETER/ TUBING INFUSION*				
(Mentor) *See ACTIVE CATH SELF-ADHERING*				
(Mentor) *See CLEAR ADVANTAGE SELF-ADHERING*				
(Mentor) *See FREEDOM CATH SELF-ADHERING*				
(Mentor) *See FREEDOM CLEAR SELF-ADHERING*				
(Mentor) *See GIZMO*				
(Mentor) *See SELF-CATH FEMALE SPECIMEN*				
(Mentor) *See SELF-CATH SOFT/STRAIGHT TIP*				
(Mentor) *See SELF-CATH STRAIGHT TIP/FEMALE*				
(Mentor) *See SELF-CATH STRAIGHT TIP/FUNNEL END*				
(Mentor) *See URO-SAN PLUS*				
(Portex) *See EPIDURAL CATHETER*				
(Portex) *See EPIDURAL CATHETER W/STYLET*				
CATHETER SUPPLIES				
(Covidien) *See PRECISION 200 URINE METER*				
(Covidien) *See PRECISION 400 ADD-A-FOLEY CATHETER TRAY*				
(Covidien) *See PRECISION 400 URINE METER CATHETERIZATION TRAY*				
(Covidien) *See PRECISION 400 URINE METER CATHETERIZATION TRAY WITH TEMPERATURE SENSOR*				
(Covidien) *See PRECISION ADD-A-FOLEY CATHETER TRAY*				
CATHETER, CENTRAL VENOUS				
(J&J Medical) *See BIOVUE MIDLINE PROCEDURE*				
(J&J Medical) *See BIOVUE MIDLINE STARTER*				
CATHETER, CENTRAL VENOUS, PERIPHERAL INSERTION				
(Becton Dickinson) *See ANGIO SET IV*				
(J&J Medical) *See BIOVUE LONG-TERM PICC PROCEDURE*				
(J&J Medical) *See BIOVUE PICC PROCEDURE*				
(J&J Medical) *See BIOVUE PICC STARTER*				
(J&J Medical) *See PROTECTIVE SAFETY INTRODUCER SYSTEM*				
CATHETER, INTRAVENOUS				
(Becton Dickinson) *See INSYTE AUTO GUARD IV*				
(Becton Dickinson) *See INSYTE-W IV*				
CATHFLO ACTIVASE (Genentech)				
alteplase, recombinant				
PDS, IV (INNER)				
2 mg, ea	**50242-0041-63**	98.24		
(VIAL)				
2 mg, ea	**50242-0041-64**	106.33		
CATHLON CLEAR IV CATHETER/FEP (J&J Medical)				
catheter				
DEV, NA (METAL HUB,14X1 1/4")				
ea	**56091-0044-18**	1.37		
(METAL HUB,14X2 1/4")				
ea	**56091-0044-28**	1.37		
(METAL HUB,16X1 1/4")				
ea	**56091-0044-12**	1.37		
(METAL HUB,16X2 1/4")				
ea	**56091-0044-22**	1.37		
(METAL HUB,18X1 1/4")				
ea	**56091-0044-25**	1.37		
(METAL HUB,18X1 3/4")				
ea	**56091-0044-24**	1.37		
(METAL HUB,20X1 1/4")				
ea	**56091-0044-26**	1.37		
(METAL HUB,20X1")				
ea	**56091-0044-27**	1.37		
(METAL HUB,RO,14X1 1/4")				
ea	**56091-0044-48**	1.37		
(METAL HUB,RO,16X1 1/4")				
ea	**56091-0044-42**	1.37		
CATHLON IV CATHETER/FEP (J&J Medical)				
catheter				
DEV, NA (METAL HUB,RO,14X2 1/4")				
ea	**56091-0044-58**	1.37		
(METAL HUB,RO,16X2 1/4")				
ea	**56091-0044-52**	1.37		
(METAL HUB,RO,18X1 1/4")				
ea	**56091-0044-55**	1.37		
(METAL HUB,RO,18X1 3/4")				
ea	**56091-0044-54**	1.37		

PROD/MFR	NDC	AWP	DP	OBC
(METAL HUB,RO,20X1 1/4")				
ea	56091-0044-56	1.37		
(METAL HUB,RO,20X1")				
ea	56091-0044-57	1.37		
CATHLON STRIPED IV CATHETER/FEP (J&J Medical)				
catheter				
DEV, NA (METAL HUB,R-0,14X2 1/4")				
ea	56091-0044-68	1.50		
(METAL HUB,R-0,16X2 1/4")				
ea	56091-0044-62	1.50		
(METAL HUB,R-0,18X1 1/4")				
ea	56091-0044-65	1.50		
(METAL HUB,R-0,18X1 3/4")				
ea	56091-0044-64	1.50		
(METAL HUB,R-0,20X1 1/4")				
ea	56091-0044-66	1.50		
(METAL HUB,R-0,20X1")				
ea	56091-0044-67	1.50		
(METAL HUB,R-0,22X1")				
ea	56091-0044-61	1.57		
CATNIP (Medisca)				
OIL, NA (1X25ML)				
25 ml	38779-1136-04	28.50		
(1X100ML)				
100 ml	38779-1136-05	58.50		
(1X500ML)				
500 ml	38779-1136-08	208.50		
(PCCA)				
OIL, NA, 1 gm	51927-1609-00	0.72		
CAUDAL ANESTHESIA TRAY (Portex)				
epinephrine/lidocaine hydrochloride				
KIT, EP (CONTINUOUS,18G QUINCKE)				
1:200000-1.5%,				
10s ea	00074-4808-20	480.70	404.80	
CAVAN ONE OMEGA (Seton)				
prenatal vitamins				
SGL, PO (SOFTGEL)				
30s ea	13925-0080-30	43.32		
CAVAN PRENATAL TAB WITH EC CALCIUM (Seton)				
prenatal vitamins				
TAB, PO (COATED TABLET)				
90s ea	13925-0106-90	126.66		
CAVAN-EC SOD DHA (Seton)				
prenatal vitamins				
KIT, PO (ENTERIC-COATED,SOFTGEL)				
60s ea	13925-0122-60	45.04		
CAVERJECT (Pfizer)				
alprostadil				
PDS, IC (VIAL)				
10 mcg, 6s ea	00009-3778-05	140.53		AP
20 mcg, 6s ea	00009-3701-05	261.59	217.99	AP
40 mcg, 6s ea	00009-7686-04	328.63	273.86	AP
SOL, IC (SYSTEM)				
0.02 mg/ml,				
2 ml 5s	00009-7650-02	198.24	165.20	
CAVERJECT IMPULSE (Pfizer)				
alprostadil				
PDS, IC (SYSTEM)				
10 mcg, 2s ea	00009-5181-01	72.46	60.38	AP
20 mcg, 2s ea	00009-5182-01	93.31	77.76	AP
(Phys Total Care)				
REPACK				
PDS, IC, 20 mcg, 2s ea	54868-4890-00	79.19		AP
CAVIRINSE (Omnii Intl)				
sodium fluoride				
SOL, PO (AF,MINT)				
0.2%, 240 ml	48878-3223-08	7.50		
CAYENNE (PCCA)				
POW, NA (90,000 HU)				
1 gm	51927-2965-00	0.23		
CAYSTON (Gilead Sciences)				
aztreonam				
PDS, IH (28-DAY KIT, W/DILUENTS)				
75 mg/vial, ea	61958-0901-01	5312.40		
CAZIANT (Watson)				
desogestrel/ethinyl estradiol				
TAB, PO, ea	52544-0959-31	87.20		
CEA-SCAN (Immunomedics, Inc.)				
arcitumomab				
PDS, IV (VIAL)				
1.25 mg, ea	55135-0007-10	1300.00	1025.00	
CEBOCAP (Forest Pharm)				
placebo				
CAP, PO (#1)				
100s ea	00456-0707-01	36.24		
(Phys Total Care)				
REPACK				
CAP, PO (#1)				
100s ea	54868-3634-00	35.87		
(#3)				
100s ea	54868-3635-00	35.87		
CECLOR (Pharma Pac)				
REPACK				
cefaclor				
PDR, PO, 250 mg/5 ml,				
150 ml	52959-0277-02	67.50		AB
(Phys Total Care)				
REPACK				
PDR, PO, 125 mg/5 ml,				
150 ml	54868-5057-01	38.09		AB
250 mg/5 ml,				
150 ml	54868-0314-01	70.22		AB
CECLOR PULVULES (Pharma Pac)				
REPACK				
cefaclor				
CAP, PO, 250 mg, 30s ea	52959-0027-30	98.27		AB
(Phys Total Care)				
REPACK				
CAP, PO, 250 mg, 15s ea	54868-0315-05	8.60		AB
30s ea	54868-0315-01	15.33		AB
500 mg, 30s ea	54868-0472-01	162.58		AB
CEDAR LEAF (PCCA)				
thuja oil				
OIL, NA (FCC)				
1 ml	51927-2473-00	1.40		
CEDAR LEAF OIL (Spectrum Pharmacy)				
thuja oil				
OIL, NA (F.C.C.)				
125 ml	49452-1845-03	171.85		
500 ml	49452-1845-04	605.50		
CEDARLEAF OIL (Amend)				
thuja oil				
OIL, NA, 120 ml	17317-0242-04	19.60		
500 ml	17317-0242-01	70.00		
CEDARWOOD OIL (Amend)				
OIL, NA, 120 ml	17317-0243-04	8.40		
500 ml	17317-0243-01	18.20		
16800 ml	17317-0243-09	318.50		
(Lorann Oil)				
OIL, NA, 9.9 ml	23535-0151-12	2.20		
(PCCA)				
OIL, NA (TEXAS)				
1 ml	51927-2026-00	0.42		
CEDAX (Shionogi)				
ceftibuten				
CAP, PO, 400 mg, 20s ea	45809-0401-20	316.19		
PDR, PO, 90 mg/5 ml,				
30 ml	45809-0801-30	37.80		
(CHERRY)				
90 mg/5 ml, 60 ml	45809-0801-60	79.91		
90 ml	45809-0801-90	127.64		
(1X120ML,CHERRY)				
90 mg/5 ml, 120 ml	45809-0801-12	161.10		
CEENU (B/M Squibb Onc/Vir)				
lomustine				
CAP, PO, 10 mg, 20s ea	00015-3030-20	211.74		
40 mg, 20s ea	00015-3031-20	637.63		
100 mg, 20s ea	00015-3032-20	1212.13		
CEFACLOR (Alvogen)				
CAP, PO (USP,HARD GELATIN)				
250 mg, 30s ea	47781-0266-03	59.69		AB
500 mg, 30s ea	47781-0267-03	116.85		AB
(Carlsbad Tech)				
CAP, PO (USP,HARD GELATIN)				
250 mg, 30s ea	61442-0171-30	59.67		AB
500 mg, 30s ea	61442-0172-30	116.84		AB
(Ranbaxy Pharm)				
CAP, PO, 250 mg, 100s ea	63304-0658-01	198.95		AB
500 mg, 100s ea	63304-0659-01	389.50		AB
PDR, PO, 125 mg/5 ml,				
75 ml	63304-0954-01	14.14		AB
150 ml	63304-0954-02	28.28		AB
250 mg/5 ml, 75 ml	63304-0956-01	28.24		AB
150 ml	63304-0956-02	51.80		AB
375 mg/5 ml, 50 ml	63304-0957-03	26.38		AB
100 ml	63304-0957-04	51.80		AB
(Teva)				
CAP, PO, 250 mg, 100s ea	00172-4770-60	198.90		AB
500 mg, 100s ea	00172-4771-60	389.45		AB
PDR, PO (BERRY)				
125 mg/5 ml, 50 ml	00172-4775-20	28.24		AB
75 ml	00172-4772-22	14.13		AB
150 ml	00172-4772-23	28.28		AB
187 mg/5 ml, 100 ml	00172-4773-21	28.28		AB
250 mg/5 ml, 75 ml	00172-4774-22	28.24		AB
150 ml	00172-4774-23	51.21		AB
375 mg/5 ml, 100 ml	00172-4775-21	51.21		AB
TER, PO, 500 mg, 100s ea	00093-1087-01	379.30		AB
(A-S Medication)				
REPACK				
CAP, PO, 250 mg, 30s ea	54569-3901-00	59.69		EE
500 mg, 30s ea	54569-3902-00	116.85		EE
PDR, PO, 125 mg/5 ml,				
150 ml	54569-4241-00	28.28		EE
250 mg/5 ml, 150 ml	54569-3904-00	51.80		EE
(Aidarex)				
REPACK				
CAP, PO, 500 mg, 7s ea	33261-0168-07	31.50		
14s ea	33261-0168-14	63.00		
21s ea	33261-0168-21	94.50		
28s ea	33261-0168-28	126.00		
30s ea	33261-0168-30	135.00		
42s ea	33261-0168-42	189.00		AB
60s ea	33261-0168-60	270.00		
(Altura)				
REPACK				
CAP, PO, 250 mg, 21s ea	63874-0119-21	70.44		EE
30s ea	63874-0119-30	100.26		EE
100s ea	63874-0119-01	335.43		EE
500 mg, 12s ea	63874-0120-12	53.62		EE
20s ea	63874-0120-20	98.37		EE
30s ea	63874-0120-30	139.40		EE
100s ea	63874-0120-01	439.47		EE
PDR, PO, 125 mg/5 ml,				
75 ml	63874-0151-75	20.24		EE
150 ml	63874-0151-15	36.18		EE
187 mg/5 ml, 50 ml	63874-0152-50	21.21		EE
100 ml	63874-0152-10	41.28		EE
250 mg/5 ml, 75 ml	63874-0153-75	35.97		EE
150 ml	63874-0153-15	67.13		EE
(Bryant Ranch)				
REPACK				
CAP, PO, 250 mg, 15s ea	63629-1305-02	41.78		
20s ea	63629-1305-03	55.71		
30s ea	63629-1305-01	83.56		
500 mg, 14s ea	63629-1320-04	76.34		
20s ea	63629-1320-02	109.06		
21s ea	63629-1320-01	114.51		
30s ea	63629-1320-03	163.59		
(Core)				
REPACK				
CAP, PO, 250 mg, 20s ea	33358-0065-20	57.10		
30s ea	33358-0065-30	85.65		
500 mg, 20s ea	33358-0066-20	111.79		
30s ea	33358-0066-30	167.68		
(Dispensing Solutions)				
REPACK				
CAP, PO, 250 mg, 15s ea	55045-2154-07	30.75		
21s ea	55045-2154-09	43.00		AB
30s ea	55045-2154-08	61.50		
30s ea	66336-0202-30	71.62		AB
500 mg, 15s ea	55045-2337-01	63.30		
15s ea	55045-2337-07	84.40		AB
20s ea	66336-0454-20	93.88		AB
28s ea	66336-0454-28	131.43		AB
30s ea	55045-2337-08	126.60		
30s ea	66336-0454-30	140.82		
PDR, PO, 125 mg/5 ml,				
150 ml	55045-2155-03	33.99		AB
(HomeMed)				
REPACK				
CAP, PO, 250 mg, 21s ea	51655-0698-28	41.99		
500 mg, 30s ea	51655-0933-24	119.99		
(Nucare Pharm)				
REPACK				
CAP, PO, 250 mg, 30s ea	66267-0262-30	109.77		EE
500 mg, 21s ea	66267-0256-21	91.99		EE
30s ea	66267-0256-30	132.36		EE
(Palmetto)				
REPACK				
CAP, PO, 250 mg, 21s ea	23490-5218-01	45.75		
28s ea	23490-5218-04	61.00		
30s ea	23490-5218-02	65.36		
500 mg, 20s ea	23490-5221-00	87.09		
28s ea	23490-5221-02	121.93		
30s ea	23490-5221-01	130.64		
PDR, PO (1X75ML)				
250 mg/5 ml, 75 ml	23490-5219-03	34.26		
150 ml	23490-5219-01	68.53		
TER, PO, 500 mg, 20s ea	23490-7012-00	86.60		

PROD/MFR	NDC	AWP	DP	OBC
(PD-Rx Pharm)				
REPACK				
CAP, PO, 250 mg, 30s ea	**55289-0749-30**	506.61		AB
(Pharma Pac)				
REPACK				
CAP, PO, 250 mg, 14s ea	**52959-0367-14**	36.05		EE
15s ea	**52959-0367-15**	38.16		EE
20s ea	**52959-0367-20**	51.45		EE
21s ea	**52959-0367-21**	54.02		EE
30s ea	**52959-0367-30**	68.25		EE
40s ea	**52959-0367-40**	89.32		EE
100s ea	**52959-0367-00**	184.80		EE
500 mg, 10s ea	**52959-0368-10**	45.60		EE
14s ea	**52959-0368-14**	62.70		EE
20s ea	**52959-0368-20**	87.10		EE
21s ea	**52959-0368-21**	91.45		EE
28s ea	**52959-0368-28**	121.53		AB
30s ea	**52959-0368-30**	128.10		EE
40s ea	**52959-0368-40**	170.83		AB
PDR, PO, 250 mg/5 ml,				
150 ml	**52959-0294-03**	51.66		EE
150 ml	**52959-0619-03**	51.66		EE
(Phys Total Care)				
REPACK				
CAP, PO, 250 mg, 10s ea	**54868-3478-03**	14.64		EE
15s ea	**54868-3478-01**	19.71		EE
20s ea	**54868-3478-02**	24.81		EE
30s ea	**54868-3478-00**	34.95		EE
500 mg, 10s ea	**54868-3511-01**	23.76		EE
15s ea	**54868-3511-04**	33.39		AB
20s ea	**54868-3511-00**	43.05		EE
30s ea	**54868-3511-02**	62.31		EE
PDR, PO, 125 mg/5 ml,				
150 ml	**54868-3472-00**	27.54		EE
250 mg/5 ml, 150 ml	**54868-3473-00**	65.07		EE
(Physician Partner)				
REPACK				
PDR, PO (1X15ML)				
250 mg/5 ml, 15 ml	**21695-0782-15**	56.48		AB
(Quality Care Prod)				
REPACK				
CAP, PO, 250 mg, 30s ea	**49999-0199-30**	111.22		EE
500 mg, 30s ea	**49999-0557-30**	142.92		
42s ea	**49999-0557-42**	200.09		AB
PDR, PO, 250 mg/5 ml,				
75 ml	**49999-0325-75**	33.86		AB
150 ml	**49999-0325-50**	67.71		AB
375 mg/5 ml, 50 ml	**49999-0556-50**	33.88		AB
100 ml	**49999-0556-00**	62.15		AB
(Southwood)				
REPACK				
CAP, PO, 250 mg, 12s ea	**58016-0872-12**	25.99		EE
15s ea	**58016-0872-15**	32.49		EE
18s ea	**58016-0872-18**	38.99		EE
20s ea	**58016-0872-20**	43.32		EE
24s ea	**58016-0872-24**	51.99		EE
30s ea	**58016-0872-30**	64.98		EE
500 mg, 12s ea	**58016-0339-12**	51.07		EE
15s ea	**58016-0339-15**	63.85		EE
18s ea	**58016-0339-18**	76.62		EE
20s ea	**58016-0339-20**	85.13		EE
24s ea	**58016-0339-24**	102.16		EE
30s ea	**58016-0339-30**	119.10		EE
PDR, PO, 125 mg/5 ml,				
150 ml	**58016-4193-05**	34.46		EE
250 mg/5 ml, 150 ml	**58016-4192-05**	55.93		EE
(Stat Rx)				
REPACK				
CAP, PO, 250 mg, 14s ea	**16590-0041-14**	48.84		
21s ea	**16590-0041-21**	73.28		
30s ea	**16590-0041-30**	104.69		
PDR, PO, 125 mg/5 ml,				
150 ml	**16590-0040-33**	29.50		
250 mg/5 ml, 150 ml	**16590-0042-33**	54.00		
(Vibranta)				
REPACK				
CAP, PO, 250 mg, 15s ea	**57866-8206-02**	51.00		AB
500 mg, 15s ea	**57866-8205-01**	73.87		
20s ea	**57866-8205-02**	99.00		
CEFACLOR ER (Bryant Ranch)				
REPACK				
cefaclor				
TER, PO, 500 mg, 30s ea	**63629-3057-01**	159.32		
CEFADROXIL				
FUL				
CAP, PO, 500 mg, 50s ea		39.15		
(Aurobindo Pharma)				
CAP, PO (USP,HARD GELATIN)				
500 mg, 50s ea	**65862-0085-50**	186.00		AB
100s ea	**65862-0085-01**	360.00		AB
(Greenstone)				
CAP, PO (USP,HARD GELATIN)				
500 mg, 50s ea	**59762-2000-01**	186.00		
100s ea	**59762-2000-04**	360.00		
(Lupin Pharma, Inc.)				
CAP, PO (USP)				
500 mg, 50s ea	**68180-0180-08**	186.00		AB
100s ea	**68180-0180-01**	360.00		AB
PDR, PO (USP,1X100ML)				
250 mg/5 ml,				
100 ml	**68180-0181-02**	60.80		AB
(USP,1X75ML)				
500 mg/5 ml, 75 ml	**68180-0182-02**	63.12		AB
(USP,1X100ML)				
500 mg/5 ml,				
100 ml	**68180-0182-03**	84.17		AB
(Northstar)				
CAP, PO (USP,HARD GELATIN)				
500 mg, 50s ea	**68820-0043-08**	186.00		AB
100s ea	**68820-0043-10**	360.00		AB
PDR, PO (USP,1X100ML,ORANGE)				
250 mg/5 ml,				
100 ml	**16714-0202-01**	60.80		AB
(USP,1X75ML,ORANGE)				
500 mg/5 ml, 75 ml	**16714-0203-01**	63.12		AB
(USP,1X100ML,ORANGE)				
500 mg/5 ml,				
100 ml	**16714-0203-02**	84.17		AB
(Ranbaxy Pharm)				
CAP, PO, 500 mg, 50s ea	**63304-0582-50**	193.42		AB
100s ea	**63304-0582-01**	414.69		AB
PDR, PO (MIXED FRUIT)				
250 mg/5 ml,				
100 ml	**63304-0973-04**	60.80		AB
500 mg/5 ml, 75 ml	**63304-0974-01**	63.12		AB
100 ml	**63304-0974-04**	84.17		AB
TAB, PO, 1 gm, 50s ea	**63304-0512-50**	357.00		AB
(Sandoz)				
CAP, PO, 500 mg, 50s ea	**00781-2938-50**	188.06		
100s ea	**00781-2938-01**	360.00		AB
(Teva)				
CAP, PO (USP)				
500 mg, 50s ea	**00093-3196-53**	186.00		AB
100s ea	**00093-3196-01**	360.00		AB
TAB, PO, 1 gm, 50s ea	**00093-4059-53**	357.08		
(West-Ward)				
CAP, PO (USP,HARD GELATIN)				
500 mg, 100s ea	**00143-9947-01**	360.00		
(4u)				
REPACK				
CAP, PO, 500 mg, 14s ea	**10544-0400-14**	74.22		AB
14s ea	**42549-0504-14**	74.22		
14s ea	**42549-0600-14**	74.22		AB
(A-S Medication)				
REPACK				
CAP, PO, 500 mg, 10s ea	**54569-4391-00**	41.47		EE
14s ea	**54569-4391-01**	58.06		EE
20s ea	**54569-4391-02**	82.94		EE
30s ea	**54569-4391-04**	124.41		EE
(Aidarex)				
REPACK				
CAP, PO, 500 mg, 7s ea	**33261-0018-07**	47.25		AB
14s ea	**33261-0018-14**	94.50		AB
20s ea	**33261-0018-20**	135.00		AB
21s ea	**33261-0018-21**	141.75		AB
28s ea	**33261-0018-28**	189.00		AB
30s ea	**33261-0018-30**	202.50		AB
40s ea	**33261-0018-40**	270.00		AB
60s ea	**33261-0018-60**	405.00		AB
90s ea	**33261-0018-90**	607.50		AB
(Altura)				
REPACK				
CAP, PO, 500 mg, 4s ea	**63874-0533-44**	7.96		AB
10s ea	**63874-0533-10**	34.66		AB
12s ea	**63874-0533-12**	54.91		AB
14s ea	**63874-0533-14**	65.23		AB
15s ea	**63874-0533-15**	50.42		AB
20s ea	**63874-0533-20**	64.08		AB
25s ea	**63874-0533-25**	114.39		AB
28s ea	**63874-0533-28**	129.32		AB
30s ea	**63874-0533-30**	91.39		AB
40s ea	**63874-0533-40**	183.02		AB
60s ea	**63874-0533-60**	274.54		AB
90s ea	**63874-0533-90**	411.80		AB
100s ea	**63874-0533-01**	457.56		AB
120s ea	**63874-0533-04**	549.07		AB
150s ea	**63874-0533-72**	686.34		AB
200s ea	**63874-0533-74**	915.12		AB
300s ea	**63874-0533-77**	1372.68		AB
(Bryant Ranch)				
REPACK				
CAP, PO, 500 mg, 10s ea	**63629-1358-01**	55.20		
20s ea	**63629-1358-02**	97.99		
(Core)				
REPACK				
CAP, PO, 500 mg, 14s ea	**33358-0067-14**	68.82		
28s ea	**33358-0067-28**	93.64		
(DHS, Inc.)				
REPACK				
CAP, PO, 500 mg, 10s ea	**55887-0893-10**	44.82		AB
14s ea	**55887-0893-14**	62.75		
15s ea	**55887-0893-15**	67.44		AB
24s ea	**55887-0893-24**	107.91		AB
30s ea	**55887-0893-30**	134.88		AB
(Dispensing Solutions)				
REPACK				
CAP, PO, 500 mg, 6s ea	**55045-2426-03**	30.42		
10s ea	**55045-2426-01**	50.70		AB
14s ea	**55045-2426-02**	70.98		AB
20s ea	**55045-2426-07**	101.40		AB
20s ea	**66336-0022-20**	89.92		AB
28s ea	**55045-2426-08**	141.96		
28s ea	**66336-0022-28**	125.89		AB
60s ea	**55045-2426-06**	304.20		AB
PDR, PO, 250 mg/5 ml,				
100 ml	**55045-3519-01**	66.00		
(Keltman Pharma., Inc.)				
REPACK				
CAP, PO, 500 mg, 14s ea	**68387-0470-14**	78.04		AB
20s ea	**68387-0470-20**	111.49		
(Nucare Pharm)				
REPACK				
CAP, PO, 500 mg, 10s ea	**66267-0045-10**	51.36		EE
14s ea	**66267-0045-14**	64.26		AB
20s ea	**66267-0045-20**	91.89		EE
24s ea	**66267-0045-24**	109.89		EE
28s ea	**66267-0045-28**	128.52		AB
(HARD GELATIN)				
500 mg, 30s ea	**66267-0045-30**	141.75		AB
(Palmetto)				
REPACK				
CAP, PO, 500 mg, 6s ea	**23490-5225-01**	47.04		
10s ea	**23490-5225-04**	56.00		
14s ea	**23490-5225-02**	78.40		
20s ea	**23490-5225-03**	112.00		
28s ea	**23490-5225-05**	156.80		
30s ea	**23490-5225-07**	168.00		
(PD-Rx Pharm)				
REPACK				
CAP, PO, 500 mg, 10s ea	**55289-0589-10**	58.33		AB
14s ea	**55289-0589-14**	80.22		AB
20s ea	**55289-0589-20**	100.00		EE
(Pharma Pac)				
REPACK				
CAP, PO, 500 mg, 4s ea	**52959-0428-04**	27.99		EE
10s ea	**52959-0428-10**	67.65		EE
14s ea	**52959-0428-14**	86.52		EE
16s ea	**52959-0428-16**	98.69		EE
18s ea	**52959-0428-18**	110.76		EE
20s ea	**52959-0428-20**	122.48		EE
28s ea	**52959-0428-28**	171.48		EE
30s ea	**52959-0428-30**	183.69		EE
(Phys Total Care)				
REPACK				
CAP, PO, 500 mg, 10s ea	**54868-3742-03**	23.94		EE
15s ea	**54868-3742-02**	34.41		EE
20s ea	**54868-3742-01**	44.85		EE
(Physician Partner)				
REPACK				
CAP, PO, 500 mg, 20s ea	**21695-0427-20**	195.16		
28s ea	**21695-0427-28**	273.22		
(Quality Care Prod)				
REPACK				
CAP, PO, 500 mg, 14s ea	**49999-0021-14**	76.44		EE
20s ea	**49999-0021-20**	131.04		EE
(Southwood)				
REPACK				
CAP, PO, 500 mg, 10s ea	**58016-0119-10**	45.76		EE
12s ea	**58016-0119-12**	54.91		EE
14s ea	**58016-0119-14**	64.06		EE
15s ea	**58016-0119-15**	68.63		EE
20s ea	**58016-0119-20**	91.51		EE

PROD/MFR	NDC	AWP	DP	OBC
25s ea	58016-0119-25	114.39		EE
30s ea	58016-0119-30	151.50		AB
40s ea	58016-0119-40	183.02		EE
60s ea	58016-0119-60	303.00		AB
90s ea	58016-0119-90	454.50		AB
100s ea	58016-0119-00	505.00		EE
120s ea	58016-0119-02	549.07		AB
150s ea	58016-0119-03	686.34		AB
200s ea	58016-0119-89	915.12		AB
300s ea	58016-0119-73	1372.68		AB
(Stat Rx)				
REPACK				
CAP, PO, 500 mg, 5s ea	16590-0043-05	20.73		AB
10s ea	16590-0043-10	41.46		AB
14s ea UD	16590-0043-14	67.50		
15s ea	16590-0043-15	62.19		AB
20s ea	16590-0043-20	96.42		
24s ea	16590-0043-24	115.70		
30s ea	16590-0043-30	144.64		
60s ea	16590-0043-60	289.00		
(Vibranta)				
REPACK				
CAP, PO, 500 mg, 20s ea	57866-7131-03	99.69		AB
CEFADROXIL MONOHYDRATE (Vibranta)				
cefadroxil				
CAP, PO, 500 mg, 14s ea	57866-7131-01	76.44		
CEFAZOLIN (Accord)				
cefazolin sodium				
PDS, IJ (USP,PF)				
1 gm, 25s ea	68330-0015-25	65.31		EE
500 mg, 25s ea	68330-0014-25	32.66		EE
(APP)				
PDS, IJ (USP,PF)				
1 gm, 25s ea	63323-0237-10	155.70		AP
CEFAZOLIN (Baxter)				
PDS, IV, 10 gm, ea	10019-0612-11	11.04		
(USP,PHARMACY BULK)				
10 gm, 10s ea	10019-0612-05	110.40		
(Hospira)				
cefazolin sodium				
PDS, IJ (SDV)				
1 gm, 25s ea	00409-0805-01	31.50	27.50	EE
CEFAZOLIN (Hospira)				
PDS, IV (SDV,ADD-VANTAGE)				
1 gm, 25s ea	00409-2585-01	66.90	58.50	AP
(PBP)				
10 gm, 10s ea	00409-0806-01	94.20	82.40	EE
(Pfizer)				
cefazolin sodium				
PDS, IJ (USP,PF)				
1 gm, 25s ea	00069-0312-20	78.00	65.00	
500 mg, 25s ea	00069-0310-20	54.00	45.00	
(Sagent)				
PDS, IJ (USP,SDV,PF)				
1 gm, 25s ea	25021-0101-10	152.19		
(USP,PF,LATEX-FREE)				
500 mg, 25s ea	25021-0100-10	48.13		AP
CEFAZOLIN (Sagent)				
PDS, IV (USP,PHARMACYBULKPKG,PF)				
10 gm, 10s ea	25021-0102-99	365.87		
(PHARMACY BULK PKG,USP)				
20 gm, 10s ea	25021-0103-99	296.82		AP
(Samson Medical)				
cefazolin sodium				
PDS, IJ, 100 gm, 100 gm	66288-1100-01	126.00	105.00	
300 gm, 300 gm	66288-1300-01	360.00	300.00	
CEFAZOLIN				
(Sandoz) *See NOVAPLUS CEFAZOLIN*				
CEFAZOLIN (Sandoz)				
cefazolin sodium				
PDS, IJ (USP)				
1 gm, 25s ea	00781-3451-96	161.43		
(INNER PACK)				
1 gm, 10 ml	00781-3451-70	6.46		
CEFAZOLIN (Sandoz)				
PDS, IV, 10 gm, ea	00781-3452-46	36.53		
(USP,PHARMACY BULK)				
10 gm, 10s ea	00781-3452-95	365.34		
CEFAZOLIN SODIUM				
(Accord) *See CEFAZOLIN*				
(Apotex Corp.)				
PDS, IJ, 1 gm, 10s ea	60505-0749-04	26.13		
25s ea	60505-0749-05	65.31		
500 mg, 10s ea	60505-0748-04	13.06		
25s ea	60505-0748-05	32.66		
(APP) *See CEFAZOLIN*				
(APP)				
PDS, IJ (P.B.,PF)				
1 gm, ea	63323-0237-65	8.87		AP
(BULK PACKAGE,PF)				
10 gm, ea	63323-0238-61	45.95		AP
20 gm, ea	63323-0446-61	33.92		AP
(VIAL,PF)				
500 mg, ea	63323-0236-10	4.06		AP
(B. Braun)				
cefazolin sodium/dextrose				
SOL, IV (DUPLEX)				
1 gm/50 ml-4%, ea	00264-3103-11	5.04		
CEFAZOLIN SODIUM (Baxter)				
PDS, IJ, 1 gm, ea	10019-0611-10	1.36		
(10ML VIAL)				
1 gm, 25s ea	10019-0611-03	33.90		
500 mg, ea	10019-0610-10	1.42		
(10ML VIAL)				
500 mg, 25s ea	10019-0610-01	35.40		
SOL, IV (GALAXY P.C.)				
1 gm/50 ml,				
50 ml 24s	00338-3503-41	161.28	134.40	
(Cura Pharm)				
PDS, IJ (VIAL)				
1 gm, 25s ea	66860-0002-03	70.00		AP
(BULK PACKAGE)				
10 gm, 10s ea	66860-0003-02	262.00		AP
(VIAL)				
500 mg, 25s ea	66860-0001-03	54.00		AP
(Hospira) *See CEFAZOLIN*				
(Hospira)				
PDS, IJ (ADD-VANTAGE,LATEX-FREE)				
1 gm, 25s ea	00074-4732-03	66.90	58.50	AP
(Pfizer) *See CEFAZOLIN*				
(Sagent) *See CEFAZOLIN*				
(Samson Medical) *See CEFAZOLIN*				
(Sandoz) *See CEFAZOLIN*				
(Sandoz) *See NOVAPLUS CEFAZOLIN*				
(Sandoz)				
PDS, IJ (VIAL)				
10 gm, ea	00781-3346-46	36.53		AP
10s ea	00781-3346-95	365.34		AP
(1X10ML VIAL)				
500 mg, ea	00781-3338-70	3.23		AP
(VIAL)				
500 mg, ea	00015-7338-12	3.23		AP
(10 VIAL PACK)				
500 mg, 10s ea	00781-3338-95	32.26		AP
(USP)				
500 mg, 10s ea	00781-3450-95	32.26		AP
(West-Ward)				
PDS, IJ (U.S.P.)				
1 gm, 25s ea	00143-9924-90	115.25		AP
(BULK PACKAGE)				
10 gm, 10s ea	00143-9983-03	240.00		AP
10s ea	00143-9983-91	240.00		AP
(U.S.P.)				
500 mg, 25s ea	00143-9923-90	87.50		AP
(Dispensing Solutions)				
REPACK				
PDS, IJ, 1 gm, ea	55045-3232-01	6.45		AP
(Phys Total Care)				
REPACK				
PDS, IJ (VIAL)				
1 gm, 10s ea	54868-0559-00	208.20		AP
(VIAL,PF)				
500 mg, 25s ea	54868-4651-00	260.13		AP
CEFAZOLIN SODIUM/DEXTROSE				
(B. Braun) *See CEFAZOLIN SODIUM*				
(PharMEDium Services)				
SOL, IV (24X100ML,USP,PF)				
2 gm/100 ml-5%/100 ml,				
100 ml 24s	61553-0211-48	15.00	12.50	
CEFDINIR				
FUL				
CAP, PO, 300 mg, 60s ea		229.59		
PDR, PO, 125 mg/5 ml,				
100 ml		62.31		
250 mg/5 ml,				
100 ml		130.79		
(Abbott Pharm) *See OMNICEF*				
(Aurobindo Pharma)				
CAP, PO (HARD GELATIN)				
300 mg, 60s ea	65862-0177-60	306.50		AB
PDR, PO (1X60ML,CREAM,STRAWBERRY)				
125 mg/5 ml, 60 ml	65862-0218-60	50.95		AB
(1X100ML,CREAM)				
125 mg/5 ml,				
100 ml	65862-0218-01	80.69		AB
(1X60ML,CREAM,STRAWBERRY)				
250 mg/5 ml, 60 ml	65862-0219-60	99.35		AB
(1X100ML,CREAM)				
250 mg/5 ml,				
100 ml	65862-0219-01	157.35		AB
(Dava Pharma)				
CAP, PO, 300 mg, 60s ea	67253-0007-60	306.83		
PDR, PO (STRAWBERRY)				
125 mg/5 ml, 60 ml	67253-0008-41	51.00		
100 ml	67253-0008-46	80.78		
250 mg/5 ml, 60 ml	67253-0009-41	99.48		
100 ml	67253-0009-46	157.54		
(Greenstone)				
CAP, PO (HARD GELATIN)				
300 mg, 60s ea	59762-2180-01	306.50		
(Lupin Pharma, Inc.)				
CAP, PO, 300 mg, 60s ea	68180-0711-60	306.83		AB
PDR, PO (STRAWBERRY)				
125 mg/5 ml, 60 ml	68180-0722-20	51.00		AB
100 ml	68180-0722-10	80.78		AB
250 mg/5 ml, 60 ml	68180-0723-20	99.48		AB
100 ml	68180-0723-10	157.54		AB
(Northstar)				
CAP, PO (3X10,USP,HARD GELATIN)				
300 mg, 30s ea	68820-0063-06	153.42		AB
(HARD GELATIN)				
300 mg, 30s ea	68820-0063-19	153.42		AB
60s ea	68820-0063-09	306.83		AB
PDR, PO, 125 mg/5 ml,				
60 ml	68820-0064-37	51.00		AB
100 ml	68820-0064-17	80.78		AB
250 mg/5 ml, 60 ml	68820-0065-37	99.48		AB
100 ml	68820-0065-17	157.54		AB
(Sandoz)				
CAP, PO (3X10)				
300 mg, 30s ea UD	00781-2176-64	153.42		AB
(5X10)				
300 mg, 50s ea UD	00781-2176-69	255.70		AB
60s ea	00781-2176-60	306.83		AB
PDR, PO (STRAWBERRY)				
125 mg/5 ml, 60 ml	00781-6077-61	51.00		AB
100 ml	00781-6077-46	80.78		AB
250 mg/5 ml, 60 ml	00781-6078-61	99.48		AB
100 ml	00781-6078-46	157.54		AB
(Teva)				
CAP, PO (HARD GELATIN)				
300 mg, 60s ea	00093-3160-06	306.86		AB
PDR, PO (CHERRY)				
125 mg/5 ml, 60 ml	00093-4136-64	51.01		AB
100 ml	00093-4136-73	80.78		AB
250 mg/5 ml, 60 ml	00093-4137-64	99.49		AB
100 ml	00093-4137-73	157.55		AB
(A-S Medication)				
REPACK				
CAP, PO, 300 mg, 20s ea	54569-5921-01	102.28		
PDR, PO, 250 mg/5 ml,				
60 ml	54569-5917-00	99.48		
100 ml	54569-5918-00	157.54		
(DHS, Inc.)				
REPACK				
CAP, PO, 300 mg, 60s ea	55887-0187-60	300.00		
(Dispensing Solutions)				
REPACK				
CAP, PO, 300 mg, 6s ea	66336-0104-06	30.68		AB
20s ea	66336-0104-20	102.28		
(PD-Rx Pharm)				
REPACK				
CAP, PO, 300 mg, 20s ea	55289-0081-20	85.86		
(Pharma Pac)				
REPACK				
CAP, PO, 300 mg, 20s ea	52959-0134-20	115.06		AB
(Phys Total Care)				
REPACK				
CAP, PO, 300 mg, 20s ea	54868-5767-00	241.44		
30s ea	54868-5767-01	209.95		AB
PDR, PO, 125 mg/5 ml,				
60 ml	54868-5768-00	111.48		
100 ml	54868-5768-01	175.71		
250 mg/5 ml, 60 ml	54868-5769-00	232.86		
100 ml	54868-5769-01	347.47		

PROD/MFR	NDC	AWP	DP	OBC
(Quality Care Prod) REPACK				
PDR, PO (1X60ML)				
125 mg/5 ml, 60 ml	**35356-0119-60**	110.08		AB
(1X100ML,STRAWBERRY) 250 mg/5 ml, 100 ml	**35356-0190-00**	327.80		
CEFDITOREN PIVOXIL (Aristos)				
TAB, PO (FILM-COATED)				
400 mg, 20s ea	**24486-0802-20**	294.81		
(Cornerstone) *See SPECTRACEF*				
CEFEPIME (Apotex Corp.)				
cefepime hydrochloride				
PDS, IJ (USP)				
1 gm, ea	**60505-0834-00**	20.33		AP
10s ea	**60505-0834-04**	203.34		AP
10s ea	**60505-6030-04**	203.34		AP
2 gm, ea	**60505-0681-00**	40.36		AP
10s ea	**60505-0681-04**	403.56		AP
10s ea	**60505-6031-04**	403.56		AP
(APP)				
PDS, IJ (USP,10X1GM)				
1 gm, 10s ea	**63323-0326-20**	203.30		
(USP,10X2GM) 2 gm, 10s ea	**63323-0340-50**	403.50		
(Baxter)				
SOL, IV (24X50ML)				
1 gm/50 ml, 50 ml 24s	**00338-1301-41**	764.93	637.44	
(12X100ML) 2 gm/100 ml, 100 ml 12s	**00338-1301-48**	613.15	510.96	
(Sagent)				
PDS, IJ (USP)				
1 gm, 10s ea	**25021-0121-20**	223.38		
2 gm, 10s ea	**25021-0122-50**	445.75		
CEFEPIME HYDROCHLORIDE				
(Apotex Corp.) *See CEFEPIME*				
(APP) *See CEFEPIME*				
(Baxter) *See CEFEPIME*				
(Elan Pharmaceuticals) *See MAXIPIME*				
(Sagent) *See CEFEPIME*				
(Sandoz)				
PDS, IJ (S.D.V,USP)				
1 gm, ea	**00781-3222-80**	20.33		
(USP) 1 gm, 10s ea	**00781-3222-95**	203.34		
(S.D.V,USP) 2 gm, ea	**00781-3223-91**	40.36		
(USP) 2 gm, 10s ea	**00781-3223-95**	403.56		
CEFIXIME				
(Lupin Pharma, Inc.) *See SUPRAX*				
CEFOTAN (Phys Total Care) REPACK				
cefotetan disodium				
PDS, IJ (VIAL)				
1 gm, 10s ea	**54868-3847-00**	135.06		
2 gm, 10s ea	**54868-3851-00**	249.80		
CEFOTAXIME (Baxter)				
cefotaxime sodium				
PDS, IJ (USP,SDV)				
1 gm, ea	**10019-0681-15**	4.36		
(S.D.V.,USP) 1 gm, 10s ea	**10019-0681-02**	43.56		
(USP,SDV) 2 gm, ea	**10019-0682-15**	8.54		
(S.D.V.,USP) 2 gm, 10s ea	**10019-0682-03**	85.44		
(USP,SDV) 500 mg, ea	**10019-0680-15**	3.65		
(S.D.V.,USP) 500 mg, 10s ea	**10019-0680-01**	36.48		
(Cura Pharm)				
PDS, IJ (USP)				
1 gm, 25s ea	**66860-0042-03**	265.00		AP
2 gm, 25s ea	**66860-0043-03**	550.00		AP
(USP,PHARMACY BULK PKG) 10 gm, ea	**66860-0044-01**	88.50		AP
(USP) 500 mg, 10s ea	**66860-0041-02**	72.00		AP
(West-Ward)				
PDS, IJ (USP)				
1 gm, 25s ea	**00143-9931-22**	162.50		AP
2 gm, 25s ea	**00143-9933-22**	325.00		AP
(USP,PHARMACY BULK) 10 gm, ea	**00143-9935-91**	65.00		AP
(USP) 500 mg, 10s ea	**00143-9930-03**	63.75		AP
(Wockhardt USA)				
PDS, IJ (USP)				
1 gm, ea	**64679-0986-01**	9.54		AP
10s ea	**64679-0986-02**	85.86		AP
25s ea	**64679-0986-03**	208.69		AP
50s ea	**64679-0986-04**	405.45		AP
CEFOTAXIME SODIUM				
(Abbott Hosp) *See CLAFORAN*				
(APP)				
PDS, IJ (S.D.V.)				
1 gm, ea	**63323-0331-15**	11.00		AP
2 gm, ea	**63323-0332-15**	22.00		AP
(BULK PAKAGE) 10 gm, ea	**63323-0333-61**	88.69		AP
(BULK PACKAGE) 20 gm, ea	**63323-0334-61**	170.00		AP
(S.D.V.) 500 mg, ea	**63323-0335-10**	7.25		AP
(Baxter) *See CEFOTAXIME*				
(Cura Pharm) *See CEFOTAXIME*				
(Hospira) *See AMERINET CLAFORAN*				
(Hospira) *See CLAFORAN*				
(Hospira) *See NOVAPLUS CLAFORAN*				
(West-Ward) *See CEFOTAXIME*				
(Wockhardt USA) *See CEFOTAXIME*				
CEFOTETAN (APP)				
cefotetan disodium				
PDS, IJ, 1 gm, 10s ea	**63323-0385-10**	142.25		
2 gm, 10s ea	**63323-0386-20**	284.50		
IV (PHARMACY BULK PACKAGE) 10 gm, ea	**63323-0396-61**	140.86		
(B. Braun)				
PDS, IJ (W/DILUENT,LATEX-FREE)				
1 gm, ea	**00264-3173-11**	17.58		
(W/ DILUENT,LATEX-FREE) 2 gm, ea	**00264-3175-11**	25.14		
CEFOTETAN DISODIUM				
(APP) *See CEFOTETAN*				
(B. Braun) *See CEFOTETAN*				
CEFOXITIN (Apotex Corp.)				
cefoxitin sodium				
PDS, IV, 1 gm, 25s ea	**60505-0759-05**	280.63		AP
2 gm, 25s ea	**60505-0760-05**	562.50		AP
(BULK PACKAGE) 10 gm, 10s ea	**60505-0761-04**	1122.50		AP
(APP)				
PDS, IJ (USP)				
1 gm, 25s ea	**63323-0341-20**	329.40		AP
(B. Braun)				
PDS, IV (DUPLEXDRUG DELIVERY SYS)				
1 gm, 24s ea	**00264-3123-11**	12.30		AP
2 gm, 24s ea	**00264-3125-11**	22.56		AP
(Sagent)				
PDS, IJ (USP,SDV,PF,LATEX-FREE)				
1 gm, 10s ea	**25021-0109-10**	131.16		
2 gm, 10s ea	**25021-0110-20**	262.80		
CEFOXITIN SODIUM				
(Apotex Corp.) *See CEFOXITIN*				
(Apotex Corp.) *See NOVAPLUS CEFOXITIN*				
(APP) *See CEFOXITIN*				
(APP)				
PDS, IJ (VIAL,PF)				
2 gm, ea	**63323-0342-20**	27.45		AP
(BULK PACKAGE,PF) 10 gm, ea	**63323-0343-61**	137.25		AP
(B. Braun) *See CEFOXITIN*				
(Sagent) *See CEFOXITIN*				
CEFPODOXIME PROFETIL (Northstar)				
cefpodoxime proxetil				
TAB, PO (USP,FILM-COATED)				
200 mg, 20s ea	**16714-0212-01**	131.63		
CEFPODOXIME PROXETIL (Aurobindo Pharma)				
PDR, PO (1X50ML,USP)				
50 mg/5 ml, 50 ml	**65862-0140-50**	28.75		AB
(1X100ML,USP) 50 mg/5 ml, 100 ml	**65862-0140-01**	54.72		AB
(1X50ML,USP) 100 mg/5 ml, 50 ml	**65862-0141-50**	54.72		AB
(1X100ML,USP) 100 mg/5 ml, 100 ml	**65862-0141-01**	104.12		AB
TAB, PO (USP,FILM-COATED)				
100 mg, 20s ea	**65862-0095-20**	97.06		AB
200 mg, 20s ea	**65862-0096-20**	128.25		AB
(Northstar) *See CEFPODOXIME PROFETIL*				
(Northstar)				
TAB, PO (USP,FILM-COATED)				
100 mg, 20s ea	**16714-0211-01**	97.06		
(Pfizer) *See VANTIN*				
(Ranbaxy Pharm)				
PDR, PO (FRUITY)				
50 mg/5 ml, 50 ml	**63304-0965-03**	28.75		AB
100 ml	**63304-0965-04**	54.72		AB
100 mg/5 ml, 50 ml	**63304-0966-03**	54.72		AB
100 ml	**63304-0966-04**	104.12		AB
TAB, PO (FILM-COATED)				
100 mg, 20s ea	**63304-0520-20**	102.17		AB
200 mg, 20s ea	**63304-0521-20**	135.00		AB
100s ea	**63304-0521-01**	674.99		AB
(Sandoz)				
PDR, PO (1 X 50ML, USP)				
50 mg/5 ml, 50 ml	**00781-6168-52**	28.75		AB
(1 X 100ML, USP) 50 mg/5 ml, 100 ml	**00781-6168-46**	54.72		AB
(1 X 50ML, USP) 100 mg/5 ml, 50 ml	**00781-6169-52**	54.72		AB
(1 X 100ML, USP) 100 mg/5 ml, 100 ml	**00781-6169-46**	104.12		AB
TAB, PO (USP,FILM-COATED)				
100 mg, 20s ea	**00781-5438-20**	102.17		AB
200 mg, 20s ea	**00781-5439-20**	128.25		AB
100s ea	**00781-5439-01**	641.25		AB
(Core) REPACK				
TAB, PO, 200 mg, 20s ea	**33358-0068-20**	125.42		
(PD-Rx Pharm) REPACK				
TAB, PO, 200 mg, 2s ea	**55289-0393-02**	18.06		
(Pharma Pac) REPACK				
TAB, PO (FILM-COATED)				
100 mg, 10s ea	**52959-0796-10**	43.55		AB
CEFPROZIL FUL				
PDR, PO, 125 mg/5 ml, 100 ml		40.80		
250 mg/5 ml, 100 ml		73.94		
TAB, PO, 250 mg, 100s ea		239.39		
500 mg, 100s ea		459.90		
(Apotex Corp.)				
TAB, PO (FILM COATED)				
250 mg, 100s ea	**60505-2532-01**	437.90		AB
500 mg, 50s ea	**60505-2533-05**	452.19		AB
100s ea	**60505-2533-01**	892.02		AB
(Aurobindo Pharma)				
PDR, PO (USP,BUBBLE-GUM)				
125 mg/5 ml, 75 ml	**65862-0099-75**	31.46		AB
100 ml	**65862-0099-01**	41.85		AB
250 mg/5 ml, 75 ml	**65862-0100-75**	57.45		AB
100 ml	**65862-0100-01**	75.83		AB
TAB, PO (USP,FILM-COATED)				
250 mg, 100s ea	**65862-0068-01**	437.90		AB
500 mg, 50s ea	**65862-0069-50**	452.19		AB
100s ea	**65862-0069-01**	892.02		AB
(Greenstone)				
TAB, PO (USP,FILM-COATED)				
250 mg, 100s ea	**59762-2220-02**	437.90		
500 mg, 50s ea	**59762-2221-01**	452.19		
100s ea	**59762-2221-02**	892.02		
(Lupin Pharma, Inc.)				
PDR, PO (BUBBLE GUM)				
125 mg/5 ml, 50 ml	**68180-0401-01**	21.05		AB
75 ml	**68180-0401-02**	31.42		AB
100 ml	**68180-0401-03**	41.80		AB
250 mg/5 ml, 50 ml	**68180-0402-01**	39.04		AB
75 ml	**68180-0402-02**	57.38		AB
100 ml	**68180-0402-03**	75.74		AB
TAB, PO (FILM-COATED)				
250 mg, 100s ea	**68180-0403-01**	437.42		AB
500 mg, 50s ea	**68180-0404-01**	451.68		AB
(Northstar)				
PDR, PO (USP,TUTTI-FRUTTI)				
125 mg/5 ml, 50 ml	**68820-0018-15**	21.07		AB

PROD/MFR	NDC	AWP	DP	OBC
75 ml	68820-0018-16	31.46		AB
100 ml	68820-0018-17	41.85		AB
250 mg/5 ml, 50 ml	68820-0019-15	39.09		AB
75 ml	68820-0019-16	57.45		AB
100 ml	68820-0019-17	75.83		AB
TAB, PO (USP,FILM-COATED)				
250 mg, 100s ea	68820-0016-10	437.90		AB
500 mg, 50s ea	68820-0017-08	452.19		AB
(Ranbaxy Pharm)				
PDR, PO, 125 mg/5 ml,				
50 ml	63304-0960-03	21.07		AB
75 ml	63304-0960-01	31.46		AB
100 ml	63304-0960-04	41.85		AB
(FRUITY)				
250 mg/5 ml, 50 ml	63304-0961-03	39.09		AB
75 ml	63304-0961-01	57.45		AB
100 ml	63304-0961-04	75.83		AB
TAB, PO (USP,FILM-COATED)				
250 mg, 100s ea	63304-0148-01	437.90		AB
500 mg, 50s ea	63304-0149-50	452.19		AB
100s ea	63304-0149-01	892.02		AB
(Sandoz)				
PDR, PO (FRUITY)				
125 mg/5 ml, 50 ml	00781-6202-91	21.07		AB
75 ml	00781-6202-57	31.46		AB
100 ml	00781-6202-46	41.85		AB
250 mg/5 ml, 50 ml	00781-6203-91	39.09		AB
75 ml	00781-6203-57	57.45		AB
100 ml	00781-6203-46	75.83		AB
TAB, PO (FILM-COATED)				
250 mg, 100s ea	00781-5043-01	437.90		AB
500 mg, 50s ea	00781-5044-50	452.19		AB
100s ea	00781-5044-01	892.02		AB
(Teva)				
PDR, PO (FRUIT-GUM)				
125 mg/5 ml, 50 ml	00093-1075-76	21.07		AB
75 ml	00093-1075-78	31.46		AB
250 mg/5 ml, 50 ml	00093-1076-76	39.09		AB
75 ml	00093-1076-78	57.45		AB
TAB, PO (FILM-COATED)				
250 mg, 100s ea	00093-1077-01	437.90		AB
500 mg, 50s ea	00093-1078-53	452.19		AB
(Wockhardt USA)				
TAB, PO (USP,FILM-COATED)				
250 mg, 100s ea	64679-0712-03	437.89		AB
500 mg, 50s ea	64679-0713-01	452.17		AB
100s ea	64679-0713-03	892.01		AB
(A-S Medication) REPACK				
PDR, PO, 250 mg/5 ml,				
100 ml	54569-5785-00	75.83		
TAB, PO (FILM COATED)				
250 mg, 20s ea	54569-5784-00	87.58		
(Palmetto) REPACK				
PDR, PO, 250 mg/5 ml,				
50 ml	23490-5231-05	46.05		
75 ml	23490-5231-07	69.08		
100 ml	23490-5231-01	92.10		
(Pharma Pac) REPACK				
TAB, PO (FILM COATED)				
500 mg, 20s ea	52959-0300-20	187.84		AB
(Phys Total Care) REPACK				
PDR, PO, 250 mg/5 ml,				
100 ml	54868-5757-00	123.81		
TAB, PO, 500 mg, 20s ea	54868-5756-00	303.39		
CEFTAZIDIME				
(Abbott Hosp) *See TAZICEF*				
(Baxter)				
PDS, IJ (SDV)				
1 gm, ea	10019-0691-27	6.38		
25s ea	10019-0691-02	159.60		
IV, 2 gm, ea	10019-0692-50	12.62		
(SDV)				
2 gm, 10s ea	10019-0692-03	126.24		
6 gm, ea	10019-0693-11	37.63		
(SDV,BULK)				
6 gm, 6s ea	10019-0693-04	225.79		
(Glaxo) *See FORTAZ*				
(Hospira) *See NOVAPLUS TAZICEF*				
(Hospira) *See TAZICEF*				
(Letco)				
POW, NA (USP, 1X1000GM)				
1000 gm	62991-2703-01	5700.00		

PROD/MFR	NDC	AWP	DP	OBC
(Sagent)				
PDS, IJ (USP,PF,LATEX-FREE)				
1 gm, 25s ea	25021-0127-20	262.50		AP
IV, 2 gm, 10s ea	25021-0128-50	200.00		AP
(USP,PHARMACYBULKPKG,PF)				
6 gm, 6s ea	25021-0129-99	575.00		AP
(Sandoz)				
PDS, IJ (USP)				
1 gm, 25s ea	00781-3177-96	261.57		AP
IV, 2 gm, ea	00781-3178-91	19.97		AP
(USP)				
2 gm, 10s ea	00781-3178-95	199.69		AP
(USP,PHARMACY BULK PKG)				
6 gm, 6s ea	00781-3179-86	582.30		AP
CEFTAZIDIME SODIUM/DEXTROSE				
(Glaxo) *See FORTAZ*				
CEFTAZIDIME WITH SODIUM CARBONATE (Medisca)				
ceftazidime/sodium carbonate				
POW, NA (1X1000GM)				
1000 gm	38779-2370-09	6150.00		
CEFTAZIDIME/SODIUM CARBONATE				
(Medisca) *See CEFTAZIDIME WITH SODIUM CARBONATE*				
CEFTIBUTEN				
(Shionogi) *See CEDAX*				
CEFTIN (Glaxo)				
cefuroxime axetil				
PDR, PO (TUTTI-FRUTTI)				
125 mg/5 ml,				
100 ml	00173-0740-00	77.16		AB
250 mg/5 ml, 50 ml	00173-0741-10	57.95		AB
100 ml	00173-0741-00	131.33		AB
TAB, PO (FILM-COATED)				
250 mg, 20s ea	00173-0387-00	230.26		AB
500 mg, 20s ea	00173-0394-00	419.58		
(A-S Medication) REPACK				
PDR, PO (TUTTI-FRUTTI)				
250 mg/5 ml,				
100 ml	54569-4737-00	136.80		AB
(AQ) REPACK				
TAB, PO, 250 mg, 10s ea	66105-0745-01	119.10		
15s ea	66105-0745-15	178.65		
30s ea	66105-0745-03	357.30		
60s ea	66105-0745-06	714.60		
90s ea	66105-0745-09	1071.90		
(Dispensing Solutions) REPACK				
TAB, PO, 250 mg, 3s ea	55045-1546-02	24.00		AB
10s ea	55045-1546-03	80.00		AB
(FILM-COATED)				
250 mg, 14s ea	55045-1546-05	112.00		AB
20s ea	55045-1546-07	160.00		AB
(PD-Rx Pharm) REPACK				
TAB, PO (FILM-COATED)				
250 mg, 10s ea	55289-0372-10	217.30		AB
14s ea	55289-0372-14	304.20		AB
(REDI-SCRIPT,FILM-COATED)				
250 mg, 20s ea	58864-0690-20	133.29		AB
(FILM-COATED)				
500 mg, 10s ea	55289-0542-10	296.97		
(Pharma Pac) REPACK				
TAB, PO, 250 mg, 20s ea	52959-0029-20	95.33		AB
24s ea	52959-0029-24	113.76		AB
(Phys Total Care) REPACK				
TAB, PO, 125 mg, 20s ea	54868-2805-00	52.21		AB
250 mg, 10s ea	54868-1080-01	80.55		AB
15s ea	54868-1080-00	119.89		AB
20s ea	54868-1080-03	150.49		AB
(Southwood) REPACK				
TAB, PO (FILM-COATED)				
250 mg, 10s ea	58016-0114-10	104.28		AB
14s ea	58016-0114-14	145.99		AB
15s ea	58016-0114-15	46.65		AB
(FILM-COATED)				
250 mg, 20s ea	58016-0114-20	208.55		AB
30s ea	58016-0114-30	312.83		AB
60s ea	58016-0114-60	625.65		AB
500 mg, 10s ea	58016-0115-10	190.29		
14s ea	58016-0115-14	266.40		
20s ea	58016-0115-20	380.57		
30s ea	58016-0115-30	570.86		
60s ea	58016-0115-60	1141.71		

PROD/MFR	NDC	AWP	DP	OBC
CEFTRIAXONE (Amer Regent)				
ceftriaxone sodium				
PDS, IJ (USP)				
1 gm, 10s ea	00517-8711-10	80.00		
2 gm, 10s ea	00517-8722-10	142.50		
250 mg, 10s ea	00517-8725-10	30.00		
500 mg, 10s ea	00517-8750-10	55.00		
(Apotex Corp.)				
PDS, IJ (1X100ML,PIGGYBACK)				
1 gm, ea	60505-0679-08	47.91		AP
(1X20ML)				
1 gm, ea	60505-0752-00	47.05		AP
(10X20ML)				
1 gm, 10s ea	60505-0752-04	459.49		AP
(1X100ML)				
2 gm, ea	60505-0679-09	94.17		AP
(1X20ML)				
2 gm, ea	60505-0753-00	93.68		AP
(10X20ML)				
2 gm, 10s ea	60505-0753-04	913.07		AP
(1X10ML)				
250 mg, ea	60505-0750-00	15.94		AP
(10X10ML)				
250 mg, 10s ea	60505-0750-04	148.16		AP
(1X10ML)				
500 mg, ea	60505-0751-00	27.99		AP
(10X10ML)				
500 mg, 10s ea	60505-0751-04	268.54		AP
IV (1X100ML,BULK PKG)				
10 gm, ea	60505-0679-05	447.93		AP
(APP)				
PDS, IJ (S.D.V.)				
1 gm, 25s ea	63323-0346-10	468.75		AP
2 gm, 10s ea	63323-0347-20	375.00		AP
250 mg, 25s ea	63323-0344-10	140.75		AP
(S.D.V.,USP)				
500 mg, 25s ea	63323-0345-10	225.00		AP
IV (BULK PACKAGE,1X100ML)				
10 gm, ea	63323-0348-61	187.50		AP
(Baxter)				
PDS, IJ (USP)				
1 gm, ea	10019-0687-71	4.63		AP
10s ea	10019-0687-03	46.32		AP
(USP)				
2 gm, ea	10019-0688-27	8.95		AP
10s ea	10019-0688-04	89.52		AP
(USP)				
250 mg, ea	10019-0685-71	2.03		AP
10s ea	10019-0685-01	20.28		AP
(USP)				
500 mg, ea	10019-0686-71	3.64		AP
10s ea	10019-0686-02	36.36		AP
IV (PHARMACYBULKPACKAGE,USP)				
10 gm, ea	10019-0689-11	41.75		
(USP,PHARMACY BULK)				
10 gm, ea	10019-0689-05	41.75		
SOL, IV, 1 gm/50 ml,				
50 ml 24s	00338-5002-41	1238.40		
2 gm/50 ml,				
50 ml 24s	00338-5003-41	2168.35		
(Bedford)				
PDS, IJ (SINGLE USE,CRYSTALLINE)				
1 gm, 10s ea	55390-0311-10	48.00		AP
2 gm, 10s ea	55390-0312-10	72.00		AP
(SDV,CRYSTALLINE)				
250 mg, 10s ea	55390-0309-10	24.00		AP
(SINGLE USE,CRYSTALLINE)				
500 mg, 10s ea	55390-0310-10	33.00		AP
IV (PHARMACY BULK)				
10 gm, ea	55390-0316-01	42.00		AP
(Cephazone)				
PDS, IJ (USP,PIGGYBACK)				
1 gm, ea	68330-0005-01	46.75		AP
(USP)				
1 gm, ea	68330-0003-01	46.75		AP
10s ea	68330-0003-10	457.50		AP
(USP,PIGGYBACK)				
2 gm, ea	68330-0006-01	91.72		AP
(USP)				
2 gm, ea	68330-0004-01	91.72		AP
10s ea	68330-0004-10	910.13		AP
250 mg, ea	68330-0001-01	15.23		AP
10s ea	68330-0001-10	148.08		AP
500 mg, ea	68330-0002-01	26.78		AP
10s ea	68330-0002-10	267.95		AP
(Cura Pharm)				
PDS, IJ, 1 gm, 10s ea	66860-0073-02	444.67		
2 gm, 10s ea	66860-0074-02	903.92		
250 mg, 10s ea	66860-0071-02	146.67		
500 mg, 10s ea	66860-0072-02	265.85		

PROD/MFR	NDC	AWP	DP	OBC
(Hospira)				
PDS, IJ (USP,ADD-VANTAGE VIAL)				
1 gm, 10s ea	**00409-7333-04**	69.48	60.80	**AP**
(USP,FLIPTOP VIAL)				
1 gm, 10s ea	**00409-7332-01**	42.84	37.50	**AP**
(USP,ADD-VANTAGE VIAL)				
2 gm, 10s ea	**00409-7336-04**	142.44	124.60	**AP**
(USP,FLIPTOP VIAL)				
2 gm, 10s ea	**00409-7335-03**	97.20	85.10	**AP**
(USP,BULK PACK)				
10 gm, ea	**00409-7334-10**	51.36	44.94	**AP**
(USP)				
250 mg, 10s ea	**00409-7337-01**	15.48	13.50	**AP**
500 mg, 10s ea	**00409-7338-01**	33.84	29.60	**AP**
(Lupin Pharma, Inc.)				
PDS, IJ, 1 gm, ea	**68180-0633-01**	47.05		**AP**
10s ea	**68180-0633-10**	460.00		**AP**
2 gm, ea	**68180-0644-01**	91.31		**AP**
10s ea	**68180-0644-10**	914.10		**AP**
250 mg, ea	**68180-0611-01**	15.94		**AP**
10s ea	**68180-0611-10**	148.30		**AP**
500 mg, ea	**68180-0622-01**	27.99		**AP**
10s ea	**68180-0622-10**	268.80		**AP**
(Pfizer)				
PDS, IJ (USP)				
1 gm, ea	**00069-4482-03**	7.56	6.30	
10s ea	**00069-4482-10**	75.60	63.00	
2 gm, ea	**00069-4483-03**	17.04	14.20	
10s ea	**00069-4483-10**	170.40	142.00	
250 mg, ea	**00069-4480-03**	2.64	2.20	
10s ea	**00069-4480-10**	26.40	22.00	
500 mg, ea	**00069-4481-03**	5.04	4.20	
10s ea	**00069-4481-10**	50.40	42.00	
(Sagent)				
PDS, IJ (USP,LATEX-FREE)				
1 gm, 25s ea	**25021-0106-10**	465.62		**AP**
2 gm, 25s ea	**25021-0107-20**	931.25		**AP**
250 mg, 25s ea	**25021-0104-10**	145.31		**AP**
500 mg, 25s ea	**25021-0105-10**	232.81		**AP**
IV (USP,PF,LATEX-FREE)				
10 gm, ea	**25021-0108-99**	42.58		
(Sandoz)				
PDS, IJ, 1 gm, ea	**00781-3208-85**	46.00		**AP**
10s ea	**00781-3208-95**	460.00		**AP**
2 gm, ea	**00781-3209-90**	91.41		**AP**
10s ea	**00781-3209-95**	914.09		**AP**
10 gm, ea	**00781-3210-46**	448.43		**AB**
250 mg, ea	**00781-3206-85**	14.83		**AP**
10s ea	**00781-3206-95**	148.32		**AP**
(INNER PACK)				
500 mg, ea	**00781-3207-85**	26.88		**AP**
10s ea	**00781-3207-95**	268.84		**AP**
(Teva)				
PDS, IJ (USP,SINGLE-DOSE)				
1 gm, ea	**00703-0335-04**	6.29		**AP**
2 gm, ea	**00703-0346-03**	14.40		**AP**
250 mg, ea	**00703-0315-03**	2.32		**AP**
500 mg, ea	**00703-0325-03**	4.16		**AP**
IV (USP,PHARMACY BULK PCKGE)				
10 gm, ea	**00703-0359-01**	57.00		**AP**
(West-Ward)				
PDS, IJ (USP)				
1 gm, 25s ea	**00143-9857-25**	437.50		**AP**
2 gm, 25s ea	**00143-9856-25**	781.25		**AP**
250 mg, 25s ea	**00143-9859-25**	125.00		**AP**
500 mg, 25s ea	**00143-9858-25**	187.50		**AP**
IV (USP,PHARMACY BULK)				
10 gm, ea	**00143-9768-01**	36.25		
(Wockhardt USA)				
PDS, IJ (USP)				
1 gm, ea	**64679-0983-01**	45.54		**AP**
10s ea	**64679-0983-02**	444.67		**AP**
2 gm, ea	**64679-0703-02**	93.22		**AP**
10s ea	**64679-0703-01**	903.92		**AP**
250 mg, ea	**64679-0701-01**	15.77		**AP**
10s ea	**64679-0701-02**	146.67		**AP**
25s ea	**64679-0701-03**	366.68		**AP**
500 mg, ea	**64679-0702-01**	27.70		**AP**
10s ea	**64679-0702-02**	265.85		**AP**
(A-S Medication)				
REPACK				
PDS, IJ, 1 gm, ea	**54569-5722-00**	47.25		
10s ea	**54569-5725-00**	454.88		
250 mg, ea	**54569-5720-00**	15.94		
10s ea	**54569-5723-00**	148.16		
500 mg, ea	**54569-5721-00**	27.99		
10s ea	**54569-5724-00**	268.54		
(Dispensing Solutions)				
REPACK				
PDS, IJ, 1 gm, ea	**55045-3511-02**	47.00		
10s ea	**55045-3511-01**	470.00		
250 mg, 10s ea	**55045-3516-01**	160.00		
500 mg, ea	**55045-3503-01**	28.00		
(PD-Rx Pharm)				
REPACK				
PDS, IJ, 250 mg, 10s ea	**43063-0002-10**	24.99		**AP**
(Phys Total Care)				
REPACK				
PDS, IJ, 250 mg, 10s ea	**54868-5589-00**	83.76		
500 mg, 10s ea	**54868-5533-00**	135.12		
(Physician Partner)				
REPACK				
PDS, IJ, 1 gm, ea	**21695-0352-01**	909.80		**AP**
(SDV,10X1GM)				
1 gm, 10s ea	**21695-0352-10**	909.80		**AP**
(SDV)				
500 mg, ea	**21695-0202-10**	59.98		
(Quality Care Prod)				
REPACK				
PDS, IJ (1X15ML)				
1 gm, 15 ml	**35356-0177-15**	49.52		**AP**
500 mg, ea	**35356-0267-01**	52.68		**AP**
(Southwood)				
REPACK				
PDS, IJ, 1 gm, ea	**58016-4786-01**	459.49		
2 gm, ea	**58016-4834-01**	94.17		
250 mg, ea	**58016-4790-01**	148.16		
CEFTRIAXONE AMERINET CHOICE (Baxter)				
ceftriaxone sodium				
PDS, IJ (PRIVATE LABEL)				
1 gm, ea	**10019-0098-71**	4.80		**AP**
10s ea	**10019-0098-01**	48.00		**AP**
CEFTRIAXONE NOVAPLUS (Hospira)				
ceftriaxone sodium				
PDS, IJ (USP,ADD-VANTAGE VIAL)				
1 gm, 10s ea	**00409-7333-49**	66.72	58.40	**AP**
2 gm, 10s ea	**00409-7336-49**	134.88	118.00	**AP**
(Sandoz)				
PDS, IJ (INNER PACK)				
1 gm, ea	**00781-9328-85**	46.00		**AP**
(PRIVATE LABEL)				
1 gm, 10s ea	**00781-9328-95**	460.00		**AP**
2 gm, ea	**00781-9329-90**	91.41		**AP**
10s ea	**00781-9329-95**	914.09		**AP**
(PRIVATE LABEL)				
10 gm, ea	**00781-9330-46**	448.43		
(INNER PACK)				
250 mg, ea	**00781-9326-85**	14.83		**AP**
(PRIVATE LABEL)				
250 mg, 10s ea	**00781-9326-95**	148.32		**AP**
500 mg, ea	**00781-9327-85**	16.88		**AP**
10s ea	**00781-9327-95**	268.84		**AP**
CEFTRIAXONE SODIUM				
(Amer Regent) *See CEFTRIAXONE*				
(Apotex Corp.) *See CEFTRIAXONE*				
(APP) *See CEFTRIAXONE*				
(B. Braun) *See CEFTRIAXONE/DEXTROSE*				
(Baxter) *See CEFTRIAXONE*				
(Baxter) *See CEFTRIAXONE AMERINET CHOICE*				
(Bedford) *See CEFTRIAXONE*				
(Cephazone) *See CEFTRIAXONE*				
(Cura Pharm) *See CEFTRIAXONE*				
(Hospira) *See AMERINET CHOICE CEFTRIAXONE*				
(Hospira) *See CEFTRIAXONE*				
(Hospira) *See CEFTRIAXONE NOVAPLUS*				
(Lupin Pharma, Inc.) *See CEFTRIAXONE*				
(Medisca)				
POW, NA (1X5000GM,USP)				
5000 gm	**38779-2383-03**	9000.00		
(Pfizer) *See CEFTRIAXONE*				
(Roche Labs) *See ROCEPHIN*				
(Sagent) *See CEFTRIAXONE*				
(Sandoz) *See CEFTRIAXONE*				
(Sandoz) *See CEFTRIAXONE NOVAPLUS*				
(Teva) *See CEFTRIAXONE*				
(West-Ward) *See CEFTRIAXONE*				
(Wockhardt USA) *See CEFTRIAXONE*				
CEFTRIAXONE/DEXTROSE (B. Braun)				
ceftriaxone sodium				
SOL, IV (DUPLEX SYSTEM)				
1 gm/50 ml, ea	**00264-3153-11**	13.92		**AP**
(DUPLEX DELIVERY SYST)				
2 gm/50 ml, ea	**00264-3155-11**	27.84		**AP**
CEFUROXIME (Cura Pharm)				
cefuroxime sodium				
PDS, IJ (PHARMACY BULK,USP)				
7.5 gm, 10s ea	**66860-0032-02**	659.50		
(Hospira)				
PDS, IV (USP)				
1.5 gm, 25s ea	**00409-0802-01**	147.30	129.00	**AP**
7.5 gm, 10s ea	**00409-0803-01**	279.12	244.20	**AP**
(Sagent)				
PDS, IJ (USP)				
750 mg, 25s ea	**25021-0118-10**	164.06		**AB**
IV, 1.5 gm, 25s ea	**25021-0119-20**	328.13		**AP**
(USP,BULK PACKAGING)				
7.5 gm, 10s ea	**25021-0120-59**	650.00		
(Bryant Ranch)				
REPACK				
cefuroxime axetil				
TAB, PO, 250 mg, 30s ea	**63629-1321-01**	120.92		
(DHS, Inc.)				
REPACK				
TAB, PO, 500 mg, 20s ea	**55887-0244-20**	160.00		
30s ea	**55887-0244-30**	240.00		
(Palmetto)				
REPACK				
PDR, PO (1X100ML)				
250 mg/5 ml, 100 ml	**23490-7075-08**	343.80		
(PD-Rx Pharm)				
REPACK				
TAB, PO, 250 mg, 4s ea	**55289-0385-04**	17.80		
CEFUROXIME AXETIL				
FUL				
TAB, PO, 250 mg, 20s ea		11.03		
500 mg, 20s ea		21.33		
(Apotex Corp.)				
TAB, PO (FILM-COATED)				
250 mg, 20s ea	**60505-1202-00**	87.97		**AB**
(USP)				
250 mg, 20s ea	**60505-2681-02**	87.97		**AB**
(FILM-COATED)				
250 mg, 60s ea	**60505-1202-03**	263.91		**AB**
(USP)				
250 mg, 60s ea	**60505-2681-06**	263.91		**AB**
(FILM-COATED)				
500 mg, 20s ea	**60505-1201-00**	160.31		**AB**
(USP)				
500 mg, 20s ea	**60505-2682-02**	160.31		**AB**
(FILM-COATED)				
500 mg, 60s ea	**60505-1201-03**	480.93		**AB**
(USP)				
500 mg, 60s ea	**60505-2682-06**	480.93		**AB**
(Aurobindo Pharma)				
TAB, PO, 250 mg, 20s ea	**65862-0034-20**	87.97		**AB**
60s ea	**65862-0034-60**	263.91		**AB**
500 mg, 20s ea	**65862-0035-20**	160.30		**AB**
60s ea	**65862-0035-60**	480.00		**AB**
(Glaxo) *See CEFTIN*				
(Greenstone)				
TAB, PO (USP,UNCOATED)				
250 mg, 20s ea	**59762-1081-01**	87.97		
60s ea	**59762-1081-02**	263.91		
500 mg, 20s ea	**59762-1083-01**	160.30		
60s ea	**59762-1083-02**	480.00		
(Lupin Pharma, Inc.)				
TAB, PO (USP,FILM-COATED)				
250 mg, 20s ea	**68180-0302-20**	87.97		**AB**
60s ea	**68180-0302-60**	263.91		**AB**
500 mg, 20s ea	**68180-0303-20**	160.31		**AB**
60s ea	**68180-0303-60**	480.93		**AB**
(Major)				
TAB, PO (10X10,USP)				
250 mg, 100s ea UD	**00904-5957-61**	438.00		**AB**
500 mg, 100s ea UD	**00904-5958-61**	788.00		**AB**
(Northstar)				
TAB, PO (USP,FILM COATED)				
250 mg, 20s ea	**16714-0232-01**	87.97		**AB**
60s ea	**16714-0232-02**	263.91		**AB**
500 mg, 20s ea	**16714-0233-01**	160.31		**AB**
60s ea	**16714-0233-02**	480.93		**AB**

PROD/MFR	NDC	AWP	DP	OBC
(Ranbaxy Pharm)				
PDR, PO (1X100ML,USP,FRUITY)				
125 mg/5 ml,				
100 ml	**63304-0963-04**	68.51		AB
(1X50ML,USP,FRUITY)				
250 mg/5 ml, 50 ml	**63304-0964-03**	51.45		AB
(1X100ML,USP,FRUITY)				
250 mg/5 ml,				
100 ml	**63304-0964-04**	116.61		AB
TAB, PO, 250 mg, 20s ea	**63304-0751-20**	87.97		AB
(USP)				
250 mg, 60s ea	**63304-0751-60**	263.91		AB
500 mg, 20s ea	**63304-0752-20**	160.31		AB
(USP)				
500 mg, 60s ea	**63304-0752-60**	480.93		AB
(Wockhardt USA)				
TAB, PO (FILM-COATED)				
250 mg, 20s ea	**64679-0921-01**	87.87		AB
60s ea	**64679-0921-02**	263.91		AB
500 mg, 20s ea	**64679-0922-01**	160.31		AB
60s ea	**64679-0922-02**	480.93		AB
(A-S Medication)				
REPACK				
TAB, PO, 250 mg, 10s ea	**54569-5386-02**	43.99		EE
14s ea	**54569-5386-03**	61.58		EE
20s ea	**54569-5386-00**	87.97		EE
500 mg, 20s ea	**54569-5418-00**	160.31		EE
(American Health)				
REPACK				
TAB, PO (USP,10X10)				
250 mg, 100s ea UD	**68084-0218-01**	421.35		
500 mg, 100s ea UD	**68084-0219-01**	758.04		
(Bryant Ranch)				
REPACK				
TAB, PO, 250 mg, 20s ea	**63629-1321-02**	142.32		AB
(DHS, Inc.)				
REPACK				
TAB, PO, 250 mg, 20s ea	**55887-0652-20**	101.88		AB
30s ea	**55887-0652-30**	152.82		AB
(Dispensing Solutions)				
REPACK				
TAB, PO, 250 mg, 20s ea	**66336-0369-20**	227.81		AB
500 mg, 20s ea	**55045-3483-02**	415.15		
(Palmetto)				
REPACK				
TAB, PO, 250 mg, 20s ea	**23490-5243-01**	101.88		
500 mg, 20s ea	**23490-5244-01**	160.31		
(Pharma Pac)				
REPACK				
TAB, PO, 500 mg, 20s ea	**52959-0939-20**	159.86		AB
30s ea	**52959-0939-30**	241.85		AB
(Phys Total Care)				
REPACK				
PDR, PO (1X100ML,FRUITY)				
125 mg/5 ml,				
100 ml	**54868-5981-00**	164.28		AB
TAB, PO, 250 mg, 20s ea	**54868-4987-00**	34.65		AB
30s ea	**54868-4987-01**	52.71		AB
(USP)				
500 mg, 15s ea	**54868-5022-02**	38.94		
20s ea	**54868-5022-01**	49.41		AB
30s ea	**54868-5022-00**	57.96		AB
(FILM-COATED)				
500 mg, 60s ea	**54868-5022-03**	87.45		AB
(Physician Partner)				
REPACK				
TAB, PO, 250 mg, 20s ea	**21695-0370-20**	175.74		AB
(FILM-COATED)				
500 mg, 20s ea	**21695-0150-20**	320.62		AB
(Quality Care Prod)				
REPACK				
TAB, PO, 250 mg, 20s ea	**49999-0309-20**	105.56		AB
30s ea	**49999-0309-30**	158.34		AB
500 mg, 20s ea	**49999-0785-20**	176.34		
(Southwood)				
REPACK				
TAB, PO, 250 mg, 30s ea	**58016-0204-30**	225.00		
60s ea	**58016-0204-60**	450.00		
90s ea	**58016-0204-90**	675.00		
100s ea	**58016-0204-00**	750.00		
500 mg, 30s ea	**58016-0964-30**	240.00		
60s ea	**58016-0964-60**	480.00		
90s ea	**58016-0964-90**	720.00		
100s ea	**58016-0964-00**	800.00		
(Stat Rx)				
REPACK				
TAB, PO, 250 mg, 20s ea	**16590-0044-20**	92.25		

PROD/MFR	NDC	AWP	DP	OBC
CEFUROXIME NOVAPLUS (Sandoz)				
cefuroxime sodium				
PDS, IJ (PRIVATE LABEL)				
1.5 gm, ea	**00781-9206-80**	13.46		AP
(PHARMACY BULK PACKAGE)				
7.5 gm, ea	**00781-9207-46**	65.94		AP
(PRIVATE LABEL)				
750 mg, ea	**00781-9205-70**	6.76		AP
CEFUROXIME SODIUM (APP)				
PDS, IJ (VIAL,PF)				
1.5 gm, ea	**63323-0353-20**	23.90		AB
(BULK PACKAGE,PF)				
7.5 gm, 10s ea	**63323-0354-61**	1167.00		AB
(VIAL,PF)				
750 mg, ea	**63323-0352-10**	12.90		AB
(B. Braun)				
SOL, IV (DUPLEX)				
1.5 gm/50 ml, ea	**00264-3114-11**	16.80		
(DUPLEX SYSTEM)				
750 mg/50 ml, ea	**00264-3112-11**	10.72		
(Baxter)				
PDS, IJ (USP)				
1.5 gm, ea	**10019-0621-20**	6.38		
(20ML VIAL)				
1.5 gm, 25s ea	**10019-0621-03**	159.60		
(USP)				
7.5 gm, ea	**10019-0622-11**	28.80		
(100ML VIAL, BULK PKG)				
7.5 gm, 10s ea	**10019-0622-05**	288.00		
750 mg, ea	**10019-0620-10**	3.01		
(10ML VIAL)				
750 mg, 25s ea	**10019-0620-01**	75.30		
(Cura Pharm) *See CEFUROXIME*				
(Cura Pharm)				
PDS, IJ, 1.5 gm, 25s ea	**66860-0031-03**	336.00		
750 mg, 25s ea	**66860-0030-03**	169.00		AB
(Glaxo) *See ZINACEF*				
(Hospira) *See CEFUROXIME*				
(Sagent) *See CEFUROXIME*				
(Sandoz) *See CEFUROXIME NOVAPLUS*				
(West-Ward)				
PDS, IJ, 750 mg, 25s ea	**00143-9979-90**	6.40		
(USP)				
750 mg, 25s ea	**00143-9979-22**	160.00		
IV, 1.5 gm, 25s ea	**00143-9977-90**	336.00		
(USP)				
1.5 gm, 25s ea	**00143-9977-22**	336.00		
(BULK PACKAGE)				
7.5 gm, 10s ea	**00143-9976-91**	65.95		AP
(USP,BULK PACKAGE)				
7.5 gm, 10s ea	**00143-9976-03**	659.50		AP
CEFZIL (A-S Medication)				
REPACK				
cefprozil				
PDR, PO, 125 mg/5 ml,				
100 ml	**54569-3743-00**	46.50		
250 mg/5 ml,				
100 ml	**54569-3630-00**	84.25		
TAB, PO, 250 mg, 20s ea	**54569-3652-00**	97.31		
(Bryant Ranch)				
REPACK				
TAB, PO, 250 mg, 20s ea	**63629-3189-01**	148.10		
(Pharma Pac)				
REPACK				
TAB, PO, 500 mg, 20s ea	**52959-0349-20**	127.12		
(Phys Total Care)				
REPACK				
PDR, PO, 250 mg/5 ml,				
50 ml	**54868-2017-01**	51.05		
100 ml	**54868-2017-00**	99.08		
TAB, PO, 250 mg, 10s ea	**54868-3343-00**	58.38		
15s ea	**54868-3343-01**	86.62		
20s ea	**54868-3343-03**	114.88		
30s ea	**54868-3343-02**	161.95		
500 mg, 10s ea	**54868-2444-00**	104.13		
(Southwood)				
REPACK				
PDR, PO, 125 mg/5 ml,				
100 ml	**58016-4148-01**	44.64		
250 mg/5 ml,				
100 ml	**58016-4147-01**	80.88		
TAB, PO, 250 mg, 12s ea	**58016-0810-12**	56.05		
15s ea	**58016-0810-15**	70.07		
30s ea	**58016-0810-30**	140.13		
60s ea	**58016-0810-60**	232.70		
100s ea	**58016-0810-00**	467.10		

PROD/MFR	NDC	AWP	DP	OBC
CELEBREX (Pfizer)				
celecoxib				
CAP, PO, 50 mg, 60s ea	**00025-1515-01**	75.74	63.12	
100 mg, 100s ea	**00025-1520-31**	270.13	225.11	
(10X10)				
100 mg, 100s ea UD	**00025-1520-34**	270.13	225.11	
500s ea	**00025-1520-51**	1350.66	1125.55	
200 mg, 100s ea	**00025-1525-31**	443.08	369.23	
(10X10)				
200 mg, 100s ea UD	**00025-1525-34**	443.08	369.23	
500s ea	**00025-1525-51**	2215.38	1846.15	
400 mg, 60s ea	**00025-1530-02**	398.77	332.31	
100s ea UD	**00025-1530-01**	664.63	553.86	
(4u)				
REPACK				
CAP, PO, 100 mg, 30s ea	**42549-0642-30**	172.68		
200 mg, 30s ea	**42549-0505-30**	246.34		
(A-S Medication)				
REPACK				
CAP, PO, 100 mg, 14s ea	**54569-4671-04**	37.52		
20s ea	**54569-4671-01**	53.60		
30s ea	**54569-4671-02**	80.40		
60s ea	**54569-4671-00**	200.67		
200 mg, 10s ea	**54569-4672-06**	43.96		
14s ea	**54569-4672-01**	61.54		
20s ea	**54569-4672-05**	87.91		
28s ea	**54569-4672-02**	123.08		
30s ea	**54569-4672-00**	131.87		
60s ea	**54569-4672-04**	329.14		
90s ea	**54569-4672-09**	493.72		
(Aidarex)				
REPACK				
CAP, PO, 100 mg, 7s ea	**33261-0653-07**	17.99		
21s ea	**33261-0653-21**	53.97		
30s ea	**33261-0653-30**	77.10		
60s ea	**33261-0653-60**	154.20		
200 mg, 14s ea	**33261-0019-14**	65.49		
30s ea	**33261-0019-30**	130.97		
60s ea	**33261-0019-60**	261.94		
90s ea	**33261-0019-90**	392.91		
(Altura)				
REPACK				
CAP, PO, 100 mg, 10s ea	**63874-0517-10**	20.80		
12s ea	**63874-0517-12**	24.96		
14s ea	**63874-0517-14**	29.12		
15s ea	**63874-0517-15**	31.20		
20s ea	**63874-0517-20**	41.60		
21s ea	**63874-0517-21**	43.68		
24s ea	**63874-0517-24**	49.92		
25s ea	**63874-0517-25**	52.00		
28s ea	**63874-0517-28**	58.24		
30s ea	**63874-0517-30**	62.40		
60s ea	**63874-0517-60**	124.80		
90s ea	**63874-0517-90**	187.20		
100s ea	**63874-0517-01**	208.00		
200 mg, 5s ea	**63874-0495-05**	17.75		
7s ea	**63874-0495-07**	24.85		
10s ea	**63874-0495-10**	35.50		
12s ea	**63874-0495-12**	42.60		
14s ea	**63874-0495-14**	61.54		
15s ea	**63874-0495-15**	53.25		
20s ea	**63874-0495-20**	87.92		
21s ea	**63874-0495-21**	74.55		
28s ea	**63874-0495-28**	99.40		
30s ea	**63874-0495-30**	131.87		
60s ea	**63874-0495-60**	213.00		
90s ea	**63874-0495-90**	319.50		
100s ea	**63874-0495-01**	355.00		
(AQ)				
REPACK				
CAP, PO, 100 mg, 100s ea	**66105-0105-10**	272.99		
200 mg, 30s ea	**66105-0106-03**	250.55		
100s ea	**66105-0106-10**	835.14		
(Bryant Ranch)				
REPACK				
CAP, PO, 200 mg, 20s ea	**63629-3021-02**	57.35		
30s ea	**63629-3021-01**	191.33		
60s ea	**63629-3021-04**	382.60		
(Core)				
REPACK				
CAP, PO, 100 mg, 14s ea	**33358-0069-14**	37.90		
20s ea	**33358-0069-20**	61.44		
30s ea	**33358-0069-30**	90.41		
60s ea	**33358-0069-60**	131.29		
200 mg, 10s ea	**33358-0070-10**	46.36		
14s ea	**33358-0070-14**	47.63		
15s ea	**33358-0070-15**	65.06		
20s ea	**33358-0070-20**	86.51		
30s ea	**33358-0070-30**	159.21		
60s ea	**33358-0070-60**	203.21		
90s ea	**33358-0070-90**	302.35		

PROD/MFR	NDC	AWP	DP	OBC
(DHS, Inc.)				
REPACK				
CAP, PO, 100 mg, 20s ea	55887-0412-20	59.09		
30s ea	55887-0412-30	88.64		
200 mg, 10s ea	55887-0736-10	49.59		
14s ea	55887-0736-14	63.42		
15s ea	55887-0736-15	65.54		
30s ea	55887-0736-30	123.00		
(Direct Pharmaceutical, Inc.)				
REPACK				
CAP, PO, 100 mg,				
30s ea UD	67801-0328-03	253.80		
200 mg, 30s ea UD	67801-0329-03	258.23		
(Dispensing Solutions)				
REPACK				
CAP, PO, 100 mg, 10s ea	55045-2671-01	30.00		
20s ea	55045-2671-07	60.00		
30s ea	55045-2671-08	90.00		
60s ea	55045-2671-06	180.00		
200 mg, 7s ea	55045-2680-02	42.00		
10s ea	55045-2680-01	60.00		
10s ea	66336-0727-10	50.74		
14s ea	66336-0727-14	71.03		
15s ea	55045-2680-06	90.00		
15s ea	66336-0727-15	76.10		
20s ea	55045-2680-07	120.00		
20s ea	66336-0727-20	101.47		
30s ea	55045-2680-08	180.00		
30s ea	66336-0727-30	152.21		
60s ea	55045-2680-09	360.00		
60s ea	66336-0727-60	304.42		
90s ea	66336-0727-90	456.63		
(HomeMed)				
REPACK				
CAP, PO, 200 mg, 14s ea	51655-0327-84	100.69		
(IPI)				
REPACK				
CAP, PO, 200 mg, 20s ea	18837-0024-20	97.81		
90s ea	18837-0024-90	395.61		
180s ea	18837-0024-96	791.21		
(Keltman Pharma., Inc.)				
REPACK				
CAP, PO, 200 mg, 15s ea	68387-0552-15	129.12		
30s ea	68387-0552-30	258.23		
60s ea	68387-0552-60	516.46		
(LWP)				
REPACK				
CAP, PO, 100 mg, 30s ea	64038-0030-30	61.96		
60s ea	64038-0030-60	118.92		
100s ea	64038-0030-01	194.86		
200 mg, 30s ea	64038-0031-30	98.43		
60s ea	64038-0031-60	191.85		
100s ea	64038-0031-01	316.41		
(Nucare Pharm)				
REPACK				
CAP, PO, 100 mg, 14s ea	66267-0046-14	74.37		
20s ea	66267-0046-20	106.25		
30s ea	66267-0046-30	159.37		
60s ea	66267-0046-60	318.74		
200 mg, 7s ea	66267-0048-07	51.34		
10s ea	66267-0048-10	73.33		
15s ea	66267-0048-15	109.99		
20s ea	66267-0048-20	146.67		
30s ea	66267-0048-30	229.83		
60s ea	66267-0048-60	440.00		
(Palmetto)				
REPACK				
CAP, PO, 100 mg, 20s ea	23490-7273-01	60.84		
20s ea	23490-9110-02	77.22		
30s ea	23490-9110-03	115.83		
200 mg, 7s ea	23490-7274-07	35.37		
10s ea	23490-7274-01	45.91		
14s ea	23490-7274-04	69.08		
15s ea	23490-7274-00	74.01		
20s ea	23490-7274-02	92.48		
30s ea	23490-7274-03	124.80		
60s ea	23490-7274-05	249.61		
(PD-Rx Pharm)				
REPACK				
CAP, PO, 100 mg, 14s ea	55289-0451-14	55.92		
20s ea	55289-0451-20	79.89		
30s ea	55289-0451-30	119.84		
(REDI-SCRIPT)				
100 mg, 30s ea	58864-0691-30	76.16		
200 mg, 10s ea	55289-0475-10	65.52		
14s ea	55289-0475-14	91.73		
20s ea	55289-0475-20	131.03		
28s ea	55289-0475-28	183.44		
30s ea	55289-0475-30	196.56		
(REDI-SCRIPT)				
200 mg, 30s ea	58864-0709-30	149.82		
60s ea	55289-0475-60	393.09		
90s ea	55289-0475-90	568.83		
180s ea	55289-0475-93	1179.30		
(Pharma Pac)				
REPACK				
CAP, PO, 100 mg, 14s ea	52959-0540-14	43.43		
15s ea	52959-0540-15	46.47		
20s ea	52959-0540-20	59.94		
21s ea	52959-0540-21	61.97		
28s ea	52959-0540-28	82.41		
30s ea	52959-0540-30	88.20		
40s ea	52959-0540-40	102.22		
60s ea	52959-0540-60	153.30		
200 mg, 5s ea	52959-0539-05	38.00		
7s ea	52959-0539-07	53.13		
10s ea	52959-0539-10	75.80		
14s ea	52959-0539-14	105.98		
15s ea	52959-0539-15	113.40		
20s ea	52959-0539-20	151.00		
21s ea	52959-0539-21	158.45		
28s ea	52959-0539-28	210.70		
30s ea	52959-0539-30	224.50		
40s ea	52959-0539-40	293.24		
45s ea	52959-0539-45	321.30		
50s ea	52959-0539-50	347.00		
60s ea	52959-0539-60	399.60		
90s ea	52959-0539-90	477.00		
100s ea	52959-0539-00	490.00		
400 mg, 30s ea	52959-0904-30	150.05		
(Phys Total Care)				
REPACK				
CAP, PO, 100 mg, 10s ea	54868-4107-03	32.67		
20s ea	54868-4107-01	63.38		
30s ea	54868-4107-00	94.09		
60s ea	54868-4107-02	175.98		
200 mg, 5s ea	54868-4101-06	30.38		
10s ea	54868-4101-04	58.15		
15s ea	54868-4101-03	85.92		
20s ea	54868-4101-02	113.68		
30s ea	54868-4101-01	159.96		
60s ea	54868-4101-00	317.31		
90s ea	54868-4101-05	474.65		
100s ea	54868-4101-07	477.04		
100s ea	54868-4101-08	509.53		
400 mg, 60s ea	54868-5506-00	401.11		
(Physician Partner)				
REPACK				
CAP, PO, 100 mg, 15s ea	21695-0022-15	95.34		
30s ea	21695-0022-30	162.08		
60s ea	21695-0022-60	324.16		
100s ea	21695-0022-00	540.26		
120s ea	21695-0022-72	762.72		
200 mg, 10s ea	21695-0023-10	92.06		
14s ea	21695-0023-14	145.96		
15s ea	21695-0023-15	156.38		
20s ea	21695-0023-20	184.11		
30s ea	21695-0023-30	265.85		
60s ea	21695-0023-60	531.70		
(Quality Care Prod)				
REPACK				
CAP, PO, 100 mg, 10s ea	49999-0383-10	84.60		
14s ea	49999-0383-14	118.44		
20s ea	49999-0383-20	169.20		
30s ea	49999-0383-30	253.80		
60s ea	49999-0383-60	507.60		
200 mg, 6s ea	49999-0004-06	55.86		
10s ea	49999-0004-10	93.06		
14s ea	49999-0004-14	118.44		
20s ea	49999-0004-20	169.20		
30s ea	49999-0004-30	279.19		
60s ea	49999-0004-60	558.38		
100s ea	49999-0004-00	931.40		
(Southwood)				
REPACK				
CAP, PO, 100 mg, 10s ea	58016-0169-10	24.50		
12s ea	58016-0169-12	29.40		
20s ea	58016-0169-20	49.00		
21s ea	58016-0169-21	51.45		
28s ea	58016-0169-28	68.61		
30s ea	58016-0169-30	73.51		
60s ea	58016-0169-60	147.01		
90s ea	58016-0169-90	220.52		
100s ea	58016-0169-00	245.02		
200 mg, 10s ea	58016-0223-10	40.19		
12s ea	58016-0223-12	48.23		
14s ea	58016-0223-14	56.26		
15s ea	58016-0223-15	60.28		
20s ea	58016-0223-20	80.38		
21s ea	58016-0223-21	84.39		
28s ea	58016-0223-28	112.53		
30s ea	58016-0223-30	120.56		
60s ea	58016-0223-60	241.13		
90s ea	58016-0223-90	361.69		
100s ea	58016-0223-00	401.88		
120s ea	58016-0223-02	482.26		
400 mg, 30s ea	58016-0724-30	180.85		
60s ea	58016-0724-60	361.70		
90s ea	58016-0724-90	542.56		
100s ea	58016-0724-00	602.84		
(St. Mary's MPP)				
REPACK				
CAP, PO, 200 mg, 20s ea	60760-0525-20	102.70		
30s ea	60760-0525-30	210.70		
60s ea	60760-0525-60	415.40		
(Stat Rx)				
REPACK				
CAP, PO, 100 mg, 30s ea	16590-0045-30	159.67		
56s ea	16590-0045-56	169.78		
60s ea	16590-0045-60	181.67		
200 mg, 10s ea	16590-0046-10	50.92		
15s ea	16590-0046-15	76.38		
20s ea	16590-0046-20	100.74		
28s ea	16590-0046-28	138.93		
30s ea	16590-0046-30	155.67		
56s ea	16590-0046-56	276.43		
60s ea	16590-0046-60	296.08		
84s ea	16590-0046-62	259.75		
90s ea	16590-0046-90	459.83		
CELECOXIB				
(Pfizer) *See CELEBREX*				
CELESTONE (Schering)				
betamethasone				
SYR, PO, 0.6 mg/5 ml,				
118 ml	00085-0942-05	70.22		
CELESTONE SOLUSPAN (Schering)				
betamethasone ace/betamethasone na phos				
SUS, IJ (M.D.V.)				
3 mg/ml-3 mg/ml,				
5 ml	00085-0566-05	40.38		
(Phys Total Care)				
REPACK				
SUS, IJ (M.D.V.)				
3 mg/ml-3 mg/ml,				
5 ml	54868-0206-00	38.79		
(Quality Care Prod)				
REPACK				
SUS, IJ, 3 mg/ml-3 mg/ml,				
ea	35356-0084-01	84.00		
(Southwood)				
REPACK				
SUS, IJ (M.D.V.)				
3 mg/ml-3 mg/ml,				
5 ml	58016-9191-01	34.95		
CELEXA (Forest Pharm)				
citalopram hydrobromide				
TAB, PO (FILM-COATED)				
10 mg, 100s ea	00456-4010-01	356.80		
20 mg, 100s ea	00456-4020-01	371.89		
40 mg, 100s ea	00456-4040-01	388.09		
(Altura)				
REPACK				
TAB, PO (FILM-COATED)				
20 mg, 10s ea	63874-0609-10	31.15		
20s ea	63874-0609-20	62.93		
30s ea	63874-0609-30	81.35		
60s ea	63874-0609-60	129.64		
90s ea	63874-0609-90	194.46		
100s ea	63874-0609-01	289.30		
(DHS, Inc.)				
REPACK				
TAB, PO (FILM-COATED)				
10 mg, 60s ea	55887-0502-60	183.30		
(Dispensing Solutions)				
REPACK				
TAB, PO (FILM-COATED)				
20 mg, 60s ea	55045-2706-09	195.00		
40 mg, 100s ea	55045-2705-00	241.00		
(Nucare Pharm)				
REPACK				
TAB, PO (FILM-COATED)				
20 mg, 30s ea	66267-0618-30	99.04		
(PD-Rx Pharm)				
REPACK				
TAB, PO (FILM-COATED)				
10 mg, 30s ea	58864-0849-30	130.60		
20 mg, 30s ea	55289-0827-30	149.96		

PROD/MFR	NDC	AWP	DP	OBC
30s ea	58864-0852-30	149.96		
(REDI-SCRIPT,FILM-COATED)				
40 mg, 15s ea	58864-0616-15	106.22		
30s ea	58864-0616-30	205.78		
(Pharma Pac)				
REPACK				
TAB, PO, 20 mg, 30s ea	52959-0010-30	86.18		
60s ea	52959-0010-60	172.35		
100s ea	52959-0010-00	287.20		
(Phys Total Care)				
REPACK				
TAB, PO (FILM-COATED)				
10 mg, 10s ea	54868-4985-01	32.34		
30s ea	54868-4985-00	93.25		
20 mg, 10s ea	54868-4159-01	49.23		
(FILM-COATED)				
20 mg, 15s ea	54868-4159-03	72.53		
30s ea	54868-4159-00	134.68		
(FILM-COATED)				
20 mg, 90s ea	54868-4159-02	385.39		
100s ea	54868-4159-04	427.99		
(FILM-COATED)				
20 mg, 100s ea	45868-4159-04	316.04		
40 mg, 10s ea	54868-4226-01	51.26		
30s ea	54868-4226-00	140.44		
50s ea	54868-4226-02	232.32		
(Quality Care Prod)				
REPACK				
TAB, PO, 10 mg, 30s ea	35356-0045-30	220.00		
20 mg, 30s ea	49999-0690-30	230.00		
40 mg, 30s ea	35356-0046-30	240.00		
(Southwood)				
REPACK				
TAB, PO (FILM-COATED)				
10 mg, 30s ea	58016-0593-30	99.11		
60s ea	58016-0593-60	198.22		
90s ea	58016-0593-90	297.33		
100s ea	58016-0593-00	330.37		
20 mg, 30s ea	58016-0598-30	103.30		
60s ea	58016-0598-60	206.60		
90s ea	58016-0598-90	309.91		
100s ea	58016-0598-00	344.34		
CELLACEFATE				
(Medisca) *See CELLULOSE ACETATE PHTHALATE*				
(PCCA)				
POW, NA (1X1GM,NF)				
1 gm	51927-1546-00	1.02		
(Spectrum Pharmacy)				
POW, NA (N.F.)				
25 gm	49452-1846-01	95.20		
100 gm	49452-1846-02	154.00		
500 gm	49452-1846-03	556.50		
CELLCEPT (Roche Labs)				
mycophenolate mofetil				
CAP, PO, 250 mg, 100s ea	00004-0259-01	511.12		
500s ea	00004-0259-43	2555.58		
1440s ea	00004-0259-05	7360.08		
PDR, PO (FRUIT)				
200 mg/ml, 175 ml	00004-0261-29	842.16		
(Roche Labs)				
mycophenolate mofetil hydrochloride				
PDS, IV (20 ML VIAL)				
500 mg, 4s ea	00004-0298-09	260.11		
(Roche Labs)				
mycophenolate mofetil				
TAB, PO (CAPLET)				
500 mg, 100s ea	00004-0260-01	1022.23		
500s ea	00004-0260-43	5111.17		
(Physician Partner)				
REPACK				
CAP, PO, 250 mg, 100s ea	21695-0171-00	763.22		
(Quality Care Prod)				
REPACK				
CAP, PO, 250 mg, 30s ea	49999-0936-30	209.86		
100s ea	49999-0936-00	457.00		
TAB, PO (CAPLET)				
500 mg, 30s ea	49999-0937-30	347.60		
CELLUGEL OVD (Alcon Surgical)				
hypromellose				
SOL, IO (SINGLE,BLUNT CANULA)				
2%, 1 ml	08065-1838-10	92.22		
CELLULASE (Medisca)				
POW, NA (1X100GM,1000IU)				
100 gm	38779-2220-05	76.50		
(1X500GM,1000IU)				
500 gm	38779-2220-08	276.00		
(PCCA)				
POW, NA, 1 gm	51927-3531-00	0.90		
(Spectrum Pharmacy)				
POW, NA (1X25GM)				
25 gm	49452-1852-01	84.00		
(1X125GM)				
125 gm	49452-1852-02	147.70		
(1X500GM)				
500 gm	49452-1852-03	476.00		
CELLULOSE				
(Baker, J.T.) *See CELLULOSE ACID WASHED*				
(Gallipot) *See CELLULOSE MICROCRYSTALLINE*				
(Medisca) *See CELLULOSE MICROCRYSTALLINE*				
(Spectrum Pharmacy) *See CELLULOSE MICROCRYSTALLINE*				
(Spectrum Pharmacy)				
POW, NA (NF)				
100 gm	49452-1875-01	72.45		
1000 gm	49452-1875-02	259.35		
CELLULOSE ACETATE PHTHALATE (Medisca)				
cellacefate				
POW, NA (1X50GM)				
50 gm	38779-1141-02	36.00		
(1X100GM)				
100 gm	38779-1141-05	76.50		
(1X500GM)				
500 gm	38779-1141-08	291.00		
CELLULOSE ACID WASHED (Baker, J.T.)				
cellulose				
POW, NA (REAGENT, ASHLESS)				
500 gm	10106-1525-01	143.84		
CELLULOSE MICROCRYSTALLINE (Gallipot)				
cellulose				
CRY, NA (U.S.P.)				
100 gm	51552-0548-05	24.08		
(Medisca)				
POW, NA (N.F.)				
100 gm	38779-0567-05	43.50		
(1X500GM)				
500 gm	38779-0567-08	61.50		
(N.F.)				
1000 gm	38779-0567-09	108.00		
(1X5000GM)				
5000 gm	38779-0567-03	459.00		
(Spectrum Pharmacy)				
CRY, NA (N.F.)				
500 gm	49452-1877-01	89.95		
2500 gm	49452-1877-02	346.50		
CELLULOSE, MICROCRYSTALLINE				
(Letco) *See MICROCRYSTALLINE CELLULOSE*				
(PCCA) *See MICROCRYSTALLINE CELLULOSE*				
CELONTIN KAPSEALS (Pfizer)				
methsuximide				
CAP, PO, 150 mg, 100s ea	00071-0537-24	62.16	51.80	
300 mg, 100s ea	00071-0525-24	152.99	127.49	
CENESTIN (Teva)				
conjugated estrogens synthetic a				
TAB, PO (FILM-COATED)				
0.3 mg, 100s ea	51285-0441-02	207.78		
0.45 mg, 100s ea	51285-0446-02	207.78		
0.625 mg, 100s ea	51285-0442-02	207.78		
0.9 mg, 100s ea	51285-0443-02	207.78		
1.25 mg, 100s ea	51285-0444-02	207.78		
(Phys Total Care)				
REPACK				
TAB, PO (FILM-COATED)				
0.45 mg, 10s ea	54868-5415-01	19.70		
30s ea	54868-5415-00	55.36		
0.625 mg, 10s ea	54868-4879-01	19.70		
30s ea	54868-4879-02	55.36		
100s ea	54868-4879-00	169.63		
1.25 mg, 10s ea	54868-1432-00	22.29		
30s ea	54868-1432-01	63.11		
CENOLATE (Hospira)				
ascorbic acid				
SOL, IJ (50X1ML,LATEX-FREE)				
500 mg/ml,				
1 ml 50s	00409-3118-31	87.00	76.00	
(50X2ML AMP,LATEX-FREE)				
500 mg/ml,				
2 ml 50s	00409-3397-32	121.20	106.00	
CENTANY (Medimetriks)				
mupirocin				
OIN, TP (1X30GM)				
2%, 30 gm	43538-0300-30	105.82		BX
CENTEX PSE (Dispensing Solutions)				
REPACK				
guaifenesin/pseudoephedrine hydrochloride				
TER, PO (CAPLET)				
600 mg-120 mg,				
12s ea	55045-2183-04	6.60		
20s ea	55045-2183-07	11.00		
CEPHADYN (Atley)				
acetaminophen/butalbital				
TAB, PO, 650 mg-50 mg,				
100s ea	59702-0650-01	54.74		EE
(Stat Rx)				
REPACK				
TAB, PO, 650 mg-50 mg,				
20s ea	16590-0351-20	40.24		
30s ea	16590-0351-30	44.31		
60s ea	16590-0351-60	56.52		
90s ea	16590-0351-90	68.73		
120s ea	16590-0351-72	81.94		
CEPHALEXIN				
FUL				
CAP, PO, 250 mg, 100s ea		16.50		
500 mg, 100s ea		27.30		
(Aurobindo Pharma)				
CAP, PO, 250 mg, 40s ea	65862-0018-40	46.33		AB
100s ea	65862-0018-01	69.50		AB
500 mg, 40s ea	65862-0019-40	90.00		AB
100s ea	65862-0019-01	133.00		AB
500s ea	65862-0019-05	605.00		AB
(Consolidated Midland)				
CAP, PO, 250 mg, 100s ea	00223-0581-01	20.95		EE
500s ea	00223-0581-05	99.50		EE
500 mg, 100s ea	00223-0582-01	46.50		EE
500s ea	00223-0582-05	225.00		EE
TAB, PO, 250 mg, 100s ea	00223-0583-01	37.50		EE
500s ea	00223-0583-05	175.00		EE
500 mg, 100s ea	00223-0584-01	72.50		EE
500s ea	00223-0584-05	352.50		EE
(Intl Ethical) *See BIO-CEF*				
(Karalex)				
CAP, PO (USP)				
250 mg, 100s ea	42043-0140-01	69.35		AB
500s ea	42043-0140-05	311.95		AB
500 mg, 100s ea	42043-0141-01	137.60		AB
500s ea	42043-0141-05	612.95		AB
PDR, PO (1X100ML, USP,ORANGE)				
125 mg/5 ml,				
100 ml	42043-0142-38	8.93		AB
(1X200ML, USP,ORANGE)				
125 mg/5 ml,				
200 ml	42043-0142-58	15.75		AB
(1X100ML, USP,ORANGE)				
250 mg/5 ml,				
100 ml	42043-0143-38	18.90		AB
(1X200ML, USP,ORANGE)				
250 mg/5 ml,				
200 ml	42043-0143-58	31.50		AB
(Lupin Pharma, Inc.)				
CAP, PO, 250 mg, 100s ea	68180-0121-01	69.35		AB
500s ea	68180-0121-02	311.95		AB
500 mg, 100s ea	68180-0122-01	137.60		AB
500s ea	68180-0122-02	612.95		AB
PDR, PO (STRAWBERRY)				
125 mg/5 ml,				
100 ml	68180-0123-01	8.93		AB
200 ml	68180-0123-02	15.75		AB
250 mg/5 ml, 100 ml	68180-0124-01	18.90		AB
200 ml	68180-0124-02	31.50		AB
(MiddleBrook) *See KEFLEX*				
(Northstar)				
CAP, PO (USP,HARD GELATIN)				
250 mg, 100s ea	16714-0641-02	69.35		AB
500s ea	16714-0641-03	311.95		AB
500 mg, 100s ea	16714-0642-02	137.60		AB
500s ea	16714-0642-03	612.95		AB
(Ranbaxy Pharm)				
CAP, PO, 250 mg, 100s ea	63304-0656-01	69.35		AB
500s ea	63304-0656-05	311.95		AB
500 mg, 100s ea	63304-0657-01	137.60		AB
500s ea	63304-0657-05	612.95		AB
PDR, PO, 125 mg/5 ml,				
100 ml	63304-0958-01	8.93		AB
200 ml	63304-0958-02	15.75		AB
250 mg/5 ml, 100 ml	63304-0959-01	18.90		AB
200 ml	63304-0959-02	31.50		AB
(Teva)				
CAP, PO, 250 mg, 100s ea	00093-3145-01	73.13		AB
500s ea	00093-3145-05	327.14		AB

PROD/MFR	NDC	AWP	DP	OBC
500 mg, 100s ea	00093-3147-01	137.60		AB
100s ea	00172-4074-60	149.55		AB
(USP)				
500 mg, 500s ea	00093-3147-05	674.15		AB
PDR, PO, 125 mg/5 ml,				
100 ml	00093-4175-73	8.93		AB
200 ml	00093-4175-74	15.75		AB
250 mg/5 ml, 100 ml	00093-4177-73	18.90		AB
200 ml	00093-4177-74	31.50		AB
TAB, PO, 250 mg, 100s ea	00093-2238-01	114.50		AB
500 mg, 100s ea	00093-2240-01	225.02		AB
(West-Ward)				
CAP, PO (USP)				
250 mg, 100s ea	00143-9898-01	68.15		
500s ea	00143-9898-05	306.40		
500 mg, 100s ea	00143-9897-01	134.75		
500s ea	00143-9897-05	600.75		
(World Gen LLC.)				
CAP, PO (POSILOK CAPS)				
250 mg, 100s ea	66814-0620-70	67.95		AB
500s ea	66814-0620-80	305.50		AB
500 mg, 100s ea	66814-0621-70	134.80		AB
500s ea	66814-0621-80	600.80		AB
(4u) REPACK				
CAP, PO, 500 mg, 4s ea	42549-0565-04	38.46		AB
10s ea	10544-0306-10	64.42		
10s ea	42549-0506-10	64.42		AB
10s ea	42549-0624-10	64.42		
28s ea	10544-0306-28	98.76		
28s ea	10544-0365-28	98.76		AB
28s ea	42549-0306-28	98.76		AB
28s ea	42549-0506-28	98.76		AB
28s ea	42549-0565-28	98.76		AB
30s ea	42549-0565-30	99.46		AB
40s ea	42549-0565-40	116.18		AB
(A-S Medication) REPACK				
CAP, PO, 250 mg, 4s ea	54569-0304-08	2.77		EE
20s ea	54569-0304-02	13.87		EE
28s ea	54569-0304-03	19.42		EE
30s ea	54569-0304-05	20.81		EE
40s ea	54569-0304-04	27.74		EE
500 mg, 6s ea	54569-3324-03	8.26		EE
8s ea	54569-0305-08	5.50		EE
10s ea	54569-0305-05	13.76		EE
14s ea	54569-0305-03	19.26		EE
20s ea	54569-0305-00	27.52		EE
28s ea	54569-0305-01	38.53		EE
30s ea	54569-0305-06	41.28		EE
40s ea	54569-0305-02	55.04		EE
100s ea	54569-0305-07	137.60		EE
PDR, PO, 125 mg/5 ml,				
200 ml	54569-1023-00	15.75		EE
250 mg/5 ml, 100 ml	54569-1024-00	18.90		EE
200 ml	54569-1025-00	31.50		EE
(Aidarex) REPACK				
CAP, PO, 500 mg, 7s ea	33261-0020-07	28.07		
10s ea	33261-0020-10	40.10		
14s ea	33261-0020-14	56.14		
20s ea	33261-0020-20	80.20		
21s ea	33261-0020-21	84.21		
28s ea	33261-0020-28	112.28		
30s ea	33261-0020-30	120.30		
40s ea	33261-0020-40	160.40		
42s ea	33261-0020-42	168.42		
48s ea	33261-0020-48	192.48		
60s ea	33261-0020-60	240.60		
(Altura) REPACK				
CAP, PO, 250 mg, 12s ea	63874-0111-12	18.00		EE
14s ea	63874-0111-14	21.00		EE
15s ea	63874-0111-15	22.50		EE
16s ea	63874-0111-16	24.00		EE
20s ea	63874-0111-20	30.00		EE
21s ea	63874-0111-21	31.50		EE
24s ea	63874-0111-24	36.00		EE
28s ea	63874-0111-28	42.00		EE
30s ea	63874-0111-30	45.00		EE
40s ea	63874-0111-40	60.00		EE
50s ea	63874-0111-50	75.00		EE
56s ea	63874-0111-56	84.00		EE
60s ea	63874-0111-60	90.00		EE
80s ea	63874-0111-80	120.00		EE
100s ea	63874-0111-01	150.00		EE
120s ea	63874-0111-04	180.00		EE
150s ea	63874-0111-72	225.00		EE
200s ea	63874-0111-74	300.00		EE
300s ea	63874-0111-77	450.00		EE
500s ea	63874-0111-03	750.00		EE
500 mg, 4s ea	63874-0112-04	11.84		EE
5s ea	63874-0112-05	14.80		EE
6s ea	63874-0112-06	17.76		EE
8s ea	63874-0112-08	23.68		EE
10s ea	63874-0112-10	29.60		EE
12s ea	63874-0112-12	35.52		EE
14s ea	63874-0112-14	41.44		EE
15s ea	63874-0112-15	44.40		EE
16s ea	63874-0112-16	47.36		EE
18s ea	63874-0112-18	53.28		EE
20s ea	63874-0112-20	59.20		EE
21s ea	63874-0112-21	62.16		EE
24s ea	63874-0112-24	71.04		EE
25s ea	63874-0112-25	74.00		EE
28s ea	63874-0112-28	82.88		EE
30s ea	63874-0112-30	88.80		EE
40s ea	63874-0112-40	118.40		EE
50s ea	63874-0112-50	148.00		EE
56s ea	63874-0112-56	165.76		EE
60s ea	63874-0112-60	177.60		EE
100s ea	63874-0112-01	296.00		EE
150s ea	63874-0112-72	444.00		EE
200s ea	63874-0112-74	592.00		EE
300s ea	63874-0112-77	888.00		EE
500s ea	63874-0112-03	1480.00		EE
PDR, PO, 125 mg/5 ml,				
100 ml	63874-0166-10	13.37		EE
200 ml	63874-0166-20	29.00		EE
250 mg/5 ml, 100 ml	63874-0155-10	25.92		EE
200 ml	63874-0155-20	52.89		EE
(American Health) REPACK				
CAP, PO (10X10)				
250 mg, 100s ea UD	62584-0235-01	170.24		AB
500 mg, 100s ea UD	62584-0236-01	348.40		AB
(Bryant Ranch) REPACK				
CAP, PO, 250 mg, 20s ea	63629-1317-03	36.32		
28s ea	63629-1317-01	42.65		
30s ea	63629-1317-04	45.48		
40s ea	63629-1317-02	72.64		
100s ea	63629-1317-05	151.60		
500 mg, 14s ea	63629-1319-06	46.03		
20s ea	63629-1319-01	66.33		
21s ea	63629-1319-05	69.04		
28s ea	63629-1319-02	92.06		
30s ea	63629-1319-04	99.49		
40s ea	63629-1319-03	132.65		
60s ea	63629-1319-07	199.99		
100s ea	63629-1319-08	270.00		
(Core) REPACK				
CAP, PO, 250 mg, 15s ea	33358-0071-15	22.11		
20s ea	33358-0071-20	37.23		
28s ea	33358-0071-28	57.17		
40s ea	33358-0071-40	78.37		
60s ea	33358-0071-60	141.58		
500 mg, 14s ea	33358-0072-14	47.18		
15s ea	33358-0072-15	60.51		
20s ea	33358-0072-20	67.99		
21s ea	33358-0072-21	68.99		
28s ea	33358-0072-28	94.36		
30s ea	33358-0072-30	101.98		
40s ea	33358-0072-40	135.97		
60s ea	33358-0072-60	204.99		
(DHS, Inc.) REPACK				
CAP, PO, 250 mg, 21s ea	55887-0991-21	28.10		AB
30s ea	55887-0991-30	40.12		AB
40s ea	55887-0991-40	53.50		AB
500 mg, 5s ea	55887-0958-05	12.75		AB
8s ea	55887-0958-08	20.40		AB
14s ea	55887-0958-14	35.70		AB
15s ea	55887-0958-15	38.25		AB
20s ea	55887-0958-20	50.40		AB
21s ea	55887-0958-21	52.92		AB
28s ea	55887-0958-28	69.40		AB
30s ea	55887-0958-30	72.00		AB
40s ea	55887-0958-40	89.00		AB
PDR, PO, 125 mg/5 ml,				
100 ml	55887-0719-01	13.91		
(1X200ML)				
125 mg/5 ml,				
200 ml	55887-0719-20	15.75		AB
(Dispensing Solutions) REPACK				
CAP, PO, 250 mg, 3s ea	66336-0441-03	5.75		AB
6s ea	55045-1170-06	9.30		AB
8s ea	66336-0441-08	15.06		AB
9s ea	55045-1170-09	13.95		AB
15s ea	55045-1170-01	23.25		AB
20s ea	55045-1170-07	31.00		AB
20s ea	66336-0441-20	30.26		AB
28s ea	66336-0441-28	42.34		AB
30s ea	55045-1170-08	46.50		AB
40s ea	55045-1170-03	62.00		AB
40s ea	66336-0441-40	60.54		AB
60s ea	55045-1170-04	93.00		AB
90s ea	55045-1170-05	139.50		AB
100s ea	55045-1170-00	155.00		AB
120s ea	55045-1170-02	186.00		AB
500 mg, 4s ea	55045-2787-04	11.96		AB
6s ea	55045-1117-01	17.94		AB
6s ea	66336-0055-06	15.57		AB
7s ea	55045-2610-07	20.93		
8s ea	55045-2610-02	23.92		AB
8s ea	66336-0055-08	20.76		AB
10s ea	55045-1117-00	29.90		AB
10s ea	66336-0055-10	25.96		AB
12s ea	55045-1117-02	35.88		AB
14s ea	55045-2610-04	41.86		AB
14s ea	66336-0055-14	36.34		AB
15s ea	55045-1117-05	44.85		AB
20s ea	55045-1117-07	59.80		
20s ea	55045-3923-01	59.80		AB
20s ea	66336-0055-20	51.91		AB
21s ea	55045-1117-09	62.79		
21s ea	66336-0055-21	54.51		AB
28s ea	55045-1117-06	83.72		AB
28s ea	66336-0055-28	72.68		AB
30s ea	55045-1117-08	89.70		AB
30s ea	66336-0055-30	77.87		AB
40s ea	55045-1117-04	119.60		AB
40s ea	66336-0055-40	103.83		AB
(POSILOK CAPS)				
500 mg, 60s ea	55045-2610-06	179.40		AB
90s ea	55045-2610-09	269.10		AB
100s ea	55045-1117-03	299.00		AB
120s ea	55045-2610-01	358.80		AB
PDR, PO, 125 mg/5 ml,				
100 ml	55045-1247-01	14.99		AB
200 ml	55045-1262-09	21.00		AB
250 mg/5 ml, 100 ml	55045-1415-01	21.00		AB
200 ml	55045-1500-09	25.05		AB
(GSMS) REPACK				
CAP, PO (UNIT OF USE)				
250 mg, 40s ea	60429-0036-40	50.00	12.50	AB
500 mg, 40s ea	60429-0037-40	100.00	25.00	AB
(HomeMed) REPACK				
CAP, PO, 250 mg, 6s ea	51655-0024-87	10.46		EE
28s ea	51655-0024-29	49.99		EE
30s ea	51655-0024-24	52.33		EE
40s ea	51655-0024-51	71.39		EE
500 mg, 10s ea	51655-0025-53	29.69		EE
14s ea	51655-0025-84	43.89		EE
20s ea	51655-0025-52	59.69		EE
28s ea	51655-0025-29	88.99		EE
30s ea	51655-0025-24	94.99		EE
40s ea	51655-0025-51	119.69		EE
(IPI) REPACK				
CAP, PO, 500 mg, 14s ea	18837-0195-14	41.50		
20s ea	18837-0195-20	58.97		AB
28s ea	18837-0195-28	79.33		
30s ea	18837-0195-30	85.00		
40s ea	18837-0195-40	113.33		
(Keltman Pharma., Inc.) REPACK				
CAP, PO, 500 mg, 20s ea	68387-0190-20	73.40		AB
21s ea	68387-0190-21	77.06		
30s ea	68387-0190-30	110.01		AB
40s ea	68387-0190-40	146.80		AB
(LWP) REPACK				
CAP, PO, 500 mg, 40s ea	64038-0033-40	55.70		AB
100s ea	64038-0033-01	139.25		AB
(Nucare Pharm) REPACK				
CAP, PO, 250 mg, 12s ea	66267-0049-12	28.22		EE
20s ea	66267-0049-20	42.00		EE
28s ea	66267-0049-28	55.78		EE
30s ea	66267-0049-30	59.23		EE
40s ea	66267-0049-40	76.46		EE
500 mg, 5s ea	66267-0050-05	15.07		EE
6s ea	66267-0050-06	18.73		
10s ea	66267-0050-10	32.80		AB
12s ea	66267-0050-12	37.47		
14s ea	66267-0050-14	45.92		AB
15s ea	66267-0050-15	49.20		AB
20s ea	66267-0050-20	65.60		AB

PROD/MFR	NDC	AWP	DP	OBC
28s ea	66267-0050-28	91.78		AB
30s ea	66267-0050-30	98.40		AB
40s ea	66267-0050-40	119.00		
60s ea	66267-0050-60	196.80		AB
PDR, PO, 250 mg/5 ml,				
100 ml	66267-0982-00	39.99		EE
200 ml	66267-0981-20	48.79		EE
(Palmetto)				
REPACK				
CAP, PO, 250 mg, 3s ea	23490-5248-01	10.07		
6s ea	23490-5248-02	16.58		
8s ea	23490-5248-03	18.95		
20s ea	23490-5248-04	39.49		
28s ea	23490-5248-05	55.28		
30s ea	23490-5248-06	59.23		
40s ea	23490-5248-07	78.97		
60s ea	23490-5248-08	118.46		
500 mg, 6s ea	23490-5251-01	26.63		
8s ea	23490-5251-02	30.43		
10s ea	23490-5251-03	31.66		
14s ea	23490-5251-04	44.33		
15s ea	23490-7843-01	47.55		
20s ea	23490-5251-05	63.33		
21s ea	23490-5251-06	66.49		
25s ea	23490-7843-02	73.24		
28s ea	23490-5251-07	88.66		
30s ea	23490-5251-08	94.99		
40s ea	23490-5251-09	126.65		
60s ea	23490-5251-00	189.98		
100s ea	23490-7843-07	317.00		
CEPHALEXIN (Palmetto)				
PDR, PO (1X100ML)				
125 mg/5 ml,				
100 ml	23490-5249-01	39.99		
CEPHALEXIN (Palmetto)				
(1X200ML,STRAWBERRY)				
125 mg/5 ml,				
200 ml	23490-5249-02	39.99		AB
250 mg/5 ml, 100 ml	23490-5250-01	39.99		
200 ml	23490-5250-02	48.79		
TAB, PO, 250 mg, 40s ea	23490-0283-04	75.55		
500 mg, 40s ea	23490-0285-04	109.97		
(PD-Rx Pharm)				
REPACK				
CAP, PO (USP)				
250 mg, 4s ea	43063-0016-04	43.50		
6s ea	43063-0016-06	86.00		
6s ea	55289-0057-06	46.00		AB
(USP)				
250 mg, 9s ea	43063-0016-09	79.10		
10s ea	55289-0057-10	54.44		AB
(USP)				
250 mg, 10s ea	43063-0016-10	94.40		
15s ea	55289-0057-15	65.00		AB
(USP)				
250 mg, 15s ea	43063-0016-15	105.00		
20s ea	55289-0057-20	75.60		AB
(USP)				
250 mg, 20s ea	43063-0016-20	115.60		
24s ea	55289-0057-24	84.00		AB
(USP)				
250 mg, 24s ea	43063-0016-24	124.00		
28s ea	55289-0057-28	92.44		AB
(USP)				
250 mg, 28s ea	43063-0016-28	132.40		
30s ea	55289-0057-30	96.67		AB
(REDI-SCRIPT)				
250 mg, 30s ea	58864-0072-30	96.67		AB
(USP)				
250 mg, 30s ea	43063-0016-30	136.70		
40s ea	55289-0057-40	117.78		AB
(REDI-SCRIPT)				
250 mg, 40s ea	58864-0072-40	117.80		AB
(USP)				
250 mg, 40s ea	43063-0016-40	157.80		
500 mg, 4s ea	43063-0047-04	100.20		
4s ea	55289-0058-04	60.20		
6s ea	43063-0047-06	46.00		
8s ea	55289-0058-08	60.20		AB
(USP)				
500 mg, 8s ea	43063-0047-08	101.80		
9s ea	43063-0047-09	79.10		
10s ea	55289-0058-10	68.89		AB
(USP)				
500 mg, 10s ea	43063-0047-10	108.90		
14s ea	55289-0058-14	83.11		AB
(USP)				
500 mg, 14s ea	43063-0047-14	123.10		
20s ea	55289-0058-20	104.44		AB
(REDI-SCRIPT)				
500 mg, 20s ea	58864-0073-20	104.40		AB
(USP)				
500 mg, 20s ea	43063-0047-20	144.40		
21s ea	55289-0058-21	108.00		AB
(USP)				
500 mg, 21s ea	43063-0047-21	148.00		
24s ea	55289-0058-24	118.67		AB
(USP)				
500 mg, 24s ea	43063-0047-24	158.70		
28s ea	55289-0058-28	132.89		AB
(REDI-SCRIPT)				
500 mg, 28s ea	58864-0073-28	140.00		AB
(USP)				
500 mg, 28s ea	43063-0047-28	172.90		
30s ea	55289-0058-30	140.00		AB
(REDI-SCRIPT)				
500 mg, 30s ea	58864-0073-30	140.00		AB
(USP)				
500 mg, 30s ea	43063-0047-30	180.00		
40s ea	55289-0058-40	175.60		AB
(REDI-SCRIPT)				
500 mg, 40s ea	58864-0073-40	175.60		AB
(USP)				
500 mg, 40s ea	43063-0047-40	215.60		
56s ea	58864-0073-56	232.44		AB
(USP)				
500 mg, 56s ea	43063-0047-56	272.40		
TAB, PO, 500 mg, 56s ea	55289-0058-56	232.44		AB
(Pharma Pac)				
REPACK				
CAP, PO, 250 mg, 8s ea	52959-0030-08	13.10		EE
12s ea	52959-0030-12	19.65		AB
20s ea	52959-0030-20	32.76		EE
24s ea	52959-0030-24	39.30		EE
28s ea	52959-0030-28	45.84		EE
30s ea	52959-0030-30	49.11		EE
40s ea	52959-0030-40	65.47		EE
56s ea	52959-0030-56	91.64		EE
100s ea	52959-0030-01	163.61		AB
500 mg, 4s ea	52959-0031-04	16.41		EE
6s ea	52959-0031-06	24.61		EE
8s ea	52959-0031-08	32.81		EE
10s ea	52959-0031-10	41.01		EE
12s ea	52959-0031-12	49.21		EE
14s ea	52959-0031-14	57.40		EE
15s ea	52959-0031-15	61.50		EE
20s ea	52959-0031-20	81.99		EE
21s ea	52959-0031-21	86.08		EE
24s ea	52959-0031-24	98.37		EE
28s ea	52959-0031-28	139.58		EE
30s ea	52959-0031-30	122.95		EE
40s ea	52959-0031-40	159.90		EE
56s ea	52959-0031-56	223.85		EE
60s ea	52959-0031-60	239.80		EE
100s ea	52959-0031-00	399.62		EE
120s ea	52959-0031-02	479.44		EE
PDR, PO (CHERI-BERI)				
125 mg/5 ml,				
100 ml	52959-0200-01	13.36		AB
200 ml	52959-0200-02	24.12		AB
250 mg/5 ml, 100 ml	52959-0620-00	32.99		AB
200 ml	52959-0620-01	47.05		AB
(Phys Total Care)				
REPACK				
CAP, PO, 250 mg, 20s ea	54868-0153-01	9.69		EE
30s ea	54868-0153-05	13.05		EE
40s ea	54868-0153-03	16.38		EE
60s ea	54868-0153-09	22.36		EE
100s ea	54868-0153-08	36.45		EE
500s ea	54868-0153-00	140.91		EE
500 mg, 10s ea	54868-0154-07	10.50		EE
14s ea	54868-0154-06	11.41		EE
20s ea	54868-0154-01	19.18		EE
28s ea	54868-0154-03	32.21		EE
30s ea	54868-0154-02	25.77		EE
40s ea	54868-0154-04	32.36		EE
60s ea	54868-0154-09	62.16		EE
500s ea	54868-0154-00	315.44		EE
PDR, PO, 125 mg/5 ml,				
100 ml	54868-0538-02	23.46		EE
200 ml	54868-0538-01	34.74		EE
250 mg/5 ml, 100 ml	54868-1385-01	25.47		EE
200 ml	54868-1385-02	49.41		EE
TAB, PO, 500 mg, 20s ea	54868-0155-01	21.04		EE
(Physician Partner)				
REPACK				
CAP, PO, 250 mg, 20s ea	21695-0316-20	32.64		
28s ea	21695-0316-28	45.69		
30s ea	21695-0316-30	48.95		
40s ea	21695-0316-40	65.27		
500 mg, 8s ea	21695-0317-08	23.08		
12s ea	21695-0317-12	40.72		AB
14s ea	21695-0317-14	47.51		
20s ea	21695-0317-20	57.69		
21s ea	21695-0317-21	60.57		
28s ea	21695-0317-28	80.76		
30s ea	21695-0317-30	86.53		
40s ea	21695-0317-40	115.38		
60s ea	21695-0317-60	165.12		
PDR, PO (1X200ML,STRAWBERRY)				
125 mg/5 ml,				
200 ml	21695-0789-20	63.00		AB
(1X20ML,STRAWBERRY)				
250 mg/5 ml, 20 ml	21695-0551-20	63.00		AB
(1X100ML,STRAWBERRY)				
250 mg/5 ml,				
100 ml	21695-0551-00	37.80		AB
(Quality Care Prod)				
REPACK				
CAP, PO, 250 mg, 4s ea	49999-0041-04	7.45		EE
10s ea	49999-0041-10	18.65		EE
20s ea	49999-0041-20	37.26		EE
28s ea	49999-0041-28	52.16		EE
30s ea	49999-0041-30	55.89		EE
40s ea	49999-0041-40	35.00		EE
500 mg, 10s ea	49999-0007-10	33.20		EE
12s ea	49999-0007-12	39.84		AB
14s ea	49999-0007-14	46.44		AB
15s ea	49999-0007-15	49.80		AB
20s ea	49999-0007-20	66.40		EE
21s ea	49999-0007-21	69.72		EE
28s ea	49999-0007-28	92.69		EE
30s ea	49999-0007-30	99.60		EE
40s ea	49999-0007-40	132.80		EE
60s ea	49999-0007-60	199.20		EE
90s ea	49999-0007-90	298.80		AB
100s ea	49999-0007-00	332.00		AB
PDR, PO, 125 mg/5 ml,				
100 ml	49999-0713-00	18.00		
(1X200ML,BUBBLE GUM)				
125 mg/5 ml,				
200 ml	49999-0713-02	46.00		
250 mg/5 ml, 100 ml	49999-0261-00	21.74		
200 ml	49999-0261-20	56.46		EE
(Southwood)				
REPACK				
CAP, PO, 250 mg, 12s ea	58016-0138-12	14.82		EE
14s ea	58016-0138-14	17.29		EE
15s ea	58016-0138-15	18.53		EE
20s ea	58016-0138-20	24.71		EE
21s ea	58016-0138-21	25.94		EE
24s ea	58016-0138-24	29.65		EE
28s ea	58016-0138-28	34.59		EE
30s ea	58016-0138-30	37.06		EE
40s ea	58016-0138-40	49.41		EE
56s ea	58016-0138-56	69.18		EE
60s ea	58016-0138-60	74.12		EE
100s ea	58016-0138-00	123.53		EE
120s ea	58016-0138-02	148.24		AB
150s ea	58016-0138-03	185.30		AB
200s ea	58016-0138-89	247.06		AB
300s ea	58016-0138-73	370.59		AB
500 mg, 4s ea	58016-0139-04	9.71		EE
5s ea	58016-0139-05	12.14		EE
6s ea	58016-0139-06	14.57		EE
8s ea	58016-0139-08	19.42		EE
10s ea	58016-0139-10	24.28		EE
12s ea	58016-0139-12	29.13		EE
14s ea	58016-0139-14	33.99		EE
15s ea	58016-0139-15	36.42		EE
18s ea	58016-0139-18	43.70		EE
20s ea	58016-0139-20	60.20		AB
21s ea	58016-0139-21	50.98		EE
24s ea	58016-0139-24	58.27		EE
28s ea	58016-0139-28	84.28		AB
30s ea	58016-0139-30	90.30		AB
40s ea	58016-0139-40	120.40		AB
50s ea	58016-0139-50	121.39		EE
56s ea	58016-0139-56	135.96		EE
60s ea	58016-0139-60	180.60		AB
90s ea	58016-0139-90	270.90		AB
100s ea	58016-0139-00	301.00		AB
120s ea	58016-0139-02	291.34		EE
150s ea	58016-0139-03	364.17		AB
200s ea	58016-0139-89	485.56		AB
300s ea	58016-0139-73	728.34		AB
PDR, PO, 125 mg/5 ml,				
100 ml	58016-1019-01	15.00		EE
200 ml	58016-1046-01	21.00		EE
250 mg/5 ml, 100 ml	58016-1021-01	21.00		EE
200 ml	58016-1045-01	24.95		EE
(Stat Rx)				
REPACK				
CAP, PO, 250 mg, 21s ea	16590-0050-21	17.50		
28s ea	16590-0050-28	23.33		

PROD/MFR	NDC	AWP	DP	OBC
30s ea	16590-0050-30	25.00		
56s ea	16590-0050-56	96.44		AB
500 mg, 4s ea	16590-0051-04	11.84		AB
8s ea	16590-0051-08	23.68		
10s ea	16590-0051-10	29.60		AB
14s ea	16590-0051-14	39.66		
16s ea	16590-0051-16	45.33		
20s ea	16590-0051-20	56.66		
21s ea	16590-0051-21	59.50		
28s ea	16590-0051-28	94.10		
30s ea	16590-0051-30	85.00		
40s ea	16590-0051-40	113.33		
56s ea	16590-0051-56	158.66		
120s ea	16590-0051-72	340.00		
PDR, PO (1X100ML,STRAWBERRY)				
250 mg/5 ml,				
100 ml	16590-0049-32	22.10		AB
200 ml	16590-0049-36	50.00		
(Vibranta)				
REPACK				
CAP, PO, 250 mg, 20s ea	57866-7216-02	37.26		
40s ea	57866-7216-03	35.00		
500 mg, 14s ea	57866-0117-04	23.16		
20s ea	57866-0117-05	30.00		
40s ea	57866-0117-03	123.48		
CEPHALEXIN HYDROCHLORIDE (Palmetto)				
REPACK				
cephalexin hydrochloride				
TAB, PO, 500 mg, 10s ea	23490-5246-00	43.44		
CEPHALEXIN MONOHYDRATE (Vibranta)				
REPACK				
cephalexin				
CAP, PO, 250 mg, 4s ea	57866-7216-07	7.45		
12s ea	57866-7216-08	18.99		
28s ea	57866-7216-01	52.16		
30s ea	57866-7216-04	55.89		
500 mg, 28s ea	57866-0117-01	74.70		
30s ea	57866-0117-06	123.75		
CEPHRADINE (Southwood)				
REPACK				
CAP, PO, 250 mg, 10s ea	58016-0154-10	8.60		EE
12s ea	58016-0154-12	10.32		EE
14s ea	58016-0154-14	12.04		EE
16s ea	58016-0154-16	13.76		EE
18s ea	58016-0154-18	15.48		EE
20s ea	58016-0154-20	17.20		EE
24s ea	58016-0154-24	20.64		EE
30s ea	58016-0154-30	25.80		EE
36s ea	58016-0154-36	30.96		EE
40s ea	58016-0154-40	34.40		EE
100s ea	58016-0154-00	85.99		EE
500 mg, 10s ea	58016-0155-10	16.89		EE
12s ea	58016-0155-12	20.27		EE
15s ea	58016-0155-15	25.33		EE
16s ea	58016-0155-16	30.08		EE
18s ea	58016-0155-18	33.84		EE
20s ea	58016-0155-20	37.60		EE
24s ea	58016-0155-24	45.12		EE
28s ea	58016-0155-28	47.29		EE
30s ea	58016-0155-30	50.67		EE
36s ea	58016-0155-36	67.68		EE
40s ea	58016-0155-40	75.20		EE
100s ea	58016-0155-00	188.00		EE
CEPROTIN (Baxter Bioscience)				
protein c, human				
PDS, IV (400-600IU)				
1 iu, ea	00944-4175-05	1.51		
(800-1200IU)				
1 iu, ea	00944-4175-10	1.51		
CEREBYX (Pfizer)				
fosphenytoin sodium				
SOL, IJ (VIAL)				
50 mg pe/ml,				
2 ml 25s	00071-4007-05	719.41	599.51	
CEREDASE (Genzyme)				
alglucerase				
SOL, IV, 80 u/ml, 5 ml	58468-1060-01	1903.20	1586.00	
CEREFOLIN (Pamlab)				
l-methylfolate/vit b12/vit b2/vit b6				
TAB, PO (SF,GLUTEN-FREE)				
1 mg-5.635 mg-50 mg-5 mg,				
90s ea	00525-0503-90	168.54		
CEREFOLIN NAC (Pamlab)				
acetylcysteine/l-methylfolate/methylcobalamin				
TAB, PO (SF,GLUTEN-FREE)				
600 mg-5.6 mg-2 mg,				
90s ea	00525-0510-90	144.92		
(A-S Medication)				
REPACK				
TAB, PO (SF,GLUTEN-FREE)				
600 mg-5.6 mg-2 mg,				
90s ea	54569-6125-00	146.56		
(Physician Partner)				
REPACK				
TAB, PO (SF,GLUTEN-FREE)				
600 mg-5.6 mg-2 mg,				
60s ea	21695-0355-60	195.41		
(Stat Rx)				
REPACK				
TAB, PO (SF,GLUTEN-FREE)				
600 mg-5.6 mg-2 mg,				
30s ea	16590-0770-30	57.02		
90s ea	16590-0770-90	168.17		
CERESIN (PCCA)				
ceresin wax				
WAX, NA, 1 gm	51927-2605-00	0.14		
CERESIN WAX				
(PCCA) *See CERESIN*				
CERETEC (GE)				
technetium tc 99m exametazime				
KIT, IJ (5 VIALS/KIT)				
ea	17156-0023-05	3728.42		
CEREZYME (Genzyme)				
imiglucerase				
PDS, IV (VIAL)				
200 u, ea	58468-1983-01	951.60	793.00	
400 u, ea	58468-4663-01	1903.20	1586.00	
CERIC AMMONIUM NITRATE (Baker, J.T.)				
ammonium ceric nitrate				
CRY, NA (A.C.S., REAGENT)				
500 gm	10106-1534-01	244.06		
CERIC AMMONIUM SULFATE DIHYDRATE (Baker, J.T.)				
ceric sulfate				
CRY, NA (A.C.S., REAGENT)				
500 gm	10106-1535-01	153.21		
CERIC SULFATE				
(Baker, J.T.) *See CERIC AMMONIUM SULFATE DIHYDRATE*				
(Baker, J.T.) *See CERIC SULFATE 0.1N VOLUMETRIC*				
CERIC SULFATE 0.1N VOLUMETRIC (Baker, J.T.)				
ceric sulfate				
SOL, NA (REAGENT)				
1000 ml	10106-5626-02	44.44		
CERON (Cypress Pharm)				
cpm/phenyleph hcl				
SOL, PO (AF,SF,RASPBERRY)				
4 mg/5 ml-12.5 mg/5 ml,				
473 ml	60258-0414-16	61.10		
(AF,SF,RASPBERRY,DROPS)				
1 mg/ml-3.5 mg/ml,				
30 ml	60258-0416-30	33.42		
CERON-DM (Cypress Pharm)				
cpm/dm/phenyleph hcl				
SOL, PO (AF,SF,GRAPE)				
118 ml	60258-0415-04	29.03		
473 ml	60258-0415-16	105.61		
(AF,SF,GRAPE,DROPS)				
30 ml	60258-0417-30	46.03		
CEROVEL (Hawthorn Pharm)				
urea				
CRE, TP, 40%, 133 gm	63717-0040-05	65.79		
GEL, TP, 40%, 25 ml	63717-0038-30	105.34		
LOT, TP, 40%, 325 ml	63717-0039-11	94.49		
CERTOLIZUMAB PEGOL				
(UCB) *See CIMZIA*				
CERTUSS (Capellon)				
carbetapentane citrate/guaifenesin				
T12, PO (DUOMATRIX RELEASE TAB)				
60 mg-1200 mg,				
90s ea	64543-0180-90	118.26		
CERTUSS-D (Capellon)				
dm/gg/phenyleph hcl				
TER, PO (FILM COATED)				
60 mg-600 mg-40 mg,				
100s ea	64543-0175-01	106.61		
CERUBIDINE (Bedford)				
daunorubicin hydrochloride				
PDS, IV (S.D.V.)				
20 mg, 10s ea	55390-0281-10	504.00		AP
CERUMENEX (Phys Total Care)				
REPACK				
triethanolamine polypeptide oleate				
SOL, OT, 10%, 6 ml	54868-0207-01	28.58		
12 ml	54868-0207-00	45.40		
(Quality Care Prod)				
REPACK				
SOL, OT, 10%, 6 ml	49999-0134-06	77.76		
12 ml	49999-0134-12	150.52		
(Southwood)				
REPACK				
SOL, OT, 10%, 6 ml	58016-6012-01	25.93		
12 ml	58016-6095-01	41.56		
CERVARIX (Glaxo)				
human papillomavirus recomb vaccine bivalent				
SUS, IM (PF)				
0.5 ml	58160-0830-32	154.35		
0.5 ml 5s	58160-0830-46	771.75		
0.5 ml 10s	58160-0830-11	1543.50		
CERVIDIL (Forest Pharm)				
dinoprostone				
ICR, VG, 0.3 mg/hr, ea	00456-4123-63	256.13		
CESIA (Prasco Labs)				
desogestrel/ethinyl estradiol				
TAB, PO (3 X 28)				
84s ea	66993-0615-28	99.99		
CESINEX (Hall)				
antidiarrheal combination				
SUS, PO (1X480ML,LEMON-LIME)				
480 ml	44411-1151-06	64.06		
CESINEX 100 (Hall)				
antidiarrheal combination				
SUS, PO (1X240ML,LEMON-LIME)				
240 ml	44411-1100-08	34.38		
CESINEX 125 (Hall)				
antidiarrheal combination				
SUS, PO (1X240ML,LEMON-LIME)				
240 ml	44411-1125-08	34.38		
CESINEX 150 (Hall)				
antidiarrheal combination				
SUS, PO (1X240ML,LEMON-LIME)				
240 ml	44411-1150-08	34.38		
CESINEX 20 (Hall)				
antidiarrheal combination				
SUS, PO (1X120ML,LEMON-LIME)				
120 ml	44411-1020-04	30.63		
CESINEX 25 (Hall)				
antidiarrheal combination				
SUS, PO (1X120ML,LEMON-LIME)				
120 ml	44411-1025-04	30.63		
CESINEX 30 (Hall)				
antidiarrheal combination				
SUS, PO (1X120ML,LEMON-LIME)				
120 ml	44411-1030-04	30.63		
CESINEX 35 (Hall)				
antidiarrheal combination				
SUS, PO (1X120ML,LEMON-LIME)				
120 ml	44411-1035-04	30.63		
CESINEX 40 (Hall)				
antidiarrheal combination				
SUS, PO (1X120ML,LEMON-LIME)				
120 ml	44411-1040-04	30.63		
CESINEX 50 (Hall)				
antidiarrheal combination				
SUS, PO (1X120ML,LEMON-LIME)				
120 ml	44411-1050-04	30.63		
CESINEX 60 (Hall)				
antidiarrheal combination				
SUS, PO (1X120ML,LEMON-LIME)				
120 ml	44411-1060-04	30.63		
CESINEX 80 (Hall)				
antidiarrheal combination				
SUS, PO (1X120ML,LEMON-LIME)				
120 ml	44411-1080-04	30.63		
CESIUM CARBONATE (PCCA)				
POW, NA, 1 gm	51927-3425-00	7.20		
CESIUM CHLORIDE (Baker, J.T.)				
POW, NA (ULTRAPURE BIOREAGENT)				
100 gm	10106-4042-04	59.69		
1000 gm	10106-4042-02	364.00		
(PCCA)				
POW, NA, 1 gm	51927-2549-00	1.65		

PROD/MFR NDC AWP DP OBC

CETACAINE (Cetylite)
benzocaine/butamben/tetracaine
GEL, TP (5GMX1)
14%-2%-2%, 5 gm . . . **10223-0215-02** 9.00
KIT, MM (1 BOT/2-J4,1-J6,1-J8CA)
14%-2%-2%, ea. **10223-0201-03** 91.00
LIQ, TP (W/LUER-LOCK DSPNSR CAP)
14%-2%-2%, 14 gm . . **10223-0202-02** 35.00
30 gm **10223-0202-04** 55.00
SPR, TP (1 BOT/I-J4)
14%-2%-2%, 56 ml . . **10223-0201-01** 79.00

(A-S Medication)
REPACK
SPR, TP, 14%-2%-2%,
56 ml. **54569-2028-00** 64.19

CETACORT (Valeant Pharm Intl)
hydrocortisone
LOT, TP, 1%, 60 ml. . . . . **00064-2000-02** 33.03 AT

CETEARETH 20/CETOSTEARYL ALCOHOL
(PCCA) *See CETEARYL ALCOHOL CETEARETH 20*

CETEARYL ALCOHOL CETEARETH 20 (PCCA)
ceteareth 20/cetostearyl alcohol
POW, NA, 1 gm **51927-2444-00** 0.54

CETETH-10
(Amend) *See BRIJ 56*

CETETH-2
(Amend) *See BRIJ 52*

CETETH-20
(PCCA) *See CETOMACROGOL 1000*
(Spectrum Pharmacy) *See BRIJ 58*

CETIRIZINE HYDROCHLORIDE (Apotex Corp.)
SYR, PO (1X120ML)
1 mg/ml, 120 ml . . . . . **60505-0385-03** 36.49 AA
(1X480ML)
1 mg/ml, 480 ml . . . . . **60505-0385-05** 145.95 AA

(Caraco)
CTB, PO (ALLERGY,TUTTI-FRUTTI)
5 mg, 30s ea. . . . . **57664-0343-83** 74.09 EE
10 mg, 30s ea. . . . . **57664-0344-83** 74.09 EE

(Cypress Pharm)
SYR, PO (1X120ML,BANANA-GRAPE)
1 mg/ml, 120 ml . . . . . **60258-0860-04** 36.50 AA
(1X480ML,BANANA-GRAPE)
1 mg/ml, 480 ml . . . . . **60258-0860-16** 145.95 AA

(Dr Reddy's)
SYR, PO (1X120ML)
1 mg/ml, 120 ml . . . . . **55111-0700-04** 36.50 AA
(1X480ML)
1 mg/ml, 480 ml . . . . . **55111-0700-16** 145.95 AA

(Perrigo)
SYR, PO (1X120ML,BANANA-GRAPE)
1 mg/ml, 120 ml . . . . . **45802-0626-26** 36.50 AA

(Qualitest)
SYR, PO (1X120ML,BANANA-GRAPE)
1 mg/ml, 120 ml **00603-9063-54** 36.50
(1X480ML,BANANA-GRAPE)
1 mg/ml, 480 ml **00603-9063-58** 145.95

(Ranbaxy Pharm)
SYR, PO (1X120ML,BANANA-GRAPE)
1 mg/ml, 120 ml . . . . . **63304-0936-04** 36.50 AA

(Teva)
SYR, PO (1X120ML,BANANA)
1 mg/ml, 120 ml . . . . . **00093-6300-12** 36.50 AA
(1X473ML,BANANA)
1 mg/ml, 473 ml . . . . . **00093-6300-16** 145.97 AA

CETOMACROGOL 1000 (PCCA)
ceteth-20
POW, NA (BP)
1 gm **51927-2526-00** 0.20

CETOSTEARYL ALCOHOL
(Spectrum Pharmacy) *See ALCOHOL CETOSTEARYL*

CETRAXAL (Wraser Pharm)
ciprofloxacin hydrochloride
SOL, OT (PF)
0.2%, 14s ea. **66992-0450-14** 99.96

CETRIMONIUM BROMIDE
(Amend) *See CETYL TRIMETHYL AMMONIUM BROMIDE*
(Medisca) *See CETYL TRIMETHYL AMMONIUM BROMIDE*
(PCCA) *See CETYL TRIMETHYL AMMONIUM BROMIDE*
(Spectrum Pharmacy) *See CETYLTRIMETHYLAMMONIUM BROMIDE*

PROD/MFR NDC AWP DP OBC

CETRORELIX ACETATE
(EMD) *See CETROTIDE*

CETROTIDE (EMD)
cetrorelix acetate
PDS, SC (M.D.V.,DILUENT/SRN,NDL)
0.25 mg, ea. **44087-1225-01** 135.28
(SDV,DILUENT/SRN,NDL)
3 mg, ea. **44087-1203-01** 676.39

CETUXIMAB
(Bristol-Myers) *See ERBITUX*

CETYL ALCOHOL
(Amend) *See ALCOHOL CETYL*
(Gallipot) *See ALCOHOL CETYL*
(Hawkins) *See ALCOHOL CETYL*
(Letco) *See ALCOHOL CETYL*
(Medisca) *See ALCOHOL CETYL*

(PCCA)
POW, NA (NF)
1 gm **51927-1353-00** 0.10

(Spectrum Pharmacy) *See ALCOHOL CETYL*

CETYL ESTERS (PCCA)
spermaceti
WAX, NA (NF)
1 gm **51927-1626-00** 0.11

CETYL MYRISTOLEATE (PCCA)
POW, NA, 1 gm **51927-3027-00** 9.00

CETYL TRIMETHYL AMMONIUM BROMIDE (Amend)
cetrimonium bromide
POW, NA, 125 gm. **17317-0244-04** 8.40
454 gm. **17317-0244-01** 26.60

(Medisca)
POW, NA, 25 gm. **38779-1150-04** 22.50
(1X500GM)
500 gm. **38779-1150-08** 87.00
(1X2500GM)
2500 gm. **38779-1150-01** 352.50

(PCCA)
POW, NA, 1 gm **51927-2249-00** 2.28

CETYLPYRIDINIUM CHLORIDE (Amend)
POW, NA (U.S.P.)
125 gm. **17317-0101-04** 11.20
500 gm. **17317-0101-01** 35.00
2270 gm. **17317-0101-05** 140.00
11350 gm **17317-0101-08** 472.50

(PCCA)
POW, NA (USP)
1 gm **51927-1743-00** 0.54

(Spectrum Pharmacy)
POW, NA (U.S.P.)
125 gm. **49452-1890-01** 85.40
500 gm. **49452-1890-02** 246.05
2500 gm. **49452-1890-03** 952.00

CETYLTRIMETHYLAMMONIUM BROMIDE (Spectrum Pharmacy)
cetrimonium bromide
POW, NA, 125 gm. **49452-1900-01** 340.90
500 gm. **49452-1900-02** 899.50
2500 gm. **49452-1900-03** 1484.00

CEVIMELINE HYDROCHLORIDE
(Daiichi Sankyo) *See EVOXAC*

CGMS SYSTEM GOLD (Medtronic Minimed)
glucose meter
DEV, NA, ea **76300-0712-01** 2493.75 1995.00

CHAMOMILE FLOWER (PCCA)
POW, NA, 1 gm **51927-3486-00** 0.45

CHAMOMILE FLOWER EXTRACT (PCCA)
SOL, NA, 1 ml **51927-3270-00** 1.50

CHAMOMILLA (CUPRO CULTA) (Weleda)
homeopathic substance
LIQ, PO (2X)
50 ml. **55946-0181-15** 9.00

CHANTIX (Pfizer)
varenicline
TAB, PO (FIRST MONTH PAK)
53s ea UD **00069-0471-97** 143.53 119.61
(FILM-COATED)
0.5 mg, 56s ea UD. . . . **00069-0468-56** 143.53 119.61
(CONTINUING MONTHS PAK)
1 mg, 14s ea UD **00069-0469-97** 143.53 119.61
(FILM-COATED)
1 mg, 56s ea. **00069-0469-56** 143.53 119.61

PROD/MFR NDC AWP DP OBC

(A-S Medication)
REPACK
TAB, PO (STARTING MONTH PAK)
53s ea. **54569-5832-00** 137.16
(CONTINUING MONTH PAK)
1 mg, 56s ea. **54569-5830-00** 137.16

(Pharma Pac)
REPACK
TAB, PO (FILM-COATED)
1 mg, 56s ea. **52959-0951-56** 138.23

(Phys Total Care)
REPACK
TAB, PO (FILM-COATED)
1 mg, 56s ea. **54868-5674-00** 171.87

(Physician Partner)
REPACK
TAB, PO (FILM-COATED)
0.5 mg, 56s ea **21695-0633-56** 287.06

(Quality Care Prod)
REPACK
TAB, PO (STARTING MONTH PACK)
53s ea. **35356-0175-53** 206.50
0.5 mg, 7s ea **35356-0011-07** 25.83
14s ea. **35356-0011-14** 51.66
(FILM-COATED)
0.5 mg, 56s ea **35356-0011-56** 206.50
1 mg, 7s ea **35356-0012-07** 25.83
14s ea. **35356-0012-14** 51.66
(CONT.MONTH PACK)
1 mg, 56s ea. **35356-0174-56** 206.50
(FILM-COATED)
1 mg, 56s ea. **35356-0012-56** 206.50

(Southwood)
REPACK
TAB, PO (FILM-COATED)
0.5 mg, 30s ea **00490-0065-30** 64.71
56s ea. **00490-0065-56** 120.80
60s ea. **00490-0065-60** 129.43
90s ea. **00490-0065-90** 194.14
100s ea. **00490-0065-00** 215.71
1 mg, 30s ea. **00490-0066-30** 64.71
56s ea. **00490-0066-56** 120.80
60s ea. **00490-0066-60** 129.43
90s ea. **00490-0066-90** 194.14
100s ea. **00490-0066-00** 215.71

CHANTIX START MONTH PAK (Phys Total Care)
REPACK
varenicline
TAB, PO, 53s ea **54868-5664-00** 171.87

CHANTIX STARTER PACK (DHS, Inc.)
REPACK
varenicline
TAB, PO, 53s ea **55887-0096-53** 117.60

CHAPARRAL
(PCCA) *See CHAPARRAL HERB*

CHAPARRAL HERB (PCCA)
chaparral
POW, NA (1X1GM)
1 gm **51927-3040-00** 0.26

CHARCOAL (Gallipot)
activated charcoal
GRA, NA (6-16 MESH TECHNICAL)
454 gm. **51552-0361-06** 20.30

CHARCOAL ACTIVATED (Baker, J.T.)
activated charcoal
POW, NA (U.S.P., F.C.C.)
125 gm. **10106-1560-04** 25.88
500 gm. **10106-1560-01** 76.83

(Mallinckrodt Lab)
POW, NA (U.S.P.)
125 gm. **00406-4394-02** 24.71
500 gm. **00406-4394-12** 61.26

(Medisca)
POW, NA (U.S.P.)
500 gm. **38779-0601-08** 58.50

(Spectrum Pharmacy)
POW, NA (U.S.P.)
125 gm. **49452-1710-03** 79.45
500 gm. **49452-1710-01** 167.30
2500 gm. **49452-1710-02** 570.50

CHARCOAL WOOD (Amend)
activated charcoal
POW, NA, 454 gm. **17317-0246-01** 7.00

CHASTEBERRY EXTRACT (PCCA)
POW, NA (4:1)
1 gm **51927-3331-00** 0.54

PROD/MFR	NDC	AWP	DP	OBC
CHEESE FLAVOR (Gallipot)				
flavoring aid				
LIQ, NA (ARTIFICIAL)				
59.14 ml	51552-0632-09	10.22		
(PCCA)				
LIQ, NA (OIL MISCIBLE)				
1 ml	51927-2899-00	0.38		
(WATER MISCIBLE)				
1 ml	51927-2900-00	0.38		
CHEESE-ADE FLAVOR (PCCA)				
flavoring aid				
POW, NA (DRY)				
1 gm	51927-3449-00	0.10		
CHEESECAKE FLAVOR (PCCA)				
flavoring aid				
SOL, NA (ARTIFICIAL,CHEESECAKE)				
1 ml	51927-3136-00	0.90		
CHELIDONIUM COMPOUND (Weleda)				
homeopathic substance				
LIQ, PO, 50 ml	55946-0183-15	9.00		
CHEMET (Lundbeck)				
succimer				
CAP, PO, 100 mg, 100s ea	67386-0201-11	819.14		
CHEMO TRANSFER PIN (APP)				
transfer unit, iv fluid				
DEV, NA, 100s ea	63323-0903-90	284.90		
CHENODAL (Manchester)				
chenodiol				
TAB, PO (FILM-COATED)				
250 mg, 100s ea	45043-0876-40	3960.00	3300.00	
CHENODEOXYCHOLIC ACID (Medisca)				
chenodiol				
POW, NA (1X25GM)				
25 gm	38779-2271-04	705.00		
(PCCA)				
POW, NA (1X1GM)				
1 gm	51927-2835-00	30.60		
CHENODIOL				
(Manchester) *See CHENODAL*				
(Medisca) *See CHENODEOXYCHOLIC ACID*				
(PCCA) *See CHENODEOXYCHOLIC ACID*				
CHERATUSSIN AC (Qualitest)				
codeine phosphate/guaifenesin				
SYR, PO, 10 mg/5 ml-100 mg/5 ml,				
120 ml, C-V	00603-1075-54	2.78		
240 ml, C-V	00603-1075-56	5.49		
480 ml, C-V	00603-1075-58	7.30		
CHERATUSSIN DAC (Vintage)				
codeine phos/gg/pse hcl				
LIQ, PO (SF)				
480 ml, C-V	00254-9065-58	11.50		
CHERRY (Medisca)				
flavoring aid				
SOL, NA (1X25ML,ARTIFICIAL)				
25 ml	38779-1153-04	21.00		
(1X100ML,ARTIFICIAL)				
100 ml	38779-1153-05	33.00		
(1X500ML,ARTIFICIAL)				
500 ml	38779-1153-08	90.00		
CHERRY FLAVOR (PCCA)				
flavoring aid				
SOL, NA (ANHYDROUS, ARTIFICIAL)				
1 ml	51927-2244-00	0.90		
(CONCENTRATE,CHERRY)				
1 ml	51927-1512-00	0.23		
1 ml	51927-2146-00	0.23		
(Spectrum Pharmacy)				
LIQ, NA (1X100ML)				
100 ml	49452-1908-02	63.70		
(1X500ML)				
500 ml	49452-1908-03	146.65		
CHERRY FLAVOR ARTIFICIAL (Gallipot)				
flavoring aid				
LIQ, NA, 59.14 ml	51552-0290-03	6.02	4.30	
CHERRY SYRUP (Humco)				
SYR, NA (N.F.)				
480 ml	00395-2662-16	6.24		
3840 ml	00802-3959-28	54.67		
(Spectrum Pharmacy)				
SYR, NA (1X480ML)				
480 ml	49452-1909-02	55.65		
500 ml	49452-1910-01	77.00		
CHERRY-ADE FLAVOR (PCCA)				
flavoring aid				
POW, NA (DRY)				
1 gm	51927-3451-00	0.10		
CHEWABLE MULTIVITAMIN WITH FLUORIDE (Major)				
multivitamin and fluoride				
CTB, PO (SF,DYE-FREE,ORANGE)				
100s ea	00904-6023-60	37.07		
100s ea	00904-6024-60	37.07		
100s ea	00904-6022-60	37.07		
CHICKEN FLAVOR (Gallipot)				
flavoring aid				
LIQ, NA (NATURAL)				
59.14 ml	51552-0569-09	10.22		
(Medisca)				
POW, NA (1X25GM,CHICKEN)				
25 gm	38779-1940-04	25.50		
(1X100GM,CHICKEN)				
100 gm	38779-1940-05	46.50		
(1X500GM,CHICKEN)				
500 gm	38779-1940-08	120.00		
(PCCA)				
LIQ, NA (GRILLED; OIL MISCIBLE)				
1 ml	51927-3605-00	0.75		
(OIL SOLUBLE)				
1 ml	51927-2901-00	0.45		
(Spectrum Pharmacy)				
LIQ, NA (1X100ML)				
100 ml	49452-1921-01	106.40		
(1X500ML)				
500 ml	49452-1921-02	325.15		
CHICKEN FLAVOR ROASTED (Medisca)				
flavoring aid				
POW, NA (1X25GM,CHICKEN)				
25 gm	38779-2417-04	22.50		
(1X100GM,CHICKEN)				
100 gm	38779-2417-05	43.50		
(1X500GM,CHICKEN)				
500 gm	38779-2417-08	105.00		
CHICKEN PROTEIN (PCCA)				
POW, NA, 1 gm	51927-2758-00	0.42		
CHICKEN-ADE FLAVOR (PCCA)				
flavoring aid				
POW, NA, 1 gm	51927-3419-00	0.12		
CHINESE GINSENG ROOT				
(PCCA) *See GINSENG ROOT*				
CHIRHOSTIM (ChiRhoClin)				
secretin				
PDS, IV, 16 mcg, ea	67066-0005-01	415.00	415.00	
CHITOSAN (PCCA)				
POW, NA, 1 gm	51927-2707-00	0.24		
CHLO TUSS (McNeil,R.A.)				
cough/cold combination				
SOL, PO (1X473ML,AF,SF)				
473 ml	12830-0760-16	49.94		
CHLOPHEDIANOL HCL/ DEXCHLORPHENIRAMINE MAL/PSE HCL				
(GM Pharm) *See VANACOF*				
CHLOPHEDIANOL HCL/GG/PSE HCL				
(GM Pharm) *See VANACOF DX*				
CHLOR-MES (Cypress Pharm)				
cpm/methscopolamine nitrate/phenyleph hcl				
TER, PO (CAPLET)				
12 mg-2.5 mg-20 mg,				
100s ea	60258-0362-01	51.95		
CHLOR-MES D (Cypress Pharm)				
cpm/methscopolamine nitrate/phenyleph hcl				
SOL, PO (AF,SF,DYE-FREE,GRAPE)				
473 ml	60258-0221-16	11.18		
CHLOR-PHEN (Truxton)				
chlorpheniramine maleate				
CER, PO, 8 mg, 1000s ea	00463-3001-10	57.60		
12 mg, 1000s ea	00463-3002-10	59.40		
CHLORAL HYDRATE (Amend)				
CRY, NA (U.S.P.)				
125 gm, C-IV	17317-0104-04	14.00		
500 gm, C-IV	17317-0104-01	37.80		
2500 gm, C-IV	17317-0104-05	179.20		
(Breckenridge Pharm) *See SOMNOTE*				
(G&W)				
SUP, RC, 500 mg,				
25s ea UD, C-IV	00713-0533-25	81.95		
100s ea UD, C-IV	00713-0533-01	281.20		
(Gallipot)				
CRY, NA (U.S.P.)				
125 gm, C-IV	51552-0528-09	29.12		
500 gm, C-IV	51552-0528-06	67.48		
(Medisca)				
POW, NA (U.S.P.)				
100 gm, C-IV	38779-0641-05	123.00		
500 gm, C-IV	38779-0641-08	202.50		
(USP,1X1000GM)				
1000 gm, C-IV	38779-0641-09	414.00		
(U.S.P.)				
2500 gm, C-IV	38779-0641-01	585.00		
(PCCA)				
POW, NA (U.S.P.)				
1 gm, C-IV	51927-1002-00	1.20		
(Pharm Assoc Inc)				
SYR, PO, 500 mg/5 ml,				
5 ml 100s UD, C-IV	00121-0532-05	100.02		
(AF,SF,LIME)				
500 mg/5 ml,				
473 ml, C-IV	00121-0532-16	24.00		
(Spectrum Pharmacy)				
CRY, NA (U.S.P.)				
125 gm, C-IV	49452-1920-03	158.90		
500 gm, C-IV	49452-1920-01	312.55		
(Southwood)				
REPACK				
SYR, PO, 500 mg/5 ml,				
30 ml, C-IV	58016-0852-06	3.90		
120 ml, C-IV	58016-0852-24	9.75		
CHLORAMBUCIL				
(Glaxo) *See LEUKERAN*				
(Medisca)				
POW, NA (U.S.P.)				
0.25 gm	38779-1156-07	111.00		
0.5 gm	38779-1156-00	202.50		
1 gm	38779-1156-06	354.00		
(PCCA)				
POW, NA, 1 gm	51927-2177-00	480.00		
(Spectrum Pharmacy)				
POW, NA (U.S.P.)				
0.25 gm	49452-1911-01	173.95		
1 gm	49452-1911-02	553.00		
CHLORAMINE T (Amend)				
chloramine-t				
POW, NA (PURIFIED)				
454 gm	17317-0105-01	210.00		
11350 gm	17317-0105-08	210.00		
(PCCA)				
POW, NA (TRIHYDRATE)				
1 gm	51927-1311-00	0.47		
CHLORAMINE-T				
(Amend) *See CHLORAMINE T*				
(PCCA) *See CHLORAMINE T*				
(Spectrum Pharmacy)				
POW, NA, 500 gm	49452-1930-05	176.75		
1000 gm	49452-1930-02	294.00		
2500 gm	49452-1930-03	584.50		
CHLORAMPHENICOL (Gallipot)				
POW, NA (U.S.P.)				
25 gm	51552-0461-04	21.84		
(Letco)				
POW, NA (U.S.P.)				
25 gm	62991-1031-02	45.00		
100 gm	62991-1031-03	120.00		
1000 gm	62991-1031-04	825.00		
(Medisca)				
POW, NA (U.S.P.)				
5 gm	38779-0203-03	28.50		
25 gm	38779-0203-04	46.50		
100 gm	38779-0203-05	123.00		
500 gm	38779-0203-08	525.00		
1000 gm	38779-0203-09	870.00		
(PCCA)				
POW, NA (U.S.P.)				
1 gm	51927-1484-00	6.60		
(Spectrum Pharmacy)				
POW, NA (1X25GM,USP)				
25 gm	49452-1945-02	200.90		
(1X100GM,USP)				
100 gm	49452-1945-03	591.50		
(1X500GM,USP)				
500 gm	49452-1945-04	941.50		

PROD/MFR	NDC	AWP	DP	OBC
CHLORAMPHENICOL PALMITATE (Gallipot)				
POW, NA (U.S.P.)				
5 gm	51552-0576-02	14.56		
25 gm	51552-0576-04	40.60		
100 gm	51552-0576-05	126.00		
(Letco)				
POW, NA (U.S.P.)				
25 gm	62991-1478-02	45.00		
100 gm	62991-1478-03	105.00		
1000 gm	62991-1478-04	870.00		
(Medisca)				
POW, NA (U.S.P.)				
5 gm	38779-0204-03	31.50		
25 gm	38779-0204-04	111.00		
100 gm	38779-0204-05	291.00		
1000 gm	38779-0204-09	1185.00		
(PCCA)				
POW, NA (U.S.P.)				
1 gm	51927-2241-00	6.60		
(Spectrum Pharmacy)				
POW, NA (U.S.P.)				
5 gm	49452-1954-01	90.65	9.95	
25 gm	49452-1954-02	211.05		
100 gm	49452-1954-03	591.50		
(1X1000GM,USP)				
1000 gm	49452-1954-04	1043.00		
CHLORAMPHENICOL SODIUM SUCCINATE (APP)				
PDS, IV (VIAL,1GMX10,PF)				
1 gm, 1 gm 10s	63323-0011-15	298.75		AP
CHLORDEX GP (Cypress Pharm)				
cpm/dm/gg/phenyleph hcl				
SYR, PO (AF,SF,GRAPE)				
473 ml	60258-0246-16	12.52		
CHLORDIAZEPOXIDE (DHS, Inc.)				
REPACK				
chlordiazepoxide hydrochloride				
CAP, PO, 10 mg,				
30s ea, C-IV	55887-0856-30	19.96		
25 mg,				
30s ea, C-IV	55887-0848-30	27.96		
(Pharma Pac)				
REPACK				
CAP, PO, 25 mg,				
30s ea, C-IV	52959-0887-30	28.20		
CHLORDIAZEPOXIDE & CLIDINIUM (Dispensing Solutions)				
REPACK				
chlordiazepoxide hydrochloride/clidinium bromide				
CAP, PO, 5 mg-2.5 mg,				
30s ea	55045-1669-08	23.40		
60s ea	55045-1669-06	46.80		
CHLORDIAZEPOXIDE AND AMITRIPTYLINE HYDROCHLORIDE (Par)				
amitriptyline hydrochloride/chlordiazepoxide				
TAB, PO (FILM COATED)				
12.5 mg-5 mg,				
100s ea, C-IV	49884-0961-01	83.95		AB
(DOUBLE STRENGTH)				
25 mg-10 mg,				
100s ea, C-IV	49884-0962-01	118.45		AB
CHLORDIAZEPOXIDE HCL (Teva)				
chlordiazepoxide hydrochloride				
CAP, PO, 5 mg,				
100s ea, C-IV	00555-0158-02	32.19		AB
500s ea, C-IV	00555-0158-04	131.86		AB
10 mg,				
100s ea, C-IV	00555-0033-02	36.33		AB
1000s ea, C-IV	00555-0033-05	240.64		AB
25 mg,				
100s ea, C-IV	00555-0159-02	39.12		AB
500s ea, C-IV	00555-0159-04	139.83		AB
(UDL)				
CAP, PO (10X10)				
5 mg,				
100s ea UD, C-IV	51079-0374-20	19.20		AB
10 mg,				
100s ea UD, C-IV	51079-0375-20	22.15		AB
25 mg,				
100s ea UD, C-IV	51079-0141-20	23.22		AB
(A-S Medication)				
REPACK				
CAP, PO, 25 mg,				
10s ea, C-IV	54569-2095-04	3.91		AB
19s ea, C-IV	54569-2095-06	7.43		AB

PROD/MFR	NDC	AWP	DP	OBC
(Altura)				
REPACK				
CAP, PO, 10 mg,				
8s ea, C-IV	63874-0256-08	4.38		AB
10s ea, C-IV	63874-0256-10	5.47		AB
12s ea, C-IV	63874-0256-12	6.58		AB
14s ea, C-IV	63874-0256-14	7.65		AB
15s ea, C-IV	63874-0256-15	8.20		AB
20s ea, C-IV	63874-0256-20	10.94		AB
21s ea, C-IV	63874-0256-21	11.49		AB
24s ea, C-IV	63874-0256-24	13.13		AB
25s ea, C-IV	63874-0256-25	13.67		AB
28s ea, C-IV	63874-0256-28	15.31		AB
30s ea, C-IV	63874-0256-30	16.40		AB
40s ea, C-IV	63874-0256-40	21.87		AB
CHLORDIAZEPOXIDE HCL (Altura)				
REPACK				
chlordiazepoxide hydrochloride				
CAP, PO, 10 mg,				
60s ea, C-IV	63874-0256-60	32.81		AB
100s ea, C-IV	63874-0256-01	54.68		AB
25 mg,				
10s ea, C-IV	63874-0274-10	5.02		AB
12s ea, C-IV	63874-0274-12	6.02		AB
30s ea, C-IV	63874-0274-30	15.06		AB
(HomeMed)				
REPACK				
CAP, PO, 10 mg,				
60s ea, C-IV	51655-0052-25	9.37		EE
90s ea, C-IV	51655-0052-26	13.56		EE
120s ea, C-IV	51655-0052-82	17.74		EE
25 mg,				
90s ea, C-IV	51655-0823-26	15.59		EE
120s ea, C-IV	51655-0823-82	20.45		EE
(Nucare Pharm)				
REPACK				
CAP, PO, 10 mg,				
60s ea, C-IV	68071-0734-60	26.06		AB
(PD-Rx Pharm)				
REPACK				
CAP, PO, 10 mg,				
6s ea, C-IV	55289-0061-06	6.02		AB
60s ea, C-IV	55289-0061-60	14.64		AB
(USP)				
25 mg, 3s ea, C-IV	43063-0046-03	13.65		AB
6s ea, C-IV	43063-0046-06	27.09		AB
15s ea, C-IV	43063-0046-15	40.95		AB
(Phys Total Care)				
REPACK				
CAP, PO, 5 mg,				
30s ea, C-IV	54868-2463-01	6.75		EE
100s ea, C-IV	54868-2463-00	8.49		EE
10 mg,				
20s ea, C-IV	54868-0070-02	10.98		EE
30s ea, C-IV	54868-0070-00	11.97		EE
25 mg,				
20s ea, C-IV	54868-2361-03	11.55		EE
100s ea, C-IV	54868-2361-00	30.69		EE
500s ea, C-IV	54868-2361-02	87.58		EE
(Quality Care Prod)				
REPACK				
CAP, PO, 25 mg,				
20s ea, C-IV	49999-0244-20	8.17		AB
(Southwood)				
REPACK				
CAP, PO, 5 mg,				
12s ea, C-IV	58016-0822-12	4.29		EE
15s ea, C-IV	58016-0822-15	5.37		EE
20s ea, C-IV	58016-0822-20	7.16		EE
30s ea, C-IV	58016-0822-30	10.73		EE
100s ea, C-IV	58016-0822-00	35.78		EE
10 mg, 8s ea, C-IV	58016-0821-08	4.17		EE
10s ea, C-IV	58016-0821-10	5.21		EE
12s ea, C-IV	58016-0821-12	6.27		EE
14s ea, C-IV	58016-0821-14	7.29		EE
15s ea, C-IV	58016-0821-15	7.81		EE
20s ea, C-IV	58016-0821-20	10.42		EE
21s ea, C-IV	58016-0821-21	10.94		EE
24s ea, C-IV	58016-0821-24	12.50		EE
25s ea, C-IV	58016-0821-25	13.02		EE
28s ea, C-IV	58016-0821-28	14.58		EE
30s ea, C-IV	58016-0821-30	15.62		EE
40s ea, C-IV	58016-0821-40	20.83		EE
50s ea, C-IV	58016-0821-50	26.04		EE
60s ea, C-IV	58016-0821-60	31.25		EE
100s ea, C-IV	58016-0821-00	52.08		EE
(Stat Rx)				
REPACK				
CAP, PO, 5 mg,				
90s ea, C-IV	16590-0766-90	16.13		AB

PROD/MFR	NDC	AWP	DP	OBC
10 mg,				
30s ea, C-IV	16590-0711-30	15.75		AB
60s ea, C-IV	16590-0711-60	30.00		AB
90s ea, C-IV	16590-0711-90	43.25		AB
CHLORDIAZEPOXIDE HYDROCHLORIDE				
FUL				
CAP, PO, 5 mg, 100s ea		11.39		
10 mg, 100s ea		8.78		
25 mg, 100s ea		9.90		
(Teva) *See CHLORDIAZEPOXIDE HCL*				
(UDL) *See CHLORDIAZEPOXIDE HCL*				
(Dispensing Solutions)				
REPACK				
CAP, PO, 25 mg,				
30s ea, C-IV	55045-1781-08	10.50		
(IPI)				
REPACK				
CAP, PO, 10 mg,				
60s ea, C-IV	18837-0328-60	23.69		
(Palmetto)				
REPACK				
CAP, PO, 10 mg,				
30s ea, C-IV	23490-5266-01	15.62		
25 mg, 6s ea, C-IV	23490-5267-01	5.09		
10s ea, C-IV	23490-5267-03	4.33		
30s ea, C-IV	23490-5267-02	12.99		
(Quality Care Prod)				
REPACK				
CAP, PO, 5 mg,				
50s ea, C-IV	49999-0214-50	18.00		
25 mg, 10s ea, C-IV	49999-0244-10	5.02		
30s ea, C-IV	49999-0244-30	12.25		
CHLORDIAZEPOXIDE HYDROCHLORIDE & CLIDINIUM BROMIDE (Excellium)				
chlordiazepoxide hydrochloride/clidinium bromide				
CAP, PO (USP)				
5 mg-2.5 mg,				
100s ea	64125-0132-01	156.94		
1000s ea	64125-0132-10	958.04		
(A-S Medication)				
REPACK				
CAP, PO, 5 mg-2.5 mg,				
30s ea	54569-0430-00	47.31		
(Phys Total Care)				
REPACK				
CAP, PO, 5 mg-2.5 mg,				
90s ea	54868-0030-07	56.59		
CHLORDIAZEPOXIDE HYDROCHLORIDE /CLIDINIUM BROMIDE (Breckenridge Pharm)				
CAP, PO, 5 mg-2.5 mg,				
100s ea	51991-0622-01	158.49		
(Excellium) *See CHLORDIAZEPOXIDE HYDROCHLORIDE & CLIDINIUM BROMIDE*				
(Oceanside)				
CAP, PO, 5 mg-2.5 mg,				
100s ea	68682-0409-10	94.80		
(Valeant Pharm Intl) *See LIBRAX*				
(Palmetto)				
REPACK				
CAP, PO, 5 mg-2.5 mg,				
28s ea	23490-5269-01	21.98		
30s ea	23490-5269-03	23.55		
56s ea	23490-5269-02	43.96		
CHLORDIAZEPOXIDE/CLIDINIUM (Altura)				
REPACK				
chlordiazepoxide hydrochloride/clidinium bromide				
CAP, PO, 5 mg-2.5 mg,				
15s ea	63874-0356-15	10.71		
20s ea	63874-0356-20	13.86		
30s ea	63874-0356-30	21.42		
100s ea	63874-0356-01	71.40		
(Bryant Ranch)				
REPACK				
CAP, PO, 5 mg-2.5 mg,				
30s ea	63629-1775-01	33.43		
(Dispensing Solutions)				
REPACK				
CAP, PO, 5 mg-2.5 mg,				
28s ea	66336-0780-28	73.19		
56s ea	66336-0780-56	145.77		
(PD-Rx Pharm)				
REPACK				
CAP, PO, 5 mg-2.5 mg,				
30s ea	55289-0062-30	41.03		

PROD/MFR	NDC	AWP	DP	OBC
(Quality Care Prod)				
REPACK				
CAP, PO, 5 mg-2.5 mg,				
30s ea	**49999-0079-30**	10.08		
CHLORDIAZEPOXIDE/CLIDINIUM BROMIDE (DHS, Inc.)				
REPACK				
chlordiazepoxide hydrochloride/clidinium bromide				
CAP, PO, 5 mg-2.5 mg,				
30s ea	**55887-0684-30**	15.00		
(PD-Rx Pharm)				
REPACK				
CAP, PO, 5 mg-2.5 mg,				
60s ea	**55289-0062-60**	87.26		
(Phys Total Care)				
REPACK				
CAP, PO, 5 mg-2.5 mg,				
15s ea	**54868-0030-06**	11.40		
30s ea	**54868-0030-05**	18.27		
40s ea	**54868-0030-00**	22.86		
60s ea	**54868-0030-04**	32.04		
100s ea	**54868-0030-02**	50.43		
200s ea	**54868-0030-03**	96.36		
(Southwood)				
REPACK				
CAP, PO, 5 mg-2.5 mg,				
15s ea	**58016-0984-15**	10.20		
20s ea	**58016-0984-20**	13.60		
30s ea	**58016-0984-30**	20.40		
60s ea	**58016-0984-60**	40.80		
90s ea	**58016-0984-90**	61.20		
100s ea	**58016-0984-00**	68.00		
CHLOREX-A (Cypress Pharm)				
cpm/phenyleph hcl/phenyltoloxamine cit				
TER, PO (CAPLET)				
4 mg-20 mg-40 mg,				
100s ea	**60258-0283-01**	54.65		
CHLORFED-A (PD-Rx Pharm)				
REPACK				
cpm/pse hcl				
CER, PO, 8 mg-120 mg,				
20s ea	**55289-0284-20**	24.75		
30s ea	**55289-0284-30**	28.37		
60s ea	**55289-0284-60**	56.73		
CHLORHEXIDENE DIACETATE (Spectrum Pharmacy)				
chlorhexidine acetate				
POW, NA, 5 gm	**49452-0128-01**	169.05		
25 gm	**49452-0128-02**	735.00		
CHLORHEXIDINE ACETATE				
(PCCA) *See CHLORHEXIDINE DIACETATE*				
(Spectrum Pharmacy) *See CHLORHEXIDENE DIACETATE*				
CHLORHEXIDINE DIACETATE (PCCA)				
chlorhexidine acetate				
POW, NA (HYDRATE)				
1 gm	**51927-2079-00**	20.40		
CHLORHEXIDINE DIGLUCONATE (PCCA)				
chlorhexidine gluconate				
SOL, NA, 20%, 1 ml	**51927-1133-00**	0.34		
CHLORHEXIDINE GLUC (Physician Partner)				
REPACK				
chlorhexidine gluconate				
LIQ, PO, 0.12%, 480 ml	**21695-0025-16**	20.80		
CHLORHEXIDINE GLUCONATE				
FUL				
LIQ, PO, 0.12%, 480 ml		5.23		
(Actavis Mid Atlantic)				
SOL, PO, 0.12%, 473 ml	**00472-0036-16**	10.50		AT
(Colgate Oral) *See PERIOGARD*				
(Gallipot) *See CHLORHEXIDINE GLUCONATE 20%*				
(Hi-Tech)				
LIQ, PO, 0.12%, 473 ml	**50383-0720-16**	10.50		AT
(Letco)				
SOL, NA, 20%, 120 ml	**62991-1030-01**	36.00		
500 ml	**62991-1030-02**	90.00		
(Medisca) *See CHLORHEXIDINE GLUCONATE 20%*				
(PCCA) *See CHLORHEXIDINE DIGLUCONATE*				
(Spectrum Pharmacy)				
SOL, NA (B.P.)				
100 ml	**49452-1947-03**	64.75		
500 ml	**49452-1947-01**	169.05		
4000 ml	**49452-1947-02**	962.50		
(Xttrium Labs)				
LIQ, PO, 0.12%, 473 ml	**00116-2001-16**	10.40		EE

PROD/MFR	NDC	AWP	DP	OBC
(Zila) *See PERIDEX*				
(A-S Medication)				
REPACK				
LIQ, PO (4X120ML)				
0.12%, 120 ml 4s	**54569-5235-01**	10.50		EE
473 ml	**54569-5235-00**	10.50		EE
(DHS, Inc.)				
REPACK				
LIQ, PO, 0.12%, 480 ml	**55887-0573-16**	12.15		EE
(Dispensing Solutions)				
REPACK				
LIQ, PO, 0.12%, 473 ml	**55045-2630-01**	10.95		AT
CHLORHEXIDINE GLUCONATE (Palmetto)				
REPACK				
SOL, PO (1X480ML)				
0.12%, 480 ml	**23490-7071-01**	19.06		
CHLORHEXIDINE GLUCONATE (Phys Total Care)				
REPACK				
LIQ, PO, 0.12%, 480 ml	**54868-3722-00**	12.36		EE
CHLORHEXIDINE GLUCONATE 20% (Gallipot)				
chlorhexidine gluconate				
SOL, NA (B.P.)				
3 ml	**51552-0078-09**	5.88		
5 ml	**51552-0078-02**	8.82		
100 ml	**51552-0078-05**	14.35		
473 ml	**51552-0078-06**	43.96		
3785 ml	**51552-0078-08**	277.20		
(Medisca)				
SOL, NA (B.P.)				
500 ml	**38779-0205-08**	112.50		
1000 ml	**38779-0205-09**	202.50		
4000 ml	**38779-0205-01**	643.50		
CHLORMEZANONE (PCCA)				
POW, NA, 1 gm	**51927-3070-00**	5.40		
CHLOROACETIC ACID				
(Amend) *See MONOCHLOROACETIC ACID*				
(Baker, J.T.)				
POW, NA (A.C.S., REAGENT)				
500 gm	**10106-0216-01**	36.64		
(PCCA) *See CHLOROACETIC ACID 99%*				
(Spectrum Pharmacy)				
CRY, NA (1X25GM)				
25 gm	**49452-4770-01**	67.90		
(1X500GM)				
500 gm	**49452-4770-02**	175.00		
CHLOROACETIC ACID 99% (PCCA)				
chloroacetic acid				
POW, NA, 1 gm	**51927-1745-00**	0.51		
CHLOROBENZENE (Baker, J.T.)				
LIQ, NA (A.C.S., REAGENT)				
500 ml	**10106-9179-01**	27.81		
4000 ml	**10106-9179-03**	162.07		
20000 ml	**10106-9179-08**	440.48		
CHLOROBUTANOL				
(Amend) *See CHLOROBUTANOL ANHYDROUS*				
(Amend) *See CHLOROBUTANOL HYDROUS*				
(Gallipot) *See CHLOROBUTANOL ANHYDROUS*				
(Gallipot) *See CHLOROBUTANOL HEMIHYDRATE*				
(Medisca)				
CRY, NA (1X25GM,ANHYDROUS)				
25 gm	**38779-1160-04**	70.50		
(1X100GM,ANHYDROUS)				
100 gm	**38779-1160-05**	255.00		
(1X500GM,ANHYDROUS)				
500 gm	**38779-1160-08**	810.00		
(PCCA)				
POW, NA (NF; ANHYDROUS)				
1 gm	**51927-1392-00**	2.88		
(NF; HYDROUS)				
1 gm	**51927-1201-00**	1.92		
(Spectrum Pharmacy) *See CHLOROBUTANOL ANHYDROUS*				
(Spectrum Pharmacy) *See CHLOROBUTANOL HEMIHYDRATE*				
CHLOROBUTANOL ANHYDROUS (Amend)				
chlorobutanol				
POW, NA (N.F.)				
125 gm	**17317-0106-04**	93.80		
454 gm	**17317-0106-01**	308.00		
2270 gm	**17317-0106-05**	1050.00		
(Gallipot)				
CRY, NA (N.F.)				
25 gm	**51552-0328-04**	21.56		

PROD/MFR	NDC	AWP	DP	OBC
(Spectrum Pharmacy)				
POW, NA (N.F.)				
25 gm	**49452-1960-01**	122.15		
125 gm	**49452-1960-04**	309.40		
500 gm	**49452-1960-03**	920.50		
CHLOROBUTANOL HEMIHYDRATE (Gallipot)				
chlorobutanol				
CRY, NA (N.F.)				
25 gm	**51552-0327-04**	21.56		
100 gm	**51552-0327-05**	62.65		
(Spectrum Pharmacy)				
POW, NA (N.F.)				
25 gm	**49452-1950-01**	101.85		
125 gm	**49452-1950-04**	189.35		
500 gm	**49452-1950-03**	612.50		
CHLOROBUTANOL HYDROUS (Amend)				
chlorobutanol				
POW, NA (N.F.)				
454 gm	**17317-0111-01**	112.00		
2270 gm	**17317-0111-05**	525.00		
CHLOROFORM (Baker, J.T.)				
LIQ, NA (PURIFIED)				
500 ml	**10106-9182-01**	13.43		
(Gallipot)				
LIQ, NA (N.F.)				
473 ml	**51552-0189-06**	16.10		
(Mallinckrodt Lab)				
LIQ, NA (PURIFIED)				
500 ml	**00406-4432-04**	12.88		
(Medisca)				
LIQ, NA (1X100ML, ACS)				
100 ml	**38779-0586-05**	28.50		
(1X500ML,ACS)				
500 ml	**38779-0586-08**	70.50		
(PCCA)				
LIQ, NA (NF)				
1 ml	**51927-1408-00**	0.14		
CHLOROMAG (Merit)				
magnesium chloride				
SOL, IJ, 200 mg/ml,				
50 ml	**30727-0304-90**	19.00	9.50	
CHLOROPHYLL (PCCA)				
POW, NA (OIL SOLUBLE)				
1 gm	**51927-1682-00**	5.76		
CHLOROPHYLLIN COPPER COMPLEX SODIUM (Medisca)				
chlorophyllin copper complex, sodium				
POW, NA (USP)				
25 gm	**38779-1163-04**	58.50		
100 gm	**38779-1163-05**	178.50		
CHLOROPHYLLIN COPPER COMPLEX, SODIUM				
(Medisca) *See CHLOROPHYLLIN COPPER COMPLEX SODIUM*				
(PCCA) *See CHLOROPHYLLIN SODIUM COPPER*				
CHLOROPHYLLIN COPPER COMPLEX, SODIUM/PAPAIN/UREA				
(Allan Pharmaceutical) *See ALLANFIL 405 OINTMENT*				
(Stratus) *See ZIOX 405*				
CHLOROPHYLLIN COPPER COMPLEX/PAPAIN/UREA				
(Allan Pharmaceutical) *See ALLANFIL*				
(Healthpoint) *See PANAFIL*				
CHLOROPHYLLIN SODIUM COPPER (PCCA)				
chlorophyllin copper complex, sodium				
POW, NA, 1 gm	**51927-1816-00**	3.12		
CHLOROPLATINIC ACID				
(Baker, J.T.) *See CHLOROPLATINIC ACID HEXAHYDRATE*				
CHLOROPLATINIC ACID HEXAHYDRATE (Baker, J.T.)				
chloroplatinic acid				
CRY, NA (A.C.S., REAGENT)				
1 gm	**10106-2890-03**	123.70		
30 gm	**10106-2890-00**	1146.96		
CHLOROPROCAINE HCL (Hospira)				
chloroprocaine hydrochloride				
SOL, IJ (25X30ML)				
2%, 30 ml 25s	**00409-4169-01**	195.90	171.50	AP
(VIAL,25X30ML)				
3%, 30 ml 25s	**00409-4170-01**	248.70	217.50	AP
CHLOROPROCAINE HYDROCHLORIDE				
(APP) *See NESACAINE*				
(APP) *See NESACAINE-MPF*				

PROD/MFR	NDC	AWP	DP	OBC
(Bedford)				
SOL, IJ (400MG/20ML, SDV, USP)				
2%, 20 ml	**55390-0403-20**	14.04		**AP**
(600MG/20ML, SDV, USP)				
3%, 20 ml	**55390-0404-20**	15.12		**AP**
(Hospira) *See CHLOROPROCAINE HCL*				
CHLOROQUINE DIPHOSPHATE (PCCA)				
chloroquine phosphate				
POW, NA, 1 gm	**51927-2586-00**	7.20		
CHLOROQUINE PHOSPHATE (Consolidated Midland)				
TAB, PO, 250 mg, 100s ea	**00223-0691-01**	37.50		**EE**
1000s ea	**00223-0691-02**	350.00		**EE**
(Gallipot)				
POW, NA (U.S.P.)				
25 gm	**51552-0373-04**	57.19		
100 gm	**51552-0373-05**	200.20		
(Global Pharm)				
TAB, PO, 250 mg, 50s ea	**00115-2790-06**	124.38		**AA**
500 mg, 25s ea	**00115-7010-09**	141.07		**AA**
(Hawkins)				
POW, NA (B.P.)				
5 gm	**63370-0053-15**	44.00		
25 gm	**63370-0053-25**	96.00		
100 gm	**63370-0053-35**	300.00		
500 gm	**63370-0053-45**	1300.00		
(Medisca)				
POW, NA (U.S.P.)				
25 gm	**38779-0115-04**	73.50		
100 gm	**38779-0115-05**	237.00		
500 gm	**38779-0115-08**	1050.00		
1000 gm	**38779-0115-09**	1912.50		
(PCCA) *See CHLOROQUINE DIPHOSPHATE*				
(Sanofi-Aventis) *See ARALEN PHOSPHATE*				
(Spectrum Pharmacy)				
CRY, NA (U.S.P.)				
5 gm	**49452-1973-01**	77.00		
25 gm	**49452-1973-02**	126.00		
100 gm	**49452-1973-03**	367.50		
500 gm	**49452-1973-04**	1463.00		
(West-Ward)				
TAB, PO, 500 mg, 25s ea	**00143-2125-22**	135.50		**AA**
(A-S Medication) REPACK				
TAB, PO, 500 mg, 6s ea	**54569-5238-02**	32.83		**EE**
8s ea	**54569-5238-01**	43.77		**EE**
10s ea	**54569-5238-00**	54.72		**EE**
60s ea	**54569-5238-03**	328.30		**AA**
(Dispensing Solutions) REPACK				
TAB, PO, 250 mg, 50s ea	**55045-1606-07**	144.00		
500 mg, 10s ea	**55045-2971-02**	66.00		
25s ea	**55045-2971-01**	165.00		
(Palmetto) REPACK				
TAB, PO, 250 mg, 50s ea	**23490-5272-05**	154.00		
500 mg, 25s ea	**23490-5273-01**	165.00		
(PD-Rx Pharm) REPACK				
TAB, PO (USP)				
500 mg, 10s ea	**55289-0856-10**	43.29		**AA**
40s ea	**55289-0856-40**	160.98		**AA**
CHLOROTHIAZIDE (Consolidated Midland)				
TAB, PO, 250 mg, 100s ea	**00223-0654-01**	4.00		**EE**
1000s ea	**00223-0654-02**	35.00		**EE**
500 mg, 100s ea	**00223-0655-01**	7.95		**EE**
1000s ea	**00223-0655-02**	75.00		**EE**
(Mylan)				
TAB, PO, 250 mg, 100s ea	**00378-0150-01**	14.81		**AB**
500 mg, 100s ea	**00378-0162-01**	26.50		**AB**
(Salix Pharm) *See DIURIL*				
(West-Ward)				
TAB, PO, 250 mg, 100s ea	**00143-1209-01**	13.63	3.15	**AB**
500 mg, 100s ea	**00143-1210-01**	25.25		**AB**
(PD-Rx Pharm) REPACK				
TAB, PO, 500 mg, 30s ea	**55289-0571-30**	14.25		**AB**
(Phys Total Care) REPACK				
TAB, PO, 500 mg, 100s ea	**54868-0672-00**	26.08		**EE**
CHLOROTHIAZIDE SODIUM (APP)				
PDS, IV (USP, SDV,LYOPHILIZED)				
0.5 gm, ea	**63323-0658-20**	357.24		**AP**
(Lundbeck) *See DIURIL SODIUM*				

PROD/MFR	NDC	AWP	DP	OBC
CHLOROTHYMOL (Medisca)				
CRY, NA (1X25GM)				
25 gm	**38779-1164-04**	61.50		
(1X100GM)				
100 gm	**38779-1164-05**	160.50		
CHLOROXYLENOL (Medisca)				
POW, NA (1X25GM,USP)				
25 gm	**38779-1165-04**	27.00		
(1X100GM,USP)				
100 gm	**38779-1165-05**	64.50		
(1X500GM,USP)				
500 gm	**38779-1165-08**	187.50		
(PCCA)				
POW, NA (USP, 4CHLORO-3,5-DIMETH)				
1 gm	**51927-1362-00**	1.05		
(Spectrum Pharmacy)				
POW, NA (U.S.P.)				
100 gm	**49452-1978-02**	120.05		
500 gm	**49452-1978-03**	497.00		
CHLOROXYLENOL/GLYCERIN/ PRAMOXINE HCL/ZN ACE				
(Arbor) *See ZINOTIC*				
(Arbor) *See ZINOTIC ES*				
CHLOROXYLENOL/HC/PRAMOXINE HCL				
(A. G. Marin) *See EXOTIC-HC*				
(Adamis) *See AERO OTIC HC*				
(Blansett) *See CORTANE-B*				
(Blansett) *See CORTANE-B AQUEOUS*				
(Breckenridge Pharm) *See OTIRX*				
(Everett) *See CORTIC*				
(Larken Labs, Inc.) *See OTO-END 10*				
(Marnel) *See OTOMAR*				
(PGD, Inc.) *See GENEXOTIC-HC*				
CHLOROXYLENOL/PRAMOXINE HYDROCHLORIDE				
(Hawthorn Pharm) *See PRAMOTIC*				
CHLORPH/PHENYL/DM (Phys Total Care) REPACK				
cpm/dm/phenyleph hcl				
SOL, PO (DROPS)				
30 ml	**54868-5818-00**	18.46		
CHLORPHENIRAMINE AND CODEINE (Breckenridge Pharm)				
chlorpheniramine maleate/codeine phosphate				
SOL, PO (1X473ML,AF,SF,DYE-FREE)				
2 mg/5 ml-10 mg/5 ml, 473 ml, C-V	**51991-0657-16**	66.06		
CHLORPHENIRAMINE MAL/PHENYLEPHRINE HCL/DM (A-S Medication) REPACK				
cpm/dm/phenyleph hcl				
SOL, PO (AF,SF)				
120 ml	**54569-5803-00**	29.04		
CHLORPHENIRAMINE MALEATE (Amend)				
POW, NA (U.S.P.)				
100 gm	**17317-0109-03**	35.00		
1000 gm	**17317-0109-06**	210.00		
(Consolidated Midland)				
INJ, IJ (VIAL)				
10 mg/ml, 10 ml	**00223-7310-10**	4.00		**EE**
30 ml	**00223-7310-30**	4.50		**EE**
(Gallipot)				
POW, NA (U.S.P.,N.F.)				
25 gm	**51552-0137-04**	18.20		
100 gm	**51552-0137-05**	66.50		
(Letco)				
POW, NA (U.S.P.,NF)				
25 gm	**62991-1032-02**	30.00		
100 gm	**62991-1032-04**	60.00		
(U.S.P., NF)				
500 gm	**62991-1032-05**	180.00		
(Medisca)				
POW, NA (U.S.P.)				
25 gm	**38779-0283-04**	70.50		
100 gm	**38779-0283-05**	177.00		
(PCCA)				
POW, NA (U.S.P.)				
1 gm	**51927-1340-00**	6.00		
(Spectrum Pharmacy)				
POW, NA (U.S.P.)				
25 gm	**49452-1980-01**	101.85		
100 gm	**49452-1980-02**	217.70		
1000 gm	**49452-1980-03**	1179.50		

PROD/MFR	NDC	AWP	DP	OBC
(Truxton) *See CHLOR-PHEN*				
(Bryant Ranch) REPACK				
TAB, PO, 4 mg, 30s ea	**63629-2745-01**	2.99		
60s ea	**63629-2745-02**	4.99		
100s ea	**63629-2745-03**	8.61		
(Palmetto) REPACK				
TAB, PO, 4 mg, 30s ea	**23490-5286-01**	7.99		
(Phys Total Care) REPACK				
CER, PO (USP)				
8 mg, 20s ea	**54868-1455-02**	8.64		
30s ea	**54868-1455-03**	10.71		
100s ea	**54868-1455-04**	29.88		
1000s ea	**54868-1455-00**	161.13		
(USP)				
12 mg, 30s ea	**54868-5599-00**	10.23		
60s ea	**54868-5599-01**	15.96		
(Southwood) REPACK				
CER, PO, 12 mg, 20s ea	**58016-0749-20**	3.22		
CHLORPHENIRAMINE MALEATE/ CODEINE PHOSPHATE				
(Breckenridge Pharm) *See CHLORPHENIRAMINE AND CODEINE*				
(CodaDose) *See ZODRYL AC 25*				
(CodaDose) *See ZODRYL AC 30*				
(CodaDose) *See ZODRYL AC 35*				
(CodaDose) *See ZODRYL AC 40*				
(CodaDose) *See ZODRYL AC 50*				
(CodaDose) *See ZODRYL AC 60*				
(CodaDose) *See ZODRYL AC 80*				
(Larken Labs, Inc.) *See ENDACOF-C*				
(MAGNA Pharm) *See Z-TUSS AC*				
(MCR American) *See COTAB A*				
(MCR American) *See COTAB AX*				
(SJ) *See NOTUSS-AC*				
CHLORPHENIRAMINE MALEATE/ METHSCOPOLAMINE NITRATE				
(Adamis) *See AEROHIST*				
(Aristos) *See RESPIVENT DOSEPACK DF*				
(Breckenridge Pharm) *See ALLERGY DN II*				
(Cornerstone) *See ALLERX DOSE PACK DF*				
(Cornerstone) *See ALLERX DOSE PACK DF 30*				
(Larken Labs, Inc.) *See NOHIST-EXT*				
CHLORPHENIRAMINE MALEATE/ PHENYLEPHRINE HCL (Phys Total Care) REPACK				
cpm/phenyleph hcl				
TER, PO (CAPLET)				
8 mg-20 mg, 20s ea	**54868-5086-01**	28.02		
60s ea	**54868-5086-00**	75.03		
CHLORPHENIRAMINE MALEATE/ SCOPOLAMINE METHONITRATE				
(SJ) *See RYNEZE*				
CHLORPHENIRAMINE PHENYLEPHRINE (PD-Rx Pharm) REPACK				
cpm/phenyleph hcl				
TER, PO, 8 mg-20 mg, 20s ea	**55289-0430-20**	12.28		
CHLORPHENIRAMINE POLISTIREX/ HYDROCODONE POLISTIREX				
(Covidien) *See TUSSICAPS*				
(UCB) *See TUSSIONEX PENNKINETIC*				
CHLORPHENIRAMINE TANNATE				
(Cypress Pharm) *See CHLORTAN*				
(Edwards) *See ED CHLORPED*				
(Edwards) *See ED-CHLOR-TAN*				
(Larken Labs, Inc.) *See TANAHIST-PD*				
(MAGNA Pharm) *See AHIST*				
CHLORPHENIRAMINE TANNATE/ HYDROCODONE TANNATE				
(SJ) *See NOVASUS*				
CHLORPHENIRAMINE TANNATE/ PHENYLEPHRINE TANNATE				
(Allegis) *See NY-TANNIC*				
(Cypress Pharm) *See CHLORTAN D*				

PROD/MFR	NDC	AWP	DP	OBC
(Edwards) *See ED CHLORPED D*				
(Larken Labs, Inc.) *See TANAHIST-D*				
(Laser Pharma) *See DALLERGY-JR*				
(Meda) *See RYNATAN*				
(Prasco Labs) *See R-TANNA*				
(Prasco Labs) *See R-TANNA PEDIATRIC*				
(Propharma) *See PRO-TANNATE PEDIATRIC*				
CHLORPHENIRAMINE TANNATE/ PSEUDOEPHEDRINE TANNATE				
(Centrix) *See DICEL*				
CHLORPHENIRAMINE/PE/DM (Dispensing Solutions)				
REPACK				
cpm/dm/phenyleph hcl				
SOL, PO, 120 ml	68258-3017-01	34.87		
CHLORPHENIRAMINE/PHENYLEPHRINE/DM (Dispensing Solutions)				
cpm/dm/phenyleph hcl				
SOL, PO, 30 ml	55045-3591-01	46.00		
CHLORPHENIRAMINE/PSEUDOEPHEDRI (HomeMed)				
REPACK				
cpm/pse hcl				
CER, PO, 8 mg-120 mg, 20s ea	51655-0545-52	14.99		
CHLORPHENIRAMINE/PSEUDOEPHEDRINE (Sandoz)				
cpm/pse hcl				
CER, PO, 8 mg-120 mg, 100s ea	00185-1304-01	138.20		
1000s ea	00185-1304-10	1382.00		
(Pharma Pac)				
REPACK				
CER, PO, 8 mg-120 mg, 20s ea	52959-0198-20	14.70		
30s ea	52959-0198-30	21.70		
(Phys Total Care)				
REPACK				
CER, PO, 8 mg-120 mg, 20s ea	54868-1022-01	74.10		
30s ea	54868-1022-04	108.90		
60s ea	54868-1022-00	213.30		
100s ea	54868-1022-03	333.17		
CHLORPHENIRAMINE/PSUEDO/DM TANNATE (Macoven)				
cpm/dm/pse hcl				
SUS, PO (BUBBLEGUM,GRAPE) 473 ml	44183-0510-16	266.36		
CHLORPROMAZINE				
(Glaxo) *See THORAZINE*				
CHLORPROMAZINE (Phys Total Care)				
REPACK				
chlorpromazine hydrochloride				
TAB, PO, 10 mg, 30s ea	54868-2684-01	20.73		
(Quality Care Prod)				
REPACK				
TAB, PO, 100 mg, 90s ea	35356-0098-90	96.30		
CHLORPROMAZINE HCL (Baxter)				
chlorpromazine hydrochloride				
SOL, IJ (USP)				
25 mg/ml, 1 ml	00641-1397-31	8.04		AP
(AMP, DOSETTE)				
25 mg/ml, 1 ml 25s	00641-1397-35	201.00		AP
(USP)				
25 mg/ml, 2 ml	00641-1398-31	8.90		AP
(AMP, DOSETTE)				
25 mg/ml, 2 ml 25s	00641-1398-35	222.60		AP
(Consolidated Midland)				
SOL, IJ (VIAL)				
25 mg/ml, 1 ml 25s	00223-7326-10	45.00		EE
(AMPULES)				
25 mg/ml, 2 ml	00223-7325-02	31.25		EE
(VIAL)				
25 mg/ml, 2 ml 25s	00223-7334-01	50.00		EE
10 ml	00223-7325-10	4.00		EE
10 ml	00223-7330-02	4.00		EE
PO, 100 mg/ml, 240 ml	00223-6246-08	22.50		EE
TAB, PO, 25 mg, 100s ea	00223-0671-01	3.00		EE
1000s ea	00223-0671-02	25.00		EE
50 mg, 100s ea	00223-0672-01	4.00		EE
1000s ea	00223-0672-02	37.50		EE
100 mg, 100s ea	00223-0673-01	7.00		EE
200 mg, 100s ea	00223-0674-01	10.00		EE
(Gallipot)				
POW, NA (U.S.P.,N.F.)				
25 gm	51552-0139-04	39.83		
100 gm	51552-0139-05	115.50		
1000 gm	51552-0139-07	623.00		
(Medisca)				
POW, NA (U.S.P.)				
10 gm	38779-0423-01	49.50		
25 gm	38779-0423-04	88.50		
100 gm	38779-0423-05	268.50		
(PCCA)				
POW, NA (U.S.P.)				
1 gm	51927-3098-00	5.40		
(Sandoz)				
TAB, PO, 10 mg, 100s ea	00781-1715-01	32.00		BP
25 mg, 100s ea	00781-1716-01	49.94		BP
50 mg, 100s ea	00781-1717-01	70.64		BP
100 mg, 100s ea	00781-1718-01	80.40		BP
200 mg, 100s ea	00781-1719-01	104.87		BP
(Spectrum Pharmacy)				
POW, NA (U.S.P.)				
25 gm	49452-1990-01	132.65		
100 gm	49452-1990-02	364.00		
1000 gm	49452-1990-03	2184.00		
(UDL)				
TAB, PO (10X10)				
10 mg, 100s ea UD	51079-0518-20	35.10		BP
25 mg, 100s ea UD	51079-0519-20	28.25		BP
50 mg, 100s ea UD	51079-0130-20	29.60		BP
100 mg, 100s ea UD	51079-0516-20	40.60		BP
200 mg, 100s ea UD	51079-0517-20	65.27		BP
(Upsher-Smith)				
TAB, PO, 10 mg, 100s ea	00832-0300-00	31.98		BP
1000s ea	00832-0300-10	284.44		BP
25 mg, 100s ea	00832-0301-00	52.96		BP
1000s ea	00832-0301-10	474.43		BP
50 mg, 100s ea	00832-0302-00	71.40		BP
1000s ea	00832-0302-10	637.54		BP
100 mg, 100s ea	00832-0303-00	81.62		BP
1000s ea	00832-0303-10	598.23		BP
200 mg, 100s ea	00832-0304-00	114.37		BP
1000s ea	00832-0304-10	1048.72		BP
(GSMS)				
REPACK				
TAB, PO (UNIT OF USE)				
50 mg, 30s ea	60429-0042-30	36.20	9.05	BP
90s ea	60429-0042-90	102.80	25.70	BP
100 mg, 30s ea	60429-0043-30	34.20	8.55	BP
90s ea	60429-0043-90	96.60	24.15	BP
(Phys Total Care)				
REPACK				
TAB, PO, 25 mg, 30s ea	54868-2464-00	19.65		EE
60s ea	54868-2464-02	34.83		EE
50 mg, 10s ea	54868-2302-00	10.17		EE
100s ea	54868-2302-02	73.18		EE
100 mg, 100s ea	54868-2347-00	57.21		EE
CHLORPROMAZINE HYDROCHLORIDE				
(Baxter) *See CHLORPROMAZINE HCL*				
(Consolidated Midland) *See CHLORPROMAZINE HCL*				
(Gallipot) *See CHLORPROMAZINE HCL*				
(Medisca) *See CHLORPROMAZINE HCL*				
(PCCA) *See CHLORPROMAZINE HCL*				
(Sandoz) *See CHLORPROMAZINE HCL*				
(Spectrum Pharmacy) *See CHLORPROMAZINE HCL*				
(UDL) *See CHLORPROMAZINE HCL*				
(Upsher-Smith) *See CHLORPROMAZINE HCL*				
CHLORPROPAMIDE				
FUL				
TAB, PO, 100 mg, 100s ea		23.25		
250 mg, 100s ea		49.17		
(Consolidated Midland)				
TAB, PO, 100 mg, 100s ea	00223-0633-01	4.50		EE
1000s ea	00223-0633-02	35.00		EE
250 mg, 100s ea	00223-0634-01	4.95		EE
1000s ea	00223-0634-02	42.50		EE
(Mylan)				
TAB, PO, 100 mg, 100s ea	00378-0197-01	33.08		AB
500s ea	00378-0197-05	154.35		AB
250 mg, 100s ea	00378-0210-01	67.31		AB
1000s ea	00378-0210-10	658.25		AB
(A-S Medication)				
REPACK				
TAB, PO, 250 mg, 50s ea	54569-0203-40	5.41		EE
(PD-Rx Pharm)				
REPACK				
TAB, PO, 250 mg, 90s ea	55289-0066-90	76.53		AB
(Phys Total Care)				
REPACK				
TAB, PO, 100 mg, 100s ea	54868-0877-01	11.70		EE
250 mg, 30s ea	54868-0036-02	25.65		EE
60s ea	54868-0036-04	46.80		EE
100s ea	54868-0036-00	75.03		EE
CHLORTAN (Cypress Pharm)				
chlorpheniramine tannate				
SUS, PO (SF,BUBBLEGUM)				
8 mg/5 ml, 473 ml	60258-0316-16	101.02		
CHLORTAN D (Cypress Pharm)				
chlorpheniramine tannate/phenylephrine tannate				
SUS, PO (SF,BUBBLEGUM)				
8 mg/5 ml-10 mg/5 ml, 473 ml	60258-0315-16	104.49		
CHLORTETRACYCLINE HCL (Medisca)				
chlortetracycline hydrochloride				
CRY, NA (U.S.P.)				
5 gm	38779-0380-03	25.50		
25 gm	38779-0380-04	108.00		
100 gm	38779-0380-05	367.50		
CHLORTETRACYCLINE HYDROCHLORIDE				
(Medisca) *See CHLORTETRACYCLINE HCL*				
CHLORTHALIDONE (Consolidated Midland)				
TAB, PO, 25 mg, 100s ea	00223-0629-01	6.75		EE
100s ea	00223-0630-01	6.75		EE
1000s ea	00223-0629-02	62.50		EE
50 mg, 100s ea	00223-0631-01	7.50		EE
1000s ea	00223-0631-02	70.00		EE
100 mg, 100s ea	00223-0632-01	8.45		
1000s ea	00223-0632-02	77.50		
(Monarch) *See THALITONE*				
(Mylan)				
TAB, PO, 25 mg, 100s ea	00378-0222-01	23.40		AB
1000s ea	00378-0222-10	234.00		AB
50 mg, 100s ea	00378-0213-01	24.55		AB
1000s ea	00378-0213-10	245.50		AB
(UDL)				
TAB, PO (10X10)				
25 mg, 100s ea UD	51079-0058-20	23.40		AB
(A-S Medication)				
REPACK				
TAB, PO, 50 mg, 30s ea	54569-0554-01	7.37		AB
(PD-Rx Pharm)				
REPACK				
TAB, PO (USP)				
25 mg, 30s ea	55289-0067-30	17.52		AB
(Phys Total Care)				
REPACK				
TAB, PO, 25 mg, 30s ea	54868-2007-00	10.83		EE
100s ea	54868-2007-01	24.15		EE
50 mg, 30s ea	54868-0138-02	22.98		EE
60s ea	54868-0138-00	41.46		EE
100s ea	54868-0138-01	64.62		EE
(Quality Care Prod)				
REPACK				
TAB, PO, 25 mg, 30s ea	49999-0650-30	9.46		AB
CHLORTHALIDONE/CLONIDINE HYDROCHLORIDE				
(Mylan) *See CLORPRES*				
(Mylan Bertek) *See CLORPRES*				
CHLORZOXAZONE				
FUL				
TAB, PO, 500 mg, 100s ea		7.57		
(Intl Ethical) *See REMULAR-S*				
(Ortho-McNeil Pharm) *See PARAFON FORTE DSC*				
(PCCA)				
POW, NA (USP)				
1 gm	51927-1596-00	1.02		
(Teva)				
TAB, PO, 500 mg, 100s ea	00555-0585-02	48.98		AA
500s ea	00555-0585-04	215.81		AA
(UDL)				
TAB, PO (10X10)				
500 mg, 100s ea UD	51079-0476-20	49.48		AA
(Watson Labs)				
TAB, PO (USP)				
500 mg, 100s ea	00591-3968-01	6.37		AA
500s ea	00591-3968-05	29.47		AA
(A-S Medication)				
REPACK				
TAB, PO, 500 mg, 10s ea	54569-1970-02	6.70		EE
16s ea	54569-1970-06	10.72		EE
20s ea	54569-1970-01	13.40		EE
28s ea	54569-1970-05	18.75		EE
30s ea	54569-1970-00	20.09		EE
40s ea	54569-1970-04	26.79		EE

PROD/MFR	NDC	AWP	DP	OBC
(Aidarex)				
REPACK				
TAB, PO, 500 mg, 7s ea	**33261-0021-07**	12.46		AA
14s ea	**33261-0021-14**	24.92		AA
20s ea	**33261-0021-20**	35.60		AA
21s ea	**33261-0021-21**	37.38		AA
28s ea	**33261-0021-28**	49.84		AA
30s ea	**33261-0021-30**	53.40		AA
60s ea	**33261-0021-60**	106.80		AA
90s ea	**33261-0021-90**	160.20		AA
(Altura)				
REPACK				
TAB, PO, 500 mg, 8s ea	**63874-0419-08**	8.35		AA
10s ea	**63874-0419-10**	10.44		AA
12s ea	**63874-0419-12**	12.53		AA
14s ea	**63874-0419-14**	23.45		AA
15s ea	**63874-0419-15**	15.66		AA
16s ea	**63874-0419-16**	16.70		AA
20s ea	**63874-0419-20**	33.50		EE
21s ea	**63874-0419-21**	35.18		EE
24s ea	**63874-0419-24**	40.20		AA
28s ea	**63874-0419-28**	49.70		EE
30s ea	**63874-0419-30**	50.25		EE
40s ea	**63874-0419-40**	67.00		EE
42s ea	**63874-0419-42**	70.35		AA
50s ea	**63874-0419-50**	83.75		AA
56s ea	**63874-0419-56**	93.80		AA
60s ea	**63874-0419-60**	100.50		AA
90s ea	**63874-0419-90**	115.66		AA
100s ea	**63874-0419-01**	167.50		EE
120s ea	**63874-0419-04**	154.21		AA
150s ea	**63874-0419-72**	192.77		AA
200s ea	**63874-0419-74**	257.02		AA
300s ea	**63874-0419-77**	385.53		AA
500s ea	**63874-0419-03**	837.50		AA
(Bryant Ranch)				
REPACK				
TAB, PO, 500 mg, 20s ea	**63629-1586-01**	19.86		
30s ea	**63629-1586-02**	53.13		
40s ea	**63629-1586-03**	24.17		
60s ea	**63629-1586-05**	99.99		
90s ea	**63629-1586-04**	138.68		
(Core)				
REPACK				
TAB, PO, 500 mg, 20s ea	**33358-0073-20**	12.39		
30s ea	**33358-0073-30**	54.46		
60s ea	**33358-0073-60**	102.49		
90s ea	**33358-0073-90**	142.15		
(DHS, Inc.)				
REPACK				
TAB, PO, 500 mg, 20s ea	**55887-0799-20**	26.09		AA
28s ea	**55887-0799-28**	42.00		
30s ea	**55887-0799-30**	45.00		AA
60s ea	**55887-0799-60**	90.00		AA
(Dispensing Solutions)				
REPACK				
TAB, PO, 500 mg, 14s ea	**55045-1594-04**	16.80		AA
15s ea	**66336-0663-15**	18.00		AA
20s ea	**55045-1594-07**	24.05		AA
30s ea	**55045-1594-08**	36.00		AA
30s ea	**66336-0663-30**	36.00		AA
40s ea	**55045-1594-09**	48.00		AA
50s ea	**55045-1594-05**	60.00		AA
60s ea	**55045-1594-06**	72.00		AA
90s ea	**55045-1594-02**	108.00		AA
100s ea	**55045-1594-01**	120.00		AA
120s ea	**55045-1594-00**	144.00		AA
(HomeMed)				
REPACK				
TAB, PO, 500 mg, 40s ea	**51655-0137-51**	66.99		
(IPI)				
REPACK				
TAB, PO, 500 mg, 16s ea	**18837-0026-16**	15.63		AA
30s ea	**18837-0026-30**	12.95		AA
60s ea	**18837-0026-60**	32.37		
(Keltman Pharma., Inc.)				
REPACK				
TAB, PO, 500 mg, 30s ea	**68387-0375-30**	34.76		AA
90s ea	**68387-0375-90**	104.28		
(LWP)				
REPACK				
TAB, PO, 500 mg, 30s ea	**64038-0034-30**	19.05		AA
100s ea	**64038-0034-01**	63.49		AA
(Nucare Pharm)				
REPACK				
TAB, PO, 500 mg, 20s ea	**66267-0055-20**	24.56		EE
30s ea	**66267-0055-30**	36.59		EE
40s ea	**66267-0055-40**	48.56		EE
60s ea	**66267-0055-60**	72.84		AA
100s ea	**68071-1365-00**	121.40		AA
120s ea	**66267-0055-91**	145.68		AA
(Palmetto)				
REPACK				
TAB, PO, 500 mg, 15s ea	**23490-5310-01**	25.35		
30s ea	**23490-5310-02**	50.69		
60s ea	**23490-5310-03**	101.38		
90s ea	**23490-5310-04**	152.07		
(PD-Rx Pharm)				
REPACK				
TAB, PO, 500 mg, 10s ea	**55289-0633-10**	20.56		AA
20s ea	**55289-0633-20**	25.56		AA
24s ea	**55289-0633-24**	29.67		AA
28s ea	**55289-0633-28**	35.22		AA
30s ea	**55289-0633-30**	35.33		AA
40s ea	**55289-0633-40**	35.78		AA
100s ea UD	**55289-0633-17**	49.85		AA
(Pharma Pac)				
REPACK				
TAB, PO, 500 mg, 10s ea	**52959-0035-10**	17.08		EE
20s ea	**52959-0035-20**	27.16		EE
21s ea	**52959-0035-21**	28.07		EE
28s ea	**52959-0035-28**	35.71		EE
30s ea	**52959-0035-30**	38.03		EE
40s ea	**52959-0035-40**	48.59		EE
56s ea	**52959-0035-56**	60.54		EE
60s ea	**52959-0035-60**	64.79		EE
70s ea	**52959-0035-70**	71.54		EE
90s ea	**52959-0035-90**	156.89		AA
100s ea	**52959-0035-00**	170.70		EE
120s ea	**52959-0035-01**	156.20		EE
(Phys Total Care)				
REPACK				
TAB, PO, 500 mg, 20s ea	**54868-0735-08**	6.66		EE
25s ea	**54868-0735-03**	7.59		EE
30s ea	**54868-0735-05**	8.49		EE
40s ea	**54868-0735-02**	9.42		EE
50s ea	**54868-0735-00**	12.15		EE
60s ea	**54868-0735-04**	13.98		EE
500s ea	**54868-0735-07**	21.99		EE
500s ea	**54868-0735-09**	71.55		EE
(Physician Partner)				
REPACK				
TAB, PO, 500 mg, 14s ea	**21695-0569-14**	27.99		AA
20s ea	**21695-0569-20**	27.99		AA
60s ea	**21695-0569-60**	101.96		
(Quality Care Prod)				
REPACK				
TAB, PO, 500 mg, 10s ea	**49999-0044-10**	14.30		AA
14s ea	**49999-0044-14**	20.03		AA
15s ea	**49999-0044-15**	21.46		EE
18s ea	**49999-0044-18**	25.74		AA
20s ea	**49999-0044-20**	28.60		EE
30s ea	**49999-0044-30**	42.90		EE
40s ea	**49999-0044-40**	57.20		AA
60s ea	**49999-0044-60**	85.80		AA
90s ea	**49999-0044-90**	128.70		AA
(Southwood)				
REPACK				
TAB, PO, 500 mg, 8s ea	**58016-0291-08**	10.28		EE
10s ea	**58016-0291-10**	12.85		EE
12s ea	**58016-0291-12**	15.42		EE
14s ea	**58016-0291-14**	17.99		EE
15s ea	**58016-0291-15**	19.28		EE
16s ea	**58016-0291-16**	20.56		EE
20s ea	**58016-0291-20**	25.70		EE
21s ea	**58016-0291-21**	26.99		EE
24s ea	**58016-0291-24**	30.84		EE
28s ea	**58016-0291-28**	35.98		EE
30s ea	**58016-0291-30**	38.55		EE
40s ea	**58016-0291-40**	51.40		EE
42s ea	**58016-0291-42**	53.97		EE
56s ea	**58016-0291-56**	71.97		EE
90s ea	**58016-0291-90**	115.66		EE
100s ea	**58016-0291-00**	128.51		EE
120s ea	**58016-0291-02**	154.21		EE
150s ea	**58016-0291-03**	192.77		AA
200s ea	**58016-0291-89**	257.02		AA
300s ea	**58016-0291-73**	385.53		AA
(Stat Rx)				
REPACK				
TAB, PO, 500 mg, 20s ea	**16590-0478-20**	15.00		AA
30s ea	**16590-0478-30**	22.50		
40s ea	**16590-0478-40**	48.79		AA
60s ea	**16590-0478-60**	73.18		AA
90s ea	**16590-0478-90**	67.50		AA
120s ea	**16590-0478-72**	90.00		AA
(Vibranta)				
REPACK				
TAB, PO, 500 mg, 30s ea	**57866-3444-01**	29.65		
60s ea	**57866-3444-04**	49.21		
90s ea	**57866-3444-06**	87.25		
CHOCOLATE (Medisca)				
flavoring aid				
SOL, NA (1X100ML,CHOCOLATE)				
100 ml	**38779-1168-05**	28.50		
(1X500ML,CHOCOLATE)				
500 ml	**38779-1168-08**	55.50		
CHOCOLATE FLAVOR (Gallipot)				
flavoring aid				
LIQ, NA (ARTIFICIAL)				
59.14 ml	**51552-0289-03**	6.02		
(PCCA)				
LIQ, NA, 1 ml	**51927-1464-00**	0.30		
POW, NA (CHOCOLATE)				
1 gm	**51927-3455-00**	0.43		
SOL, NA, 1 ml	**51927-2275-00**	0.90		
CHOCOLATE HAZELNUT FLAVOR (PCCA)				
flavoring aid				
SOL, NA, 1 ml	**51927-3314-00**	0.70		
CHOCOLATE NATURAL & ARTIFICIAL FLAVOR				
(Spectrum Pharmacy)				
flavoring aid				
LIQ, NA (1X100ML,CONCENTRATE)				
100 ml	**49452-1994-02**	58.80		
(1X500ML,CONCENTRATE)				
500 ml	**49452-1994-03**	133.70		
CHOLAN-HMB (Novartis Consumer)				
dehydrocholic acid				
TAB, PO, 250 mg, 100s ea	**00235-0728-71**	26.95		
CHOLECALCIFEROL				
(Bio-Tech Pharm) *See D3-50*				
(Letco) *See VITAMIN D3*				
(PCCA) *See VITAMIN D3*				
(Spectrum Pharmacy)				
CRY, NA (U.S.P.)				
1 gm	**49452-2000-01**	104.30		
5 gm	**49452-2000-02**	395.50		
CHOLEODORON (Weleda)				
homeopathic substance				
LIQ, PO, 50 ml	**55946-0164-15**	9.00		
CHOLESTEROL (Amend)				
POW, NA (N.F.)				
125 gm	**17317-0112-04**	21.00		
454 gm	**17317-0112-01**	70.00		
2270 gm	**17317-0112-05**	315.00		
(Baker, J.T.)				
POW, NA (N.F.)				
500 gm	**10106-1580-01**	86.86		
(PCCA)				
POW, NA (NF)				
1 gm	**51927-1203-00**	1.44		
(Spectrum Pharmacy)				
POW, NA (N.F.)				
25 gm	**49452-2010-04**	67.90		
125 gm	**49452-2010-01**	135.10		
500 gm	**49452-2010-02**	367.50		
CHOLESTERYL ACETATE (PCCA)				
POW, NA (1X1GM)				
1 gm	**51927-2011-00**	4.08		
CHOLESTYRAMINE (Medisca)				
POW, NA (U.S.P.)				
5 gm	**38779-0822-03**	82.50		
25 gm	**38779-0822-04**	285.00		
100 gm	**38779-0822-05**	945.00		
(Par) *See CHOLESTYRAMINE LIGHT*				
(Par)				
PDR, PO, 4 gm/9 gm, 60s ea	**49884-0465-65**	127.00		AB
378 gm	**49884-0465-66**	55.75		AB
(Par) *See QUESTRAN*				
(Par) *See QUESTRAN LIGHT*				
(PCCA) *See CHOLESTYRAMINE RESIN*				
(Sandoz) *See CHOLESTYRAMINE LIGHT*				
(Sandoz)				
PDR, PO (PACKET)				
4 gm/9 gm, 60s ea	**00185-0940-98**	202.15		AB
378 gm	**00185-0940-97**	88.06		AB
(Spectrum Pharmacy) *See CHOLESTYRAMINE RESIN*				
(Upsher-Smith) *See PREVALITE*				

PROD/MFR	NDC	AWP	DP	OBC
(Phys Total Care)				
REPACK				
PDR, PO, 4 gm/9 gm, 378 gm	**54868-4812-00**	149.29		AB
CHOLESTYRAMINE LIGHT (Par)				
cholestyramine				
PDR, PO, 4 gm/5 gm,				
60s ea	**49884-0466-65**	127.00		AB
210 gm	**49884-0466-67**	55.75		AB
(Sandoz)				
PDR, PO (PACKET)				
4 gm/5.7 gm,				
60s ea	**00185-0939-98**	201.06		AB
239.4 gm	**00185-0939-97**	88.56		AB
(PACKET)				
4 gm/5 gm, 60s ea	**59772-5589-01**	126.65		AB
CHOLESTYRAMINE LITE (Phys Total Care)				
REPACK				
cholestyramine				
PDR, PO, 4 gm/5.7 gm,				
60s ea	**54868-5526-00**	189.39		
CHOLESTYRAMINE RESIN (Letco)				
POW, NA (1X100GM,USP)				
100 gm	**62991-2650-01**	150.00		
(1X500GM,USP)				
500 gm	**62991-2650-02**	585.00		
(1X1000GM,USP)				
1000 gm	**62991-2650-03**	885.00		
(PCCA)				
cholestyramine				
POW, NA, 1 gm	**51927-1942-00**	21.00		
(Spectrum Pharmacy)				
POW, NA (U.S.P.)				
5 gm	**49452-2011-01**	131.60		
25 gm	**49452-2011-02**	500.50		
100 gm	**49452-2011-03**	1543.50		
CHOLETEC (Bracco Diag)				
technetium tc 99m mebrofenin				
KIT, IV (10 M.D.V.)				
ea	**00270-0083-20**	663.75	531.00	
CHOLINE BITARTRATE (Amend)				
POW, NA (N.F.)				
500 gm	**17317-0819-01**	14.00		
2270 gm	**17317-0819-05**	56.00		
11350 gm	**17317-0819-08**	227.50		
(Medisca)				
POW, NA (1X100GM, FCC)				
100 gm	**38779-2386-05**	28.50		
(1X500GM, FCC)				
500 gm	**38779-2386-08**	71.85		
(1X1000GM, FCC)				
1000 gm	**38779-2386-09**	127.50		
(PCCA)				
POW, NA (FCC)				
1 gm	**51927-3216-00**	0.20		
(USP,1X1GM)				
1 gm	**51927-3712-00**	0.46		
(Spectrum Pharmacy)				
POW, NA (F.C.C.)				
500 gm	**49452-2020-02**	126.35		
2500 gm	**49452-2020-03**	518.00		
CHOLINE CHLORIDE (Amend)				
POW, NA (F.C.C.)				
125 gm	**17317-0248-04**	7.00		
454 gm	**17317-0248-01**	14.00		
2270 gm	**17317-0248-05**	49.00		
11350 gm	**17317-0248-08**	210.00		
(Baker, J.T.)				
POW, NA (REAGENT)				
500 gm	**10106-1582-01**	30.28		
(PCCA)				
POW, NA (FCC)				
1 gm	**51927-1905-00**	0.36		
(USP,1X1GM)				
1 gm	**51927-3683-00**	0.36		
(Spectrum Pharmacy)				
POW, NA (F.C.C.)				
500 gm	**49452-2030-01**	108.85		
2500 gm	**49452-2030-02**	331.80		
12000 gm	**49452-2030-03**	1298.50		
CHOLINE DIHYDROGEN (PCCA)				
choline dihydrogen citrate				
POW, NA, 1 gm	**51927-2546-00**	0.54		
CHOLINE DIHYDROGEN CITRATE (Amend)				
POW, NA (N.F.)				
500 gm	**17317-0820-01**	15.40		
2270 gm	**17317-0820-05**	70.00		
11350 gm	**17317-0820-08**	262.50		
(PCCA) *See CHOLINE DIHYDROGEN*				
(Spectrum Pharmacy)				
POW, NA, 500 gm	**49452-2040-01**	122.15		
2500 gm	**49452-2040-02**	497.00		
CHOLINE MAG TRI (PD-Rx Pharm)				
REPACK				
choline magnesium trisalicylate				
TAB, PO, 1000 mg, 30s ea	**55289-0387-30**	44.40		
CHOLINE MAGNESIUM TRISALICYLATE (Caraco)				
TAB, PO, 500 mg, 100s ea	**57664-0219-08**	46.20		
750 mg, 100s ea	**57664-0220-08**	72.87		
1000 mg, 100s ea	**57664-0221-08**	114.91		
(Cypress Pharm)				
LIQ, PO (CHERRY)				
500 mg/5 ml,				
240 ml	**60258-0090-08**	44.05		
(PCCA)				
POW, NA, 1 gm	**51927-2399-00**	1.14		
(Silarx)				
LIQ, PO, 500 mg/5 ml,				
240 ml	**54838-0522-70**	44.05		
(Teva)				
TAB, PO, 750 mg, 500s ea	**50111-0529-02**	450.00		
(DHS, Inc.)				
REPACK				
TAB, PO, 500 mg, 30s ea	**55887-0156-30**	68.00		
60s ea	**55887-0156-60**	136.00		
90s ea	**55887-0156-90**	204.00		
750 mg, 30s ea	**55887-0155-30**	90.00		
60s ea	**55887-0155-60**	180.00		
90s ea	**55887-0155-90**	270.00		
(Dispensing Solutions)				
REPACK				
TAB, PO, 500 mg, 30s ea	**55045-2243-08**	23.10		
(Palmetto)				
REPACK				
TAB, PO, 500 mg, 120s ea	**23490-5313-07**	84.00		
750 mg, 120s ea	**23490-5314-07**	96.00		
(PD-Rx Pharm)				
REPACK				
TAB, PO, 750 mg, 28s ea	**55289-0282-28**	30.20		
(Quality Care Prod)				
REPACK				
TAB, PO, 1000 mg, 30s ea	**49999-0111-30**	25.15		
(Southwood)				
REPACK				
TAB, PO (CAPLET)				
500 mg, 30s ea	**58016-0899-30**	20.08		
60s ea	**58016-0899-60**	40.16		
90s ea	**58016-0899-90**	60.25		
100s ea	**58016-0899-00**	66.94		
120s ea	**58016-0899-02**	80.33		
750 mg, 30s ea	**58016-0911-30**	24.60		
60s ea	**58016-0911-60**	49.20		
90s ea	**58016-0911-90**	73.80		
100s ea	**58016-0911-00**	82.00		
(Vibranta)				
REPACK				
TAB, PO, 750 mg, 60s ea	**57866-1259-01**	71.00		
CHOLOGRAFIN MEGLUMINE (Bracco Diag)				
iodipamide meglumine				
SOL, IJ (VIAL)				
52%, 20 ml	**00270-0265-20**	93.75	75.00	
CHONDROCYTES, AUTOLOGOUS CULTURED				
(Genzyme) *See CARTICEL*				
CHONDROITIN SULFATE				
(Letco) *See CHONDROITIN SULFATE SODIUM*				
(Medisca) *See CHONDROITIN SULFATE SODIUM*				
(PCCA)				
POW, NA (NOT FOR INJECTION)				
1 gm	**51927-2657-00**	7.50		
(Spectrum Pharmacy) *See CHONDROITIN SULFATE SODIUM*				
CHONDROITIN SULFATE SODIUM (Letco)				
chondroitin sulfate				
POW, NA (BOVINE)				
100 gm	**62991-1588-01**	75.00		
500 gm	**62991-1588-02**	300.00		
(Medisca)				
POW, NA (1X100GM)				
100 gm	**38779-0890-05**	147.00		
(1X500GM)				
500 gm	**38779-0890-08**	567.00		
(Spectrum Pharmacy)				
POW, NA, 100 gm	**49452-2041-02**	212.10		
500 gm	**49452-2041-03**	840.00		
CHONDROITIN SULFATE/GLUCOSAMINE SULFATE (Palmetto)				
REPACK				
CAP, PO, 400 mg-500 mg,				
120s ea	**23490-7211-08**	96.00		
CHONDROITIN SULFATE/HYALURONATE SODIUM				
(Alcon Surgical) *See DISCOVISC*				
(Alcon Surgical) *See DUOVISC*				
(Alcon Surgical) *See VISCOAT*				
CHONDROITIN/GLUCOSAMINE (Altura)				
REPACK				
chondroitin sulfate/glucosamine sulfate				
CAP, PO, 1200 mg-1500 mg,				
30s ea	**63874-1107-03**	41.62		
60s ea	**63874-1107-06**	83.25		
90s ea	**63874-1107-09**	124.87		
120s ea	**63874-1107-02**	146.32		
TAB, PO, 1200 mg-1500 mg,				
30s ea	**63874-1062-03**	41.62		
60s ea	**63874-1062-06**	83.25		
90s ea	**63874-1062-09**	124.87		
120s ea	**63874-1062-02**	146.32		
CHONDROITIN/GLUCOSAMINE/PABA/ THIOCTIC ACID/VIT E				
(Deston Therapeutics, LLC) *See RELAMINE*				
(Zylera) *See PRYFLEX*				
CHORIONIC GONADOTROP (Phys Total Care)				
REPACK				
chorionic gonadotropin				
PDS, IM, 10000 u, ea	**54868-4121-00**	136.99		
CHORIONIC GONADOTROPIN (APP)				
PDS, IM (M.D.V. W/DILUENT)				
10000 u, 10s ea	**63323-0025-10**	1139.88		AP
(Consolidated Midland)				
PDS, IM (W/DILUENT)				
5000 u, ea	**00223-7760-10**	17.50		EE
10000 u, ea	**00223-7770-10**	22.50		EE
(Ferring) *See NOVAREL*				
(Organon) *See PREGNYL*				
(PCCA) *See GONADOTROPHIN, CHORIONIC EP (HUMAN)*				
CHORIONIC GONADOTROPIN ALFA, RECOMBINANT				
(EMD) *See OVIDREL*				
CHROMAGEN (Ther-RX)				
vitamin b complex, iron, and vitamin c				
TAB, PO (FILM COATED CAPLET)				
90s ea	**64011-0198-26**	121.13		
(Phys Total Care)				
REPACK				
TAB, PO (CAPLET)				
30s ea	**54868-5748-00**	42.31		
60s ea	**54868-5748-01**	82.76		
90s ea	**54868-5748-02**	121.95		
CHROMAGEN FA (Ther-RX)				
vitamin b complex, iron, and vitamin c				
TAB, PO (FILM COATED CAPLET)				
90s ea	**64011-0199-26**	121.13		
(Phys Total Care)				
REPACK				
TAB, PO (FILM COATED CAPLET)				
30s ea	**54868-5920-01**	52.57		
60s ea	**54868-5920-00**	103.17		
CHROMAGEN FORTE (Ther-RX)				
vitamin b complex, iron, and vitamin c				
TAB, PO (FILM COATED CAPLET)				
90s ea	**64011-0197-26**	121.13		
CHROMIC CHLORIDE				
(Amend) *See CHROMIUM CHLORIDE HEXAHYDRATE*				
(Amer Regent)				
SOL, IV (S.D.V.,PF)				
4 mcg/ml,				
10 ml 25s	**00517-6310-25**	62.19		EE
(Hospira) *See CHROMIUM*				
(Medisca) *See CHROMIUM TRICHLORIDE*				

PROD/MFR	NDC	AWP	DP	OBC
(PCCA) *See CHROMIUM TRICHLORIDE*				
(PCCA)				
POW, NA (USP)				
1 gm	**51927-2617-00**	1.05		
(Spectrum Pharmacy) *See CHROMIUM CHLORIDE HEXAHYDRATE*				
CHROMIC POTASSIUM SULFATE				
(Baker, J.T.) *See CHROMIUM POTASSIUM SULFATE*				
CHROMITOPE SODIUM (Bracco Diag)				
sodium chromate cr 51				
SOL, IV, 200 uci/ml,				
5 ml	**00270-0059-20**	1800.00	1440.00	
CHROMIUM (Hospira)				
chromic chloride				
SOL, IV (25X10ML,LATEX-FREE)				
4 mcg/ml,				
10 ml 25s	**00409-4093-01**	22.20	19.50	**AP**
CHROMIUM CHLORIDE				
(Baker, J.T.) *See CHROMIUM CHLORIDE HEXAHYDRATE*				
CHROMIUM CHLORIDE HEXAHYDRATE (Amend)				
chromic chloride				
CRY, NA (REAGENT, U.S.P.)				
500 gm	**17317-1681-05**	49.00		
2500 gm	**17317-1681-03**	154.00		
(Baker, J.T.)				
chromium chloride				
POW, NA (REAGENT)				
500 gm	**10106-1588-01**	127.62		
2500 gm	**10106-1588-05**	525.76		
(Spectrum Pharmacy)				
chromic chloride				
CRY, NA (U.S.P., N.F.)				
125 gm	**49452-2042-01**	207.55		
CHROMIUM GTF POLYNICOLINATE 0.2%				
(Spectrum Pharmacy)				
chromium polynicotinate				
POW, NA (1X100GM)				
100 gm	**49452-2045-01**	118.65		
(1X500GM)				
500 gm	**49452-2045-02**	249.20		
(1X2500GM)				
2500 gm	**49452-2045-03**	714.00		
CHROMIUM NITRATE				
(Baker, J.T.) *See CHROMIUM NITRATE NONAHYDRATE*				
CHROMIUM NITRATE NONAHYDRATE (Baker, J.T.)				
chromium nitrate				
CRY, NA (REAGENT)				
500 gm	**10106-1606-01**	108.25		
2500 gm	**10106-1606-05**	453.25		
CHROMIUM OXIDE (Baker, J.T.)				
POW, NA, 500 gm	**10106-1616-01**	76.99		
2500 gm	**10106-1616-05**	292.57		
CHROMIUM PICOLINATE (Medisca)				
POW, NA, 5 gm	**38779-1174-03**	269.85		
25 gm	**38779-1174-04**	1032.00		
(PCCA)				
POW, NA, 1 gm	**51927-2607-00**	90.00		
(Spectrum Pharmacy)				
POW, NA, 1 gm	**49452-2046-01**	144.90		
5 gm	**49452-2046-02**	402.50		
25 gm	**49452-2046-03**	1414.00		
(Bryant Ranch)				
REPACK				
TAB, PO, 200 mcg, 7s ea	**63629-1324-02**	5.99		
14s ea	**63629-1324-03**	7.74		
60s ea	**63629-1324-01**	10.00		
CHROMIUM PICOLINATE (Palmetto)				
REPACK				
TAB, PO, 200 mcg, 30s ea	**23490-6797-01**	4.11		
100s ea	**23490-6797-00**	13.72		
500 mcg, 60s ea	**23490-8030-06**	27.47		
CHROMIUM POLYNICOTINATE				
(Spectrum Pharmacy) *See CHROMIUM GTF POLYNICOLINATE 0.2%*				
CHROMIUM POTASSIUM SULFATE (Baker, J.T.)				
chromic potassium sulfate				
CRY, NA (ACS,REAGENT,12-HYDRATE)				
500 gm	**10106-1624-01**	150.33		
2500 gm	**10106-1624-05**	348.91		
CHROMIUM SULFATE				
(Baker, J.T.) *See CHROMIUM SULFATE N-HYDRATE*				
(PCCA)				
POW, NA, 1 gm	**51927-2207-00**	7.77		
CHROMIUM SULFATE N-HYDRATE (Baker, J.T.)				
chromium sulfate				
CRY, NA (REAGENT)				
500 gm	**10106-1630-01**	254.00		
CHROMIUM TRICHLORIDE (Medisca)				
chromic chloride				
FLA, NA, 100 gm	**38779-1177-05**	73.50		
(PCCA)				
POW, NA (SUBLIMED,ANHYDROUS)				
1 gm	**51927-2214-00**	11.40		
CHROMIUM TRIOXIDE (Baker, J.T.)				
CRY, NA (A.C.S., REAGENT)				
125 gm	**10106-1638-04**	55.72		
500 gm	**10106-1638-01**	171.03		
(PCCA)				
CRY, NA (ACS)				
1 gm	**51927-1496-00**	0.84		
CHROMIUM/COPPER/IODIDE/MANGANESE/SELENIUM/ZINC				
(APP) *See M.T.E.-6*				
(APP) *See M.T.E.-6 CONCENTRATE*				
CHROMIUM/COPPER/MANGANESE/SELENIUM/ZINC				
(Amer Regent) *See MULTITRACE-5*				
(Amer Regent) *See MULTITRACE-5 CONCENTRATE*				
(APP) *See M.T.E.-5*				
(APP) *See M.T.E.-5 CONCENTRATE*				
(APP) *See P.T.E.-5*				
CHROMIUM/COPPER/MANGANESE/ZINC				
(Amer Regent) *See MULTITRACE-4 CONCENTRATED*				
(Amer Regent) *See MULTITRACE-4 NEONATAL*				
(Amer Regent) *See MULTITRACE-4 PEDIATRIC*				
(Amer Regent) *See MULTITRACE-4 REGULAR*				
(Amer Regent) *See TRACE ELEMENT PEDIATRIC*				
(APP) *See M.T.E.-4*				
(APP) *See M.T.E.-4 CONCENTRATE*				
(APP) *See NEOTRACE-4*				
(APP) *See P.T.E.-4*				
(APP) *See PEDTRACE-4*				
(Hospira) *See TRACE METALS*				
CHRYSIN (Medisca)				
POW, NA (1X25GM)				
25 gm	**38779-2254-04**	76.50		
(1X100GM)				
100 gm	**38779-2254-05**	263.85		
(1X1000GM)				
1000 gm	**38779-2254-09**	2385.00		
(PCCA)				
POW, NA, 1 gm	**51927-3345-00**	3.72		
(Spectrum Pharmacy)				
POW, NA (1X25GM)				
25 gm	**49452-2050-02**	113.75		
(1X100GM)				
100 gm	**49452-2050-03**	353.60		
(1X1000GM)				
1000 gm	**49452-2050-04**	2362.50		
CHYMOTRYPSIN (Medisca)				
POW, NA (U.S.P., ALPHA)				
1 gm	**38779-0370-06**	120.00		
5 gm	**38779-0370-03**	478.50		
25 gm	**38779-0370-04**	2146.50		
(PCCA)				
POW, NA (U.S.P.; ALPHA)				
1 gm	**51927-3367-00**	135.00		
(Spectrum Pharmacy)				
POW, NA (U.S.P./N.F.)				
0.25 gm	**49452-2061-01**	110.95		
1 gm	**49452-2061-02**	241.50		
5 gm	**49452-2061-03**	822.50		
CIALIS (Lilly)				
tadalafil				
TAB, PO (2X15,FILM-COATED)				
2.5 mg, 30s ea	**00002-4465-34**	135.36	112.80	**EE**
5 mg, 30s ea	**00002-4462-34**	135.36	112.80	
(FILM-COATED)				
5 mg, 30s ea	**00002-4462-30**	135.36	112.80	
10 mg, 30s ea	**00002-4463-30**	588.24	490.20	
20 mg, 30s ea	**00002-4464-30**	588.24	490.20	
(A-S Medication)				
REPACK				
TAB, PO (FILM-COATED)				
10 mg, 10s ea	**54569-5544-00**	237.12		
20 mg, 5s ea	**54569-5545-02**	95.00		
10s ea	**54569-5545-00**	237.12		
(Bryant Ranch)				
REPACK				
TAB, PO, 20 mg, 2s ea	**63629-2734-05**	27.00		
5s ea	**63629-2734-01**	67.50		
7s ea	**63629-2734-02**	94.50		
10s ea	**63629-2734-03**	135.00		
30s ea	**63629-2734-04**	405.00		
(Core)				
REPACK				
TAB, PO, 5 mg, 30s ea	**33358-0076-30**	348.50		
10 mg, 30s ea	**33358-0074-30**	394.63		
20 mg, 10s ea	**33358-0075-10**	138.38		
30s ea	**33358-0075-30**	415.13		
(Dispensing Solutions)				
REPACK				
TAB, PO (FILM-COATED)				
20 mg, 30s ea	**55045-3389-03**	570.00		
(Nucare Pharm)				
REPACK				
TAB, PO (FILM-COATED)				
10 mg, 8s ea	**68071-0606-08**	212.78		
10s ea	**68071-0606-10**	265.98		
(Palmetto)				
REPACK				
TAB, PO, 5 mg, 3s ea	**23490-9386-00**	56.25		
6s ea	**23490-9386-01**	112.50		
10s ea	**23490-9386-02**	187.50		
12s ea	**23490-9386-03**	225.00		
15s ea	**23490-9386-04**	281.25		
20s ea	**23490-9386-05**	375.00		
10 mg, 3s ea	**23490-9385-00**	56.25		
6s ea	**23490-9385-01**	112.50		
10s ea	**23490-9385-02**	187.50		
12s ea	**23490-9385-03**	225.00		
15s ea	**23490-9385-04**	281.25		
20s ea	**23490-9385-05**	375.00		
20 mg, 3s ea	**23490-9387-00**	56.25		
6s ea	**23490-9387-01**	112.50		
10s ea	**23490-9387-02**	187.50		
12s ea	**23490-9387-03**	225.00		
15s ea	**23490-9387-04**	281.25		
20s ea	**23490-9387-05**	375.00		
(Phys Total Care)				
REPACK				
TAB, PO (FILM-COATED)				
5 mg, 30s ea	**54868-5956-00**	161.54		
10 mg, 3s ea	**54868-4665-03**	66.12		
5s ea	**54868-4665-01**	116.92		
10s ea	**54868-4665-02**	218.53		
30s ea	**54868-4665-00**	628.81		
20 mg, 3s ea	**54868-4968-00**	76.34		
4s ea	**54868-4968-06**	100.92		
(FILM-COATED)				
20 mg, 5s ea	**54868-4968-02**	125.50		
6s ea	**54868-4968-03**	150.07		
10s ea	**54868-4968-05**	248.38		
15s ea	**54868-4968-04**	350.78		
20s ea	**54868-4968-07**	466.83		
(FILM-COATED)				
20 mg, 30s ea	**54868-4968-01**	698.29		
(Physician Partner)				
REPACK				
TAB, PO, 10 mg, 10s ea	**21695-0028-10**	386.85		
20 mg, 10s ea	**21695-0029-10**	461.36		
(FILM-COATED)				
20 mg, 16s ea	**21695-0029-16**	686.68		
30s ea	**21695-0029-30**	1176.48		
(Quality Care Prod)				
REPACK				
TAB, PO (FILM-COATED)				
10 mg, 30s ea	**35356-0414-30**	854.40		
20 mg, 30s ea	**35356-0132-30**	833.60		
(Southwood)				
REPACK				
TAB, PO, 20 mg, 10s ea	**58016-0256-10**	138.08		
(FILM-COATED)				
20 mg, 20s ea	**58016-0256-20**	337.76		
30s ea	**58016-0256-30**	506.64		
60s ea	**58016-0256-60**	1013.28		
90s ea	**58016-0256-90**	1519.92		
100s ea	**58016-0256-00**	1688.80		

PROD/MFR	NDC	AWP	DP	OBC
(Stat Rx)				
REPACK				
TAB, PO, 20 mg, 5s ea	16590-0479-05	76.09		
10s ea	16590-0479-10	148.17		
15s ea	16590-0479-15	219.25		
20s ea	16590-0479-20	288.34		
30s ea	16590-0479-30	432.50		
CICLESONIDE				
(Sepracor) *See ALVESCO*				
(Sepracor) *See OMNARIS*				
CICLOPIROX				
FUL				
SUS, TP, 0.77%, 30 ml		45.00		
(Actavis Mid Atlantic) **ciclopirox olamine**				
CRE, TP (1X15GM)				
0.77%, 15 gm	00472-0467-15	49.18		
(1X30GM)				
0.77%, 30 gm	00472-0467-30	87.88		
(1X90GM)				
0.77%, 90 gm	00472-0467-90	212.60		
CICLOPIROX (Actavis Mid Atlantic)				
SOL, TP (NAIL LACQUER)				
8%, 6.6 ml	00472-0230-66	170.26		AT
(Apotex Corp.)				
SOL, TP (NAIL LACQUER)				
8%, 6.6 ml	60505-0379-00	170.45		AT
(Dermik) *See PENLAC*				
(Fougera)				
CRE, TP, 0.77%, 15 gm	00168-0313-15	28.65		
30 gm	00168-0313-30	51.19		
90 gm	00168-0313-90	123.81		
GEL, TP (1X30GM)				
0.77%, 30 gm	00168-0407-30	80.75		AB
(1X45GM)				
0.77%, 45 gm	00168-0407-46	121.45		AB
(1X100GM)				
0.77%, 100 gm	00168-0407-99	233.14		AB
SUS, TP (LOTION)				
0.77%, 30 ml	00168-0314-30	48.54		
60 ml	00168-0314-60	96.15		
(Harris)				
SOL, TP (1X6.6ML)				
8%, 6.6 ml	67405-0450-66	12.73		AT
(Hi-Tech)				
SOL, TP, 8%, 6.6 ml	50383-0419-06	18.00		AT
(Medicis) *See LOPROX*				
(Paddock)				
GEL, TP (1X30GM)				
0.77%, 30 gm	00574-2060-30	80.68		
(1X45GM)				
0.77%, 45 gm	00574-2060-45	121.04		
(1X100GM)				
0.77%, 100 gm	00574-2060-01	242.40		
SHA, TP (1X120ML)				
1%, 120 ml	00574-2059-12	147.35		AT
(Perrigo)				
SHA, TP (1X120ML)				
1%, 120 ml	45802-0401-09	149.79		AT
SOL, TP (1X6.6ML)				
8%, 6.6 ml	45802-0141-67	168.56		AT
SUS, TP (USP)				
0.77%, 30 ml	45802-0400-49	48.54		AB
60 ml	45802-0400-46	96.15		AB
(Sandoz)				
SOL, TP (NAIL LACQUER)				
8%, 6.6 ml	00781-7106-60	170.45		AT
(Taro) *See CICLOPIROX OLAMINE*				
(Taro)				
SOL, TP (NAIL LACQUER)				
8%, 6.6 ml	51672-4120-00	25.00		
SUS, TP, 0.77%, 30 ml	51672-1323-03	48.80		AB
60 ml	51672-1323-04	96.70		AB
(A-S Medication)				
REPACK				
SOL, TP (1X6.6ML)				
8%, 6.6 ml	54569-6109-00	168.56		AT
(Phys Total Care)				
REPACK				
CRE, TP, 0.77%, 90 gm	54868-5270-00	267.54		
SOL, TP (1X6.6ML)				
8%, 6.6 ml	54868-6064-00	30.99		AT
(Physician Partner)				
REPACK				
SOL, TP (1X6.6ML)				
8%, 6.6 ml	21695-0475-66	36.00		AT
(Quality Care Prod)				
REPACK				
CRE, TP, 0.77%, 15 gm	49999-0646-15	66.22		
CICLOPIROX OLAMINE				
FUL				
CRE, TP, 0.77%, 30 gm		49.83		
(Actavis Mid Atlantic) *See CICLOPIROX*				
(Medisca)				
POW, NA (U.S.P.)				
25 gm	38779-0313-04	256.50		
100 gm	38779-0313-05	525.00		
(PCCA)				
POW, NA (U.S.P.)				
1 gm	51927-3069-00	36.00		
(Perrigo)				
CRE, TP (1X15GM)				
0.77%, 15 gm	45802-0138-35	31.60		AB
(1X30GM)				
0.77%, 30 gm	45802-0138-11	56.50		AB
(1X90GM)				
0.77%, 90 gm	45802-0138-18	136.50		AB
(Taro) **ciclopirox**				
CRE, TP (USP)				
0.77%, 15 gm	51672-1318-01	28.60		AB
30 gm	51672-1318-02	51.10		AB
90 gm	51672-1318-08	123.75		AB
(Phys Total Care)				
REPACK				
CRE, TP (1X15GM)				
0.77%, 15 gm	54868-5270-01	28.20		AB
CICLOPIROX TOPICAL SOLUTION 8% (Acella) **ciclopirox/vitamin e**				
KIT, MR, 8%-5%, ea	42192-0705-01	166.43		
CICLOPIROX/VITAMIN E				
(Acella) *See CICLOPIROX TOPICAL SOLUTION 8%*				
CIDOFOVIR				
(Gilead Sciences) *See VISTIDE*				
CILASTATIN SODIUM/IMIPENEM				
(Merck) *See PRIMAXIN IM*				
(Merck) *See PRIMAXIN IV*				
CILOSTAZOL				
FUL				
TAB, PO, 50 mg, 60s ea		32.85		
100 mg, 60s ea		32.85		
(Apotex Corp.)				
TAB, PO, 50 mg, 60s ea	60505-2521-01	109.47		AB
100 mg, 60s ea	60505-2522-01	109.47		AB
(CorePharma)				
TAB, PO, 50 mg, 60s ea	64720-0158-06	109.47		AB
100 mg, 60s ea	64720-0159-06	109.47		AB
(Mylan)				
TAB, PO, 50 mg, 60s ea	00378-2979-91	109.50		AB
100 mg, 60s ea	00378-2980-91	109.50		AB
(Otsuka) *See PLETAL*				
(Prasco Labs)				
TAB, PO, 50 mg, 60s ea	66993-0008-60	109.47		
100 mg, 60s ea	66993-0009-60	109.47		
(Roxane)				
TAB, PO, 50 mg, 60s ea	00054-0028-21	109.47		AB
100 mg, 60s ea	00054-0044-21	109.47		AB
500s ea	00054-0044-29	912.23		AB
(Sandoz)				
TAB, PO, 50 mg, 60s ea	00185-0123-60	109.47		AB
100 mg, 60s ea	00185-0223-60	109.47		
500s ea	00185-0223-05	912.25		
(Teva)				
TAB, PO, 50 mg, 60s ea	00093-7230-06	109.47		AB
100 mg, 60s ea	00093-7231-06	109.47		AB
(10X10)				
100 mg, 100s ea UD	00172-5841-10	184.49		AB
5000s ea	00093-7231-50	9122.50		AB
(UDL)				
TAB, PO, 100 mg,				
100s ea UD	51079-0424-20	182.45		AB
(DHS, Inc.)				
REPACK				
TAB, PO, 100 mg, 100s ea	55887-0191-01	182.45		
(GSMS)				
REPACK				
TAB, PO, 50 mg, 60s ea	60429-0762-60	25.92	8.64	AB
100 mg, 60s ea	60429-0763-60	24.48	8.16	AB
(Nucare Pharm)				
REPACK				
TAB, PO, 100 mg, 60s ea	66267-1297-06	109.47		
(Phys Total Care)				
REPACK				
TAB, PO, 100 mg, 30s ea	54868-5411-01	30.69		
60s ea	54868-5411-00	56.88		
(Stat Rx)				
REPACK				
TAB, PO, 100 mg, 60s ea	16590-0285-60	131.40		
CILOXAN (Alcon Ophthalmic) **ciprofloxacin hydrochloride**				
OIN, OP, 0.3%, 3.5 gm	00065-0654-35	86.52		
SOL, OP, 0.3%, 5 ml	00065-0656-05	66.66		
(A-S Medication)				
REPACK				
SOL, OP, 0.3%, 5 ml	54569-3296-00	63.00		
(Altura)				
REPACK				
OIN, OP, 0.3%, 3.5 gm	63874-0036-04	64.95		
SOL, OP, 0.3%, 5 ml	63874-0036-05	56.16		
(Dispensing Solutions)				
REPACK				
SOL, OP, 0.3%, 5 ml	55045-2036-05	60.00		
(Pharma Pac)				
REPACK				
SOL, OP, 0.3%, 5 ml	52959-0013-00	58.73		
(Phys Total Care)				
REPACK				
OIN, OP, 0.3%, 4 gm	54868-4695-00	76.31		
SOL, OP, 0.3%, 2.5 ml	54868-2782-01	33.19		
5 ml	54868-2782-00	81.53		
(Quality Care Prod)				
REPACK				
SOL, OP (1X5ML)				
0.3%, 5 ml	35356-0435-16	115.46		
(Southwood)				
REPACK				
OIN, OP, 0.3%, 3.5 gm	58016-4744-01	74.16		
SOL, OP, 0.3%, 5 ml	58016-6285-01	52.56		
CIMETIDINE				
FUL				
TAB, PO, 200 mg, 100s ea		13.13		
300 mg, 100s ea		13.13		
400 mg, 100s ea		15.48		
800 mg, 100s ea		27.75		
(Apotex Corp.)				
TAB, PO, 200 mg, 100s ea	60505-0018-06	82.15		AB
300 mg, 100s ea	60505-0019-06	90.45		AB
500s ea	60505-0019-04	435.50		AB
400 mg, 60s ea	60505-0020-04	82.00		AB
100s ea	60505-0020-06	146.85		AB
500s ea	60505-0020-08	731.00		AB
(FILM-COATED)				
800 mg, 100s ea	60505-0021-03	256.05		AB
250s ea	60505-0021-07	640.13		AB
(Gallipot)				
POW, NA (U.S.P.)				
5 gm	51552-0531-02	13.79		
(Glaxo) *See TAGAMET*				
(Hawkins)				
POW, NA (U.S.P.)				
25 gm	63370-0054-25	60.00		
100 gm	63370-0054-35	180.00		
500 gm	63370-0054-45	740.00		
1000 gm	63370-0054-50	1320.00		
(Letco)				
POW, NA (U.S.P.)				
25 gm	62991-1456-01	45.00		
100 gm	62991-1456-02	135.00		
500 gm	62991-1456-03	555.00		
(Major)				
TAB, PO (10X10)				
300 mg, 100s ea UD	00904-5445-61	95.20		AB
400 mg, 100s ea UD	00904-5446-61	154.55		AB
(Medisca)				
POW, NA (U.S.P.)				
100 gm	38779-0325-05	145.50		
500 gm	38779-0325-08	550.50		
1000 gm	38779-0325-09	957.00		

PROD/MFR	NDC	AWP	DP	OBC
(Mylan)				
TAB, PO, 200 mg, 100s ea	**00378-0053-01**	87.00		AB
300 mg, 100s ea	**00378-0317-01**	90.40		AB
500s ea	**00378-0317-05**	452.00		AB
400 mg, 100s ea	**00378-0372-01**	147.00		AB
500s ea	**00378-0372-05**	735.00		AB
800 mg, 100s ea	**00378-0541-01**	282.35		AB
(PCCA)				
POW, NA (U.S.P.)				
1 gm	**51927-2750-00**	2.28		
(Penn Labs)				
TAB, PO, 400 mg, 60s ea	**58437-0002-18**	16.65		AB
500s ea	**58437-0002-25**	138.95		AB
(Sandoz)				
TAB, PO (FILM-COATED)				
300 mg, 100s ea	**66685-1702-00**	86.58		AB
500s ea	**66685-1702-01**	428.57		AB
1000s ea	**66685-1702-02**	839.99		AB
400 mg, 60s ea	**66685-1703-00**	86.24		AB
100s ea	**66685-1703-01**	145.76		AB
500s ea	**66685-1703-02**	718.64		AB
1000s ea	**66685-1703-03**	1408.53		AB
800 mg, 30s ea	**66685-1704-00**	76.43		AB
100s ea	**66685-1704-01**	252.22		AB
250s ea	**66685-1704-02**	624.24		AB
(Spectrum Pharmacy)				
POW, NA (U.S.P./N.F.)				
25 gm	**49452-2063-02**	79.80		
100 gm	**49452-2063-03**	239.75		
1000 gm	**49452-2063-05**	1291.50		
(Teva)				
TAB, PO (FILM-COATED)				
300 mg, 100s ea	**00172-7117-60**	83.60		AB
500s ea	**50111-0550-02**	420.00		AB
(FILM-COATED)				
300 mg, 500s ea	**00172-7117-70**	418.25		AB
400 mg, 60s ea	**00172-7171-49**	83.40		AB
100s ea	**00172-7171-60**	142.89		AB
500s ea	**00172-7171-70**	710.40		AB
800 mg, 30s ea	**00172-7711-46**	80.00		AB
100s ea	**00172-7711-60**	263.75		AB
(A-S Medication)				
REPACK				
TAB, PO, 300 mg, 30s ea	**54569-3837-00**	26.56		AB
400 mg, 30s ea	**54569-3838-00**	42.92		AB
60s ea	**54569-3838-01**	85.85		AB
800 mg, 7s ea	**54569-3839-02**	18.54		AB
30s ea	**54569-3839-00**	79.44		AB
(Aidarex)				
REPACK				
TAB, PO (FILM-COATED)				
300 mg, 30s ea	**33261-0630-30**	34.95		AB
60s ea	**33261-0630-60**	69.90		AB
90s ea	**33261-0630-90**	104.85		AB
120s ea	**33261-0630-02**	139.80		AB
(Altura)				
REPACK				
TAB, PO, 300 mg, 10s ea	**63874-0389-10**	10.10		AB
12s ea	**63874-0389-12**	12.12		AB
20s ea	**63874-0389-20**	20.21		AB
21s ea	**63874-0389-21**	21.21		AB
30s ea	**63874-0389-30**	30.31		AB
40s ea	**63874-0389-40**	40.41		AB
50s ea	**63874-0389-50**	50.52		AB
60s ea	**63874-0389-60**	60.62		AB
90s ea	**63874-0389-90**	90.93		AB
100s ea	**63874-0389-01**	101.03		AB
120s ea	**63874-0389-04**	121.24		AB
150s ea	**63874-0389-72**	151.50		AB
200s ea	**63874-0389-74**	202.00		AB
300s ea	**63874-0389-77**	303.00		AB
400 mg, 5s ea	**63874-0390-05**	8.44		AB
9s ea	**63874-0390-09**	15.20		AB
10s ea	**63874-0390-10**	16.89		AB
12s ea	**63874-0390-12**	20.27		AB
14s ea	**63874-0390-14**	23.65		AB
15s ea	**63874-0390-15**	25.34		AB
16s ea	**63874-0390-16**	27.02		AB
20s ea	**63874-0390-20**	33.78		AB
21s ea	**63874-0390-21**	35.47		AB
24s ea	**63874-0390-24**	40.54		AB
28s ea	**63874-0390-28**	47.29		AB
30s ea	**63874-0390-30**	50.67		AB
32s ea	**63874-0390-32**	54.05		AB
40s ea	**63874-0390-40**	67.56		AB
45s ea	**63874-0390-45**	76.01		AB
50s ea	**63874-0390-50**	84.45		AB
60s ea	**63874-0390-60**	101.34		AB
80s ea	**63874-0390-80**	134.13		AB
90s ea	**63874-0390-90**	152.01		AB
100s ea	**63874-0390-01**	168.90		AB
120s ea	**63874-0390-04**	202.68		AB
150s ea	**63874-0390-72**	251.50		AB
200s ea	**63874-0390-74**	335.33		AB
300s ea	**63874-0390-77**	503.00		AB
500s ea	**63874-0390-03**	731.00		AB
800 mg, 7s ea	**63874-0391-07**	20.01		AB
9s ea	**63874-0391-09**	25.84		AB
10s ea	**63874-0391-10**	28.72		AB
12s ea	**63874-0391-12**	34.46		AB
15s ea	**63874-0391-15**	43.00		AB
20s ea	**63874-0391-20**	57.43		AB
24s ea	**63874-0391-24**	68.92		AB
30s ea	**63874-0391-30**	86.15		AB
60s ea	**63874-0391-60**	172.30		AB
70s ea	**63874-0391-70**	201.02		AB
90s ea	**63874-0391-90**	258.45		AB
100s ea	**63874-0391-01**	287.17		AB
120s ea	**63874-0391-04**	344.60		AB
150s ea	**63874-0391-72**	428.75		AB
200s ea	**63874-0391-74**	571.66		AB
300s ea	**63874-0391-77**	857.49		AB
(Bryant Ranch)				
REPACK				
TAB, PO, 300 mg, 30s ea	**63629-1783-01**	26.10		
(FILM-COATED)				
300 mg, 60s ea	**63629-1783-02**	49.23		AB
400 mg, 20s ea	**63629-1497-01**	40.00		
30s ea	**63629-1497-02**	59.99		
40s ea	**63629-1497-04**	80.00		
60s ea	**63629-1497-03**	119.99		
800 mg, 30s ea	**63629-1495-01**	111.22		
(FILM-COATED)				
800 mg, 90s ea	**63629-1495-03**	301.85		AB
(Core)				
REPACK				
TAB, PO, 300 mg, 30s ea	**33358-0077-30**	26.75		
60s ea	**33358-0077-60**	37.95		
400 mg, 30s ea	**33358-0078-30**	61.49		
60s ea	**33358-0078-60**	122.99		
800 mg, 30s ea	**33358-0079-30**	114.00		
(DHS, Inc.)				
REPACK				
TAB, PO, 300 mg, 30s ea	**55887-0166-30**	27.22		
60s ea	**55887-0166-60**	54.45		
90s ea	**55887-0166-90**	81.66		
400 mg, 30s ea	**55887-0748-30**	55.00		AB
90s ea	**55887-0748-90**	112.50		AB
(Dispensing Solutions)				
REPACK				
TAB, PO, 200 mg, 30s ea	**55045-3041-08**	7.50		
(FILM-COATED)				
300 mg, 21s ea	**55045-2272-07**	21.00		AB
30s ea	**55045-2272-08**	30.00		AB
30s ea	**66336-0944-30**	30.30		AB
60s ea	**55045-2272-06**	60.00		AB
90s ea	**55045-2272-09**	90.00		AB
100s ea	**55045-2272-01**	100.00		AB
(FILM-COATED)				
300 mg, 120s ea	**55045-2272-02**	120.00		AB
400 mg, 15s ea	**55045-2135-05**	25.05		AB
30s ea	**55045-2135-08**	50.05		AB
(FILM-COATED)				
400 mg, 30s ea	**66336-0945-30**	55.00		AB
60s ea	**55045-2135-09**	100.10		AB
(FILM-COATED)				
400 mg, 60s ea	**66336-0945-60**	110.00		AB
80s ea	**55045-2135-02**	133.60		AB
90s ea	**55045-2135-06**	150.30		AB
100s ea	**55045-2135-00**	167.00		AB
(FILM-COATED)				
400 mg, 120s ea	**55045-2135-01**	200.40		AB
800 mg, 15s ea	**55045-3030-07**	42.00		AB
30s ea	**55045-3030-08**	84.00		AB
60s ea	**55045-3030-06**	168.00		AB
(FILM-COATED)				
800 mg, 90s ea	**55045-3030-09**	252.00		AB
100s ea	**55045-3030-01**	280.00		AB
120s ea	**55045-3030-02**	336.00		AB
(GSMS)				
REPACK				
TAB, PO (UNIT OF USE)				
400 mg, 30s ea	**60429-0047-30**	8.40	2.80	AB
60s ea	**60429-0047-60**	13.80	4.60	AB
90s ea	**60429-0047-90**	19.35	6.45	AB
180s ea	**60429-0047-18**	35.70	11.90	AB
(HomeMed)				
REPACK				
TAB, PO, 300 mg, 30s ea	**51655-0675-24**	34.99		
400 mg, 6s ea	**51655-0671-87**	9.40		EE
12s ea	**51655-0671-27**	17.80		EE
30s ea	**51655-0671-24**	67.89		EE
40s ea	**51655-0671-51**	57.00		EE
60s ea	**51655-0671-25**	85.00		EE
(Keltman Pharma., Inc.)				
REPACK				
TAB, PO, 400 mg, 60s ea	**68387-0290-60**	99.30		AB
(Nucare Pharm)				
REPACK				
TAB, PO, 300 mg, 30s ea	**66267-0056-30**	30.31		EE
400 mg, 30s ea	**66267-0057-30**	50.33		EE
60s ea	**66267-0057-60**	100.60		EE
800 mg, 30s ea	**66267-0258-30**	85.75		EE
(Palmetto)				
REPACK				
TAB, PO, 400 mg, 30s ea	**23490-0310-03**	57.50		
30s ea	**23490-5319-01**	68.10		
60s ea	**23490-0310-06**	115.01		
60s ea	**23490-5319-02**	136.20		
90s ea	**23490-5319-03**	204.30		
(PD-Rx Pharm)				
REPACK				
TAB, PO, 300 mg, 10s ea	**55289-0799-10**	47.41		AB
(USP)				
400 mg, 10s ea	**55289-0581-10**	37.62		AB
(FILM-COATED)				
400 mg, 20s ea	**55289-0581-20**	63.36		AB
30s ea	**55289-0581-30**	67.71		AB
60s ea	**55289-0581-60**	98.76		AB
90s ea	**55289-0581-90**	120.89		AB
(Pharma Pac)				
REPACK				
TAB, PO, 300 mg, 12s ea	**52959-0345-12**	13.06		EE
30s ea	**52959-0345-30**	30.36		EE
35s ea	**52959-0345-35**	35.37		EE
40s ea	**52959-0345-40**	40.42		EE
60s ea	**52959-0345-60**	59.59		EE
90s ea	**52959-0345-90**	88.19		EE
100s ea	**52959-0345-00**	98.02		EE
400 mg, 14s ea	**52959-0375-14**	24.20		EE
15s ea	**52959-0375-15**	25.91		EE
16s ea	**52959-0375-16**	27.48		EE
20s ea	**52959-0375-20**	34.18		EE
28s ea	**52959-0375-28**	47.35		EE
30s ea	**52959-0375-30**	50.63		EE
40s ea	**52959-0375-40**	66.91		EE
50s ea	**52959-0375-50**	83.63		EE
60s ea	**52959-0375-60**	100.79		EE
90s ea	**52959-0375-90**	138.04		EE
100s ea	**52959-0375-00**	153.35		EE
120s ea	**52959-0375-02**	183.98		EE
800 mg, 16s ea	**52959-0376-16**	45.44		EE
20s ea	**52959-0376-20**	54.99		EE
30s ea	**52959-0376-30**	82.60		EE
40s ea	**52959-0376-40**	105.50		EE
60s ea	**52959-0376-60**	142.00		EE
100s ea	**52959-0376-00**	375.65		EE
(Phys Total Care)				
REPACK				
TAB, PO, 300 mg, 30s ea	**54868-3314-01**	9.42		EE
100s ea	**54868-3314-02**	24.42		EE
400 mg, 20s ea	**54868-3315-06**	9.02		EE
30s ea	**54868-3315-02**	9.78		EE
60s ea	**54868-3315-01**	16.56		EE
100s ea	**54868-3315-03**	23.76		EE
500s ea	**54868-3315-04**	115.14		EE
1000s ea	**54868-3315-05**	228.79		EE
800 mg, 30s ea	**54868-3316-00**	34.46		EE
60s ea	**54868-3316-02**	64.43		EE
100s ea	**54868-3316-03**	102.88		EE
(Physician Partner)				
REPACK				
TAB, PO, 300 mg, 21s ea	**21695-0531-21**	44.69		AB
400 mg, 30s ea	**21695-0532-30**	85.74		AB
(Quality Care Prod)				
REPACK				
TAB, PO, 300 mg, 14s ea	**49999-0112-14**	16.94		AB
21s ea	**49999-0112-21**	25.47		AB
(FILM-COATED)				
300 mg, 30s ea	**49999-0112-30**	36.38		AB
400 mg, 30s ea	**49999-0348-30**	60.36		
60s ea	**49999-0348-60**	120.72		EE
(Southwood)				
REPACK				
TAB, PO, 300 mg, 12s ea	**58016-0510-12**	12.12		EE
20s ea	**58016-0510-20**	20.20		EE
21s ea	**58016-0510-21**	21.21		EE
30s ea	**58016-0510-30**	30.30		EE
40s ea	**58016-0510-40**	40.40		EE
50s ea	**58016-0510-50**	50.50		EE

PROD/MFR	NDC	AWP	DP	OBC
60s ea	58016-0510-60	60.60		EE
100s ea	58016-0510-00	101.00		EE
(FILM-COATED)				
300 mg, 120s ea	58016-0510-02	121.20		AB
150s ea	58016-0510-03	151.50		AB
200s ea	58016-0510-89	202.00		AB
300s ea	58016-0510-73	303.00		AB
400 mg, 9s ea	58016-0696-09	15.09		EE
10s ea	58016-0696-10	16.77		EE
12s ea	58016-0696-12	20.12		EE
14s ea	58016-0696-14	23.47		EE
15s ea	58016-0696-15	25.15		EE
16s ea	58016-0696-16	26.83		EE
20s ea	58016-0696-20	33.53		EE
21s ea	58016-0696-21	35.21		EE
24s ea	58016-0696-24	40.24		EE
28s ea	58016-0696-28	46.95		EE
30s ea	58016-0696-30	50.30		EE
32s ea	58016-0696-32	53.65		EE
40s ea	58016-0696-40	67.07		EE
60s ea	58016-0696-60	100.60		EE
80s ea	58016-0696-80	134.13		EE
(FILM-COATED)				
400 mg, 90s ea	58016-0696-90	150.90		AB
100s ea	58016-0696-00	167.67		EE
(FILM-COATED)				
400 mg, 120s ea	58016-0696-02	201.20		AB
150s ea	58016-0696-03	251.50		AB
200s ea	58016-0696-89	335.33		AB
300s ea	58016-0696-73	503.00		AB
800 mg, 7s ea	58016-0530-07	20.01		EE
9s ea	58016-0530-09	25.72		EE
12s ea	58016-0530-12	34.30		EE
15s ea	58016-0530-15	42.87		EE
20s ea	58016-0530-20	57.17		EE
24s ea	58016-0530-24	68.60		EE
30s ea	58016-0530-30	85.75		EE
100s ea	58016-0530-00	285.83		EE
120s ea	58016-0530-02	343.00		EE
150s ea	58016-0530-03	428.75		EE
200s ea	58016-0530-89	571.66		EE
300s ea	58016-0530-73	857.49		EE
(Stat Rx)				
REPACK				
TAB, PO, 300 mg, 270s ea	16590-0048-86	272.70		AB
(Vibranta)				
REPACK				
TAB, PO, 300 mg, 60s ea	57866-6747-02	75.00		AB
400 mg, 30s ea	57866-6748-01	68.10		
60s ea	57866-6748-02	105.00		
CIMETIDINE HCL (Hi-Tech)				
cimetidine hydrochloride				
SOL, PO, 300 mg/5 ml,				
237 ml	50383-0050-08	90.00		AA
(Hospira)				
SOL, IJ (LATEX-FREE)				
150 mg/ml,				
2 ml 10s	00409-7444-01	33.36	29.20	AP
(VIAL; FLIPTOP)				
150 mg/ml,				
2 ml 10s	00074-7444-01	19.20	16.80	AP
(VIAL,FLIPTOP,LATEX-FREE)				
150 mg/ml,				
8 ml 10s	00409-7445-01	96.36	84.30	AP
IV, 300 mg/50 ml,				
50 ml 48s	00409-7447-16	187.78	164.16	AP
(Morton Grove)				
SOL, PO (PEACH)				
300 mg/5 ml,				
237 ml	60432-0007-08	89.00		AA
(Pharm Assoc Inc)				
SOL, PO (SF,BERRY)				
300 mg/5 ml,				
237 ml	00121-0649-08	89.94		AA
(Teva)				
SOL, PO, 300 mg/5 ml,				
237 ml	00093-0506-87	87.50		AA
CIMETIDINE HYDROCHLORIDE				
FUL				
SOL, PO, 300 mg/5 ml,				
240 ml		27.34		
(Hi-Tech) *See CIMETIDINE HCL*				
(Hospira) *See CIMETIDINE HCL*				
(Morton Grove) *See CIMETIDINE HCL*				
(Pharm Assoc Inc) *See CIMETIDINE HCL*				

PROD/MFR	NDC	AWP	DP	OBC
(Pharm Assoc Inc)				
SOL, PO (BERRY)				
300 mg/5 ml,				
473 ml	00121-0649-16	166.90		AA
(Teva) *See CIMETIDINE HCL*				
CIMZIA (UCB)				
certolizumab pegol				
PDS, SC (PF)				
200 mg, ea	50474-0700-62	1755.19		
SOL, SC (2X1ML)				
200 mg/ml, ea	50474-0710-79	1755.19		EE
CINACALCET HYDROCHLORIDE				
(Amgen USA Inc.) *See SENSIPAR*				
CINNABAR 20X/PYRITE 3X (Weleda)				
homeopathic substance				
TAB, PO, 100s ea	55946-0186-30	6.60		
CINNAMON BARK				
(PCCA) *See CINNAMON BARK POWDER*				
CINNAMON BARK POWDER (PCCA)				
cinnamon bark				
POW, NA (1X1GM,CASSIA)				
1 gm	51927-3647-00	0.12		
CINNAMON LEAF OIL, CEYLON (PCCA)				
cinnamon oil				
OIL, NA (1X1GM)				
1 gm	51927-3154-00	0.38		
CINNAMON OIL (AmerisourceBergen)				
OIL, NA (ARTIFICIAL)				
30 ml	24385-0931-91	3.95		
(Gallipot)				
OIL, NA (F.C.C.)				
118.28 ml	51552-0425-04	10.50		
(Medisca)				
OIL, NA (LEAF NATURAL,CASSIA OIL)				
14 ml	38779-1183-03	16.50		
25 ml	38779-1183-04	31.50		
100 ml	38779-1183-05	90.00		
500 ml	38779-1183-08	261.00		
(PCCA) *See CINNAMON LEAF OIL, CEYLON*				
(PCCA)				
OIL, NA (IMITATION)				
1 ml	51927-1184-00	0.90		
(TRUE; FCC)				
1 ml	51927-1207-00	1.50		
CINRYZE (ViroPharma, Inc.)				
c1 esterase inhibitor, human				
PDS, IV, 500 u, ea	42227-0081-05	2520.38		
CIPRO (Schering)				
ciprofloxacin				
PDR, PO (W/DILUENT)				
250 mg/5 ml,				
100 ml	00085-1777-01	112.13		
500 mg/5 ml,				
100 ml	00085-1773-01	131.27		
(Schering)				
ciprofloxacin hydrochloride				
TAB, PO (FILM-COATED)				
250 mg, 100s ea	00085-1758-01	509.63		
100s ea UD	00085-1758-02	527.89		
500 mg, 100s ea	00085-1754-01	596.54		
100s ea UD	00085-1754-02	616.43		
750 mg, 50s ea	00085-1756-01	312.82		
100s ea UD	00085-1756-02	646.45		
(A-S Medication)				
REPACK				
TAB, PO, 250 mg, 6s ea	54569-1648-07	31.85		
10s ea	54569-1648-05	53.09		
500 mg, 6s ea	54569-1723-05	37.28		
10s ea	54569-1723-02	62.14		
14s ea	54569-1723-00	87.00		
20s ea	54569-1723-01	124.28		
750 mg, 14s ea	54569-2488-01	91.24		
(Altura)				
REPACK				
TAB, PO (FILM-COATED)				
500 mg, 2s ea	63874-0107-02	20.60		
4s ea	63874-0107-04	20.60		
6s ea	63874-0107-06	30.90		
8s ea	63874-0107-08	41.20		
9s ea	63874-0107-09	46.35		
10s ea	63874-0107-10	51.50		
12s ea	63874-0107-12	61.80		
14s ea	63874-0107-14	81.25		
15s ea	63874-0107-15	81.92		
16s ea	63874-0107-16	82.40		
20s ea	63874-0107-20	103.00		

PROD/MFR	NDC	AWP	DP	OBC
28s ea	63874-0107-28	144.20		
30s ea	63874-0107-30	154.50		
40s ea	63874-0107-40	206.00		
50s ea	63874-0107-50	257.50		
60s ea	63874-0107-60	309.00		
90s ea	63874-0107-90	463.50		
100s ea	63874-0107-01	515.00		
(AQ)				
REPACK				
TAB, PO, 250 mg, 100s ea	66105-0108-10	535.86		
500 mg, 10s ea	66105-0109-01	71.46		
20s ea	66105-0109-02	142.92		
30s ea	66105-0109-03	214.38		
60s ea	66105-0109-06	428.76		
100s ea	66105-0109-10	714.61		
(Dispensing Solutions)				
REPACK				
TAB, PO (FILM-COATED)				
250 mg, 20s ea	55045-1469-09	117.40		
500 mg, 10s ea	55045-1494-03	69.70		
14s ea	55045-1494-05	97.58		
20s ea	55045-1494-09	139.40		
30s ea	55045-1494-08	209.10		
750 mg, 20s ea	55045-1650-02	146.20		
(HomeMed)				
REPACK				
TAB, PO, 250 mg, 6s ea	51655-0537-87	45.40		
14s ea	51655-0537-84	99.27		
(Nucare Pharm)				
REPACK				
TAB, PO, 500 mg, 10s ea	66267-0058-10	58.59		
14s ea	66267-0058-14	80.37		
20s ea	66267-0058-20	113.30		
(PD-Rx Pharm)				
REPACK				
TAB, PO (FILM-COATED)				
250 mg, 6s ea	55289-0459-06	45.44		
10s ea	55289-0459-10	75.75		
12s ea	55289-0459-12	90.90		
14s ea	55289-0459-14	106.05		
20s ea	58864-0775-20	139.53		
500 mg, ea	55289-0371-79	8.87		
3s ea	55289-0371-03	26.60		
6s ea	55289-0371-06	53.19		
10s ea	55289-0371-10	88.67		
14s ea	55289-0371-14	124.14		
(REDI-SCRIPT,FILM-COATED)				
500 mg, 14s ea	58864-0637-14	122.28		
(FILM-COATED)				
500 mg, 15s ea	55289-0371-15	132.99		
20s ea	55289-0371-20	177.33		
(REDI-SCRIPT)				
500 mg, 20s ea	58864-0637-20	172.50		
(FILM-COATED)				
500 mg, 30s ea	55289-0371-30	266.00		
30s ea	58864-0637-30	256.20		
40s ea	55289-0371-40	414.50		
50s ea	55289-0371-50	443.33		
750 mg, 10s ea	55289-0717-10	92.99		
(Pharma Pac)				
REPACK				
TAB, PO, 250 mg, 6s ea	52959-0171-06	36.15		
10s ea	52959-0171-10	54.46		
14s ea	52959-0171-14	64.88		
20s ea	52959-0171-20	84.39		
28s ea	52959-0171-28	117.60		
500 mg, 6s ea	52959-0036-06	46.00		
10s ea	52959-0036-10	75.20		
14s ea	52959-0036-14	104.66		
15s ea	52959-0036-15	111.94		
20s ea	52959-0036-20	147.76		
28s ea	52959-0036-28	205.92		
30s ea	52959-0036-30	219.88		
750 mg, 14s ea	52959-0037-14	142.68		
20s ea	52959-0037-20	192.77		
(Phys Total Care)				
REPACK				
TAB, PO, 250 mg, 6s ea	54868-0990-05	36.86		
10s ea	54868-0990-00	60.18		
14s ea	54868-0990-02	83.50		
15s ea	54868-0990-04	89.34		
20s ea	54868-0990-01	118.49		
500 mg, 5s ea	54868-0939-05	40.00		
10s ea	54868-0939-02	77.38		
14s ea	54868-0939-00	107.29		
15s ea	54868-0939-06	114.77		
20s ea	54868-0939-01	143.85		
30s ea	54868-0939-03	214.46		
100s ea	54868-0939-07	708.12		
750 mg, 15s ea	54868-1184-03	105.80		

PROD/MFR	NDC	AWP	DP	OBC
20s ea	54868-1184-01	140.44		
50s ea	54868-1184-02	348.28		
(Quality Care Prod) REPACK				
TAB, PO (FILM-COATED)				
250 mg, 10s ea	49999-0333-10	52.80		
500 mg, 4s ea	49999-0061-04	48.33		
(FILM-COATED)				
500 mg, 6s ea	49999-0334-06	38.16		
7s ea	49999-0061-07	74.70		
(FILM-COATED)				
500 mg, 10s ea	49999-0061-10	137.50		
14s ea	49999-0061-14	192.00		
20s ea	49999-0061-20	275.00		
25s ea	49999-0061-25	229.92		
(Southwood) REPACK				
TAB, PO (FILM-COATED)				
250 mg, 10s ea	58016-0116-10	52.79		
12s ea	58016-0116-12	63.35		
14s ea	58016-0116-14	49.69		
(FILM-COATED)				
250 mg, 15s ea	58016-0116-15	79.18		
20s ea	58016-0116-20	105.58		
30s ea	58016-0116-30	158.37		
40s ea	58016-0116-40	141.96		
(FILM-COATED)				
250 mg, 60s ea	58016-0116-60	316.73		
90s ea	58016-0116-90	475.10		
100s ea	58016-0116-00	527.89		
500 mg, 10s ea	58016-0117-10	61.64		
12s ea	58016-0117-12	73.97		
14s ea	58016-0117-14	86.30		
15s ea	58016-0117-15	92.46		
20s ea	58016-0117-20	123.29		
30s ea	58016-0117-30	184.93		
60s ea	58016-0117-60	369.86		
90s ea	58016-0117-90	554.79		
100s ea	58016-0117-00	616.43		
750 mg, 10s ea	58016-0118-10	64.65		
12s ea	58016-0118-12	77.57		
14s ea	58016-0118-14	90.50		
15s ea	58016-0118-15	96.97		
20s ea	58016-0118-20	129.29		
30s ea	58016-0118-30	193.94		
50s ea	58016-0118-50	323.23		
60s ea	58016-0118-60	387.87		
90s ea	58016-0118-90	581.81		
100s ea	58016-0118-00	646.45		
CIPRO HC (Alcon Ophthalmic)				
ciprofloxacin hydrochloride/hydrocortisone				
SUS, OT, 0.2%-1%, 10 ml	00065-8531-10	126.48		
(A-S Medication) REPACK				
SUS, OT, 0.2%-1%, 10 ml	54569-4723-00	120.88		
(Dispensing Solutions) REPACK				
SUS, OT, 0.2%-1%, 10 ml	55045-3001-01	112.00		
(Pharma Pac) REPACK				
SUS, OT (1X10ML)				
0.2%-1%, 10 ml	52959-0725-10	90.15		
(Phys Total Care) REPACK				
SUS, OT (1X10ML)				
0.2%-1%, 10 ml	54868-4365-00	139.33		
(Quality Care Prod) REPACK				
SUS, OT (1X10ML)				
0.2%-1%, 10 ml	35356-0527-10	182.57		
(Southwood) REPACK				
SUS, OT, 0.2%-1%, 10 ml	58016-8716-01	88.75		
(Stat Rx) REPACK				
SUS, OT, 0.2%-1%, 10 ml	16590-0053-10	134.59		
CIPRO IV (Schering)				
ciprofloxacin				
SOL, IV (PRE-MIXED W/DEX,BAXTER)				
200 mg/100 ml,				
100 ml 24s	00085-1781-01	374.40		
(PRE-MIXED W/DEX)				
200 mg/100 ml,				
100 ml 24s	00085-1755-02	374.40		
(PRE-MIXED W/DEX,BAXTER)				
400 mg/200 ml,				
200 ml 24s	00085-1762-01	720.00		
(PRE-MIXED W/DEX)				
400 mg/200 ml,				
200 ml 24s	00085-1741-02	720.00		
(VIAL)				
10 mg/ml,				
20 ml 10s	00085-1763-03	144.00		
(Phys Total Care) REPACK				
SOL, IV (VIAL)				
10 mg/ml, 40 ml	54868-4547-00	36.36		
CIPRO XR (Schering)				
ciprofloxacin/ciprofloxacin hydrochloride				
TER, PO, 500 mg, 50s ea	00085-1775-02	523.24		
100s ea	00085-1775-01	832.20		
(FILM-COATED)				
1000 mg, 30s ea UD	00085-1778-02	357.43		
50s ea	00085-1778-03	595.72		
(A-S Medication) REPACK				
TER, PO, 500 mg, 3s ea	54569-5510-00	32.70		
(Pharma Pac) REPACK				
TER, PO, 500 mg, 7s ea	52959-0855-07	73.76		
(Phys Total Care) REPACK				
TER, PO, 500 mg, 3s ea	54868-4734-00	39.85		
7s ea	54868-4734-02	90.48		
10s ea	54868-4734-01	128.45		
15s ea	54868-4734-03	191.74		
30s ea	54868-4734-04	360.52		
(FILM-COATED)				
1000 mg, 3s ea	54868-5044-04	36.51		
5s ea	54868-5044-02	59.60		
7s ea	54868-5044-01	82.69		
15s ea	54868-5044-03	165.43		
30s ea	54868-5044-00	328.99		
CIPRODEX (Alcon Ophthalmic)				
ciprofloxacin hydrochloride/dexamethasone				
SUS, OT (DROP-TAINER SYSTEM)				
0.3%-0.1%, 7.5 ml	00065-8533-02	126.48		
(A-S Medication) REPACK				
SUS, OT, 0.3%-0.1%,				
7.5 ml	54569-5560-00	120.88		
(Phys Total Care) REPACK				
SUS, OT, 0.3%-0.1%,				
7.5 ml	54868-4928-00	139.33		
CIPROFLOXACIN (Akorn)				
ciprofloxacin hydrochloride				
SOL, OP (1X2.5ML,USP)				
0.3%, 2.5 ml	17478-0714-25	8.60		AT
(1X10ML,USP)				
0.3%, 10 ml	17478-0714-11	13.53		AT
(Apotex Corp.)				
TAB, PO (FILM-COATED)				
250 mg, 100s ea	60505-1308-01	459.35		AB
500 mg, 100s ea	60505-1309-01	537.69		AB
4500s ea	60505-1309-07	24196.05		AB
750 mg, 50s ea	60505-1310-04	281.96		AB
(USP,FILM-COATED)				
750 mg, 100s ea	60505-1310-01	563.92		AB
(Aurobindo Pharma)				
TAB, PO (USP,FILM COATED)				
250 mg, 100s ea	65862-0076-01	458.16		AB
500 mg, 100s ea	13107-0077-01	558.64		AB
100s ea	65862-0077-01	558.64		AB
CIPROFLOXACIN (Baxter)				
SOL, IV (1X100ML,USP,PREMIX,PF)				
200 mg/100 ml,				
100 ml	00338-0960-48	18.22	15.18	AP
(1X200ML,USP,PREMIX,PF)				
400 mg/200 ml,				
200 ml	00338-0960-37	26.39	21.99	AP
(Bedford)				
SOL, IV (USP,SDV)				
10 mg/ml, 20 ml	55390-0197-01	7.20		AP
40 ml	55390-0198-01	7.20		AP
(PHARMACY BULK VIAL)				
10 mg/ml, 120 ml	55390-0199-01	14.40		AP
(Carlsbad Tech)				
ciprofloxacin hydrochloride				
TAB, PO (USP,FILM-COATED)				
250 mg, 100s ea	61442-0222-01	443.55		AB
500 mg, 100s ea	61442-0223-01	519.19		AB
750 mg, 50s ea	61442-0224-50	272.26		AB
CIPROFLOXACIN (Claris)				
SOL, IV (24X100ML,USP)				
200 mg/100 ml,				
100 ml 24s	36000-0008-24	81.12		AP
(24X200ML,USP)				
400 mg/200 ml,				
200 ml 24s	36000-0009-24	157.44		AP
(Dr Reddy's)				
ciprofloxacin hydrochloride				
TAB, PO (CYSTITIS PACK)				
100 mg, 6s ea	55111-0125-06	20.22		AB
(FILM-COATED)				
250 mg, 100s ea	55111-0126-01	443.55		AB
500s ea	55111-0126-05	2106.86		AB
500 mg, 100s ea	55111-0127-01	519.19		AB
500s ea	55111-0127-05	2466.15		AB
750 mg, 50s ea	55111-0128-50	272.26		AB
(Dr Reddy's)				
ciprofloxacin/ciprofloxacin hydrochloride				
TER, PO (FILM COATED)				
500 mg, 30s ea	55111-0422-30	293.96		AB
(FILM-COATED)				
1000 mg, 30s ea	55111-0423-30	333.23		AB
(Hi-Tech)				
ciprofloxacin hydrochloride				
SOL, OP, 0.3%, 2.5 ml	50383-0282-02	24.90		AT
5 ml	50383-0282-05	47.30		AT
10 ml	50383-0282-10	94.50		AT
CIPROFLOXACIN				
(Hospira) *See AMERINET CHOICE CIPROFLOXACIN*				
(Hospira) *See NOVAPLUS CIPROFLOXACIN*				
(Hospira)				
SOL, IV (24X100ML,SINGLEDOSE,USP)				
200 mg/100 ml,				
100 ml 24s	00409-4777-23	58.75	51.36	AP
(24X200ML,SINGLEDOSE,USP)				
400 mg/200 ml,				
200 ml 24s	00409-4777-02	70.56	61.68	AP
(SINGLE-DOSE,USP)				
10 mg/ml, 20 ml	00409-4765-86	1.86	1.63	AP
40 ml	00409-4778-86	3.56	3.12	AP
(Marlex)				
ciprofloxacin hydrochloride				
TAB, PO (USP,FILM-COATED)				
500 mg, 100s ea	10135-0475-01	538.00		AB
(Martec)				
TAB, PO (FILM-COATED)				
250 mg, 100s ea	52555-0769-01	459.40		
500 mg, 100s ea	52555-0770-01	537.77		
750 mg, 50s ea	52555-0771-50	282.10		
100s ea	52555-0771-01	563.95		
(Mylan)				
TAB, PO (FILM-COATED)				
250 mg, 100s ea	00378-1322-01	458.90		
500s ea	00378-1322-05	2294.50		
500 mg, 100s ea	00378-1323-01	537.15		
(USP,FILM-COATED)				
500 mg, 100s ea	00378-7098-01	536.28		
(FILM-COATED)				
500 mg, 500s ea	00378-1323-05	2685.75		
750 mg, 50s ea	00378-1324-89	281.70		
(Mylan)				
ciprofloxacin/ciprofloxacin hydrochloride				
TER, PO (FILM COATED)				
500 mg, 50s ea	00378-1743-89	489.94		AB
1000 mg, 50s ea	00378-1745-89	557.80		AB
(Pack)				
ciprofloxacin hydrochloride				
SOL, OP (USP,1X2.5ML)				
0.3%, 2.5 ml	16571-0120-25	25.91		AT
(USP,1X5ML)				
0.3%, 5 ml	16571-0120-50	47.29		AT
TAB, PO (USP,FILM-COATED)				
250 mg, 100s ea	16571-0411-10	443.55		
500 mg, 100s ea	16571-0412-10	519.19		
750 mg, 50s ea	16571-0413-05	272.36		
CIPROFLOXACIN				
(Pfizer) *See CIPROFLOXACIN IN DEXTROSE*				
(Pfizer)				
SOL, IV (1X20ML,USP)				
10 mg/ml, 20 ml	00069-3241-15	2.58	2.15	AP
(10X20ML,USP)				
10 mg/ml,				
20 ml 10s	00069-3241-22	25.80	21.50	AP
(1X40ML,USP)				
10 mg/ml, 40 ml	00069-3342-15	3.90	3.25	AP

PROD/MFR	NDC	AWP	DP	OBC
(10X40ML,USP)				
10 mg/ml,				
40 ml 10s	**00069-3342-22**	39.00	32.50	**AP**
(PharmaForce)				
ciprofloxacin hydrochloride				
SOL, OP (1X2.5ML,USP,MULTIPLEDSE)				
0.3%, 2.5 ml	**40042-0015-52**	22.30		**AT**
(1X5ML)				
0.3%, 5 ml	**40042-0015-05**	40.44		**AT**
(1X10ML)				
0.3%, 10 ml	**40042-0015-10**	90.33		**AT**
(Ranbaxy Pharm)				
TAB, PO (FILM-COATED)				
250 mg, 100s ea	**63304-0709-01**	459.41		
500 mg, 100s ea	**63304-0710-01**	537.75		
750 mg, 50s ea	**63304-0711-50**	282.00		
100s ea	**63304-0711-01**	564.00		
CIPROFLOXACIN (Sagent)				
SOL, IV (10X100ML,USP,LATEX-FREE)				
200 mg/100 ml,				
100 ml 10s	**25021-0114-82**	161.87		**AP**
(10X200ML,USP,LATEX-FREE)				
400 mg/200 ml,				
200 ml 10s	**25021-0114-87**	311.25		**AP**
(Sandoz)				
SOL, IV (24X100ML,USP,LATEX-FREE)				
200 mg/100 ml,				
100 ml 24s	**00781-3239-09**	351.00		**AP**
(24X200ML,USP,LATEX-FREE)				
400 mg/200 ml,				
200 ml 24s	**00781-3240-09**	675.00		**AP**
(Sandoz)				
ciprofloxacin hydrochloride				
TAB, PO (FILM-COATED)				
250 mg, 100s ea	**00185-0442-01**	459.41		
500 mg, 100s ea	**00185-0451-01**	537.75		
750 mg, 50s ea	**00185-0470-53**	281.99		
CIPROFLOXACIN				
(Schering) *See CIPRO*				
(Schering) *See CIPRO IV*				
(Teva)				
SOL, IV (1X100ML,USP,LATEX-FREE)				
200 mg/100 ml,				
100 ml	**00703-0969-36**	135.12		**AP**
(1X200ML,USP,LATEX-FREE)				
400 mg/200 ml,				
200 ml	**00703-0960-36**	5.40		**AP**
(SDV,10X20ML,200MG,1%)				
10 mg/ml,				
20 ml 10s	**00703-0956-03**	99.24		**AP**
(SDV,10X40ML,400MG,1%)				
10 mg/ml,				
40 ml 10s	**00703-0958-03**	57.60		**AP**
(Teva)				
ciprofloxacin hydrochloride				
TAB, PO (FILM-COATED)				
250 mg, 100s ea UD	**00172-5311-10**	460.89		
100s ea	**00172-5311-60**	458.89		
100s ea	**00182-2631-01**	458.89		**AB**
500 mg, 100s ea UD	**00172-5312-10**	539.15		
100s ea	**00172-5312-60**	537.15		
500s ea	**00172-5312-70**	2593.60		
650s ea	**00182-2721-36**	3491.48		**AB**
750 mg, 100s ea UD	**00172-5313-10**	584.09		
100s ea	**00172-5313-60**	582.09		
(UDL)				
TAB, PO (10X10,FILM-COATED)				
250 mg, 100s ea UD	**51079-0402-20**	440.00		**AB**
500 mg, 100s ea UD	**51079-0403-20**	510.00		**AB**
(Watson Labs)				
TAB, PO (USP,FILM-COATED)				
250 mg, 100s ea	**16252-0514-01**	18.00		**AB**
500 mg, 100s ea	**16252-0515-01**	24.00		**AB**
750 mg, 50s ea	**16252-0516-05**	12.00		**AB**
(West-Ward)				
TAB, PO (FILM-COATED)				
250 mg, 100s ea	**00143-9927-01**	459.40		
500 mg, 100s ea	**00143-9928-01**	536.75		
750 mg, 50s ea	**00143-9929-50**	282.25		
(4u)				
REPACK				
TAB, PO (FILM-COATED)				
500 mg, 10s ea	**42549-0507-10**	118.88		
10s ea	**42549-0598-10**	118.88		
30s ea	**42549-0507-30**	122.46		
40s ea	**42549-0507-40**	132.52		
(A-S Medication)				
REPACK				
TAB, PO (FILM-COATED)				
250 mg, 6s ea	**54569-5584-00**	27.56		
10s ea	**54569-5584-02**	45.94		
(FILM-COATED)				
250 mg, 14s ea	**54569-5584-01**	64.31		
500 mg, ea	**54569-5574-02**	5.38		
6s ea	**54569-5574-03**	32.26		
10s ea	**54569-5574-05**	53.77		
(COATED)				
500 mg, 14s ea	**54569-5574-01**	75.28		
20s ea	**54569-5574-00**	107.54		
(FILM-COATED)				
500 mg, 28s ea	**54569-5574-04**	150.55		
(A-S Medication)				
ciprofloxacin/ciprofloxacin hydrochloride				
TER, PO, 500 mg, 3s ea	**54569-5899-00**	29.40		
(Aidarex)				
REPACK				
ciprofloxacin hydrochloride				
TAB, PO (FILM-COATED)				
250 mg, 6s ea	**33261-0399-06**	31.80		**AB**
7s ea	**33261-0399-07**	37.10		**AB**
12s ea	**33261-0399-12**	63.60		**AB**
14s ea	**33261-0399-14**	74.20		**AB**
20s ea	**33261-0399-20**	106.00		**AB**
28s ea	**33261-0399-28**	148.40		**AB**
30s ea	**33261-0399-30**	159.00		**AB**
60s ea	**33261-0399-60**	318.00		**AB**
500 mg, 7s ea	**33261-0164-07**	43.12		
14s ea	**33261-0164-14**	86.24		
20s ea	**33261-0164-20**	123.20		
21s ea	**33261-0164-21**	129.36		
28s ea	**33261-0164-28**	172.48		
30s ea	**33261-0164-30**	184.80		
40s ea	**33261-0164-40**	246.40		
60s ea	**33261-0164-60**	369.60		
750 mg, 7s ea	**33261-0367-07**	43.75		
10s ea	**33261-0367-10**	62.50		
14s ea	**33261-0367-14**	87.50		
20s ea	**33261-0367-20**	125.00		
21s ea	**33261-0367-21**	131.25		
28s ea	**33261-0367-28**	175.00		
30s ea	**33261-0367-30**	187.50		
60s ea	**33261-0367-60**	375.00		
(Altura)				
REPACK				
TAB, PO (FILM-COATED)				
500 mg, 10s ea	**63874-1086-01**	58.00		
14s ea	**63874-1086-04**	81.20		
15s ea	**63874-1086-05**	87.00		
20s ea	**63874-1086-02**	116.00		
30s ea	**63874-1086-03**	174.00		
60s ea	**63874-1086-06**	348.00		
100s ea	**63874-1086-00**	580.00		
(American Health)				
REPACK				
TAB, PO (10X10,FILM-COATED)				
250 mg, 100s ea UD	**68084-0069-01**	310.56		**AB**
(FILM-COATED)				
500 mg, 100s ea UD	**68084-0070-01**	368.55		**AB**
750 mg, 100s ea UD	**68084-0071-01**	567.00		**AB**
(Bryant Ranch)				
REPACK				
TAB, PO, 250 mg, 10s ea	**63629-1326-02**	56.70		
20s ea	**63629-1326-01**	113.40		
500 mg, 6s ea	**63629-1724-05**	35.40		
10s ea	**63629-1724-06**	74.71		
14s ea	**63629-1724-01**	104.60		
20s ea	**63629-1724-03**	143.00		
(FILM-COATED)				
500 mg, 28s ea	**63629-1724-07**	168.92		**AB**
30s ea	**63629-1724-02**	177.00		
60s ea	**63629-1724-04**	354.00		
(Core)				
REPACK				
TAB, PO, 100 mg, ea	**33358-0080-01**	4.17		
6s ea	**33358-0080-06**	21.49		
500 mg, ea	**33358-0081-01**	6.23		
6s ea	**33358-0081-06**	36.29		
10s ea	**33358-0081-10**	76.58		
14s ea	**33358-0081-14**	107.22		
20s ea	**33358-0081-20**	146.58		
28s ea	**33358-0081-28**	155.05		
30s ea	**33358-0081-30**	181.43		
60s ea	**33358-0081-60**	362.85		
(DHS, Inc.)				
REPACK				
TAB, PO, 250 mg, 20s ea	**55887-0904-20**	96.00		
30s ea	**55887-0904-30**	144.00		
60s ea	**55887-0904-60**	288.00		
500 mg, 4s ea	**55887-0584-04**	23.48		
6s ea	**55887-0584-06**	35.22		
8s ea	**55887-0584-08**	46.96		
(FILM-COATED)				
500 mg, 10s ea	**55887-0584-10**	58.70		**AB**
12s ea	**55887-0584-12**	70.44		
(FILM-COATED)				
500 mg, 14s ea	**55887-0584-14**	82.18		**AB**
20s ea	**55887-0584-20**	103.86		**AB**
21s ea	**55887-0584-21**	109.06		
25s ea	**55887-0584-25**	129.83		
28s ea	**55887-0584-28**	145.40		
(FILM-COATED)				
500 mg, 30s ea	**55887-0584-30**	162.00		**AB**
40s ea	**55887-0584-40**	190.00		**AB**
42s ea	**55887-0584-42**	199.50		
60s ea	**55887-0584-60**	285.00		
750 mg, 10s ea	**55887-0292-10**	54.50		
(FILM-COATED)				
750 mg, 28s ea	**55887-0292-28**	153.00		
(Dispensing Solutions)				
REPACK				
TAB, PO (FILM-COATED)				
250 mg, 6s ea	**66336-0433-06**	30.32		
14s ea	**66336-0433-14**	70.75		
500 mg, ea	**66336-0903-99**	6.47		
6s ea	**55045-3080-02**	35.45		**AB**
6s ea	**66336-0903-06**	38.82		
10s ea	**55045-3080-01**	59.10		**AB**
10s ea	**66336-0903-10**	64.70		
14s ea	**55045-3080-05**	82.74		**AB**
14s ea	**66336-0903-14**	90.57		
20s ea	**55045-3080-07**	118.20		**AB**
20s ea	**66336-0903-20**	129.39		
28s ea	**66336-0903-28**	181.15		
30s ea	**55045-3080-08**	177.30		**AB**
30s ea	**66336-0903-30**	194.09		
100s ea	**55045-3080-00**	591.00		
750 mg, 10s ea	**55045-3081-01**	69.00		**AB**
14s ea	**55045-3081-02**	96.60		**AB**
20s ea	**55045-3081-07**	138.00		**AB**
30s ea	**55045-3081-08**	207.00		**AB**
60s ea	**55045-3081-06**	414.00		**AB**
90s ea	**55045-3081-09**	621.00		**AB**
100s ea	**55045-3081-00**	690.00		**AB**
120s ea	**55045-3081-03**	828.00		**AB**
(GSMS)				
REPACK				
TAB, PO (FILM-COATED)				
250 mg, 100s ea	**60429-0742-01**	48.60	16.20	**AB**
500 mg, 20s ea UD	**60429-0743-20**	9.60	3.20	**AB**
100s ea	**60429-0743-01**	29.25	9.75	**AB**
500s ea	**60429-0743-05**	146.25	48.75	**AB**
750 mg, 100s ea	**60429-0744-01**	104.55	34.85	**AB**
(HomeMed)				
REPACK				
TAB, PO, 250 mg, 6s ea	**51655-0115-87**	27.56		
14s ea	**51655-0115-84**	64.32		
500 mg, ea	**51655-0118-47**	6.65		
6s ea	**51655-0118-87**	39.90		
10s ea	**51655-0118-53**	66.50		
14s ea	**51655-0118-84**	93.10		
20s ea	**51655-0118-52**	121.99		
28s ea	**51655-0118-29**	186.20		
(IPI)				
REPACK				
SOL, OP (1X5ML)				
0.3%, 5 ml	**18837-0319-05**	59.13		
TAB, PO, 500 mg, 14s ea	**18837-0245-14**	94.10		
20s ea	**18837-0245-20**	141.14		
30s ea	**18837-0245-30**	211.50		
(Keltman Pharma., Inc.)				
REPACK				
TAB, PO (FILM-COATED)				
500 mg, 10s ea	**68387-0535-10**	81.43		
15s ea	**68387-0535-15**	122.14		
20s ea	**68387-0535-20**	162.85		
750 mg, 10s ea	**68387-0534-01**	69.35		
(McKesson Packaging)				
REPACK				
TAB, PO (USP)				
250 mg, 100s ea UD	**63739-0427-10**	430.00		
500 mg, 100s ea UD	**63739-0400-10**	530.00		
(Nucare Pharm)				
REPACK				
TAB, PO (FILM-COATED)				
250 mg, 6s ea	**68071-0055-06**	29.56		**AB**
10s ea	**68071-0055-10**	49.20		**AB**

PROD/MFR	NDC	AWP	DP	OBC
14s ea	68071-0055-14	68.80		AB
20s ea	68071-0055-20	98.40		AB
28s ea	68071-0055-28	137.76		AB
30s ea	68071-0055-30	147.60		AB
500 mg, 6s ea	66267-0919-06	40.84		AB
10s ea	66267-0919-10	73.93		
14s ea	66267-0919-14	95.30		
(FILM-COATED)				
500 mg, 20s ea	66267-0919-20	148.20		
28s ea	66267-0919-28	207.49		AB
30s ea	66267-0919-30	178.85		
60s ea	66267-0919-60	440.80		AB
750 mg, 14s ea	68071-0331-14	186.99		
20s ea	68071-0331-20	285.99		
30s ea	68071-0331-30	428.98		
(Palmetto)				
REPACK				
TAB, PO, 500 mg, ea	23490-5323-01	13.68		
6s ea	23490-5323-02	43.20		
7s ea	23490-0320-07	46.58		
10s ea	23490-5323-03	72.00		
14s ea	23490-0320-04	95.30		
14s ea	23490-5323-04	100.80		
20s ea	23490-5323-05	144.00		
28s ea	23490-0320-08	186.31		
28s ea	23490-5323-06	167.99		
30s ea	23490-5323-07	216.00		
(FILM-COATED)				
500 mg, 40s ea	23490-5323-08	240.00		AB
(PD-Rx Pharm)				
REPACK				
TAB, PO, 250 mg, 6s ea	58864-0806-06	91.20		
(USP,FILM-COATED)				
250 mg, 6s ea	55289-0823-06	118.80		
(FILM-COATED)				
250 mg, 12s ea	55289-0823-12	137.20		
(REDI-SCRIPT,COATED)				
250 mg, 14s ea	58864-0806-14	114.60		
(USP,FILM-COATED)				
250 mg, 14s ea	55289-0823-14	143.40		
(FILM-COATED)				
250 mg, 20s ea	55289-0823-20	162.20		
(REDI-SCRIPT,USP)				
250 mg, 20s ea	58864-0806-20	116.00		
(USP,FILM-COATED)				
500 mg, ea	55289-0821-79	110.80		
(FILM-COATED)				
500 mg, 3s ea	55289-0821-03	113.20		
(USP,FILM-COATED)				
500 mg, 4s ea	43063-0053-04	117.80		
(FILM-COATED)				
500 mg, 6s ea	43063-0053-06	126.80		
6s ea	55289-0821-06	132.60		
(COATED)				
500 mg, 10s ea	58864-0833-10	147.80		
(FILM-COATED)				
500 mg, 10s ea	55289-0821-10	150.20		
14s ea	55289-0821-14	181.20		
(REDI-SCRIPT,FILM-COATED)				
500 mg, 20s ea	58864-0833-20	226.20		
(USP,FILM-COATED)				
500 mg, 20s ea	55289-0821-20	241.20		
30s ea	55289-0821-30	320.00		
50s ea	55289-0821-50	466.00		
(USP)				
750 mg, 10s ea	55289-0826-10	199.80		
(USP,FILM-COATED)				
750 mg, 20s ea	55289-0826-20	262.80		
(Pharma Pac)				
REPACK				
TAB, PO (FILM-COATED)				
250 mg, 6s ea	52959-0739-06	30.47		AB
10s ea	52959-0739-10	50.78		
14s ea	52959-0739-14	71.09		
20s ea	52959-0739-20	101.48		
(FILM-COATED)				
250 mg, 30s ea	52959-0739-30	152.26		
500 mg, 4s ea	52959-0730-04	23.66		
(FILM-COATED)				
500 mg, 6s ea	52959-0730-06	35.49		
10s ea	52959-0730-10	59.15		
14s ea	52959-0730-14	82.80		
15s ea	52959-0730-15	88.71		
20s ea	52959-0730-20	118.28		
21s ea	52959-0730-21	124.19		
28s ea	52959-0730-28	165.58		
30s ea	52959-0730-30	177.40		
60s ea	52959-0730-60	351.80		AB
100s ea	52959-0730-00	591.28		
750 mg, 20s ea	52959-0734-20	119.58		AB
30s ea	52959-0734-30	179.36		
60s ea	52959-0734-60	358.68		
(Phys Total Care)				
REPACK				
TAB, PO (COATED)				
250 mg, 6s ea	54868-4898-03	4.86		
10s ea	54868-4898-04	6.09		
(FILM-COATED)				
250 mg, 15s ea	54868-4898-02	7.62		AB
20s ea	54868-4898-00	9.18		AB
30s ea	54868-4898-01	12.27		AB
500 mg, 6s ea	54868-4858-04	15.21		AB
10s ea	54868-4858-01	21.35		AB
14s ea	54868-4858-08	27.48		
15s ea	54868-4858-03	29.02		AB
20s ea	54868-4858-00	36.69		AB
30s ea	54868-4858-02	52.04		AB
40s ea	54868-4858-05	67.38		
(COATED)				
500 mg, 60s ea	54868-4858-06	76.41		
(FILM-COATED)				
500 mg, 100s ea	54868-4858-07	121.85		AB
750 mg, 15s ea	54868-5023-01	15.57		AB
30s ea	54868-5023-00	26.64		AB
CIPROFLOXACIN (Physician Partner)				
REPACK				
SOL, IV (1X200ML)				
10 mg/ml, 200 ml	21695-0422-01	20.68		AP
(Physician Partner)				
ciprofloxacin hydrochloride				
TAB, PO, 250 mg, 6s ea	21695-0411-06	59.48		
10s ea	21695-0411-10	99.14		
14s ea	21695-0411-14	138.80		
500 mg, 6s ea	21695-0210-06	69.63		
(FILM-COATED)				
500 mg, 10s ea	21695-0210-10	126.47		AB
14s ea	21695-0210-14	177.05		
20s ea	21695-0210-20	252.94		
28s ea	21695-0210-28	324.95		
30s ea	21695-0210-30	326.50		
(Quality Care Prod)				
REPACK				
TAB, PO (FILM-COATED)				
250 mg, 6s ea	49999-0333-06	63.00		
14s ea	49999-0333-14	73.92		
20s ea	49999-0333-20	105.60		
(FILM-COATED)				
500 mg, ea	49999-0334-01	6.96		AB
10s ea	49999-0334-10	75.90		
14s ea	49999-0334-14	106.22		AB
(COATED)				
500 mg, 20s ea	49999-0334-20	151.80		
(FILM-COATED)				
500 mg, 28s ea	49999-0334-28	178.08		
30s ea	49999-0334-30	190.80		AB
100s ea	49999-0334-00	657.25		AB
750 mg, 10s ea	35356-0264-10	75.90		
(Southwood)				
REPACK				
SOL, OP, 0.3%, 2.5 ml	58016-4858-01	24.90		
TAB, PO, 250 mg, 10s ea	58016-0137-10	49.56		
12s ea	58016-0137-12	59.47		
15s ea	58016-0137-15	74.34		
20s ea	58016-0137-20	99.12		
30s ea	58016-0137-30	148.68		
60s ea	58016-0137-60	297.35		
90s ea	58016-0137-90	446.03		
100s ea	58016-0137-00	495.59		
120s ea	58016-0137-02	594.71		
(FILM-COATED)				
500 mg, 10s ea	58016-0953-10	58.00		
12s ea	58016-0953-12	69.60		
15s ea	58016-0953-15	87.00		
20s ea	58016-0953-20	116.00		
30s ea	58016-0953-30	174.00		
60s ea	58016-0953-60	348.00		
90s ea	58016-0953-90	522.00		
100s ea	58016-0953-00	580.00		
120s ea	58016-0953-02	696.00		
750 mg, 10s ea	58016-0957-10	60.84		
12s ea	58016-0957-12	73.01		
15s ea	58016-0957-15	91.26		
20s ea	58016-0957-20	121.68		
30s ea	58016-0957-30	182.52		
60s ea	58016-0957-60	365.04		
90s ea	58016-0957-90	547.56		
100s ea	58016-0957-00	608.40		
120s ea	58016-0957-02	730.08		
(St. Mary's MPP)				
REPACK				
TAB, PO (FILM-COATED)				
500 mg, 10s ea	60760-0815-10	67.45		AB
14s ea	60760-0815-14	88.66		
20s ea	60760-0518-20	124.09		
(Stat Rx)				
REPACK				
SOL, OP, 0.3%, 5 ml	16590-0421-05	60.00		
TAB, PO (FILM-COATED)				
250 mg, 10s ea	16590-0371-10	45.93		AB
20s ea	16590-0371-20	91.86		AB
500 mg, 14s ea	16590-0054-14	74.25		
20s ea	16590-0054-20	106.07		
(FILM-COATED)				
500 mg, 28s ea	16590-0054-28	197.68		
30s ea	16590-0054-30	195.50		
(FILM-COATED)				
500 mg, 60s ea	16590-0054-60	282.25		
750 mg, 14s ea	16590-0735-14	104.13		
20s ea	16590-0735-20	148.75		AB
(Vibranta)				
REPACK				
TAB, PO, 250 mg, 4s ea	57866-3135-01	80.25		
500 mg, 10s ea	57866-6041-03	100.25		
14s ea	57866-6041-02	106.22		
20s ea	57866-6041-01	180.99		
28s ea	57866-6041-05	184.79		
30s ea	57866-6041-04	185.00		
60s ea	57866-6041-08	190.00		
CIPROFLOXACIN HCL (Akorn)				
ciprofloxacin hydrochloride				
SOL, OP, 0.3%, 5 ml	17478-0714-10	10.20		AT
(Apotex Corp.)				
SOL, OP, 0.3%, 5 ml	60505-1000-01	47.25		AT
(Falcon Ophthalmics)				
SOL, OP, 0.3%, 2.5 ml	61314-0656-25	25.03		AT
5 ml	61314-0656-05	47.31		AT
10 ml	61314-0656-10	94.44		AT
(Hawkins)				
POW, NA (USP)				
100 gm	63370-0034-35	160.00		
500 gm	63370-0034-45	700.00		
1000 gm	63370-0034-50	1320.00		
(Medisca)				
POW, NA (U.S.P.)				
100 gm	38779-0534-05	126.00		
500 gm	38779-0534-08	585.00		
1000 gm	38779-0534-09	1125.00		
(A-S Medication)				
REPACK				
SOL, OP, 0.3%, 2.5 ml	54569-5612-00	21.92		AT
5 ml	54569-5613-00	40.94		AT
(Aidarex)				
REPACK				
SOL, OP (1X10ML)				
0.3%, 10 ml	33261-0381-01	94.44		AT
(Dispensing Solutions)				
REPACK				
SOL, OP, 0.3%, 2.5 ml	55045-3199-02	25.00		AT
(1X5ML)				
0.3%, 5 ml	55045-3199-05	47.00		AT
TAB, PO (FILM-COATED)				
250 mg, 6s ea	55045-3142-01	34.02		
14s ea	55045-3142-05	79.38		
20s ea	55045-3142-07	113.40		
(Pharma Pac)				
REPACK				
SOL, OP, 0.3%, 5 ml	52959-0557-05	45.98		AT
(Phys Total Care)				
REPACK				
SOL, OP, 0.3%, 2.5 ml 3s	54868-5130-00	73.56		AT
5 ml	54868-5130-01	105.66		AT
(Physician Partner)				
REPACK				
SOL, OP (1X2.5ML)				
0.3%, 2.5 ml	21695-0259-25	50.06		AT
(5X10ML)				
0.3%, 10 ml 5s	21695-0259-05	94.62		AT
(Quality Care Prod)				
REPACK				
SOL, OP (1X2.5ML)				
0.3%, 2.5 ml	49999-0699-25	52.30		AT
(1X5ML,DROP)				
0.3%, 5 ml	49999-0699-05	104.60		AT
CIPROFLOXACIN HYDROCHLORIDE				
FUL				
SOL, OP, 0.3%, 5 ml		37.85		
TAB, PO, 250 mg, 100s ea		37.50		
500 mg, 100s ea		45.00		
750 mg, 100s ea		48.00		
(Akorn) *See CIPROFLOXACIN*				

PROD/MFR	NDC	AWP	DP	OBC
(Akorn) *See CIPROFLOXACIN HCL*				
(Alcon Ophthalmic) *See CILOXAN*				
(Apotex Corp.) *See CIPROFLOXACIN*				
(Apotex Corp.) *See CIPROFLOXACIN HCL*				
(Aurobindo Pharma) *See CIPROFLOXACIN*				
(Carlsbad Tech) *See CIPROFLOXACIN*				
(Dr Reddy's) *See CIPROFLOXACIN*				
(Falcon Ophthalmics) *See CIPROFLOXACIN HCL*				
(Hawkins) *See CIPROFLOXACIN HCL*				
(Hi-Tech) *See CIPROFLOXACIN*				
(Marlex) *See CIPROFLOXACIN*				
(Martec) *See CIPROFLOXACIN*				
(Medisca) *See CIPROFLOXACIN HCL*				
(Medisca)				
CRY, NA (1X100GM)				
100 gm	**38779-2323-05**	117.00		
(1X500GM)				
500 gm	**38779-2323-08**	546.00		
(1X1000GM)				
1000 gm	**38779-2323-09**	1041.00		
(Mylan) *See CIPROFLOXACIN*				
(Pack) *See CIPROFLOXACIN*				
(PCCA)				
POW, NA (USP)				
1 gm	**51927-3634-00**	1.41		
(PharmaForce) *See CIPROFLOXACIN*				
(Ranbaxy Pharm) *See CIPROFLOXACIN*				
(Sandoz) *See CIPROFLOXACIN*				
(Schering) *See CIPRO*				
(Teva) *See CIPROFLOXACIN*				
(UDL) *See CIPROFLOXACIN*				
(Watson Labs) *See CIPROFLOXACIN*				
(West-Ward) *See CIPROFLOXACIN*				
(Wraser Pharm) *See CETRAXAL*				
(Altura)				
REPACK				
SOL, OP, 0.3%, 2.5 ml	**63874-0199-03**	25.03		
5 ml	**63874-0199-05**	47.31		
10 ml	**63874-0199-10**	94.50		
(Dispensing Solutions)				
REPACK				
TAB, PO, 500 mg, 7s ea	**55045-3080-03**	41.37		
100s ea	**55045-3467-01**	510.00		
(Palmetto)				
REPACK				
SOL, OP, 0.3%, 2.5 ml	**23490-5321-01**	25.00		
5 ml	**23490-5321-00**	47.50		
TAB, PO, 250 mg, 6s ea	**23490-5322-01**	41.66		
14s ea	**23490-5322-04**	69.38		
20s ea	**23490-5322-02**	99.12		
30s ea	**23490-5322-03**	148.68		
750 mg, 10s ea	**23490-5324-01**	69.00		
14s ea	**23490-5324-00**	96.60		
20s ea	**23490-5324-02**	138.00		
30s ea	**23490-5324-03**	207.00		
(Palmetto)				
ciprofloxacin/ciprofloxacin hydrochloride				
TER, PO, 500 mg, 3s ea	**23490-7664-01**	30.89		
CIPROFLOXACIN HYDROCHLORIDE (Physician Partner)				
REPACK				
SOL, OP, 0.3%, 10 ml	**21695-0259-10**	188.88		
CIPROFLOXACIN HYDROCHLORIDE/ DEXAMETHASONE				
(Alcon Ophthalmic) *See CIPRODEX*				
CIPROFLOXACIN HYDROCHLORIDE/ HYDROCORTISONE				
(Alcon Ophthalmic) *See CIPRO HC*				
CIPROFLOXACIN IN DEXTROSE (Pfizer)				
ciprofloxacin				
SOL, IV (24X100ML,SINGLE DOSE)				
200 mg/100 ml,				
100 ml 24s	**00069-4395-19**	62.40	52.00	**AP**
(24X200ML,SINGLE DOSE)				
400 mg/200 ml,				
200 ml 24s	**00069-4396-27**	123.60	103.00	**AP**
CIPROFLOXACIN/CIPROFLOXACIN HYDROCHLORIDE				
(Depomed) *See PROQUIN XR*				
(Dr Reddy's) *See CIPROFLOXACIN*				
(Mylan) *See CIPROFLOXACIN*				
(Schering) *See CIPRO XR*				
CISAPRIDE (Medisca)				
POW, NA (1X10GM)				
10 gm	**38779-1900-01**	345.00		
25 gm	**38779-1900-04**	597.00		
100 gm	**38779-1900-05**	2067.00		
500 gm	**38779-1900-08**	7350.00		
1000 gm	**38779-1900-09**	11700.00		
(PCCA)				
POW, NA, 1 gm	**51927-3346-00**	30.00		
(Spectrum Pharmacy)				
POW, NA (1X5GM)				
5 gm	**49452-2065-01**	217.35		
(1X25GM)				
25 gm	**49452-2065-02**	840.00		
(1X100GM)				
100 gm	**49452-2065-03**	2712.50		
CISATRACURIUM BESYLATE				
(Abbott Pharm) *See NIMBEX*				
CISPLATIN				
(APP) *See CISPLATIN AMERINET CHOICE*				
(APP)				
SOL, IV (M.D.V.,PF)				
1 mg/ml, 50 ml	**63323-0103-51**	22.56		**AP**
100 ml	**63323-0103-65**	45.13		**AP**
200 ml	**63323-0103-64**	90.25		**AP**
(Bedford) *See CISPLATIN NOVAPLUS*				
(Bedford)				
SOL, IV (M.D.V.)				
1 mg/ml, 50 ml	**55390-0112-50**	22.20		**AP**
100 ml	**55390-0112-99**	44.40		**AP**
200 ml	**55390-0099-01**	88.80		**AP**
(Gallipot)				
POW, NA (U.S.P.)				
0.05 gm	**51552-1076-09**	34.93	24.95	
(Spectrum Pharmacy)				
POW, NA (U.S.P.)				
0.25 gm	**49452-2078-02**	479.50		
1 gm	**49452-2078-03**	1316.00		
(Teva)				
SOL, IV (M.D.V.)				
1 mg/ml, 50 ml	**00703-5747-11**	20.40		**AP**
100 ml	**00703-5748-11**	37.20		**AP**
CISPLATIN AMERINET CHOICE (APP)				
cisplatin				
SOL, IV (M.D.V.,PRIVATE LABEL)				
1 mg/ml, 50 ml	**63323-0103-91**	22.56		**AP**
100 ml	**63323-0103-95**	45.13		**AP**
CISPLATIN NOVAPLUS (Bedford)				
cisplatin				
SOL, IV (M.D.V.,PRIVATE LABEL)				
1 mg/ml, 50 ml	**55390-0414-50**	22.20		**AP**
100 ml	**55390-0414-99**	44.40		**AP**
200 ml	**55390-0187-01**	88.80		**AP**
CITALOPRAM (Aurobindo Pharma)				
citalopram hydrobromide				
TAB, PO (USP,FILM-COATED)				
40 mg, 100s ea	**13107-0007-01**	264.45		**AB**
500s ea	**13107-0007-05**	1295.81		**AB**
(Greenstone)				
TAB, PO (USP,FILM COATED)				
10 mg, 30s ea	**59762-4800-03**	75.19		**AB**
60s ea	**59762-4800-06**	147.38		**AB**
100s ea	**59762-4800-01**	240.72		**AB**
500s ea	**59762-4800-05**	1179.52		**AB**
20 mg, 30s ea	**59762-4801-03**	78.37		**AB**
60s ea	**59762-4801-06**	153.60		**AB**
100s ea	**59762-4801-01**	250.88		**AB**
500s ea	**59762-4801-05**	1229.29		**AB**
40 mg, 30s ea	**59762-4802-03**	81.78		**AB**
60s ea	**59762-4802-06**	160.29		**AB**
100s ea	**59762-4802-01**	261.81		**AB**
500s ea	**59762-4802-05**	1282.85		**AB**
(Major)				
TAB, PO (10X10, USP,FILM-COATED)				
10 mg, 100s ea UD	**00904-6084-61**	242.71		**AB**
20 mg, 100s ea UD	**00904-6085-61**	269.31		**AB**
40 mg, 100s ea UD	**00904-6086-61**	349.20		**AB**
(Mylan)				
TAB, PO (USP,FILM-COATED)				
10 mg, 100s ea	**00378-6231-01**	244.50		**AB**
500s ea	**00378-6231-05**	1222.50		**AB**
20 mg, 100s ea	**00378-6232-01**	255.50		**AB**
500s ea	**00378-6232-05**	1277.50		**AB**
40 mg, 100s ea	**00378-6233-01**	265.50		**AB**
500s ea	**00378-6233-05**	1327.50		**AB**
(A-S Medication)				
REPACK				
TAB, PO, 20 mg, 60s ea	**54569-5626-01**	153.30		
(Aidarex)				
REPACK				
TAB, PO, 20 mg, 10s ea	**33261-0027-10**	53.30		
12s ea	**33261-0027-12**	63.96		
14s ea	**33261-0027-14**	74.62		
20s ea	**33261-0027-20**	106.60		
21s ea	**33261-0027-21**	111.93		
28s ea	**33261-0027-28**	149.24		
30s ea	**33261-0027-30**	159.75		
60s ea	**33261-0027-60**	319.80		
(Bryant Ranch)				
REPACK				
TAB, PO, 20 mg, 30s ea	**63629-1318-01**	89.94		
60s ea	**63629-1318-02**	178.89		
(Core)				
REPACK				
TAB, PO, 10 mg, 30s ea	**33358-0082-30**	88.14		
60s ea	**33358-0082-60**	176.28		
90s ea	**33358-0082-90**	224.31		
20 mg, 30s ea	**33358-0083-30**	92.19		
60s ea	**33358-0083-60**	183.46		
40 mg, 30s ea	**33358-0084-30**	97.76		
60s ea	**33358-0084-60**	245.84		
(DHS, Inc.)				
REPACK				
TAB, PO, 20 mg, 7s ea	**55887-0261-07**	14.65		
100s ea	**55887-0261-01**	209.26		
40 mg, 30s ea	**55887-0237-30**	79.00		
90s ea	**55887-0237-90**	150.00		
150s ea	**55887-0237-86**	225.00		
(IPI)				
REPACK				
TAB, PO, 20 mg, 60s ea	**18837-0253-60**	182.04		
90s ea	**18837-0253-90**	273.07		
(Physician Partner)				
REPACK				
TAB, PO, 10 mg, 30s ea	**21695-0030-30**	147.37		
(FILM-COATED)				
10 mg, 30s ea	**21695-0655-30**	147.37		
60s ea	**21695-0030-60**	294.74		
100s ea	**21695-0030-00**	491.22		
20 mg, 30s ea	**21695-0031-30**	153.58		
60s ea	**21695-0031-60**	307.16		
100s ea	**21695-0031-00**	511.96		
40 mg, 30s ea	**21695-0032-30**	159.56		
60s ea	**21695-0032-60**	319.13		
100s ea	**21695-0032-00**	531.88		
(Quality Care Prod)				
REPACK				
TAB, PO, 10 mg, 30s ea	**35356-0028-30**	84.57		
20 mg, 30s ea	**49999-0789-30**	84.57		
60s ea	**49999-0789-60**	169.14		
90s ea	**49999-0789-90**	253.71		
40 mg, 100s ea	**49999-0654-00**	317.68		
(Southwood)				
REPACK				
TAB, PO, 10 mg, 30s ea	**58016-0030-30**	72.95		
60s ea	**58016-0030-60**	145.89		
90s ea	**58016-0030-90**	218.84		
100s ea	**58016-0030-00**	243.15		
(Stat Rx)				
REPACK				
TAB, PO, 10 mg, 30s ea	**16590-0055-30**	57.00		
60s ea	**16590-0055-60**	114.00		
90s ea	**16590-0055-90**	171.00		
20 mg, 30s ea	**16590-0056-30**	60.00		
60s ea	**16590-0056-60**	120.00		
90s ea	**16590-0056-90**	160.00		
40 mg, 30s ea	**16590-0480-30**	94.58		
45s ea	**16590-0480-45**	119.67		
60s ea	**16590-0480-60**	53.00		
90s ea	**16590-0480-90**	79.50		
120s ea	**16590-0480-72**	106.00		
CITALOPRAM HYDROBROMIDE				
FUL				
SOL, PO, 10 mg/5 ml, 240 ml		74.98		
TAB, PO, 10 mg, 100s ea		16.73		
20 mg, 100s ea		17.25		
40 mg, 100s ea		17.55		

PROD/MFR	NDC	AWP	DP	OBC
(Apotex Corp.)				
TAB, PO (FILM-COATED)				
10 mg, 30s ea	60505-2518-04	73.68		
(10X10,FILM-COATED)				
10 mg, 100s ea UD	60505-2518-03	231.50		AB
(FILM-COATED)				
10 mg, 100s ea	60505-2518-01	245.61		
1000s ea	60505-2518-08	2456.10		AB
20 mg, 30s ea	60505-2519-04	76.79		
(10X10,FILM-COATED)				
20 mg, 100s ea UD	60505-2519-03	243.08		AB
(FILM-COATED)				
20 mg, 100s ea	60505-2519-01	255.98		
1000s ea	60505-2519-08	2559.80		AB
40 mg, 30s ea	60505-2520-04	80.14		
(10X10,FILM-COATED)				
40 mg, 100s ea UD	60505-2520-03	251.00		AB
(FILM-COATED)				
40 mg, 100s ea	60505-2520-01	265.94		
1000s ea	60505-2520-08	2659.40		AB
(Aurobindo Pharma) *See CITALOPRAM*				
(Aurobindo Pharma)				
SOL, PO (PEPPERMINT)				
10 mg/5 ml, 240 ml	65862-0074-24	117.50		AA
TAB, PO (FILM-COATED)				
10 mg, 100s ea	65862-0005-01	243.15		AB
(USP,FILM-COATED)				
10 mg, 100s ea	13107-0005-01	243.15		AB
(FILM-COATED)				
10 mg, 500s ea	65862-0005-05	1191.44		AB
(USP,FILM-COATED)				
10 mg, 500s ea	13107-0005-05	1191.44		AB
(FILM-COATED)				
20 mg, 100s ea	65862-0006-01	253.41		AB
(USP,FILM-COATED)				
20 mg, 100s ea	13107-0006-01	253.41		AB
(FILM-COATED)				
20 mg, 500s ea	65862-0006-05	1241.71		AB
(USP,FILM-COATED)				
20 mg, 500s ea	13107-0006-05	1241.71		AB
(FILM-COATED)				
40 mg, 100s ea	65862-0007-01	264.45		AB
500s ea	65862-0007-05	1295.81		AB
(Blu)				
TAB, PO (USP,FILM-COATED)				
10 mg, 30s ea	24658-0140-30	3.64		AB
100s ea	24658-0140-01	7.14		AB
1000s ea	24658-0140-10	70.74		AB
20 mg, 30s ea	24658-0141-30	2.53		AB
100s ea	24658-0141-01	7.14		AB
1000s ea	24658-0141-10	70.78		AB
(USP)				
40 mg, 30s ea	24658-0142-30	4.33		AB
100s ea	24658-0142-01	9.11		AB
1000s ea	24658-0142-10	89.89		AB
(Camber)				
TAB, PO (USP,FILM-COATED)				
10 mg, 100s ea	31722-0206-01	243.15		AB
20 mg, 100s ea	31722-0207-01	253.41		AB
40 mg, 100s ea	31722-0208-01	264.45		AB
(Caraco)				
TAB, PO (FILM-COATED)				
10 mg, 30s ea	57664-0507-83	73.35		
100s ea	57664-0507-88	244.50		AB
500s ea	57664-0507-13	1161.38		AB
1000s ea	57664-0507-18	2322.75		AB
20 mg, 30s ea	57664-0508-83	76.65		AB
100s ea	57664-0508-88	255.50		AB
500s ea	57664-0508-13	1213.63		AB
1000s ea	57664-0508-18	2427.25		AB
40 mg, 30s ea	57664-0509-83	79.65		AB
100s ea	57664-0509-88	265.50		AB
500s ea	57664-0509-13	1261.13		AB
1000s ea	57664-0509-18	2522.25		AB
(CorePharma)				
TAB, PO (FILM-COATED)				
10 mg, 30s ea	64720-0170-03	75.55		AB
100s ea	64720-0170-10	245.88		AB
20 mg, 30s ea	64720-0171-03	77.54		AB
100s ea	64720-0171-10	256.27		AB
40 mg, 30s ea	64720-0172-03	82.17		AB
100s ea	64720-0172-10	267.43		AB
(Cypress Pharm)				
SOL, PO (PEPPERMINT)				
10 mg/5 ml, 240 ml	60258-0830-08	135.99		AA
(Dr Reddy's)				
TAB, PO (FILM-COATED)				
10 mg, 30s ea	55111-0342-30	75.55		AB
100s ea	55111-0342-01	244.51		AB
500s ea	55111-0342-05	1161.44		AB
20 mg, 30s ea	55111-0343-30	78.75		AB
100s ea	55111-0343-01	254.84		AB
500s ea	55111-0343-05	1210.50		AB
40 mg, 30s ea	55111-0344-30	82.18		AB
100s ea	55111-0344-01	265.94		AB
500s ea	55111-0344-05	1263.22		AB
(Forest Pharm) *See CELEXA*				
(Greenstone) *See CITALOPRAM*				
(Major) *See CITALOPRAM*				
(Mylan) *See CITALOPRAM*				
(Mylan)				
TAB, PO (FILM-COATED)				
10 mg, 100s ea	00378-1921-01	232.25		AB
20 mg, 100s ea	00378-1922-01	242.05		AB
500s ea	00378-1922-05	1210.15		AB
40 mg, 100s ea	00378-1924-01	252.60		AB
500s ea	00378-1924-05	1262.90		AB
(Roxane)				
SOL, PO (PEPPERMINT)				
10 mg/5 ml, 240 ml	00054-0062-58	117.58		AA
(Sandoz)				
TAB, PO (FILM-COATED)				
10 mg, 100s ea	00185-0371-01	245.88		AB
100s ea	00781-5157-01	245.88		AB
1000s ea	00185-0371-10	2458.80		AB
20 mg, 100s ea	00185-0372-01	256.27		AB
1000s ea	00185-0372-10	2562.70		AB
40 mg, 100s ea	00185-0373-01	264.73		AB
100s ea	00781-5159-01	267.43		AB
1000s ea	00185-0373-10	2647.30		AB
(Silarx)				
SOL, PO (PEPPERMINT)				
10 mg/5 ml, 240 ml	54838-0540-70	117.50		AA
(Teva)				
TAB, PO, 10 mg, 100s ea	00093-4740-01	232.87		AB
(USP)				
10 mg, 100s ea UD	00093-4740-93	234.87		AB
1000s ea	00093-4740-10	2168.02		AB
20 mg, 100s ea	00093-4741-01	242.71		AB
(USP)				
20 mg, 100s ea UD	00093-4741-93	244.71		AB
500s ea	00093-4741-05	1189.26		AB
5000s ea	00093-4741-50	11297.97		AB
40 mg, 100s ea	00093-4742-01	253.28		AB
(USP)				
40 mg, 100s ea UD	00093-4742-93	255.28		AB
500s ea	00093-4742-05	1241.07		AB
5000s ea	00093-4742-50	11790.18		AB
(Torrent)				
TAB, PO (FILM-COATED)				
10 mg, 30s ea	13668-0009-30	85.15		AB
(10X10,FILM-COATED)				
10 mg, 100s ea UD	13668-0009-74	258.04		AB
(FILM-COATED)				
10 mg, 100s ea	13668-0009-01	258.04		AB
500s ea	13668-0009-05	1228.75		AB
9990s ea	13668-0009-09	24550.43		AB
20 mg, 30s ea	13668-0010-30	84.76		AB
(10X10,FILM-COATED)				
20 mg, 100s ea UD	13668-0010-74	273.17		AB
(FILM-COATED)				
20 mg, 100s ea	13668-0010-01	269.08		AB
500s ea	13668-0010-05	1281.35		AB
5600s ea	13668-0010-06	14351.12		AB
40 mg, 30s ea	13668-0011-30	87.56		AB
(10X10,FILM-COATED)				
40 mg, 100s ea UD	13668-0011-74	285.00		AB
(FILM-COATED)				
40 mg, 100s ea	13668-0011-01	277.97		AB
500s ea	13668-0011-05	1323.65		AB
2800s ea	13668-0011-08	7412.44		AB
(Wockhardt USA)				
TAB, PO (U.S.P.,FILM-COATED)				
10 mg, 100s ea	64679-0969-14	243.15		AB
20 mg, 100s ea	64679-0970-14	253.41		AB
40 mg, 100s ea	64679-0971-14	264.45		AB
(A-S Medication) REPACK				
TAB, PO (FILM-COATED)				
20 mg, 30s ea	54569-5626-00	76.65		AB
40 mg, 30s ea	54569-5627-00	79.65		AB
(Aidarex) REPACK				
TAB, PO (FILM-COATED)				
10 mg, 7s ea	33261-0026-07	21.00		AB
14s ea	33261-0026-14	42.00		AB
20s ea	33261-0026-20	60.00		AB
21s ea	33261-0026-21	63.00		AB
28s ea	33261-0026-28	84.00		AB
30s ea	33261-0026-30	90.00		AB
60s ea	33261-0026-60	180.00		AB
90s ea	33261-0026-90	270.00		AB
40 mg, 14s ea	33261-0028-14	49.00		AB
30s ea	33261-0028-30	105.00		AB
60s ea	33261-0028-60	210.00		AB
90s ea	33261-0028-90	315.00		AB
(Altura) REPACK				
TAB, PO (FILM COATED)				
10 mg, 30s ea	63874-1146-03	176.04		
(FILM-COATED)				
10 mg, 60s ea	63874-1146-06	176.04		AB
20 mg, 30s ea	63874-1113-03	87.76		AB
60s ea	63874-1113-06	175.52		AB
100s ea	63874-1113-01	293.00		
40 mg, 30s ea	63874-1157-03	95.58		AB
100s ea	63874-1157-00	318.60		
(DHS, Inc.) REPACK				
TAB, PO (FILM-COATED)				
10 mg, 30s ea	55887-0260-30	34.00		
90s ea	55887-0260-90	68.00		
20 mg, 30s ea	55887-0261-30	62.78		
60s ea	55887-0261-60	125.56		
90s ea	55887-0261-90	188.33		
(Dispensing Solutions) REPACK				
TAB, PO, 10 mg, 60s ea	55045-3423-02	148.20		
100s ea	55045-3423-01	247.00		
(FILM-COATED)				
20 mg, 30s ea	55045-3341-08	76.80		
30s ea	66336-0993-30	76.88		AB
60s ea	55045-3341-06	153.60		
(FILM-COATED)				
20 mg, 90s ea	66336-0993-90	230.64		AB
40 mg, 30s ea	55045-3424-08	79.20		
(FILM-COATED)				
40 mg, 30s ea	66336-0271-30	80.50		AB
100s ea	55045-3424-00	264.00		
(IPI) REPACK				
TAB, PO, 10 mg, 30s ea	18837-0242-30	91.69		
(FILM-COATED)				
20 mg, 30s ea	18837-0253-30	73.12		AB
40 mg, 30s ea	18837-0252-30	74.40		AB
(Nucare Pharm) REPACK				
TAB, PO (FILM-COATED)				
20 mg, 30s ea	68071-0231-30	95.57		AB
52s ea	68071-0231-52	153.20		AB
60s ea	68071-0231-60	153.39		
90s ea	68071-0231-90	281.26		AB
40 mg, 30s ea	68071-0222-30	99.31		AB
(Palmetto) REPACK				
TAB, PO, 10 mg, 15s ea	23490-7558-01	42.99		
30s ea	23490-7558-02	85.99		
60s ea	23490-7558-03	171.98		
20 mg, 15s ea	23490-7225-01	42.99		
28s ea	23490-7225-02	80.26		
30s ea	23490-7225-03	85.99		
56s ea	23490-7225-05	160.51		
60s ea	23490-7225-04	171.98		
90s ea	23490-7225-09	257.97		
40 mg, 30s ea	23490-7226-03	85.99		
45s ea	23490-7226-05	128.98		
60s ea	23490-7226-06	171.98		
90s ea	23490-7226-09	257.97		
(PD-Rx Pharm) REPACK				
TAB, PO (FILM-COATED)				
20 mg, 14s ea	55289-0883-14	26.72		AB
(REDI-SCRIPT,FILM-COATED)				
20 mg, 14s ea	58864-0877-14	26.70		
30s ea	55289-0883-30	32.20		
30s ea	58864-0877-30	32.20		
(FILM-COATED)				
20 mg, 60s ea	55289-0883-60	43.60		AB
90s ea	55289-0883-90	47.45		AB
(REDI-SCRIPT)				
40 mg, 15s ea	58864-0812-15	36.67		
(FILM-COATED)				
40 mg, 30s ea	58864-0812-30	56.67		AB
(Pharma Pac) REPACK				
TAB, PO (FILM-COATED)				
10 mg, 30s ea	52959-0603-30	91.90		AB
20 mg, 30s ea	52959-0773-30	73.49		AB

PROD/MFR	NDC	AWP	DP	OBC
52s ea	52959-0773-52	127.39		AB
60s ea	52959-0773-60	146.95		AB
40 mg, 30s ea	52959-0986-30	78.36		AB
(Phys Total Care)				
REPACK				
TAB, PO (FILM-COATED)				
10 mg, 30s ea	54868-5275-00	11.19		AB
60s ea	54868-5275-02	17.74		AB
90s ea	54868-5275-01	27.55		
20 mg, 15s ea	54868-5178-01	8.10		
(FILM-COATED)				
20 mg, 30s ea	54868-5178-00	13.20		AB
60s ea	54868-5178-02	23.37		
90s ea	54868-5178-04	25.06		
100s ea	54868-5178-03	21.19		
(FILM-COATED)				
40 mg, 15s ea	54868-1239-01	7.86		AB
30s ea	54868-1239-00	12.75		AB
60s ea	54868-1239-04	19.86		
90s ea	54868-1239-03	26.04		
100s ea	54868-1239-02	33.99		
(Physician Partner)				
REPACK				
TAB, PO (FILM-COATED)				
20 mg, 90s ea	21695-0031-90	460.74		AB
40 mg, 90s ea	21695-0032-90	446.40		
(Quality Care Prod)				
REPACK				
TAB, PO (FILM-COATED)				
40 mg, 30s ea	49999-0654-30	97.96		AB
(Southwood)				
REPACK				
TAB, PO (FILM-COATED)				
20 mg, 5s ea	58016-0178-05	12.78		
10s ea	58016-0178-10	25.55		
12s ea	58016-0178-12	30.66		
14s ea	58016-0178-14	35.77		
15s ea	58016-0178-15	38.33		
20s ea	58016-0178-20	51.10		
30s ea	58016-0178-30	76.65		
40s ea	58016-0178-40	102.20		
50s ea	58016-0178-50	127.75		
60s ea	58016-0178-60	153.30		
90s ea	58016-0178-90	229.95		
100s ea	58016-0178-00	255.50		
120s ea	58016-0178-02	306.60		
180s ea	58016-0178-99	459.90		
200s ea	58016-0178-89	511.00		
240s ea	58016-0178-04	613.20		
40 mg, 5s ea	58016-0224-05	12.55		
10s ea	58016-0224-10	25.10		
12s ea	58016-0224-12	30.12		
14s ea	58016-0224-14	35.14		
15s ea	58016-0224-15	37.65		
20s ea	58016-0224-20	50.20		
30s ea	58016-0224-30	75.30		
40s ea	58016-0224-40	100.40		
50s ea	58016-0224-50	125.50		
60s ea	58016-0224-60	150.60		
90s ea	58016-0224-90	225.90		
100s ea	58016-0224-00	251.00		
120s ea	58016-0224-02	301.20		
180s ea	58016-0224-99	451.80		
200s ea	58016-0224-89	502.00		
240s ea	58016-0224-04	602.40		
(Stat Rx)				
REPACK				
TAB, PO (FILM-COATED)				
20 mg, 15s ea	16590-0056-15	45.59		AB
CITANEST FORTE DENTAL (Dentsply)				
epinephrine bitartrate/prilocaine hydrochloride				
SOL, IJ (1.8MLX100)				
1:200000-4%,				
1.8 ml 100s	66312-0540-14	44.86		
CITANEST PLAIN DENTAL (Dentsply)				
prilocaine hydrochloride				
SOL, IJ (1.8MLX100)				
4%, 1.8 ml 100s	66312-0520-14	44.86		
CITRACAL PRENATE 90+DHA (Phys Total Care)				
REPACK				
prenatal vitamins				
KIT, PO, 60s ea	54868-5822-00	55.62		
CITRANATAL 90 DHA (Mission)				
prenatal vitamins				
KIT, PO (GELATIN CAPSULE)				
60s ea	00178-0829-30	51.30	38.75	
CITRANATAL ASSURE (Mission)				
prenatal vitamins				
KIT, PO (6X10,COATED)				
60s ea	00178-0893-30	54.69	43.75	
CITRANATAL B-CALM (Mission)				
ca/cholecalciferol/fe/folic acid/vit b6/vit c				
TAB, PO (COATED,UNCOATED)				
ea	00178-0866-30	45.30	37.75	
CITRANATAL DHA (Mission)				
prenatal vitamins				
KIT, PO (SIX 5X5 BLISTER PACK)				
60s ea	00178-0898-30	52.19	41.75	
CITRANATAL RX (Mission)				
prenatal vitamins				
TAB, PO, 90s ea	00178-0859-90	113.44	90.75	
CITRIC ACID				
(Baker, J.T.) *See CITRIC ACID ANHYDROUS*				
(Baker, J.T.) *See CITRIC ACID MONOHYDRATE*				
(Gallipot) *See CITRIC ACID ANHYDROUS*				
(Letco) *See CITRIC ACID ANHYDROUS*				
(Mallinckrodt Lab) *See CITRIC ACID MONOHYDRATE*				
(Medisca) *See CITRIC ACID ANHYDROUS*				
(PCCA)				
GRA, NA (USP, ANHYDROUS,FINE)				
1 gm	51927-1165-00	0.18		
POW, NA (MONOHYDRATE)				
1 gm	51927-1199-00	0.30		
(Spectrum Pharmacy) *See CITRIC ACID ANHYDROUS*				
(Spectrum Pharmacy) *See CITRIC ACID MONOHYDRATE*				
CITRIC ACID ANHYDROUS (Baker, J.T.)				
citric acid				
POW, NA (A.C.S., U.S.P.)				
500 gm	10106-0122-01	47.07		
2000 gm	10106-0122-05	174.53		
12000 gm	10106-0122-07	477.87		
(Gallipot)				
GRA, NA (U.S.P.)				
113.4 gm	51552-0048-04	5.46		
454 gm	51552-0048-06	15.26		
1000 gm	51552-0048-07	16.80		
2270 gm	51552-0048-09	39.20		
(Letco)				
POW, NA (U.S.P.)				
2500 gm	62991-1335-03	75.00		
(Medisca)				
POW, NA (USP,1X1000GM)				
1000 gm	38779-0068-09	40.50		
(Spectrum Pharmacy)				
GRA, NA (U.S.P., N.F.)				
500 gm	49452-2090-01	59.15		
2500 gm	49452-2090-02	184.80		
12000 gm	49452-2090-03	780.50		
POW, NA (U.S.P.)				
500 gm	49452-2100-01	59.15		
2500 gm	49452-2100-02	184.80		
12000 gm	49452-2100-03	780.50		
CITRIC ACID MONOHYDRATE (Baker, J.T.)				
citric acid				
GRA, NA (U.S.P., F.C.C.)				
500 gm	10106-0119-01	20.49		
2500 gm	10106-0119-05	108.55		
POW, NA, 500 gm	10106-0120-01	30.02		
2500 gm	10106-0120-05	163.56		
(Mallinckrodt Lab)				
GRA, NA (U.S.P.)				
500 gm	00406-0616-12	22.66		
(Spectrum Pharmacy)				
GRA, NA (U.S.P./N.F.)				
500 gm	49452-2110-01	99.75		
2500 gm	49452-2110-02	343.70		
12000 gm	49452-2110-03	1092.00		
POW, NA (U.S.P.)				
500 gm	49452-2119-01	99.75		
2500 gm	49452-2119-02	343.70		
12000 gm	49452-2119-03	1092.00		
CITRIC ACID/DEXTROSE/NA CIT/NA PHOS				
(Hospira) *See ANTICOAGULANT CPD*				
CITRIC ACID/DEXTROSE/SODIUM CITRATE				
(Bracco Diag) *See A-C-D MODIFIED BRACCO*				
(Citra) *See NOCLOT-50*				
CITRIC ACID/GLUCONOLACTONE/ MAGNESIUM CARBONATE				
(Guardian) *See RENACIDIN*				
CITRIC ACID/POTASSIUM BICARBONATE				
(Nomax) *See EFFER-K*				
CITRIC ACID/POTASSIUM CITRATE				
(Cypress Pharm) *See CYTRA-K*				
(Cypress Pharm) *See CYTRA-K CRYSTALS*				
(Pharm Assoc Inc)				
SOL, PO (AF,SF,BERRY,CITRUS)				
334 mg/5 ml-1100 mg/5 ml,				
473 ml	00121-0676-16	19.65		
CITRIC ACID/POTASSIUM CITRATE/SODIUM CITRATE				
(Cypress Pharm) *See CYTRA-3*				
(Pharm Assoc Inc) *See TRICITRATES*				
CITRIC ACID/SODIUM CITRATE				
(ANI) *See LIQUI-DUALCITRA*				
(Carolina) *See ORACIT*				
(Cypress Pharm) *See CYTRA-2*				
(Humco) *See SHOHL'S SOLUTION*				
(Pharm Assoc Inc)				
SOL, PO, 334 mg/5 ml-500 mg/5 ml,				
15 ml 100s UD	00121-0595-15	50.97		
30 ml 100s UD	00121-0595-30	60.70		
473 ml	00121-0595-16	14.25		
CITRONELLA (PCCA)				
citronella oil				
OIL, NA (CEYLON)				
1 ml	51927-1373-00	0.18		
CITRONELLA OIL				
(Gallipot) *See CITRONELLA OIL CEYLON*				
(Humco)				
OIL, NA (TECHNICAL)				
30 ml	00395-1943-91	3.59		
480 ml	00395-1943-16	36.06		
(Medisca)				
OIL, NA (1X14ML,JAVA,NATURAL)				
14 ml	38779-1717-03	16.50		
(1X100ML,CEYLON,NATURAL)				
100 ml	38779-1185-05	28.50		
(1X100ML,JAVA,NATURAL)				
100 ml	38779-1717-05	28.50		
(1X500ML,JAVA,NATURAL)				
500 ml	38779-1717-08	49.50		
(CEYLON,NATURAL,1X500ML)				
500 ml	38779-1185-08	49.50		
(1X4000ML,JAVA,NATURAL)				
4000 ml	38779-1717-01	82.50		
(PCCA) *See CITRONELLA*				
CITRONELLA OIL CEYLON (Gallipot)				
citronella oil				
OIL, NA, 29.57 ml	51552-0192-02	5.95		
100 ml	51552-0192-05	13.79		
473 ml	51552-0192-06	26.32		
CITRULLINE (Gallipot)				
POW, NA, 1000 gm	51552-0665-07	350.00		
(Medisca)				
POW, NA (1X25GM)				
25 gm	38779-1186-04	47.85		
(1X100GM)				
100 gm	38779-1186-05	112.50		
(1X500GM)				
500 gm	38779-1186-08	495.00		
(1X1000GM)				
1000 gm	38779-1186-09	837.00		
(PCCA)				
POW, NA (L)				
1 gm	51927-2610-00	1.17		
(Spectrum Pharmacy) *See L-CITRULLINE*				
CLADRIBINE (APP)				
SOL, IV (S.D.V.,PF)				
1 mg/ml, 10 ml	63323-0140-10	650.00		AP
(Bedford) *See CLADRIBINE NOVAPLUS*				
(Bedford)				
SOL, IV (S.D.V.,PF)				
1 mg/ml, 10 ml	55390-0124-01	540.00		AP
(Centocor) *See LEUSTATIN*				
CLADRIBINE NOVAPLUS (Bedford)				
cladribine				
SOL, IV (S.D.V.,PF,PRIVATE LABEL)				
1 mg/ml, 10 ml	55390-0115-01	342.00		AP
CLAFORAN (Abbott Hosp)				
cefotaxime sodium				
PDS, IJ (P.B.)				
1 gm, 10s ea	00039-0018-11	60.84	53.20	AP

PROD/MFR	NDC	AWP	DP	OBC
(VIAL)				
1 gm, 25s ea	**00039-0018-25**	78.00	68.25	**AP**
(ADD-VANTAGE)				
1 gm, 50s ea	**00039-0023-50**	209.40	183.00	**AP**
(VIAL)				
1 gm, 50s ea	**00039-0018-50**	156.00	136.50	**AP**
(P.B.)				
2 gm, 10s ea	**00039-0019-11**	117.60	102.90	**AP**
(VIAL)				
2 gm, 10s ea	**00039-0019-10**	58.56	51.20	**AP**
25s ea	**00039-0019-25**	155.10	135.75	**AP**
50s ea	**00039-0019-50**	310.20	271.50	**AP**
(Hospira)				
PDS, IJ (VIAL)				
1 gm, 10s ea	**00039-0018-10**	29.52	25.80	**AP**
(ADD-VANTAGE)				
1 gm, 25s ea	**00039-0023-25**	96.30	84.25	**AP**
2 gm, 25s ea	**00039-0024-25**	173.70	152.00	**AP**
50s ea	**00039-0024-50**	355.20	311.00	**AP**
(BULK VIAL)				
10 gm, ea	**00039-0020-01**	29.18	25.54	**AP**
(VIAL)				
500 mg, 10s ea	**00039-0017-10**	25.68	22.50	**AP**
(Phys Total Care)				
REPACK				
PDS, IJ (VIAL)				
1 gm, 10s ea	**54868-3429-00**	114.07		**AP**
25s ea	**54868-3429-01**	278.82		**AP**
CLARAVIS (Teva)				
isotretinoin				
SGL, PO (3X10)				
10 mg, 30s ea	**00555-1054-86**	492.06		**AB**
(10X10)				
10 mg, 100s ea	**00555-1054-56**	1577.18		**AB**
(3X10)				
20 mg, 30s ea	**00555-1055-86**	583.52		**AB**
(10X10)				
20 mg, 100s ea	**00555-1055-56**	1870.26		**AB**
(3X10)				
30 mg, 30s ea UD	**00555-1056-86**	493.55		
40 mg, 30s ea	**00555-1057-86**	677.94		**AB**
(10X10)				
40 mg, 100s ea	**00555-1057-56**	2172.87		**AB**
CLARIFOAM EF (Onset)				
sulfacetamide sodium/sulfur				
FOA, TP, 10%-5%, 60 gm	**16781-0154-60**	150.00		
CLARINEX (Schering)				
desloratadine				
SYR, PO (BUBBLE-GUM)				
0.5 mg/ml, 473 ml	**00085-1334-01**	219.08		
TAB, PO (UNIT OF USE,3X10)				
5 mg, 30s ea	**00085-1264-04**	134.41		
(10X10,HOSPITAL USE)				
5 mg, 100s ea UD	**00085-1264-03**	448.15		
(FILM-COATED)				
5 mg, 100s ea	**00085-1264-01**	448.15		
500s ea	**00085-1264-02**	2240.93		
(A-S Medication)				
REPACK				
TAB, PO (FILM-COATED)				
5 mg, 10s ea	**54569-5352-02**	44.08		
(UNIT OF USE,3X10)				
5 mg, 30s ea	**54569-5352-00**	132.24		
(AQ)				
REPACK				
TAB, PO, 5 mg, 10s ea	**66105-0807-01**	68.11		
15s ea	**66105-0807-15**	102.17		
30s ea	**66105-0807-03**	204.35		
60s ea	**66105-0807-06**	408.71		
90s ea	**66105-0807-09**	613.06		
(Core)				
REPACK				
TAB, PO, 5 mg, 30s ea	**33358-0085-30**	98.26		
(PD-Rx Pharm)				
REPACK				
TAB, PO (FILM-COATED)				
5 mg, 10s ea	**55289-0925-10**	60.04		
(REDI-SCRIPT,FILM-COATED)				
5 mg, 30s ea	**58864-0703-30**	114.25		
(Pharma Pac)				
REPACK				
TAB, PO (FILM-COATED)				
5 mg, 10s ea	**52959-0685-10**	69.90		
30s ea	**52959-0685-30**	208.57		
90s ea	**52959-0685-90**	620.95		
(Phys Total Care)				
REPACK				
TAB, PO (FILM-COATED)				
5 mg, 10s ea	**54868-4624-01**	55.64		
(UNIT OF USE,3X10)				
5 mg, 30s ea	**54868-4624-00**	152.21		
(Quality Care Prod)				
REPACK				
TAB, PO (FILM-COATED)				
5 mg, 10s ea	**49999-0410-10**	43.69		
14s ea	**49999-0410-14**	61.17		
30s ea	**49999-0410-30**	215.11		
90s ea	**49999-0410-90**	637.31		
100s ea	**49999-0410-00**	755.63		
CLARINEX REDITABS (Schering)				
desloratadine				
ODT, PO (TUTTI FRUTTI)				
2.5 mg, 30s ea	**00085-1408-01**	144.23		
5 mg, 30s ea	**00085-1384-01**	144.23		
(UNIT OF USE)				
5 mg, 30s ea	**00085-1280-01**	82.50		
CLARINEX-D (Phys Total Care)				
REPACK				
desloratadine/pseudoephedrine sulfate				
T12, PO, 2.5 mg-120 mg,				
10s ea	**54868-5708-00**	34.33		
30s ea	**54868-5708-01**	99.24		
CLARINEX-D 24 HOUR (Schering)				
desloratadine/pseudoephedrine sulfate				
T24, PO (FILM-COATED)				
5 mg-240 mg,				
100s ea	**00085-1317-01**	480.49		
CLARINEX-D 24HR (Phys Total Care)				
REPACK				
desloratadine/pseudoephedrine sulfate				
T24, PO, 5 mg-240 mg,				
10s ea	**54868-5640-00**	41.90		
30s ea	**54868-5640-01**	130.39		
CLARINEX-D12 HOUR (Schering)				
desloratadine/pseudoephedrine sulfate				
T12, PO, 2.5 mg-120 mg,				
100s ea	**00085-1322-01**	308.00		
CLARITHROMYCIN				
FUL				
TAB, PO, 250 mg, 60s ea		142.35		
500 mg, 60s ea		51.75		
(Abbott Pharm) *See BIAXIN*				
(Abbott Pharm) *See BIAXIN FILMTAB*				
(Abbott Pharm) *See BIAXIN XL*				
(Apotex Corp.)				
TAB, PO (FILM-COATED)				
250 mg, 60s ea	**60505-2616-06**	271.27		**AB**
500 mg, 60s ea	**60505-2615-06**	271.27		**AB**
(Dava Pharma)				
PDR, PO (FRUIT PUNCH)				
125 mg/5 ml, 50 ml	**68774-0302-29**	23.52		
100 ml	**68774-0302-35**	43.50		
250 mg/5 ml, 50 ml	**68774-0303-29**	44.77		
100 ml	**68774-0303-35**	82.91		
TAB, PO (FILM-COATED)				
250 mg, 60s ea	**68774-0120-60**	254.31		
500 mg, 60s ea	**68774-0122-60**	254.31		
(Letco)				
POW, NA (USP, 1X1000GM)				
1000 gm	**62991-2687-01**	2400.00		
(Mylan)				
TAB, PO (USP,FILM-COATED)				
250 mg, 60s ea	**00378-8250-91**	271.27		**AB**
500 mg, 60s ea	**00378-8500-91**	271.27		**AB**
(Ranbaxy Pharm)				
PDR, PO (1X50ML,USP)				
125 mg/5 ml, 50 ml	**63304-0821-03**	23.26		**AB**
(1X100ML,USP)				
125 mg/5 ml,				
100 ml	**63304-0821-04**	43.02		**AB**
(1X50ML,USP)				
250 mg/5 ml, 50 ml	**63304-0822-03**	44.28		**AB**
(1X100ML,USP)				
250 mg/5 ml,				
100 ml	**63304-0822-04**	81.99		**AB**
TAB, PO (FILM-COATED)				
250 mg, 60s ea	**63304-0725-60**	271.27		**AB**
100s ea	**63304-0725-01**	452.12		**AB**
500 mg, 60s ea	**63304-0726-60**	271.27		**AB**
100s ea	**63304-0726-01**	452.12		**AB**
(Roxane)				
TAB, PO (U.S.P.)				
250 mg, 60s ea	**00054-0036-21**	271.27		**AB**
(U.S.P.,FILM-COATED)				
500 mg, 60s ea	**00054-0037-21**	271.27		**AB**
(Sandoz)				
PDR, PO (USP,FRUIT PUNCH)				
125 mg/5 ml, 50 ml	**00781-6022-52**	23.53		**AB**
100 ml	**00781-6022-46**	43.51		**AB**
250 mg/5 ml, 50 ml	**00781-6023-52**	44.78		**AB**
100 ml	**00781-6023-46**	82.92		**AB**
TAB, PO (FILM-COATED)				
250 mg, 60s ea	**00781-1961-60**	271.27		**AB**
500 mg, 60s ea	**00781-1962-60**	271.27		**AB**
TER, PO, 500 mg, 60s ea	**00185-0275-60**	300.38		**AB**
(Teva)				
TAB, PO (FILM-COATED)				
250 mg, 60s ea	**00093-7157-06**	271.27		**AB**
500 mg, 60s ea	**00093-7158-06**	271.27		**AB**
TER, PO (FILM COATED)				
500 mg, 60s ea	**00093-7244-06**	300.38		**AB**
(UDL)				
TAB, PO (USP,10X10,FILM-COATED)				
250 mg, 100s ea UD	**51079-0361-20**	494.32		**AB**
(USP,5X10,FILM-COATED)				
500 mg, 50s ea UD	**51079-0673-06**	247.16		**AB**
(USP,10X10,FILM COATED)				
500 mg, 100s ea UD	**51079-0362-20**	494.32		**AB**
(Watson Labs)				
TER, PO (USP,FILM-COATED)				
500 mg, 60s ea	**62037-0777-60**	270.35		
(Wockhardt USA)				
TAB, PO (USP,FILM-COATED)				
250 mg, 60s ea	**64679-0954-01**	271.27		**AB**
500 mg, 60s ea	**64679-0949-01**	271.27		**AB**
(A-S Medication)				
REPACK				
PDR, PO, 250 mg/5 ml,				
50 ml	**54569-5829-00**	43.57		
TAB, PO (FILM-COATED)				
250 mg, 20s ea	**54569-5688-00**	90.42		**AB**
500 mg, 14s ea	**54569-5698-02**	63.30		
(FILM-COATED)				
500 mg, 20s ea	**54569-5698-00**	90.42		**AB**
30s ea	**54569-5698-01**	135.64		
(Advanced Pharm Serv, Inc.)				
REPACK				
TAB, PO, 500 mg, 10s ea	**13411-0185-01**	91.80		
15s ea	**13411-0185-15**	137.70		
30s ea	**13411-0185-03**	275.40		
40s ea	**13411-0185-04**	367.20		
60s ea	**13411-0185-06**	311.96		
(Bryant Ranch)				
REPACK				
TAB, PO, 500 mg, 14s ea	**63629-2887-02**	72.80		
20s ea	**63629-2887-01**	104.00		
(Core)				
REPACK				
TAB, PO, 500 mg, 20s ea	**33358-0086-20**	106.60		
(DHS, Inc.)				
REPACK				
TAB, PO, 500 mg, 14s ea	**55887-0147-14**	59.33		
20s ea	**55887-0147-20**	84.77		
30s ea	**55887-0147-30**	127.15		
45s ea	**55887-0147-45**	190.73		
60s ea	**55887-0147-60**	254.31		
(Dispensing Solutions)				
REPACK				
TAB, PO, 250 mg, 20s ea	**55045-3479-06**	90.40		
500 mg, 14s ea	**55045-3490-01**	63.28		
(FILM-COATED)				
500 mg, 14s ea	**66336-0347-14**	69.15		**AB**
20s ea	**66336-0347-20**	98.79		
(IPI)				
REPACK				
TAB, PO (FILM-COATED)				
500 mg, 20s ea	**18837-0340-20**	184.24		
(Nucare Pharm)				
REPACK				
TAB, PO (FILM-COATED)				
500 mg, 14s ea	**68071-0337-14**	135.42		**AB**
20s ea	**68071-0337-20**	193.45		**AB**
30s ea	**68071-0337-30**	290.18		**AB**
(Palmetto)				
REPACK				
PDR, PO, 250 mg/5 ml,				
50 ml	**23490-5330-05**	41.50		

PROD/MFR	NDC	AWP	DP	OBC
TAB, PO, 250 mg, 14s ea	23490-5329-01	64.96		
500 mg, 14s ea	23490-5331-01	62.73		
20s ea	23490-5331-04	89.61		
28s ea	23490-5331-02	125.46		
(PD-Rx Pharm) REPACK				
TAB, PO (FILM-COATED)				
500 mg, 10s ea	55289-0909-10	67.84		AB
14s ea	55289-0909-14	95.04		
(REDI-SCRIPT, U.S.P.)				
500 mg, 20s ea	58864-0837-20	185.67		
(USP)				
500 mg, 20s ea	55289-0909-20	135.68		
(USP,FILM-COATED)				
500 mg, 28s ea	55289-0909-28	190.08		
(Pharma Pac) REPACK				
TAB, PO, 500 mg, 10s ea	52959-0836-10	48.08		
14s ea	52959-0836-14	67.30		
20s ea	52959-0836-20	96.14		
(FILM-COATED)				
500 mg, 60s ea	52959-0836-60	277.05		
(Phys Total Care) REPACK				
PDR, PO (1X100ML,FRUIT PUNCH)				
250 mg/5 ml,				
100 ml	54868-0654-00	183.88		
TAB, PO (FILM-COATED)				
500 mg, 15s ea	54868-5430-00	45.69		
20s ea	54868-5430-01	59.94		
30s ea	54868-5430-02	88.38		AB
(Physician Partner) REPACK				
TAB, PO (FILM-COATED)				
250 mg, 10s ea	21695-0557-10	106.38		AB
500 mg, 10s ea	21695-0558-10	106.38		AB
14s ea	21695-0558-14	148.93		AB
20s ea	21695-0558-20	212.76		AB
28s ea	21695-0558-28	297.86		AB
(Quality Care Prod) REPACK				
TAB, PO, 250 mg, 14s ea	35356-0025-14	75.97		
500 mg, 14s ea	49999-0904-14	66.47		
20s ea	49999-0904-20	94.95		
(Southwood) REPACK				
TAB, PO (FILM-COATED)				
500 mg, 16s ea	58016-0299-16	72.34		AB
24s ea	58016-0299-24	108.51		AB
30s ea	58016-0299-30	135.64		
60s ea	58016-0299-60	271.27		
90s ea	58016-0299-90	406.91		
100s ea	58016-0299-00	452.12		
(St. Mary's MPP) REPACK				
TAB, PO (USP,FILM-COATED)				
500 mg, 20s ea	60760-0261-20	105.47		AB
(Vibranta) REPACK				
TAB, PO, 500 mg, 20s ea	57866-7071-01	91.50		
CLARITIN (Pharma Pac) REPACK				
loratadine				
TAB, PO, 10 mg, 10s ea	52959-0452-10	54.50		AB
14s ea	52959-0452-14	74.72		AB
15s ea	52959-0452-15	77.71		AB
16s ea	52959-0452-16	82.50		AB
20s ea	52959-0452-20	92.65		AB
21s ea	52959-0452-21	97.19		AB
28s ea	52959-0452-28	113.91		AB
30s ea	52959-0452-30	120.24		AB
40s ea	52959-0452-40	150.45		AB
100s ea	52959-0452-00	340.12		AB
(Phys Total Care) REPACK				
TAB, PO, 10 mg, 10s ea	54868-2646-04	38.56		AB
30s ea	54868-5247-00	27.34		AB
(Quality Care Prod) REPACK				
SYR, PO (NON-DROWSY)				
5 mg/5 ml, 120 ml	49999-0250-04	33.78		
CLARITIN REDITABS (Phys Total Care) REPACK				
loratadine				
ODT, PO (UNIT OF USE,3X10)				
10 mg, 30s ea	54868-4260-00	125.38		
CLARITIN-D (Pharma Pac) REPACK				
loratadine/pseudoephedrine sulfate				
T12, PO, 5 mg-120 mg,				
15s ea	52959-0443-15	26.58		
20s ea	52959-0443-20	36.13		
30s ea	52959-0443-30	45.60		
CLAVULANATE POTASSIUM/TICARCILLIN DISODIUM (Glaxo) *See TIMENTIN*				
CLEANSE & TREAT (Quinnova)				
benzoyl peroxide/salicylic acid				
PAD, MR, 5%-2%, 2s ea	23710-0052-02	189.00		
CLEAR ADVANTAGE SELF-ADHERING (Mentor)				
catheter				
DEV, NA (SILICONE, MALE, 23 MM)				
30s ea	81317-0061-30	63.60		
(SILICONE, MALE, 28 MM)				
30s ea	81317-0062-30	63.60		
(SILICONE, MALE, 31 MM)				
30s ea	81317-0063-30	63.60		
(SILICONE, MALE, 35 MM)				
30s ea	81317-0064-30	63.60		
(SILICONE, MALE, 40 MM)				
30s ea	81317-0065-30	63.60		
(SILICONE, MALE, 23 MM)				
100s ea	81317-0061-00	201.00		
(SILICONE, MALE, 28 MM)				
100s ea	81317-0062-00	201.00		
(SILICONE, MALE, 31 MM)				
100s ea	81317-0063-00	201.00		
(SILICONE, MALE, 35 MM)				
100s ea	81317-0064-00	201.00		
(SILICONE, MALE, 40 MM)				
100s ea	81317-0065-00	201.00		
CLEAR-CATH (Abbott Hosp)				
catheter				
DEV, NA (14G, 5-1/2" SUBCLAVIAN)				
60s ea	00074-4532-74	134.64	134.40	
(14G, 2")				
120s ea	00074-4532-14	195.84	195.60	
(16GX1-1/4")				
120s ea	00074-4532-06	195.84	195.60	
(16GX2")				
120s ea	00074-4532-16	195.84	195.60	
(18GX1-1/4")				
120s ea	00074-4532-08	195.84	195.60	
(18GX2")				
120s ea	00074-4532-18	195.84	195.60	
(20G, 1-1/4")				
120s ea	00074-4532-20	195.84	195.60	
(20G, 2")				
120s ea	00074-4532-02	195.84	195.60	
(22G, 1-1/4")				
120s ea	00074-4532-22	204.48	204.00	
(22G, 1")				
120s ea	00074-4532-32	204.48	204.00	
(24G, 3/4")				
120s ea	00074-4532-24	213.12	213.60	
CLEMASTINE FUMARATE (Major)				
SYR, PO (FRUITY)				
0.5 mg/5 ml,				
120 ml	00904-1524-00	16.75		AA
(PCCA)				
POW, NA (U.S.P.)				
1 gm	51927-2253-00	225.00		
(Qualitest)				
SYR, PO (FRUIT)				
0.5 mg/5 ml,				
120 ml	00603-1096-54	16.50		AA
(Sandoz)				
TAB, PO, 1.34 mg, 100s ea	00781-1358-01	33.00		
2.68 mg, 100s ea	00781-1359-01	86.05		AB
(Silarx)				
SYR, PO, 0.5 mg/5 ml,				
120 ml	54838-0514-40	19.50		AA
(Teva)				
SYR, PO, 0.5 mg/5 ml,				
120 ml	00093-0309-12	21.35		AA
TAB, PO, 2.68 mg, 100s ea	00093-0308-01	86.08		AB
(PD-Rx Pharm) REPACK				
TAB, PO, 1.34 mg, 30s ea	55289-0762-30	10.60		
(Pharma Pac) REPACK				
TAB, PO, 2.68 mg, 20s ea	52959-0501-20	21.57		EE
(Phys Total Care) REPACK				
TAB, PO, 1.34 mg, 100s ea	54868-5913-00	76.73		
2.68 mg, 20s ea	54868-3007-01	18.36		EE
30s ea	54868-3007-00	25.26		EE
CLENBUTEROL HYDROCHLORIDE (Medisca)				
POW, NA (1X1000GM)				
1000 gm	38779-0209-09	29850.00		
CLENIA (Upsher-Smith)				
sulfacetamide sodium/sulfur				
CRE, TP, 10%-5%, 28 gm	00245-0169-01	57.88		
SOA, TP, 10%-5%, 180 ml	00245-0168-06	67.12		
360 ml	00245-0168-12	106.59		
CLEOCIN (Phys Total Care) REPACK				
clindamycin palmitate hydrochloride				
PDS, PO (1X100ML)				
75 mg/5 ml, 100 ml	54868-5833-00	82.10		
CLEOCIN HCL (Pfizer)				
clindamycin hydrochloride				
CAP, PO, 75 mg, 100s ea	00009-0331-02	228.32	190.27	AB
150 mg, 100s ea	00009-0225-02	448.26	373.55	AB
100s ea UD	00009-0225-03	448.26	373.55	AB
300 mg, 100s ea UD	00009-0395-02	910.50	758.75	AB
100s ea	00009-0395-14	910.50	758.75	AB
CLEOCIN PEDIATRIC (Pfizer)				
clindamycin palmitate hydrochloride				
PDS, PO, 75 mg/5 ml,				
100 ml	00009-0760-04	69.70	58.08	
CLEOCIN PHOSPHATE (Pfizer)				
clindamycin phosphate				
SOL, IJ (25X2ML)				
150 mg/ml,				
2 ml 25s	00009-0870-26	122.60	102.17	AP
(25X4ML)				
150 mg/ml,				
4 ml 25s	00009-0775-26	255.24	212.70	AP
(ADD-VANTAGE,25X4ML)				
150 mg/ml,				
4 ml 25s	00009-3124-03	272.00	226.67	AP
6 ml 25s	00009-0902-18	334.50	278.75	AP
(ADD-VANTAGE,25X6ML)				
150 mg/ml,				
6 ml 25s	00009-3447-03	325.08	270.90	AP
(5X60ML)				
150 mg/ml,				
60 ml 5s	00009-0728-09	574.03	478.36	AP
IV (PREMIX)				
300 mg/50 ml,				
50 ml 24s	00009-3381-02	236.30	196.92	AP
600 mg/50 ml,				
50 ml 24s	00009-3375-02	361.76	301.47	AP
900 mg/50 ml,				
50 ml 24s	00009-3382-02	441.98	368.32	AP
(Phys Total Care) REPACK				
SOL, IJ (S.D.V.)				
150 mg/ml,				
2 ml 50s	54868-4169-00	117.39		AP
4 ml 25s	54868-4154-00	253.13		AP
CLEOCIN T (Pfizer)				
clindamycin phosphate				
GEL, TP, 1%, 30 gm	00009-3331-02	60.25	50.21	AB
60 gm	00009-3331-01	108.50	90.42	AB
LOT, TP, 1%, 60 ml	00009-3329-01	83.83	69.86	AB
PAD, TP (PLEDGET)				
1%, 60s ea	00009-3116-14	79.42	66.18	AT
SOL, TP, 1%, 30 ml	00009-3116-01	35.02	29.18	AT
60 ml	00009-3116-02	68.44	57.03	AT
(A-S Medication) REPACK				
SOL, TP, 1%, 30 ml	54569-0750-00	34.74		AT
(Pharma Pac) REPACK				
LOT, TP, 1%, 60 ml	52959-0278-01	50.25		AB
(Phys Total Care) REPACK				
GEL, TP, 1%, 30 gm	54868-0208-00	55.60		AB
LOT, TP, 1%, 60 ml	54868-0944-01	84.66		AB
PAD, TP, 1%, 60s ea	54868-5349-00	76.49		AT
SOL, TP, 1%, 60 ml	54868-0209-01	45.34		AT
(Southwood) REPACK				
SOL, TP, 1%, 30 ml	58016-3014-01	33.35		AT

PROD/MFR	NDC	AWP	DP	OBC
CLEOCIN VAGINAL (Pfizer)				
clindamycin phosphate				
CRE, VG (7 DISP APPL)				
2%, 40 gm	00009-3448-01	78.91	65.76	
(A-S Medication)				
REPACK				
CRE, VG (APPLICATORS)				
2%, 40 gm	54569-3723-00	69.83		
(Phys Total Care)				
REPACK				
CRE, VG (APPLICATORS)				
2%, 40 gm	54868-2988-00	64.75		
CLEOCIN VAGINAL OVULES (Pfizer)				
clindamycin phosphate				
SUP, VG (W/APPLICATOR)				
100 mg, 3s ea	00009-7667-01	73.80	61.50	
(Phys Total Care)				
REPACK				
SUP, VG, 100 mg, 3s ea	54868-3427-00	63.60		
CLEVIDIPINE BUTYRATE				
(Medicines Company) *See CLEVIPREX*				
CLEVIPREX (Medicines Company)				
clevidipine butyrate				
EMU, IV, 0.5 mg/ml,				
50 ml	65293-0002-50	181.25		
50 ml 10s	65293-0002-55	1812.50		
100 ml	65293-0002-00	362.50		
100 ml 10s	65293-0002-11	2900.00		
CLIDINIUM BROMIDE (PCCA)				
POW, NA (U.S.P. XXII)				
1 gm	51927-2486-00	36.00		
CLIMARA (Bayer)				
estradiol				
TDM, TD, 0.025 mg/24 hr,				
4s ea	50419-0454-04	63.06		BX
0.0375 mg/24 hr,				
4s ea	50419-0456-04	63.06		
0.05 mg/24 hr,				
4s ea	50419-0451-04	63.06		AB2
0.06 mg/24 hr,				
4s ea	50419-0459-04	63.06		
0.075 mg/24 hr,				
4s ea	50419-0453-04	63.06		BX
0.1 mg/24 hr,				
4s ea	50419-0452-04	63.06		AB2
(Dispensing Solutions)				
REPACK				
TDM, TD, 0.025 mg/24 hr,				
4s ea	55045-3134-04	46.00		
(Phys Total Care)				
REPACK				
TDM, TD, 0.025 mg/24 hr,				
4s ea	54868-5008-00	42.30		BX
0.0375 mg/24 hr,				
4s ea	54868-4900-00	42.30		
0.05 mg/24 hr,				
4s ea	54868-4089-00	52.14		AB2
0.06 mg/24 hr,				
4s ea	54868-4901-00	42.30		
0.1 mg/24 hr,				
4s ea	54868-4241-00	42.30		AB2
CLIMARA PRO (Bayer)				
estradiol/levonorgestrel				
TDM, TD, 4s ea	50419-0491-04	63.06		
(Phys Total Care)				
REPACK				
TDM, TD, 4s ea	54868-5570-00	67.84		
CLINAC BPO (Ferndale)				
benzoyl peroxide				
GEL, TP, 7%, 45 gm	00496-0857-45	78.00		
CLINACORT (Clint)				
triamcinolone diacetate				
SUS, IJ (VIAL)				
40 mg/ml, 5 ml	55553-0042-05	14.00		EE
CLINDA-DERM (Paddock)				
clindamycin phosphate				
SOL, TP, 1%, 60 ml	00574-0016-02	20.26		AT
CLINDAGEL (Galderma)				
clindamycin phosphate				
GEL, TP, 1%, 40 ml	00299-4500-40	203.75		BT
75 ml	00299-4500-75	325.00		BT
CLINDAMAX (PharmaDerm)				
clindamycin phosphate				
GEL, TP, 1%, 30 gm	00462-0390-30	56.21		AB
60 gm	00462-0390-60	101.23		AB
LOT, TP, 1%, 60 ml	00462-0391-60	78.22		AB
CLINDAMYCIN (APP)				
clindamycin phosphate				
SOL, IJ (SDV,USP,2MLX25)				
150 mg/ml,				
2 ml 25s	63323-0282-02	96.50		AP
(SDV,USP,4MLX25)				
150 mg/ml,				
4 ml 25s	63323-0282-04	115.25		AP
(SDV,USP,6MLX25)				
150 mg/ml,				
6 ml 25s	63323-0282-06	153.25		AP
IV (USP)				
150 mg/ml, 60 ml	63323-0282-60	29.33		AP
(Bedford)				
SOL, IJ (USP,PHARMACY BULK VIAL)				
150 mg/ml, 60 ml	55390-0109-01	55.58		AP
(Lannett)				
clindamycin hydrochloride				
CAP, PO, 150 mg, 100s ea	00527-1382-01	119.20		AB
(Bryant Ranch)				
REPACK				
CAP, PO, 150 mg, 12s ea	63629-2817-01	20.02		
28s ea	63629-2817-02	46.71		
42s ea	63629-2817-03	70.06		
100s ea	63629-2817-04	119.25		
300 mg, 20s ea	63629-2924-02	71.19		
30s ea	63629-2924-01	156.12		
(Core)				
REPACK				
CAP, PO, 150 mg, 12s ea	33358-0088-12	20.52		
28s ea	33358-0088-28	47.88		
30s ea	33358-0088-30	126.27		
300 mg, 20s ea	33358-0089-20	72.97		
30s ea	33358-0089-30	160.02		
(DHS, Inc.)				
REPACK				
CAP, PO, 150 mg, 8s ea	55887-0611-08	8.40		
14s ea	55887-0611-14	14.70		
30s ea	55887-0611-30	34.89		
300 mg, 28s ea	55887-0378-28	182.93		
(DHS, Inc.)				
clindamycin phosphate				
SOL, TP, 1%, 60 ml	55887-0888-60	24.25		
(Dispensing Solutions)				
REPACK				
clindamycin hydrochloride				
CAP, PO, 150 mg, 8s ea	66336-0018-08	9.53		
42s ea	66336-0018-42	50.02		
300 mg, 28s ea	66336-0906-28	104.08		
(HomeMed)				
REPACK				
CAP, PO, 150 mg, 4s ea	51655-0964-89	4.69		
20s ea	51655-0964-52	23.49		
28s ea	51655-0964-29	33.69		
30s ea	51655-0964-24	36.09		
(Keltman Pharma., Inc.)				
REPACK				
CAP, PO, 300 mg, 30s ea	68387-0117-30	127.75		
(PD-Rx Pharm)				
REPACK				
CAP, PO (USP)				
300 mg, 20s ea	55289-0890-20	53.25		
56s ea	55289-0890-56	133.20		
(Pharma Pac)				
REPACK				
CAP, PO, 150 mg, 20s ea	52959-0744-20	27.68		
30s ea	52959-0744-30	41.51		
40s ea	52959-0744-40	55.32		
42s ea	52959-0744-42	58.08		
300 mg, 4s ea	52959-0784-04	17.30		
16s ea	52959-0784-16	68.95		
21s ea	52959-0784-21	90.39		
28s ea	52959-0784-28	118.72		
30s ea	52959-0784-30	129.09		
40s ea	52959-0784-40	172.11		
(Physician Partner)				
REPACK				
CAP, PO, 150 mg, 8s ea	21695-0033-08	22.44		
12s ea	21695-0033-12	28.58		
14s ea	21695-0033-14	39.27		
21s ea	21695-0033-21	50.04		
28s ea	21695-0033-28	66.72		
(Stat Rx)				
REPACK				
CAP, PO, 150 mg, 28s ea	16590-0057-28	30.50		
30s ea	16590-0057-30	32.68		
(Vibranta)				
REPACK				
CAP, PO, 300 mg, 21s ea	57866-3148-02	97.44		
CLINDAMYCIN HCL (Gallipot)				
clindamycin hydrochloride				
POW, NA (U.S.P.)				
1 gm	51552-0394-01	6.93		
5 gm	51552-0394-02	16.80		
(Greenstone)				
CAP, PO (UNIT OF USE)				
150 mg, 100s ea	59762-3328-01	119.11		AB
300 mg, 16s ea	59762-5010-01	65.17		AB
100s ea	59762-5010-02	375.94		AB
(Hawkins)				
POW, NA, 5 gm	63370-0042-15	57.60		
25 gm	63370-0042-25	240.00		
100 gm	63370-0042-35	840.00		
(Lannett)				
CAP, PO, 300 mg, 16s ea	00527-1383-02	64.55		AB
100s ea	00527-1383-01	372.00		AB
(Letco)				
POW, NA (U.S.P.)				
25 gm	62991-1034-02	160.00		
100 gm	62991-1034-03	480.00		
(Medisca)				
POW, NA (U.S.P.)				
5 gm	38779-0005-03	37.50		
25 gm	38779-0005-04	157.50		
100 gm	38779-0005-05	531.00		
(USP,1X500GM)				
500 gm	38779-0005-08	1650.00		
(PCCA)				
POW, NA (U.S.P.: MONOHYDRATE)				
1 gm	51927-2222-00	9.60		
(Ranbaxy Pharm)				
CAP, PO, 150 mg, 100s ea	63304-0692-01	119.15		AB
300 mg, 16s ea	63304-0693-16	64.45		AB
100s ea	63304-0693-01	371.71		AB
(Sandoz)				
CAP, PO, 150 mg, 100s ea	00781-2112-01	119.22		AB
300 mg, 16s ea	00781-2113-17	64.51		AB
100s ea	00781-2113-01	372.10		AB
(Teva)				
CAP, PO, 150 mg, 100s ea	00093-3171-01	119.08		AB
300 mg, 16s ea	00093-5256-68	64.45		AB
100s ea	00093-5256-01	371.71		AB
(UDL)				
CAP, PO (ROBOT READY 25X1)				
150 mg, 25s ea UD	51079-0598-19	28.75		AB
(10X10)				
150 mg, 100s ea UD	51079-0598-20	115.00		AB
(Watson Labs)				
CAP, PO, 150 mg, 100s ea	00591-5708-01	24.37		AB
300 mg, 100s ea	00591-3120-01	162.11		AB
(A-S Medication)				
REPACK				
CAP, PO, 150 mg, 4s ea	54569-3456-03	4.77		AB
15s ea	54569-3456-01	17.88		AB
21s ea	54569-3456-06	25.04		AB
30s ea	54569-3456-00	35.77		AB
100s ea	54569-3456-04	119.22		AB
300 mg, 30s ea	54569-5774-00	111.72		AB
45s ea	54569-5774-01	167.58		AB
(Aidarex)				
REPACK				
CAP, PO, 150 mg, 28s ea	33261-0159-28	14.58		AB
30s ea	33261-0159-30	15.60		AB
40s ea	33261-0159-40	20.80		AB
60s ea	33261-0159-60	31.20		AB
90s ea	33261-0159-90	46.80		AB
100s ea	33261-0159-01	52.00		AB
120s ea	33261-0159-02	64.40		AB
180s ea	33261-0159-03	93.60		AB
(American Health)				
REPACK				
CAP, PO (10X10)				
150 mg, 100s ea UD	68084-0243-01	62.71		AB
300 mg, 100s ea UD	68084-0244-01	129.82		AB
(DHS, Inc.)				
REPACK				
CAP, PO, 150 mg, 15s ea	55887-0611-15	18.00		AB
20s ea	55887-0611-20	23.26		AB
21s ea	55887-0611-21	24.42		AB
28s ea	55887-0611-28	32.56		AB
300 mg, 21s ea	55887-0378-21	136.00		AB
30s ea	55887-0378-30	190.00		AB

PROD/MFR	NDC	AWP	DP	OBC
(Dispensing Solutions)				
REPACK				
CAP, PO, 150 mg, 4s ea	55045-2006-04	4.80		AB
12s ea	55045-2006-02	14.40		AB
14s ea	66336-0018-14	16.67		AB
20s ea	55045-2006-07	24.00		AB
20s ea	66336-0018-20	23.82		AB
21s ea	66336-0018-21	25.01		AB
28s ea	66336-0018-28	33.35		AB
30s ea	55045-2006-08	36.00		AB
80s ea	55045-2006-01	96.00		AB
300 mg, 21s ea	55045-3268-06	71.19		AB
40s ea	55045-3268-04	135.60		AB
40s ea	66336-0906-40	148.68		AB
(IPI)				
REPACK				
CAP, PO, 300 mg, 40s ea	18837-0204-40	185.86		AB
(Keltman Pharma., Inc.)				
REPACK				
CAP, PO, 150 mg, 20s ea	68387-0390-20	27.68		AB
28s ea	68387-0390-28	38.75		AB
42s ea	68387-0390-42	58.13		AB
(Nucare Pharm)				
REPACK				
CAP, PO, 150 mg, 4s ea	66267-0060-04	12.20		AB
6s ea	66267-0060-06	18.30		AB
8s ea	66267-0060-08	24.38		AB
10s ea	66267-0060-10	30.48		AB
14s ea	66267-0060-14	42.67		AB
20s ea	66267-0060-20	60.95		AB
21s ea	66267-0060-21	63.99		AB
28s ea	66267-0060-28	85.33		AB
30s ea	66267-0060-30	91.43		AB
40s ea	66267-0060-40	121.90		AB
60s ea	66267-0060-60	182.85		AB
300 mg, 6s ea	68071-0398-06	28.89		AB
14s ea	68071-0398-14	67.48		AB
20s ea	68071-0398-20	96.40		AB
30s ea	68071-0398-30	146.36		AB
40s ea	68071-0398-40	195.15		AB
90s ea	68071-0398-90	439.08		AB
(PD-Rx Pharm)				
REPACK				
CAP, PO, 150 mg, 4s ea	55289-0441-04	12.83		AB
(USP)				
150 mg, 6s ea	43063-0056-06	14.04		AB
15s ea	55289-0441-15	20.94		AB
17s ea	55289-0441-17	21.60		AB
20s ea	55289-0441-20	23.01		AB
28s ea	55289-0441-28	30.53		AB
30s ea	55289-0441-30	30.60		AB
40s ea	55289-0441-40	40.50		AB
(REDI-SCRIPT)				
150 mg, 40s ea	58864-0607-40	52.44		AB
42s ea	55289-0441-42	40.80		AB
56s ea	55289-0441-56	50.70		AB
60s ea	58864-0607-60	51.60		AB
80s ea	55289-0441-80	68.67		AB
300 mg, 30s ea	55289-0890-30	68.25		AB
(Phys Total Care)				
REPACK				
CAP, PO, 150 mg, 15s ea	54868-1857-05	8.76		AB
20s ea	54868-1857-02	10.65		EE
30s ea	54868-1857-06	14.49		EE
40s ea	54868-1857-01	18.33		EE
60s ea	54868-1857-07	25.98		EE
100s ea	54868-1857-00	39.81		EE
300 mg, 10s ea	54868-5211-00	30.42		AB
40s ea	54868-5211-02	83.79		AB
60s ea	54868-5211-01	116.82		AB
(Physician Partner)				
REPACK				
CAP, PO, 150 mg, 40s ea	21695-0033-40	95.32		AB
300 mg, 21s ea	21695-0034-21	183.86		AB
30s ea	21695-0034-30	262.66		AB
(Quality Care Prod)				
REPACK				
CAP, PO, 150 mg, 4s ea	49999-0011-04	8.46		EE
15s ea	49999-0011-15	37.16		EE
18s ea	49999-0011-18	44.59		EE
20s ea	49999-0011-20	49.54		EE
28s ea	49999-0011-28	32.22		EE
30s ea	49999-0011-30	74.10		AB
40s ea	49999-0011-40	98.80		AB
100s ea	49999-0011-00	247.70		AB
300 mg, 21s ea	49999-0290-21	97.44		AB
30s ea	49999-0290-30	139.20		AB
(Southwood)				
REPACK				
CAP, PO, 150 mg, 12s ea	58016-0453-12	13.92		EE
15s ea	58016-0453-15	17.40		EE
20s ea	58016-0453-20	23.20		EE
21s ea	58016-0453-21	24.99		EE
30s ea	58016-0453-30	34.80		EE
40s ea	58016-0453-40	46.40		EE
100s ea	58016-0453-00	116.01		EE
300 mg, 30s ea	58016-0634-30	126.72		EE
60s ea	58016-0634-60	253.44		EE
90s ea	58016-0634-90	380.16		EE
100s ea	58016-0634-00	422.40		EE
(Stat Rx)				
REPACK				
CAP, PO, 150 mg, 20s ea	16590-0057-20	21.79		AB
300 mg, 30s ea	16590-0441-30	139.39		AB
40s ea	16590-0441-40	185.85		AB
84s ea	16590-0441-62	390.28		AB
CLINDAMYCIN HYDROCHLORIDE				
FUL				
CAP, PO, 150 mg, 100s ea		21.53		
300 mg, 100s ea		119.75		
(Aurobindo Pharma)				
CAP, PO (USP,HARD GELATIN)				
150 mg, 100s ea	65862-0185-01	119.22		AB
300 mg, 100s ea	65862-0186-01	371.71		AB
(Gallipot) *See CLINDAMYCIN HCL*				
(Greenstone) *See CLINDAMYCIN HCL*				
(Hawkins) *See CLINDAMYCIN HCL*				
(Lannett) *See CLINDAMYCIN*				
(Lannett) *See CLINDAMYCIN HCL*				
(Letco) *See CLINDAMYCIN HCL*				
(Major)				
CAP, PO (USP,10X10)				
150 mg, 100s ea UD	00904-5959-61	73.05		AB
300 mg, 100s ea UD	00904-5960-61	116.84		AB
(Medisca) *See CLINDAMYCIN HCL*				
(PCCA) *See CLINDAMYCIN HCL*				
(Pfizer) *See CLEOCIN HCL*				
(Ranbaxy Pharm)				
CAP, PO (USP)				
150 mg, 500s ea	63304-0692-05	595.75		AB
(Ranbaxy Pharm) *See CLINDAMYCIN HCL*				
(Sandoz) *See CLINDAMYCIN HCL*				
(Spectrum Pharmacy)				
POW, NA (U.S.P.)				
5 gm	49452-2139-01	74.90	49.50	
25 gm	49452-2139-02	276.50	124.80	
100 gm	49452-2139-03	896.00		
(Teva) *See CLINDAMYCIN HCL*				
(UDL) *See CLINDAMYCIN HCL*				
(Watson Labs) *See CLINDAMYCIN HCL*				
(4u)				
REPACK				
CAP, PO, 150 mg, 28s ea	42549-0532-28	56.68		AB
60s ea	10544-0333-60	94.44		
60s ea	42549-0532-60	94.44		AB
(Altura)				
REPACK				
CAP, PO, 150 mg, 4s ea	63874-0235-04	4.87		
10s ea	63874-0235-10	12.18		
12s ea	63874-0235-12	14.62		
15s ea	63874-0235-15	18.27		
16s ea	63874-0235-16	19.49		
20s ea	63874-0235-20	24.36		
21s ea	63874-0235-21	24.99		
28s ea	63874-0235-28	34.11		
30s ea	63874-0235-30	36.54		
40s ea	63874-0235-40	48.73		
56s ea	63874-0235-56	68.20		
80s ea	63874-0235-80	97.46		
100s ea	63874-0235-01	121.81		
(Dispensing Solutions)				
REPACK				
CAP, PO, 150 mg, 21s ea	55045-2006-06	25.50		
25s ea	55045-2006-05	30.00		
28s ea	55045-3233-08	33.60		
30s ea	66336-0018-30	36.00		AB
40s ea	55045-3570-01	48.00		
42s ea	55045-2006-03	50.40		
56s ea	55045-2006-09	67.20		
100s ea	55045-2006-00	120.00		
300 mg, 30s ea	55045-3268-08	101.70		
(IPI)				
REPACK				
CAP, PO, 300 mg, 30s ea	18837-0204-30	139.39		
(McKesson Packaging)				
REPACK				
CAP, PO, 150 mg,				
100s ea UD	63739-0059-10	68.42		
(Palmetto)				
REPACK				
CAP, PO, 150 mg, 4s ea	23490-5332-00	12.29		
8s ea	23490-5332-01	13.82		
14s ea	23490-5332-02	16.80		
20s ea	23490-5332-03	24.00		
21s ea	23490-5332-07	25.20		
28s ea	23490-5332-04	33.60		
30s ea	23490-5332-06	36.00		
40s ea	23490-5332-08	47.20		
42s ea	23490-5332-05	50.40		
300 mg, 28s ea	23490-5333-01	140.00		
30s ea	23490-5333-03	150.00		
40s ea	23490-5333-04	200.00		
(Phys Total Care)				
REPACK				
CAP, PO, 300 mg, 20s ea	54868-5211-04	60.81		
30s ea	54868-5211-03	82.26		
(Quality Care Prod)				
REPACK				
CAP, PO, 150 mg, 60s ea	49999-0011-60	148.20		AB
300 mg, 6s ea	49999-0290-06	27.84		
10s ea	49999-0290-10	46.40		
20s ea	49999-0290-20	92.80		
(St. Mary's MPP)				
REPACK				
CAP, PO (USP)				
150 mg, 8s ea	60760-0337-08	16.48		
28s ea	60760-0337-28	42.69		
60s ea	60760-0337-60	84.62		
300 mg, 5s ea	60760-0693-05	26.44		
(Vibranta)				
REPACK				
CAP, PO, 150 mg, 18s ea	57866-0155-00	44.59		
20s ea	57866-0155-05	49.54		
CLINDAMYCIN PALMITATE HYDROCHLORIDE				
(Pfizer) *See CLEOCIN PEDIATRIC*				
CLINDAMYCIN PHOSPHATE				
FUL				
GEL, TP, 1%, 60 gm		45.88		
LOT, TP, 1%, 60 ml		47.93		
SOL, TP, 1%, 60 ml		12.36		
(APP) *See CLINDAMYCIN*				
(Bedford) *See CLINDAMYCIN*				
(Fougera)				
CRE, VG (1X40GM,W/7 APPLICATORS)				
2%, 40 gm	00168-0277-40	50.81		
GEL, TP, 1%, 30 gm	00168-0202-30	38.13		AB
60 gm	00168-0202-60	68.67		AB
LOT, TP, 1%, 60 ml	00168-0203-60	53.06		AB
SOL, TP, 1%, 30 ml	00168-0201-30	12.09		AT
60 ml	00168-0201-60	24.15		AT
(Galderma) *See CLINDAGEL*				
(Gallipot)				
CRY, NA (U.S.P., N.F.)				
5 gm	51552-0529-02	30.74		
10 gm	51552-0529-03	56.28		
(Greenstone)				
CRE, VG (W/7 APPLICATORS)				
2%, 40 gm	59762-5009-01	48.55		AB
GEL, TP, 1%, 30 gm	59762-3743-01	32.12		AB
60 gm	59762-3743-02	57.85		AB
LOT, TP, 1%, 60 ml	59762-3744-01	45.12		AB
PAD, TP (PLEDGET)				
1%, 60s ea UD	59762-3728-03	45.90		
SOL, TP, 1%, 30 ml	59762-3728-01	11.65		AT
60 ml	59762-3728-02	23.15		AT
(Hospira)				
SOL, IJ (ADD-VANTAGE,25X2ML)				
150 mg/ml,				
2 ml 25s	00409-4053-03	100.20	87.75	AP
(VIAL,FLIPTOP,LATEX-FREE)				
150 mg/ml,				
2 ml 25s	00409-4050-01	88.20	77.25	AP
(VIAL,ADD-VANTAGE)				
150 mg/ml,				
4 ml 25s	00409-4054-03	119.40	104.50	AP
(VIAL,FLIPTOP,LATEX-FREE)				
150 mg/ml,				
4 ml 25s	00409-4051-01	101.70	89.00	AP

PROD/MFR NDC AWP DP OBC

(25X6ML,LATEX-FREE)
150 mg/ml,
6 ml 25s.......... 00409-4052-01 140.70 123.00 AP
(VIAL, FLIPTOP)
150 mg/ml,
6 ml 25s.......... 00074-4052-01 135.60 118.75 AP
(VIAL,ADD-VANTAGE)
150 mg/ml,
6 ml 25s.......... 00409-4055-03 154.20 135.00 AP
(VIAL,BULK,LATEX-FREE)
150 mg/ml, 60 ml .... 00409-4197-01 25.68 22.47 AP

(Medisca)
POW, NA (U.S.P.)
5 gm............... 38779-0006-03 105.00
(1X10GM, USP)
10 gm.............. 38779-0006-01 165.00
(U.S.P.)
25 gm.............. 38779-0006-04 345.00
100 gm............. 38779-0006-05 1185.00

(Paddock) *See CLINDA-DERM*

(PCCA)
POW, NA (U.S.P.)
1 gm............... 51927-1683-00 19.80

(Perrigo)
PAD, TP (PLEDGET)
1%, 60s ea.......... 45802-0263-37 46.40 AT
69s ea.......... 45802-0263-93 53.80 AT

(Pfizer) *See CLEOCIN PHOSPHATE*

(Pfizer) *See CLEOCIN T*

(Pfizer) *See CLEOCIN VAGINAL*

(Pfizer) *See CLEOCIN VAGINAL OVULES*

(PharmaDerm) *See CLINDAMAX*

(Sirius Labs) *See CLINDAREACH*

(Stiefel Labs) *See EVOCLIN*

(Taro)
SOL, TP, 1%, 30 ml .... 51672-4081-03 11.93 AT
60 ml.......... 51672-4081-04 24.25 AT

(Ther-RX) *See CLINDESSE*

(A-S Medication)
REPACK
GEL, TP, 1%, 30 gm....... 54569-5359-00 41.49 AB
SOL, TP, 1%, 60 ml .... 54569-4349-00 23.85 AT

(Dispensing Solutions)
REPACK
GEL, TP, 1%, 30 gm....... 55045-3066-08 57.23
SOL, TP, 1%, 30 ml 55045-2127-01 33.26
60 ml.......... 55045-2127-02 25.00

(Palmetto)
REPACK
GEL, TP, 1%, 30 gm....... 23490-5334-01 104.85
PAD, TP (PLEDGETS)
1%, 60s ea.......... 23490-5335-01 125.00 AT
SOL, TP, 1%, 30 ml 23490-5336-01 33.24

(Phys Total Care)
REPACK
GEL, TP, 1%, 30 gm....... 54868-4654-01 36.15
60 gm.......... 54868-4654-00 84.57 AB
LOT, TP, 1%, 60 ml........ 54868-4806-00 68.82 AB
SOL, IJ (S.D.V.)
150 mg/ml,
2 ml 25s.......... 54868-3695-00 303.00 EE
TP (1X30ML)
1%, 30 ml.......... 54868-2875-01 16.80 AT
60 ml.......... 54868-2875-00 21.03 AT

(Physician Partner)
REPACK
SOL, TP (1X60ML)
1%, 60 ml.......... 21695-0888-60 48.30 AT

(Quality Care Prod)
REPACK
GEL, TP, 1%, 30 gm....... 49999-0280-30 33.04 AB
SOL, TP, 1%, 30 ml .... 49999-0749-30 28.94 AT

CLINDAMYCIN PHOSPHATE/TRETINOIN
(Medicis) *See ZIANA*

CLINDAMYCIN/BENZOYL PEROXIDE (Mylan)
benzoyl peroxide/clindamycin phosphate
GEL, TP (1X50GM)
5%-1%, 50 gm....... 00378-8688-54 169.63 AB

CLINDAREACH (Sirius Labs)
clindamycin phosphate
PAD, TP (2X60,SINGLE USE,PLEDGET)
1%, 120s ea.......... 65880-0503-02 194.10

CLINDESSE (Ther-RX)
clindamycin phosphate
CRE, VG, 2%, 5.8 gm 64011-0124-08 93.78

(Physician Partner)
REPACK
CRE, VG (5X5GM)
2%, 5 gm 5s......... 21695-0858-05 195.38

CLINDETS (Phys Total Care)
REPACK
clindamycin phosphate
PAD, TP, 1%, 60s ea ...... 54868-4805-00 24.01 AT

CLINICAL LAB PRODUCTS (Covidien)
device
DEV, NA (2000ML,2 BOTTLE)
4s ea.............. 08080-8472-62 125.00

CLINIMIX (Baxter)
amino acids/dextrose
SOL, IV (2B7726,6X1000ML)
4.25%-5%,
1000 ml 6s .... 00338-1133-03 289.08 240.90 EE
(CLARITY DUAL CHAMBER)
4.25%-5%,
1000 ml 6s 00338-1144-03 295.99 246.66
(CLARITY PC)
4.25%-5%,
2000 ml 4s 00338-1089-04 586.80 489.00
(CLARITY DUAL CHAMBER)
4.25%-10%,
1000 ml 6s 00338-1134-03 294.41 245.34
(CLARITY PC)
4.25%-10%,
2000 ml 4s 00338-1091-04 586.80 489.00
(CLARITY PC,SULFITE-FREE)
4.25%-20%,
1000 ml 6s 00338-1135-03 294.41 245.34
2000 ml 4s 00338-1093-04 586.80 489.00
(CLARITY DUAL CHAMBER)
4.25%-25%,
1000 ml 6s 00338-1136-03 298.01 248.34
(CLARITY PC)
4.25%-25%,
2000 ml 4s 00338-1095-04 586.80 489.00
(CLARITY PC,SULFITE-FREE)
5%-15%, 1000 ml 6s . 00338-1137-03 303.05 252.54
2000 ml 4s 00338-1099-04 601.20 501.00
5%-20%, 1000 ml 6s . 00338-1138-03 303.05 252.54
2000 ml 4s 00338-1101-04 601.20 501.00
5%-25%, 1000 ml 6s . 00338-1139-03 303.05 252.54
2000 ml 4s 00338-1103-04 601.20 501.00

CLINIMIX E 2.75/10 (Baxter)
amino acids, dextrose, and electrolytes
SOL, IV (2B7736; CLARITY PC)
1000 ml 6s 00338-1143-03 270.36 225.30
(CLARITY PC)
2000 ml 4s 00338-1109-04 579.84 483.20

CLINIMIX E 2.75/5 (Baxter)
amino acids, dextrose, and electrolytes
SOL, IV (CLARITY DUAL CHAMBER)
1000 ml 6s 00338-1132-03 266.40 222.00
1000 ml 6s 00338-1142-03 273.74 228.12
(CLARITY PC)
2000 ml 4s 00338-1107-04 578.40 482.00

CLINIMIX E 4.25/10 (Baxter)
amino acids, dextrose, and electrolytes
SOL, IV (CLARITY DUAL CHAMBER)
1000 ml 6s 00338-1145-03 297.29 247.74
(CLARITY PC)
2000 ml 4s 00338-1115-04 589.44 491.20

CLINIMIX E 4.25/25 (Baxter)
amino acids, dextrose, and electrolytes
SOL, IV (CLARITY DUAL CHAMBER)
1000 ml 6s 00338-1146-03 300.82 250.68
(CLARITY PC)
2000 ml 4s 00338-1119-04 589.44 491.20

CLINIMIX E 4.25/5 (Baxter)
amino acids, dextrose, and electrolytes
SOL, IV (CLARITY PC,SULFITE-FREE)
2000 ml 4s 00338-1113-04 589.44 491.20

CLINIMIX E 5/15 (Baxter)
amino acids, dextrose, and electrolytes
SOL, IV (CLARITY PC,SULFITE-FREE)
1000 ml 6s 00338-1147-03 307.15 255.96
2000 ml 4s 00338-1123-04 603.84 503.20

CLINIMIX E 5/20 (Baxter)
amino acids, dextrose, and electrolytes
SOL, IV (2B7741; CLARITY PC)
1000 ml 6s 00338-1148-03 307.15 255.96
(CLARITY PC,SULFITE-FREE)
2000 ml 4s 00338-1125-04 603.84 503.20

CLINIMIX E 5/25 (Baxter)
amino acids, dextrose, and electrolytes
SOL, IV (CLARITY PC,SULFITE-FREE)
1000 ml 6s 00338-1149-03 307.14 255.95
2000 ml 4s 00338-1127-04 603.84 503.20

CLINISOL (Baxter)
amino acids
SOL, IV (VIAFLEX,BULK PKG)
15%, 500 ml......... 00338-0502-03 86.40 72.00
(VIAFLEX,P.C.,BULK PKG.)
15%, 2000 ml........ 00338-0502-06 354.00 295.00

CLINORIL (Merck)
sulindac
TAB, PO, 200 mg, 100s ea . 00006-0942-68 154.54 AB

CLIOQUINOL (Amend)
POW, NA (U.S.P.)
25 gm.............. 17317-0204-02 17.50
125 gm............. 17317-0204-04 28.00
500 gm............. 17317-0204-01 98.00

(Gallipot)
POW, NA (U.S.P.,N.F.)
25 gm.............. 51552-0115-04 15.40
100 gm............. 51552-0115-05 34.24
500 gm............. 51552-0115-06 136.50

(Medisca)
POW, NA (U.S.P.)
25 gm.............. 38779-0032-04 38.85
100 gm............. 38779-0032-05 76.50
500 gm............. 38779-0032-08 289.50

(PCCA) *See IODOCHLORHYDROXYQUIN*

(Spectrum Pharmacy)
POW, NA (U.S.P.)
25 gm.............. 49452-2140-01 77.00
100 gm............. 49452-2140-02 124.60
500 gm............. 49452-2140-03 427.00

CLIOQUINOL/HYDROCORTISONE (Consolidated Midland)
CRE, TP, 3%-0.5%, 15 gm . 00223-4127-15 2.75
30 gm.............. 00223-4127-30 3.00
3%-1%, 20 gm....... 00223-4128-20 3.25
30 gm.............. 00223-4128-30 3.25
454 gm............. 00223-4128-01 34.00

(Del-Ray) *See ALA-QUIN*

(Truxton) *See DEK QUIN*

(Pharma Pac)
REPACK
CRE, TP, 3%-1%, 20 gm... 52959-0249-00 6.20

CLOBETASOL 17 PROPIONATE (Medisca)
clobetasol propionate
POW, NA (MICRONIZED)
1 gm............... 38779-0372-06 156.00
5 gm............... 38779-0372-03 630.00
10 gm.............. 38779-0372-01 1125.00
(USP,1X100GM,MICRONIZED)
100 gm............. 38779-0372-05 5955.00
(USP,1X250MG,MICRONIZED)
250 ml 38779-0372-07 61.50
(USP,1X500MG,MICRONIZED)
500 ml 38779-0372-00 105.00

CLOBETASOL 17 PROPIONATE MICRONIZED (Medisca)
clobetasol propionate, micronized
POW, NA (U.S.P.)
25 gm.............. 38779-0372-04 2250.00

CLOBETASOL PROP (Phys Total Care)
REPACK
clobetasol propionate
OIN, TP, 0.05%, 15 gm 54868-3698-02 12.25

CLOBETASOL PROPIONATE
FUL
CRE, TP, 0.05%, 30 gm 5.48
EMO, TP, 0.05%, 30 gm 13.40
FOA, TP, 100 gm 297.96
0.05%, 100 gm 297.96
GEL, TP, 0.05%, 60 gm 27.84
OIN, TP, 0.05%, 45 gm 8.73
SOL, TP, 0.05%, 50 ml 21.00

(Fougera) *See CLOBETASOL PROPIONATE EMOLLIENT*

(Fougera)
CRE, TP, 0.05%, 15 gm.... 00168-0163-15 24.71 AB1
30 gm.............. 00168-0163-30 35.86 AB1
45 gm.............. 00168-0163-46 50.21 AB1
60 gm.............. 00168-0163-60 64.17 AB1
GEL, TP, 0.05%, 15 gm.... 00168-0293-15 27.75 EE
30 gm.............. 00168-0293-30 40.69 EE
60 gm.............. 00168-0293-60 74.16 EE

PROD/MFR	NDC	AWP	DP	OBC
OIN, TP, 0.05%, 15 gm	00168-0162-15	24.71		AB
30 gm	00168-0162-30	35.86		AB
45 gm	00168-0162-46	50.21		AB
60 gm	00168-0162-60	64.17		AB
SOL, TP, 0.05%, 50 ml	00168-0269-50	53.10		AT
(Galderma) *See CLOBEX*				
(Gallipot)				
POW, NA (U.S.P.,MICRONIZED)				
0.25 gm	51552-0605-09	27.30		
1 gm	51552-0605-01	63.00		
(Glenmark Pharmaceuticals)				
CRE, TP (1X15GM,USP)				
0.05%, 15 gm	68462-0289-17	2.33		
(1X30GM,USP)				
0.05%, 30 gm	68462-0289-35	3.65		
(1X45GM,USP)				
0.05%, 45 gm	68462-0289-55	5.82		
(1X60GM,USP)				
0.05%, 60 gm	68462-0289-65	7.01		
EMO, TP (1X15GM)				
0.05%, 15 gm	68462-0363-17	5.96		
(1X30GM)				
0.05%, 30 gm	68462-0363-35	8.93		
(1X60GM)				
0.05%, 60 gm	68462-0363-65	12.92		
GEL, TP (1X15GM)				
0.05%, 15 gm	68462-0365-17	10.23		
(1X30GM)				
0.05%, 30 gm	68462-0365-35	14.83		
(1X60GM)				
0.05%, 60 gm	68462-0365-65	18.56		
OIN, TP (1X15GM,USP)				
0.05%, 15 gm	68462-0364-17	2.09		
(1X30GM,USP)				
0.05%, 30 gm	68462-0364-35	3.27		
(1X45GM,USP)				
0.05%, 45 gm	68462-0364-55	5.82		
(1X60GM,USP)				
0.05%, 60 gm	68462-0364-65	7.01		
SOL, TP (USP,1X25ML,PLASTIC)				
0.05%, 25 ml	68462-0366-28	5.09		
(USP,1X50ML,PLASTIC)				
0.05%, 50 ml	68462-0366-53	7.17		
(Medisca) *See CLOBETASOL 17 PROPIONATE*				
(Morton Grove)				
SOL, TP, 0.05%, 25 ml	60432-0133-25	20.55		AT
50 ml	60432-0133-50	39.60		AT
(Perrigo)				
FOA, TP (1X50GM)				
0.05%, 50 gm	45802-0437-32	169.86		AB
(1X100GM)				
0.05%, 100 gm	45802-0437-33	313.14		AB
GEL, TP (1X15GM)				
0.05%, 15 gm	45802-0925-14	35.89		AB
(1X30GM)				
0.05%, 30 gm	45802-0925-94	49.67		AB
(1X60GM)				
0.05%, 60 gm	45802-0925-96	90.21		AB
(PharmaDerm) *See TEMOVATE*				
(PharmaDerm) *See TEMOVATE E*				
(PharmaDerm) *See TEMOVATE SCALP APPLICATION*				
(Prasco Labs)				
FOA, TP (1X50GM)				
0.05%, 50 gm	66993-0888-49	170.24		
(1X100GM)				
0.05%, 100 gm	66993-0888-65	313.82		
(Spectrum Pharmacy)				
POW, NA (U.S.P.,MICRONIZED)				
5 gm	49452-2141-03	1015.00		
25 gm	49452-2141-04	3101.00		
(Stiefel Labs) *See OLUX*				
(Stiefel Labs) *See OLUX-E*				
(Stiefel Labs) *See OLUX/OLUX-E COMPLETE PACK*				
(Taro) *See CLOBETASOL PROPIONATE E*				
(Taro)				
CRE, TP, 0.05%, 15 gm	51672-1258-01	23.98		AB1
30 gm	51672-1258-02	33.45		AB1
45 gm	51672-1258-06	48.62		AB1
60 gm	51672-1258-03	61.68		AB1
GEL, TP, 0.05%, 15 gm	51672-1294-01	23.80		AB
30 gm	51672-1294-02	39.89		AB
60 gm	51672-1294-03	72.25		AB
OIN, TP, 0.05%, 15 gm	51672-1259-01	23.98		AB
30 gm	51672-1259-02	33.45		AB
45 gm	51672-1259-06	48.62		AB
60 gm	51672-1259-03	61.68		AB
SOL, TP, 0.05%, 25 ml	51672-1293-02	26.66		AT
50 ml	51672-1293-03	51.26		AT
(Watson) *See CORMAX*				
(Watson) *See CORMAX SCALP APPLICATION*				
(A-S Medication)				
REPACK				
CRE, TP, 0.05%, 15 gm	54569-4200-00	23.98		AB1
30 gm	54569-4550-00	35.06		AB1
(1X60GM)				
0.05%, 60 gm	54569-6065-00	64.17		AB1
OIN, TP, 0.05%, 15 gm	54569-4649-00	31.65		AB
(1X60GM)				
0.05%, 60 gm	54569-6066-00	64.17		AB
SOL, TP (1X50ML)				
0.05%, 50 ml	54569-6067-00	55.55		AT
(Altura)				
REPACK				
CRE, TP, 0.05%, 30 gm	63874-0796-30	36.69		
OIN, TP, 0.05%, 15 gm	63874-0710-15	23.17		
30 gm	63874-0710-30	32.10		
(DHS, Inc.)				
REPACK				
CRE, TP, 0.05%, 15 gm	55887-0399-15	25.05		AB1
30 gm	55887-0399-30	37.21		AB1
(Dispensing Solutions)				
REPACK				
CRE, TP, 0.05%, 15 gm	55045-2438-05	48.81		
30 gm	55045-2438-08	35.00		
45 gm	55045-2438-04	49.00		
(Keltman Pharma., Inc.)				
REPACK				
CRE, TP (1X30GM)				
0.05%, 30 gm	68387-0533-01	34.50		AB1
(Palmetto)				
REPACK				
CRE, TP, 0.05%, 15 gm	23490-5339-01	65.95		
(1X30GM)				
0.05%, 30 gm	23490-5339-02	91.98		
(1X60GM)				
0.05%, 60 gm	23490-5339-03	169.62		
CLOBETASOL PROPIONATE (Palmetto)				
OIN, TP (1X15GM)				
0.05%, 15 gm	23490-5342-00	65.94		
CLOBETASOL PROPIONATE (Pharma Pac)				
REPACK				
CRE, TP, 0.05%, 15 gm	52959-0847-15	27.95		
(Phys Total Care)				
REPACK				
CRE, TP, 0.05%, 15 gm	54868-3584-02	11.54		EE
30 gm	54868-3584-00	17.25		EE
45 gm	54868-3584-01	27.87		EE
OIN, TP, 0.05%, 30 gm	54868-3698-00	18.63		AB
45 gm	54868-3698-01	25.14		AB
SOL, TP, 0.05%, 50 ml	54868-5292-00	27.00		AT
(Physician Partner)				
REPACK				
CRE, TP (1X15GM)				
0.05%, 15 gm	21695-0201-15	49.42		AB1
60 gm	21695-0201-60	123.36		
OIN, TP (1X30GM)				
0.05%, 30 gm	21695-0483-30	71.72		AB
SOL, TP, 0.05%, 25 ml	21695-0358-25	41.10		AT
(Quality Care Prod)				
REPACK				
CRE, TP, 0.05%, 15 gm	49999-0221-15	27.93		
30 gm	49999-0221-30	39.48		
(1X45GM)				
0.05%, 45 gm	49999-0221-45	46.12		AB1
60 gm	49999-0221-60	67.85		
OIN, TP, 0.05%, 15 gm	49999-0263-15	27.92		AB
30 gm	49999-0263-30	38.63		AB
(Southwood)				
REPACK				
OIN, TP, 0.05%, 30 gm	58016-4785-01	33.33		
60 gm	58016-4837-01	64.17		
CLOBETASOL PROPIONATE E (Taro)				
clobetasol propionate				
EMO, TP, 0.05%, 15 gm	51672-1297-01	25.42		AB2
30 gm	51672-1297-02	37.23		AB2
60 gm	51672-1297-03	68.98		AB2
CLOBETASOL PROPIONATE EMOLLIENT (Fougera)				
clobetasol propionate				
EMO, TP, 0.05%, 15 gm	00168-0301-15	27.50		AB2
30 gm	00168-0301-30	42.32		AB2
60 gm	00168-0301-60	77.35		AB2
CLOBETASOL PROPIONATE MICRONIZED (Hawkins)				
clobetasol propionate, micronized				
POW, NA (USP)				
0.5 gm	63370-0055-09	112.00		
1 gm	63370-0055-10	140.00		
5 gm	63370-0055-15	640.00		
25 gm	63370-0055-25	2900.00		
(Letco)				
POW, NA (U.S.P.)				
0.5 gm	62991-1492-01	60.00		
1 gm	62991-1492-02	90.00		
5 gm	62991-1492-03	420.00		
10 gm	62991-1492-04	1125.00		
(PCCA)				
POW, NA (USP)				
1 gm	51927-2627-00	396.00		
CLOBETASOL PROPIONATE, MICRONIZED				
(Hawkins) *See CLOBETASOL PROPIONATE MICRONIZED*				
(Letco) *See CLOBETASOL PROPIONATE MICRONIZED*				
(Medisca) *See CLOBETASOL 17 PROPIONATE MICRONIZED*				
(PCCA) *See CLOBETASOL PROPIONATE MICRONIZED*				
(Spectrum Pharmacy)				
POW, NA (U.S.P.)				
0.25 gm	49452-2141-01	120.75		
1 gm	49452-2141-02	245.00		
CLOBEX (Galderma)				
clobetasol propionate				
LOT, TP, 0.05%, 59 ml	00299-3848-02	281.25		
118 ml	00299-3848-04	514.38		
SHA, TP, 0.05%, 118 ml	00299-3847-04	366.25		
SPR, TP, 0.05%, 59 ml	00299-3849-02	279.38		
125 ml	00299-3849-04	502.50		
(Phys Total Care)				
REPACK				
LOT, TP, 0.05%, 60 ml	54868-5657-01	172.61		
118 ml	54868-5657-00	312.01		
SHA, TP, 0.05%, 118 ml	54868-3967-00	272.14		
SPR, TP, 0.05%, 59 ml	54868-5510-00	287.48		
CLOCORTOLONE PIVALATE				
(Valeant Pharm Intl) *See CLODERM*				
CLODERM (Valeant Pharm Intl)				
clocortolone pivalate				
CRE, TP, 0.1%, 30 gm	13548-0031-30	113.75		
45 gm	13548-0031-45	141.90		
(1X75GM)				
0.1%, 75 gm	13548-0031-75	224.81		
90 gm	13548-0031-90	205.59		
(Phys Total Care)				
REPACK				
CRE, TP, 0.1%, 15 gm	54868-4724-00	39.65		
(Quality Care Prod)				
REPACK				
CRE, TP (1X45GM)				
0.1%, 45 gm	35356-0221-45	176.65		
CLOFARABINE				
(Genzyme) *See CLOLAR*				
CLOFIBRATE (Gallipot)				
POW, NA, 25 gm	51552-0543-04	78.40		
CLOLAR (Genzyme)				
clofarabine				
SOL, IV (SINGLE-USE VIAL,PF)				
1 mg/ml, 20 ml	58468-0100-01	2700.00	2250.00	
20 ml 4s	58468-0100-02	10800.00	9000.00	
CLOMID (Sanofi-Aventis)				
clomiphene citrate				
TAB, PO (USP)				
50 mg, 30s ea	00068-0226-30	453.18		AB
CLOMIPHENE CITRATE				
FUL				
TAB, PO, 50 mg, 30s ea		106.50		
(EMD) *See SEROPHENE*				
(Gallipot)				
POW, NA (U.S.P.)				
25 gm	51552-1070-04	404.60	289.00	
(Letco)				
POW, NA (USP)				
25 gm	62991-2702-03	435.00		
100 gm	62991-2702-02	1350.00		
(USP, 1X1000GM)				
1000 gm	62991-2702-01	13500.00		
(Medisca)				
POW, NA (U.S.P.)				
1 gm	38779-0390-06	61.50		

PROD/MFR	NDC	AWP	DP	OBC
5 gm	**38779-0390-03**	234.00		
25 gm	**38779-0390-04**	867.00		
(USP,1X100GM)				
100 gm	**38779-0390-05**	2850.00		
(USP,1X1000GM)				
1000 gm	**38779-0390-09**	16500.00		
(Par)				
TAB, PO, 50 mg, 10s ea	**49884-0701-54**	68.55		**AB**
30s ea	**49884-0701-55**	207.60		**AB**
(PCCA)				
POW, NA (USP)				
1 gm	**51927-1808-00**	63.00		
(Sanofi-Aventis) *See CLOMID*				
(Spectrum Pharmacy)				
POW, NA (U.S.P.)				
1 gm	**49452-2146-01**	106.05		
5 gm	**49452-2146-02**	337.05		
25 gm	**49452-2146-03**	1183.00		
50 gm	**49452-2146-04**	1736.00		
(Teva)				
TAB, PO, 50 mg, 10s ea	**00093-0041-03**	68.55		**AB**
(USP,3X10)				
50 mg, 30s ea	**00093-0041-65**	207.60		**AB**
(Watson Labs)				
TAB, PO, 50 mg, 30s ea	**00591-0781-30**	207.60		
(A-S Medication)				
REPACK				
TAB, PO, 50 mg, 30s ea	**54569-4943-01**	207.60		**AB**
(B&B Pharm, Inc)				
REPACK				
POW, NA, 5 gm	**63275-9964-02**	265.00		
25 gm	**63275-9964-04**	1300.00		
100 gm	**63275-9964-05**	5100.00		
500 gm	**63275-9964-08**	25000.00		
(Phys Total Care)				
REPACK				
TAB, PO, 50 mg, 5s ea	**54868-3059-00**	32.25		**EE**
10s ea	**54868-3059-01**	59.97		**EE**
(Quality Care Prod)				
REPACK				
TAB, PO, 50 mg, 5s ea	**35356-0358-05**	48.60		**AB**
10s ea	**35356-0358-10**	52.90		**AB**
CLOMIPRAMINE (Bryant Ranch)				
REPACK				
clomipramine hydrochloride				
CAP, PO, 25 mg, 30s ea	**63629-2756-01**	33.23		
CLOMIPRAMINE HCL (Gallipot)				
clomipramine hydrochloride				
POW, NA, 1 gm	**51552-0985-01**	31.50	22.50	
(Hawkins)				
POW, NA (B.P.)				
5 gm	**63370-0051-15**	220.80		
25 gm	**63370-0051-25**	984.00		
100 gm	**63370-0051-35**	2736.00		
(Medisca)				
POW, NA (1X5GM,USP)				
5 gm	**38779-2256-03**	207.00		
(B.P.)				
5 gm	**38779-2032-03**	138.00		
(1X25GM,USP)				
25 gm	**38779-2256-04**	735.00		
(B.P.)				
25 gm	**38779-2032-04**	612.00		
(1X100GM,USP)				
100 gm	**38779-2256-05**	1785.00		
(B.P.)				
100 gm	**38779-2032-05**	1530.00		
(Mylan)				
CAP, PO, 25 mg, 100s ea	**00378-3025-01**	82.85		**AB**
50 mg, 100s ea	**00378-3050-01**	111.62		**AB**
75 mg, 100s ea	**00378-3075-01**	146.90		**AB**
(PCCA)				
POW, NA, 1 gm	**51927-3024-00**	36.00		
(Sandoz)				
CAP, PO, 25 mg, 100s ea	**00781-2027-01**	78.95		**AB**
50 mg, 100s ea	**00781-2037-01**	106.45		**AB**
75 mg, 100s ea	**00781-2047-01**	140.14		**AB**
(Taro)				
CAP, PO, 25 mg, 30s ea	**51672-4011-06**	25.40		**AB**
90s ea	**51672-4011-05**	73.91		**AB**
100s ea	**51672-4011-01**	83.66		**AB**
50 mg, 30s ea	**51672-4012-06**	34.12		**AB**
90s ea	**51672-4012-05**	99.28		**AB**
100s ea	**51672-4012-01**	112.72		**AB**
75 mg, 30s ea	**51672-4013-06**	44.81		**AB**
90s ea	**51672-4013-05**	130.38		**AB**
100s ea	**51672-4013-01**	148.35		**AB**

PROD/MFR	NDC	AWP	DP	OBC
(Teva)				
CAP, PO, 25 mg, 100s ea	**00093-0956-01**	75.05		**AB**
50 mg, 100s ea	**00093-0958-01**	101.15		**AB**
75 mg, 100s ea	**00093-0960-01**	133.15		**AB**
(Phys Total Care)				
REPACK				
CAP, PO, 50 mg, 60s ea	**54868-4023-00**	33.93		**AB**
CLOMIPRAMINE HYDROCHLORIDE				
FUL				
CAP, PO, 25 mg, 100s ea		37.50		
50 mg, 100s ea		50.36		
75 mg, 100s ea		66.23		
(Covidien) *See ANAFRANIL*				
(Gallipot) *See CLOMIPRAMINE HCL*				
(Hawkins) *See CLOMIPRAMINE HCL*				
(Medisca) *See CLOMIPRAMINE HCL*				
(Mylan) *See CLOMIPRAMINE HCL*				
(PCCA) *See CLOMIPRAMINE HCL*				
(Sandoz) *See CLOMIPRAMINE HCL*				
(Spectrum Pharmacy)				
POW, NA (1X5GM,USP)				
5 gm	**49452-2149-01**	281.05		
(1X25GM,USP)				
25 gm	**49452-2149-02**	1032.50		
(1X100GM,USP)				
100 gm	**49452-2149-03**	2320.50		
(1X1000GM,USP)				
1000 gm	**49452-2149-04**	5855.50		
(Taro) *See CLOMIPRAMINE HCL*				
(Teva) *See CLOMIPRAMINE HCL*				
CLONAZEPAM				
FUL				
TAB, PO, 0.5 mg, 100s ea		6.00		
1 mg, 100s ea		7.80		
2 mg, 100s ea		10.80		
(Actavis)				
TAB, PO, 0.5 mg,				
100s ea, C-IV	**00228-3003-11**	74.91		**AB**
500s ea, C-IV	**00228-3003-50**	355.25		**AB**
1 mg, 100s ea, C-IV	**00228-3004-11**	85.51		**AB**
500s ea, C-IV	**00228-3004-50**	406.38		**AB**
2 mg, 100s ea, C-IV	**00228-3005-11**	118.41		**AB**
500s ea, C-IV	**00228-3005-50**	609.99		**AB**
(Apotex Corp.)				
TAB, PO, 0.5 mg,				
100s ea, C-IV	**60505-0066-01**	74.90		**AB**
500s ea, C-IV	**60505-0066-03**	355.25		**AB**
1 mg, 100s ea, C-IV	**60505-0067-01**	85.50		**AB**
500s ea, C-IV	**60505-0067-03**	406.38		**AB**
2 mg, 100s ea, C-IV	**60505-0068-01**	118.40		**AB**
500s ea, C-IV	**60505-0068-03**	580.70		**AB**
(Caraco)				
TAB, PO, 0.5 mg,				
100s ea, C-IV	**57664-0273-08**	74.90		**AB**
500s ea, C-IV	**57664-0273-13**	374.00		**AB**
1000s ea, C-IV	**57664-0273-18**	748.00		**AB**
1 mg, 100s ea, C-IV	**57664-0274-08**	85.50		**AB**
500s ea, C-IV	**57664-0274-13**	427.00		**AB**
1000s ea, C-IV	**57664-0274-18**	854.00		**AB**
2 mg, 100s ea, C-IV	**57664-0275-08**	118.40		**AB**
500s ea, C-IV	**57664-0275-13**	591.00		**AB**
1000s ea, C-IV	**57664-0275-18**	1182.00		**AB**
(Major)				
TAB, PO (10X10)				
0.5 mg,				
100s ea UD, C-IV	**00904-5342-61**	71.80		
(USP)				
1 mg,				
100s ea UD, C-IV	**00904-5343-61**	81.50		
(10X10,USP)				
2 mg,				
100s ea UD, C-IV	**00904-5344-61**	111.65		
(Mylan)				
TAB, PO (USP)				
0.5 mg,				
90s ea, C-IV	**00378-1910-77**	67.46		**AB**
100s ea, C-IV	**00378-1910-01**	74.95		**AB**
1000s ea, C-IV	**00378-1910-10**	735.00		**AB**
(USP)				
1 mg, 90s ea, C-IV	**00378-1912-77**	77.00		**AB**
100s ea, C-IV	**00378-1912-01**	85.55		**AB**
1000s ea, C-IV	**00378-1912-10**	837.90		**AB**
2 mg, 100s ea, C-IV	**00378-1914-01**	118.45		**AB**
500s ea, C-IV	**00378-1914-05**	580.70		**AB**

PROD/MFR	NDC	AWP	DP	OBC
(Par)				
ODT, PO, 0.125 mg,				
60s ea, C-IV	**49884-0306-02**	77.93		**AB**
0.25 mg,				
60s ea, C-IV	**49884-0307-02**	77.93		**AB**
0.5 mg, 60s ea, C-IV	**49884-0308-02**	77.80		**AB**
1 mg, 60s ea, C-IV	**49884-0309-02**	88.91		**AB**
2 mg, 60s ea, C-IV	**49884-0310-02**	123.19		**AB**
(Qualitest)				
TAB, PO (USP)				
0.5 mg,				
30s ea, C-IV	**00603-2948-16**	22.47		**AB**
60s ea, C-IV	**00603-2948-20**	44.94		**AB**
90s ea, C-IV	**00603-2948-02**	67.41		**AB**
100s ea, C-IV	**00603-2948-21**	74.90		**AB**
120s ea, C-IV	**00603-2948-22**	89.88		**AB**
(USP)				
0.5 mg,				
500s ea, C-IV	**00603-2948-28**	386.84		**AB**
1000s ea, C-IV	**00603-2948-32**	735.00		**AB**
1 mg, 30s ea, C-IV	**00603-2949-16**	25.65		**AB**
60s ea, C-IV	**00603-2949-20**	51.30		**AB**
90s ea, C-IV	**00603-2949-02**	76.95		**AB**
100s ea, C-IV	**00603-2949-21**	85.50		**AB**
120s ea, C-IV	**00603-2949-22**	102.60		**AB**
(USP)				
1 mg,				
500s ea, C-IV	**00603-2949-28**	425.44		**AB**
1000s ea, C-IV	**00603-2949-32**	837.90		**AB**
2 mg, 30s ea, C-IV	**00603-2950-16**	35.52		**AB**
60s ea, C-IV	**00603-2950-20**	71.04		**AB**
90s ea, C-IV	**00603-2950-02**	106.56		**AB**
100s ea, C-IV	**00603-2950-21**	118.40		**AB**
500s ea, C-IV	**00603-2950-28**	580.70		**AB**
(Roche Labs) *See KLONOPIN*				
(Sandoz)				
TAB, PO, 0.5 mg,				
100s ea, C-IV	**00185-0063-01**	71.37		**AB**
500s ea, C-IV	**00185-0063-05**	321.20		**AB**
1000s ea, C-IV	**00185-0063-10**	642.33		**AB**
1 mg, 100s ea, C-IV	**00185-0064-01**	81.41		**AB**
500s ea, C-IV	**00185-0064-05**	366.37		**AB**
1000s ea, C-IV	**00185-0064-10**	732.69		**AB**
2 mg, 100s ea, C-IV	**00185-0065-01**	112.82		**AB**
500s ea, C-IV	**00185-0065-05**	507.71		**AB**
1000s ea, C-IV	**00185-0065-10**	1015.38		**AB**
(Teva)				
ODT, PO (10X6,STRAWBERRY)				
0.125 mg,				
60s ea, C-IV	**00555-0094-96**	77.93		**AB**
0.25 mg,				
60s ea, C-IV	**00555-0095-96**	77.93		**AB**
0.5 mg, 60s ea, C-IV	**00555-0096-96**	77.80		**AB**
1 mg, 60s ea, C-IV	**00555-0097-96**	88.91		**AB**
2 mg, 60s ea, C-IV	**00555-0098-96**	123.19		**AB**
TAB, PO, 0.5 mg,				
100s ea, C-IV	**00093-0832-01**	74.90		**AB**
(USP)				
0.5 mg,				
100s ea UD, C-IV	**00093-0832-93**	79.75		**AB**
500s ea, C-IV	**00093-0832-05**	374.50		**AB**
1000s ea, C-IV	**00093-0832-10**	749.00		**AB**
1 mg, 100s ea, C-IV	**00093-0833-01**	85.50		**AB**
(USP)				
1 mg,				
100s ea UD, C-IV	**00093-0833-93**	90.50		**AB**
500s ea, C-IV	**00093-0833-05**	427.50		**AB**
1000s ea, C-IV	**00093-0833-10**	855.00		**AB**
2 mg, 100s ea, C-IV	**00093-0834-01**	118.40		**AB**
(USP, 10X10)				
2 mg,				
100s ea UD, C-IV	**00093-0834-93**	124.00		**AB**
500s ea, C-IV	**00093-0834-05**	592.00		**AB**
(UDL)				
TAB, PO (10X10)				
0.5 mg,				
100s ea UD, C-IV	**51079-0881-20**	79.79		**AB**
(R.N.P., 5X20)				
0.5 mg,				
100s ea UD, C-IV	**51079-0881-21**	79.79		**AB**
(10X30 PUNCH CARDS)				
0.5 mg,				
300s ea UD, C-IV	**51079-0881-56**	239.37		**AB**
(10X10)				
1 mg,				
100s ea UD, C-IV	**51079-0882-20**	90.54		**AB**
(R.N.P., 5X20)				
1 mg,				
100s ea UD, C-IV	**51079-0882-21**	90.54		**AB**

PROD/MFR	NDC	AWP	DP	OBC
(10X30 PUNCH CARDS)				
1 mg,				
300s ea UD, C-IV	51079-0882-56	271.62		AB
(10X10)				
2 mg,				
100s ea UD, C-IV	51079-0883-20	124.05		AB
(4u)				
REPACK				
TAB, PO, 1 mg,				
30s ea, C-IV	10544-0408-30	41.46		AB
30s ea, C-IV	42549-0334-30	63.28		AB
30s ea, C-IV	42549-0534-30	41.46		AB
30s ea, C-IV	42549-0608-30	41.46		AB
(A-S Medication)				
REPACK				
TAB, PO, 0.5 mg,				
30s ea, C-IV	54569-5227-00	22.47		EE
60s ea, C-IV	54569-5227-01	44.94		EE
90s ea, C-IV	54569-5227-02	67.41		EE
1 mg, 30s ea, C-IV	54569-5126-01	25.65		EE
60s ea, C-IV	54569-5126-00	51.30		EE
90s ea, C-IV	54569-5126-02	76.95		EE
2 mg, 60s ea, C-IV	54569-5503-00	71.04		
(Aidarex)				
REPACK				
TAB, PO, 0.5 mg,				
30s ea, C-IV	33261-0340-30	39.00		AB
60s ea, C-IV	33261-0340-60	78.00		AB
90s ea, C-IV	33261-0340-90	117.00		AB
120s ea, C-IV	33261-0340-02	156.00		AB
1 mg, 7s ea, C-IV	33261-0029-07	11.90		AB
14s ea, C-IV	33261-0029-14	23.80		AB
20s ea, C-IV	33261-0029-20	34.00		AB
21s ea, C-IV	33261-0029-21	35.70		AB
28s ea, C-IV	33261-0029-28	47.60		AB
30s ea, C-IV	33261-0029-30	51.00		AB
40s ea, C-IV	33261-0029-40	68.00		AB
60s ea, C-IV	33261-0029-60	102.00		AB
90s ea, C-IV	33261-0029-90	153.00		AB
100s ea, C-IV	33261-0029-00	170.00		AB
120s ea, C-IV	33261-0029-02	204.00		AB
180s ea, C-IV	33261-0029-03	306.00		AB
2 mg, 30s ea, C-IV	33261-0628-30	64.50		AB
60s ea, C-IV	33261-0628-60	129.00		AB
90s ea, C-IV	33261-0628-90	193.50		AB
120s ea, C-IV	33261-0628-02	258.00		AB
(Altura)				
REPACK				
TAB, PO, 0.5 mg,				
15s ea, C-IV	63874-0286-15	11.24		AB
20s ea, C-IV	63874-0286-20	14.99		AB
28s ea, C-IV	63874-0286-28	20.99		AB
30s ea, C-IV	63874-0286-30	22.49		AB
60s ea, C-IV	63874-0286-60	47.21		AB
90s ea, C-IV	63874-0286-90	67.47		AB
100s ea, C-IV	63874-0286-01	74.97		AB
120s ea, C-IV	63874-0286-04	89.96		AB
150s ea, C-IV	63874-0286-72	118.02		AB
200s ea, C-IV	63874-0286-74	157.36		AB
300s ea, C-IV	63874-0286-77	236.04		AB
1 mg, 10s ea, C-IV	63874-0285-10	8.56		AB
15s ea, C-IV	63874-0285-15	12.83		AB
20s ea, C-IV	63874-0285-20	17.11		AB
28s ea, C-IV	63874-0285-28	23.95		AB
30s ea, C-IV	63874-0285-30	25.67		AB
60s ea, C-IV	63874-0285-60	51.33		AB
90s ea, C-IV	63874-0285-90	77.00		AB
100s ea, C-IV	63874-0285-01	85.55		AB
120s ea, C-IV	63874-0285-04	102.66		AB
150s ea, C-IV	63874-0285-72	134.63		AB
200s ea, C-IV	63874-0285-74	179.50		AB
300s ea, C-IV	63874-0285-77	269.25		AB
2 mg, 20s ea, C-IV	63874-1002-04	23.68		
28s ea, C-IV	63874-1002-08	33.15		
30s ea, C-IV	63874-1002-03	35.52		
60s ea, C-IV	63874-1002-06	71.04		
90s ea, C-IV	63874-1002-09	106.56		
100s ea, C-IV	63874-1002-01	118.40		
(Bryant Ranch)				
REPACK				
TAB, PO, 0.5 mg,				
20s ea, C-IV	63629-1341-01	19.99		
30s ea, C-IV	63629-1341-02	26.32		
60s ea, C-IV	63629-1341-03	52.92		
90s ea, C-IV	63629-1341-04	75.32		
1 mg, 20s ea, C-IV	63629-1340-01	21.86		
30s ea, C-IV	63629-1340-02	26.65		
60s ea, C-IV	63629-1340-03	61.18		AB
2 mg, 30s ea, C-IV	63629-3339-01	36.53		
60s ea, C-IV	63629-3339-02	69.68		

PROD/MFR	NDC	AWP	DP	OBC
(Core)				
REPACK				
TAB, PO, 0.5 mg,				
20s ea, C-IV	33358-0090-20	20.49		
30s ea, C-IV	33358-0090-30	26.98		
60s ea, C-IV	33358-0090-60	54.24		
90s ea, C-IV	33358-0090-90	77.20		
1 mg, 20s ea, C-IV	33358-0091-20	22.41		
30s ea, C-IV	33358-0091-30	27.32		
60s ea, C-IV	33358-0091-60	59.34		
(DHS, Inc.)				
REPACK				
TAB, PO, 0.5 mg,				
30s ea, C-IV	55887-0523-30	35.70		AB
60s ea, C-IV	55887-0523-60	46.86		AB
90s ea, C-IV	55887-0523-90	70.29		AB
1 mg, 30s ea, C-IV	55887-0448-30	33.99		AB
60s ea, C-IV	55887-0448-60	61.92		AB
90s ea, C-IV	55887-0448-90	84.66		AB
2 mg, 30s ea, C-IV	55887-0408-30	35.05		AB
90s ea, C-IV	55887-0408-90	89.00		AB
100s ea, C-IV	55887-0408-01	116.83		
(Dispensing Solutions)				
REPACK				
TAB, PO, 0.5 mg,				
20s ea, C-IV	55045-2661-07	14.60		AB
30s ea, C-IV	55045-2661-08	21.85		AB
30s ea, C-IV	66336-0980-30	35.70		AB
60s ea, C-IV	55045-2661-06	43.80		AB
60s ea, C-IV	66336-0980-60	71.40		
90s ea, C-IV	55045-2661-09	65.70		AB
90s ea, C-IV	66336-0980-90	107.10		AB
100s ea, C-IV	55045-2661-00	73.00		AB
120s ea, C-IV	55045-2661-01	87.60		AB
1 mg, 30s ea, C-IV	55045-2681-08	42.00		AB
30s ea, C-IV	66336-0588-30	30.78		AB
60s ea, C-IV	66336-0588-60	61.92		AB
90s ea, C-IV	55045-2681-09	126.00		AB
90s ea, C-IV	66336-0588-90	84.66		
100s ea, C-IV	55045-2681-00	140.00		AB
120s ea, C-IV	55045-2681-02	168.00		AB
2 mg, 30s ea, C-IV	55045-2650-08	43.50		AB
(GSMS)				
REPACK				
TAB, PO (UNIT OF USE)				
0.5 mg,				
30s ea, C-IV	60429-0524-30	6.15	2.05	AB
60s ea, C-IV	60429-0524-60	9.75	3.25	AB
90s ea, C-IV	60429-0524-90	70.76	19.00	AB
1 mg, 30s ea, C-IV	60429-0525-30	6.75	2.25	AB
60s ea, C-IV	60429-0525-60	10.95	3.65	AB
90s ea, C-IV	60429-0525-90	57.00	19.00	AB
(HomeMed)				
REPACK				
TAB, PO, 0.5 mg,				
30s ea, C-IV	51655-0864-24	38.99		
1 mg, 30s ea, C-IV	51655-0865-24	30.99		
(IPI)				
REPACK				
TAB, PO, 0.5 mg,				
60s ea, C-IV	18837-0029-60	57.13		
90s ea, C-IV	18837-0029-90	83.69		
1 mg, 30s ea, C-IV	18837-0030-30	25.53		AB
60s ea, C-IV	18837-0030-60	60.75		
90s ea, C-IV	18837-0030-90	76.58		AB
2 mg, 30s ea, C-IV	18837-0219-30	35.49		AB
60s ea, C-IV	18837-0219-60	91.50		
(Keltman Pharma., Inc.)				
REPACK				
TAB, PO, 0.5 mg,				
24s ea, C-IV	68387-0320-24	17.63		AB
30s ea, C-IV	68387-0320-30	22.04		
90s ea, C-IV	68387-0320-90	66.22		AB
1 mg, 30s ea, C-IV	68387-0323-30	31.35		
2 mg, 30s ea, C-IV	68387-0325-30	44.83		
(McKesson Packaging)				
REPACK				
TAB, PO (USP)				
0.5 mg,				
100s ea UD, C-IV	63739-0263-10	80.45		AB
1 mg,				
100s ea UD, C-IV	63739-0264-10	91.22		AB
(Nucare Pharm)				
REPACK				
TAB, PO, 0.5 mg,				
30s ea, C-IV	66267-0708-30	29.90		AB
60s ea, C-IV	66267-0708-60	58.58		AB
90s ea, C-IV	66267-0708-90	87.87		AB
1 mg, 30s ea, C-IV	66267-0748-30	33.42		AB
60s ea, C-IV	66267-0748-60	66.83		AB

PROD/MFR	NDC	AWP	DP	OBC
90s ea, C-IV	66267-0748-90	98.97		AB
2 mg, 30s ea, C-IV	66267-0904-30	50.33		AB
60s ea, C-IV	66267-0904-60	96.08		AB
90s ea, C-IV	66267-0904-90	144.11		AB
(Palmetto)				
REPACK				
TAB, PO, 0.5 mg,				
10s ea, C-IV	23490-5346-05	13.19		
30s ea, C-IV	23490-5346-01	39.56		
60s ea, C-IV	23490-5346-02	79.12		
90s ea, C-IV	23490-5346-09	118.68		
100s ea, C-IV	23490-5346-03	131.87		
120s ea, C-IV	23490-5346-08	142.42		
180s ea, C-IV	23490-5346-04	237.36		
1 mg, 30s ea, C-IV	23490-5347-01	36.00		
60s ea, C-IV	23490-5347-06	72.00		
90s ea, C-IV	23490-5347-02	108.00		
100s ea, C-IV	23490-5347-03	120.00		
120s ea, C-IV	23490-5347-04	144.00		
180s ea, C-IV	23490-5347-05	216.00		
2 mg, 30s ea, C-IV	23490-5348-02	51.38		
60s ea, C-IV	23490-5348-06	102.76		
100s ea, C-IV	23490-5348-03	171.27		
(PD-Rx Pharm)				
REPACK				
TAB, PO, 0.5 mg,				
14s ea, C-IV	55289-0599-14	32.66		AB
21s ea, C-IV	55289-0599-21	34.96		EE
30s ea, C-IV	55289-0599-30	38.00		EE
(USP)				
0.5 mg,				
60s ea, C-IV	55289-0599-60	47.44		AB
90s ea, C-IV	55289-0599-90	61.60		AB
1 mg, 30s ea, C-IV	55289-0562-30	49.68		AB
60s ea, C-IV	55289-0562-60	58.67		AB
90s ea, C-IV	55289-0562-90	79.20		AB
120s ea, C-IV	55289-0562-98	90.64		AB
2 mg, 30s ea, C-IV	55289-0065-30	49.68		AB
(Pharma Pac)				
REPACK				
TAB, PO, 0.5 mg,				
30s ea, C-IV	52959-0009-30	31.79		AB
60s ea, C-IV	52959-0009-60	63.57		
90s ea, C-IV	52959-0009-90	95.33		
100s ea, C-IV	52959-0009-00	105.84		
120s ea, C-IV	52959-0009-12	127.05		
1 mg, 30s ea, C-IV	52959-0630-30	34.30		AB
60s ea, C-IV	52959-0630-60	67.25		AB
90s ea, C-IV	52959-0630-90	100.85		
100s ea, C-IV	52959-0630-00	112.05		
120s ea, C-IV	52959-0630-02	134.43		
180s ea, C-IV	52959-0630-18	201.59		
2 mg, 10s ea, C-IV	52959-0761-10	12.49		AB
30s ea, C-IV	52959-0761-30	37.48		AB
60s ea, C-IV	52959-0761-60	74.98		AB
100s ea, C-IV	52959-0761-00	124.50		
120s ea, C-IV	52959-0761-02	149.52		
(Phys Total Care)				
REPACK				
TAB, PO, 0.5 mg,				
30s ea, C-IV	54868-3854-02	7.41		EE
45s ea, C-IV	54868-3854-06	10.38		AB
60s ea, C-IV	54868-3854-01	10.35		EE
90s ea, C-IV	54868-3854-05	13.26		AB
100s ea, C-IV	54868-3854-04	12.75		EE
(USP)				
1 mg, 20s ea, C-IV	54868-3855-07	6.04		EE
30s ea, C-IV	54868-3855-04	9.06		EE
40s ea, C-IV	54868-3855-06	10.56		AB
60s ea, C-IV	54868-3855-05	13.62		EE
90s ea, C-IV	54868-3855-03	18.18		EE
100s ea, C-IV	54868-3855-01	19.68		EE
150s ea, C-IV	54868-3855-08	23.88		AB
2 mg, 30s ea, C-IV	54868-3861-04	10.86		
60s ea, C-IV	54868-3861-01	17.25		AB
100s ea, C-IV	54868-3861-02	24.24		AB
120s ea, C-IV	54868-3861-05	29.88		AB
1000s ea, C-IV	54868-3861-03	170.64		AB
(Physician Partner)				
REPACK				
TAB, PO, 0.5 mg,				
30s ea, C-IV	21695-0260-30	38.54		
60s ea, C-IV	21695-0260-60	77.08		
90s ea, C-IV	21695-0260-90	115.61		
100s ea, C-IV	21695-0260-00	147.74		
120s ea, C-IV	21695-0260-72	154.15		
1 mg, 30s ea, C-IV	21695-0261-30	43.96		
60s ea, C-IV	21695-0261-60	87.92		
90s ea, C-IV	21695-0261-90	131.88		
100s ea, C-IV	21695-0261-00	162.82		
120s ea, C-IV	21695-0261-72	175.84		
2 mg, 30s ea, C-IV	21695-0262-30	60.92		
60s ea, C-IV	21695-0262-60	121.84		

PROD/MFR	NDC	AWP	DP	OBC
(Quality Care Prod)				
REPACK				
TAB, PO, 0.5 mg,				
30s ea, C-IV	**49999-0328-30**	38.99		**AB**
60s ea, C-IV	**49999-0328-60**	77.98		**AB**
90s ea, C-IV	**49999-0328-90**	116.97		**AB**
120s ea, C-IV	**49999-0328-01**	155.96		**AB**
1 mg, 30s ea, C-IV	**49999-0121-30**	32.40		**AB**
60s ea, C-IV	**49999-0121-60**	64.80		**AB**
90s ea, C-IV	**49999-0121-90**	97.20		**AB**
100s ea, C-IV	**49999-0121-00**	108.00		
2 mg, 30s ea, C-IV	**49999-0518-30**	44.77		**AB**
60s ea, C-IV	**49999-0518-60**	89.54		
(Southwood)				
REPACK				
TAB, PO, 0.5 mg,				
15s ea, C-IV	**58016-0183-15**	11.80		**EE**
20s ea, C-IV	**58016-0183-20**	15.74		**EE**
28s ea, C-IV	**58016-0183-28**	22.03		**EE**
30s ea, C-IV	**58016-0183-30**	23.60		**EE**
60s ea, C-IV	**58016-0183-60**	47.21		**EE**
90s ea, C-IV	**58016-0183-90**	70.81		**EE**
100s ea, C-IV	**58016-0183-00**	78.68		**EE**
120s ea, C-IV	**58016-0183-02**	94.42		**EE**
150s ea, C-IV	**58016-0183-03**	118.02		**AB**
200s ea, C-IV	**58016-0183-89**	157.36		**AB**
300s ea, C-IV	**58016-0183-73**	236.04		**AB**
1 mg, 15s ea, C-IV	**58016-0186-15**	13.46		**AB**
20s ea, C-IV	**58016-0186-20**	17.95		**AB**
28s ea, C-IV	**58016-0186-28**	25.13		**AB**
30s ea, C-IV	**58016-0186-30**	26.93		**AB**
60s ea, C-IV	**58016-0186-60**	53.85		**AB**
90s ea, C-IV	**58016-0186-90**	80.78		**AB**
100s ea, C-IV	**58016-0186-00**	89.75		**AB**
120s ea, C-IV	**58016-0186-02**	107.70		**AB**
150s ea, C-IV	**58016-0186-03**	134.63		**AB**
200s ea, C-IV	**58016-0186-89**	179.50		**AB**
300s ea, C-IV	**58016-0186-73**	269.25		**AB**
2 mg, 10s ea, C-IV	**58016-0719-10**	12.44		**AB**
12s ea, C-IV	**58016-0719-12**	14.92		**AB**
15s ea, C-IV	**58016-0719-15**	18.65		**AB**
20s ea, C-IV	**58016-0719-20**	24.87		**AB**
25s ea, C-IV	**58016-0719-25**	31.09		**AB**
30s ea, C-IV	**58016-0719-30**	37.31		**AB**
40s ea, C-IV	**58016-0719-40**	49.74		**AB**
50s ea, C-IV	**58016-0719-50**	62.18		**AB**
60s ea, C-IV	**58016-0719-60**	74.61		**AB**
70s ea, C-IV	**58016-0719-70**	87.05		**AB**
80s ea, C-IV	**58016-0719-80**	99.48		**AB**
90s ea, C-IV	**58016-0719-90**	111.92		**AB**
100s ea, C-IV	**58016-0719-00**	124.35		**AB**
120s ea, C-IV	**58016-0719-02**	149.22		**AB**
150s ea, C-IV	**58016-0719-03**	186.53		**AB**
200s ea, C-IV	**58016-0719-89**	248.70		**AB**
300s ea, C-IV	**58016-0719-73**	373.05		**AB**
(St. Mary's MPP)				
REPACK				
TAB, PO, 0.5 mg,				
30s ea, C-IV	**60760-0273-30**	30.68		**AB**
1 mg, 30s ea, C-IV	**60760-0300-30**	32.82		**AB**
(Stat Rx)				
REPACK				
TAB, PO, 0.5 mg,				
28s ea, C-IV	**16590-0058-28**	26.06		**AB**
30s ea, C-IV	**16590-0058-30**	52.88		
56s ea, C-IV	**16590-0058-56**	53.02		**AB**
60s ea, C-IV	**16590-0058-60**	105.75		
90s ea, C-IV	**16590-0058-90**	158.62		
120s ea, C-IV	**16590-0058-72**	113.61		**AB**
1 mg, 12s ea, C-IV	**16590-0059-12**	13.70		
20s ea, C-IV	**16590-0059-20**	22.84		
28s ea, C-IV	**16590-0059-28**	28.28		**AB**
30s ea, C-IV	**16590-0059-30**	34.25		
45s ea, C-IV	**16590-0059-45**	45.45		**AB**
56s ea, C-IV	**16590-0059-56**	56.70		**AB**
60s ea, C-IV	**16590-0059-60**	68.50		
75s ea, C-IV	**16590-0059-75**	75.75		**AB**
84s ea, C-IV	**16590-0059-62**	87.98		**AB**
90s ea, C-IV	**16590-0059-90**	102.75		
120s ea, C-IV	**16590-0059-72**	126.00		**AB**
180s ea, C-IV	**16590-0059-82**	18.15		**AB**
2 mg, 12s ea, C-IV	**16590-0481-12**	13.80		
20s ea, C-IV	**16590-0481-20**	23.00		
28s ea, C-IV	**16590-0481-28**	42.23		**AB**
30s ea, C-IV	**16590-0481-30**	34.50		
45s ea, C-IV	**16590-0481-45**	68.85		**AB**
60s ea, C-IV	**16590-0481-60**	69.00		
75s ea, C-IV	**16590-0481-75**	114.75		**AB**
90s ea, C-IV	**16590-0481-90**	87.50		
120s ea, C-IV	**16590-0481-72**	92.25		
CLONIDINE				
(Boehr Ingelheim Phar) *See CATAPRES-TTS-1*				
(Boehr Ingelheim Phar) *See CATAPRES-TTS-2*				
(Boehr Ingelheim Phar) *See CATAPRES-TTS-3*				
(Par)				
TDM, TD, 0.1 mg/24 hr,				
4s ea	**49884-0774-86**	115.23		**AB**
0.2 mg/24 hr, 4s ea	**49884-0775-86**	193.99		**AB**
0.3 mg/24 hr, 4s ea	**49884-0776-86**	269.13		**AB**
(Bryant Ranch)				
REPACK				
clonidine hydrochloride				
TAB, PO, 0.2 mg, 30s ea	**63629-2753-01**	12.97		
60s ea	**63629-2753-02**	25.93		
100s ea	**63629-2753-03**	43.22		
(DHS, Inc.)				
REPACK				
TAB, PO, 0.2 mg, 100s ea	**55887-0475-01**	44.83		
(IPI)				
REPACK				
TAB, PO, 0.1 mg, 30s ea	**18837-0272-30**	17.82		
(PD-Rx Pharm)				
REPACK				
TAB, PO, 0.3 mg, 30s ea	**55289-0970-30**	30.75		
(Physician Partner)				
REPACK				
TAB, PO, 0.1 mg, 30s ea	**21695-0371-30**	25.23		
(Stat Rx)				
REPACK				
TAB, PO, 0.1 mg, 30s ea	**16590-0266-30**	12.00		
60s ea	**16590-0266-60**	24.00		
90s ea	**16590-0266-90**	36.00		
(Vibranta)				
REPACK				
TAB, PO, 0.2 mg, 180s ea	**57866-3524-04**	65.09		
CLONIDINE HCL (Actavis)				
clonidine hydrochloride				
TAB, PO, 0.1 mg, 100s ea	**00228-2127-10**	25.90		**AB**
500s ea	**00228-2127-50**	126.91		**AB**
0.2 mg, 100s ea	**00228-2128-10**	37.55		**AB**
500s ea	**00228-2128-50**	184.00		**AB**
(Consolidated Midland)				
TAB, PO, 0.1 mg, 100s ea	**00223-0660-01**	3.25		**EE**
1000s ea	**00223-0660-02**	24.50		**EE**
0.2 mg, 100s ea	**00223-0661-01**	4.25		**EE**
1000s ea	**00223-0661-02**	29.50		**EE**
0.3 mg, 100s ea	**00223-0662-01**	4.75		**EE**
1000s ea	**00223-0662-02**	32.50		**EE**
(Gallipot)				
POW, NA (U.S.P.)				
1 gm	**51552-0480-01**	30.80		
5 gm	**51552-0480-02**	117.60		
(Hawkins)				
POW, NA (USP)				
1 gm	**63370-0052-10**	100.80		
1 gm	**63370-0052-15**	384.00		
25 gm	**63370-0052-25**	1200.00		
(Letco)				
POW, NA (U.S.P.)				
1 gm	**62991-1422-01**	54.00		
5 gm	**62991-1422-02**	204.00		
(Major)				
TAB, PO (10X10)				
0.1 mg, 100s ea UD	**00904-5656-61**	23.45		
0.2 mg, 100s ea UD	**00904-5657-61**	32.13		**AB**
0.3 mg, 100s ea UD	**00904-5658-61**	47.22		**AB**
(Medisca)				
POW, NA (U.S.P.)				
1 gm	**38779-0561-06**	76.50		
5 gm	**38779-0561-03**	265.50		
10 gm	**38779-0561-01**	520.50		
25 gm	**38779-0561-04**	987.00		
(USP,1X100GM)				
100 gm	**38779-0561-05**	2475.00		
(Mutual)				
TAB, PO, 0.1 mg, 100s ea	**53489-0215-01**	25.90		**AB**
1000s ea	**53489-0215-10**	208.43		**AB**
0,2 mg, 100s ea	**53489-0216-01**	37.55		**AB**
1000s ea	**53489-0216-10**	308.70		**AB**
0.3 mg, 100s ea	**53489-0217-01**	52.40		**AB**
(Mylan)				
TAB, PO, 0.1 mg, 100s ea	**00378-0152-01**	21.60		**AB**
1000s ea	**00378-0152-10**	208.43		**AB**
0.2 mg, 100s ea	**00378-0186-01**	31.75		**AB**
1000s ea	**00378-0186-10**	308.70		**AB**
0.3 mg, 100s ea	**00378-0199-01**	46.60		**AB**
(PCCA)				
POW, NA (U.S.P.)				
1 gm	**51927-2379-00**	99.00		
(Spectrum Pharmacy)				
POW, NA (U.S.P.)				
1 gm	**49452-2147-02**	116.20		
5 gm	**49452-2147-03**	402.50		
25 gm	**49452-2147-04**	1253.00		
(UDL)				
TAB, PO (ROBOT READY 25X1)				
0.1 mg, 25s ea UD	**51079-0299-19**	5.90		**AB**
(10X10)				
0.1 mg, 100s ea UD	**51079-0299-20**	23.62		**AB**
(ROBOT READY 25X1)				
0.2 mg, 25s ea UD	**51079-0300-19**	8.11		**AB**
(10X10)				
0.2 mg, 100s ea UD	**51079-0300-20**	32.45		**AB**
(10X30 PUNCH CARDS)				
0.2 mg, 300s ea UD	**51079-0300-56**	97.35		**AB**
(10X10)				
0.3 mg, 100s ea UD	**51079-0301-20**	47.70		**AB**
(A-S Medication)				
REPACK				
TAB, PO, 0.1 mg, 30s ea	**54569-0478-00**	7.77		**EE**
60s ea	**54569-0478-01**	15.54		**EE**
90s ea	**54569-0478-07**	23.31		**EE**
100s ea	**54569-0478-02**	25.90		**EE**
0.2 mg, 15s ea	**54569-1853-04**	5.63		**EE**
30s ea	**54569-1853-00**	11.27		**EE**
60s ea	**54569-1853-01**	22.53		**EE**
(Aidarex)				
REPACK				
TAB, PO, 0.1 mg, 30s ea	**33261-0495-30**	41.10		**AB**
60s ea	**33261-0495-60**	82.20		**AB**
90s ea	**33261-0495-90**	123.30		**AB**
120s ea	**33261-0495-02**	164.40		**AB**
(American Health)				
REPACK				
TAB, PO (10X10)				
0.1 mg, 100s ea UD	**62584-0657-01**	23.30		**AB**
0.2 mg, 100s ea UD	**62584-0339-01**	32.35		**AB**
0.3 mg, 100s ea UD	**62584-0659-01**	47.50		**AB**
(B&B Pharm, Inc)				
REPACK				
POW, NA (BULK COMPOUND)				
1 gm	**63275-9974-01**	53.00		
5 gm	**63275-9974-02**	207.00		
10 gm	**63275-9974-03**	330.00		
(DHS, Inc.)				
REPACK				
TAB, PO, 0.1 mg, 30s ea	**55887-0738-30**	16.77		**AB**
60s ea	**55887-0738-60**	32.00		**AB**
90s ea	**55887-0738-90**	48.00		**AB**
0.2 mg, 10s ea	**55887-0475-10**	6.00		**AB**
30s ea	**55887-0475-30**	13.45		**AB**
60s ea	**55887-0475-60**	23.00		**AB**
90s ea	**55887-0475-90**	33.66		**AB**
(Dispensing Solutions)				
REPACK				
TAB, PO, 0.1 mg, 30s ea	**55045-1167-08**	6.00		**AB**
30s ea	**66336-0786-30**	20.23		**AB**
60s ea	**55045-1167-09**	12.00		**AB**
60s ea	**66336-0786-60**	33.72		**AB**
90s ea	**55045-1167-06**	18.00		**AB**
90s ea	**66336-0786-90**	60.70		**AB**
100s ea	**55045-1770-01**	20.00		**AB**
0.2 mg, 60s ea	**66336-0787-60**	45.55		**AB**
90s ea	**66336-0787-90**	68.33		**AB**
(HomeMed)				
REPACK				
TAB, PO, 0.1 mg, 10s ea	**51655-0353-53**	3.44		**EE**
30s ea	**51655-0353-24**	35.26		**EE**
60s ea	**51655-0353-25**	70.52		**EE**
0.2 mg, 30s ea	**51655-0362-24**	41.08		**EE**
60s ea	**51655-0362-25**	82.16		**EE**
(McKesson Packaging)				
REPACK				
TAB, PO (USP)				
0.1 mg, 100s ea UD	**63739-0060-10**	31.73		**AB**
0.2 mg, 100s ea UD	**63739-0061-10**	45.95		**AB**
(Nucare Pharm)				
REPACK				
TAB, PO, 0.1 mg, 30s ea	**66267-0061-30**	16.72		**AB**
60s ea	**66267-0061-60**	33.43		**AB**
90s ea	**66267-0061-90**	50.15		**AB**
120s ea	**66267-0061-91**	66.87		**AB**
0.2 mg, 14s ea	**66267-0062-14**	10.94		**AB**
30s ea	**66267-0062-30**	23.44		**AB**

PROD/MFR	NDC	AWP	DP	OBC
60s ea	66267-0062-60	46.89		AB
90s ea	66267-0062-90	70.33		AB
180s ea	66267-0062-92	140.66		AB
(PD-Rx Pharm)				
REPACK				
TAB, PO, 0.1 mg, 8s ea	55289-0073-08	20.67		AB
(USP)				
0.1 mg, 20s ea	55289-0073-20	26.25		AB
28s ea	58864-0633-28	30.67		AB
30s ea	55289-0073-30	30.00		AB
(REDI-SCRIPT)				
0.1 mg, 30s ea	58864-0110-30	30.00		AB
60s ea	55289-0073-60	43.33		AB
90s ea	55289-0073-90	56.67		AB
100s ea	55289-0073-01	57.50		AB
(USP)				
0.1 mg, 180s ea	55289-0073-93	84.50		AB
0.2 mg, 30s ea	55289-0074-30	32.89		AB
60s ea	55289-0074-60	50.00		AB
(USP)				
0.2 mg, 90s ea	55289-0074-90	67.00		AB
(Pharma Pac)				
REPACK				
TAB, PO, 0.1 mg, 5s ea	52959-0718-05	4.75		AB
12s ea	52959-0718-12	11.39		AB
30s ea	52959-0718-30	28.47		AB
60s ea	52959-0718-60	56.92		AB
90s ea	52959-0718-90	85.35		AB
100s ea	52959-0718-00	94.82		AB
(Phys Total Care)				
REPACK				
TAB, PO, 0.1 mg, 5s ea	54868-0048-06	3.93		EE
15s ea	54868-0048-07	5.82		AB
20s ea	54868-0048-01	6.75		EE
30s ea	54868-0048-05	8.61		EE
60s ea	54868-0048-02	14.25		EE
90s ea	54868-0048-08	19.86		AB
100s ea	54868-0048-03	21.75		EE
100s ea	54868-0048-09	38.88		EE
500s ea	54868-0048-00	80.65		EE
0.2 mg, 30s ea	54868-0049-02	11.83		EE
60s ea	54868-0049-05	18.33		EE
90s ea	54868-0049-01	26.01		AB
100s ea	54868-0049-03	32.45		EE
1000s ea	54868-0049-00	258.69		EE
0.3 mg, 30s ea	54868-1967-02	14.76		EE
60s ea	54868-1967-00	22.47		AB
90s ea	54868-1967-03	31.47		AB
100s ea	54868-1967-04	32.95		EE
(Physician Partner)				
REPACK				
TAB, PO, 0.1 mg, 15s ea	21695-0371-15	12.62		AB
90s ea	21695-0371-90	75.69		AB
100s ea	21695-0371-00	51.80		AB
0.2 mg, 30s ea	21695-0372-30	27.53		
90s ea	21695-0372-90	82.59		AB
0.3 mg, 30s ea	21695-0377-30	31.44		AB
(Quality Care Prod)				
REPACK				
TAB, PO, 0.1 mg, 4s ea	49999-0127-04	3.72		AB
12s ea	49999-0127-12	11.16		EE
20s ea	49999-0127-20	18.60		AB
30s ea	49999-0127-30	27.90		AB
90s ea	49999-0127-90	86.40		AB
100s ea	49999-0127-00	93.00		EE
0.2 mg, 90s ea	49999-0258-90	92.66		EE
0.3 mg, 30s ea	49999-0438-30	17.70		EE
100s ea	49999-0438-00	59.04		AB
(Southwood)				
REPACK				
TAB, PO, 0.1 mg, 30s ea	58016-0517-30	16.80		EE
60s ea	58016-0517-60	33.60		EE
90s ea	58016-0517-90	50.40		AB
100s ea	58016-0517-00	56.00		EE
120s ea	58016-0517-02	67.20		AB
180s ea	58016-0517-99	100.88		AB
(Vibranta)				
REPACK				
TAB, PO, 0.1 mg, 30s ea	57866-3523-01	20.25		AB
0.2 mg, 30s ea	57866-3524-01	30.89		AB
0.3 mg, 30s ea	57866-3526-01	17.70		AB
CLONIDINE HYDROCHLORIDE				
FUL				
TAB, PO, 0.1 mg, 100s ea		10.50		
0.2 mg, 100s ea		14.10		
0.3 mg, 100s ea		18.15		
(Actavis) *See CLONIDINE HCL*				
(Actavis)				
TAB, PO, 0.3 mg, 100s ea	00228-2129-10	52.40		AB

PROD/MFR	NDC	AWP	DP	OBC
(Bioniche Pharma) *See DURACLON*				
(Boehr Ingelheim Phar) *See CATAPRES*				
(Consolidated Midland) *See CLONIDINE HCL*				
(Dava Pharma)				
TAB, PO, 0.1 mg, 100s ea	67253-0263-10	25.90		
1000s ea	67253-0263-11	208.43		
0.2 mg, 100s ea	67253-0264-10	37.55		
1000s ea	67253-0264-11	308.70		
0.3 mg, 100s ea	67253-0265-10	52.40		
(Gallipot) *See CLONIDINE HCL*				
(Hawkins) *See CLONIDINE HCL*				
(Letco) *See CLONIDINE HCL*				
(Major) *See CLONIDINE HCL*				
(Medisca) *See CLONIDINE HCL*				
(Mutual) *See CLONIDINE HCL*				
(Mylan) *See CLONIDINE HCL*				
(PCCA) *See CLONIDINE HCL*				
(Qualitest)				
TAB, PO, 0.1 mg, 100s ea	00603-2957-21	25.90		AB
500s ea	00603-2957-28	123.03		AB
1000s ea	00603-2957-32	208.43		AB
0.2 mg, 100s ea	00603-2958-21	37.55		AB
500s ea	00603-2958-28	184.00		AB
1000s ea	00603-2958-32	308.70		AB
0.3 mg, 100s ea	00603-2959-21	52.40		AB
500s ea	00603-2959-28	248.90		AB
(Spectrum Pharmacy) *See CLONIDINE HCL*				
(UDL) *See CLONIDINE HCL*				
(UDL)				
TAB, PO (USP)				
0.1 mg, 30s ea	51079-0299-63	7.09		AB
0.2 mg, 30s ea	51079-0300-63	9.74		AB
0.3 mg, 30s ea	51079-0301-63	14.31		AB
(Altura)				
REPACK				
TAB, PO, 0.1 mg, 10s ea	63874-0475-10	5.88		
12s ea	63874-0475-12	7.06		
15s ea	63874-0475-15	8.82		
20s ea	63874-0475-20	11.76		
28s ea	63874-0475-28	16.46		
30s ea	63874-0475-30	17.63		
60s ea	63874-0475-60	35.39		
90s ea	63874-0475-90	85.95		
100s ea	63874-0475-01	58.98		
180s ea	63874-0475-81	106.16		
1000s ea	63874-0475-02	589.83		
0.2 mg, 10s ea	63874-0474-10	9.01		
12s ea	63874-0474-12	10.80		
14s ea	63874-0474-14	12.61		
15s ea	63874-0474-15	13.50		
20s ea	63874-0474-20	18.01		
21s ea	63874-0474-21	18.91		
24s ea	63874-0474-24	21.61		
28s ea	63874-0474-28	25.21		
30s ea	63874-0474-30	27.02		
40s ea	63874-0474-40	36.02		
60s ea	63874-0474-60	54.03		
180s ea	63874-0474-81	162.08		
1000s ea	63874-0474-02	901.00		
(Bryant Ranch)				
REPACK				
TAB, PO, 0.1 mg, 20s ea	63629-1328-03	12.84		
30s ea	63629-1328-02	18.75		
100s ea	63629-1328-01	62.18		
(Core)				
REPACK				
TAB, PO, 0.1 mg, 30s ea	33358-0092-30	19.22		
100s ea	33358-0092-00	63.73		
0.2 mg, 30s ea	33358-0093-30	13.29		
60s ea	33358-0093-60	26.58		
(Dispensing Solutions)				
REPACK				
TAB, PO, 0.2 mg, 30s ea	66336-0787-30	22.78		
100s ea	55045-1656-01	40.00		
0.3 mg, 100s ea	55045-3448-01	60.00		
(Nucare Pharm)				
REPACK				
TAB, PO, 0.3 mg, 30s ea	66267-0464-30	32.72		
60s ea	66267-0464-60	65.50		
(Palmetto)				
REPACK				
TAB, PO, 0.1 mg, 12s ea	23490-5351-01	8.40		
30s ea	23490-5351-02	21.00		
60s ea	23490-5351-03	42.00		

PROD/MFR	NDC	AWP	DP	OBC
90s ea	23490-5351-04	63.00		
0.2 mg, 30s ea	23490-5352-01	27.00		
60s ea	23490-5352-02	54.00		
90s ea	23490-5352-03	81.00		
0.3 mg, 60s ea	23490-5353-01	39.60		
(Pharma Pac)				
REPACK				
TAB, PO, 0.1 mg, 40s ea	52959-0718-40	37.95		
0.2 mg, 30s ea	52959-0788-30	29.40		
(Quality Care Prod)				
REPACK				
TAB, PO, 0.2 mg, 30s ea	49999-0258-30	30.89		
100s ea	49999-0258-00	102.97		
CLOPIDOGREL HYDROGEN SULFATE				
(Bristol-Myers) *See PLAVIX*				
CLORAZEPATE (Dispensing Solutions)				
REPACK				
clorazepate dipotassium				
TAB, PO, 3.75 mg,				
60s ea, C-IV	55045-3751-01	76.80		
7.5 mg,				
30s ea, C-IV	55045-2170-08	48.00		
60s ea, C-IV	55045-2170-06	96.00		
15 mg,				
60s ea, C-IV	55045-3744-06	130.20		
(Keltman Pharma., Inc.)				
REPACK				
TAB, PO, 7.5 mg,				
90s ea, C-IV	68387-0511-90	166.47		
(Physician Partner)				
REPACK				
TAB, PO, 3.75 mg,				
56s ea, C-IV	21695-0433-56	169.21		
60s ea, C-IV	21695-0433-60	154.10		
90s ea, C-IV	21695-0433-90	231.16		
CLORAZEPATE DIPOTASSIUM				
FUL				
TAB, PO, 3.75 mg,				
100s ea		13.77		
7.5 mg, 100s ea		19.47		
15 mg, 100s ea		27.54		
(Lundbeck) *See TRANXENE T-TAB*				
(Lundbeck) *See TRANXENE-SD*				
(Mylan)				
TAB, PO, 3.75 mg,				
100s ea, C-IV	00378-0030-01	128.42		AB
500s ea, C-IV	00378-0030-05	629.16		AB
7.5 mg,				
100s ea, C-IV	00378-0040-01	159.71		AB
500s ea, C-IV	00378-0040-05	782.78		AB
15 mg, 100s ea, C-IV	00378-0070-01	217.25		AB
(Ranbaxy Pharm)				
TAB, PO, 3.75 mg,				
100s ea, C-IV	63304-0552-01	128.45		AB
500s ea, C-IV	63304-0552-05	629.19		AB
7.5 mg,				
100s ea, C-IV	63304-0553-01	159.71		AB
500s ea, C-IV	63304-0553-05	782.18		AB
15 mg, 100s ea, C-IV	63304-0554-01	217.25		AB
(Taro)				
TAB, PO, 3.75 mg,				
100s ea, C-IV	51672-4042-01	128.41		AB
500s ea, C-IV	51672-4042-02	629.15		AB
7.5 mg,				
100s ea, C-IV	51672-4043-01	159.70		AB
500s ea, C-IV	51672-4043-02	782.77		AB
15 mg, 100s ea, C-IV	51672-4044-01	217.24		AB
(Aidarex)				
REPACK				
TAB, PO, 3.75 mg,				
7s ea, C-IV	33261-0030-07	19.25		AB
10s ea, C-IV	33261-0030-10	27.50		AB
14s ea, C-IV	33261-0030-14	38.50		AB
20s ea, C-IV	33261-0030-20	55.00		AB
21s ea, C-IV	33261-0030-21	57.75		AB
28s ea, C-IV	33261-0030-28	77.00		AB
30s ea, C-IV	33261-0030-30	82.50		AB
40s ea, C-IV	33261-0030-40	110.00		AB
60s ea, C-IV	33261-0030-60	165.00		AB
7.5 mg, 10s ea, C-IV	33261-0031-10	30.00		AB
14s ea, C-IV	33261-0031-14	42.00		AB
20s ea, C-IV	33261-0031-20	60.00		AB
21s ea, C-IV	33261-0031-21	63.00		AB
28s ea, C-IV	33261-0031-28	84.00		AB
30s ea, C-IV	33261-0031-30	90.00		AB
60s ea, C-IV	33261-0031-60	180.00		AB

PROD/MFR	NDC	AWP	DP	OBC
90s ea, C-IV	33261-0031-90	270.00		AB
15 mg, 7s ea, C-IV	33261-0032-07	25.20		AB
14s ea, C-IV	33261-0032-14	50.40		AB
20s ea, C-IV	33261-0032-20	72.00		AB
21s ea, C-IV	33261-0032-21	75.60		AB
28s ea, C-IV	33261-0032-28	100.80		AB
30s ea, C-IV	33261-0032-30	108.00		AB
40s ea, C-IV	33261-0032-40	144.00		AB
60s ea, C-IV	33261-0032-60	216.00		AB
(Altura)				
REPACK				
TAB, PO, 3.75 mg,				
30s ea, C-IV	63874-1242-03	32.30		AB
60s ea, C-IV	63874-1242-06	64.59		AB
7.5 mg, 30s ea, C-IV	63874-1239-03	63.99		AB
60s ea, C-IV	63874-1239-06	127.98		AB
(DHS, Inc.)				
REPACK				
TAB, PO, 3.75 mg,				
30s ea, C-IV	55887-0157-30	38.53		
7.5 mg, 30s ea, C-IV	55887-0158-30	47.91		
60s ea, C-IV	55887-0158-60	159.70		
15 mg, 30s ea, C-IV	55887-0159-30	65.17		
(Dispensing Solutions)				
REPACK				
TAB, PO, 7.5 mg,				
30s ea, C-IV	68258-7012-03	47.91		AB
(Keltman Pharma., Inc.)				
REPACK				
TAB, PO, 7.5 mg,				
90s ea, C-IV	68387-0510-90	143.74		AB
(Palmetto)				
REPACK				
TAB, PO, 3.75 mg,				
30s ea, C-IV	23490-5262-03	40.50		
CLORAZEPATE DIPOTASSIUM (Palmetto)				
7.5 mg,				
30s ea, C-IV	23490-5263-03	48.07		
15 mg,				
30s ea, C-IV	23490-5261-03	63.99		
CLORAZEPATE DIPOTASSIUM (PD-Rx Pharm)				
REPACK				
TAB, PO, 7.5 mg,				
12s ea, C-IV	43063-0164-12	25.26		AB
15 mg, 3s ea, C-IV	43063-0030-03	10.95		AB
6s ea, C-IV	43063-0030-06	12.96		AB
10s ea, C-IV	43063-0030-10	15.63		AB
12s ea, C-IV	46063-0030-12	18.27		AB
(Pharma Pac)				
REPACK				
TAB, PO, 3.75 mg,				
30s ea, C-IV	52959-0873-30	15.96		
60s ea, C-IV	52959-0873-60	32.16		
7.5 mg, 30s ea, C-IV	52959-0874-30	25.97		
60s ea, C-IV	52959-0874-60	52.17		
(Phys Total Care)				
REPACK				
TAB, PO, 3.75 mg,				
30s ea, C-IV	54868-2133-02	15.36		EE
50s ea, C-IV	54868-2133-01	21.57		EE
90s ea, C-IV	54868-2133-03	34.05		EE
100s ea, C-IV	54868-2133-00	37.14		EE
7.5 mg, 30s ea, C-IV	54868-0802-03	25.88		EE
50s ea, C-IV	54868-0802-00	31.74		EE
60s ea, C-IV	54868-0802-01	47.25		EE
CLORAZEPATE DIPOTASSIUM (Phys Total Care)				
REPACK				
TAB, PO, 7.5 mg,				
100s ea, C-IV	54868-0802-02	57.48		EE
(Quality Care Prod)				
REPACK				
TAB, PO, 7.5 mg,				
100s ea, C-IV	49999-0674-00	192.28		AB
(Stat Rx)				
REPACK				
TAB, PO, 7.5 mg,				
60s ea, C-IV	16590-0759-60	18.12		AB
90s ea, C-IV	16590-0759-90	25.88		AB
180s ea, C-IV	16590-0759-82	44.95		AB
270s ea, C-IV	16590-0759-86	431.19		AB
CLORPRES (Mylan)				
chlorthalidone/clonidine hydrochloride				
TAB, PO, 15 mg-0.3 mg,				
100s ea	00378-0072-01	219.53		
(Mylan Bertek)				
TAB, PO, 15 mg-0.1 mg,				
100s ea	62794-0001-01	134.17		AB
15 mg-0.2 mg,				
100s ea	62794-0027-01	179.48		AB
(Phys Total Care)				
REPACK				
TAB, PO, 15 mg-0.1 mg,				
10s ea	54868-1888-01	13.60		AB
30s ea	54868-1888-00	37.06		AB
15 mg-0.2 mg,				
10s ea	54868-5267-01	17.56		AB
30s ea	54868-5267-00	48.95		AB
CLORSULON (Spectrum Pharmacy)				
POW, NA, 100 gm	49452-2153-01	1015.00		
CLOTRIMAZOLE				
FUL				
SOL, TP, 1%, 10 ml		4.73		
(Fougera)				
CRE, TP (USP,1X15GM)				
1%, 15 gm	00168-0133-15	19.90		AB
(USP,1X30GM)				
1%, 30 gm	00168-0133-30	34.81		AB
(USP,1X45GM)				
1%, 45 gm	00168-0133-46	48.91		AB
(Gallipot)				
CRY, NA (U.S.P., N.F.,MICRONIZED)				
5 gm	51552-0138-02	10.50		
(U.S.P. ,N.F.,MICRONIZED),				
25 gm	51552-0138-04	23.10		
(U.S.P., N.F.,MICRONIZED)				
100 gm	51552-0138-05	67.20		
(Hawkins)				
POW, NA (USP)				
25 gm	63370-0048-25	52.00		
100 gm	63370-0048-35	160.00		
500 gm	63370-0048-45	560.00		
1000 gm	63370-0048-50	960.00		
(Medisca)				
POW, NA (U.S.P.)				
5 gm	38779-0019-03	25.50		
25 gm	38779-0019-04	58.50		
100 gm	38779-0019-05	232.50		
500 gm	38779-0019-08	748.50		
1000 gm	38779-0019-09	1095.00		
(Paddock)				
LOZ, MM, 10 mg, 70s ea	00574-0107-70	112.54		AB
70s ea UD	00574-0107-77	100.00		AB
140s ea	00574-0107-14	204.41		AB
(PCCA)				
POW, NA (U.S.P.)				
1 gm	51927-1348-00	4.20		
(Roxane) *See CLOTRIMAZOLE TROCHE*				
(Spectrum Pharmacy)				
POW, NA (U.S.P.)				
25 gm	49452-2148-01	109.55		
100 gm	49452-2148-02	353.50		
(1X500GM,USP)				
500 gm	49452-2148-05	1151.50		
(Taro)				
CRE, TP, 1%, 15 gm	51672-1275-01	19.94		AB
30 gm	51672-1275-02	34.85		AB
45 gm	51672-1275-06	48.95		AB
45 gm 2s	51672-1275-07	64.80		AB
SOL, TP, 1%, 10 ml	51672-2037-01	6.00		AT
30 ml	51672-1260-03	15.52		AT
(Teva)				
SOL, TP, 1%, 10 ml	00093-0248-43	7.40		AT
30 ml	00093-0248-31	15.52		AT
(Dispensing Solutions)				
REPACK				
CRE, TP, 1%, 15 gm	55045-2188-05	6.22		AB
30 gm	55045-2188-06	35.00		AB
(1X45GM)				
1%, 45 gm	55045-2188-08	49.00		AB
(Nucare Pharm)				
REPACK				
CRE, TP, 1%, 15 gm	66267-0980-15	12.56		EE
30 gm	66267-0979-30	16.99		EE
(Palmetto)				
REPACK				
CRE, TP, 1%, 15 gm	23490-5356-01	14.00		
30 gm	23490-5356-02	18.00		
45 gm	23490-5356-03	14.00		
VG, 1%, 45 gm	23490-5357-00	27.39		
(Pharma Pac)				
REPACK				
CRE, TP, 1%, 15 gm	52959-0493-15	12.60		EE
22.5 gm	52959-0493-45	25.64		EE
30 gm	52959-0493-30	17.80		EE
(Phys Total Care)				
REPACK				
CRE, TP, 1%, 30 gm	54868-3068-00	53.88		AB
LOZ, MM, 10 mg, 35s ea	54868-5463-00	139.11		
70s ea	54868-5463-01	178.90		AB
SOL, TP, 1%, 30 ml	54868-5037-00	35.31		AT
(Physician Partner)				
REPACK				
CRE, TP, 1%, 30 gm	21695-0035-30	27.16		
(Quality Care Prod)				
REPACK				
CRE, TP, 1%, 15 gm	49999-0170-15	13.38		AB
(Southwood)				
REPACK				
CRE, TP, 1%, 15 gm	58016-3503-01	11.08		AB
30 gm	58016-5602-01	17.32		
VG, 1%, 45 gm	58016-6552-01	12.00		
(Stat Rx)				
REPACK				
CRE, TP, 1%, 15 gm	16590-0060-15	13.00		
30 gm	16590-0060-30	26.00		
CLOTRIMAZOLE AND BETAMETHASONE DIPROPIONATE (Altura)				
REPACK				
betamethasone dipropionate/clotrimazole				
CRE, TP, 0.05%-1%, 15 gm	63874-0804-15	28.28		
45 gm	63874-0804-45	60.90		
(Quality Care Prod)				
REPACK				
CRE, TP, 0.05%-1%, 15 gm	49999-0223-15	49.60		
CLOTRIMAZOLE TROCHE (Roxane)				
clotrimazole				
LOZ, MM, 10 mg, 70s ea	00054-4146-22	112.54		AB
70s ea UD	00054-8146-22	120.24		AB
140s ea	00054-4146-23	204.42		AB
CLOTRIMAZOLE/BETAMETHASONE DIP (Physician Partner)				
REPACK				
betamethasone dipropionate/clotrimazole				
CRE, TP, 0.05%-1%, 15 gm	21695-0333-15	45.74		
CLOVE (PCCA)				
POW, NA, 1 gm	51927-1128-00	0.36		
CLOVE LEAF (Medisca)				
clove oil				
OIL, NA (1X14ML,NATURAL)				
14 ml	38779-0819-03	16.50		
(1X25ML,NATURAL)				
25 ml	38779-0819-04	22.50		
(1X100ML,NATURAL)				
100 ml	38779-0819-05	46.50		
(1X500ML,NATURAL)				
500 ml	38779-0819-08	160.50		
(1X4000ML,NATURAL)				
4000 ml	38779-0819-01	918.00		
CLOVE LEAF OIL (Lorann Oil)				
clove oil				
OIL, NA, 3.75 ml	23535-0080-01	0.57		
30 ml	23535-0080-05	3.75		
120 ml	23535-0080-08	11.75		
3840 ml	23535-0080-11	265.00		
CLOVE OIL				
(Lorann Oil) *See CLOVE LEAF OIL*				
(Medisca) *See CLOVE LEAF*				
(PCCA)				
OIL, NA (CLOVE)				
1 ml	51927-2789-00	1.00		
(Spectrum Pharmacy)				
OIL, NA (BUD, F.C.C.)				
25 ml	49452-2150-01	67.90		
125 ml	49452-2150-02	96.95		
500 ml	49452-2150-03	314.30		
CLOZAPINE				
(Azur Pharma, Inc.) *See FAZACLO*				
(Caraco)				
TAB, PO (USP)				
25 mg, 100s ea	57664-0345-88	129.43		AB

PROD/MFR	NDC	AWP	DP	OBC
500s ea	57664-0345-13	621.26		AB
50 mg, 100s ea	57664-0241-88	148.25		AB
(USP)				
100 mg, 100s ea	57664-0347-88	335.80		AB
500s ea	57664-0347-13	1600.05		AB
(Mylan)				
TAB, PO, 25 mg, 100s ea	00378-0825-01	131.94		AB
100 mg, 100s ea	00378-0860-01	341.86		AB
500s ea	00378-0860-05	1644.66		AB
(Novartis Pharm) *See CLOZARIL*				
(Teva)				
TAB, PO, 25 mg, 100s ea	00093-4359-01	128.47		AB
100s ea	00172-4359-60	128.47		AB
(USP,10X10)				
25 mg, 100s ea UD	00093-4359-93	132.32		AB
(USP)				
25 mg, 500s ea	00093-4359-05	624.63		AB
50 mg, 100s ea	00093-4404-01	165.00		AB
100s ea UD	00093-4404-93	167.00		AB
500s ea	00093-4404-05	825.00		AB
100 mg, 100s ea	00093-7772-01	332.80		AB
(USP)				
100 mg, 100s ea UD	00093-4360-93	342.78		AB
500s ea	00093-7772-05	1618.12		AB
200 mg, 100s ea	00093-4405-01	632.32		
100s ea UD	00093-4405-93	651.28		
500s ea	00093-4405-05	3074.43		
500s ea	00093-4405-70	3074.43		
(UDL)				
TAB, PO (10X10)				
25 mg, 100s ea UD	51079-0921-20	132.32		AB
100 mg, 100s ea UD	51079-0922-20	342.78		AB
(American Health)				
REPACK				
TAB, PO (10X10,USP)				
25 mg, 100s ea UD	68084-0233-01	121.31		
100 mg, 100s ea UD	68084-0234-01	239.78		
CLOZARIL (Novartis Pharm)				
clozapine				
TAB, PO, 25 mg, 100s ea	00078-0126-05	286.82		AB
(SANDOPAK)				
25 mg, 100s ea UD	00078-0126-06	286.82		AB
100 mg, 100s ea	00078-0127-05	743.16		AB
(SANDOPAK)				
100 mg, 100s ea UD	00078-0127-06	743.16		AB
CLUBMOSS				
(Amend) *See LYCOPODIUM*				
(Medisca) *See LYCOPODIUM*				
(PCCA) *See LYCOPODIUM*				
CMT (Phys Total Care)				
REPACK				
choline magnesium trisalicylate				
TAB, PO, 500 mg, 60s ea	54868-0806-00	4.50		
750 mg, 60s ea	54868-0820-02	90.36		
CO-GESIC (UCB)				
acetaminophen/hydrocodone bitartrate				
TAB, PO, 500 mg-5 mg,				
100s ea, C-III	00131-2104-37	92.15		AA
CO-NATAL CBF (Contract Pharmacal)				
prenatal vitamins				
TAB, PO, 100s ea	10267-2271-01	24.60		
CO-NATAL FA (Contract Pharmacal)				
prenatal vitamins				
TAB, PO, 100s ea	10267-2270-01	16.78		
COA BUTTA (Amend)				
cocoa butter				
POW, NA (IMMITATION)				
454 gm	17317-0756-01	14.00		
3178 gm	17317-0756-03	70.00		
15890 gm	17317-0756-08	294.00		
COAGULATION FACTOR IX RECOMBINANT				
(Wyeth) *See BENEFIX*				
COAGULATION FACTOR VIIA				
(Novo Nordisk) *See NOVOSEVEN*				
(Novo Nordisk) *See NOVOSEVEN RT*				
COAL TAR				
(Doak) *See DOAK TAR DISTILLATE*				
(Gallipot)				
SOL, NA (U.S.P.,N.F.)				
118.28 ml	51552-0114-04	6.23		
473 ml	51552-0114-06	15.40		
(U.S.P.N.F.)				
3785 ml	51552-0114-08	47.60		
(Medisca)				
SOL, NA (1X50GM,USP)				
50 gm	38779-0585-02	31.50		
(1X100GM,USP)				
100 gm	38779-0585-05	59.85		
(U.S.P.)				
100 ml	38779-0610-05	16.50		
(1X500GM,USP)				
500 gm	38779-0585-08	239.40		
(U.S.P.)				
500 ml	38779-0610-08	31.50		
4000 ml	38779-0610-01	135.00		
(PCCA)				
POW, NA (USP CRUDE)				
1 gm	51927-1170-00	0.36		
SOL, NA (USP)				
1 ml	51927-1051-00	0.10		
(Spectrum Pharmacy)				
LIQ, NA (U.S.P.)				
500 ml	49452-2160-01	110.60		
SOL, NA, 500 ml	49452-2172-01	60.55		
4000 ml	49452-2172-02	239.75		
COARTEM (Novartis Pharm)				
artemether/lumefantrine				
TAB, PO, 20 mg-120 mg,				
24s ea	00078-0568-45	83.52		
(A-S Medication)				
REPACK				
TAB, PO, 20 mg-120 mg,				
24s ea	54569-6146-00	83.52		
COBALT ACETATE				
(Baker, J.T.) *See COBALT ACETATE TETRAHYDRATE*				
COBALT ACETATE TETRAHYDRATE (Baker, J.T.)				
cobalt acetate				
CRY, NA (A.C.S., REAGENT)				
125 gm	10106-1658-04	63.24		
500 gm	10106-1658-01	175.98		
COBALT CARBONATE (Baker, J.T.)				
POW, NA (REAGENT)				
500 gm	10106-1666-01	296.43		
COBALT CHLORIDE				
(Baker, J.T.) *See COBALT CHLORIDE HEXAHYDRATE*				
COBALT CHLORIDE HEXAHYDRATE (Baker, J.T.)				
cobalt chloride				
CRY, NA (A.C.S., REAGENT)				
125 gm	10106-1670-04	73.80		
500 gm	10106-1670-01	159.39		
2500 gm	10106-1670-05	462.06		
COBALT GLUCONATE (PCCA)				
POW, NA, 1 gm	51927-2509-00	6.00		
COBALT NITRATE				
(Baker, J.T.) *See COBALT NITRATE HEXAHYDRATE*				
COBALT NITRATE HEXAHYDRATE (Baker, J.T.)				
cobalt nitrate				
POW, NA (A.C.S., REAGENT)				
500 gm	10106-1680-01	205.59		
2500 gm	10106-1680-05	384.40		
COBALT OXIDE (Baker, J.T.)				
POW, NA (REAGENT)				
500 gm	10106-1688-01	397.48		
COBALT SULFATE				
(Baker, J.T.) *See COBALT SULFATE HEPTAHYDRATE*				
COBALT SULFATE HEPTAHYDRATE (Baker, J.T.)				
cobalt sulfate				
CRY, NA (REAGENT)				
125 gm	10106-1696-04	79.52		
500 gm	10106-1696-01	212.64		
2500 gm	10106-1696-05	941.06		
12000 gm	10106-1696-07	2963.72		
COBALTOUS CL CO 57/ CYANOCOBALAMIN CO 57/IF/VIT B12				
(Bracco Diag) *See RUBRATOPE-57*				
COBAMAMIDE (Medisca)				
POW, NA (PHARMACEUTICAL GRADE)				
5 gm	38779-1191-03	352.50		
(PCCA)				
POW, NA (COENZYME B12)				
1 gm	51927-2649-00	285.00		
(Spectrum Pharmacy)				
POW, NA, 1 gm	49452-2175-02	374.50		
5 gm	49452-2175-03	1046.50		
COBOLIN-M (Legère)				
cyanocobalamin				
SOL, IM (VIAL)				
1000 mcg/ml, 30 ml	25332-0004-30	7.95		EE
COCA COLA (PCCA)				
cola				
SYR, NA, 1 ml	51927-2367-00	0.08		
COCAINE HCL (Covidien)				
cocaine hydrochloride				
POW, NA (U.S.P.)				
5 gm, C-II	00406-1520-53	342.19		
25 gm, C-II	00406-1520-55	1710.94		
(Medisca)				
POW, NA (U.S.P.)				
1 gm, C-II	38779-0723-06	306.00		
5 gm, C-II	38779-0723-03	1125.00		
(Roxane)				
SOL, TP, 40 mg/ml,				
4 ml, C-II	00054-8163-02	25.18		
10 ml, C-II	00054-3154-40	62.23		
(Spectrum Pharmacy)				
POW, NA (U.S.P.)				
5 gm, C-II	49452-2177-01	1708.00		
(Phys Total Care)				
REPACK				
POW, NA, 5 gm, C-II	54868-0178-00	314.31		
COCAINE HYDROCHLORIDE				
(Covidien) *See COCAINE HCL*				
(Gallipot)				
POW, NA (1X1GM,USP)				
1 gm, C-II	51552-0881-01	122.50	87.50	
(1X5GM,USP)				
5 gm, C-II	51552-0881-02	469.00	335.00	
(Lannett)				
SOL, TP (1X4ML,UNIT-OF-USE)				
40 mg/ml,				
4 ml, C-II	00527-1728-74	47.70		
(1X10ML,MULTI-DOSE)				
40 mg/ml,				
10 ml, C-II	00527-1728-73	118.80		
(1X4ML,UNIT-OF-USE)				
100 mg/ml,				
4 ml, C-II	00527-1729-74	134.40		
(Medisca) *See COCAINE HCL*				
(Roxane) *See COCAINE HCL*				
(Spectrum Pharmacy) *See COCAINE HCL*				
COCAMIDE DEA (PCCA)				
cocamide diethanolamine				
POW, NA, 1 gm	51927-2366-00	0.16		
COCAMIDE DIETHANOLAMINE				
(PCCA) *See COCAMIDE DEA*				
COCAMIDOPROPYL AMINE OXIDE (PCCA)				
cocamidopropylamine oxide				
SOL, NA (1X1ML)				
1 ml	51927-2384-00	0.08		
COCAMIDOPROPYL HYDROXYSULTAINE (PCCA)				
SOL, NA (1X1ML)				
1 ml	51927-2439-00	0.09		
COCAMIDOPROPYLAMINE OXIDE				
(PCCA) *See COCAMIDOPROPYL AMINE OXIDE*				
COCAMINE OXIDE				
(PCCA) *See DIMETHYLCOCOAMINE OXIDE*				
COCET (Poly)				
acetaminophen/codeine phosphate				
TAB, PO, 650 mg-30 mg,				
100s ea, C-III	50991-0316-01	187.49	149.99	
COCO-BETAINE				
(Medisca) *See COCOBETAINE*				
(PCCA) *See COCOBETAINE*				
COCOA BUTTER				
(Amend) *See COA BUTTA*				
(Gallipot)				
OIN, NA (NATURAL)				
28.35 gm	51552-0002-01	1.75		
454 gm	51552-0002-06	20.79		
SOA, NA, 28.35 gm	51552-0002-02	1.75		
(PCCA)				
POW, NA (NF)				
1 gm	51927-1731-00	0.10		
(Spectrum Pharmacy)				
PAS, NA (N.F.)				
500 gm	49452-2180-01	87.15		
2500 gm	49452-2180-02	353.50		

PROD/MFR	NDC	AWP	DP	OBC

COCOBETAINE (Medisca)
coco-betaine
SOL, NA (1X500ML, MACKAM CB-35)
500 ml **38779-1199-08** 46.50
(1X1000ML, MACKAM CB-35)
1000 ml **38779-1199-09** 76.50

(PCCA)
SOL, NA, 1 ml **51927-2364-00** 0.12

COCONUT FLAVOR (PCCA)
flavoring aid
SOL, NA (ARTIFICIAL)
1 ml **51927-2162-00** 0.90

COCONUT FRAGRANCE (Medisca)
coconut oil
OIL, NA (1X14ML)
14 ml **38779-1200-03** 16.50
(1X25ML)
25 ml **38779-1200-04** 31.50
(1X100ML)
100 ml **38779-1200-05** 90.00
(1X120ML)
120 ml **38779-1200-01** 67.50
(1X500ML)
500 ml **38779-1200-08** 199.50

(PCCA)
fragrance
SOL, NA (ARTIFICIAL; LIQUID)
1 gm **51927-3534-00** 0.43

COCONUT OIL
(Amend) *See NEOBEE M-5*

(Gallipot)
OIL, NA, 118.28 ml **51552-0093-04** 6.09
473 ml **51552-0093-06** 13.79

(Lorann Oil)
OIL, NA (N.F., NOT FLAVOR)
30 ml **23535-0214-05** 1.40
120 ml **23535-0214-08** 2.25
480 ml **23535-0214-01** 5.00
3840 ml **23535-0214-11** 34.00

(Medisca) *See COCONUT FRAGRANCE*

(Medisca)
OIL, NA (1X25ML)
25 ml **38779-2034-04** 16.50
(1X100ML)
100 ml **38779-2034-05** 31.50
(1X500ML)
500 ml **38779-2034-08** 46.50
(1X1000ML)
1000 ml **38779-2034-09** 75.00

(PCCA)
OIL, NA (EDIBLE,COCONUT)
1 ml **51927-1047-00** 0.09

COD LIVER OIL (Lorann Oil)
OIL, NA, 120 ml **23535-0903-08** 1.75
480 ml **23535-0903-01** 4.00
3840 ml **23535-0903-11** 23.00

(Medisca)
OIL, NA (1X500ML, USP)
500 ml **38779-2035-08** 42.00
(1X4000ML, USP)
4000 ml **38779-2035-01** 163.35

(Spectrum Pharmacy)
OIL, NA (U.S.P./N.F.)
500 ml **49452-2200-01** 76.30
4000 ml **49452-2200-02** 249.20

CODAFED EXPECTORANT (Vintage)
codeine phos/gg/pse hcl
SYR, PO (WINTERGREEN)
480 ml, C-III **00254-9073-58** 38.54

CODAL-DH (Dispensing Solutions)
REPACK
hydrocod bit/phenyleph hcl/pyril mal
SYR, PO (AF,CHERRY)
473 ml, C-III **55045-3337-01** 20.75

CODEINE PHOS/DEXCHLORPHENIRAMINE MAL/ PHENYLEPH HCL
(GM Pharm) *See VANACOF CD*

CODEINE PHOS/GG/PHENYLEPH HCL
(Gil Pharmaceutical) *See GILTUSS PED-C*
(MCR American) *See MAXIPHEN CD*
(MCR American) *See MAXIPHEN CDX*

CODEINE PHOS/GG/PSE HCL
(Axiom Pharmaceutical) *See HALOTUSSIN DAC*
(Bio-Pharm) *See BIOTUSSIN DAC*
(CodaDose) *See ZODRYL DEC 25*
(CodaDose) *See ZODRYL DEC 30*
(CodaDose) *See ZODRYL DEC 35*
(CodaDose) *See ZODRYL DEC 40*
(CodaDose) *See ZODRYL DEC 50*
(CodaDose) *See ZODRYL DEC 60*
(CodaDose) *See ZODRYL DEC 80*
(Gil Pharmaceutical) *See SUTTAR-2*
(Gil Pharmaceutical) *See SUTTAR-SF*
(MCR American) *See AMBIFED CD*
(MCR American) *See AMBIFED CDX*
(MCR American) *See AMBIFED-G CD*
(MCR American) *See AMBIFED-G CDX*
(MCR American) *See MAXIFED CD*
(MCR American) *See MAXIFED CDX*
(MCR American) *See MAXIFED-G CD*
(MCR American) *See MAXIFED-G CDX*
(Morton Grove) *See MYTUSSIN DAC*
(Pack) *See GUAIFENESIN DAC*
(PGD, Inc.) *See SUDATUSS-2*
(PGD, Inc.) *See SUDATUSS-SF*
(Poly) *See LORTUSS EX*
(Vintage) *See CHERATUSSIN DAC*
(Vintage) *See CODAFED EXPECTORANT*

CODEINE PHOS/PHENYLEPH HCL/ PROMETHAZINE HCL
(Actavis Mid Atlantic) *See PROMETHAZINE VC W/CODEINE*
(Qualitest) *See PROMETHAZINE VC WITH CODEINE*

CODEINE PHOS/PHENYLEPH HCL/PYRIL MAL
(Pro-Pharma LLC) *See PRO-RED AC*
(Vertical) *See ZOTEX-C*

CODEINE PHOS/PSE HCL/TRIPROLIDINE HCL
(Poly) *See POLY HIST NC*

CODEINE PHOSPHATE (Covidien)
POW, NA, 10 gm, C-II **00406-1548-32** 82.50
25 gm, C-II **00406-1548-35** 206.25

(Gallipot)
POW, NA (1X5GM,USP)
5 gm, C-II **51552-0688-02** 42.00 30.00
(1X10GM,USP)
10 gm, C-II **51552-0688-03** 84.00 60.00
(1X25GM,USP)
25 gm, C-II **51552-0688-04** 168.00 120.00
(1X100GM,USP)
100 gm, C-II **51552-0688-06** 525.00 375.00

(Hawkins)
POW, NA (U.S.P.)
5 gm, C-II **63370-0910-15** 124.00
25 gm, C-II **63370-0910-25** 440.00
100 gm, C-II **63370-0910-35** 1500.00

(Hospira)
SOL, IJ (LUER-LOCK,CARPUJECT)
15 mg/ml,
2 ml 10s, C-II **00409-1097-32** 27.72 24.30
(LUER LOCK,CARPUJECT)
30 mg/ml,
2 ml 10s, C-II **00409-1102-32** 29.04 25.40

(Medisca)
POW, NA (U.S.P.)
5 gm, C-II **38779-0679-03** 105.00
25 gm, C-II **38779-0679-04** 435.00
100 gm, C-II **38779-0679-05** 1197.00

(PCCA)
POW, NA (U.S.P.; CII)
1 gm, C-II **51927-1013-00** 39.60

(Ranbaxy Pharm)
TSN, IJ, 30 mg,
100s ea, C-II **63304-0748-01** 95.11
60 mg, 100s ea, C-II .. **63304-0749-01** 175.96

(Spectrum Pharmacy)
POW, NA (U.S.P.)
5 gm, C-II **49452-0027-03** 172.55
25 gm, C-II **49452-0027-02** 693.00
100 gm, C-II **49452-0027-04** 1659.00

(B&B Pharm, Inc)
REPACK
POW, NA (U.S.P.)
10 gm, C-II **63275-8100-03** 175.00
25 gm, C-II **63275-8100-04** 335.00
100 gm, C-II **63275-8100-05** 1065.00

CODEINE PHOSPHATE & ACETAMINOPHEN (Keltman Pharma., Inc.)
REPACK
acetaminophen/codeine phosphate
TAB, PO, 300 mg-30 mg,
40s ea, C-III **68387-0250-40** 26.67

CODEINE PHOSPHATE/GUAIFENESIN
(Axiom Pharmaceutical) *See HALOTUSSIN AC*
(Bio-Pharm) *See BIOTUSSIN AC*
(Boca Pharmacal) *See GUAIFENESIN AND CODEINE PHOSPHATE*
(Consolidated Midland) *See GUIATUSCON A.C.*
(Cypress Pharm) *See DEX-TUSS*
(Cypress Pharm) *See GANI-TUSS NR*
(Everett) *See TUSSO-C*
(Kenwood) *See BRONTEX*
(Larken Labs, Inc.) *See EXECLEAR-C*
(Major) *See ROBAFEN AC*
(Major) *See ROBAFEN AC COUGH SYRUP*
(McNeil,R.A.) *See M-CLEAR*
(McNeil,R.A.) *See M-CLEAR WC*
(MCR American) *See ALLFEN CD*
(MCR American) *See ALLFEN CDX*
(Morton Grove) *See MYTUSSIN AC COUGH*
(Pack) *See GUAIFENESIN AC*
(Pfeiffer) *See KOLEPHRIN #1*
(Pharm Assoc Inc) *See GUAIFENESIN AND CODEINE PHOSPHATE*
(Qualitest) *See CHERATUSSIN AC*
(Qualitest) *See IOPHEN C-NR*
(Rite Aid) *See RITE AID BRANDS*

(Palmetto)
REPACK
LIQ, PO, 10 mg/5 ml-100 mg/5 ml,
120 ml, C-V **23490-5651-01** 9.50
SYR, PO (1X120ML)
10 mg/5 ml-100 mg/5 ml,
120 ml, C-V **23490-5652-01** 7.05
180 ml, C-V **23490-5652-02** 10.75
(1X240ML)
10 mg/5 ml-100 mg/5 ml,
240 ml, C-V **23490-5652-03** 14.10
(1X480ML)
10 mg/5 ml-100 mg/5 ml,
480 ml, C-V **23490-5652-04** 28.20

(Pharma Pac)
REPACK
TAB, PO (CAPLET)
10 mg-300 mg,
15s ea, C-III **52959-0714-15** 35.35
100s ea, C-III **52959-0714-00** 76.01

CODEINE PHOSPHATE/PHENYLEPHRINE HYDROCHLORIDE
(Poly) *See ALA-HIST AC*
(SJ) *See NOTUSS-PE*

CODEINE PHOSPHATE/PROMETHAZINE HYDROCHLORIDE
FUL
SYR, PO, 10 mg/5 ml-6.25 mg/5 ml,
480 ml 18.24
(Actavis Mid Atlantic) *See CODEINE/PROMETHAZINE*
(Hi-Tech) *See CODEINE/PROMETHAZINE*
(Morton Grove) *See CODEINE/PROMETHAZINE*
(Pharm Assoc Inc) *See CODEINE/PROMETHAZINE*
(Qualitest) *See PROMETHAZINE WITH CODEINE*

CODEINE PHOSPHATE/PROMETHAZINE HYDROCHLORIDE (Palmetto)
REPACK
codeine phosphate/promethazine hydrochloride
SYR, PO (1X120ML)
10 mg/5 ml-6.25 mg/5 ml,
120 ml, C-V **23490-6188-01** 21.32

PROD/MFR NDC AWP DP OBC

CODEINE PHOSPHATE/PSEUDOEPHEDRINE HYDROCHLORIDE
(Breckenridge Pharm) *See PSEUDOEPHEDRINE AND CODEINE*
(Larken Labs, Inc.) *See ENDACOF-DC*
(SJ) *See NOTUSS-DC*

CODEINE PHOSPHATE/PYRILAMINE MALEATE
(Pro-Pharma LLC) *See PRO-CLEAR AC*

CODEINE SULFATE (Dava Pharma)
TAB, PO (USP)
30 mg,
100s ea, C-II **67253-0350-10** 46.69
60 mg, 100s ea, C-II .. **67253-0351-10** 85.52

(Glenmark Pharmaceuticals)
TAB, PO (USP)
30 mg,
100s ea, C-II **68462-0193-01** 46.69
60 mg, 100s ea, C-II .. **68462-0194-01** 85.52

(Roxane)
TAB, PO (4X25)
15 mg,
100s ea UD, C-II.... **00054-0243-24** 43.37
30 mg, 100s ea, C-II .. **00054-0244-25** 46.69
(4X25)
30 mg,
100s ea UD, C-II.... **00054-0244-24** 51.69
60 mg, 100s ea, C-II .. **00054-0245-25** 85.52

(Phys Total Care)
REPACK
TAB, PO, 60 mg,
10s ea, C-II **54868-2541-00** 33.69
30s ea, C-II **54868-2541-01** 83.06
60s ea, C-II **54868-2541-02** 122.27

CODEINE/GG/PSEUDEPH EXPECTORANT
(Phys Total Care)
codeine phos/gg/pse hcl
LIQ, PO, 120 ml, C-V **54868-1024-02** 12.81
240 ml, C-V **54868-1024-01** 19.62

CODEINE/GUAIFENESIN (A-S Medication)
REPACK
codeine phosphate/guaifenesin
SYR, PO, 10 mg/5 ml-100 mg/5 ml,
120 ml, C-V **54569-3146-00** 3.75

(Phys Total Care)
REPACK
SOL, PO (SF)
10 mg/5 ml-100 mg/5 ml,
120 ml, C-V **54868-4768-00** 14.06
473 ml, C-V **54868-4768-01** 23.25

CODEINE/PROMETHAZINE (Actavis Mid Atlantic)
codeine phosphate/promethazine hydrochloride
SYR, PO, 10 mg/5 ml-6.25 mg/5 ml,
118 ml, C-V .... **00472-1627-04** 9.05 AA
240 ml, C-V .... **00472-1627-08** 12.22 AA
473 ml, C-V .... **00472-1627-16** 32.55 AA

(Hi-Tech)
SYR, PO, 10 mg/5 ml-6.25 mg/5 ml,
473 ml, C-V .... **50383-0804-16** 32.75 AA

(Morton Grove)
SYR, PO (RASPBERRY)
10 mg/5 ml-6.25 mg/5 ml,
480 ml, C-V .... **60432-0606-16** 32.70 AA

(Pharm Assoc Inc)
SYR, PO (GRAPE)
10 mg/5 ml-6.25 mg/5 ml,
5 ml 100s UD, C-V .. **00121-0547-05** 110.32 AA

(A-S Medication)
REPACK
SYR, PO, 10 mg/5 ml-6.25 mg/5 ml,
120 ml, C-V .... **54569-1056-00** 9.20 EE
(2 X 240 ML)
10 mg/5 ml-6.25 mg/5 ml,
240 ml 2s, C-V ..... **54569-3540-02** 33.16 EE

(Altura)
REPACK
SYR, PO (1X480ML)
10 mg/5 ml-6.25 mg/5 ml,
480 ml, C-V .... **63874-0204-48** 32.55 AA

(DHS, Inc.)
REPACK
SYR, PO, 10 mg/5 ml-6.25 mg/5 ml,
120 ml, C-V .... **55887-0766-04** 22.44 AA

(Pharma Pac)
REPACK
SYR, PO, 10 mg/5 ml-6.25 mg/5 ml,
120 ml, C-V .... **52959-0118-03** 8.15 EE
180 ml, C-V .... **52959-0118-05** 9.95 EE
240 ml, C-V .... **52959-0118-06** 11.44 EE

(Phys Total Care)
REPACK
SYR, PO, 10 mg/5 ml-6.25 mg/5 ml,
120 ml, C-V .... **54868-1029-01** 18.45 EE
240 ml, C-V .... **54868-1029-00** 35.40 EE
473 ml, C-V .... **54868-1029-02** 30.30 AA

(Quality Care Prod)
REPACK
SYR, PO, 10 mg/5 ml-6.25 mg/5 ml,
120 ml, C-V .... **49999-0152-04** 20.20 AA

(Southwood)
REPACK
SYR, PO, 10 mg/5 ml-6.25 mg/5 ml,
120 ml, C-V .... **58016-0390-01** 14.23 AA

CODEINE/PSEUDOEPH/TRIPROLIDINE (Southwood)
codeine phos/pse hcl/triprolidine hcl
SYR, PO, 120 ml, C-V ..... **58016-0469-24** 7.20 EE

CODIMAL-L.A. (Phys Total Care)
REPACK
cpm/pse hcl
CER, PO, 8 mg-120 mg,
20s ea **54868-1611-01** 14.41

CODIMAL-L.A. HALF (Phys Total Care)
cpm/pse hcl
CER, PO, 4 mg-60 mg,
20s ea **54868-1958-01** 10.78

CODITUSS DH (Vintage)
hydrocod bit/phenyleph hcl/pyril mal
SYR, PO (BERRY)
473 ml, C-III **00254-9078-58** 17.98

COENZYME Q-10 (PCCA)
coenzyme q10
POW, NA, 1 gm **51927-1847-00** 43.80

COENZYME Q10
(Bio-Tech Pharm) *See COQ(10)50*

(Gallipot)
POW, NA, 25 gm **51552-0646-04** 161.00

(Letco)
POW, NA, 5 gm **62991-1343-01** 135.00
25 gm **62991-1343-02** 450.00
100 gm **62991-1343-03** 1440.00

(Medisca)
POW, NA, 5 gm **38779-0127-03** 207.00
25 gm **38779-0127-04** 855.00
100 gm **38779-0127-05** 2685.00
(1X500GM)
500 gm **38779-0127-08** 10380.00
(1X1000GM)
1000 gm **38779-0127-09** 13185.00

(PCCA) *See COENZYME Q-10*

(B&B Pharm, Inc)
REPACK
POW, NA (1X5GM)
5 gm **63275-9946-02** 75.00
(1X25GM)
25 gm **63275-9946-04** 330.00
(1X100GM)
100 gm **63275-9946-05** 1170.00
(1X1000GM)
1000 gm **63275-9946-09** 9450.00

COFEX-DM (Cypress Pharm)
dextromethorphan hydrobromide/guaifenesin
TER, PO (DYE-FREE)
55 mg-1000 mg,
100s ea **60258-0325-01** 85.30

COFFEE (Medisca)
flavoring aid
SOL, NA (1X25ML)
25 ml **38779-1201-04** 22.50
(1X100ML)
100 ml **38779-1201-05** 34.50
(1X500ML)
500 ml **38779-1201-08** 87.00

COFFEE FLAVOR (PCCA)
flavoring aid
POW, NA (ARTIFICIAL,COFFEE)
1 gm **51927-3456-00** 0.32
SOL, NA, 1 ml **51927-3299-00** 0.90

COGENTIN (Lundbeck)
benztropine mesylate
SOL, IJ (5X2ML)
1 mg/ml, 2 ml 5s **67386-0611-52** 584.12 46.03

(Phys Total Care)
REPACK
SOL, IJ (AMP)
1 mg/ml, 2 ml 6s **54868-2429-01** 51.23

COLA (Gallipot)
SYR, NA, 118.28 ml **51552-0291-04** 3.08
473 ml **51552-0291-06** 10.29
3785 ml **51552-0291-08** 27.16

(PCCA) *See COCA COLA*

COLA CONCENTRATE (Medisca)
flavoring aid
SOL, NA (1X100ML)
100 ml **38779-1202-05** 28.50
(1X500ML)
500 ml **38779-1202-08** 46.50

COLA FLAVOR (PCCA)
flavoring aid
SOL, NA (CAFFEINE-FREE)
1 ml **51927-3414-00** 0.30

COLA NUT
(PCCA) *See KOLA NUT*

COLAZAL (Salix Pharm)
balsalazide disodium
CAP, PO, 750 mg, 280s ea . **65649-0101-02** 477.67
500s ea **65649-0101-50** 853.00

COLCHICINE
(AR Scientific) *See COLCRYS*

(Consolidated Midland)
TAB, PO, 0.6 mg, 100s ea .. **00223-0703-01** 3.95
1000s ea **00223-0703-02** 19.75

(Excellium)
TAB, PO, 0.6 mg, 100s ea .. **64125-0104-01** 25.99
1000s ea **64125-0104-10** 174.99

(Gallipot)
POW, NA (1X1GM,USP)
1 gm **51552-0991-01** 54.95 39.25

(PCCA)
POW, NA (U.S.P.)
1 gm **51927-1895-00** 204.00

(Spectrum Pharmacy)
POW, NA (U.S.P.)
1 gm **49452-2210-02** 264.60
5 gm **49452-2210-03** 910.00

(Vision)
TAB, PO (USP)
0.6 mg, 100s ea **68013-0001-01** 33.32
500s ea **68013-0001-05** 166.60
1000s ea **68013-0001-10** 333.20

(Watson Labs)
TAB, PO, 0.6 mg, 100s ea .. **00591-0944-01** 10.80
1000s ea **00591-0944-10** 83.40

(West-Ward)
TAB, PO, 0.6 mg, 100s ea .. **00143-1201-01** 61.70
100s ea UD **00143-1201-25** 89.50
1000s ea **00143-1201-10** 555.50

(A-S Medication)
REPACK
TAB, PO, 0.6 mg, 30s ea ... **54569-0236-06** 17.19
60s ea **54569-0236-03** 34.39

(Bryant Ranch)
REPACK
TAB, PO, 0.6 mg, 20s ea ... **63629-2651-01** 5.00

(Core)
REPACK
TAB, PO, 0.6 mg, 20s ea ... **33358-0094-20** 5.13
30s ea **33358-0094-30** 9.73

(DHS, Inc.)
REPACK
TAB, PO, 0.6 mg, 30s ea ... **55887-0718-30** 12.09

(Dispensing Solutions)
REPACK
TAB, PO, 0.6 mg, 12s ea ... **55045-2420-04** 3.12
20s ea **55045-2420-02** 5.20
30s ea **55045-2420-08** 7.80
50s ea **66336-0401-50** 12.18
100s ea **55045-2420-01** 26.00

(HomeMed)
REPACK
TAB, PO, 0.6 mg, 10s ea ... **51655-0424-53** 2.84

PROD/MFR	NDC	AWP	DP	OBC
COLCHICINE (Palmetto)				
REPACK				
TAB, PO, 0.6 mg, 60s ea	23490-5367-04	24.18		
COLCHICINE (PD-Rx Pharm)				
REPACK				
TAB, PO, 0.6 mg, 10s ea	55289-0279-10	7.73		
(REDI-SCRIPT)				
0.6 mg, 30s ea	58864-0119-30	3.50		
(USP)				
0.6 mg, 30s ea	55289-0279-30	10.43		
(REDI-SCRIPT)				
0.6 mg, 100s ea	58864-0119-01	26.80		
(Pharma Pac)				
REPACK				
TAB, PO, 0.6 mg, 20s ea	52959-0070-20	5.85		
(Phys Total Care)				
REPACK				
TAB, PO, 0.6 mg, 10s ea	54868-0998-05	9.09		
20s ea	54868-0998-06	12.18		
25s ea	54868-0998-04	13.73		
30s ea	54868-0998-00	15.28		
60s ea	54868-0998-03	24.55		
90s ea	54868-0998-07	41.52		
100s ea	54868-0998-01	36.92		
(Physician Partner)				
REPACK				
TAB, PO, 0.6 mg, 30s ea	21695-0629-30	15.57		
(Quality Care Prod)				
REPACK				
TAB, PO, 0.6 mg, 30s ea	35356-0239-30	32.20		
(Stat Rx)				
REPACK				
TAB, PO, 0.6 mg, 20s ea	16590-0268-20	10.00		
24s ea	16590-0268-24	17.59		
30s ea	16590-0268-30	15.00		
60s ea	16590-0268-60	30.00		
COLCHICINE/PROBENECID				
(Rising) *See PROBENECID AND COLCHICINE*				
(Truxton)				
TAB, PO, 0.5 mg-500 mg,				
1000s ea	00463-6316-10	103.50		EE
(Watson Labs)				
TAB, PO, 0.5 mg-500 mg,				
100s ea	00591-5325-01	84.34		BP
(Phys Total Care)				
REPACK				
TAB, PO, 0.5 mg-500 mg,				
30s ea	54868-2179-01	86.58		EE
60s ea	54868-2179-00	168.69		EE
COLCRYS (AR Scientific)				
colchicine				
TAB, PO (FILM-COATED)				
0.6 mg, 30s ea	13310-0119-07	174.60		
100s ea	13310-0119-01	582.00		
COLD CREAM (Gallipot)				
cream base				
CRE, NA (EMMOLIENT BASE)				
454 gm	51552-0809-06	12.60	9.00	
2270 gm	51552-0809-09	50.40	36.00	
COLD CREAM UNSCENTED (Medisca)				
cream, multi ingredient				
CRE, NA (1X450GM)				
450 gm	38779-0935-08	45.00		
(1X454GM)				
454 gm	38779-0935-07	45.00		
COLDAMINE (Breckenridge Pharm)				
cpm/methscopolamine nitrate/pse hcl				
TER, PO (DYE-FREE,CAPLET)				
8 mg-2.5 mg-90 mg,				
100s ea	51991-0284-01	47.19		
COLDCOUGH (Breckenridge Pharm)				
cpm/dihydrocodeine bitartrate/pse hcl				
SOL, PO (AF,SF,DYE-FREE,GRAPE)				
473 ml, C-III	51991-0222-16	35.46		
COLDCOUGH HC (Breckenridge Pharm)				
cpm/hydrocod bit/pse hcl				
SYR, PO (AF,SF,DYE-FREE)				
480 ml, C-III	51991-0206-16	45.92		
COLDCOUGH HCM (Breckenridge Pharm)				
hydrocod bit/pse hcl				
SOL, PO (AF,SF,DYE-FREE)				
3 mg/5 ml-15 mg/5 ml,				
473 ml, C-III	51991-0306-16	28.47		
COLDCOUGH PD (Breckenridge Pharm)				
cpm/dihydrocodeine bitartrate/phenyleph hcl				
SOL, PO (AF,SF,GRAPE)				
118 ml, C-V	51991-0224-04	15.55		
COLESEVELAM HYDROCHLORIDE				
(Daiichi Sankyo) *See WELCHOL*				
COLESTID (Pfizer)				
colestipol hydrochloride				
PDR, PO, 5 gm/packet,				
30s ea	00009-0260-01	80.93	67.44	
90s ea	00009-0260-04	242.78	202.32	
5 gm/scoopful,				
300 gm	00009-0260-17	96.38	80.32	
500 gm	00009-0260-02	160.63	133.86	
TAB, PO, 1 gm, 120s ea	00009-0450-03	101.62	84.68	
COLESTID FLAVORED (Pfizer)				
colestipol hydrochloride				
PDR, PO (7.5 GM PACKET)				
5 gm/7.5 gm,				
60s ea	00009-0370-03	190.03	158.36	
450 gm	00009-0370-05	132.98	110.82	
(Phys Total Care)				
REPACK				
PDR, PO, 5 gm/7.5 gm,				
7.5 gm 30s	54868-3061-00	74.97		
COLESTID GRAN (Phys Total Care)				
colestipol hydrochloride				
PDR, PO, 5 gm/scoopful,				
500 gm	54868-3060-00	146.39		
COLESTIPOL (Phys Total Care)				
colestipol hydrochloride				
TAB, PO, 1 gm, 120s ea	54868-0610-00	203.91		
COLESTIPOL HYDROCHLORIDE (Global Pharm)				
PDR, PO, 5 gm/packet,				
30s ea	00115-5212-18	70.03		AB
(USP)				
5 gm/packet,				
90s ea	00115-5212-29	207.03		AB
(USP,W/SCOOP,TASTELESS)				
5 gm/scoopful,				
500 gm	00115-5213-02	137.69		AB
TAB, PO (FILM-COATED)				
1 gm, 120s ea	00115-5211-16	78.94		AB
(Pfizer) *See COLESTID*				
(Pfizer) *See COLESTID FLAVORED*				
COLESTIPOL HYDROCHLORIDE, MICRONIZED				
(Greenstone) *See MICRONIZED COLESTIPOL HYDROCHLORIDE*				
COLFED-A (Breckenridge Pharm)				
cpm/pse hcl				
CER, PO, 8 mg-120 mg,				
100s ea	51991-0145-01	135.00		
(Dispensing Solutions)				
REPACK				
CER, PO, 8 mg-120 mg,				
10s ea	55045-1295-03	6.90		
20s ea	55045-1295-07	13.80		
COLIDROPS PEDIATRIC (A. G. Marin)				
hyoscyamine sulfate				
LIQ, PO (AF,SF,DROPS)				
0.125 mg/ml, 30 ml	12539-0315-30	12.00		
COLISTIMETHATE (APP)				
colistimethate sodium				
PDS, IJ (USP,LYOPHILIZED CAKE)				
150 mg, ea	63323-0393-06	57.00		
(Phys Total Care)				
REPACK				
PDS, IJ, 150 mg, ea	54868-5612-00	114.18		
COLISTIMETHATE SODIUM				
(APP) *See COLISTIMETHATE*				
(JHP) *See COLY-MYCIN M PARENTERAL*				
(Medisca)				
POW, NA, 1 gm	38779-1203-06	178.50		
5 gm	38779-1203-03	693.00		
(Paddock)				
PDS, IJ (VIAL,STERILE)				
150 mg, ea	00574-0858-01	57.00		AP
(PCCA)				
POW, NA (USP)				
1 gm	51927-2101-00	225.00		
(X-Gen)				
PDS, IJ (VIAL,STERILE)				
150 mg, ea	39822-0615-01	57.00		AP
COLISTIN SULFATE (Medisca)				
POW, NA (1XBU,USP)				
1 ml	38779-0020-06	1623.00		
COLLAGEN HEMOSTAT				
(Davol) *See AVITENE MICROFIBRILLAR COLLAGEN HEMOSTAT*				
(Davol) *See AVITENE ULTRAFOAM COLLAGEN*				
(Davol) *See ENDOAVITENE*				
(Davol) *See SYRINGEAVITENE*				
COLLAGEN HYDROLYSATE (PCCA)				
collagen, bovine				
POW, NA (1X1GM)				
1 gm	51927-1132-00	0.27		
COLLAGEN NERVE ENCASEMENT				
(Integra LifeSciences Corp) *See NEURAGEN*				
(Integra LifeSciences Corp) *See NEURAWRAP*				
(Stryker) *See NEUROMATRIX*				
(Stryker) *See NEUROMEND COLLAGEN NERVE WRAP*				
COLLAGEN SCAFFOLD				
(Integra LifeSciences Corp) *See INTEGRA MOZAIK OSTEOCONDUCTIVE SCAFFOLD PUTTY*				
(Integra LifeSciences Corp) *See INTEGRA MOZAIK OSTEOCONDUCTIVE SCAFFOLD STRIP*				
(Integra LifeSciences Corp) *See INTEGRA OS OSTEOCONDUCTIVE SCAFFOLD PUTTY*				
COLLAGEN TENDON ENCASEMENT				
(Integra LifeSciences Corp) *See TENOGLIDE*				
COLLAGEN, BOVINE				
(PCCA) *See COLLAGEN HYDROLYSATE*				
(Synovis) *See VERITAS COLLAGEN MATRIX*				
(TEI Biosciences Inc.) *See PRIMATRIX DERMAL REPAIR SCAFFOLD*				
(TEI Biosciences Inc.) *See SURGIMEND COLLAGEN MATRIX*				
(TEI Biosciences Inc.) *See TISSUEMEND*				
COLLAGEN, BOVINE/GLYCOSAMINOGLYCANS				
(Integra LifeSciences Corp) *See INTEGRA BILAYER MATRIX WOUND DRESSING*				
(Integra LifeSciences Corp) *See INTEGRA DERMAL REGENERATION TEMPLATE*				
(Integra LifeSciences Corp) *See INTEGRA FLOWABLE WOUND MATRIX*				
(Integra LifeSciences Corp) *See INTEGRA MATRIX WOUND DRESSING*				
(Integra LifeSciences Corp) *See INTEGRA MESHED BILAYER WOUND MATRIX*				
COLLAGENASE				
(Healthpoint) *See SANTYL*				
(Medisca)				
POW, NA, 0.5 gm	38779-0542-00	4350.00		
1 gm	38779-0542-06	2385.00		
(PCCA)				
POW, NA, ea	51927-2877-00	2.55		
COLLAGENASE, CLOSTRIDIUM HISTOLYTICUM				
(Auxilium Pharm, Inc) *See XIAFLEX*				
COLLECTOR, URINE				
(Covidien) *See PRECISION 200 URINE METER CATHETERIZATION TRAY*				
(Covidien) *See PRECISION 400 URINE METER*				
COLLODIAN FLEXIBLE (Gallipot)				
collodion				
LIQ, NA (U.S.P.,N.F.)				
118.28 ml	51552-0117-04	12.04		
473 ml	51552-0117-06	21.98		
COLLODION				
(Amend) *See COLLODION FLEXIBLE*				
(Amend)				
LIQ, NA (U.S.P.)				
120 ml	17317-0128-04	9.80		
500 ml	17317-0128-01	21.00		
4000 ml	17317-0128-06	91.00		
20000 ml	17317-0128-08	371.00		
(Baker, J.T.) *See COLLODION FLEXIBLE*				
(Baker, J.T.)				
LIQ, NA (U.S.P.)				
100 ml	10106-9202-04	23.75		
500 ml	10106-9202-01	20.12		
(Gallipot) *See COLLODIAN FLEXIBLE*				

PROD/MFR NDC AWP DP OBC

(Gallipot)
LIQ, NA (U.S.P.,N.F.)
100 ml **51552-0203-05** 10.50
473 ml **51552-0203-06** 22.33

(Mallinckrodt Lab)
SOL, NA (U.S.P.)
120 ml **00406-4560-02** 10.05
(U.S.P.,FLEXIBLE)
150 ml **00406-4580-02** 12.79
500 ml **00406-4580-04** 19.67
(U.S.P.)
500 ml **00406-4560-09** 20.04

(Medisca) *See COLLODION FLEXIBLE*

(PCCA) *See COLLODION FLEXIBLE*

(PCCA)
SOL, NA (USP)
1 ml................ **51927-1204-00** 0.30

(Spectrum Pharmacy) *See COLLODION FLEXIBLE*

(Spectrum Pharmacy)
LIQ, NA (U.S.P.)
100 ml **49452-2220-04** 57.75
500 ml **49452-2220-02** 109.20
4000 ml **49452-2220-03** 633.50

COLLODION FLEXIBLE (Amend)
collodion
LIQ, NA (U.S.P.)
120 ml **17317-0129-04** 9.80
500 ml **17317-0129-01** 21.00
4000 ml **17317-0129-06** 91.00
20000 ml **17317-0129-08** 371.00

(Baker, J.T.)
LIQ, NA (U.S.P.)
100 ml **10106-9204-04** 36.75
500 ml **10106-9204-01** 63.25

(Medisca)
LIQ, NA (U.S.P.)
100 ml **38779-0625-05** 25.50
500 ml **38779-0625-08** 46.50
(USP,1X1000ML)
1000 ml **38779-0625-09** 76.50
(USP,1X4000ML)
4000 ml **38779-0625-01** 288.00

(PCCA)
LIQ, NA (USP)
1 ml................ **51927-1360-00** 0.44

(Spectrum Pharmacy)
LIQ, NA (U.S.P.)
100 ml **49452-2230-04** 57.75
500 ml **49452-2230-01** 109.20
4000 ml **49452-2230-02** 633.50

COLLOIDAL SULFUR
(PCCA) *See SULFUR COLLOIDAL*

COLOCORT (Paddock)
hydrocortisone
NMA, RC, 100 mg/60 ml,
60 ml............ **00574-2020-01** 12.65 AB
60 ml 7s.......... **00574-2020-07** 84.84 AB

COLOR ADDITIVE
(Amend) *See D & C GREEN #5*
(Amend) *See D & C GREEN #6*
(Amend) *See D & C GREEN #8*
(Amend) *See D & C RED #117*
(Amend) *See D & C RED #22*
(Amend) *See D & C RED #28*
(Amend) *See D & C RED #33*
(Amend) *See D & C VIOLET #2*
(Amend) *See D & C YELLOW #10*
(Amend) *See D & C YELLOW #11*
(Amend) *See D & C YELLOW #7*
(Amend) *See D & C YELLOW #8*
(Amend) *See F D & C BLUE #1*
(Amend) *See F D & C BLUE #2*
(Amend) *See F D & C GREEN #3*
(Amend) *See F D & C RED #3*
(Amend) *See F D & C RED #40*
(Amend) *See F D & C YELLOW #5*
(Amend) *See F D & C YELLOW #6*
(Gallipot) *See D&C YELLOW #10*
(Gallipot) *See F D & C BLUE #1*
(Gallipot) *See F D & C BLUE #2*
(Gallipot) *See F D & C GREEN #3*
(Gallipot) *See F D & C RED #3*
(Gallipot) *See F D & C RED #40*
(Gallipot) *See F D & C YELLOW #5*
(Gallipot) *See F D & C YELLOW #6*
(Medisca) *See BASIC FUCHSIN*
(Medisca) *See BRILLIANT GREEN*
(Medisca) *See D & C RED NO. 33*
(Medisca) *See FD&C BLUE NO. 2*
(Medisca) *See FD&C GREEN NO. 3*
(Medisca) *See FD&C RED NO. 40*
(Medisca) *See FD&C YELLOW NO. 6*
(Medisca) *See FOOD COLOR, BLUE*
(Medisca) *See FOOD COLOR, BROWN*
(Medisca) *See FOOD COLOR, GREEN*
(Medisca) *See FOOD COLOR, ORANGE*
(Medisca) *See FOOD COLOR, RED*
(Medisca) *See FOOD COLOR, VIOLET*
(Medisca) *See FOOD COLOR, YELLOW*
(PCCA) *See ACID RED 52*
(PCCA) *See BLACK FOOD COLOR*
(PCCA) *See BLUE FOOD COLOR*
(PCCA) *See BRILLIANT GREEN*
(PCCA) *See BROWN FOOD COLOR*
(PCCA) *See D & C RED NO. 28*
(PCCA) *See D & C YELLOW #10*
(PCCA) *See F D & C BLUE #1*
(PCCA) *See F D & C BLUE #2*
(PCCA) *See F D & C GREEN #3*
(PCCA) *See F D & C RED #40*
(PCCA) *See F D & C YELLOW #5*
(PCCA) *See F D & C YELLOW #6*
(PCCA) *See GREEN FOOD COLOR*
(PCCA) *See LIME GREEN FOOD COLOR*
(PCCA) *See ORANGE FOOD COLOR*
(PCCA) *See PINK FOOD COLOR*
(PCCA) *See RED FOOD COLOR*
(PCCA) *See VIOLET FOOD COLOR*
(PCCA) *See WHITE FOOD COLOR*
(PCCA) *See YELLOW FOOD COLOR*
(Spectrum Pharmacy) *See ACID RED 52*
(Spectrum Pharmacy) *See BRILLIANT GREEN*
(Spectrum Pharmacy) *See FD&C BLUE #1*

COLY-MYCIN M PARENTERAL (JHP)
colistimethate sodium
PDS, IJ (USP,PARENTERAL)
150 mg, ea .... **42023-0107-01** 72.98 AP

COLY-MYCIN S (JHP)
antibacterial/anti-inflammatory combination
SUS, OT (1X5ML,W/DROPPER)
5 ml................ **42023-0108-01** 45.38

COLY-MYCIN S OTIC (Phys Total Care)
REPACK
antibacterial/anti-inflammatory combination
SUS, OT, 5 ml **54868-0399-00** 56.15

COLYTE (Alaven)
peg electrolyte lavage solution
PDS, PO, 4000 ml......... **00091-7036-23** 35.06 AA

(Palmetto)
REPACK
k cl/na bicarb/na cl/na sulf/peg
PDR, PO, 4000 ml **23490-7890-00** 32.10

COLYTROL (Llorens Pharma Int)
atropine sulf/hyoscyamine sulf/scop hydrobrom
TAB, PO, 100s ea **54859-0704-10** 18.20

COMBIFLEX (Breckenridge Pharm)
apap/caff/phenyltoloxamine cit/salicylamide
CAP, PO, 100s ea **51991-0471-01** 60.24

COMBIFLEX ES (Breckenridge Pharm)
apap/caff/magnesium sal/phenyltoloxamine cit
TAB, PO, 100s ea **51991-0511-01** 88.75

COMBIGAN (Allergan Inc)
brimonidine tartrate/timolol maleate
SOL, OP, 0.2%-0.5%, 5 ml. **00023-9211-05** 78.64
10 ml............. **00023-9211-10** 157.27

COMBIPATCH (Novartis Pharm)
estradiol/norethindrone acetate
TDM, TD, ea............. **00078-0377-62** 7.91
(1X8)
8s ea.............. **00078-0377-42** 63.34
(3X8)
24s ea............. **00078-0377-45** 126.02
ea................. **00078-0378-62** 7.90
(1X8)
8s ea.............. **00078-0378-42** 63.25
(3X8)
24s ea............. **00078-0378-45** 125.87

(Phys Total Care)
REPACK
TDM, TD (1X8)
8s ea.............. **54868-4831-00** 46.85

COMBIVENT (Boehr Ingelheim Phar)
albuterol sulfate/ipratropium bromide
ARO, IH, 14.7 gm......... **00597-0013-14** 156.95

(A-S Medication)
REPACK
ARO, IH, 14.7 gm......... **54569-4600-00** 182.18

(Dispensing Solutions)
REPACK
ARO, IH, 14.7 gm......... **55045-3162-00** 100.00

(Phys Total Care)
REPACK
ARO, IH, 14.7 gm......... **54868-4225-00** 177.60

(Quality Care Prod)
REPACK
ARO, IH, 14.7 gm......... **49999-0990-07** 142.12

COMBIVIR (Glaxo)
lamivudine/zidovudine
TAB, PO, 150 mg-300 mg,
60s ea............. **00173-0595-00** 937.66
120s ea UD **00173-0595-02** 1875.32

(A-S Medication)
REPACK
TAB, PO, 150 mg-300 mg,
6s ea.............. **54569-4524-01** 121.90
10s ea............. **54569-4524-02** 203.16
60s ea............. **54569-4524-00** 1218.96

(Altura)
REPACK
TAB, PO, 150 mg-300 mg,
6s ea.............. **63874-0100-06** 79.98
8s ea.............. **63874-0100-08** 106.64
10s ea............. **63874-0100-10** 133.30
14s ea............. **63874-0100-14** 186.62
15s ea............. **63874-0100-15** 199.95
28s ea............. **63874-0100-28** 373.24
30s ea............. **63874-0100-30** 399.90
60s ea............. **63874-0100-60** 799.80
90s ea............. **63874-0100-90** 1199.70
100s ea............ **63874-0100-01** 1333.00

(DHS, Inc.)
REPACK
TAB, PO, 150 mg-300 mg,
10s ea............. **55887-0231-10** 187.48

(Dispensing Solutions)
REPACK
TAB, PO, 150 mg-300 mg,
6s ea.............. **55045-2856-06** 91.50

(Nucare Pharm)
REPACK
TAB, PO, 150 mg-300 mg,
6s ea.............. **66267-0509-06** 95.99

(Palmetto)
REPACK
TAB, PO, 150 mg-300 mg,
60s ea............. **23490-7087-06** 750.25

(PD-Rx Pharm)
REPACK
TAB, PO, 150 mg-300 mg,
4s ea.............. **55289-0389-04** 123.88
6s ea.............. **55289-0389-06** 185.82
14s ea............. **55289-0389-14** 433.58
20s ea............. **55289-0389-20** 619.40

PROD/MFR	NDC	AWP	DP	OBC
(Pharma Pac)				
REPACK				
TAB, PO, 150 mg-300 mg,				
2s ea	52959-0546-02	47.03		
3s ea	52959-0546-03	62.39		
4s ea	52959-0546-04	77.80		
6s ea	52959-0546-06	113.34		
8s ea	52959-0546-08	148.05		
10s ea	52959-0546-10	167.32		
14s ea	52959-0546-14	224.78		
15s ea	52959-0546-15	240.83		
20s ea	52959-0546-20	295.10		
28s ea	52959-0546-28	410.14		
(Phys Total Care)				
REPACK				
TAB, PO, 150 mg-300 mg,				
60s ea	54868-4114-00	806.49		
(Physician Partner)				
REPACK				
TAB, PO, 150 mg-300 mg,				
6s ea	21695-0846-06	216.81		
(Quality Care Prod)				
REPACK				
TAB, PO, 150 mg-300 mg,				
6s ea	49999-0062-06	248.48		
10s ea	49999-0062-10	183.36		
60s ea	49999-0062-60	2160.00		
(Southwood)				
REPACK				
TAB, PO, 150 mg-300 mg,				
30s ea	58016-0698-30	442.29		
60s ea	58016-0698-60	884.58		
90s ea	58016-0698-90	1326.87		
100s ea	58016-0698-00	1474.30		
(St. Mary's MPP)				
REPACK				
TAB, PO, 150 mg-300 mg,				
4s ea	60760-0595-04	77.63		
14s ea	60760-0595-14	256.69		
(Stat Rx)				
REPACK				
TAB, PO, 150 mg-300 mg,				
6s ea	16590-0061-06	105.25		
10s ea	16590-0061-10	173.03		
30s ea	16590-0061-30	422.00		
COMBUNOX (Forest Pharm)				
ibuprofen/oxycodone hydrochloride				
TAB, PO (FILM-COATED)				
400 mg-5 mg,				
100s ea, C-II	00456-5200-01	163.54		
COMFEEL PURILON (Coloplast)				
wound care preparation				
GEL, TP (ACCORDIAN APPLICATOR)				
8 gm 10s	11701-0855-05	65.00		
(ACCORDION APPLICATOR)				
15 gm 10s	11701-0855-10	94.30		
25 gm 10s	11701-0855-15	114.40		
COMFORT DETACHABLE INFUSION (Arkray)				
kit, administration, intravenous				
DEV, NA (27G,23" TUBING,HOSPITAL)				
10s ea	08317-9009-10	114.75	76.50	
(27G,23" TUBING,STANDARD)				
10s ea	08317-9001-10	93.75	62.50	
(27G,43" TUBING,HOSPITAL)				
10s ea	08317-9008-10	114.75	76.50	
(27G,43" TUBING,STANDARD)				
10s ea	08317-9000-10	93.75	62.50	
COMFORT PAC (PD-Rx Pharm)				
REPACK				
ibuprofen				
KIT, MR, 800 mg, ea	43063-0038-92	74.75		
COMMON PLANTAIN				
(PCCA) *See PLANTAIN LEAF*				
COMPAZINE (Pharma Pac)				
REPACK				
prochlorperazine				
SUP, RC, 25 mg, 12s ea	52959-0291-00	50.95		AB
(Pharma Pac)				
prochlorperazine maleate				
TAB, PO, 10 mg, 15s ea	52959-0391-15	24.55		AB
(Phys Total Care)				
REPACK				
prochlorperazine				
SUP, RC, 25 mg, 6s ea	54868-0622-02	28.01		AB
12s ea	54868-0622-00	54.76		AB

PROD/MFR	NDC	AWP	DP	OBC
(Phys Total Care)				
prochlorperazine maleate				
TAB, PO, 5 mg, 30s ea	54868-1284-02	26.36		AB
10 mg, 20s ea	54868-1081-02	27.01		AB
(Southwood)				
REPACK				
prochlorperazine				
SUP, RC, 5 mg, 12s ea	58016-3222-01	27.70		AB
25 mg, 12s ea	58016-3018-03	34.00		AB
COMPOUND 347 (RxElite)				
enflurane				
SOL, IH (USP)				
99.9%, 250 ml	66794-0010-25	75.00		AN
COMPOUND BENZOIN (PCCA)				
benzoin compound				
TIN, NA (USP)				
1 ml	51927-1584-00	0.12		
COMPRO (Paddock)				
prochlorperazine				
SUP, RC, 25 mg,				
12s ea UD	00574-7226-12	36.54		AB
COMTAN (Novartis Pharm)				
entacapone				
TAB, PO, 200 mg, 100s ea	00078-0327-05	346.51		
COMVAX (Merck)				
haemophilus b conjugate vac/hep b vac recombinant				
SUS, IM (SDV W/DILUENT,TAX INCL)				
0.5 ml 10s	00006-4898-00	522.68		
CONAL (Cypress Pharm)				
cpm tan/phenyleph tan/pyril tan				
SUS, PO (RASPBERRY)				
473 ml	60258-0411-16	128.43		
CONCEPT DHA (U.S. Pharm)				
prenatal vitamins				
CAP, PO, 30s ea	52747-0621-30	32.40		
CONCEPT OB (U.S. Pharm)				
prenatal vitamins				
CAP, PO, 30s ea	52747-0620-30	30.00		
CONCERTA (McNeil Consumer Healthcare)				
methylphenidate hydrochloride				
TER, PO, 36 mg,				
100s ea, C-II	50458-0586-01	526.52		EE
(Ortho-McNeil Pharm)				
TER, PO, 18 mg,				
100s ea, C-II	50458-0585-01	497.99		EE
27 mg,				
100s ea, C-II	50458-0588-01	510.47		EE
54 mg,				
100s ea, C-II	50458-0587-01	572.94		
(Palmetto)				
REPACK				
TER, PO, 18 mg,				
30s ea, C-II	23490-9415-03	135.00		
27 mg,				
30s ea, C-II	23490-9416-03	138.00		
36 mg,				
30s ea, C-II	23490-9417-03	141.00		
54 mg,				
30s ea, C-II	23490-9418-03	144.00		
(PD-Rx Pharm)				
REPACK				
TER, PO, 18 mg,				
30s ea, C-II	55289-0835-30	224.93		
90s ea, C-II	55289-0835-90	657.00		
27 mg,				
90s ea, C-II	55289-0975-90	673.01		
36 mg,				
30s ea, C-II	55289-0859-30	237.30		
90s ea, C-II	55289-0859-90	694.13		
54 mg,				
30s ea, C-II	55289-0854-30	257.43		
90s ea, C-II	55289-0854-90	754.88		
(Phys Total Care)				
REPACK				
TER, PO, 18 mg,				
10s ea, C-II	54868-4489-00	54.23		
30s ea, C-II	54868-4489-02	147.66		
60s ea, C-II	54868-4489-03	292.06		
90s ea, C-II	54868-4489-01	436.46		
27 mg,				
10s ea, C-II	54868-4957-00	67.90		
30s ea, C-II	54868-4957-01	185.20		
36 mg,				
10s ea, C-II	54868-4759-03	69.91		
20s ea, C-II	54868-4759-01	135.91		
30s ea, C-II	54868-4759-02	190.90		
60s ea, C-II	54868-4759-00	377.88		

PROD/MFR	NDC	AWP	DP	OBC
54 mg,				
10s ea, C-II	54868-4789-01	68.44		
30s ea, C-II	54868-4789-00	186.73		
(Quality Care Prod)				
REPACK				
TER, PO, 18 mg,				
30s ea, C-II	35356-0151-30	663.37		
90s ea, C-II	35356-0151-90	1982.08		
27 mg,				
30s ea, C-II	35356-0152-30	679.40		
90s ea, C-II	35356-0152-90	2030.18		
36 mg,				
30s ea, C-II	35356-0153-30	701.44		
90s ea, C-II	35356-0153-90	2096.32		
54 mg,				
30s ea, C-II	35356-0154-30	763.57		
90s ea, C-II	35356-0154-90	2282.70		
(Stat Rx)				
REPACK				
TER, PO, 18 mg,				
30s ea, C-II	16590-0787-30	166.01		EE
CONDYLOX (Watson)				
podofilox				
GEL, TP (1X3.5GM,W/APPLICATORTIP)				
0.5%, 3.5 gm	52544-0045-13	293.20		
(Watson Labs)				
SOL, TP (1X3.5ML)				
0.5%, 3.5 ml	52544-0046-13	137.88		AT
(Phys Total Care)				
REPACK				
SOL, TP, 0.5%, 3.5 ml	54868-3649-00	141.98		AT
CONGO RED (PCCA)				
POW, NA (C.I. 22120)				
1 gm	51927-2043-00	10.50		
CONIVAPTAN HYDROCHLORIDE				
(Astellas) *See VAPRISOL*				
CONJUGATED ESTROGENS				
(Wyeth) *See PREMARIN*				
(Wyeth) *See PREMARIN INTRAVENOUS*				
(Wyeth) *See PREMARIN VAGINAL*				
CONJUGATED ESTROGENS SYNTHETIC A				
(Teva) *See CENESTIN*				
CONJUGATED ESTROGENS SYNTHETIC B				
(Teva) *See ENJUVIA*				
CONJUGATED ESTROGENS/ MEDROXYPROGESTERONE ACETATE				
(Wyeth) *See PREMPHASE*				
(Wyeth) *See PREMPRO*				
CONSTULOSE (Actavis Mid Atlantic)				
lactulose				
SOL, PO, 10 gm/15 ml,				
237 ml	00472-1358-08	20.20		AA
946 ml	00472-1358-32	65.45		AA
CONTROL RX (Omnii Intl)				
sodium fluoride				
CRE, DE (MINT)				
1.1%, 56 gm	48878-3100-06	9.25		
CONTROLLER LIFECARE (Abbott Hosp)				
pump, infusion				
DEV, NA (MODEL 75,VOLUMETRIC)				
ea	00074-1924-01	2701.65	2388.82	
CONVEEN INTERMITTENT CATHETER (Coloplast)				
catheter				
DEV, NA (CURVED/TAPERED 10FR,14")				
50s ea	11701-0867-23	124.50		
(CURVED/TAPERED 12FR,14")				
50s ea	11701-0867-24	124.50		
(CURVED/TAPERED 14FR,14")				
50s ea	11701-0867-25	124.50		
(CURVED/TAPERED 16FR,14")				
50s ea	11701-0867-26	124.50		
(CURVED/TAPERED 8 FR,14")				
50s ea	11701-0867-22	124.50		
(FEMALE, 10 FR, 6")				
50s ea	11701-0867-13	40.50		
(FEMALE, 12 FR, 6")				
50s ea	11701-0867-12	40.50		
(FEMALE, 14 FR, 6")				
50s ea	11701-0867-11	40.50		
(LONG/ADOLES. 10 FR, 14")				
50s ea	11701-0867-15	49.00		
(LONG/ADOLES. 8 FR, 14")				
50s ea	11701-0867-14	49.00		
(LONG/ADULT 12 FR, 14")				
50s ea	11701-0867-16	49.00		

PROD/MFR	NDC	AWP	DP	OBC
(LONG/ADULT 14 FR, 14")				
50s ea	11701-0867-17	49.00		
(LONG/ADULT 16 FR, 14")				
50s ea	11701-0867-18	49.00		
(OLIVE TIP 14 FR, 14")				
50s ea	11701-0867-32	124.50		
CONVEEN SECURITY + CATHETER & LINER (Coloplast)				
catheter				
DEV, NA (MALE, EXTERNAL, 21MM)				
35s ea	11701-0859-10	56.00		
(MALE, EXTERNAL, 25MM)				
35s ea	11701-0859-15	56.00		
(MALE, EXTERNAL, 30MM)				
35s ea	11701-0859-20	56.00		
(MALE, EXTERNAL, 35MM)				
35s ea	11701-0859-25	56.00		
(MALE, EXTERNAL, 40MM)				
35s ea	11701-0859-30	56.00		
(MALE, EXTERNAL, 21MM)				
100s ea	11701-0859-35	144.00		
(MALE, EXTERNAL, 25 MM)				
100s ea	11701-0859-40	144.00		
(MALE, EXTERNAL, 30MM)				
100s ea	11701-0859-45	144.00		
(MALE, EXTERNAL, 35MM)				
100s ea	11701-0859-50	144.00		
(MALE, EXTERNAL, 40MM)				
100s ea	11701-0859-55	144.00		
CONVEEN SECURITY + SELF SEALING (Coloplast)				
catheter				
DEV, NA (MALE, EXTERNAL, 21MM)				
35s ea	11701-0861-10	59.15		
(MALE, EXTERNAL, 25MM)				
35s ea	11701-0861-15	59.15		
(MALE, EXTERNAL, 30MM)				
35s ea	11701-0861-20	59.15		
(MALE, EXTERNAL, 35MM)				
35s ea	11701-0861-25	59.15		
(MALE, EXTERNAL, 40MM)				
35s ea	11701-0861-30	59.15		
(MALE, EXTERNAL, 21MM)				
100s ea	11701-0861-35	162.00		
(MALE, EXTERNAL, 25MM)				
100s ea	11701-0861-40	162.00		
(MALE, EXTERNAL, 30MM)				
100s ea	11701-0861-45	162.00		
(MALE, EXTERNAL, 35MM)				
100s ea	11701-0861-50	162.00		
(MALE, EXTERNAL, 40MM)				
100s ea	11701-0861-55	162.00		
CONVEEN SECURITY + URINE LEG BAG (Coloplast)				
incontinence products				
DEV, NA (LRG W/20" TUBING)				
10s ea	11701-0870-15	65.00		
(MEDIUM W/20" TUBING)				
10s ea	11701-0870-10	65.00		
(500ML W/20" TUBING)				
15s ea	11701-0870-11	129.00		
(750ML W/20" TUBING)				
15s ea	11701-0870-16	129.00		
CONVEEN SELF SEALING URISHEATH (Coloplast)				
catheter				
DEV, NA (MALE, EXTERNAL, 20MM)				
35s ea	11701-0860-10	56.00		
(MALE, EXTERNAL, 25MM)				
35s ea	11701-0860-15	56.00		
(MALE, EXTERNAL, 30MM)				
35s ea	11701-0860-20	56.00		
(MALE, EXTERNAL, 35MM)				
35s ea	11701-0860-25	56.00		
(MALE, EXTERNAL, 40MM)				
35s ea	11701-0860-30	56.00		
(MALE, EXTERNAL, 20MM)				
100s ea	11701-0860-35	153.00		
(MALE, EXTERNAL, 25MM)				
100s ea	11701-0860-40	153.00		
(MALE, EXTERNAL, 30MM)				
100s ea	11701-0860-45	153.00		
(MALE, EXTERNAL, 35MM)				
100s ea	11701-0860-50	153.00		
(MALE, EXTERNAL, 40MM)				
100s ea	11701-0860-55	153.00		
CONVEEN ULTRA SECURE SELF-SEALING (Coloplast)				
catheter				
DEV, NA (MALE EXTERNAL,21 MM)				
35s ea	11701-0873-21	59.50		
(MALE EXTERNAL,25 MM)				
35s ea	11701-0873-25	59.50		
(MALE EXTERNAL,30 MM)				
35s ea	11701-0873-30	59.50		
(MALE EXTERNAL,35 MM)				
35s ea	11701-0873-35	59.50		
(MALE EXTERNAL,21 MM)				
100s ea	11701-0873-22	157.00		
(MALE EXTERNAL,25 MM)				
100s ea	11701-0873-26	157.00		
(MALE EXTERNAL,30 MM)				
100s ea	11701-0873-31	157.00		
(MALE EXTERNAL,35 MM)				
100s ea	11701-0873-36	157.00		
CONVEEN URISHEATH/URILINER (Coloplast)				
catheter				
DEV, NA (MALE, EXT. EX LRG-40MM)				
35s ea	11701-0858-30	41.65		
(MALE, EXT. GER/PED-20MM)				
35s ea	11701-0858-10	41.65		
(MALE, EXTERNAL LRG-35MM)				
35s ea	11701-0858-25	41.65		
(MALE, EXTERNAL MED-30MM)				
35s ea	11701-0858-20	41.65		
(MALE, EXTERNAL SM-25MM)				
35s ea	11701-0858-15	41.65		
(MALE, EXT. EX LRG-40 MM)				
100s ea	11701-0858-55	110.00		
(MALE, EXT. GER/PED-20MM)				
100s ea	11701-0858-35	110.00		
(MALE, EXTERNAL LRG-35MM)				
100s ea	11701-0858-50	110.00		
(MALE, EXTERNAL MED-30MM)				
100s ea	11701-0858-45	110.00		
(MALE, EXTERNAL SM-25MM)				
100s ea	11701-0858-40	110.00		
COPAXONE (Teva Neuroscience)				
glatiramer acetate				
KIT, MR, 20 mg/ml, ea	68546-0317-30	3303.05		
COPD (Carwin)				
dyphylline/guaifenesin				
TAB, PO, 200 mg-200 mg, 100s ea	15370-0021-10	26.75		
COPEGUS (Roche Labs)				
ribavirin				
TAB, PO (FILM COATED)				
200 mg, 168s ea	00004-0086-94	2552.35		
COPPER (Baker, J.T.)				
GRA, NA (REAGENT, 20-30 MESH)				
500 gm	10106-1720-01	113.61		
2500 gm	10106-1720-05	428.27		
12000 gm	10106-1720-07	1170.34		
POW, NA (PURIFIED)				
500 gm	10106-1728-01	82.81		
(Hospira)				
copper chloride				
SOL, IV (VIAL, 0.4 MG/ML COPPER)				
1.07 mg/ml, 10 ml 25s	00409-4092-01	23.40	20.50	
COPPER ACETATE				
(Amend) *See CUPRIC ACETATE MONOHYDRATE*				
(Baker, J.T.) *See CUPRIC ACETATE MONOHYDRATE*				
(Medisca) *See CUPRIC ACETATE*				
(PCCA) *See CUPRIC ACETATE*				
COPPER BROMIDE				
(Baker, J.T.) *See CUPRIC BROMIDE*				
COPPER CARBONATE				
(Baker, J.T.) *See CUPRIC CARBONATE*				
COPPER CHELATE (Gallipot)				
copper, chelated				
POW, NA (AMINO ACID CHELATE 20%)				
1000 gm	51552-0974-07	84.00	60.00	
COPPER CHLORIDE				
(Amend) *See CUPRIC CHLORIDE DIHYDRATE*				
(Baker, J.T.) *See CUPRIC CHLORIDE DIHYDRATE*				
(Baker, J.T.) *See CUPROUS CHLORIDE*				
(Hospira) *See COPPER*				
(Medisca) *See CUPRIC CHLORIDE*				
(PCCA) *See CUPRIC CHLORIDE*				
(Spectrum Pharmacy) *See CUPRIC CHLORIDE*				
COPPER CYANIDE				
(Baker, J.T.) *See CUPROUS CYANIDE*				
COPPER GLUCONATE (Amend)				
POW, NA (U.S.P., F.C.C.)				
454 gm	17317-0822-01	33.60		
2270 gm	17317-0822-05	133.00		
(Gallipot)				
POW, NA (U.S.P.,F.C.C.)				
113.4 gm	51552-0497-04	17.92		
(PCCA)				
POW, NA (USP)				
1 gm	51927-2218-00	0.59		
(Spectrum Pharmacy)				
POW, NA (U.S.P.)				
125 gm	49452-2267-01	94.15		
500 gm	49452-2267-02	189.00		
2500 gm	49452-2267-03	812.00		
COPPER GLYCINATE				
(PCCA) *See COPPER GLYCINATE MONOHYDRATE*				
(PCCA)				
POW, NA (ANHYDROUS; 30% COPPER)				
1 gm	51927-3182-00	1.35		
COPPER GLYCINATE MONOHYDRATE (PCCA)				
copper glycinate				
POW, NA (1X1GM)				
1 gm	51927-3562-00	0.37		
COPPER NITRATE				
(Amend) *See CUPRIC NITRATE*				
(Baker, J.T.) *See CUPRIC NITRATE 2.5-HYDRATE*				
(Baker, J.T.) *See CUPRIC NITRATE N-HYDRATE*				
(Mallinckrodt Lab) *See CUPRIC NITRATE*				
(PCCA) *See CUPRIC NITRATE TRIHYDRATE ACS*				
COPPER OXIDE				
(Amend) *See CUPRIC OXIDE ANHYDROUS*				
(Baker, J.T.) *See CUPRIC OXIDE*				
(Baker, J.T.) *See CUPROUS OXIDE*				
(Gallipot) *See CUPRIC OXIDE*				
(PCCA) *See CUPRIC OXIDE*				
COPPER OXIDE/FOLIC ACID/NIACINAMIDE/ ZINC OXIDE				
(Acella) *See NICOTINAMIDE/ZINC OXIDE/CUPRIC OXIDE/FOLIC ACID*				
(PruGen) *See NICOTINAMIDE W/ZINC AND CUPRIC OXIDES & FOLIC ACID*				
COPPER SALICYLATE (PCCA)				
POW, NA, 1 gm	51927-2532-00	8.40		
COPPER SULFATE				
(Amend) *See CUPRIC SULFATE*				
(Amend) *See CUPRIC SULFATE MONOHYDRATE*				
(Amer Regent) *See CUPRIC SULFATE*				
(Baker, J.T.) *See CUPRIC SULFATE ANHYDROUS*				
(Baker, J.T.) *See CUPRIC SULFATE PENTAHYDRATE*				
(Gallipot)				
CRY, NA (TECHNICAL)				
113.4 gm	51552-0385-04	5.95		
454 gm	51552-0385-06	14.00		
POW, NA, 56.7 gm	51552-0377-03	5.46		
454 gm	51552-0377-06	16.66		
(Humco)				
CRY, NA (TECHNICAL)				
120 gm	00395-0659-94	4.91		
454 gm	00395-0659-01	10.27		
POW, NA, 454 gm	00395-0665-01	15.26		
(Mallinckrodt Lab) *See CUPRIC SULFATE*				
(PCCA) *See CUPRIC SULFATE*				
(Spectrum Pharmacy) *See CUPRIC SULFATE PENTAHYDRATE*				
COPPER, CHELATED				
(Gallipot) *See COPPER CHELATE*				
COQ(10)50 (Bio-Tech Pharm)				
coenzyme q10				
POW, NA, 50 gm	53191-0254-05	240.00		
CORAL CALCIUM (PCCA)				
calcium carbonate				
POW, NA, 1 gm	51927-3607-00	0.55		
CORAZ (Auriga)				
hydrocortisone/salicylic acid/sulfur				
KIT, TP (USP)				
2%-2%-2%, 207 ml	14629-0516-01	75.00		
CORDARONE (Wyeth)				
amiodarone hydrochloride				
TAB, PO, 200 mg, 60s ea	00008-4188-04	281.35	234.46	AB

PROD/MFR	NDC	AWP	DP	OBC
CORDRAN (Aqua Pharmaceuticals)				
flurandrenolide				
LOT, TP, 0.05%, 15 ml	16110-0052-15	72.00		
60 ml	16110-0052-60	186.00		
(Phys Total Care)				
REPACK				
LOT, TP, 0.05%, 60 ml	54868-3227-01	45.42		AT
CORDRAN SP (Aqua Pharmaceuticals)				
flurandrenolide				
CRE, TP, 0.05%, 15 gm	16110-0035-15	72.00		
30 gm	16110-0035-30	127.20		
60 gm	16110-0035-60	186.00		
(Phys Total Care)				
REPACK				
CRE, TP, 0.05%, 15 gm	54868-1646-00	23.49		
CORDRAN TAPE (Watson)				
flurandrenolide				
TAP, TP (24X3")				
4 mcg/cm2, ea	52544-0044-24	47.06		
(80X3")				
4 mcg/cm2, ea	52544-0044-80	100.98		
COREG (Glaxo)				
carvedilol				
TAB, PO (FILM-COATED)				
3.125 mg, 100s ea	00007-4139-20	248.90		
(BLISTER CARD)				
6.25 mg, 28s ea	00007-4140-55	46.37		
(FILM-COATED)				
6.25 mg, 100s ea	00007-4140-20	248.90		
(BLISTER CARD)				
12.5 mg, 28s ea	00007-4141-55	46.37		
(FILM-COATED)				
12.5 mg, 100s ea	00007-4141-20	248.90		
(BLISTER CARD)				
25 mg, 28s ea	00007-4142-55	46.37		
(FILM-COATED)				
25 mg, 100s ea	00007-4142-20	248.90		
(DHS, Inc.)				
REPACK				
TAB, PO, 6.25 mg, 60s ea	55887-0731-60	196.50		
(PD-Rx Pharm)				
REPACK				
TAB, PO, 6.25 mg, 30s ea	55289-0986-30	102.15		
(REDI-SCRIPT,FILM-COATED)				
6.25 mg, 30s ea	58864-0737-30	89.71		
25 mg, 30s ea	58864-0727-30	89.71		
(Phys Total Care)				
REPACK				
TAB, PO (FILM-COATED)				
3.125 mg, 10s ea	54868-4421-01	33.81		
30s ea	54868-4421-00	96.21		
(FILM-COATED)				
3.125 mg, 60s ea	54868-4421-02	179.40		
6.25 mg, 10s ea	54868-4424-03	29.44		
20s ea	54868-4424-02	57.01		
30s ea	54868-4424-00	84.58		
60s ea	54868-4424-01	158.10		
12.5 mg, 10s ea	54868-4396-01	30.55		
30s ea	54868-4396-00	87.90		
(FILM-COATED)				
12.5 mg, 60s ea	54868-4396-02	164.36		
100s ea	54868-4396-03	272.06		
25 mg, 10s ea	54868-4395-03	28.82		
(FILM-COATED)				
25 mg, 20s ea	54868-4395-01	56.39		
30s ea	54868-4395-02	83.96		
(FILM-COATED)				
25 mg, 60s ea	54868-4395-00	157.48		
(Quality Care Prod)				
REPACK				
TAB, PO (FILM-COATED)				
3.125 mg, 20s ea	49999-0577-20	72.63		
6.25 mg, 30s ea	49999-0939-30	110.89		
12.5 mg, 30s ea	49999-0938-30	110.88		
25 mg, 30s ea	49999-0872-30	110.88		
COREG CR (Glaxo)				
carvedilol phosphate				
CER, PO, 10 mg, 30s ea	00007-3370-13	137.70		
20 mg, 30s ea	00007-3371-13	137.70		
40 mg, 30s ea	00007-3372-13	137.70		
80 mg, 30s ea	00007-3373-13	137.70		
(Phys Total Care)				
REPACK				
CER, PO, 10 mg, 30s ea	54868-6019-00	164.97		
90s ea	54868-6019-01	475.21		
20 mg, 30s ea	54868-0106-00	157.21		
90s ea	54868-0106-01	453.34		
40 mg, 30s ea	54868-5869-00	157.21		
90s ea	54868-5869-01	453.34		
80 mg, 30s ea	54868-5771-00	157.21		
90s ea	54868-5771-01	453.34		
(Quality Care Prod)				
REPACK				
CER, PO, 20 mg, 30s ea	35356-0518-30	244.60		
80 mg, 30s ea	35356-0490-30	236.36		
CORFEN DM (Cypress Pharm)				
cpm/dm/phenyleph hcl				
SOL, PO (AF,SF,DYE-FREE,GRAPE)				
473 ml	60258-0238-16	36.16		
CORGARD (King Pharm)				
nadolol				
TAB, PO, 20 mg, 100s ea	60793-0800-01	296.22		AB
40 mg, 100s ea	60793-0801-01	346.57		AB
80 mg, 100s ea	60793-0802-01	476.14		AB
(Phys Total Care)				
REPACK				
TAB, PO, 40 mg, 10s ea	54868-0674-01	26.06		AB
30s ea	54868-0674-00	74.43		AB
CORIANDER OIL (Medisca)				
OIL, NA (1X14ML, NATURAL)				
14 ml	38779-1214-03	16.50		
(1X25ML, NATURAL)				
25 ml	38779-1214-04	31.50		
(1X100ML, NATURAL)				
100 ml	38779-1214-05	114.00		
(1X500ML, NATURAL)				
500 ml	38779-1214-08	337.50		
(PCCA)				
OIL, NA, 1 ml	51927-1870-00	2.00		
(ARTIFICIAL)				
1 ml	51927-1871-00	1.50		
(Spectrum Pharmacy)				
OIL, NA, 100 ml	49452-2285-02	197.05		
CORLOPAM (Hospira)				
fenoldopam mesylate				
SOL, IV, 10 mg/ml, 1 ml	00409-2304-01	83.46	73.03	AP
(1X1ML,SDV,USP)				
10 mg/ml, 1 ml	00409-3373-01	75.76	66.29	AP
(1X2ML,USP,SDV)				
10 mg/ml, 2 ml	00409-3373-02	158.87	139.01	AP
(AMP,LATEX-FREE)				
10 mg/ml, 2 ml	00409-2304-02	166.92	146.06	
CORMAX (Watson)				
clobetasol propionate				
OIN, TP (1X15GM)				
0.05%, 15 gm	52544-0048-86	51.07		AB
(1X45GM)				
0.05%, 45 gm	52544-0048-89	102.89		AB
CORMAX SCALP APPLICATION (Watson)				
clobetasol propionate				
SOL, TP (1X25ML,USP)				
0.05%, 25 ml	52544-0049-83	42.29		
(1X50ML)				
0.05%, 50 ml	52544-0049-55	77.45		
CORN OIL (Medisca)				
OIL, NA (1X500ML)				
500 ml	38779-2038-08	28.50		
(1X4000ML)				
4000 ml	38779-2038-01	76.50		
(PCCA)				
OIL, NA (N.F.)				
1 ml	15927-2854-00	0.09		
(Spectrum Pharmacy)				
OIL, NA (N.F.)				
500 ml	49452-2300-01	56.35		
4000 ml	49452-2300-02	148.40		
CORN STARCH (Gallipot)				
starch, corn				
POW, NA (N.F.)				
454 gm	51552-0439-06	7.70		
2270 gm	51552-0439-09	21.98		
(Medisca)				
POW, NA (N.F.)				
500 gm	38779-0097-08	28.50		
1000 gm	38779-0097-09	46.50		
(NF)				
2500 gm	38779-0097-01	76.50		
(PCCA)				
POW, NA (NF)				
1 gm	51927-1070-00	0.06		
(Spectrum Pharmacy)				
POW, NA (N.F.)				
500 gm	49452-7250-01	49.70		
2500 gm	49452-7250-02	123.20		
CORTALO WITH ALOE (Aletheia)				
hydrocortisone acetate				
GEL, TP (1X43GM)				
2%, 43 gm	43234-0110-43	39.99		
CORTANE-B (Blansett)				
chloroxylenol/hc/pramoxine hcl				
LOT, TP, 60 ml	51674-0117-02	32.08		
SOL, OT, 10 ml	51674-0116-01	20.95		
CORTANE-B AQUEOUS (Blansett)				
chloroxylenol/hc/pramoxine hcl				
SOL, OT, 10 ml	51674-0118-01	20.95		
CORTASTAT (Clint)				
dexamethasone sodium phosphate				
SOL, IJ (VIAL)				
4 mg/ml, 5 ml	55553-0807-05	9.50		EE
CORTASTAT 10 (Clint)				
dexamethasone sodium phosphate				
SOL, IJ (VIAL)				
10 mg/ml, 10 ml	55553-0661-10	23.86		EE
CORTASTAT LA (Clint)				
dexamethasone acetate				
SUS, IJ (VIAL)				
8 mg/ml, 5 ml	55553-0092-05	27.95		EE
CORTEF (Pfizer)				
hydrocortisone				
TAB, PO, 5 mg, 50s ea	00009-0012-01	17.30	14.42	
10 mg, 100s ea	00009-0031-01	58.44	48.70	BP
20 mg, 100s ea	00009-0044-01	110.80	92.33	BP
(Dispensing Solutions)				
REPACK				
TAB, PO, 10 mg, 100s ea	55045-3458-00	50.00		
(Phys Total Care)				
REPACK				
TAB, PO, 5 mg, 100s ea	54868-3924-00	17.73		
CORTENEMA (ANI)				
hydrocortisone				
NMA, RC, 100 mg/60 ml,				
60 ml	62559-1110-01	12.42		AB
(7X60ML)				
100 mg/60 ml,				
60 ml 7s	62559-1110-07	83.89		AB
CORTIC (Everett)				
chloroxylenol/hc/pramoxine hcl				
SOL, OT, 10 ml	00642-0011-01	18.23		
CORTIC-ND (Everett)				
benzalkonium cl/chloroxylenol/hc/pramoxine hcl				
SOL, OT, 15 ml	00642-0012-15	98.63		
CORTICORELIN OVINE TRIFLUTATE				
(Ferring) *See ACTHREL*				
CORTICOTROPHIN (SYNTHETIC) (PCCA)				
corticotropin				
POW, NA (1X1GM)				
1 gm	51927-3551-00	49.80		
CORTICOTROPIN (Hawkins)				
POW, NA (ACTH)				
0.01 gm	63370-0049-04	475.20		
0.1 gm	63370-0049-06	3516.00		
0.5 gm	63370-0049-09	16132.80		
(Letco)				
POW, NA (ACTH)				
0.01 gm	62991-1657-01	372.00		
0.1 gm	62991-1657-02	2985.00		
0.5 gm	62991-1657-03	14040.00		
(Medisca)				
POW, NA (ACTH)				
0.01 gm	38779-1904-07	525.00		
0.1 gm	38779-1904-09	2445.00		
0.5 gm	38779-1904-00	10950.00		
(PCCA) *See CORTICOTROPHIN (SYNTHETIC)*				
CORTICOTROPIN, REPOSITORY				
(Questcor Pharm) *See H.P. ACTHAR*				
CORTIFOAM (Alaven)				
hydrocortisone acetate				
FOA, RC (1X15GM,WITH APPLICATOR)				
10%, 15 gm	68220-0140-15	280.65		
CORTISONE ACETATE (Consolidated Midland)				
TAB, PO, 25 mg, 100s ea	00223-0704-01	42.50		EE
1000s ea	00223-0704-02	400.00		EE
(Medisca)				
POW, NA (U.S.P.,MICRONIZED)				
1 gm	38779-0482-06	30.75		
5 gm	38779-0482-03	118.50		
25 gm	38779-0482-04	375.00		

PROD/MFR NDC AWP DP OBC

(Spectrum Pharmacy)
POW, NA (U.S.P.,MICRONIZED)
5 gm **49452-2321-02** 171.85
25 gm **49452-2321-03** 591.50

(Vita-Rx)
TAB, PO, 25 mg, 100s ea .. **49727-0092-02** 7.07 EE

(West-Ward)
TAB, PO, 25 mg, 100s ea .. **00143-1202-01** 45.75 BP

CORTISONE ACETATE MICRONIZED (PCCA)
cortisone acetate, micronized
POW, NA (USP)
1 gm **51927-1829-00** 18.00

CORTISONE ACETATE, MICRONIZED
(PCCA) *See CORTISONE ACETATE MICRONIZED*

CORTISPORIN (Monarch)
hc ace/neomycin sulf/polymyxin b sulf
CRE, TP, 0.5%-0.35%-10000 u/gm,
7.5 gm **61570-0032-75** 52.28

(Monarch)
bacitracin zn/hc/neomycin sulf/polymyxin b sulf
OIN, TP, 15 gm **61570-0031-50** 71.51

(Monarch)
hc/neomycin sulf/polymyxin b sulf
SOL, OT, 1%-0.35%-10000 u/ml,
10 ml .... **61570-0034-10** 80.02 AT

(A-S Medication)
REPACK
SUS, OP, 1%-0.35%-10000 u/ml,
7.5 ml **54569-0863-00** 76.48

(Pharma Pac)
REPACK
bacitracin zn/hc/neomycin sulf/polymyxin b sulf
OIN, OP, 3.5 gm .... **52959-0292-03** 32.80 AT

(Phys Total Care)
REPACK
hc ace/neomycin sulf/polymyxin b sulf
CRE, TP, 0.5%-0.35%-10000 u/gm,
7.5 gm **54868-1531-01** 63.13

(Phys Total Care)
hc/neomycin sulf/polymyxin b sulf
SUS, OP, 1%-0.35%-10000 u/ml,
7.5 ml **54868-0565-01** 71.52
OT, 1%-0.35%-10000 u/ml,
10 ml .... **54868-0213-01** 70.74 AT

(Quality Care Prod)
REPACK
SOL, OT (1X10ML)
1%-0.35%-10000 u/ml,
10 ml .... **35356-0517-10** 137.68 AT

(Southwood)
REPACK
SUS, OP (1X7.5ML)
1%-0.35%-10000 u/ml,
7.5 ml **58016-6443-01** 73.42

(Stat Rx)
REPACK
SOL, OT, 1%-0.35%-10000 u/ml,
10 ml **16590-0062-10** 70.00

CORTISPORIN TC (Phys Total Care)
REPACK
antibacterial/anti-inflammatory combination
SUS, OT, 10 ml **54868-0564-00** 93.19

CORTISPORIN-TC (JHP)
antibacterial/anti-inflammatory combination
SUS, OT (1X10ML,W/DROPPER)
10 ml **42023-0109-01** 82.98

CORTOMYCIN (Major)
hc/neomycin sulf/polymyxin b sulf
SOL, OT, 1%-0.35%-10000 u/ml,
10 ml .... **00904-3141-10** 16.80 AT
SUS, OT, 1%-0.35%-10000 u/ml,
10 ml .... **00904-3017-10** 30.49 AT

CORTROSYN (Amphastar)
cosyntropin
PDS, IJ (S.D.V.)
0.25 mg, 10s ea **00548-5900-00** 1278.96

CORVERT (Pfizer)
ibutilide fumarate
SOL, IV (FLIP-TOP VIAL)
0.1 mg/ml, 10 ml **00009-3794-01** 542.72 452.27

CORVITA (Trigen)
multivitamin, minerals, iron, and nutriceuticals
TAB, PO (SF,GLUTEN-FREE)
100s ea **13811-0028-10** 56.71

PROD/MFR NDC AWP DP OBC

CORVITE (Vertical)
multivitamin and minerals
TAB, PO (SF,GLUTEN-FREE)
100s ea **68025-0011-10** 76.86

CORVITE 150 (Vertical)
fe/folic acid/pyridoxine hcl/vit b12/vit c/zinc
TAB, PO (10X10,SF,GLUTEN-FREE)
100s ea UD **68025-0031-10** 144.86

CORVITE FREE (Vertical)
multivitamin, minerals, and nutriceuticals
TAB, PO (SF,DYE-FREE,GLUTEN-FREE)
100s ea **68025-0030-10** 74.81

CORYZA-D (Larken Labs, Inc.)
cough/cold combination
TER, PO, 3.5 mg-1 mg-45 mg,
100s ea **68047-0271-01** 78.35

CORYZA-DM (Larken Labs, Inc.)
dm/dexchlorpheniramine mal/phenyleph hcl/pyril mal
SYR, PO (AF,SF,DYE-FREE,GRAPE)
473 ml **68047-0270-16** 53.83

CORZALL (Hawthorn Pharm)
carbetapentane cit/pse hcl
SOL, PO (1X473ML,AF,SF,DYE-FREE)
20 mg/5 ml-30 mg/5 ml,
473 ml **63717-0552-16** 99.99

CORZALL PLUS (Hawthorn Pharm)
carbetapentane cit/pse hcl/pyril mal
SOL, PO (1X473ML,AF,SF,DYE-FREE)
473 ml **63717-0553-16** 109.99

CORZIDE (Phys Total Care)
REPACK
bendroflumethiazide/nadolol
TAB, PO, 5 mg-80 mg,
20s ea **54868-5344-02** 87.00

CORZIDE 40/5 (King Pharm)
bendroflumethiazide/nadolol
TAB, PO, 5 mg-40 mg,
100s ea .... **60793-0283-01** 334.64 EE

CORZIDE 80/5 (King Pharm)
bendroflumethiazide/nadolol
TAB, PO, 5 mg-80 mg,
100s ea **60793-0284-01** 441.54

(Phys Total Care)
REPACK
TAB, PO, 5 mg-80 mg,
10s ea **54868-5344-01** 44.44
30s ea **54868-5344-00** 122.48

COSMEGEN (Lundbeck)
dactinomycin
PDS, IV, 0.5 mg, ea **67386-0811-55** 659.30 13.43

COSOPT OCUMETER PLUS (Merck)
dorzolamide hydrochloride/timolol maleate
SOL, OP (W/CONTAINER)
2%-0.5%, 10 ml **00006-3628-36** 139.82

(Phys Total Care)
REPACK
SOL, OP, 2%-0.5%, 5 ml... **54868-4279-01** 69.80
10 ml **54868-4279-00** 156.14

(Quality Care Prod)
REPACK
SOL, OP (1X10ML)
2%-0.5%, 10 ml **35356-0100-01** 213.82

COSYNTROPIN
(Amphastar) *See CORTROSYN*

(GeneraMedix)
PDS, IJ (1X2ML,SDV,LYOPHILIZED)
0.25 mg, ea **10139-0905-02** 115.10
(1-X2ML,SDV,LYOPHILIZED)
0.25 mg, 10s ea **10139-0905-10** 1151.04

(Sandoz)
SOL, IV (NO ANTMCRBIAL&PRESRVATV)
0.25 mg/ml, 1 ml **00781-3052-71** 119.91
(10X1ML)
0.25 mg/ml,
1 ml 10s **00781-3052-95** 1199.07

COTAB A (MCR American)
chlorpheniramine maleate/codeine phosphate
TAB, PO, 4 mg-10 mg,
100s ea, C-III **58605-0436-01** 101.96

COTAB AX (MCR American)
chlorpheniramine maleate/codeine phosphate
TAB, PO, 4 mg-20 mg,
100s ea, C-III **58605-0437-01** 105.54

PROD/MFR NDC AWP DP OBC

COTABFLU (MCR American)
apap/cpm/codeine phos
TAB, PO (IMMEDIATE-RELEASE)
500 mg-4 mg-20 mg,
100s ea, C-III **58605-0438-01** 110.80

COTOLONE (Truxton)
prednisolone acetate
SUS, IJ (VIAL)
25 mg/ml, 30 ml **00463-1019-30** 10.80
50 mg/ml, 10 ml **00463-1020-10** 8.00

(Truxton)
prednisolone
TAB, PO, 5 mg, 1000s ea .. **00463-6071-10** 30.00 EE

COTTON CANDY FLAVOR (PCCA)
flavoring aid
SOL, NA, 1 ml **51927-3415-00** 0.38

COTTONSEED (Letco)
cottonseed oil
OIL, NA (NF)
500 ml **62991-1658-01** 18.75
4000 ml **62991-1658-02** 63.00

(Spectrum Pharmacy)
OIL, NA (N.F.)
500 ml **49452-2330-01** 49.35
4000 ml **49452-2330-02** 146.65

COTTONSEED OIL (Gallipot)
OIL, NA (U.S.P.,N.F.)
473 ml **51552-0258-06** 11.20

(Letco) *See COTTONSEED*

(Lorann Oil)
OIL, NA (U.S.P.)
30 ml **23535-0217-05** 1.10
120 ml **23535-0217-08** 2.10
480 ml **23535-0217-01** 5.45

(Medisca)
OIL, NA (1X500ML)
500 ml **38779-1216-08** 27.00
(1X4000ML)
4000 ml **38779-1216-01** 97.50

(PCCA)
OIL, NA (NF)
1 ml **51927-1313-00** 0.06

(Spectrum Pharmacy) *See COTTONSEED*

COUGH/COLD COMBINATION
(Auriga) *See EXTENDRYL*
(Auriga) *See ZINX COUGH*
(Breckenridge Pharm) *See HISTACOL LA*
(Breckenridge Pharm) *See HISTATAB D*
(GM Pharm) *See CARBATUSS-12*
(Hawthorn Pharm) *See DYTAN-CD*
(Hawthorn Pharm) *See DYTAN-CS*
(Hawthorn Pharm) *See DYTAN-HC*
(Larken Labs, Inc.) *See CORYZA-D*
(MAGNA Pharm) *See STAHIST*
(McNeil,R.A.) *See CHLO TUSS*
(Poly) *See POLY TAN DM*
(Respa Pharm) *See RESPA-A.R.*

COUGHTUSS (Breckenridge Pharm)
cpm/hydrocod bit/phenyleph hcl
SOL, PO (AF,SF,CANDY APPLE)
473 ml, C-III **51991-0221-16** 36.45

COUMADIN (Bristol-Myers)
warfarin sodium
PDS, IV, 5 mg, 6s ea **00590-0324-35** 204.40
TAB, PO, 1 mg, 100s ea ... **00056-0169-70** 120.14 AB
100s ea UD .... **00056-0169-75** 120.14 AB
1000s ea .... **00056-0169-90** 1201.73 AB
2 mg, 100s ea .... **00056-0170-70** 125.35 AB
100s ea UD .... **00056-0170-75** 125.35 AB
1000s ea .... **00056-0170-90** 1254.01 AB
2.5 mg, 100s ea ...... **00056-0176-70** 129.34 AB
100s ea UD .... **00056-0176-75** 129.34 AB
1000s ea .... **00056-0176-90** 1292.52 AB
3 mg, 100s ea .... **00056-0188-70** *129.84 AB
100s ea UD .... **00056-0188-75** 129.84 AB
1000s ea .... **00056-0188-90** 1298.23 AB
4 mg, 100s ea .... **00056-0168-70** 130.19 AB
100s ea UD .... **00056-0168-75** 130.19 AB
1000s ea .... **00056-0168-90** 1301.65 AB
5 mg, 100s ea .... **00056-0172-70** 134.80 AB
100s ea UD .... **00056-0172-75** 134.80 AB
1000s ea .... **00056-0172-90** 1348.22 AB

PROD/MFR	NDC	AWP	DP	OBC
6 mg, 100s ea	00056-0189-70	173.66		AB
100s ea UD	00056-0189-75	173.66		AB
1000s ea	00056-0189-90	1737.05		AB
7.5 mg, 100s ea	00056-0173-70	179.68		AB
100s ea UD	00056-0173-75	179.68		AB
(DYE-FREE)				
10 mg, 100s ea	00056-0174-70	186.38		AB
100s ea UD	00056-0174-75	186.38		AB
(A-S Medication) REPACK				
TAB, PO, 1 mg, 30s ea	54569-4443-00	34.20		AB
2 mg, 30s ea	54569-0158-00	35.68		AB
5 mg, 30s ea	54569-0159-00	38.37		AB
(AQ) REPACK				
TAB, PO, 1 mg, 100s ea	66105-0518-10	118.98		
2 mg, 100s ea	66105-0170-70	123.93		AB
2.5 mg, 100s ea	66105-0176-10	122.79		AB
3 mg, 100s ea	66105-0519-10	128.19		
5 mg, 100s ea	66105-0110-10	132.89		AB
6 mg, 100s ea	66105-0521-10	169.76		
10 mg, 100s ea	66105-0523-10	181.81		
(Nucare Pharm) REPACK				
TAB, PO, 1 mg, 100s ea	66267-0629-00	80.29		AB
2 mg, 100s ea	66267-0636-00	83.99		AB
2.5 mg, 100s ea	66267-0630-00	85.99		AB
3 mg, 100s ea	66267-0631-00	86.59		AB
4 mg, 100s ea	66267-0632-00	87.49		AB
5 mg, 100s ea	66267-0633-00	89.29		AB
6 mg, 100s ea	66267-0634-00	113.59		AB
7.5 mg, 100s ea	66267-0635-00	117.39		AB
(DYE-FREE)				
10 mg, 100s ea	66267-0628-00	121.59		AB
(PD-Rx Pharm) REPACK				
PDS, IV (REDI-SCRIPT)				
5 mg, 14s ea	58864-0223-14	21.68		
TAB, PO, 1 mg, 15s ea	58864-0357-15	18.40		AB
2 mg, 30s ea	58864-0030-30	52.30		AB
5 mg, 30s ea	55289-0286-30	54.75		AB
(REDI-SCRIPT)				
5 mg, 30s ea	58864-0223-30	41.77		AB
50s ea	55289-0286-50	91.25		AB
(Phys Total Care) REPACK				
TAB, PO, 1 mg, 10s ea	54868-2128-00	16.33		AB
30s ea	54868-2128-02	43.76		AB
90s ea	54868-2128-03	126.05		AB
2 mg, 30s ea	54868-2129-02	34.86		AB
60s ea	54868-2129-00	67.85		AB
100s ea	54868-2129-01	111.20		AB
2.5 mg, 10s ea	54868-2154-02	17.38		AB
30s ea	54868-2154-00	46.91		AB
45s ea	54868-2154-03	69.05		AB
100s ea	54868-2154-01	141.39		AB
3 mg, 10s ea	54868-4063-01	12.58		
30s ea	54868-4063-00	33.96		
4 mg, 30s ea	54868-3399-01	47.20		AB
100s ea	54868-3399-00	150.58		AB
5 mg, 10s ea	54868-1259-06	19.51		AB
20s ea	54868-1259-00	36.40		AB
30s ea	54868-1259-01	53.30		AB
60s ea	54868-1259-03	103.98		AB
90s ea	54868-1259-05	154.67		AB
100s ea	54868-1259-02	170.91		AB
7.5 mg, 30s ea	54868-2252-01	54.33		AB
(DYE-FREE)				
10 mg, 10s ea	54868-2454-02	18.22		AB
30s ea	54868-2454-01	50.92		AB
(Quality Care Prod) REPACK				
TAB, PO, 1 mg, 90s ea	35356-0540-90	186.40		AB
2.5 mg, 30s ea	49999-0411-30	70.28		AB
5 mg, 30s ea UD	49999-0093-30	57.00		AB
COUMARIN (PCCA)				
POW, NA, 1 gm	51927-1814-00	0.60		
COVARYX (Centrix)				
esterified estrogens/methyltestosterone				
TAB, PO (FILM-COATED)				
1.25 mg-2.5 mg,				
100s ea	11528-0010-01	71.94		
COVARYX HS (Centrix)				
esterified estrogens/methyltestosterone				
TAB, PO (FILM-COATED)				
0.625 mg-1.25 mg,				
100s ea	11528-0020-01	59.94		

PROD/MFR	NDC	AWP	DP	OBC
COVERA-HS (Pfizer)				
verapamil hydrochloride				
T24, PO, 180 mg, 100s ea	00025-2011-31	211.37	176.14	BC
100s ea UD	00025-2011-34	221.94	184.95	BC
240 mg, 100s ea	00025-2021-31	296.84	247.37	BC
100s ea UD	00025-2021-34	311.72	259.77	BC
COZAAR (Merck)				
losartan potassium				
TAB, PO (UNIT OF USE,FILM-COATED)				
25 mg, 90s ea	00006-0951-54	168.25		
(FILM-COATED)				
25 mg, 100s ea UD	00006-0951-28	186.94		
1000s ea	00006-0951-82	1869.46		
(BULK PACKAGE)				
25 mg, 10000s ea	00006-0951-87	18694.66		
(UNIT OF USE,FILM-COATED)				
50 mg, 30s ea	00006-0952-31	71.89		
90s ea	00006-0952-54	215.69		
(FILM-COATED)				
50 mg, 100s ea UD	00006-0952-28	239.64		
1000s ea	00006-0952-82	2396.50		
(BULK PACKAGE)				
50 mg, 10000s ea	00006-0952-87	23964.95		
(UNIT-OF-USE,FILM-COATED)				
100 mg, 30s ea	00006-0960-31	97.93		
90s ea	00006-0960-54	293.80		
(FILM-COATED)				
100 mg, 100s ea UD	00006-0960-28	326.44		
1000s ea	00006-0960-82	3264.36		
(BULK PACKAGE)				
100 mg, 5000s ea	00006-0960-86	16321.82		
(A-S Medication) REPACK				
TAB, PO (FILM-COATED)				
50 mg, 30s ea	54569-4438-00	74.89		
(Altura) REPACK				
TAB, PO (FILM COATED)				
50 mg, 10s ea	63874-0637-10	15.86		
20s ea	63874-0637-20	31.71		
30s ea	63874-0637-30	47.57		
90s ea	63874-0637-90	142.71		
100s ea	63874-0637-01	158.57		
(AQ) REPACK				
TAB, PO, 25 mg, 100s ea	66105-0552-10	194.74		
(FILM-COATED)				
50 mg, 30s ea	66105-0553-03	117.78		
100s ea	66105-0553-10	254.64		
(Bryant Ranch) REPACK				
TAB, PO, 50 mg, 30s ea	63629-1337-01	71.40		
100 mg, 30s ea	63629-2912-01	97.99		
(DHS, Inc.) REPACK				
TAB, PO (FILM-COATED)				
25 mg, 30s ea	55887-0432-30	70.00		
(Dispensing Solutions) REPACK				
TAB, PO (FILM-COATED)				
50 mg, 30s ea	55045-3401-08	64.50		
(PD-Rx Pharm) REPACK				
TAB, PO (REDI-SCRIPT,FILM-COATED)				
25 mg, 30s ea	58864-0807-30	74.00		
50 mg, 30s ea	58864-0662-30	106.86		
(FILM-COATED)				
100 mg, 30s ea	55289-0238-30	145.56		
(Phys Total Care) REPACK				
TAB, PO (FILM-COATED)				
25 mg, 30s ea	54868-5077-00	69.09		
50 mg, 30s ea	54868-3726-00	92.08		
60s ea	54868-3726-02	172.84		
(FILM-COATED)				
50 mg, 90s ea	54868-3726-01	257.29		
100 mg, 30s ea	54868-2335-00	130.73		
90s ea	54868-2335-01	367.45		
(Quality Care Prod) REPACK				
TAB, PO (FILM-COATED)				
25 mg, 90s ea	35356-0373-90	333.69		
50 mg, 30s ea	49999-0940-30	104.60		
90s ea	49999-0940-90	310.78		
100 mg, 90s ea	49999-0991-90	394.09		
(Stat Rx) REPACK				
TAB, PO, 25 mg, 30s ea	16590-0063-30	70.00		

PROD/MFR	NDC	AWP	DP	OBC
CPM 8/PE 20/MSC 1.25 (Cypress Pharm)				
cpm/methscopolamine nitrate/phenyleph hcl				
TER, PO, 8 mg-1.25 mg-20 mg,				
100s ea	60258-0250-01	57.27		
CPM 8/PSE 90/MSC 2.5 (Cypress Pharm)				
cpm/methscopolamine nitrate/pse hcl				
TER, PO (DYE-FREE)				
8 mg-2.5 mg-90 mg,				
100s ea	60258-0282-01	47.45		
CPM PSE (Boca Pharmacal)				
cpm/pse hcl				
SYR, PO (AF,DYE-FREE,GRAPE)				
2 mg/5 ml-30 mg/5 ml,				
473 ml	64376-0714-16	51.06		
CPM TAN/CARBETAPENTANE TAN/EPH TAN/PHENYLEPH TAN				
(Breckenridge Pharm) *See QUAD TANN*				
(Breckenridge Pharm) *See QUAD TANN PEDIATRIC*				
(Meda) *See RYNATUSS*				
(Unigen) *See QUADRATUSS PEDIATRIC*				
CPM TAN/CARBETAPENTANE TAN/PHENYLEPH TAN				
(Gil Pharmaceutical) *See CARBAPHEN 12*				
(Gil Pharmaceutical) *See CARBAPHEN 12 PED*				
(Hawthorn Pharm) *See XIRATUSS*				
CPM TAN/DM TAN/PSE TAN				
(Centrix) *See DICEL DM*				
CPM TAN/PHENYLEPH TAN/PYRIL TAN				
(Blansett) *See NALEX A 12*				
(Cypress Pharm) *See CONAL*				
CPM-PE-MSC (Laser Pharma)				
cpm/methscopolamine nitrate/phenyleph hcl				
SYR, PO, 473 ml	68134-0101-01	28.56		
CPM/CODEINE PHOS/PSE HCL				
(CodaDose) *See ZODRYL DAC 25*				
(CodaDose) *See ZODRYL DAC 30*				
(CodaDose) *See ZODRYL DAC 35*				
(CodaDose) *See ZODRYL DAC 40*				
(CodaDose) *See ZODRYL DAC 50*				
(CodaDose) *See ZODRYL DAC 60*				
(CodaDose) *See ZODRYL DAC 80*				
(Qualitest) *See PHENYLHISTINE DH*				
CPM/DIHYDROCODEINE BITARTRATE/PHENYLEPH HCL				
(Ballay Pharm., Inc) *See BALTUSSIN*				
(Breckenridge Pharm) *See COLDCOUGH PD*				
(Breckenridge Pharm) *See DUOHIST DH*				
(Breckenridge Pharm) *See TUSSCOUGH DHC*				
(Cypress Pharm) *See DIHYDRO-PE*				
CPM/DIHYDROCODEINE BITARTRATE/PSE HCL				
(Breckenridge Pharm) *See COLDCOUGH*				
(Cypress Pharm) *See DIHYDRO-CP*				
CPM/DM/GG/PHENYLEPH HCL				
(A. G. Marin) *See NEOTUSS-D*				
(Breckenridge Pharm) *See QUARTUSS*				
(Cypress Pharm) *See CHLORDEX GP*				
(Laser Pharma) *See DONATUSSIN*				
(PGD, Inc.) *See GENELAN*				
(PGD, Inc.) *See GENEPATUSS*				
CPM/DM/METHSCOPOLAMINE NITRATE				
(Auriga) *See EXTENDRYL DM*				
CPM/DM/PHENYLEPH HCL				
(Acella) *See DM/CHLORPHENIRAMINE MALEATE/PHENYLEPH*				
(Boca Pharmacal) *See C-PHEN DM*				
(Boca Pharmacal) *See DEX PC*				
(Breckenridge Pharm) *See MINTUSS DR*				
(Breckenridge Pharm) *See QUARTUSS DM*				
(Breckenridge Pharm) *See TRITAL DM*				
(Breckenridge Pharm) *See TUSSPLEX DM*				
(Cypress Pharm) *See CERON-DM*				
(Cypress Pharm) *See CORFEN DM*				
(Cypress Pharm) *See DE-CHLOR DM*				
(Cypress Pharm) *See DE-CHLOR DR*				

PROD/MFR NDC AWP DP OBC

(Cypress Pharm) *See RELAHIST-DM*
(Edwards) *See ED-A-HIST DM*
(Gil Pharmaceutical) *See PHENABID DM*
(Hawthorn Pharm) *See NASOHIST DM*
(Larken Labs, Inc.) *See NOHIST DMX*
(Larken Labs, Inc.) *See NOHIST-PDX*
(Larken Labs, Inc.) *See PE-HIST DM*
(Laser Pharma) *See DM-PE-CHLOR*
(Laser Pharma) *See DONATUSSIN DM*
(Laser Pharma) *See NEO DM DROPS*
(Poly) *See POLY-TUSSIN DM*
(Silarx) *See SILDEC PE-DM*
(Vertical) *See ZOTEX-12D*

CPM/DM/PHENYLEPHRINE HYDROCHLORIDE
(Pharma Pac)
REPACK
cpm/dm/phenyleph hcl
SOL, PO, 30 ml..........52959-0871-30 46.56

CPM/DM/PSE HCL
(Acella) *See ENTRE-S SUSPENSION*
(Atley) *See ATUSS DS*
(Cypress Pharm) *See NEUTRAHIST PDX*
(Macoven) *See CHLORPHENIRAMINE/PSUEDO/ DM TANNATE*
(McNeil,R.A.) *See M-END DM*
(PGD, Inc.) *See GENEDEL*
(PGD, Inc.) *See SUDATUSS DM*

CPM/GG/HYDROCOD BIT/PSE HCL
(Huckaby) *See ZHIST*

CPM/GG/PHENYLEPH HCL
(Boca Pharmacal) *See P CHLOR GG*

CPM/HYDROCOD BIT/PHENYLEPH HCL
(Blansett) *See B-TUSS*
(Breckenridge Pharm) *See COUGHTUSS*
(Breckenridge Pharm) *See LIQUICOUGH HC*
(Breckenridge Pharm) *See MINTUSS HC*
(Breckenridge Pharm) *See MINTUSS MS*
(Breckenridge Pharm) *See RINDAL HD*
(Breckenridge Pharm) *See RINDAL HD PLUS*
(Ethex) *See HISTINEX HC*
(Hawthorn Pharm) *See TRIANT-HC*
(Laser Pharma) *See NEO HC*
(Poly) *See POLY-TUSSIN HD*
(Vintage) *See H-C TUSSIVE*

CPM/HYDROCOD BIT/PHENYLEPH HCL/PYRIL MAL
(GM Pharm) *See PHENA-HC*

CPM/HYDROCOD BIT/PSE HCL
(Breckenridge Pharm) *See COLDCOUGH HC*
(Breckenridge Pharm) *See DETUSS*
(Ethex) *See HISTINEX PV*
(Ethex) *See HYDRO-TUSSIN HC*
(PGD, Inc.) *See GENECOF-HC*
(Pharmakon) *See JAYCOF-HC*
(SJ) *See NOTUSS-FORTE*

CPM/METHSCOPOLAMINE NITRATE/ PHENYLEPH HCL
(A. G. Marin) *See DRYSEC*
(Adamis) *See AEROHIST PLUS*
(Adamis) *See AEROKID*
(Auriga) *See DURAVENT*
(Auriga) *See DURAVENT-DA*
(Auriga) *See EXTENDRYL*
(Auriga) *See EXTENDRYL JR*
(Auriga) *See EXTENDRYL SR*
(Boca Pharmacal) *See PCM ALLERGY*
(Breckenridge Pharm) *See ALLERGY DN PE*
(Breckenridge Pharm) *See DURADRYL*
(Breckenridge Pharm) *See DURADRYL SR*
(Breckenridge Pharm) *See HISTATAB PH*
(Breckenridge Pharm) *See TRIALL*
(Capellon) *See RESCON*
(Capellon) *See RESCON-MX*
(Cornerstone) *See ALLERX DOSEPACK PE*
(Cypress Pharm) *See CHLOR-MES*
(Cypress Pharm) *See CHLOR-MES D*
(Cypress Pharm) *See CPM 8/PE 20/MSC 1.25*
(Cypress Pharm) *See DEHISTINE*
(Cypress Pharm) *See RALIX*
(Dexo) *See AH-CHEW*
(Dexo) *See EX-HISTINE*
(Dexo) *See OMNIHIST L.A.*
(Dexo) *See WE ALLERGY*
(Larken Labs, Inc.) *See NOHIST-PE*
(Larken Labs, Inc.) *See NOHIST-PLUS*
(Larken Labs, Inc.) *See NOHIST-PLUS JR*
(Larken Labs, Inc.) *See SCOPOHIST*
(Larken Labs, Inc.) *See SCOPOHIST-PE*
(Laser Pharma) *See CPM-PE-MSC*
(Laser Pharma) *See DALLERGY*
(Laser Pharma) *See DALLERGY PE*
(Marnel) *See PREHIST D*

CPM/METHSCOPOLAMINE NITRATE/PSE HCL
(Breckenridge Pharm) *See COLDAMINE*
(Breckenridge Pharm) *See HISTATAB*
(Cypress Pharm) *See CPM 8/PSE 90/MSC 2.5*
(Cypress Pharm) *See PCM LA*
(JayMac Pharma) *See DRYMAX*
(Larken Labs, Inc.) *See SCOPOHIST*
(Laser Pharma) *See DALLERGY PSE*

CPM/METHSCOPOLAMINE NITRATE/PSE HCL/PHENYLEPH HCL
(Cornerstone) *See ALLERX DOSE PACK*

CPM/PHENYLEPH HCL
(Boca Pharmacal) *See C-PHEN*
(Capellon) *See RESCON-JR.*
(Cypress Pharm) *See CERON*
(Edwards) *See ED A-HIST*
(Gil Pharmaceutical) *See PHENABID*
(Hawthorn Pharm) *See NASOHIST*
(Larken Labs, Inc.) *See NOHIST*
(Laser Pharma) *See DALLERGY*
(Laser Pharma) *See DALLERGY-JR*
(Silarx) *See SILDEC-PE*

CPM/PHENYLEPH HCL/PHENYLEPH TAN/PYRIL TAN
(GM Pharm) *See PHENA-S 12*

CPM/PHENYLEPH HCL/PHENYLTOLOXAMINE CIT
(Blansett) *See BLANEX-A*
(Blansett) *See NALEX-A*
(Boca Pharmacal) *See PHENYLTOLOXAMINE PE CPM*
(Breckenridge Pharm) *See RHINACON A*
(Cypress Pharm) *See CHLOREX-A*

CPM/PHENYLEPH HCL/PYRIL MAL
(Breckenridge Pharm) *See PYRICHLOR PE*
(Breckenridge Pharm) *See TRIPLEX AD*
(Carwin) *See RU-HIST FORTE*
(GM Pharm) *See PHENA-PLUS*
(GM Pharm) *See PHENA-S*
(Larken Labs, Inc.) *See MYHIST-PD*
(Poly) *See POLY HIST FORTE*
(Poly) *See POLY HIST PD*

CPM/PHENYLEPH/PPA/PHENYLTOL (Pharma Pac)
REPACK
cpm/ppa hcl/phenyleph hcl/phenyltoloxamine cit
TER, PO, 5 mg-10 mg-40 mg-15 mg,
20s ea............52959-0044-20 17.40
30s ea............52959-0044-30 27.35

CPM/PSE HCL
(Atley) *See SUDAL-12*
(Boca Pharmacal) *See CPM PSE*
(Breckenridge Pharm) *See COLFED-A*
(Breckenridge Pharm) *See DYNAHIST-ER PEDIATRIC*
(Cypress Pharm) *See NEUTRAHIST*
(Larken Labs, Inc.) *See LOHIST D*
(Larken Labs, Inc.) *See SUDAHIST*
(Sandoz) *See CHLORPHENIRAMINE/PSEU-DOEPHEDRINE*
(Truxton) *See PSEUDOCOT-C*

CPM/PSE HCL/ZINCUM ACETICUM
(Auriga) *See ZINX ALLERGY*

CR/CU/IODIDE/MN/MOLYBDENUM/SE/ZINC
(APP) *See M.T.E.-7*

CRAN-RASPBERRY FLAVOR (PCCA)
flavoring aid
SOL, NA, 1 ml............51927-3313-00 1.40

CRANBERRY (PCCA)
POW, NA (90MX)
1 gm...............51927-3288-00 0.36

CRANTEX (Breckenridge Pharm)
guaifenesin/phenylephrine hydrochloride
SYR, PO (AF,SF,DYE-FREE,ORANGE)
100 mg/5 ml-7.5 mg/5 ml,
480 ml 51991-0233-16 67.15

(Phys Total Care)
REPACK
SYR, PO (AF,SF,DYE-FREE,ORANGE)
100 mg/5 ml-7.5 mg/5 ml,
480 ml 54868-5025-00 139.77

CRANTEX HC (Breckenridge Pharm)
gg/hydrocod bit/phenyleph hcl
SYR, PO (AF,SF,DYE-FREE)
480 ml, C-III 51991-0234-16 79.65

CRATAEGUS COMPOUND (Weleda)
homeopathic substance
LIQ, PO, 50 ml............55946-0213-15 9.00

CREAM BASE
(Gallipot) *See COLD CREAM*
(Medisca) *See HRT CREAM BASE*
(Medisca) *See MEDIDERM*
(Medisca) *See NONBREAKABLE CREAM BASE*
(Medisca) *See TRANSDERMAL PAIN BASE*
(Pharmaceutica North) *See ALBA-DERM*
(Spectrum Pharmacy) *See BASE, COA*
(Spectrum Pharmacy) *See BASE, CREAM-HEAVY WITH LIPOSOME*
(Spectrum Pharmacy) *See BASE, HORMONE*
(Spectrum Pharmacy) *See BASE, HORMONE CREAM-BOTANICAL*
(Spectrum Pharmacy) *See BASE, HORMONE CREAM-HEAVY*
(Spectrum Pharmacy) *See BASE, LIPOSOME*
(Spectrum Pharmacy) *See VANISHING CREAM BASE*

CREAM, MULTI INGREDIENT
(Align) *See XCLAIR*
(Ferndale) *See ELETONE*
(Graceway) *See ATOPICLAIR*
(Medisca) *See COLD CREAM UNSCENTED*
(Medisca) *See LIPO CREAM BASE*
(Medisca) *See VANISHING CREAM*
(Ortho) *See BIAFINE*
(Promius) *See EPICERAM*
(Promius) *See PROMISEB*
(PruGen) *See PRUCLAIR*
(PruGen) *See PRUMYX*
(PruGen) *See PRUTECT*
(PruGen) *See PRUVEL*
(Stiefel Labs) *See MIMYX*
(Valeant Pharm Intl) *See TETRIX CREAM*

CREATINE
(Gallipot) *See CREATINE MONOHYDRATE*
(Medisca)
POW, NA (1X100GM,MONOHYDRATE)
100 gm.............38779-0835-05 67.50

PROD/MFR	NDC	AWP	DP	OBC
(1X250GM,MONOHYDRATE)				
250 gm	**38779-0835-07**	142.50		
(1X500GM,MONOHYDRATE)				
500 gm	**38779-0835-08**	268.50		
(1X1000GM,MONOHYDRATE)				
1000 gm	**38779-0835-09**	435.00		
(PCCA)				
POW, NA (MONOHYDRATE)				
1 gm	**51927-2571-00**	0.78		
(Spectrum Pharmacy)				
CRY, NA (1X100GM)				
100 gm	**49452-2332-02**	110.60		
(1X500GM)				
500 gm	**49452-2332-03**	420.00		
CREATINE MONOHYDRATE (Gallipot)				
creatine				
POW, NA, 25 gm	**51552-0489-04**	13.30		
100 gm	**51552-0489-05**	30.73		
1000 gm	**51552-0489-07**	273.00		
CREATININE (PCCA)				
POW, NA (NF)				
1 gm	**51927-2232-00**	7.80		
CREME DE MENTHE FLAVOR (Spectrum Pharmacy)				
flavoring aid				
LIQ, NA (1X100ML)				
100 ml	**49452-2331-02**	63.70		
(1X500ML)				
500 ml	**49452-2331-03**	146.65		
CREME DEMENTHE FLAVOR (PCCA)				
flavoring aid				
SOL, NA (NATURAL)				
1 ml	**51927-2327-00**	0.90		
CREON (Solvay)				
amylase/lipase/protease				
ECC, PO, 30000 u-6000 u-19000 u,				
100s ea	**00032-1206-01**	92.90		
250s ea	**00032-1206-07**	229.72		
60000 u-12000 u-38000 u,				
100s ea	**00032-1212-01**	173.45		
250s ea	**00032-1212-07**	429.18		
120000 u-24000 u-76000 u,				
100s ea	**00032-1224-01**	318.29		
250s ea	**00032-1224-07**	780.31		
(Phys Total Care)				
REPACK				
ECC, PO, 60000 u-12000 u-38000 u,				
10s ea	**54868-6067-00**	23.12		
60s ea	**54868-6067-01**	125.67		
CREON 10 (Solvay)				
amylase/lipase/protease				
ECC, PO (MINIMICROSPHERE)				
33200 u-10000 u-37500 u,				
100s ea	**00032-1210-01**	148.23		
250s ea	**00032-1210-07**	363.31		
(Phys Total Care)				
REPACK				
ECC, PO (MINIMICROSPHERES)				
33200 u-10000 u-37500 u,				
10s ea	**54868-5668-00**	17.24		
60s ea	**54868-5668-01**	94.08		
CREON 20 (Solvay)				
amylase/lipase/protease				
ECC, PO (MINIMICROSPHERE)				
66400 u-20000 u-75000 u,				
100s ea	**00032-1220-01**	271.99		
250s ea	**00032-1220-07**	660.57		
(Phys Total Care)				
REPACK				
ECC, PO, 66400 u-20000 u-75000 u,				
50s ea	**54868-3475-00**	116.15		
100s ea	**54868-3475-01**	217.11		
CREON 5 (Solvay)				
amylase/lipase/protease				
ECC, PO (MINIMICROSPHERE)				
16600 u-5000 u-18750 u,				
100s ea	**00032-1205-01**	79.39		
250s ea	**00032-1205-07**	194.46		
CREOSOTE (PCCA)				
SOL, NA (BEECHWOOD)				
1 ml	**51927-1485-00**	1.35		
CRESOL (PCCA)				
LIQ, NA (ACETATE)				
ea	**51927-1500-00**	3.60		
1 gm	**51927-1327-00**	0.84		
CRESTOR (AstraZeneca)				
rosuvastatin calcium				
TAB, PO, 5 mg, 90s ea	**00310-0755-90**	420.20		
10 mg, 90s ea	**00310-0751-90**	420.20		
100s ea UD	**00310-0751-39**	466.90		
20 mg, 90s ea	**00310-0752-90**	420.20		
100s ea UD	**00310-0752-39**	466.90		
40 mg, 30s ea	**00310-0754-30**	140.06		
(A-S Medication)				
REPACK				
TAB, PO, 5 mg, 30s ea	**54569-5746-00**	167.83		
10 mg, 30s ea	**54569-5600-00**	167.83		
90s ea	**54569-5600-01**	503.48		
20 mg, 30s ea	**54569-5672-00**	167.83		
(AQ)				
REPACK				
TAB, PO, 10 mg, 30s ea	**66105-0988-03**	185.25		
(Nucare Pharm)				
REPACK				
TAB, PO, 5 mg, 30s ea	**68071-0784-30**	195.00		
10 mg, 30s ea	**68071-0433-30**	195.00		
20 mg, 30s ea	**68071-0263-30**	195.00		
(PD-Rx Pharm)				
REPACK				
TAB, PO, 10 mg, 30s ea	**55289-0935-30**	191.87		
20 mg, 30s ea	**55289-0932-30**	191.87		
(Phys Total Care)				
REPACK				
TAB, PO, 5 mg, 30s ea	**54868-5341-00**	168.42		
90s ea	**54868-5341-01**	483.33		
10 mg, 15s ea	**54868-4963-02**	90.39		
30s ea	**54868-4963-00**	168.42		
60s ea	**54868-4963-03**	334.22		
90s ea	**54868-4963-01**	483.33		
20 mg, 30s ea	**54868-5085-00**	168.42		
45s ea	**54868-5085-03**	251.32		
90s ea	**54868-5085-01**	483.33		
100s ea	**54868-5085-02**	537.47		
40 mg, 30s ea	**54868-1890-00**	177.52		
90s ea	**54868-1890-01**	499.39		
(Quality Care Prod)				
REPACK				
TAB, PO, 5 mg, 30s ea	**35356-0519-30**	171.63		
10 mg, 30s ea	**49999-0873-30**	171.63		
90s ea	**49999-0873-90**	508.39		
20 mg, 30s ea	**49999-0992-30**	199.46		
90s ea	**49999-0992-90**	598.38		
40 mg, 30s ea	**35356-0413-30**	199.46		
(Southwood)				
REPACK				
TAB, PO, 10 mg, 30s ea	**58016-0037-30**	114.37		
60s ea	**58016-0037-60**	228.74		
90s ea	**58016-0037-90**	343.11		
100s ea	**58016-0037-00**	381.23		
20 mg, 30s ea	**58016-0052-30**	114.37		
60s ea	**58016-0052-60**	228.74		
90s ea	**58016-0052-90**	343.11		
100s ea	**58016-0052-00**	381.23		
40 mg, 30s ea	**58016-0071-30**	114.37		
60s ea	**58016-0071-60**	228.74		
90s ea	**58016-0071-90**	343.11		
100s ea	**58016-0071-00**	381.23		
CRESYLATE (Recsei)				
meta cresyl acetate				
SOL, OT, 25%, 15 ml	**10952-0035-13**	22.00		
CRINONE (Columbia Labs)				
progesterone				
GEL, VG (15X1.45GM)				
8%, 1.45 gm 15s	**55056-0818-05**	213.90		
CRIXIVAN (Merck)				
indinavir sulfate				
CAP, PO (UNIT OF USE)				
100 mg, 180s ea	**00006-0570-62**	137.02		
200 mg, 360s ea	**00006-0571-43**	548.11		
400 mg, 18s ea	**00006-0573-18**	54.82		
90s ea	**00006-0573-54**	274.06		
120s ea	**00006-0573-40**	365.41		
180s ea	**00006-0573-62**	548.12		
(A-S Medication)				
REPACK				
CAP, PO, 400 mg, 180s ea	**54569-8620-00**	712.56		
(DHS, Inc.)				
REPACK				
CAP, PO, 400 mg, 30s ea	**55887-0230-30**	115.50		
60s ea	**55887-0230-60**	231.00		
(Dispensing Solutions)				
REPACK				
CAP, PO, 400 mg, 30s ea	**55045-3548-01**	105.00		
(Pharma Pac)				
REPACK				
CAP, PO, 400 mg, 12s ea	**52959-0507-12**	44.10		
18s ea	**52959-0507-18**	65.80		
24s ea	**52959-0507-24**	82.25		
30s ea	**52959-0507-30**	102.60		
(Phys Total Care)				
REPACK				
CAP, PO, 400 mg, 180s ea	**54868-4113-00**	606.57		
(Physician Partner)				
REPACK				
CAP, PO, 400 mg, 18s ea	**21695-0366-18**	134.34		
(Quality Care Prod)				
REPACK				
CAP, PO, 400 mg, 60s ea	**35356-0139-60**	487.43		
180s ea	**35356-0139-18**	1316.06		
(Southwood)				
REPACK				
CAP, PO, 400 mg, 30s ea	**58016-0699-30**	91.35		
60s ea	**58016-0699-60**	182.71		
90s ea	**58016-0699-90**	274.06		
100s ea	**58016-0699-00**	304.51		
(Stat Rx)				
REPACK				
CAP, PO, 400 mg, 18s ea	**16590-0064-18**	61.20		
30s ea	**16590-0064-30**	102.00		
60s ea	**16590-0064-60**	204.00		
90s ea	**16590-0064-90**	320.35		
CROFAB (Savage)				
antivenin (crotalidae) polyvalent immune fab				
PDS, IV (VIAL)				
2s ea	**00281-0330-10**	3974.40		
CROMOLYN SODIUM				
FUL				
SOL, OP, 4%, 10 ml		33.75		
(Akorn)				
SOL, OP, 4%, 10 ml	**17478-0291-11**	37.25		AT
(Apotex Corp.)				
SOL, IH (AMP)				
10 mg/ml,				
2 ml 60s UD	**60505-0802-01**	49.80		AN
OP, 4%, 10 ml UD	**60505-0811-02**	37.25		AT
(Azur Pharma, Inc.) *See GASTROCROM*				
(Falcon Ophthalmics)				
SOL, OP, 4%, 10 ml	**61314-0237-10**	37.20		AT
(Gallipot)				
POW, NA (U.S.P.)				
5 gm	**51552-0423-02**	21.00		
25 gm	**51552-0423-04**	49.00		
100 gm	**51552-0423-05**	147.00		
1000 gm	**51552-0423-07**	1260.00		
(Hawkins)				
POW, NA (U.S.P.)				
5 gm	**63370-0050-15**	57.00		
25 gm	**63370-0050-25**	100.00		
100 gm	**63370-0050-35**	320.00		
500 gm	**63370-0050-45**	1400.00		
1000 gm	**63370-0050-50**	2600.00		
(Letco)				
POW, NA (U.S.P.)				
25 gm	**62991-1038-01**	73.50		
100 gm	**62991-1038-02**	225.00		
500 gm	**62991-1038-03**	1050.00		
1000 gm	**62991-1038-04**	1800.00		
(Medisca)				
POW, NA (U.S.P.)				
5 gm	**38779-0301-03**	46.50		
25 gm	**38779-0301-04**	116.85		
100 gm	**38779-0301-05**	357.00		
500 gm	**38779-0301-08**	1425.00		
1000 gm	**38779-0301-09**	2175.00		
(Pacific Pharma)				
SOL, OP, 4%, 10 ml	**60758-0458-10**	37.15		AT
(Spectrum Pharmacy)				
POW, NA (U.S.P.)				
5 gm	**49452-0006-02**	78.75		
25 gm	**49452-0006-03**	178.15		
100 gm	**49452-0006-04**	563.50		
(Teva)				
SOL, IH ((VIAL),USP)				
10 mg/ml,				
2 ml 60s UD	**00172-6406-49**	96.12		AN
2 ml 120s UD	**00172-6406-59**	179.28		AN
OP, 4%, 10 ml	**00093-1389-43**	36.47		EE

PROD/MFR	NDC	AWP	DP	OBC
(Phys Total Care)				
REPACK				
SOL, IH, 10 mg/ml, 2 ml 60s	54868-3555-00	13.58		AN
(Quality Care Prod)				
REPACK				
SOL, OP, 4%, 10 ml	49999-0720-10	44.64		AT
CROSCARMELLOSE SODIUM (Spectrum Pharmacy)				
POW, NA (N.F.)				
500 gm	49452-2337-01	249.55		
2500 gm	49452-2337-02	717.50		
CROTAMITON				
(Ranbaxy Labs) *See EURAX*				
CROTON OIL (Gallipot)				
OIL, NA, 10 ml	51552-0224-03	63.00		
25 ml	51552-0224-04	111.30		
100 ml	51552-0224-05	287.00		
(PCCA)				
OIL, NA, 1 gm	51927-1477-00	9.00		
(Spectrum Pharmacy)				
OIL, NA, 10 gm	49452-2340-04	220.50		
25 gm	49452-2340-01	329.35		
100 gm	49452-2340-02	980.00		
CRYSELLE (Teva)				
ethinyl estradiol/norgestrel				
TAB, PO (6X28 BLISTER PACK)				
30 mcg-0.3 mg, 168s ea	00555-9049-58	183.12		AB
(Phys Total Care)				
REPACK				
TAB, PO, 30 mcg-0.3 mg, 28s ea	54868-4851-00	43.13		AB
(Quality Care Prod)				
REPACK				
TAB, PO, 30 mcg-0.3 mg, 28s ea	35356-0370-28	56.64		AB
CUBICIN (Cubist Pharmaceuticals)				
daptomycin				
PDS, IV (PF)				
500 mg, ea	67919-0011-01	255.10		
CUCUMBER FRAGRANCE (PCCA)				
fragrance				
SOL, NA (ARTIFICIAL,LIQUID)				
1 gm	51927-3192-00	0.43		
CUPFERRON (Baker, J.T.)				
CRY, NA (A.C.S., REAGENT)				
125 gm	10106-1760-04	99.09		
500 gm	10106-1760-01	306.53		
CUPRIC ACETATE (Medisca)				
copper acetate				
CRY, NA (1X100GM)				
100 gm	38779-1221-05	43.50		
(1X500GM)				
500 gm	38779-1221-08	184.50		
(PCCA)				
POW, NA (MONOHYDRATE)				
1 gm	51927-1765-00	0.42		
CUPRIC ACETATE MONOHYDRATE (Amend)				
copper acetate				
CRY, NA, 454 gm	17317-1291-01	14.00		
2270 gm	17317-1291-05	49.00		
11350 gm	17317-1291-08	122.50		
(Baker, J.T.)				
CRY, NA (A.C.S., REAGENT)				
500 gm	10106-1766-01	93.47		
2500 gm	10106-1766-05	333.41		
CUPRIC BROMIDE (Baker, J.T.)				
copper bromide				
CRY, NA, 500 gm	10106-1780-01	186.64		
CUPRIC CARBONATE (Baker, J.T.)				
copper carbonate				
POW, NA (REAGENT)				
500 gm	10106-1786-01	170.55		
2000 gm	10106-1786-05	384.40		
CUPRIC CHLORIDE (Medisca)				
copper chloride				
CRY, NA (DIHYDRATE,USP,1X100GM)				
100 gm	38779-1222-05	70.50		
(PCCA)				
POW, NA (DIHYDRATE; CP)				
1 gm	51927-2612-00	0.75		
(Spectrum Pharmacy)				
CRY, NA, 125 gm	49452-2350-04	123.55		
(PURIFIED)				
500 gm	49452-2350-01	315.35		
CUPRIC CHLORIDE DIHYDRATE (Amend)				
copper chloride				
POW, NA (C.P.)				
500 gm	17317-0824-01	20.30		
2270 gm	17317-0824-05	56.00		
11350 gm	17317-0824-08	175.00		
(Baker, J.T.)				
CRY, NA (A.C.S., REAGENT)				
125 gm	10106-1792-04	64.74		
500 gm	10106-1792-01	129.63		
2500 gm	10106-1792-05	462.06		
CUPRIC NITRATE (Amend)				
copper nitrate				
CRY, NA (PURIFIED)				
454 gm	17317-1518-01	21.70		
(Mallinckrodt Lab)				
CRY, NA, 125 gm	00406-4828-02	31.06		
CUPRIC NITRATE 2.5-HYDRATE (Baker, J.T.)				
copper nitrate				
POW, NA (A.C.S., REAGENT)				
500 gm	10106-1800-01	122.52		
2500 gm	10106-1800-05	514.18		
12000 gm	10106-1800-07	1191.66		
CUPRIC NITRATE N-HYDRATE (Baker, J.T.)				
copper nitrate				
POW, NA (PURIFIED)				
500 gm	10106-1803-01	113.20		
CUPRIC NITRATE TRIHYDRATE ACS (PCCA)				
copper nitrate				
CRY, NA (1X1GM)				
1 gm	51927-1844-00	0.96		
CUPRIC OXIDE (Baker, J.T.)				
copper oxide				
POW, NA (A.C.S., REAGENT)				
500 gm	10106-1814-01	221.60		
2500 gm	10106-1814-05	1077.90		
(Gallipot)				
POW, NA (REAGENT)				
25 gm	51552-1001-04	10.50	7.50	
(PCCA)				
POW, NA, 1 gm	51927-2257-00	0.54		
CUPRIC OXIDE ANHYDROUS (Amend)				
copper oxide				
POW, NA (BLACK)				
454 gm	17317-0742-01	26.60		
(REAGENT, BLACK)				
500 gm	17317-1869-01	49.00		
(BLACK)				
2270 gm	17317-0742-05	105.00		
(REAGENT, BLACK)				
2270 gm	17317-1869-05	210.00		
(BLACK)				
11350 gm	17317-0742-08	472.50		
(REAGENT, BLACK)				
11350 gm	17317-1869-08	875.00		
CUPRIC SULFATE (Amend)				
copper sulfate				
CRY, NA (TECHNICAL)				
500 gm	17317-0731-01	4.90		
GRA, NA (U.S.P.)				
500 gm	17317-0130-01	21.00		
2270 gm	17317-0130-05	70.00		
11350 gm	17317-0130-08	245.00		
POW, NA (TECHNICAL)				
454 gm	17317-1628-01	7.00		
(A.C.S., REAGENT)				
500 gm	17317-1654-01	42.00		
(U.S.P.)				
500 gm	17317-0131-01	21.00		
2270 gm	17317-0131-05	70.00		
(A.C.S., REAGENT)				
2500 gm	17317-1654-05	154.00		
(U.S.P.)				
11350 gm	17317-0131-08	280.00		
(A.C.S., REAGENT)				
12000 gm	17317-1654-08	336.00		
(Amer Regent)				
SOL, IV (0.4 MG/ML COPPER,PF)				
1.57 mg/ml, 10 ml 25s	00517-6210-25	62.19		
(Mallinckrodt Lab)				
GRA, NA (U.S.P.)				
500 gm	00406-4752-10	54.36		
2500 gm	00406-4752-12	169.52		
(PCCA)				
POW, NA (USP; PENTAHYDRATE)				
1 gm	51927-3100-00	0.26		
CUPRIC SULFATE ANHYDROUS (Baker, J.T.)				
copper sulfate				
POW, NA (REAGENT)				
500 gm	10106-1850-01	178.24		
2500 gm	10106-1850-05	719.92		
CUPRIC SULFATE MONOHYDRATE (Amend)				
copper sulfate				
POW, NA (PURIFIED)				
500 gm	17317-0135-01	12.60		
2270 gm	17317-0135-05	49.00		
11350 gm	17317-0135-08	210.00		
CUPRIC SULFATE PENTAHYDRATE (Baker, J.T.)				
copper sulfate				
CRY, NA (U.S.P.)				
500 gm	10106-1844-01	34.02		
2500 gm	10106-1844-05	194.83		
(Spectrum Pharmacy)				
GRA, NA (U.S.P.)				
500 gm	49452-2380-01	199.15		
2500 gm	49452-2380-02	598.50		
POW, NA, 500 gm	49452-2390-01	199.15		
2500 gm	49452-2390-02	598.50		
CUPRIMINE (Aton)				
penicillamine				
CAP, PO, 250 mg, 100s ea	25010-0705-15	556.11		
CUPROUS CHLORIDE (Baker, J.T.)				
copper chloride				
POW, NA (A.C.S., REAGENT)				
500 gm	10106-1862-01	129.83		
CUPROUS CYANIDE (Baker, J.T.)				
copper cyanide				
POW, NA (TECHNICAL)				
500 gm	10106-1872-01	68.60		
CUPROUS OXIDE (Baker, J.T.)				
copper oxide				
POW, NA (REAGENT)				
500 gm	10106-1878-01	67.36		
CURCUMIN (PCCA)				
POW, NA, 95%, 1 gm	51927-3497-00	1.11		
CURITY BEDSIDE DRAIN BAG (Covidien)				
incontinence products				
DEV, NA (W/O ANTI-REFLUX DEVICE)				
15s ea	08080-6261-00	172.72		
CUROSURF (Cornerstone)				
poractant alfa				
SUS, IT (1X1.5ML,SDV)				
80 mg/ml, 1.5 ml	10122-0510-01	418.71	334.97	
(1X3ML, SINGLE USE)				
80 mg/ml, 3 ml	10122-0510-03	819.70	655.76	
CUTIVATE (PharmaDerm)				
fluticasone propionate				
CRE, TP, 0.05%, 30 gm	00462-0332-30	104.41		AB
60 gm	00462-0332-60	208.76		AB
LOT, TP, 0.05%, 60 ml	00462-0434-60	126.72		
120 ml	00462-0434-04	417.48		
OIN, TP, 0.005%, 30 gm	00462-0333-30	83.28		AB
60 gm	00462-0333-60	123.35		AB
(Phys Total Care)				
REPACK				
CRE, TP, 0.05%, 15 gm	54868-2446-01	28.11		
30 gm	54868-2446-02	32.48		
OIN, TP, 0.005%, 15 gm	54868-2447-01	27.28		
30 gm	54868-2447-02	41.70		
60 gm	54868-2447-00	79.47		
(Quality Care Prod)				
REPACK				
LOT, TP (1X120ML)				
0.05%, 120 ml	35356-0218-01	506.58		
CYANIDE ANTIDOTE (Akorn)				
amyl nitrite/sodium nitrite/sodium thiosulfate				
KIT, IV, ea	11098-0507-01	274.56		
CYANOCOBALAMIN (Amer Regent)				
SOL, IM, 1000 mcg/ml, 1 ml 25s	00517-0031-25	31.25		AP
(M.D.V.)				
1000 mcg/ml, 10 ml 25s	00517-0032-25	85.94		AP
30 ml 5s	00517-0130-05	23.44		AP

PROD/MFR	NDC	AWP	DP	OBC
(APP)				
SOL, IM (M.D.V.)				
1000 mcg/ml, 1 ml	**63323-0044-01**	2.21		AP
(Clint) *See VITA #12*				
(Consolidated Midland) *See HYDROXOCOBALAMIN*				
(Consolidated Midland)				
SOL, IM (VIAL)				
100 mcg/ml, 30 ml	**00223-8871-30**	4.00		EE
(AMP)				
1000 mcg/ml, 1 ml 25s	**00223-8862-25**	35.00		EE
(VIAL, DOSETTE)				
1000 mcg/ml, 1 ml 25s	**00223-8861-01**	31.25		EE
(M.D.V.)				
1000 mcg/ml, 30 ml	**00223-8860-30**	4.00		EE
(Consolidated Midland) *See VITABEE 12*				
(Fleming) *See CALOMIST*				
(Gallipot)				
CRY, NA (1X500MG,USP)				
0.5 gm	**51552-1045-09**	34.72	24.80	
(1X1GM,USP)				
1 gm	**51552-1045-01**	47.53	33.95	
(Intl Ethical) *See NEUROFORTE-R*				
(Legere) *See COBOLIN-M*				
(Legere) *See DEPO-COBOLIN*				
(Letco)				
CRY, NA (U.S.P.)				
5 gm	**62991-1039-02**	210.00		
25 gm	**62991-1039-03**	930.00		
(Medisca)				
POW, NA (U.S.P.)				
1 gm	**38779-0468-06**	88.50		
5 gm	**38779-0468-03**	345.00		
25 gm	**38779-0468-04**	1194.00		
100 gm	**38779-0468-05**	3255.00		
(Par) *See NASCOBAL*				
(PCCA)				
POW, NA (USP)				
1 gm	**51927-1662-00**	111.00		
(Spectrum Pharmacy)				
CRY, NA (U.S.P.)				
1 gm	**49452-2400-02**	148.40		
5 gm	**49452-2400-03**	497.00		
25 gm	**49452-2400-04**	1596.00		
(Truxton) *See HYDROXOCOBALAMIN*				
(Truxton) *See VITAMIN B12*				
(Vita-Rx) *See VITAMIN B12*				
(A-S Medication)				
REPACK				
SOL, IM (M.D.V.)				
1000 mcg/ml, 30 ml 5s	**54569-5533-00**	23.44		AP
(Phys Total Care)				
REPACK				
SOL, IM, 1000 mcg/ml, 1 ml 25s	**54868-0762-01**	118.35		AP
CYANOCOBALAMIN CO 57				
(Bracco Diag) *See RUBRATOPE-57*				
CYANOCOBALAMIN/FOLIC ACID				
(Poly) *See FOLTRATE*				
CYANOCOBALAMIN/FOLIC ACID/IRON				
(Seyer Pharmatec) *See HEMATRON*				
CYANOCOBALAMIN/FOLIC ACID/ IRON POLYSACCHARIDE				
(Breckenridge Pharm) *See FERREX 150 FORTE*				
(Contract Pharmacal) *See POLYSACCHARIDE IRON FORTE*				
(Cypress Pharm) *See POLY-IRON 150 FORTE*				
(ME Pharm) *See MYFERON 150 FORTE*				
(Nnodum) *See IFEREX 150 FORTE*				
CYANOCOBALAMIN/FOLIC ACID/LIVER				
(Consolidated Midland) *See FOLIC ACID/LIVER EXTRACT/VITAMIN B12*				
CYANOCOBALAMIN/FOLIC ACID/PYRIDOXINE				
(Allan Pharmaceutical) *See FOLIC ACID/ CYANOCOBALAMIN/PYRIDOXONE*				
(Breckenridge Pharm) *See FOLBEE*				
(Breckenridge Pharm) *See FOLBIC*				
(Breckenridge Pharm) *See FOLPLEX*				
(Breckenridge Pharm) *See FOLPLEX 2.2*				
(Midlothian Labs) *See FABB*				
(Midlothian Labs) *See FOLCAPS*				
(Pamlab) *See FOBALIN PLUS*				
(Pamlab) *See FOLTX*				
(Respa Pharm) *See VITA-RESPA*				
(Rising) *See NUFOL*				
(Upsher-Smith) *See FOLGARD RX*				
(Upsher-Smith)				
TAB, PO, 0.5 mg-2.2 mg-25 mg, 100s ea	**00245-0183-11**	43.40		
CYCLANDELATE (Consolidated Midland)				
CAP, PO, 200 mg, 100s ea	**00223-0706-01**	5.25		
1000s ea	**00223-0706-02**	50.00		
400 mg, 100s ea	**00223-0707-01**	7.75		
1000s ea	**00223-0707-02**	67.50		
(PCCA)				
POW, NA, 1 gm	**51927-2981-00**	3.60		
(Spectrum Pharmacy)				
POW, NA, 25 gm	**49452-2402-01**	176.40		
100 gm	**49452-2402-02**	511.00		
500 gm	**49452-2402-03**	1820.00		
CYCLESSA (Organon)				
desogestrel/ethinyl estradiol				
TAB, PO (BLISTER PACK,6X28)				
168s ea	**00052-0283-06**	306.48		AB
(Phys Total Care)				
REPACK				
TAB, PO (BLISTER PACK,6X28)				
168s ea	**54868-4911-00**	53.83		AB
CYCLOBENZ (Quality Care Prod)				
REPACK				
cyclobenzaprine hydrochloride				
TAB, PO, 5 mg, 30s ea	**49999-0791-30**	59.04		
CYCLOBENZAPRINE (4u)				
REPACK				
cyclobenzaprine hydrochloride				
TAB, PO, 10 mg, 30s ea	**10544-0308-30**	64.44		
60s ea	**10544-0308-60**	84.62		
(Bryant Ranch)				
REPACK				
TAB, PO, 10 mg, 14s ea	**63629-1339-01**	21.32		
15s ea	**63629-1339-05**	24.84		
20s ea	**63629-1339-04**	30.46		
28s ea	**63629-1339-02**	42.64		
30s ea	**63629-1339-03**	60.60		
60s ea	**63629-1339-06**	91.37		
90s ea	**63629-1339-07**	137.06		
(Core)				
REPACK				
TAB, PO, 10 mg, 15s ea	**33358-0097-15**	25.46		
20s ea	**33358-0097-20**	31.22		
28s ea	**33358-0097-28**	43.71		
30s ea	**33358-0097-30**	46.83		
60s ea	**33358-0097-60**	103.97		
90s ea	**33358-0097-90**	163.64		
100s ea	**33358-0097-00**	167.98		
120s ea	**33358-0097-01**	204.04		
(DHS, Inc.)				
REPACK				
TAB, PO, 5 mg, 10s ea	**55887-0822-10**	16.40		
30s ea	**55887-0822-30**	30.00		
(IPI)				
REPACK				
TAB, PO, 5 mg, 30s ea	**18837-0205-30**	61.52		
90s ea	**18837-0205-90**	185.12		
(Palmetto)				
REPACK				
TAB, PO, 10 mg, 9s ea	**23490-5377-01**	15.94		
12s ea	**23490-5377-02**	19.34		
14s ea	**23490-7940-02**	22.56		
15s ea	**23490-5377-03**	24.18		
20s ea	**23490-0381-02**	32.00		
20s ea	**23490-5377-04**	32.23		
21s ea	**23490-5377-00**	33.85		
25s ea	**23490-7940-01**	33.76		
30s ea	**23490-0381-03**	43.20		
30s ea	**23490-5377-06**	48.35		
40s ea	**23490-5377-05**	64.47		
60s ea	**23490-0381-06**	86.40		
60s ea	**23490-5377-07**	96.70		
90s ea	**23490-0381-09**	129.60		
90s ea	**23490-5377-08**	145.05		
120s ea	**23490-5377-09**	193.40		
(PD-Rx Pharm)				
REPACK				
TAB, PO, 5 mg, 10s ea	**55289-0236-10**	19.75		
14s ea	**55289-0236-14**	32.80		
30s ea	**55289-0236-30**	43.40		
(Pharma Pac)				
REPACK				
TAB, PO, 5 mg, 10s ea	**52959-0846-10**	17.29		
20s ea	**52959-0846-20**	34.56		
30s ea	**52959-0846-30**	51.81		
(Phys Total Care)				
REPACK				
TAB, PO (USP)				
5 mg, 30s ea	**54868-5597-00**	13.62		
(Physician Partner)				
REPACK				
TAB, PO, 10 mg, 10s ea	**21695-0037-10**	27.24		
14s ea	**21695-0037-14**	40.76		
15s ea	**21695-0037-15**	40.76		
20s ea	**21695-0037-20**	54.35		
30s ea	**21695-0037-30**	69.45		
45s ea	**21695-0037-45**	122.55		
60s ea	**21695-0037-60**	138.90		
90s ea	**21695-0037-90**	208.35		
(Southwood)				
REPACK				
TAB, PO, 5 mg, 30s ea	**58016-0076-30**	49.22		
60s ea	**58016-0076-60**	98.44		
90s ea	**58016-0076-90**	147.65		
100s ea	**58016-0076-00**	164.06		
180s ea	**58016-0076-99**	295.31		
(Stat Rx)				
REPACK				
TAB, PO, 10 mg, 15s ea	**16590-0065-15**	26.95		
20s ea	**16590-0065-20**	26.67		
30s ea	**16590-0065-30**	40.00		
40s ea	**16590-0065-40**	53.34		
120s ea	**16590-0065-12**	160.02		
CYCLOBENZAPRINE COMFORT PAC (PD-Rx Pharm)				
REPACK				
cyclobenzaprine hydrochloride				
KIT, MR, 10 mg, ea	**55289-0403-92**	74.75		
CYCLOBENZAPRINE HCL (Hawkins)				
cyclobenzaprine hydrochloride				
POW, NA (U.S.P.)				
5 gm	**63370-0058-15**	115.20		
25 gm	**63370-0058-25**	504.00		
100 gm	**63370-0058-35**	1776.00		
1000 gm	**63370-0058-50**	8640.00		
(Letco)				
POW, NA (U.S.P.)				
5 gm	**62991-1040-01**	72.00		
25 gm	**62991-1040-02**	315.00		
50 gm	**62991-1040-04**	540.00		
100 gm	**62991-1040-05**	945.00		
(Major)				
TAB, PO, 10 mg, 100s ea	**00904-7809-60**	113.75		AB
(10X10)				
10 mg, 100s ea UD	**00904-7809-61**	120.95		AB
(Medisca)				
POW, NA (U.S.P.)				
5 gm	**38779-0395-03**	105.00		
25 gm	**38779-0395-04**	429.00		
100 gm	**38779-0395-05**	1485.00		
500 gm	**38779-0395-08**	5550.00		
1000 gm	**38779-0395-09**	9450.00		
(Mutual)				
TAB, PO (FILM-COATED)				
10 mg, 100s ea	**53489-0591-01**	115.76		AB
500s ea	**53489-0591-05**	557.12		AB
1000s ea	**53489-0591-10**	1091.50		AB
(Mylan)				
TAB, PO, 10 mg, 30s ea	**00378-0751-93**	32.75		AB
100s ea	**00378-0751-01**	109.15		AB
1000s ea	**00378-0751-10**	1091.50		AB
(PCCA)				
POW, NA (U.S.P.)				
1 gm	**51927-2501-00**	36.00		
(Sandoz)				
TAB, PO (FILM-COATED)				
10 mg, 100s ea	**00781-1324-01**	115.76		AB
1000s ea	**00781-1324-10**	1099.72		AB
(Spectrum Pharmacy)				
CRY, NA (U.S.P.)				
5 gm	**49452-2407-03**	168.70		
25 gm	**49452-2407-04**	640.50		
100 gm	**49452-2407-05**	1757.00		

PROD/MFR	NDC	AWP	DP	OBC
(Teva)				
TAB, PO, 10 mg, 100s ea	50111-0563-01	114.50		AB
500s ea	50111-0563-02	543.88		AB
1000s ea	50111-0563-03	1030.50		AB
(UDL)				
TAB, PO (ROBOT READY 25X1)				
10 mg, 25s ea UD	51079-0644-19	5.08		AB
(10X10)				
10 mg, 100s ea UD	51079-0644-20	96.90		AB
(Watson Labs)				
TAB, PO, 10 mg, 100s ea	00591-5658-01	8.52		AB
500s ea	00591-5658-05	40.48		AB
1000s ea	00591-5658-10	80.95		AB
(4u) REPACK				
TAB, PO, 10 mg, 30s ea	42549-0308-30	62.28		AB
30s ea	42549-0508-30	64.44		AB
60s ea	42549-0308-60	84.62		AB
60s ea	42549-0508-60	84.62		AB
90s ea	10544-0308-90	124.28		AB
90s ea	42549-0308-90	124.28		AB
90s ea	42549-0508-90	124.28		AB
(A-S Medication) REPACK				
TAB, PO, 10 mg, 6s ea	54569-3193-08	6.91		EE
(Altura) REPACK				
TAB, PO, 10 mg, 5s ea	63874-0315-05	6.00		AB
7s ea	63874-0315-07	8.40		AB
10s ea	63874-0315-10	12.00		AB
12s ea	63874-0315-12	14.40		AB
14s ea	63874-0315-14	16.80		AB
15s ea	63874-0315-15	18.00		EE
18s ea	63874-0315-18	21.60		AB
20s ea	63874-0315-20	24.00		EE
21s ea	63874-0315-21	25.20		AB
24s ea	63874-0315-24	28.80		AB
25s ea	63874-0315-25	30.00		AB
28s ea	63874-0315-28	33.60		AB
30s ea	63874-0315-30	36.00		EE
35s ea	63874-0315-35	42.00		AB
40s ea	63874-0315-40	48.00		AB
42s ea	63874-0315-42	50.40		AB
45s ea	63874-0315-45	54.00		AB
50s ea	63874-0315-50	60.00		AB
56s ea	63874-0315-56	67.20		AB
60s ea	63874-0315-60	72.00		EE
75s ea	63874-0315-75	90.00		AB
90s ea	63874-0315-90	108.00		AB
100s ea	63874-0315-01	120.00		EE
120s ea	63874-0315-04	144.00		AB
126s ea	63874-0315-76	151.20		AB
180s ea	63874-0315-80	216.00		AB
1000s ea	63874-0315-02	811.20		EE
(B&B Pharm, Inc) REPACK				
POW, NA (U.S.P.)				
5 gm	63275-9994-02	108.00		
25 gm	63275-9994-04	405.00		
100 gm	63275-9994-05	1335.00		
(USP,1X500GM)				
500 gm	63275-9994-08	5700.00		
(DHS, Inc.) REPACK				
TAB, PO, 10 mg, 15s ea	55887-0989-15	20.25		AB
20s ea	55887-0989-20	25.60		AB
21s ea	55887-0989-21	26.02		AB
30s ea	55887-0989-30	35.21		AB
60s ea	55887-0989-60	70.42		AB
90s ea	55887-0989-90	105.63		AB
120s ea	55887-0989-82	140.84		AB
180s ea	55887-0989-92	211.26		AB
(Dispensing Solutions) REPACK				
TAB, PO, 10 mg, 7s ea	55045-1566-06	10.15		AB
9s ea	55045-1566-03	13.05		AB
9s ea	66336-0581-09	14.54		AB
10s ea	55045-1566-01	14.50		AB
15s ea	55045-1566-05	21.75		AB
15s ea	66336-0581-15	20.25		EE
20s ea	55045-1566-07	29.00		AB
20s ea	66336-0581-20	25.19		EE
21s ea	55045-1566-09	30.45		AB
21s ea	66336-0581-21	26.45		AB
30s ea	55045-1566-08	43.50		AB
30s ea	66336-0581-30	37.80		EE
40s ea	55045-3058-04	58.00		AB
42s ea	55045-1566-04	60.90		AB
45s ea	55045-1566-02	65.25		AB
56s ea	55045-3058-05	81.20		AB
60s ea	55045-3058-06	87.00		AB
60s ea	66336-0581-60	75.60		AB
90s ea	55045-3058-09	130.50		AB
100s ea	55045-1566-00	145.00		AB
120s ea	55045-3058-01	174.00		AB
(FILM-COATED)				
10 mg, 120s ea	66336-0581-94	140.84		AB
(GSMS) REPACK				
TAB, PO (UNIT OF USE)				
10 mg, 30s ea	60429-0052-30	4.29	1.43	AB
(HomeMed) REPACK				
TAB, PO, 10 mg, 4s ea	51655-0440-89	6.37		EE
9s ea	51655-0440-85	14.33		EE
15s ea	51655-0440-54	23.89		EE
20s ea	51655-0440-52	28.98		EE
20s ea	51655-0544-52	25.12		AB
30s ea	51655-0440-24	38.99		EE
60s ea	51655-0440-25	77.99		EE
(IPI) REPACK				
TAB, PO, 10 mg, 20s ea	18837-0033-20	27.28		AB
(Keltman Pharma., Inc.) REPACK				
TAB, PO, 10 mg, 30s ea	68387-0500-30	39.00		AB
45s ea	68387-0500-45	58.50		AB
60s ea	68387-0500-60	78.00		AB
90s ea	68387-0500-90	117.00		AB
(LWP) REPACK				
TAB, PO, 10 mg, 30s ea	64038-0042-30	39.35		AB
60s ea	64038-0042-60	73.70		AB
90s ea	64038-0042-90	108.05		AB
100s ea	64038-0042-01	119.50		AB
(McKesson Packaging) REPACK				
TAB, PO (USP)				
10 mg, 100s ea UD	63739-0066-10	136.41		AB
(Nucare Pharm) REPACK				
TAB, PO, 10 mg, 10s ea	66267-0064-10	19.05		EE
15s ea	66267-0064-15	28.27		AB
20s ea	66267-0064-20	30.01		AB
30s ea	66267-0064-30	56.65		AB
40s ea	66267-0064-40	45.99		EE
45s ea	66267-0064-45	59.75		AB
60s ea	66267-0064-60	84.98		AB
90s ea	66267-0064-90	121.67		AB
120s ea	66267-0064-91	159.33		AB
(PD-Rx Pharm) REPACK				
TAB, PO, 10 mg, 10s ea	55289-0567-10	27.22		AB
12s ea	55289-0567-12	29.33		AB
14s ea	55289-0567-14	31.44		AB
15s ea	55289-0567-15	32.50		AB
18s ea	55289-0567-18	35.67		AB
20s ea	55289-0567-20	37.78		AB
(REDI-SCRIPT)				
10 mg, 20s ea	58864-0128-20	37.80		AB
21s ea	55289-0567-21	38.83		AB
30s ea	55289-0567-30	48.33		AB
(REDI-SCRIPT)				
10 mg, 30s ea	58864-0128-30	48.35		AB
42s ea	55289-0567-42	61.00		AB
(REDI-SCRIPT)				
10 mg, 45s ea	58864-0128-45	64.17		AB
60s ea	55289-0567-60	80.00		AB
90s ea	55289-0567-90	111.67		AB
100s ea UD	55289-0567-17	98.15		AB
(Pharma Pac) REPACK				
TAB, PO, 10 mg, 4s ea	52959-0042-04	7.74		EE
7s ea	52959-0042-07	13.55		EE
10s ea	52959-0042-10	19.36		EE
12s ea	52959-0042-12	23.22		EE
14s ea	52959-0042-14	27.08		EE
15s ea	52959-0042-15	29.01		EE
20s ea	52959-0042-20	38.36		EE
21s ea	52959-0042-21	40.60		EE
25s ea	52959-0042-25	48.32		EE
28s ea	52959-0042-28	54.11		EE
30s ea	52959-0042-30	57.97		EE
35s ea	52959-0042-35	67.62		EE
40s ea	52959-0042-40	77.24		EE
45s ea	52959-0042-45	86.82		EE
60s ea	52959-0042-60	115.74		EE
90s ea	52959-0042-90	173.57		EE
100s ea	52959-0042-00	192.80		EE
120s ea	52959-0042-02	231.28		EE
(Phys Total Care) REPACK				
TAB, PO, 10 mg, 15s ea	54868-1110-05	8.25		EE
20s ea	54868-1110-03	9.99		EE
30s ea	54868-1110-02	13.47		EE
60s ea	54868-1110-08	18.78		EE
100s ea	54868-1110-09	29.31		EE
1000s ea	54868-1110-00	127.68		EE
(Physician Partner) REPACK				
TAB, PO, 10 mg, 12s ea	21695-0037-12	34.94		AB
(FILM COATED)				
10 mg, 21s ea	21695-0037-21	57.07		AB
100s ea	21695-0037-00	229.90		AB
(Quality Care Prod) REPACK				
TAB, PO, 10 mg, 7s ea	49999-0034-07	8.96		AB
12s ea	49999-0034-12	24.60		AB
15s ea	49999-0034-15	30.75		EE
20s ea	49999-0034-20	41.00		EE
21s ea	49999-0034-21	43.05		EE
30s ea	49999-0034-30	61.33		EE
60s ea	49999-0034-60	123.00		EE
90s ea	49999-0034-90	184.50		AB
120s ea	49999-0034-01	246.00		AB
(Southwood) REPACK				
TAB, PO, 10 mg, 7s ea	58016-0234-07	8.40		EE
10s ea	58016-0234-10	12.00		EE
12s ea	58016-0234-12	14.39		EE
14s ea	58016-0234-14	16.79		EE
15s ea	58016-0234-15	17.99		EE
18s ea	58016-0234-18	21.59		EE
20s ea	58016-0234-20	23.99		EE
21s ea	58016-0234-21	25.19		EE
24s ea	58016-0234-24	28.79		EE
28s ea	58016-0234-28	33.59		EE
(FILM-COATED)				
10 mg, 30s ea	58016-0234-30	40.50		AB
40s ea	58016-0234-40	47.98		EE
45s ea	58016-0234-45	53.98		EE
50s ea	58016-0234-50	59.98		EE
56s ea	58016-0234-56	67.17		EE
(FILM-COATED)				
10 mg, 60s ea	58016-0234-60	81.00		AB
90s ea	58016-0234-90	121.50		AB
100s ea	58016-0234-00	135.00		AB
120s ea	58016-0234-02	162.00		AB
180s ea	58016-0234-99	215.91		AB
(St. Mary's MPP) REPACK				
TAB, PO (FILM-COATED)				
10 mg, 15s ea	60760-0418-15	24.01		AB
20s ea	60760-0418-20	30.01		AB
30s ea	60760-0418-30	42.01		AB
60s ea	60760-0418-60	78.03		AB
(FILM-COATED)				
10 mg, 90s ea	60760-0418-90	114.06		AB
(Stat Rx) REPACK				
TAB, PO, 10 mg, 21s ea	16590-0065-21	49.50		AB
(FILM-COATED)				
10 mg, 28s ea	16590-0065-28	48.44		AB
45s ea	16590-0065-45	58.44		AB
50s ea	16590-0065-50	64.93		AB
56s ea	16590-0065-56	74.98		AB
60s ea	16590-0065-60	88.75		AB
84s ea	16590-0065-62	112.48		AB
90s ea	16590-0065-90	114.70		AB
(FILM-COATED)				
10 mg, 112s ea	16590-0065-73	145.70		AB
180s ea	16590-0065-82	241.02		AB
270s ea	16590-0065-86	334.14		AB
(Vibranta) REPACK				
TAB, PO, 10 mg, 20s ea	57866-4842-02	28.98		
21s ea	57866-4842-04	22.16		
30s ea	57866-4842-01	38.33		
CYCLOBENZAPRINE HYDROCHLORIDE				
FUL				
TAB, PO, 5 mg, 100s ea		15.86		
10 mg, 100s ea		10.35		
(Amneal)				
TAB, PO (USP,FILM-COATED)				
10 mg, 100s ea	65162-0541-10	114.95		AB

PROD/MFR	NDC	AWP	DP	OBC
500s ea	65162-0541-50	546.00		AB
1000s ea	65162-0541-11	1037.40		AB
(Aurobindo Pharma)				
TAB, PO (USP,FILM-COATED)				
5 mg, 100s ea	65862-0190-01	164.05		AB
10 mg, 100s ea	65862-0191-01	115.76		AB
500s ea	65862-0191-05	557.12		AB
1000s ea	65862-0191-99	1091.50		AB
(Breckenridge Pharm)				
TAB, PO (FILM-COATED)				
5 mg, 100s ea	51991-0467-01	115.76		
1000s ea	51991-0467-10	1091.50		
10 mg, 100s ea	51991-0468-01	115.76		
1000s ea	51991-0468-10	1091.50		
(Cadista)				
TAB, PO (USP,FILM COATED)				
5 mg, 100s ea	59746-0211-06	172.89		AB
1000s ea	59746-0211-10	1642.50		AB
10 mg, 100s ea	59746-0177-06	115.78		AB
1000s ea	59746-0177-10	1100.00		AB
(Cephalon) *See AMRIX*				
(Gallipot)				
POW, NA (1X5GM,USP)				
5 gm	51552-0483-02	44.80	32.00	
(1X25GM,USP)				
25 gm	51552-0483-04	182.00	130.00	
(1X100GM,USP)				
100 gm	51552-0483-05	679.00	485.00	
(Hawkins) *See CYCLOBENZAPRINE HCL*				
(Letco) *See CYCLOBENZAPRINE HCL*				
(Major) *See CYCLOBENZAPRINE HCL*				
(Medisca) *See CYCLOBENZAPRINE HCL*				
(Mutual) *See CYCLOBENZAPRINE HCL*				
(Mylan) *See CYCLOBENZAPRINE HCL*				
(Mylan)				
TAB, PO (FILM-COATED)				
5 mg, 30s ea	00378-0771-93	49.22		AB
100s ea	00378-0771-01	164.05		AB
500s ea	00378-0771-05	820.25		AB
(Ortho-McNeil Pharm) *See FLEXERIL*				
(PCCA) *See CYCLOBENZAPRINE HCL*				
(Qualitest)				
TAB, PO (FILM COATED)				
5 mg, 100s ea	00603-3078-21	164.05		AB
500s ea	00603-3078-28	787.44		AB
10 mg, 100s ea	00603-3079-21	115.75		AB
(USP,FILM COATED)				
10 mg, 500s ea	00603-3079-28	557.11		AB
(FILM COATED)				
10 mg, 1000s ea	00603-3079-32	1091.49		AB
5000s ea	00603-3079-34	5457.45		
(Sandoz) *See CYCLOBENZAPRINE HCL*				
(Sandoz)				
TAB, PO (FILM-COATED)				
5 mg, 100s ea	00781-5032-01	164.25		AB
1000s ea	00781-5032-10	1642.50		AB
(Spectrum Pharmacy) *See CYCLOBENZAPRINE HCL*				
(Teva) *See CYCLOBENZAPRINE HCL*				
(Teva)				
TAB, PO (USP,10X10,FILM-COATED)				
10 mg, 100s ea UD	00093-1919-93	40.65		AB
(UDL) *See CYCLOBENZAPRINE HCL*				
(Victory Pharma, Inc.) *See FEXMID*				
(Watson Labs) *See CYCLOBENZAPRINE HCL*				
(Watson Labs)				
TAB, PO (FILM-COATED)				
5 mg, 100s ea	00591-3256-01	20.24		AB
(4u)				
REPACK				
TAB, PO (FILM COATED)				
5 mg, 30s ea	42549-0641-30	68.76		AB
(A-S Medication)				
REPACK				
TAB, PO, 5 mg, 30s ea	54569-5782-00	46.54		
(FILM COATED)				
10 mg, 7s ea	54569-2573-06	8.07		AB
10s ea	54569-2573-09	11.52		AB
12s ea	54569-3193-01	13.83		AB
14s ea	54569-2573-07	16.13		AB
15s ea	54569-2573-00	17.29		AB
20s ea	54569-2573-01	23.05		AB
21s ea	54569-2573-08	24.20		AB
30s ea	54569-2573-02	34.57		AB
45s ea	54569-3193-05	51.86		AB
60s ea	54569-2573-03	69.14		AB
90s ea	54569-5184-00	103.72		AB
100s ea	54569-2573-04	115.24		AB
(Aidarex)				
REPACK				
TAB, PO (FILM COATED)				
5 mg, 7s ea	33261-0377-07	11.90		AB
10s ea	33261-0377-10	17.00		AB
12s ea	33261-0377-12	20.40		AB
14s ea	33261-0377-14	23.80		AB
20s ea	33261-0377-20	34.00		AB
21s ea	33261-0377-21	35.70		AB
25s ea	33261-0377-25	42.50		AB
28s ea	33261-0377-28	47.60		AB
30s ea	33261-0377-30	51.00		AB
40s ea	33261-0377-40	68.00		AB
50s ea	33261-0377-50	85.00		AB
60s ea	33261-0377-60	102.00		AB
90s ea	33261-0377-90	153.00		AB
120s ea	33261-0377-02	204.00		AB
(FILM-COATED)				
10 mg, 7s ea	33261-0033-07	14.00		AB
10s ea	33261-0033-10	20.00		AB
14s ea	33261-0033-14	28.00		AB
20s ea	33261-0033-20	40.00		AB
21s ea	33261-0033-21	42.00		AB
25s ea	33261-0033-25	50.00		AB
28s ea	33261-0033-28	56.00		AB
30s ea	33261-0033-30	60.00		AB
50s ea	33261-0033-50	100.00		AB
60s ea	33261-0033-60	120.00		AB
90s ea	33261-0033-90	180.00		AB
(Altura)				
REPACK				
TAB, PO (FILM COATED)				
5 mg, 30s ea	63874-1186-03	49.21		
60s ea	63874-1186-06	98.43		
90s ea	63874-1186-09	147.65		
120s ea	63874-1186-04	196.86		
(American Health)				
REPACK				
TAB, PO (FILM COATED)				
10 mg, 100s ea UD	68084-0397-01	7.50		AB
(Bryant Ranch)				
REPACK				
TAB, PO (FILM-COATED)				
5 mg, 30s ea	63629-3640-01	58.54		AB
90s ea	63629-3640-02	179.82		AB
(DHS, Inc.)				
REPACK				
TAB, PO (FILM COATED)				
10 mg, 40s ea	55887-0989-40	65.20		AB
(Dispensing Solutions)				
REPACK				
TAB, PO, 5 mg, 10s ea	55045-3487-01	16.50		
(FILM-COATED)				
5 mg, 10s ea	68258-7013-01	16.50		AB
20s ea	68258-7013-02	33.00		AB
30s ea	55045-3487-03	49.50		
(FILM-COATED)				
5 mg, 30s ea	68258-7013-03	49.50		AB
10 mg, 10s ea	66336-0581-10	16.15		AB
60s ea	55045-3759-06	87.00		
(FILM COATED)				
10 mg, 90s ea	66336-0581-90	113.90		AB
126s ea	55045-3717-01	182.70		
(IPI)				
REPACK				
TAB, PO (FILM-COATED)				
5 mg, 21s ea	18837-0205-21	49.50		
60s ea	18837-0205-60	123.40		AB
10 mg, 15s ea	18837-0033-15	25.70		
(FILM-COATED)				
10 mg, 21s ea	18837-0033-21	51.50		
30s ea	18837-0033-30	51.50		
(FILM-COATED)				
10 mg, 60s ea	18837-0033-60	62.25		AB
90s ea	18837-0033-90	115.88		
270s ea	18837-0033-94	368.38		
(Keltman Pharma., Inc.)				
REPACK				
TAB, PO, 5 mg, 90s ea	68387-0502-90	112.54		
10 mg, 10s ea	68387-0500-10	13.00		
15s ea	06837-0500-15	19.50		
(Nucare Pharm)				
REPACK				
TAB, PO (FILM-COATED)				
5 mg, 14s ea	68071-0462-14	31.58		AB
30s ea	68071-0462-30	67.67		AB
60s ea	68071-0462-60	129.19		AB
90s ea	68071-0462-90	193.79		AB
(Palmetto)				
REPACK				
TAB, PO, 5 mg, 14s ea	23490-7673-00	22.97		
20s ea	23490-7673-01	32.81		
30s ea	23490-7673-03	49.22		
40s ea	23490-7673-04	65.63		
(PD-Rx Pharm)				
REPACK				
TAB, PO (USP,FILM-COATED)				
10 mg, 3s ea	43063-0050-03	18.80		AB
4s ea	43063-0050-04	21.55		AB
6s ea	43063-0050-06	24.30		AB
(Pharma Pac)				
REPACK				
TAB, PO (FILM-COATED)				
5 mg, 15s ea	52959-0846-15	25.92		AB
60s ea	52959-0846-60	103.56		
90s ea	52959-0846-90	155.35		AB
100s ea	52959-0846-00	172.59		AB
(Phys Total Care)				
REPACK				
TAB, PO (FILM COATED)				
5 mg, 15s ea	54868-5597-01	8.76		AB
(FILM-COATED)				
5 mg, 90s ea	54868-5597-02	22.57		AB
10 mg, 120s ea	54868-1110-01	31.80		AB
(Physician Partner)				
REPACK				
TAB, PO (FILM-COATED)				
5 mg, 20s ea	21695-0036-20	77.20		
30s ea	21695-0036-30	98.43		
120s ea	21695-0036-72	463.20		AB
(Quality Care Prod)				
REPACK				
TAB, PO, 5 mg, 21s ea	49999-0791-21	41.33		
100s ea	49999-0791-00	196.81		
(Southwood)				
REPACK				
TAB, PO (FILM-COATED)				
5 mg, 120s ea	58016-0076-02	196.87		AB
(St. Mary's MPP)				
REPACK				
TAB, PO (USP)				
10 mg, 9s ea	60760-0418-09	16.80		
(Stat Rx)				
REPACK				
TAB, PO (FILM-COATED)				
5 mg, 15s ea	16590-0544-15	34.70		AB
20s ea	16590-0544-20	36.50		AB
21s ea	16590-0544-21	51.90		AB
30s ea	16590-0544-30	69.40		AB
40s ea	16590-0544-40	78.25		AB
45s ea	16590-0544-45	104.10		AB
60s ea	16590-0544-60	102.82		AB
90s ea	16590-0544-90	220.55		AB
120s ea	16590-0544-72	299.20		AB
(Vibranta)				
REPACK				
TAB, PO (FILM-COATED)				
10 mg, 12s ea	57866-4842-08	3.25		AB
60s ea	57866-4842-07	76.65		
90s ea	57866-4842-06	114.95		
90s ea	57866-4843-01	114.95		
CYCLOCORT (Phys Total Care)				
REPACK				
amcinonide				
CRE, TP, 0.1%, 30 gm	54868-2228-00	48.23		
CYCLODEXTRIN (PCCA)				
alfadex				
POW, NA (ALPHA)				
1 gm	51927-3351-00	35.76		
(PCCA)				
betadex				
(BETA REAGENT)				
1 gm	51927-2492-00	9.00		
CYCLOGYL (Alcon Ophthalmic)				
cyclopentolate hydrochloride				
SOL, OP, 0.5%, 15 ml	00065-0395-15	51.36		AT
1%, 2 ml	00065-0396-02	17.94		AT
5 ml	00065-0396-05	32.28		AT

PROD/MFR	NDC	AWP	DP	OBC
15 ml	00065-0396-15	54.90		AT
2%, 2 ml	00065-0397-02	23.52		AT
5 ml	00065-0397-05	38.88		AT
15 ml	00065-0397-15	64.56		AT
(A-S Medication)				
REPACK				
SOL, OP, 1%, 5 ml	54569-3087-00	67.94		AT
(Phys Total Care)				
REPACK				
SOL, OP, 1%, 5 ml	54868-0656-01	30.74		AT
15 ml	54868-0656-00	50.11		AT
2%, 2 ml	54868-1801-00	21.06		AT
5 ml	54868-1801-01	34.61		AT
(Southwood)				
REPACK				
SOL, OP, 1%, 5 ml	58016-6468-01	25.49		AT
CYCLOHEXANOL (Baker, J.T.)				
LIQ, NA (REAGENT)				
500 ml	10106-9208-01	44.81		
4000 ml	10106-9208-03	152.13		
20000 ml	10106-9208-07	485.85		
CYCLOHEXANONE (Baker, J.T.)				
LIQ, NA (PURIFIED)				
500 ml	10106-9209-01	58.35		
CYCLOMYDRIL (Alcon Ophthalmic)				
cyclopentolate hcl/phenyleph hcl				
SOL, OP, 0.2%-1%, 2 ml	00065-0359-02	18.78		
5 ml	00065-0359-05	32.94		
CYCLOPENTOLATE (DHS, Inc.)				
REPACK				
cyclopentolate hydrochloride				
SOL, OP, 2%, 15 ml	55887-0169-15	66.96		
CYCLOPENTOLATE HCL (Bausch & Lomb Inc.)				
cyclopentolate hydrochloride				
SOL, OP, 1%, 2 ml 12s	24208-0735-01	4.35		AT
15 ml	24208-0735-06	7.10		AT
(Falcon Ophthalmics)				
SOL, OP (DROP-TAINER)				
1%, 2 ml	61314-0396-01	4.40		AT
15 ml	61314-0396-03	7.20		AT
(Medisca)				
POW, NA (U.S.P.)				
25 gm	38779-0848-04	294.00		
100 gm	38779-0848-05	1125.00		
(PCCA)				
POW, NA (U.S.P.)				
1 gm	51927-3349-00	54.00		
(Dispensing Solutions)				
REPACK				
SOL, OP, 1%, 15 ml	55045-2027-02	8.00		AT
(Phys Total Care)				
REPACK				
SOL, OP, 1%, 2 ml	54868-4697-00	17.85		AT
15 ml	54868-4697-01	26.15		AT
CYCLOPENTOLATE HCL/PHENYLEPH HCL				
(Alcon Ophthalmic) *See CYCLOMYDRIL*				
CYCLOPENTOLATE HYDROCHLORIDE				
(Akorn) *See AK-PENTOLATE*				
(Alcon Ophthalmic) *See CYCLOGYL*				
(Bausch & Lomb Inc.) *See CYCLOPENTOLATE HCL*				
(Falcon Ophthalmics) *See CYCLOPENTOLATE HCL*				
(Medisca) *See CYCLOPENTOLATE HCL*				
(Ocusoft) *See CYLATE*				
(PCCA) *See CYCLOPENTOLATE HCL*				
(Palmetto)				
REPACK				
SOL, OP, 1%, 5 ml	23490-5379-01	46.75		
15 ml	23490-0384-01	7.10		
CYCLOPHOSPHAMIDE (Baxter)				
PDS, IV (PHARMACYBULKPACKAGE,USP)				
1 gm, ea	10019-0956-16	54.62		AP
(S.D.V.,PF)				
1 gm, ea	10019-0956-01	68.00		AP
2 gm, ea	10019-0957-01	122.39		
(SDV,USP,PF)				
2 gm, ea	10019-0957-11	98.30		
(S.D.V.,PF)				
500 mg, ea	10019-0955-01	37.76		AP
(SDV,USP,PF)				
500 mg, ea	10019-0955-50	30.34		AP
(Medisca)				
POW, NA (U.S.P.)				
5 gm	38779-0506-03	165.00		
25 gm	38779-0506-04	705.00		
100 gm	38779-0506-05	2055.00		
(Roxane)				
TAB, PO, 25 mg, 100s ea	00054-4129-25	209.32		AB
50 mg, 100s ea	00054-4130-25	384.15		AB
(Phys Total Care)				
REPACK				
TAB, PO, 25 mg, 10s ea	54868-5218-01	58.68		
30s ea	54868-5218-02	128.79		
100s ea	54868-5218-00	394.29		AB
50 mg, 50s ea	54868-5005-01	363.57		
100s ea	54868-5005-00	721.14		
CYCLOSERINE				
(The Chao Center) *See SEROMYCIN*				
CYCLOSPORIN A (Gallipot)				
cyclosporine				
POW, NA, 1 gm	51552-0663-01	54.60		
(Hawkins)				
POW, NA (U.S.P.)				
1 gm	63370-0057-10	168.00		
5 gm	63370-0057-15	648.00		
25 gm	63370-0057-25	2352.00		
100 gm	63370-0057-35	7200.00		
500 gm	63370-0057-45	33120.00		
(Medisca)				
POW, NA, 1 gm	38779-0660-06	112.50		
5 gm	38779-0660-03	315.00		
(USP,1X10GM)				
10 gm	38779-0660-01	495.00		
25 gm	38779-0660-04	1017.00		
100 gm	38779-0660-05	3450.00		
(PCCA)				
POW, NA (USP)				
1 gm	51927-3196-00	120.00		
CYCLOSPORINE				
(Allergan Inc) *See RESTASIS*				
(Apotex Corp.)				
CAP, PO, 25 mg, 30s ea	60505-0133-00	46.82		AB2
100 mg, 30s ea	60505-0134-00	186.97		AB2
(Apotex Corp.)				
cyclosporine, modified				
SOL, PO (U.S.P.)				
100 mg/ml, 50 ml	60505-0354-01	299.55		AB1
CYCLOSPORINE (Bedford)				
SOL, IV (S.D.V.)				
50 mg/ml, 5 ml 10s	55390-0122-10	264.00		AP
(Gallipot) *See CYCLOSPORIN A*				
(Gallipot)				
POW, NA (1X500MG,USP)				
0.5 gm	51552-0663-06	32.90	23.50	
(1X5GM,USP)				
5 gm	51552-0663-02	228.20	163.00	
(1X25GM,USP)				
25 gm	51552-0663-04	756.00	540.00	
(Hawkins) *See CYCLOSPORIN A*				
(Letco)				
POW, NA (U.S.P.,A)				
5 gm	62991-1533-01	285.00		
25 gm	62991-1533-05	825.00		
100 gm	62991-1533-02	2370.00		
(Medisca) *See CYCLOSPORIN A*				
(Morton Grove)				
SOL, PO, 100 mg/ml, 50 ml	60432-0140-50	299.61		AB2
(Novartis Pharm) *See SANDIMMUNE*				
(Paddock)				
SOL, IV, 50 mg/ml,				
5 ml 10s	00574-0866-10	272.50		
(PCCA) *See CYCLOSPORIN A*				
(Sandoz)				
SGL, PO (SOFTGEL)				
25 mg, 30s ea	00185-0932-30	41.25		AB1
100 mg, 30s ea	00185-0933-30	164.89		AB1
(Teva)				
cyclosporine, modified				
SGL, PO (USP,MODIFIED,SOFTGEL)				
25 mg, 30s ea UD	00172-7310-46	41.25		AB1
50 mg, 30s ea UD	00172-7311-46	82.15		AB1
100 mg, 30s ea UD	00172-7312-46	164.89		AB1
SOL, PO (USP,MODIFIED)				
100 mg/ml, 50 ml	00172-7313-20	299.55		AB1
CYCLOSPORINE (Watson)				
SOL, PO (1X50ML,MODIFIED)				
100 mg/ml, 50 ml	00591-2224-55	282.91		
(Watson Labs)				
SGL, PO (USP,MODIFIED)				
25 mg, 30s ea UD	00591-2222-15	39.58		
100 mg, 30s ea UD	00591-2223-15	158.27		
(American Health)				
REPACK				
CAP, PO (USP,3X10)				
100 mg, 30s ea UD	62584-0827-21	199.72		
(Phys Total Care)				
REPACK				
CAP, PO, 100 mg, 30s ea	54868-5522-00	194.04		
CYCLOSPORINE, MODIFIED				
(Abbott Pharm) *See GENGRAF*				
(Apotex Corp.) *See CYCLOSPORINE*				
(Novartis Pharm) *See NEORAL*				
(Teva) *See CYCLOSPORINE*				
CYKLOKAPRON (Pfizer)				
tranexamic acid				
SOL, IV (AMP,10X10ML)				
100 mg/ml,				
10 ml 10s	00013-1114-10	879.83	733.19	
CYLATE (Ocusoft)				
cyclopentolate hydrochloride				
SOL, OP, 1%, 2 ml	54799-0501-02	8.43		AT
15 ml	54799-0501-12	10.31		AT
CYMBALTA (Lilly)				
duloxetine hydrochloride				
ECC, PO, 20 mg, 60s ea	00002-3235-60	277.06	230.88	
30 mg, 30s ea	00002-3240-30	155.30	129.42	
(IDENTI-DOSE)				
30 mg, 100s ea UD	00002-3240-33	517.68	431.40	
60 mg, 30s ea	00002-3237-34	143.89	119.91	
(ENTERIC-COATED)				
60 mg, 30s ea	00002-3270-30	155.30	129.42	EE
(IDENTI-DOSE)				
60 mg, 100s ea UD	00002-3270-33	517.68	431.40	EE
(ENTERIC-COATED)				
60 mg, 1000s ea	00002-3270-04	5176.80	4314.00	EE
(4u)				
REPACK				
ECC, PO, 30 mg, 30s ea	42549-0646-30	268.84		
(A-S Medication)				
REPACK				
ECC, PO, 60 mg, 30s ea	54569-5678-00	149.89		
(Aidarex)				
REPACK				
ECC, PO, 30 mg, 30s ea	33261-0523-30	149.89		
60s ea	33261-0523-60	299.78		
90s ea	33261-0523-90	449.67		
120s ea	33261-0523-02	599.59		
60 mg, 7s ea	33261-0524-07	34.97		
14s ea	33261-0524-14	69.94		
30s ea	33261-0524-30	149.89		
60s ea	33261-0524-60	299.78		
90s ea	33261-0524-90	449.67		
120s ea	33261-0524-02	599.59		
(Altura)				
REPACK				
ECC, PO, 60 mg, 30s ea	63874-1253-03	111.96		
(Bryant Ranch)				
REPACK				
ECC, PO, 60 mg, 30s ea	63629-3340-01	140.04		
(Core)				
REPACK				
ECC, PO, 30 mg, 30s ea	33358-0098-30	133.47		
60s ea	33358-0098-60	257.26		
60 mg, 30s ea	33358-0099-30	144.89		
60s ea	33358-0099-60	351.78		
(DHS, Inc.)				
REPACK				
ECC, PO, 30 mg, 15s ea	55887-0271-15	75.28		
(Dispensing Solutions)				
REPACK				
ECC, PO, 30 mg, 30s ea	68258-7043-03	201.90		
60 mg, 30s ea	55045-3697-03	135.00		
30s ea	68258-7044-03	201.90		
(IPI)				
REPACK				
ECC, PO, 20 mg, 60s ea	18837-0207-60	268.85		
60 mg, 90s ea	18837-0035-90	462.20		

PROD/MFR	NDC	AWP	DP	OBC
(Keltman Pharma., Inc.)				
REPACK				
ECC, PO, 30 mg, 30s ea	68387-0554-30	192.32		
60s ea	68387-0554-60	384.64		
60 mg, 30s ea	68387-0553-30	175.89		
60s ea	68387-0553-60	351.78		
(Nucare Pharm)				
REPACK				
ECC, PO, 30 mg, 15s ea	68071-0444-15	124.00		
30s ea	68071-1312-00	217.89		
60s ea	68071-0444-60	320.18		
60 mg, 15s ea	68071-0445-15	124.00		
30s ea	68071-1313-00	217.89		
60s ea	68071-0445-60	320.18		
(PD-Rx Pharm)				
REPACK				
ECC, PO, 30 mg, 21s ea	55289-0036-21	160.76		
30s ea	55289-0036-30	229.65		
60 mg, 21s ea	55289-0028-21	160.76		
30s ea	55289-0028-30	229.65		
(Pharma Pac)				
REPACK				
ECC, PO, 30 mg, 30s ea	52959-0173-30	219.90		
60 mg, 30s ea	52959-0892-30	172.80		
60s ea	52959-0892-60	345.30		
(Phys Total Care)				
REPACK				
ECC, PO, 20 mg, 30s ea	54868-5215-02	166.59		
60s ea	54868-5215-00	329.92		
90s ea	54868-5215-01	494.55		
30 mg, 30s ea	54868-5315-00	185.81		
60s ea	54868-5315-02	370.31		
90s ea	54868-5315-01	536.37		
60 mg, 30s ea	54868-5192-00	185.81		
60s ea	54868-5192-02	370.31		
90s ea	54868-5192-01	536.37		
180s ea	54868-5192-03	1070.12		
(Physician Partner)				
REPACK				
ECC, PO, 20 mg, 60s ea	21695-0657-60	554.12		
30 mg, 15s ea	21695-0145-15	182.71		
30s ea	21695-0145-30	310.60		
60 mg, 15s ea	21695-0146-15	182.71		
30s ea	21695-0146-30	310.60		
(Quality Care Prod)				
REPACK				
ECC, PO, 20 mg, 30s ea	49999-0617-30	180.80		
30 mg, 30s ea	49999-0618-30	300.00		
60s ea	49999-0618-60	600.00		
60 mg, 30s ea	49999-0619-30	300.00		
60s ea	49999-0619-60	600.00		
(Southwood)				
REPACK				
ECC, PO, 20 mg, 30s ea	58016-0735-30	120.21		
60s ea	58016-0735-60	240.41		
90s ea	58016-0735-90	360.62		
100s ea	58016-0735-00	400.68		
30 mg, 30s ea	58016-0732-30	134.78		
60s ea	58016-0732-60	269.56		
90s ea	58016-0732-90	404.34		
100s ea	58016-0732-00	449.27		
60 mg, 30s ea	58016-0742-30	134.78		
60s ea	58016-0742-60	269.57		
90s ea	58016-0742-90	404.35		
100s ea	58016-0742-00	449.28		
(St. Mary's MPP)				
REPACK				
ECC, PO, 30 mg, 30s ea	60760-0324-30	238.95		
60 mg, 30s ea	60760-0323-30	238.95		
(Stat Rx)				
REPACK				
ECC, PO, 20 mg, 30s ea	16590-0552-30	163.38		
60s ea	16590-0552-60	323.51		
90s ea	16590-0552-90	483.64		
30 mg, 7s ea	16590-0482-07	45.14		
28s ea	16590-0066-28	156.65		
28s ea	16590-0482-28	170.79		
30s ea	16590-0066-30	135.00		
30s ea	16590-0482-30	203.31		
45s ea	16590-0482-45	266.31		
56s ea	16590-0066-56	312.14		
60s ea	16590-0066-60	270.00		
60s ea	16590-0482-60	362.28		
90s ea	16590-0482-90	541.80		
120s ea	16590-0482-72	452.00		
60 mg, 28s ea	16590-0483-28	170.79		
30s ea	16590-0067-30	135.00		
30s ea	16590-0483-30	203.31		
60s ea	16590-0067-60	270.00		

PROD/MFR	NDC	AWP	DP	OBC
60s ea	16590-0483-60	362.28		
90s ea	16590-0483-90	541.80		
120s ea	16590-0483-72	452.00		
CYPRESS OIL (Medisca)				
OIL, NA (1X14ML)				
14 ml	38779-1829-03	22.50		
(1X25ML)				
25 ml	38779-1829-04	37.50		
(1X100ML)				
100 ml	38779-1829-05	93.00		
(1X500ML)				
500 ml	38779-1829-08	273.00		
CYPROHEPTADINE (Bryant Ranch)				
REPACK				
cyproheptadine hydrochloride				
TAB, PO, 4 mg, 30s ea	63629-2982-01	17.39		
60s ea	63629-2982-02	34.78		
(HomeMed)				
REPACK				
TAB, PO, 4 mg, 20s ea	51655-0276-52	16.93		EE
CYPROHEPTADINE HCL (Consolidated Midland)				
cyproheptadine hydrochloride				
SYR, PO, 2 mg/5 ml,				
480 ml	00223-6248-01	9.00		EE
480 ml	00223-6489-01	8.50		EE
3840 ml	00223-6489-02	57.50		EE
TAB, PO, 4 mg, 100s ea	00223-0709-01	5.75		EE
1000s ea	00223-0709-02	32.50		EE
(Hawkins)				
POW, NA, 10 gm	63370-0059-20	73.00		
25 gm	63370-0059-25	170.00		
100 gm	63370-0059-35	640.00		
500 gm	63370-0059-45	3080.00		
1000 gm	63370-0059-50	5600.00		
(Letco)				
POW, NA (U.S.P.)				
25 gm	62991-1232-01	120.00		
(Major)				
TAB, PO (10X10)				
4 mg, 100s ea UD	00904-1145-61	47.67		AA
(Medisca)				
POW, NA (U.S.P.)				
10 gm	38779-1226-01	72.00		
25 gm	38779-1226-04	190.50		
100 gm	38779-1226-05	645.00		
(PCCA)				
POW, NA (U.S.P.)				
1 gm	51927-1021-00	8.70		
(Rising)				
TAB, PO, 4 mg, 100s ea	64980-0123-01	42.69		AA
1000s ea	64980-0123-10	414.09		AA
(Spectrum Pharmacy)				
POW, NA (U.S.P.)				
5 gm	49452-2409-02	97.30		
25 gm	49452-2409-03	289.45		
(PD-Rx Pharm)				
REPACK				
TAB, PO, 4 mg, 20s ea	55289-0089-20	16.93		AA
(USP)				
4 mg, 30s ea	55289-0089-30	22.06		AA
(Phys Total Care)				
REPACK				
SYR, PO, 2 mg/5 ml,				
473 ml	54868-4338-00	80.94		AA
TAB, PO, 4 mg, 15s ea	54868-1332-02	10.80		EE
24s ea	54868-1332-01	14.58		EE
30s ea	54868-1332-04	17.10		EE
50s ea	54868-1332-05	25.50		EE
90s ea	54868-1332-03	42.30		EE
100s ea	54868-1332-06	45.00		EE
(Quality Care Prod)				
REPACK				
TAB, PO, 4 mg, 18s ea	49999-0493-18	11.43		AA
(Southwood)				
REPACK				
TAB, PO, 4 mg, 30s ea	58016-0041-30	12.81		EE
60s ea	58016-0041-60	25.61		EE
90s ea	58016-0041-90	38.42		EE
100s ea	58016-0041-00	42.69		EE
CYPROHEPTADINE HYDROCHLORIDE (Actavis Mid Atlantic)				
SYR, PO (1X473ML,MINT)				
2 mg/5 ml, 473 ml	00472-1400-16	50.16		AA
(Consolidated Midland) *See CYPROHEPTADINE HCL*				

PROD/MFR	NDC	AWP	DP	OBC
(Cypress Pharm)				
TAB, PO (USP)				
4 mg, 100s ea	60258-0850-01	42.69		AA
1000s ea	60258-0850-10	414.09		AA
(Gallipot)				
POW, NA (1X25GM,USP)				
25 gm	51552-0871-04	84.00	60.00	
(1X100GM,USP)				
100 gm	51552-0871-05	266.00	190.00	
(1X500GM,USP)				
500 gm	51552-0871-06	945.00	675.00	
(Hawkins) *See CYPROHEPTADINE HCL*				
(Letco) *See CYPROHEPTADINE HCL*				
(Major) *See CYPROHEPTADINE HCL*				
(Medisca) *See CYPROHEPTADINE HCL*				
(PCCA) *See CYPROHEPTADINE HCL*				
(Rising) *See CYPROHEPTADINE HCL*				
(Rising)				
SYR, PO (MINT)				
2 mg/5 ml, 473 ml	64980-0504-48	50.16		AA
(Spectrum Pharmacy) *See CYPROHEPTADINE HCL*				
(Teva)				
TAB, PO, 4 mg, 100s ea	00172-2929-60	42.69		AA
(USP)				
4 mg, 100s ea	00093-2929-01	42.69		
100s ea UD	00093-2929-93	42.70		
1000s ea	00093-2929-10	414.09		
(Phys Total Care)				
REPACK				
TAB, PO, 4 mg, 20s ea	54868-1332-07	12.90		AA
CYSTADANE (Rare Disease)				
betaine				
PDR, PO, 1 gm/scoopful,				
180 gm	66621-4000-01	795.87	153.50	
CYSTAGON (Mylan)				
cysteamine bitartrate				
CAP, PO, 50 mg, 100s ea	00378-9040-01	43.95		
500s ea	00378-9040-05	190.90		
150 mg, 100s ea	00378-9045-01	127.95		
500s ea	00378-9045-05	557.15		
CYSTEAMINE BITARTRATE				
(Mylan) *See CYSTAGON*				
CYSTEINE (PCCA)				
POW, NA (L)				
1 gm	51927-2346-00	0.87		
(Spectrum Pharmacy) *See L-CYSTEINE*				
CYSTEINE HCL (Hospira)				
cysteine hydrochloride				
SOL, IV, 50 mg/ml,				
10 ml 10s	00409-8975-10	81.24	71.10	
CYSTEINE HYDROCHLORIDE				
(Amer Regent) *See L-CYSTEINE HYDROCHLORIDE*				
(Hospira) *See CYSTEINE HCL*				
(Parenta Pharma) *See L-CYSTEINE HYDROCHLORIDE*				
(PCCA)				
POW, NA (L, ANHYDROUS)				
1 gm	51927-3511-00	0.84		
(Spectrum Pharmacy) *See L-CYSTEINE HCL MONOHYDRATE*				
(Teva) *See L-CYSTEINE*				
CYSTEMMS-V (Truxton)				
belladonna alkaloids and analgesics				
TAB, PO, 1000s ea	00463-6259-10	60.00		
CYSTINE (Medisca)				
CRY, NA (1X25GM, L, FCC)				
25 gm	38779-2041-04	31.50		
(1X100GM, L, FCC)				
100 gm	38779-2041-05	73.50		
(1X1000GM, L, FCC)				
1000 gm	38779-2041-09	429.00		
(PCCA)				
POW, NA (L)				
1 gm	51927-2644-00	1.05		
(Spectrum Pharmacy) *See L-CYSTINE*				
CYSTOGRAFIN (Bracco Diag)				
diatrizoate meglumine				
SOL, IV, 30%, 100 ml 10s	00270-0149-60	350.00	280.00	AT
300 ml 10s	00270-0149-57	627.50	502.00	AT
CYSTOGRAFIN-DILUTE (Bracco Diag)				
diatrizoate meglumine				
SOL, IV, 18%, 300 ml 10s	00270-1410-30	367.50	294.00	

PROD/MFR	NDC	AWP	DP	OBC
CYTARABINE (APP)				
SOL, IJ (S.D.V.,LATEX-FREE)				
100 mg/ml, 20 ml	63323-0120-20	48.06		AP
(Bedford) *See CYTARABINE NOVAPLUS*				
(Bedford)				
PDS, IJ (VIAL)				
1 gm, ea	55390-0133-01	24.00		AP
2 gm, ea	55390-0134-01	48.00		AP
100 mg, 10s ea	55390-0131-10	36.00		AP
500 mg, 10s ea	55390-0132-10	102.00		AP
(Hospira)				
SOL, IJ (S.D.V. X 5,PF)				
20 mg/ml, 5 ml 5s	61703-0305-38	29.16	25.50	
(500MG/25ML,PF)				
20 mg/ml, 25 ml	61703-0304-36	10.74	9.40	
(1GM/50ML,PF)				
20 mg/ml, 50 ml	61703-0303-46	21.60	18.90	
(S.D.V.,PF)				
100 mg/ml, 20 ml	61703-0319-22	16.56	14.49	
(Mayne Pharma)				
SOL, IJ (M.D.V.)				
20 mg/ml, 25 ml 5s	61703-0304-25	143.65		
(BULK PACKAGE,PF)				
20 mg/ml, 50 ml 5s	61703-0303-50	268.95		
CYTARABINE LIPOSOME				
(Enzon Pharma, Inc.) *See DEPOCYT*				
CYTARABINE NOVAPLUS (Bedford)				
cytarabine				
PDS, IJ (VIAL,PRIVATE LABEL)				
1 gm, ea	55390-0808-01	19.20		AP
2 gm, ea	55390-0809-01	38.40		AP
100 mg, 10s ea	55390-0806-10	33.60		AP
500 mg, 10s ea	55390-0807-10	90.00		AP
CYTOGAM (CSL)				
cytomegalovirus immune globulin, human				
SOL, IV (PF)				
50 ml	44206-3101-01	1057.51		
CYTOMEGALOVIRUS IMMUNE GLOBULIN, HUMAN				
(CSL) *See CYTOGAM*				
CYTOMEL (King Pharm)				
liothyronine sodium				
TAB, PO, 0.005 mg,				
100s ea	60793-0115-01	92.36		
0.025 mg, 100s ea	60793-0116-01	121.34		
0.05 mg, 100s ea	60793-0117-01	185.36		
(A-S Medication)				
REPACK				
TAB, PO, 0.005 mg,				
60s ea	54569-2968-01	49.49		
120s ea	54569-2968-05	176.90		
0.025 mg, 30s ea	54569-2053-00	35.44		
60s ea	54569-2053-06	70.88		
(DHS, Inc.)				
REPACK				
TAB, PO, 0.05 mg, 30s ea	55887-0146-30	49.80		
60s ea	55887-0146-60	99.59		
90s ea	55887-0146-90	149.39		
(Nucare Pharm)				
REPACK				
TAB, PO, 0.05 mg, 30s ea	66267-0612-30	135.58		
(Phys Total Care)				
REPACK				
TAB, PO, 0.005 mg,				
10s ea	54868-5058-03	13.43		
30s ea	54868-5058-01	35.07		
60s ea	54868-5058-02	67.53		
100s ea	54868-5058-00	110.15		
0.025 mg, 10s ea	54868-1750-02	13.51		
30s ea	54868-1750-01	36.78		
25 mcg, 100s ea	54868-1750-00	118.23		
(Quality Care Prod)				
REPACK				
TAB, PO, 0.005 mg,				
100s ea	49999-0826-00	80.67		
CYTOTEC (Pfizer)				
misoprostol				
TAB, PO, 100 mcg, 60s ea	00025-1451-60	80.48	67.07	
100s ea UD	00025-1451-34	140.74	117.28	
120s ea	00025-1451-20	160.98	134.15	
200 mcg, 60s ea	00025-1461-60	117.24	97.70	
100s ea	00025-1461-31	195.38	162.82	
100s ea UD	00025-1461-34	205.02	170.85	
(A-S Medication)				
REPACK				
TAB, PO, 200 mcg, 60s ea	54569-2765-02	124.40		
(Nucare Pharm)				
REPACK				
TAB, PO, 200 mcg, 40s ea	66267-0428-40	60.99		
(PD-Rx Pharm)				
REPACK				
TAB, PO, 100 mcg, 28s ea	55289-0248-28	57.96		
200 mcg, 2s ea	55289-0698-02	13.08		
4s ea	55289-0698-04	18.66		
8s ea	55289-0698-08	29.81		
30s ea	55289-0698-30	91.11		
100s ea UD	55289-0698-17	299.97		
(Pharma Pac)				
REPACK				
TAB, PO, 100 mcg, 12s ea	52959-0353-12	19.90		
28s ea	52959-0353-28	28.00		
30s ea	52959-0353-30	29.55		
40s ea	52959-0353-40	38.55		
60s ea	52959-0353-60	58.00		
200 mcg, 12s ea	52959-0354-12	22.90		
30s ea	52959-0354-30	46.65		
40s ea	52959-0354-40	60.20		
120s ea	52959-0354-01	164.50		
(Phys Total Care)				
REPACK				
TAB, PO, 100 mcg, 20s ea	54868-2176-04	35.26		
30s ea	54868-2176-00	51.59		
40s ea	54868-2176-03	67.91		
(Southwood)				
REPACK				
TAB, PO, 100 mcg, 10s ea	58016-0347-10	13.01		
12s ea	58016-0347-12	15.62		
14s ea	58016-0347-14	18.22		
15s ea	58016-0347-15	19.52		
16s ea	58016-0347-16	20.82		
20s ea	58016-0347-20	26.03		
21s ea	58016-0347-21	27.33		
24s ea	58016-0347-24	31.23		
25s ea	58016-0347-25	32.53		
28s ea	58016-0347-28	21.84		
30s ea	58016-0347-30	39.04		
40s ea	58016-0347-40	52.05		
60s ea	58016-0347-60	78.08		
90s ea	58016-0347-90	117.12		
120s ea	58016-0347-00	130.13		
200 mcg, 10s ea	58016-0190-10	18.96		
12s ea	58016-0190-12	22.75		
14s ea	58016-0190-14	26.54		
15s ea	58016-0190-15	28.43		
20s ea	58016-0190-20	37.91		
30s ea	58016-0190-30	56.87		
60s ea	58016-0190-60	113.74		
90s ea	58016-0190-90	170.60		
100s ea	58016-0190-00	189.56		
120s ea	58016-0190-02	227.47		
CYTOVENE (Phys Total Care)				
REPACK				
ganciclovir				
CAP, PO, 250 mg, 180s ea	54868-3507-00	984.03		
CYTOVENE IV (Roche Labs)				
ganciclovir sodium				
PDS, IV (VIAL)				
500 mg, 25s ea	00004-6940-03	2026.56		
CYTRA-2 (Cypress Pharm)				
citric acid/sodium citrate				
SOL, PO (AF,SF,DYE-FREE,GRAPE)				
334 mg/5 ml-500 mg/5 ml,				
473 ml	60258-0001-16	9.49		
CYTRA-3 (Cypress Pharm)				
citric acid/potassium citrate/sodium citrate				
SYR, PO (VANILLA)				
473 ml	60258-0002-16	16.95		
CYTRA-K (Cypress Pharm)				
citric acid/potassium citrate				
SOL, PO (AF,SF,CHERRY)				
334 mg/5 ml-1100 mg/5 ml,				
473 ml	60258-0003-16	16.95		
CYTRA-K CRYSTALS (Cypress Pharm)				
citric acid/potassium citrate				
PDR, PO (PACKET,SF,FRUIT)				
100s ea	60258-0005-01	85.50		
D & C GREEN #5 (Amend)				
color additive				
POW, NA, 454 gm	17317-0907-01	179.20		
D & C GREEN #6 (Amend)				
color additive				
POW, NA, 454 gm	17317-0908-01	193.00		
D & C GREEN #8 (Amend)				
color additive				
POW, NA, 454 gm	17317-0909-01	154.00		
D & C RED #117 (Amend)				
color additive				
POW, NA, 454 gm	17317-0911-01	245.00		
D & C RED #22 (Amend)				
color additive				
POW, NA, 454 gm	17317-0913-01	189.00		
D & C RED #28 (Amend)				
color additive				
POW, NA, 454 gm	17317-0914-01	203.00		
D & C RED #33 (Amend)				
color additive				
POW, NA, 454 gm	17317-0915-01	210.00		
D & C RED NO. 28 (PCCA)				
color additive				
POW, NA (PHLOXINE B)				
1 gm	51927-2266-00	5.40		
D & C RED NO. 33 (Medisca)				
color additive				
POW, NA (1X25GM)				
25 gm	38779-2046-04	84.00		
(1X100GM)				
100 gm	38779-2046-05	181.50		
(1X500GM)				
500 gm	38779-2046-08	597.00		
D & C VIOLET #2 (Amend)				
color additive				
POW, NA, 454 gm	17317-0918-01	273.00		
(EXTERNAL WATER SOLUBLE)				
454 gm	17317-0917-01	273.00		
D & C YELLOW #10 (Amend)				
color additive				
POW, NA, 480 gm	17317-0921-01	203.00		
(PCCA)				
POW, NA (QUINOLINE YELLOW)				
1 gm	51927-2497-00	3.00		
D & C YELLOW #11 (Amend)				
color additive				
POW, NA, 480 gm	17317-0922-01	182.00		
500 gm	17317-0922-05	500.00		
D & C YELLOW #7 (Amend)				
color additive				
SOL, NA (EXTERNAL ALKALINE)				
480 gm	17317-0919-01	182.00		
D & C YELLOW #8 (Amend)				
color additive				
POW, NA, 480 gm	17317-0920-01	168.00		
D-2-DEOXYRIBOSE				
(PCCA) *See DEOXY-D-RIBOSE (2)*				
D-ALANINE (Spectrum Pharmacy)				
alanine				
POW, NA, 5 gm	49452-0200-01	189.70		
25 gm	49452-0200-02	602.00		
D-ALPHA TOCOPHERYL ACID SUCCINATE				
(PCCA) *See TOCOPHERYL ACID SUCCINATE*				
(Spectrum Pharmacy) *See D-VITAMIN E SUCCINATE*				
D-BIOTIN (Amend)				
biotin				
POW, NA (F.C.C.)				
1 gm	17317-0812-07	29.40		
5 gm	17317-0812-08	112.00		
(Gallipot)				
POW, NA (1X1GM,USP,FCC)				
1 gm	51552-0654-01	26.60	19.00	
(F.C.C.)				
5 gm	51552-0654-02	119.00	85.00	
(1X100GM,USP,FCC)				
100 gm	51552-0654-05	1568.00	1120.00	
(1X500MG,USP,FCC)				
500 ml	51552-0654-06	17.29	12.35	
D-CALCIUM PANTOTHENATE (Gallipot)				
calcium pantothenate				
POW, NA (1X1000GM,USP)				
1000 gm	51552-0971-07	95.20	68.00	
D-FEDA II (Dexo)				
guaifenesin/pseudoephedrine hydrochloride				
TER, PO, 600 mg-60 mg,				
100s ea	59196-0005-01	49.80		

PROD/MFR	NDC	AWP	DP	OBC
D-GLUCONOLACTONE (Spectrum Pharmacy)				
gluconolactone				
POW, NA (F.C.C.)				
100 gm	**49452-3300-01**	79.45		
1000 gm	**49452-3300-02**	229.95		
5000 gm	**49452-3300-03**	756.00		
D-GLUCOSAMINE HYDROCHLORIDE (Spectrum Pharmacy)				
glucosamine hydrochloride				
POW, NA (1X100GM)				
100 gm	**49452-3308-02**	148.75		
(1X500GM) 500 gm	**49452-3308-03**	455.00		
(1X1000GM) 1000 gm	**49452-3308-04**	742.00		
(1X5000GM) 5000 gm	**49452-3308-05**	1928.50		
D-LACTOSE MONOHYDRATE (Baker, J.T.)				
lactose				
POW, NA (A.C.S., REAGENT)				
500 gm	**10106-2248-01**	26.32		
D-MANNOSE (Spectrum Pharmacy)				
mannose				
POW, NA (1X25GM)				
25 gm	**49452-4384-01**	160.30		
(1X100GM) 100 gm	**49452-4384-02**	427.00		
D-PANTOTHENYL ALCOHOL (Consolidated Midland)				
dexpanthenol				
SOL, IM (VIAL)				
250 mg/ml, 10 ml	**00223-8235-10**	5.00		
D-PENICILLAMINE (Medisca)				
penicillamine				
POW, NA (U.S.P.)				
5 gm	**38779-0244-03**	43.50		
25 gm	**38779-0244-04**	166.50		
100 gm	**38779-0244-05**	582.00		
D-PSEUDOEPHEDRINE HYDROCHLORIDE (Amend)				
pseudoephedrine hydrochloride				
POW, NA (U.S.P.)				
25 gm	**17317-0716-02**	14.00		
100 gm	**17317-0716-03**	35.00		
1000 gm	**17317-0716-06**	210.00		
D-RIBOSE (Spectrum Pharmacy)				
ribose				
POW, NA, 25 gm	**49452-6275-03**	143.85		
100 gm	**49452-6275-04**	305.20		
D-TAB (Palm)				
guaifenesin/phenylephrine hydrochloride				
TER, PO (FILM-COATED) 1200 mg-40 mg,				
100s ea	**24518-0001-01**	68.75	55.00	
D-TARTARIC ACID (Baker, J.T.)				
tartaric acid				
CRY, NA (A.C.S., REAGENT)				
500 gm	**10106-0386-01**	88.68		
2500 gm	**10106-0386-05**	330.32		
POW, NA, 500 gm	**10106-0400-01**	100.06		
2500 gm	**10106-0400-05**	365.19		
D-USNIC ACID				
(PCCA) *See USNIC ACID*				
D-VITAMIN E SUCCINATE (Spectrum Pharmacy)				
d-alpha tocopheryl acid succinate				
POW, NA (1X25GM,USP)				
25 gm	**49452-8132-01**	88.55		
(1X100GM,USP) 100 gm	**49452-8132-02**	258.30		
(1X500GM,USP) 500 gm	**49452-8132-03**	661.50		
(1X1000GM,USP) 1000 gm	**49452-8132-04**	1141.00		
D.A. CHEWABLE (Southwood) REPACK				
cpm/methscopolamine nitrate/phenyleph hcl				
CTB, PO, 2 mg-1.25 mg-10 mg,				
30s ea	**58016-0798-30**	14.35		
60s ea	**58016-0798-60**	26.97		
100s ea	**58016-0798-00**	43.51		
D.H.E. 45 (Valeant Pharm Intl)				
dihydroergotamine mesylate				
SOL, IJ (AMP)				
1 mg/ml, 1 ml 10s	**66490-0041-01**	1259.10		**AP**
D&C GREEN NO. 6 (PCCA)				
POW, NA (QUINIZARIN GREEN SS)				
1 gm	**51927-2527-00**	3.00		
D&C RED NO. 22 (PCCA)				
POW, NA (EOSIN Y)				
1 gm	**51927-2506-00**	3.00		
D&C YELLOW #10 (Gallipot)				
color additive				
POW, NA (C147005)				
5 gm	**51552-0518-02**	14.00		
D+XYLOSE (Spectrum Pharmacy)				
xylose				
POW, NA (U.S.P.)				
25 gm	**49452-8240-01**	58.80		
100 gm	**49452-8240-02**	134.75		
D3-50 (Bio-Tech Pharm)				
cholecalciferol				
CAP, PO, 50000 iu,				
12s ea	**53191-0362-12**	9.00		
100s ea	**53191-0362-01**	15.00		
DACARBAZINE (APP)				
PDS, IV (S.D.V.)				
100 mg, ea	**63323-0127-10**	13.35		**AP**
200 mg, ea	**63323-0128-20**	26.65		**AP**
(Bayer Corp.) *See DTIC-DOME*				
(Bedford) *See DACARBAZINE NOVAPLUS*				
(Bedford)				
PDS, IV (S.D.V.)				
200 mg, 10s ea	**55390-0090-10**	226.80		**AP**
(Hospira)				
PDS, IV (SINGLE DOSE VIAL,PF)				
200 mg, ea	**61703-0327-22**	7.96	6.96	
(PCCA)				
POW, NA (U.S.P.)				
1 gm	**51927-2362-00**	63.00		
(Teva)				
PDS, IV (S.D.V.)				
200 mg, ea	**00703-5075-01**	22.21		**AP**
(VIAL) 200 mg, 10s ea	**00703-5075-03**	222.12		**AP**
DACARBAZINE NOVAPLUS (Bedford)				
dacarbazine				
PDS, IV (USP,S.D.V.)				
200 mg, 10s ea	**55390-0339-10**	226.80		**AP**
DACEX-DM (Cypress Pharm)				
dm/gg/phenyleph hcl				
SOL, PO (AF,SF,STRAWBERRY)				
473 ml	**60258-0243-16**	61.24		
DACOGEN (Eisai)				
decitabine				
PDS, IV, 50 mg, ea	**62856-0600-01**	1706.40		
DACTINOMYCIN				
(Lundbeck) *See COSMEGEN*				
DALFAMPRIDINE				
(Acorda Therapeutics) *See AMPYRA*				
DALFOPRISTIN/QUINUPRISTIN				
(Monarch) *See SYNERCID*				
DALLERGY (Laser Pharma)				
cpm/phenyleph hcl				
SOL, PO (W/DROPPER,AF,SF,PEACH) 1 mg/ml-2 mg/ml,				
30 ml	**16477-0120-30**	16.80		
(Laser Pharma)				
cpm/methscopolamine nitrate/phenyleph hcl				
SYR, PO, 473 ml	**16477-0819-01**	44.75		
TAB, PO, 4 mg-1.25 mg-10 mg, 100s ea	**00277-0160-01**	38.40		
TER, PO (DYE-FREE,CAPLET) 12 mg-2.5 mg-20 mg, 100s ea	**00277-0182-01**	69.60		
DALLERGY DM (Laser Pharma)				
bpm/dm/pse hcl				
SOL, PO (1X473ML,AF,SF)				
473 ml	**16477-0140-01**	55.00		
DALLERGY PE (Laser Pharma)				
cpm/methscopolamine nitrate/phenyleph hcl				
SYR, PO (1X473ML,GRAPE)				
473 ml	**16477-0821-01**	49.50		
DALLERGY PSE (Laser Pharma)				
cpm/methscopolamine nitrate/pse hcl				
TER, PO, 4 mg-1.25 mg-60 mg, 100s ea	**16477-0146-01**	99.95		
DALLERGY-JR (Laser Pharma)				
cpm/phenyleph hcl				
CER, PO, 4 mg-20 mg, 100s ea	**00277-0183-01**	69.90		
(Laser Pharma)				
chlorpheniramine tannate/phenylephrine tannate				
SUS, PO, 4 mg/5 ml-20 mg/5 ml, 473 ml	**00277-0186-41**	149.50		
DALMANE (Phys Total Care) REPACK				
flurazepam hydrochloride				
CAP, PO, 30 mg, 60s ea, C-IV	**54868-0675-01**	117.75		**AB**
DALTEPARIN SODIUM				
(Eisai) *See FRAGMIN*				
DAMASON-P (Mason Pharm)				
aspirin/hydrocodone bitartrate				
TAB, PO, 500 mg-5 mg,				
100s ea, C-III	**12758-0057-01**	37.68		
500s ea, C-III	**12758-0057-05**	162.18		
1000s ea, C-III	**12758-0057-10**	316.81		
DANAZOL (Lannett)				
CAP, PO, 50 mg, 100s ea	**00527-1392-01**	159.54		**AB**
100 mg, 100s ea	**00527-1368-01**	239.40		**AB**
200 mg, 60s ea	**00527-1369-06**	324.86		**AB**
100s ea	**00527-1369-01**	477.33		**AB**
(Medisca)				
POW, NA (U.S.P.)				
5 gm	**38779-0174-03**	105.00		
25 gm	**38779-0174-04**	408.00		
100 gm	**38779-0174-05**	1275.00		
(PCCA)				
POW, NA (USP)				
1 gm	**51927-1842-00**	19.80		
(Spectrum Pharmacy)				
POW, NA (U.S.P./N.F.)				
5 gm	**49452-2436-02**	159.95		
25 gm	**49452-2436-03**	591.50		
(Teva)				
CAP, PO, 50 mg, 100s ea	**00555-0633-02**	190.91		**AB**
100 mg, 100s ea	**00555-0634-02**	286.45		**AB**
200 mg, 60s ea	**00555-0635-09**	324.86		**AB**
100s ea	**00555-0635-02**	477.33		**AB**
(American Health) REPACK				
CAP, PO (USP,3X10)				
200 mg, 30s ea UD	**68084-0074-21**	144.65		**AB**
(Phys Total Care) REPACK				
CAP, PO, 200 mg, 100s ea	**54868-5280-00**	1067.40		
DANDELION				
(PCCA) *See DANDELION LEAF*				
DANDELION LEAF (PCCA)				
dandelion				
POW, NA (TARAXACUM OFFICINALE)				
1 gm	**51927-2982-00**	0.09		
DANTHRON (PCCA)				
POW, NA, 1 gm	**51927-2493-00**	2.22		
DANTRIUM (JHP)				
dantrolene sodium				
CAP, PO, 25 mg, 100s ea	**42023-0124-01**	126.02		**AB**
50 mg, 100s ea	**42023-0125-01**	188.78		**AB**
100 mg, 100s ea	**00149-0033-05**	234.84		**AB**
PDS, IV (LYOPHILIZED)				
20 mg, 6s ea	**42023-0123-06**	638.21		**AP**
(Quality Care Prod) REPACK				
CAP, PO, 100 mg, 30s ea	**35356-0439-30**	122.60		**AB**
DANTROLENE SODIUM (Global Pharm)				
CAP, PO, 25 mg, 100s ea	**00115-4411-01**	106.93		**AB**
50 mg, 100s ea	**00115-4422-01**	160.19		**AB**
100 mg, 100s ea	**00115-4433-01**	199.27		**AB**
(JHP) *See DANTRIUM*				
(Medisca)				
POW, NA (1X100GM,USP)				
100 gm	**38779-2446-05**	1725.00		
(1X100GM) 100 gm	**38779-2229-05**	1725.00		
(1X500GM,USP) 500 gm	**38779-2446-08**	7050.00		
(1X500GM) 500 gm	**38779-2229-08**	7050.00		
(1X1000GM,USP) 1000 gm	**38779-2446-09**	12600.00		
(1X1000GM) 1000 gm	**38779-2229-09**	12600.00		
(US WorldMeds)				
PDS, IV (LYOPHILIZED)				
20 mg, 6s ea	**27505-0001-65**	607.50	399.00	**AP**

PROD/MFR	NDC	AWP	DP	OBC
(American Health)				
REPACK				
CAP, PO (3X10)				
25 mg, 30s ea UD	**68084-0300-21**	35.45		AB
DANTROLENE SODIUM (Palmetto)				
REPACK				
CAP, PO, 25 mg, 60s ea	**23490-7925-06**	79.20		
DAPIPRAZOLE HYDROCHLORIDE (Medisca)				
POW, NA (1X100GM)				
100 gm	**38779-2428-05**	24000.00		
(1X1000GM)				
1000 gm	**38779-2428-09**	135000.00		
DAPSONE				
(Allergan Inc) *See ACZONE*				
(Gallipot)				
POW, NA, 5 gm	**51552-1042-02**	30.10	21.50	
(Jacobus)				
TAB, PO (2X15,USP,GLUTEN-FREE)				
25 mg, 30s ea UD	**49938-0102-30**	31.80		EE
100 mg, 30s ea UD	**49938-0101-30**	39.00		
(PCCA)				
POW, NA (U.S.P.)				
1 gm	**51927-3424-00**	5.94		
(A-S Medication)				
REPACK				
TAB, PO (GLUTEN-FREE)				
100 mg, 30s ea	**54569-6105-00**	40.63		
100s ea	**54569-2015-00**	21.35		
(PD-Rx Pharm)				
REPACK				
TAB, PO, 25 mg, 20s ea	**55289-0188-20**	20.80		
40s ea	**55289-0188-40**	31.60		
(Phys Total Care)				
REPACK				
TAB, PO (GLUTEN-FREE)				
25 mg, 30s ea	**54868-2817-00**	95.98		EE
40s ea	**54868-2817-02**	127.98		
100 mg, 30s ea	**54868-3801-01**	118.20		
DAPTACEL (Sanofi)				
dtap vaccine				
SUS, IM (10 S.D.V.,TAX INCL)				
0.5 ml 10s	**49281-0286-10**	280.58	237.57	
DAPTOMYCIN				
(Cubist Pharmaceuticals) *See CUBICIN*				
DARAPRIM (Glaxo)				
pyrimethamine				
TAB, PO, 25 mg, 100s ea	**00173-0201-55**	58.16		
(Phys Total Care)				
REPACK				
TAB, PO, 25 mg, 100s ea	**54868-3309-02**	51.98		
DARBEPOETIN ALFA				
(Amgen USA Inc.) *See ARANESP*				
DARCO G-60 (Amend)				
activated charcoal				
POW, NA, 454 gm	**17317-0983-01**	49.00		
DARIFENACIN HYDROBROMIDE				
(Novartis Pharm) *See ENABLEX*				
DARUNAVIR ETHANOLATE				
(Tibotec Therapeutics) *See PREZISTA*				
DARVOCET A500 (Xanodyne Pharma)				
acetaminophen/propoxyphene napsylate				
TAB, PO (USP,FILM COATED)				
500 mg-100 mg,				
100s ea, C-IV	**66479-0513-10**	214.49		AB
(Dispensing Solutions)				
REPACK				
TAB, PO, 500 mg-100 mg,				
12s ea, C-IV	**55045-3335-01**	17.52		
100s ea, C-IV	**55045-3335-00**	146.00		
(Phys Total Care)				
REPACK				
TAB, PO, 500 mg-100 mg,				
30s ea, C-IV	**54868-5147-00**	35.23		
(Southwood)				
REPACK				
TAB, PO, 500 mg-100 mg,				
30s ea, C-IV	**58016-0150-30**	37.41		
(FILM COATED)				
500 mg-100 mg,				
30s ea, C-IV	**58016-0151-30**	54.41		AB
60s ea, C-IV	**58016-0150-60**	74.83		
(FILM COATED)				
500 mg-100 mg,				
60s ea, C-IV	**58016-0151-60**	108.83		AB
90s ea, C-IV	**58016-0150-90**	112.24		
(FILM COATED)				
500 mg-100 mg,				
90s ea, C-IV	**58016-0151-90**	163.24		AB
100s ea, C-IV	**58016-0150-00**	124.71		
(FILM COATED)				
500 mg-100 mg,				
100s ea, C-IV	**58016-0151-00**	181.38		AB
DARVOCET-N 100 (Xanodyne Pharma)				
acetaminophen/propoxyphene napsylate				
TAB, PO (FILM COATED)				
650 mg-100 mg,				
100s ea, C-IV	**66479-0515-10**	210.66		AB
500s ea, C-IV	**66479-0515-50**	1000.50		AB
(A-S Medication)				
REPACK				
TAB, PO, 650 mg-100 mg,				
20s ea, C-IV	**54569-0007-02**	30.83		AB
30s ea, C-IV	**54569-0007-03**	46.24		AB
(PD-Rx Pharm)				
REPACK				
TAB, PO, 650 mg-100 mg,				
10s ea, C-IV	**55289-0852-10**	29.09		AB
12s ea, C-IV	**55289-0852-12**	33.68		AB
20s ea, C-IV	**55289-0852-20**	58.17		AB
(Phys Total Care)				
REPACK				
TAB, PO, 650 mg-100 mg,				
30s ea, C-IV	**54868-0676-02**	56.20		AB
100s ea, C-IV	**54868-0676-00**	182.37		AB
500s ea, C-IV	**54868-0676-03**	636.24		AB
(Southwood)				
REPACK				
TAB, PO (FILM COATED)				
650 mg-100 mg,				
30s ea, C-IV	**58016-0056-30**	53.44		AB
60s ea, C-IV	**58016-0056-60**	106.88		AB
90s ea, C-IV	**58016-0056-90**	160.33		AB
100s ea, C-IV	**58016-0056-00**	178.14		AB
(Stat Rx)				
REPACK				
TAB, PO (FILM COATED)				
650 mg-100 mg,				
120s ea, C-IV	**16590-0761-72**	275.06		AB
DARVOCET-N 50 (Xanodyne Pharma)				
acetaminophen/propoxyphene napsylate				
TAB, PO (FILM-COATED)				
325 mg-50 mg,				
100s ea, C-IV	**66479-0514-10**	113.68		AB
DARVON (Xanodyne Pharma)				
propoxyphene hydrochloride				
CAP, PO (PULVULES)				
65 mg,				
100s ea, C-IV	**66479-0510-10**	125.72		AA
DARVON-N (Xanodyne Pharma)				
propoxyphene napsylate				
TAB, PO (FILM COATED)				
100 mg,				
100s ea, C-IV	**66479-0512-10**	194.52		
(Phys Total Care)				
REPACK				
TAB, PO, 100 mg,				
100s ea, C-IV	**54868-5744-00**	158.57		
(Quality Care Prod)				
REPACK				
TAB, PO (FILM COATED)				
100 mg,				
30s ea, C-IV	**35356-0558-30**	125.84		
(Stat Rx)				
REPACK				
TAB, PO (FILM COATED)				
100 mg,				
30s ea, C-IV	**16590-0874-30**	66.31		
DASATINIB				
(Bristol-Myers) *See SPRYCEL*				
DAUNORUBICIN CITRATE LIPOSOME				
(Gilead Sciences) *See DAUNOXOME*				
DAUNORUBICIN HCL (Bedford)				
daunorubicin hydrochloride				
SOL, IV (S.D.V.,PF)				
5 mg/ml, 4 ml 10s	**55390-0108-10**	504.00		AP
10 ml	**55390-0108-01**	424.50		AP
(Teva)				
SOL, IV (S.D.V.,PF)				
5 mg/ml, 4 ml 10s	**00703-5233-13**	1630.08		AP
DAUNORUBICIN HCL NOVAPLUS (Bedford)				
daunorubicin hydrochloride				
PDS, IV (S.D.V.)				
20 mg, 10s ea	**55390-0805-10**	374.40		AP
SOL, IV (S.D.V.,PF)				
5 mg/ml, 4 ml 10s	**55390-0142-10**	374.40		AP
DAUNORUBICIN HYDROCHLORIDE (APP)				
PDS, IV (S.D.V.,PF)				
20 mg, ea	**63323-0119-08**	169.75		
SOL, IV (S.D.V.,PF,LATEX-FREE)				
5 mg/ml, 4 ml	**63323-0124-04**	44.22		
(Bedford) *See CERUBIDINE*				
(Bedford) *See DAUNORUBICIN HCL*				
(Bedford) *See DAUNORUBICIN HCL NOVAPLUS*				
(Teva) *See DAUNORUBICIN HCL*				
DAUNOXOME (Gilead Sciences)				
daunorubicin citrate liposome				
SOL, IV (S.D.V.,PF)				
2 mg/ml, 25 ml	**61958-0301-01**	340.00		
DAYPRO (Pfizer)				
oxaprozin				
TAB, PO, 600 mg, 100s ea	**00025-1381-31**	286.74	238.95	AB
(A-S Medication)				
REPACK				
TAB, PO (CAPLET)				
600 mg, 15s ea	**54569-3702-01**	41.03		AB
(DHS, Inc.)				
REPACK				
TAB, PO (CAPLET)				
600 mg, 30s ea	**55887-0114-30**	74.43		AB
60s ea	**55887-0114-60**	148.86		AB
90s ea	**55887-0114-90**	223.29		AB
(Dispensing Solutions)				
REPACK				
TAB, PO (CAPLET)				
600 mg, 15s ea	**55045-2120-06**	39.50		
30s ea	**55045-2120-08**	78.75		AB
(Nucare Pharm)				
REPACK				
TAB, PO, 600 mg, 14s ea	**66267-0065-14**	37.50		AB
30s ea	**66267-0065-30**	77.75		AB
60s ea	**66267-0065-60**	152.55		AB
(PD-Rx Pharm)				
REPACK				
TAB, PO (CAPLET)				
600 mg, 14s ea	**55289-0453-14**	49.27		AB
15s ea	**55289-0453-15**	52.41		AB
20s ea	**55289-0453-20**	68.12		AB
30s ea	**55289-0453-30**	99.53		AB
40s ea	**55289-0453-40**	130.94		AB
42s ea	**55289-0453-42**	137.22		AB
60s ea	**55289-0453-60**	193.76		AB
(Pharma Pac)				
REPACK				
TAB, PO (CAPLET)				
600 mg, 14s ea	**52959-0252-14**	39.38		AB
15s ea	**52959-0252-15**	40.85		AB
20s ea	**52959-0252-20**	54.50		AB
21s ea	**52959-0252-21**	57.23		AB
24s ea	**52959-0252-24**	65.42		AB
28s ea	**52959-0252-28**	76.23		AB
30s ea	**52959-0252-30**	81.64		AB
42s ea	**52959-0252-42**	113.40		AB
45s ea	**52959-0252-45**	121.01		AB
60s ea	**52959-0252-60**	159.00		AB
100s ea	**52959-0252-01**	263.24		AB
(Phys Total Care)				
REPACK				
TAB, PO, 600 mg, 10s ea	**54868-2997-05**	28.00		AB
(CAPLET)				
600 mg, 15s ea	**54868-2997-00**	41.05		AB
20s ea	**54868-2997-04**	54.11		AB
30s ea	**54868-2997-02**	80.24		AB
60s ea	**54868-2997-01**	149.89		AB
100s ea	**54868-2997-03**	247.93		AB
(Quality Care Prod)				
REPACK				
TAB, PO (CAPLET)				
600 mg, 30s ea	**49999-0072-30**	158.64		
60s ea	**49999-0072-60**	317.40		
DAYTRANA (Shire US Inc.)				
methylphenidate				
TDM, TD, 10 mg/9 hr,				
30s ea, C-II	**54092-0552-30**	178.82	149.02	
15 mg/9 hr,				
30s ea, C-II	**54092-0553-30**	178.82	149.02	

PROD/MFR	NDC	AWP	DP	OBC
20 mg/9 hr,				
30s ea, C-II	54092-0554-30	178.82	149.02	
30 mg/9 hr,				
30s ea, C-II	54092-0555-30	178.82	149.02	
DDAVP (Sanofi-Aventis)				
desmopressin acetate				
SOL, IJ (AMP)				
4 mcg/ml, 1 ml 10s	00075-2451-01	400.72		AP
10 ml	00075-2451-53	405.68		AP
SPR, NS, 0.01 mg/actuation,				
5 ml	00075-2452-01	234.98		AB
TAB, PO, 0.1 mg, 100s ea	00075-0016-00	413.45		
0.2 mg, 100s ea	00075-0026-00	595.66		
(Phys Total Care)				
REPACK				
SOL, IJ (VIAL)				
4 mcg/ml, 10 ml	54868-3889-00	333.76		AP
DDAVP RHINAL TUBE (Sanofi-Aventis)				
desmopressin acetate				
SOL, NS, 0.01%, 2.5 ml	00075-2450-01	135.89		BX
DE-CHLOR DM (Cypress Pharm)				
cpm/dm/phenyleph hcl				
SOL, PO (AF,SF,DYE-FREE)				
473 ml	60258-0239-16	31.39		
DE-CHLOR DR (Cypress Pharm)				
cpm/dm/phenyleph hcl				
SOL, PO (AF,SF,DYE-FREE)				
473 ml	60258-0240-16	31.59		
DEANOL BITARTRATE				
(Medisca) *See DIMETHYLAMINOETHANOL BITARTRATE*				
DECAVAC (Sanofi)				
diphtheria toxoid, adsorbed/tetanus toxoid				
SUS, IM (PRE-FILLED,TAX INCL,PF)				
0.5 ml 10s	49281-0291-10	230.92	194.93	
(TAX INCL.,PF,LATEX-FREE)				
0.5 ml 10s	49281-0291-83	230.92	194.93	
(Palmetto)				
REPACK				
SUS, IM, ea	23490-9320-00	249.87		
DECITABINE				
(Eisai) *See DACOGEN*				
DECONAMINE SR (PD-Rx Pharm)				
REPACK				
cpm/pse hcl				
CER, PO, 8 mg-120 mg,				
20s ea	55289-0575-20	58.65		
(Pharma Pac)				
REPACK				
CER, PO, 8 mg-120 mg,				
20s ea	52959-0393-20	25.88		
(Phys Total Care)				
REPACK				
CER, PO, 8 mg-120 mg,				
20s ea	54868-1014-00	101.39		
DECONSAL CT (Cornerstone)				
phenylephrine hydrochloride/pyrilamine maleate				
CTB, PO (DYE-FREE,GRAPE)				
10 mg-16 mg,				
100s ea	10122-0202-10	250.50	200.40	
DECONSAL DM (Cornerstone)				
dm/phenyleph hcl/pyril mal				
CTB, PO (DYE-FREE,GRAPE)				
15 mg-10 mg-16 mg,				
100s ea	10122-0203-10	250.50	200.40	
DECOTUSS-HD (Southwood)				
REPACK				
gg/hydrocod bit/pse hcl				
LIQ, PO, 480 ml, C-III	58016-4181-01	37.20		
DECYL METHYL SULFOXIDE (Letco)				
POW, NA, 25 gm	62991-2697-01	360.00		
(Medisca)				
POW, NA (1X5GM)				
5 gm	38779-1232-03	120.00		
(1X25GM)				
25 gm	38779-1232-04	472.50		
(1X100GM)				
100 gm	38779-1232-05	1255.50		
(PCCA) *See DECYL METHYL SULFOXIDE (N)*				
DECYL METHYL SULFOXIDE (N) (PCCA)				
decyl methyl sulfoxide				
POW, NA (1X1GM)				
1 gm	51927-2426-00	27.00		
DEFERASIROX				
(Novartis Pharm) *See EXJADE*				
DEFEROXAMINE MESYLATE (APP)				
PDS, IJ (USP,LATEX-FREE)				
2 gm, ea	63323-0599-30	49.44		AP
500 mg, ea	63323-0597-10	15.54		AP
(Bedford)				
PDS, IJ (USP,S.D.V.)				
2 gm, ea	55390-0265-01	85.84		AP
500 mg, 10s ea	55390-0263-10	220.80		AP
(Hospira)				
PDS, IJ (VIAL,LATEX-FREE)				
2 gm, 4s ea	00409-2337-25	188.50	164.92	
(LATEX-FREE)				
500 mg, 4s ea	00409-2336-10	44.93	39.32	
(Novartis Pharm) *See DESFERAL*				
(Teva)				
PDS, IJ, 2 gm, 4s ea	00555-1131-11	300.84		AP
500 mg, 4s ea	00555-1132-12	77.36		AP
(Watson Labs)				
PDS, IJ (USP,SINGLE USE)				
2 gm, ea	00591-3975-30	69.53		AP
500 mg, 4s ea	00591-3974-04	71.54		AP
DEFINITY (Lantheus)				
perflutren lipid microsphere				
SUS, IV (VIAL,GLASS)				
2 ml UD	11994-0011-04	156.00		
DEGARELIX ACETATE				
(Ferring) *See FIRMAGON*				
DEGLYCYRRHIZINATED LICORICE (PCCA)				
POW, NA, 1 gm	51927-2826-00	0.21		
DEHISTINE (Cypress Pharm)				
cpm/methscopolamine nitrate/phenyleph hcl				
SYR, PO (AF,ROOT BEER)				
473 ml	60258-0220-16	15.99		
DEHYDROCHOLIC ACID				
(Novartis Consumer) *See CHOLAN-HMB*				
(PCCA)				
POW, NA (USP)				
1 gm	51927-1499-00	2.39		
(Spectrum Pharmacy)				
POW, NA (U.S.P.)				
25 gm	49452-2441-01	105.70		
100 gm	49452-2441-02	273.35		
(USP)				
500 gm	49452-2441-03	843.50		
DEHYDROCHOLIC ACID/ENZYMES				
(Truxton) *See ZYMECOT*				
DEHYDROEPIANDRO-STEARONE, 7-KETO				
(Spectrum Pharmacy)				
7-oxodehydroepiandrosterone				
POW, NA, 5 gm	49452-2449-01	179.55		
25 gm	49452-2449-02	714.00		
100 gm	49452-2449-03	2264.50		
DEHYDROEPIANDROSTERONE (Gallipot)				
POW, NA, 5 gm	51552-0359-02	8.40		
(MICRONIZED)				
5 gm	51552-0533-02	9.80		
25 gm	51552-0359-04	33.60		
(MICRONIZED)				
25 gm	51552-0533-04	35.56		
125 gm	51552-0359-09	105.00		
(MICRONIZED)				
125 gm	51552-0533-09	115.50		
1000 gm	51552-0359-07	658.00		
(MICRONIZED)				
1000 gm	51552-0533-07	658.00		
(Letco)				
POW, NA (MICRONIZED)				
25 gm	62991-1339-01	75.00		
125 gm	62991-1339-02	225.00		
(Medisca)				
POW, NA (MICRONIZED)				
5 gm	38779-0733-03	58.50		
25 gm	38779-0733-04	195.00		
(MICRO)				
100 gm	38779-0733-05	705.00		
500 gm	38779-0733-08	2445.00		
1000 gm	38779-0733-09	3885.00		
(PCCA)				
CRY, NA (FINE)				
1 gm	51927-2931-00	15.00		
POW, NA, 1 gm	51927-2100-00	27.00		
1 gm	51927-3341-00	24.00		
(Spectrum Pharmacy) *See DEHYDROEPIANDROS-TERONE-3-ACETATE*				
DEHYDROEPIANDROSTERONE MICRO (Letco)				
dehydroepiandrosterone, micronized				
POW, NA (1X100GM)				
100 gm	62991-1339-06	225.00		
DEHYDROEPIANDROSTERONE MICRONIZED (Letco)				
dehydroepiandrosterone, micronized				
POW, NA (DHEA)				
500 gm	62991-1339-03	825.00		
1000 gm	62991-1339-04	1260.00		
(PCCA)				
POW, NA, 1 gm	51927-2960-00	12.00		
(B&B Pharm, Inc)				
REPACK				
POW, NA, 25 gm	63275-9957-04	75.00		
100 gm	63275-9957-05	300.00		
500 gm	63275-9957-08	1500.00		
1000 gm	63275-9957-09	3000.00		
(Spectrum Pharmacy)				
REPACK				
POW, NA, 5 gm	49452-2454-01	74.38		
25 gm	49452-2454-02	204.75		
100 gm	49452-2454-03	612.50		
1000 gm	49452-2454-04	2782.50		
DEHYDROEPIANDROSTERONE-3-ACETATE				
(Spectrum Pharmacy)				
dehydroepiandrosterone				
POW, NA, 5 gm	49452-2446-02	113.75		
25 gm	49452-2446-03	427.00		
100 gm	49452-2446-04	1046.50		
1000 gm	49452-2446-05	6594.00		
DEHYDROEPIANDROSTERONE, MICRONIZED				
(Letco) *See 7-KETO DHEA DEHYDROEPIANDOSTERONE*				
(Letco) *See DEHYDROEPIANDROSTERONE MICRO*				
(Letco) *See DEHYDROEPIANDROSTERONE MICRONIZED*				
(Medisca) *See 7-KETO-DHEA*				
(PCCA) *See DEHYDROEPIANDROSTERONE MICRONIZED*				
DEK-QUIN (Truxton)				
clioquinol/hydrocortisone				
CRE, TP, 3%-1%, 20 gm	00463-8003-20	3.00		
DELATESTRYL (Endo Pharm)				
testosterone enanthate				
OIL, IM (MDV,5X1ML)				
200 mg/ml,				
5 ml, C-III	67979-0501-40	99.32		AO
(Phys Total Care)				
REPACK				
OIL, IM, 200 mg/ml,				
5 ml, C-III	54868-5016-00	109.85		
DELAVIRDINE MESYLATE				
(Pfizer) *See RESCRIPTOR*				
DELBASE (Med-Derm)				
ointment base				
OIN, NA, 454 gm	00316-0180-16	12.71		
DELESTROGEN (JHP)				
estradiol valerate				
OIL, IM (1X5ML,MULTIDOSE)				
10 mg/ml, 5 ml	42023-0110-01	81.26		AO
20 mg/ml, 5 ml	42023-0111-01	114.53		AO
(1X5ML,MDV,USP)				
40 mg/ml, 5 ml	42023-0112-01	189.98		AO
DELTASONE (Phys Total Care)				
REPACK				
prednisone				
TAB, PO, 5 mg, 30s ea	54868-0923-01	3.85		AB
DEMADEX (Meda)				
torsemide				
TAB, PO, 5 mg, 100s ea	00037-5005-01	126.96		
10 mg, 100s ea	00037-5010-01	140.69		AB
20 mg, 100s ea	00037-5020-01	164.34		
100 mg, 100s ea	00037-5001-01	608.88		
(Phys Total Care)				
REPACK				
TAB, PO, 10 mg, 30s ea	54868-3835-00	35.11		AB
20 mg, 10s ea	54868-4687-01	22.39		
30s ea	54868-4687-00	61.94		
100s ea	54868-4687-02	188.71		
DEMECARIUM BROMIDE (PCCA)				
POW, NA (1X1GM,USP)				
1 gm	51927-4322-00	1149.00		
DEMECLOCYCLINE HCL (Global Pharm)				
demeclocycline hydrochloride				
TAB, PO, 150 mg, 100s ea	00115-2111-01	942.34		AB
(FILM-COATED)				
300 mg, 48s ea	00115-2122-14	818.87		AB

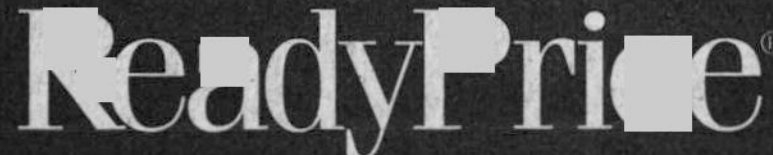

PROD/MFR	NDC	AWP	DP	OBC
(Medisca)				
POW, NA (U.S.P.)				
5 gm	**38779-0426-03**	55.50		
25 gm	**38779-0426-04**	229.50		
100 gm	**38779-0426-05**	729.00		
(PCCA)				
POW, NA (U.S.P.)				
1 gm	**51927-2461-00**	12.60		
(Teva)				
TAB, PO (FILM-COATED)				
150 mg, 100s ea	**00555-0701-02**	1057.65		**AB**
300 mg, 48s ea	**00555-0702-84**	919.07		**AB**
(American Health)				
REPACK				
TAB, PO (10X10,FILM-COATED)				
150 mg, 100s ea UD	**62584-0159-01**	1063.21		
(5X10,FILM-COATED)				
300 mg, 50s ea UD	**62584-0163-65**	1063.21		
DEMECLOCYCLINE HYDROCHLORIDE				
FUL				
TAB, PO, 150 mg, 100s ea		949.50		
300 mg, 48s ea		825.00		
(Amneal)				
TAB, PO (USP,FILM-COATED)				
150 mg, 100s ea	**65162-0554-10**	940.12		**AB**
300 mg, 48s ea	**65162-0555-48**	819.24		**AB**
(Global Pharm) *See DEMECLOCYCLINE HCL*				
(Medisca) *See DEMECLOCYCLINE HCL*				
(PCCA) *See DEMECLOCYCLINE HCL*				
(Teva) *See DEMECLOCYCLINE HCL*				
(VersaPharm)				
TAB, PO (USP,FILM COATED)				
150 mg, 100s ea	**61748-0115-01**	846.11		
300 mg, 48s ea	**61748-0113-48**	737.32		
DEMEROL (Hospira)				
meperidine hydrochloride				
SOL, IJ (25X1.5ML)				
50 mg/ml,				
1.5 ml 25s, C-II	**00409-1254-01**	27.60	24.25	**AP**
(USP,MDV)				
50 mg/ml,				
30 ml, C-II	**00409-1181-30**	24.66	21.58	**AP**
(MDV)				
100 mg/ml,				
20 ml, C-II	**00409-1201-20**	34.86	30.50	**AP**
DEMEROL HYDROCHLORIDE (Hospira)				
meperidine hydrochloride				
SOL, IJ (LLK,SLIM PK,LATEX-FREE)				
25 mg/ml,				
1 ml 10s, C-II	**00409-1176-30**	16.92	14.80	**AP**
(UNI-AMP, 5X5,LATEX-FREE)				
50 mg/ml,				
0.5 ml 25s, C-II	**00409-1203-01**	17.40	15.25	**AP**
(UNI-AMP,5X5,LATEX-FREE)				
50 mg/ml,				
0.5 ml 25s, C-II	**00074-1203-01**	17.40	15.25	**AP**
(LATEX-FREE,CARPUJECT)				
50 mg/ml,				
1 ml 10s, C-II	**00409-1178-30**	17.16	15.00	**AP**
(LATEX-FREE)				
50 mg/ml,				
1 ml 25s, C-II	**00409-1253-01**	30.60	26.75	**AP**
(UNI-AMP 5X5,LATEX-FREE)				
50 mg/ml,				
2 ml 25s, C-II	**00409-1255-02**	29.10	25.50	**AP**
(UNI-AMP,5X5,LATEX-FREE)				
50 mg/ml,				
2 ml 25s, C-II	**00074-1255-02**	29.10	25.50	**AP**
(M.D.V.,LATEX-FREE)				
50 mg/ml,				
30 ml, C-II	**00074-1181-30**	24.66	21.58	**AP**
(INTERLINK,LATEX-FREE)				
75 mg/ml,				
1 ml 10s, C-II	**00074-1179-21**	11.40	10.00	**AP**
(LATEX-FREE,CARPUJECT)				
75 mg/ml,				
1 ml 10s, C-II	**00409-1179-30**	17.40	15.20	**AP**
(LLK,SLIM PK,LATEX-FREE)				
75 mg/ml,				
1 ml 10s, C-II	**00074-1179-30**	13.80	12.10	**AP**
(CARPUJECT)				
100 mg/ml,				
1 ml 10s, C-II	**00409-1180-69**	17.40	15.20	**AP**
(25X1ML,LATEX-FREE)				
100 mg/ml,				
1 ml 25s, C-II	**00409-1256-01**	27.00	23.75	**AP**
(Sanofi-Aventis)				
TAB, PO, 50 mg,				
100s ea, C-II	**00024-0335-04**	151.96		**AA**
100 mg,				
100s ea, C-II	**00024-0337-04**	289.01		**AA**
(Phys Total Care)				
REPACK				
SOL, IJ (1MLX10)				
50 mg/ml,				
1 ml 10s, C-II	**54868-5808-00**	19.68		**AP**
(UNI-AMP)				
50 mg/ml,				
25 ml, C-II	**54868-3230-01**	14.84		**AP**
(M.D.V.)				
50 mg/ml,				
30 ml, C-II	**54868-0616-00**	27.98		**AP**
(LATEX-FREE)				
100 mg/ml,				
1 ml, C-II	**54868-4751-01**	3.28		**AP**
(CARPUJECT)				
100 mg/ml,				
1 ml 25s, C-II	**54868-4751-00**	22.56		**AP**
(M.D.V.)				
100 mg/ml,				
20 ml, C-II	**54868-3610-00**	33.89		**AP**
TAB, PO, 50 mg,				
20s ea, C-II	**54868-1071-02**	42.01		**AA**
25s ea, C-II	**54868-1071-00**	51.54		**AA**
30s ea, C-II	**54868-1071-01**	61.06		**AA**
120s ea, C-II	**54868-1071-03**	219.78		**AA**
100 mg,				
10s ea, C-II	**54868-6040-00**	40.15		**AA**
120s ea, C-II	**54868-6040-01**	414.47		**AA**
(Quality Care Prod)				
REPACK				
TAB, PO, 50 mg,				
30s ea, C-II	**35356-0559-30**	105.84		**AA**
100 mg,				
30s ea, C-II	**35356-0560-30**	198.32		**AA**
DEMSER (Aton)				
metyrosine				
CAP, PO, 250 mg, 100s ea	**25010-0305-15**	2197.55		
DEMULEN 1/35-28 (Phys Total Care)				
REPACK				
ethinyl estradiol/ethynodiol diacetate				
TAB, PO, 35 mcg-1 mg,				
28s ea	**54868-0404-00**	42.06		**AB**
DEMULEN 1/50-21 (Pfizer)				
ethinyl estradiol/ethynodiol diacetate				
TAB, PO (COMPACK, 24X21)				
50 mcg-1 mg,				
504s ea	**00025-0071-24**	840.43	700.36	**AB**
DEMULEN 1/50-28 (Phys Total Care)				
REPACK				
ethinyl estradiol/ethynodiol diacetate				
TAB, PO, 50 mcg-1 mg,				
28s ea	**54868-3790-00**	36.15		**AB**
DENATONIUM BENZOATE				
(Spectrum Pharmacy) *See BITREX*				
DENATURED ALCOHOL 190 PROOF (Gallipot)				
ethanol				
SOL, NA, 473 ml	**51552-0085-06**	4.27		
3785 ml	**51552-0085-08**	26.46		
DENATURED ALCOHOL 200 PROOF (Gallipot)				
ethanol				
SOL, NA (SDA-40-B)				
118.28 ml	**51552-0538-05**	13.65		
DENAVIR (Novartis Consumer)				
penciclovir				
CRE, TP (TUBE)				
1%, 1.5 gm	**00067-6024-15**	40.62		
(A-S Medication)				
REPACK				
CRE, TP (TUBE)				
1%, 1.5 gm	**54569-4947-00**	36.96		
(Phys Total Care)				
REPACK				
CRE, TP (TUBE)				
1%, 1.5 gm	**54868-4956-00**	52.88		
DENILEUKIN DIFTITOX				
(Eisai) *See ONTAK*				
DENTA 5000 PLUS (Rising)				
sodium fluoride				
CRE, DE (SPEARMINT)				
1.1%, 51 gm	**64980-0305-50**	7.99		
51 gm 2s	**64980-0306-50**	15.29		
(Physician Partner)				
REPACK				
CRE, DE (1X51GM,SPEARMINT)				
1.1%, 51 gm	**21695-0882-18**	31.96		
DENTAGEL (Rising)				
sodium fluoride				
GEL, DE (FRESH MINT)				
1.1%, 56 gm	**64980-0307-60**	8.23		
DEOXY-D-GLUCOSE				
(Gallipot) *See 2-DEOXY-D-GLUCOSE*				
2-DEOXY-D-GLUCOSE (Gallipot)				
deoxy-d-glucose				
POW, NA, 1 gm	**51552-0579-01**	34.65		
5 gm	**51552-0579-02**	161.00	115.00	
DEOXY-D-GLUCOSE				
(Medisca) *See 2-DEOXY-D-GLUCOSE*				
2-DEOXY-D-GLUCOSE (Medisca)				
deoxy-d-glucose				
POW, NA, 5 gm	**38779-0361-03**	330.00		
25 gm	**38779-0361-04**	1350.00		
50 gm	**38779-0361-02**	2385.00		
DEOXY-D-GLUCOSE (PCCA)				
POW, NA, 1 gm	**51927-1773-00**	72.00		
(Spectrum Pharmacy) *See 2-DEOXY-D-GLUCOSE*				
2-DEOXY-D-GLUCOSE (Spectrum Pharmacy)				
deoxy-d-glucose				
CRY, NA (1X1GM)				
1 gm	**49452-2452-01**	160.30		
(1X5GM)				
5 gm	**49452-2452-02**	511.00		
DEOXY-D-RIBOSE (2) (PCCA)				
d-2-deoxyribose				
POW, NA (1X1GM)				
1 gm	**51927-3030-00**	35.40		
DEOXYCHOLIC ACID (Letco)				
desoxycholic acid				
POW, NA, 100 gm	**62991-2689-02**	105.00		
500 gm	**62991-2689-03**	465.00		
(1X2500GM)				
2500 gm	**62991-2689-01**	2100.00		
(PCCA)				
sodium desoxycholate				
POW, NA (SODIUM SALT)				
1 gm	**51927-2805-00**	5.40		
(PCCA)				
desoxycholic acid				
99%, 1 gm	**51927-1498-00**	1.44		
DEPACON (Abbott Pharm)				
valproate sodium				
SOL, IV (S.D.V.)				
100 mg/ml,				
5 ml 10s	**00074-1564-10**	190.03	158.36	**AP**
DEPAKENE (Abbott Pharm)				
valproic acid				
SGL, PO, 250 mg, 100s ea	**00074-5681-13**	298.25	261.62	**AB**
SYR, PO, 250 mg/5 ml,				
480 ml	**00074-5682-16**	304.85	267.41	**AA**
DEPAKOTE (Abbott Pharm)				
divalproex sodium				
TCP, PO, 125 mg, 100s ea	**00074-6212-13**	106.40	93.34	
(10X10)				
125 mg, 100s ea UD	**00074-6212-11**	113.81	94.84	
250 mg, 100s ea	**00074-6214-13**	209.02	183.35	
(10X10)				
250 mg, 100s ea UD	**00074-6214-11**	221.82	184.85	
500s ea	**00074-6214-53**	1045.08	916.74	
500 mg, 100s ea	**00074-6215-13**	385.44	338.10	
(10X10)				
500 mg, 100s ea UD	**00074-6215-11**	407.52	339.60	
500s ea	**00074-6215-53**	1927.16	1690.49	
(A-S Medication)				
REPACK				
TCP, PO, 250 mg, 30s ea	**54569-0261-00**	61.62		
(Altura)				
REPACK				
TCP, PO, 250 mg, 10s ea	**63874-0535-10**	11.28		
20s ea	**63874-0535-20**	22.56		
30s ea	**63874-0535-30**	33.86		
40s ea	**63874-0535-40**	45.15		
60s ea	**63874-0535-60**	67.72		
90s ea	**63874-0535-90**	101.57		
100s ea	**63874-0535-01**	123.05		
120s ea	**63874-0535-04**	141.66		
500 mg, 10s ea	**63874-0536-10**	21.78		
20s ea	**63874-0536-20**	43.55		
30s ea	**63874-0536-30**	65.33		

PROD/MFR	NDC	AWP	DP	OBC
40s ea	63874-0536-40	87.10		
45s ea	63874-0536-45	97.99		
100s ea	63874-0536-01	217.75		
(Core)				
REPACK				
TCP, PO, 250 mg, 30s ea	33358-0100-30	49.47		
60s ea	33358-0100-60	92.52		
(Dispensing Solutions)				
REPACK				
TCP, PO, 250 mg, 30s ea	55045-2484-08	48.00		
(PD-Rx Pharm)				
REPACK				
TCP, PO (REDI-SCRIPT)				
250 mg, 60s ea	58864-0630-60	115.00		
500 mg, 30s ea	58864-0805-30	96.88		
(Pharma Pac)				
REPACK				
TCP, PO, 125 mg, 42s ea	52959-0142-42	20.50		
(Phys Total Care)				
REPACK				
TCP, PO, 250 mg, 10s ea	54868-1208-05	19.03		
30s ea	54868-1208-06	53.31		
60s ea	54868-1208-04	104.74		
90s ea	54868-1208-03	147.60		
100s ea	54868-1208-01	163.16		
500 mg, 20s ea	54868-2544-03	68.57		
60s ea	54868-2544-04	190.88		
100s ea	54868-2544-01	316.25		
(Quality Care Prod)				
REPACK				
TCP, PO, 500 mg, 60s ea	49999-0874-60	396.14		
100s ea	49999-0874-00	557.71		
(Southwood)				
REPACK				
TCP, PO, 250 mg, 30s ea	58016-0687-30	59.90		
60s ea	58016-0687-60	119.80		
90s ea	58016-0687-90	179.70		
100s ea	58016-0687-00	199.67		
500 mg, 30s ea	58016-0774-30	110.00		
60s ea	58016-0774-60	220.00		
90s ea	58016-0774-90	330.00		
100s ea	58016-0774-00	366.67		
(Stat Rx)				
REPACK				
TCP, PO, 250 mg, 30s ea	16590-0587-30	67.50		
60s ea	16590-0587-60	121.00		
90s ea	16590-0587-90	200.04		
120s ea	16590-0587-72	234.00		
DEPAKOTE ER (Abbott Pharm)				
divalproex sodium				
TER, PO, 250 mg, 100s ea	00074-3826-13	190.08	166.74	
(ABBO PAC)				
250 mg, 100s ea UD	00074-3826-11	201.89	168.24	
500 mg, 100s ea	00074-7126-13	334.36	293.29	
(ABBO-PAC,10X10)				
500 mg, 100s ea UD	00074-7126-11	353.75	294.79	
500s ea	00074-7126-53	1671.77	1466.46	
(PD-Rx Pharm)				
REPACK				
TER, PO (REDI-SCRIPT)				
250 mg, 30s ea	58864-0630-30	84.57		
120s ea	58864-0630-98	225.00		
500 mg, 30s ea	55289-0404-30	155.31		
60s ea	58864-0805-60	311.06		
(Phys Total Care)				
REPACK				
TER, PO, 250 mg, 10s ea	54868-5525-00	26.81		
30s ea	54868-5525-01	75.19		
500 mg, 20s ea	54868-4959-00	67.02		
60s ea	54868-4959-01	186.48		
(Physician Partner)				
REPACK				
TER, PO, 250 mg, 30s ea	21695-0359-30	112.08		
500 mg, 15s ea	21695-0163-15	102.32		
(Quality Care Prod)				
REPACK				
TER, PO, 250 mg, 30s ea	49999-0941-30	157.66		
100s ea	35356-0345-00	213.67		
100s ea	49999-0941-00	384.30		
500 mg, 60s ea	49999-0875-60	362.67		
100s ea	49999-0875-00	480.10		
DEPAKOTE SPRINKLES (Abbott Pharm)				
divalproex sodium				
ECC, PO, 125 mg, 100s ea	00074-6114-13	101.44	88.98	
(10X10)				
125 mg, 100s ea UD	00074-6114-11	108.58	90.48	
(PD-Rx Pharm)				
REPACK				
ECC, PO, 125 mg, 30s ea	55289-0991-30	41.12		
(Quality Care Prod)				
REPACK				
ECC, PO, 125 mg, 30s ea	49999-0942-30	84.00		
DEPEN (Meda)				
penicillamine				
TAB, PO, 250 mg, 100s ea	00037-4401-01	473.42		
DEPLIN (Pamlab)				
medical food				
TAB, PO (SF,GLUTEN-FREE)				
90s ea	00525-0450-90	234.00		
(Pamlab)				
l-methylfolate				
7.5 mg, 30s ea	00525-0410-30	78.00		
90s ea	00525-0410-90	234.00		
(Stat Rx)				
REPACK				
TAB, PO (SF,GLUTEN-FREE)				
7.5 mg, 30s ea	16590-0790-30	56.94		
DEPO MEDROL (Dispensing Solutions)				
REPACK				
methylprednisolone acetate				
SUS, IJ, 40 mg/ml, 5 ml	55045-3242-05	32.00		
10 ml	55045-3242-02	55.00		
80 mg/ml, 1 ml	55045-3243-01	15.99		
DEPO-COBOLIN (Legere)				
cyanocobalamin				
SOL, IM (VIAL)				
1000 mcg/ml, 30 ml	25332-0078-10	17.95		EE
DEPO-ESTRADIOL (Pfizer)				
estradiol cypionate				
OIL, IM (VIAL)				
5 mg/ml, 5 ml	00009-0271-01	39.44	32.87	AO
(A-S Medication)				
REPACK				
OIL, IM, 5 mg/ml, 5 ml	54569-2580-00	37.26		AO
(Phys Total Care)				
REPACK				
OIL, IM (VIAL)				
5 mg/ml, 5 ml	54868-1729-00	51.40		AO
DEPO-MEDROL (Pfizer)				
methylprednisolone acetate				
SUS, IJ (M.D.V.)				
20 mg/ml, 5 ml	00009-0274-01	18.92	15.77	BP
(S.D.V.)				
40 mg/ml, 1 ml	00009-3073-01	9.04	7.53	
(S.D.V.,25X1ML)				
40 mg/ml, 1 ml 25s	00009-3073-03	225.90	188.25	
(M.D.V.)				
40 mg/ml, 5 ml	00009-0280-02	32.04	26.70	
(M.D.V.,5X25ML)				
40 mg/ml, 5 ml 25s	00009-0280-51	801.00	667.50	
(M.D.V.)				
40 mg/ml, 10 ml	00009-0280-03	58.36	48.63	
10 ml 25s	00009-0280-52	1458.90	1215.75	
(S.D.V.)				
80 mg/ml, 1 ml	00009-3475-01	15.67	13.06	BP
(S.D.V.,25X1ML)				
80 mg/ml, 1 ml 25s	00009-3475-03	391.80	326.50	BP
(M.D.V.)				
80 mg/ml, 5 ml	00009-0306-02	58.36	48.63	BP
(M.D.V.,25X5ML)				
80 mg/ml, 5 ml 25s	00009-0306-12	1458.90	1215.75	BP
(A-S Medication)				
REPACK				
SUS, IJ (VIAL)				
40 mg/ml, 1 ml 25s	54569-3946-00	213.44		
(M.D.V.)				
40 mg/ml, 5 ml	54569-1901-01	30.28		
10 ml	54569-4265-00	55.13		
80 mg/ml, 5 ml	54569-2232-00	55.13		BP
(Phys Total Care)				
REPACK				
SUS, IJ, 40 mg/ml, 5 ml	54868-3896-02	40.21		
(M.D.V.)				
40 mg/ml, 10 ml	54868-3896-00	75.10		
25 ml	54868-3896-01	256.59		
80 mg/ml, 5 ml	54868-1185-00	64.64		BP
25 ml	54868-1185-01	407.36		BP
(Quality Care Prod)				
REPACK				
SUS, IJ (1X10ML)				
40 mg/ml, 10 ml	35356-0483-10	96.00		
(1X5ML)				
80 mg/ml, 5 ml	35356-0484-05	96.00		BP
(Southwood)				
REPACK				
SUS, IJ, 80 mg/ml, 5 ml	58016-9934-01	49.58		BP
DEPO-PROVERA (Pfizer)				
medroxyprogesterone acetate				
SUS, IM (VIAL)				
400 mg/ml, 2.5 ml	00009-0626-01	193.39	161.16	
(A-S Medication)				
REPACK				
SUS, IM (SRN, PREFILLED)				
150 mg/ml, 1 ml	54569-4904-00	75.53		
(Phys Total Care)				
REPACK				
SUS, IM (VIAL)				
400 mg/ml, 2.5 ml	54868-3348-01	124.19		
DEPO-PROVERA CONTRACEPTIVE (Pfizer)				
medroxyprogesterone acetate				
SUS, IM (VIAL)				
150 mg/ml, 1 ml	00009-0746-30	82.20	68.50	
(W/ SAFETY GLIDE NEEDLE)				
150 mg/ml, 1 ml	00009-7376-04	90.01	75.01	
(VIAL,25X1ML)				
150 mg/ml,				
1 ml 25s	00009-0746-35	2054.98	1712.48	
(A-S Medication)				
REPACK				
SUS, IM (VIAL)				
150 mg/ml, 1 ml	54569-3701-00	72.25		
1 ml 25s	54569-5527-00	1806.25		
(Dispensing Solutions)				
REPACK				
SUS, IM, 150 mg/ml, 1 ml	55045-3505-01	80.00		
(Phys Total Care)				
REPACK				
SUS, IM (SRN,PREFILLED)				
150 mg/ml, 1 ml	54868-3613-00	85.15		
1 ml	54868-4100-01	88.96		
1 ml 6s	54868-4100-00	370.05		
DEPO-SUBQ PROVERA 104 (Pfizer)				
medroxyprogesterone acetate				
SUS, SC (PRE-FILLED W/NEEDLE)				
104 mg/0.65 ml,				
0.65 ml	00009-4709-01	108.17	90.14	
(Pharmacia)				
SUS, SC (1X0.65ML,PRE-FILLED)				
104 mg/0.65 ml,				
0.65 ml	00009-4709-13	108.17	90.14	
DEPO-TESTOSTERONE (Pfizer)				
testosterone cypionate				
OIL, IM (VIAL)				
100 mg/ml,				
10 ml, C-III	00009-0347-02	76.68	63.90	AO
200 mg/ml,				
1 ml, C-III	00009-0417-01	28.63	23.86	AO
10 ml, C-III	00009-0417-02	139.37	116.14	AO
(A-S Medication)				
REPACK				
OIL, IM (VIAL)				
200 mg/ml,				
10 ml, C-III	54569-1411-00	131.68		AO
(Altura)				
REPACK				
OIL, IM, 200 mg/ml,				
10 ml, C-III	63874-1061-01	110.00		AO
(Dispensing Solutions)				
REPACK				
OIL, IM, 200 mg/ml,				
10 ml, C-III	55045-3029-02	122.00		AO
(Phys Total Care)				
REPACK				
OIL, IM, 100 mg/ml,				
10 ml, C-III	54868-0796-00	78.19		AO
(VIAL)				
200 mg/ml,				
1 ml, C-III	54868-0216-01	37.85		AO
10 ml, C-III	54868-0216-00	166.94		AO
(Quality Care Prod)				
REPACK				
OIL, IM, 100 mg/ml,				
10 ml, C-III	35356-0058-10	82.80		
DEPOCYT (Enzon Pharma, Inc.)				
cytarabine liposome				
SUS, IN (S.D.V.)				
10 mg/ml, 5 ml	57665-0331-01	2940.00	1626.56	

PROD/MFR	NDC	AWP	DP	OBC
DEPODUR (EKR)				
morphine sulfate liposome				
SER, EP (5X1ML,PF)				
10 mg/ml,				
1 ml 5s, C-II	24477-0020-04	2060.58		EE
(5X1.5ML,PF)				
10 mg/ml,				
1.5 ml 5s, C-II	24477-0020-05	3090.90		EE
DERMA-SMOOTHE/FS (Hill Derm)				
fluocinolone acetonide				
OIL, TP (BODY OIL)				
0.01%, 118.28 ml	28105-0150-04	39.38		
(SCALP OIL)				
0.01%, 118.28 ml	28105-0149-04	40.63		
(Phys Total Care)				
REPACK				
OIL, TP, 0.01%, 118 ml	54868-1572-00	44.41		
118.28 ml	54868-5351-00	45.51		
DERMAGRAFT (Advanced BioHealing)				
graftskin				
SHE, TP (W/CRYOPROTECT,5X7.5CM)				
ea	08541-0001-01	1700.00		
DERMATODORON (Weleda)				
homeopathic substance				
LIQ, PO, 50 ml	55946-0222-15	9.00		
DERMATOP (Dermik)				
prednicarbate				
EMO, TP, 0.1%, 60 gm	00066-0507-60	70.73		
OIN, TP, 0.1%, 60 gm	00066-0508-60	67.37		
(Phys Total Care)				
REPACK				
EMO, TP, 0.1%, 60 gm	54868-4457-00	66.70		
DERMAZENE (Stratus)				
hydrocortisone/iodoquinol				
CRE, TP, 1%-1%, 28.4 gm	58980-0811-10	46.00		
DERMIVIEW HYPOALLERGENIC ADHESIVE (J&J Medical)				
tape, adhesive				
DEV, NA (TRANSPARENT 3"X10YD RLL)				
4s ea	56091-0051-63	14.17		
(TRANSPARENT 2"X10YD RLL)				
6s ea	56091-0051-62	14.17		
(TRANSPARENT 1"X10YD RLL)				
12s ea	56091-0051-61	14.17		
DERMOTIC OIL (Hill Derm)				
fluocinolone acetonide				
OIL, OT (DROPS)				
0.01%, 20 ml	28105-0160-20	33.75		
DESFERAL (Novartis Pharm)				
deferoxamine mesylate				
PDS, IJ (VIAL)				
2 gm, 4s ea	00078-0347-51	455.75		
(USP)				
500 mg, 4s ea	00078-0467-91	117.24		
DESFLURANE				
(Baxter) *See AMERINET CHOICE SUPRANE*				
(Baxter) *See SUPRANE*				
DESIPRAMINE (DHS, Inc.)				
REPACK				
desipramine hydrochloride				
TAB, PO, 10 mg, 30s ea	55887-0144-30	11.93		
60s ea	55887-0144-60	23.86		
90s ea	55887-0144-90	35.78		
120s ea	55887-0144-82	47.71		
180s ea	55887-0144-92	71.57		
25 mg, 30s ea	55887-0143-30	14.63		
60s ea	55887-0143-60	29.26		
90s ea	55887-0143-90	43.88		
120s ea	55887-0143-82	58.51		
180s ea	55887-0143-92	87.77		
(Stat Rx)				
REPACK				
TAB, PO, 50 mg, 30s ea	16590-0484-30	24.00		
60s ea	16590-0484-60	48.00		
90s ea	16590-0484-90	72.00		
120s ea	16590-0484-72	86.00		
DESIPRAMINE HCL (Sandoz)				
desipramine hydrochloride				
TAB, PO, 10 mg, 100s ea	00185-0029-01	39.78		AB
100s ea	00781-1971-01	96.34		AB
25 mg, 100s ea	00185-0019-01	48.76		AB
100s ea	00781-1972-01	115.73		AB
500s ea	00185-0019-05	243.80		AB
1000s ea	00185-0019-10	463.15		AB
1000s ea	00781-1972-10	453.89		AB
50 mg, 100s ea	00185-0721-01	91.79		AB
100s ea	00781-1973-01	217.88		AB
500s ea	00185-0721-05	458.95		AB
1000s ea	00185-0721-10	871.93		AB
75 mg, 100s ea	00185-0722-01	114.50		AB
100s ea	00781-1974-01	277.30		AB
500s ea	00185-0722-05	572.50		AB
100 mg, 100s ea	00185-0736-01	150.45		AB
100s ea	00781-1975-01	364.41		AB
500s ea	00185-0736-05	752.25		AB
150 mg, 50s ea	00185-0760-53	109.00		AB
50s ea	00781-1976-50	264.01		AB
(Altura)				
REPACK				
TAB, PO, 25 mg, 10s ea	63874-0829-10	6.43		AB
14s ea	63874-0829-14	9.00		AB
15s ea	63874-0829-15	11.27		AB
20s ea	63874-0829-20	12.85		AB
28s ea	63874-0829-28	21.03		AB
30s ea	63874-0829-30	22.53		AB
42s ea	63874-0829-42	31.54		AB
50s ea	63874-0829-50	37.55		AB
60s ea	63874-0829-60	45.06		AB
100s ea	63874-0829-01	75.10		AB
(Dispensing Solutions)				
REPACK				
TAB, PO, 25 mg, 30s ea	55045-1718-08	22.50		AB
60s ea	55045-1718-06	45.00		AB
90s ea	55045-1718-09	67.50		AB
100s ea	55045-1718-00	75.00		AB
120s ea	55045-1718-02	90.00		AB
(Nucare Pharm)				
REPACK				
TAB, PO, 100 mg, 30s ea	66267-0626-30	39.99		AB
(Pharma Pac)				
REPACK				
TAB, PO, 10 mg, 30s ea	52959-0128-30	21.19		EE
60s ea	52959-0128-60	42.34		EE
25 mg, 14s ea	52959-0458-14	9.86		EE
20s ea	52959-0458-20	13.73		EE
21s ea	52959-0458-21	14.41		AB
30s ea	52959-0458-30	20.59		EE
50 mg, 12s ea	52959-0464-12	9.83		EE
14s ea	52959-0464-14	11.17		EE
20s ea	52959-0464-20	15.22		EE
100s ea	52959-0464-00	75.95		EE
(Southwood)				
REPACK				
TAB, PO, 10 mg, 15s ea	58016-0502-15	18.00		EE
28s ea	58016-0502-28	33.60		EE
30s ea	58016-0502-30	36.00		EE
50s ea	58016-0502-50	60.00		EE
60s ea	58016-0502-60	72.00		EE
100s ea	58016-0502-00	120.00		EE
25 mg, 14s ea	58016-0853-14	9.00		EE
15s ea	58016-0191-15	11.27		EE
20s ea	58016-0853-20	12.85		EE
28s ea	58016-0191-28	21.03		EE
30s ea	58016-0191-30	22.53		EE
30s ea	58016-0853-30	22.53		AB
50s ea	58016-0191-50	37.55		EE
60s ea	58016-0191-60	45.06		EE
60s ea	58016-0853-60	45.06		AB
90s ea	58016-0853-90	67.59		AB
100s ea	58016-0191-00	75.10		EE
100s ea	58016-0853-00	75.10		AB
(Stat Rx)				
REPACK				
TAB, PO, 10 mg, 30s ea	16590-0830-30	29.48		AB
25 mg, 30s ea	16590-0637-30	33.61		AB
100 mg, 30s ea	16590-0586-30	56.00		AB
60s ea	16590-0586-60	72.00		AB
90s ea	16590-0586-90	160.00		AB
120s ea	16590-0586-72	214.00		AB
DESIPRAMINE HYDROCHLORIDE				
FUL				
TAB, PO, 150 mg, 50s ea		98.09		
(Actavis)				
TAB, PO (COATED)				
10 mg, 100s ea	52152-0341-02	96.34		AB
25 mg, 100s ea	52152-0342-02	115.73		AB
500s ea	52152-0342-04	243.80		AB
1000s ea	52152-0342-05	1157.30		AB
50 mg, 100s ea	52152-0343-02	217.88		AB
500s ea	52152-0343-04	458.95		AB
1000s ea	52152-0343-05	2178.80		AB
75 mg, 100s ea	52152-0344-02	277.30		AB
500s ea	52152-0344-04	572.50		AB
100 mg, 100s ea	52152-0345-02	364.41		AB
500s ea	52152-0345-04	752.25		AB
150 mg, 50s ea	52152-0346-50	264.01		AB
(PCCA)				
POW, NA (U.S.P.)				
1 gm	51927-1897-00	14.40		
(Sandoz) *See DESIPRAMINE HCL*				
(Sanofi-Aventis) *See NORPRAMIN*				
(Spectrum Pharmacy)				
POW, NA (U.S.P./N.F.)				
5 gm	49452-2457-01	317.45	21.90	
25 gm	49452-2457-02	742.00	87.75	
(Altura)				
REPACK				
TAB, PO, 50 mg, 30s ea	63874-0766-30	22.83		
60s ea	63874-0766-60	45.66		
(Dispensing Solutions)				
REPACK				
TAB, PO (COATED)				
10 mg, 30s ea	68258-7050-03	29.29		AB
25 mg, 30s ea	68258-7051-03	35.17		AB
(Palmetto)				
REPACK				
TAB, PO, 10 mg, 60s ea	23490-5391-01	72.00		
25 mg, 30s ea	23490-5393-01	22.99		
60s ea	23490-5393-02	45.98		
50 mg, 30s ea	23490-5394-01	26.99		
60s ea	23490-5394-02	53.98		
90s ea	23490-5394-03	80.97		
100 mg, 30s ea	23490-5392-01	90.25		
(Physician Partner)				
REPACK				
TAB, PO, 25 mg, 28s ea	21695-0428-28	27.31		
30s ea	21695-0428-30	29.26		
100s ea	21695-0428-00	97.52		
(Quality Care Prod)				
REPACK				
TAB, PO (COATED)				
25 mg, 30s ea	35356-0385-30	28.40		AB
DESLORATADINE				
(Schering) *See CLARINEX*				
(Schering) *See CLARINEX REDITABS*				
DESLORATADINE/PSEUDOEPHEDRINE SULFATE				
(Schering) *See CLARINEX-D 24 HOUR*				
(Schering) *See CLARINEX-D12 HOUR*				
DESMOPRESSIN (Phys Total Care)				
REPACK				
desmopressin acetate				
SPR, NS, 0.01 mg/actuation,				
5 ml	54868-5602-00	254.13		
TAB, PO, 0.2 mg, 10s ea	54868-1129-00	73.57		
90s ea	54868-1129-01	602.85		
DESMOPRESSIN ACETATE (Apotex Corp.)				
SPR, NS, 0.01 mg/actuation,				
5 ml	60505-0815-00	143.40		AB
TAB, PO, 0.1 mg, 100s ea	60505-0257-01	302.04		AB
0.2 mg, 100s ea	60505-0258-01	435.14		AB
(Bausch & Lomb Inc.)				
SPR, NS, 0.01 mg/actuation,				
5 ml	24208-0342-05	143.34		AB
(CSL) *See STIMATE*				
(Ferring) *See DESMOPRESSIN ACETATE RHINAL TUBE*				
(Ferring) *See MINIRIN*				
(Ferring)				
SOL, IJ (AMP,PF)				
4 mcg/ml, 1 ml 10s	55566-5030-01	231.84		AP
(M.D.V.)				
4 mcg/ml, 10 ml	55566-5040-01	231.84		AP
(Hospira)				
SOL, IJ (UNI-AMP)				
4 mcg/ml, 1 ml 10s	00409-2265-01	76.44	66.90	AP
(PCCA)				
POW, NA (EP; SALT)				
ea	51927-2777-00	126.00		
(Sanofi-Aventis) *See DDAVP*				
(Sanofi-Aventis) *See DDAVP RHINAL TUBE*				
(Teva)				
SOL, IJ (VIAL)				
4 mcg/ml, 1 ml 10s	00703-5051-03	70.80		AP
(M.D.V.)				
4 mcg/ml, 10 ml	00703-5054-01	70.80		AP
TAB, PO, 0.1 mg, 100s ea	00093-7316-01	302.04		AB
0.2 mg, 100s ea	00093-7317-01	435.14		AB

PROD/MFR	NDC	AWP	DP	OBC
(UDL)				
TAB, PO (3X10)				
0.2 mg, 30s ea UD....	**51079-0446-03**	141.49		AB
(Watson Labs)				
TAB, PO, 0.1 mg, 100s ea..	**00591-2225-01**	260.96		AB
0.2 mg, 100s ea......	**00591-2226-01**	375.96		AB
(Quality Care Prod)				
REPACK				
TAB, PO, 0.2 mg, 30s ea...	**35356-0155-30**	286.59		AB
90s ea............	**35356-0155-90**	851.75		AB
DESMOPRESSIN ACETATE RHINAL TUBE (Ferring)				
desmopressin acetate				
SOL, NS, 0.01%, 2.5 ml...	**55566-5020-01**	90.42		AB
DESOGEN (Organon)				
desogestrel/ethinyl estradiol				
TAB, PO (6X28)				
0.15 mg-0.03 mg,				
168s ea...........	**00052-0261-06**	312.19		AB
(Palmetto)				
REPACK				
TAB, PO, 0.15 mg-0.03 mg,				
28s ea............	**23490-7653-01**	54.20		
(Phys Total Care)				
REPACK				
TAB, PO, 0.15 mg-0.03 mg,				
28s ea............	**54868-3863-00**	46.51		AB
DESOGESTREL/ETHINYL ESTRADIOL				
(Organon) *See CYCLESSA*				
(Organon) *See DESOGEN*				
(Ortho-McNeil Pharm) *See ORTHO-CEPT*				
(Prasco Labs) *See CESIA*				
(Prasco Labs) *See SOLIA*				
(Teva) *See APRI*				
(Teva) *See KARIVA*				
(Teva) *See MIRCETTE*				
(Teva) *See VELIVET*				
(Watson) *See AZURETTE*				
(Watson) *See CAZIANT*				
(Watson) *See RECLIPSEN*				
DESONATE (Intendis, Inc.)				
desonide				
GEL, TP, 0.05%, 60 gm....	**67402-0050-60**	238.43		
(2X60GM)				
0.05%, 60 gm 2s.....	**67402-0050-62**	406.73		
DESONIDE				
FUL				
CRE, TP, 0.05%, 60 gm........		14.02		
KIT, TP, 0.05%, 59 ml........		32.10		
60 gm........		14.02		
LOT, TP, 0.05%, 59 ml........		32.10		
OIN, TP, 0.05%, 60 gm........		24.46		
(Actavis Mid Atlantic)				
LOT, TP (1X59ML)				
0.05%, 59 ml........	**00472-0803-02**	50.94		AB
(1X118ML)				
0.05%, 118 ml.......	**00472-0803-04**	76.88		AB
(Fougera)				
LOT, TP, 0.05%, 59 ml.....	**00168-0310-02**	48.90		AB
118 ml...........	**00168-0310-04**	73.80		AB
OIN, TP, 0.05%, 15 gm....	**00168-0309-15**	15.47		AB
60 gm............	**00168-0309-60**	39.88		AB
(Galderma) *See DESOWEN*				
(Gallipot)				
POW, NA (MICRONIZED)				
1 gm..............	**51552-0451-01**	63.00		
(Intendis, Inc.) *See DESONATE*				
(Medisca)				
POW, NA (MICRONIZED)				
1 gm..............	**38779-0297-06**	178.50		
5 gm..............	**38779-0297-03**	747.00		
(Perrigo)				
CRE, TP, 0.05%, 15 gm....	**45802-0422-35**	15.45		AB
60 gm............	**45802-0422-37**	40.15		AB
OIN, TP, 0.05%, 15 gm....	**45802-0423-35**	15.45		AB
60 gm............	**45802-0423-37**	40.15		AB
(PharmaDerm) *See LOKARA*				
(Spectrum Pharmacy)				
POW, NA (MICRONIZED)				
0.25 gm............	**49452-2458-03**	124.95		
1 gm..............	**49452-2458-01**	329.35		
5 gm..............	**49452-2458-02**	1113.00		
(Stiefel Labs) *See VERDESO*				
(Taro)				
CRE, TP, 0.05%, 15 gm....	**51672-1280-01**	15.47		AB
60 gm............	**51672-1280-03**	39.88		AB
OIN, TP, 0.05%, 15 gm....	**51672-1281-01**	15.47		AB
60 gm............	**51672-1281-03**	39.88		AB
(Teva)				
CRE, TP, 0.05%, 15 gm....	**00182-5066-51**	12.10		AB
60 gm............	**00182-5066-52**	27.81		AB
(Palmetto)				
REPACK				
CRE, TP, 0.05%, 15 gm....	**23490-5397-01**	15.45		
(1X60GM)				
0.05%, 60 gm........	**23490-5397-03**	40.15		
(Phys Total Care)				
REPACK				
CRE, TP, 0.05%, 15 gm....	**54868-3284-01**	14.22		AB
60 gm............	**54868-3284-00**	20.04		EE
LOT, TP, 0.05%, 59 ml.....	**54868-5050-01**	152.47		
118 ml...........	**54868-5050-00**	262.55		AB
OIN, TP, 0.05%, 15 gm....	**54868-4453-00**	12.58		
(1X60GM)				
0.05%, 60 gm........	**54868-4453-01**	35.65		
(Physician Partner)				
REPACK				
LOT, TP (1X120GM)				
0.05%, 120 gm.......	**21695-0445-04**	147.60		AB
DESONIDE MICRONIZED (PCCA)				
desonide, micronized				
POW, NA (1X1GM)				
1 gm..............	**51927-1949-00**	138.00		
DESONIDE, MICRONIZED				
(PCCA) *See DESONIDE MICRONIZED*				
DESOWEN (Galderma)				
desonide				
KIT, TP, 0.05%, ea........	**00299-5765-00**	173.13		AB
ea...............	**00299-5765-03**	256.25		AB
ea...............	**00299-5770-01**	221.25		AB
OIN, TP, 0.05%, ea........	**00299-5775-01**	226.25		AB
(Phys Total Care)				
REPACK				
CRE, TP, 0.05%, 15 gm....	**54868-2203-01**	28.25		AB
60 gm............	**54868-2203-02**	54.96		AB
DESOXIMETASONE (Medisca)				
POW, NA (U.S.P.,MICRONIZED)				
1 gm..............	**38779-0479-06**	214.50		
5 gm..............	**38779-0479-03**	964.50		
10 gm..............	**38779-0479-01**	1830.00		
(Perrigo)				
CRE, TP (EMOLLIENT BASE)				
0.25%, 15 gm........	**45802-0495-35**	58.28		AB
60 gm............	**45802-0495-37**	199.24		AB
(Spectrum Pharmacy)				
POW, NA (U.S.P.)				
0.25 gm............	**49452-2455-01**	500.50		
1 gm..............	**49452-2455-02**	1204.00		
(Taro)				
CRE, TP, 0.05%, 15 gm....	**51672-1271-01**	46.06		AB
60 gm............	**51672-1271-03**	170.73		AB
(3X100GM,USP)				
0.05%, 100 gm 3s....	**51672-1271-08**	585.27		AB
0.25%, 15 gm........	**51672-1270-01**	57.63		AB
60 gm............	**51672-1270-03**	197.03		AB
(1X100GM,USP)				
0.25%, 100 gm.......	**51672-1270-07**	224.95		AB
(21X100GM,USP)				
0.25%, 100 gm 2s....	**51672-1270-09**	382.70		AB
GEL, TP, 0.05%, 15 gm....	**51672-1261-01**	49.10		AB
60 gm............	**51672-1261-03**	157.13		AB
OIN, TP, 0.25%, 15 gm....	**51672-1262-01**	61.97		AB
60 gm............	**51672-1262-03**	205.79		AB
(1X100GM,USP)				
0.25%, 100 gm.......	**51672-1262-07**	234.85		AB
(Taro) *See TOPICORT*				
(Taro) *See TOPICORT LP*				
(A-S Medication)				
REPACK				
CRE, TP, 0.25%, 15 gm....	**54569-4486-00**	57.63		AB
DESOXIMETASONE (Palmetto)				
REPACK				
CRE, TP (1X15GM)				
0.25%, 15 gm........	**23490-5417-01**	120.53		
(1X60GM)				
0.25%, 60 gm........	**23490-5417-02**	271.95		
DESOXIMETASONE (Pharma Pac)				
REPACK				
CRE, TP, 0.25%, 15 gm....	**52959-0154-15**	18.60		EE
(Phys Total Care)				
REPACK				
CRE, TP, 0.25%, 15 gm....	**54868-3041-00**	89.47		EE
60 gm............	**54868-3041-01**	125.86		AB
GEL, TP (1X15GM)				
0.05%, 15 gm........	**54868-2829-00**	83.29		AB
OIN, TP, 0.25%, 15 gm....	**54868-5891-00**	104.68		AB
(Quality Care Prod)				
REPACK				
CRE, TP, 0.25%, 15 gm....	**49999-0377-15**	31.03		AB
(Southwood)				
REPACK				
CRE, TP, 0.25%, 15 gm....	**58016-6228-01**	19.31		EE
DESOXIMETASONE MICRONIZED (PCCA)				
desoximetasone, micronized				
POW, NA (1X1GM, USP)				
1 gm..............	**51927-1687-00**	240.00		
DESOXIMETASONE, MICRONIZED				
(PCCA) *See DESOXIMETASONE MICRONIZED*				
DESOXYCHOLIC ACID				
(Letco) *See DEOXYCHOLIC ACID*				
(PCCA) *See DEOXYCHOLIC ACID*				
DESOXYCORTICOSTERONE ACETATE (PCCA)				
POW, NA (U.S.P. (DOCA))				
1 gm..............	**51927-1792-00**	84.00		
DESOXYN (Lundbeck)				
methamphetamine hydrochloride				
TAB, PO, 5 mg,				
100s ea, C-II.......	**67386-0102-01**	400.73		
DESPEC (Intl Ethical)				
guaifenesin/phenylephrine hydrochloride				
LIQ, PO (AF,SF,DYE-FREE,GRAPE)				
100 mg/5 ml-5 mg/5 ml,				
473 ml............	**11584-1032-06**	54.66		
DESPEC SR (Intl Ethical)				
guaifenesin/pseudoephedrine hydrochloride				
TER, PO, 800 mg-120 mg,				
100s ea...........	**11584-0442-01**	113.22		
DESPEC-SF (Intl Ethical)				
phenylephrine hydrochloride				
LIQ, PO (SF)				
5 mg/5 ml, 120 ml....	**11584-0453-04**	10.98		
DESQUAM-X 10 (Ranbaxy Labs)				
benzoyl peroxide				
GEL, TP, 10%, 42.5 gm....	**00072-6721-01**	13.33		
SOL, TP (1X150ML)				
10%, 150 ml.........	**10631-0285-05**	30.04		
DESQUAM-X 5 (Ranbaxy Labs)				
benzoyl peroxide				
SOL, TP (1X150ML)				
5%, 150 ml.........	**10631-0284-05**	28.08		
DESVENLAFAXINE SUCCINATE				
(Wyeth) *See PRISTIQ*				
DESYREL (Pharma Pac)				
REPACK				
trazodone hydrochloride				
TAB, PO, 50 mg, 20s ea...	**52959-0350-20**	42.66		AB
30s ea............	**52959-0350-30**	60.39		AB
100s ea...........	**52959-0350-00**	133.45		AB
DESYREL DIVIDOSE (Phys Total Care)				
REPACK				
trazodone hydrochloride				
TAB, PO, 150 mg, 15s ea..	**54868-2549-00**	58.15		AB
DETROL (Pfizer)				
tolterodine tartrate				
TAB, PO, 1 mg, 60s ea....	**00009-4541-02**	162.31	135.26	
(10X14)				
1 mg, 140s ea UD....	**00009-4541-01**	382.72	318.93	
500s ea...........	**00009-4541-03**	1352.56	1127.13	
2 mg, 60s ea.........	**00009-4544-02**	166.60	138.83	
(10X14)				
2 mg, 140s ea UD....	**00009-4544-01**	392.59	327.16	
500s ea...........	**00009-4544-03**	1388.27	1156.89	
(Phys Total Care)				
REPACK				
TAB, PO, 1 mg, 30s ea....	**54868-4390-00**	67.14		
2 mg, 30s ea.........	**54868-2824-01**	82.64		
60s ea............	**54868-2824-00**	153.81		
DETROL LA (Pfizer)				
tolterodine tartrate				
CER, PO, 2 mg, 30s ea....	**00009-5190-01**	144.44	120.37	

PROD/MFR	NDC	AWP	DP	OBC
90s ea	00009-5190-02	433.33	361.11	
(BLISTER PACK)				
2 mg, 100s ea UD	00009-5190-04	486.58	405.48	
500s ea	00009-5190-03	2407.39	2006.16	
4 mg, 30s ea	00009-5191-01	144.49	120.41	
90s ea	00009-5191-02	433.48	361.23	
(BLISTER PACK)				
4 mg, 100s ea UD	00009-5191-04	486.58	405.48	
500s ea	00009-5191-03	2408.20	2006.83	
(A-S Medication)				
REPACK				
CER, PO, 4 mg, 30s ea	54569-5205-01	143.35		
(PD-Rx Pharm)				
REPACK				
CER, PO, 2 mg, 30s ea	58864-0861-30	132.65		
4 mg, 21s ea	55289-0132-21	143.18		
30s ea	55289-0132-30	213.62		
(REDI-SCRIPT)				
4 mg, 30s ea	58864-0864-30	156.93		
(Phys Total Care)				
REPACK				
CER, PO, 2 mg, 30s ea	54868-5126-00	172.95		
90s ea	54868-5126-01	490.50		
4 mg, 30s ea	54868-4514-00	173.00		
90s ea	54868-4514-01	498.52		
(Quality Care Prod)				
REPACK				
CER, PO, 4 mg, 30s ea	35356-0417-30	203.34		
30s ea	49999-0910-30	203.34		
DETUSS (Breckenridge Pharm)				
cpm/hydrocod bit/pse hcl				
SYR, PO (AF,VANILLIN)				
473 ml, C-III	51991-0220-16	33.89		
DEVICE				
(Abbott Hosp) *See LIFESHIELD PLUMSET PRIMARY IV W/OL*				
(Abbott Hosp) *See LIFESHIELD PLUMSET SECONDARY IV-OL*				
(Abbott Hosp) *See NITROGLYCERIN DISTAL EXTENSION*				
(Abbott Hosp) *See PENTOTHAL DISPENSING PIN*				
(Abbott Hosp) *See PLUMSET MACRO INTEGRAL HP FILTER-OL*				
(Alaven) *See PRIMABELLA*				
(Covidien) *See CLINICAL LAB PRODUCTS*				
(J&J Medical) *See S-ENTRY DRY MAT*				
(Medtronic Minimed) *See GUARDIAN REAL-TIME STARTER*				
(Medtronic Minimed) *See MINIMED PARADIGM CGM STARTER*				
(Medtronic Minimed) *See MINIMED PARADIGM REAL-TIME TRANSMITTER*				
(Medtronic Minimed) *See PARADIGM REAL-TIME TRANSMITTER*				
(Medtronic Minimed) *See SEN-SERTER*				
(Medtronic Minimed) *See SENSOR*				
(Medtronic Minimed) *See SILHOUETTE*				
(Medtronic Minimed) *See SOF-SENSOR*				
(Owen Mumford) *See RAPPORT RING LOADING SYSTEM*				
(Pari) *See PARI TREK S PORT POWER KIT*				
(Spectrum Design Med.) *See SPECTRAGEL*				
(Teva) *See AMNISCREEN*				
(Teva) *See VIASPAN COLD STORAGE/FLUSHING*				
(Ventus) *See PROVENT SLEEP APNEA THERAPY, HR DEVICE*				
(Ventus) *See PROVENT SLEEP APNEA THERAPY, SR DEVICE*				
DEVICE, IMPOTENCE, MECHANICAL				
(Owen Mumford) *See RAPPORT VACUUM THERAPY DEVICE*				
DEVICE, INHALATION				
(Monaghan Medical) *See AEROVENT CHC*				
(Pari) *See PARI TREK S COMBO PACK*				
(Pari) *See PARI TREK S COMPACT COMPRESSOR*				
(Pari) *See PARI TREK S W/ DC ADAPTOR*				
(U.S. Pharm) *See WATCHHALER*				

PROD/MFR	NDC	AWP	DP	OBC
DEVIL'S CLAW ROOT				
(PCCA) *See DEVILS CLAW ROOT*				
DEVILS CLAW ROOT (PCCA)				
devil's claw root				
POW, NA (1X1GM)				
1 gm	51927-3041-00	0.36		
DEX PC (Boca Pharmacal)				
cpm/dm/phenyleph hcl				
SYR, PO (AF,STRAWBERRY)				
473 ml	64376-0711-16	30.07		
DEX-TUSS (Cypress Pharm)				
codeine phosphate/guaifenesin				
SOL, PO (AF,SF,GLUTEN-FREE,GRAPE)				
10 mg/5 ml-300 mg/5 ml,				
473 ml, C-V	60258-0750-16	184.34		
DEX-TUSS DM (Cypress Pharm)				
dextromethorphan hydrobromide/guaifenesin				
SOL, PO (AF,SF,GLUTEN-FREE,GRAPE)				
10 mg/5 ml-300 mg/5 ml,				
473 ml	60258-0319-16	178.75		
DEX/LACT. RINGERS/POTASSIUM CHL (Hospira)				
ca cl/dextrose/k cl/na cl/na lact				
SOL, IV (12X1000ML,LATEX-FREE)				
1000 ml 12s	00409-7111-09	41.04	35.88	AP
DEXACIDIN (Phys Total Care)				
REPACK				
dexamethasone/neomycin sulfate/polymyxin b sulfate				
SUS, OP, 5 ml	54868-1999-00	34.96		AT
DEXALL (Breckenridge Pharm)				
dm/dexbrompheniramine maleate/phenyleph hcl				
SYR, PO (1X473ML,AF,SF)				
473 ml	51991-0478-16	147.63		
DEXAMETHASONE				
(Alcon Ophthalmic) *See MAXIDEX*				
(Allergan Inc) *See OZURDEX*				
(Consolidated Midland)				
ELI, PO, 0.5 mg/5 ml,				
100 ml	00223-6496-01	7.50		EE
240 ml	00223-6496-02	17.50		EE
TAB, PO, 0.5 mg, 100s ea	00223-0790-01	6.75		EE
0.75 mg, 100s ea	00223-0791-01	7.50		EE
1000s ea	00223-0791-02	67.50		EE
1.5 mg, 100s ea	00223-0792-01	15.00		EE
(ECR) *See DEXPAK 10 DAY TAPERPAK*				
(ECR) *See DEXPAK 13 DAY TAPERPAK*				
(ECR) *See DEXPAK 6 DAY TAPERPAK*				
(Gallipot)				
POW, NA, 1 gm	51552-0430-01	14.70		
(MICRONIZED)				
5 gm	51552-0430-02	54.60		
(Letco)				
POW, NA (U.S.P.,MICRONIZED)				
5 gm	62991-2022-02	96.00		
10 gm	62991-2022-03	180.00		
25 gm	62991-2022-04	390.00		
(Macoven) *See ZEMA-PAK*				
(Medisca)				
POW, NA (U.S.P.,MICRONIZED)				
1 gm	38779-0405-06	34.50		
5 gm	38779-0405-03	127.50		
10 gm	38779-0405-01	208.50		
25 gm	38779-0405-04	538.50		
100 gm	38779-0405-05	1875.00		
(Morton Grove)				
ELI, PO (RASPBERRY)				
0.5 mg/5 ml,				
237 ml	60432-0466-08	63.69		AA
(Roxane) *See DEXAMETHASONE INTENSOL*				
(Roxane)				
SOL, PO (1X240ML)				
0.5 mg/5 ml,				
240 ml	00054-3177-57	63.69		
500 ml	00054-3177-63	23.91		
TAB, PO, 0.5 mg, 100s ea	00054-4179-25	18.87		AB
(10X10)				
0.5 mg, 100s ea UD	00054-8179-25	24.29		AB
0.75 mg, 100s ea	00054-4180-25	33.08		AB
(10X10)				
0.75 mg,				
100s ea UD	00054-8180-25	33.46		AB
1 mg, 100s ea	00054-4181-25	31.82		
(10X10)				
1 mg, 100s ea UD	00054-8174-25	34.36		
1.5 mg, 100s ea	00054-4182-25	27.14		AB

PROD/MFR	NDC	AWP	DP	OBC
(10X10)				
1.5 mg, 100s ea UD	00054-8181-25	38.85		AB
2 mg, 100s ea	00054-4183-25	62.31		
(10X10)				
2 mg, 100s ea UD	00054-8176-25	64.95		
4 mg, 100s ea	00054-4184-25	58.41		AB
(10X10)				
4 mg, 100s ea UD	00054-8175-25	62.05		AB
6 mg, 100s ea	00054-4186-25	98.88		BP
(10X10)				
6 mg, 100s ea UD	00054-8183-25	97.34		BP
(Spectrum Pharmacy) *See DEXAMETHASONE MICRONIZED*				
(Wockhardt USA) *See BAYCADRON ELIXIR*				
DEXAMETHASONE (A-S Medication)				
REPACK				
dexamethasone sodium phosphate				
SOL, OP, 0.1%, 5 ml	54569-1224-00	17.31		EE
DEXAMETHASONE (A-S Medication)				
TAB, PO, 0.75 mg, 12s ea	54569-0322-00	3.97		EE
20s ea	54569-0322-03	6.62		EE
2 mg, 6s ea	54569-0336-01	3.74		
4 mg, 6s ea	54569-0324-04	3.50		EE
28s ea	54569-5729-00	16.35		AB
(Aidarex)				
REPACK				
TAB, PO, 4 mg, 30s ea	33261-0625-30	39.00		AB
60s ea	33261-0625-60	78.00		AB
90s ea	33261-0625-90	117.00		AB
120s ea	33261-0625-02	156.00		AB
(Altura)				
REPACK				
TAB, PO (DOSE PAK)				
0.75 mg, 12s ea	63874-0444-12	8.17		EE
12s ea	63874-0444-21	14.30		EE
15s ea	63874-0444-15	10.22		EE
20s ea	63874-0444-20	13.62		EE
30s ea	63874-0444-30	20.43		EE
100s ea	63874-0444-01	68.08		EE
(Bryant Ranch)				
REPACK				
SOL, PO, 0.5 mg/5 ml,				
60 ml	63629-2696-01	4.50		
(DHS, Inc.)				
REPACK				
TAB, PO, 0.5 mg, 30s ea	55887-0165-30	7.29		
60s ea	55887-0165-60	14.57		
90s ea	55887-0165-90	21.87		
4 mg, 12s ea	55887-0377-12	21.60		
(Dispensing Solutions)				
REPACK				
dexamethasone sodium phosphate				
SOL, IJ, 4 mg/ml, 30 ml	55045-3212-03	17.00		
DEXAMETHASONE (Dispensing Solutions)				
TAB, PO, 0.5 mg, 12s ea	55045-2665-02	6.05		AB
0.75 mg, 6s ea	55045-1308-06	4.80		AB
12s ea	55045-1308-04	9.60		BP
12s ea	66336-0550-12	9.32		
15s ea	55045-1308-05	12.00		BP
20s ea	55045-1308-07	16.00		AB
30s ea	55045-1308-08	24.00		AB
36s ea	55045-1308-09	28.80		AB
60s ea	55045-1308-02	48.00		AB
90s ea	55045-1308-03	72.00		AB
100s ea	55045-1308-01	80.00		AB
4 mg, 6s ea	55045-1970-02	14.55		BP
6s ea	66336-0479-06	7.42		AB
8s ea	55045-1970-05	19.36		AB
(Nucare Pharm)				
REPACK				
TAB, PO, 0.75 mg, 12s ea	66267-0066-12	8.54		EE
30s ea	66267-0066-30	21.36		AB
4 mg, 4s ea	66267-0067-04	9.98		AB
8s ea	66267-0067-08	19.95		AB
10s ea	66267-0067-10	24.94		AB
12s ea	66267-0067-12	29.93		AB
20s ea	66267-0067-20	49.88		AB
21s ea	66267-0067-21	52.37		AB
(Palmetto)				
REPACK				
TAB, PO, 0.75 mg, 12s ea	23490-5404-01	9.60		
4 mg, 6s ea	23490-5407-01	17.98		
12s ea	23490-5407-02	25.68		

PROD/MFR	NDC	AWP	DP	OBC
(PD-Rx Pharm)				
REPACK				
TAB, PO, 0.75 mg, 10s ea	**55289-0903-10**	15.75		**BP**
20s ea	**55289-0903-20**	18.00		**BP**
4 mg, 4s ea	**55289-0582-04**	11.73		
(USP)				
4 mg, 6s ea	**55289-0582-06**	12.03		**AB**
10s ea	**55289-0582-10**	13.59		**AB**
(USP)				
4 mg, 28s ea	**55289-0582-28**	18.87		**AB**
(Pharma Pac)				
REPACK				
TAB, PO, 0.75 mg, 12s ea	**52959-0392-12**	8.95		**EE**
21s ea	**52959-0392-21**	15.12		**EE**
28s ea	**52959-0392-28**	19.54		**EE**
30s ea	**52959-0392-30**	18.76		**AB**
4 mg, 4s ea	**52959-0547-04**	9.32		**EE**
10s ea	**52959-0547-10**	23.29		**EE**
11s ea	**52959-0547-11**	25.62		**EE**
12s ea	**52959-0547-12**	27.95		**EE**
16s ea	**52959-0547-16**	37.27		**EE**
20s ea	**52959-0547-20**	46.58		**EE**
30s ea	**52959-0547-30**	69.86		**EE**
50s ea	**52959-0547-50**	116.41		**EE**
(Phys Total Care)				
REPACK				
TAB, PO, 0.5 mg, 30s ea	**54868-0927-00**	13.56		**AB**
0.75 mg, 30s ea	**54868-0916-00**	17.82		**EE**
1.5 mg, 100s ea	**54868-1744-00**	39.33		**EE**
2 mg, 10s ea	**54868-3157-00**	21.42		
(USP,GLUTEN-FREE)				
2 mg, 48s ea	**54868-3157-01**	91.42		
4 mg, 3s ea	**54868-0218-03**	4.43		**AB**
5s ea	**54868-0218-09**	6.89		**AB**
10s ea	**54868-0218-01**	7.77		**EE**
16s ea	**54868-0218-05**	10.64		**AB**
20s ea	**54868-0218-00**	12.55		**AB**
30s ea	**54868-0218-04**	17.33		**AB**
40s ea	**54868-0218-07**	22.11		**EE**
(USP)				
4 mg, 50s ea	**54868-0218-08**	26.88		**EE**
100s ea	**54868-0218-06**	49.27		**AB**
120s ea	**58468-0218-02**	60.32		**AB**
6 mg, 6s ea	**54868-5903-00**	15.88		**BP**
(Physician Partner)				
REPACK				
TAB, PO, 4 mg, 4s ea	**21695-0382-04**	14.67		
20s ea	**21695-0382-20**	23.37		**AB**
(Quality Care Prod)				
REPACK				
TAB, PO, 1 mg, 30s ea	**35356-0359-30**	24.77		
4 mg, 6s ea	**49999-0059-06**	23.40		**EE**
30s ea	**49999-0059-30**	46.60		**BP**
(Southwood)				
REPACK				
TAB, PO, 0.5 mg, 12s ea	**58016-0290-12**	6.12		**EE**
15s ea	**58016-0290-15**	7.65		**EE**
20s ea	**58016-0290-20**	10.20		**EE**
30s ea	**58016-0290-30**	15.30		**EE**
60s ea	**58016-0291-60**	30.60		**EE**
100s ea	**58016-0290-00**	51.00		**EE**
120s ea	**58016-0290-02**	61.20		**AB**
150s ea	**58016-0290-03**	76.50		**AB**
200s ea	**58016-0290-89**	102.00		**AB**
300s ea	**58016-0290-73**	153.00		**AB**
0.75 mg, 6s ea	**58016-0293-06**	4.68		**EE**
12s ea	**58016-0293-12**	9.35		**EE**
15s ea	**58016-0293-15**	11.69		**EE**
20s ea	**58016-0293-20**	15.58		**EE**
30s ea	**58016-0293-30**	23.38		**EE**
100s ea	**58016-0293-00**	77.92		**EE**
4 mg, 8s ea	**58016-0781-08**	17.12		**EE**
10s ea	**58016-0781-10**	21.40		**EE**
12s ea	**58016-0781-12**	25.68		**EE**
14s ea	**58016-0781-14**	29.96		**EE**
15s ea	**58016-0781-15**	32.10		**EE**
20s ea	**58016-0781-20**	42.80		**EE**
21s ea	**58016-0781-21**	44.94		**EE**
24s ea	**58016-0781-24**	51.36		**EE**
28s ea	**58016-0781-28**	59.92		**EE**
30s ea	**58016-0781-30**	64.20		**EE**
40s ea	**58016-0781-40**	85.60		**EE**
50s ea	**58016-0781-50**	107.00		**EE**
100s ea	**58016-0781-00**	214.00		**EE**
(Stat Rx)				
REPACK				
dexamethasone sodium phosphate				
SOL, OP, 0.1%, 5 ml	**16590-0068-05**	17.25		

PROD/MFR	NDC	AWP	DP	OBC
DEXAMETHASONE (Stat Rx)				
TAB, PO, 4 mg, 60s ea	**16590-0269-60**	58.41		**AB**
120s ea	**16590-0269-72**	116.82		**AB**
(Vibranta)				
REPACK				
TAB, PO, 4 mg, 30s ea	**57866-3581-01**	46.15		**BP**
DEXAMETHASONE 21-ISONICOTINATE MICRONIZED (PCCA)				
dexamethasone isonicotinate, micronized				
POW, NA, 1 gm	**51927-3393-00**	105.00		
DEXAMETHASONE ACETATE				
(Clint) *See CORTASTAT LA*				
(Consolidated Midland)				
SUS, IJ (VIAL)				
8 mg/ml, 5 ml	**00223-7390-05**	11.50		**EE**
(Gallipot)				
POW, NA (U.S.P.)				
1 gm	**51552-0024-01**	29.75		
5 gm	**51552-0024-02**	87.92		
10 gm	**51552-0024-03**	196.00		
(U.S.P., MICRONIZED)				
25 gm	**51552-0024-04**	329.00		
(Legere) *See DEXASONE L.A.*				
(Medisca) *See DEXAMETHASONE ACETATE ANHYDROUS*				
(Spectrum Pharmacy) *See DEXAMETHASONE ACETATE ANHYDROUS*				
DEXAMETHASONE ACETATE ANHYDROUS (Medisca)				
dexamethasone acetate				
POW, NA (U.S.P.,MICRONIZED)				
100 gm	**38779-1905-05**	2850.00		
(Spectrum Pharmacy)				
POW, NA (U.S.P,MICRONIZED)				
1 gm	**49452-2460-03**	111.30		
5 gm	**49452-2460-01**	367.50		
25 gm	**49452-2460-02**	1323.00		
DEXAMETHASONE ACETATE MICRONIZED (Medisca)				
dexamethasone acetate, micronized				
POW, NA (ANHYDROUS)				
5 gm	**38779-1905-03**	237.00		
10 gm	**38779-1905-01**	405.00		
25 gm	**38779-1905-04**	885.00		
(PCCA)				
POW, NA (U.S.P.)				
1 gm	**51927-2231-00**	75.00		
(USP)				
1 gm	**51927-3747-00**	75.00		
DEXAMETHASONE ACETATE, MICRONIZED				
(Hawkins) *See DEXAMETHASONE MICRONIZED*				
(Medisca) *See DEXAMETHASONE ACETATE MICRONIZED*				
(PCCA) *See DEXAMETHASONE ACETATE MICRONIZED*				
DEXAMETHASONE INTENSOL (Roxane)				
dexamethasone				
SOL, PO, 1 mg/ml, 30 ml	**00054-3176-44**	19.62		
DEXAMETHASONE ISONICOTINATE, MICRONIZED				
(PCCA) *See DEXAMETHASONE 21-ISONICOTINATE MICRONIZED*				
DEXAMETHASONE MICRONIZED (Hawkins)				
dexamethasone acetate, micronized				
POW, NA (U.S.P.)				
5 gm	**63370-0060-15**	150.00		
10 gm	**63370-0060-20**	280.00		
25 gm	**63370-0060-25**	580.00		
100 gm	**63370-0060-35**	2040.00		
1000 gm	**63370-0060-50**	14400.00		
(PCCA)				
dexamethasone, micronized				
POW, NA (1X1GM, USP)				
1 gm	**51927-1081-00**	39.00		
(Spectrum Pharmacy)				
dexamethasone				
POW, NA (U.S.P.)				
1 gm	**49452-2465-01**	64.40		
5 gm	**49452-2465-02**	192.85		
25 gm	**49452-2465-03**	787.50		
100 gm	**49452-2465-04**	2478.00		
DEXAMETHASONE SODIUM PHOSPHATE (Amer Regent)				
SOL, IJ (S.D.V.)				
4 mg/ml, 1 ml 25s	**00517-4901-25**	27.19		**AP**
(M.D.V.)				
4 mg/ml, 5 ml 25s	**00517-4905-25**	54.69		**AP**
30 ml 25s	**00517-4930-25**	242.19		**AP**

PROD/MFR	NDC	AWP	DP	OBC
(APP)				
SOL, IJ (VIAL)				
4 mg/ml, 1 ml	**63323-0165-01**	1.32		**AP**
(M.D.V.)				
4 mg/ml, 5 ml	**63323-0165-05**	3.12		**AP**
30 ml	**63323-0165-30**	16.80		**AP**
(LATEX-FREE)				
10 mg/ml, 1 ml 25s	**63323-0506-01**	74.75		
(10X10ML,PRESERVED)				
10 mg/ml,				
10 ml 10s	**63323-0516-10**	49.50		**AP**
(Bausch & Lomb Inc.)				
SOL, OP, 0.1%, 5 ml	**24208-0720-02**	17.31		**AT**
(Baxter)				
SOL, IJ (VIAL, DOSETTE)				
10 mg/ml, 1 ml	**00641-0367-21**	2.24		**AP**
1 ml 25s	**00641-0367-25**	56.10		**AP**
(Clint) *See CORTASTAT*				
(Clint) *See CORTASTAT 10*				
(Consolidated Midland)				
SOL, IJ (AMP)				
4 mg/ml, 1 ml 25s	**00223-7401-25**	25.00		**EE**
(DOSETTE VIAL)				
4 mg/ml, 1 ml 25s	**00223-7407-01**	31.25		**EE**
1 ml 100s	**00223-7403-01**	60.00		**EE**
(VIAL)				
4 mg/ml, 5 ml	**00223-7404-05**	2.75		**EE**
10 ml	**00223-7408-10**	4.00		**EE**
25 ml	**00223-7406-25**	7.00		**EE**
30 ml	**00223-7402-30**	5.50		**EE**
OP, 0.1%, 5 ml	**00223-6485-05**	3.75		**EE**
15 ml	**00223-6488-15**	3.50		**EE**
(Falcon Ophthalmics)				
SOL, OP, 0.1%, 5 ml	**61314-0294-05**	17.30		
(Gallipot)				
POW, NA (U.S.P.)				
1 gm	**51552-0025-01**	14.00		
5 gm	**51552-0025-02**	52.92		
10 gm	**51552-0025-03**	99.96		
25 gm	**51552-0025-04**	231.00		
(Hawkins)				
POW, NA (U.S.P.)				
1 gm	**63370-0070-10**	43.20		
5 gm	**63370-0070-15**	177.60		
10 gm	**63370-0070-20**	348.00		
25 gm	**63370-0070-25**	672.00		
100 gm	**63370-0070-35**	2400.00		
500 gm	**63370-0070-45**	7176.00		
1000 gm	**63370-0070-50**	13920.00		
(Letco)				
POW, NA (U.S.P.)				
5 gm	**62991-1041-02**	105.00		
10 gm	**62991-1041-03**	180.00		
25 gm	**62991-1041-04**	360.00		
(Medisca)				
POW, NA (USP,1X1GM)				
1 gm	**38779-0071-06**	37.50		
(U.S.P.)				
5 gm	**38779-0071-03**	147.00		
10 gm	**38779-0071-01**	208.50		
25 gm	**38779-0071-04**	597.00		
100 gm	**38779-0071-05**	1485.00		
500 gm	**38779-0071-08**	5055.00		
(USP,1X1000GM)				
1000 gm	**38779-0071-09**	9045.00		
(PCCA)				
POW, NA (U.S.P.)				
1 gm	**51927-1430-00**	42.00		
(Spectrum Pharmacy)				
POW, NA (U.S.P.)				
1 gm	**49452-2470-03**	63.70		
5 gm	**49452-2470-01**	225.70		
25 gm	**49452-2470-02**	910.00		
100 gm	**49452-2470-04**	2712.50		
(Teva)				
SOL, IJ (M.D.V.)				
10 mg/ml,				
10 ml 10s	**00703-3524-03**	49.08		**AP**
(A-S Medication)				
REPACK				
SOL, IJ (25X5ML)				
4 mg/ml, 5 ml 25s	**54569-4648-00**	81.25		**EE**
(Dispensing Solutions)				
REPACK				
SOL, OP, 0.1%, 5 ml	**55045-1755-05**	17.99		

PROD/MFR	NDC	AWP	DP	OBC
(Palmetto)				
REPACK				
SOL, IJ, 4 mg/ml, ea	23490-5413-00	6.50		
OP, 0.1%, 5 ml	23490-5411-01	18.28		
(Pharma Pac)				
REPACK				
SOL, OP, 0.1%, 5 ml	52959-0288-03	21.10		EE
(Phys Total Care)				
REPACK				
SOL, IJ (M.D.V.)				
4 mg/ml, 5 ml	54868-0871-00	64.56		EE
30 ml	54868-0871-06	67.56		EE
(1X125ML)				
4 mg/ml, 125 ml	54868-0871-01	155.88		EE
(10X10ML)				
10 mg/ml,				
10 ml 10s	54868-6099-00	143.88		AP
OP, 0.1%, 5 ml	54868-3129-00	65.91		EE
(Physician Partner)				
REPACK				
SOL, IJ (1X30ML)				
4 mg/ml, 30 ml	21695-0848-30	35.00		AP
OP (1X5ML)				
0.1%, 5 ml	21695-0847-05	34.62		
(Quality Care Prod)				
REPACK				
SOL, IJ (25X1ML)				
4 mg/ml, 1 ml 25s	49999-0434-25	43.50		AP
(Southwood)				
REPACK				
OIN, OP, 0.05%, 3.5 gm	58016-6022-01	6.34		EE
SOL, OP, 0.1%, 5 ml	58016-6024-01	15.56		EE
DEXAMETHASONE, MICRONIZED				
(PCCA) *See DEXAMETHASONE MICRONIZED*				
DEXAMETHASONE/NEOMYCIN SULFATE/ POLYMYXIN B SULFATE				
FUL				
OIN, OP, 3 gm		3.21		
(Alcon Ophthalmic) *See MAXITROL*				
(Bausch & Lomb Inc.) *See DEXAMETHASONE/NEOMYCIN/POLYMYXIN*				
(Consolidated Midland) *See DEXAMETHASONE/NEOMYCIN/POLYMYXIN*				
(Falcon Ophthalmics) *See DEXAMETHASONE/NEOMYCIN/POLYMYXIN*				
(Major) *See DEXAMETHASONE/NEOMYCIN/POLYMYXIN*				
(Major) *See METHADEX*				
(Ocusoft) *See POLY-DEX*				
(Palmetto)				
REPACK				
OIN, OP, 3.5 gm	23490-5975-01	26.50		
SUS, OP, 5 ml	23490-5976-01	26.50		
DEXAMETHASONE/NEOMYCIN/POLYMYXIN				
(Bausch & Lomb Inc.)				
dexamethasone/neomycin sulfate/polymyxin b sulfate				
OIN, OP, 3.5 gm	24208-0795-35	19.86		AT
SUS, OP, 5 ml	24208-0830-60	19.86		AT
(Consolidated Midland)				
SUS, OP, 5 ml	00223-6754-05	6.75		EE
(Falcon Ophthalmics)				
OIN, OP, 3.5 gm	61314-0631-36	18.60		AT
SUS, OP (DROP-TAINER)				
5 ml	61314-0630-06	18.60		AT
(Major)				
OIN, OP, 3.5 gm	00904-7938-38	7.25		AT
(A-S Medication)				
REPACK				
OIN, OP, 3.5 gm	54569-4360-00	8.00		EE
SUS, OP, 5 ml	54569-4359-00	8.00		EE
(Altura)				
REPACK				
OIN, OP (1X3.5GM)				
3.5 gm	63874-0845-04	27.25		AT
SUS, OP, 5 ml	63874-0745-05	27.52		AT
(DHS, Inc.)				
REPACK				
SUS, OP, 5 ml	55887-0829-05	14.02		AT
(Dispensing Solutions)				
REPACK				
SUS, OP, 5 ml	55045-1335-05	10.20		AT

PROD/MFR	NDC	AWP	DP	OBC
(Nucare Pharm)				
REPACK				
SUS, OP, 5 ml	66267-0958-05	9.04		EE
(Pharma Pac)				
REPACK				
OIN, OP, 3.5 gm	52959-0407-01	17.95		EE
SUS, OP, 5 ml	52959-0085-01	19.06		EE
(Phys Total Care)				
REPACK				
OIN, OP, 3.5 gm	54868-1192-01	18.09		AT
(Quality Care Prod)				
REPACK				
SUS, OP, 5 ml	49999-0387-05	21.87		AT
(Southwood)				
REPACK				
OIN, OP, 3.5 gm	58016-6039-03	27.25		EE
SUS, OP, 5 ml	58016-6041-01	26.50		EE
5 ml	58016-6041-05	18.95		EE
DEXAMETHASONE/TOBRAMYCIN				
(Alcon Ophthalmic) *See TOBRADEX*				
(Bausch & Lomb Inc.) *See TOBRAMYCIN AND DEXAMETHASONE*				
(Falcon Ophthalmics) *See TOBRAMYCIN AND DEXAMETHASONE*				
DEXAMETHASONE/TOBRAMYCIN (Palmetto)				
REPACK				
dexamethasone/tobramycin				
SUS, OP (1X5ML)				
0.1%-0.3%, 5 ml	23490-6397-01	55.54		
DEXASONE L.A. (Legere)				
dexamethasone acetate				
SUS, IJ (VIAL)				
8 mg/ml, 5 ml	25332-0011-05	29.95		EE
DEXASPORIN (Phys Total Care)				
REPACK				
dexamethasone/neomycin sulfate/polymyxin b sulfate				
SUS, OP, 5 ml	54868-1070-01	15.24		AT
DEXBROMPHENIRAMINE TANNATE/PHENYLEPH TAN/PYRIL MAL				
(Poly) *See POLY TAN D*				
DEXCHLORPHENIRAMINE MAL/PHENYLEPH HCL				
(Capellon) *See RESCON-MX*				
DEXCHLORPHENIRAMINE MALEATE (Actavis)				
TER, PO, 4 mg, 100s ea	52152-0014-02	42.95		
(Contract Pharmacal)				
TER, PO (SUGAR COATED)				
6 mg, 100s ea	10267-1311-01	60.50		
(Morton Grove)				
SYR, PO (ORANGE)				
2 mg/5 ml, 473 ml	60432-0539-16	83.08		AA
(PCCA)				
POW, NA (U.S.P.)				
1 gm	51927-1830-00	45.00		
(Spectrum Pharmacy)				
POW, NA (U.S.P.)				
1 gm	49452-2467-01	84.00		
5 gm	49452-2467-02	291.20		
25 gm	49452-2467-03	1015.00		
DEXCHLORPHENIRAMINE TAN/PSE TAN				
(Breckenridge Pharm) *See DUOTAN PD*				
(Cypress Pharm) *See SUTAN*				
DEXEDRINE (Phys Total Care)				
REPACK				
dextroamphetamine sulfate				
TAB, PO, 5 mg,				
10s ea, C-II	54868-3403-03	8.53		AA
50s ea, C-II	54868-3403-00	30.11		AA
90s ea, C-II	54868-3403-02	51.09		AA
100s ea, C-II	54868-3403-01	57.11		AA
DEXEDRINE SPANSULE (Glaxo)				
dextroamphetamine sulfate				
CER, PO, 5 mg,				
90s ea, C-II	00007-3512-59	207.70		AB
DEXEDRINE SPANSULES (Glaxo)				
dextroamphetamine sulfate				
CER, PO, 10 mg,				
90s ea, C-II	00007-3513-59	259.46		AB
15 mg,				
90s ea, C-II	00007-3514-59	330.82		AB

PROD/MFR	NDC	AWP	DP	OBC
(Phys Total Care)				
REPACK				
CER, PO, 5 mg,				
50s ea, C-II	54868-3402-00	64.36		
100s ea, C-II	54868-3402-01	125.61		
10 mg,				
50s ea, C-II	54868-3811-00	41.81		AB
15 mg,				
20s ea, C-II	54868-4758-00	44.25		
60s ea, C-II	54868-4758-01	126.50		
DEXFERRUM (Amer Regent)				
iron dextran				
SOL, IJ ((S.D.V.), MW267)				
50 mg/ml, 1 ml 10s	00517-0134-10	225.00		BP
2 ml 10s	00517-0234-10	450.00		BP
DEXLANSOPRAZOLE				
(Takeda) *See KAPIDEX*				
DEXMEDETOMIDINE HYDROCHLORIDE				
(Hospira) *See PRECEDEX*				
DEXMETHYLPHENIDATE HYDROCHLORIDE				
(Novartis Pharm) *See FOCALIN*				
(Novartis Pharm) *See FOCALIN XR*				
(Teva)				
TAB, PO, 2.5 mg,				
100s ea, C-II	00093-5275-01	59.81		AB
5 mg, 100s ea, C-II	00093-5276-01	85.26		AB
10 mg, 100s ea, C-II	00093-5277-01	122.59		AB
DEXPAK (Phys Total Care)				
REPACK				
dexamethasone				
TAB, PO, 1.5 mg, 35s ea	54868-5334-01	54.74		
51s ea	54868-5334-00	54.74		EE
DEXPAK 10 DAY TAPERPAK (ECR)				
dexamethasone				
TAB, PO, 1.5 mg, 35s ea	00095-0087-35	43.75		
DEXPAK 13 DAY TAPERPAK (ECR)				
dexamethasone				
TAB, PO, 1.5 mg, 51s ea	00095-0088-51	49.38		
DEXPAK 6 DAY TAPERPAK (ECR)				
dexamethasone				
TAB, PO, 1.5 mg, 21s ea	00095-0089-21	30.63		
DEXPANTHENOL				
(Amend) *See ALCOHOL D-PANTHENOL*				
(Amer Regent)				
SOL, IM (S.D.V.)				
250 mg/ml,				
2 ml 25s	00517-0131-25	101.56		
(Consolidated Midland) *See D-PANTOTHENYL ALCOHOL*				
(Consolidated Midland)				
SOL, IM (VIAL)				
250 mg/ml, 10 ml	00223-7414-10	6.00		
(Medisca) *See PANTHENOL*				
(Medisca)				
POW, NA (U.S.P.)				
25 gm	38779-1234-04	25.50		
100 gm	38779-1234-05	70.50		
500 gm	38779-1234-08	312.00		
(PCCA)				
POW, NA (USP)				
1 gm	51927-2324-00	1.19		
(Spectrum Pharmacy) *See DL-PANTHENOL*				
(Spectrum Pharmacy)				
POW, NA (U.S.P.)				
100 gm	49452-2468-02	117.25		
1000 gm	49452-2468-03	721.00		
DEXPANTHENOL/NIACINAMIDE/VIT B1/VIT B2/VIT B6				
(Bioniche Pharma) *See VITAMIN B COMPLEX 100*				
(Merit) *See B-COMPLEX*				
(Truxton) *See VITAMIN B COMPLEX 100*				
DEXRAZOXANE (Bedford)				
dexrazoxane hydrochloride				
PDS, IV (S.D.V.)				
250 mg, ea	55390-0014-02	246.28		AP
500 mg, ea	55390-0060-02	492.00		AP
DEXRAZOXANE HYDROCHLORIDE				
(Bedford) *See DEXRAZOXANE*				
(Pfizer) *See ZINECARD*				
(TopoTarget) *See TOTECT*				

PROD/MFR | NDC | AWP | DP | OBC

DEXTRAN (Hospira)
SOL, IV (VIAL, TEARTOP, HM)
32%, 100 ml 5s 00074-8085-01 135.72 118.75

(PCCA)
POW, NA (1X1GM)
1 gm 51927-3248-00 3.30

(Spectrum Pharmacy) *See DEXTRAN 40000*

(Spectrum Pharmacy) *See DEXTRAN 75000*

DEXTRAN 40/DEXTROSE
(Hospira) *See LMD IN DEXTROSE*

DEXTRAN 40/SODIUM CHLORIDE
(Hospira) *See LMD W/0.9% SODIUM CHLORIDE*

DEXTRAN 40000 (Spectrum Pharmacy)
dextran
POW, NA, 25 gm 49452-2469-01 97.30
100 gm 49452-2469-02 285.60
1000 gm 49452-2469-03 1340.50

DEXTRAN 70/DEXTROSE
(Cooper Surgical) *See HYSKON*

(Hospira) *See DEXTRAN-70/DEXTROSE*

DEXTRAN 70/SODIUM CHLORIDE
(Hospira) *See DEXTRAN-70 W/SODIUM CHLORIDE*

DEXTRAN 75000 (Spectrum Pharmacy)
dextran
POW, NA, 25 gm 49452-2474-01 149.45
100 gm 49452-2474-02 350.00
1000 gm 49452-2474-03 1578.50

DEXTRAN-70 W/SODIUM CHLORIDE (Hospira)
dextran 70/sodium chloride
SOL, IV, 6%-0.9%,
500 ml 12s 00409-1505-03 172.80 151.20

DEXTRAN-70/DEXTROSE (Hospira)
dextran 70/dextrose
SOL, IV (12X500ML)
6%-5%, 500 ml 12s .. 00074-1507-03 344.30 301.32

DEXTROAMP SAC/AMP ASPART/DEXTROAMP SULF/AMP SULF (CorePharma)
amphetamine salt combination
TAB, PO, 5 mg,
100s ea, C-II ...... 64720-0130-10 137.16 AB

(PD-Rx Pharm)
REPACK
TAB, PO, 5 mg,
30s ea, C-II ...... 55289-0700-30 17.16 AB
60s ea, C-II ...... 55289-0700-60 25.32 AB
90s ea, C-II ...... 55289-0700-90 33.47 AB

DEXTROAMPH SACC-AMPH ASP-DEXTROAM SULF-AMPHET SULF (Phys Total Care)
REPACK
amphetamine salt combination
TAB, PO, 10 mg,
120s ea, C-II 54868-4728-05 117.81

DEXTROAMPH SACC/AMPH ASP/DEXTROAM SULF/AMPHET SULF (CorePharma)
amphetamine salt combination
TAB, PO (COMPRESSED TABLET)
10 mg,
100s ea, C-II ...... 64720-0132-10 137.16 AB
20 mg,
100s ea, C-II ...... 64720-0135-10 137.16 AB
30 mg,
100s ea, C-II ...... 64720-0136-10 137.16 AB

(PD-Rx Pharm)
REPACK
TAB, PO (COMPRESSED TABLET)
10 mg,
60s ea, C-II ...... 55289-0680-60 25.32 AB
90s ea, C-II ...... 55289-0680-90 33.47 AB
20 mg,
60s ea, C-II ...... 55289-0722-60 25.32 AB
90s ea, C-II ...... 55289-0722-90 33.47 AB

DEXTROAMPHETAMINE SULFATE
FUL
TAB, PO, 10 mg, 100s ea 34.35

(Auriga) *See LIQUADD*

(Glaxo) *See DEXEDRINE SPANSULE*

(Glaxo) *See DEXEDRINE SPANSULES*

(PCCA)
POW, NA (USP)
1 gm, C-II 51927-2858-00 900.00

PROD/MFR | NDC | AWP | DP | OBC

(Teva)
CER, PO, 5 mg,
100s ea, C-II ...... 00555-0954-02 206.20 AB
10 mg, 100s ea, C-II .. 00555-0955-02 231.81 AB
15 mg, 100s ea, C-II .. 00555-0956-02 295.56 AB
TAB, PO, 5 mg,
100s ea, C-II ...... 00555-0952-02 31.95 AA
10 mg, 100s ea, C-II .. 00555-0953-02 64.47 AA

(Phys Total Care)
REPACK
CER, PO, 10 mg,
20s ea, C-II 54868-5479-01 54.75
60s ea, C-II 54868-5479-00 149.22
15 mg, 10s ea, C-II ... 54868-5388-00 32.13 AB
30s ea, C-II 54868-5388-01 81.36

(Quality Care Prod)
REPACK
TAB, PO, 5 mg,
30s ea, C-II ...... 35356-0387-30 30.63 AA

DEXTROMETHORPHAN (Spectrum Pharmacy)
POW, NA (U.S.P.)
10 gm 49452-2495-01 128.80
25 gm 49452-2495-02 235.55
100 gm 49452-2495-03 584.50

DEXTROMETHORPHAN HYDROBROMIDE (Amend)
POW, NA (U.S.P.)
10 gm 17317-0136-01 13.30
25 gm 17317-0136-02 25.20
100 gm 17317-0136-03 105.00

(Gallipot)
POW, NA (U.S.P.,N.F.)
10 gm 51552-0121-03 22.12
25 gm 51552-0121-04 45.15
100 gm 51552-0121-05 121.10

(Hawkins)
POW, NA (U.S.P.)
25 gm 63370-0072-25 112.00
100 gm 63370-0072-35 284.00
500 gm 63370-0072-45 1240.00
1000 gm 63370-0072-50 2040.00

(Letco)
POW, NA (U.S.P.)
25 gm 62991-1042-02 75.00
100 gm 62991-1042-03 195.00

(Medisca)
POW, NA (U.S.P.)
10 gm 38779-0355-01 46.50
25 gm 38779-0355-04 89.40
100 gm 38779-0355-05 232.80
500 gm 38779-0355-08 915.00
1000 gm 38779-0355-09 1561.50

(PCCA)
POW, NA (U.S.P.)
1 gm 51927-1339-00 6.00

(Spectrum Pharmacy)
POW, NA (MONOHYDRATE, U.S.P.)
10 gm 49452-2500-01 84.00
25 gm 49452-2500-02 139.30
100 gm 49452-2500-03 343.35

DEXTROMETHORPHAN HYDROBROMIDE/ GUAIFENESIN
(Breckenridge Pharm) *See GUIADRINE DX LIQUID*

(Capellon) *See TUSSI-BID*

(Cypress Pharm) *See COFEX-DM*

(Cypress Pharm) *See DEX-TUSS DM*

(Cypress Pharm) *See GANI-TUSS-DM NR*

(Cypress Pharm) *See GFN 1200/DM 60*

(Cypress Pharm) *See SIMUC-DM*

(Cypress Pharm) *See SU-TUSS DM*

(Ethex) *See GUAIFENEX DM*

(PGD, Inc.) *See GENEDOTUSS-DM*

(Qualitest) *See IOPHEN DM-NR*

(Silarx) *See GUAIFENESIN-DM NR*

(SJ) *See BIDEX-A*

(Palmetto)
REPACK
TER, PO, 30 mg-600 mg,
20s ea 23490-5654-01 11.45
30s ea 23490-5654-02 17.18
60s ea 23490-5654-03 34.36

PROD/MFR | NDC | AWP | DP | OBC

DEXTROMETHORPHAN/GUAIFENESIN (Pharma Pac)
REPACK
dextromethorphan hydrobromide/guaifenesin
TER, PO, 30 mg-600 mg,
14s ea 52959-0444-14 8.22
20s ea 52959-0444-20 10.89
28s ea 52959-0444-28 14.52
30s ea 52959-0444-30 15.26

DEXTROMETHORPHAN/PROMETHAZINE
(Actavis Mid Atlantic)
dm/promethazine hcl
SYR, PO, 15 mg/5 ml-6.25 mg/5 ml,
118 ml ...... 00472-1630-04 7.10 AA
473 ml ...... 00472-1630-16 21.40 AA

(Hi-Tech)
SYR, PO, 15 mg/5 ml-6.25 mg/5 ml,
473 ml ...... 50383-0803-16 21.65 AA

(Morton Grove)
SYR, PO (APPLE)
15 mg/5 ml-6.25 mg/5 ml,
118 ml ...... 60432-0604-04 4.79 AA
473 ml ...... 60432-0604-16 14.33 AA

(A-S Medication)
REPACK
SYR, PO, 15 mg/5 ml-6.25 mg/5 ml,
118 ml ...... 54569-1055-00 5.94 EE

(Phys Total Care)
REPACK
SYR, PO, 15 mg/5 ml-6.25 mg/5 ml,
118 ml ...... 54868-1990-00 12.24 AA
473 ml ...... 54868-1990-01 26.70 AA

(Physician Partner)
REPACK
SYR, PO (1X120ML)
15 mg/5 ml-6.25 mg/5 ml,
120 ml ...... 21695-0698-04 14.20 AA

(Quality Care Prod)
REPACK
SYR, PO, 15 mg/5 ml-6.25 mg/5 ml,
120 ml 49999-0314-04 10.80

(Southwood)
REPACK
SYR, PO, 15 mg/5 ml-6.25 mg/5 ml,
120 ml ...... 58016-0486-24 5.60 EE

DEXTROSE (Abbott Hosp)
SOL, IV (1000 ML CONTAINER)
40%, 500 ml 6s ...... 00074-5644-25 46.46 39.12 AP

(Amend) *See DEXTROSE ANHYDROUS*

(Amend) *See DEXTROSE HYDROUS MONOHYDRATE*

(Amphastar)
SOL, IV (SRN,PREFILLED,LUER-JET)
25%, 10 ml 10s 00548-3315-00 53.20
50%, 50 ml 10s ...... 00548-3301-00 53.20 EE
(MIN-I-JET,18GX1 1/2")
50%, 50 ml 25s ...... 00548-1001-00 220.12 EE
(SRN,PREFILLED,STICKGARD)
50%, 50 ml 25s ...... 00548-2001-00 230.09 EE

(B. Braun) *See DEXTROSE HYPERTONIC*

(B. Braun)
SOL, IV (100 ML PAB)
5%, 25 ml ...... 00264-1510-36 2.28 AP
50 ml ...... 00264-1510-31 1.79 AP
(150 ML PAB)
5%, 100 ml ...... 00264-1510-32 1.79 AP
(GLASS W/SS,250 ML)
5%, 150 ml ...... 00264-1102-55 1.46 AP
(EXCEL)
5%, 250 ml ...... 00264-7510-20 1.96 AP
500 ml ...... 00264-7510-10 2.05 AP
(GLASS)
5%, 500 ml ...... 00264-1101-55 2.18 AP
(EXCEL)
5%, 1000 ml ...... 00264-7510-00 2.10 AP
(1X250ML,LATEX-FREE)
10%, 250 ml ...... 00264-7520-20 1.96 AP
(EXCEL)
10%, 500 ml ...... 00264-7520-10 2.05 AP
(GLASS W/SS,1000 ML)
10%, 500 ml ...... 00264-1207-55 2.72 AP
(EXCEL)
10%, 1000 ml ...... 00264-7520-00 2.10 AP

(Baker, J.T.) *See DEXTROSE ANHYDROUS*

(Baker, J.T.) *See DEXTROSE MONOHYDRATE*

(Baxter) *See DEXTROSE*

PROD/MFR	NDC	AWP	DP	OBC
DEXTROSE (Baxter)				
SOL, IV (QUAD PACK, MINI-BAG)				
5%, 25 ml 48s	00338-0017-10	542.88		AP
(MINI-BAG PLUS)				
5%, 50 ml 80s	00338-0551-11	1160.00		AP
(MULTI PACK, MINI-BAG)				
5%, 50 ml 96s	00338-0017-31	928.51		AP
(QUAD PACK, MINI-BAG)				
5%, 50 ml 96s	00338-0017-11	928.51		AP
(SINGLE PACK MINI-BAG)				
5%, 50 ml 96s	00338-0017-41	928.51		AP
(MINI-BAG PLUS)				
5%, 100 ml 80s	00338-0551-18	1160.00		AP
(MULTI PACK, MINI-BAG)				
5%, 100 ml 96s	00338-0017-38	928.51		AP
(QUAD PACK, MINI-BAG)				
5%, 100 ml 96s	00338-0017-18	928.51		AP
(SINGLE PACK MINI-BAG)				
5%, 100 ml 96s	00338-0017-48	928.51		AP
150 ml 36s	00338-0017-01	333.08		AP
250 ml 12s	00338-0016-02	117.50		AP
250 ml 36s	00338-0017-02	333.08		AP
DEXTROSE (Baxter)				
(USP,40X250ML,AVIVA)				
5%, 250 ml 40s	00338-6346-02	532.80	444.00	AP
(USP,1X500ML)				
5%, 500 ml	00338-6346-03	14.88	12.40	AP
DEXTROSE (Baxter)				
500 ml 12s	00338-0016-03	117.50		AP
500 ml 24s	00338-0017-03	222.05		AP
DEXTROSE (Baxter)				
(USP,1X1000ML)				
5%, 1000 ml	00338-6346-04	14.21	11.84	AP
DEXTROSE (Baxter)				
1000 ml 12s	00338-0017-04	129.73		AP
10%, 250 ml 36s	00338-0023-02	382.76		AP
500 ml 24s	00338-0023-03	255.17		AP
1000 ml 12s	00338-0023-04	148.90		AP
(BULK PACKAGE)				
50%, 2000 ml 6s	00338-0031-06	331.00		AP
(12X500ML,USP)				
70%, 500 ml 12s	00338-0719-13	266.11		AP
(BULK PACKAGE)				
70%, 2000 ml 6s	00338-0719-06	386.93		EE
(Consolidated Midland)				
SOL, PO, 50%, 50 ml 25s	00223-7420-50	75.00		
(Gallipot) *See DEXTROSE ANHYDROUS*				
(Gallipot) *See DEXTROSE MONOHYDRATE*				
(Hospira)				
SOL, IV (6X1000ML)				
2.5%, 1000 ml 6s	00409-1508-05	27.79	24.30	
(THERMOJECT KIT)				
5%, 10 ml 4s	00409-1082-01	293.10	256.00	AP
(THERMOJECT,10X10ML)				
5%, 10 ml 10s	00409-1080-51	34.80	30.50	
(USP,PF)				
5%, 10 ml 25s	00409-1082-51	293.10	256.50	AP
(LIFECARE,48X25ML)				
5%, 25 ml 48s	00409-7923-20	108.29	94.56	AP
(50/150ML PART FILL)				
5%, 50 ml 12s	00409-1523-01	126.14	110.40	AP
(48X50ML,LATEX-FREE)				
5%, 50 ml 48s	00409-7923-13	111.74	97.92	AP
(ADD-VANTAGE,LATEX-FREE)				
5%, 50 ml 50s	00409-7100-66	105.00	92.00	AP
(60X50ML,SINGLE-DOSE)				
5%, 50 ml 60s	00409-7923-06	160.56	141.00	AP
(LIFECARE,QUAD PACK)				
5%, 50 ml 80s	00409-7923-36	178.56	156.00	AP
(12X100ML)				
5%, 100 ml 12s	00409-1523-11	132.19	115.68	AP
(48X100ML,LATEX-FREE)				
5%, 100 ml 48s	00409-7923-23	107.14	93.60	AP
(ADD-VANTAGE,50X100ML)				
5%, 100 ml 50s	00409-7100-67	105.00	92.00	AP
(60X100ML,SINGLE-DOSE)				
5%, 100 ml 60s	00409-7923-11	160.56	141.00	AP
(LIFECARE,80X100ML)				
5%, 100 ml 80s	00409-7923-37	178.56	156.00	AP
(12X150ML)				
5%, 150 ml 12s	00409-1522-01	57.60	50.40	AP
(LIFECARE,32X150ML)				
5%, 150 ml 32s	00409-7922-61	48.77	42.56	AP
(12X250ML)				
5%, 250 ml 12s	00409-1522-02	73.01	63.84	AP
250 ml 24s	00409-7922-02	36.58	31.92	AP
(24X250ML,VISIVCONATINER)				
5%, 250 ml 24s	00409-7922-25	48.96	42.84	AP
(ADD-VANTAGE,24X250ML)				
5%, 250 ml 24s	00409-7100-02	66.24	58.08	AP
(LIFECARE,24X250ML)				
5%, 250 ml 24s	00409-7922-53	60.77	53.28	AP
(12X500ML)				
5%, 500 ml 12s	00409-1522-03	57.60	50.40	AP
(18X500ML,LATEX-FREE)				
5%, 500 ml 18s	00409-7922-55	125.50	109.80	AP
(LIFECARE, 24X500ML)				
5%, 500 ml 24s	00409-7922-03	39.46	34.56	AP
(VISIV CONTAINER)				
5%, 500 ml 24s	00409-7922-30	35.14	30.72	AP
(LIFECARE,12X1000ML)				
5%, 1000 ml 12s	00409-7922-09	21.17	18.48	AP
(VISIV CONTAINER)				
5%, 1000 ml 12s	00409-7922-48	19.15	16.80	AP
(AMP,LATEX-FREE)				
10%, 5 ml 25s	00409-4089-02	48.00	42.00	AP
(24X250ML,LIFECARE)				
10%, 250 ml 24s	00409-7930-02	46.66	40.80	AP
(1000 ML CONTAINER)				
10%, 500 ml 6s	00074-5641-25	30.78	25.92	AP
(1000ML CONT.,12X500ML)				
10%, 500 ml 12s	00409-7938-19	62.06	54.36	AP
(LIFECARE,LATEX-FREE)				
10%, 500 ml 24s	00409-7930-03	45.50	39.84	AP
1000 ml 12s	00409-7930-09	27.22	23.76	AP
(1000ML CONTAINER)				
20%, 500 ml 12s	00409-7935-19	62.50	54.72	AP
(12X500ML)				
20%, 500 ml 12s	00409-1535-03	40.75	35.64	AP
(10X10ML, 2.5G INFANT)				
25%, 10 ml 10s	00074-1775-10	27.72	24.30	
(2.5GM INFANT ANSYR SYR)				
25%, 10 ml 10s	00409-1775-10	27.72	24.30	
(12X500ML,LATEX-FREE)				
30%, 500 ml 12s	00409-8004-15	100.94	88.32	AP
40%, 500 ml 12s	00409-7937-19	72.00	63.00	AP
(18G1-1/2,10X50ML)				
50%, 50 ml 10s	00409-4902-34	54.00	47.30	AP
(ANSYR II,LATEX-FREE)				
50%, 50 ml 10s	00074-7517-16	27.84	24.40	AP
50 ml 10s	00409-7517-16	28.80	25.20	AP
(LIFESHIELD, 18GX1-1/2)				
50%, 50 ml 10s	00074-4902-34	51.84	45.40	AP
(VIAL,FLIPTOP,ADDITIVE)				
50%, 50 ml 25s	00409-6648-02	42.00	36.75	AP
(12X500ML,LATEX-FREE)				
50%, 500 ml 12s	00409-7936-19	68.98	60.36	AP
(2000ML BAG,6X1000ML)				
50%, 1000 ml 6s	00409-7936-29	77.11	67.50	AP
(2000MLX6, PHARMCY BULK)				
50%, 2000 ml 6s	00409-7119-07	88.92	77.82	AP
(12X500ML,LATEX-FREE)				
70%, 500 ml 12s	00409-7918-19	104.69	91.56	AP
(6X2000ML,LATEX-FREE)				
70%, 2000 ml 6s	00409-7120-07	82.08	71.82	AP
(Letco) *See DEXTROSE ANHYDROUS*				
(Mallinckrodt Lab) *See DEXTROSE ANHYDROUS*				
(Mallinckrodt Lab) *See DEXTROSE MONOHYDRATE*				
(Medisca) *See DEXTROSE ANHYDROUS*				
(Medisca) *See DEXTROSE MONOHYDRATE*				
(PCCA) *See DEXTROSE ANHYDROUS*				
(Spectrum Pharmacy) *See DEXTROSE ANHYDROUS*				
(Spectrum Pharmacy) *See DEXTROSE MONOHYDRATE*				
(Phys Total Care)				
REPACK				
SOL, IV (48X100ML)				
5%, 100 ml 48s	54868-0296-04	342.03		EE
250 ml	54868-0296-02	179.37		EE
500 ml	54868-0296-01	193.59		EE
(12X1000ML)				
10%, 1000 ml 12s	54868-5727-00	112.02		
(18GX1-1/2")				
50%, 50 ml	54868-3703-00	17.19		EE
(10X50ML)				
50%, 50 ml 10s	54868-3089-00	98.07		
(1X1250ML)				
50%, 1250 ml	54868-3089-01	100.02		
DEXTROSE 5% IN RINGERS (Baxter)				
ca cl/dextrose/k cl/na cl				
SOL, IV, 500 ml 24s	00338-0111-03	274.75		AP
1000 ml 12s	00338-0111-04	179.14		AP
(Hospira)				
ca cl/dextrose/k cl/na cl/na lact				
SOL, IV (LATEX-FREE)				
500 ml 24s	00409-7929-03	43.20	37.92	AP
(LIFECARE,LATEX-FREE)				
1000 ml 12s	00409-7929-09	24.48	21.48	AP
(Hospira)				
ca cl/dextrose/k cl/na cl				
(LIFECARE, 12X1000ML)				
1000 ml 12s	00409-7933-09	27.79	24.36	AP
DEXTROSE 5%/LACTATED RINGERS (B. Braun)				
ca cl/dextrose/k cl/na cl/na lact				
SOL, IV (EXCEL)				
500 ml	00264-7751-10	2.05		AP
1000 ml	00264-7751-00	2.10		AP
DEXTROSE 5%/RINGERS (B. Braun)				
ca cl/dextrose/k cl/na cl				
SOL, IV (EXCEL)				
1000 ml	00264-7781-00	2.28		AP
DEXTROSE AND ELECTROLYTES				
(QOL Medical) *See ELLIOTTS B*				
DEXTROSE AND SODIUM CHLORIDE (Baxter)				
dextrose/sodium chloride				
SOL, IV (USP,1X500ML)				
5%-0.45%, 500 ml	00338-6308-03	14.88	12.40	
(USP,1X1000ML)				
5%-0.45%, 1000 ml	00338-6308-04	14.21	11.84	
5%-0.9%, 1000 ml	00338-6305-04	14.21	11.84	AP
(Hospira)				
SOL, IV (250MLX24,USP,LATEX-FREE)				
5%-0.9%,				
250 ml 24s	00409-7941-02	39.46	34.56	AP
(6X1000ML)				
10%-0.9%,				
1000 ml 10s	00409-1534-05	39.82	34.86	
DEXTROSE ANHYDROUS (Amend)				
dextrose				
GRA, NA (A.C.S., REAGENT)				
500 gm	17317-1506-05	42.00		
POW, NA (U.S.P.)				
454 gm	17317-0137-01	10.50		
2270 gm	17317-0137-05	30.90		
11350 gm	17317-0137-08	105.00		
(Baker, J.T.)				
POW, NA (U.S.P.)				
500 gm	10106-1919-01	16.30		
2500 gm	10106-1919-05	41.95		
(Gallipot)				
GRA, NA (U.S.P.)				
454 gm	51552-0458-06	10.15		
2270 gm	51552-0458-09	32.62		
(Letco)				
POW, NA (U.S.P.)				
500 gm	62991-2023-01	21.00		
2500 gm	62991-2023-02	60.00		
(Mallinckrodt Lab)				
GRA, NA (U.S.P.)				
500 gm	00406-4908-04	30.53		
2500 gm	00406-4908-06	77.73		
(Medisca)				
POW, NA (U.S.P.)				
500 gm	38779-0072-08	23.85		
1000 gm	38779-0072-09	38.25		
(USP,1X2500GM)				
2500 gm	38779-0072-01	70.50		
(USP,1X10000GM)				
10000 gm	38779-0072-00	229.50		
(USP,1X25000GM)				
25000 gm	38779-0072-07	496.50		
(PCCA)				
POW, NA (ACS)				
1 gm	51927-3260-00	0.57		
(U.S.P.)				
1 gm	51927-1272-00	0.07		
(Spectrum Pharmacy)				
GRA, NA (U.S.P.,E.P.,B.P.,J.P.)				
500 gm	49452-2515-01	45.15		
2500 gm	49452-2515-02	122.15		
12000 gm	49452-2515-03	427.00		
DEXTROSE HYDROUS MONOHYDRATE (Amend)				
dextrose				
POW, NA (U.S.P.)				
500 gm	17317-0138-01	9.80		
2270 gm	17317-0138-05	35.00		
11350 gm	17317-0138-08	122.50		
DEXTROSE HYPERTONIC (B. Braun)				
dextrose				
SOL, IV (GLASS W/SS,1000 ML)				
20%, 500 ml	00264-1250-55	3.53		AP
30%, 500 ml	00264-1240-55	4.22		AP
40%, 500 ml	00264-1260-55	3.91		AP
50%, 500 ml	00264-1280-50	4.36		AP

PROD/MFR	NDC	AWP	DP	OBC
(GLASS W/SOLID STOPPER)				
50%, 1000 ml	00264-1280-55	8.57		AP
2000 ml	00264-1285-55	8.82		AP
(GLASS W/SS,1000 ML)				
70%, 500 ml	00264-1290-50	5.63		AP
(GLASS W/SOLID STOPPER)				
70%, 1000 ml	00264-1290-55	7.69		AP
(GLASS W/AIR TUBE)				
70%, 2000 ml	00264-1129-50	15.00		AP
DEXTROSE MONOHYDRATE (Baker, J.T.)				
dextrose				
POW, NA (U.S.P.)				
500 gm	10106-1912-01	11.81		
2500 gm	10106-1912-05	98.63		
(Gallipot)				
POW, NA (U.S.P.,N.F.)				
454 gm	51552-0123-06	10.50		
(Mallinckrodt Lab)				
POW, NA (U.S.P.)				
500 gm	00406-8834-03	35.48		
(Medisca)				
POW, NA (U.S.P.)				
500 gm	38779-0642-08	26.85		
2500 gm	38779-0642-01	67.50	23.75	
(Spectrum Pharmacy)				
POW, NA (U.S.P.)				
500 gm	49452-2525-01	53.90		
2500 gm	49452-2525-02	131.60		
12000 gm	49452-2525-03	455.00		
DEXTROSE-MAGNESIUM SULFATE (PharMEDium Services)				
dextrose/magnesium sulfate				
SOL, IV (6X1000ML, VIAFLEX BAG)				
5%-20 gm,				
1000 ml 6s	61553-0421-04	18.76	15.63	
DEXTROSE/DILTIAZEM HYDROCHLORIDE				
(PharMEDium Services) *See DILTIAZEM/DEXTROSE*				
DEXTROSE/DOBUTAMINE (Baxter)				
dextrose/dobutamine hydrochloride				
SOL, IV, 5%-100 mg/100 ml,				
250 ml 18s	00338-1073-02	894.96		AP
5%-200 mg/100 ml,				
250 ml 18s	00338-1075-02	1549.26		AP
5%-400 mg/100 ml,				
250 ml 18s	00338-1077-02	2617.56		AP
(Hospira)				
SOL, IV (LATEX-FREE)				
5%-200 mg/100 ml,				
250 ml 12s	00409-2347-32	182.30	159.48	AP
5%-400 mg/100 ml,				
250 ml 12s	00409-3724-32	244.66	214.08	AP
DEXTROSE/DOBUTAMINE HYDROCHLORIDE				
(Baxter) *See DEXTROSE/DOBUTAMINE*				
(Hospira) *See DEXTROSE/DOBUTAMINE*				
(Hospira) *See DEXTROSE/DOBUTAMINE NOVAPLUS*				
(Hospira) *See DOBUTAMINE IN DEXTROSE*				
DEXTROSE/DOBUTAMINE NOVAPLUS (Hospira)				
dextrose/dobutamine hydrochloride				
SOL, IV (U.S.P.,PRIVATE LABEL)				
5%-200 mg/100 ml,				
250 ml 12s	00409-2347-33	168.62	147.60	AP
DEXTROSE/DOPAMINE HCL (B. Braun)				
dextrose/dopamine hydrochloride				
SOL, IV (GLASS)				
5%-80 mg/100 ml,				
500 ml	00264-1441-55	15.60		AP
(GLASS W/SOLID STOPPER)				
5%-160 mg/100 ml,				
250 ml	00264-1482-55	11.16		AP
500 ml	00264-1481-55	15.32		AP
5%-320 mg/100 ml,				
250 ml	00264-1492-55	19.58		AP
(Baxter)				
SOL, IV (PRE-MIX IN D5W)				
5%-80 mg/100 ml,				
250 ml 18s	00338-1005-02	347.33		AP
500 ml 12s	00338-1005-03	340.56		AP
5%-160 mg/100 ml,				
250 ml 18s	00338-1007-02	510.84		AP
500 ml 12s	00338-1007-03	517.68		AP
5%-320 mg/100 ml,				
250 ml 18s	00338-1009-02	776.52		AP
(Hospira)				
SOL, IV (LIFECARE,12X250ML)				
5%-80 mg/100 ml,				
250 ml 12s	00409-7808-22	153.36	134.16	AP
500 ml 12s	00074-4141-03	187.20	163.80	AP
(LIFECARE,LATEX-FREE)				
5%-80 mg/100 ml,				
500 ml 12s	00409-7808-24	204.19	178.68	AP
(LIFECARE,12X500ML)				
5%-100 mg/100 ml,				
500 ml 12s	00409-7809-24	244.08	213.60	
5%-160 mg/100 ml,				
250 ml 12s	00409-4142-02	201.74	176.52	AP
(LIFECARE,LATEX-FREE)				
5%-160 mg/100 ml,				
250 ml 12s	00409-7809-22	191.23	167.28	AP
500 ml 12s	00074-4142-03	291.31	254.88	AP
(LIFECARE,12X250ML)				
5%-320 mg/100 ml,				
250 ml 12s	00409-7810-22	255.17	223.32	AP
DEXTROSE/DOPAMINE HYDROCHLORIDE				
(B. Braun) *See DEXTROSE/DOPAMINE HCL*				
(Baxter) *See DEXTROSE/DOPAMINE HCL*				
(Hospira) *See DEXTROSE/DOPAMINE HCL*				
DEXTROSE/ELECTROLYTE 48 (Baxter)				
dextrose/k cl/k phos/mg cl/na cl/na lact				
SOL, IV, 250 ml 36s	00338-0143-02	396.36		
500 ml 24s	00338-0143-03	264.24		
DEXTROSE/EPI HCL/LIDO HCL/TETRACAINE HCL				
(Portex) *See SPINAL-22 ANESTHESIA TRAY*				
(Portex) *See SPINAL-25 ANESTHESIA TRAY*				
(Portex) *See SPINAL-26 ANESTHESIA TRAY*				
DEXTROSE/HEPARIN SODIUM (B. Braun)				
SOL, IV (EXCEL)				
5%-4000 u/100 ml,				
500 ml	00264-9567-10	6.05		AP
5%-5000 u/100 ml,				
500 ml	00264-9577-10	5.64		AP
5%-10000 u/100 ml,				
250 ml	00264-9587-20	10.00		AP
(Baxter)				
SOL, IV (VIAFLEX,AF)				
5%-4000 u/100 ml,				
500 ml 18s	00338-0549-03	129.38		AP
5%-5000 u/100 ml,				
250 ml	00338-0550-02	7.91	6.59	AP
500 ml 18s	00338-0550-03	140.18		AP
(Hospira) *See HEPARIN SODIUM IN DEXTROSE*				
(Hospira)				
SOL, IV (LATEX-FREE)				
5%-4000 u/100 ml,				
500 ml 24s	00409-7760-03	134.21	117.36	AP
(24X500ML,LATEX-FREE)				
5%-5000 u/100 ml,				
500 ml 24s	00409-7761-03	148.03	129.60	AP
(24X250ML,LATEX-FREE)				
5%-10000 u/100 ml,				
250 ml 24s	00409-7793-62	163.30	142.80	AP
DEXTROSE/K ACE/MG ACE/NA CL				
(Baxter) *See PLASMA-LYTE 56 W/DEXTROSE*				
(Hospira) *See NORMOSOL-M W/5% DEXTROSE*				
DEXTROSE/K CL/K LACT/NA CL/NA PHOS				
(Hospira) *See IONOSOL T AND 5% DEXTROSE*				
DEXTROSE/K CL/K PHOS/MG CL/NA ACE				
(B. Braun) *See ISOLYTE P W/DEXTROSE*				
DEXTROSE/K CL/K PHOS/MG CL/NA CL/NA LACT				
(Baxter) *See DEXTROSE/ELECTROLYTE 48*				
DEXTROSE/K CL/K PHOS/MG CL/NA LACT/NA PHOS				
(Hospira) *See IONOSOL MB/5% DEXTROSE*				
DEXTROSE/K CL/K PHOS/NA ACE/NA CL				
(B. Braun) *See ISOLYTE M W/DEXTROSE*				
DEXTROSE/K CL/MG CL/NA ACE/NA CL				
(B. Braun) *See ISOLYTE H W/DEXTROSE*				
DEXTROSE/K CL/MG CL/NA ACE/NA CL/ NA GLUCONATE				
(B. Braun) *See ISOLYTE S W/DEXTROSE*				
(Hospira) *See NORMOSOL-R W/5% DEXTROSE*				
DEXTROSE/K PHOS/MG CL/NA CL/NA LACT/NA PHOS				
(Hospira) *See IONOSOL B/5% DEXTROSE*				
DEXTROSE/LACTATED RINGERS/POTASSIUM CHLORIDE (Hospira)				
ca cl/dextrose/k cl/na cl/na lact				
SOL, IV (5% DEXTROSE,LATEX-FREE)				
1000 ml 12s	00409-7113-09	41.90	36.72	AP
DEXTROSE/LIDO HCL/TETRACAINE HCL				
(Portex) *See SPINAL-22 ANESTHESIA TRAY*				
(Portex) *See SPINAL-25 ANESTHESIA TRAY*				
DEXTROSE/LIDOCAINE HCL (B. Braun)				
dextrose/lidocaine hydrochloride				
SOL, IV (EXCEL)				
5%-0.4%, 250 ml	00264-9594-20	7.21		AP
500 ml	00264-9594-10	8.00		AP
5%-0.8%, 250 ml	00264-9598-20	6.40		AP
500 ml	00264-9598-10	27.12		AP
(Baxter)				
SOL, IV, 5%-0.4%,				
250 ml 24s	00338-0409-02	423.08		AP
500 ml 18s	00338-0409-03	409.32		AP
5%-0.8%,				
250 ml 24s	00338-0411-02	545.76		AP
(Hospira)				
SOL, IJ ((AMP,SPINAL)25X2ML)				
7.5%-5%, 2 ml 25s	00409-4712-01	156.30	136.75	AP
IV (LIFECARE,12X250ML)				
5%-0.4%,				
250 ml 12s	00409-7931-32	63.65	55.68	AP
(LIFECARE,24X500ML)				
5%-0.4%,				
500 ml 24s	00409-7931-24	147.74	129.36	AP
(LIFECARE,LATEX-FREE)				
5%-0.8%,				
250 ml 12s	00409-7939-32	83.95	73.44	AP
DEXTROSE/LIDOCAINE HYDROCHLORIDE				
(B. Braun) *See DEXTROSE/LIDOCAINE HCL*				
(Baxter) *See DEXTROSE/LIDOCAINE HCL*				
(Hospira) *See DEXTROSE/LIDOCAINE HCL*				
DEXTROSE/MAGNESIUM SULFATE				
(Hospira) *See MAGNESIUM SULFATE IN DEXTROSE*				
(Hospira)				
SOL, IV (PLASTIC CONTAINER)				
5%-1 gm/100 ml,				
100 ml 24s	00409-6727-23	163.58	143.04	
(PharMEDium Services) *See DEXTROSE-MAGNESIUM SULFATE*				
(PharMEDium Services) *See MAGNESIUM SULFATE IN DEXTROSE*				
DEXTROSE/MILRINONE LACTATE (Baxter)				
SOL, IV (BAG,INTRAVIA)				
5%-20 mg/100 ml,				
100 ml	00338-6010-48	145.19	120.99	AP
200 ml	00338-6011-37	283.13	235.94	AP
(Bedford) *See MILRINONE LACTATE IN DEXTROSE*				
(Hospira) *See MILRINONE LACTATE*				
DEXTROSE/MORPHINE SULFATE				
(Hospira) *See MORPHINE SULFATE IN 5% DEXTROSE*				
(Hospira)				
SOL, IV (PREMIX)				
5%-100 mg/100 ml,				
100 ml, C-II	00409-6062-11	10.26	8.98	
(PharMEDium Services)				
SOL, IV (INTRAVIA)				
5%-100 mg/100 ml,				
100 ml, C-II	61553-0183-48	26.56	22.13	
250 ml, C-II	61553-0185-02	32.04	26.70	
(SRN,35 ML)				
5%-2 mg/ml,				
25 ml, C-II	61553-0186-67	21.58	17.98	
(SRN,60 ML)				
5%-2 mg/ml,				
50 ml, C-II	61553-0187-75	23.26	19.38	
DEXTROSE/NACL/POTASSIUM CHLORIDE (Baxter)				
dextrose/potassium chloride/sodium chloride				
SOL, IV, 5%-0.075%-0.2%,				
1000 ml 12s	00338-0661-04	201.46		AP
5%-0.075%-0.45%,				
1000 ml 12s	00338-0669-04	201.46		AP
5%-0.15%-0.2%,				
500 ml 18s	00338-0663-03	273.36		AP
1000 ml 12s	00338-0663-04	201.46		AP
5%-0.15%-0.3%,				
500 ml 24s	00338-0603-03	273.36		AP
1000 ml 12s	00338-0603-04	201.46		AP
5%-0.15%-0.45%,				
500 ml 18s	00338-0671-03	273.36		AP
1000 ml 12s	00338-0671-04	201.46		AP
5%-0.15%-0.9%,				
1000 ml 12s	00338-0803-04	201.46		AP
5%-0.22%-0.45%,				
1000 ml 12s	00338-0673-04	201.46		
5%-0.3%-0.2%,				
1000 ml 12s	00338-0667-04	201.46		AP

PROD/MFR	NDC	AWP	DP	OBC
5%-0.3%-0.45%,				
1000 ml 12s	00338-0675-04	201.46		AP
5%-0.3%-0.9%,				
1000 ml 12s	00338-0807-04	201.46		AP
DEXTROSE/NICARDIPINE HYDROCHLORIDE (EKR) *See CARDENE*				
DEXTROSE/NITROGLYCERIN (Baxter)				
SOL, IV, 5%-10 mg/100 ml,				
250 ml 12s	00338-1047-02	192.08		AP
5%-20 mg/100 ml,				
250 ml 12s	00338-1049-02	196.13		AP
5%-40 mg/100 ml,				
250 ml 12s	00338-1051-02	208.47		AP
(Hospira)				
SOL, IV (LATEX-FREE)				
5%-10 mg/100 ml,				
250 ml 12s	00409-1483-02	91.44	80.04	AP
(12X500ML,LATEX-FREE)				
5%-10 mg/100 ml,				
500 ml 12s	00409-1483-03	94.03	82.32	AP
(LATEX-FREE)				
5%-20 mg/100 ml,				
250 ml 12s	00409-1482-02	85.97	75.24	AP
5%-40 mg/100 ml,				
250 ml 12s	00409-1484-02	107.71	94.20	AP
(12X500ML,LATEX-FREE)				
5%-40 mg/100 ml,				
500 ml 12s	00409-1484-03	120.53	105.48	AP
DEXTROSE/POTASSIUM CHLORIDE (B. Braun)				
SOL, IV (EXCEL)				
5%-0.15%, 1000 ml	00264-7625-00	2.80		AP
5%-0.3%, 1000 ml	00264-7628-00	2.80		AP
(Baxter)				
SOL, IV, 5%-0.15%,				
1000 ml 12s	00338-0683-04	201.46		AP
(Hospira)				
SOL, IV (LIFECARE,12X1000ML)				
5%-0.15%,				
1000 ml 12s	00409-7905-09	34.99	30.60	AP
(LATEX-FREE)				
5%-0.224%,				
1000 ml 12s	00409-7996-09	39.89	34.92	AP
(LIFECARE,12X1000ML)				
5%-0.3%,				
1000 ml 12s	00409-7906-09	34.99	30.60	AP
DEXTROSE/POTASSIUM CHLORIDE/ SODIUM CHLORIDE				
(B. Braun) *See DEXTROSE/POTASSIUM CL/SODIUM CL*				
(Baxter) *See DEXTROSE/NACL/POTASSIUM CHLORIDE*				
(Baxter) *See POTASSIUM CHLORIDE IN DEXTROSE AND SODIUM CHLORIDE*				
(Hospira) *See DEXTROSE/POTASSIUM CL/SODIUM CL*				
(Hospira)				
SOL, IV (LATEX-FREE)				
5%-0.075%-0.45%,				
1000 ml 12s	00409-7993-09	31.68	27.72	AP
(24X500ML,LATEX-FREE)				
5%-0.15%-0.3%,				
500 ml 24s	00409-7998-03	93.31	81.60	AP
(LATEX-FREE)				
5%-0.15%-0.3%,				
1000 ml 12s	00409-7998-09	35.86	31.32	AP
DEXTROSE/POTASSIUM CL/SODIUM CL (B. Braun)				
dextrose/potassium chloride/sodium chloride				
SOL, IV (EXCEL)				
5%-0.075%-0.45%,				
1000 ml	00264-7634-00	2.80		AP
5%-0.15%-0.2%,				
250 ml	00264-7645-20	2.15		AP
1000 ml	00264-7645-00	2.80		AP
5%-0.15%-0.3%,				
1000 ml	00264-7655-00	2.90		AP
5%-0.15%-0.45%,				
1000 ml	00264-7635-00	2.80		AP
5%-0.15%-0.9%,				
1000 ml	00264-7652-00	3.50		AP
5%-0.22%-0.45%,				
1000 ml	00264-7636-00	2.80		
(EXCEL,40MEQ K+/L)				
5%-0.3%-0.2%,				
1000 ml	00264-7648-00	19.06		AP
(EXCEL)				
5%-0.3%-0.45%,				
1000 ml	00264-7638-00	2.90		AP
10%-0.15%-0.2%,				
1000 ml	00264-7663-20	8.27		

PROD/MFR	NDC	AWP	DP	OBC
(Hospira)				
SOL, IV (LATEX-FREE)				
5%-0.075%-0.2%,				
1000 ml 12s	00409-7997-09	34.99	30.60	AP
(24X500ML,LATEX-FREE)				
5%-0.15%-0.2%,				
500 ml 24s	00409-7901-03	93.02	81.36	AP
(12X1000ML,LATEX-FREE)				
5%-0.15%-0.2%,				
1000 ml 12s	00409-7901-09	31.68	27.72	AP
(LATEX-FREE)				
5%-0.15%-0.45%,				
500 ml 24s	00409-7902-03	95.04	83.28	AP
1000 ml 12s	00409-7902-09	27.94	24.48	AP
5%-0.15%-0.9%,				
1000 ml 12s	00409-7107-09	37.87	33.12	AP
5%-0.22%-0.2%,				
1000 ml 12s	00409-7991-09	35.86	31.32	
5%-0.3%-0.2%,				
1000 ml 12s	00409-7992-09	33.98	29.76	AP
(12X1000ML,LATEX-FREE)				
5%-0.3%-0.45%,				
1000 ml 12s	00409-7904-09	31.68	27.72	AP
(LATEX-FREE)				
5%-0.3%-0.9%,				
1000 ml 12s	00409-7109-09	42.19	36.96	AP
DEXTROSE/POTASSIUM/SODIUM CHLORIDE				
(Hospira) *See POTASSIUM CHLORIDE*				
DEXTROSE/SODIUM CHLORIDE (B. Braun)				
SOL, IV (EXCEL)				
2.5%-0.45%, 500 ml	00264-7605-10	3.01		AP
1000 ml	00264-7605-00	2.21		AP
5%-0.2%, 250 ml	00264-7616-20	1.96		AP
500 ml	00264-7616-10	2.05		AP
1000 ml	00264-7616-00	2.10		AP
5%-0.33%, 500 ml	00264-7614-10	2.05		AP
1000 ml	00264-7614-00	2.10		AP
5%-0.45%, 250 ml	00264-7612-20	1.96		AP
500 ml	00264-7612-10	2.05		AP
1000 ml	00264-7612-00	2.10		AP
5%-0.9%, 250 ml	00264-7610-20	1.96		AP
500 ml	00264-7610-10	1.64		AP
1000 ml	00264-7610-00	2.10		AP
10%-0.2%, 250 ml	00264-7623-20	6.82		
10%-0.45%, 1000 ml	00264-7622-00	4.80		
(GLASS)				
10%-0.45%, 1000 ml	00264-1222-00	19.45		
(Baxter) *See DEXTROSE AND SODIUM CHLORIDE*				
(Baxter)				
SOL, IV, 2.5%-0.45%,				
500 ml 24s	00338-0073-03	230.98		AP
(USP,VIAFLEX PC)				
2.5%-0.45%,				
1000 ml 14s	00338-0073-04	135.50		AP
5%-0.2%, 250 ml 36s	00338-0077-02	357.69		AP
500 ml 24s	00338-0077-03	238.46		AP
(USP,VIAFLEX PC)				
5%-0.2%,				
1000 ml 14s	00338-0077-04	141.70		AP
5%-0.33%,				
500 ml 24s	00338-0081-03	238.46		AP
5%-0.45%,				
250 ml 36s	00338-0085-02	357.69		AP
500 ml 24s	00338-0085-03	238.46		AP
1000 ml 12s	00338-0085-04	141.70		AP
5%-0.9%, 250 ml 36s	00338-0089-02	357.69		AP
500 ml 24s	00338-0089-03	238.46		AP
1000 ml 12s	00338-0089-04	141.70		AP
(Hospira) *See DEXTROSE AND SODIUM CHLORIDE*				
(Hospira)				
SOL, IV (24X250ML,LATEX-FREE)				
5%-0.225%,				
250 ml 24s	00409-7924-02	35.14	30.72	
(LIFECARE, 24X500ML)				
5%-0.225%,				
500 ml 24s	00409-7924-03	38.59	33.84	
(LIFECARE, PLASTIC)				
5%-0.225%,				
1000 ml 12s	00409-7924-09	23.90	20.88	
(LIFECARE, 24X250ML)				
5%-0.3%,				
250 ml 24s	00409-7925-02	40.03	35.04	
(LIFECARE,24X500ML)				
5%-0.3%,				
500 ml 24s	00409-7925-03	47.81	41.76	
(12X1000ML)				
5%-0.3%,				
1000 ml 12s	00409-7925-09	22.90	20.04	
(LIFECARE/PLASTIC)				
5%-0.45%,				
250 ml 24s	00409-7926-02	35.14	30.72	AP

PROD/MFR	NDC	AWP	DP	OBC
(24X500ML,LATEX-FREE)				
5%-0.45%,				
500 ml 24s	00409-7926-03	38.02	33.36	AP
(VISIV CONTAINER)				
5%-0.45%,				
500 ml 24s	00409-7926-30	36.86	32.16	AP
(12X1000ML, LIFECARE)				
5%-0.45%,				
1000 ml 12s	00409-7926-09	23.62	20.64	AP
(VISIV CONTAINER)				
5%-0.45%,				
1000 ml 12s	00409-7926-48	20.02	17.52	AP
(24X500ML,LATEX-FREE)				
5%-0.9%,				
500 ml 24s	00409-7941-03	39.74	34.80	AP
(LIFECARE,12X1000ML)				
5%-0.9%,				
1000 ml 12s	00409-7941-09	25.78	22.56	AP
10%-0.225%,				
250 ml 12s	00409-4862-02	70.99	62.16	
500 ml 12s	00409-4862-03	68.83	60.24	
DEXTROSE/THEOPHYLLINE (B. Braun)				
SOL, IV (EXCEL)				
5%-80 mg/100 ml,				
500 ml	00264-9554-10	5.21		AP
1000 ml	00264-9554-00	4.91		AP
5%-160 mg/100 ml,				
500 ml	00264-9558-10	3.62		AP
(Baxter)				
SOL, IV, 5%-80 mg/100 ml,				
500 ml 18s	00338-0439-03	181.98		AP
5%-160 mg/100 ml,				
500 ml 18s	00338-0441-03	197.28		AP
(Hospira)				
SOL, IV (LATEX-FREE)				
5%-80 mg/100 ml,				
500 ml 24s	00409-7665-03	127.30	111.36	AP
1000 ml 12s	00409-7665-09	82.51	72.24	AP
(50MLX24,DEHP,LATEX-FREE)				
5%-200 mg/50 ml,				
50 ml 24s	00409-7677-13	162.72	142.32	AP
(Hospira) *See THEOPHYLLINE IN DEXTROSE*				
DEXTROSE/VANCOMYCIN HYDROCHLORIDE				
(Baxter) *See VANCOCIN HCL*				
DEXTROSTAT (Phys Total Care)				
REPACK				
dextroamphetamine sulfate				
TAB, PO, 5 mg,				
20s ea, C-II	54868-4549-00	29.19		AA
60s ea, C-II	54868-4549-01	72.60		
DI-N-PROPYL ISOCINCHOMERONATE (PCCA)				
SOL, NA (1X1ML)				
1 ml	51927-3125-00	17.40		
DIAB F.D.G. (Carrington)				
bandage				
DEV, NA (4",FREEZE-DRIED GEL)				
ea	53303-0002-04	9.19		
DIAB GEL (Carrington)				
bandage				
DEV, NA (HYDROGEL)				
85 gm	53303-0019-30	23.89		
DIABETA (Sanofi-Aventis)				
glyburide				
TAB, PO, 1.25 mg, 50s ea	00039-0053-05	16.85		BX
2.5 mg, 100s ea	00039-0051-10	65.96		BX
5 mg, 100s ea	00039-0052-10	120.97		BX
1000s ea	00039-0052-70	993.26		BX
(Phys Total Care)				
REPACK				
TAB, PO, 2.5 mg, 30s ea	54868-0373-01	18.39		BX
100s ea	54868-0373-02	56.93		BX
5 mg, 30s ea	54868-0996-02	29.41		BX
100s ea	54868-0996-01	95.23		BX
DIABETIC SUPPLIES				
(Medtronic Minimed) *See QUICK-SET PARADIGM*				
(Medtronic Minimed) *See SILHOUETTE PARADIGM*				
(Medtronic Minimed) *See SURE-T PARADIGM*				
DIACETAZONE (Stat Rx)				
REPACK				
apap/dichloralphenazone/isometheptene mucate				
CAP, PO, 325 mg-100 mg-65 mg,				
30s ea, C-IV	16590-0850-30	18.33		
60s ea, C-IV	16590-0850-60	36.66		
DIACETAZOTOL (PCCA)				
POW, NA, 1 gm	51927-2804-00	30.00		

PROD/MFR	NDC	AWP	DP	OBC
DIAL-A-FLO (Abbott Hosp)				
kit, intravenous extension tubing				
DEV, NA (IV EXTENSION,18")				
48s ea	00074-1671-02	527.25	444.00	
(LTXF,CONV PIN 78,MICDRP)				
48s ea	00074-1674-78	710.79	598.56	
DIALYVITE (Hillestad)				
vitamin b complex and vitamin c				
TAB, PO, 100s ea	10542-0010-10	15.58	14.15	
DIALYVITE 3000 (Hillestad)				
vitamin b complex, mineral, and vitamin c				
TAB, PO, 90s ea	10542-0014-09	28.73	25.34	
DIALYVITE 5000 (Hillestad)				
multivitamin, minerals, and nutriceuticals				
TAB, PO, 90s ea	10542-0011-09	47.89	42.23	
DIALYVITE WITH ZINC (Hillestad)				
vitamin b complex, mineral, and vitamin c				
TAB, PO, 100s ea	10542-0012-10	16.96	15.30	
DIAMINOPYRIDINE (PCCA)				
3,4-diaminopyridine				
POW, NA, 1 gm	51927-2569-00	134.40		
3,4-DIAMINOPYRIDINE (Spectrum Pharmacy)				
POW, NA (1X1GM)				
1 gm	49452-2527-01	171.85		
DIAMOX SEQUELS (Teva)				
acetazolamide				
CER, PO, 500 mg, 100s ea	51285-0754-02	500.97	112.16	
DIANEAL LOW CALCIUM PERITONEAL DIALYSIS W/DEXTROSE (Baxter)				
ca cl/dextrose/mg cl/na cl/na lact				
SOL, PT (ULTRABAG, 8X1500ML)				
1500 ml 8s	00941-0424-51	299.33	249.44	AT
(AMBU-FLEX III, 6X2000ML)				
2000 ml 6s	00941-0409-36	125.14	104.28	AT
(ULTRABAG, 6X2000ML)				
2000 ml 6s	00941-0424-52	209.82	174.85	AT
(ULTRABAG, 5X2500ML)				
2500 ml 5s	00941-0424-53	194.08	161.73	AT
(AMBU-FLEX III, 4X3000ML)				
3000 ml 4s	00941-0409-49	144.77	120.64	AT
(ULTRABAG, 4X3000ML)				
3000 ml 4s	00941-0424-55	171.73	143.11	AT
(AMBU-FLEX III, 2X5000ML)				
5000 ml 2s	00941-0409-27	77.83	64.86	AT
(AMBU-FLEX III, 2X6000ML)				
6000 ml 2s	00941-0409-28	93.41	77.84	AT
(ULTRABAG, 8X1500ML)				
1500 ml 8s	00941-0430-51	307.60	256.33	
(AMBU-FLEX III, 6X2000ML)				
2000 ml 6s	00941-0457-47	151.10	125.92	
(ULTRABAG, 1X2000ML)				
2000 ml 6s	00941-0430-52	234.11	195.09	
(ULTRABAG, 5X2500ML)				
2500 ml 5s	00941-0430-53	199.58	166.32	
(AMBU-FLEX III, 4X3000ML)				
3000 ml 4s	00941-0457-49	147.74	123.12	
(ULTRABAG, 4X3000ML)				
3000 ml 4s	00941-0430-55	175.51	146.26	
(AMBU-FLEX III, 2X5000ML)				
5000 ml 2s	00941-0457-25	79.90	66.58	
(AMBU-FLEX III, 2X6000ML)				
6000 ml 2s	00941-0457-28	95.87	79.89	
(ULTRABAG, 8X1500ML)				
1500 ml 8s	00941-0433-51	309.92	258.27	
(AMBU-FLEX III, 6X2000ML)				
2000 ml 6s	00941-0459-47	152.62	127.18	
(ULTRABAG, 6X2000ML)				
2000 ml 6s	00941-0433-52	236.24	196.87	
(ULTRABAG, 5X2500ML)				
2500 ml 5s	00941-0433-53	203.86	169.88	
(AMBU-FLEX III, 4X3000ML)				
3000 ml 4s	00941-0459-49	151.10	125.92	
(ULTRABAG, 4X3000ML)				
3000 ml 4s	00941-0433-55	180.89	150.74	
(AMBU-FLEX III, 2X5000ML)				
5000 ml 2s	00941-0459-25	81.86	68.22	
(AMBU-FLEX III, 2X6000ML)				
6000 ml 2s	00941-0459-28	98.23	81.86	
DIANEAL PD-2 PERITONEAL DIALYSIS SOLN W/DEXTROSE (Baxter)				
ca cl/dextrose/mg cl/na cl/na lact				
SOL, PT (AMBU-FLEX III,12X1000ML)				
1000 ml 12s	00941-0411-43	334.55	278.79	AT
(AMBU-FLEX III, 6X2000ML)				
2000 ml 6s	00941-0411-46	125.14	104.28	AT
(ULTRABAG, 6X2000ML)				
2000 ml 6s	00941-0426-52	209.82	174.85	AT
(ULTRABAG,5X2500ML)				
2500 ml 5s	00941-0426-53	194.08	161.73	AT
(AMBU-FLEX III, 4X3000ML)				
3000 ml 4s	00941-0411-49	144.77	120.64	AT
(ULTRABAG, 4X3000ML)				
3000 ml 4s	00941-0426-55	171.73	143.11	AT
(AMBU-FLEX III, 2X5000ML)				
5000 ml 2s	00941-0411-25	77.83	64.86	AT
(AMBU-FLEX III, 2X6000ML)				
6000 ml 2s	00941-0411-28	93.41	77.84	AT
(AMBU-FLEX III,12X1000ML)				
1000 ml 12s	00941-0413-43	359.64	299.70	AT
(AMBU-FLEX III, 6X2000ML)				
2000 ml 6s	00941-0413-47	151.10	125.92	AT
(ULTRABAG, 6X2000ML)				
2000 ml 6s	00941-0427-52	234.11	195.09	AT
(ULTRABAG, 5X2500ML)				
2500 ml 5s	00941-0427-53	199.58	166.32	AT
(AMBU-FLEX III, 4X3000ML)				
3000 ml 4s	00941-0413-49	147.74	123.12	AT
(ULTRABAG, 4X3000ML)				
3000 ml 4s	00941-0427-55	175.52	146.27	AT
(AMBU-FLEX III, 2X5000ML)				
5000 ml 2s	00941-0413-25	79.90	66.58	AT
(AMBU-FLEX III, 2X6000ML)				
6000 ml 2s	00941-0413-28	95.87	79.89	AT
(AMBU-FLEX III,12X1000ML)				
1000 ml 12s	00941-0415-43	358.40	298.67	AT
(AMBU-FLEX III, 6X2000ML)				
2000 ml 6s	00941-0415-47	152.62	127.18	AT
(ULTRABAG, 6X2000ML)				
2000 ml 6s	00941-0429-52	236.24	196.87	AT
(ULTRABAG, 5X2500ML)				
2500 ml 5s	00941-0429-53	203.86	169.88	AT
(AMBU-FLEX III, 4X3000ML)				
3000 ml 4s	00941-0415-49	151.10	125.92	AT
(ULTRABAG, 4X3000ML)				
3000 ml 4s	00941-0429-55	180.89	150.74	AT
(AMBU-FLEX III, 2X5000ML)				
5000 ml 2s	00941-0415-25	81.86	68.22	AT
(AMBU-FLEX III, 2X6000ML)				
6000 ml 2s	00941-0415-28	98.23	81.86	AT
DIASTAT (Dispensing Solutions)				
REPACK				
diazepam				
GEL, MR, 2.5 mg,				
ea, C-IV	55045-3706-02	270.00		
DIASTAT ACUDIAL (Valeant Pharm Intl)				
diazepam				
GEL, MR (TWIN PACK)				
10 mg, ea, C-IV	00187-0658-20	447.48		
20 mg, ea, C-IV	00187-0659-20	447.48		
(Phys Total Care)				
REPACK				
GEL, MR (TWIN PACK)				
20 mg, ea, C-IV	54868-5490-00	352.20		
DIASTAT PEDIATRIC (Valeant Pharm Intl)				
diazepam				
GEL, MR (2X2.5 MG SRNS TWIN-PACK)				
2.5 mg, ea, C-IV	66490-0650-20	377.21		
DIATRIZOATE MEGLUMINE				
(Bracco Diag) *See CYSTOGRAFIN*				
(Bracco Diag) *See CYSTOGRAFIN-DILUTE*				
(Bracco Diag) *See RENO-30*				
(Bracco Diag) *See RENO-60*				
(Bracco Diag) *See RENO-DIP*				
DIATRIZOATE MEGLUMINE/DIATRIZOATE SODIUM				
(Bracco Diag) *See GASTROGRAFIN*				
(Bracco Diag) *See RENOCAL-76*				
(Bracco Diag) *See RENOGRAFIN-60*				
(Mallinckrodt Inc.) *See MD-GASTROVIEW*				
DIATRIZOATE MEGLUMINE/ IODIPAMIDE MEGLUMINE				
(Bracco Diag) *See SINOGRAFIN*				
DIATRIZOATE SODIUM				
(GE) *See HYPAQUE SODIUM*				
DIATX ZN (Pamlab)				
vitamin b complex, mineral, and vitamin c				
TAB, PO (MEDICAL FOOD,SF)				
90s ea	00525-4281-90	71.56		
DIAZEPAM				
FUL				
TAB, PO, 2 mg, 100s ea		4.23		
5 mg, 100s ea		7.18		
10 mg, 100s ea		5.73		
(Gallipot)				
POW, NA (1X5GM,USP)				
5 gm	51552-1025-02	11.20	8.00	
(1X25GM,USP)				
25 gm	51552-1025-04	44.80	32.00	
(1X100GM,USP)				
100 gm	51552-1025-05	126.00	90.00	
(Hospira)				
SOL, IJ (10X2ML, LUER LOCK)				
5 mg/ml,				
2 ml 10s, C-IV	00409-1273-32	36.48	31.90	AP
(10X2ML,ISECURESYRINGE)				
5 mg/ml,				
2 ml 10s, C-IV	00409-1273-05	28.56	25.00	AP
(MDV,FLIPTOP)				
5 mg/ml,				
10 ml 5s, C-IV	00409-3213-02	37.02	32.40	AP
(10X10ML,USP,MDV,FLIPTOP)				
5 mg/ml,				
10 ml 10s, C-IV	00409-3213-12	58.08	50.80	AP
(Major)				
TAB, PO (USP,10X10)				
5 mg,				
100s ea UD, C-IV	00904-5880-61	31.95		EE
10 mg,				
100s ea UD, C-IV	00904-5881-61	39.86		EE
(Medisca)				
POW, NA (U.S.P.)				
100 gm	38779-0925-05	252.00		
500 gm	38779-0925-08	1020.00		
1000 gm	38779-0925-09	2356.50		
(Mylan)				
TAB, PO, 2 mg,				
100s ea, C-IV	00378-0271-01	10.45		AB
500s ea, C-IV	00378-0271-05	46.65		AB
5 mg, 100s ea, C-IV	00378-0345-01	16.35		AB
500s ea, C-IV	00378-0345-05	73.40		AB
10 mg, 100s ea, C-IV	00378-0477-01	31.25		AB
500s ea, C-IV	00378-0477-05	148.45		AB
(PCCA)				
POW, NA (U.S.P.; CIV)				
1 gm	51927-1014-00	3.84		
(Qualitest)				
TAB, PO (USP,DYE-FREE)				
2 mg, 30s ea, C-IV	00603-3213-16	4.30		AB
60s ea, C-IV	00603-3213-20	8.61		AB
100s ea, C-IV	00603-3213-21	14.35		AB
500s ea, C-IV	00603-3213-28	62.50		AB
(USP)				
5 mg, 30s ea, C-IV	00603-3214-16	6.60		AB
60s ea, C-IV	00603-3214-20	13.20		AB
90s ea, C-IV	00603-3214-02	19.80		AB
100s ea, C-IV	00603-3214-21	22.00		AB
120s ea, C-IV	00603-3214-22	26.40		AB
500s ea, C-IV	00603-3214-28	99.05		AB
1000s ea, C-IV	00603-3214-32	188.20		AB
10 mg, 30s ea, C-IV	00603-3215-16	12.63		AB
60s ea, C-IV	00603-3215-20	25.26		AB
90s ea, C-IV	00603-3215-02	37.89		AB
100s ea, C-IV	00603-3215-21	42.10		AB
120s ea, C-IV	00603-3215-22	50.52		AB
500s ea, C-IV	00603-3215-28	168.85		AB
1000s ea, C-IV	00603-3215-32	320.81		AB
(Roche Labs) *See VALIUM*				
(Roxane) *See DIAZEPAM INTENSOL*				
(Roxane)				
SOL, PO (WINTERGREEN-SPICE)				
5 mg/5 ml,				
5 ml 40s UD, C-IV	00054-8207-16	88.76		
500 ml, C-IV	00054-3188-63	50.95		
(Spectrum Pharmacy)				
CRY, NA (BP)				
100 gm, C-IV	49452-2540-01	367.50		
500 gm, C-IV	49452-2540-02	1382.50		
1000 gm, C-IV	49452-2540-03	2177.00		
(Teva)				
TAB, PO, 2 mg,				
100s ea, C-IV	00172-3925-60	12.50		AB
100s ea, C-IV	00555-0163-02	10.65		AB
500s ea, C-IV	00172-3925-70	62.50		AB
1000s ea, C-IV	00555-0163-05	95.10		AB
5 mg, 100s ea, C-IV	00172-3926-60	19.95		AB
500s ea, C-IV	00172-3926-70	99.75		AB
1000s ea, C-IV	00555-0363-05	149.70		AB
10 mg, 100s ea, C-IV	00172-3927-60	33.00		AB
100s ea, C-IV	00555-0164-02	31.85		AB
500s ea, C-IV	00172-3927-70	165.00		AB
1000s ea, C-IV	00555-0164-05	302.80		AB

PROD/MFR	NDC	AWP	DP	OBC
(UDL)				
TAB, PO (10X10)				
2 mg,				
100s ea UD, C-IV	**51079-0284-20**	24.21		AB
5 mg,				
100s ea UD, C-IV	**51079-0285-20**	32.14		AB
10 mg,				
100s ea UD, C-IV	**51079-0286-20**	42.50		AB
(Valeant Pharm Intl) *See DIASTAT ACUDIAL*				
(Valeant Pharm Intl) *See DIASTAT PEDIATRIC*				
(Watson Labs)				
TAB, PO, 2 mg,				
100s ea, C-IV	**00591-5621-01**	3.38		AB
500s ea, C-IV	**00591-5621-05**	16.42		AB
1000s ea, C-IV	**00591-5621-10**	32.20		AB
5 mg, 100s ea, C-IV	**00591-5619-01**	3.53		AB
500s ea, C-IV	**00591-5619-05**	17.11		AB
1000s ea, C-IV	**00591-5619-10**	33.53		AB
10 mg, 100s ea, C-IV	**00591-5620-01**	4.58		AB
500s ea, C-IV	**00591-5620-05**	22.24		AB
1000s ea, C-IV	**00591-5620-10**	43.58		AB
(4u)				
REPACK				
TAB, PO, 5 mg,				
30s ea, C-IV	**10544-0403-30**	34.46		AB
30s ea, C-IV	**42549-0309-30**	32.14		AB
30s ea, C-IV	**42549-0509-30**	34.46		AB
30s ea, C-IV	**42549-0603-30**	34.46		AB
90s ea, C-IV	**42549-0603-90**	103.38		AB
10 mg, 2s ea, C-IV	**42549-0554-92**	6.84		AB
30s ea, C-IV	**10544-0354-30**	54.26		AB
30s ea, C-IV	**42549-0554-30**	54.26		AB
60s ea, C-IV	**42549-0554-60**	77.46		AB
(A-S Medication)				
REPACK				
TAB, PO, 2 mg,				
30s ea, C-IV	**54569-0947-00**	4.21		EE
5 mg, 2s ea, C-IV	**54569-4764-03**	0.22		EE
6s ea, C-IV	**54569-0949-07**	1.32		EE
10s ea, C-IV	**54569-0949-04**	2.20		EE
15s ea, C-IV	**54569-0949-00**	3.30		EE
20s ea, C-IV	**54569-0949-01**	4.40		EE
30s ea, C-IV	**54569-0949-02**	6.60		EE
100s ea, C-IV	**54569-0949-05**	22.01		EE
10 mg, 2s ea, C-IV	**54569-0936-07**	0.84		EE
5s ea, C-IV	**54569-0936-05**	2.11		EE
15s ea, C-IV	**54569-0936-04**	6.33		EE
25s ea, C-IV	**54569-5354-04**	10.55		EE
30s ea, C-IV	**54569-0936-02**	12.66		EE
60s ea, C-IV	**54569-0936-03**	25.31		EE
90s ea, C-IV	**54569-0936-08**	37.97		EE
100s ea, C-IV	**54569-0936-00**	42.19		EE
(Aidarex)				
REPACK				
TAB, PO, 5 mg, 7s ea, C-IV	**33261-0034-07**	12.25		AB
14s ea, C-IV	**33261-0034-14**	24.50		AB
20s ea, C-IV	**33261-0034-20**	35.00		AB
21s ea, C-IV	**33261-0034-21**	36.75		AB
28s ea, C-IV	**33261-0034-28**	49.00		AB
30s ea, C-IV	**33261-0034-30**	52.50		AB
60s ea, C-IV	**33261-0034-60**	105.00		AB
90s ea, C-IV	**33261-0034-90**	157.50		AB
10 mg, 7s ea, C-IV	**33261-0035-07**	17.50		AB
14s ea, C-IV	**33261-0035-14**	35.00		AB
20s ea, C-IV	**33261-0035-20**	50.00		AB
21s ea, C-IV	**33261-0035-21**	52.50		AB
28s ea, C-IV	**33261-0035-28**	70.00		AB
30s ea, C-IV	**33261-0035-30**	75.00		AB
60s ea, C-IV	**33261-0035-60**	150.00		AB
90s ea, C-IV	**33261-0035-90**	225.00		AB
(Altura)				
REPACK				
TAB, PO, 2 mg,				
10s ea, C-IV	**63874-0226-10**	4.11		AB
12s ea, C-IV	**63874-0226-12**	4.94		AB
15s ea, C-IV	**63874-0226-15**	6.17		EE
20s ea, C-IV	**63874-0226-20**	8.23		EE
28s ea, C-IV	**63874-0226-28**	11.52		AB
30s ea, C-IV	**63874-0226-30**	12.34		EE
60s ea, C-IV	**63874-0226-60**	24.68		AB
90s ea, C-IV	**63874-0226-90**	37.02		AB
100s ea, C-IV	**63874-0226-01**	41.13		EE
120s ea, C-IV	**63874-0226-04**	49.36		AB
1000s ea, C-IV	**63874-0226-02**	72.80		EE
5 mg, 5s ea, C-IV	**63874-0227-05**	3.38		
6s ea, C-IV	**63874-0227-06**	4.05		
8s ea, C-IV	**63874-0227-08**	5.41		
9s ea, C-IV	**63874-0227-09**	6.08		
10s ea, C-IV	**63874-0227-10**	6.76		EE
12s ea, C-IV	**63874-0227-12**	8.11		
14s ea, C-IV	**63874-0227-14**	9.46		
15s ea, C-IV	**63874-0227-15**	10.14		AB
16s ea, C-IV	**63874-0227-16**	10.81		
18s ea, C-IV	**63874-0227-18**	12.16		
20s ea, C-IV	**63874-0227-20**	13.51		EE
21s ea, C-IV	**63874-0227-21**	14.19		
24s ea, C-IV	**63874-0227-24**	16.22		
28s ea, C-IV	**63874-0227-28**	18.92		
30s ea, C-IV	**63874-0227-30**	20.27		EE
36s ea, C-IV	**63874-0227-36**	24.33		AB
40s ea, C-IV	**63874-0227-40**	27.03		
50s ea, C-IV	**63874-0227-50**	33.78		
60s ea, C-IV	**63874-0227-60**	54.08		
90s ea, C-IV	**63874-0227-90**	60.81		
100s ea, C-IV	**63874-0227-01**	67.57		EE
120s ea, C-IV	**63874-0227-04**	81.08		
125s ea, C-IV	**63874-0227-87**	112.64		
150s ea, C-IV	**63874-0227-72**	135.17		
200s ea, C-IV	**63874-0227-74**	180.22		
300s ea, C-IV	**63874-0227-77**	270.33		
1000s ea, C-IV	**63874-0227-02**	104.00		EE
10 mg, 6s ea, C-IV	**63874-0228-06**	9.10		EE
9s ea, C-IV	**63874-0228-09**	13.65		EE
10s ea, C-IV	**63874-0228-10**	15.17		EE
12s ea, C-IV	**63874-0228-12**	18.20		EE
15s ea, C-IV	**63874-0228-15**	22.75		EE
20s ea, C-IV	**63874-0228-20**	30.34		EE
28s ea, C-IV	**63874-0228-28**	42.47		EE
30s ea, C-IV	**63874-0228-30**	45.50		EE
40s ea, C-IV	**63874-0228-40**	60.67		EE
60s ea, C-IV	**63874-0228-60**	91.00		EE
90s ea, C-IV	**63874-0228-90**	136.51		EE
100s ea, C-IV	**63874-0228-01**	151.68		EE
120s ea, C-IV	**63874-0228-04**	182.01		EE
150s ea, C-IV	**63874-0228-72**	227.51		EE
200s ea, C-IV	**63874-0228-74**	303.35		EE
300s ea, C-IV	**63874-0228-77**	455.03		EE
1000s ea, C-IV	**63874-0228-02**	185.12		EE
(American Health)				
REPACK				
TAB, PO (10X10)				
5 mg,				
100s ea UD, C-IV	**68084-0359-01**	7.50		AB
(Bryant Ranch)				
REPACK				
TAB, PO, 2 mg,				
30s ea, C-IV	**63629-2948-01**	19.65		
5 mg, 10s ea, C-IV	**63629-1523-07**	22.81		AB
12s ea, C-IV	**63629-1523-01**	25.35		
15s ea, C-IV	**63629-1523-02**	29.19		
20s ea, C-IV	**63629-1523-03**	45.59		
30s ea, C-IV	**63629-1523-04**	58.38		
60s ea, C-IV	**63629-1523-05**	118.76		
90s ea, C-IV	**63629-1523-06**	122.14		
10 mg, 20s ea, C-IV	**63629-1524-01**	39.44		
30s ea, C-IV	**63629-1524-02**	58.66		
40s ea, C-IV	**63629-1524-03**	76.88		
50s ea, C-IV	**63629-1524-04**	96.10		
60s ea, C-IV	**63629-1524-05**	188.65		
(Core)				
REPACK				
TAB, PO, 2 mg,				
30s ea, C-IV	**33358-0101-30**	20.14		
5 mg, 12s ea, C-IV	**33358-0102-12**	25.98		
15s ea, C-IV	**33358-0102-15**	29.92		
20s ea, C-IV	**33358-0102-20**	46.73		
30s ea, C-IV	**33358-0102-30**	59.84		
60s ea, C-IV	**33358-0102-60**	121.73		
90s ea, C-IV	**33358-0102-90**	125.19		
10 mg, 20s ea, C-IV	**33358-0103-20**	40.43		
30s ea, C-IV	**33358-0103-30**	60.13		
40s ea, C-IV	**33358-0103-40**	78.80		
50s ea, C-IV	**33358-0103-50**	98.50		
60s ea, C-IV	**33358-0103-60**	193.37		
90s ea, C-IV	**33358-0103-90**	203.30		
100s ea, C-IV	**33358-0103-00**	208.64		
(DHS, Inc.)				
REPACK				
TAB, PO, 5 mg, 4s ea, C-IV	**55887-0686-04**	3.60		
10s ea, C-IV	**55887-0686-10**	14.02		AB
12s ea, C-IV	**55887-0686-12**	10.80		
14s ea, C-IV	**55887-0686-14**	12.60		
15s ea, C-IV	**55887-0686-15**	13.50		
30s ea, C-IV	**55887-0686-30**	27.02		AB
40s ea, C-IV	**55887-0686-40**	36.02		
60s ea, C-IV	**55887-0686-60**	39.69		AB
90s ea, C-IV	**55887-0686-90**	51.09		AB
10 mg, 4s ea, C-IV	**55887-0522-04**	5.61		
10s ea, C-IV	**55887-0522-10**	14.03		
20s ea, C-IV	**55887-0522-20**	28.06		AB
30s ea, C-IV	**55887-0522-30**	42.09		AB
40s ea, C-IV	**55887-0522-40**	56.12		
50s ea, C-IV	**55887-0522-50**	70.15		
60s ea, C-IV	**55887-0522-60**	84.18		AB
90s ea, C-IV	**55887-0522-90**	126.77		AB
100s ea, C-IV	**55887-0522-01**	4.25		
(Dispensing Solutions)				
REPACK				
SOL, IJ, 5 mg/ml,				
10 ml, C-IV	**55045-2133-03**	15.50		AP
TAB, PO, 2 mg,				
20s ea, C-IV	**55045-1212-07**	9.20		
30s ea, C-IV	**55045-1212-08**	13.80		AB
5 mg, 2s ea, C-IV	**66336-0478-02**	4.36		AB
5s ea, C-IV	**55045-1171-02**	4.40		AB
6s ea, C-IV	**66336-0478-06**	8.50		AB
7s ea, C-IV	**55045-1171-06**	6.16		AB
10s ea, C-IV	**55045-1171-00**	8.80		AB
10s ea, C-IV	**66336-0478-10**	14.27		AB
14s ea, C-IV	**55045-3284-04**	12.32		AB
15s ea, C-IV	**55045-1171-05**	13.20		AB
15s ea, C-IV	**66336-0478-15**	21.41		AB
20s ea, C-IV	**55045-1171-07**	17.60		AB
30s ea, C-IV	**55045-1171-08**	26.40		AB
30s ea, C-IV	**66336-0478-30**	42.78		AB
40s ea, C-IV	**55045-1171-03**	35.20		AB
45s ea, C-IV	**55045-3284-03**	39.60		
50s ea, C-IV	**55045-1171-04**	44.00		AB
60s ea, C-IV	**55045-1171-09**	52.80		AB
90s ea, C-IV	**55045-3284-09**	79.20		AB
100s ea, C-IV	**55045-1171-01**	88.00		AB
120s ea, C-IV	**55045-3284-02**	105.60		AB
10 mg, 2s ea, C-IV	**55045-1624-02**	3.00		AB
3s ea, C-IV	**55045-1624-05**	3.75		AB
4s ea, C-IV	**66336-0033-44**	5.61		
10s ea, C-IV	**66336-0033-10**	14.03		AB
14s ea, C-IV	**55045-1624-06**	17.50		AB
20s ea, C-IV	**55045-1624-00**	25.00		AB
30s ea, C-IV	**55045-1624-08**	37.50		AB
30s ea, C-IV	**66336-0033-30**	42.09		AB
40s ea, C-IV	**55045-1624-04**	50.00		AB
60s ea, C-IV	**55045-1624-09**	75.00		AB
60s ea, C-IV	**66336-0033-60**	84.18		AB
90s ea, C-IV	**55045-3299-09**	112.50		AB
100s ea, C-IV	**55045-1624-01**	125.00		AB
120s ea, C-IV	**55045-3299-01**	150.00		AB
(HomeMed)				
REPACK				
TAB, PO, 2 mg, 8s ea, C-IV	**51655-0834-80**	5.06		
5 mg, 10s ea, C-IV	**51655-0801-53**	11.00		EE
30s ea, C-IV	**51655-0801-24**	65.89		EE
60s ea, C-IV	**51655-0801-25**	9.84		EE
90s ea, C-IV	**51655-0801-26**	11.26		EE
120s ea, C-IV	**51655-0801-82**	18.68		EE
10 mg, 30s ea, C-IV	**51655-0833-24**	54.99		EE
60s ea, C-IV	**51655-0833-25**	11.98		EE
90s ea, C-IV	**51655-0833-26**	17.47		EE
120s ea, C-IV	**51655-0833-82**	22.95		EE
(IPI)				
REPACK				
TAB, PO, 2 mg,				
30s ea, C-IV	**18837-0344-30**	24.69		AB
5 mg, 3s ea, C-IV	**18837-0039-03**	7.50		
30s ea, C-IV	**18837-0039-30**	27.02		
60s ea, C-IV	**18837-0039-60**	52.02		
90s ea, C-IV	**18837-0039-90**	17.83		AB
10 mg, 30s ea, C-IV	**18837-0038-30**	39.00		
60s ea, C-IV	**18837-0038-60**	78.00		
90s ea, C-IV	**18837-0038-90**	117.00		
100s ea, C-IV	**18837-0038-99**	130.00		
120s ea, C-IV	**18837-0038-98**	29.68		AB
(Keltman Pharma., Inc.)				
REPACK				
TAB, PO, 5 mg,				
30s ea, C-IV	**68387-0474-30**	33.75		AB
10 mg, ea, C-IV	**68387-0475-01**	11.65		AB
30s ea, C-IV	**68387-0475-30**	35.70		AB
90s ea, C-IV	**68387-0475-90**	107.10		
(McKesson Packaging)				
REPACK				
TAB, PO (USP)				
5 mg,				
100s ea UD, C-IV	**63739-0073-10**	22.01		AB
(Medsource)				
REPACK				
TAB, PO, 5 mg,				
30s ea, C-IV	**45865-0482-30**	6.60		AB
60s ea, C-IV	**45865-0482-60**	13.20		AB
10 mg, 30s ea, C-IV	**45865-0423-30**	12.60		AB
60s ea, C-IV	**45865-0423-60**	25.20		AB

PROD/MFR	NDC	AWP	DP	OBC
(Nucare Pharm)				
REPACK				
TAB, PO, 2 mg, 2s ea, C-IV	**66267-0550-02**	2.50		AB
12s ea, C-IV	**66267-0550-12**	13.85		AB
20s ea, C-IV	**66267-0550-20**	19.19		AB
30s ea, C-IV	**66267-0550-30**	27.16		AB
60s ea, C-IV	**66267-0550-60**	54.35		AB
90s ea, C-IV	**66267-0550-90**	81.55		AB
5 mg, 2s ea, C-IV	**66267-0069-02**	5.50		AB
2s ea, C-IV	**66267-0776-02**	5.50		AB
3s ea, C-IV	**66267-0069-03**	8.25		AB
3s ea, C-IV	**66267-0776-03**	8.25		AB
4s ea, C-IV	**66267-0069-04**	9.83		AB
4s ea, C-IV	**66267-0776-04**	9.83		AB
6s ea, C-IV	**66267-0069-06**	11.33		AB
6s ea, C-IV	**66267-0776-06**	11.33		AB
10s ea, C-IV	**66267-0069-10**	18.88		AB
10s ea, C-IV	**66267-0776-10**	18.88		AB
12s ea, C-IV	**66267-0069-12**	22.67		AB
15s ea, C-IV	**66267-0069-15**	28.32		AB
20s ea, C-IV	**66267-0069-20**	37.76		AB
30s ea, C-IV	**66267-0069-30**	56.65		AB
40s ea, C-IV	**66267-0069-40**	66.35		AB
60s ea, C-IV	**66267-0069-60**	85.80		AB
90s ea, C-IV	**66267-0069-90**	122.85		AB
120s ea, C-IV	**66267-0069-91**	163.80		AB
10 mg, ea, C-IV	**66267-0068-01**	3.45		AB
2s ea, C-IV	**66267-0068-02**	3.45		AB
4s ea, C-IV	**66267-0068-04**	11.83		AB
10s ea, C-IV	**66267-0068-10**	21.25		AB
15s ea, C-IV	**66267-0068-15**	30.48		AB
20s ea, C-IV	**66267-0068-20**	39.99		AB
28s ea, C-IV	**66267-0068-28**	55.40		AB
30s ea, C-IV	**66267-0068-30**	59.35		AB
40s ea, C-IV	**66267-0068-40**	74.20		AB
45s ea, C-IV	**66267-0068-45**	83.46		AB
60s ea, C-IV	**66267-0068-60**	109.26		AB
90s ea, C-IV	**66267-0068-90**	163.49		AB
112s ea, C-IV	**66267-0068-78**	195.45		AB
120s ea, C-IV	**66267-0068-91**	209.39		AB
(Palmetto)				
REPACK				
SOL, IJ, 5 mg/ml,				
10 ml, C-IV	**23490-7545-02**	15.00		
TAB, PO, 2 mg,				
30s ea, C-IV	**23490-5419-01**	13.83		
30s ea, C-IV	**23490-5419-02**	13.83		
100s ea, C-IV	**23490-5419-03**	46.10		
5 mg, 2s ea, C-IV	**23490-5420-01**	7.70		
6s ea, C-IV	**23490-5420-02**	10.00		
10s ea, C-IV	**23490-5420-03**	11.88		
15s ea, C-IV	**23490-5420-04**	17.82		
30s ea, C-IV	**23490-5420-05**	35.65		
60s ea, C-IV	**23490-5420-06**	71.30		
90s ea, C-IV	**23490-5420-07**	106.95		
10 mg, 4s ea, C-IV	**23490-5418-01**	18.77		
5s ea, C-IV	**23490-5418-00**	20.62		
10s ea, C-IV	**23490-5418-02**	18.33		
30s ea, C-IV	**23490-0428-03**	42.00		
30s ea, C-IV	**23490-5418-03**	54.99		
60s ea, C-IV	**23490-0428-06**	84.00		
60s ea, C-IV	**23490-5418-04**	109.98		
90s ea, C-IV	**23490-5418-05**	164.97		
100s ea, C-IV	**23490-5418-06**	183.30		
120s ea, C-IV	**23490-5418-07**	41.49		
(PD-Rx Pharm)				
REPACK				
TAB, PO, 2 mg,				
20s ea, C-IV	**55289-0979-20**	12.50		AB
30s ea, C-IV	**55289-0979-30**	13.83		AB
60s ea, C-IV	**55289-0979-60**	27.66		AB
5 mg, 6s ea, C-IV	**43063-0018-06**	11.22		AB
6s ea, C-IV	**55289-0091-06**	11.23		AB
9s ea, C-IV	**55289-0091-09**	11.87		AB
10s ea, C-IV	**55289-0091-10**	12.07		AB
(USP)				
5 mg, 12s ea, C-IV	**55289-0091-12**	12.30		AB
15s ea, C-IV	**55289-0091-15**	12.53		AB
20s ea, C-IV	**58864-0145-20**	13.60		AB
21s ea, C-IV	**55289-0091-21**	13.73		AB
30s ea, C-IV	**55289-0091-30**	15.40		AB
60s ea, C-IV	**55289-0091-60**	19.90		AB
90s ea, C-IV	**55289-0091-90**	24.83		AB
10 mg, 2s ea, C-IV	**55289-0092-02**	11.97		AB
6s ea, C-IV	**55289-0092-06**	14.37		AB
10s ea, C-IV	**55289-0092-10**	14.61		AB
20s ea, C-IV	**55289-0092-20**	14.83		AB
25s ea, C-IV	**55289-0092-25**	15.63		AB
30s ea, C-IV	**55289-0092-30**	15.80		AB
40s ea, C-IV	**55289-0092-40**	16.50		AB
60s ea, C-IV	**55289-0092-60**	21.57		AB
90s ea, C-IV	**55289-0092-90**	27.33		AB
100s ea, C-IV	**55289-0092-01**	34.08		AB
120s ea, C-IV	**55289-0092-98**	35.70		AB
(Pharma Pac)				
REPACK				
TAB, PO, 2 mg,				
10s ea, C-IV	**52959-0295-10**	7.61		EE
15s ea, C-IV	**52959-0295-15**	11.31		EE
30s ea, C-IV	**52959-0295-30**	22.99		EE
50s ea, C-IV	**52959-0295-50**	38.31		EE
120s ea, C-IV	**52959-0295-02**	60.32		EE
5 mg, ea, C-IV	**52959-0047-01**	1.20		EE
3s ea, C-IV	**52959-0047-03**	3.57		EE
5s ea, C-IV	**52959-0047-05**	5.95		EE
6s ea, C-IV	**52959-0047-06**	7.14		EE
10s ea, C-IV	**52959-0047-10**	11.89		EE
12s ea, C-IV	**52959-0047-12**	14.27		EE
15s ea, C-IV	**52959-0047-15**	17.84		EE
20s ea, C-IV	**52959-0047-20**	23.78		EE
21s ea, C-IV	**52959-0047-21**	24.96		EE
24s ea, C-IV	**52959-0047-24**	28.52		AB
25s ea, C-IV	**52959-0047-25**	29.72		EE
30s ea, C-IV	**52959-0047-30**	35.65		EE
40s ea, C-IV	**52959-0047-40**	47.53		EE
45s ea, C-IV	**52959-0047-45**	53.46		EE
50s ea, C-IV	**52959-0047-50**	59.39		EE
60s ea, C-IV	**52959-0047-60**	71.27		EE
90s ea, C-IV	**52959-0047-90**	82.05		AB
120s ea, C-IV	**52959-0047-02**	112.20		AB
10 mg, 5s ea, C-IV	**52959-0306-05**	9.90		EE
6s ea, C-IV	**52959-0306-06**	11.88		AB
10s ea, C-IV	**52959-0306-10**	19.80		EE
15s ea, C-IV	**52959-0306-15**	29.69		EE
20s ea, C-IV	**52959-0306-20**	39.58		EE
28s ea, C-IV	**52959-0306-28**	55.39		EE
30s ea, C-IV	**52959-0306-30**	59.36		EE
60s ea, C-IV	**52959-0306-60**	118.71		EE
90s ea, C-IV	**52959-0306-90**	178.04		EE
100s ea, C-IV	**52959-0306-00**	197.82		EE
(Phys Total Care)				
REPACK				
SOL, IJ (AMP)				
5 mg/ml,				
2 ml, C-IV	**54868-2320-02**	12.74		EE
2 ml 10s, C-IV	**54868-2320-01**	77.51		EE
(22GX1 1/4",CARPUJECT)				
5 mg/ml,				
2 ml 10s, C-IV	**54868-4586-00**	99.06		EE
(M.D.V.,FLIPTOP)				
5 mg/ml,				
10 ml 5s, C-IV	**54868-0617-01**	64.29		EE
(10X10ML,M.D.V)				
5 mg/ml,				
10 ml 10s, C-IV	**54868-0617-02**	89.26		AP
TAB, PO, 2 mg,				
10s ea, C-IV	**54868-2126-05**	5.75		EE
20s ea, C-IV	**54868-2126-07**	9.85		AB
30s ea, C-IV	**54868-2126-04**	8.16		EE
50s ea, C-IV	**54868-2126-01**	10.62		EE
60s ea, C-IV	**54868-2126-06**	13.34		EE
100s ea, C-IV	**54868-2126-02**	16.74		EE
5 mg, 6s ea, C-IV	**54868-0059-08**	5.22		EE
10s ea, C-IV	**54868-0059-06**	5.70		EE
15s ea, C-IV	**54868-0059-09**	6.30		EE
20s ea, C-IV	**54868-0059-01**	6.90		EE
30s ea, C-IV	**54868-0059-02**	8.10		EE
50s ea, C-IV	**54868-0059-05**	10.50		EE
60s ea, C-IV	**54868-0059-00**	11.70		EE
90s ea, C-IV	**54868-0059-03**	16.34		AB
100s ea, C-IV	**54868-0059-04**	16.50		EE
10 mg, 5s ea, C-IV	**54868-0988-07**	6.72		AB
10s ea, C-IV	**54868-0988-02**	7.41		EE
20s ea, C-IV	**54868-0988-08**	8.82		EE
30s ea, C-IV	**54868-0988-00**	10.26		EE
60s ea, C-IV	**54868-0988-06**	14.41		EE
100s ea, C-IV	**54868-0988-05**	20.16		EE
(Physician Partner)				
REPACK				
SOL, IJ (10X10ML,MDV)				
5 mg/ml,				
10 ml 10s, C-IV	**21695-0889-10**	78.80		AP
TAB, PO, 2 mg,				
90s ea, C-IV	**21695-0263-90**	53.73		AB
5 mg, 2s ea, C-IV	**21695-0264-02**	7.00		
10s ea, C-IV	**21695-0264-10**	11.79		AB
12s ea, C-IV	**21695-0264-12**	4.15		AB
15s ea, C-IV	**21695-0264-15**	17.69		
20s ea, C-IV	**21695-0264-20**	23.58		
30s ea, C-IV	**21695-0264-30**	30.06		
60s ea, C-IV	**21695-0264-60**	60.12		
90s ea, C-IV	**21695-0264-90**	90.18		
10 mg, 5s ea, C-IV	**21695-0265-05**	9.81		AB
15s ea, C-IV	**21695-0265-15**	29.41		AB
30s ea, C-IV	**21695-0265-30**	49.99		
45s ea, C-IV	**21695-0265-45**	88.22		AB
60s ea, C-IV	**21695-0265-60**	99.98		AB
(Quality Care Prod)				
REPACK				
SOL, IJ (1X2ML,LATEX-FREE)				
5 mg/ml,				
2 ml, C-IV	**35356-0371-02**	19.13		AP
(1X10ML)				
5 mg/ml,				
10 ml, C-IV	**35356-0371-10**	27.53		AP
TAB, PO, 5 mg, 2s ea, C-IV	**49999-0018-02**	4.56		AB
5s ea, C-IV	**49999-0018-05**	11.45		AB
10s ea, C-IV	**49999-0018-10**	22.90		EE
10s ea, C-IV	**58016-0018-10**	22.90		AB
15s ea, C-IV	**49999-0018-15**	34.35		EE
20s ea, C-IV	**49999-0018-20**	45.80		EE
21s ea, C-IV	**49999-0018-21**	49.20		AB
30s ea, C-IV	**49999-0018-30**	68.70		EE
60s ea, C-IV	**49999-0018-60**	137.40		EE
90s ea, C-IV	**49999-0018-90**	206.10		AB
10 mg, 2s ea, C-IV	**49999-0027-02**	6.25		AB
20s ea, C-IV	**49999-0027-20**	27.31		EE
30s ea, C-IV	**49999-0027-30**	40.97		EE
60s ea, C-IV	**49999-0027-60**	74.88		AB
90s ea, C-IV	**49999-0027-90**	122.90		AB
100s ea, C-IV	**49999-0027-00**	124.80		AB
120s ea, C-IV	**49999-0027-01**	149.76		AB
(Southwood)				
REPACK				
TAB, PO, 2 mg,				
12s ea, C-IV	**58016-0274-12**	13.66		EE
20s ea, C-IV	**58016-0274-20**	6.63		EE
30s ea, C-IV	**58016-0274-30**	9.95		EE
5 mg, 4s ea, C-IV	**58016-0275-04**	3.60		EE
6s ea, C-IV	**58016-0275-06**	5.41		EE
8s ea, C-IV	**58016-0275-08**	7.21		EE
10s ea, C-IV	**58016-0275-10**	9.01		EE
14s ea, C-IV	**58016-0275-14**	12.62		EE
15s ea, C-IV	**58016-0275-15**	13.52		EE
16s ea, C-IV	**58016-0275-16**	14.42		EE
18s ea, C-IV	**58016-0275-18**	16.22		EE
20s ea, C-IV	**58016-0275-20**	18.02		EE
21s ea, C-IV	**58016-0275-21**	18.92		EE
24s ea, C-IV	**58016-0275-24**	21.63		EE
28s ea, C-IV	**58016-0275-28**	25.23		EE
30s ea, C-IV	**58016-0275-30**	39.00		AB
36s ea, C-IV	**58016-0275-36**	32.44		EE
40s ea, C-IV	**58016-0275-40**	36.04		EE
50s ea, C-IV	**58016-0275-50**	45.06		EE
60s ea, C-IV	**58016-0275-60**	78.00		AB
90s ea, C-IV	**58016-0275-90**	117.00		AB
100s ea, C-IV	**58016-0275-00**	130.00		AB
120s ea, C-IV	**58016-0275-02**	156.00		AB
150s ea, C-IV	**58016-0275-03**	135.17		AB
200s ea, C-IV	**58016-0275-89**	180.22		AB
300s ea, C-IV	**58016-0275-73**	270.33		AB
10 mg, 6s ea, C-IV	**58016-0273-06**	9.10		EE
9s ea, C-IV	**58016-0273-09**	13.65		FF
10s ea, C-IV	**58016-0273-10**	15.17		EE
12s ea, C-IV	**58016-0273-12**	18.20		EE
15s ea, C-IV	**58016-0273-15**	22.75		EE
20s ea, C-IV	**58016-0273-20**	30.34		EE
30s ea, C-IV	**58016-0273-30**	49.50		AB
40s ea, C-IV	**58016-0273-40**	60.67		AB
60s ea, C-IV	**58016-0273-60**	99.00		AB
90s ea, C-IV	**58016-0273-90**	148.50		AB
100s ea, C-IV	**58016-0273-00**	165.00		AB
120s ea, C-IV	**58016-0273-02**	198.00		AB
150s ea, C-IV	**58016-0273-03**	227.52		AB
200s ea, C-IV	**58016-0273-89**	303.36		AB
300s ea, C-IV	**58016-0273-73**	455.04		AB
(St. Mary's MPP)				
REPACK				
TAB, PO (USP)				
5 mg, 10s ea, C-IV	**60760-0775-10**	8.19		
30s ea, C-IV	**60760-0775-30**	12.57		
(Stat Rx)				
REPACK				
TAB, PO, 2 mg,				
30s ea, C-IV	**16590-0069-30**	20.00		
60s ea, C-IV	**16590-0069-60**	40.00		
90s ea, C-IV	**16590-0069-90**	60.00		
5 mg, ea, C-IV	**16590-0070-01**	2.34		AB
2s ea, C-IV	**16590-0070-02**	2.65		AB
3s ea, C-IV	**16590-0070-03**	3.98		AB
10s ea, C-IV	**16590-0070-10**	13.00		
20s ea, C-IV	**16590-0070-20**	26.00		
30s ea, C-IV	**16590-0070-30**	39.00		
45s ea, C-IV	**16590-0070-45**	39.15		AB
60s ea, C-IV	**16590-0070-60**	78.00		

PROD/MFR	NDC	AWP	DP	OBC
75s ea, C-IV	16590-0070-75	65.25		AB
90s ea, C-IV	16590-0070-90	117.00		
100s ea, C-IV	16590-0070-71	51.50		
120s ea, C-IV	16590-0070-72	156.00		
10 mg, 10s ea, C-IV	16590-0071-10	52.24		AB
28s ea, C-IV	16590-0071-28	52.27		AB
30s ea, C-IV	16590-0071-04	7.50		AB
30s ea, C-IV	16590-0071-30	41.75		
45s ea, C-IV	16590-0071-45	83.70		AB
56s ea, C-IV	16590-0071-56	104.54		AB
60s ea, C-IV	16590-0071-60	83.50		
75s ea, C-IV	16590-0071-75	139.50		AB
84s ea, C-IV	16590-0071-62	156.81		AB
90s ea, C-IV	16590-0071-90	125.25		
120s ea, C-IV	16590-0071-72	223.20		AB
DIAZEPAM INTENSOL (Roxane)				
diazepam				
SOL, PO, 5 mg/ml,				
30 ml, C-IV	00054-3185-44	28.08		
DIAZOXIDE (Medisca)				
POW, NA (U.S.P.)				
1 gm	38779-0324-06	124.50		
5 gm	38779-0324-03	417.00		
25 gm	38779-0324-04	1035.00		
(USP,1X100GM)				
100 gm	38779-0324-05	3450.00		
(PCCA)				
POW, NA (U.S.P.)				
1 gm	51927-2742-00	123.00		
(Schering) *See HYPERSTAT*				
(Spectrum Pharmacy)				
POW, NA (U.S.P./N.F.)				
1 gm	49452-2541-02	197.05		
5 gm	49452-2541-03	612.50		
(1X25GM,USP)				
25 gm	49452-2541-04	1561.00		
(1X100GM,USP)				
100 gm	49452-2541-05	5267.50		
(Teva) *See PROGLYCEM*				
DIBENZYLINE (Wellspring Pharm)				
phenoxybenzamine hydrochloride				
CAP, PO, 10 mg, 100s ea	65197-0001-01	773.16		
DIBUCAINE				
(Amend) *See DIBUCAINE BASE*				
(Spectrum Pharmacy)				
POW, NA (U.S.P.)				
5 gm	49452-2550-01	106.40		
25 gm	49452-2550-02	240.45		
100 gm	49452-2550-03	843.50		
DIBUCAINE BASE (Amend)				
dibucaine				
POW, NA (U.S.P.)				
25 gm	17317-0142-02	28.00		
100 gm	17317-0142-03	98.00		
500 gm	17317-0142-05	420.00		
DIBUCAINE HYDROCHLORIDE (Amend)				
POW, NA (U.S.P.)				
25 gm	17317-0141-02	28.00		
500 gm	17317-0141-03	98.00		
500 gm	17317-0141-05	420.00		
(Gallipot)				
POW, NA (1X5GM,USP)				
5 gm	51552-0747-02	24.50	17.50	
(U.S.P.)				
5 gm	51552-0520-02	17.85		
(1X25GM,USP)				
25 gm	51552-0747-04	69.65	49.75	
(U.S.P.)				
25 gm	51552-0520-04	48.86		
(Medisca)				
POW, NA (U.S.P.)				
10 gm	38779-0431-01	108.00		
25 gm	38779-0431-04	195.00		
100 gm	38779-0431-05	435.00		
(USP,1X500GM)				
500 gm	38779-0431-08	2205.00		
(PCCA)				
POW, NA (U.S.P.)				
1 gm	51927-1351-00	5.40		
(Spectrum Pharmacy)				
POW, NA (U.S.P.)				
5 gm	49452-2560-01	97.30		
25 gm	49452-2560-02	193.55		
100 gm	49452-2560-03	700.00		
DIBUTYL PHTHALATE				
(Amend) *See DIBUTYLPHTHALATE*				

PROD/MFR	NDC	AWP	DP	OBC
DIBUTYL SQUARATE (Letco)				
squaric acid dibutylester				
POW, NA, 1 gm	62991-1561-01	102.00		
5 gm	62991-1561-02	270.00		
(Medisca)				
SOL, NA, 1 gm	38779-1236-06	135.00		
5 gm	38779-1236-03	315.00		
DIBUTYLPHTHALATE (Amend)				
dibutyl phthalate				
LIQ, NA, 500 ml	17317-0875-01	9.80		
3840 ml	17317-0875-06	28.00		
DICEL (Centrix)				
chlorpheniramine tannate/pseudoephedrine tannate				
SUS, PO (STRAWBERRY-BANANA)				
5 mg/5 ml-75 mg/5 ml,				
473 ml	11528-0100-16	159.47		
DICEL DM (Centrix)				
cpm tan/dm tan/pse tan				
SUS, PO (COTTON CANDY)				
473 ml	11528-0105-16	183.36		
DICHLORALPHENAZONE (PCCA)				
POW, NA (U.S.P.; CIV)				
1 gm	51927-2199-00	1.35		
DICHLOROACETIC ACID (PCCA)				
LIQ, NA, 1 gm	51927-1376-00	0.54		
DICHLOROBENZENE				
(Amend) *See P-DICHLOROBENZENE*				
(Baker, J.T.) *See O-DICHLOROBENZENE*				
DICHLOROETHANE				
(Baker, J.T.) *See ETHYLENE DICHLORIDE*				
DICHLOROINDOPHENOL SODIUM (PCCA)				
2,6-dichloroindophenol sodium				
POW, NA (2,6; REAGENT; ACS)				
1 gm	51927-3353-00	150.00		
DICHLOROPHEN				
(PCCA) *See DICHLOROPHENE*				
DICHLOROPHENE (PCCA)				
dichlorophen				
POW, NA (1X1GM)				
1 gm	51927-2890-00	2.55		
DICHLORPHENAMIDE (Medisca)				
POW, NA, 5 gm	38779-2058-03	229.50		
25 gm	38779-2058-04	612.00		
100 gm	38779-2058-05	1755.00		
(USP,1X1000GM)				
1000 gm	38779-2058-09	12240.00		
DICLOFENAC EPOLAMINE				
(King Pharm) *See FLECTOR*				
DICLOFENAC NA (Advanced Pharm Serv, Inc.)				
REPACK				
diclofenac sodium				
ECT, PO, 25 mg, 20s ea	13411-0165-02	9.20		
30s ea	13411-0165-03	13.80		
60s ea	13411-0165-06	27.60		
90s ea	13411-0165-09	41.40		
100s ea	13411-0165-10	68.92		
DICLOFENAC POT. (Stat Rx)				
REPACK				
diclofenac potassium				
TAB, PO, 50 mg, 30s ea	16590-0072-30	57.00		
30s ea	16590-0073-30	50.00		
60s ea	16590-0073-60	100.00		
90s ea	16590-0073-90	150.00		
120s ea	16590-0073-72	200.00		
DICLOFENAC POTASSIUM				
FUL				
TAB, PO, 50 mg, 100s ea		47.48		
(Apotex Corp.)				
TAB, PO (FILM-COATED)				
50 mg, 100s ea	60505-0135-00	156.55		
(Mylan)				
TAB, PO (FILM COATED)				
50 mg, 100s ea	00378-2474-01	156.60		AB
(Novartis Pharm) *See CATAFLAM*				
(Sandoz)				
TAB, PO (FILM-COATED)				
50 mg, 100s ea	00781-5017-01	155.19		AB
(Teva)				
TAB, PO, 50 mg, 100s ea	00093-0948-01	156.55		AB
500s ea	00093-0948-05	782.75		AB
(Xanodyne Pharma) *See ZIPSOR*				

PROD/MFR	NDC	AWP	DP	OBC
(A-S Medication)				
REPACK				
TAB, PO, 50 mg, 21s ea	54569-4770-01	32.81		EE
30s ea	54569-4770-00	46.87		EE
45s ea	54569-4770-03	70.30		EE
90s ea	54569-4770-04	140.60		EE
(Aidarex)				
REPACK				
TAB, PO, 50 mg, 10s ea	33261-0038-10	19.20		
20s ea	33261-0038-20	38.40		
30s ea	33261-0038-30	57.60		
40s ea	33261-0038-40	76.80		
50s ea	33261-0038-50	96.00		
60s ea	33261-0038-60	115.20		
80s ea	33261-0038-80	153.60		
90s ea	33261-0038-90	173.10		
(DHS, Inc.)				
REPACK				
TAB, PO, 50 mg, 20s ea	55887-0801-20	35.02		AB
21s ea	55887-0801-21	35.51		AB
30s ea	55887-0801-30	49.00		AB
60s ea	55887-0801-60	98.00		
(Dispensing Solutions)				
REPACK				
TAB, PO (FILM-COATED)				
50 mg, 20s ea	55045-2628-07	36.80		EE
(FILM COATED)				
50 mg, 30s ea	55045-2628-08	55.20		AB
42s ea	55045-2628-09	77.25		
60s ea	55045-2628-06	110.40		
(FILM COATED)				
50 mg, 90s ea	55045-2628-01	165.60		AB
(HomeMed)				
REPACK				
TAB, PO, 50 mg, 30s ea	51655-0755-24	55.15		
(IPI)				
REPACK				
TAB, PO, 50 mg, 90s ea	18837-0332-90	176.12		
(Keltman Pharma., Inc.)				
REPACK				
TAB, PO (FILM COATED)				
50 mg, 30s ea	68387-0280-30	56.78		AB
(LWP)				
REPACK				
TAB, PO (FILM COATED)				
50 mg, 30s ea	64038-0049-30	57.55		AB
100s ea	64038-0049-01	164.43		AB
(Nucare Pharm)				
REPACK				
TAB, PO (FILM-COATED)				
50 mg, 30s ea	66267-0070-30	64.58		AB
60s ea	66267-0070-60	123.28		AB
90s ea	66267-0070-90	184.92		AB
(Palmetto)				
REPACK				
TAB, PO, 50 mg, 30s ea	23490-6507-03	56.08		
60s ea	23490-6507-06	112.16		
90s ea	23490-6507-09	168.24		
270s ea	23490-6507-00	378.54		
(PD-Rx Pharm)				
REPACK				
TAB, PO (FILM COATED)				
50 mg, 21s ea	55289-0781-21	39.65		AB
30s ea	55289-0781-30	42.00		AB
(Pharma Pac)				
REPACK				
TAB, PO, 50 mg, 20s ea	52959-0659-20	39.25		AB
(FILM COATED)				
50 mg, 28s ea	52959-0659-28	54.60		AB
30s ea	52959-0659-30	58.49		
(FILM COATED)				
50 mg, 40s ea	52959-0659-40	75.01		AB
60s ea	52959-0659-60	112.50		
90s ea	52959-0659-90	168.57		
(Phys Total Care)				
REPACK				
TAB, PO, 50 mg, 90s ea	54868-5437-00	59.54		AB
(Physician Partner)				
REPACK				
TAB, PO (FILM-COATED)				
50 mg, 21s ea	21695-0838-21	65.18		AB
30s ea	21695-0838-30	93.11		AB
42s ea	21695-0838-42	153.36		AB
(Quality Care Prod)				
REPACK				
TAB, PO (FILM-COATED)				
50 mg, 20s ea	49999-0593-20	32.38		AB

PROD/MFR	NDC	AWP	DP	OBC
30s ea	49999-0593-30	40.57		AB
60s ea	49999-0593-60	97.13		AB
(Southwood)				
REPACK				
TAB, PO, 50 mg, 20s ea	58016-0444-20	37.39		EE
30s ea	58016-0444-30	56.08		EE
40s ea	58016-0444-40	74.77		EE
60s ea	58016-0444-60	112.16		EE
90s ea	58016-0444-90	168.23		EE
100s ea	58016-0444-00	186.93		EE
(Stat Rx)				
REPACK				
TAB, PO, 50 mg, 90s ea	16590-0072-90	171.00		AB
(Vibranta)				
REPACK				
TAB, PO, 50 mg, 20s ea	57866-6920-05	32.38		
30s ea	57866-6920-01	48.56		
60s ea	57866-6920-04	97.13		
DICLOFENAC SOD (Physician Partner)				
REPACK				
diclofenac sodium				
ECT, PO, 50 mg, 30s ea	21695-0038-30	60.56		
75 mg, 20s ea	21695-0039-20	52.71		
30s ea	21695-0039-30	67.20		
60s ea	21695-0039-60	134.40		
90s ea	21695-0039-90	201.60		
TER, PO, 100 mg, 30s ea	21695-0040-30	168.85		
60s ea	21695-0040-60	337.70		
90s ea	21695-0040-90	506.56		
DICLOFENAC SODIUM				
FUL				
SOL, OP, 0.1%, 5 ml		21.36		
TER, PO, 75 mg, 100s ea		58.50		
100 mg, 100s ea		236.18		
(Actavis) *See DICLOFENAC SODIUM DR*				
(Actavis)				
TER, PO, 100 mg, 100s ea	00228-2717-11	281.50		AB
(Akorn)				
SOL, OP, 0.1%, 2.5 ml	17478-0892-25	44.77		AT
5 ml	17478-0892-10	73.03		AT
(Bausch & Lomb Inc.)				
SOL, OP (1X2.5ML)				
0.1%, 2.5 ml	24208-0457-25	13.13		AT
(1X6ML)				
0.1%, 5 ml	24208-0457-05	17.50		AT
(Doak) *See SOLARAZE*				
(Endo Pharm) *See VOLTAREN GEL*				
(Falcon Ophthalmics)				
SOL, OP (1X2.5ML)				
0.1%, 2.5 ml	61314-0014-25	33.80		AT
(1X5ML)				
0.1%, 5 ml	61314-0014-05	55.15		AT
(Gallipot)				
POW, NA, 25 gm	51552-0482-04	22.61		
(Hawkins)				
POW, NA, 25 gm	63370-0081-25	65.00		
100 gm	63370-0081-35	220.00		
500 gm	63370-0081-45	920.00		
(Letco)				
POW, NA (U.S.P.)				
25 gm	62991-2024-01	51.00		
100 gm	62991-2024-02	171.00		
(Martec)				
ECT, PO, 75 mg, 100s ea	52555-0205-01	109.82		AB
1000s ea	52555-0205-10	1079.48		AB
(Medisca)				
POW, NA (B.P.)				
25 gm	38779-1698-04	55.50		
100 gm	38779-1698-05	187.50		
500 gm	38779-1698-08	696.00		
(Mylan)				
TER, PO, 100 mg, 100s ea	00378-0355-01	281.15		AB
(Novartis Pharm) *See VOLTAREN*				
(Novartis Pharm) *See VOLTAREN-XR*				
(Pack)				
ECT, PO (USP,DELAYED-RELEASE)				
75 mg, 60s ea	16571-0201-06	106.43		AB
100s ea	16571-0201-10	177.39		AB
500s ea	16571-0201-50	886.95		AB
1000s ea	16571-0201-11	1773.89		AB
SOL, OP (1X2.5ML)				
0.1%, 2.5 ml	16571-0101-25	44.77		AT
(1X5ML)				
0.1%, 5 ml	16571-0101-50	73.03		AT

PROD/MFR	NDC	AWP	DP	OBC
(PCCA)				
POW, NA, 1 gm	51927-1859-00	2.76		
(Sandoz)				
ECT, PO, 25 mg, 100s ea	00781-1785-01	142.18		AB
50 mg, 60s ea	00781-1787-60	88.34		AB
100s ea	00781-1787-01	147.23		AB
1000s ea	00781-1787-10	1472.33		AB
75 mg, 60s ea	00781-1789-60	106.43		AB
100s ea	00781-1789-01	177.39		AB
500s ea	00781-1789-05	886.95		AB
1000s ea	00781-1789-10	1773.89		AB
TER, PO, 100 mg, 100s ea	00781-1381-01	281.42		AB
(Spectrum Pharmacy)				
POW, NA (U.S.P.)				
25 gm	49452-2581-02	87.15		
100 gm	49452-2581-03	291.20		
500 gm	49452-2581-04	1036.00		
(Teva)				
TER, PO, 100 mg, 100s ea	00093-1041-01	281.24		AB
(Watson Labs)				
ECT, PO, 50 mg, 60s ea	00591-0338-60	54.39		EE
100s ea	00591-0338-01	100.93		EE
1000s ea	00591-0338-10	958.84		EE
75 mg, 60s ea	00591-0339-60	68.54		EE
100s ea	00591-0339-01	114.47		EE
500s ea	00591-0339-05	560.90		EE
1000s ea	00591-0339-10	1123.02		AB
TER, PO (FILM-COATED)				
100 mg, 100s ea	00591-0676-01	281.42		AB
(4u)				
REPACK				
ECT, PO, 50 mg, 60s ea	10544-0389-60	126.86		EE
60s ea	42549-0551-60	126.86		EE
60s ea	42549-0589-60	126.86		EE
75 mg, 60s ea	42549-0310-60	105.06		AB
60s ea	42549-0510-60	127.86		AB
(A-S Medication)				
REPACK				
ECT, PO, 50 mg, 30s ea	54569-4165-02	34.43		EE
75 mg, 14s ea	54569-4166-03	20.28		AB
20s ea	54569-4166-01	28.98		AB
30s ea	54569-4166-02	43.47		AB
60s ea	54569-4166-04	86.93		AB
SOL, OP (1X5ML)				
0.1%, 5 ml	54569-4753-00	17.50		AT
(Aidarex)				
REPACK				
ECT, PO, 75 mg, 10s ea	33261-0037-10	17.60		
14s ea	33261-0037-14	24.64		
20s ea	33261-0037-20	35.20		
21s ea	33261-0037-21	36.96		
28s ea	33261-0037-28	49.28		
30s ea	33261-0037-30	52.80		
40s ea	33261-0037-40	70.40		
60s ea	33261-0037-60	105.60		
80s ea	33261-0037-80	140.80		
90s ea	33261-0037-90	158.40		
100s ea	33261-0037-00	176.00		
120s ea	33261-0037-02	211.20		
(Altura)				
REPACK				
ECT, PO, 50 mg, 10s ea	63874-0334-10	12.10		EE
12s ea	63874-0334-12	14.52		EE
14s ea	63874-0334-14	16.94		EE
15s ea	63874-0334-15	18.15		EE
20s ea	63874-0334-20	24.20		EE
24s ea	63874-0334-24	29.04		EE
28s ea	63874-0334-28	33.88		EE
30s ea	63874-0334-30	36.30		EE
40s ea	63874-0334-40	48.40		EE
50s ea	63874-0334-50	60.50		EE
60s ea	63874-0334-60	80.94		EE
80s ea	63874-0334-80	107.92		EE
90s ea	63874-0334-90	108.90		EE
100s ea	63874-0334-01	121.00		EE
120s ea	63874-0334-04	145.20		EE
150s ea	63874-0334-72	202.35		EE
200s ea	63874-0334-74	269.80		EE
300s ea	63874-0334-77	404.70		EE
500s ea	63874-0334-03	530.13		EE
75 mg, 10s ea	63874-0426-10	16.30		EE
12s ea	63874-0426-12	19.56		EE
14s ea	63874-0426-14	22.82		EE
15s ea	63874-0426-15	24.45		EE
20s ea	63874-0426-20	32.60		EE
21s ea	63874-0426-21	34.23		EE
28s ea	63874-0426-28	45.64		EE
30s ea	63874-0426-30	48.90		EE
40s ea	63874-0426-40	65.20		EE
50s ea	63874-0426-50	81.50		EE

PROD/MFR	NDC	AWP	DP	OBC
60s ea	63874-0426-60	98.02		EE
80s ea	63874-0426-80	130.40		EE
90s ea	63874-0426-90	146.70		EE
100s ea	63874-0426-01	163.00		EE
120s ea	63874-0426-04	195.60		EE
150s ea	63874-0426-72	245.04		EE
200s ea	63874-0426-74	326.72		EE
300s ea	63874-0426-77	489.08		EE
500s ea	63874-0426-03	735.00		EE
TER, PO, 100 mg, 20s ea	63874-1055-02	62.40		AB
30s ea	63874-1055-03	93.60		AB
40s ea	63874-1055-04	124.80		AB
50s ea	63874-1055-05	156.00		AB
60s ea	63874-1055-06	187.20		AB
90s ea	63874-1055-09	280.80		AB
100s ea	63874-1055-01	312.00		AB
(Core)				
REPACK				
ECT, PO, 50 mg, 14s ea	33358-0104-14	36.48		
28s ea	33358-0104-28	48.84		
30s ea	33358-0104-30	53.07		
60s ea	33358-0104-60	106.15		
90s ea	33358-0104-90	178.24		
75 mg, 20s ea	33358-0105-20	45.55		
28s ea	33358-0105-28	64.08		
30s ea	33358-0105-30	68.85		
60s ea	33358-0105-60	137.69		
90s ea	33358-0105-90	194.05		
100s ea	33358-0105-00	197.14		
120s ea	33358-0105-01	201.43		
(DHS, Inc.)				
REPACK				
ECT, PO, 50 mg, 20s ea	55887-0553-20	23.28		AB
30s ea	55887-0553-30	52.00		AB
60s ea	55887-0553-60	95.00		AB
90s ea	55887-0553-90	142.50		AB
75 mg, 14s ea	55887-0542-14	26.91		AB
20s ea	55887-0542-20	36.00		AB
30s ea	55887-0542-30	53.81		AB
60s ea	55887-0542-60	106.66		AB
90s ea	55887-0542-90	126.91		AB
(Dispensing Solutions)				
REPACK				
ECT, PO, 50 mg, 15s ea	55045-2275-04	20.50		
20s ea	55045-2275-07	27.40		EE
20s ea	66336-0238-20	27.90		EE
30s ea	55045-2275-08	41.00		AB
30s ea	66336-0238-30	41.85		EE
60s ea	55045-2275-06	82.00		EE
60s ea	66336-0238-60	83.70		AB
80s ea	55045-2275-03	109.60		EE
90s ea	55045-2275-09	123.30		EE
90s ea	66336-0238-90	125.55		AB
100s ea	55045-2275-00	137.00		AB
120s ea	55045-2275-01	164.40		EE
135s ea	55045-2275-02	184.95		EE
75 mg, 14s ea	66336-0463-14	19.23		AB
15s ea	55045-2247-05	24.45		
20s ea	55045-2247-07	32.60		EE
20s ea	55045-2249-07	37.85		AB
28s ea	66336-0463-28	38.46		EE
30s ea	55045-2247-08	48.90		AB
30s ea	66336-0463-30	41.21		AB
60s ea	66336-0463-60	82.42		EE
90s ea	55045-2247-01	146.70		AB
90s ea	66336-0463-90	122.13		AB
100s ea	55045-2247-00	163.00		AB
120s ea	55045-2247-09	195.60		AB
TER, PO, 100 mg, 21s ea	66336-0383-21	64.94		AB
30s ea	55045-3266-08	85.00		
(FILM-COATED)				
100 mg, 30s ea	66336-0383-30	92.77		AB
60s ea	66336-0383-60	185.54		AB
(IPI)				
REPACK				
ECT, PO, 50 mg, 60s ea	18837-0377-60	110.42		AB
90s ea	18837-0377-90	165.63		AB
75 mg, 20s ea	18837-0041-20	35.20		
60s ea	13387-0041-60	105.75		
60s ea	18837-0041-60	67.38		EE
(Keltman Pharma., Inc.)				
REPACK				
ECT, PO, 75 mg, 20s ea	68387-0260-20	33.34		
30s ea	68387-0260-30	50.00		EE
60s ea	68387-0260-60	100.00		EE
(LWP)				
REPACK				
ECT, PO, 50 mg, 60s ea	64038-0050-60	70.92		EE
100s ea	64038-0050-01	118.20		EE
75 mg, 60s ea	64038-0051-60	72.11		EE
100s ea	64038-0051-01	120.19		EE

PROD/MFR	NDC	AWP	DP	OBC
(Medsource)				
REPACK				
TER, PO (FILM-COATED)				
100 mg, 30s ea	**45865-0364-30**	88.50		AB
60s ea	**45865-0364-60**	177.00		AB
90s ea	**45865-0364-90**	265.50		AB
100s ea	**45865-0364-00**	295.00		AB
120s ea	**45865-0364-01**	354.00		AB
150s ea	**45865-0364-02**	442.50		AB
300s ea	**45865-0364-05**	885.00		AB
(Nucare Pharm)				
REPACK				
ECT, PO, 50 mg, 30s ea	**66267-0358-30**	42.99		EE
60s ea	**66267-0358-60**	115.94		EE
90s ea	**66267-0358-90**	173.91		EE
75 mg, 20s ea	**66267-0071-20**	36.80		EE
30s ea	**66267-0071-30**	55.20		EE
60s ea	**66267-0071-60**	110.88		EE
TER, PO, 100 mg, 30s ea	**66267-0709-30**	95.60		AB
60s ea	**66267-0709-60**	197.99		AB
(Palmetto)				
REPACK				
ECT, PO, 50 mg, 20s ea	**23490-5423-00**	36.75		
30s ea	**23490-5423-01**	55.13		
60s ea	**23490-5423-06**	110.26		
90s ea	**23490-5423-09**	165.39		
75 mg, 14s ea	**23490-5424-01**	29.40		
20s ea	**23490-5424-05**	41.99		
28s ea	**23490-5424-02**	58.79		
30s ea	**23490-5424-04**	62.99		
60s ea	**23490-5424-03**	125.98		
90s ea	**23490-5424-09**	188.97		
(PD-Rx Pharm)				
REPACK				
ECT, PO, 50 mg, 10s ea	**55289-0166-10**	50.90		AB
14s ea	**55289-0166-14**	61.00		AB
20s ea	**55289-0166-20**	76.00		AB
30s ea	**55289-0166-30**	101.00		AB
75 mg, 10s ea	**55289-0150-10**	38.00		AB
15s ea	**55289-0150-15**	50.90		AB
20s ea	**55289-0150-20**	76.00		AB
30s ea	**55289-0150-30**	101.00		AB
60s ea	**55289-0150-60**	176.05		AB
(Pharma Pac)				
REPACK				
ECT, PO, 25 mg, 30s ea	**52959-0377-30**	14.75		EE
60s ea	**52959-0377-60**	27.00		EE
50 mg, 12s ea	**52959-0436-12**	17.78		EE
14s ea	**52959-0436-14**	20.75		EE
20s ea	**52959-0436-20**	29.50		EE
28s ea	**52959-0436-28**	41.16		EE
30s ea	**52959-0436-30**	43.80		EE
40s ea	**52959-0436-40**	57.55		EE
45s ea	**52959-0436-45**	64.74		EE
60s ea	**52959-0436-60**	84.00		EE
90s ea	**52959-0436-90**	124.20		EE
120s ea	**52959-0436-01**	164.29		EE
75 mg, 10s ea	**52959-0423-10**	24.23		EE
14s ea	**52959-0423-14**	33.91		EE
15s ea	**52959-0423-15**	36.33		EE
20s ea	**52959-0423-20**	48.43		EE
21s ea	**52959-0423-21**	50.84		EE
28s ea	**52959-0423-28**	67.77		EE
30s ea	**52959-0423-30**	72.59		EE
60s ea	**52959-0423-60**	145.15		EE
90s ea	**52959-0423-90**	217.15		EE
120s ea	**52959-0423-02**	200.25		EE
TER, PO, 100 mg, 15s ea	**52959-0794-15**	51.62		AB
20s ea	**52959-0794-20**	66.81		AB
30s ea	**52959-0794-30**	99.90		AB
60s ea	**52959-0794-60**	199.50		AB
(Phys Total Care)				
REPACK				
ECT, PO, 25 mg, 100s ea	**54868-3999-00**	50.55		AB
50 mg, 20s ea	**54868-3659-02**	36.87		EE
30s ea	**54868-3659-00**	53.06		EE
60s ea	**54868-3659-03**	101.62		EE
90s ea	**54868-3659-04**	117.39		EE
100s ea	**54868-3659-01**	126.78		EE
75 mg, 20s ea	**54868-3837-00**	40.53		EE
30s ea	**54868-3837-03**	58.54		EE
60s ea	**54868-3837-01**	88.57		EE
100s ea	**54868-3837-02**	140.75		EE
TER, PO, 100 mg, 10s ea	**54868-5011-01**	27.12		AB
30s ea	**54868-5011-00**	72.36		AB
100s ea	**54868-5011-02**	175.95		AB
(Physician Partner)				
REPACK				
SOL, OP (1X0.5ML)				
0.1%, 0.5 ml	**21695-0710-05**	146.06		AT
(1X2.5ML)				
0.1%, 2.5 ml	**21695-0710-25**	89.54		AT
(Quality Care Prod)				
REPACK				
ECT, PO, 25 mg, 42s ea	**49999-0492-42**	24.78		AB
50 mg, 20s ea	**49999-0233-20**	18.00		EE
28s ea	**49999-0233-28**	25.20		AB
30s ea	**49999-0233-30**	32.57		EE
42s ea	**49999-0233-42**	37.80		EE
60s ea	**49999-0233-60**	81.14		AB
90s ea	**49999-0233-90**	113.87		AB
75 mg, 14s ea	**49999-0089-14**	39.62		AB
20s ea	**49999-0089-20**	55.91		EE
28s ea	**49999-0089-28**	66.37		AB
30s ea	**49999-0089-30**	83.51		EE
60s ea	**49999-0089-60**	149.60		EE
SOL, OP (1X2.5ML)				
0.1%, 2.5 ml	**35356-0554-25**	94.19		AT
(Southwood)				
REPACK				
ECT, PO, 50 mg, 10s ea	**58016-0381-10**	13.49		EE
15s ea	**58016-0381-15**	20.24		EE
20s ea	**58016-0381-20**	26.98		EE
28s ea	**58016-0381-28**	37.77		EE
30s ea	**58016-0381-30**	40.47		EE
60s ea	**58016-0381-60**	80.94		EE
80s ea	**58016-0381-80**	107.92		EE
90s ea	**58016-0381-90**	121.41		EE
100s ea	**58016-0381-00**	134.90		EE
120s ea	**58016-0381-02**	161.88		EE
150s ea	**58016-0381-03**	202.35		EE
200s ea	**58016-0381-89**	269.80		EE
300s ea	**58016-0381-73**	404.70		EE
75 mg, 10s ea	**58016-0382-10**	16.34		EE
14s ea	**58016-0382-14**	22.87		EE
15s ea	**58016-0382-15**	24.50		EE
20s ea	**58016-0382-20**	32.67		EE
28s ea	**58016-0382-28**	45.74		EE
30s ea	**58016-0382-30**	49.01		EE
40s ea	**58016-0382-40**	65.34		EE
60s ea	**58016-0382-60**	98.02		EE
80s ea	**58016-0382-80**	130.69		EE
90s ea	**58016-0382-90**	147.02		EE
100s ea	**58016-0382-00**	163.36		EE
120s ea	**58016-0382-02**	196.03		EE
150s ea	**58016-0382-03**	245.04		EE
200s ea	**58016-0382-89**	326.72		EE
300s ea	**58016-0382-73**	490.08		EE
SOL, OP, 0.1%, 5 ml	**58016-4046-01**	35.75		EE
TER, PO, 100 mg, 10s ea	**58016-0489-10**	32.79		EE
14s ea	**58016-0489-14**	45.90		EE
15s ea	**58016-0489-15**	49.18		EE
20s ea	**58016-0489-20**	65.57		EE
21s ea	**58016-0489-21**	68.85		EE
30s ea	**58016-0489-30**	98.36		EE
40s ea	**58016-0489-40**	131.14		EE
50s ea	**58016-0489-50**	163.93		EE
60s ea	**58016-0489-60**	196.71		EE
90s ea	**58016-0489-90**	295.07		EE
100s ea	**58016-0489-00**	327.85		EE
120s ea	**58016-0489-02**	393.42		EE
150s ea	**58016-0489-03**	491.78		EE
200s ea	**58016-0489-89**	655.70		EE
300s ea	**58016-0489-73**	983.55		EE
(St. Mary's MPP)				
REPACK				
ECT, PO, 75 mg, 10s ea	**60760-0789-10**	18.35		AB
20s ea	**60760-0789-20**	30.71		AB
30s ea	**60760-0789-30**	43.06		AB
60s ea	**60760-0789-60**	80.12		AB
90s ea	**60760-0789-90**	117.18		AB
(Stat Rx)				
REPACK				
ECT, PO, 50 mg, 21s ea	**16590-0074-21**	55.48		EE
75 mg, 20s ea	**16590-0075-20**	54.75		EE
30s ea	**16590-0075-30**	82.25		EE
56s ea	**16590-0075-56**	145.50		EE
60s ea	**16590-0075-60**	155.25		EE
90s ea	**16590-0075-90**	210.25		EE
(Vibranta)				
REPACK				
ECT, PO, 50 mg, 30s ea	**57866-1182-03**	27.00		
60s ea	**57866-1182-04**	54.00		
60s ea	**57866-3067-02**	61.16		
90s ea	**57866-1182-02**	81.00		
75 mg, 14s ea	**57866-6924-03**	30.49		
20s ea	**57866-6924-04**	43.56		
30s ea	**57866-6924-01**	65.34		
60s ea	**57866-6924-02**	135.09		
TER, PO, 100 mg, 30s ea	**57866-6925-01**	137.63		
DICLOFENAC SODIUM D-R (Palmetto)				
REPACK				
diclofenac sodium				
ECT, PO, 75 mg, 30s ea	**23490-0435-03**	46.46		
60s ea	**23490-0435-06**	92.91		
DICLOFENAC SODIUM D/R (Stat Rx)				
REPACK				
diclofenac sodium				
ECT, PO, 50 mg, 30s ea	**16590-0074-30**	79.25		
60s ea	**16590-0074-60**	158.50		
90s ea	**16590-0074-90**	227.75		
DICLOFENAC SODIUM DR (Actavis)				
diclofenac sodium				
ECT, PO, 50 mg, 60s ea	**00228-2550-06**	56.82		AB
100s ea	**00228-2550-11**	94.57		AB
1000s ea	**00228-2550-96**	927.29		AB
75 mg, 60s ea	**00228-2551-06**	68.79		AB
100s ea	**00228-2551-11**	114.47		AB
1000s ea	**00228-2551-96**	1123.02		AB
(Bryant Ranch)				
REPACK				
ECT, PO, 50 mg, 30s ea	**63629-1534-01**	51.78		
60s ea	**63629-1534-02**	103.56		
TER, PO, 75 mg, 20s ea	**63629-1535-03**	44.44		
28s ea	**63629-1535-01**	62.52		
30s ea	**63629-1535-04**	67.17		
60s ea	**63629-1535-02**	134.33		
90s ea	**63629-1535-06**	189.32		
120s ea	**63629-1535-05**	196.52		
(Dispensing Solutions)				
REPACK				
ECT, PO, 75 mg, 60s ea	**55045-2247-04**	97.80		AB
(HomeMed)				
REPACK				
ECT, PO, 75 mg, 14s ea	**51655-0307-84**	29.39		
30s ea	**51655-0307-24**	62.99		
60s ea	**51655-0307-25**	124.99		
(PD-Rx Pharm)				
REPACK				
ECT, PO, 75 mg, 28s ea	**55289-0150-28**	96.00		AB
(Quality Care Prod)				
REPACK				
ECT, PO, 75 mg, 40s ea	**35356-0422-40**	111.35		AB
DICLOFENAC SODIUM ER (DHS, Inc.)				
REPACK				
diclofenac sodium				
TER, PO, 75 mg, 120s ea	**55887-0542-82**	169.22		
100 mg, 30s ea	**55887-0083-30**	85.00		
60s ea	**55887-0083-60**	170.00		
90s ea	**55887-0083-90**	255.00		
DICLOFENAC SODIUM/MISOPROSTOL (Pfizer) *See ARTHROTEC*				
DICLOFENAC SODIUM/MISOPROSTOL (Palmetto)				
REPACK				
diclofenac sodium/misoprostol				
ECT, PO, 75 mg-0.2 mg,				
60s ea	**23490-7228-01**	135.35		
DICLOFENAC-NA (4u)				
REPACK				
diclofenac sodium				
ECT, PO, 75 mg, 60s ea	**10544-0310-60**	127.86		
DICLOFENAC-NA DR (4u)				
diclofenac sodium				
ECT, PO, 50 mg, 60s ea	**10544-0351-60**	126.86		
DICLOXACILLIN (Bryant Ranch)				
REPACK				
dicloxacillin sodium				
CAP, PO, 250 mg, 20s ea	**63629-1350-01**	18.48		
30s ea	**63629-1350-03**	27.72		
40s ea	**63629-1350-02**	36.96		
500 mg, 20s ea	**63629-1351-02**	33.60		
30s ea	**63629-1351-03**	50.40		
40s ea	**63629-1351-01**	67.20		
(Core)				
REPACK				
CAP, PO, 250 mg, 14s ea	**33358-0106-14**	10.11		
20s ea	**33358-0106-20**	18.94		
30s ea	**33358-0106-30**	28.41		
40s ea	**33358-0106-40**	37.88		
500 mg, 14s ea	**33358-0107-14**	16.71		
20s ea	**33358-0107-20**	34.44		
30s ea	**33358-0107-30**	51.66		
40s ea	**33358-0107-40**	68.88		

PROD/MFR	NDC	AWP	DP	OBC
(DHS, Inc.)				
REPACK				
CAP, PO, 250 mg, 14s ea	55887-0139-14	9.24		
21s ea	55887-0139-21	13.87		
28s ea	55887-0139-28	18.49		
(IPI)				
REPACK				
CAP, PO, 500 mg, 30s ea	18837-0042-30	45.00		
DICLOXACILLIN SODIUM (Sandoz)				
CAP, PO, 250 mg, 100s ea	00781-2248-01	66.05		AB
500 mg, 100s ea	00781-2258-01	120.11		
(Teva)				
CAP, PO, 250 mg, 100s ea	00093-3123-01	66.00		AB
500 mg, 100s ea	00093-3125-01	120.00		AB
(A-S Medication)				
REPACK				
CAP, PO, 250 mg, 20s ea	54569-0384-04	13.21		EE
28s ea	54569-0384-00	18.49		EE
40s ea	54569-0384-01	26.41		EE
500 mg, 20s ea	54569-1889-04	24.01		EE
28s ea	54569-1889-00	33.62		EE
40s ea	54569-1889-01	48.02		EE
(Altura)				
REPACK				
CAP, PO, 250 mg, 12s ea	63874-0108-12	11.83		AB
14s ea	63874-0108-14	13.81		AB
15s ea	63874-0108-15	14.79		AB
18s ea	63874-0108-18	17.76		AB
20s ea	63874-0108-20	19.73		EE
24s ea	63874-0108-24	23.66		AB
28s ea	63874-0108-28	27.63		EE
30s ea	63874-0108-30	29.60		AB
40s ea	63874-0108-40	39.46		AB
60s ea	63874-0108-60	59.19		AB
100s ea	63874-0108-01	98.65		AB
500 mg, 12s ea	63874-0123-12	22.18		EE
14s ea	63874-0123-14	25.87		EE
15s ea	63874-0123-15	27.72		EE
20s ea	63874-0123-20	36.96		EE
21s ea	63874-0123-21	38.81		EE
24s ea	63874-0123-24	44.35		EE
28s ea	63874-0123-28	51.74		EE
30s ea	63874-0123-30	55.44		EE
40s ea	63874-0123-40	73.93		EE
50s ea	63874-0123-50	92.16		EE
60s ea	63874-0123-60	110.88		EE
100s ea	63874-0123-01	184.80		EE
(DHS, Inc.)				
REPACK				
CAP, PO, 500 mg, 30s ea	55887-0704-30	59.46		AB
(Dispensing Solutions)				
REPACK				
CAP, PO, 250 mg, 20s ea	55045-1918-07	18.60		AB
28s ea	55045-1918-09	26.04		AB
30s ea	55045-1918-08	27.90		AB
40s ea	55045-1918-03	37.00		AB
40s ea	66336-0480-40	38.90		AB
60s ea	55045-1918-06	55.80		AB
90s ea	55045-1918-01	83.70		AB
100s ea	55045-1918-00	93.00		AB
120s ea	55045-1918-02	111.60		AB
500 mg, 12s ea	55045-1227-02	21.48		AB
20s ea	55045-1227-07	35.80		AB
28s ea	55045-1227-09	50.00		AB
30s ea	55045-1227-08	53.70		
40s ea	55045-1227-03	71.60		AB
60s ea	55045-1227-06	107.40		
90s ea	55045-1227-01	161.10		
100s ea	55045-1227-00	179.00		
120s ea	55045-1227-04	214.80		AB
(GSMS)				
REPACK				
CAP, PO (UNIT OF USE)				
250 mg, 40s ea	60429-0059-40	61.05	20.35	AB
(HomeMed)				
REPACK				
CAP, PO, 250 mg, 28s ea	51655-0213-29	27.69		EE
40s ea	51655-0213-51	39.55		EE
(Nucare Pharm)				
REPACK				
CAP, PO, 250 mg, 20s ea	66267-0072-20	18.79		EE
28s ea	66267-0072-28	26.31		EE
40s ea	66267-0072-40	37.58		EE
500 mg, 20s ea	66267-0073-20	35.80		EE
28s ea	66267-0073-28	50.12		EE
40s ea	66267-0073-40	71.60		EE

PROD/MFR	NDC	AWP	DP	OBC
(Palmetto)				
REPACK				
CAP, PO, 250 mg, 28s ea	23490-5425-01	26.31		
40s ea	23490-5425-02	37.89		
500 mg, 28s ea	23490-5426-01	51.80		
30s ea	23490-5426-03	55.50		
40s ea	23490-5426-02	74.00		
(PD-Rx Pharm)				
REPACK				
CAP, PO (USP)				
250 mg, 6s ea	43063-0180-06	11.34		AB
10s ea	55289-0592-10	19.00		AB
20s ea	55289-0592-20	28.00		AB
28s ea	55289-0592-28	35.20		AB
28s ea	58864-0149-28	35.19		AB
40s ea	55289-0592-40	46.00		AB
(REDI-SCRIPT)				
250 mg, 40s ea	58864-0149-40	45.99		AB
500 mg, 20s ea	55289-0094-20	54.67		AB
30s ea	55289-0094-30	77.00		AB
40s ea	55289-0094-40	99.33		AB
(Pharma Pac)				
REPACK				
CAP, PO, 250 mg, 20s ea	52959-0048-20	19.06		EE
28s ea	52959-0048-28	27.27		EE
30s ea	52959-0048-30	28.13		EE
40s ea	52959-0048-40	38.25		EE
41s ea	52959-0048-41	39.08		EE
500 mg, 20s ea	52959-0049-20	54.57		EE
21s ea	52959-0049-21	57.30		EE
28s ea	52959-0049-28	74.73		EE
30s ea	52959-0049-30	79.85		EE
40s ea	52959-0049-40	103.25		EE
(Phys Total Care)				
REPACK				
CAP, PO, 250 mg, 20s ea	54868-0937-01	12.75		EE
30s ea	54868-0937-00	35.54		AB
40s ea	54868-0937-02	46.38		EE
500 mg, 20s ea	54868-1380-01	45.12		EE
30s ea	54868-1380-03	65.43		EE
40s ea	54868-1380-02	85.74		EE
60s ea	54868-1380-00	126.36		AB
(Physician Partner)				
REPACK				
CAP, PO, 250 mg, 30s ea	21695-0124-30	39.63		AB
(Quality Care Prod)				
REPACK				
CAP, PO, 250 mg, 28s ea	49999-0267-28	31.58		AB
30s ea	49999-0267-30	33.83		AB
40s ea	49999-0267-40	45.11		EE
500 mg, 20s ea	49999-0120-20	65.48		AB
28s ea	49999-0120-28	60.15		
40s ea	49999-0120-40	85.92		
(Southwood)				
REPACK				
CAP, PO, 250 mg, 10s ea	58016-0121-10	9.40		EE
12s ea	58016-0121-12	11.27		EE
14s ea	58016-0121-14	13.15		EE
15s ea	58016-0121-15	14.09		EE
18s ea	58016-0121-18	16.91		EE
20s ea	58016-0121-20	18.79		EE
24s ea	58016-0121-24	22.55		EE
28s ea	58016-0121-28	26.31		EE
30s ea	58016-0121-30	28.19		EE
40s ea	58016-0121-40	37.58		EE
100s ea	58016-0121-00	93.95		EE
500 mg, 10s ea	58016-0122-10	17.60		EE
12s ea	58016-0122-12	21.48		EE
14s ea	58016-0122-14	25.06		EE
15s ea	58016-0122-15	26.85		EE
20s ea	58016-0122-20	35.80		EE
21s ea	58016-0122-21	36.96		EE
24s ea	58016-0122-24	42.24		EE
28s ea	58016-0122-28	50.12		EE
30s ea	58016-0122-30	53.70		EE
40s ea	58016-0122-40	71.60		EE
50s ea	58016-0122-50	89.50		EE
60s ea	58016-0122-60	105.60		EE
100s ea	58016-0122-00	179.00		EE
(Stat Rx)				
REPACK				
CAP, PO, 500 mg, 21s ea	16590-0076-21	18.22		
30s ea	16590-0076-30	26.00		
DICUMAROL (PCCA)				
POW, NA, 1 gm	51927-3389-00	18.60		
4,5-DICYANOIMIDAZOLE (PCCA)				
POW, NA (1X1GM)				
1 gm	51927-3545-00	7.50		

PROD/MFR	NDC	AWP	DP	OBC
DICYCLOCOT (Truxton)				
dicyclomine hydrochloride				
SOL, IM (VIAL)				
10 mg/ml, 10 ml	00463-1104-10	9.50		EE
DICYCLOMINE (Dispensing Solutions)				
REPACK				
dicyclomine hydrochloride				
CAP, PO, 10 mg, 30s ea	66336-0911-30	12.57		
DICYCLOMINE HCL (Bedford)				
dicyclomine hydrochloride				
SOL, IM (U.S.P.)				
10 mg/ml, 2 ml 10s	55390-0066-10	171.60		AP
(Consolidated Midland)				
SOL, IM (VIAL)				
10 mg/ml, 10 ml	00223-7430-10	8.75		EE
TAB, PO, 20 mg, 100s ea	00223-0795-01	6.25		EE
1000s ea	00223-0795-02	37.50		EE
(Lannett)				
CAP, PO, 10 mg, 100s ea	00527-0586-01	26.38		AB
1000s ea	00527-0586-10	246.89		AB
TAB, PO, 20 mg, 100s ea	00527-1282-01	35.50		AB
1000s ea	00527-1282-10	277.35		AB
(Major)				
TAB, PO, 20 mg, 100s ea	00904-0195-60	29.75		EE
(Mylan)				
CAP, PO, 10 mg, 100s ea	00378-1610-01	26.38		AB
500s ea	00378-1610-05	128.00		AB
TAB, PO, 20 mg, 100s ea	00378-1620-01	35.50		AB
500s ea	00378-1620-05	165.00		AB
(Qualitest)				
CAP, PO, 10 mg, 100s ea	00603-3265-21	26.38		AB
1000s ea	00603-3265-32	246.80		AB
SYR, PO (BERRY)				
10 mg/5 ml, 473 ml	00603-1161-58	45.60		
(UDL)				
CAP, PO (10X10)				
10 mg, 100s ea UD	51079-0118-20	26.60		AB
TAB, PO, 20 mg,				
100s ea UD	51079-0119-20	34.84		AB
(Watson Labs)				
CAP, PO, 10 mg, 100s ea	00591-0794-01	7.08		AB
1000s ea	00591-0794-10	69.48		AB
TAB, PO, 20 mg, 100s ea	00591-0795-01	9.48		AB
1000s ea	00591-0795-10	88.68		AB
(West-Ward)				
CAP, PO, 10 mg, 100s ea	00143-3126-01	23.95		AB
1000s ea	00143-3126-10	215.25		AB
TAB, PO, 20 mg, 100s ea	00143-1227-01	30.50		AB
1000s ea	00143-1227-10	272.50		AB
(A-S Medication)				
REPACK				
CAP, PO, 10 mg, 30s ea	54569-0417-00	7.91		EE
60s ea	54569-0417-02	15.83		EE
TAB, PO, 20 mg, 10s ea	54569-0419-07	3.55		EE
20s ea	54569-0419-02	7.10		EE
30s ea	54569-0419-00	10.65		EE
(Altura)				
REPACK				
CAP, PO, 10 mg, 10s ea	63874-0463-10	4.84		AB
12s ea	63874-0463-12	5.80		AB
20s ea	63874-0463-20	9.67		AB
21s ea	63874-0463-21	10.16		AB
28s ea	63874-0463-28	13.54		AB
30s ea	63874-0463-30	14.51		AB
60s ea	63874-0463-60	29.02		AB
90s ea	63874-0463-90	43.53		AB
100s ea	63874-0463-01	48.37		AB
1000s ea	63874-0463-02	290.83		AB
(DHS, Inc.)				
REPACK				
CAP, PO, 10 mg, 15s ea	55887-0909-15	8.00		AB
30s ea	55887-0909-30	15.00		AB
90s ea	55887-0909-90	41.00		AB
(Dispensing Solutions)				
REPACK				
CAP, PO, 10 mg, 10s ea	55045-2045-08	5.80		AB
24s ea	55045-2197-06	13.92		AB
30s ea	55045-2197-08	17.40		AB
60s ea	55045-2197-05	34.80		AB
90s ea	55045-2197-09	52.20		AB
100s ea	55045-2197-01	58.00		AB
120s ea	55045-2197-02	69.60		AB
TAB, PO, 20 mg, 20s ea	55045-1467-02	13.60		AB
30s ea	55045-1467-08	20.40		AB
60s ea	55045-1467-09	40.80		AB
90s ea	55045-1467-06	61.20		AB
100s ea	55045-1467-01	68.00		AB

PROD/MFR	NDC	AWP	DP	OBC
120s ea	55045-1467-03	81.60		AB
(HomeMed) REPACK				
TAB, PO, 20 mg, 30s ea	51655-0293-24	21.99		EE
(Nucare Pharm) REPACK				
TAB, PO, 20 mg, 30s ea	66267-0074-30	12.89		EE
(PD-Rx Pharm) REPACK				
CAP, PO (USP)				
10 mg, 4s ea	43063-0112-04	7.50		AB
6s ea	43063-0112-06	8.40		AB
20s ea	55289-0923-20	14.00		AB
30s ea	55289-0923-30	16.00		AB
30s ea	58864-0153-30	15.99		AB
TAB, PO (USP)				
20 mg, 4s ea	43063-0045-04	10.98		AB
15s ea	55289-0095-15	12.87		AB
20s ea	55289-0095-20	14.00		AB
30s ea	55289-0095-30	15.87		AB
60s ea	55289-0095-60	21.70		AB
100s ea UD	55289-0095-17	86.00		AB
(Pharma Pac) REPACK				
CAP, PO, 10 mg, 30s ea	52959-0168-30	19.20		EE
100s ea	52959-0168-00	63.95		EE
TAB, PO, 20 mg, 20s ea	52959-0221-20	10.63		EE
30s ea	52959-0221-30	13.32		EE
100s ea	52959-0221-00	27.68		EE
(Phys Total Care) REPACK				
CAP, PO, 10 mg, 10s ea	54868-0033-06	4.44		EE
20s ea	54868-0033-00	5.85		EE
30s ea	54868-0033-03	7.29		EE
40s ea	54868-0033-05	8.73		EE
60s ea	54868-0033-07	11.58		AB
90s ea	54868-0033-08	17.38		EE
100s ea	54868-0033-02	17.31		EE
TAB, PO, 20 mg, 20s ea	54868-0818-01	7.14		EE
30s ea	54868-0818-07	9.18		EE
40s ea	54868-0818-08	11.25		EE
60s ea	54868-0818-03	15.39		EE
90s ea	54868-0818-00	19.54		AB
100s ea	54868-0818-05	22.14		EE
(Physician Partner) REPACK				
CAP, PO, 10 mg, 60s ea	21695-0218-60	28.74		AB
90s ea	21695-0218-90	43.11		AB
TAB, PO, 20 mg, 30s ea	21695-0219-30	26.64		AB
(Quality Care Prod) REPACK				
CAP, PO, 10 mg, 20s ea	49999-0291-20	13.70		
TAB, PO, 20 mg, 20s ea	49999-0081-20	19.77		AB
30s ea	49999-0081-30	29.65		EE
100s ea	49999-0081-00	98.85		AB
(Southwood) REPACK				
CAP, PO, 10 mg, 12s ea	58016-0702-12	3.32		EE
30s ea	58016-0702-30	5.36		EE
TAB, PO, 20 mg, 12s ea	58016-0703-12	5.06		EE
30s ea	58016-0703-30	12.66		EE
100s ea	58016-0703-00	42.20		EE
(Stat Rx) REPACK				
TAB, PO, 20 mg, 120s ea	16590-0324-72	40.50		AB
(Vibranta) REPACK				
CAP, PO, 10 mg, 60s ea	57866-3367-03	16.91		AB
TAB, PO, 20 mg, 60s ea	57866-3377-04	22.15		AB
DICYCLOMINE HYDROCHLORIDE FUL				
CAP, PO, 10 mg, 100s ea		8.85		
TAB, PO, 20 mg, 100s ea		4.05		
(Axcan) *See BENTYL*				
(Bedford) *See DICYCLOMINE HCL*				
(Consolidated Midland) *See DICYCLOMINE HCL*				
(Gallipot)				
POW, NA (USP)				
25 gm	51552-0741-04	23.80	17.00	
(Lannett) *See DICYCLOMINE HCL*				
(Major) *See DICYCLOMINE HCL*				
(Marlex)				
CAP, PO (USP)				
10 mg, 100s ea	10135-0520-01	26.38		AB
1000s ea	10135-0520-10	275.00		AB
TAB, PO, 20 mg, 100s ea	10135-0521-01	35.50		AB
(Mylan) *See DICYCLOMINE HCL*				
(PCCA)				
POW, NA (U.S.P.)				
1 gm	51927-1347-00	2.40		
(Qualitest) *See DICYCLOMINE HCL*				
(Truxton) *See DICYCLOCOT*				
(UDL) *See DICYCLOMINE HCL*				
(Watson Labs) *See DICYCLOMINE HCL*				
(West-Ward) *See DICYCLOMINE HCL*				
(Bryant Ranch) REPACK				
TAB, PO, 20 mg, 30s ea	63629-1299-01	14.91		
(Palmetto) REPACK				
CAP, PO, 10 mg, 6s ea	23490-5428-01	5.38		
20s ea	23490-5428-03	12.86		
30s ea	23490-5428-02	19.29		
TAB, PO, 20 mg, 20s ea	23490-5431-02	14.66		
30s ea	23490-5431-03	21.99		
60s ea	23490-5431-04	43.98		
(Physician Partner) REPACK				
CAP, PO, 10 mg, 30s ea	21695-0218-30	14.37		
(Stat Rx) REPACK				
CAP, PO, 10 mg, 30s ea	16590-0077-30	11.00		
60s ea	16590-0077-60	22.00		
90s ea	16590-0077-90	33.00		
120s ea	16590-0077-72	44.00		
DIDANOSINE (Aurobindo Pharma)				
ECC, PO (HARD GELATIN)				
125 mg, 30s ea	65862-0310-30	115.81		AB
200 mg, 30s ea	65862-0311-30	185.26		AB
250 mg, 30s ea	65862-0312-30	236.08		AB
400 mg, 30s ea	65862-0313-30	368.72		AB
(B/M Squibb Onc/Vir) *See VIDEX EC*				
(B/M Squibb Onc/Vir) *See VIDEX PEDIATRIC*				
(Teva)				
ECC, PO (ENTERIC-COATED PELLETS)				
200 mg, 30s ea	00555-0588-01	185.26		AB
250 mg, 30s ea	00555-0589-01	236.08		AB
400 mg, 30s ea	00555-0590-01	368.72		AB
(A-S Medication) REPACK				
ECC, PO, 250 mg, 30s ea	54569-5642-00	220.84		AB
400 mg, 30s ea	54569-5643-00	344.92		AB
(Advanced Pharm Serv, Inc.) REPACK				
ECC, PO, 200 mg, 20s ea	13411-0191-02	106.40		
30s ea	13411-0191-03	187.13		
60s ea	13411-0191-06	319.20		
90s ea	13411-0191-09	478.80		
100s ea	13411-0191-10	532.00		
250 mg, 20s ea	13411-0192-02	136.20		
30s ea	13411-0192-03	238.46		
60s ea	13411-0192-06	408.60		
90s ea	13411-0192-09	612.90		
100s ea	13411-0192-10	681.00		
400 mg, 20s ea	13411-0193-02	214.00		
30s ea	13411-0193-03	378.20		
60s ea	13411-0193-06	642.00		
90s ea	13411-0193-09	963.00		
100s ea	13411-0193-10	1070.00		
(American Health) REPACK				
ECC, PO (3X10)				
250 mg, 30s ea UD	62584-0046-21	283.49		AB
400 mg, 30s ea UD	62584-0048-21	449.59		AB
(Quality Care Prod) REPACK				
ECC, PO, 400 mg, 30s ea	35356-0259-30	596.00		AB
DIDANOSINE DR (Phys Total Care) REPACK				
didanosine				
ECC, PO, 250 mg, 30s ea	54868-5464-00	532.97		
DIDREX (Pfizer)				
benzphetamine hydrochloride				
TAB, PO, 50 mg,				
100s ea, C-III	00009-0024-01	176.90	147.42	
500s ea, C-III	00009-0024-02	884.52	737.10	
(A-S Medication) REPACK				
TAB, PO, 50 mg,				
30s ea, C-III	54569-0389-01	55.28		
60s ea, C-III	54569-0389-05	137.98		
90s ea, C-III	54569-0389-06	165.85		
100s ea, C-III	54569-0389-00	184.28		
(Dispensing Solutions) REPACK				
TAB, PO, 50 mg,				
21s ea, C-III	66336-0678-21	58.74		
(PD-Rx Pharm) REPACK				
TAB, PO, 50 mg,				
28s ea, C-III	55289-0432-28	73.76		
56s ea, C-III	55289-0432-56	147.36		
60s ea, C-III	55289-0432-60	158.06		
90s ea, C-III	55289-0432-90	236.94		
DIDRONEL (P & G Pharm)				
etidronate disodium				
TAB, PO (CAPLET)				
400 mg, 60s ea	00149-0406-60	488.75	407.29	
(Phys Total Care) REPACK				
TAB, PO, 400 mg, 15s ea	54868-2981-01	114.19		
60s ea	54868-2981-00	425.53		
DIENESTROL (Gallipot)				
POW, NA, 1 gm	51552-0560-01	104.30		
(PCCA)				
POW, NA (USP)				
1 gm	51927-3476-00	261.00		
(Spectrum Pharmacy)				
POW, NA (U.S.P.)				
1 gm	49452-2591-02	381.50		
5 gm	49452-2591-03	1393.00		
DIETHANOLAMINE (PCCA)				
LIQ, NA, 1 gm	51927-1302-00	0.45		
(Spectrum Pharmacy)				
LIQ, NA (N.F.)				
500 ml	49452-2585-01	149.10		
4000 ml	49452-2585-02	707.00		
DIETHYL PHTHALATE (Amend)				
LIQ, NA, 500 ml	17317-0876-01	11.20		
3840 ml	17317-0876-06	35.00		
20000 ml	17317-0876-08	140.00		
(Spectrum Pharmacy)				
LIQ, NA (N.F.)				
500 ml	49452-2595-01	116.20		
4000 ml	49452-2595-02	343.35		
20000 ml	49452-2595-03	973.00		
DIETHYL-M-TOLUAMIDE (PCCA)				
diethyltoluamide				
SOL, NA ((N,N); 98%; DEET)				
98%, 1 gm	51927-1336-00	0.53		
DIETHYLCARBAMAZINE CITRATE (PCCA)				
POW, NA, 1 gm	51927-2924-00	65.40		
DIETHYLDITHIOCARBAMIC ACID SODIUM REAGENT ACS (PCCA)				
ditiocarb sodium				
CRY, NA (1X1GM)				
1 gm	51927-1639-00	0.59		
DIETHYLENE GLYCOL MONOETHYL ETHER				
(Gallipot) *See ETHOXY DIGLYCOL*				
(PCCA) *See ETHOXY DIGLYCOL*				
(PCCA)				
SOL, NA (NF,1X1ML)				
1 ml	51927-3680-00	0.31		
DIETHYLHEXYL ADIPATE				
(Medisca) *See DIOCTYL ADIPATE*				
(PCCA) *See DIOCTYL ADIPATE*				
DIETHYLNICOTINAMIDE (N,N) (PCCA)				
nikethamide				
SOL, NA (1X1ML)				
97%, 1 ml	51927-3262-00	3.45		
DIETHYLPROPION (DHS, Inc.) REPACK				
diethylpropion hydrochloride				
TAB, PO, 25 mg,				
21s ea, C-IV	55887-0669-21	12.60		
(Dispensing Solutions) REPACK				
TAB, PO, 25 mg,				
14s ea, C-IV	66336-0864-14	7.78		
21s ea, C-IV	66336-0864-21	10.99		

PROD/MFR	NDC	AWP	DP	OBC
28s ea, C-IV	66336-0864-28	15.34		
30s ea, C-IV	66336-0864-30	17.16		
42s ea, C-IV	66336-0864-42	23.33		
60s ea, C-IV	66336-0864-60	57.98		
84s ea, C-IV	66336-0864-84	67.39		
TER, PO, 75 mg,				
7s ea, C-IV	66336-0689-07	17.04		
14s ea, C-IV	66336-0689-14	28.36		
28s ea, C-IV	66336-0689-28	44.29		
30s ea, C-IV	66336-0689-30	47.41		
DIETHYLPROPION HCL (Watson Labs)				
diethylpropion hydrochloride				
TAB, PO, 25 mg,				
100s ea, C-IV	00591-0783-01	27.50		AA
TER, PO, 75 mg,				
100s ea, C-IV	00591-0782-01	101.23		
(A-S Medication) REPACK				
TAB, PO, 25 mg,				
14s ea, C-IV	54569-2059-03	7.26		EE
28s ea, C-IV	54569-2059-04	14.52		EE
30s ea, C-IV	54569-2059-08	15.56		EE
56s ea, C-IV	54569-2059-09	29.04		EE
60s ea, C-IV	54569-2059-07	31.11		EE
90s ea, C-IV	54569-2059-05	46.67		EE
100s ea, C-IV	54569-5120-02	51.85		EE
TER, PO, 75 mg,				
15s ea, C-IV	54569-0396-01	19.53		
28s ea, C-IV	54569-0396-05	36.45		
30s ea, C-IV	54569-0396-00	39.05		
(Altura) REPACK				
TER, PO, 75 mg,				
20s ea, C-IV	63874-0265-20	26.34		
100s ea, C-IV	63874-0265-01	91.10		
(DHS, Inc.) REPACK				
TAB, PO, 25 mg,				
30s ea, C-IV	55887-0669-30	18.00		AA
60s ea, C-IV	55887-0669-60	34.00		AA
90s ea, C-IV	55887-0669-90	49.00		AA
TER, PO, 75 mg,				
30s ea, C-IV	55887-0654-30	40.00		
60s ea, C-IV	55887-0654-60	69.22		
(Dispensing Solutions) REPACK				
TAB, PO, 25 mg,				
30s ea, C-IV	55045-1283-08	13.50		AA
90s ea, C-IV	55045-1283-00	40.50		AA
TER, PO, 75 mg,				
28s ea, C-IV	55045-1284-07	36.40		
30s ea, C-IV	55045-1284-08	39.00		
(PD-Rx Pharm) REPACK				
TAB, PO (WHITE)				
25 mg, 7s ea, C-IV	55289-0794-07	7.00		AA
14s ea, C-IV	55289-0794-14	9.00		AA
21s ea, C-IV	55289-0794-21	10.98		AA
28s ea, C-IV	55289-0794-28	14.28		AA
(WHITE)				
25 mg,				
30s ea, C-IV	55289-0794-30	15.00		AA
60s ea, C-IV	55289-0794-60	23.73		AA
90s ea, C-IV	55289-0794-90	32.49		AA
100s ea, C-IV	55289-0794-01	34.47		AA
180s ea, C-IV	55289-0794-93	65.91		AA
TER, PO, 75 mg,				
7s ea, C-IV	55289-0368-07	65.91		
14s ea, C-IV	55289-0368-14	23.40		
30s ea, C-IV	55289-0368-30	42.16		
(Pharma Pac) REPACK				
TAB, PO, 25 mg,				
30s ea, C-IV	52959-0150-30	13.98		EE
90s ea, C-IV	52959-0150-90	41.67		EE
TER, PO, 75 mg,				
14s ea, C-IV	52959-0329-14	17.08		
28s ea, C-IV	52959-0329-28	34.16		
30s ea, C-IV	52959-0329-30	36.75		
90s ea, C-IV	52959-0329-90	83.25		
(Phys Total Care) REPACK				
TAB, PO, 25 mg,				
30s ea, C-IV	54868-1462-01	20.67		AA
60s ea, C-IV	54868-1462-00	35.34		AA
TER, PO, 75 mg,				
30s ea, C-IV	54868-1463-00	102.66		

PROD/MFR	NDC	AWP	DP	OBC
(Physician Partner) REPACK				
TER, PO, 75 mg,				
30s ea, C-IV	21695-0876-30	78.10		
(Quality Care Prod) REPACK				
TAB, PO, 25 mg,				
28s ea, C-IV	49999-0925-28	26.60		AA
30s ea, C-IV	49999-0925-30	27.30		AA
60s ea, C-IV	49999-0925-60	54.60		AA
90s ea, C-IV	49999-0925-90	81.90		AA
TER, PO, 75 mg,				
28s ea, C-IV	49999-0457-28	56.33		
30s ea, C-IV	49999-0457-30	87.60		
(Southwood) REPACK				
TAB, PO, 25 mg,				
15s ea, C-IV	58016-0856-15	5.05		EE
21s ea, C-IV	58016-0856-21	5.89		EE
42s ea, C-IV	58016-0856-42	7.86		EE
100s ea, C-IV	58016-0856-00	12.95		EE
TER, PO, 75 mg,				
7s ea, C-IV	58016-0836-07	9.63		
14s ea, C-IV	58016-0836-14	14.68		
15s ea, C-IV	58016-0836-15	15.37		
30s ea, C-IV	58016-0836-30	19.99		
DIETHYLPROPION HCL WITH TARTARIC ACID (PCCA)				
diethylpropion hydrochloride/tartaric acid				
POW, NA (CIV,USP)				
1%, 1 gm, C-IV	51927-1025-00	9.60		
DIETHYLPROPION HYDROCHLORIDE (CorePharma)				
TAB, PO (USP,COMPRESSED)				
25 mg,				
100s ea, C-IV	64720-0208-10	51.85		AB
(Watson Labs) *See DIETHYLPROPION HCL*				
(Palmetto) REPACK				
TAB, PO, 25 mg,				
14s ea, C-IV	23490-5434-01	8.40		
21s ea, C-IV	23490-5434-02	12.60		
28s ea, C-IV	23490-5434-03	16.80		
30s ea, C-IV	23490-5434-04	18.00		
42s ea, C-IV	23490-5434-05	25.20		
60s ea, C-IV	23490-5434-06	36.00		
84s ea, C-IV	23490-5434-07	50.40		
TER, PO, 75 mg,				
7s ea, C-IV	23490-5435-01	16.62		
14s ea, C-IV	23490-5435-02	19.67		
28s ea, C-IV	23490-5435-03	39.35		
30s ea, C-IV	23490-5435-04	42.16		
(Quality Care Prod) REPACK				
TAB, PO, 25 mg,				
100s ea, C-IV	49999-0925-00	62.00		
DIETHYLPROPION HYDROCHLORIDE/TARTARIC ACID (PCCA) *See DIETHYLPROPION HCL WITH TARTARIC ACID*				
DIETHYLSTILBESTROL (Gallipot)				
POW, NA (1X1GM,USP)				
1 gm	51552-0780-01	11.20	8.00	
(1X5GM,USP)				
5 gm	51552-0780-02	42.00	30.00	
(1X25GM,USP)				
25 gm	51552-0780-04	196.00	140.00	
(Letco)				
POW, NA (DES)				
25 gm	62991-1188-03	240.00		
100 gm	62991-1188-04	750.00		
(Medisca)				
POW, NA (U.S.P.)				
1 gm	38779-1865-06	26.85		
5 gm	38779-1865-03	67.50		
25 gm	38779-1865-04	327.00		
100 gm	38779-1865-05	840.00		
(PCCA)				
POW, NA (U.S.P.)				
1 gm	51927-3099-00	27.00		
(Spectrum Pharmacy)				
CRY, NA (U.S.P.)				
1 gm	49452-2592-01	54.25		
5 gm	49452-2592-02	111.65		
25 gm	49452-2592-03	448.00		
DIETHYLTOLUAMIDE (Medisca)				
SOL, NA (USP,1X100ML)				
100 ml	38779-1241-05	36.00		
(USP,1X1000ML)				
1000 ml	38779-1241-09	76.50		

PROD/MFR	NDC	AWP	DP	OBC
(PCCA) *See DIETHYL-M-TOLUAMIDE*				
DIFFERIN (Galderma)				
adapalene				
CRE, TP, 0.1%, 45 gm	00299-5915-45	227.50		
GEL, TP, 0.1%, 45 gm	00299-5910-45	227.50		
0.3%, 45 gm	00299-5918-45	220.00		EE
(Phys Total Care) REPACK				
CRE, TP, 0.1%, 45 gm	54868-5271-00	228.67		
GEL, TP, 0.1%, 45 gm	54868-5030-00	228.67		
(1X45GM)				
0.3%, 45 gm	54868-5958-00	251.97		EE
(Quality Care Prod) REPACK				
CRE, TP (1X45GM)				
0.1%, 45 gm	35356-0291-45	314.38		
GEL, TP, 0.1%, 45 gm	35356-0290-45	314.38		
0.3%, 45 gm	35356-0292-45	314.38		EE
DIFIL G FORTE (SJ)				
dyphylline/guaifenesin				
LIQ, PO, 240 ml	45985-0633-08	29.99		
DIFIL-G 400 (SJ)				
dyphylline/guaifenesin				
TAB, PO, 200 mg-400 mg,				
100s ea	24839-0226-01	63.73		
DIFIL-G FORTE (SJ)				
dyphylline/guaifenesin				
SOL, PO (1X480ML,MINT)				
100 mg/5 ml-100 mg/5 ml,				
480 ml	24839-0227-16	65.98		
DIFLORASONE DIACETATE (Fougera)				
CRE, TP, 0.05%, 15 gm	00168-0242-15	36.78		AB
30 gm	00168-0242-30	50.78		AB
60 gm	00168-0242-60	97.22		AB
OIN, TP, 0.05%, 15 gm	00168-0243-15	37.56		AB
30 gm	00168-0243-30	51.86		AB
60 gm	00168-0243-60	100.16		AB
(PCCA)				
POW, NA (USP)				
1 gm	51927-2933-00	1035.00		
(PharmaDerm) *See APEXICON*				
(PharmaDerm) *See APEXICON E*				
(Taro)				
CRE, TP, 0.05%, 15 gm	51672-1296-01	36.59		AB
30 gm	51672-1296-02	50.28		AB
60 gm	51672-1296-03	96.63		AB
OIN, TP, 0.05%, 15 gm	51672-1295-01	36.59		AB
30 gm	51672-1295-02	50.28		AB
60 gm	51672-1295-03	96.63		AB
(Quality Care Prod) REPACK				
CRE, TP, 0.05%, 60 gm	49999-0863-60	66.96		
(Southwood) REPACK				
CRE, TP, 0.05%, 30 gm	58016-4874-01	50.78		
DIFLORASONE DIACETATE MICRONIZED (Medisca)				
diflorasone diacetate, micronized				
POW, NA, 1 gm	38779-0857-06	1041.00		
DIFLORASONE DIACETATE, MICRONIZED (Medisca) *See DIFLORASONE DIACETATE MICRONIZED*				
DIFLUCAN (Pfizer)				
fluconazole				
PDR, PO, 50 mg/5 ml,				
35 ml	00049-3440-19	53.90	44.92	
200 mg/5 ml, 35 ml	00049-3450-19	195.82	163.18	
TAB, PO, 50 mg, 30s ea	00049-3410-30	240.24	200.20	
100 mg, 30s ea	00049-3420-30	377.50	314.58	
100s ea UD	00049-3420-41	1258.31	1048.59	
(CAPLET)				
150 mg, 12s ea	00049-3500-79	240.34	200.28	
200 mg, 30s ea	00049-3430-30	617.74	514.78	
100s ea UD	00049-3430-41	2059.09	1715.91	
(A-S Medication) REPACK				
TAB, PO (CAPLET)				
150 mg, ea	54569-3954-00	19.87		
200 mg, ea	54569-3269-00	19.46		
(Direct Pharmaceutical, Inc.) REPACK				
TAB, PO, 100 mg,				
30s ea UD	67801-0208-03	321.63		
200 mg, 30s ea UD	67801-0212-03	525.53		
(Nucare Pharm) REPACK				
TAB, PO, 150 mg, ea	66267-0978-01	18.51		

PROD/MFR	NDC	AWP	DP	OBC
(PD-Rx Pharm)				
REPACK				
TAB, PO, 200 mg, ea	**55289-0148-79**	26.07		
(Pharma Pac)				
REPACK				
TAB, PO, 150 mg, ea	**52959-0455-01**	18.71		
(Phys Total Care)				
REPACK				
TAB, PO, 100 mg, 7s ea	**54868-1863-02**	77.58		
10s ea	**54868-1863-01**	110.01		
30s ea	**54868-1863-03**	326.28		
150 mg, ea	**54868-3444-00**	20.60		
12s ea	**54868-3444-01**	216.36		
200 mg, 30s ea	**54868-1034-01**	265.98		
(Quality Care Prod)				
REPACK				
TAB, PO, 150 mg, ea UD	**49999-0158-01**	35.34		
DIFLUCAN IV (Pfizer)				
fluconazole				
SOL, IV (SODIUM CHLORIDE DILUENT)				
200 mg/100 ml,				
100 ml 6s	**00049-3371-26**	770.77	642.31	
(VIAFLEX, DEXTROSE,AF)				
200 mg/100 ml,				
100 ml 6s	**00049-3437-26**	770.77	642.31	
(VIAFLEX,SODIUM CHLORIDE)				
200 mg/100 ml,				
100 ml 6s	**00049-3435-26**	770.77	642.31	
(SODIUM CHLORIDE DILUENT)				
400 mg/200 ml,				
200 ml 6s	**00049-3372-26**	1126.51	938.76	
(VIAFLEX, DEXTROSE,AF)				
400 mg/200 ml,				
200 ml 6s	**00049-3438-26**	1126.51	938.76	
(VIAFLEX,SODIUM CHLORIDE)				
400 mg/200 ml,				
200 ml 6s	**00049-3436-26**	1126.51	938.76	
DIFLUNISAL (PCCA)				
POW, NA, 1 gm	**51927-2618-00**	1.56		
(Teva)				
TAB, PO, 500 mg, 60s ea	**00093-0755-06**	79.12		AB
100s ea	**00093-0755-01**	129.23		AB
500s ea	**00093-0755-05**	639.55		AB
(West Point)				
TAB, PO (CAPLET)				
500 mg, 500s ea	**59591-0196-74**	437.47		AB
(A-S Medication)				
REPACK				
TAB, PO, 500 mg, 10s ea	**54569-3658-00**	12.92		EE
20s ea	**54569-3658-01**	25.85		EE
30s ea	**54569-3658-02**	38.77		EE
(DHS, Inc.)				
REPACK				
TAB, PO, 500 mg, 10s ea	**55887-0608-10**	19.50		AB
20s ea	**55887-0608-20**	39.00		AB
30s ea	**55887-0608-30**	58.50		AB
(Dispensing Solutions)				
REPACK				
TAB, PO, 500 mg, 60s ea	**55045-1976-09**	78.00		AB
(PD-Rx Pharm)				
REPACK				
TAB, PO, 500 mg, 10s ea	**55289-0460-10**	24.96		AB
15s ea	**55289-0460-15**	37.44		AB
20s ea	**55289-0460-20**	49.90		AB
30s ea	**55289-0460-30**	74.86		AB
(Pharma Pac)				
REPACK				
TAB, PO, 500 mg, 15s ea	**52959-0379-15**	29.82		EE
20s ea	**52959-0379-20**	39.04		EE
30s ea	**52959-0379-30**	51.26		EE
60s ea	**52959-0379-60**	122.28		EE
(Phys Total Care)				
REPACK				
TAB, PO, 250 mg, 30s ea	**54868-3051-00**	52.33		EE
500 mg, 10s ea	**54868-3049-03**	43.32		AB
30s ea	**54868-3049-00**	117.95		EE
60s ea	**54868-3049-04**	228.39		AB
100s ea	**54868-3049-02**	301.32		AB
180s ea	**54868-3049-05**	491.10		AB
(Quality Care Prod)				
REPACK				
TAB, PO, 500 mg, 30s ea	**49999-0966-30**	68.83		
60s ea	**49999-0966-60**	137.40		
(Southwood)				
REPACK				
TAB, PO, 500 mg, 10s ea	**58016-0194-10**	11.16		EE
12s ea	**58016-0194-12**	13.39		EE
14s ea	**58016-0194-14**	15.62		EE
15s ea	**58016-0194-15**	16.73		EE
20s ea	**58016-0194-20**	22.31		EE
21s ea	**58016-0194-21**	23.43		EE
24s ea	**58016-0194-24**	26.77		EE
28s ea	**58016-0194-28**	31.24		EE
30s ea	**58016-0194-30**	33.47		EE
40s ea	**58016-0194-40**	44.62		EE
50s ea	**58016-0194-50**	55.78		AB
60s ea	**58016-0194-60**	66.94		EE
70s ea	**58016-0194-70**	78.09		AB
80s ea	**58016-0194-80**	89.25		AB
90s ea	**58016-0194-90**	100.40		AB
100s ea	**58016-0194-00**	111.56		AB
120s ea	**58016-0194-02**	133.87		AB
150s ea	**58016-0194-03**	167.34		AB
200s ea	**58016-0194-89**	223.12		AB
300s ea	**58016-0194-73**	334.68		AB
(St. Mary's MPP)				
REPACK				
TAB, PO, 500 mg, 60s ea	**60760-0196-60**	90.42		EE
(Stat Rx)				
REPACK				
TAB, PO, 500 mg, 60s ea	**16590-0797-30**	123.50		AB
(Vibranta)				
REPACK				
TAB, PO, 500 mg, 30s ea	**57866-5563-02**	78.99		
DIFLUPREDNATE				
(Sirion) *See DUREZOL*				
DIGESTANTS				
(Seyer Pharmatec) *See GASTRINEX*				
DIGESTODORON (Weleda)				
homeopathic substance				
LIQ, PO, 50 ml	**55946-0224-15**	9.00		
DIGEX NF (Pronova)				
hyoscyamine sulfate/phenyltoloxamine citrate				
CAP, PO, 0.0625 mg-15 mg,				
100s ea	**67555-0156-10**	45.00		
DIGIBIND (Glaxo)				
digoxin immune fab (ovine)				
PDS, IV (VIAL)				
38 mg, ea	**00173-0230-44**	727.91		
DIGIFAB (Savage)				
digoxin immune fab (ovine)				
PDS, IV (VIAL,PF)				
40 mg, ea	**00281-0365-10**	600.00		
DIGITEK (Mylan Bertek)				
digoxin				
TAB, PO, 0.125 mg,				
100s ea	**62794-0145-01**	21.60		AB
1000s ea	**62794-0145-10**	166.10		AB
5000s ea	**62794-0145-56**	830.50		AB
0.25 mg, 100s ea	**62794-0146-01**	21.60		AB
1000s ea	**62794-0146-10**	166.10		AB
5000s ea	**62794-0146-56**	783.90		AB
(PD-Rx Pharm)				
REPACK				
TAB, PO, 0.125 mg,				
30s ea	**58864-0769-30**	11.17		
DIGITOXIN (Gallipot)				
POW, NA (USP)				
1 gm	**51552-0950-01**	70.00	50.00	
(PCCA)				
POW, NA (U.S.P.)				
1 gm	**51927-2102-00**	372.00		
(Spectrum Pharmacy)				
POW, NA (U.S.P.)				
1 gm	**49452-2611-01**	420.00		
5 gm	**49452-2611-02**	1718.50		
DIGLYCERIDES/MONOGLYCERIDES				
(Amend) *See ARLACEL 186*				
(Amend) *See ATMOS 300*				
DIGOXIN				
FUL				
TAB, PO, 0.125 mg,				
100s ea		21.32		
0.25 mg, 100s ea		21.32		
(Baxter)				
SOL, IV (USP)				
0.25 mg/ml, 2 ml	**00641-1410-31**	1.22		AP
(AMP, DOSETTE)				
0.25 mg/ml,				
2 ml 25s	**00641-1410-35**	30.60		AP
(Caraco)				
TAB, PO, 0.125 mg, 100s ea	**57664-0437-88**	21.75		AB
1000s ea	**57664-0437-18**	171.01		AB
0.25 mg, 100s ea	**57664-0441-88**	21.75		AB
1000s ea	**57664-0441-18**	171.01		AB
(Glaxo) *See LANOXIN*				
(Glaxo) *See LANOXIN PEDIATRIC*				
(Hospira)				
SOL, IV (10X1ML,LUER LOCK)				
0.25 mg/ml,				
1 ml 10s	**00409-2169-31**	23.16	20.30	AP
(Lannett)				
TAB, PO, 0.125 mg, 100s ea	**00527-1324-01**	20.94		AB
1000s ea	**00527-1324-10**	161.04		AB
0.25 mg, 100s ea	**00527-1325-01**	20.94		AB
1000s ea	**00527-1325-10**	161.04		AB
(Major)				
TAB, PO (10X10,USP)				
0.125 mg,				
100s ea UD	**00904-5921-61**	39.18		AB
0.25 mg, 100s ea UD	**00904-5922-61**	39.18		AB
(Medisca)				
POW, NA (U.S.P.)				
0.1 gm	**38779-0215-09**	55.50		
0.5 gm	**38779-0215-00**	117.00		
1 gm	**38779-0215-06**	178.50		
(Mylan Bertek) *See DIGITEK*				
(PCCA)				
POW, NA (U.S.P.)				
1 gm	**51927-1746-00**	480.00		
(Roxane) *See DIGOXIN*				
DIGOXIN (Roxane)				
digoxin				
SOL, PO (USP,40X2.5ML,LIME)				
0.05 mg/ml,				
2.5 ml 40s UD	**00054-0057-16**	69.58		
(USP,40X5ML,LIME)				
0.05 mg/ml,				
5 ml 40s UD	**00054-0057-55**	139.16		
(USP,LIME)				
0.05 mg/ml, 60 ml	**00054-0057-46**	34.79		
DIGOXIN (Sandoz)				
SOL, IJ (USP,10X2ML)				
0.25 mg/ml,				
2 ml 10s	**00781-3059-95**	26.98		AP
(Spectrum Pharmacy)				
POW, NA (U.S.P.)				
1 gm	**49452-2612-02**	388.50		
(UDL)				
TAB, PO (10X10,USP)				
0.125 mg,				
100s ea UD	**51079-0847-20**	39.13		AB
0.25 mg, 100s ea UD	**51079-0848-20**	39.13		AB
(West-Ward)				
TAB, PO (USP)				
0.125 mg, 100s ea	**00143-1240-01**	21.70		AB
1000s ea	**00143-1240-10**	150.90		AB
5000s ea	**00143-1240-51**	654.60		AB
(USP)				
0.25 mg, 100s ea	**00143-1241-01**	21.70		AB
1000s ea	**00143-1241-10**	150.90		AB
5000s ea	**00143-1241-51**	654.60		AB
(A-S Medication)				
REPACK				
TAB, PO, 0.25 mg, 30s ea	**54569-5758-00**	7.42		AB
(American Health)				
REPACK				
TAB, PO (10X10)				
0.125 mg,				
100s ea UD	**62584-0989-01**	26.50		AB
0.25 mg, 100s ea UD	**62584-0990-01**	26.50		AB
(Bryant Ranch)				
REPACK				
TAB, PO, 0.125 mg, 30s ea	**63629-2579-01**	7.95		
(Core)				
REPACK				
TAB, PO, 0.125 mg, 30s ea	**33358-0108-30**	10.43		
(DHS, Inc.)				
REPACK				
TAB, PO, 0.125 mg, 30s ea	**55887-0703-30**	29.95		AB
60s ea	**55887-0703-60**	59.99		
90s ea	**55887-0703-90**	79.85		
(Dispensing Solutions)				
REPACK				
TAB, PO, 0.125 mg, 30s ea	**66336-0374-30**	12.00		EE
0.25 mg, 30s ea	**66336-0607-30**	17.22		EE

PROD/MFR NDC AWP DP OBC

(Palmetto)
REPACK
TAB, PO, 0.125 mg, 30s ea. 23490-5443-01 24.00
0.25 mg, 30s ea...... 23490-5445-01 23.01

(PD-Rx Pharm)
REPACK
TAB, PO, 0.125 mg, 14s ea. 58864-0870-14 17.00 EE
30s ea.......... 55289-0002-30 24.00 EE
100s ea.......... 55289-0002-01 53.49 EE
0.25 mg, 3s ea....... 55289-0626-03 14.07 EE
14s ea.......... 55289-0626-14 16.07 EE
30s ea.......... 55289-0626-30 23.00 EE
(REDI-SCRIPT)
0.25 mg, 30s ea...... 58864-0815-30 23.01
60s ea.......... 55289-0626-60 36.00 EE
100s ea.......... 55289-0626-01 52.70 EE
(REDI-SCRIPT)
0.25 mg, 100s ea..... 58864-0815-01 52.71

(Phys Total Care)
REPACK
TAB, PO, 0.125 mg, 30s ea. 54868-2134-02 15.45 EE
90s ea.......... 54868-2134-03 40.35
100s ea.......... 54868-2134-01 42.99 EE
0.25 mg, 30s ea...... 54868-0055-00 15.18 EE
100s ea.......... 54868-0055-02 43.56 EE

(Quality Care Prod)
REPACK
TAB, PO, 0.125 mg, 30s ea. 49999-0180-30 20.52
0.25 mg, 30s ea...... 49999-0181-30 20.66
100s ea.......... 49999-0181-00 68.87

(Southwood)
REPACK
TAB, PO, 0.125 mg, 30s ea. 58016-0202-30 5.07 EE
60s ea.......... 58016-0202-60 6.53 EE
100s ea.......... 58016-0202-00 9.63 EE
0.25 mg, 30s ea...... 58016-0755-30 5.07 EE
60s ea.......... 58016-0755-60 6.53 EE
100s ea.......... 58016-0755-00 9.63 EE

(Vibranta)
REPACK
TAB, PO, 0.25 mg, 30s ea.. 57866-6660-01 7.70

DIGOXIN IMMUNE FAB (OVINE)
(Glaxo) *See DIGIBIND*
(Savage) *See DIGIFAB*

DIHISTINE DH (Phys Total Care)
REPACK
cpm/codeine phos/pse hcl
ELI, PO, 120 ml, C-V...... 54868-3908-00 14.40

DIHISTINE EXPECTORANT (Dispensing Solutions)
REPACK
codeine phos/gg/pse hcl
LIQ, PO, 118 ml, C-V...... 55045-2288-08 8.30

DIHYDRO-CP (Cypress Pharm)
cpm/dihydrocodeine bitartrate/pse hcl
SOL, PO (AF,SF,DYE-FREE,GRAPE)
473 ml, C-III......... 60258-0760-16 44.56

DIHYDRO-GP (Cypress Pharm)
dihydrocodeine bitartrate/gg/pse hcl
SOL, PO (AF,SF,DYE-FREE)
473 ml, C-III......... 60258-0761-16 52.45

DIHYDRO-PE (Cypress Pharm)
cpm/dihydrocodeine bitartrate/phenyleph hcl
SOL, PO (1X118ML,GRAPE)
118 ml, C-V......... 60258-0762-04 20.99

DIHYDROCODEINE BITARTRATE/GG/PHENYLEPH HCL
(Poly) *See POLY-TUSSIN EX*

DIHYDROCODEINE BITARTRATE/GG/PSE HCL
(Cypress Pharm) *See DIHYDRO-GP*

DIHYDROCODEINE BITARTRATE/GUAIFENESIN
(JayMac Pharma) *See J-MAX DHC*

DIHYDROCODEINE BITARTRATE/PHENYLEPH HCL
(Poly) *See ALAHIST DHC*

DIHYDROCODEINE BITARTRATE/PHENYLEPH HCL/PYRIL MAL
(Poly) *See POLY HIST DHC*

DIHYDROERGOTAMINE MESYLATE (Bedford)
SOL, IJ (S.D.V.)
1 mg/ml, 1 ml 10s.... 55390-0013-10 336.00 AP

(Gallipot)
POW, NA (U.S.P.,N.F.)
1 gm.............. 51552-0233-01 70.00
5 gm.............. 51552-0233-02 294.00

PROD/MFR NDC AWP DP OBC

(Medisca)
POW, NA (U.S.P.)
1 gm.............. 38779-0303-06 135.00
5 gm.............. 38779-0303-03 597.00

(Paddock)
SOL, IJ (AMP)
1 mg/ml, 1 ml 5s..... 00574-0850-05 190.00 AP
1 ml 10s.......... 00574-0850-10 350.00 AP

(PCCA)
POW, NA (U.S.P.)
1 gm.............. 51927-1706-00 156.00

(Spectrum Pharmacy)
POW, NA (U.S.P.)
0.25 gm........... 49452-2616-01 112.00
1 gm.............. 49452-2616-02 230.65
5 gm.............. 49452-2616-03 892.50

(Valeant Pharm Intl) *See D.H.E. 45*
(Valeant Pharm Intl) *See MIGRANAL*

DIHYDROTACHYSTEROL (Medisca)
POW, NA (1X1GM)
1 gm.............. 38779-2371-06 7950.00

(PCCA)
POW, NA (1X1MG)
0.001 gm........... 51927-2329-00 21.84

DIHYDROTESTOSTERONE
(PCCA) *See 4-DIHYDROTESTOSTERONE*

4-DIHYDROTESTOSTERONE (PCCA)
dihydrotestosterone
POW, NA, 1 gm, C-III...... 51927-2524-00 147.00

DIHYDROTESTOSTERONE (Spectrum Pharmacy)
CRY, NA, 1 gm, C-III...... 49452-2617-01 455.00
5 gm, C-III.......... 49452-2617-02 959.00

DIHYDROXYACETONE (PCCA)
POW, NA, 98%, 1 gm..... 51927-1643-00 1.44

DIINDOLYLMETHANE (3,3) (PCCA)
3,3'-diindolylmethane
POW, NA (1X1GM)
1 gm.............. 51927-3365-00 13.80

DIIODO-L-THYRONINE (3,5) (PCCA)
3,5-diiodo-l-thyronine
POW, NA (1X0.001GM)
0.001 gm........... 51927-3400-00 2.55

DILACOR XR (Watson)
diltiazem hydrochloride
C24, PO (PINK)
120 mg, 100s ea..... 52544-0482-01 260.94 AB2
(LAVENDAR)
180 mg, 100s ea..... 52544-0483-01 307.22 AB2
(LIGHT BLUE)
240 mg, 100s ea..... 52544-0484-01 328.56 AB2

(Phys Total Care)
REPACK
C24, PO, 180 mg, 30s ea.. 54868-2322-02 47.04 AB2
60s ea.......... 54868-2322-01 92.88 AB2
240 mg, 30s ea...... 54868-2975-03 53.42 AB2

DILANTIN (Pfizer)
phenytoin sodium, extended
CER, PO (CONI SNAP)
30 mg, 100s ea...... 00071-3740-66 40.84 34.03 AB
(10X10,HARD)
100 mg, 100s ea UD.. 00071-0369-40 52.26 43.55 AB
(HARD)
100 mg, 100s ea..... 00071-0369-24 47.36 39.47 AB
1000s ea.......... 00071-0369-32 473.64 394.70 AB

(PD-Rx Pharm)
REPACK
CER, PO (REDI-SCRIPT,KAP)
100 mg, 42s ea...... 58864-0037-42 27.52
90s ea.......... 58864-0509-90 46.80

(Quality Care Prod)
REPACK
CER, PO, 100 mg, 30s ea.. 49999-0876-30 14.39

DILANTIN INFATABS (Pfizer)
phenytoin
CTB, PO, 50 mg, 100s ea.. 00071-0007-24 44.38 36.98
(10X10)
50 mg, 100s ea UD... 00071-0007-40 62.95 52.46

(Phys Total Care)
REPACK
CTB, PO, 50 mg, 100s ea.. 54868-2551-00 28.11

DILANTIN KAPSEALS (A-S Medication)
REPACK
phenytoin sodium, extended
CER, PO, 100 mg, 30s ea.. 54569-0161-02 12.20 AB
100s ea.......... 54569-0161-00 40.68 AB

PROD/MFR NDC AWP DP OBC

(PD-Rx Pharm)
REPACK
CER, PO, 100 mg, 10s ea.. 55289-0152-10 9.53 AB

(Phys Total Care)
REPACK
CER, PO, 30 mg, 30s ea... 54868-1486-01 17.97
100s ea.......... 54868-1486-00 53.16
100 mg, 20s ea...... 54868-0325-03 14.23 AB
30s ea.......... 54868-0325-04 16.05 AB
60s ea.......... 54868-0325-07 30.22 AB
90s ea.......... 54868-0325-02 48.87 AB
100s ea.......... 54868-0325-01 54.01 AB

(Quality Care Prod)
REPACK
CER, PO, 100 mg, 100s ea. 49999-0876-00 68.08 AB

(Southwood)
REPACK
CER, PO, 100 mg, 12s ea.. 58016-0907-12 2.61 AB
15s ea.......... 58016-0907-15 3.26 AB

DILANTIN-125 (Pfizer)
phenytoin
SUS, PO, 125 mg/5 ml,
237 ml.......... 00071-2214-20 64.36 53.63 AB

(Phys Total Care)
REPACK
SUS, PO, 125 mg/5 ml,
240 ml.......... 54868-2776-00 41.18 AB

DILATRATE-SR (UCB)
isosorbide dinitrate
CER, PO, 40 mg, 100s ea.. 00091-0920-01 148.28 BC

(Phys Total Care)
REPACK
CER, PO, 40 mg, 60s ea... 54868-3720-01 72.96 BC
100s ea.......... 54868-3720-00 119.74 BC

DILAUDID (Purdue Pharma)
hydromorphone hydrochloride
SOL, IJ (10X1ML)
1 mg/ml,
1 ml 10s, C-II..... 59011-0441-10 16.40
2 mg/ml,
1 ml 10s, C-II..... 59011-0442-10 18.08
(25X1ML)
2 mg/ml,
1 ml 25s, C-II..... 59011-0442-25 43.04
(10X1ML)
4 mg/ml,
1 ml 10s, C-II..... 59011-0444-10 21.90
PO (1X473ML)
1 mg/ml,
473 ml, C-II....... 59011-0451-01 166.21 AA
TAB, PO, 2 mg,
100s ea, C-II...... 59011-0452-10 75.78 AB
(25X4)
2 mg,
100s ea UD, C-II.... 59011-0452-01 95.82 AB
4 mg,
100s ea, C-II...... 59011-0454-10 123.71 AB
(4X25)
4 mg,
100s ea UD, C-II.... 59011-0454-01 145.74 AB
500s ea, C-II...... 59011-0454-05 589.27 AB
8 mg,
100s ea, C-II...... 59011-0458-10 225.16 AB

(Dispensing Solutions)
REPACK
TAB, PO, 4 mg,
30s ea, C-II....... 66336-0304-30 49.84 AB

(Phys Total Care)
REPACK
SOL, IJ (AMP)
4 mg/ml,
10 ml 10s, C-II..... 54868-5137-00 23.73
TAB, PO, 2 mg,
120s ea, C-II....... 54868-2413-00 72.43
4 mg, 20s ea, C-II.... 54868-2905-04 34.93
30s ea, C-II....... 54868-2905-03 50.44
60s ea, C-II....... 54868-2905-00 96.96
100s ea, C-II...... 54868-2905-01 150.37
100s ea, C-II...... 54868-2905-05 162.19 AB
120s ea, C-II...... 54868-2905-02 179.66
8 mg, 20s ea, C-II.... 54868-4147-02 49.58 AB
60s ea, C-II....... 54868-4147-00 134.74 AB
100s ea, C-II...... 54868-4147-01 221.85 AB

(Quality Care Prod)
REPACK
TAB, PO, 2 mg,
30s ea, C-II....... 35356-0514-30 54.80 AB
4 mg, 30s ea, C-II.... 35356-0007-30 79.23 AB

PROD/MFR	NDC	AWP	DP	OBC
100s ea, C-II	35356-0007-00	217.50		
(Stat Rx)				
REPACK				
TAB, PO, 2 mg,				
20s ea, C-II	16590-0768-20	22.25		AB
DILAUDID-HP (Purdue Pharma)				
hydromorphone hydrochloride				
PDS, IJ (SINGLE-DOSE,1X250MG)				
250 mg,				
250 ml, C-II	59011-0446-25	114.80		
SOL, IJ (10X1ML,PF)				
10 mg/ml,				
1 ml 10s, C-II	59011-0445-01	45.71		AP
(10X5ML,PF)				
10 mg/ml,				
5 ml 10s, C-II	59011-0445-05	217.04		AP
(SINGLE-DOSE,1X50ML,PF)				
10 mg/ml,				
50 ml, C-II	59011-0445-50	223.02		AP
DILEX-G 200 (Poly)				
dyphylline/guaifenesin				
SYR, PO (AF,SF,CHERRY,RASPBERRY)				
100 mg/5 ml-200 mg/5 ml,				
473 ml	50991-0214-16	63.47	53.98	
DILEX-G 400 (Poly)				
dyphylline/guaifenesin				
TAB, PO, 200 mg-400 mg,				
100s ea	50991-0413-01	67.47	53.98	
DILLWEED OIL (PCCA)				
OIL, NA, 1 gm	51927-1618-00	0.90		
DILT-CD (Apotex Corp.)				
diltiazem hydrochloride				
C24, PO (HARD GELATIN)				
120 mg, 90s ea	60505-0007-04	107.83		AB3
500s ea	60505-0007-08	599.06		
180 mg, 90s ea	60505-0008-04	130.12		AB3
500s ea	60505-0008-08	722.89		
240 mg, 90s ea	60505-0009-04	184.60		AB3
500s ea	60505-0009-08	1025.56		
300 mg, 90s ea	60505-0010-04	239.24		AB3
500s ea	60505-0010-08	1329.11		
DILT-XR (Apotex Corp.)				
diltiazem hydrochloride				
C24, PO, 120 mg, 100s ea	60505-0014-06	90.99		
500s ea	60505-0014-08	441.30		
180 mg, 100s ea	60505-0015-06	107.13		
500s ea	60505-0015-08	519.58		
240 mg, 100s ea	60505-0016-06	112.95		
(DHS, Inc.)				
REPACK				
C24, PO, 240 mg, 30s ea	55887-0986-30	61.00		
DILTIA XT (Watson)				
diltiazem hydrochloride				
C24, PO, 120 mg, 100s ea	62037-0548-01	52.08		AB2
1000s ea	62037-0548-10	510.38		AB2
180 mg, 100s ea	62037-0549-01	57.00		AB2
1000s ea	62037-0549-10	558.60		AB2
240 mg, 100s ea	62037-0550-01	64.18		AB2
1000s ea	62037-0550-10	628.92		AB2
DILTIAZEM (DHS, Inc.)				
REPACK				
diltiazem hydrochloride				
C24, PO, 180 mg, 30s ea	55887-0920-30	50.00		
(DHS, Inc.)				
diltiazem malate				
TER, PO, 240 mg, 30s ea	55887-0931-30	67.45		
(McKesson Packaging)				
REPACK				
diltiazem hydrochloride				
TAB, PO, 30 mg,				
100s ea UD	63739-0079-10	44.88		
60 mg, 100s ea UD	63739-0080-10	72.36		
(Palmetto)				
REPACK				
C24, PO, 240 mg, 30s ea	23490-5450-03	90.10		
(PD-Rx Pharm)				
REPACK				
CER, PO, 120 mg, 30s ea	58864-0606-30	104.09		
240 mg, 30s ea	58864-0619-30	54.85		
(Physician Partner)				
REPACK				
CER, PO, 120 mg, 30s ea	21695-0403-30	71.89		
180 mg, 30s ea	21695-0404-30	86.75		
DILTIAZEM CD (Actavis)				
diltiazem hydrochloride				
C24, PO, 120 mg, 30s ea	00228-2588-03	36.70		AB3
90s ea	00228-2588-09	107.80		AB3
500s ea	00228-2588-50	569.90		AB3
180 mg, 30s ea	00228-2577-03	45.40		AB3
90s ea	00228-2577-09	130.10		AB3
500s ea	00228-2577-50	686.60		AB3
240 mg, 30s ea	00228-2578-03	61.55		AB3
90s ea	00228-2578-09	184.55		AB3
500s ea	00228-2578-50	973.95		AB3
300 mg, 30s ea	00228-2579-03	80.65		AB3
90s ea	00228-2579-09	239.20		AB3
500s ea	00228-2579-50	1262.40		AB3
(Altura)				
REPACK				
C24, PO, 180 mg, 5s ea	63874-0605-05	10.12		AB3
10s ea	63874-0605-10	20.24		AB3
14s ea	63874-0605-14	28.28		AB3
20s ea	63874-0605-20	40.40		AB3
30s ea	63874-0605-30	60.73		AB3
(American Health)				
REPACK				
C24, PO, 120 mg, 30s ea	62584-0974-30	36.72		AB3
90s ea	62584-0974-90	107.81		AB3
(10X10)				
120 mg, 100s ea UD	62584-0974-01	119.50		AB3
(15X30)				
120 mg, 450s ea	62584-0974-85	544.00		AB3
180 mg, 30s ea	62584-0975-30	45.42		AB3
90s ea	62584-0975-90	130.11		AB3
(10X10)				
180 mg, 100s ea UD	62584-0975-01	143.75		AB3
(15X30)				
180 mg, 450s ea	62584-0975-85	650.50		AB3
240 mg, 30s ea	62584-0976-30	61.59		AB3
90s ea	62584-0976-90	184.58		AB3
(10X10)				
240 mg, 100s ea UD	62584-0976-01	204.35		AB3
(15X30)				
240 mg, 450s ea	62584-0976-85	922.75		AB3
300 mg, 30s ea	62584-0977-30	80.69		AB3
90s ea	62584-0977-90	239.22		AB3
(10X10)				
300 mg, 100s ea UD	62584-0977-01	263.31		AB3
(Dispensing Solutions)				
REPACK				
C24, PO, 180 mg, 30s ea	55045-2846-08	45.00		AB3
(McKesson Packaging)				
REPACK				
C24, PO (USP)				
120 mg, 100s ea UD	63739-0283-10	149.72		EE
180 mg, 100s ea UD	63739-0284-10	180.69		EE
240 mg, 100s ea UD	63739-0285-10	256.31		EE
(Phys Total Care)				
REPACK				
C24, PO, 120 mg, 30s ea	54868-4970-00	61.77		AB3
60s ea	54868-4970-02	101.08		AB3
90s ea	54868-4970-01	180.78		AB3
180 mg, 30s ea	54868-5081-00	81.93		AB3
240 mg, 30s ea	54868-4868-00	99.63		AB3
90s ea	54868-4868-01	292.89		AB3
300 mg, 30s ea	54868-4992-00	195.76		
(Quality Care Prod)				
REPACK				
C24, PO, 120 mg, 30s ea	35356-0511-30	40.15		AB3
(Southwood)				
REPACK				
C24, PO, 120 mg, 30s ea	58016-0504-30	32.18		AB3
100s ea	58016-0504-00	107.27		AB3
DILTIAZEM ER (Core)				
REPACK				
diltiazem hydrochloride				
C24, PO, 120 mg, 30s ea	33358-0109-30	35.88		
(Vibranta)				
REPACK				
C24, PO, 180 mg, 30s ea	57866-0230-01	105.92		
240 mg, 30s ea	57866-6126-01	128.17		
DILTIAZEM HCL (Abbott Hosp)				
diltiazem hydrochloride				
SOL, IV (VIAL,FLIPTOP)				
5 mg/ml, 10 ml 10s	00074-1172-02	78.61	66.20	AP
(Apotex Corp.)				
C24, PO, 240 mg, 500s ea	60505-0016-08	536.51		AB3
SOL, IV, 5 mg/ml,				
5 ml 10s	60505-0704-01	40.60		AP
10 ml 10s	60505-0704-02	81.20		AP
(Baxter)				
SOL, IV (SDV,1X5ML)				
5 mg/ml, 5 ml	10019-0510-79	1.62		AP
(S.D.V.)				
5 mg/ml, 5 ml 10s	10019-0510-01	16.20		AP
(SDV,1X10ML)				
5 mg/ml, 10 ml	10019-0510-78	2.83		AP
(S.D.V.)				
5 mg/ml, 10 ml 10s	10019-0510-02	28.32		AP
(SDV,1X25ML)				
5 mg/ml, 25 ml	10019-0510-35	5.82		AP
(S.D.V.)				
5 mg/ml, 25 ml 10s	10019-0510-04	58.20		AP
(Bedford)				
SOL, IV (S.D.V.)				
5 mg/ml, 5 ml 10s	55390-0565-05	24.00		AP
10 ml 10s	55390-0565-10	48.00		AP
25 ml 10s	55390-0565-30	108.00		AP
(Hawkins)				
POW, NA (U.S.P)				
5 gm	63370-0085-15	60.00		
25 gm	63370-0085-25	240.00		
(U.S.P.)				
100 gm	63370-0085-35	720.00		
(Hospira)				
SOL, IV (VIAL,FLIPTOP)				
5 mg/ml, 5 ml 10s	00074-1171-01	16.08	14.10	AP
((VIAL,FLIPTOP),10X10ML)				
5 mg/ml, 10 ml 10s	00074-1171-02	18.36	16.10	AP
(Inwood)				
C24, PO, 120 mg, 90s ea	00258-3687-90	93.31		AB4
180 mg, 90s ea	00258-3688-90	112.61		AB4
240 mg, 90s ea	00258-3689-90	159.80		AB4
300 mg, 90s ea	00258-3690-90	207.02		AB4
360 mg, 90s ea	00258-3691-90	211.01		AB4
(Ivax Corp.)				
C24, PO (10X10)				
120 mg, 100s ea UD	00182-8225-89	119.49		AB3
180 mg, 100s ea UD	00182-8226-89	143.70		AB3
240 mg, 100s ea UD	00182-8227-89	204.30		AB3
(Major)				
C24, PO (USP,10X10)				
240 mg, 100s ea UD	00904-5382-61	133.30		EE
(Medisca)				
POW, NA (U.S.P.)				
5 gm	38779-0227-03	47.85		
10 gm	38779-0227-01	82.50		
25 gm	38779-0227-04	207.00		
100 gm	38779-0227-05	597.00		
(Mylan)				
C12, PO, 60 mg, 100s ea	00378-6060-01	83.05		AB1
90 mg, 100s ea	00378-6090-01	94.95		AB1
120 mg, 100s ea	00378-6120-01	123.75		AB2
C24, PO, 120 mg, 100s ea	00378-5220-01	91.01		AB2
500s ea	00378-5220-05	443.15		AB2
180 mg, 100s ea	00378-5280-01	107.15		AB2
500s ea	00378-5280-05	521.45		AB2
240 mg, 100s ea	00378-5340-01	114.60		AB2
500s ea	00378-5340-05	557.62		AB2
TAB, PO, 30 mg, 100s ea	00378-0023-01	47.25		AB
500s ea	00378-0023-05	232.10		AB
60 mg, 100s ea	00378-0045-01	74.10		AB
500s ea	00378-0045-05	363.95		AB
(FILM COATED)				
90 mg, 100s ea	00378-0135-01	101.30		AB
500s ea	00378-0135-05	431.65		AB
(CLEAR FILM-COAT)				
120 mg, 100s ea	00378-0525-01	136.40		AB
(Spectrum Pharmacy)				
POW, NA (U.S.P.)				
5 gm	49452-4881-01	73.15		
25 gm	49452-4881-02	306.95		
100 gm	49452-4881-03	871.50		
(Teva)				
C24, PO, 120 mg, 90s ea	00093-5112-98	107.83		AB3
180 mg, 90s ea	00093-5117-98	130.12		AB3
240 mg, 90s ea	00093-5118-98	184.60		AB3
300 mg, 90s ea	00093-5119-98	239.24		AB3
SOL, IV (S.D.V.)				
5 mg/ml, 5 ml 10s	00703-1553-03	18.43		AP
10 ml 10s	00703-1554-03	26.32		AP
(SINGLE DOSE,125MG)				
5 mg/ml, 25 ml 10s	00703-1557-03	48.98		AP
TAB, PO, 30 mg, 100s ea	00093-0318-01	47.27		AB
500s ea	00093-0318-05	232.13		AB
60 mg, 100s ea	00093-0319-01	74.12		AB
500s ea	00093-0319-05	363.98		AB
90 mg, 100s ea	00093-0320-01	101.32		AB
120 mg, 100s ea	00093-0321-01	136.39		AB
(UDL)				
C12, PO (10X10)				
60 mg, 100s ea UD	51079-0924-20	83.05		AB1

PROD/MFR	NDC	AWP	DP	OBC
90 mg, 100s ea UD	51079-0925-20	94.95		AB1
120 mg, 100s ea UD	51079-0926-20	123.75		AB1
C24, PO (8X10)				
120 mg, 80s ea UD	51079-0947-08	82.00		AB2
180 mg, 80s ea UD	51079-0948-08	96.25		AB2
240 mg, 80s ea UD	51079-0949-08	103.70		AB2
TAB, PO (25X1, ROBOT READY)				
30 mg, 25s ea UD	51079-0745-19	11.25		AB
(10X10)				
30 mg, 100s ea UD	51079-0745-20	44.94		AB
(25X1, ROBOT READY)				
60 mg, 25s ea UD	51079-0746-19	17.58		AB
(10X10)				
60 mg, 100s ea UD	51079-0746-20	70.30		AB
90 mg, 100s ea UD	51079-0747-20	85.69		AB
(A-S Medication)				
REPACK				
C24, PO, 180 mg, 30s ea	54569-4913-00	43.37		EE
240 mg, 30s ea	54569-4914-00	61.53		EE
TAB, PO, 60 mg, 30s ea	54569-3667-02	22.24		EE
(Bryant Ranch)				
REPACK				
TAB, PO, 60 mg, 30s ea	63629-3649-01	22.20		AB
(DHS, Inc.)				
REPACK				
C24, PO, 120 mg, 30s ea	55887-0701-30	54.44		AB3
60s ea	55887-0701-60	108.88		AB3
240 mg, 90s ea	55887-0986-90	183.00		EE
TAB, PO, 30 mg, 30s ea	55887-0597-30	27.12		AB
60 mg, 30s ea	55887-0598-30	21.36		AB
90s ea	55887-0598-90	58.00		AB
(Dispensing Solutions)				
REPACK				
TAB, PO, 60 mg, 30s ea	55045-2357-08	22.20		AB
(PD-Rx Pharm)				
REPACK				
C24, PO, 120 mg, 30s ea	55289-0853-30	104.10		AB2
180 mg, 14s ea	55289-0770-14	90.35		AB4
240 mg, 14s ea	55289-0774-14	121.65		AB4
TAB, PO, 30 mg, 10s ea	55289-0335-10	17.40		AB
(REDI-SCRIPT)				
30 mg, 20s ea	58864-0101-20	19.80		AB
30s ea	58864-0101-30	22.10		AB
50s ea	55289-0335-50	27.00		AB
100s ea	55289-0335-01	38.95		AB
60 mg, 100s ea	55289-0329-01	53.40		AB
90 mg, 30s ea	55289-0893-30	31.50		EE
(Pharma Pac)				
REPACK				
C24, PO, 180 mg, 100s ea	52959-0072-01	48.10		EE
(Phys Total Care)				
REPACK				
C12, PO, 60 mg, 30s ea	54868-3214-01	42.75		AB1
100s ea	54868-3214-00	130.47		AB1
90 mg, 30s ea	54868-3102-00	83.40		AB1
100s ea	54868-3102-03	207.93		AB1
C24, PO, 120 mg, 30s ea	54868-3103-00	40.17		EE
60s ea	54868-3103-02	78.85		AB2
100s ea	54868-3103-03	97.76		
180 mg, 30s ea	54868-4186-00	82.24		AB2
60s ea	54868-4186-02	124.19		AB2
90s ea	54868-4186-03	183.29		AB2
100s ea	54868-4186-01	203.49		AB2
240 mg, 20s ea	54868-4184-01	81.45		AB2
30s ea	54868-4184-00	93.00		EE
100s ea	54868-4184-02	301.50		AB2
360 mg, 30s ea	54868-5208-00	120.84		
90s ea	54868-5208-01	456.18		
TAB, PO, 30 mg, 30s ea	54868-2290-03	8.46		EE
60s ea	54868-2290-00	12.39		EE
90s ea	54868-2290-04	16.35		EE
100s ea	54868-2290-02	17.64		EE
60 mg, 90s ea	54868-2276-00	29.43		AB
100s ea	54868-2276-02	32.19		EE
90 mg, 100s ea	54868-2277-00	45.95		EE
(Physician Partner)				
REPACK				
TAB, PO (FILM COATED)				
60 mg, 30s ea	21695-0408-30	44.46		AB
60s ea	21695-0408-60	88.92		AB
(CLEAR FILM-COAT)				
120 mg, 30s ea	21695-0410-30	81.84		AB
(Quality Care Prod)				
REPACK				
C24, PO, 360 mg, 10s ea	49999-0499-10	34.88		AB4
(Southwood)				
REPACK				
TAB, PO, 30 mg, 12s ea	58016-0606-12	5.22		EE
15s ea	58016-0606-15	6.53		EE
20s ea	58016-0606-20	8.70		EE
30s ea	58016-0606-30	13.05		EE
100s ea	58016-0606-00	43.50		EE
60 mg, 12s ea	58016-0607-12	8.19		EE
15s ea	58016-0607-15	10.24		EE
20s ea	58016-0607-20	13.65		EE
30s ea	58016-0607-30	20.48		EE
90s ea	58016-0607-90	61.42		EE
100s ea	58016-0607-00	68.25		EE
90 mg, 12s ea	58016-0608-12	11.51		EE
15s ea	58016-0608-15	14.38		EE
20s ea	58016-0608-20	19.18		EE
30s ea	58016-0608-30	28.76		EE
90s ea	58016-0608-90	86.29		EE
100s ea	58016-0608-00	95.88		EE
(Vibranta)				
REPACK				
CER, PO, 240 mg, 60s ea	57866-6127-01	121.74		
DILTIAZEM HCL NOVAPLUS (Bedford)				
diltiazem hydrochloride				
SOL, IV (S.D.V.,PRIVATE LABEL)				
5 mg/ml, 5 ml 10s	55390-0566-05	13.20		AP
10 ml 10s	55390-0566-10	21.60		AP
25 ml 10s	55390-0566-30	43.20		AP
DILTIAZEM HYDROCHLORIDE				
FUL				
TAB, PO, 30 mg, 100s ea		10.19		
60 mg, 100s ea		11.14		
90 mg, 100s ea		23.12		
120 mg, 100s ea		23.31		
(Abbott Hosp) *See DILTIAZEM HCL*				
(Abbott Pharm) *See CARDIZEM LA*				
(Actavis)				
CER, PO (USP)				
120 mg, 30s ea	00228-2588-73	36.70		AB3
180 mg, 30s ea	00228-2577-73	45.40		AB3
240 mg, 30s ea	00228-2578-73	61.55		AB3
(Actavis) *See DILTIAZEM CD*				
(Akorn)				
SOL, IV (10X5ML)				
5 mg/ml, 5 ml 10s	17478-0937-05	24.50		
(10X10ML)				
5 mg/ml, 10 ml 10s	17478-0937-10	49.50		
25 ml	17478-0937-25	10.68		
(Apotex Corp.) *See DILT-CD*				
(Apotex Corp.) *See DILT-XR*				
(Apotex Corp.) *See DILTIAZEM HCL*				
(Apotex Corp.) *See DILTZAC*				
(Baxter) *See DILTIAZEM HCL*				
(Bedford) *See AMERINET CHOICE DILTIAZEM HYDROCHLORIDE*				
(Bedford) *See DILTIAZEM HCL*				
(Bedford) *See DILTIAZEM HCL NOVAPLUS*				
(BTA) *See CARDIZEM*				
(BTA) *See CARDIZEM CD*				
(Ethex)				
C24, PO, 120 mg, 30s ea	58177-0061-19	34.34		AB4
90s ea	58177-0061-26	93.31		AB4
180 mg, 30s ea	58177-0062-19	41.47		AB4
90s ea	58177-0062-26	112.62		AB4
240 mg, 30s ea	58177-0063-19	58.82		AB4
90s ea	58177-0063-26	159.80		AB4
300 mg, 30s ea	58177-0064-19	76.22		AB4
90s ea	58177-0064-26	207.03		AB4
360 mg, 30s ea	58177-0065-19	77.69		AB4
90s ea	58177-0065-26	211.01		AB4
420 mg, 30s ea	58177-0066-19	91.59		AB4
90s ea	58177-0066-26	248.73		AB4
(Forest Pharm) *See TIAZAC*				
(Gallipot)				
POW, NA (1X5GM,USP)				
5 gm	51552-0740-02	21.70	15.50	
(1X25GM,USP)				
25 gm	51552-0740-04	90.65	64.75	
(Hawkins) *See DILTIAZEM HCL*				
(Hospira) *See AMERINET CHOICE DILTIAZEM HYDROCHLORIDE*				
(Hospira) *See DILTIAZEM HCL*				
(Hospira)				
PDS, IV (ADD-VANTAGE VIAL)				
100 mg, 10s ea	00409-4350-03	97.20	85.10	AP
SOL, IV (5MLX10,SDV)				
5 mg/ml, 5 ml 10s	00409-1171-01	8.88	7.80	AP
(10X10ML)				
5 mg/ml, 10 ml 10s	00409-1171-02	16.68	14.60	AP
(Inwood)				
CER, PO (USP)				
420 mg, 90s ea	00258-3692-90	221.15		
(Inwood) *See DILTIAZEM HCL*				
(Ivax Corp.) *See DILTIAZEM HCL*				
(Letco)				
POW, NA (U.S.P.)				
25 gm	62991-1046-03	135.00		
100 gm	62991-1046-01	435.00		
500 gm	62991-1046-04	1500.00		
(Major) *See DILTIAZEM HCL*				
(Medisca) *See DILTIAZEM HCL*				
(Mylan) *See DILTIAZEM HCL*				
(Spectrum Pharmacy) *See DILTIAZEM HCL*				
(Teva) *See DILTIAZEM HCL*				
(UDL) *See DILTIAZEM HCL*				
(Watson) *See CARTIA XT*				
(Watson) *See DILACOR XR*				
(Watson) *See DILTIA XT*				
(Watson) *See TAZTIA XT*				
(Altura)				
REPACK				
TAB, PO (FILM COATED)				
30 mg, 10s ea	63874-0690-10	4.56		
12s ea	63874-0690-12	5.48		
15s ea	63874-0690-15	6.86		
20s ea	63874-0690-20	9.14		
25s ea	63874-0690-25	11.42		
30s ea	63874-0690-30	13.70		
90s ea	63874-0690-90	41.10		
100s ea	63874-0690-01	45.68		
(Dispensing Solutions)				
REPACK				
TAB, PO, 30 mg, 100s ea	55045-3791-01	48.00		
90 mg, 100s ea	55045-3792-01	101.00		
120 mg, 30s ea	55045-3441-08	40.80		
(McKesson Packaging)				
REPACK				
C24, PO, 300 mg,				
100s ea UD	63739-0286-10	332.22		
(Phys Total Care)				
REPACK				
C24, PO, 300 mg, 90s ea	54868-4992-01	547.89		
420 mg, 30s ea	54868-2273-00	201.54		
(Quality Care Prod)				
REPACK				
C24, PO, 180 mg, 30s ea	49999-0496-30	55.82		
TAB, PO, 60 mg, 100s ea	35356-0026-00	88.92		
90 mg, 100s ea	35356-0027-00	121.56		
DILTIAZEM HYDROCHLORIDE ER (PD-Rx Pharm)				
REPACK				
diltiazem hydrochloride				
CER, PO (USP,REDI-SCRIPT)				
180 mg, 14s ea	58864-0873-14	21.59		
(REDI-SCRIPT,USP)				
180 mg, 30s ea	58864-0873-30	67.45		
DILTIAZEM/DEXTROSE (PharMEDium Services)				
dextrose/diltiazem hydrochloride				
SOL, IV (24X250ML,PF,LATEX-FREE)				
5%-1 mg/ml,				
250 ml 24s	61553-0718-02	102.00	85.00	
DILTZAC (Apotex Corp.)				
diltiazem hydrochloride				
CER, PO (HARD GELATIN)				
120 mg, 30s ea	60505-0210-03	34.34		AB4
90s ea	60505-0210-09	93.31		AB4
180 mg, 30s ea	60505-0211-03	41.47		AB4
90s ea	60505-0211-09	112.62		AB4
240 mg, 30s ea	60505-0212-03	58.82		AB4
90s ea	60505-0212-09	159.80		AB4
300 mg, 30s ea	60505-0213-03	76.22		AB4
90s ea	60505-0213-09	207.03		AB4
360 mg, 30s ea	60505-0214-03	77.69		AB4
90s ea	60505-0214-09	211.01		AB4
DIMENHYDRINATE (APP)				
SOL, IJ (VIAL)				
50 mg/ml, 1 ml 25s	63323-0366-01	142.50		

PROD/MFR	NDC	AWP	DP	OBC
(Consolidated Midland)				
SOL, IJ (VIAL)				
50 mg/ml, 10 ml	**00223-7475-10**	4.00		EE
(Gallipot)				
POW, NA (1X25GM,USP)				
25 gm	**51552-0676-04**	34.58	24.70	
(1X100GM,USP)				
100 gm	**51552-0676-05**	83.30	59.50	
(Medisca)				
POW, NA (U.S.P.)				
25 gm	**38779-0281-04**	31.50		
100 gm	**38779-0281-05**	76.50		
500 gm	**38779-0281-08**	270.00		
(PCCA)				
POW, NA (U.S.P.)				
1 gm	**51927-1080-00**	1.44		
(Spectrum Pharmacy)				
POW, NA (U.S.P.)				
25 gm	**49452-2615-01**	100.10		
100 gm	**49452-2615-02**	194.60		
(Truxton)				
SOL, IJ (VIAL)				
50 mg/ml, 10 ml	**00463-1086-10**	4.05		EE
DIMERCAPROL				
(Akorn) *See BAL IN OIL*				
2,3-DIMERCAPTO-1-PROPANESULFONIC ACID (Gallipot)				
POW, NA, 5 gm	**51552-0799-02**	646.80	462.00	
DIMERCAPTO-PROPANESULFONIC ACID SODIUM SALT ANHYDROUS (PCCA)				
unithiol				
POW, NA (1X1GM)				
1 gm	**51927-3684-00**	300.00		
DIMERCAPTOPROPANE SULPHONATE (Medisca)				
unithiol				
POW, NA, 10 gm	**38779-0643-01**	1125.00		
DIMERCAPTOPROPANESULFONIC ACID (PCCA)				
unithiol				
POW, NA (NA SALT (2,3))				
1 gm	**51927-3214-00**	384.00		
2,3 DIMERCAPTOSUCCINIC ACID (Gallipot)				
succimer				
POW, NA, 5 gm	**51552-0545-02**	37.10		
25 gm	**51552-0545-04**	175.00		
50 gm	**51552-0545-09**	343.00		
100 gm	**51552-0545-05**	546.00		
DIMERCAPTOSUCCINIC ACID (Hawkins)				
succimer				
POW, NA, 5 gm	**63370-0075-15**	100.00		
25 gm	**63370-0075-25**	456.00		
100 gm	**63370-0075-35**	1540.00		
1000 gm	**63370-0075-50**	7200.00		
(Letco)				
POW, NA (DMSA)				
5 gm	**62991-1416-01**	60.00		
25 gm	**62991-1416-02**	240.00		
100 gm	**62991-1416-03**	645.00		
(Medisca)				
POW, NA, 5 gm	**38779-0780-03**	76.50		
10 gm	**38779-0780-01**	147.00		
25 gm	**38779-0780-04**	343.50		
100 gm	**38779-0780-05**	1147.50		
500 gm	**38779-0780-08**	4590.00		
(PCCA)				
POW, NA (MESO-2,3; DMSA)				
1 gm	**51927-2180-00**	27.00		
DIMETHICONE				
(MPM Medical Inc.) *See RADIAPLEXRX*				
DIMETHYL BETA CYCLODEXTRIN				
(Gallipot) *See DIMETHYL-BETA-CYCLODEXTRIN*				
DIMETHYL FUMARATE (PCCA)				
POW, NA (1X1GM)				
1 gm	**51927-2929-00**	4.20		
DIMETHYL ISOSORBIDE				
(PCCA) *See ISOSORBIDE DIMETHYL ETHER*				
DIMETHYL PHTHALATE				
(Amend) *See DIMETHYLPHTHALATE*				
DIMETHYL SULFONE (Medisca)				
POW, NA (1X100GM)				
100 gm	**38779-1967-05**	41.85		
(1X500GM)				
500 gm	**38779-1967-08**	132.00		
(1X1000GM)				
1000 gm	**38779-1967-09**	225.00		
(PCCA)				
POW, NA, 1 gm	**51927-2998-00**	0.75		
DIMETHYL SULFOXIDE (Amend)				
LIQ, NA (A.C.S., REAGENT)				
500 ml	**17317-0828-01**	42.00		
(Baker, J.T.)				
LIQ, NA (A.C.S., REAGENT)				
500 ml	**10106-9224-01**	81.52		
(Bioniche Pharma) *See RIMSO-50*				
(Gallipot) *See DIMETHYLSULFOXIDE*				
(Letco)				
SOL, NA (1X500ML,USP)				
500 ml	**62991-2192-01**	225.00	75.00	
(DMSO, U.S.P.)				
500 ml	**62991-1536-01**	93.00		
(1X3840ML,USP)				
3840 ml	**62991-2192-02**	1335.00	445.00	
(DMSO, U.S.P.)				
3840 ml	**62991-1536-02**	615.00		
(Medisca)				
SOL, NA (1X100ML,REAGENT)				
100 ml	**38779-0614-05**	31.50		
(1X100ML,USP)				
100 ml	**38779-2430-05**	75.00		
(1X500ML,REAGENT)				
500 ml	**38779-0614-08**	66.00		
(1X500ML,USP)				
500 ml	**38779-2430-08**	217.50		
(1X1000ML,REAGENT)				
1000 ml	**38779-0614-09**	124.50		
(1X1000ML,USP)				
1000 ml	**38779-2430-09**	375.00		
(1X4000ML,REAGENT)				
4000 ml	**38779-0614-01**	423.00		
(1X4000ML,USP)				
4000 ml	**38779-2430-01**	1320.00		
(PCCA)				
LIQ, NA (USP)				
1 ml	**51927-1612-00**	0.50		
SOL, NA, ea	**51927-3287-00**	0.45		
(Spectrum Pharmacy)				
LIQ, NA (U.S.P.)				
100 ml	**49452-2588-04**	112.00		
500 ml	**49452-2588-01**	325.85		
4000 ml	**49452-2588-02**	1928.50		
DIMETHYL-BETA-CYCLODEXTRIN (Gallipot)				
dimethyl beta cyclodextrin				
POW, NA, 1 gm	**51552-0508-01**	133.00		
DIMETHYLACETAMIDE (PCCA)				
SOL, NA, 1 ml	**51927-2540-00**	0.23		
DIMETHYLAMINOBENZALDEHYDE-P (PCCA)				
p-dimethylaminobenzaldehyde				
POW, NA, 1 gm	**51927-3478-00**	6.96		
DIMETHYLAMINOETHANOL (PCCA)				
SOL, NA, 1 gm	**51927-1986-00**	0.56		
DIMETHYLAMINOETHANOL BITARTRATE (Medisca)				
deanol bitartrate				
CRY, NA, 100 gm	**38779-2342-05**	37.50		
500 gm	**38779-2342-08**	127.50		
5000 gm	**38779-2342-03**	1125.00		
DIMETHYLCOCOAMINE OXIDE (PCCA)				
cocamine oxide				
SOL, NA, 1 ml	**51927-2363-00**	0.10		
DIMETHYLGLYCINE HYDROCHLORIDE (PCCA)				
POW, NA (N,N)				
1 gm	**51927-2622-00**	1.14		
(Spectrum Pharmacy) *See N,N-DIMETHYLGLYCINE HCL*				
DIMETHYLGLYOXIME				
(PCCA) *See DIMETHYLGLYOXIME 99%*				
DIMETHYLGLYOXIME 99% (PCCA)				
dimethylglyoxime				
POW, NA (1X1GM)				
99%, 1 gm	**51927-2718-00**	2.25		
DIMETHYLPHTHALATE (Amend)				
dimethyl phthalate				
LIQ, NA, 500 ml	**17317-0877-01**	13.30		
3840 ml	**17317-0877-06**	42.00		
19200 ml	**17317-0877-08**	122.50		
DIMETHYLSULFOXIDE (Gallipot)				
dimethyl sulfoxide				
SOL, NA, 473 ml	**51552-1053-06**	68.32	48.80	
DINITROCHLOROBENZENE (PCCA)				
POW, NA (2,4)				
99%, 1 gm	**51927-1330-00**	2.25		
(Spectrum Pharmacy) *See 2,4-DINITROCHLOROBENZENE*				
2,4-DINITROCHLOROBENZENE (Spectrum Pharmacy)				
dinitrochlorobenzene				
CRY, NA (1X5GM)				
5 gm	**49452-2630-01**	140.70		
(1X25GM)				
25 gm	**49452-2630-02**	263.20		
(RECRYSTALLIZED)				
100 gm	**49452-2630-03**	345.10		
DINOPROSTONE				
(Forest Pharm) *See CERVIDIL*				
(Hawkins)				
POW, NA (PROSTAGLANDIN E2,USP)				
0.01 gm	**63370-0209-04**	880.00		
0.1 gm	**63370-0209-06**	4800.00		
(Pfizer) *See PREPIDIL*				
(Pfizer) *See PROSTIN E2*				
DIOCTYL ADIPATE (Medisca)				
diethylhexyl adipate				
SOL, NA (1X25ML)				
25 ml	**38779-1250-04**	22.50		
(1X100ML)				
100 ml	**38779-1250-05**	52.50		
(1X500ML)				
500 ml	**38779-1250-08**	147.00		
(PCCA)				
SOL, NA, 1 ml	**51927-2432-00**	0.90		
DIOVAN (Novartis Pharm)				
valsartan				
TAB, PO, 40 mg, 30s ea	**00078-0423-15**	68.88		
(10X10)				
40 mg, 100s ea UD	**00078-0423-06**	229.64		
80 mg, 90s ea	**00078-0358-34**	247.04		
(10X10 BLISTER PACK)				
80 mg, 100s ea UD	**00078-0358-06**	274.50		
160 mg, 90s ea	**00078-0359-34**	265.64		
(10X10 BLISTER PACK)				
160 mg, 100s ea UD	**00078-0359-06**	295.15		
320 mg, 90s ea	**00078-0360-34**	336.05		
(A-S Medication)				
REPACK				
TAB, PO, 80 mg, 30s ea	**54569-5361-00**	79.50		
160 mg, 30s ea	**54569-5362-00**	85.48		
320 mg, 30s ea	**54569-5666-00**	108.14		
(Advanced Pharm Serv, Inc.)				
REPACK				
TAB, PO, 80 mg, 10s ea	**13411-0142-01**	28.50		
20s ea	**13411-0142-02**	52.01		
30s ea	**13411-0142-03**	83.01		
60s ea	**13411-0142-06**	161.03		
90s ea	**13411-0142-09**	239.05		
160 mg, 10s ea	**13411-0143-01**	32.96		
20s ea	**13411-0143-02**	60.92		
30s ea	**13411-0143-03**	88.88		
60s ea	**13411-0143-06**	172.77		
90s ea	**13411-0143-09**	256.66		
(DHS, Inc.)				
REPACK				
TAB, PO, 80 mg, 30s ea	**55887-0307-30**	94.50		
(Dispensing Solutions)				
REPACK				
TAB, PO, 80 mg, 30s ea	**66336-0169-30**	99.84		
90s ea	**55045-3409-09**	166.50		
(Nucare Pharm)				
REPACK				
TAB, PO, 80 mg, 30s ea	**66267-0523-30**	137.00		
60s ea	**66267-0523-60**	191.00		
(Palmetto)				
REPACK				
TAB, PO, 40 mg, 30s ea	**23490-9411-03**	85.00		
90s ea	**23490-9411-09**	285.00		
80 mg, 30s ea	**23490-9412-03**	85.00		
90s ea	**23490-9412-09**	285.00		
(PD-Rx Pharm)				
REPACK				
TAB, PO, 80 mg, 30s ea	**55289-0825-30**	133.80		
(REDI-SCRIPT)				
80 mg, 30s ea	**58864-0681-30**	133.80		
160 mg, 30s ea	**55289-0817-30**	133.82		
30s ea	**58864-0605-30**	133.82		
320 mg, 30s ea	**55289-0876-30**	167.30		
(Pharma Pac)				
REPACK				
TAB, PO, 80 mg, 30s ea	**52959-0756-30**	54.89		

PROD/MFR	NDC	AWP	DP	OBC
(Phys Total Care)				
REPACK				
TAB, PO, 40 mg, 30s ea	**54868-5977-00**	80.50		
80 mg, 10s ea	**54868-4652-01**	37.02		
15s ea	**54868-4652-04**	54.22		
30s ea	**54868-4652-00**	105.83		
60s ea	**54868-4652-03**	197.57		
90s ea	**54868-4652-02**	294.39		
180s ea	**54868-4652-05**	568.61		
160 mg, 10s ea	**54868-4645-01**	36.90		
30s ea	**54868-4645-00**	105.47		
60s ea	**54868-4645-03**	196.90		
90s ea	**54868-4645-02**	293.39		
320 mg, 10s ea	**54868-5082-01**	45.99		
30s ea	**54868-5082-00**	132.73		
60s ea	**54868-5082-03**	248.39		
90s ea	**54868-5082-02**	370.63		
(Quality Care Prod)				
REPACK				
hydrochlorothiazide/valsartan				
TAB, PO, 12.5 mg-160 mg,				
90s ea	**49999-0943-90**	346.00		
(Quality Care Prod)				
valsartan				
40 mg, 30s ea	**49999-0543-30**	116.20		
100s ea	**49999-0543-00**	376.32		
80 mg, 30s ea	**49999-0878-30**	126.40		
90s ea	**49999-0878-90**	379.20		
100s ea	**49999-0878-00**	462.62		
160 mg, 30s ea	**49999-0877-30**	153.72		
90s ea	**49999-0877-90**	384.30		
100s ea	**49999-0877-00**	497.06		
320 mg, 90s ea	**35356-0101-90**	548.47		
DIOVAN HCT (Novartis Pharm)				
hydrochlorothiazide/valsartan				
TAB, PO (CAPLET)				
12.5 mg-80 mg,				
90s ea	**00078-0314-34**	265.72		
(10X10 BLISTER PACK)				
12.5 mg-80 mg,				
100s ea UD	**00078-0314-06**	295.21		
12.5 mg-160 mg,				
30s ea UD	**00078-0315-15**	96.37		EE
(CAPLET)				
12.5 mg-160 mg,				
90s ea	**00078-0315-34**	289.10		
(10X10 BLISTER PACK)				
12.5 mg-160 mg,				
100s ea UD	**00078-0315-06**	321.25		
(6X30)				
12.5 mg-160 mg,				
180s ea UD	**00078-0315-67**	578.23		EE
12.5 mg-320 mg,				
30s ea UD	**00078-0471-15**	122.09		EE
90s ea	**00078-0471-34**	366.28		EE
(6X30)				
12.5 mg-320 mg,				
180s ea UD	**00078-0471-67**	732.52		EE
25 mg-160 mg,				
30s ea UD	**00078-0383-15**	109.28		EE
90s ea	**00078-0383-34**	327.86		
(10X10 BLISTER PACK)				
25 mg-160 mg,				
100s ea UD	**00078-0383-06**	364.27		
(6X30)				
25 mg-160 mg,				
180s ea UD	**00078-0383-67**	655.69		EE
25 mg-320 mg,				
30s ea UD	**00078-0472-15**	138.52		
90s ea	**00078-0472-34**	415.54		
(6X30)				
25 mg-320 mg,				
180s ea UD	**00078-0472-67**	831.11		
(A-S Medication)				
REPACK				
TAB, PO (CAPLET)				
12.5 mg-80 mg,				
30s ea	**54569-4766-00**	85.51		
12.5 mg-160 mg,				
30s ea	**54569-4767-00**	93.03		
25 mg-160 mg,				
30s ea	**54569-5667-00**	105.51		
(Advanced Pharm Serv, Inc.)				
REPACK				
TAB, PO, 12.5 mg-80 mg,				
10s ea	**13411-0144-01**	32.97		
20s ea	**13411-0144-02**	60.94		
(CAPLET)				
12.5 mg-80 mg,				
30s ea	**13411-0144-03**	88.91		
60s ea	**13411-0144-06**	172.83		
90s ea	**13411-0144-09**	256.74		
12.5 mg-160 mg,				
10s ea	**13411-0145-01**	51.35		
20s ea	**13411-0145-02**	102.70		
(CAPLET)				
12.5 mg-160 mg,				
30s ea	**13411-0145-03**	154.07		
60s ea	**13411-0145-06**	308.14		
90s ea	**13411-0145-09**	462.21		
25 mg-160 mg,				
10s ea	**13411-0156-01**	41.40		
20s ea	**13411-0156-02**	74.03		
30s ea	**13411-0156-03**	108.54		
60s ea	**13411-0156-06**	212.09		
90s ea	**13411-0156-09**	315.63		
(AQ)				
REPACK				
TAB, PO, 12.5 mg-80 mg,				
90s ea	**66105-0544-09**	261.53		
12.5 mg-160 mg,				
10s ea	**66105-0545-01**	33.50		
30s ea	**66105-0545-03**	154.07		
60s ea	**66105-0545-06**	308.14		
90s ea	**66105-0545-09**	462.21		
100s ea	**66105-0545-10**	513.56		
(Nucare Pharm)				
REPACK				
TAB, PO (CAPLET)				
12.5 mg-80 mg,				
30s ea	**68071-0786-30**	145.00		
60s ea	**68071-0786-60**	203.00		
12.5 mg-160 mg,				
30s ea	**68071-0785-30**	155.00		
60s ea	**68071-0785-60**	223.00		
(PD-Rx Pharm)				
REPACK				
TAB, PO (CAPLET)				
12.5 mg-80 mg,				
30s ea	**55289-0815-30**	133.80		
12.5 mg-160 mg,				
30s ea	**55289-0838-30**	144.98		
25 mg-160 mg,				
30s ea	**55289-0820-30**	163.40		
(Phys Total Care)				
REPACK				
TAB, PO, 12.5 mg-80 mg,				
10s ea	**54868-4425-01**	39.62		
30s ea	**54868-4425-00**	113.63		
(CAPLET)				
12.5 mg-80 mg,				
60s ea	**54868-4425-02**	212.31		
90s ea	**54868-4425-03**	316.50		
12.5 mg-160 mg,				
10s ea	**54868-4428-01**	42.88		
30s ea	**54868-4428-00**	123.40		
(CAPLET)				
12.5 mg-160 mg,				
60s ea	**54868-4428-02**	230.76		
90s ea	**54868-4428-03**	344.18		
12.5 mg-320 mg,				
30s ea	**54868-5780-00**	147.14		
90s ea	**54868-5780-01**	421.56		EE
25 mg-160 mg,				
30s ea	**54868-5323-00**	139.59		
90s ea	**54868-5323-01**	390.07		
25 mg-320 mg,				
30s ea	**54868-5607-00**	154.57		
90s ea	**54868-5607-01**	443.12		
(Quality Care Prod)				
REPACK				
TAB, PO, 12.5 mg-80 mg,				
30s ea	**49999-0880-30**	110.60		
(CAPLET)				
12.5 mg-80 mg,				
90s ea	**49999-0880-90**	346.00		
25 mg-160 mg,				
30s ea	**35356-0060-30**	104.40		
30s ea	**49999-0879-30**	145.30		
(Stat Rx)				
REPACK				
TAB, PO (CAPLET)				
12.5 mg-80 mg,				
30s ea	**16590-0312-30**	97.05		
25 mg-160 mg,				
30s ea	**16590-0332-30**	121.50		
DIOXYBENZONE (PCCA)				
POW, NA, 1 gm	**51927-1172-00**	1.92		
DIOXYBENZONE/HYDROQUINONE/OXYBENZONE/PADIMATE O				
(Perrigo) *See HYDROQUINONE*				
DIOXYBENZONE/HYDROQUINONE/PADIMATE O				
(Perrigo) *See HYDROQUINONE SKIN BLEACHING WITH SUNSCREENS*				
DIPENTUM (Alaven)				
olsalazine sodium				
CAP, PO (HARD GELATIN)				
250 mg, 100s ea	**68220-0160-10**	241.80		
300s ea	**50474-0600-25**	654.12		
DIPHEN (Truxton)				
phenytoin sodium, prompt				
CAP, PO, 100 mg,				
1000s ea	**00463-2007-10**	35.40		
DIPHENCYPRONE (Gallipot)				
POW, NA (1X1GM)				
1 gm	**51552-0943-01**	55.30	39.50	
(1X5GM)				
5 gm	**51552-0943-02**	238.00	170.00	
(PCCA) *See DIPHENYLCYCLOPROPENONE*				
(Spectrum Pharmacy) *See DIPHENYLCYCLOPROPENONE*				
DIPHENHYDRAMINE (PCCA)				
POW, NA, 1 gm	**51927-3539-00**	0.57		
(Bryant Ranch)				
REPACK				
diphenhydramine hydrochloride				
CAP, PO, 25 mg, 20s ea	**63629-1343-02**	16.00		
24s ea	**63629-1343-04**	19.20		
30s ea	**63629-1343-01**	24.00		
42s ea	**63629-1343-03**	33.60		
50 mg, 15s ea	**63629-1349-01**	14.85		
20s ea	**63629-1349-02**	19.80		
30s ea	**63629-1349-03**	29.70		
(Core)				
REPACK				
CAP, PO, 50 mg, 20s ea	**33358-0111-20**	20.30		
30s ea	**33358-0111-30**	30.44		
(IPI)				
REPACK				
CAP, PO, 25 mg, 30s ea	**18837-0299-30**	15.50		
50 mg, 30s ea	**18837-0043-30**	15.11		
(Quality Care Prod)				
REPACK				
SOL, IJ, 50 mg/ml,				
1 ml 25s	**49999-0525-10**	10.90		
DIPHENHYDRAMINE HCL (Advance)				
diphenhydramine hydrochloride				
CAP, PO, 50 mg, 100s ea	**17714-0021-01**	3.99		EE
1000s ea	**17714-0021-10**	17.85		EE
(Amend)				
POW, NA (U.S.P.)				
100 gm	**17317-0146-03**	13.30		
500 gm	**17317-0146-05**	44.80		
1000 gm	**17317-0146-06**	86.80		
(Gallipot)				
POW, NA (U.S.P.,N.F.)				
5 gm	**51552-0124-02**	9.10		
25 gm	**51552-0124-04**	9.80		
100 gm	**51552-0124-05**	14.56		
500 gm	**51552-0124-06**	52.50		
(Hawkins)				
POW, NA (USP)				
25 gm	**63370-0071-25**	28.00		
100 gm	**63370-0071-35**	36.00		
500 gm	**63370-0071-45**	140.00		
1000 gm	**63370-0071-50**	216.00		
(Hospira)				
SOL, IJ (LUER LOCK,CARPUJECT)				
50 mg/ml, 1 ml 10s	**00409-2290-31**	14.88	13.00	AP
(Letco)				
POW, NA (U.S.P.)				
100 gm	**62991-1047-02**	30.00		
(Medisca)				
POW, NA (U.S.P.)				
25 gm	**38779-0282-04**	22.50		
100 gm	**38779-0282-05**	36.00		
500 gm	**38779-0282-08**	147.00		
1000 gm	**38779-0282-09**	206.85		
(PCCA)				
POW, NA (U.S.P.)				
1 gm	**51927-1079-00**	1.32		
(Pharm Assoc Inc)				
ELI, PO, 12.5 mg/5 ml,				
5 ml 100s UD	**00121-0489-05**	54.78		AA
10 ml 100s UD	**00121-0489-10**	62.71		AA
20 ml 100s UD	**00121-0489-20**	71.88		AA

PROD/MFR	NDC	AWP	DP	OBC
(Spectrum Pharmacy)				
POW, NA (U.S.P.)				
100 gm	**49452-2640-01**	64.75		
500 gm	**49452-2640-02**	250.60		
(Teva)				
CAP, PO, 50 mg, 100s ea	**00555-0059-02**	13.62		AA
1000s ea	**00555-0059-05**	53.90		AA
(UDL)				
CAP, PO (10X10)				
50 mg, 100s ea UD	**51079-0066-20**	13.45		AA
(A-S Medication)				
REPACK				
CAP, PO, 50 mg, 10s ea	**54569-0241-05**	0.84		EE
15s ea	**54569-0241-02**	1.25		EE
20s ea	**54569-0241-03**	1.67		EE
(Altura)				
REPACK				
CAP, PO, 50 mg, 7s ea	**63874-0006-07**	4.25		EE
10s ea	**63874-0006-10**	6.07		EE
12s ea	**63874-0006-12**	7.29		EE
14s ea	**63874-0006-14**	8.50		EE
25s ea	**63874-0006-25**	15.18		EE
28s ea	**63874-0006-28**	17.01		EE
60s ea	**63874-0006-60**	36.44		EE
100s ea	**63874-0006-01**	60.73		EE
(DHS, Inc.)				
REPACK				
CAP, PO, 25 mg, 20s ea	**55887-0973-20**	9.75		EE
50 mg, 30s ea	**55887-0885-30**	11.00		AA
(Dispensing Solutions)				
REPACK				
CAP, PO, 25 mg, 15s ea	**66336-0589-15**	8.33		AA
20s ea	**66336-0589-20**	11.11		AA
30s ea	**66336-0589-30**	16.67		AA
60s ea	**66336-0589-60**	33.33		AA
50 mg, 3s ea	**55045-1124-01**	1.83		AA
6s ea	**55045-1124-06**	3.66		AA
6s ea	**66336-0045-06**	6.25		AA
15s ea	**55045-1124-05**	9.25		AA
15s ea	**66336-0045-15**	8.99		AA
20s ea	**55045-1124-07**	12.20		AA
30s ea	**66336-0045-30**	11.31		AA
50s ea	**55045-1124-09**	30.50		AA
60s ea	**55045-1124-02**	36.60		AA
90s ea	**55045-1124-03**	54.90		AA
100s ea	**55045-1124-00**	61.00		AA
120s ea	**55045-1124-04**	73.20		AA
(HomeMed)				
REPACK				
CAP, PO, 25 mg, 12s ea	**51655-0113-27**	2.80		EE
15s ea	**51655-0133-54**	9.99		EE
60s ea	**51655-0113-25**	3.75		EE
50 mg, 20s ea	**51655-0088-52**	2.52		
30s ea	**51655-0088-24**	17.89		
TAB, PO, 25 mg, 8s ea	**51655-0113-80**	5.32		
30s ea	**51655-0113-24**	17.74		
(Nucare Pharm)				
REPACK				
ELI, PO, 12.5 mg/5 ml,				
120 ml	**66267-0977-04**	7.36		EE
(PD-Rx Pharm)				
REPACK				
CAP, PO, 25 mg, 10s ea	**55289-0479-10**	7.87		AA
12s ea	**55289-0479-12**	6.70		AA
15s ea	**55289-0479-15**	9.22		AA
20s ea	**55289-0479-20**	9.33		AA
24s ea	**55289-0479-24**	10.13		AA
30s ea	**55289-0479-30**	10.67		AA
(REDI-SCRIPT)				
25 mg, 30s ea	**58864-0162-30**	10.66		AA
56s ea	**58864-0162-56**	13.69		AA
100s ea	**55289-0479-01**	18.51		AA
50 mg, 10s ea	**55289-0100-10**	8.22		AA
15s ea	**55289-0100-15**	9.09		AA
20s ea	**55289-0100-20**	9.78		AA
30s ea	**55289-0100-30**	13.60		AA
40s ea	**55289-0100-40**	14.00		AA
100s ea	**55289-0100-01**	29.78		AA
(Pharma Pac)				
REPACK				
CAP, PO, 25 mg, 4s ea	**52959-0043-04**	3.07		EE
10s ea	**52959-0043-10**	7.48		EE
15s ea	**52959-0043-15**	10.72		EE
20s ea	**52959-0043-20**	13.45		EE
24s ea	**52959-0043-24**	15.66		EE
30s ea	**52959-0043-30**	17.92		EE
50s ea	**52959-0043-50**	22.37		EE
60s ea	**52959-0043-60**	25.14		EE
100s ea	**52959-0043-00**	21.75		EE

PROD/MFR	NDC	AWP	DP	OBC
50 mg, 6s ea	**52959-0053-06**	6.75		EE
10s ea	**52959-0053-10**	8.15		EE
12s ea	**52959-0053-12**	8.52		EE
15s ea	**52959-0053-15**	8.99		EE
20s ea	**52959-0053-20**	9.75		EE
30s ea	**52959-0053-30**	11.31		EE
52s ea	**52959-0053-52**	19.63		EE
ELI, PO, 12.5 mg/5 ml,				
120 ml	**52959-0123-03**	7.50		EE
(Phys Total Care)				
REPACK				
CAP, PO, 25 mg, 10s ea	**54868-0026-05**	3.75		EE
20s ea	**54868-0026-06**	4.50		EE
30s ea	**54868-0026-01**	5.25		EE
60s ea	**54868-0026-07**	7.57		EE
100s ea	**54868-0026-00**	9.12		EE
1000s ea	**54868-0026-04**	94.74		EE
50 mg, 15s ea	**54868-1050-06**	6.48		EE
20s ea	**54868-1050-00**	7.14		EE
30s ea	**54868-1050-01**	8.46		EE
40s ea	**54868-1050-04**	9.75		EE
100s ea	**54868-1050-05**	17.64		EE
1000s ea	**54868-1050-03**	56.43		EE
SOL, IJ (M.D.V.)				
10 mg/ml, 30 ml	**54868-3644-00**	22.27		EE
(VIAL)				
50 mg/ml, 1 ml 10s	**54868-2048-00**	51.30		EE
1 ml 25s	**54868-2048-01**	95.34		EE
(Quality Care Prod)				
REPACK				
CAP, PO, 25 mg, 60s ea	**49999-0003-60**	10.20		EE
50 mg, 4s ea	**49999-0091-04**	6.86		EE
15s ea	**49999-0091-15**	8.78		EE
20s ea	**49999-0091-20**	11.72		EE
30s ea	**49999-0091-30**	13.03		EE
60s ea	**49999-0091-60**	21.07		EE
TAB, PO, 25 mg, 6s ea	**49999-0003-06**	12.76		EE
15s ea	**49999-0003-15**	13.94		EE
24s ea	**49999-0003-24**	15.76		EE
30s ea	**49999-0003-30**	16.19		EE
40s ea	**49999-0003-40**	18.95		EE
(Southwood)				
REPACK				
CAP, PO, 50 mg, 10s ea	**58016-0409-10**	2.92		EE
12s ea	**58016-0409-12**	3.51		EE
15s ea	**58016-0409-15**	4.39		EE
20s ea	**58016-0409-20**	5.85		EE
21s ea	**58016-0409-21**	5.45		EE
24s ea	**58016-0409-24**	7.02		EE
30s ea	**58016-0409-30**	8.78		EE
40s ea	**58016-0409-40**	10.37		EE
60s ea	**58016-0409-60**	17.56		EE
90s ea	**58016-0409-90**	23.34		EE
100s ea	**58016-0409-00**	25.93		EE
(St. Mary's MPP)				
REPACK				
CAP, PO, 25 mg, 30s ea	**60760-0330-30**	6.33		EE
(Stat Rx)				
REPACK				
CAP, PO, 50 mg, 30s ea	**16590-0079-30**	16.75		EE
(Vibranta)				
REPACK				
CAP, PO, 50 mg, 15s ea	**57866-3762-05**	10.25		
20s ea	**57866-3762-02**	2.50		
30s ea	**57866-3762-01**	6.96		
90s ea	**57866-3762-04**	32.10		

DIPHENHYDRAMINE HCL/LIDO HCL/NYSTATIN
(Cutispharma) *See FIRST-BXN MOUTHWASH*

DIPHENHYDRAMINE HCL/PHENYLEPH HCL
(Poly) *See ALAHIST LQ*
(Zyber) *See ALDEX-CT*

DIPHENHYDRAMINE HCL/PSE HCL
(Capellon) *See TEKRAL*

DIPHENHYDRAMINE HYDROCHLORIDE

PROD/MFR	NDC	AWP	DP	OBC
FUL				
ELI, PO, 12.5 mg/5 ml,				
120 ml		1.64		

(Advance) *See DIPHENHYDRAMINE HCL*
(Amend) *See DIPHENHYDRAMINE HCL*

PROD/MFR	NDC	AWP	DP	OBC
(APP)				
SOL, IJ, 50 mg/ml, 1 ml	**63323-0664-01**	3.43		AP
(Baxter)				
SOL, IJ (DOSETTE VIAL)				
50 mg/ml, 1 ml	**00641-0376-21**	0.98		AP
((DOSETTE VIAL),USP)				
50 mg/ml, 1 ml 25s	**00641-0376-25**	24.60		AP
(Bioniche Pharma)				
SOL, IJ (MDV,USP,10X10ML)				
50 mg/ml,				
10 ml 10s	**67457-0124-10**	118.75		AP

(Clint) *See BANARIL*
(Gallipot) *See DIPHENHYDRAMINE HCL*
(Hawkins) *See DIPHENHYDRAMINE HCL*
(Hospira) *See DIPHENHYDRAMINE HCL*

PROD/MFR	NDC	AWP	DP	OBC
(Hospira)				
SOL, IJ (W/LUER LOCK,10X1ML,USP)				
50 mg/ml, 1 ml 10s	**00409-2290-11**	13.08	11.40	AP

(Letco) *See DIPHENHYDRAMINE HCL*
(Lunsco) *See DYTUSS*
(Medique) *See MEDI-FIRST DIPHENHYDRAMINE HYDROCHLORIDE*
(Medisca) *See DIPHENHYDRAMINE HCL*
(PCCA) *See DIPHENHYDRAMINE HCL*
(Pfizer) *See BENADRYL*
(Pharm Assoc Inc) *See DIPHENHYDRAMINE HCL*

PROD/MFR	NDC	AWP	DP	OBC
(Qualitest)				
CAP, PO (USP)				
50 mg, 100s ea	**00603-3340-21**	13.62		
1000s ea	**00603-3340-32**	83.52		

(Spectrum Pharmacy) *See DIPHENHYDRAMINE HCL*
(Teva) *See DIPHENHYDRAMINE HCL*
(Truxton) *See TRUXADRYL*
(UDL) *See DIPHENHYDRAMINE HCL*

PROD/MFR	NDC	AWP	DP	OBC
(A-S Medication)				
REPACK				
SOL, IJ (25X1ML)				
50 mg/ml, 1 ml 25s	**54569-5815-00**	57.50		
(Dispensing Solutions)				
REPACK				
CAP, PO, 25 mg, 6s ea	**55045-1125-02**	2.46		AA
24s ea	**55045-2781-06**	9.84		AA
60s ea	**55045-1125-09**	24.60		AA
90s ea	**55045-1125-03**	36.90		AA
100s ea	**55045-1125-01**	41.00		AA
120s ea	**55045-1125-00**	49.20		AA
(Keltman Pharma., Inc.)				
REPACK				
CAP, PO, 25 mg, 30s ea	**68387-0541-30**	12.63		
(Palmetto)				
REPACK				
CAP, PO, 25 mg, 6s ea	**23490-5457-01**	7.02		
15s ea	**23490-5457-02**	8.96		
20s ea	**23490-5457-03**	11.95		
24s ea	**23490-5457-00**	14.34		
30s ea	**23490-5457-04**	17.92		
60s ea	**23490-5457-05**	35.84		
50 mg, 6s ea	**23490-5459-01**	5.12		
15s ea	**23490-5459-02**	9.15		
30s ea	**23490-5459-03**	18.30		
60s ea	**23490-5459-04**	36.60		
(PD-Rx Pharm)				
REPACK				
CAP, PO (USP)				
50 mg, 6s ea	**43063-0179-06**	6.76		

DIPHENHYDRAMINE TANNATE
(Hawthorn Pharm) *See DYTAN*

DIPHENHYDRAMINE TANNATE/ PHENYLEPHRINE TANNATE
(Hawthorn Pharm) *See DYTAN-D*

DIPHENIDOL HCL **(Gallipot)**

PROD/MFR	NDC	AWP	DP	OBC
diphenidol hydrochloride				
POW, NA, 5 gm	**51552-1000-02**	20.30	14.50	
(PCCA)				
POW, NA, 1 gm	**51927-2812-00**	24.00		

DIPHENIDOL HYDROCHLORIDE
(Gallipot) *See DIPHENIDOL HCL*
(PCCA) *See DIPHENIDOL HCL*

PROD/MFR	NDC	AWP	DP	OBC
(Spectrum Pharmacy)				
POW, NA (1X5GM)				
5 gm	**49452-2647-01**	118.30		
(1X25GM)				
25 gm	**49452-2647-02**	437.50		

PROD/MFR	NDC	AWP	DP	OBC
DIPHENOX/ATROPINE (Core)				
REPACK				
atropine sulfate/diphenoxylate hydrochloride				
TAB, PO, 0.025 mg-2.5 mg,				
20s ea, C-V	33358-0112-20	21.41		
DIPHENOXYLATE HYDROCHLORIDE (PCCA)				
POW, NA (USP)				
1 gm, C-II	51927-2996-00	270.00		
DIPHENOXYLATE HYDROCHLORIDE AND ATROPINE SULFATE (Physician Partner)				
REPACK				
atropine sulfate/diphenoxylate hydrochloride				
TAB, PO, 0.025 mg-2.5 mg,				
15s ea, C-V	21695-0688-15	16.94		AA
20s ea, C-V	21695-0688-20	22.58		AA
30s ea, C-V	21695-0688-30	33.87		AA
DIPHENOXYLATE W/ ATROP (Bryant Ranch)				
REPACK				
atropine sulfate/diphenoxylate hydrochloride				
TAB, PO, 0.025 mg-2.5 mg,				
20s ea, C-V	63629-1734-01	6.00		
DIPHENOXYLATE/ATROP (Keltman Pharma., Inc.)				
REPACK				
atropine sulfate/diphenoxylate hydrochloride				
TAB, PO, 0.025 mg-2.5 mg,				
12s ea, C-V	68387-0544-12	19.50		
DIPHENOXYLATE/ATROPINE (DHS, Inc.)				
REPACK				
atropine sulfate/diphenoxylate hydrochloride				
TAB, PO, 0.025 mg-2.5 mg,				
15s ea, C-V	55887-0841-15	9.97		
25s ea, C-V	55887-0841-25	14.50		
(Stat Rx)				
REPACK				
TAB, PO, 0.025 mg-2.5 mg,				
10s ea, C-V	16590-0080-10	20.00		
15s ea, C-V	16590-0080-15	30.00		
20s ea, C-V	16590-0080-20	40.00		
30s ea, C-V	16590-0080-30	60.00		
DIPHENOXYLATE/ATROPINE SULFATE (Quality Care Prod)				
REPACK				
atropine sulfate/diphenoxylate hydrochloride				
TAB, PO, 0.025 mg-2.5 mg,				
20s ea, C-V	49999-0207-20	37.44		
30s ea, C-V	49999-0207-30	56.16		
DIPHENYLCYCLOPROPENONE (PCCA)				
diphencyprone				
POW, NA (1X1GM)				
1 gm	51927-1668-00	141.00		
(Spectrum Pharmacy)				
POW, NA (1X1GM)				
1 gm	49452-2642-01	218.75		
(1X5GM)				
5 gm	49452-2642-02	714.00		
DIPHTHERIA TOXOID, ADSORBED/TETANUS TOXOID				
(Akorn) *See TETANUS AND DIPHTHERIA TOXOIDS ADSORBED*				
(Sanofi) *See DECAVAC*				
(Sanofi) *See DIPHTHERIA/TETANUS TOXOIDS ADSORBED*				
DIPHTHERIA/TETANUS TOXOIDS ADSORBED (Sanofi)				
diphtheria toxoid, adsorbed/tetanus toxoid				
SUS, IM (SRN PREFILLED,TAX INCL)				
0.5 ml 10s	49281-0278-10	362.29	304.41	
(Phys Total Care)				
REPACK				
SUS, IM (10 DOSE VIAL,TAX INCL)				
5 ml	54868-0571-06	143.96		
DIPIVEFRIN HCL (Phys Total Care)				
dipivefrin hydrochloride				
SOL, OP, 0.1%, 10 ml	54868-3373-00	15.62		EE
DIPIVEFRIN HYDROCHLORIDE				
FUL				
SOL, OP, 0.1%, 5 ml		4.35		
DIPRIVAN (APP)				
propofol				
EMU, IV (20X25ML)				
10 mg/ml,				
20 ml 25s	63323-0269-20	187.50		
(20X50ML)				
10 mg/ml,				
50 ml 20s	63323-0269-50	375.00		
(10X100ML)				
10 mg/ml,				
100 ml 10s	63323-0269-65	375.00		

PROD/MFR	NDC	AWP	DP	OBC
DIPROLENE (Schering)				
betamethasone dipropionate, augmented				
LOT, TP, 0.05%, 30 ml	00085-0962-01	72.19		
60 ml	00085-0962-02	142.27		
OIN, TP, 0.05%, 15 gm	00085-0575-02	62.92		AB
50 gm	00085-0575-05	140.74		AB
(Phys Total Care)				
REPACK				
LOT, TP, 0.05%, 60 ml	54868-4753-00	109.69		
OIN, TP, 0.05%, 15 gm	54868-4500-00	55.59		AB
(Quality Care Prod)				
REPACK				
OIN, TP (1X50GM)				
0.05%, 50 gm	35356-0495-50	225.49		AB
DIPROLENE AF (Schering)				
betamethasone dipropionate, augmented				
CRE, TP, 0.05%, 15 gm	00085-0517-01	62.92		
50 gm	00085-0517-04	140.74		
(Dispensing Solutions)				
REPACK				
CRE, TP, 0.05%, 15 gm	55045-3039-01	49.00		
(Pharma Pac)				
REPACK				
CRE, TP, 0.05%, 15 gm	52959-0575-15	41.10		
50 gm	52959-0575-05	68.74		
(Phys Total Care)				
REPACK				
CRE, TP, 0.05%, 15 gm	54868-2851-00	55.59		
DIPROPYLENE GLYCOL (PCCA)				
SOL, NA, 1 ml	51927-3208-00	0.23		
DIPYRIDAMOLE				
FUL				
TAB, PO, 25 mg, 100s ea		29.78		
50 mg, 100s ea		47.96		
75 mg, 100s ea		64.17		
(Apotex Corp.)				
SOL, IV, 5 mg/ml, 2 ml 25s	60505-0715-00	281.25		AP
(10X10)				
5 mg/ml, 10 ml 10s	60505-0715-01	562.50		AP
(Baxter)				
SOL, IV (SDV)				
5 mg/ml, 10 ml	00641-2569-41	8.12		AP
(SDV,USP)				
5 mg/ml, 10 ml 5s	00641-2569-44	40.62		AP
(Bedford)				
SOL, IV (S.D.V.)				
5 mg/ml, 2 ml 10s	55390-0555-10	25.20		AP
(USP, SDV)				
5 mg/ml, 10 ml 10s	55390-0555-90	126.00		AP
(Boehr Ingelheim Phar) *See PERSANTINE*				
(Consolidated Midland)				
TAB, PO, 25 mg, 100s ea	00223-0837-01	4.75		EE
1000s ea	00223-0837-02	41.50		EE
(Glenmark Pharmaceuticals)				
TAB, PO (FILM-COATED)				
25 mg, 100s ea	68462-0116-01	58.40		AB
1000s ea	68462-0116-10	584.00		AB
50 mg, 100s ea	68462-0117-01	94.10		AB
1000s ea	68462-0117-10	941.00		AB
75 mg, 100s ea	68462-0118-01	125.90		AB
1000s ea	68462-0118-10	1259.00		AB
(Global Pharm)				
TAB, PO (USP,FILM-COATED)				
25 mg, 100s ea	00115-1070-01	58.40		AB
1000s ea	00115-1070-03	584.00		AB
50 mg, 100s ea	00115-1071-01	94.10		AB
1000s ea	00115-1071-03	941.00		AB
75 mg, 100s ea	00115-1072-01	125.90		AB
1000s ea	00115-1072-03	1259.00		AB
(Hospira)				
SOL, IV (AMP,UNI-NEST,LATEX-FREE)				
5 mg/ml, 2 ml 10s	00409-2043-02	30.00	26.30	AP
(Lannett)				
TAB, PO (USP,FILM-COATED)				
25 mg, 100s ea	00527-1461-01	70.08		AB
1000s ea	00527-1461-10	700.80		AB
50 mg, 100s ea	00527-1462-01	112.92		AB
1000s ea	00527-1462-10	1129.20		AB
75 mg, 100s ea	00527-1463-01	151.08		AB
1000s ea	00527-1463-10	1510.80		AB
(Major)				
TAB, PO (10X10)				
25 mg, 100s ea UD	00904-1086-61	39.00		AB
50 mg, 100s ea UD	00904-1087-61	65.65		AB
(10X10,FILM-COATED)				
75 mg, 100s ea UD	00904-1088-61	82.17		AB

PROD/MFR	NDC	AWP	DP	OBC
(PCCA)				
POW, NA (U.S.P.)				
1 gm	51927-1571-00	2.88		
(Rising)				
TAB, PO (USP,FILM-COATED)				
25 mg, 100s ea	64980-0133-01	58.40		AB
1000s ea	64980-0133-10	584.00		AB
50 mg, 100s ea	64980-0134-01	94.10		AB
1000s ea	64980-0134-10	941.00		AB
75 mg, 100s ea	64980-0135-01	125.90		AB
1000s ea	64980-0135-10	1259.00		AB
(Spectrum Pharmacy)				
CRY, NA (U.S.P.)				
25 gm	49452-2641-03	115.15		
100 gm	49452-2641-04	381.50		
500 gm	49452-2641-05	1501.50		
(Teva)				
SOL, IV (S.D.V.)				
5 mg/ml, 2 ml 5s	00703-1652-02	36.36		AP
10 ml 5s	00703-1654-02	66.00		AP
TAB, PO, 25 mg, 100s ea	00555-0252-02	55.81		AB
1000s ea	00555-0252-05	519.06		AB
50 mg, 100s ea	00555-0285-02	89.91		AB
1000s ea	00555-0285-05	836.35		AB
75 mg, 100s ea	00555-0286-02	120.30		AB
1000s ea	00555-0286-05	1118.63		AB
(Zydus Pharm.)				
TAB, PO (USP,FILM COATED)				
25 mg, 100s ea	68382-0187-01	58.40		AB
500s ea	68382-0187-05	292.00		AB
50 mg, 100s ea	68382-0188-01	94.10		AB
500s ea	68382-0188-05	470.50		AB
75 mg, 100s ea	68382-0189-01	125.90		AB
500s ea	68382-0189-05	629.50		AB
(Phys Total Care)				
REPACK				
TAB, PO (FILM-COATED)				
25 mg, 30s ea	54868-0042-02	32.02		AB
100s ea	54868-0042-04	89.73		EE
120s ea	54868-0042-01	108.57		EE
50 mg, 20s ea	54868-0043-01	30.87		AB
30s ea	54868-0043-03	41.65		EE
60s ea	54868-0043-00	86.64		AB
100s ea	54868-0043-02	142.38		EE
(FILM-COATED)				
75 mg, 30s ea	54868-0044-01	60.69		AB
90s ea	54868-0044-00	139.53		EE
100s ea	54868-0044-02	153.03		EE
DIPYRONE (Gallipot)				
POW, NA, 25 gm	51552-0989-04	35.00	25.00	
(Medisca)				
POW, NA, 25 gm	38779-1762-04	105.00		
100 gm	38779-1762-05	360.00		
DIQUINOL (Consolidated Midland)				
iodoquinol				
TAB, PO, 650 mg, 100s ea	00223-0850-01	47.50		
500s ea	00223-0850-05	225.00		
DISCOVISC (Alcon Surgical)				
chondroitin sulfate/hyaluronate sodium				
SOL, OP (27G CANNULA/LOCK)				
40 mg/ml-17 mg/ml,				
1 ml	08065-1837-10	237.36		
DISKETS DISPERSIBLE (Roxane)				
methadone hydrochloride				
TAB, PO (USP)				
40 mg,				
100s ea, C-II	00054-4538-25	33.16		AA
DISOPHENOL				
(PCCA) *See DISOPHENOL 97%*				
DISOPHENOL 97% (PCCA)				
disophenol				
POW, NA, 1 gm	51927-2555-00	20.40		
DISOPYRAMIDE (Phys Total Care)				
REPACK				
disopyramide phosphate				
CAP, PO (USP)				
100 mg, 60s ea	54868-2181-00	89.22		
DISOPYRAMIDE PHOSPHATE				
FUL				
CAP, PO, 100 mg, 100s ea		59.79		
150 mg, 100s ea		62.88		
(Consolidated Midland)				
CAP, PO, 100 mg, 100s ea	00223-0842-01	13.50		EE
500s ea	00223-0842-05	62.75		EE
150 mg, 500s ea	00223-0843-05	85.00		EE

PROD/MFR	NDC	AWP	DP	OBC
(Ethex)				
CER, PO, 150 mg, 100s ea	**58177-0002-04**	175.26		AB
(PCCA)				
POW, NA (U.S.P.)				
1 gm	**51927-2514-00**	0.90		
(Pfizer) *See NORPACE*				
(Pfizer) *See NORPACE CR*				
(Teva)				
CAP, PO, 100 mg, 100s ea	**00093-3127-01**	69.41		AB
150 mg, 100s ea	**00093-3129-01**	81.98		AB
(Watson Labs)				
CAP, PO, 100 mg, 100s ea	**00591-5560-01**	69.41		AB
150 mg, 100s ea	**00591-5561-01**	81.98		AB
(Phys Total Care)				
REPACK				
CAP, PO, 150 mg, 100s ea	**54868-3816-00**	46.82		EE
DISULFIRAM (Letco)				
POW, NA (USP)				
100 gm	**62991-1594-01**	90.00		
500 gm	**62991-1594-02**	405.00		
(Medisca)				
POW, NA, 50 gm	**38779-1971-02**	60.75		
100 gm	**38779-1971-05**	105.00		
500 gm	**38779-1971-08**	417.00		
(PCCA)				
POW, NA (U.S.P)				
1 gm	**51927-3121-00**	1.08		
(Spectrum Pharmacy)				
CRY, NA (U.S.P.)				
100 gm	**49452-2645-01**	165.90		
500 gm	**49452-2645-02**	626.50		
1000 gm	**49452-2645-03**	1018.50		
(Teva) *See ANTABUSE*				
DITIOCARB SODIUM				
(PCCA) *See DIETHYLDITHIOCARBAMIC ACID SODIUM REAGENT ACS*				
DITROPAN XL (Ortho-McNeil Pharm)				
oxybutynin chloride				
TER, PO, 5 mg, 100s ea	**50458-0805-01**	412.58	343.82	AB
10 mg, 100s ea	**50458-0810-01**	413.02	344.18	AB
15 mg, 100s ea	**50458-0815-01**	423.35	352.79	
(Phys Total Care)				
REPACK				
TER, PO, 5 mg, 10s ea	**54868-4610-01**	44.30		
30s ea	**54868-4610-00**	122.08		
60s ea	**54868-4610-02**	241.65		
100s ea	**54868-4610-03**	388.99		
10 mg, 10s ea	**54868-4502-01**	44.34		
30s ea	**54868-4502-00**	129.28		
15 mg, 10s ea	**54868-4835-01**	45.41		
30s ea	**54868-4835-00**	125.21		
100s ea	**54868-4835-02**	399.13		
DIURIL (Salix Pharm)				
chlorothiazide				
SUS, PO (1X237ML)				
250 mg/5 ml,				
237 ml	**65649-0311-12**	38.53		
DIURIL SODIUM (Lundbeck)				
chlorothiazide sodium				
PDS, IV, 0.5 gm, ea	**67386-0711-55**	433.02	12.36	
DIVALPROEX SODIUM				
FUL				
ECC, PO, 125 mg, 100s ea		82.10		
TCP, PO, 125 mg, 100s ea		26.91		
250 mg, 100s ea		52.88		
500 mg, 100s ea		97.49		
(Abbott Pharm) *See DEPAKOTE*				
(Abbott Pharm) *See DEPAKOTE ER*				
(Abbott Pharm) *See DEPAKOTE SPRINKLES*				
(Anchen)				
TER, PO (FILM COATED)				
250 mg, 100s ea	**10370-0510-10**	167.90		AB
500s ea	**10370-0510-50**	839.50		AB
(FILM-COATED)				
500 mg, 100s ea	**10370-0511-10**	295.35		AB
500s ea	**10370-0511-50**	1476.75		AB
(Apotex Corp.)				
TCP, PO (USP,ENTERIC-COATED)				
125 mg, 100s ea	**60505-3065-01**	89.72		
250 mg, 100s ea	**60505-3066-01**	176.23		
500s ea	**60505-3066-05**	881.10		
500 mg, 100s ea	**60505-3067-01**	324.97		
500s ea	**60505-3067-05**	1624.81		

PROD/MFR	NDC	AWP	DP	OBC
(Caraco)				
TCP, PO (USP,DÈLAYED RELEASE)				
125 mg, 100s ea	**62756-0796-88**	88.72		AB
500s ea	**62756-0796-13**	443.62		AB
250 mg, 100s ea	**62756-0797-88**	174.27		AB
500s ea	**62756-0797-13**	871.35		AB
500 mg, 100s ea	**62756-0798-88**	321.36		AB
500s ea	**62756-0798-13**	1606.81		AB
(Dr Reddy's)				
ECC, PO, 125 mg, 100s ea	**55111-0532-01**	89.65		AB
(SPRINKLE)				
125 mg, 500s ea	**55111-0532-05**	448.25		AB
TCP, PO (USP)				
125 mg, 100s ea	**55111-0529-01**	89.72		AB
250 mg, 100s ea	**55111-0530-01**	176.23		AB
500 mg, 100s ea	**55111-0531-01**	324.97		AB
(Global Pharm)				
TER, PO, 250 mg, 100s ea	**00115-6911-01**	168.11		AB
500s ea	**00115-6911-02**	798.52		AB
500 mg, 100s ea	**00115-6922-01**	295.36		AB
500s ea	**00115-6922-02**	1476.80		AB
(Lupin Pharma, Inc.)				
TCP, PO (USP,DELAYED RELEASE)				
125 mg, 100s ea	**68180-0265-01**	89.72		AB
(USP)				
250 mg, 100s ea	**68180-0266-01**	176.23		AB
500s ea	**68180-0266-02**	881.11		AB
500 mg, 100s ea	**68180-0267-01**	324.97		AB
500s ea	**68180-0267-02**	1624.82		AB
(Major)				
TER, PO (10X10,FILM-COATED)				
250 mg, 100s ea UD	**00904-5990-61**	212.91		AB
500 mg, 100s ea UD	**00904-6073-61**	440.62		AB
(Mylan)				
TCP, PO (FILM-COATED)				
125 mg, 100s ea	**00378-1043-01**	89.72		AB
250 mg, 100s ea	**00378-1044-01**	176.23		AB
500 mg, 100s ea	**00378-1045-01**	324.97		AB
TER, PO, 250 mg, 100s ea	**00378-0472-01**	167.91		EE
500s ea	**00378-0472-05**	839.55		EE
500 mg, 100s ea	**00378-0473-01**	295.36		AB
500s ea	**00378-0473-05**	1476.80		AB
(Northstar)				
TCP, PO (USP,ENTERIC FILM COATED)				
125 mg, 100s ea	**16714-0511-01**	89.72		EE
250 mg, 100s ea	**16714-0512-01**	176.23		EE
500s ea	**16714-0512-02**	881.10		EE
500 mg, 100s ea	**16714-0513-01**	324.97		EE
500s ea	**16714-0513-02**	1615.81		EE
(Sandoz)				
TCP, PO (USP)				
125 mg, 100s ea	**00781-1217-01**	89.72		AB
250 mg, 100s ea	**00781-1218-01**	176.23		AB
500s ea	**00781-1218-05**	881.15		AB
500 mg, 100s ea	**00781-1219-01**	324.97		AB
500s ea	**00781-1219-05**	1624.86		AB
(Teva)				
TCP, PO (USP,FILM COATED)				
125 mg, 100s ea	**00093-7439-01**	89.72		AB
250 mg, 100s ea	**00093-7440-01**	176.23		AB
500s ea	**00093-7440-05**	881.11		AB
500 mg, 100s ea	**00093-7441-01**	324.97		AB
500s ea	**00093-7441-05**	1624.82		AB
TER, PO (FILM COATED)				
500 mg, 100s ea	**00093-7340-01**	295.72		AB
500s ea	**00093-7340-05**	1478.59		AB
(UDL)				
TCP, PO (10X10,USP,FILM-COATED)				
250 mg, 100s ea UD	**51079-0474-20**	196.06		AB
(10X8,FILM-COATED)				
500 mg, 80s ea UD	**51079-0475-08**	288.08		AB
TER, PO, 250 mg, 80s ea UD	**51079-0766-08**	134.33		EE
(8X10,FILM-COATED)				
500 mg, 80s ea UD	**51079-0767-08**	236.29		EE
(30X10 PUNCH CARDS)				
500 mg, 300s ea UD	**51079-0767-56**	886.08		EE
(Upsher-Smith)				
TCP, PO (10X10,USP)				
125 mg, 100s ea UD	**00245-0180-01**	94.50		AB
(USP)				
125 mg, 100s ea	**00245-0180-11**	88.16		AB
500s ea	**00245-0180-15**	440.80		AB
(10X10,USP)				
250 mg, 100s ea UD	**00245-0181-01**	183.98		AB
(USP)				
250 mg, 100s ea	**00245-0181-11**	173.16		AB
500s ea	**00245-0181-15**	865.82		AB
(10X10,USP)				
500 mg, 100s ea UD	**00245-0182-01**	337.83		AB

PROD/MFR	NDC	AWP	DP	OBC
(USP)				
500 mg, 100s ea	**00245-0182-11**	319.32		AB
500s ea	**00245-0182-15**	1596.59		AB
(Wockhardt USA)				
TCP, PO (USP)				
125 mg, 100s ea	**64679-0973-01**	89.72		AB
250 mg, 100s ea	**64679-0974-01**	176.23		AB
500s ea	**64679-0974-02**	881.11		AB
500 mg, 100s ea	**64679-0975-01**	324.97		AB
500s ea	**64679-0975-02**	1624.82		AB
TER, PO (FILM-COATED)				
250 mg, 30s ea	**64679-0724-01**	53.09		AB
100s ea	**64679-0724-02**	168.11		AB
500s ea	**64679-0724-03**	798.52		AB
(FILM COATED)				
500 mg, 30s ea	**64679-0725-01**	88.71		AB
100s ea	**64679-0725-02**	295.70		AB
500s ea	**64679-0725-03**	1478.51		AB
(Zydus Pharm.)				
ECC, PO (SPRINKLE,HARD GELATIN)				
125 mg, 100s ea	**68382-0106-01**	89.61		AB
1000s ea	**68382-0106-10**	896.10		AB
(A-S Medication)				
REPACK				
TCP, PO, 250 mg, 30s ea	**54569-6114-00**	52.87		AB
(American Health)				
REPACK				
ECC, PO (10X10, SPRINKLE)				
125 mg, 100s ea UD	**68084-0313-01**	79.36		AB
TCP, PO, 250 mg,				
100s ea UD	**68084-0314-01**	27.50		AB
500 mg, 100s ea UD	**68084-0315-01**	85.00		AB
TER, PO (FILM-COATED)				
250 mg, 100s ea UD	**68084-0316-01**	52.50		AB
(FILM COATED)				
500 mg, 100s ea UD	**68084-0317-01**	61.25		AB
(Nucare Pharm)				
REPACK				
TCP, PO (ENTERIC-COATED)				
250 mg, 30s ea	**68071-0775-30**	58.47		
500 mg, 30s ea	**68071-0776-30**	82.00		AB
(Palmetto)				
REPACK				
TCP, PO, 250 mg, 30s ea	**23490-7663-01**	56.47		
(Phys Total Care)				
REPACK				
TCP, PO, 500 mg, 30s ea	**54868-6072-00**	23.13		AB
TER, PO (FILM-COATED)				
500 mg, 10s ea	**54868-6088-00**	25.51		AB
60s ea	**54868-6088-01**	95.53		AB
(Physician Partner)				
REPACK				
TCP, PO, 250 mg, 60s ea	**21695-0818-60**	211.48		AB
500 mg, 60s ea	**21695-0819-60**	389.97		AB
90s ea	**21695-0819-90**	584.95		AB
(Quality Care Prod)				
REPACK				
TCP, PO (DELAYED RELEASE,COATED)				
125 mg, 30s ea	**35356-0386-30**	36.70		AB
(Stat Rx)				
REPACK				
TCP, PO (DELAYED RELEASE,COATED)				
250 mg, 30s ea	**16590-0809-30**	52.69		AB
60s ea	**16590-0809-60**	105.74		AB
90s ea	**16590-0809-90**	158.40		AB
500 mg, 30s ea	**16590-0648-30**	80.00		AB
60s ea	**16590-0648-60**	160.00		AB
90s ea	**16590-0648-90**	240.00		AB
DIVIGEL (Upsher-Smith)				
estradiol				
GEL, TD, 0.25 mg/packet,				
30s ea	**00245-0880-30**	82.24		
0.5 mg/packet,				
30s ea	**00245-0881-30**	82.24		
1 mg/packet,				
1 gm 30s	**00245-0882-30**	82.24		
(Phys Total Care)				
REPACK				
GEL, TD, 1 mg/packet,				
1 ml 30s	**54868-6056-00**	96.17		
DIVISTA (U.S. Pharm)				
multivitamin, minerals, and nutriceuticals				
SGL, PO (SOFTGEL)				
60s ea	**52747-0110-60**	61.50		

PROD/MFR | NDC | AWP | DP | OBC

DL-ALANINE (Amend)
alanine
POW, NA (C.P.)
100 gm............. **17317-0723-03** 21.00
1000 gm............ **17317-0723-06** 84.00

(Spectrum Pharmacy)
POW, NA (F.C.C.)
100 gm............. **49452-0217-01** 140.70
1000 gm............ **49452-0217-02** 598.50

DL-CARNITINE HYDROCHLORIDE (Spectrum Pharmacy)
levocarnitine hydrochloride
CRY, NA (1X25GM)
25 gm.............. **49452-1780-03** 101.15
(1X100GM)
100 gm............. **49452-1780-01** 249.55

DL-LACTIC ACID (Baker, J.T.)
lactic acid
LIQ, NA (U.S.P., F.C.C.)
100 ml **10106-0196-04** 11.91
500 ml **10106-0196-01** 17.66

DL-MALIC ACID (Spectrum Pharmacy)
malic acid
POW, NA (F.C.C.)
500 gm............. **49452-4320-01** 95.55
2500 gm............ **49452-4320-02** 249.55

DL-MENTHOL (Spectrum Pharmacy)
menthol
CRY, NA (U.S.P./N.F.)
25 gm.............. **49452-4430-01** 82.95
125 gm............. **49452-4430-02** 199.15
500 gm............. **49452-4430-03** 497.00

DL-METHIONINE (Amend)
methionine
POW, NA (F.C.C.)
125 gm............. **17317-0361-04** 8.40
500 gm............. **17317-0361-01** 14.00
2500 gm............ **17317-0361-05** 50.40

(Spectrum Pharmacy)
POW, NA (F.C.C.)
500 gm............. **49452-4580-01** 169.75
2500 gm............ **49452-4580-02** 612.50

DL-PANTHENOL (Spectrum Pharmacy)
dexpanthenol
POW, NA (U.S.P.)
25 gm.............. **49452-4977-01** 74.90
100 gm............. **49452-4977-02** 164.85

DL-PHENYLALANINE (Gallipot)
phenylalanine
POW, NA (U.S.P.)
25 gm.............. **51552-0155-04** 17.85
100 gm............. **51552-0155-05** 45.92

(Spectrum Pharmacy)
CRY, NA (F.C.C.)
25 gm.............. **49452-5272-01** 75.60
100 gm............. **49452-5272-02** 184.80
1000 gm............ **49452-5272-03** 1060.50

DL-SERINE (Spectrum Pharmacy)
serine, dl-
CRY, NA (1X100GM)
100 gm............. **49452-6503-02** 156.10
(1X1000GM)
1000 gm............ **49452-6503-03** 945.00

DM TAN/DEXCHLORPHENIRAMINE TAN/ PHENYLEPH TAN
(Laser Pharma) *See DONATUSSIN DM*

DM TAN/DEXCHLORPHENIRAMINE TAN/PSE TAN
(Cypress Pharm) *See BROMATAN PLUS*
(Cypress Pharm) *See SUTAN-DM*
(Health Care Products) *See TANAFED DMX*

DM TAN/DIPHENHYDRAMINE TANNATE/ PHENYLEPH TAN
(Hawthorn Pharm) *See DYTAN-DM*

DM TAN/PHENYLEPH TAN/PYRIL TAN
(Vertical) *See ZOTEX-12*

DM-PE-CHLOR (Laser Pharma)
cpm/dm/phenyleph hcl
SOL, PO (W/CALIBRATED DROPPER,AF)
30 ml.............. **68134-0103-30** 20.63

DM/CHLORPHENIRAMINE MALEATE/PHENYLEPH (Acella)
cpm/dm/phenyleph hcl
SOL, PO (1X30ML,AF,SF)
30 ml.............. **42192-0508-30** 19.58
(1X30ML,AF,SF,BUBBLEGUM)
30 ml.............. **42192-0509-30** 20.11

DM/DEXBROMPHENIRAMINE MALEATE/GG/PHENYLEPH HCL
(Seyer Pharmatec) *See PANATUSS DXP*
(Seyer Pharmatec) *See PANATUSS DXP PEDIATRIC*

DM/DEXBROMPHENIRAMINE MALEATE/ PHENYLEPH HCL
(Breckenridge Pharm) *See DEXALL*
(Everett) *See TUSSALL*
(Everett) *See TUSSALL-ER*
(Larken Labs, Inc.) *See Y-COF DM*

DM/DEXCHLORPHENIRAMINE MAL/PHENYLEPH HCL/PYRIL MAL
(Cypress Pharm) *See RESPERAL*
(Larken Labs, Inc.) *See CORYZA-DM*

DM/GG/NA CIT
(PGD, Inc.) *See GENEXPECT-DM*

DM/GG/NA CIT/PYRIL MAL
(PGD, Inc.) *See GENEXPECT-SF*

DM/GG/PHENYLEPH HCL
(Boca Pharmacal) *See PDM GG*
(Breckenridge Pharm) *See DYNATUSS EX SYRUP*
(Capellon) *See CERTUSS-D*
(Cypress Pharm) *See ANEXTUSS*
(Cypress Pharm) *See DACEX-DM*
(Cypress Pharm) *See PHLEMEX*
(Cypress Pharm) *See PHLEMEX-PE*
(Dexo) *See SINUTUSS DM*
(Everett) *See TRITUSS*
(Everett) *See TRITUSS-ER*
(Everett) *See TUSSAFED-EX*
(Everett) *See TUSSAFED-EX PEDIATRIC*
(Everett) *See TUSSO-DM*
(Everett) *See TUSSO-DMR*
(Everett) *See TUSSO-XR*
(Gil Pharmaceutical) *See BIOTUSS*
(Gil Pharmaceutical) *See BIOTUSS PEDIATRIC*
(Gil Pharmaceutical) *See GILTUSS*
(Gil Pharmaceutical) *See GILTUSS PEDIATRIC*
(Gil Pharmaceutical) *See GILTUSS TR*
(Kramer-Novis) *See TUSSI-PRES*
(Kramer-Novis) *See TUSSI-PRES PEDIATRIC*
(MAGNA Pharm) *See Z-TUSS DM*
(PGD, Inc.) *See GENANTUSS*
(PGD, Inc.) *See GENETUSS-2*
(Vertical) *See ZOTEX-EX*

DM/GG/PHENYLEPH HYDROCHLORIDE (Pharma Pac)
REPACK
dm/gg/phenyleph hcl
SOL, PO, 118 ml.......... **52959-0883-04** 3.55

DM/GG/PSE HCL
(Acella) *See BP 8 COUGH*
(Boca Pharmacal) *See PSEUDO COUGH*
(Boca Pharmacal) *See PSEUDO DM GG*
(Breckenridge Pharm) *See LIQUICOUGH DM*
(Carwin) *See RU-TUSS DM*
(Cypress Pharm) *See GFN 600/PSE 60/DM 30*
(Ethex) *See PSEUDOVENT DM*
(Everett) *See TUSSAFED-LA*
(Larken Labs, Inc.) *See EXECLEAR-DM*
(Larken Labs, Inc.) *See SUDATEX-DM*
(Laser Pharma) *See DONATUSSIN DM*
(Llorens Pharma Int) *See TUSNEL PEDIATRIC*
(MCR American) *See AMBI 40PSE/400GFN/20DM*
(MCR American) *See AMBI 60PSE/400GFN/20DM*
(PGD, Inc.) *See GENEBRONCO-D*
(PGD, Inc.) *See GENEXPECT-PE*
(Seyer Pharmatec) *See BRONCOTRON-D*
(SJ) *See MEDENT DM*
(Zyber) *See Z-COF 8DM*

DM/K GUAI
(Blansett) *See PROLEX DM*
(Breckenridge Pharm) *See GUIADEX DM*

DM/PHENYLEPH HCL/PYRIL MAL
(Breckenridge Pharm) *See TRIPLEX DM*
(Cornerstone) *See DECONSAL DM*
(Larken Labs, Inc.) *See MYHIST-DM*
(Macoven) *See PYRIL DM*
(Poly) *See POLY HIST DM*
(Zyber) *See ALDEX DM*

DM/PROMETHAZINE HCL
(Actavis Mid Atlantic) *See DEXTROMETHORPHAN/PROMETHAZINE*
(Hi-Tech) *See DEXTROMETHORPHAN/PROMETHAZINE*
(Morton Grove) *See DEXTROMETHORPHAN/ PROMETHAZINE*
(Qualitest) *See PROMETHAZINE DM*

DM/PROMETHAZINE HYDROCHLORIDE (Palmetto)
REPACK
dm/promethazine hcl
SYR, PO (1X120ML)
15 mg/5 ml-6.25 mg/5 ml,
120 ml **23490-6178-01** 10.40
(1X180ML)
15 mg/5 ml-6.25 mg/5 ml,
180 ml **23490-6178-02** 15.60

DM/PSE HCL
(Intl Ethical) *See TUSS-DA*

DMDM HYDANTOIN (PCCA)
POW, NA, 1 gm.......... **51927-3344-00** 0.36

DOAK TAR DISTILLATE (Doak)
coal tar
LIQ, TP, 40%, 60 ml....... **10337-0410-21** 37.57

DOBUTAMINE (Hospira)
dobutamine hydrochloride
SOL, IV (10X20ML,FTV)
12.5 mg/ml,
20 ml 10s.......... **00409-2344-02** 35.88 31.40 **AP**
(10X20ML)
12.5 mg/ml,
20 ml 10s.......... **00409-2025-20** 36.60 32.00 **AP**

(Phys Total Care)
REPACK
SOL, IV, 12.5 mg/ml,
20 ml.............. **54868-5717-00** 20.88
(10X40ML)
12.5 mg/ml,
40 ml 10s.......... **54868-5717-01** 192.78
200 ml **54868-5717-02** 111.83

DOBUTAMINE HCL (Bedford)
dobutamine hydrochloride
SOL, IV (S.D.V.,PF)
12.5 mg/ml,
20 ml 10s.......... **55390-0560-90** 42.00 **AP**

(Hospira)
SOL, IV (VIAL,FLIPTOP)
12.5 mg/ml, 20 ml.... **00409-2344-01** 3.92 3.43 **AP**
(10X40ML)
12.5 mg/ml,
40 ml 10s.......... **00409-2025-54** 74.16 64.90 **AP**
(VIAL)
12.5 mg/ml, 100 ml... **00074-4729-01** 15.60 13.65 **AP**

(PCCA)
POW, NA (U.S.P.)
1 gm............... **51927-2775-00** 225.00

DOBUTAMINE HYDROCHLORIDE
(Bedford) *See DOBUTAMINE HCL*
(Hospira) *See DOBUTAMINE*
(Hospira) *See DOBUTAMINE HCL*
(Hospira) *See DOBUTAMINE NOVAPLUS*
(PCCA) *See DOBUTAMINE HCL*

DOBUTAMINE IN DEXTROSE (Hospira)
dextrose/dobutamine hydrochloride
SOL, IV (12X250ML,LATEX-FREE)
5%-100 mg/100 ml,
250 ml 12s......... **00409-2346-32** 122.69 107.40 **AP**
(12X500ML,LIFECARE)
5%-100 mg/100 ml,
500 ml 12s .... **00409-2346-34** 240.62 210.60 **AP**

PROD/MFR | NDC | AWP | DP | OBC

DOBUTAMINE NOVAPLUS (Hospira)
dobutamine hydrochloride
SOL, IV (S.D.V., U.S.P.)
12.5 mg/ml,
20 ml 10s.......... 00409-2344-88 32.76 28.70 AP

DOCETAXEL
(Sanofi-Aventis) *See TAXOTERE*

DOCOSAVIT (River's Edge)
prenatal vitamins
SGL, PO, 90s ea 68032-0280-90 80.91

DOCUSATE (Keltman Pharma., Inc.)
REPACK
docusate sodium
SGL, PO (SOFTGEL)
100 mg, 30s ea 68387-0154-30 14.75

DOCUSATE CALCIUM (DHS, Inc.)
REPACK
SGL, PO, 240 mg, 30s ea .. 55887-0964-30 10.50

(Southwood)
REPACK
SGL, PO, 240 mg, 30s ea .. 00490-0078-30 3.20
60s ea............ 00490-0078-60 6.39
90s ea............ 00490-0078-90 9.59
100s ea............ 00490-0078-00 10.65

DOCUSATE SODIUM (Gallipot)
POW, NA, 100 gm......... 51552-0267-05 38.50
454 gm............ 51552-0267-06 118.72

(Letco)
POW, NA (U.S.P., 23)
25 gm.............. 62991-1537-01 27.00

(Medisca)
POW, NA (U.S.P.)
25 gm.............. 38779-1254-04 31.50
100 gm.............. 38779-1254-05 70.50
500 gm.............. 38779-1254-08 207.00

(PCCA)
POW, NA (U.S.P.; WAX-LIKE)
1 gm.............. 51927-1379-00 1.80

(Spectrum Pharmacy)
POW, NA, 125 gm......... 49452-2665-01 106.40
(U.S.P., WAX-LIKE)
125 gm.............. 49452-2650-04 136.15
500 gm.............. 49452-2665-02 322.00
(U.S.P., WAX-LIKE)
500 gm.............. 49452-2650-02 416.50
2500 gm.............. 49452-2665-03 1123.50
(U.S.P., WAX-LIKE)
2500 gm.............. 49452-2650-03 1610.00

(A-S Medication)
REPACK
SGL, PO, 250 mg, 60s ea .. 54569-5990-00 3.94

(Bryant Ranch)
REPACK
SGL, PO, 100 mg, 30s ea .. 63629-1360-01 7.95
60s ea............ 63629-1360-03 9.89
100s ea............ 63629-1360-02 17.16
120s ea............ 63629-1360-04 17.03
250 mg, 30s ea 63629-3213-01 6.99
60s ea............ 63629-3213-02 13.89
SYR, PO, 60 mg/15 ml,
120 ml 63629-1807-02 1.53
240 ml 63629-1807-01 3.07

(Core)
REPACK
SGL, PO, 100 mg, 20s ea .. 33358-0113-20 6.13
30s ea............ 33358-0113-30 8.15
60s ea............ 33358-0113-60 10.14
90s ea............ 33358-0113-90 14.91
100s ea............ 33358-0113-00 17.59
120s ea............ 33358-0113-01 19.51
250 mg, 30s ea 33358-0114-30 7.16
60s ea............ 33358-0114-60 14.24

(IPI)
REPACK
SGL, PO, 100 mg, 30s ea .. 18837-0247-30 7.98
120s ea............ 18837-0247-98 2.95

(Palmetto)
REPACK
SGL, PO, 100 mg, 6s ea ... 23490-6654-01 3.30
60s ea............ 23490-6654-06 33.00

DOCUSATE SODIUM 85% SODIUM BENZOATE 15%
(PCCA)
docusate sodium/sodium benzoate
POW, NA (USP)
1 gm.............. 51927-2809-00 0.75

DOCUSATE SODIUM/FERROUS FUMARATE/ FOLIC ACID
(Edwards) *See ED CYTE F*

DOCUSATE SODIUM/SODIUM BENZOATE
(PCCA) *See DOCUSATE SODIUM 85% SODIUM BENZOATE 15%*

DODECYLBENZENE SODIUM SULFONATE (PCCA)
POW, NA, 1 gm.......... 51927-2195-00 0.87

DODECYLBENZYLTRIMETHYLAMMONIUM CHLORIDE
(PCCA) *See DODECYLBENZYLTRIMONIUM CHLORIDE*

DODECYLBENZYLTRIMONIUM CHLORIDE (PCCA)
dodecylbenzyltrimethylammonium chloride
SOL, NA (1X1ML)
1 ml.............. 51927-3249-00 10.95

DOFETILIDE
(Pfizer) *See TIKOSYN*

DOLASETRON MESYLATE
(Sanofi-Aventis) *See ANZEMET*

DOLGIC LQ (Athlon Pharm)
acetaminophen/butalbital/caffeine
SOL, PO, 473 ml.......... 66813-0073-16 69.14

DOLGIC PLUS (Victory Pharma, Inc.)
acetaminophen/butalbital/caffeine
TAB, PO (USP)
750 mg-50 mg-40 mg,
100s ea............ 68453-0074-10 363.65

(Stat Rx)
REPACK
TAB, PO, 750 mg-50 mg-40 mg,
60s ea............ 16590-0772-60 280.98

DOLOBID (Altura)
REPACK
diflunisal
TAB, PO, 500 mg, 10s ea .. 63874-0307-10 13.74 AB
20s ea............ 63874-0307-20 27.04 AB
60s ea............ 63874-0307-60 74.91 AB
100s ea............ 63874-0307-01 122.72 AB

DOLOGESIC (Llorens Pharma Int)
acetaminophen/phenyltoloxamine
SOL, PO, 500 mg-30 mg,
180 ml 54859-0512-06 10.35
TAB, PO (CAPLET)
500 mg-30 mg,
50s ea............ 54859-0101-50 9.00

DOLOPHINE HCL (Roxane)
methadone hydrochloride
TAB, PO, 5 mg,
100s ea, C-II .... 00054-4218-25 12.99 AA
10 mg,
100s ea, C-II .... 00054-4219-25 21.10 AA

DOLOREX (A. G. Marin)
acetaminophen/phenyltoloxamine citrate
TAB, PO, 500 mg-50 mg,
100s ea............ 12539-0590-10 36.67

DOLOREX FORTE (A. G. Marin)
acetaminophen/hydrocodone bitartrate
CAP, PO, 500 mg-5 mg,
100s ea, C-III ...... 12539-0984-01 70.20 AA

DOMPERIDONE (Gallipot)
POW, NA (1X1GM,BP)
1 gm.............. 51552-0959-01 31.50 22.50
(1X5GM,BP)
5 gm.............. 51552-0959-02 90.30 64.50
(1X25GM,BP)
25 gm.............. 51552-0959-04 385.00 275.00
(1X500GM,BP)
500 gm.............. 51552-0959-06 6916.00 4940.00

(PCCA)
POW, NA (BP)
1 gm.............. 51927-3529-00 51.60

DONATUSSIN (Laser Pharma)
guaifenesin/phenylephrine hydrochloride
SOL, PO (W/DROPPER,AF,SF)
20 mg/ml-1.5 mg/ml,
30 ml.............. 16477-0106-30 35.25

(Laser Pharma)
cpm/dm/gg/phenyleph hcl
SYR, PO, 473 ml.......... 00277-0185-41 35.00

DONATUSSIN DC (Laser Pharma)
gg/hydrocod bit/phenyleph hcl
SYR, PO (AF,CHERRY)
473 ml, C-III 16477-0956-01 56.16

DONATUSSIN DM (Laser Pharma)
cpm/dm/phenyleph hcl
SOL, PO (W/DROPPER,AF,SF)
30 ml.............. 16477-0811-30 22.60

(Laser Pharma)
dm tan/dexchlorpheniramine tan/phenyleph tan
SUS, PO (AF,SF)
473 ml 16477-0130-01 85.00

(Laser Pharma)
dm/gg/pse hcl
SYR, PO (1X473ML,AF,SF,COOL-MINT)
473 ml 16477-0132-01 59.00

DONEPEZIL HYDROCHLORIDE
(Eisai) *See ARICEPT*
(Eisai) *See ARICEPT ODT*

DONNATAL (PBM Pharmaceuticals)
atropine sulf/hyoscyamine sulf/pb/scop hydrobrom
ELI, PO (GRAPE)
118 ml 66213-0423-04 27.41
473 ml 66213-0423-16 92.14
TAB, PO, 100s ea 66213-0425-10 56.15
1000s ea 66213-0425-11 517.31

(Phys Total Care)
REPACK
TAB, PO, 20s ea 54868-1237-00 14.66
30s ea............ 54868-1237-02 20.69
100s ea............ 54868-1237-01 55.12

DONNATAL EXTENTABS (PBM Pharmaceuticals)
atropine sulf/hyoscyamine sulf/pb/scop hydrobrom
TER, PO, 100s ea 66213-0421-10 157.34
500s ea............ 66213-0421-50 765.77

DOPAMINE HCL (Amer Regent)
dopamine hydrochloride
SOL, IV (S.D.V.)
40 mg/ml, 5 ml 25s... 00517-1805-25 54.69 AP
80 mg/ml, 5 ml 25s... 00517-1905-25 102.19 AP
160 mg/ml,
5 ml 25s............ 00517-1305-25 203.44 AP

(Consolidated Midland)
SOL, IV (AMP, DOSETTE)
40 mg/ml, 5 ml 25s... 00223-7484-05 81.25 EE
(S.D.V.)
40 mg/ml, 5 ml 25s... 00223-7485-05 142.00 EE
(AMP, DOSETTE)
80 mg/ml, 5 ml 25s... 00223-7486-05 172.00 EE
(S.D.V.)
80 mg/ml, 5 ml 25s... 00223-7487-05 181.25 EE

(Hospira)
SOL, IV (FLIPTOP)
40 mg/ml, 5 ml 25s... 00409-5820-01 18.90 16.50 AP
(25X10ML)
40 mg/ml,
10 ml 25s.......... 00409-9104-20 23.40 20.50 AP
80 mg/ml,
10 ml 25s.......... 00409-4265-01 34.80 30.50 AP

(PCCA)
POW, NA, 1 gm.......... 51927-2319-00 13.80

DOPAMINE HYDROCHLORIDE
(Amer Regent) *See DOPAMINE HCL*
(Consolidated Midland) *See DOPAMINE HCL*
(Hospira) *See DOPAMINE HCL*
(PCCA) *See DOPAMINE HCL*

(Phys Total Care)
REPACK
SOL, IV, 80 mg/ml, 125 ml. 54868-0015-00 82.32

DOPRAM (Baxter)
doxapram hydrochloride
SOL, IV (M.D.V.)
20 mg/ml, 20 ml ..... 60977-0144-63 50.40 AP
20 ml 6s............ 60977-0144-02 302.40 77.90 AP

DORAL (Questcor Pharm)
quazepam
TAB, PO (USP)
15 mg,
100s ea, C-IV 63004-7734-01 460.37

(Phys Total Care)
REPACK
TAB, PO, 15 mg,
30s ea, C-IV......... 54868-2826-01 76.61

DORIBAX (Ortho-McNeil Pharm)
doripenem
PDR, IV, 500 mg, 10s ea... 50458-0401-02 459.96 383.30

DORIPENEM
(Ortho-McNeil Pharm) *See DORIBAX*

DORNASE ALFA
(Genentech) *See PULMOZYME*

DORYX (Warner Chilcott)
doxycycline hyclate
TCP, PO, 75 mg, 60s ea ... 00430-0111-20 501.93
100 mg, 100s ea 00430-0112-24 984.27
150 mg, 60s ea 00430-0113-20 1002.93

PROD/MFR	NDC	AWP	DP	OBC
DORZOLAMIDE HYDROCHLORIDE (Apotex Corp.)				
SOL, OP (1X10ML)				
2%, 10 ml	**60505-0567-01**	66.82		**AT**
(Falcon Ophthalmics)				
SOL, OP (1X10ML)				
2%, 10 ml	**61314-0019-10**	57.00		**AT**
(Hi-Tech)				
SOL, OP (1X10ML)				
2%, 10 ml	**50383-0232-10**	66.80		**AT**
(Merck) *See TRUSOPT OCUMETER PLUS*				
(Prasco Labs)				
SOL, OP (1X10ML,OCUMETER PLUS)				
2%, 10 ml	**66993-0175-20**	66.75		
(Sandoz)				
SOL, OP (1X10ML)				
2%, 10 ml	**00781-6053-70**	66.75		**AT**
(Teva)				
SOL, OP (1X10ML)				
2%, 10 ml	**00093-7618-43**	68.58		**AT**
DORZOLAMIDE HYDROCHLORIDE - TIMOLOL MALEATE (Hi-Tech)				
dorzolamide hydrochloride/timolol maleate				
SOL, OP (1X10ML)				
22.3 mg/ml-6.8 mg/ml, 10 ml..............	**50383-0233-10**	122.60		
(Phys Total Care)				
REPACK				
SOL, OP (1X10ML)				
22.3 mg/ml-6.8 mg/ml, 10 ml..............	**54868-5982-00**	228.97		
DORZOLAMIDE HYDROCHLORIDE AND TIMOLOL MALEATE (Falcon Ophthalmics)				
dorzolamide hydrochloride/timolol maleate				
SOL, OP (1X10ML)				
22.3 mg/ml-6.8 mg/ml, 10 ml..............	**61314-0030-02**	60.00		**AT**
DORZOLAMIDE HYDROCHLORIDE-TIMOLOL MALEATE (Prasco Labs)				
dorzolamide hydrochloride/timolol maleate				
SOL, OP (1X10ML,OCUMETER PLUS)				
22.3 mg/ml-6.8 mg/ml, 10 ml..............	**66993-0190-20**	122.49		
DORZOLAMIDE HYDROCHLORIDE/TIMOLOL MALEATE (Apotex Corp.)				
SOL, OP (1X10ML)				
22.3 mg/ml-6.8 mg/ml, 10 ml..............	**60505-0568-02**	122.62		**AT**
(Falcon Ophthalmics) *See DORZOLAMIDE HYDROCHLORIDE AND TIMOLOL MALEATE*				
(Hi-Tech) *See DORZOLAMIDE HYDROCHLORIDE - IMOLOL MALEATE*				
(Merck) *See COSOPT OCUMETER PLUS*				
(Prasco Labs) *See DORZOLAMIDE HYDROCHLORIDE-TIMOLOL MALEATE*				
(Sandoz)				
SOL, OP (1X10ML)				
22.3 mg/ml-6.8 mg/ml, 10 ml..............	**00781-6054-70**	122.49		**AT**
DOUBLE-NEEDLE TRANSFER DEVICE (Abbott Hosp)				
transfer unit, iv fluid				
DEV, NA (20G)				
400s ea..............	**00074-4797-02**	163.20	164.00	
DOVONEX (Warner Chilcott)				
calcipotriene				
CRE, TP, 0.005%, 60 gm...	**00430-3020-15**	264.35		
120 gm..........	**00430-3020-17**	528.72		
SOL, TP, 0.005%, 60 ml ...	**00430-3030-15**	264.35		
(Phys Total Care)				
REPACK				
CRE, TP, 0.005%, 60 gm...	**54868-4725-00**	242.67		
OIN, TP, 0.005%, 60 gm...	**54868-3240-02**	182.39		
120 gm..........	**54868-3240-00**	334.50		
SOL, TP (1X60ML)				
0.005%, 60 ml	**54868-6057-00**	302.37		
(Quality Care Prod)				
REPACK				
CRE, TP (1X120GM)				
0.005%, 120 gm	**35356-0222-01**	968.74		
DOW CORNING 9040 SILICONE ELASTOMER BLEND (PCCA)				
silicone				
GEL, NA (1X1GM)				
1 gm	**51927-3780-00**	0.60		
DOXAPRAM HCL (Bedford)				
doxapram hydrochloride				
SOL, IV (M.D.V.)				
20 mg/ml, 20 ml	**55390-0035-01**	98.43		**AP**

PROD/MFR	NDC	AWP	DP	OBC
(PCCA)				
POW, NA (U.S.P.; MONOHYDRATE)				
1 gm	**51927-3130-00**	117.00		
DOXAPRAM HYDROCHLORIDE				
(Baxter) *See DOPRAM*				
(Bedford) *See DOXAPRAM HCL*				
(PCCA) *See DOXAPRAM HCL*				
DOXAZOSIN (Core)				
REPACK				
doxazosin mesylate				
TAB, PO, 2 mg, 30s ea	**33358-0116-30**	36.17		
(Phys Total Care)				
REPACK				
TAB, PO, 2 mg, 60s ea	**54868-4801-02**	13.47		
90s ea..............	**54868-4801-03**	18.87		
DOXAZOSIN MESYLATE				
FUL				
TAB, PO, 1 mg, 100s ea..............		59.18		
2 mg, 100s ea..............		59.18		
4 mg, 100s ea..............		62.10		
8 mg, 100s ea..............		65.18		
(Apotex Corp.)				
TAB, PO (CAPLET)				
1 mg, 100s ea........	**60505-0093-00**	94.90		**AB**
1000s ea	**60505-0093-01**	833.34		**AB**
2 mg, 100s ea........	**60505-0094-00**	94.90		**AB**
1000s ea	**60505-0094-01**	877.19		**AB**
22500s ea	**60505-0094-08**	19736.78		**AB**
4 mg, 100s ea........	**60505-0095-00**	99.89		**AB**
1000s ea	**60505-0095-01**	920.75		**AB**
11500s ea	**60505-0095-05**	10588.63		
(CAPLET)				
4 mg, 13000s ea	**60505-0095-08**	11969.75		**AB**
8 mg, 100s ea........	**60505-0096-00**	104.70		**AB**
1000s ea	**60505-0096-01**	966.87		**AB**
5000s ea	**60505-0096-08**	4834.35		**AB**
(Major)				
TAB, PO (10X10)				
1 mg, 100s ea UD	**00904-5522-61**	106.97		**AB**
(CAPLET)				
2 mg, 100s ea UD	**00904-5523-61**	108.07		**AB**
4 mg, 100s ea UD	**00904-5524-61**	101.70		**AB**
(Mylan)				
TAB, PO, 1 mg, 100s ea ...	**00378-4021-01**	92.35		**AB**
2 mg, 100s ea........	**00378-4022-01**	92.35		**AB**
4 mg, 100s ea........	**00378-4024-01**	96.95		**AB**
8 mg, 100s ea........	**00378-4028-01**	101.80		**AB**
(Pfizer) *See CARDURA*				
(Pfizer) *See CARDURA XL*				
(Teva)				
TAB, PO, 1 mg, 100s ea ...	**00093-8120-01**	92.44		**AB**
100s ea..........	**00172-3685-60**	91.92		**AB**
2 mg, 100s ea........	**00093-8121-01**	92.44		**AB**
100s ea UD	**00093-8121-93**	92.44		**AB**
100s ea..........	**00172-3686-60**	91.92		**AB**
500s ea..........	**00172-3686-70**	450.43		**AB**
4 mg, 100s ea........	**00093-8122-01**	97.03		**AB**
100s ea..........	**00172-3687-60**	96.49		**AB**
500s ea..........	**00172-3687-70**	472.80		**AB**
8 mg, 100s ea........	**00093-8123-01**	101.90		**AB**
100s ea..........	**00172-3688-60**	101.32		**AB**
500s ea..........	**00172-3688-70**	496.48		**AB**
(UDL)				
TAB, PO (10X10)				
1 mg, 100s ea UD	**51079-0957-20**	92.35		**AB**
2 mg, 100s ea UD	**51079-0958-20**	92.35		**AB**
4 mg, 100s ea UD	**51079-0959-20**	96.95		**AB**
(A-S Medication)				
REPACK				
TAB, PO, 1 mg, 30s ea	**54569-5168-00**	28.47		**EE**
2 mg, 30s ea.........	**54569-5169-00**	28.47		**EE**
4 mg, 30s ea.........	**54569-5170-00**	29.97		**EE**
8 mg, 30s ea.........	**54569-5245-00**	31.54		**EE**
(Bryant Ranch)				
REPACK				
TAB, PO, 4 mg, 100s ea ...	**63629-1355-01**	99.89		
8 mg, 30s ea.........	**63629-1309-01**	31.67		
(DHS, Inc.)				
REPACK				
TAB, PO, 2 mg, 30s ea	**55887-0506-30**	26.05		**AB**
90s ea..........	**55887-0506-90**	72.00		**AB**
4 mg, 30s ea.........	**55887-0507-30**	29.95		**AB**
90s ea..........	**55887-0507-90**	75.00		**AB**

PROD/MFR	NDC	AWP	DP	OBC
(Dispensing Solutions)				
REPACK				
TAB, PO, 1 mg, 30s ea	**55045-3161-08**	27.60		**AB**
100s ea..........	**55045-3161-00**	92.00		**AB**
2 mg, 30s ea.........	**55045-3130-08**	27.60		**AB**
100s ea..........	**55045-3130-00**	92.00		**AB**
(GSMS)				
REPACK				
TAB, PO (CAPLET)				
1 mg, 100s ea........	**60429-0053-01**	8.55	2.85	**AB**
1000s ea	**60429-0053-10**	81.45	27.15	**AB**
2 mg, 100s ea........	**60429-0054-01**	8.25	2.75	**AB**
1000s ea	**60429-0054-10**	78.45	26.15	**AB**
4 mg, 100s ea........	**60429-0055-01**	11.55	3.85	
1000s ea	**60429-0055-10**	111.45	37.15	
(CAPLET)				
8 mg, 100s ea........	**60429-0056-01**	15.15	5.05	**AB**
1000s ea	**60429-0056-10**	147.45	49.15	**AB**
DOXAZOSIN MESYLATE (Palmetto)				
REPACK				
TAB, PO, 4 mg, 30s ea	**23490-5475-03**	34.27		
DOXAZOSIN MESYLATE (Palmetto)				
8 mg, 100s ea........	**23490-5476-01**	119.97		
(PD-Rx Pharm)				
REPACK				
TAB, PO, 2 mg, 90s ea	**55289-0022-90**	40.20		**AB**
(REDI-SCRIPT)				
2 mg, 90s ea.........	**58864-0809-90**	39.56		
4 mg, 30s ea.........	**55289-0600-30**	28.68		**AB**
90s ea..........	**55289-0600-90**	49.00		**AB**
(Phys Total Care)				
REPACK				
TAB, PO (CAPLET)				
1 mg, 30s ea.........	**54868-4895-00**	8.22		**AB**
100s ea..........	**54868-4895-01**	18.96		
2 mg, 30s ea.........	**54868-4801-00**	8.22		**AB**
100s ea..........	**54868-4801-01**	18.96		**AB**
4 mg, 25s ea.........	**54868-4802-03**	8.97		**AB**
30s ea..........	**54868-4802-00**	10.17		**AB**
60s ea..........	**54868-4802-02**	17.31		**AB**
90s ea..........	**54868-4802-04**	24.48		
100s ea..........	**54868-4802-01**	25.35		
(CAPLET)				
8 mg, 30s ea.........	**54868-4767-00**	10.80		**AB**
90s ea..........	**54868-4767-02**	26.40		**AB**
100s ea..........	**54868-4767-01**	27.48		**AB**
(Quality Care Prod)				
REPACK				
TAB, PO, 2 mg, 30s ea	**49999-0206-30**	22.19		
(Southwood)				
REPACK				
TAB, PO, 2 mg, 30s ea	**58016-0997-30**	32.66		**AB**
60s ea..........	**58016-0997-60**	65.31		**AB**
90s ea..........	**58016-0997-90**	97.97		**AB**
100s ea..........	**58016-0997-00**	108.85		**AB**
120s ea..........	**58016-0997-02**	130.62		**AB**
4 mg, 30s ea.........	**58016-0625-30**	34.27		**AB**
60s ea..........	**58016-0625-60**	68.54		**AB**
90s ea..........	**58016-0625-90**	102.82		**AB**
100s ea..........	**58016-0625-00**	114.24		**AB**
120s ea..........	**58016-0625-02**	137.09		**AB**
8 mg, 30s ea.........	**58016-0644-30**	35.99		**AB**
60s ea..........	**58016-0644-60**	71.98		**AB**
90s ea..........	**58016-0644-90**	107.97		**AB**
100s ea..........	**58016-0644-00**	119.97		**AB**
120s ea..........	**58016-0644-02**	143.96		**AB**
(Vibranta)				
REPACK				
TAB, PO, 1 mg, 30s ea	**57866-6310-01**	28.10		**AB**
60s ea..........	**57866-6310-02**	56.54		**AB**
90s ea..........	**57866-6310-03**	84.26		**AB**
120s ea..........	**57866-6310-04**	111.98		**AB**
2 mg, 30s ea.........	**57866-6311-01**	30.72		**AB**
60s ea..........	**57866-6311-02**	56.54		**AB**
90s ea..........	**57866-6311-03**	84.26		**AB**
120s ea..........	**57866-6311-04**	111.98		**AB**
4 mg, 30s ea.........	**57866-6312-01**	31.42		**AB**
60s ea..........	**57866-6312-02**	59.30		**AB**
90s ea..........	**57866-6312-03**	88.40		**AB**
120s ea..........	**57866-6312-04**	117.50		**AB**
8 mg, 30s ea.........	**57866-6619-01**	31.67		**AB**
60s ea..........	**57866-6619-02**	62.20		**AB**
90s ea..........	**57866-6619-03**	92.81		**AB**
120s ea..........	**57866-6619-04**	123.80		**AB**
DOXEPIN (Bryant Ranch)				
REPACK				
doxepin hydrochloride				
CAP, PO, 10 mg, 30s ea ...	**63629-3221-01**	8.70		

PROD/MFR	NDC	AWP	DP	OBC
(Core)				
REPACK				
CAP, PO, 10 mg, 30s ea	**33358-0117-30**	8.92		
60s ea	**33358-0117-60**	26.30		
25 mg, 30s ea	**33358-0118-30**	20.05		
60s ea	**33358-0118-60**	31.43		
50 mg, 30s ea	**33358-0119-30**	21.01		
60s ea	**33358-0119-60**	42.03		
(DHS, Inc.)				
REPACK				
CAP, PO, 10 mg, 30s ea	**55887-0101-30**	10.90		
60s ea	**55887-0101-60**	21.84		
90s ea	**55887-0101-90**	32.70		
100 mg, 30s ea	**55887-0095-30**	29.95		
60s ea	**55887-0095-60**	59.89		
90s ea	**55887-0095-90**	89.85		
(Phys Total Care)				
REPACK				
CAP, PO, 150 mg, 100s ea	**54868-3533-01**	89.14		
(Southwood)				
REPACK				
CAP, PO, 75 mg, 30s ea	**58016-0797-30**	27.60		
60s ea	**58016-0797-60**	55.20		
90s ea	**58016-0797-90**	82.80		
100s ea	**58016-0797-00**	92.00		
(Stat Rx)				
REPACK				
CAP, PO, 50 mg, 30s ea	**16590-0081-30**	20.50		
60s ea	**16590-0081-60**	41.00		
90s ea	**16590-0081-90**	61.50		
120s ea	**16590-0081-72**	82.00		
DOXEPIN HCL (Major)				
doxepin hydrochloride				
CAP, PO (10X10)				
25 mg, 100s ea UD	**00904-1261-61**	36.50		AB
(Medisca)				
POW, NA (U.S.P.)				
5 gm	**38779-0218-03**	43.50		
25 gm	**38779-0218-04**	142.50		
100 gm	**38779-0218-05**	367.50		
(Morton Grove)				
SOL, PO (PEPPERMINT)				
10 mg/ml, 118 ml	**60432-0651-04**	18.25		AA
(Mylan)				
CAP, PO, 10 mg, 100s ea	**00378-1049-01**	31.60		AB
1000s ea	**00378-1049-10**	308.00		AB
25 mg, 100s ea	**00378-3125-01**	41.60		AB
1000s ea	**00378-3125-10**	416.00		AB
50 mg, 100s ea	**00378-4250-01**	55.20		AB
1000s ea	**00378-4250-10**	595.85		AB
75 mg, 100s ea	**00378-5375-01**	91.60		AB
1000s ea	**00378-5375-10**	896.00		AB
100 mg, 100s ea	**00378-6410-01**	99.80		AB
1000s ea	**00378-6410-10**	978.00		AB
(Par)				
CAP, PO, 150 mg, 50s ea	**49884-0222-03**	169.78		AB
100s ea	**49884-0222-01**	332.77		AB
500s ea	**49884-0222-05**	1580.61		AB
(PCCA)				
POW, NA (U.S.P.)				
1 gm	**51927-2227-00**	10.20		
(Silarx)				
SOL, PO (CONCENTRATE,PEPPERMINT)				
10 mg/ml, 120 ml	**54838-0512-40**	23.70		AA
(Spectrum Pharmacy)				
POW, NA (U.S.P.)				
5 gm	**49452-2692-01**	73.50		
25 gm	**49452-2692-02**	245.35		
100 gm	**49452-2692-03**	539.00		
(Teva)				
SOL, PO (BLUEBERRY MINT)				
10 mg/ml, 120 ml	**00093-9612-12**	23.70		AA
(UDL)				
CAP, PO (10X10)				
10 mg, 100s ea UD	**51079-0436-20**	32.45		AB
25 mg, 100s ea UD	**51079-0437-20**	42.85		AB
50 mg, 100s ea UD	**51079-0438-20**	56.86		AB
100 mg, 100s ea UD	**51079-0651-20**	102.79		AB
(A-S Medication)				
REPACK				
CAP, PO, 50 mg, 30s ea	**54569-1696-01**	19.83		EE
(DHS, Inc.)				
REPACK				
CAP, PO, 25 mg, 30s ea	**55887-0356-30**	21.49		AB
60s ea	**55887-0356-60**	42.97		AB
50 mg, 30s ea	**55887-0289-30**	20.98		AB
60s ea	**55887-0289-60**	41.06		AB
(Dispensing Solutions)				
REPACK				
CAP, PO, 10 mg, 30s ea	**55045-1837-08**	8.70		AB
60s ea	**55045-1837-06**	17.40		AB
90s ea	**55045-1837-09**	26.10		AB
100s ea	**55045-1837-01**	29.00		AB
120s ea	**55045-1837-02**	34.80		AB
25 mg, 30s ea	**55045-1884-08**	15.30		AB
30s ea	**66336-0553-30**	17.50		AB
60s ea	**55045-1884-06**	30.60		AB
90s ea	**55045-1884-09**	45.90		AB
100s ea	**55045-1884-01**	51.00		AB
120s ea	**55045-1884-02**	61.20		AB
50 mg, 100s ea	**55045-2084-01**	70.00		AB
(Nucare Pharm)				
REPACK				
CAP, PO, 25 mg, 30s ea	**66267-0084-30**	18.79		AB
50 mg, 30s ea	**66267-0680-30**	24.58		AB
(PD-Rx Pharm)				
REPACK				
CAP, PO, 50 mg, 30s ea	**55289-0018-30**	27.40		AB
100s ea	**55289-0018-01**	60.44		AB
75 mg, 30s ea	**55289-0258-30**	52.36		AB
(Pharma Pac)				
REPACK				
CAP, PO, 10 mg, 10s ea	**52959-0541-10**	5.26		EE
20s ea	**52959-0541-20**	9.99		EE
30s ea	**52959-0537-30**	10.90		EE
30s ea	**52959-0541-30**	13.81		EE
60s ea	**52959-0541-60**	31.20		EE
90s ea	**52959-0537-90**	28.40		EE
50 mg, 30s ea	**52959-0662-30**	21.75		AB
(Phys Total Care)				
REPACK				
CAP, PO, 10 mg, 30s ea	**54868-2317-03**	8.19		EE
60s ea	**54868-2317-02**	13.38		EE
100s ea	**54868-2317-04**	20.31		EE
25 mg, 15s ea	**54868-0062-04**	6.45		EE
30s ea	**54868-0062-02**	9.93		EE
100s ea	**54868-0062-00**	26.07		EE
50 mg, 30s ea	**54868-1964-02**	13.50		EE
100s ea	**54868-1964-03**	34.50		EE
75 mg, 30s ea	**54868-2552-02**	15.72		EE
100s ea	**54868-2552-00**	41.88		EE
100 mg, 30s ea	**54868-2284-06**	18.06		EE
100s ea	**54868-2284-02**	49.68		EE
150 mg, 30s ea	**54868-3533-00**	36.13		AB
(Physician Partner)				
REPACK				
CAP, PO, 10 mg, 30s ea	**21695-0441-30**	21.84		AB
(Quality Care Prod)				
REPACK				
CAP, PO, 25 mg, 30s ea	**35356-0484-30**	21.30		AB
60s ea	**35356-0424-60**	15.40		AB
(Southwood)				
REPACK				
CAP, PO, 10 mg, 30s ea	**58016-0663-30**	9.45		EE
60s ea	**58016-0663-60**	18.90		EE
90s ea	**58016-0663-90**	28.35		EE
100s ea	**58016-0663-00**	31.50		EE
25 mg, 10s ea	**58016-0833-10**	5.05		EE
14s ea	**58016-0833-14**	7.07		EE
15s ea	**58016-0833-15**	7.58		EE
20s ea	**58016-0833-20**	10.10		EE
30s ea	**58016-0833-30**	15.15		EE
32s ea	**58016-0833-21**	10.61		EE
40s ea	**58016-0833-40**	20.20		EE
50s ea	**58016-0833-50**	25.25		EE
50 mg, 10s ea	**58016-0834-10**	7.10		EE
14s ea	**58016-0834-14**	9.94		EE
15s ea	**58016-0834-15**	10.65		EE
20s ea	**58016-0834-20**	14.20		EE
21s ea	**58016-0834-21**	14.91		EE
30s ea	**58016-0834-30**	21.30		EE
40s ea	**58016-0834-40**	28.40		EE
50s ea	**58016-0834-50**	35.50		EE
60s ea	**58016-0834-60**	42.60		EE
90s ea	**58016-0834-90**	63.90		EE
100s ea	**58016-0834-00**	71,00		EE
(Stat Rx)				
REPACK				
CAP, PO, 10 mg, 30s ea	**16590-0631-30**	10.15		AB
60s ea	**16590-0631-60**	20.30		AB
25 mg, 30s ea	**16590-0567-30**	38.50		AB
60s ea	**16590-0567-60**	70.00		AB
90s ea	**16590-0567-90**	89.75		AB
50 mg, 28s ea	**16590-0081-28**	20.85		AB
75 mg, 30s ea	**16590-0485-30**	27.50		AB
60s ea	**16590-0485-60**	53.86		AB
100 mg, 30s ea	**16590-0764-30**	7.98		AB
150 mg, 30s ea	**16590-0820-30**	99.83		AB
(Vibranta)				
REPACK				
CAP, PO, 25 mg, 30s ea	**57866-4564-01**	13.46		AB
50 mg, 30s ea	**57866-4565-01**	17.29		
60s ea	**57866-4565-02**	36.50		
90s ea	**57866-4565-03**	54.20		
120s ea	**57866-4565-04**	71.90		
100 mg, 30s ea	**57866-4566-01**	41.00		AB
DOXEPIN HYDROCHLORIDE				
FUL				
CAP, PO, 10 mg, 100s ea		8.91		
25 mg, 100s ea		18.22		
50 mg, 100s ea		14.47		
75 mg, 100s ea		20.52		
100 mg, 100s ea		41.74		
SOL, PO, 10 mg/ml, 120 ml		13.74		
(Doak) *See ZONALON*				
(Gallipot)				
POW, NA (1X5GM,USP)				
5 gm	**51552-0982-04**	21.28	15.20	
(1X100GM,USP)				
100 gm	**51552-0982-05**	231.00	165.00	
(Healthpoint) *See PRUDOXIN*				
(Major) *See DOXEPIN HCL*				
(Medisca) *See DOXEPIN HCL*				
(Morton Grove) *See DOXEPIN HCL*				
(Mylan) *See DOXEPIN HCL*				
(Par) *See DOXEPIN HCL*				
(PCCA) *See DOXEPIN HCL*				
(Silarx) *See DOXEPIN HCL*				
(Spectrum Pharmacy) *See DOXEPIN HCL*				
(Teva) *See DOXEPIN HCL*				
(UDL) *See DOXEPIN HCL*				
(Altura)				
REPACK				
CAP, PO, 25 mg, 10s ea	**63874-0579-10**	5.05		
12s ea	**63874-0579-12**	6.06		
14s ea	**63874-0579-14**	7.07		
15s ea	**63874-0579-15**	7.58		
20s ea	**63874-0579-20**	10.10		
28s ea	**63874-0579-28**	14.14		
30s ea	**63874-0579-30**	15.15		
32s ea	**63874-0579-32**	16.16		
40s ea	**63874-0579-40**	20.20		
50s ea	**63874-0579-50**	25.25		
60s ea	**63874-0579-60**	30.30		
90s ea	**63874-0579-90**	45.45		
100s ea	**63874-0579-01**	50.50		
120s ea	**63874-0579-04**	60.60		
50 mg, 10s ea	**63874-0638-10**	7.10		
14s ea	**63874-0638-14**	9.94		
15s ea	**63874-0638-15**	10.65		
20s ea	**63874-0638-20**	14.20		
21s ea	**63874-0638-21**	14.91		
28s ea	**63874-0638-28**	19.88		
30s ea	**63874-0638-30**	21.30		
40s ea	**63874-0638-40**	28.40		
50s ea	**63874-0638-50**	35.50		
60s ea	**63874-0638-60**	42.60		
90s ea	**63874-0638-90**	63.90		
100s ea	**63874-0638-01**	71.00		
120s ea	**63874-0638-04**	85.20		
(Dispensing Solutions)				
REPACK				
CAP, PO, 50 mg, 30s ea	**55045-2084-03**	21.00		
60s ea	**55045-2084-06**	42.00		
(IPI)				
REPACK				
CAP, PO, 25 mg, 30s ea	**18837-0044-30**	17.08		
50 mg, 30s ea	**18837-0045-30**	22.34		
(Palmetto)				
REPACK				
CAP, PO, 25 mg, 30s ea	**23490-5480-03**	18.00		
(PD-Rx Pharm)				
REPACK				
CAP, PO (USP)				
25 mg, 30s ea	**55289-0370-30**	11.96		
(Quality Care Prod)				
REPACK				
CAP, PO, 50 mg, 30s ea	**49999-0190-30**	25.56		
DOXERCALCIFEROL				
(Genzyme) *See HECTOROL*				

PROD/MFR	NDC	AWP	DP	OBC
DOXIL (Centocor)				
doxorubicin hydrochloride liposome				
SOL, IV (STEALTH LIPOSOME)				
2 mg/ml, 10 ml	17314-9600-01	1157.76		
25 ml	17314-9600-02	2894.40		
DOXORUBICIN HCL NOVAPLUS (Bedford)				
doxorubicin hydrochloride				
PDS, IV (S.D.V.,PF)				
10 mg, 10s ea	55390-0241-10	78.00		AP
50 mg, ea	55390-0243-01	36.00		AP
SOL, IV, 2 mg/ml,				
5 ml 10s	55390-0245-10	68.40		AP
10 ml 10s	55390-0246-10	162.00		AP
25 ml	55390-0247-01	30.00		AP
(M.D.V.)				
2 mg/ml, 100 ml	55390-0248-01	93.60		AP
DOXORUBICIN HYDROCHLORIDE (APP)				
SOL, IV (USP,STERILE,SDV,PF)				
2 mg/ml, 5 ml	63323-0883-05	13.75		AP
10 ml	63323-0883-10	27.50		AP
25 ml	63323-0883-30	67.50		AP
(USP,STERILE,MDV,PF)				
2 mg/ml, 100 ml	63323-0101-61	275.00		AP
(Bedford) *See ADRIAMYCIN*				
(Bedford) *See DOXORUBICIN HCL NOVAPLUS*				
(Teva)				
SOL, IV (S.D.V., 10X5ML,PF)				
2 mg/ml, 5 ml 10s	00703-5043-03	145.20		AP
(S.D.V. POLYMER,PF)				
2 mg/ml, 25 ml	00703-5046-01	56.40		AP
(M.D.V. POLYMER,PF)				
2 mg/ml, 100 ml	00703-5040-01	168.98		AP
DOXORUBICIN HYDROCHLORIDE LIPOSOME				
(Centocor) *See DOXIL*				
DOXY 100 (APP)				
doxycycline hyclate				
PDS, IV (VIAL,PF)				
100 mg, 10s ea	63323-0130-11	185.52		AP
DOXYCYCLINE				
(Aqua Pharmaceuticals) *See MONODOX*				
(Avidas) *See AVIDOXY*				
(Doak) *See ADOXA*				
(Doak) *See ADOXA CK*				
(Doak) *See ADOXA PAK 1/150*				
(Doak) *See ADOXA PAK 1/75*				
(Doak) *See ADOXA TT*				
(Galderma) *See ORACEA*				
(Lannett) *See DOXYCYLINE*				
(Lannett)				
TAB, PO (FILM COATED)				
75 mg, 100s ea	00527-1535-01	598.02		AB
(FILM-COATED CAPLET)				
100 mg, 50s ea	00527-1338-50	211.55		AB
250s ea	00527-1338-25	1016.65		AB
(FILM COATED)				
150 mg, 30s ea	00527-1537-30	329.00		AB
(Major)				
doxycycline hyclate				
CAP, PO, 100 mg, 20s ea	00904-0428-95	4.40		AB
TAB, PO, 100 mg,				
100s ea UD	00904-0430-61	138.40		AB
DOXYCYCLINE (Medisca)				
POW, NA (1X100GM,USP)				
100 gm	38779-1982-05	450.00		
(1X500GM,USP)				
500 gm	38779-1982-08	1875.00		
(1X1000GM,USP)				
1000 gm	38779-1982-09	3150.00		
(Mylan)				
TAB, PO (FILM-COATED)				
50 mg, 100s ea	00378-6021-01	372.25		AB
75 mg, 100s ea	00378-6022-01	498.35		AB
(Mylan)				
doxycycline hyclate				
100 mg, 50s ea	00378-6023-89	272.75		AB
DOXYCYCLINE (Mylan)				
150 mg, 30s ea	00378-6124-93	273.87		AB
(Par) *See DOXYCYCLINE MONOHYDRATE*				
(Par)				
TAB, PO (MONOHYDRATE,FILM-COATED)				
50 mg, 100s ea	49884-0091-01	335.71		AB
(FILM-COATED)				
75 mg, 100s ea	49884-0092-01	498.92		AB
(MONOHYDRATE,FILM-COATED)				
100 mg, 50s ea	49884-0093-03	246.02		AB
250s ea	49884-0093-04	1182.23		AB
(FILM-COATED)				
150 mg, 30s ea	49884-0236-11	274.18		AB
(Pfizer) *See VIBRAMYCIN MONOHYDRATE*				
(Ranbaxy Pharm)				
TAB, PO (FILM COATED)				
75 mg, 100s ea	63304-0131-01	493.40		AB
100 mg, 50s ea	63304-0132-50	270.07		AB
250s ea	63304-0132-04	1297.77		AB
(Sandoz) *See DOXYCYCLINE MONOHYDRATE*				
(Sandoz)				
TAB, PO (FILM-COATED)				
50 mg, 100s ea	00185-0036-01	417.38		AB
75 mg, 100s ea	00185-0106-01	573.79		AB
100 mg, 50s ea	00185-0216-53	311.35		AB
250s ea	00185-0216-52	1496.08		AB
(Watson Labs) *See DOXYCYCLINE MONOHYDRATE*				
(Bryant Ranch)				
REPACK				
CAP, PO, 100 mg, 10s ea	63629-1531-01	16.23		
20s ea	63629-1531-02	32.45		
30s ea	63629-1531-03	48.68		
40s ea	63629-1531-04	64.90		
60s ea	63629-1531-05	97.36		
TAB, PO, 100 mg, 20s ea	63629-1357-01	32.45		
30s ea	63629-1357-03	48.68		
40s ea	63629-1357-02	64.90		
(Core)				
REPACK				
doxycycline hyclate				
CAP, PO, 100 mg, 14s ea	33358-0120-14	21.88		
20s ea	33358-0120-20	33.26		
30s ea	33358-0120-30	49.90		
40s ea	33358-0120-40	66.52		
60s ea	33358-0120-60	99.79		
TAB, PO, 100 mg, 20s ea	33358-0121-20	33.26		
30s ea	33358-0121-30	49.90		
(Physician Partner)				
REPACK				
CAP, PO, 100 mg, 14s ea	21695-0044-14	34.51		
20s ea	21695-0044-20	49.30		
28s ea	21695-0044-28	69.02		
40s ea	21695-0044-40	98.60		
42s ea	21695-0044-42	103.53		
(Southwood)				
REPACK				
TAB, PO, 20 mg, 30s ea	58016-0075-30	35.69		
60s ea	58016-0075-60	71.39		
90s ea	58016-0075-90	107.08		
100s ea	58016-0075-00	118.98		
DOXYCYCLINE CALCIUM				
(Pfizer) *See VIBRAMYCIN CALCIUM*				
DOXYCYCLINE HYCLATE				
FUL				
CAP, PO, 50 mg, 50s ea		6.59		
100 mg, 50s ea		7.46		
TAB, PO, 100 mg, 50s ea		6.44		
(Actavis Mid Atlantic)				
TAB, PO, 20 mg, 100s ea	00472-0850-10	118.98		
(Apace)				
CAP, PO (USP,HARD GELATIN)				
100 mg, 14s ea	15338-0100-14	19.25		
(APP) *See DOXY 100*				
(Axiom Pharmaceutical)				
CAP, PO, 50 mg, 50s ea	67870-0109-50	37.50		
100 mg, 50s ea	67870-0110-50	68.40		
500s ea	67870-0110-05	579.00		
TAB, PO (FILM-COATING)				
100 mg, 50s ea	67870-0112-50	67.00		
500s ea	67870-0112-05	569.00		
(Bedford)				
PDS, IV, 100 mg, 10s ea	55390-0110-10	141.60		AP
(Blu)				
TAB, PO (USP,FILM COATED)				
100 mg, 20s ea	24658-0220-20	3.83		AB
500s ea	24658-0220-05	40.14		AB
(Consolidated Midland)				
CAP, PO, 50 mg, 50s ea UD	00223-0871-00	10.00		EE
100s ea	00223-0871-01	19.50		EE
TAB, PO, 100 mg, 50s ea	00223-0872-05	12.50		EE
500s ea	00223-0872-50	107.50		EE
(E5) *See ORAXYL*				
(Galderma) *See PERIOSTAT*				
(Gallipot)				
POW, NA (1X25GM,USP)				
25 gm	51552-0852-04	55.30	39.50	
(1X100GM,USP)				
100 gm	51552-0852-05	210.00	150.00	
(Hawkins)				
POW, NA (USP)				
25 gm	63370-0074-25	100.80		
100 gm	63370-0074-35	384.00		
1000 gm	63370-0074-50	2880.00		
(Lannett)				
TAB, PO (USP,FILM COATED)				
20 mg, 100s ea	00527-1336-01	115.14		AB
(Major)				
CAP, PO, 50 mg, 50s ea	00904-0427-51	36.50		AB
100 mg, 50s ea	00904-0428-51	65.75		AB
(10X10)				
100 mg, 100s ea UD	00904-0428-61	141.38		AB
500s ea	00904-0428-40	574.20		AB
(Major) *See DOXYCYCLINE*				
(Major)				
TAB, PO, 100 mg, 50s ea	00904-0430-51	63.75		AB
500s ea	00904-0430-40	574.20		AB
(Medisca)				
POW, NA (U.S.P.)				
25 gm	38779-0434-04	62.85		
100 gm	38779-0434-05	240.00		
(USP,1X500GM)				
500 gm	38779-0434-08	795.00		
(USP,1X1000GM)				
1000 gm	38779-0434-09	1425.00		
(Mutual)				
CAP, PO, 50 mg, 50s ea	53489-0118-02	37.80		AB
500s ea	53489-0118-05	336.00		AB
100 mg, 50s ea	53489-0119-02	67.10		AB
500s ea	53489-0119-05	580.00		AB
TAB, PO (FILM-COATED)				
20 mg, 100s ea	53489-0647-01	118.98		AB
100 mg, 50s ea	53489-0120-02	67.10		AB
500s ea	53489-0120-05	580.00		AB
(Mylan) *See DOXYCYCLINE*				
(Ocusoft) *See ALODOX*				
(PCCA)				
POW, NA (U.S.P.)				
1 gm	51927-3129-00	4.20		
(Pfizer) *See VIBRA-TABS*				
(Pfizer) *See VIBRAMYCIN HYCLATE*				
(Qualitest)				
CAP, PO, 100 mg, 50s ea	00603-3481-19	70.21		AB
500s ea	00603-3481-28	616.41		AB
TAB, PO, 100 mg, 500s ea	00603-3482-28	580.00		AB
(Sandoz)				
ECC, PO, 75 mg, 60s ea	00185-0814-60	296.75		
60s ea	00781-2268-60	267.07		EE
100 mg, 50s ea	00185-0815-53	290.96		
50s ea	00781-2269-50	261.86		
TAB, PO (USP,FILM-COATED)				
20 mg, 100s ea	00781-5115-01	118.98		AB
(Teva)				
TAB, PO (FILM-COATED)				
20 mg, 100s ea	00172-4626-60	118.98		AB
500s ea	00172-4626-70	565.16		AB
100 mg, 50s ea	00172-3626-48	31.21		AB
(10X10)				
100 mg, 100s ea UD	00182-1535-89	52.15		AB
500s ea	00172-3626-70	291.69		AB
(VersaPharm)				
CAP, PO, 100 mg, 14s ea	61748-0111-14	3.00		AB
(Warner Chilcott) *See DORYX*				
(Watson Labs)				
CAP, PO, 50 mg, 50s ea	00591-5535-50	37.35		AB
100 mg, 50s ea	00591-5440-50	68.47		AB
500s ea	00591-5440-05	580.00		AB
TAB, PO, 100 mg, 50s ea	00591-5553-50	68.47		AB
500s ea	00591-5553-05	580.00		AB
(West-Ward)				
CAP, PO, 50 mg, 50s ea	00143-3141-50	36.60		AB
100 mg, 14s ea UD	00143-3142-14	6.60		AB
50s ea	00143-3142-50	67.50		AB
100s ea UD	00143-3142-25	55.50		AB
500s ea	00143-3142-05	569.50		AB
TAB, PO (FILM COATED)				
100 mg, 50s ea	00143-2112-50	67.50		
500s ea	00143-2112-05	569.50		
(A-S Medication)				
REPACK				
CAP, PO, 50 mg, 20s ea	54569-0147-02	15.12		AB
100 mg, 20s ea	54569-1840-01	23.20		EE
40s ea	54569-1840-00	46.40		EE
TAB, PO, 100 mg, 2s ea	54569-3074-06	2.70		EE
6s ea	54569-3074-00	8.10		EE
7s ea	54569-0118-02	9.45		EE
10s ea	54569-0118-00	13.50		EE
14s ea	54569-0118-01	18.90		EE
20s ea	54569-0118-03	27.00		EE
28s ea	54569-0118-05	37.80		EE

PROD/MFR	NDC	AWP	DP	OBC
DOXYCYCLINE HYCLATE (A-S Medication)				
REPACK				
TAB, PO, 100 mg, 30s ea	54569-0118-06	40.50		EE
50s ea	54569-3074-08	67.50		EE
60s ea	54569-0118-08	81.00		EE
100s ea	54569-0118-09	135.00		EE
(Aidarex)				
REPACK				
TAB, PO, 100 mg, 7s ea	33261-0143-07	35.00		AB
14s ea	33261-0143-14	70.00		AB
20s ea	33261-0143-20	100.00		AB
21s ea	33261-0143-21	105.00		AB
28s ea	33261-0143-28	140.00		AB
30s ea	33261-0143-30	150.00		AB
60s ea	33261-0143-60	300.00		AB
90s ea	33261-0143-90	450.00		AB
(Altura)				
REPACK				
CAP, PO, 100 mg, 10s ea	63874-0109-10	9.31		AB
12s ea	63874-0109-12	11.17		AB
14s ea	63874-0109-14	13.03		AB
15s ea	63874-0109-15	13.95		AB
16s ea	63874-0109-16	14.90		AB
18s ea	63874-0109-18	16.76		AB
20s ea	63874-0109-20	18.62		AB
21s ea	63874-0109-21	19.54		AB
24s ea	63874-0109-24	19.55		AB
28s ea	63874-0109-28	26.06		AB
30s ea	63874-0109-30	27.92		AB
40s ea	63874-0109-40	37.23		AB
50s ea	63874-0109-50	46.55		AB
60s ea	63874-0109-60	66.86		AB
500s ea	63874-0109-03	465.50		AB
TAB, PO (FILM COATED)				
100 mg, 5s ea	63874-0237-05	4.65		AB
6s ea	63874-0237-06	5.32		AB
7s ea	63874-0237-07	6.20		AB
10s ea	63874-0237-10	9.31		AB
12s ea	63874-0237-12	11.17		AB
14s ea	63874-0237-14	13.06		AB
15s ea	63874-0237-15	13.97		AB
16s ea	63874-0237-16	14.18		AB
20s ea	63874-0237-20	18.62		AB
21s ea	63874-0237-21	19.55		AB
24s ea	63874-0237-24	22.34		AB
28s ea	63874-0237-28	26.06		AB
30s ea	63874-0237-30	27.93		AB
40s ea	63874-0237-40	37.23		AB
(FILM COATED)				
100 mg, 50s ea	63874-0237-50	46.55		AB
60s ea	63874-0237-60	55.86		AB
100s ea	63874-0237-01	93.10		AB
120s ea	63874-0237-04	106.32		AB
150s ea	63874-0237-72	132.90		AB
200s ea	63874-0237-74	177.20		AB
300s ea	63874-0237-77	265.80		AB
(DHS, Inc.)				
REPACK				
CAP, PO, 100 mg, 3s ea	55887-0979-03	2.84		AB
4s ea	55887-0979-04	3.78		AB
10s ea	55887-0979-10	9.47		AB
11s ea	55887-0979-11	10.42		AB
12s ea	55887-0979-12	11.36		AB
14s ea	55887-0979-14	13.26		AB
16s ea	55887-0979-16	15.15		AB
20s ea	55887-0979-20	18.26		AB
21s ea	55887-0979-21	19.07		AB
24s ea	55887-0979-24	21.79		AB
28s ea	55887-0979-28	25.43		AB
30s ea	55887-0979-30	27.24		AB
60s ea	55887-0979-60	48.00		AB
120s ea	55887-0979-82	108.96		AB
(Dispensing Solutions)				
REPACK				
CAP, PO, 100 mg, 14s ea	66336-0109-14	19.61		AB
20s ea	66336-0109-20	28.00		AB
28s ea	66336-0109-28	47.73		AB
30s ea	66336-0109-30	51.00		AB
42s ea	66336-0109-42	58.80		AB
50s ea	66336-0109-50	70.00		AB
60s ea	66336-0109-60	84.00		AB
TAB, PO (FILM COATED)				
100 mg, ea	66336-0449-10	11.18		
ea	66336-0449-14	15.65		
ea	66336-0449-20	24.44		
6s ea	55045-1207-06	7.85		AB
8s ea	55045-1207-02	10.48		AB
10s ea	55045-1207-05	13.10		AB
12s ea	55045-1207-01	15.72		AB
14s ea	55045-1207-04	18.34		AB
20s ea	55045-1207-07	26.20		AB
(FILM COATED)				
100 mg, 20s ea	55045-3932-01	26.20		
28s ea	55045-1207-08	36.68		AB
30s ea	55045-3306-08	39.30		AB
40s ea	55045-3306-04	52.40		
(USP)				
100 mg, 42s ea	55045-1207-03	55.02		
50s ea	55045-3306-05	65.50		AB
60s ea	55045-3306-06	78.60		
100s ea	55045-1207-00	131.00		AB
(GSMS)				
REPACK				
TAB, PO (UNIT OF USE)				
100 mg, 20s ea	60429-0069-20	16.35	5.45	AB
(FILM COATED)				
100 mg, 92s ea	60429-0069-92	28.20	9.40	
(HomeMed)				
REPACK				
CAP, PO, 100 mg, 14s ea	51655-0186-84	26.99		EE
20s ea	51655-0186-52	28.99		EE
28s ea	51655-0186-29	31.72		EE
TAB, PO, 100 mg, 30s ea	51655-0412-24	33.99		
(Keltman Pharma., Inc.)				
REPACK				
CAP, PO, 100 mg, 20s ea	68387-0380-20	21.43		AB
TAB, PO (FILM COATED)				
100 mg, 20s ea	68387-0381-20	21.43		
(Nucare Pharm)				
REPACK				
CAP, PO, 100 mg, 6s ea	66267-0085-06	7.89		EE
10s ea	66267-0085-10	11.49		EE
14s ea	66267-0085-14	15.56		EE
20s ea	66267-0085-20	19.99		EE
30s ea	66267-0085-30	17.88		EE
TAB, PO (FILM COATED)				
100 mg, 400s ea	68071-0014-83	455.60		
(Palmetto)				
REPACK				
CAP, PO, 100 mg, 4s ea	23490-5483-01	7.23		
14s ea	23490-5483-02	15.86		
20s ea	23490-5483-03	22.66		
28s ea	23490-5483-04	31.72		
30s ea	23490-0490-03	39.60		
30s ea	23490-5483-05	33.99		
40s ea	23490-5483-08	67.98		
50s ea	23490-5483-06	56.65		
60s ea	23490-0490-06	79.20		
60s ea	23490-5483-07	67.98		
TAB, PO, 100 mg, 10s ea	23490-5485-01	13.50		
14s ea	23490-5485-02	18.70		
20s ea	23490-5485-03	27.00		
30s ea	23490-5485-05	40.50		
40s ea	23490-5485-04	54.00		
100s ea	23490-5485-06	135.00		
(PD-Rx Pharm)				
REPACK				
CAP, PO, 50 mg, 16s ea	55289-0502-16	19.10		AB
30s ea	55289-0502-30	20.25		AB
60s ea	55289-0502-60	37.67		AB
(USP)				
100 mg, ea	55289-0107-79	10.37		AB
2s ea	55289-0107-02	10.73		AB
6s ea	43063-0019-06	12.21		AB
6s ea	55289-0107-06	12.20		AB
10s ea	55289-0107-10	13.67		AB
12s ea	55289-0107-12	14.40		AB
(REDI-SCRIPT)				
100 mg, 12s ea	58864-0190-12	14.40		AB
14s ea	55289-0107-14	15.09		AB
20s ea	55289-0107-20	17.33		AB
(REDI-SCRIPT)				
100 mg, 20s ea	58864-0190-20	17.34		AB
28s ea	55289-0107-28	20.27		AB
28s ea	58864-0190-28	20.28		AB
30s ea	55289-0107-30	21.00		AB
(REDI-SCRIPT)				
100 mg, 30s ea	58864-0190-30	21.00		AB
40s ea	55289-0107-40	24.67		AB
56s ea	55289-0107-56	30.53		AB
60s ea	55289-0107-60	32.00		AB
(USP)				
100 mg, 180s ea	55289-0107-93	56.67		AB
TAB, PO, 100 mg, 2s ea	55289-0866-02	10.58		AB
4s ea	55289-0866-04	11.20		AB
(USP,FILM COATED)				
100 mg, 6s ea	55289-0866-06	12.06		
8s ea	55289-0866-08	12.40		AB
(REDI-SCRIPT)				
100 mg, 10s ea	58864-0189-10	13.68		AB
14s ea	55289-0866-14	14.19		AB
20s ea	55289-0866-20	16.00		AB
(REDI-SCRIPT)				
100 mg, 20s ea	58864-0189-20	15.99		AB
28s ea	55289-0866-28	18.40		AB
(REDI-SCRIPT)				
100 mg, 28s ea	58864-0189-28	18.39		AB
(USP,FILM COATED)				
100 mg, 30s ea	55289-0866-30	21.54		
60s ea	55289-0866-60	25.92		
90s ea	55289-0866-90	27.84		
180s ea	55289-0866-93	54.99		
(FILM COATED)				
100 mg, 360s ea	55289-0866-86	73.89		
(USP,FILM COATED)				
100 mg, 400s ea	55289-0866-74	79.74		
(Pharma Pac)				
REPACK				
CAP, PO, 100 mg, 6s ea	52959-0055-06	10.27		EE
7s ea	52959-0055-07	11.98		AB
10s ea	52959-0055-10	17.11		EE
12s ea	52959-0055-12	20.43		AB
14s ea	52959-0055-14	23.82		EE
15s ea	52959-0055-15	25.50		EE
20s ea	52959-0055-20	33.90		EE
28s ea	52959-0055-28	47.16		EE
30s ea	52959-0055-30	49.98		EE
90s ea	52959-0055-90	148.58		EE
100s ea	52959-0055-00	165.14		EE
120s ea	52959-0055-02	198.30		EE
TAB, PO, 100 mg, 14s ea	52959-0474-14	19.15		AB
20s ea	52959-0474-20	27.34		EE
30s ea	52959-0474-30	40.98		AB
(Phys Total Care)				
REPACK				
CAP, PO, 50 mg, 20s ea	54868-3169-01	10.23		EE
30s ea	54868-3169-04	13.08		EE
40s ea	54868-3169-02	15.96		EE
60s ea	54868-3169-00	21.66		EE
100s ea	54868-3169-05	31.62		AB
100 mg, 10s ea	54868-0023-06	8.64		EE
14s ea	54868-0023-14	10.89		EE
20s ea	54868-0023-08	14.28		EE
30s ea	54868-0023-05	19.92		EE
40s ea	54868-0023-09	25.56		EE
60s ea	54868-0023-08	36.84		EE
100s ea	54868-0023-00	59.40		EE
500s ea	54868-0023-03	217.14		EE
TAB, PO (FILM-COATED)				
20 mg, 60s ea	54868-5269-00	150.60		AB
100 mg, 11s ea	54868-0191-02	10.10		EE
14s ea	54868-0191-03	10.64		EE
20s ea	54868-0191-01	15.90		EE
(USP)				
100 mg, 30s ea	54868-0191-05	13.66		EE
50s ea	54868-0191-06	21.69		EE
60s ea	54868-0191-04	41.71		EE
500s ea	54868-0191-07	97.41		AB
(Physician Partner)				
REPACK				
CAP, PO, 100 mg, 6s ea	21695-0044-06	14.79		AB
TAB, PO (FILM-COATED)				
100 mg, 14s ea	21695-0581-14	29.22		
(FILM COATED)				
100 mg, 20s ea	21695-0581-20	41.74		
30s ea	21695-0581-30	62.62		AB
(Quality Care Prod)				
REPACK				
CAP, PO, 100 mg, 11s ea	49999-0126-11	28.24		AB
14s ea	49999-0126-14	35.95		
20s ea	49999-0126-20	51.35		
30s ea	49999-0126-30	77.03		AB
56s ea	49999-0126-56	143.78		AB
TAB, PO, 100 mg, 14s ea	49999-0020-14	15.95		EE
20s ea	49999-0020-20	22.33		EE
28s ea	49999-0020-28	31.90		EE
30s ea	49999-0020-30	33.50		EE
100s ea	49999-0020-00	107.00		EE
(Southwood)				
REPACK				
CAP, PO, 100 mg, 10s ea	58016-0161-10	8.87		EE
12s ea	58016-0161-12	10.64		EE
14s ea	58016-0161-14	12.40		EE
15s ea	58016-0161-15	13.29		EE
16s ea	58016-0161-16	14.19		EE
18s ea	58016-0161-18	15.96		EE
20s ea	58016-0161-20	17.73		EE
21s ea	58016-0161-21	18.61		EE
24s ea	58016-0161-24	21.28		EE
28s ea	58016-0161-28	24.82		EE
30s ea	58016-0161-30	26.58		EE
40s ea	58016-0161-40	35.46		EE
50s ea	58016-0161-50	44.33		EE

PROD/MFR	NDC	AWP	DP	OBC
60s ea	58016-0161-60	53.20		EE
90s ea	58016-0156-90	103.50		AB
TAB, PO, 100 mg, 6s ea	58016-0156-06	5.32		EE
7s ea	58016-0156-07	6.20		EE
10s ea	58016-0156-10	8.86		EE
12s ea	58016-0156-12	10.63		EE
14s ea	58016-0156-14	12.40		EE
15s ea	58016-0156-15	13.29		EE
16s ea	58016-0156-16	14.18		EE
20s ea	58016-0156-20	23.00		EE
21s ea	58016-0156-21	18.61		EE
24s ea	58016-0156-24	21.26		EE
28s ea	58016-0156-28	32.20		EE
30s ea	58016-0156-30	34.50		EE
40s ea	58016-0156-40	46.00		EE
60s ea	58016-0156-60	69.00		EE
100s ea	58016-0156-00	115.00		EE
120s ea	58016-0156-02	138.00		EE
150s ea	58016-0156-03	132.90		EE
200s ea	58016-0156-89	177.20		EE
300s ea	58016-0156-73	265.80		EE
(St. Mary's MPP)				
REPACK				
CAP, PO, 100 mg, 20s ea	60760-0562-20	31.06		AB
(Stat Rx)				
REPACK				
CAP, PO, 100 mg, 14s ea	16590-0082-14	11.50		AB
20s ea	16590-0082-20	25.00		
21s ea	16590-0082-21	25.55		
28s ea	16590-0082-28	34.16		
30s ea	16590-0082-30	36.50		
(Vibranta)				
REPACK				
TAB, PO, 100 mg, 6s ea	57866-0340-05	8.90		
14s ea	57866-0340-01	17.34		
20s ea	57866-0340-02	28.30		
DOXYCYCLINE MONOHYDRATE (Par)				
doxycycline				
CAP, PO, 50 mg, 100s ea	49884-0726-01	145.10		AB
100 mg, 50s ea	49884-0727-03	118.45		AB
250s ea	49884-0727-04	569.29		AB
(Sandoz)				
CAP, PO, 50 mg, 100s ea	00185-0805-01	130.61		AB
100 mg, 50s ea	00185-0810-53	106.61		AB
100s ea	00185-0810-01	213.23		AB
250s ea	00185-0810-52	512.39		AB
(Watson Labs)				
CAP, PO, 50 mg, 100s ea	00591-0410-01	118.74		
100 mg, 50s ea	00591-0411-50	96.92		AB
(Vibranta)				
REPACK				
CAP, PO, 50 mg, 30s ea	57866-0343-01	40.43		AB
100 mg, 14s ea	57866-0341-02	18.52		AB
30s ea	57866-0341-04	62.74		AB
DOXYCYCLINE/FLAXSEED OIL/ OMEGA-3 FATTY ACIDS/VIT E				
(Advanced Vision) *See NUTRIDOX CONVENIENCE*				
DOXYCYCLINE/OCTINOXATE/SALICYLIC ACID/ ZINC OXIDE				
(Avidas) *See AVIDOXY DK*				
DOXYCYLINE (Lannett)				
doxycycline				
TAB, PO (FILM-COATED)				
50 mg, 100s ea	00527-1335-01	288.70		AB
DOXYLAMINE SUCCINATE (Gallipot)				
POW, NA, 25 gm	51552-0251-04	52.15		
100 gm	51552-0251-05	175.00		
(PCCA)				
POW, NA (U.S.P.)				
1 gm	51927-1094-00	7.20		
(Spectrum Pharmacy)				
POW, NA (U.S.P./N.F.)				
5 gm	49452-2695-03	80.15		
(U.S.P.)				
25 gm	49452-2695-01	205.45		
100 gm	49452-2695-02	626.50		
(Zyber) *See ALDEX AN*				
DPT, HEPATITIS B, AND POLIO VACCINE				
(Glaxo) *See PEDIARIX*				
DRESSING				
(King Pharm) *See THROMBI-GEL*				
(Medline) *See TENDERWET CAVITY SYSTEM*				
DREXOPHED SR (Phys Total Care)				
REPACK				
dexbrompheniramine maleate/pseudoephedrine sulfate				
TER, PO, 6 mg-120 mg,				
20s ea	54868-2874-01	11.82		
DRISDOL (Sanofi-Aventis)				
ergocalciferol				
SGL, PO, 50000 iu,				
50s ea	00024-0392-02	106.34		AA
(Pharma Pac)				
REPACK				
SGL, PO, 50000 iu,				
25s ea	52959-0528-25	34.75		AA
DRITHO-SCALP (Summers)				
anthralin				
CRE, TP, 0.5%, 50 gm	11086-0035-01	112.94		
DRITHOCREME (Summers)				
anthralin				
CRE, TP, 1%, 50 gm	11086-0037-01	112.94		
DRONABINOL (Par)				
SGL, PO (USP,SOFT GELATIN)				
2.5 mg,				
60s ea, C-III	49884-0867-02	353.57		AB
5 mg, 60s ea, C-III	49884-0868-02	735.85		AB
10 mg, 60s ea, C-III	49884-0869-02	1351.30		AB
(Unimed Pharm) *See MARINOL*				
(Watson)				
SGL, PO (SOFT GELATIN)				
2.5 mg,				
60s ea, C-III	00591-3591-60	339.44		
5 mg, 60s ea, C-III	00591-3592-60	706.45		
10 mg, 60s ea, C-III	00591-3593-60	1297.32		
(Phys Total Care)				
REPACK				
SGL, PO (SOFT GELATIN)				
5 mg,				
60s ea, C-III	54868-5929-00	1337.38		AB
(Stat Rx)				
REPACK				
SGL, PO (SOFT GELATIN)				
2.5 mg,				
60s ea, C-III	16590-0750-60	303.45		
DRONEDARONE HYDROCHLORIDE				
(Sanofi-Aventis) *See MULTAQ*				
DROPERIDOL (Amer Regent)				
SOL, IJ (S.D.V.)				
2.5 mg/ml,				
2 ml 25s	00517-9702-25	106.25		AP
(Hospira)				
SOL, IJ (10X2ML AMP,LATEX-FREE)				
2.5 mg/ml,				
2 ml 10s	00409-1187-01	13.32	11.70	AP
(Medisca)				
POW, NA (U.S.P.)				
0.5 gm	38779-0501-00	276.00		
1 gm	38779-0501-06	735.00		
(PCCA)				
POW, NA (USP)				
1 gm	51927-2182-00	648.00		
(Spectrum Pharmacy)				
POW, NA (U.S.P.)				
1 gm	49452-2696-02	1274.00		
(Phys Total Care)				
REPACK				
SOL, IJ (AMP)				
2.5 mg/ml,				
1 ml 10s	54868-3890-00	23.33		EE
DROSPIRENONE/ESTRADIOL				
(Bayer) *See ANGELIQ*				
DROSPIRENONE/ETHINYL ESTRADIOL				
(Bayer) *See YASMIN*				
(Bayer) *See YAZ*				
(Teva) *See OCELLA*				
(Palmetto)				
REPACK				
TAB, PO, 3 mg-0.03 mg,				
28s ea	23490-7564-01	44.90		
DROTRECOGIN ALFA				
(Lilly) *See XIGRIS*				
DROXIA (B/M Squibb Onc/Vir)				
hydroxyurea				
CAP, PO, 200 mg, 60s ea	00003-6335-17	56.76		
300 mg, 60s ea	00003-6336-17	56.76		
400 mg, 60s ea	00003-6337-17	58.31		
DRYMAX (JayMac Pharma)				
cpm/methscopolamine nitrate/pse hcl				
SYR, PO (1X118ML,AF,GLUTEN-FREE)				
118 ml	64661-0090-04	55.37	41.53	
DRYSEC (A. G. Marin)				
cpm/methscopolamine nitrate/phenyleph hcl				
TER, PO (DYE-FREE)				
8 mg-2.5 mg-20 mg,				
100s ea	12539-0727-01	76.80		
DRYSOL (Person & Covey)				
aluminum chloride				
SOL, TP (DAB-O-MATIC)				
20%, 35 ml	00096-0707-35	6.33		
37.5 ml	00096-0707-37	5.87		
(DAB-O-MATIC)				
20%, 60 ml	00096-0707-60	8.62		
(Quality Care Prod)				
REPACK				
SOL, TP (1X37.5ML)				
20%, 37.5 ml	35356-0247-37	34.50		
DSS/FE/FOLIC ACID/IF/VIT B12/VIT C/VIT E				
(PGD, Inc.) *See GENHEMAT*				
DSS/FE/FOLIC ACID/VIT B12/VIT C				
(Mission) *See FERRALET 90*				
DTAP AND HAEMOPHILUS B VACCINE				
(Sanofi) *See TRIHIBIT*				
DTAP AND POLIO VACCINE				
(Glaxo) *See KINRIX*				
DTAP VACCINE				
(Glaxo) *See INFANRIX*				
(Sanofi) *See DAPTACEL*				
(Sanofi) *See TRIPEDIA*				
DTIC-DOME (Bayer Corp.)				
dacarbazine				
PDS, IV (VIAL)				
200 mg, 12s ea	00026-8151-20	332.72		AP
DUAC CS (Stiefel Labs)				
benzoyl peroxide/clindamycin phosphate				
KIT, TP (SOAP-FREE)				
5%-1%, ea	00145-2367-01	181.15		BT
DUANE READE PRESTIGE SMART SYSTEM				
(Home Diag)				
glucose, blood test				
DEV, NA (STRIP)				
50s ea	56151-0306-50	28.60		
DUET (Xanodyne Pharma)				
prenatal vitamins				
TAB, PO, 100s ea	66479-0828-01	56.50		
DUET DHA (Xanodyne Pharma)				
prenatal vitamins				
KIT, PO (ENTERIC-COATED,SOFTGEL)				
60s ea	66479-0880-30	48.59		
DUET DHA COMPLETE (Xanodyne Pharma)				
prenatal vitamins				
KIT, PO (ENTERIC-COATED,SOFTGEL)				
60s ea	66479-0885-30	48.59		
DUET STUARTNATAL (Xanodyne Pharma)				
prenatal vitamins				
CTB, PO, 90s ea	64731-0830-90	49.67		
DUETACT (Takeda)				
glimepiride/pioglitazone hydrochloride				
TAB, PO, 2 mg-30 mg,				
30s ea	64764-0302-30	242.76		
4 mg-30 mg, 30s ea	64764-0304-30	242.76		
DUETDHA STUARTNATAL (Xanodyne Pharma)				
prenatal vitamins				
KIT, PO (5X12,SOFTGEL)				
60s ea UD	66479-0855-30	39.60		
DULOXETINE HYDROCHLORIDE				
(Lilly) *See CYMBALTA*				
DULSE FLAKES (PCCA)				
rhodymenia palmetta				
POW, NA (1X1GM)				
1 gm	51927-2969-00	0.36		

PROD/MFR	NDC	AWP	DP	OBC
DUO-VIL 2-10 (Phys Total Care)				
REPACK				
amitriptyline hydrochloride/perphenazine				
TAB, PO, 10 mg-2 mg,				
50s ea	54868-0124-02	18.75		EE
100s ea	54868-0124-03	32.97		EE
DUO-VIL 2-25 (Phys Total Care)				
amitriptyline hydrochloride/perphenazine				
TAB, PO, 25 mg-2 mg,				
30s ea	54868-0125-02	23.40		EE
50s ea	54868-0125-03	36.00		EE
100s ea	54868-0125-04	66.00		EE
DUOHIST DH (Breckenridge Pharm)				
cpm/dihydrocodeine bitartrate/phenyleph hcl				
SOL, PO (1X473ML,AF,SF,DYE-FREE)				
473 ml, C-III	51991-0598-16	143.81		
DUOMAX (Capellon)				
guaifenesin/phenylephrine hydrochloride				
TER, PO, 1200 mg-40 mg,				
100s ea	64543-0142-01	62.94		
DUONEB (Dey, L.P.)				
albuterol sulfate/ipratropium bromide				
SOL, IH (VIAL,U.D.)				
3 mg/3 ml-0.5 mg/3 ml,				
3 ml 30s UD	49502-0672-30	76.66		
3 ml 60s UD	49502-0672-60	153.32		
(Phys Total Care)				
REPACK				
SOL, IH, 3 mg/3 ml-0.5 mg/3 ml,				
3 ml 30s	54868-0948-00	83.76		
DUOTAN PD (Breckenridge Pharm)				
dexchlorpheniramine tan/pse tan				
SUS, PO (BANANA-STRAWBERRY)				
2.5 mg/5 ml-75 mg/5 ml,				
118 ml	51991-0189-04	33.68		
473 ml	51991-0189-16	123.68		
DUOVISC (Alcon Surgical)				
chondroitin sulfate/hyaluronate sodium				
KIT, OP (0.35ML VISC/0.4ML PROV)				
ea	08065-1831-35	187.14		
(0.5ML VISC/0.55ML PROV)				
ea	08065-1831-50	198.00		
DURA-TAP/PD (Southwood)				
REPACK				
cpm/pse hcl				
CER, PO, 4 mg-60 mg,				
30s ea	58016-0799-30	18.45		
60s ea	58016-0799-60	34.67		
100s ea	58016-0799-00	55.92		
DURABAC (Poly)				
apap/caff/phenyltoloxamine cit/salicylamide				
CAP, PO, 100s ea	66869-0826-10	92.24	73.79	
(Phys Total Care)				
REPACK				
CAP, PO, 20s ea	54868-5557-01	19.20		
60s ea	54868-5557-00	53.86		
DURABAC FORTE (Poly)				
apap/caff/magnesium sal/phenyltoloxamine cit				
TAB, PO (CLEAR COATED)				
100s ea	66869-0827-10	109.70	87.76	
(Stat Rx)				
REPACK				
TAB, PO (CLEAR COATED)				
60s ea	16590-0801-60	112.00		
DURACLON (Bioniche Pharma)				
clonidine hydrochloride				
SOL, EP (SDV,PF)				
0.1 mg/ml, 10 ml	66479-0520-01	150.00		EE
0.5 mg/ml, 10 ml	66479-0521-01	494.00		
DURADRYL (Breckenridge Pharm)				
cpm/methscopolamine nitrate/phenyleph hcl				
CTB, PO (GRAPE)				
2 mg-1.25 mg-10 mg,				
100s ea	51991-0591-01	25.75		
SYR, PO (CHERRY)				
480 ml	51991-0016-16	16.75		
(A-S Medication)				
REPACK				
SYR, PO, 120 ml 4s	54569-4668-00	16.75		
DURADRYL SR (Breckenridge Pharm)				
cpm/methscopolamine nitrate/phenyleph hcl				
TER, PO, 8 mg-2.5 mg-20 mg,				
100s ea	51991-0592-01	65.50		
DURAFLU (Kowa)				
apap/dm/gg/pse hcl				
TAB, PO (DYE-FREE)				
100s ea	66869-0723-30	113.51	90.80	
(Phys Total Care)				
REPACK				
TAB, PO (DYE-FREE)				
20s ea	54868-5155-00	21.38		
DURAGESIC (PriCara)				
fentanyl				
TDM, TD, 12.5 mcg/hr,				
5s ea, C-II	50458-0090-05	97.86	81.55	AB
25 mcg/hr,				
5s ea, C-II	50458-0091-05	118.15	98.46	AB
50 mcg/hr,				
5s ea, C-II	50458-0092-05	216.01	180.01	AB
75 mcg/hr,				
5s ea, C-II	50458-0093-05	329.48	274.57	AB
100 mcg/hr,				
5s ea, C-II	50458-0094-05	437.29	364.41	AB
(Phys Total Care)				
REPACK				
TDM, TD, 12.5 mcg/hr,				
5s ea, C-II	54868-5706-00	88.05		
25 mcg/hr,				
5s ea, C-II	54868-3074-00	104.83		
50 mcg/hr,				
5s ea, C-II	54868-3076-00	179.56		
75 mcg/hr,				
5s ea, C-II	54868-3073-00	273.20		
100 mcg/hr,				
5s ea, C-II	54868-3075-00	377.60		
(Stat Rx)				
REPACK				
TDM, TD, 50 mcg/hr,				
5s ea, C-II	16590-0730-05	235.26		
100 mcg/hr,				
5s ea, C-II	16590-0716-05	471.65		
DURAMORPH (Baxter)				
morphine sulfate				
SOL, IJ (PF)				
0.5 mg/ml,				
10 ml, C-II	60977-0016-73	13.10		AP
(AMP,DOSETTE,PF)				
0.5 mg/ml,				
10 ml 10s, C-II	60977-0016-02	131.04		AP
(PF)				
1 mg/ml,				
10 ml, C-II	60977-0017-73	9.12		AP
(AMP,DOSETTE,PF)				
1 mg/ml,				
10 ml 10s, C-II	60977-0017-01	91.20		AP
DURAPATITE				
(PCCA) *See CALCIUM HYDROXYAPATITE*				
DURATUSS (Phys Total Care)				
REPACK				
guaifenesin/pseudoephedrine hydrochloride				
TER, PO (DYE-FREE)				
600 mg-120 mg,				
20s ea	54868-3943-00	23.39		
DURAVENT (Auriga)				
cpm/methscopolamine nitrate/phenyleph hcl				
CTB, PO (ROOT BEER)				
2 mg-1.25 mg-10 mg,				
100s ea	33753-0103-01	25.75		
DURAVENT DPB (Auriga)				
bpm/dm/phenyleph hcl				
SYR, PO (1X473ML,AF,SF)				
473 ml	33753-0105-16	80.96		
DURAVENT-DA (Auriga)				
cpm/methscopolamine nitrate/phenyleph hcl				
TER, PO, 8 mg-2.5 mg-20 mg,				
100s ea	33753-0101-01	31.76		
DUREZOL (Sirion)				
difluprednate				
EMU, OP, 0.05%, 5 ml	42826-0601-05	112.14		
DURICEF (Pharma Pac)				
REPACK				
cefadroxil				
CAP, PO, 500 mg, 10s ea	52959-0056-10	46.51		AB
14s ea	52959-0056-14	65.17		AB
20s ea	52959-0056-20	85.36		AB
(Phys Total Care)				
REPACK				
CAP, PO, 500 mg, 10s ea	54868-0407-04	53.80		AB
20s ea	54868-0407-01	106.37		AB
PDR, PO, 250 mg/5 ml,				
100 ml	54868-1392-00	97.74		
500 mg/5 ml,				
100 ml	54868-2910-00	125.53		
(Quality Care Prod)				
REPACK				
CAP, PO, 500 mg, 14s ea	49999-0809-14	135.17		
DUTASTERIDE				
(Glaxo) *See AVODART*				
DY-G (Cypress Pharm)				
dyphylline/guaifenesin				
LIQ, PO (AF,DYE-FREE,MINT)				
100 mg/5 ml-100 mg/5 ml,				
473 ml	60258-0371-16	25.68		
DYAZIDE (Glaxo)				
hydrochlorothiazide/triamterene				
CAP, PO (PATIENT-PAK)				
25 mg-37.5 mg,				
100s ea	00007-3650-22	121.14		AB
1000s ea	00007-3650-30	1163.93		AB
(PD-Rx Pharm)				
REPACK				
CAP, PO, 25 mg-37.5 mg,				
30s ea	55289-0454-30	30.13		AB
30s ea	58864-0660-30	30.13		AB
(Phys Total Care)				
REPACK				
CAP, PO, 25 mg-37.5 mg,				
10s ea	54868-3366-02	9.16		AB
30s ea	54868-3366-01	23.73		AB
60s ea	54868-3366-00	45.59		AB
DYCLONINE HCL (Medisca)				
dyclonine hydrochloride				
POW, NA (U.S.P.)				
25 gm	38779-0500-04	90.00		
100 gm	38779-0500-05	291.00		
500 gm	38779-0500-08	1185.00		
(PCCA)				
POW, NA (U.S.P.)				
1 gm	52927-1748-00	7.80		
(Spectrum Pharmacy)				
POW, NA (U.S.P.)				
100 gm	49452-2586-02	430.50		
500 gm	49452-2586-03	1683.50		
DYCLONINE HYDROCHLORIDE (Gallipot)				
POW, NA (1X5GM,USP)				
5 gm	51552-1037-02	24.50	17.50	
(Medisca) *See DYCLONINE HCL*				
(PCCA) *See DYCLONINE HCL*				
(Spectrum Pharmacy) *See DYCLONINE HCL*				
DYGASE (Cypress Pharm)				
amylase/lipase/protease				
CAP, PO, 30000 u-2400 u-30000 u,				
100s ea	60258-0811-01	72.32		
DYLIX (Lunsco)				
dyphylline				
ELI, PO, 100 mg/15 ml,				
480 ml	10892-0150-65	46.68		
DYNACIN (Medicis)				
minocycline hydrochloride				
TAB, PO (FILM-COATED)				
50 mg, 100s ea	99207-0490-10	834.42		
(FILM COATED)				
75 mg, 100s ea	99207-0491-10	1225.06		
100 mg, 50s ea	99207-0492-50	731.27		
DYNACIRC (Phys Total Care)				
REPACK				
isradipine				
CAP, PO, 2.5 mg, 30s ea	54868-2469-01	55.45		
100s ea	54868-2469-00	169.90		
5 mg, 60s ea	54868-4064-01	148.84		
100s ea	54868-4064-00	247.24		
DYNACIRC CR (Glaxo)				
isradipine				
TER, PO (FILM-COATED)				
5 mg, 30s ea	65726-0235-10	86.45		
10 mg, 30s ea	65726-0236-10	132.43		
(Phys Total Care)				
REPACK				
TER, PO, 5 mg, 30s ea	54868-5476-00	92.25		

PROD/MFR	NDC	AWP	DP	OBC
DYNAHIST-ER PEDIATRIC (Breckenridge Pharm)				
cpm/pse hcl				
CER, PO (DYE-FREE)				
4 mg-60 mg,				
100s ea	**51991-0217-01**	43.75		
DYNATUSS EX SYRUP (Breckenridge Pharm)				
dm/gg/phenyleph hcl				
SYR, PO (AF,CHERRY-VANILLA)				
473 ml	**51991-0211-16**	51.00		
DYNATUSS HC (Breckenridge Pharm)				
gg/hydrocod bit/phenyleph hcl				
SOL, PO (AF,SF,CHERRY)				
473 ml, C-III	**51991-0212-16**	48.95		
DYNEX 12 (Athlon Pharm)				
carbetapentane tannate/phenylephrine tannate				
SUS, PO (GRAPE)				
22.5 mg/5 ml-9 mg/5 ml,				
473 ml	**66813-0038-16**	198.05		
DYNEX HD (Athlon Pharm)				
gg/hydrocod bit/pse hcl				
SYR, PO (GRAPE)				
480 ml, C-III	**66813-0933-16**	94.30		
DYNEX LA (Athlon Pharm)				
guaifenesin/phenylephrine hydrochloride				
TER, PO, 800 mg-30 mg,				
100s ea	**66813-0036-01**	147.11		
DYNEX VR (Athlon Pharm)				
carbetapentane citrate/guaifenesin				
C12, PO, 30 mg-400 mg,				
100s ea	**66813-0034-01**	116.08		
DYPHYLLINE				
(Lunsco) *See DYLIX*				
(Meda) *See LUFYLLIN*				
(Meda) *See LUFYLLIN-400*				
(PCCA)				
POW, NA, 1 gm	**51927-1659-00**	1.38		
(Spectrum Pharmacy)				
POW, NA (1X25GM)				
25 gm	**49452-2589-01**	107.80		
(1X100GM)				
100 gm	**49452-2589-02**	360.50		
(1X500GM)				
500 gm	**49452-2589-03**	892.50		
DYPHYLLINE GG (Cypress Pharm)				
dyphylline/guaifenesin				
TAB, PO (USP)				
200 mg-200 mg,				
100s ea	**60258-0336-01**	67.99		
DYPHYLLINE GG ES (Breckenridge Pharm)				
dyphylline/guaifenesin				
TAB, PO, 200 mg-300 mg,				
100s ea	**51991-0536-01**	77.87		
DYPHYLLINE-GG (Cypress Pharm)				
dyphylline/guaifenesin				
ELI, PO (WINE)				
473 ml	**60258-0335-16**	15.95		
(Silarx)				
ELI, PO, 473 ml	**54838-0513-80**	15.95		
DYPHYLLINE/GG (Breckenridge Pharm)				
dyphylline/guaifenesin				
TAB, PO, 200 mg-200 mg,				
100s ea	**51991-0375-01**	68.95		
DYPHYLLINE/GUAIFENESIN				
(Breckenridge Pharm) *See DYPHYLLINE GG ES*				
(Breckenridge Pharm) *See DYPHYLLINE/GG*				
(Carwin) *See COPD*				
(Cypress Pharm) *See DY-G*				
(Cypress Pharm) *See DYPHYLLINE GG*				
(Cypress Pharm) *See DYPHYLLINE-GG*				
(JayMac Pharma) *See JAY-PHYL*				
(Meda) *See LUFYLLIN-GG*				
(Pharmakon) *See JAY-PHYL*				
(Poly) *See DILEX-G 200*				
(Poly) *See DILEX-G 400*				
(Silarx) *See DYPHYLLINE-GG*				
(SJ) *See DIFIL G FORTE*				
(SJ) *See DIFIL-G 400*				
(SJ) *See DIFIL-G FORTE*				

PROD/MFR	NDC	AWP	DP	OBC
DYRENIUM (Wellspring Pharm)				
triamterene				
CAP, PO, 50 mg, 100s ea	**65197-0002-01**	133.08		
100 mg, 100s ea	**65197-0003-01**	231.00		
(Phys Total Care)				
REPACK				
CAP, PO, 100 mg, 10s ea	**54868-5092-01**	24.51		
30s ea	**54868-5092-00**	69.77		
(Southwood)				
REPACK				
CAP, PO, 100 mg, 30s ea	**58016-0087-30**	58.47		
60s ea	**58016-0087-60**	116.93		
90s ea	**58016-0087-90**	175.40		
100s ea	**58016-0087-00**	194.89		
DYSPORT (Tercica)				
abobotulinumtoxina				
PDS, IM, 500 u, ea	**15054-0500-01**	852.00		
DYTAN (Hawthorn Pharm)				
diphenhydramine tannate				
CTB, PO (BERRY)				
25 mg, 60s ea	**63717-0571-06**	82.49		
SUS, PO, 25 mg/5 ml,				
120 ml	**63717-0570-04**	34.38		
DYTAN-AT (Hawthorn Pharm)				
carbetapentane tannate/diphenhydramine tannate				
SUS, PO (COTTON CANDY)				
30 mg/5 ml-25 mg/5 ml,				
118 ml	**63717-0590-04**	49.99		
DYTAN-CD (Hawthorn Pharm)				
cough/cold combination				
SUS, PO (STRAWBERRY)				
118 ml	**63717-0585-04**	43.74		
DYTAN-CS (Hawthorn Pharm)				
cough/cold combination				
SUS, PO (BANANA-STRAWBERRY)				
118 ml	**63717-0580-04**	45.39		
TER, PO (AF,SF,DYE-FREE)				
30 mg-25 mg-10 mg,				
60s ea	**63717-0581-06**	108.14		
DYTAN-D (Hawthorn Pharm)				
diphenhydramine tannate/phenylephrine tannate				
CTB, PO (BERRY)				
25 mg-10 mg,				
60s ea	**63717-0577-06**	94.89		
SUS, PO (BUBBLEGUM)				
25 mg/5 ml-7.5 mg/5 ml,				
118 ml	**63717-0576-04**	54.99		
DYTAN-DM (Hawthorn Pharm)				
dm tan/diphenhydramine tannate/phenyleph tan				
SUS, PO (BLACK CHERRY)				
118 ml	**63717-0591-04**	49.99		
DYTAN-HC (Hawthorn Pharm)				
cough/cold combination				
SUS, PO (AF,SF,GRAPE)				
118 ml, C-III	**63717-0710-04**	66.89		
DYTUSS (Lunsco)				
diphenhydramine hydrochloride				
SYR, PO, 12.5 mg/5 ml,				
480 ml	**10892-0112-65**	4.20		
E-Z SPACER (FSC Laboratories)				
spacer, inhalation				
DEV, NA (SINGLE-PATIENT USE)				
ea	**13551-0601-01**	36.00		
E-Z SPACER & MASK COMBO (Dexo)				
spacer, inhalation				
DEV, NA (DRUG DEL. SYSTEM W/MASK)				
ea	**59196-0029-01**	27.60		
E-Z SPACER MASK (Dexo)				
mask, face				
DEV, NA (SMALL)				
ea	**59196-0020-01**	8.40		
E-Z-DISK (E-Z-EM)				
barium sulfate				
TAB, PO, 648 mg, 100s ea	**10361-0778-01**	268.84	224.03	
E.E.S. 200 (Nucare Pharm)				
REPACK				
erythromycin ethylsuccinate				
SUS, PO, 200 mg/5 ml,				
100 ml	**66267-0927-00**	18.29		**AB**
(Quality Care Prod)				
REPACK				
SUS, PO, 200 mg/5 ml,				
100 ml	**49999-0516-00**	9.97		**AB**
E.E.S. 400 FILMTAB (Abbott Pharm)				
erythromycin ethylsuccinate				
TAB, PO, 400 mg, 100s ea	**00074-5729-13**	25.30	22.19	**AB**

PROD/MFR	NDC	AWP	DP	OBC
(A-S Medication)				
REPACK				
TAB, PO, 400 mg, 40s ea	**54569-0127-03**	10.78		**AB**
(Dispensing Solutions)				
REPACK				
TAB, PO, 400 mg, 30s ea	**66336-0617-30**	17.52		**AB**
40s ea	**66336-0617-40**	23.36		**AB**
(Nucare Pharm)				
REPACK				
TAB, PO, 400 mg, 28s ea	**66267-0086-28**	16.89		**AB**
40s ea	**66267-0086-40**	23.59		**AB**
(PD-Rx Pharm)				
REPACK				
TAB, PO (USP)				
400 mg, 6s ea	**43063-0110-06**	5.79		**AB**
(Phys Total Care)				
REPACK				
TAB, PO, 400 mg, 20s ea	**54868-0333-07**	7.91		**AB**
30s ea	**54868-0333-01**	10.94		**AB**
40s ea	**54868-0333-02**	13.95		**AB**
50s ea	**54868-0333-04**	16.98		**AB**
60s ea	**54868-0333-06**	19.99		**AB**
(Quality Care Prod)				
REPACK				
TAB, PO, 400 mg, 28s ea	**49999-0080-28**	23.04		**AB**
30s ea	**49999-0080-30**	27.45		**AB**
40s ea	**49999-0080-40**	36.80		**AB**
(Southwood)				
REPACK				
TAB, PO, 400 mg, 12s ea	**58016-0167-12**	2.59		**AB**
15s ea	**58016-0167-15**	3.24		**AB**
20s ea	**58016-0167-20**	4.68		**AB**
30s ea	**58016-0167-30**	7.02		**AB**
40s ea	**58016-0167-40**	9.36		**AB**
60s ea	**58016-0167-60**	14.04		**AB**
90s ea	**58016-0167-90**	21.06		**AB**
100s ea	**58016-0167-00**	23.40		**AB**
E.E.S. GRANULE (Quality Care Prod)				
REPACK				
erythromycin ethylsuccinate				
PDR, PO, 200 mg/5 ml,				
100 ml	**49999-0810-00**	16.48		
E.E.S. GRANULES (Abbott Pharm)				
erythromycin ethylsuccinate				
PDR, PO, 200 mg/5 ml,				
100 ml	**00074-6369-02**	9.12	8.00	**AB**
200 ml	**00074-6369-10**	16.99	14.90	**AB**
(A-S Medication)				
REPACK				
PDR, PO (1X100ML)				
200 mg/5 ml,				
100 ml	**54569-0126-00**	9.23		**AB**
(Phys Total Care)				
REPACK				
PDR, PO, 200 mg/5 ml,				
200 ml	**54868-1146-00**	17.68		**AB**
E.S.P (Altura)				
REPACK				
erythromycin ethylsuccinate/sulfisoxazole acetyl				
PDR, PO, 200 mg/5 ml-600 mg/5 ml,				
100 ml	**63874-0156-10**	16.86		
150 ml	**63874-0156-15**	20.95		
200 ml	**63874-0156-20**	28.83		
E.S.P. (Teva)				
erythromycin ethylsuccinate/sulfisoxazole acetyl				
PDR, PO (USP)				
200 mg/5 ml-600 mg/5 ml,				
100 ml	**51285-0445-22**	19.37		**AB**
150 ml	**51285-0445-21**	28.79		**AB**
200 ml	**51285-0445-23**	37.79		**AB**
(A-S Medication)				
REPACK				
PDR, PO (1X100ML)				
200 mg/5 ml-600 mg/5 ml,				
100 ml	**54569-6083-00**	19.37		**AB**
(1X200ML)				
200 mg/5 ml-600 mg/5 ml,				
200 ml	**54569-6084-00**	37.79		**AB**
(Physician Partner)				
REPACK				
PDR, PO, 200 mg/5 ml-600 mg/5 ml,				
100 ml	**21695-0690-00**	17.75		**AB**

PROD/MFR NDC AWP DP OBC

EAR DROPS (A-S Medication)
REPACK
antipyrine/benzocaine
SOL, OT, 54 mg/ml-14 mg/ml,
15 ml.............. **54569-2113-00** 16.72

(Southwood)
REPACK
SOL, OT, 54 mg/ml-14 mg/ml,
10 ml.............. **58016-6444-01** 5.05

EAR WAX DROPS (Physician Partner)
REPACK
carbamide peroxide
SOL, OT, 6.5%, 15 ml **21695-0334-15** 14.96

EASIVENT MASK (Dey, L.P.)
mask, face
DEV, NA (LARGE)
ea................... **49502-0208-03** 8.63
(MEDIUM)
ea................... **49502-0208-02** 8.63
(SMALL)
ea................... **49502-0208-01** 8.63

EASIVENT VALVED HOLDING CHAMBER (Dey, L.P.)
spacer, inhalation
DEV, NA (RETAIL)
ea................... **49502-0207-01** 19.55
(HOSPITAL)
25s ea............... **49502-0207-25** 460.00

EASPRIN (Rosedale)
aspirin
ECT, PO, 975 mg, 100s ea . **10802-9757-01** 59.15

EC NAPROSYN (Roche Labs)
naproxen
ECT, PO (BOTTLE,CAPLET)
375 mg, 100s ea ..... **00004-6415-01** 178.99 AB
500 mg, 100s ea ..... **00004-6416-01** 218.59 AB

(PD-Rx Pharm)
REPACK
ECT, PO (CAPLET)
500 mg, 14s ea ...... **55289-0693-14** 37.20 AB
15s ea............ **55289-0693-15** 39.50 AB
30s ea............ **55289-0693-30** 74.00 AB

(Pharma Pac)
REPACK
ECT, PO (BOTTLE,CAPLET)
500 mg, 30s ea ...... **52959-0456-30** 68.58 AB
40s ea............ **52959-0456-40** 87.59 AB
60s ea............ **52959-0456-60** 119.88 AB

EC NAPROXEN (Dispensing Solutions)
REPACK
naproxen
ECT, PO, 375 mg, 15s ea .. **55045-3046-06** 27.00
60s ea............ **55045-3046-07** 108.00

ECALLANTIDE
(Dyax) *See KALBITOR*

ECHINACEA ANGUSTIFOLIAE (PCCA)
TIN, NA, 1 ml............. **51927-3461-00** 0.30

ECHINACEA PURPUREA ROOT (Gallipot)
POW, NA, 500 gm......... **51552-0833-06** 77.00 55.00

(PCCA)
POW, NA, 1 gm........... **51927-3036-00** 1.09

ECHINACEA ROOT (PCCA)
POW, NA (ANGUSTIFOLIA)
1 gm................. **51927-2966-00** 1.09

ECHOTHIOPHATE IODIDE
(Wyeth) *See PHOSPHOLINE IODIDE*

ECONAZOLE NITRATE (Fougera)
CRE, TP, 1%, 15 gm....... **00168-0312-15** 17.50 AB
30 gm............ **00168-0312-30** 30.92 AB
85 gm............ **00168-0312-85** 63.06 AB

(Medisca)
POW, NA (U.S.P.)
5 gm................ **38779-0789-03** 38.85
25 gm............... **38779-0789-04** 141.00
100 gm.............. **38779-0789-05** 447.00
500 gm.............. **38779-0789-08** 1275.00
1000 gm............. **38779-0789-09** 2065.50

(PCCA)
POW, NA (U.S.P.)
1 gm................ **51927-2658-00** 10.80

(Perrigo)
CRE, TP, 1%, 15 gm....... **45802-0466-35** 19.65
30 gm............ **45802-0466-11** 34.70
85 gm............ **45802-0466-53** 70.80

(Prasco Labs)
CRE, TP, 1%, 15 gm....... **66993-0879-15** 17.50 AB
30 gm............ **66993-0879-31** 30.92 AB
85 gm............ **66993-0879-85** 63.06 AB

(Spectrum Pharmacy)
POW, NA (B.P.)
5 gm................ **49452-2699-01** 74.90
25 gm............... **49452-2699-02** 211.75
100 gm.............. **49452-2699-03** 658.00

(Taro) *See ECONAZOLE NITRATE 1%*

(Altura)
REPACK
CRE, TP, 1%, 15 gm....... **63874-0854-15** 16.28
30 gm............ **63874-0854-30** 28.76

(Physician Partner)
REPACK
CRE, TP (1X15GM)
1%, 15 gm........... **21695-0892-15** 39.30
(1X30GM)
1%, 30 gm........... **21695-0892-30** 69.40
(1X85GM)
1%, 85 gm........... **21695-0892-85** 141.60

(Quality Care Prod)
REPACK
CRE, TP (1X30GM)
1%, 30 gm........... **35356-0191-30** 40.60 AB

ECONAZOLE NITRATE 1% (Taro)
econazole nitrate
CRE, TP, 1%, 15 gm....... **51672-1303-01** 17.60
30 gm............ **51672-1303-02** 30.93
85 gm............ **51672-1303-08** 63.06

(A-S Medication)
REPACK
CRE, TP, 1%, 30 gm....... **54569-5708-00** 30.93

(Phys Total Care)
REPACK
CRE, TP, 1%, 30 gm....... **54868-5042-00** 36.45

(Quality Care Prod)
REPACK
CRE, TP, 1%, 15 gm....... **49999-0299-15** 26.66

ECONOPRED PLUS (Phys Total Care)
REPACK
prednisolone acetate
SUS, OP, 1%, 5 ml........ **54868-1152-00** 37.36 AB
10 ml............. **54868-1152-01** 60.51 AB

ECULIZUMAB
(Alexion Pharmaceuticals) *See SOLIRIS*

ECZEMOL (Loma Lux)
kali bromatum/niccolum sulphuricum/sulfur
TAB, PO, 1 x-1 x-1 x,
100s ea........... **61480-0127-05** 81.25

ED A-HIST (Edwards)
cpm/phenyleph hcl
LIQ, PO (GRAPE)
4 mg/5 ml-10 mg/5 ml,
473 ml **00485-0055-16** 19.00
TER, PO (CAPLET)
8 mg-20 mg,
100s ea........... **00485-0054-01** 27.00

ED CHLORPED (Edwards)
chlorpheniramine tannate
SUS, PO (DROPS,COTTON CANDY)
2 mg/ml, 60 ml......... **00485-0074-02** 21.00

ED CHLORPED D (Edwards)
chlorpheniramine tannate/phenylephrine tannate
SUS, PO (APPLE SAUCE,DROPS)
2 mg/ml-6 mg/ml,
60 ml............. **00485-0076-02** 40.00

ED CYTE F (Edwards)
docusate sodium/ferrous fumarate/folic acid
TAB, PO (FILM-COATED)
50 mg-324 mg-1 mg,
100s ea........... **00485-0065-01** 18.00

ED-A-HIST DM (Edwards)
cpm/dm/phenyleph hcl
SOL, PO (AF,SF,BANANA)
473 ml **00485-0071-16** 32.75

ED-BRON G (Edwards)
guaifenesin/theophylline sodium glycinate
LIQ, PO (ORANGE)
473 ml **00485-0059-16** 28.00

ED-CHLOR-TAN (Edwards)
chlorpheniramine tannate
TAB, PO, 8 mg, 100s ea ... **00485-0072-01** 60.00

ED-FLEX (Edwards)
apap/phenyltoloxamine cit/salicylamide
CAP, PO, 300 mg-20 mg-200 mg,
100s ea........... **00485-0066-01** 45.00

EDECRIN (Aton)
ethacrynic acid
TAB, PO, 25 mg, 100s ea .. **25010-0205-15** 296.16

EDECRIN SODIUM (Aton)
ethacrynate sodium
PDS, IV, 50 mg, ea........ **00006-3620-50** 118.75

EDETATE ACID (PCCA)
edetic acid
POW, NA (EDTA)
1 gm................ **51927-1431-00** 0.36

EDETATE CALCIUM DISODIUM (Amend)
POW, NA (U.S.P.)
4540 gm............. **17317-2409-02** 182.00

(Gallipot)
POW, NA (U.S.P.,F.C.C.)
100 gm.............. **51552-0435-05** 24.50

(Graceway) *See CALCIUM DISODIUM VERSENATE*

(PCCA)
POW, NA (USP, HYDRATE)
1 gm................ **51927-2059-00** 0.60

(Spectrum Pharmacy)
POW, NA (U.S.P.)
125 gm.............. **49452-2697-01** 67.90
500 gm.............. **49452-2697-02** 190.40
2500 gm............. **49452-2697-03** 735.00

EDETATE DISODIUM
(Amend) *See EDETATE DISODIUM DIHYDRATE*

(Amend)
POW, NA (A.C.S., REAGENT)
125 gm.............. **17317-1485-04** 10.00
454 gm.............. **17317-1565-01** 14.00
(A.C.S., REAGENT)
500 gm.............. **17317-1485-01** 30.80
2270 gm............. **17317-1565-05** 49.00
(A.C.S., REAGENT)
2500 gm............. **17317-1485-05** 105.00
11350 gm **17317-1565-08** 175.00

(Baker, J.T.)
CRY, NA (U.S.P.)
500 gm.............. **10106-8994-01** 56.94

(Consolidated Midland)
SOL, IV (VIAL)
150 mg/ml, 20 ml .... **00223-7494-20** 9.95 EE

(Gallipot)
POW, NA (U.S.P.)
454 gm.............. **51552-0588-06** 69.58

(Hospira) *See ENDRATE*

(Letco)
POW, NA (U.S.P./N.F.)
100 gm.............. **62991-2026-02** 27.00
500 gm.............. **62991-2026-03** 51.00
(DIHYDRATE)
1000 gm............. **62991-2026-04** 81.00

(Mallinckrodt Lab)
POW, NA (U.S.P.)
500 gm.............. **00406-1395-04** 101.74

(Medisca)
POW, NA (USP,1X100GM)
100 gm.............. **38779-0545-05** 24.00
(USP,1X500GM)
500 gm.............. **38779-0545-08** 58.50
(USP,1X1000GM)
1000 gm............. **38779-0545-09** 87.00
(USP,1X2500GM)
2500 gm............. **38779-0545-01** 202.50
(USP,1X5000GM)
5000 gm............. **38779-0545-03** 375.00
(USP,1X25000GM)
25000 gm **38779-0545-07** 1305.00

(PCCA)
POW, NA (USP; DIHYDRATE)
1 gm................ **51927-1317-00** 1.32

(Spectrum Pharmacy) *See EDETATE DISODIUM DIHYDRATE*

EDETATE DISODIUM DIHYDRATE (Amend)
edetate disodium
POW, NA (U.S.P.)
454 gm.............. **17317-0829-01** 21.00
2270 gm............. **17317-0829-05** 91.00
11350 gm **17317-0829-08** 315.00

PROD/MFR NDC AWP DP OBC

(Spectrum Pharmacy)
POW, NA (U.S.P.)
125 gm 49452-2702-03 54.25
500 gm 49452-2702-01 92.75
2500 gm 49452-2702-02 402.50

EDETATE SODIUM
(PCCA) *See EDETATE TETRASODIUM*

(Spectrum Pharmacy) *See ETHYLENEDIAMINETE-TRAACETIC ACID TETRASODIUM SALT*

EDETATE TETRASODIUM (PCCA)
edetate sodium
POW, NA (TETRAHYDRATE)
1 gm 51927-1664-00 0.36

EDETATE TRISODIUM (PCCA)
POW, NA, 1 gm 51927-2403-00 0.45

EDETIC ACID
(Baker, J.T.) *See EDTA*

(Baker, J.T.) *See EDTA DISODIUM SALT*

(Baker, J.T.) *See EDTA DISODIUM SALT DIHYDRATE 0.1M*

(Baker, J.T.) *See EDTA STANDARD*

(Medisca) *See ETHYLENE DIAMINE TETRA ACETIC ACID*

(Medisca)
POW, NA (1X100GM)
100 gm 38779-0169-05 58.50
(1X500GM)
500 gm 38779-0169-08 208.50
(1X1000GM)
1000 gm 38779-0169-09 367.50

(PCCA) *See EDETATE ACID*

(Spectrum Pharmacy) *See ETHYLENEDIAMINETE-TRAACETIC ACID*

(Spectrum Pharmacy)
POW, NA (N.F.)
100 gm 49452-2703-01 88.55
500 gm 49452-2703-02 199.15

EDEX (UCB)
alprostadil
KIT, MR (2 CARTRIDGES)
10 mcg, ea .... 00091-1110-16 69.98 AP
(6 CARTRIDGES)
10 mcg, ea .... 00091-1110-20 209.96 AP
(2 CARTRIDGES)
20 mcg, ea .... 00091-1120-16 90.16 AP
(6 CARTRIDGES)
20 mcg, ea .... 00091-1120-20 270.48 AP
(2 CARTRIDGES)
40 mcg, ea .... 00091-1140-16 123.53 AP
(6 CARTRIDGES)
40 mcg, ea .... 00091-1140-20 370.60 AP

EDLUAR (Meda)
zolpidem tartrate
TAB, SL, 5 mg,
30s ea, C-IV .... 00037-6050-30 150.00 120.00 EE
10 mg,
30s ea, C-IV .... 00037-6010-30 150.00 120.00 EE

EDROPHONIUM CHLORIDE
(Bioniche Pharma) *See ENLON*

EDTA (Baker, J.T.)
edetic acid
POW, NA (A.C.S., REAGENT)
500 gm 10106-8991-01 121.75

EDTA DISODIUM SALT (Baker, J.T.)
edetic acid
CRY, NA (ULTRAPURE BIOREAGENT)
100 gm 10106-4040-00 33.11
(A.C.S,REAGENT,DIHYDRATE)
500 gm 10106-8993-01 130.40
(ULTRAPURE BIOREAGENT)
500 gm 10106-4040-01 80.70
1000 gm 10106-4040-04 111.24
5000 gm 10106-4040-06 375.33
(A.C.S,REAGENT,DIHYDRATE)
12000 gm 10106-8993-07 1163.85

EDTA DISODIUM SALT DIHYDRATE 0.1M (Baker, J.T.)
edetic acid
SOL, NA (REAGENT, VOLUMETRIC)
1000 ml 10106-5632-02 45.53

EDTA STANDARD (Baker, J.T.)
edetic acid
SOL, NA (REAGENT)
1000 ml 10106-5648-02 24.41
4000 ml 10106-5648-03 49.13
20000 ml 10106-5648-07 144.25

EEMT (Creekwood Pharma)
esterified estrogens/methyltestosterone
TAB, PO (FILM-COATED)
1.25 mg-2.5 mg,
100s ea 15310-0010-01 192.95

EEMT HS (Creekwood Pharma)
esterified estrogens/methyltestosterone
TAB, PO (FILM-COATED)
0.625 mg-1.25 mg,
100s ea 15310-0020-01 157.95

EFAVIRENZ
(B/M Squibb Onc/Vir) *See SUSTIVA*

EFAVIRENZ/EMTRICITABINE/ TENOFOVIR DISOPROXIL FUM
(Bristol-Myers Squibb) *See ATRIPLA*

EFFER-K (Nomax)
citric acid/potassium bicarbonate
TEF, PO (CHERRY VANILLA)
10 meq, 30s ea 51801-0014-30 12.60
(DYE-FREE,UNFLAVORED)
10 meq, 30s ea 51801-0013-30 12.60
20 meq, 30s ea 51801-0011-30 15.00
(ORANGE CREAM)
20 meq, 30s ea 51801-0012-30 15.00
(CHERRY BERRY)
25 meq, 30s ea 51801-0006-30 6.64 5.31
(LEMON CITRUS)
25 meq, 30s ea 51801-0005-30 6.64 5.31
(LIME,ORANGE)
25 meq, 30s ea 51801-0002-30 6.64 5.31
(ORANGE,ORANGE)
25 meq, 30s ea 51801-0001-30 6.64 5.31
(UNFLAVORED)
25 meq, 30s ea 51801-0007-30 6.64 5.31
(ORANGE,ORANGE)
25 meq, 100s ea 51801-0001-40 21.80 17.50

EFFERVESCENT POTASSIUM (TOWER)
potassium bicarbonate/potassium citrate
TEF, PO (ORANGE)
25 meq, 30s ea 50201-2400-02 10.47
100s ea 50201-2400-04 27.96
250s ea 50201-2400-06 69.23

EFFERVESCENT POTASSIUM/CHLORIDE (TOWER)
potassium bicarbonate/potassium chloride
TEF, PO (FRUIT PUNCH)
25 meq, 30s ea 50201-1300-02 23.81
100s ea 50201-1300-04 75.16
250s ea 50201-1300-06 176.99

EFFEXOR (Wyeth)
venlafaxine hydrochloride
TAB, PO, 50 mg, 30s ea ... 00008-0703-07 76.49 63.74

(A-S Medication)
REPACK
TAB, PO, 37.5 mg, 30s ea .. 54569-4131-01 77.32

(Altura)
REPACK
TAB, PO, 37.5 mg, 60s ea .. 63874-1130-06 133.80
75 mg, 10s ea 63874-0599-10 24.20
14s ea 63874-0599-14 33.88
15s ea 63874-0599-15 36.30
20s ea 63874-0599-20 48.40
21s ea 63874-0599-21 50.82
28s ea 63874-0599-28 67.76
30s ea 63874-0599-30 72.60
40s ea 63874-0599-40 96.80
50s ea 63874-0599-50 121.00
60s ea 63874-0599-60 145.20
90s ea 63874-0599-90 217.80
100s ea 63874-0599-01 242.00

(Core)
REPACK
TAB, PO, 37.5 mg, 30s ea .. 33358-0124-30 96.71
60s ea 33358-0124-60 194.32
90s ea 33358-0124-90 290.98
75 mg, 30s ea 33358-0125-30 113.11
60s ea 33358-0125-60 214.75
90s ea 33358-0125-90 318.28

(DHS, Inc.)
REPACK
TAB, PO, 75 mg, 30s ea ... 55887-0660-30 114.99

(Dispensing Solutions)
REPACK
TAB, PO, 25 mg, 30s ea ... 55045-3088-08 57.50
37.5 mg, 60s ea 55045-3220-09 153.00
75 mg, 30s ea 55045-3387-08 78.00

(PD-Rx Pharm)
REPACK
TAB, PO, 75 mg, 30s ea ... 55289-0830-30 125.86

(Pharma Pac)
REPACK
TAB, PO, 75 mg, 30s ea ... 52959-0818-30 104.10
60s ea 52959-0818-60 208.19

(Phys Total Care)
REPACK
TAB, PO, 37.5 mg, 10s ea .. 54868-3414-04 30.14
20s ea 54868-3414-02 61.73
30s ea 54868-3414-00 91.66
60s ea 54868-3414-03 171.48
90s ea 54868-3414-05 256.28
100s ea 54868-3414-01 284.54
75 mg, 10s ea 54868-3523-03 31.30
30s ea 54868-3523-01 89.54
60s ea 54868-3523-00 168.01
100s ea 54868-3523-02 278.57

(Quality Care Prod)
REPACK
TAB, PO, 37.5 mg, 30s ea .. 49999-0595-30 86.25
75 mg, 30s ea 49999-0596-30 122.47

(Southwood)
REPACK
TAB, PO, 25 mg, 10s ea ... 58016-0350-10 24.03
14s ea 58016-0350-14 33.64
15s ea 58016-0350-15 36.05
20s ea 58016-0350-20 48.06
20s ea 58016-0350-21 50.47
28s ea 58016-0350-28 67.29
40s ea 58016-0350-40 96.13
50s ea 58016-0350-50 120.16
37.5 mg, 10s ea 58016-0349-10 24.74
14s ea 58016-0349-14 34.64
15s ea 58016-0349-15 37.11
20s ea 58016-0349-20 49.48
21s ea 58016-0349-21 51.96
30s ea 58016-0349-30 74.23
40s ea 58016-0349-40 98.97
50s ea 58016-0349-50 123.71
60s ea 58016-0349-60 148.45
90s ea 58016-0349-90 222.68
100s ea 58016-0349-00 247.42
50 mg, 10s ea 58016-0351-10 25.50
14s ea 58016-0351-14 35.70
15s ea 58016-0351-15 38.25
20s ea 58016-0351-20 50.99
21s ea 58016-0351-21 53.54
28s ea 58016-0351-28 71.39
30s ea 58016-0351-30 76.49
40s ea 58016-0351-40 101.99
50s ea 58016-0351-50 127.48
60s ea 58016-0351-60 152.98
90s ea 58016-0351-90 229.47
100s ea 58016-0351-00 254.97
75 mg, 10s ea 58016-0323-10 27.02
14s ea 58016-0323-14 37.83
15s ea 58016-0323-15 40.54
20s ea 58016-0323-20 54.05
21s ea 58016-0323-21 56.75
28s ea 58016-0323-28 75.67
30s ea 58016-0323-30 81.07
40s ea 58016-0323-40 108.09
50s ea 58016-0323-50 102.88
60s ea 58016-0323-60 162.14
90s ea 58016-0323-90 243.21
100s ea 58016-0323-00 270.23
100 mg, 10s ea 58016-0352-10 17.32
14s ea 58016-0352-14 24.25
15s ea 58016-0352-15 25.98
20s ea 58016-0220-20 57.28
20s ea 58016-0352-20 34.64
21s ea 58016-0352-21 36.37
28s ea 58016-0352-28 48.58
30s ea 58016-0220-30 85.92
30s ea 58016-0352-30 51.96
40s ea 58016-0352-40 69.28
50s ea 58016-0352-50 86.60
60s ea 58016-0220-60 171.84
60s ea 58016-0352-60 103.92
90s ea 58016-0220-90 257.76
90s ea 58016-0352-90 155.88
100s ea 58016-0220-00 286.40
100s ea 58016-0352-00 173.20

(Stat Rx)
REPACK
TAB, PO, 37.5 mg, 30s ea .. 16590-0083-30 72.75
60s ea 16590-0083-60 145.50
75 mg, 30s ea 16590-0084-30 85.50
60s ea 16590-0084-60 171.00

PROD/MFR	NDC	AWP	DP	OBC
EFFEXOR XR (Advanced Pharm Serv, Inc.) REPACK				
venlafaxine hydrochloride				
CER, PO, 37.5 mg, 10s ea	13411-0109-01	47.21		
60s ea	13411-0109-06	258.27		
90s ea	13411-0109-09	402.91		
100s ea	13411-0109-10	427.12		
75 mg, 10s ea	13411-0110-01	74.60		
60s ea	13411-0110-06	324.21		
90s ea	13411-0110-09	491.31		
100s ea	13411-0110-10	540.35		
(Core) REPACK				
CER, PO, 150 mg, 30s ea	33358-0123-30	126.40		
60s ea	33358-0123-60	231.29		
90s ea	33358-0123-90	352.56		
(Direct Pharmaceutical, Inc.) REPACK				
CER, PO, 37.5 mg,				
30s ea UD	67801-0321-03	208.70		
75 mg, 30s ea UD	67801-0411-03	270.80		
150 mg, 30s ea UD	67801-0312-03	233.88		
(Dispensing Solutions) REPACK				
CER, PO, 75 mg, 90s ea	55045-3196-09	382.50		
(Keltman Pharma., Inc.) REPACK				
CER, PO, 150 mg, 15s ea	68387-0349-15	85.63		
30s ea	68387-0349-30	171.25		
(Pharma Pac) REPACK				
CER, PO, 37.5 mg, 60s ea	52959-0771-60	188.95		
(Phys Total Care) REPACK				
CER, PO, 75 mg, 100s ea	54868-4253-04	595.82		
(Physician Partner) REPACK				
CER, PO, 37.5 mg, 15s ea	21695-0045-15	134.05		
75 mg, 15s ea	21695-0046-15	174.86		
15s ea	21695-0096-15	135.24		
15s ea	21695-0296-15	156.08		
30s ea	21695-0046-30	311.04		
45s ea	21695-0046-45	431.68		
45s ea	21695-0296-45	450.90		
60s ea	21695-0046-60	489.24		
90s ea	21695-0046-90	933.12		
150 mg, 15s ea	21695-0047-15	190.46		
45s ea	21695-0047-45	490.86		
(Quality Care Prod) REPACK				
CER, PO, 150 mg, 30s ea	49999-0599-30	261.50		
60s ea	49999-0599-60	540.00		
(Stat Rx) REPACK				
CER, PO, 75 mg, 30s ea	16590-0486-30	131.00		
60s ea	16590-0486-60	231.00		
90s ea	16590-0486-90	390.00		
120s ea	16590-0486-72	504.00		
150 mg, 90s ea	16590-0487-90	390.75		
120s ea	16590-0487-72	520.00		
EFFEXOR-XR (Wyeth)				
venlafaxine hydrochloride				
CER, PO (UNIT-OF-USE)				
37.5 mg, 15s ea	00008-0837-20	69.38	57.82	
30s ea	00008-0837-21	138.78	115.65	
90s ea	00008-0837-22	416.38	346.98	
(REDIPAK,10X10)				
37.5 mg, 100s ea	00008-0837-03	462.61	385.51	
(UNIT-OF-USE)				
75 mg, 15s ea	00008-0833-20	77.76	64.80	
30s ea	00008-0833-21	155.52	129.60	
90s ea	00008-0833-22	466.56	388.80	
(REDIPAK,10X10)				
75 mg, 100s ea	00008-0833-03	518.40	432.00	
(UNIT-OF-USE)				
150 mg, 15s ea	00008-0836-20	84.70	70.58	
30s ea	00008-0836-21	169.40	141.17	
90s ea	00008-0836-22	508.20	423.50	
(REDIPAK,10X10)				
150 mg, 100s ea	00008-0836-03	564.65	470.54	
(A-S Medication) REPACK				
CER, PO, 75 mg, 30s ea	54569-4659-00	148.63		
150 mg, 30s ea	54569-5231-00	161.89		
(Advanced Pharm Serv, Inc.) REPACK				
CER, PO, 37.5 mg, 30s ea	13411-0109-03	131.60		
75 mg, 30s ea	13411-0110-03	167.10		

PROD/MFR	NDC	AWP	DP	OBC
(Aidarex) REPACK				
CER, PO, 75 mg, 30s ea	33261-0654-30	142.00		
60s ea	33261-0654-60	284.00		
90s ea	33261-0654-90	426.00		
120s ea	33261-0654-02	568.00		
(AQ) REPACK				
CER, PO, 37.5 mg,				
100s ea	66105-0111-10	447.06		
75 mg, 10s ea	66105-0112-01	54.03		
15s ea	66105-0112-15	81.05		
30s ea	66105-0112-03	162.11		
60s ea	66105-0112-06	324.21		
100s ea	66105-0112-10	540.35		
(DHS, Inc.) REPACK				
CER, PO, 37.5 mg, 60s ea	55887-0662-60	357.96		
75 mg, 60s ea	55887-0665-60	251.69		
120s ea	55887-0665-82	502.57		
150 mg, 30s ea	55887-0193-30	142.75		
60s ea	55887-0193-60	272.69		
(Dispensing Solutions) REPACK				
CER, PO, 75 mg, 30s ea	55045-3196-08	127.50		
60s ea	55045-3196-06	255.00		
150 mg, 30s ea	55045-3368-08	139.50		
(IPI) REPACK				
CER, PO, 75 mg, 60s ea	18837-0049-60	278.07		
150 mg, 90s ea	18837-0048-90	485.66		
(Nucare Pharm) REPACK				
CER, PO, 37.5 mg, 30s ea	68071-0333-30	128.44		
75 mg, 30s ea	68071-0322-30	160.59		
40s ea	68071-0322-40	210.05		
60s ea	68071-0322-60	315.07		
90s ea	68071-0322-90	446.56		
150 mg, 15s ea	68071-0412-15	131.50		
30s ea	68071-0412-30	174.91		
60s ea	68071-0412-60	315.00		
90s ea	68071-1314-00	496.59		
(Palmetto) REPACK				
CER, PO, 75 mg, 30s ea	23490-9012-01	120.00		
45s ea	23490-9012-00	180.00		
120s ea	23490-9012-02	480.00		
(PD-Rx Pharm) REPACK				
CER, PO, 37.5 mg, 30s ea	55289-0869-30	273.98		
30s ea	58864-0696-30	273.98		
75 mg, 30s ea	55289-0277-30	305.78		
(REDI-SCRIPT)				
75 mg, 30s ea	58864-0629-30	210.54		
150 mg, 30s ea	55289-0756-30	332.18		
30s ea	55289-0897-30	332.18		
(REDI-SCRIPT)				
150 mg, 30s ea	58864-0756-30	332.18		
(Pharma Pac) REPACK				
CER, PO, 75 mg, 30s ea	52959-0550-30	104.10		
60s ea	52959-0550-60	208.18		
150 mg, 30s ea	52959-0388-30	140.65		
60s ea	52959-0388-60	226.20		
(Phys Total Care) REPACK				
CER, PO, 37.5 mg, 10s ea	54868-4504-01	55.81		
30s ea	54868-4504-00	153.33		
75 mg, 10s ea	54868-4253-01	67.59		
30s ea	54868-4253-00	186.71		
60s ea	54868-4253-02	370.81		
90s ea	54868-4253-03	554.90		
150 mg, 10s ea	54868-4252-01	67.54		
30s ea	54868-4252-00	186.58		
60s ea	54868-4252-02	370.55		
90s ea	54868-4252-04	536.72		
100s ea	54868-4252-03	595.41		
(Quality Care Prod) REPACK				
CER, PO, 75 mg, 15s ea	49999-0249-15	116.00		
30s ea	49999-0249-30	248.00		
150 mg, 15s ea	49999-0599-15	132.50		
90s ea	49999-0599-90	793.70		
(Southwood) REPACK				
CER, PO, 37.5 mg, 30s ea	58016-0765-30	119.11		
60s ea	58016-0765-60	238.21		
90s ea	58016-0765-90	357.32		

PROD/MFR	NDC	AWP	DP	OBC
100s ea	58016-0765-00	397.02		
75 mg, 30s ea	58016-0615-30	133.47		
60s ea	58016-0615-60	266.94		
90s ea	58016-0615-90	400.41		
100s ea	58016-0615-00	444.90		
150 mg, 30s ea	58016-0616-30	145.38		
60s ea	58016-0616-60	290.76		
90s ea	58016-0616-90	436.14		
100s ea	58016-0616-00	484.60		
(Stat Rx) REPACK				
CER, PO, 37.5 mg, 28s ea	16590-0085-28	146.58		
30s ea	16590-0085-30	156.73		
60s ea	16590-0085-60	312.03		
75 mg, 30s ea	16590-0086-30	168.18		
56s ea	16590-0086-56	309.74		
60s ea	16590-0086-60	333.19		
90s ea	16590-0086-90	496.93		
150 mg, 30s ea	16590-0087-30	181.09		
30s ea	16590-0487-30	156.00		
56s ea	16590-0087-56	336.82		
60s ea	16590-0087-60	360.76		
60s ea	16590-0487-60	285.50		
90s ea	16590-0087-90	540.44		
EFFIENT (Lilly)				
prasugrel hydrochloride				
TAB, PO (FILM-COATED)				
5 mg, 7s ea	00002-4760-76	45.78	38.15	
30s ea	00002-4760-30	196.20	163.50	
10 mg, 30s ea	00002-4759-30	196.20	163.50	
90s ea	00002-4759-77	588.60	490.50	
EFLORNITHINE HYDROCHLORIDE (SkinMedica) *See VANIQA*				
EFUDEX (Valeant Pharm Intl)				
fluorouracil				
CRE, TP, 5%, 40 gm	00187-3204-47	428.19		
(Phys Total Care) REPACK				
CRE, TP, 5%, 25 gm	54868-0951-01	125.00		
40 gm	54868-0951-00	248.93		
EGCG (PCCA)				
epigallocatechin gallate				
POW, NA (1X1GM)				
1 gm	51927-3876-00	13.80		
EGGNOG (Medisca)				
flavoring aid				
SOL, NA (1X25ML)				
25 ml	38779-1258-04	22.50		
(1X100ML)				
100 ml	38779-1258-05	31.50		
(1X500ML)				
500 ml	38779-1258-08	105.00		
EGGNOG FLAVOR (PCCA)				
flavoring aid				
SOL, NA (ARTIFICIAL)				
1 ml	51927-2160-00	0.90		
ELAPRASE (Shire HGT, Inc.)				
idursulfase				
SOL, IV (PF)				
2 mg/ml, 3 ml	54092-0700-01	3153.84		
ELASTIN (Medisca)				
SOL, NA, 5 gm	38779-1259-03	28.50		
25 gm	38779-1259-04	135.00		
ELAVIL (Pharma Pac) REPACK				
amitriptyline hydrochloride				
TAB, PO, 10 mg, 30s ea	52959-0396-30	15.38		AB
(Phys Total Care) REPACK				
TAB, PO, 25 mg, 15s ea	54868-0409-00	11.56		AB
ELDEPRYL (Somerset)				
selegiline hydrochloride				
CAP, PO, 5 mg, 60s ea	39506-0022-60	178.20		AB
ELDERBERRY EXTRACT MALTODEXTRIN (PCCA)				
elderberry extract/maltodextrin				
POW, NA, 75%-25%, 1 gm	51927-3507-00	1.35		
ELDERBERRY EXTRACT/MALTODEXTRIN (PCCA) *See ELDERBERRY EXTRACT MALTODEXTRIN*				
ELDOPAQUE FORTE (Valeant Pharm Intl)				
hydroquinone				
CRE, TP, 4%, 28.35 gm	00187-0395-31	61.75		
ELDOQUIN FORTE (Valeant Pharm Intl)				
hydroquinone				
CRE, TP, 4%, 28.35 gm	00187-0394-31	61.75		

PROD/MFR	NDC	AWP	DP	OBC
(Phys Total Care)				
REPACK				
CRE, TP, 4%, 30 gm	54868-0953-00	47.38		
ELECTROLYTES				
(B. Braun) See *ISOLYTE S PH 7.4*				
ELECTROLYTES, ADENINE, AND INOSINE				
(enCyte) See *REJUVESOL*				
ELECTROLYTES/MULTIMINERAL				
(B. Braun) See *HYPERLITE*				
ELESTAT (Allergan Inc)				
epinastine hydrochloride				
SOL, OP, 0.05%, 5 ml	00023-9201-05	114.68		
(Phys Total Care)				
REPACK				
SOL, OP, 0.05%, 5 ml	54868-5563-00	99.27		
ELESTRIN (Azur Pharma, Inc.)				
estradiol				
GEL, TD (1X144GM)				
0.06%, 144 gm	18860-0490-02	157.49		
ELETONE (Ferndale)				
cream, multi ingredient				
CRE, TP, 100 gm	00496-0598-01	80.40		
ELETRIPTAN HYDROBROMIDE				
(Pfizer) See *RELPAX*				
ELEUTHEROCOCCUS SENTICOSUS (PCCA)				
ginseng, siberian				
POW, NA, 1 gm	51927-3231-00	0.15		
ELIDEL (Novartis Pharm)				
pimecrolimus				
CRE, TP, 1%, 30 gm	00078-0375-46	96.18		
60 gm	00078-0375-49	192.36		
100 gm	00078-0375-63	303.62		
(A-S Medication)				
REPACK				
CRE, TP, 1%, 30 gm	54569-5502-00	91.16		
(Phys Total Care)				
REPACK				
CRE, TP, 1%, 30 gm	54868-4878-00	122.51		
(1X60GM)				
1%, 60 gm	54868-4878-02	189.83		
100 gm	54868-4878-01	243.71		
(Quality Care Prod)				
REPACK				
CRE, TP (1X100GM)				
1%, 100 gm	35356-0223-00	515.29		
ELIGARD (Sanofi-Aventis)				
leuprolide acetate				
PI1, SC (SRN,PREFILLED,W/NDL)				
7.5 mg, ea	00024-0793-75	493.20		
PI3, SC, 22.5 mg, ea	00024-0222-05	1479.60		
PI4, SC (SINGLE-USE)				
30 mg, ea	00024-0610-30	1972.80		
PI6, SC (SINGLE-USE KIT)				
45 mg, ea	00024-0605-45	2959.20		
ELIPHOS (Hawthorn Pharm)				
calcium acetate				
TAB, PO, 667 mg, 200s ea	63717-0910-02	112.49		
ELITE OB WITH DHA (Trigen)				
prenatal vitamins				
SGL, PO (SOFTGEL)				
60s ea	13811-0029-60	99.29		
ELITE-OB (Trigen)				
multimineral/multivitamin				
TAB, PO (10X10,SF,GLUTEN-FREE)				
1000s ea UD	13811-0027-10	112.64		
ELITEK (Sanofi-Aventis)				
rasburicase				
PDS, IV (3 S.D.V. W/DILUENT,PF)				
1.5 mg, 3s ea	00024-5150-10	1844.78		
(SDV,W/DILUENT)				
7.5 mg, ea	00024-5151-75	3074.69		
ELIXOPHYLLIN (Forest Pharm)				
theophylline				
ELI, PO, 80 mg/15 ml,				
473 ml	00456-0644-16	91.25		AA
ELLENCE (Pfizer)				
epirubicin hydrochloride				
SOL, IV (S.D.V.,PF)				
2 mg/ml, 25 ml	00009-5091-01	755.17	629.31	
100 ml	00009-5093-01	3020.69	2517.24	
ELLIOTTS B (QOL Medical)				
dextrose and electrolytes				
SOL, IN (FOR INTRATHECAL USE,PF)				
10 ml 10s	67871-0007-10	470.59	126.30	

PROD/MFR	NDC	AWP	DP	OBC
ELM BARK (PCCA)				
slippery elm bark				
POW, NA (1X1GM)				
1 gm	51927-2030-00	0.56		
ELMIRON (Ortho-McNeil Pharm)				
pentosan polysulfate sodium				
CAP, PO (HARD GELATIN)				
100 mg, 100s ea	50458-0098-01	401.21	334.34	
(A-S Medication)				
REPACK				
CAP, PO, 100 mg, 90s ea	54569-5123-01	427.12		
(Phys Total Care)				
REPACK				
CAP, PO, 100 mg, 10s ea	54868-4525-02	48.37		
30s ea	54868-4525-01	139.88		
100s ea	54868-4525-00	434.10		
ELOCON (Schering)				
mometasone furoate				
CRE, TP, 0.1%, 15 gm	00085-0567-01	40.32		
45 gm	00085-0567-02	73.84		
LOT, TP, 0.1%, 30 ml	00085-0854-01	43.69		
60 ml	00085-0854-02	83.50		
OIN, TP, 0.1%, 15 gm	00085-0370-01	40.32		
45 gm	00085-0370-02	73.84		
(A-S Medication)				
REPACK				
CRE, TP, 0.1%, 45 gm	54569-2619-00	76.91		
OIN, TP, 0.1%, 15 gm	54569-5208-00	38.75		AB
(Dispensing Solutions)				
REPACK				
CRE, TP, 0.1%, 15 gm	55045-1572-05	32.00		
(Pharma Pac)				
REPACK				
CRE, TP, 0.1%, 15 gm	52959-0736-01	33.90		
45 gm	52959-0736-02	52.85		
(Phys Total Care)				
REPACK				
CRE, TP, 0.1%, 15 gm	54868-2223-00	52.50		
45 gm	54868-2223-01	94.51		
LOT, TP, 0.1%, 30 ml	54868-2224-00	30.75		
OIN, TP, 0.1%, 15 gm	54868-2225-00	37.89		AB
(Southwood)				
REPACK				
CRE, TP, 0.1%, 15 gm	58016-3241-01	40.32		
45 gm	58016-5605-01	73.84		
ELOXATIN (Sanofi-Aventis)				
oxaliplatin				
SOL, IV (S.D.V.,PF)				
5 mg/ml, 10 ml	00024-0590-10	1177.20		
20 ml	00024-0591-20	2354.39		
(SDV,PF)				
5 mg/ml, 40 ml	00024-0592-40	4708.76		
ELSPAR (Lundbeck)				
asparaginase				
PDS, IJ, 10000 iu, ea	67386-0411-51	70.42	52.73	
ELTROMBOPAG OLAMINE				
(Glaxo) See *PROMACTA*				
EMADINE (Alcon Ophthalmic)				
emedastine difumarate				
SOL, OP (DROP-TAINER)				
0.05%, 5 ml	00065-0325-05	77.88		
EMBEDA (King Pharm)				
morphine sulfate/naltrexone hydrochloride				
CER, PO, 20 mg-0.8 mg,				
100s ea, C-II	60793-0430-01	471.70		
30 mg-1.2 mg,				
100s ea, C-II	60793-0431-01	513.02		
50 mg-2 mg,				
100s ea, C-II	60793-0433-01	857.34		
60 mg-2.4 mg,				
100s ea, C-II	60793-0434-01	1026.05		
80 mg-3.2 mg,				
100s ea, C-II	60793-0435-01	1366.92		
100 mg-4 mg,				
100s ea, C-II	60793-0437-01	1714.67		
(Quality Care Prod)				
REPACK				
CER, PO, 20 mg-0.8 mg,				
30s ea, C-II	35356-0551-30	246.28		
30 mg-1.2 mg,				
30s ea, C-II	35356-0552-30	267.62		
60 mg-2.4 mg,				
30s ea, C-II	35356-0549-30	432.06		
100 mg-4 mg,				
30s ea, C-II	35356-0550-30	720.10		

PROD/MFR	NDC	AWP	DP	OBC
(Stat Rx)				
REPACK				
CER, PO, 20 mg-0.8 mg,				
30s ea, C-II	16590-0897-30	169.81		
60s ea, C-II	16590-0897-60	339.62		
EMBELINE SCALP APPLICATION (Altura)				
REPACK				
clobetasol propionate				
SOL, TP, 0.05%, 25 ml	63874-1161-05	32.56		
EMCYT (Pfizer)				
estramustine phosphate sodium				
CAP, PO (RX PAK)				
140 mg, 100s ea	00013-0132-02	642.05	535.04	
EMEDASTINE DIFUMARATE				
(Alcon Ophthalmic) See *EMADINE*				
EMEND (Merck)				
aprepitant				
CAP, PO (COMBO PACK)				
3s ea	00006-3862-03	390.97		
40 mg, ea	00006-0464-10	52.74		
5s ea UD	00006-0464-05	263.70		
(BI-PACK)				
80 mg, 2s ea	00006-0461-02	209.35		
6s ea UD	00006-0461-06	628.02		
125 mg, 6s ea UD	00006-0462-06	968.03		
(Merck)				
fosaprepitant dimeglumine				
PDS, IV, 115 mg, ea	00006-3884-32	223.87		
(A-S Medication)				
REPACK				
aprepitant				
CAP, PO, 3s ea	54569-5741-00	485.91		
(Pharma Pac)				
REPACK				
CAP, PO, 40 mg, ea	52959-0748-01	55.61		
(Phys Total Care)				
REPACK				
CAP, PO, 3s ea	54868-5325-00	449.85		
80 mg, 2s ea	54868-5231-02	259.45		
6s ea	54868-5231-01	749.46		
EMLA (APP)				
lidocaine/prilocaine				
CRE, TP (1X30GM)				
2.5%-2.5%, 30 gm	63323-0290-30	53.90		AB
(A-S Medication)				
REPACK				
CRE, TP, 2.5%-2.5%,				
30 gm	54569-4323-00	56.15		
(Dispensing Solutions)				
REPACK				
CRE, TP, 2.5%-2.5%, 5 gm	55045-2480-02	15.55		
(Phys Total Care)				
REPACK				
CRE, TP, 2.5%-2.5%, 5 gm	54868-3824-00	12.41		
5 gm 5s	54868-3824-01	56.95		
(Quality Care Prod)				
REPACK				
CRE, TP, 2.5%-2.5%,				
30 gm	35356-0041-30	87.40		
(Southwood)				
REPACK				
CRE, TP, 2.5%-2.5%,				
30 gm	58016-3529-01	53.90		AB
EMPTY STERILIZED VIAL (APP)				
vial, medication				
DEV, NA (10 ML SEALED CLEAR VIAL)				
ea	63323-0001-10	1.24		
(100ML SEALED CLEAR VIAL)				
ea	63323-0001-00	9.97		
(30 ML SEALED CLEAR VIAL)				
ea	63323-0001-30	1.86		
(5 ML SEALED CLEAR VIAL)				
ea	63323-0001-05	1.24		
EMSAM (Dey, L.P.)				
selegiline				
TDM, TD, 6 mg/24 hr,				
30s ea	49502-0900-30	602.98		
9 mg/24 hr, 30s ea	49502-0901-30	602.98		
12 mg/24 hr,				
30s ea	49502-0902-30	602.98		EE
EMTRICITABINE				
(Gilead Sciences) See *EMTRIVA*				
EMTRICITABINE/TENOFOVIR DISOPROXIL FUMARATE				
(Gilead Sciences) See *TRUVADA*				

PROD/MFR	NDC	AWP	DP	OBC
EMTRIVA (Gilead Sciences)				
emtricitabine				
CAP, PO, 200 mg, 30s ea	**61958-0601-01**	437.28		
SOL, PO (W/MARKED DOSE CUP)				
10 mg/ml, 170 ml	**61958-0602-01**	103.25		
(A-S Medication)				
REPACK				
CAP, PO, 200 mg, 30s ea	**54569-5521-00**	410.81		
(Phys Total Care)				
REPACK				
CAP, PO, 200 mg, 30s ea	**54868-4853-00**	451.78		
(Quality Care Prod)				
REPACK				
CAP, PO, 200 mg, 30s ea	**35356-0205-30**	818.59		
EMU (Medisca)				
emu oil				
OIL, NA, 500 ml	**38779-1969-08**	229.50		
EMU OIL				
(Medisca) *See EMU*				
(PCCA)				
OIL, NA, 1 ml	**51927-2925-00**	0.47		
ENABLEX (Novartis Pharm)				
darifenacin hydrobromide				
TER, PO, 7.5 mg, 30s ea	**00078-0419-15**	150.59		
90s ea	**00078-0419-34**	451.76		
15 mg, 30s ea	**00078-0420-15**	150.59		
90s ea	**00078-0420-34**	451.76		
(Nucare Pharm)				
REPACK				
TER, PO, 15 mg, 30s ea	**68071-1315-00**	250.55		
(Phys Total Care)				
REPACK				
TER, PO, 7.5 mg, 30s ea	**54868-5704-00**	180.22		
15 mg, 30s ea	**54868-5363-00**	151.49		
(Quality Care Prod)				
REPACK				
TER, PO, 7.5 mg, 30s ea	**35356-0273-30**	248.55		
15 mg, 30s ea	**35356-0272-30**	248.55		
ENALAPRIL (Core)				
REPACK				
enalapril maleate				
TAB, PO, 5 mg, 30s ea	**33358-0126-30**	44.09		
10 mg, 30s ea	**33358-0127-30**	46.16		
60s ea	**33358-0127-60**	92.31		
20 mg, 30s ea	**33358-0128-30**	65.67		
60s ea	**33358-0128-60**	131.33		
(DHS, Inc.)				
REPACK				
TAB, PO, 2.5 mg, 30s ea	**55887-0099-30**	24.11		
20 mg, 30s ea	**55887-0227-30**	45.76		
60s ea	**55887-0227-60**	91.52		
90s ea	**55887-0227-90**	137.28		
(Dispensing Solutions)				
REPACK				
TAB, PO, 10 mg, 30s ea	**66336-0389-30**	39.51		
(PD-Rx Pharm)				
REPACK				
TAB, PO, 5 mg, 90s ea	**55289-0694-90**	22.50		
ENALAPRIL MALEATE				
FUL				
TAB, PO, 2.5 mg, 100s ea		4.73		
5 mg, 100s ea		5.70		
10 mg, 100s ea		7.32		
20 mg, 100s ea		8.55		
(Apotex Corp.)				
TAB, PO (USP)				
2.5 mg, 100s ea	**60505-0049-07**	80.36		
1000s ea	**60505-0049-09**	803.60		
5 mg, 100s ea	**60505-0050-07**	102.10		
1000s ea	**60505-0050-09**	1021.00		
10 mg, 100s ea	**60505-0051-07**	107.21		
1000s ea	**60505-0051-09**	1072.10		
20 mg, 100s ea	**60505-0052-07**	152.54		
1000s ea	**60505-0052-09**	1525.40		
(BTA) *See VASOTEC*				
(Gallipot)				
POW, NA (1X25GM,USP)				
25 gm	**51552-0944-04**	91.00	65.00	
(1X100GM,USP)				
100 gm	**51552-0944-05**	315.00	225.00	
(1X500GM,USP)				
500 gm	**51552-0944-06**	1414.00	1010.00	
(Major)				
TAB, PO, 2.5 mg,				
100s ea UD	**00904-5609-61**	89.29		AB
5 mg, 100s ea UD	**00904-5502-61**	106.37		AB
10 mg, 100s ea UD	**00904-5610-61**	119.12		AB
20 mg, 100s ea UD	**00904-5611-61**	169.49		AB
(Medisca)				
POW, NA (U.S.P.)				
25 gm	**38779-0514-04**	225.00		
100 gm	**38779-0514-05**	765.00		
(Mylan)				
TAB, PO, 2.5 mg, 100s ea	**00378-1051-01**	80.30		AB
500s ea	**00378-1051-05**	401.50		AB
5 mg, 100s ea	**00378-1052-01**	102.00		AB
1000s ea	**00378-1052-10**	1020.00		AB
10 mg, 100s ea	**00378-1053-01**	107.10		AB
1000s ea	**00378-1053-10**	1071.00		AB
20 mg, 100s ea	**00378-1054-01**	152.40		AB
500s ea	**00378-1054-05**	762.00		AB
(PCCA)				
POW, NA (U.S.P.)				
1 gm	**51927-3336-00**	14.40		
(Ranbaxy Pharm)				
TAB, PO (WHITE)				
2.5 mg, 100s ea	**63304-0834-01**	80.36		AB
5 mg, 100s ea	**63304-0835-01**	102.10		AB
(Sandoz)				
TAB, PO, 2.5 mg, 100s ea	**00185-0114-01**	80.37		AB
(U.S.P.)				
2.5 mg, 100s ea	**66685-0301-00**	80.35		AB
(USP)				
2.5 mg, 100s ea	**00781-5441-01**	80.37		AB
1000s ea	**00185-0114-10**	803.70		AB
(U.S.P.)				
2.5 mg, 1000s ea	**66685-0301-02**	803.50		AB
(USP)				
2.5 mg, 1000s ea	**00781-5441-10**	803.70		AB
5000s ea	**00185-0114-50**	4018.50		AB
5 mg, 100s ea	**00185-0127-01**	102.11		AB
(U.S.P.)				
5 mg, 100s ea	**66685-0302-00**	102.07		AB
(USP)				
5 mg, 100s ea	**00781-5442-01**	102.11		AB
1000s ea	**00185-0127-10**	1021.17		AB
(U.S.P.)				
5 mg, 1000s ea	**66685-0302-02**	1020.70		AB
(USP)				
5 mg, 1000s ea	**00781-5442-10**	1021.10		AB
5000s ea	**00185-0127-50**	5105.85		AB
10 mg, 100s ea	**00185-0147-01**	107.22		AB
(U.S.P.)				
10 mg, 100s ea	**66685-0303-00**	107.18		AB
(USP)				
10 mg, 100s ea	**00781-5443-01**	107.21		AB
1000s ea	**00185-0147-10**	1072.13		AB
(U.S.P.)				
10 mg, 1000s ea	**66685-0303-02**	1071.80		AB
(USP)				
10 mg, 1000s ea	**00781-5443-10**	1072.10		AB
5000s ea	**00185-0147-50**	5360.63		AB
20 mg, 100s ea	**00185-0214-01**	152.54		AB
(U.S.P.)				
20 mg, 100s ea	**66685-0304-00**	152.49		AB
(USP)				
20 mg, 100s ea	**00781-5444-01**	152.54		AB
1000s ea	**00185-0214-10**	1525.39		AB
(U.S.P.)				
20 mg, 1000s ea	**66685-0304-02**	1524.90		AB
(USP)				
20 mg, 1000s ea	**00781-5444-10**	1525.38		AB
5000s ea	**00185-0214-50**	7626.96		AB
(Taro)				
TAB, PO (USP)				
2.5 mg, 100s ea	**51672-4037-01**	80.90		AB
1000s ea	**51672-4037-03**	768.55		AB
5 mg, 100s ea	**51672-4038-01**	102.72		AB
1000s ea	**51672-4038-03**	975.84		AB
10 mg, 100s ea	**51672-4039-01**	107.85		AB
1000s ea	**51672-4039-03**	1024.58		AB
20 mg, 100s ea	**51672-4040-01**	153.37		AB
1000s ea	**51672-4040-03**	1457.02		AB
(Teva)				
TAB, PO, 2.5 mg, 100s ea	**00093-0026-01**	80.37		AB
(10X10)				
2.5 mg, 100s ea UD	**00172-4195-10**	78.86		AB
(USP)				
2.5 mg, 1000s ea	**00093-0026-10**	803.75		AB
5 mg, 100s ea	**00093-0027-01**	102.11		AB
100s ea UD	**00172-4196-10**	99.64		AB
(USP)				
5 mg, 5000s ea	**00093-0027-50**	4728.97		AB
10 mg, 100s ea	**00093-0028-01**	107.21		AB
(10X10)				
10 mg, 100s ea UD	**00172-4197-10**	104.52		AB
1000s ea	**00093-0028-10**	1072.10		AB
(USP)				
10 mg, 5000s ea	**00093-0028-50**	5226.49		AB
20 mg, 100s ea	**00093-0029-01**	152.54		AB
(10X10)				
20 mg, 100s ea UD	**00172-4198-10**	147.87		AB
1000s ea	**00093-0029-10**	1525.38		AB
(USP)				
20 mg, 5000s ea	**00093-0029-50**	7436.23		AB
(UDL)				
TAB, PO (10X10)				
2.5 mg, 100s ea UD	**51079-0950-20**	80.30		AB
5 mg, 100s ea UD	**51079-0951-20**	102.00		AB
10 mg, 100s ea UD	**51079-0952-20**	107.10		AB
20 mg, 100s ea UD	**51079-0953-20**	152.40		AB
(Wockhardt USA)				
TAB, PO (USP)				
2.5 mg, 100s ea	**64679-0923-02**	80.37		AB
1000s ea	**64679-0923-03**	803.70		AB
(5X8000,USP)				
2.5 mg, 40000s ea	**64679-0923-09**	32148.00		AB
(USP)				
5 mg, 100s ea	**64679-0924-02**	102.11		AB
1000s ea	**64679-0924-03**	1024.10		AB
(5X8000,USP)				
5 mg, 40000s ea	**64679-0924-09**	40964.00		AB
(USP)				
10 mg, 100s ea	**64679-0925-02**	107.21		AB
1000s ea	**64679-0925-03**	1072.10		AB
(5X8000,USP)				
10 mg, 40000s ea	**64679-0925-09**	42884.00		AB
(USP)				
20 mg, 100s ea	**64679-0926-02**	152.54		AB
1000s ea	**64679-0926-03**	1525.38		AB
(5X8000,USP)				
20 mg, 40000s ea	**64679-0926-09**	61015.20		AB
(A-S Medication)				
REPACK				
TAB, PO, 5 mg, 30s ea	**54569-5133-00**	30.65		EE
100s ea	**54569-5133-01**	102.15		EE
10 mg, 30s ea	**54569-5134-00**	32.18		EE
60s ea	**54569-5134-02**	64.35		EE
100s ea	**54569-5134-01**	107.25		EE
20 mg, 30s ea	**54569-5135-00**	45.78		EE
60s ea	**54569-5135-01**	91.55		EE
(Altura)				
REPACK				
TAB, PO, 5 mg, 7s ea	**63874-0423-07**	8.86		AB
10s ea	**63874-0423-10**	12.40		AB
14s ea	**63874-0423-14**	17.36		AB
20s ea	**63874-0423-20**	24.80		AB
30s ea	**63874-0423-30**	37.20		AB
60s ea	**63874-0423-60**	74.40		AB
100s ea	**63874-0423-01**	124.00		AB
10 mg, 10s ea	**63874-0655-10**	12.90		AB
14s ea	**63874-0655-14**	18.06		AB
20s ea	**63874-0655-20**	25.80		AB
30s ea	**63874-0655-30**	38.70		AB
60s ea	**63874-0655-60**	77.40		AB
100s ea	**63874-0655-01**	129.00		AB
20 mg, 10s ea	**63874-0987-10**	15.00		AB
14s ea	**63874-0987-14**	21.00		AB
20s ea	**63874-0987-20**	30.00		AB
30s ea	**63874-0987-30**	45.00		AB
60s ea	**63874-0987-60**	90.00		AB
100s ea	**63874-0987-01**	150.00		AB
(American Health)				
REPACK				
TAB, PO, 5 mg, 100s ea UD	**68084-0390-01**	7.98		AB
10 mg, 100s ea UD	**68084-0391-01**	8.52		AB
20 mg, 100s ea UD	**68084-0392-01**	12.50		AB
(Apace)				
REPACK				
TAB, PO (USP,COMPRESSED TABLET)				
2.5 mg, 30s ea	**15338-0200-30**	289.32		AB
5 mg, 30s ea	**15338-0211-30**	368.64		AB
10 mg, 30s ea	**15338-0220-30**	385.92		AB
20 mg, 30s ea	**15338-0233-30**	549.12		AB
(Bryant Ranch)				
REPACK				
TAB, PO, 5 mg, 30s ea	**63629-1522-03**	43.01		
100s ea	**63629-1522-02**	143.37		
150s ea	**63629-1522-01**	215.06		
10 mg, 30s ea	**63629-1526-02**	45.03		
60s ea	**63629-1526-01**	90.06		
20 mg, 30s ea	**63629-1525-03**	64.07		
60s ea	**63629-1525-02**	128.13		
100s ea	**63629-1525-01**	213.55		

PROD/MFR	NDC	AWP	DP	OBC
(DHS, Inc.)				
REPACK				
TAB, PO, 5 mg, 30s ea	55887-0596-30	30.03		AB
60s ea	55887-0596-60	60.06		AB
90s ea	55887-0596-90	88.44		AB
10 mg, 30s ea	55887-0612-30	29.95		AB
60s ea	55887-0612-60	58.99		AB
90s ea	55887-0612-90	88.88		AB
20 mg, 30s ea	55887-0558-30	40.05		AB
90s ea	55887-0558-90	101.00		AB
(Dispensing Solutions)				
REPACK				
TAB, PO, 5 mg, 30s ea	55045-2799-00	30.10		AB
30s ea	66336-0391-30	36.03		AB
60s ea	55045-2799-06	60.00		AB
60s ea	66336-0391-60	71.45		AB
90s ea	55045-2799-09	90.00		AB
100s ea	55045-2799-01	100.00		AB
120s ea	55045-2799-02	120.00		AB
10 mg, 30s ea	55045-2827-08	37.50		AB
60s ea	55045-2827-06	75.00		AB
60s ea	66336-0389-60	78.53		AB
90s ea	55045-2827-09	112.50		AB
100s ea	55045-2827-00	125.00		AB
120s ea	55045-2827-04	150.00		AB
20 mg, 30s ea	55045-2832-08	44.45		AB
30s ea	66336-0393-30	54.00		AB
60s ea	66336-0393-60	108.00		AB
(HomeMed)				
REPACK				
TAB, PO, 5 mg, 30s ea	51655-0636-24	30.69		
60s ea	51655-0636-25	60.39		
10 mg, 30s ea	51655-0620-24	32.39		
20 mg, 30s ea	51655-0279-24	45.99		
(Nucare Pharm)				
REPACK				
TAB, PO, 5 mg, 30s ea	66267-0413-30	25.80		AB
60s ea	66267-0413-60	51.60		AB
90s ea	66267-0413-90	77.40		AB
180s ea	66267-0413-92	154.80		AB
10 mg, 30s ea	66267-0323-30	32.10		AB
60s ea	66267-0323-60	64.20		AB
90s ea	66267-0323-90	94.50		AB
120s ea	66267-0323-91	124.80		AB
20 mg, 30s ea	66267-0380-30	39.90		AB
60s ea	66267-0380-60	79.80		AB
90s ea	66267-0380-90	119.72		AB
120s ea	66267-0380-91	159.61		AB
(Palmetto)				
REPACK				
TAB, PO, 5 mg, 30s ea	23490-5494-01	35.12		
60s ea	23490-5494-02	70.24		
10 mg, 30s ea	23490-5491-01	37.50		
60s ea	23490-5491-02	75.00		
90s ea	23490-5491-09	112.50		
180s ea	23490-5491-08	225.00		
20 mg, 30s ea	23490-5492-01	45.99		
60s ea	23490-5492-02	91.98		
(PD-Rx Pharm)				
REPACK				
TAB, PO, 5 mg, 10s ea	55289-0694-10	11.80		EE
30s ea	55289-0694-30	15.77		EE
30s ea	58864-0754-30	15.77		AB
10 mg, 30s ea	55289-0591-30	15.90		EE
30s ea	58864-0755-30	15.90		
90s ea	55289-0591-90	24.84		
20 mg, 30s ea	55289-0984-30	16.47		AB
30s ea	58864-0762-30	16.40		AB
(Pharma Pac)				
REPACK				
TAB, PO, 20 mg, 30s ea	52959-0942-30	46.78		AB
(Phys Total Care)				
REPACK				
TAB, PO, 2.5 mg, 30s ea	54868-4332-01	6.24		AB
60s ea	54868-4332-00	9.51		AB
100s ea	54868-4332-02	12.36		AB
5 mg, 30s ea	54868-4357-00	8.55		EE
60s ea	54868-4357-01	16.80		EE
90s ea	54868-4357-03	14.58		EE
100s ea	54868-4357-02	24.48		EE
10 mg, 30s ea	54868-4358-00	6.66		EE
60s ea	54868-4358-01	10.35		EE
90s ea	54868-4358-03	15.72		AB
100s ea	54868-4358-02	13.74		EE
20 mg, 30s ea	54868-4331-01	8.46		EE
60s ea	54868-4331-02	13.95		EE
100s ea	54868-4331-00	19.74		EE
(Physician Partner)				
REPACK				
TAB, PO, 5 mg, 30s ea	21695-0487-30	61.27		AB
10 mg, 30s ea	21695-0488-30	64.32		AB
60s ea	21695-0488-60	128.64		AB
20 mg, 90s ea	21695-0489-90	262.26		AB
(Quality Care Prod)				
REPACK				
TAB, PO, 2.5 mg, 30s ea	35356-0541-30	31.02		AB
5 mg, 30s ea	49999-0239-30	37.08		
60s ea	49999-0239-60	74.16		AB
100s ea	49999-0239-00	123.60		
10 mg, 30s ea	49999-0240-30	38.88		
100s ea	49999-0240-00	129.60		
20 mg, 30s ea	49999-0345-30	53.99		AB
100s ea	49999-0345-00	179.98		
(Southwood)				
REPACK				
TAB, PO, 5 mg, 20s ea	58016-0579-20	20.08		EE
30s ea	58016-0579-30	30.13		EE
60s ea	58016-0579-60	60.25		EE
100s ea	58016-0579-00	100.42		EE
10 mg, 20s ea	58016-0580-20	21.08		EE
30s ea	58016-0580-30	31.63		EE
60s ea	58016-0530-60	63.25		EE
60s ea	58016-0580-60	63.25		EE
100s ea	58016-0580-00	105.42		EE
20 mg, 20s ea	58016-0581-20	30.00		EE
30s ea	58016-0581-30	45.00		EE
60s ea	58016-0581-60	89.99		EE
100s ea	58016-0581-00	149.98		EE
(Stat Rx)				
REPACK				
TAB, PO, 10 mg, 30s ea	16590-0277-30	30.25		AB
60s ea	16590-0277-60	60.50		AB
90s ea	16590-0277-90	85.50		AB
20 mg, 30s ea	16590-0392-30	35.50		AB
60s ea	16590-0392-60	71.00		AB
90s ea	16590-0392-90	87.50		AB
(Vibranta)				
REPACK				
TAB, PO, 5 mg, 30s ea	57866-6859-01	35.12		AB
60s ea	57866-6859-02	89.18		AB
90s ea	57866-6859-03	103.16		AB
120s ea	57866-6859-04	137.18		AB
ENALAPRIL MALEATE AND HYDROCHLOROTHIAZIDE				
(Apotex Corp.)				
enalapril maleate/hydrochlorothiazide				
TAB, PO (USP)				
5 mg-12.5 mg,				
100s ea	60505-0208-01	128.69		AB
10 mg-25 mg,				
100s ea	60505-0209-01	143.34		AB
(Phys Total Care)				
REPACK				
TAB, PO, 5 mg-12.5 mg,				
30s ea	54868-5503-00	16.77		
90s ea	54868-5503-01	44.34		
10 mg-25 mg,				
90s ea	54868-5100-02	43.34		AB
ENALAPRIL MALEATE/HYDROCHLOROTHIAZIDE				
(Apotex Corp.) *See ENALAPRIL MALEATE AND HYDROCHLOROTHIAZIDE*				
(BTA) *See VASERETIC*				
(Dr Reddy's) *See ENALAPRIL/HCTZ*				
(Mylan) *See ENALAPRIL/HCTZ*				
(Par) *See ENALAPRIL/HCTZ*				
(Sandoz) *See ENALAPRIL/HCTZ*				
(Taro) *See ENALAPRIL/HCTZ*				
(Teva) *See ENALAPRIL/HCTZ*				
ENALAPRIL/HCT (Quality Care Prod)				
REPACK				
enalapril maleate/hydrochlorothiazide				
TAB, PO, 10 mg-25 mg,				
100s ea	49999-0823-00	131.51		
ENALAPRIL/HCTZ (Dr Reddy's)				
enalapril maleate/hydrochlorothiazide				
TAB, PO, 5 mg-12.5 mg,				
100s ea	55111-0133-01	107.20		AB
10 mg-25 mg,				
100s ea	55111-0134-01	119.40		AB
(Mylan)				
TAB, PO, 5 mg-12.5 mg,				
100s ea	00378-0712-01	107.10		AB
100s ea	55390-0712-01	107.10		AB
10 mg-25 mg,				
100s ea	00378-0723-01	119.30		AB
(Par)				
TAB, PO, 5 mg-12.5 mg,				
100s ea	49884-0686-01	107.20		AB
10 mg-25 mg,				
100s ea	49884-0687-01	119.40		AB
(Sandoz)				
TAB, PO, 5 mg-12.5 mg,				
100s ea	00185-0151-01	107.22		AB
10 mg-25 mg,				
100s ea	00185-0172-01	119.39		AB
1000s ea	00185-0172-10	1193.90		AB
(Taro)				
TAB, PO, 5 mg-12.5 mg,				
100s ea	51672-4045-01	109.60		AB
10 mg-25 mg,				
100s ea	51672-4046-01	122.05		AB
(Teva)				
TAB, PO, 5 mg-12.5 mg,				
100s ea	00093-1044-01	107.21		AB
10 mg-25 mg,				
100s ea	00093-1052-01	119.40		AB
(DHS, Inc.)				
REPACK				
TAB, PO, 5 mg-12.5 mg,				
30s ea	55887-0594-30	25.04		AB
90s ea	55887-0594-90	72.91		AB
10 mg-25 mg,				
30s ea	55887-0595-30	25.44		AB
90s ea	55887-0595-90	73.05		AB
(Dispensing Solutions)				
REPACK				
TAB, PO, 5 mg-12.5 mg,				
30s ea	55045-3373-08	32.70		AB
(Phys Total Care)				
REPACK				
TAB, PO, 10 mg-25 mg,				
30s ea	54868-5100-01	15.45		AB
100s ea	54868-5100-00	42.99		AB
(Physician Partner)				
REPACK				
TAB, PO, 10 mg-25 mg,				
30s ea	21695-0780-30	73.23		AB
(Southwood)				
REPACK				
TAB, PO, 5 mg-12.5 mg,				
30s ea	00490-7030-30	32.88		
60s ea	00490-7030-60	65.76		
90s ea	00490-7030-90	98.64		
100s ea	00490-7030-00	109.60		
10 mg-25 mg,				
30s ea	00490-0067-30	36.62		
60s ea	00490-0067-60	73.23		
90s ea	00490-0067-90	109.85		
100s ea	00490-0067-00	122.05		
ENALAPRILAT (Bedford)				
SOL, IV (S.D.V.)				
1.25 mg/ml,				
1 ml 10s	55390-0010-10	36.00		AP
2 ml 10s	55390-0011-10	72.00		AP
(Hospira) *See ENALAPRILAT NOVAPLUS*				
(Hospira)				
SOL, IV, 1.25 mg/ml, 1 ml (VIAL,LATEX-FREE)	00409-2122-01	2.05	1.80	AP
1.25 mg/ml, 1 ml (VIAL)	00074-2122-01	2.05	1.80	AP
1.25 mg/ml, 1 ml (LATEX-FREE)	61703-0237-44	3.41	2.98	AP
1.25 mg/ml, 2 ml (VIAL)	00409-2122-02	3.72	3.26	AP
1.25 mg/ml, 2 ml	61703-0237-16	6.02	5.27	AP
(Teva)				
SOL, IV (25X1ML)				
1.25 mg/ml,				
1 ml 25s (25X2ML)	00703-8401-04	60.00		AP
1.25 mg/ml,				
2 ml 25s	00703-8411-04	105.00		AP
(West-Ward)				
SOL, IV (10X1ML)				
1.25 mg/ml,				
1 ml 10s (10X2ML)	00143-9787-10	36.00		AP
1.25 mg/ml,				
2 ml 10s	00143-9786-10	72.00		AP

PROD/MFR	NDC	AWP	DP	OBC
ENALAPRILAT NOVAPLUS (Hospira)				
enalaprilat				
SOL, IV (PRIVATE LABEL)				
1.25 mg/ml, 1 ml	**00409-2122-13**	2.04	1.79	**AP**
2 ml	**00409-2122-88**	3.50	3.07	**AP**
ENBREL (Amgen USA Inc.)				
etanercept				
PDS, SC (S.D. TRAY,PF)				
25 mg, ea	**58406-0425-41**	232.96		
4s ea	**58406-0425-34**	931.82		
SOL, SC (27G,1/2",PF)				
50 mg/ml, 0.51 ml	**58406-0455-01**	232.96		
(4X0.51ML,27G,1/2",PF)				
50 mg/ml,				
0.51 ml 4s	**58406-0455-04**	931.82		
(ACTUAL FILL 50MG/0.98ML)				
50 mg/ml, 0.98 ml	**58406-0435-01**	465.91		
(SURECLICK AUTOINJECTOR)				
50 mg/ml, 0.98 ml	**58406-0445-01**	465.91		
(ACTUAL FILL 50MG/0.98ML)				
50 mg/ml,				
0.98 ml 4s	**58406-0435-04**	1863.65		
(SURECLICK AUTOINJECTOR)				
50 mg/ml,				
0.98 ml 4s	**58406-0445-04**	1863.65		
(Phys Total Care)				
REPACK				
PDS, SC (PF)				
25 mg, 4s ea	**54868-4782-00**	912.41		
SOL, SC (4X0.98ML,PF)				
50 mg/ml,				
0.98 ml 4s	**54868-5444-00**	2001.00		
ENCORA (Ther-RX)				
multivitamin and minerals/nutriceutical				
KIT, PO (30-DAY SUPPLY)				
60s ea	**64011-0166-36**	56.10		
ENDACOF-AC (Larken Labs, Inc.)				
brompheniramine maleate/codeine phosphate				
SOL, PO (1X118ML,AF,SF)				
2 mg/5 ml-10 mg/5 ml,				
118 ml, C-V	**68047-0138-04**	29.52		
ENDACOF-C (Larken Labs, Inc.)				
chlorpheniramine maleate/codeine phosphate				
SOL, PO (1X480ML,AF,SF,DYE-FREE)				
2 mg/5 ml-10 mg/5 ml,				
480 ml, C-V	**68047-0145-16**	58.30		
ENDACOF-DC (Larken Labs, Inc.)				
codeine phosphate/pseudoephedrine hydrochloride				
SOL, PO (1X473ML,AF,SF,DYE-FREE)				
10 mg/5 ml-30 mg/5 ml,				
480 ml, C-V	**68047-0146-16**	61.05		
ENDACOF-DH (Larken Labs, Inc.)				
bpm/dihydrocodeine bitartrate/phenyleph hcl				
SOL, PO (1X473ML,AF,SF,DYE-FREE)				
473 ml, C-V	**68047-0139-16**	76.32		
ENDACOF-PD (Larken Labs, Inc.)				
bpm/dm/pse hcl				
SOL, PO (PEDIATRIC DROPS,SF)				
30 ml	**68047-0010-30**	30.15		
ENDITUSSIN-HD (Southwood)				
REPACK				
cpm/hydrocod bit/phenyleph hcl				
SYR, PO, 120 ml, C-III	**58016-4177-04**	11.00		
ENDOAVITENE (Davol)				
collagen hemostat				
POW, NA (50MMX15MMX1MM PRELOAD)				
6s ea	**03031-0101-50**	848.70	707.25	
(50MMX5MMX1MM PRE-LOADED)				
6s ea	**03031-0102-60**	499.62	416.35	
ENDOCET (Endo Generics)				
acetaminophen/oxycodone hydrochloride				
TAB, PO, 325 mg-5 mg,				
100s ea, C-II	**60951-0602-70**	57.67		**AA**
500s ea, C-II	**60951-0602-85**	288.34		**AA**
325 mg-7.5 mg,				
100s ea, C-II	**60951-0700-70**	136.07		
325 mg-10 mg,				
100s ea, C-II	**60951-0712-70**	177.92		
(CAPLET)				
500 mg-7.5 mg,				
100s ea, C-II	**60951-0796-70**	145.30		**AA**
650 mg-10 mg,				
100s ea, C-II	**60951-0797-70**	190.02		**AA**
(4u)				
REPACK				
TAB, PO, 325 mg-5 mg,				
28s ea, C-II	**10544-0382-28**	64.22		**AA**
28s ea, C-II	**42549-0582-28**	64.22		**AA**
30s ea, C-II	**42549-0582-30**	66.94		**AA**
60s ea, C-II	**42549-0582-60**	120.22		**AA**
84s ea, C-II	**10544-0382-84**	162.42		**AA**
84s ea, C-II	**42549-0582-84**	162.42		**AA**
120s ea, C-II	**10544-0382-03**	218.22		**AA**
120s ea, C-II	**42549-0582-03**	218.22		**AA**
325 mg-7.5 mg,				
28s ea, C-II	**42549-0583-28**	118.86		
30s ea, C-II	**42549-0583-30**	123.46		
60s ea, C-II	**42549-0583-60**	216.72		
84s ea, C-II	**42549-0583-84**	358.34		
168s ea, C-II	**42549-0583-08**	462.22		
325 mg-10 mg,				
28s ea, C-II	**42549-0584-28**	101.76		
30s ea, C-II	**42549-0584-30**	104.44		
84s ea, C-II	**42549-0584-84**	278.14		
112s ea, C-II	**42549-0584-02**	326.86		
(CAPLET)				
500 mg-7.5 mg,				
60s ea, C-II	**42549-0595-60**	238.16		**AA**
650 mg-10 mg,				
30s ea, C-II	**42549-0585-30**	138.36		**AA**
60s ea, C-II	**42549-0585-60**	248.78		**AA**
168s ea, C-II	**42549-0585-08**	462.92		**AA**
(Core)				
REPACK				
TAB, PO, 325 mg-10 mg,				
20s ea, C-II	**33358-0130-20**	41.29		
40s ea, C-II	**33358-0130-40**	80.84		
60s ea, C-II	**33358-0130-60**	113.21		
500 mg-7.5 mg,				
30s ea, C-II	**33358-0129-30**	50.52		
60s ea, C-II	**33358-0129-60**	94.29		
650 mg-10 mg,				
30s ea, C-II	**33358-0131-30**	67.39		
60s ea, C-II	**33358-0131-60**	123.77		
(Nucare Pharm)				
REPACK				
TAB, PO, 650 mg-10 mg,				
30s ea, C-II	**68071-0489-30**	82.30		**AA**
(Palmetto)				
REPACK				
TAB, PO, 325 mg-7.5 mg,				
30s ea, C-II	**23490-7827-03**	112.25		
60s ea, C-II	**23490-7827-06**	224.51		
90s ea, C-II	**23490-7827-09**	336.77		
500 mg-7.5 mg,				
30s ea, C-II	**23490-7835-03**	93.43		
90s ea, C-II	**23490-7835-09**	280.29		
120s ea, C-II	**23490-7835-07**	373.72		
650 mg-10 mg,				
30s ea, C-II	**23490-7812-03**	122.18		
60s ea, C-II	**23490-7812-06**	175.20		
90s ea, C-II	**23490-7812-09**	262.80		
120s ea, C-II	**23490-7812-07**	488.73		
(Quality Care Prod)				
REPACK				
TAB, PO, 500 mg-7.5 mg,				
30s ea, C-II	**49999-0830-30**	86.89		
ENDODAN (Endo Pharm)				
aspirin/oxycodone hydrochloride				
TAB, PO (USP)				
325 mg-4.8355 mg,				
100s ea, C-II	**60951-0310-70**	118.16		
ENDOMETRIN (Ferring)				
progesterone				
TAB, VG (INSERT)				
100 mg, 21s ea	**55566-6500-03**	148.32		**EE**
ENDRATE (Hospira)				
edetate disodium				
SOL, IV (25X20ML)				
150 mg/ml,				
20 ml 25s	**00409-6940-03**	746.70	653.25	**AP**
ENDURON (Phys Total Care)				
REPACK				
methyclothiazide				
TAB, PO, 5 mg, 30s ea	**54868-3785-00**	23.00		**AB**
ENFLURANE				
(Baxter) *See ETHRANE*				
(RxElite) *See COMPOUND 347*				
ENFUVIRTIDE				
(Roche Labs) *See FUZEON*				
ENGERIX-B (Glaxo)				
hepatitis b vaccine recombinant				
SUS, IM (10X0.5ML,SD,TAXINCL,PF)				
10 mcg/0.5 ml,				
0.5 ml 10s	**58160-0820-51**	254.90		
(5X1ML,TAXINCL,PF)				
20 mcg/ml, 1 ml 5s	**58160-0821-46**	314.25		
(SDV,TAXINCL,PF)				
20 mcg/ml,				
1 ml 10s	**58160-0821-11**	628.50		
(A-S Medication)				
REPACK				
SUS, IM (TIP-LOK W/O NDL,TAX,PF)				
20 mcg/ml, 1 ml 5s	**54569-5408-00**	313.78		
(Dispensing Solutions)				
REPACK				
SUS, IM (1X1ML,PF)				
20 mcg/ml, 1 ml	**68258-3042-01**	81.71		
(Phys Total Care)				
REPACK				
SUS, IM (S.D.V.,PF)				
20 mcg/ml, 1 ml	**54868-0734-00**	75.82		
ENGERIX-B PEDIATRIC (Glaxo)				
hepatitis b vaccine recombinant				
SUS, IM (TIPLOK,23GX1,TAX INC,PF)				
10 mcg/0.5 ml,				
0.5 ml 5s	**58160-0856-35**	128.21		
(10X0.5ML,SDV,TAXINCL,PF)				
10 mcg/0.5 ml,				
0.5 ml 10s	**58160-0820-11**	254.90		
(A-S Medication)				
REPACK				
SUS, IM (S.D.V.,TAX INCL.,PF)				
10 mcg/0.5 ml,				
0.5 ml 10s	**54569-5311-00**	265.21		
(Phys Total Care)				
REPACK				
SUS, IM, 10 mcg/0.5 ml,				
0.5 ml	**54868-3236-00**	31.66		
(PEDIATRIC,PF)				
10 mcg/0.5 ml,				
0.5 ml	**54868-4781-00**	32.51		
ENGLISH TOFFEE FLAVOR (PCCA)				
flavoring aid				
SOL, NA (ARTIFICIAL)				
1 ml	**51927-2698-00**	0.90		
ENGYSTOL N (Heel/BHI)				
homeopathic substance				
INJ, IJ (AMP)				
20 ml 10s	**50114-7010-01**	29.00	29.00	
ENJUVIA (Teva)				
conjugated estrogens synthetic b				
TAB, PO (FILM-COATED)				
0.3 mg, 100s ea	**51285-0406-02**	194.02		
0.45 mg, 100s ea	**51285-0407-02**	194.02		
0.625 mg, 100s ea	**51285-0408-02**	194.02		
0.9 mg, 100s ea	**51285-0409-02**	194.02		**EE**
1.25 mg, 100s ea	**51285-0410-02**	194.02		
ENLON (Bioniche Pharma)				
edrophonium chloride				
SOL, IJ (MDV)				
10 mg/ml, 15 ml	**67457-0190-15**	30.00		**EE**
ENLON-PLUS (Bioniche Pharma)				
atropine sulfate/edrophonium chloride				
SOL, IV (SINGLE DOSE)				
0.14 mg/ml-10 mg/ml,				
5 ml 10s	**67457-0192-05**	137.50		**EE**
(MDV)				
0.14 mg/ml-10 mg/ml,				
15 ml	**67457-0191-15**	30.00		**EE**
ENOXAPARIN SODIUM				
(Sanofi-Aventis) *See LOVENOX*				
(Sanofi-Aventis) *See NOVAPLUS LOVENOX*				
ENPRESSE (Dispensing Solutions)				
REPACK				
ethinyl estradiol/levonorgestrel				
TAB, PO, 168s ea	**55045-3782-06**	165.00		
ENPRESSE-28 (Teva)				
ethinyl estradiol/levonorgestrel				
TAB, PO, 168s ea	**00555-9047-58**	164.92		**AB**
(Phys Total Care)				
REPACK				
TAB, PO, 28s ea	**54868-4860-00**	30.21		**AB**
(Physician Partner)				
REPACK				
TAB, PO, 28s ea	**21695-0855-01**	54.97		**AB**
ENROFLOXACIN (Letco)				
POW, NA (U.S.P.)				
50 gm	**62991-2300-01**	225.00		
(VET USE ONLY)				
1000 gm	**62991-2300-02**	1350.00		

PROD/MFR NDC AWP DP OBC

(Medisca)
POW, NA (U.S.P.)
25 gm............38779-1787-04 165.00
100 gm............38779-1787-05 495.00
500 gm............38779-1787-08 1455.00
(PCCA)
POW, NA (1X1GM)
1 gm............51927-3666-00 7.44
ENTACAPONE
(Novartis Pharm) *See COMTAN*
ENTECAVIR
(Bristol-Myers) *See BARACLUDE*
ENTERAL PUMP (Abbott Hosp)
kit, feeding (enteral)
DEV, NA (98",W/40MM SCREW CAP)
24s ea............00074-1765-01 251.14 251.28
ENTEREG (Glaxo)
alvimopan
CAP, PO (HARD-GELATIN)
12 mg, 30s ea UD....11227-0010-30 2250.00
ENTEROCOCCUS FAECIUM (PCCA)
streptococcus
POW, NA (STREPTOCOCCUS)
1 gm............51927-3505-00 1.20
ENTEX (Athlon Pharm)
pseudoephedrine tannate
SUS, PO (1X473ML,GRAPE)
22.5 mg/5 ml,
473 ml............66813-0555-16 172.90
ENTEX LA (Athlon Pharm)
guaifenesin/phenylephrine hydrochloride
TER, PO (BILAYERED)
800 mg-30 mg,
100s ea............66813-0535-01 147.11
(Quality Care Prod)
REPACK
CER, PO, 400 mg-30 mg,
20s ea............49999-0364-20 68.58
ENTEX PSE (Athlon Pharm)
guaifenesin/pseudoephedrine hydrochloride
TER, PO (DYE-FREE)
525 mg-50 mg,
100s ea............66813-0525-01 103.32
(Quality Care Prod)
REPACK
CER, PO, 400 mg-120 mg,
20s ea............49999-0398-20 33.84
ENTOCORT EC (Prometheus Labs)
budesonide
ECC, PO, 3 mg, 100s ea...65483-0702-10 1222.26
(Phys Total Care)
REPACK
ECC, PO, 3 mg, 10s ea....54868-4910-00 52.11
90s ea............54868-4910-01 454.03
100s ea............54868-4910-02 723.75
ENTRE-S SUSPENSION (Acella)
cpm/dm/pse hcl
SUS, PO (1X473ML,GRAPE BUBBLEGUM)
473 ml............42192-0514-16 261.50
ENULOSE (Actavis Mid Atlantic)
lactulose
SOL, PO, 10 gm/15 ml,
473 ml............00472-1360-16 36.35 AA
EOVIST (Bayer)
gadoxetate disodium
SOL, IV, 181.43 mg/ml,
10 ml............50419-0320-01 156.00
(5X10ML,SINGLE DOSE)
181.43 mg/ml,
10 ml 5s............50419-0320-05 156.00
EPH HCL/GG/PB/THEOPH
(Consolidated Midland) *See GUIAPHED*
EPHEDRA HERB (PCCA)
ma huang
POW, NA (EPHEDRA SINICA)
1 gm............51927-2855-00 0.07
EPHEDRINE HYDROCHLORIDE (Amend)
POW, NA (U.S.P.)
25 gm............17317-0153-02 17.15
125 gm............17317-0153-04 49.00
454 gm............17317-0153-01 154.00
(Gallipot)
POW, NA (U.S.P.,N.F.)
100 gm............51552-0229-05 58.80

(PCCA)
POW, NA (U.S.P.)
1 gm............51927-1381-00 1.80
EPHEDRINE SULFATE (Akorn)
SOL, IJ (USP,10X1ML,SINGLE DOSE)
50 mg/ml, 1 ml 10s...17478-0515-00 36.78
(Consolidated Midland)
CAP, PO, 50 mg, 100s ea..00223-0621-01 5.95
1000s ea............00223-0621-02 55.50
(Gallipot)
POW, NA (U.S.P.)
25 gm............51552-0260-04 25.55
100 gm............51552-0260-05 97.72
1000 gm............51552-0260-07 630.00
(Hospira)
SOL, IJ (AMP,LATEX-FREE)
50 mg/ml, 1 ml 50s...00409-3073-31 37.80 33.00
(Parenta Pharma)
SOL, IJ (PF)
50 mg/ml, 1 ml............66758-0008-01 0.84 0.70
1 ml 25s............66758-0008-02 43.75 35.00
(PCCA)
POW, NA (U.S.P.)
1 gm............51927-1471-00 8.00
EPI-PEN (Dispensing Solutions)
REPACK
epinephrine
KIT, MR (DELIVERY 0.3MG)
1 mg/ml, ea............55045-3207-01 61.00
2s ea............55045-3207-02 114.00
EPI-PEN JR (Dispensing Solutions)
epinephrine
KIT, MR (DELIVERY 0.15MG)
0.5 mg/ml, ea............55045-3780-01 61.00
2s ea............55045-3598-01 114.00
EPICERAM (Promius)
cream, multi ingredient
CRE, TP (1X90GM,FRAGRANCE-FREE)
90 gm............67857-0800-90 69.34
EPIDRIN (Excellium)
apap/dichloralphenazone/isometheptene mucate
CAP, PO, 325 mg-100 mg-65 mg,
100s ea, C-IV............64125-0101-01 66.74
250s ea, C-IV............64125-0101-02 139.75
(DHS, Inc.)
REPACK
CAP, PO, 325 mg-100 mg-65 mg,
20s ea, C-IV............55887-0265-20 22.00
30s ea, C-IV............55887-0265-30 33.00
60s ea, C-IV............55887-0265-60 66.00
90s ea, C-IV............55887-0265-90 99.00
(IPI)
REPACK
CAP, PO, 325 mg-100 mg-65 mg,
30s ea, C-IV............18837-0263-30 25.60
(Nucare Pharm)
REPACK
CAP, PO, 325 mg-100 mg-65 mg,
60s ea, C-IV............66267-0354-60 79.20
EPIDUO (Galderma)
adapalene/benzoyl peroxide
GEL, TP (1X45GM)
0.1%-2.5%, 45 gm...00299-5908-45 230.63
(Phys Total Care)
REPACK
GEL, TP (1X45GM)
0.1%-2.5%, 45 gm...54868-5991-00 264.05
EPIDURAL ANESTHESIA TRAY (Portex)
kit, anesthesia, epidural
DEV, NA (CONTINUOUS,18G HUSTEAD)
10s ea............00074-4889-20 508.49 428.20
(Portex)
epinephrine/lidocaine hydrochloride
KIT, EP (CONTINUOUS,17G TUOHY)
1:200000-1.5%,
10s ea............00074-8284-20 559.55 471.20
(CONTINUOUS,18G HUSTEAD)
1:200000-1.5%,
10s ea............00074-3093-20 620.71 522.70
10s ea............00074-3096-20 583.18 491.10
10s ea............00074-4775-20 613.46 516.60
10s ea............00074-4810-20 576.06 485.10
(SINGLE-SHOT,CRAWFORD)
1:200000-1.5%,
10s ea............00074-4769-20 566.32 476.90

EPIDURAL CATHETER (Portex)
catheter
DEV, NA (NYLON)
25s ea............00074-1193-01 392.17 330.25
EPIDURAL CATHETER W/STYLET (Portex)
catheter
DEV, NA (20G, RADIOPAQUE)
25s ea............00074-6947-02 392.17 330.25
EPIFOAM (Alaven)
hydrocortisone acetate/pramoxine hydrochloride
FOA, TP (1X10GM)
1%-1%, 10 gm............68220-0144-10 37.74 BX
EPIGALLOCATECHIN GALLATE
(PCCA) *See EGCG*
EPINASTINE HYDROCHLORIDE
(Allergan Inc) *See ELESTAT*
EPINEPHRINE (Adamis)
SOL, IJ (USP,1X0.3ML,SINGLE-DOSE)
1 mg/ml, ea............38739-0030-01 50.57 42.14
(Amer Regent)
SOL, IJ (AMP)
1 mg/ml, 1 ml 25s....00517-1071-25 109.38
(M.D.V.)
1 mg/ml, 30 ml 5s....00517-1130-05 46.25
(Dey, L.P.) *See EPIPEN 2-PAK AUTO-INJECTOR*
(Dey, L.P.) *See EPIPEN AUTO-INJECTOR*
(Dey, L.P.) *See EPIPEN JR 2-PAK AUTO-INJECTOR*
(Dey, L.P.) *See EPIPEN JR AUTO-INJECTOR*
(Gallipot)
POW, NA (U.S.P. ,N.F.)
100 gm............51552-0526-05 516.60
(Hawkins)
POW, NA (U.S.P.)
0.18 gm............63370-0088-07 36.00
5 gm............63370-0088-15 108.00
25 gm............63370-0088-25 440.00
(JHP) *See ADRENALIN CHLORIDE*
(Medisca)
POW, NA (U.S.P.)
25 gm............38779-0436-04 382.50
100 gm............38779-0436-05 1485.00
(PCCA)
POW, NA (BASE)
1 gm............15927-3220-00 42.00
(Shionogi) *See ADRENACLICK*
(Shionogi) *See TWINJECT*
(Spectrum Pharmacy)
POW, NA (U.S.P.)
100 gm............49452-2740-01 3241.00
(Verus) *See TWINJECT*
EPINEPHRINE (Phys Total Care)
REPACK
epinephrine hydrochloride
SOL, IJ (10X10ML)
0.1 mg/ml,
10 ml 10s............54868-5725-00 100.38
EPINEPHRINE 1:1000 (Cura Pharm)
epinephrine hydrochloride
SOL, IJ (10X1ML AMPS,PF)
1 mg/ml, 1 ml 10s....66860-0021-02 43.60
EPINEPHRINE BITARTRATE (Gallipot)
POW, NA (U.S.P.)
0.1 gm............51552-0454-05 11.90
0.18 gm............51552-0454-09 12.60
5 gm............51552-0454-02 31.50
(PCCA)
POW, NA (U.S.P.)
1 gm............51927-2395-00 240.00
(Spectrum Pharmacy)
POW, NA (U.S.P.)
5 gm............49452-2750-01 221.55
25 gm............49452-2750-02 777.00
EPINEPHRINE BITARTRATE/
PRILOCAINE HYDROCHLORIDE
(Dentsply) *See CITANEST FORTE DENTAL*
EPINEPHRINE HCL (Amphastar)
epinephrine hydrochloride
SOL, IJ (SRN,PREFILLED,LUER-JET)
0.1 mg/ml,
10 ml 10s............00548-3316-00 53.20

PROD/MFR NDC AWP DP OBC

(MIN-I-JET,21GX1 1/2")
0.1 mg/ml,
10 ml 25s.......... **00548-1016-00** 129.68
(SRN,PREFILLED,STICKGARD)
0.1 mg/ml,
10 ml 25s.......... **00548-2016-00** 139.65
(M.D.V.)
1 mg/ml, 30 ml....... **00548-9061-00** 5.99

(Consolidated Midland)
SOL, IJ (VIAL, AQUEOUS)
1 mg/ml, 1 ml 25s.... **00223-7520-05** 20.00
(VIAL)
1 mg/ml, 1 ml 100s... **00223-7520-01** 60.00

(Hospira)
SOL, IJ (18GX3-1/2,10X10ML)
0.1 mg/ml,
10 ml 10s.......... **00409-4901-18** 51.48 45.00
(LIFE,21GX1-1/2)
0.1 mg/ml,
10 ml 10s.......... **00074-4921-34** 23.28 20.40
10 ml 10s.......... **00409-4921-34** 24.48 21.40
(AMP)
1 mg/ml, 1 ml 25s.... **00074-7241-01** 36.30 31.75
1 ml 25s.......... **00409-7241-01** 38.40 33.50

(Medisca)
POW, NA, 1 gm.......... **38779-2065-06** 169.50
5 gm................ **38779-2065-03** 643.50

(PCCA)
POW, NA (USP)
1 gm................ **51927-1715-00** 171.00

(West-Ward)
SOL, IJ (10X30ML,M.D.V.)
1 mg/ml, 30 ml 10s... **00143-9984-90** 55.00

(Dispensing Solutions)
REPACK
SOL, IJ (SYRINGE,LATEX-FREE)
0.1 mg/ml, 10 ml..... **55045-9903-03** 6.95

(Phys Total Care)
REPACK
SOL, IJ, 1 mg/ml, 1 ml.... **54868-2065-00** 8.19
1 ml 25s.......... **54868-2065-01** 106.24
(M.D.V.)
1 mg/ml, 30 ml....... **54868-3641-00** 14.64

(Physician Partner)
REPACK
SOL, IJ (1X30ML)
1 mg/ml, 30 ml....... **21695-0845-30** 13.00

EPINEPHRINE HYDROCHLORIDE
(Amphastar) *See EPINEPHRINE HCL*
(Consolidated Midland) *See EPINEPHRINE HCL*
(Cura Pharm) *See EPINEPHRINE 1:1000*
(Hospira) *See EPINEPHRINE HCL*
(JHP) *See ADRENALIN*
(Medisca) *See EPINEPHRINE HCL*
(PCCA) *See EPINEPHRINE HCL*
(West-Ward) *See EPINEPHRINE HCL*

(Palmetto)
REPACK
SOL, IJ, 1 mg/ml, 1 ml.... **23490-5497-02** 3.00

EPINEPHRINE/LIDOCAINE HCL (Hospira)
epinephrine/lidocaine hydrochloride
SOL, EP (VIAL,FLIPTOP)
1:200000-1.5%,
30 ml 5s.......... **00409-3181-01** 46.56 40.75 **AP**
IJ (VIAL, FLIPTOP)
1:200000-0.5%,
50 ml 25s.......... **00074-3177-01** 72.90 63.75 **AP**
(VIAL,FLIPTOP)
1:200000-0.5%,
50 ml 25s.......... **00409-3177-01** 80.10 70.00 **AP**
(AMP,LATEX-FREE)
1:200000-1%,
30 ml 5s.......... **00074-3179-01** 30.96 27.10 **AP**
(5X20ML)
1:200000-2%,
20 ml 5s.......... **00409-3183-01** 60.06 52.55 **AP**
(VIAL, FLIPTOP)
1:100000-1%,
20 ml 25s.......... **00409-3178-01** 61.20 53.50 **AP**
(FTV,25X30ML)
1:100000-1%,
30 ml 25s.......... **00409-3178-02** 95.10 83.25 **AP**
(FTV,25X50ML)
1:100000-1%,
50 ml 25s.......... **00409-3178-03** 83.10 72.75 **AP**

PROD/MFR NDC AWP DP OBC

(FTV,25X20ML)
1:100000-2%,
20 ml 25s.......... **00409-3182-01** 71.40 62.50 **AP**
(VIAL, FLIPTOP)
1:100000-2%,
30 ml 25s.......... **00409-3182-02** 91.20 79.75 **AP**
50 ml 25s.......... **00074-3182-03** 81.90 71.75 **AP**
(VIAL,FLIPTOP,25X50ML)
1:100000-2%,
50 ml 25s.......... **00409-3182-03** 116.10 101.50 **AP**

(Dispensing Solutions)
REPACK
SOL, IJ, 1:100000-1%,
30 ml.............. **55045-3250-03** 3.10 **AP**
30 ml.............. **55045-3338-03** 3.00 **AP**

(Southwood)
REPACK
SOL, IJ (M.D.V.)
1:100000-1%, 30 ml.. **58016-9332-01** 1.41 **AP**

EPINEPHRINE/LIDOCAINE HYDROCHLORIDE
(APP) *See XYLOCAINE W/EPINEPHRINE*
(APP) *See XYLOCAINE WITH EPINEPHRINE*
(APP) *See XYLOCAINE-MPF W/EPINEPHRINE*
(APP) *See XYLOCAINE-MPF WITH EPINEPHRINE*
(Dentsply) *See XYLOCAINE DENTAL W/EPINEPHRINE*
(Hospira) *See EPINEPHRINE/LIDOCAINE HCL*
(Hospira) *See LIDOCAINE HCL AND EPINEPHRINE*
(Hospira) *See LIDOCAINE HYDROCHLORIDE AND EPINEPHRINE*
(Portex) *See CAUDAL ANESTHESIA TRAY*
(Portex) *See EPIDURAL ANESTHESIA TRAY*

EPIPEN (Phys Total Care)
REPACK
epinephrine
KIT, MR, 1 mg/ml, ea...... **54868-2804-00** 83.18
2s ea.............. **54868-2804-01** 178.39

EPIPEN 2-PAK AUTO-INJECTOR (Dey, L.P.)
epinephrine
KIT, MR (0.3 MG/DELIVERY)
1 mg/ml, 2s ea....... **49502-0500-02** 149.16

(Quality Care Prod)
REPACK
KIT, MR, 1 mg/ml, 2s ea... **49999-0718-02** 237.20

EPIPEN AUTO-INJECTOR (Dey, L.P.)
epinephrine
KIT, MR (0.3 MG/DELIVERY)
1 mg/ml, ea.......... **49502-0500-01** 74.58

(A-S Medication)
REPACK
KIT, MR (0.3 MG/DELIVERY)
1 mg/ml, ea.......... **54569-1392-00** 64.83

(Quality Care Prod)
REPACK
KIT, MR, 1 mg/ml, ea...... **49999-0718-03** 62.73

EPIPEN JR 2-PAK AUTO-INJECTOR (Dey, L.P.)
epinephrine
KIT, MR (0.15 MG/DELIVERY)
0.5 mg/ml, 2s ea..... **49502-0501-02** 149.16

(Phys Total Care)
REPACK
KIT, MR (0.15 MG/DELIVERY)
0.5 mg/ml, 2s ea..... **54868-4819-00** 178.39

EPIPEN JR AUTO-INJECTOR (Dey, L.P.)
epinephrine
KIT, MR (0.15 MG/DELIVERY)
0.5 mg/ml, ea........ **49502-0501-01** 74.58

(A-S Medication)
REPACK
KIT, MR (0.15 MG/DELIVERY)
0.5 mg/ml, ea........ **54569-1391-00** 64.83

(Phys Total Care)
REPACK
KIT, MR, 0.5 mg/ml, ea.... **54868-4819-01** 95.37

EPIPEN TRAINER (Dey, L.P.)
trainer, injection
DEV, NA, ea.............. **49502-0500-00** 5.94

EPIQUIN MICRO (SkinMedica)
hydroquinone
CRE, TP, 4%, 30 gm....... **67402-0010-30** 118.75 95.00

(Pharma Pac)
REPACK
CRE, TP, 4%, 30 gm....... **52959-0808-03** 88.58

PROD/MFR NDC AWP DP OBC

EPIRUBICIN HYDROCHLORIDE (APP)
SOL, IV (1X25ML,PF)
2 mg/ml, 25 ml....... **63323-0151-25** 719.21 100.10 **AP**
(1X100ML,PF)
2 mg/ml, 100 ml..... **63323-0151-00** 2876.82 525.00 **AP**

(Bedford)
SOL, IV (S.D.V.,PF)
2 mg/ml, 25 ml....... **55390-0207-01** 204.00 **AP**
100 ml............ **55390-0208-01** 840.00 **AP**

(Greenstone)
SOL, IV (SINGLE USE,PF)
2 mg/ml, 25 ml....... **59762-5091-01** 673.51
100 ml............ **59762-5093-01** 2694.02

(Hospira) *See NOVAPLUS EPIRUBICIN HYDROCHLORIDE*

(Hospira)
PDS, IV (S.D.V.)
50 mg, ea........... **61703-0347-35** 67.86 59.38
200 mg, ea.......... **61703-0348-59** 2845.85 2490.12
SOL, IV (1X5ML,SINGLE USE,PF)
2 mg/ml, 5 ml........ **61703-0359-92** 19.74 17.27 **AP**
(PF)
2 mg/ml, 25 ml....... **61703-0359-93** 86.20 75.42 **AP**
(1X75ML,SINGLE USE,PF)
2 mg/ml, 75 ml....... **61703-0359-91** 282.16 246.89 **AP**
(PF)
2 mg/ml, 100 ml..... **61703-0359-59** 336.00 294.00 **AP**

(Pfizer) *See ELLENCE*

(Sagent)
SOL, IV (1X25ML,SINGLE-DOSE,PF)
2 mg/ml, 25 ml....... **25021-0203-25** 212.50 **AP**
(1X100ML,SINGLE-DOSE,PF)
2 mg/ml, 100 ml..... **25021-0203-51** 875.00 **AP**

(Teva)
SOL, IV (SDV,PF)
2 mg/ml, 25 ml....... **00703-3067-11** 180.00 **AP**
100 ml............ **00703-3069-11** 660.00 **AP**

EPITESTOSTERONE (PCCA)
POW, NA (1X0.001GM)
1 gm................ **51927-3430-00** 3.90

EPITOL (Teva)
carbamazepine
TAB, PO, 200 mg, 100s ea. **00093-0090-01** 30.17 **AB**

EPIVIR (Glaxo)
lamivudine
SOL, PO (AF,BANANA-STRAWBERRY)
10 mg/ml, 240 ml.... **00173-0471-00** 115.33
TAB, PO (FILM-COATED)
150 mg, 60s ea...... **00173-0470-01** 432.46
(FILM-COATED TABLET)
300 mg, 30s ea...... **00173-0714-00** 432.46

(A-S Medication)
REPACK
SOL, PO (AF,BANANA-STRAWBERRY)
10 mg/ml, 240 ml.... **54569-4333-00** 149.93
TAB, PO (FILM-COATED)
150 mg, 60s ea...... **54569-4221-00** 450.48
(FILM-COATED TABLET)
300 mg, 30s ea...... **54569-5501-00** 562.20

(DHS, Inc.)
REPACK
TAB, PO, 300 mg, 10s ea.. **55887-0750-10** 173.98
20s ea............ **55887-0750-20** 347.96
30s ea............ **55887-0750-30** 521.94

(Dispensing Solutions)
REPACK
TAB, PO, 150 mg, 6s ea... **55045-2308-02** 42.00
10s ea............ **55045-2308-04** 70.00
(FILM-COATED)
150 mg, 14s ea...... **55045-2308-03** 98.00
60s ea............ **55045-2308-01** 420.00

(Pharma Pac)
REPACK
TAB, PO, 150 mg, 2s ea... **52959-0508-02** 13.16
4s ea............. **52959-0508-04** 23.65
6s ea............. **52959-0508-06** 31.55
8s ea............. **52959-0508-08** 39.40
14s ea............ **52959-0508-14** 64.37
15s ea............ **52959-0508-15** 68.96
60s ea............ **52959-0508-60** 275.45

(Phys Total Care)
REPACK
TAB, PO, 150 mg, 30s ea.. **54868-3693-02** 243.43
60s ea............ **54868-3693-00** 468.67
300 mg, 30s ea...... **54868-5416-00** 429.00

PROD/MFR	NDC	AWP	DP	OBC
(Physician Partner)				
REPACK				
TAB, PO (FILM-COATED)				
150 mg, 6s ea	21695-0367-06	199.99		
(Quality Care Prod)				
REPACK				
TAB, PO, 150 mg, 6s ea	49999-0119-06	80.58		
(FILM-COATED)				
150 mg, 60s ea	49999-0119-60	762.05		
300 mg, 30s ea	35356-0065-30	731.20		
(Southwood)				
REPACK				
TAB, PO (FILM-COATED)				
150 mg, 30s ea	58016-0689-30	203.99		
60s ea	58016-0689-60	407.98		
90s ea	58016-0689-90	611.97		
100s ea	58016-0689-00	679.97		
(FILM-COATED TABLET)				
300 mg, 30s ea	58016-0795-30	407.98		
60s ea	58016-0795-60	815.96		
90s ea	58016-0795-90	1223.94		
100s ea	58016-0795-00	1359.93		
EPIVIR A/F (Quality Care Prod)				
REPACK				
lamivudine				
SOL, PO (1X240ML)				
10 mg/ml, 240 ml	35356-0066-24	141.00		
EPIVIR HBV (Glaxo)				
lamivudine				
SOL, PO (BANANA-STRAWBERRY)				
5 mg/ml, 240 ml	00173-0663-00	163.97		
TAB, PO, 100 mg, 60s ea	00173-0662-00	819.84		
EPLERENONE (Apotex Corp.)				
TAB, PO (FILM-COATED)				
25 mg, 30s ea	60505-2651-03	123.07		AB
90s ea	60505-2651-09	369.22		AB
500s ea	60505-2651-05	2051.22		AB
50 mg, 30s ea	60505-2652-03	123.07		AB
90s ea	60505-2652-09	369.22		AB
(Greenstone)				
TAB, PO (FILM-COATED)				
25 mg, 30s ea	59762-1710-02	122.94		
90s ea	59762-1710-03	368.81		
(10X10,FILM-COATED)				
25 mg, 100s ea UD	59762-1710-01	409.80		
(FILM-COATED)				
50 mg, 30s ea	59762-1720-01	122.94		
90s ea	59762-1720-02	368.81		
(Pfizer) *See INSPRA*				
(Sandoz)				
TAB, PO (FILM-COATED)				
25 mg, 30s ea	00185-5368-30	123.08		AB
90s ea	00185-5368-09	369.23		AB
50 mg, 30s ea	00185-5369-30	123.08		AB
90s ea	00185-5369-09	369.23		AB
(Phys Total Care)				
REPACK				
TAB, PO (FILM-COATED)				
25 mg, 30s ea	54868-6065-00	197.31		AB
90s ea	54868-6065-01	542.76		AB
EPOETIN ALFA				
(Amgen USA Inc.) *See EPOGEN*				
(Centocor) *See PROCRIT*				
EPOGEN (Amgen USA Inc.)				
epoetin alfa				
SOL, IJ (S.D.V.,S2,PF)				
2000 u/ml, 1 ml	55513-0126-01	30.36		
1 ml 10s	55513-0126-10	303.60		
(S.D.V.,S3,PF)				
3000 u/ml, 1 ml	55513-0267-01	45.54		
1 ml 10s	55513-0267-10	455.40		
(S.D.V.,S4,PF)				
4000 u/ml, 1 ml	55513-0148-01	60.72		
1 ml 10s	55513-0148-10	607.20		
(S.D.V.,S10,PF)				
10000 u/ml, 1 ml	55513-0144-01	151.80		
1 ml 10s	55513-0144-10	1518.00		
(M.D.V.,M10)				
10000 u/ml, 2 ml	55513-0283-01	303.60		
2 ml 10s	55513-0283-10	3036.00		
(M.D.V.,M20)				
20000 u/ml, 1 ml	55513-0478-01	303.60		
1 ml 10s	55513-0478-10	3036.00		
(S.D.V.,S40,PF)				
40000 u/ml, 1 ml	55513-0823-01	640.37		
1 ml 10s	55513-0823-10	6403.68		
EPOPROSTENOL SODIUM (Teva)				
PDS, IV, 0.5 mg, ea	00703-1985-01	13.88		AP
1.5 mg, ea	00703-1995-01	33.53		AP

PROD/MFR	NDC	AWP	DP	OBC
EPOPROSTENOL SODIUM DILUENT (Teva)				
glycine/sodium chloride				
SOL, IV (2X50ML)				
50 ml 2s	00703-9258-09	20.16		
EPROSARTAN MESYLATE				
(Abbott Pharm) *See TEVETEN*				
EPROSARTAN MESYLATE/HYDROCHLOROTHIAZIDE				
(Abbott Pharm) *See TEVETEN HCT*				
EPSOM SALT (Cardinal Health)				
magnesium sulfate				
PDR, NA (U.S.P.,PRIVATE LABEL)				
480 gm	37205-0602-43	1.13		
1920 gm	37205-0602-07	2.59		
(Gallipot)				
PDR, NA (U.S.P.)				
113.4 gm	51552-0376-04	3.15		
480 gm	51552-0376-06	9.10		
11350 gm	51552-0376-08	66.50		
22700 gm	51552-0376-09	111.30		
(McKesson)				
PDR, NA, 480 gm	52297-0721-43	1.43		
1810 gm	52297-0721-07	2.99		
(Phys Total Care)				
REPACK				
PDR, NA, 480 gm	54868-3241-01	3.72		
EPTIFIBATIDE				
(Schering) *See INTEGRILIN*				
EPZICOM (Glaxo)				
abacavir sulfate/lamivudine				
TAB, PO (FILM-COATED)				
600 mg-300 mg,				
30s ea	00173-0742-00	1013.56		
(A-S Medication)				
REPACK				
TAB, PO (FILM-COATED)				
600 mg-300 mg,				
30s ea	54569-5594-00	1317.63		
(Phys Total Care)				
REPACK				
TAB, PO, 600 mg-300 mg,				
30s ea	54868-5600-00	1163.04		
(Quality Care Prod)				
REPACK				
TAB, PO (FILM-COATED)				
600 mg-300 mg,				
6s ea	35356-0109-06	370.66		
30s ea	35356-0109-30	1900.31		
EQUAGESIC (Caraco)				
aspirin/meprobamate				
TAB, PO, 325 mg-200 mg,				
100s ea, C-IV	10551-0091-10	208.34		
EQUETRO (Validus)				
carbamazepine				
CER, PO (HARD GELATIN)				
100 mg, 120s ea	30698-0419-12	208.80		EE
200 mg, 120s ea	30698-0421-12	258.00		EE
300 mg, 120s ea	30698-0423-12	318.00		
ERAXIS (Pfizer)				
anidulafungin				
PDS, IV (SINGLE-USE VIAL,PF)				
50 mg, ea	00049-0114-28	108.00	90.00	
(W/ DILUENT,PF)				
50 mg, ea	00049-1010-28	108.00	90.00	
(PF)				
100 mg, ea	00049-0115-28	216.00	180.00	
(SINGLE-USE VIAL,PF)				
100 mg, ea	00049-0116-28	216.00	180.00	
ERBITUX (Bristol-Myers)				
cetuximab				
SOL, IV (PF)				
2 mg/ml, 50 ml	66733-0948-23	576.00		
100 ml	66733-0958-23	1152.00		EE
ERGOCALCIFEROL				
(Breckenridge Pharm) *See VITAMIN D*				
(Consolidated Midland) *See VITAMIN D*				
(Gallipot)				
POW, NA (1X1GM,USP)				
1 gm	51552-0861-01	80.50	57.50	
(1X5GM,USP)				
5 gm	51552-0861-02	315.00	225.00	
(PCCA)				
POW, NA (U.S.P.)				
1 gm	51927-2722-00	144.00		
(Sanofi-Aventis) *See DRISDOL*				

PROD/MFR	NDC	AWP	DP	OBC
(Spectrum Pharmacy)				
POW, NA (U.S.P.)				
1 gm	49452-2760-01	220.85		
5 gm	49452-2760-02	777.00		
(Teva) *See VITAMIN D*				
(Winthrop)				
CAP, PO, 50000 iu, 50s ea	00955-0250-50	95.60		
ERGOLOID MESYLATES (Gallipot)				
POW, NA (1X1GM,USP)				
1 gm	51552-0798-01	68.53	48.95	
(1X5GM,USP)				
5 gm	51552-0798-02	315.70	225.50	
(Medisca)				
POW, NA (U.S.P.)				
1 gm	38779-0860-06	105.00		
5 gm	38779-0860-03	420.00		
10 gm	38779-0860-01	811.50		
(Mutual)				
TAB, PO, 1 mg, 100s ea	53489-0281-01	466.31		AB
(PCCA)				
POW, NA (U.S.P.)				
1 gm	51927-2481-00	138.00		
(Spectrum Pharmacy)				
POW, NA (U.S.P.)				
1 gm	49452-2764-01	190.05		
5 gm	49452-2764-02	700.00		
(Phys Total Care)				
REPACK				
TAB, PO, 1 mg, 10s ea	54868-0899-01	69.46		
30s ea	54868-0899-00	202.38		
ERGOMAR (Rosedale)				
ergotamine tartrate				
TAB, SL (5-2X2INDVL FOIL STRIP)				
2 mg, 20s ea	10802-1202-00	179.40		
ERGONOVINE MALEATE (Gallipot)				
POW, NA (U.S.P.,N.F.)				
0.1 gm	51552-0188-07	42.00		
1 gm	51552-0188-01	266.00		
100 gm	51552-0188-05	3500.00		
(PCCA)				
POW, NA, 1 gm	51927-2099-00	900.00		
(Spectrum Pharmacy)				
POW, NA (U.S.P.)				
0.5 gm	49452-2762-02	388.50		
1 gm	49452-2762-03	605.50		
(A-S Medication)				
REPACK				
TAB, PO, 0.2 mg, 12s ea	54569-4456-02	6.00		
(PD-Rx Pharm)				
REPACK				
TAB, PO, 0.2 mg, 3s ea	55289-0458-03	6.80		
4s ea	55289-0458-04	7.40		
6s ea	55289-0458-06	8.60		
8s ea	55289-0458-08	9.80		
9s ea	55289-0458-09	10.40		
10s ea	55289-0458-10	11.00		
12s ea	55289-0458-12	12.20		
18s ea	55289-0458-18	15.80		
20s ea	55289-0458-20	17.00		
28s ea	55289-0458-28	21.80		
100s ea	55289-0458-01	65.00		
ERGOTAMINE TARTRATE (Gallipot)				
POW, NA, 1 gm	51552-0181-01	69.44		
5 gm	51552-0181-02	170.80		
(Medisca)				
POW, NA (U.S.P.)				
25 gm	38779-0219-04	1209.00		
(PCCA)				
POW, NA (U.S.P.)				
1 gm	51927-1955-00	108.00		
(Rosedale) *See ERGOMAR*				
(Spectrum Pharmacy)				
POW, NA (U.S.P.)				
1 gm	49452-2763-01	200.90		
5 gm	49452-2763-02	693.00		
ERGOTAMINE TARTRATE AND CAFFEINE (Cypress Pharm)				
caffeine/ergotamine tartrate				
TAB, PO (FILM-COATED)				
100 mg-1 mg,				
100s ea	60258-0070-01	120.79		
ERLOTINIB				
(Genentech) *See TARCEVA*				

PROD/MFR	NDC	AWP	DP	OBC
ERRIN (Teva)				
norethindrone				
TAB, PO (6 BLISTER PAKS OF 28EA)				
0.35 mg, 168s ea	**00555-0344-58**	221.49		**AB2**
(Dispensing Solutions)				
REPACK				
TAB, PO (6X28)				
0.35 mg, 168s ea	**55045-3498-01**	222.00		
ERTACZO (Ortho)				
sertaconazole nitrate				
CRE, TP, 2%, 30 gm	**00062-1650-03**	87.48	72.90	
60 gm	**00062-1650-02**	156.00	130.00	
(Physician Partner)				
REPACK				
CRE, TP (1X30GM)				
2%, 30 gm	**21695-0454-30**	165.08		
(Quality Care Prod)				
REPACK				
CRE, TP (1X30GM)				
2%, 30 gm	**35356-0224-30**	150.19		
ERTAPENEM SODIUM				
(Merck) *See INVANZ*				
ERVOL LIGHT (Amend)				
mineral oil				
OIL, NA (N.F.)				
480 ml	**17317-1064-01**	4.90		
3840 ml	**17317-1064-06**	21.00		
19200 ml	**17317-1064-08**	70.00		
ERY (Perrigo)				
erythromycin				
PAD, TP, 2%, 60s ea	**45802-0962-72**	94.86		
(A-S Medication)				
REPACK				
PAD, TP, 2%, 60s ea	**54569-5364-00**	84.43		
ERY TABS (Stat Rx)				
REPACK				
erythromycin				
ECT, PO, 333 mg, 21s ea	**16590-0089-21**	27.50		
30s ea	**16590-0089-30**	39.29		
40s ea	**16590-0089-40**	52.38		
ERY-TAB (Abbott Pharm)				
erythromycin				
ECT, PO, 250 mg, 100s ea	**00074-6304-13**	27.40	24.03	**AB**
333 mg, 100s ea	**00074-6320-13**	40.32	35.37	**AB**
500 mg, 100s ea	**00074-6321-13**	46.24	40.56	**AB**
(A-S Medication)				
REPACK				
ECT, PO, 250 mg, 28s ea	**54569-3563-05**	8.12		**AB**
40s ea	**54569-3563-04**	11.60		**AB**
500 mg, 20s ea	**54569-2508-01**	9.35		**AB**
28s ea	**54569-2508-00**	13.09		**AB**
40s ea	**54569-2508-03**	18.70		**AB**
(Altura)				
REPACK				
ECT, PO, 333 mg, 18s ea	**63874-0127-18**	6.24		**AB**
20s ea	**63874-0127-20**	10.64		**AB**
21s ea	**63874-0127-21**	11.17		**AB**
28s ea	**63874-0127-28**	14.90		**AB**
30s ea	**63874-0127-30**	15.96		**AB**
40s ea	**63874-0127-40**	21.28		
42s ea	**63874-0127-42**	22.34		**AB**
100s ea	**63874-0127-01**	53.20		**AB**
500s ea	**63874-0127-05**	266.00		**AB**
(Core)				
REPACK				
ECT, PO, 250 mg, 30s ea	**33358-0377-30**	12.40		
333 mg, 30s ea	**33358-0132-30**	15.90		
500 mg, 28s ea	**33358-0133-28**	23.46		
(DHS, Inc.)				
REPACK				
ECT, PO, 250 mg, 28s ea	**55887-0787-28**	15.50		**AB**
333 mg, 21s ea	**55887-0955-21**	21.00		**AB**
30s ea	**55887-0955-30**	29.00		**AB**
(Dispensing Solutions)				
REPACK				
ECT, PO, 250 mg, 20s ea	**55045-2012-05**	10.00		**AB**
28s ea	**55045-2012-08**	14.00		**AB**
30s ea	**55045-2012-02**	15.00		**AB**
40s ea	**55045-2012-09**	20.00		**AB**
333 mg, 9s ea	**55045-1270-06**	5.40		**AB**
15s ea	**55045-1270-05**	9.05		**AB**
21s ea	**55045-1270-09**	12.60		**AB**
21s ea	**66336-0098-21**	17.83		**AB**
28s ea	**55045-1270-04**	16.80		**AB**
28s ea	**66336-0098-28**	20.87		**AB**
30s ea	**55045-1270-08**	18.00		**AB**
30s ea	**55045-3922-01**	18.00		**AB**
30s ea	**66336-0098-30**	22.36		**AB**
40s ea	**55045-1270-03**	24.00		**AB**
500 mg, 20s ea	**55045-2162-07**	17.50		**AB**
30s ea	**55045-2162-08**	26.40		**AB**
40s ea	**55045-2162-04**	35.20		**AB**
TCP, PO (ENTERIC-COATED)				
500 mg, 40s ea	**66336-0644-40**	30.80		**AB**
(HomeMed)				
REPACK				
ECT, PO, 333 mg, 30s ea	**51655-0480-24**	30.34		
(Nucare Pharm)				
REPACK				
ECT, PO, 333 mg, 15s ea	**66267-0088-15**	8.56		**AB**
21s ea	**66267-0088-21**	10.76		**AB**
30s ea	**66267-0088-30**	15.36		**AB**
500 mg, 20s ea	**66267-0089-20**	14.98		**AB**
28s ea	**66267-0089-28**	20.97		**AB**
(PD-Rx Pharm)				
REPACK				
ECT, PO (REDI-SCRIPT)				
250 mg, 40s ea	**58864-0632-40**	48.67		**AB**
333 mg, 21s ea	**55289-0525-21**	33.30		**AB**
30s ea	**55289-0525-30**	41.49		**AB**
(REDI-SCRIPT)				
333 mg, 30s ea	**58864-0615-30**	41.49		**AB**
40s ea	**55289-0525-40**	52.00		**AB**
42s ea	**55289-0525-42**	54.72		**AB**
63s ea	**55289-0525-63**	83.23		**AB**
500 mg, 28s ea	**55289-0217-28**	37.35		**AB**
(REDI-SCRIPT)				
500 mg, 30s ea	**58864-0845-30**	45.00		**AB**
40s ea	**55289-0217-40**	53.37		**AB**
(FILM COATED)				
500 mg, 40s ea	**58864-0845-40**	57.93		
(Pharma Pac)				
REPACK				
ECT, PO, 250 mg, 20s ea	**52959-0060-20**	10.02		**AB**
28s ea	**52959-0060-28**	14.02		**AB**
30s ea	**52959-0060-30**	15.01		**AB**
40s ea	**52959-0060-40**	19.98		**AB**
56s ea	**52959-0060-56**	27.98		**AB**
333 mg, 15s ea	**52959-0061-15**	17.50		**AB**
18s ea	**52959-0061-18**	20.32		**AB**
20s ea	**52959-0061-20**	21.86		**AB**
21s ea	**52959-0061-21**	22.96		**AB**
24s ea	**52959-0061-24**	25.92		**AB**
28s ea	**52959-0061-28**	28.42		**AB**
30s ea	**52959-0061-30**	30.34		**AB**
40s ea	**52959-0061-40**	36.56		**AB**
42s ea	**52959-0061-42**	41.12		**AB**
500 mg, 10s ea	**52959-0062-10**	15.52		**AB**
20s ea	**52959-0062-20**	31.08		**AB**
21s ea	**52959-0062-21**	32.63		**AB**
28s ea	**52959-0062-28**	35.26		**AB**
30s ea	**52959-0062-30**	38.44		**AB**
40s ea	**52959-0062-40**	48.02		**AB**
56s ea	**52959-0062-56**	64.66		**AB**
(Phys Total Care)				
REPACK				
ECT, PO, 333 mg, 15s ea	**54868-0840-04**	27.18		**AB**
20s ea	**54868-0840-00**	34.71		**AB**
30s ea	**54868-0840-02**	49.83		**AB**
40s ea	**54868-0840-01**	64.95		**AB**
100s ea	**54868-0840-03**	118.56		**AB**
500 mg, 30s ea	**54868-2840-00**	18.44		**AB**
TCP, PO (ENTERIC-COATED)				
500 mg, 20s ea	**54868-2840-01**	12.91		**AB**
(Quality Care Prod)				
REPACK				
ECT, PO, 333 mg, 10s ea	**49999-0014-10**	10.98		**AB**
21s ea	**49999-0014-21**	23.06		**AB**
30s ea	**49999-0014-30**	32.94		**AB**
100s ea	**49999-0014-00**	109.80		**AB**
500 mg, 28s ea	**49999-0067-28**	17.29		**AB**
40s ea	**49999-0067-40**	24.70		**AB**
(Southwood)				
REPACK				
ECT, PO, 250 mg, 28s ea	**58016-0162-28**	5.06		**AB**
30s ea	**58016-0162-30**	7.61		**AB**
40s ea	**58016-0162-40**	6.30		**AB**
60s ea	**58016-0162-60**	15.22		**AB**
90s ea	**58016-0162-90**	22.82		**AB**
100s ea	**58016-0162-00**	25.36		**AB**
333 mg, 15s ea	**58016-0126-15**	5.60		**AB**
18s ea	**58016-0126-18**	6.72		**AB**
20s ea	**58016-0126-20**	7.46		**AB**
21s ea	**58016-0126-21**	7.84		**AB**
28s ea	**58016-0126-28**	10.45		**AB**
30s ea	**58016-0126-30**	11.20		**AB**
42s ea	**58016-0126-42**	15.67		**AB**
60s ea	**58016-0126-60**	22.39		**AB**
90s ea	**58016-0126-90**	33.59		**AB**
100s ea	**58016-0126-00**	37.32		**AB**
180s ea	**58016-0126-99**	67.18		**AB**
(St. Mary's MPP)				
REPACK				
ECT, PO, 333 mg, 30s ea	**60760-0320-30**	18.83		**AB**
ERY-TABS (DHS, Inc.)				
REPACK				
erythromycin				
ECT, PO, 250 mg, 20s ea	**55887-0787-20**	11.07		
40s ea	**55887-0787-40**	19.37		
ERYC (PD-Rx Pharm)				
REPACK				
erythromycin				
ECC, PO, 250 mg, 20s ea	**55289-0111-20**	161.70		**AB**
28s ea	**55289-0111-28**	214.62		**AB**
40s ea	**55289-0111-40**	290.89		**AB**
56s ea	**55289-0111-56**	411.16		**AB**
80s ea	**55289-0111-80**	545.11		**AB**
ERYCETTE (Southwood)				
REPACK				
erythromycin				
SWA, TP, 2%, 60s ea	**58016-3205-01**	26.04		**AT**
ERYPED (Phys Total Care)				
REPACK				
erythromycin ethylsuccinate				
PDR, PO (DROPS)				
100 mg/2.5 ml,				
50 ml	**54868-1886-00**	8.90		
ERYPED 200 (Abbott Pharm)				
erythromycin ethylsuccinate				
PDR, PO, 200 mg/5 ml,				
100 ml	**00074-6302-13**	9.50	8.34	**AB**
(Phys Total Care)				
REPACK				
PDR, PO, 200 mg/5 ml,				
100 ml	**54868-1426-01**	10.95		**AB**
(Southwood)				
REPACK				
PDR, PO, 200 mg/5 ml,				
100 ml	**58016-1036-01**	7.70		**AB**
200 ml	**58016-1037-06**	14.02		**AB**
ERYPED 400 (Abbott Pharm)				
erythromycin ethylsuccinate				
PDR, PO, 400 mg/5 ml,				
100 ml	**00074-6305-13**	14.62	12.82	
(Phys Total Care)				
REPACK				
PDR, PO, 400 mg/5 ml,				
100 ml	**54868-1887-01**	17.39		
200 ml	**54868-1887-00**	30.89		
(Southwood)				
REPACK				
PDR, PO, 400 mg/5 ml,				
100 ml	**58016-1038-01**	11.85		
200 ml	**58016-1039-06**	21.62		
ERYSIDORON 1 (Weleda)				
homeopathic substance				
LIQ, PO, 20 ml	**55946-0230-10**	4.65		
ERYSIDORON 2 (Weleda)				
homeopathic substance				
TAB, PO, 100s ea	**55946-0240-30**	6.60		
ERYTHORBIC ACID (Spectrum Pharmacy)				
POW, NA (F.C.C.)				
100 gm	**49452-2767-01**	128.80		
500 gm	**49452-2767-02**	308.00		
ERYTHROCIN LACTOBIONATE (Hospira)				
erythromycin lactobionate				
PDS, IV (ADD-VANTAGE,LATEX-FREE)				
1 gm, 10s ea	**00074-6478-44**	216.60	189.50	**AP**
(ADD-VANTAGE VIAL)				
1 gm, 1 gm 10s	**00409-6478-44**	258.00	225.80	**AP**
(ADD-VANTAGE VIAL,PF)				
500 mg, 10s ea	**00409-6476-44**	154.80	135.50	**AP**
(ADD-VANTAGE,LATEX-FREE)				
500 mg, 10s ea	**00074-6476-44**	154.80	135.50	**AP**
(LATEX-FREE)				
500 mg, 10s ea	**00409-6482-01**	136.32	119.30	**AP**
ERYTHROCIN STEARATE (Altura)				
REPACK				
erythromycin stearate				
TAB, PO (FILM-COATED)				
250 mg, 8s ea	**63874-0129-08**	1.23		
10s ea	**63874-0129-10**	1.45		
12s ea	**63874-0129-12**	1.73		

PROD/MFR	NDC	AWP	DP	OBC
14s ea	63874-0129-14	2.03		
15s ea	63874-0129-15	2.16		
16s ea	63874-0129-16	2.47		
20s ea	63874-0129-20	2.89		
21s ea	63874-0129-21	3.03		
24s ea	63874-0129-24	3.47		
28s ea	63874-0129-28	11.86		
30s ea	63874-0129-30	12.70		
40s ea	63874-0129-40	16.93		
56s ea	63874-0129-56	23.70		
60s ea	63874-0129-60	25.39		
100s ea	63874-0129-01	42.33		
120s ea	63874-0129-04	50.80		
500s ea	63874-0129-50	211.79		
(FILM COATED)				
500 mg, 3s ea	63874-0130-03	1.67		
6s ea	63874-0130-06	3.36		
9s ea	63874-0130-09	5.04		
10s ea	63874-0130-10	5.59		
12s ea	63874-0130-12	6.70		
14s ea	63874-0130-14	7.82		
15s ea	63874-0130-15	8.38		
20s ea	63874-0130-20	11.18		
21s ea	63874-0130-21	11.74		
24s ea	63874-0130-24	13.42		
28s ea	63874-0130-28	15.65		
30s ea	63874-0130-30	16.77		
40s ea	63874-0130-40	22.36		
60s ea	63874-0130-60	33.54		
100s ea	63874-0130-01	55.90		
ERYTHROCIN STEARATE FILMTAB (Abbott Pharm)				
erythromycin stearate				
TAB, PO (FILMTAB)				
250 mg, 100s ea	00074-6346-20	15.86	13.92	AB
500 mg, 100s ea	00074-6316-13	28.67	25.15	AB
(A-S Medication)				
REPACK				
TAB, PO (FILMTAB)				
250 mg, 20s ea	54569-0124-01	3.21		AB
28s ea	54569-0124-02	4.49		AB
40s ea	54569-0124-03	6.42		AB
500 mg, 20s ea	54569-3347-01	5.80		AB
28s ea	54569-0125-05	8.12		AB
40s ea	54569-0125-02	11.60		AB
(Dispensing Solutions)				
REPACK				
TAB, PO (FILMTAB)				
250 mg, 10s ea	55045-1113-01	7.00		AB
20s ea	55045-1113-07	9.00		AB
28s ea	55045-1113-09	14.00		AB
30s ea	66336-0580-30	13.88		AB
40s ea	55045-1113-03	19.60		AB
100s ea	55045-1113-00	28.00		AB
500 mg, 12s ea	55045-1381-04	9.45		AB
20s ea	55045-1381-05	15.80		AB
30s ea	55045-1381-08	23.70		AB
60s ea	55045-1381-09	47.40		AB
90s ea	55045-1381-06	71.10		AB
(PD-Rx Pharm)				
REPACK				
TAB, PO, 250 mg, 40s ea	55289-0050-40	14.60		AB
(Pharma Pac)				
REPACK				
TAB, PO (FILMTAB)				
500 mg, 28s ea	52959-0504-28	13.93		AB
(Phys Total Care)				
REPACK				
TAB, PO, 250 mg, 100s ea	54868-0985-01	12.75		AB
(Quality Care Prod)				
REPACK				
TAB, PO (FILMTAB)				
250 mg, 28s ea	49999-0743-28	9.15		AB
500 mg, 21s ea	49999-0101-21	14.10		AB
(FILMTAB)				
500 mg, 40s ea	49999-0101-40	26.86		AB
ERYTHROMYCIN				
FUL				
GEL, TP, 2%, 30 gm		18.75		
(Abbott Pharm) *See ERY-TAB*				
(Abbott Pharm) *See ERYTHROMYCIN DELAYED-RELEASE*				
(Abbott Pharm) *See PCE DISPERTAB*				
(Abbott Pharm)				
TAB, PO, 250 mg, 100s ea	00074-6326-13	16.08	14.11	
500 mg, 100s ea	00074-6227-13	29.53	25.91	
(Bausch & Lomb Inc.)				
OIN, OP, 5 mg/gm,				
1 gm 50s UD	24208-0910-19	459.80		AT
3.5 gm	24208-0910-55	19.00		AT

PROD/MFR	NDC	AWP	DP	OBC
(Consolidated Midland)				
OIN, OP, 5 mg/gm, 3.5 gm	00223-4288-03	2.75		EE
SOL, TP, 1.5%, 60 ml	00223-6145-01	6.25		EE
2%, 60 ml	00223-6146-01	4.80		EE
(Fera)				
OIN, OP (USP,50X1GM)				
5 mg/gm,				
1 gm 50s UD	48102-0008-11	434.78		
(USP,24X3.5GM)				
5 mg/gm,				
3.5 gm 24s	48102-0008-39	431.14		
(Fougera)				
GEL, TP, 2%, 30 gm	00168-0216-30	25.19		AT
(W/APPLICATOR)				
2%, 60 gm	00168-0216-60	44.34		AT
SOL, TP, 2%, 60 ml	00168-0215-60	16.41		AT
(Gallipot)				
POW, NA (U.S.P.)				
25 gm	51552-0555-04	27.02	19.30	
(Medisca)				
POW, NA (U.S.P.)				
25 gm	38779-0842-04	59.25		
100 gm	38779-0842-05	210.00		
500 gm	38779-0842-08	855.00		
(Morton Grove)				
SOL, TP, 2%, 60 ml	60432-0671-60	17.44		AT
(Ocusoft) *See ROMYCIN*				
(PCCA)				
POW, NA (U.S.P.)				
1 gm	51927-1440-00	2.04		
(Perrigo) *See ERY*				
(Perrigo)				
GEL, TP (1X30GM,USP)				
2%, 30 gm	45802-0966-94	25.20		AT
(USP,1X60GM)				
2%, 60 gm	45802-0966-96	45.00		AT
(Valeant Pharm Intl) *See AKNE-MYCIN*				
(Wilson Ophthalmic)				
OIN, OP (PF)				
5 mg/gm, 3.5 gm	51394-0479-35	5.52		EE
(A-S Medication)				
REPACK				
GEL, TP, 2%, 30 gm	54569-4810-00	25.20		EE
OIN, OP, 5 mg/gm, 3.5 gm	54569-1193-00	13.09		AT
SOL, TP, 2%, 60 ml	54569-1883-02	16.93		AT
TAB, PO, 250 mg, 40s ea	54569-2433-00	8.22		
500 mg, 12s ea	54569-2502-03	3.59		
28s ea	54569-2502-00	8.37		
(Altura)				
REPACK				
OIN, OP, 5 mg/gm, 3.5 gm	63874-0181-04	6.81		
TAB, PO, 500 mg, 10s ea	63874-0231-10	16.90		
12s ea	63874-0231-12	23.89		
14s ea	63874-0231-14	27.68		
15s ea	63874-0231-15	29.05		
20s ea	63874-0231-20	38.73		
21s ea	63874-0231-21	40.67		
28s ea	63874-0231-28	47.88		
30s ea	63874-0231-30	50.77		
40s ea	63874-0231-40	57.26		
100s ea	63874-0231-01	169.23		
(Bryant Ranch)				
REPACK				
erythromycin ethylsuccinate				
SUS, PO, 400 mg/5 ml,				
120 ml	63629-2755-01	238.80		
240 ml	63629-2755-02	477.60		
ERYTHROMYCIN (Bryant Ranch)				
TCP, PO, 333 mg, 20s ea	63629-1883-01	10.34		
30s ea	63629-1883-02	15.51		
(Core)				
REPACK				
OIN, OP, 5 mg/gm, 3.5 gm	33358-0134-35	10.25		
(DHS, Inc.)				
REPACK				
ECC, PO, 250 mg, 20s ea	55887-0855-20	24.25		AB
GEL, TP, 2%, 60 gm	55887-0403-60	45.66		AT
OIN, OP, 5 mg/gm, 3.5 gm	55887-0626-35	8.04		AT
SOL, TP, 2%, 60 ml	55887-0241-60	18.25		
TAB, PO, 250 mg, 20s ea	55887-0586-20	11.66		
28s ea	55887-0586-28	16.33		
500 mg, 21s ea	55887-0768-21	19.66		
30s ea	55887-0768-30	28.08		
(Dispensing Solutions)				
REPACK				
GEL, TP, 2%, 30 gm	55045-2415-08	25.00		

PROD/MFR	NDC	AWP	DP	OBC
OIN, OP, 5 mg/gm, 3.5 gm	55045-1350-09	8.05		AT
TAB, PO, 250 mg, 3s ea	66336-0037-03	7.38		
20s ea	66336-0037-20	11.72		
28s ea	66336-0037-28	13.53		
28s ea	66336-0580-28	14.89		
40s ea	66336-0037-40	15.05		
500 mg, 20s ea	66336-0077-20	18.62		
40s ea	66336-0077-40	25.60		
(GSMS)				
REPACK				
TAB, PO (UNIT OF USE)				
250 mg, 40s ea	60429-0070-40	27.00	9.00	
(HomeMed)				
REPACK				
ECC, PO, 250 mg, 28s ea	51655-0674-29	27.73		EE
40s ea	51655-0674-51	11.49		EE
TAB, PO, 250 mg, 28s ea	51655-0519-29	10.30		
40s ea	51655-0519-51	15.67		
500 mg, 40s ea	51655-0297-51	23.10		
(Keltman Pharma., Inc.)				
REPACK				
OIN, OP, 5 mg/gm, 3.5 gm	68387-0540-01	11.11		
(Nucare Pharm)				
REPACK				
OIN, OP, 5 mg/gm, 3.5 gm	66267-0975-35	8.00		EE
TAB, PO, 250 mg, 20s ea	66267-0090-20	11.23		
28s ea	66267-0090-28	14.98		
40s ea	66267-0090-40	16.98		
500 mg, 20s ea	66267-0091-20	12.89		
28s ea	66267-0091-28	15.89		
30s ea	66267-0091-30	16.35		
40s ea	66267-0091-40	21.86		
(Palmetto)				
REPACK				
ECC, PO, 250 mg, 20s ea	23490-5503-01	24.25		
28s ea	23490-5503-02	33.96		
ECT, PO, 250 mg, 40s ea	23490-5504-01	23.97		
333 mg, 6s ea	23490-5509-01	11.62		
21s ea	23490-5509-02	29.04		
30s ea	23490-5509-03	41.49		
40s ea	23490-5509-04	55.32		
500 mg, 30s ea	23490-5512-01	45.00		
40s ea	23490-5512-02	60.00		
OIN, OP, 5 mg/gm, 3.5 gm	23490-5511-01	8.49		
SOL, TP, 2%, 60 ml	23490-5507-01	16.47		
TAB, PO, 250 mg, 3s ea	23490-5505-01	5.49		
6s ea	23490-5505-02	8.26		
20s ea	23490-5505-03	27.38		
28s ea	23490-5505-04	38.25		
500 mg, 6s ea	23490-5513-01	9.07		
20s ea	23490-5513-02	21.59		
28s ea	23490-5513-03	30.23		
30s ea	23490-5513-05	32.39		
40s ea	23490-5513-04	43.19		
(PD-Rx Pharm)				
REPACK				
ECT, PO, 250 mg, 20s ea	55289-0645-20	17.81		AB
28s ea	55289-0645-28	17.95		AB
30s ea	55289-0645-30	17.98		AB
40s ea	55289-0645-40	22.26		AB
56s ea	55289-0645-56	30.77		AB
80s ea	55289-0645-80	39.41		AB
333 mg, 15s ea	55289-0915-15	15.42		AB
24s ea	55289-0915-24	20.66		AB
30s ea	55289-0915-30	20.75		AB
TAB, PO, 250 mg, 40s ea	55289-0075-40	15.80		
56s ea	55289-0075-56	21.12		
500 mg, 4s ea	55289-0025-04	8.80		
20s ea	55289-0025-20	14.05		
28s ea	55289-0025-28	18.55		
30s ea	55289-0025-30	18.58		
40s ea	55289-0025-40	23.10		
(REDI-SCRIPT, FILMTAB)				
500 mg, 40s ea	58864-0195-40	19.63		
(Pharma Pac)				
REPACK				
ECC, PO, 250 mg, 20s ea	52959-0064-20	11.00		EE
28s ea	52959-0064-28	14.95		EE
40s ea	52959-0064-40	16.95		EE
OIN, OP, 5 mg/gm, 3.5 gm	52959-0301-00	8.49		EE
TAB, PO, 500 mg, 20s ea	52959-0816-20	23.02		
28s ea	52959-0816-28	32.21		
30s ea	52959-0816-30	34.50		
(Phys Total Care)				
REPACK				
ECC, PO, 250 mg, 20s ea	54868-0224-04	12.06		EE
30s ea	54868-0224-06	16.58		EE
40s ea	54868-0224-01	21.11		EE
60s ea	54868-0224-03	30.17		EE
GEL, TP, 2%, 30 gm	54868-4461-00	12.11		AT

PROD/MFR	NDC	AWP	DP	OBC
OIN, OP, 5 mg/gm, 3.5 gm	54868-0644-01	8.22		EE
SOL, TP, 2%, 60 ml	54868-0946-00	11.64		EE
TAB, PO (FILM-COATED)				
250 mg, 20s ea	54868-1386-05	16.56		
30s ea	54868-1386-03	22.59		
40s ea	54868-1386-01	28.62		
60s ea	54868-1386-04	40.68		
500s ea	54868-1386-02	173.22		
500 mg, 15s ea	54868-1387-02	23.07		
20s ea	54868-1387-00	28.76		
30s ea	54868-1387-01	40.14		
(Physician Partner) REPACK				
ECT, PO (DELAYED ACTION)				
333 mg, 15s ea	21695-0457-15	16.67		
30s ea	21695-0457-30	43.33		
OIN, OP, 5 mg/gm, 3.5 gm	21695-0173-18	38.00		
TAB, PO, 250 mg, 30s ea	21695-0387-30	16.31		
500 mg, 30s ea	21695-0389-30	47.09		
(Quality Care Prod) REPACK				
GEL, TP, 2%, 30 gm	49999-0887-30	32.75		
OIN, OP, 5 mg/gm, 3.5 gm	35356-0535-01	21.80		AT
3.5 gm	49999-0136-35	8.18		AT
SOL, TP, 2%, 60 ml	49999-0217-60	11.36		
60 ml	49999-0752-60	11.58		AT
TAB, PO, 250 mg, 20s ea	49999-0023-20	8.01		
28s ea	49999-0023-28	17.57		
30s ea	49999-0023-30	18.82		
40s ea	49999-0023-40	25.08		
100s ea	49999-0023-00	62.70		
500 mg, 20s ea	49999-0012-20	19.18		
28s ea	49999-0012-28	28.45		
30s ea	49999-0012-30	32.24		
40s ea	49999-0012-40	43.12		
100s ea	49999-0012-00	107.80		
(Southwood) REPACK				
ECC, PO, 250 mg, 12s ea	58016-0123-12	6.27		EE
15s ea	58016-0123-15	7.83		EE
20s ea	58016-0123-20	10.45		EE
24s ea	58016-0123-24	12.54		EE
28s ea	58016-0123-28	14.63		EE
30s ea	58016-0123-30	15.68		EE
40s ea	58016-0123-40	20.90		EE
100s ea	58016-0123-00	52.25		EE
GEL, TP, 2%, 60 gm	58016-4876-01	44.34		
OIN, OP, 5 mg/gm, 3.5 gm	58016-6086-01	6.81		EE
SOL, TP, 2%, 60 ml	58016-3129-01	9.65		EE
(Stat Rx) REPACK				
OIN, OP, 5 mg/gm, 3.5 gm	16590-0090-35	9.00		
ERYTHROMYCIN BASE (DHS, Inc.) REPACK				
erythromycin				
TAB, PO, 500 mg, 14s ea	55887-0768-14	14.00		
20s ea	55887-0768-20	18.75		
28s ea	55887-0768-28	26.10		
32s ea	55887-0768-32	29.95		
(Dispensing Solutions) REPACK				
TAB, PO, 500 mg, 28s ea	66336-0077-28	19.98		
(Physician Partner) REPACK				
TAB, PO, 250 mg, 28s ea	21695-0387-28	15.22		
(Stat Rx) REPACK				
ECT, PO, 250 mg, 21s ea	16590-0091-21	27.75		
30s ea	16590-0091-30	39.64		
40s ea	16590-0091-40	52.86		
ERYTHROMYCIN D/R (Stat Rx)				
erythromycin				
ECC, PO, 250 mg, 28s ea	16590-0088-28	18.00		
30s ea	16590-0088-30	19.29		
40s ea	16590-0088-40	25.71		
ERYTHROMYCIN DELAYED-RELEASE (Abbott Pharm)				
erythromycin				
ECC, PO, 250 mg, 100s ea	00074-6301-13	28.04	24.60	AB
(A-S Medication) REPACK				
ECC, PO, 250 mg, 28s ea	54569-2281-00	7.94		AB
40s ea	54569-2281-01	11.34		AB
(Dispensing Solutions) REPACK				
ECC, PO, 250 mg, 12s ea	55045-2076-04	6.75		AB
28s ea	55045-2076-06	15.68		AB
30s ea	55045-2076-02	16.80		AB
40s ea	55045-2076-03	22.40		AB
ERYTHROMYCIN ESTOLATE (Consolidated Midland)				
SUS, PO, 125 mg/5 ml,				
480 ml	00223-6140-01	27.50		EE
250 mg/5 ml, 480 ml	00223-6141-01	42.50		EE
(PCCA)				
POW, NA (USP)				
1 gm	51927-3285-00	5.16		
(Southwood) REPACK				
SUS, PO, 250 mg/5 ml,				
150 ml	58016-0175-30	17.06		EE
200 ml	58016-0175-40	20.48		EE
ERYTHROMYCIN ETHYLSUCCINATE				
(Abbott Pharm) *See E.E.S. 400 FILMTAB*				
(Abbott Pharm) *See E.E.S. GRANULES*				
(Abbott Pharm) *See ERYPED 200*				
(Abbott Pharm) *See ERYPED 400*				
(Abbott Pharm)				
TAB, PO, 400 mg, 100s ea	00074-2589-13	25.30	22.19	AB
(Consolidated Midland)				
SUS, PO, 200 mg/5 ml,				
100 ml	00223-6142-10	6.95		EE
480 ml	00223-6142-01	23.50		EE
400 mg/5 ml, 100 ml	00223-6143-10	10.95		EE
480 ml	00223-6143-01	42.50		EE
TAB, PO, 400 mg, 100s ea	00223-0912-01	27.50		EE
500s ea	00223-0912-05	112.50		EE
(Hawkins)				
POW, NA (USP,CITRATE WASHED)				
25 gm	63370-0079-25	92.00		
100 gm	63370-0079-35	220.00		
500 gm	63370-0079-45	760.00		
1000 gm	63370-0079-50	1080.00		
(Letco)				
POW, NA (U.S.P.)				
25 gm	62991-2027-01	45.00		
500 gm	62991-2027-03	525.00		
(Medisca)				
POW, NA (U.S.P.)				
25 gm	38779-0023-04	58.50		
100 gm	38779-0023-05	165.00		
500 gm	38779-0023-08	567.00		
1000 gm	38779-0023-09	795.00		
(Mylan)				
TAB, PO, 400 mg, 500s ea	00378-6400-05	143.10		AB
(PCCA)				
POW, NA (U.S.P.; NONMICRONIZED)				
1 gm	51927-3116-00	4.32		
(A-S Medication) REPACK				
TAB, PO, 400 mg, 20s ea	54569-2507-07	5.12		AB
30s ea	54569-2507-04	7.67		AB
40s ea	54569-2507-02	10.23		AB
(Altura) REPACK				
SUS, PO, 200 mg/5 ml,				
100 ml	63874-0159-10	16.75		EE
200 ml	63874-0159-20	34.10		EE
400 mg/5 ml, 100 ml	63874-0160-10	18.52		EE
200 ml	63874-0160-20	28.33		EE
480 ml	63874-0160-48	39.05		EE
TAB, PO, 400 mg, 28s ea	63874-0110-28	12.35		EE
40s ea	63874-0110-40	16.32		EE
100s ea	63874-0110-01	31.20		EE
500s ea	63874-0110-50	109.13		EE
(Bryant Ranch) REPACK				
SUS, PO, 200 mg/5 ml,				
120 ml	63629-2685-01	18.60		
240 ml	63629-2685-02	37.20		
TAB, PO (FILM-COATED)				
400 mg, 30s ea	63629-1835-02	7.02		
40s ea	63629-1835-01	9.36		
(DHS, Inc.) REPACK				
TAB, PO, 400 mg, 28s ea	55887-0849-28	12.66		AB
30s ea	55887-0071-30	17.35		AB
30s ea	55887-0849-30	13.59		AB
40s ea	55887-0071-40	23.13		AB
(Dispensing Solutions) REPACK				
TAB, PO, 400 mg, 20s ea	55045-1168-06	11.60		AB
28s ea	55045-1168-07	16.24		AB
30s ea	55045-1168-08	17.40		AB
40s ea	55045-1168-03	23.20		AB
(HomeMed) REPACK				
TAB, PO, 400 mg, 28s ea	51655-0120-29	18.19		EE
(Palmetto) REPACK				
SUS, PO, 200 mg/5 ml,				
100 ml	23490-5522-02	12.00		
TAB, PO, 400 mg, 6s ea	23490-5523-01	5.02		
30s ea	23490-5523-02	17.93		
40s ea	23490-5523-03	23.91		
(PD-Rx Pharm) REPACK				
TAB, PO, 400 mg, 3s ea	55289-0110-03	9.20		AB
9s ea	55289-0110-09	9.30		AB
20s ea	55289-0110-20	13.63		AB
28s ea	55289-0110-28	17.90		AB
30s ea	55289-0110-30	17.93		AB
40s ea	55289-0110-40	22.25		AB
56s ea	55289-0110-56	30.80		AB
(Pharma Pac) REPACK				
SUS, PO, 200 mg/5 ml,				
100 ml	52959-0310-01	15.50		EE
200 ml	52959-0310-02	19.25		EE
TAB, PO, 400 mg, 21s ea	52959-0063-21	11.72		EE
28s ea	52959-0063-28	14.43		EE
30s ea	52959-0063-30	15.12		EE
40s ea	52959-0063-40	17.49		EE
(Phys Total Care) REPACK				
SUS, PO, 200 mg/5 ml,				
100 ml	54868-0971-01	29.73		EE
200 ml	54868-0971-00	55.73		EE
TAB, PO, 400 mg, 15s ea	54868-0018-05	18.72		EE
20s ea	54868-0018-03	23.46		EE
30s ea	54868-0018-04	32.94		EE
40s ea	54868-0018-01	42.39		EE
60s ea	54868-0018-09	61.35		AB
100s ea	54868-0018-07	99.24		EE
120s ea	54868-0018-06	93.84		EE
500s ea	54868-0018-00	262.68		EE
(Physician Partner) REPACK				
TAB, PO, 400 mg, 28s ea	21695-0388-28	26.06		AB
(Southwood) REPACK				
SUS, PO, 200 mg/5 ml,				
100 ml	58016-1017-03	7.70		EE
200 ml	58016-1018-06	14.02		EE
TAB, PO, 400 mg, 6s ea	58016-0127-06	3.47		EE
8s ea	58016-0127-08	4.62		EE
10s ea	58016-0127-10	5.78		EE
14s ea	58016-0127-14	8.09		EE
20s ea	58016-0127-20	11.55		EE
21s ea	58016-0127-21	12.13		EE
24s ea	58016-0127-24	13.86		EE
28s ea	58016-0127-28	16.17		EE
30s ea	58016-0127-30	17.32		EE
40s ea	58016-0127-40	23.10		EE
42s ea	58016-0127-42	24.26		EE
50s ea	58016-0127-50	28.88		EE
60s ea	58016-0127-60	34.65		EE
ERYTHROMYCIN ETHYLSUCCINATE/ SULFISOXAZOLE ACETYL				
(Teva) *See E.S.P.*				
(Palmetto) REPACK				
PDR, PO, 200 mg/5 ml-600 mg/5 ml,				
100 ml	23490-5526-01	20.33		
200 ml	23490-5526-02	34.82		
ERYTHROMYCIN LACTOBIONATE				
(Hospira) *See ERYTHROCIN LACTOBIONATE*				
ERYTHROMYCIN PLEDGETS (Phys Total Care) REPACK				
erythromycin				
SWA, TP, 2%, 60s ea	54868-2187-01	27.73		AT
ERYTHROMYCIN STEARATE				
(Abbott Pharm) *See ERYTHROCIN STEARATE FILMTAB*				
(Consolidated Midland)				
TAB, PO, 250 mg, 100s ea	00223-0914-01	13.25		EE
500s ea	00223-0914-05	70.00		EE
(Bryant Ranch) REPACK				
TAB, PO, 250 mg, 28s ea	63629-1834-03	5.70		
(FILM COATED)				
250 mg, 28s ea	63629-2940-01	14.32		
30s ea	63629-1834-01	6.11		

PROD/MFR	NDC	AWP	DP	OBC
40s ea	63629-1834-02	8.14		
500 mg, 14s ea	63629-1374-04	5.42		
20s ea	63629-1374-03	7.74		
30s ea	63629-1374-02	11.61		
30s ea	63629-2938-01	23.90		
40s ea	63629-1374-01	15.48		
(Core)				
REPACK				
TAB, PO, 250 mg, 15s ea	33358-0135-15	5.16		
28s ea	33358-0135-28	18.43		
40s ea	33358-0135-40	20.05		
500 mg, 15s ea	33358-0136-15	6.12		
20s ea	33358-0136-20	16.29		
28s ea	33358-0136-28	18.34		
30s ea	33358-0136-30	19.83		
40s ea	33358-0136-40	22.20		
60s ea	33358-0136-60	36.27		
(Dispensing Solutions)				
REPACK				
TAB, PO, 500 mg, 28s ea	55045-3466-08	22.12		
(HomeMed)				
REPACK				
TAB, PO, 250 mg, 6s ea	51655-0098-87	8.00		EE
28s ea	51655-0098-29	12.47		EE
40s ea	51655-0098-51	15.67		EE
56s ea	51655-0098-95	13.00		EE
500 mg, 28s ea	51655-0152-29	18.55		EE
(Keltman Pharma., Inc.)				
REPACK				
TAB, PO, 500 mg, 28s ea	68387-0548-28	36.45		
(Palmetto)				
REPACK				
TAB, PO, 250 mg, 30s ea	23490-5516-01	8.09		
500 mg, 28s ea	23490-5517-01	17.34		
30s ea	23490-5517-02	18.58		
40s ea	23490-5517-03	24.77		
(PD-Rx Pharm)				
REPACK				
TAB, PO, 250 mg, 28s ea	55289-0112-28	12.47		AB
500 mg, 56s ea	55289-0705-56	32.09		AB
(Pharma Pac)				
REPACK				
TAB, PO, 500 mg, 20s ea	52959-0504-20	9.99		EE
30s ea	52959-0504-30	14.99		EE
40s ea	52959-0504-40	15.99		EE
(Phys Total Care)				
REPACK				
TAB, PO, 250 mg, 30s ea	54868-0413-04	22.32		EE
40s ea	54868-0413-02	28.29		EE
60s ea	54868-0413-00	40.17		EE
100s ea	54868-0413-07	63.96		EE
500 mg, 30s ea	54868-0225-00	48.36		EE
40s ea	54868-0225-01	49.23		EE
(Southwood)				
REPACK				
TAB, PO, 250 mg, 8s ea	58016-0124-08	2.16		EE
10s ea	58016-0124-10	2.70		EE
12s ea	58016-0124-12	3.23		EE
14s ea	58016-0124-14	2.16		EE
15s ea	58016-0124-15	2.31		EE
16s ea	58016-0124-16	4.31		EE
20s ea	58016-0124-20	5.39		EE
21s ea	58016-0124-21	3.24		EE
24s ea	58016-0124-24	6.47		EE
28s ea	58016-0124-28	7.55		EE
30s ea	58016-0124-30	8.09		EE
40s ea	58016-0124-40	10.78		EE
50s ea	58016-0124-50	13.48		EE
56s ea	58016-0124-56	15.09		EE
60s ea	58016-0124-60	16.17		EE
90s ea	58016-0124-90	24.26		EE
100s ea	58016-0124-00	26.95		EE
120s ea	58016-0124-02	32.34		EE
120s ea	58016-0124-99	18.49		EE
500 mg, 3s ea	58016-0125-03	2.93		EE
6s ea	58016-0125-06	3.36		EE
9s ea	58016-0125-09	5.04		EE
10s ea	58016-0125-10	5.60		EE
12s ea	58016-0125-12	6.72		EE
14s ea	58016-0125-14	7.84		EE
15s ea	58016-0125-15	8.40		EE
20s ea	58016-0125-20	11.20		EE
21s ea	58016-0125-21	11.76		EE
24s ea	58016-0125-24	13.44		EE
28s ea	58016-0125-28	16.80		EE
30s ea	58016-0125-30	17.95		EE
40s ea	58016-0125-40	22.40		EE
60s ea	58016-0125-60	33.60		EE
100s ea	58016-0125-00	56.00		EE
ERYTHROMYCIN STEARATE FILMTAB (DHS, Inc.)				
REPACK				
erythromycin stearate				
TAB, PO, 250 mg, 20s ea	55887-0138-20	9.25		
30s ea	55887-0138-30	11.00		
60s ea	55887-0138-60	22.55		
90s ea	55887-0138-90	24.50		
ERYTHROMYCIN/SULFISOXAZOLE (A-S Medication)				
REPACK				
erythromycin ethylsuccinate/sulfisoxazole acetyl				
PDR, PO, 200 mg/5 ml-600 mg/5 ml,				
100 ml	54569-2000-00	15.97		EE
200 ml	54569-2002-00	31.16		EE
(Dispensing Solutions)				
REPACK				
PDR, PO, 200 mg/5 ml-600 mg/5 ml,				
100 ml	55045-1442-01	13.00		AB
200 ml	55045-1471-00	28.40		AB
(Pharma Pac)				
REPACK				
PDR, PO, 200 mg/5 ml-600 mg/5 ml,				
150 ml	52959-0164-06	20.95		EE
200 ml	52959-0164-03	25.50		EE
(Phys Total Care)				
REPACK				
PDR, PO, 200 mg/5 ml-600 mg/5 ml,				
100 ml	54868-1865-01	56.04		EE
150 ml	54868-1865-02	80.33		EE
200 ml	54868-1865-03	80.67		EE
(Quality Care Prod)				
REPACK				
PDR, PO, 200 mg/5 ml-600 mg/5 ml,				
100 ml	49999-0315-00	22.97		AB
(Southwood)				
REPACK				
PDR, PO, 200 mg/5 ml-600 mg/5 ml,				
100 ml	58016-1023-03	15.95		EE
150 ml	58016-1024-01	23.03		EE
200 ml	58016-1025-01	32.48		EE
ESCITALOPRAM OXALATE				
(Forest Pharm) *See LEXAPRO*				
ESGIC (Forest Pharm)				
acetaminophen/butalbital/caffeine				
CAP, PO, 325 mg-50 mg-40 mg,				
100s ea	00535-0012-01	215.74		AB
TAB, PO, 325 mg-50 mg-40 mg,				
100s ea	00535-0011-01	227.22		AB
(Quality Care Prod)				
REPACK				
CAP, PO, 325 mg-50 mg-40 mg,				
100s ea	35356-0005-00	245.00		
ESGIC-PLUS (Forest Pharm)				
acetaminophen/butalbital/caffeine				
CAP, PO, 500 mg-50 mg-40 mg,				
100s ea	00456-0679-01	183.89		AB
TAB, PO, 500 mg-50 mg-40 mg,				
100s ea	00456-0678-01	184.51		AB
(A-S Medication)				
REPACK				
TAB, PO, 500 mg-50 mg-40 mg,				
8s ea	54569-3441-00	13.95		AB
(PD-Rx Pharm)				
REPACK				
TAB, PO, 500 mg-50 mg-40 mg,				
12s ea	55289-0264-12	44.45		AB
(Phys Total Care)				
REPACK				
TAB, PO, 500 mg-50 mg-40 mg,				
20s ea	54868-2778-02	36.70		AB
30s ea	54868-2778-01	54.11		AB
60s ea	54868-2778-03	105.73		AB
100s ea	54868-2778-00	165.70		AB
ESKALITH (Phys Total Care)				
lithium carbonate				
CAP, PO, 300 mg, 100s ea	54868-1336-00	26.74		AB
ESKALITH-CR (Phys Total Care)				
lithium carbonate				
TER, PO, 450 mg, 100s ea	54868-2557-00	75.97		
ESMOLOL HCL (Baxter)				
esmolol hydrochloride				
SOL, IV (S.D.V.,PF)				
10 mg/ml, 10 ml	00641-2965-41	12.60		
(S.D.V. X 25,PF)				
10 mg/ml,				
10 ml 25s	00641-2965-45	315.00		
(Bedford)				
SOL, IV (S.D.V.,PF)				
10 mg/ml,				
10 ml 10s	55390-0062-10	220.68		AP
ESMOLOL HYDROCHLORIDE (APP)				
SOL, IV (25X10ML,PF)				
10 mg/ml,				
10 ml 25s	63323-0652-10	404.75		
(Baxter) *See BREVIBLOC*				
(Baxter) *See ESMOLOL HCL*				
(Bedford) *See ESMOLOL HCL*				
(Bedford) *See NOVAPLUS ESMOLOL HYDROCHLORIDE*				
(Bioniche Pharma)				
SOL, IV (10X10ML)				
10 mg/ml,				
10 ml 10s	67457-0182-10	87.50		AP
ESOMEPRAZOLE MAGNESIUM				
(AstraZeneca) *See NEXIUM*				
(Palmetto)				
REPACK				
ECC, PO, 40 mg, 30s ea	23490-7534-01	161.27		
ESOMEPRAZOLE SODIUM				
(AstraZeneca) *See NEXIUM I.V.*				
ESSIAN (Prasco Labs)				
esterified estrogens/methyltestosterone				
TAB, PO (USP,FILM-COATED)				
1.25 mg-2.5 mg,				
100s ea	66993-0920-02	192.95		
ESSIAN HS (Prasco Labs)				
esterified estrogens/methyltestosterone				
TAB, PO (USP,HALF-STRENGTH)				
0.625 mg-1.25 mg,				
100s ea	66993-0921-02	157.95		
ESTAZOLAM				
FUL				
TAB, PO, 1 mg, 100s ea		59.25		
2 mg, 100s ea		64.49		
(Teva)				
TAB, PO, 1 mg,				
100s ea, C-IV	00093-0129-01	89.00		AB
2 mg, 100s ea, C-IV	00093-0130-01	99.00		AB
(Watson Labs)				
TAB, PO, 1 mg,				
100s ea, C-IV	00591-0744-01	88.78		AB
2 mg, 100s ea, C-IV	00591-0745-01	98.92		AB
(Pharma Pac)				
REPACK				
TAB, PO, 1 mg,				
30s ea, C-IV	52959-0970-30	35.10		AB
(Physician Partner)				
REPACK				
TAB, PO, 2 mg,				
30s ea, C-IV	21695-0220-30	59.35		
(Quality Care Prod)				
REPACK				
TAB, PO, 1 mg,				
15s ea, C-IV	49999-0317-15	16.02		AB
(Southwood)				
REPACK				
TAB, PO, 2 mg,				
30s ea, C-IV	58016-0791-30	25.82		AB
60s ea, C-IV	58016-0791-60	51.64		AB
90s ea, C-IV	58016-0791-90	77.45		AB
100s ea, C-IV	58016-0791-00	86.06		AB
ESTERIFIED ESTROGEN/METHYLTESTOSTERONE				
(Glenmark Pharmaceuticals)				
esterified estrogens/methyltestosterone				
TAB, PO, 0.625 mg-1.25 mg,				
100s ea	68462-0173-01	157.95		
1.25 mg-2.5 mg,				
100s ea	68462-0174-01	192.95		
(Lannett)				
TAB, PO (HALF-STRENGTH)				
0.625 mg-1.25 mg,				
100s ea	00527-1410-01	157.95		
1000s ea	00527-1410-10	1532.11		
(FILM-COATED)				
1.25 mg-2.5 mg,				
100s ea	00527-1409-01	192.95		
1000s ea	00527-1409-10	1871.62		
ESTERIFIED ESTROGENS				
(Monarch) *See MENEST*				

PROD/MFR	NDC	AWP	DP	OBC
ESTERIFIED ESTROGENS AND METHYLTESTOSTERONE (Amneal)				
esterified estrogens/methyltestosterone				
TAB, PO (HALF STRENGTH,USP)				
0.625 mg-1.25 mg, 100s ea	**53746-0077-01**	157.95		
(USP,FILM-COATED)				
1.25 mg-2.5 mg, 100s ea	**53746-0078-01**	192.95		
ESTERIFIED ESTROGENS/METHYLTESTOSTERONE				
(Amneal) *See ESTERIFIED ESTROGENS AND METHYLTESTOSTERONE*				
(Breckenridge Pharm) *See ESTERIFIED ESTROGENS/METHYLTESTOSTERONE DS*				
(Breckenridge Pharm) *See ESTERIFIED ESTROGENS/METHYLTESTOSTERONE HS*				
(Centrix) *See COVARYX*				
(Centrix) *See COVARYX HS*				
(Creekwood Pharma) *See EEMT*				
(Creekwood Pharma) *See EEMT HS*				
(Glenmark Pharmaceuticals) *See ESTERIFIED ESTROGEN/METHYLTESTOSTERONE*				
(Lannett) *See ESTERIFIED ESTROGEN/ METHYLTESTOSTERONE*				
(Prasco Labs) *See ESSIAN*				
(Prasco Labs) *See ESSIAN HS*				
(Solvay) *See ESTRATEST*				
(Solvay) *See ESTRATEST H.S.*				
(Dispensing Solutions)				
REPACK				
TAB, PO, 1.25 mg-2.5 mg, 100s ea	**55045-3480-01**	193.00		
ESTERIFIED ESTROGENS/METHYLTESTOSTERONE DS (Breckenridge Pharm)				
esterified estrogens/methyltestosterone				
TAB, PO (FILM-COATED)				
1.25 mg-2.5 mg, 100s ea	**51991-0079-01**	192.95		
ESTERIFIED ESTROGENS/METHYLTESTOSTERONE HS (Breckenridge Pharm)				
esterified estrogens/methyltestosterone				
TAB, PO (FILM-COATED)				
0.625 mg-1.25 mg, 100s ea	**51991-0078-01**	157.95		
ESTRACE (Warner Chilcott)				
estradiol				
CRE, VG (W/APPLICATOR)				
0.1 mg/gm, 42.5 gm	**00430-3754-14**	127.23		
TAB, PO (USP)				
0.5 mg, 100s ea	**00430-0720-24**	217.73		
1 mg, 100s ea	**00430-0721-24**	217.73		
2 mg, 100s ea	**00430-0722-24**	279.52		
(PD-Rx Pharm)				
REPACK				
TAB, PO, 1 mg, 30s ea	**55289-0101-30**	87.02		AB
50s ea	**55289-0101-50**	145.05		AB
2 mg, 30s ea	**55289-0396-30**	111.72		AB
(Phys Total Care)				
REPACK				
CRE, VG, 0.1 mg/gm, 42.5 gm	**54868-0496-00**	155.06		
TAB, PO, 1 mg, 10s ea	**54868-0494-03**	22.93		
25s ea	**54868-0494-02**	54.39		AB
30s ea	**54868-0494-01**	70.88		AB
100s ea	**54868-0494-00**	216.86		AB
2 mg, 25s ea	**54868-0495-00**	29.20		AB
30s ea	**54868-0495-01**	34.66		AB
(Southwood)				
REPACK				
CRE, VG, 0.1 mg/gm, 42.5 gm	**58016-3389-01**	108.88		
TAB, PO, 1 mg, 30s ea	**58016-0039-30**	38.37		
60s ea	**58016-0039-60**	76.73		
90s ea	**58016-0039-90**	115.10		
100s ea	**58016-0039-00**	127.89		
ESTRADERM (Novartis Pharm)				
estradiol				
TDM, TD, 0.05 mg/24 hr, ea	**00078-0480-62**	8.08		BX
8s ea	**00078-0480-42**	64.57		BX
0.1 mg/24 hr, ea	**00078-0481-62**	8.65		BX
8s ea	**00078-0481-42**	69.24		BX
(Southwood)				
REPACK				
TDM, TD, 0.05 mg/24 hr, 8s ea	**58016-3182-01**	20.64		BX
ESTRADIOL				
FUL				
TAB, PO, 0.5 mg, 100s ea		17.91		
1 mg, 100s ea		21.75		
2 mg, 100s ea		30.60		
(Ascend) *See ESTROGEL*				
(Azur Pharma, Inc.) *See ELESTRIN*				
(Bayer) *See CLIMARA*				
(Bayer) *See MENOSTAR*				
(Gallipot) *See ESTRADIOL HEMIHYDRATE*				
(Graceway) *See ESTRASORB*				
(Letco)				
POW, NA (U.S.P.,MICRONIZED)				
1 gm	**62991-1049-01**	28.20		
5 gm	**62991-1049-02**	105.00		
25 gm	**62991-1049-03**	298.50		
(U.S.P., MICRONIZED)				
100 gm	**62991-1049-04**	825.00		
(Medisca)				
POW, NA (U.S.P.,MICRONIZED)				
1 gm	**38779-0869-06**	31.50		
5 gm	**38779-0869-03**	135.00		
10 gm	**38779-0869-01**	220.50		
25 gm	**38779-0869-04**	397.50		
100 gm	**38779-0869-05**	1335.00		
(Mylan)				
TAB, PO, 0.5 mg, 100s ea	**00378-1452-01**	25.50		AB
500s ea	**00378-1452-05**	125.00		AB
1 mg, 100s ea	**00378-1454-01**	34.50		AB
500s ea	**00378-1454-05**	170.00		AB
2 mg, 100s ea	**00378-1458-01**	49.50		AB
500s ea	**00378-1458-05**	235.00		AB
TDM, TD, 0.025 mg/24 hr, 4s ea	**00378-3349-99**	39.35		AB2
0.0375 mg/24 hr, 4s ea	**00378-3360-99**	39.35		AB
0.05 mg/24 hr, 4s ea	**00378-3350-99**	39.35		AB2
0.06 mg/24 hr, 4s ea	**00378-3361-99**	39.35		AB
0.075 mg/24 hr, 4s ea	**00378-3351-99**	39.35		AB2
0.1 mg/24 hr, 4s ea	**00378-3352-99**	39.35		AB2
(Novartis Pharm) *See ESTRADERM*				
(Novartis Pharm) *See VIVELLE-DOT*				
(Novavax) *See GYNODIOL*				
(Novo Nordisk) *See VAGIFEM*				
(PCCA)				
POW, NA (U.S.P.; NON-MICRONIZED)				
1 gm	**51927-3609-00**	45.00		
(U.S.P.)				
1 gm	**51927-1959-00**	45.00		
(Pfizer) *See ESTRING*				
ESTRADIOL (Spectrum Pharmacy)				
estradiol, micronized				
POW, NA (1X1GM)				
1 gm	**49452-2801-01**	54.95		
ESTRADIOL (Spectrum Pharmacy)				
(U.S.P.,MICRONIZED)				
1 gm	**49452-2780-01**	54.95		
(Spectrum Pharmacy)				
estradiol, micronized				
(1X5GM)				
5 gm	**49452-2801-02**	201.95		
ESTRADIOL (Spectrum Pharmacy)				
(U.S.P.,MICRONIZED)				
5 gm	**49452-2780-02**	201.95		
(Spectrum Pharmacy)				
estradiol, micronized				
(1X25GM)				
25 gm	**49452-2801-03**	619.50		
ESTRADIOL (Spectrum Pharmacy)				
(U.S.P.,MICRONIZED)				
25 gm	**49452-2780-03**	619.50		
(Spectrum Pharmacy)				
estradiol, micronized				
(1X100GM)				
100 gm	**49452-2801-04**	1638.00		
ESTRADIOL (Spectrum Pharmacy)				
(U.S.P.,MICRONIZED)				
100 gm	**49452-2780-04**	1638.00		
(Teva)				
TAB, PO, 0.5 mg, 100s ea	**00555-0899-02**	24.35		AB
1 mg, 100s ea	**00555-0886-02**	32.47		AB
500s ea	**00555-0886-04**	154.40		AB
2 mg, 100s ea	**00555-0887-02**	47.45		AB
500s ea	**00555-0887-04**	225.40		AB
(Ther-RX) *See EVAMIST*				
(Upsher-Smith) *See DIVIGEL*				
(Warner Chilcott) *See ESTRACE*				
(Watson) *See ALORA*				
(Watson Labs)				
TAB, PO, 0.5 mg, 100s ea	**00591-0528-01**	25.50		AB
1 mg, 100s ea	**00591-0487-01**	34.50		AB
500s ea	**00591-0487-05**	170.00		AB
2 mg, 100s ea	**00591-0488-01**	49.50		AB
500s ea	**00591-0488-05**	235.00		AB
(A-S Medication)				
REPACK				
TAB, PO, 1 mg, 30s ea	**54569-4907-00**	10.34		EE
(DHS, Inc.)				
REPACK				
TAB, PO, 0.5 mg, 30s ea	**55887-0266-30**	15.75		AB
90s ea	**55887-0266-90**	31.50		AB
1 mg, 30s ea	**55887-0342-30**	8.96		
90s ea	**55887-0342-90**	26.87		
(Dispensing Solutions)				
REPACK				
TAB, PO, 1 mg, 100s ea	**55045-2739-00**	33.10		AB
2 mg, 100s ea	**55045-2850-00**	45.00		AB
(Palmetto)				
REPACK				
TDM, TD, 0.025 mg/24 hr, 4s ea	**23490-7794-01**	26.25		
0.05 mg/24 hr, 4s ea	**23490-5528-02**	26.25		
0.1 mg/24 hr, 4s ea	**23490-5529-02**	28.00		
(PD-Rx Pharm)				
REPACK				
TAB, PO, 0.5 mg, 7s ea	**55289-0603-07**	6.40		AB
21s ea	**55289-0603-21**	6.63		AB
30s ea	**58864-0803-30**	6.78		AB
1 mg, 30s ea	**55289-0761-30**	8.05		AB
(REDI-SCRIPT)				
1 mg, 30s ea	**58864-0804-30**	8.05		AB
100s ea	**55289-0761-01**	44.45		AB
2 mg, 100s ea	**43063-0201-01**	48.90		AB
(Pharma Pac)				
REPACK				
TAB, PO, 2 mg, 30s ea	**52959-0323-30**	14.70		EE
100s ea	**52959-0323-00**	49.95		EE
(Phys Total Care)				
REPACK				
TAB, PO, 0.5 mg, 30s ea	**54868-4370-00**	6.63		
100s ea	**54868-4370-01**	13.59		AB
1 mg, 30s ea	**54868-4030-00**	7.56		EE
90s ea	**54868-4030-02**	16.01		AB
100s ea	**54868-4030-01**	14.28		EE
2 mg, 15s ea	**54868-4031-02**	5.31		AB
30s ea	**54868-4031-00**	7.62		AB
90s ea	**54868-4031-03**	22.99		AB
100s ea	**54868-4031-01**	16.92		AB
TDM, TD, 0.025 mg/24 hr, 4s ea	**54868-5009-00**	98.95		AB2
0.05 mg/24 hr, 4s ea	**54868-4811-00**	97.44		AB2
0.1 mg/24 hr, 4s ea	**54868-4813-00**	126.51		AB2
(Quality Care Prod)				
REPACK				
TAB, PO, 1 mg, 30s ea	**49999-0083-30**	12.42		EE
ESTRADIOL ACETATE				
(Warner Chilcott) *See FEMRING*				
(Warner Chilcott) *See FEMTRACE*				
ESTRADIOL BENZOATE (Gallipot)				
POW, NA, 5 gm	**51552-0491-02**	64.75		
(Medisca)				
POW, NA, 1 gm	**38779-0329-06**	31.50		
5 gm	**38779-0329-03**	126.00		
(PCCA)				
POW, NA, 1 gm	**51927-1457-00**	33.00		
(1X1GM,USP)				
1 gm	**51927-4360-00**	72.00		
ESTRADIOL CYPIONATE (Consolidated Midland)				
OIL, IM (VIAL)				
5 mg/ml, 10 ml	**00223-7602-10**	8.50		EE

PROD/MFR	NDC	AWP	DP	OBC
(Hawkins)				
POW, NA (USP)				
1 gm	63370-0084-10	60.00		
5 gm	63370-0084-15	248.00		
25 gm	63370-0084-25	1100.00		
(Medisca)				
POW, NA (U.S.P.)				
5 gm	38779-1901-03	435.00		
25 gm	38779-1901-04	1275.00		
100 gm	38779-1901-05	3510.00		
(PCCA)				
POW, NA (U.S.P.)				
1 gm	51927-3163-00	165.00		
(Pfizer) *See DEPO-ESTRADIOL*				
(Spectrum Pharmacy)				
POW, NA (1X1GM,USP)				
1 gm	49452-2789-01	161.35		
(1X5GM,USP)				
5 gm	49452-2789-02	668.50		
(1X25GM,USP)				
25 gm	49452-2789-03	2054.50		
ESTRADIOL HEMIHYDRATE (Gallipot)				
estradiol				
POW, NA (U.S.P.,MICRONIZED)				
1 gm	51552-0384-01	13.23		
(U.S.P., MICRONIZED)				
5 gm	51552-0384-02	51.03		
(U.S.P.,MICRONIZED)				
25 gm	51552-0384-04	168.00		
100 gm	51552-0384-05	595.00		
ESTRADIOL MICRONIZED (Hawkins)				
estradiol, micronized				
POW, NA (U.S.P.)				
1 gm	63370-0078-10	43.20		
5 gm	63370-0078-15	168.00		
(USP)				
25 gm	63370-0078-25	576.00		
(U.S.P.)				
100 gm	63370-0078-35	1680.00		
1000 gm	63370-0078-50	9360.00		
(PCCA)				
POW, NA (U.S.P.; E2)				
1 gm	51927-1778-00	42.00		
(B&B Pharm, Inc)				
REPACK				
POW, NA (U.S.P.)				
1 gm	63275-9987-01	42.00		
5 gm	63275-9987-02	210.00		
25 gm	63275-9987-04	1050.00		
100 gm	63275-9987-05	4200.00		
ESTRADIOL VALERATE (Consolidated Midland)				
OIL, IM (VIAL)				
20 mg/ml, 10 ml	00223-7606-10	13.95		EE
40 mg/ml, 10 ml	00223-7607-10	16.95		EE
(Gallipot)				
POW, NA (1X1GM,USP)				
1 gm	51552-0888-01	16.73	11.95	
(1X5GM,USP)				
5 gm	51552-0888-02	65.52	46.80	
(1X25GM,USP)				
25 gm	51552-0888-04	259.00	185.00	
(Hawkins)				
POW, NA (U.S.P.)				
1 gm	63370-0086-10	48.00		
5 gm	63370-0086-15	184.00		
25 gm	63370-0086-25	716.00		
(JHP) *See DELESTROGEN*				
(Letco)				
POW, NA, 5 gm	62991-1662-02	120.00		
25 gm	62991-1662-03	450.00		
100 gm	62991-1662-04	1500.00		
(Medisca)				
POW, NA (U.S.P.)				
1 gm	38779-0568-06	40.50		
5 gm	38779-0568-03	157.50		
25 gm	38779-0568-04	597.00		
(PCCA)				
POW, NA (U.S.P.)				
1 gm	51927-1698-00	42.00		
(Sandoz)				
OIL, IM, 10 mg/ml, 5 ml	00781-3030-75	76.19		AO
20 mg/ml, 5 ml	00781-3029-75	107.37		AO
40 mg/ml, 5 ml	00781-3031-75	178.11		AO
(Spectrum Pharmacy)				
POW, NA (U.S.P.)				
1 gm	49452-2791-01	85.75		
5 gm	49452-2791-02	254.80		
25 gm	49452-2791-03	766.50		
ESTRADIOL, MICRONIZED				
(Hawkins) *See ESTRADIOL MICRONIZED*				
(PCCA) *See ESTRADIOL MICRONIZED*				
(Spectrum Pharmacy) *See ESTRADIOL*				
ESTRADIOL/LEVONORGESTREL				
(Bayer) *See CLIMARA PRO*				
ESTRADIOL/NORETHINDRONE ACETATE				
(Breckenridge Pharm)				
TAB, PO (FILM-COATED)				
1 mg-0.5 mg,				
28s ea	51991-0474-28	61.51		AB
(Novartis Pharm) *See COMBIPATCH*				
(Novo Nordisk) *See ACTIVELLA*				
ESTRADIOL/NORGESTIMATE				
(Teva) *See PREFEST*				
ESTRAGYN 5 (Clint)				
estrone				
SUS, IM (VIAL)				
5 mg/ml, 10 ml	55553-0041-10	18.50		
ESTRAMUSTINE PHOSPHATE SODIUM				
(Pfizer) *See EMCYT*				
ESTRASORB (Graceway)				
estradiol				
EMU, TD (56X1.74GM)				
2.5 mg/gm,				
1.74 gm 56s	15456-0325-56	67.72		
ESTRATEST (Solvay)				
esterified estrogens/methyltestosterone				
TAB, PO, 1.25 mg-2.5 mg,				
100s ea	00032-1026-01	395.53		
1000s ea	00032-1026-10	3936.02		
(Phys Total Care)				
REPACK				
TAB, PO, 1.25 mg-2.5 mg,				
10s ea	54868-3565-02	49.55		
30s ea	54868-3565-01	144.73		
100s ea	54868-3565-00	450.78		
ESTRATEST H.S. (Solvay)				
esterified estrogens/methyltestosterone				
TAB, PO, 0.625 mg-1.25 mg,				
100s ea	00032-1023-01	323.07		
(Phys Total Care)				
REPACK				
TAB, PO, 0.625 mg-1.25 mg,				
10s ea	54868-3564-02	20.86		
30s ea	54868-3564-01	58.83		
100s ea	54868-3564-00	191.08		
ESTRING (Pfizer)				
estradiol				
ICR, VG, 0.0075 mg/24 hr,				
ea	00013-2150-36	202.30	168.58	
ESTRING RING (Phys Total Care)				
REPACK				
estradiol				
ICR, VG, 0.0075 mg/24 hr,				
ea	54868-5538-00	138.74		
ESTRIOL (Gallipot)				
POW, NA (U.S.P., MICRONIZED)				
0.5 gm	51552-0381-08	42.00		
(U.S.P.,MICRONIZED)				
1 gm	51552-0381-01	59.50		
5 gm	51552-0381-02	252.00		
(U.S.P., MICRONIZED)				
25 gm	51552-0381-04	1015.00		
(U.S.P.,MICRONIZED)				
100 gm	51552-0381-05	2030.00		
(Letco)				
POW, NA (U.S.P.,MICRONIZED)				
1 gm	62991-2159-01	105.00		
(Medisca)				
POW, NA (U.S.P.,MICRONIZED)				
0.5 gm	38779-0732-00	76.50		
1 gm	38779-0732-06	129.00		
5 gm	38779-0732-03	534.00		
10 gm	38779-0732-01	975.00		
25 gm	38779-0732-04	1785.00		
100 gm	38779-0732-05	3300.00		
ESTRIOL MICRONIZED (Hawkins)				
estriol, micronized				
POW, NA (U.S.P.)				
1 gm	63370-0080-10	163.20		
(YAM, U.S.P.)				
1 gm	63370-0087-10	100.00		
(U.S.P.)				
5 gm	63370-0080-15	696.00		
(YAM, U.S.P.)				
5 gm	63370-0087-15	480.00		
(U.S.P.)				
25 gm	63370-0080-25	2160.00		
(YAM, U.S.P.)				
25 gm	63370-0087-25	1160.00		
(U.S.P.)				
100 gm	63370-0080-35	4800.00		
(YAM, U.S.P.)				
100 gm	63370-0087-35	3500.00		
(U.S.P.)				
1000 gm	63370-0080-504	3200.00		
(YAM, U.S.P.)				
1000 gm	63370-0087-50	34400.00		
(Letco)				
POW, NA, 5 gm	62991-2159-02	435.00		
(U.S.P.)				
25 gm	62991-2159-03	1350.00		
100 gm	62991-2159-04	2550.00		
(PCCA)				
POW, NA (U.S.P.; E3)				
1 gm	51927-1714-00	276.00		
(B&B Pharm, Inc)				
REPACK				
POW, NA, 1 gm	63275-9985-01	276.00		
5 gm	63275-9985-02	1380.00		
25 gm	63275-9985-04	6900.00		
100 gm	63275-9985-05	27600.00		
ESTRIOL, MICRONIZED				
(Hawkins) *See ESTRIOL MICRONIZED*				
(Letco) *See ESTRIOL MICRONIZED*				
(PCCA) *See ESTRIOL MICRONIZED*				
ESTROGEL (Ascend)				
estradiol				
GEL, TD (METERED DOSE PUMP)				
0.06%, 50 gm	17139-0617-40	81.52		
93 gm	00051-1028-58	102.22		
ESTRONE				
(Clint) *See ESTRAGYN 5*				
(Consolidated Midland)				
SUS, IM (VIAL, AQUEOUS)				
2 mg/ml, 10 ml	00223-7660-10	14.95		
5 mg/ml, 10 ml	00223-7670-10	14.95		
(Gallipot)				
CRY, NA (U.S.P.)				
1 gm	51552-0445-01	11.76		
5 gm	51552-0445-02	44.80		
25 gm	51552-0445-04	182.00		
(Hawkins)				
POW, NA (USP,1X1GM)				
1 gm	63370-0090-10	36.00		
(USP,1X5GM)				
5 gm	63370-0090-15	132.00		
(USP,1X25GM)				
25 gm	63370-0090-25	604.00		
(USP,1X100GM)				
100 gm	63370-0090-35	1344.00		
(Letco)				
POW, NA (U.S.P.)				
1 gm	62991-1051-01	27.00		
5 gm	62991-1051-02	99.00		
25 gm	62991-1051-03	360.00		
100 gm	62991-1051-04	915.00		
(Medisca)				
POW, NA (U.S.P.)				
1 gm	38779-0891-06	27.75		
5 gm	38779-0891-03	105.00		
25 gm	38779-0891-04	417.00		
100 gm	38779-0891-05	960.00		
(PCCA)				
POW, NA (U.S.P. E-1)				
1 gm	51927-1709-00	36.00		
(Spectrum Pharmacy)				
POW, NA (1X1GM,USP)				
1 gm	49452-2802-01	48.30		
(U.S.P.)				
1 gm	49452-2795-01	48.30		
(1X5GM,USP)				
5 gm	49452-2802-02	163.45		
(U.S.P.)				
5 gm	49452-2795-02	163.45		
(1X25GM,USP)				
25 gm	49452-2802-03	654.50		

PROD/MFR NDC AWP DP OBC

(U.S.P.)
25 gm 49452-2795-04 654.50
(1X100GM,USP)
100 gm 49452-2795-03 1554.00
100 gm 49452-2802-04 1554.00

(Truxton)
SUS, IM (VIAL, AQUEOUS)
5 mg/ml, 30 ml 00463-1029-30 8.00

(B&B Pharm, Inc)
REPACK
POW, NA (U.S.P.)
1 gm 63275-9986-01 36.00
5 gm 63275-9986-02 180.00
25 gm 63275-9986-04 900.00

ESTRONE SULFATE PIPERAZINE (Spectrum Pharmacy)
estropipate
CRY, NA, 1 gm 49452-2796-02 306.25
5 gm 49452-2796-03 1141.00

ESTRONE SULFATE PIPERAZINE SALT (PCCA)
estropipate
POW, NA (USP XXII)
1 gm 51927-1978-00 102.00

ESTROPIPATE
FUL
TAB, PO, 0.75 mg,
100s ea 27.54
1.5 mg, 100s ea 34.50
3 mg, 100s ea 86.22

(Mylan)
TAB, PO, 0.75 mg, 100s ea 00378-4551-01 47.00 AB
1.5 mg, 100s ea . . . . . 00378-4553-01 65.00 AB

(PCCA) *See ESTRONE SULFATE PIPERAZINE SALT*

(Spectrum Pharmacy) *See ESTRONE SULFATE PIPERAZINE*

(Teva)
TAB, PO, 0.75 mg, 100s ea. 00555-0727-02 41.28 AB
1.5 mg, 100s ea . . . . . 00555-0728-02 57.67 AB
3 mg, 100s ea . . . . . 00555-0729-02 100.39 AB

(Watson Labs)
TAB, PO, 0.75 mg, 100s ea. 00591-0414-01 43.15 AB
1.5 mg, 100s ea . . . . . 00591-0415-01 62.00 AB
3 mg, 100s ea . . . . . 00591-0416-01 100.39 AB

(Dispensing Solutions)
REPACK
TAB, PO, 0.75 mg, 30s ea. . 66336-0977-30 15.23 AB

(Palmetto)
REPACK
TAB, PO, 0.75 mg, 30s ea. . 23490-6906-01 12.69

(Pharma Pac)
REPACK
TAB, PO, 0.75 mg, 100s ea. 52959-0326-10 70.15 EE

(Phys Total Care)
REPACK
TAB, PO, 0.75 mg, 30s ea. . 54868-3114-00 13.05
100s ea . . . . . 54868-3114-01 34.96 AB
1.5 mg, 30s ea 54868-4149-00 17.52
100s ea 54868-4149-01 46.38
3 mg, 30s ea 54868-4761-01 33.57
60s ea 54868-4761-02 62.64

ESTROSTEP FE (Warner Chilcott)
ethinyl estradiol/ferrous fum/norethindrone ace
TAB, PO (3X28)
84s ea 00430-0570-45 245.83

(Phys Total Care)
REPACK
TAB, PO, 28s ea 54868-3948-00 51.76

ESZOPICLONE
(Sepracor) *See LUNESTA*

ETANERCEPT
(Amgen USA Inc.) *See ENBREL*

ETH-OXYDOSE (Quality Care Prod)
REPACK
oxycodone hydrochloride
SOL, PO, 20 mg/ml,
30 ml, C-II 35356-0009-30 41.30

ETHACRYNATE SODIUM
(Aton) *See EDECRIN SODIUM*

(Aton) *See SODIUM EDECRIN*

ETHACRYNIC ACID
(Aton) *See EDECRIN*

(PCCA)
POW, NA, 1 gm 51927-3515-00 26.40

ETHAMBUTOL HCL (Medisca)
ethambutol hydrochloride
POW, NA (U.S.P.)
100 gm 38779-0118-05 495.00
500 gm 38779-0118-08 1836.00

(Teva)
TAB, PO, 400 mg, 100s ea . 00555-0923-02 178.63 AB

(VersaPharm)
TAB, PO (FILM-COATED)
100 mg, 100s ea . . . . . 61748-0011-01 59.21 AB
400 mg, 60s ea . . . . . 61748-0014-06 106.68 AB
90s ea . . . . . 61748-0014-09 160.02 AB
100s ea . . . . . 61748-0014-01 177.92 AB
(10X10)
400 mg, 100s ea UD . . 61748-0014-11 177.92 AB
1000s ea . . . . . 61748-0014-10 1779.26 AB

ETHAMBUTOL HYDROCHLORIDE (Heritage)
TAB, PO (USP,FILM COATED)
100 mg, 100s ea 23155-0100-01 59.19
400 mg, 100s ea 23155-0101-01 178.59

(Lupin Pharma, Inc.)
TAB, PO (USP,FILM-COATED)
100 mg, 100s ea . . . . . 68180-0280-01 59.20 AB
400 mg, 100s ea . . . . . 68180-0281-01 178.60 AB

(Medisca) *See ETHAMBUTOL HCL*

(Teva) *See ETHAMBUTOL HCL*

(VersaPharm) *See ETHAMBUTOL HCL*

(X-Gen) *See MYAMBUTOL*

(American Health)
REPACK
TAB, PO (FILM-COATED)
400 mg, 100s ea UD . . 68084-0280-01 162.50 AB

ETHAMOLIN (QOL Medical)
ethanolamine oleate
SOL, IV (10X2ML AMP)
50 mg/ml, 2 ml 10s . . . 67871-4790-06 923.94

ETHANOL
(Abbott Hosp) *See ALCOHOL ABSOLUTE*

(Amer Regent) *See ALCOHOL DEHYDRATED*

(Consolidated Midland) *See ALCOHOL ABSOLUTE*

(Gallipot) *See ALCOHOL ETHYL 200% ANHYDROUS*

(Gallipot) *See DENATURED ALCOHOL 190 PROOF*

(Gallipot) *See DENATURED ALCOHOL 200 PROOF*

(Letco) *See ALCOHOL ETHYL 95%*

(Mallinckrodt Lab) *See ALCOHOL ABSOLUTE*

(Medisca)
SOL, NA (DENATURED,1X500ML)
500 ml 38779-0616-08 31.50
(DENATURED,1X1000ML)
1000 ml 38779-0616-09 54.00
(DENATURED,1X4000ML)
4000 ml 38779-0616-01 186.00

(PCCA) *See ETHYL ALCOHOL*

(Spectrum Pharmacy) *See ALCOHOL DENATURED*

(Spectrum Pharmacy) *See ALCOHOL DENATURED ANHYDROUS*

(Spectrum Pharmacy) *See ALCOHOL ETHYL ANHYDROUS 190 PROOF*

(Spectrum Pharmacy) *See ALCOHOL ETHYL ANHYDROUS 200 PROOF*

(Spectrum Pharmacy) *See BASE, ALCOHOL GEL*

(Spectrum Pharmacy)
SOL, NA (REAGENT)
1000 ml 49452-2808-01 133.70
4000 ml 49452-2808-02 294.35
20000 ml 49452-2808-03 892.50

ETHANOLAMINE
(Baker, J.T.) *See MONOETHANOLAMINE*

(Medisca) *See MONOETHANOLAMINE*

(PCCA)
SOL, NA (MONOETHANOLAMINE)
1 gm 51927-1597-00 0.17

(Spectrum Pharmacy) *See MONOETHANOLAMINE*

ETHANOLAMINE OLEATE
(QOL Medical) *See ETHAMOLIN*

ETHER
(Baker, J.T.) *See ETHER ANHYDROUS*

(Baker, J.T.)
LIQ, NA (U.S.P., FOR ANESTHESIA)
250 ml 10106-9249-02 12.62

(Humco)
LIQ, NA (C.P., SOLVENT GRADE)
480 ml 00395-0819-16 15.86

(Mallinckrodt Lab)
LIQ, NA (U.S.P.)
500 gm 00406-0812-10 27.66

(Medisca)
LIQ, NA (USP,1X500ML)
500 ml 38779-0620-08 126.00
(U.S.P.)
1000 ml 38779-0620-09 210.00 44.10
(USP,1X4000ML)
4000 ml 38779-0620-01 475.50

(PCCA)
POW, NA (USP)
1 gm 51927-1452-00 0.28

(Spectrum Pharmacy)
LIQ, NA (1X500GM)
500 gm 49452-2805-01 348.25
(U.S.P.)
500 ml 49452-2820-02 207.90
(U.S.P., FOR ANESTHESIA)
2500 gm 49452-2805-02 1277.50 95.50
(U.S.P.)
4000 ml 49452-2820-03 861.00

ETHER ANHYDROUS (Baker, J.T.)
ether
LIQ, NA (A.C.S., REAGENT)
250 ml 10106-9244-01 38.26
500 ml 10106-9244-06 42.75

ETHEZYME 650 (Ethex)
papain/urea
OIN, TP, 650000 u/gm-10%,
30 gm 58177-0868-02 44.62

ETHEZYME 830 PAPAIN (Altura)
REPACK
papain/urea
OIN, TP, 830000 u/gm-100 mg/gm,
30 gm 63874-1147-03 59.10

ETHIDIUM BROMIDE (Baker, J.T.)
homidium bromide
POW, NA (ULTRAPURE, BIOREAGENT)
1 gm 10106-4007-00 22.25
5 gm 10106-4007-01 78.49
25 gm 10106-4007-02 324.76

ETHINYL ESTRADIOL (PCCA)
POW, NA (USP)
1 gm 51927-1856-00 78.00

(Spectrum Pharmacy)
POW, NA (U.S.P.)
1 gm 49452-2825-01 120.75
5 gm 49452-2825-02 504.00
25 gm 49452-2825-03 1764.00

ETHINYL ESTRADIOL-NORGESTREL (PD-Rx Pharm)
REPACK
ethinyl estradiol/norgestrel
TAB, PO, 50 mcg-0.5 mg,
4s ea 55289-0887-04 22.31

ETHINYL ESTRADIOL/ETHYNODIOL DIACETATE
(Pfizer) *See DEMULEN 1/50-21*

(Teva) *See KELNOR 1/35*

(Watson) *See ZOVIA 1/35E*

(Watson) *See ZOVIA 1/50E*

ETHINYL ESTRADIOL/ETONOGESTREL
(Organon) *See NUVARING*

ETHINYL ESTRADIOL/FERROUS FUM/NORETHIN-DRONE ACE
(Qualitest) *See GILDESS FE 1.5/30*

(Qualitest) *See GILDESS FE 1/20*

(Teva) *See JUNEL FE 1.5/30*

(Teva) *See JUNEL FE 1/20*

(Teva) *See LOESTRIN FE 1.5/30*

(Teva) *See LOESTRIN FE 1/20*

(Teva) *See TRI-LEGEST FE 28*

(Warner Chilcott) *See ESTROSTEP FE*

(Warner Chilcott) *See LOESTRIN 24 FE*

(Watson) *See MICROGESTIN FE 1.5/30*

(Watson) *See MICROGESTIN FE 1/20*

(Watson) *See TILIA FE*

PROD/MFR	NDC	AWP	DP	OBC
ETHINYL ESTRADIOL/FERROUS FUMARATE/NORETHINDRONE				
(Warner Chilcott) *See FEMCON FE*				
ETHINYL ESTRADIOL/LEVONORGESTREL				
(Bayer) *See LEVLEN*				
(Duramed) *See LOSEASONIQUE*				
(Duramed) *See SEASONALE*				
(Duramed) *See SEASONIQUE*				
(Teva) *See AVIANE*				
(Teva) *See ENPRESSE-28*				
(Teva) *See JOLESSA*				
(Teva) *See LESSINA 28*				
(Teva) *See NORDETTE-28*				
(Teva) *See PORTIA-28*				
(Watson) *See LEVORA-28*				
(Watson) *See LUTERA*				
(Watson) *See QUASENSE*				
(Watson) *See SRONYX*				
(Watson) *See TRIVORA-28*				
(Wyeth) *See LYBREL*				
ETHINYL ESTRADIOL/NORELGESTROMIN				
(Ortho-McNeil Pharm) *See ORTHO EVRA*				
(Palmetto)				
REPACK				
TDM, TD, ea	**23490-7615-01**	47.80		
ETHINYL ESTRADIOL/NORETHINDRONE				
(Ortho-McNeil Pharm) *See MODICON*				
(Ortho-McNeil Pharm) *See ORTHO-NOVUM 1/35*				
(Ortho-McNeil Pharm) *See ORTHO-NOVUM 7/7/7*				
(Teva) *See ARANELLE*				
(Teva) *See BALZIVA*				
(Teva) *See NORTREL*				
(Teva) *See NORTREL 7/7/7*				
(Warner Chilcott) *See OVCON 35*				
(Warner Chilcott) *See OVCON 50*				
(Watson) *See BREVICON*				
(Watson) *See LEENA*				
(Watson) *See NECON 0.5/35*				
(Watson) *See NECON 1/35*				
(Watson) *See NECON 10/11*				
(Watson) *See NECON 7/7/7*				
(Watson) *See NORINYL 1/35*				
(Watson) *See TRI-NORINYL*				
(Watson) *See ZENCHENT*				
ETHINYL ESTRADIOL/NORETHINDRONE ACETATE				
(Teva) *See JUNEL 1.5/30*				
(Teva) *See JUNEL 1/20*				
(Teva) *See LOESTRIN 21 1.5/30*				
(Teva) *See LOESTRIN 21 1/20*				
(Warner Chilcott) *See FEMHRT 1/5*				
(Warner Chilcott) *See FEMHRT LO*				
(Watson) *See MICROGESTIN 1.5/30*				
(Watson) *See MICROGESTIN 1/20*				
ETHINYL ESTRADIOL/NORGESTIMATE				
FUL				
TAB, PO; 35 mcg-0.25 mg, 28s ea		32.58		
(Ortho-McNeil Pharm) *See ORTHO TRI-CYCLEN*				
(Ortho-McNeil Pharm) *See ORTHO TRI-CYCLEN LO*				
(Ortho-McNeil Pharm) *See ORTHO-CYCLEN*				
(Qualitest) *See PREVIFEM*				
(Qualitest) *See TRI-PREVIFEM*				
(Teva) *See SPRINTEC*				
(Teva) *See TRI-LO-SPRINTEC*				
(Teva) *See TRI-SPRINTEC 28*				
(Watson) *See MONONESSA*				
(Watson Labs) *See TRINESSA*				
ETHINYL ESTRADIOL/NORGESTREL				
(Akrimax) *See LO/OVRAL-28*				
(Rouses) *See NORGESTREL/ETHINYL ESTRADIOL*				
(Teva) *See CRYSELLE*				
(Watson) *See LOW-OGESTREL 28*				
(Watson) *See OGESTREL-28*				
ETHIONAMIDE				
(Wyeth) *See TRECATOR*				
ETHOPROPAZINE HCL (PCCA)				
ethopropazine hydrochloride				
POW, NA (USP)				
1 gm	**51927-2744-00**	25.20		
(Spectrum Pharmacy)				
POW, NA, 5 gm	**49452-2804-01**	285.60		
25 gm	**49452-2804-02**	1095.50		
ETHOPROPAZINE HYDROCHLORIDE				
(PCCA) *See ETHOPROPAZINE HCL*				
(Spectrum Pharmacy) *See ETHOPROPAZINE HCL*				
ETHOSUXIMIDE (PCCA)				
POW, NA (USP)				
1 gm	**51927-3436-00**	5.40		
(Pfizer) *See ZARONTIN*				
(Pharm Assoc Inc)				
SYR, PO (AF,CHERRY,RASPBERRY) 250 mg/5 ml,				
474 ml	**00121-0670-16**	107.60		AA
(Teva)				
SGL, PO (SOFTGEL)				
250 mg, 100s ea	**50111-0901-01**	132.77		AB
SYR, PO, 250 mg/5 ml,				
474 ml	**00093-9660-16**	80.95		AA
(VersaPharm)				
SGL, PO (USP,SOFTGEL)				
250 mg, 100s ea	**61748-0025-01**	132.75		AB
SYR, PO (USP,RASPBERRY) 250 mg/5 ml,				
473 ml	**61748-0024-16**	78.90		AA
ETHOTOIN				
(Lundbeck) *See PEGANONE*				
ETHOXY DIGLYCOL (Gallipot)				
diethylene glycol monoethyl ether				
LIQ, NA (REAGENT)				
100 ml	**51552-0575-05**	11.20	8.00	
(1X500ML,REAGENT)				
500 ml	**51552-0575-06**	27.86	19.90	
(1X4000ML,REAGENT)				
4000 ml	**51552-0575-08**	105.00	75.00	
(PCCA)				
SOL, NA, 1 gm	**51927-3573-00**	0.13		
2-ETHOXYBENZOIC ACID (PCCA)				
SOL, NA (1X1ML)				
1 ml	**51927-3630-00**	1.74		
ETHOXYDIGLYCOL (Medisca)				
SOL, NA (1X500ML)				
500 ml	**38779-1903-08**	82.50		
(1X4000ML)				
4000 ml	**38779-1903-01**	285.00		
ETHOXYETHANOL (Medisca)				
ethylene glycol monoethyl ether				
SOL, NA (1X500ML)				
500 ml	**38779-1263-08**	31.50		
ETHRANE (Baxter)				
enflurane				
SOL, IH (ANESTHETIC)				
99.9%, 250 ml 6s	**10019-0350-60**	822.24		AN
ETHYL ACETATE (Amend)				
LIQ, NA (A.C.S., REAGENT)				
500 ml	**17317-1380-01**	11.20		
(N.F.)				
500 ml	**17317-0264-01**	10.50		
(A.C.S., REAGENT)				
4000 ml	**17317-1380-06**	49.00		
(N.F.)				
4000 ml	**17317-0264-06**	42.00		
19200 ml	**17317-0264-08**	140.00		
(Baker, J.T.)				
LIQ, NA (A.C.S., REAGENT)				
500 ml	**10106-9280-01**	29.97		
4000 ml	**10106-9280-03**	149.71		
(PCCA)				
LIQ, NA (N.F.)				
1 ml	**51927-1676-00**	0.11		
(Spectrum Pharmacy)				
LIQ, NA (N.F.)				
500 ml	**49452-2830-01**	75.60		
4000 ml	**49452-2830-02**	333.20		
20000 ml	**49452-2830-03**	994.00		
ETHYL ALCOHOL (PCCA)				
ethanol				
SOL, NA (ANHYDROUS;USP)				
1 ml	**51927-2999-00**	0.23		
(USP; 190 PROOF)				
1 ml	**51927-3161-00**	0.23		
ETHYL CHLORIDE				
(Gebauer) *See GEBAUER'S ETHYL CHLORIDE*				
(Medisca)				
SPR, NA (1X100ML)				
100 ml	**38779-0583-05**	60.00		
ETHYL OLEATE (Medisca)				
SOL, NA (1X4000ML, NF)				
4000 ml	**38779-1267-01**	1350.00		
(PCCA) *See ETHYL OLEATE NF*				
(Spectrum Pharmacy)				
CRY, NA (N.F.)				
500 gm	**49452-2885-02**	430.50		
ETHYL OLEATE NF (PCCA)				
ethyl oleate				
SOL, NA, 1 ml	**51927-3549-00**	0.60		
ETHYL VANILLIN (Amend)				
POW, NA (N.F.)				
454 gm	**17317-0754-01**	37.80		
2270 gm	**17317-0754-05**	147.00		
(PCCA)				
POW, NA (NF)				
1 gm	**51927-3173-00**	0.42		
(Spectrum Pharmacy)				
POW, NA (N.F.)				
125 gm	**49452-2900-01**	150.50		
500 gm	**49452-2900-02**	331.45		
ETHYLCELLULOSE (PCCA)				
POW, NA (AQUEOUS DISPERSION; NF)				
1 gm	**51927-3490-00**	0.51		
(Spectrum Pharmacy)				
POW, NA (N.F.)				
125 gm	**49452-2860-01**	104.65		
500 gm	**49452-2860-02**	277.90		
2500 gm	**49452-2860-03**	1018.50		
ETHYLENE DIAMINE TETRA ACETIC ACID (Medisca)				
edetic acid				
POW, NA (1X100GM)				
100 gm	**38779-1271-05**	37.50		
(1X500GM)				
500 gm	**38779-1271-08**	120.00		
ETHYLENE DICHLORIDE (Baker, J.T.)				
dichloroethane				
LIQ, NA (F.C.C.)				
150 ml	**10106-9301-04**	5.23		
500 ml	**10106-9301-01**	17.07		
ETHYLENE GLYCOL (Amend)				
SOL, NA (PURIFIED)				
454 gm	**17317-0834-01**	7.00		
3840 ml	**17317-0834-06**	19.60		
22700 gm	**17317-0834-08**	90.00		
(Baker, J.T.)				
LIQ, NA (REAGENT)				
500 ml	**10106-9300-01**	40.02		
(Spectrum Pharmacy)				
LIQ, NA (1X1000ML)				
1000 ml	**49452-2881-02**	114.80		
(1X4000ML)				
4000 ml	**49452-2881-03**	309.40		
ETHYLENE GLYCOL MONOBUTYL ETHER (Medisca)				
SOL, NA, 500 ml	**38779-1273-08**	46.50		
1000 ml	**38779-1273-09**	76.50		
ETHYLENE GLYCOL MONOETHYL ETHER				
(Medisca) *See ETHOXYETHANOL*				
ETHYLENE GLYCOL MONOMETHYL ETHER (PCCA)				
SOL, NA, 1 ml	**51927-1632-00**	0.24		
ETHYLENEDIAMINE (Baker, J.T.)				
LIQ, NA (REAGENT)				
500 ml	**10106-9299-01**	40.53		
4000 ml	**10106-9299-03**	94.71		
(PCCA) *See ETHYLENEDIAMINE 99%*				
ETHYLENEDIAMINE 99% (PCCA)				
ethylenediamine				
LIQ, NA, 1 gm	**51927-1749-00**	0.60		

PROD/MFR	NDC	AWP	DP	OBC
ETHYLENEDIAMINETETRAACETIC ACID (Spectrum Pharmacy)				
edetic acid				
CRY, NA (1X100GM)				
100 gm	49452-2879-01	160.30		
(1X250GM)				
250 gm	49452-2879-02	304.50		
(TRISODIUM, EDTA)				
500 gm	49452-2877-02	219.80		
(1X1000GM)				
1000 gm	49452-2879-04	798.00		
(TRISODIUM,EDTA)				
3000 gm	49452-2877-03	539.00		
POW, NA (A.C.S.,REAGENT)				
125 gm	49452-2876-01	118.30		
500 gm	49452-2876-02	252.70		
ETHYLENEDIAMINETETRAACETIC ACID TETRASODIUM SALT (Spectrum Pharmacy)				
edetate sodium				
CRY, NA (1X500GM)				
500 gm	49452-2878-01	117.25		
(1X3000GM)				
3000 gm	49452-2878-02	402.50		
ETHYLHEXYL SALICYLATE (Gallipot)				
LIQ, NA, 473 ml	51552-0113-06	53.20		
ETHYLPARABEN (Amend)				
POW, NA (N.F.)				
125 gm	17317-0833-04	7.70		
(U.S.P.)				
500 gm	17317-0833-01	18.20		
(N.F.)				
2270 gm	17317-0833-05	70.00		
(Spectrum Pharmacy)				
LIQ, NA (N.F.)				
2500 ml	49452-2890-02	584.50		
POW, NA, 125 gm	49452-2890-03	79.45		
500 gm	49452-2890-01	172.90		
ETHYOL (Medimmune Oncology)				
amifostine				
PDS, IV (S.D.V.)				
500 mg, ea	58178-0017-01	558.04		
3s ea	58178-0017-03	1817.63		
ETIDRONATE DISODIUM (Mylan)				
TAB, PO (USP)				
200 mg, 60s ea	00378-3286-91	209.82		AB
400 mg, 60s ea	00378-3288-91	419.55		AB
(P & G Pharm) *See DIDRONEL*				
ETILEFRINE HYDROCHLORIDE (PCCA)				
POW, NA, 1 gm	51927-3165-00	19.20		
ETODOLAC				
FUL				
CAP, PO, 200 mg, 100s ea		58.50		
TAB, PO, 400 mg, 100s ea		39.23		
500 mg, 100s ea		75.00		
(Actavis)				
TAB, PO, 400 mg, 100s ea	00228-2599-11	146.70		AB
500s ea	00228-2599-50	702.35		AB
500 mg, 100s ea	00228-2632-11	146.50		AB
(Apotex Corp.)				
CAP, PO (HARD GELATIN CAPSULE)				
200 mg, 100s ea	60505-0039-01	125.63		AB
300 mg, 100s ea	60505-0040-01	142.54		AB
TAB, PO, 400 mg, 100s ea	60505-0041-01	146.25		AB
500 mg, 100s ea	60505-0102-01	148.00		AB
(Gallipot)				
POW, NA (1X25GM,USP)				
25 gm	51552-0945-04	44.80	32.00	
(1X100GM,USP)				
100 gm	51552-0945-05	161.00	115.00	
(1X500GM,USP)				
500 gm	51552-0945-06	682.50	487.50	
(PCCA)				
POW, NA, 1 gm	51927-3010-00	5.76		
(Ranbaxy Pharm)				
TAB, PO, 400 mg, 100s ea	63304-0701-01	146.78		AB
(Sandoz)				
TAB, PO, 400 mg, 100s ea	00185-0140-01	132.37		AB
500s ea	00185-0140-05	628.75		AB
1000s ea	00185-0140-10	1231.04		AB
500 mg, 100s ea	00185-0139-01	140.62		AB
500s ea	00185-0139-05	703.12		AB
1000s ea	00185-0139-10	1406.24		AB
(Taro)				
CAP, PO, 200 mg, 100s ea	51672-4016-01	125.62		AB
300 mg, 100s ea	51672-4017-01	142.53		AB
TAB, PO (FILM-COATED)				
400 mg, 100s ea	51672-4018-01	146.78		AB
500 mg, 100s ea	51672-4036-01	150.14		AB
TER, PO (FILM COATED)				
400 mg, 60s ea	51672-4051-04	88.31		AB
100s ea	51672-4051-01	147.18		AB
500 mg, 60s ea	51672-4052-04	92.28		AB
100s ea	51672-4052-01	153.80		AB
600 mg, 60s ea	51672-4053-04	167.08		AB
100s ea	51672-4053-01	278.47		AB
(Teva)				
CAP, PO, 300 mg, 100s ea	00093-8397-01	126.38		AB
TAB, PO, 400 mg, 100s ea	00093-0892-01	146.80		AB
(USP,FILM-COATED)				
500 mg, 100s ea	00093-1893-01	150.14		AB
TER, PO (FILM-COATED)				
400 mg, 100s ea	00093-1122-01	140.17		AB
500 mg, 100s ea	00093-7172-01	146.48		AB
600 mg, 100s ea	00093-1118-01	265.21		AB
(4u)				
REPACK				
TAB, PO, 400 mg, 30s ea	42549-0511-30	94.92		AB
60s ea	10544-0311-60	106.12		
60s ea	42549-0511-60	106.12		AB
(A-S Medication)				
REPACK				
CAP, PO, 300 mg, 21s ea	54569-4545-01	29.93		EE
30s ea	54569-4545-00	42.76		EE
60s ea	54569-4545-03	85.52		EE
TAB, PO, 400 mg, 14s ea	54569-4468-00	20.55		EE
20s ea	54569-4468-01	29.36		EE
30s ea	54569-4460-02	44.03		EE
60s ea	54569-4468-05	88.07		EE
500 mg, 14s ea	54569-4630-04	21.02		EE
20s ea	54569-4630-00	30.03		EE
30s ea	54569-4630-03	45.04		EE
60s ea	54569-4630-05	90.08		EE
(Aidarex)				
REPACK				
CAP, PO, 300 mg, 30s ea	33261-0042-30	59.60		AB
60s ea	33261-0042-60	119.20		AB
90s ea	33261-0042-90	178.80		AB
120s ea	33261-0042-02	238.40		AB
TAB, PO, 400 mg, 14s ea	33261-0043-14	38.36		AB
20s ea	33261-0043-20	54.80		AB
21s ea	33261-0043-21	57.54		AB
28s ea	33261-0043-28	76.72		AB
30s ea	33261-0043-30	82.20		AB
40s ea	33261-0043-40	109.60		AB
60s ea	33261-0043-60	164.40		AB
90s ea	33261-0043-90	246.60		AB
100s ea	33261-0043-00	274.00		AB
120s ea	33261-0043-02	328.80		AB
180s ea	33261-0043-03	493.20		AB
500 mg, 30s ea	33261-0044-30	92.20		AB
60s ea	33261-0044-60	184.40		AB
90s ea	33261-0044-90	276.60		AB
120s ea	33261-0044-02	368.80		AB
(Altura)				
REPACK				
CAP, PO, 300 mg, 10s ea	63874-0401-10	16.05		
12s ea	63874-0401-12	19.26		
14s ea	63874-0401-14	22.47		
15s ea	63874-0401-15	24.08		
20s ea	63874-0401-20	32.10		
21s ea	63874-0401-21	33.71		
30s ea	63874-0401-30	48.15		
40s ea	63874-0401-40	64.20		
42s ea	63874-0401-42	67.41		
60s ea	63874-0401-60	96.30		
90s ea	63874-0401-90	144.45		
100s ea	63874-0401-01	160.50		
120s ea	63874-0401-04	192.60		
TAB, PO (FILM-COATED)				
400 mg, 10s ea	63874-0402-10	19.48		AB
14s ea	63874-0402-14	27.27		AB
15s ea	63874-0402-15	29.22		AB
20s ea	63874-0402-20	38.96		AB
21s ea	63874-0402-21	35.64		AB
28s ea	63874-0402-28	54.54		AB
30s ea	63874-0402-30	58.44		AB
40s ea	63874-0402-40	77.92		AB
42s ea	63874-0402-42	71.27		AB
90s ea	63874-0402-90	175.32		AB
100s ea	63874-0402-01	194.80		AB
120s ea	63874-0402-04	233.76		AB
500 mg, 14s ea	63874-0644-14	23.91		EE
20s ea	63874-0644-20	34.16		EE
21s ea	63874-0644-21	35.87		EE
28s ea	63874-0644-28	47.82		EE
30s ea	63874-0644-30	51.24		EE
40s ea	63874-0644-40	68.32		EE
50s ea	63874-0644-50	85.40		EE
60s ea	63874-0644-60	102.48		EE
90s ea	63874-0644-90	153.72		EE
100s ea	63874-0644-01	170.80		EE
120s ea	63874-0644-04	204.96		EE
TER, PO, 400 mg, 60s ea	63874-0402-60	116.88		EE
(Bryant Ranch)				
REPACK				
CAP, PO, 300 mg, 20s ea	63629-1376-01	31.09		
(HARD GELATIN CAPSULE)				
300 mg, 30s ea	63629-1376-03	46.63		AB
60s ea	63629-1376-02	100.18		AB
TAB, PO, 400 mg, 14s ea	63629-1377-02	29.92		
20s ea	63629-1377-01	42.60		
30s ea	63629-1377-03	63.40		
60s ea	63629-1377-05	106.32		
90s ea	63629-1377-06	159.99		
100s ea	63629-1377-04	177.65		
500 mg, 60s ea	63629-3198-01	106.99		
(Core)				
REPACK				
TAB, PO, 400 mg, 20s ea	33358-0138-20	43.67		
30s ea	33358-0138-30	64.99		
60s ea	33358-0138-60	108.98		
90s ea	33358-0138-90	163.99		
100s ea	33358-0138-00	182.09		
500 mg, 60s ea	33358-0139-60	109.66		
(DHS, Inc.)				
REPACK				
CAP, PO, 300 mg, 14s ea	55887-0172-14	19.95		
15s ea	55887-0172-15	21.37		
20s ea	55887-0172-20	28.50		
21s ea	55887-0172-21	29.92		
30s ea	55887-0172-30	42.75		
42s ea	55887-0172-42	59.85		
60s ea	55887-0172-60	85.51		
90s ea	55887-0172-90	128.27		
100s ea	55887-0172-01	142.50		
TAB, PO, 400 mg, 20s ea	55887-0808-20	33.69		AB
30s ea	55887-0808-30	49.66		AB
40s ea	55887-0808-40	65.00		AB
60s ea	55887-0808-60	99.32		AB
90s ea	55887-0808-90	146.25		AB
(Dispensing Solutions)				
REPACK				
CAP, PO, 300 mg, 15s ea	55045-2592-07	24.00		AB
30s ea	55045-2592-08	48.00		AB
60s ea	55045-2592-06	96.00		AB
60s ea	66336-0376-60	102.86		AB
90s ea	55045-2592-09	144.00		AB
(HARD GELATIN CAPSULE)				
300 mg, 90s ea	66336-0376-90	154.29		AB
100s ea	55045-2592-01	160.00		AB
120s ea	55045-2592-02	192.00		AB
TAB, PO (FILM-COATED)				
400 mg, 14s ea	55045-2490-03	23.80		AB
20s ea	55045-2490-02	34.00		AB
30s ea	55045-2490-08	51.00		AB
30s ea	66336-0878-30	53.45		AB
(FILM-COATED)				
400 mg, 30s ea	55045-3924-01	51.00		AB
40s ea	55045-2490-04	68.00		AB
60s ea	66336-0878-60	106.30		AB
(FILM-COATED)				
400 mg, 60s ea	55045-2490-06	102.00		AB
90s ea	55045-2490-01	153.00		AB
100s ea	55045-2490-00	170.00		AB
120s ea	55045-2490-05	204.00		AB
500 mg, 10s ea	55045-2894-01	19.50		AB
15s ea	55045-2894-03	29.25		AB
21s ea	55045-2894-02	40.95		AB
30s ea	55045-2894-08	58.50		AB
30s ea	66336-0076-30	53.88		
60s ea	55045-2900-06	117.00		AB
60s ea	66336-0076-60	107.16		
80s ea	55045-2894-04	156.00		AB
90s ea	55045-2894-09	175.50		AB
90s ea	66336-0076-90	160.74		AB
100s ea	55045-2894-05	195.00		AB
120s ea	55045-2894-06	234.00		AB
TER, PO (FILM COATED)				
400 mg, 30s ea	55045-3283-08	55.50		AB
(FILM-COATED)				
400 mg, 60s ea	55045-3283-06	111.00		AB
(IPI)				
REPACK				
TAB, PO, 400 mg, 30s ea	18837-0050-30	55.13		AB
90s ea	18837-0050-90	165.37		
500 mg, 30s ea	18837-0051-30	55.13		
60s ea	18837-0051-60	110.25		

PROD/MFR	NDC	AWP	DP	OBC
(Keltman Pharma., Inc.)				
REPACK				
CAP, PO, 300 mg, 30s ea	**68387-0152-30**	49.18		
60s ea	**68387-0152-60**	98.36		
TAB, PO (FILM-COATED)				
400 mg, 30s ea	**68387-0150-30**	52.50		AB
60s ea	**68387-0150-60**	105.00		
90s ea	**68387-0150-90**	157.50		
(Medsource)				
REPACK				
CAP, PO (HARD GELATIN CAPSULE)				
300 mg, 30s ea	**45865-0362-30**	45.00		AB
60s ea	**45865-0362-60**	90.00		AB
90s ea	**45865-0362-90**	135.00		AB
100s ea	**45865-0362-00**	150.00		AB
120s ea	**45865-0362-01**	180.00		AB
150s ea	**45865-0362-02**	225.00		AB
300s ea	**45865-0362-05**	450.00		AB
(Nucare Pharm)				
REPACK				
TAB, PO, 400 mg, 28s ea	**66267-0095-28**	49.89		EE
30s ea	**66267-0095-30**	109.39		AB
40s ea	**66267-0095-40**	68.56		EE
60s ea	**66267-0095-60**	200.53		AB
90s ea	**66267-0095-90**	119.83		AB
100s ea	**68071-1364-00**	170.60		AB
120s ea	**66267-0095-91**	159.54		AB
TER, PO (FILM-COATED)				
400 mg, 60s ea	**68071-0542-60**	88.41		AB
500 mg, 30s ea	**66267-0520-30**	64.99		AB
60s ea	**66267-0520-60**	115.76		AB
(Palmetto)				
REPACK				
CAP, PO, 300 mg, 21s ea	**23490-5556-00**	33.60		
30s ea	**23490-5556-01**	48.00		
60s ea	**23490-5556-02**	96.00		
90s ea	**23490-5556-09**	144.00		
TAB, PO, 400 mg, 30s ea	**23490-5557-01**	51.00		
60s ea	**23490-5557-02**	102.00		
90s ea	**23490-5557-03**	153.00		
500 mg, 30s ea	**23490-6991-01**	58.50		
60s ea	**23490-6991-02**	117.00		
ETODOLAC (Palmetto)				
TER, PO, 400 mg, 30s ea	**23490-7020-03**	121.42		
ETODOLAC (Palmetto)				
500 mg, 30s ea	**23490-7124-03**	64.99		
60s ea	**23490-7124-01**	129.98		
ETODOLAC (Palmetto)				
600 mg, 30s ea	**23490-7021-03**	229.73		
ETODOLAC (PD-Rx Pharm)				
REPACK				
CAP, PO, 300 mg, 30s ea	**55289-0501-30**	63.83		AB
(USP)				
300 mg, 60s ea	**55289-0501-60**	100.04		AB
TAB, PO, 400 mg, 12s ea	**55289-0239-12**	34.67		AB
20s ea	**55289-0239-20**	49.45		AB
21s ea	**55289-0239-21**	50.67		AB
28s ea	**58864-0665-28**	60.65		AB
30s ea	**55289-0239-30**	66.67		AB
45s ea	**55289-0239-45**	93.33		AB
60s ea	**55289-0239-60**	120.00		AB
500 mg, 14s ea	**55289-0418-14**	37.47		AB
20s ea	**55289-0418-20**	38.22		AB
30s ea	**55289-0418-30**	50.67		AB
(Pharma Pac)				
REPACK				
CAP, PO, 300 mg, 20s ea	**52959-0483-20**	33.40		AB
21s ea	**52959-0483-21**	35.07		AB
28s ea	**52959-0483-28**	46.76		AB
30s ea	**52959-0483-30**	50.09		AB
42s ea	**52959-0483-42**	68.35		AB
45s ea	**52959-0483-45**	75.13		AB
60s ea	**52959-0483-60**	100.17		AB
90s ea	**52959-0483-90**	150.23		AB
120s ea	**52959-0483-02**	200.26		AB
TAB, PO, 400 mg, 12s ea	**52959-0471-12**	21.36		AB
14s ea	**52959-0471-14**	24.92		AB
15s ea	**52959-0471-15**	26.69		AB
20s ea	**52959-0471-20**	35.59		AB
25s ea	**52959-0471-25**	44.46		AB
28s ea	**52959-0471-28**	49.81		AB
30s ea	**52959-0471-30**	53.37		AB
60s ea	**52959-0471-60**	106.72		AB
90s ea	**52959-0471-90**	160.05		AB
120s ea	**52959-0471-02**	213.36		AB
500 mg, 14s ea	**52959-0530-14**	24.94		AB
20s ea	**52959-0530-20**	35.62		AB
28s ea	**52959-0530-28**	49.87		AB
30s ea	**52959-0530-30**	53.42		AB
30s ea	**52959-0649-30**	57.00		AB
45s ea	**52959-0530-45**	80.12		AB
60s ea	**52959-0530-60**	106.81		AB
90s ea	**52959-0530-90**	160.20		AB
120s ea	**52959-0530-02**	213.54		AB
TER, PO, 600 mg, 60s ea	**52959-0821-60**	169.75		AB
(Phys Total Care)				
REPACK				
CAP, PO (HARD GELATIN CAPSULE)				
200 mg, 20s ea	**54868-5274-01**	33.75		AB
30s ea	**54868-5274-02**	48.39		AB
60s ea	**54868-5274-00**	92.25		AB
90s ea	**54868-5274-03**	105.15		AB
TAB, PO, 400 mg, 30s ea	**54868-3955-00**	22.38		EE
60s ea	**54868-3955-01**	41.73		EE
90s ea	**54868-3955-02**	61.11		EE
100s ea	**54868-3955-04**	62.77		EE
120s ea	**54868-3955-03**	80.49		EE
500 mg, 10s ea	**54868-4059-00**	12.69		EE
15s ea	**54868-4059-01**	17.54		
60s ea	**54868-4059-03**	61.15		EE
100s ea	**54868-4059-02**	75.62		
TER, PO (FILM COATED)				
400 mg, 30s ea	**54868-1978-00**	79.05		AB
500 mg, 30s ea	**54868-1852-00**	88.14		AB
60s ea	**54868-1852-01**	170.28		
(Physician Partner)				
REPACK				
CAP, PO, 300 mg, 21s ea	**21695-0049-21**	70.43		
30s ea	**21695-0049-30**	85.52		
42s ea	**21695-0049-42**	140.86		AB
60s ea	**21695-0049-60**	171.04		
90s ea	**21695-0049-90**	256.56		
TAB, PO, 400 mg, 21s ea	**21695-0050-21**	72.52		
30s ea	**21695-0050-30**	88.06		
60s ea	**21695-0050-60**	176.12		
90s ea	**21695-0050-90**	264.18		
(Quality Care Prod)				
REPACK				
TAB, PO, 400 mg, 14s ea	**49999-0038-14**	45.43		EE
28s ea	**49999-0038-28**	90.86		EE
(FILM-COATED)				
400 mg, 30s ea	**49999-0038-30**	97.33		AB
40s ea	**49999-0038-40**	129.79		AB
60s ea	**49999-0038-60**	194.69		AB
90s ea	**49999-0038-90**	292.30		AB
100s ea	**49999-0038-00**	325.00		AB
TER, PO, 500 mg, 60s ea	**35356-0324-60**	158.60		AB
(Southwood)				
REPACK				
CAP, PO, 200 mg, 14s ea	**58016-0206-14**	17.95		EE
15s ea	**58016-0206-15**	19.23		EE
20s ea	**58016-0206-20**	25.64		EE
21s ea	**58016-0206-21**	26.92		EE
30s ea	**58016-0206-30**	38.46		EE
42s ea	**58016-0206-42**	53.84		EE
100s ea	**58016-0206-00**	128.20		EE
300 mg, 14s ea	**58016-0209-14**	22.47		EE
15s ea	**58016-0209-15**	24.08		EE
20s ea	**58016-0209-20**	32.10		EE
21s ea	**58016-0209-21**	33.71		EE
(HARD GELATIN CAPSULE)				
300 mg, 30s ea	**58016-0209-30**	52.50		AB
42s ea	**58016-0209-42**	67.41		EE
(HARD GELATIN CAPSULE)				
300 mg, 60s ea	**58016-0209-60**	105.00		AB
90s ea	**58016-0209-90**	157.50		AB
100s ea	**58016-0209-00**	175.00		AB
120s ea	**58016-0209-02**	210.00		AB
TAB, PO, 400 mg, 14s ea	**58016-0208-14**	23.76		EE
15s ea	**58016-0208-15**	25.46		EE
20s ea	**58016-0208-20**	33.94		EE
21s ea	**58016-0208-21**	35.64		EE
30s ea	**58016-0208-30**	57.60		AB
42s ea	**58016-0208-42**	71.27		EE
60s ea	**58016-0208-60**	115.20		AB
90s ea	**58016-0208-90**	172.80		AB
100s ea	**58016-0208-00**	192.00		AB
120s ea	**58016-0208-02**	230.40		AB
500 mg, 14s ea	**58016-0375-14**	23.91		EE
20s ea	**58016-0375-20**	34.16		EE
21s ea	**58016-0375-21**	35.87		EE
28s ea	**58016-0375-28**	47.82		EE
30s ea	**58016-0375-30**	51.24		EE
40s ea	**58016-0375-40**	68.32		EE
60s ea	**58016-0375-60**	102.48		EE
90s ea	**58016-0375-90**	153.72		EE
100s ea	**58016-0375-00**	170.80		EE
TER, PO (FILM COATED)				
400 mg, 30s ea	**58016-0867-30**	44.15		AB
60s ea	**58016-0867-60**	88.31		AB
90s ea	**58016-0867-90**	132.46		AB
100s ea	**58016-0867-00**	147.18		AB
120s ea	**58016-0867-02**	176.62		AB
500 mg, 30s ea	**58016-0647-30**	51.32		AB
60s ea	**58016-0647-60**	102.64		AB
90s ea	**58016-0647-90**	153.96		AB
100s ea	**58016-0647-00**	171.07		AB
120s ea	**58016-0647-02**	205.28		AB
(St. Mary's MPP)				
REPACK				
TAB, PO, 400 mg, 20s ea	**60760-0552-20**	36.90		AB
30s ea	**60760-0552-30**	52.36		AB
60s ea	**60760-0552-60**	98.71		AB
90s ea	**60760-0552-90**	145.07		AB
(Stat Rx)				
REPACK				
CAP, PO, 300 mg, 30s ea	**16590-0488-30**	48.00		
60s ea	**16590-0488-60**	96.00		
90s ea	**16590-0488-90**	144.00		
120s ea	**16590-0488-72**	192.00		
TAB, PO, 400 mg, 30s ea	**16590-0092-30**	47.25		
(FILM-COATED)				
400 mg, 56s ea	**16590-0092-56**	103.88		AB
60s ea	**16590-0092-60**	94.50		
90s ea	**16590-0092-90**	141.75		
500 mg, 30s ea	**16590-0574-30**	55.13		AB
60s ea	**16590-0574-60**	110.26		AB
90s ea	**16590-0574-90**	135.00		AB
120s ea	**16590-0574-72**	170.00		AB
TER, PO (FILM-COATED)				
400 mg, 30s ea	**16590-0549-30**	60.00		AB
60s ea	**16590-0549-60**	115.00		AB
90s ea	**16590-0549-90**	169.00		AB
(Vibranta)				
REPACK				
CAP, PO, 300 mg, 20s ea	**57866-0264-02**	30.10		EE
30s ea	**57866-0264-01**	46.30		EE
TAB, PO, 400 mg, 15s ea	**57866-0262-01**	26.29		EE
28s ea	**57866-0262-03**	47.02		EE
30s ea	**57866-0262-02**	65.48		
60s ea	**57866-0262-04**	194.69		
90s ea	**57866-0262-05**	243.90		
180s ea	**57866-0262-07**	93.93		
500 mg, 30s ea	**57866-7137-01**	56.11		EE
ETODOLAC E/R (Stat Rx)				
REPACK				
etodolac				
TER, PO, 500 mg, 30s ea	**16590-0093-30**	68.50		
60s ea	**16590-0093-60**	137.00		
90s ea	**16590-0093-90**	205.50		
ETODOLAC ER (Altura)				
REPACK				
etodolac				
TER, PO, 500 mg, 30s ea	**63874-1116-03**	68.32		
(Pharma Pac)				
REPACK				
TER, PO, 400 mg, 30s ea	**52959-0785-30**	48.38		
500 mg, 20s ea	**52959-0649-20**	38.01		
60s ea	**52959-0649-60**	113.99		
(Phys Total Care)				
REPACK				
TER, PO, 400 mg, 60s ea	**54868-1978-01**	164.58		
ETOLDOLAC (HomeMed)				
REPACK				
etodolac				
TAB, PO, 400 mg, 30s ea	**51655-0877-24**	98.99		
ETOMIDATE (Bedford)				
SOL, IV (S.D.V.)				
2 mg/ml, 10 ml 10s	**55390-0762-10**	118.20		AP
20 ml 10s	**55390-0763-20**	121.80		AP
(Hospira) *See AMIDATE*				
ETOPOPHOS (B/M Squibb Onc/Vir)				
etoposide phosphate				
PDS, IV (S.D.V.)				
100 mg, ea	**00015-3404-20**	159.55		
ETOPOSIDE (APP)				
SOL, IV (M.D.V.)				
20 mg/ml, 5 ml	**63323-0104-05**	157.60		AP
25 ml	**63323-0104-25**	665.30		AP
50 ml	**63323-0104-50**	1393.40		AP
(Bedford) *See ETOPOSIDE NOVAPLUS*				
(Bedford)				
SOL, IV (M.D.V.)				
20 mg/ml, 5 ml	**55390-0291-01**	9.00		AP
25 ml	**55390-0292-01**	45.00		AP
50 ml	**55390-0293-01**	90.60		AP

PROD/MFR	NDC	AWP	DP	OBC
(Medisca)				
POW, NA (U.S.P.)				
1 gm	38779-0784-06	918.00		
5 gm	38779-0784-03	4071.00		
(Mylan)				
SGL, PO (BLISTER PACK,SOFTGEL)				
50 mg, 20s ea	00378-3266-94	952.75		AB
(PCCA)				
POW, NA (U.S.P.)				
1 gm	51927-2772-00	1050.00		
(Teva) *See TOPOSAR*				
(Phys Total Care) REPACK				
SGL, PO, 50 mg, ea	54868-5355-02	55.79		
7s ea	54868-5355-01	358.26		
20s ea	54868-5355-00	965.91		
ETOPOSIDE NOVAPLUS (Bedford)				
etoposide				
SOL, IV (M.D.V.,PRIVATE LABEL)				
20 mg/ml, 5 ml	55390-0491-01	7.20		AP
25 ml	55390-0492-01	28.80		AP
50 ml	55390-0493-01	54.00		AP
ETOPOSIDE PHOSPHATE				
(B/M Squibb Onc/Vir) *See ETOPOPHOS*				
ETRAVIRINE				
(Tibotec Therapeutics) *See INTELENCE*				
EUCALYPTOL (Gallipot)				
LIQ, NA, 25 ml	51552-0770-04	38.50	27.50	
(Lorann Oil)				
OIL, NA (N.F.)				
30 ml	23535-0707-05	2.50		
120 ml	23535-0707-08	7.00		
480 ml	23535-0707-01	20.00		
(PCCA)				
LIQ, NA (USP,1X1ML)				
1 ml	51927-3628-00	0.55		
EUCALYPTOL FLAVOR (PCCA)				
flavoring aid				
SOL, NA, 1 ml	51927-1415-00	0.38		
EUCALYPTUS (Medisca)				
eucalyptus oil				
OIL, NA (1X14ML,NATURAL)				
14 ml	38779-0820-03	15.00		
(1X25ML,NATURAL)				
25 ml	38779-0820-04	22.50		
(1X100ML,NATURAL)				
100 ml	38779-0820-05	42.00		
(1X500ML,NATURAL)				
500 ml	38779-0820-08	97.50		
EUCALYPTUS FLAVOR OIL (PCCA)				
eucalyptus oil				
OIL, NA, 1 ml	51927-1137-00	0.25		
EUCALYPTUS OIL (Gallipot)				
OIL, NA, 29.57 ml	51552-0182-02	4.55		
59.14 ml	51552-0182-03	6.44		
100 ml	51552-0182-05	9.80		
473 ml	51552-0182-06	30.80		
(Lorann Oil) *See EUCALYPTUS OIL 70/75%*				
(Lorann Oil)				
OIL, NA, 9.9 ml	23535-0151-15	2.25		
(Medisca) *See EUCALYPTUS*				
(PCCA) *See EUCALYPTUS FLAVOR OIL*				
(Spectrum Pharmacy)				
OIL, NA (F.C.C.)				
100 ml	49452-2915-01	54.25		
500 ml	49452-2915-02	120.40		
4000 ml	49452-2915-03	532.00		
EUCALYPTUS OIL 70/75% (Lorann Oil)				
eucalyptus oil				
OIL, NA (N.F.)				
30 ml	23535-0219-05	2.00		
120 ml	23535-0219-08	5.00		
480 ml	23535-0219-01	16.80		
EUDAGRIT L-100 (PCCA)				
methacrylic acid copolymer a				
POW, NA (1X1GM)				
1 gm	51927-3180-00	0.87		
EUDRAGIT S-100 (PCCA)				
acrylates copolymer				
POW, NA, 1 gm	51927-2651-00	0.75		
EUFLEXXA (Ferring)				
hyaluronate sodium				
SOL, IJ, 10 mg/ml,				
2 ml 3s	55566-4100-01	618.19		
EUGENOL (Lorann Oil)				
OIL, NA (U.S.P.)				
30 ml	23535-0708-05	2.00		
120 ml	23535-0708-08	5.90		
480 ml	23535-0708-01	21.10		
(Medisca)				
SOL, NA (1X50ML)				
50 ml	38779-0871-02	22.50		
(1X100ML)				
100 ml	38779-0871-05	37.50		
(1X500ML)				
500 ml	38779-0871-08	70.50		
(Spectrum Pharmacy)				
LIQ, NA (U.S.P.)				
100 ml	49452-2920-01	64.75		
500 ml	49452-2920-02	125.30		
EUGENOL FLAVOR (PCCA)				
flavoring aid				
SOL, NA (USP)				
1 ml	51927-1136-00	0.45		
EURAX (Ranbaxy Labs)				
crotamiton				
CRE, TP (1X60GM)				
10%, 60 gm	10631-0091-60	48.90		
LOT, TP (1X60GM,USP)				
10%, 60 gm	10631-0092-60	52.13		AT
(1X454GM,USP)				
10%, 454 gm	10631-0092-16	339.45		AT
(A-S Medication) REPACK				
CRE, TP, 10%, 60 gm	54569-1926-00	16.29		
EVAMIST (Ther-RX)				
estradiol				
SPR, TD, 1.53 mg/actuation,				
8.1 ml	64011-0215-41	76.58		
EVEN CARE (Medline)				
glucose, blood test				
DEV, NA (STRIP)				
50s ea	08327-0486-29	46.12		
EVEN CARE CONTROL (Medline)				
glucose meter test control				
DEV, NA (HIGH/LOW)				
ea	08327-0486-92	15.44		
EVEN CARE MONITORING SYSTEM (Medline)				
glucose meter				
DEV, NA, ea	08327-0486-09	93.67		
EVENING PRIMROSE OIL (PCCA)				
OIL, NA, 1 ml	51927-3468-00	0.88		
EVEROLIMUS				
(Novartis Pharm) *See AFINITOR*				
EVISTA (Lilly)				
raloxifene hydrochloride				
TAB, PO (UNIT OF USE,FILM COATED)				
60 mg, 30s ea	00002-4165-30	121.03	100.86	EE
(UNIT OF USE)				
60 mg, 100s ea UD	00002-4165-02	403.44	336.20	
2000s ea	00002-4165-07	8068.80	6724.00	
(A-S Medication) REPACK				
TAB, PO, 60 mg, 30s ea	54569-4628-00	157.34		
(AQ) REPACK				
TAB, PO, 60 mg, 30s ea	66105-0538-03	181.16		
(PD-Rx Pharm) REPACK				
TAB, PO, 60 mg, 30s ea	55289-0266-30	179.90		
(Phys Total Care) REPACK				
TAB, PO, 60 mg, 30s ea	54868-4170-00	145.24		
60s ea	54868-4170-01	289.18		
(Quality Care Prod) REPACK				
TAB, PO, 60 mg, 30s ea	49999-0458-30	178.26		
EVOCLIN (Stiefel Labs)				
clindamycin phosphate				
FOA, TP (VERSAFOAM CAN)				
1%, 50 gm	63032-0061-50	184.88		
100 gm	63032-0061-00	282.97		
(Quality Care Prod) REPACK				
FOA, TP (1X50GM)				
1%, 50 gm	35356-0225-50	331.84		
(1X100GM)				
1%, 100 gm	35356-0225-00	490.18		
EVOXAC (Daiichi Sankyo)				
cevimeline hydrochloride				
CAP, PO, 30 mg, 100s ea	63395-0201-13	252.00		
(Bryant Ranch) REPACK				
CAP, PO, 30 mg, 100s ea	63629-1379-01	193.99		
(Nucare Pharm) REPACK				
CAP, PO, 30 mg, 100s ea	66267-1298-00	259.36		
(Stat Rx) REPACK				
CAP, PO, 30 mg, 100s ea	16590-0859-71	292.72		
EX-HISTINE (Dexo)				
cpm/methscopolamine nitrate/phenyleph hcl				
SYR, PO, 480 ml	59196-0013-48	12.20		
EXACTACAIN (Healthpoint)				
benzocaine/butamben/tetracaine hydrochloride				
SPR, MM (W/APPLICATORS,CHERRY)				
14%-2%-2%, 60 gm	00064-1070-60	58.50		
(Onset)				
benzocaine/butamben/tetracaine				
SPR, TP (1X60GM)				
14%-2%-2%, 60 gm	16781-0113-60	58.50		
EXALL (Hawthorn Pharm)				
carbetapentane citrate/guaifenesin				
SOL, PO (1X473ML,AF,SF,DYE-FREE)				
10 mg/5 ml-100 mg/5 ml,				
473 ml	63717-0554-16	99.99		
EXALL-D (Hawthorn Pharm)				
carbetapentane cit/gg/pse hcl				
SOL, PO (1X473ML,AF,SF,DYE-FREE)				
473 ml	63717-0555-16	109.99		
EXECLEAR-C (Larken Labs, Inc.)				
codeine phosphate/guaifenesin				
SOL, PO (1X473ML,AF,SF,DYE-FREE)				
10 mg/5 ml-200 mg/5 ml,				
473 ml, C-V	68047-0222-16	77.35		
EXECLEAR-DM (Larken Labs, Inc.)				
dm/gg/pse hcl				
SOL, PO (1X473ML,AF,SF,RASPBERRY)				
473 ml	68047-0223-16	47.63		
EXEFEN-IR (Larken Labs, Inc.)				
guaifenesin/pseudoephedrine hydrochloride				
TAB, PO, 400 mg-60 mg,				
100s ea	68047-0154-01	67.88		
EXELDERM (Ranbaxy Labs)				
sulconazole nitrate				
CRE, TP (1X15GM)				
1%, 15 gm	10631-0101-15	36.69		
30 gm	00072-8200-30	64.54		
60 gm	00072-8200-60	106.92		
SOL, TP (1X30ML)				
1%, 30 ml	10631-0100-30	64.55		
(Phys Total Care) REPACK				
CRE, TP, 1%, 15 gm	54868-3292-00	13.43		
EXELON (Novartis Pharm)				
rivastigmine tartrate				
CAP, PO, 1.5 mg, 60s ea	00078-0323-44	264.64		
100s ea UD	00078-0323-06	441.04		
3 mg, 60s ea	00078-0324-44	264.64		
100s ea UD	00078-0324-06	441.04		
4.5 mg, 60s ea	00078-0325-44	264.64		
100s ea UD	00078-0325-06	441.04		
6 mg, 60s ea	00078-0326-44	264.64		
100s ea UD	00078-0326-06	441.04		
SOL, PO (W/DISPENSER)				
2 mg/ml, 120 ml	00078-0339-31	475.76		
(Novartis Pharm)				
rivastigmine				
TDM, TD, 4.6 mg/24 hr,				
ea	00078-0501-61	7.49		
30s ea	00078-0501-15	242.48		
9.5 mg/24 hr, ea	00078-0502-61	7.49		
30s ea	00078-0502-15	242.48		
(Phys Total Care) REPACK				
rivastigmine tartrate				
CAP, PO, 1.5 mg, 30s ea	54868-4512-01	127.85		
60s ea	54868-4512-00	253.21		
3 mg, 60s ea	54868-5839-00	315.22		
4.5 mg, 30s ea	54868-5240-00	103.11		
6 mg, 60s ea	54868-5339-00	292.01		

PROD/MFR	NDC	AWP	DP	OBC
(Phys Total Care)				
rivastigmine				
TDM, TD, 4.6 mg/24 hr,				
30s ea	54868-6070-00	267.74		
9.5 mg/24 hr,				
30s ea	54868-5954-00	267.74		
(Physician Partner)				
REPACK				
TDM, TD, 4.6 mg/24 hr,				
30s ea	21695-0357-30	467.76		
(Quality Care Prod)				
REPACK				
TDM, TD, 4.6 mg/24 hr,				
30s ea	35356-0394-30	236.43		
EXEMESTANE				
(Pfizer) *See AROMASIN*				
EXENATIDE				
(Amylin) *See BYETTA*				
EXFORGE (Novartis Pharm)				
amlodipine besylate/valsartan				
TAB, PO (FILM-COATED)				
5 mg-160 mg,				
30s ea	00078-0488-15	97.06		
5 mg-320 mg,				
30s ea	00078-0490-15	123.12		
10 mg-160 mg,				
30s ea	00078-0489-15	110.10		
10 mg-320 mg,				
30s ea	00078-0491-15	139.76		
(Phys Total Care)				
REPACK				
TAB, PO (FILM-COATED)				
5 mg-160 mg,				
30s ea	54868-5997-00	123.61		
90s ea	54868-5997-01	347.28		
5 mg-320 mg,				
30s ea	54868-5996-00	147.71		
90s ea	54868-5996-01	425.76		
10 mg-160 mg,				
30s ea	54868-5804-00	129.85		
(FILM-COATED)				
10 mg-320 mg,				
30s ea	54868-5983-00	155.29		
90s ea	54868-5983-01	447.78		
EXFORGE HCT (Novartis Pharm)				
amlodipine besylate/hydrochlorothiazide/valsartan				
TAB, PO (FILM-COATED)				
5 mg-12.5 mg-160 mg,				
30s ea	00078-0559-15	97.06		
5 mg-25 mg-160 mg,				
30s ea	00078-0560-15	97.06		
10 mg-12.5 mg-160 mg,				
30s ea	00078-0561-15	110.10		
10 mg-25 mg-160 mg,				
30s ea	00078-0562-15	110.10		
10 mg-25 mg-320 mg,				
30s ea	00078-0563-15	139.76		
EXJADE (Novartis Pharm)				
deferasirox				
TBS, PO, 125 mg, 30s ea	00078-0468-15	589.58		
250 mg, 30s ea	00078-0469-15	1179.14		
500 mg, 30s ea	00078-0470-15	2358.25		
EXODERM (A. G. Marin)				
salicylic acid/sodium thiosulfate				
LOT, TP, 1%-25%, 120 ml	12539-0531-04	22.02		
EXOTIC-HC (A. G. Marin)				
chloroxylenol/hc/pramoxine hcl				
SOL, OT, 10 ml	12539-0623-10	22.75		
EXPECTUSS (Centurion)				
carbetapentane citrate/guaifenesin				
SOL, PO (AF,SF,CHERRY)				
20 mg/5 ml-75 mg/5 ml,				
473 ml	23359-0003-16	66.38		
EXTAVIA (Novartis Pharm)				
interferon beta-1b				
PDS, SC (LYOPHILIZED)				
0.3 mg, 15s ea	00078-0569-12	2951.42		
EXTENDED PHENYTOIN SODIUM (Amneal)				
phenytoin sodium, extended				
CER, PO (USP,HARD GELATIN)				
100 mg, 100s ea	65162-0212-10	33.90		AB
500s ea	65162-0212-50	169.50		AB
1000s ea	65162-0212-11	339.00		AB
(Caraco)				
CER, PO, 100 mg, 100s ea	62756-0402-01	33.90		AB
1000s ea	62756-0402-03	322.95		AB
(USP,HARD GELATIN)				
200 mg, 30s ea	62756-0299-83	24.00		AB
100s ea	62756-0299-88	79.97		AB
300 mg, 30s ea	62756-0432-83	35.94		AB
100s ea	62756-0432-88	119.81		AB
(Taro)				
CER, PO, 100 mg, 100s ea	51672-4111-01	33.90		AB
1000s ea	51672-4111-03	339.00		AB
(Altura)				
REPACK				
CER, PO, 100 mg, 12s ea	63874-0453-12	2.74		
15s ea	63874-0453-15	3.42		
20s ea	63874-0453-20	4.56		
25s ea	63874-0453-25	5.70		
28s ea	63874-0453-28	6.38		
30s ea	63874-0453-30	6.85		
40s ea	63874-0453-40	9.12		
45s ea	63874-0453-45	10.26		
60s ea	63874-0453-60	13.68		
90s ea	63874-0453-90	20.52		
100s ea	63874-0453-01	22.81		
120s ea	63874-0453-04	65.32		
(Bryant Ranch)				
REPACK				
CER, PO, 100 mg, 30s ea	63629-2552-02	12.53		
90s ea	63629-2552-04	27.00		
100s ea	63629-2552-01	41.77		
180s ea	63629-2552-03	75.19		
(Dispensing Solutions)				
REPACK				
CER, PO, 100 mg, 60s ea	66336-0732-60	38.49		AB
90s ea	66336-0732-90	57.74		
(Phys Total Care)				
REPACK				
CER, PO, 100 mg, 60s ea	54868-5534-03	56.53		AB
(Physician Partner)				
REPACK				
CER, PO, 100 mg, 30s ea	21695-0167-30	20.34		
90s ea	21695-0167-90	61.02		
120s ea	21695-0167-72	95.72		AB
EXTENDRYL (Auriga)				
cpm/methscopolamine nitrate/phenyleph hcl				
CTB, PO (ROOT BEER)				
2 mg-1.25 mg-10 mg,				
100s ea	14629-0103-01	58.59		
(Auriga)				
cough/cold combination				
SYR, PO, 473 ml	14629-0114-16	64.38		
EXTENDRYL DM (Auriga)				
cpm/dm/methscopolamine nitrate				
TER, PO, 8 mg-30 mg-2.5 mg,				
100s ea	14629-0202-01	111.18		
EXTENDRYL G (Auriga)				
guaifenesin/phenylephrine hydrochloride				
TER, PO (DYE-FREE,CAPLET)				
1000 mg-30 mg,				
100s ea	14629-0204-01	101.06		
EXTENDRYL GCP (Auriga)				
carbetapentane cit/gg/phenyleph hcl				
SOL, PO (1X473ML,AF,STRAWBERRY)				
473 ml	14629-0105-16	112.21		
EXTENDRYL JR (Auriga)				
cpm/methscopolamine nitrate/phenyleph hcl				
TER, PO, 4 mg-1.25 mg-10 mg,				
100s ea	14629-0102-01	62.54		
EXTENDRYL PEM (Auriga)				
methscopolamine nitrate/phenyleph hcl				
TER, PO, 1.25 mg-30 mg,				
100s ea	14629-0205-01	157.81		
EXTENDRYL PSE (Auriga)				
methscopolamine nitrate/pse hcl				
TER, PO, 2.5 mg-120 mg,				
100s ea	14629-0201-01	111.18		
EXTENDRYL SR (Auriga)				
cpm/methscopolamine nitrate/phenyleph hcl				
TER, PO, 8 mg-2.5 mg-20 mg,				
100s ea	14629-0101-01	73.60		
(Dispensing Solutions)				
REPACK				
CER, PO, 8 mg-2.5 mg-20 mg,				
20s ea	55045-2601-07	10.85		
TER, PO, 8 mg-2.5 mg-20 mg,				
20s ea	55045-3468-07	14.00		
(Phys Total Care)				
REPACK				
CER, PO, 8 mg-2.5 mg-20 mg,				
30s ea	54868-0524-02	27.51		
EXTINA (Stiefel Labs)				
ketoconazole				
FOA, TP, 2%, 50 gm	63032-0051-50	184.55		
100 gm	63032-0051-00	343.80		
EXTRANEAL (Baxter)				
ca cl/icodextrin/mg cl/na cl/na lact				
SOL, PT (6X2000ML,AMBU-FLEX III)				
2000 ml 6s	00941-0679-47	544.63	453.86	
(6X2000ML,ULTRABAG)				
2000 ml 6s	00941-0679-52	665.66	554.72	
(5X2500ML,AMBU-FLEX III)				
2500 ml 5s	00941-0679-48	579.94	483.28	
(5X2500ML,ULTRABAG)				
2500 ml 5s	00941-0679-53	693.40	577.83	
EYE WASH (Physician Partner)				
REPACK				
boric acid/sodium borate/sodium chloride				
SOL, OP, 120 ml	21695-0311-04	17.50		
EZETIMIBE				
(Merck/Schering-Plough) *See ZETIA*				
(Palmetto)				
REPACK				
TAB, PO, 10 mg, 30s ea	23490-7645-01	92.22		
EZETIMIBE/SIMVASTATIN				
(Merck/Schering-Plough) *See VYTORIN*				
EZFE 200 (McNeil,R.A.)				
iron				
CAP, PO, 200 mg, 100s ea	12830-0824-01	31.45		
F D & C BLUE #1 (Amend)				
color additive				
POW, NA, 454 gm	17317-0847-01	154.00		
(Gallipot)				
POW, NA (ALUM LAKE)				
25 gm	51552-0651-04	17.64		
(C.I. ERIOGLAUCINE)				
25 gm	51552-0108-04	16.80		
454 gm	51552-0108-06	94.92		
(PCCA)				
POW, NA, 1 gm	51927-1542-00	2.28		
F D & C BLUE #2 (Amend)				
color additive				
POW, NA, 454 gm	17317-0849-01	175.00		
(Gallipot)				
POW, NA (C.I. 73015)				
25 gm	51552-0247-04	16.80		
454 gm	51552-0247-06	113.05		
(PCCA)				
POW, NA (INDIGO CARMINE)				
1 gm	51927-2388-00	2.28		
F D & C GREEN #3 (Amend)				
color additive				
POW, NA, 454 gm	61972-0850-01	231.00		
(Gallipot)				
POW, NA (C.I. 42053 FAST GRN FCF)				
25 gm	51552-0109-04	20.16		
(C.I. FAST GREEN)				
454 gm	51552-0109-06	249.20		
(PCCA)				
POW, NA, 1 gm	51927-1836-00	2.76		
F D & C RED #3 (Amend)				
color additive				
POW, NA, 454 gm	17317-0851-01	154.00		
(Gallipot)				
POW, NA (C.I. 4543)				
25 gm	51552-0341-04	16.80		
(C.I. 45430)				
454 gm	51552-0341-06	111.30		
F D & C RED #40 (Amend)				
color additive				
POW, NA, 454 gm	17317-0853-01	154.00		
(Gallipot)				
POW, NA (ALUM LAKE)				
25 gm	51552-0577-04	16.80		
(C.I. 16035)				
25 gm	51552-0248-04	11.34		
454 gm	51552-0248-06	62.72		
(PCCA)				
POW, NA, 1 gm	51927-2415-00	1.80		

PROD/MFR	NDC	AWP	DP	OBC
F D & C YELLOW #5 (Amend)				
color additive				
POW, NA, 454 gm	17317-0855-01	154.00		
(Gallipot)				
POW, NA (C.I. 19140)				
25 gm	51552-0249-04	11.20		
454 gm	51552-0249-06	48.72		
(PCCA)				
POW, NA (TARTRAZINE)				
1 gm	51927-1350-00	1.44		
F D & C YELLOW #6 (Amend)				
color additive				
POW, NA, 454 gm	17317-0857-01	154.00		
(Gallipot)				
POW, NA (C.I. 15985)				
25 gm	51552-0322-04	11.06		
454 gm	51552-0322-06	48.72		
(PCCA)				
POW, NA, 1 gm	51927-2422-00	0.75		
FABB (Midlothian Labs)				
cyanocobalamin/folic acid/pyridoxine				
TAB, PO (FILM-COATED)				
1 mg-2.2 mg-25 mg, 100s ea	68308-0326-10	57.05		
FABRAZYME (Genzyme)				
agalsidase beta				
PDS, IV (PF)				
5 mg, ea	58468-0041-01	771.60	643.00	
35 mg, ea	58468-0040-01	5403.60	4503.00	
FACTIVE (Cornerstone)				
gemifloxacin mesylate				
TAB, PO (BLISTER PACK)				
320 mg, 5s ea	67707-0320-05	148.31	118.65	
7s ea	67707-0320-07	207.64	166.11	
FACTOR IX COMPLEX HUMAN				
(Baxter Bioscience) *See BEBULIN VH*				
(Grifols USA, Inc.) *See PROFILNINE SD*				
FACTOR IX HUMAN, PURIFIED				
(CSL) *See MONONINE*				
(Grifols USA, Inc.) *See ALPHANINE SD*				
FAMCICLOVIR				
(Novartis Pharm) *See FAMVIR*				
(Teva)				
TAB, PO (FILM-COATED)				
125 mg, 30s ea	00093-8117-56	139.30		AB
250 mg, 30s ea	00093-8118-56	151.45		AB
500 mg, 30s ea	00093-8119-56	304.15		AB
(A-S Medication)				
REPACK				
TAB, PO (FILM-COATED)				
500 mg, 30s ea	54569-6046-00	304.15		AB
(PD-Rx Pharm)				
REPACK				
TAB, PO (FILM-COATED)				
500 mg, 3s ea	55289-0168-03	47.25		AB
(Pharma Pac)				
REPACK				
TAB, PO (FILM-COATED)				
500 mg, 4s ea	52959-0946-04	35.69		AB
21s ea	52959-0946-21	261.26		AB
(Phys Total Care)				
REPACK				
TAB, PO (FILM-COATED)				
500 mg, 10s ea	54868-5905-03	252.55		AB
20s ea	54868-5905-00	470.21		AB
21s ea	54868-5905-01	495.00		AB
FAMOTIDINE				
FUL				
TAB, PO, 20 mg, 100s ea		15.00		
40 mg, 100s ea		30.00		
(APP)				
SOL, IV (S.D.V.,25X2ML)				
10 mg/ml, 2 ml 25s	63323-0739-12	102.50		AP
(M.D.V.,CONCENTRATED)				
10 mg/ml, 4 ml	63323-0738-04	8.20		AP
((M.D.V.),10X20ML)				
10 mg/ml, 20 ml 10s	63323-0738-20	413.00		AP
(Baxter)				
SOL, IV (GALAXY PC,PF)				
0.4 mg/ml, 50 ml	00338-5197-41	6.54	5.45	AP
(SDV,PF)				
10 mg/ml, 2 ml	10019-0045-17	0.71		AP
(S.D.V.,PF)				
10 mg/ml, 2 ml 25s	10019-0045-02	17.70	75.00	AP
(MDV)				
10 mg/ml, 4 ml	10019-0046-14	1.97		AP
(M.D.V.)				
10 mg/ml, 4 ml 25s	10019-0046-04	49.20	150.00	AP
(MDV)				
10 mg/ml, 20 ml	10019-0046-63	5.52		AP
(M.D.V.)				
10 mg/ml, 20 ml 10s	10019-0046-03	55.20	300.00	AP
(Bedford)				
SOL, IV (S.D.V.,PF)				
10 mg/ml, 2 ml 10s	55390-0029-10	14.30		AP
(TWO DOSE VIAL,PF)				
10 mg/ml, 4 ml 10s	55390-0028-10	28.48		AP
(M.D.V.,PF)				
10 mg/ml, 20 ml	55390-0027-01	14.28		AP
(PHARMACY BULK VIAL)				
10 mg/ml, 50 ml	55390-0026-01	35.70		AP
(Carlsbad Tech)				
TAB, PO (USP)				
20 mg, 100s ea	61442-0121-01	173.00		
1000s ea	61442-0121-10	1730.00		
40 mg, 100s ea	61442-0122-01	334.40		
1000s ea	61442-0122-10	3349.00		
(Dr Reddy's)				
TAB, PO (FILM-COATED)				
20 mg, 30s ea	55111-0119-30	52.05		AB
100s ea	55111-0119-01	173.50		AB
1000s ea	55111-0119-10	1734.00		AB
40 mg, 30s ea	55111-0120-30	100.50		AB
100s ea	55111-0120-01	335.00		AB
1000s ea	55111-0120-10	3350.00		AB
(Hawkins)				
POW, NA (USP)				
25 gm	63370-0091-25	80.00		
100 gm	63370-0091-35	300.00		
500 gm	63370-0091-45	1400.00		
(Major)				
TAB, PO (FILM-COATED)				
20 mg, 100s ea UD	00904-5553-61	191.32		AB
(10X10,FILM-COATED)				
40 mg, 100s ea UD	00904-5554-61	497.80		AB
(Medisca)				
POW, NA (U.S.P.)				
25 gm	38779-0655-04	76.50		
100 gm	38779-0655-05	268.50		
500 gm	38779-0655-08	1215.00		
(Merck) *See PEPCID*				
(Mylan)				
TAB, PO, 20 mg, 100s ea	00378-3020-01	173.90		AB
500s ea	00378-3020-05	869.50		AB
40 mg, 100s ea	00378-3040-01	336.10		AB
(Northstar)				
TAB, PO (FILM-COATED)				
20 mg, 30s ea	16714-0361-01	52.20		AB
100s ea	16714-0361-04	173.50		AB
500s ea	16714-0361-05	867.25		AB
1000s ea	16714-0361-06	1734.00		AB
40 mg, 30s ea	16714-0362-01	100.89		AB
100s ea	16714-0362-04	355.55		AB
500s ea	16714-0362-05	1672.00		AB
1000s ea	16714-0362-06	3356.00		AB
(PCCA)				
POW, NA (U.S.P.)				
1 gm	51927-3408-00	3.48		
(Salix Pharm) *See PEPCID*				
(Spectrum Pharmacy)				
POW, NA (U.S.P.)				
25 gm	49452-3038-03	117.60		
100 gm	49452-3038-04	406.00		
500 gm	49452-3038-05	1683.50		
(Teva)				
TAB, PO (BLISTER PACK,10X10)				
20 mg, 100s ea UD	00172-5728-10	173.00		AB
(FILM COATED)				
20 mg, 100s ea	00172-5728-60	173.00		AB
500s ea	00172-5728-70	865.00		AB
(FILM-COATED)				
20 mg, 1000s ea	00172-5728-80	1730.00		AB
(BLISTER PACK,10X10)				
40 mg, 100s ea UD	00172-5729-10	334.40		AB
(FILM COATED)				
40 mg, 100s ea	00172-5729-60	334.40		AB
500s ea	00172-5729-70	1672.00		AB
(UDL)				
TAB, PO (ROBOT READY,25X1)				
20 mg, 25s ea UD	51079-0966-19	43.47		AB
(10X10)				
20 mg, 100s ea UD	51079-0966-20	173.90		AB
(Watson)				
TAB, PO, 20 mg, 100s ea	62037-0955-01	8.62		AB
1000s ea	62037-0955-10	78.55		AB
40 mg, 100s ea	62037-0956-01	15.55		AB
1000s ea	62037-0956-10	147.76		AB
(Wockhardt USA)				
TAB, PO (FILM-COATED)				
20 mg, 30s ea	64679-0936-01	52.20		AB
100s ea	64679-0936-02	173.99		AB
1000s ea	64679-0936-03	1739.99		AB
40 mg, 30s ea	64679-0937-01	100.89		AB
100s ea	64679-0937-02	336.30		AB
1000s ea	64679-0937-03	3362.99		AB
(A-S Medication)				
REPACK				
TAB, PO, 20 mg, 30s ea	54569-5942-00	52.20		
(Altura)				
REPACK				
TAB, PO, 20 mg, 10s ea	63874-0526-10	17.00		AB
20s ea	63874-0526-20	34.00		AB
30s ea	63874-0526-30	51.00		AB
60s ea	63874-0526-60	102.00		AB
92s ea	63874-0526-92	153.00		AB
100s ea	63874-0526-01	170.00		AB
(American Health)				
REPACK				
TAB, PO (10X10,FILM-COATED)				
20 mg, 100s ea UD	68084-0172-01	17.40		AB
(10X10)				
20 mg, 100s ea UD	68084-0171-01	17.40		
(Bryant Ranch)				
REPACK				
TAB, PO, 20 mg, 20s ea	63629-2904-03	34.99		
30s ea	63629-2904-01	50.99		
60s ea	63629-2904-02	99.89		
40 mg, 30s ea	63629-2782-01	141.25		
60s ea	63629-2782-02	282.49		
100s ea	63629-2782-03	470.82		
(Core)				
REPACK				
TAB, PO, 20 mg, 20s ea	33358-0140-20	35.86		
30s ea	33358-0140-30	52.26		
60s ea	33358-0140-60	102.39		
40 mg, 30s ea	33358-0141-30	144.78		
60s ea	33358-0141-60	289.55		
(DHS, Inc.)				
REPACK				
TAB, PO, 20 mg, 10s ea	55887-0428-10	16.94		
(FILM-COATED)				
20 mg, 30s ea	55887-0428-30	50.84		AB
60s ea	55887-0428-60	100.04		AB
40 mg, 15s ea	55887-0152-15	26.10		
30s ea	55887-0152-30	52.20		
60s ea	55887-0152-60	104.40		
90s ea	55887-0152-90	156.60		
(Dispensing Solutions)				
REPACK				
TAB, PO, 10 mg, 18s ea	55045-3183-08	5.94		
20 mg, 10s ea	55045-3072-01	16.70		
20s ea	66336-0355-20	37.10		
(FILM-COATED)				
20 mg, 30s ea	55045-3072-08	50.10		AB
40s ea	55045-3072-04	66.80		AB
60s ea	66336-0355-60	104.10		AB
(FILM-COATED)				
20 mg, 60s ea	55045-3072-06	100.20		AB
90s ea	55045-3072-09	150.30		
(FILM-COATED)				
40 mg, 30s ea	55045-3073-08	98.75		AB
(GSMS)				
REPACK				
TAB, PO (UNIT OF USE)				
20 mg, 60s ea	60429-0720-60	36.60	12.20	EE
(HomeMed)				
REPACK				
TAB, PO, 20 mg, 30s ea	51655-0288-24	50.99		
(McKesson Packaging)				
REPACK				
TAB, PO (USP)				
20 mg, 100s ea UD	63739-0325-10	212.50		
(Nucare Pharm)				
REPACK				
TAB, PO, 20 mg, 20s ea	66267-0543-20	49.99		EE
(Palmetto)				
REPACK				
TAB, PO, 20 mg, 20s ea	23490-5559-01	50.00		
60s ea	23490-5559-06	150.00		

PROD/MFR	NDC	AWP	DP	OBC
FAMOTIDINE (Palmetto)				
40 mg, 60s ea	**23490-5560-06**	261.30		
FAMOTIDINE (PD-Rx Pharm)				
REPACK				
TAB, PO (FILM COATED)				
20 mg, 6s ea	**43063-0086-06**	7.42		AB
30s ea	**55289-0765-30**	48.70		AB
(USP)				
20 mg, 30s ea	**58864-0955-30**	48.69		
(Pharma Pac)				
REPACK				
TAB, PO, 20 mg, 20s ea	**52959-0758-20**	40.30		AB
30s ea	**52959-0758-30**	60.45		
40s ea	**52959-0758-40**	80.59		
60s ea	**52959-0758-60**	120.87		
100s ea	**52959-0758-00**	202.59		AB
40 mg, 30s ea	**52959-0116-30**	82.48		AB
60s ea	**52959-0116-60**	164.94		
(Phys Total Care)				
REPACK				
TAB, PO, 20 mg, 30s ea	**54868-4563-00**	9.84		EE
60s ea	**54868-4563-02**	14.08		EE
(FILM-COATED)				
20 mg, 100s ea	**54868-4563-01**	24.35		AB
40 mg, 30s ea	**54868-4567-00**	21.45		EE
60s ea	**54868-4567-01**	41.40		EE
100s ea	**54868-4567-02**	44.54		EE
(Physician Partner)				
REPACK				
TAB, PO, 20 mg, 30s ea	**21695-0297-30**	104.40		
60s ea	**21695-0297-60**	208.80		
40 mg, 30s ea	**21695-0582-30**	201.77		
60s ea	**21695-0582-60**	403.55		
(Quality Care Prod)				
REPACK				
TAB, PO, 20 mg, 30s ea	**49999-0237-30**	134.52		
90s ea	**49999-0238-90**	188.10		
40 mg, 30s ea	**49999-0230-30**	69.60		
(Southwood)				
REPACK				
TAB, PO, 20 mg, 30s ea	**58016-0635-30**	51.00		EE
60s ea	**58016-0635-60**	102.00		EE
92s ea	**58016-0635-90**	153.00		EE
100s ea	**58016-0635-00**	170.00		EE
40 mg, 30s ea	**58016-0751-30**	78.78		
60s ea	**58016-0751-60**	157.56		
90s ea	**58016-0751-90**	236.34		
100s ea	**58016-0751-00**	262.60		
120s ea	**58016-0751-02**	315.12		
150s ea	**58016-0751-03**	393.90		
200s ea	**58016-0751-89**	525.20		
300s ea	**58016-0751-73**	787.80		
(Stat Rx)				
REPACK				
TAB, PO (FILM-COATED)				
20 mg, 20s ea	**16590-0281-20**	34.80		AB
28s ea	**16590-0281-28**	48.55		AB
30s ea	**16590-0281-30**	52.20		AB
60s ea	**16590-0281-60**	104.40		AB
90s ea	**16590-0281-90**	156.60		AB
(Vibranta)				
REPACK				
TAB, PO, 20 mg, 60s ea	**57866-7371-01**	105.00		
FAMVIR (Novartis Pharm)				
famciclovir				
TAB, PO (FILM COATED)				
125 mg, 30s ea	**00078-0366-15**	193.82		
250 mg, 30s ea	**00078-0367-15**	210.72		
500 mg, 30s ea	**00078-0368-15**	423.19		
(Phys Total Care)				
REPACK				
TAB, PO, 125 mg, 10s ea	**54868-3882-01**	49.18		
15s ea	**54868-3882-00**	72.81		
250 mg, 10s ea	**54868-3969-01**	61.15		
20s ea	**54868-3969-00**	119.79		
(FILM COATED)				
500 mg, 10s ea	**54868-4009-01**	140.21		
20s ea	**54868-4009-00**	278.47		
(Quality Care Prod)				
REPACK				
TAB, PO (FILM COATED)				
500 mg, 21s ea	**49999-0308-21**	329.63		
30s ea	**49999-0308-30**	470.99		
(Southwood)				
REPACK				
TAB, PO, 250 mg, 30s ea	**58016-0350-30**	168.28		
60s ea	**58016-0350-60**	336.56		
90s ea	**58016-0350-90**	504.84		
100s ea	**58016-0350-00**	560.93		
FANAPT (Novartis Pharm)				
iloperidone				
TAB, PO (UNCOATED)				
1 mg, 60s ea	**43068-0101-02**	630.00		EE
2 mg, 60s ea	**43068-0102-02**	630.00		EE
4 mg, 60s ea	**43068-0104-02**	630.00		EE
6 mg, 60s ea	**43068-0106-02**	630.00		EE
8 mg, 60s ea	**43068-0108-02**	630.00		EE
10 mg, 60s ea	**43068-0110-02**	630.00		EE
12 mg, 60s ea	**43068-0112-02**	630.00		
FANAPT TITRATION PACK (Novartis Pharm)				
iloperidone				
TAB, PO (UNCOATED)				
8s ea	**43068-0113-04**	84.00		
FARESTON (GTX)				
toremifene citrate				
TAB, PO, 60 mg, 30s ea	**11399-0005-30**	540.00		
FASLODEX (AstraZeneca)				
fulvestrant				
SOL, IM (SRN,PREFILL,SAFETYGUIDE)				
50 mg/ml, 5 ml	**00310-0720-50**	972.94		
FAT EMULSION IV (Abbott Hosp)				
tubing, fluid delivery				
DEV, NA (LTXF,CNVT PIN,80" W/INJ)				
48s ea	**00074-4065-68**	297.79	297.60	
(72 IN MICROBORE -SL)				
50s ea	**00074-6464-01**	169.80	170.00	
FATTY ACID BASE (Gallipot)				
ointment base				
OIN, NA (GRATED)				
2270 gm	**51552-0007-07**	71.40		
FAZACLO (Azur Pharma, Inc.)				
clozapine				
ODT, PO (MINT)				
12.5 mg, 100s ea	**18860-0101-10**	178.58		
25 mg, 100s ea	**18860-0102-10**	218.63		
100 mg, 100s ea	**18860-0104-10**	596.29		
FD&C BLUE #1 (Spectrum Pharmacy)				
color additive				
POW, NA (1X100GM)				
100 gm	**49452-3045-01**	191.10		
(1X500GM)				
500 gm	**49452-3045-02**	532.00		
FD&C BLUE NO. 2 (Medisca)				
color additive				
POW, NA (1X25GM,INDIGO CARMINE)				
25 gm	**38779-1276-04**	55.50		
(1X100GM,INDIGO CARMINE)				
100 gm	**38779-1276-05**	111.00		
(1X500GM,INDIGO CARMINE)				
500 gm	**38779-1276-08**	297.00		
FD&C GREEN NO. 3 (Medisca)				
color additive				
POW, NA (1X5GM)				
5 gm	**38779-1277-03**	22.50		
(1X25GM)				
25 gm	**38779-1277-04**	76.50		
(1X100GM)				
100 gm	**38779-1277-05**	165.00		
(1X500GM)				
500 gm	**38779-1277-08**	535.50		
FD&C RED NO. 3 (Medisca)				
POW, NA (1X25GM)				
25 gm	**38779-1278-04**	52.50		
(1X100GM)				
100 gm	**38779-1278-05**	99.00		
(1X500GM)				
500 gm	**38779-1278-08**	240.00		
(PCCA)				
POW, NA, 1 gm	**51927-1835-00**	2.40		
FD&C RED NO. 40 (Medisca)				
color additive				
POW, NA (1X25GM)				
25 gm	**38779-1279-04**	34.50		
(1X100GM)				
100 gm	**38779-1279-05**	178.50		
FD&C YELLOW NO. 6 (Medisca)				
color additive				
POW, NA (1X100GM,SUNSET YELLOW)				
100 gm	**38779-1281-05**	43.50		
(1X500GM,SUNSET YELLOW)				
500 gm	**38779-1281-08**	120.00		
FE C TAB PLUS (Boca Pharmacal)				
fe pentacarbonyl/folic acid/vit b12/vit c				
TAB, PO, 100s ea	**64376-0802-01**	30.81		
FE PENTACARBONYL/FOLIC ACID/VIT B12/VIT C				
(Boca Pharmacal) *See FE C TAB PLUS*				
(Hawthorn Pharm) *See ICAR-C PLUS*				
FE/FOLIC ACID/PYRIDOXINE HCL/VIT B12/ VIT C/ZINC				
(Vertical) *See CORVITE 150*				
FE/FOLIC ACID/SUCCINIC ACID/VIT B12/VIT C				
(Ther-RX) *See NIFEREX-150 FORTE*				
(Ther-RX) *See REPLIVA 21/7*				
FE/NA FLUORIDE/VIT A/VIT C/VIT D				
(Hi-Tech) *See TRI-VITAMIN W/FLUORIDE & IRON*				
(NextWave) *See MYKIDZ IRON FL*				
(Qualitest) *See TRI-VIT WITH FLUORIDE AND IRON*				
FEBUXOSTAT				
(Takeda) *See ULORIC*				
FEIBA-VH IMMUNO (Baxter Bioscience)				
anti-inhibitor coagulant complex				
PDS, IV (1750-3250IU)				
1 iu, ea	**64193-0222-05**	2.12		
(400-650IU)				
1 iu, ea	**64193-0222-03**	2.12		
(651-1200IU)				
1 iu, ea	**64193-0222-04**	2.12		
FELBAMATE				
(Meda) *See FELBATOL*				
FELBATOL (Meda)				
felbamate				
SUS, PO, 600 mg/5 ml,				
237 ml	**00037-0442-67**	326.25		
960 ml	**00037-0442-17**	1258.02		
TAB, PO (CAPLET)				
400 mg, 100s ea	**00037-0430-01**	265.47		
600 mg, 100s ea	**00037-0431-01**	304.23		
FELDENE (Pfizer)				
piroxicam				
CAP, PO, 10 mg, 100s ea	**00069-3220-66**	282.44	235.37	AB
20 mg, 100s ea	**00069-3230-66**	483.36	402.80	AB
(PD-Rx Pharm)				
REPACK				
CAP, PO, 20 mg, 7s ea	**55289-0471-07**	49.55		AB
10s ea	**55289-0471-10**	68.65		AB
14s ea	**55289-0471-14**	94.10		AB
30s ea	**55289-0471-30**	144.50		AB
(Pharma Pac)				
REPACK				
CAP, PO, 20 mg, 7s ea	**52959-0066-07**	27.40		AB
10s ea	**52959-0066-10**	39.80		AB
18s ea	**52959-0066-18**	59.15		AB
20s ea	**52959-0066-20**	64.30		AB
30s ea	**52959-0066-30**	85.93		AB
100s ea	**52959-0066-00**	259.95		AB
(Phys Total Care)				
REPACK				
CAP, PO, 20 mg, 10s ea	**54868-0474-01**	43.80		AB
FELODIPINE (Mutual)				
TER, PO (FILM-COATED)				
2.5 mg, 100s ea	**53489-0368-01**	151.09		AB
5 mg, 100s ea	**53489-0369-01**	151.09		AB
10 mg, 100s ea	**53489-0370-01**	271.52		AB
(Mylan)				
TER, PO (USP,FILM-COATED)				
2.5 mg, 100s ea	**00378-5011-01**	151.09		
500s ea	**00378-5011-05**	755.45		
5 mg, 100s ea	**00378-5012-01**	151.09		
500s ea	**00378-5012-05**	755.45		
10 mg, 100s ea	**00378-5013-01**	271.52		
500s ea	**00378-5013-05**	1357.60		
(Ranbaxy Pharm)				
TER, PO, 2.5 mg, 100s ea	**63304-0435-01**	158.01		
5 mg, 100s ea	**63304-0436-01**	158.01		
10 mg, 100s ea	**63304-0437-01**	283.96		
(UDL)				
TER, PO (10X10,USP,FILM-COATED)				
5 mg, 100s ea UD	**51079-0467-20**	151.09		AB
10 mg, 100s ea UD	**51079-0468-20**	271.52		AB
(A-S Medication)				
REPACK				
TER, PO, 10 mg, 30s ea	**54569-6117-00**	85.19		
(PD-Rx Pharm)				
REPACK				
TER, PO (REDI-SCRIPT)				
5 mg, 30s ea	**58864-0810-30**	58.43		
(USP,FILM-COATED)				
5 mg, 30s ea	**55289-0306-30**	43.67		AB
(REDI-SCRIPT)				
5 mg, 90s ea	**58864-0810-90**	165.30		
(Phys Total Care)				
REPACK				
TER, PO, 5 mg, 10s ea	**54868-5197-01**	43.86		
30s ea	**54868-5197-00**	94.80		
90s ea	**54868-5197-02**	275.43		
(FILM-COATED)				
10 mg, 10s ea	**54868-0826-01**	87.34		AB
30s ea	**54868-0826-00**	194.54		AB
90s ea	**54868-0826-02**	542.94		

PROD/MFR	NDC	AWP	DP	OBC
(Quality Care Prod)				
REPACK				
TER, PO, 5 mg, 10s ea	49999-0821-10	13.59		
(FILM-COATED)				
10 mg, 10s ea	49999-0572-10	23.21		AB
FELODIPINE ER (Phys Total Care)				
REPACK				
felodipine				
TER, PO, 2.5 mg, 30s ea	54868-0823-00	119.37		
FEM PH (Pharmics)				
acetic acid glacial/oxyquinoline sulfate				
GEL, VG, 0.9%-0.025%,				
50 gm	00813-0799-55	27.56		
FEMARA (Novartis Pharm)				
letrozole				
TAB, PO (FILM-COATED)				
2.5 mg, 30s ea	00078-0249-15	473.06		
(A-S Medication)				
REPACK				
TAB, PO (FILM-COATED)				
2.5 mg, 30s ea	54569-5714-00	559.59		
(Phys Total Care)				
REPACK				
TAB, PO (FILM-COATED)				
2.5 mg, 30s ea	54868-4151-00	543.88		
(Quality Care Prod)				
REPACK				
TAB, PO (FILM-COATED)				
2.5 mg, 30s ea	35356-0409-30	716.70		
FEMCON FE (Warner Chilcott)				
ethinyl estradiol/ferrous fumarate/norethindrone				
KIT, PO (5X28,SPEARMINT)				
35 mcg-0.4 mg,				
140s ea	00430-0482-14	370.68		
FEMHRT 1/5 (Warner Chilcott)				
ethinyl estradiol/norethindrone acetate				
TAB, PO, 5 mcg-1 mg,				
90s ea	00430-0544-23	213.63		
(DAY DISPENSER, 5X28)				
5 mcg-1 mg,				
140s ea	00430-0544-14	332.33		
(Phys Total Care)				
REPACK				
TAB, PO, 5 mcg-1 mg,				
28s ea	54868-4679-00	50.89		
(Quality Care Prod)				
REPACK				
TAB, PO, 5 mcg-1 mg,				
90s ea	35356-0404-90	238.48		
FEMHRT LO (Warner Chilcott)				
ethinyl estradiol/norethindrone acetate				
TAB, PO, 2.5 mcg-0.5 mg,				
90s ea	00430-0145-23	213.63		
(5X28)				
2.5 mcg-0.5 mg,				
140s ea	00430-0145-14	332.33		
FEMRING (Warner Chilcott)				
estradiol acetate				
ICR, VG (RING)				
0.05 mg/24 hr, ea	00430-6201-40	195.89		
0.1 mg/24 hr, ea	00430-6202-40	208.73		
(Phys Total Care)				
REPACK				
ICR, VG (RING)				
0.1 mg/24 hr, ea	54868-6030-00	239.16		
FEMTABS (Azur Pharma, Inc.)				
multivitamin and minerals				
TAB, PO (CAPLET)				
90s ea	66663-0517-01	59.40		
FEMTRACE (Warner Chilcott)				
estradiol acetate				
TAB, PO, 0.45 mg,				
100s ea	00430-0389-24	200.68		
0.9 mg, 100s ea	00430-0390-24	200.68		
1.8 mg, 100s ea	00430-0391-24	257.65		
FENBENDAZOLE (Medisca)				
POW, NA (1X500GM,VET USE ONLY)				
500 gm	38779-1979-08	337.50		
FENNEL OIL (Lorann Oil)				
OIL, NA, 9.9 ml	23535-0151-18	3.50		
(PCCA)				
OIL, NA (F.C.C.)				
1 ml	51927-3019-00	1.17		
(Spectrum Pharmacy)				
OIL, NA (F.C.C.)				
100 ml	49452-3037-01	183.05		
500 ml	49452-3037-02	458.50		
FENOFIBRATE				
(Abbott Pharm) *See TRICOR*				
(Gate) *See LOFIBRA*				
(Global Pharm)				
TAB, PO (FILM-COATED)				
54 mg, 90s ea	00115-5511-10	71.29		AB
160 mg, 90s ea	00115-5522-10	213.88		AB
(Kowa) *See LIPOFEN*				
(Mylan)				
TAB, PO (FILM-COATED)				
54 mg, 90s ea	00378-7100-77	71.29		AB
160 mg, 90s ea	00378-7101-77	213.88		AB
(Ranbaxy Pharm)				
TAB, PO (FILM COATED)				
54 mg, 90s ea	63304-0900-90	71.29		AB
160 mg, 90s ea	63304-0901-90	213.88		AB
(Shionogi) *See FENOGLIDE*				
(Shionogi) *See TRIGLIDE*				
(American Health)				
REPACK				
TAB, PO (3X10,FILM-COATED)				
160 mg, 30s ea UD	68084-0328-21	213.88		AB
(Phys Total Care)				
REPACK				
TAB, PO, 54 mg, 90s ea	54868-5697-00	186.15		
160 mg, 30s ea	54868-5660-00	185.10		
90s ea	54868-5660-01	514.71		
FENOFIBRATE MICRONIZED (Global Pharm)				
fenofibrate, micronized				
CAP, PO, 67 mg, 100s ea	00115-0511-01	93.26		AB
134 mg, 100s ea	00115-0522-01	171.70		AB
200 mg, 100s ea	00115-0533-01	266.58		AB
(American Health)				
REPACK				
CAP, PO (3X10)				
200 mg, 30s ea	68084-0329-21	242.51		AB
(Phys Total Care)				
REPACK				
CAP, PO, 134 mg, 10s ea	54868-5994-00	59.73		AB
30s ea	54868-5994-01	129.27		AB
200 mg, 10s ea	54868-5575-01	69.18		
30s ea	54868-5575-00	190.11		
90s ea	54868-5575-02	574.59		
FENOFIBRATE, MICRONIZED				
(Gate) *See LOFIBRA*				
(Global Pharm) *See FENOFIBRATE MICRONIZED*				
(Lupin Pharma, Inc.) *See ANTARA*				
FENOFIBRIC ACID				
(Abbott Pharm) *See TRILIPIX*				
(AR Scientific) *See FIBRICOR*				
(Mutual)				
TAB, PO, 35 mg, 30s ea	53489-0677-07	30.03		
105 mg, 30s ea	53489-0678-07	90.10		
90s ea	53489-0678-90	270.29		
FENOGLIDE (Shionogi)				
fenofibrate				
TAB, PO, 40 mg, 90s ea	59630-0490-90	155.11		
120 mg, 90s ea	59630-0495-90	465.31		
FENOLDOPAM MESYLATE (Bedford)				
SOL, IV (S.D.V.)				
10 mg/ml, 1 ml	55390-0071-01	96.00		AP
2 ml	55390-0072-01	192.00		AP
(Hospira) *See CORLOPAM*				
(Sandoz)				
SOL, IV, 10 mg/ml, 1 ml	00781-3005-71	213.75		
2 ml	00781-3005-92	411.47		
FENOPROFEN CALCIUM (Mylan)				
TAB, PO, 600 mg, 100s ea	00378-0471-01	69.71		AB
(PCCA)				
POW, NA (USP)				
1 gm	51927-1853-00	1.59		
(Pedinol) *See NALFON*				
(A-S Medication)				
REPACK				
TAB, PO, 600 mg, 20s ea	54569-2105-01	13.94		AB
(Altura)				
REPACK				
TAB, PO, 600 mg, 20s ea	63874-0416-20	15.76		EE
28s ea	63874-0416-28	18.53		EE
30s ea	63874-0416-30	21.28		EE
100s ea	63874-0416-01	70.66		EE
500s ea	63874-0416-50	286.66		EE
(Dispensing Solutions)				
REPACK				
TAB, PO, 600 mg, 30s ea	55045-1571-08	19.00		AB
(PD-Rx Pharm)				
REPACK				
TAB, PO, 600 mg, 20s ea	55289-0334-20	16.04		AB
30s ea	55289-0334-30	28.38		AB
(Pharma Pac)				
REPACK				
TAB, PO, 600 mg, 20s ea	52959-0067-20	14.20		EE
30s ea	52959-0067-30	19.15		EE
(Phys Total Care)				
REPACK				
TAB, PO, 600 mg, 60s ea	54868-0775-03	64.05		EE
(Quality Care Prod)				
REPACK				
TAB, PO, 600 mg, 30s ea	35356-0332-30	41.60		AB
(Southwood)				
REPACK				
TAB, PO, 600 mg, 6s ea	58016-0244-06	5.13		EE
20s ea	58016-0244-20	14.04		EE
21s ea	58016-0244-21	14.63		EE
30s ea	58016-0244-30	19.11		EE
60s ea	58016-0244-60	25.49		EE
FENTANYL				
(Actavis) *See FENTANYL TRANSDERMAL SYSTEM*				
(Mylan)				
TDM, TD, 12.5 mcg/hr,				
5s ea, C-II	00378-9119-98	69.00		AB
25 mcg/hr,				
5s ea, C-II	00378-9121-98	72.10		
50 mcg/hr,				
5s ea, C-II	00378-9122-98	131.80		
75 mcg/hr,				
5s ea, C-II	00378-9123-98	201.05		
100 mcg/hr,				
5s ea, C-II	00378-9124-98	266.80		
(PriCara) *See DURAGESIC*				
(Sandoz) *See FENTANYL TRANSDERMAL SYSTEM*				
(Sandoz)				
TDM, TD, 25 mcg/hr,				
5s ea, C-II	00781-7111-55	72.17		
50 mcg/hr,				
5s ea, C-II	00781-7112-55	131.92		
75 mcg/hr,				
5s ea, C-II	00781-7113-55	201.23		
100 mcg/hr,				
5s ea, C-II	00781-7114-55	267.07		
(Teva) *See FENTANYL TRANSDERMAL SYSTEM*				
(Watson Labs) *See FENTANYL TRANSDERMAL SYSTEM*				
(Watson Labs) *See NOVAPLUS FENTANYL*				
(DHS, Inc.)				
REPACK				
TDM, TD, 25 mcg/hr,				
5s ea, C-II	55887-0895-05	139.28		
50 mcg/hr,				
5s ea, C-II	55887-0089-05	230.64		
75 mcg/hr,				
5s ea, C-II	55887-0890-05	397.03		
100 mcg/hr,				
5s ea, C-II	55887-0088-05	455.68		
(Dispensing Solutions)				
REPACK				
TDM, TD, 12.5 mcg/hr,				
5s ea, C-II	68258-3040-01	149.04		AB
(Palmetto)				
REPACK				
TDM, TD, 25 mcg/hr,				
5s ea, C-II	23490-5567-01	126.26		
50 mcg/hr,				
5s ea, C-II	23490-5568-01	221.52		
75 mcg/hr,				
5s ea, C-II	23490-5569-01	326.32		
100 mcg/hr,				
5s ea, C-II	23490-5566-01	432.63		
(Phys Total Care)				
REPACK				
TDM, TD, 25 mcg/hr,				
5s ea, C-II	54868-0162-00	132.06		
10s ea, C-II	54868-0162-01	232.02		
50 mcg/hr,				
5s ea, C-II	54868-0244-00	236.43		
10s ea, C-II	54868-0244-01	441.27		
75 mcg/hr,				
5s ea, C-II	54868-0287-00	337.98		
10s ea, C-II	54868-0287-01	593.40		
100 mcg/hr,				
5s ea, C-II	54868-1523-00	448.11		
10s ea, C-II	54868-1523-01	887.20		
(Quality Care Prod)				
REPACK				
TDM, TD, 12.5 mcg/hr,				
5s ea, C-II	35356-0062-05	296.00		
25 mcg/hr, ea, C-II	49999-0831-01	37.55		

PROD/MFR	NDC	AWP	DP	OBC
FENTANYL (Quality Care Prod)				
REPACK				
TDM, TD, 25 mcg/hr,				
5s ea, C-II	**49999-0831-05**	187.75		
50 mcg/hr, ea, C-II	**49999-0832-01**	64.92		
5s ea, C-II	**49999-0832-05**	324.60		
75 mcg/hr, ea, C-II	**49999-0833-01**	105.36		
5s ea, C-II	**49999-0833-05**	526.80		
100 mcg/hr, ea, C-II	**49999-0834-01**	138.44		
5s ea, C-II	**49999-0834-05**	692.20		
(Stat Rx)				
REPACK				
TDM, TD, 12.5 mcg/hr,				
5s ea, C-II	**16590-0732-05**	85.28		AB
FENTANYL CITRATE				
(Akorn) *See SUBLIMAZE*				
(Baxter)				
SOL, IJ (1X2ML,USP,PF)				
0.05 mg/ml,				
2 ml, C-II	**10019-0038-39**	7.08		AP
((AMP),DOSETTE)				
0.05 mg/ml,				
2 ml 10s, C-II	**10019-0038-67**	7.08		AP
(1X5ML,USP,PF)				
0.05 mg/ml,				
5 ml, C-II	**10019-0033-39**	0.96		AP
((AMP),DOSETTE)				
0.05 mg/ml,				
5 ml 10s, C-II	**10019-0033-72**	9.60		AP
10 ml 5s, C-II	**10019-0034-73**	21.00		AP
(1X20ML,USP,PF)				
0.05 mg/ml,				
20 ml, C-II	**10019-0035-39**	18.00		AP
((AMP),DOSETTE,PF)				
0.05 mg/ml,				
20 ml 5s, C-II	**10019-0035-74**	18.00		AP
(1X50ML,SDV,USP,PF)				
0.05 mg/ml,				
50 ml, C-II	**10019-0037-39**	6.52		AP
(S.D.V.)				
0.05 mg/ml,				
50 ml, C-II	**10019-0037-83**	6.52		AP
(Cephalon) *See ACTIQ*				
(Cephalon) *See FENTORA*				
(Covidien)				
LOZ, MM, 0.2 mg,				
30s ea, C-II	**00406-9202-30**	564.12		AB
0.4 mg, 30s ea, C-II	**00406-9204-30**	714.71		AB
0.6 mg, 30s ea, C-II	**00406-9206-30**	875.40		AB
0.8 mg, 30s ea, C-II	**00406-9208-30**	1037.22		AB
1.2 mg, 30s ea, C-II	**00406-9212-30**	1348.50		AB
1.6 mg, 30s ea, C-II	**00406-9216-30**	1663.15		AB
POW, NA, 1 gm, C-II	**00406-1130-52**	1350.00		
(Gallipot)				
POW, NA (1X1GM,USP)				
1 gm, C-II	**51552-0687-01**	966.00	690.00	
(1X500MG,USP)				
500 ml, C-II	**51552-0687-09**	560.00	400.00	
(Hawkins)				
POW, NA (U.S.P.)				
0.1 gm, C-II	**63370-0920-06**	480.00		
0.5 gm, C-II	**63370-0920-09**	1632.00		
1 gm, C-II	**63370-0920-10**	2880.00		
5 gm, C-II	**63370-0920-15**	10560.00		
(Hospira)				
SOL, IJ (10X2ML,LATEX-FREE)				
0.05 mg/ml,				
2 ml 10s, C-II	**00409-9093-32**	4.08	3.60	AP
(AMP,LATEX-FREE)				
0.05 mg/ml,				
2 ml 10s, C-II	**00074-9093-32**	3.72	3.30	AP
(LUER LOCK,10X2ML,PF)				
0.05 mg/ml,				
2 ml 10s, C-II	**00409-1276-32**	14.76	12.90	AP
(FTV,25X2ML,LATEX-FREE)				
0.05 mg/ml,				
2 ml 25s, C-II	**00409-9094-22**	27.00	23.75	AP
(AMP,LATEX-FREE)				
0.05 mg/ml,				
5 ml 10s, C-II	**00074-9093-35**	4.44	3.90	AP
5 ml 10s, C-II	**00409-9093-35**	5.40	4.70	AP
(VIAL,FLIPTOP,LATEX-FREE)				
0.05 mg/ml,				
5 ml 25s, C-II	**00409-9094-25**	38.40	33.50	AP
(AMP,LATEX-FREE)				
0.05 mg/ml,				
10 ml 5s, C-II	**00074-9093-36**	4.86	4.25	AP
(SINGLE-DOSE,5X10ML)				
0.05 mg/ml,				
10 ml 5s, C-II	**00409-9093-36**	5.64	4.95	AP
(25X10ML,FTV)				
0.05 mg/ml,				
10 ml 25s, C-II	**00409-9094-28**	69.90	61.25	AP
(VIAL,FLIPTOP,LATEX-FREE)				
0.05 mg/ml,				
10 ml 25s, C-II	**00074-9094-28**	63.30	55.50	AP
(5X20ML)				
0.05 mg/ml,				
20 ml 5s, C-II	**00409-9093-38**	9.90	8.65	AP
(AMP,LATEX-FREE)				
0.05 mg/ml,				
20 ml 5s, C-II	**00074-9093-38**	8.88	7.75	AP
(FTV,LATEX-FREE)				
0.05 mg/ml,				
20 ml 25s, C-II	**00409-9094-31**	134.10	117.25	AP
(VIAL,FLIPTOP,LATEX-FREE)				
0.05 mg/ml,				
20 ml 25s, C-II	**00074-9094-31**	120.60	105.50	AP
(VIAL, FLIPTOP)				
0.05 mg/ml,				
50 ml 25s, C-II	**00409-9094-61**	168.60	147.50	AP
(Meda) *See ONSOLIS*				
(Medisca)				
POW, NA (U.S.P.)				
0.1 gm, C-II	**38779-1756-09**	387.00		
0.5 gm, C-II	**38779-1756-00**	1215.00		
1 gm, C-II	**38779-1756-06**	1950.00		
5 gm, C-II	**38779-1756-03**	6450.00		
(PCCA)				
POW, NA (U.S.P.)				
1 gm, C-II	**51927-1019-00**	5250.00		
(PharMEDium Services)				
SOL, IJ (5X100ML)				
0.05 mg/ml,				
100 ml 5s, C-II	**61553-0273-48**	57.00	47.50	AP
IV (INTRAVIA)				
0.05 mg/ml,				
50 ml, C-II	**61553-0118-41**	39.02	32.52	EE
(10X30ML, PCA VIAL)				
50 mcg/ml,				
30 ml 10s, C-II	**61553-0795-68**	58.50	48.75	
(Spectrum Pharmacy)				
POW, NA (U.S.P.)				
0.1 gm, C-II	**49452-0032-02**	535.50		
1 gm, C-II	**49452-0032-01**	2282.00		
(1X5GM,USP)				
5 gm, C-II	**49452-0032-03**	5659.50		
(Teva) *See ORAL TRANSMUCOSAL FENTANYL CITRATE*				
(Watson Labs) *See ORAL TRANSMUCOSAL FENTANYL CITRATE*				
(B&B Pharm, Inc)				
REPACK				
POW, NA (U.S.P.)				
0.1 gm, C-II	**63275-5100-06**	525.00		
1 gm, C-II	**63275-5100-01**	5250.00		
5 gm, C-II	**63275-5100-02**	26250.00		
(Phys Total Care)				
REPACK				
SOL, IJ (AMP)				
0.05 mg/ml,				
2 ml, C-II	**54868-3738-01**	3.15		EE
2 ml 10s, C-II	**54868-3738-00**	9.78		EE
FENTANYL CITRATE-SODIUM CHLORIDE				
(PharMEDium Services)				
fentanyl citrate/sodium chloride				
SOL, IV (10X30ML, PCA VIAL)				
10 mcg/ml-0.9%,				
30 ml 10s, C-II	**61553-0791-68**	46.50	38.75	
20 mcg/ml-0.9%,				
30 ml 10s, C-II	**61553-0792-68**	49.50	41.25	
(5X100ML, CASSETTE,PF)				
20 mcg/ml-0.9%,				
100 ml 5s, C-II	**61553-0852-48**	396.60	330.50	
(10X30ML, PCA VIAL)				
25 mcg/ml-0.9%,				
30 ml 10s, C-II	**61553-0730-68**	54.00	45.00	
30 mcg/ml-0.9%,				
30 ml 10s, C-II	**61553-0793-68**	52.50	43.75	
40 mcg/ml-0.9%,				
30 ml 10s, C-II	**61553-0794-68**	55.50	46.25	
FENTANYL CITRATE/SODIUM CHLORIDE				
(PharMEDium Services) *See FENTANYL CITRATE-SODIUM CHLORIDE*				
(PharMEDium Services)				
SOL, IV (INTRAVIA)				
0.2 mg/100 ml-0.9%,				
100 ml, C-II	**61553-0602-48**	24.42	20.35	
(SRN,12 ML)				
0.5 mg/100 ml-0.9%,				
10 ml, C-II	**61553-0109-72**	20.26	16.88	
(INTRAVIA)				
0.5 mg/100 ml-0.9%,				
250 ml, C-II	**61553-0107-02**	31.21	26.01	
1 mg/100 ml-0.9%,				
100 ml, C-II	**61553-0111-48**	29.90	24.92	
(IPUMP BAG)				
1 mg/100 ml-0.9%,				
100 ml, C-II	**61553-0112-48**	43.82	36.52	
(INTRAVIA)				
1 mg/100 ml-0.9%,				
250 ml, C-II	**61553-0113-02**	38.84	32.36	
(IPUMP BAG)				
1 mg/100 ml-0.9%,				
250 ml, C-II	**61553-0114-02**	54.77	45.65	
(INTRAVIA)				
2 mg/100 ml-0.9%,				
100 ml, C-II	**61553-0116-48**	35.86	29.89	
FENTANYL TRANSDERMAL SYSTEM (Actavis)				
fentanyl				
TDM, TD, 25 mcg/hr,				
5s ea, C-II	**67767-0120-18**	83.26		AB
50 mcg/hr,				
5s ea, C-II	**67767-0121-18**	152.41		AB
75 mcg/hr,				
5s ea, C-II	**67767-0122-18**	232.46		AB
100 mcg/hr,				
5s ea, C-II	**67767-0123-18**	308.52		AB
(Sandoz)				
TDM, TD, 12.5 mcg/hr,				
5s ea, C-II	**00781-7109-55**	69.00		
5s ea, C-II	**00781-7240-55**	69.00		
25 mcg/hr,				
5s ea, C-II	**00781-7241-55**	72.17		
50 mcg/hr,				
5s ea, C-II	**00781-7242-55**	131.92		
75 mcg/hr,				
5s ea, C-II	**00781-7243-55**	201.23		
100 mcg/hr,				
5s ea, C-II	**00781-7244-55**	267.07		
(Teva)				
TDM, TD, 25 mcg/hr,				
5s ea, C-II	**00093-6900-45**	83.34		AB
50 mcg/hr,				
5s ea, C-II	**00093-6901-45**	152.37		AB
75 mcg/hr,				
5s ea, C-II	**00093-6902-45**	232.40		AB
100 mcg/hr,				
5s ea, C-II	**00093-6903-45**	308.45		AB
(Watson Labs)				
TDM, TD (INNER PACK)				
25 mcg/hr,				
ea, C-II	**00591-3198-54**	13.00		AB
5s ea, C-II	**00591-3198-72**	64.96		AB
(INNER PACK)				
50 mcg/hr,				
ea, C-II	**00591-3212-54**	23.75		AB
5s ea, C-II	**00591-3212-72**	118.73		AB
(INNER PACK)				
75 mcg/hr,				
ea, C-II	**00591-3213-54**	36.22		AB
5s ea, C-II	**00591-3213-72**	181.10		AB
(INNER PACK)				
100 mcg/hr,				
ea, C-II	**00591-3214-54**	48.07		AB
5s ea, C-II	**00591-3214-72**	240.36		AB
(4u)				
REPACK				
TDM, TD, 25 mcg/hr,				
5s ea, C-II	**10544-0373-05**	152.26		AB
5s ea, C-II	**42549-0573-05**	152.26		AB
50 mcg/hr,				
5s ea, C-II	**42549-0628-05**	219.54		AB
(Altura)				
REPACK				
TDM, TD, 25 mcg/hr,				
5s ea, C-II	**63874-1277-05**	77.16		AB
50 mcg/hr,				
5s ea, C-II	**63874-1278-05**	126.74		AB
75 mcg/hr,				
5s ea, C-II	**63874-1279-05**	184.27		AB
100 mcg/hr,				
5s ea, C-II	**63874-1280-05**	238.92		AB

PROD/MFR NDC AWP DP OBC

(Dispensing Solutions)
REPACK
TDM, TD, 25 mcg/hr,
5s ea, C-II .... 68258-3023-01 108.01 AB
50 mcg/hr,
5s ea, C-II .... 68258-3010-01 157.37 AB
75 mcg/hr,
5s ea, C-II .... 68258-3024-01 237.37 AB
100 mcg/hr,
5s ea, C-II .... 68258-3025-01 313.40 AB

(Phys Total Care)
REPACK
TDM, TD, 12.5 mcg/hr,
5s ea, C-II 54868-5963-00 194.52

(St. Mary's MPP)
REPACK
TDM, TD, 25 mcg/hr,
5s ea, C-II .... 60760-0911-05 114.26 AB
50 mcg/hr,
5s ea, C-II .... 60760-0912-05 203.70 AB

(Stat Rx)
REPACK
TDM, TD, 25 mcg/hr,
5s ea, C-II .... 16590-0602-05 155.32 AB
50 mcg/hr,
5s ea, C-II .... 16590-0603-05 158.25 AB
75 mcg/hr,
5s ea, C-II .... 16590-0604-05 239.01 AB
100 mcg/hr,
5s ea, C-II .... 16590-0605-05 345.00 AB

FENTANYL TROCHE (Stat Rx)
fentanyl citrate
LOZ, MM, 1.6 mg,
30s ea, C-II 16590-0887-30 1995.84

FENTORA (Cephalon)
fentanyl citrate
TAB, BC (7X4 BLISTER CARDS)
100 mcg,
28s ea, C-II 63459-0541-28 522.00
200 mcg,
28s ea, C-II 63459-0542-28 660.00
(7X4)
300 mcg,
28s ea, C-II .... 63459-0543-28 807.60 EE
(7X4 BLISTER CARDS)
400 mcg,
28s ea, C-II 63459-0544-28 958.80
600 mcg,
28s ea, C-II 63459-0546-28 1245.60
800 mcg,
28s ea, C-II 63459-0548-28 1533.60

(Quality Care Prod)
REPACK
TAB, BC, 600 mcg,
28s ea, C-II 35356-0378-28 1326.32
60s ea, C-II 35356-0378-60 3346.25

(Stat Rx)
REPACK
TAB, BC, 200 mcg,
28s ea, C-II 16590-0857-28 696.80
800 mcg,
28s ea, C-II 16590-0888-28 1673.28

FEOGEN (Phys Total Care)
REPACK
vitamin b complex, iron, and vitamin c
SGL, PO, 20s ea 54868-5253-02 15.27
30s ea 54868-5253-00 25.65
60s ea 54868-5253-01 46.80

FERAHEME (Amag)
ferumoxytol
SOL, IV, 30 mg/ml, 17 ml .. 59338-0775-01 476.14
17 ml 10s 59338-0775-10 4761.36

FERBEE (Truxton)
vitamin b complex and mineral
SOL, IJ, 30 ml 00463-1031-30 18.00

FERIDEX IV (Bayer)
ferumoxides
SOL, IV (S.D.V.)
11.2 mg/ml,
5 ml 5s 59338-7035-05 731.75
5 ml 10s 59338-7035-00 1463.50

FEROCON (Breckenridge Pharm)
ferrous fum/folic acid/if/vit b12/vit c
CAP, PO, 100s ea 51991-0635-01 43.95

FEROTRIN (Boca Pharmacal)
multivitamin and nutriceuticals
CAP, PO, 60s ea UD 64376-0805-06 43.08

PROD/MFR NDC AWP DP OBC

FEROTRINSIC (Contract Pharmacal)
multivitamin and nutriceuticals
CAP, PO, 100s ea 10267-0464-01 32.50

FERRAGEN (Contract Pharmacal)
ferrous fum/stomach, desiccated/vit b12/vit c
CAP, PO, 100s ea 10267-1439-01 21.50

FERRALET 90 (Mission)
dss/fe/folic acid/vit b12/vit c
TAB, PO (DUAL-IRON DELIVERY)
90s ea 00178-0089-90 79.20 66.00

FERREX 150 FORTE (Breckenridge Pharm)
cyanocobalamin/folic acid/iron polysaccharide
CAP, PO (BLISTER PACK)
25 mcg-1 mg-150 mg,
100s ea UD 51991-0198-11 27.50

FERREX 150 FORTE PLUS (Breckenridge Pharm)
vitamin b complex, iron, and vitamin c
CAP, PO, 90s ea 51991-0798-90 114.35

FERREX 28 (Breckenridge Pharm)
multivitamin and iron
TAB, PO, 28s ea 51991-0588-28 28.95

FERRIC AMMONIUM CITRATE
(Amend) *See FERRIC AMMONIUM CITRATE BROWN*
(Amend) *See FERRIC AMMONIUM CITRATE GREEN*
(Baker, J.T.) *See FERRIC AMMONIUM CITRATE BROWN*
(Baker, J.T.) *See FERRIC AMMONIUM CITRATE GREEN*
(Gallipot) *See FERRIC AMMONIUM CITRATE BROWN*
(PCCA) *See FERRIC AMMONIUM CITRATE BROWN*
(Spectrum Pharmacy) *See FERRIC AMMONIUM CITRATE BROWN*
(Spectrum Pharmacy) *See FERRIC AMMONIUM CITRATE GREEN*

FERRIC AMMONIUM CITRATE BROWN (Amend)
ferric ammonium citrate
POW, NA (F.C.C.)
454 gm 17317-0162-01 17.50
2270 gm 17317-0162-05 56.00
11350 gm 17317-0162-08 210.00

(Baker, J.T.)
POW, NA (F.C.C.)
500 gm 10106-1980-01 23.40

(Gallipot)
POW, NA (F.C.C.)
454 gm 51552-0593-06 23.45

(PCCA)
POW, NA (F.C.C.)
1 gm 51927-2508-00 0.18

(Spectrum Pharmacy)
POW, NA (F.C.C.)
125 gm 49452-3040-03 88.55
500 gm 49452-3040-01 145.25
2500 gm 49452-3040-02 553.00

FERRIC AMMONIUM CITRATE GREEN (Amend)
ferric ammonium citrate
POW, NA (F.C.C.)
454 gm 17317-0163-01 17.50
2270 gm 17317-0163-05 56.00
11350 gm 17317-0163-08 210.00

(Baker, J.T.)
POW, NA (F.C.C.)
500 gm 10106-1977-01 39.60

(Spectrum Pharmacy)
POW, NA (F.C.C.)
125 gm 49452-3050-03 88.55
500 gm 49452-3050-01 145.25
2500 gm 49452-3050-02 553.00

FERRIC AMMONIUM OXALATE
(PCCA) *See FERRIC AMMONIUM OXALATE REAGENT GRADE*

FERRIC AMMONIUM OXALATE REAGENT GRADE (PCCA)
ferric ammonium oxalate
CRY, NA (1X1GM)
1 gm 51927-2297-00 36.00

FERRIC AMMONIUM SULFATE 12-HYDRATE (Baker, J.T.)
ammonium ferric sulfate
CRY, NA (A.C.S., REAGENT)
500 gm 10106-1988-01 84.77
2500 gm 10106-1988-05 303.08

FERRIC CHLORIDE (Amend)
LUM, NA (PURIFIED)
500 gm 17317-0165-01 13.30

PROD/MFR NDC AWP DP OBC

2270 gm 17317-0165-05 42.00
11350 gm 17317-0165-08 210.00

(Baker, J.T.) *See FERRIC CHLORIDE HEXAHYDRATE*

(Gallipot)
LUM, NA (PURIFIED)
454 gm 51552-0644-06 29.40
2270 gm 51552-0644-09 97.65

(PCCA)
POW, NA, 1 gm 51927-1125-00 0.36

(Spectrum Pharmacy) *See FERRIC CHLORIDE HEXAHYDRATE*

FERRIC CHLORIDE HEXAHYDRATE (Baker, J.T.)
ferric chloride
LUM, NA (PURIFIED)
500 gm 10106-2000-01 60.51
2500 gm 10106-2000-05 190.76

(Spectrum Pharmacy)
LUM, NA (A.C.S. REAGENT)
125 gm 49452-3060-01 74.90
500 gm 49452-3060-02 114.10
2500 gm 49452-3060-03 331.10

FERRIC NITRATE
(Baker, J.T.) *See FERRIC NITRATE NONOHYDRATE*

FERRIC NITRATE NONOHYDRATE (Baker, J.T.)
ferric nitrate
CRY, NA (A.C.S., REAGENT)
500 gm 10106-2018-01 70.14
2500 gm 10106-2018-05 234.48
12000 gm 10106-2018-07 523.96

FERRIC OXIDE
(Amend) *See FERRIC OXIDE RED*

(Baker, J.T.)
POW, NA (REAGENT)
500 gm 10106-2024-01 48.67
2500 gm 10106-2024-05 140.29

(Medisca)
POW, NA (N.F.,RED)
100 gm 38779-1283-05 34.50
500 gm 38779-1283-08 55.50

(PCCA) *See FERRIC OXIDE RED*
(PCCA) *See FERROSOFERRIC OXIDE, BLACK POWDER*
(PCCA) *See IRON OXIDE, BLACK*
(PCCA) *See IRON OXIDE, RED*
(PCCA) *See IRON OXIDE, YELLOW*

FERRIC OXIDE RED (Amend)
ferric oxide
POW, NA (COSMETIC GRADE)
500 gm 17317-1207-01 8.40
2500 gm 17317-1207-05 29.40
12000 gm 17317-1207-08 111.80

(PCCA)
POW, NA (COSMETIC)
1 gm 51927-2104-00 0.36

FERRIC PHOSPHATE (Spectrum Pharmacy)
POW, NA (F.C.C.)
500 gm 49452-3072-01 117.60
2500 gm 49452-3072-02 427.00

FERRIC PYROPHOSPHATE (Spectrum Pharmacy)
POW, NA (F.C.C.)
500 gm 49452-3075-01 220.85
2500 gm 49452-3075-02 794.50

FERRIC SUBSULFATE (Amend)
SOL, NA (PURIFIED)
500 ml 17317-0171-01 18.90
3840 ml 17317-0171-06 125.00

(Baker, J.T.)
SOL, NA (PURIFIED)
500 ml 10106-2041-01 22.73

(Cooper Surgical) *See ASTRINGYN*

(Gallipot)
POW, NA (PURIFIED)
113.4 gm 51552-0296-04 19.81
454 gm 51552-0296-06 53.41
SOL, NA (MONSEL'S)
60 ml 51552-0357-03 8.82

(Mallinckrodt Lab)
SOL, NA (PURIFIED)
500 ml 00406-5548-04 22.64

(Medisca)
POW, NA, 100 gm 38779-0938-05 37.50
500 gm 38779-0938-08 114.00
1000 gm 38779-0938-09 208.50

PROD/MFR | NDC | AWP | DP | OBC

(1X2500GM)
2500 gm............38779-0938-01 459.00
SOL, NA (USP,1X100ML)
100 ml..............38779-1284-05 28.50
(N.F.,MONSEL'S SOLUTION)
500 ml..............38779-1284-08 67.50

(PCCA)
POW, NA (PURIFIED)
1 gm................51927-1328-00 0.48
SOL, NA (USP; MONSEL'S SOLUTION)
1 ml................51927-3361-00 0.02

(Spectrum Pharmacy)
POW, NA (PURIFIED)
125 gm..............49452-3080-01 85.40
500 gm..............49452-3080-02 212.10
2500 gm.............49452-3080-03 924.00
SOL, NA (U.S.P.)
500 ml..............49452-3081-02 123.55

FERRIC SULFATE
(Baker, J.T.) *See FERRIC SULFATE N-HYDRATE*
(PCCA) *See FERRIC SULFATE HYDRATE*

FERRIC SULFATE HYDRATE (PCCA)
ferric sulfate
POW, NA, 1 gm...........51927-2267-00 0.75

FERRIC SULFATE N-HYDRATE (Baker, J.T.)
ferric sulfate
POW, NA, 500 gm.........10106-2046-01 137.30
2500 gm.............10106-2046-05 378.73

FERRLECIT (Sanofi-Aventis)
sodium ferric gluconate complex
SOL, IV (10X5ML,SINGLE-USE)
62.5 mg/5 ml,
5 ml 10s...........00024-2791-50 381.60

(Watson)
SOL, IV (SINGLE USE AMP)
62.5 mg/5 ml,
5 ml 10s...........52544-0922-26 430.00

FERROCITE F (Breckenridge Pharm)
ferrous fumarate/folic acid
TAB, PO (10X10,AF,SF,FILM COATED)
324 mg-1 mg,
100s ea UD.........51991-0183-11 22.25

FERROCITE PLUS (Breckenridge Pharm)
multivitamin and minerals
CAP, PO, 30s ea..........51991-0682-33 14.70
100s ea.............51991-0682-01 49.00

(Breckenridge Pharm)
multivitamin, minerals, and iron
TAB, PO (10X10,AF,SF,FILM COATED)
100s ea UD..........51991-0182-11 39.50

FERROGELS FORTE (Cypress Pharm)
ferrous fum/folic acid/vit b12/vit c
SGL, PO (10X10,SOFTGEL)
100s ea UD..........60258-0189-01 61.65

FERROSOFERRIC OXIDE, BLACK POWDER (PCCA)
ferric oxide
POW, NA (1X1GM)
1 gm................51927-2973-00 0.18

FERROUS AMMONIUM SULFATE (Amend)
CRY, NA (A.C.S., REAGENT)
454 gm..............17317-0837-01 43.40
2270 gm.............17317-0837-05 168.00

(Baker, J.T.) *See FERROUS AMMONIUM SULFATE 6-HYDRATE*

FERROUS AMMONIUM SULFATE 6-HYDRATE
(Baker, J.T.)
ferrous ammonium sulfate
CRY, NA (FINE, A.C.S., REAGENT)
500 gm..............10106-2054-01 119.74
2500 gm.............10106-2054-05 464.43

FERROUS CHLORIDE
(Baker, J.T.) *See FERROUS CHLORIDE TETRAHYDRATE*

FERROUS CHLORIDE TETRAHYDRATE (Baker, J.T.)
ferrous chloride
CRY, NA (REAGENT)
500 gm..............10106-2064-01 107.53
2500 gm.............10106-2064-05 383.88

FERROUS FUM/FOLIC ACID/IF/VIT B12/VIT C
(Breckenridge Pharm) *See FEROCON*
(Marlop) *See MARTINIC*
(Marlop) *See PROMAR*
(Nnodum) *See TRICON*
(Sandoz) *See FOLTRIN*

FERROUS FUM/FOLIC ACID/VIT B12/VIT C
(Cypress Pharm) *See FERROGELS FORTE*
(Nnodum) *See ZIKS HEMATOGEN FA*
(Nnodum) *See ZIKS HEMATOGEN FORTE*

FERROUS FUM/STOMACH, DESICCATED/ VIT B12/VIT C
(Contract Pharmacal) *See FERRAGEN*
(Nnodum) *See ZIKS HEMATOGEN*

FERROUS FUMARATE (Amend)
POW, NA (U.S.P.)
454 gm..............17317-0773-01 10.50
2270 gm.............17317-0773-05 37.80
11350 gm............17317-0773-08 112.50

(Cypress Pharm)
TAB, PO, 324 mg, 100s ea.60258-0182-01 20.58

(Medisca)
POW, NA (U.S.P.)
500 gm..............38779-2076-08 46.50
2500 gm.............38779-2076-01 160.50

(PCCA)
POW, NA (USP)
1 gm................51927-1834-00 0.15

(Spectrum Pharmacy)
POW, NA (U.S.P.)
500 gm..............49452-3110-01 121.80
2500 gm.............49452-3110-02 364.00

FERROUS FUMARATE/FOLIC ACID
(Breckenridge Pharm) *See FERROCITE F*
(Contract Pharmacal) *See HEMOPLEX F*
(Cypress Pharm) *See HEMATINIC W/FOLIC ACID*
(U.S. Pharm) *See HEMOCYTE-F*

FERROUS FUMARATE/FOLIC ACID/ IRON POLYSACCHARIDE
(U.S. Pharm) *See TANDEM F*

FERROUS GLUCONATE (Amend)
GRA, NA (U.S.P.)
454 gm..............17317-0164-01 8.40
2270 gm.............17317-0164-05 42.00
11350 gm............17317-0164-08 140.00

(PCCA)
GRA, NA (USP, DIHYDRATE,GRANULAR)
1 gm................51927-2179-00 0.30

(Spectrum Pharmacy)
POW, NA (U.S.P.)
500 gm..............49452-3120-01 79.80
2500 gm.............49452-3120-02 344.75

(Palmetto)
REPACK
TAB, PO, 325 mg, 100s ea.23490-6664-07 8.56

(Phys Total Care)
REPACK
TAB, PO, 324 mg, 100s ea.54868-4246-00 21.67

FERROUS SULFATE
(Baker, J.T.) *See FERROUS SULFATE HEPTAHYDRATE*

(Gallipot)
GRA, NA (U.S.P.)
454 gm..............51552-0310-06 14.00
POW, NA, 454 gm.........51552-0586-06 27.79

(Mallinckrodt Lab)
SOL, NA, 500 gm.........00406-5572-04 45.93

(Medisca)
GRA, NA (U.S.P.)
500 gm..............38779-1288-08 31.50

(PCCA)
GRA, NA (USP; HEPTAHYDRATE)
1 gm................51927-1378-00 0.33
POW, NA (USP; ANHYDROUS)
1 gm................51927-3160-00 0.30

(Spectrum Pharmacy)
GRA, NA (U.S.P.)
500 gm..............49452-3140-01 84.00
2500 gm.............49452-3140-02 254.10
12000 gm............49452-3140-03 735.00
POW, NA, 500 gm.........49452-3150-01 81.90
2500 gm.............49452-3150-02 245.00
12000 gm............49452-3150-03 693.00

(Bryant Ranch)
REPACK
TAB, PO, 325 mg, 50s ea..63629-1754-02 1.99
100s ea.............63629-1754-01 2.50

(Southwood)
REPACK
LIQ, PO (DROPS)
75 mg/0.6 ml,
50 ml...............58016-4819-01 5.75

FERROUS SULFATE HEPTAHYDRATE (Baker, J.T.)
ferrous sulfate
CRY, NA (U.S.P./F.C.C.)
500 gm..............10106-2074-01 14.69
2500 gm.............10106-2074-05 132.23

FERUMOXIDES
(Bayer) *See FERIDEX IV*

FERUMOXYTOL
(Amag) *See FERAHEME*

FESOTERODINE FUMARATE
(Pfizer) *See TOVIAZ*

FETRIN (Lunsco)
ascorbic acid/cyanocobalamin/ferrous fumarate
CER, PO, 60 mg-5 mcg-200 mg,
100s ea.............10892-0114-10 47.88

FEVERFEW
(PCCA) *See FEVERFEW EXTRACT 4:1*

FEVERFEW EXTRACT 4:1 (PCCA)
feverfew
POW, NA (1X1GM)
1 gm................51927-3235-00 0.45

FEXMID (Victory Pharma, Inc.)
cyclobenzaprine hydrochloride
TAB, PO (USP,FILM-COATED)
7.5 mg, 100s ea......68453-0950-10 398.48

(IPI)
REPACK
TAB, PO, 7.5 mg, 90s ea...18837-0285-90 394.50

(Stat Rx)
REPACK
TAB, PO (FILM-COATED)
7.5 mg, 28s ea.......16590-0699-28 122.72
90s ea..............16590-0699-90 394.47

FEXOFENADINE (Bryant Ranch)
REPACK
fexofenadine hydrochloride
TAB, PO, 180 mg, 30s ea..63629-3190-01 203.13

(Core)
REPACK
TAB, PO, 180 mg, 30s ea..33358-0142-30 82.50

(DHS, Inc.)
REPACK
TAB, PO, 180 mg, 15s ea..55887-0666-15 36.39
30s ea..............55887-0666-30 72.78
60s ea..............55887-0666-60 145.57
90s ea..............55887-0666-90 218.36

(Pharma Pac)
REPACK
TAB, PO, 60 mg, 10s ea...52959-0848-10 16.05
30s ea..............52959-0848-30 48.20

(Southwood)
REPACK
TAB, PO, 60 mg, 30s ea...58016-0238-30 41.96
60s ea..............58016-0238-60 83.92
90s ea..............58016-0238-90 125.88
100s ea.............58016-0238-00 139.87

(Stat Rx)
REPACK
TAB, PO, 180 mg, 20s ea..16590-0536-20 58.00
30s ea..............16590-0536-30 87.00
60s ea..............16590-0536-60 174.00
90s ea..............16590-0536-90 261.00
120s ea.............16590-0536-72 300.00

(Vibranta)
REPACK
TAB, PO, 180 mg, 30s ea..57866-7072-01 154.71

FEXOFENADINE HCL (Prasco Labs)
fexofenadine hydrochloride
TAB, PO (FILM-COATED)
30 mg, 100s ea......66993-0106-02 69.76
60 mg, 100s ea......66993-0107-02 139.87
500s ea.............66993-0107-04 699.35
180 mg, 100s ea.....66993-0109-02 242.63
500s ea.............66993-0109-04 1213.15

(Teva)
TAB, PO (FILM-COATED)
30 mg, 100s ea......00093-7251-01 69.76 AB

PROD/MFR	NDC	AWP	DP	OBC
60 mg, 100s ea	00093-7252-01	139.87		AB
500s ea	00093-7252-05	699.35		AB
180 mg, 100s ea	00093-7253-01	242.63		AB
500s ea	00093-7253-05	1213.15		AB
(A-S Medication)				
REPACK				
TAB, PO, 60 mg, 10s ea	54569-5737-00	13.99		
30s ea	54569-5737-01	41.96		
180 mg, 10s ea	54569-5738-00	72.79		
(Altura)				
REPACK				
TAB, PO (FILM-COATED)				
60 mg, 30s ea	63874-1231-03	45.00		
100s ea	63874-1231-01	150.00		
(Palmetto)				
REPACK				
TAB, PO (FILM-COATED)				
30 mg, 14s ea	23490-7428-01	21.00		AB
28s ea	23490-7428-02	42.00		AB
30s ea	23490-7428-03	45.00		AB
(PD-Rx Pharm)				
REPACK				
TAB, PO (FILM-COATED)				
180 mg, 90s ea	55289-0957-90	297.36		
(Phys Total Care)				
REPACK				
TAB, PO, 180 mg, 10s ea	54868-5409-00	58.26		
30s ea	54868-5409-01	132.06		
60s ea	54868-5409-03	256.47		
90s ea	54868-5409-02	362.10		
100s ea	54868-5409-04	400.50		
(Quality Care Prod)				
REPACK				
TAB, PO (FILM-COATED)				
30 mg, 30s ea	35356-0156-30	25.39		
90s ea	35356-0156-90	68.14		
60 mg, 30s ea	49999-0771-30	45.90		
60s ea	49999-0771-60	91.80		
90s ea	49999-0771-90	137.70		
180 mg, 30s ea	49999-0772-30	84.63		
60s ea	49999-0772-60	169.26		
90s ea	49999-0772-90	253.89		
FEXOFENADINE HCL AND PSEUDOEPHEDRINE HCL				
(Sanofi-Aventis)				
fexofenadine hcl/pse hcl				
TER, PO (FILM COATED)				
60 mg-120 mg,				
100s ea	00955-1705-10	223.74		
500s ea	00955-1705-50	1118.71		
(Teva)				
TER, PO (FILM COATED)				
60 mg-120 mg,				
100s ea	00093-1130-01	223.98		
500s ea	00093-1130-05	1119.96		
(Phys Total Care)				
REPACK				
TER, PO (FILM COATED)				
60 mg-120 mg,				
10s ea	54868-6087-01	65.24		
30s ea	54868-6087-02	138.72		
60s ea	54868-6087-00	280.82		
FEXOFENADINE HCL/PSE HCL				
(Sanofi-Aventis) *See ALLEGRA-D 12 HOUR*				
(Sanofi-Aventis) *See ALLEGRA-D 24HOUR*				
(Sanofi-Aventis) *See FEXOFENADINE HCL AND PSEUDOEPHEDRINE HCL*				
(Teva) *See FEXOFENADINE HCL AND PSEUDOEPHEDRINE HCL*				
FEXOFENADINE HYDROCHLORIDE				
FUL				
CAP, PO, 60 mg, 100s ea		115.40		
TAB, PO, 30 mg, 100s ea		57.56		
60 mg, 100s ea		115.40		
180 mg, 100s ea		200.18		
(Dr Reddy's)				
TAB, PO, 30 mg, 90s ea	55111-0192-90	62.78		AB
100s ea	55111-0192-01	69.76		AB
500s ea	55111-0192-05	348.80		AB
60 mg, 90s ea	55111-0193-90	125.88		AB
100s ea	55111-0193-01	139.87		AB
500s ea	55111-0193-05	699.35		AB
180 mg, 90s ea	55111-0194-90	218.36		AB
100s ea	55111-0194-01	242.63		AB
500s ea	55111-0194-05	1213.15		AB

PROD/MFR	NDC	AWP	DP	OBC
(Major)				
TAB, PO (10X10)				
30 mg, 100s ea UD	00904-5961-61	89.63		AB
60 mg, 100s ea UD	00904-5962-61	90.88		AB
180 mg, 100s ea UD	00904-5963-61	218.37		AB
(Mylan)				
TAB, PO (USP,FILM-COATED)				
30 mg, 100s ea	00378-0752-01	69.76		
60 mg, 100s ea	00378-0753-01	139.87		
500s ea	00378-0753-05	699.35		
(FILM-COATED)				
180 mg, 100s ea	00378-0755-01	242.63		AB
500s ea	00378-0755-05	1213.15		AB
(Prasco Labs) *See FEXOFENADINE HCL*				
(Prasco Labs)				
TAB, PO (FILM-COATED)				
180 mg, 90s ea	66993-0109-90	218.37		
(Sanofi-Aventis) *See ALLEGRA*				
(Sanofi-Aventis) *See ALLEGRA ODT*				
(Teva) *See FEXOFENADINE HCL*				
(UDL)				
TAB, PO (10X10,FILM-COATED)				
60 mg, 100s ea UD	51079-0529-20	151.46		AB
(USP,10X10,FILM-COATED)				
180 mg, 100s ea UD	51079-0526-20	242.63		AB
(Bryant Ranch)				
REPACK				
TAB, PO, 60 mg, 30s ea	63629-3973-01	41.98		AB
(DHS, Inc.)				
REPACK				
TAB, PO, 60 mg, 10s ea	55887-0137-10	15.00		
20s ea	55887-0137-20	28.00		
30s ea	55887-0137-30	42.00		
60s ea	55887-0137-60	84.00		
(Dispensing Solutions)				
REPACK				
TAB, PO, 60 mg, 14s ea	55045-3437-04	21.00		
30s ea	55045-3437-08	45.00		
100s ea	55045-3437-00	150.00		
180 mg, 30s ea	66336-0710-30	78.27		AB
(Nucare Pharm)				
REPACK				
TAB, PO (FILM-COATED)				
60 mg, 30s ea	68071-0402-30	56.71		
(Palmetto)				
REPACK				
TAB, PO, 60 mg, 14s ea	23490-7429-00	21.00		
30s ea	23490-7429-01	50.79		
30s ea	23490-7429-03	45.00		
180 mg, 30s ea	23490-7410-01	73.22		
(PD-Rx Pharm)				
REPACK				
TAB, PO, 60 mg, 28s ea	55289-0941-28	67.55		
180 mg, 5s ea	55289-0957-05	21.44		
30s ea	55289-0957-30	73.22		
(Phys Total Care)				
REPACK				
TAB, PO, 30 mg, 30s ea	54868-5468-00	59.79		
60s ea	54868-5468-01	89.07		
60 mg, 10s ea	54868-5417-02	35.31		
30s ea	54868-5417-00	77.13		
60s ea	54868-5417-01	151.23		
(Physician Partner)				
REPACK				
TAB, PO, 60 mg, 20s ea	21695-0461-20	65.82		
180 mg, 10s ea	21695-0462-10	57.09		AB
30s ea	21695-0462-30	145.58		AB
60s ea	21695-0492-60	291.16		AB
(Quality Care Prod)				
REPACK				
TAB, PO, 60 mg, 8s ea	49999-0771-08	12.25		
20s ea	49999-0771-20	30.60		
(St. Mary's MPP)				
REPACK				
TAB, PO (USP)				
60 mg, 20s ea	60760-0103-20	36.77		
60s ea	60760-0103-60	98.31		AB
90s ea	60760-0103-90	144.47		AB
FIBRICOR (AR Scientific)				
fenofibric acid				
TAB, PO, 35 mg, 30s ea	13310-0101-07	41.18		EE
105 mg, 30s ea	13310-0102-07	123.56		EE
90s ea	13310-0102-90	370.68		EE
FIBRINOGEN				
(CSL) *See RIASTAP*				

PROD/MFR	NDC	AWP	DP	OBC
FILGRASTIM				
(Amgen USA Inc.) *See NEUPOGEN*				
FILTER, INTRAVENOUS TUBING				
(Abbott Hosp) *See LIFESHIELD EXTENSION PEDIATRIC*				
(Abbott Hosp) *See PLUMSET MACRO INTEGRAL HP FILTER-OL*				
FILTER, SYRINGE				
(Abbott Hosp) *See SYRINGE FILTER 1.0 MICRON*				
FINACEA (Intendis, Inc.)				
azelaic acid				
GEL, TP, 15%, 50 gm	10922-0825-02	143.15		
(Phys Total Care)				
REPACK				
GEL, TP, 15%, 30 gm	54868-5236-00	161.44		
50 gm	54868-5236-01	171.42		
(Quality Care Prod)				
REPACK				
GEL, TP (1X50GM)				
15%, 50 gm	35356-0227-50	244.48		
FINACEA PLUS (Intendis, Inc.)				
azelaic acid				
KIT, TP, 15%, ea	10922-0826-10	143.15		EE
FINASTERIDE				
FUL				
TAB, PO, 5 mg, 100s ea		173.03		
(Actavis)				
TAB, PO (USP,FILM-COATED)				
5 mg, 30s ea	52152-0500-30	93.92		AB
90s ea	52152-0500-08	281.76		AB
100s ea	52152-0500-02	313.07		AB
(Aurobindo Pharma)				
TAB, PO (USP,FILM-COATED)				
5 mg, 30s ea	65862-0149-30	93.80		AB
90s ea	65862-0149-90	281.40		AB
100s ea	65862-0149-01	312.65		AB
(Dr Reddy's)				
TAB, PO (USP,FILM-COATED)				
5 mg, 80s ea	55111-0172-30	93.39		AB
30s ea	55111-0554-30	93.39		AB
90s ea	55111-0172-90	280.14		AB
90s ea	55111-0554-90	280.14		AB
(Greenstone)				
TAB, PO (USP,FILM-COATED)				
5 mg, 30s ea	59762-0850-02	93.80		
90s ea	59762-0850-03	281.40		
500s ea	59762-0850-07	1563.33		
(Medisca)				
CRY, NA (USP,1X25GM)				
25 gm	38779-2410-04	1335.00		
(USP,1X100GM)				
100 gm	38779-2410-05	3825.00		
(USP,1X500GM)				
500 gm	38779-2410-08	15600.00		
(USP,1X1000GM)				
1000 gm	38779-2410-09	24750.00		
(Merck) *See PROPECIA*				
(Merck) *See PROSCAR*				
(Mylan)				
TAB, PO (USP,FILM-COATED)				
5 mg, 30s ea	00378-3151-93	93.80		AB
90s ea	00378-3151-77	281.39		AB
100s ea	00378-3151-01	312.65		AB
(Northstar)				
TAB, PO (FILM-COATED)				
5 mg, 30s ea	16714-0522-01	93.80		
90s ea	16714-0522-03	281.39		
100s ea	16714-0522-04	312.98		
(Teva)				
TAB, PO (USP,FILM-COATED)				
5 mg, 30s ea	00093-7355-56	93.90		AB
90s ea	00093-7355-98	281.76		AB
(FILM-COATED)				
5 mg, 100s ea	00093-7355-01	313.07		AB
(USP,FILM-COATED)				
5 mg, 500s ea	00093-7355-05	1565.33		AB
(UDL)				
TAB, PO (10X10,USP,FILM-COATED)				
5 mg, 100s ea UD	51079-0520-20	312.66		AB
(10X30,USP,FILM-COATED)				
5 mg, 300s ea UD	51079-0520-56	937.99		AB
(A-S Medication)				
REPACK				
TAB, PO (FILM-COATED)				
5 mg, 30s ea	54569-6048-00	93.92		AB

PROD/MFR	NDC	AWP	DP	OBC
(American Health)				
REPACK				
TAB, PO (10X10,FILM-COATED)				
5 mg, 100s ea UD	**68084-0247-01**	333.07		AB
(Dispensing Solutions)				
REPACK				
TAB, PO, 5 mg, 30s ea	**55045-3674-08**	94.50		
90s ea	**55045-3674-09**	283.50		
(Phys Total Care)				
REPACK				
TAB, PO, 5 mg, 30s ea	**54868-5636-00**	202.64		
FIORICET (Watson)				
acetaminophen/butalbital/caffeine				
TAB, PO, 325 mg-50 mg-40 mg,				
100s ea	**52544-0957-01**	188.20		AB
500s ea	**52544-0957-05**	896.24		AB
(PD-Rx Pharm)				
REPACK				
TAB, PO, 325 mg-50 mg-40 mg,				
12s ea	**55289-0690-12**	34.85		AB
(Phys Total Care)				
REPACK				
TAB, PO, 325 mg-50 mg-40 mg,				
10s ea	**54868-1053-01**	18.75		AB
30s ea	**54868-1053-02**	52.49		AB
(USP)				
325 mg-50 mg-40 mg,				
40s ea	**54868-1053-05**	69.35		AB
100s ea	**54868-1053-00**	161.20		AB
120s ea	**54868-1053-04**	193.06		AB
(Southwood)				
REPACK				
TAB, PO, 325 mg-50 mg-40 mg,				
30s ea	**58016-0089-30**	51.21		AB
60s ea	**58016-0089-60**	102.42		AB
90s ea	**58016-0089-90**	153.63		AB
100s ea	**58016-0089-00**	170.70		AB
FIORICET W/CODEINE (Phys Total Care)				
REPACK				
apap/butalbital/caff/codeine phos				
CAP, PO				
325 mg-50 mg-40 mg-30 mg,				
30s ea, C-III	**54868-3317-00**	51.03		AB
FIORICET WITH CODEINE (Watson)				
apap/butalbital/caff/codeine phos				
CAP, PO				
325 mg-50 mg-40 mg-30 mg,				
100s ea, C-III	**52544-0958-01**	394.43		AB
(Southwood)				
REPACK				
CAP, PO				
325 mg-50 mg-40 mg-30 mg,				
30s ea, C-III	**58016-0093-30**	107.33		AB
60s ea, C-III	**58016-0093-60**	214.66		AB
90s ea, C-III	**58016-0093-90**	321.98		AB
100s ea, C-III	**58016-0093-00**	357.76		AB
FIORINAL (Watson)				
aspirin/butalbital/caffeine				
CAP, PO, 325 mg-50 mg-40 mg,				
100s ea, C-III	**52544-0955-01**	188.20		AB
(Dispensing Solutions)				
REPACK				
CAP, PO, 325 mg-50 mg-40 mg,				
100s ea, C-III	**55045-3129-01**	150.00		AB
(Phys Total Care)				
REPACK				
CAP, PO, 325 mg-50 mg-40 mg,				
120s ea, C-III	**54868-1031-00**	159.59		AB
TAB, PO, 325 mg-50 mg-40 mg,				
30s ea, C-III	**54868-1031-02**	44.08		AB
(Southwood)				
REPACK				
CAP, PO, 325 mg-50 mg-40 mg,				
30s ea, C-III	**58016-0092-30**	51.21		AB
60s ea, C-III	**58016-0092-60**	102.42		AB
90s ea, C-III	**58016-0092-90**	153.63		AB
100s ea, C-III	**58016-0092-00**	170.70		AB
FIORINAL W/CODEINE (Watson)				
aspirin/butalbital/caffeine/codeine phosphate				
CAP, PO				
325 mg-50 mg-40 mg-30 mg,				
100s ea, C-III	**52544-0956-01**	394.43		AB
(PD-Rx Pharm)				
REPACK				
CAP, PO				
325 mg-50 mg-40 mg-30 mg,				
20s ea, C-III	**55289-0026-20**	111.66		AB
(Phys Total Care)				
REPACK				
CAP, PO				
325 mg-50 mg-40 mg-30 mg,				
20s ea, C-III	**54868-0530-03**	54.21		AB
25s ea, C-III	**54868-0530-02**	67.14		AB
30s ea, C-III	**54868-0530-04**	80.06		AB
50s ea, C-III	**54868-0530-00**	131.78		AB
(Southwood)				
REPACK				
CAP, PO				
325 mg-50 mg-40 mg-30 mg,				
30s ea, C-III	**58016-0091-30**	107.33		AB
60s ea, C-III	**58016-0091-60**	214.66		AB
90s ea, C-III	**58016-0091-90**	321.98		AB
100s ea, C-III	**58016-0091-00**	357.76		AB
FIR NEEDLE OIL				
(Spectrum Pharmacy) *See FIR NEEDLE OIL CANADIAN*				
FIR NEEDLE OIL CANADIAN (Spectrum Pharmacy)				
fir needle oil				
OIL, NA (F.C.C.)				
100 ml	**49452-3158-01**	214.20		
500 ml	**49452-3158-02**	532.00		
FIRMAGON (Ferring)				
degarelix acetate				
PDS, SC (80MGX1,LYOPHILIZED)				
80 mg, ea	**55566-8301-01**	373.20		EE
(120MGX2,LYOPHILIZED)				
120 mg, 2s ea	**55566-8401-01**	1119.60		
FIRST-BXN MOUTHWASH (Cutispharma)				
diphenhydramine hcl/lido hcl/nystatin				
KIT, MR, 0.2 gm-1.6 gm-1.6 gm,				
ea	**65628-0051-01**	38.30		
FIRST-HYDROCORTISONE (Cutispharma)				
hydrocortisone				
KIT, TP (FOR COMPOUNDING)				
10%, 60 gm	**65628-0010-01**	71.00		
FIRST-MOUTHWASH BLM (Cutispharma)				
antacid combination				
KIT, MR, 237 ml	**65628-0050-01**	34.00		
FIRST-PROGESTERONE VGS 100 (Cutispharma)				
progesterone, wettable				
KIT, VG (USP,SUPP COMPOUND KIT)				
100 mg, 30s ea	**65628-0062-01**	90.00		
FIRST-PROGESTERONE VGS 200 (Cutispharma)				
progesterone, wettable				
KIT, VG (USP,SUPP COMPOUND KIT)				
200 mg, 30s ea	**65628-0063-01**	94.60		
FIRST-PROGESTERONE VGS 25 (Cutispharma)				
progesterone, wettable				
KIT, VG (USP,SUPP COMPOUND KIT)				
25 mg, 30s ea	**65628-0060-01**	86.30		
FIRST-PROGESTERONE VGS 400 (Cutispharma)				
progesterone, wettable				
KIT, VG (USP,SUPP COMPOUND KIT)				
400 mg, 30s ea	**65628-0064-01**	99.80		
FIRST-PROGESTERONE VGS 50 (Cutispharma)				
progesterone, wettable				
KIT, VG (USP,SUPP COMPOUND KIT)				
50 mg, 30s ea	**65628-0061-01**	88.00		
FIRST-TESTOSTERONE (Cutispharma)				
testosterone propionate				
KIT, TP (FOR COMPOUNDING)				
2%, 60 gm, C-III	**65628-0020-01**	52.60		
FIRST-TESTOSTERONE MC (Cutispharma)				
testosterone propionate				
KIT, TP (FOR COMPOUNDING)				
2%, 60 gm, C-III	**65628-0021-01**	54.40		
FISH #1 FLAVOR (PCCA)				
flavoring aid				
LIQ, NA (OIL SOLUBLE)				
1 ml	**51927-2903-00**	0.38		
FISH MEAL (PCCA)				
POW, NA (1X1GM)				
1 gm	**51927-3238-00**	0.06		
FISH OIL (PCCA)				
POW, NA, 1 gm	**51927-3373-00**	0.24		
FLAGYL (Pfizer)				
metronidazole				
TAB, PO, 250 mg, 50s ea	**00025-1831-50**	171.18	142.65	AB
100s ea	**00025-1831-31**	342.35	285.29	AB
2500s ea	**00025-1831-55**	8558.78	7132.32	AB
500 mg, 50s ea	**00025-1821-50**	305.80	254.83	AB
100s ea	**00025-1821-31**	611.59	509.66	AB
500s ea	**00025-1821-51**	2284.20	1903.50	AB
FLAGYL 375 (Pfizer)				
metronidazole				
CAP, PO, 375 mg, 50s ea	**00025-1942-50**	261.85	218.21	
FLAGYL ER (Pfizer)				
metronidazole				
TER, PO, 750 mg, 30s ea	**00025-1961-30**	380.86	317.38	
FLAREX (Alcon Ophthalmic)				
fluorometholone acetate				
SUS, OP, 0.1%, 5 ml	**00065-0096-05**	40.56		
FLAVOCOXID				
(Primus Pharma) *See LIMBREL*				
FLAVOCOXID/ZINC, CHELATED				
(Primus Pharma) *See LIMBREL 250*				
(Primus Pharma) *See LIMBREL 500*				
FLAVOR, BACON NATURAL (PCCA)				
flavoring aid				
LIQ, NA (1X1ML)				
1 ml	**51927-3676-00**	1.40		
FLAVOR, CHICKEN BROTH, SPRAY DRIED (PCCA)				
flavoring aid				
POW, NA (1X1GM)				
1 gm	**51927-3646-00**	0.42		
FLAVOR, HAM NATURAL (PCCA)				
flavoring aid				
LIQ, NA (1X1ML)				
1 ml	**51927-3677-00**	1.40		
FLAVOR, IRISH CREAM POWDER (PCCA)				
flavoring aid				
POW, NA (1X1GM)				
1 gm	**51927-3659-00**	0.75		
FLAVOR, PASSION FRUIT NATURAL (PCCA)				
flavoring aid				
POW, NA (1X1GM)				
1 gm	**51927-3661-00**	0.78		
FLAVOR, PIZZA NATURAL (PCCA)				
flavoring aid				
LIQ, NA (1X1ML)				
1 ml	**51927-3675-00**	1.30		
FLAVOR, SHRIMP NATURAL (PCCA)				
flavoring aid				
LIQ, NA (1X1ML)				
1 ml	**51927-3674-00**	1.50		
FLAVOR, WINE (SHERRY) NATURAL (PCCA)				
flavoring aid				
POW, NA (1X1GM)				
1 gm	**51927-3662-00**	0.75		
FLAVORING AID				
(Gallipot) *See APPLE FLAVOR*				
(Gallipot) *See APPLE FLAVORING*				
(Gallipot) *See BACON FLAVOR*				
(Gallipot) *See BANANA FLAVOR*				
(Gallipot) *See BEEF FLAVOR*				
(Gallipot) *See BUBBLE GUM SYRUP*				
(Gallipot) *See CHEESE FLAVOR*				
(Gallipot) *See CHERRY FLAVOR ARTIFICIAL*				
(Gallipot) *See CHICKEN FLAVOR*				
(Gallipot) *See CHOCOLATE FLAVOR*				
(Gallipot) *See GRAPE FLAVOR*				
(Gallipot) *See RASPBERRY FLAVOR*				
(Gallipot) *See SARDINE FLAVOR*				
(Gallipot) *See STRAWBERRY FLAVOR*				
(Gallipot) *See TUTTI-FRUTTI CONCENTRATE*				
(Gallipot) *See WILD CHERRY FLAVOR*				
(Medisca) *See APPLE*				
(Medisca) *See APPLE POWDER*				
(Medisca) *See BACON FLAVOR*				
(Medisca) *See BANANA*				
(Medisca) *See BANANA CREAM*				
(Medisca) *See BANANA DAIQUIRI*				
(Medisca) *See BEEF*				
(Medisca) *See BLACKBERRY*				
(Medisca) *See BLUEBERRY*				
(Medisca) *See BUBBLE GUM*				
(Medisca) *See BUTTER*				
(Medisca) *See BUTTERSCOTCH*				

PROD/MFR | NDC | AWP | DP | OBC

(Medisca) *See CHERRY*

(Medisca) *See CHICKEN FLAVOR*

(Medisca) *See CHICKEN FLAVOR ROASTED*

(Medisca) *See CHOCOLATE*

(Medisca) *See COFFEE*

(Medisca) *See COLA CONCENTRATE*

(Medisca) *See EGGNOG*

(Medisca) *See GRAPE*

(Medisca) *See HOREHOUND*

(Medisca) *See KAHLUA*

(Medisca) *See LEMON EXTRACT, PURE*

(Medisca) *See MAPLE FLAVOR*

(Medisca) *See MARGARITA FLAVOR*

(Medisca) *See MARSHMALLOW FLAVOR*

(Medisca) *See ORANGE FLAVOR*

(Medisca) *See PEACH FLAVOR*

(Medisca) *See PEANUT BUTTER FLAVOR*

(Medisca) *See PINA COLADA FLAVOR*

(Medisca) *See PINEAPPLE FLAVOR*

(Medisca) *See PUMPKIN FLAVOR*

(Medisca) *See RASPBERRY FLAVOR*

(Medisca) *See ROOT BEER FLAVOR*

(Medisca) *See STRAWBERRY*

(Medisca) *See TROPICAL PUNCH*

(Medisca) *See TUNA*

(Medisca) *See TUTTI-FRUTTI*

(Medisca) *See VANILLA BUTTERNUT*

(Medisca) *See WATERMELON*

(Medisca) *See WILD CHERRY*

(PCCA) *See APPLE FLAVOR*

(PCCA) *See APPLE POWDER FLAVOR*

(PCCA) *See APPLE-ADE FLAVOR*

(PCCA) *See APRICOT FLAVOR*

(PCCA) *See BANANA CREME FLAVOR*

(PCCA) *See BANANA FLAVOR*

(PCCA) *See BEEF FLAVOR*

(PCCA) *See BEEF-ADE FLAVOR*

(PCCA) *See BITTER STOP FLAVOR*

(PCCA) *See BLACK WALNUT FLAVOR*

(PCCA) *See BLACKBERRY FLAVOR*

(PCCA) *See BLUEBERRY FLAVOR*

(PCCA) *See BUBBLE GUM FLAVOR*

(PCCA) *See BUTTER FLAVOR*

(PCCA) *See BUTTER RUM FLAVOR*

(PCCA) *See BUTTERSCOTCH FLAVOR*

(PCCA) *See CARAMEL FLAVOR*

(PCCA) *See CHEESE FLAVOR*

(PCCA) *See CHEESE-ADE FLAVOR*

(PCCA) *See CHEESECAKE FLAVOR*

(PCCA) *See CHERRY FLAVOR*

(PCCA) *See CHERRY-ADE FLAVOR*

(PCCA) *See CHICKEN FLAVOR*

(PCCA) *See CHICKEN-ADE FLAVOR*

(PCCA) *See CHOCOLATE FLAVOR*

(PCCA) *See CHOCOLATE HAZELNUT FLAVOR*

(PCCA) *See COCONUT FLAVOR*

(PCCA) *See COFFEE FLAVOR*

(PCCA) *See COLA FLAVOR*

(PCCA) *See COTTON CANDY FLAVOR*

(PCCA) *See CRAN-RASPBERRY FLAVOR*

(PCCA) *See CREME DEMENTHE FLAVOR*

(PCCA) *See EGGNOG FLAVOR*

(PCCA) *See ENGLISH TOFFEE FLAVOR*

(PCCA) *See EUCALYPTOL FLAVOR*

(PCCA) *See EUGENOL FLAVOR*

(PCCA) *See FISH #1 FLAVOR*

(PCCA) *See FLAVOR, BACON NATURAL*

(PCCA) *See FLAVOR, CHICKEN BROTH, SPRAY DRIED*

(PCCA) *See FLAVOR, HAM NATURAL*

(PCCA) *See FLAVOR, IRISH CREAM POWDER*

(PCCA) *See FLAVOR, PASSION FRUIT NATURAL*

(PCCA) *See FLAVOR, PIZZA NATURAL*

(PCCA) *See FLAVOR, SHRIMP NATURAL*

(PCCA) *See FLAVOR, WINE (SHERRY) NATURAL*

(PCCA) *See GRAPE FLAVOR*

(PCCA) *See GUAVA FLAVOR*

(PCCA) *See HONEY FLAVOR*

(PCCA) *See HOREHOUND FLAVOR*

(PCCA) *See KAHLUA FLAVOR*

(PCCA) *See LEMON EXTRACT FLAVOR*

(PCCA) *See LEMON FLAVOR*

(PCCA) *See LEMONADE OIL FLAVOR*

(PCCA) *See LIVER FLAVOR*

(PCCA) *See MAGNASWEET 110*

(PCCA) *See MAGNASWEET 135*

(PCCA) *See MANGO FLAVOR*

(PCCA) *See MAPLE FLAVOR*

(PCCA) *See MARGARITA FLAVOR*

(PCCA) *See MARSHMALLOW FLAVOR*

(PCCA) *See MENTHOL EUCALYPTUS FLAVOR*

(PCCA) *See METHYL SALICYLATE FLAVOR*

(PCCA) *See MINT CHOCOLATE CHIP FLAVOR SOLN*

(PCCA) *See MOLASSES-ADE FLAVOR*

(PCCA) *See ORANGE CREAM FLAVOR*

(PCCA) *See ORANGE FLAVOR*

(PCCA) *See PEACH FLAVOR*

(PCCA) *See PEANUT BUTTER FLAVOR*

(PCCA) *See PINA COLADA FLAVOR*

(PCCA) *See PINEAPPLE FLAVOR*

(PCCA) *See PRALINES AND CREAM FLAVOR*

(PCCA) *See PUMPKIN FLAVOR*

(PCCA) *See RASPBERRY FLAVOR*

(PCCA) *See ROOT BEER FLAVOR*

(PCCA) *See ROOT BEER FLAVOR SOLN*

(PCCA) *See SARSAPARILLA FLAVOR*

(PCCA) *See STRAWBERRY FLAVOR*

(PCCA) *See SUPER SYNERSWEET FLAVOR*

(PCCA) *See SWEETNESS ENHANCE FLAVOR*

(PCCA) *See TANGERINE FLAVOR*

(PCCA) *See TEABERRY OIL FLAVOR*

(PCCA) *See TEQUILA SUNRISE FLAVOR*

(PCCA) *See TROPICAL PUNCH FLAVOR*

(PCCA) *See TUNA FLAVOR*

(PCCA) *See TUTTI FRUTTI FLAVOR*

(PCCA) *See VANILLA BUTTERNUT FLAVOR*

(PCCA) *See VANILLA EXTRACT FLAVOR*

(PCCA) *See WATERMELON FLAVOR*

(PCCA) *See WILD CHERRY FLAVOR*

(Spectrum Pharmacy) *See APPLE FLAVOR*

(Spectrum Pharmacy) *See BANANA ARTIFICIAL FLAVOR*

(Spectrum Pharmacy) *See BANANA CREAM*

(Spectrum Pharmacy) *See BUBBLE GUM ARTIFICIAL FLAVOR*

(Spectrum Pharmacy) *See BUTTERSCOTCH FLAVOR*

(Spectrum Pharmacy) *See CHERRY FLAVOR*

(Spectrum Pharmacy) *See CHICKEN FLAVOR*

(Spectrum Pharmacy) *See CHOCOLATE NATURAL & ARTIFICIAL FLAVOR*

(Spectrum Pharmacy) *See CREME DE MENTHE FLAVOR*

(Spectrum Pharmacy) *See GRAPE ARTIFICIAL FLAVOR*

(Spectrum Pharmacy) *See GREEN APPLE*

(Spectrum Pharmacy) *See LEMON FLAVOR EXTRACT*

(Spectrum Pharmacy) *See MARSHMALLOW*

(Spectrum Pharmacy) *See MOLASSES FLAVOR*

(Spectrum Pharmacy) *See ORANGE FLAVOR*

(Spectrum Pharmacy) *See PEANUT BUTTER FLAVOR*

(Spectrum Pharmacy) *See PINEAPPLE FLAVOR*

(Spectrum Pharmacy) *See RASPBERRY ARTIFICIAL FLAVOR*

(Spectrum Pharmacy) *See ROOTBEER ARTIFICIAL FLAVOR*

(Spectrum Pharmacy) *See STRAWBERRY FLAVOR*

(Spectrum Pharmacy) *See TROPICAL PUNCH*

(Spectrum Pharmacy) *See TUTTI FRUTTI ARTIFICIAL FLAVOR*

(Spectrum Pharmacy) *See VANILLA BUTTERNUT ARTIFICIAL FLAVOR*

(Spectrum Pharmacy) *See WATERMELON ARTIFICIAL FLAVOR*

FLAVOXATE HCL (Global Pharm)
flavoxate hydrochloride
TAB, PO (FILM COATED)
100 mg, 100s ea ..... **00115-1811-01** 146.32 **AB**

(Paddock)
TAB, PO (FILM-COATED)
100 mg, 100s ea ..... **00574-0115-01** 146.32 **AB**

FLAVOXATE HYDROCHLORIDE
(Global Pharm) *See FLAVOXATE HCL*

(Paddock) *See FLAVOXATE HCL*

FLAXSEED (PCCA)
POW, NA (WHOLE FLAXSEED)
1 gm **51927-3190-00** 0.10

FLAXSEED OIL
(Medisca) *See LINSEED OIL*

(PCCA) *See LINSEED OIL*

FLEBOGAMMA (Grifols USA, Inc.)
immune globulin
SOL, IV (DIF,PF)
5 gm/100 ml,
400 ml **61953-0004-05** 1935.36 1612.80

FLEBOGAMMA 5% (Grifols USA, Inc.)
immune globulin
SOL, IV (0.5 GM/VIAL,PF)
50 mg/ml, 10 ml **61953-0003-01** 48.38 40.32
(2.5 GM/VIAL,PF)
50 mg/ml, 50 ml **61953-0003-02** 241.92 201.60
(5 GM/VIAL,PF)
50 mg/ml, 100 ml **61953-0003-03** 483.84 403.20
(10 GM/VIAL,PF)
50 mg/ml, 200 ml **61953-0003-04** 967.68 806.40

FLEBOGAMMA 5% DIF (Grifols USA, Inc.)
immune globulin
SOL, IV (PF)
5 gm/100 ml, 10 ml .. **61953-0004-01** 48.38 40.32
50 ml.............. **61953-0004-02** 241.92 201.60
100 ml **61953-0004-03** 483.84 403.20
200 ml **61953-0004-04** 967.68 806.40

FLECAINIDE (Phys Total Care)
REPACK
flecainide acetate
TAB, PO, 150 mg, 60s ea .. **54868-5586-00** 161.79

FLECAINIDE ACETATE
FUL
TAB, PO, 50 mg, 100s ea.......................... 86.10
100 mg, 100s ea.......................... 140.70
150 mg, 100s ea.......................... 193.28

(Amneal)
TAB, PO (USP)
50 mg, 100s ea ...... **65162-0641-10** 174.05 **AB**
100 mg, 100s ea ..... **65162-0642-10** 273.05 **AB**
150 mg, 100s ea ..... **65162-0643-10** 375.80 **AB**

(Graceway) *See TAMBOCOR*

(Mylan)
TAB, PO, 150 mg, 100s ea . **00378-8515-01** 375.45 **AB**

(Ranbaxy Pharm)
TAB, PO, 50 mg, 100s ea .. **63304-0794-01** 174.09 **AB**
100 mg, 100s ea ..... **63304-0795-01** 273.08 **AB**
150 mg, 100s ea ..... **63304-0796-01** 375.84 **AB**

(Roxane)
TAB, PO, 50 mg, 60s ea ... **00054-0010-21** 104.46 **AB**
100s ea............ **00054-0010-25** 174.10 **AB**
100 mg, 60s ea ...... **00054-0011-21** 163.85 **AB**

PROD/MFR	NDC	AWP	DP	OBC
100s ea	00054-0011-25	273.08		AB
150 mg, 60s ea	00054-0012-21	225.50		AB
100s ea	00054-0012-25	375.84		AB
(Teva)				
TAB, PO, 50 mg, 100s ea	00555-0859-02	174.08		AB
100 mg, 100s ea	00555-0860-02	273.06		AB
150 mg, 100s ea	00555-0861-02	375.81		AB
(A-S Medication)				
REPACK				
TAB, PO, 50 mg, 60s ea	54569-6131-00	104.46		AB
100 mg, 60s ea	54569-6132-00	163.85		AB
(Dispensing Solutions)				
REPACK				
TAB, PO, 50 mg, 100s ea	55045-3819-01	170.00		
(Phys Total Care)				
REPACK				
TAB, PO, 50 mg, 20s ea	54868-5074-01	28.32		AB
60s ea	54868-5074-00	59.13		AB
100 mg, 60s ea	54868-5405-00	93.54		AB
150 mg, 30s ea	54868-5586-01	83.56		AB
(Southwood)				
REPACK				
TAB, PO, 100 mg, 30s ea	58016-0962-30	81.92		AB
40s ea	58016-0962-40	109.22		AB
56s ea	58016-0962-56	152.91		AB
60s ea	58016-0962-60	163.84		AB
90s ea	58016-0962-90	245.75		AB
120s ea	58016-0962-02	327.67		AB
150s ea	58016-0962-03	409.59		AB
240s ea	58016-0962-04	655.34		AB
FLECTOR (King Pharm)				
diclofenac epolamine				
TDM, TP, 1.3%, 30s ea	63857-0111-33	183.65		
(4u)				
REPACK				
TDM, TP, 1.3%, ea	42549-0606-01	11.55		
5s ea	42549-0606-05	57.75		
30s ea	42549-0606-30	288.72		
(Dispensing Solutions)				
REPACK				
TDM, TP, 1.3%, 30s ea	68258-3018-03	220.37		
(IPI)				
REPACK				
TDM, TP, 1.3%, 30s ea	18837-0311-30	179.52		
(Keltman Pharma., Inc.)				
REPACK				
TDM, TP, 1.3%, 30s ea	68387-0641-30	184.30		
(Nucare Pharm)				
REPACK				
TDM, TP, 1.3%, ea	68071-0797-01	8.55		
30s ea	66267-1257-03	318.39		
(Pharma Pac)				
REPACK				
TDM, TP, 1.3%, 30s ea	52959-0518-30	289.90		
(Phys Total Care)				
REPACK				
TDM, TP, 1.3%, 30s ea	54868-5962-00	210.99		
(Physician Partner)				
REPACK				
TDM, TP, 1.3%, ea	21695-0707-01	13.24		
30s ea	21695-0707-30	397.20		
(Quality Care Prod)				
REPACK				
TDM, TP, 1.3%, 30s ea	35356-0077-30	383.00		
(St. Mary's MPP)				
REPACK				
TDM, TP, 1.3%, 30s ea	60760-0111-30	270.87		
(Stat Rx)				
REPACK				
TDM, TP, 1.3%, 30s ea	16590-0566-30	221.91		
FLEET (Southwood)				
REPACK				
na phos, dibasic/na phos, monobasic				
NMA, RC, 135 ml	58016-4895-01	1.07		
FLEXBUMIN (Baxter Bioscience)				
albumin human				
SOL, IV (SINGLE DOSE GALAXY,PF)				
25%, 50 ml	00944-0493-01	115.90		
100 ml	00944-0493-02	231.79		
FLEXERIL (Ortho-McNeil Pharm)				
cyclobenzaprine hydrochloride				
TAB, PO (FILM-COATED)				
5 mg, 100s ea	50580-0280-10	189.13	157.61	
10 mg, 100s ea	50580-0874-11	209.86	174.88	AB

PROD/MFR	NDC	AWP	DP	OBC
(A-S Medication)				
REPACK				
TAB, PO, 10 mg, 12s ea	54569-0835-08	24.30		AB
(DHS, Inc.)				
REPACK				
TAB, PO (FILM-COATED)				
5 mg, 30s ea	55887-0435-30	92.62		
(PD-Rx Pharm)				
REPACK				
TAB, PO (FILM-COATED)				
5 mg, 10s ea	55289-0745-10	26.06		
20s ea	55289-0745-20	52.08		
10 mg, 15s ea	55289-0115-15	52.40		AB
20s ea	55289-0115-20	67.38		AB
21s ea	55289-0115-21	70.37		AB
30s ea	55289-0115-30	97.31		AB
(Pharma Pac)				
REPACK				
TAB, PO (FILM-COATED)				
5 mg, 10s ea	52959-0006-10	16.82		
20s ea	52959-0006-20	33.62		
30s ea	52959-0006-30	49.59		
90s ea	52959-0006-90	148.73		
10 mg, 10s ea	52959-0069-10	19.16		AB
15s ea	52959-0069-15	27.05		AB
20s ea	52959-0069-20	34.60		AB
21s ea	52959-0069-21	35.66		AB
30s ea	52959-0069-30	50.11		AB
(Phys Total Care)				
REPACK				
TAB, PO (FILM-COATED)				
5 mg, 10s ea	54868-5375-01	21.64		
30s ea	54868-5375-00	61.16		
10 mg, 20s ea	54868-0318-04	48.27		AB
30s ea	54868-0318-02	71.79		AB
(FILM-COATED)				
10 mg, 60s ea	54868-0318-01	142.33		AB
90s ea	54868-0318-00	212.88		AB
(FILM-COATED)				
10 mg, 100s ea	54868-0318-03	222.70		AB
(Quality Care Prod)				
REPACK				
TAB, PO (FILM-COATED)				
5 mg, 10s ea	49999-0274-10	34.70		
21s ea	49999-0274-21	35.30		
(FILM-COATED)				
10 mg, 15s ea	35356-0265-15	58.91		AB
20s ea	35356-0265-20	79.55		AB
(Southwood)				
REPACK				
TAB, PO (FILM-COATED)				
5 mg, 30s ea	58016-0987-30	52.56		
60s ea	58016-0987-60	105.12		
90s ea	58016-0987-90	157.68		
100s ea	58016-0987-00	175.20		
120s ea	58016-0987-02	210.24		
150s ea	58016-0987-03	183.00		
150s ea	58016-0987-05	262.80		
10 mg, 30s ea	58016-0070-30	58.32		
(FILM-COATED)				
10 mg, 60s ea	58016-0070-60	116.64		AB
90s ea	58016-0070-90	174.96		AB
100s ea	58016-0070-00	194.40		AB
(Stat Rx)				
REPACK				
TAB, PO, 5 mg, 30s ea	16590-0095-30	62.00		
60s ea	16590-0095-60	114.00		
(FILM-COATED)				
10 mg, 56s ea	16590-0656-56	150.00		AB
84s ea	16590-0656-62	225.00		AB
90s ea	16590-0656-90	241.07		AB
FLEXTRA (Poly)				
acetaminophen/caffeine/phenyltoloxamine citrate				
CAP, PO, 425 mg-35 mg-45 mg,				
100s ea	50991-0436-01	92.49	73.99	
FLEXTRA-650 (Poly)				
acetaminophen/phenyltoloxamine citrate				
TAB, PO, 650 mg-60 mg,				
100s ea	50991-0650-01	64.68	52.87	
FLEXTRA-DS (Poly)				
acetaminophen/phenyltoloxamine citrate				
TAB, PO, 500 mg-50 mg,				
100s ea	50991-0830-01	26.24	20.99	
FLOMAX (Boehr Ingelheim Phar)				
tamsulosin hydrochloride				
CAP, PO, 0.4 mg, 100s ea	00597-0058-01	468.70		

PROD/MFR	NDC	AWP	DP	OBC
(A-S Medication)				
REPACK				
CAP, PO, 0.4 mg, 30s ea	54569-4768-00	123.28		
90s ea	54569-4768-02	462.15		
(AQ)				
REPACK				
CAP, PO, 0.4 mg, 30s ea	66105-0992-03	185.25		
(DHS, Inc.)				
REPACK				
CAP, PO, 0.4 mg, 30s ea	55887-0305-30	126.00		
60s ea	55887-0305-60	246.00		
(Nucare Pharm)				
REPACK				
CAP, PO, 0.4 mg, 30s ea	66267-0693-30	209.00		
60s ea	66267-0693-60	253.00		
(PD-Rx Pharm)				
REPACK				
CAP, PO (REDI-SCRIPT)				
0.4 mg, 30s ea	58864-0882-30	208.08		
(Pharma Pac)				
REPACK				
CAP, PO, 0.4 mg, 10s ea	52959-0947-10	259.81		
(Phys Total Care)				
REPACK				
CAP, PO, 0.4 mg, 4s ea	54868-4356-02	22.39		
10s ea	54868-4356-01	52.06		
30s ea	54868-4356-00	142.71		
60s ea	54868-4356-03	282.80		
90s ea	54868-4356-04	422.89		
(Quality Care Prod)				
REPACK				
CAP, PO, 0.4 mg, 30s ea	49999-0881-30	144.33		
100s ea	49999-0881-00	189.94		
(Southwood)				
REPACK				
CAP, PO, 0.4 mg, 30s ea	58016-0410-30	108.58		
60s ea	58016-0410-60	217.15		
90s ea	58016-0410-90	325.73		
100s ea	58016-0410-00	361.92		
(Stat Rx)				
REPACK				
CAP, PO, 0.4 mg, 4s ea	16590-0489-04	24.50		
30s ea	16590-0489-30	153.10		
60s ea	16590-0489-60	303.17		
90s ea	16590-0489-90	453.25		
100s ea	16590-0489-71	503.30		
FLONASE (Glaxo)				
fluticasone propionate				
SPR, NS, 0.05 mg/actuation,				
16 gm	00173-0453-01	90.95		AB
(A-S Medication)				
REPACK				
SPR, NS, 0.05 mg/actuation,				
16 gm	54569-4120-00	94.74		
(Dispensing Solutions)				
REPACK				
SPR, NS, 0.05 mg/actuation,				
16 gm	55045-2248-08	86.00		
(Phys Total Care)				
REPACK				
SPR, NS, 0.05 mg/actuation,				
16 gm	54868-3718-00	111.26		
(Southwood)				
REPACK				
SPR, NS, 0.05 mg/actuation,				
16 gm	58016-6533-01	90.95		AB
FLOR-DAC TRI-VITAMIN (Perry Med)				
ascorbic acid/sodium fluoride/vitamin a/vitamin d				
CTB, PO, 100s ea	11763-0530-01	3.74		
FLORINEF ACETATE (Phys Total Care)				
REPACK				
fludrocortisone acetate				
TAB, PO, 0.1 mg, 10s ea	54868-1742-00	13.63		AB
60s ea	54868-1742-02	71.75		AB
FLOVENT (Dispensing Solutions)				
REPACK				
fluticasone propionate				
ARO, IH, 0.044 mg/actuation,				
13 gm	55045-3054-01	62.50		
0.11 mg/actuation,				
13 gm	55045-2819-00	84.25		
0.22 mg/actuation,				
13 gm	55045-2919-01	128.00		

PROD/MFR	NDC	AWP	DP	OBC
FLOVENT DISKUS (Glaxo)				
fluticasone propionate				
POW, IH, 50 mcg/actuation,				
60s ea	**00173-0600-02**	104.22		
100 mcg/actuation,				
60s ea	**00173-0602-02**	109.88		
250 mcg/actuation,				
60s ea	**00173-0601-02**	147.13		
(Quality Care Prod)				
REPACK				
POW, IH, 50 mcg/actuation,				
ea	**35356-0494-01**	187.80		
FLOVENT HFA (Glaxo)				
fluticasone propionate				
ARO, IH (WITH DOSE COUNTER)				
0.044 mg/actuation,				
10.6 gm	**00173-0718-20**	109.88		
0.11 mg/actuation,				
12 gm	**00173-0719-20**	147.13		
0.22 mg/actuation,				
12 gm	**00173-0720-20**	228.53		
(A-S Medication)				
REPACK				
ARO, IH, 0.044 mg/actuation,				
10.6 gm	**54569-5671-00**	93.39		
0.11 mg/actuation,				
12 gm	**54569-5663-00**	125.04		
0.22 mg/actuation,				
12 gm	**54569-5702-00**	282.93		
(Dispensing Solutions)				
REPACK				
ARO, IH, 0.044 mg/actuation,				
10.6 gm	**55045-3416-00**	95.00		
0.11 mg/actuation,				
12 gm	**55045-3351-00**	130.00		
0.22 mg/actuation,				
12 gm	**55045-3354-00**	197.00		
(Phys Total Care)				
REPACK				
ARO, IH (1X10.6GM)				
0.044 mg/actuation,				
10.6 gm	**54868-5995-00**	139.69		
0.11 mg/actuation,				
12 gm	**54868-5362-00**	167.84		
0.22 mg/actuation,				
12 gm	**54868-5637-00**	272.48		
(Quality Care Prod)				
REPACK				
ARO, IH, 0.044 mg/actuation,				
ea	**35356-0157-01**	155.14		
0.11 mg/actuation,				
12 gm	**49999-0614-12**	123.28		
FLOW-EZE VENTED (APP)				
needle and/or syringe supplies				
DEV, NA (VENTED PLASTIC NEEDLE)				
500s ea	**63323-0904-90**	247.50		
FLOXIN (A-S Medication)				
REPACK				
ofloxacin				
SOL, OT, 0.3%, 5 ml	**54569-4687-00**	86.63		
(AQ)				
REPACK				
TAB, PO, 200 mg, 50s ea	**66105-0473-05**	270.19		
300 mg, 50s ea	**66105-0474-05**	321.55		
400 mg, 100s ea	**66105-0475-10**	420.56		
(Dispensing Solutions)				
REPACK				
SOL, OT, 0.3%, 5 ml	**55045-2743-05**	82.00		
(Phys Total Care)				
REPACK				
SOL, OT, 0.3%, 5 ml	**54868-4327-00**	106.20		
TAB, PO, 200 mg, 6s ea	**54868-2641-00**	35.38		
25s ea	**54868-2641-02**	144.08		
50s ea	**54868-2641-03**	269.86		
300 mg, 20s ea	**54868-1772-00**	150.00		
50s ea	**54868-1772-02**	371.55		
400 mg, 20s ea	**54868-2201-01**	136.73		
(Quality Care Prod)				
REPACK				
SOL, OT, 0.3%, 10 ml	**49999-0545-10**	169.50		
FLOXIN OTIC SINGLES (Daiichi Sankyo)				
ofloxacin				
SOL, OT, 0.3%, 20s ea	**63395-0101-11**	85.68		
FLOXURIDINE (APP)				
PDS, IJ, 0.5 gm, ea	**63323-0145-07**	150.00		AP
(Bedford)				
PDS, IJ (VIAL)				
0.5 gm, ea	**55390-0135-01**	144.00		AP
(Hospira) *See FUDR*				
FLUARIX (Glaxo)				
influenza virus vaccine (subvirion)				
SOL, IM (2006-2007,PF)				
45 mcg/0.5 ml,				
0.5 ml 5s	**58160-0873-46**	78.75		
(2007-2008,TAX INCL,PF)				
45 mcg/0.5 ml,				
0.5 ml 5s	**58160-0874-46**	78.75		
(Glaxo)				
influenza virus vaccine, inactivated				
(2008-09,TAXINC,5X.5ML)				
45 mcg/0.5 ml,				
0.5 ml 5s	**58160-0875-46**	78.75		
(2009-2010, TAX INC,PF)				
45 mcg/0.5 ml,				
0.5 ml 5s	**58160-0876-46**	78.75		
FLUCAINE (Ocusoft)				
fluorescein sodium/proparacaine hydrochloride				
SOL, OP, 0.25%-0.5%,				
5 ml	**54799-0507-21**	11.87		AT
FLUCONAZOLE				
FUL				
TAB, PO, 50 mg, 30s ea		15.00		
100 mg, 30s ea		26.48		
200 mg, 30s ea		42.23		
(Apotex Corp.)				
SOL, IV (FLEXBAG,DEXTROSE)				
200 mg/100 ml,				
100 ml 10s	**60505-0734-01**	595.50		AP
(FLEXBAG)				
200 mg/100 ml,				
100 ml 10s	**60505-0733-01**	568.50		AP
(FLEXBAG,DEXTROSE)				
400 mg/200 ml,				
200 ml 10s	**60505-0734-02**	882.88		
(FLEXBAG)				
400 mg/200 ml,				
200 ml 10s	**60505-0733-02**	842.88		
TAB, PO, 50 mg, 30s ea	**60505-0119-01**	167.88		
100 mg, 30s ea	**60505-0120-01**	263.79		
150 mg, 12s ea UD	**60505-0121-03**	167.94		
200 mg, 30s ea	**60505-0122-01**	431.66		
(APP)				
SOL, IV (GLASS BOTTLE,10X100ML)				
200 mg/100 ml,				
100 ml 10s	**63323-0308-61**	600.00		
(GLASS BOTTLE,10X200ML)				
400 mg/200 ml,				
200 ml 10s	**63323-0308-63**	875.00		
(Baxter)				
SOL, IV (INTRAVIA CONTAINERS)				
200 mg/100 ml,				
100 ml 10s	**00338-6046-48**	545.76	454.80	
(INTRAVIA CONTAINER)				
400 mg/200 ml,				
200 ml 10s	**00338-6045-37**	809.16	674.30	
(Bedford)				
SOL, IV (1X50ML)				
100 mg/50 ml,				
50 ml	**55390-0194-01**	12.00		EE
200 mg/100 ml,				
100 ml	**55390-0012-01**	18.00		AP
(10X100ML)				
200 mg/100 ml,				
100 ml 10s	**55390-0227-01**	120.00		AP
400 mg/200 ml,				
200 ml	**55390-0046-01**	24.00		AP
(10X200ML)				
400 mg/200 ml,				
200 ml 10s	**55390-0228-01**	180.00		AP
(Gallipot)				
POW, NA (1X1GM)				
1 gm	**51552-1031-01**	12.95	9.25	
(1X5GM)				
5 gm	**51552-1031-02**	49.00	35.00	
(1X25GM)				
25 gm	**51552-1031-04**	175.00	125.00	
(Glenmark Pharmaceuticals)				
TAB, PO, 50 mg, 30s ea	**68462-0101-30**	168.06		AB
100 mg, 30s ea	**68462-0102-30**	264.09		AB
(1X12)				
150 mg, 12s ea UD	**68462-0103-40**	168.13		AB
200 mg, 30s ea	**68462-0104-30**	432.14		AB
(Greenstone)				
PDR, PO (ORANGE)				
50 mg/5 ml, 35 ml	**59762-5029-01**	35.80		
200 mg/5 ml, 35 ml	**59762-5030-01**	130.03		
TAB, PO, 50 mg, 30s ea	**59762-5015-01**	167.13		
100 mg, 30s ea	**59762-5016-01**	262.62		
(BLISTER PAK)				
150 mg, 12s ea UD	**59762-5017-01**	167.20		
200 mg, 30s ea	**59762-5018-01**	429.75		
(Hawkins)				
POW, NA (USP)				
25 gm	**63370-0089-25**	600.00		
100 gm	**63370-0089-35**	1680.00		
500 gm	**63370-0089-45**	3600.00		
1000 gm	**63370-0089-50**	4320.00		
(Hospira) *See AMERINET CHOICE FLUCONAZOLE*				
(Hospira) *See NOVAPLUS FLUCONAZOLE*				
(Hospira)				
SOL, IV (6X100ML,LATEX FREE)				
200 mg/100 ml,				
100 ml 6s	**00409-4688-23**	60.05	52.56	AP
(6X100ML)				
200 mg/100 ml,				
100 ml 6s	**00409-4684-23**	196.27	171.72	AP
(PVC FLEXIBLE BAGS)				
200 mg/100 ml,				
100 ml 10s	**61703-0414-63**	174.72	152.90	
(6X200ML,LATEX-FREE)				
400 mg/200 ml,				
200 ml 6s	**00409-4684-02**	259.20	226.80	
(6X200ML)				
400 mg/200 ml,				
200 ml 6s	**00409-4688-02**	86.40	75.60	AP
(PVC FLEXIBLE BAGS)				
400 mg/200 ml,				
200 ml 10s	**61703-0414-64**	257.76	225.50	
(Medisca)				
POW, NA (1X25GM,USP)				
25 gm	**38779-2442-04**	345.00		
(1X25GM)				
25 gm	**38779-0794-04**	345.00		
(1X100GM,USP)				
100 gm	**38779-2442-05**	900.00		
(1X100GM)				
100 gm	**38779-0794-05**	900.00		
(1X1000GM,USP)				
1000 gm	**38779-2442-09**	2250.00		
(1X1000GM)				
1000 gm	**38779-0794-09**	2250.00		
(Mylan)				
TAB, PO, 50 mg, 30s ea	**00378-2514-93**	167.90		AB
100 mg, 30s ea	**00378-2516-93**	263.80		AB
150 mg, 12s ea UD	**00378-2518-96**	167.90		AB
200 mg, 30s ea	**00378-2520-93**	431.70		AB
(Pfizer) *See DIFLUCAN*				
(Pfizer) *See DIFLUCAN IV*				
(Ranbaxy Pharm)				
PDR, PO (CHERRY)				
50 mg/5 ml, 35 ml	**63304-0975-05**	35.80		AB
200 mg/5 ml, 35 ml	**63304-0976-05**	130.04		AB
TAB, PO, 50 mg, 30s ea	**63304-0803-30**	167.13		AB
100 mg, 30s ea	**63304-0804-30**	262.62		AB
100s ea	**63304-0804-01**	875.40		AB
150 mg, 12s ea UD	**63304-0805-12**	167.20		AB
200 mg, 30s ea	**63304-0806-30**	429.74		AB
100s ea	**63304-0806-01**	1432.46		AB
(Roxane)				
PDR, PO (ORANGE)				
10 mg/ml, 35 ml	**00054-0002-85**	36.00		AB
40 mg/ml, 35 ml	**00054-0003-85**	130.76		AB
(Sagent)				
SOL, IV (10X100ML,PF,LATEX-FREE)				
200 mg/100 ml,				
100 ml 10s	**25021-0113-82**	250.00		AP
(10X200ML,PF,LATEX-FREE)				
400 mg/200 ml,				
200 ml 10s	**25021-0113-87**	312.50		AP
(Sandoz)				
TAB, PO, 50 mg, 30s ea	**00781-1927-31**	168.06		AB
200 mg, 30s ea	**00781-1931-31**	432.14		AB
(Teva) *See FLUCONAZOLE IV*				
(Teva) *See FLUONAZOLE*				
(Teva)				
SOL, IV (6X200ML)				
400 mg/200 ml,				
200 ml 6s	**00703-1020-30**	168.00		AP
TAB, PO, 50 mg, 30s ea	**00172-5410-46**	167.13		AB

PROD/MFR	NDC	AWP	DP	OBC
100s ea UD	00172-5410-10	531.25		AB
100s ea	00172-5410-60	529.25		AB
100 mg, 30s ea	00172-5411-46	262.62		AB
100s ea UD	00172-5411-10	875.39		AB
100s ea	00172-5411-60	831.63		AB
150 mg, 12s ea UD	00093-7204-22	168.13		
12s ea UD	00172-5412-11	167.19		AB
200 mg, 30s ea	00093-7205-56	432.14		
30s ea	00172-5413-46	429.74		AB
100s ea UD	00172-5413-10	1362.85		AB
100s ea	00172-5413-60	1360.85		AB
(West-Ward)				
SOL, IV (6X100ML)				
200 mg/100 ml,				
100 ml 6s	00143-9899-06	112.10		AP
(A-S Medication)				
REPACK				
TAB, PO, 150 mg, ea	54569-5585-00	13.93		
200 mg, 28s ea	54569-5730-00	402.10		AB
30s ea	54569-5730-01	430.82		AB
(B&B Pharm, Inc)				
REPACK				
POW, NA, 1 gm	63275-9960-01	74.00		
5 gm	63275-9960-02	365.00		
25 gm	63275-9960-04	1800.00		
100 gm	63275-9960-05	7100.00		
1000 gm	63275-9960-09	69000.00		
(Core)				
REPACK				
TAB, PO, 150 mg, ea	33358-0143-01	20.39		
12s ea	33358-0143-12	306.63		
(DHS, Inc.)				
REPACK				
TAB, PO, 100 mg, 30s ea	55887-0374-30	50.25		
150 mg, ea	55887-0379-01	7.01		
2s ea	55887-0379-02	13.58		
3s ea	55887-0379-03	20.37		
4s ea	55887-0379-04	27.16		
5s ea	55887-0379-05	31.42		
6s ea	55887-0379-06	37.00		
10s ea	55887-0379-10	56.00		AB
200 mg, ea	55887-0383-01	8.02		
2s ea	55887-0383-02	14.00		
(Dispensing Solutions)				
REPACK				
TAB, PO, 100 mg, 30s ea	55045-3238-08	262.50		
150 mg, ea	55045-3200-01	12.99		
12s ea	55045-3200-02	155.88		
200 mg, 2s ea	55045-3453-02	33.00		
(Keltman Pharma., Inc.)				
REPACK				
TAB, PO, 150 mg, ea	68387-0566-02	35.75		AB
(Nucare Pharm)				
REPACK				
TAB, PO, 150 mg, ea	66267-1307-01	33.78		AB
12s ea	66267-1308-01	173.15		AB
(Palmetto)				
REPACK				
PDR, PO, 10 mg/ml, 35 ml	23490-5580-01	51.72		
40 mg/ml, 35 ml	23490-5579-01	162.78		
TAB, PO, 150 mg, ea	23490-5577-01	18.41		
2s ea	23490-5577-02	36.00		
200 mg, ea	23490-5578-01	27.29		
(PD-Rx Pharm)				
REPACK				
TAB, PO, 150 mg, 12s ea	43063-0028-01	167.20		AB
(REDI-SCRIPT)				
200 mg, 10s ea	58864-0835-10	10.97		AB
20s ea	55289-0824-20	19.78		AB
30s ea	55289-0824-30	23.10		AB
(Pharma Pac)				
REPACK				
TAB, PO, 150 mg, ea	52959-0799-01	15.55		
2s ea	52959-0799-02	35.18		AB
12s ea	52959-0799-12	181.67		
200 mg, 2s ea	52959-0745-02	37.04		
30s ea	52959-0745-30	357.59		
(Phys Total Care)				
REPACK				
PDR, PO (ORANGE)				
10 mg/ml, 35 ml	54868-5248-00	37.86		AB
TAB, PO, 100 mg, ea	54868-5345-04	3.80		
7s ea	54868-5345-01	8.63		
10s ea	54868-5345-00	11.04		
15s ea	54868-5345-03	15.07		
20s ea	54868-5345-05	19.09		
30s ea	54868-5345-02	27.13		
150 mg, ea	54868-5129-00	3.94		

PROD/MFR	NDC	AWP	DP	OBC
12s ea	54868-5129-01	74.73		
200 mg, ea	54868-5144-01	4.26		
3s ea	54868-5144-02	6.81		
7s ea	54868-5144-05	12.92		
10s ea	54868-5144-00	15.66		
14s ea	54868-5144-03	20.73		
20s ea	54868-5144-04	28.32		
30s ea	54868-5144-06	43.98		AB
(Physician Partner)				
REPACK				
TAB, PO, 100 mg, 30s ea	21695-0131-30	528.18		AB
150 mg, ea UD	21695-0193-01	32.78		
2s ea UD	21695-0193-02	55.72		AB
12s ea UD	21695-0193-12	334.32		AB
200 mg, 7s ea	21695-0560-07	235.94		
30s ea	21695-0560-30	859.48		AB
(Quality Care Prod)				
REPACK				
TAB, PO, 100 mg, 2s ea	49999-0765-02	5.59		
150 mg, ea UD	49999-0520-01	4.84		
(Southwood)				
REPACK				
TAB, PO, 100 mg, 30s ea	58016-0061-30	262.62		
60s ea	58016-0061-60	525.24		
90s ea	58016-0061-90	787.86		
100s ea	58016-0061-00	875.40		
200 mg, 30s ea	58016-0494-30	356.68		
60s ea	58016-0494-60	713.36		
90s ea	58016-0494-90	1070.04		
100s ea	58016-0494-00	1188.93		
120s ea	58016-0494-02	1426.72		
(Stat Rx)				
REPACK				
TAB, PO, 150 mg, ea	16590-0282-01	13.75		
2s ea	16590-0282-02	27.50		
3s ea	16590-0282-03	41.25		
(Vibranta)				
REPACK				
TAB, PO, 200 mg, 3s ea	57866-0267-02	62.13		
14s ea	57866-0267-03	68.11		
FLUCONAZOLE IV (Teva)				
fluconazole				
SOL, IV, 200 mg/100 ml,				
100 ml 6s	00703-1019-09	114.00		
(6X100ML)				
200 mg/100 ml,				
100 ml 6s	00703-1029-30	126.00		
400 mg/200 ml,				
200 ml 6s	00703-1010-09	245.00		
FLUCYTOSINE				
(Valeant Pharm Intl) *See ANCOBON*				
FLUDARA (Genzyme)				
fludarabine phosphate				
PDS, IV, 50 mg, ea	50419-0511-06	367.02	305.85	
FLUDARABINE PHOSPHATE (APP)				
PDS, IV (USP)				
50 mg, ea	63323-0196-06	344.09		AP
SOL, IV (SDV, 1X2ML)				
25 mg/ml, 2 ml	63323-0192-02	344.00		AP
(Genzyme) *See FLUDARA*				
(Hospira)				
PDS, IV (USP,LYOPHILIZED)				
50 mg, ea	61703-0344-18	166.93	146.07	AP
(Parenta Pharma)				
SOL, IV (SDV,PF)				
25 mg/ml, 2 ml	66758-0046-01	350.00		AP
(Sagent)				
PDS, IV (USP,SINGLE-DOSE,PF)				
50 mg, ea	25021-0205-05	344.09		AP
(Sanofi-Aventis) *See OFORTA*				
(Teva) *See NOVAPLUS FLUDARABINE PHOSPHATE*				
(Teva) *See OTN FLUDARABINE PHOSPHATE*				
(Teva)				
PDS, IV, 50 mg, ea	00703-5854-01	289.07		AP
SOL, IV (SDV)				
25 mg/ml, 2 ml	00703-4852-11	289.07		
FLUDROCORTISONE ACETATE (Gallipot)				
POW, NA (U.S.P.,MICRONIZED)				
1 gm	51552-0912-01	54.60	39.00	
(Global Pharm)				
TAB, PO, 0.1 mg, 100s ea	00115-7033-01	74.77		AB
500s ea	00115-7033-02	373.85		AB
(Medisca)				
POW, NA (U.S.P.,MICRONIZED)				
1 gm	38779-0129-06	118.50		

PROD/MFR	NDC	AWP	DP	OBC
5 gm	38779-0129-03	358.50		
25 gm	38779-0129-04	1455.00		
100 gm	38779-0129-05	4470.00		
(Spectrum Pharmacy)				
POW, NA (U.S.P./N.F.,MICRONIZED)				
1 gm	49452-3155-01	207.20		
5 gm	49452-3155-02	605.50		
(Teva)				
TAB, PO (USP)				
0.1 mg, 100s ea	00555-0997-02	79.35		
(American Health)				
REPACK				
TAB, PO (10X10)				
0.1 mg, 100s ea UD	68084-0288-01	80.25		AB
(Phys Total Care)				
REPACK				
TAB, PO, 0.1 mg, 10s ea	54868-5446-03	26.19		
15s ea	54868-5446-00	37.05		
20s ea	54868-5446-02	47.88		
30s ea	54868-5446-04	69.58		
60s ea	54868-5446-01	104.04		
FLUDROCORTISONE ACETATE MICRONIZED				
(Hawkins)				
fludrocortisone acetate, micronized				
POW, NA (USP)				
1 gm	63370-0092-10	128.00		
5 gm	63370-0092-15	420.00		
25 gm	63370-0092-25	1960.00		
(PCCA)				
POW, NA (USP)				
1 gm	51927-2408-00	162.00		
FLUDROCORTISONE ACETATE, MICRONIZED				
(Hawkins) *See FLUDROCORTISONE ACETATE MICRONIZED*				
(PCCA) *See FLUDROCORTISONE ACETATE MICRONIZED*				
FLULAVAL (Glaxo)				
influenza virus vaccine (subvirion)				
SOL, IM (GSK 888-822-2749 OPT 1)				
45 mcg/0.5 ml,				
5 ml	19515-0884-07			
5 ml	19515-0885-07			
5 ml	19515-0886-07			
FLUMADINE (Forest Pharm)				
rimantadine hydrochloride				
TAB, PO, 100 mg, 100s ea	00456-0521-01	262.36		AB
(Pharma Pac)				
REPACK				
TAB, PO, 100 mg, 10s ea	52959-0490-10	25.60		
14s ea	52959-0490-14	32.62		
20s ea	52959-0490-20	44.60		
(Phys Total Care)				
REPACK				
TAB, PO, 100 mg, 20s ea	54868-3441-00	57.68		AB
FLUMAZENIL (Akorn)				
SOL, IV (USP,MDV,10X5ML)				
0.1 mg/ml,				
5 ml 10s	23360-0031-05	92.80		AP
(USP,MDV,10X10ML)				
0.1 mg/ml,				
10 ml 10s	23360-0031-10	185.70		AP
(Apotex Corp.)				
SOL, IV, 0.1 mg/ml,				
5 ml 10s	60505-0667-01	886.85		AP
10 ml 10s	60505-0667-02	1410.85		AP
(APP)				
SOL, IV (M.D.V.,10X5ML)				
0.1 mg/ml,				
5 ml 10s	63323-0424-05	512.50		
(M.D.V.)				
0.1 mg/ml, 10 ml	63323-0424-10	78.00		
(Baxter)				
SOL, IV (MDV)				
0.1 mg/ml, 5 ml	10019-0321-54	18.60		AP
(M.D.V.)				
0.1 mg/ml,				
5 ml 10s	10019-0321-01	123.00		AP
(MDV)				
0.1 mg/ml, 10 ml	10019-0321-62	28.62		AP
(M.D.V.)				
0.1 mg/ml,				
10 ml 10s	10019-0321-02	286.20		AP
(Bedford)				
SOL, IV (M.D.V.)				
0.1 mg/ml,				
5 ml 10s	55390-0092-10	90.00		AP
10 ml 10s	55390-0093-10	180.00		AP

PROD/MFR	NDC	AWP	DP	OBC
(Roche Labs) *See ROMAZICON*				
(Sandoz)				
SOL, IV (1X5ML)				
0.1 mg/ml, 5 ml	**00781-3003-75**	93.22		**AP**
(10X5ML)				
0.1 mg/ml, 5 ml 10s	**00781-3003-92**	932.22		**AP**
(1X10ML,MULTI-DOSE)				
0.1 mg/ml, 10 ml	**00781-3003-70**	148.31		**AP**
(10X10ML)				
0.1 mg/ml, 10 ml 10s	**00781-3003-95**	1483.05		**AP**
(Teva) *See NOVAPLUS FLUMAZENIL*				
(West-Ward)				
SOL, IV (10X5ML,MULTIPLE-DOSE)				
0.1 mg/ml, 5 ml 10s	**00143-9784-10**	81.25		
(10X10ML,MULTIPLE-DOSE)				
0.1 mg/ml, 10 ml 10s	**00143-9783-10**	162.50		
(Phys Total Care) REPACK				
SOL, IV (10X5ML)				
0.1 mg/ml, 5 ml 10s	**54868-5715-00**	351.54		
FLUMIST (Medimmune)				
influenza virus vaccine, live				
SOL, NS (2006-2007, TAX INCL,PF)				
10s ea	**66019-0104-01**	222.90		
(2007-2008, TAX INCL,PF)				
10s ea	**66019-0105-01**	231.90		
(2008-2009,TAX INCL,PF)				
10s ea	**66019-0106-01**	234.90		
(2009-2010, TAX INCL)				
10s ea	**66019-0107-01**	234.90		
FLUNISOLIDE (Apotex Corp.)				
SPR, NS, 29 mcg/actuation, 25 ml	**60505-0824-00**	54.96		**AB**
(Bausch & Lomb Inc.)				
SPR, NS, 0.025 mg/actuation, 25 ml	**24208-0344-25**	46.49		
(Forest Pharm) *See AEROBID*				
(Forest Pharm) *See AEROBID-M*				
(Gallipot) *See FLUNISOLIDE ANHYDROUS*				
(Medisca) *See FLUNISOLIDE ANHYDROUS*				
(PCCA) *See FLUNISOLIDE ANHYDROUS*				
(Rising)				
SPR, NS (W/PUMP AND ACTUATOR)				
0.025 mg/actuation, 25 ml	**64980-0506-25**	46.49		**AB**
(Spectrum Pharmacy) *See FLUNISOLIDE ANHYDROUS*				
(Phys Total Care) REPACK				
SPR, NS, 0.025 mg/actuation, 25 ml	**54868-4799-00**	123.78		
(Southwood) REPACK				
SPR, NS, 0.025 mg/actuation, 25 ml	**58018-4878-01**	46.49		
FLUNISOLIDE ANHYDROUS (Gallipot)				
flunisolide				
POW, NA (U.S.P.,MICRONIZED)				
1 gm	**51552-0611-01**	302.40		
5 gm	**51552-0611-02**	1162.00		
(Medisca)				
POW, NA (U.S.P.,MICRONIZED)				
0.1 gm	**38779-0406-09**	165.00		
0.5 gm	**38779-0406-00**	480.00		
1 gm	**38779-0406-06**	795.00		
(PCCA)				
POW, NA (U.S.P.)				
1 gm	**51927-1794-00**	900.00		
(Spectrum Pharmacy)				
POW, NA (MICRONIZED)				
0.1 gm	**49452-3162-01**	260.40		
0.5 gm	**49452-3162-02**	927.50		
1 gm	**49452-3162-03**	1015.00		
FLUNIXIN MEGLUMINE (Gallipot)				
POW, NA (U.S.P.)				
25 gm	**51552-0993-04**	168.00	120.00	
(Letco)				
POW, NA (U.S.P., VET USE ONLY)				
100 gm	**62991-1604-02**	375.00		
1000 gm	**62991-1604-04**	2250.00		
(Medisca)				
POW, NA (U.S.P.)				
25 gm	**38779-1934-04**	477.00		
100 gm	**38779-1934-05**	1650.00		
1000 gm	**38779-1934-09**	5550.00		
(PCCA)				
POW, NA (U.S.P.)				
1 gm	**51927-3254-00**	34.56		
(Spectrum Pharmacy)				
CRY, NA (U.S.P.)				
25 gm	**49452-3153-01**	731.50		
100 gm	**49452-3153-02**	2226.00		
FLUOBORIC ACID				
(Baker, J.T.) *See FLUOBORIC ACID 48-50%*				
FLUOBORIC ACID 48-50% (Baker, J.T.)				
fluoboric acid				
LIQ, NA (PURIFIED)				
500 ml	**10106-9528-01**	83.40		
FLUOCINOLONE (Southwood) REPACK				
fluocinolone acetonide				
SOL, TP, 0.01%, 60 ml	**58016-4787-01**	11.00		
(Stat Rx) REPACK				
CRE, TP, 0.01%, 30 gm	**16590-0097-30**	10.25		
FLUOCINOLONE ACETONIDE				
(Bausch & Lomb Inc.) *See RETISERT*				
(Consolidated Midland)				
CRE, TP, 0.01%, 15 gm	**00223-4297-15**	1.95		**EE**
60 gm	**00223-4297-60**	4.25		**EE**
425 gm	**00223-4297-13**	17.50		**EE**
0.025%, 15 gm	**00223-4296-15**	2.50		**EE**
60 gm	**00223-4296-60**	7.25		**EE**
425 gm	**00223-4296-13**	45.00		**EE**
OIN, TP, 0.025%, 15 gm	**00223-4290-15**	4.95		**EE**
30 gm	**00223-4290-60**	10.75		**EE**
SOL, TP, 0.01%, 20 ml	**00223-6180-20**	5.00		**EE**
60 ml	**00223-6180-60**	11.50		**EE**
(Fougera)				
CRE, TP, 0.01%, 15 gm	**00168-0058-15**	9.90		**AT**
60 gm	**00168-0058-60**	29.70		**AT**
0.025%, 15 gm	**00168-0060-15**	7.50		**AT**
60 gm	**00168-0060-60**	22.50		**AT**
OIN, TP, 0.025%, 15 gm	**00168-0064-15**	7.50		**AT**
60 gm	**00168-0064-60**	22.50		**AT**
SOL, TP, 0.01%, 60 ml	**00168-0059-60**	14.40		**AT**
(Galderma) *See CAPEX*				
(Gallipot)				
POW, NA (U.S.P.)				
1 gm	**51552-0134-01**	37.03		
(U.S.P., MICRONIZED)				
5 gm	**51552-0134-02**	154.00		
(Hill Derm) *See DERMA-SMOOTHE/FS*				
(Hill Derm) *See DERMOTIC OIL*				
(Medisca) *See FLUOCINOLONE ACETONIDE ANHYDROUS*				
(Spectrum Pharmacy) *See FLUOCINOLONE ACETONIDE ANHYDROUS*				
(A-S Medication) REPACK				
CRE, TP, 0.01%, 15 gm	**54569-1544-00**	10.31		**AT**
FLUOCINOLONE ACETONIDE (Palmetto) REPACK				
CRE, TP (1X15GM)				
0.01%, 15 gm	**23490-5583-00**	24.78		
FLUOCINOLONE ACETONIDE (Pharma Pac) REPACK				
CRE, TP, 0.01%, 15 gm	**52959-0314-00**	12.95		**EE**
0.025%, 15 gm	**52959-0184-01**	4.69		
(Phys Total Care) REPACK				
CRE, TP, 0.01%, 15 gm	**54868-3660-01**	4.73		**EE**
60 gm	**54868-3660-00**	8.33		**EE**
0.025%, 15 gm	**54868-0978-01**	7.20		**EE**
60 gm	**54868-0978-00**	9.30		**AT**
SOL, TP, 0.01%, 20 ml	**54868-2264-00**	12.81		**EE**
(1X60ML)				
0.01%, 60 ml	**54868-2264-01**	14.49		**AT**
(Southwood) REPACK				
CRE, TP, 0.01%, 15 gm	**58016-3083-01**	4.78		**EE**
0.025%, 15 gm	**58016-3104-01**	4.64		**EE**
FLUOCINOLONE ACETONIDE ANHYDROUS (Medisca)				
fluocinolone acetonide				
POW, NA (U.S.P.,MICRONIZED)				
1 gm	**38779-0022-06**	174.00		
5 gm	**38779-0022-03**	615.00		
(MICRONIZED)				
10 gm	**38779-0022-01**	754.50		
25 gm	**38779-0022-04**	1696.50		
(USP,1X250MG,MICRONIZED)				
250 ml	**38779-0022-07**	72.00		
(USP,1X500MG,MICRONIZED)				
500 ml	**38779-0022-00**	120.00		
(Spectrum Pharmacy)				
POW, NA (U.S.P./N.F.,MICRONIZED)				
0.25 gm	**49452-3156-01**	130.55		
1 gm	**49452-3156-02**	244.30		
5 gm	**49452-3156-03**	1081.50		
FLUOCINOLONE ACETONIDE/HYDROQUINONE/TRETINOIN				
(Galderma) *See TRI-LUMA*				
FLUOCINONIDE				
FUL				
CRE, TP, 0.05%, 60 gm		7.12		
EMO, TP, 0.05%, 60 gm		14.72		
GEL, TP, 0.05%, 60 gm		29.79		
SOL, TP, 0.05%, 60 ml		15.84		
(Fougera)				
CRE, TP, 0.05%, 15 gm	**00168-0139-15**	10.61		**AB**
30 gm	**00168-0139-30**	14.75		**AB**
60 gm	**00168-0139-60**	24.03		**AB**
EMO, TP (EMOLLIENT BASE)				
0.05%, 15 gm	**00168-0246-15**	19.45		
30 gm	**00168-0246-30**	26.82		
60 gm	**00168-0246-60**	45.00		
GEL, TP, 0.05%, 15 gm	**00168-0135-15**	21.01		**AB**
60 gm	**00168-0135-60**	48.83		**AB**
SOL, TP, 0.05%, 60 ml	**00168-0134-60**	27.27		**AT**
(Gallipot)				
POW, NA (U.S.P.,MICRONIZED)				
1 gm	**51552-0056-01**	41.30		
(U.S.P.)				
5 gm	**51552-0056-02**	185.85		
(Medicis) *See VANOS*				
(Medisca)				
POW, NA (U.S.P.,MICRONIZED)				
1 gm	**38779-0018-06**	79.50		
5 gm	**38779-0018-03**	352.50		
10 gm	**38779-0018-01**	616.50		
25 gm	**38779-0018-04**	1377.00		
(Spectrum Pharmacy)				
POW, NA (U.S.P./N.F.,MICRONIZED)				
0.25 gm	**49452-3161-01**	95.20		
1 gm	**49452-3161-02**	183.75		
5 gm	**49452-3161-03**	798.00		
(Taro)				
CRE, TP, 0.05%, 15 gm	**51672-1253-01**	9.00		**AB**
30 gm	**51672-1253-02**	13.90		**AB**
60 gm	**51672-1253-03**	23.72		**AB**
120 gm	**51672-1253-04**	42.00		**AB**
(Taro) *See FLUOCINONIDE E*				
(Taro)				
GEL, TP, 0.05%, 15 gm	**51672-1279-01**	20.87		**AB**
30 gm	**51672-1279-02**	28.94		**AB**
60 gm	**51672-1279-03**	48.55		**AB**
OIN, TP, 0.05%, 15 gm	**51672-1264-01**	21.04		**AB**
30 gm	**51672-1264-02**	29.19		**AB**
60 gm	**51672-1264-03**	49.00		**AB**
SOL, TP, 0.05%, 20 ml	**51672-1273-02**	16.88		**AT**
60 ml	**51672-1273-04**	27.00		**AT**
(Teva)				
CRE, TP, 0.05%, 15 gm	**00093-0262-15**	8.97		**AB**
30 gm	**00093-0262-30**	13.02		**AB**
60 gm	**00093-0262-92**	21.84		**AB**
(Teva) *See FLUOCINONIDE E*				
(Teva)				
GEL, TP, 0.05%, 60 gm	**00093-0265-92**	46.01		**AB**
OIN, TP, 0.05%, 15 gm	**00093-0264-15**	19.91		**AB**
30 gm	**00093-0264-30**	27.51		**AB**
60 gm	**00093-0264-92**	46.01		**AB**
SOL, TP, 0.05%, 60 ml	**00093-0266-39**	26.18		**AT**
(A-S Medication) REPACK				
CRE, TP, 0.05%, 15 gm	**54569-2177-00**	9.53		**EE**
30 gm	**54569-3887-00**	13.90		**EE**
60 gm	**54569-2275-00**	23.72		**EE**
OIN, TP, 0.05%, 15 gm	**54569-4210-00**	21.04		**EE**

PROD/MFR	NDC	AWP	DP	OBC
(Altura)				
REPACK				
CRE, TP, 0.05%, 15 gm	63874-0811-15	25.41		AB
30 gm	63874-0811-30	30.35		AB
60 gm	63874-0811-60	35.26		AB
OIN, TP, 0.05%, 15 gm	63874-0864-15	22.15		
(DHS, Inc.)				
REPACK				
CRE, TP, 0.05%, 15 gm	55887-0777-15	12.09		AB
30 gm	55887-0777-30	23.66		AB
(Dispensing Solutions)				
REPACK				
CRE, TP, 0.05%, 15 gm	55045-2047-05	23.25		AB
(1X15GM)				
0.05%, 15 gm	55045-3936-01	23.25		AB
30 gm	55045-2047-06	30.50		AB
GEL, TP, 0.05%, 15 gm	55045-3787-05	24.00		
(IPI)				
REPACK				
CRE, TP (1X15GM)				
0.05%, 15 gm	18837-0331-15	24.91		
(Keltman Pharma., Inc.)				
REPACK				
CRE, TP (1X30GM)				
0.05%, 30 gm	68387-0627-01	26.50		AB
(Nucare Pharm)				
REPACK				
CRE, TP, 0.05%, 15 gm	66267-0973-15	27.40		AB
(Palmetto)				
REPACK				
CRE, TP, 0.05%, 15 gm	23490-5588-01	25.36		
30 gm	23490-5588-02	46.65		
(1X60GM)				
0.05%, 60 gm	23490-5588-03	77.99		
(Pharma Pac)				
REPACK				
CRE, TP, 0.05%, 15 gm	52959-0093-01	25.36		EE
15 gm	52959-0299-05	15.66		AB
30 gm	52959-0093-03	30.35		EE
30 gm	52959-0299-30	29.32		AB
60 gm	52959-0093-02	48.98		EE
60 gm	52959-0299-60	51.65		AB
GEL, TP, 0.05%, 60 gm	52959-0652-60	60.50		AB
OIN, TP, 0.05%, 15 gm	52959-0315-01	22.15		EE
30 gm	52959-0315-03	46.65		EE
(Phys Total Care)				
REPACK				
CRE, TP, 0.05%, 15 gm	54868-0431-02	6.48		EE
30 gm	54868-0431-03	8.16		EE
60 gm	54868-0431-01	11.34		EE
GEL, TP, 0.05%, 60 gm	54868-3023-00	44.25		AB
OIN, TP (1X15GM)				
0.05%, 15 gm	54868-3435-02	21.46		AB
30 gm	54868-3435-00	42.21		EE
60 gm	54868-3435-01	80.88		EE
SOL, TP, 0.05%, 60 ml	54868-2451-01	25.11		EE
(Physician Partner)				
REPACK				
EMO, TP, 0.05%, 15 gm	21695-0207-15	38.80		
60 gm	21695-0207-60	90.12		
(Quality Care Prod)				
REPACK				
CRE, TP, 0.05%, 15 gm	49999-0172-15	28.98		AB
30 gm	49999-0172-30	57.96		AB
(Southwood)				
REPACK				
CRE, TP, 0.05%, 15 gm	58016-3042-01	23.29		EE
30 gm	58016-3121-01	24.90		EE
GEL, TP, 0.05%, 15 gm	58016-4879-01	21.01		EE
60 gm	58016-3274-01	52.55		EE
(Stat Rx)				
REPACK				
CRE, TP, 0.05%, 15 gm	16590-0368-15	24.00		
30 gm	16590-0368-30	22.00		
(1X30GM)				
0.05%, 30 gm	16590-0398-30	7.00		
60 gm	16590-0368-60	29.00		
(1X60GM)				
0.05%, 60 gm	16590-0398-60	14.00		
FLUOCINONIDE E (Taro)				
fluocinonide				
EMO, TP (EMULSIFIED BASE)				
0.05%, 15 gm	51672-1254-01	19.40		AB
30 gm	51672-1254-02	26.88		AB
60 gm	51672-1254-03	45.06		AB
(Teva)				
EMO, TP (EMULSIFIED BASE)				
0.05%, 15 gm	00093-0263-15	19.90		AB
30 gm	00093-0263-30	27.50		AB
60 gm	00093-0263-92	46.00		AB
(Phys Total Care)				
REPACK				
EMO, TP, 0.05%, 30 gm	54868-3408-00	28.59		EE
60 gm	54868-3408-01	49.96		EE
(Physician Partner)				
REPACK				
EMO, TP, 0.05%, 30 gm	21695-0207-30	77.60		AB
FLUOCINONIDE MICRONIZED (PCCA)				
fluocinonide, micronized				
POW, NA (USP, 1X1GM)				
1 gm	51927-1616-00	78.00		
FLUOCINONIDE, MICRONIZED				
(PCCA) *See FLUOCINONIDE MICRONIZED*				
FLUONAZOLE (Teva)				
fluconazole				
PDR, PO (1X35ML,ORANGE)				
10 mg/ml, 35 ml	00093-5414-95	36.46		
40 mg/ml, 35 ml	00093-5415-95	132.45		
FLUOR-A-DAY (Pharmascience Labs)				
sodium fluoride				
CTB, PO (SF,RASPBERRY)				
0.25 mg, 120s ea	51817-0602-16	9.33		
0.5 mg, 120s ea	51817-0611-16	9.63		
1 mg, 120s ea	51817-0622-16	9.93		
LIQ, PO (DROPS)				
0.125 mg/drp,				
30 ml	51817-0656-61	6.32		
FLUOR-I-STRIP A.T. (Phys Total Care)				
REPACK				
fluorescein sodium				
TES, OP, 1 mg, 300s ea	54868-5127-00	98.00		
FLUORABON (Perry Med)				
sodium fluoride				
CTB, PO (ORANGE)				
1 mg, 100s ea	11763-0525-01	2.31		
100s ea	11763-0526-01	2.31		
LIQ, PO (DROPS)				
0.25 mg/0.6 ml,				
60 ml	11763-0524-20	3.08		
FLUORACAINE (Akorn)				
fluorescein sodium/proparacaine hydrochloride				
SOL, OP (GLASS BOTTLE)				
0.25%-0.5%, 5 ml	17478-0320-10	9.15		
FLUORES/BENOX (Phys Total Care)				
REPACK				
benoxinate hydrochloride/fluorescein sodium				
SOL, OP, 0.4%-0.25%,				
5 ml	54868-3957-00	31.41		
FLUORESCEIN (HUB Pharma)				
fluorescein sodium				
SOL, IV (SDV,5MLX12,USP,STERILE)				
10%, 5 ml 12s	17238-0301-05	56.25		
(SDV,2MLX12,USP,STERILE)				
25%, 2 ml 12s	17238-0401-02	56.25		
FLUORESCEIN (PCCA)				
POW, NA (C.I. 45350)				
1 gm	51927-1852-00	0.78		
FLUORESCEIN LITE (Altaire)				
fluorescein sodium				
SOL, IV (S.D.V.)				
10%, 5 ml	59390-0188-05	4.68		
25%, 2 ml	59390-0187-02	4.68		
FLUORESCEIN SODIUM				
(Akorn) *See AK-FLUOR*				
(Akorn) *See FUL-GLO*				
(Alcon Ophthalmic) *See FLUORESCITE*				
(Altaire) *See FLUORESCEIN LITE*				
(Altaire)				
SOL, IV (SDV,12X5ML,BURGANDY DYE)				
10%, 5 ml 12s	59390-0199-05	7.80		
(SDV,12X2ML,DARKBURGANDY)				
25%, 2 ml 12s	59390-0200-02	7.80		
(Bausch & Lomb Inc.) *See FLUORETS*				
(Eyesupply USA) *See ANGIOSCEIN*				
(Gallipot)				
POW, NA (USP,1X25GM)				
25 gm	51552-0968-04	15.05	10.75	
(USP,1X100GM)				
100 gm	51552-0968-05	38.50	27.50	
(HUB Pharma) *See BIO GLO*				
(HUB Pharma) *See FLUORESCEIN*				
(PCCA)				
POW, NA (U.S.P.)				
1 gm	51927-1681-00	0.96		
(Spectrum Pharmacy)				
POW, NA (U.S.P.)				
25 gm	49452-3160-03	121.45		
100 gm	49452-3160-01	235.55		
1000 gm	49452-3160-02	1477.00		
FLUORESCEIN SODIUM AND BENOXINATE HYDROCHLORIDE (HUB Pharma)				
benoxinate hydrochloride/fluorescein sodium				
SOL, OP (DROPS)				
0.4%-0.25%, 5 ml	17238-0501-05	8.19		
FLUORESCEIN SODIUM/PROPARACAINE HYDROCHLORIDE				
(Akorn) *See FLUORACAINE*				
(Altaire) *See FLUOROCAINE SOD/PROPARACAINE HCL*				
(Ocusoft) *See FLUCAINE*				
FLUORESCEIN/BENOXINATE (DHS, Inc.)				
REPACK				
benoxinate hydrochloride/fluorescein sodium				
SOL, OP, 0.4%-0.25%,				
5 ml	55887-0778-05	14.75		
(Southwood)				
REPACK				
SOL, OP, 0.4%-0.25%,				
5 ml	58016-4994-01	11.81		
FLUORESCITE (Alcon Ophthalmic)				
fluorescein sodium				
SOL, IV (1X5ML,LATEX-FREE)				
10%, 5 ml	00065-0092-65	31.44		AP
FLUORETS (Bausch & Lomb Inc.)				
fluorescein sodium				
TES, OP (STRIP)				
1 mg, 100s ea	24208-0391-82	22.97		
(Quality Care Prod)				
REPACK				
TES, OP, 1 mg, 100s ea	35356-0179-00	56.40		
FLUORI-METHANE (Phys Total Care)				
REPACK				
dichlorodifluoromethane/trichlorofluoromethane				
SPR, TP (FINE)				
15%-85%, 103 ml	54868-4156-00	39.30		
FLUORIDE (Cypress Pharm)				
sodium fluoride				
CTB, PO (SF,SACCHARIN-FREE,LEMON)				
0.25 mg, 120s ea	60258-0155-20	6.65		
(SF,SACCHARIN-FREE,GRAPE)				
0.5 mg, 120s ea	60258-0156-20	6.89		
1000s ea	60258-0156-10	55.44		
1 mg, 120s ea	60258-0157-20	6.65		
FLUORIDEX DAILY DEFENSE (Discus Dental)				
sodium fluoride				
GEL, DE (1X113GM)				
1.1%, 113 gm	64854-0020-01	11.99		
FLUORIDEX DAILY DEFENSE ENHANCED WHITENING (Discus Dental)				
sodium fluoride				
GEL, DE (ENHANCED WHITENING,MINT)				
1.1%, 113 gm	64854-0016-01	9.99		
FLUORIDEX DAILY DEFENSE SENSITIVITY RELIEF (Discus Dental)				
potassium nitrate/sodium fluoride				
GEL, MM (1X112GM)				
5%-1.1%, 112 gm	64854-0031-01	13.99		
FLUORINSE (Oral B Lab)				
sodium fluoride				
SOL, PO (AF,CINNAMON)				
0.2%, 480 ml	00041-0351-07	7.49		
(AF,MINT)				
0.2%, 480 ml	00041-0350-07	7.49		
FLUORITAB (Fluoritab)				
sodium fluoride				
CTB, PO (CHERRY)				
0.5 mg, 100s ea	00288-1106-01	4.60		
1000s ea	00288-1106-10	22.00		
5000s ea	00288-1106-02	48.00		
1 mg, 100s ea	00288-2203-01	4.60		
1000s ea	00288-2203-10	22.00		
5000s ea	00288-2203-02	48.00		
LIQ, PO (DYE-FREE,DROPS)				
0.25 mg/drp, 23 ml	00288-5523-23	4.60		

PROD/MFR	NDC	AWP	DP	OBC
FLUORO/GLY GEL (Topix)				
glycolic acid				
GEL, TP (OFFICE USE ONLY)				
120 gm	51326-0025-04	15.00		
120 gm	51326-0027-04	25.00		
120 gm	51326-0029-04	35.00		
FLUORO/GLY PADS (Topix)				
glycolic acid				
PAD, TP (OFFICE USE ONLY)				
30s ea	51326-0006-30	30.00		
30s ea	51326-0008-30	50.00		
30s ea	51326-0010-30	70.00		
FLUOROCAINE SOD/PROPARACAINE HCL (Altaire)				
fluorescein sodium/proparacaine hydrochloride				
SOL, OP (STERILE)				
0.25%-0.5%, 5 ml	59390-0205-05	9.15		
FLUOROMETHOLONE				
(Allergan Inc) *See FML FORTE LIQUIFILM*				
(Allergan Inc) *See FML LIQUIFILM*				
(Allergan Inc) *See FML S.O.P.*				
(Pacific Pharma)				
SUS, OP, 0.1%, 5 ml	60758-0880-05	10.05		AB
10 ml	60758-0880-10	16.01		AB
15 ml	60758-0880-15	22.39		AB
(PCCA)				
POW, NA (U.S.P.)				
ea	51927-2773-00	2.18		
(Spectrum Pharmacy)				
POW, NA (U.S.P.)				
0.5 gm	49452-3170-02	696.50		
(A-S Medication)				
REPACK				
SUS, OP, 0.1%, 5 ml	54569-4371-00	10.05		EE
(Pharma Pac)				
REPACK				
SUS, OP, 0.1%, 5 ml	52959-0316-05	16.25		EE
(Phys Total Care)				
REPACK				
SUS, OP, 0.1%, 5 ml	54868-4012-00	40.92		EE
10 ml	54868-4012-01	78.07		AB
15 ml	54868-4012-02	78.07		AB
FLUOROMETHOLONE ACETATE				
(Alcon Ophthalmic) *See FLAREX*				
FLUOROPLEX (Allergan Inc)				
fluorouracil				
CRE, TP, 1%, 30 gm	00023-0812-30	235.46		
SOL, TP, 1%, 30 ml	00023-0810-30	75.61		
FLUOROURACIL				
FUL				
SOL, TP, 5%, 10 ml		116.90		
(Allergan Inc) *See FLUOROPLEX*				
(APP)				
SOL, IV (S.D.V.,PF)				
50 mg/ml, 10 ml	63323-0117-10	3.75		AP
20 ml	63323-0117-20	7.50		AP
(BULK PACKAGE,PF)				
50 mg/ml, 50 ml	63323-0117-51	16.06		AP
100 ml	63323-0117-61	32.12		AP
(Dermik) *See CARAC*				
(Gallipot)				
POW, NA (1X1GM,USP)				
1 gm	51552-0733-01	9.59	6.85	
(1X5GM,USP)				
5 gm	51552-0733-02	21.35	15.25	
(1X25GM,USP)				
25 gm	51552-0733-04	87.92	62.80	
(1X100GM,USP)				
100 gm	51552-0733-05	266.00	190.00	
(GeneraMedix)				
SOL, IV (1X10ML,USP,SDV)				
50 mg/ml, 10 ml	10139-0063-10	3.30		AP
(USP,SDV,10MLX10)				
50 mg/ml, 10 ml 10s UD	10139-0063-11	33.00		AP
(1X20ML,USP,SDV)				
50 mg/ml, 20 ml	10139-0063-20	6.60		AP
(USP,SDV,20MLX10)				
50 mg/ml, 20 ml 10s UD	10139-0063-12	66.00		AP
(USP,PBP(VIAL))				
50 mg/ml, 50 ml	10139-0063-50	15.30		AP
(USP,BULK)				
50 mg/ml, 100 ml	10139-0063-01	27.54		AP
(Hawkins) *See 5-FLUOROURACIL*				
5-FLUOROURACIL (Hawkins)				
fluorouracil				
POW, NA (U.S.P.)				
5 gm	63370-0095-15	56.00		
25 gm	63370-0095-25	244.00		
100 gm	63370-0095-35	760.00		
FLUOROURACIL (Letco)				
POW, NA (U.S.P.)				
10 gm	62991-1486-03	60.00		
25 gm	62991-1486-02	105.00		
(Medisca)				
POW, NA (U.S.P., 5-FU)				
10 gm	38779-0025-01	99.00		
(U.S.P.)				
25 gm	38779-0025-04	207.00		
100 gm	38779-0025-05	615.00		
(Oceanside)				
CRE, TP (1X40GM)				
5%, 40 gm	68682-0004-31	247.09		
(Parenta Pharma)				
SOL, IV (10X10ML,SDV,USP)				
50 mg/ml, 10 ml 10s	66758-0044-03	50.00		AP
(PCCA)				
POW, NA (U.S.P., -5 FU)				
1 gm	51927-1085-00	13.20		
(Spear Dermatology)				
CRE, TP (USP,1X40GM)				
5%, 40 gm	66530-0249-40	247.09		AB
(Spectrum Pharmacy) *See 5-FLUOROURACIL*				
5-FLUOROURACIL (Spectrum Pharmacy)				
fluorouracil				
POW, NA (U.S.P.)				
1 gm	49452-3175-01	67.90		
5 gm	49452-3175-02	88.55		
25 gm	49452-3175-03	331.80		
100 gm	49452-3175-04	885.50		
FLUOROURACIL (Taro)				
SOL, TP, 2%, 10 ml	51672-4062-01	75.61		AT
5%, 10 ml	51672-4063-01	111.33		AT
(Teva) *See ADRUCIL*				
(Valeant Pharm Intl) *See EFUDEX*				
FLUOXETINE (Aurobindo Pharma)				
fluoxetine hydrochloride				
CAP, PO (USP,HARD GELATIN)				
10 mg, 100s ea	65862-0192-01	259.83		AB1
500s ea	65862-0192-05	1286.16		AB1
1000s ea	65862-0192-99	2546.33		AB1
20 mg, 100s ea	65862-0193-01	266.81		AB1
500s ea	65862-0193-05	1320.71		AB1
1000s ea	65862-0193-99	2614.74		AB1
40 mg, 30s ea	65862-0194-30	160.09		AB
100s ea	65862-0194-01	508.83		AB
(Major)				
CAP, PO (10X10,USP)				
10 mg, 100s ea UD	00904-5784-61	241.90		AB
20 mg, 100s ea UD	00904-5785-61	248.40		AB
(Mylan)				
CAP, PO (USP,HARD SHELL GELATIN)				
10 mg, 28s ea	00378-5410-28	172.98		AB2
(HARD GELATIN)				
10 mg, 100s ea	00378-4210-01	259.85		AB
(USP,HARD SHELL GELATIN)				
20 mg, 28s ea	00378-5420-28	177.44		AB2
(HARD GELATIN)				
20 mg, 100s ea	00378-4220-01	266.55		AB
40 mg, 30s ea	00378-4350-93	160.09		AB
(Northstar)				
CAP, PO (USP)				
10 mg, 100s ea	16714-0351-03	259.84		AB1
1000s ea	16714-0351-02	2546.33		AB1
20 mg, 100s ea	16714-0352-03	266.55		AB1
1000s ea	16714-0352-02	2614.74		AB1
40 mg, 30s ea	16714-0353-01	160.09		AB
100s ea	16714-0353-03	519.94		AB
500s ea	16714-0353-04	2407.42		AB
1000s ea	16714-0353-02	5063.98		AB
(Par)				
CAP, PO (USP)				
40 mg, 30s ea	49884-0872-11	160.09		
100s ea	49884-0872-01	533.56		
(USP)				
40 mg, 500s ea	49884-0872-05	2668.00		
(Ranbaxy Pharm)				
CAP, PO, 10 mg, 30s ea	63304-0686-30	77.97		
90s ea	63304-0686-90	234.00		
20 mg, 30s ea	63304-0687-30	79.92		
90s ea	63304-0687-90	239.76		
(Sandoz)				
CAP, PO, 10 mg,				
28s ea UD	00781-2827-08	172.98		AB1
20 mg, 28s ea UD	00781-2828-08	177.44		AB1
(Silarx)				
SYR, PO (USP,MINT)				
20 mg/5 ml, 120 ml	54838-0523-40	118.00		AA
(Teva)				
CAP, PO (USP,HARD GELATIN)				
10 mg, 100s ea	00093-1042-01	259.83		AB2
1000s ea	00093-1042-10	2586.50		AB2
(USP)				
20 mg, 500s ea	00555-0877-04	1320.71		AB
1000s ea	00555-0877-05	2614.74		AB
(USP,10X10,HARD GELATIN)				
40 mg, 100s ea UD	00093-7198-93	508.83		AB
(USP,HARD GELATIN)				
40 mg, 100s ea	00093-7198-01	506.83		AB
500s ea	00093-7198-05	2407.42		AB
(Advanced Pharm Serv, Inc.)				
REPACK				
CAP, PO, 10 mg, 10s ea	13411-0172-01	26.50		
30s ea	13411-0172-03	79.50		
60s ea	13411-0172-06	159.00		
90s ea	13411-0172-09	238.50		
100s ea	13411-0172-10	298.83		
20 mg, 10s ea	13411-0173-01	28.60		
30s ea	13411-0173-03	85.80		
60s ea	13411-0173-06	171.60		
90s ea	13411-0173-09	257.40		
100s ea	13411-0173-10	306.53		
(Bryant Ranch)				
REPACK				
CAP, PO, 10 mg, 30s ea	63629-1609-01	77.79		
90s ea	63629-1609-02	149.99		
20 mg, 15s ea	63629-1610-04	41.44		
30s ea	63629-1610-01	111.43		
60s ea	63629-1610-03	157.99		
100s ea	63629-1610-02	371.42		
(Core)				
REPACK				
CAP, PO, 10 mg, 30s ea	33358-0144-30	79.73		
60s ea	33358-0144-60	160.52		
90s ea	33358-0144-90	153.74		
20 mg, 30s ea	33358-0145-30	114.22		
60s ea	33358-0145-60	161.94		
(DHS, Inc.)				
REPACK				
CAP, PO, 10 mg, 40s ea	55887-0458-40	100.58		
20 mg, 7s ea	55887-0947-07	20.30		
30s ea	55887-0947-30	87.00		
100s ea	55887-0661-01	292.40		
40 mg, 30s ea	55887-0075-30	160.05		
(Dispensing Solutions)				
REPACK				
CAP, PO, 10 mg, 30s ea	55045-3766-08	81.00		
90s ea	55045-2907-09	243.00		
100s ea	55045-2907-00	270.00		
120s ea	55045-2907-02	324.00		
20 mg, 60s ea	55045-2908-06	166.84		
90s ea	55045-2908-09	250.20		
100s ea	55045-2908-00	278.00		
120s ea	55045-2908-02	333.60		
TAB, PO, 20 mg, 30s ea	66336-0418-30	101.37		
(HomeMed)				
REPACK				
CAP, PO, 20 mg, 30s ea	51655-0243-24	79.99		
(IPI)				
REPACK				
CAP, PO, 10 mg, 30s ea	18837-0304-30	77.60		
20 mg, 30s ea	18837-0054-30	99.38		
60s ea	18837-0054-60	198.75		
(Keltman Pharma., Inc.)				
REPACK				
TAB, PO, 10 mg, 30s ea	68387-0125-30	91.72		
(PD-Rx Pharm)				
REPACK				
CAP, PO (USP)				
40 mg, 30s ea	43063-0197-30	150.08		
TAB, PO, 10 mg, 60s ea	55289-0613-60	47.04		
(Phys Total Care)				
REPACK				
CAP, PO, 10 mg, 30s ea	54868-5663-00	8.94		
60s ea	54868-5663-02	12.23		
100s ea	54868-5663-01	17.76		

PROD/MFR	NDC	AWP	DP	OBC
(Physician Partner)				
REPACK				
CAP, PO, 10 mg, 20s ea	21695-0052-20	311.78		
30s ea	21695-0052-30	155.89		
60s ea	21695-0052-60	311.78		
90s ea	21695-0052-90	467.69		
20 mg, 30s ea	21695-0053-30	156.87		
60s ea	21695-0053-60	313.74		
90s ea	21695-0053-90	470.61		
40 mg, 7s ea	21695-0054-07	87.89		
30s ea	21695-0054-30	320.18		
60s ea	21695-0054-60	640.36		
90s ea	21695-0054-90	960.53		
TAB, PO, 10 mg, 90s ea	21695-0320-90	491.58		
100s ea	21695-0320-00	546.20		
20 mg, 30s ea	21695-0321-30	168.04		
(FILM COATED)				
20 mg, 30s ea	21695-0596-30	168.04		
60s ea	21695-0321-60	336.08		
90s ea	21695-0321-90	470.61		
100s ea	21695-0321-00	560.12		
(Quality Care Prod)				
REPACK				
CAP, PO, 40 mg, 30s ea	49999-0886-30	207.00		
(Stat Rx)				
REPACK				
CAP, PO, 10 mg, 60s ea	16590-0099-60	165.00		
40 mg, 30s ea	16590-0490-30	190.06		
60s ea	16590-0490-60	165.50		
90s ea	16590-0490-90	227.50		
120s ea	16590-0490-72	303.25		
FLUOXETINE HCL (Apotex Corp.)				
fluoxetine hydrochloride				
SOL, PO (MINT)				
20 mg/5 ml, 120 ml	60505-0352-01	118.35		AA
(Covidien)				
CAP, PO, 10 mg, 5000s ea	00406-0661-91	12350.00		AB
20 mg, 5000s ea	00406-0663-91	12650.00		AB
(Dr Reddy's)				
CAP, PO, 10 mg, 100s ea	55111-0147-01	259.85		AB
20 mg, 100s ea	55111-0148-01	266.55		AB
1000s ea	55111-0148-10	2614.74		AB
40 mg, 30s ea	55111-0149-30	160.05		AB
100s ea	55111-0149-01	506.83		AB
(Morton Grove)				
SOL, PO (USP,MINT)				
20 mg/5 ml, 120 ml	60432-0162-04	31.55		AA
(Par)				
TAB, PO, 10 mg, 30s ea	49884-0734-11	81.93		AB
100s ea	49884-0734-01	273.10		AB
1000s ea	49884-0734-10	2730.41		AB
20 mg, 30s ea	49884-0735-11	84.02		
100s ea	49884-0735-01	280.06		
1000s ea	49884-0735-10	2800.09		
(Pharm Assoc Inc)				
SOL, PO (40X5ML,SPEARMINT)				
20 mg/5 ml, 5 ml 40s	00121-4721-05	234.00		AA
(SPEARMINT)				
20 mg/5 ml, 120 ml UD	00121-0721-04	123.03		AA
(Ranbaxy Pharm)				
CAP, PO, 40 mg, 30s ea	63304-0632-30	160.09		AB
100s ea	63304-0632-01	533.05		AB
(Sandoz)				
CAP, PO, 10 mg, 100s ea	00185-0080-01	260.12		AB
100s ea	00781-2823-01	259.83		AB
1000s ea	00185-0080-10	2601.18		AB
1000s ea	00781-2823-10	2468.39		AB
20 mg, 100s ea	00185-0085-01	266.81		AB
100s ea	00781-2822-01	266.52		AB
1000s ea	00185-0085-10	2668.14		AB
1000s ea	00781-2822-10	2531.94		AB
40 mg, 30s ea	00781-2824-31	160.09		AB
100s ea	00781-2824-01	533.05		AB
1000s ea	00781-2824-10	5063.98		AB
(Spectrum Pharmacy)				
CRY, NA (U.S.P.)				
25 gm	49452-3176-01	186.20		
100 gm	49452-3176-02	455.00		
500 gm	49452-3176-03	1722.00		
(Teva)				
CAP, PO, 10 mg, 100s ea	00555-0876-02	260.09		AB
100s ea	50111-0647-01	259.83		AB
500s ea	50111-0647-02	1286.16		AB
1000s ea	50111-0647-03	2546.33		AB
20 mg, 100s ea	00555-0877-02	266.81		AB
100s ea	50111-0648-01	266.81		AB
(USP,HARD GELATIN)				
20 mg, 100s ea	00093-4356-01	266.81		AB1
500s ea	50111-0648-02	1320.71		AB
(USP,HARD GELATIN)				
20 mg, 500s ea	00093-4356-05	1326.50		AB1
1000s ea	50111-0648-03	2614.74		AB
2000s ea	00555-0877-07	5336.20		AB
2000s ea	50111-0648-44	5176.11		AB
(HARDGELATIN)				
40 mg, 30s ea	00093-7198-56	160.05		AB
SOL, PO (MINT)				
20 mg/5 ml, 120 ml	00093-6108-12	118.49		AA
(UDL)				
CAP, PO (10X10)				
10 mg, 100s ea UD	51079-0997-20	259.85		AB
(ROBOT READY,25X1)				
20 mg, 25s ea UD	51079-0971-19	66.74		AB
(10X10)				
20 mg, 100s ea UD	51079-0971-20	266.95		AB
(4u)				
REPACK				
CAP, PO, 20 mg, 30s ea	10544-0399-30	104.84		AB
30s ea	42549-0599-30	104.84		AB
(A-S Medication)				
REPACK				
CAP, PO, 10 mg, 30s ea	54569-5319-00	77.98		AB
60s ea	54569-5319-01	155.95		AB
20 mg, 30s ea	54569-5291-00	80.04		EE
60s ea	54569-5291-01	160.09		EE
90s ea	54569-5291-03	240.13		AB
40 mg, 30s ea	54569-5320-00	160.09		EE
(Aidarex)				
REPACK				
CAP, PO, 10 mg, 7s ea	33261-0184-07	31.50		AB
14s ea	33261-0184-14	63.00		AB
20s ea	33261-0184-20	90.00		AB
21s ea	33261-0184-21	94.50		AB
28s ea	33261-0184-28	126.00		AB
30s ea	33261-0184-30	135.00		AB
40s ea	33261-0184-40	180.00		AB
60s ea	33261-0184-60	270.00		AB
90s ea	33261-0184-90	405.00		AB
100s ea	33261-0184-00	450.00		AB
120s ea	33261-0184-02	540.00		AB
180s ea	33261-0184-03	810.00		AB
(HARD GELATIN)				
20 mg, 7s ea	33261-0045-07	38.50		AB1
14s ea	33261-0045-14	77.00		AB1
20s ea	33261-0045-20	110.00		AB1
21s ea	33261-0045-21	115.50		AB1
28s ea	33261-0045-28	154.00		AB1
30s ea	33261-0045-30	165.00		AB1
40s ea	33261-0045-40	220.00		AB1
60s ea	33261-0045-60	330.00		AB1
90s ea	33261-0045-90	495.00		AB1
100s ea	33261-0045-00	550.00		AB1
120s ea	33261-0045-02	660.00		AB1
180s ea	33261-0045-03	990.00		AB1
(Altura)				
REPACK				
CAP, PO, 10 mg, 10s ea	63874-0574-10	30.35		AB
14s ea	63874-0574-14	42.49		AB
20s ea	63874-0574-20	60.70		AB
21s ea	63874-0574-21	63.74		AB
28s ea	63874-0574-28	84.98		AB
30s ea	63874-0574-30	91.05		AB
60s ea	63874-0574-60	182.10		AB
90s ea	63874-0574-90	273.15		AB
100s ea	63874-0574-01	303.50		AB
120s ea	63874-0574-04	364.20		AB
150s ea	63874-0574-72	455.19		AB
200s ea	63874-0574-74	606.10		AB
300s ea	63874-0574-77	909.15		AB
20 mg, 10s ea	63874-0573-10	29.60		AB
14s ea	63874-0573-14	41.44		AB
15s ea	63874-0573-15	44.40		AB
20s ea	63874-0573-20	59.20		AB
21s ea	63874-0573-21	62.16		AB
28s ea	63874-0573-28	82.88		AB
30s ea	63874-0573-30	88.80		AB
60s ea	63874-0573-60	177.60		AB
90s ea	63874-0573-90	266.40		AB
100s ea	63874-0573-01	296.00		AB
120s ea	63874-0573-04	355.20		AB
150s ea	63874-0573-72	444.00		AB
200s ea	63874-0573-74	592.00		AB
300s ea	63874-0573-77	888.00		AB
40 mg, 30s ea	63874-1080-03	159.90		AB
60s ea	63874-1080-06	330.06		AB
TAB, PO, 20 mg, 14s ea	63874-0828-14	41.44		
20s ea	63874-0828-20	59.20		
21s ea	63874-0828-21	62.16		
28s ea	63874-0828-28	82.88		
30s ea	63874-0828-30	88.80		
60s ea	63874-0828-60	177.60		
90s ea	63874-0828-90	266.40		
100s ea	63874-0828-01	296.00		
120s ea	63874-0828-04	355.00		
(DHS, Inc.)				
REPACK				
CAP, PO, 10 mg, 30s ea	55887-0458-30	75.44		AB
60s ea	55887-0458-60	150.87		AB
90s ea	55887-0458-90	219.32		AB
20 mg, 30s ea	55887-0661-30	87.72		AB
60s ea	55887-0661-60	175.44		AB
90s ea	55887-0661-90	263.16		AB
(Dispensing Solutions)				
REPACK				
CAP, PO, 10 mg, 30s ea	55045-2907-08	81.00		AB
30s ea	66336-0844-30	77.95		AB
60s ea	55045-2907-06	162.00		AB
90s ea	66336-0844-90	233.85		AB
20 mg, 30s ea	55045-2908-08	83.42		AB
30s ea	66336-0004-30	87.72		
90s ea	66336-0004-90	263.16		AB
40 mg, 30s ea	68258-7003-03	162.05		AB
(HARDGELATIN)				
40 mg, 30s ea	55045-3137-08	160.00		AB
(GSMS)				
REPACK				
CAP, PO (UNIT OF USE)				
10 mg, 30s ea	60429-0718-30	9.00	3.00	EE
60s ea	60429-0718-60	15.60	5.20	EE
90s ea	60429-0718-90	21.90	7.30	EE
180s ea	60429-0718-18	41.25	13.75	EE
20 mg, 30s ea	60429-0719-30	9.30	3.10	EE
60s ea	60429-0719-60	16.20	5.40	EE
90s ea	60429-0719-90	22.80	7.60	EE
180s ea	60429-0719-18	43.05	14.35	EE
(Keltman Pharma., Inc.)				
REPACK				
CAP, PO, 20 mg, 30s ea	68387-0120-30	88.56		AB
60s ea	68387-0120-60	177.12		AB
90s ea	68387-0120-90	265.68		AB
(Medsource)				
REPACK				
CAP, PO, 10 mg, 30s ea	45865-0368-30	22.50		AB
60s ea	45865-0368-60	45.00		AB
90s ea	45865-0368-90	67.50		AB
100s ea	45865-0368-00	75.00		AB
(Nucare Pharm)				
REPACK				
CAP, PO, 20 mg, 30s ea	66267-0488-30	104.34		AB
60s ea	66267-0488-60	208.69		AB
90s ea	66267-0488-90	314.31		AB
40 mg, 30s ea	66267-0587-30	199.56		AB
TAB, PO, 10 mg, 30s ea	66267-0576-30	104.46		AB
(PD-Rx Pharm)				
REPACK				
CAP, PO, 10 mg, 14s ea	55289-0613-14	34.13		AB
30s ea	55289-0613-30	44.27		AB
20 mg, 14s ea	55289-0610-14	36.89		AB
(REDI-SCRIPT)				
20 mg, 15s ea	58864-0103-15	37.60		AB
(HARD GELATIN)				
20 mg, 28s ea	55289-0610-28	47.08		AB
30s ea	55289-0610-30	48.53		AB
30s ea	58864-0103-30	48.56		AB
60s ea	55289-0610-60	49.68		AB
60s ea	58864-0103-60	51.20		AB
90s ea	55289-0610-90	63.47		AB
100s ea	43063-0009-01	266.52		AB
(Pharma Pac)				
REPACK				
CAP, PO, 40 mg, 30s ea	52959-0717-30	170.00		AB
TAB, PO, 10 mg, 30s ea	52959-0669-30	95.01		
30s ea	52959-0991-30	79.10		AB
59s ea	52959-0669-59	153.92		
60s ea	52959-0669-60	156.53		
(Phys Total Care)				
REPACK				
CAP, PO, 10 mg, 100s ea	54868-4560-01	32.10		AB
20 mg, 30s ea	54868-4537-00	8.31		EE
60s ea	54868-4537-01	14.70		EE
100s ea	54868-4537-02	20.97		EE
240s ea	54868-4537-04	46.92		AB
40 mg, 30s ea	54868-4562-00	69.60		AB
90s ea	54868-4562-01	168.63		AB
TAB, PO, 10 mg, 30s ea	54868-4560-00	12.18		AB

PROD/MFR	NDC	AWP	DP	OBC
(Quality Care Prod)				
REPACK				
CAP, PO, 20 mg, 20s ea	49999-0128-20	28.47		AB
30s ea	49999-0128-30	77.24		AB
60s ea	49999-0128-60	85.40		
100s ea	49999-0128-00	355.20		AB
TAB, PO, 10 mg, 14s ea	49999-0362-14	50.98		AB
30s ea	49999-0362-30	109.25		AB
(Southwood)				
REPACK				
CAP, PO, 10 mg, 30s ea	58016-0906-30	90.92		AB
60s ea	58016-0906-60	181.83		AB
90s ea	58016-0906-90	272.75		EE
100s ea	58016-0906-00	303.05		AB
120s ea	58016-0906-02	363.66		AB
150s ea	58016-0906-03	454.58		AB
200s ea	58016-0906-89	606.10		AB
300s ea	58016-0906-73	909.15		AB
20 mg, 10s ea	58016-0905-10	29.60		AB
20s ea	58016-0905-20	59.20		EE
30s ea	58016-0905-30	88.80		AB
60s ea	58016-0905-60	177.60		EE
100s ea	58016-0905-00	296.00		EE
120s ea	58016-0905-02	355.20		AB
150s ea	58016-0905-03	444.00		AB
200s ea	58016-0905-89	592.00		AB
300s ea	58016-0905-73	888.00		AB
40 mg, 30s ea	58016-0704-30	165.00		AB
60s ea	58016-0704-60	330.00		AB
90s ea	58016-0704-90	495.00		AB
100s ea	58016-0704-00	550.00		AB
120s ea	58016-0704-02	660.00		AB
150s ea	58016-0704-03	825.00		AB
200s ea	58016-0704-89	1100.00		AB
300s ea	58016-0704-73	1650.00		AB
(St. Mary's MPP)				
REPACK				
CAP, PO, 20 mg, 30s ea	60760-0647-30	92.29		AB
(Stat Rx)				
REPACK				
CAP, PO, 10 mg, 30s ea	16590-0099-30	99.38		AB
(Vibranta)				
REPACK				
CAP, PO, 20 mg, 30s ea	57866-0922-01	77.02		AB
60s ea	57866-0922-02	152.94		AB
90s ea	57866-0922-03	228.87		AB
TAB, PO, 20 mg, 30s ea	57866-0920-01	77.25		
60s ea	57866-0920-02	104.65		
90s ea	57866-0920-03	156.97		
FLUOXETINE HYDROCHLORIDE				
FUL				
CAP, PO, 10 mg, 100s ea		13.86		
20 mg, 100s ea		14.54		
40 mg, 30s ea		34.88		
SOL, PO, 20 mg/5 ml, 120 ml		27.00		
TAB, PO, 10 mg, 30s ea		18.00		
(Apotex Corp.) *See FLUOXETINE HCL*				
(Aurobindo Pharma) *See FLUOXETINE*				
(Covidien) *See FLUOXETINE HCL*				
(Dista) *See PROZAC*				
(Dr Reddy's) *See FLUOXETINE HCL*				
(Lilly) *See PROZAC WEEKLY*				
(Major) *See FLUOXETINE*				
(Medisca)				
POW, NA (USP,1X100GM)				
100 gm	38779-0013-05	267.00		
(USP,1X500GM)				
500 gm	38779-0013-08	1170.00		
(Morton Grove) *See FLUOXETINE HCL*				
(Mylan) *See FLUOXETINE*				
(Northstar) *See FLUOXETINE*				
(Par) *See FLUOXETINE*				
(Par) *See FLUOXETINE HCL*				
(PCCA)				
POW, NA (USP)				
1 gm	51927-3409-00	39.00		
(Pharm Assoc Inc) *See FLUOXETINE HCL*				
(PRX) *See RAPIFLUX*				
(Ranbaxy Pharm) *See FLUOXETINE*				
(Ranbaxy Pharm) *See FLUOXETINE HCL*				
(Sandoz) *See FLUOXETINE*				
(Sandoz) *See FLUOXETINE HCL*				
(Silarx) *See FLUOXETINE*				
(Spectrum Pharmacy) *See FLUOXETINE HCL*				
(Teva)				
CAP, PO, 10 mg, 100s ea	00172-4363-10	259.89		AB
500s ea	00172-4363-70	1293.25		AB
20 mg, 100s ea	00172-4356-10	266.99		AB
1000s ea	00093-4356-10	2653.00		AB
(Teva) *See FLUOXETINE*				
(Teva) *See FLUOXETINE HCL*				
(Teva) *See SELFEMRA*				
(Teva)				
TAB, PO (FILM-COATED)				
10 mg, 30s ea	00093-7188-56	78.04		AB
500s ea	00172-4510-70	1293.25		AB
(FILM-COATED)				
10 mg, 1000s ea	00093-7188-10	2586.50		AB
(UDL) *See FLUOXETINE HCL*				
(Warner Chilcott) *See SARAFEM*				
(4u)				
REPACK				
CAP, PO, 20 mg, 30s ea	42549-0336-30	98.46		AB
30s ea	42549-0536-30	104.84		AB
(Altura)				
REPACK				
TAB, PO, 10 mg, 20s ea	63874-1053-02	60.69		AB
21s ea	63874-1053-05	63.73		AB
28s ea	63874-1053-08	84.97		AB
30s ea	63874-1053-03	91.04		AB
60s ea	63874-1053-06	182.08		AB
90s ea	63874-1053-09	273.12		AB
100s ea	63874-1053-01	303.47		AB
120s ea	63874-1053-04	364.16		AB
(DHS, Inc.)				
REPACK				
TAB, PO, 10 mg, 30s ea	55887-0664-30	90.98		AB
90s ea	55887-0664-90	272.93		AB
(Dispensing Solutions)				
REPACK				
CAP, PO, 20 mg, 60s ea	66336-0004-60	169.30		AB
FLUOXETINE HYDROCHLORIDE (Palmetto)				
REPACK				
CAP, PO, 10 mg, 30s ea	23490-5601-03	90.92		
FLUOXETINE HYDROCHLORIDE (Palmetto)				
20 mg, 30s ea	23490-5602-01	88.80		
60s ea	23490-5602-02	177.60		
100s ea	23490-5602-03	296.00		
40 mg, 30s ea	23490-7327-03	166.50		
(Pharma Pac)				
REPACK				
CAP, PO, 20 mg, 10s ea	52959-0732-10	38.82		AB
14s ea	52959-0732-14	47.35		AB
15s ea	52959-0732-15	50.37		
20s ea	52959-0732-20	65.00		AB
30s ea	52959-0732-30	95.39		AB
40s ea	52959-0732-40	127.18		AB
50s ea	52959-0732-50	158.95		AB
60s ea	52959-0732-60	190.71		AB
100s ea	52959-0732-00	294.35		AB
(Phys Total Care)				
REPACK				
CAP, PO, 20 mg, 90s ea	54868-4537-03	20.52		AB
(Quality Care Prod)				
REPACK				
CAP, PO, 10 mg, 90s ea	49999-0362-90	327.75		AB
20 mg, 14s ea	49999-0128-14	37.56		
90s ea	49999-0128-90	319.68		
(Stat Rx)				
REPACK				
CAP, PO, 20 mg, 30s ea	16590-0100-30	101.72		AB
56s ea	16590-0100-56	189.88		AB
60s ea	16590-0100-60	203.44		AB
90s ea	16590-0100-90	305.16		AB
FLUOXETINE HYDROCHLORIDE/OLANZAPINE				
(Lilly) *See SYMBYAX*				
FLUOXYMESTERONE (PCCA)				
POW, NA (U.S.P.; CIII)				
1 gm, C-III	51927-2515-00	555.00		
(Spectrum Pharmacy)				
POW, NA (U.S.P.)				
1 gm, C-III	49452-3177-01	476.00		
5 gm, C-III	49452-3177-02	1802.50		
(Upsher-Smith) *See ANDROXY*				
FLUPHENAZINE DECANOATE (APP)				
OIL, IJ (M.D.V.)				
25 mg/ml, 5 ml	63323-0272-05	74.18		AO
(Bedford)				
OIL, IJ (M.D.V.)				
25 mg/ml, 5 ml	55390-0465-05	9.60		AO
(PCCA)				
POW, NA (U.S.P.)				
1 gm	51927-2234-00	120.00		
FLUPHENAZINE HCL (Mylan) fluphenazine hydrochloride				
TAB, PO, 1 mg, 100s ea	00378-6004-01	54.90		AB
500s ea	00378-6004-05	268.80		AB
2.5 mg, 100s ea	00378-6009-01	83.50		AB
500s ea	00378-6009-05	375.60		AB
5 mg, 100s ea	00378-6074-01	97.10		AB
500s ea	00378-6074-05	475.90		AB
10 mg, 100s ea	00378-6097-01	125.00		AB
500s ea	00378-6097-05	612.20		AB
(PCCA)				
POW, NA (U.S.P.)				
1 gm	51927-2293-00	78.00		
(Pharm Assoc Inc)				
ELI, PO (RASPBERRY)				
2.5 mg/5 ml, 60 ml	00121-0654-02	29.52		AA
473 ml	00121-0654-16	192.00		AA
SOL, PO (W/DROPPER,SF,DYE-FREE)				
5 mg/ml, 120 ml	00121-0653-04	154.15		AA
(Sandoz)				
TAB, PO (FILM-COATED)				
1 mg, 100s ea	00781-1436-01	49.75		AB
100s ea UD	00781-1436-13	62.99		AB
2.5 mg, 100s ea	00781-1437-01	75.75		AB
5 mg, 100s ea	00781-1438-01	89.95		AB
10 mg, 100s ea	00781-1439-01	114.75		AB
(UDL)				
TAB, PO (10X10)				
1 mg, 100s ea UD	51079-0485-20	62.40		AB
2.5 mg, 100s ea UD	51079-0486-20	89.60		AB
5 mg, 100s ea UD	51079-0487-20	132.74		AB
10 mg, 100s ea UD	51079-0488-20	168.50		AB
(PD-Rx Pharm)				
REPACK				
TAB, PO, 2.5 mg, 40s ea	58864-0802-40	14.09		AB
(Phys Total Care)				
REPACK				
TAB, PO, 1 mg, 30s ea	54868-2156-00	11.97		EE
60s ea	54868-2156-01	19.44		EE
2.5 mg, 30s ea	54868-1354-01	13.68		EE
5 mg, 30s ea	54868-2303-00	13.68		EE
(Vibranta)				
REPACK				
TAB, PO, 1 mg, 30s ea	57866-4406-01	17.57		AB
60s ea	57866-4406-02	34.04		AB
90s ea	57866-4406-03	50.51		AB
120s ea	57866-4406-04	66.98		AB
2.5 mg, 30s ea	57866-4407-01	26.15		AB
60s ea	57866-4407-02	51.20		AB
90s ea	57866-4407-03	76.25		AB
120s ea	57866-4407-04	101.30		AB
(FILM-COATED)				
5 mg, 30s ea	57866-4405-01	30.23		AB
60s ea	57866-4405-02	59.36		AB
90s ea	57866-4405-03	88.49		AB
120s ea	57866-4405-04	117.62		AB
10 mg, 30s ea	57866-4408-01	38.60		AB
60s ea	57866-4408-02	76.10		AB
90s ea	57866-4408-03	113.60		AB
120s ea	57866-4408-04	151.10		AB
FLUPHENAZINE HYDROCHLORIDE				
FUL				
TAB, PO, 1 mg, 100s ea		22.73		
5 mg, 100s ea		35.46		
10 mg, 100s ea		50.99		
(APP)				
SOL, IM (M.D.V.,AMBER)				
2.5 mg/ml, 10 ml	63323-0281-10	81.44		AP
(Mylan) *See FLUPHENAZINE HCL*				
(PCCA) *See FLUPHENAZINE HCL*				
(Pharm Assoc Inc) *See FLUPHENAZINE HCL*				
(Sandoz) *See FLUPHENAZINE HCL*				
(UDL) *See FLUPHENAZINE HCL*				

PROD/MFR	NDC	AWP	DP	OBC
FLURA-DROPS (Kirkman Labs)				
sodium fluoride				
LIQ, PO, 0.125 mg/drp,				
30 ml	58223-0684-30	2.76		
0.25 mg/drp, 24 ml	58223-0684-24	2.64		
FLURA-LOZ (Kirkman Labs)				
sodium fluoride				
CTB, PO, 1 mg, 100s ea	58223-0672-01	2.52		
1000s ea	58223-0672-04	12.00		
FLURA-SAFE (Altaire)				
benoxinate hydrochloride/fluorexon disodium				
SOL, OP, 0.4%-0.35%,				
6 ml	59390-0172-06	3.90		
FLURANDRENOLIDE				
(Aqua Pharmaceuticals) *See CORDRAN*				
(Aqua Pharmaceuticals) *See CORDRAN SP*				
(Watson) *See CORDRAN TAPE*				
FLURAZEPAM (Bryant Ranch)				
REPACK				
flurazepam hydrochloride				
CAP, PO, 15 mg,				
30s ea, C-IV	63629-3034-01	22.54		
60s ea, C-IV	63629-3034-02	43.98		
30 mg,				
30s ea, C-IV	63629-3200-01	37.10		
(Core)				
REPACK				
CAP, PO, 15 mg,				
30s ea, C-IV	33358-0146-30	23.10		
60s ea, C-IV	33358-0146-60	45.08		
30 mg,				
30s ea, C-IV	33358-0147-30	38.03		
60s ea, C-IV	33358-0147-60	60.83		
FLURAZEPAM HCL (Mylan)				
flurazepam hydrochloride				
CAP, PO, 15 mg,				
100s ea, C-IV	00378-4415-01	28.75		AB
500s ea, C-IV	00378-4415-05	139.40		AB
30 mg,				
100s ea, C-IV	00378-4430-01	34.65		AB
500s ea, C-IV	00378-4430-05	168.75		AB
(West-Ward)				
CAP, PO, 15 mg,				
100s ea, C-IV	00143-3367-01	28.25		AB
500s ea, C-IV	00143-3367-05	138.50		AB
30 mg,				
100s ea, C-IV	00143-3370-01	34.25		AB
500s ea, C-IV	00143-3370-05	167.10		AB
(A-S Medication)				
REPACK				
CAP, PO, 15 mg,				
30s ea, C-IV	54569-2376-02	8.55		EE
30 mg,				
30s ea, C-IV	54569-0898-00	10.34		EE
(Altura)				
REPACK				
CAP, PO, 15 mg,				
5s ea, C-IV	63874-0213-05	3.75		AB
12s ea, C-IV	63874-0213-12	9.00		AB
15s ea, C-IV	63874-0213-15	11.25		AB
20s ea, C-IV	63874-0213-20	15.00		AB
30s ea, C-IV	63874-0213-30	22.50		EE
40s ea, C-IV	63874-0213-40	30.00		AB
60s ea, C-IV	63874-0213-60	45.00		AB
100s ea, C-IV	63874-0213-01	75.00		EE
30 mg, 6s ea, C-IV	63874-0214-06	4.98		AB
9s ea, C-IV	63874-0214-09	7.47		AB
10s ea, C-IV	63874-0214-10	8.30		AB
12s ea, C-IV	63874-0214-12	9.96		AB
14s ea, C-IV	63874-0214-14	11.62		AB
15s ea, C-IV	63874-0214-15	12.45		AB
20s ea, C-IV	63874-0214-20	16.60		EE
21s ea, C-IV	63874-0214-21	17.43		AB
24s ea, C-IV	63874-0214-24	19.92		AB
30s ea, C-IV	63874-0214-30	24.90		EE
60s ea, C-IV	63874-0214-60	49.80		AB
100s ea, C-IV	63874-0214-01	83.00		EE
(DHS, Inc.)				
REPACK				
CAP, PO, 30 mg,				
30s ea, C-IV	55887-0185-30	26.20		AB
60s ea, C-IV	55887-0185-60	52.40		AB
90s ea, C-IV	55887-0185-90	78.60		AB
(Dispensing Solutions)				
REPACK				
CAP, PO, 15 mg,				
14s ea, C-IV	55045-1477-03	11.20		AB
20s ea, C-IV	55045-1477-07	16.00		AB

PROD/MFR	NDC	AWP	DP	OBC
30s ea, C-IV	55045-1477-08	24.00		AB
40s ea, C-IV	55045-1477-04	32.00		AB
60s ea, C-IV	55045-1477-06	48.00		AB
90s ea, C-IV	55045-1477-09	72.00		AB
100s ea, C-IV	55045-1477-00	80.00		AB
120s ea, C-IV	55045-1477-01	96.00		AB
30 mg,				
30s ea, C-IV	55045-1922-08	25.50		AB
40s ea, C-IV	55045-1922-04	34.00		AB
60s ea, C-IV	55045-1922-06	51.00		AB
90s ea, C-IV	55045-1922-09	76.50		AB
100s ea, C-IV	55045-1922-00	85.00		AB
120s ea, C-IV	55045-1922-02	102.00		AB
(HomeMed)				
REPACK				
CAP, PO, 15 mg,				
30s ea, C-IV	51655-0825-24	9.35		EE
30 mg,				
30s ea, C-IV	51655-0842-24	9.35		EE
60s ea, C-IV	51655-0842-25	17.70		EE
(Nucare Pharm)				
REPACK				
CAP, PO, 15 mg,				
20s ea, C-IV	68071-0220-20	14.76		AB
30s ea, C-IV	68071-0220-30	22.15		AB
30 mg,				
15s ea, C-IV	66267-0331-15	19.62		AB
30s ea, C-IV	66267-0331-30	26.62		AB
45s ea, C-IV	66267-0331-45	39.93		AB
(PD-Rx Pharm)				
REPACK				
CAP, PO, 30 mg,				
30s ea, C-IV	55289-0038-30	24.19		AB
(Pharma Pac)				
REPACK				
CAP, PO, 15 mg,				
6s ea, C-IV	52959-0369-06	4.27		EE
30s ea, C-IV	52959-0369-30	19.35		EE
40s ea, C-IV	52959-0369-40	25.00		EE
60s ea, C-IV	52959-0369-60	38.69		AB
100s ea, C-IV	52959-0369-00	55.10		EE
30 mg, ea, C-IV	52959-0236-60	73.77		AB
14s ea, C-IV	52959-0236-14	19.64		EE
15s ea, C-IV	52959-0236-15	20.66		EE
20s ea, C-IV	52959-0236-20	25.89		EE
24s ea, C-IV	52959-0236-24	31.08		AB
30s ea, C-IV	52959-0236-30	36.89		EE
(Phys Total Care)				
REPACK				
CAP, PO, 15 mg,				
20s ea, C-IV	54868-0092-02	10.80		EE
30s ea, C-IV	54868-0092-01	13.20		EE
30 mg,				
10s ea, C-IV	54868-0093-00	7.50		EE
30s ea, C-IV	54868-0093-01	13.50		EE
(Physician Partner)				
REPACK				
CAP, PO, 30 mg,				
30s ea, C-IV	21695-0363-30	23.55		AB
(Quality Care Prod)				
REPACK				
CAP, PO, 30 mg,				
30s ea, C-IV	35356-0430-30	36.15		AB
(Southwood)				
REPACK				
CAP, PO, 15 mg,				
5s ea, C-IV	58016-0811-05	3.75		EE
14s ea, C-IV	58016-0811-14	10.50		EE
15s ea, C-IV	58016-0811-15	11.25		EE
30s ea, C-IV	58016-0811-30	22.50		EE
40s ea, C-IV	58016-0811-40	30.00		EE
60s ea, C-IV	58016-0811-60	45.00		EE
30 mg, 6s ea, C-IV	58016-0812-06	7.45		EE
9s ea, C-IV	58016-0812-09	11.17		EE
10s ea, C-IV	58016-0812-10	12.41		EE
12s ea, C-IV	58016-0812-12	14.89		EE
14s ea, C-IV	58016-0812-14	17.38		EE
15s ea, C-IV	58016-0812-15	18.62		EE
20s ea, C-IV	58016-0812-20	24.82		EE
21s ea, C-IV	58016-0812-21	26.06		EE
24s ea, C-IV	58016-0812-24	29.79		EE
30s ea, C-IV	58016-0812-30	37.23		EE
60s ea, C-IV	58016-0812-60	74.47		EE
100s ea, C-IV	58016-0812-00	124.11		EE
120s ea, C-IV	58016-0812-02	148.93		AB
150s ea, C-IV	58016-0812-03	186.17		AB
200s ea, C-IV	58016-0812-89	248.22		AB
300s ea, C-IV	58016-0812-73	372.33		AB

PROD/MFR	NDC	AWP	DP	OBC
FLURAZEPAM HYDROCHLORIDE				
FUL				
CAP, PO, 15 mg, 100s ea		9.75		
30 mg, 100s ea		11.48		
(Mylan) *See FLURAZEPAM HCL*				
(West-Ward) *See FLURAZEPAM HCL*				
(Keltman Pharma., Inc.)				
REPACK				
CAP, PO, 30 mg,				
15s ea, C-IV	68387-0610-15	19.27		
30s ea, C-IV	68387-0610-30	38.54		
(Palmetto)				
REPACK				
CAP, PO, 15 mg,				
30s ea, C-IV	23490-5610-03	22.50		
60s ea, C-IV	23490-5610-06	45.00		
30 mg, 30s ea, C-IV	23490-5611-03	27.00		
60s ea, C-IV	23490-5611-06	54.00		
FLURBIPROFEN				
FUL				
TAB, PO, 100 mg, 100s ea		24.38		
(Caraco)				
TAB, PO, 50 mg, 100s ea	57664-0164-08	78.80		AB
100 mg, 100s ea	57664-0165-08	118.65		AB
500s ea	57664-0165-13	573.25		AB
(Gallipot)				
POW, NA (B.P.,U.S.P.)				
5 gm	51552-0818-02	43.05	30.75	
(Medisca)				
POW, NA (1X5GM)				
5 gm	38779-0362-03	97.50		
(1X10GM)				
10 gm	38779-0362-01	157.50		
(B.P.)				
25 gm	38779-0362-04	315.00		
100 gm	38779-0362-05	658.50		
500 gm	38779-0362-08	2985.00		
(Mylan)				
TAB, PO, 50 mg, 100s ea	00378-0076-01	78.80		AB
100 mg, 100s ea	00378-0093-01	118.70		AB
500s ea	00378-0093-05	573.30		AB
(PCCA)				
POW, NA (U.S.P.)				
1 gm	51927-2701-00	12.60		
(Spectrum Pharmacy)				
POW, NA (U.S.P./N.F.)				
5 gm	49452-3178-02	147.00		
25 gm	49452-3178-03	518.00		
(Teva)				
TAB, PO, 100 mg, 100s ea	00093-0711-01	108.25		AB
500s ea	00093-0711-05	521.76		AB
(A-S Medication)				
REPACK				
TAB, PO, 100 mg, 10s ea	54569-3858-04	11.87		AB
30s ea	54569-3858-00	35.60		AB
60s ea	54569-3858-03	71.19		AB
(Altura)				
REPACK				
TAB, PO, 100 mg, 20s ea	63874-0340-20	25.85		EE
30s ea	63874-0340-30	38.78		EE
500s ea	63874-0340-50	520.00		EE
(Bryant Ranch)				
REPACK				
TAB, PO, 100 mg, 20s ea	63629-1250-01	30.21		
30s ea	63629-1250-02	42.00		
(Core)				
REPACK				
TAB, PO, 100 mg, 20s ea	33358-0148-20	30.97		
30s ea	33358-0148-30	43.05		
(Dispensing Solutions)				
REPACK				
TAB, PO, 100 mg, 10s ea	55045-2142-01	14.00		AB
14s ea	55045-2142-02	19.60		AB
20s ea	55045-2142-07	28.00		AB
30s ea	55045-2142-08	42.00		AB
60s ea	55045-2142-06	84.00		AB
(Nucare Pharm)				
REPACK				
TAB, PO, 100 mg, 30s ea	66267-0486-30	38.95		EE
(PD-Rx Pharm)				
REPACK				
TAB, PO, 100 mg, 10s ea	55289-0561-10	22.44		AB
15s ea	55289-0561-15	27.02		AB
30s ea	55289-0561-30	35.45		AB

PROD/MFR	NDC	AWP	DP	OBC
(Pharma Pac)				
REPACK				
TAB, PO, 100 mg, 14s ea	**52959-0346-14**	19.99		EE
20s ea	**52959-0346-20**	28.93		EE
21s ea	**52959-0346-21**	30.37		EE
30s ea	**52959-0346-30**	42.99		EE
(Phys Total Care)				
REPACK				
TAB, PO, 100 mg, 20s ea	**54868-3362-00**	14.43		EE
60s ea	**54868-3362-01**	34.29		
100s ea	**54868-3362-02**	52.65		AB
(Physician Partner)				
REPACK				
TAB, PO, 100 mg, 15s ea	**21695-0419-15**	41.89		AB
30s ea	**21695-0419-30**	71.19		AB
(Quality Care Prod)				
REPACK				
TAB, PO, 100 mg, 60s ea	**49999-0311-60**	85.40		
(Southwood)				
REPACK				
TAB, PO, 50 mg, 10s ea	**58016-0340-10**	8.25		EE
15s ea	**58016-0340-15**	12.38		EE
20s ea	**58016-0340-20**	16.50		EE
28s ea	**58016-0340-28**	23.10		EE
30s ea	**58016-0340-30**	24.75		EE
40s ea	**58016-0340-40**	33.00		EE
100s ea	**58016-0340-00**	82.50		EE
120s ea	**58016-0340-02**	99.00		EE
150s ea	**58016-0340-03**	123.75		EE
200s ea	**58016-0340-89**	165.00		EE
300s ea	**58016-0340-73**	247.50		EE
100 mg, 10s ea	**58016-0750-10**	14.23		EE
12s ea	**58016-0750-12**	17.08		EE
14s ea	**58016-0750-14**	19.92		EE
15s ea	**58016-0750-15**	21.35		EE
20s ea	**58016-0750-20**	28.47		EE
28s ea	**58016-0750-28**	39.85		EE
30s ea	**58016-0750-30**	42.70		EE
40s ea	**58016-0750-40**	56.93		EE
100s ea	**58016-0750-00**	142.33		EE
(Stat Rx)				
REPACK				
TAB, PO, 100 mg, 10s ea	**16590-0096-10**	16.00		
20s ea	**16590-0096-20**	32.00		
30s ea	**16590-0096-30**	48.00		
60s ea	**16590-0096-60**	71.22		AB
(Vibranta)				
REPACK				
TAB, PO, 100 mg, 30s ea	**57866-6011-01**	60.58		AB
FLURBIPROFEN MICRONIZED (Hawkins)				
flurbiprofen, micronized				
POW, NA (USP)				
5 gm	**63370-0096-15**	72.00		
25 gm	**63370-0096-25**	276.00		
100 gm	**63370-0096-35**	932.00		
500 gm	**63370-0096-45**	4320.00		
FLURBIPROFEN SODIUM				
FUL				
SOL, OP, 0.03%, 2 ml		8.14		
(Allergan Inc) *See OCUFEN*				
(Bausch & Lomb Inc.)				
SOL, OP, 0.03%, 2.5 ml	**24208-0314-25**	8.73		AT
(Pacific Pharma)				
SOL, OP, 0.03%, 2.5 ml	**60758-0910-03**	9.48		AT
(A-S Medication)				
REPACK				
SOL, OP, 0.03%, 2.5 ml	**54569-4626-00**	9.11		EE
(Dispensing Solutions)				
REPACK				
SOL, OP, 0.03%, 2.5 ml	**55045-2714-02**	11.99		
FLURBIPROFEN, MICRONIZED				
(Hawkins) *See FLURBIPROFEN MICRONIZED*				
FLURESS (Akorn)				
benoxinate hydrochloride/fluorescein sodium				
SOL, OP, 0.4%-0.25%,				
5 ml	**17478-0640-10**	11.44		
(Phys Total Care)				
REPACK				
SOL, OP, 0.4%-0.25%,				
5 ml	**54868-3802-00**	13.71		
FLUROX (Ocusoft)				
benoxinate hydrochloride/fluorescein sodium				
SOL, OP, 0.4%-0.25%,				
5 ml	**54799-0508-05**	12.43		
(1X5ML)				
0.4%-0.25%, 5 ml	**54799-0506-05**	11.18		
(Southwood)				
REPACK				
SOL, OP, 0.4%-0.25%,				
5 ml	**58016-4792-01**	12.44		
FLURZEPAM (DHS, Inc.)				
REPACK				
flurazepam hydrochloride				
CAP, PO, 15 mg,				
30s ea, C-IV	**55887-0170-30**	8.62		
60s ea, C-IV	**55887-0170-60**	17.23		
90s ea, C-IV	**55887-0170-90**	25.84		
FLUTABS (Breckenridge Pharm)				
apap/dm/gg/pse hcl				
TAB, PO (DYE-FREE)				
100s ea	**51991-0442-01**	101.02		
FLUTAMIDE (Par)				
CAP, PO, 125 mg, 180s ea	**49884-0753-13**	376.60		AB
(Sandoz)				
CAP, PO (BLISTER PACK,10X10)				
125 mg, 100s ea UD	**00185-1125-88**	209.22		AB
180s ea	**00185-1125-18**	376.60		AB
500s ea	**00185-1125-05**	1046.29		AB
(Teva)				
CAP, PO, 125 mg, 180s ea	**00172-4960-58**	374.60		AB
500s ea	**00172-4960-70**	1040.45		AB
(Watson Labs)				
CAP, PO (USP)				
125 mg, 180s ea	**00591-2227-18**	334.75		AB
(Phys Total Care)				
REPACK				
CAP, PO, 125 mg, 180s ea	**54868-4628-00**	466.14		AB
(Southwood)				
REPACK				
CAP, PO, 125 mg, 30s ea	**58016-0170-30**	62.43		
60s ea	**58016-0170-60**	124.87		
90s ea	**58016-0170-90**	187.30		
100s ea	**58016-0170-00**	208.11		
180s ea	**58016-0170-99**	374.60		
FLUTICASONE (Palmetto)				
REPACK				
fluticasone propionate				
SPR, NS, 0.05 mg/actuation,				
16 gm	**23490-5615-01**	96.84		
(Quality Care Prod)				
REPACK				
SPR, NS, 0.05 mg/actuation,				
16 gm	**49999-0982-16**	90.32		
FLUTICASONE FUROATE				
(Glaxo) *See VERAMYST*				
FLUTICASONE PROP (Phys Total Care)				
REPACK				
fluticasone propionate				
SPR, NS, 0.05 mg/actuation,				
16 gm	**54868-5545-00**	119.70		
FLUTICASONE PROPIONATE				
FUL				
CRE, TP, 0.05%, 30 gm		33.33		
OIN, TP, 0.005%, 30 gm		33.33		
(Apotex Corp.) *See NOVAPLUS FLUTICASONE PROPIONATE*				
(Apotex Corp.)				
SPR, NS (120 METERED SPRAYS)				
0.05 mg/actuation,				
15 ml	**60505-0829-01**	85.26		AB
(Fougera)				
CRE, TP, 0.05%, 15 gm	**00168-0332-15**	22.18		
30 gm	**00168-0332-30**	34.18		
60 gm	**00168-0332-60**	53.88		
OIN, TP, 0.005%, 15 gm	**00168-0333-15**	22.18		
30 gm	**00168-0333-30**	34.18		
60 gm	**00168-0333-60**	53.88		
(G&W)				
CRE, TP, 0.05%, 15 gm	**00713-0631-15**	22.18		AB
30 gm	**00713-0631-31**	34.18		AB
60 gm	**00713-0631-60**	53.88		AB
OIN, TP, 0.005%, 15 gm	**00713-0632-15**	22.18		AB
30 gm	**00713-0632-31**	34.18		AB
60 gm	**00713-0632-60**	53.88		AB
(Glaxo) *See FLONASE*				
(Glaxo) *See FLOVENT DISKUS*				
(Glaxo) *See FLOVENT HFA*				
(Glaxo)				
SPR, NS (1X16GM,120 DOSES)				
0.05 mg/actuation,				
16 gm	**00173-3001-01**	23.82		AB
(Hi-Tech)				
SPR, NS (1X16GM)				
0.05 mg/actuation,				
16 gm	**50383-0700-16**	84.32		AB
(PCCA)				
POW, NA (1X1GM)				
1 gm	**51927-4309-00**	600.00		
(Perrigo)				
CRE, TP, 0.05%, 15 gm	**45802-0222-35**	22.25		
30 gm	**45802-0222-11**	34.30		
60 gm	**45802-0222-37**	54.10		
OIN, TP, 0.005%, 15 gm	**45802-0221-35**	22.25		
30 gm	**45802-0221-11**	34.30		
60 gm	**45802-0221-37**	54.10		
(PharmaDerm) *See CUTIVATE*				
(Roxane)				
SPR, NS, 0.05 mg/actuation,				
16 gm	**00054-3270-99**	75.27		AB
(Sandoz)				
CRE, TP, 0.05%, 15 gm	**00781-7069-27**	22.31		AT
30 gm	**00781-7069-03**	34.37		AT
60 gm	**00781-7069-35**	54.19		AT
(A-S Medication)				
REPACK				
SPR, NS, 0.05 mg/actuation,				
16 gm	**54569-5780-00**	75.26		AB
(Aidarex)				
REPACK				
SPR, NS (120 METERED SPRAYS)				
0.05 mg/actuation,				
15 gm	**33261-0446-01**	89.70		AB
FLUTICASONE PROPIONATE (Palmetto)				
REPACK				
CRE, TP (1X15GM)				
0.05%, 15 gm	**23490-5616-01**	61.00		
(1X30GM)				
0.05%, 30 gm	**23490-5616-03**	94.00		
(1X60GM)				
0.05%, 60 gm	**23490-5616-06**	148.17		
FLUTICASONE PROPIONATE (Pharma Pac)				
REPACK				
SPR, NS (1X16GM)				
0.05 mg/actuation,				
16 gm	**52959-0956-16**	61.26		AB
(Phys Total Care)				
REPACK				
CRE, TP, 0.05%, 30 gm	**54868-5337-00**	39.45		
OIN, TP, 0.005%, 60 gm	**54868-5458-00**	63.69		
(Physician Partner)				
REPACK				
SPR, NS (1X16GM)				
0.05 mg/actuation,				
16 gm	**21695-0704-16**	150.54		
(Quality Care Prod)				
REPACK				
CRE, TP (1X15GM)				
0.05%, 15 gm	**35356-0246-15**	36.40		
(Southwood)				
REPACK				
SPR, NS, 0.05 mg/actuation,				
ea	**58016-4875-01**	75.26		
FLUTICASONE PROPIONATE MICRO (Letco)				
fluticasone propionate, micronized				
POW, NA, 100 gm	**62991-2698-02**	74250.00		
FLUTICASONE PROPIONATE, MICRONIZED				
(Letco) *See FLUTICASONE PROPIONATE MICRO*				
FLUTICASONE PROPIONATE/SALMETEROL XINAFOATE				
(Glaxo) *See ADVAIR DISKUS 100/50*				
(Glaxo) *See ADVAIR DISKUS 250/50*				
(Glaxo) *See ADVAIR DISKUS 500/50*				
(Glaxo) *See ADVAIR HFA*				
FLUVASTATIN SODIUM				
(Novartis Pharm) *See LESCOL*				
(Novartis Pharm) *See LESCOL XL*				

PROD/MFR	NDC	AWP	DP	OBC
FLUVIRIN (Novartis)				
influenza virus vaccine (subvirion)				
SOL, IM (2006-2007,PF)				
45 mcg/0.5 ml,				
0.5 ml 10s	66521-0109-01	182.40		
(2007-2008,TAX INCL,PF)				
45 mcg/0.5 ml,				
0.5 ml 10s	66521-0110-01	184.94		
(2006-2007,MDV)				
45 mcg/0.5 ml,				
5 ml	66521-0109-10	148.10		
(2007-2008,TAX INCL,PF)				
45 mcg/0.5 ml,				
5 ml	66521-0110-10	148.22		
(Novartis)				
influenza virus vaccine				
SUS, IM (10X0.5ML,2008-2009)				
45 mcg/0.5 ml,				
0.5 ml 10s	66521-0111-01	184.94		
0.5 ml 10s	66521-0111-02	184.94		
(2009-2010,TAX INCL)				
45 mcg/0.5 ml,				
0.5 ml 10s	66521-0112-02	136.50	115.00	
(1X5ML,2008-2009,MDV)				
45 mcg/0.5 ml,				
5 ml	66521-0111-10	148.22		
(2009-2010,TAX INCL, MDV)				
45 mcg/0.5 ml,				
5 ml	66521-0112-10	117.30	99.00	
(A-S Medication) REPACK				
influenza virus vaccine (subvirion)				
SOL, IM (10X5ML,2006-2007)				
45 mcg/0.5 ml,				
5 ml 10s	54569-5821-00	140.60		
(Phys Total Care) REPACK				
SOL, IM (2005-06)				
45 mcg/0.5 ml,				
5 ml	54868-5495-00	203.96		
(2006-07)				
45 mcg/0.5 ml,				
5 ml	54868-5665-00	179.79		
(2007-08)				
45 mcg/0.5 ml,				
5 ml	54868-5813-00	171.76		
(Physician Partner) REPACK				
SOL, IM (MULTI-DOSE)				
45 mcg/0.5 ml,				
5 ml	21695-0632-05	296.44		
FLUVOXAMINE (Quality Care Prod) REPACK				
fluvoxamine maleate				
TAB, PO, 25 mg, 30s ea	35356-0029-30	168.00		
50 mg, 30s ea	35356-0030-30	186.00		
100 mg, 30s ea	35356-0031-30	189.00		
FLUVOXAMINE MALEATE FUL				
TAB, PO, 25 mg, 100s ea		108.83		
50 mg, 100s ea		108.30		
100 mg, 100s ea		117.75		
(Apotex Corp.)				
TAB, PO (FILM-COATED)				
25 mg, 100s ea	60505-0164-01	230.30		AB
50 mg, 100s ea	60505-0165-01	257.35		AB
100 mg, 100s ea	60505-0166-01	264.14		AB
(BayPharma)				
TAB, PO (USP,FILM-COATED)				
25 mg, 100s ea	42769-1222-00	230.00		
50 mg, 100s ea	42769-1225-00	257.00		
100 mg, 100s ea	42769-1221-00	263.00		
(Caraco)				
TAB, PO (FILM-COATED)				
25 mg, 100s ea	57664-0357-88	230.30		AB
50 mg, 100s ea	57664-0361-88	257.35		AB
500s ea	57664-0361-13	1286.75		AB
100 mg, 100s ea	57664-0362-88	263.95		AB
500s ea	57664-0362-13	1319.75		AB
(Jazz) *See LUVOX CR*				
(Mylan)				
TAB, PO, 25 mg, 100s ea	00378-0407-01	230.30		AB
50 mg, 100s ea	00378-0412-01	257.35		AB
100 mg, 100s ea	00378-0414-01	263.95		AB
(Sandoz)				
TAB, PO, 25 mg, 100s ea	00185-0017-01	230.30		AB
50 mg, 100s ea	00185-0027-01	257.35		AB
500s ea	00185-0027-05	1286.75		AB

PROD/MFR	NDC	AWP	DP	OBC
100 mg, 100s ea	00185-0157-01	263.95		AB
500s ea	00185-0157-05	1319.75		AB
(Teva)				
TAB, PO, 25 mg, 100s ea	00555-0967-02	230.30		AB
(USP)				
25 mg, 100s ea	00093-0072-01	229.18		AB
50 mg, 100s ea	00555-0968-02	257.35		AB
(USP,FILM-COATED)				
50 mg, 100s ea	00093-0056-01	256.10		AB
100 mg, 100s ea	00555-0969-02	263.95		AB
(USP,FILM-COATED)				
100 mg, 100s ea	00093-0057-01	262.67		AB
(UDL)				
TAB, PO (10X10)				
50 mg, 100s ea UD	51079-0992-20	257.35		AB
100 mg, 100s ea UD	51079-0993-20	263.95		AB
(GSMS) REPACK				
TAB, PO (USP,FILM-COATED)				
25 mg, 100s ea	60429-0758-01	58.50	19.50	AB
50 mg, 30s ea	60429-0759-30	21.24	7.08	AB
90s ea	60429-0759-90	55.80	18.60	AB
100s ea	60429-0759-01	61.92	20.64	AB
100 mg, 30s ea	60429-0760-30	24.30	8.10	AB
90s ea	60429-0760-90	64.80	21.60	AB
100s ea	60429-0760-01	72.00	24.00	AB
(Phys Total Care) REPACK				
TAB, PO, 50 mg, 30s ea	54868-5635-00	52.53		
(Stat Rx) REPACK				
TAB, PO (FILM-COATED)				
25 mg, 30s ea	16590-0270-30	79.00		
FLUZONE (Sanofi)				
influenza virus vaccine, inactivated				
SOL, IM (2009-2010,TAX INC)				
22.5 mcg/0.25 ml,				
0.25 ml 10s	49281-0009-25	156.40	131.58	
(2009-10,TAX INC)				
45 mcg/0.5 ml,				
0.5 ml 10s	49281-0009-10	127.03	107.11	
0.5 ml 10s	49281-0009-50	127.03	107.11	
(2009-2010,TAX INC)				
45 mcg/0.5 ml,				
5 ml	49281-0384-15	115.18	97.23	
(A-S Medication) REPACK				
influenza virus vaccine (subvirion)				
SOL, IM (10X0.25ML)				
45 mcg/0.5 ml,				
0.25 ml 10s	54569-5971-00	176.33		
(Phys Total Care) REPACK				
influenza virus vaccine, inactivated				
SOL, IM (2008-2009,1X5ML)				
45 mcg/0.5 ml,				
5 ml	54868-5941-00	175.53		
(Sanofi) REPACK				
SOL, IM (1X5ML,LATEX-FREE)				
45 mcg/0.5 ml,				
5 ml	54868-6059-00	136.96		
FLUZONE HIGH-DOSE (Sanofi)				
influenza virus vaccine (subvirion)				
SUS, IM (2009-2010, TAX INC,PF)				
180 mcg/0.5 ml,				
0.5 ml 10s	49281-0385-65	307.50	257.50	
FML FORTE LIQUIFILM (Allergan Inc)				
fluorometholone				
SUS, OP, 0.25%, 2 ml	11980-0228-02	8.54		
5 ml	11980-0228-05	25.45		
10 ml	11980-0228-10	44.69		
FML LIQUIFILM (Allergan Inc)				
fluorometholone				
SUS, OP, 0.1%, 5 ml	11980-0211-05	31.34		AB
10 ml	11980-0211-10	57.12		AB
15 ml	11980-0211-15	79.87		AB
(Southwood) REPACK				
SUS, OP, 0.1%, 5 ml	58016-6096-01	18.44		AB
FML S.O.P. (Allergan Inc)				
fluorometholone				
OIN, OP, 0.1%, 3.5 gm	00023-0316-04	40.42		
(Southwood) REPACK				
OIN, OP, 0.1%, 3.5 gm	58016-6561-03	21.00		

PROD/MFR	NDC	AWP	DP	OBC
FOAM, MULTI INGREDIENT				
(Onset) *See HYLATOPIC EMOLLIENT FOAM*				
(Quinnova) *See NEOSALUS*				
FOBALIN PLUS (Pamlab)				
cyanocobalamin/folic acid/pyridoxine				
TAB, PO (SF,DYE-FREE)				
2 mg-2.5 mg-25 mg,				
90s ea	12593-0047-90	41.34	29.53	
FOCALIN (Novartis Pharm)				
dexmethylphenidate hydrochloride				
TAB, PO, 2.5 mg,				
100s ea, C-II	00078-0380-05	75.92		
5 mg,				
100s ea, C-II	00078-0381-05	108.23		
10 mg,				
100s ea, C-II	00078-0382-05	155.65		
FOCALIN XR (Novartis Pharm)				
dexmethylphenidate hydrochloride				
CER, PO, 5 mg,				
100s ea, C-II	00078-0430-05	494.66		
10 mg,				
100s ea, C-II	00078-0431-05	501.80		
15 mg,				
100s ea, C-II	00078-0493-05	516.07		
20 mg,				
100s ea, C-II	00078-0432-05	516.07		
30 mg,				
100s ea, C-II	00078-0433-05	541.87		EE
(Quality Care Prod) REPACK				
CER, PO, 5 mg,				
30s ea, C-II	35356-0158-30	224.46		
90s ea, C-II	35356-0158-90	665.37		
10 mg,				
30s ea, C-II	35356-0159-30	227.80		
90s ea, C-II	35356-0159-90	675.39		
20 mg,				
30s ea, C-II	35356-0160-30	234.48		
90s ea, C-II	35356-0160-90	695.43		
(Stat Rx) REPACK				
CER, PO, 15 mg,				
30s ea, C-II	16590-0649-30	146.90		
60s ea, C-II	16590-0649-60	292.00		
90s ea, C-II	16590-0649-90	435.50		
FOLAST (Acella)				
l-methylfolate/methylcobalamin/pyridoxal phosphate				
TAB, PO (COATED)				
2.8 mg-2 mg-25 mg,				
90s ea	42192-0311-90	79.22		
FOLBECAL (Breckenridge Pharm)				
calcium/cyanocobalamin/folic acid/pyridoxine				
TAB, PO (FILM-COATED)				
30s ea	51991-0077-33	32.79		
FOLBEE (Breckenridge Pharm)				
cyanocobalamin/folic acid/pyridoxine				
TAB, PO (SF,DYE-FREE)				
1 mg-2.5 mg-25 mg,				
90s ea	51991-0084-90	52.37		
FOLBEE PLUS (Breckenridge Pharm)				
vitamin b complex and vitamin c				
TAB, PO (SF,DYE-FREE)				
90s ea	51991-0082-90	47.77		
FOLBEE PLUS CZ (Breckenridge Pharm)				
medical food				
TAB, PO (SF,GLUTEN-FREE)				
90s ea	51991-0528-90	63.69		
FOLBIC (Breckenridge Pharm)				
cyanocobalamin/folic acid/pyridoxine				
TAB, PO (AF,GLUTEN-FREE,SOY-FREE)				
2 mg-2.5 mg-25 mg,				
90s ea	51991-0384-90	65.42		
FOLCAL DHA (Midlothian Labs)				
prenatal vitamins				
SGL, PO (SOFTGEL)				
30s ea	68308-0350-30	46.59		
FOLCAPS (Midlothian Labs)				
cyanocobalamin/folic acid/pyridoxine				
TAB, PO (FILM-COATED)				
0.5 mg-2.2 mg-25 mg,				
100s ea	68308-0324-10	43.46		
FOLCAPS CARE ONE (Midlothian Labs)				
prenatal vitamins				
SGL, PO (SOFT GEL)				
30s ea	68308-0167-30	43.02		

PROD/MFR	NDC	AWP	DP	OBC
FOLEY CATHETER				
(Covidien) *See PRECISION ADD-A-FOLEY DRAINAGE BAG TRAY*				
(Mentor) *See SELF-CATH COUDE/OLIVE TIP*				
(Mentor) *See SELF-CATH COUDE/TAPERED TIP*				
(Mentor) *See SELF-CATH PEDIATRIC STRAIGHT TIP*				
FOLGARD OS (Upsher-Smith)				
b/ca/folic acid/mg/vit b12/vit b6/vit d				
TAB, PO, 60s ea	00245-0155-60	24.75		
FOLGARD RX (Upsher-Smith)				
cyanocobalamin/folic acid/pyridoxine				
TAB, PO (FILM-COATED)				
1 mg-2.2 mg-25 mg,				
100s ea	00245-0191-11	63.46		
FOLI-IRON & C (Contract Pharmacal)				
ascorbic acid/ferrous sulfate/folic acid				
TER, PO (CAPLET)				
500 mg-105 mg-0.8 mg,				
60s ea UD	10267-2465-07	28.73		
100s ea UD	10267-2465-01	45.94		
FOLIC ACID				
FUL				
TAB, PO, 1 mg, 100s ea		3.78		
(Allan Pharmaceutical)				
TAB, PO, 1 mg, 100s ea	13279-0600-10	34.45		
1000s ea	13279-0600-11	88.95		
(Amend)				
POW, NA (U.S.P.)				
5 gm	17317-0175-08	5.60		
10 gm	17317-0175-01	8.70		
25 gm	17317-0175-02	17.50		
100 gm	17317-0175-03	49.00		
500 gm	17317-0175-05	224.00		
(Amneal)				
TAB, PO, 1 mg, 100s ea	65162-0361-10	33.15		
1000s ea	65162-0361-11	78.00		
(APP)				
SOL, IJ (M.D.V.)				
5 mg/ml, 10 ml	63323-0184-10	22.25		AP
(Blu)				
TAB, PO (USP,COMPRESSED TABLET)				
1 mg, 100s ea	24658-0110-01	4.20		AA
1000s ea	24658-0110-10	33.66		AA
(Breckenridge Pharm)				
TAB, PO (USP)				
1 mg, 1000s ea	51991-0201-10	78.00		AA
(Cadista)				
TAB, PO, 1 mg, 100s ea	59746-0012-06	34.50		AA
1000s ea	59746-0012-10	79.50		AA
(Consolidated Midland)				
TAB, PO, 1 mg, 100s ea	00223-1002-01	2.75		EE
1000s ea	00223-1002-02	9.75		EE
(Contract Pharmacal)				
TAB, PO, 1 mg, 100s ea	10267-0120-01	11.70		EE
1000s ea	10267-0120-04	79.62		EE
(Deca Pharm)				
TAB, PO (USP)				
1 mg, 100s ea	68552-0529-01	36.20		AA
1000s ea	68552-0529-10	99.74		AA
(Excellium)				
TAB, PO (USP)				
1 mg, 100s ea	64125-0127-01	36.00		AA
1000s ea	64125-0127-10	79.00		AA
(Gallipot)				
POW, NA (U.S.P.)				
10 gm	51552-0418-03	15.19		
25 gm	51552-0418-04	25.90		
(Major)				
TAB, PO, 1 mg, 1000s ea	00904-0625-80	77.81		AA
(Marlex)				
TAB, PO, 1 mg, 100s ea	10135-0182-01	2.95		
1000s ea	10135-0182-10	9.33		
(Medisca)				
POW, NA (U.S.P.)				
10 gm	38779-0224-01	32.85		
25 gm	38779-0224-04	59.85		
100 gm	38779-0224-05	179.85		
(USP,1X500GM)				
500 gm	38779-0224-08	394.50		
(U.S.P.)				
1000 gm	38779-0224-09	687.00		
(PCCA)				
POW, NA (U.S.P.)				
1 gm	51927-1341-00	4.50		
(Prasco Labs)				
TAB, PO, 1 mg, 1000s ea	66993-0425-05	78.60		
(Qualitest)				
TAB, PO, 1 mg, 1000s ea	00603-3714-32	78.00		AA
(Spectrum Pharmacy)				
POW, NA (U.S.P.)				
10 gm	49452-3180-01	64.75		
25 gm	49452-3180-02	110.95		
100 gm	49452-3180-03	281.75		
1000 gm	49452-3180-04	1039.50		
(Teva)				
TAB, PO (USP,10X10)				
1 mg, 100s ea UD	00093-0507-93	22.67		AA
(TriMarc Labs)				
TAB, PO (USP,COMPRESSED TABLET)				
1 mg, 100s ea	68752-0001-01	14.75		AA
1000s ea	68752-0001-10	77.50		AA
(Truxton)				
TAB, PO, 1 mg, 1000s ea	00463-6096-10	8.50		EE
(UDL)				
TAB, PO (ROBOT READY 25X1)				
1 mg, 25s ea UD	51079-0041-19	5.70		AA
(10X10)				
1 mg, 100s ea UD	51079-0041-20	15.95		AA
(West-Ward)				
TAB, PO, 1 mg, 100s ea	00143-1248-01	34.50		AA
1000s ea	00143-1248-10	78.60		AA
(A-S Medication)				
REPACK				
TAB, PO, 1 mg, 30s ea	54569-0958-02	10.80		EE
100s ea	54569-0958-00	36.00		EE
(American Health)				
REPACK				
TAB, PO (10X10)				
1 mg, 100s ea UD	62584-0897-01	36.20		AA
(15X30)				
1 mg, 450s ea	62584-0897-85	56.88		AA
(Apace)				
REPACK				
TAB, PO (USP)				
1 mg, 100s ea	15338-0170-00	36.00		AA
(Bryant Ranch)				
REPACK				
TAB, PO, 1 mg, 30s ea	63629-2816-01	10.80		
(DHS, Inc.)				
REPACK				
TAB, PO, 1 mg, 30s ea	55887-0298-30	10.00		
(Dispensing Solutions)				
REPACK				
TAB, PO, 1 mg, 30s ea	66336-0697-30	9.00		AA
100s ea	55045-1166-01	36.00		
(GSMS)				
REPACK				
TAB, PO (UNIT OF USE)				
1 mg, 90s ea	60429-0212-90	31.50	10.50	AA
(HomeMed)				
REPACK				
TAB, PO, 1 mg, 30s ea	51655-0008-24	4.17		EE
90s ea	51655-0008-26	3.70		EE
(McKesson Packaging)				
REPACK				
TAB, PO (USP)				
1 mg, 100s ea UD	63739-0110-10	29.63		EE
(BLISTER PACK)				
1 mg, 750s ea UD	63739-0110-01	222.24		EE
(Palmetto)				
REPACK				
TAB, PO, 1 mg, 30s ea	23490-5617-01	11.40		
(PD-Rx Pharm)				
REPACK				
TAB, PO, 1 mg, 30s ea	55289-0492-30	26.23		AA
30s ea	58864-0217-30	26.22		EE
90s ea	55289-0492-90	37.50		AA
(Phys Total Care)				
REPACK				
TAB, PO, 1 mg, 30s ea	54868-2314-02	15.78		
30s ea	54868-5098-01	58.88		EE
60s ea	54868-2314-03	26.51		EE
90s ea	54868-2314-04	33.83		EE
100s ea	54868-2314-00	40.68		EE
(Quality Care Prod)				
REPACK				
TAB, PO, 1 mg, 60s ea	49999-0433-60	70.48		AA
(Southwood)				
REPACK				
TAB, PO, 0.4 mg, 30s ea	58016-0079-30	0.65		
60s ea	58016-0079-60	1.30		
90s ea	58016-0079-90	1.95		
100s ea	58016-0079-00	2.17		
FOLIC ACID/CYANOCOBALAMIN/PYRIDOXINE				
(Phys Total Care)				
REPACK				
cyanocobalamin/folic acid/pyridoxine				
TAB, PO, 1 mg-2.5 mg-25 mg,				
60s ea	54868-5098-00	86.87		
90s ea	54868-5098-02	125.81		
FOLIC ACID/CYANOCOBALAMIN/PYRIDOXONE				
(Allan Pharmaceutical)				
cyanocobalamin/folic acid/pyridoxine				
TAB, PO (FILM-COATED)				
0.5 mg-2.2 mg-25 mg,				
100s ea	13279-0601-10	43.50		
FOLIC ACID/HYDROXOCOBALAMIN/MG/VIT B6/VIT E				
(Alaven) *See FOLPACE RX*				
FOLIC ACID/IRON				
(Colorado Biolabs) *See PROFERRIN-FORTE*				
FOLIC ACID/LIVER EXTRACT/VITAMIN B12				
(Consolidated Midland)				
cyanocobalamin/folic acid/liver				
SOL, IJ (VIAL)				
10 ml	00223-7956-10	25.00		
FOLIC ACID/OMEGA-3 FATTY ACIDS/VIT B12/VIT B6				
(PBM Pharmaceuticals) *See ANIMI-3*				
FOLITAB 500 (Rising)				
ascorbic acid/ferrous sulfate/folic acid				
TER, PO (BLISTER PACK,CAPLET)				
500 mg-525 mg-0.8 mg,				
30s ea UD	64980-0105-03	19.68		
FOLLICLE STIMULATING HORMONE/LUTEINIZING HORMONE				
(Ferring) *See MENOPUR*				
(Ferring) *See REPRONEX*				
FOLLISTIM AQ (Organon)				
follitropin beta				
SOL, IJ, 75 iu/0.5 ml,				
0.5 ml	00052-0308-02	109.51		
150 iu/0.5 ml,				
0.5 ml	00052-0309-02	219.02		
SC, 300 iu/0.36 ml,				
0.42 ml	00052-0313-01	438.05		
600 iu/0.72 ml,				
0.78 ml	00052-0316-01	876.10		
(DELIVERS 900IU,BLUECAP)				
900 iu/1.08 ml,				
1.17 ml	00052-0326-01	1314.14		
FOLLITROPIN ALFA				
(EMD) *See GONAL-F*				
(EMD) *See GONAL-F RFF*				
FOLLITROPIN BETA				
(Organon) *See FOLLISTIM AQ*				
FOLOTYN (Allos)				
pralatrexate				
SOL, IV (PF)				
20 mg/ml, 1 ml	48818-0001-01	3750.00		
2 ml	48818-0001-02	7500.00		
FOLPACE RX (Alaven)				
folic acid/hydroxocobalamin/mg/vit b6/vit e				
TAB, PO (SF,DYE-FREE)				
90s ea	68220-0018-90	67.53		
FOLPLEX (Breckenridge Pharm)				
cyanocobalamin/folic acid/pyridoxine				
TAB, PO, 1 mg-2.2 mg-25 mg,				
100s ea	51991-0352-01	49.95		
FOLPLEX 2.2 (Breckenridge Pharm)				
cyanocobalamin/folic acid/pyridoxine				
TAB, PO (AF,SF,GLUTEN-FREE)				
0.5 mg-2.2 mg-25 mg,				
100s ea	51991-0252-01	38.76		
FOLTABS 90 PLUS DHA (Midlothian Labs)				
prenatal vitamins				
KIT, PO, 6s ea	68308-0190-30	42.70	29.46	
FOLTABS PRENATAL (Midlothian Labs)				
prenatal vitamins				
TAB, PO, 90s ea	68308-0165-90	42.49	31.45	

PROD/MFR | NDC | AWP | DP | OBC

FOLTABS PRENATAL PLUS DHA (Midlothian Labs)
prenatal vitamins
KIT, PO, 60s ea 68308-0160-30 42.42

FOLTRATE (Poly)
cyanocobalamin/folic acid
TAB, PO (FILM-COATED)
0.5 mg-1 mg,
100s ea 66869-0122-10 84.99 67.99

FOLTRIN (Sandoz)
ferrous fum/folic acid/if/vit b12/vit c
CAP, PO (6X10,BLISTER PACK)
60s ea UD 00185-5380-76 45.35
(10X10,BLISTER PACK)
100s ea UD 00185-5380-88 57.93

FOLTX (Pamlab)
cyanocobalamin/folic acid/pyridoxine
TAB, PO (SF,LACTOSE-FREE,COATED)
2 mg-2.5 mg-25 mg,
90s ea 00525-0906-90 84.53

(DHS, Inc.)
REPACK
TAB, PO, 1 mg-2.5 mg-25 mg,
30s ea 55887-0724-30 32.00
60s ea 55887-0724-60 64.00
90s ea 55887-0724-90 96.00
100s ea 55887-0724-01 106.67

(Phys Total Care)
REPACK
TAB, PO (SF,DYE-FREE)
2 mg-2.5 mg-25 mg,
30s ea 54868-5096-00 31.51
60s ea 54868-5096-01 61.15
90s ea 54868-5096-02 90.16

FOMEPIZOLE (GeneraMedix)
SOL, IV (1X1.5ML,PF)
1 gm/ml, 1.5 ml .... 10139-0910-15 1197.60 AP
(Jazz) *See ANTIZOL*
(PCCA) *See METHYLPYRAZOLE*
(Sandoz)
SOL, IV (1X1.5ML,PF)
1 gm/ml, 1.5 ml 00781-3182-73 1364.85
(4X1.5ML,PF)
1 gm/ml, 1.5 ml 4s 00781-3182-84 5459.40
(X-Gen)
SOL, IV (1X1.5ML,PF)
1 gm/ml, 1.5 ml 39822-0710-01 1312.00

FONDAPARINUX SODIUM
(Glaxo) *See ARIXTRA*

FOOD COLOR, BLUE (Medisca)
color additive
POW, NA (1X5GM,FD&C BLUE NO.1)
5 gm 38779-1293-03 16.50
(1X100GM,FD&C BLUE NO.1)
100 gm 38779-1293-05 66.00
SOL, NA (1X14ML)
14 ml 38779-1292-03 8.25

FOOD COLOR, BROWN (Medisca)
color additive
POW, NA (1X5GM)
5 gm 38779-1294-03 13.50

FOOD COLOR, GREEN (Medisca)
color additive
POW, NA (1X5GM,FD&C GREEN NO.3)
5 gm 38779-1296-03 16.50
(1X100GM,FD&C GREEN NO.3)
100 gm 38779-1296-05 66.00

FOOD COLOR, ORANGE (Medisca)
color additive
POW, NA (1X5GM,D&C ORANGE NO.4)
5 gm 38779-1298-03 16.50
(1X100GM,D&C ORANGE NO.4)
100 gm 38779-1298-05 123.00

FOOD COLOR, RED (Medisca)
color additive
SOL, NA (1X14ML)
14 ml 38779-1300-03 16.50
(1X500ML)
500 ml 38779-1300-08 48.00

FOOD COLOR, VIOLET (Medisca)
color additive
POW, NA (1X5GM)
5 gm 38779-1302-03 13.50
(1X100GM)
100 gm 38779-1302-05 61.50

FOOD COLOR, YELLOW (Medisca)
color additive
POW, NA (1X5GM,FD&C YELLOW NO.6)
5 gm 38779-1305-03 13.50
SOL, NA (1X14ML)
14 ml 38779-1304-03 3.00
(1X500ML)
500 ml 38779-1304-08 48.00

FORADIL AEROLIZER (Phys Total Care)
REPACK
formoterol fumarate
CAP, IH, 0.012 mg,
12s ea 54868-4972-00 38.81
60s ea 54868-4972-01 176.59

FORANE (Baxter)
isoflurane
LIQ, IH, 99.9%,
100 ml 6s .... 10019-0360-40 144.00 AN
250 ml 6s .... 10019-0360-60 345.60 AN

FORMA-RAY (Gordon)
formaldehyde
SOL, TP (W/DAUBER)
20%, 60 ml 10481-3015-05 15.35
120 ml 10481-3015-02 17.40

FORMADON (Gordon)
formaldehyde
SOL, TP (W/DAUBER)
10%, 60 ml 10481-1050-05 12.00
120 ml 10481-1050-02 14.90

FORMALDEHYDE
(Baker, J.T.) *See FORMALDEHYDE 37%*
(Breckenridge Pharm)
SOL, TP (W/ ROLL-ON APPLICATOR)
10%, 85.05 gm 51991-0512-19 53.06
(Gallipot) *See FORMALDEHYDE 10%*
(Gordon) *See FORMA-RAY*
(Gordon) *See FORMADON*
(Mallinckrodt Lab)
SOL, NA (U.S.P.)
500 ml 00406-5014-04 9.85
4000 ml 00406-5014-10 274.08
(Medisca)
SOL, NA (1X100ML,37%)
100 ml 38779-0605-05 43.50
(1X500ML,37%)
500 ml 38779-0605-08 52.50
(1X1000ML,37%)
1000 ml 38779-0605-09 87.00
(1X4000ML,37%)
4000 ml 38779-0605-01 255.00
(PCCA)
SOL, NA (USP)
1 ml 51927-3097-00 0.17
(Pedinol) *See LAZERFORMALYDE*
(Spectrum Pharmacy) *See FORMALDEHYDE 10%*
(Spectrum Pharmacy) *See FORMALDEHYDE 37%*

FORMALDEHYDE 10% (Gallipot)
formaldehyde
SOL, NA (HISTOLOGY)
473 ml 51552-0427-06 14.00
(Spectrum Pharmacy)
SOL, NA (1X1000ML,FRAGRANCE-FREE)
1000 ml 49452-3195-04 149.45
(NEUTRALIZED/BUFFERED)
4000 ml 49452-3195-02 280.00

FORMALDEHYDE 37% (Baker, J.T.)
formaldehyde
SOL, NA (A.C.S., REAGENT)
150 ml 10106-2106-04 21.06
(A.C.S., REAGENT, GLASS)
500 ml 10106-2106-01 33.06
(A.C.S., REAGENT, POLY)
500 ml 10106-2106-02 33.06
4000 ml 10106-2106-05 94.35
(Spectrum Pharmacy)
SOL, NA (U.S.P., N.F.)
120 ml 49452-3191-01 77.35
500 ml 49452-3191-02 106.40
1000 ml 49452-3191-03 170.45
4000 ml 49452-3191-04 348.60

FORMAMIDE (Baker, J.T.)
LIQ, NA, 100 ml 10106-4028-00 26.78
500 ml 10106-4028-01 59.69

FORMIC ACID
(Baker, J.T.) *See FORMIC ACID 88%*
(Baker, J.T.) *See FORMIC ACID 90%*
(PCCA)
POW, NA, 98%, 1 gm 51927-2089-00 0.31

FORMIC ACID 88% (Baker, J.T.)
formic acid
LIQ, NA (A.C.S., REAGENT)
500 ml 10106-0128-01 56.80
2500 ml 10106-0128-05 130.24

FORMIC ACID 90% (Baker, J.T.)
formic acid
LIQ, NA (REAGENT)
500 ml 10106-0129-01 76.79
2500 ml 10106-0129-05 350.41

FORMOTEROL FUMARATE
(Dey, L.P.) *See PERFOROMIST*
(Hawkins) *See FORMOTEROL FUMARATE DIHYDRATE*
(Letco)
POW, NA, 0.5 gm 62991-2516-03 900.00
1 gm 62991-2516-01 1440.00
(Medisca)
POW, NA (1X1GM)
1 gm 38779-2295-06 1500.00
(1X5GM)
5 gm 38779-2295-03 6600.00
(1X25GM)
25 gm 38779-2295-04 33990.00
(1X500MG)
500 ml 38779-2295-00 825.00
(PCCA)
POW, NA (DIHYDRATE)
1 gm 51927-3643-00 1800.00

FORMOTEROL FUMARATE DIHYDRATE (Hawkins)
formoterol fumarate
POW, NA (1X0.5GM)
0.5 gm 63370-0069-09 1324.00
(1X1GM)
1 gm 63370-0069-10 1940.00

FORMULA B PLUS (Major)
multivitamin and minerals
TAB, PO, 100s ea 00904-7929-60 19.94

FORTAMET (Shionogi)
metformin hydrochloride
TER, PO (FILM-COATED)
500 mg, 60s ea .... 59630-0574-60 146.94 BX
1000 mg, 60s ea .... 59630-0575-60 346.77 BX
(Phys Total Care)
REPACK
TER, PO, 500 mg, 60s ea 54868-5558-00 148.78
(FILM-COATED)
500 mg, 90s ea .... 54868-5558-01 210.61 BX

FORTAZ (Glaxo)
ceftazidime
PDS, IJ, 1 gm, 10s ea .... 00173-0378-10 142.32 AP
(ADD-VANTAGE)
1 gm, 25s ea .... 00173-0434-00 367.68 AP
2 gm, 10s ea .... 00173-0435-00 289.34 AP
(VIAL)
2 gm, 10s ea .... 00173-0379-34 284.53 AP
(BULK VIAL)
6 gm, 6s ea .... 00173-0382-37 496.80 AP
500 mg, 10s ea .... 00173-0377-10 71.16 AP
(Glaxo)
ceftazidime sodium/dextrose
SOL, IV (PREMIX,PC)
1 gm/50 ml-2.2 gm/50 ml,
50 ml 24s .... 00173-0412-00 406.24 AP
2 gm/50 ml-1.6 gm/50 ml,
50 ml 24s .... 00173-0413-00 747.67 AP

FORTEO (Lilly)
teriparatide
SOL, SC (1X2.4ML)
250 mcg/ml, 2.4 ml 00002-8400-01 1042.74 868.95
(Phys Total Care)
REPACK
SOL, SC (RDNA ORIGIN)
250 mcg/ml, 3 ml 54868-5406-00 1016.01

FORTICAL (Upsher-Smith)
calcitonin (salmon)
SPR, NS (W/PUMP)
200 iu/actuation,
3.7 ml 00245-0008-35 102.89

PROD/MFR	NDC	AWP	DP	OBC
(Phys Total Care)				
REPACK				
SPR, NS, 200 iu/actuation,				
3.7 ml	54868-5499-00	183.96		
FOSAMAX (Merck)				
alendronate sodium				
SOL, PO (RASPBERRY)				
70 mg/75 ml,				
75 ml 4s	00006-3833-34	102.46		
TAB, PO (UNIT OF USE)				
5 mg, 30s ea	00006-0925-31	100.13		
100s ea	00006-0925-58	333.73		
10 mg, 30s ea	00006-0936-31	100.13		
100s ea	00006-0936-58	333.73		
(BULK PACKAGE)				
10 mg, 1000s ea	00006-0936-82	3337.36		
(UNIT OF USE,BLISTER PK)				
35 mg, 4s ea	00006-0077-44	93.46		
20s ea UD	00006-0077-21	467.23		
(UNIT OF USE)				
40 mg, 30s ea	00006-0212-31	225.73		
(UNIT OF USE,BLISTER PCK)				
70 mg, 4s ea	00006-0031-44	93.46		
20s ea UD	00006-0031-21	467.23		
(A-S Medication)				
REPACK				
TAB, PO (UNIT OF USE,BLISTER PK)				
70 mg, 4s ea	54569-5218-00	121.50		
(Altura)				
REPACK				
TAB, PO, 10 mg, 100s ea	63874-0089-01	231.29		
(Direct Pharmaceutical, Inc.)				
REPACK				
TAB, PO, 10 mg,				
30s ea UD	67801-0320-03	106.54		
(Palmetto)				
REPACK				
TAB, PO, 35 mg, 4s ea	23490-9174-01	96.00		
(Phys Total Care)				
REPACK				
TAB, PO, 5 mg, 30s ea	54868-4384-00	79.63		
10 mg, 30s ea	54868-3857-00	111.25		
(UNIT OF USE,BLISTER PK)				
35 mg, 4s ea	54868-4463-00	99.72		
70 mg, 4s ea	54868-4462-00	97.59		
(Quality Care Prod)				
REPACK				
TAB, PO, 70 mg, 4s ea	49999-0501-04	137.60		
(Southwood)				
REPACK				
TAB, PO, 10 mg, 30s ea	58016-0788-30	93.66		
60s ea	58016-0788-60	187.32		
90s ea	58016-0788-90	280.98		
100s ea	58016-0788-00	312.20		
70 mg, 4s ea	58016-0613-04	87.42		
20s ea	58016-0613-20	437.08		
30s ea	58016-0613-30	655.62		
60s ea	58016-0613-60	1311.24		
90s ea	58016-0613-90	1966.86		
100s ea	58016-0613-00	2185.40		
(Stat Rx)				
REPACK				
TAB, PO, 70 mg, 4s ea	16590-0491-04	114.25		
FOSAMAX PLUS D (Merck)				
alendronate sodium/cholecalciferol				
TAB, PO, 70 mg-2800 iu,				
4s ea	00006-0710-44	98.12		
20s ea UD	00006-0710-21	437.08		
70 mg-5600 iu,				
4s ea	00006-0270-44	98.12		
(Phys Total Care)				
REPACK				
TAB, PO, 70 mg-2800 iu,				
4s ea	54868-5480-00	124.96		
FOSAMPRENAVIR CALCIUM				
(Glaxo) *See LEXIVA*				
FOSAPREPITANT DIMEGLUMINE				
(Merck) *See EMEND*				
FOSCARNET SODIUM (Hospira)				
SOL, IV (12X250ML,PF)				
24 mg/ml,				
250 ml 12s	00409-3863-02	1088.64	952.56	
(12X500ML,PF)				
24 mg/ml,				
500 ml 12s	00409-3863-05	2094.34	1832.52	
FOSFOMYCIN TROMETHAMINE				
(Forest Pharm) *See MONUROL*				
FOSINOPRIL (DHS, Inc.)				
REPACK				
fosinopril sodium				
TAB, PO, 40 mg, 30s ea	55887-0304-30	35.80		
60s ea	55887-0304-60	55.80		
90s ea	55887-0304-90	80.00		
(Phys Total Care)				
REPACK				
TAB, PO, 40 mg, 60s ea	54868-5182-02	49.16		
(Vibranta)				
REPACK				
TAB, PO, 10 mg, 30s ea	57866-0275-02	76.50		
20 mg, 30s ea	57866-3138-01	77.00		
40 mg, 30s ea	57866-0274-01	77.00		
FOSINOPRIL SODIUM				
FUL				
TAB, PO, 10 mg, 90s ea		53.82		
20 mg, 90s ea		53.82		
40 mg, 90s ea		53.82		
(Apotex Corp.)				
TAB, PO, 10 mg, 90s ea	60505-2510-02	107.08		AB
1000s ea	60505-2510-04	1261.13		AB
20 mg, 90s ea	60505-2511-02	107.08		AB
1000s ea	60505-2511-04	1261.13		AB
40 mg, 90s ea	60505-2512-02	107.08		AB
1000s ea	60505-2512-08	1261.13		AB
(Bristol-Myers) *See MONOPRIL*				
(Deca Pharm)				
TAB, PO, 10 mg, 90s ea	68552-0221-90	113.50		AB
1000s ea	68552-0221-10	1261.13		AB
20 mg, 90s ea	68552-0222-90	113.50		AB
1000s ea	68552-0222-10	1261.13		AB
40 mg, 90s ea	68552-0223-90	113.50		AB
1000s ea	68552-0223-10	1261.13		AB
(Glenmark Pharmaceuticals)				
TAB, PO, 10 mg, 90s ea	68462-0367-90	113.50		AB
1000s ea	68462-0367-10	1261.13		AB
20 mg, 90s ea	68462-0368-90	113.50		AB
1000s ea	68462-0368-10	1261.13		AB
40 mg, 90s ea	68462-0369-90	113.50		AB
1000s ea	68462-0369-10	1261.13		AB
(Ranbaxy Pharm)				
TAB, PO, 10 mg, 90s ea	63304-0775-90	113.50		
1000s ea	63304-0775-10	1261.13		
20 mg, 90s ea	63304-0776-90	113.50		
1000s ea	63304-0776-10	1261.13		
40 mg, 90s ea	63304-0777-90	113.50		
1000s ea	63304-0777-10	1261.13		
(Sandoz)				
TAB, PO, 10 mg, 90s ea	00185-0041-09	107.08		
90s ea	00781-5083-92	107.08		
1000s ea	00185-0041-10	1189.75		
1000s ea	00781-5083-10	1130.31		
20 mg, 90s ea	00185-0042-09	107.08		
90s ea	00781-5084-92	107.08		
1000s ea	00185-0042-10	1189.75		
1000s ea	00781-5084-10	1130.31		
40 mg, 90s ea	00185-0047-09	107.08		
90s ea	00781-5085-92	107.08		
1000s ea	00185-0047-10	1189.75		
(Teva)				
TAB, PO, 10 mg, 90s ea	00093-7222-98	107.08		
1000s ea	00093-7222-10	1189.75		
20 mg, 90s ea	00093-7223-98	107.08		
1000s ea	00093-7223-10	1189.75		
40 mg, 90s ea	00093-7224-98	107.08		
1000s ea	00093-7224-10	1189.75		
(A-S Medication)				
REPACK				
TAB, PO, 10 mg, 30s ea	54569-5621-00	37.83		
40 mg, 30s ea	54569-6098-00	35.69		
(GSMS)				
REPACK				
TAB, PO (UNIT-OF-USE)				
10 mg, 45s ea	60429-0755-45	43.56	14.52	AB
90s ea	60429-0755-90	87.09	29.03	AB
1000s ea	60429-0755-10	939.75	313.25	AB
(UNIT-OF-USE)				
20 mg, 45s ea	60429-0756-45	43.56	14.52	AB
90s ea	60429-0756-90	87.09	29.03	AB
180s ea	60429-0756-18	174.18	58.06	AB
1000s ea	60429-0756-10	939.75	313.25	AB
(UNIT-OF-USE)				
40 mg, 45s ea	60429-0757-45	43.56	14.52	AB
90s ea	60429-0757-90	87.09	29.03	AB
180s ea	60429-0757-18	174.18	58.06	AB
1000s ea	60429-0757-10	939.75	313.25	AB
(Phys Total Care)				
REPACK				
TAB, PO, 10 mg, 30s ea	54868-5064-01	29.07		
90s ea	54868-5064-00	79.68		
20 mg, 30s ea	54868-5055-00	26.07		
40 mg, 30s ea	54868-5182-00	26.07		
90s ea	54868-5182-01	72.24		
FOSINOPRIL SODIUM AND HYDROCHLOROTHIAZIDE				
(Aurobindo Pharma)				
fosinopril sodium/hydrochlorothiazide				
TAB, PO (USP)				
10 mg-12.5 mg,				
100s ea	65862-0308-01	148.05		AB
20 mg-12.5 mg,				
100s ea	65862-0309-01	148.05		AB
FOSINOPRIL SODIUM-HYDROCHLOROTHIAZIDE				
(Ranbaxy Pharm)				
fosinopril sodium/hydrochlorothiazide				
TAB, PO, 10 mg-12.5 mg,				
100s ea	63304-0403-01	126.13		AB
20 mg-12.5 mg,				
100s ea	63304-0404-01	126.13		AB
FOSINOPRIL SODIUM/HYDROCHLOROTHIAZIDE				
FUL				
TAB, PO, 10 mg-12.5 mg,				
100s ea		134.54		
20 mg-12.5 mg,				
100s ea		134.54		
(Aurobindo Pharma) *See FOSINOPRIL SODIUM AND HYDROCHLOROTHIAZIDE*				
(Ranbaxy Pharm) *See FOSINOPRIL SODIUM-HYDROCHLOROTHIAZIDE*				
(Sandoz)				
TAB, PO, 10 mg-12.5 mg,				
100s ea	00185-0341-01	154.39		AB
20 mg-12.5 mg,				
100s ea	00185-0342-01	154.39		AB
FOSINOPRIL/HCTZ (Phys Total Care)				
REPACK				
fosinopril sodium/hydrochlorothiazide				
TAB, PO, 20 mg-12.5 mg,				
10s ea	54868-5469-01	39.54		
30s ea	54868-5469-00	84.90		
FOSPHENYTOIN SODIUM (Akorn)				
SOL, IJ (USP,25X2ML,SDV)				
50 mg pe/ml,				
2 ml 25s	23360-0021-02	53.25		AP
(USP,10X10ML,SDV)				
50 mg pe/ml,				
10 ml 10s	23360-0021-10	70.20		AP
(Apotex Corp.)				
phenytoin sodium, prompt				
SOL, IV (25X2ML)				
50 mg/ml, 2 ml 24s	60505-0746-05	642.26		AP
(10X10ML)				
50 mg/ml,				
10 ml 10s	60505-0765-04	770.73		AP
FOSPHENYTOIN SODIUM (APP)				
SOL, IJ (USP,25X2ML)				
75 mg/ml, 2 ml 25s	63323-0403-02	76.50		AP
(USP,10X10ML)				
75 mg/ml,				
10 ml 10s	63323-0403-10	90.10		AP
(Bedford)				
SOL, IJ (SDV,USP,10X2ML)				
50 mg pe/ml,				
2 ml 10s	55390-0175-10	54.00		AP
(SDV,USP,10X10ML)				
50 mg pe/ml,				
10 ml 10s	55390-0176-10	222.00		AP
(Hospira) *See NOVAPLUS FOSPHENYTOIN SODIUM*				
(Hospira)				
SOL, IJ (USP,2MLX25)				
75 mg/ml, 2 ml 25s	00409-4857-02	43.20	37.75	AP
(USP,10MLX10)				
75 mg/ml,				
10 ml 10s	00409-4857-10	60.48	52.90	AP
(Pfizer) *See CEREBYX*				
FOSPHENYTOIN SODIUM (Teva)				
phenytoin sodium, prompt				
SOL, IV (USP,25X2ML)				
50 mg/ml, 2 ml 25s	00703-7101-04	43.20		AP
(USP,10X10ML)				
50 mg/ml,				
10 ml 10s	00703-7105-03	79.20		AP

PROD/MFR	NDC	AWP	DP	OBC
FOSPHENYTOIN SODIUM (Wockhardt USA)				
SOL, IJ (SDV,USP,25X2ML)				
75 mg/ml, 2 ml 25s	64679-0729-01	665.16		AP
(SDV,USP,10X10ML) 75 mg/ml, 10 ml 10s	64679-0730-01	799.29		AP
FOSPROPOFOL DISODIUM (Eisai) *See LUSEDRA*				
FOSRENOL (Shire US Inc.)				
lanthanum carbonate				
CTB, PO (2X45)				
500 mg, 90s ea	54092-0252-90	674.47	562.06	
(6 X 15) 750 mg, 90s ea	54092-0253-90	674.47	562.06	
(9 X 10) 1000 mg, 90s ea	54092-0254-90	674.47	562.06	
FRAGMIN (Eisai)				
dalteparin sodium				
SOL, SC (27GX1/2", 10X1ML,PF)				
10000 iu/ml, 1 ml 10s	62856-0101-10	733.82		
(10X0.2ML,PF) 2500 iu/0.2 ml, 0.2 ml 10s	62856-0250-10	226.18		
(27GX1/2",10X0.2ML,PF) 5000 iu/0.2 ml, 0.2 ml 10s	62856-0500-10	366.91		
(PREFILLED) 7500 iu/0.3 ml, 0.3 ml 10s	62856-0750-10	550.39		
(SINGLE DOSE,PF) 12500 iu/0.5 ml, 0.5 ml 10s	62856-0125-10	917.28		
15000 iu/0.6 ml, 0.6 ml 10s	62856-0150-10	1100.74		
18000 iu/0.72 ml, 0.72 ml 10s	62856-0180-10	1320.86		
(MDV) 25000 iu/ml, 3.8 ml	62856-0251-01	630.73		
FRAGRANCE				
(Medisca) *See POWDER SCENT*				
(Medisca) *See RAIN FRAGRANCE*				
(PCCA) *See COCONUT FRAGRANCE*				
(PCCA) *See CUCUMBER FRAGRANCE*				
(PCCA) *See GARDENIA OIL FRAGRANCE*				
(PCCA) *See HONEY ALMOND FRAGRANCE*				
(PCCA) *See HONEYSUCKLE FRAGRANCE*				
(PCCA) *See KIWI FRAGRANCE*				
(PCCA) *See MUSK OIL*				
(PCCA) *See PATCHOULY OIL FRAGRANCE*				
(PCCA) *See POWDER SCENT FRAGRANCE*				
(PCCA) *See SKIN SOFT FRAGRANCE*				
FRANKINCENSE OIL (Lorann Oil)				
OIL, NA, 9.9 ml	23535-0151-21	10.00		
(PCCA)				
OIL, NA, 1 ml	51927-2980-00	4.50		
FREAMINE HBC (B. Braun)				
amino acids				
SOL, IV (GLASS,1000 ML)				
6.9%, 750 ml	00264-9350-55	78.90		
FREAMINE III (B. Braun)				
amino acids				
SOL, IV (GLASS W/SOLID STOPPER)				
8.5%, 500 ml	00264-9031-55	14.00		
1000 ml	00264-9030-55	24.00		
10%, 500 ml	00264-9011-55	13.00		
1000 ml	00264-9010-55	15.40		
FREAMINE III W/ELECTROLYTES (B. Braun)				
amino acids and electrolytes				
SOL, IV (GLASS W/SOLID STOPPER)				
1000 ml	00264-9040-55	12.00		
FREEDOM CATH SELF-ADHERING (Mentor)				
catheter				
DEV, NA (MALE EXTERNAL, 23 MM)				
30s ea	81317-0080-30	54.60		
(MALE EXTERNAL, 28 MM) 30s ea	81317-0082-30	54.60		
(MALE EXTERNAL, 31 MM) 30s ea	81317-0082-35	54.60		
(MALE EXTERNAL, 35 MM) 30s ea	81317-0084-30	54.60		
(MALE EXTENAL, 31 MM) 100s ea	81317-0082-05	166.00		
(MALE EXTERNAL, 23 MM) 100s ea	81317-0080-00	166.00		
(MALE EXTERNAL, 28 MM) 100s ea	81317-0082-00	166.00		
(MALE EXTERNAL, 35 MM) 100s ea	81317-0084-00	166.00		
FREEDOM CLEAR SELF-ADHERING (Mentor)				
catheter				
DEV, NA (MALE, 23 MM)				
30s ea	81317-0051-30	54.60		
(MALE, 28 MM) 30s ea	81317-0052-30	54.60		
(MALE, 31 MM) 30s ea	81317-0053-30	54.60		
(MALE, 35 MM) 30s ea	81317-0054-30	54.60		
(MALE, 40 MM) 30s ea	81317-0055-30	54.60		
(MALE, 23 MM) 100s ea	81317-0051-00	166.00		
(MALE, 28 MM) 100s ea	81317-0052-00	166.00		
(MALE, 31 MM) 100s ea	81317-0053-00	166.00		
(MALE, 35 MM) 100s ea	81317-0540-00	166.00		
(MALE, 40 MM) 100s ea	81317-0055-00	166.00		
FRENADOL (A. G. Marin)				
acetaminophen/salicylamide				
TAB, PO, 250 mg-600 mg, 100s ea	12539-0850-10	36.66		
FRESHKOTE (Focus Labs, Inc.)				
polyvinyl alcohol/povidone				
SOL, OP (W/ CONTROL DROPPER)				
2.7%-2%, 15 ml	15821-0101-15	27.10		
FROVA (Endo Labs)				
frovatriptan succinate				
TAB, PO (BLISTER PACK)				
2.5 mg, 9s ea	63481-0025-09	252.22		
(Physician Partner) REPACK				
TAB, PO, 2.5 mg, 9s ea	21695-0222-09	397.06		
(Quality Care Prod) REPACK				
TAB, PO (FILM-COATED)				
2.5 mg, 9s ea	35356-0169-09	380.60		
(Southwood) REPACK				
TAB, PO (FILM-COATED)				
2.5 mg, 9s ea	58016-0838-01	210.13		
FROVATRIPTAN SUCCINATE (Endo Labs) *See FROVA*				
FRUCTOOLIGOSACCHARIDE (PCCA) *See FRUCTOOLIGOSACCHARIDES*				
FRUCTOOLIGOSACCHARIDES (PCCA)				
fructooligosaccharide				
POW, NA, 1 gm	51927-2730-00	0.50		
FRUCTOSE (Amend)				
CRY, NA (U.S.P.)				
500 gm	17317-0177-01	10.50		
2270 gm	17317-0177-05	28.00		
11350 gm	17317-0177-08	105.00		
(Gallipot)				
CRY, NA (U.S.P.)				
454 gm	51552-0367-06	11.90		
2270 gm	51552-0367-08	45.99		
(PCCA)				
POW, NA (U.S.P.)				
1 gm	51927-1271-00	0.07		
(Spectrum Pharmacy)				
GRA, NA (U.S.P.)				
500 gm	49452-3205-01	64.75		
2500 gm	49452-3205-02	173.25		
FUCHSIN, BASIC				
(PCCA) *See BASIC FUCHSIN HYDROCHLORIDE*				
(Spectrum Pharmacy) *See BASIC FUCHSIN*				
(Spectrum Pharmacy) *See BASIC FUCHSIN HYDROCHLORIDE*				
FUDR (Hospira)				
floxuridine				
PDS, IJ (INTRA-ARTERIAL INFUSION)				
0.5 gm, ea	61703-0331-09	121.06	105.92	AP
FUL-GLO (Akorn)				
fluorescein sodium				
TES, OP (STRIP)				
0.6 mg, 300s ea	17478-0403-03	36.88		
1 mg, 100s ea	17478-0404-01	14.25		
FULLER'S EARTH (Amend)				
POW, NA, 500 gm	17317-0178-01	9.80		
2270 gm	17317-0178-05	28.00		
11350 gm	17317-0178-08	96.25		
(Gallipot)				
POW, NA (TECHNICAL)				
454 gm	51552-0409-06	9.73		
(Humco)				
POW, NA (TECHNICAL)				
120 gm	00395-0967-94	6.95		
360 gm	00395-0967-12	9.05		
(PCCA)				
POW, NA, 1 gm	51927-1636-00	0.08		
FULVESTRANT (AstraZeneca) *See FASLODEX*				
FULVICIN P/G (Phys Total Care) REPACK				
griseofulvin, ultramicrocrystalline				
TAB, PO, 330 mg, 60s ea	54868-2245-01	80.43		AB
FUMARIC ACID (Amend)				
POW, NA (N.F., F.C.C.)				
454 gm	17317-1883-01	9.80		
2270 gm	17317-1883-05	35.00		
11350 gm	17317-1883-08	131.25		
(PCCA)				
POW, NA (NF)				
1 gm	51927-2780-00	0.15		
(Spectrum Pharmacy)				
POW, NA (N.F.)				
500 gm	49452-3215-01	152.60		
2500 gm	49452-3215-02	423.50		
FUMATINIC (Laser Pharma)				
ascorbic acid/cyanocobalamin/ferrous fumarate				
CER, PO, 60 mg-5 mcg-200 mg, 100s ea	00277-0181-01	47.00		
FURADANTIN (Shionogi)				
nitrofurantoin				
SUS, PO (1X230ML)				
25 mg/5 ml, 230 ml	59630-0450-08	490.63		
FURAZOLIDONE (PCCA)				
POW, NA (U.S.P.)				
1 gm	51927-3151-00	2.04		
FUROCOT (Truxton)				
furosemide				
TAB, PO, 20 mg, 1000s ea	00463-6102-10	15.60		EE
40 mg, 1000s ea	00463-6283-10	24.00		EE
FUROSEMIDE FUL				
SOL, PO, 10 mg/ml, 60 ml		7.80		
TAB, PO, 20 mg, 100s ea		5.63		
40 mg, 100s ea		5.99		
80 mg, 100s ea		10.43		
(Amer Regent)				
SOL, IJ (S.D.V.)				
10 mg/ml, 2 ml 25s	00517-5702-25	22.19		AP
4 ml 25s	00517-5704-25	35.94		AP
10 ml 25s	00517-5710-25	57.19		AP
(APP)				
SOL, IJ (25X2ML,SDV,PF)				
10 mg/ml, 2 ml 25s	63323-0280-02	118.50		AP
(25X4ML,SDV,PF) 10 mg/ml, 4 ml 25s	63323-0280-04	238.50		AP
(25X10ML,SDV,PF) 10 mg/ml, 10 ml 25s	63323-0280-10	448.50		AP
(Consolidated Midland)				
SOL, IJ (AMP, DOSETTE)				
10 mg/ml, 2 ml 25s	00223-7700-02	27.25		EE
(VIAL) 10 mg/ml, 2 ml 25s	00223-7701-02	40.00		EE
(AMP, DOSETTE) 10 mg/ml, 4 ml 25s	00223-7704-04	37.50		EE
(VIAL) 10 mg/ml, 4 ml 25s	00223-7705-04	55.00		EE
10 ml	00223-7708-20	6.25		EE
(AMP, DOSETTE) 10 mg/ml, 10 ml 25s	00223-7707-10	125.00		EE
TAB, PO, 20 mg, 100s ea	00223-1012-01	2.00		EE

PROD/MFR	NDC	AWP	DP	OBC
1000s ea	00223-1012-02	17.50		EE
40 mg, 100s ea	00223-1013-01	2.50		EE
1000s ea	00223-1013-02	22.50		EE
(Dava Pharma)				
TAB, PO, 20 mg, 100s ea	67253-0540-10	14.25		
1000s ea	67253-0540-11	139.70		
40 mg, 100s ea	67253-0541-10	16.25		
1000s ea	67253-0541-11	159.30		
80 mg, 100s ea	67253-0542-10	43.65		
500s ea	67253-0542-50	213.70		
(Excellium)				
TAB, PO (USP)				
20 mg, 100s ea	64125-0116-01	14.30		AB
1000s ea	64125-0116-10	139.90		AB
40 mg, 100s ea	64125-0117-01	16.30		AB
1000s ea	64125-0117-10	159.50		AB
80 mg, 100s ea	64125-0118-01	43.70		AB
500s ea	64125-0118-05	213.90		AB
(Gallipot)				
POW, NA (U.S.P.)				
5 gm	51552-0940-02	25.55	18.25	
(Hospira)				
SOL, IJ (CARPUJECT W/LUER LOCK)				
10 mg/ml, 2 ml 10s	00409-1275-32	20.04	17.50	AP
(VIAL,FLIPTOP,ABBOJECT)				
10 mg/ml, 2 ml 25s	00409-6102-02	10.80	9.50	AP
(ANSYR,LATEX-FREE)				
10 mg/ml, 4 ml 10s	00074-9631-04	25.44	22.30	AP
(PF)				
10 mg/ml, 4 ml 10s	00409-9631-04	26.40	23.10	AP
(VIAL,FLIPTOP,ABBOJECT)				
10 mg/ml, 4 ml 25s	00409-6102-04	12.90	11.25	AP
(10X10ML, ANSYR)				
10 mg/ml, 10 ml 10s	00409-1639-10	38.76	33.90	AP
(VIAL,FLIPTOP,ABBOJECT)				
10 mg/ml, 10 ml 25s	00409-6102-10	15.90	14.00	AP
(Major)				
TAB, PO (10X10,USP)				
20 mg, 100s ea UD	00904-5796-61	11.67		AB
40 mg, 100s ea UD	00904-5797-61	13.33		AB
80 mg, 100s ea UD	00904-5798-61	26.66		AB
(Medisca)				
POW, NA (U.S.P.)				
25 gm	38779-0226-04	40.50		
100 gm	38779-0226-05	135.00		
500 gm	38779-0226-08	606.00		
(Morton Grove)				
SOL, PO (ORANGE)				
10 mg/ml, 60 ml	60432-0613-60	10.40		AA
120 ml	60432-0613-04	14.28		AA
(Mylan)				
TAB, PO, 20 mg, 30s ea	00378-0208-93	4.29		AB
100s ea	00378-0208-01	14.30		AB
1000s ea	00378-0208-10	139.90		AB
40 mg, 30s ea	00378-0216-93	4.89		AB
100s ea	00378-0216-01	16.30		AB
1000s ea	00378-0216-10	159.50		AB
80 mg, 30s ea	00378-0232-93	13.11		AB
100s ea	00378-0232-01	43.70		AB
500s ea	00378-0232-05	213.90		AB
(PCCA)				
POW, NA (U.S.P.)				
1 gm	51927-1784-00	2.16		
(Precision Dose)				
SOL, PO (30X4ML,ORANGE)				
10 mg/ml, 4 ml 30s UD	68094-0742-62	48.60		AA
(Qualitest)				
TAB, PO, 20 mg, 100s ea	00603-3739-21	15.43		
1000s ea	00603-3739-32	151.21		
5000s ea	00603-3739-34	740.93		
40 mg, 100s ea	00603-3740-21	17.58		
1000s ea	00603-3740-32	172.38		
5000s ea	00603-3740-34	844.66		
80 mg, 100s ea	00603-3741-21	43.70		
500s ea	00603-3741-28	213.90		
1000s ea	00603-3741-32	419.24		
(Ranbaxy Pharm)				
TAB, PO (USP)				
20 mg, 100s ea	63304-0624-01	14.30		AB
1000s ea	63304-0624-10	139.90		AB
40 mg, 100s ea	63304-0625-01	16.30		AB
1000s ea	63304-0625-10	159.50		AB
80 mg, 100s ea	63304-0626-01	43.70		AB
500s ea	63304-0626-05	213.90		AB

PROD/MFR	NDC	AWP	DP	OBC
(Roxane)				
SOL, PO, 40 mg/5 ml,				
5 ml 40s UD	00054-8298-16	64.87		
500 ml	00054-3298-63	39.66		
10 mg/ml, 60 ml	00054-3294-46	10.40		AA
120 ml	00054-3294-50	20.10		AA
TAB, PO, 20 mg, 100s ea	00054-4297-25	14.30		AB
(10X10)				
20 mg, 100s ea UD	00054-8297-25	17.16		AB
1000s ea	00054-4297-31	139.90		AB
40 mg, 100s ea	00054-4299-25	16.30		AB
(10X10)				
40 mg, 100s ea UD	00054-8299-25	19.56		AB
1000s ea	00054-4299-31	159.50		AB
80 mg, 100s ea	00054-4301-25	43.70		AB
(10X10)				
80 mg, 100s ea UD	00054-8301-25	52.44		AB
500s ea	00054-4301-29	213.69		AB
(Sandoz)				
TAB, PO, 20 mg, 100s ea	00781-1818-01	13.58		AB
1000s ea	00781-1818-10	122.78		AB
40 mg, 100s ea	00781-1966-01	15.50		AB
1000s ea	00781-1966-10	140.30		AB
80 mg, 100s ea	00781-1446-01	41.60		AB
500s ea	00781-1446-05	198.00		AB
(Sanofi-Aventis) *See LASIX*				
(Spectrum Pharmacy)				
CRY, NA (U.S.P./N.F.)				
500 gm	49452-3222-03	962.50		
POW, NA, 25 gm	49452-3222-01	78.40		
100 gm	49452-3222-02	243.95		
(Teva)				
TAB, PO, 20 mg, 100s ea	00172-2908-60	15.38		AB
(10X10)				
20 mg, 100s ea UD	00182-1170-89	16.27		AB
1000s ea	00172-2908-80	140.00		AB
40 mg, 100s ea UD	00172-2907-10	21.67		AB
100s ea	00172-2907-60	17.49		AB
1000s ea	00172-2907-80	160.00		AB
(Truxton) *See FUROCOT*				
(UDL)				
TAB, PO (ROBOT READY 25X1)				
20 mg, 25s ea UD	51079-0072-19	4.03		AB
(10X10)				
20 mg, 100s ea UD	51079-0072-20	14.73		AB
(USP,PUNCH CARDS,10X30)				
20 mg, 300s ea UD	51079-0072-56	44.19		AB
(ROBOT READY 25X1)				
40 mg, 25s ea UD	51079-0073-19	4.20		AB
(10X10)				
40 mg, 100s ea UD	51079-0073-20	16.79		AB
(USP,PUNCH CARDS,10X30)				
40 mg, 300s ea UD	51079-0073-56	50.37		AB
(ROBOT READY 25X1)				
80 mg, 25s ea UD	51079-0527-19	11.25		AB
(10X10)				
80 mg, 100s ea UD	51079-0527-20	45.01		AB
(Watson Labs)				
TAB, PO (USP)				
20 mg, 100s ea	00591-0300-01	4.56		AB
(Wockhardt USA)				
SOL, IJ (USP,SDV)				
10 mg/ml, 2 ml	64679-0759-04	1.03		AP
(USP,SDV,10X2ML)				
10 mg/ml, 2 ml 10s	64679-0759-07	10.30		AP
(USP,SDV,25X2ML)				
10 mg/ml, 2 ml 25s	64679-0759-01	25.75		AP
(USP,SDV)				
10 mg/ml, 4 ml	64679-0759-05	1.38		AP
(USP,SDV,10X4ML)				
10 mg/ml, 4 ml 10s	64679-0759-08	13.80		AP
(USP,SDV,4X25ML)				
10 mg/ml, 4 ml 25s	64679-0759-02	34.50		AP
(USP,SDV)				
10 mg/ml, 10 ml	64679-0759-06	2.18		AP
(USP,SDV,10X10ML)				
10 mg/ml, 10 ml 10s	64679-0759-09	21.80		AP
(USP,SDV,10X25ML)				
10 mg/ml, 10 ml 25s	64679-0759-03	54.50		AP
(A-S Medication)				
REPACK				
TAB, PO, 20 mg, 30s ea	54569-0572-00	4.34		EE
100s ea	54569-0572-01	14.46		
200s ea	54569-0572-07	28.92		
40 mg, 15s ea	54569-0574-02	2.47		
30s ea	54569-0574-00	4.94		

PROD/MFR	NDC	AWP	DP	OBC
60s ea	54569-0574-03	9.89		
100s ea	54569-0574-01	16.50		
(Aidarex)				
REPACK				
TAB, PO, 40 mg, 7s ea	33261-0374-07	3.01		AB
14s ea	33261-0374-14	6.02		AB
20s ea	33261-0374-20	8.60		AB
21s ea	33261-0374-21	9.03		AB
28s ea	33261-0374-28	12.04		AB
30s ea	33261-0374-30	12.90		AB
40s ea	33261-0374-40	17.20		AB
60s ea	33261-0374-60	25.80		AB
(Altura)				
REPACK				
TAB, PO, 20 mg, 10s ea	63874-0400-10	1.16		
12s ea	63874-0400-12	2.28		
14s ea	63874-0400-14	2.66		
15s ea	63874-0400-15	2.85		
20s ea	63874-0400-20	3.31		
21s ea	63874-0400-21	3.47		
30s ea	63874-0400-30	4.97		
50s ea	63874-0400-50	5.82		
60s ea	63874-0400-60	6.98		
90s ea	63874-0400-90	10.48		
100s ea	63874-0400-01	16.54		
1000s ea	63874-0400-02	116.40		
40 mg, 10s ea	63874-0358-10	2.32		
12s ea	63874-0358-12	2.78		
14s ea	63874-0358-14	3.24		
15s ea	63874-0358-15	3.49		
20s ea	63874-0358-20	4.64		
21s ea	63874-0358-21	4.87		
24s ea	63874-0358-24	5.57		
25s ea	63874-0358-25	5.81		
28s ea	63874-0358-28	6.50		
30s ea	63874-0358-30	6.96		
60s ea	63874-0358-60	13.92		
90s ea	63874-0358-90	20.88		
100s ea	63874-0358-01	23.20		
1000s ea	63874-0358-02	232.00		
80 mg, 30s ea	63874-1121-03	11.66		
100s ea	63874-1121-01	38.87		
(American Health)				
REPACK				
TAB, PO (10X10)				
20 mg, 100s ea UD	68084-0014-01	17.01		AB
(15X30)				
20 mg, 450s ea	68084-0014-85	63.20		AB
(10X10)				
40 mg, 100s ea UD	68084-0016-01	21.03		AB
(15X30)				
40 mg, 450s ea	68084-0016-85	71.79		AB
(10X10)				
80 mg, 100s ea UD	68084-0017-01	44.99		AB
(Bryant Ranch)				
REPACK				
TAB, PO, 20 mg, 30s ea	63629-2683-01	14.40		
40 mg, 30s ea	63629-1434-02	6.69		
40s ea	63629-1434-01	8.92		
100s ea	63629-1434-03	22.30		
80 mg, 30s ea	63629-1435-02	18.92		
100s ea	63629-1435-01	59.52		
(Core)				
REPACK				
TAB, PO, 20 mg, 20s ea	33358-0149-20	8.88		
30s ea	33358-0149-30	14.76		
40 mg, 30s ea	33358-0150-30	16.97		
40s ea	33358-0150-40	19.80		
80 mg, 30s ea	33358-0151-30	19.39		
(DHS, Inc.)				
REPACK				
TAB, PO, 20 mg, 30s ea	55887-0997-30	10.09		AB
90s ea	55887-0997-90	29.88		AB
40 mg, 30s ea	55887-0574-30	8.36		AB
60s ea	55887-0574-60	18.74		AB
90s ea	55887-0574-90	26.98		
100s ea	55887-0574-01	27.86		
80 mg, 30s ea	55887-0978-30	17.75		
90s ea	55887-0978-90	35.25		
(Dispensing Solutions)				
REPACK				
TAB, PO, 20 mg, 30s ea	66336-0761-30	7.71		AB
100s ea	55045-1553-00	22.00		AB
40 mg, 10s ea	55045-1217-03	3.40		AB
30s ea	66336-0487-30	10.55		AB
(USP)				
40 mg, 30s ea	55045-1217-08	10.20		AB
60s ea	55045-1217-06	20.40		
90s ea	55045-1217-09	30.60		AB
90s ea	66336-0487-90	31.65		

PROD/MFR	NDC	AWP	DP	OBC
100s ea	55045-1217-00	34.00		AB
120s ea	55045-1217-02	40.80		AB
80 mg, 30s ea	55045-2200-08	12.90		
60s ea	55045-2200-06	25.80		
100s ea	55045-2200-01	43.00		
(GSMS)				
REPACK				
TAB, PO (UNIT OF USE)				
20 mg, 90s ea	60429-0078-90	9.00	3.00	AB
180s ea	60429-0078-18	14.55	4.85	AB
40 mg, 90s ea	60429-0079-90	21.75	7.25	AB
(HomeMed)				
REPACK				
TAB, PO, 20 mg, 30s ea	51655-0193-24	13.99		EE
90s ea	51655-0193-26	12.05		EE
40 mg, 30s ea	51655-0081-24	10.99		EE
60s ea	51655-0081-25	9.40		EE
90s ea	51655-0081-26	13.60		EE
100s ea	51655-0081-21	15.05		EE
180s ea	51655-0081-83	26.40		EE
(Keltman Pharma., Inc.)				
REPACK				
TAB, PO, 20 mg, 30s ea	68387-0365-30	5.20		AB
(McKesson Packaging)				
REPACK				
TAB, PO, 20 mg, 100s ea UD	63739-0111-10	15.35		AB
(BLISTER PACK)				
20 mg, 750s ea UD	63739-0111-01	115.11		AB
(PUNCH CARD 25X30)				
20 mg, 750s ea	63739-0111-03	115.11		AB
40 mg, 100s ea UD	63739-0112-10	17.72		AB
(BLISTER PACK)				
40 mg, 750s ea UD	63739-0112-01	132.90		AB
80 mg, 100s ea UD	63739-0113-10	49.50		AB
(Nucare Pharm)				
REPACK				
TAB, PO, 20 mg, 30s ea	66267-0097-30	8.51		AB
60s ea	66267-0097-60	16.99		AB
90s ea	66267-0097-90	25.50		AB
40 mg, 30s ea	66267-0098-30	9.73		AB
60s ea	66267-0098-60	16.46		AB
90s ea	66267-0098-90	29.20		AB
(Palmetto)				
REPACK				
SOL, IJ, 10 mg/ml, 2 ml	23490-5621-02	1.55		
TAB, PO, 20 mg, 6s ea	23490-5622-01	3.95		
15s ea	23490-5622-04	6.99		
30s ea	23490-5622-02	13.99		
90s ea	23490-5622-03	41.97		
40 mg, 20s ea	23490-5623-01	7.33		
30s ea	23490-5623-02	10.99		
FUROSEMIDE (Palmetto)				
80 mg, 30s ea	23490-5624-03	16.78		
FUROSEMIDE (PD-Rx Pharm)				
REPACK				
TAB, PO, 20 mg, 20s ea	58864-0220-01	19.44		AB
30s ea	55289-0593-30	10.50		AB
30s ea	58864-0220-30	10.50		
(USP)				
20 mg, 90s ea	55289-0593-90	13.50		AB
100s ea	55289-0593-01	19.44		AB
40 mg, 4s ea	55289-0118-04	7.11		AB
10s ea	55289-0118-10	7.60		
14s ea	55289-0118-14	10.27		AB
30s ea	55289-0118-30	10.47		AB
(REDI-SCRIPT)				
40 mg, 30s ea	58864-0221-30	10.46		AB
60s ea	55289-0118-60	14.27		AB
90s ea	55289-0118-90	16.67		AB
100s ea	55289-0118-01	17.80		AB
(Pharma Pac)				
REPACK				
TAB, PO, 20 mg, 30s ea	52959-0499-30	6.25		EE
40 mg, 15s ea	52959-0751-15	4.68		AB
30s ea	52959-0751-30	9.30		
100s ea	52959-0751-00	30.90		
(Phys Total Care)				
REPACK				
SOL, IJ (CARPUJECT)				
10 mg/ml, 2 ml 10s	54868-3645-00	28.87		EE
(VIAL,FLIPTOP,ABBOJECT)				
10 mg/ml, 2 ml 25s	54868-4998-00	71.85		AP
(ABBOJECT)				
10 mg/ml, 250 ml	54868-2299-00	24.09		AP
PO, 10 mg/ml, 60 ml	54868-2188-00	22.73		EE
TAB, PO, 20 mg, 10s ea	54868-0057-07	4.20		EE
30s ea	54868-0057-03	6.60		EE
60s ea	54868-0057-06	10.23		EE
90s ea	54868-0057-00	13.83		EE

PROD/MFR	NDC	AWP	DP	OBC
100s ea	54868-0057-04	13.56		EE
40 mg, 15s ea	54868-0058-08	4.86		AB
20s ea	54868-0058-00	5.49		EE
30s ea	54868-0058-02	6.75		EE
50s ea	54868-0058-05	9.24		EE
60s ea	54868-0058-06	10.47		EE
90s ea	54868-0058-09	14.22		EE
100s ea	54868-0058-03	15.45		EE
80 mg, 30s ea	54868-2180-01	8.58		EE
60s ea	54868-2180-00	14.19		EE
90s ea	54868-2180-03	21.61		EE
100s ea	54868-2180-02	21.66		EE
(Physician Partner)				
REPACK				
SOL, IJ (25X2ML)				
10 mg/ml, 2 ml 25s	21695-0721-25	44.50		AP
TAB, PO, 20 mg, 30s ea	21695-0490-30	14.52		AB
90s ea	21695-0490-90	43.56		AB
40 mg, 30s ea	21695-0491-30	17.98		AB
90s ea	21695-0491-90	53.94		AB
100s ea	21695-0491-00	59.94		AB
(Quality Care Prod)				
REPACK				
TAB, PO, 20 mg, ea	49999-0149-30	6.84		EE
10s ea	49999-0179-10	2.28		EE
30s ea	49999-0179-30	12.36		AB
40s ea	49999-0179-40	9.20		AB
60s ea	49999-0179-60	24.72		AB
90s ea	49999-0179-90	37.08		EE
40 mg, 10s ea	49999-0030-10	4.00		AB
30s ea	49999-0030-30	16.60		EE
60s ea	49999-0030-60	33.20		
90s ea	49999-0030-90	48.60		AB
100s ea	49999-0030-00	31.80		EE
80 mg, 30s ea	49999-0225-30	19.86		AB
60s ea	49999-0255-60	39.72		
(Southwood)				
REPACK				
TAB, PO, 20 mg, 12s ea	58016-0538-12	2.28		EE
15s ea	58016-0538-15	2.85		EE
20s ea	58016-0538-20	3.80		EE
30s ea	58016-0538-30	5.70		EE
50s ea	58016-0538-50	9.50		EE
100s ea	58016-0538-00	19.00		EE
40 mg, 10s ea	58016-0539-10	2.65		EE
12s ea	58016-0539-12	3.18		EE
14s ea	58016-0539-14	3.71		EE
15s ea	58016-0539-15	3.98		EE
20s ea	58016-0539-20	5.30		EE
21s ea	58016-0539-21	5.57		EE
24s ea	58016-0539-24	6.36		EE
25s ea	58016-0539-25	6.63		EE
28s ea	58016-0539-28	7.42		EE
30s ea	58016-0539-30	7.95		EE
60s ea	58016-0539-60	15.90		EE
100s ea	58016-0539-00	26.50		EE
80 mg, 10s ea	58016-0576-10	3.85		EE
12s ea	58016-0576-12	4.62		EE
14s ea	58016-0576-14	5.39		EE
15s ea	58016-0576-15	5.77		EE
18s ea	58016-0576-18	6.93		EE
20s ea	58016-0576-20	7.70		EE
21s ea	58016-0576-21	8.08		EE
24s ea	58016-0576-24	9.24		EE
25s ea	58016-0576-25	9.62		EE
28s ea	58016-0576-28	10.77		EE
30s ea	58016-0576-30	11.54		EE
40s ea	58016-0576-40	15.39		EE
50s ea	58016-0576-50	19.24		EE
60s ea	58016-0576-60	23.09		EE
100s ea	58016-0576-00	38.48		EE
120s ea	58016-0576-02	46.18		AB
150s ea	58016-0576-03	57.72		AB
200s ea	58016-0576-89	76.96		AB
300s ea	58016-0576-73	115.44		AB
(Stat Rx)				
REPACK				
TAB, PO, 20 mg, 14s ea	16590-0442-14	2.60		
40 mg, 20s ea	16590-0284-20	12.25		
30s ea	16590-0284-30	18.40		
60s ea	16590-0284-60	36.75		
(Vibranta)				
REPACK				
TAB, PO, 20 mg, 30s ea	57866-3840-01	4.78		
40 mg, 30s ea	57866-3841-01	56.47		
60s ea	57866-3841-02	16.90		
90s ea	57866-3841-03	32.56		
FURSULTIAMINE HCL (PCCA)				
fursultiamine hydrochloride				
POW, NA, 1 gm	51927-3567-00	8.40		

PROD/MFR	NDC	AWP	DP	OBC
FURSULTIAMINE HYDROCHLORIDE (PCCA) *See FURSULTIAMINE HCL*				
FUSILEV (Spectrum)				
levoleucovorin calcium				
PDS, IV (LYOPHILIZED)				
50 mg, ea	68152-0101-00	160.48		
FUTURA SAFETY SCALPEL (Arkray)				
surgical instrument, disposable				
DEV, NA (NO. 10 BLADE,LATEX-FREE)				
20s ea	08317-6802-10	37.50	25.00	
(NO. 11 BLADE,LATEX-FREE)				
20s ea	08317-6802-11	37.50	25.00	
(NO. 15 BLADE,LATEX-FREE)				
20s ea	08317-6802-15	37.50	25.00	
FUZEON (Roche Labs)				
enfuvirtide				
PDS, SC (90MG)				
90 mg, ea	00004-0380-39	2973.04		
(A-S Medication)				
REPACK				
PDS, SC (90MG)				
90 mg, ea	54569-5781-00	2841.20		
(Quality Care Prod)				
REPACK				
PDS, SC, 90 mg, 60s ea	35356-0206-60	4663.42		
G-PHED (DHS, Inc.)				
REPACK				
guaifenesin/pseudoephedrine hydrochloride				
CER, PO, 250 mg-120 mg,				
28s ea	55887-0931-28	12.05		
G-PHED-PD (Dispensing Solutions)				
REPACK				
guaifenesin/pseudoephedrine hydrochloride				
CER, PO, 300 mg-60 mg,				
20s ea	55045-2476-06	12.00		
GABADONE (Physician Thera, LLC)				
amino acids and nutriceuticals				
CAP, PO (PF,SF,DYE-FREE)				
60s ea	68405-1004-02	194.30		
(Altura)				
REPACK				
CAP, PO, 60s ea	63874-1179-06	151.80		
(Dispensing Solutions)				
REPACK				
CAP, PO (PF,SF,DYE-FREE)				
60s ea	55045-3398-06	151.80		
GABAPENTIN				
FUL				
CAP, PO, 100 mg, 100s ea		8.25		
300 mg, 100s ea		12.38		
400 mg, 100s ea		15.38		
TAB, PO, 600 mg, 100s ea		97.38		
800 mg, 100s ea		117.56		
(Actavis)				
CAP, PO, 100 mg, 100s ea	00228-2665-11	53.18		AB
500s ea	00228-2665-50	265.90		AB
300 mg, 100s ea	00228-2666-11	8.25		AB
500s ea	00228-2666-50	664.80		AB
400 mg, 100s ea	00228-2667-11	159.53		AB
500s ea	00228-2667-50	797.65		AB
TAB, PO (FILM-COATED)				
600 mg, 100s ea	00228-2636-11	252.62		AB
500s ea	00228-2636-50	1263.10		AB
800 mg, 100s ea	00228-2637-11	303.10		AB
500s ea	00228-2637-50	1515.50		AB
(Amneal)				
CAP, PO (HARD GELATIN)				
100 mg, 100s ea	53746-0101-01	53.69		AB
500s ea	53746-0101-05	268.45		AB
1000s ea	53746-0101-10	533.25		AB
300 mg, 100s ea	53746-0102-01	134.18		AB
500s ea	53746-0102-05	670.90		AB
1000s ea	53746-0102-10	1332.00		AB
400 mg, 100s ea	53746-0103-01	159.71		AB
500s ea	53746-0103-05	798.55		AB
(Apotex Corp.)				
CAP, PO, 100 mg, 100s ea	60505-0112-01	53.24		AB
(10X10)				
100 mg, 100s ea UD	60505-0112-00	55.24		AB
1000s ea	60505-0112-08	532.40		AB
8500s ea	60505-0112-07	4525.40		AB
300 mg, 100s ea	60505-0113-01	133.11		AB
(10X10)				
300 mg, 100s ea UD	60505-0113-00	135.11		AB
1000s ea	60505-0113-08	1331.10		AB
3500s ea	60505-0113-07	4658.85		AB
400 mg, 100s ea	60505-0114-01	159.71		AB

PROD/MFR	NDC	AWP	DP	OBC
(10X10)				
400 mg, 100s ea UD	60505-0114-00	161.71		AB
500s ea	60505-0114-05	798.55		AB
2500s ea	60505-0114-07	3992.75		AB
TAB, PO (FILM-COATED)				
600 mg, 100s ea	60505-2551-01	252.62		AB
500s ea	60505-2551-05	1263.25		AB
800 mg, 100s ea	60505-2552-01	303.10		AB
500s ea	60505-2552-05	1515.50		AB
(Caraco)				
CAP, PO (HARD GELATIN CAPSULE)				
100 mg, 100s ea	62756-0137-02	53.30		AB
500s ea	62756-0137-05	266.50		AB
300 mg, 100s ea	62756-0138-02	133.20		AB
500s ea	62756-0138-05	665.95		AB
400 mg, 100s ea	62756-0139-02	159.80		AB
500s ea	62756-0139-05	799.00		AB
TAB, PO (FILM COATED)				
600 mg, 100s ea	62756-0202-01	252.90		AB
500s ea	62756-0202-03	1264.50		AB
800 mg, 100s ea	62756-0204-01	303.20		AB
500s ea	62756-0204-03	1516.00		AB
(Gallipot)				
CRY, NA (1X5GM)				
5 gm	51552-0902-02	27.30	19.50	
(1X25GM)				
25 gm	51552-0902-04	89.60	64.00	
(1X100GM)				
100 gm	51552-0902-05	322.00	230.00	
(1X500GM)				
500 gm	51552-0902-06	1050.00	750.00	
(1X1000GM)				
1000 gm	51552-0902-07	2660.00	1900.00	
(Glenmark Pharmaceuticals)				
TAB, PO (FILM-COATED)				
600 mg, 100s ea	68462-0126-01	252.90		AB
500s ea	68462-0126-05	1264.50		AB
800 mg, 100s ea	68462-0127-01	303.44		AB
500s ea	68462-0127-05	1517.20		AB
(Greenstone)				
CAP, PO, 100 mg, 100s ea	59762-5026-01	53.18		
300 mg, 100s ea	59762-5027-01	132.96		
(HARD-GELATIN)				
300 mg, 500s ea	59762-5027-02	664.80		
400 mg, 100s ea	59762-5028-01	159.53		
TAB, PO (FILM-COATED)				
600 mg, 100s ea	59762-5023-01	252.62		
800 mg, 100s ea	59762-5024-01	303.10		
(Hawkins)				
POW, NA, 25 gm	63370-0099-25	312.00		
100 gm	63370-0099-35	864.00		
500 gm	63370-0099-45	3600.00		
1000 gm	63370-0099-50	6720.00		
(Letco)				
POW, NA, 25 gm	62991-2204-01	198.00		
100 gm	62991-2204-02	564.00		
500 gm	62991-2204-03	1560.00		
(Major)				
CAP, PO, 100 mg, 90s ea	00904-5631-89	57.65		AB
(10X10)				
100 mg, 100s ea UD	00904-5631-61	58.79		AB
300 mg, 30s ea	00904-5632-46	56.22		AB
(10X10)				
300 mg, 100s ea UD	00904-5632-61	192.65		AB
400 mg, 100s ea UD	00904-5633-61	184.76		AB
(Medisca)				
CRY, NA (USP,1X10GM)				
10 gm	38779-2461-01	129.00		
(USP,1X25GM)				
25 gm	38779-2461-04	229.50		
(USP,1X100GM)				
100 gm	38779-2461-05	765.00		
(USP,1X500GM)				
500 gm	38779-2461-08	1950.00		
(USP,1X1000GM)				
1000 gm	38779-2461-09	2835.00		
(USP,1X5000GM)				
5000 gm	38779-2461-03	11250.00		
POW, NA, 10 gm	38779-1980-01	129.00		
25 gm	38779-1980-04	229.50		
100 gm	38779-1980-05	765.00		
(1X500GM)				
500 gm	38779-1980-08	1950.00		
(1X1000GM)				
1000 gm	38779-1980-09	2835.00		
(1X5000GM)				
5000 gm	38779-1980-03	11250.00		
(PCCA)				
CRY, NA (USP)				
1 gm	51927-4213-00	33.00		
POW, NA, 1 gm	51927-3301-00	30.00		
(Pfizer) *See NEURONTIN*				
(Ranbaxy Pharm)				
CAP, PO, 100 mg, 100s ea	63304-0627-01	53.24		AB
500s ea	63304-0627-05	266.20		AB
300 mg, 100s ea	63304-0628-01	133.11		AB
500s ea	63304-0628-05	665.55		AB
400 mg, 100s ea	63304-0629-01	159.71		AB
500s ea	63304-0629-05	798.55		AB
TAB, PO (FILM-COATED)				
600 mg, 100s ea	63304-0592-01	252.90		AB
500s ea	63304-0592-05	1264.50		AB
800 mg, 100s ea	63304-0593-01	303.44		AB
500s ea	63304-0593-05	1517.20		AB
(Sandoz)				
CAP, PO, 100 mg, 100s ea	00185-0091-01	53.67		AB
500s ea	00185-0091-05	268.35		AB
1000s ea	00185-0091-10	536.70		AB
300 mg, 100s ea	00185-0093-01	134.18		AB
500s ea	00185-0093-05	670.91		AB
1000s ea	00185-0093-10	1341.80		AB
400 mg, 100s ea	00185-0094-01	160.98		AB
500s ea	00185-0094-05	804.92		AB
1000s ea	00185-0094-10	1609.80		AB
TAB, PO (FILM-COATED)				
600 mg, 100s ea	00185-0107-01	254.65		AB
800 mg, 100s ea	00185-0113-01	305.15		AB
(Spectrum Pharmacy)				
CRY, NA, 25 gm	49452-3240-02	331.52		
(1X25GM,USP)				
25 gm	49452-3241-01	331.45		
100 gm	49452-3240-03	1127.00		
(1X100GM,USP)				
100 gm	49452-3241-02	1127.00		
(1X500GM,USP)				
500 gm	49452-3241-03	2362.50		
(1X1000GM,USP)				
1000 gm	49452-3241-04	3377.50		
(Teva)				
CAP, PO (10X10)				
100 mg, 100s ea UD	00172-4381-10	55.15		
300 mg, 100s ea UD	00172-4382-10	134.95		
400 mg, 100s ea UD	00172-4383-10	161.50		
(Teva) *See GABARONE*				
(Teva)				
TAB, PO, 600 mg, 100s ea	00093-4443-01	252.65		AB
100s ea UD	00172-4443-10	254.65		AB
500s ea	00093-4443-05	1200.09		AB
1000s ea	00093-4443-10	2280.17		AB
800 mg, 10s ea UD	00172-4444-10	305.15		AB
100s ea	00093-4444-01	303.15		AB
500s ea	00093-4444-05	1439.96		AB
(UDL)				
CAP, PO (ROBOT READY 25X1,GRAY)				
100 mg, 25s ea UD	51079-0785-19	14.78		AB
(10X10)				
100 mg, 100s ea UD	51079-0785-20	59.10		AB
(ROBOT READY 25X1,ORANGE)				
300 mg, 25s ea UD	51079-0786-19	34.90		AB
(10X10)				
300 mg, 100s ea UD	51079-0786-20	139.60		AB
(West-Ward)				
CAP, PO, 300 mg, 100s ea	00143-9993-01	133.00		AB
400 mg, 100s ea	00143-9994-01	159.65		AB
(4u)				
REPACK				
CAP, PO, 100 mg, 28s ea	10544-0312-28	44.18		AB
28s ea	42549-0512-28	44.18		AB
60s ea	10544-0312-60	64.46		
60s ea	42549-0512-60	64.46		AB
90s ea	42549-0512-90	90.24		AB
300 mg, 28s ea	10544-0313-28	90.22		AB
28s ea	42549-0513-28	90.22		AB
30s ea	10544-0313-30	94.44		
30s ea	42549-0513-30	94.44		AB
60s ea	10544-0313-60	124.88		
60s ea	42549-0513-60	124.88		AB
90s ea	10544-0313-90	185.56		
90s ea	42549-0513-90	186.56		AB
(HARD GELATIN CAPSULE)				
300 mg, 90s ea	42549-0313-90	186.56		AB
112s ea	10544-0313-02	214.92		AB
112s ea	42549-0513-02	214.92		AB
TAB, PO, 600 mg, 60s ea	10544-0337-60	204.84		
(FILM-COATED)				
600 mg, 60s ea	42549-0337-60	204.84		AB
60s ea	42549-0537-60	204.84		AB
90s ea	10544-0337-90	288.62		AB
90s ea	42549-0537-90	288.62		AB
(A-S Medication)				
REPACK				
CAP, PO (HARD GELATIN)				
100 mg, 30s ea	54569-5734-00	16.00		AB
90s ea	54569-5734-02	48.01		AB
100s ea	54569-5734-01	53.34		AB
300 mg, 30s ea	54569-5633-01	40.00		AB
60s ea	54569-5633-02	80.00		AB
90s ea	54569-5633-04	120.01		AB
100s ea	54569-5633-00	133.34		AB
120s ea	54569-5633-03	160.01		AB
400 mg, 90s ea	54569-5981-00	143.83		AB
TAB, PO (FILM-COATED)				
600 mg, 30s ea	54569-5956-02	75.79		AB
60s ea	54569-5956-01	151.57		AB
90s ea	54569-5956-00	227.36		
(Aidarex)				
REPACK				
CAP, PO, 100 mg, 10s ea	33261-0048-10	13.20		
12s ea	33261-0048-12	15.84		
14s ea	33261-0048-14	18.48		
20s ea	33261-0048-20	26.40		
21s ea	33261-0048-21	27.72		
28s ea	33261-0048-28	36.96		
30s ea	33261-0048-30	40.80		
40s ea	33261-0048-40	52.80		
60s ea	33261-0048-60	79.20		
90s ea	33261-0048-90	118.80		
120s ea	33261-0048-02	158.40		
300 mg, 10s ea	33261-0049-10	19.00		
12s ea	33261-0049-12	22.80		
14s ea	33261-0049-14	26.60		
20s ea	33261-0049-20	38.00		
21s ea	33261-0049-21	39.90		
28s ea	33261-0049-28	53.20		
30s ea	33261-0049-30	57.00		
40s ea	33261-0049-40	76.00		
(HARD GELATIN)				
300 mg, 42s ea	33261-0049-42	79.80		AB
60s ea	33261-0049-60	114.00		
90s ea	33261-0049-90	171.00		
120s ea	33261-0049-02	228.00		
(HARD GELATIN)				
300 mg, 180s ea	33261-0049-03	342.00		AB
180s ea	33261-0049-99	342.00		AB
400 mg, 7s ea	33261-0050-07	14.00		AB
14s ea	33261-0050-14	28.00		AB
28s ea	33261-0050-28	56.00		AB
30s ea	33261-0050-30	60.00		AB
40s ea	33261-0050-40	80.00		AB
60s ea	33261-0050-60	120.00		AB
90s ea	33261-0050-90	180.00		AB
120s ea	33261-0050-02	240.00		AB
TAB, PO, 600 mg, 10s ea	33261-0051-10	23.70		
14s ea	33261-0051-14	33.18		
20s ea	33261-0051-20	47.40		
21s ea	33261-0051-21	49.77		
28s ea	33261-0051-28	66.36		
30s ea	33261-0051-30	71.10		
40s ea	33261-0051-40	94.80		
60s ea	33261-0051-60	142.00		
90s ea	33261-0051-90	213.30		
120s ea	33261-0051-02	284.40		
(FILM-COATED)				
800 mg, 30s ea	33261-0116-30	129.00		AB
60s ea	33261-0116-60	252.00		AB
90s ea	33261-0116-90	387.00		AB
120s ea	33261-0116-02	516.00		AB
(Altura)				
REPACK				
CAP, PO, 100 mg, 30s ea	63874-1102-03	16.20		AB
40s ea	63874-1102-04	21.60		AB
60s ea	63874-1102-06	32.40		AB
90s ea	63874-1102-09	48.60		AB
100s ea	63874-1102-01	54.00		AB
120s ea	63874-1102-02	64.80		AB
180s ea	63874-1102-08	97.20		AB
300 mg, 30s ea	63874-1103-03	42.55		AB
40s ea	63874-1103-04	56.72		AB
60s ea	63874-1103-06	85.09		AB
90s ea	63874-1103-09	127.63		AB
100s ea	63874-1103-01	141.80		AB
120s ea	63874-1103-02	170.17		AB
180s ea	63874-1103-08	255.25		AB
400 mg, 30s ea	63874-1104-03	52.50		
40s ea	63874-1104-04	70.00		
60s ea	63874-1104-06	105.00		
90s ea	63874-1104-09	157.50		
100s ea	63874-1104-01	175.00		

PROD/MFR	NDC	AWP	DP	OBC
120s ea	63874-1104-02	210.00		
180s ea	63874-1104-08	315.00		
TAB, PO (FILM-COATED)				
600 mg, 30s ea	63874-1131-03	90.94		
60s ea	63874-1131-06	181.88		
90s ea	63874-1131-09	252.60		
100s ea	63874-1131-01	280.66		
800 mg, 30s ea	63874-1129-03	109.11		
60s ea	63874-1129-06	208.78		
90s ea	63874-1129-09	327.34		
100s ea	63874-1129-01	363.70		
(American Health)				
REPACK				
CAP, PO (5X10)				
100 mg, 50s ea UD	68084-0079-65	30.71		AB
90s ea	68084-0079-90	47.86		AB
(10X10)				
100 mg, 100s ea UD	68084-0079-01	58.35		AB
180s ea	68084-0079-08	98.75		AB
(5X10)				
300 mg, 50s ea UD	68084-0080-65	72.46		AB
90s ea	68084-0080-90	119.66		AB
(10X10)				
300 mg, 100s ea UD	68084-0080-01	137.67		AB
180s ea	68084-0080-08	239.33		AB
(5X10)				
400 mg, 50s ea UD	68084-0081-65	84.15		AB
90s ea	68084-0081-90	143.58		AB
(10X10)				
400 mg, 100s ea UD	68084-0081-01	159.89		AB
180s ea	68084-0081-08	287.15		AB
TAB, PO (10X10)				
600 mg, 100s ea UD	68084-0122-01	242.19		
800 mg, 100s ea	68084-0123-01	290.56		
(B&B Pharm, Inc)				
REPACK				
POW, NA (BULK COMPOUND)				
25 gm	63275-9970-04	123.00		
100 gm	63275-9970-05	426.00		
500 gm	63275-9970-08	1911.00		
1000 gm	63275-9970-09	3025.00		
(Bryant Ranch)				
REPACK				
CAP, PO, 100 mg, 20s ea	63629-1572-01	14.89		
30s ea	63629-1572-03	19.99		
60s ea	63629-1572-04	46.16		AB
90s ea	63629-1572-02	67.01		
300 mg, 30s ea	63629-3056-01	49.90		
60s ea	63629-3056-03	95.89		
90s ea	63629-3056-02	129.70		
100s ea	63629-3056-05	148.22		AB
120s ea	63629-3056-04	186.32		AB
400 mg, 20s ea	63629-2593-01	49.65		
TAB, PO, 600 mg, 30s ea	63629-3063-01	75.00		
60s ea	63629-3063-02	150.00		
(FILM-COATED)				
600 mg, 90s ea	63629-3063-04	262.32		AB
100s ea	63629-3063-05	262.32		AB
120s ea	63629-3063-06	299.54		AB
180s ea	63629-3063-03	450.00		
(FILM-COATED)				
800 mg, 30s ea	63629-3375-01	101.32		AB
60s ea	63629-3375-02	206.32		AB
90s ea	63629-3375-03	303.10		AB
100s ea	63629-3375-06	303.10		AB
120s ea	63629-3375-05	365.25		AB
180s ea	63629-3375-04	506.21		AB
(Core)				
REPACK				
CAP, PO, 100 mg, 20s ea	33358-0152-20	15.26		
30s ea	33358-0152-30	41.65		
60s ea	33358-0152-60	94.98		
90s ea	33358-0152-90	101.94		
120s ea	33358-0152-01	107.86		
300 mg, 30s ea	33358-0153-30	51.15		
60s ea	33358-0153-60	98.29		
90s ea	33358-0153-90	132.94		
120s ea	33358-0153-01	174.69		
(DHS, Inc.)				
REPACK				
CAP, PO, 100 mg, 30s ea	55887-0329-30	16.05		
60s ea	55887-0329-60	32.10		
90s ea	55887-0329-90	48.15		
100s ea	55887-0329-01	53.50		
150s ea	55887-0329-86	80.25		
200s ea	55887-0329-83	107.00		
300s ea	55887-0329-84	160.50		
300 mg, 30s ea	55887-0338-30	46.91		AB
45s ea	55887-0338-45	70.36		
60s ea	55887-0338-60	92.82		AB
90s ea	55887-0338-90	124.44		AB
100s ea	55887-0338-01	156.36		
120s ea	55887-0338-82	165.92		AB
180s ea	55887-0338-92	248.88		
240s ea	55887-0338-91	331.84		
400 mg, 30s ea	55887-0177-30	48.29		
60s ea	55887-0177-60	96.58		
TAB, PO, 400 mg, 60s ea	55887-0276-60	110.30		
(FILM-COATED)				
600 mg, 30s ea	55887-0282-30	84.46		AB
90s ea	55887-0282-90	194.95		AB
800 mg, 30s ea	55887-0281-30	90.96		
60s ea	55887-0281-60	181.94		
90s ea	55887-0281-90	194.95		
100s ea	55887-0281-01	216.61		
120s ea	55887-0281-82	363.84		
150s ea	55887-0281-86	342.92		
(Dispensing Solutions)				
REPACK				
CAP, PO, 100 mg, 30s ea	55045-3264-08	36.00		
30s ea	66336-0567-30	18.36		
60s ea	55045-3264-06	72.00		AB
60s ea	66336-0567-60	36.72		
90s ea	55045-3264-09	108.00		
90s ea	66336-0567-90	55.08		
100s ea	55045-3264-01	120.00		
120s ea	55045-3264-02	144.00		
300 mg, 30s ea	55045-3234-08	39.90		
30s ea	66336-0439-30	45.00		
60s ea	55045-3234-06	79.80		
60s ea	55045-3765-06	79.80		
60s ea	66336-0439-60	89.41		
90s ea	55045-3234-09	119.70		
90s ea	66336-0439-90	134.12		AB
100s ea	55045-3234-01	133.00		
120s ea	55045-3234-02	159.60		AB
(HARD GELATIN)				
300 mg, 120s ea	66336-0439-94	178.82		AB
126s ea	55045-3723-01	167.58		
400 mg, 30s ea	55045-3421-08	48.00		AB
30s ea	66336-0266-30	53.87		
60s ea	55045-3421-06	96.00		
90s ea	55045-3421-09	144.00		AB
90s ea	66336-0266-90	161.61		AB
120s ea	66336-0266-94	215.48		AB
180s ea	55045-3421-01	288.00		
TAB, PO (FILM-COATED)				
600 mg, 30s ea	55045-3322-08	75.60		AB
30s ea	66336-0471-30	79.58		AB
60s ea	55045-3322-06	151.20		AB
90s ea	55045-3322-09	226.80		AB
90s ea	66336-0471-90	238.73		AB
100s ea	55045-3322-00	252.00		AB
(FILM-COATED)				
600 mg, 120s ea	55045-3322-01	302.40		AB
120s ea	66336-0471-94	318.31		AB
800 mg, 30s ea	55045-3422-08	91.50		AB
90s ea	55045-3422-09	274.50		AB
90s ea	66336-0762-90	286.43		AB
100s ea	55045-3422-00	305.00		
(FILM-COATED)				
800 mg, 120s ea	66336-0762-94	381.91		AB
(GSMS)				
REPACK				
CAP, PO (HARD GELATIN CAPSULE)				
100 mg, 500s ea	60429-0738-05	93.60	31.20	AB
300 mg, 500s ea	60429-0739-05	232.05	77.35	AB
400 mg, 500s ea	60429-0740-05	354.00	118.00	AB
(HomeMed)				
REPACK				
CAP, PO, 300 mg, 30s ea	51655-0246-24	39.90		
(IPI)				
REPACK				
CAP, PO, 100 mg, 30s ea	18837-0055-30	19.97		
90s ea	18837-0055-90	59.90		
300 mg, 30s ea	18837-0056-30	50.32		
60s ea	18837-0056-60	79.87		AB
90s ea	18837-0056-90	119.80		AB
120s ea	18837-0056-98	199.67		
270s ea	18837-0056-94	448.86		
400 mg, 30s ea	18837-0057-30	59.89		AB
60s ea	18837-0057-60	95.83		
90s ea	18837-0057-90	143.74		AB
TAB, PO (FILM-COATED)				
600 mg, 30s ea	18837-0058-30	94.84		AB
60s ea	18837-0058-60	151.74		AB
120s ea	18837-0058-98	303.48		AB
180s ea	18837-0058-96	570.03		AB
270s ea	18837-0058-94	853.54		AB
800 mg, 60s ea	18837-0059-60	227.58		
(FILM-COATED)				
800 mg, 90s ea	18837-0059-90	273.10		AB
100s ea	18837-0059-99	379.30		
(FILM-COATED)				
800 mg, 120s ea	18837-0059-98	182.06		AB
(Keltman Pharma., Inc.)				
REPACK				
CAP, PO, 100 mg, 30s ea	68387-0420-30	28.00		
45s ea	68387-0420-45	42.00		AB
90s ea	68387-0420-90	84.00		AB
120s ea	68387-0420-12	112.00		
300 mg, 30s ea	68387-0410-10	165.00		
30s ea	68387-0410-30	49.50		
45s ea	68387-0410-45	74.25		AB
60s ea	68387-0410-60	99.00		
90s ea	68387-0410-90	148.50		AB
180s ea	68387-0410-18	297.00		
400 mg, 90s ea	68387-0404-90	143.85		
TAB, PO, 600 mg, 90s ea	68387-0405-90	253.66		
(FILM-COATED)				
600 mg, 90s ea	68387-0421-90	253.66		AB
120s ea	68387-0421-12	338.21		AB
800 mg, 90s ea	68387-0408-90	294.50		
(FILM-COATED)				
800 mg, 120s ea	68387-0408-12	392.66		AB
(LWP)				
REPACK				
POW, NA (1X30GM)				
30 gm	64038-0490-30	390.01		
(1X33GM)				
33 gm	64038-0490-33	429.02		
(1X90GM)				
90 gm	64038-0490-90	1170.04		
(1X99GM)				
99 gm	64038-0490-99	1287.04		
(1X165GM)				
165 gm	64038-0490-16	1991.85		
(1X198GM)				
198 gm	64038-0490-19	2574.08		
(1X396GM)				
396 gm	64038-0490-39	5148.15		
(1X660GM)				
660 gm	64038-0490-06	8580.26		
(1X780GM)				
780 gm	64038-0490-78	13182.40		
(1X1300GM)				
1300 gm	64038-0490-13	16900.52		
(McKesson Packaging)				
REPACK				
CAP, PO, 100 mg,				
100s ea UD	63739-0374-10	66.47		
300 mg, 100s ea UD	63739-0375-10	166.00		
400 mg, 100s ea UD	63739-0376-10	199.25		
TAB, PO, 600 mg,				
100s ea UD	63739-0391-10	315.75		
800 mg, 100s ea UD	63739-0392-10	378.75		
(Medsource)				
REPACK				
CAP, PO, 300 mg, 30s ea	45865-0347-30	47.70		AB
60s ea	45865-0347-60	95.40		AB
90s ea	45865-0347-90	143.10		AB
100s ea	45865-0347-00	159.00		AB
120s ea	45865-0347-01	190.80		AB
150s ea	45865-0347-02	238.50		AB
300s ea	45865-0347-05	477.00		AB
TAB, PO (FILM-COATED)				
600 mg, 30s ea	45865-0356-30	82.50		AB
60s ea	45865-0356-60	165.00		AB
90s ea	45865-0356-90	247.50		AB
100s ea	45865-0356-00	275.00		AB
120s ea	45865-0356-01	330.00		AB
150s ea	45865-0356-02	412.50		AB
300s ea	45865-0356-05	825.00		AB
800 mg, 30s ea	45865-0405-30	105.00		AB
60s ea	45865-0405-60	210.00		AB
90s ea	45865-0405-90	315.00		AB
100s ea	45865-0405-00	350.00		AB
120s ea	45865-0405-01	420.00		AB
150s ea	45865-0405-02	525.00		AB
300s ea	45865-0405-05	1050.00		AB
(Nucare Pharm)				
REPACK				
CAP, PO, 100 mg, 30s ea	68071-0228-30	21.97		AB
45s ea	68071-0228-45	32.95		AB
90s ea	68071-0228-90	65.89		AB
(HARD GELATIN)				
300 mg, 30s ea	68071-0212-30	55.35		AB
45s ea	68071-0212-45	59.63		AB
(HARD GELATIN)				
300 mg, 60s ea	68071-0212-60	105.87		AB
90s ea	68701-0212-90	108.23		AB
100s ea	66267-1259-00	174.71		AB
(HARD GELATIN)				
300 mg, 120s ea	68071-0212-91	209.65		AB

PROD/MFR	NDC	AWP	DP	OBC
180s ea	68071-0212-92	216.46		
(HARD GELATIN)				
400 mg, 30s ea	68071-0291-30	65.88		AB
60s ea	68071-0291-60	125.77		AB
90s ea	68071-0291-90	190.16		AB
TAB, PO, 600 mg, 30s ea	68071-0292-30	99.58		AB
60s ea	68071-0292-60	200.21		AB
90s ea	68071-0292-90	294.08		AB
120s ea	68071-0292-91	391.76		AB
(FILM-COATED)				
800 mg, 30s ea	68071-0293-30	93.83		AB
60s ea	68071-0293-60	234.41		AB
90s ea	68071-0293-90	351.61		AB
120s ea	68071-0293-91	464.26		AB
(Palmetto) REPACK				
CAP, PO, 100 mg, 30s ea	23490-6513-01	21.00		
60s ea	23490-6513-06	42.00		
90s ea	23490-6513-02	63.00		
120s ea	23490-6513-07	71.40		
270s ea	23490-6513-08	141.75		
300 mg, 100s ea	23490-6514-07	156.37		
120s ea	23490-6514-04	159.50		
180s ea	23490-6514-05	211.10		
240s ea	23490-6514-06	281.47		
400 mg, 30s ea	23490-6515-01	53.82		
60s ea	23490-6515-06	107.64		
90s ea	23490-6515-09	161.46		
135s ea	23490-6515-07	214.38		
180s ea	23490-6515-02	242.19		
TAB, PO, 300 mg, 30s ea	23490-0626-03	75.81		
30s ea	23490-6514-01	46.91		
60s ea	23490-0626-06	151.62		
60s ea	23490-6514-02	93.82		
90s ea	23490-0626-09	227.43		
90s ea	23490-6514-03	140.73		
100s ea	23490-7738-01	156.00		
600 mg, 20s ea	23490-7325-02	56.00		
30s ea	23490-0628-03	80.24		
30s ea	23490-7325-03	84.00		
45s ea	23490-7325-04	126.00		
60s ea	23490-0628-06	160.48		
60s ea	23490-7325-06	168.00		
90s ea	23490-0628-09	240.71		
90s ea	23490-7325-09	252.00		
120s ea	23490-7325-00	300.00		
800 mg, 20s ea	23490-7326-02	66.00		
30s ea	23490-7326-03	99.00		
45s ea	23490-7326-04	148.50		
60s ea	23490-7326-06	198.00		
90s ea	23490-7326-09	297.00		
120s ea	23490-7326-00	356.40		
(PD-Rx Pharm) REPACK				
CAP, PO, 100 mg, 30s ea	55289-0939-30	30.00		
45s ea	55289-0939-45	36.00		
90s ea	55289-0939-90	74.10		
(HARD GELATIN)				
100 mg, 270s ea	55289-0939-94	144.00		AB
360s ea	55289-0939-86	178.98		AB
300 mg, 30s ea	55289-0898-30	45.00		
45s ea	55289-0898-45	54.00		
90s ea	55289-0898-90	105.00		
(HARD GELATIN)				
300 mg, 180s ea	55289-0898-93	170.34		AB
240s ea	55289-0898-99	220.14		AB
240s ea	55289-0939-99	220.14		AB
270s ea	55289-0898-94	245.04		AB
360s ea	55289-0898-86	319.56		AB
540s ea	55289-0898-83	469.08		AB
TAB, PO, 600 mg, 60s ea	55289-0959-60	119.58		
90s ea	55289-0959-90	177.42		AB
120s ea	55289-0959-98	239.16		AB
(Pharma Pac) REPACK				
CAP, PO, 100 mg, 3s ea	52959-0757-03	6.10		AB
20s ea	52959-0757-20	11.25		AB
21s ea	52959-0757-21	11.81		
30s ea	52959-0757-30	16.88		AB
60s ea	52959-0757-60	33.75		AB
80s ea	52959-0757-80	44.96		AB
90s ea	52959-0757-90	50.56		AB
100s ea	52959-0757-01	56.30		
120s ea	52959-0757-02	67.47		AB
270s ea	52959-0757-27	151.56		AB
300 mg, 20s ea	52959-0754-20	31.62		AB
30s ea	52959-0754-30	47.18		AB
45s ea	52959-0754-45	70.73		AB
60s ea	52959-0754-60	93.60		AB
63s ea	52959-0754-63	98.55		AB
75s ea	52959-0754-75	116.77		AB
90s ea	52959-0754-90	140.05		AB
100s ea	52959-0754-00	155.90		AB
120s ea	52959-0754-02	187.15		AB
180s ea	52959-0754-08	280.71		AB
400 mg, 30s ea	52959-0810-30	53.10		AB
60s ea	52959-0810-60	106.25		AB
80s ea	52959-0810-80	141.60		AB
90s ea	52959-0810-90	159.30		
120s ea	52959-0810-02	193.57		AB
TAB, PO (FILM-COATED)				
600 mg, 30s ea	52959-0789-30	84.09		AB
60s ea	52959-0789-60	168.15		
(FILM-COATED)				
600 mg, 63s ea	52959-0789-63	176.54		AB
90s ea	52959-0789-90	252.05		
120s ea	52959-0789-12	335.95		
800 mg, 30s ea	52959-0772-30	100.09		
(FILM-COATED)				
800 mg, 60s ea	52959-0772-60	199.35		AB
90s ea	52959-0772-90	299.01		
120s ea	52959-0772-02	398.25		
(Phys Total Care) REPACK				
CAP, PO, 100 mg, 30s ea	54868-5226-01	9.21		AB
60s ea	54868-5226-02	15.42		AB
90s ea	54868-5226-03	21.66		
100s ea	54868-5226-00	17.34		AB
100s ea	54868-5226-04	113.01		
150s ea	54868-5226-05	30.37		AB
300 mg, 20s ea	54868-5166-04	21.90		AB
30s ea	54868-5166-02	30.60		AB
60s ea	54868-5166-00	56.70		AB
90s ea	54868-5166-03	82.80		AB
100s ea	54868-5166-01	90.00		AB
120s ea	54868-5166-05	45.60		
(HARD GELATIN)				
300 mg, 180s ea	54868-5166-07	88.08		AB
270s ea	54868-5166-06	113.54		AB
400 mg, 30s ea	54868-5164-03	16.29		
30s ea	54868-5901-03	17.89		AB
60s ea	54868-5901-00	28.29		AB
90s ea	54868-5901-01	42.01		AB
100s ea	54868-5901-02	44.68		AB
120s ea	54868-5901-04	53.58		AB
TAB, PO, 400 mg, 10s ea	54868-5164-01	7.44		
60s ea	54868-5164-04	29.55		
90s ea	54868-5164-02	42.84		
100s ea	54868-5164-00	45.75		
(FILM-COATED)				
600 mg, 10s ea	54868-5219-03	16.65		AB
90s ea	54868-5219-02	96.94		AB
120s ea	54868-5219-04	121.35		AB
800 mg, 10s ea	54868-5195-01	18.81		
30s ea	54868-5195-02	47.43		
90s ea	54868-5195-03	102.97		
100s ea	54868-5195-00	112.41		
(FILM-COATED)				
800 mg, 120s ea	54868-5195-05	130.94		AB
(Physician Partner) REPACK				
CAP, PO, 100 mg, 30s ea	21695-8055-30	33.09		
(COATED,HARD GELATIN)				
100 mg, 60s ea	21695-0055-60	66.18		
90s ea	21695-0055-90	99.27		
100s ea	21695-0055-00	110.30		
300 mg, 30s ea	21695-0056-30	79.87		
42s ea	21695-0056-42	131.53		
60s ea	21695-0056-60	159.72		
90s ea	21695-0056-90	239.59		
100s ea	21695-0056-00	266.21		
120s ea	21695-0056-72	319.46		AB
180s ea	21695-0056-78	479.18		
270s ea	21695-0056-87	718.77		
400 mg, 60s ea	21695-0344-60	191.44		
90s ea	21695-0344-90	287.15		
TAB, PO, 400 mg, 90s ea	21695-0057-90	285.87		
100s ea	21695-0057-00	317.64		
(FILM-COATED)				
600 mg, 30s ea	21695-0058-30	151.74		AB
42s ea	21695-0058-42	106.22		AB
60s ea	21695-0058-60	303.48		
90s ea	21695-0058-90	455.22		
100s ea	21695-0058-00	505.80		
800 mg, 30s ea	21695-0059-30	182.06		
60s ea	21695-0059-60	364.12		
90s ea	21695-0059-90	546.19		
100s ea	21695-0059-00	606.88		
(Quality Care Prod) REPACK				
CAP, PO, 100 mg, 30s ea	49999-0568-30	15.60		AB
60s ea	49999-0586-60	31.00		
90s ea	49999-0568-90	46.80		
100s ea	49999-0568-00	52.00		
300 mg, 30s ea	49999-0539-30	81.18		AB
90s ea	49999-0539-90	243.54		
120s ea	49999-0539-01	324.72		
180s ea	49999-0539-18	487.08		
400 mg, 30s ea	49999-0540-30	57.60		AB
90s ea	49999-0540-90	172.80		
150s ea	49999-0540-15	288.00		
TAB, PO, 100 mg, 60s ea	49999-0568-60	31.00		
300 mg, 60s ea	49999-0539-60	162.36		
600 mg, 30s ea	49999-0784-30	75.90		
60s ea	49999-0784-60	151.80		
90s ea	49999-0784-90	227.70		
120s ea	49999-0784-01	303.60		
800 mg, 60s ea	49999-0799-60	181.86		
90s ea	49999-0799-90	272.79		
120s ea	49999-0799-01	363.72		
(Southwood) REPACK				
CAP, PO, 100 mg, 10s ea	58016-0134-10	5.30		AB
14s ea	58016-0134-14	7.41		AB
15s ea	58016-0134-15	7.94		AB
20s ea	58016-0134-20	10.59		AB
21s ea	58016-0134-21	11.12		AB
28s ea	58016-0134-28	14.83		AB
30s ea	58016-0134-30	22.80		AB
40s ea	58016-0134-40	21.18		AB
50s ea	58016-0134-50	26.48		AB
60s ea	58016-0134-60	45.60		AB
90s ea	58016-0134-90	68.40		AB
100s ea	58016-0134-00	76.00		AB
120s ea	58016-0134-02	91.20		AB
150s ea	58016-0134-03	79.43		AB
180s ea	58016-0134-99	95.32		AB
300 mg, 10s ea	58016-0298-10	15.53		AB
14s ea	58016-0298-14	21.74		AB
15s ea	58016-0298-15	23.30		AB
20s ea	58016-0298-20	31.06		AB
21s ea	58016-0298-21	32.61		AB
28s ea	58016-0298-28	43.48		AB
30s ea	58016-0298-30	50.40		AB
40s ea	58016-0298-40	62.12		AB
50s ea	58016-0298-50	77.65		AB
60s ea	58016-0298-60	100.80		AB
63s ea	58016-0298-63	97.84		
90s ea	58016-0298-90	151.20		AB
100s ea	58016-0298-00	168.00		AB
120s ea	58016-0298-02	201.60		AB
135s ea	58016-0298-67	209.66		AB
150s ea	58016-0298-03	232.35		AB
180s ea	58016-0298-99	279.54		AB
200s ea	58016-0298-89	310.60		AB
224s ea	58016-0298-91	347.87		AB
240s ea	58016-0298-04	372.72		AB
(HARD GELATIN CAPSULE)				
300 mg, 300s ea	58016-0298-73	465.90		AB
400 mg, 10s ea	58016-0133-10	15.88		AB
14s ea	58016-0133-14	22.23		AB
15s ea	58016-0133-15	23.82		AB
20s ea	58016-0133-20	31.76		AB
21s ea	58016-0133-21	33.35		AB
28s ea	58016-0133-28	44.47		AB
30s ea	58016-0133-30	57.60		AB
40s ea	58016-0133-40	63.53		AB
50s ea	58016-0133-50	79.41		AB
60s ea	58016-0133-60	115.20		AB
90s ea	58016-0133-90	172.80		AB
100s ea	58016-0133-00	192.00		AB
120s ea	58016-0133-02	230.40		AB
150s ea	58016-0133-03	238.23		AB
180s ea	58016-0133-99	285.88		AB
TAB, PO, 100 mg, 10s ea	58016-0301-10	5.30		
14s ea	58016-0301-14	7.41		
15s ea	58016-0301-15	7.94		
20s ea	58016-0301-20	10.59		
21s ea	58016-0301-21	11.12		
28s ea	58016-0301-28	14.83		
30s ea	58016-0301-30	15.89		
40s ea	58016-0301-40	21.18		
50s ea	58016-0301-50	26.48		
60s ea	58016-0301-60	31.77		
90s ea	58016-0301-90	47.66		
100s ea	58016-0301-00	52.95		
120s ea	58016-0301-02	63.54		
150s ea	58016-0301-03	79.43		
300 mg, 10s ea	58016-0285-10	13.24		
14s ea	58016-0285-14	18.53		
15s ea	58016-0285-15	19.86		
20s ea	58016-0285-20	26.47		
21s ea	58016-0285-21	27.80		
28s ea	58016-0285-28	37.06		
30s ea	58016-0285-30	39.71		
40s ea	58016-0285-40	52.95		
50s ea	58016-0285-50	66.19		

PROD/MFR	NDC	AWP	DP	OBC
60s ea	58016-0285-60	79.42		
90s ea	58016-0285-90	119.13		
100s ea	58016-0285-00	132.37		
120s ea	58016-0285-02	158.84		
150s ea	58016-0285-03	198.56		
400 mg, 10s ea	58016-0295-10	15.88		
14s ea	58016-0295-14	22.23		
15s ea	58016-0295-15	23.82		
20s ea	58016-0295-20	31.76		
21s ea	58016-0295-21	33.35		
28s ea	58016-0295-28	44.47		
30s ea	58016-0295-30	47.65		
40s ea	58016-0295-40	63.53		
50s ea	58016-0295-50	79.41		
60s ea	58016-0295-60	95.29		
90s ea	58016-0295-90	142.94		
100s ea	58016-0295-00	158.82		
120s ea	58016-0295-02	190.58		
150s ea	58016-0295-03	238.23		
(FILM-COATED)				
600 mg, 10s ea	58016-0312-10	27.50		AB
14s ea	58016-0312-14	38.50		AB
15s ea	58016-0312-15	41.25		AB
20s ea	58016-0312-20	55.00		AB
21s ea	58016-0312-21	57.75		AB
28s ea	58016-0312-28	77.00		AB
30s ea	58016-0312-30	82.50		AB
40s ea	58016-0312-40	110.00		AB
50s ea	58016-0312-50	137.50		AB
60s ea	58016-0312-60	165.00		AB
63s ea	58016-0312-88	173.25		AB
90s ea	58016-0312-90	247.50		AB
100s ea	58016-0312-00	275.00		AB
120s ea	58016-0312-02	330.00		AB
150s ea	58016-0312-03	412.50		AB
180s ea	58016-0312-99	495.00		AB
300s ea	58016-0312-73	825.00		AB
800 mg, 10s ea	58016-0320-10	33.00		AB
14s ea	58016-0320-14	46.20		AB
15s ea	58016-0320-15	49.50		AB
20s ea	58016-0320-20	66.00		AB
21s ea	58016-0320-21	69.30		AB
28s ea	58016-0320-28	92.40		AB
30s ea	58016-0320-30	99.00		AB
40s ea	58016-0320-40	132.00		AB
50s ea	58016-0320-50	165.00		AB
60s ea	58016-0320-60	198.00		AB
90s ea	58016-0320-90	297.00		AB
100s ea	58016-0320-00	330.00		AB
120s ea	58016-0320-02	396.00		AB
150s ea	58016-0320-03	495.00		AB
180s ea	58016-0320-99	594.00		AB
(St. Mary's MPP)				
REPACK				
CAP, PO, 100 mg, 60s ea	60760-0627-60	41.14		
300 mg, 30s ea	60760-0039-30	49.93		AB
60s ea	60760-0039-60	93.85		AB
90s ea	60760-0039-90	137.78		
(HARD GELATIN)				
400 mg, 90s ea	60760-0035-90	164.11		AB
TAB, PO (FILM-COATED)				
600 mg, 30s ea	60760-0173-30	09.46		AB
60s ea	60760-0173-60	172.91		
(FILM COATED)				
600 mg, 90s ea	60760-0173-90	256.45		AB
(FILM-COATED)				
600 mg, 120s ea	60760-0173-92	339.50		AB
(FILM COATED)				
800 mg, 60s ea	60760-0038-60	206.11		AB
(Stat Rx)				
REPACK				
CAP, PO, 100 mg, 30s ea	16590-0101-30	20.77		
45s ea	16590-0101-45	29.00		AB
60s ea	16590-0101-60	38.67		
84s ea	16590-0101-62	55.94		AB
90s ea	16590-0101-90	58.00		
112s ea	16590-0101-73	72.38		AB
120s ea	16590-0101-72	77.55		AB
270s ea	16590-0101-86	180.90		AB
300 mg, 28s ea	16590-0102-28	47.07		AB
(HARD GELATIN)				
300 mg, 30s ea	16590-0102-30	50.32		AB
45s ea	16590-0102-45	75.63		AB
50s ea	16590-0102-50	84.03		AB
56s ea	16590-0102-56	94.14		AB
60s ea	16590-0102-60	100.84		AB
84s ea	16590-0102-62	141.17		AB
90s ea	16590-0102-90	149.76		AB
100s ea	16590-0102-71	168.06		AB
112s ea	16590-0102-73	188.23		AB
120s ea	16590-0102-72	201.67		AB
150s ea	16590-0102-83	195.00		
180s ea	16590-0102-82	302.51		AB
270s ea	16590-0102-86	448.86		AB
400 mg, 30s ea	16590-0492-30	51.00		

PROD/MFR	NDC	AWP	DP	OBC
40s ea	16590-0492-40	68.00		
60s ea	16590-0492-60	102.00		
84s ea	16590-0492-62	142.80		AB
90s ea	16590-0492-90	181.10		
112s ea	16590-0492-73	190.40		AB
120s ea	16590-0492-72	204.00		
150s ea	16590-0492-83	255.00		
180s ea	16590-0492-82	300.00		
TAB, PO, 600 mg, 28s ea	16590-0103-28	93.94		AB
30s ea	16590-0103-30	64.67		
42s ea	16590-0103-42	90.50		
56s ea	16590-0103-56	187.88		AB
60s ea	16590-0103-60	129.34		
(FILM-COATED)				
600 mg, 84s ea	16590-0103-62	234.61		AB
90s ea	16590-0103-90	285.52		AB
100s ea	16590-0103-71	201.56		
120s ea	16590-0103-72	380.35		AB
150s ea	16590-0103-83	303.00		
180s ea	16590-0103-82	343.50		
(FILM-COATED)				
600 mg, 270s ea	16590-0103-86	855.79		AB
800 mg, 15s ea	16590-0104-15	32.50		
30s ea	16590-0104-30	65.00		
60s ea	16590-0104-60	227.58		AB
(FILM-COATED)				
800 mg, 84s ea	16590-0104-62	401.95		AB
90s ea	16590-0104-90	341.37		AB
112s ea	16590-0104-73	422.18		AB
120s ea	16590-0104-72	259.00		
150s ea	16590-0104-83	313.50		
180s ea	16590-0104-82	355.00		
(Vibranta)				
REPACK				
CAP, PO, 100 mg, 30s ea	57866-1263-01	15.50		
60s ea	57866-1263-02	31.00		
TAB, PO, 300 mg, 30s ea	57866-7285-01	38.40		
60s ea	57866-7285-02	132.30		
90s ea	57866-7285-04	115.02		
120s ea	57866-7285-05	153.36		
400 mg, 90s ea	57866-0177-01	162.94		
600 mg, 90s ea	57866-3011-01	226.80		
800 mg, 90s ea	57866-3905-01	272.79		
GABAPENTIN TAB 600MG (Phys Total Care)				
REPACK				
gabapentin				
TAB, PO, 600 mg, 20s ea	54868-5219-01	30.30		
30s ea	54868-5219-06	43.98		
60s ea	54868-5219-00	65.67		
100s ea	54868-5219-05	105.93		
GABARONE (Teva)				
gabapentin				
TAB, PO, 100 mg, 100s ea	00182-2718-01	59.15		
300 mg, 100s ea	00182-2719-01	147.89		
400 mg, 100s ea	00182-2720-01	177.40		
GABITRIL (Cephalon)				
tiagabine hydrochloride				
TAB, PO, 2 mg, 30s ea	63459-0402-30	146.40		
100s ea	63459-0402-01	486.00		
4 mg, 30s ea	63459-0404-30	146.40		
100s ea	63459-0404-01	486.00		
12 mg, 30s ea	63459-0412-30	188.40		
100s ea	63459-0412-01	627.60		
16 mg, 30s ea	63459-0416-30	247.20		
100s ea	63459-0416-01	823.20		
(DHS, Inc.)				
REPACK				
TAB, PO, 2 mg, 30s ea	55887-0497-30	55.06		
90s ea	55887-0497-90	165.18		
4 mg, 30s ea	55887-0499-30	66.20		
90s ea	55887-0499-90	195.52		
(IPI)				
REPACK				
TAB, PO, 4 mg, 30s ea	18837-0060-30	138.00		
(Keltman Pharma., Inc.)				
REPACK				
TAB, PO, 4 mg, 30s ea	68387-0490-30	63.24		
60s ea	68387-0490-60	116.47		
90s ea	68387-0490-90	161.32		
(Nucare Pharm)				
REPACK				
TAB, PO, 4 mg, 30s ea	68071-0312-30	176.78		
60s ea	68071-0312-60	346.82		
12 mg, 45s ea	68071-0446-45	294.68		
(Pharma Pac)				
REPACK				
TAB, PO, 2 mg, 60s ea	52959-0878-60	189.03		
4 mg, 14s ea	52959-0684-14	26.49		
30s ea	52959-0684-30	56.76		
100s ea	52959-0684-00	160.49		

PROD/MFR	NDC	AWP	DP	OBC
(Phys Total Care)				
REPACK				
TAB, PO, 2 mg, 10s ea	54868-5145-01	25.29		
30s ea	54868-5145-00	72.11		
60s ea	54868-5145-02	142.35		
4 mg, 10s ea	54868-4545-02	23.23		
30s ea	54868-4545-00	62.89		
60s ea	54868-4545-01	123.90		
(Physician Partner)				
REPACK				
TAB, PO, 4 mg, 30s ea	21695-0293-30	291.60		
16 mg, 30s ea	21695-0660-30	407.25		
(Quality Care Prod)				
REPACK				
TAB, PO, 4 mg, 60s ea	49999-0692-60	480.30		
(Southwood)				
REPACK				
TAB, PO, 2 mg, 30s ea	58016-0739-30	132.48		
30s ea	58016-0739-60	264.96		
90s ea	58016-0739-90	397.44		
100s ea	58016-0739-00	441.60		
4 mg, 30s ea	58016-0753-30	132.48		
60s ea	58016-0753-60	264.96		
90s ea	58016-0753-90	397.44		
100s ea	58016-0753-00	441.60		
(Stat Rx)				
REPACK				
TAB, PO, 2 mg, 30s ea	16590-0626-30	156.23		
60s ea	16590-0626-60	312.46		
84s ea	16590-0626-62	436.85		
90s ea	16590-0626-90	468.69		
4 mg, 30s ea	16590-0105-30	171.78		
60s ea	16590-0105-60	340.31		
90s ea	16590-0105-90	508.84		
120s ea	16590-0105-72	677.37		
12 mg, 30s ea	16590-0832-30	199.20		
(Vibranta)				
REPACK				
TAB, PO, 4 mg, 90s ea	57866-3143-01	157.49		

GADOBENATE DIMEGLUMINE
(Bracco Diag) *See MULTIHANCE*

GADODIAMIDE
(GE) *See NOVAPLUS OMNISCAN*
(GE) *See OMNISCAN*

GADODIAMIDE/SODIUM CHLORIDE
(GE) *See OMNISCAN PREFILL PLUS*

GADOFOSVESET TRISODIUM
(Lantheus) *See ABLAVAR*

GADOPENTETATE DIMEGLUMINE
(Bayer) *See MAGNEVIST*

GADOTERIDOL
(Bracco Diag) *See PROHANCE*

GADOVERSETAMIDE
(Mallinckrodt Inc.) *See OPTIMARK*

GADOXETATE DISODIUM
(Bayer) *See EOVIST*

PROD/MFR	NDC	AWP	DP	OBC
GALACTOSE (PCCA)				
POW, NA ((D) ANHYDROUS)				
1 gm	51927-2537-00	0.63		
GALANTAMINE (Dr Reddy's)				
galantamine hydrobromide				
TAB, PO (USP,FILM-COATED)				
4 mg, 60s ea	55111-0407-60	190.84		AB
8 mg, 60s ea	55111-0408-60	190.84		AB
12 mg, 60s ea	55111-0409-60	190.84		AB
(Mylan)				
TAB, PO (USP,FILM-COATED)				
4 mg, 60s ea	00378-2721-91	190.73		AB
8 mg, 60s ea	00378-2722-91	190.73		AB
60s ea	00378-2723-91	190.73		AB
(Teva)				
TAB, PO (USP,FILM-COATED)				
4 mg, 60s ea	00555-0138-09	190.94		AB
8 mg, 60s ea	00555-0139-09	190.94		AB
12 mg, 60s ea	00555-0140-09	190.94		AB
(UDL)				
TAB, PO (3X10,FILM-COATED)				
4 mg, 30s ea UD	51079-0852-03	95.37		AB

PROD/MFR | NDC | AWP | DP | OBC

GALANTAMINE (UDL)
galantamine hydrobromide
TAB, PO (3X10,FILM-COATED)
8 mg, 30s ea UD ..... **51079-0853-03** 95.37 AB
30s ea UD .... **51079-0854-03** 95.37 AB

GALANTAMINE HBR (Patriot Pharmaceuticals)
galantamine hydrobromide
CER, PO (HARD GELATIN)
8 mg, 30s ea......... **10147-0891-03** 183.12
16 mg, 30s ea........ **10147-0892-03** 183.12
24 mg, 30s ea........ **10147-0893-03** 183.12

GALANTAMINE HYDROBROMIDE
(Dr Reddy's) *See GALANTAMINE*
(Global)
CER, PO, 8 mg, 30s ea .... **00115-1120-08** 190.94 AB
16 mg, 30s ea........ **00115-1121-08** 190.94 AB
24 mg, 30s ea........ **00115-1122-08** 190.94 AB
(Mylan) *See GALANTAMINE*
(Ortho-McNeil Neuro) *See RAZADYNE*
(Ortho-McNeil Neuro) *See RAZADYNE ER*
(Patriot Pharmaceuticals) *See GALANTAMINE HBR*
(Patriot Pharmaceuticals)
TAB, PO (FILM-COATED)
4 mg, 60s ea......... **10147-0881-06** 183.12
8 mg, 60s ea......... **10147-0882-06** 183.12
12 mg, 60s ea........ **10147-0883-06** 183.12
(Roxane)
SOL, PO (1X100ML)
4 mg/ml, 100 ml ..... **00054-0137-49** 220.45 AA
(Teva)
CER, PO (TWO-PIECE HARD GELATIN)
8 mg, 30s ea......... **00555-1020-01** 190.94 AB
16 mg, 30s ea........ **00555-1021-01** 190.94 AB
24 mg, 30s ea........ **00555-1022-01** 190.94 AB
(Teva) *See GALANTAMINE*
(UDL) *See GALANTAMINE*
(UDL)
TAB, PO (3X10,FILM-COATED)
4 mg, 30s ea UD ..... **51079-0469-03** 95.37 AB
8 mg, 30s ea UD ..... **51079-0470-03** 95.37 AB
12 mg, 30s ea UD .... **51079-0471-03** 95.37 AB
(Watson Labs)
CER, PO (HARD GELATIN)
8 mg, 30s ea......... **00591-3496-30** 164.98
16 mg, 30s ea........ **00591-3497-30** 164.98
24 mg, 30s ea........ **00591-3498-30** 164.98

GALLIC ACID (Amend)
POW, NA (PURIFIED)
125 gm.............. **17317-0180-04** 10.50
454 gm.............. **17317-0180-01** 28.00
(Medisca)
POW, NA (PURIFIED,1X100GM)
100 gm.............. **38779-1310-05** 37.50
(PURIFIED,1X500GM)
500 gm.............. **38779-1310-08** 169.50
(PCCA)
POW, NA, 1 gm.......... **51927-3328-00** 0.90

GALLIUM CITRATE GA 67
(Lantheus) *See GALLIUM CITRATE GA-67*

GALLIUM CITRATE GA-67 (Lantheus)
gallium citrate ga 67
SOL, IJ, 2 mci/ml,
1.65 ml.............. **11994-0121-03** 111.30 BS
3.3 ml............... **11994-0121-06** 248.68 BS
4.95 ml.............. **11994-0121-09** 347.63 BS
6.6 ml............... **11994-0121-13** 430.96 BS
8.25 ml.............. **11994-0121-16** 516.89 BS
9.9 ml............... **11994-0121-19** 596.32 BS

GALLIUM NITRATE
(Genta Inc.) *See GANITE*
(PCCA)
POW, NA (HYDRATE (III))
1 gm................ **51927-3256-00** 219.00

GALSULFASE
(Biomarin) *See NAGLAZYME*

GALZIN (Gate)
zinc acetate
CAP, PO, 25 mg, 250s ea .. **57844-0215-52** 251.11
50 mg, 250s ea **57844-0208-52** 418.51

GAMASTAN S/D (Talecris)
immune globulin
SOL, IM (1X2ML,PF,LATEX-FREE)
2 ml................ **13533-0635-03** 32.14
(S.D.V.,PF,LATEX-FREE)
2 ml................ **13533-0635-04** 48.88
10 ml............... **13533-0635-12** 223.30
(A-S Medication)
REPACK
SOL, IM (SDV)
2 ml................ **54569-5828-00** 31.88

GAMMA AMINOBUTYRIC ACID
(PCCA) *See AMINOBUTYRIC ACID*
(Spectrum Pharmacy) *See 4-AMINOBUTYRIC ACID*

GAMMA ORYZANOL (PCCA)
POW, NA, 1 gm.......... **51927-2894-00** 2.55

GAMMAGARD LIQUID (Baxter Bioscience)
immune globulin
SOL, IV (PF,LATEX-FREE)
100 mg/ml, 10 ml **00944-2700-02** 137.92
25 ml............... **00944-2700-03** 344.80
50 ml............... **00944-2700-04** 689.58
100 ml **00944-2700-05** 1379.16
200 ml **00944-2700-06** 2758.32

GAMMAGARD S/D (Baxter Bioscience)
immune globulin
PDS, IV, 0.5 gm, ea **00944-2620-01** 92.71
2.5 gm, ea **00944-2620-02** 321.72
5 gm, ea............. **00944-2620-03** 643.44
10 gm, ea............ **00944-2620-04** 1286.88

GAMMAGARD S/D (IGA<1UG/ML) (Baxter Bioscience)
immune globulin
PDS, IV (W/TRANSFER SET,PF)
5 gm, ea............. **00944-2655-03** 712.38
10 gm, ea............ **00944-2655-04** 1424.77

GAMUNEX (Talecris)
immune globulin
SOL, IV (PF)
100 mg/ml, 10 ml **13533-0645-12** 115.99
25 ml............... **13533-0645-15** 289.98
50 ml............... **13533-0645-20** 579.96
100 ml **13533-0645-71** 1159.92
200 ml **13533-0645-24** 2319.84

GANCICLOVIR
(Bausch & Lomb Inc.) *See VITRASERT*
(Ranbaxy Pharm)
CAP, PO, 250 mg, 180s ea . **63304-0636-28** 849.63 AB
500 mg, 180s ea ..... **63304-0637-28** 1699.24 AB
(Phys Total Care)
REPACK
CAP, PO, 500 mg, 60s ea .. **54868-5460-00** 1181.22 AB

GANCICLOVIR SODIUM
(Roche Labs) *See CYTOVENE IV*

GANI-TUSS NR (Cypress Pharm)
codeine phosphate/guaifenesin
LIQ, PO (AF,SF,RASPBERRY)
10 mg/5 ml-100 mg/5 ml,
473 ml, C-V......... **60258-0261-16** 39.95

GANI-TUSS-DM NR (Cypress Pharm)
dextromethorphan hydrobromide/guaifenesin
LIQ, PO (AF,SF,RASPBERRY)
10 mg/5 ml-100 mg/5 ml,
473 ml **60258-0262-16** 39.95

GANIDIN NR (Cypress Pharm)
guaifenesin
LIQ, PO (A.F,S.F,AF,SF,DYE-FREE)
100 mg/5 ml,
473 ml **60258-0256-16** 36.95

GANIRELIX ACETATE
(Organon) *See GANIRELIX ACETATE*

GANIRELIX ACETATE (Organon)
ganirelix acetate
SOL, SC, 250 mcg/0.5 ml,
0.5 ml.............. **00052-0301-51** 117.31

GANITE (Genta Inc.)
gallium nitrate
SOL, IV (PF)
25 mg/ml, 20 ml 5s... **66657-0301-05** 4680.00

GARAMYCIN (Phys Total Care)
REPACK
gentamicin sulfate
SOL, OP, 3 mg/ml, 5 ml ... **54868-0259-00** 26.95 AT
(Southwood)
REPACK
OIN, OP, 3 mg/gm, 3.5 gm . **58016-6433-00** 21.64 AT
SOL, OP, 3 mg/ml, 5 ml ... **58016-6441-05** 21.64 AT

GARDASIL (Merck)
human papillomavirus recomb vaccine quadrivalent
SUS, IM (SDV, TAX INCL,PF)
0.5 ml.............. **00006-4045-00** 156.50
(6X0.5ML,TAX INCL,PF)
0.5 ml 6s........... **00006-4109-09** 948.00
(10 X 0.5ML, TAX INCL,PF)
0.5 ml 10s.......... **00006-4045-41** 1561.76

GARDENIA
(Medisca) *See GARDENIA OIL*

GARDENIA OIL (Medisca)
gardenia
OIL, NA (1X14ML)
14 ml............... **38779-1722-03** 16.50
(1X25ML)
25 ml............... **38779-1722-04** 31.50
(1X100ML)
100 ml **38779-1722-05** 76.50
(1X500ML)
500 ml **38779-1722-08** 273.00

GARDENIA OIL FRAGRANCE (PCCA)
fragrance
SOL, NA (ARTIFICIAL)
1 ml................ **51927-3555-00** 0.75

GARLIC (PCCA)
POW, NA (ALLIUM SATIVUM)
1 gm................ **51927-2967-00** 0.17

GASTRINEX (Seyer Pharmatec)
digestants
CAP, PO, 100s ea **11026-2614-01** 46.20

GASTROCROM (Azur Pharma, Inc.)
cromolyn sodium
SOL, PO (USP,96X5ML)
100 mg/5 ml,
5 ml 96s UD **18860-0678-70** 372.64

GASTROGRAFIN (Bracco Diag)
diatrizoate meglumine/diatrizoate sodium
SOL, PO (24X30ML)
66%-10%, 30 ml 24s . **00270-0445-35** 628.75 503.00 AA
120 ml 12s .... **00270-0445-40** 906.25 725.00 AA

GATIFLOXACIN
(Allergan Inc) *See ZYMAR*

GEBAUER'S ETHYL CHLORIDE (Gebauer)
ethyl chloride
SPR, TP (MIST)
100%, 103.5 ml **00386-0001-02** 27.50
(STREAM)
100%, 103.5 ml **00386-0001-06** 27.50
(FINE PINPOINT)
100%, 105 ml........ **00386-0001-04** 34.25
(MEDIUM JET STREAM)
100%, 105 ml........ **00386-0001-03** 32.50

GEBAUER'S PAIN EASE (Gebauer)
1,1,1,3,3-pentafluoropropane/norflurane
SPR, TP (MEDIUM STREAM SPRAY)
.... **00386-0008-03** 27.50
(MIST SPRAY)
.... **00386-0008-02** 27.50

GEFITINIB
(AstraZeneca) *See IRESSA*

GEL BASE
(Gallipot) *See CARBOGEL*
(Gallipot) *See CARBOHOL*
(Medisca) *See HRT GEL BASE*
(Medisca) *See MEDIHOL GEL BASE*
(Spectrum Pharmacy) *See BASE, PLURONIC*
(Spectrum Pharmacy) *See BASE, WATER*

GEL-KAM (Colgate Oral)
stannous fluoride
SOL, DE (MINT)
0.63%, 300 ml **00126-2310-68** 15.75
300 ml **00126-2312-68** 15.75

GEL, MULTI INGREDIENT
(MCR American) *See RADIGEL*
(Medisca) *See JET*
(MPM Medical Inc.) *See RADIAPLEXRX*
(PCCA) *See VERSABASE GEL*

GELATIN (Amend)
POW, NA (N.F., 175 BLOOM)
454 gm.............. **17317-0181-01** 14.00
2270 gm............. **17317-0181-05** 49.00
11350 gm **17317-0181-08** 227.50

PROD/MFR NDC AWP DP OBC

(Baker, J.T.)
POW, NA (N.F.)
500 gm............. **10106-2124-01** 24.99
2500 gm............. **10106-2124-05** 149.43

(Gallipot)
POW, NA (U.S.P.,N.F.)
113.4 gm............. **51552-0095-04** 9.10
454 gm............. **51552-0095-06** 22.12

(Medisca)
POW, NA (1X250GM)
250 gm............. **38779-1311-07** 27.00
(1X500GM)
500 gm............. **38779-1311-08** 48.00

(PCCA) *See PCCA GELATIN*

(PCCA)
POW, NA (NF, TYPE A)
1 gm............. **51927-1101-00** 0.36

(Spectrum Pharmacy)
POW, NA (N.F.)
500 gm............. **49452-3250-01** 98.70
2500 gm............. **49452-3250-02** 374.50

GELATIN SPONGE
(Pfizer) *See GELFILM*

(Pfizer) *See GELFILM OPHTHALMIC*

(Pfizer) *See GELFOAM*

(Phys Total Care) *See GELFOAM*

GELCLAIR (EKR)
hyaluronate sodium/povidone
GEL, MM (SINGLE-USE,15X15ML)
15 ml 15s............. **24477-0010-15** 165.60

(OSI Pharmaceuticals)
GEL, MM (15 ML GEL DOSE PACK)
21s ea............. **65231-0021-01** 68.25
(12X21 15 ML GEL DOSE PK)
252s ea............. **65231-0021-12** 819.00

(Phys Total Care)
REPACK
GEL, MM, 15s ea **54868-5366-01** 158.90
21s ea............. **54868-5366-00** 168.18

GELFILM (Pfizer)
gelatin sponge
SHE, NA (100X125MM)
ea............. **00009-0283-01** 697.07 580.89

GELFILM OPHTHALMIC (Pfizer)
gelatin sponge
SHE, NA (25X50MM)
6s ea............. **00009-0297-03** 442.13 368.44

GELFOAM (Pfizer)
gelatin sponge
POW, NA (PACKET,6X1GM)
1 gm 6s............. **00009-0433-04** 545.20 454.33
SPG, NA (SIZE 50)
4s ea............. **00009-0323-01** 133.76 111.47
(COMPRESSED SIZE 100)
6s ea............. **00009-0353-01** 299.33 249.44
(SIZE 100)
6s ea............. **00009-0342-01** 299.93 249.94
(SIZE 200,STERILE)
6s ea............. **00009-0349-03** 558.34 465.28
(SIZE 12-7 MM,STERILE)
12s ea............. **00009-0315-08** 123.77 103.14
(SIZE 4)
12s ea............. **00009-0396-05** 72.98 60.82

(Phys Total Care)
SPG, NA (SIZE 100)
6s ea............. **54868-4197-00** 290.33

GELNIQUE (Watson)
oxybutynin chloride
GEL, TD, 100 mg/gm,
1 gm 30s............. **52544-0084-30** 146.18

GEMCITABINE HYDROCHLORIDE
(Lilly) *See GEMZAR*

GEMFIBROZIL
FUL
TAB, PO, 600 mg, 500s ea......................... 67.50

(Apotex Corp.)
TAB, PO (FILM-COATED)
600 mg, 60s ea ...... **60505-0034-04** 74.75 AB
100s ea............. **60505-0034-01** 122.11 AB
(USP,10X10,FILM COATED)
600 mg, 100s ea UD.. **60505-0034-00** 109.25
(FILM-COATED)
600 mg, 200s ea ..... **60505-0034-02** 244.15 AB
500s ea............. **60505-0034-08** 593.65 AB
(USP,FILM COATED)
600 mg, 2500s ea **60505-0034-06** 2968.25

(Blu)
TAB, PO (USP,FILM COATED)
600 mg, 60s ea ...... **24658-0130-60** 10.09 AB
180s ea............. **24658-0130-18** 29.33 AB
500s ea............. **24658-0130-05** 84.04 AB

(Camber)
TAB, PO (FILM COATED)
600 mg, 60s ea ...... **31722-0225-60** 74.80 AB
500s ea............. **31722-0225-05** 593.60 AB

(Caraco)
TAB, PO (USP,FILM-COATED)
600 mg, 60s ea ...... **57664-0115-86** 74.80 AB
500s ea............. **57664-0115-13** 593.69 AB

(Global Pharm)
TAB, PO (USP,FILM-COATED)
600 mg, 60s ea **00115-9911-13** 74.80

(Major)
TAB, PO (FILM COATED)
600 mg, 60s ea ...... **00904-5988-52** 134.55 AB
500s ea............. **00904-5988-40** 1187.30 AB

(Medisca)
POW, NA (U.S.P.)
100 gm............. **38779-0373-05** 123.00
500 gm............. **38779-0373-08** 502.50
1000 gm............. **38779-0373-09** 918.00

(PCCA)
POW, NA (U.S.P.)
1 gm............. **51927-2643-00** 1.56

(Pfizer) *See LOPID*

(Spectrum Pharmacy)
POW, NA (U.S.P.)
25 gm............. **49452-3263-01** 98.00
100 gm............. **49452-3263-02** 255.15

(Teva)
TAB, PO, 600 mg, 60s ea .. **00093-0670-06** 74.80 AB
(10X10,FILM-COATED)
600 mg, 100s ea UD.. **00093-0670-93** 109.25 AB
500s ea............. **00093-0670-05** 593.69 AB

(UDL)
TAB, PO (ROBOT READY 25X1)
600 mg, 25s ea UD... **51079-0787-19** 25.95 AB

(West-Ward)
TAB, PO (USP,FILM COATED)
600 mg, 100s ea ..... **00143-9130-60** 74.80 AB
(FILM COATED)
600 mg, 500s ea ..... **00143-9130-05** 593.69 AB

(A-S Medication)
REPACK
TAB, PO, 600 mg, 60s ea .. **54569-3695-00** 71.24 AB

(Altura)
REPACK
TAB, PO (FILM-COATED)
600 mg, 20s ea **63874-0408-20** 23.01
30s ea............. **63874-0408-30** 34.51
60s ea............. **63874-0408-60** 69.03
100s ea............. **63874-0408-01** 95.57
500s ea............. **63874-0408-03** 477.85

(Bryant Ranch)
REPACK
TAB, PO, 600 mg, 30s ea .. **63629-1390-02** 49.87
60s ea............. **63629-1390-01** 99.73
100s ea............. **63629-1390-03** 166.22

(Core)
REPACK
TAB, PO, 600 mg, 30s ea .. **33358-0155-30** 51.12
60s ea............. **33358-0155-60** 102.22

(DHS, Inc.)
REPACK
TAB, PO, 600 mg, 30s ea .. **55887-0335-30** 33.20 AB
60s ea............. **55887-0335-60** 59.00 AB
90s ea............. **55887-0335-90** 87.00 AB

(Dispensing Solutions)
REPACK
TAB, PO (FILM-COATED)
600 mg, 30s ea ...... **55045-2323-08** 37.50 AB
60s ea............. **55045-2323-06** 75.00 AB
(USP)
600 mg, 60s ea **66336-0367-60** 140.79
(FILM-COATED)
600 mg, 90s ea ...... **55045-2323-09** 112.50 AB
100s ea............. **55045-2323-01** 125.00 AB
120s ea............. **55045-2323-02** 150.00 AB

(GSMS)
REPACK
TAB, PO (UNIT OF USE)
600 mg, 60s ea ...... **60429-0081-60** 22.74 7.58 AB
180s ea............. **60429-0081-18** 148.41 49.47 AB
500s ea............. **60429-0081-05** 152.73 50.91 AB

(Palmetto)
REPACK
TAB, PO, 600 mg, 30s ea .. **23490-5626-02** 56.18
60s ea............. **23490-5626-01** 112.36

(PD-Rx Pharm)
REPACK
TAB, PO, 600 mg, 60s ea .. **55289-0411-60** 82.35 AB
60s ea............. **58864-0710-60** 99.13 AB
(USP)
600 mg, 180s ea ..... **55289-0411-93** 213.71 AB

(Pharma Pac)
REPACK
TAB, PO (FILM-COATED)
600 mg, 30s ea ...... **52959-0937-30** 37.15 AB

(Phys Total Care)
REPACK
TAB, PO, 600 mg, 30s ea .. **54868-2353-03** 21.24 EE
60s ea............. **54868-2353-01** 38.01 EE
(FILM-COATED)
600 mg, 90s ea ...... **54868-2353-05** 39.06 AB
100s ea............. **54868-2353-02** 63.84 EE
500s ea............. **54868-2353-00** 179.82 AB

(Physician Partner)
REPACK
TAB, PO (FILM-COATED)
600 mg, 30s ea ...... **21695-0732-30** 74.75 AB
60s ea............. **21695-0732-60** 149.50 AB
90s ea............. **21695-0732-90** 224.25 AB

(Quality Care Prod)
REPACK
TAB, PO, 600 mg, 30s ea .. **49999-0114-30** 49.92 AB
60s ea............. **49999-0114-60** 99.84 AB

(Southwood)
REPACK
TAB, PO, 600 mg, 60s ea .. **58016-0540-60** 83.20 EE
100s ea............. **58016-0540-00** 138.66 EE

(Vibranta)
REPACK
TAB, PO, 600 mg, 30s ea .. **57866-6540-02** 56.18
60s ea............. **57866-6540-04** 72.36

GEMIFLOXACIN MESYLATE
(Cornerstone) *See FACTIVE*

GEMTUZUMAB OZOGAMICIN
(Wyeth) *See MYLOTARG*

GEMZAR (Lilly)
gemcitabine hydrochloride
PDS, IV (VIAL)
1 gm, ea............. **00002-7502-01** 869.16 724.30
200 mg, ea **00002-7501-01** 173.83 144.86

GENANTUSS (PGD, Inc.)
dm/gg/phenyleph hcl
LIQ, PO (MENTHOL-PEACH)
473 ml **55422-0420-16** 14.88

GENEBROM DM (PGD, Inc.)
bpm/dm/pse hcl
SYR, PO (CHERRY)
473 ml .... **55422-0410-16** 19.50 EE

GENEBRONCO-D (PGD, Inc.)
dm/gg/pse hcl
LIQ, PO (AF,SF,DYE-FREE,CHERRY)
473 ml **65615-0401-16** 25.92

GENECAR (PGD, Inc.)
acetaminophen/phenyltoloxamine citrate
TAB, PO, 500 mg-30 mg,
100s ea............. **55422-0111-10** 10.38

GENECOF-HC (PGD, Inc.)
cpm/hydrocod bit/pse hcl
LIQ, PO (AF,SF,DYE-FREE)
473 ml, C-III **55422-0421-16** 12.00
473 ml, C-III **65615-0423-16** 31.33

GENECOF-XP (PGD, Inc.)
gg/hydrocod bit/pse hcl
LIQ, PO (AF,SF,DYE-FREE)
473 ml, C-III **55422-0422-16** 12.00
SYR, PO, 473 ml, C-III **65615-0424-16** 33.53

GENEDEL (PGD, Inc.)
cpm/dm/pse hcl
SYR, PO (AF,SF,GRAPE)
473 ml **65615-0408-16** 18.38

PROD/MFR	NDC	AWP	DP	OBC
GENEDOTUSS-DM (PGD, Inc.)				
dextromethorphan hydrobromide/guaifenesin				
LIQ, PO (AF,SF,DYE-FREE,GRAPE)				
20 mg/5 ml-200 mg/5 ml,				
473 ml	**65615-0416-16**	17.40		
GENELAN (PGD, Inc.)				
cpm/dm/gg/phenyleph hcl				
LIQ, PO (SF,DYE-FREE)				
473 ml	**65615-0414-16**	17.40		
GENEPATUSS (PGD, Inc.)				
cpm/dm/gg/phenyleph hcl				
LIQ, PO (AF,SF,DYE-FREE,GRAPE)				
473 ml	**65615-0403-16**	27.36		
GENERLAC (Morton Grove)				
lactulose				
SOL, PO, 10 gm/15 ml,				
473 ml	**60432-0038-16**	25.85		**AA**
1892 ml	**60432-0038-64**	98.77		**AA**
GENESUPP-500 (PGD, Inc.)				
multivitamin and minerals				
LIQ, PO (AF,SF,DYE-FREE)				
473 ml	**65615-0418-16**	15.20		
GENETECT PLUS (PGD, Inc.)				
multivitamin and minerals				
LIQ, PO (AF,SF,DYE-FREE,CHERRY)				
473 ml	**55422-0413-16**	18.60		
GENETICAL (PGD, Inc.)				
bioflavonoid/calcium/magnesium/vitamin d				
SGL, PO (SOFTGEL)				
60s ea	**65615-0110-60**	6.00		
GENETUSS-2 (PGD, Inc.)				
dm/gg/phenyleph hcl				
LIQ, PO (AF,SF,DYE-FREE,GRAPE)				
473 ml	**65615-0426-16**	14.30		
GENEVIT PLUS (PGD, Inc.)				
multivitamin, minerals, and nutriceuticals				
SYR, PO (SF)				
473 ml	**55422-0415-16**	15.60		
GENEXOTIC-HC (PGD, Inc.)				
chloroxylenol/hc/pramoxine hcl				
SOL, OT, 10 ml	**65615-0430-10**	9.45		
GENEXPECT-DM (PGD, Inc.)				
dm/gg/na cit				
LIQ, PO (AF,SF,CHERRY,RASPBERRY)				
473 ml	**65615-0407-16**	17.71		
GENEXPECT-PE (PGD, Inc.)				
dm/gg/pse hcl				
LIQ, PO (AF,SF,DYE-FREE,GRAPE)				
473 ml	**65615-0428-16**	18.38		
GENEXPECT-SF (PGD, Inc.)				
dm/gg/na cit/pyril mal				
LIQ, PO (AF,SF,DYE-FREE)				
473 ml	**65615-0427-16**	18.38		
GENGRAF (Abbott Pharm)				
cyclosporine, modified				
SGL, PO (BLISTER PACK)				
25 mg, 30s ea UD	**00074-6463-32**	39.62	34.76	**AB1**
100 mg, 30s ea UD	**00074-6479-32**	158.29	138.85	**AB1**
SOL, PO, 100 mg/ml,				
50 ml	**00074-7269-50**	298.88	261.52	**AB**
GENHEMAT (PGD, Inc.)				
dss/fe/folic acid/if/vit b12/vit c/vit e				
TAB, PO (CAPLET)				
60s ea	**65615-0220-60**	26.85		
GENOPTIC (Allergan Inc)				
gentamicin sulfate				
SOL, OP, 3 mg/ml, 5 ml	**11980-0117-05**	17.93		**AT**
(Phys Total Care)				
REPACK				
SOL, OP, 3 mg/ml, 5 ml	**54868-1659-00**	18.72		**AT**
GENOPTIC S.O.P. (Allergan Inc)				
gentamicin sulfate				
OIN, OP, 3 mg/gm, 3.5 gm	**00023-0320-04**	18.03		**AT**
GENOTROPIN (Pfizer)				
somatropin, e-coli derived				
PDS, SC, 5.8 mg, ea	**00013-2626-81**	376.16	313.47	
13.8 mg, ea	**00013-2646-81**	902.81	752.34	**BX**
(Southwood)				
REPACK				
PDS, SC, 13.8 mg, ea	**58016-4771-01**	694.53		
GENOTROPIN MINIQUICK (Pfizer)				
somatropin, e-coli derived				
PDS, SC (SRN,PREFILLED,PF)				
0.2 mg, 7s ea	**00013-2649-02**	105.32	87.77	
0.4 mg, 7s ea	**00013-2650-02**	210.65	175.54	

PROD/MFR	NDC	AWP	DP	OBC
0.6 mg, 7s ea	**00013-2651-02**	315.96	263.30	
0.8 mg, 7s ea	**00013-2652-02**	421.30	351.08	
1 mg, 7s ea	**00013-2653-02**	526.62	438.85	
(SRN,PF)				
1.2 mg, 7s ea	**00013-2654-02**	631.94	526.62	
1.4 mg, 7s ea	**00013-2655-02**	737.27	614.39	
1.6 mg, 7s ea	**00013-2656-02**	842.58	702.15	
1.8 mg, 7s ea	**00013-2657-02**	947.90	789.92	
2 mg, 7s ea	**00013-2658-02**	1053.23	877.69	
(Phys Total Care)				
REPACK				
PDS, SC, 0.2 mg, 7s ea	**54868-5601-00**	95.34		
0.4 mg, 7s ea	**54868-5634-00**	226.86		
(PF)				
0.6 mg, 7s ea	**54868-5917-00**	322.59		
0.8 mg, 7s ea	**54868-5760-00**	451.75		
GENTAK (Akorn)				
gentamicin sulfate				
OIN, OP, 3 mg/gm, 3.5 gm	**17478-0284-35**	19.67		**AT**
SOL, OP, 3 mg/ml, 5 ml	**17478-0283-10**	9.54		**AT**
(Dispensing Solutions)				
REPACK				
OIN, OP, 3 mg/gm, 3.5 gm	**55045-1267-09**	28.80		**AT**
(1X3.5GM)				
3 mg/gm, 3.5 gm	**68258-3015-01**	28.80		**AT**
(IPI)				
REPACK				
SOL, OP, 3 mg/ml, 5 ml	**18837-0300-05**	11.93		**AT**
(Quality Care Prod)				
REPACK				
OIN, OP, 3 mg/gm, 3.5 gm	**49999-0159-35**	32.60		**AT**
GENTAMICIN (Core)				
REPACK				
gentamicin sulfate				
OIN, OP, 3 mg/gm, 3.5 gm	**33358-0156-35**	88.15		
SOL, OP, 3 mg/ml, 5 ml	**33358-0156-05**	22.50		
15 ml	**33358-0156-15**	31.66		
(DHS, Inc.)				
REPACK				
OIN, OP, 3 mg/gm, 3.5 gm	**55887-0870-35**	43.98		**AT**
(Physician Partner)				
REPACK				
OIN, OP, 3 mg/gm, 3.5 gm	**21695-0691-35**	35.40		**AT**
GENTAMICIN SULF (Physician Partner)				
gentamicin sulfate				
SOL, OP, 3 mg/ml, 5 ml	**21695-0187-05**	16.34		
15 ml	**21695-0187-15**	49.02		
GENTAMICIN SULFATE				
FUL				
CRE, TP, 0.1%, 15 gm		3.00		
OIN, TP, 0.1%, 15 gm		3.00		
SOL, OP, 3 mg/ml, 5 ml		2.85		
(Akorn) *See GENTAK*				
(Allergan Inc) *See GENOPTIC*				
(Allergan Inc) *See GENOPTIC S.O.P.*				
(APP) *See GENTAMICIN SULFATE PEDIATRIC*				
(APP)				
SOL, IJ (M.D.V.)				
40 mg/ml, 2 ml	**63323-0010-02**	5.30		**AP**
(M.D.V.25X20ML)				
40 mg/ml,				
20 ml 25s	**63323-0010-20**	405.00		**AP**
(Bausch & Lomb Inc.)				
SOL, OP, 3 mg/ml, 5 ml	**24208-0580-60**	8.17		**AT**
15 ml	**24208-0580-64**	10.78		**AT**
(Baxter)				
gentamicin sulfate/sodium chloride				
SOL, IV, 60 mg/100 ml-0.9%,				
100 ml 24s	**00338-0501-48**	222.91		**AP**
(VIAFLEX)				
0.8 mg/ml-0.9%,				
100 ml 24s	**00338-0503-48**	237.89		**AP**
100 mg/100 ml-0.9%,				
100 ml 24s	**00338-0505-48**	258.62		**AP**
(24X50ML)				
1.2 mg/ml-0.9%,				
50 ml 24s	**00338-0507-41**	222.91		**AP**
(24X100ML)				
1.2 mg/ml-0.9%,				
100 ml 24s	**00338-0507-48**	263.94		**AP**
1.6 mg/ml-0.9%,				
50 ml 24s	**00338-0509-41**	237.89		**AP**
2 mg/ml-0.9%,				
50 ml 24s	**00338-0511-41**	258.62		**AP**
GENTAMICIN SULFATE (Consolidated Midland)				
CRE, TP, 0.1%, 15 gm	**00223-4304-15**	3.25		**EE**

PROD/MFR	NDC	AWP	DP	OBC
OIN, TP, 0.1%, 15 gm	**00223-4306-15**	3.25		**EE**
SOL, IJ (VIAL)				
10 mg/ml, 2 ml	**00223-7715-02**	1.75		**EE**
2 ml 25s	**00223-7714-02**	37.50		**EE**
40 mg/ml, 2 ml	**00223-7719-02**	2.25		**EE**
2 ml 25s	**00223-7719-25**	52.50		**EE**
2 ml 25s	**00223-7721-02**	50.00		**EE**
20 ml	**00223-7717-20**	8.25		**EE**
OP, 3 mg/ml, 5 ml	**00223-6651-05**	4.75		**EE**
15 ml	**00223-6651-15**	5.50		**EE**
(Falcon Ophthalmics)				
SOL, OP (DROP-TAINER)				
3 mg/ml, 5 ml	**61314-0633-05**	9.50		**AT**
(Fougera)				
CRE, TP, 0.1%, 15 gm	**00168-0071-15**	3.72		**AT**
OIN, TP, 0.1%, 15 gm	**00168-0078-15**	3.72		**AT**
(Gallipot) *See GENTAMYCIN SULFATE*				
(Hawkins)				
POW, NA (U.S.P.)				
5 gm	**63370-0098-15**	52.80		
25 gm	**63370-0098-25**	115.20		
100 gm	**63370-0098-35**	432.00		
1000 gm	**63370-0098-50**	1440.00		
5000 gm	**63370-0098-55**	6840.00		
(Hospira)				
SOL, IJ (VIAL-ADD-VANTAGE)				
10 mg/ml, 8 ml 25s	**00409-3401-01**	46.20	40.50	**AP**
(VIAL,FLIPTOP)				
40 mg/ml, 2 ml 25s	**00409-1207-03**	21.30	18.75	**AP**
IV (25X6ML,ADD-VANTAGE)				
10 mg/ml, 6 ml 25s	**00409-3400-01**	37.80	33.00	**AP**
(SD, USP, 25X10ML)				
10 mg/ml,				
10 ml 25s	**00409-3402-01**	47.10	41.25	**AP**
(Letco)				
POW, NA (U.S.P.)				
25 gm	**62991-1072-01**	72.00		
100 gm	**62991-1072-02**	270.00		
(Major)				
SOL, OP, 3 mg/ml, 5 ml	**00904-1907-05**	9.44		**EE**
15 ml	**00904-1907-35**	11.67		**EE**
(Medisca)				
POW, NA (USP,1X5GM)				
5 gm	**38779-0632-02**	37.50		
(U.S.P.,MICRONIZED)				
25 gm	**38779-0029-04**	135.00		
(U.S.P.)				
25 gm	**38779-0632-04**	117.00		
(U.S.P.,MICRONIZED)				
100 gm	**38779-0029-05**	345.00		
(U.S.P.)				
100 gm	**38779-0632-05**	330.00		
(U.S.P.,MICRONIZED)				
500 gm	**38779-0029-08**	1935.00		
(U.S.P.)				
500 gm	**38779-0632-08**	585.00		
(MICRONIZED)				
1000 gm	**38779-0029-09**	1560.00		
(U.S.P.)				
1000 gm	**38779-0632-09**	900.00		
(Ocusoft) *See GENTASOL*				
(Pacific Pharma)				
SOL, OP, 3 mg/ml, 5 ml	**60758-0188-05**	8.75		**AT**
(PCCA)				
POW, NA (U.S.P.)				
1 gm	**51927-1610-00**	8.40		
(Perrigo)				
CRE, TP, 0.1%, 15 gm	**45802-0056-35**	3.60		**AT**
30 gm	**45802-0056-11**	4.90		**AT**
OIN, TP, 0.1%, 15 gm	**45802-0046-35**	3.60		**AT**
30 gm	**45802-0046-11**	4.90		**AT**
(Spectrum Pharmacy)				
POW, NA (U.S.P.,CRYSTALLINE)				
5 gm	**49452-3261-01**	73.50		
25 gm	**49452-3261-02**	201.95		
100 gm	**49452-3261-03**	518.00		
(A-S Medication)				
REPACK				
OIN, OP, 3 mg/gm, 3.5 gm	**54569-1229-00**	19.67		**EE**
TP, 0.1%, 15 gm	**54569-1144-00**	3.66		**EE**
SOL, OP, 3 mg/ml, 5 ml	**54569-4355-00**	8.73		**AT**
15 ml	**54569-1218-00**	11.23		**EE**
(Altura)				
REPACK				
CRE, TP, 0.1%, 15 gm	**63874-0132-15**	13.07		**EE**
30 gm	**63874-0132-30**	26.10		**EE**
OIN, OP, 3 mg/gm, 3.5 gm	**63874-0173-04**	21.15		**AT**

PROD/MFR	NDC	AWP	DP	OBC
TP, 0.1%, 15 gm	63874-0172-15	17.47		EE
30 gm	63874-0172-30	33.54		EE
SOL, OP, 3 mg/ml, 5 ml	63874-0133-05	23.07		EE
(DHS, Inc.) REPACK				
CRE, TP, 0.1%, 15 gm	55887-0876-15	12.91		AT
SOL, OP, 3 mg/ml, 5 ml	55887-0949-05	26.76		AT
(Dispensing Solutions) REPACK				
SOL, OP, 3 mg/ml, 5 ml	55045-1240-05	18.95		AT
15 ml	55045-1240-06	27.55		AT
(Keltman Pharma., Inc.) REPACK				
OIN, OP (1X3.5GM)				
3 mg/gm, 3.5 gm	68387-0448-01	31.75		
SOL, OP, 3 mg/ml, 5 ml	68387-0455-01	13.75		AT
(Nucare Pharm) REPACK				
OIN, OP, 3 mg/gm, 3.5 gm	66267-0972-35	20.99		EE
SOL, OP, 3 mg/ml, 5 ml	66267-0971-05	18.95		EE
15 ml	66267-0970-15	27.80		EE
(Palmetto) REPACK				
OIN, OP, 3 mg/gm, 3.5 gm	23490-5629-01	25.00		
SOL, OP, 3 mg/ml, 5 ml	23490-0637-01	8.75		
5 ml	23490-5630-02	21.73		
15 ml	23490-0637-02	10.78		
15 ml	23490-5630-01	28.22		
(Pharma Pac) REPACK				
OIN, OP, 3 mg/gm, 3.5 gm	52959-0078-03	21.12		EE
SOL, OP, 3 mg/ml, 5 ml	52959-0103-00	28.94		EE
15 ml	52959-0103-01	47.39		EE
(Phys Total Care) REPACK				
CRE, TP, 0.1%, 15 gm	54868-3524-00	8.46		EE
OIN, OP, 3 mg/gm, 3.5 gm	54868-1040-01	55.14		EE
SOL, IJ (FLIPTOP VIAL)				
40 mg/ml, 2 ml 25s	54868-4103-00	74.46		AP
OP, 3 mg/ml, 5 ml	54868-6745-01	13.35		EE
15 ml	54868-6745-02	20.34		EE
(Physician Partner) REPACK				
OIN, TP (1X15GM)				
0.1%, 15 gm	21695-0785-15	17.20		AT
(Quality Care Prod) REPACK				
OIN, TP, 0.1%, 15 gm	49999-0137-15	24.72		AT
SOL, OP, 3 mg/ml, 5 ml	49999-0138-05	35.48		AT
15 ml	49999-0138-15	74.46		AT
(Southwood) REPACK				
CRE, TP, 0.1%, 15 gm	58016-3026-01	3.05		AT
30 gm	58016-4696-01	4.02		AT
OIN, OP, 3 mg/gm, 3.5 gm	58016-6026-01	24.95		EE
TP, 0.1%, 15 gm	58016 3027 02	3.05		AT
30 gm	58016-4708-01	4.02		AT
SOL, OP, 3 mg/ml, 5 ml	58016-6027-01	18.60		EE
(Vibranta) REPACK				
SOL, OP, 3 mg/ml, 5 ml	57866-7061-01	10.60		
GENTAMICIN SULFATE IN SODIUM CHLORIDE				
(Hospira)				
gentamicin sulfate/sodium chloride				
SOL, IV (LIFECARE,24X100ML)				
90 mg/100 ml-0.9%,				
100 ml 24s	00409-7886-23	118.08	103.44	AP
(LATEX-FREE)				
1.2 mg/ml-0.9%,				
50 ml 24s	00409-7879-13	116.93	102.24	
GENTAMICIN SULFATE PEDIATRIC (APP)				
gentamicin sulfate				
SOL, IJ (PEDIATRIC,M.D.V,25X2ML)				
10 mg/ml, 2 ml 25s	63323-0513-02	125.00		AP
(PEDIATRIC,S.D.V,25X2ML)				
10 mg/ml, 2 ml 25s	63323-0173-02	124.69		AP
GENTAMICIN SULFATE/PREDNISOLONE ACETATE				
(Allergan Inc) *See PRED-G*				
(Allergan Inc) *See PRED-G S.O.P.*				
GENTAMICIN SULFATE/SODIUM CHLORIDE				
(B. Braun)				
SOL, IV (150 ML PAB CONTAINER)				
60 mg/100 ml-0.9%,				
100 ml	00264-5806-32	3.64		AP
80 mg/100 ml-0.9%,				
100 ml	00264-5808-32	3.24		AP

PROD/MFR	NDC	AWP	DP	OBC
100 mg/100 ml-0.9%,				
100 ml	00264-5810-32	3.43		AP
(100 ML PAB CONTAINER)				
1.2 mg/ml-0.9%,				
50 ml	00264-5812-38	5.16		AP
1.6 mg/ml-0.9%,				
50 ml	00264-5816-38	3.05		AP
(Baxter) *See GENTAMICIN SULFATE*				
(Hospira) *See GENTAMICIN SULFATE IN SODIUM CHLORIDE*				
(Hospira)				
SOL, IV (LIFECARE,24X100ML)				
80 mg/100 ml-0.9%,				
100 ml 24s	00409-7884-23	94.18	82.32	AP
100 mg/100 ml-0.9%,				
100 ml 24s	00409-7889-23	114.62	100.32	AP
(LIFECARE, 24X50ML)				
1.4 mg/ml-0.9%,				
50 ml 24s	00409-7881-13	114.05	99.84	AP
(LIFECARE,LATEX-FREE)				
1.6 mg/ml-0.9%,				
50 ml 24s	00409-7883-13	97.63	85.44	AP
GENTAMYCIN (Stat Rx) REPACK				
gentamicin sulfate				
CRE, TP, 0.1%, 15 gm	16590-0107-15	12.75		
OIN, OP, 3 mg/gm, 3.5 gm	16590-0108-35	40.00		
TP, 0.1%, 15 gm	16590-0109-15	17.25		
30 gm	16590-0109-30	33.25		
SOL, OP, 3 mg/ml, 5 ml	16590-0106-05	18.25		
GENTAMYCIN SULFATE (Gallipot)				
gentamicin sulfate				
POW, NA (1X1GM,USP)				
1 gm	51552-0775-01	12.60	9.00	
(1X5GM,USP)				
5 gm	51552-0775-02	16.80	12.00	
(1X25GM,USP)				
25 gm	51552-0775-04	33.60	24.00	
(1X100GM,USP)				
100 gm	51552-0775-05	126.00	90.00	
GENTASOL (Ocusoft)				
gentamicin sulfate				
SOL, OP, 3 mg/ml, 5 ml	54799-0510-05	7.00		AT
GENTEX 30 (Gentex Pharma)				
carbetapentane cit/gg/phenyleph hcl				
SOL, PO (1X120ML,CHERRY)				
120 ml	15014-0888-04	37.40		
GENTEX ADE (Gentex Pharma)				
prenatal vitamins				
TAB, PO, 100s ea	15014-0100-10	54.71		
GENTEX HC (Gentex Pharma)				
gg/hydrocod bit/phenyleph hcl				
SOL, PO (CHERRY)				
473 ml, C-III	15014-0003-16	119.99		
GENTEX LA (Gentex Pharma)				
guaifenesin/phenylephrine hydrochloride				
TER, PO, 650 mg-23.75 mg,				
100s ea	15014-0002-01	116.00		
GENTEX-LQ (Gentex Pharma)				
carbetapentane cit/gg/phenyleph hcl				
SYR, PO (SPEARMINT)				
473 ml	15014-0001-16	77.39		
GENTIAN VIOLET (Gallipot)				
CRY, NA (U.S.P.)				
25 gm	51552-0297-04	13.30		
POW, NA, 125 gm	51552-0297-09	27.37		
(Medisca)				
CRY, NA (U.S.P.)				
25 gm	38779-0073-04	40.50		
100 gm	38779-0073-05	67.50		
(USP,1X500GM)				
500 gm	38779-0073-08	199.50		
(PCCA)				
POW, NA (USP)				
1 gm	51927-1210-00	1.68		
(Spectrum Pharmacy) *See GENTIAN VIOLET 1% AQUEOUS*				
(Spectrum Pharmacy) *See GENTIAN VIOLET 2% AQUEOUS*				
(Spectrum Pharmacy)				
POW, NA (U.S.P.)				
125 gm	49452-3270-01	191.45		
GENTIAN VIOLET 1% AQUEOUS (Spectrum Pharmacy)				
gentian violet				
SOL, NA, 100 ml	49452-3276-01	63.70		
500 ml	49452-3276-02	136.15		

PROD/MFR	NDC	AWP	DP	OBC
GENTIAN VIOLET 2% AQUEOUS (Spectrum Pharmacy)				
gentian violet				
SOL, NA, 100 ml	49452-3277-01	63.70		
500 ml	49452-3277-02	136.15		
GEODON (Pfizer)				
ziprasidone hydrochloride				
CAP, PO, 20 mg, 60s ea	00049-3960-60	479.00	399.17	
(8X10)				
20 mg, 80s ea UD	00049-3960-41	638.68	532.23	
40 mg, 60s ea	00049-3970-60	479.00	399.17	
(8X10)				
40 mg, 80s ea UD	00049-3970-41	638.68	532.23	
60 mg, 60s ea	00049-3980-60	581.30	484.42	
(8X10)				
60 mg, 80s ea UD	00049-3980-41	775.04	645.87	
80 mg, 60s ea	00049-3990-60	581.30	484.42	
(8X10)				
80 mg, 80s ea UD	00049-3990-41	775.04	645.87	
(Pfizer)				
ziprasidone mesylate				
PDS, IM, 20 mg, 10s ea	00049-3920-83	162.23	135.19	
(Nucare Pharm) REPACK				
ziprasidone hydrochloride				
CAP, PO, 20 mg, 15s ea	68071-0608-15	159.00		
40 mg, 15s ea	68071-0795-15	159.00		
(PD-Rx Pharm) REPACK				
CAP, PO, 20 mg, 30s ea	58864-0960-30	196.72		
40 mg, 30s ea	58864-0962-30	196.72		
60 mg, 30s ea	58864-0958-30	214.22		
80 mg, 30s ea	58864-0964-30	214.22		
(Phys Total Care) REPACK				
CAP, PO, 20 mg, 60s ea	54868-4544-00	472.45		
40 mg, 90s ea	54868-5605-00	541.63		
60 mg, 60s ea	54868-5485-00	572.93		
80 mg, 30s ea	54868-5606-00	210.23		
60s ea	54868-5606-01	429.96		
(Physician Partner) REPACK				
CAP, PO, 20 mg, 10s ea	21695-0060-10	187.84		
15s ea	21695-0060-15	274.31		
45s ea	21695-0060-45	822.94		
40 mg, 15s ea	21695-0061-15	274.31		
45s ea	21695-0061-45	822.94		
60 mg, 60s ea	21695-0062-60	1162.60		
80 mg, 60s ea	21695-0063-60	1162.60		
(Quality Care Prod) REPACK				
CAP, PO, 20 mg, 60s ea	49999-0620-60	742.68		
40 mg, 60s ea	35356-0274-60	742.68		
60 mg, 60s ea	49999-0621-60	786.63		
80 mg, 60s ea	35356-0097-60	786.63		
(Stat Rx) REPACK				
CAP, PO, 20 mg, 30s ea	16590-0895-30	262.00		
60s ea	16590-0895-60	520.74		
40 mg, 60s ea	16590-0816-60	476.76		
80 mg, 30s ea	16590-0758-30	317.24		
60s ea	16590-0758-60	631.23		
GEONE (Alphagen)				
acetaminophen/butalbital/caffeine				
CAP, PO, 325 mg-50 mg-40 mg,				
100s ea	59743-0004-01	41.50		AB
(DHS, Inc.) REPACK				
CAP, PO, 325 mg-50 mg-40 mg,				
20s ea	55887-0355-20	13.56		AB
GERANIOL (PCCA)				
POW, NA, 1 gm	51927-1337-00	5.16		
GERANIUM OIL (PCCA)				
OIL, NA (ARTIFICIAL)				
1 ml	51927-2650-00	0.90		
GERMANIUM SESQUIOXIDE (PCCA)				
POW, NA, 1 gm	51927-2592-00	24.00		
GESTICARE (Azur Pharma, Inc.)				
prenatal vitamins				
TAB, PO (BI-PHASIC RELEASE)				
90s ea	18860-0215-01	157.12		
GESTICARE DHA (Azur Pharma, Inc.)				
prenatal vitamins				
KIT, PO (SOFTGEL)				
60s ea	18860-0253-30	56.93		

PROD/MFR NDC AWP DP OBC

GFN 1200/DM 60 (Cypress Pharm)
dextromethorphan hydrobromide/guaifenesin
TER, PO, 60 mg-1200 mg,
100s ea........... 60258-0263-01 85.99

GFN 1200/PHENYLEPHRINE 40 (Cypress Pharm)
guaifenesin/phenylephrine hydrochloride
TER, PO, 1200 mg-40 mg,
100s ea........... 60258-0284-01 76.07

GFN 600/PHENYLEPHRINE 20 (Cypress Pharm)
guaifenesin/phenylephrine hydrochloride
TER, PO (DYE-FREE)
600 mg-20 mg,
100s ea........... 60258-0269-01 48.75

GFN 600/PSE 60/DM 30 (Cypress Pharm)
dm/gg/pse hcl
TER, PO (DYE-FREE,CAPLET)
30 mg-600 mg-60 mg,
100s ea........... 60258-0264-01 57.17

GG-200 NR (Alphagen)
guaifenesin
TAB, PO, 200 mg, 100s ea . 59743-0019-01 24.92

GG/HYDROCOD BIT/PHENYLEPH HCL
(Breckenridge Pharm) *See CRANTEX HC*
(Breckenridge Pharm) *See DYNATUSS HC*
(Breckenridge Pharm) *See GUIAPLEX HC*
(Breckenridge Pharm) *See MINTUSS G*
(Everett) *See TUSSAFED-HC*
(Everett) *See TUSSAFED-HCG*
(Gentex Pharma) *See GENTEX HC*
(Gil Pharmaceutical) *See GILTUSS HC*
(Hawthorn Pharm) *See NARIZ-HC*
(Laser Pharma) *See DONATUSSIN DC*
(Monte Sano) *See MONTEFLU HC*
(Poly) *See POLY-TUSSIN XP*

GG/HYDROCOD BIT/PSE HCL
(Athlon Pharm) *See DYNEX HD*
(Blansett) *See NALEX EXPECTORANT*
(Breckenridge Pharm) *See PSEUDATEX HC*
(Ethex) *See HYDRO-TUSSIN HD*
(Ethex) *See HYDRO-TUSSIN XP*
(GM Pharm) *See VANACON*
(PGD, Inc.) *See GENECOF-XP*
(Pharmakon) *See JAYCOF-XP*

GG/PHENYLEPH HCL/ZINCUM ACETICUM
(Auriga) *See ZINX CONGESTION*

GG/PHENYLEPH TAN/PYRIL TAN
(Meda) *See RYNA-12X*

GG/PSE HCL/THEOPH
(Marlop) *See BRONCOMAR*

GG/PSEUDOEPH HCL (Pharma Pac)
REPACK
guaifenesin/pseudoephedrine hydrochloride
TER, PO, 600 mg-120 mg,
14s ea........... 52959-0397-14 13.45
15s ea........... 52959-0397-15 14.40
20s ea........... 52959-0397-20 18.25
30s ea........... 52959-0397-30 26.15

GIBBERELLIC ACID (PCCA)
POW, NA, 1 gm........... 51927-2410-00 147.00

GILDESS FE 1.5/30 (Qualitest)
ethinyl estradiol/ferrous fum/norethindrone ace
TAB, PO (6X28,FILM-COATED)
30 mcg-75 mg-1.5 mg,
168s ea........... 00603-7608-17 173.60

GILDESS FE 1/20 (Qualitest)
ethinyl estradiol/ferrous fum/norethindrone ace
TAB, PO (6X28,FILM-COATED)
20 mcg-75 mg-1 mg,
168s ea........... 00603-7609-17 171.93

GILPHEX TR (Gil Pharmaceutical)
guaifenesin/phenylephrine hydrochloride
TAB, PO (PF,SF,DYE-FREE)
388 mg-10 mg,
100s ea........... 58552-0313-01 79.76
TER, PO (SF,DYE-FREE)
600 mg-25 mg,
100s ea........... 58552-0304-01 80.87

GILTUSS (Gil Pharmaceutical)
dm/gg/phenyleph hcl
LIQ, PO (AF,SF,GRAPE)
237 ml........... 58552-0108-08 19.93

GILTUSS HC (Gil Pharmaceutical)
gg/hydrocod bit/phenyleph hcl
SYR, PO (BANANA-STRAWBERRY)
473 ml, C-III........... 58552-0110-16 106.38

GILTUSS PED-C (Gil Pharmaceutical)
codeine phos/gg/phenyleph hcl
SOL, PO (AF,SF,DYE-FREE)
60 ml, C-V........... 58552-0116-02 28.63

GILTUSS PEDIATRIC (Gil Pharmaceutical)
dm/gg/phenyleph hcl
LIQ, PO (SRN,AF,SF,GRAPE)
60 ml........... 58552-0107-02 17.96

GILTUSS TR (Gil Pharmaceutical)
dm/gg/phenyleph hcl
CAP, PO (PF,SF)
14 mg-288 mg-7 mg,
100s ea........... 58552-0312-01 89.28
TER, PO (SF,DYE-FREE)
30 mg-600 mg-20 mg,
100s ea........... 58552-0303-01 90.40

GINGER (Spectrum Pharmacy)
ginger oil
OIL, NA (F.C.C.)
25 ml........... 49452-3295-01 79.45
100 ml........... 49452-3295-02 221.20

GINGER OIL (Lorann Oil)
OIL, NA, 9.9 ml........... 23535-0151-24 6.00

(Medisca)
OIL, NA (1X14ML)
14 ml........... 38779-1317-03 16.50
(1X25ML)
25 ml........... 38779-1317-04 34.50
(1X100ML)
100 ml........... 38779-1317-05 105.00
(1X500ML)
500 ml........... 38779-1317-08 459.00
(1X1000ML)
1000 ml........... 38779-1317-09 871.50
(1X4000ML)
4000 ml........... 38779-1317-01 3289.50

(PCCA)
OIL, NA, 1 gm........... 51927-1617-00 1.80

(Spectrum Pharmacy) *See GINGER*

GINGER ROOT (Medisca)
POW, NA (1X500GM,5% EXTRACT)
500 gm........... 38779-2347-08 285.00
(1X500GM)
500 gm........... 38779-1318-08 37.50
(1X1000GM,5% EXTRACT)
1000 gm........... 38779-2347-09 390.00
(1X1000GM)
1000 gm........... 38779-1318-09 67.50

(PCCA)
POW, NA, 1 gm........... 51927-2252-00 0.11

GINKGO BILOBA (PCCA)
LIQ, PO, 1 ml........... 51927-2485-00 1.80
POW, NA, 1 gm........... 51927-3062-00 5.40

GINKGO BILOBA LEAF (PCCA)
POW, NA, 1 gm........... 51927-2962-00 0.12

GINSENG ROOT (PCCA)
chinese ginseng root
POW, NA (PANAX GINSENG)
1 gm........... 51927-2495-00 0.75

GINSENG, SIBERIAN
(PCCA) *See ELEUTHEROCOCCUS SENTICOSUS*

GIZMO (Mentor)
catheter
DEV, NA (MALE, 2 PIECE, LARGE)
144s ea........... 81317-0072-00 135.36
(MALE, 2 PIECE, MEDIUM)
144s ea........... 81317-0072-50 135.36
(MALE, 2 PIECE, SMALL)
144s ea........... 81317-0072-75 135.36

GLACIAL ACETIC ACID (PCCA)
acetic acid
SOL, NA (U.S.P)
1 ml........... 51927-1297-00 0.12

GLATIRAMER ACETATE
(Teva Neuroscience) *See COPAXONE*

GLEEVEC (Novartis Pharm)
imatinib mesylate
TAB, PO (FILM COATED)
100 mg, 90s ea 00078-0401-34 4165.88
(FILM-COATED)
400 mg, 30s ea 00078-0438-15 5003.75

(Phys Total Care)
REPACK
TAB, PO, 100 mg, 10s ea .. 54868-5289-01 452.88
30s ea........... 54868-5289-00 1353.40
(FILM COATED)
100 mg, 60s ea 54868-5289-04 2836.55
90s ea........... 54868-5289-02 3971.42
100s ea........... 54868-5289-03 4412.40
400 mg, 15s ea 54868-5427-01 2808.30
30s ea........... 54868-5427-00 5497.63
45s ea........... 54868-5427-02 8246.11

GLIADEL (Eisai)
carmustine
IMP, IP (WAFER)
7.7 mg, 8s ea........ 58063-0100-01 29343.60 18118.00

GLIMEPIRIDE
FUL
TAB, PO, 1 mg, 100s ea........... 13.41
2 mg, 100s ea........... 21.74
4 mg, 100s ea........... 41.00

(Accord)
TAB, PO, 1 mg, 100s ea ... 16729-0001-01 40.15 AB
2 mg, 100s ea........ 16729-0002-01 65.09 AB
4 mg, 100s ea........ 16729-0003-01 122.80 AB

(Dr Reddy's)
TAB, PO, 1 mg, 100s ea ... 55111-0320-01 40.18 AB
500s ea........... 55111-0320-05 194.86 AB
2 mg, 100s ea........ 55111-0321-01 65.12 AB
500s ea........... 55111-0321-05 315.85 AB
4 mg, 100s ea........ 55111-0322-01 122.83 AB
500s ea........... 55111-0322-05 595.73 AB

(Mylan)
TAB, PO, 1 mg, 100s ea ... 00378-4011-01 40.15 AB
2 mg, 100s ea........ 00378-4012-01 65.10 AB
4 mg, 100s ea........ 00378-4013-01 122.80 AB

(Perrigo)
TAB, PO, 1 mg, 100s ea ... 45802-0770-78 39.77 AB
2 mg, 100s ea........ 45802-0822-78 64.47 AB
4 mg, 100s ea........ 45802-0947-78 121.60 AB

(Prasco Labs)
TAB, PO, 1 mg, 100s ea ... 66993-0162-02 40.18
2 mg, 100s ea........ 66993-0163-02 65.12
4 mg, 100s ea........ 66993-0164-02 122.83

(Ranbaxy Pharm)
TAB, PO, 1 mg, 100s ea ... 63304-0425-01 40.22 AB
2 mg, 100s ea........ 63304-0426-01 65.20 AB
4 mg, 100s ea........ 63304-0427-01 122.97 AB

(Sandoz)
TAB, PO, 1 mg, 100s ea ... 00781-5045-01 40.22 AB
2 mg, 100s ea........ 00781-5046-01 65.20 AB
4 mg, 100s ea........ 00781-5047-01 122.97 AB

(Sanofi-Aventis) *See AMARYL*

(Teva)
TAB, PO, 1 mg, 100s ea ... 00093-7254-01 40.22 AB
2 mg, 100s ea........ 00093-7255-01 65.20 AB
4 mg, 100s ea........ 00093-7256-01 122.97 AB
250s ea........... 00093-7256-52 307.42 AB

(UDL)
TAB, PO (10X10)
2 mg, 100s ea UD .... 51079-0425-20 65.20 AB
4 mg, 100s ea UD .... 51079-0426-20 122.97 AB

(A-S Medication)
REPACK
TAB, PO, 2 mg, 30s ea .... 54569-6072-00 19.56 AB
4 mg, 30s ea........ 54569-5855-00 36.85

(American Health)
REPACK
TAB, PO, 2 mg, 100s ea UD. 68084-0326-01 88.20 AB
4 mg, 100s ea UD .... 68084-0327-01 121.97 AB

(Bryant Ranch)
REPACK
TAB, PO, 2 mg, 30s ea 63629-3043-01 19.12
4 mg, 30s ea........ 63629-1255-01 43.38
60s ea........... 63629-1255-02 86.76 AB

(DHS, Inc.)
REPACK
TAB, PO, 2 mg, 30s ea 55887-0222-30 19.56
60s ea........... 55887-0222-60 39.12
90s ea........... 55887-0222-90 58.68

PROD/MFR	NDC	AWP	DP	OBC
(PD-Rx Pharm)				
REPACK				
TAB, PO, 1 mg, 30s ea	**43063-0121-30**	25.16		
90s ea	**43063-0121-90**	28.40		
2 mg, 30s ea	**43063-0034-30**	26.04		
90s ea	**43063-0034-90**	31.10		
4 mg, 30s ea	**43063-0122-30**	27.52		
90s ea	**43063-0122-90**	35.52		
(Pharma Pac)				
REPACK				
TAB, PO, 2 mg, 30s ea	**52959-0936-30**	21.58		AB
4 mg, 30s ea	**52959-0888-30**	38.95		AB
100s ea	**52959-0888-00**	134.15		
(Phys Total Care)				
REPACK				
TAB, PO, 1 mg, 30s ea	**54868-3327-00**	7.14		
2 mg, 30s ea	**54868-5457-00**	9.93		
60s ea	**54868-5457-02**	16.08		AB
90s ea	**54868-5457-01**	20.82		
4 mg, 30s ea	**54868-3377-00**	14.76		
60s ea	**54868-3377-01**	23.91		
90s ea	**54868-3377-02**	30.75		
(Physician Partner)				
REPACK				
TAB, PO, 2 mg, 30s ea	**21695-0746-30**	39.12		AB
90s ea	**21695-0746-90**	117.36		AB
4 mg, 30s ea	**21695-0747-30**	73.78		AB
60s ea	**21695-0747-60**	147.56		AB
90s ea	**21695-0747-90**	221.34		AB
(Quality Care Prod)				
REPACK				
TAB, PO, 2 mg, 100s ea	**49999-0781-00**	26.05		
4 mg, 100s ea	**49999-0807-00**	49.19		
(Southwood)				
REPACK				
TAB, PO, 2 mg, 30s ea	**58016-0005-30**	19.56		
60s ea	**58016-0005-60**	39.12		
90s ea	**58016-0005-90**	58.68		
100s ea	**58016-0005-00**	65.20		
4 mg, 30s ea	**58016-0467-30**	36.89		
30s ea	**58016-0844-30**	36.89		
60s ea	**58016-0467-60**	73.78		
60s ea	**58016-0844-60**	73.78		
90s ea	**58016-0467-90**	110.66		
90s ea	**58016-0844-90**	110.67		
100s ea	**58016-0467-00**	122.96		
100s ea	**58016-0844-00**	122.97		
(Vibranta)				
REPACK				
TAB, PO, 2 mg, 30s ea	**57866-7073-01**	45.05		
90s ea	**57866-7073-02**	53.04		
4 mg, 30s ea	**57866-7074-01**	54.74		
90s ea	**57866-7074-02**	58.21		

GLIMEPIRIDE/PIOGLITAZONE HYDROCHLORIDE
(Takeda) *See DUETACT*

GLIMEPIRIDE/ROSIGLITAZONE MALEATE
(Glaxo) *See AVANDARYL*

GLIPIZIDE

PROD/MFR	NDC	AWP	DP	OBC
FUL				
TAB, PO, 5 mg, 100s ea		6.99		
10 mg, 100s ea		11.92		
(Actavis)				
TER, PO (FILM-COATED)				
2.5 mg, 30s ea	**00228-2898-03**	12.20		AB
5 mg, 100s ea	**00228-2899-10**	40.71		AB
500s ea	**00228-2899-50**	203.50		AB
(FILM-COATED)				
5 mg, 1000s ea	**00228-2899-96**	407.00		AB
10 mg, 100s ea	**00228-2900-10**	80.62		
500s ea	**00228-2900-50**	403.07		
(FILM-COATED)				
10 mg, 1000s ea	**00228-2900-96**	806.14		AB
(Apotex Corp.)				
TAB, PO, 5 mg, 100s ea	**60505-0141-00**	36.35		AB
500s ea	**60505-0141-02**	175.12		AB
1000s ea	**60505-0141-01**	316.40		AB
18000s ea	**60505-0141-08**	5695.20		AB
10 mg, 100s ea	**60505-0142-00**	66.90		AB
500s ea	**60505-0142-02**	323.32		AB
1000s ea	**60505-0142-01**	565.75		AB
10000s ea	**60505-0142-04**	5657.50		AB
(Caraco)				
TAB, PO (USP)				
5 mg, 100s ea	**57664-0398-88**	43.50		AB
500s ea	**57664-0398-13**	217.50		AB
1000s ea	**57664-0398-18**	435.00		AB
10 mg, 100s ea	**57664-0399-88**	74.50		AB
500s ea	**57664-0399-13**	372.50		AB
1000s ea	**57664-0399-18**	745.00		AB
(Greenstone) *See GLIPIZIDE XL*				
(Major)				
TAB, PO, 5 mg, 100s ea UD	**00904-7924-61**	38.50		AB
10 mg, 100s ea UD	**00904-7925-61**	71.50		AB
(Medisca)				
POW, NA (U.S.P.)				
1 gm	**38779-0765-06**	49.50		
5 gm	**38779-0765-03**	177.00		
25 gm	**38779-0765-04**	735.00		
(Mylan)				
TAB, PO, 5 mg, 100s ea	**00378-1105-01**	34.75		AB
500s ea	**00378-1105-05**	165.15		AB
10 mg, 100s ea	**00378-1110-01**	59.75		AB
500s ea	**00378-1110-05**	292.75		AB
(PCCA)				
POW, NA (U.S.P.)				
1 gm	**51927-3111-00**	45.00		
(Pfizer) *See GLUCOTROL*				
(Pfizer) *See GLUCOTROL XL*				
(Sandoz)				
TAB, PO, 5 mg, 100s ea	**00781-1452-01**	33.60		AB
1000s ea	**00781-1452-10**	316.40		AB
10 mg, 100s ea	**00781-1453-01**	58.50		AB
1000s ea	**00781-1453-10**	555.75		AB
(Spectrum Pharmacy)				
POW, NA (U.S.P./N.F.)				
1 gm	**49452-3299-01**	81.20		
5 gm	**49452-3299-02**	274.40		
25 gm	**49452-3299-03**	1053.50		
(Teva)				
TAB, PO, 5 mg, 100s ea	**00172-3649-60**	35.00		AB
(10X10,USP)				
5 mg, 100s ea UD	**00172-3649-10**	36.35		AB
10 mg, 100s ea	**00172-3650-60**	63.00		AB
(USP)				
10 mg, 100s ea UD	**00172-3650-10**	66.90		AB
500s ea	**00172-3650-70**	323.40		AB
(UDL)				
TAB, PO (ROBOT READY 25X1)				
5 mg, 25s ea UD	**51079-0810-19**	9.37		AB
(10X10)				
5 mg, 100s ea UD	**51079-0810-20**	37.49		AB
(ROBOT READY 25X1)				
10 mg, 25s ea UD	**51079-0811-19**	17.25		AB
(10X10)				
10 mg, 100s ea UD	**51079-0811-20**	69.01		AB
(Watson)				
TER, PO (USP,FILM-COATED)				
2.5 mg, 30s ea	**00591-0900-30**	10.42		AB
(Watson Labs)				
TAB, PO, 5 mg, 100s ea	**00591-0460-01**	5.71		AB
500s ea	**00591-0460-05**	27.14		AB
1000s ea	**00591-0460-10**	54.29		AB
10 mg, 100s ea	**00591-0461-01**	8.38		AB
500s ea	**00591-0461-05**	39.76		AB
1000s ea	**00591-0461-10**	79.51		AB
TER, PO (FILM-COATED)				
5 mg, 30s ea	**00591-0844-15**	10.44		AB
100s ea	**00591-0844-01**	34.80		AB
1000s ea	**00591-0844-10**	330.60		AB
(1X30,FILM-COATED)				
10 mg, 30s ea	**00591-0845-15**	20.62		AB
(FILM-COATED)				
10 mg, 100s ea	**00591-0845-01**	68.70		AB
1000s ea	**00591-0845-10**	652.66		AB
(A-S Medication)				
REPACK				
TAB, PO, 5 mg, 30s ea	**54569-3841-00**	11.31		EE
60s ea	**54569-3841-01**	22.62		EE
100s ea	**54569-3841-02**	37.70		EE
10 mg, 30s ea	**54569-3842-00**	19.12		EE
60s ea	**54569-3842-01**	38.24		EE
100s ea	**54569-3842-02**	63.73		EE
200s ea	**54569-3842-04**	127.46		EE
TER, PO (FILM-COATED)				
5 mg, 30s ea	**54569-5547-00**	12.21		AB
10 mg, 30s ea	**54569-5548-00**	24.18		AB
(Altura)				
REPACK				
TAB, PO, 5 mg, 5s ea	**63874-0316-05**	1.89		AB
10s ea	**63874-0316-10**	3.77		AB
12s ea	**63874-0316-12**	4.52		AB
14s ea	**63874-0316-14**	5.28		AB
15s ea	**63874-0316-15**	5.65		AB
20s ea	**63874-0316-20**	7.54		AB
21s ea	**63874-0316-21**	7.92		AB
24s ea	**63874-0316-24**	9.05		AB
28s ea	**63874-0316-28**	10.56		AB
30s ea	**63874-0316-30**	11.31		AB
50s ea	**63874-0316-50**	18.85		AB
60s ea	**63874-0316-60**	22.63		AB
90s ea	**63874-0316-90**	33.94		AB
100s ea	**63874-0316-01**	37.72		AB
120s ea	**63874-0316-04**	45.26		AB
180s ea	**63874-0316-81**	67.89		AB
1000s ea	**63874-0316-02**	377.20		AB
10 mg, 10s ea	**63874-0432-10**	7.68		
14s ea	**63874-0432-14**	10.75		
20s ea	**63874-0432-20**	15.36		
21s ea	**63874-0432-21**	16.13		
24s ea	**63874-0432-24**	18.44		
28s ea	**63874-0432-28**	21.51		
30s ea	**63874-0432-30**	23.04		
60s ea	**63874-0432-60**	46.09		
90s ea	**63874-0432-90**	69.13		
100s ea	**63874-0432-01**	76.82		
120s ea	**63874-0432-04**	92.18		
180s ea	**63874-0432-81**	138.27		
500s ea	**63874-0432-50**	384.05		
1000s ea	**63874-0432-02**	768.10		
(American Health)				
REPACK				
TER, PO (3X10,FILM-COATED)				
2.5 mg, 30s ea	**68084-0295-21**	20.02		AB
(10X10,FILM-COATED)				
5 mg, 100s ea UD	**68084-0111-01**	48.32		AB
10 mg, 100s ea UD	**68084-0112-01**	69.82		AB
(Bryant Ranch)				
REPACK				
TAB, PO, 5 mg, 30s ea	**63629-1398-02**	19.91		
60s ea	**63629-1398-03**	39.82		
100s ea	**63629-1398-01**	65.70		
10 mg, 30s ea	**63629-1394-02**	27.36		
60s ea	**63629-1394-01**	54.72		
100s ea	**63629-1394-03**	91.20		
(Core)				
REPACK				
TAB, PO, 5 mg, 30s ea	**33358-0158-30**	20.41		
60s ea	**33358-0158-60**	49.82		
100s ea	**33358-0158-00**	67.34		
10 mg, 30s ea	**33358-0157-30**	28.04		
60s ea	**33358-0157-60**	56.09		
(DHS, Inc.)				
REPACK				
TAB, PO, 5 mg, 30s ea	**55887-0727-30**	11.01		AB
60s ea	**55887-0727-60**	20.00		AB
90s ea	**55887-0727-90**	29.09		
10 mg, 30s ea	**55887-0693-30**	21.01		AB
60s ea	**55887-0693-60**	39.88		AB
90s ea	**55887-0693-90**	48.96		AB
(Dispensing Solutions)				
REPACK				
TAB, PO, 5 mg, 30s ea	**66336-0730-30**	11.04		AB
60s ea	**66336-0730-60**	21.47		AB
90s ea	**66336-0730-90**	32.20		AB
100s ea	**55045-2265-01**	33.00		AB
10 mg, 30s ea	**55045-2266-08**	18.90		AB
30s ea	**66336-0662-30**	19.40		AB
60s ea	**55045-2266-06**	37.80		AB
60s ea	**66336-0662-60**	38.81		AB
90s ea	**55045-2266-09**	56.70		AB
90s ea	**66336-0662-90**	58.22		AB
100s ea	**55045-2266-01**	63.00		AB
120s ea	**55045-2266-02**	75.60		AB
TER, PO (FILM-COATED)				
10 mg, 100s ea	**55045-3300-01**	85.00		AB
(GSMS)				
REPACK				
TAB, PO (UNIT OF USE)				
5 mg, 30s ea	**60429-0082-30**	10.50	3.50	AB
60s ea	**60429-0082-60**	18.75	6.25	AB
10 mg, 30s ea	**60429-0083-30**	12.30	4.10	AB
60s ea	**60429-0083-60**	22.50	7.50	AB
120s ea	**60429-0083-12**	42.75	14.25	AB
(HomeMed)				
REPACK				
TAB, PO, 5 mg, 30s ea	**51655-0961-24**	17.99		
60s ea	**51655-0961-25**	22.89		
10 mg, 30s ea	**51655-0962-24**	21.69		
(McKesson Packaging)				
REPACK				
TAB, PO, 5 mg, 100s ea UD	**63739-0116-10**	34.09		AB
(Nucare Pharm)				
REPACK				
TAB, PO, 5 mg, 30s ea	**66267-0100-30**	14.21		AB
60s ea	**66267-0100-60**	28.45		AB

PROD/MFR	NDC	AWP	DP	OBC
90s ea	66267-0100-90	42.65		AB
120s ea	66267-0100-91	57.89		AB
180s ea	66267-0100-92	86.30		AB
(Palmetto)				
REPACK				
TAB, PO, 5 mg, 30s ea	23490-5634-03	12.00		
10 mg, 30s ea	23490-5632-01	24.16		
60s ea	23490-5632-02	48.32		
90s ea	23490-5632-03	72.48		
TER, PO, 5 mg, 30s ea	23490-5635-03	13.50		
10 mg, 30s ea	23490-5633-01	67.50		
(PD-Rx Pharm)				
REPACK				
TAB, PO, 5 mg, 14s ea	55289-0806-14	12.27		AB
14s ea	58864-0027-14	12.27		AB
30s ea	55289-0806-30	17.34		AB
30s ea	58854-0027-30	17.34		AB
60s ea	55289-0806-60	20.04		AB
(REDI-SCRIPT)				
5 mg, 60s ea	58864-0027-60	24.60		AB
90s ea	58864-0027-90	23.81		AB
(USP)				
5 mg, 90s ea	55289-0806-90	34.80		AB
360s ea	55289-0806-86	50.61		AB
10 mg, 14s ea	55289-0976-14	15.53		AB
30s ea	55289-0976-30	21.16		AB
30s ea	58864-0161-30	21.18		AB
60s ea	58864-0161-60	23.50		AB
(USP)				
10 mg, 60s ea	55289-0976-60	30.57		AB
100s ea	55289-0976-01	35.91		AB
(USP)				
10 mg, 180s ea	55289-0976-93	40.89		AB
TER, PO (FILM-COATED)				
5 mg, 7s ea	55289-0779-07	17.47		AB
(USP,FILM-COATED)				
10 mg, 180s ea	55289-0301-93	187.50		AB
(Pharma Pac)				
REPACK				
TAB, PO, 5 mg, 20s ea	52959-0823-20	9.94		AB
60s ea	52959-0823-60	26.10		AB
10 mg, 30s ea	52959-0822-30	28.01		AB
60s ea	52959-0822-60	55.60		
100s ea	52959-0822-00	121.09		AB
(Phys Total Care)				
REPACK				
TAB, PO, 5 mg, 30s ea	54868-3318-01	7.29		EE
60s ea	54868-3318-03	11.55		EE
90s ea	54868-3318-05	17.58		EE
100s ea	54868-3318-02	17.25		EE
1000s ea	54868-3318-04	145,62		EE
10 mg, 30s ea	54868-3319-02	9.06		EE
60s ea	54868-3319-04	15.12		EE
90s ea	54868-3319-05	21.18		EE
100s ea	54868-3319-01	25.14		EE
(USP)				
10 mg, 120s ea	54868-3319-06	27.26		EE
1000s ea	54868-3319-03	150.58		EE
TER, PO (FILM-COATED)				
10 mg, 90s ea	54868-4988-04	83.56		AB
(Physician Partner)				
REPACK				
TAB, PO, 5 mg, 30s ea	21695-0469-30	22.62		AB
90s ea	21695-0469-90	67.89		AB
10 mg, 60s ea	21695-0470-60	71.70		AB
90s ea	21695-0470-90	107.55		AB
100s ea	21695-0470-00	133.80		AB
(Quality Care Prod)				
REPACK				
TAB, PO, 5 mg, 30s ea	49999-0108-30	21.60		AB
60s ea	49999-0108-60	43.20		AB
100s ea	49999-0108-00	42.67		EE
10 mg, 20s ea	49999-0107-20	14.58		AB
30s ea	49999-0107-30	21.87		AB
60s ea	49999-0107-60	43.74		AB
90s ea	49999-0107-90	65.61		AB
100s ea	49999-0107-00	72.90		AB
TER, PO, 2.5 mg, 30s ea	49999-0514-30	20.35		
(Southwood)				
REPACK				
TAB, PO, 5 mg, 5s ea	58016-0876-40	12.27		EE
10s ea	58016-0876-10	3.07		EE
12s ea	58016-0876-12	3.68		EE
14s ea	58016-0876-14	4.30		EE
15s ea	58016-0876-15	4.60		EE
20s ea	58016-0876-20	6.14		EE
21s ea	58016-0876-21	6.44		EE
24s ea	58016-0876-24	7.36		EE
28s ea	58016-0876-28	8.59		EE
28s ea	58016-0876-30	9.20		EE
50s ea	58016-0876-50	15.34		EE
60s ea	58016-0876-60	18.41		EE
100s ea	58016-0876-00	30.68		AB
10 mg, 30s ea	58016-0376-30	24.16		
60s ea	58016-0376-60	48.32		
90s ea	58016-0376-90	72.48		
100s ea	58016-0376-00	80.53		
120s ea	58016-0376-02	96.64		
180s ea	58016-0376-99	144.95		
TER, PO, 5 mg, 30s ea	58016-0344-30	12.77		
60s ea	58016-0334-60	25.53		
90s ea	58016-0344-90	38.30		
100s ea	58016-0334-00	42.55		
120s ea	58016-0334-02	51.06		
(FILM-COATED)				
10 mg, 30s ea	58016-0691-30	24.16		AB
60s ea	58016-0691-60	48.32		AB
90s ea	58016-0691-90	72.48		AB
100s ea	58016-0691-00	80.53		AB
(Stat Rx)				
REPACK				
TAB, PO, 10 mg, 30s ea	16590-0287-30	22.00		
60s ea	16590-0287-60	44.00		
90s ea	16590-0287-90	66.00		
(Vibranta)				
REPACK				
TAB, PO, 5 mg, 30s ea	57866-6463-01	11.75		AB
60s ea	57866-6463-02	21.25		AB
10 mg, 30s ea	57866-6462-01	22.85		AB
GLIPIZIDE AND METFORMIN HYDROCHLORIDE (Mylan)				
glipizide/metformin hydrochloride				
TAB, PO (FILM-COATED)				
2.5 mg-250 mg, 100s ea	00378-3131-01	82.90		AB
2.5 mg-500 mg, 100s ea	00378-3132-01	98.90		AB
5 mg-500 mg, 100s ea	00378-3133-01	98.90		AB
(Watson Labs)				
TAB, PO (FILM-COATED)				
2.5 mg-250 mg, 100s ea	00591-3971-01	74.60		AB
2.5 mg-500 mg, 100s ea	00591-3972-01	89.00		AB
5 mg-500 mg, 100s ea	00591-3973-01	89.00		AB
GLIPIZIDE ER (Bryant Ranch)				
REPACK				
glipizide				
TER, PO, 10 mg, 30s ea	63629-3158-01	51.90		
60s ea	63629-3158-02	103.80		
100s ea	63629-3158-03	173.00		
(DHS, Inc.)				
REPACK				
TER, PO, 5 mg, 30s ea	55887-0212-30	21.75		
10 mg, 30s ea	55887-0179-30	38.00		
(PD-Rx Pharm)				
REPACK				
TER, PO (REDI-SCRIPT)				
5 mg, 30s ea	58864-0957-30	15.80		
(USP)				
10 mg, 30s ea	58864-0956-30	22.58		
(Phys Total Care)				
REPACK				
TER, PO, 2.5 mg, 30s ea	54868-5364-02	39.57		
60s ea	54868-5364-00	74.64		
90s ea	54868-5364-01	84.96		
5 mg, 30s ea	54868-5210-00	25.14		
60s ea	54868-5210-01	47.28		
90s ea	54868-5210-02	69.42		
100s ea	54868-5210-03	76.80		
10 mg, 30s ea	54868-4988-00	45.93		
60s ea	54868-4988-02	68.64		
100s ea	54868-4988-01	110.91		
120s ea	54868-4988-03	116.48		
GLIPIZIDE XL (Greenstone)				
glipizide				
TER, PO, 2.5 mg, 30s ea	59762-5031-01	12.20		
5 mg, 100s ea	59762-5032-01	40.71		
500s ea	59762-5032-02	203.50		
10 mg, 100s ea	59762-5033-01	80.62		
500s ea	59762-5033-02	403.07		
(A-S Medication)				
REPACK				
TER, PO, 10 mg, 60s ea	54569-5548-01	48.35		
(Dispensing Solutions)				
REPACK				
TER, PO, 10 mg, 30s ea	66336-0269-30	29.59		
GLIPIZIDE/METFORMIN (Teva)				
glipizide/metformin hydrochloride				
TAB, PO (FILM-COATED)				
2.5 mg-250 mg, 100s ea	00093-7455-01	82.90		AB
2.5 mg-500 mg, 100s ea	00093-7456-01	98.89		AB
5 mg-500 mg, 100s ea	00093-7457-01	98.89		AB
(Phys Total Care)				
REPACK				
TAB, PO, 2.5 mg-250 mg, 100s ea	54868-0795-00	190.59		
GLIPIZIDE/METFORMIN HCL (Sandoz)				
glipizide/metformin hydrochloride				
TAB, PO (FILM-COATED)				
2.5 mg-250 mg, 100s ea	00781-5304-01	82.90		AB
2.5 mg-500 mg, 100s ea	00781-5305-01	98.89		AB
5 mg-500 mg, 100s ea	00781-5306-01	98.89		AB
(A-S Medication)				
REPACK				
TAB, PO (FILM-COATED)				
5 mg-500 mg, 60s ea	54569-5993-01	59.33		AB
(Phys Total Care)				
REPACK				
TAB, PO, 2.5 mg-500 mg,				
10s ea	54868-5188-01	33.78		
30s ea	54868-5188-00	92.31		
60s ea	54868-5188-02	138.78		
5 mg-500 mg,				
10s ea	54868-5467-01	33.78		
30s ea	54868-5467-00	92.31		
60s ea	54868-5467-02	138.78		
GLIPIZIDE/METFORMIN HYDROCHLORIDE (Bristol-Myers) *See METAGLIP*				
(Caraco)				
TAB, PO (FILM COATED)				
2.5 mg-250 mg, 100s ea	57664-0727-88	82.90		AB
2.5 mg-500 mg, 100s ea	57664-0725-88	98.89		AB
5 mg-500 mg, 100s ea	57664-0724-88	98.89		AB
(Mylan) *See GLIPIZIDE AND METFORMIN HYDROCHLORIDE*				
(Sandoz) *See GLIPIZIDE/METFORMIN HCL*				
(Teva) *See GLIPIZIDE/METFORMIN*				
(Watson Labs) *See GLIPIZIDE AND METFORMIN HYDROCHLORIDE*				
GLORIA (Amend)				
mineral oil				
OIL, NA (U.S.P.)				
480 ml	17317-1062-01	4.90		
3840 ml	17317-1062-06	21.00		
19200 ml	17317-1062-08	70.00		
GLUCAGEN (Bedford)				
glucagon hydrochloride				
PDS, IJ (VIAL)				
1 mg, 10s ea	55390-0004-10	840.00		
GLUCAGEN DIAGNOSTIC KIT (Bedford)				
glucagon hydrochloride				
PDS, IJ (VIAL W/STERILE WATER)				
1 mg, ea	55390-0004-01	84.00		
GLUCAGEN HYPOKIT (Novo Nordisk)				
glucagon hydrochloride				
PDS, IJ (1ML STERLE WATER SYRNGE)				
1 mg, ea	00169-7065-15	120.36		
GLUCAGON EMERGENCY KIT (Lilly)				
glucagon hydrochloride				
PDS, IJ (HYPORET DISPOSABLE SRN)				
1 mg, ea	00002-8031-01	119.28	99.40	
(A-S Medication)				
REPACK				
PDS, IJ, 1 mg, ea	54569-4734-00	103.30		
(Phys Total Care)				
REPACK				
PDS, IJ, 1 mg, ea	54868-5070-00	122.10		
GLUCAGON HYDROCHLORIDE (Bedford) *See GLUCAGEN*				
(Bedford) *See GLUCAGEN DIAGNOSTIC KIT*				
(Lilly) *See GLUCAGON EMERGENCY KIT*				

PROD/MFR	NDC	AWP	DP	OBC
(Novo Nordisk) *See GLUCAGEN HYPOKIT*				
GLUCOLET 2 UNITIZED (Bayer Diabetes Care)				
lancet device				
DEV, NA (AUTOMATIC LANCING)				
ea	00193-5979-01	14.04		
GLUCONIC ACID LACTONE (PCCA)				
gluconolactone				
POW, NA (FCC)				
1 gm	51927-1188-00	0.48		
GLUCONO DELTA LACTONE (Spectrum Pharmacy)				
gluconolactone				
POW, NA (U.S.P.)				
100 gm	49452-3285-01	79.45		
1000 gm	49452-3285-02	229.95		
5000 gm	49452-3285-03	749.00		
GLUCONOLACTONE (Gallipot)				
POW, NA (U.S.P.)				
25 gm	51552-0760-04	18.48	13.20	
(PCCA) *See GLUCONIC ACID LACTONE*				
(Spectrum Pharmacy) *See D-GLUCONOLACTONE*				
(Spectrum Pharmacy) *See GLUCONO DELTA LACTONE*				
GLUCOPHAGE (Bristol-Myers)				
metformin hydrochloride				
TAB, PO, 500 mg, 100s ea	00087-6060-05	111.77		AB
500s ea	00087-6060-10	558.80		AB
850 mg, 100s ea	00087-6070-05	190.01		AB
1000 mg, 100s ea	00087-6071-11	230.23		AB
(A-S Medication)				
REPACK				
TAB, PO, 500 mg, 30s ea	54569-4202-02	34.93		AB
850 mg, 60s ea	54569-4740-00	118.76		AB
(Dispensing Solutions)				
REPACK				
TAB, PO, 500 mg, 30s ea	55045-3045-08	25.00		AB
60s ea	55045-3045-06	49.00		AB
100s ea	55045-3045-01	81.00		AB
850 mg, 100s ea	55045-2504-01	137.00		AB
(PD-Rx Pharm)				
REPACK				
TAB, PO, 500 mg, 60s ea	55289-0211-60	74.53		AB
(Phys Total Care)				
REPACK				
TAB, PO, 500 mg, 30s ea	54868-3545-02	34.26		
60s ea	54868-3545-03	66.65		
100s ea	54868-3545-00	97.84		
120s ea	54868-3545-01	131.43		
850 mg, 30s ea	54868-3546-01	55.24		AB
100s ea	54868-3546-00	169.25		AB
1000 mg, 30s ea	54868-4160-00	66.54		
60s ea	54868-4160-01	124.01		
(Southwood)				
REPACK				
TAB, PO, 500 mg, 10s ea	58016-0213-10	7.40		
30s ea	58016-0213-30	22.19		
60s ea	58016-0213-60	44.37		
100s ea	58016-0213-00	73.95		
850 mg, 10s ea	58016-0457-10	11.90		
30s ea	58016-0457-30	35.70		
60s ea	58016-0457-60	71.40		
100s ea	58016-0457-00	119.00		
1000 mg, 10s ea	58016-0553-10	15.00		
30s ea	58016-0553-30	44.99		
60s ea	58016-0553-60	89.97		
100s ea	58016-0553-00	149.95		
(Vibranta)				
REPACK				
TAB, PO, 500 mg, 60s ea	57866-9059-01	55.75		AB
120s ea	57866-9059-02	110.90		AB
1000 mg, 30s ea	57866-9057-02	50.74		AB
60s ea	57866-9057-01	100.88		AB
GLUCOPHAGE XR (Bristol-Myers)				
metformin hydrochloride				
TER, PO (FILM-COATED)				
500 mg, 100s ea	00087-6063-13	114.08		
750 mg, 100s ea	00087-6064-13	171.14		
(Dispensing Solutions)				
REPACK				
TER, PO, 500 mg, 60s ea	66336-0292-60	74.75		
(PD-Rx Pharm)				
REPACK				
TER, PO (REDI-SCRIPT,FILM-COATED)				
500 mg, 30s ea	58864-0507-30	40.48		

PROD/MFR	NDC	AWP	DP	OBC
(Phys Total Care)				
REPACK				
TER, PO (FILM-COATED)				
500 mg, 10s ea	54868-4569-01	12.55		
30s ea	54868-4569-00	33.91		
(FILM-COATED)				
500 mg, 60s ea	54868-4569-02	65.96		
GLUCOSAMINE (Southwood)				
REPACK				
glucosamine sulfate				
CAP, PO, 500 mg, 30s ea	58016-0003-30	1.69		
60s ea	58016-0003-60	3.38		
90s ea	58016-0003-90	5.07		
100s ea	58016-0003-00	5.63		
120s ea	58016-0003-02	6.76		
GLUCOSAMINE HCL (Letco)				
glucosamine hydrochloride				
POW, NA, 500 gm	62991-1194-01	150.00		
1000 gm	62991-1194-02	240.00		
(PCCA)				
POW, NA, 1 gm	51927-2727-00	0.90		
GLUCOSAMINE HYDROCHLORIDE (Gallipot)				
POW, NA, 100 gm	51552-0544-05	38.92		
(Letco) *See GLUCOSAMINE HCL*				
(Medisca)				
POW, NA (1X25GM)				
25 gm	38779-1966-04	37.50		
(1X100GM)				
100 gm	38779-1966-05	96.00		
(1X500GM)				
500 gm	38779-1966-08	297.00		
(PCCA) *See GLUCOSAMINE HCL*				
(Spectrum Pharmacy) *See D-GLUCOSAMINE HYDROCHLORIDE*				
GLUCOSAMINE SULF (Core)				
REPACK				
glucosamine sulfate				
CAP, PO, 500 mg, 60s ea	33358-0159-60	56.36		
90s ea	33358-0159-90	87.11		
120s ea	33358-0159-01	111.71		
GLUCOSAMINE SULFATE (Gallipot)				
POW, NA, 25 gm	51552-0592-04	20.16		
100 gm	51552-0592-05	32.34		
(Letco)				
POW, NA, 100 gm	62991-1670-01	60.00		
1000 gm	62991-1670-02	240.00		
(Medisca)				
POW, NA, 25 gm	38779-0868-04	37.50		
100 gm	38779-0868-05	82.50		
500 gm	38779-0868-08	267.00		
1000 gm	38779-0868-09	454.50		
5000 gm	38779-0868-03	1194.00		
(PCCA)				
POW, NA, 1 gm	51927-2682-00	1.74		
(Spectrum Pharmacy)				
POW, NA, 100 gm	49452-3304-02	144.20		
500 gm	49452-3304-03	413.00		
2500 gm	49452-3304-04	1102.50		
(Palmetto)				
REPACK				
CAP, PO, 500 mg, 60s ea	23490-6993-06	12.00		
(Vibranta)				
REPACK				
CAP, PO, 750 mg, 180s ea	57866-3056-01	125.00		
GLUCOSAMINE SULFATE/POTASSIUM CHLORIDE (Medisca)				
POW, NA (1X25GM,USP)				
25 gm	38779-2463-04	37.50		
(1X100GM,USP)				
100 gm	38779-2463-05	82.50		
(1X500GM,USP)				
500 gm	38779-2463-08	267.00		
(1X1000GM,USP)				
1000 gm	38779-2463-09	454.50		
(1X5000GM,USP)				
5000 gm	38779-2463-03	1194.00		
GLUCOSAMINE/CHONDROITIN (Bryant Ranch)				
REPACK				
chondroitin sulfate/glucosamine hydrochloride				
TAB, PO, 400 mg-500 mg,				
60s ea	63629-3143-01	54.99		
120s ea	63629-3143-02	108.99		

PROD/MFR	NDC	AWP	DP	OBC
(DHS, Inc.)				
REPACK				
CAP, PO, 400 mg-500 mg,				
100s ea	55887-0520-01	42.50		
(Vibranta)				
REPACK				
chondroitin sulfate/glucosamine sulfate				
CAP, PO, 400 mg-500 mg,				
90s ea	57866-3054-01	72.00		
120s ea	57866-3054-02	96.00		
240s ea	57866-3054-03	192.00		
GLUCOSE DATA MANAGEMENT				
(DexCom) *See SEVEN PLUS CONTINUOUS GLUCOSE MONITORING SYSTEM*				
(DexCom) *See SEVEN SYSTEM SENSOR PACK*				
(Medtronic Minimed) *See GUARDIAN REAL-TIME SYSTEM*				
(Medtronic Minimed) *See GUARDIAN REAL-TIME SYSTEM PEDIATRIC*				
GLUCOSE METER				
(Medline) *See EVEN CARE MONITORING SYSTEM*				
(Medtronic Minimed) *See CGMS SYSTEM GOLD*				
(Medtronic Minimed) *See REPLACEMENT PEDIATRIC MONITOR*				
GLUCOSE METER TEST CONTROL				
(Medline) *See EVEN CARE CONTROL*				
GLUCOSE, BLOOD TEST				
(Home Diag) *See DUANE READE PRESTIGE SMART SYSTEM*				
(Medline) *See EVEN CARE*				
GLUCOTROL (Pfizer)				
glipizide				
TAB, PO (DYE-FREE)				
5 mg, 100s ea	00049-4110-66	64.07	53.39	AB
10 mg, 100s ea	00049-4120-66	117.58	97.98	AB
(DHS, Inc.)				
REPACK				
TER, PO, 5 mg, 30s ea	55887-0969-30	30.00		
(PD-Rx Pharm)				
REPACK				
TAB, PO, 5 mg, 30s ea	55289-0424-30	26.54		AB
10 mg, 30s ea	55289-0125-30	40.13		AB
(Phys Total Care)				
REPACK				
TAB, PO, 5 mg, 30s ea	54868-0997-01	19.21		AB
60s ea	54868-0997-04	36.55		AB
100s ea	54868-0997-02	59.68		AB
10 mg, 30s ea	54868-1089-01	33.70		AB
60s ea	54868-1089-03	65.54		AB
100s ea	54868-1089-02	107.98		AB
GLUCOTROL XL (Pfizer)				
glipizide				
TER, PO, 2.5 mg, 30s ea	00049-1620-30	20.70	17.25	
5 mg, 100s ea	00049-1550-66	69.04	57.53	
500s ea	00049-1550-73	345.18	287.65	
10 mg, 100s ea	00049-1560-66	136.81	114.01	
500s ea	00049-1560-73	684.11	570.09	
(A-S Medication)				
REPACK				
TER, PO, 5 mg, 30s ea	54569-3937-00	18.85		
10 mg, 30s ea	54569-3938-00	37.36		
(PD-Rx Pharm)				
REPACK				
TER, PO, 2.5 mg, 30s ea	58864-0858-30	24.77		
(REDI-SCRIPT)				
5 mg, 30s ea	58864-0705-30	24.77		
10 mg, 30s ea	58864-0689-30	43.67		
60s ea	58864-0689-60	81.23		
(Phys Total Care)				
REPACK				
TER, PO, 2.5 mg, 30s ea	54868-4420-00	20.16		
5 mg, 15s ea	54868-3335-01	14.52		
30s ea	54868-3335-00	26.43		
60s ea	54868-3335-03	50.25		
100s ea	54868-3335-02	82.00		
10 mg, 10s ea	54868-3334-03	14.36		
30s ea	54868-3334-00	39.35		
60s ea	54868-3334-02	76.81		
90s ea	54868-3334-04	114.29		
100s ea	54868-3334-01	126.15		
(Quality Care Prod)				
REPACK				
TER, PO, 5 mg, 90s ea	35356-0121-90	41.40		

PROD/MFR	NDC	AWP	DP	OBC
GLUCOVANCE (Bristol-Myers)				
glyburide/metformin hydrochloride				
TAB, PO (CAPLET,FILM-COATED)				
2.5 mg-500 mg,				
100s ea	**00087-6073-11**	146.99		
(FILM-COATED CAPLET)				
5 mg-500 mg,				
100s ea	**00087-6074-11**	146.99		
(Dispensing Solutions)				
REPACK				
TAB, PO, 5 mg-500 mg,				
30s ea	**66336-0319-30**	49.92		
(Phys Total Care)				
REPACK				
TAB, PO (CAPLET,FILM-COATED)				
1.25 mg-250 mg,				
100s ea	**54868-4906-00**	116.61		
(CAPLET)				
2.5 mg-500 mg,				
60s ea	**54868-4609-00**	100.67		
(CAPLET,FILM-COATED)				
2.5 mg-500 mg,				
100s ea	**54868-4609-01**	158.19		
(CAPLET)				
5 mg-500 mg,				
10s ea	**54868-4529-02**	16.08		
(FILM-COATED CAPLET)				
5 mg-500 mg,				
30s ea	**54868-4529-03**	44.46		
(CAPLET)				
5 mg-500 mg,				
60s ea	**54868-4529-01**	87.06		
100s ea	**54868-4529-00**	135.34		
(Quality Care Prod)				
REPACK				
TAB, PO (FILM-COATED CAPLET)				
5 mg-500 mg,				
30s ea	**49999-0660-30**	51.98		
60s ea	**49999-0660-60**	103.96		
GLUMETZA (Depomed)				
metformin hydrochloride				
TER, PO (FILM-COATED)				
500 mg, 100s ea	**13913-0002-13**	167.76	139.80	BX
1000 mg, 90s ea	**13913-0003-16**	367.40	306.17	BX
(Phys Total Care)				
REPACK				
TER, PO, 500 mg, 10s ea	**54868-0830-00**	17.98		
30s ea	**54868-0830-01**	50.20		
GLUTAMIC ACID				
(Amend) *See L-GLUTAMIC ACID HYDROCHLORIDE*				
(Gallipot) *See GLUTAMIC-L ACID*				
(Spectrum Pharmacy) *See L-GLUTAMIC ACID*				
(Spectrum Pharmacy) *See L-GLUTAMIC ACID HCL*				
(Spectrum Pharmacy) *See L-GLUTAMIC ACID MONOSODIUM SALT*				
GLUTAMIC ACID HYDROCHLORIDE (PCCA)				
POW, NA (FCC)				
1 gm	**51927-1367-00**	0.36		
GLUTAMIC-L ACID (Gallipot)				
glutamic acid				
POW, NA, 100 gm	**51552-0443-05**	13.72		
GLUTAMINE				
See NUTRESTORE				
(Gallipot) *See L-GLUTAMINE*				
(Medisca) *See L-GLUTAMINE*				
(PCCA)				
POW, NA, 1 gm	**51927-3601-00**	1.68		
(L)				
1 gm	**51927-2080-00**	1.19		
(Spectrum Pharmacy) *See L-GLUTAMINE*				
GLUTARAL				
(Baker, J.T.) *See GLUTARALDEHYDE 25% AQUEOUS*				
(Gallipot) *See GLUTARALDEHYDE 25% AQUEOUS*				
(Medisca) *See GLUTARALDEHYDE 25% AQUEOUS*				
(PCCA) *See GLUTARALDEHYDE 25% AQUEOUS*				
(PCCA) *See GLUTARALDEHYDE 50% IN WATER*				
(Spectrum Pharmacy) *See GLUTARALDEHYDE 24%*				
GLUTARALDEHYDE 24% (Spectrum Pharmacy)				
glutaral				
SOL, NA, 100 ml	**49452-3350-01**	67.90		
1000 ml	**49452-3350-02**	275.80		
4000 ml	**49452-3350-03**	609.00		
GLUTARALDEHYDE 25% AQUEOUS (Baker, J.T.)				
glutaral				
SOL, NA (REAGENT)				
500 ml	**10106-2127-01**	106.91		
(Gallipot)				
SOL, NA, 100 ml	**51552-0197-05**	13.30		
1000 ml	**51552-0197-07**	33.53		
(Medisca)				
SOL, NA, 500 ml	**38779-0597-08**	58.50		
1000 ml	**38779-0597-09**	99.00		
(PCCA)				
SOL, NA, 1 ml	**51927-1211-00**	0.11		
GLUTARALDEHYDE 50% IN WATER (PCCA)				
glutaral				
SOL, NA, 1 ml	**51927-2787-00**	0.78		
GLUTATHIONE				
(Gallipot) *See GLUTATHIONE-L*				
(PCCA)				
POW, NA ((L) REDUCED)				
1 gm	**51927-2284-00**	12.00		
(Spectrum Pharmacy) *See L-GLUTATHIONE REDUCED FORM*				
GLUTATHIONE-L (Gallipot)				
glutathione				
CRY, NA, 1000 gm	**51552-0554-07**	1379.00		
GLUTOFAC-MX (Kenwood)				
multivitamin, minerals, and iron				
TAB, PO (6X10,BLISTER PK,CAPLET)				
60s ea	**00482-0157-06**	78.67		
GLUTOFAC-ZX (Kenwood)				
multivitamin, minerals, and nutriceuticals				
TAB, PO (FILM-COATED CAPLET)				
60s ea	**00482-0159-06**	104.74		
GLYBURIDE				
FUL				
TAB, PO, 1.25 mg,				
100s ea		12.44		
2.5 mg, 100s ea		18.93		
5 mg, 100s ea		28.31		
(Greenstone)				
TAB, PO (UNIT OF USE)				
1.25 mg, 100s ea	**59762-3725-01**	27.56		AB
2.5 mg, 100s ea	**59762-3726-03**	45.93		AB
5 mg, 100s ea	**59762-3727-04**	77.68		AB
500s ea	**59762-3727-06**	341.29		AB
1000s ea	**59762-3727-07**	660.51		AB
(Major)				
TAB, PO (COMPRESSED)				
1.25 mg, 100s ea	**00904-6137-60**	15.00		AB
2.5 mg, 100s ea	**00904-6138-60**	15.00		AB
500s ea	**00904-6138-40**	55.00		AB
5 mg, 100s ea	**00904-6139-60**	15.00		AB
1000s ea	**00904-6139-80**	62.50		AB
(PCCA)				
POW, NA (U.S.P.)				
1 gm	**51927-2678-00**	54.00		
(Pfizer) *See MICRONASE*				
(Sandoz)				
TAB, PO, 1.25 mg, 100s ea	**00781-1138-01**	27.56		AB
2.5 mg, 100s ea	**00781-1146-01**	45.93		AB
5 mg, 100s ea	**00781-1191-01**	77.70		AB
1000s ea	**00781-1191-10**	738.15		AB
(Sanofi-Aventis) *See DIABETA*				
(Teva)				
TAB, PO, 1.25 mg, 50s ea	**00093-9477-53**	13.78		BX
100s ea	**00093-8342-01**	27.56		AB
2.5 mg, 100s ea	**00093-8343-01**	45.93		AB
100s ea	**00093-9433-01**	45.93		AB
100s ea UD	**00182-2646-89**	30.58		AB
500s ea	**00093-8343-05**	229.65		AB
500s ea	**00093-9433-05**	229.65		AB
1000s ea	**00093-8343-10**	459.30		AB
5 mg, 100s ea	**00093-8344-01**	77.70		AB
100s ea	**00093-9364-01**	77.70		BX
(10X10,USP)				
5 mg, 100s ea UD	**00093-8344-93**	52.59		AB
500s ea	**00093-8344-05**	341.32		AB
500s ea	**00093-9364-05**	341.32		BX
1000s ea	**00093-8344-10**	660.54		AB
1000s ea	**00093-9364-10**	660.54		BX
(UDL)				
TAB, PO (10X10)				
2.5 mg, 100s ea UD	**51079-0872-20**	30.60		AB
(ROBOT READY 25X1)				
5 mg, 25s ea UD	**51079-0873-19**	13.15		AB
(10X10)				
5 mg, 100s ea UD	**51079-0873-20**	52.60		AB
(A-S Medication)				
REPACK				
TAB, PO, 2.5 mg, 30s ea	**54569-3830-00**	13.78		AB
200s ea	**54569-3830-02**	91.86		AB
5 mg, 30s ea	**54569-3831-00**	23.31		AB
60s ea	**54569-3831-02**	46.62		AB
100s ea	**54569-3831-01**	77.70		AB
200s ea	**54569-3831-08**	155.40		AB
(Altura)				
REPACK				
TAB, PO, 1.25 mg, 10s ea	**63874-0665-10**	2.76		
14s ea	**63874-0665-14**	3.86		
30s ea	**63874-0665-30**	8.27		
60s ea	**63874-0665-60**	16.54		
90s ea	**63874-0665-90**	24.81		
100s ea	**63874-0665-01**	27.57		
120s ea	**63874-0665-04**	33.08		
2.5 mg, 10s ea	**63874-0588-10**	4.59		BX
14s ea	**63874-0588-14**	6.43		BX
20s ea	**63874-0588-20**	9.19		BX
30s ea	**63874-0588-30**	13.78		BX
60s ea	**63874-0588-60**	27.56		BX
80s ea	**63874-0588-80**	36.75		BX
90s ea	**63874-0588-90**	41.34		BX
100s ea	**63874-0588-01**	45.93		BX
120s ea	**63874-0588-04**	55.12		BX
5 mg, 10s ea	**63874-0317-10**	11.28		
12s ea	**63874-0317-12**	13.54		
14s ea	**63874-0317-14**	15.79		
15s ea	**63874-0317-15**	16.92		
20s ea	**63874-0317-20**	22.56		
24s ea	**63874-0317-24**	27.07		
28s ea	**63874-0317-28**	31.58		
30s ea	**63874-0317-30**	33.84		
40s ea	**63874-0317-40**	45.12		
50s ea	**63874-0317-50**	56.40		
60s ea	**63874-0317-60**	67.68		
90s ea	**63874-0317-90**	101.52		
100s ea	**63874-0317-01**	112.80		
120s ea	**63874-0317-04**	135.36		
1000s ea	**63874-0317-02**	1128.00		
(AQ)				
REPACK				
TAB, PO, 1.25 mg, 30s ea	**66105-0984-03**	11.10		
60s ea	**66105-0984-06**	20.15		
100s ea	**66105-0984-10**	32.33		
500s ea	**66105-0984-50**	153.58		
1000s ea	**66105-0984-11**	305.16		
2.5 mg, 30s ea	**66105-0985-03**	17.14		
60s ea	**66105-0985-06**	32.29		
100s ea	**66105-0985-10**	52.52		
500s ea	**66105-0985-50**	254.61		
1000s ea	**66105-0985-11**	507.23		
5 mg, 30s ea	**66105-0986-03**	27.64		
60s ea	**66105-0986-06**	53.28		
100s ea	**66105-0986-10**	87.47		
500s ea	**66105-0986-50**	377.45		
1000s ea	**66105-0986-11**	728.59		
(Bryant Ranch)				
REPACK				
TAB, PO, 2.5 mg, 30s ea	**63629-2907-01**	19.29		
60s ea	**63629-2907-02**	38.58		
5 mg, 30s ea	**63629-1393-01**	27.74		
100s ea	**63629-1393-03**	92.48		
120s ea	**63629-1393-02**	110.97		
(Core)				
REPACK				
TAB, PO, 2.5 mg, 30s ea	**33358-0160-30**	19.77		
60s ea	**33358-0160-60**	39.54		
5 mg, 30s ea	**33358-0161-30**	28.43		
60s ea	**33358-0161-60**	74.83		
(CorePharma)				
REPACK				
TAB, PO (USP,NONMICRONIZED)				
1.25 mg, 100s ea	**64720-0123-10**	30.30		AB
2.5 mg, 100s ea	**64720-0124-10**	50.50		AB
5 mg, 100s ea	**64720-0125-10**	85.50		AB
1000s ea	**64720-0125-11**	811.96		AB
(DHS, Inc.)				
REPACK				
TAB, PO, 1.25 mg, 30s ea	**55887-0965-30**	8.27		
2.5 mg, 30s ea	**55887-0535-30**	13.59		BX
60s ea	**55887-0535-60**	25.98		BX
90s ea	**55887-0535-90**	39.89		BX
5 mg, 30s ea	**55887-0536-30**	22.14		
60s ea	**55887-0536-60**	44.28		
90s ea	**55887-0536-90**	66.42		

PROD/MFR	NDC	AWP	DP	OBC
(Dispensing Solutions)				
REPACK				
TAB, PO, 2.5 mg, 30s ea	**66336-0028-30**	14.38		BX
5 mg, 30s ea	**66336-0938-30**	10.73		
60s ea	**66336-0938-60**	19.20		
180s ea	**55045-2138-01**	138.60		AB
(GSMS)				
REPACK				
TAB, PO (UNIT OF USE)				
5 mg, 30s ea	**60429-0085-30**	15.90	5.30	AB
60s ea	**60429-0085-60**	28.80	9.60	AB
90s ea	**60429-0085-90**	42.00	14.00	AB
120s ea	**60429-0085-12**	54.90	18.30	AB
180s ea	**60429-0085-18**	81.00	27.00	AB
270s ea	**60429-0085-27**	119.70	39.90	AB
360s ea	**60429-0085-36**	158.40	52.80	AB
(HomeMed)				
REPACK				
TAB, PO, 1.25 mg, 50s ea	**51655-0758-77**	10.86		EE
2.5 mg, 30s ea	**51655-0753-24**	13.59		EE
5 mg, 30s ea	**51655-0904-24**	30.99		
60s ea	**51655-0904-25**	54.99		
(McKesson Packaging)				
REPACK				
TAB, PO (USP)				
2.5 mg, 100s ea UD	**63739-0118-10**	57.25		AB
5 mg, 100s ea UD	**63739-0119-10**	82.50		AB
(Palmetto)				
REPACK				
TAB, PO, 2.5 mg, 30s ea	**23490-5638-01**	16.50		
60s ea	**23490-5638-02**	16.50		AB
5 mg, 30s ea	**23490-5639-01**	31.83		
60s ea	**23490-5639-02**	63.66		
(PD-Rx Pharm)				
REPACK				
TAB, PO, 2.5 mg, 30s ea	**55289-0606-30**	19.13		EE
(USP)				
2.5 mg, 90s ea	**55289-0606-90**	37.50		AB
5 mg, 14s ea	**55289-0892-14**	19.93		BX
15s ea	**55289-0892-15**	20.91		AB
30s ea	**55289-0892-30**	31.81		AB
30s ea	**58864-0224-30**	31.83		BX
60s ea	**55289-0892-60**	53.62		AB
60s ea	**58864-0224-60**	53.64		AB
(USP)				
5 mg, 90s ea	**55289-0892-90**	59.10		AB
100s ea	**55289-0892-01**	82.70		AB
120s ea	**55289-0892-98**	98.91		AB
(REDI-SCRIPT)				
5 mg, 180s ea	**58864-0224-93**	140.79		AB
(USP)				
5 mg, 180s ea	**55289-0892-93**	98.91		AB
360s ea	**55289-0892-86**	271.60		AB
(Pharma Pac)				
REPACK				
TAB, PO, 1.25 mg, 90s ea	**52959-0598-90**	27.95		AB
5 mg, 30s ea	**52959-0449-30**	28.25		AB
60s ea	**52959-0449-60**	56.49		AB
100s ea	**52959-0449-01**	58.35		AB
(Phys Total Care)				
REPACK				
TAB, PO, 1.25 mg, 30s ea	**54868-3426-01**	9.21		AB
100s ea	**54868-3426-00**	22.17		EE
(Phys Total Care)				
glyburide, micronized				
1.5 mg, 30s ea	**54868-5712-00**	9.00		
GLYBURIDE (Phys Total Care)				
2.5 mg, 30s ea	**54868-3266-02**	9.90		EE
60s ea	**54868-3266-04**	16.52		EE
90s ea	**54868-3266-03**	23.73		EE
100s ea	**54868-3266-01**	26.04		EE
5 mg, 30s ea	**54868-3265-01**	8.79		EE
60s ea	**54868-3265-03**	14.58		EE
90s ea	**54868-3265-04**	20.37		EE
100s ea	**54868-3265-00**	22.29		EE
(Physician Partner)				
REPACK				
TAB, PO, 2.5 mg, 30s ea	**21695-0467-30**	27.56		AB
60s ea	**21695-0467-60**	55.12		AB
5 mg, 60s ea	**21695-0468-60**	93.24		AB
(Quality Care Prod)				
REPACK				
TAB, PO, 2.5 mg, 30s ea	**35356-0360-30**	26.90		AB
5 mg, 30s ea	**49999-0113-30**	31.06		EE
60s ea	**49999-0113-60**	55.80		BX
90s ea	**49999-0113-90**	93.18		BX
100s ea	**49999-0113-00**	103.53		EE
120s ea	**49999-0113-01**	124.24		BX

PROD/MFR	NDC	AWP	DP	OBC
(Southwood)				
REPACK				
TAB, PO, 5 mg, 30s ea	**58016-0378-30**	23.31		
60s ea	**58016-0378-60**	46.62		
90s ea	**58016-0378-90**	69.93		
100s ea	**58016-0378-00**	77.70		
120s ea	**58016-0378-02**	93.24		
180s ea	**58016-0378-99**	139.86		
(Vibranta)				
REPACK				
TAB, PO, 5 mg, 30s ea	**57866-6409-01**	29.75		
60s ea	**57866-6409-02**	39.85		
90s ea	**57866-6409-03**	61.40		
120s ea	**57866-6409-04**	81.50		
180s ea	**57866-6409-05**	121.70		
360s ea	**57866-6409-06**	213.14		
GLYBURIDE AND METFORMIN HYDROCHLORIDE				
(Aurobindo Pharma)				
glyburide/metformin hydrochloride				
TAB, PO (FILM-COATED)				
1.25 mg-250 mg,				
100s ea	**65862-0080-01**	88.60		AB
2.5 mg-500 mg,				
100s ea	**65862-0081-01**	105.69		AB
5 mg-500 mg,				
100s ea	**65862-0082-01**	105.69		AB
(Dr Reddy's)				
TAB, PO (USP,FILM COATED)				
1.25 mg-250 mg,				
100s ea	**55111-0695-01**	86.20		AB
2.5 mg-500 mg,				
100s ea	**55111-0696-01**	102.83		AB
1000s ea	**55111-0696-10**	976.89		AB
5 mg-500 mg,				
100s ea	**55111-0697-01**	102.83		AB
1000s ea	**55111-0697-10**	976.89		AB
(Teva)				
TAB, PO (USP,FILM-COATED)				
1.25 mg-250 mg,				
100s ea	**00093-5710-01**	86.15		AB
100s ea UD	**00093-5710-93**	88.15		AB
(FILM-COATED)				
1.25 mg-250 mg,				
500s ea	**00093-5710-05**	409.21		AB
2.5 mg-500 mg,				
100s ea	**00093-5711-01**	102.79		AB
(USP,FILM-COATED)				
2.5 mg-500 mg,				
100s ea UD	**00093-5711-93**	104.79		AB
(FILM-COATED)				
2.5 mg-500 mg,				
500s ea	**00093-5711-05**	488.25		AB
5 mg-500 mg,				
100s ea	**00093-5712-01**	102.79		AB
(USP,FILM-COATED)				
5 mg-500 mg,				
100s ea UD	**00093-5712-93**	104.79		AB
(FILM-COATED)				
5 mg-500 mg,				
500s ea	**00093-5712-05**	484.49		AB
(A-S Medication)				
REPACK				
TAB, PO (FILM-COATED)				
2.5 mg-500 mg,				
30s ea	**54569-5618-01**	31.13		AB
60s ea	**54569-5618-00**	62.27		AB
5 mg-500 mg,				
30s ea	**54569-5619-01**	31.19		AB
60s ea	**54569-5619-00**	62.38		AB
(American Health)				
REPACK				
TAB, PO (MICRONIZED,10X10)				
1.25 mg-250 mg,				
100s ea UD	**68084-0136-01**	88.19		AB
2.5 mg-500 mg,				
100s ea UD	**68084-0137-01**	104.83		AB
5 mg-500 mg,				
100s ea UD	**68084-0138-01**	104.83		AB
(PD-Rx Pharm)				
REPACK				
TAB, PO (FILM-COATED)				
5 mg-500 mg,				
30s ea	**55289-0281-30**	20.16		AB
60s ea	**55289-0281-60**	28.35		AB
360s ea	**55289-0281-86**	235.65		AB
(Phys Total Care)				
REPACK				
TAB, PO (FILM-COATED)				
2.5 mg-500 mg,				
90s ea	**54868-5148-03**	44.67		AB

PROD/MFR	NDC	AWP	DP	OBC
GLYBURIDE MICRONIZED (Dava Pharma)				
glyburide, micronized				
TAB, PO, 1.5 mg, 100s ea	**67253-0460-10**	37.78		AB
3 mg, 100s ea	**67253-0461-10**	63.88		AB
500s ea	**67253-0461-50**	280.24		AB
1000s ea	**67253-0461-11**	618.49		AB
6 mg, 100s ea	**67253-0462-10**	107.32		AB
500s ea	**67253-0462-50**	475.00		AB
1000s ea	**67253-0462-11**	802.08		AB
(Mylan)				
TAB, PO, 1.5 mg, 100s ea	**00378-1113-01**	37.40		AB
3 mg, 100s ea	**00378-1125-01**	63.20		AB
1000s ea	**00378-1125-10**	618.50		AB
6 mg, 100s ea	**00378-1142-01**	106.70		AB
(Teva)				
TAB, PO, 1.5 mg, 100s ea	**00093-8034-01**	35.65		AB
3 mg, 100s ea	**00093-8035-01**	60.20		AB
500s ea	**00093-8035-05**	264.35		AB
6 mg, 100s ea	**00093-8036-01**	84.09		AB
(West-Ward)				
TAB, PO, 1.5 mg, 100s ea	**00143-9918-01**	37.50		AB
3 mg, 100s ea	**00143-9919-01**	60.50		AB
500s ea	**00143-9919-05**	260.20		AB
6 mg, 100s ea	**00143-9920-01**	107.50		AB
500s ea	**00143-9920-05**	445.60		AB
1000s ea	**00143-9920-10**	802.10		AB
(DHS, Inc.)				
REPACK				
TAB, PO, 3 mg, 30s ea	**55887-0339-30**	15.15		AB
60s ea	**55887-0339-60**	28.95		AB
90s ea	**55887-0339-90**	57.00		AB
(PD-Rx Pharm)				
REPACK				
TAB, PO (MICRONIZED)				
3 mg, 90s ea	**43063-0119-90**	53.50		AB
6 mg, 90s ea	**43063-0120-90**	67.00		AB
(Phys Total Care)				
REPACK				
TAB, PO, 3 mg, 30s ea	**54868-4091-02**	6.96		EE
(USP)				
3 mg, 60s ea	**54868-4091-01**	10.75		EE
100s ea	**54868-4091-00**	14.43		EE
6 mg, 60s ea	**54868-4842-02**	21.24		
90s ea	**54868-4842-01**	29.64		AB
100s ea	**54868-4842-00**	30.93		AB
(Quality Care Prod)				
REPACK				
TAB, PO, 3 mg, 100s ea	**49999-0808-00**	76.66		
6 mg, 60s ea	**49999-0571-60**	60.54		AB
GLYBURIDE MICRONIZED/METFORMIN HCL (Sandoz)				
glyburide/metformin hydrochloride				
TAB, PO (FILM-COATED)				
1.25 mg-250 mg,				
100s ea	**00781-5170-01**	86.20		AB
2.5 mg-500 mg,				
100s ea	**00781-5171-01**	102.83		AB
500s ea	**00781-5171-05**	501.30		AB
5 mg-500 mg,				
100s ea	**00781-5172-01**	102.83		AB
500s ea	**00781-5172-05**	501.30		AB
(Teva)				
TAB, PO (FILM-COATED)				
1.25 mg-250 mg,				
100s ea	**00093-7260-01**	86.20		AB
2.5 mg-500 mg,				
100s ea	**00093-7261-01**	102.83		AB
500s ea	**00093-7261-05**	498.73		AB
5 mg-500 mg,				
500s ea	**00093-7262-05**	498.73		AB
(Phys Total Care)				
REPACK				
TAB, PO (FILM-COATED)				
1.25 mg-250 mg,				
20s ea	**54868-5185-02**	13.20		AB
60s ea	**54868-5185-01**	33.57		AB
2.5 mg-500 mg,				
100s ea	**54868-5148-02**	75.63		AB
5 mg-500 mg,				
30s ea	**54868-5243-03**	25.22		AB
90s ea	**54868-5243-04**	69.72		AB
120s ea	**54868-5243-02**	91.95		AB
(Quality Care Prod)				
REPACK				
TAB, PO (FILM-COATED)				
5 mg-500 mg,				
30s ea	**49999-0401-30**	37.20		AB

PROD/MFR | NDC | AWP | DP | OBC

GLYBURIDE MICRONIZED/ METFORMIN HYDROCHLORIDE (DHS, Inc.)
REPACK
glyburide/metformin hydrochloride
TAB, PO (FILM-COATED)
5 mg-500 mg,
60s ea............ **55887-0368-60** 61.80 **AB**
90s ea............ **55887-0368-90** 92.70 **AB**

(Dispensing Solutions)
REPACK
TAB, PO (FILM-COATED)
5 mg-500 mg,
60s ea............ **66336-0784-60** 62.87 **AB**
90s ea............ **66336-0784-90** 94.31 **AB**

(Phys Total Care)
REPACK
TAB, PO (FILM COATED)
1.25 mg-250 mg,
100s ea............ **54868-5185-00** 52.44 **AB**
(FILM-COATED)
2.5 mg-500 mg,
30s ea............ **54868-5148-01** 25.23 **AB**
60s ea............ **54868-5148-00** 39.90 **AB**
5 mg-500 mg,
60s ea............ **54868-5243-00** 47.47 **AB**
100s ea............ **54868-5243-01** 74.34 **AB**

GLYBURIDE, MICRONIZED
(Dava Pharma) *See GLYBURIDE MICRONIZED*
(Mylan) *See GLYBURIDE MICRONIZED*
(Pfizer) *See GLYNASE PRES-TAB*
(Teva) *See GLYBURIDE MICRONIZED*
(West-Ward) *See GLYBURIDE MICRONIZED*

GLYBURIDE/METFORMIN (Bryant Ranch)
REPACK
glyburide/metformin hydrochloride
TAB, PO, 2.5 mg-500 mg,
30s ea............ **63629-1392-02** 43.18
60s ea............ **63629-1392-03** 86.36
100s ea............ **63629-1392-01** 143.93
5 mg-500 mg,
30s ea............ **63629-2793-01** 42.32
30s ea............ **63629-2793-02** 42.32
60s ea............ **63629-2793-03** 84.63
90s ea............ **63629-2793-04** 126.95

(DHS, Inc.)
REPACK
TAB, PO, 1.25 mg-250 mg,
30s ea............ **55887-0173-30** 25.86

(Dispensing Solutions)
REPACK
TAB, PO, 5 mg-500 mg,
30s ea............ **66336-0784-30** 35.76

(Phys Total Care)
REPACK
TAB, PO, 1.25 mg-250 mg,
30s ea............ **54868-5185-03** 18.29

(Physician Partner)
REPACK
TAB, PO, 5 mg-500 mg,
30s ea............ **21695-0568-30** 61.70

(Southwood)
REPACK
TAB, PO, 1.25 mg-250 mg,
30s ea............ **58016-0058-30** 26.58
60s ea............ **58016-0058-60** 53.16
90s ea............ **58016-0058-90** 79.74
100s ea............ **58016-0058-00** 88.60

GLYBURIDE/METFORMIN HCL (Actavis)
glyburide/metformin hydrochloride
TAB, PO (FILM-COATED)
1.25 mg-250 mg,
100s ea............ **00228-2751-11** 88.60 **AB**
500s ea............ **00228-2751-50** 420.85 **AB**
2.5 mg-500 mg,
100s ea............ **00228-2752-11** 105.69 **AB**
500s ea............ **00228-2752-50** 502.03 **AB**
5 mg-500 mg,
100s ea............ **00228-2753-11** 105.69 **AB**
500s ea............ **00228-2753-50** 502.03 **AB**

(Southwood)
REPACK
TAB, PO (FILM-COATED)
5 mg-500 mg,
30s ea............ **58016-0411-30** 29.27
60s ea............ **58016-0411-60** 58.54
90s ea............ **58016-0411-90** 87.81
100s ea............ **58016-0411-00** 97.57
120s ea............ **58016-0411-02** 117.08

GLYBURIDE/METFORMIN HYDROCHLORIDE
FUL
TAB, PO, 1.25 mg-250 mg,
100s ea............ 84.05
2.5 mg-500 mg,
100s ea............ 100.26
5 mg-500 mg,
100s ea............ 100.26

(Actavis) *See GLYBURIDE/METFORMIN HCL*
(Aurobindo Pharma) *See GLYBURIDE AND METFORMIN HYDROCHLORIDE*
(Bristol-Myers) *See GLUCOVANCE*
(Dr Reddy's) *See GLYBURIDE AND METFORMIN HYDROCHLORIDE*
(Sandoz) *See GLYBURIDE MICRONIZED/ METFORMIN HCL*
(Teva) *See GLYBURIDE AND METFORMIN HYDROCHLORIDE*
(Teva) *See GLYBURIDE MICRONIZED/METFORMIN HCL*

(Altura)
REPACK
TAB, PO (FILM-COATED)
5 mg-500 mg,
10s ea............ **63874-0939-10** 10.68
30s ea............ **63874-0939-30** 32.34
60s ea............ **63874-0939-60** 64.68
100s ea............ **63874-0939-01** 106.78

(DHS, Inc.)
REPACK
TAB, PO (FILM-COATED)
5 mg-500 mg,
30s ea............ **55887-0368-30** 30.90 **AB**

(Palmetto)
REPACK
TAB, PO, 5 mg-500 mg,
30s ea............ **23490-7449-01** 37.31

(PD-Rx Pharm)
REPACK
TAB, PO, 2.5 mg-500 mg,
30s ea............ **58864-0952-30** 11.63
5 mg-500 mg, 30s ea . **58864-0953-30** 37.31
90s ea............ **55289-0281-90** 115.00

(Quality Care Prod)
REPACK
TAB, PO (FILM-COATED)
5 mg-500 mg,
60s ea............ **49999-0401-60** 74.16 **AB**

GLYCERIN
(Baker, J.T.) *See GLYCEROL ANHYDROUS*

(Baker, J.T.)
LIQ, NA (U.S.P., F.C.C.)
500 ml **10106-2140-01** 24.41
4000 ml **10106-2140-03** 226.17

(Gallipot) *See GLYCERIN 99.5%*

(Gallipot)
LIQ, NA (NATURAL,USP,EP,BP,JP)
473 ml **51552-1026-06** 27.72 19.80

(Letco)
LIQ, NA (U.S.P., SYNTHETIC)
500 ml **62991-2151-01** 36.00
3840 ml **62991-1195-02** 180.00

(Lorann Oil) *See GLYCERINE SYNTHETIC 99.5%*

(Mallinckrodt Lab)
LIQ, NA (U.S.P.)
500 ml **00406-5100-04** 41.91

(Marlex)
LIQ, NA (U.S.P.)
120 ml **10135-0104-04** 1.51
480 ml **10135-0104-08** 2.97
3785 ml **10135-0104-18** 30.00

(Medisca) *See GLYCEROL FORMAL*

(Medisca)
LIQ, NA (USP,1X100ML)
100 ml **38779-0613-05** 10.50
(U.S.P.)
500 ml **38779-0613-08** 31.50
(USP,1X4000ML)
4000 ml **38779-0613-01** 135.00
(USP,20000MLX1EA)
20000 ml **38779-0613-07** 441.00

(PCCA) *See GLYCEROL*

(PCCA)
LIQ, NA (U.S.P.; NATURAL)
1 ml............ **51927-2865-00** 0.12
(U.S.P.; SYNTHETIC)
1 ml............ **51927-9025-00** 0.07

(Spectrum Pharmacy)
LIQ, NA (U.S.P., NATURAL,E.P.,B.)
500 ml **49452-3359-01** 77.35
(U.S.P., SYNTHETIC,E.P.)
500 ml **49452-3360-01** 56.35
(U.S.P., NATURAL,E.P.,B.)
4000 ml **49452-3359-02** 247.10
(U.S.P., SYNTHET,E.P.)
4000 ml **49452-3360-02** 199.15
(U.S.P., NATURAL,E.P.,B.)
20000 ml **49452-3359-03** 941.50
(U.S.P., SYNTHETIC)
20000 ml **49452-3360-03** 847.00

(Palmetto)
REPACK
SUP, RC, 12s ea **23490-6675-01** 4.82
12s ea............ **23490-6675-02** 4.80

GLYCERIN 99.5% (Gallipot)
glycerin
LIQ, NA (U.S.P.)
60 ml............ **51552-0094-03** 2.94
118.28 ml **51552-0094-04** 5.60
236.56 ml **51552-0094-05** 9.73
473 ml **51552-0094-06** 15.19
3785 ml **51552-0094-08** 46.06

GLYCERIN/WITCH HAZEL
(Walker Pharmacal) *See SUCCUS CINERARIA MARITIMA*

GLYCERINE SYNTHETIC 99.5% (Lorann Oil)
glycerin
LIQ, NA (U.S.P.)
120 ml **23535-0711-08** 1.40
480 ml **23535-0711-01** 4.10
3840 ml **23535-0721-11** 25.00

GLYCEROL (PCCA)
glycerin
LIQ, NA (ACS)
1 ml............ **51927-2397-00** 0.17

GLYCEROL ANHYDROUS (Baker, J.T.)
glycerin
LIQ, NA (A.C.S., REAGENT)
500 ml **10106-2136-01** 58.97
4000 ml **10106-2136-03** 283.20

GLYCEROL FORMAL (Letco)
SOL, NA, 500 ml............ **62991-1480-01** 153.00
3840 ml **62991-1480-02** 300.00

(Medisca)
glycerin
LIQ, NA, 500 ml **38779-0931-08** 195.00
(1X1000ML)
1000 ml **38779-0931-09** 285.00
(1X4000ML)
4000 ml **38779-0931-01** 465.00

GLYCEROL FORMAL (PCCA)
SOL, NA, 1 ml............ **51927-2869-00** 0.57

GLYCEROL MONOOLEATE (PCCA)
glyceryl monooleate
POW, NA, 1 gm............ **51927-2621-00** 0.90

GLYCERYL HYDROGENATED ROSINATE
(PCCA) *See STAYBELITE ESTER 5*

GLYCERYL MONOOLEATE
(PCCA) *See GLYCEROL MONOOLEATE*

GLYCERYL MONOSTEARATE
(Amend) *See ATMUL 84*

(Amend)
POW, NA, 454 gm............ **17317-0627-01** 12.60
(PURE)
454 gm............ **17317-0273-01** 11.20
2270 gm............ **17317-0627-05** 49.00
(PURE)
2270 gm............ **17317-0273-05** 44.80
11350 gm **17317-0627-08** 140.00
(PURE)
11350 gm **17317-0273-08** 122.50

(Gallipot)
FLA, NA (COSMETIC GRADE)
454 gm............ **51552-0320-06** 31.50

(Medisca)
FLA, NA (PURE,1X100GM)
100 gm............ **38779-2086-05** 31.50
(PURE,1X500GM)
500 gm............ **38779-2086-08** 52.50

PROD/MFR	NDC	AWP	DP	OBC
(PCCA)				
POW, NA (PURE)				
1 gm	51927-1604-00	0.30		
GLYCERYL MONOSTEARATE/PEG-100 STEARATE				
(PCCA) *See ARLACEL 165*				
GLYCINE				
(Amend) *See AMINO ACETIC ACID*				
(B. Braun) *See GLYCINE IRRIGATION*				
(Baker, J.T.)				
POW, NA (U.S.P./F.C.C.)				
500 gm	10106-0581-01	28.43		
2000 gm	10106-0581-05	143.50		
(Baxter) *See GLYCINE IRRIGATION*				
(Gallipot)				
POW, NA (U.S.P.)				
100 gm	51552-0492-05	13.30		
2270 gm	51552-0492-09	74.90		
(Hospira) *See GLYCINE IRRIGATION*				
(Mallinckrodt Lab)				
POW, NA (U.S.P.)				
500 gm	00406-5104-12	19.15		
(Medisca)				
POW, NA (1X100GM)				
100 gm	38779-1923-05	37.50		
(1X500GM)				
500 gm	38779-1923-08	65.25		
(1X2500GM)				
2500 gm	38779-1923-01	211.50		
(PCCA)				
POW, NA (AMINOACETIC ACID)				
1 gm	51927-1287-00	0.42		
(Spectrum Pharmacy) *See AMINOACETIC ACID*				
GLYCINE IRRIGATION (B. Braun)				
glycine				
SOL, IL, 1.5%, 2000 ml	00264-2302-50	7.04		AT
4000 ml	00264-2302-70	12.62		AT
(Baxter)				
SOL, IL, 1.5%,				
3000 ml 4s	00338-0289-47	65.14		AT
5000 ml 2s	00338-0289-49	52.60		AT
(Hospira)				
SOL, IL (AQUALITE,PF,LATEX-FREE)				
1.5%, 1500 ml 9s	00074-6142-36	52.60	45.99	AT
(FLEX CONTAINER,PF)				
1.5%, 3000 ml 4s	00409-7974-08	51.36	44.96	AT
GLYCINE/SODIUM CHLORIDE				
(Teva) *See EPOPROSTENOL SODIUM DILUENT*				
GLYCO TREATMENT PADS (Topix)				
glycolic acid				
PAD, TP (OFFICE USE ONLY)				
30s ea	51326-0019-30	30.00		
30s ea	51326-0020-30	70.00		
30s ea	51326-0021-30	50.00		
GLYCOLAX (Kremers Urban)				
polyethylene glycol 3350				
PDS, PO, 17 gm/dose,				
255 gm	62175-0442-15	19.54		AA
(IPI)				
REPACK				
PDS, PO, 17 gm/dose,				
527 gm	18837-0241-27	48.83		
(Palmetto)				
REPACK				
PDS, PO (1X255GM)				
17 gm/dose, 255 gm	23490-7971-01	53.73		
(Stat Rx)				
REPACK				
PKT, PO, 17 gm/packet,				
17 gm	16590-0493-17	22.50		
GLYCOLIC ACID (Gallipot)				
CRY, NA (HIGH PURITY)				
25 gm	51552-0183-04	27.16		
(PURIFIED)				
100 gm	51552-0183-05	34.79		
(Gallipot) *See GLYCOLIC ACID 70%*				
(Medisca)				
CRY, NA, 25 gm	38779-0030-04	91.80		
100 gm	38779-0030-05	210.45		
500 gm	38779-0030-08	495.00		
1000 gm	38779-0030-09	825.00		
(Medisca) *See GLYCOLIC ACID 70%*				
(Neurovites)				
CRY, NA, 100 gm	93595-2040-01	25.10		

PROD/MFR	NDC	AWP	DP	OBC
(Neurovites) *See GLYCOLIC ACID 70%*				
(PCCA) *See GLYCOLIC ACID 70%*				
(PCCA)				
GRA, NA, 1 gm	51927-1733-00	1.68		
(Spectrum Pharmacy)				
CRY, NA (1X25GM)				
25 gm	49452-3384-01	73.50		
(1X100GM)				
100 gm	49452-3384-02	155.40		
(1X1000GM)				
1000 gm	49452-3384-04	1099.00		
(Spectrum Pharmacy) *See GLYCOLIC ACID 70%*				
(Topix) *See FLUORO/GLY GEL*				
(Topix) *See FLUORO/GLY PADS*				
(Topix) *See GLYCO TREATMENT PADS*				
GLYCOLIC ACID 70% (Gallipot)				
glycolic acid				
SOL, NA (HIGH PURITY)				
118.28 ml	51552-0369-04	21.00		
473 ml	51552-0369-06	33.60		
3785 ml	51552-0369-08	273.00		
(Medisca)				
SOL, NA (1X100ML)				
100 ml	38779-0353-05	37.50		
500 ml	38779-0353-08	73.50		
1000 ml	38779-0353-09	138.00		
(Neurovites)				
SOL, NA, 480 ml	93595-2039-01	37.62		
(PCCA)				
SOL, NA, 1 ml	51927-2705-00	0.23		
(Spectrum Pharmacy)				
LIQ, NA (HIGH PURITY)				
100 ml	49452-3387-01	95.20		
500 ml	49452-3387-02	172.90		
4000 ml	49452-3387-03	644.00		
20000 ml	49452-3387-04	2054.50		
GLYCOPYRROLATE (Amer Regent)				
SOL, IJ (S.D.V.)				
0.2 mg/ml,				
1 ml 25s	00517-4601-25	22.19		AP
2 ml 25s	00517-4602-25	35.94		AP
(M.D.V.)				
0.2 mg/ml,				
5 ml 25s	00517-4605-25	78.44		AP
20 ml 25s	00517-4620-25	155.94		AP
(Baxter) *See ROBINUL*				
(Baxter)				
SOL, IJ (1X1ML,SDV,USP)				
0.2 mg/ml, 1 ml	10019-0016-39	0.64		AP
((S.D.V.),USP)				
0.2 mg/ml,				
1 ml 25s	10019-0016-81	15.90		AP
(1X2ML,SDV,USP)				
0.2 mg/ml, 2 ml	10019-0016-37	0.78		AP
(S.D.V.)				
0.2 mg/ml,				
2 ml 25s	10019-0016-17	19.50		
(1X5ML,MDV,USP)				
0.2 mg/ml, 5 ml	10019-0016-36	1.02		AP
(M.D.V.)				
0.2 mg/ml,				
5 ml 25s	10019-0016-54	25.50		
(MDV)				
0.2 mg/ml, 20 ml	10019-0016-29	4.80		AP
(M.D.V.)				
0.2 mg/ml,				
20 ml 10s	10019-0016-02	48.00		
(Consolidated Midland)				
SOL, IJ (VIAL)				
0.2 mg/ml,				
5 ml 25s	00223-7722-05	125.00		EE
20 ml	00223-7723-20	6.00		EE
(Dr Reddy's)				
TAB, PO, 1 mg, 100s ea	55111-0648-01	131.29		
2 mg, 100s ea	55111-0649-01	219.96		
(Gallipot)				
POW, NA (U.S.P.)				
1 gm	51552-0042-01	75.46		
(Medisca)				
POW, NA (U.S.P.)				
1 gm	38779-2087-06	375.00		
5 gm	38779-2087-03	1365.00		

PROD/MFR	NDC	AWP	DP	OBC
(Par)				
TAB, PO (USP)				
1 mg, 100s ea	49884-0065-01	131.25		
2 mg, 100s ea	49884-0066-01	219.90		
(PCCA)				
POW, NA (U.S.P.)				
1 gm	51927-1575-00	294.00		
(Qualitest)				
TAB, PO (USP,DYE-FREE)				
1 mg, 100s ea	00603-3180-21	131.29		
2 mg, 100s ea	00603-3181-21	219.96		
(Rising)				
TAB, PO, 1 mg, 100s ea	64980-0131-01	131.30		AA
2 mg, 100s ea	64980-0132-01	219.97		AA
(Shionogi) *See ROBINUL*				
(Shionogi) *See ROBINUL FORTE*				
(Spectrum Pharmacy)				
CRY, NA (U.S.P.)				
1 gm	49452-3358-01	423.50		
5 gm	49452-3358-02	1449.00		
(United Research)				
TAB, PO, 1 mg, 100s ea	00677-1931-01	131.29		
2 mg, 100s ea	00677-1932-01	219.96		
(American Health)				
REPACK				
TAB, PO, 1 mg, 100s ea UD	68084-0231-01	131.30		AA
2 mg, 100s ea UD	68084-0232-01	219.95		AA
(Dispensing Solutions)				
REPACK				
TAB, PO, 1 mg, 100s ea	55045-3486-01	150.00		
(Phys Total Care)				
REPACK				
TAB, PO, 2 mg, 10s ea	54868-5329-00	58.26		AA
30s ea	54868-5329-01	127.86		AA
GLYCYRRHIZIC ACID (PCCA)				
POW, NA (GLYCYRRHIZIN)				
1 gm	51927-2702-00	27.00		
GLYNASE PRES-TAB (Pfizer)				
glyburide, micronized				
TAB, PO, 1.5 mg, 100s ea	00009-0341-01	82.25	68.54	AB
3 mg, 100s ea	00009-0352-01	139.07	115.89	AB
1000s ea	00009-0352-04	1390.68	1158.90	AB
6 mg, 100s ea	00009-3449-01	219.29	182.74	AB
500s ea	00009-3449-03	1096.44	913.70	AB
(Phys Total Care)				
REPACK				
TAB, PO, 3 mg, 30s ea	54868-3017-00	28.05		AB
6 mg, 15s ea	54868-3711-00	34.61		AB
60s ea	54868-3711-01	132.81		AB
GLYSET (Pfizer)				
miglitol				
TAB, PO (FILM-COATED)				
25 mg, 100s ea	00009-5012-01	110.33	91.94	
50 mg, 100s ea	00009-5013-01	121.32	101.10	
100 mg, 100s ea	00009-5014-01	143.12	119.27	
(Phys Total Care)				
REPACK				
TAB, PO, 50 mg, 100s ea	54868-4203-00	102.53		
GOLD CHLORIDE				
(Baker, J.T.) *See GOLD CHLORIDE TRIHYDRATE*				
GOLD CHLORIDE TRIHYDRATE (Baker, J.T.)				
gold chloride				
CRY, NA (A.C.S., REAGENT)				
0.1 gm	10106-2146-03	76.22		
30 gm	10106-2146-00	1370.16		
GOLD SODIUM THIOMALATE				
(Akorn) *See MYOCHRYSINE*				
(PCCA)				
POW, NA, 1 gm	51927-2895-00	480.00		
(Sabex)				
SOL, IM (M.D.V.)				
50 mg/ml, 1 ml 10s	54643-1006-00	175.00		
10 ml	54643-1007-00	175.00		
GOLDENSEAL				
(PCCA) *See GOLDENSEAL HERB*				
GOLDENSEAL HERB (PCCA)				
goldenseal				
POW, NA (HYDRASTIS CANADENSIS)				
1 gm	51927-3199-00	0.66		
GOLIMUMAB				
(Centocor) *See SIMPONI*				

PROD/MFR NDC AWP DP OBC

GOLYTELY (Braintree)
k cl/na bicarb/na cl/na sulf/peg
PDR, PO (PACKET)
ea.................52268-0700-01 11.44 AA

(Braintree)
peg electrolyte lavage solution
PDS, PO, 4000 ml.........52268-0100-01 21.11 AA
4000 ml ....52268-0101-01 22.54 AA

GONADOTROPHIN, CHORIONIC EP (HUMAN) (PCCA)
chorionic gonadotropin
POW, NA (1X1GM)
1 gm 51927-3560-00 22000.00

GONAL-F (EMD)
follitropin alfa
PDS, SC (M.D.V.)
450 iu, ea............44087-9030-01 704.81
(MDV)
1200 iu, ea...........44087-9070-01 1644.55

GONAL-F RFF (EMD)
follitropin alfa
PDS, SC, 75 iu, ea 44087-9005-01 117.47
10s ea............44087-9005-06 1174.68
SOL, SC (29GX1/2,PEN)
300 iu/0.5 ml,
0.5 ml.............44087-1113-01 469.87
(29GX1/2 NEEDLE,PEN)
450 iu/0.75 ml,
0.75 ml...........44087-1112-01 704.81
(29GX1/2,PEN)
900 iu/1.5 ml,
1.5 ml............44087-1114-01 1409.62

GORDON'S UREA (Gordon)
urea
CRE, TP, 40%, 30 gm 10481-3005-01 51.25

GOSERELIN ACETATE
(AstraZeneca) *See ZOLADEX*

GOTU KOLA
(PCCA) *See GOTU KOLA HERB*

GOTU KOLA HERB (PCCA)
gotu kola
POW, NA, 1 gm...........51927-2914-00 0.23

GRAFTJACKET (Wright Medical Tech)
graftskin
SHE, TP (HAND SURGERY,8SQ CM)
ea..............08121-8602-04 925.00
(MAX FORCE,25SQ CM)
ea.................08121-8600-55 2525.00
(MAXFORCEEXTREME28SQ CM)
ea.................08121-8604-07 3250.00
(MAXIMUM FORCE,28SQ CM)
ea.................08121-8600-47 2835.00
(TISSUE MATRIX 16SQ CM)
ea.................08121-8604-04 1295.00
(TISSUE MATRIX,25SQ CM)
ea.................08121-8605-05 1975.00
(TISSUE MATRIX,50SQ CM)
ea.................08121-8605-10 2480.00

GRAFTJACKET SLR (Wright Medical Tech)
graftskin
SHE, TP (SMALL LIGAMENT,1.5SQ CM)
ea.................08121-8605-30 995.00

GRAFTJACKET XPRESS (Wright Medical Tech)
graftskin
PDR, TP, ea 08121-8602-00 1795.00

GRAFTSKIN
(Advanced BioHealing) *See DERMAGRAFT*
(Novartis Pharm) *See APLIGRAF*
(Ortec Int'l) *See ORCEL*
(Wright Medical Tech) *See GRAFTJACKET*
(Wright Medical Tech) *See GRAFTJACKET SLR*
(Wright Medical Tech) *See GRAFTJACKET XPRESS*

GRAMICIDIN (Medisca)
POW, NA (GRAMICIDIN D)
1 gm 38779-2088-06 214.50
5 gm 38779-2088-03 811.50

(PCCA)
POW, NA (USP)
1 gm 51927-1174-00 234.00

GRAMICIDIN/NEOMYCIN SULFATE/ POLYMYXIN B SULFATE
FUL
SOL, OP, 10 ml.. 20.25

(Bausch & Lomb Inc.) *See GRAMICIDIN/NEOMYCIN/POLYMYXIN B*

(Consolidated Midland) *See GRAMICIDIN/NEOMYCIN/POLYMYXIN B*
(Major) *See NEOCIDIN*
(Monarch) *See NEOSPORIN*
(Paddock) *See NEOMYCIN AND POLYMYXIN B SULFATES AND GRAMICIDIN*

GRAMICIDIN/NEOMYCIN/POLYMYXIN B (Bausch & Lomb Inc.)
gramicidin/neomycin sulfate/polymyxin b sulfate
SOL, OP, 10 ml ....24208-0790-62 30.03 AT

(Consolidated Midland)
SOL, OP, 2 ml ....00223-6755-02 3.75 EE
15 ml...............00223-6755-15 4.50 EE

(A-S Medication)
REPACK
SOL, OP, 10 ml ....54569-1188-00 30.03 EE

(Dispensing Solutions)
REPACK
SOL, OP, 10 ml ....55045-1194-02 28.80 AT

(Nucare Pharm)
REPACK
SOL, OP, 10 ml ....66267-0956-10 27.43 AT

(Pharma Pac)
REPACK
SOL, OP, 10 ml ....52959-0254-00 36.05 EE

(Phys Total Care)
REPACK
SOL, OP, 10 ml ....54868-6662-01 86.58 EE

(Southwood)
REPACK
SOL, OP, 10 ml ....58016-6048-01 26.60 EE

GRANISETRON
(ProStrakan) *See SANCUSO*

GRANISETRON HYDROCHLORIDE (Apotex Corp.)
SOL, IV (5X1ML,SINGLE-USE,PF)
0.1 mg/ml, 1 ml 5s ...60505-0764-02 54.11 AP
(1X1ML,SINGLE-USE)
1 mg/ml, 1 ml.......60505-0692-00 77.65 AP
(1X4ML,MULTI-USE)
1 mg/ml, 4 ml.......60505-0693-00 281.25 AP

(APP)
SOL, IV (10X1ML,S.D.V,PF)
0.1 mg/ml,
1 ml 10s..........63323-0317-01 108.25 AP
(1X1ML,SDV,PF)
1 mg/ml, 1 ml.......63323-0318-01 77.65 EE
(1X4ML,MDV)
1 mg/ml, 4 ml.......63323-0319-04 281.25 EE

(Baxter)
SOL, IV (1X4ML,INNER,LATEX-FREE)
1 mg/ml, 4 ml........10019-0053-14 210.00 AP
(1X4ML,LATEX-FREE)
1 mg/ml, 4 ml........10019-0053-03 210.00 AP

(Bedford)
SOL, IV (10X1ML,SDV)
0.1 mg/ml,
1 ml 10s..........55390-0250-10 36.00 AP

(CorePharma)
TAB, PO (FILM-COATED)
1 mg, 2s ea.........64720-0198-98 116.71 AB
20s ea.........64720-0198-02 1167.07 AB

(Cura Pharm)
SOL, IV (SDV,5X1ML)
0.1 mg/ml, 1 ml 5s ...66860-0081-06 53.03
1 mg/ml, 1 ml 5s.....66860-0082-06 388.15
(MDV,1X4ML)
1 mg/ml, 4 ml........66860-0083-01 221.43

(Dava Pharma)
TAB, PO (FILM-COATED)
1 mg, 2s ea UD ......67253-0417-12 118.02 AB

(Hawthorn Pharm) *See GRANISOL*

(Northstar)
TAB, PO (FILM-COATED)
1 mg, 2s ea..........16714-0221-30 117.00 AB

(Parenta Pharma)
SOL, IV (5X1ML)
0.1 mg/ml, 1 ml 5s ...66758-0037-02 25.00 AP
(1X1ML,SINGLE-USE)
1 mg/ml, 1 ml........66758-0035-01 50.00
(1X4ML,MULTI-USE)
1 mg/ml, 4 ml........66758-0036-01 200.00

(Roche Labs) *See KYTRIL*

(Roxane)
TAB, PO, 1 mg, 2s ea......00054-0143-87 118.04 AB
(2X10)
1 mg, 20s ea UD .....00054-0143-08 1180.18 AB

(Teva) *See GRANISTERON HYDROCHLORIDE*

(Teva)
SOL, IV (5X1ML,SINGLE-USE,PF)
0.1 mg/ml, 1 ml 5s ...00703-7891-02 36.00 AP
(10X1ML,SINGLE-USE)
1 mg/ml, 1 ml 10s....00703-7971-03 276.00 AP
(1X4ML)
1 mg/ml, 4 ml........00703-7973-01 96.00 AP

(UDL)
TAB, PO (2CARDSX10,FILM-COATED)
1 mg, 20s ea UD .....51079-0472-05 1178.70 AB

(Wockhardt USA)
SOL, IV (5X1ML,PF)
0.1 mg/ml, 1 ml 5s ...64679-0662-01 53.03 AP
(1X1ML)
1 mg/ml, 1 ml........64679-0661-03 77.63 AP
(1X4ML)
1 mg/ml, 4 ml........64679-0661-02 281.23 AP

GRANISOL (Hawthorn Pharm)
granisetron hydrochloride
SOL, PO (1X30ML,AMBER GLASS)
2 mg/10 ml, 30 ml....63717-0801-30 373.74

GRANISTERON HYDROCHLORIDE (Teva)
granisetron hydrochloride
TAB, PO (2X1,FILM COATED)
1 mg, 2s ea UD ......00093-7485-12 118.02 AB
(5X4,FILM COATED)
1 mg, 20s ea UD .....00093-7485-20 1180.05 AB

GRANULEX (UDL)
castor oil/peru balsam/trypsin
SPR, TP, 56.7 gm.........51079-0621-81 15.15
113.4 gm...........51079-0621-82 19.41

GRAPE (Medisca)
flavoring aid
SOL, NA (ARTIFICIAL FLAVOR)
25 ml...............38779-1327-04 22.50
100 ml 38779-1327-05 34.50
(CONCENTRATE)
100 ml 38779-1329-05 22.50
500 ml 38779-1329-08 39.00

GRAPE ARTIFICIAL FLAVOR (Spectrum Pharmacy)
flavoring aid
LIQ, NA (1X100ML,CONCENTRATE)
100 ml 49452-3388-02 53.20
(1X500ML,CONCENTRATE)
500 ml 49452-3388-03 118.30

GRAPE FLAVOR (Gallipot)
flavoring aid
LIQ, NA (ARTIFICIAL)
59.14 ml............51552-0165-03 6.02

(PCCA)
SOL, NA (ARTIFICIAL)
1 ml................51927-2243-00 0.90
(CONCENTRATE)
1 ml................51927-1279-00 0.23
1 ml................51927-2145-00 0.33

GRAPE SEED EXTRACT (Gallipot)
POW, NA (FCC)
1000 gm.............51552-0986-07 315.00 225.00

GRAPE SEED OIL
(Medisca) *See GRAPESEED OIL*
(PCCA) *See GRAPESEED OIL*

GRAPEFRUIT OIL (PCCA)
OIL, NA, 1 ml............51927-3011-00 0.70

GRAPEFRUIT SEED EXTRACT (PCCA)
SOL, NA, 60%, 1 ml.......51927-3146-00 1.20

GRAPESEED OIL (Medisca)
grape seed oil
OIL, NA (1X500ML)
500 ml 38779-2089-08 58.50

(PCCA)
OIL, NA, 1 ml............51927-3046-00 0.13

GRAPHITE
(Baker, J.T.) *See CARBON ACID WASHED*

GREEN APPLE (Spectrum Pharmacy)
flavoring aid
SOL, NA (1X100ML)
100 ml 49452-3390-01 59.50
(1X500ML)
500 ml 49452-3390-02 131.95

PROD/MFR	NDC	AWP	DP	OBC
GREEN FOOD COLOR (PCCA)				
color additive				
POW, NA, 1 gm	51927-1278-00	6.50		
SOL, NA, 1 ml	51927-1487-00	3.86		
GREEN LIPPED MUSSEL (PCCA)				
POW, NA, 1 gm	51927-3492-00	1.20		
GREEN SOAP (Gallipot)				
TIN, NA, 118.28 ml	51552-0151-04	4.34		
473 ml	51552-0151-06	10.15		
3785 ml	51552-0151-08	46.55		
(PCCA)				
POW, NA (USP; SOFT SOAP)				
1 gm	51927-2005-00	0.10		
(Spectrum Pharmacy)				
TIN, NA (U.S.P./N.F.)				
500 ml	49452-3400-01	78.75		
4000 ml	49452-3400-02	226.45		
GREEN TEA EXTRACT (PCCA)				
POW, NA (90% POLYPHENOLS)				
1 gm	51927-3570-00	1.05		
GRIFULVIN V (Ortho)				
griseofulvin, microcrystalline				
TAB, PO, 500 mg, 100s ea	00062-0214-60	468.47	390.39	
(Dispensing Solutions)				
REPACK				
SUS, PO, 125 mg/5 ml, 120 ml	55045-1565-09	60.00		
(PD-Rx Pharm)				
REPACK				
TAB, PO, 500 mg, 42s ea	55289-0857-42	144.58		AB
(Phys Total Care)				
REPACK				
SUS, PO, 125 mg/5 ml, 120 ml	54868-2050-00	69.40		
TAB, PO, 500 mg, 10s ea	54868-5402-00	31.13		
45s ea	54868-5402-01	126.21		
GRIS-PEG (Pedinol)				
griseofulvin, ultramicrocrystalline				
TAB, PO, 125 mg, 100s ea	00884-0763-04	214.50		AB
250 mg, 100s ea	00884-0773-04	274.75		AB
500s ea	00884-0773-50	1310.13		AB
(Dispensing Solutions)				
REPACK				
TAB, PO, 250 mg, 100s ea	55045-3111-00	165.00		AB
(PD-Rx Pharm)				
REPACK				
TAB, PO, 250 mg, 30s ea	55289-0358-30	71.88		AB
(Phys Total Care)				
REPACK				
TAB, PO, 250 mg, 200s ea	54868-2560-00	226.59		AB
(Quality Care Prod)				
REPACK				
TAB, PO, 125 mg, 30s ea	49999-0726-30	90.35		AB
250 mg, 30s ea	49999-0373-30	142.45		AB
60s ea	49999-0373-60	284.90		AB
GRISEOFULVIN (Actavis Mid Atlantic)				
griseofulvin, microcrystalline				
SUS, PO (USP,MICROSIZE) 125 mg/5 ml, 120 ml	00472-0013-04	61.98		AB
(Gallipot)				
griseofulvin, micronized				
POW, NA (1X25GM,USP) 25 gm	51552-0987-04	59.50	42.50	
(1X100GM,USP) 100 gm	51552-0987-05	126.00	90.00	
(Medisca)				
griseofulvin, microcrystalline				
POW, NA (U.S.P.)				
100 gm	38779-0119-05	184.50		
500 gm	38779-0119-08	628.50		
1000 gm	38779-0119-09	994.50		
(Patriot Pharmaceuticals)				
SUS, PO (MICROSIZE) 125 mg/5 ml, 120 ml	10147-0810-04	41.73		
(Perrigo)				
SUS, PO (USP,1X120ML,MICROSIZE) 125 mg/5 ml, 120 ml	45802-0968-26	41.69		AB
(Teva)				
SUS, PO (1X120ML,USP) 125 mg/5 ml, 120 ml	00093-7102-12	62.06		
(Bryant Ranch)				
REPACK				
CAP, PO, 250 mg, 30s ea	63629-2930-01	72.32		
TAB, PO, 500 mg, 30s ea	63629-2929-01	99.65		
(Phys Total Care)				
REPACK				
SUS, PO, 125 mg/5 ml, 120 ml	54868-5234-00	93.78		
(Phys Total Care)				
griseofulvin, ultramicrocrystalline				
TAB, PO, 250 mg, 100s ea	54868-3636-01	157.22		EE
GRISEOFULVIN MICROCRYSTALLINE (Letco)				
griseofulvin, microcrystalline				
POW, NA (U.S.P.)				
100 gm	62991-1074-02	195.00		
500 gm	62991-1074-03	825.00		
1000 gm	62991-1074-04	1350.00		
(Medisca)				
POW, NA (U.S.P.,MICRONIZED)				
100 gm	38779-0321-05	216.00		
500 gm	38779-0321-08	889.50		
1000 gm	38779-0321-09	1455.00		
(USP,1X5000GM,MICRONIZED) 5000 gm	38779-0321-03	5550.00		
(USP,1X25000GM) 25000 gm	38779-0321-07	39780.00		
(Spectrum Pharmacy)				
POW, NA (1X100GM) 100 gm	49452-3363-01	367.50		
GRISEOFULVIN MICRONIZED (Hawkins)				
griseofulvin, micronized				
POW, NA (U.S.P.)				
25 gm	63370-0093-25	80.00		
100 gm	63370-0093-35	280.00		
500 gm	63370-0093-45	1120.00		
1000 gm	63370-0093-50	2000.00		
5000 gm	63370-0093-55	9200.00		
(PCCA)				
POW, NA (U.S.P.) 1 gm	51927-3084-00	3.12		
(Spectrum Pharmacy)				
POW, NA (B.P.,E.P.) 1000 gm	49452-3363-03	2047.50		
GRISEOFULVIN, MICROCRYSTALLINE				
(Actavis Mid Atlantic) *See GRISEOFULVIN*				
(Letco) *See GRISEOFULVIN MICROCRYSTALLINE*				
(Medisca) *See GRISEOFULVIN*				
(Medisca) *See GRISEOFULVIN MICROCRYSTALLINE*				
(Ortho) *See GRIFULVIN V*				
(Patriot Pharmaceuticals) *See GRISEOFULVIN*				
(Perrigo) *See GRISEOFULVIN*				
(Spectrum Pharmacy) *See GRISEOFULVIN MICROCRYSTALLINE*				
(Teva) *See GRISEOFULVIN*				
(Palmetto)				
REPACK				
SUS, PO, 125 mg/5 ml, 120 ml	23490-5644-01	51.87		
GRISEOFULVIN, MICRONIZED				
(Gallipot) *See GRISEOFULVIN*				
(Hawkins) *See GRISEOFULVIN MICRONIZED*				
(PCCA) *See GRISEOFULVIN MICRONIZED*				
(Spectrum Pharmacy) *See GRISEOFULVIN MICRONIZED*				
GRISEOFULVIN, ULTRAMICROCRYSTALLINE				
(Pedinol) *See GRIS-PEG*				
GUAIAC GUM (Medisca)				
POW, NA (1X25GM) 25 gm	38779-1331-04	58.50		
(1X100GM) 100 gm	38779-1331-05	163.50		
GUAIACOL (Amend)				
LIQ, NA (PURIFIED) 500 ml	17317-0194-01	28.00		
(Gallipot)				
LIQ, NA (PURIFIED)				
100 ml	51552-0176-05	20.72		
473 ml	51552-0176-06	55.16		
(PCCA)				
LIQ, NA (PURIFIED) 1 ml	51927-1209-00	0.45		
(Spectrum Pharmacy)				
LIQ, NA (PURIFIED)				
100 ml	49452-3410-01	85.75		
500 ml	49452-3410-02	224.70		
GUAIBID LA (Bryant Ranch)				
REPACK				
guaifenesin				
TER, PO, 600 mg, 20s ea	63629-1409-01	20.52		
40s ea	63629-1409-02	40.65		
GUAIFEN AC (DHS, Inc.)				
REPACK				
codeine phosphate/guaifenesin				
SYR, PO, 10 mg/5 ml-100 mg/5 ml, 120 ml, C-V	55887-0804-04	9.50		
GUAIFEN PSE (Vintage)				
guaifenesin/pseudoephedrine hydrochloride				
TER, PO (CAPLET) 600 mg-120 mg, 100s ea	00254-6211-28	55.99		
(Dispensing Solutions)				
REPACK				
TER, PO, 600 mg-120 mg, 14s ea	66336-0933-14	8.84		
20s ea	66336-0933-20	11.78		
(Quality Care Prod)				
REPACK				
TER, PO, 600 mg-120 mg, 30s ea	49999-0243-30	13.70		
GUAIFEN PSEUDOPHED (Quality Care Prod)				
guaifenesin/pseudoephedrine hydrochloride				
TER, PO, 600 mg-60 mg, 28s ea	49999-0031-28	17.26		
GUAIFEN-PSE (Quality Care Prod)				
guaifenesin/pseudoephedrine hydrochloride				
TER, PO, 600 mg-120 mg, 14s ea	49999-0243-14	6.44		
90s ea	49999-0243-90	41.40		
GUAIFEN/CODEINE (Stat Rx)				
REPACK				
codeine phosphate/guaifenesin				
SYR, PO, 10 mg/5 ml-100 mg/5 ml, 120 ml, C-V	16590-0110-04	7.25		
GUAIFENESIN				
(Alphagen) *See GG-200 NR*				
(Amend)				
POW, NA (U.S.P.)				
125 gm	17317-0190-04	7.00		
500 gm	17317-0190-01	21.00		
2270 gm	17317-0190-05	84.00		
11350 gm	17317-0190-08	350.00		
(Cypress Pharm) *See GANIDIN NR*				
(Dexo) *See HUMAVENT LA*				
(Gallipot)				
POW, NA (U.S.P.,N.F.)				
100 gm	51552-0140-05	11.20		
454 gm	51552-0140-06	28.00		
(Hawkins)				
POW, NA (U.S.P.)				
500 gm	63370-0097-45	80.00		
1000 gm	63370-0097-50	140.00		
2500 gm	63370-0097-53	320.00		
(Letco)				
POW, NA (U.S.P.)				
100 gm	62991-1075-01	27.00		
500 gm	62991-1075-02	60.00		
2500 gm	62991-1075-03	210.00		
(Meda) *See ORGANIDIN NR*				
(Medisca)				
POW, NA (U.S.P.)				
100 gm	38779-0696-05	36.00		
500 gm	38779-0696-08	73.50		
1000 gm	38779-0696-09	133.50		
2500 gm	38779-0696-01	285.00		
(PCCA)				
POW, NA (U.S.P.) 1 gm	51927-1147-00	0.24		
(Qualitest) *See IOPHEN-NR*				
(Qualitest) *See ORGAN-1 NR*				
(Silarx) *See GUAIFENESIN NR*				
(Spectrum Pharmacy)				
POW, NA (U.S.P.)				
500 gm	49452-3420-02	106.40		
2500 gm	49452-3420-03	423.50		

PROD/MFR	NDC	AWP	DP	OBC

(Bryant Ranch)
REPACK
TAB, PO, 200 mg, 100s ea . 63629-1399-01 16.98

(DHS, Inc.)
REPACK
SYR, PO, 100 mg/5 ml,
120 ml 55887-0221-82 4.79
TAB, PO, 400 mg, 40s ea . . 55887-0186-40 13.12

(HomeMed)
REPACK
TER, PO, 600 mg, 10s ea . . 51655-0948-53 3.87
20s ea............ 51655-0948-52 6.69

(Palmetto)
REPACK
SYR, PO, 100 mg/5 ml,
120 ml 23490-6676-00 5.50

(Physician Partner)
REPACK
SYR, PO (1X120ML)
100 mg/5 ml,
120 ml 21695-0705-04 9.98

(Quality Care Prod)
REPACK
TER, PO, 600 mg, 20s ea . . 49999-0078-20 11.83

GUAIFENESIN AC (Pack)
codeine phosphate/guaifenesin
SOL, PO (1X473ML)
10 mg/5 ml-100 mg/5 ml,
473 ml, C-V........ 16571-0302-16 11.72

(Dispensing Solutions)
REPACK
SYR, PO, 10 mg/5 ml-100 mg/5 ml,
118 ml, C-V........ 55045-1495-09 7.05

GUAIFENESIN AND CODEINE PHOSPHATE
(Boca Pharmacal)
codeine phosphate/guaifenesin
SOL, PO (1X118ML,SF)
10 mg/5 ml-100 mg/5 ml,
118 ml, C-V........ 64376-0435-40 3.20
(1X473ML,SF)
10 mg/5 ml-100 mg/5 ml,
473 ml, C-V........ 64376-0435-16 8.90

(Pharm Assoc Inc)
SOL, PO (USP,AF,SF,CHERRY)
10 mg/5 ml-100 mg/5 ml,
118 ml, C-V........ 00121-0775-04 4.76
473 ml, C-V........ 00121-0775-16 11.72

(Altura)
REPACK
SOL, PO (1X120ML,AF,SF,CHERRY)
10 mg/5 ml-100 mg/5 ml,
120 ml, C-V........ 63874-0211-12 6.66
(1X240ML,AF,SF,CHERRY)
10 mg/5 ml-100 mg/5 ml,
240 ml, C-V........ 63874-0211-24 13.32
(1X480ML,AF,SF,CHERRY)
10 mg/5 ml-100 mg/5 ml,
480 ml, C-V........ 63874-0211-48 40.40

(Nucare Pharm)
REPACK
SOL, PO (AF,SF,CHERRY)
10 mg/5 ml-100 mg/5 ml,
120 ml, C-V........ 68071-1350-04 11.50

GUAIFENESIN DAC (Pack)
codeine phos/gg/pse hcl
SOL, PO (1X473ML)
473 ml, C-V.......... 16571-0301-16 39.66

GUAIFENESIN DM (Dispensing Solutions)
REPACK
dextromethorphan hydrobromide/guaifenesin
TER, PO, 30 mg-600 mg,
20s ea............ 66336-0182-20 10.31
(CAPLET)
30 mg-600 mg,
30s ea............ 55045-2096-08 16.50

(HomeMed)
REPACK
TER, PO, 30 mg-600 mg,
20s ea............ 51655-0766-52 12.22

(Pharma Pac)
REPACK
SYR, PO, 10 mg/5 ml-100 mg/5 ml,
120 ml 52959-0750-04 6.89
240 ml 52959-0750-08 14.10

(Vibranta)
REPACK
SYR, PO, 10 mg/5 ml-100 mg/5 ml,
120 ml 57866-0870-97 5.70

GUAIFENESIN LA (Core)
REPACK
guaifenesin
TER, PO, 600 mg, 20s ea . . 33358-0162-20 23.37

(Nucare Pharm)
REPACK
TER, PO, 600 mg, 14s ea . . 66267-0105-14 5.56
28s ea............ 66267-0105-28 8.99

(Pharma Pac)
REPACK
TER, PO, 600 mg, 14s ea . . 52959-0438-14 7.75
20s ea............ 52959-0438-20 10.50
28s ea............ 52959-0438-28 14.40
40s ea............ 52959-0438-40 18.46

(Quality Care Prod)
REPACK
TER, PO, 600 mg, 28s ea . . 49999-0098-28 14.98

GUAIFENESIN NR (Silarx)
guaifenesin
SYR, PO (AF,SF)
100 mg/5 ml,
473 ml 54838-0123-80 37.25

GUAIFENESIN W/ CODEINE (Southwood)
REPACK
codeine phosphate/guaifenesin
SYR, PO, 10 mg/5 ml-100 mg/5 ml,
120 ml, C-V........ 58016-5593-01 4.76

GUAIFENESIN W/CODEINE (Quality Care Prod)
REPACK
codeine phosphate/guaifenesin
SYR, PO, 10 mg/5 ml-100 mg/5 ml,
120 ml, C-V........ 49999-0610-04 15.06

GUAIFENESIN WITH CODEINE (A-S Medication)
REPACK
codeine phosphate/guaifenesin
SYR, PO (1X236ML,SF)
10 mg/5 ml-100 mg/5 ml,
236 ml, C-V........ 54569-6164-00 5.49

GUAIFENESIN-DM (Southwood)
REPACK
dextromethorphan hydrobromide/guaifenesin
TAB, PO, 20 mg-400 mg,
30s ea............ 58016-0141-30 7.61
60s ea............ 58016-0141-60 15.22
90s ea............ 58016-0141-90 22.82
100s ea........... 58016-0141-00 25.36

GUAIFENESIN-DM NR (Silarx)
dextromethorphan hydrobromide/guaifenesin
LIQ, PO (AF,SF,RASPBERRY)
10 mg/5 ml-100 mg/5 ml,
473 ml 54838-0124-80 45.25

GUAIFENESIN-HYDROCODONE BITARTRATE
(DHS, Inc.)
REPACK
guaifenesin/hydrocodone bitartrate
SYR, PO, 100 mg/5 ml-5 mg/5 ml,
120 ml, C-III 55887-0336-04 19.06

GUAIFENESIN/CODEINE (Bryant Ranch)
REPACK
codeine phosphate/guaifenesin
SYR, PO, 10 mg/5 ml-100 mg/5 ml,
120 ml, C-V........ 63629-2961-01 38.04

(Southwood)
REPACK
SOL, PO, 10 mg/5 ml-100 mg/5 ml,
473 ml, C-V........ 58016-4862-01 47.10

GUAIFENESIN/DM (Southwood)
dextromethorphan hydrobromide/guaifenesin
LIQ, PO, 10 mg/5 ml-100 mg/5 ml,
473 ml 58016-4861-01 45.25

GUAIFENESIN/HYDROCODONE BITARTRATE
(Endo Labs) *See HYCOTUSS EXPECTORANT*

(Ethex)
LIQ, PO (AF,SF,DYE-FREE)
100 mg/5 ml-5 mg/5 ml,
480 ml, C-III 58177-0881-07 43.43
960 ml, C-III 58177-0881-12 86.87

(Everett) *See TUSSO-DF*
(Everett) *See TUSSO-HC*
(Hawthorn Pharm) *See XPECT-HC*
(Monte Sano) *See MONTE-G HC*

(Pharmakon) *See PHANATUSS-HC DIABETIC CHOICE*

(Palmetto)
REPACK
SYR, PO, 100 mg/5 ml-5 mg/5 ml,
118 ml, C-III 23490-5687-02 12.51
118 ml, C-III 23490-5688-03 16.05
120 ml, C-III 23490-5687-00 12.51
177 ml, C-III 23490-5687-03 18.76
177 ml, C-III 23490-5688-04 24.07
(1X180ML)
100 mg/5 ml-5 mg/5 ml,
180 ml, C-III 23490-5687-04 18.76
473 ml, C-III 23490-5688-05 48.28
(1X480ML)
100 mg/5 ml-5 mg/5 ml,
480 ml, C-III 23490-5687-01 49.97

GUAIFENESIN/PHENYLEPHRINE
(JayMac Pharma) *See J-MAX*

GUAIFENESIN/PHENYLEPHRINE (Palmetto)
REPACK
guaifenesin/phenylephrine hydrochloride
TER, PO, 600 mg-40 mg,
20s ea............ 23490-7946-02 22.00
30s ea............ 23490-7946-03 29.50

(Pharma Pac)
REPACK
TER, PO, 600 mg-30 mg,
15s ea............ 52959-0695-15 22.50
30s ea............ 52959-0695-30 45.00

GUAIFENESIN/PHENYLEPHRINE HCL (Prasco Labs)
guaifenesin/phenylephrine hydrochloride
TER, PO (CAPLET)
1200 mg-25 mg,
100s ea........... 66993-0325-02 169.33

GUAIFENESIN/PHENYLEPHRINE HYDROCHLORIDE
(Acella) *See PHENYLEPHRINE HYDROCHLORIDE/GUAIFENESIN*
(Actavis) *See NEW AMI-TEX LA*
(Athlon Pharm) *See DYNEX LA*
(Athlon Pharm) *See ENTEX LA*
(Auriga) *See EXTENDRYL G*
(Blansett) *See PROLEX PD*
(Blansett) *See PROLEX-D*
(Breckenridge Pharm) *See CRANTEX*
(Breckenridge Pharm) *See GUIATEX PE*
(Capellon) *See DUOMAX*
(Capellon) *See LIQUIBID-D*
(Capellon) *See LIQUIBID-D 1200*
(Capellon) *See LIQUIBID-PD*
(Centurion) *See MYDOCS*
(Cypress Pharm) *See GFN 1200/PHENYLEPHRINE 40*
(Cypress Pharm) *See GFN 600/PHENYLEPHRINE 20*
(Cypress Pharm) *See PENDEX*
(Cypress Pharm) *See RELURI*
(Cypress Pharm) *See SIMUC*
(Cypress Pharm) *See XEDEC II*
(Dexo) *See SINUVENT PE*
(Ethex) *See PHENAVENT D*
(Gentex Pharma) *See GENTEX LA*
(Gil Pharmaceutical) *See GILPHEX TR*
(Hawthorn Pharm) *See NARIZ*
(Hawthorn Pharm) *See XPECT-PE*
(Intl Ethical) *See DESPEC*
(JayMac Pharma) *See J-MAX*
(Laser Pharma) *See DONATUSSIN*
(Laser Pharma) *See PE-GUAI*
(Monte Sano) *See MONTEPHEN*
(Palm) *See D-TAB*
(Prasco Labs) *See GUAIFENESIN/PHENYLEPHRINE HCL*
(SJ) *See MEDENT-PE*
(Vindex Pharma Inc) *See SITREX PD*

(Keltman Pharma., Inc.)
REPACK
TER, PO, 600 mg-20 mg,
20s ea............ 68387-0631-20 15.58

PROD/MFR NDC AWP DP OBC

(Quality Care Prod)
REPACK
TER, PO, 600 mg-20 mg,
20s ea............49999-0893-20 65.74

GUAIFENESIN/PHENYLEPHRINE TANNATE
(Meda) *See SINA-12X*

GUAIFENESIN/PSE (Dispensing Solutions)
REPACK
guaifenesin/pseudoephedrine hydrochloride
TER, PO, 600 mg-60 mg,
20s ea............66336-0870-20 12.89

(Southwood)
REPACK
TER, PO, 600 mg-120 mg,
20s ea............58016-0693-20 17.40
30s ea............58016-0693-30 26.10
60s ea............58016-0693-60 52.20
90s ea............58016-0693-90 78.30
100s ea...........58016-0693-00 87.00

GUAIFENESIN/PSEUDOEPHEDRINE (Altura)
REPACK
guaifenesin/pseudoephedrine hydrochloride
TER, PO (FILM-COATED)
600 mg-120 mg,
15s ea............63874-0320-15 13.74
20s ea............63874-0320-20 18.32
30s ea............63874-0320-30 30.79
60s ea............63874-0320-60 57.83
100s ea...........63874-0320-01 93.29

(Dispensing Solutions)
REPACK
TER, PO (CAPLET)
600 mg-60 mg,
14s ea............55045-2098-04 5.04
20s ea............55045-2098-07 7.20
600 mg-120 mg,
30s ea............55045-2183-08 16.50
100s ea...........55045-2183-00 55.00

(HomeMed)
REPACK
TER, PO, 600 mg-120 mg,
20s ea............51655-0768-52 22.85

(Nucare Pharm)
REPACK
TER, PO, 600 mg-120 mg,
20s ea............66267-0220-20 12.99

(Pharma Pac)
REPACK
TER, PO (CAPLET)
600 mg-60 mg,
28s ea............52959-0715-28 15.25

(Quality Care Prod)
REPACK
TER, PO, 600 mg-60 mg,
20s ea............49999-0031-20 12.33

GUAIFENESIN/PSEUDOEPHEDRINE HYDROCHLORIDE
(Athlon Pharm) *See ENTEX PSE*
(Auriga) *See LEVALL G*
(Boca Pharmacal) *See PSEUDOEPHEDRINE GG*
(Cypress Pharm) *See NOMUC-PE*
(Dexo) *See D-FEDA II*
(Dexo) *See WE MIST II LA*
(Dexo) *See WE MIST LA*
(Ethex) *See GUAIFENEX GP*
(Ethex) *See GUAIFENEX PSE 120*
(Ethex) *See GUAIFENEX PSE 60*
(Ethex) *See GUAIFENEX PSE 80*
(Ethex) *See GUAIFENEX PSE 85*
(Intl Ethical) *See DESPEC SR*
(Larken Labs, Inc.) *See EXEFEN-IR*
(Laser Pharma) *See RESPAIRE-120 SR*
(Laser Pharma) *See RESPAIRE-30*
(Laser Pharma) *See RESPAIRE-60 SR*
(Llorens Pharma Int) *See TUSNEL PEDIATRIC*
(MCR American) *See AMBI 40PSE/400GFN*
(MCR American) *See AMBI 60PSE/400GFN*
(Truxton) *See PSEUDOCOT-G*
(Vintage) *See GUAIFEN PSE*

PROD/MFR NDC AWP DP OBC

(Palmetto)
REPACK
CER, PO, 300 mg-60 mg,
20s ea............23490-6221-02 11.83
30s ea............23490-6221-03 17.75
60s ea............23490-6221-06 35.50
TER, PO, 600 mg-60 mg,
14s ea............23490-6222-00 12.22
20s ea............23490-6222-01 12.89
600 mg-120 mg, 6s ea 23490-6224-01 7.98
10s ea............23490-6224-05 9.50
12s ea............23490-6224-00 11.40
14s ea............23490-6224-02 13.30
20s ea............23490-6224-03 19.00
30s ea............23490-6224-04 28.50

GUAIFENESIN/PSEUDOEPHEDRINE/CODEINE (Altura)
REPACK
codeine phos/gg/pse hcl
SYR, PO, 120 ml, C-V.....63874-0210-12 12.03

GUAIFENESIN/PSEUDOEPHEDRINE/DEXTROMETHORPHAN (Pharma Pac)
REPACK
dm/gg/pse hcl
SOL, PO, 120 ml..........52959-0866-04 3.97

GUAIFENESIN/PSEUDOPHEDRINE (Quality Care Prod)
REPACK
guaifenesin/pseudoephedrine hydrochloride
TER, PO, 600 mg-120 mg,
20s ea............49999-0243-20 9.13
60s ea............49999-0243-60 27.40

GUAIFENESIN/THEOPHYLLINE
(Consolidated Midland) *See THEOCON*
(Tarmac) *See NEOASMA*

GUAIFENESIN/THEOPHYLLINE SODIUM GLYCINATE
(Edwards) *See ED-BRON G*

GUAIFENEX DM (Ethex)
dextromethorphan hydrobromide/guaifenesin
TER, PO, 30 mg-600 mg,
100s ea...........58177-0213-04 42.95

GUAIFENEX GP (Ethex)
guaifenesin/pseudoephedrine hydrochloride
TER, PO (DYE-FREE,FILM-COATED)
1200 mg-120 mg,
100s ea...........58177-0373-04 77.02

GUAIFENEX PSE 120 (Ethex)
guaifenesin/pseudoephedrine hydrochloride
TER, PO (DYE-FREE)
600 mg-120 mg,
100s ea...........58177-0208-04 53.15

GUAIFENEX PSE 60 (Ethex)
guaifenesin/pseudoephedrine hydrochloride
TER, PO, 600 mg-60 mg,
100s ea...........58177-0214-04 35.90

GUAIFENEX PSE 80 (Ethex)
guaifenesin/pseudoephedrine hydrochloride
TER, PO (CAPLET)
800 mg-80 mg,
100s ea...........58177-0413-04 44.46

GUAIFENEX PSE 85 (Ethex)
guaifenesin/pseudoephedrine hydrochloride
TER, PO, 795 mg-85 mg,
100s ea...........58177-0478-04 44.46

GUANABENZ ACETATE (PCCA)
POW, NA (U.S.P.)
1 gm..............51927-2747-00 123.00

(Spectrum Pharmacy)
POW, NA (U.S.P.)
1 gm..............49452-3421-01 174.48
5 gm..............49452-3421-02 682.60

(Teva)
TAB, PO, 4 mg, 100s ea...00172-4226-60 97.99 AB
8 mg, 100s ea........00172-4227-60 190.57 AB

GUANETHIDINE MONOSULFATE (Gallipot)
POW, NA, 5 gm..........51552-0602-02 182.70
(Medisca) *See GUANETHIDINE SULFATE*

(PCCA)
POW, NA (U.S.P.)
1 gm..............51927-1990-00 102.00

GUANETHIDINE SULFATE (Medisca)
guanethidine monosulfate
POW, NA (1X100GM)
100 gm............38779-2361-05 2925.00

PROD/MFR NDC AWP DP OBC

GUANFACINE (Amneal)
guanfacine hydrochloride
TAB, PO (USP)
1 mg, 100s ea........65162-0711-10 87.20 AB
2 mg, 100s ea........65162-0713-10 133.97 AB

(Altura)
REPACK
TAB, PO, 1 mg, 100s ea...63874-1159-01 122.10

(Palmetto)
REPACK
TAB, PO, 1 mg, 30s ea....23490-7952-03 33.48

GUANFACINE HCL (Mylan)
guanfacine hydrochloride
TAB, PO, 1 mg, 100s ea...00378-1160-01 87.20 AB
2 mg, 100s ea........00378-1190-01 117.60 AB

(PCCA)
POW, NA, 0.001 gm.......51927-3639-00 28.50

(Watson Labs)
TAB, PO, 1 mg, 100s ea...00591-0444-01 87.20 AB
2 mg, 100s ea........00591-0453-01 117.60 AB

(Pharma Pac)
REPACK
TAB, PO, 1 mg, 100s ea...52959-0945-00 102.05 AB

(Phys Total Care)
REPACK
TAB, PO, 2 mg, 30s ea....54868-4876-00 19.05 AB
60s ea............54868-4876-01 33.57 AB
100s ea...........54868-4876-02 51.45 AB

(Quality Care Prod)
REPACK
TAB, PO, 1 mg, 30s ea....35356-0161-30 13.56 AB
90s ea............35356-0161-90 29.06 AB

GUANFACINE HYDROCHLORIDE
FUL
TAB, PO, 1 mg, 100s ea............................ 12.42
2 mg, 100s ea.................................... 70.11
(Amneal) *See GUANFACINE*
(Mylan) *See GUANFACINE HCL*
(PCCA) *See GUANFACINE HCL*
(Promius) *See TENEX*
(Shire US Inc.) *See INTUNIV*
(Watson Labs) *See GUANFACINE HCL*

GUANIDINE HYDROCHLORIDE (Baker, J.T.)
POW, NA (ULTRAPURE BIOREAGENT)
100 gm............10106-4076-00 31.26
500 gm............10106-4076-01 104.55
2500 gm...........10106-4076-05 407.93
2500 gm...........10106-4168-05 407.93
12000 gm..........10106-4076-07 1621.17

(PCCA)
POW, NA, 1 gm..........51927-2683-00 1.44
(Schering) *See GUANIDINE HYDROCHLORIDE*

GUANIDINE HYDROCHLORIDE (Schering)
guanidine hydrochloride
TAB, PO, 125 mg, 100s ea.00085-0492-01 25.32

GUANIDINE HYDROCHLORIDE (Spectrum Pharmacy)
CRY, NA (1X100GM)
100 gm............49452-3425-01 132.65
(1X500GM)
500 gm............49452-3425-02 472.50
(1X2500GM)
2500 gm...........49452-3425-03 1452.50

GUAR GUM (Amend)
POW, NA, 500 gm.........17317-0839-01 9.80
2500 gm...........17317-0839-05 42.00

(Medisca)
POW, NA (1X500GM)
500 gm............38779-1333-08 33.00
(1X1000GM)
1000 gm...........38779-1333-09 60.00

(PCCA)
POW, NA (FOOD GRADE)
1 gm..............51927-1443-00 0.12
(NF)
1 gm..............51927-3614-00 0.12

(Spectrum Pharmacy)
POW, NA (F.C.C.)
500 gm............49452-3430-01 72.10
(N.F.)
500 gm............49452-3435-01 72.10
(F.C.C.)
2500 gm...........49452-3430-02 236.25
(N.F.)
2500 gm...........49452-3435-02 236.25

PROD/MFR	NDC	AWP	DP	OBC
GUARANA EXTRACT (PCCA)				
POW, NA (22% CAFFEINE)				
1 gm	51927-3483-00	0.42		
GUARDIAN REAL-TIME STARTER (Medtronic Minimed)				
device				
DEV, NA, ea	76300-0007-01	1606.80	999.00	
GUARDIAN REAL-TIME SYSTEM (Medtronic Minimed)				
glucose data management				
DEV, NA, ea	76300-0072-01	1432.80	1194.00	
GUARDIAN REAL-TIME SYSTEM PEDIATRIC (Medtronic Minimed)				
glucose data management				
DEV, NA, ea	76300-0072-02	1432.80	1194.00	
GUAVA FLAVOR (PCCA)				
flavoring aid				
POW, NA (NATURAL,GUAVA)				
1 gm	51927-3454-00	1.95		
SOL, NA (GUAVA)				
1 ml	51927-3137-00	0.90		
GUIADEX DM (Breckenridge Pharm)				
dm/k guai				
SOL, PO (AF,SF,ORANGE,PINEAPPLE)				
15 mg/5 ml-300 mg/5 ml,				
473 ml	51991-0087-16	36.45		
GUIADRINE DX LIQUID (Breckenridge Pharm)				
dextromethorphan hydrobromide/guaifenesin				
SOL, PO (1X473ML,AF,SF,GRAPE)				
25 mg/5 ml-225 mg/5 ml,				
473 ml	51991-0633-16	120.48		
GUIAFENESIN/PSE (Core)				
REPACK				
guaifenesin/pseudoephedrine hydrochloride				
TER, PO, 600 mg-120 mg,				
20s ea	33358-0163-20	15.58		
30s ea	33358-0163-30	18.84		
GUIAPHED (Consolidated Midland)				
eph hcl/gg/pb/theoph				
ELI, PO, 480 ml	00223-6513-01	15.50		
GUIAPLEX HC (Breckenridge Pharm)				
gg/hydrocod bit/phenyleph hcl				
SOL, PO (AF,SF,GRAPE)				
473 ml, C-III	51991-0444-16	58.62		
GUIATEX PE (Breckenridge Pharm)				
guaifenesin/phenylephrine hydrochloride				
SOL, PO (1X473ML,AF,SF)				
200 mg/5 ml-5 mg/5 ml,				
473 ml	51991-0597-16	87.01		
GUIATUSCON A.C. (Consolidated Midland)				
codeine phosphate/guaifenesin				
SYR, PO, 10 mg/5 ml-100 mg/5 ml,				
120 ml, C-V	00223-6515-01	2.85		
480 ml, C-V	00223-6515-02	8.50		
GUIATUSS AC (Pharma Pac)				
REPACK				
codeine phosphate/guaifenesin				
SYR, PO, 10 mg/5 ml-100 mg/5 ml,				
120 ml, C-V	52959-0169-03	6.50		
180 ml, C-V	52959-0169-05	7.95		
240 ml, C-V	52959-0169-06	10.95		
(Phys Total Care)				
REPACK				
SYR, PO, 10 mg/5 ml-100 mg/5 ml,				
120 ml, C-V	54868-0576-01	11.97		
240 ml, C-V	54868-0576-02	17.97		
(Physician Partner)				
REPACK				
SYR, PO, 10 mg/5 ml-100 mg/5 ml,				
120 ml, C-V	21695-0421-04	16.38		
(Quality Care Prod)				
REPACK				
SYR, PO, 10 mg/5 ml-100 mg/5 ml,				
120 ml, C-V	49999-0186-04	11.16		
(Southwood)				
REPACK				
SYR, PO, 10 mg/5 ml-100 mg/5 ml,				
120 ml, C-V	58016-0420-24	6.34		
GUIATUSS DAC (Altura)				
REPACK				
codeine phos/gg/pse hcl				
SYR, PO, 240 ml, C-V	63874-0210-24	24.06		
(Pharma Pac)				
REPACK				
SYR, PO, 120 ml, C-V	52959-0083-03	7.75		
480 ml, C-V	52959-0083-06	21.79		
(Quality Care Prod)				
REPACK				
SYR, PO, 480 ml, C-V	49999-0898-01	28.33		
GYMNEMA SYLVESTRE				
(PCCA) *See GYMNEMA SYLVESTRIS*				
GYMNEMA SYLVESTRIS (PCCA)				
gymnema sylvestre				
POW, NA, 1 gm	51927-3463-00	0.30		
GYNAZOLE-1 (Ther-RX)				
butoconazole nitrate				
CRE, VG (PREFILLED APPLICATOR)				
2%, 5.8 gm	64011-0001-08	69.67		
(A-S Medication)				
REPACK				
CRE, VG, 2%, 5.8 gm	54569-5452-00	54.45		
(Phys Total Care)				
REPACK				
CRE, VG, 2%, 5.8 gm	54868-4838-00	59.86		
GYNODIOL (Novavax)				
estradiol				
TAB, PO, 0.5 mg, 100s ea	66500-0768-01	27.34		AB
1 mg, 100s ea	66500-0259-01	36.69		AB
1.5 mg, 100s ea	66500-0158-01	52.35		
2 mg, 100s ea	66500-0748-01	53.25		AB
H-C TUSSIVE (Vintage)				
cpm/hydrocod bit/phenyleph hcl				
SYR, PO (AF,SF,ORANGE)				
480 ml, C-III	00254-9188-58	27.95		
H.P. ACTHAR (Questcor Pharm)				
corticotropin, repository				
GEL, IJ (M.D.V.)				
80 u/ml, 5 ml	63004-7731-01	29086.25		
HABITROL (Southwood)				
REPACK				
nicotine				
TDM, TD, 21 mg/24 hr,				
30s ea	58016-9323-01	149.38		AB
HAEMOPHILUS B CONJUGATE VAC/HEP B VAC RECOMBINANT				
(Merck) *See COMVAX*				
HAEMOPHILUS B CONJUGATE VACCINE				
(Glaxo) *See HIBERIX*				
(Merck) *See PEDVAXHIB*				
(Sanofi) *See ACTHIB*				
HALAZONE (PCCA)				
POW, NA, 1 gm	51927-2251-00	60.00		
HALCINONIDE				
(Ranbaxy Labs) *See HALOG*				
HALCION (Pfizer)				
triazolam				
TAB, PO (R.N.P.)				
0.25 mg,				
100s ea UD, C-IV	00009-0017-55	198.72	165.60	AB
(UNIT OF USE,10X10)				
0.25 mg,				
100s ea, C-IV	00009-0017-59	198.72	165.60	AB
(Phys Total Care)				
REPACK				
TAB, PO, 0.125 mg,				
30s ea, C-IV	54868-0828-01	40.04		AB
60s ea, C-IV	54868-0828-02	74.03		AB
0.25 mg,				
20s ea, C-IV	54868-0829-02	29.67		AB
30s ea, C-IV	54868-0829-01	43.61		AB
60s ea, C-IV	54868-0829-03	80.76		AB
100s ea, C-IV	54868-0829-04	132.80		AB
(Quality Care Prod)				
REPACK				
TAB, PO, 0.25 mg,				
10s ea, C-IV	49999-0175-10	33.66		
30s ea, C-IV	49999-0175-30	100.98		AB
60s ea, C-IV	49999-0175-60	201.96		AB
90s ea, C-IV	49999-0175-90	302.94		AB
HALDOL (Ortho-McNeil Pharm)				
haloperidol lactate				
SOL, IM (AMP)				
5 mg/ml, 1 ml 10s	00045-0255-01	133.98	111.65	AP
HALDOL DECANOATE (Ortho-McNeil Pharm)				
haloperidol decanoate				
SUS, IM (AMP)				
50 mg/ml, 1 ml 3s	00045-0253-03	169.61	141.34	AO
1 ml 10s	00045-0253-01	565.34	471.12	AO
100 mg/ml, 1 ml 5s	00045-0254-14	538.86	449.05	AO
(Phys Total Care)				
REPACK				
SUS, IM (AMP)				
50 mg/ml, 1 ml	54868-2889-01	42.03		AO
1 ml 3s	54868-2889-00	124.90		AO
HALFLYTELY & BISACODYL TABLETS BOWEL PREP (Braintree)				
KIT, PO (W/LEMON-LIME PACK)				
ea	52268-0522-01	58.39		
(WITH 3 FLAVOR PACKS)				
ea	52268-0521-01	58.39		
HALFLYTELY AND BISACODYL TABLET BOWEL PREP KIT (Braintree)				
KIT, PO (LEMON LIME)				
ea	52268-0502-01	51.01		
(W/3 FLAVOR PACKS)				
ea	52268-0520-01	51.01		
HALOBETASOL PROPIONATE				
FUL				
CRE, TP, 0.05%, 50 gm		24.00		
OIN, TP, 0.05%, 50 gm		26.63		
(Actavis Mid Atlantic)				
OIN, TP, 0.05%, 15 gm	00472-0261-15	32.54		AB
50 gm	00472-0261-50	78.26		AB
(Fougera)				
CRE, TP, 0.05%, 15 gm	00168-0355-15	31.49		AB
50 gm	00168-0355-50	75.72		AB
OIN, TP, 0.05%, 15 gm	00168-0356-15	31.49		AB
50 gm	00168-0356-50	75.72		AB
(G&W)				
OIN, TP, 0.05%, 15 gm	00713-0639-15	15.75		AB
50 gm	00713-0639-86	27.25		AB
(Perrigo)				
CRE, TP, 0.05%, 15 gm	45802-0129-35	31.65		AB
50 gm	45802-0129-32	76.10		AB
OIN, TP, 0.05%, 15 gm	45802-0131-35	31.65		AB
50 gm	45802-0131-32	76.10		AB
(Ranbaxy Labs) *See ULTRAVATE*				
(Taro)				
CRE, TP, 0.05%, 15 gm	51672-1321-01	31.49		AB
50 gm	51672-1321-03	75.72		AB
OIN, TP, 0.05%, 15 gm	51672-1322-01	31.49		AB
50 gm	51672-1322-03	75.72		AB
(A-S Medication)				
REPACK				
CRE, TP, 0.05%, 15 gm	54569-5783-00	31.65		
(Pharma Pac)				
REPACK				
OIN, TP (1X50GM)				
0.05%, 50 gm	52959-0961-50	74.59		AB
(Phys Total Care)				
REPACK				
CRE, TP, 0.05%, 50 gm	54868-4907-00	108.72		AB
OIN, TP, 0.05%, 15 gm	54868-5482-00	73.62		
(1X50GM)				
0.05%, 50 gm	54868-5482-01	107.22		
(Quality Care Prod)				
REPACK				
OIN, TP (1X15GM)				
0.05%, 15 gm	35356-0245-15	137.66		AB
HALOG (Ranbaxy Labs)				
halcinonide				
CRE, TP (1X30GM)				
0.1%, 30 gm	10631-0094-20	90.19		EE
(1X60GM,USP)				
0.1%, 60 gm	10631-0094-30	153.37		EE
(1X216GM)				
0.1%, 216 gm	10631-0094-76	460.10		EE
OIN, TP (1X30GM)				
0.1%, 30 gm	10631-0096-20	90.19		
(1X60GM)				
0.1%, 60 gm	10631-0096-30	153.37		
(Phys Total Care)				
REPACK				
CRE, TP, 0.1%, 15 gm	54868-1084-01	28.38		
30 gm	54868-1084-02	39.91		
60 gm	54868-1084-00	78.10		
(Quality Care Prod)				
REPACK				
OIN, TP (1X60GM)				
0.1%, 60 gm	35356-0228-60	180.57		

PROD/MFR	NDC	AWP	DP	OBC
HALOPERIDOL (Apotex Corp.)				
haloperidol lactate				
SOL, IM (PF)				
5 mg/ml, 1 ml 10s	60505-0727-03	76.00		AP
HALOPERIDOL (Consolidated Midland)				
TAB, PO, 0.5 mg, 100s ea	00223-1020-01	6.75		EE
1000s ea	00223-1020-02	42.50		EE
1 mg, 100s ea	00223-1021-01	7.95		EE
1000s ea	00223-1021-02	54.50		EE
2 mg, 100s ea	00223-1022-01	10.95		EE
1000s ea	00223-1022-02	72.50		EE
5 mg, 100s ea	00223-1023-01	16.00		EE
1000s ea	00223-1023-02	99.50		EE
10 mg, 100s ea	00223-1024-01	22.50		EE
1000s ea	00223-1024-02	175.00		EE
(Gallipot)				
POW, NA (U.S.P.)				
1 gm	51552-0519-01	21.28		
5 gm	51552-0519-02	45.50		
(Hawkins)				
POW, NA (U.S.P.,BASE)				
5 gm	63370-0102-15	144.00		
25 gm	63370-0102-25	576.00		
100 gm	63370-0102-35	2112.00		
(Letco)				
POW, NA (U.S.P.)				
1 gm	62991-2031-01	43.50		
5 gm	62991-2031-02	90.00		
10 gm	62991-2031-03	135.00		
25 gm	62991-2031-04	225.00		
(Major)				
TAB, PO (10X10)				
1 mg, 100s ea UD	00904-5923-61	43.16		AB
2 mg, 100s ea UD	00904-5924-61	59.12		AB
5 mg, 100s ea UD	00904-5925-61	92.62		AB
(Medisca)				
POW, NA (U.S.P.)				
1 gm	38779-0330-06	52.50		
5 gm	38779-0330-03	117.00		
10 gm	38779-0330-01	210.00		
25 gm	38779-0330-04	405.00		
100 gm	38779-0330-05	1425.00		
(Mylan)				
TAB, PO, 0.5 mg, 100s ea	00378-0351-01	24.80		AB
1000s ea	00378-0351-10	223.20		AB
1 mg, 100s ea	00378-0257-01	35.15		AB
1000s ea	00378-0257-10	351.50		AB
2 mg, 100s ea	00378-0214-01	48.15		AB
1000s ea	00378-0214-10	481.50		AB
5 mg, 100s ea	00378-0327-01	78.00		AB
1000s ea	00378-0327-10	780.00		AB
(USP)				
10 mg, 100s ea	00378-0334-01	143.45		
20 mg, 100s ea	00378-0335-01	275.70		
(PCCA)				
POW, NA (U.S.P.)				
1 gm	51927-1433-00	63.00		
(Sandoz)				
TAB, PO, 0.5 mg, 100s ea	00781-1391-01	23.59		AB
100s ea UD	00781-1391-13	29.49		AB
1 mg, 100s ea	00781-1392-01	35.18		AB
100s ea UD	00781-1392-13	45.43		AB
2 mg, 100s ea	00781-1393-01	48.15		AB
100s ea UD	00781-1393-13	60.19		AB
5 mg, 100s ea	00781-1396-01	77.99		AB
100s ea UD	00781-1396-13	97.49		AB
1000s ea	00781-1396-10	740.91		AB
10 mg, 100s ea	00781-1397-01	143.45		AB
100s ea UD	00781-1397-13	179.31		AB
20 mg, 100s ea	00781-1398-01	275.70		AB
(Spectrum Pharmacy)				
POW, NA (U.S.P.)				
5 gm	49452-3446-01	229.95		
25 gm	49452-3446-02	735.00		
(UDL)				
TAB, PO (10X10)				
0.5 mg, 100s ea UD	51079-0733-20	24.80		AB
1 mg, 100s ea UD	51079-0734-20	35.15		AB
2 mg, 100s ea UD	51079-0735-20	48.15		AB
5 mg, 100s ea UD	51079-0736-20	78.00		AB
(10X30,PUNCH CARDS,USP)				
5 mg, 300s ea UD	51079-0736-56	234.00		AB
(10X10,USP)				
10 mg, 100s ea UD	51079-0431-20	143.45		AB
(Zydus Pharm.)				
TAB, PO (USP)				
10 mg, 100s ea	68382-0080-01	143.45		AB
20 mg, 100s ea	68382-0081-01	275.70		AB
(American Health)				
REPACK				
TAB, PO (10X10)				
10 mg, 100s ea UD	68084-0249-01	174.53		AB
(3X10)				
20 mg, 30s ea UD	68084-0250-21	105.20		AB
(GSMS)				
REPACK				
TAB, PO (UNIT OF USE)				
1 mg, 60s ea	60429-0087-60	24.00	8.00	AB
2 mg, 60s ea	60429-0088-60	31.80	10.60	AB
90s ea	60429-0088-90	45.00	15.00	AB
5 mg, 60s ea	60429-0089-60	34.05	11.35	AB
10 mg, 60s ea	60429-0090-60	295.65	98.55	AB
90s ea	60429-0090-90	442.05	147.35	AB
(McKesson Packaging)				
REPACK				
TAB, PO (USP)				
1 mg, 100s ea UD	63739-0121-10	41.77		AB
5 mg, 100s ea UD	63739-0123-10	92.61		AB
(Nucare Pharm)				
REPACK				
TAB, PO, 0.5 mg, 30s ea	68071-0494-30	36.83		AB
2 mg, 30s ea	66267-0847-30	79.45		AB
(PD-Rx Pharm)				
REPACK				
TAB, PO (REDI-SCRIPT)				
1 mg, 15s ea	58864-0222-15	12.86		AB
2 mg, 42s ea	58864-0731-42	13.90		
(Phys Total Care)				
REPACK				
TAB, PO, 0.5 mg, 30s ea	54868-2570-01	11.19		EE
100s ea	54868-2570-00	25.35		EE
1 mg, 30s ea	54868-0091-01	15.15		EE
60s ea	54868-0091-03	25.80		AB
100s ea	54868-0091-02	39.94		EE
5 mg, 30s ea	54868-2296-02	20.55		EE
60s ea	54868-2296-03	36.60		AB
100s ea	54868-2296-00	56.49		EE
10 mg, 100s ea	54868-2306-00	20.12		EE
(Physician Partner)				
REPACK				
TAB, PO, 5 mg, 60s ea	21695-0653-60	93.60		
(Quality Care Prod)				
REPACK				
TAB, PO, 5 mg, 60s ea	35356-0095-60	41.06		
(Southwood)				
REPACK				
TAB, PO, 2 mg, 30s ea	58016-0029-30	14.45		EE
60s ea	58016-0029-60	28.89		EE
90s ea	58016-0029-90	43.34		EE
100s ea	58016-0029-00	48.15		EE
(Vibranta)				
REPACK				
TAB, PO, 2 mg, 30s ea	57866-3878-01	20.35		AB
5 mg, 30s ea	57866-3879-01	28.20		
10 mg, 30s ea	57866-3880-01	30.28		
60s ea	57866-3880-02	65.00		
20 mg, 30s ea	57866-3881-01	47.78		
HALOPERIDOL AMERINET CHOICE (APP)				
haloperidol lactate				
SOL, IM (VIAL)				
5 mg/ml, 1 ml	63323-0474-91	7.70		AP
(APP)				
haloperidol decanoate				
SUS, IM (VIAL,FLIP-TOP)				
50 mg/ml, 1 ml	63323-0469-51	28.80		
100 mg/ml, 1 ml	63323-0471-51	52.80		
(M.D.V.,FLIP-TOP)				
100 mg/ml, 5 ml	63323-0471-55	264.00		
HALOPERIDOL DECANOATE				
(Apotex Corp.) *See NOVAPLUS HALOPERIDOL DECANOATE*				
(Apotex Corp.)				
SUS, IM (M.D.V.)				
50 mg/ml, 5 ml	60505-0702-01	140.00		AO
100 mg/ml, 5 ml	60505-0703-01	247.25		AO
(APP) *See HALOPERIDOL AMERINET CHOICE*				
(APP)				
SUS, IM (VIAL)				
50 mg/ml, 1 ml	63323-0469-01	28.80		AO
(M.D.V.)				
50 mg/ml, 5 ml	63323-0469-05	144.00		AO
(VIAL)				
100 mg/ml, 1 ml	63323-0471-01	52.80		AO
(M.D.V.)				
100 mg/ml, 5 ml	63323-0471-05	264.00		AO
(Bedford)				
SOL, IM (S.D.V.)				
50 mg/ml, 1 ml 10s	55390-0412-01	55.20		AO
(M.D.V.)				
50 mg/ml, 5 ml	55390-0412-05	19.20		AO
(S.D.V.)				
100 mg/ml, 1 ml 10s	55390-0413-01	110.40		AO
(M.D.V.)				
100 mg/ml, 5 ml	55390-0413-05	48.00		AO
(Ortho-McNeil Pharm) *See HALDOL DECANOATE*				
(Teva)				
SUS, IM ((VIAL),10X1ML)				
50 mg/ml, 1 ml 10s	00703-7011-03	76.25		AO
(M.D.V.)				
50 mg/ml, 5 ml	00703-7013-01	31.88		AO
((VIAL),10X1ML)				
100 mg/ml, 1 ml 10s	00703-7021-03	72.00		AO
((M.D.V.),1X5ML)				
100 mg/ml, 5 ml	00703-7023-01	22.80		AO
HALOPERIDOL LACTATE				
FUL				
SOL, PO, 2 mg/ml, 120 ml		16.43		
(Apotex Corp.) *See HALOPERIDOL*				
(APP) *See HALOPERIDOL AMERINET CHOICE*				
(APP)				
SOL, IM (25X1ML)				
5 mg/ml, 1 ml 25s	63323-0474-01	192.50		AP
(M.D.V.)				
5 mg/ml, 10 ml	63323-0474-10	75.00		AP
(Bedford) *See HALOPERIDOL LACTATE NOVAPLUS*				
(Bedford)				
SOL, IM (S.D.V.)				
5 mg/ml, 1 ml 10s	55390-0147-10	25.80		AP
(M.D.V.)				
5 mg/ml, 10 ml	55390-0147-01	25.20		AP
(Consolidated Midland)				
SOL, PO, 2 mg/ml, 15 ml	00223-6525-15	7.75		EE
120 ml	00223-6525-04	32.00		EE
(Ortho-McNeil Pharm) *See HALDOL*				
(Pharm Assoc Inc)				
SOL, PO (AF,SF,DYE-FREE)				
2 mg/ml,				
5 ml 100s UD	00121-0581-05	373.34		AA
(W/DROPPER,AF,SF)				
2 mg/ml, 120 ml	00121-0581-04	42.30		AA
(Qualitest)				
SOL, PO, 2 mg/ml, 120 ml	00603-1290-54	32.75		AA
(Silarx)				
SOL, PO, 2 mg/ml, 120 ml	54838-0501-40	54.32		AA
(Teva)				
SOL, IM ((S.D.V.),10X1ML)				
5 mg/ml, 1 ml 10s	00703-7041-03	36.88		AP
((M.D.V.),1X10ML)				
5 mg/ml, 10 ml	00703-7045-01	76.25		AP
PO, 2 mg/ml, 15 ml	00093-9604-23	13.00		AA
120 ml	00093-9604-12	54.32		AA
(W/DROPPER)				
2 mg/ml, 120 ml	00182-6059-71	54.32		AA
(Phys Total Care)				
REPACK				
SOL, IM (S.D.V.)				
5 mg/ml, 1 ml 10s	54868-3459-00	32.10		EE
HALOPERIDOL LACTATE NOVAPLUS (Bedford)				
haloperidol lactate				
SOL, IM (S.D.V.)				
5 mg/ml, 1 ml 10s	55390-0447-10	13.20		AP
(M.D.V.)				
5 mg/ml, 10 ml	55390-0447-01	13.20		AP
HALOTHANE (Hospira)				
LIQ, IH, 99.9%, 250 ml 6s	00074-4894-02	358.06	313.32	AN
HALOTUSSIN AC (Axiom Pharmaceutical)				
codeine phosphate/guaifenesin				
SOL, PO (SF,CHERRY,RASPBERRY)				
10 mg/5 ml-100 mg/5 ml,				
118 ml, C-V	67870-0100-04	24.20		
473 ml, C-V	67870-0100-16	47.80		
3785 ml, C-V	67870-0100-28	79.75		
HALOTUSSIN DAC (Axiom Pharmaceutical)				
codeine phos/gg/pse hcl				
SOL, PO (SF,CHERRY,RASPBERRY)				
473 ml, C-V	67870-0101-16	18.80		

PROD/MFR	NDC	AWP	DP	OBC
HAVRIX (Glaxo)				
hepatitis a vaccine, inactivated				
SUS, IM (TIP-LOK,TAXINCL,PF)				
1440 el u/ml,				
1 ml 5s	**58160-0826-46**	377.85		
(SDV,TAXINCL,PF)				
1440 el u/ml,				
1 ml 10s	**58160-0826-11**	755.70		
(A-S Medication)				
REPACK				
SUS, IM (TIP-LOK SYR W/O NEEDLE)				
1440 el u/ml,				
1 ml 5s	**54569-5475-00**	359.61		
(Phys Total Care)				
REPACK				
SUS, IM, 1440 el u/ml,				
5 ml	**54868-4056-01**	400.78		
(1X10ML)				
1440 el u/ml,				
10 ml	**54868-4056-02**	751.59		
(Quality Care Prod)				
REPACK				
SUS, IM (S.D.V.)				
1440 el u/ml, 1 ml	**49999-0412-01**	79.80		
HAVRIX PEDIATRIC (Glaxo)				
hepatitis a vaccine, inactivated				
SUS, IM (S.D.V.)				
720 el u/0.5 ml,				
0.5 ml	**58160-0837-01**	34.34		
(0.5X10,TIP-LOK,PF)				
720 el u/0.5 ml,				
0.5 ml 10s	**58160-0825-51**	335.88		
(SDV,0.5MLX10,TAXINCL,PF)				
720 el u/0.5 ml,				
0.5 ml 10s	**58160-0825-11**	343.38		
(A-S Medication)				
REPACK				
SUS, IM (5X0.5ML)				
720 el u/0.5 ml,				
0.5 ml 5s	**54569-5888-00**	178.69		
HAWTHORN BERRY				
(PCCA) *See HAWTHORNE BERRY*				
HAWTHORNE BERRY (PCCA)				
hawthorn berry				
POW, NA (1X1GM)				
1 gm	**51927-3079-00**	0.33		
HC ACE/LIDO HCL/PSYLLIUM				
(Auriga) *See XYRALID RC*				
HC ACE/NEOMYCIN SULF/POLYMYXIN B SULF				
(Monarch) *See CORTISPORIN*				
HC TUSSIVE (Bryant Ranch)				
REPACK				
cpm/hydrocod bit/phenyleph hcl				
SYR, PO, 120 ml, C-III	**63629-1408-01**	9.78		
(DHS, Inc.)				
REPACK				
SYR, PO, 120 ml, C-III	**55887-0194-04**	17.95		
HC W/BACITRACIN-NEOMYCIN-POLYMYXIN				
(Consolidated Midland)				
bacitracin zn/hc/neomycin sulf/polymyxin b sulf				
OIN, OP, 3.75 gm	**00223-4111-03**	3.00		EE
HC/NEOMYCIN SULF/POLYMYXIN B SULF				
(Bausch & Lomb Inc.) *See HYDROCORTISONE/NEOMYCIN/POLYMYXIN B*				
(Consolidated Midland) *See HC/NEOMYCIN/POLYMYXIN*				
(Falcon Ophthalmics) *See HC/NEOMYCIN/POLYMYXIN*				
(Falcon Ophthalmics) *See HYDROCORTISONE/NEOMYCIN/POLYMYXIN B*				
(Major) *See CORTOMYCIN*				
(Monarch) *See CORTISPORIN*				
(Paddock) *See NEOMYCIN/POLYMYXIN B SULFATES/HYDROCORTISONE*				
(Palmetto)				
REPACK				
SOL, OT, 1%-0.35%-10000 u/ml,				
10 ml	**23490-6859-01**	52.22		
SUS, OT, 1%-0.35%-10000 u/ml,				
10 ml	**23490-6860-01**	35.00		
HC/NEOMYCIN/POLYMYXIN (Consolidated Midland)				
hc/neomycin sulf/polymyxin b sulf				
SOL, OT, 1%-0.35%-10000 u/ml,				
10 ml	**00223-6750-10**	4.00		EE
SUS, OT, 1%-0.35%-10000 u/ml,				
10 ml	**00223-6751-10**	4.50		EE

PROD/MFR	NDC	AWP	DP	OBC
(Falcon Ophthalmics)				
SOL, OT, 1%-0.35%-10000 u/ml,				
10 ml	**61314-0646-10**	30.80		AT
SUS, OT (1X10ML,USP)				
1%-0.35%-10000 u/ml,				
10 ml	**61314-0645-11**	18.16		AT
(Altura)				
REPACK				
SOL, OT, 1%-0.35%-10000 u/ml,				
10 ml	**63874-0141-10**	32.24		AT
SUS, OT, 1%-0.35%-10000 u/ml,				
10 ml	**63874-0135-10**	31.20		EE
(DHS, Inc.)				
REPACK				
SOL, OT, 1%-0.35%-10000 u/ml,				
10 ml	**55887-0905-10**	52.22		AT
(Nucare Pharm)				
REPACK				
SOL, OT, 1%-0.35%-10000 u/ml,				
10 ml	**66267-0954-10**	20.58		EE
(Pharma Pac)				
REPACK				
SOL, OT, 1%-0.35%-10000 u/ml,				
10 ml	**52959-0098-00**	35.88		EE
10 ml	**52959-0098-10**	73.27		EE
SUS, OT, 1%-0.35%-10000 u/ml,				
10 ml	**52959-0084-00**	35.88		EE
(Phys Total Care)				
REPACK				
SUS, OP, 1%-0.35%-10000 u/ml,				
7.5 ml	**54868-3250-01**	235.89		EE
(Southwood)				
REPACK				
SOL, OT, 1%-0.35%-10000 u/ml,				
10 ml	**58016-6087-01**	35.00		EE
SUS, OT, 1%-0.35%-10000 u/ml,				
10 ml	**58016-6091-01**	35.00		EE
HCTZ-METOPROLOL (Mylan)				
hydrochlorothiazide/metoprolol tartrate				
TAB, PO, 25 mg-50 mg,				
100s ea	**00378-0424-01**	113.40		
25 mg-100 mg,				
100s ea	**00378-0434-01**	177.25		
50 mg-100 mg,				
100s ea	**00378-0445-01**	187.95		
(Phys Total Care)				
REPACK				
TAB, PO, 25 mg-50 mg,				
10s ea	**54868-5400-01**	39.84		
30s ea	**54868-5400-00**	85.59		
HCTZ/LISINOPRIL (Apotex Corp.)				
hydrochlorothiazide/lisinopril				
TAB, PO, 12.5 mg-10 mg,				
100s ea	**60505-0205-03**	111.00		
18000s ea	**60505-0205-07**	19980.00		
12.5 mg-20 mg,				
100s ea	**60505-0206-03**	121.15		
17000s ea	**60505-0206-07**	20595.50		
25 mg-20 mg,				
100s ea	**60505-0207-03**	121.60		
15600s ea	**60505-0207-07**	18969.60		
(Mylan)				
TAB, PO, 12.5 mg-10 mg,				
100s ea	**00378-1012-01**	110.90		AB
12.5 mg-20 mg,				
100s ea	**00378-2012-01**	120.05		AB
25 mg-20 mg,				
100s ea	**00378-2025-01**	121.50		AB
(Ranbaxy Pharm)				
TAB, PO, 12.5 mg-10 mg,				
100s ea	**63304-0536-01**	46.62		AB
500s ea	**63304-0536-05**	552.25		AB
12.5 mg-20 mg,				
100s ea	**63304-0537-01**	48.88		AB
500s ea	**63304-0537-05**	598.00		AB
25 mg-20 mg,				
100s ea	**63304-0538-01**	49.46		AB
500s ea	**63304-0538-05**	607.00		AB
(Sandoz)				
TAB, PO, 12.5 mg-10 mg,				
100s ea	**00185-7100-01**	111.00		AB
100s ea	**00781-1848-01**	112.04		AB
1000s ea	**00185-7100-10**	1109.97		AB
12.5 mg-20 mg,				
100s ea	**00185-0152-01**	120.15		AB
100s ea	**00781-1176-01**	121.28		AB
1000s ea	**00185-0152-10**	1201.50		AB

PROD/MFR	NDC	AWP	DP	OBC
25 mg-20 mg,				
100s ea	**00185-0173-01**	121.60		AB
100s ea	**00781-1178-01**	122.75		AB
1000s ea	**00185-0173-10**	1215.99		AB
(Teva)				
TAB, PO, 12.5 mg-10 mg,				
100s ea	**00172-5033-60**	110.40		AB
(10X10)				
12.5 mg-10 mg,				
100s ea UD	**00172-5033-10**	112.40		AB
500s ea	**00172-5033-70**	540.85		AB
12.5 mg-20 mg,				
100s ea	**00172-5034-60**	119.50		AB
(10X10)				
12.5 mg-20 mg,				
100s ea UD	**00172-5034-10**	121.50		AB
500s ea	**00172-5034-70**	585.45		AB
25 mg-20 mg,				
100s ea	**00172-5032-60**	120.90		AB
(10X10)				
25 mg-20 mg,				
100s ea UD	**00172-5032-10**	122.90		AB
500s ea	**00172-5032-70**	592.55		AB
(Watson Labs)				
TAB, PO, 12.5 mg-10 mg,				
100s ea	**00591-0860-01**	18.65		AB
500s ea	**00591-0860-05**	88.58		AB
12.5 mg-20 mg,				
100s ea	**00591-0861-01**	20.18		AB
500s ea	**00591-0861-05**	95.86		AB
25 mg-20 mg,				
100s ea	**00591-0862-01**	20.44		AB
500s ea	**00591-0862-05**	97.06		AB
(West-Ward)				
TAB, PO, 12.5 mg-10 mg,				
100s ea	**00143-1262-01**	110.50	72.50	AB
1000s ea	**00143-1262-10**	1060.25	165.10	AB
12.5 mg-20 mg,				
100s ea	**00143-1263-01**	119.75	78.80	AB
1000s ea	**00143-1263-10**	1160.25	177.50	AB
25 mg-20 mg,				
100s ea	**00143-1264-01**	120.95	81.00	AB
1000s ea	**00143-1264-10**	1180.25	180.00	AB
(A-S Medication)				
REPACK				
TAB, PO, 12.5 mg-10 mg,				
30s ea	**54569-6091-00**	46.54		AB
12.5 mg-20 mg,				
30s ea	**54569-6092-00**	50.42		AB
(DHS, Inc.)				
REPACK				
TAB, PO, 12.5 mg-10 mg,				
30s ea	**55887-0425-30**	21.44		AB
60s ea	**55887-0425-60**	40.69		AB
90s ea	**55887-0425-90**	59.42		AB
12.5 mg-20 mg,				
30s ea	**55887-0426-30**	24.90		AB
60s ea	**55887-0426-60**	46.00		AB
90s ea	**55887-0426-90**	60.00		AB
(Dispensing Solutions)				
REPACK				
TAB, PO, 12.5 mg-10 mg,				
30s ea	**66336-0572-30**	36.50		AB
12.5 mg-20 mg,				
30s ea	**66336-0805-30**	38.27		AB
90s ea	**66336-0805-90**	114.82		AB
25 mg-20 mg,				
30s ea	**66336-0810-30**	40.13		AB
90s ea	**66336-0810-90**	120.38		AB
(PD-Rx Pharm)				
REPACK				
TAB, PO, 12.5 mg-10 mg,				
30s ea	**43063-0118-30**	17.70		AB
90s ea	**43063-0118-90**	26.80		AB
12.5 mg-20 mg,				
30s ea	**43063-0065-30**	18.00		AB
(USP)				
12.5 mg-20 mg,				
90s ea	**43063-0065-90**	28.60		AB
25 mg-20 mg,				
30s ea	**55289-0878-30**	18.18		AB
90s ea	**43063-0130-90**	34.00		AB
(Pharma Pac)				
REPACK				
TAB, PO, 25 mg-20 mg,				
30s ea	**52959-0997-30**	44.55		AB

PROD/MFR	NDC	AWP	DP	OBC
(Phys Total Care)				
REPACK				
TAB, PO, 12.5 mg-10 mg,				
30s ea	**54868-4977-01**	14.13		**AB**
90s ea	**54868-4977-02**	33.36		
100s ea	**54868-4977-00**	35.07		**AB**
12.5 mg-20 mg,				
30s ea	**54868-4637-00**	17.07		**AB**
60s ea	**54868-4637-02**	31.17		**AB**
90s ea	**54868-4637-03**	31.04		**AB**
100s ea	**54868-4637-01**	48.45		**AB**
180s ea	**54868-4637-04**	57.51		**AB**
25 mg-20 mg,				
30s ea	**54868-4785-00**	19.20		**AB**
60s ea	**54868-4785-01**	35.40		**AB**
(Physician Partner)				
REPACK				
TAB, PO, 12.5 mg-10 mg,				
30s ea	**21695-0733-30**	66.27		**AB**
12.5 mg-20 mg,				
30s ea	**21695-0734-30**	71.76		**AB**
(Quality Care Prod)				
REPACK				
TAB, PO, 25 mg-20 mg,				
30s ea	**49999-0321-30**	29.51		**AB**
100s ea	**49999-0321-00**	98.37		**AB**
(Southwood)				
REPACK				
TAB, PO, 12.5 mg-20 mg,				
30s ea	**58016-0228-30**	36.99		**AB**
60s ea	**58016-0228-60**	73.99		**AB**
90s ea	**58016-0228-90**	110.98		**AB**
100s ea	**58016-0228-00**	123.31		**AB**
120s ea	**58016-0228-02**	147.97		**AB**
HCTZ/METHYLDOPA (Consolidated Midland)				
hydrochlorothiazide/methyldopa				
TAB, PO, 15 mg-250 mg,				
100s ea	**00223-1587-01**	27.00		**EE**
500s ea	**00223-1587-05**	107.50		**EE**
1000s ea	**00223-1587-02**	212.50		**EE**
25 mg-250 mg,				
100s ea	**00223-1588-01**	25.00		**EE**
500s ea	**00223-1588-05**	122.50		**EE**
1000s ea	**00223-1588-02**	240.00		**EE**
30 mg-500 mg,				
100s ea	**00223-1589-01**	42.75		**EE**
500s ea	**00223-1589-05**	197.50		**EE**
(Mylan)				
TAB, PO, 15 mg-250 mg,				
100s ea	**00378-0507-01**	51.45		**AB**
25 mg-250 mg,				
100s ea	**00378-0711-01**	57.70		**AB**
1000s ea	**00378-0711-10**	564.90		**AB**
(Phys Total Care)				
REPACK				
TAB, PO, 25 mg-250 mg,				
100s ea	**54868-1310-01**	82.50		**EE**
(Quality Care Prod)				
REPACK				
TAB, PO, 25 mg-250 mg,				
60s ea	**49999-0082-60**	17.96		**AB**
HCTZ/PROPRANOLOL (Mylan)				
hydrochlorothiazide/propranolol hydrochloride				
TAB, PO, 25 mg-40 mg,				
100s ea	**00378-0731-01**	53.26		**AB**
25 mg-80 mg,				
100s ea	**00378-0347-01**	65.41		**AB**
HCTZ/QUINAPRIL (Phys Total Care)				
REPACK				
hydrochlorothiazide/quinapril hydrochloride				
TAB, PO, 25 mg-20 mg,				
30s ea	**54868-5475-00**	90.36		
HCTZ/SPIRONOLACTONE (Greenstone)				
hydrochlorothiazide/spironolactone				
TAB, PO, 25 mg-25 mg,				
100s ea	**59762-5014-01**	50.48		**AB**
(Mutual)				
TAB, PO, 25 mg-25 mg,				
100s ea	**53489-0144-01**	50.40		**AB**
500s ea	**53489-0144-05**	239.40		**AB**
1000s ea	**53489-0144-10**	454.86		**AB**
(Mylan)				
TAB, PO, 25 mg-25 mg,				
100s ea	**00378-0141-01**	50.40		**AB**
500s ea	**00378-0141-05**	239.40		**AB**
(UDL)				
TAB, PO (10X10)				
25 mg-25 mg,				
100s ea UD	**51079-0104-20**	46.04		**AB**
(A-S Medication)				
REPACK				
TAB, PO, 25 mg-25 mg,				
30s ea	**54569-0502-00**	15.14		**EE**
(Dispensing Solutions)				
REPACK				
TAB, PO, 25 mg-25 mg,				
14s ea	**66336-0984-14**	8.40		**AB**
28s ea	**66336-0984-28**	16.80		**AB**
(PD-Rx Pharm)				
REPACK				
TAB, PO, 25 mg-25 mg,				
30s ea	**58864-0785-30**	29.41		**AB**
(Phys Total Care)				
REPACK				
TAB, PO, 25 mg-25 mg,				
30s ea	**54868-0699-02**	29.55		**EE**
100s ea	**54868-0699-01**	88.05		**EE**
(Vibranta)				
REPACK				
TAB, PO, 25 mg-25 mg,				
30s ea	**57866-6111-01**	18.89		
HCTZ/TRIAMTERENE (Mylan)				
hydrochlorothiazide/triamterene				
CAP, PO, 25 mg-37.5 mg,				
100s ea	**00378-2537-01**	39.40		**AB**
1000s ea	**00378-2537-10**	382.20		**AB**
TAB, PO, 25 mg-37.5 mg,				
100s ea	**00378-1352-01**	35.70		**AB**
500s ea	**00378-1352-05**	176.30		**AB**
50 mg-75 mg,				
100s ea	**00378-1355-01**	88.70		**AB**
500s ea	**00378-1355-05**	430.20		**AB**
(Sandoz)				
CAP, PO, 25 mg-37.5 mg,				
100s ea	**00781-2074-01**	37.53		**AB**
1000s ea	**00781-2074-10**	360.68		**AB**
25 mg-50 mg,				
100s ea	**00781-2715-01**	207.68		**AB**
TAB, PO, 25 mg-37.5 mg,				
100s ea	**00781-1123-01**	33.95		**AB**
500s ea	**00781-1123-05**	161.26		**AB**
50 mg-75 mg,				
100s ea	**00781-1008-01**	88.70		**AB**
500s ea	**00781-1008-05**	430.20		**AB**
(Teva)				
CAP, PO, 25 mg-37.5 mg,				
1000s ea	**00555-0488-05**	360.68		**AB**
(UDL)				
CAP, PO (10X10)				
25 mg-37.5 mg,				
100s ea UD	**51079-0935-20**	45.20		**AB**
TAB, PO, 50 mg-75 mg,				
100s ea UD	**51079-0433-20**	91.36		**AB**
(Watson Labs)				
TAB, PO, 25 mg-37.5 mg,				
100s ea	**00591-0424-01**	35.70		**AB**
500s ea	**00591-0424-05**	176.30		**AB**
50 mg-75 mg,				
100s ea	**00591-0348-01**	91.68		**AB**
500s ea	**00591-0348-05**	468.92		**AB**
1000s ea	**00591-0348-10**	673.62		**AB**
(A-S Medication)				
REPACK				
CAP, PO, 25 mg-37.5 mg,				
30s ea	**54569-3967-00**	11.45		**EE**
100s ea	**54569-3967-01**	38.15		**EE**
25 mg-50 mg,				
30s ea	**54569-0543-01**	17.51		**AB**
TAB, PO, 50 mg-75 mg,				
14s ea	**54569-2545-04**	12.83		**EE**
30s ea	**54569-2545-00**	27.49		**EE**
100s ea	**54569-2545-02**	91.63		**EE**
(Dispensing Solutions)				
REPACK				
CAP, PO, 25 mg-50 mg,				
30s ea	**66336-0771-30**	21.00		**AB**
100s ea	**55045-1216-01**	75.00		**AB**
TAB, PO, 25 mg-37.5 mg,				
30s ea	**55045-2958-08**	12.00		**AB**
30s ea	**66336-0790-30**	19.04		**AB**
60s ea	**55045-2958-06**	24.00		**AB**
90s ea	**66336-0790-90**	38.09		**AB**
100s ea	**55045-2958-01**	40.00		**AB**
50 mg-75 mg,				
30s ea	**55045-1901-08**	22.50		**AB**
30s ea	**66336-0704-30**	42.71		**AB**
(GSMS)				
REPACK				
CAP, PO (UNIT OF USE)				
25 mg-50 mg,				
30s ea	**60429-0190-30**	7.65	2.55	**AB**
TAB, PO, 50 mg-75 mg,				
30s ea	**60429-0191-30**	8.10	2.70	**AB**
45s ea	**60429-0191-45**	8.40	2.80	**AB**
90s ea	**60429-0191-90**	19.35	6.45	**AB**
(PD-Rx Pharm)				
REPACK				
CAP, PO (REDI-SCRIPT)				
25 mg-37.5 mg,				
30s ea	**58864-0766-30**	10.96		**AB**
25 mg-50 mg,				
30s ea	**55289-0725-30**	26.07		**AB**
TAB, PO, 25 mg-37.5 mg,				
30s ea	**55289-0090-30**	10.97		**AB**
90s ea	**55289-0090-90**	25.50		**AB**
50 mg-75 mg,				
15s ea	**55289-0488-15**	7.42		**AB**
30s ea	**55289-0488-30**	7.67		**AB**
100s ea	**55289-0488-01**	13.22		**AB**
(Pharma Pac)				
REPACK				
CAP, PO, 25 mg-50 mg,				
30s ea	**52959-0719-30**	19.49		**EE**
90s ea	**52959-0719-90**	46.20		**EE**
(Phys Total Care)				
REPACK				
CAP, PO, 25 mg-37.5 mg,				
30s ea	**54868-5113-01**	10.16		**AB**
100s ea	**54868-5113-00**	20.64		**AB**
25 mg-50 mg,				
10s ea	**54868-0932-07**	34.74		**EE**
30s ea	**54868-0932-01**	118.76		**EE**
60s ea	**54868-0932-06**	178.46		**EE**
100s ea	**54868-0932-04**	291.94		**EE**
TAB, PO, 25 mg-37.5 mg,				
10s ea	**54868-2679-00**	6.09		**EE**
30s ea	**54868-2679-02**	9.30		**EE**
60s ea	**54868-2679-04**	14.07		**EE**
(USP)				
25 mg-37.5 mg,				
90s ea	**54868-2679-05**	18.87		**EE**
100s ea	**54868-2679-01**	20.46		**EE**
500s ea	**54868-2679-03**	66.27		**EE**
50 mg-75 mg,				
15s ea	**54868-1866-03**	6.66		**EE**
30s ea	**54868-1866-01**	8.82		**EE**
60s ea	**54868-1866-04**	13.11		**EE**
100s ea	**54868-1866-02**	18.84		**EE**
500s ea	**54868-1866-06**	76.14		**EE**
(Physician Partner)				
REPACK				
CAP, PO, 25 mg-37.5 mg,				
90s ea	**21695-0839-90**	67.55		**AB**
TAB, PO, 25 mg-37.5 mg,				
30s ea	**21695-0496-30**	21.42		**AB**
90s ea	**21695-0496-90**	64.26		**AB**
(Quality Care Prod)				
REPACK				
CAP, PO, 25 mg-37.5 mg,				
30s ea	**49999-0066-30**	17.80		**AB**
100s ea	**49999-0066-00**	98.02		**AB**
TAB, PO, 50 mg-75 mg,				
30s ea	**49999-0094-30**	29.40		**AB**
60s ea	**49999-0094-60**	58.81		**EE**
100s ea	**49999-0094-00**	99.00		**EE**
(Southwood)				
REPACK				
CAP, PO, 25 mg-37.5 mg,				
30s ea	**58016-0394-30**	26.40		**AB**
60s ea	**58016-0394-60**	52.80		**AB**
90s ea	**58016-0394-90**	79.20		**AB**
100s ea	**58016-0394-00**	88.00		**AB**
25 mg-50 mg,				
12s ea	**58016-0520-12**	9.61		**EE**
15s ea	**58016-0520-15**	12.02		**EE**
20s ea	**58016-0520-20**	16.02		**EE**
30s ea	**58016-0520-30**	24.03		**EE**
60s ea	**58016-0520-60**	48.06		**EE**
100s ea	**58016-0520-00**	80.10		**EE**
120s ea	**58016-0520-99**	96.12		**EE**
TAB, PO, 25 mg-37.5 mg,				
ea	**58016-0368-15**	6.18		**EE**
30s ea	**58016-0368-30**	12.37		**EE**

PROD/MFR | NDC | AWP | DP | OBC

60s ea............58016-0368-60 24.75 EE
100s ea...........58016-0368-00 41.26 EE
50 mg-75 mg,
15s ea............58016-0545-15 12.50 EE
20s ea............58016-0545-20 16.50 EE
30s ea............58016-0545-30 24.50 EE
50s ea............58016-0545-50 41.25 EE
100s ea...........58016-0545-00 82.50 EE

(Vibranta)
REPACK
CAP, PO, 25 mg-37.5 mg,
30s ea............57866-6809-01 34.50
TAB, PO, 50 mg-75 mg,
15s ea............57866-6811-02 17.33 AB
30s ea............57866-6811-01 61.60 AB

HECTOROL (Genzyme)
doxercalciferol
CAP, PO (SOFT GELATIN)
0.5 mcg, 50s ea......58468-0120-01 372.08 310.07 EE
(SOFTGEL)
1 mcg, 50s ea........58468-0124-01 744.16 620.13
(SOFT GELATIN)
2.5 mcg, 50s ea......58468-0121-01 1293.06 1077.55
SOL, IV (50X2ML)
2 mcg/ml, 2 ml 50s...58468-0122-01 1496.40 1247.00
2 ml 50s..........58468-0123-01 1639.20 1366.00

HELIDAC THERAPY (Prometheus Labs)
bi subsalicylate/metronidazole/tetracycline hcl
KIT, PO, 262.4 mg-250 mg-500 mg,
56s ea............65483-0495-14 373.55

HELIXATE FS (CSL)
ahf viii (recombinant) sucrose formulated
PDS, IV (1000IU,SINGLE-USE,PF)
1 iu, ea............00053-8133-02 1.56
(2000IU,SINGLE-USE,PF)
1 iu, ea............00053-8134-02 1.56
(2000IU,ULTRA HIGH,PF)
1 iu, ea............00053-8130-05 1.44
(250IU,SINGLE-USE,PF)
1 iu, ea............00053-8131-02 1.56
(3000IU,PF)
1 iu, ea............00053-8135-02 1.56
(500IU,SINGLE-USE,PF)
1 iu, ea............00053-8132-02 1.56

(CSL)
antihemophilic factor viii (recombinant)
(APPROX. 1000 IU/VIAL)
1 iu, ea............00053-8130-04 1.44
(APPROX. 250 IU/VIAL)
1 iu, ea............00053-8130-01 1.44
(APPROX. 500 IU/VIAL)
1 iu, ea............00053-8130-02 1.44

HEMABATE (Pfizer)
carboprost tromethamine
SOL, IM (AMP,10X1ML)
250 mcg/ml,
1 ml 10s..........00009-0856-08 1113.73 928.11

HEMATINIC PLUS COMPLEX (Phys Total Care)
REPACK
multivitamin, minerals, and iron
TAB, PO, 60s ea..........54868-5532-00 75.09

HEMATINIC PLUS VITAMINS & MINERALS (Cypress Pharm)
multivitamin, minerals, and iron
TAB, PO (CAPLET)
100s ea............60258-0180-01 37.59

HEMATINIC W/FOLIC ACID (Cypress Pharm)
ferrous fumarate/folic acid
TAB, PO (PRENATAL)
324 mg-1 mg,
100s ea............60258-0181-01 21.48

HEMATOPORPHYRIN (PCCA)
POW, NA (1X1GM)
1 gm..............51927-2881-00 177.00

HEMATOXYLIN (PCCA)
POW, NA, 1 gm..........51927-3059-00 9.60

HEMATRON (Seyer Pharmatec)
cyanocobalamin/folic acid/iron
LIQ, PO (DROPS)
30 ml..............11026-2747-01 13.20

(Seyer Pharmatec)
multivitamin and minerals
237 ml............11026-2746-08 25.80

HEMATRON-AF (Seyer Pharmatec)
multivitamin, minerals, and iron
TER, PO (LAYERED CAPLET)
90s ea UD..........11026-2755-09 74.40

HEMAX (Pronova)
biotin/cu/dss/fe/folic acid/vit b12/vit c/vit e
TAB, PO (LAYERED CAPLET)
90s ea..............67555-0135-90 68.75

HEMIN
(Lundbeck) *See PANHEMATIN*

HEMLOCK OIL (Medisca)
OIL, NA (SPRUCE,CONIUM FRUIT)
14 ml..............38779-1335-03 16.50
25 ml..............38779-1335-04 28.50
100 ml.............38779-1335-05 61.50
500 ml.............38779-1335-08 214.50

(PCCA)
OIL, NA (SPRUCE)
1 ml..............51927-2626-00 1.20

HEMOCYTE PLUS (U.S. Pharm)
multivitamin and minerals
CAP, PO, 30s ea UD.......52747-0800-30 16.74
100s ea UD..........52747-0800-60 55.77

(Phys Total Care)
REPACK
CAP, PO, 30s ea..........54868-3223-00 21.07

HEMOCYTE-F (U.S. Pharm)
ferrous fumarate/folic acid
TAB, PO (CHILD PROOF PACKAGING)
324 mg-1 mg,
30s ea............52747-0306-30 9.99
(10X10)
324 mg-1 mg,
100s ea UD........52747-0306-70 33.26

(Phys Total Care)
REPACK
TAB, PO, 324 mg-1 mg,
30s ea............54868-3788-00 7.01

HEMOFIL M (Baxter Bioscience)
antihemophilic factor viii:c human
PDS, IV (1000IU)
1 iu, ea............00944-2932-01 1.34
(1700IU)
1 iu, ea............00944-2933-01 1.34
(250IU)
1 iu, ea............00944-2930-01 1.34
(500IU)
1 iu, ea............00944-2931-01 1.34

HEMOPLEX F (Contract Pharmacal)
ferrous fumarate/folic acid
TAB, PO, 106 mg-1 mg,
100s ea............10267-1327-01 16.00

HEMOPLEX PLUS (Contract Pharmacal)
multivitamin, minerals, and iron
TAB, PO (10X10, CHILD PROOF PKG)
100s ea UD..........10267-1325-01 22.00

HEMORRHOIDAL HC (Actavis Mid Atlantic)
hydrocortisone acetate
SUP, RC, 25 mg, 12s ea...00472-0511-12 11.25
24s ea............00472-0511-24 21.50

(Consolidated Midland)
SUP, RC, 25 mg, 12s ea...00223-5555-12 10.95
100s ea............00223-5555-01 89.50

(A-S Medication)
REPACK
SUP, RC, 25 mg, 12s ea...54569-2586-00 10.86

HEMRIL-30 (Upsher-Smith)
hydrocortisone acetate
SUP, RC, 30 mg, 12s ea...00245-0112-12 75.44
24s ea............00245-0112-24 141.45

HEP A VAC, INACTIVATED/
HEP B VAC RECOMBINANT
(Glaxo) *See TWINRIX*

HEP-LOCK (Baxter)
heparin sodium
SOL, IV (MDV)
100 u/ml, 10 ml......00641-2436-41 0.80 AP
(M.D.V.)
100 u/ml,
10 ml 25s..........00641-2436-45 20.10 AP

(Phys Total Care)
REPACK
SOL, IV (VIAL,DOSETTE)
100 u/ml, 1 ml 25s...54868-2526-00 15.26 AP

HEP-LOCK U/P (Phys Total Care)
heparin sodium
SOL, IV (VIAL,DOSETTE,PF)
100 u/ml, 1 ml 25s...54868-3615-00 16.93 AP

HEPAGAM B (Apotex Corp.)
hepatitis b immune globulin
SOL, IM (SDV,PF)
1 ml..............60492-0052-01 182.80
5 ml..............60492-0051-01 800.00

HEPARIN LOCK FLUSH (AMSINO)
heparin sodium
SOL, IV (IN 3ML SD SYRINGE,PF)
10 u/ml,
2.5 ml 180s........68883-0010-06 522.00
(IN 6ML SD SYRINGE,PF)
10 u/ml, 3 ml 180s...68883-0010-03 556.20
(IN 12ML SD SYRINGE,PF)
10 u/ml, 5 ml 180s...68883-0010-05 703.80
100 u/ml,
3 ml 180s..........68883-0100-04 628.20
(IN 6ML SD SYRINGE,PF)
100 u/ml,
3 ml 180s..........68883-0100-03 556.20
(IN 12ML SD SYRINGE,PF)
100 u/ml,
5 ml 180s..........68883-0100-05 703.80
(IN 6ML SD SYRINGE,PF)
100 u/ml,
5 ml 180s..........68883-0100-06 646.20

(APP)
SOL, IV (M.D.V.,P.C.)
10 u/ml, 1 ml 25s....63323-0544-01 50.31 AP
(M.D.V.)
10 u/ml, 10 ml 25s...63323-0544-11 52.18 AP
(M.D.V.,P.C.)
100 u/ml, 1 ml 25s...63323-0545-01 50.31 AP
(M.D.V.)
100 u/ml, 5 ml 25s...63323-0545-05 62.18 AP

(BD Dickinson Hosp Prod)
SOL, IV (3ML SRN, 30X2ML)
10 u/ml, 2 ml 30s....08290-0340-02 19.05 EE
(10ML SRN, 3X30ML)
10 u/ml, 3 ml 30s....08290-0360-03 20.10 EE
(3ML SRN,30X3ML)
10 u/ml, 3 ml 30s....08290-0340-03 20.10 EE
(10ML SRN W/CANNULA)
10 u/ml, 5 ml 30s....08290-0361-05 27.83 EE
(10ML SRN,30X5ML)
10 u/ml, 5 ml 30s....08290-0360-05 21.23 EE
(5ML SRN,30X5ML)
10 u/ml, 5 ml 30s....08290-0350-05 20.10 EE
(10ML SRN, 30X6ML)
10 u/ml, 6 ml 30s....08290-0360-06 21.23 EE
(3ML SRN,30X2ML)
100 u/ml, 2 ml 30s...08290-0370-02 19.05 EE
(10ML SRN,30X3ML)
100 u/ml, 3 ml 30s...08290-0390-03 21.23 EE
(3 ML SRN,30X3ML)
100 u/ml, 3 ml 30s...08290-0370-03 19.05 EE
(5ML SRN,30X3ML)
100 u/ml, 3 ml 30s...08290-0380-03 20.10 EE
(10ML SRN W/CANNULA)
100 u/ml, 5 ml 30s...08290-0391-05 27.83 EE
(10ML SRN,30X5ML)
100 u/ml, 5 ml 30s...08290-0390-05 21.23 EE
(5ML SRN,30X5ML)
100 u/ml, 5 ml 30s...08290-0380-05 20.10 EE

(Consolidated Midland)
SOL, IV (VIAL, DOSETTE)
10 u/ml, 1 ml 25s....00223-7861-01 37.50 EE
2 ml 25s..........00223-7863-02 25.00 EE
100 u/ml, 1 ml 25s...00223-7865-01 13.75 EE
2 ml 25s..........00223-7867-02 20.00 EE

(Deen Pre-Fld Syr LLC)
SOL, IV (6ML W/CANNULA)
10 u/ml, 3 ml........08450-6034-03 3.84 3.20
(6ML,PRE-FILLED SYRINGE)
10 u/ml, 3 ml........08450-6026-03 3.05 2.54
(12ML W/CANNULA)
10 u/ml, 5 ml........08450-6037-05 4.10 3.42
(12ML,PRE-FILLED SYRINGE)
10 u/ml, 5 ml........08450-6030-05 3.30 2.75
100 u/ml, 3 ml.......08450-6049-03 3.30 2.75
(6ML W/CANNULA)
100 u/ml, 3 ml.......08450-6055-03 3.84 3.20
(6ML,PRE-FILLED SYRINGE)
100 u/ml, 3 ml.......08450-6046-03 3.05 2.54
(12ML W/CANNULA)
100 u/ml, 5 ml.......08450-6058-05 4.10 3.42
(12ML,PRE-FILLED SYRINGE)
100 u/ml, 5 ml.......08450-6050-05 3.30 2.75

(Excelsior)
SOL, IV (1X3ML,LATEX-FREE)
1 u/ml, 3 ml.........63807-0360-31 3.59

PROD/MFR	NDC	AWP	DP	OBC
(LATEX-FREE)				
1 u/ml, 3 ml	63807-0300-31	3.59		
2 u/ml, 5 ml	63807-0400-31	3.59		
10 u/ml, 3 ml	63807-0500-31	3.50		
(1X5ML,LATEX-FREE)				
10 u/ml, 5 ml	63807-0560-51	3.50		
(LATEX-FREE)				
10 u/ml, 5 ml	63807-0500-51	3.50		
100 u/ml, 3 ml	63807-0600-31	3.50		
(1X5ML,LATEX-FREE)				
100 u/ml, 5 ml	63807-0660-51	3.50		
(LATEX-FREE)				
100 u/ml, 5 ml	63807-0600-51	3.50		
(Hospira)				
SOL, IV (USP,3MLX100,PF)				
1 u/ml, 3 ml 100s	63807-0300-35	57.60	50.00	
2 u/ml, 3 ml 100s	63807-0400-35	57.60	50.00	
(LUER LOCK)				
10 u/ml, 1 ml 50s	00409-1280-31	74.40	65.00	
2 ml 50s	00409-1280-32	69.60	61.00	
3 ml 25s	00409-1280-33	38.40	33.50	
5 ml 25s	00409-1280-35	36.90	32.25	
(LATEX-FREE)				
10 u/ml, 5 ml 100s	63807-0500-55	57.60	50.00	
(25X10ML)				
10 u/ml, 10 ml 25s	00409-1151-12	24.00	21.00	
(FTV,25X10ML)				
10 u/ml, 10 ml 25s	00409-1151-70	19.80	17.25	
(FTV,25X30ML)				
10 u/ml, 30 ml 25s	00409-1151-78	20.70	18.00	
(LUER LOCK,50X1ML)				
100 u/ml, 1 ml 50s	00409-1281-31	70.20	61.50	AP
(LUER LOCK,CARPUJECT)				
100 u/ml, 2 ml 50s	00409-1281-32	73.80	64.50	AP
(LUER LOCK,25X3ML)				
100 u/ml, 3 ml 25s	00409-1281-33	38.10	33.25	AP
(LUER LOCK,CARPUJECT)				
100 u/ml, 5 ml 25s	00409-1281-35	43.80	38.25	AP
(ANSYR,LATEX-FREE)				
100 u/ml, 5 ml 50s	00074-3454-25	45.00	39.50	AP
5 ml 100s	63807-0600-55	57.60	50.00	AP
(VIAL, FLIPTOP)				
100 u/ml,				
10 ml 25s	00409-1152-70	17.70	15.50	AP
(VIAL,FLIPTOP,LIFESHIELD)				
100 u/ml,				
10 ml 25s	00409-1152-12	24.90	21.75	AP
(VIAL,FLIPTOP)				
100 u/ml,				
30 ml 25s	00409-1152-78	26.70	23.25	AP
(Medefil)				
SOL, IV (6ML PRE-FILLED SYRINGE)				
1 u/ml, 1 ml 120s	64253-0444-21	3.01		
2 ml 120s	64253-0444-22	3.25		
(12ML PRE-FILLED SYRINGE)				
1 u/ml, 3 ml 120s	64253-0444-33	3.75		
(6ML PRE-FILLED SYRINGE)				
1 u/ml, 3 ml 120s	64253-0444-23	3.49		
(12ML PRE-FILLED SYRINGE)				
1 u/ml, 5 ml 120s	64253-0444-35	4.05		
(6ML PRE-FILLED SYRINGE)				
1 u/ml, 5 ml 120s	64253-0444-25	3.79		
(12ML PRE-FILLED SYRINGE)				
1 u/ml, 10 ml 120s	64253-0444-30	4.55		
(Medefil)				
heparin sodium/sodium chloride				
(SRN,6 ML W/LUER LOCK,PF)				
10 u/ml-0.9%, 1 ml	64253-0222-21	2.61		
2 ml	64253-0222-22	2.85		
(SRN,12 ML W/LUER LOCK)				
10 u/ml-0.9%, 3 ml	64253-0222-33	3.29		
(SRN,6 ML W/LUER LOCK,PF)				
10 u/ml-0.9%, 3 ml	64253-0222-23	2.99		
(SRN,12 ML W/LUER LOCK)				
10 u/ml-0.9%, 5 ml	64253-0222-35	3.61		
(SRN,6 ML W/LUER LOCK,PF)				
10 u/ml-0.9%, 5 ml	64253-0222-25	3.39		
(SRN W/LUER LOCK,PF)				
10 u/ml-0.9%,				
10 ml	64253-0222-30	3.85		
(SRN,6 ML W/LUER LOCK,PF)				
100 u/ml-0.9%,				
1 ml	64253-0333-21	2.71		
2 ml	64253-0333-22	2.95		
(SRN,12 ML W/LUER LOCK)				
100 u/ml-0.9%,				
3 ml	64253-0333-33	3.39		
(SRN,6 ML W/LUER LOCK,PF)				
100 u/ml-0.9%,				
3 ml	64253-0333-23	3.09		
(SRN,12 ML W/LUER LOCK)				
100 u/ml-0.9%,				
5 ml	64253-0333-35	3.71		
(SRN,6 ML W/LUER LOCK,PF)				
100 u/ml-0.9%,				
5 ml	64253-0333-25	3.49		
(SRN W/LUER LOCK,PF)				
100 u/ml-0.9%,				
10 ml	64253-0333-30	3.95		
(Sierra)				
heparin sodium				
SOL, IV (1X3ML,USP,PF,LATEX-FREE)				
10 u/ml, 3 ml	64054-3003-02	3.60		
(1X5ML,USP,PF,LATEX-FREE)				
10 u/ml, 5 ml	64054-3005-02	3.60		
(PF,LATEX-FREE)				
100 u/ml, 3 ml UD	64054-1003-01	3.60	3.60	
5 ml UD	64054-1003-02	3.60	3.60	
HEPARIN SODIUM				
(AMSINO) *See HEPARIN LOCK FLUSH*				
(APP) *See HEPARIN LOCK FLUSH*				
(APP) *See HEPFLUSH-10*				
(APP) *See NOVAPLUS HEPARIN SODIUM*				
(APP)				
SOL, IJ (M.D.V.,P.C.)				
1000 u/ml,				
1 ml 25s	63323-0540-01	120.31		AP
(S.D.V.)				
1000 u/ml,				
2 ml 25s	63323-0276-02	412.18		AP
(M.D.V.)				
1000 u/ml,				
10 ml 25s	63323-0540-11	227.18		AP
30 ml 25s	63323-0540-31	379.06		AP
(M.D.V.,P.C.)				
5000 u/ml,				
1 ml 25s	63323-0262-01	130.00		AP
(M.D.V.)				
5000 u/ml,				
10 ml 25s	63323-0047-10	498.43		AP
(M.D.V.,P.C.)				
10000 u/ml,				
1 ml 25s	63323-0542-01	218.75		AP
(M.D.V.)				
10000 u/ml,				
5 ml 25s	63323-0542-07	588.75		AP
(M.D.V.,P.C.)				
20000 u/ml,				
1 ml 25s	63323-0915-01	523.75		AP
(Baxter) *See HEP-LOCK*				
(Baxter)				
SOL, IJ, 5000 u/ml, 1 ml	00641-0400-64	1.09		AP
1 ml 25s	00641-0400-02	27.30		AP
(M.D.V.)				
5000 u/ml, 10 ml	00641-2460-41	3.00		AP
10 ml 25s	00641-2460-45	75.00		AP
10000 u/ml, 1 ml	00641-0410-64	1.40		AP
1 ml 25s	00641-0410-02	35.10		AP
(M.D.V.)				
10000 u/ml, 4 ml	00641-2470-41	2.88		AP
4 ml 25s	00641-2470-45	72.00		AP
(BD Dickinson Hosp Prod) *See HEPARIN LOCK FLUSH*				
(BD Dickinson Hosp Prod) *See POSIFLUSH HEPARIN*				
(Consolidated Midland) *See HEPARIN LOCK FLUSH*				
(Consolidated Midland)				
SOL, IJ (VIAL)				
1000 u/ml,				
1 ml 25s	00223-7801-01	20.00		EE
(M.D.V.)				
1000 u/ml, 10 ml	00223-7843-10	4.50		EE
(VIAL, PORK)				
1000 u/ml, 10 ml	00223-7810-10	4.75		EE
(M.D.V.)				
1000 u/ml, 30 ml	00223-7844-30	12.50		EE
(VIAL, PORK)				
5000 u/ml,				
1 ml 25s	00223-7811-30	22.50		EE
1 ml 25s UD	00223-7845-25	25.00		EE
(VIAL)				
5000 u/ml,				
1 ml 25s	00223-7818-01	25.00		EE
(VIAL, PORK)				
5000 u/ml, 10 ml	00223-7820-10	17.50		EE
(VIAL)				
10000 u/ml,				
1 ml UD	00223-7846-01	4.75		EE
(VIAL, PORK)				
10000 u/ml,				
1 ml 25s	00223-7828-01	35.00		EE
(M.D.V.)				
10000 u/ml, 4 ml	00223-7847-04	5.00		EE
(VIAL, PORK)				
10000 u/ml,				
4 ml 25s	00223-7830-04	90.00		EE
(VIAL)				
10000 u/ml,				
4 ml 25s	00223-7847-25	100.00		EE
5 ml	00223-7831-05	3.90		EE
(VIAL, PORK)				
10000 u/ml, 10 ml	00223-7832-10	11.50		EE
20000 u/ml, 5 ml	00223-7840-05	11.95		EE
(VIAL)				
20000 u/ml, 5 ml	00223-7840-01	14.95		EE
(Covidien) *See MONOJECT PREFILL ADVANCED HEPARIN LOCK FLUSH*				
(Covidien) *See MONOJECT PREFILL HEPARIN LOCK FLUSH*				
(Deen Pre-Fld Syr LLC) *See HEPARIN LOCK FLUSH*				
(Excelsior) *See HEPARIN LOCK FLUSH*				
(Hospira) *See HEPARIN LOCK FLUSH*				
(Hospira)				
SOL, IJ (25X1ML,SDV,USP)				
1000 u/ml,				
1 ml 25s	00409-2720-01	55.80	48.75	AP
(25X10ML,MDV,USP)				
1000 u/ml,				
10 ml 25s	00409-2720-02	107.40	94.00	AP
(25X30ML,MDV,USP)				
1000 u/ml,				
30 ml 25s	00409-2720-03	185.40	162.25	AP
(25X10ML,PF,LATEX-FREE)				
2500 u/ml,				
10 ml 25s	00409-2584-02	225.90	197.75	AP
(LUER LOCK,CARPUJECT)				
5000 u/ml,				
1 ml 10s	00409-1402-31	22.44	19.60	AP
(25X1ML,SDV,USP)				
5000 u/ml,				
1 ml 25s	00409-2723-01	60.90	53.25	AP
(25X10ML,MDV,USP)				
5000 u/ml,				
10 ml 25s	00409-2723-02	243.00	212.75	AP
(10X0.5ML,W/ LUER LOCK)				
5000 u/0.5 ml,				
0.5 ml 10s	00409-1316-25	19.80	17.30	AP
(PF,CARPUJECT)				
10000 u/ml,				
0.5 ml 10s	00409-1316-66	22.44	19.60	AP
(CARPUJECT W/LUER LOCK)				
10000 u/ml,				
0.5 ml 50s	00409-1316-32	112.20	98.00	AP
(25X1ML,SDV,USP)				
10000 u/ml,				
1 ml 25s	00409-2721-01	101.10	88.50	AP
IV (ADD-VANTAGE VIAL)				
2000 u/ml,				
5 ml 25s	00409-2581-02	124.80	109.25	
(Intl Tech)				
SOL, IJ (HEMOCHRON RXDX,VIAL)				
1000 u/ml, 10 ml	11743-0210-02	4.50		EE
(Medefil) *See HEPARIN LOCK FLUSH*				
(Medisca)				
POW, NA (USP,1X1MU)				
1 ml	38779-2090-06	555.00		
(USP,1X10000U)				
10000 ml	38779-2090-01	19.50		
(USP,1X25000U)				
25000 ml	38779-2090-07	37.50		
(PCCA)				
POW, NA (USP)				
1 gm	51927-3286-00	132.00		
(Sierra) *See HEPARIN LOCK FLUSH*				
(Spectrum Pharmacy)				
POW, NA (USP, 160 UNITS/MG)				
0.6 gm	49452-3450-02	221.38		
(U.S.P., 160 UNITS/MG)				
1.6 gm	49452-3450-01	103.25		
(USP, 160 UNITS/MG)				
6.3 gm	49452-3450-03	1137.50		
(Vital Signs) *See VASCEZE HEPARIN LOCK FLUSH*				

PROD/MFR NDC AWP DP OBC

HEPARIN SODIUM IN DEXTROSE (Hospira)
dextrose/heparin sodium
SOL, IV (24X250ML,USP,LATEX-FREE)
5%-5000 u/100 ml,
250 ml 24s ....**00409-7794-62** 133.06 116.40 EE
(USP, SD, 100MLX24)
5%-10000 u/100 ml,
100 ml 24s ....**00409-7793-23** 141.98 124.32 AP

HEPARIN SODIUM/SODIUM CHLORIDE (B. Braun)
SOL, IV, 200 u/100 ml-0.9%,
500 ml ....**00264-9872-10** 3.72 AP

(Baxter)
SOL, IV, 200 u/100 ml-0.9%,
500 ml 18s ....**00338-0431-03** 123.66 AP
1000 ml 12s ....**00338-0433-04** 87.84 AP

(Hospira)
SOL, IV (18X500ML,LATEX-FREE)
200 u/100 ml-0.9%,
500 ml 18s ....**00409-7620-03** 72.14 63.18 AP
(LATEX-FREE)
200 u/100 ml-0.9%,
1000 ml 12s ....**00409-7620-59** 47.52 41.64 AP
(24X250ML,LATEX-FREE)
5000 u/100 ml-0.45%,
250 ml 24s ....**00409-7651-62** 124.13 108.72 AP
(24X500ML,LATEX-FREE)
5000 u/100 ml-0.45%,
500 ml 24s ....**00409-7651-03** 125.28 109.68 AP
(24X250ML,LATEX-FREE)
10000 u/100 ml-0.45%,
250 ml 24s ....**00409-7650-62** 125.28 109.68 AP

(Medefil) *See HEPARIN LOCK FLUSH*

HEPATAMINE (B. Braun)
amino acids
SOL, IV (GLASS W/SOLID STOPPER)
8%, 500 ml **00264-9371-55** 93.71

HEPATASOL (Baxter)
amino acids
SOL, IV (VIAFLEX,SULFITE-FREE)
8%, 500 ml 24s **00338-0504-03** 3110.40 2160.00

HEPATITIS A VACCINE, INACTIVATED
(Glaxo) *See HAVRIX*
(Glaxo) *See HAVRIX PEDIATRIC*
(Merck) *See VAQTA*
(Merck) *See VAQTA PEDIATRIC*

HEPATITIS B IMMUNE GLOBULIN
(Apotex Corp.) *See HEPAGAM B*
(Apotex Corp.) *See NOVAPLUS HEPAGAM B*
(Biotest) *See NABI-HB*
(Talecris) *See HYPERHEP B S/D*

HEPATITIS B VACCINE RECOMBINANT
(Glaxo) *See ENGERIX-B*
(Glaxo) *See ENGERIX-B PEDIATRIC*
(Merck) *See RECOMBIVAX HB*
(Merck) *See RECOMBIVAX HB PEDIATRIC/ADOLESCENT*

HEPATOLITE (Pharmlucence)
technetium tc 99m disofenin
KIT, IV (5 VIALS,PF)
ea....................**45567-0475-01** 228.60 190.50
(5 VLS/KIT,PF)
6s ea.................**45567-0475-02** 1371.60 1143.00

HEPES
(Baker, J.T.) *See HEPES FREE ACID*
(Baker, J.T.) *See HEPES SODIUM SALT*

HEPES FREE ACID (Baker, J.T.)
hepes
POW, NA (ULTRAPURE, BIOREAGENT)
25 gm...............**10106-4018-00** 19.36
100 gm.............**10106-4018-01** 51.71
500 gm.............**10106-4018-04** 206.88
5000 gm............**10106-4018-06** 1166.84
12000 gm **10106-4018-07** 2659.46

HEPES SODIUM SALT (Baker, J.T.)
hepes
POW, NA (ULTRAPURE, BIOREAGENT)
25 gm...............**10106-4153-00** 22.15
100 gm.............**10106-4153-01** 50.21
1000 gm............**10106-4153-05** 355.14

HEPFLUSH-10 (APP)
heparin sodium
SOL, IV (S.D.V.,PF)
10 u/ml, 10 ml 25s ...**63323-0017-10** 238.18 AP

HEPSERA (Gilead Sciences)
adefovir dipivoxil
TAB, PO, 10 mg, 30s ea ...**61958-0501-01** 975.73

HEPTAMINOL (PCCA)
SOL, NA (1X1ML)
1 ml..................**51927-3438-00** 45.00

HEPTANE
(Baker, J.T.) *See N-HEPTANE*

HERCEPTIN (Genentech)
trastuzumab
PDS, IV (M.D.V.,W/DILUENT 20ML)
440 mg, ea **50242-0134-68** 3359.47

HESPAN (B. Braun)
hetastarch/sodium chloride
SOL, IV (EXCEL CONTAINER)
6 gm/100 ml-0.9%,
500 ml **00264-1965-10** 15.43

HESPERIDIN
(PCCA) *See HESPERIDIN 98%*

HESPERIDIN 98% (PCCA)
hesperidin
POW, NA, 1 gm...........**51927-3083-00** 1.05

HETASTARCH/SODIUM CHLORIDE
(B. Braun) *See HESPAN*

(Baxter)
SOL, IV (P.C.)
6 gm/100 ml-0.9%,
500 ml 12s **10019-0999-59** 216.00

(Hospira) *See HETASTARCH/ SODIUM CHLORIDE AMERINET*

(Hospira)
SOL, IV (LATEX-FREE)
6 gm/100 ml-0.9%,
500 ml 12s **00409-7248-03** 281.95 246.72
(VHA+,LATEX-FREE)
6 gm/100 ml-0.9%,
500 ml 12s **00409-7248-49** 186.48 163.20

(Teva)
SOL, IV (12X500ML)
6 gm/100 ml-0.9%,
500 ml 12s **00703-5079-37** 243.90

HETASTARCH/SODIUM CHLORIDE AMERINET
(Hospira)
hetastarch/sodium chloride
SOL, IV (LATEX-FREE)
6 gm/100 ml-0.9%,
500 ml 12s **00074-7248-61** 281.95 246.72

HEXACHLOROPHENE
(Sanofi-Aventis) *See PHISOHEX*

(Spectrum Pharmacy)
POW, NA (U.S.P.)
5 gm..................**49452-3460-03** 107.80
25 gm................**49452-3460-01** 247.45
100 gm..............**49452-3460-02** 815.50

HEXALEN (Eisai)
altretamine
CAP, PO, 50 mg, 100s ea ..**58063-0001-70** 1180.00

HEXANE
(Baker, J.T.) *See HEXANES*
(Baker, J.T.) *See HEXANES 85%*
(Baker, J.T.) *See HEXANES 95%*

HEXANES (Baker, J.T.)
hexane
LIQ, NA (A.C.S., REAGENT)
500 ml **10106-9309-01** 28.07
4000 ml **10106-9309-03** 96.67
4000 ml **10106-9309-05** 106.09
20000 ml **10106-9309-07** 209.19

HEXANES 85% (Baker, J.T.)
hexane
LIQ, NA (HPLC)
4000 ml **10106-9308-03** 80.75

HEXANES 95% (Baker, J.T.)
hexane
LIQ, NA (HPLC)
1000 ml **10106-9304-02** 54.64
(ULTRA RESI-ANALYZED)
1000 ml **10106-9262-02** 34.71
(HPLC)
4000 ml **10106-9304-03** 126.33
(ULTRA RESI-ANALYZED)
4000 ml **10106-9262-03** 90.38

1-HEXANOL (Baker, J.T.)
hexyl alcohol
LIQ, NA (PURIFIED)
500 ml **10106-9307-01** 45.84
4000 ml **10106-9307-03** 164.18

HEXTEND (Hospira)
ca cl/dextrose/hetastarch/k cl/mg cl/na cl/na lact
SOL, IV (P.C.,FLEXIBLE)
500 ml 12s **00409-1555-54** 479.81 419.88

HEXYL ALCOHOL
(Baker, J.T.) *See 1-HEXANOL*

HEXYL NICOTINATE
(PCCA) *See NICOTINIC ACID N-HEXYL ESTER*

HEXYLENE GLYCOL (Amend)
SOL, NA, 500 ml..........**17317-0873-01** 9.80
3840 ml **17317-0873-06** 42.00
19249.5996 gm **17317-0873-03** 178.08

(Medisca)
SOL, NA (1X100ML)
100 ml **38779-1339-05** 37.50
(1X500ML)
500 ml **38779-1339-08** 87.00

(PCCA)
SOL, NA (NF)
1 ml..................**51927-2465-00** 0.31

HEXYLRESORCINOL (Medisca)
POW, NA (4-HEXYLRESORCINOL)
10 gm **38779-1340-01** 105.00

(PCCA)
POW, NA, 1 gm...........**51927-3434-00** 10.80

HI-VOLUME PUMPING CHAMBER SET (APP)
kit, administration, intravenous
DEV, NA (PLASTIC TUBING)
ea.....................**63323-0906-90** 13.43

HIBERIX (Glaxo)
haemophilus b conjugate vaccine
PDS, IM (W/DILUENT SYRINGE)
10 mcg, 10s ea.......**58160-0806-05** 272.46

HIPREX (Sanofi-Aventis)
methenamine hippurate
TAB, PO, 1 gm, 100s ea ...**00068-0277-61** 215.42 AB

HISTA-VENT DA (Phys Total Care)
REPACK
cpm/methscopolamine nitrate/phenyleph hcl
TER, PO, 8 mg-2.5 mg-20 mg,
20s ea.............**54868-4487-00** 20.49
100s ea...........**54868-4487-01** 82.95

HISTACOL DM PEDIATRIC (Breckenridge Pharm)
bpm/dm/gg/pse hcl
SYR, PO (AF,GRAPE)
473 ml **51991-0163-16** 35.75

HISTACOL LA (Breckenridge Pharm)
cough/cold combination
TER, PO (DYE-FREE)
100s ea...............**51991-0164-01** 85.48

HISTAMINE DIHYDROCHLORIDE (PCCA)
POW, NA (REAGENT)
1 gm **51927-2510-00** 12.60

HISTAMINE DIPHOSPHATE (Gallipot)
histamine phosphate
POW, NA, 5 gm...........**51552-0585-02** 37.45
25 gm..............**51552-0585-04** 108.36

(PCCA)
POW, NA (USP; ANHYDROUS)
1 gm **51927-3078-00** 54.00

(Spectrum Pharmacy)
POW, NA (U.S.P.)
0.5 gm **49452-0044-03** 66.50
5 gm **49452-0044-01** 116.55
25 gm **49452-0044-02** 455.00

HISTAMINE PHOSPHATE
(Alk-Abello) *See HISTATROL*
(Gallipot) *See HISTAMINE DIPHOSPHATE*

(Medisca)
POW, NA (U.S.P.)
5 gm **38779-1341-03** 76.50
25 gm **38779-1341-04** 285.00
100 gm **38779-1341-05** 1071.00

(PCCA) *See HISTAMINE DIPHOSPHATE*
(Spectrum Pharmacy) *See HISTAMINE DIPHOSPHATE*

PROD/MFR NDC AWP DP OBC

HISTATAB (Breckenridge Pharm)
cpm/methscopolamine nitrate/pse hcl
TER, PO, 8 mg-1.25 mg-60 mg,
100s ea............51991-0423-01 64.64

HISTATAB D (Breckenridge Pharm)
cough/cold combination
TER, PO, 3.5 mg-1 mg-45 mg,
100s ea............51991-0583-01 82.95

HISTATAB PH (Breckenridge Pharm)
cpm/methscopolamine nitrate/phenyleph hcl
TER, PO, 8 mg-1.25 mg-20 mg,
100s ea............51991-0424-01 64.64

HISTATROL (Alk-Abello)
histamine phosphate
SOL, ID (M.D.V.)
0.275 mg/ml, 5 ml....00268-0248-05 71.16 52.30
TP (SCRATCH)
2.75 mg/ml, 5 ml.....00268-0247-05 74.16 54.50

HISTEX SR (Tiber)
bpm/pse hcl
TER, PO (CAPLET)
10 mg-120 mg,
100s ea............23589-0003-10 152.78

HISTIDINE
(Spectrum Pharmacy) *See L-HISTIDINE*
(Spectrum Pharmacy) *See L-HISTIDINE MONOHYDROCHLORIDE*

HISTIDINE MONOHYDROCHLORIDE (Medisca)
POW, NA, 100 gm.........38779-1342-05 126.00
(1X1000GM)
1000 gm.............38779-1342-09 765.00
(PCCA)
POW, NA (L,FCC, MONOHYDRATE)
1 gm................51927-1787-00 1.02

HISTINEX HC (Ethex)
cpm/hydrocod bit/phenyleph hcl
SYR, PO (AF,SF)
480 ml, C-III.........58177-0877-07 27.95
960 ml, C-III.........58177-0877-12 55.90
(Altura)
REPACK
SYR, PO (1X120ML,AF,SF)
120 ml, C-III.........63874-0275-12 9.78
(Pharma Pac)
REPACK
SYR, PO, 180 ml, C-III....52959-0889-06 19.80

HISTINEX PV (Ethex)
cpm/hydrocod bit/pse hcl
SYR, PO (AF,SF,FRUIT)
480 ml, C-III.........58177-0883-07 38.84

HISTRELIN ACETATE
(Endo Pharm) *See SUPPRELIN LA*
(Endo Pharm) *See VANTAS*

HOMATROPAIRE (Altaire)
homatropine hydrobromide
SOL, OP (STERILE)
5%, 5 ml 59390-0192-05 17.34

HOMATROPINE HYDROBROMIDE
(Alcon Ophthalmic) *See ISOPTO HOMATROPINE*
(Altaire) *See HOMATROPAIRE*
(Amend)
POW, NA (U.S.P.)
25 gm...............17317-0348-02 42.00
(PCCA)
POW, NA (USP,1X1GM)
1 gm................51927-3668-00 36.30
(Spectrum Pharmacy)
CRY, NA (U.S.P.)
5 gm................49452-3530-01 115.50
25 gm...............49452-3530-02 324.10
(Southwood)
REPACK
SOL, OP, 2%, 1 ml 12s....58016-6324-01 33.44

HOMATROPINE METHYLBROMIDE (PCCA)
POW, NA (U.S.P.)
1 gm................51927-9007-00 8.10
(Spectrum Pharmacy)
POW, NA (U.S.P.)
5 gm................49452-3540-01 125.65
25 gm...............49452-3540-02 348.25

HOMATROPINE METHYLBROMIDE/HYDROCODONE BITARTRATE
(Actavis Mid Atlantic) *See HYDROMET*
(Endo Labs) *See HYCODAN*
(Hi-Tech) *See HYDROCODONE BITARTRATE & HOMATROPINE METHYLBROMIDE*
(Monarch) *See TUSSIGON*
(Morton Grove) *See HOMATROPINE/HYDROCODONE*
(Pharm Assoc Inc)
SYR, PO (40X5ML,CHERRY)
1.5 mg/5 ml-5 mg/5 ml,
5 ml 40s UD, C-III..00121-4811-05 150.00 AA

HOMATROPINE/HYDROCODONE (Morton Grove)
homatropine methylbromide/hydrocodone bitartrate
SYR, PO (CHERRY)
1.5 mg/5 ml-5 mg/5 ml,
473 ml, C-III.......60432-0455-16 87.44 AA
(A-S Medication)
REPACK
SYR, PO, 1.5 mg/5 ml-5 mg/5 ml,
480 ml, C-III.......54569-3515-00 23.34 EE
(Dispensing Solutions)
REPACK
TAB, PO, 1.5 mg-5 mg,
20s ea, C-III.......55045-3228-07 15.00
(Quality Care Prod)
REPACK
SYR, PO (1X480ML,CHERRY)
1.5 mg/5 ml-5 mg/5 ml,
480 ml, C-III.......35356-0436-16 172.65 AA

HOMEOPATHIC
(Gensco) *See TRANZGEL*
(Gensco) *See TRAUMANIL*
(Loma Lux) *See ACUNOL*
(Loma Lux) *See PSORIZIDE FORTE*

HOMEOPATHIC SUBSTANCE
(Heel/BHI) *See AURUMHEEL*
(Heel/BHI) *See ENGYSTOL N*
(Heel/BHI) *See VERTIGOHEEL*
(Weleda) *See ANAEMODORON*
(Weleda) *See ANISE PYRITE*
(Weleda) *See AURUM*
(Weleda) *See BRYOPHYLLUM (ARGENTO CULTUM)*
(Weleda) *See CALCON II*
(Weleda) *See CALCON-AM*
(Weleda) *See CARDIODORON*
(Weleda) *See CARDIODORON/MAGNESIA PHOSPHORICA 6X*
(Weleda) *See CHAMOMILLA (CUPRO CULTA)*
(Weleda) *See CHELIDONIUM COMPOUND*
(Weleda) *See CHOLEODORON*
(Weleda) *See CINNABAR 20X/PYRITE 3X*
(Weleda) *See CRATAEGUS COMPOUND*
(Weleda) *See DERMATODORON*
(Weleda) *See DIGESTODORON*
(Weleda) *See ERYSIDORON 1*
(Weleda) *See ERYSIDORON 2*
(Weleda) *See INFLUDO*
(Weleda) *See KALIUM ACETICUM COMPOUND*
(Weleda) *See LEVISTICUM*
(Weleda) *See MANDRAGORA COMPOUND*
(Weleda) *See ONOPORDON COMPOUND*
(Weleda) *See PERTUDORON 1*
(Weleda) *See PERTUDORON 2 (CUPRUM ACETICUM)*
(Weleda) *See PNEUMODORON 1*
(Weleda) *See PNEUMODORON 2*
(Weleda) *See RAUWOLFIA*
(Weleda) *See RHEUMADORON 1*
(Weleda) *See RHEUMADORON 102A*
(Weleda) *See RHEUMADORON 2*
(Weleda) *See SCLERON*
(Weleda) *See TARAXACUM (STANNO CULTUM)*
(Weleda) *See URTICA DIOICA (FERRO CULTA)*
(Weleda) *See VITIS COMPOUND*

HOMIDIUM BROMIDE
(Baker, J.T.) *See ETHIDIUM BROMIDE*

HONEY ALMOND FRAGRANCE (PCCA)
fragrance
SOL, NA, 1 ml............51927-3266-00 0.90

HONEY BEE TREATMENT (Alk-Abello)
bee venom
PDS, IJ (KIT (6X1ML))
0.1 mg, ea...........52709-0801-01 97.80 81.70
(MDV)
0.1 mg, ea...........52709-0801-02 142.68 105.80

HONEY BEE VENOM PROTEIN (Hollister-Stier)
bee venom
PDS, IJ (M.D.V.)
0.55 mg, ea..........65044-9940-05 54.80
1.3 mg, ea...........65044-9940-06 118.10

HONEY FLAVOR (PCCA)
flavoring aid
SOL, NA (ARTIFICIAL,HONEY)
1 ml.................51927-3138-00 0.90

HONEYSUCKLE FRAGRANCE (PCCA)
fragrance
SOL, NA, 1 ml............51927-3255-00 1.63

HOP FLOWER
(PCCA) *See HOPS FLOWER*

HOPS FLOWER (PCCA)
hop flower
POW, NA (1X1GM)
1 gm.................51927-3185-00 0.21

HOREHOUND (Medisca)
flavoring aid
SOL, NA (1X25ML)
25 ml................38779-1345-04 21.00
(1X100ML)
100 ml 38779-1345-05 39.00

HOREHOUND FLAVOR (PCCA)
flavoring aid
SOL, NA, 1 ml............51927-2159-00 1.20

HORSE CHESTNUT EXTRACT
(PCCA) *See HORSECHESTNUT SPRAY DRIED EXTRACT*

HORSECHESTNUT SPRAY DRIED EXTRACT (PCCA)
horse chestnut extract
POW, NA (1X1GM)
1 gm.................51927-3202-00 1.80

HORSETAIL
(PCCA) *See SHAVEGRASS*

HRT CREAM BASE (Medisca)
cream base
CRE, NA (WOMEN,1X100GM)
100 gm...............38779-0701-05 36.30
(WOMEN,1X500GM)
500 gm...............38779-0701-08 207.00
(WOMEN,1X1000GM)
1000 gm..............38779-0701-09 387.00
(WOMEN,1X2500GM)
2500 gm..............38779-0701-01 675.00
(WOMEN,1X5000GM)
5000 gm..............38779-0701-03 1437.00
(WOMEN,1X10000GM)
10000 gm 38779-0701-00 2397.00

HRT GEL BASE (Medisca)
gel base
GEL, NA (MEN,1X100GM)
100 gm...............38779-2257-05 55.00
(MEN,1X500GM)
500 gm...............38779-2257-08 240.00
(MEN,1X1000GM)
1000 gm..............38779-2257-09 435.00
(MEN,1X5000GM)
5000 gm..............38779-2257-03 1950.00
(MEN,1X10000GM)
10000 gm 38779-2257-00 3450.00

HUMALOG (Lilly)
insulin lispro, recombinant
SUS, SC (1X3ML)
100 u/ml, 3 ml.......00002-7510-17 35.88 29.90
(CARTRIDGE)
100 u/ml, 3 ml 5s....00002-7516-59 222.12 185.10
(KWIKPEN,5X3ML)
100 u/ml, 3 ml 5s....00002-8799-59 230.94 192.45
(VIAL)
100 u/ml, 10 ml......00002-7510-01 119.58 99.65
(Phys Total Care)
REPACK
SUS, SC, 100 u/ml, 10 ml .54868-5108-00 133.64

PROD/MFR | NDC | AWP | DP | OBC

(Quality Care Prod)
REPACK
SUS, SC (10X10ML)
100 u/ml,
10 ml 10s.......... 35356-0102-00 189.15

HUMALOG MIX 50/50 (Lilly)
insulin lispro/insulin lispro protamine
SUS, SC (KWIKPEN,5X3ML)
50 u/ml-50 u/ml,
3 ml 5s........... 00002-8798-59 230.94 192.45
(PEN,5X3ML)
50 u/ml-50 u/ml,
3 ml 5s........... 00002-8793-59 230.94 192.45
10 ml........... 00002-7512-01 119.58 99.65

HUMALOG MIX 75/25 (Lilly)
insulin lispro/insulin lispro protamine
SUS, SC (VIAL)
75 u/ml-25 u/ml,
10 ml............. 00002-7511-01 119.58 99.65

(Phys Total Care)
REPACK
SUS, SC (VIAL)
75 u/ml-25 u/ml,
10 ml............. 54868-4381-00 141.38

HUMALOG MIX 75/25 PEN (Lilly)
insulin lispro/insulin lispro protamine
SUS, SC (PREFILLED DISPOSABLE)
75 u/ml-25 u/ml,
3 ml 5s........... 00002-8794-59 230.94 192.45

HUMALOG MIX75/25 (Lilly)
insulin lispro/insulin lispro protamine
SUS, SC (KWIKPEN,5X3ML)
75 u/ml-25 u/ml,
3 ml 5s........... 00002-8797-59 230.94 192.45

HUMALOG PEN (Lilly)
insulin lispro, recombinant
SUS, SC (PREFILLED DISPOSABLE)
100 u/ml, 3 ml 5s 00002-8725-59 230.94 192.45

(Phys Total Care)
REPACK
SUS, SC (1X15ML)
100 u/ml, 15 ml 54868-5899-00 223.83

HUMAN PAPILLOMAVIRUS RECOMB VACCINE BIVALENT
(Glaxo) *See CERVARIX*

HUMAN PAPILLOMAVIRUS RECOMB VACCINE QUADRIVALENT
(Merck) *See GARDASIL*

HUMAPEN LUXURA HD (Lilly)
insulin syringe/needle
DEV, NA, ea 00002-9673-01 56.25 45.00

HUMAPEN MEMOIR (Lilly)
insulin syringe/needle
DEV, NA, ea 00002-9660-01 125.00 100.00

HUMATE-P (CSL)
ahf human/von willebrand factor
PDS, IV (1200IU, W/LOW DILUENT)
1 iu-1 iu, ea.......... 00053-7615-10 1.00
(2400IU, W/ LOW DILUENT)
1 iu-1 iu, ea.......... 00053-7615-20 1.00
(600IU, W/LOW DILUENT)
1 iu-1 iu, ea.......... 00053-7615-05 1.00

HUMATROPE (Lilly)
somatropin, e-coli derived
PDS, IJ (CARTRIDGE W/DILUENT)
6 mg, ea............ 00002-8147-01 455.72 379.77 BX
12 mg, ea........... 00002-8148-01 911.45 759.54
24 mg, ea........... 00002-8149-01 1822.90 1519.08
SC (WITH STERILE DILUENT)
5 mg, ea............ 00002-7335-11 354.92 234.28 BX
(W/DILUENT)
5 mg, 6s ea......... 00002-7335-16 2278.62 1898.85 BX

HUMAVENT LA (Dexo)
guaifenesin
TER, PO, 600 mg, 100s ea . 59196-0008-01 25.00
500s ea........... 59196-0008-05 129.29

HUMIBID L.A. (PD-Rx Pharm)
REPACK
guaifenesin/potassium guaiacolsulfonate
TER, PO (REDI-SCRIPT)
600 mg-300 mg,
20s ea............ 58864-0656-20 26.39

HUMIRA (Abbott Pharm)
adalimumab
KIT, MR (2X1ML,PF)
40 mg/0.8 ml,
2s ea.............. 00074-4339-02 1828.76 1604.18
(PF,PREFILLED SYRINGE)
40 mg/0.8 ml,
2s ea.............. 00074-3799-02 1828.76 1604.18
(SINGLE-USE,6X1ML,,PF)
40 mg/0.8 ml,
6s ea.............. 00074-4339-06 5486.29 4812.54
SOL, SC (SINGLE-DOSE,PF)
20 mg/0.4 ml,
2s ea.............. 00074-9374-02 1828.76 1604.18
(PSORIASIS STARTER KIT)
40 mg/0.8 ml,
4s ea.............. 00074-4339-07 3657.53 3208.36 EE

(Phys Total Care)
REPACK
KIT, MR (KIT,PF)
40 mg/0.8 ml,
2s ea.............. 54868-4822-00 1436.81

HUMULIN (Quality Care Prod)
REPACK
insulin human isophane (nph)/insulin human regular
SUS, SC, 70 u/ml-30 u/ml,
10 ml.............. 49999-0993-10 143.34

HUMULIN N (Southwood)
REPACK
insulin human isophane (nph)
SUS, SC, 100 u/ml, 10 ml . 58016-4788-01 33.20

HUMULIN R CONCENTRATED U-500 (Lilly)
insulin human regular
SOL, IJ (VIAL)
500 u/ml, 20 ml 00002-8501-01 309.54 257.95

HUMULIN R U-100 (Dispensing Solutions)
REPACK
insulin human regular
SOL, IJ, 100 u/ml, 10 ml .. 55045-3506-01 38.00

HYALGAN (Sanofi-Aventis)
hyaluronate sodium
SOL, IJ (SRN,PREFILLED,LUER LOCK)
10 mg/ml, 2 ml....... 08024-0724-20 145.78
(VIAL)
10 mg/ml, 2 ml....... 08024-0724-12 145.78

(IPI)
REPACK
SOL, IJ, 10 mg/ml, ea 18837-0265-02 173.44

(Physician Partner)
REPACK
SOL, IJ, 10 mg/ml, 2 ml ... 21695-0374-02 303.70

(Quality Care Prod)
REPACK
SOL, IJ, 10 mg/ml, ea 35356-0219-01 312.85

HYALURONATE SODIUM
(Alcon Surgical) *See PROVISC*
(Aletheia) *See HYGEL*
(Bausch & Lomb Inc.) *See AMVISC PLUS*
(Cypress Pharm) *See SODIUM HYALURONATE*
(Cypress Pharm) *See SODIUM HYALURONATE HYDRATING LOTION*
(Cytosol Ophth) *See SHELLGEL*
(Ferring) *See EUFLEXXA*
(Hawthorn Pharm) *See HYLIRA*
(JSJ Pharma) *See BIONECT*
(Letco) *See HYALURONIC ACID*
(Sanofi-Aventis) *See HYALGAN*
(Smith & Nephew) *See SUPARTZ*

HYALURONATE SODIUM/POVIDONE
(EKR) *See GELCLAIR*
(OSI Pharmaceuticals) *See GELCLAIR*

HYALURONIC ACID
(DePuy) *See ORTHOVISC*

HYALURONIC ACID (Letco)
hyaluronate sodium
POW, NA, 0.2 gm 62991-1352-01 150.00
1 gm 62991-1352-02 525.00
10 gm 62991-1352-04 3000.00

HYALURONIC ACID (Spectrum Pharmacy)
CRY, NA, 0.2 gm 49452-3543-01 385.00
1 gm 49452-3543-02 1036.00

HYALURONIDASE
(Amphastar) *See AMPHADASE*
(ISTA Pharm.) *See VITRASE*

(PCCA)
POW, NA (SALT-FREE,LYOPHILIZED)
1 gm 51927-3038-00 900.00

HYALURONIDASE HUMAN, RECOMBINANT
(Baxter) *See HYLENEX*

HYAMINE 1622 (Amend)
benzethonium chloride
CRY, NA, 454 gm 17317-1204-01 70.00
2270 gm.............. 17317-1204-05 315.00
11350 gm 17317-1204-08 875.00

HYCAMTIN (Glaxo)
topotecan hydrochloride
CAP, PO, 0.25 mg, 10s ea .. 00007-4205-11 869.05
1 mg, 10s ea......... 00007-4207-11 3476.22
PDS, IV (S.D.V.)
4 mg, ea............. 00007-4201-01 1264.99
5s ea.............. 00007-4201-05 6324.97

HYCET (Xanodyne Pharma)
acetaminophen/hydrocodone bitartrate
ELI, PO (TROPICAL FRUIT PUNCH)
473 ml, C-III 66479-0574-16 143.12

HYCODAN (Endo Labs)
homatropine methylbromide/hydrocodone bitartrate
SYR, PO, 1.5 mg/5 ml-5 mg/5 ml,
480 ml, C-III .... 63481-0234-16 105.06 AA
TAB, PO, 1.5 mg-5 mg,
100s ea, C-III ...... 63481-0042-70 99.12 AA

(Dispensing Solutions)
REPACK
TAB, PO, 1.5 mg-5 mg,
20s ea, C-III 55045-2728-07 28.00

(Quality Care Prod)
REPACK
SYR, PO (1X480ML)
1.5 mg/5 ml-5 mg/5 ml,
480 ml, C-III .... 35356-0122-16 164.60 AA

HYCOTUSS EXPECTORANT (Endo Labs)
guaifenesin/hydrocodone bitartrate
SYR, PO, 100 mg/5 ml-5 mg/5 ml,
480 ml, C-III 63481-0235-16 102.84

HYDRALAZINE (Dispensing Solutions)
REPACK
hydralazine hydrochloride
TAB, PO, 50 mg, 100s ea .. 55045-3793-01 60.00

(Phys Total Care)
REPACK
TAB, PO, 10 mg, 30s ea ... 54868-5788-00 21.28
90s ea.............. 54868-5788-01 59.33
100 mg, 30s ea 54868-0536-01 67.98
90s ea.............. 54868-0536-02 150.03
100s ea............. 54868-0536-00 164.82

HYDRALAZINE HCL (Consolidated Midland)
hydralazine hydrochloride
TAB, PO, 10 mg, 100s ea .. 00223-1060-01 2.75 EE
1000s ea .... 00223-1060-02 17.50 EE
25 mg, 100s ea ...... 00223-1061-01 3.25 EE
1000s ea .... 00223-1061-02 19.50 EE
50 mg, 100s ea ...... 00223-1062-01 3.50 EE
1000s ea .... 00223-1062-02 24.50 EE

(Gallipot)
POW, NA (U.S.P.)
5 gm 51552-0802-02 27.30 19.50

(Par)
TAB, PO, 10 mg, 100s ea .. 49884-0029-01 41.13 AA
1000s ea .... 49884-0029-10 410.47 AA
25 mg, 100s ea ...... 49884-0027-01 50.83 AA
1000s ea .... 49884-0027-10 507.28 AA
50 mg, 100s ea ...... 49884-0028-01 56.32 AA
1000s ea .... 49884-0028-10 562.07 AA
100 mg, 100s ea ..... 49884-0121-01 101.28 AA
1000s ea .... 49884-0121-10 1010.77 AA

(PCCA)
POW, NA (U.S.P.)
1 gm 51927-1979-00 30.00

(Spectrum Pharmacy)
POW, NA (U.S.P.)
5 gm 49452-3544-01 132.30
25 gm 49452-3544-02 353.50
100 gm 49452-3544-03 857.50

(Teva)
TAB, PO, 10 mg, 100s ea .. 50111-0398-01 41.15 AA
1000s ea .... 50111-0398-03 403.23 AA

PROD/MFR	NDC	AWP	DP	OBC
25 mg, 100s ea	50111-0327-01	50.84		AA
1000s ea	50111-0327-03	498.28		AA
50 mg, 100s ea	50111-0328-01	56.33		AA
1000s ea	50111-0328-03	552.04		AA
100 mg, 100s ea	50111-0397-01	101.30		AA
(A-S Medication)				
REPACK				
TAB, PO, 50 mg, 60s ea	54569-0517-01	33.80		EE
(McKesson Packaging)				
REPACK				
TAB, PO (10X10,USP)				
25 mg, 100s ea UD	63739-0126-10	62.29		AA
50 mg, 100s ea UD	63739-0127-10	69.01		AA
(PD-Rx Pharm)				
REPACK				
TAB, PO (REDI-SCRIPT)				
10 mg, 28s ea	58864-0641-28	11.53		AA
100s ea	55289-0325-01	27.32		AA
25 mg, 90s ea	55289-0133-90	11.84		AA
100s ea	55289-0133-01	33.78		AA
50 mg, 90s ea	55289-0134-90	14.00		AA
(Phys Total Care)				
REPACK				
TAB, PO, 25 mg, 30s ea	54868-1949-03	29.37		AA
60s ea	54868-1949-01	54.09		EE
90s ea	54868-1949-02	82.80		EE
100s ea	54868-1949-00	91.50		EE
50 mg, 100s ea	54868-2893-00	84.84		AA
(Southwood)				
REPACK				
TAB, PO, 10 mg, 12s ea	58016-0505-12	2.47		EE
15s ea	58016-0505-15	3.09		EE
20s ea	58016-0505-20	4.12		EE
30s ea	58016-0505-30	6.18		EE
100s ea	58016-0505-00	20.60		EE
25 mg, 12s ea	58016-0506-12	3.53		EE
15s ea	58016-0506-15	4.42		EE
20s ea	58016-0506-20	5.89		EE
30s ea	58016-0506-30	8.83		EE
100s ea	58016-0506-00	29.44		EE
50 mg, 12s ea	58016-0507-12	5.22		EE
15s ea	58016-0507-15	6.53		EE
20s ea	58016-0507-20	8.70		EE
30s ea	58016-0036-30	16.90		EE
30s ea	58016-0507-30	13.05		EE
60s ea	58016-0036-60	33.79		EE
90s ea	58016-0036-90	50.69		EE
100s ea	58016-0036-00	56.32		EE
100s ea	58016-0507-00	43.50		EE
HYDRALAZINE HYDROCHLORIDE				
FUL				
TAB, PO, 10 mg, 100s ea		25.56		
25 mg, 100s ea		32.84		
50 mg, 100s ea		42.00		
100 mg, 100s ea		78.38		
(Akorn)				
SOL, IJ (10X1ML,SDV)				
20 mg/ml, 1 ml 10s	17478-0934-01	148.50		AP
(Amer Regent)				
SOL, IJ (S.D.V.)				
20 mg/ml, 1 ml 25s	00517-0901-25	468.75		AP
(APP) *See NOVAPLUS HYDRALAZINE HYDROCHLORIDE*				
(APP)				
SOL, IJ (S.D.V.)				
20 mg/ml, 1 ml	63323-0614-01	15.00		AP
(Camber)				
TAB, PO (USP)				
10 mg, 100s ea	31722-0519-01	41.13		AA
25 mg, 100s ea	31722-0520-01	50.80		AA
1000s ea	31722-0520-10	507.00		AA
50 mg, 100s ea	31722-0521-01	56.30		AA
1000s ea	31722-0521-10	562.00		AA
100 mg, 100s ea	31722-0522-01	101.28		AA
(Consolidated Midland) *See HYDRALAZINE HCL*				
(Gallipot) *See HYDRALAZINE HCL*				
(Heritage)				
TAB, PO (USP,FILM COATED)				
10 mg, 100s ea	23155-0001-01	41.15		
1000s ea	23155-0001-10	403.23		
(USP,FILM-COATED)				
25 mg, 100s ea	23155-0002-01	50.80		
1000s ea	23155-0002-10	507.00		
50 mg, 100s ea	23155-0003-01	56.30		
1000s ea	23155-0003-10	562.00		
(USP,FILM COATED)				
100 mg, 100s ea	23155-0004-01	101.30		
(Par) *See HYDRALAZINE HCL*				
(PCCA) *See HYDRALAZINE HCL*				
(Spectrum Pharmacy) *See HYDRALAZINE HCL*				
(Teva) *See HYDRALAZINE HCL*				
(Teva)				
TAB, PO ((10X10),USP)				
10 mg, 100s ea UD	00182-0905-89	21.79		AA
(10X10)				
25 mg, 100s ea UD	00182-0554-89	35.38		AA
((10X10),USP)				
50 mg, 100s ea UD	00182-0555-89	43.98		AA
(UDL)				
TAB, PO (10X10)				
10 mg, 100s ea UD	51079-0074-20	41.45		AA
(ROBOT READY 25X1)				
25 mg, 25s ea	51079-0075-19	12.71		AA
(10X10)				
25 mg, 100s ea UD	51079-0075-20	50.84		AA
50 mg, 100s ea UD	51079-0076-20	56.33		AA
(American Health)				
REPACK				
TAB, PO (10X10,USP,FILM-COATED)				
25 mg, 100s ea UD	62584-0733-01	25.38		
50 mg, 100s ea UD	62584-0734-01	43.98		
(GSMS)				
REPACK				
TAB, PO (USP)				
10 mg, 100s ea	60429-0064-01	27.36	9.12	AA
1000s ea	60429-0064-10	272.58	90.86	AA
25 mg, 100s ea	60429-0065-01	35.82	11.94	AA
1000s ea	60429-0065-10	358.20	119.40	AA
50 mg, 100s ea	60429-0066-01	47.88	15.96	AA
1000s ea	60429-0066-10	477.27	159.09	AA
100 mg, 100s ea	60429-0067-01	79.20	26.40	AA
1000s ea	60429-0067-10	774.00	258.00	AA
(Phys Total Care)				
REPACK				
TAB, PO, 50 mg, 60s ea	54868-2893-01	68.37		
90s ea	54868-2893-02	107.72		
(Quality Care Prod)				
REPACK				
TAB, PO, 50 mg, 100s ea	49999-0777-00	53.07		
HYDRALAZINE HYDROCHLORIDE/ ISOSORBIDE DINITRATE				
(Nitromed) *See BIDIL*				
HYDRAZINE SULFATE (Baker, J.T.)				
CRY, NA (A.C.S., REAGENT)				
125 gm	10106-2177-04	50.32		
500 gm	10106-2177-01	78.33		
(Gallipot)				
POW, NA (REAGENT)				
125 gm	51552-0577-09	38.92		
(Medisca)				
POW, NA (CRYSTAL)				
25 gm	38779-1346-04	49.35		
(1X100GM,CRYSTAL)				
100 gm	38779-1346-05	81.00		
(1X500GM,CRYSTAL)				
500 gm	38779-1346-08	267.00		
(PCCA)				
CRY, NA (ACS)				
1 gm	51927-1876-00	1.80		
HYDREA (B/M Squibb Onc/Vir)				
hydroxyurea				
CAP, PO, 500 mg, 100s ea	00003-0830-50	145.79		AB
(Phys Total Care)				
REPACK				
CAP, PO, 500 mg, 100s ea	54868-1367-00	156.90		AB
HYDRIODIC ACID				
(Baker, J.T.) *See HYDRIODIC ACID 47-51%*				
(Baker, J.T.) *See HYDRIODIC ACID 55% UNSTABILIZED*				
(PCCA)				
POW, NA (55-58%)				
1 gm	51927-1541-00	2.28		
HYDRIODIC ACID 47-51% (Baker, J.T.)				
hydriodic acid				
LIQ, NA (A.C.S., REAGENT)				
120 ml	10106-0150-04	92.75		
500 ml	10106-0150-01	248.49		
HYDRIODIC ACID 55% UNSTABILIZED (Baker, J.T.)				
hydriodic acid				
POW, NA (A.C.S., REAGENT)				
500 gm	10106-0152-01	113.45		
HYDRO 35 (Quinnova)				
urea				
FOA, TP (1X150GM)				
35%, 150 gm	23710-0035-15	175.00		
HYDRO 40 (Quinnova)				
urea				
FOA, TP (1X70GM)				
40%, 70 gm	23710-0040-75	125.18		
(1X150GM)				
40%, 150 gm	23710-0040-15	162.50		
HYDRO-TUSSIN HC (Ethex)				
cpm/hydrocod bit/pse hcl				
SYR, PO (AF,SF,DYE-FREE)				
473 ml, C-III	58177-0915-07	40.87		
HYDRO-TUSSIN HD (Ethex)				
gg/hydrocod bit/pse hcl				
LIQ, PO (AF,SF,FRUIT)				
480 ml, C-III	58177-0890-07	31.69		
HYDRO-TUSSIN XP (Ethex)				
gg/hydrocod bit/pse hcl				
SYR, PO (AF,SF,DYE-FREE)				
480 ml, C-III	58177-0916-07	42.24		
HYDROBROMIC ACID				
(Baker, J.T.) *See HYDROBROMIC ACID 47-49%*				
HYDROBROMIC ACID 47-49% (Baker, J.T.)				
hydrobromic acid				
LIQ, NA (A.C.S., REAGENT)				
500 ml	10106-0160-01	104.29		
4000 ml	10106-0160-03	266.05		
HYDROCHLORIC ACID (Baker, J.T.)				
LIQ, NA (N.F., F.C.C.)				
2500 ml	10106-9544-03	33.37		
(Mallinckrodt Lab)				
LIQ, NA (N.F., DILUTED)				
500 ml	00406-2608-02	18.28		
SOL, NA (N.F.)				
500 ml	00406-2612-14	19.68		
(Medisca)				
SOL, NA (1X500ML)				
500 ml	38779-0584-08	73.50		
(PCCA)				
SOL, NA (ACS)				
1 ml	51927-1647-00	0.24		
(Spectrum Pharmacy) *See HYDROCHLORIC ACID 37%*				
(Spectrum Pharmacy) *See HYDROCHLORIC ACID DILUTED 10%*				
(Spectrum Pharmacy)				
LIQ, NA (1X500ML)				
500 ml	49452-3550-02	130.55		
(1X2500ML)				
2500 ml	49452-3550-01	258.65		
HYDROCHLORIC ACID 37% (Spectrum Pharmacy)				
hydrochloric acid				
SOL, NA (N.F.)				
500 ml	49452-3560-01	103.95		
2500 ml	49452-3560-02	206.85		
HYDROCHLORIC ACID DILUTED 10% (Spectrum Pharmacy)				
hydrochloric acid				
SOL, NA (N.F.)				
500 ml	49452-3570-01	96.25		
2500 ml	49452-3570-02	175.00		
HYDROCHLOROTHIAZIDE				
FUL				
CAP, PO, 12.5 mg, 100s ea		12.00		
TAB, PO, 25 mg, 1000s ea		18.00		
50 mg, 1000s ea		49.90		
(Actavis)				
TAB, PO, 12.5 mg, 100s ea	00228-2820-11	82.43		AB
25 mg, 1000s ea	00228-2221-96	79.44		AB
50 mg, 1000s ea	00228-2222-96	133.00		AB
(Apotex Corp.)				
TAB, PO (USP)				
25 mg, 100s ea	60505-2640-01	8.48		AB
1000s ea	60505-2640-08	79.25		AB
28000s ea	60505-2640-07	2219.00		AB
50 mg, 100s ea	60505-2641-01	16.45		AB
1000s ea	60505-2641-08	132.99		AB
14000s ea	60505-2641-07	1861.86		AB
(Aurobindo Pharma)				
CAP, PO, 12.5 mg, 100s ea	65862-0113-01	42.45		AB
TAB, PO (USP)				
25 mg, 100s ea	65862-0133-01	7.92		AB
1000s ea	65862-0133-99	79.20		AB

PROD/MFR	NDC	AWP	DP	OBC
50 mg, 100s ea	65862-0134-01	13.30		AB
1000s ea	65862-0134-99	133.00		AB
(Cadista)				
CAP, PO (HARD GELATIN)				
12.5 mg, 100s ea	59746-0382-06	42.40		AB
1000s ea	59746-0382-10	402.80		AB
TAB, PO (USP)				
25 mg, 100s ea	59746-0125-01	8.48		AB
1000s ea	59746-0125-10	79.44		AB
50 mg, 100s ea	59746-0127-01	16.45		AB
1000s ea	59746-0127-10	133.00		AB
(Caraco)				
TAB, PO (USP)				
25 mg, 100s ea	57664-0428-88	8.45		AB
1000s ea	57664-0428-18	79.40		AB
50 mg, 100s ea	57664-0429-88	16.35		AB
1000s ea	57664-0429-18	132.90		AB
(Consolidated Midland)				
TAB, PO, 25 mg, 100s ea	00223-1069-01	1.75		EE
1000s ea	00223-1069-02	9.95		EE
50 mg, 100s ea	00223-1070-01	2.75		EE
1000s ea	00223-1070-02	11.25		EE
100 mg, 100s ea	00223-1068-01	2.75		EE
1000s ea	00223-1068-02	14.95		EE
(Dava Pharma)				
TAB, PO, 25 mg, 100s ea	67253-0820-10	8.45		
1000s ea	67253-0820-11	79.20		
50 mg, 100s ea	67253-0821-10	16.40		
1000s ea	67253-0821-11	132.95		
(Excellium)				
TAB, PO (USP)				
25 mg, 100s ea	64125-0131-01	8.48		AB
1000s ea	64125-0131-10	79.44		AB
50 mg, 100s ea	64125-0130-01	16.45		AB
1000s ea	64125-0130-10	133.00		AB
(Greenstone)				
CAP, PO (HARD GELATIN)				
12.5 mg, 100s ea	59762-1735-02	82.43		
TAB, PO (UNCOATED)				
25 mg, 100s ea	59762-1736-02	7.92		
1000s ea	59762-1736-07	79.20		
50 mg, 100s ea	59762-1737-02	13.30		
1000s ea	59762-1737-07	133.00		
(Heritage)				
CAP, PO (HARD-GELATIN)				
12.5 mg, 500s ea	23155-0140-05	60.00		AB
TAB, PO (USP,UNCOATED)				
25 mg, 100s ea	23155-0138-01	8.48		AB
1000s ea	23155-0138-10	79.44		AB
50 mg, 100s ea	23155-0139-01	16.45		AB
1000s ea	23155-0139-10	133.00		AB
(Lannett)				
TAB, PO (USP)				
25 mg, 100s ea	00527-1413-01	4.74		AB
1000s ea	00527-1413-10	21.90		AB
50 mg, 100s ea	00527-1414-01	7.80		AB
1000s ea	00527-1414-10	43.20		AB
(Major)				
CAP, PO (10X10,HARD GELATIN)				
12.5 mg,				
100s ea UD	00904-5967-61	40.94		AB
(Medisca)				
POW, NA (U.S.P.)				
25 gm	38779-0314-04	27.00		
100 gm	38779-0314-05	64.50		
500 gm	38779-0314-08	237.00		
1000 gm	38779-0314-09	429.00		
(Mylan)				
CAP, PO, 12.5 mg, 30s ea	00378-0810-93	12.74		AB
100s ea	00378-0810-01	42.45		AB
500s ea	00378-0810-05	212.25		AB
TAB, PO (USP)				
25 mg, 100s ea	00378-3601-01	8.48		AB
1000s ea	00378-3601-10	79.20		AB
50 mg, 100s ea	00378-3602-01	16.45		AB
1000s ea	00378-3602-10	133.00		AB
(PCCA)				
POW, NA (U.S.P.)				
1 gm	51927-1611-00	1.20		
(Qualitest)				
CAP, PO, 12.5 mg, 100s ea	00603-3855-21	42.45		AB
300s ea	00603-3855-25	123.53		AB
1000s ea	00603-3855-32	403.11		AB
TAB, PO, 25 mg, 100s ea	00603-3856-21	8.48		AB
1000s ea	00603-3856-32	79.44		AB
5000s ea	00603-3856-34	377.34		AB
50 mg, 100s ea	00603-3857-21	16.45		AB
1000s ea	00603-3857-32	133.00		AB
(Ranbaxy Pharm)				
TAB, PO (USP)				
25 mg, 100s ea	63304-0914-01	8.48		
1000s ea	63304-0914-10	79.44		
50 mg, 100s ea	63304-0915-01	16.45		
1000s ea	63304-0915-10	133.00		
(Spectrum Pharmacy)				
POW, NA (U.S.P., N.F.)				
25 gm	49452-3575-01	64.75		
500 gm	49452-3575-03	367.50		
(Teva)				
CAP, PO, 12.5 mg, 100s ea	00172-4870-10	45.49		
100s ea	00172-4870-60	42.49		
1000s ea	00172-4870-80	403.15		
TAB, PO, 25 mg, 100s ea	00172-2083-60	8.48		AB
(10X10)				
25 mg, 100s ea UD	00182-0556-89	14.82		AB
1000s ea	00172-2083-80	79.25		AB
50 mg, 100s ea	00172-2089-60	16.45		AB
(10X10)				
50 mg, 100s ea UD	00182-0557-89	17.54		AB
1000s ea	00172-2089-80	132.99		AB
5000s ea	00172-2089-85	819.59		AB
(Truxton) *See HYDROCOT*				
(UDL)				
CAP, PO, 12.5 mg,				
100s ea UD	51079-0776-20	42.45		AB
(Unichem)				
TAB, PO (USP)				
25 mg, 100s ea	29300-0128-01	8.48		AB
1000s ea	29300-0128-10	79.40		AB
50 mg, 100s ea	29300-0129-01	16.45		AB
1000s ea	29300-0129-10	132.95		AB
(Watson) *See MICROZIDE*				
(Watson Labs)				
CAP, PO, 12.5 mg, 100s ea	00591-0347-01	9.60		AB
500s ea	00591-0347-05	45.60		AB
(West-Ward)				
CAP, PO (HARD-GELATIN)				
12.5 mg, 100s ea	00143-3125-01	42.45		AB
TAB, PO (USP)				
25 mg, 100s ea	00143-1256-01	8.48		AB
1000s ea	00143-1256-10	79.30	6.30	AB
5000s ea	00143-1256-51	345.00		AB
50 mg, 100s ea	00143-1257-01	16.45	1.25	AB
1000s ea	00143-1257-10	132.99	7.00	AB
5000s ea	00143-1257-51	610.00		AB
(A-S Medication)				
REPACK				
CAP, PO, 12.5 mg, 30s ea	54569-5236-00	14.24		AB
TAB, PO, 12.5 mg, 30s ea	54569-6040-00	24.73		
35s ea	54569-6040-01	28.85		AB
25 mg, 30s ea	54569-0547-00	2.54		EE
35s ea	54569-0547-09	2.97		AB
100s ea	54569-0547-01	8.48		EE
200s ea	54569-0547-08	16.96		EE
50 mg, 30s ea	54569-0549-00	4.94		EE
100s ea	54569-0549-01	16.45		EE
(Aidarex)				
REPACK				
TAB, PO, 25 mg, 30s ea	33261-0158-30	9.95		AB
60s ea	33261-0158-60	19.90		AB
90s ea	33261-0158-90	29.85		AB
120s ea	33261-0158-02	39.80		AB
(Altura)				
REPACK				
TAB, PO, 25 mg, 7s ea	63874-0364-07	0.99		
10s ea	63874-0364-10	1.41		
12s ea	63874-0364-12	1.70		
14s ea	63874-0364-14	1.98		
15s ea	63874-0364-15	2.12		
20s ea	63874-0364-20	2.83		
30s ea	63874-0364-30	4.24		
60s ea	63874-0364-60	8.48		
90s ea	63874-0364-90	12.72		
100s ea	63874-0364-01	14.13		
120s ea	63874-0364-04	16.69		
1000s ea	63874-0364-02	141.16		
50 mg, 10s ea	63874-0365-10	2.24		AB
12s ea	63874-0365-12	2.69		AB
14s ea	63874-0365-14	3.14		AB
15s ea	63874-0365-15	3.36		AB
20s ea	63874-0365-20	4.49		AB
30s ea	63874-0365-30	6.73		AB
60s ea	63874-0365-60	13.46		AB
90s ea	63874-0365-90	20.19		AB
100s ea	63874-0365-01	22.43		AB
120s ea	63874-0365-04	26.92		AB
1000s ea	63874-0365-02	224.20		AB
(American Health)				
REPACK				
TAB, PO, 25 mg,				
100s ea UD	68084-0086-01	14.79		AB
50 mg, 100s ea UD	68084-0087-01	17.43		AB
(Bryant Ranch)				
REPACK				
CAP, PO, 12.5 mg, 30s ea	63629-2926-01	1.80		
TAB, PO, 25 mg, 7s ea	63629-1400-03	1.99		
14s ea	63629-1400-04	3.31		
30s ea	63629-1400-02	7.37		
60s ea	63629-1400-05	14.75		
100s ea	63629-1400-01	24.91		
50 mg, 30s ea	63629-1413-01	7.23		
(Core)				
REPACK				
TAB, PO, 25 mg, 20s ea	33358-0164-20	4.25		
30s ea	33358-0164-30	6.45		
(DHS, Inc.)				
REPACK				
CAP, PO, 12.5 mg, 30s ea	55887-0865-30	31.96		
TAB, PO, 25 mg, 7s ea	55887-0839-07	2.00		
30s ea	55887-0839-30	8.00		AB
60s ea	55887-0839-60	12.00		AB
90s ea	55887-0839-90	16.00		AB
100s ea	55887-0839-01	18.00		AB
50 mg, 30s ea	55887-0579-30	8.56		AB
60s ea	55887-0579-60	15.98		AB
90s ea	55887-0579-90	23.71		AB
(Dispensing Solutions)				
REPACK				
CAP, PO, 12.5 mg, 30s ea	66336-0823-30	17.04		AB
TAB, PO, 25 mg, 30s ea	55045-1298-08	4.20		AB
30s ea	66336-0184-30	7.90		AB
60s ea	55045-1298-09	8.40		AB
60s ea	66336-0184-60	14.75		AB
90s ea	66336-0184-90	22.13		AB
100s ea	55045-1298-01	14.00		AB
50 mg, 30s ea	55045-1431-08	7.20		AB
30s ea	66336-0675-30	7.25		AB
60s ea	66336-0675-60	14.50		AB
90s ea	66336-0675-90	21.75		AB
100s ea	55045-1431-00	24.00		AB
(GSMS)				
REPACK				
TAB, PO (UNIT OF USE)				
25 mg, 90s ea	60429-0218-90	11.55	3.85	EE
50 mg, 90s ea	60429-0213-90	24.75	8.25	AB
(HomeMed)				
REPACK				
CAP, PO, 12.5 mg, 30s ea	51655-0314-24	15.65		
TAB, PO, 25 mg, 30s ea	51655-0126-24	7.69		AB
60s ea	51655-0126-25	2.64		AB
90s ea	51655-0126-26	4.00		AB
100s ea	51655-0126-21	5.15		AB
120s ea	51655-0126-82	4.89		AB
50 mg, 30s ea	51655-0077-24	2.25		AB
60s ea	51655-0077-25	2.50		AB
90s ea	51655-0077-26	3.60		AB
100s ea	51655-0077-21	3.80		AB
120s ea	51655-0077-82	3.90		AB
(Keltman Pharma., Inc.)				
REPACK				
TAB, PO, 25 mg, 30s ea	68387-0537-30	9.89		
(McKesson Packaging)				
REPACK				
TAB, PO, 25 mg,				
100s ea UD	63739-0128-10	12.73		AB
(Nucare Pharm)				
REPACK				
CAP, PO (HARD-GELATIN)				
12.5 mg, 30s ea	68071-0255-30	19.25		AB
(Palmetto)				
REPACK				
CAP, PO, 12.5 mg, 30s ea	23490-7038-01	15.65		
TAB, PO, 12.5 mg, 30s ea	23490-7037-01	29.73		
25 mg, 14s ea	23490-5682-01	3.73		
30s ea	23490-5682-02	8.00		
60s ea	23490-5682-03	16.00		
90s ea	23490-5682-04	24.00		
100s ea	23490-5682-05	26.67		
50 mg, 30s ea	23490-5683-03	7.50		
60s ea	23490-5683-06	15.00		
(PD-Rx Pharm)				
REPACK				
CAP, PO, 12.5 mg, 30s ea	55289-0565-30	9.66		AB
30s ea	58864-0792-30	15.65		AB
TAB, PO, 25 mg, 6s ea	55289-0136-06	6.05		AB

PROD/MFR	NDC	AWP	DP	OBC
12s ea	55289-0136-12	6.27		AB
16s ea	55289-0136-16	6.50		AB
20s ea	55289-0136-20	6.87		AB
30s ea	55289-0136-30	7.82		AB
(REDI-SCRIPT)				
25 mg, 30s ea	58864-0250-30	7.81		AB
(USP)				
25 mg, 45s ea	55289-0136-45	9.15		
(REDI-SCRIPT)				
25 mg, 60s ea	58864-0250-60	9.60		AB
90s ea	55289-0136-90	10.40		AB
(REDI-SCRIPT)				
25 mg, 90s ea	58864-0250-90	10.40		AB
100s ea	43063-0010-01	79.44		AB
100s ea	55289-0136-01	10.98		AB
(REDI-SCRIPT)				
25 mg, 100s ea	58864-0250-01	10.98		AB
120s ea	55289-0136-98	11.73		AB
50 mg, 14s ea	55289-0135-14	6.40		AB
30s ea	55289-0135-30	8.02		AB
30s ea	58864-0251-30	8.01		AB
45s ea	55289-0135-45	9.66		AB
90s ea	55289-0135-90	13.20		AB
100s ea	55289-0135-01	15.06		AB
100s ea UD	58864-0251-17	33.63		AB
(Pharma Pac)				
REPACK				
TAB, PO, 25 mg, 30s ea	52959-0132-30	4.15		EE
60s ea	52959-0132-60	8.19		EE
100s ea	52959-0132-00	13.17		EE
50 mg, 30s ea	52959-0133-30	7.25		EE
90s ea	52959-0133-90	20.03		EE
100s ea	52959-0133-00	22.25		EE
(Phys Total Care)				
REPACK				
CAP, PO, 12.5 mg, 30s ea	54868-4438-00	17.25		EE
90s ea	54868-4438-02	45.78		EE
100s ea	54868-4438-01	49.05		AB
TAB, PO, 25 mg, 15s ea	54868-0792-07	6.24		AB
30s ea	54868-0792-01	7.95		EE
40s ea	54868-0792-03	9.12		EE
60s ea	54868-0792-06	11.42		AB
90s ea	54868-0792-05	14.88		AB
100s ea	54868-0792-02	16.05		EE
1000s ea	54868-0792-00	110.43		EE
50 mg, 30s ea	54868-0056-02	11.17		EE
40s ea	54868-0056-04	13.89		EE
60s ea	54868-0056-06	14.64		EE
100s ea	54868-0056-03	30.23		EE
1000s ea	54868-0056-00	273.81		EE
100 mg, 30s ea	54868-2494-01	6.86		EE
(Physician Partner)				
REPACK				
TAB, PO, 25 mg, 30s ea	21695-0538-30	20.09		AB
90s ea	21695-0538-90	60.27		AB
50 mg, 30s ea	21695-0539-30	24.87		
50s ea	21695-0539-50	48.76		AB
90s ea	21695-0539-90	74.61		AB
(Quality Care Prod)				
REPACK				
CAP, PO, 12.5 mg, 30s ea	49999-0388-30	42.73		AB
60s ea	49999-0388-60	85.46		AB
90s ea	49999-0388-90	128.19		AB
TAB, PO, 25 mg, 10s ea	49999-0167-10	3.35		EE
28s ea	49999-0167-28	13.30		AB
30s ea	49999-0167-30	10.06		EE
60s ea	49999-0167-60	20.12		AB
100s ea	49999-0167-00	40.80		AB
50 mg, 30s ea	49999-0279-30	11.99		EE
(Southwood)				
REPACK				
TAB, PO, 25 mg, 12s ea	58016-0523-12	1.62		EE
15s ea	58016-0523-15	2.02		EE
20s ea	58016-0523-20	2.70		EE
30s ea	58016-0523-30	4.04		EE
100s ea	58016-0523-00	13.48		EE
50 mg, 12s ea	58016-0524-12	2.56		EE
15s ea	58016-0524-15	3.20		EE
20s ea	58016-0524-20	4.27		EE
30s ea	58016-0524-30	6.41		EE
100s ea	58016-0524-00	21.35		EE
(Stat Rx)				
REPACK				
CAP, PO, 12.5 mg, 30s ea	16590-0580-30	10.00		AB
60s ea	16590-0580-60	20.00		AB
90s ea	16590-0580-90	27.00		AB

PROD/MFR	NDC	AWP	DP	OBC
(Vibranta)				
REPACK				
CAP, PO, 12.5 mg, 30s ea	57866-6733-01	51.58		
TAB, PO, 25 mg, 30s ea	57866-3922-01	46.37		
50 mg, 30s ea	57866-3919-01	6.10		
HYDROCHLOROTHIAZIDE/IRBESARTAN				
(Bristol-Myers) *See AVALIDE*				
HYDROCHLOROTHIAZIDE/LISINOPRIL				
FUL				
TAB, PO, 12.5 mg-10 mg, 100s ea		20.97		
12.5 mg-20 mg, 100s ea		21.99		
25 mg-20 mg, 100s ea		22.25		
(Apotex Corp.) *See HCTZ/LISINOPRIL*				
(Apotex Corp.) *See LISINOPRIL AND HYDROCHLOROTHIAZIDE*				
(AstraZeneca) *See ZESTORETIC*				
(Aurobindo Pharma) *See LISINOPRIL-HYDROCHLOROTHIAZIDE*				
(Greenstone) *See LISINOPRIL-HYDROCHLOROTHIAZIDE*				
(Lupin Pharma, Inc.) *See LISINOPRIL AND HYDROCHLOROTHIAZIDE*				
(Merck) *See PRINZIDE*				
(Mylan) *See HCTZ/LISINOPRIL*				
(Ranbaxy Pharm) *See HCTZ/LISINOPRIL*				
(Sandoz) *See HCTZ/LISINOPRIL*				
(Teva) *See HCTZ/LISINOPRIL*				
(Watson Labs) *See HCTZ/LISINOPRIL*				
(West-Ward) *See HCTZ/LISINOPRIL*				
(Dispensing Solutions)				
REPACK				
TAB, PO, 25 mg-20 mg, 60s ea	55045-3225-06	72.00		
(Palmetto)				
REPACK				
TAB, PO, 12.5 mg-10 mg, 30s ea	23490-5820-01	46.00		
12.5 mg-20 mg, 30s ea	23490-5821-01	46.47		
25 mg-20 mg, 30s ea	23490-5822-01	43.99		
HYDROCHLOROTHIAZIDE/LOSARTAN POTASSIUM				
(Merck) *See HYZAAR*				
HYDROCHLOROTHIAZIDE/METHYLDOPA				
(Consolidated Midland) *See HCTZ/METHYLDOPA*				
(Mylan) *See HCTZ/METHYLDOPA*				
HYDROCHLOROTHIAZIDE/METOPROLOL TARTRATE				
(Mylan) *See HCTZ-METOPROLOL*				
(Novartis Pharm) *See LOPRESSOR HCT*				
(Sandoz) *See METOPROLOL TARTRATE AND HYDROCHLOROTHIAZIDE*				
HYDROCHLOROTHIAZIDE/MOEXIPRIL HYDROCHLORIDE				
FUL				
TAB, PO, 12.5 mg-7.5 mg, 100s ea		121.11		
12.5 mg-15 mg, 100s ea		121.11		
25 mg-15 mg, 100s ea		121.11		
(Kremers Urban) *See MOEXIPRIL HYDROCHLORIDE AND HYDROCHLOROTHIAZIDE*				
(Paddock) *See MOEXIPRIL HYDROCHLORIDE AND HYDROCHLOROTHIAZIDE*				
(Teva) *See MOEXIPRIL HYDROCHLORIDE AND HYDROCHLOROTHIAZIDE*				
(UCB) *See UNIRETIC*				
(Watson Labs) *See MOEXIPRIL HYDROCHLORIDE/HYDROCHLOROTHIAZIDE*				
HYDROCHLOROTHIAZIDE/OLMESARTAN MEDOXOMIL				
(Daiichi Sankyo) *See BENICAR HCT*				
HYDROCHLOROTHIAZIDE/PROPRANOLOL HYDROCHLORIDE				
FUL				
TAB, PO, 25 mg-40 mg, 100s ea		8.77		
25 mg-80 mg, 100s ea		13.20		

PROD/MFR	NDC	AWP	DP	OBC
(Mylan) *See HCTZ/PROPRANOLOL*				
HYDROCHLOROTHIAZIDE/QUINAPRIL HYDROCHLORIDE				
(Aurobindo Pharma) *See QUINAPRIL HYDROCHLORIDE AND HYDROCHLOROTHIAZIDE*				
(Greenstone) *See QUINAPRIL HYDROCHLORIDE/HYDROCHLOROTHIAZIDE*				
(Mylan) *See QUINAPRIL HYDROCHLORIDE AND HYDROCHLOROTHIAZIDE*				
(Pfizer) *See ACCURETIC*				
HYDROCHLOROTHIAZIDE/SPIRONOLACTONE				
FUL				
TAB, PO, 25 mg-25 mg, 100s ea		34.63		
(Greenstone) *See HCTZ/SPIRONOLACTONE*				
(Mutual) *See HCTZ/SPIRONOLACTONE*				
(Mylan) *See HCTZ/SPIRONOLACTONE*				
(Pfizer) *See ALDACTAZIDE*				
(UDL) *See HCTZ/SPIRONOLACTONE*				
(Palmetto)				
REPACK				
TAB, PO, 25 mg-25 mg, 30s ea	23490-6300-02	29.41		
100s ea	23490-6300-00	98.03		
HYDROCHLOROTHIAZIDE/TELMISARTAN				
(Boehr Ingelheim Phar) *See MICARDIS HCT*				
HYDROCHLOROTHIAZIDE/TRIAMTERENE				
FUL				
CAP, PO, 25 mg-37.5 mg, 100s ea		31.77		
TAB, PO, 25 mg-37.5 mg, 100s ea		16.83		
50 mg-75 mg, 100s ea		4.88		
(Apotex Corp.) *See TRIAMTERENE AND HYDROCHLOROTHIAZIDE*				
(Glaxo) *See DYAZIDE*				
(Mylan) *See HCTZ/TRIAMTERENE*				
(Mylan) *See MAXZIDE*				
(Mylan) *See MAXZIDE-25*				
(Mylan Bertek) *See MAXZIDE*				
(Sandoz) *See HCTZ/TRIAMTERENE*				
(Teva) *See HCTZ/TRIAMTERENE*				
(UDL) *See HCTZ/TRIAMTERENE*				
(Watson Labs) *See HCTZ/TRIAMTERENE*				
(Altura)				
REPACK				
CAP, PO, 25 mg-37.5 mg, 5s ea	63874-0508-05	2.05		
10s ea	63874-0508-10	4.10		
14s ea	63874-0508-14	5.74		
20s ea	63874-0508-20	8.20		
30s ea	63874-0508-30	12.30		
90s ea	63874-0508-90	37.13		
100s ea	63874-0508-01	41.00		
(Palmetto)				
REPACK				
CAP, PO, 25 mg-50 mg, 30s ea	23490-6427-01	26.07		
60s ea	23490-6427-02	52.14		
TAB, PO, 25 mg-37.5 mg, 30s ea	23490-6430-01	19.04		
90s ea	23490-6430-02	57.12		
50 mg-75 mg, 30s ea	23490-6428-01	45.00		
HYDROCHLOROTHIAZIDE/VALSARTAN				
(Novartis Pharm) *See DIOVAN HCT*				
HYDROCOD BIT & ACET (Pharma Pac)				
REPACK				
acetaminophen/hydrocodone bitartrate				
ELI, PO, 120 ml, C-III	52959-0797-04	22.45		
TAB, PO, 500 mg-2.5 mg, 30s ea, C-III	52959-0795-30	25.50		
HYDROCOD BIT/PHENYLEPH HCL/PYRIL MAL				
(Breckenridge Pharm) *See MINTUSS MR*				
(Breckenridge Pharm) *See TUSSPLEX*				
(Poly) *See POLY HIST HC*				
(Poly) *See POLY-TUSSIN*				
(Vintage) *See CODITUSS DH*				

PROD/MFR	NDC	AWP	DP	OBC
HYDROCOD BIT/PSE HCL				
(Breckenridge Pharm) *See COLDCOUGH HCM*				
HYDROCODONE BIT & ACET (Pharma Pac)				
REPACK				
acetaminophen/hydrocodone bitartrate				
TAB, PO, 750 mg-7.5 mg,				
16s ea, C-III	**52959-0415-16**	11.52		
HYDROCODONE BIT AND ACET (Pharma Pac)				
acetaminophen/hydrocodone bitartrate				
TAB, PO, 500 mg-5 mg,				
42s ea, C-III	**52959-0312-42**	30.08		
HYDROCODONE BIT/GUAIFENESIN (Altura)				
REPACK				
guaifenesin/hydrocodone bitartrate				
LIQ, PO, 100 mg/5 ml-5 mg/5 ml,				
120 ml, C-III	**63874-0298-12**	12.33		
HYDROCODONE BIT/PHENY HYDROCHLORIDE/CHLOR MAL (Palmetto)				
REPACK				
cpm/hydrocod bit/phenyleph hcl				
SYR, PO, 120 ml, C-III	**23490-1944-01**	18.00		
180 ml, C-III	**23490-1944-02**	27.00		
HYDROCODONE BITART/ACET (Phys Total Care)				
REPACK				
acetaminophen/hydrocodone bitartrate				
ELI, PO, 120 ml, C-III	**54868-4747-00**	28.74		
473 ml, C-III	**54868-4747-01**	58.02		
TAB, PO, 325 mg-5 mg,				
30s ea, C-III	**54868-5146-00**	33.54		
(USP)				
325 mg-5 mg,				
40s ea, C-III	**54868-5146-02**	54.14		
60s ea, C-III	**54868-5146-03**	77.46		
90s ea, C-III	**54868-5146-04**	77.32		
100s ea, C-III	**54868-5146-01**	78.54		
(USP)				
325 mg-7.5 mg,				
20s ea, C-III	**54868-5167-06**	32.55		
40s ea, C-III	**54868-5167-04**	62.21		
(USP)				
325 mg-7.5 mg,				
60s ea, C-III	**54868-5167-05**	88.66		
90s ea, C-III	**54868-5167-07**	90.81		
100s ea, C-III	**54868-5167-01**	111.75		
120s ea, C-III	**54868-5167-03**	133.20		
200s ea, C-III	**54868-5167-02**	166.86		
(USP)				
325 mg-10 mg,				
20s ea, C-III	**54868-4974-05**	20.43		
30s ea, C-III	**54868-4974-01**	28.38		
(USP)				
325 mg-10 mg,				
40s ea, C-III	**54868-4974-04**	37.86		
60s ea, C-III	**54868-4974-00**	52.26		
90s ea, C-III	**54868-4974-03**	76.14		
100s ea, C-III	**54868-4974-06**	84.12		
120s ea, C-III	**54868-4974-07**	96.00		
500s ea, C-III	**54868-4974-02**	307.41		
(USP)				
500 mg-2.5 mg,				
40s ea, C-III	**54868-4360-01**	22.77		
60s ea, C-III	**54868-4360-00**	31.17		
500 mg-5 mg,				
10s ea, C-III	**54868-0071-03**	6.60		
15s ea, C-III	**54868-0071-05**	7.65		
20s ea, C-III	**54868-0071-02**	10.08		
30s ea, C-III	**54868-0071-01**	14.37		
40s ea, C-III	**54868-0071-04**	15.66		
50s ea, C-III	**54868-0071-07**	18.45		
60s ea, C-III	**54868-0071-00**	21.24		
100s ea, C-III	**54868-0071-08**	32.43		
500 mg-7.5 mg,				
20s ea, C-III	**54868-3038-02**	9.66		
30s ea, C-III	**54868-3038-01**	12.24		
40s ea, C-III	**54868-3038-05**	14.84		
50s ea, C-III	**54868-3038-07**	17.42		
60s ea, C-III	**54868-3038-04**	20.01		
90s ea, C-III	**54868-3038-03**	27.75		
100s ea, C-III	**54868-3038-00**	28.85		
120s ea, C-III	**54868-3038-06**	35.52		
500 mg-10 mg,				
20s ea, C-III	**54868-4237-00**	14.64		
30s ea, C-III	**54868-4237-04**	23.64		
(USP)				
500 mg-10 mg,				
40s ea, C-III	**54868-4237-06**	26.31		
60s ea, C-III	**54868-4237-03**	41.31		
90s ea, C-III	**54868-4237-02**	58.95		
100s ea, C-III	**54868-4237-01**	64.86		
120s ea, C-III	**54868-4237-07**	76.62		
500s ea, C-III	**54868-4237-05**	215.49		
650 mg-7.5 mg,				
20s ea, C-III	**54868-3585-00**	10.14		
40s ea, C-III	**54868-3585-02**	15.78		
60s ea, C-III	**54868-3585-03**	21.42		
100s ea, C-III	**54868-3585-01**	32.70		
650 mg-10 mg,				
20s ea, C-III	**54868-3729-02**	12.00		
30s ea, C-III	**54868-3729-01**	15.78		
40s ea, C-III	**54868-3729-08**	21.03		
60s ea, C-III	**54868-3729-03**	27.03		
90s ea, C-III	**54868-3729-05**	38.31		
100s ea, C-III	**54868-3729-04**	42.06		
120s ea, C-III	**54868-3729-06**	49.59		
500s ea, C-III	**54868-3729-07**	100.59		
660 mg-10 mg,				
30s ea, C-III	**54868-5059-01**	25.89		
40s ea, C-III	**54868-5059-03**	35.31		
75s ea, C-III	**54868-5059-00**	55.74		
100s ea, C-III	**54868-5059-02**	72.33		
750 mg-7.5 mg,				
10s ea, C-III	**54868-2281-04**	6.90		
15s ea, C-III	**54868-2281-02**	8.10		
20s ea, C-III	**54868-2281-03**	9.30		
30s ea, C-III	**54868-2281-01**	11.70		
40s ea, C-III	**54868-2281-06**	14.13		
60s ea, C-III	**54868-2281-05**	18.93		
90s ea, C-III	**54868-2281-08**	26.14		
100s ea, C-III	**54868-2281-00**	28.56		
120s ea, C-III	**54868-2281-07**	33.36		
HYDROCODONE BITART/IBU (Phys Total Care)				
hydrocodone bitartrate/ibuprofen				
TAB, PO (USP)				
7.5 mg-200 mg,				
40s ea, C-III	**54868-4976-03**	71.64		
100s ea, C-III	**54868-4976-04**	170.13		
HYDROCODONE BITARTRATE (Covidien)				
POW, NA, 5 gm, C-II	**00406-1582-53**	240.13		
(Elge, Inc.)				
POW, NA (USP)				
100 gm, C-II	**58298-0535-02**	2000.00		
(Gallipot)				
POW, NA (1X1GM,USP)				
1 gm, C-II	**51552-0677-01**	25.90	18.50	
(1X5GM,USP)				
5 gm, C-II	**51552-0677-02**	63.00	45.00	
(1X25GM,USP)				
25 gm, C-II	**51552-0677-04**	266.00	190.00	
(1X100GM,USP)				
100 gm, C-II	**51552-0677-06**	896.00	640.00	
(Hawkins)				
POW, NA (U.S.P.)				
5 gm, C-II	**63370-0925-15**	240.00		
100 gm, C-II	**63370-0925-35**	3600.00		
(Letco)				
POW, NA (1X5GM,USP)				
5 gm, C-II	**62991-1406-02**	232.00	58.00	
(1X25GM,USP)				
25 gm, C-II	**62991-1406-03**	808.00	202.00	
(1X100GM,USP)				
100 gm, C-II	**62991-1406-04**	2728.00	682.00	
(1X1000GM,USP)				
1000 gm, C-II	**62991-1406-05**	24000.00	6000.00	
(Medisca)				
POW, NA (U.S.P.)				
1 gm, C-II	**38779-0764-06**	57.00		
5 gm, C-II	**38779-0764-03**	138.00		
25 gm, C-II	**38779-0764-04**	573.00		
100 gm, C-II	**38779-0764-05**	1959.00		
500 gm, C-II	**38779-0764-08**	8550.00		
(PCCA)				
POW, NA (U.S.P.; CII)				
1 gm, C-II	**51927-1010-00**	84.00		
(Spectrum Pharmacy)				
POW, NA (U.S.P.)				
1 gm, C-II	**49452-0033-02**	122.50		
5 gm, C-II	**49452-0033-01**	218.05		
25 gm, C-II	**49452-0033-03**	896.00		
100 gm, C-II	**49452-0033-04**	2569.00		
(B&B Pharm, Inc)				
REPACK				
POW, NA (U.S.P.)				
5 gm, C-II	**63275-4100-02**	420.00		
25 gm, C-II	**63275-4100-04**	2100.00		
100 gm, C-II	**63275-4100-05**	8400.00		
(Hawkins)				
REPACK				
POW, NA (U.S.P.)				
25 gm, C-II	**63370-0925-25**	912.00		
HYDROCODONE BITARTRATE & ACET (Pharma Pac)				
REPACK				
acetaminophen/hydrocodone bitartrate				
TAB, PO, 660 mg-10 mg,				
60s ea, C-III	**52959-0071-60**	27.57		
90s ea, C-III	**52959-0071-90**	41.33		
HYDROCODONE BITARTRATE & ACETAMINOPHEN (Keltman Pharma., Inc.)				
REPACK				
acetaminophen/hydrocodone bitartrate				
TAB, PO, 325 mg-10 mg,				
30s ea, C-III	**68387-0235-30**	34.23		
60s ea, C-III	**68387-0235-60**	68.45		
180s ea, C-III	**68387-0235-18**	205.35		
500 mg-5 mg,				
12s ea, C-III	**68387-0300-02**	9.50		
40s ea, C-III	**68387-0300-40**	28.33		
650 mg-7.5 mg,				
40s ea, C-III	**68387-0201-40**	25.30		
660 mg-10 mg,				
60s ea, C-III	**68387-0401-60**	68.56		
(Pharma Pac)				
REPACK				
TAB, PO, 325 mg-7.5 mg,				
40s ea, C-III	**52959-0735-40**	51.62		
50s ea, C-III	**52959-0735-50**	64.44		
80s ea, C-III	**52959-0735-80**	102.32		
84s ea, C-III	**52959-0735-84**	107.39		
120s ea, C-III	**52959-0735-02**	152.88		
HYDROCODONE BITARTRATE & HOMATROPINE METHYLBROMIDE (Hi-Tech)				
homatropine methylbromide/hydrocodone bitartrate				
SYR, PO (1X473ML,CHERRY)				
1.5 mg/5 ml-5 mg/5 ml,				
473 ml, C-III	**50383-0043-16**	87.44		AA
(Altura)				
REPACK				
SYR, PO (1X180ML,CHERRY)				
1.5 mg/5 ml-5 mg/5 ml,				
180 ml, C-III	**63874-0255-18**	16.34		AA
(1X240ML,CHERRY)				
1.5 mg/5 ml-5 mg/5 ml,				
240 ml, C-III	**63874-0255-24**	19.31		AA
(Quality Care Prod)				
REPACK				
SYR, PO (1X473ML,CHERRY)				
1.5 mg/5 ml-5 mg/5 ml,				
473 ml, C-III	**35356-0200-73**	187.40		AA
HYDROCODONE BITARTRATE & IBUPROFEN (Keltman Pharma., Inc.)				
REPACK				
hydrocodone bitartrate/ibuprofen				
TAB, PO, 7.5 mg-200 mg,				
30s ea, C-III	**68387-0562-30**	46.18		
60s ea, C-III	**68387-0562-60**	92.35		
HYDROCODONE BITARTRATE AND ACETAMINOPHEN (Amneal)				
acetaminophen/hydrocodone bitartrate				
TAB, PO (USP)				
325 mg-5 mg,				
100s ea, C-III	**53746-0109-01**	54.22		AA
500s ea, C-III	**53746-0109-05**	271.10		AA
325 mg-10 mg,				
100s ea, C-III	**53746-0110-01**	69.89		AA
500s ea, C-III	**53746-0110-05**	337.28		AA
500 mg-5 mg,				
100s ea, C-III	**53746-0111-01**	48.12		AA
500s ea, C-III	**53746-0111-05**	220.82		AA
500 mg-7.5 mg,				
100s ea, C-III	**53746-0112-01**	57.21		AA
500s ea, C-III	**53746-0112-05**	257.46		AA
500 mg-10 mg,				
100s ea, C-III	**53746-0119-01**	53.27		AA
500s ea, C-III	**53746-0119-05**	253.03		AA
650 mg-7.5 mg,				
100s ea, C-III	**53746-0113-01**	69.50		AA
500s ea, C-III	**53746-0113-05**	292.51		AA
650 mg-10 mg,				
100s ea, C-III	**53746-0114-01**	97.76		AA
500s ea, C-III	**53746-0114-05**	454.58		AA
750 mg-7.5 mg,				
100s ea, C-III	**53746-0118-01**	43.78		AA
500s ea, C-III	**53746-0118-05**	204.53		AA
(Caraco)				
TAB, PO (USP,UNCOATED)				
325 mg-5 mg,				
100s ea, C-III	**57664-0126-88**	54.20		AA
500s ea, C-III	**57664-0126-13**	271.00		AA
325 mg-7.5 mg,				
100s ea, C-III	**57664-0170-88**	61.85		AA

PROD/MFR	NDC	AWP	DP	OBC
500s ea, C-III	57664-0170-13	309.75		AA
325 mg-10 mg,				
100s ea, C-III	57664-0176-88	70.25		AA
500s ea, C-III	57664-0176-13	351.25		AA
(USP)				
660 mg-10 mg,				
100s ea, C-III	57664-0111-88	71.50		AA
500s ea, C-III	57664-0111-13	345.00		AA
(Pharm Assoc Inc)				
SOL, PO (10X15ML,FRUIT)				
325 mg/15 ml-10 mg/15 ml,				
15 ml 10s UD, C-III	00121-4771-15	56.82		
(10X7.5ML,FRUIT)				
7.5 ml 10s UD, C-III	00121-4771-07	35.66		
167 mg/5 ml-2.5 mg/5 ml,				
5 ml 40s UD, C-III	00121-4655-05	122.67		AA
10 ml 40s UD, C-III	00121-4655-10	138.86		AA
15 ml 40s UD, C-III	00121-4655-15	155.00		AA
118 ml, C-III	00121-0655-04	17.78		AA
473 ml, C-III	00121-0655-16	58.24		AA
(Qualitest)				
TAB, PO, 325 mg-5 mg,				
100s ea, C-III	00603-3890-21	54.22		AA
500s ea, C-III	00603-3890-28	271.09		
325 mg-7.5 mg,				
100s ea, C-III	00603-3891-21	61.86		AA
500s ea, C-III	00603-3891-28	309.30		
(UDL)				
TAB, PO (USP,5X20)				
325 mg-5 mg,				
100s ea UD, C-III	51079-0777-21	54.20		AA
325 mg-7.5 mg,				
100s ea UD, C-III	51079-0778-21	61.83		AA
325 mg-10 mg,				
100s ea UD, C-III	51079-0779-21	110.00		AA
(USP,15X6EA)				
500 mg-5 mg,				
90s ea, C-III	51079-0780-99	60.00		
(5X20, USP)				
500 mg-10 mg,				
100s ea UD, C-III	51079-0254-21	130.80		
(4u)				
REPACK				
TAB, PO, 325 mg-5 mg,				
28s ea, C-III	42549-0556-28	47.16		AA
500 mg-5 mg,				
28s ea, C-III	10544-0315-28	46.88		AA
28s ea, C-III	42549-0515-28	46.88		AA
30s ea, C-III	42549-0315-30	46.92		AA
30s ea, C-III	42549-0515-30	48.22		AA
60s ea, C-III	42549-0515-60	86.26		AA
84s ea, C-III	10544-0315-84	122.24		AA
84s ea, C-III	42549-0515-84	122.24		AA
112s ea, C-III	10544-0315-02	154.76		AA
112s ea, C-III	42549-0515-02	154.76		AA
140s ea, C-III	42549-0515-04	204.58		AA
500 mg-7.5 mg,				
15s ea, C-III	42549-0516-15	39.24		AA
30s ea, C-III	42549-0316-30	48.22		AA
30s ea, C-III	42549-0516-30	58.82		AA
40s ea, C-III	42549-0516-40	62.34		AA
60s ea, C-III	42549-0316-60	64.12		AA
60s ea, C-III	42549-0516-60	74.44		AA
84s ea, C-III	10544-0316-84	87.34		AA
84s ea, C-III	42549-0516-84	87.34		AA
90s ea, C-III	42549-0516-90	89.56		AA
112s ea, C-III	10544-0316-02	109.72		AA
112s ea, C-III	42549-0516-02	109.72		AA
750 mg-7.5 mg,				
42s ea, C-III	10544-0386-42	65.24		AA
42s ea, C-III	42549-0586-42	65.24		AA
84s ea, C-III	10544-0386-84	87.34		AA
84s ea, C-III	42549-0586-84	87.34		AA
(A-S Medication)				
REPACK				
TAB, PO, 325 mg-10 mg,				
20s ea, C-III	54569-5240-01	14.00		AA
30s ea, C-III	54569-5240-04	21.00		AA
60s ea, C-III	54569-5240-00	42.01		AA
100s ea, C-III	54569-5240-02	70.01		AA
120s ea, C-III	54569-5240-05	84.01		AA
180s ea, C-III	54569-5240-03	125.93		AA
(American Health)				
REPACK				
TAB, PO, 325 mg-5 mg,				
100s ea UD, C-III	68084-0368-01	40.00		AA
(Bryant Ranch)				
REPACK				
TAB, PO, 325 mg-5 mg,				
40s ea, C-III	63629-2946-06	40.00		AA
500 mg-7.5 mg,				
30s ea, C-III	63629-3178-02	42.10		AA
40s ea, C-III	63629-3178-00	54.99		AA
650 mg-7.5 mg,				
20s ea, C-III	63629-3944-04	12.32		AA
30s ea, C-III	63629-3944-05	18.01		AA
60s ea, C-III	63629-3944-03	36.21		AA
90s ea, C-III	63629-3944-02	54.11		AA
120s ea, C-III	63629-3944-01	70.20		AA
(Dispensing Solutions)				
REPACK				
TAB, PO, 325 mg-5 mg,				
20s ea, C-III	66336-0670-20	18.35		AA
40s ea, C-III	66336-0670-40	36.67		AA
(GSMS)				
REPACK				
TAB, PO, 500 mg-5 mg,				
30s ea, C-III	60429-0509-30	4.14	1.38	AA
60s ea, C-III	60429-0509-60	6.87	2.29	AA
90s ea, C-III	60429-0509-90	9.54	3.18	AA
120s ea, C-III	60429-0509-12	12.24	4.08	AA
180s ea, C-III	60429-0509-18	18.00	6.00	AA
240s ea, C-III	60429-0509-24	24.48	8.16	AA
(IPI)				
REPACK				
TAB, PO, 325 mg-5 mg,				
30s ea, C-III	18837-0067-30	20.32		
40s ea, C-III	18837-0067-40	27.00		
90s ea, C-III	18837-0067-90	60.75		
325 mg-7.5 mg,				
30s ea, C-III	18837-0068-30	23.20		
40s ea, C-III	18837-0068-40	30.92		
325 mg-10 mg,				
30s ea, C-III	18837-0066-30	52.87		
40s ea, C-III	18837-0066-40	70.50		
60s ea, C-III	18837-0066-60	105.75		
120s ea, C-III	18837-0066-98	81.35		AA
500 mg-5 mg,				
15s ea, C-III	18837-0064-15	26.28		
30s ea, C-III	18837-0064-30	41.00		
40s ea, C-III	18837-0064-40	58.37		
45s ea, C-III	18837-0064-45	65.56		
50s ea, C-III	18837-0064-50	23.24		
60s ea, C-III	18837-0064-60	87.55		
90s ea, C-III	18837-0064-90	131.33		
100s ea, C-III	18837-0064-99	145.92		
120s ea, C-III	18837-0064-98	175.11		
500 mg-7.5 mg,				
15s ea, C-III	18837-0065-15	19.17		AA
60s ea, C-III	18837-0065-60	42.50		
90s ea, C-III	18837-0065-90	65.61		
120s ea, C-III	18837-0065-98	86.52		
150s ea, C-III	18837-0065-94	108.15		
500 mg-10 mg,				
30s ea, C-III	18837-0063-30	40.78		
60s ea, C-III	18837-0063-60	61.20		
90s ea, C-III	18837-0063-90	91.80		
100s ea, C-III	18837-0063-99	101.21		
150s ea, C-III	18837-0063-94	151.82		
650 mg-7.5 mg,				
60s ea, C-III	18837-0062-60	35.10		AA
650 mg-10 mg,				
15s ea, C-III	18837-0061-15	17.05		
30s ea, C-III	18837-0061-30	34.08		
50s ea, C-III	18837-0061-50	56.82		
60s ea, C-III	18837-0061-60	68.25		
90s ea, C-III	18837-0061-90	102.38		
120s ea, C-III	18837-0061-98	136.50		
750 mg-7.5 mg,				
30s ea, C-III	18837-0069-30	20.03		
60s ea, C-III	18837-0069-60	35.07		
90s ea, C-III	18837-0069-90	50.10		
(Medsource)				
REPACK				
TAB, PO, 500 mg-7.5 mg,				
30s ea, C-III	45865-0454-30	15.60		AA
60s ea, C-III	45865-0454-60	31.20		AA
84s ea, C-III	45865-0454-84	43.68		AA
90s ea, C-III	45865-0454-90	46.80		AA
100s ea, C-III	45865-0454-49	52.00		AA
120s ea, C-III	45865-0454-51	62.40		AA
252s ea, C-III	45865-0454-59	131.04		AA
650 mg-7.5 mg,				
30s ea, C-III	45865-0412-30	20.70		AA
60s ea, C-III	45865-0412-60	41.40		AA
84s ea, C-III	45865-0412-84	57.96		AA
90s ea, C-III	45865-0412-90	62.10		AA
100s ea, C-III	45865-0412-49	69.00		AA
120s ea, C-III	45865-0412-51	82.80		AA
252s ea, C-III	45865-0412-59	173.88		AA
650 mg-10 mg,				
30s ea, C-III	45865-0480-30	29.33		AA
60s ea, C-III	45865-0480-60	58.66		AA
84s ea, C-III	45865-0480-84	82.12		AA
90s ea, C-III	45865-0480-90	87.98		AA
100s ea, C-III	45865-0480-49	97.76		AA
120s ea, C-III	45865-0480-51	117.31		AA
252s ea, C-III	45865-0480-59	246.36		AA
(Nucare Pharm)				
REPACK				
TAB, PO, 500 mg-10 mg,				
100s ea, C-III	66267-1013-00	106.27		AA
750 mg-7.5 mg,				
100s ea, C-III	68071-1362-00	76.00		AA
(PD-Rx Pharm)				
REPACK				
TAB, PO, 325 mg-5 mg,				
6s ea, C-III	43063-0091-06	18.05		AA
15s ea, C-III	55289-0997-15	36.90		AA
30s ea, C-III	55289-0997-30	45.80		AA
40s ea, C-III	55289-0997-40	61.45		AA
60s ea, C-III	55289-0997-60	79.75		AA
325 mg-10 mg,				
21s ea, C-III	55289-0737-21	47.00		AA
500 mg-5 mg,				
2s ea, C-III	43063-0004-02	17.75		AA
4s ea, C-III	43063-0004-04	18.00		AA
6s ea, C-III	43063-0004-06	18.65		AA
12s ea, C-III	43063-0004-12	20.15		AA
100s ea, C-III	43063-0004-01	50.65		AA
500 mg-7.5 mg,				
6s ea, C-III	43063-0031-06	19.90		AA
120s ea, C-III	55289-0268-98	78.20		AA
650 mg-10 mg,				
30s ea, C-III	55289-0311-30	34.45		AA
50s ea, C-III	55289-0311-50	43.45		AA
100s ea, C-III	55289-0311-01	62.00		AA
(Pharma Pac)				
REPACK				
TAB, PO, 500 mg-10 mg,				
12s ea, C-III	52959-0521-12	12.58		AA
(Phys Total Care)				
REPACK				
TAB, PO, 750 mg-7.5 mg,				
150s ea, C-III	54868-2281-09	35.33		AA
(Physician Partner)				
REPACK				
TAB, PO, 650 mg-7.5 mg,				
60s ea, C-III	21695-0436-60	83.40		AA
(St. Mary's MPP)				
REPACK				
TAB, PO, 325 mg-5 mg,				
30s ea, C-III	60760-0202-30	23.89		AA
60s ea, C-III	60760-0202-60	41.78		
90s ea, C-III	60760-0202-90	59.67		AA
325 mg-10 mg,				
15s ea, C-III	60760-0388-15	17.13		
500 mg-10 mg,				
90s ea, C-III	60760-0540-90	56.01		AA
(Stat Rx)				
REPACK				
TAB, PO, 325 mg-5 mg,				
28s ea, C-III	16590-0494-28	37.32		AA
40s ea, C-III	16590-0494-40	53.33		AA
56s ea, C-III	16590-0494-56	74.65		AA
HYDROCODONE BITARTRATE AND IBUPROFEN				
(Amneal)				
hydrocodone bitartrate/ibuprofen				
TAB, PO (FILM-COATED)				
7.5 mg-200 mg,				
100s ea, C-III	53746-0145-01	114.65		AB
(Qualitest)				
TAB, PO (FILM-COATED)				
7.5 mg-200 mg,				
100s ea, C-III	00603-3897-21	114.65		AB
500s ea, C-III	00603-3897-28	515.93		AB
(A-S Medication)				
REPACK				
TAB, PO (FILM-COATED)				
7.5 mg-200 mg,				
60s ea, C-III	54569-6121-00	61.91		AB
(American Health)				
REPACK				
TAB, PO (10X10)				
7.5 mg-200 mg,				
100s ea UD, C-III	68084-0227-01	125.64		

PROD/MFR	NDC	AWP	DP	OBC
(Medsource) REPACK				
TAB, PO (FILM-COATED)				
7.5 mg-200 mg,				
30s ea, C-III	**45865-0500-30**	34.35		AB
60s ea, C-III	**45865-0500-60**	68.70		AB
90s ea, C-III	**45865-0500-90**	103.05		AB
100s ea, C-III	**45865-0500-49**	114.50		AB
120s ea, C-III	**45865-0500-51**	137.40		AB
150s ea, C-III	**45865-0500-62**	171.75		AB
(Physician Partner) REPACK				
TAB, PO (FILM-COATED)				
7.5 mg-200 mg,				
20s ea, C-III	**21695-0631-20**	53.95		AB
60s ea, C-III	**21695-0631-60**	137.58		AB
(Southwood) REPACK				
TAB, PO (FILM-COATED)				
7.5 mg-200 mg,				
30s ea, C-III	**58016-0944-30**	47.70		AB
60s ea, C-III	**58016-0944-60**	95.40		AB
90s ea, C-III	**58016-0944-90**	143.10		AB
100s ea, C-III	**58016-0944-00**	159.00		AB
120s ea, C-III	**58016-0944-02**	190.80		AB
(Stat Rx) REPACK				
TAB, PO (FILM-COATED)				
7.5 mg-200 mg,				
84s ea, C-III	**16590-0296-62**	150.65		AB
HYDROCODONE BITARTRATE/ACETAMINOPHEN				
(A-S Medication) REPACK				
acetaminophen/hydrocodone bitartrate				
ELI, PO, 120 ml, C-III	**54569-5800-00**	18.08		
(American Health) REPACK				
TAB, PO (10X10)				
325 mg-10 mg,				
100s ea UD, C-III	**68084-0353-01**	87.50		AA
500 mg-7.5 mg,				
100s ea UD, C-III	**68084-0145-01**	23.75		AA
500 mg-10 mg,				
100s ea UD, C-III	**68084-0362-01**	50.00		AA
(Palmetto) REPACK				
TAB, PO, 325 mg-7.5 mg,				
30s ea, C-III	**23490-0108-03**	21.99		
30s ea, C-III	**23490-7486-03**	27.00		
40s ea, C-III	**23490-7486-04**	30.80		
60s ea, C-III	**23490-0108-06**	43.99		
90s ea, C-III	**23490-7486-09**	69.30		
120s ea, C-III	**23490-7486-07**	92.40		
325 mg-10 mg,				
30s ea, C-III	**23490-0106-03**	31.49		
30s ea, C-III	**23490-7053-01**	34.80		
40s ea, C-III	**23490-7053-05**	46.40		
60s ea, C-III	**23490-0106-06**	62.98		
60s ea, C-III	**23490-7053-02**	69.60		
90s ea, C-III	**23490-7053-03**	104.40		
100s ea, C-III	**23490-7053-04**	116.00		
120s ea, C-III	**23490-7053-00**	118.32		
HYDROCODONE BITARTRATE/APAP (Ranbaxy Pharm)				
acetaminophen/hydrocodone bitartrate				
TAB, PO (USP)				
325 mg-10 mg,				
100s ea, C-III	**63304-0497-01**	69.89		AA
500s ea, C-III	**63304-0497-05**	337.27		AA
500 mg-5 mg,				
100s ea, C-III	**63304-0560-01**	50.65		AA
500s ea, C-III	**63304-0560-05**	232.44		AA
500 mg-10 mg,				
100s ea, C-III	**63304-0498-01**	53.27		AA
500s ea, C-III	**63304-0498-05**	253.03		AA
750 mg-7.5 mg,				
100s ea, C-III	**63304-0496-01**	43.78		AA
500s ea, C-III	**63304-0496-05**	204.53		AA
(Aidarex) REPACK				
TAB, PO, 325 mg-10 mg,				
7s ea, C-III	**33261-0058-07**	24.15		
10s ea, C-III	**33261-0058-10**	34.50		
12s ea, C-III	**33261-0058-12**	41.40		
14s ea, C-III	**33261-0058-14**	48.30		
20s ea, C-III	**33261-0058-20**	29.00		
21s ea, C-III	**33261-0058-21**	30.45		
28s ea, C-III	**33261-0058-28**	40.60		
30s ea, C-III	**33261-0058-30**	43.50		
40s ea, C-III	**33261-0058-40**	58.00		
42s ea, C-III	**33261-0058-42**	60.90		
48s ea, C-III	**33261-0058-48**	69.60		
60s ea, C-III	**33261-0058-60**	87.00		
90s ea, C-III	**33261-0058-90**	130.50		
100s ea, C-III	**33261-0058-00**	145.00		
120s ea, C-III	**33261-0058-02**	174.00		
180s ea, C-III	**33261-0058-05**	261.00		
500 mg-5 mg,				
7s ea, C-III	**33261-0054-07**	8.54		
10s ea, C-III	**33261-0054-10**	12.20		
12s ea, C-III	**33261-0054-12**	14.64		
14s ea, C-III	**33261-0054-14**	17.08		
20s ea, C-III	**33261-0054-20**	24.40		
21s ea, C-III	**33261-0054-21**	25.62		
28s ea, C-III	**33261-0054-28**	34.16		
30s ea, C-III	**33261-0054-30**	36.60		
40s ea, C-III	**33261-0054-40**	48.80		
42s ea, C-III	**33261-0054-42**	51.24		
48s ea, C-III	**33261-0054-48**	58.56		
60s ea, C-III	**33261-0054-60**	73.20		
80s ea, C-III	**33261-0054-80**	97.60		
82s ea, C-III	**33261-0054-82**	100.04		
84s ea, C-III	**33261-0054-84**	102.48		
90s ea, C-III	**33261-0054-90**	109.80		
100s ea, C-III	**33261-0054-00**	122.00		
120s ea, C-III	**33261-0054-02**	146.40		
180s ea, C-III	**33261-0054-05**	219.60		
650 mg-10 mg,				
7s ea, C-III	**33261-0059-07**	11.90		
10s ea, C-III	**33261-0059-10**	17.00		
12s ea, C-III	**33261-0059-12**	20.40		
14s ea, C-III	**33261-0059-14**	23.80		
20s ea, C-III	**33261-0059-20**	34.00		
21s ea, C-III	**33261-0059-21**	35.70		
28s ea, C-III	**33261-0059-28**	47.60		
30s ea, C-III	**33261-0059-30**	51.00		
40s ea, C-III	**33261-0059-40**	68.00		
HYDROCODONE BITARTRATE/APAP (Aidarex) REPACK				
acetaminophen/hydrocodone bitartrate				
TAB, PO, 650 mg-10 mg,				
42s ea, C-III	**33261-0059-42**	71.40		
48s ea, C-III	**33261-0059-48**	81.60		
60s ea, C-III	**33261-0059-60**	102.00		
82s ea, C-III	**33261-0059-82**	106.60		
90s ea, C-III	**33261-0059-90**	153.00		
100s ea, C-III	**33261-0059-00**	170.00		
120s ea, C-III	**33261-0059-02**	204.00		
(Altura) REPACK				
TAB, PO, 325 mg-5 mg,				
30s ea, C-III	**63874-1092-03**	19.80		
40s ea, C-III	**63874-1092-04**	26.40		
60s ea, C-III	**63874-1092-06**	39.60		
325 mg-7.5 mg,				
30s ea, C-III	**63874-1105-03**	22.25		
40s ea, C-III	**63874-1105-04**	29.67		
60s ea, C-III	**63874-1105-06**	44.50		
90s ea, C-III	**63874-1105-09**	66.74		
660 mg-10 mg,				
10s ea, C-III	**63874-0279-10**	16.60		
15s ea, C-III	**63874-0279-15**	24.90		
20s ea, C-III	**63874-0279-20**	33.20		
28s ea, C-III	**63874-0279-28**	46.48		
30s ea, C-III	**63874-0279-30**	49.80		
40s ea, C-III	**63874-0279-40**	66.40		
42s ea, C-III	**63874-0279-42**	69.72		
50s ea, C-III	**63874-0279-50**	83.00		
56s ea, C-III	**63874-0279-56**	92.96		
60s ea, C-III	**63874-0279-60**	99.60		
80s ea, C-III	**63874-0279-80**	132.80		
84s ea, C-III	**63874-0279-84**	139.44		
90s ea, C-III	**63874-0279-90**	149.40		
100s ea, C-III	**63874-0279-01**	166.00		
120s ea, C-III	**63874-0279-04**	199.20		
180s ea, C-III	**63874-0279-88**	298.80		
(Dispensing Solutions) REPACK				
TAB, PO, 500 mg-5 mg,				
30s ea, C-III	**55045-3755-08**	16.40		
84s ea, C-III	**55045-3125-08**	46.20		
126s ea, C-III	**55045-3715-01**	69.30		
(McKesson Packaging) REPACK				
TAB, PO (USP)				
325 mg-5 mg,				
100s ea UD, C-III	**63739-0384-10**	54.22		
HYDROCODONE BITARTRATE/IBUPROFEN				
(Abbott Pharm) *See VICOPROFEN*				
(Amneal) *See HYDROCODONE BITARTRATE AND IBUPROFEN*				
(Centrix) *See REPREXAIN*				
(Hawthorn Pharm) *See REPREXAIN*				
(Poly) *See IBUDONE*				
(Qualitest) *See HYDROCODONE BITARTRATE AND IBUPROFEN*				
(Teva)				
TAB, PO (FILM-COATED)				
7.5 mg-200 mg,				
100s ea, C-III	**00093-5161-01**	114.65		
(Watson)				
TAB, PO (FILM-COATED)				
7.5 mg-200 mg,				
100s ea, C-III	**62037-0524-01**	101.94		
500s ea, C-III	**62037-0524-05**	458.72		
(Aidarex) REPACK				
TAB, PO (FILM-COATED)				
7.5 mg-200 mg,				
10s ea, C-III	**33261-0378-10**	24.30		
14s ea, C-III	**33261-0378-14**	34.02		
20s ea, C-III	**33261-0378-20**	48.60		
21s ea, C-III	**33261-0378-21**	51.03		
25s ea, C-III	**33261-0378-25**	60.75		
28s ea, C-III	**33261-0378-28**	68.04		
30s ea, C-III	**33261-0378-30**	72.90		
50s ea, C-III	**33261-0378-50**	121.50		
60s ea, C-III	**33261-0378-60**	145.80		
90s ea, C-III	**33261-0378-90**	218.70		
120s ea, C-III	**33261-0378-02**	291.60		
(Altura) REPACK				
TAB, PO (FILM COATED)				
7.5 mg-200 mg,				
15s ea, C-III	**63874-1106-08**	19.89		
20s ea, C-III	**63874-1106-02**	26.52		
30s ea, C-III	**63874-1106-03**	39.80		
40s ea, C-III	**63874-1106-04**	53.04		
50s ea, C-III	**63874-1106-05**	66.30		
60s ea, C-III	**63874-1106-06**	79.56		
90s ea, C-III	**63874-1106-09**	119.34		
100s ea, C-III	**63874-1106-01**	132.60		
(Bryant Ranch) REPACK				
TAB, PO (FILM-COATED)				
7.5 mg-200 mg,				
60s ea, C-III	**63629-2958-02**	219.32		
120s ea, C-III	**63629-2958-03**	454.20		
(DHS, Inc.) REPACK				
TAB, PO (FILM-COATED)				
7.5 mg-200 mg,				
30s ea, C-III	**55887-0290-30**	49.00		
60s ea, C-III	**55887-0290-60**	98.00		
90s ea, C-III	**55887-0290-90**	146.99		
(Dispensing Solutions) REPACK				
TAB, PO (FILM-COATED)				
7.5 mg-200 mg,				
10s ea, C-III	**66336-0893-10**	13.76		
12s ea, C-III	**55045-3065-03**	18.00		
(FILM-COATED)				
7.5 mg-200 mg,				
20s ea, C-III	**55045-3065-07**	25.00		
30s ea, C-III	**55045-3065-08**	37.50		
30s ea, C-III	**66336-0893-30**	41.27		
40s ea, C-III	**55045-3065-04**	50.00		
(FILM-COATED)				
7.5 mg-200 mg,				
60s ea, C-III	**55045-3065-06**	75.00		
60s ea, C-III	**66336-0893-60**	82.55		
90s ea, C-III	**55045-3065-02**	112.50		
(FILM-COATED)				
7.5 mg-200 mg,				
100s ea, C-III	**55045-3065-01**	125.00		
120s ea, C-III	**55045-3065-09**	150.00		
120s ea, C-III	**66336-0893-94**	165.10		
(IPI) REPACK				
TAB, PO (FILM-COATED)				
7.5 mg-200 mg,				
30s ea, C-III	**18837-0196-30**	38.69		
90s ea, C-III	**18837-0196-90**	92.87		
(Nucare Pharm) REPACK				
TAB, PO (FILM-COATED)				
7.5 mg-200 mg,				
30s ea, C-III	**68071-0274-30**	42.56		
90s ea, C-III	**68071-0274-90**	121.88		

PROD/MFR	NDC	AWP	DP	OBC
(Palmetto)				
REPACK				
TAB, PO, 7.5 mg-200 mg,				
20s ea, C-III	**23490-7086-02**	44.19		
30s ea, C-III	**23490-7086-03**	66.28		
120s ea, C-III	**23490-7086-00**	265.12		
(PD-Rx Pharm)				
REPACK				
TAB, PO (FILM-COATED)				
7.5 mg-200 mg,				
60s ea, C-III	**55289-0944-60**	96.50		
(Pharma Pac)				
REPACK				
TAB, PO (FILM-COATED)				
7.5 mg-200 mg,				
12s ea, C-III	**52959-0738-12**	19.79		
15s ea, C-III	**52959-0738-15**	24.73		
20s ea, C-III	**52959-0738-20**	32.97		
30s ea, C-III	**52959-0738-30**	49.44		
40s ea, C-III	**52959-0738-40**	65.90		
50s ea, C-III	**52959-0738-50**	82.36		
60s ea, C-III	**52959-0738-60**	98.81		
90s ea, C-III	**52959-0738-90**	148.18		
120s ea, C-III	**52959-0738-02**	197.43		
(Phys Total Care)				
REPACK				
TAB, PO (FILM-COATED)				
7.5 mg-200 mg,				
20s ea, C-III	**54868-4976-01**	48.93		
30s ea, C-III	**54868-4976-00**	70.38		
60s ea, C-III	**54868-4976-05**	90.03		
90s ea, C-III	**54868-4976-07**	102.16		
120s ea, C-III	**54868-4976-02**	192.00		
180s ea, C-III	**54868-4976-06**	196.82		
(Quality Care Prod)				
REPACK				
TAB, PO (FILM-COATED)				
7.5 mg-200 mg,				
15s ea, C-III	**49999-0588-15**	31.95		
30s ea, C-III	**49999-0588-30**	63.90		
60s ea, C-III	**49999-0588-60**	127.80		
90s ea, C-III	**49999-0588-90**	191.70		
120s ea, C-III	**49999-0588-01**	255.60		
(Southwood)				
REPACK				
TAB, PO (FILM-COATED)				
7.5 mg-200 mg,				
15s ea, C-III	**58016-0944-15**	16.20		
20s ea, C-III	**58016-0944-20**	21.60		
40s ea, C-III	**58016-0944-40**	43.20		
50s ea, C-III	**58016-0944-50**	54.00		
(Stat Rx)				
REPACK				
TAB, PO (FILM-COATED)				
7.5 mg-200 mg,				
60s ea, C-III	**16590-0296-60**	114.75		
90s ea, C-III	**16590-0296-90**	161.41		
HYDROCODONE BITARTRATE/ PHENYLEPHRINE HYDROCHLORIDE				
(Blansett) *See NALEX DH*				
HYDROCODONE BITARTRATE/ POTASSIUM GUAIACOLSULFONATE				
(Blansett) *See PROLEX DH*				
(Breckenridge Pharm) *See MINTUSS NX*				
(Marnel) *See MARCOF EXPECTORANT*				
(Pharmakon) *See JAYCOF EXPECTORANT*				
HYDROCODONE COMPOUND (Pharma Pac)				
REPACK				
homatropine methylbromide/hydrocodone bitartrate				
SYR, PO, 1.5 mg/5 ml-5 mg/5 ml,				
120 ml, C-III	**52959-0580-03**	8.95		EE
HYDROCODONE TANNATE/ PSEUDOEPHEDRINE TANNATE				
(Athlon Pharm) *See SYMTAN*				
HYDROCODONE W/ APAP (HomeMed)				
REPACK				
acetaminophen/hydrocodone bitartrate				
TAB, PO, 325 mg-10 mg,				
30s ea, C-III	**51655-0835-24**	21.07		
500 mg-5 mg,				
10s ea, C-III	**51655-0812-53**	16.32		
15s ea, C-III	**51655-0812-54**	20.70		
30s ea, C-III	**51655-0812-24**	13.51		
60s ea, C-III	**51655-0812-25**	26.99		
500 mg-7.5 mg,				
20s ea, C-III	**51655-0871-52**	30.02		
30s ea, C-III	**51655-0871-24**	33.94		
650 mg-7.5 mg,				
12s ea, C-III	**51655-0866-27**	12.90		
20s ea, C-III	**51655-0866-52**	19.09		
750 mg-7.5 mg,				
12s ea, C-III	**51655-0836-27**	12.01		
20s ea, C-III	**51655-0836-52**	16.02		
30s ea, C-III	**51655-0836-24**	24.03		
HYDROCODONE-APAP (Quality Care Prod)				
REPACK				
acetaminophen/hydrocodone bitartrate				
TAB, PO, 325 mg-5 mg,				
30s ea, C-III	**49999-0608-30**	45.47		
60s ea, C-III	**49999-0608-60**	133.09		
90s ea, C-III	**49999-0608-90**	196.44		
120s ea, C-III	**49999-0608-01**	262.87		
325 mg-10 mg,				
90s ea, C-III	**49999-0169-90**	171.81		
650 mg-10 mg,				
150s ea, C-III	**49999-0277-15**	239.06		
HYDROCODONE/ACET (Physician Partner)				
REPACK				
acetaminophen/hydrocodone bitartrate				
TAB, PO, 325 mg-5 mg,				
28s ea, C-III	**21695-0268-28**	30.36		
60s ea, C-III	**21695-0268-60**	65.06		
325 mg-7.5 mg,				
10s ea, C-III	**21695-0386-10**	12.37		
60s ea, C-III	**21695-0386-60**	74.24		
325 mg-10 mg,				
10s ea, C-III	**21695-0272-10**	13.49		
30s ea, C-III	**21695-0272-30**	40.97		
60s ea, C-III	**21695-0272-60**	80.94		
90s ea, C-III	**21695-0272-90**	121.41		
100s ea, C-III	**21695-0272-00**	139.78		
500 mg-5 mg,				
15s ea, C-III	**21695-0269-15**	16.40		
20s ea, C-III	**21695-0269-20**	21.87		
28s ea, C-III	**21695-0269-28**	26.03		
30s ea, C-III	**21695-0269-30**	27.89		
60s ea, C-III	**21695-0269-60**	55.78		
90s ea, C-III	**21695-0269-90**	83.67		
120s ea, C-III	**21695-0269-72**	131.24		
500 mg-7.5 mg,				
20s ea, C-III	**21695-0270-20**	24.23		
28s ea, C-III	**21695-0270-28**	28.83		
30s ea, C-III	**21695-0270-30**	30.89		
60s ea, C-III	**21695-0270-60**	61.78		
500 mg-10 mg,				
28s ea, C-III	**21695-0273-28**	28.34		
30s ea, C-III	**21695-0273-30**	30.36		
60s ea, C-III	**21695-0273-60**	60.72		
90s ea, C-III	**21695-0273-90**	91.08		
650 mg-10 mg,				
15s ea, C-III	**21695-0274-15**	27.28		
30s ea, C-III	**21695-0274-30**	54.55		
60s ea, C-III	**21695-0274-60**	109.10		
90s ea, C-III	**21695-0274-90**	163.65		
100s ea, C-III	**21695-0274-00**	195.52		
120s ea, C-III	**21695-0274-72**	256.70		
660 mg-10 mg,				
60s ea, C-III	**21695-0508-60**	85.84		
750 mg-7.5 mg,				
15s ea, C-III	**21695-0271-15**	14.44		
20s ea, C-III	**21695-0271-20**	19.25		
28s ea, C-III	**21695-0271-28**	22.90		
30s ea, C-III	**21695-0271-30**	24.54		
40s ea, C-III	**21695-0271-40**	38.50		
60s ea, C-III	**21695-0271-60**	49.09		
90s ea, C-III	**21695-0271-90**	73.62		
100s ea, C-III	**21695-0271-00**	87.56		
120s ea, C-III	**21695-0271-72**	115.48		
HYDROCODONE/ACETAMINOPHEN (Bryant Ranch)				
REPACK				
acetaminophen/hydrocodone bitartrate				
TAB, PO, 325 mg-7.5 mg,				
60s ea, C-III	**63629-3342-02**	52.08		
100s ea, C-III	**63629-3342-01**	86.80		
(Physician Partner)				
REPACK				
TAB, PO, 500 mg-2.5 mg,				
60s ea, C-III	**21695-0579-60**	40.02		
HYDROCODONE/APAP (4u)				
REPACK				
acetaminophen/hydrocodone bitartrate				
TAB, PO, 325 mg-10 mg,				
30s ea, C-III	**10544-0314-30**	59.96		
90s ea, C-III	**10544-0314-90**	106.88		
500 mg-5 mg,				
30s ea, C-III	**10544-0315-30**	48.22		
60s ea, C-III	**10544-0315-60**	86.26		
500 mg-7.5 mg,				
30s ea, C-III	**10544-0316-30**	58.82		
60s ea, C-III	**10544-0316-60**	74.44		
(Bryant Ranch)				
REPACK				
TAB, PO, 325 mg-5 mg,				
30s ea, C-III	**63629-2946-01**	27.99		
60s ea, C-III	**63629-2946-03**	55.98		
120s ea, C-III	**63629-2946-02**	111.96		
325 mg-10 mg,				
20s ea, C-III	**63629-2947-03**	38.40		
30s ea, C-III	**63629-2947-01**	57.60		
60s ea, C-III	**63629-2947-06**	115.20		
90s ea, C-III	**63629-2947-02**	172.80		
100s ea, C-III	**63629-2947-05**	107.68		
120s ea, C-III	**63629-2947-04**	230.40		
500 mg-5 mg,				
10s ea, C-III	**63629-1532-05**	30.76		
15s ea, C-III	**63629-1532-04**	73.83		
20s ea, C-III	**63629-1532-01**	17.56		
24s ea, C-III	**63629-1532-02**	14.61		
30s ea, C-III	**63629-1532-03**	25.89		
45s ea, C-III	**63629-1532-06**	26.40		
60s ea, C-III	**63629-1532-07**	35.54		
90s ea, C-III	**63629-1532-08**	52.65		
100s ea, C-III	**63629-1532-09**	111.32		
500 mg-7.5 mg,				
20s ea, C-III	**63629-3178-01**	17.99		
60s ea, C-III	**63629-3178-03**	53.85		
90s ea, C-III	**63629-3178-04**	79.98		
120s ea, C-III	**63629-3178-05**	119.97		
500 mg-10 mg,				
30s ea, C-III	**63629-3092-01**	31.25		
50s ea, C-III	**63629-3092-05**	53.32		
60s ea, C-III	**63629-3092-02**	62.51		
90s ea, C-III	**63629-3092-03**	89.32		
650 mg-10 mg,				
20s ea, C-III	**63629-3115-01**	30.70		
30s ea, C-III	**63629-3115-02**	43.56		
60s ea, C-III	**63629-3115-03**	86.11		
90s ea, C-III	**63629-3115-05**	124.98		
120s ea, C-III	**63629-3115-04**	163.01		
750 mg-7.5 mg,				
20s ea, C-III	**63629-1529-03**	19.95		
30s ea, C-III	**63629-1529-02**	24.93		
40s ea, C-III	**63629-1529-04**	29.91		
50s ea, C-III	**63629-1529-09**	42.32		
60s ea, C-III	**63629-1529-01**	49.86		
70s ea, C-III	**63629-1529-07**	43.32		
90s ea, C-III	**63629-1529-05**	74.79		
100s ea, C-III	**63629-1529-08**	72.98		
120s ea, C-III	**63629-1529-06**	59.72		
(Core)				
REPACK				
TAB, PO, 325 mg-5 mg,				
90s ea, C-III	**33358-0165-90**	52.79		
325 mg-7.5 mg,				
30s ea, C-III	**33358-0167-30**	19.74		
60s ea, C-III	**33358-0167-60**	48.45		
90s ea, C-III	**33358-0167-90**	57.79		
325 mg-10 mg,				
30s ea, C-III	**33358-0170-30**	59.04		
60s ea, C-III	**33358-0170-60**	90.61		
90s ea, C-III	**33358-0170-90**	177.12		
120s ea, C-III	**33358-0170-01**	236.16		
500 mg-5 mg,				
10s ea, C-III	**33358-0166-10**	25.69		
20s ea, C-III	**33358-0166-20**	29.86		
24s ea, C-III	**33358-0166-24**	34.12		
30s ea, C-III	**33358-0166-30**	44.87		
500 mg-7.5 mg,				
30s ea, C-III	**33358-0168-30**	26.33		
60s ea, C-III	**33358-0168-60**	71.80		
90s ea, C-III	**33358-0168-90**	110.70		
100s ea, C-III	**33358-0168-00**	119.68		
120s ea, C-III	**33358-0168-01**	143.61		
500 mg-10 mg,				
4s ea, C-III	**33358-0171-04**	5.45		
30s ea, C-III	**33358-0171-30**	32.03		
40s ea, C-III	**33358-0171-40**	46.46		
50s ea, C-III	**33358-0171-50**	56.99		
60s ea, C-III	**33358-0171-60**	72.99		
90s ea, C-III	**33358-0171-90**	118.24		
100s ea, C-III	**33358-0171-00**	126.64		
120s ea, C-III	**33358-0171-01**	158.91		
650 mg-10 mg,				
20s ea, C-III	**33358-0172-20**	31.47		
30s ea, C-III	**33358-0172-30**	44.65		
60s ea, C-III	**33358-0172-60**	88.26		
90s ea, C-III	**33358-0172-90**	128.10		
100s ea, C-III	**33358-0172-00**	139.45		
120s ea, C-III	**33358-0172-01**	167.09		

PROD/MFR	NDC	AWP	DP	OBC
750 mg-7.5 mg,				
15s ea, C-III	33358-0169-15	13.99		
20s ea, C-III	33358-0169-20	20.45		
30s ea, C-III	33358-0169-30	25.55		
50s ea, C-III	33358-0169-50	36.82		
60s ea, C-III	33358-0169-60	51.11		
(DHS, Inc.)				
REPACK				
TAB, PO, 325 mg-5 mg,				
10s ea, C-III	55887-0295-10	9.16		
12s ea, C-III	55887-0295-12	10.99		
15s ea, C-III	55887-0295-15	13.74		
20s ea, C-III	55887-0295-20	18.33		
25s ea, C-III	55887-0295-25	22.91		
30s ea, C-III	55887-0295-30	27.49		
40s ea, C-III	55887-0295-40	40.00		
50s ea, C-III	55887-0295-50	45.83		
60s ea, C-III	55887-0295-60	55.00		
70s ea, C-III	55887-0295-70	64.16		
80s ea, C-III	55887-0295-80	73.33		
90s ea, C-III	55887-0295-90	82.49		
120s ea, C-III	55887-0295-82	109.99		
325 mg-10 mg,				
21s ea, C-III	55887-0443-21	26.59		
25s ea, C-III	55887-0443-25	31.66		
40s ea, C-III	55887-0443-40	50.66		
45s ea, C-III	55887-0443-45	69.89		
50s ea, C-III	55887-0443-50	63.33		
100s ea, C-III	55887-0443-01	90.00		
180s ea, C-III	55887-0443-92	164.00		
500 mg-7.5 mg,				
12s ea, C-III	55887-0447-12	10.80		
14s ea, C-III	55887-0447-14	14.00		
45s ea, C-III	55887-0447-45	40.50		
50s ea, C-III	55887-0447-50	28.60		
500 mg-10 mg,				
28s ea, C-III	55887-0538-28	29.00		
32s ea, C-III	55887-0538-32	33.06		
50s ea, C-III	55887-0538-50	26.63		
100s ea, C-III	55887-0538-01	88.12		
180s ea, C-III	55887-0538-92	158.62		
650 mg-7.5 mg,				
16s ea, C-III	55887-0680-16	16.00		
750 mg-7.5 mg,				
15s ea, C-III	55887-0623-15	14.00		
16s ea, C-III	55887-0623-16	15.00		
24s ea, C-III	55887-0623-24	23.00		
40s ea, C-III	55887-0623-40	36.00		
50s ea, C-III	55887-0623-50	45.00		
(Dispensing Solutions)				
REPACK				
ELI, PO, 118 ml, C-III	55045-3831-01	17.00		
TAB, PO, 650 mg-10 mg,				
20s ea, C-III	66336-0406-20	23.64		
30s ea, C-III	66336-0406-30	35.47		
750 mg-7.5 mg,				
16s ea, C-III	66336-0106-16	12.55		
120s ea, C-III	66336-0106-94	94.12		
(Keltman Pharma., Inc.)				
REPACK				
TAB, PO, 325 mg-5 mg,				
30s ea, C-III	68387-0236-30	27.15		
500 mg-10 mg,				
120s ea, C-III	68387-0220-12	157.20		
180s ea, C-III	68387-0220-18	235.80		
650 mg-10 mg,				
40s ea, C-III	68387-0200-40	49.04		
180s ea, C-III	68387-0200-18	220.68		
(Nucare Pharm)				
REPACK				
TAB, PO, 500 mg-5 mg,				
10s ea, C-III	68071-0659-10	14.59		
(Palmetto)				
REPACK				
TAB, PO, 500 mg-5 mg,				
6s ea, C-III	23490-5691-01	17.16		
10s ea, C-III	23490-5691-02	14.59		
12s ea, C-III	23490-5691-03	17.51		
15s ea, C-III	23490-5691-04	21.89		
16s ea, C-III	23490-5691-05	23.35		
20s ea, C-III	23490-5691-06	29.19		
24s ea, C-III	23490-5691-07	35.02		
30s ea, C-III	23490-5691-08	43.78		
40s ea, C-III	23490-5691-09	58.37		
60s ea, C-III	23490-0111-06	128.11		
60s ea, C-III	23490-5691-00	87.56		
500 mg-7.5 mg,				
6s ea, C-III	23490-5693-01	8.40		
12s ea, C-III	23490-5693-00	12.00		
15s ea, C-III	23490-5693-02	15.00		
20s ea, C-III	23490-5693-03	20.00		
30s ea, C-III	23490-0112-03	26.24		
30s ea, C-III	23490-5693-04	30.00		
60s ea, C-III	23490-5693-05	60.00		
90s ea, C-III	23490-5693-06	90.00		
100s ea, C-III	23490-5693-08	100.00		
120s ea, C-III	23490-5693-07	120.00		
180s ea, C-III	23490-5693-09	180.00		
(Stat Rx)				
REPACK				
TAB, PO, 325 mg-5 mg,				
20s ea, C-III	16590-0494-20	20.00		
30s ea, C-III	16590-0494-30	40.00		
60s ea, C-III	16590-0494-60	80.00		
90s ea, C-III	16590-0494-90	120.00		
120s ea, C-III	16590-0494-72	160.00		
325 mg-7.5 mg,				
30s ea, C-III	16590-0114-30	22.00		
60s ea, C-III	16590-0114-60	44.00		
90s ea, C-III	16590-0114-90	66.00		
120s ea, C-III	16590-0114-72	88.00		
325 mg-10 mg,				
30s ea, C-III	16590-0118-30	22.00		
60s ea, C-III	16590-0118-60	88.50		
90s ea, C-III	16590-0118-90	115.00		
120s ea, C-III	16590-0118-72	158.92		
500 mg-2.5 mg,				
30s ea, C-III	16590-0112-30	23.00		
60s ea, C-III	16590-0112-60	46.00		
90s ea, C-III	16590-0112-90	69.00		
120s ea, C-III	16590-0112-72	92.00		
500 mg-5 mg,				
10s ea, C-III	16590-0113-10	11.75		
20s ea, C-III	16590-0113-20	23.50		
30s ea, C-III	16590-0113-30	35.00		
40s ea, C-III	16590-0113-40	46.66		
60s ea, C-III	16590-0113-60	62.50		
90s ea, C-III	16590-0113-90	105.00		
120s ea, C-III	16590-0113-72	95.50		
500 mg-7.5 mg,				
10s ea, C-III	16590-0115-10	7.75		
80s ea, C-III	16590-0105-80	61.68		
500 mg-10 mg,				
10s ea, C-III	16590-0119-10	8.33		
20s ea, C-III	16590-0119-20	16.67		
30s ea, C-III	16590-0119-30	25.00		
45s ea, C-III	16590-0119-45	37.50		
60s ea, C-III	16590-0119-60	50.00		
80s ea, C-III	16590-0119-80	66.66		
90s ea, C-III	16590-0119-90	75.00		
100s ea, C-III	16590-0119-71	83.33		
120s ea, C-III	16590-0119-72	112.50		
650 mg-7.5 mg,				
20s ea, C-III	16590-0116-20	14.63		
30s ea, C-III	16590-0116-30	21.94		
60s ea, C-III	16590-0116-60	43.88		
90s ea, C-III	16590-0116-90	65.82		
100s ea, C-III	16590-0116-71	87.17		
120s ea, C-III	16590-0116-72	87.76		
650 mg-10 mg,				
30s ea, C-III	16590-0120-30	57.92		
60s ea, C-III	16590-0120-60	72.00		
90s ea, C-III	16590-0120-90	108.00		
120s ea, C-III	16590-0120-72	144.00		
150s ea, C-III	16590-0120-83	170.00		
750 mg-7.5 mg,				
10s ea, C-III	16590-0117-10	7.85		
20s ea, C-III	16590-0117-20	15.70		
30s ea, C-III	16590-0117-30	23.00		
90s ea, C-III	16590-0117-90	69.00		
120s ea, C-III	16590-0117-72	92.00		
HYDROCODONE/GUAIFENESIN (Dispensing Solutions)				
REPACK				
guaifenesin/hydrocodone bitartrate				
SYR, PO, 100 mg/5 ml-5 mg/5 ml,				
118 ml, C-III	55045-3500-02	12.00		
473 ml, C-III	55045-1783-01	48.00		
473 ml, C-III	55045-3500-01	48.00		
(Southwood)				
REPACK				
SOL, PO, 100 mg/5 ml-5 mg/5 ml,				
480 ml, C-III	58016-5680-01	43.43		
HYDROCODONE/HOMATROPINE (Phys Total Care)				
REPACK				
homatropine methylbromide/hydrocodone bitartrate				
SYR, PO (1X473ML)				
1.5 mg/5 ml-5 mg/5 ml,				
473 ml, C-III	54868-5168-00	273.14		
(Southwood)				
REPACK				
TAB, PO, 1.5 mg-5 mg,				
30s ea, C-III	58016-0080-30	20.54		
60s ea, C-III	58016-0080-60	41.07		
90s ea, C-III	58016-0080-90	61.61		
100s ea, C-III	58016-0080-00	68.45		
HYDROCODONE/IBU (Pharma Pac)				
REPACK				
hydrocodone bitartrate/ibuprofen				
TAB, PO, 7.5 mg-200 mg,				
10s ea, C-III	52959-0738-10	16.50		
100s ea, C-III	52959-0738-00	164.60		
HYDROCODONE/IBUPROFEN (Bryant Ranch)				
REPACK				
hydrocodone bitartrate/ibuprofen				
TAB, PO, 7.5 mg-200 mg,				
20s ea, C-III	63629-2958-01	75.80		
(Core)				
REPACK				
TAB, PO, 7.5 mg-200 mg,				
12s ea, C-III	33358-0173-12	26.55		
(DHS, Inc.)				
REPACK				
TAB, PO, 7.5 mg-200 mg,				
15s ea, C-III	55887-0290-15	24.50		
100s ea, C-III	55887-0290-01	163.33		
120s ea, C-III	55887-0290-82	196.00		
HYDROCORT ACET (Pharma Pac)				
REPACK				
hydrocortisone acetate				
SUP, RC, 25 mg, 24s ea	52959-0250-24	18.72		
HYDROCORT/CHLOROXY/PRAM (Phys Total Care)				
REPACK				
chloroxylenol/hc/pramoxine hcl				
SOL, OT (DROP)				
10 ml	54868-5733-00	40.14		
HYDROCORTISONE				
FUL				
CRE, TP, 0.5%, 30 gm		1.53		
1%, 30 gm		1.68		
2.5%, 30 gm		4.95		
LOT, TP, 1%, 120 ml		6.86		
2.5%, 59 ml		44.25		
OIN, TP, 1%, 30 gm		1.68		
(Actavis Mid Atlantic)				
CRE, TP, 1%, 28.4 gm	00472-0321-26	4.10		AT
2.5%, 20 gm	00472-0337-20	6.75		AT
30 gm	00472-0337-30	8.95		AT
OIN, TP, 1%, 28.4 gm	00472-1326-26	4.10		AT
(Alaven) *See PROCTOCREAM-HC*				
(Amend)				
POW, NA (U.S.P.)				
5 gm	17317-0198-08	14.00		EE
10 gm	17317-0198-01	24.50		EE
25 gm	17317-0198-02	49.00		EE
100 gm	17317-0198-03	175.00		EE
(ANI) *See CORTENEMA*				
(Arbor) *See PEDIADERM HC KIT*				
(Avidas) *See SCALACORT*				
(BayPharma)				
NMA, RC (1X60ML,USP,RETENTION,SD)				
100 mg/60 ml,				
60 ml	42769-1380-01	11.05		
(7X60ML,USP,RETENTION,SD)				
100 mg/60 ml,				
60 ml 7s	42769-1380-07	74.66		
(Carolina) *See HYDROCORTISONE 1% IN ABSORBASE*				
(Consolidated Midland)				
CRE, TP, 1%, 5 gm	00223-4124-05	1.40		EE
15 gm	00223-4124-15	2.00		EE
20 gm	00223-4124-20	2.40		EE
30 gm	00223-4124-30	2.50		EE
120 gm	00223-4124-11	8.75		EE
454 gm	00223-4124-04	30.00		EE
2.5%, 5 gm	00223-4159-05	2.25		EE
20 gm	00223-4159-20	4.75		EE
120 gm	00223-4159-03	16.50		EE
454 gm	00223-4159-13	77.50		EE
OIN, TP, 1%, 15 gm	00223-4161-15	1.95		EE
20 gm	00223-4161-20	2.25		EE
30 gm	00223-4161-30	2.50		EE
454 gm	00223-4161-13	29.50		EE
2.5%, 5 gm	00223-4125-05	2.25		EE
20 gm	00223-4125-20	4.95		EE
454 gm	00223-4125-13	77.50		EE
TAB, PO, 20 mg, 100s ea	00223-1063-01	42.50		EE
1000s ea	00223-1063-02	57.50		EE
(Cutispharma) *See FIRST-HYDROCORTISONE*				

PROD/MFR	NDC	AWP	DP	OBC
(Del-Ray) *See ALA-CORT*				
(Del-Ray) *See ALA-SCALP HP*				
(Fougera)				
CRE, TP, 1%, 28.35 gm	**00168-0015-31**	3.60		AT
453.6 gm	**00168-0015-16**	31.45		AT
2.5%, 30 gm	**00168-0080-31**	11.00		AT
453.6 gm	**00168-0080-16**	90.00		AT
LOT, TP, 2.5%, 59 ml	**00168-0288-02**	52.03		AT
OIN, TP, 1%, 28.35 gm	**00168-0020-31**	3.72		AT
453.6 gm	**00168-0020-16**	31.87		AT
2.5%, 28.35 gm	**00168-0146-30**	11.00		AT
453.6 gm	**00168-0146-16**	90.00		AT
(Gallipot)				
POW, NA (U.S.P.,MICRONIZED)				
1 gm	**51552-0020-01**	5.60		
5 gm	**51552-0020-02**	16.80		
10 gm	**51552-0020-03**	23.10		
25 gm	**51552-0020-04**	49.00		
100 gm	**51552-0020-05**	175.00		
1000 gm	**51552-0020-07**	1274.00		
(Humco)				
POW, NA (U.S.P.)				
10 gm	**00802-3953-18**	32.03		
25 gm	**00802-3953-19**	70.63		
(JSJ Pharma) *See TEXACORT*				
(Major)				
TAB, PO, 20 mg, 100s ea	**00904-2674-60**	30.26		BP
(Mallinckrodt Lab)				
POW, NA (U.S.P.,MICRONIZED)				
5 gm	**00406-8830-03**	41.11		EE
10 gm	**00406-8830-05**	70.43		EE
(Medisca)				
POW, NA (U.S.P.,MICRONIZED)				
10 gm	**38779-0009-01**	82.50		EE
25 gm	**38779-0009-04**	147.00		EE
100 gm	**38779-0009-05**	435.00		EE
500 gm	**38779-0009-08**	2025.00		EE
1000 gm	**38779-0009-09**	3420.00		EE
(Paddock) *See COLOCORT*				
(Paddock)				
POW, NA (U.S.P.,MICRONIZED)				
10 gm	**00574-0420-10**	42.50		
25 gm	**00574-0420-25**	82.50		
100 gm	**00574-0420-01**	315.00		
(Perrigo)				
CRE, TP, 2.5%, 20 gm	**45802-0004-02**	4.90		AT
28 gm	**45802-0004-03**	10.80		AT
LOT, TP (USP,1X118ML)				
1%, 118 ml	**45802-0933-26**	20.20		
120 ml	**45802-0283-06**	9.98		EE
(1X59ML,USP)				
2.5%, 59 ml	**45802-0937-16**	53.47		
(USP,1X118ML)				
2.5%, 118 ml	**45802-0937-26**	76.49		
OIN, TP, 2.5%, 20 gm	**45802-0014-02**	4.96		AT
454 gm	**45802-0014-05**	58.32		AT
(Pfizer) *See CORTEF*				
(Qualitest)				
CRE, TP, 2.5%, 30 gm	**00603-7781-78**	11.00		AT
LOT, TP, 2.5%, 60 ml	**00603-7785-52**	45.64		AT
TAB, PO (USP)				
5 mg, 50s ea	**00603-3899-19**	15.22		AB
10 mg, 100s ea	**00603-3900-21**	51.43		AB
20 mg, 100s ea	**00603-3901-21**	94.18		AB
(Ranbaxy Labs) *See PROCTO-KIT 1%*				
(Ranbaxy Labs) *See PROCTO-KIT 2.5%*				
(Ranbaxy Labs) *See PROCTOSOL-HC*				
(Rising) *See PROCTO-PAK*				
(Rising) *See PROCTOZONE-HC*				
(Salix Pharm) *See ANUSOL-HC*				
(Salix Pharm) *See PROCTOCORT*				
(Spectrum Pharmacy)				
POW, NA (U.S.P.,MICRONIZED)				
5 gm	**49452-3580-01**	66.50		
25 gm	**49452-3580-02**	174.30		
100 gm	**49452-3580-03**	637.00		
500 gm	**49452-3580-05**	2184.00		EE
1000 gm	**49452-3580-04**	4060.00		EE
(Taro)				
CRE, TP, 1%, 28.35 gm	**51672-3004-02**	3.25		AT
(Teva) *See HYDROCORTISONE ENEMA*				
(Valeant Pharm Intl) *See CETACORT*				

PROD/MFR	NDC	AWP	DP	OBC
(West-Ward)				
TAB, PO, 20 mg, 100s ea	**00143-1254-01**	20.50		BP
(X-Gen)				
POW, NA (U.S.P.)				
10 gm	**39822-5000-01**	24.25		AA
25 gm	**39822-5000-03**	58.75		AA
50 gm	**39822-5000-05**	105.50		AA
100 gm	**39822-5000-07**	199.75		AA
(A-S Medication)				
REPACK				
CRE, TP, 2.5%, 20 gm	**54569-2299-00**	5.83		EE
30 gm	**54569-1154-00**	11.57		AT
LOT, TP, 1%, 120 ml	**54569-2830-00**	10.15		EE
OIN, TP, 1%, 30 gm	**54569-1118-00**	3.99		EE
2.5%, 20 gm	**54569-4030-00**	4.96		EE
(Aidarex)				
REPACK				
CRE, TP (1X30GM)				
1%, 30 gm	**33261-0359-01**	8.40		AT
(Altura)				
REPACK				
CRE, TP (1X45GM)				
1%, 45 gm	**63874-0049-45**	37.37		AT
2.5%, 20 gm	**63874-0037-20**	11.04		
30 gm	**63874-0037-30**	12.81		
(American Health)				
REPACK				
TAB, PO (3X10)				
20 mg, 30s ea UD	**68084-0224-21**	15.50		
(DHS, Inc.)				
REPACK				
CRE, TP, 1%, 30 gm	**55887-0913-30**	8.29		
2.5%, 15 gm	**55887-0059-15**	15.50		
30 gm	**55887-0898-30**	10.10		
OIN, TP, 2.5%, 20 gm	**55887-0836-20**	7.50		
(Dispensing Solutions)				
REPACK				
CRE, TP, 2.5%, 20 gm	**55045-1600-07**	25.80		AT
30 gm	**55045-1600-06**	10.55		AT
(Keltman Pharma., Inc.)				
REPACK				
CRE, TP, 2.5%, 30 gm	**68387-0532-01**	16.18		AT
(Nucare Pharm)				
REPACK				
CRE, TP, 1%, 20 gm	**66267-0968-20**	8.56		EE
30 gm	**66267-0969-01**	9.89		EE
2.5%, 20 gm	**66267-0966-20**	9.64		EE
30 gm	**66267-0967-01**	10.22		EE
(Palmetto)				
REPACK				
CRE, RC, 2.5%, 20 gm	**23490-5714-00**	19.60		
30 gm	**23490-5714-01**	36.76		
TP, 1%, 30 gm	**23490-5710-02**	9.90		
2.5%, 20 gm	**23490-5715-02**	9.78		
30 gm	**23490-5715-01**	10.00		
(PD-Rx Pharm)				
REPACK				
TAB, PO, 10 mg, 30s ea	**43063-0208-30**	31.92		AB
60s ea	**43063-0208-60**	56.33		AB
100s ea	**43063-0208-01**	88.88		AB
(Pharma Pac)				
REPACK				
CRE, TP, 1%, 30 gm	**52959-0039-03**	10.13		EE
2.5%, 3.5 gm	**52959-0019-03**	7.13		AT
20 gm	**52959-0019-01**	10.02		EE
30 gm	**52959-0019-02**	10.18		EE
OIN, TP, 1%, 30 gm	**52959-0631-00**	9.35		
(Phys Total Care)				
REPACK				
CRE, TP, 2.5%, 20 gm	**54868-2143-00**	8.76		EE
30 gm	**54868-2143-01**	11.37		EE
454 gm	**54868-2143-02**	8.64		EE
LOT, TP (1X118ML)				
2.5%, 118 ml	**54868-5893-00**	97.41		AT
OIN, TP (1X28.35GM)				
2.5%, 28.35 gm	**54868-5834-00**	11.72		
TAB, PO, 20 mg, 30s ea	**54868-1743-03**	16.68		EE
50s ea	**54868-1743-00**	23.28		EE
60s ea	**54868-1743-02**	27.33		BP
(USP)				
20 mg, 90s ea	**54868-1743-04**	42.51		BP
100s ea	**54868-1743-01**	42.06		BP
(Physician Partner)				
REPACK				
CRE, TP, 1%, 30 gm	**21695-0529-01**	7.20		
2.5%, 30 gm	**21695-0206-30**	22.00		

PROD/MFR	NDC	AWP	DP	OBC
(Quality Care Prod)				
REPACK				
CRE, TP, 2.5%, 20 gm	**49999-0162-20**	8.54		
28 gm	**49999-0162-28**	6.29		
30 gm	**49999-0162-01**	12.40		AT
30 gm	**49999-0162-30**	51.04		AT
(Southwood)				
REPACK				
CRE, TP, 0.5%, 30 gm	**58016-3141-01**	5.07		EE
1%, 30 gm	**58016-3017-01**	8.41		EE
120 gm	**58016-3179-01**	10.94		EE
454 gm	**58016-3118-01**	35.59		EE
2.5%, 30 gm	**58016-3186-01**	9.54		EE
LOT, TP, 1%, 120 ml	**58016-3223-01**	15.46		EE
OIN, TP, 1%, 30 gm	**58016-3131-01**	5.25		EE
2.5%, 30 gm	**58016-4991-01**	11.00		
(Southwood)				
hydrocortisone acetate				
SUP, RC, 25 mg, 24s ea	**58016-4823-01**	13.97		
HYDROCORTISONE (Stat Rx)				
REPACK				
CRE, TP, 1%, 30 gm	**16590-0121-30**	10.00		
(1X30GM)				
2.5%, 30 gm	**16590-0364-30**	12.48		AT
HYDROCORTISONE 1% IN ABSORBASE (Carolina)				
hydrocortisone				
OIN, TP, 1%, 25 gm	**46287-0003-01**	64.20	48.00	AT
110 gm	**46287-0003-04**	120.00	90.00	AT
454 gm	**46287-0003-16**	31.80	23.85	AT
HYDROCORTISONE ACETATE				
(Actavis Mid Atlantic) *See HEMORRHOIDAL HC*				
(Alaven) *See CORTIFOAM*				
(Aletheia) *See CORTALO WITH ALOE*				
(Amend)				
POW, NA (U.S.P.,MICRONIZED)				
5 gm	**17317-0199-08**	14.00		
(U.S.P,MICRONIZED)				
10 gm	**17317-0199-01**	24.50		
(U.S.P.,MICRONIZED)				
25 gm	**17317-0199-02**	49.00		
100 gm	**17317-0199-03**	175.00		
(Bio-Pharm) *See RECTASOL-HC*				
(Breckenridge Pharm) *See KERATOL HC*				
(Consolidated Midland) *See HEMORRHOIDAL HC*				
(Cypress Pharm) *See HYDROCORTISONE ACETATE WITH ALOE*				
(G&W) *See ANUCORT-HC*				
(Gallipot)				
POW, NA (U.S.P.)				
1 gm	**51552-0021-01**	5.60		
5 gm	**51552-0021-02**	18.13		
10 gm	**51552-0021-03**	30.80		
25 gm	**51552-0021-04**	52.50		
100 gm	**51552-0021-05**	175.00		
(Letco)				
POW, NA (U.S.P.,MICRONIZED)				
10 gm	**62991-1078-02**	63.00		
25 gm	**62991-1078-03**	105.00		
100 gm	**62991-1078-04**	375.00		
500 gm	**62991-1078-05**	1440.00		
(Major) *See ANU-MED HC*				
(Medisca)				
POW, NA (U.S.P.,MICRONIZED)				
5 gm	**38779-0008-15**	76.50		
10 gm	**38779-0008-01**	64.50		
25 gm	**38779-0008-04**	135.00		
100 gm	**38779-0008-05**	435.00		
500 gm	**38779-0008-08**	1515.00		
(Paddock)				
POW, NA (U.S.P.,MICRONIZED)				
25 gm	**00574-0421-25**	82.50		
100 gm	**00574-0421-01**	315.00		
SUP, RC, 25 mg,				
12s ea UD	**00574-7090-12**	10.46		
30 mg, 12s ea UD	**00574-7093-12**	45.75	45.75	
(PCCA) *See HYDROCORTISONE ACETATE MICRONIZED*				
(Salix Pharm) *See ANUSOL-HC*				
(Salix Pharm) *See PROCTOCORT*				
(Spectrum Pharmacy)				
POW, NA (U.S.P.,MICRONIZED)				
5 gm	**49452-3590-01**	71.40		
25 gm	**49452-3590-02**	204.75		
100 gm	**49452-3590-03**	658.00		
500 gm	**49452-3590-06**	2418.50		
1000 gm	**49452-3590-04**	4448.50		

PROD/MFR NDC AWP DP OBC

(Taro) *See U-CORT*

(Truxton)
SUS, IJ (VIAL)
25 mg/ml, 10 ml ..... **00463-1036-10** 3.60 EE

(Upsher-Smith) *See HEMRIL-30*

(Wraser Pharm) *See NUCORT*

(Wraser Pharm) *See NUZON*

(X-Gen)
POW, NA (U.S.P., MICRONIZED)
10 gm **39822-5090-01** 24.25
(U.S.P.,MICRONIZED)
25 gm **39822-5090-03** 58.75
(U.S.P., MICRONIZED)
50 gm **39822-5090-05** 105.50

(Altura)
REPACK
hydrocortisone
OIN, TP, 2.5%, 30 gm **63874-0043-30** 12.81

HYDROCORTISONE ACETATE (Altura)
SUP, RC, 25 mg, 12s ea ... **63874-0847-12** 9.72

(Dispensing Solutions)
REPACK
SUP, RC, 25 mg, 12s ea ... **55045-1277-04** 12.00

(Phys Total Care)
REPACK
SUP, RC, 25 mg, 6s ea **54868-2138-01** 7.05
12s ea............. **54868-2138-00** 8.07

HYDROCORTISONE ACETATE AND PRAMOXINE HYDROCHLORIDE (Ferndale)
hydrocortisone acetate/pramoxine hydrochloride
CRE, TP (1X30GM,PARABEN-FREE)
2.5%-1%, 30 gm **00496-0953-05** 48.85

(Phys Total Care)
REPACK
CRE, TP (1X30GM,PARABEN-FREE)
2.5%-1%, 30 gm **54868-2661-00** 127.61

HYDROCORTISONE ACETATE MICRONIZED (Hawkins)
hydrocortisone acetate, micronized
POW, NA (USP)
5 gm **63370-0108-15** 44.00
25 gm **63370-0108-25** 144.00
100 gm.............. **63370-0108-35** 540.00
500 gm.............. **63370-0108-45** 1980.00
1000 gm............. **63370-0108-50** 3840.00

(Medisca)
POW, NA (U.S.P.)
1000 gm............. **38779-0008-09** 3075.00

(PCCA)
hydrocortisone acetate
POW, NA (U.S.P.)
1 gm **51927-1110-00** 8.70

HYDROCORTISONE ACETATE WITH ALOE (Cypress Pharm)
hydrocortisone acetate
GEL, TP, 2%, 43 gm....... **60258-0048-43** 39.99

HYDROCORTISONE ACETATE-PRAMOXINE HYDROCHLORIDE (Acella)
hydrocortisone acetate/pramoxine hydrochloride
CRE, TP, 2.5%-1%, 30 gm . **42192-0107-01** 62.26

HYDROCORTISONE ACETATE, MICRONIZED
(Hawkins) *See HYDROCORTISONE ACETATE MICRONIZED*

(Medisca) *See HYDROCORTISONE ACETATE MICRONIZED*

HYDROCORTISONE ACETATE/LIDOCAINE HYDROCHLORIDE
(Aristos) *See LIDOCORT*

(Auriga) *See XYRALID*

(Auriga) *See XYRALID LP*

(Azur Pharma, Inc.) *See RECTAGEL HC*

(Cypress Pharm) *See LIDOCAINE/HC*

(Doak) *See LIDA MANTLE HC*

(Doak) *See LIDAMANTLE HC RELIEF*

(Fougera) *See LIDOCAINE HYDROCHLORIDE AND HYDROCORTISONE ACETATE*

(Kenwood) *See ANAMANTLE HC*

(Kenwood) *See ANAMANTLE HC FORTE*

(Kenwood) *See PERANEX HC*

PROD/MFR NDC AWP DP OBC

(Rising) *See LIDAZONE HC*

(River's Edge) *See LIDOCAINE HYDROCHLORIDE - HYDROCORTISONE ACETATE*

HYDROCORTISONE ACETATE/PRAMOXINE HYDROCHLORIDE (Acella)
CRE, TP (1X30GM)
1%-1%, 30 gm **42192-0109-01** 62.26
(30X4GM,SINGLES)
2.5%-1%, 4 gm 30s .. **42192-0108-04** 152.83

(Acella) *See HYDROCORTISONE ACETATE-PRAMOXINE HYDROCHLORIDE*

(Alaven) *See EPIFOAM*

(Alaven) *See PROCTOFOAM-HC*

(Ferndale) *See ANALPRAM E*

(Ferndale) *See ANALPRAM HC*

(Ferndale) *See ANALPRAM-HC*

(Ferndale) *See HYDROCORTISONE ACETATE AND PRAMOXINE HYDROCHLORIDE*

(Ferndale) *See PRAMOSONE*

(Major)
CRE, TP (1X30GM)
2.5%-1%, 30 gm **00904-6015-31** 62.26

(Vertical) *See ZYPRAM*

HYDROCORTISONE ACETATE/UREA
(Doak) *See CARMOL HC*

HYDROCORTISONE AND ACETIC ACID (Actavis)
acetic acid/hydrocortisone
SOL, OT (1X10ML,USP)
2%-1%, 10 ml .... **45963-0412-61** 203.43 AT

(Hi-Tech)
SOL, OT (1X10ML,USP)
2%-1%, 10 ml **50383-0901-10** 201.40

HYDROCORTISONE BUTYRATE
FUL
CRE, TP, 0.1%, 45 gm 50.30
SOL, TP, 0.1%, 20 ml 7.58

(Rouses)
CRE, TP (1X15GM)
0.1%, 15 gm **43478-0270-15** 19.69
(1X45GM)
0.1%, 45 gm **43478-0270-45** 42.25
OIN, TP (1X15GM)
0.1%, 15 gm **43478-0271-15** 10.52
(1X45GM)
0.1%, 45 gm **43478-0271-45** 22.38

(Taro)
CRE, TP (U.S.P.)
0.1%, 15 gm .... **51672-4074-01** 22.25 AB
45 gm .... **51672-4074-06** 47.53 AB
OIN, TP, 0.1%, 15 gm ..... **51672-4083-01** 11.15 AB
45 gm .... **51672-4083-06** 23.69 AB
SOL, TP, 0.1%, 20 ml ..... **51672-4061-02** 6.96 AT
60 ml............. **51672-4061-04** 14.34 AT

(Triax Pharm)
CRE, TP (1X15GM)
0.1%, 15 gm **14290-0270-15** 20.51
(1X45GM)
0.1%, 45 gm **14290-0270-45** 44.01

(Triax Pharm) *See LOCOID*

(Triax Pharm) *See LOCOID LIPOCREAM*

(Triax Pharm)
OIN, TP (1X15GM)
0.1%, 15 gm **14290-0271-15** 10.96
(1X45GM)
0.1%, 45 gm **14290-0271-45** 23.31
SOL, TP (1X20ML)
0.1%, 20 ml **14290-0273-62** 31.14
(1X60ML)
0.1%, 60 ml **14290-0273-61** 93.41

(Pharma Pac)
REPACK
CRE, TP (1X15GM)
0.1%, 15 gm .... **52959-0955-15** 28.56 AB

HYDROCORTISONE ENEMA (Teva)
hydrocortisone
NMA, RC, 100 mg/60 ml,
60 ml 7s............ **00093-9168-71** 84.84 AB

HYDROCORTISONE HEMISUCCINATE (Medisca)
POW, NA (U.S.P.,MONOHYDRATE)
10 gm **38779-0136-01** 90.00
25 gm **38779-0136-04** 175.50
100 gm.............. **38779-0136-05** 658.50
500 gm.............. **38779-0136-08** 3045.00
1000 gm............. **38779-0136-09** 7800.00

PROD/MFR NDC AWP DP OBC

(PCCA) *See HYDROCORTISONE HEMISUCCINATE .H20*

(Spectrum Pharmacy)
POW, NA (U.S.P.)
5 gm **49452-3595-01** 123.90
25 gm **49452-3595-02** 281.05
100 gm.............. **49452-3595-03** 994.00

HYDROCORTISONE HEMISUCCINATE .H20 (PCCA)
hydrocortisone hemisuccinate
POW, NA (USP)
1 gm **51927-1296-00** 9.90

HYDROCORTISONE MICRONIZED (Hawkins)
hydrocortisone, micronized
POW, NA (U.S.P.)
10 gm **63370-0100-20** 79.20
25 gm **63370-0100-25** 134.40
100 gm.............. **63370-0100-35** 504.00
500 gm.............. **63370-0100-45** 2400.00
1000 gm............. **63370-0100-50** 4368.00

(Letco)
POW, NA (U.S.P.)
25 gm **62991-1673-02** 105.00
100 gm.............. **62991-1673-03** 375.00
500 gm.............. **62991-1673-04** 1425.00

(PCCA)
POW, NA (USP)
1 gm **51927-9028-00** 10.20

HYDROCORTISONE PROBUTATE
(PharmaDerm) *See PANDEL*

HYDROCORTISONE SODIUM SUCCINATE
(Consolidated Midland)
PDS, IJ, 1 gm, ea .... **00223-7899-08** 30.00 EE
100 mg, ea .... **00223-7893-02** 3.75 EE
250 mg, ea .... **00223-7894-02** 9.50 EE
500 mg, ea .... **00223-7898-08** 15.00 EE

(Hospira) *See A-HYDROCORT*

(Pfizer) *See SOLU-CORTEF*

HYDROCORTISONE VALERATE
FUL
CRE, TP, 0.2%, 45 gm 29.62
OIN, TP, 0.2%, 45 gm 29.62

(Perrigo)
CRE, TP, 0.2%, 15 gm ..... **45802-0455-35** 15.50 AB
45 gm .... **45802-0455-42** 32.15 AB
60 gm .... **45802-0455-37** 38.70 AB

(Ranbaxy Labs) *See WESTCORT*

(Sandoz)
CRE, TP, 0.2%, 15 gm ..... **59772-8100-07** 15.25 EE

(Taro)
CRE, TP, 0.2%, 15 gm ..... **51672-1290-01** 15.52 AB
45 gm .... **51672-1290-06** 32.20 AB
60 gm .... **51672-1290-03** 38.73 AB
OIN, TP, 0.2%, 15 gm ..... **51672-1292-01** 22.60 AB
45 gm .... **51672-1292-06** 46.86 AB
60 gm .... **51672-1292-03** 56.36 AB

(A-S Medication)
REPACK
CRE, TP, 0.2%, 15 gm ..... **54569-4814-00** 15.50 EE
OIN, TP, 0.2%, 15 gm ..... **54569-4906-00** 22.60 AB

(Palmetto)
REPACK
CRE, TP, 0.2%, 15 gm **23490-5706-01** 15.50

(Phys Total Care)
REPACK
CRE, TP, 0.2%, 15 gm ..... **54868-4451-00** 19.50 EE
45 gm .... **54868-4451-01** 53.16 EE
60 gm .... **54868-4451-02** 33.57 AB
OIN, TP (1X60GM)
0.2%, 60 gm .... **54868-5251-01** 81.67 AB

(Physician Partner)
REPACK
CRE, TP (1X15GM)
0.2%, 15 gm .... **21695-0730-15** 31.04 AB

(Quality Care Prod)
REPACK
CRE, TP (1X15GM)
0.2%, 15 gm .... **35356-0266-15** 21.60 AB

(Southwood)
REPACK
CRE, TP, 0.2%, 45 gm **58016-4839-01** 32.15
OIN, TP, 0.2%, 15 gm **58016-4864-01** 15.52

HYDROCORTISONE W/ ALOE (Pharma Pac)
REPACK
hydrocortisone
CRE, TP, 1%, 15 gm....... **52959-0830-05** 7.75

PROD/MFR	NDC	AWP	DP	OBC
HYDROCORTISONE, MICRONIZED				
(Hawkins) *See HYDROCORTISONE MICRONIZED*				
(Letco) *See HYDROCORTISONE MICRONIZED*				
(PCCA) *See HYDROCORTISONE MICRONIZED*				
HYDROCORTISONE/IODOCHLORHYDROXYQUIN				
(Phys Total Care)				
REPACK				
clioquinol/hydrocortisone				
CRE, TP, 3%-1%, 20 gm	**54868-0969-01**	10.18		
30 gm	**54868-0969-02**	81.87		
(Southwood)				
REPACK				
CRE, TP, 3%-1%, 20 gm	**58016-3101-01**	5.64		
HYDROCORTISONE/IODOQUINOL (Perrigo)				
CRE, TP (1X28.4GM,GREASELESS)				
1%-1%, 28.4 gm	**45802-0930-64**	61.40		
(Stratus) *See DERMAZENE*				
(Pharma Pac)				
REPACK				
CRE, TP (GREASELESS)				
1%-1%, 30 gm	**52959-0963-01**	60.91		
(Phys Total Care)				
REPACK				
CRE, TP, 1%-1%, 30 gm	**54868-5066-00**	35.00		
HYDROCORTISONE/KETOCONAZOLE				
(Stiefel Labs) *See XOLEGEL COREPAK*				
HYDROCORTISONE/NEOMYCIN (Phys Total Care)				
REPACK				
hydrocortisone acetate/neomycin sulfate				
OIN, TP, 1%-0.5%, 20 gm	**54868-1858-01**	15.39		
HYDROCORTISONE/NEOMYCIN/POLYMYXIN B				
(Bausch & Lomb Inc.)				
hc/neomycin sulf/polymyxin b sulf				
SOL, OT, 1%-0.35%-10000 u/ml,				
10 ml	**24208-0631-10**	30.80		**AT**
SUS, OT, 1%-0.35%-10000 u/ml,				
10 ml	**24208-0635-62**	30.80		**AT**
(Falcon Ophthalmics)				
SUS, OP (USP)				
1%-0.35%-10000 u/ml,				
7.5 ml	**61314-0641-75**	67.24		
(A-S Medication)				
REPACK				
SUS, OP, 1%-0.35%-10000 u/ml,				
7.5 ml	**54569-5706-00**	76.74		
(Altura)				
REPACK				
SUS, OP, 1%-0.35%-10000 u/ml,				
7.5 ml	**63874-0169-75**	52.75		
10 ml	**63874-0169-10**	36.99		
(DHS, Inc.)				
REPACK				
SUS, OP, 1%-0.35%-10000 u/ml,				
7.5 ml	**55887-0427-75**	72.00		
(Dispensing Solutions)				
REPACK				
SOL, OT, 1%-0.35%-10000 u/ml,				
10 ml	**55045-1156-02**	35.40		**AT**
SUS, OT, 1%-0.35%-10000 u/ml,				
10 ml	**55045-2075-02**	32.10		**AT**
(1X10ML)				
1%-0.35%-10000 u/ml,				
10 ml	**55045-3938-01**	32.10		**AT**
(Pharma Pac)				
REPACK				
SUS, OP, 1%-0.35%-10000 u/ml,				
7.5 ml	**52959-0790-03**	52.75		
HYDROCORTISONE/SALICYLIC ACID/SULFUR				
(Auriga) *See CORAZ*				
(Avidas) *See SCALACORT DK*				
HYDROCOT (Truxton)				
hydrochlorothiazide				
TAB, PO, 25 mg, 1000s ea	**00463-6105-10**	14.40		**EE**
50 mg, 1000s ea	**00463-6268-10**	18.00		**EE**
HYDROFLUORIC ACID				
(Baker, J.T.) *See HYDROFLUORIC ACID 47-52%*				
(PCCA)				
POW, NA (ACS)				
49%, 1 gm	**51927-1593-00**	0.30		

PROD/MFR	NDC	AWP	DP	OBC
HYDROFLUORIC ACID 47-52% (Baker, J.T.)				
hydrofluoric acid				
SOL, NA (TECHNICAL)				
500 ml	**10106-9572-01**	50.57		
4000 ml	**10106-9572-06**	202.09		
HYDROGEL (Medisca)				
GEL, NA (1X100GM)				
100 gm	**38779-2298-05**	35.85		
(1X500GM)				
500 gm	**38779-2298-08**	118.50		
(1X3000GM)				
3000 gm	**38779-2298-03**	525.00		
HYDROGEL, ALOE VERA BASE				
(Carrington) *See SALICEPT FDG*				
HYDROGEN PEROXIDE				
(Baker, J.T.) *See HYDROGEN PEROXIDE 2.5%-3.5%*				
(Baker, J.T.) *See HYDROGEN PEROXIDE 30%*				
(Humco) *See HYDROGEN PEROXIDE 3%*				
(Mallinckrodt Lab)				
SOL, NA (TOPICAL)				
500 ml	**00406-5232-12**	21.29		
4000 ml	**00406-5232-10**	36.32		
(Medisca)				
SOL, NA (35%)				
500 ml	**38779-0849-08**	52.50		
4000 ml	**38779-0849-01**	157.50		
(PCCA) *See HYDROGEN PEROXIDE 35%*				
(PCCA)				
SOL, NA (ACS)				
1 ml	**51927-2755-00**	0.39		
(Spectrum Pharmacy) *See HYDROGEN PEROXIDE 3%*				
(Spectrum Pharmacy) *See HYDROGEN PEROXIDE 30%*				
(Spectrum Pharmacy) *See HYDROGEN PEROXIDE 35%*				
HYDROGEN PEROXIDE 2.5%-3.5% (Baker, J.T.)				
hydrogen peroxide				
SOL, NA (U.S.P.)				
500 ml	**10106-2182-01**	14.60		
4000 ml	**10106-2182-03**	89.41		
HYDROGEN PEROXIDE 3% (Humco)				
hydrogen peroxide				
SOL, NA, 120 ml	**00395-1113-94**	0.52		
240 ml	**00395-1113-98**	0.60		
480 ml	**00395-1113-16**	0.66		
960 ml	**00395-1113-32**	1.20		
3840 ml	**00395-1113-28**	8.36		
(Spectrum Pharmacy)				
SOL, NA (U.S.P.)				
500 ml	**49452-3600-01**	53.90		
4000 ml	**49452-3600-02**	171.85		
HYDROGEN PEROXIDE 30% (Baker, J.T.)				
hydrogen peroxide				
SOL, NA (BAKER)				
500 ml	**10106-2189-01**	76.32		
4000 ml	**10106-2189-03**	348.40		
(Spectrum Pharmacy)				
SOL, NA (A.C.S.,REAGENT)				
100 ml	**49452-3610-01**	102.55		
500 ml	**49452-3610-02**	257.25		
4000 ml	**49452-3610-03**	822.50		
HYDROGEN PEROXIDE 35% (PCCA)				
hydrogen peroxide				
SOL, NA (F.C.C.)				
1 ml	**51927-3029-00**	0.21		
(Spectrum Pharmacy)				
SOL, NA (F.C.C.)				
500 ml	**49452-3605-01**	111.65		
4000 ml	**49452-3605-02**	420.00		
HYDROGENATED VEGETABLE OIL (PCCA)				
vegetable oil				
OIL, NA (BASE X)				
1 gm	**51927-1116-00**	0.11		
HYDROGESIC (Edwards)				
acetaminophen/hydrocodone bitartrate				
CAP, PO, 500 mg-5 mg,				
100s ea, C-III	**00485-0050-01**	65.00	40.00	**AA**
HYDROLYZED SILK				
(PCCA) *See SOLU-SILK PROTEIN 20*				
HYDROMET (Actavis Mid Atlantic)				
homatropine methylbromide/hydrocodone bitartrate				
SYR, PO, 1.5 mg/5 ml-5 mg/5 ml,				
473 ml, C-III	**00472-1030-16**	87.44		**AA**

PROD/MFR	NDC	AWP	DP	OBC
(Altura)				
REPACK				
SYR, PO, 1.5 mg/5 ml-5 mg/5 ml,				
120 ml, C-III	**63874-0255-12**	11.44		**AA**
480 ml, C-III	**63874-0255-48**	31.20		**AA**
3840 ml, C-III	**63874-0255-38**	62.00		**AA**
(Bryant Ranch)				
REPACK				
SYR, PO, 1.5 mg/5 ml-5 mg/5 ml,				
120 ml, C-III	**63629-2962-01**	6.99		
HYDROMORPHONE (Core)				
REPACK				
hydromorphone hydrochloride				
TAB, PO, 2 mg,				
6s ea, C-II	**33358-0178-06**	5.80		
100s ea, C-II	**33358-0178-00**	46.36		
(Quality Care Prod)				
REPACK				
TAB, PO, 4 mg,				
30s ea, C-II	**49999-0835-30**	61.75		
60s ea, C-II	**49999-0835-60**	86.40		
90s ea, C-II	**49999-0835-90**	185.25		
120s ea, C-II	**49999-0835-01**	160.55		
8 mg, 90s ea, C-II	**49999-0836-90**	180.00		
120s ea, C-II	**49999-0836-01**	240.00		
HYDROMORPHONE HCL (Baxter)				
hydromorphone hydrochloride				
SOL, IJ (USP)				
2 mg/ml,				
1 ml, C-II	**00641-2341-39**	6.60		
(Covidien)				
POW, NA, 1 gm, C-II	**00406-3245-52**	166.25		
TAB, PO, 2 mg,				
100s ea, C-II	**00406-3243-01**	48.04		
4 mg,				
100s ea, C-II	**00406-3244-01**	69.06		
(Ethex)				
TAB, PO, 2 mg,				
100s ea, C-II	**58177-0298-04**	42.64		
100s ea UD, C-II	**58177-0298-11**	47.17		
4 mg,				
100s ea, C-II	**58177-0299-04**	69.61		
100s ea UD, C-II	**58177-0299-11**	71.71		
(Hawkins)				
POW, NA (U.S.P.)				
1 gm, C-II	**63370-0930-10**	408.00		
5 gm, C-II	**63370-0930-15**	2016.00		
10 gm, C-II	**63370-0930-20**	3264.00		
25 gm, C-II	**63370-0930-25**	7680.00		
100 gm, C-II	**63370-0930-35**	24000.00		
(Hospira)				
SOL, IJ (22GX1-1/4")				
1 mg/ml,				
1 ml 10s, C-II	**00074-1283-01**	9.12	8.00	
(LUER LOCK,10X1ML)				
1 mg/ml,				
1 ml 10s, C-II	**00409-1283-31**	12.72	11.10	
(USP,10X1ML)				
1 mg/ml,				
1 ml 10s, C-II	**00409-2552-01**	11.76	10.30	
(10X1ML,LLK,SLIM PK)				
2 mg/ml,				
1 ml 10s, C-II	**00409-1312-30**	14.16	12.40	
(10X1ML,USP)				
2 mg/ml,				
1 ml 10s, C-II	**00409-3356-01**	12.00	10.50	
(SDV,25X1ML)				
2 mg/ml,				
1 ml 25s, C-II	**00409-3365-01**	27.60	24.25	
(LUER LOCK,10X1ML)				
4 mg/ml,				
1 ml 10s, C-II	**00409-1304-31**	13.68	12.00	
(USP,10X1ML)				
4 mg/ml,				
1 ml 10s, C-II	**00409-2540-01**	17.40	15.20	
(HIGH POTENCY)				
10 mg/ml,				
1 ml 25s, C-II	**00409-2172-01**	79.80	69.75	**AP**
5 ml 10s, C-II	**00409-2172-05**	111.48	97.50	**AP**
(Medisca)				
POW, NA (U.S.P.)				
1 gm, C-II	**38779-0731-06**	261.00		
5 gm, C-II	**38779-0731-03**	1147.50		
10 gm, C-II	**38779-0731-01**	1845.00		
25 gm, C-II	**38779-0731-04**	3897.00		
(1X100GM)				
100 gm, C-II	**38779-0731-05**	13245.00		

PROD/MFR	NDC	AWP	DP	OBC
(Paddock)				
POW, NA, 0.972 gm, C-II	**00574-2017-01**	181.53		
SUP, RC, 3 mg,				
6s ea UD, C-II	**00574-7224-06**	66.65		
(PCCA)				
POW, NA (U.S.P.; CII)				
1 gm, C-II	**51927-1003-00**	315.00		
(Spectrum Pharmacy)				
POW, NA (U.S.P.)				
1 gm, C-II	**49452-0029-01**	353.50		
5 gm, C-II	**49452-0029-02**	1529.50		
10 gm, C-II	**49452-0029-03**	2835.00		
25 gm, C-II	**49452-0029-04**	4280.50		
(Vintage)				
TAB, PO, 2 mg,				
100s ea, C-II	**00254-3611-28**	28.12		
(4u)				
REPACK				
TAB, PO, 2 mg,				
28s ea, C-II	**10544-0394-28**	68.26		
28s ea, C-II	**42549-0594-28**	68.26		
4 mg, 28s ea, C-II	**10544-0374-28**	72.22		
28s ea, C-II	**42549-0574-28**	72.22		
30s ea, C-II	**42549-0574-30**	75.86		
56s ea, C-II	**10544-0374-56**	118.84		
56s ea, C-II	**42549-0574-56**	118.84		
60s ea, C-II	**42549-0574-60**	122.92		
140s ea, C-II	**10544-0374-04**	238.48		
140s ea, C-II	**42549-0574-04**	238.48		
168s ea, C-II	**42549-0574-08**	266.98		
(B&B Pharm, Inc)				
REPACK				
POW, NA (U.S.P.)				
1 gm, C-II	**63275-2001-01**	315.00		
5 gm, C-II	**63275-2005-02**	1575.00		
10 gm, C-II	**63275-2010-03**	3150.00		
100 gm, C-II	**63275-2100-05**	31500.00		
1000 gm, C-II	**63275-2100-09**	91000.00		
(Bryant Ranch)				
REPACK				
TAB, PO, 4 mg,				
30s ea, C-II	**63629-3798-01**	19.32		
180s ea, C-II	**63629-3798-02**	113.52		
(PD-Rx Pharm)				
REPACK				
TAB, PO (USP)				
2 mg, 6s ea, C-II	**43063-0051-06**	8.28		
(Phys Total Care)				
REPACK				
SOL, IJ (25X1ML)				
2 mg/ml,				
1 ml 25s, C-II	**54868-5319-00**	91.86		
TAB, PO, 2 mg,				
10s ea, C-II	**54868-3165-01**	11.22		
20s ea, C-II	**54868-3165-00**	14.94		
50s ea, C-II	**54868-3165-02**	26.07		
60s ea, C-II	**54868-3165-07**	38.66		
90s ea, C-II	**54868-3165-04**	40.95		
100s ea, C-II	**54868-3165-03**	44.64		
120s ea, C-II	**54868-3165-06**	49.08		
4 mg, 30s ea, C-II	**54868-4969-04**	22.05		
60s ea, C-II	**54868-4969-00**	36.60		
90s ea, C-II	**54868-4969-02**	51.15		
100s ea, C-II	**54868-4969-03**	56.01		
120s ea, C-II	**54868-4969-01**	65.70		
8 mg, 30s ea, C-II	**54868-4598-04**	87.16		AB
60s ea, C-II	**54868-4598-00**	143.28		AB
100s ea, C-II	**54868-4598-01**	234.81		AB
120s ea, C-II	**54868-4598-02**	280.56		AB
(Quality Care Prod)				
REPACK				
TAB, PO, 8 mg,				
30s ea, C-II	**49999-0836-30**	87.30		AB
(Stat Rx)				
REPACK				
TAB, PO, 2 mg,				
20s ea, C-II	**16590-0827-20**	9.60		
30s ea, C-II	**16590-0827-30**	14.40		
56s ea, C-II	**16590-0827-56**	26.88		
60s ea, C-II	**16590-0827-60**	28.80		
4 mg, 15s ea, C-II	**16590-0715-15**	9.49		
20s ea, C-II	**16590-0715-20**	12.65		
28s ea, C-II	**16590-0715-28**	17.16		
30s ea, C-II	**16590-0715-30**	18.39		
56s ea, C-II	**16590-0715-56**	34.33		
60s ea, C-II	**16590-0715-60**	36.79		
90s ea, C-II	**16590-0715-90**	55.18		
112s ea, C-II	**16590-0715-73**	77.28		
120s ea, C-II	**16590-0715-72**	73.57		
180s ea, C-II	**16590-0715-82**	110.36		
HYDROMORPHONE HCL/SODIUM CHLORIDE				
(PharMEDium Services)				
hydromorphone hydrochloride/sodium chloride				
SOL, IV (SRN,35 ML)				
1 mg/5 ml-0.9%,				
25 ml, C-II	**61553-0162-67**	20.68	17.23	
(INTRAVIA)				
10 mg/50 ml-0.9%,				
50 ml, C-II	**61553-0161-41**	26.07	21.73	
(SRN,60 ML)				
1 mg/5 ml-0.9%,				
50 ml, C-II	**61553-0163-75**	21.82	18.18	
(IPUMP BAG)				
20 mg/100 ml-0.9%,				
100 ml, C-II	**61553-0624-48**	38.26	31.88	
(SRN,35 ML)				
1 mg/ml-0.9%,				
25 ml, C-II	**61553-0166-67**	25.24	21.03	
(INTRAVIA)				
50 mg/50 ml-0.9%,				
50 ml, C-II	**61553-0165-41**	35.37	29.48	
(SRN,50 ML)				
1 mg/ml-0.9%,				
50 ml, C-II	**61553-0167-75**	30.94	25.78	
HYDROMORPHONE HYDROCHLORIDE				
FUL				
TAB, PO, 2 mg, 100s ea		21.84		
(Baxter) *See HYDROMORPHONE HCL*				
(Baxter)				
SOL, IJ (VIAL,DOSETTE,USP)				
2 mg/ml,				
1 ml, C-II	**00641-0121-21**	1.02		
1 ml 25s, C-II	**00641-0121-25**	25.50		
((M.D.V.),USP)				
2 mg/ml,				
20 ml, C-II	**00641-2341-41**	6.60		
(Covidien) *See HYDROMORPHONE HCL*				
(Covidien)				
TAB, PO, 8 mg,				
100s ea, C-II	**00406-3249-01**	138.42		AB
(Ethex) *See HYDROMORPHONE HCL*				
(Ethex)				
TAB, PO (10X10)				
2 mg,				
10s ea UD, C-II	**58177-0620-11**	40.90		
100s ea, C-II	**58177-0620-04**	37.18		
(10X10)				
4 mg,				
10s ea UD, C-II	**58177-0621-11**	67.44		
100s ea, C-II	**58177-0621-04**	61.31		
8 mg, 100s ea, C-II	**58177-0449-04**	131.30		AB
(Gallipot)				
POW, NA (1X1GM,USP)				
1 gm, C-II	**51552-0682-01**	119.00	85.00	
(1X5GM,USP)				
5 gm, C-II	**51552-0682-02**	588.00	420.00	
(1X10GM,USP)				
10 gm, C-II	**51552-0682-03**	910.00	650.00	
(1X25GM,USP)				
25 gm, C-II	**51552-0682-04**	2275.00	1625.00	
(Hawkins) *See HYDROMORPHONE HCL*				
(Hospira) *See HYDROMORPHONE HCL*				
(Hospira)				
SOL, IJ (10X1ML,SDA,USP)				
10 mg/ml,				
1 ml 10s, C-II	**00409-2634-01**	29.04	25.40	AP
(10X5ML,SDA,USP)				
10 mg/ml,				
5 ml 10s, C-II	**00409-2634-05**	83.52	73.10	AP
(1X50ML,SDA,USP)				
10 mg/ml,				
50 ml, C-II	**00409-2634-50**	123.65	108.19	AP
(Lannett)				
TAB, PO (USP)				
2 mg,				
100s ea, C-II	**00527-1353-01**	44.70		AB
4 mg, 100s ea, C-II	**00527-1354-01**	73.62		AB
8 mg, 100s ea, C-II	**00527-1355-01**	158.40		AB
(Medisca) *See HYDROMORPHONE HCL*				
(Paddock) *See HYDROMORPHONE HCL*				
(PCCA) *See HYDROMORPHONE HCL*				
(PharMEDium Services)				
SOL, IV (10X30ML, PCA VIAL)				
2 mg/ml,	**61553-0780-68**	65.40	54.50	
(Purdue Pharma) *See DILAUDID*				
(Purdue Pharma) *See DILAUDID-HP*				
(Rhodes)				
TAB, PO (4X25,USP)				
2 mg,				
100s ea UD, C-II	**42858-0301-25**	49.88		
(USP)				
2 mg,				
100s ea, C-II	**42858-0301-01**	49.88		
(4X25,USP)				
4 mg,				
100s ea UD, C-II	**42858-0302-25**	72.81		
(USP)				
4 mg,				
100s ea, C-II	**42858-0302-01**	72.81		
500s ea, C-II	**42858-0302-50**	196.80		
8 mg, 100s ea, C-II	**42858-0303-01**	140.31		
(Roxane)				
TAB, PO (USP, 4X25)				
4 mg,				
100s ea UD, C-II	**00054-0264-24**	71.71		AB
(USP)				
4 mg,				
100s ea, C-II	**00054-0264-25**	61.31		AB
8 mg, 100s ea, C-II	**00054-0265-25**	131.93		AB
(Spectrum Pharmacy) *See HYDROMORPHONE HCL*				
(Teva)				
SOL, IJ (10X1ML,PF)				
10 mg/ml,				
1 ml 10s, C-II	**00555-1117-05**	31.26		AP
(10X5ML,PF)				
10 mg/ml,				
5 ml 10s, C-II	**00555-1117-06**	117.75		AP
(SDV,PF)				
10 mg/ml,				
50 ml, C-II	**00555-1117-07**	187.50		AP
(Vintage) *See HYDROMORPHONE HCL*				
(Dispensing Solutions)				
REPACK				
TAB, PO, 4 mg,				
30s ea, C-II	**66336-0303-30**	22.09		AB
(Palmetto)				
REPACK				
TAB, PO, 2 mg, 6s ea, C-II	**23490-7778-01**	10.50		
30s ea, C-II	**23490-7778-03**	52.50		
60s ea, C-II	**23490-7778-06**	105.00		
90s ea, C-II	**23490-7778-09**	157.50		
4 mg, 30s ea, C-II	**23490-7779-03**	64.50		
60s ea, C-II	**23490-7779-06**	129.00		
90s ea, C-II	**23490-7779-09**	193.50		
100s ea, C-II	**23490-7779-08**	215.00		
(Phys Total Care)				
REPACK				
TAB, PO (USP)				
2 mg, 30s ea, C-II	**54868-3165-05**	15.66		
4 mg, 50s ea, C-II	**54868-4969-05**	31.74		
100s ea, C-II	**54868-4969-06**	101.19		
8 mg, 20s ea, C-II	**54868-4598-03**	61.11		AB
150s ea, C-II	**54868-4598-05**	307.85		AB
(Stat Rx)				
REPACK				
TAB, PO, 8 mg,				
30s ea, C-II	**16590-0774-30**	37.69		AB
60s ea, C-II	**16590-0774-60**	73.15		AB
120s ea, C-II	**16590-0774-72**	166.80		AB
HYDROMORPHONE HYDROCHLORIDE-SODIUM CHLORIDE (PharMEDium Services)				
hydromorphone hydrochloride/sodium chloride				
SOL, IV (10X30ML, PCA VIAL)				
0.1 mg/ml-0.9%,				
30 ml 10s, C-II	**61553-0701-68**	49.50	41.25	
0.2 mg/ml-0.9%,				
30 ml 10s, C-II	**61553-0702-68**	46.50	38.75	
(5X55ML, BD SYRINGES)				
0.2 mg/ml-0.9%,				
55 ml 5s, C-II	**61553-0681-76**	25.50	21.25	
(5X100ML, CASSETTE)				
0.2 mg/ml-0.9%,				
100 ml 5s, C-II	**61553-0890-48**	187.50	156.25	
(10X30ML, PCA VIAL)				
0.4 mg/ml-0.9%,				
30 ml 10s, C-II	**61553-0704-68**	52.50	43.75	
0.5 mg/ml-0.9%,				
30 ml 10s, C-II	**61553-0705-68**	49.50	41.25	
0.6 mg/ml-0.9%,				
30 ml 10s, C-II	**61553-0706-68**	53.26	44.38	

PROD/MFR	NDC	AWP	DP	OBC
1 mg/ml-0.9%,				
30 ml 10s, C-II	61553-0710-68	52.50	43.75	
1.2 mg/ml-0.9%,				
30 ml 10s, C-II	61553-0712-68	55.50	46.25	
HYDROMORPHONE HYDROCHLORIDE/ SODIUM CHLORIDE				
(PharMEDium Services) *See HYDROMORPHONE HCL/SODIUM CHLORIDE*				
(PharMEDium Services) *See HYDROMORPHONE HYDROCHLORIDE-SODIUM CHLORIDE*				
HYDROPHYLLIC PETROLATUM (Medisca)				
petrolatum, hydrophilic				
OIN, NA (1X500GM)				
500 gm	38779-0649-08	46.50		
(1X1000GM)				
1000 gm	38779-0649-09	70.50		
HYDROQUINONE (Amend)				
POW, NA (U.S.P.)				
125 gm	17317-0292-04	15.75		
500 gm	17317-0292-01	35.00		
2500 gm	17317-0292-05	140.00		
11350 gm	17317-0292-08	647.50		
(Consolidated Midland)				
CRE, TP, 4%, 60 gm	00223-4330-02	2.75		
120 gm	00223-4330-04	4.00		
(Gallipot)				
POW, NA (U.S.P.)				
113.4 gm	51552-0066-04	14.00		
454 gm	51552-0066-06	44.80		
2270 gm	51552-0066-09	187.11		
(JSJ Pharma) *See ACLARO*				
(Letco)				
POW, NA (U.S.P.)				
100 gm	62991-1196-02	30.00		
500 gm	62991-1196-03	105.00		
(Medisca)				
POW, NA (U.S.P.)				
100 gm	38779-0075-05	37.50		
500 gm	38779-0075-08	111.00		
1000 gm	38779-0075-09	214.50		
(U.S.P.)				
2500 gm	38779-0075-01	495.00		
(Neutrogena) *See MELANEX*				
(PCCA)				
POW, NA (MONO BENZYL ETHER)				
1 gm	51927-3200-00	5.28		
(U.S.P.)				
1 gm	51927-1124-00	4.50		
(Perrigo)				
dioxybenzone/hydroquinone/oxybenzone/padimate o				
CRE, TP (1X28.35GM,USP)				
3%-4%-2%-8%,				
28.35 gm	45802-0975-64	45.03		
HYDROQUINONE (Perrigo)				
(USP,1X28.35GM)				
4%, 28.35 gm	45802-0980-64	45.03		
(1X30GM,USP,TIME-RELEASE)				
4%, 30 gm	45802-0338-94	106.88		
(SkinMedica) *See EPIQUIN MICRO*				
(Spectrum Pharmacy)				
POW, NA (U.S.P.)				
125 gm	49452-3620-01	71.40		
500 gm	49452-3620-02	185.50		
2500 gm	49452-3620-03	766.50		
(Stratus) *See ALPHAQUIN HP*				
(Stratus) *See MELPAQUE HP*				
(Stratus) *See MELQUIN HP*				
(Stratus) *See MELQUIN-3*				
(Stratus) *See NUQUIN HP*				
(Taro) *See LUSTRA*				
(Taro) *See LUSTRA-AF*				
(Taro) *See LUSTRA-ULTRA*				
(Valeant Pharm Intl) *See ELDOPAQUE FORTE*				
(Valeant Pharm Intl) *See ELDOQUIN FORTE*				
(Pharma Pac)				
REPACK				
CRE, TP, 4%, 28.35 gm	52959-0850-02	32.79		
(Phys Total Care)				
REPACK				
CRE, TP, 4%, 28.35 gm	54868-5633-00	38.42		
HYDROQUINONE SKIN BLEACHING MOISTURIZING (Perrigo)				
hydroquinone/octinoxate/oxybenzone/padimate o				
CRE, TP (1X28.4GM,USP)				
28.4 gm	45802-0984-64	48.25		
HYDROQUINONE SKIN BLEACHING WITH SUNSCREENS (Perrigo)				
dioxybenzone/hydroquinone/padimate o				
GEL, TP (1X28.35GM)				
28.35 gm	45802-0982-64	45.03		
HYDROQUINONE/OCTINOXATE/OXYBENZONE/ PADIMATE O				
(Perrigo) *See HYDROQUINONE SKIN BLEACHING MOISTURIZING*				
HYDROXOCOBALAMIN (Consolidated Midland)				
cyanocobalamin				
SOL, IM (VIAL)				
1000 mcg/ml, 10 ml	00223-7912-10	7.50		EE
30 ml	00223-7912-30	9.75		EE
HYDROXOCOBALAMIN (Letco)				
POW, NA, 1 gm	62991-1674-02	240.00		
5 gm	62991-1674-03	1050.00		
(Medisca)				
POW, NA (USP)				
0.5 gm	38779-0472-00	231.00		
1 gm	38779-0472-06	397.50		
5 gm	38779-0472-03	1257.00		
25 gm	38779-0472-04	4197.00		
(Spectrum Pharmacy)				
POW, NA (U.S.P.)				
0.1 gm	49452-3623-01	175.70		
0.5 gm	49452-3623-02	360.50		
1 gm	49452-3623-04	549.50		
5 gm	49452-3623-05	1659.00		
25 gm	49452-3623-06	5834.50		
(Truxton)				
cyanocobalamin				
SOL, IM (VIAL)				
1000 mcg/ml, 30 ml	00463-1094-30	5.62		EE
HYDROXOCOBALAMIN (Watson Labs)				
SOL, IM (MDV)				
1000 mcg/ml, 30 ml	00591-2888-30	38.26		
HYDROXOCOBALAMIN HCL (PCCA)				
hydroxocobalamin hydrochloride				
POW, NA (VITAMIN B12A)				
1 gm	51927-2185-00	576.00		
HYDROXOCOBALAMIN HYDROCHLORIDE (PCCA) *See HYDROXOCOBALAMIN HCL*				
HYDROXY CITRATE EXTRACT (NLT 50%) (PCCA)				
hydroxycitric acid extract				
POW, NA (1X1GM)				
1 gm	51927-2852-00	0.75		
5-HYDROXY-L-TRYPTOPHAN (Letco)				
tryptophan				
POW, NA, 100 gm	62991-1333-03	112.50		
500 gm	62991-1333-04	435.00		
HYDROXYAMPHETAMINE HYDROBROMIDE (PCCA)				
POW, NA, 1 gm	51927-2239-00	168.00		
(Spectrum Pharmacy)				
CRY, NA (U.S.P.)				
1 gm	49452-3624-01	324.10		
HYDROXYAMPHETAMINE HYDROBROMIDE/ TROPICAMIDE				
(Akorn) *See PAREMYD*				
HYDROXYCHLOROQUINE (Palmetto)				
REPACK				
hydroxychloroquine sulfate				
TAB, PO, 200 mg, 30s ea	23490-5724-03	47.23		
60s ea	23490-5724-06	94.46		
90s ea	23490-5724-09	141.69		
HYDROXYCHLOROQUINE SULFATE				
FUL				
TAB, PO, 200 mg, 100s ea		22.50		
(Gallipot)				
POW, NA (USP,1X25GM)				
25 gm	51552-0756-04	42.00	30.00	
(USP,1X100GM)				
100 gm	51552-0756-05	141.68	101.20	
(Hawkins)				
POW, NA (U.S.P.)				
25 gm	63370-0104-25	112.00		
100 gm	63370-0104-35	392.00		
500 gm	63370-0104-45	1820.00		
(Medisca)				
POW, NA (U.S.P.)				
25 gm	38779-1352-04	111.00		
100 gm	38779-1352-05	375.00		
500 gm	38779-1352-08	1393.50		
(Mylan)				
TAB, PO, 200 mg, 100s ea	00378-0373-01	123.20		AB
(PCCA)				
POW, NA (U.S.P.; NO. 6 SIEVE)				
1 gm	51927-2136-00	4.44		
(Ranbaxy Labs)				
TAB, PO (USP)				
200 mg, 100s ea	63304-0296-01	123.20		
500s ea	63304-0296-05	585.20		
(Sandoz)				
TAB, PO, 200 mg, 100s ea	00781-1407-01	109.55		AB
500s ea	00781-1407-05	514.65		AB
(Sanofi-Aventis) *See PLAQUENIL*				
(Spectrum Pharmacy)				
CRY, NA (U.S.P.)				
25 gm	49452-3625-02	183.75		
100 gm	49452-3625-03	623.00		
(Teva)				
TAB, PO (FILM-COATED)				
200 mg, 100s ea	00093-9774-01	117.35		AB
500s ea	00093-9774-05	575.00		AB
(Watson Labs)				
TAB, PO, 200 mg, 100s ea	00591-0698-01	24.00		AB
500s ea	00591-0698-05	114.00		AB
(Winthrop)				
TAB, PO, 200 mg, 100s ea	00955-0790-01	121.78		
500s ea	00955-0790-05	608.89		
(Zydus Pharm.)				
TAB, PO (USP,FILM COATED)				
200 mg, 100s ea	68382-0096-01	123.20		AB
(A-S Medication)				
REPACK				
TAB, PO, 200 mg, 60s ea	54569-4981-01	73.92		EE
(American Health)				
REPACK				
TAB, PO (10X10,FILM COATED)				
200 mg, 100s ea UD	68084-0026-01	59.10		AB
100s ea UD	68084-0269-01	59.10		AB
(Pharma Pac)				
REPACK				
TAB, PO, 200 mg, 60s ea	52959-0176-60	75.50		EE
100s ea	52959-0176-00	125.80		EE
(Phys Total Care)				
REPACK				
TAB, PO, 200 mg, 30s ea	54868-3821-02	24.15		AB
60s ea	54868-3821-01	43.80		EE
100s ea	54868-3821-00	68.49		EE
(FILM-COATED)				
200 mg, 500s ea	54868-3821-03	253.41		AB
(Quality Care Prod)				
REPACK				
TAB, PO (FILM-COATED)				
200 mg, 60s ea	49999-0372-60	89.40		AB
(Vibranta)				
REPACK				
TAB, PO, 200 mg, 60s ea	57866-9027-01	74.50		
HYDROXYCITRIC ACID EXTRACT (PCCA) *See HYDROXY CITRATE EXTRACT (NLT 50%)*				
HYDROXYETHYL CELLULOSE (Gallipot)				
POW, NA, 454 gm	51552-0591-06	55.65		
(Letco)				
POW, NA (5000 CPS,N.F.)				
100 gm	62991-1282-01	42.00		
500 gm	62991-1282-02	105.00		
(Medisca)				
POW, NA (1X100GM)				
100 gm	38779-2101-05	67.50		
(1X500GM)				
500 gm	38779-2101-08	195.00		
(1X1000GM)				
1000 gm	38779-2101-09	345.00		
(PCCA)				
POW, NA (NF)				
1 gm	51927-1766-00	0.45		
(Spectrum Pharmacy)				
POW, NA (1X100GM)				
100 gm	49452-3637-01	69.30		
(1X500GM)				
500 gm	49452-3637-02	194.60		

PROD/MFR	NDC	AWP	DP	OBC
(N.F.,75-150 CPS)				
500 gm	49452-3640-02	180.60		
(1X2500GM)				
2500 gm	49452-3637-03	798.00		
(N.F.,75-150 CPS)				
2500 gm	49452-3640-03	756.00		
HYDROXYETHYL METHACRYLATE				
(PCCA) *See HYDROXYETHYL METHACRYLATE (2)*				
(Spectrum Pharmacy) *See 2-HYDROXYETHYL METHACRYLATE*				
2-HYDROXYETHYL METHACRYLATE (Spectrum Pharmacy)				
hydroxyethyl methacrylate				
SOL, NA (1X100GM)				
96%, 100 gm	49452-3658-01	218.50		
(1X500GM)				
96%, 500 gm	49452-3658-02	388.50		
HYDROXYETHYL METHACRYLATE (2) (PCCA)				
hydroxyethyl methacrylate				
SOL, NA (1X1ML)				
96%, 1 ml	51927-2936-00	3.60		
HYDROXYLAMINE HYDROCHLORIDE (Baker, J.T.)				
CRY, NA (A.C.S., REAGENT)				
125 gm	10106-2195-04	62.21		
500 gm	10106-2195-01	168.41		
HYDROXYPROGESTERONE CAPROATE				
(Consolidated Midland)				
OIL, IM (VIAL)				
250 mg/ml, 5 ml	00223-7896-05	13.50		EE
5 ml	00223-7915-05	15.00		EE
(Gallipot)				
POW, NA, 25 gm	51552-1028-04	84.00	60.00	
(Hawkins)				
POW, NA (U.S.P.)				
5 gm	63370-0105-15	60.00		
25 gm	63370-0105-25	240.00		
100 gm	63370-0105-35	920.00		
500 gm	63370-0105-45	4400.00		
1000 gm	63370-0105-50	7200.00		
(Legere) *See PRODROX*				
(Letco)				
POW, NA, 25 gm	62991-2034-02	90.00		
100 gm	62991-2034-03	240.00		
500 gm	62991-2034-04	990.00		
(Medisca)				
POW, NA, 5 gm	38779-2102-03	63.00		
25 gm	38779-2102-04	261.00		
100 gm	38779-2102-05	918.00		
(PCCA)				
POW, NA (U.S.P.)				
1 gm	51927-2733-00	13.20		
(Spectrum Pharmacy)				
CRY, NA (U.S.P.)				
5 gm	49452-3639-01	94.15		
25 gm	49452-3639-02	364.00		
100 gm	49452-3639-03	1267.00		
500 gm	49452-3639-04	4662.00		
HYDROXYPROPYL BETA CYCLODEXTRIN				
(PCCA) *See HYDROXYPROPYL-BETA-CYCLODEXTRIN*				
HYDROXYPROPYL CELLULOSE				
(Aton) *See LACRISERT*				
(Gallipot)				
POW, NA (1500-3000 C.P.S.)				
100 gm	51552-0299-05	14.00		
454 gm	51552-0299-06	52.50		
(Letco)				
POW, NA, 100 gm	62991-1591-01	51.00		
500 gm	62991-1591-02	147.00		
(PCCA)				
POW, NA (NF,(1500 CPS))				
1 gm	51927-1996-00	0.48		
(Spectrum Pharmacy)				
POW, NA (N.F.,150-400 CPS)				
125 gm	49452-3642-01	90.30		
(N.F.,75-100 CPS)				
125 gm	49452-3641-01	90.30		
(NF,4000-6500 CPS)				
125 gm	49452-3643-04	90.30		
(N.F., 75-100 CPS)				
500 gm	49452-3641-02	236.95		
(N.F.,150-400 CPS)				
500 gm	49452-3642-02	236.95		
(NF,4000-6500 CPS)				
500 gm	49452-3643-01	236.95		
(N.F., 75-100 CPS)				
2500 gm	49452-3641-03	707.00		
(N.F.,150-400 CPS)				
2500 gm	49452-3642-03	707.00		
(NF,4000-6500 CPS)				
2500 gm	49452-3643-02	707.00		
HYDROXYPROPYL METHYLCELLULOSE 2208				
(Spectrum Pharmacy)				
hypromellose				
POW, NA (100,000CPS,U.S.P.)				
125 gm	49452-3646-01	72.45		
500 gm	49452-3646-02	178.15		
2500 gm	49452-3646-03	570.50		
HYDROXYPROPYL-BETA-CYCLODEXTRIN (PCCA)				
hydroxypropyl beta cyclodextrin				
POW, NA (1X1GM)				
1 gm	51927-3081-00	34.68		
HYDROXYQUINOLINE (PCCA)				
oxyquinoline				
POW, NA (PURE; OXYQUINOLINE BASE)				
1 gm	51927-1553-00	0.99		
HYDROXYQUINOLINE SULFATE (PCCA)				
oxyquinoline sulfate				
POW, NA (MONOHYDRATE)				
1 gm	51927-1918-00	2.16		
HYDROXYTRYPTOPHAN (Medisca)				
POW, NA, 5 gm	38779-0719-03	108.00		
25 gm	38779-0719-04	429.00		
100 gm	38779-0719-05	1300.50		
500 gm	38779-0719-08	4650.00		
(PCCA)				
POW, NA (DIHYDRATE)				
1 gm	51927-2939-00	30.00		
(L-5)				
1 gm	51927-2024-00	27.00		
HYDROXYUREA				
(B/M Squibb Onc/Vir) *See DROXIA*				
(B/M Squibb Onc/Vir) *See HYDREA*				
(Medisca)				
POW, NA (U.S.P.)				
25 gm	38779-1354-04	102.00		
(USP,1X50GM)				
50 gm	38779-1354-02	156.00		
(U.S.P.)				
100 gm	38779-1354-05	345.00		
250 gm	38779-1354-07	765.00		
500 gm	38779-1354-08	1350.00		
(Par)				
CAP, PO, 500 mg, 100s ea	49884-0724-01	127.73		AB
(PCCA)				
POW, NA (U.S.P.)				
1 gm	51927-2655-00	3.84		
(Spectrum Pharmacy)				
POW, NA (U.S.P.)				
25 gm	49452-3650-01	164.85		
100 gm	49452-3650-02	539.00		
500 gm	49452-3650-03	1904.00		
(Teva)				
CAP, PO, 500 mg, 100s ea	00555-0882-02	127.73		AB
(A-S Medication)				
REPACK				
CAP, PO, 500 mg, 100s ea	54569-5715-00	127.73		AB
(American Health)				
REPACK				
CAP, PO (10X10)				
500 mg, 100s ea UD	68084-0284-01	88.11		AB
(Phys Total Care)				
REPACK				
CAP, PO, 500 mg, 30s ea	54868-4773-00	35.55		AB
50s ea	54868-4773-02	57.24		AB
60s ea	54868-4773-03	68.07		AB
100s ea	54868-4773-01	84.45		AB
HYDROXYYZINE PAMOATE (Bryant Ranch)				
REPACK				
hydroxyzine pamoate				
CAP, PO, 25 mg, 20s ea	63629-1533-01	61.40		
30s ea	63629-1533-02	72.10		
30s ea	63629-1856-01	31.65		
60s ea	63629-1856-02	63.89		
HYDROXYZINE (Bryant Ranch)				
hydroxyzine hydrochloride				
SYR, PO, 10 mg/5 ml,				
120 ml	63629-1855-01	8.45		
240 ml	63629-1855-02	16.90		
TAB, PO, 10 mg, 30s ea	63629-1751-01	23.57		
100s ea	63629-1751-02	78.58		
(DHS, Inc.)				
REPACK				
TAB, PO, 10 mg, 20s ea	55887-0232-20	21.50		
60s ea	55887-0232-60	64.50		
90s ea	55887-0232-90	96.75		
100s ea	55887-0232-01	107.50		
50 mg, 15s ea	55887-0942-15	28.00		
(Dispensing Solutions)				
REPACK				
TAB, PO, 10 mg, 15s ea	66336-0795-15	12.47		
50 mg, 30s ea	66336-0796-30	40.22		
(IPI)				
REPACK				
TAB, PO, 10 mg, 40s ea	18837-0315-40	28.06		
(Palmetto)				
REPACK				
SYR, PO, 10 mg/5 ml,				
120 ml	23490-5728-01	11.52		
(Pharma Pac)				
REPACK				
TAB, PO, 50 mg, 30s ea	52959-0882-30	49.99		
(Southwood)				
REPACK				
SYR, PO, 10 mg/5 ml,				
480 ml	58016-4845-01	3.94		EE
HYDROXYZINE HCL (Amer Regent)				
hydroxyzine hydrochloride				
SOL, IM (S.D.V.)				
25 mg/ml, 1 ml 25s	00517-4201-25	93.75		AP
50 mg/ml, 1 ml 25s	00517-5601-25	103.13		AP
2 ml 25s	00517-5602-25	125.00		AP
(M.D.V.)				
50 mg/ml,				
10 ml 25s	00517-5610-25	265.63		AP
(Consolidated Midland)				
SOL, IM (VIAL, DOSETTE)				
25 mg/ml, 1 ml 25s	00223-7885-01	25.00		EE
(VIAL)				
25 mg/ml, 10 ml	00223-7877-10	3.00		EE
(VIAL, DOSETTE)				
50 mg/ml, 1 ml 25s	00223-7883-01	25.00		EE
(VIAL)				
50 mg/ml, 2 ml 25s	00223-7884-02	25.00		EE
10 ml	00223-7878-10	3.50		EE
10 ml	00223-7882-10	5.50		EE
SYR, PO, 10 mg/5 ml,				
480 ml	00223-6525-01	11.50		EE
3840 ml	00223-6525-02	75.00		EE
TAB, PO, 10 mg, 100s ea	00223-1006-01	5.25		EE
1000s ea	00223-1006-02	47.50		EE
25 mg, 100s ea	00223-1007-01	6.95		EE
500s ea	00223-1007-05	32.50		EE
1000s ea	00223-1007-02	69.50		EE
50 mg, 100s ea	00223-1008-01	8.75		EE
1000s ea	00223-1008-02	75.00		EE
100 mg, 100s ea	00223-1009-01	22.50		EE
(Hawkins)				
POW, NA (U.S.P.)				
25 gm	63370-0107-25	74.00		
100 gm	63370-0107-35	224.00		
1000 gm	63370-0107-50	1280.00		
5000 gm	63370-0107-55	6000.00		
(Hi-Tech)				
SYR, PO, 10 mg/5 ml,				
473 ml	50383-0796-16	39.94		AA
(Medisca)				
POW, NA (U.S.P.)				
25 gm	38779-0298-04	67.50		
100 gm	38779-0298-05	207.00		
(USP,1X500GM)				
500 gm	38779-0298-08	660.00		
(USP,1X1000GM)				
1000 gm	38779-0298-09	1050.00		
(Morton Grove)				
SYR, PO (PEPPERMINT)				
10 mg/5 ml, 118 ml	60432-0150-04	19.94		AA
473 ml	60432-0150-16	39.94		AA
(PCCA)				
POW, NA (U.S.P.)				
1 gm	51927-1400-00	3.24		
(Spectrum Pharmacy)				
POW, NA (U.S.P.)				
25 gm	49452-3652-02	152.60		
100 gm	49452-3652-03	623.00		
(Teva)				
TAB, PO (FILM-COATED)				
10 mg, 100s ea	50111-0307-01	62.36		AB

PROD/MFR	NDC	AWP	DP	OBC
500s ea	50111-0307-02	289.99		AB
1000s ea	50111-0307-03	561.27		AB
25 mg, 100s ea	50111-0308-01	91.46		AB
500s ea	50111-0308-02	425.29		AB
1000s ea	50111-0308-03	823.14		AB
50 mg, 100s ea	50111-0309-01	111.50		AB
500s ea	50111-0309-02	518.47		AB
1000s ea	50111-0309-03	998.50		AB
(A-S Medication)				
REPACK				
SYR, PO, 10 mg/5 ml,				
120 ml	54569-1640-01	12.92		EE
TAB, PO (FILM-COATED)				
10 mg, 20s ea	54569-0406-03	12.49		AB
30s ea	54569-0406-00	18.73		AB
25 mg, 6s ea	54569-0413-08	5.52		EE
15s ea	54569-0413-06	13.79		EE
20s ea	54569-0413-00	18.39		EE
30s ea	54569-0413-01	27.59		EE
60s ea	54569-0413-04	55.17		EE
50 mg, 17s ea	54569-0409-03	19.06		EE
25s ea	54569-0409-04	28.03		EE
30s ea	54569-0409-01	33.63		EE
(Altura)				
REPACK				
SYR, PO, 10 mg/5 ml,				
120 ml	63874-0718-12	13.65		EE
TAB, PO, 10 mg, 30s ea	63874-0303-30	42.12		EE
25 mg, 20s ea	63874-0303-20	28.08		EE
30s ea	63874-0304-30	29.12		EE
60s ea	63874-0304-60	54.36		EE
1000s ea	63874-0304-02	170.12		EE
50 mg, 30s ea	63874-0077-30	33.80		EE
500s ea	63874-0077-50	123.73		EE
(DHS, Inc.)				
REPACK				
TAB, PO, 25 mg, 10s ea	55887-0985-10	15.00		AB
15s ea	55887-0985-15	20.00		AB
30s ea	55887-0985-30	36.00		AB
(Dispensing Solutions)				
REPACK				
SYR, PO (PEPPERMINT)				
10 mg/5 ml, 118 ml	55045-1417-02	20.00		AA
TAB, PO (FILM-COATED)				
10 mg, 30s ea	55045-1805-08	26.55		AB
25 mg, 15s ea	55045-1446-05	14.10		AB
20s ea	55045-1446-07	18.80		AB
(FILM-COATED)				
25 mg, 20s ea	66336-0086-20	27.08		AB
30s ea	55045-1446-08	28.20		AB
(FILM-COATED)				
25 mg, 30s ea	66336-0086-30	40.15		AB
(HomeMed)				
REPACK				
TAB, PO, 10 mg, 15s ea	51655-0078-54	21.99		EE
24s ea	51655-0078-30	3.26		EE
30s ea	51655-0078-24	4.05		EE
25 mg, 8s ea	51655-0079-80	15.00		EE
12s ea	51655-0079-27	2.90		EE
30s ea	51655-0079-24	70.69		EE
(Nucare Pharm)				
REPACK				
TAB, PO, 10 mg, 15s ea	66267-0112-15	10.23		
30s ea	66267-0112-30	18.99		
40s ea	66267-0112-40	30.87		AB
60s ea	66267-0112-60	40.93		
(FILM-COATED)				
25 mg, 20s ea	66267-0113-20	25.15		AB
30s ea	66267-0113-30	37.73		AB
(PD-Rx Pharm)				
REPACK				
TAB, PO, 10 mg, 10s ea	55289-0912-10	10.50		AB
30s ea	55289-0912-30	21.50		AB
60s ea	55289-0912-60	38.00		AB
(FILM-COATED)				
25 mg, 6s ea	43063-0095-06	9.42		AB
6s ea	55289-0139-06	9.42		AB
10s ea	55289-0139-10	10.68		AB
12s ea	55289-0139-12	11.31		AB
20s ea	55289-0139-20	13.85		AB
(REDI-SCRIPT,FILM-COATED)				
25 mg, 20s ea	58864-0045-20	20.00		AB
(FILM-COATED)				
25 mg, 30s ea	55289-0139-30	17.03		AB
30s ea	58864-0045-30	27.50		AB
40s ea	55289-0139-40	20.19		AB
(REDI-SCRIPT,FILM-COATED)				
25 mg, 42s ea	58864-0045-42	36.50		AB
60s ea	58864-0045-60	49.77		AB
50 mg, 12s ea	55289-0138-12	17.60		AB
20s ea	55289-0138-20	26.00		AB
30s ea	55289-0138-30	36.50		AB
(Pharma Pac)				
REPACK				
SYR, PO, 10 mg/5 ml,				
120 ml	52959-0582-03	7.90		EE
TAB, PO, 10 mg, 10s ea	52959-0481-10	12.32		AB
12s ea	52959-0481-12	14.77		AB
20s ea	52959-0481-20	24.38		AB
30s ea	52959-0481-30	36.60		AB
25 mg, 12s ea	52959-0074-12	18.68		EE
13s ea	52959-0074-13	20.22		EE
15s ea	52959-0074-15	22.49		EE
16s ea	52959-0074-16	23.96		EE
20s ea	52959-0074-20	27.08		EE
21s ea	52959-0074-21	28.35		EE
24s ea	52959-0074-24	32.15		EE
30s ea	52959-0074-30	49.90		EE
40s ea	52959-0074-40	51.90		EE
50s ea	52959-0074-50	64.87		EE
60s ea	52959-0074-60	77.82		EE
(Phys Total Care)				
REPACK				
SOL, IM (VIAL)				
25 mg/ml, 1 ml 25s (M.D.V.)	54868-0858-00	78.54		EE
50 mg/ml, 10 ml	54868-0231-00	8.33		EE
SYR, PO, 10 mg/5 ml,				
120 ml	54868-4336-00	62.84		EE
480 ml	54868-2032-00	117.23		EE
TAB, PO, 10 mg, 20s ea	54868-0229-01	20.79		EE
30s ea	54868-0229-02	28.95		EE
60s ea	54868-0229-04	53.40		EE
100s ea	54868-0229-03	65.34		EE
25 mg, 10s ea	54868-0063-09	12.78		EE
20s ea	54868-0063-02	22.59		EE
30s ea	54868-0063-03	32.37		EE
40s ea	54868-0063-07	42.15		EE
90s ea	54868-0063-00	70.38		EE
100s ea	54868-0063-05	76.35		EE
500s ea	54868-0063-01	325.89		EE
50 mg, 20s ea	54868-1804-02	56.55		EE
30s ea	54868-1804-04	40.08		EE
500s ea	54868-1804-00	595.86		EE
(Physician Partner)				
REPACK				
TAB, PO (FILM-COATED)				
10 mg, 30s ea	21695-0378-30	37.42		AB
25 mg, 15s ea	21695-0208-15	32.12		AB
20s ea	21695-0208-20	42.82		AB
(Quality Care Prod)				
REPACK				
TAB, PO, 10 mg, 60s ea	35356-0123-60	84.00		AB
25 mg, 12s ea	49999-0024-12	12.95		EE
20s ea	49999-0024-20	24.30		AB
(FILM-COATED)				
25 mg, 24s ea	49999-0024-24	25.89		AB
30s ea	49999-0024-30	32.36		EE
60s ea	49999-0024-60	64.72		EE
(FILM-COATED)				
25 mg, 90s ea	49999-0024-90	97.08		AB
100s ea	49999-0024-00	107.92		AB
50 mg, 24s ea	49999-0035-24	42.00		AB
30s ea	49999-0035-30	52.50		EE
60s ea	49999-0035-60	41.76		EE
(Southwood)				
REPACK				
SOL, IM, 50 mg/ml, 10 ml	58016-9299-01	4.75		EE
TAB, PO, 10 mg, 6s ea	58016-0405-06	3.79		EE
10s ea	58016-0405-10	6.31		EE
15s ea	58016-0405-15	9.47		EE
20s ea	58016-0405-20	12.62		EE
30s ea	58016-0405-30	18.93		EE
100s ea	58016-0405-00	63.10		EE
25 mg, 9s ea	58016-0406-09	8.09		EE
12s ea	58016-0406-12	16.90		EE
15s ea	58016-0406-15	13.49		EE
20s ea	58016-0406-20	17.98		EE
30s ea	58016-0406-30	26.97		EE
40s ea	58016-0406-40	35.96		EE
(FILM-COATED)				
25 mg, 60s ea	58016-0406-60	53.94		AB
100s ea	58016-0406-00	89.90		EE
50 mg, 20s ea	58016-0452-20	11.32		EE
30s ea	58016-0452-30	16.98		EE
100s ea	58016-0452-00	56.60		EE
(St. Mary's MPP)				
REPACK				
TAB, PO, 10 mg, 20s ea	60760-0307-20	19.95		AB
25 mg, 30s ea	60760-0971-30	34.07		EE
(Stat Rx)				
REPACK				
TAB, PO, 25 mg, 12s ea	16590-0122-12	14.10		AB
15s ea	16590-0122-15	17.68		AB
(Vibranta)				
REPACK				
TAB, PO (FILM-COATED)				
10 mg, 20s ea	57866-3875-04	8.11		AB
30s ea	57866-3875-01	9.54		AB
25 mg, 20s ea	57866-3874-04	16.00		
30s ea	57866-3874-01	26.16		
60s ea	57866-3874-03	51.50		
90s ea	57866-3874-06	78.34		
50 mg, 30s ea	57866-3876-02	34.90		
60s ea	57866-3876-03	69.89		
90s ea	57866-3876-04	104.70		
HYDROXYZINE HYDROCHLORIDE				
FUL				
TAB, PO, 10 mg, 100s ea		48.65		
25 mg, 100s ea		71.34		
(Amer Regent) *See HYDROXYZINE HCL*				
(Clint) *See RESTALL*				
(Consolidated Midland) *See HYDROXYZINE HCL*				
(Glenmark Pharmaceuticals)				
TAB, PO (USP,FILM-COATED)				
10 mg, 100s ea	68462-0360-01	65.00		AB
500s ea	68462-0360-05	289.99		AB
25 mg, 100s ea	68462-0361-01	91.97		AB
500s ea	68462-0361-05	425.29		AB
50 mg, 100s ea	68462-0362-01	112.12		AB
500s ea	68462-0362-05	532.50		AB
(Harris)				
TAB, PO (USP,FILM COATED)				
10 mg, 100s ea	67405-0575-10	26.64		AB
500s ea	67405-0575-50	133.20		AB
1000s ea	67405-0575-96	241.02		AB
25 mg, 100s ea	67405-0671-10	37.92		AB
500s ea	67405-0671-50	189.60		AB
1000s ea	67405-0671-96	379.20		AB
50 mg, 100s ea	67405-0577-10	45.70		AB
500s ea	67405-0577-50	228.48		AB
(Hawkins) *See HYDROXYZINE HCL*				
(Heritage)				
TAB, PO (USP,FILM-COATED)				
10 mg, 100s ea	23155-0105-01	62.36		AB
500s ea	23155-0105-05	290.99		AB
25 mg, 100s ea	23155-0106-01	91.46		AB
(FILM-COATED)				
25 mg, 500s ea	23155-0106-05	425.29		AB
50 mg, 100s ea	23155-0107-01	111.50		AB
500s ea	23155-0107-05	518.47		AB
(Hi-Tech) *See HYDROXYZINE HCL*				
(KVK)				
SYR, PO (1X473ML,USP)				
10 mg/5 ml, 473 ml	10702-0052-16	40.20		AA
TAB, PO (USP,FILM-COATED)				
10 mg, 100s ea	10702-0010-01	63.40		AB
500s ea	10702-0010-50	290.99		AB
1000s ea	10702-0010-10	578.10		AB
25 mg, 100s ea	10702-0011-01	91.97		AB
500s ea	10702-0011-50	427.10		AB
1000s ea	10702-0011-10	845.26		AB
50 mg, 100s ea	10702-0012-01	111.50		AB
500s ea	10702-0012-50	513.47		AB
1000s ea	10702-0012-10	1025.10		AB
(Major)				
TAB, PO (USP,FILM-COATED)				
10 mg, 100s ea	00904-0357-60	56.79		AB
500s ea	00904-0357-40	291.08		AB
25 mg, 100s ea	00904-0358-60	86.40		AB
500s ea	00904-0358-40	426.97		AB
50 mg, 100s ea	00904-0359-60	112.05		AB
500s ea	00904-0359-40	479.25		AB
(Medisca) *See HYDROXYZINE HCL*				
(Morton Grove) *See HYDROXYZINE HCL*				
(Northstar)				
TAB, PO (USP)				
10 mg, 100s ea	16714-0081-04	62.36		AB
500s ea	16714-0081-05	289.99		AB
25 mg, 100s ea	16714-0082-04	91.71		AB
500s ea	16714-0082-05	425.29		AB
1000s ea	16714-0082-06	823.14		AB
50 mg, 100s ea	16714-0083-04	112.10		AB
500s ea	16714-0083-05	532.50		AB
(PCCA) *See HYDROXYZINE HCL*				
(Spectrum Pharmacy) *See HYDROXYZINE HCL*				

PROD/MFR	NDC	AWP	DP	OBC
(Teva) *See HYDROXYZINE HCL*				
(Truxton) *See VISTACOT*				
(UDL)				
TAB, PO (10X10,USP,FILM COATED)				
10 mg, 100s ea UD	**51079-0413-20**	62.36		AB
(Watson Labs)				
TAB, PO (FILM-COATED)				
10 mg, 100s ea	**00591-5522-01**	26.64		AB
500s ea	**00591-5522-05**	126.54		AB
25 mg, 100s ea	**00591-5523-01**	37.92		AB
500s ea	**00591-5523-05**	183.91		AB
1000s ea	**00591-5523-10**	360.24		AB
(USP,FILM-COATED)				
50 mg, 100s ea	**00591-3423-01**	45.70		AB
500s ea	**00591-3423-05**	221.63		AB
1000s ea	**00591-3423-10**	434.11		AB
(American Health) REPACK				
TAB, PO (10X10,USP,FILM-COATED)				
10 mg, 100s ea	**68084-0253-01**	27.74		AB
25 mg, 100s ea	**68084-0254-01**	39.49		AB
50 mg, 100s ea	**68084-0255-01**	47.49		AB
(Core) REPACK				
SYR, PO, 10 mg/5 ml,				
120 ml	**33358-0180-01**	8.66		
TAB, PO, 10 mg, 30s ea	**33358-0179-30**	24.16		
25 mg, 20s ea	**33358-0181-20**	22.54		
30s ea	**33358-0181-30**	31.76		
(IPI) REPACK				
TAB, PO, 25 mg, 30s ea	**18837-0070-30**	34.30		
(Palmetto) REPACK				
TAB, PO, 10 mg, 15s ea	**23490-5727-01**	13.50		
20s ea	**23490-5727-02**	18.00		
25 mg, 6s ea	**23490-5729-01**	11.34		
15s ea	**23490-5729-02**	20.25		
20s ea	**23490-5729-03**	27.00		
25s ea	**23490-5729-05**	33.75		
30s ea	**23490-5729-04**	40.50		
60s ea	**23490-5729-06**	81.00		
50 mg, 17s ea	**23490-5731-00**	29.46		
30s ea	**23490-5731-01**	51.99		
(Physician Partner) REPACK				
TAB, PO, 25 mg, 30s ea	**21695-0208-30**	54.60		
60s ea	**21695-0208-60**	109.20		
90s ea	**21695-0208-90**	163.80		
50 mg, 60s ea	**21695-0356-60**	133.80		
(Stat Rx) REPACK				
TAB, PO (FILM-COATED)				
10 mg, 30s ea	**16590-0646-30**	21.00		AB
40s ea	**16590-0646-40**	28.00		AB
60s ea	**16590-0646-60**	38.00		AB
90s ea	**16590-0646-90**	55.00		AB
25 mg, 20s ea	**16590-0122-20**	65.75		
30s ea	**16590-0122-30**	98.70		
40s ea	**16590-0122-40**	131.50		
60s ea	**16590-0122-60**	197.26		
90s ea	**16590-0122-90**	280.00		
(FILM-COATED)				
50 mg, 120s ea	**16590-0680-72**	141.93		AB
HYDROXYZINE PAM (Core) REPACK				
hydroxyzine pamoate				
CAP, PO, 25 mg, 20s ea	**33358-0182-20**	62.94		
30s ea	**33358-0182-30**	73.90		
HYDROXYZINE PAMOATE FUL				
CAP, PO, 25 mg, 100s ea		11.50		
50 mg, 100s ea		15.72		
(Consolidated Midland)				
CAP, PO, 25 mg, 100s ea	**00223-1049-01**	7.95		EE
1000s ea	**00223-1049-02**	67.50		EE
50 mg, 100s ea	**00223-1050-01**	11.25		EE
1000s ea	**00223-1050-02**	97.50		EE
100 mg, 100s ea	**00223-1051-01**	18.95		EE
1000s ea	**00223-1051-02**	167.50		EE
(Gallipot)				
POW, NA (U.S.P.)				
25 gm	**51552-0979-04**	35.70	25.50	
(Medisca)				
POW, NA (U.S.P.)				
25 gm	**38779-0228-04**	103.50		
100 gm	**38779-0228-05**	327.00		

PROD/MFR	NDC	AWP	DP	OBC
(Monument Pharmaceuti)				
SUS, PO (BANANA)				
25 mg/5 ml, 120 ml	**62927-0621-04**	28.00	20.00	
480 ml	**62927-0621-16**	100.00	75.00	
(PCCA)				
POW, NA (U.S.P.)				
1 gm	**51927-2316-00**	4.56		
(Pfizer) *See VISTARIL*				
(Sandoz)				
CAP, PO, 25 mg, 100s ea	**00185-0613-01**	29.94		AB
500s ea	**00185-0613-05**	145.20		AB
50 mg, 100s ea	**00185-0615-01**	32.19		AB
500s ea	**00185-0615-05**	156.12		AB
(Spectrum Pharmacy)				
POW, NA (U.S.P./N.F.)				
25 gm	**49452-3659-01**	176.40		
100 gm	**49452-3659-02**	630.00		
(Teva)				
CAP, PO, 25 mg, 100s ea	**00555-0323-02**	29.94		AB
500s ea	**00555-0323-04**	145.20		AB
50 mg, 100s ea	**00555-0302-02**	32.19		AB
500s ea	**00555-0302-04**	156.12		AB
100 mg, 100s ea	**00555-0324-02**	62.69		AB
(UDL)				
CAP, PO (10X10)				
25 mg, 100s ea UD	**51079-0077-20**	29.94		AB
50 mg, 100s ea UD	**51079-0078-20**	32.19		AB
(Watson)				
CAP, PO, 50 mg, 100s ea	**00591-0801-01**	12.58	8.25	AB
500s ea	**00591-0801-05**	61.00	38.50	AB
(Watson Labs)				
CAP, PO (USP)				
25 mg, 100s ea	**00591-0800-01**	9.20		AB
500s ea	**00591-0800-05**	44.64		AB
(4u) REPACK				
CAP, PO, 25 mg, 30s ea	**10544-0328-30**	48.22		
30s ea	**42549-0528-30**	48.22		AB
(A-S Medication) REPACK				
CAP, PO, 25 mg, 30s ea	**54569-2353-05**	7.34		EE
50 mg, 20s ea	**54569-2571-01**	5.25		EE
(Altura) REPACK				
CAP, PO, 25 mg, 5s ea	**63874-0442-05**	5.24		AB
9s ea	**63874-0442-09**	9.43		AB
10s ea	**63874-0442-10**	10.48		AB
14s ea	**63874-0442-14**	14.68		AB
15s ea	**63874-0442-15**	15.72		AB
20s ea	**63874-0442-20**	20.97		AB
25s ea	**63874-0442-25**	26.21		AB
28s ea	**63874-0442-28**	29.35		AB
30s ea	**63874-0442-30**	31.45		AB
40s ea	**63874-0442-40**	41.93		AB
45s ea	**63874-0442-45**	47.17		AB
60s ea	**63874-0442-60**	62.90		AB
90s ea	**63874-0442-90**	94.35		AB
100s ea	**63874-0442-01**	104.83		AB
120s ea	**63874-0442-04**	125.80		AB
500s ea	**63874-0442-03**	524.16		AB
1000s ea	**63874-0442-02**	1048.30		AB
50 mg, 10s ea	**63874-0757-10**	28.63		
15s ea	**63874-0757-15**	42.95		
20s ea	**63874-0757-20**	57.27		
21s ea	**63874-0757-21**	60.13		
24s ea	**63874-0757-24**	68.71		
28s ea	**63874-0757-28**	80.17		
30s ea	**63874-0757-30**	85.90		
60s ea	**63874-0757-60**	171.80		
90s ea	**63874-0757-90**	257.70		
100s ea	**63874-0757-01**	286.33		
120s ea	**63874-0757-04**	343.60		
(DHS, Inc.) REPACK				
CAP, PO, 25 mg, 30s ea	**55887-0422-30**	30.87		AB
60s ea	**55887-0422-60**	61.74		
(Dispensing Solutions) REPACK				
CAP, PO, 25 mg, 9s ea	**55045-2195-04**	6.30		AB
15s ea	**55045-2195-05**	10.50		AB
20s ea	**55045-2195-07**	14.00		AB
20s ea	**66336-0208-20**	9.00		
30s ea	**55045-2195-08**	21.00		AB
30s ea	**55045-3933-01**	21.00		AB
30s ea	**66336-0208-30**	12.78		
60s ea	**55045-2195-06**	42.00		AB
90s ea	**55045-2195-09**	63.00		AB
120s ea	**55045-2195-02**	84.00		AB

PROD/MFR	NDC	AWP	DP	OBC
50 mg, 20s ea	**55045-1661-02**	28.00		AB
30s ea	**55045-1661-08**	42.00		AB
40s ea	**55045-1661-03**	56.00		AB
60s ea	**55045-1661-06**	84.00		AB
60s ea	**66336-0797-60**	83.95		AB
90s ea	**55045-1661-09**	126.00		AB
100s ea	**55045-1661-00**	140.00		AB
120s ea	**55045-1661-01**	168.00		AB
(HomeMed) REPACK				
CAP, PO, 25 mg, 20s ea	**51655-0533-52**	20.97		
(IPI) REPACK				
CAP, PO, 25 mg, 30s ea	**18837-0355-30**	24.50		AB
(Keltman Pharma., Inc.) REPACK				
CAP, PO, 50 mg, 30s ea	**68387-0468-30**	44.25		
100 mg, 30s ea	**68387-0469-30**	67.30		
(Nucare Pharm) REPACK				
CAP, PO, 25 mg, 30s ea	**66267-0114-30**	26.95		AB
(Palmetto) REPACK				
CAP, PO, 25 mg, 20s ea	**23490-5733-01**	21.00		
30s ea	**23490-5733-02**	31.50		
(PD-Rx Pharm) REPACK				
CAP, PO, 25 mg, 4s ea	**43063-0172-04**	6.36		AB
10s ea	**55289-0226-10**	5.93		AB
15s ea	**55289-0226-15**	6.60		AB
(USP)				
25 mg, 100s ea	**43063-0172-01**	23.22		AB
50 mg, 10s ea	**55289-0354-10**	6.00		AB
(Pharma Pac) REPACK				
CAP, PO, 25 mg, 10s ea	**52959-0433-10**	3.75		EE
15s ea	**52959-0433-15**	5.55		EE
20s ea	**52959-0433-20**	7.10		EE
30s ea	**52959-0433-30**	10.65		EE
40s ea	**52959-0433-40**	13.75		EE
60s ea	**52959-0433-60**	20.61		EE
50 mg, 6s ea	**52959-0833-06**	8.40		
20s ea	**52959-0833-20**	27.99		
(Phys Total Care) REPACK				
CAP, PO, 25 mg, 15s ea	**54868-2892-04**	6.80		EE
20s ea	**54868-2892-05**	9.57		AB
30s ea	**54868-2892-03**	10.60		AB
100s ea	**54868-2892-00**	26.85		EE
500s ea	**54868-2892-02**	130.27		EE
50 mg, 30s ea	**54868-1854-01**	10.89		EE
60s ea	**54868-1854-03**	18.78		EE
100s ea	**54868-1854-00**	27.81		EE
500s ea	**54868-1854-04**	134.55		EE
100 mg, 100s ea	**54868-4109-00**	60.48		EE
(Physician Partner) REPACK				
CAP, PO, 25 mg, 20s ea	**21695-0573-20**	14.69		AB
30s ea	**21695-0573-30**	22.04		AB
40s ea	**21695-0573-40**	34.57		AB
(Quality Care Prod) REPACK				
CAP, PO, 25 mg, 30s ea	**49999-0701-30**	45.60		AB
100 mg, 12s ea	**49999-0036-12**	7.92		AB
60s ea	**49999-0036-60**	39.60		EE
(Southwood) REPACK				
CAP, PO, 25 mg, 10s ea	**58016-0259-10**	10.50		EE
20s ea	**58016-0259-20**	21.00		EE
30s ea	**58016-0259-30**	31.50		EE
50s ea	**58016-0259-50**	52.50		EE
60s ea	**58016-0259-60**	63.00		EE
90s ea	**58016-0259-90**	94.50		EE
100s ea	**58016-0259-00**	105.00		EE
120s ea	**58016-0259-02**	126.00		EE
50 mg, 10s ea	**58016-0464-10**	28.63		EE
15s ea	**58016-0464-15**	42.95		EE
20s ea	**58016-0464-20**	57.27		EE
30s ea	**58016-0464-30**	85.90		EE
(Stat Rx) REPACK				
CAP, PO, 25 mg, 9s ea	**16590-0357-09**	8.05		
12s ea	**16590-0357-12**	10.75		
20s ea	**16590-0357-20**	17.85		
30s ea	**16590-0357-30**	26.75		
120s ea	**16590-0357-72**	98.75		AB
50 mg, 30s ea	**16590-0737-30**	33.75		AB
120s ea	**16590-0737-72**	123.60		AB

PROD/MFR NDC AWP DP OBC

(Vibranta)
REPACK
CAP, PO, 25 mg, 30s ea ... **57866-3893-01** 26.16
60s ea **57866-3893-02** 32.10
90s ea **57866-3893-03** 38.90
50 mg, 30s ea **57866-3894-01** 28.32
60s ea **57866-3894-02** 37.45
90s ea **57866-3894-03** 42.10

HYFLEX-DS (Breckenridge Pharm)
acetaminophen/phenyltoloxamine citrate
TAB, PO, 500 mg-50 mg,
100s ea **51991-0056-01** 47.00

(Southwood)
REPACK
TAB, PO, 500 mg-50 mg,
30s ea **58016-0057-30** 14.10
60s ea **58016-0057-60** 28.20
90s ea **58016-0057-90** 42.30
100s ea **58016-0057-00** 47.00

HYGEL (Aletheia)
hyaluronate sodium
GEL, TP (1X340GM)
0.2%, 340 gm **43234-0105-12** 101.12

HYLAN POLYMERS A AND B
(Genzyme) *See SYNVISC*
(Genzyme) *See SYNVISC ONE*

HYLATOPIC EMOLLIENT FOAM (Onset)
foam, multi ingredient
FOA, TP, 100 gm **16781-0189-96** 118.20 98.50

HYLENEX (Baxter)
hyaluronidase human, recombinant
SOL, IJ (PF)
150 u/ml, 1 ml **60977-0319-44** 108.00
(4X1ML VIALS,PF)
150 u/ml, 1 ml 4s **60977-0319-03** 432.00

HYLIRA (Hawthorn Pharm)
hyaluronate sodium
GEL, TP (1X340GM)
0.2%, 340 gm **63717-0034-12** 124.99
LOT, TP (HYPOALLERGENIC)
1000 gm **63717-0036-10** 156.25
0.1%, 340 gm **63717-0036-12** 87.49

(Phys Total Care)
REPACK
GEL, TP (1X340GM)
0.2%, 340 gm **54868-5892-00** 129.14

HYMENOPTERA VENOM DIAGNOSTIC KIT (Alk-Abello)
hymenoptera venom, mixed
PDS, IJ (5X1ML)
0.1 mg/ml, ea **52709-1401-01** 172.80 133.10

HYMENOPTERA VENOM, MIXED
(Alk-Abello) *See HYMENOPTERA VENOM DIAGNOSTIC KIT*

HYOMAX (Aristos)
hyoscyamine sulfate
TAB, PO, 0.125 mg,
100s ea **24486-0605-10** 91.65

HYOMAX-DT (Aristos)
hyoscyamine sulfate
TER, PO (BILAYERED)
0.375 mg, 90s ea **24486-0604-90** 153.53

HYOMAX-FT (Aristos)
hyoscyamine sulfate
CTB, PO (DISINTEGRATING)
0.125 mg, 100s ea **24486-0603-10** 84.41

HYOMAX-SL (Aristos)
hyoscyamine sulfate
TAB, SL (PEPPERMINT)
0.125 mg, 100s ea **24486-0601-10** 85.95

HYOMAX-SR (Aristos)
hyoscyamine sulfate
TER, PO, 0.375 mg,
100s ea **24486-0602-10** 161.48

HYOSCYAMINE (Breckenridge Pharm)
hyoscyamine sulfate
TAB, SL (USP)
0.125 mg, 100s ea **51991-0656-01** 91.14

(Seton)
TER, PO, 0.375 mg,
100s ea **13925-0108-01** 160.50

(Core)
REPACK
TAB, PO, 0.125 mg,
30s ea **33358-0183-30** 14.84

(HomeMed)
REPACK
TAB, PO, 0.125 mg,
20s ea **51655-0371-52** 6.95

(Phys Total Care)
REPACK
LIQ, PO (DROP)
0.125 mg/ml, 15 ml ... **54868-5661-00** 17.49

HYOSCYAMINE SULFATE
(A. G. Marin) *See COLIDROPS PEDIATRIC*
(Alaven) *See LEVBID*
(Alaven) *See LEVSIN*
(Alaven) *See LEVSIN/SL*
(Alaven) *See LEVSINEX*
(Alaven) *See NULEV*
(Aristos) *See HYOMAX*
(Aristos) *See HYOMAX-DT*
(Aristos) *See HYOMAX-FT*
(Aristos) *See HYOMAX-SL*
(Aristos) *See HYOMAX-SR*
(Ascher) *See ANASPAZ*
(Breckenridge Pharm) *See HYOSCYAMINE*

(Breckenridge Pharm)
TAB, PO, 0.125 mg, 100s ea. **51991-0325-01** 91.14

(Capellon) *See SYMAX DUOTAB*
(Capellon) *See SYMAX FASTABS*
(Capellon) *See SYMAX-SL*
(Capellon) *See SYMAX-SR*

(Contract Pharmacal)
TAB, SL (SPEARMINT)
0.125 mg, 100s ea **10267-2734-01** 12.95

(County Line)
ODT, PO (MINT)
0.125 mg, 100s ea **43199-0012-01** 113.57
TAB, PO, 0.125 mg, 100s ea. **43199-0013-01** 101.42
SL (MINT)
0.125 mg, 100s ea **43199-0011-01** 109.64
TER, PO, 0.375 mg, 100s ea. **43199-0014-01** 160.00

(Cypress Pharm)
ELI, PO (ORANGE)
0.125 mg/5 ml,
473 ml **60258-0801-16** 107.99
LIQ, PO (ORANGE,DROPS)
0.125 mg/ml, 15 ml ... **60258-0802-15** 41.99

(Gallipot)
POW, NA (U.S.P.,N.F.)
5 gm **51552-0141-02** 27.44
25 gm **51552-0141-04** 123.20

(Kremers Urban)
TER, PO, 0.375 mg, 100s ea. **62175-0108-01** 69.15

(Paddock)
ODT, PO (MINT)
0.125 mg, 100s ea **00574-0247-01** 85.00
TAB, PO, 0.125 mg, 100s ea. **00574-0246-01** 85.00
SL, 0.125 mg, 100s ea .. **00574-0250-01** 85.00
TER, PO, 0.375 mg, 100s ea. **00574-0251-01** 160.00

(PCCA)
POW, NA (U.S.P.)
1 gm **51927-1831-00** 63.00

(Prasco Labs)
TAB, PO, 0.15 mg, 100s ea. **66993-0402-02** 38.82

(Seton) *See HYOSCYAMINE*
(Silarx) *See HYOSYNE*

(Spectrum Pharmacy)
POW, NA (U.S.P.)
5 gm **49452-3656-01** 208.25
25 gm **49452-3656-02** 770.00

(Teva)
CER, PO, 0.375 mg,
100s ea **00182-1993-01** 53.20

(Vintage)
LIQ, PO (DRPS,ORANGE)
0.125 mg/ml, 15 ml ... **00254-9216-43** 14.60

(Vision)
ODT, PO (MINT)
0.125 mg, 100s ea **68013-0005-01** 113.62
TAB, SL, 0.125 mg,
100s ea **68013-0018-01** 109.69

(A-S Medication)
REPACK
TAB, PO, 0.125 mg, 20s ea. **54569-3763-02** 6.95

(DHS, Inc.)
REPACK
TAB, PO, 0.125 mg, 10s ea. **55887-0483-10** 7.28
21s ea **55887-0483-21** 15.29
30s ea **55887-0483-30** 22.30

(Dispensing Solutions)
REPACK
TAB, SL, 0.125 mg, 100s ea. **55045-2675-00** 84.00

(Palmetto)
REPACK
LIQ, PO, 0.125 mg/ml,
15 ml **23490-5740-01** 19.93

(PD-Rx Pharm)
REPACK
TAB, PO, 0.125 mg, 20s ea. **55289-0956-20** 7.68

(Pharma Pac)
REPACK
TAB, PO, 0.125 mg, 2s ea .. **52959-0175-02** 2.00
30s ea **52959-0175-30** 24.00

(Phys Total Care)
REPACK
CER, PO, 0.375 mg, 20s ea. **54868-3215-01** 10.14
30s ea **54868-3215-03** 12.96
60s ea **54868-3215-02** 21.45
ODT, PO (DYE-FREE,MINT)
0.125 mg, 50s ea **54868-3116-00** 9.09
TAB, PO, 0.125 mg, 10s ea. **54868-2209-04** 5.34
20s ea **54868-2209-02** 46.90
30s ea **54868-2209-06** 68.10
40s ea **54868-2209-00** 89.29
50s ea **54868-2209-07** 85.55
60s ea **54868-2209-05** 101.76
100s ea **54868-2209-03** 165.11
TER, PO, 0.375 mg, 10s ea. **54868-5277-01** 41.50
(CAPLET)
0.375 mg, 30s ea **54868-5277-00** 80.05
60s ea **54868-5277-02** 168.89

(Physician Partner)
REPACK
TAB, PO, 0.125 mg, 10s ea . **21695-0442-10** 21.44

(Southwood)
REPACK
CER, PO, 0.375 mg, 30s ea . **58016-0032-30** 16.19
60s ea **58016-0032-60** 32.37
90s ea **58016-0032-90** 48.56
100s ea **58016-0032-00** 53.95

(Stat Rx)
REPACK
TAB, PO, 0.125 mg, 20s ea. **16590-0297-20** 20.77
30s ea **16590-0297-30** 30.06

(Vibranta)
REPACK
TAB, PO, 0.15 mg, 30s ea .. **57866-9028-01** 18.04

HYOSCYAMINE SULFATE/ PHENYLTOLOXAMINE CITRATE
(Pronova) *See DIGEX NF*

HYOSYNE (Silarx)
hyoscyamine sulfate
ELI, PO, 0.125 mg/5 ml,
473 ml **54838-0511-80** 105.49
LIQ, PO (DROPS,DROPS)
0.125 mg/ml, 15 ml ... **54838-0506-15** 39.99

(Phys Total Care)
REPACK
LIQ, PO (1X15ML,DROPS,DROPS)
0.125 mg/ml, 15 ml ... **54868-5959-00** 69.85

HYPAQUE SODIUM (GE)
diatrizoate sodium
PDR, PO (CAN)
100%, 250 gm **00407-0769-01** 171.01

HYPER-SAL (Pari)
sodium chloride
SOL, IH (4MLX60,PF)
7%, 4 ml 60s **83490-0107-60** 73.50

HYPERCARE (Stratus)
aluminum chloride
SOL, TP (DAB-O-MATIC APPLICATOR)
20%, 35 ml **58980-0150-11** 5.95
37.5 ml **58980-0150-10** 5.55
(DAB-O-MATIC APPLICATOR)
20%, 60 ml **58980-0150-20** 8.05

PROD/MFR	NDC	AWP	DP	OBC
(Phys Total Care)				
REPACK				
SOL, TP, 20%, 60 ml	54868-0123-01	34.78		
HYPERHEP B S/D (Talecris)				
hepatitis b immune globulin				
SOL, IM (NEONATAL SINGLE DOSE,PF)				
0.5 ml	13533-0636-03	87.52		
(PF)				
1 ml	13533-0636-01	165.04		
(SINGLE DOSE,PF)				
1 ml	13533-0636-02	165.04		
(SDV,PF)				
5 ml	13533-0636-05	791.82		
HYPERLITE (B. Braun)				
electrolytes/multimineral				
SOL, IV (VIAL,PF)				
250 ml	00264-1943-20	25.00		
HYPERRAB S/D (Talecris)				
rabies immune globulin				
SOL, IM (1X2ML,PF,LATEX-FREE)				
150 iu/ml, 2 ml	13533-0618-03	199.58		
(PF,LATEX-FREE)				
150 iu/ml, 2 ml	13533-0618-02	448.13		
10 ml	13533-0618-10	2045.39		
HYPERRHO S/D (Talecris)				
rho(d) immune globulin				
SOL, IM (MINI-,SINGLE DOSE SYR)				
0.17 ml 10s	13533-0631-06	392.45		
(FULL DOSE,PF)				
1 ml	13533-0631-02	110.27		
(A-S Medication)				
REPACK				
SOL, IM (FULL DOSE)				
1 ml	54569-5764-00	114.51		
HYPERSTAT (Schering)				
diazoxide				
SOL, IV (AMP)				
15 mg/ml, 20 ml	00085-0201-05	129.42		
HYPERTENSA (Physician Thera, LLC)				
amino acids and nutriceuticals				
CAP, PO, 60s ea	68405-1007-02	188.80		
(PF,SF,STARCH-FREE)				
90s ea	68405-1007-03	226.56		
(Altura)				
REPACK				
CAP, PO, 60s ea	63874-1180-06	99.98		
(Dispensing Solutions)				
REPACK				
CAP, PO, 60s ea	55045-3400-06	147.40		
HYPERTET S/D (Talecris)				
tetanus immune globulin				
SOL, IM (PF)				
250 u, 1 ml	13533-0634-02	324.23		
HYPOPHOSPHOROUS ACID				
(Baker, J.T.) *See HYPOPHOSPHORUS ACID 50%*				
(PCCA)				
LIQ, NA (30-32%(W/V) SOLUTION)				
1 ml	51927-2272-00	1.00		
HYPOPHOSPHORUS ACID 50% (Baker, J.T.)				
hypophosphorous acid				
LIQ, NA (PURIFIED)				
500 ml	10106-0178-01	102.49		
HYPROMELLOSE				
(Alcon Surgical) *See CELLUGEL OVD*				
(Medisca)				
POW, NA (METHOCEL E4M,USP)				
100 gm	38779-0483-05	37.50		
(METHOCEL K4M(4000MPA.S))				
100 gm	38779-2262-05	34.50		
(USP(100000MPA.S))				
100 gm	38779-2237-05	34.50		
(USP(100MPA.S),1X100GM)				
100 gm	38779-1985-05	31.50		
(METHOCEL E4M,USP)				
500 gm	38779-0483-08	97.50		
(METHOCEL K4M(4000MPA.S))				
500 gm	38779-2262-08	97.50		
(USP(100000MPA.S))				
500 gm	38779-2237-08	117.00		
(USP(100MPA.S),1X500GM)				
500 gm	38779-1985-08	99.00		
(METHOCEL E4M,USP)				
1000 gm	38779-0483-09	166.50		
(METHOCEL K4M(4000MPA.S))				
1000 gm	38779-2262-09	166.50		
(USP(100000MPA.S))				
1000 gm	38779-2237-09	184.50		
(METHOCEL E4M)				
2500 gm	38779-0483-01	315.00		
(USP(100000MPA.S))				
2500 gm	38779-2237-01	382.50		
(USP(100MPA.S))				
2500 gm	38779-1985-01	328.50		
(METHOCEL E4M,USP)				
12000 gm	38779-0483-07	1300.50		
(PCCA) *See METHOCEL << E4M*				
(PCCA) *See METHOCEL K100M*				
(Spectrum Pharmacy) *See HYDROXYPROPYL METHYLCELLULOSE 2208*				
(Spectrum Pharmacy)				
POW, NA (U.S.P.)				
125 gm	49452-3663-01	62.65		
500 gm	49452-3663-02	160.65		
2500 gm	49452-3663-03	486.50		
HYSKON (Cooper Surgical)				
dextran 70/dextrose				
SOL, VG, 32%-10%, 100 ml	61563-0231-61	32.88		
HYTONE (Phys Total Care)				
REPACK				
hydrocortisone				
CRE, TP, 2.5%, 30 gm	54868-2234-00	46.84		AT
HYTRIN (Phys Total Care)				
terazosin hydrochloride				
CAP, PO, 2 mg, 30s ea	54868-3842-00	76.39		AB
5 mg, 10s ea	54868-3662-03	31.33		AB
30s ea	54868-3662-00	89.61		AB
60s ea	54868-3662-02	168.79		AB
10 mg, 10s ea	54868-4228-01	31.33		AB
30s ea	54868-4228-00	90.24		AB
60s ea	54868-4228-02	154.16		AB
HYZAAR (Merck)				
hydrochlorothiazide/losartan potassium				
TAB, PO (UNIT OF USE,FILM-COATED)				
12.5 mg-50 mg,				
30s ea	00006-0717-31	79.50		
90s ea	00006-0717-54	238.49		
(FILM-COATED)				
12.5 mg-50 mg,				
100s ea UD	00006-0717-28	265.00		
(BULK PACKAGE)				
12.5 mg-50 mg,				
1000s ea	00006-0717-82	2649.91		
5000s ea	00006-0717-86	13249.56		
12.5 mg-100 mg,				
30s ea UD	00006-0745-31	108.29		
90s ea	00006-0745-54	324.86		
100s ea UD	00006-0745-28	360.96		
(BULK PACKAGE)				
12.5 mg-100 mg,				
1000s ea	00006-0745-82	3609.55		
5000s ea	00006-0745-86	18047.76		
(UNIT OF USE,FILM-COATED)				
25 mg-100 mg,				
30s ea	00006-0747-31	108.29		
90s ea	00006-0747-54	324.86		
(FILM-COATED)				
25 mg-100 mg,				
100s ea UD	00006-0747-28	360.96		
1000s ea	00006-0747-82	3609.55		
(BULK PACKAGE)				
25 mg-100 mg,				
4000s ea	00006-0747-81	14438.22		
(A-S Medication)				
REPACK				
TAB, PO (FILM-COATED)				
12.5 mg-50 mg,				
30s ea	54569-4722-01	103.35		
12.5 mg-100 mg,				
30s ea	54569-5999-00	140.78		
(FILM-COATED)				
25 mg-100 mg,				
30s ea	54569-5880-01	140.78		
(AQ)				
REPACK				
TAB, PO (FILM-COATED)				
12.5 mg-50 mg,				
30s ea	66105-0669-03	126.48		
25 mg-100 mg,				
30s ea	66105-0663-03	142.96		
(Bryant Ranch)				
REPACK				
TAB, PO, 12.5 mg-50 mg,				
30s ea	63629-3183-01	61.46		
(Nucare Pharm)				
REPACK				
TAB, PO (FILM-COATED)				
12.5 mg-50 mg,				
60s ea	68071-0787-60	194.00		
(PD-Rx Pharm)				
REPACK				
TAB, PO (FILM-COATED)				
25 mg-100 mg,				
30s ea	55289-0522-30	160.94		
(REDI-SCRIPT,FILM-COATED)				
25 mg-100 mg,				
30s ea	58864-0659-30	152.01		
(Phys Total Care)				
REPACK				
TAB, PO, 12.5 mg-50 mg,				
30s ea	54868-3866-00	91.65		
(FILM-COATED)				
12.5 mg-50 mg,				
90s ea	54868-3866-01	255.42		
12.5 mg-100 mg,				
30s ea	54868-5705-00	123.49		
25 mg-100 mg,				
30s ea	54868-4341-00	144.34		
(FILM-COATED)				
25 mg-100 mg,				
90s ea	54868-4341-01	405.36		
(Quality Care Prod)				
REPACK				
TAB, PO (FILM-COATED)				
12.5 mg-50 mg,				
30s ea	35356-0416-30	133.14		
I-PORT (Patton)				
cannula, injection				
DEV, NA (6MM)				
10s ea	85190-0101-10	174.60		
(9MM)				
10s ea	85190-0102-10	174.60		
IBANDRONATE SODIUM				
(Roche Labs) *See BONIVA*				
IBRITUMOMAB TIUXETAN/SODIUM ACETATE				
(Spectrum) *See ZEVALIN IN-111*				
(Spectrum) *See ZEVALIN Y-90*				
IBU (Ascend)				
ibuprofen				
TAB, PO (USP)				
400 mg, 100s ea	67877-0119-01	20.65		AB
500s ea	67877-0119-05	85.50		AB
25000s ea	67877-0119-95	3850.00		AB
(USP,CAPLET)				
600 mg, 100s ea	67877-0120-01	29.50		AB
500s ea	67877-0120-05	121.10		AB
(CAPLET)				
600 mg, 15000s ea	67877-0120-93	3269.70		AB
(USP,CAPLET)				
800 mg, 100s ea	67877-0121-01	38.45		AB
500s ea	67877-0121-05	152.94		AB
(CAPLET)				
800 mg, 12000s ea	67877-0121-91	3303.55		AB
(Dr Reddy's)				
TAB, PO, 400 mg, 100s ea	55111-0682-01	20.50		AB
500s ea	55111-0682-05	84.86		AB
(CAPLET)				
600 mg, 100s ea	55111-0683-01	29.04		AB
500s ea	55111-0683-05	120.15		AB
800 mg, 100s ea	55111-0684-01	38.10		AB
500s ea	55111-0684-05	152.38		AB
(McKesson Packaging)				
REPACK				
TAB, PO, 400 mg,				
100s ea UD	63739-0442-10	22.10		AB
750s ea UD	63739-0442-01	159.11		AB
(CAPLET)				
600 mg, 100s ea UD	63739-0443-10	30.04		AB
750s ea UD	63739-0443-01	225.28		AB
800 mg, 100s ea UD	63739-0444-10	38.10		AB
750s ea UD	63739-0444-01	285.71		AB
750s ea	63739-0444-03	285.71		AB
(PD-Rx Pharm)				
REPACK				
TAB, PO (CAPLET)				
800 mg, 4s ea	43063-0013-04	21.84		AB
6s ea	43063-0013-06	22.14		AB
IBU-4 (Truxton)				
ibuprofen				
TAB, PO, 400 mg, 500s ea	00463-6311-05	35.40		EE

PROD/MFR	NDC	AWP	DP	OBC
IBU-6 (Truxton)				
ibuprofen				
TAB, PO, 600 mg, 500s ea	00463-6113-05	39.00		EE
IBU-8 (Truxton)				
ibuprofen				
TAB, PO, 800 mg, 500s ea	00463-6114-05	42.00		EE
IBUDONE (Poly)				
hydrocodone bitartrate/ibuprofen				
TAB, PO (FILM-COATED)				
5 mg-200 mg,				
100s ea, C-III	66869-0118-10	86.88	69.50	
(FILM COATED)				
10 mg-200 mg,				
100s ea, C-III	66869-0128-10	114.38	91.50	
IBUPROFEN				
FUL				
TAB, PO, 400 mg, 100s ea		3.45		
600 mg, 100s ea		4.17		
800 mg, 100s ea		6.38		
(Actavis Mid Atlantic)				
SUS, PO (BERRY)				
100 mg/5 ml,				
120 ml	00472-1270-94	7.26		AB
473 ml	00472-1270-16	24.28		AB
(Amneal)				
TAB, PO (USP,AQUEOUS FILM-COATED)				
400 mg, 100s ea	53746-0464-01	20.48		AB
500s ea	53746-0464-05	84.84		AB
10000s ea	53746-0464-00	929.25		AB
(USP,FILM-COATED)				
400 mg, 10000s ea	53746-0131-00	885.00		AB
(FILM-COATED)				
600 mg, 30s ea	53746-0132-30	8.40		AB
(USP,AQUEOUS FILM-COATED)				
600 mg, 30s ea	53746-0465-30	8.82		AB
(FILM-COATED)				
600 mg, 50s ea	53746-0132-50	14.00		AB
(USP,AQUEOUS FILM-COATED)				
600 mg, 50s ea	53746-0465-50	14.70		AB
(FILM-COATED)				
600 mg, 60s ea	53746-0132-60	16.80		AB
(USP,AQUEOUS FILM-COATED)				
600 mg, 60s ea	53746-0465-60	17.64		AB
(FILM-COATED)				
600 mg, 90s ea	53746-0132-90	25.20		AB
(USP,AQUEOUS FILM-COATED)				
600 mg, 90s ea	53746-0465-90	26.46		AB
100s ea	53746-0465-01	29.02		AB
500s ea	53746-0465-05	120.13		AB
10000s ea	53746-0465-00	1315.65		AB
(USP,FILM-COATED)				
600 mg, 10000s ea	53746-0132-00	1253.50		AB
(FILM-COATED)				
800 mg, 30s ea	53746-0137-30	12.00		AB
(USP,AQUEOUS FILM-COATED)				
800 mg, 30s ea	53746-0466-30	12.60		AB
(FILM-COATED)				
800 mg, 50s ea	53746-0137-50	20.00		AB
(USP,AQUEOUS FILM-COATED)				
800 mg, 50s ea	53746-0466-50	21.00		AB
(FILM-COATED)				
800 mg, 60s ea	53746-0137-60	24.00		AB
(USP,AQUEOUS FILM-COATED)				
800 mg, 60s ea	53746-0466-60	25.20		AB
(FILM-COATED)				
800 mg, 90s ea	53746-0137-90	36.00		AB
(USP,AQUEOUS FILM-COATED)				
800 mg, 90s ea	53746-0466-90	37.80		AB
100s ea	53746-0466-01	38.08		AB
500s ea	53746-0466-05	152.36		AB
10000s ea	53746-0466-00	1667.40		AB
(Asafi Pharmaceutical)				
TAB, PO, 400 mg, 500s ea	65557-0401-05	17.56	11.81	EE
600 mg, 500s ea	65557-0402-05	18.70	14.94	EE
800 mg, 500s ea	65557-0400-05	36.41	21.19	EE
(Ascend) *See IBU*				
(Consolidated Midland)				
TAB, PO, 400 mg, 500s ea	00223-1091-05	27.50		EE
600 mg, 100s ea	00223-1092-01	7.75		EE
500s ea	00223-1092-05	29.75		EE
800 mg, 100s ea	00223-1093-01	13.25		EE
500s ea	00223-1093-05	44.50		EE
(Cumberland Pharma) *See CALDOLOR*				
(Dr Reddy's) *See IBU*				
(Dr Reddy's)				
TAB, PO (FILM COATED)				
400 mg, 100s ea	55111-0101-01	20.55		AB
500s ea	55111-0101-05	85.79		AB
600 mg, 100s ea	55111-0102-01	29.02		AB
500s ea	55111-0102-05	120.12		AB
800 mg, 100s ea	55111-0103-01	38.45		AB
500s ea	55111-0103-05	152.30		AB
(Gallipot)				
POW, NA (U.S.P.)				
25 gm	51552-0378-04	10.08		
100 gm	51552-0378-05	16.38		
1000 gm	51552-0378-07	70.00		
(Hawkins)				
POW, NA (U.S.P.)				
500 gm	63370-0110-45	132.00		
1000 gm	63370-0110-50	200.00		
5000 gm	63370-0110-55	880.00		
(Letco)				
POW, NA (U.S.P.)				
100 gm	62991-1081-02	30.00		
500 gm	62991-1081-03	90.00		
1000 gm	62991-1081-04	147.00		
(Major)				
TAB, PO, 400 mg, 100s ea	00904-1748-60	19.39		AB
(10X10,USP,FILM-COATED)				
400 mg, 100s ea UD	00904-5853-61	21.55		AB
500s ea	00904-1748-40	79.99		AB
(10X10,CAPLET)				
600 mg, 100s ea UD	00904-5854-61	30.45		
(FILM-COATED)				
600 mg, 100s ea	00904-5186-60	27.39		AB
500s ea	00904-5186-40	113.29		AB
(10X10,CAPLET)				
800 mg, 100s ea UD	00904-5855-61	39.95		
(FILM-COATED)				
800 mg, 100s ea	00904-5187-60	35.95		AB
500s ea	00904-5187-40	143.69		AB
(Medisca)				
POW, NA (U.S.P.)				
25 gm	38779-0299-04	25.50		
100 gm	38779-0299-05	37.50		
500 gm	38779-0299-08	127.50		
1000 gm	38779-0299-09	190.50		
(Par)				
TAB, PO, 400 mg, 100s ea	49884-0777-01	20.50		AB
500s ea	49884-0777-05	84.86		AB
600 mg, 100s ea	49884-0778-01	29.04		AB
500s ea	49884-0778-05	120.15		AB
800 mg, 100s ea	49884-0779-01	38.10		AB
500s ea	49884-0779-05	152.38		AB
(PCCA)				
POW, NA (U.S.P.)				
1 gm	51927-1192-00	1.32		
(Perrigo)				
SUS, PO (USP,BERRY)				
100 mg/5 ml,				
120 ml	45802-0952-26	7.22		AB
473 ml	45802-0952-43	24.21		AB
(Qualitest)				
TAB, PO (USP,AQUEOUS FILM-COATED)				
400 mg, 100s ea	00603-4021-21	20.50		AB
500s ea	00603-4021-28	85.85		AB
(AQUEOUS FILM-COATED)				
600 mg, 100s ea	00603-4022-21	29.04		AB
(USP,AQUEOUS FILM-COATED)				
600 mg, 500s ea	00603-4022-28	120.15		AB
(USP,FILM-COATED)				
800 mg, 100s ea	00603-4023-21	38.54		AB
(USP,AQUEOUS FILM-COATED)				
800 mg, 500s ea	00603-4023-28	152.37		AB
(Spectrum Pharmacy)				
CRY, NA (U.S.P.)				
100 gm	49452-3657-02	68.25		
500 gm	49452-3657-03	189.70		
1000 gm	49452-3657-04	287.00		
5000 gm	49452-3657-05	1060.50		
(Truxton) *See IBU-4*				
(Truxton) *See IBU-6*				
(Truxton) *See IBU-8*				
(UDL)				
TAB, PO (ROBOT READY 25X1)				
800 mg, 25s ea UD	51079-0596-19	5.19		AB
(10X10)				
800 mg, 100s ea UD	51079-0596-20	31.60		AB
(VistaPharm, Inc.)				
SUS, PO (5MLX50,USP,BERRY)				
100 mg/5 ml,				
5 ml 50s UD	66689-0009-50	42.00		
(4u)				
REPACK				
TAB, PO, 600 mg, 40s ea	10544-0317-40	22.86		
(AQUEOUS FILM-COATED)				
600 mg, 40s ea	42549-0517-40	22.86		AB
60s ea	10544-0317-60	26.34		
(AQUEOUS FILM-COATED)				
600 mg, 60s ea	42549-0517-60	26.34		AB
(FILM-COATED)				
600 mg, 60s ea	42549-0317-60	26.34		AB
800 mg, 30s ea	10544-0318-30	20.86		
30s ea	10544-0388-30	20.86		AB
30s ea	42549-0518-30	20.86		AB
30s ea	42549-0588-30	20.86		AB
60s ea	10544-0318-60	37.74		
60s ea	42549-0518-60	37.74		AB
60s ea	42549-0588-60	37.74		AB
90s ea	42549-0518-90	54.22		AB
100s ea	10544-0388-00	47.76		AB
100s ea	42549-0518-00	47.76		AB
100s ea	42549-0588-00	47.76		AB
(FILM-COATED)				
800 mg, 100s ea	42549-0318-00	56.46		AB
(A-S Medication)				
REPACK				
SUS, PO, 100 mg/5 ml,				
120 ml	54569-5174-00	7.24		EE
TAB, PO (AQUEOUS FILM-COATED)				
400 mg, 12s ea	54569-0285-07	2.91		AB
15s ea	54569-0285-09	3.64		AB
16s ea	54569-0285-00	3.88		AB
20s ea	54569-0285-04	4.85		AB
21s ea	54569-0285-06	5.09		AB
28s ea	54569-3820-02	6.79		AB
30s ea	54569-0285-01	7.28		AB
40s ea	54569-0285-05	9.70		AB
50s ea	54569-0285-02	12.13		AB
60s ea	54569-0285-08	14.56		AB
90s ea	54569-3820-00	21.83		AB
100s ea	54569-0285-03	24.26		AB
600 mg, 4s ea	54569-4002-02	1.17		AB
10s ea	54569-0287-00	2.93		AB
12s ea	54569-0287-01	3.51		AB
15s ea	54569-4002-00	4.39		AB
16s ea	54569-0287-02	4.68		AB
20s ea	54569-0287-08	5.85		AB
21s ea	54569-4002-01	6.14		AB
24s ea	54569-0287-09	7.02		AB
28s ea	54569-4002-04	8.19		AB
30s ea	54569-0287-03	8.78		AB
40s ea	54569-0287-07	11.70		AB
60s ea	54569-0287-04	17.55		AB
90s ea	54569-4002-05	26.33		AB
100s ea	54569-0287-05	29.25		AB
800 mg, 4s ea	54569-3332-00	1.49		EE
(AQUEOUS FILM-COATED)				
800 mg, 6s ea	54569-3332-06	2.24		AB
10s ea	54569-0289-00	3.73		AB
12s ea	54569-0289-08	4.47		AB
15s ea	54569-0289-01	5.59		AB
20s ea	54569-3332-07	7.46		AB
21s ea	54569-0289-07	7.83		AB
28s ea	54569-3332-04	10.44		AB
30s ea	54569-0289-02	11.19		AB
40s ea	54569-0289-09	14.92		AB
42s ea	54569-3332-02	15.66		AB
45s ea	54569-0289-03	16.78		AB
50s ea	54569-0289-06	18.65		AB
60s ea	54569-0289-04	22.37		AB
90s ea	54569-3332-05	33.56		AB
100s ea	54569-0289-05	37.29		AB
500s ea	54569-3332-08	186.45		AB
(Aidarex)				
REPACK				
TAB, PO, 400 mg, 7s ea	33261-0155-07	2.17		AB
14s ea	33261-0155-14	4.34		AB
20s ea	33261-0155-20	6.20		AB
21s ea	33261-0155-21	6.51		AB
28s ea	33261-0155-28	8.68		AB
30s ea	33261-0155-30	9.30		AB
40s ea	33261-0155-40	12.40		AB
60s ea	33261-0155-60	18.60		AB
90s ea	33261-0155-90	27.90		AB
100s ea	33261-0155-00	31.00		AB
120s ea	33261-0155-02	37.20		AB
180s ea	33261-0155-03	55.80		AB
(FILM-COATED)				
600 mg, 7s ea	33261-0061-07	2.80		AB
14s ea	33261-0061-14	5.60		AB
20s ea	33261-0061-20	8.00		AB
21s ea	33261-0061-21	8.40		AB
28s ea	33261-0061-28	11.20		AB
30s ea	33261-0061-30	12.00		AB
40s ea	33261-0061-40	16.00		AB
60s ea	33261-0061-60	24.00		AB

PROD/MFR	NDC	AWP	DP	OBC
90s ea	33261-0061-90	36.00		AB
120s ea	33261-0061-02	48.00		AB
180s ea	33261-0061-03	72.00		AB
360s ea	33261-0061-04	144.00		AB
800 mg, 7s ea	33261-0062-07	4.55		AB
14s ea	33261-0062-14	9.10		AB
20s ea	33261-0062-20	13.00		AB
21s ea	33261-0062-21	13.65		AB
28s ea	33261-0062-28	18.20		AB
30s ea	33261-0062-30	19.50		AB
40s ea	33261-0062-40	26.00		AB
60s ea	33261-0062-60	39.00		AB
84s ea	33261-0062-84	54.60		AB
90s ea	33261-0062-90	58.50		AB
100s ea	33261-0062-01	65.00		AB
120s ea	33261-0062-02	78.00		AB
(Altura)				
REPACK				
TAB, PO, 400 mg, 8s ea	63874-0322-08	3.28		AB
12s ea	63874-0322-12	4.92		AB
14s ea	63874-0322-14	5.74		AB
15s ea	63874-0322-15	6.15		AB
16s ea	63874-0322-16	6.56		AB
20s ea	63874-0322-20	8.20		AB
21s ea	63874-0322-21	8.61		AB
24s ea	63874-0322-24	9.84		AB
25s ea	63874-0322-25	10.25		AB
28s ea	63874-0322-28	11.48		AB
30s ea	63874-0322-30	12.30		AB
40s ea	63874-0322-40	16.40		AB
45s ea	63874-0322-45	18.45		AB
50s ea	63874-0322-50	20.50		AB
56s ea	63874-0322-56	22.96		AB
60s ea	63874-0322-60	24.60		AB
90s ea	63874-0322-90	36.90		AB
100s ea	63874-0322-01	41.00		AB
500s ea	63874-0322-03	163.75		AB
(FILM-COATED)				
600 mg, 6s ea	63874-0324-06	2.82		AB
8s ea	63874-0324-08	3.36		AB
10s ea	63874-0324-10	3.87		AB
12s ea	63874-0324-12	5.25		AB
(FILM-COATED)				
600 mg, 14s ea	63874-0324-14	6.13		AB
15s ea	63874-0324-15	6.56		AB
(FILM-COATED)				
600 mg, 16s ea	63874-0324-16	7.00		AB
20s ea	63874-0324-20	8.75		AB
21s ea	63874-0324-21	9.19		AB
24s ea	63874-0324-24	10.50		AB
(FILM-COATED)				
600 mg, 25s ea	63874-0324-25	10.94		AB
28s ea	63874-0324-28	12.25		AB
30s ea	63874-0324-30	13.13		AB
40s ea	63874-0324-40	17.50		AB
(FILM-COATED)				
600 mg, 45s ea	63874-0324-45	19.69		AB
50s ea	63874-0324-50	21.88		AB
60s ea	63874-0324-60	26.26		AB
(FILM-COATED)				
600 mg, 80s ea	63874-0324-80	22.49		AB
90s ea	63874-0324-90	39.39		AB
100s ea	63874-0324-01	45.90		AB
(FILM-COATED)				
600 mg, 120s ea	63874-0324-04	52.52		AB
500s ea	63874-0324-03	95.19		AB
800 mg, 12s ea	63874-0323-12	5.42		AB
14s ea	63874-0323-14	6.33		AB
15s ea	63874-0323-15	6.61		AB
16s ea	63874-0323-16	7.23		AB
20s ea	63874-0323-20	8.84		AB
21s ea	63874-0323-21	9.50		AB
24s ea	63874-0323-24	10.86		AB
25s ea	63874-0323-25	11.31		AB
28s ea	63874-0323-28	12.68		AB
30s ea	63874-0323-30	13.58		AB
40s ea	63874-0323-40	20.45		AB
42s ea	63874-0323-42	19.04		AB
45s ea	63874-0323-45	23.00		AB
50s ea	63874-0323-50	25.66		AB
56s ea	63874-0323-56	25.39		AB
60s ea	63874-0323-60	28.51		AB
80s ea	63874-0323-80	36.27		AB
84s ea	63874-0323-84	38.09		AB
90s ea	63874-0323-90	40.81		AB
100s ea	63874-0323-01	45.27		AB
120s ea	63874-0323-04	57.02		AB
500s ea	63874-0323-03	143.95		AB
(American Health)				
REPACK				
TAB, PO (10X10)				
400 mg, 100s ea UD	62584-0746-01	26.02		AB

PROD/MFR	NDC	AWP	DP	OBC
(15X30)				
400 mg, 450s ea	62584-0746-85	76.37		AB
(10X10)				
600 mg, 100s ea UD	62584-0747-01	36.15		AB
800 mg, 100s ea UD	62584-0748-01	42.79		AB
(15X30)				
800 mg, 450s ea	62584-0748-85	137.14		AB
(B&B Pharm, Inc)				
REPACK				
POW, NA (U.S.P.)				
500 gm	63275-9995-08	80.00		
1000 gm	63275-9995-09	135.00		
(Bryant Ranch)				
REPACK				
TAB, PO, 200 mg, 15s ea	63629-1467-02	8.99		
20s ea	63629-1467-01	10.99		
30s ea	63629-1467-03	14.99		
50s ea	63629-1467-06	19.99		
60s ea	63629-1467-05	25.80		
100s ea	63629-1467-04	43.99		
400 mg, 20s ea	63629-1468-01	9.75		
30s ea	63629-1468-02	14.13		
40s ea	63629-1468-03	19.50		
60s ea	63629-1468-04	26.65		
600 mg, 15s ea	63629-1469-02	7.55		
20s ea	63629-1469-01	11.73		
30s ea	63629-1469-03	15.09		
40s ea	63629-1469-04	20.46		
50s ea	63629-1469-08	24.32		
60s ea	63629-1469-05	30.19		
90s ea	63629-1469-06	44.28		
120s ea	63629-1469-07	53.87		
800 mg, 20s ea	63629-1470-01	8.86		
21s ea	63629-1470-04	9.96		
30s ea	63629-1470-05	12.80		
40s ea	63629-1470-03	17.61		
42s ea	63629-1470-02	18.92		
60s ea	63629-1470-09	29.99		
90s ea	63629-1470-06	39.40		
100s ea	63629-1470-07	39.65		
120s ea	63629-1470-08	50.65		
(Core)				
REPACK				
SUS, PO, 100 mg/5 ml,				
120 ml	33358-0184-04	8.56		
TAB, PO, 400 mg, 15s ea	33358-0186-15	6.59		
20s ea	33358-0186-20	9.99		
30s ea	33358-0186-30	14.48		
40s ea	33358-0186-40	19.99		
60s ea	33358-0186-60	30.94		
90s ea	33358-0186-90	45.39		
120s ea	33358-0186-01	50.90		
600 mg, 15s ea	33358-0187-15	7.74		
20s ea	33358-0187-20	12.02		
30s ea	33358-0187-30	15.47		
40s ea	33358-0187-40	20.97		
50s ea	33358-0187-50	25.99		
60s ea	33358-0187-60	30.94		
90s ea	33358-0187-90	45.39		
120s ea	33358-0187-01	55.22		
800 mg, 10s ea	33358-0188-10	5.89		
15s ea	33358-0188-15	10.99		
20s ea	33358-0188-20	11.90		
21s ea	33358-0188-21	13.33		
30s ea	33358-0188-30	15.82		
40s ea	33358-0188-40	20.14		
60s ea	33358-0188-60	29.99		
100s ea	33358-0188-00	46.95		
120s ea	33358-0188-01	48.45		
(DHS, Inc.)				
REPACK				
TAB, PO, 400 mg, 20s ea	55887-0896-20	8.17		
30s ea	55887-0896-30	12.25		AB
90s ea	55887-0896-90	36.74		
600 mg, 30s ea	55887-0995-30	18.00		AB
(FILM-COATED)				
600 mg, 60s ea	55887-0995-60	36.00		AB
90s ea	55887-0995-90	50.00		AB
800 mg, 20s ea	55887-0976-20	12.00		AB
21s ea	55887-0976-21	12.60		AB
30s ea	55887-0976-30	18.00		AB
42s ea	55887-0976-42	25.00		AB
50s ea	55887-0976-50	29.75		AB
(FILM-COATED)				
800 mg, 60s ea	55887-0976-60	36.00		AB
90s ea	55887-0976-90	50.00		AB
(Dispensing Solutions)				
REPACK				
TAB, PO (FILM-COATED)				
400 mg, 6s ea	55045-1421-03	2.70		AB
12s ea	55045-1421-02	5.40		AB

PROD/MFR	NDC	AWP	DP	OBC
15s ea	66336-0430-15	6.12		
(FILM-COATED)				
400 mg, 20s ea	55045-1421-07	9.00		AB
20s ea	66336-0430-20	8.16		AB
30s ea	55045-1421-08	13.55		AB
(USP)				
400 mg, 30s ea	66336-0430-30	12.25		AB
(FILM-COATED)				
400 mg, 40s ea	55045-1421-04	18.00		AB
40s ea	66336-0430-40	16.33		AB
60s ea	66336-0430-60	24.50		AB
(FILM-COATED)				
400 mg, 60s ea	55045-1421-09	27.00		AB
90s ea	55045-1421-06	40.50		AB
100s ea	55045-1421-00	45.00		AB
120s ea	55045-1421-01	54.00		AB
600 mg, 6s ea	55045-1173-00	2.82		AB
10s ea	66336-0556-10	6.00		AB
15s ea	66336-0556-15	9.00		EE
(FILM-COATED)				
600 mg, 15s ea	55045-1173-05	7.00		AB
16s ea	66336-0556-16	9.60		AB
20s ea	66336-0556-20	12.00		EE
(FILM-COATED)				
600 mg, 20s ea	55045-1173-07	9.40		AB
21s ea	66336-0556-21	12.60		AB
28s ea	66336-0556-28	16.80		EE
30s ea	66336-0556-30	18.00		EE
(FILM-COATED)				
600 mg, 30s ea	55045-1173-08	14.10		AB
40s ea	66336-0556-40	24.00		EE
(FILM-COATED)				
600 mg, 40s ea	55045-1173-03	18.80		AB
60s ea	55045-3763-06	28.20		
(FILM-COATED)				
600 mg, 60s ea	55045-1173-09	28.20		AB
60s ea	66336-0556-60	36.00		AB
90s ea	55045-1173-06	42.30		AB
90s ea	66336-0556-90	50.00		AB
100s ea	55045-1173-01	47.00		AB
120s ea	55045-1173-02	56.40		AB
135s ea	55045-1173-04	63.45		AB
800 mg, 6s ea	55045-1257-00	3.60		AB
12s ea	66336-0030-12	7.20		AB
15s ea	55045-1257-05	9.05		AB
15s ea	66336-0030-15	9.00		AB
16s ea	66336-0030-16	9.60		EE
20s ea	55045-1257-07	12.00		
(FILM-COATED)				
800 mg, 20s ea	66336-0030-20	12.00		AB
21s ea	55045-1257-02	12.60		
21s ea	66336-0030-21	12.60		EE
30s ea	55045-1257-08	18.00		
30s ea	66336-0030-30	18.00		EE
(FILM-COATED)				
800 mg, 30s ea	55045-3925-01	18.00		AB
40s ea	55045-1257-06	24.00		
40s ea	66336-0030-40	24.00		EE
45s ea	55045-1257-03	27.00		
50s ea	55045-3193-05	30.00		
60s ea	55045-1257-09	36.00		
60s ea	66336-0030-60	36.00		EE
90s ea	55045-1257-04	54.00		
90s ea	66336-0030-90	54.00		EE
100s ea	55045-1257-01	60.00		
(FILM-COATED)				
800 mg, 100s ea	66336-0030-00	60.00		AB
120s ea	55045-3193-01	72.00		AB
135s ea	55045-3193-04	81.00		
(GSMS)				
REPACK				
TAB, PO (UNIT OF USE)				
400 mg, 30s ea	60429-0092-30	9.30	3.10	AB
60s ea	60429-0092-60	18.60	6.20	AB
90s ea	60429-0092-90	27.90	9.30	AB
600 mg, 30s ea	60429-0093-30	12.45	4.15	AB
60s ea	60429-0093-60	13.50	4.50	AB
90s ea	60429-0093-90	14.70	4.90	AB
800 mg, 30s ea	60429-0094-30	15.15	5.05	AB
90s ea	60429-0094-90	19.80	6.60	AB
270s ea	60429-0094-27	69.00	23.00	AB
(HomeMed)				
REPACK				
TAB, PO, 400 mg, 2s ea	51655-0049-31	2.80		EE
6s ea	51655-0049-87	3.80		EE
20s ea	51655-0049-52	15.99		EE
30s ea	51655-0049-24	16.99		EE
40s ea	51655-0049-51	19.99		EE
60s ea	51655-0049-25	10.70		EE
90s ea	51655-0049-26	15.54		EE
120s ea	51655-0049-82	20.39		EE
600 mg, 20s ea	51655-0050-52	15.99		EE

PROD/MFR	NDC	AWP	DP	OBC
30s ea	51655-0050-24	16.99		EE
40s ea	51655-0050-51	18.99		EE
60s ea	51655-0050-25	26.99		EE
90s ea	51655-0050-26	21.59		EE
120s ea	51655-0050-82	28.71		EE
180s ea	51655-0050-83	35.83		EE
270s ea	51655-0050-92	63.03		EE
800 mg, 15s ea	51655-0051-54	5.35		EE
20s ea	51655-0051-52	8.99		EE
21s ea	51655-0051-28	9.99		EE
30s ea	51655-0051-24	18.99		EE
40s ea	51655-0051-51	17.99		EE
60s ea	51655-0051-25	24.99		EE
90s ea	51655-0051-26	27.12		EE
180s ea	51655-0051-83	53.24		EE
270s ea	51655-0051-92	79.85		EE
(IPI)				
REPACK				
TAB, PO, 600 mg, 40s ea	18837-0071-40	13.44		
50s ea	18837-0071-50	12.05		AB
60s ea	18837-0071-60	18.02		
90s ea	18837-0071-90	35.74		
(FILM-COATED)				
800 mg, 21s ea	18837-0072-21	17.62		AB
(AQUEOUS FILM-COATED)				
800 mg, 30s ea	18837-0072-30	8.14		AB
60s ea	18837-0072-60	26.50		
(AQUEOUS FILM-COATED)				
800 mg, 90s ea	18837-0072-90	27.42		AB
100s ea	18837-0072-99	56.50		
(AQUEOUS FILM-COATED)				
800 mg, 120s ea	18837-0072-98	36.57		AB
(Keltman Pharma., Inc.)				
REPACK				
TAB, PO, 600 mg, 21s ea	68387-0208-21	9.92		
90s ea	68387-0208-90	42.51		
(FILM-COATED)				
800 mg, 30s ea	68387-0210-30	13.33		AB
60s ea	68387-0210-60	26.66		AB
90s ea	68387-0210-90	40.00		AB
100s ea	68387-0210-10	44.43		AB
(LWP)				
REPACK				
TAB, PO, 400 mg, 60s ea	64038-0072-60	17.30		AB
100s ea	64038-0072-01	25.50		AB
600 mg, 60s ea	64038-0076-60	22.42		AB
100s ea	64038-0076-01	34.04		AB
800 mg, 60s ea	64038-0071-60	27.86		AB
90s ea	64038-0071-90	39.29		
100s ea	64038-0071-01	43.10		AB
(McKesson Packaging)				
REPACK				
TAB, PO, 400 mg,				
100s ea UD	63739-0135-10	22.05		AB
(BLISTER PACK)				
400 mg, 750s ea UD	63739-0135-01	165.38		AB
600 mg, 100s ea UD	63739-0136-10	30.61		
(BLISTER PACK)				
600 mg, 750s ea UD	63739-0136-01	229.58		
(PUNCH CARD 25X30)				
600 mg, 750s ea	63739-0136-03	229.58		
800 mg, 100s ea UD	63739-0137-10	32.21		AB
(BLISTER PACK)				
800 mg, 750s ea UD	63739-0137-01	241.58		AB
(PUNCH CARD 25X30)				
800 mg, 750s ea	63739-0137-03	241.58		AB
(Medsource)				
REPACK				
TAB, PO (FILM-COATED)				
800 mg, 30s ea	45865-0373-30	16.50		AB
60s ea	45865-0373-60	33.00		AB
90s ea	45865-0373-90	49.50		AB
100s ea	45865-0373-00	55.00		AB
120s ea	45865-0373-01	66.00		AB
150s ea	45865-0373-02	82.50		AB
(Nucare Pharm)				
REPACK				
TAB, PO, 400 mg, 15s ea	66267-0116-15	6.45		EE
20s ea	66267-0116-20	8.45		EE
30s ea	66267-0116-30	12.89		EE
40s ea	66267-0116-40	16.95		EE
60s ea	66267-0116-60	24.98		EE
90s ea	66267-0116-90	29.89		EE
600 mg, 15s ea	66267-0117-15	7.36		EE
20s ea	66267-0117-20	8.81		EE
30s ea	66267-0117-30	15.49		EE
40s ea	66267-0117-40	17.55		EE
60s ea	66267-0117-60	25.89		EE
90s ea	66267-0117-90	39.89		EE
100s ea	66267-0964-00	44.45		EE
800 mg, 15s ea	66267-0118-15	8.72		EE
20s ea	66267-0118-20	10.61		EE
21s ea	66267-0118-21	11.00		EE
(AQUEOUS FILM-COATED)				
800 mg, 30s ea	66267-0118-30	21.01		AB
40s ea	66267-0118-40	23.49		EE
(AQUEOUS FILM-COATED)				
800 mg, 50s ea	66267-0118-50	24.45		AB
60s ea	66267-0118-60	27.89		EE
(AQUEOUS FILM-COATED)				
800 mg, 90s ea	66267-0118-90	50.99		AB
100s ea	66267-0963-00	62.15		EE
(AQUEOUS FILM-COATED)				
800 mg, 120s ea	66267-0118-91	71.50		AB
(Palmetto)				
REPACK				
SUS, PO, 100 mg/5 ml,				
120 ml	23490-5741-00	7.15		
480 ml	23490-5741-01	9.99		
TAB, PO, 200 mg, 6s ea	23490-5742-01	2.94		
20s ea	23490-5742-02	7.00		
30s ea	23490-5742-03	10.50		
40s ea	23490-5742-06	14.00		
50s ea	23490-5742-00	46.67		
60s ea	23490-5742-04	21.00		
90s ea	23490-1482-09	4.99		
90s ea	23490-5742-05	31.50		
100s ea	23490-5742-07	35.00		
400 mg, 6s ea	23490-5743-01	4.20		
15s ea	23490-5743-02	7.50		
20s ea	23490-5743-03	10.00		
30s ea	23490-5743-04	15.00		
40s ea	23490-5743-05	20.00		
60s ea	23490-5743-08	30.00		
90s ea	23490-5743-07	45.00		
100s ea	23490-5743-06	50.00		
600 mg, 6s ea	23490-5744-01	4.62		
10s ea	23490-5744-02	5.50		
15s ea	23490-5744-03	8.25		
16s ea	23490-5744-04	8.80		
20s ea	23490-5744-05	11.00		
21s ea	23490-5744-06	11.55		
28s ea	23490-5744-07	15.40		
30s ea	23490-5744-08	16.50		
40s ea	23490-5744-09	22.00		
60s ea	23490-5744-00	33.00		
90s ea	23490-7865-00	49.50		
800 mg, 6s ea	23490-5745-01	5.04		
12s ea	23490-5745-02	7.20		
15s ea	23490-5745-03	9.00		
16s ea	23490-5745-04	9.60		
20s ea	23490-5745-05	12.00		
21s ea	23490-5745-06	12.60		
25s ea	23490-7866-02	15.00		
28s ea	23490-5745-00	16.80		
30s ea	23490-0722-03	18.71		
30s ea	23490-5745-07	18.00		
40s ea	23490-5745-08	24.00		
60s ea	23490-0722-06	37.41		
60s ea	23490-5745-09	36.00		
90s ea	23490-0722-09	56.12		
90s ea	23490-7866-00	54.00		
100s ea	23490-7866-01	60.00		
(PD-Rx Pharm)				
REPACK				
TAB, PO, 400 mg, 8s ea	55289-0590-08	22.13		AB
10s ea	55289-0590-10	22.67		AB
12s ea	55289-0590-12	23.20		AB
15s ea	55289-0590-15	24.00		AB
16s ea	55289-0590-16	24.60		AB
20s ea	55289-0590-20	25.33		AB
21s ea	55289-0590-21	25.60		AB
30s ea	55289-0590-30	28.00		AB
(REDI-SCRIPT)				
400 mg, 30s ea	58864-0285-30	28.08		AB
36s ea	55289-0590-36	29.60		AB
40s ea	55289-0590-40	30.67		AB
(REDI-SCRIPT,FILM-COATED)				
400 mg, 56s ea	58864-0285-56	34.93		AB
60s ea	55289-0590-60	36.00		AB
(REDI-SCRIPT, U.S.P.)				
400 mg, 60s ea	58864-0285-60	36.00		AB
90s ea	55289-0590-90	44.00		AB
100s ea UD	55289-0590-17	46.68		AB
600 mg, 6s ea	55289-0142-06	22.00		AB
10s ea	55289-0142-10	23.33		AB
12s ea	55289-0142-12	24.00		AB
14s ea	55289-0142-14	24.67		AB
15s ea	55289-0142-15	25.00		AB
18s ea	55289-0142-18	26.00		AB
20s ea	55289-0142-20	26.67		AB
21s ea	55289-0142-21	27.00		AB
24s ea	55289-0142-24	28.00		AB
28s ea	55289-0142-28	29.33		AB
30s ea	55289-0142-30	30.00		AB
(REDI-SCRIPT)				
600 mg, 30s ea	58864-0286-30	30.00		AB
40s ea	55289-0142-40	33.33		AB
60s ea	55289-0142-60	40.00		AB
(REDI-SCRIPT)				
600 mg, 60s ea	58864-0286-60	40.02		AB
(FILM-COATED)				
600 mg, 90s ea	58864-0286-90	44.00		AB
(USP)				
600 mg, 90s ea	55289-0142-90	43.44		AB
100s ea	55289-0142-01	47.22		AB
800 mg, 10s ea	55289-0140-10	24.00		AB
12s ea	55289-0140-12	25.50		AB
15s ea	55289-0140-15	26.00		AB
20s ea	55289-0140-20	28.00		AB
21s ea	55289-0140-21	28.40		AB
(USP,FILM-COATED)				
800 mg, 24s ea	55289-0140-24	29.64		AB
30s ea	55289-0140-30	32.00		AB
(REDI-SCRIPT)				
800 mg, 30s ea	58864-0287-30	31.98		AB
40s ea	55289-0140-40	36.00		AB
42s ea	55289-0140-42	36.80		AB
(REDI-SCRIPT)				
800 mg, 45s ea	58864-0287-45	38.00		AB
50s ea	55289-0140-50	40.00		AB
60s ea	55289-0140-60	44.00		AB
(REDI-SCRIPT)				
800 mg, 60s ea	58864-0287-60	43.98		AB
(FILM-COATED)				
800 mg, 90s ea	55289-0140-90	56.00		AB
(REDI-SCRIPT)				
800 mg, 90s ea	58864-0287-90	56.00		AB
100s ea	55289-0140-01	56.53		AB
180s ea	55289-0140-93	95.94		AB
(USP,FILM-COATED)				
800 mg, 270s ea	55289-0140-94	117.06		AB
(Pharma Pac)				
REPACK				
SUS, PO (1X120ML,BERRY)				
100 mg/5 ml,				
120 ml	52959-0948-04	7.35		AB
TAB, PO, 400 mg, 20s ea	52959-0075-20	6.13		EE
21s ea	52959-0075-21	6.43		EE
30s ea	52959-0075-30	9.18		EE
40s ea	52959-0075-40	12.22		EE
60s ea	52959-0075-60	18.31		EE
90s ea	52959-0075-90	27.42		EE
100s ea	52959-0075-00	30.45		EE
120s ea	52959-0075-02	36.50		EE
600 mg, 4s ea	52959-0076-04	1.63		EE
10s ea	52959-0076-10	4.08		EE
12s ea	52959-0076-12	4.90		EE
15s ea	52959-0076-15	6.12		EE
16s ea	52959-0076-16	6.52		EE
20s ea	52959-0076-20	8.15		EE
21s ea	52959-0076-21	8.56		EE
24s ea	52959-0076-24	9.77		EE
25s ea	52959-0076-25	10.18		EE
28s ea	52959-0076-28	11.39		EE
30s ea	52959-0076-30	12.20		EE
40s ea	52959-0076-40	16.26		EE
45s ea	52959-0076-45	18.28		EE
50s ea	52959-0076-50	20.31		EE
60s ea	52959-0076-60	24.35		EE
90s ea	52959-0076-90	36.47		EE
100s ea	52959-0076-00	40.51		EE
120s ea	52959-0076-02	48.58		EE
800 mg, 4s ea	52959-0077-04	2.07		EE
6s ea	52959-0077-06	3.10		AB
10s ea	52959-0077-10	5.18		EE
12s ea	52959-0077-12	6.21		EE
14s ea	52959-0077-14	7.25		EE
15s ea	52959-0077-15	7.76		EE
16s ea	52959-0077-16	8.28		EE
18s ea	52959-0077-18	9.31		EE
20s ea	52959-0077-20	10.34		EE
21s ea	52959-0077-21	10.86		EE
24s ea	52959-0077-24	12.40		EE
25s ea	52959-0077-25	12.92		EE
28s ea	52959-0077-28	14.46		EE
30s ea	52959-0077-30	15.49		EE
40s ea	52959-0077-40	20.64		EE
42s ea	52959-0077-42	21.66		EE
45s ea	52959-0077-45	23.20		EE
50s ea	52959-0077-50	25.77		EE
60s ea	52959-0077-60	30.90		EE
90s ea	52959-0077-90	46.32		EE
100s ea	52959-0077-00	51.45		EE
120s ea	52959-0077-02	61.72		EE

PROD/MFR	NDC	AWP	DP	OBC
(Phys Total Care)				
REPACK				
SUS, PO (BERRY)				
100 mg/5 ml,				
118 ml	**54868-4342-00**	14.01		AB
TAB, PO, 400 mg, 15s ea	**54868-0079-00**	6.03		EE
20s ea	**54868-0079-05**	6.54		EE
30s ea	**54868-0079-07**	7.56		EE
60s ea	**54868-0079-02**	10.62		EE
100s ea	**54868-0079-04**	12.15		EE
500s ea	**54868-0079-09**	41.31		EE
1000s ea	**54868-0079-08**	79.62		EE
600 mg, 15s ea	**54868-0080-04**	5.10		EE
20s ea	**54868-0080-02**	5.82		EE
30s ea	**54868-0080-08**	7.23		EE
40s ea	**54868-0080-03**	8.64		EE
60s ea	**54868-0080-05**	11.46		EE
90s ea	**54868-0080-00**	15.66		EE
100s ea	**54868-0080-06**	17.07		EE
120s ea	**54868-0080-01**	19.89		EE
500s ea	**54868-0080-09**	71.88		EE
800 mg, 15s ea	**54868-0133-01**	5.67		EE
20s ea	**54868-0133-05**	7.02		EE
30s ea	**54868-0133-06**	9.03		EE
40s ea	**54868-0133-02**	11.04		EE
60s ea	**54868-0133-04**	15.06		EE
90s ea	**54868-0133-03**	21.06		EE
100s ea	**54868-0133-00**	23.07		EE
500s ea	**54868-0133-08**	101.88		EE
(Physician Partner)				
REPACK				
SUS, PO, 100 mg/5 ml,				
120 ml	**21695-0420-12**	24.44		
TAB, PO, 400 mg, 20s ea	**21695-0066-20**	8.20		
30s ea	**21695-0066-30**	12.30		
(FILM-COATED)				
400 mg, 40s ea	**21695-0066-40**	19.29		
60s ea	**21695-0066-60**	24.60		
(FILM COATED)				
400 mg, 90s ea	**21695-0066-90**	36.90		
600 mg, 20s ea	**21695-0067-20**	11.60		
21s ea	**21695-0067-21**	12.18		
30s ea	**21695-0067-30**	17.42		
40s ea	**21695-0067-40**	23.22		
42s ea	**21695-0067-42**	24.38		
60s ea	**21695-0067-60**	34.84		
90s ea	**21695-0067-90**	52.62		
100s ea	**21695-0067-00**	58.46		
120s ea	**21695-0067-72**	69.68		
800 mg, 20s ea	**21695-0068-20**	14.33		
21s ea	**21695-0068-21**	15.05		
(FILM-COATED)				
800 mg, 28s ea	**21695-0068-28**	20.07		AB
30s ea	**21695-0068-30**	21.50		
40s ea	**21695-0068-40**	28.66		
42s ea	**21695-0068-42**	30.09		
45s ea	**21695-0068-45**	32.25		
60s ea	**21695-0068-60**	43.00		
90s ea	**21695-0068-90**	64.50		
100s ea	**21695-0068-00**	71.66		
120s ea	**21695-0068-72**	86.00		
(Quality Care Prod)				
REPACK				
TAB, PO, 400 mg, 16s ea	**49999-0097-16**	10.18		EE
18s ea	**49999-0097-18**	8.86		EE
20s ea	**49999-0097-20**	12.95		EE
28s ea	**49999-0097-28**	17.92		EE
30s ea	**49999-0097-30**	14.76		EE
(FILM-COATED)				
400 mg, 50s ea	**49999-0097-50**	24.50		AB
60s ea	**49999-0097-60**	29.52		EE
90s ea	**49999-0097-90**	44.28		AB
600 mg, 6s ea	**49999-0006-06**	5.68		EE
15s ea	**49999-0006-15**	6.89		EE
20s ea	**49999-0006-20**	15.99		EE
21s ea	**49999-0006-21**	7.38		EE
28s ea	**49999-0006-28**	9.99		EE
30s ea	**49999-0006-30**	16.99		EE
40s ea	**49999-0006-40**	18.75		EE
60s ea	**49999-0006-60**	26.99		EE
90s ea	**49999-0006-90**	32.40		EE
100s ea	**49999-0006-00**	36.00		AB
120s ea	**49999-0006-01**	43.20		EE
800 mg, 6s ea	**49999-0042-06**	4.26		EE
10s ea	**49999-0042-10**	7.10		AB
15s ea	**49999-0042-15**	8.16		EE
18s ea	**49999-0042-18**	10.22		EE
20s ea	**49999-0042-20**	10.88		EE
21s ea	**49999-0042-21**	11.43		EE
25s ea	**49999-0042-25**	14.27		EE
30s ea	**49999-0042-30**	16.32		EE
40s ea	**49999-0042-40**	21.77		EE
45s ea	**49999-0042-45**	24.49		AB
50s ea	**49999-0042-50**	27.21		AB
60s ea	**49999-0042-60**	32.65		EE
90s ea	**49999-0042-90**	49.50		EE
100s ea	**49999-0042-00**	54.41		AB
120s ea	**49999-0042-01**	65.30		EE
(Southwood)				
REPACK				
CTB, PO, 100 mg, 24s ea	**58016-0097-24**	3.65		
24s ea	**58016-4844-01**	2.30		
30s ea	**58016-0097-30**	4.56		
60s ea	**58016-0097-60**	9.13		
90s ea	**58016-0097-90**	13.69		
100s ea	**58016-0097-00**	15.21		
TAB, PO, 400 mg, 8s ea	**58016-0241-08**	3.28		EE
12s ea	**58016-0241-12**	4.92		EE
14s ea	**58016-0241-14**	5.74		EE
15s ea	**58016-0241-15**	6.15		EE
16s ea	**58016-0241-16**	6.56		EE
20s ea	**58016-0241-20**	8.20		EE
21s ea	**58016-0241-21**	8.61		EE
(AQUEOUS FILM-COATED)				
400 mg, 30s ea	**58016-0241-30**	15.30		AB
40s ea	**58016-0241-40**	16.40		EE
50s ea	**58016-0241-50**	20.50		EE
56s ea	**58016-0241-56**	22.96		EE
(AQUEOUS FILM-COATED)				
400 mg, 60s ea	**58016-0241-60**	30.60		AB
90s ea	**58016-0241-90**	45.90		AB
100s ea	**58016-0241-00**	51.00		AB
120s ea	**58016-0241-02**	61.20		AB
600 mg, 6s ea	**58016-0242-06**	2.69		EE
8s ea	**58016-0242-08**	3.20		EE
10s ea	**58016-0242-10**	3.69		EE
12s ea	**58016-0242-12**	4.08		EE
15s ea	**58016-0242-15**	4.84		EE
20s ea	**58016-0242-20**	5.62		EE
21s ea	**58016-0242-21**	5.90		EE
28s ea	**58016-0242-28**	11.80		EE
(AQUEOUS FILM-COATED)				
600 mg, 30s ea	**58016-0242-30**	16.50		AB
40s ea	**58016-0242-40**	11.24		EE
(FILM-COATED)				
600 mg, 42s ea	**58016-0242-42**	11.80		AB
50s ea	**58016-0242-50**	14.05		EE
(AQUEOUS FILM-COATED)				
600 mg, 60s ea	**58016-0242-60**	33.00		AB
80s ea	**58016-0242-80**	22.49		EE
(AQUEOUS FILM-COATED)				
600 mg, 90s ea	**58016-0242-90**	49.50		AB
100s ea	**58016-0242-00**	55.00		AB
120s ea	**58016-0242-02**	66.00		AB
135s ea	**58016-0242-67**	60.61		EE
800 mg, 12s ea	**58016-0243-12**	5.44		EE
14s ea	**58016-0243-14**	6.35		EE
15s ea	**58016-0243-15**	6.80		EE
16s ea	**58016-0243-16**	7.25		EE
20s ea	**58016-0243-20**	9.07		EE
21s ea	**58016-0243-21**	9.52		EE
24s ea	**58016-0243-24**	10.88		EE
28s ea	**58016-0243-28**	12.70		EE
(AQUEOUS FILM-COATED)				
800 mg, 30s ea	**58016-0243-30**	17.10		AB
40s ea	**58016-0243-40**	18.14		EE
42s ea	**58016-0243-42**	19.04		EE
45s ea	**58016-0243-45**	20.40		EE
50s ea	**58016-0243-50**	22.67		EE
56s ea	**58016-0243-56**	25.39		EE
(AQUEOUS FILM-COATED)				
800 mg, 60s ea	**58016-0243-60**	34.20		AB
80s ea	**58016-0243-80**	36.27		EE
84s ea	**58016-0243-84**	38.09		EE
(AQUEOUS FILM-COATED)				
800 mg, 90s ea	**58016-0243-90**	51.30		AB
100s ea	**58016-0243-00**	57.00		AB
120s ea	**58016-0243-02**	68.40		AB
135s ea	**58016-0243-67**	93.19		EE
150s ea	**58016-0243-03**	68.01		EE
(St. Mary's MPP)				
REPACK				
TAB, PO (USP,FILM-COATED)				
600 mg, 20s ea	**60760-0076-20**	11.03		AB
40s ea	**60760-0076-40**	16.57		AB
(FILM-COATED)				
600 mg, 60s ea	**60760-0076-60**	21.86		AB
100s ea	**60760-0076-00**	32.43		AB
(USP)				
800 mg, 9s ea	**60760-0135-09**	9.02		
(USP,FILM-COATED)				
800 mg, 20s ea	**60760-0135-20**	12.38		AB
30s ea	**60760-0135-30**	16.06		AB
60s ea	**60760-0135-60**	26.12		AB
100s ea	**60760-0135-00**	39.53		AB
(Stat Rx)				
REPACK				
TAB, PO, 400 mg, 20s ea	**16590-0124-20**	11.43		
30s ea	**16590-0124-30**	17.10		
40s ea	**16590-0124-40**	19.50		
60s ea	**16590-0124-60**	48.53		AB
90s ea	**16590-0124-90**	72.28		AB
120s ea	**16590-0124-72**	51.30		
600 mg, 20s ea	**16590-0125-20**	11.50		
(FILM-COATED)				
600 mg, 28s ea	**16590-0125-28**	16.10		AB
30s ea	**16590-0125-30**	17.25		
40s ea	**16590-0125-40**	23.00		
(FILM-COATED)				
600 mg, 50s ea	**16590-0125-50**	28.75		AB
56s ea	**16590-0125-56**	32.20		AB
60s ea	**16590-0125-60**	34.50		AB
90s ea	**16590-0125-90**	50.25		
(FILM-COATED)				
600 mg, 100s ea	**16590-0125-71**	57.50		AB
120s ea	**16590-0125-72**	69.00		AB
800 mg, 20s ea	**16590-0126-20**	16.54		AB
28s ea	**16590-0126-28**	18.26		AB
30s ea	**16590-0126-30**	15.00		
40s ea	**16590-0126-40**	20.00		
56s ea	**16590-0126-56**	36.51		AB
60s ea	**16590-0126-60**	30.00		
84s ea	**16590-0126-62**	43.40		AB
90s ea	**16590-0126-90**	55.80		
100s ea	**16590-0126-71**	50.00		
120s ea	**16590-0126-72**	52.50		
180s ea	**16590-0126-82**	93.00		AB
(Vibranta)				
REPACK				
TAB, PO, 400 mg, 16s ea	**57866-4604-08**	4.10		
30s ea	**57866-4604-01**	15.99		
40s ea	**57866-4604-06**	18.54		AB
60s ea	**57866-4604-02**	25.60		
90s ea	**57866-4604-05**	34.10		
270s ea	**57866-4604-09**	46.91		
600 mg, 12s ea	**57866-4605-00**	8.28		AB
20s ea	**57866-4605-05**	25.09		AB
24s ea	**57866-4605-09**	11.25		AB
30s ea	**57866-4605-01**	16.99		AB
60s ea	**57866-4605-02**	26.99		AB
90s ea	**57866-4607-02**	27.24		AB
100s ea	**57866-4605-03**	36.00		
270s ea	**57866-4607-01**	85.69		AB
800 mg, 10s ea	**57866-4606-07**	4.10		
15s ea	**57866-4606-05**	7.56		
21s ea	**57866-4606-03**	10.10		
30s ea	**57866-4606-01**	16.32		
40s ea	**57866-4606-06**	17.99		
60s ea	**57866-4606-02**	49.20		
90s ea	**57866-4606-09**	49.50		
100s ea	**57866-4606-00**	54.41		
270s ea	**57866-4606-08**	83.09		

IBUPROFEN LYSINE

(Lundbeck) *See NEOPROFEN*

IBUPROFEN W/ HYDROCODONE (PD-Rx Pharm)

PROD/MFR	NDC	AWP	DP	OBC
REPACK				
hydrocodone bitartrate/ibuprofen				
TAB, PO, 7.5 mg-200 mg,				
15s ea, C-III	**55289-0944-15**	88.30		

IBUPROFEN/OXYCODONE HYDROCHLORIDE

(Actavis) *See OXYCODONE HYDROCHLORIDE AND IBUPROFEN*

(Forest Pharm) *See COMBUNOX*

(Teva) *See OXYCODONE HYDROCHLORIDE AND IBUPROFEN*

(Watson Labs) *See OXYCODONE HYDROCHLORIDE AND IBUPROFEN*

IBUTILIDE FUMARATE (Paddock)

PROD/MFR	NDC	AWP	DP	OBC
SOL, IV (1X10ML,SDV)				
0.1 mg/ml, 10 ml	**00574-0840-01**	336.00		AP

(Pfizer) *See AMERINET CHOICE CORVERT*

(Pfizer) *See CORVERT*

(Pfizer) *See NOVAPLUS CORVERT*

IC-GREEN ANGIOGRAPHY (Akorn)

PROD/MFR	NDC	AWP	DP	OBC
indocyanine green				
KIT, NA (6 VIALS EA IC& DILUENT)				
25 mg, ea	**17478-0701-02**	635.95		

IC400 (GM Pharm)

PROD/MFR	NDC	AWP	DP	OBC
caff/ibuprofen/vit b1/vit b12/vit b2/vit b6				
KIT, PO, ea	**58809-0640-60**	21.19	17.30	

PROD/MFR	NDC	AWP	DP	OBC
IC800 (GM Pharm)				
caff/ibuprofen/vit b1/vit b12/vit b2/vit b6				
KIT, PO (CAPLET)				
ea	58809-0680-60	25.45	20.36	
ICAR PRENATAL (Hawthorn Pharm)				
prenatal vitamins				
KIT, PO (ORANGE,SOFTGEL)				
120s ea	63717-0150-03	24.99		
ICAR-C PLUS (Hawthorn Pharm)				
fe pentacarbonyl/folic acid/vit b12/vit c				
TAB, PO, 100s ea	63717-0100-01	59.99		
ICAR-C PLUS SR (Hawthorn Pharm)				
ascorbic acid/cyanocobalamin/folic acid/iron				
CER, PO, 100s ea UD	63717-0112-01	62.49		
ICHTHAMMOL (Gallipot)				
POW, NA (U.S.P.,N.F.)				
113.4 gm	51552-0314-04	23.80		
454 gm	51552-0314-06	52.01		
(Medisca)				
POW, NA (U.S.P.)				
25 gm	38779-0327-04	25.50		
100 gm	38779-0327-05	48.00		
500 gm	38779-0327-08	118.50		
(PCCA)				
POW, NA (U.S.P.)				
1 gm	51927-1273-00	0.96		
(Spectrum Pharmacy)				
POW, NA (U.S.P.)				
125 gm	49452-3660-01	102.90		
500 gm	49452-3660-02	237.65		
2500 gm	49452-3660-03	756.00		
IDAMYCIN PFS (Pfizer)				
idarubicin hydrochloride				
SOL, IV (SDV,PF,CYTOSAFE VIAL,PF)				
1 mg/ml, 5 ml	00013-2576-91	495.08	412.57	AP
(SDV.PF,CYTOSAFE VIAL,PF)				
1 mg/ml, 10 ml	00013-2586-91	990.17	825.14	AP
(SDV,PF,CYTOSAFE VIAL,PF)				
1 mg/ml, 20 ml	00013-2596-91	1980.34	1650.28	AP
IDARUBICIN HYDROCHLORIDE (APP)				
SOL, IV (1X5ML,SINGLE-USE,PF)				
1 mg/ml, 5 ml	63323-0194-05	92.70		AP
(1X10ML,SINGLE-USE,PF)				
1 mg/ml, 10 ml	63323-0194-10	160.66		AP
(1X20ML,SINGLE-USE,PF)				
1 mg/ml, 20 ml	63323-0194-20	275.63		AP
(Bedford)				
SOL, IV (S.D.V.,PF)				
1 mg/ml, 5 ml	55390-0215-01	360.00		AP
10 ml	55390-0216-01	720.00		AP
20 ml	55390-0217-01	1440.00		AP
(Greenstone)				
SOL, IV (PF)				
1 mg/ml, 5 ml	59762-2576-01	442.04		
10 ml	59762-2586-01	884.06		
20 ml	59762-2596-01	1767.81		
(Pfizer) *See IDAMYCIN PFS*				
(Teva) *See NOVAPLUS IDARUBICIN HYDROCHLORIDE*				
(Teva)				
SOL, IV (S.D.V.)				
1 mg/ml, 5 ml	00703-4154-11	144.00		AP
10 ml	00703-4155-11	288.00		AP
20 ml	00703-4156-11	576.00		AP
IDEBENONE (PCCA)				
POW, NA (1X1GM)				
1 gm	51927-3808-00	16.20		
IDOXURIDINE (Gallipot)				
POW, NA (U.S.P.)				
1 gm	51552-0890-01	80.15	57.25	
(Medisca)				
POW, NA (U.S.P.)				
1 gm	38779-1356-06	268.50		
5 gm	38779-1356-03	885.00		
(PCCA)				
POW, NA (USP)				
1 gm	51927-1633-00	207.00		
(Spectrum Pharmacy)				
POW, NA (U.S.P.)				
1 gm	49452-3661-03	490.00		
IDURSULFASE				
(Shire HGT, Inc.) *See ELAPRASE*				
IFEREX 150 FORTE (Nnodum)				
cyanocobalamin/folic acid/iron polysaccharide				
CAP, PO (10X10)				
25 mcg-1 mg-150 mg,				
100s ea UD	63044-0198-62	19.99		
IFEX (Baxter)				
ifosfamide				
PDS, IV (USP,SDV)				
1 gm, ea	00338-3991-01	79.66		
3 gm, ea	00338-3993-01	125.56		
IFOSFAMIDE (APP)				
PDS, IV (S.D.V.)				
1 gm, ea	63323-0142-10	72.56		
(SDV,PRIVATE LABEL)				
1 gm, ea	63323-0142-12	72.56		
(Baxter) *See IFEX*				
(Baxter)				
PDS, IV (SDV,30ML VIAL)				
1 gm, ea	10019-0925-01	56.40		
(SDV,30ML)				
1 gm, ea	10019-0925-82	56.40		
(SDV,75ML VIAL)				
3 gm, ea	10019-0926-02	114.00		
(SDV,75ML)				
3 gm, ea	10019-0926-16	114.00		
(Teva)				
SOL, IV (1X20ML)				
1 gm/20 ml, 20 ml	00703-3427-11	48.00		
(1X60ML)				
3 gm/60 ml, 60 ml	00703-3429-11	180.00		
IFOSFAMIDE/MESNA (Teva)				
KIT, IV (COMBO-PACK)				
5 gm-3 gm, ea	00703-4100-48	787.50		
6 gm-6 gm, ea	00703-4100-68	1170.00		
10 gm-10 gm, ea	00703-4100-58	1200.00		
ILARIS (Novartis Pharm)				
canakinumab				
PDS, SC (PF,LYOPHILIZED POWDER)				
180 mg, ea	00078-0582-61	19000.01		
ILOPERIDONE				
(Novartis Pharm) *See FANAPT*				
(Novartis Pharm) *See FANAPT TITRATION PACK*				
ILOPROST				
(Actelion Pharm) *See VENTAVIS*				
(CoTherix, Inc) *See VENTAVIS*				
IMATINIB MESYLATE				
(Novartis Pharm) *See GLEEVEC*				
IMDUR (Schering)				
isosorbide mononitrate				
TER, PO, 30 mg, 100s ea	00085-1374-01	284.51		AB
60 mg, 100s ea	00085-2028-01	299.42		AB
120 mg, 100s ea	00085-0091-01	419.16		AB
(10X10)				
120 mg, 100s ea UD	00085-1153-04	333.48		AB
(Phys Total Care) REPACK				
TER, PO, 60 mg, 10s ea	54868-3245-01	34.65		AB
30s ea	54868-3245-00	100.04		AB
IMDUR ER (Phys Total Care)				
isosorbide mononitrate				
TER, PO, 30 mg, 10s ea	54868-4353-01	29.50		
30s ea	54868-4353-00	84.76		
IMIDAZOLIDINYL UREA (Medisca)				
imidurea				
POW, NA (1X100GM)				
100 gm	38779-1357-05	31.50		
(1X500GM)				
500 gm	38779-1357-08	126.00		
IMIDUREA (Letco)				
POW, NA (1X100GM)				
100 gm	62991-2675-01	45.00		
(1X500GM)				
500 gm	62991-2675-02	150.00		
(Medisca) *See IMIDAZOLIDINYL UREA*				
(PCCA)				
POW, NA (N.F.)				
1 gm	51927-2370-00	0.60		
(Spectrum Pharmacy)				
POW, NA (N.F.)				
125 gm	49452-3664-01	93.10		
500 gm	49452-3664-02	264.60		
2500 gm	49452-3664-03	857.60		
IMIGLUCERASE				
(Genzyme) *See CEREZYME*				
IMIPRAMINE (Core) REPACK				
imipramine pamoate				
CAP, PO, 75 mg, 30s ea	33358-0191-30	328.55		
(Core)				
imipramine hydrochloride				
TAB, PO, 25 mg, 30s ea	33358-0189-30	15.47		
60s ea	33358-0189-60	48.95		
50 mg, 30s ea	33358-0190-30	41.21		
60s ea	33358-0190-60	80.67		
IMIPRAMINE HCL (Consolidated Midland)				
imipramine hydrochloride				
TAB, PO, 10 mg, 100s ea	00223-1103-01	3.25		EE
1000s ea	00223-1103-02	25.95		EE
25 mg, 100s ea	00223-1102-01	4.50		EE
1000s ea	00223-1102-02	34.50		EE
50 mg, 100s ea	00223-1104-01	5.75		EE
1000s ea	00223-1104-02	43.50		EE
(Gallipot)				
POW, NA (U.S.P.)				
25 gm	51552-0886-04	69.72	49.80	
(Medisca)				
POW, NA (U.S.P.)				
25 gm	38779-0443-04	67.50		
100 gm	38779-0443-05	229.50		
(USP,1X1000GM)				
1000 gm	38779-0443-09	2142.00		
(Mutual)				
TAB, PO, 10 mg, 100s ea	53489-0330-01	42.96		AB
25 mg, 100s ea	53489-0331-01	71.75		AB
50 mg, 100s ea	53489-0332-01	121.65		AB
(Par)				
TAB, PO, 10 mg, 100s ea	49884-0054-01	42.95		AB
1000s ea	49884-0054-10	408.00		AB
25 mg, 100s ea	49884-0055-01	71.75		AB
1000s ea	49884-0055-10	681.70		AB
50 mg, 100s ea	49884-0056-01	121.85		AB
1000s ea	49884-0056-10	1157.80		AB
(PCCA)				
POW, NA (U.S.P.)				
1 gm	51927-1625-00	2.76		
(Sandoz)				
TAB, PO, 10 mg, 100s ea	00781-1762-01	42.95		AB
25 mg, 100s ea	00781-1764-01	71.76		AB
100s ea UD	00781-1764-13	87.30		AB
1000s ea	00781-1764-10	681.72		AB
50 mg, 100s ea	00781-1766-01	121.88		AB
100s ea UD	00781-1766-13	146.26		AB
1000s ea	00781-1766-10	1157.86		AB
(A-S Medication) REPACK				
TAB, PO, 25 mg, 30s ea	54569-0194-00	21.53		EE
(DHS, Inc.) REPACK				
TAB, PO, 50 mg, 30s ea	55887-0288-30	67.05		AB
(HomeMed) REPACK				
TAB, PO, 25 mg, 40s ea	51655-0148-51	9.30		EE
50s ea	51655-0148-77	11.05		EE
50 mg, 40s ea	51655-0223-51	10.80		EE
(PD-Rx Pharm) REPACK				
TAB, PO, 25 mg, 14s ea	55289-0144-14	16.31		AB
30s ea	55289-0144-30	27.33		AB
90s ea	55289-0144-90	68.67		AB
(Pharma Pac) REPACK				
TAB, PO, 25 mg, 30s ea	52959-0791-30	22.50		AB
(Phys Total Care) REPACK				
TAB, PO, 10 mg, 30s ea	54868-2571-00	22.29		AB
60s ea	54868-2571-01	40.08		
25 mg, 30s ea	54868-1344-00	30.90		EE
50s ea	54868-1344-02	49.50		EE
60s ea	54868-1344-04	58.80		AB
100s ea	54868-1344-03	96.00		EE
50 mg, 15s ea	54868-2221-05	18.64		AB
30s ea	54868-2221-03	34.28		EE
60s ea	54868-2221-01	65.56		EE
100s ea	54868-2221-00	81.23		EE
1000s ea	54868-2221-04	798.79		EE
(Quality Care Prod) REPACK				
TAB, PO, 25 mg, 30s ea	49999-0400-30	15.71		AB

PROD/MFR	NDC	AWP	DP	OBC
(Southwood)				
REPACK				
TAB, PO, 10 mg, 12s ea	**58016-0839-12**	5.16		EE
15s ea	**58016-0839-15**	6.44		EE
20s ea	**58016-0839-20**	8.59		EE
30s ea	**58016-0839-30**	12.89		EE
60s ea	**58016-0839-60**	25.78		EE
90s ea	**58016-0839-90**	38.66		EE
100s ea	**58016-0839-00**	42.96		EE
120s ea	**58016-0839-02**	51.55		EE
25 mg, 12s ea	**58016-0841-12**	8.61		EE
15s ea	**58016-0841-15**	10.76		EE
20s ea	**58016-0841-20**	14.35		EE
30s ea	**58016-0841-30**	21.53		EE
60s ea	**58016-0841-60**	43.05		EE
90s ea	**58016-0841-90**	64.58		EE
100s ea	**58016-0841-00**	71.75		EE
120s ea	**58016-0841-02**	86.10		EE
50 mg, 12s ea	**58016-0866-12**	13.89		EE
15s ea	**58016-0866-15**	17.36		EE
20s ea	**58016-0866-20**	23.15		EE
30s ea	**58016-0866-30**	34.73		EE
60s ea	**58016-0866-60**	69.46		EE
90s ea	**58016-0866-90**	104.18		EE
100s ea	**58016-0866-00**	115.76		EE
120s ea	**58016-0866-02**	138.91		EE
(Stat Rx)				
REPACK				
TAB, PO, 25 mg, 30s ea	**16590-0577-30**	42.00		AB
60s ea	**16590-0577-60**	75.00		AB
90s ea	**16590-0577-90**	100.00		AB
(Vibranta)				
REPACK				
TAB, PO, 25 mg, 30s ea	**57866-3930-01**	14.72		AB
50 mg, 30s ea	**57866-3931-01**	20.77		AB
IMIPRAMINE HYDROCHLORIDE				
FUL				
TAB, PO, 10 mg, 100s ea		26.43		
25 mg, 100s ea		35.51		
50 mg, 100s ea		46.04		
(Consolidated Midland) *See IMIPRAMINE HCL*				
(Covidien) *See TOFRANIL*				
(Gallipot) *See IMIPRAMINE HCL*				
(Medisca) *See IMIPRAMINE HCL*				
(Mutual) *See IMIPRAMINE HCL*				
(Par) *See IMIPRAMINE HCL*				
(PCCA) *See IMIPRAMINE HCL*				
(Sandoz) *See IMIPRAMINE HCL*				
(Bryant Ranch)				
REPACK				
TAB, PO, 50 mg, 100s ea	**63629-1510-01**	98.65		
(Dispensing Solutions)				
REPACK				
TAB, PO, 10 mg, 30s ea	**55045-1794-08**	13.50		
100s ea	**55045-3799-01**	45.00		
25 mg, 30s ea	**55045-1721-08**	20.55		
100s ea	**55045-1721-00**	68.50		
50 mg, 30s ea	**55045-1722-08**	36.60		
100s ea	**55045-1722-01**	122.00		
IMIPRAMINE PAMOATE (Covidien)				
CAP, PO, 75 mg, 30s ea	**00406-9931-03**	505.73		
100 mg, 30s ea	**00406-9932-03**	505.73		
125 mg, 30s ea	**00406-9933-03**	505.73		
150 mg, 30s ea	**00406-9934-03**	505.73		
(Covidien) *See TOFRANIL-PM*				
IMIPRAMINE PM (Pharma Pac)				
REPACK				
imipramine pamoate				
CAP, PO, 75 mg, 30s ea	**52959-0900-30**	389.98		
IMIQUIMOD				
(Graceway) *See ALDARA*				
IMITREX (Glaxo)				
sumatriptan succinate				
SOL, SC (SRN,PREFILLED,UNIT/USE)				
6 mg/0.5 ml, 0.5 ml 2s	**68115-0770-02**	183.74		
(S.D.V.,5X0.5ML)				
6 mg/0.5 ml, 0.5 ml 5s	**00173-0449-02**	534.16		
(Glaxo)				
sumatriptan				
SPR, NS (SINGLE USE)				
5 mg, 6s ea	**00173-0524-00**	274.38		
20 mg, 6s ea	**00173-0523-00**	274.38		

PROD/MFR	NDC	AWP	DP	OBC
(Glaxo)				
sumatriptan succinate				
TAB, PO (FILM-COATED)				
25 mg, 9s ea	**00173-0735-00**	286.34		
50 mg, 9s ea	**00173-0736-01**	266.11		
100 mg, 9s ea	**00173-0737-01**	266.11		
(A-S Medication)				
REPACK				
SOL, SC (S.D.V.)				
6 mg/0.5 ml, 0.5 ml 5s	**54569-3704-00**	425.25		
TAB, PO (FILM-COATED)				
50 mg, 9s ea	**54569-4191-00**	329.47		
(Altura)				
REPACK				
sumatriptan				
SPR, NS (SINGLE USE)				
20 mg, 6s ea	**63874-0897-06**	131.09		
(Altura)				
sumatriptan succinate				
TAB, PO, 25 mg, 9s ea	**63874-0898-09**	151.26		
(DHS, Inc.)				
REPACK				
TAB, PO, 25 mg, 18s ea	**55887-0513-18**	359.01		
100 mg, 9s ea	**55887-0148-09**	201.69		
(Dispensing Solutions)				
REPACK				
SOL, SC (5X0.5ML)				
6 mg/0.5 ml, 0.5 ml 5s	**55045-3512-01**	390.00		
(Dispensing Solutions)				
sumatriptan				
SPR, NS, 5 mg, 6s ea	**55045-3732-06**	207.00		
20 mg, 6s ea	**55045-3502-01**	207.00		
(Dispensing Solutions)				
sumatriptan succinate				
TAB, PO, 50 mg, 9s ea	**55045-3040-09**	211.50		
100 mg, 9s ea	**55045-3731-09**	211.50		
(Pharma Pac)				
REPACK				
TAB, PO, 25 mg, 9s ea	**52959-0422-09**	173.62		
50 mg, 9s ea	**52959-0477-09**	152.80		
100 mg, 9s ea	**52959-0909-09**	212.75		
(Phys Total Care)				
REPACK				
KIT, SC (SRN, SELF DOSE SYSTEM)				
6 mg/0.5 ml, ea	**54868-3180-00**	225.98		
SOL, SC (S.D.V.)				
6 mg/0.5 ml, 0.5 ml 2s	**54868-2652-00**	82.83		
(SRN)				
6 mg/0.5 ml, 2 ml	**54868-3181-00**	190.65		
(SDV)				
6 mg/0.5 ml, 5 ml	**54868-2652-01**	409.13		
(Phys Total Care)				
sumatriptan				
SPR, NS, 5 mg, 0.1 ml 6s	**54868-4764-00**	222.16		
(SINGLE USE)				
20 mg, 6s ea	**54868-4606-00**	172.70		
(Phys Total Care)				
sumatriptan succinate				
TAB, PO, 25 mg, 9s ea	**54868-3777-00**	200.98		
50 mg, 9s ea	**54868-3852-00**	262.38		
(FILM-COATED)				
100 mg, 9s ea	**54868-5118-00**	287.03		
(Physician Partner)				
REPACK				
TAB, PO (FILM-COATED)				
50 mg, 9s ea	**21695-0154-09**	459.48		
(Quality Care Prod)				
REPACK				
sumatriptan				
SPR, NS, 20 mg, 6s ea	**49999-0822-06**	229.28		
(Quality Care Prod)				
sumatriptan succinate				
TAB, PO (FILM-COATED)				
50 mg, 9s ea	**35356-0253-09**	498.60		
90s ea	**35356-0253-18**	825.20		
100 mg, 9s ea	**35356-0254-09**	498.60		
(Southwood)				
REPACK				
sumatriptan				
SPR, NS, 20 mg, 0.1 ml 6s	**58016-1231-01**	248.87		

PROD/MFR	NDC	AWP	DP	OBC
(Southwood)				
sumatriptan succinate				
TAB, PO (FILM-COATED)				
25 mg, 9s ea	**58016-0246-09**	259.73		
50 mg, 9s ea	**58016-5574-09**	241.37		
(Stat Rx)				
REPACK				
TAB, PO, 25 mg, 9s ea	**16590-0127-09**	175.00		
100 mg, 9s ea	**16590-0128-09**	175.00		
IMITREX STAT DOSE REFILL (Dispensing Solutions)				
REPACK				
sumatriptan succinate				
KIT, SC, 6 mg/0.5 ml, ea	**55045-3271-01**	170.00		
IMITREX STATDOSE (Glaxo)				
sumatriptan succinate				
SOL, SC (PEN & 2 SYRINGES)				
4 mg/0.5 ml, ea	**00173-0739-00**	229.02		
(REFILL W/2 SYRINGES)				
4 mg/0.5 ml, ea	**00173-0739-02**	216.92		
IMITREX STATDOSE REFILL (Glaxo)				
sumatriptan succinate				
KIT, SC (2 SRN CARTRIDGES)				
6 mg/0.5 ml, ea	**00173-0478-00**	216.92		
IMITREX STATDOSE SYSTEM (Glaxo)				
sumatriptan succinate				
KIT, SC (2 SRN CARTRIDGES & PEN)				
6 mg/0.5 ml, ea	**00173-0479-00**	229.02		
IMMUNE GLOBULIN				
(Amer Red Cross-Blood) *See PANGLOBULIN NF*				
(Baxter Bioscience) *See GAMMAGARD LIQUID*				
(Baxter Bioscience) *See GAMMAGARD S/D*				
(Baxter Bioscience) *See GAMMAGARD S/D (IGA<1UG/ML)*				
(CSL) *See CARIMUNE NF*				
(CSL) *See PRIVIGEN*				
(CSL) *See VIVAGLOBIN*				
(Grifols USA, Inc.) *See FLEBOGAMMA*				
(Grifols USA, Inc.) *See FLEBOGAMMA 5%*				
(Grifols USA, Inc.) *See FLEBOGAMMA 5% DIF*				
(Octapharma USA) *See OCTAGAM*				
(Talecris) *See GAMASTAN S/D*				
(Talecris) *See GAMUNEX*				
IMOGAM RABIES-HT (Sanofi)				
rabies immune globulin				
SOL, IM (VIAL,PF)				
150 iu/ml, 2 ml	**49281-0190-20**	358.80	299.00	
10 ml	**49281-0190-10**	1794.00	1495.00	
IMOGEN (PGD, Inc.)				
loperamide hydrochloride				
LIQ, PO (AF,SF)				
1 mg/5 ml, 473 ml	**55422-0419-16**	8.00		
IMOVAX RABIES (Sanofi)				
rabies vaccine				
PDR, IM (SRNDLUENT,PLNGR,SDV,PF)				
2.5 iu, ea	**49281-0250-51**	234.00	195.00	
(Quality Care Prod)				
REPACK				
PDR, IM (SDV W/DILUENT,SRN,PF)				
2.5 iu, ea	**49999-0414-01**	190.56		
IMPLANT INSERTION DEVICE				
(AxoGen) *See AVANCE NERVE GRAFT*				
(AxoGen) *See AXOGUARD NERVE CONNECTOR*				
(AxoGen) *See AXOGUARD NERVE PROTECTOR*				
(Covidien) *See PERMACOL*				
IMURAN (Prometheus Labs)				
azathioprine				
TAB, PO, 50 mg, 100s ea	**65483-0590-10**	385.22		AB
(Pharma Pac)				
REPACK				
TAB, PO, 50 mg, 100s ea	**52959-0079-00**	163.03		AB
(Phys Total Care)				
REPACK				
TAB, PO, 50 mg, 20s ea	**54868-0921-02**	60.31		AB
30s ea	**54868-0921-01**	89.54		AB
50s ea	**54868-0921-04**	147.98		AB
INAMRINONE (Bedford)				
inamrinone lactate				
SOL, IV (S.D.V.)				
5 mg/ml, 20 ml	**55390-0042-10**	126.00		

PROD/MFR	NDC	AWP	DP	OBC
INAMRINONE LACTATE				
(Bedford) *See INAMRINONE*				
INATAL ADVANCE (Nnodum)				
prenatal vitamins				
TAB, PO (9X10,DYE-FREE)				
90s ea UD	**63044-0153-64**	13.99		
INATAL GT (Nnodum)				
prenatal vitamins				
TAB, PO (10X9)				
90s ea	**63044-0159-10**	50.99		
INATAL ULTRA TAB (Nnodum)				
prenatal vitamins				
TAB, PO (10X10)				
100s ea UD	**63044-0154-63**	20.99		
INCONTINENCE PRODUCTS				
(Coloplast) *See CONVEEN SECURITY + URINE LEG BAG*				
(Covidien) *See CURITY BEDSIDE DRAIN BAG*				
(Covidien) *See KENGUARD URINARY DRAINAGE BAG*				
INCRELEX (Tercica)				
mecasermin				
SOL, SC (10X4ML,M.D.V.)				
10 mg/ml, 4 ml 10s	**15054-1040-05**	8785.20		
INDAPAMIDE				
FUL				
TAB, PO, 1.25 mg,				
100s ea		10.35		
2.5 mg, 100s ea		11.25		
(Actavis)				
TAB, PO, 1.25 mg, 100s ea	**00228-2597-11**	67.95		AB
1000s ea	**00228-2597-96**	613.00		AB
2.5 mg, 100s ea	**00228-2571-11**	83.05		AB
1000s ea	**00228-2571-96**	811.75		AB
(Mylan)				
TAB, PO (FILM-COATED)				
1.25 mg, 100s ea	**00378-0069-01**	67.95		AB
500s ea	**00378-0069-05**	380.90		AB
(USP,FILM-COATED)				
2.5 mg, 90s ea	**00378-0080-77**	74.75		AB
(FILM-COATED)				
2.5 mg, 100s ea	**00378-0080-01**	83.05		AB
1000s ea	**00378-0080-10**	811.75		AB
(PCCA)				
POW, NA (U.S.P.)				
1 gm	**51927-2685-00**	99.00		
(UDL)				
TAB, PO (10X10)				
2.5 mg, 100s ea UD	**51079-0868-20**	85.28		AB
(A-S Medication)				
REPACK				
TAB, PO, 2.5 mg, 90s ea	**54569-8604-00**	74.75		EE
(DHS, Inc.)				
REPACK				
TAB, PO, 1.25 mg, 30s ea	**55887-0359-30**	15.56		AB
2.5 mg, 30s ea	**55887-0358-30**	16.05		AB
60s ea	**55887-0358-60**	49.83		
(PD-Rx Pharm)				
REPACK				
TAB, PO (USP,FILM-COATED)				
1.25 mg, 90s ea	**43063-0124-90**	21.40		AB
2.5 mg, 90s ea	**43063-0123-90**	23.20		AB
(Phys Total Care)				
REPACK				
TAB, PO, 1.25 mg, 30s ea	**54868-3885-00**	6.87		EE
100s ea	**54868-3885-01**	14.37		AB
2.5 mg, 30s ea	**54868-3106-00**	9.81		EE
60s ea	**54868-3106-02**	15.12		EE
100s ea	**54868-3106-03**	20.67		AB
(Quality Care Prod)				
REPACK				
TAB, PO (FILM-COATED)				
1.25 mg, 30s ea	**35356-0227-30**	31.88		AB
100s ea	**35356-0226-00**	106.00		AB
(Southwood)				
REPACK				
TAB, PO, 2.5 mg, 30s ea	**58016-0088-30**	30.54		
60s ea	**58016-0088-60**	61.08		
90s ea	**58016-0088-90**	91.62		
100s ea	**58016-0088-00**	101.80		
(Vibranta)				
REPACK				
TAB, PO, 2.5 mg, 30s ea	**57866-3971-01**	25.45		AB
INDERAL LA (Akrimax)				
propranolol hydrochloride				
CER, PO, 60 mg, 100s ea	**24090-0470-88**	461.62		AB
80 mg, 100s ea	**24090-0471-88**	539.19		AB
120 mg, 100s ea	**24090-0473-88**	668.83		AB
160 mg, 100s ea	**24090-0479-88**	875.66		AB
(Phys Total Care)				
REPACK				
CER, PO, 60 mg, 10s ea	**54868-1441-01**	19.00		
30s ea	**54868-1441-00**	53.26		
80 mg, 10s ea	**54868-0680-01**	21.89		
30s ea	**54868-0680-00**	61.90		
120 mg, 10s ea	**54868-1442-02**	26.69		
30s ea	**54868-1442-01**	76.31		
100s ea	**54868-1442-00**	235.60		
160 mg, 10s ea	**54868-2572-01**	34.36		
30s ea	**54868-2572-00**	99.32		
100s ea	**54868-2572-02**	308.04		
(Southwood)				
REPACK				
CER, PO, 80 mg, 30s ea	**58016-0859-30**	134.91		AB
60s ea	**58016-0859-60**	269.81		AB
90s ea	**58016-0859-90**	404.72		AB
100s ea	**58016-0859-00**	449.69		AB
INDICLOR (GE)				
indium in 111 chloride				
SOL, IJ, 5 mci/0.5 ml,				
0.5 ml	**17156-0523-01**	613.92		
INDIGO CARMINE (Akorn)				
indigotindisulfonate sodium				
SOL, IJ (10X5ML)				
8 mg/ml, 5 ml 10s	**17478-0508-01**	83.50		
(Amer Regent)				
SOL, IJ (AMP)				
8 mg/ml, 5 ml 10s	**00517-0375-10**	90.00		
(Consolidated Midland)				
SOL, IJ (AMP)				
8 mg/ml, 5 ml 10s	**00223-7902-05**	150.00		
INDIGOTINDISULFONATE SODIUM				
(Akorn) *See INDIGO CARMINE*				
(Amer Regent) *See INDIGO CARMINE*				
(Consolidated Midland) *See INDIGO CARMINE*				
INDINAVIR SULFATE				
(Merck) *See CRIXIVAN*				
INDIUM IN 111 CAPROMAB PENDETIDE				
(EUSA) *See PROSTASCINT*				
INDIUM IN 111 CHLORIDE				
(GE) *See INDICLOR*				
INDIUM IN 111 OXYQUINOLINE				
(GE) *See INDIUM IN-111 OXYQUINOLINE*				
INDIUM IN 111 PENTETATE DISODIUM				
(GE) *See INDIUM IN-111 DTPA*				
INDIUM IN 111 PENTETREOTIDE				
(Mallinckrodt Inc.) *See OCTREOSCAN*				
INDIUM IN-111 DTPA (GE)				
indium in 111 pentetate disodium				
SOL, IN (S.D.V.)				
1 mci/ml, 1.5 ml	**17156-0251-08**	1011.77		
INDIUM IN-111 OXYQUINOLINE (GE)				
indium in 111 oxyquinoline				
SOL, IJ, 1 mci/ml, 1 ml	**17156-0021-01**	637.44		
INDIUM SULFATE (PCCA)				
POW, NA, 1 gm	**51927-3452-00**	60.00		
INDOCIN (Iroko)				
indomethacin				
SUP, RC, 50 mg, 30s ea	**42211-0102-43**	259.88		EE
SUS, PO (1X237ML)				
25 mg/5 ml, 237 ml	**42211-0101-11**	195.56		
(Lundbeck)				
indomethacin sodium				
PDS, IV, 1 mg, 3s ea	**67386-0511-51**	1927.80	108.88	
(Phys Total Care)				
REPACK				
indomethacin				
CAP, P.O, 25 mg, 20s ea	**54868-0738-02**	17.68		AB
INDOCIN SR (Forte Pharma)				
indomethacin				
CER, PO (UNIT OF USE)				
75 mg, 60s ea	**64814-0695-60**	167.01		AB
(Phys Total Care)				
REPACK				
CER, PO, 75 mg, 30s ea	**54868-0878-00**	83.18		AB
INDOCYANINE GREEN				
(Akorn) *See IC-GREEN ANGIOGRAPHY*				
(HUB Pharma)				
PDS, IV (W/ DILUENT,USP)				
25 mg, ea	**25431-0424-02**	635.95		AP
(PCCA)				
POW, NA, ea	**51927-3354-00**	15.00		
INDOLE 3 CARBINOL (PCCA)				
indole-3-carbinol				
POW, NA (1X1GM)				
1 gm	**51927-3203-00**	5.85		
INDOLE-3-CARBINOL				
(PCCA) *See INDOLE 3 CARBINOL*				
INDOMETHACIN (Bedford)				
indomethacin sodium				
PDS, IV (SDV, USP,LYOPHILIZED)				
1 mg, ea	**55390-0299-01**	600.00		AP
INDOMETHACIN (Consolidated Midland)				
CAP, PO, 25 mg, 100s ea	**00223-1195-01**	6.50		EE
500s ea	**00223-1195-05**	29.50		EE
50 mg, 100s ea	**00223-1196-01**	7.50		EE
500s ea	**00223-1196-05**	31.95		EE
(Forte Pharma) *See INDOCIN SR*				
(G&W)				
SUP, RC, 50 mg, 30s ea	**00713-0176-30**	75.00		
(Gallipot)				
POW, NA (U.S.P.,N.F.)				
5 gm	**51552-0262-02**	10.15		
25 gm	**51552-0262-04**	26.32		
100 gm	**51552-0262-05**	88.20		
(Hawkins)				
POW, NA (USP)				
5 gm	**63370-0114-15**	36.00		
25 gm	**63370-0114-25**	72.00		
100 gm	**63370-0114-35**	236.00		
500 gm	**63370-0114-45**	900.00		
1000 gm	**63370-0114-50**	1500.00		
(Iroko) *See INDOCIN*				
(KVK)				
CER, PO, 75 mg, 60s ea	**10702-0016-06**	182.12		
100s ea	**10702-0016-01**	303.53		
500s ea	**10702-0016-50**	1517.65		
1000s ea	**10702-0016-10**	3003.68		
(Letco)				
POW, NA (U.S.P.)				
25 gm	**62991-1239-02**	54.00		
100 gm	**62991-1239-01**	177.00		
(Major)				
CAP, PO (USP,10X10)				
25 mg, 100s ea UD	**00904-5926-61**	54.49		EE
50 mg, 100s ea UD	**00904-5927-61**	64.14		EE
CER, PO (10X10)				
75 mg, 100s ea UD	**00904-5966-61**	442.92		
(USP)				
75 mg, 100s ea	**00904-5966-60**	288.35		
500s ea	**00904-5966-40**	1441.76		
(Medisca)				
POW, NA (U.S.P.)				
5 gm	**38779-0076-03**	25.50		
25 gm	**38779-0076-04**	63.00		
100 gm	**38779-0076-05**	202.50		
500 gm	**38779-0076-08**	705.00		
1000 gm	**38779-0076-09**	1185.00		
(Mylan)				
CAP, PO, 25 mg, 100s ea	**00378-0143-01**	38.00		AB
1000s ea	**00378-0143-10**	379.80		AB
50 mg, 100s ea	**00378-0147-01**	63.50		AB
500s ea	**00378-0147-05**	317.50		AB
(PCCA)				
POW, NA (U.S.P.)				
1 gm	**51927-1083-00**	3.00		
(Sandoz)				
CAP, PO, 25 mg, 100s ea	**00781-2325-01**	38.00		AB
1000s ea	**00781-2325-10**	379.80		AB
50 mg, 100s ea	**00781-2350-01**	63.50		AB
CER, PO, 75 mg, 60s ea	**00185-0720-60**	180.22		AB
100s ea	**00185-0720-01**	300.37		AB
500s ea	**00185-0720-05**	1501.84		AB
(Spectrum Pharmacy)				
POW, NA (U.S.P.)				
25 gm	**49452-3670-02**	100.45		
100 gm	**49452-3670-03**	310.45		
(1X1000GM,USP)				
1000 gm	**49452-3670-05**	1704.50		
(Teva)				
CAP, PO (USP)				
25 mg, 100s ea	**00093-4029-01**	38.20		
1000s ea	**00093-4029-10**	362.90		
50 mg, 100s ea	**00093-4030-01**	63.75		
500s ea	**00093-4030-05**	310.78		

PROD/MFR	NDC	AWP	DP	OBC
(UDL)				
CAP, PO (10X10)				
25 mg, 100s ea UD	51079-0190-20	40.17		AB
(USP,10X30 PUNCH CARDS)				
25 mg, 300s ea UD	51079-0190-56	120.51		EE
(10X10)				
50 mg, 100s ea UD	51079-0191-20	67.88		AB
(USP,10X30)				
50 mg, 300s ea UD	51079-0191-56	203.64		AB
(A-S Medication)				
REPACK				
CAP, PO, 25 mg, 15s ea	54569-0277-04	5.72		EE
28s ea	54569-4123-02	10.67		EE
30s ea	54569-0277-01	11.43		EE
100s ea	54569-0277-03	38.10		EE
50 mg, 15s ea	54569-0275-05	9.54		EE
21s ea	54569-0275-00	13.36		EE
30s ea	54569-0275-01	19.09		EE
CER, PO, 75 mg, 14s ea	54569-1518-02	42.27		AB
20s ea	54569-1518-03	60.39		AB
30s ea	54569-1518-00	90.59		AB
(Altura)				
REPACK				
CAP, PO, 25 mg, 8s ea	63874-0318-08	4.53		AB
20s ea	63874-0318-20	11.33		AB
21s ea	63874-0318-21	19.08		AB
22s ea	63874-0318-22	19.99		AB
25s ea	63874-0318-25	22.71		EE
28s ea	63874-0318-28	25.44		AB
30s ea	63874-0318-30	27.26		EE
40s ea	63874-0318-40	36.34		AB
50s ea	63874-0318-50	45.42		AB
60s ea	63874-0318-60	54.51		AB
75s ea	63874-0318-75	68.13		AB
90s ea	63874-0318-90	81.77		AB
100s ea	63874-0318-01	90.85		AB
1000s ea	63874-0318-02	908.57		EE
50 mg, 14s ea	63874-0394-14	13.35		AB
15s ea	63874-0394-15	16.54		EE
20s ea	63874-0394-20	22.05		AB
21s ea	63874-0394-21	23.16		AB
30s ea	63874-0394-30	28.61		EE
40s ea	63874-0394-40	36.96		AB
50s ea	63874-0394-50	46.20		AB
60s ea	63874-0394-60	55.44		AB
100s ea	63874-0394-01	92.40		AB
1000s ea	63874-0394-02	1102.67		EE
(Bryant Ranch)				
REPACK				
CAP, PO, 25 mg, 20s ea	63629-1780-01	23.59		
30s ea	63629-1780-02	28.38		
50 mg, 21s ea	63629-1418-01	21.38		
30s ea	63629-1418-03	30.54		
42s ea	63629-1418-02	42.76		
(Core)				
REPACK				
CAP, PO, 25 mg, 20s ea	33358-0195-20	24.18		
30s ea	33358-0195-30	29.10		
50 mg, 21s ea	33358-0196-21	21.91		
30s ea	33358-0196-30	31.30		
60s ea	33358-0196-60	46.46		
(DHS, Inc.)				
REPACK				
CAP, PO, 25 mg, 20s ea	55887-0917-20	12.21		AB
21s ea	55887-0917-21	12.82		AB
30s ea	55887-0917-30	28.38		AB
90s ea	55887-0917-90	34.00		AB
50 mg, 15s ea	55887-0928-15	15.03		
20s ea	55887-0928-20	20.05		AB
21s ea	55887-0928-21	21.04		
30s ea	55887-0928-30	30.98		AB
(Dispensing Solutions)				
REPACK				
CAP, PO, 25 mg, 20s ea	55045-1163-02	15.00		AB
30s ea	55045-1163-08	22.50		AB
30s ea	66336-0684-30	24.69		AB
40s ea	55045-1163-04	30.00		AB
60s ea	55045-1163-06	45.00		
90s ea	55045-1163-09	67.50		AB
100s ea	55045-1163-01	75.00		AB
50 mg, 21s ea	55045-1385-07	22.89		AB
30s ea	55045-1385-08	32.70		AB
60s ea	55045-1385-02	65.40		AB
100s ea	55045-1385-01	109.00		
CER, PO, 75 mg, 15s ea	55045-1437-06	32.10		AB
30s ea	55045-1437-08	64.20		AB
(GSMS)				
REPACK				
CAP, PO (UNIT OF USE)				
25 mg, 21s ea	60429-0098-21	7.65	2.55	AB
(HomeMed)				
REPACK				
CAP, PO, 25 mg, 15s ea	51655-0128-54	4.15		EE
30s ea	51655-0128-24	27.69		EE
90s ea	51655-0128-26	19.90		EE
50 mg, 21s ea	51655-0230-28	20.69		EE
30s ea	51655-0230-24	27.99		EE
CER, PO, 75 mg, 14s ea	51655-0582-84	23.50		
(Keltman Pharma., Inc.)				
REPACK				
CAP, PO, 25 mg, 30s ea	68387-0344-30	27.12		
CER, PO, 75 mg, 30s ea	68387-0345-30	160.92		
(Nucare Pharm)				
REPACK				
CAP, PO, 25 mg, 30s ea	66267-0119-30	19.19		EE
50 mg, 20s ea	66267-0120-20	18.97		EE
30s ea	66267-0120-30	28.46		EE
100s ea	66267-0926-00	65.80		EE
CER, PO, 75 mg, 14s ea	66267-0121-14	24.45		EE
15s ea	66267-0121-15	26.89		EE
20s ea	66267-0121-20	34.93		EE
(Palmetto)				
REPACK				
CAP, PO, 25 mg, 30s ea	23490-5755-01	22.50		
60s ea	23490-5755-02	45.00		
90s ea	23490-5755-03	67.50		
50 mg, 6s ea	23490-5756-06	6.86		
20s ea	23490-5756-01	22.88		
21s ea	23490-5756-03	24.02		
30s ea	23490-5756-02	34.32		
60s ea	23490-5756-09	68.64		
CER, PO, 75 mg, 30s ea	23490-5758-01	79.50		
60s ea	23490-5758-02	159.00		
(PD-Rx Pharm)				
REPACK				
CAP, PO, 25 mg, 15s ea	55289-0147-15	18.00		AB
20s ea	55289-0147-20	19.50		AB
21s ea	55289-0147-21	19.80		AB
30s ea	55289-0147-30	24.00		AB
(REDI-SCRIPT)				
25 mg, 42s ea	58864-0296-42	18.40		AB
90s ea	58864-0296-90	20.89		AB
50 mg, 20s ea	55289-0663-20	25.50		AB
30s ea	55289-0663-30	32.97		AB
100s ea	55289-0663-01	88.65		AB
CER, PO, 75 mg, 10s ea	55289-0469-10	61.57		AB
14s ea	55289-0469-14	82.33		AB
15s ea	55289-0469-15	87.50		AB
20s ea	55289-0469-20	113.10		AB
30s ea	55289-0469-30	164.63		AB
(Pharma Pac)				
REPACK				
CAP, PO, 25 mg, 20s ea	52959-0080-20	13.59		EE
21s ea	52959-0080-21	14.27		EE
25s ea	52959-0080-25	16.98		EE
30s ea	52959-0080-30	20.37		EE
40s ea	52959-0080-40	27.15		EE
90s ea	52959-0080-90	60.84		EE
50 mg, 20s ea	52959-0081-20	20.36		EE
21s ea	52959-0081-21	21.35		EE
30s ea	52959-0081-30	29.57		EE
40s ea	52959-0081-40	37.70		EE
90s ea	52959-0081-90	62.17		EE
100s ea	52959-0081-00	69.09		EE
CER, PO, 75 mg, 7s ea	52959-0082-07	16.54		EE
14s ea	52959-0082-14	33.08		EE
15s ea	52959-0082-15	35.45		EE
20s ea	52959-0082-20	54.80		EE
21s ea	52959-0082-21	49.62		EE
30s ea	52959-0082-30	81.87		EE
60s ea	52959-0082-60	162.89		EE
(Phys Total Care)				
REPACK				
CAP, PO, 25 mg, 15s ea	54868-0074-08	21.69		EE
20s ea	54868-0074-09	27.91		EE
30s ea	54868-0074-03	40.38		EE
40s ea	54868-0074-04	52.83		EE
60s ea	54868-0074-05	77.74		EE
90s ea	54868-0074-07	88.74		EE
100s ea	54868-0074-02	98.25		EE
1000s ea	54868-0074-00	872.16		EE
50 mg, 15s ea	54868-0875-07	16.82		EE
20s ea	54868-0875-06	20.93		EE
30s ea	54868-0875-02	29.15		EE
40s ea	54868-0875-04	37.36		EE
60s ea	54868-0875-00	53.79		EE
90s ea	54868-0875-05	78.44		EE
100s ea	54868-0875-01	86.65		EE
CER, PO, 75 mg, 15s ea	54868-0922-07	87.11		EE
20s ea	54868-0922-03	115.14		EE
30s ea	54868-0922-01	171.22		EE
40s ea	54868-0922-06	227.29		EE
60s ea	54868-0922-02	319.24		EE
100s ea	54868-0922-00	532.57		EE
(Physician Partner)				
REPACK				
CAP, PO (HARD GELATIN)				
25 mg, 30s ea	21695-0522-30	22.80		
60s ea	21695-0522-60	45.60		AB
50 mg, 21s ea	21695-0523-21	26.67		AB
(Quality Care Prod)				
REPACK				
CAP, PO, 25 mg, 15s ea	49999-0234-15	11.16		AB
20s ea	49999-0234-20	14.88		AB
30s ea	49999-0234-30	22.32		AB
60s ea	49999-0234-60	44.64		AB
90s ea	49999-0234-90	66.96		EE
50 mg, 15s ea	49999-0100-15	17.16		AB
21s ea	49999-0100-21	24.02		EE
30s ea	49999-0100-30	34.32		EE
50s ea	49999-0100-50	57.20		AB
60s ea	49999-0100-60	68.64		AB
90s ea	49999-0100-90	102.94		EE
CER, PO, 75 mg, 30s ea	49999-0371-30	162.34		AB
(Southwood)				
REPACK				
CAP, PO, 25 mg, 8s ea	58016-0235-08	4.94		EE
20s ea	58016-0235-20	12.36		EE
30s ea	58016-0235-30	18.54		EE
60s ea	58016-0235-60	37.08		EE
75s ea	58016-0235-75	46.35		EE
100s ea	58016-0235-00	61.80		EE
50 mg, 14s ea	58016-0236-14	13.35		EE
20s ea	58016-0236-20	19.07		EE
21s ea	58016-0236-21	20.02		EE
30s ea	58016-0236-30	28.60		EE
40s ea	58016-0236-40	38.13		EE
60s ea	58016-0236-60	57.20		EE
100s ea	58016-0236-00	95.33		EE
CER, PO, 75 mg, 7s ea	58016-0237-07	11.43		EE
10s ea	58016-0237-10	16.33		EE
12s ea	58016-0237-12	19.60		EE
14s ea	58016-0237-14	22.86		EE
15s ea	58016-0237-15	24.50		EE
20s ea	58016-0237-20	54.00		EE
21s ea	58016-0237-21	34.30		EE
24s ea	58016-0237-24	39.20		EE
28s ea	58016-0237-28	45.73		EE
40s ea	58016-0237-40	65.33		EE
(St. Mary's MPP)				
REPACK				
CAP, PO (USP)				
25 mg, 30s ea	60760-0402-30	17.98		AB
CER, PO, 75 mg, 14s ea	60760-0607-14	38.91		AB
(Stat Rx)				
REPACK				
CAP, PO, 25 mg, 20s ea	16590-0129-20	20.25		
30s ea	16590-0129-30	28.50		AB
120s ea	16590-0129-72	100.15		
50 mg, 20s ea	16590-0130-20	20.25		
28s ea	16590-0130-28	27.53		AB
60s ea	16590-0130-60	59.00		AB
CER, PO, 75 mg, 20s ea	16590-0131-20	115.51		AB
30s ea	16590-0131-30	113.53		AB
(Vibranta)				
REPACK				
CAP, PO, 25 mg, 30s ea	57866-3981-01	22.32		
60s ea	57866-3981-02	59.19		
50 mg, 21s ea	57866-3982-03	30.58		
30s ea	57866-3982-01	34.32		AB
40s ea	57866-3982-06	59.49		
90s ea	57866-3982-05	102.94		
CER, PO, 75 mg, 30s ea	57866-4939-02	62.17		AB
INDOMETHACIN ER (Core)				
REPACK				
indomethacin				
CER, PO, 75 mg, 30s ea	33358-0197-30	70.53		
(Southwood)				
REPACK				
CER, PO, 75 mg, 30s ea	58016-0237-30	102.60		
60s ea	58016-0237-60	205.20		
90s ea	58016-0237-90	307.80		
100s ea	58016-0237-00	342.00		

INDOMETHACIN SODIUM

(Bedford) *See INDOMETHACIN*

(Lundbeck) *See INDOCIN*

PROD/MFR NDC AWP DP OBC

INDOMETHACIN SR (Bryant Ranch)
REPACK
indomethacin
CER, PO, 75 mg, 30s ea ... 63629-3201-01 59.99
60s ea ... 63629-3201-02 115.65

INFANRIX (Glaxo)
dtap vaccine
SUS, IM (SD,TIP-LOK)
0.5 ml 5s ... 58160-0810-46 115.13
(10X0.5ML,SDV,TAX INCLD)
0.5 ml 10s ... 58160-0810-11 246.96

(A-S Medication)
REPACK
SUS, IM (S.D.V.,TAX INCL)
0.5 ml 10s ... 54569-4969-00 256.31

INFASURF (ONY)
calfactant
SUS, IT (1X3ML,SINGLE-USE)
35 mg/ml, 3 ml UD ... 61938-0456-03 413.64
(1X6ML,SINGLE-USE)
35 mg/ml, 6 ml UD ... 61938-0456-06 732.12

INFED (Watson)
iron dextran
SOL, IJ (INNER PACK,USP)
50 mg/ml, 2 ml ... 52544-0931-07 BP
(MW 165, S.D.V.)
50 mg/ml, 2 ml 10s ... 52544-0931-02 377.04 BP

(Phys Total Care)
REPACK
SOL, IJ (2MLX10)
50 mg/ml, 2 ml 10s ... 54868-4319-00 331.00

INFERGEN (Three Rivers Pharm)
interferon alfacon-1
SOL, SC (1X0.3ML,PF)
30 mcg/ml, 0.3 ml ... 66435-0201-95 140.56
(6X0.3ML,SDV,PF)
30 mcg/ml,
0.3 ml 6s ... 66435-0201-99 843.38
(1X0.5ML,PF)
30 mcg/ml, 0.5 ml ... 66435-0201-96 140.56
(6X0.5ML,SDV,PF)
30 mcg/ml,
0.5 ml 6s ... 66435-0201-15 843.38

INFERROUS (Clint)
vitamin b complex and iron
INJ, IJ (VIAL)
10 ml ... 55553-0010-10 24.95

INFLAMASE FORTE (Novartis Pharm)
prednisolone sodium phosphate
SOL, OP, 1%, 10 ml ... 58768-0877-10 27.03 AT

INFLIXIMAB
(Centocor) *See REMICADE*

INFLUDO (Weleda)
homeopathic substance
LIQ, PO, 20 ml ... 55946-0280-10 4.65

INFLUENZA A VIRUS VACCINE, H1N1, INACTIVATED
(CSL Biotherapies)
SUS, IM (2009,PF)
15 mcg/0.5 ml,
0.5 ml 10s ... 33332-0519-01
(2009, 1X5 MDVIAL)
15 mcg/0.5 ml,
5 ml ... 33332-0629-10

(Novartis)
SUS, IM (2009,PF)
15 mcg/0.5 ml,
0.5 ml 10s ... 66521-0200-02
(2009, 1X5 MDVIAL)
15 mcg/0.5 ml,
5 ml ... 66521-0200-10
(2009, 25X5ML MDVIAL)
15 mcg/0.5 ml,
5 ml 25s ... 66521-0200-25

(Sanofi)
SUS, IM (2009)
15 mcg/0.5 ml,
0.25 ml 10s ... 49281-0650-25
0.25 ml 25s ... 49281-0650-70
0.5 ml 10s ... 49281-0650-10
0.5 ml 10s ... 49281-0650-50
0.5 ml 25s ... 49281-0650-90
(2009, 1X5ML MDVIAL)
15 mcg/0.5 ml,
5 ml ... 49281-0640-15

PROD/MFR NDC AWP DP OBC

INFLUENZA A VIRUS VACCINE, H1N1, LIVE
(Medimmune)
SPR, NS (2009,PF)
10s ea ... 66019-0200-10

INFLUENZA VIRUS VACCINE
(CSL Biotherapies) *See AFLURIA*
(Novartis) *See AGRIFLU*
(Novartis) *See FLUVIRIN*

INFLUENZA VIRUS VACCINE (SUBVIRION)
(Glaxo) *See FLUARIX*
(Glaxo) *See FLULAVAL*
(Novartis) *See FLUVIRIN*
(Sanofi) *See FLUZONE HIGH-DOSE*

INFLUENZA VIRUS VACCINE, INACTIVATED
(Glaxo) *See FLUARIX*
(Sanofi) *See FLUZONE*

INFLUENZA VIRUS VACCINE, LIVE
(Medimmune) *See FLUMIST*

INFUMORPH 200 (Baxter)
morphine sulfate
SOL, IJ (PF)
10 mg/ml,
1 ml, C-II ... 60977-0114-74 156.00
(AMP, DOSETTE,PF)
10 mg/ml,
20 ml, C-II ... 60977-0114-01 156.00

INFUMORPH 500 (Baxter)
morphine sulfate
SOL, IJ (PF)
25 mg/ml,
1 ml, C-II ... 60977-0115-74 264.00
(AMP, DOSETTE,PF)
25 mg/ml,
20 ml, C-II ... 60977-0115-01 264.00

INFUSION PUMP, INSULIN
(Medtronic Minimed) *See PARADIGM 515*
(Medtronic Minimed) *See PARADIGM 522*
(Medtronic Minimed) *See PARADIGM 712*
(Medtronic Minimed) *See PARADIGM 715*
(Medtronic Minimed) *See PARADIGM 722*
(Medtronic Minimed) *See PARADIGM INSULIN PUMP PATHWAY PROGRAM*
(Medtronic Minimed) *See PARADIGM SURE-T INFUSION SET*
(Medtronic Minimed) *See SILHOUETTE PARADIGM INFUSION SET*

INFUSION PUMP, PARENTERAL
(Animas Corp.) *See ANIMAS INSULIN PUMP R1000*
(Medtronic Minimed) *See MINIMED SYRINGE RESERVOIR*
(Medtronic Minimed) *See PARADIGM POLYFIN QR WITH WINGS*
(Medtronic Minimed) *See PARADIGM RESERVOIR*
(Medtronic Minimed) *See SOF-SET MICRO NON-NEEDLE INFUSION*

INFUSION SET W/DRIP CHAMBER (GE)
kit, administration, intravenous
DEV, NA (VENTED)
10s ea ... 08024-3900-01 15.00

INFUVITE (Baxter)
multivitamin
SOL, IV (#1-5 MLX5,#2-5 MLX5,SDV)
10 ml 5s ... 54643-5649-01 40.99 34.16
(PHARMACY BULK PACK)
100 ml 10s ... 54643-5649-02 648.72 540.60

INFUVITE PEDIATRIC (Baxter)
multivitamin
SOL, IV (#1-4 MLX5,#2-1 MLX5,SDV)
5 ml 5s ... 54643-5646-01 64.50 53.75
(PHARMACY BULK PACKAGE)
50 ml ... 54643-5647-00 110.88 92.40

INJECTION DEVICE
(Novo Nordisk) *See INNOVO*

INJECTOR, MEDICATION (INOCULATOR)
(INJEX-Equidyne Systems) *See INJEX 30 AMPULES*
(INJEX-Equidyne Systems) *See INJEX 30 INJECTOR SYSTEM*
(INJEX-Equidyne Systems) *See INJEX 30 VIAL ADAPTERS*
(Novo Nordisk) *See NORDIPEN 15 DELIVERY SYSTEM*

PROD/MFR NDC AWP DP OBC

(Novo Nordisk) *See NORDIPEN 5 DELIVERY SYSTEM*

INJEX 30 AMPULES (INJEX-Equidyne Systems)
injector, medication (inoculator)
DEV, NA (0.3 ML, SINGLE USE)
100s ea ... 18270-0100-30 50.00 37.50

INJEX 30 INJECTOR SYSTEM (INJEX-Equidyne Systems)
injector, medication (inoculator)
DEV, NA (NEEDLE-FREE, STARTER)
ea ... 18270-0000-30 260.00 180.00

INJEX 30 VIAL ADAPTERS (INJEX-Equidyne Systems)
injector, medication (inoculator)
DEV, NA (SINGLE USE)
10s ea ... 18270-0201-10 10.00 8.00

INNOHEP (Celgene Corp)
tinzaparin sodium
SOL, SC (M.D.V.)
20000 iu/ml, 2 ml ... 67211-0342-08 181.44
2 ml 10s ... 67211-0342-53 1814.40

INNOPRAN XL (Glaxo)
propranolol hydrochloride
CER, PO, 80 mg, 30s ea ... 65726-0250-10 72.18
100s ea ... 65726-0250-25 240.62
120 mg, 30s ea ... 65726-0251-10 72.18
100s ea ... 65726-0251-25 240.62

(Phys Total Care)
REPACK
CER, PO, 120 mg, 30s ea ... 54868-5395-00 57.72

(Stat Rx)
REPACK
CER, PO, 80 mg, 30s ea ... 16590-0132-30 80.00
60s ea ... 16590-0132-60 160.00
120 mg, 30s ea ... 16590-0133-30 80.00
60s ea ... 16590-0133-60 160.00

INNOVO (Novo Nordisk)
injection device
DEV, NA (INSULIN DELIVERY SYSTEM)
ea ... 00169-1852-74 59.00

INOMAX (Ikaria / Ino)
nitric oxide
GAS, IH ($131.00/HOUR OF USE)
100 ppm, ea ... 64693-0001-01 137.50
ea ... 64693-0001-02 137.50
800 ppm, ea ... 64693-0002-01 137.50
ea ... 64693-0002-02 137.50

INOSINE (Medisca)
POW, NA (F.C.C.,ORAL)
25 gm ... 38779-0229-04 43.50
100 gm ... 38779-0229-05 147.00

(PCCA)
POW, NA, 1 gm ... 51927-1678-00 2.28

INOSITOL (Medisca)
POW, NA (1X25GM)
25 gm ... 38779-0284-04 28.50
(N.F.)
100 gm ... 38779-0284-05 58.50
500 gm ... 38779-0284-08 177.00

(PCCA)
POW, NA (PURIFIED)
1 gm ... 51927-1342-00 1.44

(Spectrum Pharmacy)
POW, NA (F.C.C.)
100 gm ... 49452-3692-01 97.30
500 gm ... 49452-3692-02 264.95

INOSITOL HEXANICOTINATE (Gallipot)
inositol niacinate
POW, NA, 1000 gm ... 51552-1005-07 138.60 99.00

(PCCA)
POW, NA, 1 gm ... 51927-2847-00 2.10

INOSITOL HEXAPHOSPHATE SODIUM SALT (PCCA)
phytic acid sodium
POW, NA (1X1GM)
1 gm ... 51927-3298-00 1.80

INOSITOL NIACINATE
(Gallipot) *See INOSITOL HEXANICOTINATE*
(PCCA) *See INOSITOL HEXANICOTINATE*

INPERSOL ADMINISTRATION SET (Abbott Hosp)
catheter
DEV, NA (11FR 11" W/L-CONNECTOR)
6s ea ... 00074-4711-01 109.30 109.32

INPERSOL PERITONEAL DIALYSIS TRAY (Abbott Hosp)
kit, administration, peritoneal dialysis, disp
DEV, NA, 4s ea ... 00074-4354-03 466.12 392.52

PROD/MFR	NDC	AWP	DP	OBC
INSPIRATION COMPRESSOR/NEBULIZER				
(Respironics)				
nebulizer, direct patient interface				
DEV, NA, ea	**83730-0006-26**	71.25		
INSPIREASE (Schering)				
spacer, inhalation				
DEV, NA (DRUG DEL. SYSTEM)				
ea	**00085-4602-02**	29.54		
(REPLACEMENT MOUTHPIECE)				
ea	**00085-4604-02**	21.38		
(RESERVOIR BAGS)				
3s ea	**00085-4602-03**	15.98		
(MOUTHPIECE)				
144s ea	**00085-4604-01**	1055.60		
(REPLACEMENT BAGS)				
144s ea	**00085-4602-70**	511.84		
INSPRA (Pfizer)				
eplerenone				
TAB, PO (FILM-COATED)				
25 mg, 30s ea	**00025-1710-01**	143.35	119.46	
90s ea	**00025-1710-02**	430.06	358.38	
(10X10,FILM-COATED)				
25 mg, 100s ea UD	**00025-1710-03**	477.86	398.22	
(FILM-COATED)				
50 mg, 30s ea	**00025-1720-03**	143.35	119.46	
90s ea	**00025-1720-01**	430.06	358.38	
(A-S Medication)				
REPACK				
TAB, PO (FILM-COATED)				
50 mg, 30s ea	**54569-6120-00**	143.59		
(Phys Total Care)				
REPACK				
TAB, PO (FILM-COATED)				
50 mg, 30s ea	**54868-5051-00**	126.25		
INSUFLON (Arkray)				
catheter				
DEV, NA (23GX19MM, INDWELLING)				
10s ea	**08317-9900-02**	72.30	48.20	
INSULIN ASPART, RECOMBINANT				
(Novo Nordisk) *See NOVOLOG*				
(Novo Nordisk) *See NOVOLOG FLEXPEN*				
INSULIN ASPART/INSULIN ASPART PROTAMINE				
(Novo Nordisk) *See NOVOLOG MIX 70/30*				
INSULIN BOVINE (Medisca)				
POW, NA, 1 gm	**38779-1932-06**	2385.00		
(PCCA)				
CRY, NA (PURIFIED BEEF)				
1 ml	**51927-3371-00**	0.11		
INSULIN DETEMIR				
(Novo Nordisk) *See LEVEMIR*				
INSULIN GLARGINE, RECOMBINANT				
(Sanofi-Aventis) *See LANTUS*				
(Sanofi-Aventis) *See LANTUS SOLOSTAR*				
INSULIN GLULISINE				
(Sanofi-Aventis) *See APIDRA*				
(Sanofi-Aventis) *See APIDRA SOLOSTAR*				
INSULIN HUMAN REGULAR				
(Lilly) *See HUMULIN R CONCENTRATED U-500*				
(Palmetto)				
REPACK				
SOL, IJ, 100 u/ml, 10 ml	**23490-6687-00**	38.00		
INSULIN LISPRO, RECOMBINANT				
(Lilly) *See HUMALOG*				
(Lilly) *See HUMALOG PEN*				
(Midwest IV) *See LISPRO-PFC*				
INSULIN LISPRO/INSULIN LISPRO PROTAMINE				
(Lilly) *See HUMALOG MIX 50/50*				
(Lilly) *See HUMALOG MIX 75/25*				
(Lilly) *See HUMALOG MIX 75/25 PEN*				
(Lilly) *See HUMALOG MIX75/25*				
INSULIN SYRINGE (Albertson's)				
insulin syringe/needle				
DEV, NA (29GX1/2",3/10CC)				
100s ea	**41163-4022-02**	17.50		
(AmerisourceBergen)				
DEV, NA (28GX1/2",1/2CC)				
100s ea	**36652-4000-01**	12.34		
100s ea	**36652-4009-01**	12.34		
(28GX1/2",1CC)				
100s ea	**36652-4000-04**	12.34		
100s ea	**36652-4009-04**	12.34		
(29GX1/2",1/2CC)				
100s ea	**36652-4000-03**	17.73		
100s ea	**36652-4009-03**	14.08		
(29GX1/2",1CC)				
100s ea	**36652-4000-05**	11.73		
100s ea	**36652-4009-05**	14.08		
(29GX1/2",3/10CC)				
100s ea	**36652-4000-02**	11.73		
100s ea	**36652-4009-02**	14.08		
(30GX5/16",1/2CC,SHT NDL)				
100s ea	**36652-4000-08**	14.15		
100s ea	**36652-4009-07**	14.08		
(30GX5/16",1CC,SHT NDL)				
100s ea	**36652-4000-06**	15.72		
100s ea	**36652-4009-06**	12.73		
(30GX5/16",3/10CC,SHT ND)				
100s ea	**36652-4000-07**	14.15		
100s ea	**36652-4009-08**	12.67		
(McKesson)				
DEV, NA (0.3 CC, 29GX1/2")				
100s ea	**49348-0908-10**	15.99		
(0.3 CC,29GX1/2")				
100s ea	**52297-0867-78**	15.99		
(0.3CC,30GX1/2")				
100s ea	**49348-0368-10**	15.98		
(0.5 CC, 28GX1/2")				
100s ea	**49348-0906-10**	14.49		
100s ea	**52297-0865-78**	14.49		
(0.5 CC, 29GX1/2")				
100s ea	**49348-0909-10**	15.99		
100s ea	**52297-0868-78**	15.99		
(0.5CC,30GX1/2")				
100s ea	**49348-0370-10**	15.98		
(1 CC, 28GX1/2")				
100s ea	**49348-0907-10**	14.49		
100s ea	**52297-0866-78**	14.49		
(1 CC, 29GX1/2")				
100s ea	**49348-0910-10**	15.99		
100s ea	**52297-0869-78**	15.99		
(1CC,30GX1/2")				
100s ea	**49348-0369-10**	15.98		
(Rugby)				
DEV, NA (28GX1/2",1/2CC,U100)				
100s ea	**00536-9916-01**	23.85		
(28GX1/2",1CC,U100)				
100s ea	**00536-9915-01**	23.85		
(Specialty Medical)				
DEV, NA (28GX1",1/2CC)				
100s ea	**08415-0051-28**	23.00		
(28GX1",1CC)				
100s ea	**08415-0011-28**	23.00		
(28GX1/2",1/2CC)				
100s ea	**08415-0055-28**	23.00		
(29GX1",1/2CC)				
100s ea	**08415-0051-29**	23.00		
(29GX1",1CC)				
100s ea	**08415-0011-29**	23.00		
(29GX1",3/10CC)				
100s ea	**08415-0031-29**	23.00		
(29GX1/2",1/2CC)				
100s ea	**08415-0055-29**	23.00		
(29GX1/2",1CC)				
100s ea	**08415-0015-28**	23.00		
(29GX1/2",3/10CC)				
100s ea	**08415-0035-29**	23.00		
(29GX1/2"1CC)				
100s ea	**08415-0015-29**	23.00		
(29GX5/16",1/2CC)				
100s ea	**08415-0056-29**	23.00		
(29GX5/16",1CC)				
100s ea	**08415-0016-29**	23.00		
(29GX5/16",3/10CC)				
100s ea	**08415-0036-29**	23.00		
(30GX1",3/10CC)				
100s ea	**08415-0031-30**	23.00		
(30GX1/2",1/2CC)				
100s ea	**08415-0055-30**	23.00		
(30GX1/2",1CC)				
100s ea	**08415-0015-30**	23.00		
(30GX1/2",3/10CC)				
100s ea	**08415-0035-30**	23.00		
(30GX5/16",1/2CC)				
100s ea	**08415-0056-30**	23.00		
(30GX5/16",1CC)				
100s ea	**08415-0016-30**	23.00		
(30GX5/16",3/10CC)				
100s ea	**08415-0036-30**	23.00		
(31GX5/16",1/2CC)				
100s ea	**08415-0056-31**	23.00		
(31GX5/16",1CC)				
100s ea	**08415-0016-31**	23.00		
(31GX5/16",3/10CC)				
100s ea	**08415-0035-31**	23.00		
(A-S Medication)				
REPACK				
DEV, NA (1CC, 28G X 1/2")				
100s ea	**54569-2505-00**	27.30		
INSULIN SYRINGE/NEEDLE				
(Abbott) *See PRECISION SURE-DOSE*				
(Albertson's) *See INSULIN SYRINGE*				
(AmerisourceBergen) *See INSULIN SYRINGE*				
(BD Consumer) *See B-D SAFETY GLIDE*				
(BD Consumer) *See B-D SYRINGE LUER-LOK*				
(BD Consumer) *See BD INSULIN SYRINGE*				
(BD Consumer) *See BD MICRO-FINE*				
(BD Consumer) *See BD MICRO-FINE IV*				
(BD Consumer) *See BD ULTRA-FINE*				
(BD Consumer) *See BD ULTRA-FINE PEN*				
(BD Dickinson Hosp Prod) *See B-D INSULIN LO-DOSE BLISTER PACKAGE*				
(BD Dickinson Hosp Prod) *See B-D INSULIN SYRINGE BLISTER PACKAGE*				
(BD Dickinson Hosp Prod) *See B-D INSULIN SYRINGE SELF-CONTAINED*				
(BD Dickinson Hosp Prod) *See B-D INSULIN W/DETACHABLE NEEDLE*				
(BD Dickinson Hosp Prod) *See B-D LO-DOSE MICRO-FINE IV*				
(BD Dickinson Hosp Prod) *See B-D SAFETY-LOK W/ATTACHED NEEDLE*				
(BD Dickinson Hosp Prod) *See B-D SYRINGE ECCENTRIC TIP*				
(BD Dickinson Hosp Prod) *See B-D SYRINGE/NEEDLE COMBO LUER-LOK*				
(BD Dickinson Hosp Prod) *See B-D TUBERCULIN COMBINATION SLIP TIP*				
(BD Dickinson Hosp Prod) *See B-D TUBERCULIN SYRINGE*				
(BD Dickinson Hosp Prod) *See B-D TUBERCULIN W/DETACHABLE NEEDLE*				
(Can-Am Care) *See LEADER INSULIN SYRINGE*				
(Can-Am Care) *See RELI ON INSULIN SYRINGE*				
(Cardinal Health) *See ULTRA COMFORT*				
(Delta Hi-Tech) *See AIMSCO*				
(Delta Hi-Tech) *See AIMSCO ULTRA-THIN II*				
(Lilly) *See HUMAPEN LUXURA HD*				
(Lilly) *See HUMAPEN MEMOIR*				
(McKesson) *See INSULIN SYRINGE*				
(Medicore) *See LITE TOUCH*				
(Novo Nordisk) *See NOVOFINE 30*				
(Owen Mumford) *See UNIFINE PENTIPS*				
(Rugby) *See INSULIN SYRINGE*				
(Specialty Medical) *See INSULIN SYRINGE*				
(Terumo) *See TERUMO INSULIN*				
(Terumo) *See TERUMO SURE DOSE*				
(Terumo) *See TERUMO SURE DOSE PLUS*				
(UltiMed) *See ULTICARE*				
(UltiMed) *See ULTIGUARD*				
(Walgreens) *See SUPER THIN COMFORT ASSURED*				
(Walgreens) *See SUPER THIN II COMFORT ASSURED*				
INSULIN-HUMALOG (Phys Total Care)				
REPACK				
insulin lispro, recombinant				
SUS, SC (1X15ML)				
100 u/ml, 15 ml	**54868-5836-00**	207.78		
INSYTE AUTO GUARD IV (Becton Dickinson)				
catheter, intravenous				
DEV, NA (14GX2", RADIOPAQUE)				
50s ea	**08290-3812-67**	2.29		
(16GX1-1/4", RADIOPAQUE)				
50s ea	**08290-3812-54**	2.29		
(16GX2", RADIOPAQUE)				
50s ea	**08290-3812-57**	2.29		
(18GX1-1/4", RADIOPAQUE)				
50s ea	**08290-3812-44**	2.29		

PROD/MFR NDC AWP DP OBC

(18GX2", RADIOPAQUE)
50s ea..............08290-3812-47 2.29
(20GX1-1/4", RADIOPAQUE)
50s ea..............08290-3812-34 2.29
(20GX1", RADIOPAQUE)
50s ea..............08290-3812-33 2.29
(20GX2", RADIOPAQUE)
50s ea..............08290-3812-37 2.29
(22GX1" RADIOPAQUE)
50s ea..............08290-3812-23 2.41
(24GX3/4", RADIOPAQUE)
50s ea..............08290-3812-12 2.62

INSYTE-W IV (Becton Dickinson)
catheter, intravenous
DEV, NA (20GX1-1/4", VIALON)
ea..................08290-3813-34 2.29
(22GX1", VIALON)
ea..................08290-3813-23 2.41
(22GX1", W/WINGS)
ea..................08290-3884-22 2.35
(24GX3/4", VIALON)
ea..................08290-3813-12 2.62
(24GX3/4", W/WINGS)
ea..................08290-3883-24 2.56
(16GX1-1/4", VIALON)
50s ea..............08290-3813-54 2.29
(16GX2", VIALON)
50s ea..............08290-3813-57 2.29
(18GX1-1/4, VIALON)
50s ea..............08290-3813-44 2.29
(18GX2", VIALON)
50s ea..............08290-3813-47 2.29
(20GX1", VIALON)
50s ea..............08290-3813-33 2.29
(20GX2", VIALON)
50s ea..............08290-3813-37 2.29

INTEGRA BILAYER MATRIX WOUND DRESSING (Integra LifeSciences Corp)
collagen, bovine/glycosaminoglycans
SHE, TP (2"X2")
ea..................08478-4004-02 1525.00
(4"X10")
ea..................08478-4004-06 3325.00
(4"X5")
ea..................08478-4004-05 2415.00
(8"X10")
ea..................08478-4004-08 4600.00

INTEGRA DERMAL REGENERATION TEMPLATE (Integra LifeSciences Corp)
collagen, bovine/glycosaminoglycans
SHE, TP (2"X2")
ea..................08478-8004-02 1525.00
(4"X10")
ea..................08478-8004-06 3325.00
(4"X5")
ea..................08478-8004-05 2415.00
(8"X10")
ea..................08478-8004-08 4600.00

INTEGRA FLOWABLE WOUND MATRIX (Integra LifeSciences Corp)
collagen, bovine/glycosaminoglycans
PDS, IP (LATEX-FREE)
ea..................08478-4016-01 2775.00

INTEGRA MATRIX WOUND DRESSING (Integra LifeSciences Corp)
collagen, bovine/glycosaminoglycans
SHE, TP (2"X2")
ea..................08478-4014-02 1525.00
(4"X10")
ea..................08478-4014-06 3325.00
(4"X5")
ea..................08478-4014-05 2415.00
(8"X10")
ea..................08478-4014-08 4600.00

INTEGRA MESHED BILAYER WOUND MATRIX (Integra LifeSciences Corp)
collagen, bovine/glycosaminoglycans
SHE, TP (2X2",SINGLE USE)
ea..................08478-4003-02 1750.00
(4X10",SINGLE USE)
ea..................08478-4003-06 3825.00
(4X5",SINGLE USE)
ea..................08478-4003-05 2775.00
(8X10",SINGLE USE)
ea..................08478-4003-08 5250.00

INTEGRA MOZAIK OSTEOCONDUCTIVE SCAFFOLD PUTTY (Integra LifeSciences Corp)
collagen scaffold
DEV, NA (SINGLEUSE,10CC)
ea..................08478-4018-10 1625.00
(SINGLEUSE,15CC)
ea..................08478-4018-15 1950.00
(SINGLEUSE,2.5CC)
ea..................08478-4018-02 600.00
(SINGLEUSE,5CC)
ea..................08478-4018-05 975.00

INTEGRA MOZAIK OSTEOCONDUCTIVE SCAFFOLD STRIP (Integra LifeSciences Corp)
collagen scaffold
DEV, NA (SINGLE USE,10CC)
ea..................08478-4019-10 1625.00
(SINGLE USE,15CC)
ea..................08478-4019-15 1950.00

INTEGRA OS OSTEOCONDUCTIVE SCAFFOLD PUTTY (Integra LifeSciences Corp)
collagen scaffold
DEV, NA (SINGLE-USE, 5CC)
ea..................08478-4017-05 876.00
(SINGLEUSE,2.5CC)
ea..................08478-4017-02 515.00

INTEGRA PLUS (U.S. Pharm)
multivitamin, minerals, and iron
CAP, PO (GLUTEN-FREE)
90s ea..............52747-0712-60 59.70

INTEGRA-F (U.S. Pharm)
multivitamin and iron
CAP, PO (GLUTEN-FREE)
90s ea..............52747-0711-60 47.70

INTEGRILIN (Schering)
eptifibatide
SOL, IV (VIAL)
0.75 mg/ml, 100 ml...00085-1136-01 388.42
2 mg/ml, 10 ml.......00085-1177-01 124.12
100 ml...........00085-1177-02 1073.66

INTELENCE (Tibotec Therapeutics)
etravirine
TAB, PO, 100 mg, 120s ea.59676-0570-01 876.82

(A-S Medication)
REPACK
TAB, PO, 100 mg, 120s ea.54569-6102-00 1075.33

(Phys Total Care)
REPACK
TAB, PO, 100 mg, 120s ea.54868-5864-00 949.55

INTERFERON ALFA-2B
(Schering) *See INTRON A*

INTERFERON ALFA-N3
(Hemispherx) *See ALFERON N*

INTERFERON ALFACON-1
(Three Rivers Pharm) *See INFERGEN*

INTERFERON BETA-1A
(Biogen Idec) *See AVONEX*
(EMD) *See REBIF*

INTERFERON BETA-1B
(Bayer) *See BETASERON*
(Novartis Pharm) *See EXTAVIA*

INTERFERON BETA-1B/SODIUM CHLORIDE
(Bayer) *See BETASERON*

INTERFERON GAMMA-1B
(Intermune) *See ACTIMMUNE*

INTRALIPID (Baxter)
soybean oil
EMU, IV (EXCEL,10X10ML)
20%, 100 ml 10s.....00338-0519-48 288.96 240.80 AP
(EXCEL,10X250ML)
20%, 250 ml 10s.....00338-0519-02 341.88 284.90 AP
(EXCEL,10X500ML)
20%, 500 ml 12s.....00338-0519-03 790.70 658.92 AP
(EXCEL,6X1000ML)
20%, 1000 ml 6s.....00338-0519-04 869.77 724.81 AP
(EXCEL)
30%, 500 ml 12s.....00338-0520-03 1186.30 988.38 AP

INTRAUTERINE DEVICE, CONTRACEPTIVE & INTRODUCER
(FEI Products LLC) *See PARAGARD T380A*
(Teva) *See PARAGARD T380A*

INTRON A (Schering)
interferon alfa-2b
PDS, IJ (W/DILUENT IN VIAL)
10 million iu, ea......00085-0571-02 178.00
18 million iu, ea......00085-1110-01 320.41
50 million iu, ea......00085-0539-01 890.10
SOL, IJ (M.D.V.,AF)
6 million iu/ml,
3.8 ml...........00085-1168-01 394.21
10 million iu/ml,
3.2 ml...........00085-1133-01 547.56
(M.D. PEN,6 DOSE UNIT)
3 million iu/0.2 ml,
1.5 ml...........00085-1242-01 394.21
5 million iu/0.2 ml,
1.5 ml...........00085-1235-01 657.06
10 million iu/0.2 ml,
1.5 ml...........00085-1254-01 1068.12

(Phys Total Care)
REPACK
PDS, IJ, 50 million iu,
ea................54868-3341-00 907.51

INTUNIV (Shire US Inc.)
guanfacine hydrochloride
TER, PO, 1 mg, 100s ea...54092-0513-02 549.60
2 mg, 100s ea........54092-0515-02 549.60
3 mg, 100s ea........54092-0517-02 549.60
4 mg, 100s ea........54092-0519-02 549.60

INVANZ (Merck)
ertapenem sodium
PDS, IJ (S.D.V.)
1 gm, 10s ea.........00006-3843-71 693.92
(SD,ADD-VANTAGE)
1 gm, 10s ea.........00006-3845-71 728.56

INVEGA (Janssen)
paliperidone
TER, PO, 1.5 mg, 30s ea..50458-0554-01 429.23 357.69 EE
3 mg, 30s ea.........50458-0550-01 429.23 357.69
100s ea UD.........50458-0550-10 1430.75 1192.29
6 mg, 30s ea.........50458-0551-01 429.23 357.69
100s ea UD.........50458-0551-10 1430.75 1192.29
9 mg, 30s ea.........50458-0552-01 643.84 536.53
100s ea UD.........50458-0552-10 2146.14 1788.45

(Physician Partner)
REPACK
TER, PO, 6 mg, 30s ea....21695-0455-30 858.46

(Quality Care Prod)
REPACK
TER, PO, 3 mg, 30s ea....35356-0450-30 692.60
6 mg, 30s ea.........35356-0502-30 692.60

INVEGA SUSTENNA (Janssen)
paliperidone palmitate
SER, IM, 39 mg, 0.25 ml..50458-0560-01 296.45 247.04 EE
78 mg, 0.5 ml........50458-0561-01 592.92 494.10 EE
117 mg, 0.75 ml.....50458-0562-01 889.37 741.14 EE
156 mg, 1 ml........50458-0563-01 1185.86 988.22 EE
234 mg, 1.5 ml.......50458-0564-01 1778.80 1482.33 EE

INVIRASE (Roche Labs)
saquinavir mesylate
CAP, PO, 200 mg, 270s ea.00004-0245-15 975.06
TAB, PO (FILM-COATED)
500 mg, 120s ea.....00004-0244-51 996.44

(A-S Medication)
REPACK
TAB, PO (FILM-COATED)
500 mg, 120s ea.....54569-5664-00 1037.96

(Phys Total Care)
REPACK
CAP, PO, 200 mg, 30s ea..54868-3699-02 89.53
60s ea............54868-3699-01 167.44
270s ea...........54868-3699-00 722.76

IOBENGUANE I 123
(GE) *See ADREVIEW*

IODIC ACID (Baker, J.T.)
CRY, NA (A.C.S., REAGENT)
500 gm.............10106-0186-01 295.15

IODINE
(Baker, J.T.) *See IODINE 2%*
(Baker, J.T.) *See IODINE SUBLIMED*
(Baker, J.T.)
POW, NA (U.S.P.)
30 gm..............10106-2211-00 18.69
125 gm.............10106-2211-04 28.40
500 gm.............10106-2211-01 172.76
(Gallipot) *See IODINE 7%*
(Gallipot) *See IODINE RESUBLIMED*
(Libby)
TIN, TP (IPA)
480 ml.............00492-0076-16 26.00
(Mallinckrodt Lab)
CRY, NA (U.S.P.)
30 gm..............00406-0984-34 39.37
125 gm.............00406-0984-02 20.75
500 gm.............00406-0984-12 69.53

PROD/MFR	NDC	AWP	DP	OBC
(Medisca) *See IODINE RESUBLIMED*				
(Medisca) *See IODINE TINCTURE 7%*				
(PCCA)				
POW, NA (USP; RESUBLIMED)				
1 gm	**51927-1252-00**	1.25		
(Spectrum Pharmacy) *See STRONG IODINE TINCTURE*				
IODINE 2% (Baker, J.T.)				
iodine				
TIN, NA (U.S.P.)				
500 ml	**10106-2214-01**	39.41		
IODINE 5% (Gallipot)				
iodine/potassium iodide				
SOL, NA (STRONG)				
118.28 ml	**51552-0194-04**	13.16		
473 ml	**51552-0194-06**	27.72		
IODINE 7% (Gallipot)				
iodine				
TIN, NA (STRONG,U.S.P.)				
473 ml	**51552-0647-06**	40.63	32.50	
IODINE I 131 TOSITUMOMAB				
(Glaxo) *See BEXXAR*				
IODINE RESUBLIMED (Gallipot)				
iodine				
CRY, NA (U.S.P.)				
25 gm	**51552-0184-04**	9.80		
100 gm	**51552-0184-05**	33.04		
454 gm	**51552-0184-06**	67.20		
(Medisca)				
CRY, NA (U.S.P.)				
25 gm	**38779-0077-04**	22.50		
100 gm	**38779-0077-05**	49.50		
(USP,1X1000GM)				
1000 gm	**38779-0077-09**	367.50		
IODINE STRONG (Marlex)				
iodine/potassium iodide				
SOL, PO (LUGOL'S SOLUTION)				
5%-10%, 120 ml	**10135-0107-04**	2.17		
480 ml	**10135-0107-08**	7.22		
IODINE SUBLIMED (Baker, J.T.)				
iodine				
POW, NA (A.C.S., REAGENT)				
125 gm	**10106-2208-04**	107.64		
500 gm	**10106-2208-01**	213.11		
2500 gm	**10106-2208-05**	755.35		
IODINE TINCTURE 7% (Medisca)				
iodine				
TIN, NA (USP,(STRONG),1X100ML)				
7%, 100 ml	**38779-2108-05**	28.50		
(USP,(STRONG),1X500ML)				
7%, 500 ml	**38779-2108-08**	49.50		
(USP,(STRONG),1X4000ML)				
7%, 4000 ml	**38779-2108-01**	313.50		
IODINE/POTASSIUM IODIDE				
(Cooper Surgical) *See LUGOL'S STRONG IODINE*				
(Gallipot) *See IODINE 5%*				
(Humco) *See LUGOL'S SOLUTION*				
(Marlex) *See IODINE STRONG*				
(Medisca) *See LUGOL'S SOLUTION*				
(PCCA) *See LUGOL'S SOLUTION*				
(Safecor) *See LUGOL'S SOLUTION*				
IODIPAMIDE MEGLUMINE				
(Bracco Diag) *See CHOLOGRAFIN MEGLUMINE*				
IODIXANOL				
(GE) *See VISIPAQUE*				
IODOCHLORHYDROXYQUIN (PCCA)				
clioquinol				
POW, NA (USP)				
1 gm	**51927-1052-00**	2.04		
IODOFLEX (Smith & Nephew)				
cadexomer iodine				
DRE, TP, 0.9%, 5 gm 5s	**40565-0122-51**	54.24		
10 gm 3s	**40565-0122-53**	65.96		
IODOFORM (Amend)				
POW, NA (PURIFIED)				
25 gm	**17317-0298-02**	8.40		
125 gm	**17317-0298-04**	23.80		
500 gm	**17317-0298-01**	70.00		
2270 gm	**17317-0298-05**	280.00		
(Baker, J.T.)				
POW, NA (PURIFIED)				
125 gm	**10106-2220-04**	78.42		
500 gm	**10106-2220-01**	98.22		
(Gallipot)				
POW, NA (PURIFIED,REAGENT)				
25 gm	**51552-0230-04**	18.20		
125 gm	**51552-0230-09**	58.10		
(Mallinckrodt Lab)				
POW, NA (PURIFIED)				
125 gm	**00406-1026-01**	122.12		
500 gm	**00406-1026-03**	226.10		
(Medisca)				
POW, NA (PURIFIED)				
25 gm	**38779-1360-04**	43.50		
100 gm	**38779-1360-05**	142.50		
500 gm	**38779-1360-08**	357.00		
(PCCA)				
POW, NA (PURIFIED)				
1 gm	**51927-1127-00**	1.92		
(USP,1X1GM)				
1 gm	**51927-3615-00**	1.92		
(Spectrum Pharmacy)				
POW, NA (1X25GM)				
25 gm	**49452-3775-01**	77.00		
(1X100GM)				
100 gm	**49452-3775-02**	215.95		
(1X500GM)				
500 gm	**49452-3775-03**	528.50		
IODOPEN (APP)				
sodium iodide				
SOL, IJ (S.D.V.,25X10ML,PF)				
118 mcg/ml,				
10 ml 25s	**63323-0019-10**	312.19		
IODOQUINOL				
(Consolidated Midland) *See DIQUINOL*				
(Consolidated Midland)				
TAB, PO, 650 mg, 100s ea	**00223-0851-01**	47.50		
500s ea	**00223-0851-05**	225.00		
(Glenwood) *See YODOXIN*				
(Spectrum Pharmacy)				
POW, NA (U.S.P.)				
25 gm	**49452-3770-01**	70.70		
100 gm	**49452-3770-02**	162.05		
IODOQUINOL MICRONIZED (PCCA)				
iodoquinol, micronized				
POW, NA (USP)				
1 gm	**51927-1690-00**	1.32		
IODOQUINOL, MICRONIZED				
(PCCA) *See IODOQUINOL MICRONIZED*				
IODOSORB (Smith & Nephew)				
cadexomer iodine				
GEL, TP, 0.9%, 40 gm	**40565-0122-49**	77.18		
IODOTOPE (Bracco Diag)				
sodium iodide i 131				
CAP, PO, ea	**00270-0072-00**	212.50	170.00	
IOFED (Phys Total Care)				
REPACK				
bpm/pse hcl				
CER, PO, 12 mg-120 mg,				
20s ea	**54868-3989-00**	12.36		
IOHEXOL				
(GE) *See OMNIPAQUE 140*				
(GE) *See OMNIPAQUE 180*				
(GE) *See OMNIPAQUE 240*				
(GE) *See OMNIPAQUE 300*				
(GE) *See OMNIPAQUE 350*				
IONOSOL B/5% DEXTROSE (Hospira)				
dextrose/k phos/mg cl/na cl/na lact/na phos				
SOL, IV (LIFECARE,LATEX-FREE)				
500 ml 24s	**00409-7371-03**	70.27	61.44	
(LIFECARE, 12X1000ML)				
1000 ml 12s	**00409-7371-09**	41.04	35.88	
IONOSOL MB/5% DEXTROSE (Hospira)				
dextrose/k cl/k phos/mg cl/na lact/na phos				
SOL, IV (LIFECARE,24X250ML)				
250 ml 24s	**00409-7372-62**	62.21	54.48	
(LIFECARE,LATEX-FREE)				
500 ml 24s	**00409-7372-03**	58.18	50.88	
1000 ml 12s	**00409-7372-09**	34.70	30.36	
IONOSOL T AND 5% DEXTROSE (Hospira)				
dextrose/k cl/k lact/na cl/na phos				
SOL, IV (LIFECARE,24X500ML)				
500 ml 24s	**00409-7373-03**	87.84	76.80	
(LIFECARE,12X1000ML)				
1000 ml 12s	**00409-7373-09**	37.01	32.40	
IOPAMIDOL				
(Bracco Diag) *See ISOVUE MULTIPACK-250*				
(Bracco Diag) *See ISOVUE MULTIPACK-300*				
(Bracco Diag) *See ISOVUE MULTIPACK-370*				
(Bracco Diag) *See ISOVUE-200*				
(Bracco Diag) *See ISOVUE-250*				
(Bracco Diag) *See ISOVUE-300*				
(Bracco Diag) *See ISOVUE-370*				
(Bracco Diag) *See ISOVUE-M 200*				
(Bracco Diag) *See ISOVUE-M 300*				
IOPANOIC ACID (Medisca)				
POW, NA (1X5GM)				
5 gm	**38779-2312-03**	196.50		
(1X25GM)				
25 gm	**38779-2312-04**	837.00		
(1X100GM)				
100 gm	**38779-2312-05**	2055.00		
(PCCA)				
POW, NA, 1 gm	**51927-3580-00**	54.00		
(Spectrum Pharmacy)				
POW, NA (1X25GM)				
25 gm	**49452-3780-01**	1456.00		
(1X100GM)				
100 gm	**49452-3780-02**	4448.50		
IOPHEN C-NR (Qualitest)				
codeine phosphate/guaifenesin				
LIQ, PO (RASPBERRY)				
10 mg/5 ml-100 mg/5 ml,				
473 ml, C-V	**00603-1329-58**	40.40		
IOPHEN DM-NR (Qualitest)				
dextromethorphan hydrobromide/guaifenesin				
LIQ, PO (ORANGE-RASPBERRY)				
10 mg/5 ml-100 mg/5 ml,				
473 ml	**00603-1330-58**	45.15		
IOPHEN-NR (Qualitest)				
guaifenesin				
LIQ, PO (RASPBERRY)				
100 mg/5 ml,				
480 ml	**00603-1328-58**	37.15		
IOPIDINE (Alcon Ophthalmic)				
apraclonidine hydrochloride				
SOL, OP, 0.5%, 5 ml	**00065-0665-05**	95.04		
10 ml	**00065-0665-10**	188.82		
1%, 24s ea UD	**00065-0660-10**	379.44		
(Phys Total Care)				
REPACK				
SOL, OP, 0.5%, 5 ml	**54868-4002-00**	82.31		
IOPROMIDE				
(Bayer) *See ULTRAVIST*				
(Hospira) *See ULTRAVIST*				
IOVERSOL				
(Mallinckrodt Inc.) *See OPTIRAY 160*				
(Mallinckrodt Inc.) *See OPTIRAY 240*				
(Mallinckrodt Inc.) *See OPTIRAY 300*				
(Mallinckrodt Inc.) *See OPTIRAY 320*				
(Mallinckrodt Inc.) *See OPTIRAY 350*				
IOXILAN				
(Cook Inc) *See OXILAN-300*				
(Cook Inc) *See OXILAN-350*				
IPECAC (Medisca)				
ipecac syrup				
SYR, NA (USP,1X500ML)				
500 ml	**38779-0608-08**	37.50		
(USP,1X4000ML)				
4000 ml	**38779-0608-01**	240.00		
IPECAC SYRUP				
(Medisca) *See IPECAC*				
IPOL (Sanofi)				
poliovirus vaccine, inactivated				
SUS, IJ, 80 d antigen u/0.5 ml,				
0.5 ml	**49281-0860-55**	295.01	247.09	
(10 DOSE VIAL,TAX INCL)				
80 d antigen u/0.5 ml,				
5 ml	**49281-0860-10**	295.01	247.09	
IPRATROPIUM (Southwood)				
REPACK				
ipratropium bromide				
SOL, IH (2.5MLX25)				
0.02%, 2.5 ml 25s	**58016-4849-01**	15.65		

PROD/MFR	NDC	AWP	DP	OBC
IPRATROPIUM BROM (Phys Total Care)				
REPACK				
ipratropium bromide				
SPR, NS, 0.03%, 30 ml	54868-5751-00	167.55		
IPRATROPIUM BROMIDE				
FUL				
SOL, IH, 0.02%,				
2.5 ml 25s		6.75		
(Apotex Corp.)				
SOL, IH (AMP)				
0.02%, 2.5 ml 25s	60505-0806-01	56.00		AN
SPR, NS (METERED DOSE SPRAY)				
0.03%, 30 ml	60505-0826-01	51.75		AB
0.06%, 15 ml	60505-0827-01	44.37		AB
(Bausch & Lomb Inc.)				
SPR, NS (WITH METERED SPRAY PUMP)				
0.03%, 30 ml	24208-0398-30	44.69		
0.06%, 15 ml	24208-0399-15	37.19		AB
(Boehr Ingelheim Phar) *See ATROVENT*				
(Boehr Ingelheim Phar) *See ATROVENT HFA*				
(Dey, L.P.)				
SOL, IH (2.5X25)				
0.02%,				
2.5 ml 25s UD	49502-0685-26	44.10		AN
(SINGLE-PAK)				
0.02%,				
2.5 ml 30s UD	49502-0685-30	53.40		AN
(VIAL)				
0.02%,				
2.5 ml 30s UD	49502-0685-31	52.80		AN
2.5 ml 60s UD	49502-0685-62	105.60		AN
(Gallipot)				
POW, NA (B.P.)				
1 gm	51552-0393-01	63.00		
5 gm	51552-0393-02	231.00		
25 gm	51552-0393-04	1010.80		
100 gm	51552-0393-05	1960.00		
(Hawkins)				
POW, NA (EP)				
1 gm	63370-0120-10	120.00		
5 gm	63370-0120-15	508.80		
25 gm	63370-0120-25	2064.00		
100 gm	63370-0120-35	7200.00		
1000 gm	63370-0120-50	43200.00		
(Letco)				
POW, NA, 1 gm	62991-1085-01	73.50		
5 gm	62991-1085-02	318.00		
(PH. EUR)				
25 gm	62991-1085-03	1170.00		
100 gm	62991-1085-04	2910.00		
1000 gm	62991-1085-06	22500.00		
(Medisca)				
POW, NA, 1 gm	38779-0230-06	148.50		
5 gm	38779-0230-03	490.50		
25 gm	38779-0230-04	1650.00		
100 gm	38779-0230-05	3555.00		
(Mylan)				
SOL, IH (25X2.5ML,PF)				
0.02%,				
2.5 ml 25s UD	00378-6989-62	47.52		AN
(30X2.5ML,PF)				
0.02%,				
2.5 ml 30s UD	00378-6989-64	57.02		AN
2.5 ml 30s UD	00378-6989-93	67.09		AN
(60X2.5ML,PF)				
0.02%,				
2.5 ml 60s UD	00378-6989-66	114.05		AN
(Nephron)				
SOL, IH (PF)				
0.02%,				
2.5 ml 25s UD	00487-9801-25	33.00		AN
2.5 ml 30s UD	00487-9801-01	39.60		AN
2.5 ml 30s UD	00487-9801-30	39.60		AN
(ROBOT READY,PF)				
0.02%,				
2.5 ml 30s UD	00487-9801-02	39.60		AN
(PF)				
0.02%,				
2.5 ml 60s UD	00487-9801-60	79.20		AN
(PCCA)				
POW, NA, 1 gm	51927-1648-00	300.00		
(Roxane)				
SPR, NS (WITH SPRAY PUMP)				
0.03%, 30 ml	00054-0045-44	51.80		
0.06%, 15 ml	00054-0046-41	44.42		
(Spectrum Pharmacy)				
POW, NA (B.P.,E.P.)				
1 gm	49452-3791-02	237.50		
5 gm	49452-3791-03	714.00		
(Watson Labs)				
SOL, IH (25X2.5ML,LDPE)				
0.02%,				
2.5 ml 25s UD	16252-0098-22	4.50		
(30X2.5ML,LDPE)				
0.02%,				
2.5 ml 30s UD	16252-0098-33	5.40		
(60X2.5ML,LDPE)				
0.02%,				
2.5 ml 60s UD	16252-0098-66	10.80		
(A-S Medication)				
REPACK				
SOL, IH (VIAL)				
0.02%,				
2.5 ml 25s UD	54569-4910-00	18.51		AN
(B&B Pharm, Inc)				
REPACK				
POW, NA (U.S.P.)				
1 gm	63275-9998-01	81.00		
5 gm	63275-9998-02	365.00		
25 gm	63275-9998-04	1605.00		
100 gm	63275-9998-05	4925.00		
(Palmetto)				
REPACK				
SOL, IH (25X2.5ML)				
0.02%,				
2.5 ml 25s UD	23490-5761-01	17.50		
(Phys Total Care)				
REPACK				
SOL, IH (VIAL)				
0.02%,				
2.5 ml 25s UD	54868-4082-01	5.06		EE
2.5 ml 60s UD	54868-4082-00	10.96		EE
SPR, NS, 0.06%, 15 ml	54868-5049-00	142.57		AB
(Physician Partner)				
REPACK				
SOL, IH, 0.02%, 25s ea UD	21695-0911-25	88.20		
(Quality Care Prod)				
REPACK				
SOL, IH (30X2.5ML,PF)				
0.02%,				
2.5 ml 30s UD	35356-0124-30	219.02		AN
SPR, NS, 0.03%, 30 ml	49999-0389-30	61.48		
IPRATROPIUM BROMIDE AND ALBUTEROL SULFATE (Mylan)				
albuterol sulfate/ipratropium bromide				
SOL, IH (30X3ML,1 VIAL/POUCH)				
3 mg/3 ml-0.5 mg/3 ml,				
3 ml 30s UD	00378-6988-93	69.04		
(30X3ML,5 VIALS/POUCH)				
3 mg/3 ml-0.5 mg/3 ml,				
3 ml 30s UD	00378-6988-58	65.54		
(60X3ML 5 VIALS/POUCH)				
3 mg/3 ml-0.5 mg/3 ml,				
3 ml 60s UD	00378-6988-91	131.07		
(Nephron)				
SOL, IH (30X3ML, ROBOT READY)				
3 mg/3 ml-0.5 mg/3 ml,				
3 ml 30s	00487-0201-02	69.84		AN
(30X3ML)				
3 mg/3 ml-0.5 mg/3 ml,				
3 ml 30s UD	00487-0201-01	66.24		AN
3 ml 30s UD	00487-0201-03	65.71		AN
(60X3ML)				
3 mg/3 ml-0.5 mg/3 ml,				
3 ml 60s	00487-0201-60	126.16		AN
(Sandoz)				
SOL, IH (30X3ML)				
3 mg/3 ml-0.5 mg/3 ml,				
3 ml 30s	00185-7322-13	69.12		AN
3 ml 30s	00185-7322-30	65.61		AN
(60X3ML)				
3 mg/3 ml-0.5 mg/3 ml,				
3 ml 60s	00185-7322-60	131.22		AN
(Teva)				
SOL, IH (30X3ML)				
3 mg/3 ml-0.5 mg/3 ml,				
3 ml 30s UD	00093-6723-73	65.61		AN
(60X3ML)				
3 mg/3 ml-0.5 mg/3 ml,				
3 ml 60s UD	00093-6723-74	131.22		AN
(Watson Labs)				
SOL, IH (30X3ML)				
3 mg/3 ml-0.5 mg/3 ml,				
3 ml 30s UD	00591-3433-30	27.55		AN
(60X3ML)				
3 mg/3 ml-0.5 mg/3 ml,				
3 ml 60s UD	00591-3433-60	55.12		AN
(Phys Total Care)				
REPACK				
SOL, IH (90X3ML)				
3 mg/3 ml-0.5 mg/3 ml,				
3 ml 90s	54868-5974-00	55.04		AN
IPRATROPIUM BROMIDE/ALBUTEROL SULFATE (Watson Labs)				
albuterol sulfate/ipratropium bromide				
SOL, IH (30X3ML)				
3 mg/3 ml-0.5 mg/3 ml,				
3 ml 30s UD	16252-0547-33	14.40		
(60X3ML)				
3 mg/3 ml-0.5 mg/3 ml,				
3 ml 60s UD	16252-0547-66	28.80		
IPRIFLAVONE (Medisca)				
POW, NA (1X1000GM)				
1000 gm	38779-2240-09	337.50		
(PCCA)				
POW, NA, 1 gm	51927-3339-00	4.80		
IQUIX (Vistakon)				
levofloxacin				
SOL, OP, 1.5%, 5 ml	68669-0145-05	78.54		
IRBESARTAN				
(Bristol-Myers) *See AVAPRO*				
IRESSA (AstraZeneca)				
gefitinib				
TAB, PO, 250 mg, 30s ea	00310-0482-30	2042.26		
IRINOTECAN HYDROCHLORIDE (Actavis)				
SOL, IV (1X2ML)				
20 mg/ml, 2 ml	18111-0002-02	275.84		AP
(1X5ML)				
20 mg/ml, 5 ml	18111-0002-03	689.59		AP
(APP)				
SOL, IV (1X2ML,SINGLE DOSE)				
20 mg/ml, 2 ml	63323-0193-02	265.07	41.50	
(1X5ML,SINGLE DOSE)				
20 mg/ml, 5 ml	63323-0193-05	662.67	101.00	
(Baxter)				
SOL, IV (1X2ML,SDV,AMBER GLASS)				
20 mg/ml, 2 ml	10019-0934-01	63.00		
(1X2ML,SDV,INNER NDC)				
20 mg/ml, 2 ml	10019-0934-17	63.00		
(1X5ML,SDV,AMBER GLASS)				
20 mg/ml, 5 ml	10019-0934-02	157.42		
(1X5ML,SDV,INNER NDC)				
20 mg/ml, 5 ml	10019-0934-79	157.42		
(Bedford)				
SOL, IV (1X2ML,SINGLE DOSE)				
20 mg/ml, 2 ml	55390-0295-01	60.00		AP
(1X5ML,SINGLE DOSE)				
20 mg/ml, 5 ml	55390-0296-01	156.00		AP
(Greenstone)				
SOL, IV (1X2ML,SDV)				
20 mg/ml, 2 ml	59762-7529-01	275.84		
(1X5ML,SDV)				
20 mg/ml, 5 ml	59762-7529-02	689.59		
(Hospira) *See AMERINET CHOICE IRINOTECAN HYDROCHLORIDE*				
(Hospira)				
SOL, IV (1X2ML)				
20 mg/ml, 2 ml	61703-0349-16	28.84	25.23	AP
(1X5ML)				
20 mg/ml, 5 ml	61703-0349-09	54.58	47.75	AP
(1X25ML,SDV)				
20 mg/ml, 25 ml	61703-0349-36	263.86	230.87	AP
(Pfizer) *See CAMPTOSAR*				
(Sagent)				
SOL, IV (1X2ML,SINGLE DOSE,PF)				
20 mg/ml, 2 ml	25021-0200-02	65.58		AP
(1X5ML,SINGLE DOSE,PF)				
20 mg/ml, 5 ml	25021-0200-05	158.50		AP
(Sandoz)				
SOL, IV (1X2ML,S.D.V)				
20 mg/ml, 2 ml	00781-3066-72	276.15		AP
(1X2ML,SINGLE-DOSE)				
20 mg/ml, 2 ml	66758-0048-01	276.15		AP
(1X5ML,S.D.V)				
20 mg/ml, 5 ml	00781-3066-75	690.35		AP

PROD/MFR	NDC	AWP	DP	OBC
(1X5ML,SINGLE-DOSE)				
20 mg/ml, 5 ml	66758-0048-02	690.35		AP
(Teva) *See NOVAPLUS IRINOTECAN HYDROCHLORIDE*				
(Teva)				
SOL, IV (1X2ML,SINGLE DOSE)				
20 mg/ml, 2 ml	00703-4432-11	44.40		AP
(1X5ML,SINGLE DOSE)				
20 mg/ml, 5 ml	00703-4434-11	106.80		AP
(1X25ML,SINGLE DOSE)				
20 mg/ml, 25 ml	00703-4437-11	596.75		AP
IRISH MOSS (PCCA)				
carrageenan				
POW, NA, 1 gm	51927-1497-00	0.13		
IRON (Baker, J.T.)				
POW, NA (REAGENT)				
500 gm	10106-2226-01	71.22		
(REDUCED, F.C.C.)				
500 gm	10106-2228-01	22.20		
2500 gm	10106-2228-05	198.99		
(McNeil,R.A.) *See EZFE 200*				
IRON DEXTRAN				
(Amer Regent) *See DEXFERRUM*				
(Watson) *See INFED*				
(Phys Total Care)				
REPACK				
SOL, IJ, 50 mg/ml, 20 ml	54868-4715-00	762.96		
IRON OXIDE (PCCA)				
synthetic iron oxide				
POW, NA (SYNTHETIC)				
1 gm	51927-1779-00	1.20		
IRON OXIDE, BLACK (PCCA)				
ferric oxide				
PAS, NA (1X1GM)				
1 gm	51927-3821-00	1.56		
IRON OXIDE, RED (PCCA)				
ferric oxide				
PAS, NA (1X1GM)				
1 gm	51927-3822-00	1.56		
IRON OXIDE, YELLOW (PCCA)				
ferric oxide				
PAS, NA (1X1GM)				
1 gm	51927-3823-00	1.50		
IRON POLYSACCHARIDE				
(ME Pharm) *See MYFERON 150*				
IRON SUCROSE				
(Amer Regent) *See VENOFER*				
(Fresenius) *See VENOFER*				
IRON/LIVER EXTRACT/VITAMINS				
(Consolidated Midland)				
vitamin b complex and mineral				
SOL, IJ (VIAL)				
30 ml	00223-7950-30	25.00		
ISENTRESS (Merck)				
raltegravir potassium				
TAB, PO (FILM-COATED)				
400 mg, 60s ea	00006-0227-61	1074.64		
(A-S Medication)				
REPACK				
TAB, PO (FILM-COATED)				
400 mg, 60s ea	54569-6034-00	1338.16		
(Phys Total Care)				
REPACK				
TAB, PO (FILM-COATED)				
400 mg, 60s ea	54868-0117-00	1180.48		
(Quality Care Prod)				
REPACK				
TAB, PO (FILM-COATED)				
400 mg, 6s ea	35356-0110-06	223.10		
60s ea	35356-0110-60	2201.20		
ISMO (Promius)				
isosorbide mononitrate				
TAB, PO (FILM-COATED)				
20 mg, 100s ea	67857-0702-01	198.22	114.33	AB
(Phys Total Care)				
REPACK				
TAB, PO, 20 mg, 30s ea	54868-3001-03	62.10		AB
60s ea	54868-3001-01	122.33		AB
100s ea	54868-3001-04	202.00		AB
120s ea	54868-3001-02	242.78		AB
ISO-ACETAZONE (HomeMed)				
REPACK				
apap/dichloralphenazone/isometheptene mucate				
CAP, PO, 325 mg-100 mg-65 mg,				
10s ea, C-IV	51655-0451-53	5.50		
28s ea, C-IV	51655-0451-29	11.51		
ISOBUTYL ALCOHOL				
(Baker, J.T.) *See ALCOHOL ISOBUTYL*				
ISOCARBOXAZID				
(Validus) *See MARPLAN*				
ISOCHRON (Forest Pharm)				
isosorbide dinitrate				
TER, PO, 40 mg, 100s ea	00456-0637-01	107.32		
ISOFLAVONE				
(PCCA) *See ISOFLAVONE COMPOUND*				
ISOFLAVONE COMPOUND (PCCA)				
isoflavone				
POW, NA, 1 gm	51927-3364-00	4.20		
ISOFLUPREDONE ACETATE MICRONIZED (PCCA)				
isoflupredone acetate, micronized				
POW, NA (1X1GM)				
1 gm	51927-3559-00	177.00		
ISOFLUPREDONE ACETATE, MICRONIZED				
(PCCA) *See ISOFLUPREDONE ACETATE MICRONIZED*				
ISOFLURANE				
(Baxter) *See FORANE*				
(Halocarbon)				
LIQ, IH, 99.9%, 100 ml	12164-0002-10	26.25		AN
250 ml	12164-0002-25	63.95		AN
(Hospira)				
LIQ, IH (LATEX-FREE)				
99.9%, 250 ml	00409-3292-02	44.44	38.88	AN
SOL, IH, 99.9%, 100 ml	00409-3292-01	19.27	16.86	AN
(RxElite) *See TERRELL*				
ISOLEUCINE				
(Medisca) *See L-ISOLEUCINE*				
(PCCA)				
POW, NA (FCC)				
1 gm	51927-1880-00	2.04		
(L,USP)				
1 gm	51927-3640-00	2.04		
(Spectrum Pharmacy)				
POW, NA (U.S.P.)				
25 gm	49452-3793-01	71.75		
100 gm	49452-3793-02	224.70		
1000 gm	49452-3793-03	1536.50		
ISOLYTE H W/DEXTROSE (B. Braun)				
dextrose/k cl/mg cl/na ace/na cl				
SOL, IV (EXCEL, 5% DEX)				
1000 ml	00264-7719-00	4.60		
ISOLYTE M W/DEXTROSE (B. Braun)				
dextrose/k cl/k phos/na ace/na cl				
SOL, IV (EXCEL, 5% DEX)				
1000 ml	00264-7720-00	3.50		
ISOLYTE P W/DEXTROSE (B. Braun)				
dextrose/k cl/k phos/mg cl/na ace				
SOL, IV (EXCEL, 5% DEX)				
500 ml	00264-7730-10	7.64		
ISOLYTE S (B. Braun)				
k cl/mg cl/na ace/na cl/na gluconate				
SOL, IV (EXCEL)				
1000 ml	00264-7703-00	3.10		AP
ISOLYTE S PH 7.4 (B. Braun)				
electrolytes				
SOL, IV (EXCEL)				
500 ml	00264-7707-10	4.00		
1000 ml	00264-7707-00	4.00		
ISOLYTE S W/DEXTROSE (B. Braun)				
dextrose/k cl/mg cl/na ace/na cl/na gluconate				
SOL, IV (5% DEX, EXCEL)				
1000 ml	00264-7704-00	3.50		AP
ISOMETH/DICHLOR/APAP (Dispensing Solutions)				
REPACK				
apap/dichloralphenazone/isometheptene mucate				
CAP, PO, 325 mg-100 mg-65 mg,				
20s ea, C-IV	55045-2888-07	11.00		
30s ea, C-IV	55045-2888-08	16.50		
50s ea, C-IV	55045-2888-05	27.50		
60s ea, C-IV	55045-2888-06	33.00		
90s ea, C-IV	55045-2888-09	49.50		
100s ea, C-IV	55045-2888-01	55.00		
120s ea, C-IV	55045-2888-02	66.00		
ISOMETHEPTENE MUCATE (PCCA)				
POW, NA (USP)				
1 gm	51927-2200-00	3.24		
ISOMETHEPTENE/DICHLORALPHENAZONE/ACETAMINOPHEN (Quality Care Prod)				
REPACK				
apap/dichloralphenazone/isometheptene mucate				
CAP, PO, 325 mg-100 mg-65 mg,				
30s ea, C-IV	49999-0802-30	15.19		
ISONARIF (VersaPharm)				
isoniazid/rifampin				
CAP, PO, 150 mg-300 mg,				
60s ea	61748-0017-60	143.62		AB
ISONIAZID				
FUL				
TAB, PO, 100 mg, 100s ea		5.61		
300 mg, 100s ea		8.90		
(Amneal)				
TAB, PO, 300 mg, 35s ea	65162-0182-35	9.92		AA
(Carolina)				
SOL, PO (USP)				
50 mg/5 ml, 473 ml	46287-0009-01	58.00	42.00	
(Consolidated Midland)				
TAB, PO, 100 mg, 100s ea	00223-1150-01	4.95		EE
1000s ea	00223-1150-02	32.50		EE
300 mg, 30s ea	00223-1151-30	4.75		EE
100s ea	00223-1151-01	6.95		EE
1000s ea	00223-1151-02	62.50		EE
(Gallipot)				
POW, NA (U.S.P.)				
100 gm	51552-0860-05	48.30	34.50	
(Medisca)				
POW, NA (U.S.P.)				
25 gm	38779-0120-04	21.00		
100 gm	38779-0120-05	88.50		
500 gm	38779-0120-08	364.50		
(PCCA)				
POW, NA (U.S.P.)				
1 gm	51927-1883-00	1.56		
(Sandoz) *See NYDRAZID*				
(Sandoz)				
SOL, IM (USP,MDV)				
100 mg/ml, 10 ml	00781-3056-70	273.65		AP
TAB, PO, 100 mg, 30s ea	00185-4351-30	3.10		AA
100s ea	00185-4351-01	8.19		AA
1000s ea	00185-4351-10	48.46		AA
300 mg, 30s ea	00185-4350-30	9.06		AA
100s ea	00185-4350-01	13.06		AA
1000s ea	00185-4350-10	87.38		AA
(Spectrum Pharmacy)				
POW, NA (U.S.P.)				
100 gm	49452-3800-01	136.85		
500 gm	49452-3800-02	539.00		
(Teva)				
TAB, PO, 100 mg, 100s ea	00555-0066-02	9.83		AA
1000s ea	00555-0066-05	93.38		AA
300 mg, 30s ea	00555-0071-01	10.15		AA
100s ea	00555-0071-02	20.63		AA
1000s ea	00555-0071-05	157.28		AA
(UDL)				
TAB, PO (10X10)				
300 mg, 100s ea UD	51079-0083-20	15.10		AA
(VersaPharm)				
TAB, PO, 100 mg, 100s ea	61748-0016-01	6.67		AA
300 mg, 30s ea	61748-0013-30	4.06		AA
100s ea	61748-0013-01	10.96		AA
1000s ea	61748-0013-10	86.80		AA
(West-Ward)				
TAB, PO, 100 mg, 100s ea	00143-1260-01	9.65		AA
1000s ea	00143-1260-10	89.75		AA
300 mg, 30s ea	00143-1261-30	6.43		AA
100s ea	00143-1261-01	14.15		AA
1000s ea	00143-1261-10	115.75		AA
(A-S Medication)				
REPACK				
SYR, PO, 50 mg/5 ml,				
480 ml	54569-2900-00	33.75		
TAB, PO, 100 mg, 30s ea	54569-2942-01	2.95		EE
100s ea	54569-2942-00	9.83		EE
300 mg, 30s ea	54569-2509-03	4.41		AA
100s ea	54569-2509-01	14.70		AA
(Altura)				
REPACK				
TAB, PO, 300 mg, 30s ea	63874-0366-30	4.01		EE
100s ea	63874-0366-01	13.38		EE

PROD/MFR	NDC	AWP	DP	OBC
(Bryant Ranch)				
REPACK				
TAB, PO, 300 mg, 30s ea	63629-1422-02	25.20		
60s ea	63629-1422-03	50.40		
100s ea	63629-1422-01	84.00		
(Dispensing Solutions)				
REPACK				
TAB, PO, 300 mg, 30s ea	55045-1855-08	4.20		
30s ea	66336-0097-30	8.03		AA
60s ea	66336-0097-60	10.87		AA
(GSMS)				
REPACK				
TAB, PO (UNIT OF USE)				
300 mg, 30s ea	60429-0115-30	12.87	4.29	AA
(HomeMed)				
REPACK				
TAB, PO, 300 mg, 30s ea	51655-0391-24	4.53		EE
35s ea	51655-0391-81	5.29		EE
(Nucare Pharm)				
REPACK				
TAB, PO, 300 mg, 30s ea	66267-0124-30	25.25		AA
60s ea	66267-0124-60	48.75		AA
100s ea	68071-1326-00	81.25		AA
(Palmetto)				
REPACK				
TAB, PO, 100 mg, 100s ea	23490-5766-01	15.00		
300 mg, 30s ea	23490-5767-01	13.50		
60s ea	23490-5767-02	27.00		
100s ea	23490-5767-03	45.00		
(PD-Rx Pharm)				
REPACK				
TAB, PO, 100 mg, 30s ea	55289-0055-30	20.00		AA
45s ea	55289-0055-45	23.33		AA
60s ea	55289-0055-60	26.67		AA
75s ea	55289-0055-75	30.00		AA
100s ea	55289-0055-01	35.56		AA
300 mg, 30s ea	55289-0742-30	22.67		AA
35s ea	55289-0742-35	24.22		AA
ISONIAZID (PD-Rx Pharm)				
REPACK				
TAB, PO, 300 mg, 50s ea	55289-0742-50	28.89		AA
60s ea	55289-0742-60	32.00		AA
100s ea	55289-0742-01	44.44		AA
(Pharma Pac)				
REPACK				
TAB, PO, 300 mg, 30s ea	52959-0145-30	11.44		AA
30s ea	52959-0419-30	25.20		AA
50s ea	52959-0145-50	18.00		AA
60s ea	52959-0145-60	21.50		AA
100s ea	52959-0145-00	25.70		AA
180s ea	52959-0145-81	39.68		AA
180s ea	52959-0419-81	87.30		AA
(Phys Total Care)				
REPACK				
TAB, PO, 300 mg, 30s ea	54868-2416-02	16.41		EE
100s ea	54868-2416-00	44.19		EE
(Quality Care Prod)				
REPACK				
TAB, PO, 300 mg, 100s ea	49999-0703-00	24.76		
(Southwood)				
REPACK				
TAB, PO, 100 mg, 100s ea	58016-0912-00	9.93		EE
300 mg, 10s ea	58016-0913-10	1.27		EE
14s ea	58016-0913-14	1.78		EE
15s ea	58016-0913-15	1.91		EE
20s ea	58016-0913-20	2.55		EE
21s ea	58016-0913-21	2.68		EE
24s ea	58016-0913-24	3.06		EE
28s ea	58016-0913-28	3.57		EE
30s ea	58016-0913-30	3.82		EE
40s ea	58016-0913-40	5.10		EE
60s ea	58016-0913-60	7.64		EE
100s ea	58016-0913-00	12.74		EE
(Vibranta)				
REPACK				
TAB, PO, 300 mg, 30s ea	57866-3941-01	14.67		
ISONIAZID/PYRAZINAMIDE/RIFAMPIN				
(Sanofi-Aventis) *See RIFATER*				
ISONIAZID/RIFAMPIN				
(Sanofi-Aventis) *See RIFAMATE*				
(VersaPharm) *See ISONARIF*				
ISOPROPAMIDE IODIDE (Gallipot)				
POW, NA, 10 gm	51552-0075-03	52.50		
(PCCA)				
POW, NA (U.S.P.)				
1 gm	51927-1402-00	9.00		

PROD/MFR	NDC	AWP	DP	OBC
(Spectrum Pharmacy)				
POW, NA (U.S.P./N.F.)				
10 gm	49452-3803-01	237.30		
ISOPROPYL ALCOHOL				
(Baker, J.T.) *See ALCOHOL ISOPROPYL*				
(Gallipot) *See ALCOHOL ISOPROPYL 50%*				
(Gallipot) *See ALCOHOL ISOPROPYL 70%*				
(Gallipot) *See ALCOHOL ISOPROPYL 91%*				
(Humco) *See ALCOHOL ISOPROPYL 70%*				
(Mallinckrodt Lab) *See ALCOHOL ISOPROPYL*				
(Medisca)				
SOL, NA (USP,1X500ML)				
500 ml	38779-0810-08	27.75		
(USP,1X1000ML)				
1000 ml	38779-0810-09	34.50		
(USP,1X4000ML)				
4000 ml	38779-0810-01	117.00		
(Medisca) *See STERILE 70% ISOPROPANOL*				
(PCCA) *See ISOPROPYL ALCOHOL 70%*				
(PCCA)				
LIQ, NA (USP)				
1 ml	51927-3305-00	0.03		
(Spectrum Pharmacy) *See ALCOHOL ISOPROPYL 70%*				
(Spectrum Pharmacy) *See ALCOHOL ISOPROPYL 99%*				
ISOPROPYL ALCOHOL 70% (PCCA)				
isopropyl alcohol				
LIQ, NA (STERILE)				
1 ml	51927-3608-00	0.16		
ISOPROPYL MYRISTATE (Amend)				
LIQ, NA (COSMETIC GRADE)				
500 ml	17317-0695-01	12.60		
(N.F.)				
500 ml	61972-1095-01	12.60		
(COSMETIC GRADE)				
3840 ml	17317-0695-06	42.00		
(N.F.)				
3840 ml	61972-1095-06	42.00		
(COSMETIC GRADE)				
20000 ml	17317-0695-08	175.00		
(N.F.)				
20000 ml	61972-1095-08	175.00		
(Gallipot)				
LIQ, NA (N.F.)				
473 ml	51552-0612-06	15.75		
(Letco)				
LIQ, NA (N.F.)				
500 ml	62991-2037-01	36.00		
(Medisca)				
SOL, NA (1X500ML)				
500 ml	38779-0906-08	37.50		
(1X1000ML)				
1000 ml	38779-0906-09	61.50		
4000 ml	38779-0906-01	156.00		
(PCCA)				
LIQ, NA (NF)				
1 ml	51927-1131-00	0.12		
(Spectrum Pharmacy)				
LIQ, NA (N.F.)				
500 ml	49452-3830-01	68.25		
4000 ml	49452-3830-02	246.40		
20000 ml	49452-3830-03	1071.00		
ISOPROPYL PALMITATE (Amend)				
LIQ, NA (COSMETIC GRADE)				
500 ml	17317-1097-01	12.60		
3840 ml	17317-1097-06	42.00		
(N.F.)				
3840 ml	17317-0696-06	42.00		
(COSMETIC GRADE)				
20000 ml	17317-1097-08	175.00		
(N.F.)				
20000 ml	17317-0696-08	175.00		
(Gallipot)				
LIQ, NA (N.F.)				
473 ml	51552-0277-06	15.75		
(Letco)				
LIQ, NA (N.F.)				
1000 ml	62991-1281-01	69.00		
3840 ml	62991-1281-02	123.00		
(Medisca)				
SOL, NA (1X500ML)				
500 ml	38779-0832-08	37.50		
(1X1000ML)				
1000 ml	38779-0832-09	64.50		

PROD/MFR	NDC	AWP	DP	OBC
(1X4000ML)				
4000 ml	38779-0832-01	127.50		
(PCCA)				
LIQ, NA (N.F.)				
1 ml	51927-1665-00	0.09		
(Spectrum Pharmacy)				
LIQ, NA (N.F.)				
500 ml	49452-3840-01	64.75		
4000 ml	49452-3840-02	191.10		
20000 ml	49452-3840-03	889.00		
ISOPROPYL PALMITATE/LECITHIN				
(Gallipot) *See LIPOIL*				
(Medisca) *See LIPMAX*				
ISOPROPYL PALMITATE/LECITHIN/SORBIC ACID				
(Letco) *See LECITHIN*				
ISOPROTERENOL HCL (PCCA)				
isoproterenol hydrochloride				
POW, NA (U.S.P.)				
1 gm	51927-1940-00	10.20		
ISOPROTERENOL HYDROCHLORIDE				
(Hospira) *See ISUPREL*				
(PCCA) *See ISOPROTERENOL HCL*				
ISOPROTERENOL SULFATE (Gallipot)				
POW, NA (U.S.P.)				
25 gm	51552-0517-04	103.88		
(PCCA)				
POW, NA (USP)				
1 gm	51927-1935-00	315.00		
ISOPTIN SR (Ranbaxy Labs)				
verapamil hydrochloride				
TER, PO (FILM-COATED)				
120 mg, 100s ea	10631-0488-01	228.73	123.27	
180 mg, 100s ea	10631-0489-01	289.91	156.23	
240 mg, 100s ea	10631-0490-01	331.65	178.75	
500s ea	10631-0490-05	1658.24	884.84	
(Phys Total Care)				
REPACK				
TER, PO, 240 mg, 20s ea	54868-1283-01	71.90		
60s ea	54868-1283-00	200.26		
ISOPTO ATROPINE (Alcon Ophthalmic)				
atropine sulfate				
SOL, OP, 1%, 5 ml	00998-0303-05	25.32		
15 ml	00998-0303-15	34.32		
ISOPTO CARBACHOL (Alcon Ophthalmic)				
carbachol				
SOL, OP, 1.5%, 15 ml	00998-0223-15	46.08		
3%, 15 ml	00998-0225-15	52.68		
(Phys Total Care)				
REPACK				
SOL, OP, 3%, 30 ml	54868-0630-02	60.40		
ISOPTO CARPINE (Alcon Ophthalmic)				
pilocarpine hydrochloride				
SOL, OP, 1%, 15 ml	00998-0203-15	33.18		
2%, 15 ml	00998-0204-15	33.90		
4%, 15 ml	00998-0206-15	35.58		
(Phys Total Care)				
REPACK				
SOL, OP, 0.25%, 15 ml	54868-3401-00	17.67		
ISOPTO HOMATROPINE (Alcon Ophthalmic)				
homatropine hydrobromide				
SOL, OP, 2%, 5 ml	00998-0311-05	27.84		
5%, 5 ml	00998-0315-05	32.04		
(Dispensing Solutions)				
REPACK				
SOL, OP, 5%, 5 ml	55045-2594-05	32.00		
(Phys Total Care)				
REPACK				
SOL, OP, 2%, 5 ml	54868-3400-00	17.21		
(Quality Care Prod)				
REPACK				
SOL, OP, 5%, 5 ml	49999-0534-05	33.53		
(Southwood)				
REPACK				
SOL, OP, 5%, 5 ml	58016-6532-01	25.06		
ISOPTO HYOSCINE (Alcon Ophthalmic)				
scopolamine hydrobromide				
SOL, OP, 0.25%, 5 ml	00998-0331-05	27.96		
(Phys Total Care)				
REPACK				
SOL, OP, 0.25%, 5 ml	54868-0658-01	26.85		

PROD/MFR	NDC	AWP	DP	OBC
(Southwood)				
REPACK				
SOL, OP, 0.25%, 5 ml	58016-6473-01	15.56		
ISORDIL TITRADOSE (BTA)				
isosorbide dinitrate				
TAB, PO, 5 mg, 100s ea	64455-0152-01	71.75	59.79	
40 mg, 100s ea	64455-0192-01	157.94	131.62	AB
(Phys Total Care)				
REPACK				
TAB, PO, 10 mg, 100s ea	54868-0682-01	46.86		AB
ISOSORBIDE (PCCA)				
POW, NA, 1 gm	51927-3324-00	2.16		
(Bryant Ranch)				
REPACK				
isosorbide mononitrate				
TER, PO, 30 mg, 30s ea	63629-1424-01	60.82		
ISOSORBIDE DIMETHYL ETHER (PCCA)				
dimethyl isosorbide				
POW, NA, 1 gm	51927-3420-00	11.40		
ISOSORBIDE DINITRATE				
FUL				
TAB, PO, 5 mg, 100s ea		4.88		
10 mg, 100s ea		5.25		
20 mg, 100s ea		5.63		
(BTA) *See ISORDIL TITRADOSE*				
(Caraco)				
TER, PO, 40 mg, 100s ea	00258-3613-01	84.56		AB
(Consolidated Midland)				
TAB, PO, 2.5 mg, 100s ea	00223-1091-01	2.00		EE
5 mg, 100s ea	00223-1095-01	2.60		EE
1000s ea	00223-1095-02	12.50		EE
10 mg, 100s ea	00223-1096-01	2.95		EE
1000s ea	00223-1096-02	11.25		EE
20 mg, 100s ea	00223-1099-01	4.25		EE
1000s ea	00223-1099-02	18.75		EE
SL, 2.5 mg, 1000s ea	00223-1091-02	8.75		EE
5 mg, 100s ea	00223-1094-01	2.50		EE
1000s ea	00223-1094-02	11.00		EE
(Forest Pharm) *See ISOCHRON*				
(Major)				
TAB, PO (10X10)				
5 mg, 100s ea UD	00904-2150-61	14.25		AB
10 mg, 100s ea UD	00904-2151-61	16.98		AB
20 mg, 100s ea UD	00904-2154-61	20.94		AB
(Par)				
TAB, PO, 5 mg, 100s ea	49884-0020-01	17.05		AB
1000s ea	49884-0020-10	161.98		AB
10 mg, 100s ea	49884-0021-01	18.00		AB
1000s ea	49884-0021-10	171.00		AB
20 mg, 100s ea	49884-0022-01	21.00		AB
1000s ea	49884-0022-10	199.50		AB
30 mg, 100s ea	49884-0009-01	53.15		AB
1000s ea	49884-0009-10	478.35		AB
(Qualitest)				
TAB, PO, 5 mg, 100s ea	00603-4116-21	17.04		AB
1000s ea	00603-4116-32	161.98		AB
20 mg, 100s ea	00603-4118-21	24.80		AB
SL, 2.5 mg, 100s ea	00603-4122-21	10.28		AB
5 mg, 100s ea	00603-4123-21	10.28		AB
(Rising)				
TER, PO (USP,COMPRESSED TABLET)				
40 mg, 100s ea	64980-0144-01	84.56		AB
(Sandoz)				
TAB, PO, 5 mg, 100s ea	00781-1635-01	13.74		AB
1000s ea	00781-1635-10	130.53		AB
10 mg, 100s ea	00781-1556-01	15.37		AB
100s ea UD	00781-1556-13	19.56		AB
1000s ea	00781-1556-10	146.02		AB
20 mg, 100s ea	00781-1695-01	24.80		AB
100s ea UD	00781-1695-13	29.76		AB
1000s ea	00781-1695-10	235.60		AB
(UCB) *See DILATRATE-SR*				
(West-Ward)				
TAB, PO, 2.5 mg, 100s ea	00143-1765-01	20.65		AB
5 mg, 100s ea	00143-1767-01	20.65		AB
100s ea	00143-1769-01	16.50		AB
100s ea UD	00143-1769-25	21.35		AB
1000s ea	00143-1769-10	156.75		AB
10 mg, 100s ea	00143-1771-01	17.15		AB
100s ea UD	00143-1771-25	24.45		AB
1000s ea	00143-1771-10	162.93		AB
20 mg, 100s ea	00143-1772-01	20.05		AB
100s ea UD	00143-1772-25	26.85		AB
1000s ea	00143-1772-10	190.45		AB
(USP)				
30 mg, 100s ea	00143-1773-01	53.00		AB
1000s ea	00143-1773-10	443.00		AB
(Bryant Ranch)				
REPACK				
TAB, PO, 10 mg, 30s ea	63629-2573-01	6.84		
90s ea	63629-2573-02	20.53		
(DHS, Inc.)				
REPACK				
TAB, PO, 10 mg, 30s ea	55887-0360-30	6.99		AB
(GSMS)				
REPACK				
TAB, PO (UNIT OF USE)				
10 mg, 90s ea	60429-0101-90	9.75	3.25	AB
270s ea	60429-0101-27	22.80	7.60	AB
360s ea	60429-0101-36	29.25	9.75	AB
20 mg, 270s ea	60429-0102-27	34.95	11.65	AB
360s ea	60429-0102-36	45.60	15.20	AB
(HomeMed)				
REPACK				
TAB, PO, 10 mg, 90s ea	51655-0406-26	6.07		EE
100s ea	51655-0406-21	6.75		EE
20 mg, 90s ea	51655-0544-26	6.40		EE
100s ea	51655-0544-21	9.00		EE
270s ea	51655-0544-92	17.82		EE
(Palmetto)				
REPACK				
TAB, PO, 10 mg, 90s ea	23490-6875-01	24.75		
20 mg, 90s ea	23490-5771-01	53.97		
(PD-Rx Pharm)				
REPACK				
TAB, PO, 10 mg, 8s ea	55289-0667-08	5.68		AB
30s ea	58864-0642-30	7.50		AB
(REDI-SCRIPT)				
10 mg, 56s ea	58864-0642-56	9.67		AB
100s ea	55289-0667-01	12.17		AB
(REDI-SCRIPT)				
20 mg, 56s ea	58864-0304-56	8.75		AB
60s ea	55289-0174-60	11.37		AB
90s ea	58864-0304-90	19.33		EE
(REDI-SCRIPT)				
30 mg, 90s ea	58864-0816-90	18.05		AB
100s ea	43063-0128-01	26.46		AB
(Pharma Pac)				
REPACK				
TAB, PO, 10 mg, 90s ea	52959-0884-90	20.70		
20 mg, 180s ea	52959-0966-18	10.80		AB
(Phys Total Care)				
REPACK				
TAB, PO, 5 mg, 100s ea	54868-2297-00	16.35		EE
10 mg, 30s ea	54868-0681-00	7.26		EE
90s ea	54868-0681-03	15.75		AB
100s ea	54868-0681-01	17.16		EE
20 mg, 30s ea	54868-2127-03	7.89		AB
90s ea	54868-2127-02	14.67		EE
100s ea	54868-2127-01	15.81		EE
30 mg, 15s ea	54868-2590-04	14.31		EE
200s ea	54868-2590-02	135.12		EE
500s ea	54868-2590-03	331.05		EE
TER, PO, 40 mg, 30s ea	54868-2711-01	66.96		EE
60s ea	54868-2711-02	100.05		AB
100s ea	54868-2711-00	212.76		EE
(Quality Care Prod)				
REPACK				
TAB, PO, 10 mg, 60s ea	49999-0396-60	20.38		AB
30 mg, 30s ea	49999-0513-30	19.13		AB
TER, PO, 40 mg, 30s ea	49999-0440-30	60.24		AB
(Southwood)				
REPACK				
TAB, PO, 2.5 mg, 30s ea	00490-0059-30	6.20		
60s ea	00490-0059-60	12.39		
90s ea	00490-0059-90	18.59		
100s ea	00490-0059-00	20.65		
20 mg, 30s ea	58016-0707-30	17.99		EE
60s ea	58016-0707-60	35.98		EE
90s ea	58016-0707-90	53.96		EE
100s ea	58016-0707-00	59.96		EE
(Vibranta)				
REPACK				
TAB, PO, 10 mg, 90s ea	57866-3943-02	18.22		
180s ea	57866-3943-04	35.35		
360s ea	57866-3943-05	69.61		
ISOSORBIDE MONONITRATE				
FUL				
TAB, PO, 10 mg, 100s ea		61.10		
20 mg, 100s ea		49.50		
TER, PO, 60 mg, 100s ea		60.00		
(Actavis)				
TAB, PO, 10 mg, 100s ea	00228-2631-11	70.81		AB
20 mg, 100s ea	00228-2620-11	74.52		AB
(Ethex)				
TER, PO, 30 mg, 100s ea UD	58177-0222-11	132.85		AB
60 mg, 100s ea UD	58177-0238-11	136.25		AB
(Kremers Urban)				
TAB, PO, 10 mg, 100s ea	62175-0106-01	50.91		AB
20 mg, 100s ea	62175-0107-01	41.25		AB
TER, PO, 30 mg, 100s ea	62175-0128-37	51.64		AB
1000s ea	62175-0128-43	500.89		AB
60 mg, 100s ea	62175-0119-37	54.34		AB
1000s ea	62175-0119-43	527.08		AB
120 mg, 100s ea	62175-0129-37	76.08		AB
(Promius) *See ISMO*				
(Schering) *See IMDUR*				
(UCB) *See MONOKET*				
(West-Ward)				
TAB, PO (WHITE)				
20 mg, 100s ea	00143-1333-01	73.50		AB
1000s ea	00143-1333-10	450.56		AB
TER, PO (FILM-COATED)				
30 mg, 100s ea	00143-2230-01	111.56		AB
60 mg, 100s ea	00143-2260-01	142.50	5.25	AB
(A-S Medication)				
REPACK				
TER, PO, 60 mg, 30s ea	54569-5341-00	43.08		EE
(DHS, Inc.)				
REPACK				
TER, PO, 60 mg, 30s ea	55887-0950-30	14.00		
(Dispensing Solutions)				
REPACK				
TER, PO, 30 mg, 100s ea	55045-3105-00	112.00		AB
(McKesson Packaging)				
REPACK				
TER, PO, 30 mg, 100s ea UD	63739-0417-10	33.19		EE
60 mg, 100s ea UD	63739-0418-10	29.38		EE
(PD-Rx Pharm)				
REPACK				
TER, PO (REDI-SCRIPT)				
30 mg, 30s ea	58864-0721-30	13.65		
60 mg, 30s ea	58864-0725-30	8.42		AB
(Phys Total Care)				
REPACK				
TAB, PO, 20 mg, 60s ea	54868-3822-02	32.88		AB
100s ea	54868-3822-01	39.18		EE
TER, PO, 30 mg, 15s ea	54868-4416-02	24.62		EE
30s ea	54868-4416-00	43.23		EE
60s ea	54868-4416-01	80.46		EE
90s ea	54868-4416-04	91.42		EE
100s ea	54868-4416-03	99.41		AB
60 mg, 15s ea	54868-4417-03	24.65		AB
30s ea	54868-4417-00	43.30		EE
60s ea	54868-4417-01	80.60		EE
100s ea	54868-4417-02	99.58		AB
120 mg, 30s ea	54868-5543-00	19.23		
(Quality Care Prod)				
REPACK				
TER, PO, 30 mg, 30s ea	49999-0760-30	19.11		
(Southwood)				
REPACK				
TAB, PO, 10 mg, 30s ea	58016-0882-30	21.15		AB
60s ea	58016-0882-60	42.29		AB
90s ea	58016-0882-90	63.44		AB
100s ea	58016-0882-00	70.49		AB
(Stat Rx)				
REPACK				
TAB, PO, 20 mg, 30s ea	16590-0654-30	25.00		AB
60s ea	16590-0654-60	50.00		AB
90s ea	16590-0654-90	75.00		AB
(Vibranta)				
REPACK				
TER, PO, 30 mg, 30s ea	57866-3944-01	51.72		
60 mg, 30s ea	57866-3945-01	54.38		
120 mg, 30s ea	57866-3946-01	75.68		
ISOSORBIDE MONONITRATE ER (DHS, Inc.)				
REPACK				
isosorbide mononitrate				
TER, PO, 30 mg, 30s ea	55887-0296-30	11.93		
ISOSULFAN BLUE				
(Covidien) *See LYMPHAZURIN*				
ISOTRETINOIN (Medisca)				
POW, NA (U.S.P.)				
1 gm	38779-0911-06	105.00		
5 gm	38779-0911-03	450.00		

PROD/MFR | NDC | AWP | DP | OBC

(Mylan Bertek) *See AMNESTEEM*
(Ranbaxy Labs) *See SOTRET*
(Teva) *See CLARAVIS*
(Phys Total Care)
REPACK
SGL, PO, 20 mg, 30s ea . . . **54868-5163-00** 759.03
40 mg, 30s ea. **54868-5128-01** 788.87

ISOVUE MULTIPACK-250 (Bracco Diag)
iopamidol
SOL, IJ (BOTTLE)
51%, 200 ml 10s . . . . . **00270-1317-41** 1839.00 1471.20 **AP**

ISOVUE MULTIPACK-300 (Bracco Diag)
iopamidol
SOL, IJ (BOTTLE)
61%, 200 ml 10s . . . . . **00270-1315-41** 2062.50 1650.00 **AP**
500 ml 6s. . . . . **00270-1315-98** 2992.50 2394.00 **AP**

ISOVUE MULTIPACK-370 (Bracco Diag)
iopamidol
SOL, IJ (BOTTLE)
76%, 200 ml 10s . . . . . **00270-1316-41** 2200.00 1760.00 **AP**
500 ml 6s. . . . . **00270-1316-98** 3112.50 2490.00 **AP**

ISOVUE-200 (Bracco Diag)
iopamidol
SOL, IJ (VIAL)
41%, 50 ml 10s . . . . . . **00270-1314-30** 537.50 430.00 **AP**
(BOTTLE)
41%, 100 ml 10s . . . . . **00270-1314-34** 875.00 700.00 **AP**
(S.D. BOTTLE)
41%, 200 ml 10s . . . . . **00270-1314-15** 1562.50 1250.00 **AP**

ISOVUE-250 (Bracco Diag)
iopamidol
SOL, IJ (VIAL)
51%, 50 ml 10s . . . . . . **00270-1317-05** 553.12 442.50 **AP**
(BOTTLE)
51%, 100 ml 10s . . . . . **00270-1317-02** 981.50 785.20 **AP**
(INJECTOR SRN,PREFILLED)
51%, 150 ml 10s . . . . . **00270-1317-43** 1425.00 1140.00 **AP**
(S.D. BOTTLE)
51%, 150 ml 10s . . . . . **00270-1317-09** 1274.12 1019.30 **AP**
200 ml 10s . . . . **00270-1317-39** 1826.50 1461.20 **AP**

ISOVUE-300 (Bracco Diag)
iopamidol
SOL, IJ (VIAL)
61%, 30 ml 10s . . . . . . **00270-1315-25** 540.75 432.60 **AP**
50 ml 10s. . . . . **00270-1315-30** 574.88 459.90 **AP**
(S.D. BOTTLE)
61%, 75 ml 10s . . . . . . **00270-1315-47** 931.88 745.50 **AP**
(INJECTOR SRN,PREFILLED)
61%, 100 ml 10s . . . . . **00270-1315-57** 1199.52 1020.00 **AP**
(S.D. BOTTLE)
61%, 100 ml 10s . . . . . **00270-1315-35** 1123.50 898.80 **AP**
(INJECTOR SRN,PREFILLED)
61%, 125 ml 10s . . . . . **00270-1315-59** 1458.24 1240.00 **AP**
150 ml 10s . . . . **00270-1315-58** 1664.04 1415.00 **AP**
(S.D.BOTTLE)
61%, 150 ml 10s . . . . . **00270-1315-50** 1637.50 1310.00 **AP**

ISOVUE-370 (Bracco Diag)
iopamidol
SOL, IJ (S.D. BOTTLE)
76%, 50 ml 10s . . . . . . **00270-1316-01** 625.00 500.00 **AP**
(VIAL)
76%, 50 ml 10s . . . . . . **00270-1316-30** 625.00 500.00 **AP**
(INJECTOR SRN,PREFILLED)
76%, 75 ml 10s . . . . . . **00270-1316-56** 1046.64 890.00 **AP**
(S.D. BOTTLE)
76%, 75 ml 10s . . . . . . **00270-1316-52** 937.50 750.00 **AP**
(INJECTOR SRN,PREFILLED)
76%, 100 ml 10s . . . . . **00270-1316-57** 1293.60 1100.00 **AP**
(S.D.BOTTLE)
76%, 100 ml 10s . . . . . **00270-1316-35** 1246.88 997.50 **AP**
(INJECTOR SRN,PREFILLED)
76%, 125 ml 10s . . . . . **00270-1316-59** 1531.741302.50 **AP**
(S.D. BOTTLE)
76%, 125 ml 10s . . . . . **00270-1316-04** 1473.62 1178.90 **AP**
150 ml 10s . . . . **00270-1316-37** 1725.00 1380.00 **AP**
175 ml 10s . . . . **00270-1316-44** 2009.44 1607.55 **AP**
200 ml 10s . . . . **00270-1316-40** 2200.00 1760.00 **AP**

ISOVUE-M 200 (Bracco Diag)
iopamidol
SOL, IJ (VIAL)
41%, 10 ml 10s **00270-1411-11** 738.56 628.03
20 ml 10s. **00270-1411-25** 1011.89 860.44

ISOVUE-M 300 (Bracco Diag)
iopamidol
SOL, IJ (VIAL)
61%, 15 ml 10s **00270-1412-15** 981.36 834.49

ISOXSUPRINE HCL (Hawkins)
isoxsuprine hydrochloride
POW, NA (USP)
5 gm **63370-0119-15** 72.00
25 gm **63370-0119-25** 336.00
100 gm. **63370-0119-35** 1008.00
500 gm. **63370-0119-45** 4320.00
1000 gm. **63370-0119-50** 7920.00

(Medisca)
POW, NA (U.S.P.)
5 gm **38779-0234-03** 76.50
(USP,1X25GM)
25 gm **38779-0234-04** 315.00
(U.S.P.)
100 gm. **38779-0234-05** 750.00
1000 gm. **38779-0234-09** 2565.00

(PCCA)
POW, NA (U.S.P.)
1 gm **51927-3056-00** 23.40

(Sandoz)
TAB, PO, 10 mg, 100s ea . . **00781-1840-01** 115.56
20 mg, 100s ea **00781-1842-01** 186.37

(Spectrum Pharmacy)
POW, NA (U.S.P.)
5 gm **49452-3821-01** 152.60
25 gm **49452-3821-02** 598.50
100 gm. **49452-3821-03** 1326.50

(Phys Total Care)
REPACK
TAB, PO, 20 mg, 100s ea . . **54868-1464-00** 17.63

ISOXSUPRINE HYDROCHLORIDE
(Hawkins) *See ISOXSUPRINE HCL*
(Medisca) *See ISOXSUPRINE HCL*
(PCCA) *See ISOXSUPRINE HCL*
(Sandoz) *See ISOXSUPRINE HCL*
(Spectrum Pharmacy) *See ISOXSUPRINE HCL*

ISRADIPINE
(Glaxo) *See DYNACIRC CR*
(Watson Labs)
CAP, PO, 2.5 mg, 100s ea. . **16252-0539-01** 116.28 **AB**
5 mg, 100s ea. . . . . **16252-0540-01** 170.05 **AB**
(Phys Total Care)
REPACK
CAP, PO (USP)
5 mg, 20s ea. **54868-5561-01** 103.23
60s ea **54868-5561-00** 300.69

ISTALOL (ISTA Pharm.)
timolol maleate
SOL, OP, 0.5%, 2.5 ml. **67425-0003-12** 69.00
5 ml. **67425-0003-50** 136.56

ISUPREL (Hospira)
isoproterenol hydrochloride
SOL, IV (25X1ML, AMP,LATEX-FREE)
0.2 mg/ml,
1 ml 25s. . . . . **00074-1410-01** 282.00 246.75 **AP**
(AMP,25X1ML,LATEX-FREE)
0.2 mg/ml,
1 ml 25s. . . . . **00409-1410-01** 352.20 308.25 **AP**
(10X5ML,AMP,LATEX-FREE)
0.2 mg/ml,
5 ml 10s. . . . . **00409-1410-05** 164.04 143.50 **AP**

ITRACONAZOLE (B&B Pharm, Inc)
POW, NA, 5 gm **63275-9963-02** 315.00
25 gm **63275-9963-04** 1575.00
100 gm. **63275-9963-05** 6200.00
1000 gm. **63275-9963-09** 59000.00
(Centocor) *See SPORANOX*
(Gallipot)
POW, NA (1X5GM)
5 gm **51552-0920-02** 68.60 49.00
(1X25GM)
25 gm **51552-0920-04** 266.00 190.00
(1X100GM)
100 gm. **51552-0920-05** 1015.00 725.00
(1X500GM)
500 gm. **51552-0920-06** 4550.00 3250.00
(Janssen) *See SPORANOX*
(Letco)
POW, NA, 5 gm **62991-2562-03** 105.00
25 gm **62991-2562-02** 450.00
100 gm. **62991-2562-01** 1200.00
(Medisca)
POW, NA, 10 gm. **38779-1931-01** 315.00
(1X10GM, BP)
10 gm **38779-2467-01** 315.00
(1X25GM, BP)
25 gm **38779-2467-04** 645.00
(1X25GM)
25 gm **38779-1931-04** 645.00
(1X100GM, BP)
100 gm. **38779-2467-05** 2040.00
(1X100GM)
100 gm. **38779-1931-05** 2040.00
(1X1000GM, BP)
1000 gm. **38779-2467-09** 7260.00
(1X1000GM)
1000 gm. **38779-1931-09** 7260.00
(Patriot Pharmaceuticals)
CAP, PO, 100 mg,
28s ea UD **10147-1700-07** 250.08
30s ea. **10147-1700-03** 278.31
(Sandoz)
CAP, PO (7X4)
100 mg, 28s ea UD . . . **00185-0550-83** 278.33 **AB**
30s ea. . . . . **00185-0550-30** 260.50 **AB**
(Spectrum Pharmacy)
CRY, NA, 1 gm. **49452-3845-01** 156.10
5 gm **49452-3845-02** 511.00
25 gm **49452-3845-03** 808.50
100 gm. **49452-3845-04** 2712.50
POW, NA (1X1GM)
1 gm **49452-3847-01** 156.10
(1X5GM)
5 gm **49452-3847-02** 511.00
(1X25GM)
25 gm **49452-3847-03** 808.50
(1X100GM)
100 gm. **49452-3847-04** 2712.50
(Phys Total Care)
REPACK
CAP, PO (7-DAY PACK)
100 mg, 28s ea . . . . . . **54868-5328-00** 609.03 **AB**

ITRACONAZOLE EP MICRONIZED (PCCA)
itraconazole, micronized
POW, NA (1X1GM)
1 gm **51927-4325-00** 135.00

ITRACONAZOLE MICRONIZED (Hawkins)
itraconazole, micronized
POW, NA, 5 gm **63370-0122-15** 240.00
25 gm **63370-0122-25** 960.00
100 gm. **63370-0122-35** 2880.00
(PCCA)
POW, NA, 1 gm **51927-3306-00** 87.00

ITRACONAZOLE, MICRONIZED
(Hawkins) *See ITRACONAZOLE MICRONIZED*
(PCCA) *See ITRACONAZOLE EP MICRONIZED*
(PCCA) *See ITRACONAZOLE MICRONIZED*

IV TRANSFER SPIKE (APP)
transfer unit, iv fluid
DEV, NA (PLASTIC DBL-PNT SPIKE)
100s ea. **63323-0001-31** 173.69

IVERMECTIN (Gallipot)
POW, NA, 5 gm **51552-0619-02** 70.00
(Hawkins)
POW, NA (U.S.P.,B.P.)
5 gm **63370-0123-15** 120.00
25 gm **63370-0123-25** 560.00
100 gm. **63370-0123-35** 1920.00
500 gm. **63370-0123-50** 6800.00
(Medisca)
POW, NA, 5 gm **38779-0948-03** 177.00
(1X5GM)
5 gm **38779-2485-03** 177.00
25 gm **38779-0948-04** 675.00
(1X25GM)
25 gm **38779-2485-04** 675.00
100 gm. **38779-0948-05** 1365.00
(1X100GM)
100 gm. **38779-2485-05** 1365.00
500 gm. **38779-0948-08** 5202.00
1000 gm. **38779-0948-09** 5265.00
(1X100GM)
1000 gm. **38779-2485-09** 5265.00
(Merck) *See STROMECTOL*
(PCCA)
POW, NA, 1 gm **51927-3197-00** 39.60
(Spectrum Pharmacy)
POW, NA (1X1GM, USP)
1 gm **49452-3855-01** 111.65

PROD/MFR NDC AWP DP OBC

(1X5GM, USP)
5 gm 49452-3855-02 281.05
(1X25GM, USP)
25 gm 49452-3855-03 1081.50
(1X100GM, USP)
100 gm............... 49452-3855-04 2446.50

IVITES RX (Breckenridge Pharm)
vitamin b complex, mineral, and vitamin c
TAB, PO (FILM-COATED)
100s ea............. 51991-0593-01 25.87

IXABEPILONE
(B/M Squibb Onc/Vir) *See IXEMPRA*

IXEMPRA (B/M Squibb Onc/Vir)
ixabepilone
PDS, IV (W/DILUENT)
15 mg, ea........... 00015-1910-12 1106.35
45 mg, ea........... 00015-1911-13 3319.07

IXIARO (Novartis)
japanese encephalitis vaccine, inactivated adsorb
SUS, IM (TAX INCL.)
6 mcg/0.5 ml,
0.5 ml 42515-0001-01 234.75 195.75

J-COF DHC (JayMac Pharma)
bpm/dihydrocodeine bitartrate/pse hcl
SOL, PO (1X473ML,AF,SF,DYE-FREE)
473 ml, C-III 64661-0060-16 105.98 79.69

J-MAX (JayMac Pharma)
guaifenesin/phenylephrine hydrochloride
SYR, PO (DYE-FREE,GLUTEN-FREE)
200 mg/5 ml-5 mg/5 ml,
473 ml 64661-0011-16 110.85 83.35

(JayMac Pharma)
guaifenesin/phenylephrine
T12, PO, 1200 mg-35 mg,
100s ea........... 64661-0010-01 136.86 102.90

J-MAX DHC (JayMac Pharma)
dihydrocodeine bitartrate/guaifenesin
SOL, PO (1X473ML,AF,GRAPE)
7.5 mg/5 ml-100 mg/5 ml,
473 ml, C-III 64661-0070-16 105.98 79.69

J-TAN (JayMac Pharma)
brompheniramine tannate
SUS, PO (STRAWBERRY CREAM)
4 mg/5 ml, 473 ml.... 64661-0020-16 131.97 99.23

J-TAN D (JayMac Pharma)
brompheniramine tannate/phenylephrine tannate
CTB, PO, 1.58 mg-2.2 mg,
100s ea........... 64661-0021-01 158.07 118.85
SUS, PO (STRAWBERRY CREAM)
5 mg/5 ml-5 mg/5 ml,
473 ml 64661-0022-16 158.07 118.85

J-TAN D HC (JayMac Pharma)
bpm/hydrocod bit/pse hcl
SOL, PO (AF,SF,DYE-FREE)
473 ml, C-III 64661-0040-16 91.77 69.00

J-TAN D PD (JayMac Pharma)
bpm/pse hcl
SOL, PO (W/DROPPER,AF,SF)
1 mg/ml-7.5 mg/ml,
30 ml.............. 64661-0032-30 38.67 29.07

J-TAN D SR (JayMac Pharma)
bpm/phenyleph hcl
TER, PO, 6 mg-30 mg,
100s ea........... 64661-0050-01 150.87 110.45

J-TAN PD (JayMac Pharma)
brompheniramine maleate
SOL, PO (W/DROPPER,AF,SF)
1 mg/ml, 30 ml....... 64661-0031-30 38.67 29.07

JANTOVEN (Upsher-Smith)
warfarin sodium
TAB, PO, 1 mg, ea .... 00832-1211-89 0.49 AB
100s ea........... 00832-1211-00 49.19 AB
100s ea UD .... 00832-1211-01 49.19 AB
1000s ea .... 00832-1211-10 491.91 AB
2 mg, ea............ 00832-1212-89 0.51 AB
100s ea........... 00832-1212-00 51.36 AB
100s ea UD .... 00832-1212-01 51.36 AB
1000s ea .... 00832-1212-10 513.61 AB
2.5 mg, ea.......... 00832-1213-89 0.53 AB
100s ea........... 00832-1213-00 52.81 AB
100s ea UD .... 00832-1213-01 52.81 AB
1000s ea .... 00832-1213-10 528.08 AB
3 mg, ea............ 00832-1214-89 0.53 AB
100s ea........... 00832-1214-00 52.81 AB
100s ea UD .... 00832-1214-01 52.81 AB
1000s ea .... 00832-1214-10 528.08 AB
4 mg, ea............ 00832-1215-89 0.53 AB
100s ea........... 00832-1215-00 52.81 AB
100s ea UD .... 00832-1215-01 52.81 AB
1000s ea .... 00832-1215-10 528.08 AB
5 mg, ea............ 00832-1216-89 0.55 AB
100s ea........... 00832-1216-00 54.98 AB
100s ea UD .... 00832-1216-01 54.98 AB
1000s ea .... 00832-1216-10 549.78 AB
6 mg, ea............ 00832-1217-89 0.71 AB
100s ea........... 00832-1217-00 70.89 AB
100s ea UD .... 00832-1217-01 70.89 AB
1000s ea .... 00832-1217-10 708.93 AB
7.5 mg, ea.......... 00832-1218-89 0.74 AB
100s ea........... 00832-1218-00 73.79 AB
100s ea UD .... 00832-1218-01 73.79 AB
500s ea........... 00832-1218-50 368.93 AB
(DYE-FREE)
10 mg, ea........... 00832-1219-89 0.76 AB
100s ea........... 00832-1219-00 75.96 AB
100s ea UD .... 00832-1219-01 75.96 AB
500s ea........... 00832-1219-50 379.79 AB

(Phys Total Care)
REPACK
TAB, PO, 2 mg, 30s ea .... 54868-0822-00 20.59 AB
3 mg, 30s ea......... 54868-5425-00 23.42 AB
4 mg, 30s ea......... 54868-0825-00 23.43
5 mg, 30s ea......... 54868-5207-00 32.10 AB
100s ea........... 54868-5207-01 101.76
6 mg, 30s ea......... 54868-1216-00 32.24 AB

JANUMET (Merck)
metformin hydrochloride/sitagliptin phosphate
TAB, PO (FILM-COATED)
500 mg-50 mg,
50s ea UD 00006-0575-52 171.50
60s ea........... 00006-0575-61 205.80
180s ea........... 00006-0575-62 617.36
1000s ea 00006-0575-82 3429.86
1000 mg-50 mg,
50s ea UD 00006-0577-52 171.50
60s ea........... 00006-0577-61 205.80
180s ea........... 00006-0577-62 617.36
1000s ea 00006-0577-82 3429.86

(Phys Total Care)
REPACK
TAB, PO (FILM-COATED)
500 mg-50 mg,
60s ea........... 54868-5973-00 229.85
1000 mg-50 mg,
60s ea........... 54868-1097-00 245.58
180s ea........... 54868-1097-01 709.89

(Quality Care Prod)
REPACK
TAB, PO (FILM-COATED)
500 mg-50 mg,
60s ea........... 35356-0136-60 315.20

JANUVIA (Merck)
sitagliptin phosphate
TAB, PO (FILM-COATED)
25 mg, 30s ea........ 00006-0221-31 205.80
90s ea........... 00006-0221-54 617.36
100s ea UD 00006-0221-28 685.97
50 mg, 30s ea........ 00006-0112-31 205.80
90s ea........... 00006-0112-54 617.36
100s ea UD 00006-0112-28 685.97
100 mg, 30s ea 00006-0277-31 205.80
90s ea........... 00006-0277-54 617.36
100s ea UD 00006-0277-28 685.97
1000s ea 00006-0277-82 6859.72

(A-S Medication)
REPACK
TAB, PO (FILM-COATED)
100 mg, 30s ea 54569-5925-00 267.54

(AQ)
REPACK
TAB, PO (FILM-COATED)
100 mg, 30s ea 66105-0652-03 300.40

(Phys Total Care)
REPACK
TAB, PO (FILM-COATED)
50 mg, 30s ea........ 54868-6031-00 245.58
90s ea........... 54868-6031-01 709.89
100 mg, 30s ea 54868-5840-00 245.58

(Quality Care Prod)
REPACK
TAB, PO (FILM-COATED)
100 mg, 30s ea 35356-0103-30 313.21

JAPANESE ENCEPHALITIS VACCINE, INACTIVATED ADSORB
(Novartis) *See IXIARO*

JAPANESE ENCEPHALITIS VIRUS VACCINE, INACTIVATED
(Sanofi) *See JE-VAX*

JASMINE (PCCA)
jasmine oil
OIL, NA (ARTIFICIAL)
1 ml............... 51927-1257-00 1.20

JASMINE OIL (Amend)
OIL, NA (ARTIFICIAL)
120 ml 17317-0304-04 12.60
500 ml 17317-0304-01 42.00

(Gallipot)
OIL, NA (ARTIFICIAL)
100 ml 51552-0609-05 27.30

(Medisca)
OIL, NA (1X14ML,SYNTHETIC)
14 ml............... 38779-1364-03 13.50
(1X25ML,SYNTHETIC)
25 ml............... 38779-1364-04 22.50
(1X100ML,SYNTHETIC)
100 ml 38779-1364-05 49.50
(1X500ML,SYNTHETIC)
500 ml 38779-1364-08 223.50

(PCCA) *See JASMINE*

JAY-PHYL (JayMac Pharma)
dyphylline/guaifenesin
SYR, PO (AF,SF,ORANGE,VANILLA)
100 mg/5 ml-50 mg/5 ml,
473 ml 64661-0814-16 112.90 84.89

(Pharmakon)
SYR, PO (A.F,AF,SF,ORANGE)
100 mg/5 ml-50 mg/5 ml,
473 ml 55422-0814-16 36.00

JAYCOF EXPECTORANT (Pharmakon)
hydrocodone bitartrate/potassium guaiacolsulfonate
SYR, PO (AF,SF,CHERRY)
5 mg/5 ml-350 mg/5 ml,
473 ml, C-III 55422-0811-16 48.95

JAYCOF-HC (Pharmakon)
cpm/hydrocod bit/pse hcl
LIQ, PO (AF,SF,DYE-FREE)
473 ml, C-III 55422-0813-16 48.95

JAYCOF-XP (Pharmakon)
gg/hydrocod bit/pse hcl
SYR, PO (D.F,AF,SF,DYE-FREE)
473 ml, C-III 55422-0812-16 49.50

JE-VAX (Sanofi)
japanese encephalitis virus vaccine, inactivated
PDR, SC (S.D.V. W/DILUENT)
3s ea.............. 49281-0680-30 346.68 288.90

JELCO IV CATHETER/FEP (J&J Medical)
catheter
DEV, NA (PLASTIC HUB,RO,20X1")
ea................. 56091-0040-57 1.04
(PLASTIC HUB,RO,22X1")
ea................. 56091-0040-50 1.11
(PLASTIC HUB,RO,24X3/4")
ea................. 56091-0040-53 1.50
(PLSTC HUB,RO,14X1 1/4")
ea................. 56091-0040-48 1.04
(PLSTC HUB,RO,14X2 1/4")
ea................. 56091-0040-58 1.04
(PLSTC HUB,RO,16X1 1/4")
ea................. 56091-0040-42 1.04
(PLSTC HUB,RO,16X2 1/4")
ea................. 56091-0040-52 1.04
(PLSTC HUB,RO,18X1 1/4")
ea................. 56091-0040-55 1.04
(PLSTC HUB,RO,18X1 3/4")
ea................. 56091-0040-54 1.04
(PLSTC HUB,RO,20X1 1/4")
ea................. 56091-0040-56 1.04
(PLSTC HUB,RO,20X1 3/4")
ea................. 56091-0040-59 1.04

JELCO STRIPED IV CATHETER/FEP (J&J Medical)
catheter
DEV, NA (PLASTIC HUB,RO,20X1")
ea................. 56091-0040-67 1.17
(PLASTIC HUB,RO,22X1")
ea................. 56091-0040-60 1.24
(PLASTIC HUB,RO,24X3/4")
ea................. 56091-0040-63 1.63
(PLSTC HUB,RO,14X2 1/4")
ea................. 56091-0040-68 1.17

PROD/MFR | NDC | AWP | DP | OBC

(PLSTC HUB,RO,16X2 1/4")
ea.................. 56091-0040-62 1.17
(PLSTC HUB,RO,18X1 1/4")
ea.................. 56091-0040-65 1.17
(PLSTC HUB,RO,18X1 3/4")
ea.................. 56091-0040-64 1.17
(PLSTC HUB,RO,20X1 1/4")
ea.................. 56091-0040-66 1.17
(PLSTC HUB,RO,20X1 3/4")
ea.................. 56091-0040-69 1.17

JELCO WINGED IV CATHETER/FEP (J&J Medical)
catheter
DEV, NA (PLASTIC HUB,RO,20X1")
ea.................. 56091-0040-77 1.25
(PLASTIC HUB,RO,22X1")
ea.................. 56091-0040-70 1.32
(PLASTIC HUB,RO,24X5/8")
ea.................. 56091-0040-73 1.74
(PLSTC HUB,RO,14X1 1/4")
ea.................. 56091-0040-78 1.25
(PLSTC HUB,RO,16X1 1/4")
ea.................. 56091-0040-72 1.25
(PLSTC HUB,RO,18X1 1/4")
ea.................. 56091-0040-75 1.25
(PLSTC HUB,RO,18X1 3/4")
ea.................. 56091-0040-74 1.25
(PLSTC HUB,RO,20X1 1/4")
ea.................. 56091-0040-76 1.25

JET (Medisca)
gel, multi ingredient
GEL, NA (1X500GM)
500 gm............. 38779-2299-08 87.00

JOJOBA (PCCA)
jojoba oil
OIL, NA, 1 ml............ 51927-2374-00 1.20

JOJOBA OIL (Medisca)
OIL, NA (1X14ML)
14 ml............... 38779-1365-03 16.50
(1X25ML)
25 ml............... 38779-1365-04 25.50
(1X100ML)
100 ml 38779-1365-05 58.50
(1X500ML)
500 ml 38779-1365-08 258.00

(PCCA) *See JOJOBA*

JOLESSA (Teva)
ethinyl estradiol/levonorgestrel
TAB, PO (3X91,FILM COATED)
30 mcg-0.15 mg,
273s ea........... 00555-9123-66 482.02

(Phys Total Care)
REPACK
TAB, PO (FILM COATED)
30 mcg-0.15 mg,
91s ea............ 54868-6044-00 321.22

JOLIVETTE (Watson)
norethindrone
TAB, PO (6 X 28)
0.35 mg, 168s ea..... 52544-0892-28 221.52

JUNEL 1.5/30 (Teva)
ethinyl estradiol/norethindrone acetate
TAB, PO (3X21,USP)
30 mcg-1.5 mg,
63s ea............ 00555-9027-42 86.81

JUNEL 1/20 (Teva)
ethinyl estradiol/norethindrone acetate
TAB, PO (3X21)
20 mcg-1 mg,
63s ea............ 00555-9025-42 85.97

(Southwood)
REPACK
TAB, PO, 20 mcg-1 mg,
21s ea............ 58016-4747-01 171.94

JUNEL FE 1.5/30 (Teva)
ethinyl estradiol/ferrous fum/norethindrone ace
TAB, PO (BLISTER CARD, 6X28)
30 mcg-75 mg-1.5 mg,
168s ea........... 00555-9028-58 173.61

(Phys Total Care)
REPACK
TAB, PO, 30 mcg-75 mg-1.5 mg,
28s ea............ 54868-5935-00 66.03

JUNEL FE 1/20 (Teva)
ethinyl estradiol/ferrous fum/norethindrone ace
TAB, PO (BLISTER CARD, 6X28)
20 mcg-75 mg-1 mg,
168s ea........... 00555-9026-58 171.94

(Phys Total Care)
REPACK
TAB, PO, 20 mcg-75 mg-1 mg,
28s ea............ 54868-5326-00 67.97

JUNIPER BERRY OIL (Lorann Oil)
OIL, NA, 9.9 ml.......... 23535-0151-27 7.00

(Medisca)
OIL, NA (1X14ML,NATURAL)
14 ml............... 38779-1727-03 28.50
(1X25ML,NATURAL)
25 ml............... 38779-1727-04 43.50
(1X100ML,NATURAL)
100 ml 38779-1727-05 120.00
(1X500ML,NATURAL)
500 ml 38779-1727-08 567.00

JUNIPER TAR (Lorann Oil)
juniper tar oil
SOL, NA, 30 ml.......... 23535-0713-05 2.00
480 ml 23535-0713-01 14.00
3840 ml 23535-0713-11 80.00

(Medisca)
OIL, NA (NATURAL,CADE OIL)
100 ml 38779-1366-05 82.50
500 ml 38779-1366-08 178.50

(PCCA)
OIL, NA (USP (CADE OIL))
1 ml................ 51927-1439-00 0.62

JUNIPER TAR OIL (Amend)
OIL, NA (U.S.P./F.C.C.)
30 ml............... 17317-0306-02 4.20
(U.S.P./ F.C.C.)
120 ml 17317-0306-04 7.00
(U.S.P./F.C.C.)
500 ml 17317-0306-01 20.30

(Gallipot)
OIL, NA (U.S.P.,N.F.)
100 ml 51552-0363-05 20.93
500 ml 51552-0363-06 83.65

(Lorann Oil) *See JUNIPER TAR*

(Medisca) *See JUNIPER TAR*

(PCCA) *See JUNIPER TAR*

K CL/K PHOS/MG SULF/NA CL/NA PHOS
(Baxter) *See TIS-U-SOL*

K CL/MG CL/NA ACE/NA CL/NA GLUCONATE
(B. Braun) *See ISOLYTE S*

(B. Braun) *See PHYSIOLYTE*

(Baxter) *See PLASMA-LYTE 148*

(Baxter) *See PLASMA-LYTE A PH-7.4*

(Hospira) *See NORMOSOL-R*

(Hospira) *See NORMOSOL-R PH 7.4*

(Hospira) *See PHYSIOSOL*

K CL/NA BICARB/NA CL/NA SULF/PEG
(Braintree) *See GOLYTELY*

(Kremers Urban) *See PEG 3350 & ELECTROLYTES*

K CL/NA BICARB/NA CL/
POLYETHYLENE GLYCOL 3350
(Alaven) *See TRILYTE W/FLAVOR PACKS*

(Braintree) *See NULYTELY*

K PHOS, MONOBASIC/NA PHOS, MONOBASIC
(Beach Pharm) *See K-PHOS MF*

(Beach Pharm) *See K-PHOS NO. 2*

K PHOS/NA PHOS, DIBASIC/NA PHOS, MONOBASIC
(Beach Pharm) *See K-PHOS NEUTRAL*

(Rising) *See PHOSPHA 250 NEUTRAL*

K-DUR (PD-Rx Pharm)
REPACK
potassium chloride
TER, PO, 20 meq, 30s ea .. 58864-0361-40 32.25

K-DUR 20 (Phys Total Care)
REPACK
potassium chloride
TER, PO, 20 meq, 30s ea .. 54868-0354-01 22.06 AB
60s ea............ 54868-0354-00 42.88 AB
100s ea........... 54868-0354-02 62.09 AB

K-EFFERVESCENT (Qualitest)
potassium bicarbonate
TEF, PO, 25 meq, 30s ea... 00603-4170-16 10.05

K-LYTE (Southwood)
REPACK
potassium bicarbonate/potassium citrate
TEF, PO (ORANGE)
25 meq, 100s ea 58016-0595-00 112.48

K-LYTE CL (Phys Total Care)
REPACK
potassium bicarbonate/potassium chloride
TEF, PO (CITRUS)
25 meq, 60s ea....... 54868-3238-02 80.58

K-PHOS MF (Beach Pharm)
k phos, monobasic/na phos, monobasic
TAB, PO, 155 mg-350 mg,
100s ea........... 00486-1135-01 15.25
500s ea........... 00486-1135-05 73.10

K-PHOS NEUTRAL (Beach Pharm)
k phos/na phos, dibasic/na phos, monobasic
TAB, PO (CAPLET)
155 mg-852 mg-130 mg,
100s ea........... 00486-1125-01 23.00
500s ea........... 00486-1125-05 112.15

K-PHOS NO. 2 (Beach Pharm)
k phos, monobasic/na phos, monobasic
TAB, PO (CAPLET)
305 mg-700 mg,
100s ea........... 00486-1134-01 23.75

K-PHOS ORIGINAL (Beach Pharm)
potassium phosphate, monobasic
TAB, PO, 500 mg, 100s ea . 00486-1111-01 15.25
500s ea........... 00486-1111-05 73.75

K-TAB (Abbott Pharm)
potassium chloride
TER, PO (CAPLET)
10 meq, 100s ea ..... 00074-7804-13 65.75 57.67 BC
1000s ea .... 00074-7804-19 624.58 547.87 BC

(PD-Rx Pharm)
REPACK
TER, PO (REDI-SCRIPT,CAPLET)
10 meq, 30s ea....... 58864-0801-30 35.44 BC

(Phys Total Care)
REPACK
TER, PO, 10 meq, 100s ea . 54868-1304-01 64.45 BC

K-TAN (Prasco Labs)
phenylephrine tannate/pyrilamine tannate
TER, PO, 25 mg-60 mg,
100s ea........... 66993-0525-02 124.35

K-VESCENT (Major)
potassium bicarbonate
TEF, PO, 25 meq, 30s ea... 00904-2720-46 9.95
100s ea........... 00904-2720-60 27.25

KADIAN (Actavis)
morphine sulfate
CER, PO, 10 mg,
100s ea, C-II .... 46987-0410-11 459.48 EE
20 mg,
100s ea, C-II 46987-0322-11 507.63
30 mg,
100s ea, C-II .... 46987-0325-11 552.11 BX
50 mg,
100s ea, C-II 46987-0323-11 922.65
60 mg,
100s ea, C-II .... 46987-0326-11 1104.20 BX
80 mg,
100s ea, C-II 46987-0412-11 1471.04
100 mg,
100s ea, C-II 46987-0324-11 1845.28
200 mg,
100s ea, C-II 46987-0377-11 3690.58

(Phys Total Care)
REPACK
CER, PO, 10 mg,
10s ea, C-II .... 54868-5964-00 54.64 EE
30s ea, C-II .... 54868-5964-02 156.09 EE
60s ea, C-II .... 54868-5964-01 291.35 EE
20 mg,
20s ea, C-II 54868-4571-01 116.00
30s ea, C-II 54868-4571-02 162.69
60s ea, C-II 54868-4571-00 321.46
30 mg,
10s ea, C-II 54868-4981-01 64.87
60s ea, C-II 54868-4981-00 348.64
90s ea, C-II 54868-4981-02 505.26
50 mg,
20s ea, C-II 54868-4572-02 180.42
30s ea, C-II 54868-4572-01 268.67
60s ea, C-II 54868-4572-00 533.42
60 mg,
20s ea, C-II 54868-5850-00 234.16

PROD/MFR	NDC	AWP	DP	OBC
30s ea, C-II	54868-5850-02	349.28		
60s ea, C-II	54868-5850-01	672.36		
100 mg,				
10s ea, C-II	54868-4573-02	196.30		
30s ea, C-II	54868-4573-01	581.07		
60s ea, C-II	54868-4573-00	1120.98		
(Quality Care Prod) REPACK				
CER, PO, 10 mg,				
30s ea, C-II	35356-0047-30	207.00		
60s ea, C-II	35356-0047-60	414.40		EE
100s ea, C-II	35356-0047-00	634.80		
20 mg,				
30s ea, C-II	35356-0048-30	220.00		
60s ea, C-II	35356-0048-60	440.00		
100s ea, C-II	35356-0048-00	660.00		
30 mg,				
30s ea, C-II	35356-0049-30	237.50		
60s ea, C-II	35356-0049-60	475.00		
100s ea, C-II	35356-0049-00	712.50		
50 mg,				
30s ea, C-II	35356-0050-30	392.50		
60s ea, C-II	35356-0050-60	785.00		
100s ea, C-II	35356-0050-00	1175.50		
60 mg,				
30s ea, C-II	35356-0051-30	477.00		
60s ea, C-II	35356-0051-60	858.60		
100s ea, C-II	35356-0051-00	1431.00		
80 mg,				
30s ea, C-II	35356-0076-30	621.99		
100s ea, C-II	35356-0076-00	1865.70		
100 mg,				
30s ea, C-II	35356-0052-30	767.00		
60s ea, C-II	35356-0052-60	1534.00		
100s ea, C-II	35356-0052-00	2301.00		
(St. Mary's MPP) REPACK				
CER, PO, 50 mg,				
30s ea, C-II	60760-0023-30	355.46		
(Stat Rx) REPACK				
CER, PO, 50 mg,				
30s ea, C-II	16590-0606-30	285.04		
60s ea, C-II	16590-0606-60	566.84		
90s ea, C-II	16590-0606-90	848.63		
60 mg,				
30s ea, C-II	16590-0598-30	340.50		
56s ea, C-II	16590-0598-56	632.77		
60s ea, C-II	16590-0598-60	677.74		
90s ea, C-II	16590-0598-90	1014.99		
100 mg,				
60s ea, C-II	16590-0740-60	1130.40		
112s ea, C-II	16590-0740-73	2107.27		
KAHLUA (Medisca)				
flavoring aid				
SOL, NA (1X25ML)				
25 ml	38779-1367-04	22.50		
(1X100ML)				
100 ml	38779-1367-05	37.50		
KAHLUA FLAVOR (PCCA)				
flavoring aid				
SOL, NA (KEOKE COFFEE,ARTIFICIAL)				
1 ml	51927-2158-00	0.90		
KALBITOR (Dyax)				
ecallantide				
SOL, SC (SINGLE-USE VIAL,PF)				
10 mg/ml, 1 ml 3s	47783-0101-01	9540.00		
KALETRA (Abbott Pharm)				
lopinavir/ritonavir				
SOL, PO, 80 mg/ml-20 mg/ml,				
160 ml	00074-3956-46	420.95	369.25	
TAB, PO (FILM-COATED)				
100 mg-25 mg,				
60s ea	00074-0522-60	210.48	184.63	
200 mg-50 mg,				
120s ea	00074-6799-22	841.90	738.50	
(A-S Medication) REPACK				
SOL, PO, 80 mg/ml-20 mg/ml,				
160 ml	54569-5525-00	547.24		
TAB, PO, 200 mg-50 mg,				
120s ea	54569-5752-00	1094.47		
(Dispensing Solutions) REPACK				
TAB, PO, 200 mg-50 mg,				
10s ea	55045-3482-01	76.70		
(PD-Rx Pharm) REPACK				
TAB, PO (FILM-COATED)				
200 mg-50 mg,				
12s ea	55289-0947-12	125.12		
(Pharma Pac) REPACK				
TAB, PO (FILM-COATED)				
100 mg-25 mg,				
12s ea	52959-0968-12	70.16		
200 mg-50 mg,				
18s ea	52959-0134-18	129.90		
(Phys Total Care) REPACK				
TAB, PO, 200 mg-50 mg,				
120s ea	54868-5566-00	1039.33		
(Physician Partner) REPACK				
TAB, PO (FILM-COATED)				
200 mg-50 mg,				
12s ea	21695-0362-12	206.35		
(Quality Care Prod) REPACK				
TAB, PO (FILM-COATED)				
100 mg-25 mg,				
60s ea	35356-0111-60	275.82		
200 mg-50 mg,				
30s ea	35356-0112-30	485.52		
120s ea	35356-0112-01	1941.60		
(Southwood) REPACK				
TAB, PO (FILM-COATED)				
200 mg-50 mg,				
30s ea	00490-7028-30	210.48		
60s ea	00490-7028-60	420.95		
90s ea	00490-7028-90	631.43		
100s ea	00490-7028-00	701.58		
120s ea	00490-7028-02	841.90		
KALEXATE (KVK)				
sodium polystyrene sulfonate				
PDR, PO (USP,1X454GM)				
454 gm	10702-0036-45	175.00		AA
KALI BROMATUM/NICCOLUM SULPHURICUM/ SULFUR				
(Loma Lux) *See ECZEMOL*				
KALI BROMATUM/NICCOLUM SULPHURICUM/ ZINCUM BROMATUM				
(Loma Lux) *See PSORIZIDE ULTRA*				
KALIUM ACETICUM COMPOUND (Weleda)				
homeopathic substance				
POW, PO (6X)				
30 gm	55946-0290-40	5.70		
KANAMYCIN ACID SULFATE				
(Medisca) *See KANAMYCIN SULFATE*				
KANAMYCIN SULFATE (APP)				
SOL, IJ (10X3ML)				
1 gm/3 ml,				
3 ml 10s	63323-0359-03	181.25		AP
(Gallipot)				
POW, NA (1X1GM,USP)				
1 gm	51552-0913-01	19.32	13.80	
(1X5GM,USP)				
5 gm	51552-0913-02	50.68	36.20	
(Hawkins)				
POW, NA (U.S.P.)				
10 gm	63370-0124-20	96.00		
25 gm	63370-0124-25	192.00		
100 gm	63370-0124-35	576.00		
(Medisca)				
kanamycin acid sulfate				
POW, NA (DRIED)				
10 gm	38779-0872-01	81.00		
KANAMYCIN SULFATE (Medisca)				
(XXX U/MG)				
10 gm	38779-1981-01	81.00		
(Medisca)				
kanamycin acid sulfate				
(DRIED)				
25 gm	38779-0872-04	184.50		
KANAMYCIN SULFATE (Medisca)				
(XXX U/MG)				
25 gm	38779-1981-04	184.50		
(Medisca)				
kanamycin acid sulfate				
(DRIED)				
100 gm	38779-0872-05	535.50		
KANAMYCIN SULFATE (Medisca)				
(XXX U/MG)				
100 gm	38779-1981-05	535.50		
(Medisca)				
kanamycin acid sulfate				
(DRIED)				
500 gm	38779-0872-08	1989.00		
KANAMYCIN SULFATE (Medisca)				
(XXX U/MG)				
500 gm	38779-1981-08	1680.00		
(Medisca)				
kanamycin acid sulfate				
(DRIED)				
1000 gm	38779-0872-09	3366.00		
KANAMYCIN SULFATE (PCCA)				
POW, NA (U.S.P.)				
1 gm	51927-3158-00	8.70		
(Spectrum Pharmacy)				
POW, NA (U.S.P.)				
10 gm	49452-3885-01	133.70		
25 gm	49452-3885-02	289.10		
100 gm	49452-3885-03	843.50		
KAOLIN				
(Amend) *See KAOLIN COLLOIDAL*				
(Baker, J.T.)				
POW, NA (U.S.P., F.C.C.)				
500 gm	10106-2242-01	19.22		
1500 gm	10106-2242-05	39.72		
(Gallipot)				
POW, NA (U.S.P.,N.F.)				
454 gm	51552-0195-06	11.90		
2270 gm	51552-0195-09	42.00		
(Letco)				
POW, NA, 500 gm	62991-1518-01	30.00		
2500 gm	62991-1518-02	75.00		
(Mallinckrodt Lab)				
POW, NA (U.S.P., COLLOIDAL)				
500 gm	00406-5645-12	28.52		
(Medisca)				
POW, NA (USP,1X500GM)				
500 gm	38779-0079-08	21.00		
(USP,1X10500GM)				
1000 gm	38779-0079-09	37.50		
(USP,1X2500GM)				
2500 gm	38779-0079-01	84.00		
(PCCA)				
POW, NA (USP)				
1 gm	51927-1212-00	0.07		
(Spectrum Pharmacy)				
POW, NA (B.P.,E.P.,U.S.P.)				
500 gm	49452-3890-01	63.00		
2500 gm	49452-3890-02	193.55		
KAOLIN COLLOIDAL (Amend)				
kaolin				
POW, NA (U.S.P.)				
500 gm	17317-0694-01	9.80		
2270 gm	17317-0694-05	30.80		
11350 gm	17317-0694-08	87.50		
KAON-CL 10 (Savage)				
potassium chloride				
TER, PO, 10 meq, 100s ea	00281-3131-17	24.15		BC
(STAT-PAK, 10X10)				
10 meq, 100s ea UD	00281-3131-18	26.83		BC
1000s ea	00281-3131-23	229.23		BC
KAPIDEX (Takeda)				
dexlansoprazole				
ECC, PO, 30 mg, 30s ea	64764-0905-30	131.40		
60 mg, 30s ea	64764-0915-30	131.40		
(ENTERIC-COATED GRANULES)				
60 mg, 90s ea	64764-0915-90	394.20		
(Phys Total Care) REPACK				
ECC, PO, 30 mg, 30s ea	54868-5998-00	157.52		
90s ea	54868-5998-01	454.23		
KARAYA GUM (Gallipot)				
POW, NA (F.C.C.)				
454 gm	51552-0152-06	17.36		
(Medisca)				
POW, NA (1X500GM)				
500 gm	38779-1368-08	34.50		
(1X1000GM)				
1000 gm	38779-1368-09	64.50		
(1X2500GM)				
2500 gm	38779-1368-01	129.00		

PROD/MFR NDC AWP DP OBC

(PCCA)
POW, NA (NF)(STERCULIA GUM)
1 gm 51927-1811-00 0.10

(Spectrum Pharmacy)
POW, NA (F.C.C.)
500 gm 49452-3910-01 86.45
2500 gm 49452-3910-02 302.75

KARIVA (Teva)
desogestrel/ethinyl estradiol
TAB, PO (6 X 28)
168s ea .... 00555-9050-58 359.88 AB

(A-S Medication)
REPACK
TAB, PO, 28s ea 54569-5826-00 57.67

(Palmetto)
REPACK
TAB, PO, 28s ea .... 23490-9400-00 49.00 AB

(Quality Care Prod)
REPACK
TAB, PO, 28s ea .... 35356-0361-28 98.98 AB

KAVA KAVA ROOT (PCCA)
kava root
POW, NA, 1 gm 51927-3005-00 0.46

KAVA ROOT
(PCCA) *See KAVA KAVA ROOT*

KAYDOL (Amend)
mineral oil
OIL, NA (U.S.P.)
480 ml 17317-1061-01 4.90
3840 ml 17317-1061-06 21.00
19200 ml 17317-1061-08 70.00

KAYEXALATE (Sanofi-Aventis)
sodium polystyrene sulfonate
PDR, PO, 453.6 gm ...... 00024-1075-01 362.47 AA

KEFLEX (MiddleBrook)
cephalexin
CAP, PO, 250 mg, 20s ea .. 11042-0112-97 65.93 AB
100s ea .... 11042-0112-96 289.40 AB
500 mg, 20s ea 11042-0113-97 129.73
100s ea 11042-0113-96 568.85
750 mg, 50s ea 11042-0115-40 163.48

(Pharma Pac)
REPACK
CAP, PO, 250 mg, 20s ea .. 52959-0660-20 57.56 AB
30s ea .... 52959-0660-30 86.22 AB
500 mg, 20s ea ...... 52959-0087-20 68.77 AB
40s ea .... 52959-0087-40 115.85 AB

(Phys Total Care)
REPACK
CAP, PO, 500 mg, 20s ea .. 54868-0425-01 80.82 AB
40s ea .... 54868-0425-00 150.99 AB

(Southwood)
REPACK
CAP, PO, 500 mg, 30s ea .. 58016-0633-30 156.56
60s ea 58016-0633-60 313.13
90s ea 58016-0633-90 469.69
100s ea 58016-0633-00 521.88

(Stat Rx)
REPACK
CAP, PO, 750 mg, 30s ea .. 16590-0553-30 108.25
60s ea 16590-0553-60 216.50
90s ea 16590-0553-90 324.00

KELNOR 1/35 (Teva)
ethinyl estradiol/ethynodiol diacetate
TAB, PO, 35 mcg-1 mg,
168s ea .... 00555-9064-58 179.28 AB

(Phys Total Care)
REPACK
TAB, PO, 35 mcg-1 mg,
28s ea .... 54868-5942-00 80.86 AB

KENALOG (Ranbaxy Labs)
triamcinolone acetonide
SPR, TP (WITH SPRAY TUBE)
0.147 mg/gm, 63 gm . 10631-0093-62 136.21

(Phys Total Care)
REPACK
SPR, TP, 0.147 mg/gm,
63 gm 54868-3255-00 33.77

(Quality Care Prod)
REPACK
SUS, IJ, 10 mg/ml, ea 35356-0082-01 24.60

KENALOG 40 (Dispensing Solutions)
REPACK
triamcinolone acetonide
SUS, IJ, 40 mg/ml, 1 ml ... 55045-3248-01 12.00

KENALOG IN ORABASE (Phys Total Care)
REPACK
triamcinolone acetonide
PAS, MM, 0.1%, 5 gm ..... 54868-5276-00 21.98 AT

KENALOG-10 (Bristol-Myers Squibb Mature Brands)
triamcinolone acetonide
SUS, IJ (VIAL)
10 mg/ml, 5 ml 00003-0494-20 11.60

(A-S Medication)
REPACK
SUS, IJ (VIAL)
10 mg/ml, 5 ml 54569-1827-01 10.29

(Phys Total Care)
REPACK
SUS, IJ (VIAL)
10 mg/ml, 5 ml 54868-0234-00 15.83

KENALOG-40 (Bristol-Myers Squibb Mature Brands)
triamcinolone acetonide
SUS, IJ (VIAL)
40 mg/ml, 1 ml .... 00003-0293-05 8.99 BP
5 ml .... 00003-0293-20 45.62 BP
10 ml .... 00003-0293-28 68.14 BP

(A-S Medication)
REPACK
SUS, IJ (VIAL)
40 mg/ml, 5 ml .... 54569-1398-00 40.41 BP
10 ml .... 54569-5465-00 60.36 BP

(Phys Total Care)
REPACK
SUS, IJ (VIAL)
40 mg/ml, 1 ml .... 54868-0235-00 9.00 BP
5 ml .... 54868-0235-01 44.70 BP
10 ml .... 54868-0235-02 70.72 BP

(Physician Partner)
REPACK
SUS, IJ (1X1ML)
40 mg/ml, 1 ml .... 21695-0360-01 28.72 BP

(Quality Care Prod)
REPACK
SUS, IJ (VIAL)
40 mg/ml, 5 ml .... 49999-0415-05 93.80 BP

(Southwood)
REPACK
SUS, IJ, 40 mg/ml, 1 ml ... 58016-9799-01 6.20 BP

KENDALL AMD ANTIMICROBIAL FENESTRATED FOAMDRESSING (Covidien)
polihexanide
SHE, TP (3.5"X3",SINGLE-USE)
0.5%, 50s ea 08080-0555-35 360.94
(W/TOPSHEET,3.5"X3")
0.5%, 50s ea 08080-5553-52 393.75

KENDALL AMD ANTIMICROBIAL FOAM DRESSING (Covidien)
polihexanide
SHE, TP (4"X4",SINGLE-USE)
0.5%, 50s ea 08080-0555-44 393.75
(4"X8",SINGLE-USE)
0.5%, 50s ea 08080-0555-48 721.88
(6"X6",SINGLE-USE)
0.5%, 50s ea 08080-0555-66 984.37
(8"X8",SINGLE-USE)
0.5%, 50s ea 08080-0555-88 1050.00
(2"X2",SINGLE-USE)
0.5%, 100s ea 08080-0555-22 525.00

KENDALL AMD ANTIMICROBIAL FOAM DRESSING W/TOPSHEET (Covidien)
polihexanide
SHE, TP (4"X4",SINGLE-USE)
0.5%, 50s ea 08080-5554-43 459.38

KENGUARD URINARY DRAINAGE BAG (Covidien)
incontinence products
DEV, NA (2000CC)
20s ea 08080-3502-00 58.10

KEPIVANCE (Biovitrum)
palifermin
PDS, IV (PF)
6.25 mg, ea 55513-0520-01 1650.00
6s ea 55513-0520-06 9900.00

KEPPRA (UCB)
levetiracetam
SOL, IV (10X5ML)
100 mg/ml,
5 ml 10s 50474-0002-63 464.02
PO (GRAPE)
100 mg/ml, 473 ml ... 50474-0001-48 404.41
TAB, PO (FILM COATED)
250 mg, 120s ea ..... 50474-0594-40 435.29 EE
500 mg, 120s ea ..... 50474-0595-40 532.02 EE
750 mg, 120s ea ..... 50474-0596-40 720.77 EE
1000 mg, 60s ea 50474-0597-66 532.02

(IPI)
REPACK
TAB, PO (FILM COATED)
250 mg, 30s ea ...... 18837-0343-30 98.11 EE
500 mg, 60s ea 18837-0074-60 239.82

(Nucare Pharm)
REPACK
TAB, PO (FILM COATED)
250 mg, 60s ea ...... 68071-0499-60 206.02 EE
500 mg, 60s ea ...... 68071-0298-60 247.01 EE

(PD-Rx Pharm)
REPACK
TAB, PO, 500 mg, 30s ea .. 55289-0097-30 167.93

(Phys Total Care)
REPACK
TAB, PO (FILM-COATED)
500 mg, 30s ea 54868-4947-00 135.22
60s ea 54868-4947-02 268.49
90s ea 54868-4947-01 401.75
750 mg, 30s ea 54868-5266-01 168.36
(FILM-COATED)
750 mg, 60s ea 54868-5266-00 334.76
150s ea 54868-5266-02 833.97

(Physician Partner)
REPACK
TAB, PO (FILM COATED)
500 mg, 15s ea ...... 21695-0070-15 131.40 EE

(Quality Care Prod)
REPACK
TAB, PO, 500 mg, 30s ea .. 49999-0944-30 192.90
60s ea 49999-0944-60 385.80
(FILM COATED)
1000 mg, 30s ea 35356-0393-30 244.36

(Stat Rx)
REPACK
TAB, PO (FILM COATED)
250 mg, 30s ea ...... 16590-0583-30 110.25 EE
60s ea .... 16590-0583-60 220.25 EE
90s ea .... 16590-0583-90 330.75 EE
(FILM-COATED)
500 mg, 30s ea 16590-0134-30 133.58
60s ea 16590-0134-60 265.69
750 mg, 30s ea 16590-0135-30 135.00
60s ea 16590-0135-60 270.00

KEPPRA XR (UCB)
levetiracetam
TER, PO (FILM COATED)
500 mg, 60s ea 50474-0598-66 241.14
750 mg, 60s ea 50474-0599-66 362.09

(Quality Care Prod)
REPACK
TER, PO (FILM COATED)
500 mg, 60s ea 35355-0492-60 385.80

KERAFOAM (Onset)
urea
FOA, TP, 30%, 60 gm 16781-0157-60 118.80

KERAFOAM 42 (Onset)
urea
FOA, TP (1X60GM)
42%, 60 gm 16781-0181-60 118.80

KERALAC (Doak)
urea
CRE, TP, 50%, 142 gm 10337-0658-05 176.70
255 gm 10337-0658-09 251.21
GEL, TP (NAIL)
50%, 18 ml 10337-0659-15 267.88
LOT, TP, 35%, 207 ml 10337-0663-49 256.21
325 ml 10337-0663-11 308.74
OIN, TP, 50%, 45 gm 10337-0647-45 124.04
SOL, TP (6X2.4ML)
50%, 2.4 ml 6s 10337-0648-10 231.88

(Quality Care Prod)
REPACK
CRE, TP, 50%, 150 gm 49999-0727-05 79.41
GEL, TP, 50%, 18 ml 49999-0728-18 115.00

KERALYT GEL (Summers)
salicylic acid
GEL, TP (1X40GM)
6%, 40 gm 11086-0030-40 48.72
(1X100GM)
6%, 100 gm 11086-0030-10 50.40

PROD/MFR	NDC	AWP	DP	OBC
(Phys Total Care) REPACK				
GEL, TP (1X40GM)				
6%, 40 gm	54868-1400-00	63.03		
KERALYT SCALP (Summers)				
salicylic acid				
KIT, MR (COMPLETE KIT)				
ea	11086-0047-01	56.50		
KERATOL 40 (Breckenridge Pharm)				
urea				
CRE, TP, 40%, 28.3 gm	51991-0268-41	27.42		
85 gm	51991-0268-19	44.22		
198.4 gm	51991-0268-37	82.88		
GEL, TP (AF,SF,DYE-FREE)				
40%, 15 ml	51991-0269-15	79.93		
LOT, TP, 40%, 237 ml	51991-0270-18	81.08		
KERATOL HC (Breckenridge Pharm)				
hydrocortisone acetate				
CRE, TP (PARABEN-FREE)				
1%, 28.3 gm	51991-0271-41	27.71		
(NONOCCLUSIVE,USP)				
1%, 85.2 gm	51991-0271-19	82.68		
KERATOL PLUS (Breckenridge Pharm)				
urea				
GEL, TP, 50%, 18 ml	51991-0460-81	89.95		
LOT, TP, 35%, 207 ml	51991-0459-37	82.66		
325 ml	51991-0459-27	100.98		
KERLONE (Sanofi-Aventis)				
betaxolol hydrochloride				
TAB, PO (FILM COATED)				
10 mg, 100s ea	00024-2301-10	156.89		AB
20 mg, 100s ea	00024-2300-20	235.25		AB
KEROL (Doak)				
urea				
EMU, TP (1X283.5GM)				
50%, 283.5 gm	10337-0646-10	232.66		
SUS, TP, 50%, 284 gm	10337-0645-10	215.80		
KEROL AD (PharmaDerm)				
urea				
EMU, TP (1X240ML, ACCU-DOSE)				
45%, 240 ml	10337-0643-24	215.42		
KEROL REDI-CLOTHS (Doak)				
urea				
PAD, TP, 42%, 30s ea	10337-0649-10	215.53		
KEROL ZX (Doak)				
urea				
FIL, TP (1X12ML)				
50%, 12 ml	10337-0644-97	290.82		
KETALAR (JHP)				
ketamine hydrochloride				
SOL, IJ (MULTI-DOSE VIAL,20MLX10)				
10 mg/ml,				
20 ml 10s, C-III	42023-0113-10	197.98		
(MDV,10X10ML)				
50 mg/ml,				
10 ml 10s, C-III	42023-0114-10	75.00		AP
(10X5ML)				
100 mg/ml,				
5 ml 10s, C-III	42023-0115-10	97.50		AP
KETAMINE HCL (Bedford)				
ketamine hydrochloride				
SOL, IJ (VIAL)				
50 mg/ml,				
10 ml 10s, C-III	55390-0475-10	156.00		AP
(Bioniche Pharma)				
SOL, IJ (10X10ML,S.D.V.)				
50 mg/ml,				
10 ml 10s, C-III	67457-0001-10	75.00		AP
100 mg/ml,				
10 ml 10s, C-III	67457-0108-10	142.50		AP
(Hawkins)				
POW, NA (U.S.P.)				
5 gm, C-III	63370-0125-15	129.60		
25 gm, C-III	63370-0125-25	260.00		
100 gm, C-III	63370-0125-35	1152.00		
1000 gm, C-III	63370-0125-50	8160.00		
(Hospira)				
SOL, IJ (VIAL)				
50 mg/ml,				
10 ml 10s, C-III	00409-2053-10	72.00	63.00	AP
100 mg/ml,				
5 ml 10s, C-III	00409-2051-05	120.24	105.20	AP
(Letco)				
POW, NA (U.S.P.)				
25 gm, C-III	62991-1087-01	195.00		
50 gm, C-III	62991-1087-03	360.00		
100 gm, C-III	62991-1087-02	615.00		
(Medisca)				
POW, NA, 5 gm, C-III	38779-1754-03	90.00		
(U.S.P.)				
25 gm, C-III	38779-1754-04	177.00		
100 gm, C-III	38779-1754-05	660.00		
250 gm, C-III	38779-1754-07	1425.00		
(USP,1X500GM)				
500 gm, C-III	38779-1754-08	2550.00		
(U.S.P.)				
1000 gm, C-III	38779-1754-09	4080.00		
(Spectrum Pharmacy)				
CRY, NA (U.S.P.)				
5 gm, C-III	49452-3912-01	119.00		
25 gm, C-III	49452-3912-02	298.20		
100 gm, C-III	49452-3912-03	1022.00		
(1X250GM,USP)				
250 gm, C-III	49452-3912-06	2012.50		
(B&B Pharm, Inc) REPACK				
POW, NA (U.S.P.)				
25 gm, C-III	63275-9980-04	202.00		
100 gm, C-III	63275-9980-05	648.00		
1000 gm, C-III	63275-9980-09	4590.00		
(Phys Total Care) REPACK				
SOL, IJ (VIAL)				
50 mg/ml,				
10 ml 10s, C-III	54868-4399-00	205.63		AP
100 mg/ml,				
5 ml 10s, C-III	54868-5093-00	108.78		AP
KETAMINE HYDROCHLORIDE				
(Bedford) *See KETAMINE HCL*				
(Bioniche Pharma) *See KETAMINE HCL*				
(Bioniche Pharma)				
SOL, IJ (20MLX10)				
10 mg/ml,				
20 ml 10s, C-III	67457-0181-20	206.23		AP
(Gallipot)				
POW, NA (1X5GM,USP)				
5 gm, C-III	51552-0697-02	39.20	28.00	
(1X25GM,USP)				
25 gm, C-III	51552-0697-04	112.00	80.00	
(1X100GM,USP)				
100 gm, C-III	51552-0697-05	336.00	240.00	
(Hawkins) *See KETAMINE HCL*				
(Hospira) *See KETAMINE HCL*				
(JHP) *See KETALAR*				
(Letco) *See KETAMINE HCL*				
(Medisca) *See KETAMINE HCL*				
(PCCA)				
POW, NA (U.S.P.; CIII)				
1 gm, C-III	51927-2790-00	19.20		
(Spectrum Pharmacy) *See KETAMINE HCL*				
KETEK (Sanofi-Aventis)				
telithromycin				
TAB, PO (FILM-COATED)				
300 mg, 20s ea	00088-2223-20	115.19		
400 mg, 60s ea	00088-2225-41	345.58		
(Phys Total Care) REPACK				
TAB, PO (FILM-COATED)				
400 mg, 20s ea	54868-5171-01	132.84		
(Southwood) REPACK				
TAB, PO (FILM-COATED)				
400 mg, 30s ea	00490-0056-30	172.79		
60s ea	00490-0056-60	345.58		
90s ea	00490-0056-90	518.37		
100s ea	00490-0056-00	575.97		
KETEK PAK (Phys Total Care) REPACK				
telithromycin				
TAB, PO (FILM-COATED)				
400 mg, 10s ea	54868-5171-00	70.91		
7-KETO DHEA DEHYDROEPIANDOSTERONE (Letco)				
dehydroepiandrosterone, micronized				
POW, NA (1X25GM,MICRONIZED)				
25 gm	62991-2505-01	195.00		
(1X100GM,MICRONIZED)				
100 gm	62991-2505-02	720.00		
(1X500GM,MICRONIZED)				
500 gm	62991-2505-05	2250.00		
7-KETO-DHEA (Medisca)				
dehydroepiandrosterone, micronized				
POW, NA, 25 gm	38779-2418-04	465.00		
100 gm	38779-2418-05	1425.00		
500 gm	38779-2418-08	5655.00		
KETOCONAZOLE				
FUL				
TAB, PO, 200 mg, 100s ea		225.00		
(Apotex Corp.)				
TAB, PO, 200 mg, 30s ea	60505-0092-02	94.80		AB
100s ea	60505-0092-00	316.00		AB
(Fougera)				
CRE, TP, 2%, 15 gm	00168-0099-15	16.43		AB
30 gm	00168-0099-30	27.60		AB
60 gm	00168-0099-60	42.04		AB
(Gallipot)				
CRY, NA (U.S.P.)				
5 gm	51552-0627-02	35.00		
(Hawkins)				
POW, NA (U.S.P.)				
5 gm	63370-0127-15	56.00		
25 gm	63370-0127-25	120.00		
100 gm	63370-0127-35	440.00		
500 gm	63370-0127-45	1600.00		
1000 gm	63370-0127-50	3120.00		
(Janssen) *See NIZORAL*				
(JSJ Pharma) *See KURIC*				
(Letco)				
POW, NA, 25 gm	62991-1461-02	90.00		
100 gm	62991-1461-03	255.00		
(Medisca)				
POW, NA (U.S.P.)				
5 gm	38779-0279-03	73.50		
10 gm	38779-0279-01	132.00		
25 gm	38779-0279-04	297.00		
100 gm	38779-0279-05	927.00		
500 gm	38779-0279-08	1995.00		
(USP, 1X1000GM)				
1000 gm	38779-0279-09	2955.00		
(Mylan)				
TAB, PO, 200 mg, 100s ea	00378-0261-01	315.80		AB
(Patriot Pharmaceuticals)				
SHA, TP, 2%, 120 ml	10147-0750-04	27.78		
(PCCA)				
POW, NA (U.S.P.)				
1 gm	51927-3194-00	18.00		
(Perrigo)				
SHA, TP, 2%, 120 ml	45802-0465-64	27.75		
(Sandoz) *See KETOCONAZOLE SHAMPOO*				
(Spectrum Pharmacy)				
POW, NA (U.S.P.)				
5 gm	49452-3913-01	129.85		
25 gm	49452-3913-02	465.50		
100 gm	49452-3913-03	1305.50		
(1X1000GM,U.S.P.)				
1000 gm	49452-3913-04	4410.00		
(Stiefel Labs) *See EXTINA*				
(Stiefel Labs) *See XOLEGEL*				
(Taro)				
CRE, TP, 2%, 15 gm	51672-1298-01	16.45		AB
30 gm	51672-1298-02	27.68		AB
60 gm	51672-1298-03	42.05		AB
TAB, PO, 200 mg, 30s ea	51672-4026-06	94.80		AB
100s ea	51672-4026-01	316.00		AB
(Teva)				
CRE, TP, 2%, 15 gm	00093-0840-15	16.46		AB
30 gm	00093-0840-30	27.70		AB
60 gm	00093-0840-92	42.08		AB
TAB, PO, 200 mg, 100s ea	00093-0900-01	313.98		AB
500s ea	00093-0900-05	1519.20		AB
(A-S Medication) REPACK				
CRE, TP, 2%, 15 gm	54569-5220-00	16.59		EE
30 gm	54569-5221-00	27.89		EE
TAB, PO, 200 mg, 30s ea	54569-5237-00	93.94		AB
(Altura) REPACK				
TAB, PO, 200 mg, 20s ea	63874-0452-20	64.97		
30s ea	63874-0452-30	94.54		
60s ea	63874-0452-60	53.16		
100s ea	63874-0452-01	324.85		
(Bryant Ranch) REPACK				
TAB, PO, 200 mg, 10s ea	63629-1485-01	42.54		
30s ea	63629-1485-02	127.61		

PROD/MFR	NDC	AWP	DP	OBC
(DHS, Inc.)				
REPACK				
CRE, TP, 2%, 15 gm	**55887-0400-15**	37.84		AB
30 gm	**55887-0400-30**	60.44		AB
60 gm	**55887-0400-60**	43.00		
TAB, PO, 200 mg, 30s ea	**55887-0932-30**	94.80		AB
30s ea	**55887-0994-30**	94.80		
(Dispensing Solutions)				
REPACK				
CRE, TP, 2%, 15 gm	**55045-2945-05**	16.85		
SHA, TP, 2%, 120 ml	**55045-3779-04**	28.00		
(PD-Rx Pharm)				
REPACK				
TAB, PO (USP)				
200 mg, 30s ea	**43063-0036-30**	26.58		AB
(Pharma Pac)				
REPACK				
CRE, TP, 2%, 15 gm	**52959-0497-15**	26.75		EE
30 gm	**52959-0497-30**	53.49		EE
60 gm	**52959-0497-60**	106.96		EE
TAB, PO, 200 mg, 2s ea	**52959-0699-02**	11.00		AB
20s ea	**52959-0699-20**	89.50		AB
30s ea	**52959-0699-30**	130.00		AB
100s ea	**52959-0699-00**	318.20		AB
(Phys Total Care)				
REPACK				
CRE, TP, 2%, 15 gm	**54868-4448-01**	35.25		AB
30 gm	**54868-4448-00**	67.96		AB
60 gm	**54868-4448-02**	75.09		AB
TAB, PO, 200 mg, 4s ea	**54868-5071-03**	9.02		AB
6s ea	**54868-5071-01**	11.40		AB
15s ea	**54868-5071-02**	21.78		AB
30s ea	**54868-5071-00**	37.56		AB
(Physician Partner)				
REPACK				
CRE, TP, 2%, 15 gm	**21695-0554-15**	32.90		AB
30 gm	**21695-0555-30**	55.36		AB
(1X60GM)				
2%, 60 gm	**21695-0556-60**	84.10		AB
(Quality Care Prod)				
REPACK				
CRE, TP, 2%, 15 gm	**49999-0748-15**	32.10		AB
30 gm	**49999-0748-30**	46.81		
TAB, PO, 200 mg, 20s ea	**49999-0301-20**	75.80		AB
30s ea	**49999-0301-30**	113.76		AB
(Southwood)				
REPACK				
CRE, TP, 2%, 60 gm	**58016-4846-01**	43.00		
(Vibranta)				
REPACK				
CRE, TP, 2%, 30 gm	**57866-3092-07**	46.81		
KETOCONAZOLE SHAMPOO (Sandoz)				
ketoconazole				
SHA, TP, 2%, 120 ml	**00781-7090-04**	27.79		
KETOCONAZOLE/PYRITHIONE ZINC				
(Stiefel Labs) *See XOLEGEL DUO*				
KETOGLUTARIC ACID (PCCA)				
alpha ketoglutaric acid				
POW, NA (ALPHA)				
1 gm	**51927-2309-00**	1.80		
KETOPROFEN (Gallipot)				
POW, NA (U.S.P.)				
25 gm	**51552-0307-04**	21.00		
100 gm	**51552-0307-05**	74.20		
500 gm	**51552-0307-06**	280.00		
1000 gm	**51552-0307-07**	525.00		
(Hawkins)				
POW, NA (U.S.P.)				
ea	**63370-0130-61**	27840.00		
25 gm	**63370-0130-25**	60.00		
100 gm	**63370-0130-35**	192.00		
500 gm	**63370-0130-45**	936.00		
1000 gm	**63370-0130-50**	1680.00		
5000 gm	**63370-0130-55**	7080.00		
(Letco)				
POW, NA (1X25GM,USP,MICRONIZED)				
25 gm	**62991-2733-01**	40.50		
(U.S.P.)				
25 gm	**62991-1088-01**	40.50		
(1X100GM,USP,MICRONIZED)				
100 gm	**62991-2733-02**	123.00		
(U.S.P.)				
100 gm	**62991-1088-02**	123.00		
(1X500GM,USP,MICRONIZED)				
500 gm	**62991-2733-03**	495.00		
(U.S.P., 25)				
500 gm	**62991-1088-03**	510.00		
(1X1000GM,USP,MICRONIZED)				
1000 gm	**62991-2733-04**	780.00		
(U.S.P., 25)				
1000 gm	**62991-1088-04**	780.00		
(1X2500GM,USP,MICRONIZED)				
2500 gm	**62991-2733-05**	1740.00		
(1X5000GM,USP,MICRONIZED)				
5000 gm	**62991-2733-06**	3300.00		
(U.S.P., 25)				
5000 gm	**62991-1088-05**	4200.00		
(1X25000GM,USP)				
25000 gm	**62991-2733-07**	16500.00		
(Medisca)				
POW, NA (U.S.P.)				
25 gm	**38779-0078-04**	46.50		
100 gm	**38779-0078-05**	163.50		
500 gm	**38779-0078-08**	643.50		
1000 gm	**38779-0078-09**	1125.00		
(Mylan)				
CAP, PO, 50 mg, 100s ea	**00378-4070-01**	96.50		AB
75 mg, 100s ea	**00378-5750-01**	107.30		AB
CER, PO, 200 mg, 100s ea	**00378-8200-01**	280.25		AB
(PCCA)				
POW, NA (U.S.P.)				
1 gm	**51927-2352-00**	3.12		
(Spectrum Pharmacy)				
POW, NA (B.P.)				
25 gm	**49452-3916-03**	69.65		
(U.S.P.)				
25 gm	**49452-3917-03**	77.00		
(B.P.)				
100 gm	**49452-3916-04**	246.05		
(U.S.P.)				
100 gm	**49452-3917-04**	256.55		
(B.P.)				
1000 gm	**49452-3916-06**	1456.00		
(U.S.P.)				
1000 gm	**49452-3917-05**	1477.00		
(Teva)				
CAP, PO, 50 mg, 100s ea	**00093-3193-01**	96.50		AB
75 mg, 100s ea	**00093-3195-01**	107.30		AB
500s ea	**00093-3195-05**	472.40		AB
(A-S Medication)				
REPACK				
CAP, PO, 75 mg, 20s ea	**54569-3688-01**	21.46		EE
21s ea	**54569-3688-04**	22.53		EE
30s ea	**54569-3688-00**	32.19		EE
60s ea	**54569-3688-05**	64.38		EE
(Aidarex)				
REPACK				
CAP, PO, 75 mg, 10s ea	**33261-0064-10**	14.11		
20s ea	**33261-0064-20**	28.22		
21s ea	**33261-0064-21**	29.61		
28s ea	**33261-0064-28**	39.48		
30s ea	**33261-0064-30**	42.30		
40s ea	**33261-0064-40**	56.40		
42s ea	**33261-0064-42**	59.26		EE
60s ea	**33261-0064-60**	84.60		
90s ea	**33261-0064-90**	127.00		
(Altura)				
REPACK				
CAP, PO, 50 mg, 15s ea	**63874-1108-05**	16.69		AB
21s ea	**63874-1108-02**	26.04		AB
28s ea	**63874-1108-08**	31.15		AB
30s ea	**63874-1108-03**	33.38		AB
40s ea	**63874-1108-04**	38.58		AB
60s ea	**63874-1108-06**	66.75		AB
100s ea	**63874-1108-00**	111.25		AB
120s ea	**63874-1108-01**	133.50		AB
75 mg, 12s ea	**63874-0418-12**	15.62		EE
14s ea	**63874-0418-14**	16.19		EE
15s ea	**63874-0418-15**	19.53		EE
20s ea	**63874-0418-20**	26.04		EE
21s ea	**63874-0418-21**	27.34		EE
24s ea	**63874-0418-24**	27.75		EE
28s ea	**63874-0418-28**	36.46		EE
30s ea	**63874-0418-30**	39.06		EE
40s ea	**63874-0418-40**	52.08		EE
50s ea	**63874-0418-50**	57.81		EE
60s ea	**63874-0418-60**	78.12		EE
90s ea	**63874-0418-90**	117.18		EE
100s ea	**63874-0418-01**	130.20		EE
(B&B Pharm, Inc)				
REPACK				
POW, NA (U.S.P.)				
100 gm	**63275-9996-05**	135.00		
500 gm	**63275-9996-08**	608.00		
1000 gm	**63275-9996-09**	1080.00		
(Bryant Ranch)				
REPACK				
CAP, PO, 75 mg, 20s ea	**63629-1836-01**	26.45		
30s ea	**63629-1836-02**	39.68		
60s ea	**63629-1836-03**	79.23		AB
(Core)				
REPACK				
CAP, PO, 50 mg, 30s ea	**33358-0198-30**	36.58		
(DHS, Inc.)				
REPACK				
CAP, PO, 50 mg, 30s ea	**55887-0208-30**	28.95		AB
60s ea	**55887-0208-60**	57.90		AB
75 mg, 30s ea	**55887-0912-30**	43.00		AB
60s ea	**55887-0912-60**	84.50		AB
90s ea	**55887-0912-90**	126.74		AB
(Dispensing Solutions)				
REPACK				
CAP, PO, 50 mg, 20s ea	**55045-2011-07**	22.20		
30s ea	**55045-2011-08**	33.30		
30s ea	**66336-0856-30**	28.95		AB
60s ea	**55045-2011-06**	66.60		
90s ea	**55045-2011-09**	99.90		
100s ea	**55045-2011-01**	111.00		
120s ea	**55045-2011-00**	133.20		
75 mg, 20s ea	**55045-2005-07**	25.00		
30s ea	**55045-2005-08**	37.50		
30s ea	**55045-3927-01**	37.50		AB
30s ea	**66336-0667-30**	43.00		AB
60s ea	**55045-2005-06**	75.00		
90s ea	**55045-2005-09**	112.50		
90s ea	**66336-0667-90**	126.75		AB
100s ea	**55045-2005-01**	125.00		
120s ea	**55045-2005-02**	150.00		
(IPI)				
REPACK				
CAP, PO, 75 mg, 30s ea	**18837-0075-30**	54.54		AB
60s ea	**18837-0075-60**	80.25		
(Medsource)				
REPACK				
CAP, PO, 75 mg, 30s ea	**45865-0379-30**	37.50		AB
60s ea	**45865-0379-60**	75.00		AB
90s ea	**45865-0379-90**	112.50		AB
100s ea	**45865-0379-00**	125.00		AB
120s ea	**45865-0379-01**	150.00		AB
150s ea	**45865-0379-02**	187.50		AB
300s ea	**45865-0379-05**	375.00		AB
(Nucare Pharm)				
REPACK				
CAP, PO, 50 mg, 21s ea	**66267-0125-21**	22.32		EE
75 mg, 21s ea	**66267-0126-21**	24.42		EE
30s ea	**66267-0126-30**	59.99		AB
60s ea	**66267-0126-60**	88.28		AB
(Palmetto)				
REPACK				
CAP, PO, 75 mg, 30s ea	**23490-5789-03**	43.00		
60s ea	**23490-5789-06**	86.00		
90s ea	**23490-5789-09**	129.00		
(PD-Rx Pharm)				
REPACK				
CAP, PO, 50 mg, 30s ea	**55289-0287-30**	24.62		AB
75 mg, 15s ea	**55289-0181-15**	20.00		AB
20s ea	**55289-0181-20**	22.22		AB
21s ea	**55289-0181-21**	22.67		AB
30s ea	**55289-0181-30**	26.67		AB
60s ea	**55289-0181-60**	35.76		AB
(Pharma Pac)				
REPACK				
CAP, PO, 50 mg, 21s ea	**52959-0503-21**	23.44		EE
30s ea	**52959-0503-30**	34.08		AB
40s ea	**52959-0503-40**	38.58		EE
75 mg, 14s ea	**52959-0245-14**	19.74		EE
15s ea	**52959-0245-15**	21.15		AB
20s ea	**52959-0245-20**	27.44		EE
21s ea	**52959-0245-21**	28.85		EE
30s ea	**52959-0245-30**	39.22		EE
60s ea	**52959-0245-60**	78.30		EE
90s ea	**52959-0245-90**	118.25		AB
CER, PO, 200 mg, 10s ea	**52959-0520-10**	33.39		AB
15s ea	**52959-0520-15**	50.08		AB
20s ea	**52959-0520-20**	66.77		AB
30s ea	**52959-0520-30**	100.15		AB
60s ea	**52959-0520-60**	200.28		AB
(Phys Total Care)				
REPACK				
CAP, PO, 50 mg, 30s ea	**54868-2414-00**	19.71		EE
75 mg, 10s ea	**54868-2415-06**	10.19		AB
20s ea	**54868-2415-00**	17.19		EE
30s ea	**54868-2415-02**	23.55		EE
60s ea	**54868-2415-01**	42.57		EE

PROD/MFR	NDC	AWP	DP	OBC
90s ea	54868-2415-03	61.62		EE
100s ea	54868-2415-04	67.95		AB
500s ea	54868-2415-05	146.21		AB
CER, PO, 200 mg, 10s ea	54868-4826-01	64.48		AB
30s ea	54868-4826-00	184.45		AB
60s ea	54868-4826-03	345.90		AB
100s ea	54868-4826-02	569.50		AB
(Physician Partner)				
REPACK				
CAP, PO, 50 mg, 120s ea	21695-0340-72	272.47		
75 mg, 21s ea	21695-0341-21	53.02		
30s ea	21695-0341-30	26.72		AB
42s ea	21695-0341-42	106.04		AB
60s ea	21695-0341-60	128.76		
(Quality Care Prod)				
REPACK				
CAP, PO, 75 mg, 30s ea	49999-0132-30	47.21		EE
60s ea	49999-0132-60	89.28		EE
(Southwood)				
REPACK				
CAP, PO, 50 mg, 10s ea	58016-0262-10	11.13		EE
15s ea	58016-0262-15	16.69		EE
20s ea	58016-0262-20	22.25		EE
28s ea	58016-0262-28	31.15		EE
30s ea	58016-0262-30	33.38		EE
60s ea	58016-0262-60	66.75		EE
100s ea	58016-0262-00	111.25		EE
120s ea	58016-0262-02	133.50		EE
75 mg, 10s ea	58016-0380-10	12.40		EE
12s ea	58016-0380-12	14.88		EE
14s ea	58016-0380-14	17.36		EE
15s ea	58016-0380-15	18.60		EE
20s ea	58016-0380-20	24.80		EE
21s ea	58016-0380-21	26.04		EE
24s ea	58016-0380-24	29.76		EE
28s ea	58016-0380-28	34.72		EE
30s ea	58016-0380-30	41.70		AB
40s ea	58016-0380-40	49.60		EE
50s ea	58016-0380-50	62.00		EE
60s ea	58016-0380-60	83.40		AB
90s ea	58016-0380-90	125.10		AB
100s ea	58016-0380-00	139.00		AB
120s ea	58016-0380-02	166.80		AB
CER, PO, 100 mg, 15s ea	58016-0496-15	33.83		EE
20s ea	58016-0496-20	45.10		EE
30s ea	58016-0496-30	67.65		EE
40s ea	58016-0496-40	90.20		EE
50s ea	58016-0496-50	112.75		EE
60s ea	58016-0496-60	135.30		EE
100s ea	58016-0496-00	225.50		EE
200 mg, 30s ea	58016-0754-30	84.07		EE
(Stat Rx)				
REPACK				
CAP, PO, 50 mg, 30s ea	16590-0136-30	32.58		
60s ea	16590-0136-60	65.17		
90s ea	16590-0136-90	97.75		
75 mg, 30s ea	16590-0137-30	43.00		
60s ea	16590-0137-60	86.00		
90s ea	16590-0137-90	129.00		
(Vibranta)				
REPACK				
CAP, PO, 75 mg, 20s ea	57866-4639-02	26.68		AB
30s ea	57866-4639-01	38.44		AB
KETOROLAC (Bryant Ranch)				
REPACK				
ketorolac tromethamine				
TAB, PO, 10 mg, 10s ea	63629-2974-02	14.35		
20s ea	63629-2974-03	32.00		
30s ea	63629-2974-01	43.05		
(Core)				
REPACK				
TAB, PO, 10 mg, 30s ea	33358-0199-30	34.43		
(Dispensing Solutions)				
REPACK				
TAB, PO, 10 mg, 10s ea	55045-2530-03	16.00		
15s ea	55045-2530-04	32.00		
20s ea	55045-2530-05	32.00		
(HomeMed)				
REPACK				
TAB, PO, 10 mg, 15s ea	51655-0889-54	26.38		
20s ea	51655-0889-52	34.28		
(Physician Partner)				
REPACK				
SOL, IJ (1MLX25)				
30 mg/ml, 1 ml 25s	21695-0588-25	78.00		
(Stat Rx)				
REPACK				
TAB, PO, 10 mg, 10s ea	16590-0138-10	17.00		
20s ea	16590-0138-20	34.00		
30s ea	16590-0138-30	51.00		
40s ea	16590-0138-40	68.00		
KETOROLAC TROMETHAMINE				
FUL				
TAB, PO, 10 mg, 100s ea		67.73		
(Akorn)				
SOL, OP (1X5ML)				
0.4%, 5 ml	17478-0208-10	106.87		AT
(1X3ML)				
0.5%, 3 ml	17478-0209-19	48.73		AT
(1X5ML)				
0.5%, 5 ml	17478-0209-10	106.87		AT
(1X10ML)				
0.5%, 10 ml	17478-0209-11	213.73		AT
(Allergan Inc) *See ACULAR*				
(Allergan Inc) *See ACULAR LS*				
(Allergan Inc) *See ACUVAIL*				
(Amer Regent)				
SOL, IJ (USP,25X1ML,SDV)				
15 mg/ml, 1 ml 25s	00517-0601-25	43.75		
(USP,25X2ML,SDV)				
30 mg/ml, 2 ml 25s	00517-0801-25	47.00		
IM, 30 mg/ml, 2 ml 25s	00517-0902-25	50.00		
(Apotex Corp.)				
SOL, IJ (10X1ML PREFILLED SYR)				
15 mg/ml, 1 ml 10s	60505-0725-01	87.35		AP
(SDV)				
15 mg/ml, 1 ml 25s	60505-0705-00	87.35		AP
(10X1ML PREFILLED SYR)				
30 mg/ml, 1 ml 10s	60505-0726-01	91.35		AP
(SDV)				
30 mg/ml, 1 ml 25s	60505-0706-00	91.35		AP
(10X2ML PREFILLED SYR)				
30 mg/ml, 2 ml 10s	60505-0726-02	96.97		AP
IM (S.D.V.)				
30 mg/ml, 2 ml 25s	60505-0706-01	96.97		AP
OP (1X5ML)				
0.4%, 5 ml	60505-0570-01	106.87		AT
0.5%, 5 ml	60505-1003-01	106.87		AT
(1X10ML)				
0.5%, 10 ml	60505-1003-02	213.73		AT
(APP)				
SOL, IJ (S.D.V.)				
15 mg/ml, 1 ml	63323-0161-01	8.39		AP
30 mg/ml, 1 ml	63323-0162-01	8.79		AP
IM, 30 mg/ml, 2 ml	63323-0162-02	8.34		AP
(Baxter)				
SOL, IJ, 15 mg/ml, 1 ml	10019-0029-12	1.27		AP
(1X25)				
15 mg/ml, 1 ml 25s	10019-0029-02	31.80		AP
(USP)				
30 mg/ml, 1 ml	10019-0030-12	1.50		AP
(1X25)				
30 mg/ml, 1 ml 25s	10019-0030-03	33.90		AP
2 ml	10019-0030-17	1.50		AP
(1X25)				
30 mg/ml, 2 ml 25s	10019-0030-04	37.50		AP
(Bedford)				
SOL, IJ (S.D.V.)				
15 mg/ml, 1 ml 10s	55390-0480-01	16.80		AP
30 mg/ml, 1 ml 10s	55390-0481-01	18.00		AP
(M.D.V.)				
30 mg/ml, 10 ml 10s	55390-0481-10	96.00		AP
IM (S.D.V.)				
30 mg/ml, 2 ml 10s	55390-0481-02	19.20		AP
(Caraco)				
SOL, OP (1X3ML)				
0.5%, 3 ml	41616-0219-90	52.25		AT
(1X5ML)				
0.5%, 5 ml	41616-0220-90	106.28		AT
(1X10ML)				
0.5%, 10 ml	41616-0221-90	212.54		AT
(Cura Pharm)				
SOL, IJ (SDV,USP,25X1ML)				
15 mg/ml, 1 ml 25s	66860-0084-03	43.75		AP
30 mg/ml, 1 ml 25s	66860-0085-03	50.00		AP
IM (25X2ML,SDV,USP)				
30 mg/ml, 2 ml 25s	66860-0086-03	60.00		AP
(Ethex)				
TAB, PO, 10 mg, 100s ea	58177-0301-04	92.98		AB
(Falcon Ophthalmics)				
SOL, OP (1X5ML)				
0.4%, 5 ml	61314-0018-05	33.60		AT
0.5%, 5 ml	61314-0126-05	33.60		AT
(1X10ML)				
0.5%, 10 ml	61314-0126-10	67.20		AT
(Hospira) *See KETOROLAC TROMETHAMINE AMERINET*				
(Hospira) *See KETOROLAC TROMETHAMINE NOVAPLUS*				
(Hospira)				
SOL, IJ (10X1ML)				
15 mg/ml, 1 ml 10s	00409-2288-21	13.44	11.80	AP
(LUER LOCK,LATEX-FREE)				
15 mg/ml, 1 ml 10s	00409-2288-31	18.36	16.10	AP
(USP,FLIPTOP VIAL)				
15 mg/ml, 1 ml 25s	00409-3793-01	26.40	23.00	AP
(10X1ML, USP)				
30 mg/ml, 1 ml 10s	00409-2287-21	13.44	11.80	AP
(LUER LOCK,CARPUJECT)				
30 mg/ml, 1 ml 10s	00409-2287-31	18.84	16.50	AP
(LATEX-FREE)				
30 mg/ml, 1 ml 25s	00409-3795-01	24.00	21.00	AP
(10X2ML)				
30 mg/ml, 2 ml 10s	00409-2287-22	14.16	12.40	AP
IM ((LUER LOCK),10X2ML)				
30 mg/ml, 2 ml 10s	00409-2287-61	19.92	17.40	AP
(VIAL, FLIPTOP)				
30 mg/ml, 2 ml 25s	00409-3796-01	24.90	21.75	AP
(VIAL,FLIPTOP,LATEX-FREE)				
30 mg/ml, 2 ml 25s	00074-3796-01	24.90	21.75	AP
(Mylan)				
TAB, PO, 10 mg, 100s ea	00378-1134-01	102.00		AB
(PCCA)				
POW, NA (USP)				
1 gm	51927-3443-00	60.00		
(Spectrum Pharmacy)				
CRY, NA (U.S.P.)				
5 gm	49452-3919-05	317.80		
25 gm	49452-3919-01	990.50		
100 gm	49452-3919-02	3272.50		
500 gm	49452-3919-03	8183.00		
(Teva)				
TAB, PO, 10 mg, 100s ea	00093-0314-01	92.97		AB
(Wockhardt USA)				
SOL, IJ (USP,SDV)				
15 mg/ml, 1 ml 10s	64679-0757-02	17.50		AP
1 ml 25s	64679-0757-01	43.75		AP
30 mg/ml, 1 ml 10s	64679-0758-04	18.80		AP
1 ml 25s	64679-0758-01	45.00		AP
(USP,S.D.V.)				
30 mg/ml, 2 ml	64679-0758-05	2.00		AP
(USP,SDV,2X10ML)				
30 mg/ml, 2 ml 10s	64679-0758-06	20.00		AP
(USP,SDV,25X2ML)				
30 mg/ml, 2 ml 25s	64679-0758-02	50.00		AP
(4u)				
REPACK				
TAB, PO, 10 mg, 12s ea	10544-0387-12	29.84		AB
12s ea	42549-0538-12	29.84		AB
12s ea	42549-0587-12	29.84		AB
20s ea	10544-0338-20	38.12		
20s ea	42549-0538-20	38.12		AB
20s ea	42549-0587-20	38.12		AB
20s ea	42549-0622-20	38.12		AB
(A-S Medication)				
REPACK				
SOL, OP (1X5ML)				
0.5%, 5 ml	54569-6148-00	106.87		AT
TAB, PO, 10 mg, 15s ea	54569-4494-02	14.64		AB
20s ea	54569-4494-00	19.52		AB
(Aidarex)				
REPACK				
TAB, PO, 10 mg, 7s ea	33261-0065-07	7.14		AB
14s ea	33261-0065-14	14.28		AB
20s ea	33261-0065-20	20.40		AB
21s ea	33261-0065-21	21.42		AB
28s ea	33261-0065-28	28.56		AB
30s ea	33261-0065-30	30.60		AB
40s ea	33261-0065-40	40.80		AB
60s ea	33261-0065-60	61.20		AB
(Altura)				
REPACK				
TAB, PO, 10 mg, 8s ea	63874-0472-08	10.74		EE
10s ea	63874-0472-10	13.43		AB
12s ea	63874-0472-12	20.67		AB
15s ea	63874-0472-15	25.84		EE
16s ea	63874-0472-16	27.56		AB
20s ea	63874-0472-20	28.36		EE
21s ea	63874-0472-21	29.78		AB
30s ea	63874-0472-30	40.29		EE
50s ea	63874-0472-50	55.10		AB
100s ea	63874-0472-01	116.00		EE
500s ea	63874-0472-03	551.00		AB

PROD/MFR	NDC	AWP	DP	OBC
(DHS, Inc.) REPACK				
TAB, PO, 10 mg, 20s ea	**55887-0880-20**	26.98		AB
30s ea	**55887-0880-30**	38.06		AB
60s ea	**55887-0880-60**	76.12		AB
(Dispensing Solutions) REPACK				
TAB, PO, 10 mg, 8s ea	**66336-0446-08**	10.39		AB
10s ea	**66336-0446-10**	12.85		AB
(Keltman Pharma., Inc.) REPACK				
TAB, PO, 10 mg, 20s ea	**68387-0440-20**	27.48		
30s ea	**68387-0440-30**	41.22		
(Nucare Pharm) REPACK				
TAB, PO, 10 mg, 20s ea	**66267-0418-20**	34.99		EE
60s ea	**66267-0418-60**	76.70		AB
(Palmetto) REPACK				
SOL, IJ, 30 mg/ml, 1 ml 10s	**23490-5792-04**	59.55		
TAB, PO, 10 mg, 8s ea	**23490-5791-01**	13.63		
10s ea	**23490-5791-02**	14.22		
20s ea	**23490-5791-03**	28.45		
90s ea	**23490-5791-04**	128.01		
(PD-Rx Pharm) REPACK				
TAB, PO, 10 mg, 4s ea	**43063-0174-04**	19.40		AB
10s ea	**55289-0328-10**	30.84		AB
12s ea	**55289-0328-12**	31.56		AB
15s ea	**55289-0328-15**	32.27		AB
20s ea	**55289-0328-20**	32.49		AB
30s ea	**55289-0328-30**	42.67		AB
(Pharma Pac) REPACK				
TAB, PO, 10 mg, 8s ea	**52959-0512-08**	14.08		AB
9s ea	**52959-0512-09**	15.84		AB
10s ea	**52959-0512-10**	17.22		AB
12s ea	**52959-0512-12**	20.64		AB
14s ea	**52959-0512-14**	23.98		AB
15s ea	**52959-0512-15**	25.65		AB
20s ea	**52959-0512-20**	34.15		AB
30s ea	**52959-0512-30**	50.99		AB
40s ea	**52959-0512-40**	65.16		AB
60s ea	**52959-0512-60**	94.80		AB
(Phys Total Care) REPACK				
SOL, IM, 30 mg/ml, 2 ml (S.D.V.)	**54868-4419-01**	9.81		AP
30 mg/ml, 2 ml 10s	**54868-4419-00**	65.04		AP
TAB, PO, 10 mg, 15s ea	**54868-4171-02**	22.10		AB
20s ea	**54868-4171-00**	27.47		AB
30s ea	**54868-4171-01**	38.21		AB
(Physician Partner) REPACK				
SOL, IJ, 30 mg/ml, 10s ea	**21695-0588-10**	40.60		AP
(1X1ML) 30 mg/ml, 1 ml	**21695-0588-01**	14.00		AP
TAB, PO, 10 mg, 15s ea	**21695-0432-15**	32.81		AB
20s ea	**21695-0432-20**	43.75		AB
(FILM-COATED) 10 mg, 30s ea	**21695-0432-30**	55.79		
(Quality Care Prod) REPACK				
SOL, IJ (1X1ML) 30 mg/ml, 1 ml	**49999-0670-01**	27.00		AP
IM (1X2ML,LATEX-FREE) 30 mg/ml, 2 ml	**49999-0416-01**	54.00		AP
TAB, PO, 10 mg, 10s ea	**49999-0130-10**	12.60		AB
10s ea	**49999-0130-15**	18.90		AB
20s ea	**49999-0130-20**	25.23		
21s ea	**49999-0130-21**	26.48		
30s ea	**49999-0130-30**	37.85		
(Southwood) REPACK				
SOL, IM (SDV) 30 mg/ml, 2 ml	**58016-9413-01**	116.64		EE
TAB, PO, 10 mg, 10s ea	**58016-0247-10**	10.80		AB
12s ea	**58016-0247-12**	12.96		AB
15s ea	**58016-0247-15**	16.20		AB
20s ea	**58016-0247-20**	21.60		AB
21s ea	**58016-0247-21**	22.68		AB
30s ea	**58016-0247-30**	32.40		AB
40s ea	**58016-0247-40**	43.20		AB
60s ea	**58016-0247-60**	64.80		AB
90s ea	**58016-0247-90**	97.20		AB
100s ea	**58016-0247-00**	108.00		AB
120s ea	**58016-0247-02**	129.60		AB
150s ea	**58016-0247-03**	162.00		AB
200s ea	**58016-0247-89**	216.00		AB
300s ea	**58016-0247-73**	324.00		AB
(St. Mary's MPP) REPACK				
TAB, PO, 10 mg, 20s ea	**60760-0314-20**	26.45		AB
(Stat Rx) REPACK				
TAB, PO, 10 mg, 15s ea	**16590-0138-15**	34.80		AB
60s ea	**16590-0138-60**	84.00		AB
(Vibranta) REPACK				
TAB, PO, 10 mg, 15s ea	**57866-7382-01**	18.90		AB
20s ea	**57866-7382-03**	34.28		AB
KETOROLAC TROMETHAMINE AMERINET (Hospira) ketorolac tromethamine				
SOL, IM (FTV,AMERINET,LATEX-FREE) 30 mg/ml, 2 ml 25s	**00409-3796-61**	21.00	18.50	AP
KETOROLAC TROMETHAMINE NOVAPLUS (Hospira) ketorolac tromethamine				
SOL, IJ (U.S.P.,25X1ML) 15 mg/ml, 1 ml 25s	**00409-3793-49**	22.80	20.00	AP
KETOTIFEN FUMARATE (Apotex Corp.)				
SOL, OP, 0.025%, 5 ml	**60505-0569-01**	64.86		AT
(PCCA)				
POW, NA (1X1GM) 1 gm	**51927-3880-00**	1245.00		
1 gm	**51927-4345-00**	66.00		
(Pharma Pac) REPACK				
SOL, OP, 0.025%, 5 ml	**52959-0858-05**	63.79		
KINERET (Amgen USA Inc.) anakinra				
SOL, SC (SRN,W/27G NDL,PF) 100 mg/0.67 ml, 0.67 ml 7s	**55513-0177-07**	361.03		
(Biovitrum)				
SOL, SC (SRN,W/27G NDL,PF) 100 mg/0.67 ml, 0.67 ml	**55513-0177-01**	54.11		
0.67 ml 28s	**55513-0177-28**	1515.02		
KINETIN (Medisca)				
POW, NA (1X5GM) 5 gm	**38779-2234-03**	180.00		
(1X25GM) 25 gm	**38779-2234-04**	597.00		
(1X100GM) 1000 gm	**38779-2234-05**	1530.00		
(PCCA)				
POW, NA, 1 gm	**51927-3209-00**	99.00		
KINEVAC (Bracco Diag) sincalide				
PDS, IV (VIAL) 5 mcg, 10s ea	**00270-0556-15**	700.00	560.00	
KINLYTIC (ImaRx) urokinase				
PDS; IV (LYOPHILIZED) 250000 iu, ea	**24430-1003-01**	539.78		
KINRIX (Glaxo) dtap and polio vaccine				
SUS, IM (5X0.05ML,TAX INCL,PF) 0.5 ml 5s	**58160-0812-46**	285.00		
(SDV,10X0.05ML,TAX INCL) 0.5 ml 10s	**58160-0812-11**	570.00		
KIONEX (Paddock) sodium polystyrene sulfonate				
PDR, PO, 454 gm	**00574-2004-16**	201.90		AA
SUS, NA (RASPBERRY) 15 gm/60 ml, 60 ml 10s UD	**00574-2002-02**	87.50		AA
(1X480ML,RASPBERRY) 15 gm/60 ml, 480 ml	**00574-2002-16**	60.00		AA
KIT FOR PREPARATION OF TECHNETIUM TC 99M MEDRONATE (Pharmlucence) technetium tc 99m medronate				
KIT, IV, ea	**45567-0040-01**	93.00	77.50	
ea	**45567-0040-02**	558.00	465.00	
KIT FOR PREPARATION OF TECHNETIUM TC 99M PENTETATE (Pharmlucence) technetium tc 99m pentetate				
KIT, IV, ea	**45567-0010-01**	79.50	66.25	AP
ea	**45567-0010-02**	477.00	397.50	AP
KIT FOR PREPARATION OF TECHNETIUM TC 99M SESTAMIBI (Pharmlucence) technetium tc 99m sestamibi				
KIT, IV, ea	**45567-0555-01**	1770.00	1475.00	AP
ea	**45567-0555-02**	10620.00	8850.00	AP
KIT PREPARATION OF TECHNETIUM 99M SULFUR COLLOID (Pharmlucence) technetium tc 99m sulfurcolloid				
KIT, NA, ea	**45567-0030-01**	894.00	745.00	
KIT PREPARATION OF TECHNETIUM TC 99M MEBROFENIN (Pharmlucence) technetium tc 99m mebrofenin				
KIT, IV (M.D.V) ea	**45567-0455-01**	259.50	216.25	AP
ea	**45567-0455-02**	1557.00	1297.50	AP
KIT PREPARATION OF TECHNETIUM TC 99M PYROPHOSPHATE (Pharmlucence) technetium tc 99m pyrophosphate				
KIT, IV, ea	**45567-0060-01**	136.20	113.50	
ea	**45567-0060-02**	817.20	681.00	

KIT, ADMINISTRATION, BLOOD

(Abbott Hosp) *See BLOOD ADMINISTRATION W/CAIR CLAMP*

(Abbott Hosp) *See BLOOD SECONDARY*

KIT, ADMINISTRATION, INTRAVENOUS

(Abbott Hosp) *See LIFECARE 75 FLOW DETECTOR*

(Abbott Hosp) *See LIFESHIELD PLUMSET PRIMARY IV W/OL*

(Abbott Hosp) *See NITROGLYCERIN PRIMARY PUMP*

(Abbott Hosp) *See PCA CONTINUOUS INFUSION-OL*

(Abbott Hosp) *See PCA INJECTOR*

(Abbott Hosp) *See PCA LONG W/INJECTOR-OL*

(Abbott Hosp) *See PCA MINIBORE*

(Abbott Hosp) *See PCA W/INJECTOR-OL*

(Abbott Hosp) *See PLUM LC 5000*

(Abbott Hosp) *See PLUM LC 5000 LATEX-FREE*

(Abbott Hosp) *See PLUMSET LIFESHIELD H-FLOW*

(Abbott Hosp) *See PLUMSET MICRO SECONDARY MIDLENGTH*

(Abbott Hosp) *See PLUMSET MICRODRIP NITROGLYCERIN-OL*

(Abbott Hosp) *See PLUMSET MICRODRIP PRIMARY IV W/OL*

(Abbott Hosp) *See PLUMSET MICRODRIP VENTED*

(Abbott Hosp) *See PLUMSET PRIMARY IV W/OL*

(Abbott Hosp) *See PLUMSET SPECIALTY MICROBORE PUMP-OL*

(Abbott Hosp) *See PRIMARY CONVERTABLE PIN LATEX FREE*

(Abbott Hosp) *See PRIMARY IV SET-SL W/IVEX-HP*

(Abbott Hosp) *See PRIMARY MACRO IV PUMP*

(Abbott Hosp) *See PRIMARY NONVENTED IV SET-OL*

(Abbott Hosp) *See PROVIDER PUMP*

(Abbott Hosp) *See VENOSET*

(Animas Corp.) *See ANIMAS INFUSION*

(APP) *See HI-VOLUME PUMPING CHAMBER SET*

(Arkray) *See COMFORT DETACHABLE INFUSION*

(Bracco Diag) *See SOLUTION ADMINISTRATION SET*

(GE) *See INFUSION SET W/DRIP CHAMBER*

(Medtronic Minimed) *See PARADIGM QUICK-SET INFUSION*

(Medtronic Minimed) *See POLYFIN NEEDLE INFUSION*

(Medtronic Minimed) *See POLYFIN QR NEEDLE INFUSION*

(Medtronic Minimed) *See QUICK-SET INFUSION*

(Medtronic Minimed) *See SOF-SERTER INFUSION/INSERTION SYST*

KIT, ADMINISTRATION, PERITONEAL DIALYSIS, DISP

(Abbott Hosp) *See INPERSOL PERITONEAL DIALYSIS TRAY*

KIT, ANESTHESIA, EPIDURAL

(Portex) *See EPIDURAL ANESTHESIA TRAY*

KIT, BLOOD COLLECTION, PHLEBOTOMY

(Abbott Hosp) *See BLOOD COLLECTION*

PROD/MFR	NDC	AWP	DP	OBC
KIT, CATHETERIZATION, INTRAVENOUS, WINGED				
(Abbott Hosp) *See BUTTERFLY INFUSION*				
(Abbott Hosp) *See BUTTERFLY INFUSION PEDIATRIC*				
(Abbott Hosp) *See BUTTERFLY INT INFUSION*				
(J&J Medical) *See PROTECTIV PLUS-W IV CATH SAFETY SYS*				
(J&J Medical) *See PROTECTIV-W IV CATHETER SAFETY SYST*				
KIT, DISPOSABLE PROCEDURE				
(Cooper Surgical) *See LEEP REDIKIT*				
KIT, FEEDING (ENTERAL)				
(Abbott) *See PATROL EASY-FEED*				
(Abbott) *See PATROL PUMP SET*				
(Abbott Hosp) *See ENTERAL PUMP*				
(Abbott Hosp) *See PLUM LC 5000*				
(Hospira) *See NUTRIMIX*				
KIT, INTRAVENOUS EXTENSION TUBING				
(Abbott Hosp) *See DIAL-A-FLO*				
(Abbott Hosp) *See MINIBORE EXTENSION*				
(Abbott Hosp) *See PCA EXTENSION*				
(Medtronic Minimed) *See POLYFIN TUBING EXTENSION*				
KIWI FRAGRANCE (PCCA)				
fragrance				
SOL, NA, 1 ml	51927-3224-00	1.00		
KLARON (Dermik)				
sulfacetamide sodium				
LOT, TP, 10%, 118 ml	00066-7500-04	152.77		
(Phys Total Care) REPACK				
LOT, TP, 10%, 118 ml	54868-5401-00	128.23		
KLEAROL LIGHT (Amend)				
mineral oil				
OIL, NA (N.F.) 480 ml	17317-1068-01	4.90		
3840 ml	17317-1068-06	21.00		
19200 ml	17317-1068-08	70.00		
KLONOPIN (Roche Labs)				
clonazepam				
TAB, PO, 0.5 mg, 100s ea, C-IV	00004-0068-01	173.90		AB
10000s ea, C-IV	00004-0068-32	16870.42		AB
1 mg, 100s ea, C-IV	00004-0058-01	198.37		AB
10000s ea, C-IV	00004-0058-32	19241.05		AB
2 mg, 100s ea, C-IV	00004-0098-01	274.87		AB
10000s ea, C-IV	00004-0098-32	19193.82		AB
(Phys Total Care) REPACK				
TAB, PO, 0.5 mg, 60s ea, C-IV	54868-2574-00	79.18		AB
90s ea, C-IV	54868-2574-02	117.81		AB
1 mg, 30s ea, C-IV	54868-1694-00	53.60		AB
90s ea, C-IV	54868-1694-03	149.05		AB
100s ea, C-IV	54868-1694-02	174.91		AB
(Southwood) REPACK				
TAB, PO, 1 mg, 30s ea, C-IV	58016-0035-30	47.09		AB
60s ea, C-IV	58016-0035-60	94.18		AB
90s ea, C-IV	58016-0035-90	141.26		AB
100s ea, C-IV	58016-0035-00	156.96		AB
2 mg, 30s ea, C-IV	00490-0043-30	65.25		AB
60s ea, C-IV	00490-0043-60	130.49		AB
90s ea, C-IV	00490-0043-90	195.74		AB
100s ea, C-IV	00490-0043-00	217.49		AB
KLOR-CON (Upsher-Smith)				
potassium chloride				
PDS, PO, 20 meq, 30s ea UD	00245-0035-30	30.80		
100s ea UD	00245-0035-01	102.66		
(Phys Total Care) REPACK				
PDS, PO, 20 meq, 100s ea	54868-1504-00	16.84		
KLOR-CON 10 (Upsher-Smith)				
potassium chloride				
TER, PO, 10 meq, 100s ea UD	00245-0041-01	50.22		BC
100s ea	00245-0041-11	43.61		BC
500s ea	00245-0041-15	213.27		BC
5000s ea	00245-0041-55	2031.00		BC
(PD-Rx Pharm) REPACK				
TER, PO (REDI-SCRIPT) 10 meq, 30s ea	58864-0729-30	11.92		BC
(Phys Total Care) REPACK				
TER, PO, 10 meq, 30s ea	54868-1302-01	26.64		BC
100s ea	54868-1302-02	59.43		BC
KLOR-CON 8 (Upsher-Smith)				
potassium chloride				
TER, PO, 8 meq, ea	00245-0040-89	0.28		AB
100s ea UD	00245-0040-01	28.16		AB
100s ea	00245-0040-11	22.88		AB
500s ea	00245-0040-15	112.26		AB
5000s ea	00245-0040-55	1122.31		AB
KLOR-CON M10 (Upsher-Smith)				
potassium chloride				
TER, PO, 10 meq, ea	00245-0057-89	0.30		AB
(USP) 10 meq, 90s ea	00245-0057-90	27.09		AB
100s ea UD	00245-0057-01	30.10		AB
100s ea	00245-0057-11	29.05		AB
1000s ea	00245-0057-10	•278.99		AB
(Apace) REPACK				
TER, PO (USP) 10 meq, 30s ea	15338-0122-30	73.05		AB
KLOR-CON M15 (Upsher-Smith)				
potassium chloride				
TER, PO, 15 meq, ea	00245-0150-89	0.50		
100s ea	00245-0150-11	45.94		
KLOR-CON M20 (Upsher-Smith)				
potassium chloride				
TER, PO, 20 meq, ea	00245-0058-89	0.57		AB
90s ea	00245-0058-90	48.57		AB
100s ea UD	00245-0058-01	57.35		AB
100s ea	00245-0058-11	52.91		AB
500s ea	00245-0058-15	262.49		AB
1000s ea	00245-0058-10	516.10		AB
(Apace) REPACK				
TER, PO (USP) 20 meq, 30s ea	15338-0133-30	135.30		AB
(Phys Total Care) REPACK				
TER, PO, 20 meq, 100s ea	54868-5383-00	130.32		AB
KLOR-CON/25 (Upsher-Smith)				
potassium chloride				
PDS, PO, 25 meq, 30s ea UD	00245-0037-30	36.61		
100s ea UD	00245-0037-01	122.04		
KLOR-CON/EF (Upsher-Smith)				
potassium bicarbonate/potassium citrate				
TEF, PO, 25 meq, 30s ea UD	00245-0039-30	12.65		
100s ea UD	00245-0039-01	39.64		
KOATE-DVI (Talecris)				
antihemophilic factor viii human				
PDS, IV (1000IU) 1 iu, ea	13533-0665-50	1.31		
(250IU) 1 iu, ea	13533-0665-20	1.31		
(500IU) 1 iu, ea	13533-0665-30	1.31		
KOGENATE FS (Bayer)				
antihemophilic factor viii (recombinant)				
PDS, IV (1000IU) 1 iu, ea	00026-3785-50	1.68		
(250IU) 1 iu, ea	00026-3782-20	1.68		
(3000IU,PF) 1 iu, ea	00026-3787-70	1.68		
(500IU) 1 iu, ea	00026-3783-30	1.68		
(Bayer Corp.)				
PDS, IV (2000IU) 1 iu, ea	00026-3786-60	1.68		
KOGENATE FS WITH BIO-SET (Bayer)				
antihemophilic factor viii (recombinant)				
PDS, IV (1000IU) 1 iu, ea	00026-3795-50	1.68		
(250IU) 1 iu, ea	00026-3792-20	1.68		
(3000IU,PF) 1 iu, ea	00026-3797-70	1.68		
(500IU) 1 iu, ea	00026-3793-30	1.68		
(Bayer Corp.)				
PDS, IV (2000IU) 1 iu, ea	00026-3796-60	1.68		
KOJIC ACID				
(Gallipot) *See KOJIC ACID 98%*				
(Medisca)				
POW, NA (1X5GM) 5 gm	38779-1768-03	75.00		
(1X25GM) 25 gm	38779-1768-04	186.00		
(1X100GM) 100 gm	38779-1768-05	582.00		
(1X500GM) 500 gm	38779-1768-08	2601.00		
(PCCA)				
POW, NA, 1 gm	51927-2749-00	8.28		
(Spectrum Pharmacy)				
POW, NA (1X5GM) 5 gm	49452-3915-02	126.70		
(1X25GM) 25 gm	49452-3915-03	291.90		
(1X100GM) 100 gm	49452-3915-04	857.50		
KOJIC ACID 98% (Gallipot)				
kojic acid				
POW, NA, 25 gm	51552-0552-04	82.95		
KOLA NUT (PCCA)				
cola nut				
POW, NA, 1 gm	51927-2970-00	0.26		
KOLEPHRIN #1 (Pfeiffer)				
codeine phosphate/guaifenesin				
LIQ, PO, 10 mg/5 ml-100 mg/5 ml, 120 ml, C-V	00927-0153-12	3.10		
KOVIA (Stratus)				
papain/urea				
OIN, TP, 830000 u/gm-100 mg/gm, 3.5 gm 100s UD	58980-0711-35	580.00		
30 gm	58980-0711-11	44.62		
KRISTALOSE (Cumberland Pharma)				
lactulose				
PDR, PO (SINGLE DOSE) 10 gm/packet, 30s ea	66220-0719-30	49.06		
20 gm/packet, 30s ea	66220-0729-30	76.13		
(Stat Rx) REPACK				
PDR, PO, 20 gm/packet, ea	16590-0495-01	15.50		
30s ea	16590-0495-30	70.75		
KRONOFED-A (Southwood) REPACK				
cpm/pse hcl				
CER, PO, 8 mg-120 mg, 20s ea	58016-0642-20	5.63		
KURIC (JSJ Pharma)				
ketoconazole				
CRE, TP, 2%, 25 gm	68712-0006-01	37.50		
75 gm	68712-0006-03	75.00		
KUVAN (Biomarin)				
sapropterin dihydrochloride				
ODT, PO, 100 mg, 120s ea	68135-0300-02	4380.00		
KYTRIL (Roche Labs)				
granisetron hydrochloride				
SOL, IV (S.D.V.) 1 mg/ml, 1 ml	00004-0239-09	187.39		
(M.D.V.) 1 mg/ml, 4 ml	00004-0240-09	749.57		
PO (ORANGE) 2 mg/10 ml, 30 ml	00004-0237-09	359.72		
TAB, PO (UNIT OF USE) 1 mg, 2s ea	00004-0241-33	125.90		
(Phys Total Care) REPACK				
TAB, PO, 1 mg, 2s ea	54868-4139-00	150.36		
3s ea	54868-4139-04	225.53		
6s ea	54868-4139-02	449.11		
8s ea	54868-4139-03	578.92		
10s ea	54868-4139-01	729.64		
20s ea	54868-4139-05	1426.03		
30s ea	54868-4139-06	2139.05		
L-4-THIAZOLIDINECARBOXYLIC ACID				
(PCCA) *See TIMONACIC*				
L-5-HYDROXYTRYPTOPHAN (Gallipot)				
tryptophan				
POW, NA, 5 gm	51552-0630-02	43.05		

PROD/MFR	NDC	AWP	DP	OBC
25 gm	51552-0630-04	189.00		
100 gm	51552-0630-05	511.00		
L-ALANINE (Amend)				
alanine				
POW, NA (C.P.)				
100 gm	17317-1856-03	21.00		
(Spectrum Pharmacy)				
POW, NA (U.S.P.)				
100 gm	49452-0212-02	210.35		
1000 gm	49452-0212-03	1235.50		
L-ARGININE (Spectrum Pharmacy)				
arginine				
POW, NA (U.S.P.)				
100 gm	49452-0702-01	68.60		
1000 gm	49452-0702-02	504.00		
L-ARGININE MONOHYDROCHLORIDE (Amend)				
arginine hydrochloride				
POW, NA (U.S.P.)				
25 gm	17317-0209-02	8.40		
L-ASPARAGINE MONOHYDRATE (Spectrum Pharmacy)				
asparagine monohydrate				
POW, NA (F.C.C.)				
100 gm	49452-0759-01	187.25		
1000 gm	49452-0759-02	854.00		
L-ASPARTIC ACID (Spectrum Pharmacy)				
aspartic acid				
POW, NA (F.C.C.)				
100 gm	49452-0758-01	98.00		
1000 gm	49452-0758-02	406.00		
L-ASPARTIC ACID SODIUM SALT (Spectrum Pharmacy)				
aspartic acid sodium				
POW, NA, 100 gm	49452-0757-01	212.10		
1000 gm	49452-0757-02	1064.00		
L-CARNITINE (Gallipot)				
levocarnitine hydrochloride				
POW, NA, 100 gm	51552-0649-05	75.60		
(U.S.P.)				
1000 gm	51552-0649-07	546.00		
L-CARNITINE FREE BASE (Spectrum Pharmacy)				
levocarnitine				
POW, NA, 25 gm	49452-1775-01	107.10		
100 gm	49452-1775-02	325.50		
500 gm	49452-1775-03	1032.50		
L-CARNITINE HYDROCHLORIDE (Spectrum Pharmacy)				
levocarnitine				
POW, NA, 25 gm	49452-1776-01	174.65		
100 gm	49452-1776-02	514.50		
L-CARNOSINE (Letco)				
carnosine				
POW, NA (1X25GM)				
25 gm	62991-2610-01	225.00		
(1X100GM)				
100 gm	62991-2610-02	450.00		
L-CITRULLINE (Spectrum Pharmacy)				
citrulline				
POW, NA, 25 gm	49452-2111-02	86.45		
100 gm	49452-2111-03	173.25		
1000 gm	49452-2111-04	1151.50		
L-CYSTEINE (Spectrum Pharmacy)				
cysteine				
POW, NA, 100 gm	49452-2410-02	142.45		
1000 gm	49452-2410-04	847.00		
(Teva)				
cysteine hydrochloride				
SOL, IV (S.D.V.)				
50 mg/ml,				
10 ml 10s	00703-5324-03	31.25		
(BULK PACKAGE)				
50 mg/ml,				
50 ml 10s	00703-5328-03	144.00		
L-CYSTEINE HCL MONOHYDRATE				
(Spectrum Pharmacy)				
cysteine hydrochloride				
POW, NA (U.S.P.)				
100 gm	49452-2412-03	143.50		
1000 gm	49452-2412-05	787.50		
L-CYSTEINE HYDROCHLORIDE (Amer Regent)				
cysteine hydrochloride				
SOL, IV (S.D.V.,PF)				
50 mg/ml,				
10 ml 25s	00517-2064-25	221.90		
((VIAL),50MLX5)				
50 mg/ml, 50 ml 5s	00517-2050-05	103.00		
(Parenta Pharma)				
SOL, IV (USP, S.D.V.)				
50 mg/ml, 10 ml	66758-0004-01	5.83	4.80	
10 ml 10s	66758-0004-02	58.30	48.00	
(USP, BULK PACKAGE)				
50 mg/ml, 50 ml	66758-0005-01	19.80	16.50	
50 ml 5s	66758-0005-02	99.00	82.50	
L-CYSTINE (Spectrum Pharmacy)				
cystine				
CRY, NA (F.C.C.)				
100 gm	49452-2435-02	145.95		
(FCC)				
1000 gm	49452-2435-03	819.00		
L-DOPA (Spectrum Pharmacy)				
levodopa				
POW, NA (U.S.P.)				
5 gm	49452-2680-01	67.90		
25 gm	49452-2680-02	183.05		
100 gm	49452-2680-03	591.50		
L-GLUTAMIC ACID (Spectrum Pharmacy)				
glutamic acid				
POW, NA (F.C.C.)				
1000 gm	49452-3315-02	210.35		
L-GLUTAMIC ACID HCL (Spectrum Pharmacy)				
glutamic acid				
POW, NA (F.C.C.)				
1000 gm	49452-3335-02	210.35		
L-GLUTAMIC ACID HYDROCHLORIDE (Amend)				
glutamic acid				
POW, NA (N.F.)				
125 gm	17317-0187-04	7.00		
500 gm	17317-0187-01	14.00		
2500 gm	17317-0187-05	56.00		
11350 gm	17317-0187-08	210.00		
L-GLUTAMIC ACID MONOSODIUM SALT (Spectrum Pharmacy)				
glutamic acid				
POW, NA (F.C.C.)				
500 gm	49452-3338-02	114.10		
(N.F.)				
500 gm	49452-3337-02	103.95		
(F.C.C.)				
2500 gm	49452-3338-03	250.60		
(N.F.)				
2500 gm	49452-3337-03	236.25		
(F.C.C.)				
12000 gm	49452-3338-04	574.00		
(N.F.)				
12000 gm	49452-3337-04	570.50		
L-GLUTAMINE (Gallipot)				
glutamine				
POW, NA (F.C.C.)				
25 gm	51552-0285-04	11.34		
100 gm	51552-0285-05	23.52		
1000 gm	51552-0285-07	149.94		
(Medisca)				
POW, NA, 25 gm	38779-1104-04	27.00		
100 gm	38779-1104-05	67.50		
500 gm	38779-1104-08	171.00		
1000 gm	38779-1104-09	297.00		
(Spectrum Pharmacy)				
CRY, NA (F.C.C.)				
100 gm	49452-3342-02	101.50		
1000 gm	49452-3342-03	458.50		
L-GLUTATHIONE REDUCED FORM				
(Spectrum Pharmacy)				
glutathione				
POW, NA (1X5GM)				
5 gm	49452-3352-02	95.20		
(1X25GM)				
25 gm	49452-3352-03	319.55		
(1X100GM)				
100 gm	49452-3352-04	987.00		
(1X500GM)				
500 gm	49452-3352-06	2712.50		
L-HISTIDINE (Spectrum Pharmacy)				
histidine				
POW, NA (U.S.P.)				
100 gm	49452-3502-01	219.80		
1000 gm	49452-3502-02	1533.00		
L-HISTIDINE MONOHYDROCHLORIDE (Spectrum Pharmacy)				
histidine				
POW, NA (F.C.C.)				
100 gm	49452-3515-02	170.80		
1000 gm	49452-3515-03	1060.50		
L-ISOLEUCINE (Medisca)				
isoleucine				
POW, NA (U.S.P.)				
25 gm	38779-0359-04	46.50		
100 gm	38779-0359-05	147.00		
500 gm	38779-0359-08	652.50		
L-LEUCINE (Gallipot)				
leucine				
POW, NA (U.S.P.)				
1000 gm	51552-0400-07	188.30		
(Medisca)				
POW, NA (U.S.P.)				
100 gm	38779-0333-05	57.00		
500 gm	38779-0333-08	213.00		
1000 gm	38779-0333-09	315.00		
(Spectrum Pharmacy)				
POW, NA (U.S.P.)				
100 gm	49452-4033-01	97.30		
1000 gm	49452-4033-02	584.50		
L-LYSINE MONOHYDROCHLORIDE (Amend)				
lysine hydrochloride				
POW, NA (U.S.P./F.C.C.)				
125 gm	17317-0336-04	7.70		
500 gm	17317-0336-01	14.00		
2270 gm	17317-0336-05	56.00		
11350 gm	17317-0336-08	255.00		
(Gallipot)				
POW, NA, 100 gm	51552-0300-05	10.50		
(Lorann Oil)				
CRY, NA, 454 gm	23535-0608-01	12.25		
2270 gm	23535-0130-00	60.50		
4540 gm	23535-0140-00	110.00		
(Spectrum Pharmacy)				
POW, NA (F.C.C.)				
100 gm	49452-4159-01	64.75		
(U.S.P.)				
100 gm	49452-4158-01	64.75		
(F.C.C.)				
1000 gm	49452-4159-03	227.50		
(U.S.P.)				
1000 gm	49452-4158-03	227.50		
(1X5000GM,USP)				
5000 gm	49452-4159-04	756.00		
(U.S.P.)				
5000 gm	49452-4158-04	756.00		
L-MENTHOL (Amend)				
menthol				
CRY, NA (U.S.P.)				
30 gm	17317-0352-02	11.90		
125 gm	17317-0352-04	27.60		
500 gm	17317-0352-01	77.00		
2270 gm	17317-0352-05	294.00		
(Spectrum Pharmacy)				
CRY, NA (U.S.P.)				
25 gm	49452-4440-01	63.35		
125 gm	49452-4440-02	133.70		
500 gm	49452-4440-03	332.50		
L-METHIONINE (Gallipot)				
methionine				
POW, NA, 100 gm	51552-0610-05	35.91		
(Spectrum Pharmacy)				
POW, NA (U.S.P.)				
25 gm	49452-4581-01	113.05		
(F.C.C.)				
100 gm	49452-4582-02	181.30		
(U.S.P.)				
100 gm	49452-4581-02	150.85		
(F.C.C.)				
500 gm	49452-4582-03	497.00		
(U.S.P.)				
500 gm	49452-4581-03	423.50		
(F.C.C.)				
1000 gm	49452-4582-04	871.50		
(U.S.P.)				
1000 gm	49452-4581-04	756.00		
L-METHYLFOLATE				
(Pamlab) *See DEPLIN*				
(Pamlab) *See ZERVALX*				
L-METHYLFOLATE/METHYLCOBALAMIN/ PYRIDOXAL PHOSPHATE				
(Acella) *See FOLAST*				
(Pamlab) *See METANX*				
L-METHYLFOLATE/VIT B12/VIT B2/VIT B6				
(Pamlab) *See CEREFOLIN*				

PROD/MFR	NDC	AWP	DP	OBC
L-ORNITHINE HYDROCHLORIDE (Medisca)				
ornithine hydrochloride				
POW, NA (1X25GM)				
25 gm	38779-1370-04	36.00		
(1X100GM)				
100 gm	38779-1370-05	87.00		
(1X500GM)				
500 gm	38779-1370-08	375.00		
(1X1000GM)				
1000 gm	38779-1370-09	630.00		
L-ORNITHINE MONOHYDROCHLORIDE (Amend)				
ornithine				
POW, NA, 100 gm	17317-1579-01	19.60		
(Gallipot)				
POW, NA, 1000 gm	51552-0988-07	240.80	172.00	
L-PHENYLALANINE (Spectrum Pharmacy)				
phenylalanine				
POW, NA (U.S.P.)				
25 gm	49452-5275-01	79.45		
100 gm	49452-5275-02	190.75		
1000 gm	49452-5275-03	983.50		
L-PROLINE (Spectrum Pharmacy)				
proline				
CRY, NA (U.S.P.)				
25 gm	49452-6082-01	103.25		
100 gm	49452-6082-02	189.70		
1000 gm	49452-6082-03	1123.50		
L-SELENOME-THIONINE BLEND (Spectrum Pharmacy)				
calcium phosphate, dibasic/selenomethionine				
POW, NA, 5 gm	49452-6499-01	141.75		
25 gm	49452-6499-02	284.90		
100 gm	49452-6499-03	518.00		
L-SERINE (Spectrum Pharmacy)				
serine				
POW, NA (U.S.P.)				
100 gm	49452-6501-02	176.40		
1000 gm	49452-6501-03	1060.50		
L-THREONINE (Gallipot)				
threonine				
POW, NA, 100 gm	51552-0746-05	46.90	33.50	
(Medisca)				
POW, NA (U.S.P.)				
25 gm	38779-0308-04	31.50		
100 gm	38779-0308-05	82.50		
500 gm	38779-0308-08	352.50		
(Spectrum Pharmacy)				
POW, NA (U.S.P.)				
100 gm	49452-7762-02	171.85		
L-THYROXINE SODIUM (Gallipot)				
levothyroxine sodium				
POW, NA (1X1GM)				
1 gm	51552-0742-01	168.00	120.00	
(1X5GM)				
5 gm	51552-0742-02	268.80	192.00	
(Spectrum Pharmacy)				
POW, NA (1X1GM,U.S.P.)				
1 gm	49452-4156-02	266.00		
(1X5GM,U.S.P.)				
5 gm	49452-4156-03	931.00		
(1X0.25GM,U.S.P.)				
25 gm	49452-4156-01	128.80		
(1X25GM,U.S.P.)				
25 gm	49452-4156-04	3241.00		
(HomeMed)				
REPACK				
TAB, PO, 0.1 mg, 30s ea	51655-0091-24	24.99		
100s ea	51655-0091-21	5.49		
0.15 mg, 100s ea	51655-0209-21	6.09		
0.2 mg, 100s ea	51655-0477-01	6.28		
L-TRYPTOPHAN (Letco)				
tryptophan				
POW, NA (U.S.P.)				
100 gm	62991-1266-02	112.50		
500 gm	62991-1266-03	435.00		
1000 gm	62991-1266-04	750.00		
L-TYROSINE (Gallipot)				
tyrosine				
POW, NA (USP)				
100 gm	52552-0788-05	19.53	13.95	
(Medisca)				
POW, NA (U.S.P.)				
25 gm	38779-0883-04	28.50		
100 gm	38779-0883-05	46.50		
500 gm	38779-0883-08	195.00		
(USP)				
1000 gm	38779-0883-09	357.00		
L-VALINE (Gallipot)				
valine				
POW, NA (U.S.P.)				
1000 gm	51552-0398-07	195.30		
(Medisca)				
POW, NA, 100 gm	38779-0358-05	58.50		
500 gm	38779-0358-08	285.00		
(U.S.P.)				
1000 gm	38779-0358-09	477.00		
(Spectrum Pharmacy)				
CRY, NA (U.S.P.)				
25 gm	49452-8091-01	71.40		
100 gm	49452-8091-02	117.95		
1000 gm	49452-8091-03	731.50		
LABETALOL (DHS, Inc.)				
REPACK				
labetalol hydrochloride				
TAB, PO, 100 mg, 100s ea	55887-0180-01	52.95		
(Phys Total Care)				
REPACK				
TAB, PO, 300 mg, 100s ea	54868-4903-02	69.54		
(Southwood)				
REPACK				
SOL, IV, 5 mg/ml, 20 ml	58016-4810-01	3.26		
LABETALOL HCL (Akorn)				
labetalol hydrochloride				
SOL, IV (M.D.V.)				
5 mg/ml, 20 ml	17478-0420-20	4.95		
40 ml	17478-0420-40	9.50		
(Apotex Corp.)				
SOL, IV (S.D.V.)				
5 mg/ml, 4 ml 10s	60505-0717-00	47.62		AP
(Bedford)				
SOL, IV (M.D.V.)				
5 mg/ml, 20 ml	55390-0130-20	4.80		AP
40 ml	55390-0130-40	9.60		AP
(Hospira)				
SOL, IV (LUER LOCK,LATEX-FREE)				
5 mg/ml, 4 ml 10s	00074-2339-34	36.36	31.80	AP
4 ml 10s	00409-2339-34	36.96	32.30	AP
(100MG/20ML)				
5 mg/ml, 20 ml	61703-0233-47	2.96	2.59	AP
(200MG/40ML)				
5 mg/ml, 40 ml	61703-0233-48	5.24	4.59	AP
(M.D.V.,LATEX-FREE)				
5 mg/ml, 40 ml	00409-2267-54	3.85	3.37	AP
(Mayne Pharma)				
SOL, IV (M.D.V.)				
5 mg/ml, 20 ml 10s	61703-0233-22	350.00		AP
40 ml 10s	61703-0233-41	650.00		AP
(Sandoz)				
TAB, PO, 100 mg, 100s ea	00185-0010-01	50.28		AB
500s ea	00185-0010-05	238.59		AB
200 mg, 100s ea	00185-0117-01	71.33		AB
500s ea	00185-0117-05	338.87		AB
(FILM-COATED)				
300 mg, 100s ea	00185-0118-01	94.89		AB
500s ea	00185-0118-05	474.45		AB
(Spectrum Pharmacy)				
POW, NA (U.S.P.)				
5 gm	49452-3911-01	179.90		
25 gm	49452-3911-02	584.50		
100 gm	49452-3911-03	1554.00		
(UDL)				
TAB, PO (10X10)				
100 mg, 100s ea UD	51079-0928-20	48.20		AB
200 mg, 100s ea UD	51079-0929-20	68.20		AB
(Watson Labs)				
TAB, PO, 100 mg, 100s ea	00591-0605-01	17.26		AB
500s ea	00591-0605-05	84.53		AB
200 mg, 100s ea	00591-0606-01	25.03		AB
500s ea	00591-0606-05	122.66		AB
300 mg, 100s ea	00591-0607-01	39.67		AB
(Phys Total Care)				
REPACK				
SOL, IV (M.D.V.)				
5 mg/ml, 20 ml	54868-4486-00	17.10		AP
(Quality Care Prod)				
REPACK				
TAB, PO, 100 mg, 60s ea	35356-0362-60	61.33		AB
LABETALOL HYDROCHLORIDE				
FUL				
TAB, PO, 100 mg, 100s ea		21.57		
200 mg, 100s ea		35.82		
300 mg, 100s ea		53.63		
(Akorn) *See LABETALOL HCL*				
(Apotex Corp.) *See LABETALOL HCL*				
(Bedford) *See LABETALOL HCL*				
(Hospira) *See LABETALOL HCL*				
(Hospira)				
SOL, IV (USP,MDV)				
5 mg/ml, 20 ml	00409-2267-20	1.93	1.69	AP
(Major)				
TAB, PO (10X10,USP)				
100 mg, 100s ea UD	00904-5928-61	67.42		AB
200 mg, 100s ea UD	00904-5929-61	76.98		AB
300 mg, 100s ea UD	00904-5930-61	109.50		AB
(Mayne Pharma) *See LABETALOL HCL*				
(Prometheus Labs) *See TRANDATE*				
(Sandoz) *See LABETALOL HCL*				
(Spectrum Pharmacy) *See LABETALOL HCL*				
(Teva)				
TAB, PO, 100 mg, 100s ea	00172-4364-60	53.39		AB
100s ea UD	00182-8202-89	48.19		AB
500s ea	00172-4364-70	250.44		AB
(FILM COATED)				
200 mg, 100s ea	00172-4365-60	77.98		AB
100s ea UD	00182-8203-89	68.19		AB
500s ea	00172-4365-70	367.86		AB
300 mg, 100s ea	00172-4366-60	105.64		AB
(UDL) *See LABETALOL HCL*				
(Watson Labs) *See LABETALOL HCL*				
(DHS, Inc.)				
REPACK				
TAB, PO (FILM COATED)				
200 mg, 30s ea	55887-0259-30	34.50		AB
(McKesson Packaging)				
REPACK				
TAB, PO, 200 mg,				
100s ea UD	63739-0366-10	71.33		
(Phys Total Care)				
REPACK				
TAB, PO, 100 mg, 30s ea	54868-4921-00	16.26		AB
60s ea	54868-4921-02	30.45		AB
100s ea	54868-4921-01	45.72		AB
(FILM COATED)				
200 mg, 30s ea	54868-4844-00	24.99		AB
60s ea	54868-4844-01	45.48		AB
90s ea	54868-4844-02	65.97		
(FILM COATED)				
200 mg, 120s ea	54868-4844-03	75.84		AB
300 mg, 30s ea	54868-4903-00	30.60		AB
(FILM-COATED)				
300 mg, 60s ea	54868-4903-01	56.70		
LABORATORY TESTS AND/OR SUPPLIES				
(Bracco Diag) *See CARDIOGEN-82 INFUSION SYSTEM*				
(Bracco Diag) *See CARDIOGEN-82 WASTE BOTTLE*				
LAC-HYDRIN (Ranbaxy Labs)				
ammonium lactate				
CRE, TP (2X140GM)				
12%, 140 gm 2s	10631-0099-28	51.28		AB
(1X385GM)				
12%, 385 gm	10631-0099-38	67.13		AB
LOT, TP (1X225GM)				
12%, 225 gm	10631-0098-08	48.97		AB
(1X400GM)				
12%, 400 gm	10631-0098-14	77.08		AB
(Phys Total Care)				
REPACK				
LOT, TP, 12%, 225 gm	54868-2262-03	52.28		
400 gm	54868-2262-00	77.70		
LAC-LOTION (Paddock)				
ammonium lactate				
LOT, TP, 12%, 225 gm	00574-2021-08	38.12		AB
400 gm	00574-2021-16	60.00		AB
LACOSAMIDE				
(UCB) *See VIMPAT*				
LACRISERT (Aton)				
hydroxypropyl cellulose				
DEV, OP (PF)				
5 mg, 60s ea UD	25010-0805-68	248.75		
LACTASE				
(PCCA) *See LACTASE 5000*				
LACTASE 5000 (PCCA)				
lactase				
POW, NA (FOOD GRADE)				
1 gm	51927-2530-00	1.05		

PROD/MFR	NDC	AWP	DP	OBC
LACTATED RINGER'S (B. Braun)				
ca cl/k cl/na cl/na lact				
SOL, IR (PIC CONTAINER)				
1000 ml	00264-2203-00	6.60		AT
2000 ml	00264-2203-50	12.31		AT
4000 ml	00264-2203-70	15.30		AT
IV (EXCEL)				
250 ml	00264-7750-20	1.96		AP
500 ml	00264-7750-10	2.05		AP
1000 ml	00264-7750-00	1.90		AP
(Baxter)				
SOL, IR, 1000 ml 12s	00338-0114-04	205.46		AT
3000 ml 4s	00338-0137-27	53.24		AT
5000 ml 2s	00338-0137-29	44.04		AT
IV, 250 ml 36s	00338-0117-02	396.15		AP
(USP,1X500ML)				
500 ml	00338-6307-03	14.88	12.40	AP
500 ml 24s	00338-0117-03	264.10		AP
(USP,1X1000ML)				
1000 ml	00338-6307-04	14.21	11.84	AP
1000 ml 12s	00338-0117-04	148.32		AP
(Bristol-Myers)				
lactated ringer's solution				
SOL, IV (USP,LATEX-FREE)				
250 ml	00338-6307-02	1.96	1.63	
(Hospira)				
ca cl/k cl/na cl/na lact				
SOL, IR (FLEX CONTAINER,4X3000ML)				
3000 ml 4s	00409-7828-08	47.86	41.88	AT
IV (LIFECARE,LATEX-FREE)				
250 ml 24s	00409-7953-02	38.59	33.84	AP
(LIFECARE,24X500ML)				
500 ml 24s	00409-7953-03	39.46	34.56	AP
(VISIV CONTAINER)				
500 ml 24s	00409-7953-30	38.30	33.60	AP
(LIFECARE,LATEX-FREE)				
1000 ml 12s	00409-7953-09	19.73	17.28	AP
(VISIV, 12X1000ML)				
1000 ml 12s	00409-7953-48	22.18	19.44	AP
(Phys Total Care)				
REPACK				
SOL, IV (12X1000ML)				
1000 ml 12s	54868-0102-00	30.08		
LACTATED RINGER'S AND DEXTROSE (Baxter)				
ca cl/dextrose/k cl/na cl/na lact				
SOL, IV (USP,1X1000ML)				
1000 ml	00338-6306-04	14.21	11.84	AP
LACTATED RINGER'S IRRIGATION (Baxter)				
ca cl/k cl/na cl/na lact				
SOL, IR (FOR STERILE SLUSH)				
1000 ml 6s	00338-0118-44	307.20		AT
LACTATED RINGER'S SOLUTION				
(Bristol-Myers) *See LACTATED RINGER'S*				
LACTATED RINGER'S SOLUTION/ MAGNESIUM SULFATE				
(PharMEDium Services) *See MAGNESIUM SULFATE-LACTATED RINGER'S*				
LACTATED RINGER'S SOLUTION/OXYTOCIN				
(PharMEDium Services) *See OXYTOCIN-LACTATED RINGERS*				
LACTATED RINGER'S/DEXTROSE 5% (Baxter)				
ca cl/dextrose/k cl/na cl/na lact				
SOL, IV, 500 ml 24s	00338-0125-03	267.84		AP
1000 ml 12s	00338-0125-04	161.42		AP
LACTIC ACID				
(Baker, J.T.) *See DL-LACTIC ACID*				
(Baker, J.T.) *See LACTIC ACID 85%*				
(Gallipot) *See LACTIC ACID 85%*				
(Letco)				
SOL, NA (U.S.P.)				
85%, 500 ml	62991-1579-01	42.00		
(Mallinckrodt Lab) *See LACTIC ACID 86%*				
(Medisca) *See LACTIC ACID 85%*				
(PCCA)				
LIQ, NA (USP; 88%)				
1 ml	51927-3110-00	0.31		
(Rising)				
LOT, TP, 10%, 354.84 ml	64980-0310-36	36.00		
(1X473.12ML)				
10%, 473.12 ml	64980-0310-48	69.95		
(Spectrum Pharmacy) *See LACTIC ACID 85%*				

PROD/MFR	NDC	AWP	DP	OBC
LACTIC ACID 85% (Baker, J.T.)				
lactic acid				
LIQ, NA (A.C.S., REAGENT)				
500 ml	10106-0194-01	83.38		
4000 ml	10106-0194-03	352.21		
(Gallipot)				
LIQ, NA (U.S.P.,N.F.)				
118.28 ml	51552-0116-04	14.35		
473 ml	51552-0116-06	22.75		
(Medisca)				
LIQ, NA (USP,RACEMIC,1X100ML)				
100 ml	38779-0565-05	34.50		
(U.S.P., RACEMIC)				
500 ml	38779-0565-08	58.50		
(USP,RACEMIC,1X1000ML)				
1000 ml	38779-0565-09	105.00		
(Spectrum Pharmacy)				
LIQ, NA (U.S.P.)				
125 ml	49452-3920-01	55.65		
500 ml	49452-3920-02	98.35		
4000 ml	49452-3920-03	493.50		
LACTIC ACID 86% (Mallinckrodt Lab)				
lactic acid				
POW, NA (U.S.P.)				
500 gm	00406-2672-06	27.06		
LACTIC ACID E (Rising)				
lactic acid/vitamin e				
CRE, TP, 10%-3500 iu/30 gm,				
113.4 gm	64980-0309-12	19.80		
226.8 gm	64980-0309-24	56.55		
(Quality Care Prod)				
REPACK				
CRE, TP, 10%-3500 iu/30 gm,				
120 gm	49999-0927-01	23.76		
LACTIC ACID/VITAMIN E				
(Rising) *See LACTIC ACID E*				
LACTINOL-E (Quality Care Prod)				
REPACK				
lactic acid/vitamin e				
CRE, TP, 10%-3500 iu/30 gm,				
120 gm	49999-0729-01	78.00		
LACTOBACILLUS ACIDOPHILUS				
(Letco) *See ACIDOPHILUS LACTOBACILLUS*				
(Medisca) *See ACIDOPHILUS LACTOBACILLUS*				
(PCCA) *See ACIDOPHILUS LACTOBACILLUS*				
(Spectrum Pharmacy) *See ACIDOPHILUS LACTOBACILLUS*				
LACTOBACILLUS COMBINATION				
(Kenwood) *See PAMINE FQ*				
(PCCA) *See ACIDOPHILUS LACTOBACILLUS PLANTARUM*				
LACTOCAL-F (Laser Pharma)				
prenatal vitamins				
TAB, PO, 100s ea	00277-0179-01	39.90		
LACTOSE				
(Amend) *See LACTOSE ANHYDROUS*				
(Amend) *See LACTOSE MONOHYDRATE*				
(Baker, J.T.) *See D-LACTOSE MONOHYDRATE*				
(Baker, J.T.) *See LACTOSE MONOHYDRATE*				
(Gallipot) *See LACTOSE ANHYDROUS*				
(Gallipot) *See LACTOSE MONOHYDRATE*				
(Letco) *See LACTOSE ANHYDROUS*				
(Letco) *See LACTOSE HYDROUS*				
(Letco) *See LACTOSE MONOHYDRATE*				
(Mallinckrodt Lab) *See LACTOSE HYDROUS*				
(Medisca) *See LACTOSE ANHYDROUS*				
(Medisca)				
POW, NA (1X500GM)				
500 gm	38779-0315-08	28.50		
(MONOHYDRATE,NF,SPRY DRY)				
500 gm	38779-0316-08	28.50		
(1X1000GM)				
1000 gm	38779-0315-09	51.00		
(MONOHYDRATE,NF,SPRY DRY)				
1000 gm	38779-0316-09	54.00		
(1X2500GM)				
2500 gm	38779-0315-01	87.00		
(MONOHYDRATE,NF,SPRY DRY)				
2500 gm	38779-0316-01	87.00		

PROD/MFR	NDC	AWP	DP	OBC
10000 gm	38779-0316-00	270.00		
(1X25000GM)				
25000 gm	38779-0315-07	660.00		
(MONOHYDRATE,NF,SPRY DRY)				
25000 gm	38779-0316-07	495.00		
(PCCA) *See LACTOSE ANHYDROUS*				
(PCCA) *See LACTOSE MONOHYDRATE*				
(Spectrum Pharmacy) *See LACTOSE ANHYDROUS*				
(Spectrum Pharmacy) *See LACTOSE MONOHYDRATE*				
(Phys Total Care)				
REPACK				
POW, NA, 454 gm	54868-2412-02	12.03		
LACTOSE ANHYDROUS (Amend)				
lactose				
POW, NA (N.F.)				
454 gm	17317-1537-01	9.80		
2270 gm	17317-1537-05	35.00		
11350 gm	17317-1537-08	122.50		
(Gallipot)				
POW, NA (U.S.P.,N.F.)				
454 gm	51552-0618-06	12.60		
(Letco)				
POW, NA (N.F.)				
500 gm	62991-1279-02	37.50		
2500 gm	62991-1279-01	105.00		
(Medisca)				
POW, NA (N.F.)				
500 gm	38779-0080-08	31.50		
(NF, 1X1000GM)				
1000 gm	38779-0080-09	54.00		
(N.F.)				
2500 gm	38779-0080-01	117.00		
(NF, 1X10000GM)				
10000 gm	38779-0080-00	360.00		
(PCCA)				
POW, NA (N.F.)				
1 gm	51927-2338-00	0.08		
(Spectrum Pharmacy)				
POW, NA (N.F.)				
500 gm	49452-3925-01	59.50		
2500 gm	49452-3925-02	187.60		
12000 gm	49452-3925-03	661.50		
LACTOSE HYDROUS (Letco)				
lactose				
POW, NA (N.F.)				
500 gm	62991-1336-01	29.50		
2500 gm	62991-1336-02	75.00		
(Mallinckrodt Lab)				
POW, NA (N.F.)				
500 gm	00406-6270-04	12.26		
LACTOSE MONOHYDRATE (Amend)				
lactose				
POW, NA (N.F.)				
500 gm	17317-0313-01	11.20		
2270 gm	17317-0313-05	30.80		
11350 gm	17317-0313-08	105.00		
(Baker, J.T.)				
POW, NA (N.F.)				
500 gm	10106-2249-01	13.52		
2500 gm	10106-2249-05	73.81		
(Gallipot)				
POW, NA (N.F.,SPRAY-DRIED)				
454 gm	51552-0136-06	12.46		
(U.S.P.,N.F.)				
454 gm	51552-0090-06	11.20		
(N.F.,SPRAY-DRIED)				
2270 gm	51552-0136-02	52.50		
(Letco)				
POW, NA (N.F.,SPRAY-DRIED)				
2500 gm	62991-1384-02	75.00		
(PCCA)				
POW, NA (NF, SPRAY-DRIED)				
1 gm	51927-3329-00	0.07		
(NF)				
1 gm	51927-1067-00	0.07		
(Spectrum Pharmacy)				
POW, NA (N.F.,SPRAY-DRIED)				
500 gm	49452-3930-01	54.95		
(N.F.)				
500 gm	49452-3931-01	54.95		
(N.F.,SPRAY-DRIED)				
2500 gm	49452-3930-02	140.35		
(N.F.)				
2500 gm	49452-3931-02	140.35		

PROD/MFR	NDC	AWP	DP	OBC
(N.F.,SPRAY-DRIED)				
12000 gm	49452-3930-03	567.00		
(N.F.)				
12000 gm	49452-3931-03	567.00		
LACTULOSE				
FUL				
SOL, PO, 10 gm/15 ml,				
480 ml		10.61		
(Actavis Mid Atlantic) *See CONSTULOSE*				
(Actavis Mid Atlantic) *See ENULOSE*				
(Actavis Mid Atlantic)				
SOL, PO (5X10)				
10 gm/15 ml,				
15 ml 50s UD	00472-5000-60	75.00		AA
30 ml 50s UD	00472-5001-60	150.00		AA
(ANI)				
SOL, PO (USP)				
10 gm/15 ml,				
237 ml	62559-5501-08	20.10		AA
473 ml	62559-5501-06	36.30		AA
946 ml	62559-5501-03	65.40		AA
(Apotex Corp.)				
SOL, PO, 10 gm/15 ml,				
237 ml	60505-0360-00	14.40		AA
473 ml	60505-0360-01	32.40		AA
946 ml	60505-0360-02	58.00		AA
(BayPharma)				
SOL, NA (USP,1X237ML,UNFLAVORED)				
10 gm/15 ml,				
237 ml	42769-1340-08	20.10		
(USP,1X473ML,UNFLAVORED)				
10 gm/15 ml,				
473 ml	42769-1340-06	36.30		
(USP,1X946ML,UNFLAVORED)				
10 gm/15 ml,				
946 ml	42769-1340-03	65.40		
(Cumberland Pharma) *See KRISTALOSE*				
(Hi-Tech)				
SOL, PO, 10 gm/15 ml,				
237 ml	50383-0779-08	20.45		AA
473 ml	50383-0795-16	36.50		AA
(USP)				
10 gm/15 ml,				
473 ml	50383-0779-16	36.50		AA
946 ml	50383-0779-32	65.65		AA
(Morton Grove) *See GENERLAC*				
(Morton Grove)				
SOL, PO, 10 gm/15 ml,				
237 ml	60432-0037-08	13.91		AA
946 ml	60432-0037-32	49.95		AA
(Pharm Assoc Inc)				
SOL, PO (15ML-4X10)				
10 gm/15 ml,				
15 ml 40s UD	00121-4577-15	100.46		AA
(ORANGE PINEAPPLE)				
10 gm/15 ml,				
30 ml 40s UD	00121-4577-30	119.20		
(30ML-10X10)				
10 gm/15 ml,				
30 ml 100s UD	00121-4577-35	298.00		AA
(ORANGE PINEAPPLE)				
10 gm/15 ml,				
237 ml	00121-0577-08	6.55		AA
473 ml	00121-0577-16	34.70		AA
946 ml	00121-0577-32	55.20		AA
(Qualitest)				
SOL, PO, 10 gm/15 ml,				
236 ml	00603-1378-56	18.28		AA
473 ml	00603-1378-58	34.75		AA
946 ml	00603-1378-59	67.41		AA
1892 ml	00603-1378-65	134.82		AA
(Roxane)				
SOL, PO, 10 gm/15 ml,				
30 ml 40s UD	00054-8486-16	115.60		AA
500 ml	00054-3486-63	54.98		AA
(Spectrum Pharmacy)				
SOL, NA (U.S.P.)				
500 ml	49452-3922-01	191.80		
1000 ml	49452-3922-03	269.15		
4000 ml	49452-3922-02	640.50		
(A-S Medication)				
REPACK				
SOL, PO, 10 gm/15 ml,				
237 ml	54569-4952-00	18.36		EE
(DHS, Inc.)				
REPACK				
SOL, PO, 10 gm/15 ml,				
473 ml	55887-0937-16	47,25		
(Dispensing Solutions)				
REPACK				
SOL, PO, 10 gm/15 ml,				
473 ml	55045-3106-00	35.00		
960 ml	55045-3106-01	55.00		
(Pharma Pac)				
REPACK				
SOL, PO, 10 gm/15 ml,				
960 ml	52959-0764-02	67.25		
(Phys Total Care)				
REPACK				
SOL, PO, 10 gm/15 ml,				
473 ml	54868-3101-01	17.19		AA
(ORANGE PINEAPPLE)				
10 gm/15 ml,				
946 ml	54868-3101-02	33.12		AA
SYR, PO, 10 gm/15 ml,				
240 ml	54868-3101-00	13.41		EE
(Quality Care Prod)				
REPACK				
SYR, PO, 10 gm/15 ml,				
946 ml	49999-0800-32	69.60		
(Southwood)				
REPACK				
SOL, PO, 10 gm/15 ml,				
960 ml	58016-5455-01	39.12		AA
(Stat Rx)				
REPACK				
SOL, PO, 10 gm/15 ml,				
30 ml	16590-0496-30	9.50		
(1X236ML)				
10 gm/15 ml,				
236 ml	16590-0496-08	9.30		AA
473 ml	16590-0496-16	6.54		AA
LAGESIC (Laser Pharma)				
acetaminophen/phenyltoloxamine citrate				
TER, PO (CAPLET)				
600 mg-66 mg,				
100s ea	00277-0187-01	60.50		
LAMICTAL (Glaxo)				
lamotrigine				
TAB, PO (STARTER KIT)				
49s ea	00173-0594-02	267.65		
98s ea	00173-0594-01	535.28		
25 mg, 35s ea	00173-0633-10	187.37		
100s ea	00173-0633-02	535.33		
100 mg, 100s ea	00173-0642-55	611.50		
150 mg, 60s ea	00173-0643-60	402.12		
200 mg, 60s ea	00173-0644-60	437.76		
(PD-Rx Pharm)				
REPACK				
TAB, PO, 100 mg, 30s ea	55289-0410-30	259.67		
(Phys Total Care)				
REPACK				
TAB, PO, 100 mg, 20s ea	54868-4675-01	141.65		
30s ea	54868-4675-02	199.58		
60s ea	54868-4675-00	396.54		
100s ea	54868-4675-03	637.33		
200 mg, 30s ea	54868-4916-01	236.97		
60s ea	54868-4916-02	471.33		
90s ea	54868-4916-00	684.25		
(Physician Partner)				
REPACK				
TAB, PO, 100 mg, 15s ea	21695-0223-15	161.41		
30s ea	21695-0223-30	363.98		
60s ea	21695-0223-60	633.49		
150 mg, 15s ea	21695-0224-15	204.21		
(Quality Care Prod)				
REPACK				
TAB, PO, 25 mg, 100s ea	35356-0172-00	875.85		
100 mg, 30s ea	35356-0162-30	277.24		
90s ea	35356-0162-90	823.70		
100s ea	35356-0162-00	999.73		
150 mg, 60s ea	35356-0203-60	717.10		
200 mg, 60s ea	35356-0173-60	1192.41		
LAMICTAL CD (Glaxo)				
lamotrigine				
CTB, PO (DISPERSABLE)				
5 mg, 100s ea	00173-0526-00	518.00		
25 mg, 100s ea	00173-0527-00	556.09		
LAMICTAL ODT (Glaxo)				
lamotrigine				
ODT, MM, 25 mg, 30s ea	00173-0772-02	152.95		EE
50 mg, 30s ea	00173-0774-02	163.84		EE
100 mg, 30s ea	00173-0776-02	174.71		EE
200 mg, 30s ea	00173-0777-02	208.46		EE
LAMICTAL ODT PATIENT TITRATION (Glaxo)				
lamotrigine				
ODT, MM, 28s ea	00173-0779-00	178.44		EE
35s ea	00173-0778-00	254.90		EE
56s ea	00173-0780-00	509.80		EE
LAMICTAL XR (Glaxo)				
lamotrigine				
TER, PO (FILM-COATED)				
25 mg, 30s ea	00173-0754-00	152.95		
50 mg, 30s ea	00173-0755-00	305.90		
100 mg, 30s ea	00173-0756-00	327.66		
200 mg, 30s ea	00173-0757-00	349.43		
LAMICTAL XR PATIENT TITRATION (Glaxo)				
lamotrigine				
TER, PO (FILM-COATED)				
28s ea	00173-0758-00	178.44		
35s ea	00173-0759-00	509.80		
35s ea	00173-0760-00	254.90		
LAMISIL (Novartis Pharm)				
terbinafine hydrochloride				
PKT, PO, 125 mg/packet,				
ea	00078-0499-62	9.25		
14s ea	00078-0499-58	129.59		
(3X14)				
125 mg/packet,				
42s ea	00078-0499-59	388.75		
187.5 mg/packet,				
ea	00078-0500-62	13.88		
14s ea	00078-0500-58	194.39		
(3X14)				
187.5 mg/packet,				
42s ea	00078-0500-59	583.15		
SPR, TP, 1%, 30 ml	00078-0328-82	84.79		
TAB, PO, 250 mg, 30s ea	00078-0179-15	505.36		
(Core)				
REPACK				
TAB, PO, 250 mg, 30s ea	33358-0266-30	399.20		
(PD-Rx Pharm)				
REPACK				
TAB, PO, 250 mg, 14s ea	55289-0513-14	350.51		
(Pharma Pac)				
REPACK				
CRE, TP, 1%, 15 gm	52959-0439-15	37.61		
30 gm	52959-0439-30	53.23		
(Phys Total Care)				
REPACK				
TAB, PO, 250 mg, 15s ea	54868-4008-01	240.86		
30s ea	54868-4008-00	463.18		
(Quality Care Prod)				
REPACK				
TAB, PO, 250 mg, 30s ea	49999-0466-30	373.61		
(Southwood)				
REPACK				
CRE, TP, 1%, 15 gm	58016-3416-01	32.00		
LAMISIL AT (Dispensing Solutions)				
REPACK				
terbinafine hydrochloride				
CRE, TP, 1%, 15 gm	55045-3507-07	12.99		
LAMIVUDINE				
(Glaxo) *See EPIVIR*				
(Glaxo) *See EPIVIR HBV*				
LAMIVUDINE/ZIDOVUDINE				
(Glaxo) *See COMBIVIR*				
LAMOTRIGINE				
FUL				
CTB, PO, 5 mg, 100s ea		66.09		
25 mg, 100s ea		69.23		
TAB, PO, 25 mg, 100s ea		30.35		
100 mg, 100s ea		34.67		
150 mg, 60s ea		22.80		
200 mg, 60s ea		24.81		
(Apotex Corp.)				
TAB, PO, 25 mg, 100s ea	60505-2663-01	415.96		AB
500s ea	60505-2663-05	2017.41		AB
100 mg, 100s ea	60505-2664-01	475.12		AB
500s ea	60505-2664-05	2304.33		AB
150 mg, 60s ea	60505-2665-06	312.44		AB
500s ea	60505-2665-05	2525.40		AB
200 mg, 60s ea	60505-2680-06	340.15		AB
500s ea	60505-2680-05	2749.47		AB
(Aurobindo Pharma)				
TAB, PO, 25 mg, 100s ea	65862-0227-01	415.96		AB
100 mg, 100s ea	65862-0228-01	475.12		AB

PROD/MFR	NDC	AWP	DP	OBC
150 mg, 60s ea	65862-0229-60	312.44		AB
100s ea	65862-0229-01	520.73		AB
200 mg, 60s ea	65862-0230-60	340.15		AB
100s ea	65862-0230-01	566.92		AB
(Cadista)				
TAB, PO, 25 mg, 100s ea	59746-0245-01	414.76		
500s ea	59746-0245-05	2073.80		
100 mg, 100s ea	59746-0246-01	473.76		
1000s ea	59746-0246-10	4737.60		
150 mg, 60s ea	59746-0247-60	311.54		
500s ea	59746-0247-05	2596.17		
200 mg, 60s ea	59746-0248-60	339.16		
500s ea	59746-0248-05	2826.33		
(Dr Reddy's)				
CTB, PO (UNCOATED)				
5 mg, 100s ea	55111-0225-01	305.33		AB
25 mg, 100s ea	55111-0226-01	319.80		AB
500s ea	55111-0226-05	1551.03		AB
TAB, PO, 25 mg, 100s ea	55111-0220-01	415.96		AB
500s ea	55111-0220-05	2017.41		AB
100 mg, 100s ea	55111-0221-01	475.12		AB
500s ea	55111-0221-05	2304.33		AB
150 mg, 60s ea	55111-0222-60	312.44		AB
500s ea	55111-0222-05	2525.56		AB
200 mg, 60s ea	55111-0223-60	340.15		AB
500s ea	55111-0223-05	2749.55		AB
(Glaxo) *See LAMICTAL*				
(Glaxo) *See LAMICTAL CD*				
(Glaxo) *See LAMICTAL ODT*				
(Glaxo) *See LAMICTAL ODT PATIENT TITRATION*				
(Glaxo) *See LAMICTAL XR*				
(Glaxo) *See LAMICTAL XR PATIENT TITRATION*				
(Greenstone)				
CTB, PO, 5 mg, 100s ea	59762-2460-02	305.33		
500s ea	59762-2460-05	1526.65		
1000s ea	59762-2460-08	3053.30		
25 mg, 100s ea	59762-2461-02	319.80		
500s ea	59762-2461-05	1599.00		
1000s ea	59762-2461-08	3198.00		
TAB, PO, 25 mg, 100s ea	59762-2040-02	415.96		
1000s ea	59762-2040-08	831.92		
100 mg, 100s ea	59762-2041-02	475.12		
1000s ea	59762-2041-08	4751.20		
150 mg, 100s ea	59762-2042-02	520.73		
1000s ea	59762-2042-08	5207.33		
200 mg, 100s ea	59762-2043-02	566.92		
1000s ea	59762-2043-08	5669.17		
(Mylan)				
CTB, PO (DISPERSIBLE)				
5 mg, 100s ea	00378-6905-01	305.33		
25 mg, 100s ea	00378-6925-01	319.80		
TAB, PO, 25 mg, 100s ea	00378-4251-01	415.96		AB
500s ea	00378-4251-05	2079.80		AB
100 mg, 100s ea	00378-4252-01	475.12		AB
500s ea	00378-4252-05	2375.60		AB
150 mg, 60s ea	00378-4253-91	312.44		AB
500s ea	00378-4253-05	2603.67		AB
200 mg, 60s ea	00378-4254-91	340.15		AB
500s ea	00378-4254-05	2834.58		AB
(Taro)				
CTB, PO, 5 mg, 100s ea	51672-4139-01	435.58		AB
25 mg, 100s ea	51672-4140-01	467.61		AB
TAB, PO, 25 mg, 100s ea	51672-4130-01	450.16		EE
1000s ea	51672-4130-03	4501.00		EE
100 mg, 100s ea	51672-4131-01	514.20		EE
1000s ea	51672-4131-03	5142.00		EE
150 mg, 60s ea	51672-4132-04	338.13		EE
1000s ea	51672-4132-03	5635.00		EE
200 mg, 60s ea	51672-4133-04	368.13		EE
1000s ea	51672-4133-03	6135.00		EE
(Teva)				
CTB, PO (CHERRY)				
5 mg, 100s ea	00093-0688-01	305.33		AB
25 mg, 100s ea	00093-0132-01	319.80		AB
TAB, PO, 25 mg, 100s ea	00093-0039-01	415.96		AB
500s ea	00093-0039-05	2079.80		AB
100 mg, 100s ea	00093-0463-01	475.12		AB
500s ea	00093-0463-05	2375.60		AB
150 mg, 60s ea	00093-7247-06	312.44		AB
500s ea	00093-7247-05	2603.67		AB
200 mg, 60s ea	00093-7248-06	340.15		AB
500s ea	00093-7248-05	2834.58		AB
(Torrent) *See LAMOTRIGINE STARTER KIT*				
(Torrent)				
TAB, PO (UNCOATED)				
25 mg, 30s ea	13668-0045-30	124.50		AB
(STARTER KIT,5X7)				
25 mg, 35s ea UD	13668-0045-29	145.25		AB
(UNCOATED)				
25 mg, 100s ea	13668-0045-01	415.00		AB
500s ea	13668-0045-05	2075.00		AB
100 mg, 30s ea	13668-0047-30	142.50		AB
100s ea	13668-0047-01	475.00		AB
500s ea	13668-0047-05	2375.00		AB
150 mg, 30s ea	13668-0048-30	156.00		AB
60s ea	13668-0048-60	312.00		AB
100s ea	13668-0048-01	520.00		AB
500s ea	13668-0048-05	2600.00		AB
200 mg, 30s ea	13668-0049-30	169.80		AB
60s ea	13668-0049-60	339.60		AB
100s ea	13668-0049-01	566.00		AB
500s ea	13668-0049-05	2830.00		AB
(UDL)				
TAB, PO (10X10)				
25 mg, 100s ea UD	51079-0498-20	415.96		AB
100 mg, 100s ea UD	51079-0499-20	475.12		AB
150 mg, 100s ea UD	51079-0865-20	597.73		AB
200 mg, 100s ea UD	51079-0866-20	650.71		AB
(Watson Labs)				
CTB, PO, 5 mg, 100s ea	16252-0597-01	36.00		AB
25 mg, 100s ea	16252-0598-01	37.80		AB
(Zydus Pharm.)				
CTB, PO, 5 mg, 100s ea	68382-0108-01	439.98		AB
25 mg, 100s ea	68382-0109-01	472.33		AB
TAB, PO, 25 mg, 100s ea	68382-0006-01	454.71		AB
1000s ea	68382-0006-10	4547.10		AB
100 mg, 100s ea	68382-0008-01	519.40		AB
1000s ea	68382-0008-10	5194.00		AB
150 mg, 60s ea	68382-0009-14	341.56		AB
500s ea	68382-0009-05	2846.33		AB
200 mg, 60s ea	68382-0010-14	371.84		AB
500s ea	68382-0010-05	3098.66		AB
(American Health)				
REPACK				
CTB, PO (3X10)				
5 mg, 30s ea UD	68084-0334-21	118.68		AB
25 mg, 30s ea UD	68084-0335-21	131.88		AB
TAB, PO (10X10)				
25 mg, 100s ea UD	68084-0318-01	14.86		AB
100 mg, 100s ea UD	68084-0319-01	20.31		AB
(3X10)				
150 mg, 30s ea UD	68084-0320-01	23.13		AB
200 mg, 30s ea UD	68084-0321-21	27.50		AB
(McKesson Packaging)				
REPACK				
TAB, PO (10X10,UNCOATED)				
25 mg, 100s ea UD	63739-0448-10	504.35		AB
(PD-Rx Pharm)				
REPACK				
TAB, PO (UNCOATED)				
100 mg, 30s ea	43063-0203-30	164.00		AB
200 mg, 30s ea	43063-0202-30	160.50		AB
(Phys Total Care)				
REPACK				
TAB, PO, 25 mg, 30s ea	54868-6078-00	19.68		AB
60s ea	54868-6078-01	25.80		AB
100 mg, 10s ea	54868-5921-01	115.36		AB
30s ea	54868-5921-00	318.59		AB
60s ea	54868-5921-02	632.68		AB
200 mg, 30s ea	54868-5955-01	380.76		AB
90s ea	54868-5955-00	1092.54		AB
(Physician Partner)				
REPACK				
TAB, PO, 25 mg, 60s ea	21695-0227-60	540.19		AB
100 mg, 30s ea	21695-0228-30	308.52		EE
60s ea	21695-0228-60	617.04		EE
150 mg, 60s ea	21695-0107-60	676.26		AB
200 mg, 60s ea	21695-0229-60	736.24		AB
(Quality Care Prod)				
REPACK				
TAB, PO, 100 mg, 100s ea	35356-0448-00	369.41		AB
(Stat Rx)				
REPACK				
TAB, PO (UNCOATED)				
25 mg, 30s ea	16590-0822-30	124.50		AB
60s ea	16590-0822-60	249.00		AB
120s ea	16590-0822-72	498.00		AB
100 mg, 30s ea	16590-0802-30	142.50		AB
45s ea	16590-0802-45	213.80		AB
60s ea	16590-0802-60	285.00		AB
200 mg, 30s ea	16590-0777-30	220.36		AB
60s ea	16590-0777-60	439.23		AB
LAMOTRIGINE STARTER KIT (Torrent)				
lamotrigine				
TAB, PO (UNCOATED)				
49s ea UD	13668-0266-99	207.55		AB
98s ea UD	13668-0266-28	415.10		AB
LAMP BLACK POWDER (Amend)				
activated charcoal				
POW, NA, 454 gm	17317-1397-01	12.60		
LAMPRENE (Phys Total Care)				
REPACK				
clofazimine				
CAP, PO, 50 mg, 60s ea	54868-3417-00	16.33		
LANCET				
(Medicore) *See AURORA HEALTH CARE LANCETS*				
(Medicore) *See LITE TOUCH LANCETS*				
(Nova) *See NOVA SUREFLEX*				
LANCET (Specialty Medical)				
lancet				
DEV, NA (28G,PULL TOP)				
100s ea	08415-2000-28	6.50	6.00	
(28G,TWIST TOP)				
100s ea	38415-0100-28	6.50	6.00	
LANCET				
(Specialty Medical) *See LANCET*				
LANCET DEVICE				
(Bayer Diabetes Care) *See GLUCOLET 2 UNITIZED*				
(BD Consumer) *See BD LANCET*				
(Kendall) *See MONOLETTOR SAFETY LANCET*				
(Specialty Medical) *See LANCING DEVICE*				
LANCING DEVICE (Specialty Medical)				
lancet device				
DEV, NA, ea	38415-0203-03	16.80		
ea	38415-0510-02	16.80		
(ADJUSTABLE COMFORT TIP)				
ea	38415-0510-01	15.00	14.00	
LANOLIN				
(Amend) *See LANTROL*				
(Baker, J.T.)				
POW, NA (U.S.P.)				
454 gm	10106-2252-01	27.03		
(Gallipot)				
GEL, NA (HYDROUS,USP)				
454 gm	51552-1013-06	13.79	9.85	
(Gallipot) *See LANOLIN ANHYDROUS*				
(Gallipot) *See LANOLIN OIL*				
(Gallipot)				
POW, NA (ALCOHOL)				
113.4 gm	51552-0874-04	17.50	12.50	
(Lorann Oil) *See LANOLIN ANHYDROUS*				
(PCCA) *See LANOLIN OIL*				
(PCCA)				
POW, NA (USP, ANHYDROUS)				
1 gm	51927-1023-00	0.12		
(Spectrum Pharmacy)				
OIN, NA (1X430GM,U.S.P.)				
430 gm	49452-3940-05	95.20		
LANOLIN ALCOHOL (Letco)				
lanolin alcohols				
POW, NA (1X500GM)				
500 gm	62991-2669-01	105.00		
(PCCA)				
POW, NA, 1 gm	51927-2028-00	0.45		
LANOLIN ALCOHOLS				
(Letco) *See LANOLIN ALCOHOL*				
(PCCA) *See LANOLIN ALCOHOL*				
LANOLIN ANHYDROUS (Gallipot)				
lanolin				
POW, NA (U.S.P.,N.F.)				
454 gm	51552-0243-06	15.40		
18160 gm	51552-0243-09	282.24		
(Lorann Oil)				
OIN, NA (U.S.P.)				
480 gm	23535-0905-01	5.50		
LANOLIN OIL (Gallipot)				
lanolin				
OIL, NA, 25 ml	51552-0864-04	4.90	3.50	
(PCCA)				
OIL, NA, 1 gm	51927-1817-00	0.51		

PROD/MFR	NDC	AWP	DP	OBC
LANOXICAPS (Phys Total Care)				
REPACK				
digoxin				
SGL, PO, 0.1 mg, 20s ea	54868-2160-01	9.71		
30s ea	54868-2160-02	17.25		
60s ea	54868-2160-00	25.40		
100s ea	54868-2160-03	40.45		
(Vibranta)				
REPACK				
SGL, PO, 0.1 mg, 30s ea	57866-1257-01	11.01		
0.2 mg, 30s ea	57866-1258-01	12.70		
LANOXIN (Glaxo)				
digoxin				
SOL, IV (AMP)				
0.25 mg/ml,				
2 ml 10s	00173-0260-10	28.78		AP
2 ml 50s	00173-0260-35	117.52		AP
TAB, PO, 0.125 mg,				
100s ea	00173-0242-55	29.93		AB
(2X5X10)				
0.125 mg,				
100s ea UD	00173-0242-56	41.78		AB
1000s ea	00173-0242-75	230.04		AB
0.25 mg, 100s ea	00173-0249-55	29.93		AB
(2X5X10)				
0.25 mg,				
100s ea UD	00173-0249-56	41.78		AB
1000s ea	00173-0249-75	230.04		AB
5000s ea	00173-0249-80	1085.78		AB
(A-S Medication)				
REPACK				
TAB, PO, 0.125 mg,				
30s ea	54569-0483-00	9.35		AB
0.25 mg, 30s ea	54569-0484-00	9.35		AB
(PD-Rx Pharm)				
REPACK				
TAB, PO, 0.125 mg,				
14s ea	58864-0634-14	11.92		AB
(REDI-SCRIPT)				
0.125 mg, 20s ea	58864-0634-20	11.90		AB
30s ea	55289-0098-30	13.35		AB
30s ea	55289-0927-30	13.35		AB
30s ea	58864-0634-30	15.50		AB
60s ea	55289-0098-60	26.69		AB
100s ea	55289-0098-01	44.49		AB
100s ea	55289-0927-01	44.49		AB
0.25 mg, 20s ea	58864-0068-20	11.75		AB
(REDI-SCRIPT)				
0.25 mg, 30s ea	58864-0068-30	15.50		AB
(Phys Total Care)				
REPACK				
TAB, PO, 0.125 mg,				
30s ea	54868-0790-02	13.87		AB
60s ea	54868-0790-05	25.13		AB
100s ea	54868-0790-03	40.14		AB
0.25 mg, 30s ea	54868-0683-02	13.87		AB
60s ea	54868-0683-04	25.12		AB
100s ea	54868-0683-01	40.12		AB
(Quality Care Prod)				
REPACK				
TAB, PO, 0.125 mg,				
30s ea	49999-0073-30	16.50		AB
0.25 mg, 30s ea	49999-0945-30	21.90		
(Southwood)				
REPACK				
TAB, PO, 0.25 mg, 3s ea	58016-0537-03	1.25		AB
10s ea	58016-0537-10	4.18		AB
12s ea	58016-0537-12	5.01		AB
15s ea	58016-0537-15	6.27		AB
30s ea	58016-0537-30	12.53		AB
60s ea	58016-0537-60	25.07		AB
90s ea	58016-0537-90	37.60		AB
100s ea	58016-0537-00	41.78		AB
LANOXIN PEDIATRIC (Glaxo)				
digoxin				
SOL, IV (AMP)				
0.1 mg/ml,				
1 ml 10s	00173-0262-10	69.11		AP
LANREOTIDE ACETATE				
(Tercica) *See SOMATULINE DEPOT*				
LANSOPRAZOLE (Medisca)				
POW, NA (USP,1X5GM)				
5 gm	38779-2289-03	180.00		
(USP,1X25GM)				
25 gm	38779-2289-04	675.00		
(USP,1X100GM)				
100 gm	38779-2289-05	2355.00		
(Mylan)				
ECC, PO (HARD GELATIN)				
15 mg, 30s ea	00378-8015-93	176.93		AB
1000s ea	00378-8015-10	5897.74		AB
30 mg, 90s ea	00378-8030-77	530.80		AB
500s ea	00378-8030-05	2948.90		AB
(Sandoz)				
ECC, PO (HARD GELATIN)				
15 mg, 30s ea	00781-2353-31	170.05		
1000s ea	00781-2353-10	5668.20		
30 mg, 100s ea	00781-2355-01	566.82		
1000s ea	00781-2355-10	5668.20		
(Takeda) *See PREVACID*				
(Takeda) *See PREVACID I.V.*				
(Takeda) *See PREVACID SOLUTAB*				
(Teva)				
ECC, PO (USP,HARD GELATIN)				
15 mg, 30s ea	00093-7350-56	170.05		AB
30 mg, 30s ea	00093-7351-56	170.05		AB
(UDL)				
ECC, PO (8X10,HARD GELATIN)				
30 mg, 80s ea UD	51079-0121-08	452.95		AB
(A-S Medication)				
REPACK				
ECC, PO (HARD GELATIN)				
30 mg, 30s ea	54569-6149-00	566.82		
(Palmetto)				
REPACK				
ECC, PO, 30 mg, 40s ea	23490-6855-01	228.47		
(Phys Total Care)				
REPACK				
ECC, PO (HARD GELATIN)				
30 mg, 30s ea	54868-6086-00	202.82		AB
60s ea	54868-6086-01	380.60		AB
(Physician Partner)				
REPACK				
ECC, PO (HARD GELATIN)				
15 mg, 30s ea	21695-0474-30	340.10		
(Quality Care Prod)				
REPACK				
ECC, PO (HARD GELATIN)				
30 mg, 30s ea	35356-0557-30	169.80		AB
LANSOPRAZOLE/NAPROXEN				
(Takeda) *See PREVACID NAPRAPAC 375*				
LANTHANUM CARBONATE				
(Shire US Inc.) *See FOSRENOL*				
LANTROL (Amend)				
lanolin				
OIL, NA, 480 ml	17317-1234-01	15.40		
3840 ml	17317-1234-06	86.80		
20640 ml	17317-1234-08	361.20		
LANTUS (Sanofi-Aventis)				
insulin glargine, recombinant				
SOL, SC (U-100,5X3ML)				
100 u/ml, 3 ml 5s	00088-2220-52	215.28		
10 ml	00088-2220-33	111.42		
(A-S Medication)				
REPACK				
SOL, SC, 100 u/ml, 10 ml	54569-5605-00	107.46		
(Dispensing Solutions)				
REPACK				
SOL, SC, 100 u/ml, 10 ml	55045-3685-01	85.00		
(Phys Total Care)				
REPACK				
SOL, SC, 100 u/ml,				
5 ml 3s	54868-5765-00	223.83		
(VIAL)				
100 u/ml, 10 ml	54868-4626-00	131.26		
(Quality Care Prod)				
REPACK				
SOL, SC, 100 u/ml, 10 ml	49999-0994-10	137.37		
LANTUS SOLOSTAR (Sanofi-Aventis)				
insulin glargine, recombinant				
SOL, SC, 100 u/ml,				
3 ml 5s	00088-2220-60	215.28		
LAP J LAPAROSCOPIC JEJUNOSTOMY (Abbott)				
tube, gastrointestinal				
DEV, NA (10 FR, W/T-FASTENER SET)				
ea	70074-0514-43	237.60	198.00	
LAP J REPLACEMENT JEJUNOSTOMY TUBE (Abbott)				
tube, gastrointestinal				
DEV, NA (10 FR)				
ea	70074-0519-97	71.88	59.90	
LAPASE (Cypress Pharm)				
amylase/lipase/protease				
CAP, PO, 15000 u-1200 u-15000 u,				
100s ea	60258-0810-01	64.69		
LAPATINIB DITOSYLATE				
(Glaxo) *See TYKERB*				
LARIAM (Roche Labs)				
mefloquine hydrochloride				
TAB, PO (BLISTER CARD)				
250 mg, 25s ea	00004-0172-02	310.36		AB
(A-S Medication)				
REPACK				
TAB, PO, 250 mg, ea	54569-2965-05	12.93		
6s ea	54569-2965-04	77.59		
8s ea	54569-2965-03	103.45		
10s ea	54569-2965-00	129.32		
(PD-Rx Pharm)				
REPACK				
TAB, PO, 250 mg, 5s ea	55289-0780-05	90.17		AB
(Pharma Pac)				
REPACK				
TAB, PO, 250 mg, 25s ea	52959-0583-00	229.42		AB
(Phys Total Care)				
REPACK				
TAB, PO, 250 mg, 6s ea	54868-3178-01	92.70		AB
25s ea	54868-3178-00	347.14		AB
(Quality Care Prod)				
REPACK				
TAB, PO, 250 mg, 10s ea	49999-0655-10	94.23		AB
LARONIDASE				
(Genzyme) *See ALDURAZYME*				
LARYNG-O-JET (Amphastar)				
lidocaine hydrochloride				
KIT, MM (SRN,PREFILLED,CANNULA)				
4%, 25s ea	00548-6300-00	235.41		AT
LASIX (Sanofi-Aventis)				
furosemide				
TAB, PO, 20 mg, 100s ea	00039-0067-10	32.74		AB
1000s ea	00039-0067-70	321.07		AB
(UNIT OF USE)				
40 mg, 100s ea	00039-0060-13	45.86		AB
500s ea	00039-0060-50	229.37		AB
1000s ea	00039-0060-70	452.14		AB
80 mg, 50s ea	00039-0066-05	37.09		AB
500s ea	00039-0066-50	370.74		AB
(Phys Total Care)				
REPACK				
TAB, PO, 40 mg, 30s ea	54868-0788-02	17.78		AB
60s ea	54868-0788-03	33.60		AB
100s ea	54868-0788-00	54.04		AB
LATANOPROST				
(Pfizer) *See XALATAN*				
LATISSE (Allergan Inc)				
bimatoprost				
SOL, OP (3ML IN A 5ML BOTTLE)				
0.03%, 3 ml	00023-3616-03	108.00	72.00	
(A-S Medication)				
REPACK				
SOL, OP, 0.03%, 3 ml	54569-6142-00	140.40		
(Phys Total Care)				
REPACK				
SOL, OP (1X3ML+60APPLICATORS)				
0.03%, 3 ml	54868-6053-00	129.80		
LAURETH-23				
(Amend) *See BRIJ 35*				
(Amend) *See BRIJ 35 SP*				
(Gallipot) *See BRIJ 35*				
(PCCA) *See BRIJ 35*				
LAURETH-4				
(Amend) *See BRIJ 30*				
(PCCA)				
POW, NA (BRIJ<<30)				
1 gm	51927-3143-00	0.24		
LAURIC ACID (PCCA)				
CRY, NA (1X1GM)				
1 gm	51927-1642-00	0.18		
LAVANDIN OIL				
(Spectrum Pharmacy) *See LAVANDIN OIL ABRIAL*				
LAVANDIN OIL ABRIAL (Spectrum Pharmacy)				
lavandin oil				
OIL, NA (1X100ML,F.C.C.)				
100 ml	49452-3957-01	147.35		
500 ml	49452-3957-02	430.50		

PROD/MFR	NDC	AWP	DP	OBC
LAVENDER OIL (Gallipot)				
OIL, NA, 29.57 ml	51552-0413-02	10.92		
100 ml	51552-0413-05	38.50		
(Lorann Oil)				
OIL, NA, 9.9 ml	23535-0151-30	3.45		
(N.F.)				
30 ml	23535-0227-05	4.20		
120 ml	23535-0227-08	13.50		
480 ml	23535-0227-01	47.00		
3840 ml	23535-0227-11	265.00		
(Medisca)				
OIL, NA (1X14ML,NATURAL)				
14 ml	38779-0914-03	16.50		
(1X25ML,NATURAL)				
25 ml	38779-0914-04	28.50		
(1X100ML,NATURAL)				
100 ml	38779-0914-05	64.50		
(1X500ML,NATURAL)				
500 ml	38779-0914-08	202.50		
(PCCA)				
OIL, NA, 1 ml	51927-1265-00	1.20		
1 ml	51927-2556-00	1.20		
LAVOCLEN-4 (Prasco Labs)				
benzoyl peroxide				
KIT, TP, 4%, ea	66993-0923-98	62.25		
LAVOCLEN-4 ACNE WASH (Prasco Labs)				
benzoyl peroxide				
KIT, TP (SOAP-FREE)				
4%, ea	66993-0928-98	62.25		
LAVOCLEN-4 CREAMY WASH (Prasco Labs)				
benzoyl peroxide				
SOA, TP, 4%, 170.1 gm	66993-0913-06	55.03		
(1X170.1GM)				
4%, 170.1 gm	66993-0926-06	55.03		
LAVOCLEN-8 (Prasco Labs)				
benzoyl peroxide				
KIT, TP, 8%, ea	66993-0924-98	64.58		
LAVOCLEN-8 ACNE WASH (Prasco Labs)				
benzoyl peroxide				
KIT, TP (SOAP-FREE)				
8%, ea	66993-0929-98	64.58		
LAVOCLEN-8 CREAMY WASH (Prasco Labs)				
benzoyl peroxide				
SOA, TP, 8%, 170.1 gm	66993-0914-06	57.25		
(1X170.1GM)				
8%, 170.1 gm	66993-0927-06	57.25		
LAZERFORMALYDE (Pedinol)				
formaldehyde				
SOL, TP, 10%, 90 ml	00884-3986-03	59.62		
LEAD (Baker, J.T.)				
GRA, NA (A.C.S., REAGENT)				
500 gm	10106-2256-01	69.94		
2500 gm	10106-2256-05	276.25		
LEAD ACETATE				
(Baker, J.T.) *See LEAD ACETATE TRIHYDRATE*				
(PCCA)				
POW, NA (ACS; TRIHYDRATE)				
1 gm	51927-1516-00	0.45		
(Spectrum Pharmacy) *See LEAD ACETATE TRIHYDRATE*				
LEAD ACETATE TRIHYDRATE (Baker, J.T.)				
lead acetate				
GRA, NA (REAGENT)				
500 gm	10106-2271-01	87.29		
2500 gm	10106-2271-05	293.96		
(Spectrum Pharmacy)				
CRY, NA (1X500GM,ACS)				
500 gm	49452-5960-02	250.60		
LEAD CHLORIDE (Baker, J.T.)				
POW, NA (REAGENT)				
125 gm	10106-2308-04	48.20		
500 gm	10106-2308-01	98.93		
LEAD CHROMATE (Baker, J.T.)				
POW, NA (A.C.S., REAGENT)				
125 gm	10106-2314-04	46.66		
500 gm	10106-2314-01	66.59		
LEAD DIOXIDE (Baker, J.T.)				
POW, NA (A.C.S., REAGENT)				
125 gm	10106-2348-04	46.87		
500 gm	10106-2348-01	86.88		
LEAD NITRATE (Baker, J.T.)				
CRY, NA (A.C.S., REAGENT)				
125 gm	10106-2322-04	34.66		
500 gm	10106-2322-01	100.99		
LEAD OXIDE				
(Baker, J.T.) *See LEAD OXIDE RED*				
(Baker, J.T.)				
POW, NA (A.C.S., REAGENT)				
125 gm	10106-2338-04	31.21		
500 gm	10106-2338-01	42.13		
(Gallipot) *See LEAD OXIDE YELLOW*				
LEAD OXIDE RED (Baker, J.T.)				
lead oxide				
POW, NA (REAGENT)				
500 gm	10106-2334-01	59.84		
LEAD OXIDE YELLOW (Gallipot)				
lead oxide				
POW, NA (REAGENT)				
454 gm	51552-0542-06	41.30		
LEAD SULFATE (Baker, J.T.)				
POW, NA (REAGENT)				
125 gm	10106-2356-04	67.26		
500 gm	10106-2356-01	141.11		
LEAD TETROXIDE				
(PCCA) *See LEAD TETROXIDE 99% PURE*				
LEAD TETROXIDE 99% PURE (PCCA)				
lead tetroxide				
POW, NA (1X1GM)				
1 gm	51927-1151-00	2.16		
LEADER INSULIN SYRINGE (Can-Am Care)				
insulin syringe/needle				
DEV, NA (28G,1/2CC,1/2")				
100s ea	38396-0401-08	15.50		
(28G,1CC,1/2")				
100s ea	38396-0402-08	15.50		
(29G,1/2CC,1/2")				
100s ea	38396-0404-08	17.50		
(29G,1CC,1/2")				
100s ea	38396-0405-08	17.50		
(29G,3/10CC,1/2")				
100s ea	38396-0403-08	17.50		
(30G,1/2CC,5/16")				
100s ea	38396-0407-08	17.50		
(30G,1CC,ULTRA COMFORT)				
100s ea	38396-0418-08	17.50		
(30G,3/10CC,5/16")				
100s ea	38396-0406-08	17.50		
(31G,1/2CC,5/16")				
100s ea	38396-0420-08	17.50		
(31G,1CC,5/16")				
100s ea	38396-0421-08	17.50		
(31G,3/10CC,5/16")				
100s ea	38396-0419-08	17.50		
LEADER NEEDLES (Cardinal Health)				
needle				
DEV, NA (PEN, 29G, 1/2", 12MM)				
100s ea	37205-0417-78	18.40		
(PEN, 31G, 5/16", 8MM)				
100s ea	37205-0418-78	18.40		
LECITHIN (Gallipot)				
GRA, NA (F.C.C.)				
454 gm	51552-0265-06	12.60		
2270 gm	51552-0265-01	49.00		
11350 gm	51552-0265-09	269.22		
POW, NA (EGG)				
25 gm	51552-0578-04	37.52		
(Letco)				
isopropyl palmitate/lecithin/sorbic acid				
SOL, NA (ORGANOGEL)				
480 ml	62991-1567-01	63.00		
3840 ml	62991-1567-02	330.00		
LECITHIN (Lorann Oil)				
LIQ, NA (N.F.)				
120 ml	23535-0608-58	1.00		
480 ml	23535-0608-51	2.50		
3840 ml	23535-0608-55	12.00		
(Medisca)				
GRA, NA (1X500GM)				
500 gm	38779-0947-08	36.75		
(1X1000GM)				
1000 gm	38779-0947-09	64.50		
(1X2500GM)				
2500 gm	38779-0947-01	135.00		
(1X10000GM)				
10000 gm	38779-0947-00	382.50		
(Spectrum Pharmacy)				
GRA, NA (F.C.C.)				
500 gm	49452-4000-01	64.75		
(N.F.)				
500 gm	49452-3999-01	59.50		
(F.C.C.)				
2500 gm	49452-4000-02	228.90		
(N.F.)				
2500 gm	49452-3999-02	209.65		
(F.C.C.)				
12000 gm	49452-4000-03	857.50		
(N.F.)				
12000 gm	49452-3999-03	787.50		
LECITHIN IN SOYA OIL (PCCA)				
lecithin/soybean oil				
OIL, NA, 1 gm	51927-2631-00	0.36		
LECITHIN SOYA (PCCA)				
soybean lecithin				
POW, NA (FINE)				
1 gm	51927-3538-00	0.10		
(GRANULAR)				
1 gm	51927-1309-00	0.24		
LECITHIN/SOYBEAN OIL				
(PCCA) *See LECITHIN IN SOYA OIL*				
LEENA (Watson)				
ethinyl estradiol/norethindrone				
TAB, PO (6X28)				
168s ea	52544-0219-28	236.10		AB
LEEP REDIKIT (Cooper Surgical)				
kit, disposable procedure				
DEV, NA (CARTRIDGES W/SWABS)				
ea	59365-0606-01	32.14		
LEFLUNOMIDE				
FUL				
TAB, PO, 10 mg, 30s ea		75.00		
20 mg, 30s ea		75.00		
(Apotex Corp.)				
TAB, PO, 10 mg, 30s ea	60505-2502-01	492.17		AB
1000s ea	60505-2502-03	16405.67		AB
20 mg, 30s ea	60505-2503-01	492.17		AB
1000s ea	60505-2503-03	16405.67		AB
(Prasco Labs)				
TAB, PO (FILM-COATED)				
10 mg, 30s ea	66993-0160-30	492.17		
20 mg, 30s ea	66993-0161-30	492.17		
(Sandoz)				
TAB, PO (FILM-COATED)				
10 mg, 30s ea	00781-5056-31	492.71		AB
20 mg, 30s ea	00781-5057-31	492.71		AB
(Sanofi-Aventis) *See ARAVA*				
(Teva)				
TAB, PO (FILM-COATED)				
10 mg, 30s ea	00093-0173-56	492.71		AB
30s ea	00555-0351-01	492.66		AB
20 mg, 30s ea	00093-0174-56	492.71		AB
30s ea	00555-0352-01	492.66		AB
(Phys Total Care)				
REPACK				
TAB, PO, 20 mg, 30s ea	54868-2319-00	65.34		
LEMON BALM (PCCA)				
POW, NA, 1 gm	51927-3327-00	0.21		
LEMON EXTRACT FLAVOR (PCCA)				
flavoring aid				
SOL, NA (PURE)				
1 ml	51927-1479-00	0.23		
LEMON EXTRACT, PURE (Medisca)				
flavoring aid				
SOL, NA (1X100ML,LEMON)				
100 ml	38779-1385-05	25.50		
(1X500ML,LEMON)				
500 ml	38779-1385-08	46.50		
LEMON FLAVOR (PCCA)				
flavoring aid				
SOL, NA (CONCENTRATE; NATURAL)				
1 ml	51927-2270-00	0.23		
LEMON FLAVOR EXTRACT (Spectrum Pharmacy)				
flavoring aid				
SOL, NA (1X100ML)				
100 ml	49452-1035-01	56.70		
LEMON GRASS OIL (Lorann Oil)				
lemongrass oil				
OIL, NA, 9.9 ml	23535-0151-36	2.50		
LEMON OIL				
(Lorann Oil) *See LEMON OIL NATURAL*				
(Lorann Oil)				
OIL, NA, 9.9 ml	23535-0151-33	2.75		
(Medisca)				
OIL, NA (CA TYPE, NATURAL)				
100 ml	38779-0831-05	43.50		
500 ml	38779-0831-08	135.00		

PROD/MFR	NDC	AWP	DP	OBC
(PCCA) *See LEMON OIL FLAVOR*				
LEMON OIL FLAVOR (PCCA)				
lemon oil				
OIL, NA, 1 ml	51927-1627-00	0.47		
(NATURAL)				
1 ml	51927-2322-00	1.50		
LEMON OIL NATURAL (Lorann Oil)				
lemon oil				
OIL, NA (U.S.P.)				
30 ml	23535-0020-05	3.75		
120 ml	23535-0020-08	11.75		
480 ml	23535-0020-10	40.00		
LEMONADE OIL FLAVOR (PCCA)				
flavoring aid				
SOL, NA, 1 ml	51927-3312-00	0.70		
LEMONGRASS OIL				
(Lorann Oil) *See LEMON GRASS OIL*				
(Medisca)				
OIL, NA ((NATURAL),1X14ML)				
14 ml	38779-1387-03	12.00		
((NATURAL),1X100ML)				
100 ml	38779-1387-05	52.50		
((NATURAL),1X500ML)				
500 ml	38779-1387-08	181.50		
LENALIDOMIDE				
(Celgene Corp) *See REVLIMID*				
LEPIRUDIN				
(Bayer) *See REFLUDAN*				
LESCOL (Novartis Pharm)				
fluvastatin sodium				
CAP, PO, 20 mg, 30s ea	00078-0176-15	99.35		
100s ea	00078-0176-05	330.61		
40 mg, 30s ea	00078-0234-15	99.35		
100s ea	00078-0234-05	330.61		
(A-S Medication)				
REPACK				
CAP, PO, 20 mg, 30s ea	54569-3821-00	85.68		
(Advanced Pharm Serv, Inc.)				
REPACK				
CAP, PO, 20 mg, 10s ea	13411-0111-01	31.88		
20s ea	13411-0111-02	63.76		
30s ea	13411-0111-03	95.66		
60s ea	13411-0111-06	191.32		
100s ea	13411-0111-10	318.87		
(AQ)				
REPACK				
CAP, PO, 20 mg, 10s ea	66105-0147-01	31.88		
30s ea	66105-0147-03	95.66		
60s ea	66105-0147-06	191.32		
90s ea	66105-0147-09	286.98		
100s ea	66105-0147-10	318.87		
(Phys Total Care)				
REPACK				
CAP, PO, 20 mg, 30s ea	54868-3329-00	84.24		
40 mg, 30s ea	54868-4224-00	100.74		
60s ea	54868-4224-01	189.79		
LESCOL XL (Novartis Pharm)				
fluvastatin sodium				
TER, PO (FILM-COATED)				
80 mg, 30s ea	00078-0354-15	127.25		
100s ea	00078-0354-05	424.14		
(Phys Total Care)				
REPACK				
TER, PO, 80 mg, 30s ea	54868-4601-00	133.36		
LESSINA 28 (Teva)				
ethinyl estradiol/levonorgestrel				
TAB, PO (3X28)				
0.02 mg-0.1 mg,				
84s ea	00555-9014-67	104.89		AB
LETAIRIS (Gilead Sciences)				
ambrisentan				
TAB, PO (FILM-COATED)				
5 mg, 30s ea	61958-0801-02	6516.00		
10 mg, 30s ea	61958-0802-02	6516.00		
LETROZOLE				
(Novartis Pharm) *See FEMARA*				
LEUCINE				
(Gallipot) *See L-LEUCINE*				
(Medisca) *See L-LEUCINE*				
(PCCA)				
POW, NA (FCC)				
1 gm	51927-1878-00	0.66		
(Spectrum Pharmacy) *See L-LEUCINE*				
LEUCOVORIN CALCIUM				
(Bedford) *See LEUCOVORIN CALCIUM NOVAPLUS*				
(Bedford)				
PDS, IJ (S.D.V.,USP)				
50 mg, 10s ea	55390-0051-10	36.00		AP
100 mg, 10s ea	55390-0052-10	48.00		AP
200 mg, ea	55390-0053-01	14.40		AP
(S.D.V.,PF)				
350 mg, ea	55390-0054-01	13.80		AP
SOL, IJ, 10 mg/ml, 50 ml	55390-0009-01	18.30		AP
(PCCA)				
POW, NA (USP; ANHYDROUS)				
1 gm	51927-2692-00	450.00		
(Roxane)				
TAB, PO, 5 mg, 30s ea	00054-4496-13	61.48		AB
(5X10)				
5 mg, 50s ea UD	00054-8496-19	140.00		AB
100s ea	00054-4496-25	202.60		AB
10 mg, 12s ea	00054-4497-05	90.93		AB
24s ea	00054-4497-10	180.05		AB
15 mg, 24s ea	00054-4498-10	254.62		AB
25 mg, 25s ea	00054-4499-11	618.35		AB
(Spectrum Pharmacy)				
POW, NA (U.S.P.)				
0.1 gm	49452-4036-04	112.00		
0.5 gm	49452-4036-01	357.00		
1 gm	49452-4036-02	577.50		
(Teva)				
PDS, IJ (VIAL,PF)				
100 mg, ea	00703-5140-01	6.00		AP
(PF)				
350 mg, ea	00703-5145-01	8.28		AP
TAB, PO, 5 mg, 30s ea	00555-0484-01	70.81		AB
100s ea	00555-0484-02	235.20		AB
25 mg, 25s ea	00555-0485-27	600.00		AB
(UDL)				
TAB, PO (5X10)				
5 mg, 50s ea UD	51079-0581-06	162.50		AB
(2X10)				
25 mg, 20s ea UD	51079-0582-05	273.75		AB
(Phys Total Care)				
REPACK				
TAB, PO, 5 mg, 10s ea	54868-3310-02	47.07		EE
50s ea	54868-3310-01	158.22		EE
60s ea	54868-3310-00	188.97		EE
15 mg, 24s ea	54868-5915-00	384.60		AB
LEUCOVORIN CALCIUM NOVAPLUS (Bedford)				
leucovorin calcium				
PDS, IJ (S.D.V.,PRIVATE LABEL)				
100 mg, 10s ea	55390-0818-10	38.40		AP
200 mg, ea	55390-0824-01	7.20		AP
(S.D.V.,PF,PRIVATE LABEL)				
350 mg, ea	55390-0825-01	9.60		AP
SOL, IJ, 10 mg/ml, 50 ml	55390-0826-01	12.00		AP
LEUKERAN (Glaxo)				
chlorambucil				
TAB, PO, 2 mg, 50s ea	00173-0635-35	193.13		
(Phys Total Care)				
REPACK				
TAB, PO, 2 mg, 5s ea	54868-1126-04	18.16		
10s ea	54868-1126-02	34.45		
25s ea	54868-1126-03	83.30		
30s ea	54868-1126-01	99.59		
50s ea	54868-1126-00	155.68		
100s ea	54868-1126-05	308.86		
LEUKINE (Genzyme)				
sargramostim				
PDS, IV (VIAL)				
250 mcg, 5s ea	50419-0002-33	1023.96	853.30	
SOL, IJ (M.D.V.)				
500 mcg/ml,				
1 ml 5s	50419-0050-30	1879.98	1566.65	
(Phys Total Care)				
REPACK				
SOL, IV, 500 mcg/ml,				
5 ml	54868-3188-00	1815.39		
LEUPROLIDE ACETATE				
(Abbott Pharm) *See LUPRON DEPOT*				
(Abbott Pharm) *See LUPRON DEPOT-PED*				
(Bayer Corp.) *See VIADUR*				
(Caraco)				
SOL, SC (MDV, 1X2.8ML)				
5 mg/ml, ea	41616-0936-40	385.30		AP
(Covidien)				
POW, NA, 0.005 gm	00406-8050-03	1242.00		
(Sandoz)				
KIT, SC (2 WEEK ADMINISTRATION)				
5 mg/ml, ea	00185-7400-85	385.33		AP
(Sanofi-Aventis) *See ELIGARD*				
(Teva)				
KIT, SC (2 WEEK ADMINISTRATION)				
5 mg/ml, ea	00703-4014-18	144.00		AP
SOL, SC (M.D.V.)				
5 mg/ml, 2.8 ml 6s	00703-4014-19	2219.47		AP
(A-S Medication)				
REPACK				
KIT, SC, 5 mg/ml, ea	54569-6136-00	306.15		AP
LEUSTATIN (Centocor)				
cladribine				
SOL, IV (S.D.V.)				
1 mg/ml, 10 ml	59676-0201-01	1027.81		AP
LEVACET (Wraser Pharm)				
acetaminophen/aspirin/caffeine/salicylamide				
TAB, PO (CAPLET)				
50s ea	66992-0160-50	55.79		
LEVALBUTEROL (Mylan)				
levalbuterol hydrochloride				
SOL, IH (USP,PF)				
1.25 mg/0.5 ml,				
0.5 ml 30s	00378-6993-93	119.75		AN
LEVALBUTEROL HYDROCHLORIDE (Letco)				
POW, NA, 100%, 25 gm	62991-2549-01	2250.00		
100 gm	62991-2549-02	8100.00		
(Mylan) *See LEVALBUTEROL*				
(Sepracor) *See XOPENEX*				
(Sepracor) *See XOPENEX PEDIATRIC*				
LEVALBUTEROL TARTRATE				
(Sepracor) *See XOPENEX HFA*				
LEVALL (Auriga)				
carbetapentane cit/gg/phenyleph hcl				
SOL, PO (1X473ML,AF,STRAWBERRY)				
473 ml	14629-0305-16	104.33		
LEVALL G (Auriga)				
guaifenesin/pseudoephedrine hydrochloride				
CER, PO, 400 mg-90 mg,				
100s ea	66813-0035-01	157.81		
LEVALL-12 (Auriga)				
carbetapentane tannate/phenylephrine tannate				
SUS, PO (4X118ML,STRAWBERRY)				
30 mg/5 ml-25 mg/5 ml,				
118 ml 4s	14629-0304-04	193.22		
LEVAMISOLE HCL (PCCA)				
levamisole hydrochloride				
POW, NA (U.S.P.)				
1 gm	51927-1732-00	6.60		
(Spectrum Pharmacy)				
POW, NA (U.S.P./N.F.)				
5 gm	49452-4029-01	67.90		
25 gm	49452-4029-02	180.60		
100 gm	49452-4029-03	472.50		
(1X1000GM,U.S.P.)				
1000 gm	49452-4029-04	1984.50		
LEVAMISOLE HYDROCHLORIDE (Gallipot)				
POW, NA (USP,1X5GM)				
5 gm	51552-0941-02	23.45	16.75	
(USP,1X25GM)				
25 gm	51552-0941-04	47.88	34.20	
(USP,1X100GM)				
100 gm	51552-0941-05	127.26	90.90	
(USP,1X1000GM)				
1000 gm	51552-0941-07	315.00	225.00	
(PCCA) *See LEVAMISOLE HCL*				
(Spectrum Pharmacy) *See LEVAMISOLE HCL*				
LEVAQUIN (Ortho-McNeil Pharm)				
levofloxacin				
SOL, IV (PREMIXED W/DEXTROSE)				
5 mg/ml, 50 ml	00045-0067-01	21.91	18.26	
100 ml	00045-0068-01	43.82	36.52	
150 ml	00045-0066-01	58.16	48.47	
(1X20ML,SINGLE-USE,PF)				
25 mg/ml, 20 ml	50458-0164-20	43.82	36.52	
(1X30ML,SINGLE-USE,PF)				
25 mg/ml, 30 ml	50458-0165-30	58.16	48.47	
PO (1X480ML)				
25 mg/ml, 480 ml	50458-0170-01	483.65	403.04	

PROD/MFR	NDC	AWP	DP	OBC
TAB, PO (FILM-COATED)				
250 mg, 50s ea	50458-0920-50	704.39	586.99	EE
500 mg, 50s ea	50458-0925-50	807.29	672.74	EE
(10X10,FILM-COATED)				
500 mg, 100s ea UD	50458-0925-10	1614.59	1345.49	EE
750 mg, 100s ea UD	50458-0930-10	3023.36	2519.47	
(PriCara)				
TAB, PO (FILM-COATED)				
250 mg, 100s ea UD	50458-0920-10	1408.78	1173.98	EE
750 mg, 20s ea	50458-0930-20	604.67	503.89	
(A-S Medication) REPACK				
TAB, PO (FILM-COATED)				
250 mg, 3s ea	54569-4915-01	40.06		
10s ea	54569-4915-00	166.64		
500 mg, 3s ea	54569-4489-02	45.91		
7s ea	54569-4489-03	107.13		
10s ea	54569-4489-00	153.04		
750 mg, 5s ea	54569-6115-01	143.28		
(Advanced Pharm Serv, Inc.) REPACK				
TAB, PO, 250 mg, 10s ea	13411-0154-01	146.87		
20s ea	13411-0154-02	293.74		
(FILM-COATED)				
250 mg, 30s ea	13411-0154-03	440.61		
50s ea	13411-0154-05	734.40		
60s ea	13411-0154-06	881.23		
500 mg, 10s ea	13411-0112-01	168.33		
20s ea	13411-0112-02	336.66		
(FILM-COATED)				
500 mg, 30s ea	13411-0112-03	504.99		
50s ea	13411-0112-05	841.69		
60s ea	13411-0112-06	1009.99		
(Altura) REPACK				
TAB, PO, 250 mg, 3s ea	63874-0523-03	24.67		
5s ea	63874-0523-05	41.12		
6s ea	63874-0523-06	49.34		
7s ea	63874-0523-07	57.57		
10s ea	63874-0523-10	82.24		
14s ea	63874-0523-14	115.13		
20s ea	63874-0523-20	164.48		
30s ea	63874-0523-30	246.72		
100s ea	63874-0523-01	822.40		
(AQ) REPACK				
TAB, PO, 250 mg, 50s ea	66105-0477-05	672.69		
500 mg, 50s ea	66105-0478-05	770.18		
(Core) REPACK				
TAB, PO, 500 mg, 10s ea	33358-0202-10	118.27		
30s ea	33358-0202-30	368.97		
60s ea	33358-0202-60	729.01		
100s ea UD	33358-0202-00	1231.67		
(DHS, Inc.) REPACK				
TAB, PO, 500 mg, 7s ea	55887-0810-07	127.48		
(Dispensing Solutions) REPACK				
SOL, IV, 25 mg/ml, 20 ml	55045-3532-01	51.00		
TAB, PO, 250 mg, 30s ea	55045-3310-08	299.10		
(FILM-COATED)				
500 mg, 5s ea	55045-2597-02	73.35		
7s ea	55045-2597-03	117.36		
7s ea	55045-2597-05	87.50		
7s ea	66336-0386-07	121.71		
10s ea	55045-2597-01	146.70		
10s ea	66336-0386-10	168.95		EE
14s ea	55045-2597-06	205.38		
30s ea	55045-2597-08	440.10		
750 mg, 5s ea	66336-0830-05	132.41		
(Nucare Pharm) REPACK				
TAB, PO, 500 mg, 10s ea	66267-0363-10	147.60		
(FILM-COATED)				
500 mg, 14s ea	66267-0363-14	206.64		
(Palmetto) REPACK				
TAB, PO, 500 mg, 7s ea	23490-9260-01	87.50		
10s ea	23490-9260-00	125.00		
30s ea	23490-9260-03	375.00		
50s ea	23490-9260-05	625.00		
(PD-Rx Pharm) REPACK				
TAB, PO (FILM-COATED)				
250 mg, 3s ea	55289-0841-03	62.81		
10s ea	55289-0841-10	209.39		
500 mg, 3s ea	43063-0113-03	72.00		
7s ea	55289-0711-07	167.99		
10s ea	55289-0711-10	199.76		
(FILM-COATED)				
500 mg, 10s ea	58864-0034-10	199.76		
14s ea	55289-0711-14	335.97		
14s ea	58864-0034-14	236.13		
750 mg, 5s ea	55289-0394-05	224.67		
7s ea	55289-0394-07	314.55		
(Pharma Pac) REPACK				
TAB, PO (FILM-COATED)				
250 mg, 3s ea	52959-0690-03	42.82		
5s ea	52959-0690-05	71.36		
7s ea	52959-0690-07	99.90		
14s ea	52959-0690-14	199.78		
30s ea	52959-0690-30	428.09		
500 mg, ea	52959-0492-01	14.90		
2s ea	52959-0492-02	29.08		
4s ea	52959-0492-04	59.55		
6s ea	52959-0492-06	89.25		
7s ea	52959-0492-07	104.10		
10s ea	52959-0492-10	148.65		
12s ea	52959-0492-12	178.32		
14s ea	52959-0492-14	207.98		
30s ea	52959-0492-30	444.90		
(FILM-COATED)				
750 mg, 7s ea	52959-0782-07	214.67		
10s ea	52959-0782-10	266.28		
20s ea	52959-0782-20	438.95		
(Phys Total Care) REPACK				
TAB, PO, 250 mg, 3s ea	54868-4175-01	50.81		
5s ea	54868-4175-03	82.95		
7s ea	54868-4175-02	115.08		
10s ea	54868-4175-00	154.35		
(FILM-COATED)				
250 mg, 14s ea	54868-4175-05	215.05		
30s ea	54868-4175-04	457.83		
(FILM-COATED)				
500 mg, 3s ea	54868-3923-02	63.32		
5s ea	54868-3923-03	103.80		
7s ea	54868-3923-01	136.40		
10s ea	54868-3923-00	187.57		
(FILM-COATED)				
500 mg, 15s ea	54868-3923-05	280.05		
30s ea	54868-3923-04	557.49		
750 mg, 5s ea	54868-4971-00	180.90		
10s ea	54868-4971-01	360.50		
(Physician Partner) REPACK				
TAB, PO (FILM-COATED)				
500 mg, 7s ea	21695-0464-07	265.93		
750 mg, 7s ea	21695-0519-07	497.96		
90s ea	21695-0519-90	273.24		
(Quality Care Prod) REPACK				
TAB, PO (FILM-COATED)				
250 mg, 10s ea	49999-0417-10	234.15		
500 mg, 2s ea	49999-0418-02	47.20		
7s ea	49999-0418-07	187.20		
10s ea	49999-0418-10	238.00		
30s ea	49999-0418-30	804.00		
50s ea	49999-0418-50	1340.00		
(Southwood) REPACK				
TAB, PO (FILM-COATED)				
250 mg, 30s ea	58016-0924-30	349.92		
50s ea	58016-0924-50	583.20		
60s ea	58016-0924-60	699.84		
90s ea	58016-0924-90	1049.76		
100s ea	58016-0924-00	1166.40		
500 mg, 7s ea	58016-0573-07	77.61		
10s ea	58016-0573-10	110.88		
20s ea	58016-0573-20	221.76		
30s ea	58016-0573-30	332.63		
60s ea	58016-0573-60	665.27		
90s ea	58016-0573-90	997.90		
100s ea	58016-0573-00	1108.78		
(FILM-COATED)				
750 mg, 30s ea	58016-0975-30	750.96		
60s ea	58016-0975-60	1501.92		
90s ea	58016-0975-90	2252.88		
100s ea	58016-0975-00	2503.20		
(Stat Rx) REPACK				
TAB, PO (FILM-COATED)				
250 mg, 14s ea	16590-0559-14	158.75		
20s ea	16590-0559-20	228.50		
30s ea	16590-0559-30	330.00		
500 mg, 4s ea	16590-0554-04	69.82		
7s ea	16590-0554-07	120.32		
14s ea	16590-0554-14	240.64		
20s ea	16590-0554-20	343.77		
30s ea	16590-0554-30	389.50		
60s ea	16590-0554-60	779.00		
90s ea	16590-0554-90	1168.00		
750 mg, 5s ea	16590-0578-05	161.50		
7s ea	16590-0578-07	225.52		
30s ea	16590-0578-30	966.53		
LEVAQUIN LEVA-PAK (A-S Medication) REPACK				
levofloxacin				
TAB, PO (FILM-COATED)				
750 mg, 5s ea	54569-5557-01	130.38		
LEVATOL (UCB)				
penbutolol sulfate				
TAB, PO, 20 mg, 100s ea	00091-4500-15	285.23		
LEVBID (Alaven)				
hyoscyamine sulfate				
TER, PO, 0.375 mg,				
100s ea	68220-0115-10	209.48		
500s ea	68220-0115-50	742.21		
(Phys Total Care) REPACK				
TER, PO, 0.375 mg,				
20s ea	54868-3939-00	33.09		
60s ea	54868-3939-01	95.51		
LEVEMIR (Novo Nordisk)				
insulin detemir				
SOL, SC (5X3ML,FLEXPEN)				
100 u/ml, 3 ml 5s	00169-6439-10	214.20		
10 ml	00169-3687-12	110.88		
(Phys Total Care) REPACK				
SOL, SC (1X10ML)				
100 u/ml, 10 ml	54868-0112-00	123.96		
(1X15ML,FLEX PEN)				
100 u/ml, 15 ml	54868-5883-00	204.06		
LEVETIRACETAM FUL				
SOL, PO, 100 mg/ml,				
473 ml		164.98		
TAB, PO, 250 mg, 120s ea		51.76		
500 mg, 120s ea		63.25		
750 mg, 120s ea		85.69		
1000 mg, 60s ea		84.43		
(Actavis Mid Atlantic)				
SOL, PO (1X473ML,GRAPE)				
100 mg/ml, 473 ml	00472-0235-16	307.74		AA
(Aurobindo Pharma)				
SOL, PO (1X473ML,GRAPE)				
100 mg/ml, 473 ml	65862-0250-47	307.74		AA
TAB, PO (FILM-COATED)				
250 mg, 120s ea	65862-0245-08	345.04		AB
500 mg, 120s ea	65862-0246-08	421.71		AB
750 mg, 120s ea	65862-0247-08	571.31		AB
1000 mg, 60s ea	65862-0315-60	422.18		AB
(Boca Pharmacal)				
TAB, PO (FILM COATED)				
250 mg, 60s ea	64376-0136-61	176.04		AB
90s ea	64376-0136-90	264.06		AB
120s ea	64376-0136-12	345.04		AB
500s ea	64376-0136-05	1437.65		AB
(FILM-COATED)				
500 mg, 60s ea	64376-0137-61	215.16		AB
90s ea	64376-0137-90	322.74		AB
120s ea	64376-0137-12	419.12		AB
500s ea	64376-0137-05	1757.13		AB
(FILM COATED)				
750 mg, 60s ea	64376-0138-61	291.49		AB
90s ea	64376-0138-90	437.23		AB
120s ea	64376-0138-12	571.31		AB
500s ea	64376-0138-05	2380.48		AB
(Cypress Pharm)				
SOL, PO (1X473ML,DYE-FREE,GRAPE)				
100 mg/ml, 473 ml	60258-0865-16	292.99		AA
(Dr Reddy's)				
TAB, PO (FILM COATED)				
250 mg, 120s ea	55111-0181-04	345.38		
500 mg, 120s ea	55111-0182-04	422.13		
750 mg, 120s ea	55111-0183-04	571.89		
1000 mg, 60s ea	55111-0248-60	422.13		
(Glenmark Pharmaceuticals)				
TAB, PO (FILM COATED)				
250 mg, 120s ea	68462-0545-08	345.04		
500 mg, 120s ea	68462-0546-08	421.71		
750 mg, 120s ea	68462-0547-08	571.31		

PROD/MFR	NDC	AWP	DP	OBC
(Greenstone)				
TAB, PO (FILM-COATED)				
250 mg, 120s ea	**59762-0060-02**	345.04		
500s ea	**59762-0060-05**	1437.65		
500 mg, 120s ea	**59762-0061-02**	421.71		
500s ea	**59762-0061-05**	1757.13		
750 mg, 120s ea	**59762-0062-02**	571.31		
500s ea	**59762-0062-05**	2380.48		
1000 mg, 30s ea	**59762-0063-03**	211.09		
60s ea	**59762-0063-01**	422.18		
500s ea	**59762-0063-05**	3518.18		
(Lupin Pharma, Inc.)				
TAB, PO (FILM-COATED)				
250 mg, 90s ea	**68180-0112-09**	258.78		AB
(FILM COATED)				
250 mg, 120s ea	**68180-0112-16**	331.60		AB
(FILM-COATED)				
250 mg, 500s ea	**68180-0112-02**	1437.65		AB
500 mg, 90s ea	**68180-0113-09**	316.28		AB
(FILM COATED)				
500 mg, 120s ea	**68180-0113-16**	405.29		AB
(FILM-COATED)				
500 mg, 500s ea	**68180-0113-02**	1757.13		AB
750 mg, 90s ea	**68180-0114-09**	428.48		AB
(FILM COATED)				
750 mg, 120s ea	**68180-0114-16**	549.07		AB
(FILM-COATED)				
750 mg, 500s ea	**68180-0114-02**	2308.48		AB
(FILM COATED)				
1000 mg, 60s ea	**68180-0115-07**	405.29		AB
500s ea	**68180-0115-02**	3518.18		AB
(Major)				
TAB, PO (10X10,FILM COATED)				
250 mg, 100s ea UD	**00904-6001-61**	258.78		AB
(10X10,FILM-COATED)				
500 mg, 100s ea UD	**00904-6052-61**	316.29		AB
(10X10,FILM COATED)				
750 mg, 100s ea UD	**00904-6002-61**	428.48		AB
1000 mg, 100s ea UD	**00904-6003-61**	476.10		AB
(Mylan)				
TAB, PO (FILM COATED)				
250 mg, 120s ea	**00378-5613-78**	345.04		AB
500s ea	**00378-5613-05**	1437.65		AB
500 mg, 120s ea	**00378-5615-78**	421.71		AB
500s ea	**00378-5615-05**	1757.13		AB
750 mg, 120s ea	**00378-5617-78**	571.31		AB
500s ea	**00378-5617-05**	2380.48		AB
(FILM-COATED)				
1000 mg, 60s ea	**00378-5619-91**	421.67		AB
(Pharm Assoc Inc)				
SOL, PO (10X5ML,DYE-FREE,GRAPE)				
100 mg/ml,				
5 ml 10s UD	**00121-4802-05**	93.46		AA
(Roxane)				
SOL, PO (1X500ML,DYE-FREE,CHERRY)				
100 mg/ml, 500 ml	**00054-0224-63**	320.92		
TAB, PO (FILM COATED)				
250 mg, 120s ea	**00054-0150-23**	391.76		
250s ea	**00054-0150-27**	719.63		
500 mg, 120s ea	**00054-0151-23**	478.82		
500s ea	**00054-0151-29**	1759.09		
750 mg, 120s ea	**00054-0152-23**	648.69		
250s ea	**00054-0152-27**	1191.56		
1000 mg, 60s ea	**00054-0257-21**	422.18		
(Sandoz)				
SOL, PO (1X473ML,GRAPE)				
100 mg/ml, 473 ml	**00781-6141-16**	320.92		
TAB, PO (FILM-COATED)				
250 mg, 120s ea	**00781-5111-72**	345.04		EE
500 mg, 120s ea	**00781-5112-72**	421.71		EE
750 mg, 120s ea	**00781-5113-72**	571.31		EE
1000 mg, 60s ea	**00781-5114-60**	422.18		EE
(Silarx)				
SOL, PO (1X473ML,GRAPE)				
100 mg/ml, 473 ml	**54838-0548-80**	290.45		AA
(Taro)				
SOL, PO (1X473ML,GRAPE)				
100 mg/ml, 473 ml	**51672-4136-09**	344.59		AA
(Teva)				
TAB, PO (FILM COATED)				
250 mg, 120s ea	**00093-7285-89**	345.42		AB
500 mg, 120s ea	**00093-7286-89**	422.18		AB
750 mg, 120s ea	**00093-7287-89**	571.95		AB
1000 mg, 60s ea	**00093-7493-06**	422.18		AB
(Torrent)				
TAB, PO (FILM-COATED)				
250 mg, 60s ea	**13668-0014-60**	172.52		AB
(8X10,FILM-COATED)				
250 mg, 80s ea UD	**13668-0014-77**	230.02		AB
(FILM-COATED)				
250 mg, 120s ea	**13668-0014-12**	345.04		AB
250s ea	**13668-0014-25**	718.83		AB
500s ea	**13668-0014-05**	1437.65		AB
(6X10,FILM-COATED)				
500 mg, 60s ea UD	**13668-0015-62**	210.86		AB
(FILM-COATED)				
500 mg, 60s ea	**13668-0015-60**	210.86		AB
120s ea	**13668-0015-12**	421.71		AB
250s ea	**13668-0015-25**	878.56		AB
500s ea	**13668-0015-05**	1757.13		AB
(5X10,FILM-COATED)				
750 mg, 50s ea UD	**13668-0016-61**	238.05		AB
(FILM-COATED)				
750 mg, 60s ea	**13668-0016-60**	285.65		AB
120s ea	**13668-0016-12**	571.31		AB
250s ea	**13668-0016-25**	1190.23		AB
500s ea	**13668-0016-05**	2380.45		AB
(5X10,FILM-COATED)				
1000 mg, 50s ea UD	**13668-0017-61**	238.05		AB
(FILM-COATED)				
1000 mg, 60s ea	**13668-0017-60**	285.65		AB
120s ea	**13668-0017-12**	571.31		AB
250s ea	**13668-0017-25**	1190.23		AB
500s ea	**13668-0017-05**	2380.45		AB
(UCB) *See KEPPRA*				
(UCB) *See KEPPRA XR*				
(UDL)				
TAB, PO (10X10,FILM COATED)				
250 mg, 100s ea UD	**51079-0820-20**	287.53		AB
500 mg, 100s ea UD	**51079-0821-20**	351.43		AB
(10X30 PUNCH CARDS)				
500 mg, 300s ea UD	**51079-0821-56**	1054.28		AB
(10X10,FILM COATED)				
750 mg, 100s ea UD	**51079-0822-20**	476.09		AB
(Watson Labs)				
TAB, PO (FILM-COATED)				
250 mg, 100s ea	**16252-0577-01**	49.20		AB
500 mg, 100s ea	**16252-0578-01**	61.20		AB
750 mg, 100s ea	**16252-0579-01**	72.00		AB
1000 mg, 100s ea	**16252-0580-01**	90.00		AB
(American Health)				
REPACK				
TAB, PO (10X10,FILM-COATED)				
250 mg, 100s ea UD	**68084-0336-01**	59.88		AB
500 mg, 100s ea UD	**68084-0337-01**	71.88		AB
750 mg, 100s ea UD	**68084-0338-01**	83.88		AB
1000 mg, 100s ea UD	**68084-0356-01**	167.88		AB
(IPI)				
REPACK				
TAB, PO (FILM COATED)				
500 mg, 60s ea	**18837-0378-60**	210.86		AB
(Phys Total Care)				
REPACK				
TAB, PO (FILM-COATED)				
500 mg, 30s ea	**54868-6075-01**	44.20		AB
60s ea	**54868-6075-00**	82.29		AB
1000 mg, 60s ea	**54868-6076-00**	118.18		AB
(Physician Partner)				
REPACK				
TAB, PO (FILM-COATED)				
250 mg, 60s ea	**21695-0071-60**	327.92		AB
500 mg, 60s ea	**21695-0006-60**	400.79		AB
90s ea	**21695-0006-90**	601.18		AB
750 mg, 60s ea	**21695-0136-60**	542.98		AB
1000 mg, 60s ea	**21695-0016-60**	400.78		AB
(Quality Care Prod)				
REPACK				
TAB, PO (FILM COATED)				
250 mg, 60s ea	**35356-0429-60**	320.39		AB
500 mg, 60s ea	**35356-0533-60**	182.60		AB
(Stat Rx)				
REPACK				
TAB, PO (FILM-COATED)				
250 mg, 30s ea	**16590-0320-30**	103.68		AB
60s ea	**16590-0320-60**	207.36		AB
(FILM COATED)				
500 mg, 60s ea	**16590-0685-60**	233.31		AB
(FILM-COATED)				
750 mg, 30s ea	**16590-0867-30**	142.80		AB
60s ea	**16590-0867-60**	285.65		AB
LEVISTICUM (Weleda)				
homeopathic substance				
LIQ, PO (3X)				
20 ml	**55946-0300-10**	4.65		
LEVITRA (Schering)				
vardenafil hydrochloride				
TAB, PO, 2.5 mg, 30s ea	**00085-1923-01**	523.76		
5 mg, 30s ea	**00085-1945-01**	523.76		
10 mg, 30s ea	**00085-1901-01**	523.76		
20 mg, 30s ea	**00085-1934-01**	523.76		
(A-S Medication)				
REPACK				
TAB, PO, 20 mg, 5s ea	**54569-5529-04**	86.60		
10s ea	**54569-5529-00**	226.96		
30s ea	**54569-5529-03**	479.35		
(Core)				
REPACK				
TAB, PO, 20 mg, 10s ea	**33358-0203-10**	133.54		
(Palmetto)				
REPACK				
TAB, PO, 5 mg, 3s ea	**23490-9392-00**	56.25		
6s ea	**23490-9392-01**	112.50		
10s ea	**23490-9392-02**	187.50		
12s ea	**23490-9392-03**	225.00		
15s ea	**23490-9392-04**	281.25		
20s ea	**23490-9392-05**	375.00		
10 mg, 3s ea	**23490-9391-00**	56.25		
6s ea	**23490-9391-01**	112.50		
10s ea	**23490-9391-02**	187.50		
12s ea	**23490-9391-03**	225.00		
15s ea	**23490-9391-04**	281.25		
20s ea	**23490-9391-05**	375.00		
20 mg, 3s ea	**23490-9390-00**	56.25		
6s ea	**23490-9390-01**	112.50		
10s ea	**23490-9390-02**	187.50		
12s ea	**23490-9390-03**	225.00		
15s ea	**23490-9390-04**	281.25		
20s ea	**23490-9390-05**	375.00		
(PD-Rx Pharm)				
REPACK				
TAB, PO, 10 mg, 6s ea	**55289-0194-06**	155.69		
20 mg, 6s ea	**55289-0193-06**	155.69		
(Phys Total Care)				
REPACK				
TAB, PO, 10 mg, 3s ea	**54868-4984-01**	59.64		
4s ea	**54868-4984-02**	78.86		
5s ea	**54868-4984-00**	98.09		
10s ea	**54868-4984-03**	194.22		
20 mg, 3s ea	**54868-4967-02**	64.48		
4s ea	**54868-4967-01**	85.98		
5s ea	**54868-4967-00**	106.82		
6s ea	**54868-4967-03**	127.66		
10s ea	**54868-4967-04**	211.02		
15s ea	**54868-4967-05**	297.86		
30s ea	**54868-4967-06**	573.40		
(Quality Care Prod)				
REPACK				
TAB, PO, 20 mg, 30s ea	**49999-0625-30**	383.28		
(Southwood)				
REPACK				
TAB, PO, 20 mg, 30s ea	**58016-0021-30**	460.18		
60s ea	**58016-0021-60**	920.36		
90s ea	**58016-0021-90**	1380.54		
100s ea	**58016-0021-00**	1533.93		
LEVLEN (Bayer)				
ethinyl estradiol/levonorgestrel				
TAB, PO (UNIT OF USE, 3X28)				
30 mcg-0.15 mg,				
84s ea	**50419-0411-12**	109.50		AB
LEVLITE 28 (Phys Total Care)				
REPACK				
ethinyl estradiol/levonorgestrel				
TAB, PO, 0.02 mg-0.1 mg,				
28s ea	**54868-4368-00**	46.73		AB
LEVO-DROMORAN (Valeant Pharm Intl)				
levorphanol tartrate				
SOL, IJ (AMP)				
2 mg/ml,				
1 ml 10s, C-II	**00187-3072-10**	39.63		
(M.D.V.)				
2 mg/ml,				
10 ml, C-II	**00004-1911-06**	45.38		
LEVO-MENTHOL (Baker, J.T.)				
menthol				
CRY, NA (U.S.P., F.C.C.)				
30 gm	**10106-2688-00**	35.07		
125 gm	**10106-2688-04**	38.44		
1000 gm	**10106-2688-02**	684.22		
LEVOBUNOLOL HCL (Apotex Corp.)				
levobunolol hydrochloride				
SOL, OP, 0.5%, 5 ml	**60505-0553-01**	16.63		AT
10 ml	**60505-0553-02**	32.25		AT
15 ml	**60505-0553-03**	48.20		AT
(Bausch & Lomb Inc.)				
SOL, OP, 0.5%, 5 ml	**24208-0505-05**	16.64		AT

PROD/MFR	NDC	AWP	DP	OBC
10 ml	24208-0505-10	32.29		AT
15 ml	24208-0505-15	48.32		AT
(Falcon Ophthalmics)				
SOL, OP, 0.5%, 5 ml	61314-0229-05	16.60		AT
10 ml	61314-0229-10	32.25		AT
15 ml	61314-0229-15	48.25		AT
(Pacific Pharma)				
SOL, OP, 0.25%, 5 ml	60758-0063-05	14.06		AT
10 ml	60758-0063-10	27.18		AT
0.5%, 5 ml	60758-0060-05	16.64		AT
10 ml	60758-0060-10	32.29		AT
15 ml	60758-0060-15	48.32		AT
(Phys Total Care) REPACK				
SOL, OP, 0.5%, 5 ml	54868-3363-01	16.05		EE
10 ml	54868-3363-00	18.98		EE
LEVOBUNOLOL HYDROCHLORIDE FUL				
SOL, OP, 0.25%, 10 ml		12.75		
0.5%, 10 ml		14.93		
(Allergan Inc) *See BETAGAN*				
(Apotex Corp.) *See LEVOBUNOLOL HCL*				
(Bausch & Lomb Inc.) *See LEVOBUNOLOL HCL*				
(Falcon Ophthalmics) *See LEVOBUNOLOL HCL*				
(Pacific Pharma) *See LEVOBUNOLOL HCL*				
LEVOCARNITINE (Amer Regent)				
SOL, IV (S.D.V.) 200 mg/ml, 5 ml 25s	00517-1045-25	343.75		AP
(Bedford)				
SOL, IV (S.D.V.) 200 mg/ml, 5 ml 10s	55390-0136-05	384.00		AP
(Hi-Tech)				
SOL, PO (USP,CHERRY) 100 mg/ml, 118 ml	50383-0171-04	29.75		
TAB, PO, 330 mg, 90s ea	50383-0172-90	77.45		
(Medisca) *See CARNITINE*				
(PCCA)				
POW, NA (USP) 1 gm	51927-1865-00	3.00		
(Rising)				
SOL, PO (USP,CHERRY) 100 mg/ml, 118 ml	64980-0503-12	29.45		AA
TAB, PO (9X10,USP) 330 mg, 90s ea UD	64980-0130-09	77.50		AB
(Sigma-Tau) *See CARNITOR*				
(Sigma-Tau) *See CARNITOR SF*				
(Spectrum Pharmacy) *See L-CARNITINE FREE BASE*				
(Spectrum Pharmacy) *See L-CARNITINE HYDROCHLORIDE*				
(Teva)				
SOL, IV (VIAL) 200 mg/ml, 5 ml 5s	00703-0404-02	63.60		AP
12.5 ml 5s	00703-0405-02	144.00		AP
LEVOCARNITINE HYDROCHLORIDE				
(Gallipot) *See ACETYL-L-CARNITINE HCL*				
(Gallipot) *See L-CARNITINE*				
(Medisca) *See ACETYL-L-CARNITINE HCL*				
(PCCA) *See ACETYL-L-CARNITINE HCL*				
(Spectrum Pharmacy) *See ACETYL-L-CARNITINE HCL*				
(Spectrum Pharmacy) *See DL-CARNITINE HYDROCHLORIDE*				
LEVOCETIRIZINE DIHYDROCHLORIDE				
(Sanofi-Aventis) *See XYZAL*				
LEVODOPA (Medisca)				
POW, NA (U.S.P.) 5 gm	38779-0235-03	35.85		
25 gm	38779-0235-04	127.50		
100 gm	38779-0235-05	570.00		
(USP,1X500GM) 500 gm	38779-0235-08	1875.00		
(PCCA)				
POW, NA (USP) 1 gm	51927-2139-00	9.00		
(Spectrum Pharmacy) *See L-DOPA*				
(Spectrum Pharmacy)				
POW, NA (1X500GM,U.S.P.) 500 gm	49452-2680-04	2443.00		

PROD/MFR	NDC	AWP	DP	OBC
LEVOFLOXACIN (Letco)				
POW, NA, 100 gm	62991-2707-02	195.00		
500 gm	62991-2707-03	780.00		
(Medisca) *See LEVOFLOXACIN HEMIHYDRATE*				
(Ortho-McNeil Pharm) *See LEVAQUIN*				
(PCCA) *See LEVOFLOXACIN HEMIHYDRATE*				
(PriCara) *See LEVAQUIN*				
(Vistakon) *See IQUIX*				
(Vistakon) *See QUIXIN*				
(Palmetto) REPACK				
TAB, PO, 500 mg, 10s ea	23490-7032-02	117.20		
LEVOFLOXACIN HEMIHYDRATE (Medisca) levofloxacin				
POW, NA (1X1GM) 1 gm	38779-2363-06	179.85		
(1X25GM) 25 gm	38779-2363-04	1335.00		
(1X100GM) 100 gm	38779-2363-05	4185.00		
(PCCA)				
POW, NA (1X1GM) 1 gm	51927-4385-00	100.00		
LEVOLEUCOVORIN CALCIUM				
(Spectrum) *See FUSILEV*				
LEVONORGESTREL				
(Bayer) *See MIRENA*				
(Medisca)				
POW, NA (U.S.P.) 5 gm	38779-2224-03	1683.00		
(Teva) *See PLAN B*				
(Teva) *See PLAN B ONE-STEP*				
(Watson) *See NEXT CHOICE*				
LEVOPHED (Hospira) norepinephrine bitartrate				
SOL, IV (10X4ML,USP) 1 mg/ml, 4 ml 10s	00409-3375-04	30.72	26.90	AP
LEVOPHED BITARTRATE (Hospira) norepinephrine bitartrate				
SOL, IV (10X4ML, AMP,LATEX-FREE) 1 mg/ml, 4 ml 10s	00409-1443-04	62.88	55.00	
LEVORA-28 (Watson) ethinyl estradiol/levonorgestrel				
TAB, PO (6X28) 30 mcg-0.15 mg, 168s ea	52544-0279-28	185.58		AB
(A-S Medication) REPACK				
TAB, PO, 30 mcg-0.15 mg, 28s ea	54569-4997-00	30.93		AB
(Phys Total Care) REPACK				
TAB, PO, 30 mcg-0.15 mg, 28s ea	54868-4607-00	34.95		AB
LEVORPHANOL TARTRATE (Covidien)				
POW, NA (U.S.P.) 1 gm, C-II	00406-0735-52	910.80		
(Medisca)				
POW, NA (U.S.P.) 1 gm, C-II	38779-0885-06	1350.00		
5 gm, C-II	38779-0885-03	5085.00		
25 gm, C-II	38779-0885-04	11250.00		
(PCCA)				
POW, NA (U.S.P.; CII) 1 gm, C-II	51927-1007-00	1800.00		
(Roxane)				
TAB, PO, 2 mg, 100s ea, C-II	00054-4494-25	107.24		AB
(Spectrum Pharmacy)				
CRY, NA (U.S.P.) 0.5 gm, C-II	49452-9201-06	1211.00		
1 gm, C-II	49452-9201-05	1855.00		
5 gm, C-II	49452-9201-01	6909.00		
(Valeant Pharm Intl) *See LEVO-DROMORAN*				
(B&B Pharm, Inc) REPACK				
POW, NA (U.S.P.) 0.5 gm, C-II	63275-1200-07	1265.00		
1 gm, C-II	63275-1200-01	1909.00		
5 gm, C-II	63275-1200-02	8280.00		
25 gm, C-II	63275-1200-04	41400.00		

PROD/MFR	NDC	AWP	DP	OBC
LEVOTHROID (Forest Pharm) levothyroxine sodium				
TAB, PO (NEW FORMULATION,CAPLET) 0.025 mg, 100s ea	00456-1320-01	13.16		
(CAPLET) 0.025 mg, 1000s ea	00456-1320-00	129.01		
(NEW FORMULATION,CAPLET) 0.05 mg, 100s ea	00456-1321-01	14.52		
(CAPLET) 0.05 mg, 1000s ea	00456-1321-00	142.18		
(NEW FORMULATION,CAPLET) 0.075 mg, 100s ea	00456-1322-01	16.00		
1000s ea	00456-1322-00	156.76		
0.088 mg, 100s ea	00456-1329-01	16.39		
1000s ea	00456-1329-00	160.64		
(CAPLET) 0.1 mg, 100s ea	00456-1323-01	16.56		
1000s ea	00456-1323-00	162.31		
(NEW FORMULATION,CAPLET) 0.112 mg, 100s ea	00456-1330-01	17.95		
1000s ea	00456-1330-00	175.93		
(CAPLET) 0.125 mg, 100s ea	00456-1324-01	19.20		
1000s ea	00456-1324-00	188.16		
(GLUTEN-FREE) 0.137 mg, 100s ea	00456-1331-01	19.54		
1000s ea	00456-1331-00	191.45		
(CAPLET) 0.15 mg, 100s ea	00456-1325-01	19.78		
1000s ea	00456-1325-00	193.81		
(NEW FORMULATION,CAPLET) 0.175 mg, 100s ea	00456-1326-01	22.34		
1000s ea	00456-1326-00	218.98		
0.2 mg, 100s ea	00456-1327-01	24.50		
1000s ea	00456-1327-00	240.07		
0.3 mg, 100s ea	00456-1328-01	34.07		
1000s ea	00456-1328-00	333.86		
(Bryant Ranch) REPACK				
TAB, PO, 0.025 mg, 30s ea	63629-1437-01	9.78		
(DHS, Inc.) REPACK				
TAB, PO (CAPLET) 0.025 mg, 60s ea	55887-0604-60	19.96		
0.1 mg, 60s ea	55887-0628-60	40.40		
(CAPLET) 0.125 mg, 60s ea	55887-0556-60	54.82		
90s ea	55887-0556-90	80.00		
(Dispensing Solutions) REPACK				
TAB, PO, 0.05 mg, 30s ea	55045-1784-02	9.00		
0.1 mg, 30s ea	55045-1341-08	9.00		
(PD-Rx Pharm) REPACK				
TAB, PO (CAPLET) 0.05 mg, 30s ea	55289-0782-30	23.01		
0.075 mg, 30s ea	55289-0772-30	24.50		
(CAPLET) 0.1 mg, 30s ea	55289-0786-30	24.63		
0.125 mg, 30s ea	55289-0777-30	26.80		
0.2 mg, 30s ea	55289-0764-30	31.17		
(Phys Total Care) REPACK				
TAB, PO (CAPLET) 0.05 mg, 100s ea	54868-4922-01	58.14		
0.075 mg, 10s ea	54868-4936-01	10.56		
30s ea	54868-4936-00	22.71		
(CAPLET) 0.075 mg, 100s ea	54868-4936-02	63.75		
0.088 mg, 30s ea	54868-5193-01	21.69		
90s ea	54868-5193-02	59.04		
(CAPLET) 0.088 mg, 100s ea	54868-5193-00	63.75		
0.1 mg, 30s ea	54868-2706-01	21.87		
100s ea	54868-2706-00	64.35		
(CAPLET) 0.112 mg, 30s ea	54868-4441-01	23.46		
90s ea	54868-4441-00	64.35		
100s ea	54868-4441-02	69.66		
0.125 mg, 30s ea	54868-4922-00	21.06		
30s ea	54868-4923-00	26.37		
(CAPLET) 0.125 mg, 100s ea	54868-4923-01	75.73		
0.15 mg, 30s ea	54868-4602-01	27.03		
90s ea	54868-4602-02	72.09		
100s ea	54868-4602-00	78.09		
(USP) 0.175 mg, 30s ea	54868-4918-02	29.94		
90s ea	54868-4918-01	80.85		
100s ea	54868-4918-00	87.84		

PROD/MFR	NDC	AWP	DP	OBC
(CAPLET)				
0.2 mg, 30s ea	54868-5312-02	32.41		
90s ea	54868-5312-00	88.23		
100s ea	54868-5312-01	74.16		
LEVOTHROID SODIUM (Quality Care Prod)				
REPACK				
levothyroxine sodium				
TAB, PO, 0.05 mg, 30s ea	49999-0235-30	13.80		
0.1 mg, 30s ea	49999-0238-30	15.60		
0.15 mg, 30s ea	49999-0236-30	9.72		
LEVOTHYROXINE (Bryant Ranch)				
REPACK				
levothyroxine sodium				
TAB, PO, 0.025 mg,				
30s ea	63629-2806-01	9.78		
0.05 mg, 30s ea	63629-2712-01	11.11		
0.075 mg, 30s ea	63629-1838-01	12.52		
0.1 mg, 30s ea	63629-1839-02	12.57		
60s ea	63629-1839-03	48.65		
100s ea	63629-1839-01	41.92		
0.15 mg, 30s ea	63629-2727-01	18.92		
0.2 mg, 30s ea	63629-2697-02	19.03		
100s ea	63629-2697-01	63.42		
(Core)				
REPACK				
TAB, PO, 0.025 mg,				
30s ea	33358-0204-30	10.02		
0.05 mg, 30s ea	33358-0205-30	11.39		
0.1 mg, 30s ea	33358-0206-30	12.88		
100s ea	33358-0206-00	42.92		
0.125 mg, 30s ea	33358-0207-30	15.11		
(DHS, Inc.)				
REPACK				
TAB, PO, 0.025 mg,				
30s ea	55887-0503-30	16.00		
90s ea	55887-0503-90	44.00		
0.1 mg, 30s ea	55887-0504-30	18.00		
90s ea	55887-0504-90	49.00		
100s ea	55887-0504-01	54.00		
0.125 mg, 30s ea	55887-0971-30	15.83		
(Pharma Pac)				
REPACK				
TAB, PO, 0.05 mg,				
100s ea	52959-0921-00	36.18		
0.075 mg, 100s ea	52959-0922-00	45.06		
0.125 mg, 100s ea	52959-0920-00	47.08		
(Southwood)				
REPACK				
TAB, PO, 0.088 mg,				
30s ea	58016-0983-30	9.09		
60s ea	58016-0983-60	18.18		
90s ea	58016-0983-90	27.27		
100s ea	58016-0983-00	30.30		
0.112 mg, 30s ea	58016-0025-30	35.30		
60s ea	58016-0025-60	70.60		
90s ea	58016-0025-90	105.90		
100s ea	58016-0025-00	117.67		
LEVOTHYROXINE SODIUM				
FUL				
TAB, PO, 0.025 mg,				
100s ea		23.18		
0.05 mg, 100s ea		26.33		
0.075 mg, 100s ea		29.10		
0.088 mg, 100s ea		29.55		
0.1 mg, 100s ea		29.85		
0.112 mg, 100s ea		34.43		
0.125 mg, 100s ea		34.95		
0.15 mg, 100s ea		36.00		
0.175 mg, 100s ea		42.75		
0.2 mg, 100s ea		44.18		
0.3 mg, 100s ea		60.23		
(Abbott Pharm) *See SYNTHROID*				
(APP)				
PDS, IJ (S.D.V.,PF)				
0.2 mg, ea	63323-0247-10	40.74		
0.5 mg, ea	63323-0248-10	44.34		
(Bedford)				
PDS, IJ (S.D.V.,PF)				
0.2 mg, ea	55390-0880-10	24.00		
0.5 mg, ea	55390-0881-10	24.00		
(Forest Pharm) *See LEVOTHROID*				
(Gallipot) *See L-THYROXINE SODIUM*				
(King Pharm) *See LEVOXYL*				
(Lannett)				
TAB, PO, 0.025 mg, 100s ea	00527-1341-01	23.71		AB1
1000s ea	00527-1341-10	222.25		AB1
0.05 mg, 100s ea	00527-1342-01	26.94		AB1
1000s ea	00527-1342-10	252.48		AB1
0.075 mg, 100s ea	00527-1343-01	29.75		AB1
1000s ea	00527-1343-10	278.88		AB1
0.088 mg, 100s ea	00527-1344-01	30.27		AB1
1000s ea	00527-1344-10	283.75		AB1
0.1 mg, 100s ea	00527-1345-01	30.50		AB1
1000s ea	00527-1345-10	285.85		AB1
0.112 mg, 100s ea	00527-1346-01	35.27		AB1
1000s ea	00527-1346-10	330.49		AB1
0.125 mg, 100s ea	00527-1347-01	35.74		AB1
1000s ea	00527-1347-10	335.01		AB1
(USP)				
0.137 mg, 100s ea	00527-1638-01	35.10		AB1
1000s ea	00527-1638-10	326.40		AB1
0.15 mg, 100s ea	00527-1349-01	36.80		AB1
1000s ea	00527-1349-10	344.90		AB1
0.175 mg, 100s ea	00527-1350-01	43.74		AB1
1000s ea	00527-1350-10	409.87		AB1
0.2 mg, 100s ea	00527-1351-01	43.83		AB1
1000s ea	00527-1351-10	410.82		AB1
0.3 mg, 100s ea	00527-1352-01	58.68		AB1
1000s ea	00527-1352-10	559.36		AB1
(Lannett) *See UNITHROID*				
(Medisca)				
POW, NA (U.S.P.)				
0.5 gm	38779-1657-00	87.00		
1 gm	38779-1657-06	156.00		
(USP)				
5 gm	38779-1657-03	555.00		
25 gm	38779-1657-04	1845.00		
(Mylan)				
TAB, PO, 0.025 mg, 100s ea	00378-1800-01	29.57		AB
500s ea	00378-1800-05	147.84		AB
(USP)				
0.025 mg, 1000s ea	00378-1800-10	295.70		AB1
0.05 mg, 100s ea	00378-1803-01	33.57		AB
1000s ea	00378-1803-10	335.69		AB
0.075 mg, 100s ea	00378-1805-01	37.08		AB
1000s ea	00378-1805-10	370.84		AB
0.088 mg, 100s ea	00378-1807-01	37.72		AB
500s ea	00378-1807-05	188.61		AB
1000s ea	00378-1807-10	377.20		AB
0.1 mg, 100s ea	00378-1809-01	38.02		AB
1000s ea	00378-1809-10	380.19		AB
0.112 mg, 100s ea	00378-1811-01	43.96		AB
500s ea	00378-1811-05	219.81		AB
(USP)				
0.112 mg, 1000s ea	00378-1811-10	439.60		AB1
0.125 mg, 100s ea	00378-1813-01	44.55		AB
1000s ea	00378-1813-10	445.54		AB
(USP,CAPLET)				
0.137 mg, 100s ea	00378-1823-01	45.18		AB1
500s ea	00378-1823-05	225.92		AB1
1000s ea	00378-1823-10	451.84		AB1
0.15 mg, 100s ea	00378-1815-01	45.86		AB
1000s ea	00378-1815-10	458.58		AB
0.175 mg, 100s ea	00378-1817-01	54.52		AB
500s ea	00378-1817-05	272.58		AB
(USP)				
0.175 mg, 1000s ea	00378-1817-10	545.20		AB
0.2 mg, 100s ea	00378-1819-01	54.64		AB
1000s ea	00378-1819-10	546.41		AB
0.3 mg, 100s ea	00378-1821-01	74.38		AB
500s ea	00378-1821-05	308.50		AB
(PCCA) *See THYROXINE SODIUM PENTAHYDRATE*				
(Sandoz)				
TAB, PO, 0.025 mg, 100s ea	00781-5180-01	26.09		
1000s ea	00781-5180-10	260.90		
0.05 mg, 100s ea	00781-5181-01	29.63		
1000s ea	00781-5181-10	296.30		
0.075 mg, 100s ea	00781-5182-01	32.73		
1000s ea	00781-5182-10	327.30		
0.088 mg, 100s ea	00781-5183-01	33.29		
0.1 mg, 100s ea	00781-5184-01	33.55		
1000s ea	00781-5184-10	335.50		
0.112 mg, 100s ea	00781-5185-01	38.80		
0.125 mg, 100s ea	00781-5186-01	39.31		
1000s ea	00781-5186-10	393.10		
0.137 mg, 100s ea	00781-5191-01	39.88		
0.15 mg, 100s ea	00781-5187-01	40.48		
1000s ea	00781-5187-10	404.80		
0.175 mg, 100s ea	00781-5188-01	48.11		
0.2 mg, 100s ea	00781-5189-01	48.21		
0.3 mg, 100s ea	00781-5190-01	65.65		
(Spectrum Pharmacy) *See L-THYROXINE SODIUM*				
(UDL)				
TAB, PO (USP,10X10)				
0.025 mg,				
100s ea UD	51079-0444-20	29.57		AB1
0.05 mg, 100s ea UD	51079-0440-20	33.57		AB
0.075 mg, 100s ea UD	51079-0441-20	37.08		AB
0.1 mg, 100s ea UD	51079-0442-20	38.02		AB
0.125 mg, 100s ea UD	51079-0443-20	44.55		AB
0.15 mg, 100s ea UD	51079-0445-20	45.86		AB1
(A-S Medication)				
REPACK				
TAB, PO, 0.05 mg, 30s ea	54569-5617-00	10.07		AB
0.075 mg, 30s ea	54569-5653-00	11.12		AB
0.1 mg, 30s ea	54569-5620-00	11.41		AB
0.125 mg, 30s ea	54569-5654-00	13.37		AB
0.15 mg, 30s ea	54569-5655-00	13.76		AB
(Altura)				
REPACK				
TAB, PO, 0.025 mg, 10s ea	63874-0386-10	3.27		AB1
30s ea	63874-0386-30	9.80		AB1
90s ea	63874-0386-90	29.41		AB1
100s ea	63874-0386-01	32.68		AB1
1000s ea	63874-0386-02	326.80		AB1
0.05 mg, 15s ea	63874-0385-15	3.84		
20s ea	63874-0385-20	5.12		
30s ea	63874-0385-30	7.68		
60s ea	63874-0385-60	15.36		
100s ea	63874-0385-01	25.60		
0.075 mg, 30s ea	63874-0387-30	1.42		
90s ea	63874-0387-90	51.45		
100s ea	63874-0387-01	4.74		
0.1 mg, 12s ea	63874-0331-12	3.50		
15s ea	63874-0331-15	4.37		
20s ea	63874-0331-20	5.83		
30s ea	63874-0331-30	8.75		
90s ea	63874-0331-90	26.24		
100s ea	63874-0331-01	29.17		
1000s ea	63874-0331-02	265.40		
(American Health)				
REPACK				
TAB, PO (USP,10X10)				
0.025 mg,				
100s ea UD	62584-0146-01	23.71		
0.05 mg, 100s ea UD	62584-0154-01	26.94		
0.075 mg, 100s ea UD	62584-0155-01	29.75		
0.1 mg, 100s ea UD	62584-0218-01	30.50		
0.125 mg, 100s ea UD	62584-0232-01	35.74		
0.15 mg, 100s ea UD	62584-0241-01	36.80		
(Bryant Ranch)				
REPACK				
TAB, PO, 0.125 mg, 30s ea	63629-2718-01	14.74		
100s ea	63629-2718-02	49.12		
(DHS, Inc.)				
REPACK				
TAB, PO, 0.05 mg, 30s ea	55887-0602-30	11.00		AB1
90s ea	55887-0602-90	23.05		AB1
0.075 mg, 30s ea	55887-0601-30	15.00		AB1
90s ea	55887-0601-90	30.15		AB1
(Dispensing Solutions)				
REPACK				
TAB, PO, 0.025 mg, 30s ea	55045-1487-07	9.00		
60s ea	55045-1487-06	18.00		
90s ea	55045-1487-09	27.00		
100s ea	55045-1487-01	30.00		
120s ea	55045-1487-02	36.00		
0.075 mg, 30s ea	66336-0849-30	14.99		
0.112 mg, 30s ea	55045-2873-03	12.60		
100s ea	55045-2873-00	42.00		
0.125 mg, 30s ea	66336-0752-30	17.87		
0.15 mg, 30s ea	66336-0801-30	18.82		
(HomeMed)				
REPACK				
TAB, PO, 0.05 mg, 30s ea	51655-0749-24	8.99		
0.075 mg, 30s ea	51655-0092-24	16.99		
0.125 mg, 30s ea	51655-0290-24	14.99		
0.15 mg, 30s ea	51655-0298-24	12.99		
0.2 mg, 30s ea	51655-0085-24	29.82		
(Palmetto)				
REPACK				
TAB, PO, 0.025 mg, 30s ea	23490-6378-01	23.12		
100s ea	23490-6378-02	77.07		
0.05 mg, 30s ea	23490-6379-01	23.10		
0.075 mg, 30s ea	23490-6380-01	25.48		
100s ea	23490-6380-02	84.93		
0.088 mg, 30s ea	23490-6381-01	25.90		
0.1 mg, 30s ea	23490-6382-01	26.12		
0.112 mg, 30s ea	23490-6383-01	30.18		
0.125 mg, 30s ea	23490-6384-01	30.61		
0.15 mg, 30s ea	23490-6385-01	23.10		
(PD-Rx Pharm)				
REPACK				
TAB, PO, 0.025 mg, 30s ea	55289-0076-30	20.57		
100s ea	55289-0076-01	45.20		

PROD/MFR	NDC	AWP	DP	OBC
(REDI-SCRIPT)				
0.025 mg, 100s ea....	58864-0818-01	45.21		
0.05 mg, 30s ea......	58864-0950-30	64.13		
100s ea...........	55289-0085-01	53.13		
0.075 mg, 30s ea.....	55289-0082-30	24.48		
100s ea...........	55289-0082-01	57.17		
(USP)				
0.088 mg, 100s ea....	43063-0209-01	52.47		AB
0.1 mg, 30s ea.......	55289-0153-30	24.63		
(REDI-SCRIPT)				
0.1 mg, 30s ea.......	58864-0820-30	24.63		
100s ea...........	55289-0153-01	58.70		
(REDI-SCRIPT)				
0.1 mg, 100s ea......	58864-0820-01	58.71		
0.125 mg, 30s ea.....	55289-0858-30	28.23		
30s ea...........	58864-0897-30	28.23		
100s ea...........	55289-0858-01	70.70		
0.15 mg, 100s ea.....	55289-0084-01	67.50		
0.2 mg, 90s ea.......	55289-0154-90	73.43		
100s ea...........	55289-0154-01	80.47		
(Pharma Pac)				
REPACK				
TAB, PO, 0.075 mg, 30s ea.	52959-0922-30	45.50		AB1
0.125 mg, 30s ea....	52959-0920-30	55.36		AB1
(Phys Total Care)				
REPACK				
TAB, PO, 0.025 mg, 30s ea.	54868-3388-02	16.44		AB1
90s ea...........	54868-3388-03	43.29		
100s ea...........	54868-3388-00	47.76		
0.05 mg, 30s ea......	54868-2131-00	39.91		
45s ea...........	54868-2131-04	58.37		AB1
(USP)				
0.05 mg, 60s ea......	54868-2131-05	76.83		
90s ea...........	54868-2131-03	87.68		
100s ea...........	54868-2131-01	95.59		
0.075 mg, 30s ea.....	54868-2539-00	19.26		
60s ea...........	54868-2539-02	32.70		AB1
100s ea...........	54868-2539-01	55.74		
0.088 mg, 30s ea.....	54868-0935-01	17.99		AB1
90s ea...........	54868-0935-02	44.96		AB1
100s ea...........	54868-0935-00	57.42		
0.1 mg, 30s ea.......	54868-0805-01	19.05		
90s ea...........	54868-0805-00	52.68		
100s ea...........	54868-0805-02	55.05		
0.112 mg, 10s ea.....	54868-6097-00	12.46		AB
90s ea...........	54868-6097-01	64.11		AB
0.125 mg, 30s ea.....	54868-3390-02	24.87		
90s ea...........	54868-3390-03	61.37		
100s ea...........	54868-3390-00	75.93		
0.137 mg, 30s ea.....	54868-5477-00	24.87		
100s ea...........	54868-5477-01	74.43		
0.15 mg, 30s ea......	54868-1093-01	53.43		
50s ea...........	54868-1093-00	87.05		
60s ea...........	54868-1093-05	80.12		
90s ea...........	54868-1093-06	67.06		
100s ea...........	54868-1093-02	130.04		
0.175 mg, 30s ea.....	54868-4507-00	29.31		
100s ea...........	54868-4507-01	85.71		AB1
0.2 mg, 30s ea.......	54868-0890-01	24.45		
60s ea...........	54868-0890-00	45.93		
100s ea...........	54868-0890-02	56.22		
0.3 mg, 30s ea.......	54868-2271-02	40.26		
100s ea...........	54868-2271-00	96.51		
1000s ea	54868-2271-01	1243.95		
(Physician Partner)				
REPACK				
TAB, PO, 0.025 mg, 30s ea.	21695-0748-30	14.25		AB1
0.05 mg, 30s ea......	21695-0749-30	16.20		AB1
90s ea...........	21695-0749-90	48.60		AB1
0.075 mg, 30s ea.....	21695-0750-30	17.88		AB1
90s ea...........	21695-0750-90	53.64		AB1
0.1 mg, 30s ea.......	21695-0752-30	18.33		AB1
90s ea...........	21695-0752-90	54.99		AB1
100s ea...........	21695-0752-00	61.00		AB1
0.112 mg, 30s ea.....	21695-0753-30	21.16		AB1
0.125 mg, 100s ea....	21695-0754-00	71.60		AB1
0.137 mg, 30s ea.....	21695-0755-30	21.90		AB1
0.15 mg, 30s ea......	21695-0756-30	22.11		AB1
90s ea...........	21695-0756-90	66.33		AB1
0.175 mg, 30s ea.....	21695-0757-30	28.87		
0.2 mg, 30s ea.......	21695-0758-30	28.93		
90s ea...........	21695-0758-90	86.79		
(Quality Care Prod)				
REPACK				
TAB, PO, 0.05 mg, 30s ea..	49999-0792-30	10.52		
100s ea...........	49999-0792-00	35.07		
0.075 mg, 30s ea.....	49999-0793-30	11.21		
0.1 mg, ea...........	49999-0794-01	0.40		
30s ea...........	49999-0794-30	11.91		
100s ea...........	49999-0794-00	39.70		
0.125 mg, ea.........	49999-0795-01	0.42		
30s ea...........	49999-0795-30	12.61		
100s ea...........	49999-0795-00	42.00		
0.137 mg, 30s ea.....	35356-0515-30	26.40		
0.15 mg, ea..........	49999-0796-01	0.44		
30s ea...........	49999-0796-30	13.31		
100s ea...........	49999-0796-00	44.37		
0.175 mg, 30s ea.....	49999-0797-30	14.01		
(Southwood)				
REPACK				
TAB, PO, 0.05 mg, 15s ea..	58016-0249-15	3.89		
20s ea...........	58016-0249-20	5.18		
30s ea...........	58016-0249-30	7.77		
100s ea...........	58016-0249-00	25.90		
0.075 mg, 100s ea....	58016-0185-00	4.74		
0.1 mg, 12s ea.......	58016-0931-12	3.50		
15s ea...........	58016-0931-15	4.37		
20s ea...........	58016-0931-20	5.83		
30s ea...........	58016-0931-30	8.75		
100s ea...........	58016-0931-00	29.15		
0.125 mg, 30s ea.....	58016-0176-30	8.91		
60s ea...........	58016-0176-60	17.83		
90s ea...........	58016-0176-90	26.74		
100s ea...........	58016-0176-00	29.71		
120s ea...........	58016-0176-02	35.65		
0.15 mg, 30s ea......	58016-0135-30	9.17		
60s ea...........	58016-0135-60	18.35		
90s ea...........	58016-0135-90	27.52		
100s ea...........	58016-0135-00	30.58		
120s ea...........	58016-0135-02	36.70		
0.2 mg, 15s ea.......	58016-0932-15	6.23		
20s ea...........	58016-0932-20	8.30		
30s ea...........	58016-0932-30	12.45		
100s ea...........	58016-0932-00	41.50		
0.3 mg, 15s ea.......	58016-0769-15	6.27		
20s ea...........	58016-0769-20	8.36		
30s ea...........	58016-0769-30	12.54		
100s ea...........	58016-0769-00	41.80		
(Vibranta)				
REPACK				
TAB, PO, 0.025 mg, 30s ea.	57866-5503-01	10.55		AB1
0.1 mg, 30s ea.......	57866-3953-02	11.35		AB1
0.15 mg, 30s ea......	57866-4380-01	12.87		
LEVOTHYROXINE SODIUM/LIOTHYRONINE SODIUM				
(Forest Pharm) *See THYROLAR*				
LEVOXYL (King Pharm)				
levothyroxine sodium				
TAB, PO, 0.025 mg,				
100s ea...........	60793-0850-01	35.51		AB1
(USP)				
0.025 mg, 1000s ea ..	60793-0850-10	332.78		AB1
0.05 mg, 100s ea.....	60793-0851-01	40.31		AB1
(USP)				
0.05 mg, 1000s ea....	60793-0851-10	378.05		AB1
0.075 mg, 100s ea....	60793-0852-01	44.54		AB1
1000s ea	60793-0852-10	417.54		AB1
0.088 mg, 100s ea....	60793-0853-01	45.31		AB1
1000s ea	60793-0853-10	424.87		AB1
0.1 mg, 100s ea......	60793-0854-01	45.66		AB1
(USP)				
0.1 mg, 1000s ea.....	60793-0854-10	428.00		AB1
0.112 mg, 100s ea....	60793-0855-01	52.80		AB1
1000s ea	60793-0855-10	494.82		AB1
0.125 mg, 100s ea....	60793-0856-01	53.53		AB1
(USP)				
0.125 mg, 1000s ea ..	60793-0856-10	501.61		AB1
0.137 mg, 100s ea....	60793-0857-01	54.28		AB1
(USP)				
0.137 mg, 1000s ea ..	60793-0857-10	508.76		AB1
0.15 mg, 100s ea.....	60793-0858-01	55.09		AB1
(USP)				
0.15 mg, 1000s ea....	60793-0858-10	516.40		AB1
0.175 mg, 100s ea....	60793-0859-01	65.48		AB1
(USP)				
0.175 mg, 1000s ea ..	60793-0859-10	613.70		AB1
0.2 mg, 100s ea......	60793-0860-01	65.62		AB1
(USP)				
0.2 mg, 1000s ea.....	60793-0860-10	615.13		AB1
(A-S Medication)				
REPACK				
TAB, PO, 0.05 mg, 30s ea..	54569-5300-01	11.65		BX
100s ea...........	54569-5300-00	38.83		BX
0.075 mg, 30s ea.....	54569-5383-00	12.87		BX
0.1 mg, 30s ea.......	54569-5297-00	13.19		BX
100s ea...........	54569-5297-01	43.98		BX
0.2 mg, 30s ea.......	54569-5298-00	18.96		BX
(Dispensing Solutions)				
REPACK				
TAB, PO, 0.025 mg,				
30s ea...........	66336-0254-30	23.12		
0.05 mg, 30s ea......	66336-0979-30	13.64		
0.1 mg, 30s ea.......	66336-0578-30	19.76		
(PD-Rx Pharm)				
REPACK				
TAB, PO, 0.025 mg,				
30s ea...........	55289-0758-30	17.58		
30s ea...........	58864-0800-30	17.58		
0.05 mg, 14s ea......	55289-0771-14	13.82		
30s ea...........	58864-0610-30	17.32		
0.075 mg, 30s ea.....	58864-0850-30	19.72		
0.1 mg, 14s ea.......	55289-0805-14	14.15		
30s ea...........	58864-0624-30	24.60		
0.125 mg, 14s ea.....	55289-0760-14	15.68		
(REDI-SCRIPT)				
0.125 mg, 30s ea.....	58864-0613-30	24.09		
0.15 mg, 14s ea......	55289-0775-14	16.00		
(Phys Total Care)				
REPACK				
TAB, PO, 0.025 mg,				
30s ea...........	54868-4087-01	15.93		BX
100s ea...........	54868-4087-00	46.36		BX
0.05 mg, 30s ea......	54868-4092-02	17.73		BX
90s ea...........	54868-4092-01	47.96		BX
100s ea...........	54868-4092-00	52.34		BX
0.075 mg, 30s ea.....	54868-4534-01	19.30		BX
100s ea...........	54868-4534-00	57.57		BX
0.088 mg, 30s ea.....	54868-4177-01	19.59		BX
90s ea UD	54868-4177-02	53.53		BX
100s ea...........	54868-4177-00	58.54		BX
0.1 mg, 30s ea.......	54868-4176-01	19.71		BX
90s ea...........	54868-4176-02	53.91		AB1
100s ea...........	54868-4176-00	58.95		BX
0.112 mg, 30s ea.....	54868-3849-01	19.51		BX
100s ea...........	54868-3849-00	60.06		BX
0.125 mg, 10s ea.....	54868-4536-02	9.32		AB1
30s ea...........	54868-4536-01	22.74		BX
100s ea...........	54868-4536-00	69.06		BX
0.137 mg, 10s ea.....	54868-5519-01	9.41		AB1
30s ea...........	54868-5519-00	23.02		AB1
0.15 mg, 30s ea......	54868-4535-01	23.25		BX
90s ea...........	54868-4535-02	64.51		BX
100s ea...........	54868-4535-00	70.73		BX
0.175 mg, 30s ea.....	54868-4821-01	24.63		BX
100s ea...........	54868-4821-00	77.09		BX
0.2 mg, 30s ea.......	54868-4542-01	24.68		BX
100s ea...........	54868-4542-00	77.90		BX
0.3 mg, 100s ea......	54868-5603-00	235.08		
(Southwood)				
REPACK				
TAB, PO, 0.125 mg,				
30s ea...........	58016-0621-30	16.06		AB1
60s ea...........	58016-0621-60	32.12		AB1
90s ea...........	58016-0621-90	48.18		AB1
100s ea...........	58016-0621-00	53.53		AB1
LEVSIN (Alaven)				
hyoscyamine sulfate				
SOL, IJ (5X1ML,(AMP))				
0.5 mg/ml, 1 ml 5s...	68220-0111-05	157.50		
TAB, PO, 0.125 mg,				
100s ea...........	68220-0112-10	118.39		
500s ea...........	68220-0112-50	455.25		
(Phys Total Care)				
REPACK				
TAB, PO, 0.125 mg,				
100s ea...........	54868-1555-02	90.51		
LEVSIN/SL (Alaven)				
hyoscyamine sulfate				
TAB, SL, 0.125 mg,				
100s ea...........	68220-0113-10	122.59		
500s ea...........	68220-0113-50	438.83		
(Phys Total Care)				
REPACK				
TAB, SL, 0.125 mg,				
30s ea...........	54868-1767-00	36.82		
LEVSINEX (Alaven)				
hyoscyamine sulfate				
CER, PO, 0.375 mg,				
100s ea...........	00091-3537-01	168.65		
500s ea...........	00091-3537-05	795.09		
LEVULAN KERASTICK (Dusa Pharmaceuticals)				
aminolevulinic acid				
STI, TP, 20%, ea.........	67308-0101-01	170.25		
6s ea...........	67308-0101-06	1072.59		
LEXAPRO (Forest Pharm)				
escitalopram oxalate				
SOL, PO (PEPPERMINT)				
5 mg/5 ml, 240 ml....	00456-2101-08	166.10		
TAB, PO (FILM-COATED)				
5 mg, 100s ea........	00456-2005-01	332.98		
10 mg, 100s ea	00456-2010-01	348.16		

PROD/MFR	NDC	AWP	DP	OBC
(10X10)				
10 mg, 100s ea UD	**00456-2010-63**	355.14		
20 mg, 100s ea	**00456-2020-01**	363.30		
(10X10)				
20 mg, 100s ea UD	**00456-2020-63**	370.56		
(A-S Medication)				
REPACK				
TAB, PO, 10 mg, 30s ea	**54569-5483-00**	101.21		
20 mg, 30s ea	**54569-5484-00**	105.61		
(Altura)				
REPACK				
TAB, PO (FILM COATED)				
10 mg, 30s ea	**63874-1009-03**	116.10		
60s ea	**63874-1009-06**	232.20		
90s ea	**63874-1009-09**	348.30		
100s ea	**63874-1009-01**	387.00		
(AQ)				
REPACK				
TAB, PO, 10 mg, 30s ea	**66105-0969-03**	192.30		
20 mg, 30s ea	**66105-0977-03**	200.66		
(Bryant Ranch)				
REPACK				
TAB, PO, 20 mg, 30s ea	**63629-2981-01**	82.50		
(Core)				
REPACK				
TAB, PO, 5 mg, 30s ea	**33358-0208-30**	92.51		
20 mg, 30s ea	**33358-0209-30**	104.60		
(Direct Pharmaceutical, Inc.)				
REPACK				
TAB, PO, 10 mg,				
30s ea UD	**67801-0409-30**	150.86		
20 mg, 30s ea UD	**67801-0310-30**	175.68		
(Dispensing Solutions)				
REPACK				
TAB, PO, 10 mg, 30s ea	**55045-2934-08**	102.60		
100s ea	**55045-2934-00**	342.00		
20 mg, 30s ea	**55045-2985-08**	108.00		
100s ea	**55045-2985-00**	360.00		
(IPI)				
REPACK				
TAB, PO, 10 mg, 90s ea	**18837-0076-90**	307.51		
20 mg, 60s ea	**18837-0077-60**	206.15		
(Keltman Pharma., Inc.)				
REPACK				
TAB, PO, 10 mg, 30s ea	**68387-0127-30**	107.55		
20 mg, 30s ea	**68387-0128-30**	112.75		
(Nucare Pharm)				
REPACK				
TAB, PO, 10 mg, 30s ea	**68071-0294-30**	167.00		
60s ea	**68071-0294-60**	211.16		
20 mg, 30s ea	**66267-0728-30**	172.00		
60s ea	**66267-0728-60**	220.35		
(PD-Rx Pharm)				
REPACK				
TAB, PO, 10 mg, 30s ea	**55289-0768-30**	146.07		
20 mg, 30s ea	**55289-0828-30**	151.07		
(Pharma Pac)				
REPACK				
TAB, PO, 10 mg, 30s ea	**52959-0703-30**	128.90		
60s ea	**52959-0703-60**	257.40		
100s ea	**52959-0703-00**	232.93		
20 mg, 30s ea	**52959-0704-30**	134.80		
60s ea	**52959-0704-60**	255.65		
100s ea	**52959-0704-00**	275.11		
(Phys Total Care)				
REPACK				
TAB, PO (FILM-COATED)				
5 mg, 10s ea	**54868-5951-01**	41.44		
30s ea	**54868-5951-02**	119.08		
90s ea	**54868-5951-00**	332.61		
10 mg, 10s ea	**54868-4700-00**	46.25		
20s ea	**54868-4700-04**	89.89		
30s ea	**54868-4700-01**	133.53		
45s ea	**54868-4700-05**	188.07		
60s ea	**54868-4700-02**	249.89		
90s ea	**54868-4700-06**	373.53		
100s ea	**54868-4700-03**	414.09		
20 mg, 10s ea	**54868-4775-00**	48.15		
30s ea	**54868-4775-01**	139.22		
45s ea	**54868-4775-03**	196.14		
60s ea	**54868-4775-04**	260.64		
90s ea	**54868-4775-05**	389.66		
100s ea	**54868-4775-02**	432.01		
(Physician Partner)				
REPACK				
TAB, PO, 10 mg, 15s ea	**21695-0073-15**	119.07		
30s ea	**21695-0073-30**	202.42		
45s ea	**21695-0073-45**	336.98		
20 mg, 15s ea	**21695-0074-15**	117.22		
30s ea	**21695-0074-30**	211.22		
(Quality Care Prod)				
REPACK				
TAB, PO, 10 mg, 15s ea	**49999-0600-15**	76.18		
30s ea	**49999-0600-30**	154.32		
90s ea	**49999-0600-90**	476.99		
100s ea	**49999-0600-00**	461.30		
20 mg, 30s ea	**49999-0627-30**	171.90		
60s ea	**49999-0627-60**	314.14		
100s ea	**49999-0627-00**	426.93		
(Southwood)				
REPACK				
TAB, PO (FILM-COATED)				
5 mg, 30s ea	**58016-0027-30**	87.66		
60s ea	**58016-0027-60**	175.33		
90s ea	**58016-0027-90**	262.99		
100s ea	**58016-0027-00**	292.21		
10 mg, 30s ea	**58016-0977-30**	91.66		
60s ea	**58016-0977-60**	183.32		
90s ea	**58016-0977-90**	274.98		
100s ea	**58016-0977-00**	305.53		
120s ea	**58016-0977-02**	291.37		
(Stat Rx)				
REPACK				
TAB, PO (FILM-COATED)				
5 mg, 30s ea	**16590-0833-30**	102.14		
45s ea	**16590-0833-45**	146.24		
90s ea	**16590-0833-90**	324.47		
10 mg, 28s ea	**16590-0139-28**	108.29		
30s ea	**16590-0139-30**	113.83		
45s ea	**16590-0139-45**	170.02		
60s ea	**16590-0139-60**	226.23		
90s ea	**16590-0139-90**	340.17		
20 mg, 28s ea	**16590-0497-28**	111.54		
30s ea	**16590-0497-30**	120.45		
60s ea	**16590-0497-60**	237.38		
90s ea	**16590-0497-90**	354.83		
120s ea	**16590-0497-72**	375.75		
LEXISCAN (Astellas)				
regadenoson				
SOL, IV (1X5ML,PF)				
0.08 mg/ml, 5 ml	**00469-6501-89**	247.68		
LEXIVA (Glaxo)				
fosamprenavir calcium				
SUS, PO (GRAPE-BUBBLE-PEPPERMINT)				
50 mg/ml, 225 ml	**00173-0727-00**	125.78		
TAB, PO (FILM COATED)				
700 mg, 60s ea	**00173-0721-00**	820.99		
(A-S Medication)				
REPACK				
TAB, PO (FILM COATED)				
700 mg, 60s ea	**54569-5550-00**	1067.29		
(Phys Total Care)				
REPACK				
TAB, PO (FILM COATED)				
700 mg, 60s ea	**54868-4954-00**	738.68		
(Quality Care Prod)				
REPACK				
TAB, PO (FILM COATED)				
700 mg, 6s ea	**35356-0067-06**	256.08		
60s ea	**35356-0067-60**	2280.00		
LIALDA (Shire US Inc.)				
mesalamine				
TCP, PO (FILM-COATED)				
1.2 gm, 120s ea	**54092-0476-12**	674.41	562.01	
LIBRAX (Valeant Pharm Intl)				
chlordiazepoxide hydrochloride/clidinium bromide				
CAP, PO, 5 mg-2.5 mg,				
100s ea	**00187-4100-10**	602.24		
LIBRIUM (Southwood)				
REPACK				
chlordiazepoxide hydrochloride				
CAP, PO, 10 mg,				
30s ea, C-IV	**58016-0996-30**	49.34		AB
60s ea, C-IV	**58016-0996-60**	98.67		AB
90s ea, C-IV	**58016-0996-90**	148.01		AB
100s ea, C-IV	**58016-0996-00**	164.45		AB
25 mg,				
30s ea, C-IV	**58016-0064-30**	65.09		
60s ea, C-IV	**58016-0064-60**	130.18		
90s ea, C-IV	**58016-0064-90**	195.27		
100s ea, C-IV	**58016-0064-00**	216.97		
LICORICE (PCCA)				
LIQ, NA (ARTIFICIAL)				
1 ml	**51927-3412-00**	0.90		
(NF)				
1 ml	**51927-2376-00**	0.19		
LICORICE EXTRACT (Amend)				
LIQ, NA (N.F.)				
120 ml	**17317-0325-04**	3.15		
480 ml	**17317-0325-01**	8.40		
4000 ml	**17317-0325-06**	43.40		
LICORICE ROOT (Amend)				
POW, NA, 454 gm	**17317-0322-01**	10.50		
11350 gm	**17317-0322-08**	175.00		
(PCCA)				
POW, NA (GLYCYRRHIZA GLABRA)				
1 gm	**51927-1256-00**	0.36		
LIDA MANTLE (Doak)				
lidocaine hydrochloride				
CRE, TP, 3%, 85 gm	**10337-0700-19**	172.33		
LOT, TP, 3%, 177 ml	**10337-0705-10**	246.32		
(Quality Care Prod)				
REPACK				
LOT, TP, 3%, 177 ml	**49999-0731-77**	160.45		
LIDA MANTLE HC (Doak)				
hydrocortisone acetate/lidocaine hydrochloride				
CRE, TP, 0.5%-3%, 85 gm	**10337-0710-19**	191.53		
LOT, TP, 0.5%-3%, 177 ml	**10337-0715-10**	273.82		
(Quality Care Prod)				
REPACK				
LOT, TP, 0.5%-3%, 177 ml	**49999-0730-77**	178.36		
LIDAMANTLE HC RELIEF (Doak)				
hydrocortisone acetate/lidocaine hydrochloride				
PAD, TP, 2%-2%, 60s ea	**10337-0716-60**	282.61		
LIDAZONE HC (Rising)				
hydrocortisone acetate/lidocaine hydrochloride				
CRE, TP, 0.5%-3%,				
7 gm 14s	**64980-0319-14**	75.50		
KIT, MR, 0.5%-3%, ea	**64980-0319-20**	129.18		
(Physician Partner)				
REPACK				
CRE, TP (14X7GM)				
0.5%-3%, 7 gm 14s	**21695-0824-14**	150.92		
LIDEX (Quality Care Prod)				
REPACK				
fluocinonide				
CRE, TP, 0.05%, 30 gm	**49999-0212-30**	107.08		
LIDOCAINE (Amend)				
POW, NA (U.S.P.)				
25 gm	**17317-0326-02**	9.10		
125 gm	**17317-0326-04**	25.20		
1000 gm	**17317-0326-09**	140.00		
5000 gm	**17317-0326-05**	595.00		
(Endo Labs) *See LIDODERM*				
(Fougera)				
OIN, TP, 5%, 35.44 gm	**00168-0204-37**	12.00		AT
(Gallipot)				
POW, NA (U.S.P.,N.F.)				
25 gm	**51552-0145-04**	12.60		
100 gm	**51552-0145-05**	32.34		
454 gm	**51552-0145-06**	119.00		
(Hawkins)				
POW, NA (U.S.P.)				
25 gm	**63370-0144-25**	39.60		
100 gm	**63370-0144-35**	115.20		
1000 gm	**63370-0144-45**	408.00		
(Letco)				
POW, NA (U.S.P.)				
25 gm	**62991-1094-01**	27.75		
100 gm	**62991-1094-02**	66.00		
500 gm	**62991-1094-03**	225.00		
1000 gm	**62991-1094-04**	345.00		
(Medisca)				
POW, NA (U.S.P.)				
25 gm	**38779-0081-04**	31.50		
100 gm	**38779-0081-05**	96.00		
500 gm	**38779-0081-08**	267.00		
1000 gm	**38779-0081-09**	447.00		
(PCCA)				
POW, NA (U.S.P.)				
1 gm	**51927-1031-00**	1.56		
(Spectrum Pharmacy)				
POW, NA (U.S.P.)				
25 gm	**49452-4040-01**	63.00		
100 gm	**49452-4040-02**	147.70		
500 gm	**49452-4040-03**	395.50		

PROD/MFR	NDC	AWP	DP	OBC
(Aidarex)				
REPACK				
OIN, TP (1X50GM,SPEARMINT)				
5%, 50 gm	**33261-0564-01**	37.25		AT
(Altura)				
REPACK				
OIN, TP, 5%, 50 gm	**63874-1064-05**	26.99		
(Pharma Pac)				
REPACK				
OIN, TP (1X37.5GM)				
5%, 37.5 gm	**52959-0993-01**	19.90		AT
(Phys Total Care)				
REPACK				
lidocaine hydrochloride				
CRE, TP, 3%, 28.35 gm	**54868-5537-00**	82.95		
LIDOCAINE (Phys Total Care)				
OIN, TP, 5%, 37.5 gm	**54868-3282-00**	16.08		EE
(Phys Total Care)				
lidocaine hydrochloride				
SOL, IV (10X5ML)				
2%, 5 ml 10s	**54868-5719-00**	81.45		
LIDOCAINE (Physician Partner)				
REPACK				
OIN, TP (1X35.44GM)				
5%, 35.44 gm	**21695-0826-15**	30.38		AT
(Quality Care Prod)				
REPACK				
OIN, TP, 5%, 35 gm	**49999-0751-35**	21.27		AT
(Southwood)				
REPACK				
lidocaine hydrochloride				
SOL, EP (SDA)				
1%, 5 ml 5s	**58016-4840-01**	3.38		
LIDOCAINE (Stat Rx)				
REPACK				
OIN, TP (1X37.5GM)				
5%, 37.5 gm	**16590-0865-12**	10.69		AT
LIDOCAINE 2% W/ EPI (Southwood)				
REPACK				
epinephrine/lidocaine hydrochloride				
SOL, IJ, 1:100000-2%,				
20 ml	**58016-4806-01**	43.13		
LIDOCAINE HCL (Abbott Hosp)				
lidocaine hydrochloride				
SOL, IV (VIAL, PINTOP)				
20%, 10 ml 25s	**00074-6217-02**	238.39	200.75	AP
(Akorn)				
GEL, TP (USP)				
2%, 5 ml 10s	**17478-0711-10**	78.01		AT
30 ml	**17478-0711-30**	16.67		AT
(Amend)				
POW, NA (U.S.P.)				
25 gm	**17317-0735-02**	9.40		
125 gm	**17317-0735-04**	26.00		
500 gm	**17317-0735-01**	77.00		
1000 gm	**17317-0735-06**	140.00		
5000 gm	**17317-0735-03**	595.00		
(Amer Regent)				
SOL, EP (M.D.V.)				
1%, 50 ml 25s	**00517-0625-25**	27.19		AP
IJ, 2%, 50 ml 25s	**00517-0626-25**	30.94		AP
(Amphastar)				
GEL, TP (SRN,PREFILLED,URO-JET)				
2%, 5 ml 25s	**00548-3012-00**	191.19		AT
(SRN,PREFILLED,UROJET AC)				
2%, 5 ml 25s	**00548-3011-00**	199.50		AT
(SRN,PREFILLED,URO-JET)				
2%, 10 ml 25s	**00548-3013-00**	213.13		AT
20 ml 25s	**00548-3015-00**	256.69		AT
SOL, IV (SRN,PREFILLED,LUER-JET)				
2%, 5 ml 10s	**00548-3390-00**	33.25		AP
(MINIJET,21GX1 1/2")				
2%, 5 ml 25s	**00548-1190-00**	133.67		AP
(SRN,PREFILLED,STICKGARD)				
2%, 5 ml 25s	**00548-2190-00**	143.64		AP
(Cypress Pharm)				
CRE, TP, 3%, 28.35 gm	**60258-0040-01**	35.11		
85 gm	**60258-0040-03**	55.32		
(Gallipot)				
POW, NA (U.S.P.)				
4 gm	**51552-0106-09**	8.82		
(U.S.P.,N.F.)				
25 gm	**51552-0106-04**	12.60		
100 gm	**51552-0106-05**	32.34		
454 gm	**51552-0106-06**	127.19		
(Hawkins)				
POW, NA (U.S.P.)				
4 gm	**63370-0145-14**	28.80		
25 gm	**63370-0145-25**	43.20		
100 gm	**63370-0145-35**	105.60		
1000 gm	**63370-0145-50**	624.00		
5000 gm	**63370-0145-55**	1560.00		
(Hi-Tech)				
SOL, MM (VISCOUS)				
2%, 100 ml	**50383-0775-04**	5.99		AT
(Hospira)				
SOL, EP (LATEX-FREE)				
1%, 2 ml 50s	**00409-4713-32**	72.60	63.50	AP
(10X5ML,LATEX-FREE)				
1%, 5 ml 10s	**00409-4904-34**	43.56	38.10	AP
(ANSYR,10X5ML,LATEX-FREE)				
1%, 5 ml 10s	**00409-9137-05**	21.48	18.80	AP
(25X5ML,LATEX-FREE)				
1%, 5 ml 25s	**00409-4713-02**	29.10	25.50	AP
(FTV,25X20ML)				
1%, 20 ml 25s	**00409-4276-01**	33.90	29.75	AP
(STERILE,SDV,EPIDURAL,PF)				
1%, 30 ml 25s	**00409-4270-01**	184.50	161.50	AP
(TEARDROP BOTTLE)				
1%, 30 ml 25s	**00409-4279-02**	67.50	59.00	AP
(25X50ML)				
1%, 50 ml 25s	**00409-4276-02**	65.70	57.50	AP
IJ, 0.5%, 50 ml 25s	**00409-4278-01**	87.00	76.25	AP
(VIAL, FLIPTOP)				
0.5%, 50 ml 25s	**00409-4275-01**	94.50	82.75	AP
(AMP,25X2ML,LATEX-FREE)				
2%, 2 ml 25s	**00409-4282-01**	30.60	26.75	AP
(10X5ML, ANSYR)				
2%, 5 ml 10s	**00074-1323-05**	18.60	16.30	AP
5 ml 10s	**00409-1323-05**	20.88	18.30	AP
(21GX1-1/2",LATEX-FREE)				
2%, 5 ml 10s	**00074-4903-34**	36.72	32.10	AP
5 ml 10s	**00409-4903-34**	39.36	34.40	AP
(VIAL,LATEX-FREE)				
2%, 5 ml 10s	**00409-2066-05**	22.44	19.60	AP
(25X20ML,LATEX-FREE)				
2%, 20 ml 25s	**00409-4277-01**	48.30	42.25	AP
(FTV,25X50ML,LATEX-FREE)				
2%, 50 ml 25s	**00409-4277-02**	72.30	63.25	AP
(AMP,LATEX-FREE)				
4%, 5 ml 25s	**00409-4283-01**	100.50	88.00	AP
(Letco)				
POW, NA (U.S.P., B.P.)				
25 gm	**62991-1095-01**	24.00		
100 gm	**62991-1095-02**	63.00		
500 gm	**62991-1095-03**	237.00		
1000 gm	**62991-1095-04**	315.00		
(USP)				
2500 gm	**62991-1095-06**	447.00		
(Medisca)				
POW, NA (U.S.P.)				
25 gm	**38779-0082-04**	31.50		
100 gm	**38779-0082-05**	96.00		
500 gm	**38779-0082-08**	267.00		
1000 gm	**38779-0082-09**	447.00		
(Morton Grove)				
SOL, TP, 4%, 50 ml	**60432-0465-50**	15.78		AT
(PCCA)				
POW, NA (U.S.P.)				
1 gm	**51927-1213-00**	1.68		
(Roxane)				
SOL, TP, 4%, 50 ml	**00054-3505-47**	9.16		AT
(Teva)				
GEL, TP, 2%, 30 gm	**00093-9200-31**	15.52		AT
(A-S Medication)				
REPACK				
GEL, TP, 2%, 5 ml	**54569-5645-00**	7.80		AT
30 gm	**54569-4258-00**	15.52		
SOL, IJ (5X5ML)				
2%, 5 ml 5s	**54569-5312-01**	3.05		EE
5 ml 10s	**54569-5312-00**	30.49		EE
TP, 4%, 50 ml	**54569-1923-01**	15.78		EE
(B&B Pharm, Inc)				
REPACK				
POW, NA, 25 gm	**63275-9991-04**	22.00		
100 gm	**63275-9991-05**	59.00		
500 gm	**63275-9991-08**	216.00		
(USP,1X1000GM)				
1000 gm	**63275-9991-09**	378.00		
(DHS, Inc.)				
REPACK				
SOL, MM (VISCOUS)				
2%, 100 ml	**55887-0751-01**	17.85		AT
(Dispensing Solutions)				
REPACK				
SOL, EP, 1%, 50 ml	**55045-3231-01**	3.75		AP
(Pharma Pac)				
REPACK				
SOL, MM, 2%, 100 ml	**52959-0251-00**	8.87		EE
(Phys Total Care)				
REPACK				
GEL, TP, 2%, 30 gm	**54868-4195-00**	46.62		EE
SOL, IJ (M.D.V.)				
2%, 50 ml	**54868-2064-00**	5.40		EE
1250 ml	**54868-2064-01**	63.00		EE
(Physician Partner)				
REPACK				
SOL, IJ (1X50ML,LATEX-FREE)				
2%, 50 ml	**21695-0362-01**	13.16		AP
MM (1X100ML)				
2%, 100 ml	**21695-0783-00**	21.98		AT
(Quality Care Prod)				
REPACK				
SOL, EP (1X50ML)				
1%, 50 ml	**49999-0671-50**	6.90		AP
IJ (1X50ML,LATEX-FREE)				
2%, 50 ml	**35356-0180-50**	10.41		AP
(Southwood)				
REPACK				
SOL, EP (M.D.V.)				
1%, 50 ml	**58016-9331-01**	0.86		AP
(Stat Rx)				
REPACK				
CRE, TP, 3%, 85 gm	**16590-0722-03**	64.50		
LIDOCAINE HCL AND EPINEPHRINE (Hospira)				
epinephrine/lidocaine hydrochloride				
SOL, EP (EPIDURAL TEST DOSE)				
1:200000-1.5%,				
5 ml 10s	**00409-1209-01**	32.64	28.60	AP
LIDOCAINE HCL MONOHYDRATE (Spectrum Pharmacy)				
lidocaine hydrochloride				
POW, NA (U.S.P.)				
25 gm	**49452-4050-01**	63.00		
100 gm	**49452-4050-02**	147.70		
500 gm	**49452-4050-03**	395.50		
(1X5000GM,U.S.P.)				
5000 gm	**49452-4050-09**	2243.50		
LIDOCAINE HCL VISCOUS (Morton Grove)				
lidocaine hydrochloride				
SOL, MM (SLIGHT,CHERRY)				
2%, 100 ml	**60432-0464-00**	14.20		AT
(Roxane)				
SOL, MM, 2%,				
20 ml 40s UD	**00054-8500-16**	50.50		AT
100 ml	**00054-3500-49**	3.42		AT
(A-S Medication)				
REPACK				
SOL, MM, 2%, 100 ml	**54569-1285-00**	8.92		EE
(Dispensing Solutions)				
REPACK				
SOL, MM, 2%, 100 ml	**55045-1249-01**	17.00		AT
(Nucare Pharm)				
REPACK				
SOL, MM, 2%, 100 ml	**66267-0962-00**	9.38		EE
(Phys Total Care)				
REPACK				
SOL, MM, 2%, 100 ml	**54868-1827-01**	12.45		EE
(Quality Care Prod)				
REPACK				
SOL, MM, 2%, 100 ml	**49999-0140-00**	20.78		EE
(Southwood)				
REPACK				
SOL, MM, 2%, 100 ml	**58016-9018-01**	17.31		EE
LIDOCAINE HYDROCHLORIDE				
FUL				
SOL, MM, 2%, 100 ml		5.13		

(Abbott Hosp) *See LIDOCAINE HCL*
(Abbott Hosp) *See LTA PEDIATRIC*
(Akorn) *See AKTEN*
(Akorn) *See LIDOCAINE HCL*
(Amend) *See LIDOCAINE HCL*
(Amer Regent) *See LIDOCAINE HCL*
(Amphastar) *See LARYNG-O-JET*
(Amphastar) *See LIDOCAINE HCL*

PROD/MFR	NDC	AWP	DP	OBC
(APP)				
SOL, EP (S.D.V.,P.C.)				
1%, 2 ml	**63323-0201-02**	2.00		**AP**
(M.D.V.)				
1%, 10 ml	**63323-0201-10**	1.63		**AP**
IJ (S.D.V.)				
2%, 2 ml	**63323-0202-02**	2.00		**AP**
IV (S.D.V.,PF)				
2%, 5 ml	**63323-0208-05**	2.10		**AP**
(APP) *See XYLOCAINE*				
(APP) *See XYLOCAINE-MPF*				
(Breckenridge Pharm) *See SENATEC*				
(Clint) *See ANESTACAINE*				
(Covidien) *See PARACENTESIS TRAY*				
(Cypress Pharm) *See LIDOCAINE HCL*				
(Dentsply) *See XYLOCAINE DENTAL*				
(Doak) *See LIDA MANTLE*				
(Gallipot) *See LIDOCAINE HCL*				
(Hawkins) *See LIDOCAINE HCL*				
(Hi-Tech) *See LIDOCAINE HCL*				
(Hospira) *See LIDOCAINE HCL*				
(Hospira) *See LTA PREATTACHED*				
(Hospira)				
SOL, IJ (AMP,PF)				
1.5%, 20 ml 5s	**00409-4056-01**	49.68	43.45	
(25X20ML,PF)				
1.5%, 20 ml 25s	**00409-4776-01**	185.10	162.00	
(USP,25X10ML,SDA,PF)				
2%, 10 ml 25s	**00409-4282-02**	72.30	63.25	**AP**
(Letco) *See LIDOCAINE HCL*				
(Medisca) *See LIDOCAINE HCL*				
(Morton Grove) *See LIDOCAINE HCL*				
(Morton Grove) *See LIDOCAINE HCL VISCOUS*				
(PCCA) *See LIDOCAINE HCL*				
(Portex) *See AMNIOCENTESIS TRAY*				
(Portex) *See LUMBAR PUNCTURE TRAY*				
(Portex) *See PERITONEAL LAVAGE TRAY*				
(Qualitest)				
SOL, MM (USP,CHERRY)				
2%, 100 ml	**00603-1393-64**	14.20		
(USP)				
4%, 50 ml	**00603-1394-47**	15.75		**AT**
(Roxane) *See LIDOCAINE HCL*				
(Roxane) *See LIDOCAINE HCL VISCOUS*				
(Spectrum Pharmacy) *See LIDOCAINE HCL MONOHYDRATE*				
(Teva) *See LIDOCAINE HCL*				
(Dispensing Solutions)				
REPACK				
SOL, IJ, 2%, 50 ml	**55045-3249-05**	3.75		
(Palmetto)				
REPACK				
GEL, TP, 2%, 30 ml	**23490-5804-01**	21.34		
SOL, MM, 2%, 100 ml	**23490-5806-01**	17.85		
LIDOCAINE HYDROCHLORIDE - HYDROCORTISONE ACETATE (River's Edge)				
hydrocortisone acetate/lidocaine hydrochloride				
GEL, TP (20X7GM)				
2.5%-3%, ea	**68032-0193-20**	182.83		
(Quality Care Prod)				
REPACK				
GEL, TP, 2.5%-3%, 7 gm	**35356-0486-07**	28.00		
LIDOCAINE HYDROCHLORIDE AND EPINEPHRINE (Hospira)				
epinephrine/lidocaine hydrochloride				
SOL, IJ (USP)				
1:100000-2%,				
1.8 ml 50s	**00409-0996-01**	18.60	16.50	
(USP, FOR DENTAL USE)				
1:50000-2%,				
1.8 ml 50s	**00409-7263-01**	18.60	16.50	
LIDOCAINE HYDROCHLORIDE AND HYDROCORTISONE ACETATE (Fougera)				
hydrocortisone acetate/lidocaine hydrochloride				
CRE, RC (W/APPLICATOR)				
0.5%-3%, 7 gm 14s	**18754-0480-14**	74.91		
1%-3%, 7 gm 20s	**18754-0481-20**	167.47		
GEL, TP, 2.5%-3%, ea	**18754-0482-20**	188.43		
LIDOCAINE VISCOUS (Altura)				
REPACK				
lidocaine hydrochloride				
SOL, TP, 2%, 100 ml	**63874-0740-10**	16.53		
(Stat Rx)				
REPACK				
SOL, MM, 2%, 100 ml	**16590-0140-32**	17.75		
LIDOCAINE W/ EPI (Southwood)				
REPACK				
epinephrine/lidocaine hydrochloride				
SOL, IJ, 1:100000-2%,				
5 ml 25s	**58016-4828-01**	43.13		
LIDOCAINE/EPI (Phys Total Care)				
REPACK				
epinephrine/lidocaine hydrochloride				
SOL, IJ (25X30ML)				
1:100000-1%,				
30 ml 25s	**54868-2068-00**	131.13		
LIDOCAINE/HC (Cypress Pharm)				
hydrocortisone acetate/lidocaine hydrochloride				
CRE, TP, 0.5%-3%,				
28.35 gm	**60258-0041-01**	38.60		
85 gm	**60258-0041-03**	60.35		
LIDOCAINE/PRILOCAINE				
(APP) *See EMLA*				
(Dentsply) *See ORAQIX*				
(Fougera)				
CRE, TP (PF)				
2.5%-2.5%, 30 gm	**00168-0357-30**	45.82		**AB**
(Hi-Tech)				
CRE, TP (PF)				
2.5%-2.5%, 30 gm	**50383-0667-30**	45.95		**AB**
(Sandoz)				
CRE, TP (W/2 TEGADERM DRESSINGS)				
2.5%-2.5%, 5 gm	**00781-7058-39**	8.04		
(W/12 TEGADERM DRESSINGS)				
2.5%-2.5%, 5 gm 5s	**00781-7058-05**	40.20		
(PF)				
2.5%-2.5%, 30 gm	**00781-7058-03**	46.07		
(DHS, Inc.)				
REPACK				
CRE, TP (PF)				
2.5%-2.5%, 30 gm	**55887-0209-30**	26.00		**AB**
(Phys Total Care)				
REPACK				
CRE, TP (PF)				
2.5%-2.5%, 5 gm 5s	**54868-5194-00**	108.87		**AB**
30 gm	**54868-5194-02**	32.64		
(Physician Partner)				
REPACK				
CRE, TP (1X30GM,PF)				
2.5%-2.5%, 30 gm	**21695-0388-30**	91.64		**AB**
(Quality Care Prod)				
REPACK				
CRE, TP (PF)				
2.5%-2.5%, 30 gm	**49999-0523-30**	54.98		**AB**
(Stat Rx)				
REPACK				
CRE, TP, 2.5%-2.5%, 5 gm	**16590-0498-05**	40.00		
30 gm	**16590-0498-30**	47.75		
LIDOCAINE/TETRACAINE				
(Zars) *See SYNERA*				
LIDOCORT (Aristos)				
hydrocortisone acetate/lidocaine hydrochloride				
GEL, TP (20X7GM)				
2.5%-3%, 7 gm 20s	**24486-0401-20**	188.43		
LIDODERM (Endo Labs)				
lidocaine				
TDM, TP (6X5)				
5%, 30s ea	**63481-0687-06**	231.58		
(4u)				
REPACK				
TDM, TP, 5%, ea	**42549-0576-01**	15.11		
30s ea	**42549-0576-30**	377.64		
(A-S Medication)				
REPACK				
TDM, TP, 5%, 30s ea	**54569-5469-01**	211.40		
30s ea	**54569-6094-00**	286.72		
30s ea	**54569-6094-01**	286.72		
(Aidarex)				
REPACK				
TDM, TP, 5%, 30s ea	**33261-0672-01**	447.66		
(Altura)				
REPACK				
TDM, TP (6X5)				
5%, 30s ea	**63874-0831-30**	200.06		
(Core)				
REPACK				
TDM, TP, 5%, 30s ea	**33358-0419-05**	407.00		
(DHS, Inc.)				
REPACK				
TDM, TP, 5%, 30s ea	**55887-0485-30**	274.50		
(Dispensing Solutions)				
REPACK				
TDM, TP, 5%, ea	**68258-3016-01**	10.05		
30s ea	**68258-3016-03**	243.20		
(6X5)				
5%, 30s ea	**55045-3060-00**	200.00		
(Keltman Pharma., Inc.)				
REPACK				
TDM, TP, 5%, 30s ea	**68387-0590-30**	288.00		
(Nucare Pharm)				
REPACK				
TDM, TP, 5%, ea	**68071-0796-01**	10.07		
30s ea	**66267-1014-03**	254.41		
(Pharma Pac)				
REPACK				
TDM, TP, 5%, ea	**52959-0694-01**	10.08		
30s ea	**52959-0694-30**	299.56		
(Phys Total Care)				
REPACK				
TDM, TP, 5%, 30s ea	**54868-4146-00**	263.04		
(Physician Partner)				
REPACK				
TDM, TP, 5%, ea	**21695-0075-01**	16.58		
(30 PATCHES/BOX)				
5%, 30s ea	**21695-0075-30**	497.40		
(Quality Care Prod)				
REPACK				
TDM, TP, 5%, ea	**49999-0419-01**	10.00		
(6X5)				
5%, 30s ea	**49999-0419-30**	412.80		
(Southwood)				
REPACK				
TDM, TP (6X5)				
5%, 30s ea	**58016-5611-01**	184.40		
(St. Mary's MPP)				
REPACK				
TDM, TP, 5%, 30s ea	**60760-0687-30**	350.61		
(Stat Rx)				
REPACK				
TDM, TP, 5%, 30s ea	**16590-0141-30**	278.00		
LIFECARE 75 FLOW DETECTOR (Abbott Hosp)				
kit, administration, intravenous				
DEV, NA, ea	**00074-1976-01**	300.18	252.78	
LIFECARE PUMP MODEL 4 PIGGYBACK (Abbott Hosp)				
pump, infusion				
DEV, NA (W/RS485)				
ea	**00074-2506-04**	4479.73	3772.40	
LIFESHIELD EXTENSION PEDIATRIC (Abbott Hosp)				
filter, intravenous tubing				
DEV, NA (HP FILTER, PP-Y, OL,PF)				
48s ea	**00074-2694-68**	391.68	342.72	
LIFESHIELD PLUMSET PRIMARY IV W/OL (Abbott Hosp)				
kit, administration, intravenous				
DEV, NA (CONV PIN, 1-LAV-Y)				
48s ea	**00074-1646-48**	466.56	466.56	
(Abbott Hosp)				
device				
(CONV PIN, DUAL CH, 1-Y)				
48s ea	**00074-1648-48**	529.92	441.60	
(Abbott Hosp)				
kit, administration, intravenous				
(CONV PIN, LOWER PP, 1-Y)				
48s ea	**00074-1642-48**	456.77	761.28	

PROD/MFR	NDC	AWP	DP	OBC
(Abbott Hosp)				
device				
(CONV PIN,104" D-CHANN)				
48s ea	00074-1650-48	528.19	528.00	
LIFESHIELD PLUMSET SECONDARY IV-OL (Abbott Hosp)				
device				
DEV, NA (CONV PIN,32")				
48s ea	00074-1643-48	328.32	273.60	
LILAC OIL (Medisca)				
OIL, NA, 14 ml	38779-0899-03	16.50		
25 ml	38779-0899-04	31.50		
100 ml	38779-0899-05	90.00		
500 ml	38779-0899-08	261.00		
LILY OF THE VALLEY				
(Medisca) *See LILY OF THE VALLEY OIL*				
LILY OF THE VALLEY OIL (Medisca)				
lily of the valley				
OIL, NA (1X14ML)				
14 ml	38779-0900-03	16.50		
(1X25ML)				
25 ml	38779-0900-04	31.50		
(1X100ML)				
100 ml	38779-0900-05	90.00		
(1X500ML)				
500 ml	38779-0900-08	261.00		
LIMBITROL (Phys Total Care)				
REPACK				
amitriptyline hydrochloride/chlordiazepoxide				
TAB, PO, 12.5 mg-5 mg,				
100s ea, C-IV	54868-0501-00	135.61		AB
LIMBITROL DS (Phys Total Care)				
amitriptyline hydrochloride/chlordiazepoxide				
TAB, PO, 25 mg-10 mg,				
100s ea, C-IV	54868-0426-00	188.63		AB
LIMBREL (Primus Pharma)				
flavocoxid				
CAP, PO, 250 mg, 60s ea	68040-0601-16	100.25		
500 mg, 60s ea	68040-0602-16	115.31	85.40	
(Pharma Pac)				
REPACK				
CAP, PO, 250 mg, 60s ea	52959-0807-60	92.98		
(Phys Total Care)				
REPACK				
CAP, PO, 250 mg, 60s ea	54868-5324-00	104.70		
(Quality Care Prod)				
REPACK				
CAP, PO, 500 mg, 60s ea	35356-0421-60	203.63		
(Stat Rx)				
REPACK				
CAP, PO, 250 mg, 60s ea	16590-0630-60	112.68		
500 mg, 60s ea	16590-0540-60	120.75		
LIMBREL 250 (Primus Pharma)				
flavocoxid/zinc, chelated				
CAP, PO, 250 mg-50 mg,				
60s ea	68040-0605-16	100.25		
LIMBREL 500 (Primus Pharma)				
flavocoxid/zinc, chelated				
CAP, PO, 500 mg-50 mg,				
60s ea	68040-0606-16	115.31		
(Stat Rx)				
REPACK				
CAP, PO, 500 mg-50 mg,				
60s ea	16590-0331-60	121.00		
LIME (Amend)				
calcium hydroxide				
POW, NA, 500 gm	17317-0328-01	9.80		
LIME GREEN FOOD COLOR (PCCA)				
color additive				
POW, NA, 1 gm	51927-1739-00	6.50		
LIME OIL (Lorann Oil)				
OIL, NA, 9.9 ml	23535-0151-39	2.75		
(Medisca)				
OIL, NA (NATURAL,1X14ML)				
14 ml	38779-1389-03	22.50		
(NATURAL,1X25ML)				
25 ml	38779-1389-04	37.50		
(NATURAL,1X100ML)				
100 ml	38779-1389-05	64.50		
(NATURAL,1X500ML)				
500 ml	38779-1389-08	153.00		
(PCCA) *See LIME OIL FLAVOR*				
LIME OIL FLAVOR (PCCA)				
lime oil				
OIL, NA (NATURAL)				
1 ml	51927-2157-00	1.40		
LIME SOLUTION, SULFURATED (Amend)				
calcium hydroxide				
SOL, NA, 500 ml	17317-0329-01	14.00		
LIMONENE (D) (PCCA)				
limonene, d-				
SOL, NA (1X1ML)				
1 ml	51927-3259-00	0.27		
LIMONENE, D-				
(PCCA) *See LIMONENE (D)*				
LINALYL ACETATE (Medisca)				
SOL, NA (1X25ML)				
25 ml	38779-1391-04	37.50		
(1X100ML)				
100 ml	38779-1391-05	117.00		
(PCCA)				
SOL, NA (1X1ML)				
1 ml	51927-2129-00	1.50		
LINCOCIN (Pfizer)				
lincomycin hydrochloride				
SOL, IJ (VIAL)				
300 mg/ml, 2 ml	00009-0555-01	15.58	12.98	
10 ml	00009-0555-02	58.96	49.13	
(A-S Medication)				
REPACK				
SOL, IJ (VIAL)				
300 mg/ml, 10 ml	54569-1387-00	50.75		
(Dispensing Solutions)				
REPACK				
SOL, IJ (1X10ML)				
300 mg/ml, 10 ml	55045-3535-01	65.00		
LINCOMYCIN HCL (Medisca)				
lincomycin hydrochloride				
POW, NA (U.S.P.)				
25 gm	38779-0034-04	80.55		
100 gm	38779-0034-05	247.50		
500 gm	38779-0034-08	885.00		
(USP, 1X1000GM)				
1000 gm	38779-0034-09	1410.00		
(PCCA)				
POW, NA (U.S.P.)				
1 gm	51927-3177-00	2.40		
LINCOMYCIN HYDROCHLORIDE (Gallipot)				
POW, NA (USP,1X100GM)				
100 gm	51552-0674-05	95.90	68.50	
(USP,1X1000GM)				
1000 gm	51552-0674-07	672.00	480.00	
(Medisca) *See LINCOMYCIN HCL*				
(PCCA) *See LINCOMYCIN HCL*				
(Pfizer) *See LINCOCIN*				
LINDANE (Consolidated Midland)				
LOT, TP, 1%, 60 ml	00223-6546-02	2.75		EE
480 ml	00223-6546-16	17.00		EE
SHA, TP, 1%, 60 ml	00223-6562-02	3.00		EE
480 ml	00223-6562-16	22.50		EE
(Morton Grove)				
LOT, TP (USP)				
1%, 60 ml	60432-0833-60	136.86		AT
SHA, TP, 1%, 60 ml	60432-0834-60	136.86		AT
(PCCA)				
POW, NA, ea	51927-1701-00	3.90		
(Spectrum Pharmacy)				
POW, NA (1X100GM)				
100 gm	49452-4055-02	626.50		
(1X500GM)				
500 gm	49452-4055-03	2054.50		
(Altura)				
REPACK				
LOT, TP, 1%, 60 ml	63874-0704-60	14.37		EE
SHA, TP, 1%, 60 ml	63874-0705-60	14.72		EE
(Dispensing Solutions)				
REPACK				
LOT, TP, 1%, 60 ml	55045-1412-09	123.00		AT
SHA, TP, 1%, 60 ml	55045-1223-09	123.00		AT
(Phys Total Care)				
REPACK				
LOT, TP, 1%, 60 ml	54868-0188-02	373.23		EE
SHA, TP, 1%, 60 ml	54868-0572-01	77.79		EE
480 ml	54868-0572-00	121.36		EE
(Southwood)				
REPACK				
LOT, TP, 1%, 60 ml	58016-3039-01	2.75		EE
SHA, TP, 1%, 60 ml	58016-3041-01	3.00		EE
LINEZOLID				
(Pfizer) *See ZYVOX*				
LINOLEIC ACID (PCCA)				
SOL, NA (HIGH PURITY)				
1 gm	51927-2552-00	18.00		
LINOLEIC ACID METHYL ESTER (PCCA)				
methyl linoleate				
SOL, NA (1X1ML)				
1 ml	51927-3320-00	87.00		
LINOLENIC ACID (PCCA)				
SOL, NA, 1 gm	51927-1514-00	12.00		
(1X1ML)				
55%, 1 ml	51927-3657-00	10.20		
LINSEED OIL (Medisca)				
flaxseed oil				
OIL, NA (RAW,1X500ML)				
500 ml	38779-1392-08	28.50		
(RAW,1X4000ML)				
4000 ml	38779-1392-01	99.00		
(PCCA)				
OIL, NA (RAW)				
1 ml	51927-1438-00	0.09		
LIORESAL INTRATHECAL REFILL KIT				
(Medtronic Neurologic)				
baclofen				
KIT, MR, 0.5 mg/ml,				
20 ml 2s	58281-0560-02	516.00	430.00	
(1X20ML AMP)				
2 mg/ml, 20 ml	58281-0563-01	1032.00	860.00	
20 ml 2s	58281-0563-02	2064.00	1720.00	
SOL, IN, 0.5 mg/ml,				
20 ml	58281-0560-01	258.00	215.00	
2 mg/ml, 5 ml 2s	58281-0561-02	516.00	430.00	
LIORESAL INTRATHECAL SCREENING KIT				
(Medtronic Neurologic)				
baclofen				
SOL, IN, 0.05 mg/ml,				
1 ml	58281-0562-01	84.00	70.00	
LIOTHYRONINE SODIUM (Gallipot)				
POW, NA (U.S.P.)				
0.25 gm	51552-0354-09	35.00		
1 gm	51552-0354-01	70.00		
5 gm	51552-0354-02	315.00		
(Hawkins)				
POW, NA (USP)				
0.5 gm	63370-0139-09	108.00		
1 gm	63370-0139-10	180.00		
(JHP) *See TRIOSTAT*				
(King Pharm) *See CYTOMEL*				
(Letco)				
POW, NA (U.S.P.)				
0.25 gm	62991-1096-02	63.00	21.00	
1 gm	62991-1096-01	135.00	45.00	
(Medisca)				
POW, NA (U.S.P.)				
1 gm	38779-0031-06	330.00		
5 gm	38779-0031-03	1095.00		
(USP, 1X500MG)				
500 ml	38779-0031-00	210.00		
(Mylan)				
TAB, PO (USP)				
5 mcg, 100s ea	00378-3611-01	80.82		AB
1000s ea	00378-3611-10	808.20		AB
25 mcg, 100s ea	00378-3612-01	106.19		AB
1000s ea	00378-3612-10	1061.87		AB
(USP,CAPLET)				
50 mcg, 100s ea	00378-3613-01	162.21		AB
(Paddock)				
TAB, PO, 5 mcg, 100s ea	00574-0220-01	80.02		
25 mcg, 100s ea	00574-0222-01	105.14		
50 mcg, 100s ea	00574-0223-01	160.60		
(PCCA) *See TRIIODO-L-THYRONINE SODIUM*				
(Spectrum Pharmacy)				
POW, NA (U.S.P./N.F.)				
0.25 gm	49452-4082-03	128.45		
1 gm	49452-4082-01	301.70		

PROD/MFR	NDC	AWP	DP	OBC
5 gm	49452-4082-02	1018.50		
(1X25GM,U.S.P.) 25 gm	49452-4082-04	3566.50		
(X-Gen)				
SOL, IV (AQUEOUS)				
0.01 mg/ml, 1 ml	39822-0151-01	460.00		AP
(Stat Rx)				
REPACK				
TAB, PO, 50 mcg, 30s ea	16590-0303-30	57.82		
LIP BALM BASE (Gallipot)				
ointment base				
OIN, NA, 90 gm	51552-0318-09	5.74		
454 gm	51552-0318-06	15.61		
LIPASE				
(PCCA) *See LIPASE 16*				
(Spectrum Pharmacy)				
POW, NA, 100 gm	49452-4085-01	131.60		
500 gm	49452-4085-02	451.50		
LIPASE 16 (PCCA)				
lipase				
POW, NA (PORCINE)				
1 gm	51927-2951-00	0.75		
LIPITOR (Pfizer)				
atorvastatin calcium				
TAB, PO, 10 mg, 90s ea	00071-0155-23	309.24	257.70	
(10X10,HOSPITAL USE)				
10 mg, 100s ea UD	00071-0155-40	360.77	300.64	
5000s ea	00071-0155-34	17180.00	14316.67	
20 mg, 90s ea	00071-0156-23	441.11	367.59	
(10X10,HOSPITAL USE)				
20 mg, 100s ea UD	00071-0156-40	514.64	428.87	
5000s ea	00071-0156-94	24506.00	20421.67	
40 mg, 90s ea	00071-0157-23	441.11	367.59	
(10X10)				
40 mg, 100s ea UD	00071-0157-40	514.64	428.87	
500s ea	00071-0157-73	2450.59	2042.16	
2500s ea	00071-0157-88	12253.00	10210.83	
(8X8)				
80 mg, 64s ea UD	00071-0158-92	329.38	274.48	
90s ea	00071-0158-23	441.11	367.59	
500s ea	00071-0158-73	2450.59	2042.16	
2500s ea	00071-0158-88	12253.00	10210.83	
(A-S Medication)				
REPACK				
TAB, PO, 10 mg, 30s ea	54569-4466-00	100.35		
90s ea	54569-4466-02	375.71		
100s ea	54569-4466-01	417.46		
20 mg, 30s ea	54569-4467-00	143.14		
90s ea	54569-4467-01	535.93		
40 mg, 30s ea	54569-4587-00	143.14		
90s ea	54569-4587-01	535.93		
80 mg, 30s ea	54569-5382-00	143.14		
(Advanced Pharm Serv, Inc.)				
REPACK				
TAB, PO, 10 mg, 10s ea	13411-0113-01	38.45		
15s ea	13411-0113-15	55.17		
30s ea	13411-0113-03	105.35		
60s ea	13411-0113-06	205.70		
90s ea	13411-0113-09	306.05		
20 mg, 10s ea	13411-0114-01	52.71		
15s ea	13411-0114-15	76.57		
30s ea	13411-0114-03	148.14		
60s ea	13411-0114-06	291.29		
90s ea	13411-0114-09	434.43		
40 mg, 10s ea	13411-0115-01	52.71		
15s ea	13411-0115-15	76.57		
30s ea	13411-0115-03	148.14		
60s ea	13411-0115-06	291.29		
LIPITOR (Advanced Pharm Serv, Inc.)				
REPACK				
atorvastatin calcium				
TAB, PO, 40 mg, 90s ea	13411-0115-09	434.43		
(AQ)				
REPACK				
TAB, PO, 10 mg, 90s ea	66105-0113-09	306.05		
20 mg, 90s ea	66105-0114-09	434.43		
40 mg, 90s ea	66105-0115-09	434.43		
(Bryant Ranch)				
REPACK				
TAB, PO, 10 mg, 30s ea	63629-1446-02	72.68		
90s ea	63629-1446-01	338.23		
20 mg, 30s ea	63629-1447-01	119.65		
(Core)				
REPACK				
TAB, PO, 10 mg, 30s ea	33358-0210-30	91.36		
60s ea	33358-0210-60	184.58		
90s ea	33358-0210-90	277.52		
120s ea	33358-0210-01	368.42		
(DHS, Inc.)				
REPACK				
TAB, PO, 10 mg, 90s ea	55887-0624-90	290.00		
20 mg, 30s ea	55887-0730-30	172.50		
60s ea	55887-0730-60	345.00		
90s ea	55887-0730-90	517.50		
(Direct Pharmaceutical, Inc.)				
REPACK				
TAB, PO, 10 mg, 30s ea UD	67801-0301-03	215.88		
20 mg, 30s ea UD	67801-0402-30	177.33		
40 mg, 30s ea UD	67801-0314-03	207.23		
(Dispensing Solutions)				
REPACK				
TAB, PO, 10 mg, 90s ea	68258-6000-09	345.60		
20 mg, 90s ea	68258-6001-09	489.89		
40 mg, 90s ea	68258-6002-09	480.89		
(HomeMed)				
REPACK				
TAB, PO, 10 mg, 30s ea	51655-0226-24	72.56		
(Nucare Pharm)				
REPACK				
TAB, PO, 10 mg, 30s ea	68071-0399-30	151.00		
20 mg, 30s ea	68071-0154-30	215.00		
40 mg, 30s ea	68071-0310-30	215.00		
(PD-Rx Pharm)				
REPACK				
TAB, PO, 10 mg, 30s ea	55289-0870-30	154.53		
30s ea	58864-0608-30	125.85		
20 mg, 30s ea	55289-0800-30	195.51		
30s ea	58864-0685-30	195.51		
40 mg, 15s ea	58864-0623-15	105.67		
30s ea	55289-0861-30	195.51		
(REDI-SCRIPT)				
40 mg, 30s ea	58864-0623-30	177.33		
80 mg, 30s ea	58864-0834-30	204.24		
(Pharma Pac)				
REPACK				
TAB, PO, 10 mg, 90s ea	52959-0759-90	232.55		
20 mg, 90s ea	52959-0760-90	337.43		
40 mg, 30s ea	52959-0046-30	109.92		
(Phys Total Care)				
REPACK				
TAB, PO, 10 mg, 10s ea	54868-3934-03	45.68		
30s ea	54868-3934-00	131.81		
60s ea	54868-3934-02	246.65		
90s ea	54868-3934-01	368.01		
20 mg, 15s ea	54868-3946-01	94.76		
30s ea	54868-3946-00	176.67		
60s ea	54868-3946-03	350.73		
90s ea	54868-3946-02	507.29		
40 mg, 15s ea	54868-4229-02	94.76		
30s ea	54868-4229-00	176.67		
45s ea	54868-4229-03	263.70		
90s ea	54868-4229-01	507.29		
80 mg, 30s ea	54868-4934-00	176.67		
90s ea	54868-4934-01	507.29		
(Quality Care Prod)				
REPACK				
TAB, PO, 10 mg, 30s ea	49999-0392-30	160.50		
90s ea	49999-0392-90	481.50		
20 mg, 30s ea	49999-0467-30	228.00		
90s ea	49999-0467-90	684.00		
40 mg, 30s ea	49999-0468-30	228.00		
90s ea	49999-0468-90	684.00		
80 mg, 30s ea	49999-0882-30	401.94		
90s ea	49999-0882-90	1205.82		
(Southwood)				
REPACK				
TAB, PO, 80 mg, 30s ea	58016-0051-30	130.87		
60s ea	58016-0051-60	261.75		
90s ea	58016-0051-90	392.62		
100s ea	58016-0051-00	436.24		
LIPMAX (Medisca)				
isopropyl palmitate/lecithin				
SOL, NA (1X100ML)				
100 ml	38779-2301-05	19.50		
(1X500ML) 500 ml	38779-2301-08	58.50		
(1X1000ML) 1000 ml	38779-2301-09	109.50		
(1X4000ML) 4000 ml	38779-2301-01	405.00		
LIPO CREAM BASE (Medisca)				
cream, multi ingredient				
CRE, NA (1X100GM)				
100 gm	38779-2259-05	76.50		
(1X500GM) 500 gm	38779-2259-08	229.50		
(1X5000GM) 5000 gm	38779-2259-03	1845.00		
(1X10000GM) 10000 gm	38779-2259-00	3285.00		
LIPOFEN (Kowa)				
fenofibrate				
CAP, PO (HARD GELATIN)				
50 mg, 90s ea	66869-0137-30	140.21	116.84	
150 mg, 90s ea	66869-0147-30	307.46	256.22	
LIPOIC ACID (Medisca)				
thioctic acid				
POW, NA (1X1GM,REAGENT)				
1 gm	38779-2113-06	37.50		
(1X5GM,REAGENT) 5 gm	38779-2113-03	114.00		
(1X25GM,REAGENT) 25 gm	38779-2113-04	459.00		
(1X100GM,REAGENT) 100 gm	38779-2113-05	1215.00		
(PCCA)				
POW, NA (DL-ALPHA)				
1 gm	51927-2781-00	25.20		
(Spectrum Pharmacy)				
POW, NA (REAGENT)				
5 gm	49452-4083-02	185.15		
25 gm	49452-4083-03	735.00		
(1X100GM) 100 gm	49452-4083-04	1820.00		
LIPOIL (Gallipot)				
isopropyl palmitate/lecithin				
OIL, NA (PRESERVED)				
100 ml	51552-0550-04	9.80		
473 ml	51552-0550-06	18.20		
LIPOSYN II (Abbott Hosp)				
safflower oil/soybean oil				
EMU, IV (W/ADMIN. SET)				
10%-10%, 500 ml 8s	00074-9793-01	280.44	236.16	
(Hospira)				
EMU, IV, 5%-5%, 200 ml 6s	00409-9786-01	181.44	158.76	
(12X250ML,SINGLE-DOSE) 5%-5%, 250 ml 12s	00409-9786-02	201.89	176.64	
(12X500ML) 5%-5%, 500 ml 12s	00409-9786-03	153.07	133.92	
(12X200ML,SINGLE-DOSE) 10%-10%, 200 ml 12s	00409-9789-01	181.44	158.76	
(12X250ML,SINGLE-DOSE) 10%-10%, 250 ml 12s	00409-9789-02	194.40	170.16	
(SINGLE DOSE,12X500ML) 10%-10%, 500 ml 12s	00409-9789-03	289.01	252.84	
LIPOSYN III (Hospira)				
soybean oil				
EMU, IV (12X250ML)				
10%, 250 ml 12s	00409-9790-02	192.67	168.60	AP
500 ml 12s	00409-9790-03	170.64	149.28	AP
(12X500ML,SINGLE DOSE) 10%, 500 ml 12s	00409-9790-01	181.44	158.76	AP
(12X200ML,SINGLE-DOSE) 20%, 200 ml 12s	00409-9791-01	155.23	135.84	AP
(12X250ML,SINGLE-DOSE) 20%, 250 ml 12s	00409-9791-02	173.66	151.92	AP
(12X500ML,SINGLE DOSE) 20%, 500 ml 12s	00409-9791-03	272.59	238.56	AP
(12X500ML) 30%, 500 ml 12s	00409-6892-03	390.96	342.12	AP
LIPOVAN BASE (Gallipot)				
paste base				
PAS, NA, 454 gm	51552-1022-06	81.90	58.50	
LIPRAM 4500 (Global Pharm)				
amylase/lipase/protease				
ECC, PO (MICROSPHERES,DYE-FREE)				
20000 u-4500 u-25000 u, 100s ea	00115-7035-01	60.03		
LIPRAM-PN10 (Global Pharm)				
amylase/lipase/protease				
ECC, PO (MICROSPHERES)				
30000 u-10000 u-30000 u, 100s ea	00115-7040-01	119.23		
LIPRAM-PN16 (Global Pharm)				
amylase/lipase/protease				
ECC, PO (MICROSPHERES)				
48000 u-16000 u-48000 u, 100s ea	00115-7023-01	191.44		

PROD/MFR	NDC	AWP	DP	OBC
LIPRAM-PN20 (Global Pharm)				
amylase/lipase/protease				
ECC, PO (MICROSPHERES)				
56000 u-20000 u-44000 u,				
100s ea	00115-7055-01	226.66		
LIQUADD (Auriga)				
dextroamphetamine sulfate				
SOL, PO (1X473ML,BUBBLE GUM)				
5 mg/5 ml,				
473 ml, C-II	14629-0117-16	174.99		
LIQUI-DUALCITRA (ANI)				
citric acid/sodium citrate				
SOL, PO (SF,GRAPE)				
334 mg/5 ml-500 mg/5 ml,				
473 ml	62559-8041-06	9.60		
LIQUIBID-D (Capellon)				
guaifenesin/phenylephrine hydrochloride				
TER, PO (DUOMATRIX,BI-LAYERED)				
650 mg-40 mg,				
90s ea	64543-0150-90	99.38		
LIQUIBID-D 1200 (Capellon)				
guaifenesin/phenylephrine hydrochloride				
TER, PO (DUOMATRIX,BIPHASIC)				
1200 mg-40 mg,				
90s ea	64543-0240-90	112.63		
100s ea	64543-0140-01	93.71		
LIQUIBID-PD (Capellon)				
guaifenesin/phenylephrine hydrochloride				
TER, PO, 275 mg-25 mg,				
100s ea	64543-0146-01	71.62		
(DUOMATRIX SYSTEM)				
315 mg-20 mg,				
90s ea	64543-0246-90	92.75		
LIQUICOUGH DM (Breckenridge Pharm)				
dm/gg/pse hcl				
SOL, PO (AF,SF,GRAPE)				
473 ml	51991-0646-16	50.54		
LIQUICOUGH HC (Breckenridge Pharm)				
cpm/hydrocod bit/phenyleph hcl				
SOL, PO (AF,SF,RASPBERRY)				
473 ml, C-III	51991-0372-16	42.81		
LIQUID BASE				
(PCCA) *See BASE, PCCA FIXED OIL SUSPENSION VEHICLE*				
(PCCA) *See PCCA LECITHIN ISOPROPYL PALMITATE*				
(PCCA) *See PCCA SWEET-SF*				
(PCCA) *See PCCA SYRUP VEHICLE*				
(PCCA) *See PCCA-PLUS*				
LIRAGLUTIDE				
(Novo Nordisk) *See VICTOZA*				
LISDEXAMFETAMINE DIMESYLATE				
(Shire US Inc.) *See VYVANSE*				
LISINOPRIL				
FUL				
TAB, PO, 2.5 mg, 100s ea		3.68		
5 mg, 100s ea		4.83		
10 mg, 100s ea		6.75		
20 mg, 100s ea		7.95		
30 mg, 100s ea		16.31		
40 mg, 100s ea		15.00		
(Apotex Corp.)				
TAB, PO, 2.5 mg, 100s ea	60505-0184-00	64.25		AB
(USP)				
2.5 mg, 100s ea	60505-2683-01	64.25		AB
1000s ea	60505-0184-01	636.08		AB
5 mg, 90s ea	60505-0185-09	86.70		AB
(USP)				
5 mg, 90s ea	60505-2684-09	86.70		AB
100s ea	60505-0185-00	96.33		AB
(USP)				
5 mg, 100s ea	60505-2684-01	96.33		AB
1000s ea	60505-0185-01	953.19		AB
1000s ea	60505-2684-08	953.19		AB
22500s ea	60505-0185-07	21446.78		AB
10 mg, 90s ea	60505-0186-09	89.52		AB
(USP)				
10 mg, 90s ea	60505-2685-09	89.52		AB
100s ea	60505-0186-00	99.47		AB
(USP)				
10 mg, 100s ea	60505-2685-01	99.47		AB
1000s ea	60505-0186-01	985.37		AB
(USP)				
10 mg, 1000s ea	60505-2685-08	985.37		AB
15500s ea	60505-0186-07	15273.24		AB
20 mg, 90s ea	60505-0187-09	95.84		AB
(USP)				
20 mg, 90s ea	60505-2686-09	95.84		AB
100s ea	60505-0187-00	106.49		AB
(USP)				
20 mg, 100s ea	60505-2686-01	106.49		AB
1000s ea	60505-0187-01	1054.58		AB
(USP)				
20 mg, 1000s ea	60505-2686-08	1054.58		AB
17500s ea	60505-0187-07	18455.15		AB
30 mg, 100s ea	60505-0188-00	150.75		AB
1000s ea	60505-0188-01	1492.51		AB
40 mg, 90s ea	60505-0189-09	140.16		AB
(USP)				
40 mg, 90s ea	60505-2688-09	140.16		AB
100s ea	60505-0189-00	155.73		AB
(USP)				
40 mg, 100s ea	60505-2688-01	155.73		AB
1000s ea	60505-0189-01	1541.78		AB
(USP)				
40 mg, 1000s ea	60505-2688-08	1541.78		AB
10100s ea	60505-0189-08	15571.98		AB
(AstraZeneca) *See ZESTRIL*				
(Aurobindo Pharma)				
TAB, PO (USP)				
2.5 mg, 100s ea	65862-0037-01	64.20		AB
500s ea	65862-0037-05	315.00		AB
(USP)				
5 mg, 100s ea	65862-0038-01	95.20		AB
500s ea	65862-0038-05	472.05		AB
(USP)				
10 mg, 100s ea	65862-0039-01	97.90		AB
500s ea	65862-0039-05	487.45		AB
(USP)				
20 mg, 100s ea	65862-0040-01	105.60		AB
500s ea	65862-0040-05	528.00		AB
30 mg, 100s ea	65862-0041-01	149.05		AB
40 mg, 100s ea	65862-0042-01	153.95		AB
500s ea	65862-0042-05	769.75		AB
(Blu)				
TAB, PO (USP)				
2.5 mg, 90s ea	24658-0240-90	3.04		AB
1000s ea	24658-0240-10	27.41		AB
5 mg, 30s ea	24658-0241-30	1.34		AB
45s ea	24658-0241-45	1.69		AB
90s ea	24658-0241-90	2.76		AB
1000s ea	24658-0241-10	23.63		AB
10 mg, 15s ea	24658-0242-15	1.15		AB
30s ea	24658-0242-30	1.67		AB
45s ea	24658-0242-45	2.19		AB
90s ea	24658-0242-90	3.75		AB
180s ea	24658-0242-18	6.87		AB
1000s ea	24658-0242-10	34.65		AB
20 mg, 15s ea	24658-0243-15	1.58		AB
30s ea	24658-0243-30	2.52		AB
45s ea	24658-0243-45	3.47		AB
90s ea	24658-0243-90	6.30		AB
180s ea	24658-0243-18	11.97		AB
1000s ea	24658-0243-10	63.00		AB
30 mg, 100s ea	24658-0244-01	9.14		AB
1000s ea	24658-0244-10	94.50		AB
40 mg, 15s ea	24658-0245-15	1.83		AB
30s ea	24658-0245-30	3.04		AB
45s ea	24658-0245-45	4.24		AB
60s ea	24658-0245-60	5.45		AB
90s ea	24658-0245-90	7.86		AB
180s ea	24658-0245-18	15.09		AB
1000s ea	24658-0245-10	80.33		AB
(Greenstone)				
TAB, PO (USP)				
2.5 mg, 30s ea	59762-2270-01	19.26		
100s ea	59762-2270-03	64.20		
500s ea	59762-2270-07	315.00		
5 mg, 30s ea	59762-2271-01	28.56		
100s ea	59762-2271-03	95.20		
500s ea	59762-2271-07	472.05		
10 mg, 30s ea	59762-2272-01	29.37		
100s ea	59762-2272-03	97.90		
500s ea	59762-2272-07	487.45		
20 mg, 30s ea	59762-2273-01	31.68		
100s ea	59762-2273-03	105.60		
500s ea	59762-2273-07	528.00		
30 mg, 30s ea	59762-2274-01	44.72		
100s ea	59762-2274-03	149.05		
500s ea	59762-2274-07	745.25		
(Lupin Pharma, Inc.)				
TAB, PO, 2.5 mg, 100s ea	68180-0512-01	64.83		
500s ea	68180-0512-02	320.91		
5 mg, 100s ea	68180-0513-01	96.23		
1000s ea	68180-0513-03	952.29		
10 mg, 100s ea	68180-0514-01	99.37		
1000s ea	68180-0514-03	984.48		
20 mg, 100s ea	68180-0515-01	106.37		
1000s ea	68180-0515-03	1053.41		
30 mg, 100s ea	68180-0516-01	150.70		
500s ea	68180-0516-02	745.90		
40 mg, 100s ea	68180-0517-01	155.71		
1000s ea	68180-0517-03	1541.58		
(Major)				
TAB, PO (USP)				
2.5 mg, 90s ea	00904-5812-89	56.67		AB
500s ea	00904-5812-40	304.86		AB
5 mg, 30s ea	00904-5811-46	11.22		AB
45s ea	00904-5811-43	16.83		AB
90s ea	00904-5811-89	33.66		AB
(USP,10X10)				
5 mg, 100s ea UD	00904-5811-61	48.00		AB
(USP)				
5 mg, 1000s ea	00904-5811-80	1078.31		AB
10 mg, 15s ea	00904-5808-48	5.79		AB
30s ea	00904-5808-46	11.58		AB
45s ea	00904-5808-43	17.38		AB
90s ea	00904-5808-89	34.75		AB
(USP,10X10)				
10 mg, 100s ea UD	00904-5808-61	51.00		AB
(USP)				
10 mg, 180s ea	00904-5808-93	69.51		AB
1000s ea	00904-5808-80	1050.04		AB
20 mg, 15s ea	00904-5809-48	23.32		AB
30s ea	00904-5809-46	12.40		AB
45s ea	00904-5809-43	18.60		AB
90s ea	00904-5809-89	37.20		AB
(USP,10X10)				
20 mg, 100s ea UD	00904-5809-61	57.00		AB
(USP)				
20 mg, 180s ea	00904-5809-93	74.90		AB
1000s ea	00904-5809-80	1123.78		AB
(USP,SF)				
40 mg, 15s ea	00904-5810-48	8.79		AB
30s ea	00904-5810-46	17.58		AB
(USP)				
40 mg, 45s ea	00904-5810-43	26.37		AB
(USP,SF)				
40 mg, 60s ea	00904-5810-52	35.16		AB
90s ea	00904-5810-89	52.73		AB
(USP,10X10)				
40 mg, 100s ea UD	00904-5810-61	77.00		AB
(USP,SF)				
40 mg, 180s ea	00904-5810-93	105.47		AB
(USP)				
40 mg, 1000s ea	00904-5810-80	1493.51		AB
(Merck) *See PRINIVIL*				
(Mylan)				
TAB, PO, 2.5 mg, 100s ea	00378-2072-01	64.20		AB
5 mg, 100s ea	00378-2073-01	96.25		AB
1000s ea	00378-2073-10	952.15		AB
10 mg, 100s ea	00378-2074-01	99.40		AB
1000s ea	00378-2074-10	984.30		AB
20 mg, 100s ea	00378-2075-01	106.40		AB
1000s ea	00378-2075-10	1053.45		AB
30 mg, 100s ea	00378-2077-01	150.60		EE
40 mg, 100s ea	00378-2076-01	155.60		AB
(USP)				
40 mg, 500s ea	00378-2076-05	778.00		AB
(PCCA)				
POW, NA (USP)				
1 gm	51927-3471-00	21.60		
(Ranbaxy Pharm)				
TAB, PO, 2.5 mg, 100s ea	63304-0531-01	64.85		AB
5 mg, 100s ea	63304-0532-01	97.25		AB
1000s ea	63304-0532-10	962.27		AB
10 mg, 100s ea	63304-0533-01	100.42		AB
1000s ea	63304-0533-10	994.77		AB
20 mg, 100s ea	63304-0534-01	107.51		AB
1000s ea	63304-0534-10	1064.64		AB
(USP)				
30 mg, 100s ea	63304-0599-01	150.76		AB
40 mg, 100s ea	63304-0535-01	157.21		AB
1000s ea	63304-0535-10	1556.40		AB
(Sandoz)				
TAB, PO, 2.5 mg, 100s ea	00185-0025-01	64.85		AB
100s ea	66685-0701-01	64.20		AB
1000s ea	00185-0025-10	648.54		AB
1000s ea	66685-0701-02	641.36		AB
5 mg, 100s ea	00185-5400-01	97.25		AB
100s ea	66685-0702-01	96.25		AB
1000s ea	00185-5400-10	972.50		AB
1000s ea	66685-0702-02	961.53		AB
5000s ea	66685-0702-03	4807.65		AB
10 mg, 100s ea	00185-0101-01	100.42		AB
100s ea	00781-1666-01	100.42		AB
100s ea	66685-0703-01	99.40		AB
1000s ea	00185-0101-10	1004.20		AB

PROD/MFR	NDC	AWP	DP	OBC
1000s ea	66685-0703-02	993.00		AB
3000s ea	00185-0101-33	3012.66		AB
5000s ea	66685-0703-03	4965.00		AB
20 mg, 100s ea	00185-0102-01	107.51		AB
100s ea	66685-0704-01	106.40		AB
1000s ea	00185-0102-10	1075.10		AB
1000s ea	66685-0704-02	1062.94		AB
3000s ea	00185-0102-33	3225.15		AB
5000s ea	66685-0704-03	5314.70		AB
30 mg, 100s ea	00185-0103-01	150.76		AB
100s ea	66685-0705-01	150.60		AB
500s ea	66685-0705-02	752.25		AB
1000s ea	00185-0103-10	1507.59		AB
40 mg, 100s ea	00185-0104-01	157.21		AB
100s ea	66685-0706-01	155.60		AB
1000s ea	00185-0104-10	1572.12		AB
1000s ea	66685-0706-03	1554.44		AB
2000s ea	66685-0706-04	3108.88		AB
(Teva)				
TAB, PO, 2.5 mg, 100s ea (10X10)	00172-3757-60	63.55		AB
2.5 mg, 100s ea UD	00172-3757-10	65.55		AB
500s ea	00172-3757-70	314.50		AB
5 mg, 100s ea (10X10)	00172-3758-60	95.25		AB
5 mg, 100s ea UD	00172-3758-10	97.25		AB
500s ea	00172-3758-70	471.55		AB
1000s ea	00172-3758-80	942.60		AB
10 mg, 100s ea (10X10)	00172-3759-60	98.35		AB
10 mg, 100s ea UD	00172-3759-10	100.35		AB
500s ea	00172-3759-70	486.95		AB
1000s ea	00172-3759-80	974.45		AB
20 mg, 100s ea (10X10)	00172-3760-60	105.30		AB
20 mg, 100s ea UD	00172-3760-10	107.30		AB
500s ea	00172-3760-70	521.30		AB
1000s ea	00172-3760-80	1042.85		AB
30 mg, 100s ea (10X10)	00172-3762-60	149.10		AB
30 mg, 100s ea UD	00172-3762-10	151.10		AB
500s ea	00172-3762-70	737.95		AB
40 mg, 100s ea (10X10)	00172-3761-60	154.00		AB
40 mg, 100s ea UD	00172-3761-10	156.00		AB
500s ea	00172-3761-70	762.30		AB
1000s ea	00172-3761-80	1524.65		AB
(UDL) *See LISINOPRIL*				
(UDL)				
TAB, PO (10X10)				
5 mg, 100s ea UD	51079-0981-20	91.44		AB
LISINOPRIL (UDL) (USP,PUNCH CARDS,10X30)				
5 mg, 300s ea UD	51079-0981-56	274.32		AB
LISINOPRIL (UDL) (10X10)				
10 mg, 100s ea UD	51079-0982-20	94.43		AB
LISINOPRIL (UDL) (USP,PUNCH CARDS,10X30)				
10 mg, 300s ea UD	51079-0982-56	283.29		AB
LISINOPRIL (UDL) (10X10)				
20 mg, 100s ea UD	51079-0983-20	101.10		AB
LISINOPRIL (UDL) (USP,PUNCH CARDS,10X30)				
20 mg, 300s ea UD	51079-0983-56	303.30		AB
LISINOPRIL (UDL) (10X10)				
40 mg, 100s ea UD	51079-0984-20	147.84		AB
(Watson Labs)				
TAB, PO, 2.5 mg, 100s ea	00591-0405-01	2.94		AB
500s ea	00591-0405-05	14.70		AB
5 mg, 100s ea	00591-0406-01	3.86		AB
1000s ea	00591-0406-10	36.73		AB
10 mg, 100s ea	00591-0407-01	5.44		AB
1000s ea	00591-0407-10	51.65		AB
20 mg, 100s ea	00591-0408-01	8.15		AB
1000s ea	00591-0408-10	77.36		AB
30 mg, 100s ea	00591-0885-01	13.04		AB
40 mg, 100s ea	00591-0409-01	14.69		AB
500s ea	00591-0409-05	73.44		AB
(USP)				
40 mg, 500s ea	00591-0409-75	73.44		AB
(West-Ward)				
TAB, PO, 2.5 mg, 100s ea	00143-1265-01	64.15		AB
1000s ea	00143-1265-10	639.78		AB
5 mg, 100s ea	00143-1266-01	96.20		AB
1000s ea	00143-1266-10	953.10		AB
10 mg, 100s ea	00143-1267-01	99.45		AB
1000s ea	00143-1267-10	987.45		AB
20 mg, 100s ea	00143-1268-01	106.80		AB
1000s ea	00143-1268-10	1055.50		AB
(USP)				
30 mg, 100s ea	00143-1280-01	150.76		AB
1000s ea	00143-1280-10	1492.51		AB
40 mg, 100s ea	00143-1270-01	125.50		AB
1000s ea	00143-1270-10	1542.24		AB
(Wockhardt USA)				
TAB, PO, 2.5 mg, 100s ea	64679-0927-01	64.80		AB
500s ea	64679-0927-05	314.52		AB
1000s ea	64679-0927-02	629.04		AB
5 mg, 100s ea	64679-0928-01	97.20		AB
500s ea	64679-0928-05	471.42		AB
1000s ea	64679-0928-06	942.84		AB
10 mg, 100s ea	64679-0929-01	94.40		AB
500s ea	64679-0929-05	457.84		AB
1000s ea	64679-0929-06	915.68		AB
20 mg, 100s ea	64679-0941-01	101.05		AB
500s ea	64679-0941-05	490.09		AB
1000s ea	64679-0941-06	980.19		AB
30 mg, 100s ea	64679-0953-01	148.95		AB
500s ea	64679-0953-05	722.41		AB
1000s ea	64679-0953-02	1444.82		AB
40 mg, 100s ea	64679-0942-01	153.95		AB
500s ea	64679-0942-05	746.66		AB
1000s ea	64679-0942-02	1493.32		AB
(A-S Medication) REPACK				
TAB, PO, 2.5 mg, 30s ea	54569-5437-00	19.46		AB
5 mg, 30s ea	54569-5438-00	29.18		AB
10 mg, 30s ea	54569-5434-00	30.13		AB
60s ea	54569-5434-03	60.25		AB
200s ea	54569-5434-04	200.84		AB
20 mg, 30s ea	54569-5435-00	32.25		AB
60s ea	54569-5435-03	64.51		AB
200s ea	54569-5435-04	215.02		AB
30 mg, 30s ea	54569-5728-00	45.23		EE
40 mg, 30s ea	54569-5472-00	47.16		AB
(Aidarex) REPACK				
TAB, PO, 10 mg, 7s ea	33261-0332-07	7.00		AB
14s ea	33261-0332-14	14.00		AB
20s ea	33261-0332-20	20.00		AB
21s ea	33261-0332-21	21.00		AB
28s ea	33261-0332-28	28.00		AB
30s ea	33261-0332-30	30.00		AB
60s ea	33261-0332-60	60.00		AB
90s ea	33261-0332-90	90.00		AB
20 mg, 7s ea	33261-0110-07	11.20		AB
14s ea	33261-0110-14	22.40		AB
20s ea	33261-0110-20	32.00		AB
21s ea	33261-0110-21	33.60		AB
28s ea	33261-0110-28	44.80		AB
30s ea	33261-0110-30	48.00		AB
60s ea	33261-0110-60	96.00		AB
90s ea	33261-0110-90	144.00		AB
(Altura) REPACK				
TAB, PO, 5 mg, 10s ea	63874-0558-10	8.51		
14s ea	63874-0558-14	13.61		
16s ea	63874-0558-16	15.55		
28s ea	63874-0558-28	23.81		
30s ea	63874-0558-30	25.52		
60s ea	63874-0558-60	51.03		
90s ea	63874-0558-90	76.55		
100s ea	63874-0558-01	85.05		
30 mg, 90s ea	63874-1114-09	159.39		
40 mg, 10s ea	63874-0618-10	15.40		AB
15s ea	63874-0618-15	23.10		AB
30s ea	63874-0618-30	46.20		AB
40s ea	63874-0618-40	61.60		AB
60s ea	63874-0618-60	92.40		AB
(American Health) REPACK				
TAB, PO (USP,10X10)				
2.5 mg, 100s ea UD	68084-0058-01	62.95		
5 mg, 100s ea UD	68084-0060-01	87.20		
10 mg, 100s ea UD	68084-0061-01	92.60		
20 mg, 100s ea UD	68084-0062-01	98.86		
40 mg, 100s ea UD	68084-0064-01	142.20		
(Bryant Ranch) REPACK				
TAB, PO, 10 mg, 30s ea	63629-2688-01	30.85		
20 mg, 30s ea	63629-2908-01	51.00		
60s ea	63629-2908-02	102.00		
90s ea	63629-2908-03	153.00		
40 mg, 30s ea	63629-2935-01	75.00		
(Core) REPACK				
TAB, PO, 5 mg, 30s ea	33358-0211-30	30.74		
10 mg, 30s ea	33358-0212-30	31.62		
20 mg, 30s ea	33358-0213-30	52.28		
(DHS, Inc.) REPACK				
TAB, PO, 2.5 mg, 30s ea	55887-0590-30	18.91		AB
60s ea	55887-0590-60	36.82		AB
90s ea	55887-0590-90	52.00		AB
5 mg, 30s ea	55887-0589-30	30.09		AB
90s ea	55887-0589-90	88.71		AB
10 mg, 20s ea	55887-0591-20	19.97		
30s ea	55887-0591-30	29.95		AB
60s ea	55887-0591-60	58.90		AB
90s ea	55887-0591-90	86.09		AB
100s ea	55887-0591-01	99.85		
20 mg, 30s ea	55887-0581-30	32.09		AB
60s ea	55887-0581-60	61.58		AB
90s ea	55887-0581-90	90.05		AB
40 mg, 30s ea	55887-0569-30	35.00		AB
60s ea	55887-0569-60	65.00		AB
90s ea	55887-0569-90	80.05		AB
(Dispensing Solutions) REPACK				
TAB, PO, 2.5 mg, 30s ea	55045-3059-08	22.50		
100s ea	55045-3059-00	75.00		
5 mg, 30s ea	55045-2938-08	28.80		
100s ea	55045-2938-00	96.00		
10 mg, 30s ea	55045-2929-08	29.70		
30s ea	66336-0972-30	35.67		AB
60s ea	55045-2929-06	59.40		
90s ea	66336-0972-90	89.51		AB
100s ea	55045-2937-00	99.00		
20 mg, 30s ea	55045-2936-08	31.80		
30s ea	55045-3772-08	31.80		
30s ea	66336-0741-30	32.25		
90s ea	66336-0741-90	96.76		AB
100s ea	55045-2936-00	106.00		
40 mg, 30s ea	55045-2975-08	46.50		
30s ea	66336-0867-30	46.50		
60s ea	55045-2975-06	93.00		
90s ea	66336-0867-90	139.50		
100s ea	55045-2975-00	155.00		
(GSMS) REPACK				
TAB, PO, 2.5 mg, 30s ea	60429-0728-30	5.10	1.70	AB
100s ea	60429-0728-01	9.00	3.00	AB
1000s ea	60429-0728-10	66.60	22.20	AB
5 mg, 30s ea	60429-0729-30	5.40	1.80	AB
(USP)				
5 mg, 45s ea	60429-0729-45	7.02	2.34	AB
90s ea	60429-0729-90	13.35	4.45	AB
100s ea	60429-0729-01	13.35	4.45	AB
1000s ea	60429-0729-10	71.97	23.99	AB
10 mg, 30s ea	60429-0730-30	6.12	2.04	AB
(USP)				
10 mg, 45s ea	60429-0730-45	8.10	2.70	AB
90s ea	60429-0730-90	13.86	4.62	AB
100s ea	60429-0730-01	13.65	4.55	AB
1000s ea	60429-0730-10	99.75	33.25	AB
20 mg, 30s ea	60429-0731-30	7.92	2.64	AB
(USP)				
20 mg, 45s ea	60429-0731-45	10.80	3.60	AB
90s ea	60429-0731-90	19.26	6.42	AB
100s ea	60429-0731-01	20.55	6.85	AB
1000s ea	60429-0731-10	201.51	67.17	AB
30 mg, 30s ea	60429-0732-30	10.08	3.36	AB
90s ea	60429-0732-90	24.30	8.10	AB
1000s ea	60429-0732-10	218.58	72.86	AB
40 mg, 30s ea	60429-0733-30	11.70	3.90	AB
(USP)				
40 mg, 45s ea	60429-0733-45	16.38	5.46	AB
90s ea	60429-0733-90	30.24	10.08	AB
100s ea	60429-0733-01	38.55	12.85	AB
1000s ea	60429-0733-10	213.57	71.19	AB
(HomeMed) REPACK				
TAB, PO, 5 mg, 30s ea	51655-0231-24	29.99		
10 mg, 30s ea	51655-0244-24	29.99		
20 mg, 30s ea	51655-0280-24	30.99		
40 mg, 30s ea	51655-0292-24	39.99		
(IPI) REPACK				
TAB, PO, 5 mg, 30s ea	18837-0277-30	35.71		
(Keltman Pharma., Inc.) REPACK				
TAB, PO, 10 mg, 30s ea	68387-0543-30	31.16		

PROD/MFR	NDC	AWP	DP	OBC
(McKesson Packaging)				
REPACK				
TAB, PO, 10 mg,				
100s ea UD	63739-0349-10	123.65		
(USP)				
20 mg, 100s ea UD	63739-0350-10	132.37		
(Nucare Pharm)				
REPACK				
TAB, PO, 10 mg, 30s ea	66267-0577-30	31.63		AB
60s ea	66267-0577-60	63.24		AB
90s ea	66267-0577-90	94.86		AB
20 mg, 30s ea	66267-0570-30	34.90		AB
60s ea	66267-0570-60	69.79		AB
90s ea	66267-0570-90	97.84		AB
40 mg, 30s ea	66267-0583-30	47.25		AB
60s ea	66267-0583-60	94.50		AB
90s ea	66267-0583-90	141.75		AB
(Palmetto)				
REPACK				
TAB, PO, 2.5 mg, 30s ea	23490-5817-02	22.50		
5 mg, 30s ea	23490-5819-02	30.09		
10 mg, 10s ea	23490-5815-00	10.40		
30s ea	23490-5815-01	31.21		
20 mg, 30s ea	23490-5816-01	33.42		
60s ea	23490-5816-06	67.30		
90s ea	23490-5816-02	100.26		
40 mg, 30s ea	23490-5818-02	55.52		
(PD-Rx Pharm)				
REPACK				
TAB, PO (USP)				
2.5 mg, 90s ea	43063-0138-90	32.68		AB
(REDI-SCRIPT)				
5 mg, 30s ea	58864-0753-30	12.78		AB
(USP)				
5 mg, 30s ea	55289-0884-30	14.08		AB
90s ea	58864-0753-90	25.00		AB
(USP)				
5 mg, 90s ea	55289-0884-90	21.40		AB
10 mg, 12s ea	55289-0638-12	9.00		
14s ea	55289-0638-14	13.20		AB
15s ea	58864-0603-15	13.67		AB
30s ea	55289-0638-30	20.67		AB
30s ea	58864-0603-30	20.66		AB
90s ea	55289-0638-90	48.67		AB
(REDI-SCRIPT)				
10 mg, 90s ea	58864-0603-90	48.66		AB
100s ea	55289-0638-01	53.33		AB
120s ea	55289-0638-98	61.38		
20 mg, 14s ea	55289-0696-14	16.24		AB
30s ea	55289-0696-30	25.33		AB
30s ea	58864-0000-63	25.34		
(USP)				
20 mg, 30s ea	58864-0006-30	25.34		AB
90s ea	55289-0696-90	58.67		
100s ea	43063-0007-01	105.30		AB
120s ea	55289-0696-98	92.00		
30 mg, 30s ea	58864-0750-30	24.00		AB
40 mg, 15s ea	58864-0618-15	7.95		
(REDI-SCRIPT)				
40 mg, 30s ea	58864-0618-30	20.67		AB
(USP)				
40 mg, 30s ea	55289-0917-30	27.00		
90s ea	55289-0917-90	63.00		AB
100s ea	43063-0032-01	155.60		AB
(Pharma Pac)				
REPACK				
TAB, PO, 2.5 mg, 30s ea	52959-0973-30	23.10		AB
5 mg, 20s ea	52959-0854-20	21.15		
30s ea	52959-0854-30	31.41		AB
30s ea	52959-0975-30	25.45		AB
10 mg, 15s ea	52959-0728-15	17.60		
20s ea	52959-0728-20	23.46		
30s ea	52959-0728-30	35.18		AB
90s ea	52959-0728-90	81.59		AB
20 mg, 30s ea	52959-0729-30	33.48		AB
90s ea	52959-0729-90	41.26		
40 mg, 30s ea	52959-0753-30	52.31		AB
100s ea	52959-0753-00	174.30		AB
(Phys Total Care)				
REPACK				
TAB, PO, 2.5 mg, 30s ea	54868-4656-00	5.64		AB
60s ea	54868-4656-02	10.74		AB
100s ea	54868-4656-01	10.32		
5 mg, 30s ea	54868-4678-00	6.84		
90s ea	54868-4678-02	16.05		AB
100s ea	54868-4678-01	14.34		AB
10 mg, 30s ea	54868-4657-00	11.25		AB
45s ea	54868-4657-03	14.64		AB
60s ea	54868-4657-02	18.00		AB
(USP)				
10 mg, 90s ea	54868-4657-04	24.78		AB
100s ea	54868-4657-01	25.53		AB
180s ea	54868-4657-06	40.31		
1000s ea	54868-4657-05	92.08		AB
20 mg, 30s ea	54868-4658-00	12.60		AB
60s ea	54868-4658-02	21.00		AB
90s ea	54868-4658-03	28.51		AB
100s ea	54868-4658-01	33.54		AB
30 mg, 30s ea	54868-4780-00	21.93		AB
100s ea	54868-4780-01	61.11		
40 mg, 30s ea	54868-4646-00	19.41		AB
60s ea	54868-4646-02	35.85		
(USP)				
40 mg, 90s ea	54868-4646-03	52.26		
100s ea	54868-4646-01	56.25		
180s ea	54868-4646-04	58.92		AB
(Physician Partner)				
REPACK				
TAB, PO, 5 mg, 30s ea	21695-0328-30	58.35		
90s ea	21695-0328-90	175.05		AB
10 mg, 30s ea	21695-0329-30	60.25		
90s ea	21695-0329-90	180.75		
20 mg, 20s ea	21695-0330-20	50.59		AB
30s ea	21695-0330-30	64.51		
90s ea	21695-0330-90	193.54		
40 mg, 30s ea	21695-0331-30	94.99		AB
90s ea	21695-0331-90	284.97		AB
(Quality Care Prod)				
REPACK				
TAB, PO, 5 mg, 10s ea	49999-0295-10	5.35		
30s ea	49999-0295-30	16.06		AB
100s ea	49999-0295-00	106.98		
10 mg, 10s ea	49999-0182-10	16.90		
30s ea	49999-0182-30	50.76		
60s ea	49999-0182-60	92.16		
20 mg, 10s ea	49999-0183-10	17.98		
30s ea	49999-0183-30	53.95		
60s ea	49999-0183-60	84.88		
90s ea	49999-0183-90	161.85		AB
30 mg, 100s ea	49999-0870-00	225.90		
40 mg, 10s ea	49999-0469-10	12.67		AB
30s ea	49999-0469-30	50.68		
60s ea	49999-0469-60	101.36		AB
90s ea	49999-0469-90	152.04		AB
(Southwood)				
REPACK				
TAB, PO, 5 mg, 30s ea	58016-0917-30	24.22		AB
60s ea	58016-0917-60	48.43		AB
90s ea	58018-0917-90	72.65		AB
100s ea	58016-0917-00	80.72		AB
10 mg, 30s ea	58016-0963-30	25.01		AB
60s ea	58016-0963-60	50.03		AB
90s ea	58016-0963-90	75.04		AB
100s ea	58016-0963-00	83.38		AB
20 mg, 30s ea	58016-0998-30	26.77		AB
60s ea	58016-0998-60	53.54		AB
90s ea	58016-0998-90	80.31		AB
100s ea	58016-0998-00	89.23		AB
30 mg, 30s ea	58016-0069-30	44.98		
60s ea	58016-0069-60	89.95		
90s ea	58016-0069-90	134.93		
100s ea	58016-0069-00	149.92		
(Stat Rx)				
REPACK				
TAB, PO, 40 mg, 30s ea	16590-0356-30	40.25		
(Vibranta)				
REPACK				
TAB, PO, 10 mg, 30s ea	57866-4000-01	65.25		
20 mg, 30s ea	57866-5000-01	75.00		
40 mg, 30s ea	57866-8700-01	85.00		
LISINOPRIL AND HYDROCHLOROTHIAZIDE (Apotex Corp.)				
hydrochlorothiazide/lisinopril				
TAB, PO, 12.5 mg-10 mg,				
100s ea	60505-2689-01	111.00		AB
12.5 mg-20 mg,				
100s ea	60505-2690-01	121.15		AB
25 mg-20 mg,				
100s ea	60505-2691-01	121.60		AB
(Lupin Pharma, Inc.)				
TAB, PO, 12.5 mg-10 mg,				
100s ea	68180-0518-01	112.04		AB
500s ea	68180-0518-02	560.20		AB
12.5 mg-20 mg,				
100s ea	68180-0519-01	121.28		AB
500s ea	68180-0519-02	606.40		AB
25 mg-20 mg,				
100s ea	68180-0520-01	122.75		AB
500s ea	68180-0520-02	613.75		AB
(Pharma Pac)				
REPACK				
TAB, PO, 12.5 mg-10 mg,				
15s ea	52959-0137-15	20.38		
LISINOPRIL HCTZ (Phys Total Care)				
REPACK				
hydrochlorothiazide/lisinopril				
TAB, PO, 25 mg-20 mg,				
90s ea	54868-4785-03	49.24		
100s ea	54868-4785-02	55.50		
LISINOPRIL-HYDROCHLOROTHIAZIDE (Aurobindo Pharma)				
hydrochlorothiazide/lisinopril				
TAB, PO, 12.5 mg-10 mg,				
100s ea	65862-0043-01	110.45		AB
500s ea	65862-0043-05	552.25		AB
12.5 mg-20 mg,				
100s ea	65862-0044-01	119.60		AB
500s ea	65862-0044-05	598.00		AB
25 mg-20 mg,				
100s ea	65862-0045-01	121.40		AB
500s ea	65862-0045-05	607.00		AB
(Greenstone)				
TAB, PO, 12.5 mg-10 mg,				
30s ea	59762-3293-01	32.80		
100s ea	59762-3293-02	109.35		
500s ea	59762-3293-03	546.73		
1000s ea	59762-3293-04	1093.46		
12.5 mg-20 mg,				
30s ea	59762-3294-01	35.52		
100s ea	59762-3294-02	118.40		
500s ea	59762-3294-03	592.02		
1000s ea	59762-3294-04	1184.04		
25 mg-20 mg,				
30s ea	59762-3295-01	36.06		
100s ea	59762-3295-02	120.19		
500s ea	59762-3295-03	600.93		
1000s ea	59762-3295-04	1201.86		
LISINOPRIL/HCTZ (Bryant Ranch)				
REPACK				
hydrochlorothiazide/lisinopril				
TAB, PO, 12.5 mg-10 mg,				
30s ea	63629-1679-03	45.43		
60s ea	63629-1679-02	90.86		
90s ea	63629-1679-01	136.29		
(Core)				
REPACK				
TAB, PO, 12.5 mg-10 mg,				
30s ea	33358-0214-30	46.57		
60s ea	33358-0214-60	93.13		
(DHS, Inc.)				
REPACK				
TAB, PO, 25 mg-20 mg,				
30s ea	55887-0532-30	30.02		
60s ea	55887-0532-60	60.03		
90s ea	55887-0532-90	90.05		
100s ea	55887-0532-01	100.06		
(Quality Care Prod)				
REPACK				
TAB, PO, 12.5 mg-20 mg,				
10s ea	49999-0924-10	14.39		
30s ea	49999-0924-30	43.20		
60s ea	49999-0924-60	86.40		
100s ea	49999-0924-00	143.90		
25 mg-20 mg,				
60s ea	49999-0321-60	59.02		
(Stat Rx)				
REPACK				
TAB, PO, 25 mg-20 mg,				
30s ea	16590-0309-30	30.25		
60s ea	16590-0309-60	60.50		
90s ea	16590-0309-90	90.75		
120s ea	16590-0309-72	121.00		
LISINOPRIL/HYDROCHLOROTHIAZIDE (Quality Care Prod)				
REPACK				
hydrochlorothiazide/lisinopril				
TAB, PO, 12.5 mg-10 mg,				
30s ea	49999-0761-30	28.54		
100s ea	49999-0761-00	95.00		
LISPRO-PFC (Midwest IV)				
insulin lispro, recombinant				
SUS, SC (RDNA ORIGIN)				
100 u/ml,				
3.15 ml 5s	66143-7510-05	155.46	132.14	

PROD/MFR	NDC	AWP	DP	OBC
LISSAMINE GREEN B (PCCA)				
acid brilliant green bs				
POW, NA (1X1GM)				
1 gm	**51927-2825-00**	19.20		
LITE TOUCH (Medicore)				
insulin syringe/needle				
DEV, NA (29GX1/2",3/10 CC)				
ea	**32671-0005-06**	2.20		
(30GX5/16",3/10CC)				
ea	**32671-0005-07**	2.20		
(28GX1/2",1 CC)				
10s ea	**32671-0005-01**	2.00		
(28GX1/2",1/2 CC)				
10s ea	**32671-0005-00**	2.00		
(29GX1/2",1 CC)				
10s ea	**32671-0005-03**	2.00		
(29GX1/2",1/2 CC)				
10s ea	**32671-0005-02**	2.00		
(30GX5/16",1/2 CC)				
10s ea	**32671-0005-04**	2.10	0.90	
(30GX5/16",1CC)				
10s ea	**32671-0005-05**	2.10	0.90	
(31GX5/16",1/2ML)				
10s ea	**32671-0005-09**	2.30	1.19	
(31GX5/16",1ML)				
10s ea	**32671-0005-20**	2.30	1.19	
(31GX5/16",3/10ML)				
10s ea	**32671-0005-08**	2.50	1.39	
LITE TOUCH LANCETS (Medicore)				
lancet				
DEV, NA, 100s ea	**32671-0201-33**	7.00	3.00	
200s ea	**32671-0202-33**	12.00	4.50	
LITHIUM (Roxane)				
SOL, PO (USP,100X5ML)				
8 meq/5 ml,				
5 ml 100s UD	**00054-8529-04**	71.56		
LITHIUM BORATE				
(Baker, J.T.) *See LITHIUM META-BORATE*				
LITHIUM BROMIDE (PCCA)				
POW, NA, 1 gm	**51927-2048-00**	1.44		
LITHIUM CARB (Physician Partner)				
REPACK				
lithium carbonate				
TER, PO, 300 mg, 30s ea	**21695-0412-30**	27.91		
90s ea	**21695-0412-90**	83.74		
100s ea	**21695-0412-00**	93.04		
LITHIUM CARBONATE				
FUL				
CAP, PO, 300 mg, 100s ea		13.82		
(Apotex Corp.)				
CAP, PO (10X10)				
300 mg, 100s ea UD	**60505-2504-03**	18.30		AB
(U.S.P)				
300 mg, 100s ea	**60505-2504-01**	17.91		AB
1000s ea	**60505-2504-02**	179.10		AB
(Baker, J.T.)				
POW, NA (A.C.S., REAGENT)				
500 gm	**10106-2362-01**	125.71		
2500 gm	**10106-2362-05**	565.26		
(Glenmark Pharmaceuticals)				
CAP, PO (USP,HARD GELATIN)				
150 mg, 100s ea	**68462-0220-01**	15.00		
300 mg, 100s ea	**68462-0221-01**	17.91		
600 mg, 100s ea	**68462-0222-01**	35.82		
(Noven) *See LITHOBID*				
(PCCA)				
POW, NA (USP)				
1 gm	**51927-3126-00**	0.69		
(Roxane)				
CAP, PO, 150 mg, 100s ea	**00054-2526-25**	13.97		
(10X10)				
150 mg, 100s ea UD	**00054-8526-25**	18.77		
300 mg, 100s ea	**00054-2527-25**	17.46		AB
(10X10)				
300 mg, 100s ea UD	**00054-8527-25**	20.95		AB
1000s ea	**00054-2527-31**	161.73		AB
600 mg, 100s ea	**00054-2531-25**	39.11		
(10X10)				
600 mg, 100s ea UD	**00054-8531-25**	46.93		
TAB, PO, 300 mg, 100s ea	**00054-4527-25**	21.52		AB
(10X10)				
300 mg, 100s ea UD	**00054-8528-25**	25.82		AB
1000s ea	**00054-4527-31**	215.04		AB
TER, PO (FILM-COATED)				
300 mg, 100s ea	**00054-0021-25**	46.52		AB
500s ea	**00054-0021-29**	232.60		AB
450 mg, 100s ea	**00054-0020-25**	53.69		

PROD/MFR	NDC	AWP	DP	OBC
(Spectrum Pharmacy)				
POW, NA (1X125GM,ACS)				
125 gm	**49452-4090-02**	139.30		
(1X500GM,ACS)				
500 gm	**49452-4090-03**	388.50		
(West-Ward)				
CAP, PO, 150 mg, 100s ea	**00143-3188-01**	13.25		AB
300 mg, 100s ea	**00143-3189-01**	17.40		EE
1000s ea	**00143-3189-10**	160.50		EE
TER, PO, 450 mg, 100s ea	**00143-1277-01**	52.10	38.64	AB
(American Health)				
REPACK				
TER, PO (10X10,USP)				
450 mg, 100s ea UD	**68084-0043-01**	75.56		
(Core)				
REPACK				
CAP, PO, 300 mg, 30s ea	**33358-0215-30**	8.76		
60s ea	**33358-0215-60**	15.84		
(HomeMed)				
REPACK				
CAP, PO, 300 mg, 12s ea	**51655-0490-27**	4.23		EE
(McKesson Packaging)				
REPACK				
CAP, PO, 300 mg,				
100s ea UD	**63739-0265-10**	20.06		
(PD-Rx Pharm)				
REPACK				
CAP, PO (REDI-SCRIPT)				
150 mg, 60s ea	**58864-0821-60**	23.56		
300 mg, 30s ea	**58864-0668-30**	12.67		AB
42s ea	**58864-0668-42**	15.07		AB
(USP)				
300 mg, 60s ea	**43063-0196-60**	14.24		EE
TER, PO, 300 mg, 60s ea	**58864-0819-60**	18.67		
(Phys Total Care)				
REPACK				
CAP, PO, 150 mg, 100s ea	**54868-3632-00**	51.69		
300 mg, 30s ea	**54868-1335-04**	9.72		EE
(USP)				
300 mg, 60s ea	**54868-1335-05**	14.97		EE
100s ea	**54868-1335-02**	20.46		EE
TER, PO, 300 mg, 30s ea	**54868-5239-01**	39.36		
60s ea	**54868-5239-00**	74.22		AB
450 mg, 20s ea	**54868-5340-01**	30.81		AB
60s ea	**54868-5340-00**	83.43		AB
(Quality Care Prod)				
REPACK				
CAP, PO, 300 mg, 120s ea	**49999-0736-01**	60.82		AB
TER, PO, 450 mg, 30s ea	**35356-0506-30**	42.30		AB
(Stat Rx)				
REPACK				
CAP, PO, 300 mg, 30s ea	**16590-0781-30**	10.37		EE
90s ea	**16590-0781-90**	9.18		EE
(Vibranta)				
REPACK				
CAP, PO, 300 mg, 30s ea	**57866-6523-01**	34.16		
60s ea	**57866-6523-02**	20.20		
90s ea	**57866-6523-04**	29.91		
120s ea	**57866-6523-05**	39.64		
LITHIUM CHLORIDE (Baker, J.T.)				
GRA, NA (A.C.S., REAGENT)				
500 gm	**10106-2370-01**	72.92		
(PURIFIED)				
500 gm	**10106-2374-01**	88.99		
(A.C.S, REAGENT)				
2500 gm	**10106-2370-05**	469.94		
(PCCA)				
POW, NA, 1 gm	**51927-2615-00**	1.26		
LITHIUM CITRATE (Morton Grove)				
SYR, PO (SF,RASPBERRY)				
300 mg/5 ml,				
473 ml	**60432-0616-16**	69.90		AA
(PCCA)				
POW, NA (TETRAHYDRATE)				
1 gm	**51927-1288-00**	1.05		
(Precision Dose)				
SOL, PO (1X5ML,USP,SF,RASPBERRY)				
8 meq/5 ml,				
5 ml UD	**68094-0767-59**	0.66		AA
(30X5ML,USP,SF,RASPBERRY)				
8 meq/5 ml,				
5 ml 30s UD	**68094-0767-62**	19.70		AA

PROD/MFR	NDC	AWP	DP	OBC
(Spectrum Pharmacy)				
POW, NA (1X125GM)				
125 gm	**49452-4089-01**	176.40		
(1X500GM)				
500 gm	**49452-4089-02**	518.00		
LITHIUM META-BORATE (Baker, J.T.)				
lithium borate				
POW, NA (A.C.S., REAGENT)				
100 gm	**10106-2382-05**	334.49		
LITHIUM NITRATE (Baker, J.T.)				
CRY, NA (REAGENT)				
500 gm	**10106-2384-01**	112.12		
2500 gm	**10106-2384-05**	421.79		
12000 gm	**10106-2384-07**	1089.28		
LITHIUM PERCHLORATE				
(Baker, J.T.) *See LITHIUM PERCHLORATE ANHYDROUS*				
LITHIUM PERCHLORATE ANHYDROUS (Baker, J.T.)				
lithium perchlorate				
POW, NA (A.C.S., REAGENT)				
100 gm	**10106-2385-01**	99.50		
LITHIUM SULFATE				
(Baker, J.T.) *See LITHIUM SULFATE MONOHYDRATE*				
LITHIUM SULFATE MONOHYDRATE (Baker, J.T.)				
lithium sulfate				
GRA, NA (A.C.S., REAGENT)				
500 gm	**10106-2388-01**	115.98		
2500 gm	**10106-2388-05**	395.98		
LITHOBID (Noven)				
lithium carbonate				
TER, PO (FILM-COATED)				
300 mg, 100s ea	**68968-4492-01**	228.74		AB
LITHOSTAT (Mission)				
acetohydroxamic acid				
TAB, PO, 250 mg, 100s ea	**00178-0500-01**	172.50		
LIVER (Gallipot)				
LIQ, NA (ARTIFICIAL)				
59.14 ml	**51552-0568-03**	10.22		
(Medisca)				
POW, NA (1X25GM)				
25 gm	**38779-1941-04**	22.50		
(1X100GM)				
100 gm	**38779-1941-05**	43.50		
(1X5100GM)				
500 gm	**38779-1941-08**	105.00		
(PCCA) *See LIVER ANIMAL TREAT*				
(PCCA) *See LIVER BEEF*				
(PCCA) *See LIVER FLAVOR*				
LIVER ANIMAL TREAT (PCCA)				
liver				
POW, NA (BASE (TM))				
1 gm	**51927-3246-00**	0.45		
LIVER BEEF (PCCA)				
liver				
POW, NA (EDIBLE-SPRAY DRIED)				
1 gm	**51927-2111-00**	0.26		
LIVER FLAVOR (PCCA)				
liver				
POW, NA (SOLUBLE;PORCINE,LIVER)				
1 gm	**51927-2694-00**	1.44		
(PCCA)				
flavoring aid				
SOL, NA (OIL MISCIBLE)				
1 ml	**51927-2904-00**	0.38		
(WATER MISCIBLE)				
1 ml	**51927-2905-00**	0.45		
LIVOSTIN (Pharma Pac)				
REPACK				
levocabastine hydrochloride				
SUS, OP, 0.05%, 5 ml	**52959-0328-03**	39.98		
(Phys Total Care)				
REPACK				
SUS, OP, 0.05%, 10 ml	**54868-3376-00**	96.40		
LMD IN DEXTROSE (Hospira)				
dextran 40/dextrose				
SOL, IV (12X500ML,LATEX-FREE)				
10%-5%, 500 ml 12s	**00409-7418-03**	305.28	267.12	
LMD W/0.9% SODIUM CHLORIDE (Hospira)				
dextran 40/sodium chloride				
SOL, IV (LATEX-FREE)				
10%-0.9%,				
500 ml 12s	**00409-7419-03**	332.21	290.64	

PROD/MFR	NDC	AWP	DP	OBC
LO/OVRAL (Dispensing Solutions)				
REPACK				
ethinyl estradiol/norgestrel				
TAB, PO (6X28)				
30 mcg-0.3 mg,				
168s ea	**55045-3485-06**	282.00		
(Palmetto)				
REPACK				
TAB, PO, 30 mcg-0.3 mg,				
28s ea	**23490-7699-01**	32.03		
LO/OVRAL-28 (Akrimax)				
ethinyl estradiol/norgestrel				
TAB, PO (PILPAK, 6X28)				
30 mcg-0.3 mg,				
168s ea	**00008-2514-02**	367.54		**AB**
(A-S Medication)				
REPACK				
TAB, PO, 30 mcg-0.3 mg,				
28s ea	**54569-0679-00**	40.84		**AB**
(PD-Rx Pharm)				
REPACK				
TAB, PO, 30 mcg-0.3 mg,				
8s ea	**55289-0246-08**	22.77		**AB**
(Phys Total Care)				
REPACK				
TAB, PO (PILPAK)				
30 mcg-0.3 mg,				
28s ea	**54868-0428-00**	49.05		**AB**
LOCOID (Triax Pharm)				
hydrocortisone butyrate				
CRE, TP (1X15GM)				
0.1%, 15 gm	**14290-0310-15**	58.80		**AB**
(1X45GM)				
0.1%, 45 gm	**14290-0310-45**	176.76		**AB**
LOT, TP (1X59ML)				
0.1%, 59 ml	**14290-0314-61**	234.06		
(1X118ML)				
0.1%, 118 ml	**14290-0314-63**	460.31		
OIN, TP (1X15GM)				
0.1%, 15 gm	**14290-0311-15**	56.05		
(1X45GM)				
0.1%, 45 gm	**14290-0311-45**	168.14		
SOL, TP (1X20ML)				
0.1%, 20 ml	**14290-0312-62**	74.74		**AT**
(1X60ML)				
0.1%, 60 ml	**14290-0312-61**	224.18		**AT**
(Phys Total Care)				
REPACK				
CRE, TP, 0.1%, 45 gm	**54868-2231-00**	174.54		
(Quality Care Prod)				
REPACK				
OIN, TP (1X15GM)				
0.1%, 15 gm	**35356-0229-15**	108.40		
LOCOID LIPOCREAM (Triax Pharm)				
hydrocortisone butyrate				
CRE, TP (1X15GM)				
0.1%, 15 gm	**14290-0313-15**	84.67		
(1X45GM)				
0.1%, 45 gm	**14290-0313-45**	241.84		
(1X60GM)				
0.1%, 60 gm	**14290-0313-60**	322.46		
LOCUST BEAN GUM (PCCA)				
POW, NA (CAROB FLOUR)				
1 gm	**51927-1862-00**	0.30		
LODINE (Pharma Pac)				
REPACK				
etodolac				
CAP, PO, 300 mg, 20s ea	**52959-0211-20**	43.63		**AB**
21s ea	**52959-0211-21**	45.61		**AB**
30s ea	**52959-0211-30**	64.28		**AB**
42s ea	**52959-0211-42**	84.40		**AB**
TAB, PO, 400 mg, 14s ea	**52959-0281-14**	31.05		**AB**
20s ea	**52959-0281-20**	44.10		**AB**
30s ea	**52959-0281-30**	63.19		**AB**
60s ea	**52959-0281-60**	101.82		**AB**
500 mg, 20s ea	**52959-0445-20**	48.40		**AB**
30s ea	**52959-0445-30**	57.56		**AB**
(Phys Total Care)				
REPACK				
CAP, PO, 200 mg, 60s ea	**54868-1813-00**	110.91		**AB**
300 mg, 30s ea	**54868-2018-01**	58.27		**AB**
40s ea	**54868-2018-03**	73.06		**AB**
60s ea	**54868-2018-04**	115.33		**AB**
TAB, PO, 400 mg, 12s ea	**54868-2987-01**	27.99		**AB**
60s ea	**54868-2987-00**	125.16		**AB**
500 mg, 10s ea	**54868-3856-00**	23.78		**AB**

PROD/MFR	NDC	AWP	DP	OBC
(Quality Care Prod)				
REPACK				
TAB, PO, 400 mg, 14s ea	**49999-0013-14**	54.75		**AB**
28s ea	**49999-0013-28**	109.50		**AB**
LODINE XL (Pharma Pac)				
REPACK				
etodolac				
TER, PO, 400 mg, 14s ea	**52959-0467-14**	30.29		**AB**
30s ea	**52959-0467-30**	61.82		**AB**
500 mg, 28s ea	**52959-0095-28**	45.36		**AB**
30s ea	**52959-0095-30**	48.60		**AB**
(Phys Total Care)				
REPACK				
TER, PO, 400 mg, 20s ea	**54868-3901-00**	41.80		**AB**
30s ea	**54868-3901-01**	61.76		**AB**
60s ea	**54868-3901-02**	121.65		**AB**
LODOSYN (Bristol-Myers)				
carbidopa				
TAB, PO, 25 mg, 100s ea	**00056-0511-68**	80.50		
LODOXAMIDE TROMETHAMINE				
(Alcon Ophthalmic) *See ALOMIDE*				
LODRANE 12D (ECR)				
bpm/pse hcl				
TER, PO (DYE-FREE)				
6 mg-45 mg,				
100s ea	**00095-0645-01**	50.00		
LODRANE 24 (ECR)				
brompheniramine maleate				
CER, PO (DYE-FREE)				
12 mg, 60s ea	**00095-1200-06**	72.60		
LODRANE 24D (ECR)				
bpm/pse hcl				
C24, PO, 12 mg-90 mg,				
60s ea	**00095-1290-06**	81.68		
LODRANE D (ECR)				
brompheniramine tannate/pseudoephedrine tannate				
SUS, PO (AF,SF,STRAWBERRY)				
8 mg/5 ml-90 mg/5 ml,				
480 ml	**00095-9008-16**	87.00		
LODRANE XR (Phys Total Care)				
REPACK				
brompheniramine tannate				
SUS, PO (AF,SF,STRAWBERRY)				
8 mg/5 ml, 480 ml	**54868-5221-00**	89.05		
LOESTRIN 21 1.5/30 (Teva)				
ethinyl estradiol/norethindrone acetate				
TAB, PO (COMPACK, 5X21)				
30 mcg-1.5 mg,				
105s ea	**51285-0082-97**	367.50		**AB**
LOESTRIN 21 1/20 (Teva)				
ethinyl estradiol/norethindrone acetate				
TAB, PO (COMPACK,5X21)				
20 mcg-1 mg,				
105s ea	**51285-0079-97**	367.50		**AB**
LOESTRIN 24 FE (Warner Chilcott)				
ethinyl estradiol/ferrous fum/norethindrone ace				
TAB, PO (5X28)				
20 mcg-75 mg-1 mg,				
140s ea	**00430-0530-14**	370.68		
(Phys Total Care)				
REPACK				
TAB, PO (5X28)				
20 mcg-75 mg-1 mg,				
140s ea	**54868-6100-00**	91.17		
(Quality Care Prod)				
REPACK				
TAB, PO (5X28)				
20 mcg-75 mg-1 mg,				
28s ea	**35356-0476-28**	118.28		
LOESTRIN FE 1.5/30 (Teva)				
ethinyl estradiol/ferrous fum/norethindrone ace				
TAB, PO (5X28)				
30 mcg-75 mg-1.5 mg,				
140s ea	**51285-0083-70**	367.50		**AB**
(COMPACK, 30X28)				
30 mcg-75 mg-1.5 mg,				
840s ea	**51285-0084-98**	2205.00		**AB**
(Phys Total Care)				
REPACK				
TAB, PO (COMPACK)				
30 mcg-75 mg-1.5 mg,				
28s ea	**54868-0502-00**	65.46		**AB**

PROD/MFR	NDC	AWP	DP	OBC
LOESTRIN FE 1/20 (Teva)				
ethinyl estradiol/ferrous fum/norethindrone ace				
TAB, PO (COMPACK, 5X28)				
20 mcg-75 mg-1 mg,				
140s ea	**51285-0080-70**	367.50		**AB**
(Phys Total Care)				
REPACK				
TAB, PO (COMPACK)				
20 mcg-75 mg-1 mg,				
28s ea	**54868-1512-00**	65.46		**AB**
(Quality Care Prod)				
REPACK				
TAB, PO, 20 mcg-75 mg-1 mg,				
28s ea	**35356-0363-28**	146.30		**AB**
LOFIBRA (Gate)				
fenofibrate, micronized				
CAP, PO, 67 mg, 100s ea	**57844-0322-01**	104.21		
134 mg, 100s ea	**57844-0323-01**	200.73		**AB**
200 mg, 100s ea	**57844-0324-01**	312.62		**AB**
(Gate)				
fenofibrate				
TAB, PO (FILM-COATED)				
54 mg, 90s ea	**57844-0691-98**	93.78		**AB**
160 mg, 90s ea	**57844-0692-98**	281.36		**AB**
(Phys Total Care)				
REPACK				
fenofibrate, micronized				
CAP, PO, 200 mg, 10s ea	**54868-5512-01**	32.84		
30s ea	**54868-5512-00**	94.77		
LOHIST D (Larken Labs, Inc.)				
cpm/pse hcl				
SYR, PO (AF,DYE-FREE,PEACH)				
2 mg/5 ml-30 mg/5 ml,				
473 ml	**68047-0120-16**	37.22		
LOHIST-12 (Larken Labs, Inc.)				
brompheniramine maleate				
TER, PO (DYE-FREE)				
6 mg, 100s ea	**68047-0121-01**	35.88		
LOHIST-12D (Larken Labs, Inc.)				
bpm/pse hcl				
TER, PO (DYE-FREE)				
6 mg-45 mg,				
100s ea	**68047-0122-01**	35.88		
LOHIST-DM (Larken Labs, Inc.)				
bpm/dm/phenyleph hcl				
SYR, PO (1X473ML,AF,SF)				
473 ml	**68047-0129-16**	63.90		
LOHIST-PD (Larken Labs, Inc.)				
bpm/pse hcl				
SOL, PO (PEDIATRIC DROPS,SF)				
1 mg/ml-12.5 mg/ml,				
30 ml	**68047-0011-30**	27.70		
LOKARA (PharmaDerm)				
desonide				
LOT, TP, 0.05%, 59 ml	**00462-0392-02**	98.36		**AB**
118 ml	**00462-0392-04**	146.06		**AB**
LOMOCOT (Truxton)				
atropine sulfate/diphenoxylate hydrochloride				
TAB, PO, 0.025 mg-2.5 mg,				
1000s ea, C-V	**00463-6286-10**	24.00		**EE**
LOMOTIL (Pfizer)				
atropine sulfate/diphenoxylate hydrochloride				
TAB, PO, 0.025 mg-2.5 mg,				
100s ea, C-V	**00025-0061-31**	112.00	93.33	**AA**
(PD-Rx Pharm)				
REPACK				
TAB, PO, 0.025 mg-2.5 mg,				
10s ea, C-V	**55289-0230-10**	77.33		**AA**
(Phys Total Care)				
REPACK				
SOL, PO, 60 ml, C-V	**54868-1511-01**	21.11		**AA**
TAB, PO, 0.025 mg-2.5 mg,				
6s ea, C-V	**54868-0427-02**	11.29		**AA**
10s ea, C-V	**54868-0427-05**	16.64		**AA**
12s ea, C-V	**54868-0427-04**	19.31		**AA**
20s ea, C-V	**54868-0427-01**	30.01		**AA**
30s ea, C-V	**54868-0427-03**	43.38		**AA**
100s ea, C-V	**54868-0427-00**	135.66		**AA**
LOMUSTINE				
(B/M Squibb Onc/Vir) *See CEENU*				
LONOX (Sandoz)				
atropine sulfate/diphenoxylate hydrochloride				
TAB, PO, 0.025 mg-2.5 mg,				
100s ea, C-V	**00781-1262-01**	47.90		**AA**
100s ea UD, C-V	**00781-1262-13**	50.73		**AA**

PROD/MFR	NDC	AWP	DP	OBC
500s ea, C-V	00781-1262-05	227.36		AA
1000s ea, C-V	00781-1262-10	420.78		AA
LOPERAMIDE (DHS, Inc.)				
REPACK				
loperamide hydrochloride				
CAP, PO, 2 mg, 10s ea	55887-0999-10	10.00		
20s ea	55887-0999-20	15.00		
(Southwood)				
REPACK				
LIQ, PO, 1 mg/5 ml, 120 ml	58016-4854-01	5.60		
LOPERAMIDE HCL (Hawkins)				
loperamide hydrochloride				
POW, NA (U.S.P.)				
1 gm	63370-0147-10	40.00		
5 gm	63370-0147-15	120.00		
25 gm	63370-0147-25	380.00		
100 gm	63370-0147-35	1400.00		
(Medisca)				
POW, NA (U.S.P.)				
5 gm	38779-0446-03	127.50		
25 gm	38779-0446-04	321.00		
(Mylan)				
CAP, PO, 2 mg, 100s ea	00378-2100-01	68.20		AB
500s ea	00378-2100-05	313.70		AB
(PCCA)				
POW, NA (U.S.P.)				
1 gm	51927-2357-00	32.40		
(Spectrum Pharmacy)				
POW, NA (U.S.P./N.F.)				
5 gm	49452-4133-01	212.10		
25 gm	49452-4133-02	539.00		
(1X100GM, U.S.P.)				
100 gm	49452-4133-03	1596.00		
(Teva)				
CAP, PO, 2 mg, 100s ea	00093-0311-01	61.10		AB
500s ea	00093-0311-05	298.10		AB
(UDL)				
CAP, PO (ROBOT READY 25X1)				
2 mg, 25s ea UD	51079-0690-19	17.56		AB
(10X10)				
2 mg, 100s ea UD	51079-0690-20	70.25		AB
(A-S Medication)				
REPACK				
CAP, PO, 2 mg, 15s ea	54569-3707-00	9.70		EE
(Dispensing Solutions)				
REPACK				
CAP, PO, 2 mg, 6s ea	66336-0046-06	5.05		AB
12s ea	66336-0046-12	10.12		AB
(HomeMed)				
REPACK				
CAP, PO, 2 mg, 12s ea	51655-0547-27	7.18		AB
(Nucare Pharm)				
REPACK				
CAP, PO, 2 mg, 12s ea	66267-0132-12	8.89		AB
(PD-Rx Pharm)				
REPACK				
CAP, PO, 2 mg, 6s ea	55289-0315-06	8.78		AB
(USP)				
2 mg, 8s ea	55289-0315-08	8.96		AB
10s ea	55289-0315-10	9.14		AB
12s ea	55289-0315-12	10.87		AB
(USP)				
2 mg, 12s ea	43063-0020-12	10.86		AB
15s ea	55289-0315-15	11.78		AB
(USP)				
2 mg, 20s ea	55289-0315-20	14.98		AB
30s ea	55289-0315-30	17.20		AB
(REDI-SCRIPT)				
2 mg, 30s ea	58864-0798-30	17.20		AB
(Pharma Pac)				
REPACK				
CAP, PO, 2 mg, 15s ea	52959-0905-15	9.29		AB
(Phys Total Care)				
REPACK				
CAP, PO, 2 mg, 10s ea	54868-2118-00	5.52		EE
15s ea	54868-2118-06	6.81		AB
20s ea	54868-2118-01	8.07		EE
(USP)				
2 mg, 30s ea	54868-2118-08	10.59		EE
40s ea	54868-2118-05	13.14		EE
50s ea	54868-2118-07	15.66		AB
100s ea	54868-2118-04	30.54		EE
(Physician Partner)				
REPACK				
CAP, PO, 2 mg, 10s ea	21695-0692-10	14.38		AB
(Quality Care Prod)				
REPACK				
CAP, PO, 2 mg, 20s ea	49999-0155-20	21.08		AB
(Southwood)				
REPACK				
CAP, PO, 2 mg, 12s ea	58016-0254-12	8.57		EE
15s ea	58016-0254-15	10.71		EE
20s ea	58016-0254-20	14.28		EE
30s ea	58016-0254-30	21.42		EE
100s ea	58016-0254-00	71.39		EE
LOPERAMIDE HYDROCHLORIDE				
(Hawkins) *See LOPERAMIDE HCL*				
(Medisca) *See LOPERAMIDE HCL*				
(Mylan) *See LOPERAMIDE HCL*				
(PCCA) *See LOPERAMIDE HCL*				
(PGD, Inc.) *See IMOGEN*				
(Spectrum Pharmacy) *See LOPERAMIDE HCL*				
(Teva) *See LOPERAMIDE HCL*				
(UDL) *See LOPERAMIDE HCL*				
(Altura)				
REPACK				
CAP, PO, 2 mg, 12s ea	63874-0433-12	9.00		
15s ea	63874-0433-15	11.25		
16s ea	63874-0433-16	10.35		
20s ea	63874-0433-20	15.01		
24s ea	63874-0433-24	18.01		
30s ea	63874-0433-30	22.49		
100s ea	63874-0433-01	74.96		
(Bryant Ranch)				
REPACK				
CAP, PO, 2 mg, 15s ea	63629-1452-01	12.52		
20s ea	63629-1452-03	16.69		
30s ea	63629-1452-02	25.04		
(Core)				
REPACK				
CAP, PO, 2 mg, 15s ea	33358-0216-15	12.83		
20s ea	33358-0216-20	17.11		
30s ea	33358-0216-30	25.67		
(Palmetto)				
REPACK				
CAP, PO, 2 mg, 6s ea	23490-5828-01	8.48		
12s ea	23490-5828-02	12.12		
(Pharma Pac)				
REPACK				
CAP, PO, 2 mg, 20s ea	52959-0905-20	6.20		
(Quality Care Prod)				
REPACK				
CAP, PO, 2 mg, 12s ea	49999-0155-12	12.65		
15s ea	49999-0155-15	15.84		
LOPID (Pfizer)				
gemfibrozil				
TAB, PO, 600 mg, 60s ea	00071-0737-20	148.22	123.52	AB
500s ea	00071-0737-30	1235.22	1029.35	AB
(Phys Total Care)				
REPACK				
TAB, PO, 600 mg, 30s ea	54868-1418-00	65.70		AB
60s ea	54868-1418-01	128.90		AB
LOPINAVIR/RITONAVIR				
(Abbott Pharm) *See KALETRA*				
LOPRESSOR (Novartis Pharm)				
metoprolol tartrate				
SOL, IV (AMP)				
1 mg/ml, 5 ml 10s	00078-0400-01	192.74		AP
TAB, PO, 50 mg, 100s ea	00078-0458-05	179.40		AB
100 mg, 100s ea	00078-0459-05	269.36		AB
(PD-Rx Pharm)				
REPACK				
TAB, PO, 50 mg, 30s ea	55289-0627-30	72.78		AB
(Phys Total Care)				
REPACK				
TAB, PO, 50 mg, 30s ea	54868-0685-01	40.51		AB
100 mg, 20s ea	54868-1063-02	52.45		AB
30s ea	54868-1063-01	59.90		AB
60s ea	54868-1063-00	117.91		AB
LOPRESSOR HCT (Novartis Pharm)				
hydrochlorothiazide/metoprolol tartrate				
TAB, PO (CAPLET)				
25 mg-50 mg, 100s ea	00078-0460-05	205.72		
25 mg-100 mg, 100s ea	00078-0461-05	321.48		
LOPROX (Medicis)				
ciclopirox				
GEL, TP, 0.77%, 30 gm	99207-0013-30	131.28		
45 gm	99207-0013-45	196.92		
100 gm	99207-0013-01	394.40		
SHA, TP, 1%, 120 ml	99207-0010-10	179.75		
(Dispensing Solutions)				
REPACK				
CRE, TP, 0.77%, 15 gm	55045-2684-05	52.00		
(Pharma Pac)				
REPACK				
CRE, TP, 0.77%, 15 gm	52959-0381-01	28.20		
(Phys Total Care)				
REPACK				
ciclopirox olamine				
CRE, TP, 1%, 15 gm	54868-0372-02	24.34		
30 gm	54868-0372-03	41.36		
90 gm	54868-0372-01	81.26		
(Phys Total Care)				
ciclopirox				
SHA, TP, 1%, 120 ml	54868-5403-00	99.60		
(Quality Care Prod)				
REPACK				
CRE, TP, 0.77%, 15 gm	49999-0319-15	66.22		
GEL, TP (1X100GM)				
0.77%, 100 gm	35356-0230-00	612.60		
LORATADINE (PCCA)				
POW, NA (1X1GM)				
1 gm	51927-4219-00	33.60		
(Bryant Ranch)				
REPACK				
TAB, PO, 10 mg, 20s ea	63629-1329-01	21.40		
(Core)				
REPACK				
TAB, PO, 10 mg, 20s ea	33358-0217-20	21.94		
30s ea	33358-0217-30	28.09		
(IPI)				
REPACK				
TAB, PO, 10 mg, 30s ea	18837-0301-30	30.94		
(Keltman Pharma., Inc.)				
REPACK				
TAB, PO, 10 mg, 10s ea	68387-0620-10	10.27		
(Palmetto)				
REPACK				
SYR, PO, 5 mg/5 ml, 120 ml	23490-5832-01	12.64		
TAB, PO, 10 mg, 3s ea	23490-5833-01	6.22		
4s ea	23490-5833-00	7.81		
10s ea	23490-5833-03	12.23		
14s ea	23490-7847-00	41.75		
30s ea	23490-5833-02	36.69		
(Pharma Pac)				
REPACK				
TAB, PO, 10 mg, 15s ea	52959-0740-15	17.68		
(Southwood)				
REPACK				
TAB, PO, 10 mg, 20s ea	58016-4797-01	1.73		
LORATADINE D (Palmetto)				
REPACK				
loratadine/pseudoephedrine sulfate				
T24, PO, 10 mg-240 mg,				
14s ea	23490-7868-00	17.90		
15s ea	23490-7868-01	19.17		
LORATADINE-D (DHS, Inc.)				
REPACK				
loratadine/pseudoephedrine sulfate				
T24, PO, 10 mg-240 mg,				
15s ea	55887-0122-15	37.92		
LORAZEPAM				
FUL				
TAB, PO, 0.5 mg, 100s ea		7.40		
1 mg, 100s ea		8.22		
2 mg, 100s ea		14.67		
(Actavis)				
TAB, PO, 0.5 mg,				
100s ea, C-IV	00228-2057-10	67.75		AB
500s ea, C-IV	00228-2057-50	331.05		AB
1 mg, 100s ea, C-IV	00228-2059-10	88.25		AB
500s ea, C-IV	00228-2059-50	430.75		AB
2 mg, 100s ea, C-IV	00228-2063-10	128.45		AB
500s ea, C-IV	00228-2063-50	628.15		AB
(Akorn)				
SOL, IJ (S.D.V.)				
2 mg/ml,				
1 ml 10s, C-IV	17478-0040-01	12.62		AP

PROD/MFR	NDC	AWP	DP	OBC
(Baxter) *See ATIVAN*				
(Baxter) *See NOVAPLUS LORAZEPAM*				
(Baxter)				
SOL, IJ, 2 mg/ml,				
1 ml, C-IV	**10019-0102-39**	0.90		**AP**
(S.D.V.)				
2 mg/ml,				
1 ml 25s, C-IV	**10019-0102-01**	22.50		**AP**
10 ml, C-IV	**10019-0102-37**	8.14		**AP**
(M.D.V.)				
2 mg/ml,				
10 ml 10s, C-IV	**10019-0102-10**	81.36		**AP**
(S.D.V.)				
4 mg/ml,				
1 ml 25s, C-IV	**10019-0103-01**	54.00		**AP**
10 ml, C-IV	**10019-0103-37**	11.06		**AP**
(M.D.V.)				
4 mg/ml,				
10 ml 10s, C-IV	**10019-0103-10**	110.64		**AP**
25 ml, C-IV	**10019-0103-39**	2.16		**AP**
(Bedford)				
SOL, IJ (USP,SDV,1MLX10,PF)				
2 mg/ml,				
1 ml 10s, C-IV	**55390-0168-10**	12.24		**AP**
(USP,MDV,10MLX10)				
2 mg/ml,				
10 ml 10s, C-IV	**55390-0170-10**	93.60		**AP**
(USP,SDV,1MLX10,PF)				
4 mg/ml,				
1 ml 10s, C-IV	**55390-0169-10**	48.00		**AP**
(USP,MDV,10MLX10)				
4 mg/ml,				
10 ml 10s, C-IV	**55390-0171-10**	133.32		**AP**
(BTA) *See ATIVAN*				
(Excellium)				
TAB, PO, 0.5 mg,				
100s ea, C-IV	**64125-0904-01**	64.31		**AB**
500s ea, C-IV	**64125-0904-05**	312.59		**AB**
1000s ea, C-IV	**64125-0904-10**	640.00		**AB**
1 mg, 100s ea, C-IV	**64125-0905-01**	83.77		**AB**
500s ea, C-IV	**64125-0905-05**	405.24		**AB**
1000s ea, C-IV	**64125-0905-10**	843.20		**AB**
2 mg, 100s ea, C-IV	**64125-0906-01**	122.11		**AB**
500s ea, C-IV	**64125-0906-05**	594.11		**AB**
1000s ea, C-IV	**64125-0906-10**	1152.57		**AB**
(Gallipot)				
POW, NA (1X500MG,USP)				
0.5 gm, C-IV	**51552-0729-09**	16.80	12.00	
(1X1GM,USP)				
1 gm, C-IV	**51552-0729-01**	28.00	20.00	
(1X5GM,USP)				
5 gm, C-IV	**51552-0729-02**	48.65	34.75	
(1X25GM,USP)				
25 gm, C-IV	**51552-0729-04**	170.10	121.50	
(1X100GM,USP)				
100 gm, C-IV	**51552-0729-05**	440.93	314.95	
(Hawkins)				
POW, NA (U.S.P.)				
1 gm, C-IV	**63370-0935-10**	16.00		
5 gm, C-IV	**63370-0935-15**	56.00		
25 gm, C-IV	**63370-0935-25**	260.00		
100 gm, C-IV	**63370-0935-35**	960.00		
(Hospira)				
SOL, IJ (10X1ML)				
2 mg/ml,				
1 ml 10s, C-IV	**00409-1985-05**	20.40	17.90	**AP**
1 ml 10s, C-IV	**00409-6778-02**	11.76	10.30	**AP**
1 ml 10s, C-IV	**00409-6778-62**	8.88	7.80	**AP**
(LUER LOCK,CARPUJECT)				
2 mg/ml,				
1 ml 10s, C-IV	**00409-1985-30**	26.40	23.10	**AP**
10 ml, C-IV	**00409-1985-10**	11.26	9.85	**AP**
(VIAL,FLIPTOP)				
2 mg/ml,				
10 ml 10s, C-IV	**00409-6780-02**	91.20	79.80	**AP**
(10X1ML, LUER LOCK)				
4 mg/ml,				
1 ml 10s, C-IV	**00409-1539-31**	35.76	31.30	**AP**
(U.S.P., 10X10ML)				
4 mg/ml,				
10 ml 10s, C-IV	**00409-6781-02**	134.88	118.00	**AP**
(VIAL, FLIPTOP)				
4 mg/ml,				
10 ml 10s, C-IV	**00409-6779-02**	27.00	23.60	**AP**
(Letco)				
POW, NA, 25 gm, C-IV	**62991-1682-01**	216.00		
(Major)				
TAB, PO, 0.5 mg,				
100s ea, C-IV	**00904-6007-60**	63.69		**AB**
500s ea, C-IV	**00904-6007-40**	311.85		**AB**
1 mg, 100s ea, C-IV	**00904-6008-60**	82.95		**AB**
(USP)				
2 mg,				
100s ea, C-IV	**00904-6009-60**	127.36		**AB**
(Medisca)				
POW, NA (U.S.P.)				
1 gm, C-IV	**38779-0927-06**	70.50		
5 gm, C-IV	**38779-0927-03**	124.50		
10 gm, C-IV	**38779-0927-01**	204.00		
25 gm, C-IV	**38779-0927-04**	459.00		
100 gm, C-IV	**38779-0927-05**	1125.00		
500 gm, C-IV	**38779-0927-08**	3567.00		
(Mylan)				
TAB, PO, 0.5 mg,				
100s ea, C-IV	**00378-0321-01**	67.75		**AB**
(USP)				
0.5 mg,				
100s ea, C-IV	**00378-2321-01**	67.75		**AB**
500s ea, C-IV	**00378-0321-05**	331.05		**AB**
(USP)				
0.5 mg,				
500s ea, C-IV	**00378-2321-05**	331.05		**AB**
1 mg, 100s ea, C-IV	**00378-0457-01**	88.25		**AB**
(USP)				
1 mg,				
100s ea, C-IV	**00378-2457-01**	88.25		**AB**
500s ea, C-IV	**00378-0457-05**	430.75		**AB**
1000s ea, C-IV	**00378-2457-10**	843.20		**AB**
2 mg, 100s ea, C-IV	**00378-2777-01**	128.45		**AB**
500s ea, C-IV	**00378-0777-05**	628.15		**AB**
(USP)				
2 mg,				
500s ea, C-IV	**00378-2777-05**	628.15		**AB**
(Paddock)				
SOL, PO (1X30ML, USP)				
2 mg/ml,				
30 ml, C-IV	**00574-0163-30**	39.60		**AA**
(PCCA)				
POW, NA (U.S.P.; CIV)				
1 gm, C-IV	**51927-1005-00**	165.00		
(Ranbaxy Pharm)				
TAB, PO (USP)				
0.5 mg,				
90s ea, C-IV	**63304-0772-90**	60.98		**AB**
100s ea, C-IV	**63304-0772-01**	67.75		**AB**
500s ea, C-IV	**63304-0772-05**	331.05		**AB**
(USP)				
1 mg, 90s ea, C-IV	**63304-0773-90**	79.43		**AB**
100s ea, C-IV	**63304-0773-01**	88.25		**AB**
500s ea, C-IV	**63304-0773-05**	430.75		**AB**
1000s ea, C-IV	**63304-0773-10**	843.20		**AB**
(USP)				
2 mg, 90s ea, C-IV	**63304-0774-90**	115.61		**AB**
100s ea, C-IV	**63304-0774-01**	128.45		**AB**
500s ea, C-IV	**63304-0774-05**	628.15		**AB**
(Roxane) *See LORAZEPAM INTENSOL*				
(Sandoz)				
TAB, PO, 0.5 mg,				
100s ea, C-IV	**00781-1403-01**	64.31		**AB**
500s ea, C-IV	**00781-1403-05**	312.59		**AB**
1 mg, 100s ea, C-IV	**00781-1404-01**	83.77		**AB**
500s ea, C-IV	**00781-1404-05**	405.24		**AB**
2 mg, 100s ea, C-IV	**00781-1405-01**	122.11		**AB**
500s ea, C-IV	**00781-1405-05**	594.11		**AB**
(Spectrum Pharmacy)				
POW, NA (U.S.P.)				
5 gm, C-IV	**49452-4140-01**	197.75		
25 gm, C-IV	**49452-4140-02**	693.00		
100 gm, C-IV	**49452-4140-03**	1610.00		
500 gm, C-IV	**49452-4140-04**	4994.50		
(Teva)				
TAB, PO (USP)				
0.5 mg,				
100s ea, C-IV	**00093-4820-01**	64.31		**AB**
500s ea, C-IV	**00093-4820-05**	312.59		**AB**
1000s ea, C-IV	**00093-4820-10**	640.00		**AB**
1 mg, 100s ea, C-IV	**00093-4821-01**	88.25		**AB**
500s ea, C-IV	**00093-4821-05**	430.21		**AB**
1000s ea, C-IV	**00093-4821-10**	843.20		**AB**
2 mg, 100s ea, C-IV	**00093-4822-01**	128.20		**AB**
500s ea, C-IV	**00093-4822-05**	627.90		**AB**
1000s ea, C-IV	**00093-4822-10**	1152.57		**AB**
(UDL)				
TAB, PO (10X10)				
0.5 mg,				
100s ea UD, C-IV	**51079-0417-20**	69.53		**AB**
(R.N.P., 5X20)				
0.5 mg,				
100s ea UD, C-IV	**51079-0417-21**	69.53		**AB**
(10X30)				
0.5 mg,				
300s ea UD, C-IV	**51079-0417-56**	208.59		**AB**
(10X10)				
1 mg,				
100s ea UD, C-IV	**51079-0386-20**	90.64		**AB**
(R.N.P., 5X20)				
1 mg,				
100s ea UD, C-IV	**51079-0386-21**	90.64		**AB**
(10X30)				
1 mg,				
300s ea UD, C-IV	**51079-0386-56**	271.92		**AB**
(10X10)				
2 mg,				
100s ea UD, C-IV	**51079-0387-20**	132.05		**AB**
(R.N.P., 5X20)				
2 mg,				
100s ea UD, C-IV	**51079-0387-21**	132.05		**AB**
(Watson Labs)				
TAB, PO, 0.5 mg,				
100s ea, C-IV	**00591-0240-01**	6.18		**AB**
500s ea, C-IV	**00591-0240-05**	30.13		**AB**
1000s ea, C-IV	**00591-0240-10**	60.26		**AB**
1 mg, 100s ea, C-IV	**00591-0241-01**	7.60		**AB**
500s ea, C-IV	**00591-0241-05**	37.03		**AB**
1000s ea, C-IV	**00591-0241-10**	74.06		**AB**
2 mg, 100s ea, C-IV	**00591-0242-01**	11.74		**AB**
500s ea, C-IV	**00591-0242-05**	57.22		**AB**
1000s ea, C-IV	**00591-0242-10**	114.43		**AB**
(4u) REPACK				
TAB, PO, 2 mg,				
30s ea, C-IV	**10544-0358-30**	46.82		**AB**
30s ea, C-IV	**42549-0558-30**	46.82		**AB**
(A-S Medication) REPACK				
TAB, PO, 0.5 mg,				
30s ea, C-IV	**54569-2687-00**	20.33		**EE**
1 mg, 10s ea, C-IV	**54569-5401-00**	8.83		**EE**
20s ea, C-IV	**54569-1585-05**	17.65		**EE**
30s ea, C-IV	**54569-1585-00**	26.48		**EE**
60s ea, C-IV	**54569-1585-02**	52.95		**EE**
100s ea, C-IV	**54569-1585-01**	88.25		**EE**
2 mg, 30s ea, C-IV	**54569-2173-00**	38.54		**EE**
(Aidarex) REPACK				
TAB, PO, 1 mg, 7s ea, C-IV	**33261-0068-07**	9.73		
14s ea, C-IV	**33261-0068-14**	19.46		
21s ea, C-IV	**33261-0068-21**	29.19		
28s ea, C-IV	**33261-0068-28**	38.92		
30s ea, C-IV	**33261-0068-30**	41.70		
60s ea, C-IV	**33261-0068-60**	83.20		
90s ea, C-IV	**33261-0068-90**	125.10		
2 mg, 7s ea, C-IV	**33261-0069-07**	10.99		
14s ea, C-IV	**33261-0069-14**	21.96		
21s ea, C-IV	**33261-0069-21**	32.97		
28s ea, C-IV	**33261-0069-28**	43.96		
30s ea, C-IV	**33261-0069-30**	47.00		
60s ea, C-IV	**33261-0069-60**	94.20		
90s ea, C-IV	**33261-0069-90**	141.30		
(Altura) REPACK				
TAB, PO, 0.5 mg,				
10s ea, C-IV	**63874-0208-10**	9.35		**AB**
15s ea, C-IV	**63874-0208-15**	14.03		**AB**
20s ea, C-IV	**63874-0208-20**	18.70		**AB**
30s ea, C-IV	**63874-0208-30**	28.05		**AB**
36s ea, C-IV	**63874-0208-36**	33.66		**AB**
60s ea, C-IV	**63874-0208-60**	56.10		**AB**
90s ea, C-IV	**63874-0208-90**	84.15		**AB**
100s ea, C-IV	**63874-0208-01**	93.50		**AB**
1 mg, 4s ea, C-IV	**63874-0205-04**	3.43		**AB**
6s ea, C-IV	**63874-0205-06**	5.15		**AB**
10s ea, C-IV	**63874-0205-10**	8.59		**AB**
12s ea, C-IV	**63874-0205-12**	10.31		**AB**
15s ea, C-IV	**63874-0205-15**	12.88		**AB**
20s ea, C-IV	**63874-0205-20**	17.18		**AB**
30s ea, C-IV	**63874-0205-30**	25.76		**AB**
50s ea, C-IV	**63874-0205-50**	153.58		**AB**
60s ea, C-IV	**63874-0205-60**	51.53		**AB**
90s ea, C-IV	**63874-0205-90**	77.29		**AB**
100s ea, C-IV	**63874-0205-01**	85.88		**AB**
150s ea, C-IV	**63874-0205-72**	136.97		**AB**
200s ea, C-IV	**63874-0205-74**	182.62		**AB**
300s ea, C-IV	**63874-0205-77**	273.93		**AB**
500s ea, C-IV	**63874-0205-03**	429.33		**AB**
1000s ea, C-IV	**63874-0205-02**	278.74		**EE**
2 mg, 12s ea, C-IV	**63874-0207-12**	15.41		**AB**

PROD/MFR	NDC	AWP	DP	OBC
15s ea, C-IV	63874-0207-15	19.27		AB
20s ea, C-IV	63874-0207-20	25.69		AB
30s ea, C-IV	63874-0207-30	38.54		AB
60s ea, C-IV	63874-0207-60	77.07		AB
90s ea, C-IV	63874-0207-90	115.61		AB
100s ea, C-IV	63874-0207-01	128.45		AB
120s ea, C-IV	63874-0207-04	154.14		AB
150s ea, C-IV	63874-0207-72	199.70		AB
200s ea, C-IV	63874-0207-74	266.26		AB
300s ea, C-IV	63874-0207-77	399.39		AB
(American Health)				
REPACK				
TAB, PO (10X10)				
0.5 mg,				
100s ea UD, C-IV	68084-0088-01	69.45		AB
(USP,10X10)				
1 mg,				
100s ea UD, C-IV	68084-0089-01	90.50		AB
2 mg,				
100s ea UD, C-IV	68084-0090-01	132.00		AB
(B&B Pharm, Inc)				
REPACK				
POW, NA (U.S.P.)				
5 gm, C-IV	63275-9979-02	140.00		
25 gm, C-IV	63275-9979-04	425.00		
100 gm, C-IV	63275-9979-05	1350.00		
(Bryant Ranch)				
REPACK				
TAB, PO, 0.5 mg,				
30s ea, C-IV	63629-2953-01	24.31		
1 mg, 14s ea, C-IV	63629-1233-04	16.53		
15s ea, C-IV	63629-1233-03	17.71		
30s ea, C-IV	63629-1233-01	35.41		
50s ea, C-IV	63629-1233-06	59.02		
60s ea, C-IV	63629-1233-07	69.58		AB
90s ea, C-IV	63629-1233-05	106.24		
100s ea, C-IV	63629-1233-09	117.77		AB
2 mg, 30s ea, C-IV	63629-2954-01	45.00		
60s ea, C-IV	63629-2954-02	44.10		
(Core)				
REPACK				
TAB, PO, 0.5 mg,				
30s ea, C-IV	33358-0219-30	30.74		
60s ea, C-IV	33358-0219-60	45.46		
1 mg, 3s ea, C-IV	33358-0220-03	10.25		
14s ea, C-IV	33358-0220-14	16.94		
15s ea, C-IV	33358-0220-15	18.15		
30s ea, C-IV	33358-0220-30	36.30		
50s ea, C-IV	33358-0220-50	60.50		
60s ea, C-IV	33358-0220-60	62.74		
90s ea, C-IV	33358-0220-90	108.90		
2 mg, 30s ea, C-IV	33358-0221-30	46.13		
60s ea, C-IV	33358-0221-60	53.33		
(DHS, Inc.)				
REPACK				
TAB, PO, 0.5 mg,				
15s ea, C-IV	55887-0633-15	12.95		AB
30s ea, C-IV	55887-0633-30	23.00		AB
60s ea, C-IV	55887-0633-60	46.00		AB
90s ea, C-IV	55887-0633-90	69.00		AB
1 mg, 30s ea, C-IV	55887-0250-30	24.75		AB
60s ea, C-IV	55887-0250-60	31.00		AB
90s ea, C-IV	55887-0250-90	38.75		AB
120s ea, C-IV	55887-0250-82	97.44		AB
2 mg, 30s ea, C-IV	55887-0948-30	35.00		
60s ea, C-IV	55887-0948-60	70.00		
90s ea, C-IV	55887-0948-90	105.00		
(Dispensing Solutions)				
REPACK				
TAB, PO, 0.5 mg,				
6s ea, C-IV	55045-1372-06	4.86		
15s ea, C-IV	55045-1372-03	12.15		AB
20s ea, C-IV	55045-1372-07	16.20		
30s ea, C-IV	55045-1372-08	24.30		
30s ea, C-IV	66336-0363-30	32.65		AB
50s ea, C-IV	55045-1372-04	40.50		
60s ea, C-IV	55045-1372-05	48.60		
90s ea, C-IV	55045-1372-09	72.00		
100s ea, C-IV	55045-1372-01	81.00		
120s ea, C-IV	55045-1372-02	97.20		
1 mg, 2s ea, C-IV	55045-1123-05	3.04		
3s ea, C-IV	55045-1123-03	4.55		
4s ea, C-IV	55045-1123-01	6.08		
6s ea, C-IV	55045-1123-06	9.12		
8s ea, C-IV	55045-1123-02	12.16		
10s ea, C-IV	66336-0047-10	14.72		AB
14s ea, C-IV	55045-3286-04	21.28		
15s ea, C-IV	55045-3286-05	22.80		
20s ea, C-IV	55045-1123-07	30.40		
28s ea, C-IV	55045-3286-08	42.56		
30s ea, C-IV	55045-1123-08	45.60		AB
30s ea, C-IV	66336-0047-30	40.43		AB
50s ea, C-IV	55045-1123-04	76.00		
60s ea, C-IV	55045-3286-06	91.20		
90s ea, C-IV	55045-3286-09	136.80		
100s ea, C-IV	55045-1123-00	152.00		
120s ea, C-IV	55045-3286-02	182.40		
2 mg, 2s ea, C-IV	66336-0800-99	2.48		
30s ea, C-IV	55045-1255-08	46.50		
30s ea, C-IV	66336-0800-30	45.60		
60s ea, C-IV	55045-1255-06	93.00		
(GSMS)				
REPACK				
TAB, PO (UNIT OF USE)				
1 mg, 30s ea, C-IV	60429-0512-30	28.50	9.50	AB
90s ea, C-IV	60429-0512-90	81.15	27.05	AB
(HomeMed)				
REPACK				
TAB, PO, 0.5 mg,				
30s ea, C-IV	51655-0824-24	19.75		EE
60s ea, C-IV	51655-0824-25	38.51		EE
90s ea, C-IV	51655-0824-26	57.26		EE
120s ea, C-IV	51655-0824-82	76.27		EE
1 mg, 30s ea, C-IV	51655-0822-24	33.69		EE
60s ea, C-IV	51655-0822-25	49.73		EE
90s ea, C-IV	51655-0822-26	73.95		EE
120s ea, C-IV	51655-0822-82	99.51		EE
2 mg, 30s ea, C-IV	51655-0831-24	34.99		EE
(IPI)				
REPACK				
TAB, PO, 0.5 mg,				
60s ea, C-IV	18837-0279-60	48.00		
1 mg, 30s ea, C-IV	18837-0281-30	31.62		
60s ea, C-IV	18837-0281-60	63.24		
2 mg, 30s ea, C-IV	18837-0078-30	47.11		
(McKesson Packaging)				
REPACK				
TAB, PO, 0.5 mg,				
100s ea UD, C-IV	63739-0154-10	64.67		AB
(BLISTER PACK)				
0.5 mg,				
750s ea UD, C-IV	63739-0154-01	484.99		AB
(PUNCH CARD 25X30)				
0.5 mg,				
750s ea, C-IV	63739-0154-03	484.90		AB
1 mg,				
100s ea UD, C-IV	63739-0155-10	84.67		AB
2 mg,				
100s ea UD, C-IV	63739-0156-10	118.51		AB
(Medsource)				
REPACK				
TAB, PO, 0.5 mg,				
30s ea, C-IV	45865-0499-30	20.10		AB
60s ea, C-IV	45865-0499-60	40.20		AB
90s ea, C-IV	45865-0499-90	60.30		AB
100s ea, C-IV	45865-0499-49	67.00		AB
1 mg, 30s ea, C-IV	45865-0470-30	26.40		AB
60s ea, C-IV	45865-0470-60	52.80		AB
90s ea, C-IV	45865-0470-90	79.20		AB
100s ea, C-IV	45865-0470-49	88.00		AB
2 mg, 30s ea, C-IV	45865-0422-30	38.40		AB
60s ea, C-IV	45865-0422-60	76.80		AB
90s ea, C-IV	45865-0422-90	115.20		AB
100s ea, C-IV	45865-0422-49	128.00		AB
(Nucare Pharm)				
REPACK				
TAB, PO, 0.5 mg,				
30s ea, C-IV	66267-0133-30	24.99		AB
60s ea, C-IV	66267-0133-60	52.80		AB
1 mg, 20s ea, C-IV	66267-0427-20	23.99		EE
30s ea, C-IV	66267-0427-30	34.78		AB
60s ea, C-IV	66267-0427-60	52.80		AB
90s ea, C-IV	66267-0427-90	115.36		AB
2 mg, 30s ea, C-IV	66267-0608-30	51.82		AB
(Palmetto)				
REPACK				
TAB, PO, 0.5 mg,				
15s ea, C-IV	23490-5834-00	14.85		
30s ea, C-IV	23490-5834-01	29.69		
1 mg, 6s ea, C-IV	23490-5835-01	9.66		
10s ea, C-IV	23490-5835-02	11.50		
30s ea, C-IV	23490-5835-03	34.50		
60s ea, C-IV	23490-5835-04	69.00		
2 mg, ea, C-IV	23490-5836-01	2.57		
2s ea, C-IV	23490-5836-00	4.86		
30s ea, C-IV	23490-5836-02	40.50		
(PD-Rx Pharm)				
REPACK				
TAB, PO (USP)				
0.5 mg,				
6s ea, C-IV	43063-0057-06	18.65		AB
15s ea, C-IV	58864-0701-15	22.50		AB
30s ea, C-IV	55289-0402-30	6.00		
(USP)				
0.5 mg,				
90s ea, C-IV	55289-0402-90	11.10		AB
1 mg, ea, C-IV	55289-0487-79	25.15		AB
2s ea, C-IV	55289-0487-02	25.35		AB
4s ea, C-IV	43063-0048-04	25.95		AB
4s ea, C-IV	55289-0487-04	25.75		AB
6s ea, C-IV	55289-0487-06	26.60		AB
(USP)				
1 mg, 6s ea, C-IV	43063-0048-06	26.60		AB
15s ea, C-IV	43063-0048-15	27.85		AB
15s ea, C-IV	55289-0487-15	27.85		AB
20s ea, C-IV	55289-0487-20	30.10		AB
30s ea, C-IV	55289-0487-30	30.72		AB
60s ea, C-IV	55289-0487-60	44.78		AB
90s ea, C-IV	55289-0487-90	58.83		AB
120s ea, C-IV	55289-0487-98	72.89		AB
2 mg, 30s ea, C-IV	55289-0594-30	29.55		AB
60s ea, C-IV	55289-0594-60	50.72		AB
90s ea, C-IV	55289-0594-90	100.00		AB
(Pharma Pac)				
REPACK				
TAB, PO, 0.5 mg,				
10s ea, C-IV	52959-0538-10	9.70		EE
20s ea, C-IV	52959-0538-20	19.39		EE
30s ea, C-IV	52959-0538-30	29.08		EE
40s ea, C-IV	52959-0538-40	38.76		EE
60s ea, C-IV	52959-0538-60	58.13		EE
90s ea, C-IV	52959-0538-90	87.16		EE
100s ea, C-IV	52959-0538-00	96.80		EE
1 mg, 4s ea, C-IV	52959-0331-04	5.20		EE
5s ea, C-IV	52959-0331-05	6.52		EE
10s ea, C-IV	52959-0331-10	13.03		EE
14s ea, C-IV	52959-0331-14	18.24		EE
15s ea, C-IV	52959-0331-15	19.54		EE
20s ea, C-IV	52959-0331-20	26.05		EE
21s ea, C-IV	52959-0331-21	27.35		EE
30s ea, C-IV	52959-0331-30	39.06		EE
40s ea, C-IV	52959-0331-40	52.07		EE
45s ea, C-IV	52959-0331-45	58.59		EE
60s ea, C-IV	52959-0331-60	78.10		EE
90s ea, C-IV	52959-0331-90	117.14		EE
100s ea, C-IV	52959-0331-00	130.10		EE
2 mg, 5s ea, C-IV	52959-0365-05	8.89		EE
15s ea, C-IV	52959-0365-15	26.66		EE
30s ea, C-IV	52959-0365-30	53.31		EE
60s ea, C-IV	52959-0365-60	106.61		EE
90s ea, C-IV	52959-0365-90	159.84		EE
120s ea, C-IV	52959-0365-01	212.40		EE
(Phys Total Care)				
REPACK				
SOL, IJ (M.D.V.)				
2 mg/ml,				
1 ml, C-IV	54868-3566-01	13.80		EE
10 ml, C-IV	54868-3566-00	123.54		EE
25 ml, C-IV	54868-3566-02	277.46		EE
TAB, PO, 0.5 mg,				
3s ea, C-IV	54868-2145-07	5.01		EE
10s ea, C-IV	54868-2145-00	6.24		EE
15s ea, C-IV	54868-2145-08	7.11		AB
20s ea, C-IV	54868-2145-02	7.98		EE
30s ea, C-IV	54868-2145-03	9.72		EE
50s ea, C-IV	54868-2145-05	13.20		EE
60s ea, C-IV	54868-2145-06	14.94		EE
100s ea, C-IV	54868-2145-04	20.40		EE
1 mg, 3s ea, C-IV	54868-1338-06	6.60		AB
(USP)				
1 mg, 10s ea, C-IV	54868-1338-07	8.04		EE
15s ea, C-IV	54868-1338-00	9.06		AB
20s ea, C-IV	54868-1338-01	10.08		EE
30s ea, C-IV	54868-1338-03	12.12		EE
60s ea, C-IV	54868-1338-04	18.24		EE
(USP)				
1 mg, 90s ea, C-IV	54868-1338-08	24.36		EE
100s ea, C-IV	54868-1338-02	26.40		EE
120s ea, C-IV	54868-1338-09	26.99		EE
2 mg, 30s ea, C-IV	54868-0061-03	11.79		EE
60s ea, C-IV	54868-0061-05	20.58		EE
90s ea, C-IV	54868-0061-04	30.87		EE
100s ea, C-IV	54868-0061-02	33.81		EE
(Physician Partner)				
REPACK				
TAB, PO, 0.5 mg,				
30s ea, C-IV	21695-0238-30	38.40		
90s ea, C-IV	21695-0238-90	115.20		
100s ea, C-IV	21695-0238-00	128.62		
1 mg, 3s ea, C-IV	21695-0239-03	5.95		
30s ea, C-IV	21695-0239-30	50.59		
60s ea, C-IV	21695-0239-60	101.18		
90s ea, C-IV	21695-0239-90	151.78		

PROD/MFR	NDC	AWP	DP	OBC
100s ea, C-IV	21695-0239-00	167.54		
2 mg, 3s ea, C-IV	21695-0240-03	8.14		
30s ea, C-IV	21695-0240-30	69.16		
60s ea, C-IV	21695-0240-60	138.31		
(Quality Care Prod)				
REPACK				
TAB, PO, 0.5 mg,				
30s ea, C-IV	49999-0805-30	31.06		AB
1 mg, 14s ea, C-IV	49999-0122-14	22.97		AB
20s ea, C-IV	49999-0122-20	28.91		EE
30s ea, C-IV	49999-0122-30	42.50		AB
60s ea, C-IV	49999-0122-60	98.42		AB
90s ea, C-IV	49999-0122-90	147.63		AB
100s ea, C-IV	49999-0122-01	164.00		AB
2 mg, 30s ea, C-IV	49999-0266-30	53.10		EE
(Southwood)				
REPACK				
TAB, PO, 0.5 mg,				
30s ea, C-IV	58016-0805-30	27.26		EE
60s ea, C-IV	58016-0805-60	54.52		AB
90s ea, C-IV	58016-0805-90	81.78		AB
100s ea, C-IV	58016-0805-00	90.87		AB
120s ea, C-IV	58016-0805-02	109.04		AB
1 mg, 5s ea, C-IV	58016-0803-05	4.57		EE
12s ea, C-IV	58016-0803-12	10.96		EE
15s ea, C-IV	58016-0803-15	13.70		EE
20s ea, C-IV	58016-0803-20	18.26		EE
30s ea, C-IV	58016-0803-30	35.10		AB
60s ea, C-IV	58016-0803-60	70.20		AB
90s ea, C-IV	58016-0803-90	105.30		AB
100s ea, C-IV	58016-0803-00	117.00		AB
120s ea, C-IV	58016-0803-02	140.40		AB
150s ea, C-IV	58016-0803-03	136.97		AB
200s ea, C-IV	58016-0803-89	182.62		AB
300s ea, C-IV	58016-0803-73	273.93		AB
2 mg, 12s ea, C-IV	58016-0804-12	15.98		EE
15s ea, C-IV	58016-0804-15	19.97		EE
20s ea, C-IV	58016-0804-20	26.63		EE
30s ea, C-IV	58016-0804-30	39.94		EE
100s ea, C-IV	58016-0804-00	133.13		EE
120s ea, C-IV	58016-0804-02	159.76		AB
150s ea, C-IV	58016-0804-03	199.70		AB
200s ea, C-IV	58016-0804-89	266.26		AB
300s ea, C-IV	58016-0804-73	399.39		AB
(St. Mary's MPP)				
REPACK				
TAB, PO, 1 mg,				
10s ea, C-IV	60760-0457-10	15.28		AB
(USP)				
1 mg, 30s ea, C-IV	60760-0457-30	33.83		AB
(Stat Rx)				
REPACK				
TAB, PO, 0.5 mg,				
15s ea, C-IV	16590-0143-15	7.00		
30s ea, C-IV	16590-0143-30	23.88		AB
60s ea, C-IV	16590-0143-60	28.00		
1 mg, 30s ea, C-IV	16590-0584-30	42.00		AB
60s ea, C-IV	16590-0584-60	94.19		AB
90s ea, C-IV	16590-0584-90	126.00		AB
120s ea, C-IV	16590-0584-72	168.00		AB
2 mg, 30s ea, C-IV	16590-0499-30	37.50		
60s ea, C-IV	16590-0499-60	75.00		
90s ea, C-IV	16590-0499-90	112.50		
120s ea, C-IV	16590-0499-72	150.00		
LORAZEPAM INTENSOL (Roxane)				
lorazepam				
SOL, PO, 2 mg/ml,				
30 ml, C-IV*	00054-3532-44	48.03		
(Phys Total Care)				
REPACK				
SOL, PO, 2 mg/ml,				
30 ml, C-IV	54868-6010-00	133.11		
LORCET 10/650 (Forest Pharm)				
acetaminophen/hydrocodone bitartrate				
TAB, PO (CAPLET)				
650 mg-10 mg,				
100s ea, C-III	00785-6350-01	183.54		AA
500s ea, C-III	00785-6350-50	853.42		AA
(Dispensing Solutions)				
REPACK				
TAB, PO, 650 mg-10 mg,				
30s ea, C-III	55045-2122-08	54.00		
(PD-Rx Pharm)				
REPACK				
TAB, PO, 650 mg-10 mg,				
20s ea, C-III	55289-0407-20	45.12		AA
(Pharma Pac)				
REPACK				
TAB, PO, 650 mg-10 mg,				
20s ea, C-III	52959-0403-20	31.17		AA
30s ea, C-III	52959-0403-30	46.77		AA
(Phys Total Care)				
REPACK				
TAB, PO (CAPLET)				
650 mg-10 mg,				
10s ea, C-III	54868-2986-04	23.33		AA
20s ea, C-III	54868-2986-02	49.28		AA
30s ea, C-III	54868-2986-01	72.28		AA
(CAPLET)				
650 mg-10 mg,				
60s ea, C-III	54868-2986-06	141.30		AA
90s ea, C-III	54868-2986-00	198.81		AA
100s ea, C-III	54868-2986-03	220.54		AA
(CAPLET)				
650 mg-10 mg,				
500s ea, C-III	54868-2986-05	1054.57		AA
(Southwood)				
REPACK				
TAB, PO (CAPLET)				
650 mg-10 mg,				
30s ea, C-III	58016-0094-30	51.95		AA
60s ea, C-III	58016-0094-60	103.89		AA
90s ea, C-III	58016-0094-90	155.84		AA
100s ea, C-III	58016-0094-00	173.15		AA
(Stat Rx)				
REPACK				
TAB, PO (CAPLET)				
650 mg-10 mg,				
84s ea, C-III	16590-0623-62	181.46		AA
112s ea, C-III	16590-0623-73	240.86		AA
LORCET PLUS (Forest Pharm)				
acetaminophen/hydrocodone bitartrate				
TAB, PO, 650 mg-7.5 mg,*				
100s ea, C-III	00785-1122-01	130.45		AA
500s ea, C-III	00785-1122-50	549.19		AA
(Phys Total Care)				
REPACK				
TAB, PO, 650 mg-7.5 mg,				
20s ea, C-III	54868-1844-02	28.81		AA
30s ea, C-III	54868-1844-01	42.28		AA
60s ea, C-III	54868-1844-00	82.68		AA
90s ea, C-III	54868-1844-04	123.09		AA
100s ea, C-III	54868-1844-03	129.08		AA
500s ea, C-III	54868-1844-05	530.83		AA
(Southwood)				
REPACK				
TAB, PO, 650 mg-7.5 mg,				
30s ea, C-III	58016-0077-30	36.92		AA
60s ea, C-III	58016-0077-60	73.84		AA
90s ea, C-III	58016-0077-90	110.76		AA
100s ea, C-III	58016-0077-00	123.07		AA
(Stat Rx)				
REPACK				
TAB, PO, 650 mg-7.5 mg,				
84s ea, C-III	16590-0676-62	121.80		AA
LORCET-HD (PD-Rx Pharm)				
REPACK				
acetaminophen/hydrocodone bitartrate				
CAP, PO, 500 mg-5 mg,				
6s ea, C-III	55289-0514-06	9.80		AA
12s ea, C-III	55289-0514-12	14.60		AA
15s ea, C-III	55289-0514-15	17.02		AA
LORTAB (UCB)				
acetaminophen/hydrocodone bitartrate				
ELI, PO, 473 ml, C-III	50474-0909-16	150.47		
(Phys Total Care)				
REPACK				
ELI, PO, 16 ml, C-III	54868-2908-00	166.03		
TAB, PO, 500 mg-10 mg,				
30s ea, C-III	54868-3812-02	40.56		
(Southwood)				
REPACK				
TAB, PO, 500 mg-7.5 mg,				
30s ea, C-III	58016-0095-30	30.94		
60s ea, C-III	58016-0095-60	61.87		
90s ea, C-III	58016-0095-90	92.81		
100s ea, C-III	58016-0095-00	103.12		
500 mg-10 mg,				
30s ea, C-III	58016-0793-30	33.78		
60s ea, C-III	58016-0793-60	67.56		
90s ea, C-III	58016-0793-90	101.34		
100s ea, C-III	58016-0793-00	112.60		
LORTAB 10/500 (UCB)				
acetaminophen/hydrocodone bitartrate				
TAB, PO (4X25,CAPLET)				
500 mg-10 mg,				
100s ea UD, C-III	50474-0910-60	158.58		AA
(CAPLET)				
500 mg-10 mg,				
100s ea, C-III	50474-0910-01	158.58		AA
500s ea, C-III	50474-0910-50	713.57		AA
(A-S Medication)				
REPACK				
TAB, PO (CAPLET)				
500 mg-10 mg,				
4s ea, C-III	54569-4347-01	5.82		AA
40s ea, C-III	54569-4347-00	49.49		AA
(Phys Total Care)				
REPACK				
TAB, PO (CAPLET)				
500 mg-10 mg,				
100s ea, C-III	54868-3812-01	131.48		
500s ea, C-III	54868-3812-00	511.12		AA
(Quality Care Prod)				
REPACK				
TAB, PO (CAPLET)				
500 mg-10 mg,				
30s ea, C-III	35356-0452-30	125.05		AA
90s ea, C-III	35356-0452-90	364.90		AA
(Stat Rx)				
REPACK				
TAB, PO (CAPLET)				
500 mg-10 mg,				
112s ea, C-III	16590-0628-73	187.75		AA
120s ea, C-III	16590-0628-72	205.05		AA
180s ea, C-III	16590-0628-82	305.95		AA
LORTAB 5/500 (UCB)				
acetaminophen/hydrocodone bitartrate				
TAB, PO (CAPLET)				
500 mg-5 mg,				
100s ea, C-III	50474-0902-01	136.55		AA
500s ea, C-III	50474-0902-50	614.53		AA
(Phys Total Care)				
REPACK				
TAB, PO, 500 mg-5 mg,				
30s ea, C-III	54868-1111-01	35.88		AA
100s ea, C-III	54868-1111-00	98.93		AA
120s ea, C-III	54868-1111-02	135.99		AA
LORTAB 7.5/500 (UCB)				
acetaminophen/hydrocodone bitartrate				
TAB, PO (4X25,CAPLET)				
500 mg-7.5 mg,				
100s ea UD, C-III	50474-0907-60	151.26		AA
(CAPLET)				
500 mg-7.5 mg,				
100s ea, C-III	50474-0907-01	151.26		AA
500s ea, C-III	50474-0907-50	680.69		AA
(A-S Medication)				
REPACK				
TAB, PO (CAPLET)				
500 mg-7.5 mg,				
12s ea, C-III	54569-0957-01	16.65		AA
(PD-Rx Pharm)				
REPACK				
TAB, PO, 500 mg-7.5 mg,				
10s ea, C-III	55289-0849-10	19.04		AA
20s ea, C-III	55289-0849-20	32.97		AA
(Phys Total Care)				
REPACK				
TAB, PO, 500 mg-7.5 mg,				
30s ea, C-III	54868-1845-01	55.45		AA
(CAPLET)				
500 mg-7.5 mg,				
100s ea, C-III	54868-1845-00	167.54		AA
(Stat Rx)				
REPACK				
TAB, PO (CAPLET)				
500 mg-7.5 mg,				
84s ea, C-III	16590-0636-62	137.98		AA
LORTUSS EX (Poly)				
codeine phos/gg/pse hcl				
SOL, PO (1X473ML,AF,SF,DYE-FREE)				
473 ml, C-V	50991-0515-16	86.46		
LOSARTAN POTASSIUM				
(Merck) *See COZAAR*				
LOSEASONIQUE (Duramed)				
ethinyl estradiol/levonorgestrel				
TAB, PO, 182s ea	51285-0092-87	436.80		EE

PROD/MFR	NDC	AWP	DP	OBC
LOTEMAX (Bausch & Lomb Inc.)				
loteprednol etabonate				
SUS, OP, 0.5%, 2.5 ml	24208-0299-25	34.03		
5 ml	24208-0299-05	68.02		
10 ml	24208-0299-10	135.26		
15 ml	24208-0299-15	181.21		
(Phys Total Care) REPACK				
SUS, OP, 0.5%, 5 ml	54868-4278-01	68.76		
15 ml	54868-4278-00	86.43		
LOTENSIN (Novartis Pharm)				
benazepril hydrochloride				
TAB, PO, 5 mg, 100s ea	00078-0447-05	190.40		
10 mg, 100s ea	00078-0448-05	190.40		
20 mg, 100s ea	00078-0449-05	190.40		
40 mg, 100s ea	00078-0450-05	190.40		
(PD-Rx Pharm) REPACK				
TAB, PO, 20 mg, 30s ea	55289-0086-30	51.57		
(Phys Total Care) REPACK				
TAB, PO, 5 mg, 30s ea	54868-3690-01	33.73		
10 mg, 10s ea	54868-2350-04	15.55		
30s ea	54868-2350-03	42.89		
60s ea	54868-2350-01	83.90		
100s ea	54868-2350-02	137.95		
20 mg, 10s ea	54868-2351-02	16.63		
30s ea	54868-2351-00	46.12		
100s ea	54868-2351-03	140.58		
40 mg, 10s ea	54868-2352-01	16.63		
30s ea	54868-2352-00	46.12		
(Quality Care Prod) REPACK				
TAB, PO, 20 mg, 30s ea	49999-0287-30	87.70		
(Southwood) REPACK				
TAB, PO, 10 mg, 10s ea	58016-0420-10	8.90		
30s ea	58016-0420-30	47.29		
60s ea	58016-0420-60	94.58		
90s ea	58016-0420-90	141.88		
100s ea	58016-0420-00	157.64		
20 mg, 10s ea	58016-0685-10	8.90		
30s ea	58016-0685-30	47.29		
60s ea	58016-0685-60	94.58		
90s ea	58016-0685-90	141.88		
100s ea	58016-0685-00	157.64		
40 mg, 10s ea	58016-0686-10	8.90		
30s ea	58016-0686-30	47.29		
60s ea	58016-0686-60	94.58		
90s ea	58016-0686-90	141.88		
100s ea	58016-0686-00	157.64		
LOTENSIN HCT (Novartis Pharm)				
benazepril hydrochloride/hydrochlorothiazide				
TAB, PO, 5 mg-6.25 mg, 100s ea	00078-0451-05	190.40		
10 mg-12.5 mg, 100s ea	00078-0452-05	190.40		
20 mg-12.5 mg, 100s ea	00078-0453-05	190.40		
20 mg-25 mg, 100s ea	00078-0454-05	190.40		
(Phys Total Care) REPACK				
TAB, PO, 20 mg-12.5 mg, 10s ea	54868-4904-01	15.55		
30s ea	54868-4904-00	42.89		
20 mg-25 mg, 10s ea	54868-5313-01	16.63		
30s ea	54868-5313-00	46.12		
LOTEPREDNOL ETABONATE				
(Bausch & Lomb Inc.) *See ALREX*				
(Bausch & Lomb Inc.) *See LOTEMAX*				
LOTEPREDNOL ETABONATE/TOBRAMYCIN				
(Bausch & Lomb Inc.) *See ZYLET*				
LOTION, MULTI INGREDIENT				
(ECR) *See TROPAZONE*				
(PCCA) *See VERSABASE LOTION*				
LOTREL (Novartis Pharm)				
amlodipine besylate/benazepril hydrochloride				
CAP, PO, 2.5 mg-10 mg, 100s ea	00078-0404-05	375.83		
5 mg-10 mg, 100s ea	00078-0405-05	383.28		
5 mg-20 mg, 100s ea	00078-0406-05	404.75		
5 mg-40 mg, 100s ea	00078-0384-05	428.90		EE
10 mg-20 mg, 100s ea	00078-0364-05	470.23		
10 mg-40 mg, 100s ea	00078-0379-05	518.15		
(A-S Medication) REPACK				
CAP, PO, 5 mg-10 mg, 30s ea	54569-4696-00	136.02		
5 mg-20 mg, 30s ea	54569-5232-00	143.63		
10 mg-20 mg, 30s ea	54569-5878-00	121.67		
(Bryant Ranch) REPACK				
CAP, PO, 5 mg-20 mg, 30s ea	63629-1454-01	82.09		
(Core) REPACK				
CAP, PO, 5 mg-20 mg, 100s ea	33358-0222-00	300.03		
(Direct Pharmaceutical, Inc.) REPACK				
CAP, PO, 2.5 mg-10 mg, 30s ea UD	67801-0340-03	91.20		
5 mg-10 mg, 30s ea	67801-0441-03	94.01		
5 mg-20 mg, 30s ea UD	67801-0342-03	98.22		
10 mg-20 mg, 30s ea UD	67801-0343-03	114.10		
(PD-Rx Pharm) REPACK				
CAP, PO, 5 mg-10 mg, 30s ea	55289-0096-30	155.51		
5 mg-20 mg, 30s ea	55289-0039-30	164.22		
10 mg-20 mg, 30s ea	55289-0981-30	190.80		
(Phys Total Care) REPACK				
CAP, PO, 2.5 mg-10 mg, 10s ea	54868-4066-01	36.12		
30s ea	54868-4066-00	104.61		
5 mg-10 mg, 10s ea	54868-4073-01	46.33		
30s ea	54868-4073-00	126.47		
60s ea	54868-4073-02	250.32		
100s ea	54868-4073-03	414.80		
5 mg-20 mg, 10s ea	54868-4074-02	43.96		
30s ea	54868-4074-00	127.97		
60s ea	54868-4074-04	239.97		
90s ea	54868-4074-01	358.98		
100s ea	54868-4074-03	398.00		
5 mg-40 mg, 10s ea	54868-5783-00	40.33		
30s ea	54868-5783-01	118.50		
10 mg-20 mg, 10s ea	54868-4870-01	44.73		
30s ea	54868-4870-00	123.28		
90s ea	54868-4870-02	365.48		
10 mg-40 mg, 10s ea	54868-5690-00	61.71		
30s ea	54868-5690-01	170.04		
90s ea	54868-5690-03	488.70		
100s ea	54868-5690-02	542.05		
(Quality Care Prod) REPACK				
CAP, PO, 5 mg-10 mg, 30s ea	49999-0947-30	146.50		
5 mg-20 mg, 30s ea	49999-0948-30	150.89		
10 mg-20 mg, 30s ea	49999-0946-30	178.60		
LOTRIMIN (Phys Total Care) REPACK				
clotrimazole				
CRE, TP, 1%, 15 gm	54868-0613-01	19.20		AB
30 gm	54868-0613-02	32.17		AB
SOL, TP, 1%, 10 ml	54868-0963-00	17.41		AT
(Southwood) REPACK				
CRE, TP, 1%, 30 gm	58016-3105-01	23.69		AB
LOTRISONE (Schering)				
betamethasone dipropionate/clotrimazole				
CRE, TP, 0.05%-1%, 15 gm	00085-0924-01	40.70		AB
45 gm	00085-0924-02	87.64		AB
LOT, TP, 0.05%-1%, 30 ml	00085-0809-01	84.41		
(Pharma Pac) REPACK				
CRE, TP, 0.05%-1%, 15 gm	52959-0385-00	36.58		AB
45 gm	52959-0385-03	61.99		AB
(Phys Total Care) REPACK				
LOT, TP, 0.05%-1%, 30 ml	54868-4622-00	88.07		
(Southwood) REPACK				
CRE, TP, 0.05%-1%, 15 gm	58016-3046-01	40.70		AB
45 gm	58016-3252-01	87.64		AB
LOTRONEX (Prometheus Labs)				
alosetron hydrochloride				
TAB, PO (FILM-COATED)				
0.5 mg, 30s ea	65483-0894-03	472.06		
1 mg, 30s ea	65483-0895-03	649.49		
LOVASTATIN				
FUL				
TAB, PO, 10 mg, 60s ea		19.71		
20 mg, 60s ea		27.73		
40 mg, 60s ea		47.53		
(Actavis)				
TAB, PO, 10 mg, 60s ea	00228-2633-06	80.70		AB
500s ea	00228-2633-50	672.50		AB
20 mg, 60s ea	00228-2634-06	142.30		AB
500s ea	00228-2634-50	1162.10		AB
40 mg, 60s ea	00228-2635-06	256.10		AB
500s ea	00228-2635-50	2134.15		AB
(Apotex Corp.)				
TAB, PO (USP)				
10 mg, 60s ea	60505-0177-00	80.73		AB
20 mg, 60s ea	60505-0178-00	142.37		AB
40 mg, 60s ea	60505-0179-00	256.29		AB
(Carlsbad Tech)				
TAB, PO, 10 mg, 60s ea	61442-0141-60	79.89		AB
100s ea	61442-0141-01	134.51		AB
1000s ea	61442-0141-10	1278.23		AB
20 mg, 60s ea	61442-0142-60	141.59		AB
100s ea	61442-0142-01	237.25		AB
500s ea	61442-0142-05	1162.10		AB
1000s ea	61442-0142-10	2254.25		AB
40 mg, 60s ea	61442-0143-60	254.82		AB
100s ea	61442-0143-01	427.10		AB
500s ea	61442-0143-05	2134.15		AB
1000s ea	61442-0143-10	4057.23		AB
(Lupin Pharma, Inc.)				
TAB, PO (USP)				
10 mg, 60s ea	68180-0467-07	80.73		AB
100s ea	68180-0467-01	134.55		AB
20 mg, 60s ea	68180-0468-07	142.37		AB
100s ea	68180-0468-01	237.28		AB
1000s ea	68180-0468-03	2372.83		AB
40 mg, 60s ea	68180-0469-07	256.29		AB
100s ea	68180-0469-01	427.15		AB
1000s ea	68180-0469-03	4271.50		AB
(Major)				
TAB, PO (USP)				
10 mg, 60s ea	00904-5581-52	79.89		
20 mg, 60s ea	00904-5582-52	141.59		
40 mg, 60s ea	00904-5583-52	254.82		
(Merck) *See MEVACOR*				
(Mutual)				
TAB, PO (USP)				
10 mg, 60s ea	53489-0607-06	80.73		AB
100s ea	53489-0607-01	134.51		AB
20 mg, 60s ea	53489-0608-06	142.37		AB
100s ea	53489-0608-01	237.25		AB
1000s ea	53489-0608-10	2254.25		AB
40 mg, 60s ea	53489-0609-06	256.29		AB
100s ea	53489-0609-01	427.11		AB
1000s ea	53489-0609-10	4057.84		AB
(Mylan)				
TAB, PO, 10 mg, 60s ea	00378-6510-91	80.65		AB
20 mg, 60s ea	00378-6520-91	142.25		AB
500s ea	00378-6520-05	1185.40		AB
40 mg, 60s ea	00378-6540-91	256.10		AB
500s ea	00378-6540-05	2134.15		AB
(Sandoz)				
TAB, PO, 10 mg, 60s ea	00185-0070-60	80.73		AB
100s ea	00185-0070-01	134.55		AB
500s ea	00185-0070-05	672.75		AB
1000s ea	00185-0070-10	1345.50		AB
20 mg, 60s ea	00185-0072-60	142.37		AB
100s ea	00185-0072-01	237.28		AB
1000s ea	00185-0072-10	2372.81		AB
40 mg, 60s ea	00185-0074-60	256.28		AB
100s ea	00185-0074-01	427.14		AB
1000s ea	00185-0074-10	4271.43		AB
(Shionogi) *See ALTOPREV*				
(Teva)				
TAB, PO, 10 mg, 60s ea (10X10S)	00093-0926-06	80.73		AB
10 mg, 100s ea UD	00093-0926-93	134.55		AB
1000s ea	00093-0926-10	1278.23		AB
20 mg, 60s ea	00093-0576-06	142.37		AB

PROD/MFR	NDC	AWP	DP	OBC
(10X10S)				
20 mg, 100s ea UD	00093-0576-93	237.28		AB
1000s ea	00093-0576-10	2254.21		AB
40 mg, 60s ea	00093-0928-06	256.28		AB
(10X10)				
40 mg, 100s ea UD	00093-0928-93	427.13		AB
1000s ea	00093-0928-10	4057.83		AB
(UDL)				
TAB, PO (10X10)				
10 mg, 100s ea UD	51079-0974-20	134.42		AB
20 mg, 100s ea UD	51079-0975-20	237.08		AB
(USP,10X30)				
20 mg, 300s ea UD	51079-0975-56	711.24		AB
(10X10)				
40 mg, 100s ea UD	51079-0976-20	426.83		AB
(Watson)				
TAB, PO, 20 mg, 60s ea	62037-0792-60	22.19		AB
40 mg, 60s ea	62037-0793-60	38.03		AB
(A-S Medication) REPACK				
TAB, PO, 10 mg, 30s ea	54569-5345-00	40.37		EE
20 mg, 30s ea	54569-5346-00	71.18		EE
40 mg, 30s ea	54569-5347-00	128.14		EE
(Altura) REPACK				
TAB, PO, 20 mg, 10s ea	63874-0363-10	23.70		AB
20s ea	63874-0363-20	47.40		AB
30s ea	63874-0363-30	71.11		AB
60s ea	63874-0363-60	142.21		AB
90s ea	63874-0363-90	213.33		AB
100s ea	63874-0363-01	237.03		
(American Health) REPACK				
TAB, PO (USP,10X10)				
10 mg, 100s ea UD	68084-0131-01	70.63		
20 mg, 100s ea UD	68084-0132-01	126.13		
40 mg, 100s ea UD	68084-0133-01	220.63		
(Bryant Ranch) REPACK				
TAB, PO, 20 mg, 30s ea	63629-1464-01	99.65		
60s ea	63629-1464-03	143.65		
100s ea	63629-1464-02	332.17		
40 mg, 30s ea	63629-1784-01	179.40		
(Core) REPACK				
TAB, PO, 10 mg, 30s ea	33358-0223-30	67.66		
20 mg, 30s ea	33358-0225-30	102.14		
60s ea	33358-0225-60	147.24		
100s ea	33358-0225-00	340.47		
40 mg, 30s ea	33358-0226-30	183.89		
(DHS, Inc.) REPACK				
TAB, PO, 10 mg, 30s ea	55887-0350-30	40.04		
20 mg, 30s ea	55887-0974-30	63.00		
40 mg, 30s ea	55887-0369-30	89.58		AB
60s ea	55887-0369-60	170.82		AB
90s ea	55887-0369-90	268.74		AB
(Dispensing Solutions) REPACK				
TAB, PO, 20 mg, 30s ea	55045-3014-08	71.10		
60s ea	55045-3014-09	142.20		
60s ea	66336-0310-60	142.97		
90s ea	55045-3014-06	213.30		
100s ea	55045-3014-01	237.00		
120s ea	55045-3014-02	280.80		
40 mg, 30s ea	55045-3015-08	128.13		
100s ea	55045-3015-01	427.00		
(McKesson Packaging) REPACK				
TAB, PO (USP)				
20 mg, 100s ea UD	63739-0281-10	290.53		
40 mg, 100s ea UD	63739-0282-10	284.26		
(Palmetto) REPACK				
TAB, PO, 10 mg, 30s ea	23490-5838-02	45.00		
60s ea	23490-5838-06	90.00		
90s ea	23490-5838-09	135.00		
20 mg, 30s ea	23490-5839-00	71.89		
60s ea	23490-5839-01	143.78		
40 mg, 5s ea	23490-5840-01	32.03		
30s ea	23490-5840-02	128.14		
(PD-Rx Pharm) REPACK				
TAB, PO, 10 mg, 30s ea	58864-0781-30	32.93		AB
20 mg, 30s ea	55289-0881-30	39.76		AB
30s ea	58864-0780-30	52.12		AB
60s ea	58864-0780-60	97.56		
40 mg, 14s ea	55289-0692-14	36.92		AB
30s ea	55289-0692-30	40.74		AB
(Pharma Pac) REPACK				
TAB, PO, 10 mg, 30s ea	52959-0974-30	45.02		AB
100s ea	52959-0974-00	138.59		AB
20 mg, 30s ea	52959-0720-30	82.77		
60s ea	52959-0720-60	139.15		AB
(Phys Total Care) REPACK				
TAB, PO, 10 mg, 30s ea	54868-4593-00	29.76		EE
90s ea	54868-4593-02	80.81		EE
100s ea	54868-4593-01	86.28		AB
20 mg, 30s ea	54868-4585-00	39.00		EE
60s ea	54868-4585-01	73.50		EE
40 mg, 30s ea	54868-4774-00	57.27		AB
60s ea	54868-4774-03	85.23		AB
90s ea	54868-4774-01	125.58		AB
100s ea	54868-4774-02	137.55		AB
(Physician Partner) REPACK				
TAB, PO, 10 mg, 30s ea	21695-0534-30	80.70		
20 mg, 30s ea	21695-0535-30	142.35		
90s ea	21695-0535-90	427.05		AB
40 mg, 30s ea	21695-0536-30	256.27		AB
90s ea	21695-0536-90	768.81		AB
(Quality Care Prod) REPACK				
TAB, PO, 10 mg, 30s ea	49999-0293-30	71.17		
20 mg, 30s ea	49999-0470-30	86.70		AB
60s ea	49999-0470-60	173.40		AB
90s ea	49999-0470-90	260.10		AB
40 mg, 30s ea	49999-0471-30	154.97		AB
60s ea	49999-0471-60	299.94		AB
100s ea	49999-0471-00	499.90		
(Southwood) REPACK				
TAB, PO, 10 mg, 20s ea	58016-0979-20	23.41		AB
30s ea	58016-0979-30	40.35		AB
60s ea	58016-0979-60	80.70		AB
90s ea	58016-0979-90	121.05		AB
100s ea	58016-0979-00	134.50		AB
120s ea	58016-0979-02	161.40		
20 mg, 30s ea	58016-0900-30	65.65		
60s ea	58016-0900-60	131.29		
90s ea	58016-0900-90	196.94		
100s ea	58016-0900-00	218.82		
120s ea	58016-0900-02	262.58		
40 mg, 30s ea	58016-0922-30	118.18		
60s ea	58016-0922-60	236.35		
90s ea	58016-0922-90	354.53		
100s ea	58016-0922-00	393.92		
120s ea	58016-0922-02	472.70		
(Stat Rx) REPACK				
TAB, PO, 20 mg, 30s ea	16590-0547-30	72.45		AB
60s ea	16590-0547-60	144.90		AB
90s ea	16590-0547-90	210.35		AB
120s ea	16590-0547-72	259.25		AB
(Vibranta) REPACK				
TAB, PO, 10 mg, 30s ea	57866-6400-01	45.80		
20 mg, 30s ea	57866-6601-01	82.58		
40 mg, 30s ea	57866-6500-01	104.60		
LOVASTATIN/NIACIN				
(Abbott Pharm) *See ADVICOR*				
LOVAZA (Glaxo)				
omega-3-acid ethyl esters				
SGL, PO (SOFTGEL)				
1 gm, 120s ea	00173-0783-02	183.56		
(A-S Medication) REPACK				
SGL, PO (SOFT GELATIN)				
1 gm, 120s ea	54569-5947-02	173.44		
(Phys Total Care) REPACK				
SGL, PO (SOFT GELATIN)				
1 gm, 30s ea	54868-5816-02	57.39		
60s ea	54868-5816-00	111.52		
(SOFT GELATIN)				
1 gm, 90s ea	54868-5816-03	157.82		
120s ea	54868-5816-01	209.57		
(SOFTGEL)				
1 gm, 360s ea	54868-5816-04	602.80		
(Quality Care Prod) REPACK				
SGL, PO (SOFT GELATIN)				
1 gm, 60s ea	35356-0104-60	143.08		
100s ea	35356-0104-00	147.31		
120s ea	35356-0104-01	281.78		
LOVENOX (Sanofi-Aventis)				
enoxaparin sodium				
SOL, IJ (W/AUTO SAFETY DEVICE)				
30 mg/0.3 ml, 0.3 ml 10s	00075-0624-30	270.64		
40 mg/0.4 ml, 0.4 ml 10s	00075-0620-40	360.83		
(SRN,PREFILLED)				
60 mg/0.6 ml, 0.6 ml 10s	00075-0621-60	541.88		
80 mg/0.8 ml, 0.8 ml 10s	00075-0622-80	722.52		
100 mg/ml, 1 ml 10s	00075-0623-00	903.13		
(W/AUTO SAFETY DEVICE)				
120 mg/0.8 ml, 0.8 ml 10s	00075-2912-01	1084.12		
150 mg/ml, 1 ml 10s	00075-2915-01	1355.16		
SC (VIAL,MULTIPLE DOSE VIAL)				
100 mg/ml, 3 ml	00075-0626-03	270.64		
(Phys Total Care) REPACK				
SOL, IJ (10X1ML)				
100 mg/ml, 1 ml 10s	54868-5835-00	987.29		
(8X0.8ML)				
120 mg/0.8 ml, 0.8 ml 8s	54868-5837-00	1184.73		
SC, 40 mg/0.4 ml, 0.4 ml	54868-5440-00	40.84		
0.4 ml 10s	54868-5440-01	375.12		
60 mg/0.6 ml, 0.6 ml	54868-5587-00	62.91		
80 mg/0.8 ml, 0.8 ml	54868-5112-01	85.38		
0.8 ml 10s	54868-5112-00	790.24		
60 mg/0.6 ml, 6 ml	54868-5587-01	564.35		
(Quality Care Prod) REPACK				
SOL, IJ (10X0.3ML)				
30 mg/0.3 ml, 0.3 ml 10s	35356-0481-10	456.04		
SC (10X0.6ML)				
60 mg/0.6 ml, 0.6 ml 10s	35356-0019-10	763.02		
(10X0.8ML)				
80 mg/0.8 ml, 0.8 ml 10s	35356-0020-10	1016.69		
(Southwood) REPACK				
SOL, SC, 40 mg/0.4 ml, 0.4 ml 10s	58016-4872-01	309.21		
LOW-OGESTREL (Dispensing Solutions) REPACK				
ethinyl estradiol/norgestrel				
TAB, PO (6X28)				
30 mcg-0.3 mg, 168s ea	55045-3497-01	186.00		
LOW-OGESTREL 28 (Watson)				
ethinyl estradiol/norgestrel				
TAB, PO (6X28)				
30 mcg-0.3 mg, 168s ea	52544-0847-28	183.12		AB
(A-S Medication) REPACK				
TAB, PO, 30 mcg-0.3 mg, 28s ea	54569-4998-00	30.52		AB
LOXAPINE (UDL)				
loxapine succinate				
CAP, PO (10X10)				
10 mg, 100s ea UD	51079-0901-20	127.20		AB
25 mg, 100s ea UD	51079-0902-20	192.45		AB
50 mg, 100s ea UD	51079-0903-20	257.15		AB
LOXAPINE SUCCINATE (Gallipot)				
POW, NA (U.S.P.)				
25 gm	51552-1038-04	581.00	415.00	
(Medisca)				
POW, NA (U.S.P.)				
5 gm	38779-0477-03	142.50		
25 gm	38779-0477-04	495.00		
(Mylan)				
CAP, PO, 5 mg, 100s ea	00378-7005-01	99.30		
10 mg, 100s ea	00378-7010-01	127.20		
25 mg, 100s ea	00378-7025-01	192.45		
50 mg, 100s ea	00378-7050-01	257.15		

PROD/MFR	NDC	AWP	DP	OBC
(PCCA)				
POW, NA (USP)				
1 gm	51927-1889-00	58.20		
(UDL) *See LOXAPINE*				
(Watson) *See LOXITANE*				
(Watson Labs)				
CAP, PO, 5 mg, 100s ea	00591-0369-01	99.32		AB
10 mg, 100s ea	00591-0370-01	127.23		AB
25 mg, 100s ea	00591-0371-01	192.45		AB
50 mg, 100s ea	00591-0372-01	257.18		AB
(Phys Total Care) REPACK				
CAP, PO, 10 mg, 100s ea	54868-2327-00	175.64		EE
LOXITANE (Watson) loxapine succinate				
CAP, PO, 5 mg, 100s ea	52544-0494-01	154.98		AB
10 mg, 100s ea	52544-0495-01	200.26		AB
25 mg, 100s ea	52544-0496-01	302.59		AB
50 mg, 100s ea	52544-0497-01	403.73		AB
LOZOL (Phys Total Care) REPACK indapamide				
TAB, PO, 2.5 mg, 30s ea	54868-1295-01	41.57		AB
LTA PEDIATRIC (Abbott Hosp) lidocaine hydrochloride				
KIT, MM (LATEX-FREE)				
2%, 24s ea	00074-5648-01	233.57	233.52	AT
LTA PREATTACHED (Hospira) lidocaine hydrochloride				
KIT, MM, 4%, 25s ea	00074-4698-01	151.20	132.25	AT
25s ea	00409-4698-01	156.30	136.75	AT
LUBIPROSTONE				
(Takeda) *See AMITIZA*				
LUCENTIS (Genentech) ranibizumab				
SOL, IO (INTRAVITREAL INJECTION)				
0.5 mg/0.05 ml,				
0.05 ml	50242-0080-01	2437.50		
LUDENT FLUORIDE (Sancilio) sodium fluoride				
CTB, PO (SF,DYE-FREE,ORANGE)				
0.25 mg, 120s ea	44946-1015-03	9.00		
0.5 mg, 120s ea	44946-1016-03	9.00		
1 mg, 120s ea	44946-1017-03	9.00		
LUFYLLIN (Meda) dyphylline				
TAB, PO, 200 mg, 100s ea	00037-0521-92	314.81		BP
LUFYLLIN-400 (Meda) dyphylline				
TAB, PO, 400 mg, 100s ea	00037-0731-92	462.27		BP
LUFYLLIN-GG (Meda) dyphylline/guaifenesin				
ELI, PO, 473 ml	00037-0545-68	274.75		
LUGOL'S SOLUTION (Humco) iodine/potassium iodide				
SOL, NA, 480 ml	00395-2775-16	16.56		
(Medisca)				
SOL, NA, 500 ml	38779-0598-08	48.00		
(PCCA)				
SOL, NA (USP)				
1 ml	51927-1547-00	0.17		
(Safecor)				
SOL, NA, 15 ml	48433-0230-15	21.12	17.60	
LUGOL'S STRONG IODINE (Cooper Surgical) iodine/potassium iodide				
SOL, TP (12-8ML VIALS,PF)				
5%-10%, 8 ml 12s	59365-6064-01	74.98		
LUMBAR PUNCTURE TRAY (Portex) lidocaine hydrochloride				
KIT, IJ (ADULT,20G,3-1/2"QUINCKE)				
1%, 10s ea	00074-4824-20	390.81	329.10	
(ADULT,22G,3-1/2"QUINCKE)				
1%, 10s ea	00074-4825-20	390.81	329.10	
LUMIGAN (Allergan Inc) bimatoprost				
SOL, OP, 0.03%, 2.5 ml	00023-9187-03	84.56		
5 ml	00023-9187-05	169.07		
7.5 ml	00023-9187-07	253.60		
(Phys Total Care) REPACK				
SOL, OP, 0.03%, 3 ml	54868-4575-02	102.91		
5 ml	54868-4575-00	176.43		
7.5 ml	54868-4575-01	273.61		
(Quality Care Prod) REPACK				
SOL, OP (1X2.5ML,DROP)				
0.03%, 2.5 ml	35356-0405-25	155.48		
LUMINAL SODIUM (Hospira) phenobarbital sodium				
SOL, IJ (LUER LOCK,10X1ML)				
60 mg/ml,				
1 ml 10s, C-IV	00409-2343-31	34.32	30.00	
(LUER LOCK,CARPUJECT)				
130 mg/ml,				
1 ml 10s, C-IV	00409-2349-31	46.32	40.50	
LUNESTA (Sepracor) eszopiclone				
TAB, PO (FILM-COATED)				
1 mg, 30s ea, C-IV	63402-0190-30	200.88		
100s ea, C-IV	63402-0190-10	555.60		
2 mg, 90s ea, C-IV	63402-0191-09	455.76		
100s ea, C-IV	63402-0191-10	669.60		
3 mg, 90s ea, C-IV	63402-0193-09	455.76		
100s ea, C-IV	63402-0193-10	669.60		
(A-S Medication) REPACK				
TAB, PO (FILM-COATED)				
2 mg, 30s ea, C-IV	54569-5696-00	237.74		
3 mg, 30s ea, C-IV	54569-5684-00	237.74		
(Aidarex) REPACK				
TAB, PO (FILM-COATED)				
3 mg, 14s ea, C-IV	33261-0530-14	81.02		
30s ea, C-IV	33261-0530-30	173.62		
60s ea, C-IV	33261-0530-60	347.24		
90s ea, C-IV	33261-0530-90	520.86		
(Altura) REPACK				
TAB, PO, 1 mg,				
30s ea, C-IV	63874-1152-03	133.36		
(FILM-COATED)				
3 mg, 30s ea, C-IV	63874-1153-03	133.36		
(Bryant Ranch) REPACK				
TAB, PO, 3 mg,				
30s ea, C-IV	63629-3142-01	132.90		
(Core) REPACK				
TAB, PO, 3 mg,				
30s ea, C-IV	33358-0227-30	126.94		
(Dispensing Solutions) REPACK				
TAB, PO, 2 mg,				
30s ea, C-IV	55045-3461-08	150.00		
(FILM-COATED)				
2 mg, 30s ea, C-IV	68258-7048-03	210.31		
3 mg, 30s ea, C-IV	55045-3462-08	178.40		
(FILM-COATED)				
3 mg, 30s ea, C-IV	68258-7049-03	220.97		
(IPI) REPACK				
TAB, PO, 3 mg,				
60s ea, C-IV	18837-0081-60	381.98		
90s ea, C-IV	18837-0081-90	572.96		
(Keltman Pharma., Inc.) REPACK				
TAB, PO, 3 mg,				
30s ea, C-IV	68387-0487-30	151.00		
(Nucare Pharm) REPACK				
TAB, PO (FILM-COATED)				
2 mg, 30s ea, C-IV	68071-0304-30	200.54		
3 mg, 30s ea, C-IV	68071-0305-30	200.54		
(PD-Rx Pharm) REPACK				
TAB, PO (FILM-COATED)				
3 mg, 30s ea, C-IV	55289-0014-30	276.41		
(Pharma Pac) REPACK				
TAB, PO, 2 mg,				
30s ea, C-IV	52959-0919-30	215.20		
(FILM-COATED)				
2 mg, 60s ea, C-IV	52959-0919-60	419.90		
100s ea, C-IV	52959-0919-00	616.80		
3 mg, 10s ea, C-IV	52959-0852-10	53.80		
12s ea, C-IV	52959-0852-12	64.58		
30s ea, C-IV	52959-0852-30	146.13		
(FILM-COATED)				
3 mg, 60s ea, C-IV	52959-0852-60	419.90		
100s ea, C-IV	52959-0852-00	537.99		
(Phys Total Care) REPACK				
TAB, PO, 1 mg,				
20s ea, C-IV	54868-5439-01	155.43		
(FILM-COATED)				
1 mg, 60s ea, C-IV	54868-5439-00	436.24		
2 mg, 10s ea, C-IV	54868-5273-01	79.02		
20s ea, C-IV	54868-5273-02	156.08		
(FILM-COATED)				
2 mg, 30s ea, C-IV	54868-5273-00	219.75		
3 mg, 10s ea, C-IV	54868-5394-00	86.54		
15s ea, C-IV	54868-5394-02	128.50		
(FILM-COATED)				
3 mg, 30s ea, C-IV	54868-5394-01	241.06		
90s ea, C-IV	54868-5394-03	692.97		
(Physician Partner) REPACK				
TAB, PO, 2 mg,				
30s ea, C-IV	21695-0225-30	401.76		
3 mg, 15s ea, C-IV	21695-0226-15	169.41		
30s ea, C-IV	21695-0226-30	401.76		
(Quality Care Prod) REPACK				
TAB, PO (FILM-COATED)				
1 mg, 30s ea, C-IV	49999-0778-30	133.37		
2 mg, 15s ea, C-IV	49999-0779-15	177.65		
30s ea, C-IV	49999-0779-30	323.00		
(FILM-COATED)				
3 mg, 14s ea, C-IV	49999-0737-14	165.81		
15s ea, C-IV	49999-0737-15	177.65		
30s ea, C-IV	49999-0737-30	323.00		
60s ea, C-IV	49999-0737-60	646.00		
90s ea, C-IV	49999-0737-90	969.00		
(FILM-COATED)				
3 mg,				
100s ea, C-IV	49999-0737-00	866.83		
(Southwood) REPACK				
TAB, PO (FILM-COATED)				
2 mg, 30s ea, C-IV	58016-0040-30	166.68		
60s ea, C-IV	58016-0040-60	333.36		
90s ea, C-IV	58016-0040-90	500.04		
100s ea, C-IV	58016-0040-00	555.60		
3 mg, 30s ea, C-IV	58016-0292-30	166.68		
60s ea, C-IV	58016-0292-60	333.36		
90s ea, C-IV	58016-0292-90	500.04		
100s ea, C-IV	58016-0292-00	555.60		
(St. Mary's MPP) REPACK				
TAB, PO (FILM-COATED)				
2 mg, 30s ea, C-IV	60760-0191-30	315.36		
3 mg, 30s ea, C-IV	60760-0193-30	315.36		
(Stat Rx) REPACK				
TAB, PO (FILM-COATED)				
1 mg, 30s ea, C-IV	16590-0502-30	214.64		
60s ea, C-IV	16590-0502-60	426.04		
90s ea, C-IV	16590-0502-90	415.50		
120s ea, C-IV	16590-0502-72	535.00		
(FILM-COATED)				
2 mg, 25s ea, C-IV	16590-0501-25	179.41		
28s ea, C-IV	16590-0501-28	200.55		
30s ea, C-IV	16590-0501-30	214.64		
60s ea, C-IV	16590-0501-60	283.55		
90s ea, C-IV	16590-0501-90	415.50		
120s ea, C-IV	16590-0501-72	535.00		
(FILM-COATED)				
3 mg, 25s ea, C-IV	16590-0500-25	179.41		
28s ea, C-IV	16590-0500-28	200.55		
30s ea, C-IV	16590-0500-30	222.52		
60s ea, C-IV	16590-0500-60	426.04		
90s ea, C-IV	16590-0500-90	476.89		
120s ea, C-IV	16590-0500-72	627.40		
LUPRON DEPOT (Abbott Pharm) leuprolide acetate				
PI1, IM, 3.75 mg, ea	00074-3641-03	729.58	607.98	
(STERILE,1X75MG)				
7.5 mg, ea	00074-3642-03	869.42	724.52	
PI3, IM (DUAL-CHAMBER SYRINGE)				
11.25 mg, ea	00074-3663-03	2188.78	1823.98	
(STERILE,1X22.5MG)				
22.5 mg, ea	00074-3346-03	2608.24	2173.53	
PI4, IM (LYOPHILIZED)				
30 mg, ea	00074-3683-03	3477.66	2898.05	
(Phys Total Care) REPACK				
PI1, IM, 3.75 mg, ea	54868-2825-00	685.56		
7.5 mg, 1 ml	54868-3277-00	785.29		
PI4, IM, 30 mg, ea	54868-5568-00	3071.33		

PROD/MFR	NDC	AWP	DP	OBC
LUPRON DEPOT-PED (Abbott Pharm)				
leuprolide acetate				
PI1, IM (LYOPHILIZED)				
7.5 mg, ea	**00074-2108-03**	877.69	731.41	
11.25 mg, ea	**00074-2282-03**	1593.46	1327.88	
15 mg, ea	**00074-2440-03**	1755.01	1462.51	
LURIDE (Colgate Oral)				
sodium fluoride				
CTB, PO (VANILLA)				
0.25 mg, 120s ea	**00126-0186-21**	7.40		
(GRAPE)				
0.5 mg, 120s ea	**00126-0014-21**	7.40		
(CHERRY)				
1 mg, 120s ea	**00126-0006-21**	7.40		
LIQ, PO (W/DROPPER,PEACH,DROPS)				
0.5 mg/ml, 50 ml	**00126-0002-62**	9.06		
(Quality Care Prod)				
REPACK				
CTB, PO (GRAPE)				
0.5 mg, 30s ea	**49999-0689-30**	7.50		
(CHERRY)				
1 mg, 30s ea	**49999-0560-30**	7.25		
LUSEDRA (Eisai)				
fospropofol disodium				
SOL, IV (8X30ML,SINGLE-USE)				
35 mg/ml, 30 ml 8s	**62856-0350-08**	345.60		
LUSONAL (Wraser Pharm)				
phenylephrine hydrochloride				
SOL, PO (STRAWBERRY)				
7.5 mg/5 ml,				
473 ml	**66992-0146-16**	68.01		
LUSTRA (Taro)				
hydroquinone				
CRE, TP, 4%, 56.8 gm	**51672-1326-03**	137.40		
LUSTRA-AF (Taro)				
hydroquinone				
CRE, TP, 4%, 56.8 gm	**51672-1327-03**	151.11		
(Phys Total Care)				
REPACK				
CRE, TP, 4%, 56.8 gm	**54868-5238-00**	166.96		
LUSTRA-ULTRA (Taro)				
hydroquinone				
CRE, TP (1X28.4GM)				
4%, 28.4 gm	**51672-1328-02**	90.58		
56.8 gm	**51672-1328-03**	146.71		
LUTEIN (PCCA)				
BEA, NA, 1 gm	**51927-3396-00**	3.75		
LUTERA (Watson)				
ethinyl estradiol/levonorgestrel				
TAB, PO (6X28)				
0.02 mg-0.1 mg,				
168s ea	**52544-0949-28**	210.96		**AB**
(A-S Medication)				
REPACK				
TAB, PO, 0.02 mg-0.1 mg,				
28s ea	**54569-5798-00**	31.47		
LUTROPIN ALFA				
(EMD) *See LUVERIS*				
LUVERIS (EMD)				
lutropin alfa				
PDS, SC (W/DILUENT)				
75 iu, ea	**44087-1375-01**	38.88		
LUVOX CR (Jazz)				
fluvoxamine maleate				
CER, PO (GLUTEN-FREE)				
100 mg, 30s ea	**68727-0600-01**	162.00		
150 mg, 30s ea	**68727-0601-01**	172.80		
LUXIQ (Stiefel Labs)				
betamethasone valerate				
FOA, TP, 0.12%, 50 gm	**63032-0021-50**	155.53		
100 gm	**63032-0021-00**	289.50		
(Phys Total Care)				
REPACK				
FOA, TP, 0.12%, 100 gm	**54868-5424-00**	305.26		
(Quality Care Prod)				
REPACK				
FOA, TP (1X100GM)				
0.12%, 100 gm	**35356-0231-00**	501.38		
LYBREL (Wyeth)				
ethinyl estradiol/levonorgestrel				
TAB, PO (FILM-COATED)				
20 mcg-90 mcg,				
28s ea	**00008-1117-30**	55.44	46.20	
LYCOPENE (PCCA)				
BEA, NA, 1 gm	**51927-3277-00**	1.14		
1 gm	**51927-3302-00**	1.74		
(PCCA) *See LYCOPENE BEADLETS*				
LYCOPENE BEADLETS (PCCA)				
lycopene				
SOL, NA (1X1ML)				
10%, 1 ml	**51927-4221-00**	1.02		
LYCOPODIUM (Amend)				
clubmoss				
POW, NA, 454 gm	**17317-0335-01**	39.20		
(Medisca)				
POW, NA (1X100GM)				
100 gm	**38779-1398-05**	37.50		
(1X500GM)				
500 gm	**38779-1398-08**	123.00		
(PCCA)				
POW, NA, 1 gm	**51927-2013-00**	0.75		
LYMPHAZURIN (Covidien)				
isosulfan blue				
SOL, SC (6X5ML VIAL)				
10 mg/ml, 5 ml 6s	**63261-0250-21**	3952.80		
LYPHOLYTE (APP)				
ca ace/k ace/k cl/mg ace/na ace/na gluconate				
SOL, IV (S.D.V.)				
20 ml	**63323-0009-20**	6.60		
(MAXIVIAL,BULK PACK)				
200 ml	**63323-0009-63**	53.13		
LYPHOLYTE-II (APP)				
ca cl/k cl/mg cl/na ace/na cl				
SOL, IV (S.D.V.)				
20 ml	**63323-0146-20**	5.51		
40 ml	**63323-0146-40**	11.17		
(MAXIVIAL,BULK PACK)				
100 ml	**63323-0146-61**	24.41		
200 ml	**63323-0146-63**	41.83		
LYRICA (Pfizer)				
pregabalin				
CAP, PO, 25 mg,				
90s ea, C-V	**00071-1012-68**	242.89	202.41	
50 mg, 90s ea, C-V	**00071-1013-68**	242.89	202.41	
100s ea UD, C-V	**00071-1013-41**	296.86	247.38	
75 mg, 90s ea, C-V	**00071-1014-68**	242.89	202.41	
100s ea UD, C-V	**00071-1014-41**	296.86	247.38	
100 mg,				
90s ea, C-V	**00071-1015-68**	242.89	202.41	
100s ea UD, C-V	**00071-1015-41**	296.86	247.38	
150 mg,				
90s ea, C-V	**00071-1016-68**	242.89	202.41	
100s ea UD, C-V	**00071-1016-41**	296.86	247.38	
200 mg,				
90s ea, C-V	**00071-1017-68**	242.89	202.41	
225 mg,				
90s ea, C-V	**00071-1019-68**	242.89	202.41	
300 mg,				
90s ea, C-V	**00071-1018-68**	242.89	202.41	
(4u)				
REPACK				
CAP, PO, 75 mg,				
60s ea, C-V	**42549-0612-60**	292.86		
90s ea, C-V	**42549-0612-90**	432.14		
(A-S Medication)				
REPACK				
CAP, PO, 75 mg,				
30s ea, C-V	**54569-5825-00**	80.32		
(Aidarex)				
REPACK				
CAP, PO, 50 mg,				
30s ea, C-V	**33261-0521-30**	80.31		
60s ea, C-V	**33261-0521-60**	160.64		
90s ea, C-V	**33261-0521-90**	240.96		
120s ea, C-V	**33261-0521-02**	321.28		
100 mg,				
30s ea, C-V	**33261-0522-30**	80.31		
60s ea, C-V	**33261-0522-60**	160.64		
90s ea, C-V	**33261-0522-90**	240.96		
120s ea, C-V	**33261-0522-02**	321.28		
(Bryant Ranch)				
REPACK				
CAP, PO, 50 mg,				
60s ea, C-V	**63629-3367-02**	238.80		
75 mg, 90s ea, C-V	**63629-3368-03**	221.06		
(Core)				
REPACK				
CAP, PO, 50 mg,				
60s ea, C-V	**33358-0228-60**	158.11		
90s ea, C-V	**33358-0228-90**	204.31		
75 mg, 60s ea, C-V	**33358-0229-60**	159.13		
100 mg,				
60s ea, C-V	**33358-0230-60**	177.58		
(DHS, Inc.)				
REPACK				
CAP, PO, 50 mg,				
30s ea, C-V	**55887-0164-30**	64.01		
45s ea, C-V	**55887-0164-45**	96.01		
50s ea, C-V	**55887-0164-50**	106.68		
60s ea, C-V	**55887-0164-60**	128.01		
90s ea, C-V	**55887-0164-90**	192.04		
75 mg, 30s ea, C-V	**55887-0163-30**	64.01		
45s ea, C-V	**55887-0163-45**	96.02		
50s ea, C-V	**55887-0163-50**	106.69		
60s ea, C-V	**55887-0163-60**	128.03		
90s ea, C-V	**55887-0163-90**	192.04		
100 mg,				
30s ea, C-V	**55887-0162-30**	70.41		
45s ea, C-V	**55887-0162-45**	96.02		
50s ea, C-V	**55887-0162-50**	117.36		
60s ea, C-V	**55887-0162-60**	128.03		
90s ea, C-V	**55887-0162-90**	192.04		
(Dispensing Solutions)				
REPACK				
CAP, PO, 50 mg,				
30s ea, C-V	**68258-7045-03**	112.13		
60s ea, C-V	**68258-7045-06**	198.40		
75 mg, 30s ea, C-V	**68258-7046-03**	112.13		
60s ea, C-V	**55045-3460-06**	147.00		
60s ea, C-V	**68258-7046-06**	198.40		
90s ea, C-V	**68258-7046-09**	297.60		
100 mg,				
60s ea, C-V	**68258-7052-06**	169.63		
150 mg,				
60s ea, C-V	**68258-7047-06**	169.63		
200 mg,				
60s ea, C-V	**55045-3439-06**	147.00		
(IPI)				
REPACK				
CAP, PO, 25 mg,				
60s ea, C-V	**18837-0199-60**	156.79		
50 mg,				
100s ea, C-V	**18837-0083-99**	261.31		
180s ea, C-V	**18837-0083-96**	540.91		
75 mg,				
120s ea, C-V	**18837-0084-98**	369.47		
180s ea, C-V	**18837-0084-96**	554.21		
270s ea, C-V	**18837-0084-94**	831.31		
100 mg,				
180s ea, C-V	**18837-0198-96**	496.25		
150 mg,				
120s ea, C-V	**18837-0082-98**	360.61		
180s ea, C-V	**18837-0082-96**	470.36		
200 mg,				
270s ea, C-V	**18837-0254-94**	744.37		
(Keltman Pharma., Inc.)				
REPACK				
CAP, PO, 50 mg,				
30s ea, C-V	**68387-0660-30**	70.42		
90s ea, C-V	**68387-0660-90**	211.25		
75 mg, 90s ea, C-V	**68387-0661-90**	211.25		
100 mg,				
90s ea, C-V	**68387-0662-90**	211.25		
150 mg,				
90s ea, C-V	**68387-0663-90**	211.25		
(Nucare Pharm)				
REPACK				
CAP, PO, 50 mg,				
30s ea, C-V	**68071-0365-30**	94.66		
60s ea, C-V	**68071-0365-60**	189.32		
90s ea, C-V	**68071-1353-00**	278.57		
75 mg, 30s ea, C-V	**68071-0353-30**	96.99		
60s ea, C-V	**68071-0353-60**	193.98		
90s ea, C-V	**68071-0353-90**	285.41		
90s ea, C-V	**68071-1355-00**	285.41		
100 mg,				
30s ea, C-V	**68071-0476-30**	86.85		
60s ea, C-V	**68071-0476-60**	173.69		
90s ea, C-V	**68071-1354-00**	255.56		
150 mg,				
30s ea, C-V	**68071-0389-30**	95.25		
60s ea, C-V	**68071-0389-60**	189.32		
90s ea, C-V	**68071-1356-00**	278.57		
200 mg,				
60s ea, C-V	**68071-0740-60**	173.69		
90s ea, C-V	**68071-1358-00**	255.56		
270s ea, C-V	**68071-0740-93**	759.26		
300 mg,				
60s ea, C-V	**68071-0662-60**	173.69		
90s ea, C-V	**68071-1357-00**	255.56		

PROD/MFR	NDC	AWP	DP	OBC
(PD-Rx Pharm)				
REPACK				
CAP, PO, 50 mg,				
30s ea, C-V	**55289-0969-30**	123.00		
75 mg, 15s ea, C-V	**55289-0569-15**	65.24		
60s ea, C-V	**55289-0569-60**	238.49		
100 mg,				
30s ea, C-V	**55289-0257-30**	123.00		
150 mg,				
30s ea, C-V	**55289-0214-30**	123.00		
300 mg,				
30s ea, C-V	**55289-0255-30**	123.00		
(Pharma Pac)				
REPACK				
CAP, PO, 50 mg,				
60s ea, C-V	**52959-0891-60**	254.50		
90s ea, C-V	**52959-0891-90**	369.90		
120s ea, C-V	**52959-0891-02**	378.00		
75 mg, 30s ea, C-V	**52959-0747-30**	135.40		
60s ea, C-V	**52959-0747-60**	249.50		
90s ea, C-V	**52959-0747-90**	369.90		
120s ea, C-V	**52959-0747-01**	378.00		
100 mg,				
30s ea, C-V	**52959-0746-30**	135.40		
60s ea, C-V	**52959-0746-60**	249.50		
90s ea, C-V	**52959-0746-90**	369.90		
150 mg,				
30s ea, C-V	**52959-0897-30**	135.40		
60s ea, C-V	**52959-0897-60**	249.50		
(Phys Total Care)				
REPACK				
CAP, PO, 25 mg,				
30s ea, C-V	**54868-5662-01**	74.35		
60s ea, C-V	**54868-5662-00**	138.21		
50 mg, 30s ea, C-V	**54868-5494-01**	99.91		
60s ea, C-V	**54868-5494-02**	185.17		
90s ea, C-V	**54868-5494-00**	277.10		
75 mg, 30s ea, C-V	**54868-5550-01**	104.10		
60s ea, C-V	**54868-5550-00**	194.30		
90s ea, C-V	**54868-5550-02**	289.49		
100 mg,				
30s ea, C-V	**54868-5530-00**	99.91		
60s ea, C-V	**54868-5530-01**	185.82		
90s ea, C-V	**54868-5530-03**	227.10		
100s ea, C-V	**54868-5530-02**	284.71		
150 mg,				
15s ea, C-V	**54868-5456-03**	53.35		
30s ea, C-V	**54868-5456-04**	98.46		
60s ea, C-V	**54868-5456-01**	194.30		
90s ea, C-V	**54868-5456-00**	289.49		
120s ea, C-V	**54868-5456-02**	385.99		
200 mg,				
270s ea, C-V	**54868-6063-00**	838.03		
(Physician Partner)				
REPACK				
CAP, PO, 25 mg,				
15s ea, C-V	**21695-0276-15**	95.25		
30s ea, C-V	**21695-0276-30**	161.93		
50 mg, 15s ea, C-V	**21695-0277-15**	94.49		
30s ea, C-V	**21695-0277-30**	161.93		
90s ea, C-V	**21695-0277-90**	485.78		
75 mg, 30s ea, C-V	**21695-0278-30**	161.93		
60s ea, C-V	**21695-0278-60**	323.86		
90s ea, C-V	**21695-0278-90**	485.78		
(HARD GELATIN)				
100 mg,				
60s ea, C-V	**21695-0661-60**	323.86		
90s ea, C-V	**21695-0661-90**	485.78		
150 mg,				
30s ea, C-V	**21695-0662-30**	161.93		
60s ea, C-V	**21695-0662-60**	323.86		
90s ea, C-V	**21695-0662-90**	485.78		
200 mg,				
90s ea, C-V	**21695-0663-90**	485.78		
(HARD GELATIN)				
300 mg,				
90s ea, C-V	**21695-0664-90**	485.78		
(Quality Care Prod)				
REPACK				
CAP, PO, 25 mg,				
30s ea, C-V	**35356-0053-30**	175.00		
90s ea, C-V	**35356-0053-90**	393.00		
50 mg, 30s ea, C-V	**49999-0949-30**	418.00		
90s ea, C-V	**49999-0949-90**	453.00		
75 mg, 4s ea, C-V	**49999-0895-04**	28.92		
30s ea, C-V	**49999-0895-30**	217.00		
60s ea, C-V	**49999-0895-60**	302.00		
90s ea, C-V	**49999-0895-90**	435.00		
100 mg,				
30s ea, C-V	**49999-0905-30**	225.00		
60s ea, C-V	**49999-0905-60**	450.00		
90s ea, C-V	**49999-0905-90**	463.00		
150 mg,				
30s ea, C-V	**35356-0054-30**	235.00		
60s ea, C-V	**35356-0054-60**	368.00		
90s ea, C-V	**35356-0054-90**	478.00		
200 mg, 2s ea, C-V	**49999-0906-02**	16.34		
30s ea, C-V	**49999-0906-30**	245.00		
60s ea, C-V	**49999-0906-60**	490.00		
90s ea, C-V	**49999-0906-90**	485.00		
300 mg,				
60s ea, C-V	**35356-0398-60**	489.44		
(Southwood)				
REPACK				
CAP, PO, 50 mg,				
30s ea, C-V	**58016-0362-30**	77.81		
60s ea, C-V	**58016-0362-60**	155.63		
90s ea, C-V	**58016-0362-90**	233.44		
100s ea, C-V	**58016-0362-00**	259.38		
75 mg, 30s ea, C-V	**58016-0318-30**	77.81		
60s ea, C-V	**58016-0318-60**	155.63		
90s ea, C-V	**58016-0318-90**	233.44		
100s ea, C-V	**58016-0318-00**	259.38		
100 mg,				
30s ea, C-V	**58016-0059-30**	77.81		
60s ea, C-V	**58016-0059-60**	155.63		
90s ea, C-V	**58016-0059-90**	233.44		
100s ea, C-V	**58016-0059-00**	259.38		
150 mg,				
30s ea, C-V	**00490-0038-30**	77.81		
60s ea, C-V	**00490-0038-60**	155.63		
90s ea, C-V	**00490-0038-90**	233.44		
100s ea, C-V	**00490-0038-00**	259.38		
200 mg,				
30s ea, C-V	**58016-0015-30**	70.74		
60s ea, C-V	**58016-0015-60**	141.48		
90s ea, C-V	**58016-0015-90**	212.22		
100s ea, C-V	**58016-0015-00**	235.80		
(St. Mary's MPP)				
REPACK				
CAP, PO, 25 mg,				
30s ea, C-V	**60760-0012-30**	126.48		
60s ea, C-V	**60760-0012-60**	246.96		
90s ea, C-V	**60760-0012-90**	367.44		
50 mg, 30s ea, C-V	**60760-0101-30**	126.48		
60s ea, C-V	**60760-0101-60**	246.96		
90s ea, C-V	**60760-0101-90**	367.44		
75 mg, 30s ea, C-V	**60760-0014-30**	130.68		
60s ea, C-V	**60760-0014-60**	255.37		
90s ea, C-V	**60760-0014-90**	367.44		
100 mg,				
60s ea, C-V	**60760-0106-60**	255.37		
90s ea, C-V	**60760-0106-90**	380.05		
150 mg,				
30s ea, C-V	**60760-0016-30**	126.48		
60s ea, C-V	**60760-0016-60**	246.96		
90s ea, C-V	**60760-0016-90**	380.05		
200 mg,				
90s ea, C-V	**60760-0018-90**	380.05		
(Stat Rx)				
REPACK				
CAP, PO, 25 mg,				
30s ea, C-V	**16590-0550-30**	92.38		
60s ea, C-V	**16590-0550-60**	250.60		
90s ea, C-V	**16590-0550-90**	292.66		
50 mg, 28s ea, C-V	**16590-0503-28**	79.12		
30s ea, C-V	**16590-0503-30**	91.18		
56s ea, C-V	**16590-0503-56**	156.47		
60s ea, C-V	**16590-0503-60**	180.93		
90s ea, C-V	**16590-0503-90**	270.41		
120s ea, C-V	**16590-0503-72**	300.25		
120s ea, C-V	**16590-0506-72**	360.07		
180s ea, C-V	**16590-0503-82**	538.06		
75 mg, 28s ea, C-V	**16590-0504-28**	113.54		
30s ea, C-V	**16590-0504-30**	92.37		
56s ea, C-V	**16590-0504-56**	168.96		
60s ea, C-V	**16590-0504-60**	180.93		
84s ea, C-V	**16590-0504-62**	252.73		
90s ea, C-V	**16590-0504-90**	299.68		
120s ea, C-V	**16590-0504-72**	369.47		
100 mg,				
30s ea, C-V	**16590-0505-30**	91.09		
60s ea, C-V	**16590-0505-60**	197.91		
90s ea, C-V	**16590-0505-90**	296.15		
120s ea, C-V	**16590-0505-72**	394.39		
150 mg,				
30s ea, C-V	**16590-0506-30**	91.18		
56s ea, C-V	**16590-0506-56**	171.36		
60s ea, C-V	**16590-0506-60**	180.93		
90s ea, C-V	**16590-0506-90**	270.67		
200 mg,				
30s ea, C-V	**16590-0507-30**	124.06		
60s ea, C-V	**16590-0507-60**	248.12		
90s ea, C-V	**16590-0507-90**	372.18		
120s ea, C-V	**16590-0507-72**	300.25		
300 mg,				
28s ea, C-V	**16590-0508-28**	84.72		
30s ea, C-V	**16590-0508-30**	92.38		
60s ea, C-V	**16590-0508-60**	180.93		
90s ea, C-V	**16590-0508-90**	270.67		
120s ea, C-V	**16590-0508-72**	360.43		
180s ea, C-V	**16590-0508-82**	544.55		
LYSINE ACETATE (Spectrum Pharmacy)				
POW, NA (U.S.P.)				
100 gm	**49452-4163-02**	314.65		
1000 gm	**49452-4163-03**	1410.65		
LYSINE HYDROCHLORIDE				
(Amend) *See L-LYSINE MONOHYDROCHLORIDE*				
(Gallipot) *See L-LYSINE MONOHYDROCHLORIDE*				
(Lorann Oil) *See L-LYSINE MONOHYDROCHLORIDE*				
(Medisca)				
POW, NA (USP,1X100GM)				
100 gm	**38779-0823-05**	31.50		
(1X500GM,USP)				
500 gm	**38779-0823-08**	79.50		
(1X1000GM,USP)				
1000 gm	**38779-0823-09**	136.50		
(PCCA)				
POW, NA (USP; L)				
1 gm	**51927-1122-00**	0.42		
(Spectrum Pharmacy) *See L-LYSINE MONOHYDROCHLORIDE*				
LYSIPLEX PLUS (Kramer-Novis)				
multivitamin, minerals, and iron				
TAB, PO, 90s ea	**52083-0841-90**	30.00		
LYSODREN (B/M Squibb Onc/Vir)				
mitotane				
TAB, PO, 500 mg, 100s ea	**00015-3080-60**	479.05	399.21	
LYSOZYME (PCCA)				
POW, NA (MURAMIDASE)				
1 gm	**51927-2365-00**	225.00		
M-CLEAR (McNeil,R.A.)				
codeine phosphate/guaifenesin				
CAP, PO, 9 mg-200 mg,				
100s ea, C-V	**12830-0714-01**	36.25		
M-CLEAR WC (McNeil,R.A.)				
codeine phosphate/guaifenesin				
SOL, PO (1X473ML,AF,SF,DYE-FREE)				
6.33 mg/5 ml-100 mg/5 ml,				
473 ml, C-V	**12830-0717-16**	25.94		
M-END DM (McNeil,R.A.)				
cpm/dm/pse hcl				
LIQ, PO (FRUIT)				
473 ml	**12830-0810-16**	34.65		
M-END PE (McNeil,R.A.)				
bpm/codeine phos/phenyleph hcl				
SOL, PO (COTTON CANDY)				
354 ml, C-V	**12830-0754-12**	24.49		
M-END WC (McNeil,R.A.)				
bpm/codeine phos/pse hcl				
SOL, PO (1X473ML,AF,SF)				
473 ml, C-V	**12830-0735-16**	35.04		
M-M-R II (Merck)				
measles, mumps, and rubella virus vaccine, live				
PDS, SC (SDV W/DILUENT,TAX INCL)				
10s ea	**00006-4681-00**	575.27		
(A-S Medication)				
REPACK				
PDS, SC (VIAL,TAX INCL)				
10s ea	**54569-1588-00**	539.86		
(Phys Total Care)				
REPACK				
PDS, SC (SDV W/DILUENT,TAX INCL)				
ea	**54868-0980-00**	63.09		
(Quality Care Prod)				
REPACK				
PDS, SC (SDV W/DILUENT,TAX INCL)				
ea	**49999-0422-01**	58.51		
10s ea	**49999-0422-10**	507.04		
M-VIT (McNeil,R.A.)				
multivitamin, minerals, and iron				
TAB, PO (CAPLET)				
100s ea	**12830-0800-01**	31.94		
M.T.E.-4 (APP)				
chromium/copper/manganese/zinc				
SOL, IV (S.D.V.,PF)				
3 ml	**63323-0081-03**	2.39		
10 ml	**63323-0081-10**	7.90		
(M.D.V.,PF)				
30 ml	**63323-0087-30**	17.22		

PROD/MFR	NDC	AWP	DP	OBC
M.T.E.-4 CONCENTRATE (APP)				
chromium/copper/manganese/zinc				
SOL, IV (S.D.V.,PF)				
1 ml	63323-0094-01	2.74		
(M.D.V.,PF)				
10 ml	63323-0098-10	17.96		
M.T.E.-5 (APP)				
chromium/copper/manganese/selenium/zinc				
SOL, IV (S.D.V.,PF)				
10 ml	63323-0018-10	16.96		
M.T.E.-5 CONCENTRATE (APP)				
chromium/copper/manganese/selenium/zinc				
SOL, IV (M.D.V.)				
10 ml	63323-0029-10	25.94		
(S.D.V.,PF)				
1 ml	63323-0028-01	3.50		
M.T.E.-6 (APP)				
chromium/copper/iodide/manganese/selenium/zinc				
SOL, IV (S.D.V.,PF)				
10 ml	63323-0020-10	19.76		
M.T.E.-6 CONCENTRATE (APP)				
chromium/copper/iodide/manganese/selenium/zinc				
SOL, IV (M.D.V.)				
10 ml	63323-0036-10	31.12		
M.T.E.-7 (APP)				
cr/cu/iodide/mn/molybdenum/se/zinc				
SOL, IV (S.D.V.,PF)				
10 ml	63323-0014-10	23.02		
M.V.I-12 (Mayne Pharma)				
multivitamin and minerals				
SOL, IV (2X5 ML S.D.V.,#1 & #2)				
10 ml 10s	66591-0199-38	88.20		AP
(TWO-CHAMBERED S.D.V.)				
10 ml 10s	66591-0199-41	96.70		AP
(2 X 50ML M.D.V.,#1)				
100 ml 10s	66591-0199-71	619.98		AP
M.V.I.-12 W/O VITAMIN K (Hospira)				
multivitamin				
SOL, IV (10X10ML,2 CHAMBER SDV)				
10 ml 10s	61703-0423-81	103.44	90.50	
(20X50ML)				
50 ml 20s	61703-0423-83	647.16	566.30	
M.V.I.ADULT (Hospira)				
multivitamin				
SOL, IV (2X50ML,PHARMACY BULK)				
ea	61703-0422-83	554.64	485.30	
(10MLX10)				
10 ml 10s	61703-0422-81	99.12	86.70	
(SD VIAL #1 AND #2,2X5ML)				
10 ml 10s	61703-0422-82	63.84	55.90	
MA HUANG				
(PCCA) *See EPHEDRA HERB*				
MACK'S SAFE SOUND FOAM EARPLUGS (McKeon)				
plug, ear				
DEV, NA (SOFT,ORIGINAL,3PAIRS)				
6s ea	33732-0009-03	0.96		
(SOFT,ORIGINAL,5PAIRS)				
10s ea	33732-0009-05	1.34		
MACROBID (P & G Pharm)				
nitrofurantoin monohydrate/nitrofurantoin, macro				
CAP, PO, 100 mg, 100s ea	00149-0710-01	285.26	237.72	
(A-S Medication)				
REPACK				
CAP, PO, 100 mg, 10s ea	54569-3544-02	29.72		
14s ea	54569-3544-01	41.60		
20s ea	54569-3544-00	59.43		
(AQ)				
REPACK				
nitrofurantoin, macrocrystals				
CAP, PO, 100 mg, 100s ea	66105-0450-10	302.15		
(Dispensing Solutions)				
REPACK				
nitrofurantoin monohydrate/nitrofurantoin, macro				
CAP, PO, 100 mg, 14s ea	55045-2341-05	38.05		
(PD-Rx Pharm)				
REPACK				
CAP, PO, 100 mg, 6s ea	55289-0031-06	34.88		
10s ea	55289-0031-10	55.17		
14s ea	55289-0031-14	64.78		
(REDI-SCRIPT)				
100 mg, 14s ea	58864-0323-14	64.79		
20s ea	55289-0031-20	78.91		
(Pharma Pac)				
REPACK				
CAP, PO, 100 mg, 10s ea	52959-0404-10	25.05		
14s ea	52959-0404-14	35.25		
20s ea	52959-0404-20	50.20		
(Phys Total Care)				
REPACK				
CAP, PO, 100 mg, 6s ea	54868-2366-06	20.31		
10s ea	54868-2366-01	32.60		
14s ea	54868-2366-02	44.89		
15s ea	54868-2366-03	47.95		
20s ea	54868-2366-04	63.31		
30s ea	54868-2366-05	94.04		
50s ea	54868-2366-07	146.94		
60s ea	54868-2366-00	175.95		
(Quality Care Prod)				
REPACK				
CAP, PO, 100 mg, 14s ea	49999-0675-14	92.30		
MACRODANTIN (P & G Pharm)				
nitrofurantoin, macrocrystals				
CAP, PO, 25 mg, 100s ea	00149-0007-05	116.83	97.36	AB
50 mg, 100s ea	00149-0008-05	153.85	128.21	AB
100 mg, 100s ea	00149-0009-05	261.29	217.74	AB
(PD-Rx Pharm)				
REPACK				
CAP, PO, 50 mg, 12s ea	55289-0179-12	27.44		AB
28s ea	55289-0179-28	64.02		AB
40s ea	55289-0179-40	91.47		AB
100 mg, 12s ea	55289-0914-12	46.61		AB
14s ea	55289-0914-14	54.36		AB
(REDI-SCRIPT)				
100 mg, 14s ea	58864-0651-14	46.53		AB
15s ea	55289-0914-15	58.26		AB
20s ea	55289-0914-20	77.67		AB
28s ea	55289-0914-28	108.74		AB
30s ea	55289-0914-30	116.51		AB
40s ea	55289-0914-40	155.34		AB
(Phys Total Care)				
REPACK				
CAP, PO, 50 mg, 40s ea	54868-0429-03	61.26		AB
MACROTEC (Bracco Diag)				
technetium tc 99m albumin aggregated				
KIT, IV (TECHNETIUM PREPARATION)				
ea	00270-0076-08	534.54	427.63	BS
MACUGEN (Eyetech)				
pegaptanib octasodium				
SOL, IO (1X0.09MLLUERLOK30GX1/2")				
0.3 mg/0.09 ml,				
0.09 ml	68782-0001-02	1194.00	995.00	
(PF)				
0.3 mg/0.09 ml,				
0.09 ml	68782-0001-01	1194.00	995.00	
MACUTEK (Zyber)				
medical food				
ODT, PO (ORANGE)				
90s ea	65224-0570-01	45.00		
MAFENIDE ACETATE (Letco)				
POW, NA (U.S.P.)				
1000 gm	62991-1739-03	1950.00		
5000 gm	62991-1739-04	7305.00		
(Mylan Bertek) *See SULFAMYLON*				
(UDL) *See SULFAMYLON*				
MAFENIDE HYDROCHLORIDE				
(Spectrum Pharmacy) *See P-(AMINOMETHYL) BENZENESULFONAMIDE HYDROCHLORIDE*				
MAGNACET (Victory Pharma, Inc.)				
acetaminophen/oxycodone hydrochloride				
TAB, PO, 400 mg-2.5 mg,				
100s ea, C-II	23635-0991-01	356.97		
400 mg-5 mg,				
100s ea, C-II	23635-0992-01	356.97		
400 mg-7.5 mg,				
100s ea, C-II	23635-0993-01	356.97		
400 mg-10 mg,				
100s ea, C-II	23635-0994-01	392.66		
(Stat Rx)				
REPACK				
TAB, PO, 400 mg-5 mg,				
60s ea, C-II	16590-0763-60	229.32		
400 mg-10 mg,				
30s ea, C-II	16590-0814-30	114.61		
60s ea, C-II	16590-0814-60	229.22		
MAGNASWEET 110 (PCCA)				
flavoring aid				
SOL, NA, 1 gm	51927-2628-00	1.44		
MAGNASWEET 135 (PCCA)				
flavoring aid				
POW, NA, 1 gm	51927-2629-00	1.80		
(Spectrum Pharmacy)				
ammoniated glycyrrhizin				
POW, NA (1X25GM)				
25 gm	49452-4164-01	85.75		
(1X100GM)				
100 gm	49452-4164-02	183.75		
MAGNEBIND 400 RX (Nephro-Tech)				
calcium carbonate/folic acid/magnesium carbonate				
TAB, PO, 200 mg-1 mg-400 mg,				
150s ea	59528-0416-05	38.50		
MAGNES SULF (Phys Total Care)				
REPACK				
magnesium sulfate				
SOL, IJ (25X10ML)				
500 mg/ml,				
10 ml 25s	54868-5724-00	230.22		
MAGNESIUM ACETATE (Amend)				
CRY, NA (A.C.S., REAGENT)				
500 gm	17317-1888-01	38.50		
2500 gm	17317-1888-05	100.80		
(Baker, J.T.) *See MAGNESIUM ACETATE TETRAHYDRATE*				
(Medisca)				
CRY, NA (1X100GM)				
100 gm	38779-1403-05	31.50		
(1X500GM)				
500 gm	38779-1403-08	102.00		
(1X2500GM)				
2500 gm	38779-1403-01	313.50		
(PCCA)				
CRY, NA (ACS, REAGENT)				
1 gm	51927-2147-00	0.50		
MAGNESIUM ACETATE TETRAHYDRATE (Baker, J.T.)				
magnesium acetate				
CRY, NA (A.C.S., REAGENT)				
500 gm	10106-2424-01	102.74		
2500 gm	10106-2424-05	241.33		
MAGNESIUM ALUMINUM SILICATE				
(Gallipot) *See VEEGUM*				
(PCCA)				
POW, NA (NF)				
1 gm	51927-1153-00	0.36		
(Spectrum Pharmacy)				
POW, NA (1X500GM,NF)				
500 gm	49452-4175-01	163.10		
MAGNESIUM ASCORBATE (PCCA)				
POW, NA, 1 gm	51927-2820-00	0.20		
MAGNESIUM ASPARTATE				
(PCCA) *See ASPARTIC ACID MAGNESIUM SALT*				
MAGNESIUM CARBONATE (Baker, J.T.)				
POW, NA (U.S.P.)				
500 gm	10106-2436-01	16.69		
(Gallipot) *See MAGNESIUM CARBONATE HEAVY*				
(Gallipot) *See MAGNESIUM CARBONATE LIGHT*				
(Medisca)				
POW, NA (1X1000GM,USP,HEAVY)				
1 gm 1000s	38779-1405-09	81.00		
(1X100GM,USP,HEAVY)				
100 gm	38779-1405-05	498.75		
(1X500GM,USP,HEAVY)				
500 gm	38779-1405-08	47.85		
(1X500GM,USP,LIGHT)				
500 gm	38779-1406-08	47.85		
(1X2500GM,USP,LIGHT)				
2500 gm	38779-1406-01	117.00		
(USP,1X2500GM)				
2500 gm	38779-1405-01	171.00		
(PCCA) *See MAGNESIUM CARBONATE LIGHT*				
(PCCA)				
POW, NA (USP)				
1 gm	51927-1304-00	0.10		
(Spectrum Pharmacy) *See MAGNESIUM CARBONATE HEAVY*				
(Spectrum Pharmacy) *See MAGNESIUM CARBONATE LIGHT*				
MAGNESIUM CARBONATE HEAVY (Gallipot)				
magnesium carbonate				
POW, NA (U.S.P.)				
454 gm	51552-0368-06	14.00		
2270 gm	51552-0368-09	55.58		
(Spectrum Pharmacy)				
POW, NA (U.S.P.)				
500 gm	49452-4180-01	85.05		
2500 gm	49452-4180-02	261.10		

PROD/MFR | NDC | AWP | DP | OBC

MAGNESIUM CARBONATE LIGHT (Gallipot)
magnesium carbonate
POW, NA (U.S.P.)
454 gm 51552-0507-06 14.00
2270 gm 51552-0507-09 53.83

(PCCA)
POW, NA (USP)
1 gm 51927-2067-00 0.10

(Spectrum Pharmacy)
POW, NA (U.S.P.)
500 gm 49452-4170-01 85.05
2500 gm 49452-4170-02 261.10

MAGNESIUM CHLORIDE (Amend)
POW, NA (U.S.P./F.C.C.)
454 gm 17317-1890-01 11.20
2270 gm 17317-1890-05 42.00
11350 gm 17317-1890-08 157.50

(Amer Regent)
SOL, IJ (M.D.V.)
200 mg/ml, 50 ml 00517-5034-01 12.50

(Baker, J.T.) *See MAGNESIUM CHLORIDE HEXAHYDRATE*

(Bioniche Pharma)
SOL, IJ (M.D.V.)
200 mg/ml, 50 ml 67457-0134-50 17.38

(Gallipot)
CRY, NA (U.S.P.,N.F.)
454 gm 51552-0213-06 14.00
2270 gm 51552-0213-09 55.16

(McGuff)
SOL, IJ (M.D.V.)
200 mg/ml, 50 ml 67157-0102-50 11.95

(Merit) *See CHLOROMAG*

(PCCA)
POW, NA (USP; HEXAHYDRATE)
1 gm 51927-1259-00 0.10

(Spectrum Pharmacy) *See MAGNESIUM CHLORIDE HEXAHYDRATE*

MAGNESIUM CHLORIDE HEXAHYDRATE (Baker, J.T.)
magnesium chloride
CRY, NA (U.S.P., F.C.C.)
500 gm 10106-2448-01 24.29
(ULTRAPURE BIOREAGENT)
500 gm 10106-4003-01 37.70
(U.S.P., F.C.C.)
2500 gm 10106-2448-05 166.36
(ULTRAPURE BIOREAGENT)
2500 gm 10106-4003-05 146.88

(Spectrum Pharmacy)
CRY, NA (B.P.,E.P.,U.S.P.)
500 gm 49452-4190-01 63.70
2500 gm 49452-4190-02 220.15
12000 gm 49452-4190-03 829.50
FLA, NA (F.C.C.)
500 gm 49452-4200-01 67.90
2500 gm 49452-4200-02 236.25
12000 gm 49452-4200-03 934.50

MAGNESIUM CITRATE
(Gallipot) *See MAGNESIUM CITRATE DIBASIC*

(Gallipot) *See MAGNESIUM CITRATE TRIBASIC*

(PCCA)
POW, NA (TRIBASIC; PURIFIED)
1 gm 51927-2957-00 0.60
(USP; TRIBASIC HYDRATE)
1 gm 51927-3326-00 0.60

MAGNESIUM CITRATE DIBASIC (Gallipot)
magnesium citrate
POW, NA, 113.4 gm 51552-0472-04 29.26
454 gm 51552-0472-06 69.30

MAGNESIUM CITRATE TRIBASIC (Gallipot)
magnesium citrate
POW, NA, 454 gm 51552-0642-06 82.88

MAGNESIUM FLUORIDE (Medisca)
CRY, NA, 100 gm 38779-1408-05 31.50
500 gm 38779-1408-08 108.00

MAGNESIUM GLUCONATE (Amend)
POW, NA (U.S.P.)
454 gm 17317-0340-01 23.10
2270 gm 17317-0340-05 84.00
11350 gm 17317-0340-08 350.00

(Gallipot)
POW, NA (U.S.P.)
454 gm 51552-1020-06 55.72 39.80

(Medisca)
POW, NA (1X100GM,USP,ODOR-FREE)
100 gm 38779-2115-05 37.50
(1X500GM,USP,ODOR-FREE)
500 gm 38779-2115-08 88.50
(1X2500GM,USP,ODOR-FREE)
2500 gm 38779-2115-01 261.00

(PCCA)
POW, NA (USP (HYDRATE))
1 gm 51927-1563-00 0.36

(Spectrum Pharmacy)
POW, NA (U.S.P.)
100 gm 49452-4220-03 74.90
500 gm 49452-4220-01 138.95
2500 gm 49452-4220-02 514.50

MAGNESIUM GLYCINATE (Letco)
POW, NA, 14%, 500 gm ... 62991-2674-02 105.00
(1X2500GM)
14%, 2500 gm 62991-2674-01 345.00

(Medisca)
POW, NA (1X500GM,15%)
500 gm 38779-2489-08 90.00
(1X1000GM,15%)
1000 gm 38779-2489-09 165.00

(PCCA)
POW, NA (15% MAGNESIUM)
1 gm 51927-2861-00 0.21

(Spectrum Pharmacy) *See MAGNESIUM GLYCINATE DIHYDRATE 11.7%*

MAGNESIUM GLYCINATE DIHYDRATE 11.7%
(Spectrum Pharmacy)
magnesium glycinate
POW, NA (1X500GM)
500 gm 49452-4225-02 145.95
(1X2500GM)
2500 gm 49452-4225-03 476.00

MAGNESIUM HYDROXIDE (Amend)
POW, NA (U.S.P.)
500 gm 17317-0341-01 8.40
2270 gm 17317-0341-05 28.00

(Medisca)
POW, NA (1X500GM,USP)
500 gm 38779-2116-08 46.50
(1X2500GM,USP)
2500 gm 38779-2116-01 132.00

(PCCA)
POW, NA (USP)
1 gm 51927-1924-00 0.10

(Spectrum Pharmacy)
POW, NA (U.S.P.)
500 gm 49452-4240-01 79.10
2500 gm 49452-4240-02 243.60

MAGNESIUM MALATE (PCCA)
POW, NA, 1 gm 51927-3620-00 0.18

MAGNESIUM NITRATE
(Baker, J.T.) *See MAGNESIUM NITRATE HEXAHYDRATE*

MAGNESIUM NITRATE HEXAHYDRATE (Baker, J.T.)
magnesium nitrate
FLA, NA (TECHNICAL)
11300 gm 10106-2473-07 271.92

MAGNESIUM OXIDE
(Baker, J.T.) *See MAGNESIUM OXIDE HEAVY*

(Baker, J.T.) *See MAGNESIUM OXIDE LIGHT*

(Baker, J.T.)
POW, NA (A.C.S., REAGENT)
500 gm 10106-2476-01 415.86

(Gallipot) *See MAGNESIUM OXIDE HEAVY*

(Mallinckrodt Lab)
POW, NA (U.S.P.)
500 gm 00406-6010-12 59.79

(Medisca)
POW, NA (1X500GM,USP,HEAVY)
500 gm 38779-2118-08 55.50
(1X500GM,USP,LIGHT)
500 gm 38779-2119-08 55.50
(1X2500GM,USP,HEAVY)
2500 gm 38779-2118-01 181.50
(1X2500GM,USP,LIGHT)
2500 gm 38779-2119-01 135.00

(PCCA)
POW, NA (USP)
1 gm 51927-1214-00 0.36
1 gm 51927-1586-00 0.13

(Spectrum Pharmacy) *See MAGNESIUM OXIDE HEAVY*

(Spectrum Pharmacy) *See MAGNESIUM OXIDE LIGHT*

MAGNESIUM OXIDE HEAVY (Baker, J.T.)
magnesium oxide
POW, NA (U.S.P., F.C.C.)
500 gm 10106-2484-01 16.74
2500 gm 10106-2484-05 118.91

(Gallipot)
POW, NA (U.S.P.)
454 gm 51552-0506-06 16.94

(Spectrum Pharmacy)
POW, NA (U.S.P.)
500 gm 49452-4260-01 85.40
2500 gm 49452-4260-02 259.35

MAGNESIUM OXIDE LIGHT (Baker, J.T.)
magnesium oxide
POW, NA (U.S.P., F.C.C.)
500 gm 10106-2480-01 23.20
2000 gm 10106-2480-05 147.90

(Spectrum Pharmacy)
POW, NA (U.S.P.)
500 gm 49452-4250-01 88.90
2500 gm 49452-4250-02 272.30

MAGNESIUM PHOSPHATE (PCCA)
POW, NA, 1 gm 51927-2927-00 0.27

(Spectrum Pharmacy) *See MAGNESIUM PHOSPHATE DIBASIC TRIHYDRATE*

MAGNESIUM PHOSPHATE DIBASIC TRIHYDRATE
(Spectrum Pharmacy)
magnesium phosphate
POW, NA (F.C.C.)
500 gm 49452-4270-01 274.40
2500 gm 49452-4270-02 567.00
12000 gm 49452-4270-03 1802.50

MAGNESIUM SALICYLATE
(Cypress Pharm) *See MST 600*

(PCCA)
POW, NA (USP)
1 gm 51927-2796-00 0.24

MAGNESIUM STEARATE (Gallipot)
POW, NA (N.F.)
454 gm 51552-0887-06 16.80 12.00

(Medisca)
POW, NA (N.F.)
500 gm 38779-0382-08 52.50
1000 gm 38779-0382-09 55.50

(PCCA)
POW, NA (NF)
1 gm 51927-1129-00 0.30

(Spectrum Pharmacy)
POW, NA (N.F.)
500 gm 49452-4290-01 93.10
2500 gm 49452-4290-02 204.40

MAGNESIUM SULFATE (Amer Regent)
SOL, IJ (S.D.V.,PF)
500 mg/ml,
2 ml 25s .... 00517-2602-25 14.69 EE
10 ml 25s .... 00517-2610-25 23.44 EE
50 ml 25s .... 00517-2650-25 60.94 EE

(APP)
SOL, IJ (S.D.V.,P.C.)
500 mg/ml, 2 ml ..... 63323-0064-02 1.18 AP
(S.D.V.,P.C.,PF)
500 mg/ml, 10 ml .... 63323-0064-10 3.91 AP
(S.D.V.)
500 mg/ml, 20 ml .... 63323-0064-20 7.95 AP
50 ml .... 63323-0064-50 16.74 AP

(Baker, J.T.) *See MAGNESIUM SULFATE ANHYDROUS*

(Baker, J.T.) *See MAGNESIUM SULFATE HEPTAHYDRATE*

(Cardinal Health) *See EPSOM SALT*

(Gallipot) *See EPSOM SALT*

(Hospira)
SOL, IJ (10X10ML,SINGLE-DOSE,USP)
500 mg/ml,
10 ml 10s .... 00409-1754-10 40.32 35.30 AP
(VIAL, FLIPTOP)
500 mg/ml,
20 ml 25s .... 00409-2168-02 29.70 26.00 AP
50 ml 25s .... 00409-2168-03 44.40 38.75 AP
IV (SINGLE DOSE,LATEX-FREE)
40 mg/ml,
50 ml 24s 00409-6729-24 177.98 155.76
(24X100ML,LATEX-FREE)
40 mg/ml,
100 ml 24s 00409-6729-23 171.36 150.00

PROD/MFR	NDC	AWP	DP	OBC
(24X500ML,LATEX-FREE)				
40 mg/ml,				
500 ml 24s	00409-6729-03	138.24	120.96	
(PLASTIC,12X1000ML)				
40 mg/ml,				
1000 ml 12s	00409-6729-09	104.54	91.44	
(LATEX-FREE)				
80 mg/ml,				
50 ml 24s	00409-6730-13	172.51	150.96	
(Lorann Oil)				
POW, NA, 120 gm	23535-0608-68	1.10		
480 gm	23535-0608-61	3.25		
(Mallinckrodt Lab)				
POW, NA (U.S.P.)				
500 gm	00406-4200-12	11.93		
(McKesson) *See EPSOM SALT*				
(Medisca)				
CRY, NA (1X100GM,USP)				
100 gm	38779-0792-05	12.00		
(1X500GM,USP)				
500 gm	38779-0792-08	21.00		
(1X2500GM,USP)				
2500 gm	38779-0792-01	34.50		
(PCCA)				
POW, NA (ANHYDROUS REAGENT)				
1 gm	51927-2298-00	0.42		
(USP; HEPTAHYDRATE)				
1 gm	51927-2732-00	0.07		
(Spectrum Pharmacy) *See MAGNESIUM SULFATE HEPTAHYDRATE*				
(Phys Total Care)				
REPACK				
SOL, IJ (1X50ML,PF)				
500 mg/ml, 50 ml	54868-5949-00	60.18		EE
MAGNESIUM SULFATE ANHYDROUS (Baker, J.T.)				
magnesium sulfate				
POW, NA (REAGENT)				
500 gm	10106-2506-01	70.40		
2500 gm	10106-2506-05	253.53		
MAGNESIUM SULFATE HEPTAHYDRATE (Baker, J.T.)				
magnesium sulfate				
CRY, NA (U.S.P.)				
500 gm	10106-2504-01	68.08		
2500 gm	10106-2504-05	141.53		
(Spectrum Pharmacy)				
POW, NA (U.S.P.,E.P.,B.P.,J.P.)				
500 gm	49452-4300-01	67.55		
2500 gm	49452-4300-02	96.25		
12000 gm	49452-4300-03	249.90		
MAGNESIUM SULFATE IN DEXTROSE (Hospira)				
dextrose/magnesium sulfate				
SOL, IV (SINGLE DOSE,LATEX-FREE)				
5%-2 gm/100 ml,				
500 ml 24s	00409-6728-03	181.44	158.88	
(PharMEDium Services)				
SOL, IV (24X250ML)				
5%-8 gm/100 ml,				
250 ml 24s	61553-0423-02	15.71	13.09	
MAGNESIUM SULFATE-LACTATED RINGER'S (PharMEDium Services)				
lactated ringer's solution/magnesium sulfate				
SOL, IV (VIAFLEX BAG,PF)				
40 gm, 1000 ml	61553-0408-04	19.44	16.20	
MAGNESIUM SULFATE-SODIUM CHLORIDE (PharMEDium Services)				
magnesium sulfate/sodium chloride				
SOL, IV (VIAFLEX BAG,PF)				
2 gm-0.9%, 50 ml	61553-0432-41	12.46	10.38	
(24X100ML, VIAFLEX BAG)				
6 gm-0.9%,				
100 ml 24s	61553-0443-48	388.80	324.00	
MAGNESIUM SULFATE/SODIUM CHLORIDE (PharMEDium Services) *See MAGNESIUM SULFATE-SODIUM CHLORIDE*				
MAGNESIUM TRISILICATE (Gallipot)				
POW, NA (U.S.P.)				
454 gm	51552-0629-06	14.98	10.70	
(Medisca) *See MAGNESIUM TRISILICATE ANHYDROUS*				
(PCCA)				
POW, NA ((U.S.P.); HYDRATE)				
1 gm	51927-9008-00	0.10		
(Spectrum Pharmacy)				
POW, NA (U.S.P.)				
500 gm	49452-4310-01	87.85		
2500 gm	49452-4310-02	266.70		
MAGNESIUM TRISILICATE ANHYDROUS (Medisca)				
magnesium trisilicate				
POW, NA (U.S.P.)				
454 gm	38779-0334-08	31.50		
(1X2500GM,USP)				
2500 gm	38779-0334-01	105.00		
MAGNEVIST (Bayer)				
gadopentetate dimeglumine				
SOL, IV (VIAL)				
496.01 mg/ml,				
5 ml 20s	50419-0188-05	554.40		
(SRN)				
496.01 mg/ml,				
10 ml 5s	50419-0188-36	288.00		
(S.D.V.)				
496.01 mg/ml,				
10 ml 20s	50419-0188-01	1032.00		
(SRN)				
496.01 mg/ml,				
15 ml 5s	50419-0188-37	414.00		
(S.D.V.)				
496.01 mg/ml,				
15 ml 20s	50419-0188-15	1512.00		
(SRN)				
496.01 mg/ml,				
20 ml 5s	50419-0188-38	540.00		
(S.D.V.)				
496.01 mg/ml,				
20 ml 20s	50419-0188-02	1992.00		
50 ml 10s	50419-0188-58	2490.00		
100 ml 10s	50419-0188-11	4980.00		
MAITAKE MUSHROOM (PCCA)				
POW, NA, 1 gm	51927-3401-00	1.50		
MALACHITE GREEN				
(Amend) *See MALACHITE GREEN HYDROCHLORIDE*				
(Gallipot) *See MALACHITE GREEN OXALATE*				
(PCCA) *See MALACHITE GREEN OXALATE*				
MALACHITE GREEN HYDROCHLORIDE (Amend)				
malachite green				
CRY, NA, 100 gm	17317-1728-01	75.00		
MALACHITE GREEN OXALATE (Gallipot)				
malachite green				
POW, NA, 10 gm	51552-0606-02	13.65		
(PCCA)				
POW, NA (CI 42000; STAIN)				
1 gm	51927-1562-00	3.24		
MALARONE (Glaxo)				
atovaquone/proguanil hydrochloride				
TAB, PO (BLISTER PACK,2X12)				
250 mg-100 mg,				
24s ea	00173-0675-02	179.78		
100s ea	00173-0675-01	734.16		
(A-S Medication)				
REPACK				
TAB, PO, 250 mg-100 mg,				
7s ea	54569-5129-09	50.27		
12s ea	54569-5762-00	86.17		
14s ea	54569-5129-05	100.53		
16s ea	54569-5129-01	114.89		
24s ea	54569-5129-02	172.34		
100s ea	54569-5129-00	896.16		
(Dispensing Solutions)				
REPACK				
TAB, PO, 250 mg-100 mg,				
10s ea	55045-3201-02	67.00		
24s ea	55045-3201-04	160.80		
(Nucare Pharm)				
REPACK				
TAB, PO, 250 mg-100 mg,				
100s ea	68071-1347-00	710.92		
(PD-Rx Pharm)				
REPACK				
TAB, PO, 250 mg-100 mg,				
20s ea	55289-0747-20	216.96		
MALARONE PEDIATRIC (Glaxo)				
atovaquone/proguanil hydrochloride				
TAB, PO, 62.5 mg-25 mg,				
100s ea	00173-0676-01	271.55		
(Nucare Pharm)				
REPACK				
TAB, PO, 62.5 mg-25 mg,				
100s ea	68071-1346-00	364.26		
MALATHION (Karalex)				
LOT, TP (USP,1X59ML)				
0.5%, 59 ml	42043-0150-23	156.45		
(PCCA)				
SOL, NA, 1 gm	51927-2948-00	11.40		
(Taro)				
LOT, TP (USP,1X59ML)				
0.5%, 59 ml	51672-5277-04	165.14		
(Taro) *See OVIDE*				
MALDEMAR (Hawthorn Pharm)				
scopolamine hydrobromide				
TAB, PO, 0.4 mg, 100s ea.	63717-0840-01	34.95		
MALEIC ACID (PCCA)				
maleic acid, bis(2-ethylhexyl) ester				
POW, NA, 1 gm	51927-3247-00	4.50		
MALEIC ACID (PCCA)				
(1X1GM)				
1 gm	51927-2752-00	2.88		
MALEIC ACID, BIS(2-ETHYLHEXYL) ESTER (PCCA) *See MALEIC ACID*				
MALIC ACIC (PCCA)				
malic acid				
POW, NA (FCC; DL)				
1 gm	51927-1991-00	0.29		
MALIC ACID				
(Gallipot) *See MALIC ACID DL*				
(PCCA) *See MALIC ACIC*				
(Spectrum Pharmacy)				
CRY, NA (1X500GM)				
500 gm	49452-4319-01	129.15		
(1X2500GM)				
2500 gm	49452-4319-02	385.00		
(Spectrum Pharmacy) *See DL-MALIC ACID*				
MALIC ACID DL (Gallipot)				
malic acid				
POW, NA (F.C.C.)				
454 gm	51552-0583-06	14.40		
MALTODEXTRIN (PCCA)				
POW, NA (NF)				
1 gm	51927-3066-00	0.12		
(Spectrum Pharmacy)				
POW, NA (F.C.C.)				
500 gm	49452-4325-01	93.10		
2500 gm	49452-4325-02	299.95		
12000 gm	49452-4325-03	805.00		
MANDELIC ACID				
(PCCA) *See MANDELIC ACID (DL)*				
MANDELIC ACID (DL) (PCCA)				
mandelic acid				
POW, NA (1X1GM)				
1 gm	51927-1175-00	1.80		
MANDRAGORA COMPOUND (Weleda)				
homeopathic substance				
LIQ, PO, 50 ml	55946-0303-15	9.00		
MANGANESE (Hospira)				
manganese chloride				
SOL, IV (VIAL,FLIPTOP,LATEX-FREE)				
0.1 mg/ml,				
10 ml 25s	00409-4091-01	17.70	15.50	
MANGANESE CARBONATE (Amend)				
POW, NA (REAGENT)				
500 gm	17317-0698-01	26.60		
2500 gm	17317-0698-05	84.00		
12000 gm	17317-0698-08	268.80		
(Baker, J.T.) *See MANGANOUS CARBONATE*				
MANGANESE CHLORIDE				
(Baker, J.T.) *See MANGANOUS CHLORIDE TETRAHYDRATE*				
(Hospira) *See MANGANESE*				
(Medisca)				
CRY, NA (1X100GM,USP)				
100 gm	38779-1413-05	27.00		
(1X500GM,USP)				
500 gm	38779-1413-08	93.00		
(1X2500GM,USP)				
2500 gm	38779-1413-01	373.50		
(PCCA)				
CRY, NA (ANHYDROUS)				
1 gm	51927-2746-00	10.80		
POW, NA (USP; TETRAHYDRATE)				
1 gm	51927-1521-00	0.60		
(Spectrum Pharmacy) *See MANGANESE CHLORIDE TETRAHYDRATE*				

PROD/MFR	NDC	AWP	DP	OBC
MANGANESE CHLORIDE TETRAHYDRATE (Spectrum Pharmacy)				
manganese chloride				
CRY, NA (U.S.P.)				
125 gm	**49452-7397-01**	89.95		
500 gm	**49452-7397-02**	220.15		
2500 gm	**49452-7397-03**	812.00		
MANGANESE DIOXIDE (Baker, J.T.)				
POW, NA (REAGENT)				
500 gm	**10106-8392-01**	95.48		
2500 gm	**10106-8392-05**	317.91		
(TECHNICAL)				
2500 gm	**10106-2526-05**	98.06		
MANGANESE GLUCONATE (PCCA)				
POW, NA (USP; DIHYDRATE)				
1 gm	**51927-2219-00**	0.60		
(Spectrum Pharmacy) *See MANGANESE GLUCONATE ANHYDROUS*				
MANGANESE GLUCONATE ANHYDROUS (Spectrum Pharmacy)				
manganese gluconate				
POW, NA (U.S.P.)				
500 gm	**49452-4351-01**	126.70		
2500 gm	**49452-4351-02**	472.50		
12000 gm	**49452-4351-03**	1452.50		
MANGANESE NITRATE				
(Baker, J.T.) *See MANGANOUS NITRATE 50-52%*				
MANGANESE SULFATE				
(Amend) *See MANGANESE SULFATE MONOHYDRATE*				
(Amer Regent)				
SOL, IV (S.D.V.)				
0.1 mg/ml,				
10 ml 25s	**00517-6410-25**	62.19		
(Baker, J.T.) *See MANGANOUS SULFATE MONOHYDRATE*				
(PCCA)				
POW, NA (U.S.P.; MONOHYDRATE)				
1 gm	**51927-1345-00**	0.13		
(Spectrum Pharmacy) *See MANGANESE SULFATE MONOHYDRATE*				
MANGANESE SULFATE MONOHYDRATE (Amend)				
manganese sulfate				
POW, NA (U.S.P./F.C.C.)				
454 gm	**17317-0700-01**	14.35		
2270 gm	**17317-0700-05**	44.10		
(U.S.P./F.C.C.)				
11350 gm	**17317-0700-08**	210.00		
(Spectrum Pharmacy)				
POW, NA (U.S.P.)				
500 gm	**49452-4365-01**	85.40		
2500 gm	**49452-4365-02**	304.15		
MANGANOUS CARBONATE (Baker, J.T.)				
manganese carbonate				
POW, NA (REAGENT)				
500 gm	**10106-2536-01**	63.35		
2500 gm	**10106-2536-05**	225.47		
MANGANOUS CHLORIDE TETRAHYDRATE (Baker, J.T.)				
manganese chloride				
CRY, NA (A.C.S., REAGENT)				
125 gm	**10106-2540-04**	30.13		
500 gm	**10106-2540-01**	91.26		
MANGANOUS NITRATE 50-52% (Baker, J.T.)				
manganese nitrate				
SOL, NA (REAGENT)				
500 ml	**10106-2544-01**	49.44		
2500 ml	**10106-2544-05**	226.81		
MANGANOUS SULFATE MONOHYDRATE (Baker, J.T.)				
manganese sulfate				
POW, NA (A.C.S., REAGENT)				
500 gm	**10106-2550-01**	112.32		
2500 gm	**10106-2550-05**	407.26		
MANGO FLAVOR (PCCA)				
flavoring aid				
POW, NA (1X1GM,MANGO)				
1 gm	**51927-3660-00**	0.75		
(NATURAL,MANGO)				
1 gm	**51927-3457-00**	0.36		
MANNITOL (Amend)				
GRA, NA (U.S.P.)				
500 gm	**17317-1011-01**	28.00		
2270 gm	**17317-1011-05**	84.00		
11350 gm	**17317-1011-08**	315.00		
22700 gm	**17317-1011-09**	560.00		
POW, NA (REAGENT)				
454 gm	**17317-1012-01**	28.00		
(U.S.P.)				
500 gm	**17317-1010-01**	28.00		
2270 gm	**17317-1010-05**	84.00		
(REAGENT)				
11350 gm	**17317-1012-08**	350.00		
(U.S.P.)				
11350 gm	**17317-1010-08**	315.00		
(REAGENT)				
22700 gm	**17317-1012-03**	630.00		
(U.S.P.)				
22700 gm	**17317-1010-03**	560.00		
(Amer Regent)				
SOL, IV (S.D.V.,PF)				
25%, 50 ml 25s	**00517-4050-25**	85.94		AP
(APP)				
SOL, IV (FLIPOFF TOP,PF)				
25%, 50 ml	**63323-0024-25**	3.56		AP
(B. Braun) *See RESECTISOL*				
(B. Braun)				
SOL, IV (EXCEL)				
20%, 250 ml	**00264-7578-20**	17.57		AP
500 ml	**00264-7578-10**	18.01		AP
(Baker, J.T.)				
POW, NA (U.S.P.)				
2500 gm	**10106-2555-05**	120.37		
(Baxter) *See OSMITROL*				
(Consolidated Midland)				
SOL, IV (VIAL)				
25%, 50 ml	**00223-8105-50**	5.50		EE
(Gallipot)				
POW, NA (U.S.P.,N.F.)				
0.8 gm	**51552-0380-01**	5.88		
100 gm	**51552-0380-05**	13.23		
454 gm	**51552-0380-06**	29.40		
(U.S.P.)				
2270 gm	**51552-0380-08**	110.11		
11350 gm	**51552-0380-09**	553.00		
(Hospira)				
SOL, IV (LATEX-FREE)				
5%, 1000 ml 12s	**00409-7712-09**	189.36	165.72	AP
(USP,LATEX-FREE)				
10%, 1000 ml 12s	**00409-7713-09**	277.20	242.52	
(LATEX-FREE)				
15%, 500 ml 12s	**00409-7714-03**	196.70	172.08	AP
(FLEX CONTAINER,24X250ML)				
20%, 250 ml 24s	**00409-7715-02**	487.58	426.72	AP
(FLEX CONTAINER,12X500ML)				
20%, 500 ml 12s	**00409-7715-03**	242.78	212.40	AP
(VIAL, FLIPTOP)				
25%, 50 ml 25s	**00409-4031-01**	32.70	28.50	AP
(Letco)				
POW, NA (U.S.P.)				
500 gm	**62991-1568-01**	60.00		
(Mallinckrodt Lab)				
mannitol/sorbitol				
POW, NA (U.S.P.)				
500 gm	**00406-6208-04**	78.87		
2500 gm	**00406-6208-05**	291.84		
MANNITOL (Medisca)				
POW, NA (U.S.P.)				
500 gm	**38779-0599-08**	70.50		
(USP,D-MANNITOL)				
1000 gm	**38779-0599-09**	126.00		
(U.S.P.)				
2500 gm	**38779-0599-01**	258.00		
(PCCA)				
POW, NA (USP)				
1 gm	**51927-1781-00**	0.17		
(Spectrum Pharmacy)				
POW, NA (U.S.P.)				
500 gm	**49452-4380-01**	119.35		
2500 gm	**49452-4380-02**	535.50		
12000 gm	**49452-4380-03**	1764.00		
MANNITOL-SINCALIDE (PCCA)				
mannitol/sincalide				
POW, NA (U.S.P.)				
1 gm-100 mcg,				
0.001 gm	**51927-3416-00**	15000.00		
MANNITOL/SECRETIN				
(PCCA) *See SECRETIN, 99% MANNITOL*				
MANNITOL/SINCALIDE				
(PCCA) *See MANNITOL-SINCALIDE*				
MANNITOL/SORBITOL				
(Hospira) *See SORBITOL-MANNITOL*				
(Mallinckrodt Lab) *See MANNITOL*				
MANNOSE (PCCA)				
POW, NA, 1 gm	**51927-2977-00**	3.00		
(Spectrum Pharmacy) *See D-MANNOSE*				
MAPLE FLAVOR (Medisca)				
flavoring aid				
SOL, NA (1X100ML)				
100 ml	**38779-1417-05**	37.50		
(PCCA)				
SOL, NA (ARTIFICIAL)				
1 ml	**51927-2156-00**	0.90		
MAPROTILINE HCL (Mylan)				
maprotiline hydrochloride				
TAB, PO, 25 mg, 100s ea	**00378-0060-01**	56.00		AB
50 mg, 100s ea	**00378-0087-01**	82.90		AB
75 mg, 100s ea	**00378-0092-01**	113.75		AB
MAPROTILINE HYDROCHLORIDE				
(Mylan) *See MAPROTILINE HCL*				
MARAVIROC				
(Pfizer) *See SELZENTRY*				
MARCAINE (Phys Total Care)				
REPACK				
bupivacaine hydrochloride				
SOL, IJ, 0.25%, 50 ml	**54868-3437-00**	10.28		
MARCAINE EPI (Phys Total Care)				
bupivacaine hydrochloride/epinephrine bitartrate				
SOL, IJ, 0.25%-1:200000,				
50 ml	**54868-3438-00**	12.09		
0.5%-1:200000,				
50 ml	**54868-3439-00**	17.84		
MARCAINE HCL (Hospira)				
bupivacaine hydrochloride				
SOL, IJ (10X10ML, S.D.V.)				
0.25%, 10 ml 10s	**00409-1559-10**	25.80	22.60	AP
(S.D.V.,LATEX-FREE)				
0.25%, 30 ml 10s	**00409-1559-30**	29.64	25.90	AP
(M.D.V.,LATEX-FREE)				
0.25%, 50 ml	**00409-1587-50**	4.60	4.02	AP
(S.D.V.)				
0.5%, 10 ml 10s	**00074-1560-10**	29.28	25.60	AP
10 ml 10s	**00409-1560-10**	30.96	27.10	AP
30 ml 10s	**00409-1560-29**	27.60	24.20	AP
(M.D.V.)				
0.5%, 50 ml	**00074-1610-50**	3.43	3.00	AP
50 ml	**00409-1610-50**	3.43	3.00	AP
(10X10ML, S.D.V.)				
0.75%, 10 ml 10s	**00409-1582-10**	31.56	27.60	AP
(10X30ML,LATEX-FREE)				
0.75%, 30 ml 10s	**00409-1582-29**	48.72	42.60	AP
(A-S Medication)				
REPACK				
SOL, IJ (M.D.V.)				
0.25%, 50 ml	**54569-3260-00**	4.83		AP
(Phys Total Care)				
REPACK				
SOL, IJ (S.D.V.)				
0.5%, 30 ml 10s	**54868-3134-00**	43.26		AP
50 ml	**54868-3134-01**	8.28		AP
(Physician Partner)				
REPACK				
SOL, IJ (1X50ML)				
0.5%, 50 ml	**21695-0850-50**	17.40		AP
(Southwood)				
REPACK				
SOL, IJ (M.D.V.)				
0.5%, 50 ml	**58016-9343-01**	7.48		AP
MARCAINE HCL/EPINEPHRINE (Abbott Hosp)				
bupivacaine hydrochloride/epinephrine bitartrate				
SOL, IJ (AMP,LATEX-FREE)				
0.75%-1:200000,				
30 ml 5s	**00074-1750-30**	46.67	39.30	AP
(Hospira)				
SOL, IJ (10X10ML, S.D.V.)				
0.25%-1:200000,				
10 ml 10s	**00409-1746-10**	31.92	27.90	AP
(S.D.V.,10X30ML)				
0.25%-1:200000,				
30 ml 10s	**00409-1746-30**	75.24	65.80	AP
(M.D.V.)				
0.25%-1:200000,				
50 ml	**00074-1752-50**	5.51	4.82	AP
(FTV,10X10ML,LATEX-FREE)				
0.5%-1:200000,				
10 ml 10s	**00409-1749-10**	31.56	27.60	AP

PROD/MFR NDC AWP DP OBC

(AMP,LATEX-FREE)
0.5%-1:200000,
30 ml 5s.......... 00074-1749-30 49.16 41.40 AP
(10X30ML, S.D.V.)
0.5%-1:200000,
30 ml 10s......... 00409-1749-29 42.36 37.10 AP

(Quality Care Prod)
REPACK
SOL, IJ (M.D.V.)
0.5%-1:200000,
50 ml.......... 49999-0420-50 12.88 AP

MARCAINE HYDROCHLORIDE (Dispensing Solutions)
REPACK
bupivacaine hydrochloride
SOL, IJ, 0.25%, 50 ml..... 55045-3252-02 6.00
0.5%, 50 ml 55045-3251-05 7.00

MARCAINE SPINAL (Hospira)
bupivacaine hydrochloride
SOL, IJ (AMP,W/DEXTROSE,PF)
0.75%, 2 ml 10s ..... 00409-1761-02 17.76 15.50 AP

MARCAINE W/ EPINEPHRINE (Hospira)
bupivacaine hydrochloride/epinephrine bitartrate
SOL, IJ, 0.25%-1:200000,
50 ml............. 00409-1752-50 6.13 5.37 AP

MARCAINE WITH EPINEPHRINE (Hospira)
bupivacaine hydrochloride/epinephrine bitartrate
SOL, IJ (10X3ML,USP,PF)
0.5%-1:200000,
3 ml 10s.......... 00409-1749-03 29.04 25.40 AP
(FOR NERVE BLOCK)
0.5%-1:200000,
50 ml............. 00409-1755-50 9.78 8.56 AP

MARCOF EXPECTORANT (Marnel)
hydrocodone bitartrate/potassium guaiacolsulfonate
SYR, PO (AF,SF,DYE-FREE)
5 mg/5 ml-350 mg/5 ml,
480 ml, C-III 00682-0420-16 40.08

MARGARITA FLAVOR (Medisca)
flavoring aid
SOL, NA (1X100ML,CONCENTRATE)
100 ml 38779-1418-05 34.50
(1X500ML,CONCENTRATE)
500 ml 38779-1418-08 58.50

(PCCA)
SOL, NA (CONCENTRATE)
1 ml................ 51927-2603-00 0.30

MARGESIC (Marnel)
acetaminophen/butalbital/caffeine
CAP, PO, 325 mg-50 mg-40 mg,
100s ea.......... 00682-0804-01 62.70 AB

MARGESIC-H (Marnel)
acetaminophen/hydrocodone bitartrate
CAP, PO, 500 mg-5 mg,
100s ea, C-III ...... 00682-0808-01 62.40 AA

MARIGOLD EXTRACT (PCCA)
LIQ, NA (CALENDULA)
1 ml................ 51927-2470-00 1.80

MARINOL (Unimed Pharm)
dronabinol
CAP, PO (SOFTGEL)
2.5 mg,
60s ea, C-III 00051-0021-21 486.96
SGL, PO (SOFT GELATIN)
5 mg,
60s ea, C-III 00051-0022-21 1013.46
(SOFTGEL)
10 mg,
60s ea, C-III 00051-0023-21 1861.08

(Phys Total Care)
REPACK
CAP, PO (SOFTGEL)
2.5 mg,
30s ea, C-III 54868-3084-01 283.75
60s ea, C-III 54868-3084-00 545.52
90s ea, C-III 54868-3084-02 815.67
SGL, PO, 5 mg,
15s ea, C-III 54868-3189-03 208.16
(SOFTGEL)
5 mg,
25s ea, C-III 54868-3189-00 334.85
60s ea, C-III 54868-3189-02 798.62
100s ea, C-III 54868-3189-01 1301.45

(Southwood)
REPACK
SGL, PO (SOFTGEL)
5 mg,
30s ea, C-III 58016-0951-30 445.63
60s ea, C-III 58016-0951-60 891.25
90s ea, C-III 58016-0951-90 1336.88
100s ea, C-III 58016-0951-00 1485.42

MARJORAM OIL (Lorann Oil)
OIL, NA, 9.9 ml 23535-0151-42 4.00

MARNATAL-F (Marnel)
prenatal vitamins
CAP, PO, 30s ea 00682-1570-01 11.95

MARNATAL-F PLUS (Marnel)
nutriceutical/prenatal vitamins
KIT, PO (90EA,LICAP)
ea.................. 00682-2500-01 41.85

MARPLAN (Validus)
isocarboxazid
TAB, PO, 10 mg, 100s ea .. 30698-0032-01 331.20

MARSHMALLOW (Spectrum Pharmacy)
flavoring aid
SOL, NA (1X100ML)
100 ml 49452-4387-02 63.70
(1X500ML)
500 ml 49452-4387-03 146.65

MARSHMALLOW FLAVOR (Medisca)
flavoring aid
SOL, NA (1X25ML)
25 ml............... 38779-2125-04 22.50
(1X100ML)
100 ml 38779-2125-05 37.50
(1X500ML)
500 ml 38779-2125-08 76.50

(PCCA)
POW, NA (SPRAY DRIED, ARTIFICIAL)
1 gm 51927-3458-00 0.23
SOL, NA (ARTIFICIAL)
1 ml 51927-2699-00 0.90

MARTEN-TAB (Marnel)
acetaminophen/butalbital
TAB, PO, 325 mg-50 mg,
100s ea........... 00682-1400-01 55.16 AB

MARTINIC (Marlop)
ferrous fum/folic acid/if/vit b12/vit c
CAP, PO, 60s ea 12939-0305-41 20.85

MASK, FACE
(Dexo) *See E-Z SPACER MASK*
(Dey, L.P.) *See EASIVENT MASK*
(Pari) *See NEBULIZER AEROSOL MASK ADULT*
(Pari) *See PARI BABY*
(Respironics) *See OPTICHAMBER FACE MASK*
(Respironics) *See PEDIATRIC MASK OPTICHAMBER*

MASTIC GUM
(PCCA) *See MASTIC GUM TEARS*

MASTIC GUM TEARS (PCCA)
mastic gum
FLA, NA, 1 gm 51927-1887-00 6.00

MATERNITY VITAMIN LOW IRON (Contract Pharmacal)
prenatal vitamins
TAB, PO, 100s ea 10267-1991-01 23.00

MATHYLENE BLUE (Medisca)
methylene blue
POW, NA (U.S.P.)
25 gm.............. 38779-0825-04 28.50
100 gm............. 38779-0825-05 81.00
(USP, 1X500GM)
500 gm............. 38779-0825-08 246.00

MATRISTEM MICROMATRIX (ACell)
wound and/or dressing supplies
DEV, NA (100MG)
ea.................. 08619-0102-10 322.80
(200MG)
ea.................. 08619-0102-20 550.80
(20MG)
5s ea............... 08619-0502-02 322.80
(30MG)
5s ea............... 08619-0502-03 540.00
(60MG)
5s ea............... 08619-0502-06 900.00

MATRISTEM WOUND SHEET (ACell)
wound and/or dressing supplies
DEV, NA (10CMX15CM)
ea.................. 08619-0101-07 474.00
(3CMX3.5CM)
ea.................. 08619-0101-06 129.52
(3CMX7CM)
ea.................. 08619-0101-04 184.01
(7CMX10CM)
ea.................. 08619-0101-01 357.60
(10CMX15CM)
5s ea............... 08619-0501-07 1950.00
(3CMX3.5CM)
5s ea............... 08619-0501-06 504.00
(3CMX7CM)
5s ea............... 08619-0501-04 894.00
(7CMX10CM)
5s ea............... 08619-0501-01 1788.00

MATULANE (Sigma-Tau)
procarbazine hydrochloride
CAP, PO, 50 mg, 100s ea .. 54482-0053-01 5568.00

(Phys Total Care)
REPACK
CAP, PO, 50 mg, 100s ea .. 54868-1366-00 5980.64

MAVIK (Abbott Pharm)
trandolapril
TAB, PO, 1 mg, 100s ea ... 00074-2278-13 144.44 126.71
2 mg, 100s ea........ 00074-2279-13 144.44 126.71
4 mg, 100s ea........ 00074-2280-13 144.44 126.71

(Phys Total Care)
REPACK
TAB, PO, 4 mg, 10s ea 54868-5099-01 21.53
30s ea............ 54868-5099-00 59.37

(Quality Care Prod)
REPACK
TAB, PO, 4 mg, 30s ea 49999-0294-30 76.90

MAXAIR (Phys Total Care)
REPACK
pirbuterol acetate
ARO, IH, 0.2 mg/actuation,
14 gm 54868-2821-01 108.50

MAXAIR AUTOHALER (Graceway)
pirbuterol acetate
ARO, IH (1X14GM,400ACTUATIONS)
0.2 mg/actuation,
14 gm 29336-0815-21 119.27

MAXALT (Merck)
rizatriptan benzoate
TAB, PO (UNIT OF USE,CAPLET)
5 mg, 9s ea 00006-0266-09 206.83
12s ea............ 00006-0266-12 303.74 EE
(UNIT OF USE,CAPLET)
10 mg, 9s ea......... 00006-0267-09 227.80
12s ea............ 00006-0267-12 303.74

(DHS, Inc.)
REPACK
TAB, PO (CAPLET)
10 mg, 9s ea......... 55887-0210-09 199.00

(Dispensing Solutions)
REPACK
TAB, PO, 10 mg, 9s ea 55045-3688-01 195.30

(Nucare Pharm)
REPACK
TAB, PO (CAPLET)
10 mg, 6s ea......... 68071-0262-06 158.87

(Pharma Pac)
REPACK
TAB, PO (CAPLET)
10 mg, 6s ea......... 52959-0786-06 118.50

(Phys Total Care)
REPACK
TAB, PO, 10 mg, 3s ea 54868-4251-01 97.79
6s ea 54868-4251-03 182.40
(CAPLET)
10 mg, 9s ea......... 54868-4251-00 271.63
12s ea............ 54868-4251-02 361.53

(Quality Care Prod)
REPACK
TAB, PO, 10 mg, 12s ea ... 35356-0252-12 489.66

(Southwood)
REPACK
TAB, PO (CAPLET)
5 mg, 6s ea.......... 58016-0938-06 137.89
9s ea 58016-0938-09 206.83
12s ea............ 58016-0938-12 275.77
30s ea............ 58016-0938-30 689.43
60s ea............ 58016-0938-60 1378.87
90s ea............ 58016-0938-90 2068.30
100s ea........... 58016-0938-00 2298.11
(UNIT OF USE)
10 mg, 6s ea......... 58016-5712-06 146.03
9s ea 58016-5712-01 219.05

PROD/MFR	NDC	AWP	DP	OBC
(Stat Rx)				
REPACK				
TAB, PO, 5 mg, 9s ea	**16590-0144-09**	220.50		
MAXALT MLT (Stat Rx)				
rizatriptan benzoate				
ODT, PO, 5 mg, 9s ea	**16590-0145-09**	220.50		
MAXALT-MLT (Merck)				
rizatriptan benzoate				
ODT, PO (UNIT OF USE,PEPPERMINT)				
5 mg, 9s ea	**00006-3800-09**	227.80		
(4X3,PEPPERMINT)				
5 mg, 12s ea	**00006-3800-12**	303.74		EE
(UNIT OF USE,PEPPERMINT)				
10 mg, 9s ea	**00006-3801-09**	227.80		
(4X3,PEPPERMINT)				
10 mg, 12s ea	**00006-3801-12**	303.74		
(Phys Total Care)				
REPACK				
ODT, PO (UNIT OF USE,PEPPERMINT)				
10 mg, 3s ea	**54868-4499-00**	97.14		
(PEPPERMINT,LYOPHILIZED)				
10 mg, 6s ea	**54868-4499-02**	182.40		
12s ea	**54868-4499-01**	361.53		
(Quality Care Prod)				
REPACK				
ODT, PO (PEPPERMINT,LYOPHILIZED)				
10 mg, 12s ea	**35356-0275-12**	534.55		
MAXARON FORTE (Centrix)				
vitamin b complex, iron, and vitamin c				
CAP, PO, 100s ea	**11528-0135-01**	83.94		
MAXIDEX (Alcon Ophthalmic)				
dexamethasone				
SUS, OP, 0.1%, 5 ml	**00998-0615-05**	48.66		
(Quality Care Prod)				
REPACK				
SUS, OP, 0.1%, 5 ml	**49999-0722-05**	52.79		
MAXIDONE (Watson)				
acetaminophen/hydrocodone bitartrate				
TAB, PO, 750 mg-10 mg,				
100s ea, C-III	**52544-0634-01**	185.92		
MAXIFED CD (MCR American)				
codeine phos/gg/pse hcl				
TAB, PO, 10 mg-400 mg-60 mg,				
100s ea, C-III	**58605-0410-01**	109.84		
MAXIFED CDX (MCR American)				
codeine phos/gg/pse hcl				
TAB, PO, 20 mg-400 mg-60 mg,				
100s ea, C-III	**58605-0411-01**	113.83		
MAXIFED-G CD (MCR American)				
codeine phos/gg/pse hcl				
TAB, PO, 10 mg-400 mg-40 mg,				
100s ea, C-III	**58605-0412-01**	108.49		
MAXIFED-G CDX (MCR American)				
codeine phos/gg/pse hcl				
TAB, PO, 20 mg-400 mg-40 mg,				
100s ea, C-III	**58605-0413-01**	112.21		
MAXIFILL TRANSFER SET (APP)				
transfer unit, iv fluid				
DEV, NA (PLASTIC TUBING)				
12s ea	**63323-0001-21**	74.88		
MAXIFLU CD (MCR American)				
apap/codeine phos/gg/pse hcl				
TAB, PO, 100s ea, C-III	**58605-0430-01**	112.49		
MAXIFLU CDX (MCR American)				
apap/codeine phos/gg/pse hcl				
TAB, PO, 100s ea, C-III	**58605-0431-01**	115.18		
MAXIPHEN CD (MCR American)				
codeine phos/gg/phenyleph hcl				
TAB, PO, 10 mg-400 mg-10 mg,				
100s ea, C-III	**58605-0426-01**	113.60		
MAXIPHEN CDX (MCR American)				
codeine phos/gg/phenyleph hcl				
TAB, PO, 20 mg-400 mg-10 mg,				
100s ea, C-III	**58605-0427-01**	115.24		
MAXIPIME (Elan Pharmaceuticals)				
cefepime hydrochloride				
PDS, IJ (ADD-VANTAGE)				
1 gm, ea	**51479-0054-02**	21.26		
(P.B.)				
1 gm, ea	**51479-0054-01**	21.90		
(VIAL)				
1 gm, ea	**51479-0054-03**	20.46		
(ADD-VANTAGE,ADD-VANTAGE)				
1 gm, 10s ea	**51479-0054-20**	225.44		
(VIAL)				
1 gm, 10s ea	**51479-0054-30**	216.90		
(ADD-VANTAGE)				
2 gm, ea	**51479-0055-01**	36.59		
(P.B.)				
2 gm, ea	**51479-0055-02**	42.06		
(VIAL)				
2 gm, ea	**51479-0055-03**	40.61		
(ADD-VANTAGE)				
2 gm, 10s ea	**51479-0055-10**	439.14		
(VIAL)				
2 gm, 10s ea	**51479-0055-30**	430.48		
500 mg, ea	**51479-0053-01**	10.26		
10s ea	**51479-0053-10**	108.85		
MAXITROL (Alcon Ophthalmic)				
dexamethasone/neomycin sulfate/polymyxin b sulfate				
OIN, OP, 3.5 gm	**00065-0631-36**	83.94		AT
SUS, OP, 5 ml	**00998-0630-06**	72.96		AT
(Quality Care Prod)				
REPACK				
OIN, OP (1X3.5GM)				
3.5 gm	**35356-0449-35**	134.84		AT
SUS, OP, 5 ml	**49999-0723-05**	73.90		AT
MAXZIDE (Mylan)				
hydrochlorothiazide/triamterene				
TAB, PO, 50 mg-75 mg,				
100s ea	**00378-0460-01**	205.47		AB
(Mylan Bertek)				
TAB, PO (10X10)				
25 mg-37.5 mg,				
100s ea UD	**62794-0464-88**	77.30		AB
500s ea	**62794-0464-05**	351.14		AB
(Phys Total Care)				
REPACK				
TAB, PO, 25 mg-37.5 mg,				
30s ea	**54868-0907-01**	24.16		AB
60s ea	**54868-0907-02**	46.46		AB
50 mg-75 mg,				
30s ea	**54868-0866-02**	33.14		AB
60s ea	**54868-0866-03**	68.82		AB
MAXZIDE-25 (Mylan)				
hydrochlorothiazide/triamterene				
TAB, PO, 25 mg-37.5 mg,				
100s ea	**00378-0464-01**	91.62		AB
MD-GASTROVIEW (Mallinckrodt Inc.)				
diatrizoate meglumine/diatrizoate sodium				
SOL, PO (25X30ML,LEMON VANILLA)				
66%-10%, 30 ml 25s	**00019-4816-04**	495.00		AA
(12X120ML,LEMON VANILLA)				
66%-10%,				
120 ml 12s	**00019-4816-05**	480.00		AA
(12X240ML,LEMON VANILLA)				
66%-10%,				
240 ml 12s	**00019-4816-06**	900.00		AA
MEASLES VIRUS VACCINE, LIVE				
(Merck) *See ATTENUVAX*				
MEASLES, MUMPS, AND RUBELLA VIRUS VACCINE, LIVE				
(Merck) *See M-M-R II*				
MEASLES, MUMPS, RUBELLA AND VARICELLA VACCINE LIVE				
(Merck) *See PROQUAD*				
MEBARAL (Lundbeck)				
mephobarbital				
TAB, PO, 32 mg,				
250s ea, C-IV	**67386-0801-02**	221.75		
50 mg,				
250s ea, C-IV	**67386-0802-02**	317.54		
100 mg,				
250s ea, C-IV	**67386-0803-02**	425.60		
(Phys Total Care)				
REPACK				
TAB, PO, 32 mg,				
60s ea, C-IV	**54868-4072-00**	44.39		
MEBENDAZOLE (Medisca)				
POW, NA (U.S.P.)				
25 gm	**38779-0121-04**	55.50		
100 gm	**38779-0121-05**	160.50		
500 gm	**38779-0121-08**	673.50		
(PCCA)				
POW, NA (USP)				
1 gm	**51927-2021-00**	2.76		
(Spectrum Pharmacy)				
POW, NA (U.S.P.)				
25 gm	**49452-4395-01**	108.50		
100 gm	**49452-4395-02**	313.95		
500 gm	**49452-4395-03**	1197.00		
(Teva)				
CTB, PO, 100 mg, 12s ea	**00093-9107-29**	63.85		AB
(Advanced Pharm Serv, Inc.)				
REPACK				
CTB, PO, 100 mg, 10s ea	**13411-0175-01**	127.20		
12s ea	**13411-0175-12**	73.43		
20s ea	**13411-0175-02**	254.40		
30s ea	**13411-0175-03**	381.60		
60s ea	**13411-0175-06**	763.20		
(Bryant Ranch)				
REPACK				
CTB, PO, 100 mg, 2s ea	**63629-1528-01**	14.90		
3s ea	**63629-1528-02**	22.35		
12s ea	**63629-1528-03**	89.39		
(DHS, Inc.)				
REPACK				
CTB, PO, 100 mg, ea	**55887-0121-01**	73.43		
(Pharma Pac)				
REPACK				
CTB, PO, 100 mg, ea	**52959-0383-01**	6.75		EE
(Phys Total Care)				
REPACK				
CTB, PO, 100 mg, 2s ea	**54868-3732-03**	35.34		AB
6s ea	**54868-3732-02**	97.50		EE
12s ea	**54868-3732-00**	153.83		EE
MECASERMIN				
(Tercica) *See INCRELEX*				
MECHLORETHAMINE HYDROCHLORIDE				
(Lundbeck) *See MUSTARGEN*				
(PCCA)				
POW, NA (1X0.001GM)				
0.001 gm	**51927-3824-00**	15.00		
MECLICOT (Truxton)				
meclizine hydrochloride				
TAB, PO, 12.5 mg,				
1000s ea	**00463-7015-10**	15.00		EE
25 mg, 1000s ea	**00463-6310-10**	19.20		EE
MECLIZINE (DHS, Inc.)				
REPACK				
meclizine hydrochloride				
TAB, PO, 12.5 mg, 20s ea	**55887-0992-20**	5.71		
30s ea	**55887-0992-30**	8.57		
42s ea	**55887-0992-42**	12.00		
(Dispensing Solutions)				
REPACK				
TAB, PO, 25 mg, 20s ea	**55045-1451-07**	13.20		
50s ea	**55045-1451-01**	33.00		
(IPI)				
REPACK				
CTB, PO, 25 mg, 30s ea	**18837-0283-30**	23.85		
90s ea	**18837-0283-90**	45.15		
(Palmetto)				
REPACK				
TAB, PO, 12.5 mg, 6s ea	**23490-5849-01**	5.97		
30s ea	**23490-0881-03**	13.06		
30s ea	**23490-5849-03**	29.86		
60s ea	**23490-5849-06**	59.72		
90s ea	**23490-0881-09**	39.19		
90s ea	**23490-5849-09**	89.59		
(PD-Rx Pharm)				
REPACK				
CTB, PO, 25 mg, 6s ea	**43063-0073-06**	17.24		
8s ea	**43063-0073-08**	18.04		
10s ea	**43063-0073-10**	18.28		
12s ea	**43063-0073-12**	18.56		
20s ea	**43063-0073-20**	19.56		
30s ea	**43063-0073-30**	20.84		
(Stat Rx)				
REPACK				
TAB, PO, 25 mg, 20s ea	**16590-0146-20**	13.94		
30s ea	**16590-0146-30**	20.01		
60s ea	**16590-0146-60**	40.02		
MECLIZINE HCL (Consolidated Midland)				
meclizine hydrochloride				
TAB, PO, 12.5 mg,				
100s ea	**00223-1162-01**	2.75		EE
1000s ea	**00223-1162-02**	12.95		EE
25 mg, 100s ea	**00223-1163-01**	3.25		EE
100s ea	**00223-1164-01**	3.50		EE
1000s ea	**00223-1163-02**	17.95		EE
1000s ea	**00223-1164-02**	21.00		EE
(Medisca)				
POW, NA (U.S.P.)				
100 gm	**38779-0236-05**	102.00		
500 gm	**38779-0236-08**	435.00		

PROD/MFR	NDC	AWP	DP	OBC
(Par)				
TAB, PO, 25 mg, 100s ea	**49884-0035-01**	40.14		AA
1000s ea	**49884-0035-10**	401.32		AA
(PCCA)				
POW, NA (U.S.P.)				
1 gm	**51927-2394-00**	1.92		
(Sandoz)				
TAB, PO, 12.5 mg,				
1000s ea	**00781-1542-10**	71.34		AA
(A-S Medication)				
REPACK				
TAB, PO, 25 mg, 8s ea	**54569-5759-00**	3.21		AA
10s ea	**54569-0349-04**	4.01		AA
20s ea	**54569-0349-00**	8.03		AA
30s ea	**54569-0349-01**	12.04		AA
(Aidarex)				
REPACK				
CTB, PO, 25 mg, 7s ea	**33261-0165-07**	7.07		
14s ea	**33261-0165-14**	14.14		
20s ea	**33261-0165-20**	20.20		
21s ea	**33261-0165-21**	21.21		
28s ea	**33261-0165-28**	28.28		
30s ea	**33261-0165-30**	30.30		
40s ea	**33261-0165-40**	40.40		
60s ea	**33261-0165-60**	60.60		
(Altura)				
REPACK				
TAB, PO, 25 mg, 8s ea	**63874-0014-08**	2.93		AA
10s ea	**63874-0014-10**	3.66		AA
12s ea	**63874-0014-12**	7.10		AA
14s ea	**63874-0014-14**	8.28		AA
15s ea	**63874-0014-15**	8.87		AA
20s ea	**63874-0014-20**	11.83		AA
24s ea	**63874-0014-24**	14.20		AA
25s ea	**63874-0014-25**	14.79		AA
30s ea	**63874-0014-30**	17.59		AA
60s ea	**63874-0014-60**	35.18		AA
90s ea	**63874-0014-90**	52.77		AA
100s ea	**63874-0014-01**	58.63		AA
120s ea	**63874-0014-04**	66.65		AA
150s ea	**63874-0014-72**	83.31		AA
200s ea	**63874-0014-74**	111.08		AA
300s ea	**63874-0014-77**	166.62		AA
1000s ea	**63874-0014-02**	832.77		AA
(DHS, Inc.)				
REPACK				
TAB, PO, 25 mg, 20s ea	**55887-0939-20**	11.53		AA
21s ea	**55887-0939-21**	12.11		AA
30s ea	**55887-0939-30**	17.31		AA
60s ea	**55887-0939-60**	32.00		AA
90s ea	**55887-0939-90**	45.00		AA
(Dispensing Solutions)				
REPACK				
TAB, PO, 25 mg, 15s ea	**55045-1451-05**	9.90		AA
30s ea	**55045-1451-08**	19.85		AA
30s ea	**66336-0694-30**	24.16		EE
(HomeMed)				
REPACK				
TAB, PO, 12.5 mg, 30s ea	**51655-0318-24**	17.59		EE
25 mg, 20s ea	**51655-0107-52**	4.23		EE
30s ea	**51655-0107-24**	21.99		EE
(Nucare Pharm)				
REPACK				
TAB, PO, 12.5 mg, 30s ea	**66267-0138-30**	13.75		EE
25 mg, 20s ea	**66267-0139-20**	14.99		EE
30s ea	**66267-0139-30**	26.24		AA
90s ea	**66267-0139-90**	49.67		AA
(PD-Rx Pharm)				
REPACK				
TAB, PO, 25 mg, 20s ea	**58864-0159-20**	19.56		AA
(REDI-SCRIPT)				
25 mg, 30s ea	**58864-0159-30**	22.68		AA
56s ea	**58864-0159-56**	29.51		AA
60s ea	**58864-0159-60**	29.69		AA
(Pharma Pac)				
REPACK				
TAB, PO, 25 mg, 4s ea	**52959-0033-04**	3.92		EE
10s ea	**52959-0033-10**	8.30		EE
20s ea	**52959-0033-20**	15.67		EE
20s ea	**52959-0327-20**	19.80		EE
21s ea	**52959-0033-21**	16.45		EE
25s ea	**52959-0033-25**	19.25		EE
30s ea	**52959-0033-30**	29.59		EE
30s ea	**52959-0327-30**	29.70		EE
60s ea	**52959-0033-60**	57.67		EE
90s ea	**52959-0033-90**	86.49		EE
100s ea	**52959-0033-00**	95.90		AA
(Phys Total Care)				
REPACK				
TAB, PO, 12.5 mg, 15s ea	**54868-0089-00**	5.28		AA
30s ea	**54868-0089-02**	7.56		EE
50s ea	**54868-0089-07**	10.62		EE
100s ea	**54868-0089-04**	18.24		EE
25 mg, 15s ea	**54868-0077-01**	10.73		EE
20s ea	**54868-0077-07**	32.34		EE
30s ea	**54868-0077-04**	46.26		EE
40s ea	**54868-0077-03**	60.18		EE
60s ea	**54868-0077-08**	68.37		EE
90s ea	**54868-0077-02**	100.30		EE
100s ea	**54868-0077-05**	110.95		EE
(Physician Partner)				
REPACK				
TAB, PO, 25 mg, 10s ea	**21695-0237-10**	13.06		AA
15s ea	**21695-0237-15**	19.59		AA
30s ea	**21695-0237-30**	33.30		AA
40s ea	**21695-0237-40**	44.40		AA
90s ea	**21695-0237-90**	99.90		AA
(Quality Care Prod)				
REPACK				
TAB, PO, 12.5 mg, 15s ea	**49999-0087-15**	6.45		AA
30s ea	**49999-0087-30**	12.85		EE
100s ea	**49999-0087-00**	43.00		AA
25 mg, 5s ea	**49999-0029-05**	6.81		EE
20s ea	**49999-0029-20**	24.80		AA
30s ea	**49999-0029-30**	37.20		AA
(Southwood)				
REPACK				
TAB, PO, 12.5 mg, 12s ea	**58016-0801-12**	4.28		EE
15s ea	**58016-0801-15**	5.35		EE
20s ea	**58016-0801-20**	7.13		EE
30s ea	**58016-0801-30**	10.70		EE
100s ea	**58016-0801-00**	35.65		EE
25 mg, 8s ea	**58016-0802-08**	4.44		EE
12s ea	**58016-0802-12**	6.76		EE
15s ea	**58016-0802-15**	8.45		EE
20s ea	**58016-0802-20**	11.11		EE
30s ea	**58016-0802-30**	16.66		EE
60s ea	**58016-0802-60**	33.32		EE
90s ea	**58016-0802-90**	49.99		AA
100s ea	**58016-0802-00**	55.54		EE
120s ea	**58016-0802-02**	66.65		AA
150s ea	**58016-0802-03**	83.31		AA
200s ea	**58016-0802-89**	111.08		AA
300s ea	**58016-0802-73**	166.62		AA
(Vibranta)				
REPACK				
TAB, PO, 12.5 mg, 30s ea	**57866-3986-01**	17.59		AA
MECLIZINE HYDROCHLORIDE				
FUL				
TAB, PO, 12.5 mg,				
100s ea		5.99		
(Consolidated Midland) *See MECLIZINE HCL*				
(Medisca) *See MECLIZINE HCL*				
(Par) *See MECLIZINE HCL*				
(Par)				
TAB, PO, 12.5 mg, 100s ea	**49884-0034-01**	32.56		AA
1000s ea	**49884-0034-10**	325.60		AA
(PCCA) *See MECLIZINE HCL*				
(Pfizer) *See ANTIVERT*				
(Pfizer) *See ANTIVERT/25*				
(Pfizer) *See ANTIVERT/50*				
(Sandoz) *See MECLIZINE HCL*				
(Truxton) *See MECLICOT*				
(UDL)				
TAB, PO (10X10)				
12.5 mg,				
100s ea UD	**51079-0089-20**	71.39		AA
25 mg, 100s ea UD	**51079-0090-20**	86.51		AA
(A-S Medication)				
REPACK				
TAB, PO, 12.5 mg, 30s ea	**54569-0347-03**	9.77		AA
(Bryant Ranch)				
REPACK				
TAB, PO, 25 mg, 20s ea	**63629-1266-04**	15.74		
25s ea	**63629-1266-03**	18.43		
30s ea	**63629-1266-02**	22.12		
(Core)				
REPACK				
TAB, PO, 25 mg, 20s ea	**33358-0231-20**	16.13		
25s ea	**33358-0231-25**	18.89		
30s ea	**33358-0231-30**	22.67		
100s ea	**33358-0231-00**	25.96		
(Dispensing Solutions)				
REPACK				
TAB, PO, 12.5 mg, 30s ea	**55045-1230-08**	19.50		AA
(Keltman Pharma., Inc.)				
REPACK				
TAB, PO, 25 mg, 30s ea	**68387-0542-30**	19.91		
(Palmetto)				
REPACK				
TAB, PO, 25 mg, 5s ea	**23490-6877-04**	5.70		
6s ea	**23490-6877-01**	6.38		
20s ea	**23490-6877-00**	15.12		
30s ea	**23490-6877-02**	22.68		
60s ea	**23490-6877-06**	45.36		
90s ea	**23490-6877-03**	68.04		
(Pharma Pac)				
REPACK				
TAB, PO, 12.5 mg, 60s ea	**52959-0225-60**	29.40		AA
90s ea	**52959-0225-90**	45.02		AA
(Physician Partner)				
REPACK				
TAB, PO, 12.5 mg, 30s ea	**21695-0383-30**	19.54		AA
MECLOCYCLINE SULFOSALICYLATE (PCCA)				
POW, NA (U.S.P.)				
1 gm	**51927-2874-00**	54.00		
MECLOFENAMATE SODIUM (Medisca)				
POW, NA (U.S.P.)				
5 gm	**38779-0237-03**	90.00		
25 gm	**38779-0237-04**	225.00		
100 gm	**38779-0237-05**	705.00		
(USP, 1X500GM)				
500 gm	**38779-0237-08**	2670.00		
(USP, 1X1000GM)				
1000 gm	**38779-0237-09**	4545.00		
(Mylan)				
CAP, PO, 50 mg, 100s ea	**00378-2150-01**	192.15		AB
100 mg, 100s ea	**00378-3000-01**	356.70		AB
500s ea	**00378-3000-05**	1783.50		AB
(PCCA)				
POW, NA (U.S.P.)				
1 gm	**51927-1866-00**	5.04		
(Spectrum Pharmacy)				
POW, NA (U.S.P.)				
5 gm	**49452-4397-01**	145.95		
25 gm	**49452-4397-02**	292.25		
MECLOFENOXATE HYDROCHLORIDE (PCCA)				
POW, NA, 1 gm	**51927-2926-00**	11.40		
MEDENT DM (SJ)				
dm/gg/pse hcl				
TER, PO (DYE-FREE)				
30 mg-800 mg-60 mg,				
100s ea	**45985-0641-01**	102.29		
MEDENT-PE (SJ)				
guaifenesin/phenylephrine hydrochloride				
TER, PO (DYE-FREE)				
600 mg-12.5 mg,				
100s ea	**24839-0224-01**	100.79		
MEDI-FIRST DIPHENHYDRAMINE HYDROCHLORIDE (Medique)				
diphenhydramine hydrochloride				
CAP, PO (PRIVATE LABEL)				
25 mg, 100s ea	**47682-0858-87**	8.34		
MEDIBASE C (Medisca)				
peg-6				
SOL, NA, 500 ml	**38779-0750-08**	31.50		
1000 ml	**38779-0750-09**	52.50		
4000 ml	**38779-0750-01**	165.00		
MEDICAL FOOD				
(Accera) *See AXONA*				
(Arbor) *See XYLAREX*				
(Breckenridge Pharm) *See FOLBEE PLUS CZ*				
(Fleming) *See PROBARIMIN QT*				
(Pamlab) *See DEPLIN*				
(Pamlab) *See NEEVODHA*				
(Physician Thera, LLC) *See TREPADONE*				
(Zyber) *See MACUTEK*				
(Zyber) *See QUINZYME*				
(Zyber) *See REZYST IM*				
MEDIDERM (Medisca)				
cream base				
CRE, NA (1X100GM)				
100 gm	**38779-0738-05**	22.50		

PROD/MFR	NDC	AWP	DP	OBC
(1X500GM)				
500 gm	38779-0738-08	34.50		
(1X2500GM)				
2500 gm	38779-0738-01	157.50		
(1X5000GM)				
5000 gm	38779-0738-03	285.00		
MEDIHOL GEL BASE (Medisca)				
gel base				
GEL, NA (1X500GM,ALCOHOL)				
500 gm	38779-2258-08	117.00		
MEDROL (Pfizer)				
methylprednisolone				
TAB, PO, 2 mg, 100s ea	00009-0049-02	83.95	69.96	
(UNIT OF USE)				
4 mg, 21s ea	00009-0056-04	33.35	27.79	AB
100s ea	00009-0056-02	158.81	132.34	AB
8 mg, 25s ea	00009-0022-01	55.76	46.47	AB
16 mg, 50s ea	00009-0073-01	172.26	143.55	AB
32 mg, 25s ea	00009-0176-01	128.26	106.88	AB
(A-S Medication)				
REPACK				
TAB, PO (UNIT OF USE)				
4 mg, 21s ea	54569-0327-00	33.40		AB
(Phys Total Care)				
REPACK				
TAB, PO, 2 mg, 10s ea	54868-4952-01	9.16		
30s ea	54868-4952-00	23.73		
(DOSE PACK)				
4 mg, 21s ea	54868-0776-01	30.19		AB
(Quality Care Prod)				
REPACK				
TAB, PO (DOSE PACK)				
4 mg, 21s ea	35356-0194-21	76.20		AB
MEDROXYPROGESTERONE (Bryant Ranch)				
REPACK				
medroxyprogesterone acetate				
TAB, PO, 2.5 mg, 30s ea	63629-2613-01	13.14		
60s ea	63629-2613-02	26.28		
100s ea	63629-2613-03	43.81		
(DHS, Inc.)				
REPACK				
TAB, PO, 10 mg, 10s ea	55887-0472-10	8.50		
30s ea	55887-0472-30	22.00		
90s ea	55887-0472-90	44.00		
MEDROXYPROGESTERONE ACETATE				
FUL				
TAB, PO, 2.5 mg, 100s ea		20.25		
5 mg, 100s ea		30.61		
10 mg, 100s ea		37.87		
(Greenstone)				
SUS, IM, 150 mg/ml, 1 ml	59762-4537-01	53.05		AB
(PREFILLED SYRINGE,USP)				
150 mg/ml, 1 ml	59762-4538-01	58.23		
1 ml 25s	59762-4537-02	1326.25		AB
TAB, PO (UNIT OF USE)				
2.5 mg, 100s ea	59762-3740-01	29.83		AB
1000s ea	59762-3740-05	298.30		AB
(UNIT OF USE)				
5 mg, 100s ea	59762-3741-01	45.01		AB
1000s ea	59762-3741-04	450.10		AB
(UNIT OF USE)				
10 mg, 100s ea	59762-3742-02	46.75		AB
1000s ea	59762-3742-08	467.50		AB
(Medisca)				
POW, NA (U.S.P.,MICRONIZED)				
5 gm	38779-1422-03	93.00		
25 gm	38779-1422-04	414.00		
100 gm	38779-1422-05	1485.00		
(USP, 1X500GM,MICRONIZED)				
500 gm	38779-1422-08	3825.00		
(USP, 1X1000GM)				
1000 gm	38779-1422-09	6750.00		
(PCCA)				
POW, NA (U.S.P. (MICRONIZED))				
1 gm	51927-1490-00	30.00		
(Pfizer) *See DEPO-PROVERA*				
(Pfizer) *See DEPO-PROVERA CONTRACEPTIVE*				
(Pfizer) *See DEPO-SUBQ PROVERA 104*				
(Pfizer) *See PROVERA*				
(Pharmacia) *See DEPO-SUBQ PROVERA 104*				
(Teva)				
SUS, IM (ODOR-FREE)				
150 mg/ml, 1 ml	00703-6801-01	44.40		
1 ml	00703-6811-21	46.80		
1 ml 25s	00703-6801-04	1080.00		
TAB, PO, 2.5 mg, 100s ea	00555-0872-02	31.29		AB
500s ea	00555-0872-04	151.76		AB
5 mg, 100s ea	00555-0873-02	47.25		AB
500s ea	00555-0873-04	229.16		AB
10 mg, 100s ea	00555-0779-02	49.14		AB
500s ea	00555-0779-04	238.33		AB
(A-S Medication)				
REPACK				
TAB, PO, 2.5 mg, 30s ea	54569-3806-02	9.17		EE
5 mg, 30s ea	54569-3807-01	13.84		EE
10 mg, 5s ea	54569-0809-01	2.46		EE
10s ea	54569-0809-00	4.91		EE
30s ea	54569-0809-02	14.74		EE
(DHS, Inc.)				
REPACK				
TAB, PO, 2.5 mg, 10s ea	55887-0291-10	7.50		AB
30s ea	55887-0291-30	11.50		AB
60s ea	55887-0291-60	18.95		AB
90s ea	55887-0291-90	28.00		AB
(Dispensing Solutions)				
REPACK				
TAB, PO, 2.5 mg, 30s ea	66336-0213-30	22.29		AB
5 mg, 30s ea	66336-0603-30	33.22		AB
(Palmetto)				
REPACK				
SUS, IM, 150 mg/ml, 1 ml	23490-5854-01	70.24		
TAB, PO, 2.5 mg, 30s ea	23490-5855-03	30.00		
5 mg, 30s ea	23490-5857-01	29.33		
10 mg, 10s ea	23490-5853-00	7.33		
30s ea	23490-5853-02	22.00		
(PD-Rx Pharm)				
REPACK				
TAB, PO, 2.5 mg, 30s ea	55289-0816-30	17.36		AB
5 mg, 15s ea	58864-0744-15	7.85		AB
30s ea	55289-0908-30	26.64		AB
(REDI-SCRIPT,USP)				
5 mg, 30s ea	58864-0744-30	26.64		AB
42s ea	55289-0908-42	34.00		AB
10 mg, 5s ea	55289-0160-05	11.03		AB
7s ea	55289-0160-07	11.08		AB
10s ea	55289-0160-10	11.39		AB
13s ea	55289-0160-13	13.78		AB
30s ea	55289-0160-30	17.50		AB
40s ea	55289-0160-40	20.56		AB
42s ea	55289-0160-42	21.17		AB
50s ea	55289-0160-50	23.67		AB
(Pharma Pac)				
REPACK				
TAB, PO, 10 mg, 10s ea	52959-0943-10	6.95		AB
(Phys Total Care)				
REPACK				
SUS, IM, 150 mg/ml, 1 ml	54868-5257-00	111.57		
TAB, PO, 2.5 mg, 30s ea	54868-2984-00	11.16		EE
40s ea	54868-2984-02	13.41		EE
100s ea	54868-2984-03	26.76		EE
5 mg, 30s ea	54868-2985-00	13.86		EE
40s ea	54868-2985-01	16.95		EE
90s ea	54868-2985-03	32.55		AB
100s ea	54868-2985-02	35.64		EE
10 mg, 5s ea	54868-0109-06	5.46		EE
10s ea	54868-0109-01	7.92		EE
20s ea	54868-0109-07	12.84		AB
25s ea	54868-0109-00	15.30		AB
30s ea	54868-0109-02	17.76		EE
40s ea	54868-0109-05	22.65		EE
60s ea	54868-0109-08	33.99		EE
100s ea	54868-0109-03	52.14		EE
(Physician Partner)				
REPACK				
TAB, PO, 10 mg, 10s ea	21695-0896-10	11.56		AB
(Quality Care Prod)				
REPACK				
TAB, PO, 5 mg, 10s ea	49999-0494-10	5.44		AB
10 mg, 5s ea	49999-0092-05	7.09		EE
10s ea	49999-0092-10	14.18		AB
14s ea	35356-0364-14	14.18		AB
(Southwood)				
REPACK				
TAB, PO, 10 mg, 10s ea	58016-0926-10	6.62		EE
14s ea	58016-0926-14	9.27		EE
15s ea	58016-0926-15	9.93		EE
20s ea	58016-0926-20	13.25		EE
30s ea	58016-0926-30	19.87		EE
40s ea	58016-0926-40	26.49		EE
50s ea	58016-0926-50	33.12		EE
100s ea	58016-0926-00	66.23		EE
MEDROXYPROGESTERONE ACETATE MICRONIZED (Letco)				
medroxyprogesterone acetate, micronized				
POW, NA (U.S.P.)				
5 gm	62991-1474-01	81.00		
25 gm	62991-1474-02	345.00		
100 gm	62991-1474-03	1050.00		
(Spectrum Pharmacy)				
POW, NA (U.S.P.)				
5 gm	49452-4725-02	145.95		
25 gm	49452-4725-03	630.00		
100 gm	49452-4725-05	2128.00		
MEDROXYPROGESTERONE ACETATE, MICRONIZED (Letco) *See MEDROXYPROGESTERONE ACETATE MICRONIZED*				
(Spectrum Pharmacy) *See MEDROXYPROGESTERONE. ACETATE MICRONIZED*				
MEFENAMIC ACID (PCCA)				
POW, NA, 1 gm	51927-2082-00	1.68		
(Shionogi) *See PONSTEL*				
(Spectrum Pharmacy)				
CRY, NA (B.P.)				
100 gm	49452-4398-02	239.40		
500 gm	49452-4398-03	693.00		
MEFLOQUINE HCL (Sandoz)				
mefloquine hydrochloride				
TAB, PO, 250 mg, 25s ea	00781-5076-86	264.74		AB
(Teva)				
TAB, PO (5X5 BLISTER)				
250 mg, 25s ea	00555-0171-78	264.74		AB
(A-S Medication)				
REPACK				
TAB, PO, 250 mg, 8s ea	54569-5407-04	84.72		
10s ea	54569-5407-01	105.90		
25s ea	54569-5407-02	264.74		
(Dispensing Solutions)				
REPACK				
TAB, PO, 250 mg, 25s ea	55045-3321-02	300.00		AB
(Pharma Pac)				
REPACK				
TAB, PO, 250 mg, 25s ea	52959-0803-25	268.75		AB
(Phys Total Care)				
REPACK				
TAB, PO, 250 mg, 6s ea	54868-5434-00	61.20		AB
8s ea	54868-5434-01	61.67		AB
(Physician Partner)				
REPACK				
TAB, PO, 250 mg, 25s ea	21695-0449-25	529.48		AB
MEFLOQUINE HYDROCHLORIDE (Roche Labs) *See LARIAM*				
(Roxane)				
TAB, PO, 250 mg, 25s ea	00054-0025-11	264.74		AB
(Sandoz) *See MEFLOQUINE HCL*				
(Teva) *See MEFLOQUINE HCL*				
(Palmetto)				
REPACK				
TAB, PO, 250 mg, 5s ea	23490-5858-01	135.26		
10s ea	23490-5858-02	180.34		
25s ea	23490-5858-04	450.85		
MEGA-C/A PLUS (Merit)				
ascorbic acid				
SOL, IJ, 500 mg/ml,				
50 ml	30727-0339-90	15.95		
MEGACE (B/M Squibb Onc/Vir)				
megestrol acetate				
SUS, PO, 40 mg/ml,				
240 ml	00015-0508-42	170.32	141.93	AB
(Phys Total Care)				
REPACK				
SUS, PO, 40 mg/ml,				
240 ml	54868-3099-01	195.82		AB
MEGACE ES (Par)				
megestrol acetate				
SUS, PO (LEMON-LIME)				
625 mg/5 ml,				
150 ml	49884-0949-69	656.40		
(A-S Medication)				
REPACK				
SUS, PO (LEMON-LIME)				
625 mg/5 ml,				
150 ml	54569-5858-00	683.75		

PROD/MFR	NDC	AWP	DP	OBC
(Phys Total Care)				
REPACK				
SUS, PO, 625 mg/5 ml,				
150 ml	**54868-5572-00**	753.90		
(Stat Rx)				
REPACK				
SUS, PO (1X150ML,LEMON-LIME)				
625 mg/5 ml,				
150 ml	**16590-0254-33**	760.18		
MEGAVITE RX (Breckenridge Pharm)				
multivitamin, minerals, iron, and nutriceuticals				
TAB, PO (FILM-COATED, CAPLET)				
100s ea	**51991-0594-01**	32.40		
MEGESTROL ACETATE				
FUL				
TAB, PO, 20 mg, 100s ea		34.89		
40 mg, 100s ea		67.55		
(Apotex Corp.)				
SUS, PO (USP,LEMON-LIME)				
40 mg/ml, 240 ml	**60505-0368-01**	143.95		AB
(B/M Squibb Onc/Vir) *See MEGACE*				
(Gallipot)				
POW, NA (MICRONIZED)				
1 gm	**51552-0667-01**	26.25		
25 gm	**51552-0667-04**	147.00		
100 gm	**51552-0667-05**	490.00		
(Letco)				
POW, NA (BP98)				
25 gm	**62991-1496-03**	240.00		
100 gm	**62991-1496-04**	825.00		
(Major)				
TAB, PO (10X10)				
40 mg, 100s ea UD	**00904-3571-61**	136.75		AB
(Medisca)				
POW, NA (U.S.P.,MICRONIZED)				
5 gm	**38779-0140-05**	1107.00		
(USP, 1X5GM,MICRONIZED)				
5 gm	**38779-0140-03**	117.00		
(USP, 1X25GM,MICRONIZED)				
25 gm	**38779-0140-04**	327.00		
(Morton Grove)				
SUS, PO (LEMON-LIME)				
40 mg/ml, 240 ml	**60432-0126-08**	143.95		AB
480 ml	**60432-0126-16**	286.46		AB
(Par) *See MEGACE ES*				
(Par)				
SUS, PO, 40 mg/ml, 240 ml	**49884-0907-38**	143.95		AB
480 ml	**49884-0907-61**	286.46		AB
TAB, PO, 20 mg, 100s ea	**49884-0289-01**	69.20		AB
40 mg, 100s ea	**49884-0290-01**	123.00		AB
250s ea	**49884-0290-04**	270.60		AB
500s ea	**49884-0290-05**	530.38		AB
(Pharm Assoc Inc)				
SUS, PO (40X10ML CUPS,APRICOT)				
40 mg/ml,				
10 ml 40s UD	**00121-4776-10**	389.20		AB
(40X20ML,APRICOT)				
40 mg/ml,				
20 ml 40s UD	**00121-4776-20**	125.34		AB
(Precision Dose)				
SUS, PO (1X10ML,LEMON-LIME)				
40 mg/ml, 10 ml UD	**68094-0528-59**	4.23		AB
(LEMON-LIME)				
40 mg/ml,				
10 ml 30s UD	**68094-0528-62**	126.79		AB
(10X10,LEMON-LIME)				
40 mg/ml,				
10 ml 100s UD	**68094-0528-61**	422.64		AB
(1X20ML,LEMON-LIME)				
40 mg/ml, 20 ml UD	**68094-0518-59**	8.35		AB
(30X20ML,LEMON-LIME)				
40 mg/ml,				
20 ml 30s UD	**68094-0518-62**	250.50		AB
(Roxane)				
SUS, PO (LEMON,LIME)				
40 mg/ml, 240 ml	**00054-3542-58**	143.95		AB
TAB, PO, 20 mg, 100s ea	**00054-4603-25**	65.48		AB
(10X10)				
20 mg, 100s ea UD	**00054-8603-25**	90.88		AB
40 mg, 100s ea	**00054-4604-25**	116.80		AB
(10X10)				
40 mg, 100s ea UD	**00054-8604-25**	128.48		AB
(Spectrum Pharmacy)				
POW, NA (U.S.P.,N.F.,MICRONIZED)				
1 gm	**49452-4401-01**	108.85		
5 gm	**49452-4401-02**	200.90		
25 gm	**49452-4401-03**	539.00		
100 gm	**49452-4401-04**	1568.00		
(Teva)				
SUS, PO (APRICOT)				
40 mg/ml, 240 ml	**00093-9634-87**	143.95		
TAB, PO, 20 mg, 100s ea	**00555-0606-02**	67.12		AB
40 mg, 100s ea	**00555-0607-02**	110.21		AB
500s ea	**00555-0607-04**	529.39		AB
(UDL)				
TAB, PO (10X10)				
20 mg, 100s ea UD	**51079-0434-20**	65.65		AB
40 mg, 100s ea UD	**51079-0435-20**	106.95		AB
(VistaPharm, Inc.)				
SUS, PO (50X10ML)				
40 mg/ml,				
10 ml 50s	**66689-0020-50**	223.20		AB
(McKesson Packaging)				
REPACK				
TAB, PO (USP)				
40 mg, 100s ea UD	**63739-0165-10**	104.61		AB
(Pharma Pac)				
REPACK				
TAB, PO, 20 mg, 30s ea	**52959-0928-30**	43.89		AB
(Phys Total Care)				
REPACK				
SUS, PO, 40 mg/ml, 240 ml	**54868-5389-00**	87.96		AB
480 ml	**54868-5389-01**	284.79		
TAB, PO, 40 mg, 14s ea	**54868-1629-01**	17.40		AB
30s ea	**54868-1629-02**	32.13		
100s ea	**54868-1629-00**	73.41		AB
(Stat Rx)				
REPACK				
SUS, PO (1X240ML)				
40 mg/ml, 24 ml	**16590-0898-08**	172.74		AB
(1X480ML)				
40 mg/ml, 480 ml	**16590-0898-16**	345.48		AB
(Vibranta)				
REPACK				
TAB, PO, 20 mg, 30s ea	**57866-4822-01**	42.64		AB
MEGESTROL ACETATE MICRONIZED (PCCA)				
megestrol acetate, micronized				
POW, NA (U.S.P.)				
1 gm	**51927-1670-00**	30.60		
(B&B Pharm, Inc)				
REPACK				
POW, NA (U.S.P.)				
25 gm	**63275-9975-04**	297.00		
100 gm	**63275-9975-05**	878.00		
1000 gm	**63275-9975-09**	7560.00		
(Hawkins)				
REPACK				
POW, NA (U.S.P.)				
5 gm	**63370-0149-15**	120.00		
25 gm	**63370-0149-25**	398.00		
100 gm	**63370-0149-35**	1356.00		
500 gm	**63370-0149-45**	6600.00		
MEGESTROL ACETATE, MICRONIZED (PCCA) *See MEGESTROL ACETATE MICRONIZED*				
MEGLUMINE (Spectrum Pharmacy)				
POW, NA (U.S.P.)				
100 gm	**49452-4405-03**	138.95		
500 gm	**49452-4405-02**	336.35		
2500 gm	**49452-4405-01**	1015.00		
MELANEX (Neutrogena)				
hydroquinone				
SOL, TP, 3%, 30 ml	**10812-0930-01**	13.66		
MELATONIN (Medisca)				
POW, NA, 1 gm	**38779-0687-06**	49.50		
5 gm	**38779-0687-03**	223.50		
25 gm	**38779-0687-04**	615.00		
(1X100GM)				
100 gm	**38779-0687-05**	1920.00		
(PCCA)				
POW, NA, 1 gm	**51927-2220-00**	90.00		
(Spectrum Pharmacy)				
POW, NA, 1 gm	**49452-4407-02**	77.00		
5 gm	**49452-4407-03**	331.80		
25 gm	**49452-4407-04**	962.50		
100 gm	**49452-4407-05**	1967.00		
MELOXICAM				
FUL				
TAB, PO, 7.5 mg, 100s ea		14.25		
15 mg, 100s ea		20.93		
(Apotex Corp.)				
TAB, PO, 7.5 mg, 100s ea	**60505-2553-01**	316.84		AB
1000s ea	**60505-2553-08**	3168.40		AB
15 mg, 100s ea	**60505-2554-01**	484.44		AB
1000s ea	**60505-2554-08**	4844.40		AB
(Aurobindo Pharma)				
TAB, PO, 7.5 mg, 100s ea	**65862-0097-01**	316.45		AB
15 mg, 100s ea	**65862-0098-01**	484.44		AB
(Boehr Ingelheim Phar) *See MOBIC*				
(Breckenridge Pharm)				
TAB, PO, 7.5 mg, 100s ea	**51991-0404-01**	278.53		AB
1000s ea	**51991-0404-10**	2785.30		AB
15 mg, 100s ea	**51991-0419-01**	425.87		AB
1000s ea	**51991-0419-10**	4258.70		AB
(Caraco)				
TAB, PO, 7.5 mg, 100s ea	**57664-0512-88**	316.52		AB
500s ea	**57664-0512-13**	1582.60		AB
1000s ea	**57664-0512-18**	3165.20		AB
15 mg, 100s ea	**57664-0513-88**	483.96		AB
500s ea	**57664-0513-13**	2419.80		AB
1000s ea	**57664-0513-18**	4839.60		AB
(Carlsbad Tech)				
TAB, PO (USP)				
7.5 mg, 100s ea	**61442-0126-01**	278.53		AB
15 mg, 100s ea	**61442-0127-01**	425.87		AB
(Glenmark Pharmaceuticals)				
TAB, PO, 7.5 mg, 100s ea	**68462-0140-01**	311.59		AB
15 mg, 100s ea	**68462-0141-01**	476.42		AB
(Lannett)				
TAB, PO, 7.5 mg, 100s ea	**00527-1419-01**	11.40		AB
1000s ea	**00527-1419-10**	109.20		AB
15 mg, 100s ea	**00527-1420-01**	15.90		AB
1000s ea	**00527-1420-10**	153.60		AB
(Lupin Pharma, Inc.)				
TAB, PO, 7.5 mg, 100s ea	**68180-0501-01**	316.84		AB
1000s ea	**68180-0501-03**	3168.40		AB
15 mg, 100s ea	**68180-0502-01**	484.44		AB
1000s ea	**68180-0502-03**	4844.40		AB
(Medisca)				
POW, NA (1X10GM)				
10 gm	**38779-1991-01**	555.00		
(1X25GM)				
25 gm	**38779-1991-04**	945.00		
(Mylan)				
TAB, PO, 7.5 mg, 100s ea	**00378-1066-01**	316.45		AB
500s ea	**00378-1066-05**	1582.25		AB
15 mg, 100s ea	**00378-1089-01**	483.90		AB
500s ea	**00378-1089-05**	2419.50		AB
(Roxane)				
SUS, PO (RASPBERRY)				
7.5 mg/5 ml,				
100 ml	**00054-0228-49**	86.91		
(Sandoz)				
TAB, PO, 7.5 mg, 100s ea	**00781-5195-01**	316.87		AB
1000s ea	**00781-5195-10**	3168.70		AB
15 mg, 100s ea	**00781-5196-01**	484.50		AB
1000s ea	**00781-5196-10**	4845.00		AB
(Teva)				
TAB, PO, 7.5 mg, 100s ea	**00093-7234-01**	316.87		AB
15 mg, 100s ea	**00093-7299-01**	484.50		AB
(UDL)				
TAB, PO (10X10)				
7.5 mg, 100s ea UD	**51079-0457-20**	313.35		AB
(10 X 10)				
15 mg, 100s ea UD	**51079-0459-20**	479.11		AB
(Unichem)				
TAB, PO (USP)				
7.5 mg, 100s ea	**29300-0124-01**	316.87		AB
1000s ea	**29300-0124-10**	3168.70		AB
15 mg, 100s ea	**29300-0125-01**	484.50		AB
1000s ea	**29300-0125-10**	4845.00		AB
(Zydus Pharm.)				
TAB, PO, 7.5 mg, 100s ea	**68382-0050-01**	316.87		AB
500s ea	**68382-0050-05**	1584.35		AB
15 mg, 100s ea	**68382-0051-01**	484.49		AB
500s ea	**68382-0051-05**	2422.45		AB
(4u)				
REPACK				
TAB, PO, 7.5 mg, 30s ea	**10544-0391-30**	136.46		AB
30s ea	**42549-0320-30**	156.36		AB
30s ea	**42549-0520-30**	136.46		AB
30s ea	**42549-0562-30**	136.46		AB
30s ea	**42549-0591-30**	136.46		AB
30s ea	**42549-0604-30**	136.46		AB
15 mg, 30s ea	**10544-0390-30**	188.86		AB
30s ea	**42549-0319-30**	188.86		AB
30s ea	**42549-0519-30**	188.86		AB
30s ea	**42549-0590-30**	188.86		AB

PROD/MFR	NDC	AWP	DP	OBC
(A-S Medication)				
REPACK				
TAB, PO, 7.5 mg, 14s ea	**54569-5811-01**	44.36		
30s ea	**54569-5811-02**	95.06		
60s ea	**54569-5811-03**	190.12		
15 mg, 7s ea	**54569-5812-00**	33.92		
14s ea	**54569-5812-01**	67.83		
30s ea	**54569-5812-02**	145.35		
60s ea	**54569-5812-03**	290.70		
(Aidarex)				
REPACK				
TAB, PO, 7.5 mg, 7s ea	**33261-0070-07**	23.80		**AB**
14s ea	**33261-0070-14**	47.60		**AB**
20s ea	**33261-0070-20**	68.00		**AB**
21s ea	**33261-0070-21**	71.40		**AB**
28s ea	**33261-0070-28**	95.20		**AB**
30s ea	**33261-0070-30**	102.00		**AB**
60s ea	**33261-0070-60**	204.00		**AB**
90s ea	**33261-0070-90**	306.00		**AB**
100s ea	**33261-0070-00**	340.00		**AB**
120s ea	**33261-0070-02**	408.00		**AB**
15 mg, 7s ea	**33261-0071-07**	29.75		**AB**
14s ea	**33261-0071-14**	59.50		**AB**
20s ea	**33261-0071-20**	85.00		**AB**
21s ea	**33261-0071-21**	89.25		**AB**
30s ea	**33261-0071-30**	127.50		**AB**
40s ea	**33261-0071-40**	170.00		**AB**
60s ea	**33261-0071-60**	255.00		**AB**
90s ea	**33261-0071-90**	382.50		**AB**
(Altura)				
REPACK				
TAB, PO, 7.5 mg, 14s ea	**63874-1203-07**	46.79		
15s ea	**63874-1203-05**	44.85		
30s ea	**63874-1203-03**	89.70		
60s ea	**63874-1203-06**	179.40		
90s ea	**63874-1203-09**	269.10		
100s ea	**63874-1203-01**	299.00		
15 mg, 14s ea	**63874-1204-07**	63.98		
15s ea	**63874-1204-05**	68.55		
30s ea	**63874-1204-03**	153.31		
60s ea	**63874-1204-06**	274.20		
90s ea	**63874-1204-09**	411.30		
100s ea	**63874-1204-01**	457.00		
(Bryant Ranch)				
REPACK				
TAB, PO, 7.5 mg, 30s ea	**63629-3248-01**	172.36		
60s ea	**63629-3248-02**	289.30		
15 mg, 30s ea	**63629-3328-01**	209.70		
60s ea	**63629-3328-02**	415.32		
90s ea	**63629-3328-03**	629.13		
(Core)				
REPACK				
TAB, PO, 7.5 mg, 15s ea	**33358-0232-15**	54.13		
20s ea	**33358-0232-20**	72.17		
30s ea	**33358-0232-30**	108.26		
60s ea	**33358-0232-60**	298.30		
90s ea	**33358-0232-90**	447.44		
120s ea	**33358-0232-01**	596.59		
15 mg, 15s ea	**33358-0233-15**	54.80		
20s ea	**33358-0233-20**	109.59		
30s ea	**33358-0233-30**	164.66		
60s ea	**33358-0233-60**	329.31		
90s ea	**33358-0233-90**	493.96		
120s ea	**33358-0233-01**	658.62		
(DHS, Inc.)				
REPACK				
TAB, PO, 7.5 mg, 14s ea	**55887-0297-14**	42.00		
20s ea	**55887-0297-20**	60.00		
30s ea	**55887-0297-30**	90.00		
40s ea	**55887-0297-40**	120.00		
60s ea	**55887-0297-60**	180.00		
90s ea	**55887-0297-90**	270.00		
15 mg, 14s ea	**55887-0682-14**	64.17		
30s ea	**55887-0682-30**	137.50		
60s ea	**55887-0682-60**	275.00		
90s ea	**55887-0682-90**	412.50		
(Dispensing Solutions)				
REPACK				
TAB, PO, 7.5 mg, 30s ea	**55045-3545-01**	94.80		
30s ea	**66336-0099-30**	100.41		
60s ea	**55045-3545-06**	189.60		
60s ea	**66336-0099-60**	200.82		**AB**
100s ea	**55045-3545-00**	316.00		
15 mg, 7s ea	**66336-0774-07**	33.87		**AB**
30s ea	**55045-3531-01**	145.50		
30s ea	**66336-0774-30**	153.22		
60s ea	**66336-0774-60**	290.70		**AB**
100s ea	**55045-3531-00**	485.00		
(IPI)				
REPACK				
TAB, PO, 7.5 mg, 20s ea	**18837-0239-20**	80.13		**AB**
30s ea	**18837-0239-30**	120.67		**AB**
60s ea	**18837-0239-60**	189.91		**AB**
90s ea	**18837-0239-90**	284.81		**AB**
180s ea	**18837-0239-96**	714.01		**AB**
15 mg, 30s ea	**18837-0240-30**	145.33		**AB**
60s ea	**18837-0240-60**	362.93		
90s ea	**18837-0240-90**	544.39		
(Keltman Pharma., Inc.)				
REPACK				
TAB, PO, 7.5 mg, 30s ea	**68387-0480-30**	105.00		
60s ea	**68387-0480-60**	210.00		
90s ea	**68387-0480-90**	315.00		
15 mg, 30s ea	**68387-0481-30**	158.50		
90s ea	**68387-0481-90**	475.50		
(Nucare Pharm)				
REPACK				
TAB, PO, 7.5 mg, 7s ea	**68071-0528-07**	32.66		**AB**
15s ea	**68071-0528-15**	64.98		**AB**
20s ea	**68071-0528-20**	88.14		**AB**
30s ea	**68071-0528-30**	126.70		**AB**
40s ea	**68071-0528-40**	168.24		**AB**
60s ea	**68071-0528-60**	247.55		**AB**
90s ea	**68071-0528-90**	368.75		**AB**
15 mg, 30s ea	**68071-0529-30**	190.53		**AB**
60s ea	**68071-0529-60**	373.82		**AB**
(Palmetto)				
REPACK				
TAB, PO, 7.5 mg, 15s ea	**23490-7423-00**	52.67		
30s ea	**23490-7423-03**	105.34		
60s ea	**23490-7423-06**	210.68		
90s ea	**23490-7423-09**	316.02		
15 mg, 30s ea	**23490-7474-03**	188.94		
60s ea	**23490-7474-06**	377.88		
(PD-Rx Pharm)				
REPACK				
TAB, PO, 7.5 mg, 14s ea	**55289-0272-14**	68.76		**AB**
20s ea	**55289-0272-20**	90.00		**AB**
30s ea	**55289-0272-30**	125.00		**AB**
60s ea	**55289-0272-60**	156.28		**AB**
90s ea	**55289-0272-90**	187.52		**AB**
15 mg, 30s ea	**55289-0376-30**	129.92		**AB**
60s ea	**55289-0376-60**	162.48		**AB**
90s ea	**55289-0376-90**	195.00		**AB**
(Pharma Pac)				
REPACK				
TAB, PO, 7.5 mg, 14s ea	**52959-0856-14**	59.62		**AB**
15s ea	**52959-0856-15**	63.87		
20s ea	**52959-0856-20**	85.15		
21s ea	**52959-0856-21**	89.39		**AB**
30s ea	**52959-0856-30**	127.70		
45s ea	**52959-0856-45**	191.52		
60s ea	**52959-0856-60**	255.30		
90s ea	**52959-0856-90**	382.86		
120s ea	**52959-0856-01**	510.42		
15 mg, 15s ea	**52959-0857-15**	75.89		
20s ea	**52959-0857-20**	101.04		
21s ea	**52959-0857-21**	106.08		**AB**
30s ea	**52959-0857-30**	151.76		
45s ea	**52959-0857-45**	227.60		**AB**
60s ea	**52959-0857-60**	303.45		
90s ea	**52959-0857-90**	455.08		**AB**
(Phys Total Care)				
REPACK				
TAB, PO, 7.5 mg, 30s ea	**54868-5650-00**	26.43		
60s ea	**54868-5650-01**	49.86		
90s ea	**54868-5650-03**	17.26		**AB**
100s ea	**54868-5650-02**	81.09		
15 mg, 30s ea	**54868-5651-00**	9.66		
60s ea	**54868-5651-02**	17.82		
100s ea	**54868-5651-01**	211.80		
(Physician Partner)				
REPACK				
TAB, PO, 7.5 mg, 14s ea	**21695-0076-14**	104.26		**AB**
15s ea	**21695-0076-15**	111.71		
30s ea	**21695-0076-30**	189.90		
60s ea	**21695-0076-60**	379.80		
90s ea	**21695-0076-90**	569.70		
15 mg, 14s ea	**21695-0077-14**	159.42		**AB**
15s ea	**21695-0077-15**	170.81		
30s ea	**21695-0077-30**	290.37		
60s ea	**21695-0077-60**	552.50		
90s ea	**21695-0077-90**	871.11		
(Quality Care Prod)				
REPACK				
TAB, PO, 7.5 mg, 10s ea	**49999-0868-10**	72.90		**AB**
15s ea	**49999-0868-15**	109.35		**AB**
30s ea	**49999-0868-30**	89.38		
60s ea	**49999-0868-60**	178.76		
90s ea	**49999-0868-90**	268.14		
15 mg, 10s ea	**49999-0869-10**	29.80		**AB**
15s ea	**49999-0869-15**	44.70		**AB**
30s ea	**49999-0869-30**	218.74		
60s ea	**49999-0869-60**	437.48		
90s ea	**49999-0869-90**	656.22		
(Southwood)				
REPACK				
TAB, PO, 7.5 mg, 21s ea	**58016-0022-21**	76.65		**AB**
30s ea	**58016-0022-30**	109.50		**AB**
60s ea	**58016-0022-60**	219.00		**AB**
63s ea	**58016-0022-88**	188.37		**AB**
90s ea	**58016-0022-90**	328.50		**AB**
100s ea	**58016-0022-00**	365.00		**AB**
120s ea	**58016-0022-02**	438.00		**AB**
15 mg, 21s ea	**58016-0023-21**	117.60		**AB**
30s ea	**58016-0023-30**	168.00		**AB**
60s ea	**58016-0023-60**	336.00		**AB**
63s ea	**58016-0023-88**	283.50		**AB**
90s ea	**58016-0023-90**	504.00		**AB**
100s ea	**58016-0023-00**	560.00		**AB**
120s ea	**58016-0023-02**	672.00		**AB**
(St. Mary's MPP)				
REPACK				
TAB, PO (USP)				
7.5 mg, 10s ea	**60760-0404-10**	40.86		
30s ea	**60760-0404-30**	109.41		
60s ea	**60760-0404-60**	215.13		**AB**
(USP)				
15 mg, 30s ea	**60760-0419-30**	164.11		
60s ea	**60760-0419-60**	322.22		**AB**
(Stat Rx)				
REPACK				
TAB, PO, 7.5 mg, 20s ea	**16590-0434-20**	80.13		**AB**
28s ea	**16590-0434-28**	110.77		**AB**
30s ea	**16590-0434-30**	105.06		**AB**
40s ea	**16590-0434-40**	158.23		**AB**
56s ea	**16590-0434-56**	177.45		**AB**
60s ea	**16590-0434-60**	207.86		**AB**
90s ea	**16590-0434-90**	284.81		**AB**
100s ea	**16590-0434-71**	92.12		
120s ea	**16590-0434-72**	110.55		
15 mg, 15s ea	**16590-0469-15**	90.74		**AB**
20s ea	**16590-0469-20**	36.85		
28s ea	**16590-0469-28**	135.10		**AB**
30s ea	**16590-0469-30**	181.46		**AB**
56s ea	**16590-0469-56**	338.74		**AB**
60s ea	**16590-0469-60**	362.93		**AB**
90s ea	**16590-0469-90**	544.40		**AB**
(Vibranta)				
REPACK				
TAB, PO, 15 mg, 30s ea	**57866-9787-01**	8.55		**AB**
MELPAQUE HP (Stratus)				
hydroquinone				
CRE, TP (W/SUNBLOCK)				
4%, 14.2 gm	**58980-0473-05**	18.00		
28.4 gm	**58980-0473-10**	35.50		
MELPHALAN				
(Celgene Corp) *See ALKERAN*				
(Glaxo) *See ALKERAN*				
MELPHALAN HYDROCHLORIDE				
(Celgene Corp) *See ALKERAN IV*				
(Glaxo) *See ALKERAN*				
MELQUIN HP (Stratus)				
hydroquinone				
CRE, TP, 4%, 14.2 gm	**58980-0472-05**	18.00		
28.4 gm	**58980-0472-10**	35.50		
MELQUIN-3 (Stratus)				
hydroquinone				
SOL, TP, 3%, 30 ml	**58980-0476-10**	11.50		
MEMANTINE HYDROCHLORIDE				
(Forest Pharm) *See NAMENDA*				
MEMBRANEBLUE (Dutch Ophthalmic USA)				
trypan blue				
SOL, IO, 0.15%,				
0.5 ml 5s	**68803-0672-05**	475.00	475.00	
MENACTRA (Sanofi)				
meningococcal polysaccharide vac diphtheria conj				
SUS, IM (0.5MLX5,TAX INCL,PF)				
16 mcg/0.5 ml,				
0.5 ml 5s	**49281-0589-05**	619.72	517.06	
(0.5MLX5,W/TAX,LATEXFREE)				
16 mcg/0.5 ml,				
0.5 ml 5s	**49281-0589-15**	619.72	517.06	

PROD/MFR	NDC	AWP	DP	OBC
MENADIONE (PCCA)				
POW, NA (USP)				
1 gm	51927-1722-00	2.52		
(Spectrum Pharmacy)				
POW, NA (U.S.P.)				
25 gm	49452-4410-01	120.40		
100 gm	49452-4410-02	276.85		
MENEST (Monarch)				
esterified estrogens				
TAB, PO (FILM-COATED)				
0.3 mg, 100s ea	61570-0072-01	69.47		
0.625 mg, 100s ea	61570-0073-01	98.69		
1.25 mg, 100s ea	61570-0074-01	137.68		
2.5 mg, 50s ea	61570-0075-50	128.20		
(Dispensing Solutions)				
REPACK				
TAB, PO, 1.25 mg,				
100s ea	55045-3484-01	118.00		
(PD-Rx Pharm)				
REPACK				
TAB, PO, 0.625 mg,				
30s ea	58864-0951-30	34.89		
(Phys Total Care)				
REPACK				
TAB, PO (FILM-COATED)				
0.625 mg, 10s ea	54868-5934-00	14.17		
30s ea	54868-5934-01	37.29		
MENINGOCOCCAL OLIGOSACCHARIDE VAC DIPHTHERIA CONJ				
(Novartis) *See MENVEO*				
MENINGOCOCCAL POLYSACCHARIDE VAC DIPHTHERIA CONJ				
(Sanofi) *See MENACTRA*				
MENINGOCOCCAL POLYSACCHARIDE VACCINE				
(Sanofi) *See MENOMUNE-A/C/Y/W-135*				
MENOMUNE-A/C/Y/W-135 (Sanofi)				
meningococcal polysaccharide vaccine				
PDS, SC (S.D.V. W/DILUENT)				
0.05 mg, ea	49281-0489-01	126.34	105.41	
(10DOSE W/DILUENT)				
0.5 mg, ea	49281-0489-91	1239.44	1034.12	
MENOPUR (Ferring)				
follicle stimulating hormone/luteinizing hormone				
PDS, SC, 75 iu-75 iu,				
5s ea	55566-7501-02	469.27		
(WITH DILUENTS)				
75 iu-75 iu, 5s ea	55566-7501-01	427.86		
MENOSTAR (Bayer)				
estradiol				
TDM, TD (LATEX-FREE)				
0.014 mg/24 hr,				
4s ea	50419-0455-04	69.84		
(Phys Total Care)				
REPACK				
TDM, TD (LATEX-FREE)				
0.014 mg/24 hr,				
4s ea	54868-5371-00	61.64		
MENTAX (Mylan)				
butenafine hydrochloride				
CRE, TP, 1%, 15 gm	00378-6151-46	54.48		
30 gm	00378-6151-49	109.00		
MENTHOL				
(Amend) *See L-MENTHOL*				
(Baker, J.T.) *See LEVO-MENTHOL*				
(Gallipot)				
CRY, NA (U.S.P.)				
25 gm	51552-0045-04	9.59		
100 gm	51552-0045-05	14.70		
(Letco)				
CRY, NA (U.S.P.)				
100 gm	62991-1098-02	45.00		
500 gm	62991-1098-03	126.00		
(Lorann Oil)				
CRY, NA, 30 gm	23535-0609-05	3.00		
120 gm	23535-0609-08	10.20		
480 gm	23535-0609-01	36.30		
(Mallinckrodt Lab)				
CRY, NA (U.S.P.)				
30 gm	00406-6222-12	17.12		
125 gm	00406-6222-02	36.49		
(Medisca)				
CRY, NA (U.S.P.)				
25 gm	38779-0521-04	34.50		
100 gm	38779-0521-05	84.00		
500 gm	38779-0521-08	255.00		
(USP, 1X1000GM)				
1000 gm	38779-0521-09	465.00		
(USP, 1X5000GM)				
5000 gm	38779-0521-03	1725.00		
(PCCA)				
CRY, NA (USP; L NATURAL)				
1 gm	51927-1138-00	0.99		
(Spectrum Pharmacy) *See DL-MENTHOL*				
(Spectrum Pharmacy) *See L-MENTHOL*				
MENTHOL EUCALYPTUS FLAVOR (PCCA)				
flavoring aid				
SOL, NA, 1 ml	51927-3432-00	1.40		
MENVEO (Novartis)				
meningococcal oligosaccharide vac diphtheria conj				
KIT, IM (TAX INCLUDED,LATEX-FREE)				
ea	46028-0208-01	619.71	517.05	
MEPENZOLATE BROMIDE				
(Sanofi-Aventis) *See CANTIL*				
MEPEREDINE (Quality Care Prod)				
REPACK				
meperidine hydrochloride				
TAB, PO, 50 mg,				
30s ea, C-II	49999-0837-30	63.20		
100 mg,				
30s ea, C-II	49999-0838-30	84.30		
120s ea, C-II	49999-0838-01	187.20		
MEPERGAN (Phys Total Care)				
REPACK				
meperidine hcl/promethazine hcl				
SOL, IJ (TUBEX,22GX1 1/4")				
25 mg/ml-25 mg/ml,				
2 ml 10s, C-II	54868-4136-00	99.35		
MEPERIDINE (Palmetto)				
REPACK				
meperidine hydrochloride				
TAB, PO, 50 mg,				
30s ea, C-II	23490-9300-03	25.50		
60s ea, C-II	23490-9300-06	51.00		
90s ea, C-II	23490-9300-09	76.50		
MEPERIDINE HCL (Baxter)				
meperidine hydrochloride				
SOL, IJ (SRN,PREFILLED,GLASS)				
10 mg/ml,				
50 ml 10s, C-II	00338-2691-75	311.40	259.50	EE
25 mg/ml,				
1 ml, C-II	10019-0159-44	0.78		EE
(SDV (DOSETTE))				
25 mg/ml,				
1 ml 25s, C-II	10019-0159-01	19.50		EE
50 mg/ml,				
1 ml, C-II	10019-0160-44	0.84		EE
(SDV (DOSETTE))				
50 mg/ml,				
1 ml 25s, C-II	10019-0160-01	21.00		EE
100 mg/ml,				
1 ml, C-II	10019-0162-44	0.86		EE
(SDV (DOSETTE))				
100 mg/ml,				
1 ml 25s, C-II	10019-0162-01	21.60		EE
(Covidien)				
POW, NA (U.S.P.)				
25 gm, C-II	00406-1585-55	262.81		
(Hawkins)				
POW, NA (U.S.P.)				
5 gm, C-II	63370-0937-15	104.00		
25 gm, C-II	63370-0937-25	380.00		
100 gm, C-II	63370-0937-35	1396.00		
(Medisca)				
POW, NA (U.S.P.)				
5 gm, C-II	38779-1766-03	450.00		
25 gm, C-II	38779-1766-04	1485.00		
100 gm, C-II	38779-1766-05	4350.00		
(PCCA)				
POW, NA (U.S.P.; CII)				
1 gm, C-II	51927-1018-00	15.00		
(Roxane)				
TAB, PO (R.N.P.)				
50 mg,				
25s ea UD, C-II	00054-8595-11	17.35		AA
100s ea, C-II	00054-4595-25	68.63		AA
100 mg,				
100s ea, C-II	00054-4596-25	130.55		AA
(Spectrum Pharmacy)				
POW, NA (U.S.P.)				
5 gm, C-II	49452-0031-03	177.45		
25 gm, C-II	49452-0031-01	518.00		
(Teva)				
TAB, PO, 50 mg,				
100s ea, C-II	00555-0381-02	68.12		AA
100 mg,				
100s ea, C-II	00555-0382-02	129.57		AA
(B&B Pharm, Inc)				
REPACK				
POW, NA (U.S.P.)				
25 gm, C-II	63275-7100-04	552.00		
100 gm, C-II	63275-7100-05	2208.00		
(Dispensing Solutions)				
REPACK				
TAB, PO, 50 mg,				
30s ea, C-II	66336-0302-30	26.50		AA
(Nucare Pharm)				
REPACK				
TAB, PO, 50 mg,				
30s ea, C-II	68071-0760-30	27.50		AA
(Phys Total Care)				
REPACK				
TAB, PO, 50 mg,				
10s ea, C-II	54868-1233-01	17.82		EE
30s ea, C-II	54868-1233-03	38.49		EE
(USP)				
50 mg,				
40s ea, C-II	54868-1233-02	48.84		EE
MEPERIDINE HCL/SODIUM CHLORIDE				
(PharMEDium Services)				
meperidine hydrochloride/sodium chloride				
SOL, IV (INTRAVIA)				
1 gm/100 ml-0.9%,				
100 ml, C-II	61553-0172-48	46.06	38.38	
(IPUMP BAG)				
1 gm/100 ml-0.9%,				
100 ml, C-II	61553-0173-48	59.74	49.78	
(INTRAVIA)				
500 mg/50 ml-0.9%,				
50 ml, C-II	61553-0170-41	35.19	29.33	
MEPERIDINE HYDROCHLORIDE				
FUL				
TAB, PO, 50 mg, 100s ea		31.88		
100 mg, 100s ea		62.93		
(Baxter) *See MEPERIDINE HCL*				
(Caraco)				
TAB, PO (USP)				
50 mg,				
100s ea, C-II	57664-0467-08	68.50		AA
100 mg,				
100s ea, C-II	57664-0471-08	129.90		AA
(Covidien) *See MEPERIDINE HCL*				
(Gallipot)				
POW, NA (USP,1X1GM)				
1 gm, C-II	51552-0686-01	25.20	18.00	
(USP,1X5GM)				
5 gm, C-II	51552-0686-02	46.20	33.00	
(USP,1X25GM)				
25 gm, C-II	51552-0686-04	133.00	95.00	
(USP,1X100GM)				
100 gm, C-II	51552-0686-06	511.00	365.00	
(Hawkins) *See MEPERIDINE HCL*				
(Hospira) *See DEMEROL*				
(Hospira) *See DEMEROL HYDROCHLORIDE*				
(Hospira)				
SOL, IV (SDV,USP,10X30ML)				
10 mg/ml,				
30 ml 10s, C-II	00409-6030-04	98.40	86.10	AP
(Medisca) *See MEPERIDINE HCL*				
(PCCA) *See MEPERIDINE HCL*				
(Qualitest) *See MEPERITAB*				
(Roxane) *See MEPERIDINE HCL*				
(Roxane)				
SOL, PO (USP,UNFLAVRED,COLORLESS)				
50 mg/5 ml,				
500 ml, C-II	00054-3545-63	94.09		
(Sanofi-Aventis) *See DEMEROL HYDROCHLORIDE*				
(Spectrum Pharmacy) *See MEPERIDINE HCL*				
(Teva) *See MEPERIDINE HCL*				
MEPERIDINE HYDROCHLORIDE/PROMETHAZINE HCL				
(Palmetto)				
REPACK				
meperidine hcl/promethazine hcl				
CAP, PO, 50 mg-25 mg,				
4s ea, C-II	23490-7775-01	2.51		

PROD/MFR NDC AWP DP OBC

20s ea, C-II 23490-7775-02 12.55
30s ea, C-II 23490-7775-03 18.82
40s ea, C-II 23490-7775-04 24.28

MEPERIDINE HYDROCHLORIDE/SODIUM CHLORIDE
(PharMEDium Services) *See MEPERIDINE HCL/SODIUM CHLORIDE*

MEPERIDINE-PROMETHAZINE (Phys Total Care)
REPACK
meperidine hcl/promethazine hcl
CAP, PO, 50 mg-25 mg,
10s ea, C-II 54868-5151-01 19.89
20s ea, C-II 54868-5151-02 32.28
30s ea, C-II 54868-5151-00 44.68
40s ea, C-II 54868-5151-03 55.57
100s ea, C-II 54868-5151-04 102.26

MEPERITAB (Qualitest)
meperidine hydrochloride
TAB, PO, 50 mg,
100s ea, C-II ....00603-4415-21 68.60 AA
100 mg,
100s ea, C-II ....00603-4416-21 130.50 AA

(Phys Total Care)
REPACK
TAB, PO, 50 mg,
20s ea, C-II ....54868-1233-06 24.66 AA
100s ea, C-II ....54868-1233-04 76.52 AA
120s ea, C-II ....54868-1233-05 101.43 AA

(Stat Rx)
REPACK
TAB, PO, 50 mg,
30s ea, C-II ....16590-0640-30 32.25 AA
60s ea, C-II ....16590-0640-60 42.75 AA
90s ea, C-II ....16590-0640-90 53.50 AA
100s ea, C-II ....16590-0640-71 57.00 AA

MEPHOBARBITAL (Breckenridge Pharm)
TAB, PO (USP)
32 mg,
250s ea, C-IV 51991-0416-02 128.65
50 mg, 250s ea, C-IV .51991-0417-02 184.23
100 mg,
250s ea, C-IV 51991-0418-02 246.92

(Lundbeck) *See MEBARAL*

MEPHYTON (Aton)
phytonadione
TAB, PO, 5 mg, 100s ea ...25010-0405-15 506.63

(Dispensing Solutions)
REPACK
TAB, PO, 5 mg, 10s ea 55045-2840-00 22.00

(PD-Rx Pharm)
REPACK
TAB, PO, 5 mg, 2s ea......55289-0793-02 13.94
10s ea..............55289-0793-10 72.30
12s ea..............55289-0793-12 86.75

(Phys Total Care)
REPACK
TAB, PO, 5 mg, 5s ea......54868-5438-01 13.85
30s ea..............54868-5438-00 73.72

(Physician Partner)
REPACK
TAB, PO, 5 mg, 10s ea 21695-0168-10 48.53

(Quality Care Prod)
REPACK
TAB, PO, 5 mg, 2s ea......49999-0573-02 8.34

MEPIVACAINE HCL (Medisca)
mepivacaine hydrochloride
POW, NA (U.S.P.)
5 gm 38779-0557-03 61.50
25 gm...............38779-0557-04 214.50
100 gm..............38779-0557-05 399.00

(PCCA)
POW, NA (U.S.P.)
1 gm 51927-2283-00 12.60

(Spectrum Pharmacy)
POW, NA (U.S.P.)
5 gm 49452-0061-02 111.65
25 gm 49452-0061-03 364.00

MEPIVACAINE HYDROCHLORIDE
(APP) *See POLOCAINE*
(APP) *See POLOCAINE-MPF*
(Dentsply) *See POLOCAINE DENTAL*
(Hospira) *See CARBOCAINE*
(Hospira) *See CARBOCAINE HCL*
(Hospira)
SOL, IJ (50X1.8ML,DENTALCARPULE)
3%, 1.8 ml 50s.........00409-7551-01 22.80 20.00 AP

PROD/MFR NDC AWP DP OBC

(Medisca) *See MEPIVACAINE HCL*
(PCCA) *See MEPIVACAINE HCL*
(Spectrum Pharmacy) *See MEPIVACAINE HCL*

MEPROBAMATE (Dr Reddy's)
TAB, PO (USP)
200 mg,
100s ea, C-IV ......55111-0640-01 140.02 AA
400 mg,
100s ea, C-IV ......55111-0641-01 183.11 AA

(Heritage)
TAB, PO (USP,UNCOATED TABLET)
200 mg,
100s ea, C-IV ......23155-0128-01 140.02 AA
(USP,UNCOATED)
400 mg,
100s ea, C-IV ......23155-0129-01 183.11 AA

(Truxton) *See TRANCOT*

(Watson Labs)
TAB, PO, 200 mg,
100s ea, C-IV ......00591-5239-01 134.41 AA
400 mg,
100s ea, C-IV ......00591-5238-01 175.79 AA

(PD-Rx Pharm)
REPACK
TAB, PO, 400 mg,
30s ea, C-IV.........55289-0983-30 63.01 EE

MEPRON (Glaxo)
atovaquone
SUS, PO, 750 mg/5 ml,
5 ml 42s UD 00173-0547-00 1039.46
210 ml 00173-0665-18 1091.41

(Phys Total Care)
REPACK
SUS, PO, 750 mg/5 ml,
210 ml 54868-3705-00 817.86

MEPROZINE (Phys Total Care)
meperidine hcl/promethazine hcl
CAP, PO, 50 mg-25 mg,
90s ea, C-II 54868-5151-05 119.03

MEQUINOL (PCCA)
POW, NA, 1 gm..............51927-3544-00 1.44

MEQUINOL/TRETINOIN
(Stiefel Labs) *See SOLAGE*

MERBROMIN (Amend)
POW, NA (PURIFIED)
25 gm..............17317-0622-02 7.35
100 gm.............17317-0622-03 17.50
1000 gm............17317-0622-06 98.00

(Spectrum Pharmacy)
POW, NA, 25 gm..........49452-4460-01 85.05
100 gm.............49452-4460-02 176.40
(PURIFIED)
1000 gm............49452-4460-04 836.50

MERCAPTOACETIC ACID SODIUM SALT (PCCA)
sodium thioglycolate
POW, NA (1X1GM)
1 gm 51927-3405-00 7.20

MERCAPTOBENZOTHIAZOLE (PCCA)
POW, NA (-2,REAGENT)
1 gm 51927-2217-00 2.97

MERCAPTOETHANOL (PCCA)
2-mercaptoethanol
SOL, NA (2)
1 gm 51927-2619-00 0.66

MERCAPTOPURINE
(Gate) *See PURINETHOL*
(Medisca) *See MERCAPTOPURINE MONOHYDRATE*
(Mylan)
TAB, PO (U.S.P.)
50 mg, 25s ea........00378-3547-52 102.25 AB
250s ea...........00378-3547-25 1022.45 AB

(Par)
TAB, PO, 50 mg, 60s ea ...49884-0922-02 245.53
250s ea...........49884-0922-04 1022.48

(PCCA) *See MERCAPTOPURINE MONOHYDRATE*

(Roxane)
TAB, PO (USP)
50 mg, 25s ea........00054-4581-11 102.31
250s ea...........00054-4581-27 897.37

(Spectrum Pharmacy) *See MERCAPTOPURINE MONOHYDRATE*

(Teva)
TAB, PO (USP)
50 mg, 60s ea........00093-5510-06 245.53 AB

PROD/MFR NDC AWP DP OBC

(American Health)
REPACK
TAB, PO, 50 mg, 30s ea UD.68084-0325-21 62.50

(Phys Total Care)
REPACK
TAB, PO, 50 mg, 25s ea ...54868-5282-01 114.45
60s ea.............54868-5282-00 453.00

MERCAPTOPURINE MONOHYDRATE (Medisca)
mercaptopurine
POW, NA (U.S.P.)
1 gm 38779-1427-06 40.50
5 gm 38779-1427-03 166.50
25 gm 38779-1427-04 658.50

(PCCA)
POW, NA (U.S.P.)(6)
1 gm 51927-2000-00 42.00

(Spectrum Pharmacy)
POW, NA, 1 gm..........49452-4463-01 70.70
5 gm 49452-4463-02 246.40

MERCURIC ACETATE (Baker, J.T.)
POW, NA (A.C.S., REAGENT)
125 gm.............10106-2584-04 128.49
500 gm.............10106-2584-01 324.40

MERCURIC BROMIDE (Baker, J.T.)
POW, NA (A.C.S., REAGENT)
125 gm.............10106-2590-04 133.13
500 gm.............10106-2590-01 253.48

MERCURIC CHLORIDE
(Baker, J.T.) *See MERCURY BICHLORIDE*
(Baker, J.T.)
POW, NA (A.C.S., REAGENT)
125 gm.............10106-2594-04 127.00
500 gm.............10106-2594-01 272.02

(Medisca)
CRY, NA (REAGENT)
10 gm 38779-1428-01 22.50
25 gm 38779-1428-04 39.00
100 gm.............38779-1428-05 52.50
500 gm.............38779-1428-08 175.50

(Spectrum Pharmacy)
CRY, NA (A.C.S.,REAGENT)
125 gm.............49452-4465-02 143.85
500 gm.............49452-4465-03 472.50
2500 gm............49452-4465-04 2012.50

MERCURIC IODIDE
(Baker, J.T.) *See MERCURIC IODIDE RED*
(PCCA)
POW, NA (RED ACS)
1 gm 51927-2665-00 3.72

(Spectrum Pharmacy) *See MERCURIC IODIDE RED*

MERCURIC IODIDE RED (Baker, J.T.)
mercuric iodide
POW, NA (A.C.S., REAGENT)
125 gm.............10106-2608-04 81.47
500 gm.............10106-2608-01 305.60

(Spectrum Pharmacy)
POW, NA (A.C.S. REAGENT)
25 gm 49452-4490-01 169.05
(A.S.C.,REAGENT)
125 gm.............49452-4490-02 336.00
(A.C.S.,REAGENT)
500 gm.............49452-4490-03 955.50

MERCURIC NITRATE
(Baker, J.T.) *See MERCURIC NITRATE MONOHYDRATE*

MERCURIC NITRATE MONOHYDRATE (Baker, J.T.)
mercuric nitrate
POW, NA (A.C.S., REAGENT)
125 gm.............10106-2614-04 137.97
500 gm.............10106-2614-01 213.21

MERCURIC OXIDE
(Baker, J.T.) *See MERCURIC OXIDE RED*
(Baker, J.T.) *See MERCURIC OXIDE YELLOW*
(PCCA)
POW, NA (ACS)
1 gm 51927-3356-00 2.28

MERCURIC OXIDE RED (Baker, J.T.)
mercuric oxide
POW, NA (A.C.S., REAGENT)
125 gm.............10106-2620-04 139.77
500 gm.............10106-2620-01 294.37

MERCURIC OXIDE YELLOW (Baker, J.T.)
mercuric oxide
POW, NA (A.C.S., REAGENT)
125 gm.............10106-2630-04 133.02
500 gm.............10106-2630-01 306.68

PROD/MFR	NDC	AWP	DP	OBC
MERCURIC SULFATE (Baker, J.T.)				
POW, NA (A.C.S., REAGENT)				
125 gm	10106-2640-04	128.80		
500 gm	10106-2640-01	319.97		
MERCUROUS CHLORIDE				
(Amend) *See CALOMEL*				
(Baker, J.T.) *See CALOMEL MILD*				
(Baker, J.T.) *See MERCUROUS NITRATE DIHYDRATE*				
(Baker, J.T.)				
POW, NA (A.C.S., REAGENT)				
125 gm	10106-2654-04	115.82		
500 gm	10106-2654-01	256.52		
(Medisca) *See CALOMEL*				
(Spectrum Pharmacy)				
POW, NA (A.C.S.,REAGENT)				
25 gm	49452-4530-01	126.70		
125 gm	49452-4530-02	286.65		
500 gm	49452-4530-03	770.00		
MERCUROUS NITRATE DIHYDRATE (Baker, J.T.)				
mercurous chloride				
CRY, NA (A.C.S., REAGENT)				
125 gm	10106-2660-04	116.65		
500 gm	10106-2660-01	218.67		
MERCURY				
(Baker, J.T.) *See MERCURY TRIPLE DISTILLED*				
(Mallinckrodt Lab)				
LIQ, NA (TRIPLE DISTILLED)				
480 ml	00406-1278-03	184.85		
POW, NA (PURIFIED)				
120 gm	00406-1280-01	66.08		
454 gm	00406-1280-03	79.30		
(Medisca)				
ammoniated mercury				
POW, NA (1X25GM,USP,AMMONIATED)				
25 gm	38779-0591-04	27.00		
(1X100GM,USP,AMMONIATED)				
100 gm	38779-0591-05	64.50		
MERCURY (PCCA)				
POW, NA, 1 gm	51927-2348-00	1.06		
MERCURY AMMONIATED (Amend)				
ammoniated mercury				
POW, NA (U.S.P.)				
30 gm	17317-0024-02	8.05		
125 gm	17317-0024-04	25.20		
500 gm	17317-0024-01	84.00		
2500 gm	17317-0024-05	329.00		
(Baker, J.T.)				
POW, NA (PURIFIED)				
125 gm	10106-2563-04	38.57		
454 gm	10106-2563-01	143.32		
(Gallipot)				
POW, NA (1X25GM)				
25 gm	51552-0546-04	12.53	8.95	
(U.S.P.,N.F.)				
113.4 gm	51552-0546-09	30.10		
(1X454GM)				
454 gm	51552-0546-06	125.30	89.50	
(Spectrum Pharmacy)				
POW, NA (U.S.P.)				
125 gm	49452-0470-01	149.45		
500 gm	49452-0470-02	493.50		
MERCURY BICHLORIDE (Baker, J.T.)				
mercuric chloride				
GRA, NA (PURIFIED)				
500 gm	10106-2578-01	196.42		
MERCURY TRIPLE DISTILLED (Baker, J.T.)				
mercury				
POW, NA (INSTRA-ANALYZED)				
125 gm	10106-2567-01	154.50		
(PURIFIED)				
125 gm	10106-2569-04	64.89		
454 gm	10106-2569-01	183.75		
MERIDIA (Abbott Pharm)				
sibutramine hydrochloride				
CAP, PO, 5 mg,				
90s ea, C-IV	00074-2456-12	375.49	329.38	
100s ea, C-IV	00074-2456-13	417.23	365.99	
10 mg,				
90s ea, C-IV	00074-2457-12	375.49	329.38	
100s ea, C-IV	00074-2457-13	417.23	365.99	
15 mg,				
90s ea, C-IV	00074-2458-12	485.57	425.94	
100s ea, C-IV	00074-2458-13	539.51	473.25	

PROD/MFR	NDC	AWP	DP	OBC
(A-S Medication)				
REPACK				
CAP, PO, 15 mg,				
30s ea, C-IV	54569-4556-00	163.69		
(Bryant Ranch)				
REPACK				
CAP, PO, 10 mg,				
30s ea, C-IV	63629-2966-01	120.00		
15 mg,				
30s ea, C-IV	63629-1456-01	132.00		
(PD-Rx Pharm)				
REPACK				
CAP, PO, 5 mg,				
7s ea, C-IV	55289-0377-07	53.57		
14s ea, C-IV	55289-0377-14	102.03		
10 mg, 7s ea, C-IV	55289-0375-07	53.59		
14s ea, C-IV	55289-0375-14	102.07		
28s ea, C-IV	55289-0375-28	150.66		
15 mg, 7s ea, C-IV	55289-0380-07	67.74		
14s ea, C-IV	55289-0380-14	130.36		
(Pharma Pac)				
REPACK				
CAP, PO, 15 mg,				
30s ea, C-IV	52959-0106-30	158.40		
(Phys Total Care)				
REPACK				
CAP, PO, 10 mg,				
10s ea, C-IV	54868-4027-01	50.24		
30s ea, C-IV	54868-4027-00	139.53		
15 mg,				
10s ea, C-IV	54868-4896-01	58.80		
30s ea, C-IV	54868-4896-00	163.18		
(Quality Care Prod)				
REPACK				
CAP, PO, 5 mg,				
30s ea, C-IV	35356-0508-30	167.40		
10 mg,				
30s ea, C-IV	49999-0421-30	167.40		
90s ea, C-IV	49999-0421-90	502.20		
15 mg,				
30s ea, C-IV	35356-0509-30	289.37		
60s ea, C-IV	35356-0352-60	571.20		
MEROPENEM				
(AstraZeneca) *See MERREM IV*				
(AstraZeneca) *See NOVAPLUS MERREM*				
MERREM IV (AstraZeneca)				
meropenem				
PDS, IV (VIAL)				
1 gm, 10s ea	00310-0321-30	781.90		
500 mg, 10s ea	00310-0325-20	390.95		
MERUVAX II (Merck)				
rubella virus vaccine, live				
PDS, SC (SDV W/DILUENT,TAX INCL)				
1000 tcid50,				
10s ea	00006-4673-00	228.31		
MESALAMINE				
(Alaven) *See ROWASA*				
(Alaven) *See SFROWASA*				
(Axcan) *See CANASA*				
MESALAMINE (Hawkins)				
aminosalicylic acid				
POW, NA (U.S.P.)				
25 gm	63370-0150-25	40.00		
100 gm	63370-0150-35	94.00		
500 gm	63370-0150-45	368.00		
2500 gm	63370-0150-53	1360.00		
5000 gm	63370-0150-55	2560.00		
MESALAMINE				
(P & G Pharm) *See ASACOL*				
(P & G Pharm) *See ASACOL HD*				
(Perrigo)				
NMA, RC, 4 gm/60 ml,				
60 ml 7s	45802-0098-51	116.35		
(7X60ML,USP)				
4 gm/60 ml,				
60 ml 7s UD	45802-0923-41	171.05		
60 ml 28s	45802-0098-28	442.20		
(28X60ML,USP)				
4 gm/60 ml,				
60 ml 28s UD	45802-0923-49	669.38		
(Prasco Labs)				
NMA, RC (7X60ML,W/APPLICATOR)				
4 gm/60 ml,				
60 ml 7s UD	66993-0950-77	111.13		
(Salix Pharm) *See APRISO*				

PROD/MFR	NDC	AWP	DP	OBC
(Shire US Inc.) *See LIALDA*				
(Shire US Inc.) *See PENTASA*				
(Spectrum Pharmacy)				
POW, NA (U.S.P.)				
100 gm	49452-0450-01	127.05		
500 gm	49452-0450-02	437.50		
2500 gm	49452-0450-05	1543.50		
(Teva)				
NMA, RC, 4 gm/60 ml,				
60 ml 7s	00093-6888-71	105.90		AB
MESNA (APP)				
SOL, IV (M.D.V.)				
100 mg/ml, 10 ml	63323-0733-11	132.44		AP
(M.D.V.,10MLX10)				
100 mg/ml,				
10 ml 10s	63323-0733-10	1324.40		AP
(Baxter) *See MESNEX*				
(Baxter)				
SOL, IV, 100 mg/ml, 1 ml	10019-0953-62	42.00		
(S.D.V.)				
100 mg/ml, 10 ml	10019-0953-01	42.00		
10 ml 10s	10019-0953-02	420.00		
(Bedford) *See MESNA AMERINET CHOICE*				
(Bedford) *See MESNA NOVAPLUS*				
(Bedford)				
SOL, IV (M.D.V.)				
100 mg/ml, 10 ml	55390-0045-01	56.40		AP
(Teva)				
SOL, IV (M.D.V.)				
100 mg/ml,				
10 ml 10s	00703-4805-03	480.00		AP
MESNA AMERINET CHOICE (Bedford)				
mesna				
SOL, IV (M.D.V.,PRIVATE LABEL)				
100 mg/ml, 10 ml	55390-0266-01	177.60		
MESNA NOVAPLUS (Bedford)				
mesna				
SOL, IV (M.D.V.,PRIVATE LABEL)				
100 mg/ml, 10 ml	55390-0347-01	56.40		AP
MESNEX (Baxter)				
mesna				
SOL, IV (M.D.V,1X10ML)				
100 mg/ml, 10 ml	00338-1305-01	99.90		AP
(M.D.V,10X10ML)				
100 mg/ml,				
10 ml 10s	00338-1305-03	999.00		AP
TAB, PO (10X10,FILM-COATED)				
400 mg, 100s ea	67108-3565-09	890.40		
MESO-2,3-DIMERCAPTO-SUCCINIC ACID				
(Spectrum Pharmacy)				
succimer				
POW, NA, 5 gm	49452-2620-02	165.90		
25 gm	49452-2620-03	640.50		
100 gm	49452-2620-04	1711.50		
MESTINON (Valeant Pharm Intl)				
pyridostigmine bromide				
SYR, PO, 60 mg/5 ml,				
473 ml	00187-3012-20	146.95		
TAB, PO, 60 mg, 100s ea	00187-3010-30	203.54		
(Phys Total Care)				
REPACK				
TAB, PO, 60 mg, 100s ea	54868-3936-00	79.66		
MESTINON TIMESPAN (Valeant Pharm Intl)				
pyridostigmine bromide				
TER, PO, 180 mg, 30s ea	00187-3013-30	102.94		
MESTRANOL/NORETHINDRONE				
(Watson) *See NECON 1/50*				
(Watson) *See NORINYL 1/50*				
META CRESYL ACETATE				
(Recsei) *See CRESYLATE*				
METADATE CD (UCB)				
methylphenidate hydrochloride				
CER, PO, 10 mg,				
100s ea, C-II	53014-0579-07	420.37		
20 mg,				
100s ea, C-II	53014-0580-07	420.37		
30 mg,				
100s ea, C-II	53014-0581-07	420.37		
(USP)				
40 mg,				
100s ea, C-II	53014-0582-07	576.61		BX
50 mg,				
100s ea, C-II	53014-0583-07	708.48		EE
60 mg,				
100s ea, C-II	53014-0584-07	708.48		

PROD/MFR	NDC	AWP	DP	OBC
(Phys Total Care)				
REPACK				
CER, PO, 10 mg,				
10s ea, C-II	**54868-5397-01**	37.84		
30s ea, C-II	**54868-5397-00**	107.28		
20 mg,				
10s ea, C-II	**54868-4718-01**	46.52		
30s ea, C-II	**54868-4718-00**	126.09		
30 mg,				
10s ea, C-II	**54868-0668-01**	37.84		
30s ea, C-II	**54868-0668-00**	107.28		
METADATE ER (UCB)				
methylphenidate hydrochloride				
TER, PO, 20 mg,				
100s ea, C-II	**53014-0594-07**	132.10		AB
METAGLIP (Bristol-Myers)				
glipizide/metformin hydrochloride				
TAB, PO, 2.5 mg-500 mg,				
100s ea	**00087-6077-31**	132.10		
5 mg-500 mg,				
100s ea	**00087-6078-31**	132.10		
(Phys Total Care)				
REPACK				
TAB, PO, 2.5 mg-500 mg,				
10s ea	**54868-5399-01**	14.74		
30s ea	**54868-5399-00**	40.46		
5 mg-500 mg,				
10s ea	**54868-5288-01**	14.74		
30s ea	**54868-5288-00**	40.46		
60s ea	**54868-5288-02**	79.05		
METANX (Pamlab)				
l-methylfolate/methylcobalamin/pyridoxal phosphate				
TAB, PO (MEDICAL FOOD,SF)				
2.8 mg-2 mg-25 mg,				
90s ea	**00525-8019-90**	88.02		
(SF,GLUTEN-FREE)				
2.8 mg-2 mg-25 mg,				
500s ea	**00525-8019-50**	489.00		
(Phys Total Care)				
REPACK				
TAB, PO (MEDICAL FOOD)				
2.8 mg-2 mg-25 mg,				
30s ea	**54868-5556-00**	34.86		
(Quality Care Prod)				
REPACK				
TAB, PO (SF,GLUTEN-FREE)				
2.8 mg-2 mg-25 mg,				
60s ea	**35356-0379-60**	109.53		
90s ea	**35356-0379-90**	164.30		
METAPROTERENOL (Altura)				
REPACK				
metaproterenol sulfate				
SYR, PO, 10 mg/5 ml,				
120 ml	**63874-0701-12**	12.65		
473 ml	**63874-0701-48**	31.87		
(Bryant Ranch)				
REPACK				
SYR, PO, 10 mg/5 ml,				
120 ml	**63629-1866-01**	11.17		
240 ml	**63629-1866-02**	22.33		
METAPROTERENOL SULFATE (Apotex Corp.)				
SOL, IH (AMP)				
0.4%, 2.5 ml 25s	**60505-0807-01**	34.83		AN
0.6%, 2.5 ml 25s	**60505-0808-01**	34.83		AN
(Gallipot)				
POW, NA (U.S.P.,N.F.)				
25 gm	**51552-0079-04**	105.00		
100 gm	**51552-0079-02**	33.60		
100 gm	**51552-0079-05**	322.00		
1000 gm	**51552-0079-07**	2870.00		
(Hawkins)				
POW, NA (U.S.P.)				
10 gm	**63370-0153-20**	140.00		
25 gm	**63370-0153-25**	280.00		
100 gm	**63370-0153-35**	800.00		
500 gm	**63370-0153-45**	3800.00		
(Letco)				
POW, NA (U.S.P.)				
25 gm	**62991-1099-02**	210.00		
100 gm	**62991-1099-03**	585.00		
(Medisca)				
POW, NA (U.S.P.)				
10 gm	**38779-0171-01**	117.00		
25 gm	**38779-0171-04**	229.50		
100 gm	**38779-0171-05**	675.00		
500 gm	**38779-0171-08**	2550.00		
1000 gm	**38779-0171-09**	4335.00		
(Par)				
TAB, PO, 10 mg, 100s ea	**49884-0258-01**	99.95		AB
20 mg, 100s ea	**49884-0259-01**	139.28		AB
(PCCA)				
POW, NA (U.S.P.)				
1 gm	**51927-1370-00**	16.50		
(Qualitest)				
SYR, PO (CHERRY)				
10 mg/5 ml, 473 ml	**00603-1422-58**	31.87		AA
(Silarx)				
SYR, PO, 10 mg/5 ml,				
473 ml	**54838-0507-80**	31.90		AA
(Spectrum Pharmacy)				
POW, NA (U.S.P.)				
5 gm	**49452-4555-02**	132.30		
25 gm	**49452-4555-03**	388.50		
100 gm	**49452-4555-05**	1116.50		
(PD-Rx Pharm)				
REPACK				
TAB, PO, 10 mg, 8s ea	**55289-0544-08**	9.88		AB
60s ea	**55289-0544-60**	38.00		AB
(Pharma Pac)				
REPACK				
TAB, PO, 10 mg, 60s ea	**52959-0952-60**	59.45		AB
(Southwood)				
REPACK				
SYR, PO, 10 mg/5 ml,				
120 ml	**58016-4021-04**	14.80		EE
TAB, PO, 10 mg, 12s ea	**58016-0402-12**	4.10		EE
20s ea	**58016-0402-20**	6.84		EE
30s ea	**58016-0402-30**	10.26		EE
100s ea	**58016-0402-00**	34.20		EE
20 mg, 30s ea	**58016-0403-30**	15.31		EE
100s ea	**58016-0403-00**	48.59		EE
METASTRON (GE)				
strontium chloride sr 89				
SOL, IV, 1 mci/ml, 4 ml	**17156-0524-01**	4088.70		
METAXALONE				
(King Pharm) *See SKELAXIN*				
(Palmetto)				
REPACK				
TAB, PO, 800 mg, 15s ea	**23490-7641-01**	45.77		
METER, PEAK FLOW, SPIROMETRY				
(Monaghan Medical) *See TRUZONE PEAK FLOW METER*				
(Respironics) *See ASSESS PEAK FLOW METER ZONE SYSTEM*				
(Respironics) *See ASTHMA PACK II PEAK FLOW METER*				
(Respironics) *See ASTHMA PACK III PEAK FLOW METER*				
(Respironics) *See ASTHMA PACK PEAK FLOW METER*				
(Respironics) *See PERSONAL BEST PEAK FLOW METER*				
METFOMIN HYDROCHLORIDE (Bryant Ranch)				
REPACK				
metformin hydrochloride				
TAB, PO, 850 mg, 30s ea	**63629-1396-02**	36.00		
60s ea	**63629-1396-01**	72.00		
METFORMIN (Zydus Pharm.)				
metformin hydrochloride				
TAB, PO (FILM-COATED)				
500 mg, 100s ea	**68382-0028-01**	70.42		AB
500s ea	**68382-0028-05**	352.13		AB
1000s ea	**68382-0028-10**	703.78		AB
850 mg, 100s ea	**68382-0029-01**	119.69		AB
500s ea	**68382-0029-05**	598.43		AB
1000s ea	**68382-0029-10**	1196.90		AB
1000 mg, 100s ea	**68382-0030-01**	144.99		AB
500s ea	**68382-0030-05**	721.24		AB
1000s ea	**68382-0030-10**	1442.48		AB
(Aidarex)				
REPACK				
TAB, PO (FILM-COATED)				
500 mg, 30s ea	**33261-0157-30**	33.30		AB
60s ea	**33261-0157-60**	66.60		AB
90s ea	**33261-0157-90**	99.90		AB
120s ea	**33261-0157-02**	133.20		AB
(Bryant Ranch)				
REPACK				
TAB, PO, 500 mg, 30s ea	**63629-1395-01**	21.60		
60s ea	**63629-1395-02**	43.20		
100s ea	**63629-1395-03**	72.00		
(Core)				
REPACK				
TAB, PO, 500 mg, 30s ea	**33358-0234-30**	22.14		
60s ea	**33358-0234-60**	44.28		
100s ea	**33358-0234-00**	73.80		
850 mg, 30s ea	**33358-0236-30**	36.90		
60s ea	**33358-0236-60**	73.80		
1000 mg, 30s ea	**33358-0237-30**	51.35		
60s ea	**33358-0237-60**	102.71		
(DHS, Inc.)				
REPACK				
TAB, PO, 500 mg, 180s ea	**55887-0627-92**	131.22		
850 mg, 30s ea	**55887-0614-30**	37.50		
90s ea	**55887-0614-90**	99.00		
TER, PO, 750 mg, 60s ea	**55887-0940-60**	50.00		
(Dispensing Solutions)				
REPACK				
TAB, PO, 500 mg, 30s ea	**55045-2904-08**	21.60		
90s ea	**55045-2904-09**	64.80		
100s ea	**55045-2904-00**	72.00		
850 mg, 30s ea	**55045-2905-08**	36.00		
60s ea	**55045-2905-06**	72.00		
100s ea	**55045-2905-00**	120.00		
(HomeMed)				
REPACK				
TAB, PO, 500 mg, 30s ea	**51655-0245-24**	25.39		
METFORMIN (HomeMed)				
REPACK				
metformin hydrochloride				
TAB, PO, 500 mg, 60s ea	**51655-0245-25**	43.99		
1000 mg, 30s ea	**51655-0404-24**	49.99		
60s ea	**51655-0404-25**	86.99		
(Palmetto)				
REPACK				
TAB, PO, 1000 mg, 30s ea	**23490-0900-03**	44.77		
30s ea	**23490-7260-01**	49.99		
60s ea	**23490-0900-06**	89.54		
60s ea	**23490-7260-02**	99.98		
90s ea	**23490-7260-03**	149.97		
100s ea	**23490-7260-04**	166.63		
(PD-Rx Pharm)				
REPACK				
TAB, PO, 1000 mg, 60s ea	**55289-0919-60**	49.64		
(Stat Rx)				
REPACK				
TAB, PO, 1000 mg, 30s ea	**16590-0397-30**	27.00		
60s ea	**16590-0397-60**	45.00		
90s ea	**16590-0397-90**	55.00		
METFORMIN ER (Sandoz)				
metformin hydrochloride				
TER, PO, 500 mg, 100s ea	**00185-4416-01**	74.50		AB
500s ea	**00185-4416-05**	372.50		AB
(Teva)				
TER, PO, 500 mg, 100s ea	**00093-7267-01**	74.50		
100s ea	**00172-4435-60**	74.18		AB
(10X10)				
500 mg, 100s ea UD	**00172-4435-10**	76.18		AB
1000s ea	**00093-7267-10**	725.69		
(A-S Medication)				
REPACK				
TER, PO, 500 mg, 30s ea	**54569-5546-01**	22.37		
60s ea	**54569-5546-00**	44.75		
(DHS, Inc.)				
REPACK				
TER, PO, 500 mg, 30s ea	**55887-0414-30**	22.35		
60s ea	**55887-0414-60**	44.70		
90s ea	**55887-0414-90**	67.05		
(Palmetto)				
REPACK				
TER, PO, 500 mg, 60s ea	**23490-7458-06**	56.82		
(Phys Total Care)				
REPACK				
TER, PO, 500 mg, 30s ea	**54868-5217-01**	10.74		
60s ea	**54868-5217-00**	18.48		
100s ea	**54868-5217-02**	27.30		
(Quality Care Prod)				
REPACK				
TER, PO, 500 mg, 28s ea	**49999-0106-28**	29.60		
60s ea	**49999-0820-60**	34.24		
(Southwood)				
REPACK				
TER, PO, 500 mg, 30s ea	**58016-0883-30**	23.35		
60s ea	**58016-0883-60**	46.69		
90s ea	**58016-0883-90**	70.04		
100s ea	**58016-0883-00**	77.82		
METFORMIN HCL (Actavis)				
metformin hydrochloride				
TER, PO (FILM-COATED)				
750 mg, 100s ea	**00228-2728-11**	123.06		AB
(Apotex Corp.)				
TAB, PO, 500 mg, 100s ea	**60505-0190-00**	70.43		AB

PROD/MFR	NDC	AWP	DP	OBC
500s ea	**60505-0190-01**	352.14		AB
4500s ea	**60505-0190-04**	3169.26		AB
850 mg, 100s ea	**60505-0191-00**	119.73		AB
500s ea	**60505-0191-01**	598.60		AB
2500s ea	**60505-0191-04**	2993.00		AB
1000 mg, 100s ea	**60505-0192-00**	144.90		AB
500s ea	**60505-0192-01**	724.50		AB
2000s ea	**60505-0192-04**	2898.00		AB
TER, PO, 500 mg, 100s ea	**60505-0260-01**	74.50		AB
500s ea	**60505-0260-02**	372.50		AB
2500s ea	**60505-0260-07**	1862.50		AB
(Aurobindo Pharma)				
TAB, PO (FILM-COATED)				
500 mg, 100s ea	**65862-0008-01**	71.00		AB
500s ea	**65862-0008-05**	344.00		AB
850 mg, 100s ea	**65862-0009-01**	120.00		AB
500s ea	**65862-0009-05**	582.00		AB
1000 mg, 100s ea	**65862-0010-01**	145.00		AB
500s ea	**65862-0010-05**	703.00		AB
(Caraco)				
TAB, PO (FILM-COATED)				
500 mg, 100s ea	**57664-0397-51**	70.40		AB
100s ea	**57664-0397-88**	70.40		AB
500s ea	**57664-0397-13**	351.90		AB
500s ea	**57664-0397-53**	351.90		AB
1000s ea	**57664-0397-18**	703.78		AB
1000s ea	**57664-0397-58**	703.78		AB
850 mg, 100s ea	**57664-0435-51**	119.70		AB
100s ea	**57664-0435-88**	119.70		AB
500s ea	**57664-0435-13**	598.48		AB
500s ea	**57664-0435-53**	598.48		AB
1000s ea	**57664-0435-18**	1196.90		AB
1000s ea	**57664-0435-58**	1196.90		AB
1000 mg, 100s ea	**57664-0474-51**	144.01		AB
100s ea	**57664-0474-88**	144.01		AB
500s ea	**57664-0474-13**	720.05		AB
500s ea	**57664-0474-53**	720.05		AB
1000s ea	**57664-0474-18**	1440.00		AB
1000s ea	**57664-0474-58**	1440.00		AB
(Major)				
TAB, PO (FILM COATED)				
850 mg, 100s ea UD	**00904-5602-61**	132.29		
(FILM-COATED)				
1000 mg,				
100s ea UD	**00904-5603-61**	160.30		AB
(Medisca)				
POW, NA (B.P.)				
25 gm	**38779-2126-04**	52.50		
(U.S.P.)				
100 gm	**38779-2126-05**	157.50		
500 gm	**38779-2126-08**	673.50		
(Mutual)				
TAB, PO, 500 mg, 100s ea	**53489-0467-01**	70.43		AB
500s ea	**53489-0467-05**	352.13		AB
1000s ea	**53489-0467-10**	700.00		AB
850 mg, 100s ea	**53489-0468-01**	119.69		AB
500s ea	**53489-0468-05**	590.43		AB
1000s ea	**53489-0468-10**	1190.48		AB
(FILM-COATED)				
1000 mg, 100s ea	**53489-0469-01**	144.99		AB
500s ea	**53489-0469-05**	721.24		AB
1000s ea	**53489-0469-10**	1442.00		AB
(Mylan)				
TAB, PO, 500 mg, 100s ea	**00378-0234-01**	70.35		AB
500s ea	**00378-0234-05**	351.75		AB
850 mg, 100s ea	**00378-0240-01**	119.65		AB
1000 mg, 100s ea	**00378-0244-01**	145.00		AB
TER, PO, 500 mg, 100s ea	**00378-0352-01**	74.50		AB
500s ea	**00378-0352-05**	372.50		AB
750 mg, 100s ea	**00378-0350-01**	119.70		AB
(PCCA)				
POW, NA, 1 gm	**51927-3105-00**	2.40		
(Ranbaxy Pharm)				
TER, PO (CAPLET)				
500 mg, 100s ea	**63304-0860-01**	74.58		
500s ea	**63304-0860-05**	372.90		
750 mg, 100s ea	**63304-0767-01**	119.70		AB
(Sandoz)				
TAB, PO, 500 mg, 100s ea	**00185-0213-01**	70.43		AB
100s ea	**00781-5050-01**	70.36		AB
500s ea	**00185-0213-05**	352.17		AB
500s ea	**00781-5050-05**	351.80		AB
1000s ea	**00781-5050-10**	668.38		AB
850 mg, 100s ea	**00185-0215-01**	119.74		AB
100s ea	**00781-5051-01**	119.60		AB
500s ea	**00185-0215-05**	586.73		AB
500s ea	**00781-5051-05**	580.07		AB
1000 mg, 100s ea	**00185-0221-01**	145.10		AB
100s ea	**00781-5052-01**	144.94		AB
500s ea	**00185-0221-05**	710.99		AB
500s ea	**00781-5052-05**	702.94		AB
(Spectrum Pharmacy)				
POW, NA (B.P.)				
25 gm	**49452-4545-01**	95.20		
100 gm	**49452-4545-02**	247.10		
500 gm	**49452-4545-03**	969.50		
(Teva)				
TAB, PO (10X10,USP,FILM-COATED)				
500 mg, 100s ea UD	**00093-1048-93**	72.00		AB
(FILM-COATED)				
500 mg, 100s ea	**00093-1048-01**	70.43		AB
1000s ea	**00093-1048-10**	704.30		AB
850 mg, 100s ea	**00093-1049-01**	119.73		AB
1000s ea	**00093-1049-10**	1197.30		AB
1000 mg, 100s ea	**00093-7214-01**	145.06		AB
1000s ea	**00093-7214-10**	1450.60		AB
TER, PO, 750 mg, 100s ea	**00093-7212-01**	119.70		AB
(UDL)				
TAB, PO (USP,25X1,ROBOT READY)				
500 mg, 25s ea UD	**51079-0972-19**	17.59		AB
(10X10)				
500 mg, 100s ea UD	**51079-0972-20**	70.35		AB
850 mg, 100s ea UD	**51079-0973-20**	119.65		AB
1000 mg,				
100s ea UD	**51079-0995-20**	144.40		AB
(Watson)				
TER, PO, 500 mg, 100s ea	**62037-0571-01**	10.45		BX
1000s ea	**62037-0571-10**	99.30		BX
750 mg, 100s ea	**62037-0577-01**	26.94		AB
1000s ea	**62037-0577-10**	255.94		AB
(Wockhardt USA)				
TAB, PO (U.S.P.,FILM-COATED)				
500 mg, 100s ea	**64679-0528-04**	71.00		AB
500s ea	**64679-0528-05**	344.00		AB
850 mg, 100s ea	**64679-0529-04**	120.00		AB
500s ea	**64679-0529-05**	582.00		AB
1000 mg, 100s ea	**64679-0530-04**	145.00		AB
500s ea	**64679-0530-05**	703.00		AB
(A-S Medication)				
REPACK				
TAB, PO (FILM-COATED)				
500 mg, 60s ea	**54569-5360-00**	42.51		AB
100s ea	**54569-5360-03**	70.85		AB
850 mg, 30s ea	**54569-5353-03**	35.91		AB
60s ea	**54569-5353-00**	71.81		EE
100s ea	**54569-5353-02**	119.69		EE
1000 mg, 60s ea	**54569-5373-00**	86.99		EE
(Aidarex)				
REPACK				
TAB, PO (FILM-COATED)				
1000 mg, 30s ea	**33261-0145-30**	69.00		AB
60s ea	**33261-0145-60**	138.00		AB
90s ea	**33261-0145-90**	207.00		AB
120s ea	**33261-0145-02**	276.00		AB
(Altura)				
REPACK				
TAB, PO (FILM-COATED)				
500 mg, 10s ea	**63874-0501-10**	8.53		AB
14s ea	**63874-0501-14**	11.94		AB
20s ea	**63874-0501-20**	17.05		AB
24s ea	**63874-0501-24**	20.46		AB
28s ea	**63874-0501-28**	23.87		AB
30s ea	**63874-0501-30**	25.58		AB
60s ea	**63874-0501-60**	51.16		AB
90s ea	**63874-0501-90**	76.73		AB
100s ea	**63874-0501-01**	85.26		AB
120s ea	**63874-0501-04**	102.31		AB
850 mg, 10s ea	**63874-0635-10**	11.96		AB
20s ea	**63874-0635-20**	23.92		AB
28s ea	**63874-0635-28**	33.49		AB
30s ea	**63874-0635-30**	35.89		AB
60s ea	**63874-0635-60**	71.77		AB
90s ea	**63874-0635-90**	107.65		AB
100s ea	**63874-0635-01**	119.62		AB
1000 mg, 30s ea	**63874-0974-30**	43.30		AB
60s ea	**63874-0974-60**	86.59		AB
(FILM-COATED)				
1000 mg, 100s ea	**63874-0974-01**	144.33		AB
(American Health)				
REPACK				
TAB, PO (10X10)				
500 mg, 100s ea UD	**62584-0259-01**	70.12		AB
(15X30)				
500 mg, 450s ea	**62584-0259-85**	316.92		AB
(10X10,FILM-COATED)				
1000 mg,				
100s ea UD	**62584-0452-01**	152.35		AB
(15X30,FILM-COATED)				
1000 mg, 450s ea	**62584-0452-85**	649.12		AB
(DHS, Inc.)				
REPACK				
TAB, PO, 500 mg, 30s ea	**55887-0627-30**	21.88		AB
60s ea	**55887-0627-60**	43.75		AB
90s ea	**55887-0627-90**	65.61		AB
120s ea	**55887-0627-82**	87.48		AB
1000 mg, 30s ea	**55887-0571-30**	42.50		AB
60s ea	**55887-0571-60**	84.06		AB
90s ea	**55887-0571-90**	119.29		AB
120s ea	**55887-0571-82**	159.09		AB
TER, PO, 750 mg, 30s ea	**55887-0940-30**	30.00		AB
90s ea	**55887-0940-90**	75.00		AB
(Dispensing Solutions)				
REPACK				
TAB, PO, 500 mg, 14s ea	**66336-0884-14**	11.89		AB
28s ea	**66336-0884-28**	23.18		AB
30s ea	**55045-3761-08**	21.60		
60s ea	**55045-2904-06**	43.20		
60s ea	**66336-0884-60**	48.99		AB
90s ea	**66336-0884-90**	65.61		AB
120s ea	**55045-2904-02**	86.40		
(FILM-COATED)				
500 mg, 180s ea	**66336-0884-62**	131.22		AB
850 mg, 30s ea	**66336-0883-30**	43.27		AB
60s ea	**66336-0883-60**	85.94		AB
1000 mg, 30s ea	**55045-2906-08**	43.50		AB
(FILM-COATED)				
1000 mg, 30s ea	**66336-0358-30**	43.28		AB
60s ea	**55045-2906-06**	87.00		AB
(FILM-COATED)				
1000 mg, 60s ea	**66336-0358-60**	86.55		AB
90s ea	**55045-2906-09**	130.50		AB
90s ea	**66336-0358-90**	129.83		AB
100s ea	**55045-2906-00**	145.00		AB
120s ea	**55045-2906-02**	174.00		AB
180s ea	**55045-2906-01**	261.00		AB
TER, PO, 500 mg, 60s ea	**66336-0270-60**	49.02		BX
90s ea	**66336-0270-90**	73.52		BX
(GSMS)				
REPACK				
TAB, PO, 500 mg, 120s ea	**60429-0723-12**	60.00	20.00	AB
180s ea	**60429-0723-18**	90.03	30.01	AB
(UNIT OF USE)				
1000 mg, 180s ea	**60429-0722-18**	122.28	40.76	EE
TER, PO (UNIT-OF-USE)				
500 mg, 60s ea	**60429-0725-60**	13.14	4.38	BX
90s ea	**60429-0725-90**	21.45	6.60	BX
180s ea	**60429-0725-18**	39.60	13.20	BX
500s ea	**60429-0725-05**	67.20	22.40	BX
(Nucare Pharm)				
REPACK				
TAB, PO (FILM-COATED)				
500 mg, 60s ea	**66267-0493-60**	51.28		AB
(PD-Rx Pharm)				
REPACK				
TAB, PO, 500 mg, 14s ea	**55289-0615-14**	14.13		AB
(REDI-SCRIPT)				
500 mg, 28s ea	**58864-0015-28**	22.00		AB
30s ea	**55289-0615-30**	22.67		AB
(REDI-SCRIPT,FILM-COATED)				
500 mg, 30s ea	**58864-0015-30**	22.68		AB
(REDI-SCRIPT)				
500 mg, 60s ea	**58864-0015-60**	38.66		AB
(USP)				
500 mg, 60s ea	**55289-0615-60**	38.67		AB
90s ea	**55289-0615-90**	57.98		AB
(REDI-SCRIPT,FILM-COATED)				
500 mg, 90s ea	**58864-0015-90**	54.67		AB
(FILM-COATED)				
500 mg, 100s ea	**43063-0012-01**	74.58		AB
120s ea	**55289-0615-98**	77.32		AB
180s ea	**55289-0615-93**	99.98		AB
(FILM-COATED)				
500 mg, 270s ea	**55289-0615-94**	133.96		AB
360s ea	**55289-0615-86**	157.96		AB
850 mg, 30s ea	**58864-0789-30**	14.80		AB
(USP,FILM-COATED)				
850 mg, 30s ea	**55289-0934-30**	24.98		AB
(FILM-COATED)				
850 mg, 60s ea	**55289-0934-60**	44.78		AB
120s ea	**55289-0934-98**	89.96		AB
180s ea	**55289-0934-93**	131.98		AB
270s ea	**55289-0934-94**	169.96		AB
1000 mg, 30s ea	**55289-0919-30**	26.82		AB
(REDI-SCRIPT,FILM-COATED)				
1000 mg, 30s ea	**58864-0693-30**	16.76		AB

PROD/MFR	NDC	AWP	DP	OBC
60s ea	58864-0693-60	17.58		AB
90s ea	55289-0919-90	73.64		AB
120s ea	55289-0919-98	95.78		AB
(FILM-COATED)				
1000 mg, 180s ea	55289-0919-93	141.98		AB
270s ea	55289-0919-94	189.98		AB
TER, PO (CAPLET)				
500 mg, 60s ea	55289-0384-60	49.98		
90s ea	55289-0384-90	65.98		
270s ea	55289-0384-94	193.96		
360s ea	55289-0384-86	247.98		
(Pharma Pac)				
REPACK				
TAB, PO, 500 mg, 30s ea	52959-0207-30	24.45		AB
60s ea	52959-0207-60	48.89		AB
100s ea	52959-0207-00	81.44		AB
1000 mg, 120s ea	52959-0860-02	179.70		AB
(Phys Total Care)				
REPACK				
TAB, PO, 500 mg, 15s ea	54868-4564-03	5.55		AB
30s ea	54868-4564-02	8.10		AB
60s ea	54868-4564-01	13.20		AB
90s ea	54868-4564-04	18.00		AB
100s ea	54868-4564-00	18.48		AB
850 mg, 30s ea	54868-4561-01	11.16		AB
60s ea	54868-4561-02	19.35		AB
90s ea	54868-4561-03	25.44		AB
100s ea	54868-4561-00	30.24		AB
1000 mg, 30s ea	54868-4566-00	11.52		EE
60s ea	54868-4566-01	20.04		EE
90s ea	54868-4566-03	28.56		EE
100s ea	54868-4566-02	29.88		AB
180s ea	54868-4566-04	51.77		EE
TER, PO, 500 mg, 90s ea	54868-5217-05	25.73		BX
(CAPLET)				
500 mg, 120s ea	54868-5217-04	32.03		
180s ea	54868-5217-03	45.05		
750 mg, 10s ea	54868-5505-01	10.59		
30s ea	54868-5505-00	22.77		
90s ea	54868-5505-02	51.07		
(Physician Partner)				
REPACK				
TAB, PO (FILM-COATED)				
850 mg, 30s ea	21695-0472-30	71.82		AB
60s ea	21695-0472-60	143.63		AB
1000 mg, 30s ea	21695-0473-30	86.40		AB
(FILM COATED)				
1000 mg, 60s ea	21695-0473-60	172.80		AB
90s ea	21695-0473-90	259.20		AB
(Quality Care Prod)				
REPACK				
TAB, PO, 500 mg, 30s ea	49999-0106-30	30.55		
60s ea	49999-0106-60	59.68		AB
90s ea	49999-0106-90	91.65		
100s ea	49999-0106-00	82.90		AB
120s ea	49999-0106-01	119.36		
850 mg, 30s ea	49999-0495-30	42.86		
60s ea	49999-0495-60	85.72		AB
1000 mg, 30s ea	49999-0116-30	42.69		AB
60s ea	49999-0116-60	85.38		AB
100s ea	49999-0116-00	170.76		AB
(Southwood)				
REPACK				
TAB, PO, 500 mg, 30s ea	58016-0772-30	17.54		AB
60s ea	58016-0772-60	35.08		AB
90s ea	58016-0772-90	52.61		AB
100s ea	58016-0772-00	58.46		AB
850 mg, 30s ea	58016-0536-30	29.81		AB
60s ea	58016-0536-60	59.61		AB
90s ea	58016-0536-90	89.42		AB
100s ea	58016-0536-00	99.35		AB
(FILM-COATED)				
1000 mg, 30s ea	58016-0466-30	36.10		AB
60s ea	58016-0466-60	72.20		AB
90s ea	58016-0466-90	108.31		AB
100s ea	58016-0466-00	120.34		AB
(Vibranta)				
REPACK				
TAB, PO, 500 mg, 30s ea	57866-9056-01	47.25		
60s ea	57866-9056-02	44.00		
90s ea	57866-9056-03	64.88		
120s ea	57866-9056-04	86.00		
180s ea	57866-9056-05	59.00		
850 mg, 30s ea	57866-9055-01	33.20		
60s ea	57866-9055-02	64.90		
90s ea	57866-9055-03	96.60		
120s ea	57866-9055-04	128.30		
1000 mg, 30s ea	57866-9054-01	39.91		AB
60s ea	57866-9054-02	78.33		AB
90s ea	57866-9054-03	116.75		AB
120s ea	57866-9054-04	155.16		AB
METFORMIN HYDROCHLORIDE				
HCFA				
TAB, PO, 500 mg, 100s ea		7.50		
850 mg, 100s ea		14.64		
1000 mg, 100s ea		16.58		
TER, PO, 500 mg, 100s ea		13.07		
750 mg, 100s ea		33.68		
(Actavis) *See METFORMIN HCL*				
(Amneal)				
TAB, PO (USP,FILM-COATED)				
500 mg, 100s ea	65162-0175-10	70.43		AB
500s ea	65162-0175-50	352.00		AB
850 mg, 100s ea	65162-0174-10	119.70		AB
500s ea	65162-0174-50	598.50		AB
1000 mg, 100s ea	65162-0177-10	144.95		AB
500s ea	65162-0177-50	721.00		AB
TER, PO, 500 mg, 90s ea	53746-0178-90	67.05		AB
100s ea	53746-0178-01	74.50		AB
500s ea	53746-0178-05	372.90		AB
750 mg, 100s ea	53746-0179-01	119.70		AB
500s ea	53746-0179-05	538.65		AB
(Apotex Corp.) *See METFORMIN HCL*				
(Apotex Corp.)				
TAB, PO (FILM-COATED)				
500 mg, 1000s ea	60505-0190-08	704.28		AB
850 mg, 1000s ea	60505-0191-08	1197.20		
(FILM COATED)				
1000 mg, 1000s ea	60505-0192-08	1449.00		
TER, PO, 750 mg, 100s ea	60505-1329-01	123.06		
(Aurobindo Pharma) *See METFORMIN HCL*				
(Bristol-Myers) *See GLUCOPHAGE*				
(Bristol-Myers) *See GLUCOPHAGE XR*				
(Caraco) *See METFORMIN HCL*				
(Caraco)				
TER, PO, 500 mg, 100s ea	62756-0142-01	74.50		AB
500s ea	62756-0142-02	372.50		AB
750 mg, 100s ea	62756-0143-01	119.70		AB
(Depomed) *See GLUMETZA*				
(Glenmark Pharmaceuticals)				
TAB, PO (USP,FILM COATED)				
500 mg, 100s ea	68462-0159-01	70.43		AB
500s ea	68462-0159-05	352.14		AB
850 mg, 100s ea	68462-0160-01	119.74		AB
1000 mg, 100s ea	68462-0161-01	145.10		AB
(Greenstone)				
TAB, PO (FILM COATED)				
500 mg, 60s ea	59762-4320-06	42.60		
100s ea	59762-4320-00	71.00		
500s ea	59762-4320-02	344.00		
850 mg, 60s ea	59762-4321-06	72.00		
100s ea	59762-4321-00	120.00		
500s ea	59762-4321-02	582.00		
1000 mg, 60s ea	59762-4322-06	87.00		
100s ea	59762-4322-00	145.00		
500s ea	59762-4322-02	703.00		
(Major) *See METFORMIN HCL*				
(Major)				
TAB, PO (FILM-COATED)				
500 mg, 60s ea	00904-5849-52	40.53		AB
90s ea	00904-5849-89	62.69		AB
(10X10,USP,FILM-COATED)				
500 mg, 100s ea UD	00904-6090-61	77.82		AB
(FILM-COATED)				
500 mg, 100s ea	00904-5634-61	77.82		
120s ea	00904-5849-18	81.05		AB
180s ea	00904-5849-93	121.58		AB
270s ea	00904-5849-53	182.36		AB
360s ea	00904-5849-14	243.15		AB
450s ea	00904-5849-54	303.94		AB
500s ea	00904-5849-40	334.53		AB
1000s ea	00904-5849-80	665.00		AB
850 mg, 90s ea	00904-5850-89	84.95		AB
100s ea	00904-5635-61	146.73		
180s ea	00904-5850-93	199.79		AB
270s ea	00904-5850-53	299.68		AB
500s ea	00904-5850-40	568.67		AB
1000 mg, 60s ea	00904-5851-52	97.95		AB
90s ea	00904-5851-89	123.83		AB
(FILM COATED)				
1000 mg,				
100s ea UD	00904-5636-61	160.30		
(FILM-COATED)				
1000 mg, 180s ea	00904-5851-93	246.58		AB
500s ea	00904-5851-40	712.85		AB
TER, PO (10X10)				
750 mg, 100s ea UD	00904-5795-61	116.91		AB
(Medisca) *See METFORMIN HCL*				
(Mutual) *See METFORMIN HCL*				
(Mylan) *See METFORMIN HCL*				
(PCCA) *See METFORMIN HCL*				
(Provident)				
TAB, PO (FILM-COATED)				
500 mg, 100s ea	20091-0531-01	76.45		AB
500s ea	20091-0531-05	348.09		AB
1000s ea	20091-0531-10	686.34		AB
850 mg, 100s ea	20091-0533-01	119.53		AB
500s ea	20091-0533-05	589.34		AB
1000s ea	20091-0533-10	1193.89		AB
1000 mg, 100s ea	20091-0535-01	145.55		AB
500s ea	20091-0535-05	714.12		AB
1000s ea	20091-0535-10	1445.30		AB
(Ranbaxy Labs) *See RIOMET*				
(Ranbaxy Pharm) *See METFORMIN HCL*				
(Sandoz) *See METFORMIN ER*				
(Sandoz) *See METFORMIN HCL*				
(Sandoz)				
TAB, PO (12X60,USP,FILM-COATED)				
500 mg, 720s ea	00781-5050-61	506.64		AB
850 mg, 720s ea	00781-5051-61	861.12		AB
1000 mg, 720s ea	00781-5052-61	1043.52		AB
(Shionogi) *See FORTAMET*				
(Solco)				
TAB, PO (USP,FILM-COATED)				
500 mg, 100s ea	43547-0248-10	70.46		AB
500s ea	43547-0248-50	352.30		AB
850 mg, 100s ea	43547-0249-10	119.50		AB
500s ea	43547-0249-50	597.50		AB
1000 mg, 100s ea	43547-0250-10	144.87		AB
500s ea	43547-0250-50	724.35		AB
(Spectrum Pharmacy) *See METFORMIN HCL*				
(Teva) *See METFORMIN ER*				
(Teva) *See METFORMIN HCL*				
(Teva)				
TAB, PO (10X10,FILM-COATED)				
850 mg, 100s ea UD	00172-4330-10	121.05		AB
(FILM-COATED)				
1000 mg,				
100s ea UD	00172-4432-10	146.25		AB
(UDL) *See METFORMIN HCL*				
(UDL) *See METFORMIN HYDROCHLORIDE*				
METFORMIN HYDROCHLORIDE (UDL)				
metformin hydrochloride				
TAB, PO (USP,PUNCH CARDS,10X30)				
500 mg, 300s ea UD	51079-0972-56	211.05		AB
METFORMIN HYDROCHLORIDE				
(Watson) *See METFORMIN HCL*				
(Watson)				
TAB, PO (FILM-COATED)				
500 mg, 100s ea	62037-0674-01	7.51		AB
1000s ea	62037-0674-10	67.31		AB
850 mg, 100s ea	62037-0675-01	11.71		AB
1000s ea	62037-0675-10	110.08		AB
1000 mg, 100s ea	62037-0676-01	13.26		AB
1000s ea	62037-0676-10	119.15		AB
(Wockhardt USA) *See METFORMIN HCL*				
(Zydus Pharm.) *See METFORMIN*				
(A-S Medication)				
REPACK				
TAB, PO (FILM-COATED)				
1000 mg, 100s ea	54569-5373-02	144.99		AB
(Advanced Pharm Serv, Inc.)				
REPACK				
TAB, PO, 500 mg, 20s ea	13411-0163-02	18.40		
30s ea	13411-0163-03	27.60		
60s ea	13411-0163-06	55.20		
90s ea	13411-0163-09	82.80		
100s ea	13411-0163-10	80.99		
850 mg, 20s ea	13411-0164-02	26.60		
30s ea	13411-0164-03	39.90		
60s ea	13411-0164-06	79.80		
90s ea	13411-0164-09	119.70		
100s ea	13411-0164-10	137.69		
(American Health)				
REPACK				
TAB, PO (USP,10X10)				
850 mg, 100s ea UD	62584-0332-01	120.35		

PROD/MFR	NDC	AWP	DP	OBC
(Bryant Ranch)				
REPACK				
TAB, PO, 1000 mg, 30s ea	**63629-1397-03**	50.10		
60s ea	**63629-1397-01**	100.20		
100s ea	**63629-1397-02**	167.00		
(Dispensing Solutions)				
REPACK				
TAB, PO, 500 mg, 30s ea	**66336-0270-30**	24.51		
30s ea	**66336-0884-30**	24.83		
(HomeMed)				
REPACK				
TAB, PO, 850 mg, 30s ea	**51655-0291-24**	33.89		
(McKesson Packaging)				
REPACK				
TAB, PO, 500 mg,				
100s ea UD	**63739-0299-10**	15.63		
850 mg, 100s ea UD	**63739-0300-10**	21.88		
1000 mg, 100s ea UD	**63739-0301-10**	25.00		
(Nucare Pharm)				
REPACK				
TAB, PO (FILM-COATED)				
500 mg, 14s ea	**66267-0493-14**	12.66		**AB**
30s ea	**66267-0493-30**	25.64		**AB**
90s ea	**66267-0493-90**	77.95		**AB**
120s ea	**66267-0493-91**	103.55		**AB**
180s ea	**66267-0493-92**	134.84		**AB**
270s ea	**66267-0493-93**	193.96		**AB**
(Palmetto)				
REPACK				
TAB, PO, 500 mg, 14s ea	**23490-6838-01**	11.85		
28s ea	**23490-6838-02**	23.70		
30s ea	**23490-6838-04**	25.39		
60s ea	**23490-6838-03**	50.78		
850 mg, 30s ea	**23490-6839-01**	38.92		
60s ea	**23490-6839-02**	77.84		
(PD-Rx Pharm)				
REPACK				
TER, PO, 500 mg, 30s ea	**55289-0384-30**	29.98		**AB**
180s ea	**55289-0384-93**	127.98		
(Pharma Pac)				
REPACK				
TAB, PO, 500 mg, 28s ea	**52959-0207-28**	22.68		
850 mg, 60s ea	**52959-0896-60**	66.16		
100s ea	**52959-0896-01**	110.20		
1000 mg, 30s ea	**52959-0860-30**	44.88		
60s ea	**52959-0860-60**	89.70		
90s ea	**52959-0860-90**	134.10		
(Physician Partner)				
REPACK				
TAB, PO (FILM-COATED)				
500 mg, 30s ea	**21695-0471-30**	42.26		**AB**
90s ea	**21695-0471-90**	126.78		**AB**
100s ea	**21695-0471-00**	140.80		**AB**
180s ea	**21695-0471-78**	298.16		**AB**

METFORMIN HYDROCHLORIDE/PIOGLITAZONE HYDROCHLORIDE
(Takeda) *See ACTOPLUS MET*

METFORMIN HYDROCHLORIDE/REPAGLINIDE
(Novo Nordisk) *See PRANDIMET*

METFORMIN HYDROCHLORIDE/ ROSIGLITAZONE MALEATE
(Glaxo) *See AVANDAMET*

METFORMIN HYDROCHLORIDE/ SITAGLIPTIN PHOSPHATE
(Merck) *See JANUMET*

PROD/MFR	NDC	AWP	DP	OBC
METFORMIN XR (Bryant Ranch)				
REPACK				
metformin hydrochloride				
TER, PO, 500 mg, 60s ea	**63629-2883-01**	44.40		
(Core)				
REPACK				
TER, PO, 500 mg, 60s ea	**33358-0235-60**	45.51		
METHACHOLINE CHLORIDE (Gallipot)				
CRY, NA, 0.1 gm	**51552-0301-09**	12.60		
(U.S.P.)				
1 gm	**51552-0234-01**	29.40		
POW, NA, 1 gm	**51552-0301-01**	25.90		
5 gm	**51552-0301-02**	59.22		
25 gm	**51552-0301-04**	238.00		
(Medisca)				
POW, NA, 5 gm	**38779-1430-03**	405.00		
25 gm	**38779-1430-04**	1725.00		

(Methapharm) *See PROVOCHOLINE*

PROD/MFR	NDC	AWP	DP	OBC
(PCCA)				
POW, NA (USP)				
1 gm	**51927-3086-00**	45.00		
(Spectrum Pharmacy)				
CRY, NA, 25 gm	**49452-4550-03**	1165.50		
POW, NA, 1 gm	**49452-4550-01**	147.35		
5 gm	**49452-4550-02**	336.35		

METHACRYLIC ACID COPOLYMER A
(PCCA) *See EUDAGRIT L-100*

PROD/MFR	NDC	AWP	DP	OBC
METHADEX (Major)				
dexamethasone/neomycin sulfate/polymyxin b sulfate				
SUS, OP, 5 ml	**00904-3003-05**	19.86		
METHADONE (DHS, Inc.)				
REPACK				
methadone hydrochloride				
TAB, PO, 5 mg,				
90s ea, C-II	**55887-0090-90**	14.85		
120s ea, C-II	**55887-0090-82**	19.80		
10 mg,				
42s ea, C-II	**55887-0200-42**	18.35		
56s ea, C-II	**55887-0200-56**	24.47		
90s ea, C-II	**55887-0200-90**	21.00		
120s ea, C-II	**55887-0200-82**	28.00		
40 mg,				
60s ea, C-II	**55887-0134-60**	64.50		
90s ea, C-II	**55887-0134-90**	96.75		
(Dispensing Solutions)				
REPACK				
TAB, PO, 5 mg,				
90s ea, C-II	**66336-0170-90**	14.85		
120s ea, C-II	**66336-0170-94**	18.14		
180s ea, C-II	**66336-0170-62**	22.41		
10 mg,				
60s ea, C-II	**66336-0171-60**	26.22		
(Phys Total Care)				
REPACK				
TAB, PO (USP)				
5 mg, 60s ea, C-II	**54868-5701-00**	20.34		
90s ea, C-II	**54868-5701-01**	26.76		
120s ea, C-II	**54868-5701-02**	33.21		
10 mg,				
30s ea, C-II	**54868-4948-05**	15.42		
90s ea, C-II	**54868-4948-06**	34.26		
300s ea, C-II	**54868-4948-04**	82.77		
(Quality Care Prod)				
REPACK				
TAB, PO, 5 mg,				
30s ea, C-II	**49999-0963-30**	13.50		
60s ea, C-II	**49999-0963-60**	27.00		
90s ea, C-II	**49999-0963-90**	40.50		
10 mg,				
30s ea, C-II	**49999-0839-30**	70.50		
60s ea, C-II	**49999-0839-60**	141.00		
90s ea, C-II	**49999-0839-90**	211.50		
METHADONE HCL (Cebert Pharm)				
methadone hydrochloride				
POW, NA, 50 gm, C-II	**64019-0750-85**	295.31		
100 gm, C-II	**64019-0750-88**	695.63		
(Covidien)				
POW, NA, 50 gm, C-II	**00406-1510-56**	532.00		
100 gm, C-II	**00406-1510-57**	1064.00		
500 gm, C-II	**00406-1510-59**	5320.00		
(Gallipot)				
POW, NA (U.S.P.)				
1 gm, C-II	**51552-0728-01**	42.70	30.50	
5 gm, C-II	**51552-0728-02**	154.00	110.00	
25 gm, C-II	**51552-0728-04**	623.00	445.00	
(Hawkins)				
POW, NA (U.S.P.)				
5 gm, C-II	**63370-0939-15**	556.80		
25 gm, C-II	**63370-0939-25**	2299.20		
100 gm, C-II	**63370-0939-35**	8232.00		
(Medisca)				
POW, NA (USP, 1X1GM)				
1 gm, C-II	**38779-0104-06**	18.00		
(U.S.P.)				
5 gm, C-II	**38779-0104-03**	367.50		
25 gm, C-II	**38779-0104-04**	1285.50		
100 gm, C-II	**38779-0104-05**	4269.00		
(PCCA)				
POW, NA (U.S.P.; CII)				
1 gm, C-II	**51927-1017-00**	90.00		
(Roxane)				
SOL, PO (LEMON)				
5 mg/5 ml,				
500 ml, C-II	**00054-3555-63**	39.88		

PROD/MFR	NDC	AWP	DP	OBC
10 mg/5 ml,				
500 ml, C-II	**00054-3556-63**	69.07		
(CHERRY)				
10 mg/ml,				
946 ml, C-II	**00054-3554-67**	79.88		**AA**
TAB, PO, 5 mg,				
100s ea, C-II	**00054-4570-25**	8.87		**AA**
(R.N.P., 4X25)				
5 mg,				
100s ea UD, C-II	**00054-8553-24**	38.45		**AA**
10 mg,				
100s ea, C-II	**00054-4571-25**	14.74		**AA**
(R.N.P., 4X25)				
10 mg,				
100s ea UD, C-II	**00054-8554-24**	43.74		**AA**
(Spectrum Pharmacy)				
POW, NA (U.S.P.)				
5 gm, C-II	**49452-4553-01**	521.50		
25 gm, C-II	**49452-4553-02**	1921.50		
100 gm, C-II	**49452-4553-03**	6555.50		
(VistaPharm, Inc.)				
POW, NA, 100 gm, C-II	**66689-0681-55**	600.00		
TBS, PO, 40 mg,				
100s ea, C-II	**66689-0898-40**	29.76		**AA**
(B&B Pharm, Inc)				
REPACK				
POW, NA (U.S.P.)				
25 gm, C-II	**63275-9100-04**	2250.00		
100 gm, C-II	**63275-9100-05**	9000.00		
(Bryant Ranch)				
REPACK				
TAB, PO, 5 mg,				
90s ea, C-II	**63629-3788-01**	8.23		**AA**
10 mg,				
30s ea, C-II	**63629-3771-02**	4.89		**AA**
90s ea, C-II	**63629-3771-03**	14.55		**AA**
120s ea, C-II	**63629-3771-04**	18.33		**AA**
150s ea, C-II	**63629-3771-01**	24.31		**AA**
180s ea, C-II	**63629-3771-05**	27.29		**AA**
(Dispensing Solutions)				
REPACK				
TAB, PO, 5 mg,				
60s ea, C-II	**66336-0170-60**	14.06		**AA**
(PD-Rx Pharm)				
REPACK				
TAB, PO, 10 mg,				
90s ea, C-II	**55289-0814-90**	28.00		**AA**
120s ea, C-II	**55289-0814-98**	33.34		**AA**
(Phys Total Care)				
REPACK				
TAB, PO, 5 mg,				
30s ea, C-II	**54868-5701-03**	15.42		**AA**
10 mg,				
50s ea, C-II	**54868-4948-03**	22.74		**AA**
60s ea, C-II	**54868-4948-00**	26.07		**AA**
100s ea, C-II	**54868-4948-01**	39.45		**AA**
120s ea, C-II	**54868-4948-02**	43.65		**AA**
150s ea, C-II	**54868-4948-07**	52.96		**AA**
(Quality Care Prod)				
REPACK				
TAB, PO, 10 mg,				
120s ea, C-II	**49999-0839-01**	282.00		**AA**
(Stat Rx)				
REPACK				
TAB, PO, 10 mg,				
7s ea, C-II	**16590-0670-07**	3.38		**AA**
30s ea, C-II	**16590-0670-30**	14.49		**AA**
60s ea, C-II	**16590-0670-60**	28.97		**AA**
90s ea, C-II	**16590-0670-90**	28.75		**AA**
120s ea, C-II	**16590-0670-72**	57.94		**AA**
180s ea, C-II	**16590-0670-82**	579.43		**AA**
240s ea, C-II	**16590-0670-84**	76.67		**AA**
270s ea, C-II	**16590-0670-86**	87.48		**AA**
TBS, PO, 40 mg,				
60s ea, C-II	**16590-0836-60**	25.64		**AA**
METHADONE HCL CONCENTRATE (VistaPharm, Inc.)				
methadone hydrochloride				
SOL, PO (1X1000ML,CHERRY,U.S.P.)				
10 mg/ml,				
1000 ml, C-II	**66689-0694-79**	81.20		
METHADONE HCL INTENSOL (Roxane)				
methadone hydrochloride				
SOL, PO, 10 mg/ml,				
30 ml, C-II	**00054-3553-44**	25.35		**AA**
METHADONE HYDROCHLORIDE (Bioniche Pharma)				
SOL, IJ (USP,MDV)				
10 mg/ml,				
20 ml, C-II	**66479-0530-02**	135.00		

PROD/MFR	NDC	AWP	DP	OBC
(Cebert Pharm) *See METHADONE HCL*				
(Covidien) *See METHADONE HCL*				
(Covidien) *See METHADOSE*				
(Covidien)				
TAB, PO (USP,10X10)				
5 mg,				
100s ea UD, C-II	**00406-5755-62**	38.40		AA
(USP)				
5 mg,				
100s ea, C-II	**00406-5755-01**	8.68		AA
10 mg, 100s ea, C-II	**00406-5771-01**	14.10		AA
(10X10,USP)				
10 mg,				
100s ea UD, C-II	**00406-5771-62**	43.70		AA
TBS, PO (USP,ORANGE,DISPERSIBLE)				
40 mg,				
100s ea, C-II	**00406-2540-01**	33.16		AA
(Gallipot) *See METHADONE HCL*				
(Hawkins) *See METHADONE HCL*				
(Medisca) *See METHADONE HCL*				
(PCCA) *See METHADONE HCL*				
(Roxane) *See DISKETS DISPERSIBLE*				
(Roxane) *See DOLOPHINE HCL*				
(Roxane) *See METHADONE HCL*				
(Roxane) *See METHADONE HCL INTENSOL*				
(Roxane)				
SOL, PO (SF,DYE-FREE,UNFLAVORED)				
10 mg/ml,				
946 ml, C-II	**00054-3553-67**	79.88		AA
(Spectrum Pharmacy) *See METHADONE HCL*				
(VistaPharm, Inc.) *See METHADONE HCL*				
(VistaPharm, Inc.) *See METHADONE HCL CONCENTRATE*				
(4u)				
REPACK				
TAB, PO, 5 mg,				
28s ea, C-II	**10544-0377-28**	29.92		AA
28s ea, C-II	**42549-0577-28**	29.92		AA
112s ea, C-II	**10544-0377-02**	72.88		AA
112s ea, C-II	**42549-0577-02**	72.88		AA
10 mg, 28s ea, C-II	**10544-0378-28**	59.48		AA
28s ea, C-II	**42549-0578-28**	59.48		AA
30s ea, C-II	**10544-0378-30**	61.18		AA
30s ea, C-II	**42549-0578-30**	61.18		AA
56s ea, C-II	**10544-0378-56**	108.98		AA
56s ea, C-II	**42549-0578-56**	108.98		AA
60s ea, C-II	**10544-0378-60**	114.62		AA
60s ea, C-II	**42549-0578-60**	114.62		AA
112s ea, C-II	**10544-0378-02**	164.36		AA
112s ea, C-II	**42549-0578-02**	164.36		AA
168s ea, C-II	**10544-0378-08**	198.52		AA
168s ea, C-II	**42549-0578-08**	198.52		AA
(Altura)				
REPACK				
TAB, PO, 10 mg,				
30s ea, C-II	**63874-1265-03**	71.13		AA
60s ea, C-II	**63874-1265-06**	142.26		AA
(DHS, Inc.)				
REPACK				
TAB, PO, 10 mg,				
60s ea, C-II	**55887-0200-60**	60.35		AA
(Dispensing Solutions)				
REPACK				
TAB, PO, 5 mg,				
30s ea, C-II	**66336-0170-30**	10.55		AA
10 mg, 30s ea, C-II	**66336-0171-30**	13.11		AA
42s ea, C-II	**66336-0171-42**	18.35		AA
56s ea, C-II	**66336-0171-56**	24.47		AA
(Palmetto)				
REPACK				
TAB, PO, 5 mg,				
30s ea, C-II	**23490-5878-03**	15.00		
60s ea, C-II	**23490-5878-01**	17.93		
90s ea, C-II	**23490-5878-09**	45.00		
100s ea, C-II	**23490-5878-02**	29.38		
10 mg, 30s ea, C-II	**23490-5877-03**	30.00		
60s ea, C-II	**23490-5877-06**	60.00		
90s ea, C-II	**23490-5877-09**	90.00		
100s ea, C-II	**23490-5877-07**	100.00		
40 mg, 30s ea, C-II	**23490-7798-03**	37.50		
100s ea, C-II	**23490-7798-01**	125.00		
METHADOSE (Covidien)				
methadone hydrochloride				
SOL, PO (CHERRY)				
10 mg/ml,				
1000 ml, C-II	**00406-0527-10**	104.59		AA
(SF,DYE-FREE)				
10 mg/ml,				
1000 ml, C-II	**00406-8725-10**	104.59		AA
TAB, PO (DISPERSABLE)				
40 mg,				
100s ea, C-II	**00406-0540-34**	33.00		AA
(Phys Total Care)				
REPACK				
TAB, PO, 5 mg,				
20s ea, C-II	**54868-4408-01**	4.91		AA
60s ea, C-II	**54868-4408-00**	8.48		AA
10 mg,				
30s ea, C-II	**54868-2854-01**	6.69		AA
60s ea, C-II	**54868-2854-02**	10.86		AA
100s ea, C-II	**54868-2854-00**	16.44		AA
(USP)				
10 mg,				
300s ea, C-II	**54868-2854-03**	44.33		
(Quality Care Prod)				
REPACK				
TAB, PO, 10 mg,				
30s ea, C-II	**49999-0840-30**	20.98		
60s ea, C-II	**49999-0840-60**	41.96		
40 mg,				
30s ea, C-II	**49999-0841-30**	36.65		
60s ea, C-II	**49999-0841-60**	73.30		
METHAMPHETAMINE HYDROCHLORIDE				
(Lundbeck) *See DESOXYN*				
METHANESULFONIC ACID (Gallipot)				
LIQ, NA, 25 ml	**51552-0284-04**	13.86		
(Medisca)				
SOL, NA (1X25ML,99%)				
25 gm	**38779-1431-04**	76.50		
(1X100ML,99%)				
100 gm	**38779-1431-05**	229.50		
(PCCA)				
LIQ, NA (99+%)				
1 gm	**51927-2563-00**	3.24		
METHANOL (Baker, J.T.)				
methyl alcohol				
LIQ, NA (A.C.S., REAGENT)				
500 ml	**10106-9070-01**	14.37		
(A.C.S., REAGENT, GLASS)				
4000 ml	**10106-9070-03**	60.36		
(A.C.S., REAGENT, POLY)				
4000 ml	**10106-9070-05**	60.36		
(Medisca)				
SOL, NA (1X500ML,NF)				
500 ml	**38779-2127-08**	29.25		
(1X4000ML,NF)				
4000 ml	**38779-2127-01**	81.00		
(1X20000ML,NF)				
20000 ml	**38779-2127-07**	261.00		
(PCCA)				
LIQ, NA (ACS)				
1 ml	**51927-2778-00**	0.17		
METHANOL ANHYDROUS (Baker, J.T.)				
methyl alcohol				
LIQ, NA (A.C.S., REAGENT)				
1000 ml	**10106-9049-02**	43.36		
(A.C.S., REAGENT, GLASS)				
4000 ml	**10106-9049-03**	77.40		
METHAZOLAMIDE				
FUL				
TAB, PO, 25 mg, 100s ea		31.50		
50 mg, 100s ea		46.50		
(PCCA)				
POW, NA (U.S.P.)				
1 gm	**51927-1900-00**	26.40		
(Sandoz)				
TAB, PO, 25 mg, 100s ea	**00781-1072-01**	53.20		AB
50 mg, 100s ea	**00781-1071-01**	78.90		AB
(Teva)				
TAB, PO, 25 mg, 100s ea	**00093-9411-01**	48.00		AB
50 mg, 100s ea	**00093-9424-01**	72.00		AB
(Phys Total Care)				
REPACK				
TAB, PO, 50 mg, 100s ea	**54868-2996-00**	61.11		
METHENAMINE (Amend)				
GRA, NA (U.S.P.)				
500 gm	**17317-0360-01**	11.20		
2500 gm	**17317-0360-05**	37.80		
12000 gm	**17317-0360-08**	163.80		
(Gallipot)				
POW, NA, 500 gm	**51552-0824-06**	24.99	17.85	
(Mallinckrodt Lab)				
GRA, NA (U.S.P.)				
500 gm	**00406-5180-12**	31.57		
(PCCA)				
POW, NA (USP)				
1 gm	**51927-1113-00**	0.36		
(Spectrum Pharmacy)				
POW, NA (U.S.P.)				
500 gm	**49452-4558-01**	190.05		
METHENAMINE HIPPURATE (CorePharma)				
TAB, PO (USP)				
1 gm, 100s ea	**64720-0139-10**	200.84		
(Rising)				
TAB, PO (K29/32)				
1 gm, 100s ea	**64980-0119-01**	178.82		
(Sanofi-Aventis) *See HIPREX*				
METHENAMINE MANDELATE				
FUL				
TAB, PO, 1 gm, 100s ea		29.23		
(Consolidated Midland)				
TAB, PO, 0.5 gm, 100s ea	**00223-1043-01**	5.25		
1000s ea	**00223-1043-02**	39.50		
1 gm, 100s ea	**00223-1044-01**	6.95		
1000s ea	**00223-1044-02**	49.50		
(Edenbridge)				
TAB, PO (USP,FILM COATED)				
0.5 gm, 100s ea	**42799-0105-01**	88.63		
1 gm, 100s ea	**42799-0106-01**	166.59		
(PCCA)				
POW, NA, 1 gm	**51927-1972-00**	0.60		
(Seton)				
TAB, PO (USP,FILM COATED)				
1 gm, 100s ea	**13925-0107-01**	165.00		
METHENAMINE MANDELATE/SODIUM PHOSPHATE, MONOBASIC				
(Beach Pharm) *See UROQID-ACID NO. 2*				
(Breckenridge Pharm) *See UTAC*				
METHERGINE (Novartis Pharm)				
methylergonovine maleate				
SOL, IJ (AMP)				
0.2 mg/ml,				
1 ml 20s	**00078-0053-03**	156.35		
TAB, PO, 0.2 mg, 100s ea	**00078-0054-05**	141.71		
(A-S Medication)				
REPACK				
TAB, PO, 0.2 mg, 6s ea	**54569-0973-01**	8.06		
12s ea	**54569-0973-03**	16.12		
100s ea	**54569-0973-08**	167.62		
(Core)				
REPACK				
TAB, PO, 0.2 mg, 100s ea	**33358-0238-00**	107.09		
(DHS, Inc.)				
REPACK				
TAB, PO, 0.2 mg, 6s ea	**55887-0790-06**	14.98		
(Dispensing Solutions)				
REPACK				
TAB, PO, 0.2 mg, 3s ea	**55045-1707-03**	6.00		
6s ea	**55045-1707-02**	12.00		
6s ea	**66336-0402-06**	12.30		
8s ea	**55045-1707-08**	16.00		
9s ea	**55045-1707-09**	18.00		
12s ea	**55045-1707-04**	24.00		
15s ea	**55045-1707-05**	30.00		
18s ea	**55045-1707-07**	36.00		
(PD-Rx Pharm)				
REPACK				
TAB, PO, 0.2 mg, 3s ea	**55289-0708-03**	13.58		
4s ea	**55289-0708-04**	15.59		
6s ea	**55289-0708-06**	19.62		
(USP)				
0.2 mg, 6s ea	**43063-0147-06**	16.77		
8s ea	**55289-0708-08**	23.67		
9s ea	**55289-0708-09**	25.70		

PROD/MFR	NDC	AWP	DP	OBC
10s ea	55289-0708-10	27.72		
12s ea	55289-0708-12	31.77		
18s ea	55289-0708-18	43.89		
20s ea	55289-0708-20	47.93		
28s ea	55289-0708-28	64.10		
(Phys Total Care)				
REPACK				
TAB, PO, 0.2 mg, 10s ea	54868-4880-00	11.43		
METHIMAZOLE				
FUL				
TAB, PO, 5 mg, 100s ea		42.12		
15 mg, 100s ea		71.76		
(Caraco)				
TAB, PO (USP)				
5 mg, 100s ea	57664-0458-88	44.40		AB
1000s ea	57664-0458-18	444.00		AB
10 mg, 100s ea	57664-0459-88	76.75		AB
1000s ea	57664-0459-18	767.50		AB
(Centrix) *See NORTHYX*				
(Gallipot)				
POW, NA (USP,1X5GM)				
5 gm	51552-0822-02	28.35	20.25	
(USP,1X25GM)				
25 gm	51552-0822-04	86.66	61.90	
(Hawkins)				
POW, NA (U.S.P.)				
5 gm	63370-0151-15	50.40		
25 gm	63370-0151-25	158.40		
100 gm	63370-0151-35	576.00		
(King Pharm) *See TAPAZOLE*				
(Letco)				
POW, NA (U.S.P.)				
5 gm	62991-1515-01	34.50		
25 gm	62991-1515-02	90.00		
100 gm	62991-1515-03	315.00		
(Medisca)				
POW, NA (U.S.P.)				
5 gm	38779-0360-03	46.50		
25 gm	38779-0360-04	168.00		
100 gm	38779-0360-05	435.00		
(USP, 1X500GM)				
500 gm	38779-0360-08	1500.00		
(USP, 1X1000GM)				
1000 gm	38779-0360-09	2700.00		
(Par)				
TAB, PO, 5 mg, 100s ea	49884-0640-01	44.44		AB
10 mg, 100s ea	49884-0641-01	76.78		AB
(PCCA)				
POW, NA (U.S.P.)				
1 gm	51927-1943-00	13.20		
(Sandoz)				
TAB, PO, 5 mg, 100s ea	00185-0205-01	44.44		AB
1000s ea	00185-0205-10	435.55		AB
10 mg, 100s ea	00185-0210-01	76.78		AB
1000s ea	00185-0210-10	752.44		AB
(Spectrum Pharmacy)				
CRY, NA (U.S.P.)				
5 gm	49452-4573-01	93.10		
25 gm	49452-4573-02	278.95		
(U.S.P./N.F.)				
100 gm	49452-4573-03	756.00		
(United Research)				
TAB, PO, 5 mg, 100s ea	00677-1945-01	44.25		AB
10 mg, 100s ea	00677-1946-01	76.25		AB
(American Health)				
REPACK				
TAB, PO (10X10)				
5 mg, 100s ea UD	68084-0275-01	44.40		AB
10 mg, 100s ea UD	68084-0276-01	76.75		AB
(Dispensing Solutions)				
REPACK				
TAB, PO, 5 mg, 30s ea	55045-3455-08	15.30		
(Phys Total Care)				
REPACK				
TAB, PO, 5 mg, 30s ea	54868-6071-00	23.70		AB
10 mg, 100s ea	54868-5135-00	121.32		AB
METHIONINE				
(Amend) *See DL-METHIONINE*				
(Gallipot) *See L-METHIONINE*				
(Medisca)				
CRY, NA (1X25GM,L-METHIONINE)				
25 gm	38779-1805-04	37.50		
(1X100GM,L-METHIONINE)				
100 gm	38779-1805-05	93.00		
(USP,L-METHIONINE)				
500 gm	38779-1805-08	285.00		
(PCCA)				
POW, NA (DL,FCC)				
1 gm	51927-1121-00	0.36		
(USP, L)				
1 gm	51927-3524-00	1.05		
(Spectrum Pharmacy) *See DL-METHIONINE*				
(Spectrum Pharmacy) *See L-METHIONINE*				
METHITEST (Global Pharm)				
methyltestosterone				
TAB, PO, 10 mg,				
100s ea, C-III	00115-7037-01	484.34		BP
METHOCARBAMOL				
FUL				
TAB, PO, 500 mg, 100s ea		19.43		
750 mg, 100s ea		25.20		
(Baxter) *See ROBAXIN*				
(Consolidated Midland)				
SOL, IJ (VIAL)				
100 mg/ml, 10 ml	00223-8150-10	4.00		EE
TAB, PO, 500 mg, 100s ea	00223-1277-01	8.50		EE
500s ea	00223-1277-05	34.50		EE
1000s ea	00223-1277-02	59.00		EE
750 mg, 100s ea	00223-1278-01	11.95		EE
500s ea	00223-1278-05	49.50		EE
1000s ea	00223-1278-02	87.50		EE
(Gallipot)				
POW, NA (USP,1X100GM)				
100 gm	51552-1018-05	35.70	25.50	
(Hawkins)				
POW, NA (U.S.P.)				
100 gm	63370-0143-35	100.00		
500 gm	63370-0143-45	372.00		
1000 gm	63370-0143-50	640.00		
(Lannett)				
TAB, PO, 500 mg, 100s ea	00527-1302-01	37.65		AA
500s ea	00527-1302-05	170.59		AA
750 mg, 100s ea	00527-1152-01	49.41		AA
500s ea	00527-1152-05	235.29		AA
(Medisca)				
POW, NA (U.S.P.)				
100 gm	38779-1943-05	93.00		
500 gm	38779-1943-08	337.50		
1000 gm	38779-1943-09	585.00		
(PCCA)				
POW, NA (U.S.P.)				
1 gm	51927-2519-00	0.99		
(Qualitest)				
TAB, PO, 500 mg, 100s ea	00603-4485-21	37.64		AA
500s ea	00603-4485-28	170.55		AA
750 mg, 100s ea	00603-4486-21	49.40		AA
500s ea	00603-4486-28	235.25		AA
(Sandoz)				
TAB, PO, 500 mg, 100s ea	00781-1760-01	50.80		AA
750 mg, 100s ea	00781-1750-01	72.61		AA
(UCB) *See ROBAXIN*				
(UCB) *See ROBAXIN-750*				
(Watson Labs)				
TAB, PO, 500 mg, 100s ea	00591-5381-01	9.30		AA
500s ea	00591-5381-05	44.17		AA
750 mg, 100s ea	00591-5382-01	9.60		AA
500s ea	00591-5382-05	45.60		AA
(West-Ward)				
TAB, PO, 500 mg, 100s ea	00143-1290-01	36.85		AA
500s ea	00143-1290-05	168.75		AA
750 mg, 100s ea	00143-1292-01	46.80		AA
500s ea	00143-1292-05	233.75		AA
(4u)				
REPACK				
TAB, PO, 750 mg, 30s ea	10544-0321-30	42.46		AA
30s ea	42549-0521-30	42.46		AA
40s ea	10544-0321-40	42.46		
40s ea	42549-0321-40	42.46		AA
40s ea	42549-0521-40	52.34		AA
60s ea	10544-0321-60	68.82		AA
60s ea	42549-0521-60	68.82		AA
90s ea	42549-0521-90	94.50		AA
120s ea	42549-0521-12	116.38		AA
180s ea	10544-0321-81	156.74		AA
180s ea	42549-0521-81	156.74		AA
(A-S Medication)				
REPACK				
TAB, PO, 500 mg, 7s ea	54569-4614-02	2.81		AA
10s ea	54569-4614-00	4.01		EE
14s ea	54569-0852-05	5.62		EE
20s ea	54569-0852-01	8.02		EE
30s ea	54569-0852-04	12.04		EE
40s ea	54569-0852-00	16.05		EE
60s ea	54569-0852-03	24.07		EE
750 mg, 7s ea	54569-4048-04	3.75		AA
12s ea	54569-0843-07	6.42		EE
20s ea	54569-0843-00	10.71		EE
28s ea	54569-0843-02	14.99		EE
30s ea	54569-0843-03	16.06		EE
40s ea	54569-0843-01	21.41		EE
60s ea	54569-0843-04	32.12		EE
90s ea	54569-5966-00	48.18		EE
100s ea	54569-0843-06	53.53		EE
(Aidarex)				
REPACK				
TAB, PO, 750 mg, 100s ea	33261-0072-00	126.00		AA
(Altura)				
REPACK				
TAB, PO, 500 mg, 12s ea	63874-0371-12	7.32		AA
14s ea	63874-0371-14	8.54		AA
15s ea	63874-0371-15	9.15		AA
20s ea	63874-0371-20	12.20		AA
24s ea	63874-0371-24	14.64		AA
30s ea	63874-0371-30	18.30		AA
40s ea	63874-0371-40	24.40		AA
50s ea	63874-0371-50	42.05		AA
60s ea	63874-0371-60	50.46		AA
84s ea	63874-0371-84	51.24		AA
100s ea	63874-0371-01	61.00		AA
120s ea	63874-0371-04	73.20		AA
168s ea	63874-0371-73	102.48		AA
500s ea	63874-0371-03	420.50		AA
750 mg, 8s ea	63874-0372-08	7.14		AA
10s ea	63874-0372-10	8.93		AA
12s ea	63874-0372-12	10.71		AA
14s ea	63874-0372-14	12.50		AA
15s ea	63874-0372-15	13.39		AA
20s ea	63874-0372-20	17.85		AA
21s ea	63874-0372-21	18.74		AA
24s ea	63874-0372-24	21.42		AA
28s ea	63874-0372-28	24.99		AA
30s ea	63874-0372-30	26.78		AA
40s ea	63874-0372-40	35.70		AA
42s ea	63874-0372-42	37.49		AA
50s ea	63874-0372-50	44.63		AA
56s ea	63874-0372-56	49.98		AA
60s ea	63874-0372-60	53.55		AA
90s ea	63874-0372-90	80.33		AA
100s ea	63874-0372-01	89.25		AA
120s ea	63874-0372-04	107.10		AA
500s ea	63874-0372-03	450.25		AA
(Bryant Ranch)				
REPACK				
TAB, PO, 500 mg, 14s ea	63629-1622-01	11.61		
20s ea	63629-1622-03	17.45		
30s ea	63629-1622-02	25.17		
40s ea	63629-1622-06	33.56		AA
60s ea	63629-1622-04	46.99		
90s ea	63629-1622-07	75.71		AA
750 mg, 20s ea	63629-1623-01	24.09		
30s ea	63629-1623-02	34.64		
40s ea	63629-1623-03	46.18		
50s ea	63629-1623-07	59.65		
60s ea	63629-1623-05	63.99		
90s ea	63629-1623-06	105.40		
120s ea	63629-1623-04	106.99		
(Core)				
REPACK				
TAB, PO, 500 mg, 14s ea	33358-0239-14	11.90		
20s ea	33358-0239-20	17.89		
30s ea	33358-0239-30	25.81		
60s ea	33358-0239-60	48.16		
90s ea	33358-0239-90	64.46		
750 mg, 20s ea	33358-0240-20	24.69		
30s ea	33358-0240-30	35.51		
40s ea	33358-0240-40	47.33		
60s ea	33358-0240-60	65.59		
90s ea	33358-0240-90	97.36		
120s ea	33358-0240-01	109.66		

PROD/MFR	NDC	AWP	DP	OBC
(DHS, Inc.)				
REPACK				
TAB, PO, 500 mg, 20s ea	**55887-0907-20**	16.33		AA
28s ea	**55887-0907-28**	22.86		
30s ea	**55887-0907-30**	24.49		AA
60s ea	**55887-0907-60**	47.00		AA
120s ea	**55887-0907-82**	97.95		
750 mg, 20s ea	**55887-0860-20**	24.00		AA
30s ea	**55887-0860-30**	36.95		AA
40s ea	**55887-0860-40**	45.00		AA
50s ea	**55887-0860-50**	57.00		AA
60s ea	**55887-0860-60**	68.90		AA
90s ea	**55887-0860-90**	82.80		AA
(Dispensing Solutions)				
REPACK				
TAB, PO, 500 mg, 20s ea	**55045-1531-09**	16.80		AA
20s ea	**66336-0080-20**	19.08		AA
24s ea	**55045-1531-06**	20.16		
30s ea	**55045-1531-08**	25.20		AA
30s ea	**66336-0080-30**	28.33		AA
40s ea	**55045-1531-03**	33.60		AA
40s ea	**66336-0080-40**	37.57		AA
60s ea	**55045-1531-02**	50.40		AA
84s ea	**55045-3718-04**	70.56		
90s ea	**55045-1531-04**	75.60		AA
100s ea	**55045-1531-01**	84.00		AA
120s ea	**55045-1531-00**	100.80		
750 mg, 12s ea	**55045-1386-02**	11.88		AA
20s ea	**55045-1386-07**	19.80		AA
20s ea	**66336-0063-20**	19.80		AA
28s ea	**55045-1386-06**	27.72		
28s ea	**66336-0063-28**	27.72		AA
30s ea	**55045-1386-08**	29.70		AA
30s ea	**66336-0063-30**	29.70		AA
40s ea	**55045-1386-09**	39.60		AA
40s ea	**55045-3930-01**	39.60		AA
40s ea	**66336-0063-40**	39.60		AA
45s ea	**55045-1386-03**	44.55		
50s ea	**55045-1386-05**	49.50		
60s ea	**55045-1386-04**	59.40		AA
60s ea	**66336-0063-60**	59.40		AA
80s ea	**55045-3229-08**	79.20		
90s ea	**55045-1386-00**	89.10		AA
90s ea	**66336-0063-90**	89.10		AA
100s ea	**55045-1386-01**	99.00		AA
120s ea	**55045-3229-01**	118.80		
180s ea	**55045-3229-09**	178.20		AA
(GSMS)				
REPACK				
TAB, PO (UNIT OF USE)				
500 mg, 40s ea	**60429-0118-40**	15.66	5.22	AA
90s ea	**60429-0118-90**	45.30	15.10	AA
(UNIT OF USE)				
750 mg, 90s ea	**60429-0119-90**	62.10		AA
(HomeMed)				
REPACK				
TAB, PO, 500 mg, 20s ea	**51655-0576-52**	17.99		EE
30s ea	**51655-0576-24**	24.99		EE
40s ea	**51655-0576-51**	16.06		EE
60s ea	**51655-0576-25**	25.59		EE
750 mg, 20s ea	**51655-0141-52**	21.99		EE
40s ea	**51655-0141-51**	37.50		EE
(IPI)				
REPACK				
TAB, PO, 500 mg, 30s ea	**18837-0087-30**	22.78		
40s ea	**18837-0087-40**	30.06		
42s ea	**18837-0087-42**	32.50		AA
60s ea	**18837-0087-60**	45.56		
90s ea	**18837-0087-90**	67.38		
750 mg, 30s ea	**18837-0088-30**	35.50		
60s ea	**18837-0088-60**	28.05		AA
90s ea	**18837-0088-90**	66.05		
120s ea	**18837-0088-98**	56.46		AA
270s ea	**18837-0088-94**	195.50		
(Keltman Pharma., Inc.)				
REPACK				
TAB, PO, 500 mg, 60s ea	**68387-0342-60**	56.72		
750 mg, 30s ea	**68387-0340-30**	30.00		AA
45s ea	**68387-0340-45**	45.00		AA
60s ea	**68387-0340-60**	60.00		AA
90s ea	**68387-0340-90**	90.00		AA
(McKesson Packaging)				
REPACK				
TAB, PO, 500 mg,				
100s ea UD	**63739-0166-10**	42.64		
750 mg, 100s ea UD	**63739-0167-10**	58.81		
(Nucare Pharm)				
REPACK				
TAB, PO, 500 mg, 20s ea	**66267-0145-20**	15.99		EE
30s ea	**66267-0145-30**	23.56		EE
40s ea	**66267-0145-40**	30.99		EE
60s ea	**66267-0145-60**	72.66		AA
90s ea	**66267-0145-90**	108.99		AA
750 mg, 12s ea	**66267-0146-12**	13.89		EE
20s ea	**66267-0146-20**	18.95		EE
30s ea	**66267-0146-30**	28.43		AA
40s ea	**66267-0146-40**	36.87		EE
60s ea	**66267-0146-60**	55.30		EE
90s ea	**66267-0146-90**	100.12		AA
120s ea	**66267-0146-91**	133.50		AA
(Palmetto)				
REPACK				
TAB, PO, 500 mg, 20s ea	**23490-5882-01**	17.00		
30s ea	**23490-5882-02**	25.50		
40s ea	**23490-5882-03**	34.00		
60s ea	**23490-5882-06**	51.00		
90s ea	**23490-5882-05**	76.50		
100s ea	**23490-5882-04**	85.00		
750 mg, 20s ea	**23490-5883-01**	28.85		
28s ea	**23490-5883-02**	40.38		
30s ea	**23490-5883-03**	43.27		
40s ea	**23490-5883-04**	57.69		
60s ea	**23490-5883-05**	86.54		
90s ea	**23490-5883-06**	129.81		
(PD-Rx Pharm)				
REPACK				
TAB, PO, 500 mg, 10s ea	**55289-0670-10**	27.27		AA
12s ea	**55289-0670-12**	28.14		
14s ea	**55289-0670-14**	28.40		AA
20s ea	**55289-0670-20**	34.47		AA
24s ea	**55289-0670-24**	36.24		AA
28s ea	**55289-0670-28**	36.92		AA
30s ea	**55289-0670-30**	37.68		
40s ea	**55289-0670-40**	48.93		AA
(REDI-SCRIPT)				
500 mg, 56s ea	**58864-0043-56**	57.36		AA
(USP)				
500 mg, 60s ea	**55289-0670-60**	64.50		AA
90s ea	**55289-0670-90**	75.00		
100s ea	**55289-0670-01**	78.40		AA
180s ea	**55289-0670-93**	137.88		AA
750 mg, 10s ea	**55289-0164-10**	27.80		AA
15s ea	**55289-0164-15**	31.67		AA
20s ea	**55289-0164-20**	35.60		AA
20s ea	**58864-0652-20**	35.58		AA
28s ea	**55289-0164-28**	41.20		AA
30s ea	**55289-0164-30**	43.27		AA
(REDI-SCRIPT)				
750 mg, 30s ea	**58864-0652-30**	43.26		AA
40s ea	**55289-0164-40**	51.00		AA
60s ea	**55289-0164-60**	60.00		AA
90s ea	**55289-0164-90**	78.06		AA
100s ea	**55289-0164-01**	83.64		AA
180s ea	**55289-0164-93**	131.94		AA
(Pharma Pac)				
REPACK				
TAB, PO, 500 mg, 10s ea	**52959-0167-10**	8.68		EE
12s ea	**52959-0167-12**	10.30		EE
15s ea	**52959-0167-15**	12.74		EE
20s ea	**52959-0167-20**	16.79		EE
21s ea	**52959-0167-21**	17.50		EE
24s ea	**52959-0167-24**	20.04		EE
30s ea	**52959-0167-30**	24.58		EE
40s ea	**52959-0167-40**	32.43		EE
60s ea	**52959-0167-60**	47.01		EE
90s ea	**52959-0167-90**	70.49		EE
100s ea	**52959-0167-00**	66.98		EE
120s ea	**52959-0167-03**	78.75		EE
750 mg, 10s ea	**52959-0099-10**	14.65		EE
15s ea	**52959-0099-15**	21.68		EE
20s ea	**52959-0099-20**	28.90		EE
21s ea	**52959-0099-21**	30.34		EE
28s ea	**52959-0099-28**	40.44		EE
30s ea	**52959-0099-30**	43.32		EE
40s ea	**52959-0099-40**	57.74		EE
45s ea	**52959-0099-45**	64.93		EE
50s ea	**52959-0099-50**	72.12		EE
60s ea	**52959-0099-60**	86.51		EE
90s ea	**52959-0099-90**	129.69		EE
100s ea	**52959-0099-00**	144.03		EE
120s ea	**52959-0099-03**	172.74		EE
(Phys Total Care)				
REPACK				
TAB, PO, 500 mg, 15s ea	**54868-0586-01**	7.29		EE
20s ea	**54868-0586-02**	9.00		EE
30s ea	**54868-0586-03**	12.00		EE
40s ea	**54868-0586-05**	15.00		EE
60s ea	**54868-0586-07**	20.16		AA
90s ea	**54868-0586-08**	28.14		AA
100s ea	**54868-0586-06**	31.50		EE
750 mg, 15s ea	**54868-1103-08**	7.59		EE
28s ea	**54868-1103-01**	28.97		AA
30s ea	**54868-1103-06**	12.21		EE
40s ea	**54868-1103-03**	14.94		EE
60s ea	**54868-1103-09**	21.42		EE
100s ea	**54868-1103-07**	31.35		EE
(Physician Partner)				
REPACK				
TAB, PO, 500 mg, 20s ea	**21695-0078-20**	21.26		
30s ea	**21695-0078-30**	27.11		
60s ea	**21695-0078-60**	54.22		
90s ea	**21695-0078-90**	81.32		
750 mg, 7s ea	**21695-0079-07**	11.26		AA
12s ea	**21695-0079-12**	16.41		AA
20s ea	**21695-0079-20**	27.35		AA
30s ea	**21695-0079-30**	34.87		
60s ea	**21695-0079-60**	69.74		
90s ea	**21695-0079-90**	104.61		
100s ea	**21695-0079-00**	126.24		AA
(Quality Care Prod)				
REPACK				
TAB, PO, 500 mg, 20s ea	**49999-0048-20**	14.64		EE
30s ea	**49999-0048-30**	23.52		AA
40s ea	**49999-0048-40**	29.08		EE
60s ea	**49999-0048-60**	56.17		AA
90s ea	**49999-0048-90**	84.26		EE
120s ea	**49999-0048-01**	112.34		EE
750 mg, 12s ea	**49999-0065-12**	12.84		EE
20s ea	**49999-0065-20**	21.42		EE
30s ea	**49999-0065-30**	32.14		EE
40s ea	**49999-0065-40**	42.84		EE
60s ea	**49999-0065-60**	64.26		EE
90s ea	**49999-0065-90**	97.20		EE
120s ea	**49999-0065-01**	128.52		EE
(Southwood)				
REPACK				
TAB, PO, 500 mg, 12s ea	**58016-0257-12**	7.32		EE
14s ea	**58016-0257-14**	8.54		EE
15s ea	**58016-0257-15**	9.15		EE
20s ea	**58016-0257-20**	12.20		EE
24s ea	**58016-0257-24**	14.64		EE
30s ea	**58016-0257-30**	25.20		AA
40s ea	**58016-0257-40**	24.40		EE
50s ea	**58016-0257-50**	30.50		EE
60s ea	**58016-0257-60**	50.40		AA
84s ea	**58016-0257-84**	51.24		EE
90s ea	**58016-0257-90**	75.60		AA
100s ea	**58016-0257-00**	84.00		AA
120s ea	**58016-0257-02**	100.80		AA
150s ea	**58016-0257-03**	91.50		AA
180s ea	**58016-0257-99**	109.80		AA
200s ea	**58016-0257-89**	122.00		AA
300s ea	**58016-0257-73**	183.00		AA
750 mg, 8s ea	**58016-0258-08**	7.14		EE
10s ea	**58016-0258-10**	8.93		EE
12s ea	**58016-0258-12**	10.71		EE
14s ea	**58016-0258-14**	12.50		EE
15s ea	**58016-0258-15**	13.39		EE
20s ea	**58016-0258-20**	17.85		EE
21s ea	**58016-0258-21**	18.74		EE
24s ea	**58016-0258-24**	21.42		EE
28s ea	**58016-0258-28**	24.99		EE
30s ea	**58016-0258-30**	33.90		AA
40s ea	**58016-0258-40**	35.70		EE
42s ea	**58016-0258-42**	37.49		EE
46s ea	**58016-0258-46**	41.06		EE
50s ea	**58016-0258-50**	44.63		EE
56s ea	**58016-0258-56**	49.98		EE
60s ea	**58016-0258-60**	67.80		AA
80s ea	**58016-0258-80**	71.40		EE
90s ea	**58016-0258-90**	101.70		AA
100s ea	**58016-0258-00**	113.00		AA
112s ea	**58016-0258-92**	99.96		EE
120s ea	**58016-0258-02**	135.60		AA
150s ea	**58016-0258-03**	133.88		EE
180s ea	**58016-0258-99**	160.65		AA
200s ea	**58016-0258-89**	178.50		AA
300s ea	**58016-0258-73**	267.75		AA
(St. Mary's MPP)				
REPACK				
TAB, PO, 750 mg, 40s ea	**60760-0347-40**	26.57		AA
120s ea	**60760-0347-92**	67.71		AA
(Stat Rx)				
REPACK				
TAB, PO, 500 mg, 30s ea	**16590-0147-30**	22.78		AA
40s ea	**16590-0147-40**	30.37		AA
45s ea	**16590-0147-45**	35.00		
60s ea	**16590-0147-60**	45.56		AA
90s ea	**16590-0147-90**	68.34		AA
120s ea	**16590-0147-72**	132.73		AA
180s ea	**16590-0147-82**	199.10		AA
750 mg, 20s ea	**16590-0018-20**	24.00		AA
30s ea	**16590-0148-30**	36.00		AA

PROD/MFR	NDC	AWP	DP	OBC
40s ea	16590-0148-40	54.22		AA
45s ea	16590-0148-45	54.00		AA
60s ea	16590-0148-60	79.90		AA
84s ea	16590-0148-62	100.80		AA
90s ea	16590-0148-90	108.00		AA
112s ea	16590-0148-73	134.40		AA
120s ea	16590-0148-72	144.00		AA
150s ea	16590-0148-83	180.00		AA
180s ea	16590-0148-82	216.00		AA
(Vibranta)				
REPACK				
TAB, PO, 500 mg, 40s ea	57866-4026-02	27.45		AA
750 mg, 20s ea	57866-4027-02	19.51		
30s ea	57866-4027-01	28.22		
40s ea	57866-4027-04	37.50		
METHOCEL << E4M (PCCA)				
hypromellose				
POW, NA (USP)				
1 gm	51927-1186-00	0.96		
METHOCEL E4M PREMIUM (Gallipot)				
methylcellulose				
POW, NA, 100 gm	51552-0037-05	13.23		
454 gm	51552-0037-06	37.52		
(Letco)				
POW, NA (U.S.P.)				
500 gm	62991-1278-03	81.00		
1000 gm	62991-1278-04	147.00		
2500 gm	62991-1278-05	294.00		
METHOCEL K100M (PCCA)				
hypromellose				
POW, NA (USP)				
1 gm	51927-2123-00	0.36		
METHOCEL K100M PREMIUM (Gallipot)				
methylcellulose				
POW, NA (U.S.P.,N.F.)				
100 gm	51552-0217-05	11.76		
454 gm	51552-0217-06	47.04		
(Letco)				
POW, NA (U.S.P.)				
500 gm	62991-1280-02	96.00		
1000 gm	62991-1280-03	144.00		
2500 gm	62991-1280-04	327.00		
METHOHEXITAL SODIUM				
(JHP) *See BREVITAL SODIUM*				
METHOTREXATE (Dava Pharma)				
TAB, PO (USP)				
2.5 mg, 36s ea	67253-0320-36	145.80		
100s ea	67253-0320-10	356.40		
(Gallipot)				
POW, NA (USP,1X100MG)				
0.1 gm	51552-1054-09	20.72	14.80	
(USP,1X1GM)				
1 gm	51552-1054-01	137.90	98.50	
(GeneraMedix)				
methotrexate sodium				
SOL, IJ (USP,SDV,PF)				
25 mg/ml, 2 ml	10139-0062-02	4.70		AP
10 ml UD	10139-0062-10	11.17		AP
40 ml UD	10139-0062-40	41.16		AP
METHOTREXATE (Hawkins)				
POW, NA (U.S.P.)				
1 gm	63370-0154-10	160.00		
5 gm	63370-0154-15	680.00		
25 gm	63370-0154-25	2600.00		
(Major)				
TAB, PO (USP)				
2.5 mg, 100s ea	00904-6012-60	365.40		
(Parenta Pharma)				
methotrexate sodium				
SOL, IJ (USP,SINGLE DOSE VIAL,PF)				
25 mg/ml, 2 ml 10s	66758-0040-02	49.00		
10 ml 10s	66758-0040-08	145.38		
(USP, SINGLE DOSE VIAL)				
25 mg/ml, 40 ml	66758-0041-01	56.18		
METHOTREXATE (PCCA)				
POW, NA (U.S.P.)				
1 gm	51927-1565-00	300.00		
(Bryant Ranch)				
REPACK				
methotrexate sodium				
TAB, PO, 2.5 mg, 30s ea	63629-1472-01	46.76		
(Palmetto)				
REPACK				
TAB, PO, 2.5 mg, 24s ea	23490-5889-00	114.00		
METHOTREXATE (PD-Rx Pharm)				
REPACK				
TAB, PO, 2.5 mg, 30s ea	55289-0924-30	46.76		
(Phys Total Care)				
REPACK				
TAB, PO, 2.5 mg, 12s ea	54868-3826-01	63.95		
16s ea	54868-3826-00	60.42		
24s ea	54868-3826-02	93.26		
30s ea	54868-3826-07	32.79		
(Quality Care Prod)				
REPACK				
TAB, PO, 2.5 mg, 36s ea	49999-0380-36	154.08		
METHOTREXATE SODIUM				
FUL				
TAB, PO, 2.5 mg, 100s ea		126.37		
(APP)				
PDS, IJ (S.D.V.,PF)				
1 gm, ea	63323-0122-50	61.39		
SOL, IJ, 25 mg/ml, 2 ml	63323-0121-02	5.00		
(VIAL)				
25 mg/ml, 2 ml	63323-0123-02	5.60		
(S.D.V.,PF)				
25 mg/ml, 4 ml	63323-0121-04	7.63		
8 ml	63323-0121-08	10.63		
10 ml	63323-0121-10	11.88		
(VIAL)				
25 mg/ml, 10 ml	63323-0123-10	13.25		
(VIAL,PF)				
25 mg/ml, 40 ml	63323-0121-40	43.75		
(Bedford)				
PDS, IJ (S.D.V.,30ML VIAL,PF)				
1 gm, ea	55390-0143-01	51.60		
SOL, IJ (S.D.V.,PF)				
25 mg/ml, 2 ml 10s	55390-0031-10	48.00		AP
4 ml 10s	55390-0032-10	60.00		AP
8 ml 10s	55390-0033-10	90.00		AP
10 ml 10s	55390-0034-10	114.00		AP
(Dava Pharma) *See RHEUMATREX DOSE PACK*				
(GeneraMedix) *See METHOTREXATE*				
(Hospira)				
SOL, IJ (MDV,5X2ML)				
25 mg/ml, 2 ml 5s	61703-0350-38	23.64	20.70	AP
(SDV,PF)				
25 mg/ml, 40 ml	61703-0408-41	44.46	38.90	AP
(Mylan)				
TAB, PO, 2.5 mg, 100s ea	00378-0014-01	356.40		AB
5000s ea	00378-0014-50	17820.00		AB
(Parenta Pharma) *See METHOTREXATE*				
(Roxane)				
TAB, PO, 2.5 mg, 36s ea	00054-4550-15	133.88		AB
100s ea	00054-4550-25	305.16		AB
(10X10)				
2.5 mg, 100s ea UD	00054-8550-25	353.77		AB
(Teva)				
TAB, PO, 2.5 mg, 36s ea	00555-0572-35	145.80		AB
100s ea	00555-0572-02	356.40		AB
(Teva) *See TREXALL*				
(UDL)				
TAB, PO (2X10)				
2.5 mg, 20s ea UD	51079-0670-05	78.63		AB
(A-S Medication)				
REPACK				
TAB, PO, 2.5 mg, 32s ea	54569-1818-08	114.05		EE
36s ea	54569-1818-09	128.30		AB
(Pharma Pac)				
REPACK				
TAB, PO, 2.5 mg, 100s ea	52959-0244-00	325.55		EE
(Phys Total Care)				
REPACK				
SOL, IJ (PF)				
25 mg/ml, 2 ml 2s	54868-0173-00	187.56		AP
10 ml	54868-4809-00	50.49		AP
(P.F.V.,PF)				
25 mg/ml, 10 ml	54868-4716-00	60.24		
TAB, PO, 2.5 mg, 20s ea	54868-3826-03	22.86		AB
28s ea	54868-3826-04	30.81		AB
50s ea	54868-3826-06	52.65		AB
100s ea	54868-3826-05	77.43		AB
(Physician Partner)				
REPACK				
TAB, PO, 2.5 mg, 100s ea	21695-0111-00	712.80		AB
(Quality Care Prod)				
REPACK				
TAB, PO, 2.5 mg, 24s ea	49999-0380-24	102.65		AB
METHOXSALEN (Gallipot)				
POW, NA, 1 gm	51552-0636-01	69.65		
(Medisca)				
CRY, NA (U.S.P.)				
1 gm	38779-0039-06	138.00		
5 gm	38779-0039-03	405.00		
10 gm	38779-0039-01	841.50		
25 gm	38779-0039-04	1782.00		
100 gm	38779-0039-05	5985.00		
(PCCA)				
POW, NA (USP)				
1 gm	51927-1685-00	150.00		
(Spectrum Pharmacy)				
POW, NA (U.S.P./N.F.)				
1 gm	49452-4603-01	208.95		
5 gm	49452-4603-02	605.50		
(U.S.P.)				
25 gm	49452-4603-04	2527.00		
(Therakos) *See UVADEX*				
(Valeant Pharm Intl) *See 8-MOP*				
(Valeant Pharm Intl) *See OXSORALEN*				
(Valeant Pharm Intl) *See OXSORALEN-ULTRA*				
METHSCOPOLAMINE BROMIDE (Boca Pharmacal)				
TAB, PO (USP,LACTOSE-FREE)				
2.5 mg, 100s ea	64376-0603-01	160.77		AA
5 mg, 60s ea	64376-0604-61	125.24		AA
(Fougera)				
TAB, PO (LACTOSE-FREE)				
2.5 mg, 100s ea	18754-0061-01	160.57		
(5X12,LACTOSE-FREE)				
5 mg, 60s ea UD	18754-0062-06	125.14		
(Kenwood) *See PAMINE*				
(Kenwood) *See PAMINE FORTE*				
(PCCA)				
POW, NA, 1 gm	51927-1513-00	75.00		
(Spectrum Pharmacy) *See SCOPOLAMINE METHYL BROMIDE*				
METHSCOPOLAMINE NITRATE				
(PCCA) *See SCOPOLAMINE METHYL NITRATE*				
METHSCOPOLAMINE NITRATE/PHENYLEPH HCL				
(Auriga) *See EXTENDRYL PEM*				
METHSCOPOLAMINE NITRATE/PSE HCL				
(Aristos) *See RESPIVENT-D*				
(Auriga) *See EXTENDRYL PSE*				
(Cornerstone) *See ALLERX-D*				
(Larken Labs, Inc.) *See SUDATRATE*				
(Prasco Labs) *See AMDRY-D*				
METHSUXIMIDE				
(Pfizer) *See CELONTIN KAPSEALS*				
METHYCLOTHIAZIDE (Medisca)				
POW, NA (U.S.P.)				
5 gm	38779-0336-03	55.50		
25 gm	38779-0336-04	237.00		
(Mylan)				
TAB, PO, 5 mg, 100s ea	00378-0160-01	73.17		AB
(PCCA)				
POW, NA (U.S.P.)				
1 gm	51927-2250-00	10.80		
METHYL 2-PYRROLIDINONE (PCCA)				
methyl pyrrolidone				
SOL, NA, 1 ml	51927-2041-00	0.66		
METHYL ACETATE (PCCA)				
SOL, NA (1X1ML)				
1 ml	51927-1455-00	0.29		
METHYL ALCOHOL				
(Amend) *See ALCOHOL METHYL*				
(Baker, J.T.) *See METHANOL*				
(Baker, J.T.) *See METHANOL ANHYDROUS*				
(Mallinckrodt Lab) *See ALCOHOL METHYL*				
(Mallinckrodt Lab) *See ALCOHOL METHYL ANHYDROUS*				
(Medisca) *See METHANOL*				
(PCCA) *See METHANOL*				
METHYL BENZOATE (Medisca)				
SOL, NA (1X100ML)				
100 ml	38779-1435-05	25.50		
(1X500ML)				
500 ml	38779-1435-08	52.50		
(PCCA) *See METHYL BENZOATE 99%*				

PROD/MFR	NDC	AWP	DP	OBC
METHYL BENZOATE 99% (PCCA)				
methyl benzoate				
LIQ, NA, 1 gm	**51927-1614-00**	0.31		
METHYL ETHYL KETONE (Baker, J.T.)				
LIQ, NA (A.C.S., REAGENT)				
500 ml	**10106-9319-01**	32.24		
(A.C.S., REAGENT, GLASS)				
4000 ml	**10106-9319-03**	123.91		
(PCCA)				
LIQ, NA (REAGENT)				
1 ml	**51927-2184-00**	0.27		
METHYL LINOLEATE				
(PCCA) *See LINOLEIC ACID METHYL ESTER*				
METHYL METHACRYLATE (PCCA)				
SOL, NA, 1 gm	**51927-2566-00**	0.18		
METHYL NICOTINATE (Medisca)				
POW, NA (BP, 1X25GM)				
25 gm	**38779-0693-04**	28.50		
(B.P.)				
100 gm	**38779-0693-05**	81.00		
500 gm	**38779-0693-08**	294.00		
(PCCA)				
POW, NA, 1 gm	**51927-1108-00**	1.80		
(Spectrum Pharmacy)				
POW, NA (REAGENT)				
100 gm	**49452-4670-01**	189.70		
500 gm	**49452-4670-02**	623.00		
METHYL ORANGE				
(Baker, J.T.) *See METHYL ORANGE SODIUM SALT*				
METHYL ORANGE SODIUM SALT (Baker, J.T.)				
methyl orange				
POW, NA (A.C.S., REAGENT)				
30 gm	**10106-2694-00**	38.01		
125 gm	**10106-2694-04**	63.45		
500 gm	**10106-2694-01**	194.57		
METHYL PYRROLIDONE				
(PCCA) *See METHYL 2-PYRROLIDINONE*				
METHYL SALICYLATE (Baker, J.T.)				
LIQ, NA (N.F., F.C.C., SYNTHETIC)				
500 ml	**10106-2700-01**	24.77		
4000 ml	**10106-2700-03**	165.91		
(Gallipot)				
LIQ, NA (U.S.P.,N.F.)				
59.14 ml	**51552-0326-03**	4.62		
473 ml	**51552-0326-06**	14.70		
(Mallinckrodt Lab)				
LIQ, NA (N.F.)				
500 ml	**00406-2064-04**	17.85		
(Medisca) *See METHYL SALICYLATE WINTERGREEN*				
(Medisca) *See WINTERGREEN OIL*				
(Spectrum Pharmacy)				
LIQ, NA (N.F.)				
500 ml	**49452-4690-01**	78.75		
4000 ml	**49452-4690-02**	413.00		
20000 ml	**49452-4690-03**	1480.50		
METHYL SALICYLATE FLAVOR (PCCA)				
flavoring aid				
SOL, NA (NF,WINTERGREEN)				
1 ml	**51927-1140-00**	0.25		
METHYL SALICYLATE WINTERGREEN (Medisca)				
methyl salicylate				
OIL, NA (N.F.,SYNTHETIC)				
100 ml	**38779-0942-05**	46.50		
500 ml	**38779-0942-08**	67.50		
(NF, 1X4000ML)				
4000 ml	**38779-0942-01**	285.00		
METHYLAMINE HYDROCHLORIDE				
(PCCA) *See AMINOMETHANE HYDROCHLORIDE*				
METHYLCELLULOSE				
(Gallipot) *See METHOCEL E4M PREMIUM*				
(Gallipot) *See METHOCEL K100M PREMIUM*				
(Gallipot)				
POW, NA (4000 CPS,U.S.P.,N.F.)				
0.15 gm	**51552-0210-09**	8.82		
(1500CPS,U.S.P.)				
10 gm	**51552-0462-02**	5.81		
(400 CPS,U.S.P.,N.F.)				
113.4 gm	**51552-0212-04**	14.91		
(4000 CPS,U.S.P.,N.F.)				
113.4 gm	**51552-0210-04**	11.90		
(1500CPS,U.S.P.)				
454 gm	**51552-0462-06**	30.10		
(400 CPS,U.S.P.,N.F.)				
454 gm	**51552-0212-06**	30.10		
(4000 CPS,U.S.P.,N.F.)				
454 gm	**51552-0210-06**	30.10		
(Letco) *See METHOCEL E4M PREMIUM*				
(Letco) *See METHOCEL K100M PREMIUM*				
(Medisca)				
POW, NA (1500 CPS, U.S.P.)				
100 gm	**38779-0085-05**	31.50		
(4000 CPS, U.S.P.)				
100 gm	**38779-0084-05**	31.50		
(1500 CPS, U.S.P.)				
500 gm	**38779-0085-08**	76.50		
(4000 CPS, U.S.P.)				
500 gm	**38779-0084-08**	88.50		
(4000 CPS,USP,1X1000GM)				
1000 gm	**38779-0084-09**	157.50		
(1500 CPS, U.S.P.)				
2500 gm	**38779-0085-01**	315.00		
(4000 CPS, U.S.P.)				
2500 gm	**38779-0084-01**	345.00		
(PCCA)				
POW, NA (USP; (4000 CPS))				
1 gm	**51927-1423-00**	0.36		
(USP)				
1 gm	**51927-1020-00**	0.36		
(Spectrum Pharmacy)				
POW, NA (15 CPS,U.S.P.)				
500 gm	**49452-4655-02**	121.80		
(1500 CPS, U.S.P.)				
500 gm	**49452-4645-02**	121.80		
(400 CPS,U.S.P.)				
500 gm	**49452-4640-01**	121.80		
(4000 CPS, U.S.P.)				
500 gm	**49452-4650-02**	121.80		
(1500 CPS, U.S.P.)				
2500 gm	**49452-4645-03**	514.50		
(4000 CPS, U.S.P.)				
2500 gm	**49452-4650-03**	514.50		
(U.S.P.)				
2500 gm	**49452-4640-02**	514.50		
(1500 CPS, U.S.P.)				
12000 gm	**49452-4645-04**	1967.00		
(400 CPS,U.S.P.)				
12000 gm	**49452-4640-03**	1967.00		
(4000 CPS, U.S.P.)				
12000 gm	**49452-4650-04**	1967.00		
METHYLCOBALAMIN (Letco)				
POW, NA, 5 gm	**62991-2561-03**	600.00		
10 gm	**62991-2561-02**	1035.00		
25 gm	**62991-2561-01**	2250.00		
(Medisca)				
POW, NA, 0.5 gm	**38779-1974-00**	375.00		
1 gm	**38779-1974-06**	585.00		
5 gm	**38779-1974-03**	2085.00		
10 gm	**38779-1974-01**	3150.00		
(1X25GM)				
25 gm	**38779-1974-04**	5250.00		
(1X100GM)				
100 gm	**38779-1974-05**	9885.00		
(PCCA)				
POW, NA, 1 gm	**51927-2963-00**	1170.00		
(Spectrum Pharmacy)				
POW, NA, 0.25 gm	**49452-4658-03**	591.50		
1 gm	**49452-4658-04**	987.00		
5 gm	**49452-4658-05**	3570.00		
METHYLDOPA (Consolidated Midland)				
TAB, PO, 125 mg, 100s ea	**00223-1584-01**	9.75		EE
1000s ea	**00223-1584-02**	87.50		EE
250 mg, 100s ea	**00223-1585-01**	12.50		EE
1000s ea	**00223-1585-02**	92.50		EE
500 mg, 100s ea	**00223-1586-01**	22.50		EE
500s ea	**00223-1586-05**	92.50		EE
1000s ea	**00223-1586-02**	210.00		EE
(Mylan)				
TAB, PO, 250 mg, 100s ea	**00378-0611-01**	35.70		AB
1000s ea	**00378-0611-10**	346.50		AB
500 mg, 100s ea	**00378-0421-01**	63.30		AB
500s ea	**00378-0421-05**	316.50		AB
(PCCA)				
POW, NA (L)				
1 gm	**51927-3359-00**	38.76		
(Teva)				
TAB, PO (FILM-COATED)				
250 mg, 100s ea	**00093-2931-01**	38.40		
(USP,FILM-COATED)				
250 mg, 1000s ea	**00093-2931-10**	365.52		
500 mg, 100s ea	**00093-2932-01**	68.49		EE
500s ea	**00093-2932-05**	334.73		EE
(UDL)				
TAB, PO (10X10)				
250 mg, 100s ea UD	**51079-0200-20**	36.77		AB
500 mg, 100s ea UD	**51079-0201-20**	67.26		AB
(A-S Medication)				
REPACK				
TAB, PO, 250 mg, 30s ea	**54569-0508-01**	11.52		EE
(DHS, Inc.)				
REPACK				
TAB, PO, 250 mg, 30s ea	**55887-0262-30**	31.00		AB
60s ea	**55887-0262-60**	21.42		AB
90s ea	**55887-0262-90**	32.13		AB
(PD-Rx Pharm)				
REPACK				
TAB, PO, 250 mg, 30s ea	**55289-0734-30**	11.58		AB
100s ea	**55289-0734-01**	26.93		AB
(Phys Total Care)				
REPACK				
TAB, PO, 250 mg, 30s ea	**54868-0050-04**	22.44		EE
60s ea	**54868-0050-01**	30.73		AB
90s ea	**54868-0050-03**	62.82		EE
100s ea	**54868-0050-02**	69.30		EE
500 mg, 30s ea	**54868-1328-00**	32.13		EE
(FILM-COATED)				
500 mg, 60s ea	**54868-1328-02**	59.76		AB
100s ea	**54868-1328-01**	95.07		EE
(Physician Partner)				
REPACK				
TAB, PO, 250 mg, 60s ea	**21695-0879-60**	46.08		AB
(FILM-COATED)				
500 mg, 60s ea	**21695-0880-60**	82.18		AB
(Quality Care Prod)				
REPACK				
TAB, PO, 250 mg, 60s ea	**49999-0098-60**	31.96		EE
METHYLDOPATE HCL (Amer Regent)				
methyldopate hydrochloride				
SOL, IV (S.D.V.)				
50 mg/ml, 5 ml 10s	**00517-8905-10**	500.00		AP
METHYLDOPATE HYDROCHLORIDE				
(Amer Regent) *See METHYLDOPATE HCL*				
METHYLENE BLUE (Akorn)				
SOL, IV (VIAL)				
10 mg/ml, 1 ml 10s	**11098-0504-01**	47.40		
(10X10ML,USP)				
10 mg/ml, 10 ml 10s	**17478-0504-10**	60.30		
(Amend)				
POW, NA (U.S.P.)				
25 gm	**17317-0365-02**	9.45		
125 gm	**17317-0365-04**	22.40		
(Amer Regent)				
SOL, IV (S.D.V.)				
10 mg/ml, 1 ml 10s	**00517-0301-10**	78.13		
(AMP)				
10 mg/ml, 1 ml 25s	**00517-0372-71**	175.00		
(S.D.V.,PF)				
10 mg/ml, 10 ml 10s	**00517-0310-10**	101.75		
(AMP)				
10 mg/ml, 10 ml 25s	**00517-0373-70**	293.75		
(Baker, J.T.)				
POW, NA (PURIFIED)				
125 gm	**10106-2702-04**	73.65		
500 gm	**10106-2702-01**	182.83		
(Consolidated Midland)				
SOL, IV (AMP)				
10 mg/ml, 1 ml 25s	**00223-8174-01**	400.00		
10 ml 25s	**00223-8175-10**	450.00		
(Mayne Pharma)				
SOL, IV (S.D.V.,PF)				
10 mg/ml, 1 ml 10s	**61703-0402-42**	30.24	26.46	
10 ml 10s	**61703-0402-32**	41.40	36.23	
(Medisca) *See MATHYLENE BLUE*				
(PCCA)				
POW, NA (U.S.P.)				
1 gm	**51927-1115-00**	1.32		

PROD/MFR	NDC	AWP	DP	OBC
(Spectrum Pharmacy)				
POW, NA (U.S.P.)				
25 gm	**49452-4660-01**	77.00		
125 gm	**49452-4660-02**	173.60		
500 gm	**49452-4660-03**	479.50		
METHYLENE CHLORIDE (PCCA)				
SOL, NA (NF, DICHLOROMETHANE)				
1 ml	**51927-2074-00**	0.19		
(Spectrum Pharmacy)				
SOL, NA (NF)				
100 ml	**49452-4667-01**	67.90		
500 ml	**49452-4667-02**	139.30		
METHYLENE IODIDE (PCCA)				
POW, NA, 1 gm	**51927-3503-00**	4.20		
METHYLERGONOVINE MALEATE				
(Novartis Pharm) *See METHERGINE*				
(PharmaForce)				
SOL, IJ (20X1ML,USP)				
0.2 mg/ml,				
1 ml 20s	**40042-0051-01**	110.03		AP
METHYLIN (Covidien)				
methylphenidate hydrochloride				
TAB, PO, 5 mg,				
100s ea, C-II	**00406-1121-01**	33.39		AB
1000s ea, C-II	**00406-1121-10**	333.90		AB
10 mg,				
100s ea, C-II	**00406-1122-01**	47.72		AB
1000s ea, C-II	**00406-1122-10**	477.20		AB
20 mg,				
100s ea, C-II	**00406-1124-01**	68.61		AB
1000s ea, C-II	**00406-1124-10**	686.10		AB
(Shionogi)				
CTB, PO (GRAPE)				
2.5 mg,				
100s ea, C-II	**68188-0132-01**	179.71		EE
5 mg,				
100s ea, C-II	**59630-0761-10**	256.70		EE
10 mg,				
100s ea, C-II	**68188-0137-01**	365.95		
SOL, PO (1X500ML,GRAPE)				
5 mg/5 ml,				
500 ml, C-II	**59630-0750-50**	295.44		
10 mg/5 ml,				
500 ml, C-II	**59630-0755-50**	421.18		
(Phys Total Care)				
REPACK				
TAB, PO, 10 mg,				
10s ea, C-II	**54868-5073-02**	11.52		AB
30s ea, C-II	**54868-5073-01**	19.53		AB
60s ea, C-II	**54868-5073-03**	31.56		AB
90s ea, C-II	**54868-5073-00**	43.59		AB
METHYLIN ER (Covidien)				
methylphenidate hydrochloride				
TER, PO, 10 mg,				
100s ea, C-II	**00406-1423-01**	83.59		AB
20 mg,				
100s ea, C-II	**00406-1451-01**	111.95		AB
METHYLNALTREXONE BROMIDE				
(Wyeth) *See RELISTOR*				
METHYLPARABEN (Gallipot)				
POW, NA (U.S.P.,N.F.)				
56.7 gm	**51552-0101-03**	11.76		
113.4 gm	**51552-0101-04**	13.93		
454 gm	**51552-0101-06**	25.20		
(Letco)				
POW, NA (U.S.P./N.F.)				
100 gm	**62991-1311-01**	33.00		
500 gm	**62991-1311-02**	54.00		
(Medisca)				
POW, NA (N.F.)				
25 gm	**38779-1439-04**	22.50		
100 gm	**38779-1439-05**	37.50		
500 gm	**38779-1439-08**	53.25		
(PCCA)				
POW, NA (NF)				
1 gm	**51927-1163-00**	1.08		
(Spectrum Pharmacy)				
POW, NA (NF)				
100 gm	**49452-4680-06**	64.75		
(N.F.)				
500 gm	**49452-4680-02**	97.30		
METHYLPARABEN SODIUM (Spectrum Pharmacy)				
POW, NA (N.F.)				
125 gm	**49452-4684-01**	189.35		
500 gm	**49452-4684-02**	472.50		
2500 gm	**49452-4684-03**	1183.00		
METHYLPHENIDATE				
(Shire US Inc.) *See DAYTRANA*				
METHYLPHENIDATE (Bryant Ranch)				
REPACK				
methylphenidate hydrochloride				
TAB, PO, 20 mg,				
30s ea, C-II	**63629-3166-01**	66.93		
100s ea, C-II	**63629-3166-02**	161.29		
(Palmetto)				
REPACK				
TAB, PO, 5 mg,				
30s ea, C-II	**23490-7954-03**	12.82		
(Phys Total Care)				
REPACK				
TAB, PO, 20 mg,				
10s ea, C-II	**54868-2974-03**	31.96		
TER, PO, 10 mg,				
10s ea, C-II	**54868-5832-00**	32.41		
90s ea, C-II	**54868-5832-01**	178.97		
METHYLPHENIDATE ER (Bryant Ranch)				
REPACK				
methylphenidate hydrochloride				
TER, PO, 20 mg,				
30s ea, C-II	**63629-3065-01**	51.82		
(Palmetto)				
REPACK				
TER, PO, 20 mg,				
30s ea, C-II	**23490-7955-03**	67.50		
METHYLPHENIDATE HCL (Hawkins)				
methylphenidate hydrochloride				
POW, NA (U.S.P.)				
5 gm, C-II	**63370-0938-15**	400.00		
25 gm, C-II	**63370-0938-25**	1600.00		
100 gm, C-II	**63370-0938-35**	5000.00		
(Medisca)				
POW, NA (U.S.P.)				
5 gm, C-II	**38779-0851-03**	555.00		
25 gm, C-II	**38779-0851-04**	1875.00		
(PCCA)				
POW, NA (U.S.P.; CII)				
1 gm, C-II	**51927-3076-00**	90.00		
(Sandoz)				
TAB, PO, 5 mg,				
100s ea, C-II	**00781-8840-01**	34.85		AB
1000s ea, C-II	**00781-8840-10**	334.00		AB
10 mg,				
100s ea, C-II	**00781-5749-01**	49.68		AB
100s ea, C-II	**00781-8841-01**	49.68		AB
1000s ea, C-II	**00781-1749-10**	477.20		AB
20 mg,				
100s ea, C-II	**00781-8842-01**	71.43		AB
1000s ea, C-II	**00781-1753-10**	686.10		AB
TER, PO, 20 mg,				
100s ea, C-II	**00781-8843-01**	110.95		AB
(Spectrum Pharmacy)				
CRY, NA (U.S.P.)				
1 gm	**49452-4682-04**	416.50		
5 gm	**49452-4682-05**	1116.50		
(UCB)				
TAB, PO, 5 mg,				
100s ea, C-II	**53014-0531-07**	34.10		AB
10 mg,				
100s ea, C-II	**53014-0530-07**	47.69		AB
20 mg,				
100s ea, C-II	**53014-0532-07**	69.76		AB
(Watson Labs)				
TAB, PO, 5 mg,				
100s ea, C-II	**00591-5882-01**	18.02		AB
10 mg,				
100s ea, C-II	**00591-5883-01**	24.05		AB
20 mg,				
100s ea, C-II	**00591-5884-01**	26.47		AB
(PD-Rx Pharm)				
REPACK				
TAB, PO (USP)				
5 mg, 30s ea, C-II	**55289-0819-30**	12.41		AB
60s ea, C-II	**55289-0819-60**	15.81		AB
90s ea, C-II	**55289-0819-90**	19.22		AB
10 mg,				
30s ea, C-II	**55289-0829-30**	13.47		AB
60s ea, C-II	**55289-0829-60**	17.94		AB
90s ea, C-II	**55289-0829-90**	22.41		AB
(Phys Total Care)				
REPACK				
TAB, PO, 5 mg,				
20s ea, C-II	**54868-1704-02**	17.64		AB
25s ea, C-II	**54868-1704-01**	20.16		AB
30s ea, C-II	**54868-1704-03**	22.68		AB
45s ea, C-II	**54868-1704-05**	30.27		AB
60s ea, C-II	**54868-1704-00**	37.89		EE
90s ea, C-II	**54868-1704-04**	42.36		AB
100s ea, C-II	**54868-1704-06**	39.65		AB
10 mg,				
20s ea, C-II	**54868-0733-02**	15.51		EE
30s ea, C-II	**54868-0733-04**	19.53		EE
60s ea, C-II	**54868-0733-01**	31.56		EE
90s ea, C-II	**54868-0733-03**	43.59		AB
100s ea, C-II	**54868-0733-00**	38.16		EE
20 mg,				
20s ea, C-II	**54868-2974-01**	51.99		AB
30s ea, C-II	**54868-2974-02**	71.25		AB
60s ea, C-II	**54868-2974-00**	109.56		AB
TER, PO, 20 mg,				
10s ea, C-II	**54868-3454-05**	18.57		EE
30s ea, C-II	**54868-3454-04**	50.91		EE
50s ea, C-II	**54868-3454-00**	62.82		EE
90s ea, C-II	**54868-3454-06**	107.07		EE
100s ea, C-II	**54868-3454-03**	118.14		EE
(Stat Rx)				
REPACK				
TAB, PO, 5 mg,				
30s ea, C-II	**16590-0837-30**	10.02		AB
10 mg,				
30s ea, C-II	**16590-0886-30**	18.90		AB
METHYLPHENIDATE HYDROCHLORIDE				
FUL				
TAB, PO, 5 mg, 100s ea		22.53		
10 mg, 100s ea		30.06		
20 mg, 100s ea		33.09		
(Covidien) *See METHYLIN*				
(Covidien) *See METHYLIN ER*				
(Hawkins) *See METHYLPHENIDATE HCL*				
(McNeil Consumer Healthcare) *See CONCERTA*				
(Medisca) *See METHYLPHENIDATE HCL*				
(Novartis Pharm) *See RITALIN*				
(Novartis Pharm) *See RITALIN LA*				
(Novartis Pharm) *See RITALIN-SR*				
(Ortho-McNeil Pharm) *See CONCERTA*				
(PCCA) *See METHYLPHENIDATE HCL*				
(Sandoz) *See METHYLPHENIDATE HCL*				
(Sandoz)				
TAB, PO, 5 mg,				
100s ea, C-II	**00781-5748-01**	34.85		AB
20 mg, 100s ea, C-II	**00781-5753-01**	71.43		
TER, PO (FILM-COATED)				
20 mg,				
100s ea, C-II	**00781-5754-01**	110.95		
(Shionogi) *See METHYLIN*				
(Spectrum Pharmacy) *See METHYLPHENIDATE HCL*				
(UCB) *See METADATE CD*				
(UCB) *See METADATE ER*				
(UCB) *See METHYLPHENIDATE HCL*				
(Watson Labs) *See METHYLPHENIDATE HCL*				
(Phys Total Care)				
REPACK				
TER, PO, 20 mg,				
20s ea, C-II	**54868-3454-02**	29.64		
60s ea, C-II	**54868-3454-01**	73.89		
(Quality Care Prod)				
REPACK				
TAB, PO, 5 mg,				
30s ea, C-II	**49999-0842-30**	20.02		
10 mg, 30s ea, C-II	**49999-0843-30**	24.79		
20 mg, 30s ea, C-II	**49999-0844-30**	51.90		
METHYLPRED DP (DHS, Inc.)				
REPACK				
methylprednisolone				
TAB, PO, 4 mg, 21s ea	**55887-0953-21**	22.75		AB
METHYLPRED-DP (Stat Rx)				
REPACK				
methylprednisolone				
TAB, PO, 4 mg, 21s ea	**16590-0149-21**	14.00		
METHYLPREDNISOLONE				
FUL				
TAB, PO, 4 mg, 100s ea		43.04		
(Breckenridge Pharm)				
TAB, PO (UNIT OF USE)				
4 mg, 21s ea	**51991-0188-31**	11.00		AB
100s ea	**51991-0188-01**	54.00		AB

PROD/MFR	NDC	AWP	DP	OBC
(Cadista)				
TAB, PO, 4 mg, 21s ea	**59746-0001-03**	14.25		AB
100s ea	**59746-0001-06**	67.86		AB
(USP)				
8 mg, 25s ea	**59746-0002-04**	50.26		AB
16 mg, 50s ea	**59746-0003-14**	155.29		
32 mg, 25s ea	**59746-0015-04**	115.62		
(Gallipot)				
POW, NA (U.S.P.,MICRONIZED)				
5 gm	**51552-0603-02**	69.30		
(Major)				
TAB, PO (UNIPAK)				
4 mg, 21s ea	**00904-2175-19**	10.99		AB
(Medisca)				
POW, NA (U.S.P.,MICRONIZED)				
1 gm	**38779-0142-06**	40.50		
5 gm	**38779-0142-03**	160.50		
25 gm	**38779-0142-04**	664.50		
(Pfizer) *See MEDROL*				
(Qualitest)				
TAB, PO (DOSE PACK)				
4 mg, 21s ea	**00603-4593-15**	10.65		AB
100s ea	**00603-4593-21**	48.40		AB
(Sandoz)				
TAB, PO (UNIT OF USE)				
4 mg, 21s ea	**00781-5022-07**	14.09	9.26	AB
100s ea	**00781-5022-01**	69.41	45.47	AB
(Spectrum Pharmacy)				
POW, NA (U.S.P.,MICRONIZED)				
1 gm	**49452-4686-01**	88.55		
5 gm	**49452-4686-02**	297.50		
25 gm	**49452-4686-03**	1081.50		
(Teva)				
TAB, PO, 4 mg, 21s ea	**00555-0301-38**	11.00		AB
100s ea	**00555-0301-02**	54.00		AB
(4u) REPACK				
TAB, PO, 4 mg, 21s ea	**10544-0322-21**	24.84		
21s ea	**42549-0522-21**	24.84		AB
(A-S Medication) REPACK				
TAB, PO, 4 mg, 21s ea	**54569-1036-00**	12.64		AB
(Aidarex) REPACK				
TAB, PO (DOSE PACK)				
4 mg, 21s ea	**33261-0335-21**	27.00		AB
(Altura) REPACK				
TAB, PO, 4 mg, 21s ea	**63874-0413-21**	16.78		EE
(Core) REPACK				
TAB, PO, 4 mg, 21s ea	**33358-0241-21**	38.85		
(Dispensing Solutions) REPACK				
TAB, PO (DOSEPAK)				
4 mg, 21s ea	**55045-1259-09**	19.76		AB
30s ea	**55045-1811-08**	22.50		
40s ea	**55045-1811-03**	30.00		
8 mg, 25s ea	**55045-3513-01**	41.00		
(Keltman Pharma., Inc.) REPACK				
TAB, PO, 4 mg, 21s ea	**68387-0170-01**	20.77		
(McKesson Packaging) REPACK				
TAB, PO (USP)				
4 mg, 100s ea UD	**63739-0161-10**	60.50		
(Nucare Pharm) REPACK				
TAB, PO, 4 mg, 21s ea	**66267-0961-21**	38.85		EE
(Palmetto) REPACK				
TAB, PO, 4 mg, 21s ea	**23490-1911-02**	10.83		
21s ea	**23490-5902-01**	25.20		
(PD-Rx Pharm) REPACK				
TAB, PO, 4 mg, 30s ea	**55289-0649-30**	33.17		AB
120s ea	**55289-0649-98**	87.56		AB
(Pharma Pac) REPACK				
TAB, PO (DOSE PACK)				
4 mg, 21s ea	**52959-0100-00**	29.95		EE
(Phys Total Care) REPACK				
TAB, PO, 4 mg, 20s ea	**54868-2913-03**	11.15		AB

PROD/MFR	NDC	AWP	DP	OBC
(DOSE PACK)				
4 mg, 21s ea	**54868-6624-01**	11.07		EE
30s ea	**54868-2913-01**	15.51		EE
60s ea	**54868-2913-02**	26.55		AB
100s ea	**54868-2913-00**	31.08		EE
(Physician Partner) REPACK				
methylprednisolone sodium succinate				
PDS, IJ, 125 mg, 10s ea	**21695-0587-10**	100.00		
(Quality Care Prod) REPACK				
methylprednisolone acetate				
SUS, IJ, 40 mg/ml, ea	**35356-0083-01**	96.00		
METHYLPREDNISOLONE (Quality Care Prod)				
TAB, PO, 4 mg, 21s ea	**49999-0153-21**	27.47		AB
(Southwood) REPACK				
TAB, PO, 4 mg, 21s ea	**58016-2001-01**	15.90		EE
(DOSE PACK)				
4 mg, 21s ea	**58016-2004-01**	22.39		AB
8 mg, 25s ea	**58016-4719-01**	34.59		AB
(Vibranta) REPACK				
TAB, PO, 4 mg, 21s ea	**57866-4037-01**	32.58		
8 mg, 25s ea	**57866-7100-01**	95.90		
METHYLPREDNISOLONE ACETATE (Gallipot)				
methylprednisolone acetate, micronized				
POW, NA (USP,1X5GM,MICRONIZED)				
5 gm	**51552-0958-02**	66.50	47.50	
(USP,1X25GM,MICRONIZED)				
25 gm	**51552-0958-04**	308.00	220.00	
(USP,1X100GM,MICRONIZED)				
100 gm	**51552-0958-05**	1155.00	825.00	
(USP,1X500GM,MICRONIZED)				
500 gm	**51552-0958-06**	5250.00	3750.00	
METHYLPREDNISOLONE ACETATE (Medisca)				
POW, NA (U.S.P.,MICRONIZED)				
1 gm	**38779-0144-06**	49.50		
5 gm	**38779-0144-03**	196.50		
25 gm	**38779-0144-04**	795.00		
(Pfizer) *See DEPO-MEDROL*				
(Pfizer) *See NOVAPLUS DEPO-MEDROL*				
(Sandoz)				
SUS, IJ (USP,SINGLE-DOSE)				
40 mg/ml, 1 ml	**00781-3131-71**	7.25		AB
1 ml 10s	**00781-3131-95**	72.50		AB
(1X10ML,USP,MDV)				
40 mg/ml, 10 ml	**00781-3136-70**	49.61		AB
(1X1ML,USP,SINGLE-DOSE)				
80 mg/ml, 1 ml	**00781-3132-71**	11.94		EE
(10X1ML,USP,SINGLE-DOSE)				
80 mg/ml, 1 ml 10s	**00781-3132-95**	119.40		EE
(1X5ML,USP,MDV)				
80 mg/ml, 5 ml	**00781-3137-75**	49.61		AB
(Spectrum Pharmacy)				
POW, NA (U.S.P.,MICRONIZED)				
1 gm	**49452-4688-01**	101.85		
5 gm	**49452-4688-02**	307.30		
25 gm	**49452-4688-03**	1162.00		
(Teva)				
SUS, IJ (SDV)				
40 mg/ml, 1 ml	**00703-0031-01**	5.70		AB
1 ml 25s	**00703-0031-04**	142.50		AB
(MDV,USP)				
40 mg/ml, 5 ml	**00703-0043-01**	21.60		AB
10 ml	**00703-0045-01**	43.20		AB
(SDV)				
80 mg/ml, 1 ml	**00703-0051-01**	10.20		AB
1 ml 25s	**00703-0051-04**	255.00		AB
(MDV,USP)				
80 mg/ml, 5 ml	**00703-0063-01**	43.20		AB
(Physician Partner) REPACK				
SUS, IJ (1X10ML)				
40 mg/ml, 10 ml	**21695-0849-10**	99.22		AB
(Quality Care Prod) REPACK				
SUS, IJ (1X5ML)				
80 mg/ml, 5 ml	**35356-0178-05**	94.00		AB
(Southwood) REPACK				
SUS, IJ, 80 mg/ml, 1 ml	**58016-4893-01**	11.94		

PROD/MFR	NDC	AWP	DP	OBC
METHYLPREDNISOLONE ACETATE MICRONIZED				
(Letco)				
methylprednisolone acetate, micronized				
POW, NA (U.S.P.)				
5 gm	**62991-1635-02**	144.00		
25 gm	**62991-1635-03**	687.00		
100 gm	**62991-1635-04**	2520.00		
250 gm	**62991-1635-05**	5700.00		
1000 gm	**62991-1635-06**	18600.00		
(Medisca)				
POW, NA (U.S.P.)				
100 gm	**38779-0144-05**	2550.00		
(USP)				
500 gm	**38779-0144-08**	10155.00		
(1X1000GM,USP)				
1000 gm	**38779-0144-09**	18690.00		
(PCCA)				
POW, NA (U.S.P.)				
1 gm	**51927-1332-00**	66.00		
METHYLPREDNISOLONE ACETATE, MICRONIZED				
(Gallipot) *See METHYLPREDNISOLONE ACETATE*				
(Letco) *See METHYLPREDNISOLONE ACETATE MICRONIZED*				
(Medisca) *See METHYLPREDNISOLONE ACETATE MICRONIZED*				
(PCCA) *See METHYLPREDNISOLONE ACETATE MICRONIZED*				
METHYLPREDNISOLONE MICRONIZED (PCCA)				
methylprednisolone, micronized				
POW, NA (1X1GM)				
1 gm	**51927-2287-00**	51.00		
METHYLPREDNISOLONE SODIUM SUCCINATE (APP)				
PDS, IJ (PF)				
1 gm, ea	**63323-0265-30**	32.90		
40 mg, 25s ea	**63323-0255-03**	146.25		
125 mg, 25s ea	**63323-0258-03**	280.00		
(Bedford)				
PDS, IJ (USP,MDV,LYOPHILIZED)				
1 gm, ea	**55390-0259-01**	31.20		AP
(SDV)				
40 mg, 10s ea	**55390-0209-10**	30.00		AP
125 mg, 10s ea	**55390-0210-10**	48.00		AP
(USP,MDV,LYOPHILIZED)				
500 mg, ea	**55390-0258-01**	15.60		AP
(Consolidated Midland)				
PDS, IJ, 1 gm, ea	**00223-8163-04**	65.00		EE
(VIAL)				
40 mg, ea	**00223-8160-01**	4.00		EE
125 mg, ea	**00223-8160-02**	12.50		EE
ea	**00223-8161-02**	12.00		EE
500 mg, ea	**00223-8162-03**	37.50		EE
(Hospira) *See A-METHAPRED*				
(PCCA)				
POW, NA (BUFFERED)				
1 gm	**51927-3552-00**	72.00		
(Pfizer) *See SOLU-MEDROL*				
(Pharmacia) *See NOVAPLUS SOLU-MEDROL*				
(Pharmacia) *See SOLU-MEDROL*				
METHYLPREDNISOLONE, MICRONIZED				
(PCCA) *See METHYLPREDNISOLONE MICRONIZED*				
METHYLPREDNISONE (Physician Partner) REPACK				
methylprednisolone				
TAB, PO, 4 mg, 21s ea	**21695-0080-21**	36.24		
METHYLPYRAZOLE (PCCA)				
fomepizole				
SOL, NA (REAGENT)				
1 ml	**51927-2541-00**	345.00		
METHYLTESTOSTERONE (Gallipot)				
POW, NA (U.S.P.)				
1 gm, C-III	**51552-0031-01**	7.35		
5 gm, C-III	**51552-0031-02**	21.70		
10 gm, C-III	**51552-0031-03**	38.08		
25 gm, C-III	**51552-0031-04**	56.00		
100 gm, C-III	**51552-0031-05**	196.00		
(Global Pharm) *See METHITEST*				
(Medisca)				
POW, NA (U.S.P.,MICRONIZED)				
5 gm, C-III	**38779-0086-03**	41.85		
25 gm, C-III	**38779-0086-04**	151.80		
100 gm, C-III	**38779-0086-05**	498.00		
(Spectrum Pharmacy)				
POW, NA (U.S.P.,MICRONIZED)				
5 gm, C-III	**49452-4710-01**	90.30		

PROD/MFR	NDC	AWP	DP	OBC
25 gm, C-III	**49452-4710-02**	273.35		
100 gm, C-III	**49452-4710-03**	843.50		
(Valeant Pharm Intl) *See ANDROID*				
(Valeant Pharm Intl) *See TESTRED*				
METHYLTESTOSTERONE MICRONIZED (Hawkins)				
methyltestosterone, micronized				
POW, NA (U.S.P.)				
5 gm, C-III	**63370-0940-15**	56.00		
25 gm, C-III	**63370-0940-25**	192.00		
100 gm, C-III	**63370-0940-35**	628.00		
1000 gm, C-III	**63370-0940-50**	5700.00		
(Medisca)				
POW, NA (U.S.P.)				
500 gm, C-III	**38779-0086-08**	3060.00		
(PCCA)				
POW, NA (U.S.P.; CIII)				
1 gm, C-III	**51927-1028-00**	11.40		
METHYLTESTOSTERONE, MICRONIZED				
(Hawkins) *See METHYLTESTOSTERONE MICRONIZED*				
(Medisca) *See METHYLTESTOSTERONE MICRONIZED*				
(PCCA) *See METHYLTESTOSTERONE MICRONIZED*				
METHYSERGIDE MALEATE (Medisca)				
POW, NA (1X1GM,USP)				
1 gm	**38779-2306-06**	1425.00		
(1X5GM,USP)				
5 gm	**38779-2306-03**	4785.00		
(1X25GM,USP)				
25 gm	**38779-2306-04**	26700.00		
(PCCA)				
POW, NA, 1 gm	**51927-3526-00**	2580.00		
(Spectrum Pharmacy)				
POW, NA, 0.5 gm	**49452-4694-01**	1431.50		
1 gm	**49452-4694-02**	2282.00		
5 gm	**49452-4694-03**	7220.50		
METIMYD (Pharma Pac)				
REPACK				
prednisolone acetate/sulfacetamide sodium				
SUS, OP, 0.5%-10%, 5 ml	**52959-0448-03**	34.05		
METIPRANOLOL				
(Bausch & Lomb Inc.) *See OPTIPRANOLOL*				
(Bausch & Lomb Inc.)				
SOL, OP, 0.3%, 5 ml	**24208-0402-05**	17.75		AT
10 ml	**24208-0402-10**	30.00		AT
(Falcon Ophthalmics)				
SOL, OP, 0.3%, 5 ml	**61314-0447-05**	17.04		AT
10 ml	**61314-0447-10**	28.80		AT
METOCLOPRAMIDE (Actavis)				
metoclopramide hydrochloride				
TAB, PO, 10 mg, 100s ea	**00228-2269-10**	27.75		AB
500s ea	**00228-2269-50**	130.25		AB
(ANI)				
SOL, PO (1X473ML,USP,AF,SF)				
5 mg/5 ml, 473 ml	**62559-1106-06**	18.70		AA
(Hospira)				
SOL, IV (LEUR LOCK,CARPUJECT)				
5 mg/ml, 2 ml 10s	**00409-2173-32**	11.40	10.00	AP
(AMP,25X2ML)				
5 mg/ml, 2 ml 25s	**00409-3413-01**	13.80	12.00	AP
(Major)				
TAB, PO, 10 mg, 100s ea	**00904-1070-60**	27.25		AB
(10X10)				
10 mg, 100s ea UD	**00904-1070-61**	35.80		AB
1000s ea	**00904-1070-80**	212.85		AB
(Mayne Pharma)				
SOL, IV (S.D.V.,PF)				
5 mg/ml, 20 ml 10s	**61703-0210-21**	60.00	52.50	AP
(150MG/30ML,PF)				
5 mg/ml, 30 ml	**61703-0210-35**	6.76	5.91	AP
(S.D.V.,PF)				
5 mg/ml, 30 ml 10s	**61703-0210-31**	203.00		AP
(Morton Grove)				
SOL, PO (BUTTERSCOTCH)				
5 mg/5 ml, 473 ml	**60432-0622-16**	19.25		AA
(Mutual)				
TAB, PO, 5 mg, 100s ea	**53489-0384-01**	33.20		AB
500s ea	**53489-0384-05**	164.95		AB
(Northstar)				
TAB, PO (USP)				
5 mg, 100s ea	**16714-0061-04**	32.00		AB
500s ea	**16714-0061-05**	138.00		AB
10 mg, 100s ea	**16714-0062-04**	27.50		AB
500s ea	**16714-0062-05**	130.00		AB
1000s ea	**16714-0062-06**	215.00		AB
(Pharm Assoc Inc)				
SOL, PO (10ML-10X10)				
5 mg/5 ml,				
10 ml 100s UD	**00121-1576-10**	60.66		AA
473 ml	**00121-0576-16**	19.27		AA
(Precision Dose)				
SOL, PO (USP,50X0.9ML,SF)				
5 mg/5 ml,				
0.9 ml 50s UD	**68094-0680-58**	63.00		
(1X10ML,USP,SF)				
5 mg/5 ml,				
10 ml UD	**68094-0676-59**	0.50		
(30X10ML,SF)				
5 mg/5 ml,				
10 ml 30s UD	**68094-0676-62**	15.12		
(Qualitest)				
TAB, PO (USP)				
5 mg, 100s ea	**00603-4614-21**	33.21		AB
500s ea	**00603-4614-28**	164.96		AB
1000s ea	**00603-4614-32**	320.02		AB
10 mg, 60s ea	**00603-4615-20**	16.65		AB
(USP)				
10 mg, 100s ea	**00603-4615-21**	27.75		AB
500s ea	**00603-4615-28**	130.24		AB
1000s ea	**00603-4615-32**	252.67		AB
(Ranbaxy Pharm)				
TAB, PO (USP)				
5 mg, 100s ea	**63304-0845-01**	32.00		AB
500s ea	**63304-0845-05**	138.00		AB
10 mg, 100s ea	**63304-0846-01**	27.50		AB
500s ea	**63304-0846-05**	130.00		AB
1000s ea	**63304-0846-10**	247.10		AB
(Silarx)				
SOL, PO, 5 mg/5 ml,				
473 ml	**54838-0508-80**	16.70		AA
(Teva)				
SOL, IV (S.D.V.)				
5 mg/ml, 2 ml 25s	**00703-4502-04**	15.60		AP
TAB, PO, 5 mg, 100s ea	**00093-2204-01**	33.25		AB
(10X10)				
5 mg, 100s ea UD	**00182-1898-89**	42.53		AB
500s ea	**00093-2204-05**	165.00		AB
10 mg, 100s ea	**00093-2203-01**	27.75		AB
(10X10)				
10 mg, 100s ea UD	**00182-1789-89**	31.32		AB
500s ea	**00093-2203-05**	130.25		AB
1000s ea	**00093-2203-10**	215.00		AB
(UDL)				
TAB, PO (10X10)				
5 mg, 100s ea UD	**51079-0629-20**	40.40		AB
(ROBOT READY 25X1)				
10 mg, 25s ea UD	**51079-0283-19**	7.15		AB
(10X10)				
10 mg, 100s ea UD	**51079-0283-20**	28.54		AB
(Watson Labs)				
TAB, PO (USP)				
5 mg, 100s ea	**00591-2228-01**	8.64		
500s ea	**00591-2228-05**	37.92		
10 mg, 100s ea	**00591-2229-01**	9.54		AB
500s ea	**00591-2229-05**	45.30		AB
1000s ea	**00591-2229-10**	85.86		AB
(Altura)				
REPACK				
TAB, PO, 10 mg, 10s ea	**63874-0355-10**	6.46		AB
12s ea	**63874-0355-12**	7.75		AB
15s ea	**63874-0355-15**	9.72		AB
20s ea	**63874-0355-20**	12.97		AB
30s ea	**63874-0355-30**	19.46		AB
56s ea	**63874-0355-56**	36.33		AB
60s ea	**63874-0355-60**	38.92		AB
90s ea	**63874-0355-90**	58.38		AB
100s ea	**63874-0355-01**	64.85		AB
120s ea	**63874-0355-04**	77.50		AB
(American Health)				
REPACK				
TAB, PO (10X10)				
10 mg, 100s ea UD	**68084-0091-01**	28.50		AB
(Bryant Ranch)				
REPACK				
TAB, PO, 10 mg, 30s ea	**63629-1618-01**	9.03		
60s ea	**63629-1618-03**	18.06		
100s ea	**63629-1618-02**	45.93		
(DHS, Inc.)				
REPACK				
TAB, PO, 10 mg, 20s ea	**55887-0653-20**	12.49		
90s ea	**55887-0653-90**	50.00		
120s ea	**55887-0653-82**	65.00		
(Dispensing Solutions)				
REPACK				
TAB, PO, 10 mg, 30s ea	**66336-0802-30**	17.25		
90s ea	**55045-1169-09**	25.20		AB
(HomeMed)				
REPACK				
TAB, PO, 10 mg, 30s ea	**51655-0407-24**	22.69		
(IPI)				
REPACK				
TAB, PO, 5 mg, 30s ea	**18837-0089-30**	10.35		
(McKesson Packaging)				
REPACK				
TAB, PO, 10 mg,				
100s ea UD	**63739-0172-10**	29.51		
(PUNCH CARD 25X30)				
10 mg, 750s ea	**63739-0172-03**	221.33		AB
(Nucare Pharm)				
REPACK				
TAB, PO, 5 mg, 30s ea	**66267-0500-30**	13.61		AB
(Palmetto)				
REPACK				
SYR, PO, 5 mg/5 ml,				
120 ml	**23490-9366-01**	5.75		
180 ml	**23490-9366-02**	8.62		
240 ml	**23490-9366-03**	11.49		
480 ml	**23490-9366-04**	22.99		
(Pharma Pac)				
REPACK				
TAB, PO, 5 mg, 30s ea	**52959-0849-30**	13.20		
10 mg, 60s ea	**52959-0480-60**	72.53		AB
(Phys Total Care)				
REPACK				
TAB, PO, 5 mg, 30s ea	**54868-1873-02**	9.39		
60s ea	**54868-1873-03**	15.78		
10 mg, 90s ea	**54868-0034-00**	22.23		AB
(Physician Partner)				
REPACK				
TAB, PO, 10 mg, 15s ea	**21695-0346-15**	15.05		AB
20s ea	**21695-0346-20**	20.08		AB
30s ea	**21695-0346-30**	25.60		AB
60s ea	**21695-0346-60**	51.20		AB
(Quality Care Prod)				
REPACK				
TAB, PO, 10 mg, 30s ea	**49999-0057-30**	22.24		AB
(Southwood)				
REPACK				
TAB, PO, 5 mg, 12s ea	**58016-0729-12**	4.74		EE
15s ea	**58016-0729-15**	5.93		EE
20s ea	**58016-0729-20**	7.91		EE
30s ea	**58016-0729-30**	11.86		EE
100s ea	**58016-0729-00**	39.53		EE
10 mg, 12s ea	**58016-0733-12**	7.41		EE
15s ea	**58016-0733-15**	9.26		EE
20s ea	**58016-0733-20**	12.35		EE
30s ea	**58016-0733-30**	18.53		EE
60s ea	**58016-0733-60**	37.06		EE
100s ea	**58016-0733-00**	61.76		EE
(Stat Rx)				
REPACK				
TAB, PO, 10 mg, 120s ea	**16590-0151-72**	25.80		AB
(Vibranta)				
REPACK				
TAB, PO, 10 mg, 90s ea	**57866-4042-04**	28.45		AB
METOCLOPRAMIDE HCL (Actavis Mid Atlantic)				
metoclopramide hydrochloride				
SOL, PO (5X10,SF)				
5 mg/5 ml,				
10 ml 50s UD	**00472-5006-60**	54.13		AA
(Baxter)				
SOL, IV, 5 mg/ml, 2 ml	**10019-0450-39**	0.54		AP
(S.D.V.)				
5 mg/ml, 2 ml 25s	**10019-0450-02**	13.50		AP
(Hawkins)				
POW, NA (U.S.P., MONOHYDRATE)				
5 gm	**63370-0141-15**	52.80		
25 gm	**63370-0141-25**	153.60		
100 gm	**63370-0141-35**	456.00		
(Letco)				
POW, NA (U.S.P.)				
5 gm	**62991-2042-01**	30.00		

PROD/MFR	NDC	AWP	DP	OBC
25 gm	62991-2042-02	93.00		
100 gm	62991-2042-03	240.00		
(Medisca)				
POW, NA (U.S.P.)				
10 gm	38779-0403-01	75.00		
25 gm	38779-0403-04	118.50		
100 gm	38779-0403-05	315.00		
(PCCA)				
POW, NA (U.S.P.)				
1 gm	51927-1082-00	9.00		
(A-S Medication)				
REPACK				
TAB, PO, 10 mg, 30s ea	54569-0434-00	8.25		EE
(Altura)				
REPACK				
TAB, PO, 5 mg, 30s ea	63874-1038-03	15.00		AB
100s ea	63874-1038-01	50.00		AB
(DHS, Inc.)				
REPACK				
TAB, PO, 5 mg, 30s ea	55887-0249-30	17.25		AB
(Dispensing Solutions)				
REPACK				
TAB, PO, 5 mg, 90s ea	66336-0880-90	39.19		AB
(McKesson Packaging)				
REPACK				
TAB, PO (USP)				
5 mg, 100s ea UD	63739-0171-10	29.51		AB
(BLISTER PACK)				
10 mg, 750s ea UD	63739-0172-01	221.33		AB
(Pharma Pac)				
REPACK				
TAB, PO, 10 mg, 30s ea	52959-0480-30	36.53		AB
100s ea	52959-0480-00	121.72		AB
(Phys Total Care)				
REPACK				
SOL, IV (S.D.V.)				
5 mg/ml, 2 ml 25s	54868-4167-00	75.09		EE
PO, 5 mg/5 ml,				
480 ml	54868-3485-00	24.27		EE
TAB, PO, 5 mg, 20s ea	54868-1873-00	7.26		AB
90s ea	54868-1873-04	25.65		AB
100s ea	54868-1873-01	24.27		AB
10 mg, 20s ea	54868-0034-09	8.43		EE
30s ea	54868-0034-04	10.41		EE
40s ea	54868-0034-07	12.39		EE
50s ea	54868-0034-05	14.34		EE
60s ea	54868-0034-02	16.32		EE
100s ea	54868-0034-03	24.21		EE
120s ea	54868-0034-08	29.37		EE
(Quality Care Prod)				
REPACK				
TAB, PO, 10 mg, 10s ea	49999-0057-10	7.44		AB
100s ea	49999-0057-00	74.40		AB
120s ea	49999-0057-12	89.28		AB
(Vibranta)				
REPACK				
TAB, PO, 5 mg, 90s ea	57866-4041-01	38.16		AB
METOCLOPRAMIDE HCL MONOHYDRATE (Gallipot)				
metoclopramide hydrochloride				
POW, NA (U.S.P.)				
10 gm	51552-0180-03	34.30		
25 gm	51552-0180-04	54.60		
100 gm	51552-0180-05	132.86		
(Spectrum Pharmacy)				
POW, NA (U.S.P.)				
10 gm	49452-4715-01	127.75		
25 gm	49452-4715-02	203.00		
100 gm	49452-4715-03	486.50		
METOCLOPRAMIDE HYDROCHLORIDE				
FUL				
SOL, PO, 5 mg/5 ml,				
480 ml		7.44		
TAB, PO, 5 mg, 100s ea		18.42		
10 mg, 100s ea		10.95		
(Actavis) *See METOCLOPRAMIDE*				
(Actavis Mid Atlantic) *See METOCLOPRAMIDE HCL*				
(Alaven) *See REGLAN*				
(ANI) *See METOCLOPRAMIDE*				
(Baxter) *See METOCLOPRAMIDE HCL*				
(Baxter) *See REGLAN*				
(Gallipot) *See METOCLOPRAMIDE HCL MONOHYDRATE*				
(Hawkins) *See METOCLOPRAMIDE HCL*				
(Hospira) *See AMERINET CHOICE METOCLOPRAMIDE*				

PROD/MFR	NDC	AWP	DP	OBC
(Hospira) *See METOCLOPRAMIDE*				
(Hospira)				
SOL, IJ (25X2ML,PF)				
5 mg/ml, 2 ml 25s	00409-3414-01	12.60	11.00	AP
(Letco) *See METOCLOPRAMIDE HCL*				
(Major) *See METOCLOPRAMIDE*				
(Mayne Pharma) *See METOCLOPRAMIDE*				
(Medisca) *See METOCLOPRAMIDE HCL*				
(Morton Grove) *See METOCLOPRAMIDE*				
(Mutual) *See METOCLOPRAMIDE*				
(Northstar) *See METOCLOPRAMIDE*				
(PCCA) *See METOCLOPRAMIDE HCL*				
(Pharm Assoc Inc) *See METOCLOPRAMIDE*				
(Precision Dose) *See METOCLOPRAMIDE*				
(Qualitest) *See METOCLOPRAMIDE*				
(Ranbaxy Pharm) *See METOCLOPRAMIDE*				
(Salix Pharm) *See METOZOLV ODT*				
(Silarx) *See METOCLOPRAMIDE*				
(Spectrum Pharmacy) *See METOCLOPRAMIDE HCL MONOHYDRATE*				
(Teva) *See METOCLOPRAMIDE*				
(UDL) *See METOCLOPRAMIDE*				
(Watson Labs) *See METOCLOPRAMIDE*				
(Palmetto)				
REPACK				
SOL, IV, 5 mg/ml, 2 ml	23490-5914-01	54.50		
TAB, PO, 5 mg, 30s ea	23490-5913-03	15.00		
60s ea	23490-5913-06	30.00		
90s ea	23490-5913-09	45.00		
10 mg, 12s ea	23490-5913-00	6.00		
20s ea	23490-5912-00	21.09		
30s ea	23490-5912-01	31.63		
60s ea	23490-5912-06	63.26		
90s ea	23490-5912-09	94.89		
(Quality Care Prod)				
REPACK				
TAB, PO, 5 mg, 30s ea	49999-0758-30	15.31		
(Stat Rx)				
REPACK				
TAB, PO, 5 mg, 30s ea	16590-0150-30	16.00		
60s ea	16590-0150-60	32.00		
90s ea	16590-0150-90	48.00		
10 mg, 30s ea	16590-0151-30	15.00		
60s ea	16590-0151-60	30.00		
90s ea	16590-0151-90	45.00		
METOLAZONE				
FUL				
TAB, PO, 2.5 mg, 100s ea		89.10		
5 mg, 100s ea		106.80		
10 mg, 100s ea		134.25		
(Mylan)				
TAB, PO, 2.5 mg, 100s ea	00378-6172-01	130.25		
5 mg, 100s ea	00378-6173-01	148.00		AB
10 mg, 100s ea	00378-6174-01	177.25		AB
(Sandoz)				
TAB, PO, 2.5 mg, 100s ea	00185-5050-01	130.37		AB
1000s ea	00185-5050-10	1303.70		AB
5 mg, 100s ea	00185-0055-01	148.15		AB
1000s ea	00185-0055-10	1481.50		AB
10 mg, 100s ea	00185-5600-01	177.38		AB
(UCB) *See ZAROXOLYN*				
(UDL)				
TAB, PO (USP, 10X10)				
2.5 mg, 100s ea UD	51079-0023-20	148.25		AB
(10X10)				
5 mg, 100s ea UD	51079-0024-20	168.50		AB
(Upstate Pharma)				
TAB, PO, 2.5 mg, 100s ea	65580-0643-71	128.92		
5 mg, 100s ea	65580-0644-71	146.50		
10 mg, 100s ea	65580-0645-71	175.41		
(DHS, Inc.)				
REPACK				
TAB, PO, 2.5 mg, 30s ea	55887-0328-30	79.96		
5 mg, 30s ea	55887-0864-30	133.32		
(McKesson Packaging)				
REPACK				
TAB, PO (USP)				
5 mg, 100s ea UD	63739-0404-10	148.15		

PROD/MFR	NDC	AWP	DP	OBC
(PD-Rx Pharm)				
REPACK				
TAB, PO, 2.5 mg, 30s ea	58864-0894-30	43.14		
(Phys Total Care)				
REPACK				
TAB, PO, 2.5 mg, 30s ea	54868-5104-00	56.85		
90s ea	54868-5104-01	126.57		
5 mg, 10s ea	54868-5056-00	32.73		
30s ea	54868-5056-02	71.22		
60s ea	54868-5056-01	139.41		
10 mg, 15s ea	54868-5119-00	78.57		
20s ea	54868-5119-01	80.04		AB
30s ea	54868-5119-02	117.78		
METOPIRONE (Novartis Pharm)				
metyrapone				
TAB, PO, 250 mg, 18s ea	00083-0133-11	60.97		
METOPROLOL (Core)				
REPACK				
metoprolol tartrate				
TAB, PO, 50 mg, 30s ea	33358-0242-30	23.43		
60s ea	33358-0242-60	46.86		
90s ea	33358-0242-90	56.88		
100s ea	33358-0242-00	78.11		
100 mg, 30s ea	33358-0243-30	32.77		
100s ea	33358-0243-00	93.60		
(DHS, Inc.)				
REPACK				
TAB, PO, 50 mg, 30s ea	55887-0474-30	13.26		
60s ea	55887-0474-60	26.52		
90s ea	55887-0474-90	39.78		
180s ea	55887-0474-92	75.00		
100 mg, 30s ea	55887-0274-30	20.70		
90s ea	55887-0274-90	62.11		
(HomeMed)				
REPACK				
TAB, PO, 50 mg, 30s ea	51655-0384-24	17.99		
60s ea	51655-0928-25	32.99		
(PD-Rx Pharm)				
REPACK				
TAB, PO, 25 mg, 30s ea	55289-0382-30	13.50		
(Phys Total Care)				
REPACK				
SOL, IV (SDV,10X5ML)				
1 mg/ml, 5 ml 10s	54868-5726-00	88.38		
(Quality Care Prod)				
REPACK				
TAB, PO, 25 mg, 30s ea	49999-0575-30	6.30		
(Southwood)				
REPACK				
SOL, IV (5MLX3)				
1 mg/ml, 5 ml 3s	58016-4996-01	28.80		
METOPROLOL SR (Vibranta)				
REPACK				
metoprolol succinate				
TER, PO, 25 mg, 30s ea	57866-7053-01	100.15		
50 mg, 30s ea	57866-7054-01	110.25		
100 mg, 30s ea	57866-7056-01	125.00		
METOPROLOL SUCCINATE				
(AstraZeneca) *See TOPROL XL*				
(Ethex)				
TER, PO (USP,10X10,FILM COATED)				
25 mg, 100s ea UD	58177-0293-11	95.50		AB
(USP,FILM COATED)				
25 mg, 100s ea	58177-0293-04	87.14		AB
1000s ea	58177-0293-09	871.40		AB
(USP,10X10,FILM COATED)				
50 mg, 100s ea UD	58177-0369-11	95.50		
(USP,FILM COATED)				
50 mg, 100s ea	58177-0369-04	90.13		
1000s ea	58177-0369-09	901.80		
(USP,10X10 CARDS)				
100 mg, 100s ea UD	58177-0368-11	135.37		AB
(USP,FILM COATED)				
100 mg, 100s ea	58177-0368-04	135.37		AB
1000s ea	58177-0368-09	1286.03		AB
200 mg, 100s ea	58177-0358-04	215.38		AB
1000s ea	58177-0358-09	2046.13		AB
(Par)				
TER, PO (FILM COATED)				
25 mg, 100s ea	49884-0404-01	105.38		
(USP,FILM COATED)				
25 mg, 1000s ea	49884-0404-10	1053.80		
(FILM COATED)				
50 mg, 100s ea	49884-0405-01	105.38		
(USP,FILM COATED)				
50 mg, 1000s ea	49884-0405-10	1053.80		

PROD/MFR	NDC	AWP	DP	OBC
(FILM COATED)				
100 mg, 100s ea	49884-0406-01	158.35		
(USP,FILM COATED)				
100 mg, 1000s ea	49884-0406-10	1583.51		
(FILM COATED)				
200 mg, 100s ea	49884-0407-01	251.95		
(USP,FILM COATED)				
200 mg, 1000s ea	49884-0407-10	2519.46		
(Sandoz)				
TER, PO (USP,FILM COATED)				
25 mg, 100s ea	00185-0281-01	87.14		AB
1000s ea	00185-0281-10	871.40		AB
(USP,FILM-COATED)				
50 mg, 100s ea	00185-0282-01	90.18		AB
1000s ea	00185-0282-10	901.80		AB
100 mg, 100s ea	00185-0283-01	143.65		AB
1000s ea	00185-0283-10	1436.49		AB
200 mg, 100s ea	00185-0284-01	228.56		AB
1000s ea	00185-0284-10	2285.55		AB
(Watson)				
TER, PO (USP,COATED)				
25 mg, 100s ea	62037-0830-01	89.93		AB
1000s ea	62037-0830-10	854.32		AB
50 mg, 100s ea	62037-0831-01	89.93		AB
1000s ea	62037-0831-10	854.32		AB
(A-S Medication)				
REPACK				
TER, PO (FILM COATED)				
25 mg, 30s ea	54569-5870-00	31.61		
50 mg, 30s ea	54569-5954-00	31.61		
100 mg, 30s ea	54569-5961-00	47.51		
(Dispensing Solutions)				
REPACK				
TER, PO, 25 mg, 100s ea	55045-3798-01	90.00		
(PD-Rx Pharm)				
REPACK				
TER, PO (FILM COATED)				
25 mg, 30s ea	43063-0210-30	108.60		
50 mg, 30s ea	43063-0211-30	116.34		
(Phys Total Care)				
REPACK				
TER, PO, 25 mg, 10s ea	54868-5729-04	40.58		
30s ea	54868-5729-00	85.34		
60s ea	54868-5729-01	164.68		
90s ea	54868-5729-02	244.01		
100s ea	54868-5729-03	268.96		
(FILM COATED)				
50 mg, 10s ea	54868-5730-05	40.58		
100s ea	54868-5730-04	186.56		
100 mg, 10s ea	54868-5731-04	57.97		
200 mg, 10s ea	54868-5732-01	35.33		AB
METOPROLOL SUCCINATE XL (Phys Total Care)				
metoprolol succinate				
TER, PO, 50 mg, 30s ea	54868-5730-00	88.28		
50s ea	54868-5730-02	104.75		
60s ea	54868-5730-01	172.07		
90s ea	54868-5730-03	169.71		
100 mg, 30s ea	54868-5731-00	115.41		
60s ea	54868-5731-01	148.65		
90s ea	54868-5731-02	220.72		
100s ea	54868-5731-03	243.25		
200 mg, 30s ea	54868-5732-00	140.64		
METOPROLOL TARTRATE				
FUL				
TAB, PO, 25 mg, 100s ea		7.20		
50 mg, 100s ea		5.00		
100 mg, 100s ea		6.90		
(Amer Regent)				
SOL, IV (25X5ML,USP,SDV)				
1 mg/ml, 5 ml 25s	00517-1355-25	31.25		
(Aurobindo Pharma)				
TAB, PO (USP,FILM-COATED)				
25 mg, 100s ea	65862-0062-01	24.25		AB
1000s ea	65862-0062-99	242.50		AB
50 mg, 100s ea	65862-0063-01	55.50		AB
1000s ea	65862-0063-99	544.30		AB
100 mg, 100s ea	65862-0064-01	80.10		AB
1000s ea	65862-0064-99	761.30		AB
(Bedford) *See AMERINET CHOICE METOPROLOL TARTRATE*				
(Bedford) *See METOPROLOL TARTRATE NOVAPLUS*				
(Bedford)				
SOL, IV (U.S.P.,S.D.V.)				
1 mg/ml, 5 ml 10s	55390-0073-10	24.00		AP
(Caraco)				
TAB, PO (FILM-COATED)				
25 mg, 100s ea	57664-0506-08	27.00		AB

PROD/MFR	NDC	AWP	DP	OBC
100s ea	57664-0506-52	27.00		AB
1000s ea	57664-0506-18	270.00		AB
1000s ea	57664-0506-58	270.00		AB
50 mg, 100s ea	57664-0166-08	55.50		AB
100s ea	57664-0166-52	55.50		AB
(FILM-COATED)				
50 mg, 100s ea	57664-0477-08	55.50		AB
100s ea	57664-0477-52	55.50		AB
1000s ea	57664-0166-18	544.30		AB
1000s ea	57664-0166-58	544.30		AB
(FILM-COATED)				
50 mg, 1000s ea	57664-0477-18	544.30		AB
1000s ea	57664-0477-58	544.30		AB
100 mg, 100s ea	57664-0167-08	80.10		AB
100s ea	57664-0167-52	80.10		AB
1000s ea	57664-0167-18	761.30		AB
1000s ea	57664-0167-58	761.30		AB
(Gallipot)				
POW, NA (U.S.P.)				
5 gm	51552-0915-02	19.25	13.75	
(Greenstone)				
TAB, PO (USP,FILM COATED)				
25 mg, 100s ea	59762-1300-01	24.25		
1000s ea	59762-1300-03	242.50		
50 mg, 100s ea	59762-1301-01	55.50		
1000s ea	59762-1301-03	544.30		
100 mg, 100s ea	59762-1302-01	80.10		
1000s ea	59762-1302-03	761.30		
(Hospira)				
SOL, IV (LUER LOCK,CARPUJECT)				
1 mg/ml, 5 ml 3s	00074-1778-35	14.26	12.48	AP
5 ml 3s	00409-1778-35	14.26	12.48	AP
(10X5ML,SDV,CARPUJECT)				
1 mg/ml, 5 ml 10s	00409-1778-05	11.16	9.80	AP
(12X5ML,LATEX-FREE)				
1 mg/ml, 5 ml 12s	00409-2285-05	17.86	15.60	AP
(AMP,LATEX-FREE)				
1 mg/ml, 5 ml 12s	00074-2285-05	16.99	14.88	AP
(Major)				
TAB, PO (10X10,USP,FILM-COATED)				
50 mg, 100s ea UD	00904-6033-61	57.00		AB
(USP,FILM-COATED)				
50 mg, 100s ea	00904-6033-60	50.65		AB
1000s ea	00904-6033-80	430.70		AB
(10X10,USP,FILM-COATED)				
100 mg, 100s ea UD	00904-6034-61	79.00		AB
(USP,FILM-COATED)				
100 mg, 100s ea	00904-6034-60	65.40		AB
1000s ea	00904-7947-80	647.25		AB
(USP,FILM-COATED)				
100 mg, 1000s ea	00904-6034-80	647.25		AB
(Medisca)				
POW, NA (U.S.P.)				
25 gm	38779-0578-04	135.00		
100 gm	38779-0578-05	459.00		
500 gm	38779-0578-08	1395.00		
(Mylan)				
TAB, PO (FILM-COATED)				
25 mg, 60s ea	00378-0018-91	14.55		
100s ea	00378-0018-01	24.25		
500s ea	00378-0018-05	121.25		
50 mg, 100s ea	00378-0032-01	55.50		AB
1000s ea	00378-0032-10	544.30		AB
100 mg, 100s ea	00378-0047-01	80.10		AB
1000s ea	00378-0047-10	761.30		AB
(Novartis Pharm) *See LOPRESSOR*				
(PCCA)				
POW, NA (U.S.P.)				
1 gm	51927-2697-00	5.52		
(Ranbaxy Pharm)				
TAB, PO (USP,FILM COATED)				
25 mg, 100s ea	63304-0579-01	24.25		AB
1000s ea	63304-0579-10	235.22		AB
50 mg, 100s ea	63304-0580-01	55.50		AB
1000s ea	63304-0580-10	544.30		AB
100 mg, 100s ea	63304-0581-01	80.10		AB
1000s ea	63304-0581-10	761.30		AB
(Sandoz)				
SOL, IV, 1 mg/ml, 5 ml 10s	00781-3070-95	45.83		AP
(10X5ML)				
1 mg/ml, 5 ml 10s	00781-3071-95	45.83		AP
TAB, PO (CAPLET)				
50 mg, 1000s ea	00781-1223-10	527.25		AB
100 mg, 100s ea	00781-1228-01	80.10		AB
1000s ea	00781-1228-10	760.95		AB

PROD/MFR	NDC	AWP	DP	OBC
(Spectrum Pharmacy)				
POW, NA (U.S.P.)				
5 gm	49452-4718-01	88.55		
25 gm	49452-4718-02	239.05		
100 gm	49452-4718-03	714.00	102.50	
(UDL) *See METOPROLOL TARTRATE*				
(UDL)				
TAB, PO (USP,25X1,ROBOT READY)				
25 mg, 25s ea UD	51079-0255-19	6.06		AB
(USP, 10X10,FILM-COATED)				
25 mg, 100s ea UD	51079-0255-20	24.25		AB
(25X1, ROBOT READY)				
50 mg, 25s ea UD	51079-0801-19	14.29		AB
(10X10)				
50 mg, 100s ea UD	51079-0801-20	57.17		AB
METOPROLOL TARTRATE (UDL)				
(USP,PUNCH CARDS,10X30)				
50 mg, 300s ea UD	51079-0801-56	171.51		AB
METOPROLOL TARTRATE (UDL)				
(ROBOT READY 25X1)				
100 mg, 25s ea UD	51079-0802-19	20.63		AB
(10X10)				
100 mg, 100s ea UD	51079-0802-20	82.50		AB
(Watson Labs)				
TAB, PO, 50 mg, 100s ea	00591-0462-01	55.50		AB
1000s ea	00591-0462-10	544.30		AB
100 mg, 100s ea	00591-0463-01	80.10		AB
1000s ea	00591-0463-10	761.30		AB
(West-Ward)				
SOL, IV (1X5ML,USP)				
1 mg/ml, 5 ml	00143-9873-10	24.05		
(A-S Medication)				
REPACK				
TAB, PO, 50 mg, 30s ea	54569-3787-00	16.53		AB
60s ea	54569-3787-01	33.06		AB
(CAPLET)				
100 mg, 30s ea	54569-3788-00	23.59		AB
60s ea	54569-3788-01	47.18		AB
(Altura)				
REPACK				
TAB, PO, 50 mg, 10s ea	63874-0406-10	5.90		
14s ea	63874-0406-14	8.26		
15s ea	63874-0406-15	8.85		
20s ea	63874-0406-20	11.80		
28s ea	63874-0406-28	16.52		
30s ea	63874-0406-30	17.70		
60s ea	63874-0406-60	35.40		
100s ea	63874-0406-01	59.00		
100 mg, 10s ea	63874-0407-10	8.70		AB
15s ea	63874-0407-15	13.05		AB
20s ea	63874-0407-20	17.40		AB
30s ea	63874-0407-30	26.10		AB
60s ea	63874-0407-60	52.20		AB
90s ea	63874-0407-90	78.30		AB
100s ea	63874-0407-01	87.00		AB
(American Health)				
REPACK				
TAB, PO (10X10,USP)				
25 mg, 100s ea UD	62584-0265-01	10.78		
50 mg, 100s ea UD	62584-0266-01	7.35		AB
100 mg, 100s ea UD	62584-0267-01	10.92		AB
(AQ)				
REPACK				
TAB, PO, 50 mg, 15s ea	66105-0994-15	8.33		
30s ea	66105-0994-03	16.65		
60s ea	66105-0994-06	33.30		
100s ea	66105-0994-10	55.50		
1000s ea	66105-0994-11	544.30		
100 mg, 15s ea	66105-0996-15	12.02		
30s ea	66105-0996-03	24.03		
60s ea	66105-0996-06	48.06		
100s ea	66105-0996-10	80.10		
1000s ea	66105-0996-11	761.30		
(Bryant Ranch)				
REPACK				
TAB, PO, 50 mg, 30s ea	63629-1463-02	22.86		
60s ea	63629-1463-03	45.72		
100s ea	63629-1463-01	76.20		
120s ea	63629-1463-04	69.99		
100 mg, 30s ea	63629-1462-01	31.97		
100s ea	63629-1462-02	91.32		
(Dispensing Solutions)				
REPACK				
TAB, PO, 50 mg, 30s ea	55045-2282-08	15.00		
30s ea	55045-3762-08	15.00		
30s ea	66336-0523-30	19.98		AB
50s ea	55045-2282-07	25.00		
60s ea	55045-2282-09	30.00		

PROD/MFR	NDC	AWP	DP	OBC
60s ea	66336-0523-60	39.96		AB
90s ea	55045-2282-06	45.00		
90s ea	66336-0523-90	59.94		AB
100s ea	55045-2282-00	50.00		AB
120s ea	55045-2282-02	60.00		
100 mg, 30s ea	55045-2217-08	24.00		
30s ea	66336-0514-30	28.84		AB
60s ea	55045-2217-09	48.00		
60s ea	66336-0514-60	57.67		
90s ea	55045-2217-06	72.00		
90s ea	66336-0514-90	86.51		AB
100s ea	55045-2217-00	80.00		
120s ea	55045-2217-02	96.00		
(GSMS)				
REPACK				
TAB, PO (UNIT OF USE)				
50 mg, 30s ea	60429-0126-30	5.88	1.96	AB
60s ea	60429-0126-60	9.63	3.21	AB
100 mg, 30s ea	60429-0127-30	8.73	2.91	AB
(McKesson Packaging)				
REPACK				
TAB, PO (USP)				
25 mg, 100s ea UD	63739-0405-10	27.00		
50 mg, 100s ea UD	63739-0428-10	9.60		AB
(Palmetto)				
REPACK				
TAB, PO, 50 mg, 30s ea	23490-5921-01	28.99		
60s ea	23490-5921-02	57.98		
100 mg, 30s ea	23490-5920-00	43.53		
90s ea	23490-5920-01	130.59		
(PD-Rx Pharm)				
REPACK				
TAB, PO (USP,FILM-COATED)				
25 mg, 180s ea	55289-0382-93	40.20		
(REDI-SCRIPT)				
50 mg, 28s ea	58864-0016-28	21.42		AB
30s ea	55289-0413-30	22.03		AB
(REDI-SCRIPT)				
50 mg, 30s ea	58864-0016-30	22.02		AB
(FILM-COATED)				
50 mg, 60s ea	55289-0413-60	32.67		AB
(USP)				
50 mg, 60s ea	58864-0016-60	7.99		AB
90s ea	55289-0413-90	42.99		AB
(REDI-SCRIPT)				
50 mg, 100s ea	58864-0016-01	50.01		AB
180s ea	55289-0413-93	75.99		AB
(FILM-COATED)				
50 mg, 270s ea	55289-0413-94	106.98		AB
100 mg, 30s ea	55289-0093-30	18.60		AB
(REDI-SCRIPT)				
100 mg, 30s ea	58864-0695-30	18.60		AB
90s ea	55289-0093-90	36.87		AB
100s ea	43063-0006-01	80.10		AB
(USP)				
100 mg, 180s ea	55289-0093-93	93.00		AB
(Pharma Pac)				
REPACK				
TAB, PO (FILM-COATED)				
50 mg, 30s ea	52959-0839-30	30.70		AB
60s ea	52959-0839-60	58.05		
(Phys Total Care)				
REPACK				
TAB, PO (FILM-COATED)				
25 mg, 30s ea	54868-5021-00	7.08		AB
60s ea	54868-5021-01	11.16		AB
100s ea	54868-5021-02	15.12		AB
50 mg, 10s ea	54868-2989-04	4.38		EE
15s ea	54868-2989-06	5.07		AB
30s ea	54868-2989-02	7.17		EE
60s ea	54868-2989-03	11.34		EE
90s ea	54868-2989-05	15.51		EE
100s ea	54868-2989-00	15.39		EE
100 mg, 30s ea	54868-2990-00	8.73		EE
45s ea	54868-2990-04	12.60		EE
60s ea	54868-2990-03	14.46		EE
100s ea	54868-2990-02	22.11		EE
(Physician Partner)				
REPACK				
TAB, PO (FILM-COATED)				
25 mg, 180s ea	21695-0494-78	102.71		AB
50 mg, 30s ea	21695-0298-30	31.63		
(CAPLET)				
50 mg, 90s ea	21695-0298-90	94.89		AB
180s ea	21695-0298-78	235.06		AB
100 mg, 30s ea	21695-0299-30	48.06		
(CAPLET)				
100 mg, 90s ea	21695-0299-90	144.18		AB
100s ea	21695-0299-00	160.20		

PROD/MFR	NDC	AWP	DP	OBC
(Quality Care Prod)				
REPACK				
TAB, PO, 25 mg, 10s ea	49999-0575-10	2.10		
(FILM-COATED)				
25 mg, 20s ea	49999-0575-20	4.20		AB
50 mg, 30s ea	35356-0415-30	20.16		AB
30s ea	49999-0010-30	20.16		EE
60s ea	49999-0010-60	39.96		EE
100s ea	49999-0010-00	68.60		EE
100 mg, 30s ea	49999-0226-30	28.50		AB
60s ea	49999-0226-60	57.10		
100s ea	49999-0226-00	95.17		AB
(Southwood)				
REPACK				
TAB, PO, 50 mg, 30s ea	58016-0442-30	16.65		EE
60s ea	58016-0442-60	33.30		EE
90s ea	58016-0442-90	49.95		EE
100s ea	58016-0442-00	55.50		EE
120s ea	58016-0442-02	66.60		EE
180s ea	58016-0442-99	99.90		EE
(Stat Rx)				
REPACK				
TAB, PO, 50 mg, 30s ea	16590-0317-30	25.75		AB
60s ea	16590-0317-60	51.50		AB
90s ea	16590-0317-90	68.50		AB
120s ea	16590-0317-72	79.00		AB
100 mg, 30s ea	16590-0428-30	23.50		AB
60s ea	16590-0428-60	47.00		AB
90s ea	16590-0428-90	62.00		AB
120s ea	16590-0428-72	75.00		AB
(Vibranta)				
REPACK				
TAB, PO, 25 mg, 60s ea	57866-3155-01	46.50		
50 mg, 30s ea	57866-6578-01	17.70		
60s ea	57866-6578-02	7.55		AB
(CAPLET)				
100 mg, 30s ea	57866-6579-01	26.10		
90s ea	57866-6579-03	14.10		AB
METOPROLOL TARTRATE AND HYDROCHLOROTHIAZIDE (Sandoz)				
hydrochlorothiazide/metoprolol tartrate				
TAB, PO (USP)				
25 mg-50 mg,				
100s ea	00781-5630-01	113.40		
25 mg-100 mg,				
100s ea	00781-5631-01	177.25		
(Phys Total Care)				
REPACK				
TAB, PO (USP)				
25 mg-100 mg,				
10s ea	54868-5524-01	59.73		
30s ea	54868-5524-00	131.19		
METOPROLOL TARTRATE NOVAPLUS (Bedford)				
metoprolol tartrate				
SOL, IV (USP,SDV,PRIVATE LABEL)				
1 mg/ml, 5 ml 10s	55390-0348-10	15.60		AP
METOZOLV ODT (Salix Pharm)				
metoclopramide hydrochloride				
ODT, PO (10X10,MINT)				
5 mg, 100s ea UD	65649-0431-02	132.00		
10 mg, 100s ea UD	65649-0432-02	132.00		
METROCREAM (Galderma)				
metronidazole				
CRE, TP, 0.75%, 45 gm	00299-3836-45	280.63		
(Phys Total Care)				
REPACK				
CRE, TP, 0.75%, 45 gm	54868-3825-00	76.18		
METROGEL (Galderma)				
metronidazole				
GEL, TP, 1%, ea	00299-3820-04	201.25		
60 gm	00299-3820-60	201.25		
(A-S Medication)				
REPACK				
GEL, TP (1X60GM)				
1%, 60 gm	54569-6108-00	230.41		
(Phys Total Care)				
REPACK				
GEL, TP, 0.75%, 30 gm	54868-0943-00	47.19		
45 gm	54868-0943-01	93.69		
(1X60GM)				
1%, 60 gm	54868-5585-01	230.66		
60 gm	54868-5948-00	230.66		
(Quality Care Prod)				
REPACK				
GEL, VG (WITH APPLICATOR)				
0.75%, 70 gm	49999-0208-70	143.07		

PROD/MFR	NDC	AWP	DP	OBC
METROGEL-VAGINAL (Graceway)				
metronidazole				
GEL, VG (1X70GM)				
0.75%, 70 gm	29336-0200-25	36.00		AB
(A-S Medication)				
REPACK				
GEL, VG, 0.75%, 70 gm	54569-3660-00	37.50		
(Phys Total Care)				
REPACK				
GEL, VG, 0.75%, 70 gm	54868-3110-00	96.25		
(Southwood)				
REPACK				
GEL, VG, 0.75%, 70 gm	58016-3517-01	36.00		AB
METROLOTION (Galderma)				
metronidazole				
LOT, TP, 0.75%, 59 ml	00299-3838-02	293.13		
(Phys Total Care)				
REPACK				
LOT, TP, 0.75%, 60 ml	54868-4454-00	124.63		
METRONIDAZOLE				
FUL				
CRE, TP, 0.75%, 45 gm		73.18		
GEL, TP, 0.75%, 45 gm		69.38		
LOT, TP, 0.75%, 59 ml		69.00		
TAB, PO, 250 mg, 100s ea		8.49		
500 mg, 100s ea		21.84		
(Actavis Mid Atlantic)				
CRE, TP (1X45GM)				
0.75%, 45 gm	00472-0911-45	84.57		AB
LOT, TP (1X59ML)				
0.75%, 59 ml	00472-0912-02	98.99		AB
(B. Braun) *See METRONIDAZOLE*				
METRONIDAZOLE (B. Braun)				
metronidazole				
SOL, IV (150 ML PAB CONTAINER)				
500 mg/100 ml,				
100 ml	00264-5535-32	2.50		AP
METRONIDAZOLE (Baxter)				
SOL, IV, 500 mg/100 ml,				
100 ml 24s	00338-1055-48	368.16		AP
(Claris)				
SOL, IV (24X100ML,SINGLEDOSE,USP)				
500 mg/100 ml,				
100 ml 24s	36000-0001-24	61.44		AP
(Dermik) *See NORITATE*				
(Fougera)				
CRE, TP, 0.75%, 45 gm	00168-0323-46	70.37		
GEL, TP (USP)				
0.75%, 45 gm	00168-0275-45	71.15		AB
LOT, TP, 0.75%, 59 ml	00168-0383-60	90.00		
(Galderma) *See METROCREAM*				
(Galderma) *See METROGEL*				
(Galderma) *See METROLOTION*				
(Gallipot)				
POW, NA (U.S.P.)				
10 gm	51552-0038-03	11.76		
25 gm	51552-0038-04	16.45		
100 gm	51552-0038-05	44.10		
500 gm	51552-0038-06	182.00		
(Graceway) *See METROGEL-VAGINAL*				
(Harris)				
CRE, TP (1X45GM)				
0.75%, 45 gm	67405-0110-45	30.19		AB
(Hawkins)				
POW, NA (U.S.P.)				
25 gm	63370-0152-25	49.20		
100 gm	63370-0152-35	148.80		
500 gm	63370-0152-45	633.60		
(Hospira)				
SOL, IV (S.D.V.,LATEX-FREE)				
500 mg/100 ml,				
100 ml 24s	00409-7811-24	71.71	62.64	AP
(LIFECARE,QUAD PACK)				
500 mg/100 ml,				
100 ml 80s	00409-7811-37	205.44	180.00	AP
(Letco)				
POW, NA (U.S.P.)				
25 gm	62991-1685-01	30.00		
100 gm	62991-1685-02	75.00		
500 gm	62991-1685-03	270.00		
(Major)				
TAB, PO (10X10)				
250 mg, 100s ea UD	00904-1453-61	47.81		AB

PROD/MFR	NDC	AWP	DP	OBC
(Medisca)				
POW, NA (U.S.P.)				
25 gm	**38779-0146-04**	40.50		
100 gm	**38779-0146-05**	105.00		
500 gm	**38779-0146-08**	435.00		
1000 gm	**38779-0146-09**	780.00		
(PCCA)				
POW, NA (U.S.P.)				
1 gm	**51927-1449-00**	1.80		
(Pfizer) *See FLAGYL*				
(Pfizer) *See FLAGYL 375*				
(Pfizer) *See FLAGYL ER*				
(Pfizer)				
SOL, IV (24X100ML,USP)				
500 mg/100 ml,				
100 ml 24s	**00069-2390-01**	62.40	52.00	EE
(Prasco Labs)				
GEL, VG (W/5 APPLICATORS)				
0.75%, 70 gm	**66993-0935-70**	33.71		
(Sagent)				
SOL, IV (USP,24X100ML,PF)				
500 mg/100 ml,				
100 ml 24s	**25021-0131-82**	74.70		**AP**
(Sandoz)				
GEL, TP (USP)				
0.75%, 45 gm	**00781-7078-19**	71.15		**AB**
VG (W/ 5 VAG APPLICATORS)				
0.75%, 70 gm	**00781-7077-87**	65.90		**AB**
(Spectrum Pharmacy)				
POW, NA (U.S.P.)				
25 gm	**49452-4726-01**	69.65		
100 gm	**49452-4726-02**	164.50		
500 gm	**49452-4726-03**	682.50		
(Taro)				
GEL, TP (USP)				
0.75%, 45 gm	**51672-4116-06**	71.15		**AB**
(Teva)				
CAP, PO, 375 mg, 50s ea	**50111-0884-05**	234.46		**AB**
TAB, PO, 250 mg, 100s ea	**50111-0333-01**	43.39		**AB**
(10X10)				
250 mg, 100s ea UD	**00182-1330-89**	62.63		**AB**
250s ea	**50111-0333-06**	105.22		**AB**
500s ea	**50111-0333-02**	206.10		**AB**
500 mg, 100s ea	**50111-0334-01**	72.79		**AB**
(10X10)				
500 mg, 100s ea UD	**00182-1517-89**	114.01		**AB**
500s ea	**50111-0334-02**	345.75		**AB**
(UDL)				
TAB, PO (ROBOT READY 25X1)				
250 mg, 25s ea UD	**51079-0122-19**	13.86		**AB**
(10X10)				
250 mg, 100s ea UD	**51079-0122-20**	55.45		**AB**
(ROBOT READY 25X1)				
500 mg, 25s ea UD	**51079-0126-19**	20.74		**AB**
(10X10)				
500 mg, 100s ea UD	**51079-0126-20**	82.94		**AB**
(Upsher-Smith) *See VANDAZOLE*				
(Watson Labs)				
TAB, PO (USP)				
250 mg, 100s ea	**00591-3969-01**	10.06		**AB**
250s ea	**00591-3969-25**	24.66		**AB**
500s ea	**00591-3969-05**	47.76		**AB**
500 mg, 50s ea	**00591-3970-50**	10.06		**AB**
500s ea	**00591-3970-05**	98.94		**AB**
(West-Ward)				
SOL, IV (24X100ML,USP)				
500 mg/100 ml,				
100 ml 24s	**00143-9772-26**	60.00		**AP**
(A-S Medication)				
REPACK				
GEL, VG, 0.75%, 70 gm	**54569-5871-00**	65.90		
TAB, PO, 250 mg, 14s ea	**54569-0965-08**	6.08		**AB**
21s ea	**54569-0965-00**	9.12		**AB**
28s ea	**54569-0965-01**	12.15		**EE**
30s ea	**54569-0965-02**	13.02		**EE**
500 mg, 4s ea	**54569-0967-00**	2.91		**EE**
14s ea	**54569-0967-03**	10.19		**EE**
20s ea	**54569-0967-09**	14.56		**EE**
21s ea	**54569-0967-04**	15.29		**EE**
28s ea	**54569-0967-06**	20.38		**EE**
42s ea	**54569-3354-02**	30.57		**AB**
(Altura)				
REPACK				
TAB, PO, 250 mg, 5s ea	**63874-0313-05**	6.85		**AB**
8s ea	**63874-0313-08**	10.44		**AB**
9s ea	**63874-0313-09**	12.34		**AB**

PROD/MFR	NDC	AWP	DP	OBC
10s ea	**63874-0313-10**	13.70		**AB**
12s ea	**63874-0313-12**	16.45		**AB**
14s ea	**63874-0313-14**	19.19		**AB**
20s ea	**63874-0313-20**	27.43		**AB**
21s ea	**63874-0313-21**	28.79		**AB**
25s ea	**63874-0313-25**	34.28		**AB**
28s ea	**63874-0313-28**	38.39		**AB**
30s ea	**63874-0313-30**	41.13		**AB**
40s ea	**63874-0313-40**	54.84		**AB**
42s ea	**63874-0313-42**	57.58		**AB**
50s ea	**63874-0313-50**	65.55		**AB**
56s ea	**63874-0313-56**	76.77		**AB**
60s ea	**63874-0313-60**	82.25		**AB**
100s ea	**63874-0313-01**	137.11		**AB**
250s ea	**63874-0313-06**	342.80		**AB**
500 mg, 7s ea	**63874-0314-07**	17.38		
9s ea	**63874-0314-09**	22.35		
10s ea	**63874-0314-10**	24.83		
12s ea	**63874-0314-12**	29.80		
14s ea	**63874-0314-14**	33.11		
15s ea	**63874-0314-15**	37.25		
18s ea	**63874-0314-18**	44.70		
20s ea	**63874-0314-20**	49.67		
21s ea	**63874-0314-21**	52.15		
24s ea	**63874-0314-24**	59.60		
28s ea	**63874-0314-28**	69.51		
30s ea	**63874-0314-30**	74.50		
40s ea	**63874-0314-40**	99.33		
50s ea	**63874-0314-50**	124.16		
100s ea	**63874-0314-01**	248.33		
(American Health)				
REPACK				
TAB, PO (USP,10X10)				
250 mg, 100s ea UD	**68084-0130-01**	15.37		**AB**
(Apace)				
REPACK				
TAB, PO, 500 mg, 4s ea	**15338-0150-04**	2.76		**AB**
14s ea	**15338-0150-14**	7.90		**AB**
(Bryant Ranch)				
REPACK				
TAB, PO, 250 mg, 20s ea	**63629-1388-03**	11.54		
21s ea	**63629-1388-01**	12.12		
30s ea	**63629-1388-02**	17.31		
60s ea	**63629-1388-04**	33.89		
500 mg, 14s ea	**63629-1386-03**	13.55		
20s ea	**63629-1386-01**	19.36		
21s ea	**63629-1386-05**	20.33		
30s ea	**63629-1386-02**	29.04		
56s ea	**63629-1386-04**	54.21		
(Core)				
REPACK				
CAP, PO, 375 mg, 50s ea	**33358-0245-50**	173.90		
TAB, PO, 250 mg, 5s ea	**33358-0244-05**	6.69		
10s ea	**33358-0244-10**	13.38		
14s ea	**33358-0244-14**	18.74		
20s ea	**33358-0244-20**	26.77		
21s ea	**33358-0244-21**	28.11		
25s ea	**33358-0244-25**	33.47		
28s ea	**33358-0244-28**	37.47		
30s ea	**33358-0244-30**	40.15		
500 mg, 7s ea	**33358-0246-07**	17.41		
10s ea	**33358-0246-10**	24.24		
14s ea	**33358-0246-14**	33.93		
15s ea	**33358-0246-15**	36.37		
18s ea	**33358-0246-18**	43.63		
20s ea	**33358-0246-20**	48.48		
21s ea	**33358-0246-21**	48.86		
24s ea	**33358-0246-24**	58.18		
28s ea	**33358-0246-28**	67.86		
30s ea	**33358-0246-30**	72.72		
(DHS, Inc.)				
REPACK				
TAB, PO, 250 mg, 9s ea	**55887-0788-09**	11.96		
14s ea	**55887-0788-14**	18.06		
21s ea	**55887-0788-21**	27.09		
30s ea	**55887-0788-30**	38.70		**AB**
500 mg, 4s ea	**55887-0789-04**	9.17		
9s ea	**55887-0789-09**	20.89		
14s ea	**55887-0789-14**	32.09		**AB**
20s ea	**55887-0789-20**	45.84		**AB**
21s ea	**55887-0789-21**	48.13		
28s ea	**55887-0789-28**	64.18		
30s ea	**55887-0789-30**	68.76		**AB**
(Dispensing Solutions)				
REPACK				
TAB, PO, 250 mg, 14s ea	**66336-0592-14**	10.51		**AB**
21s ea	**55045-1128-09**	26.67		**AB**
21s ea	**66336-0592-21**	15.77		**AB**
28s ea	**55045-1128-07**	35.55		**AB**
28s ea	**66336-0592-28**	21.05		**AB**
40s ea	**55045-1128-08**	50.80		

PROD/MFR	NDC	AWP	DP	OBC
500 mg, 4s ea	**55045-1220-04**	9.35		**AB**
4s ea	**66336-0507-44**	5.47		**AB**
14s ea	**55045-1220-05**	32.76		**AB**
14s ea	**66336-0507-14**	19.15		**AB**
20s ea	**55045-3307-07**	46.80		
21s ea	**55045-1220-00**	49.14		
21s ea	**66336-0507-21**	28.73		**AB**
28s ea	**55045-1220-09**	65.52		**AB**
30s ea	**55045-1220-07**	70.20		
30s ea	**66336-0507-30**	41.04		**AB**
40s ea	**55045-1220-08**	93.60		
60s ea	**55045-3307-06**	140.40		
90s ea	**55045-3307-09**	210.60		
100s ea	**55045-3307-01**	234.00		
120s ea	**55045-3307-02**	280.80		
(GSMS)				
REPACK				
TAB, PO (UNIT OF USE)				
250 mg, 28s ea	**60429-0128-28**	11.40	3.80	**AB**
(HomeMed)				
REPACK				
TAB, PO, 250 mg, 21s ea	**51655-0123-28**	27.39		**EE**
28s ea	**51655-0123-29**	6.40		**EE**
30s ea	**51655-0123-24**	39.29		**EE**
500 mg, 4s ea	**51655-0189-89**	9.76		**EE**
14s ea	**51655-0189-84**	39.89		**EE**
28s ea	**51655-0189-29**	64.95		**EE**
(Keltman Pharma., Inc.)				
REPACK				
TAB, PO, 500 mg, 20s ea	**68387-0191-20**	15.70		
(McKesson Packaging)				
REPACK				
TAB, PO (USP)				
250 mg, 100s ea UD	**63739-0175-10**	43.39		**AB**
500 mg, 100s ea UD	**63739-0176-10**	72.79		
(Palmetto)				
REPACK				
GEL, VG, 0.75%, 70 gm	**23490-5923-01**	73.63		
TAB, PO, 250 mg, 4s ea	**23490-5924-05**	8.38		
8s ea	**23490-5924-01**	12.58		
14s ea	**23490-5924-02**	18.34		
21s ea	**23490-5924-03**	27.50		
28s ea	**23490-5924-04**	36.67		
500 mg, 2s ea	**23490-5925-01**	8.52		
4s ea	**23490-5925-04**	9.47		
14s ea	**23490-5925-02**	33.13		
20s ea	**23490-5925-06**	47.32		
21s ea	**23490-5925-05**	49.69		
30s ea	**23490-5925-03**	70.99		
40s ea	**23490-5925-07**	94.64		
(PD-Rx Pharm)				
REPACK				
TAB, PO (USP)				
250 mg, 6s ea	**43063-0108-06**	5.78		**AB**
8s ea	**55289-0172-08**	8.18		**AB**
20s ea	**58864-0354-20**	10.44		**AB**
21s ea	**55289-0172-21**	10.62		**AB**
21s ea	**58864-0354-21**	10.62		**AB**
28s ea	**55289-0172-28**	11.94		**AB**
30s ea	**55289-0172-30**	12.31		**AB**
56s ea	**55289-0172-56**	17.20		**AB**
500 mg, 4s ea	**43063-0021-04**	9.76		**AB**
4s ea	**55289-0521-04**	9.76		**AB**
8s ea	**55289-0521-08**	9.84		**AB**
10s ea	**55289-0521-10**	9.89		**AB**
14s ea	**55289-0521-14**	12.98		**AB**
(REDI-SCRIPT)				
500 mg, 14s ea	**58864-0355-14**	12.98		**AB**
20s ea	**58864-0355-20**	15.56		**AB**
21s ea	**55289-0521-21**	16.13		**AB**
28s ea	**55289-0521-28**	16.29		**AB**
30s ea	**55289-0521-30**	16.33		**AB**
30s ea	**58864-0355-30**	16.34		**AB**
40s ea	**55289-0521-40**	19.56		**AB**
(REDI-SCRIPT)				
500 mg, 40s ea	**58864-0355-40**	19.56		**AB**
100s ea UD	**55289-0521-17**	67.02		**AB**
(Pharma Pac)				
REPACK				
TAB, PO, 250 mg, 15s ea	**52959-0400-15**	20.69		**EE**
21s ea	**52959-0400-21**	28.56		**EE**
28s ea	**52959-0400-28**	37.49		**EE**
30s ea	**52959-0400-30**	40.18		**EE**
40s ea	**52959-0400-40**	53.03		**EE**
56s ea	**52959-0400-56**	73.36		**EE**
500 mg, 4s ea	**52959-0102-04**	9.77		**EE**
8s ea	**52959-0102-08**	19.53		**EE**
14s ea	**52959-0102-14**	34.18		**EE**
15s ea	**52959-0102-15**	36.62		**EE**
20s ea	**52959-0102-20**	48.82		**EE**

PROD/MFR	NDC	AWP	DP	OBC
21s ea	52959-0102-21	51.26		EE
28s ea	52959-0102-28	68.35		EE
30s ea	52959-0102-30	73.23		EE
42s ea	52959-0102-42	102.51		EE
(Phys Total Care)				
REPACK				
CRE, TP, 0.75%, 45 gm	54868-5655-00	115.92		
LOT, TP (1X59ML)				
0.75%, 59 ml	54868-5882-00	158.26		
TAB, PO, 250 mg, 10s ea	54868-0108-02	4.65		EE
(USP)				
250 mg, 14s ea	54868-0108-08	7.05		EE
20s ea	54868-0108-03	6.30		EE
21s ea	54868-0108-01	6.45		EE
30s ea	54868-0108-06	7.92		EE
100s ea	54868-0108-07	19.44		EE
500s ea	54868-0108-00	87.78		EE
500 mg, 10s ea	54868-0158-03	13.86		EE
14s ea	54868-0158-01	17.61		EE
20s ea	54868-0158-05	23.22		EE
30s ea	54868-0158-08	32.58		EE
40s ea	54868-0158-06	41.97		EE
500s ea	54868-0158-09	146.88		EE
(Physician Partner)				
REPACK				
TAB, PO, 250 mg, 21s ea	21695-0308-21	21.44		
28s ea	21695-0308-28	24.30		
30s ea	21695-0308-30	26.03		AB
500 mg, 14s ea	21695-0309-14	22.78		
21s ea	21695-0309-21	34.17		
30s ea	21695-0309-30	41.49		AB
56s ea	21695-0309-56	77.44		AB
(Quality Care Prod)				
REPACK				
TAB, PO, 250 mg, 21s ea	49999-0313-21	32.91		AB
28s ea	49999-0313-28	43.88		AB
30s ea	49999-0313-30	47.01		AB
100s ea	49999-0313-00	156.70		AB
500 mg, 4s ea	49999-0095-04	7.57		EE
14s ea	49999-0095-14	39.72		AB
20s ea	49999-0095-20	37.83		EE
21s ea	49999-0095-21	59.73		AB
28s ea	49999-0095-28	79.44		AB
30s ea	49999-0095-30	85.11		EE
100s ea	49999-0095-00	283.71		AB
(Southwood)				
REPACK				
TAB, PO, 250 mg, 5s ea	58016-0129-05	6.53		EE
8s ea	58016-0129-08	10.45		EE
9s ea	58016-0129-09	11.75		EE
10s ea	58016-0129-10	13.05		EE
12s ea	58016-0129-12	15.67		EE
14s ea	58016-0129-14	18.28		EE
20s ea	58016-0129-20	26.12		EE
21s ea	58016-0129-21	27.42		EE
25s ea	58016-0129-25	32.65		EE
28s ea	58016-0129-28	36.56		EE
30s ea	58016-0129-30	39.17		EE
100s ea	58016-0129-00	130.58		EE
500 mg, 7s ea	58016-0725-07	16.55		EE
9s ea	58016-0725-09	21.29		EE
10s ea	58016-0725-10	23.65		EE
12s ea	58016-0725-12	28.38		EE
14s ea	58016-0725-14	33.10		EE
15s ea	58016-0725-15	35.48		EE
18s ea	58016-0725-18	42.57		EE
20s ea	58016-0725-20	47.30		EE
21s ea	58016-0725-21	49.67		EE
24s ea	58016-0725-24	56.76		EE
28s ea	58016-0725-28	66.20		EE
30s ea	58016-0725-30	70.95		EE
100s ea	58016-0725-00	236.50		EE
(Stat Rx)				
REPACK				
TAB, PO, 500 mg, 4s ea	16590-0152-04	2.78		AB
10s ea	16590-0152-10	14.50		
14s ea	16590-0152-14	20.30		
20s ea	16590-0152-20	28.50		
28s ea	16590-0152-28	39.76		
30s ea	16590-0152-30	42.50		
(Vibranta)				
REPACK				
TAB, PO, 500 mg, 4s ea	57866-4033-03	5.85		AB
14s ea	57866-4033-01	20.81		AB
20s ea	57866-4033-06	34.40		
METRONIDAZOLE BENZOATE (Gallipot)				
POW, NA, 25 gm	51552-0465-04	35.00		
100 gm	51552-0465-05	98.00		

PROD/MFR	NDC	AWP	DP	OBC
(Hawkins)				
POW, NA (B.P.)				
10 gm	63370-0155-20	57.60		
25 gm	63370-0155-25	120.00		
100 gm	63370-0155-35	336.00		
500 gm	63370-0155-45	1104.00		
1000 gm	63370-0155-50	1824.00		
(Letco)				
POW, NA, 25 gm	62991-1103-02	57.00		
100 gm	62991-1103-03	150.00		
1000 gm	62991-1103-04	900.00		
(Medisca)				
POW, NA (B.P.)				
10 gm	38779-0238-01	46.50		
25 gm	38779-0238-04	82.50		
100 gm	38779-0238-05	232.50		
500 gm	38779-0238-08	780.00		
1000 gm	38779-0238-09	1230.00		
(PCCA)				
POW, NA (BP)				
1 gm	51927-1559-00	5.10		
(Spectrum Pharmacy)				
POW, NA (BP)				
10 gm	49452-4727-04	89.60		
(B.P.)				
25 gm	49452-4727-02	124.60		
100 gm	49452-4727-03	333.20		
(BP)				
1000 gm	49452-4727-05	1582.00		
METYRAPONE				
(Novartis Pharm) *See METOPIRONE*				
METYROSINE				
(Aton) *See DEMSER*				
MEVACOR (Merck)				
lovastatin				
TAB, PO (UNIT OF USE)				
20 mg, 60s ea	00006-0731-61	162.34		
40 mg, 60s ea	00006-0732-61	292.24		AB
(PD-Rx Pharm)				
REPACK				
TAB, PO, 20 mg, 30s ea	55289-0400-30	120.65		
40 mg, 30s ea	55289-0548-30	217.17		AB
(Phys Total Care)				
REPACK				
TAB, PO, 10 mg, 30s ea	54868-1968-00	54.38		AB
20 mg, 30s ea	54868-0686-01	94.46		
60s ea	54868-0686-03	176.76		
90s ea	54868-0686-04	264.21		
90s ea	54868-4585-02	85.95		AB
100s ea	54868-0686-02	294.37		
100s ea	54868-4585-03	93.27		AB
40 mg, 30s ea	54868-1087-01	159.29		
60s ea	54868-1087-00	316.69		
MEXAR (Hawthorn Pharm)				
sulfacetamide sodium				
SOA, TP (WASH)				
10%, 170 ml	63717-0035-06	41.79		
MEXILETINE (Quality Care Prod)				
REPACK				
mexiletine hydrochloride				
CAP, PO, 150 mg, 90s ea	49999-0916-90	97.73		
250 mg, 90s ea	49999-0917-90	133.74		
MEXILETINE HCL (Medisca)				
mexiletine hydrochloride				
POW, NA (U.S.P.)				
25 gm	38779-2134-04	255.00		
100 gm	38779-2134-05	780.00		
(PCCA)				
POW, NA (U.S.P.)				
1 gm	51927-2953-00	7.44		
(Teva)				
CAP, PO, 150 mg, 100s ea	00093-8739-01	90.49		AB
180s ea	58016-0740-99	133.56		AB
200 mg, 100s ea	00093-8740-01	107.15		AB
250 mg, 100s ea	00093-8741-01	123.83		AB
(Phys Total Care)				
REPACK				
CAP, PO, 150 mg, 60s ea	54868-3776-01	42.99		EE
100s ea	54868-3776-00	67.14		EE
(Southwood)				
REPACK				
CAP, PO, 150 mg, 20s ea	58016-0740-20	14.84		AB

PROD/MFR	NDC	AWP	DP	OBC
30s ea	58016-0740-30	22.26		AB
60s ea	58016-0740-60	44.52		AB
90s ea	58016-0740-90	66.78		AB
100s ea	58016-0740-00	74.20		AB
120s ea	58016-0740-02	89.04		AB
240s ea	58016-0740-04	178.08		AB
MEXILETINE HYDROCHLORIDE				
FUL				
CAP, PO, 200 mg, 100s ea		97.12		
(Medisca) *See MEXILETINE HCL*				
(PCCA) *See MEXILETINE HCL*				
(Teva) *See MEXILETINE HCL*				
(Altura)				
REPACK				
CAP, PO, 150 mg, 90s ea	63874-1078-09	100.17		
(Dispensing Solutions)				
REPACK				
CAP, PO, 150 mg, 90s ea	55045-3634-01	81.90		
100s ea	55045-3634-02	91.00		
200 mg, 100s ea	55045-3651-01	107.00		
250 mg, 90s ea	55045-3635-01	111.60		
100s ea	55045-3635-02	124.00		
MI-OMEGA NF (Midlothian Labs)				
nutriceutical				
CAP, PO, 60s ea	68308-0502-60	65.83	46.08	
MIACALCIN (Novartis Pharm)				
calcitonin (salmon)				
SOL, IJ (VIAL)				
200 iu/ml, 2 ml	00078-0149-23	61.46		AP
SPR, NS, 200 iu/actuation,				
3.7 ml	00078-0311-54	134.03		
(Phys Total Care)				
REPACK				
SPR, NS, 200 iu/actuation,				
3.7 ml	54868-3827-01	106.79		
MIBOLERONE (Medisca)				
POW, NA (1X1GM)				
1 gm, C-III	38779-2331-06	1125.00		
(1X5GM)				
5 gm, C-III	38779-2331-03	4485.00		
(1X500MG)				
500 ml, C-III	38779-2331-00	735.00		
MICAFUNGIN SODIUM				
(Astellas) *See MYCAMINE*				
MICARDIS (Boehr Ingelheim Phar)				
telmisartan				
TAB, PO (BLISTER CARD,4X7)				
20 mg, 28s ea	00597-0039-28	50.98		
(3X10)				
20 mg, 30s ea UD	00597-0039-37	98.64		
(BLISTER CARD,3X10)				
40 mg, 30s ea	00597-0040-37	98.64		
80 mg, 30s ea	00597-0041-37	98.64		
(AQ)				
REPACK				
TAB, PO, 40 mg, 28s ea	66105-0842-28	59.92		
30s ea	66105-0842-03	64.20		
60s ea	66105-0842-06	128.40		
90s ea	66105-0842-09	192.60		
100s ea	66105-0842-10	214.00		
(Phys Total Care)				
REPACK				
TAB, PO, 40 mg, 30s ea	54868-4539-01	114.76		
80 mg, 30s ea	54868-4605-01	114.76		
90s ea	54868-4605-02	322.22		
(Quality Care Prod)				
REPACK				
TAB, PO, 20 mg, 30s ea	35356-0295-30	127.00		
40 mg, 30s ea	35356-0296-30	127.21		
80 mg, 30s ea	35356-0298-30	149.76		
MICARDIS HCT (Boehr Ingelheim Phar)				
hydrochlorothiazide/telmisartan				
TAB, PO (BLISTER CARD,3X10)				
12.5 mg-40 mg,				
30s ea	00597-0043-37	98.64		
12.5 mg-80 mg,				
30s ea	00597-0044-37	98.64		
25 mg-80 mg,				
30s ea	00597-0042-37	98.64		
(A-S Medication)				
REPACK				
TAB, PO, 12.5 mg-80 mg,				
30s ea UD	54569-5665-00	93.75		

PROD/MFR	NDC	AWP	DP	OBC

(Phys Total Care)
REPACK
TAB, PO, 12.5 mg-40 mg,
30s ea 54868-5418-00 114.76
12.5 mg-80 mg,
30s ea 54868-4540-01 114.76
25 mg-80 mg,
30s ea 54868-5297-00 127.88

(Southwood)
REPACK
TAB, PO, 12.5 mg-80 mg,
28s ea 58016-4631-01 81.16

MICONAZOLE (Medisca)
POW, NA (1X5GM,USP)
5 gm 38779-0239-03 32.55
(U.S.P.)
25 gm 38779-0239-04 112.50
100 gm 38779-0239-05 387.00

(PCCA)
POW, NA (BASE; U.S.P.)
1 gm 51927-2094-00 6.30

(Spectrum Pharmacy)
CRY, NA (U.S.P.)
5 gm 49452-4723-01 82.95
25 gm 49452-4723-02 176.40
100 gm 49452-4723-03 581.00

MICONAZOLE NIT (Vibranta)
REPACK
miconazole nitrate
CRE, TP, 2%, 30 gm 57866-7016-01 64.80

MICONAZOLE NITRATE
(Actavis Mid Atlantic) *See MICONAZOLE-3*

(Gallipot)
POW, NA (U.S.P.,N.F.)
5 gm 51552-0122-02 27.93
25 gm 51552-0122-04 50.40
100 gm 51552-0122-05 165.20

(Hawkins)
POW, NA (U.S.P.)
25 gm 63370-0156-25 104.00
100 gm 63370-0156-35 340.00

(Medisca)
POW, NA (U.S.P.)
10 gm 38779-0038-01 52.50
25 gm 38779-0038-04 87.00
100 gm 38779-0038-05 297.00
500 gm 38779-0038-08 1125.00

(PCCA)
POW, NA (USP)
1 gm 51927-1154-00 5.10

(Spectrum Pharmacy)
POW, NA (U.S.P.)
5 gm 49452-4775-01 86.45
25 gm 49452-4775-02 141.05
100 gm 49452-4775-03 455.00
1000 gm 49452-4775-06 1582.00

(A-S Medication)
REPACK
CRE, TP, 2%, 15 gm 54569-5980-00 3.50

MICONAZOLE NITRATE/PETROLATUM, WHITE/ZINC OXIDE
(Stiefel Labs) *See VUSION*

MICONAZOLE-3 (Actavis Mid Atlantic)
miconazole nitrate
SUP, VG, 200 mg, 3s ea ... 00472-1738-03 49.23 AB

MICRHOGAM ULTRA-FILTERED (Ortho-Clinical)
rho(d) immune globulin
SOL, IM (PF)
1 ml 00562-7808-01 54.36
(SRN,~50MCG ANTI-RHO,PF)
1 ml 5s 00562-7808-06 271.80
1 ml 25s 00562-7808-26 1359.00

MICRHOGAM ULTRA-FILTERED PLUS (Ortho-Clinical)
rho(d) immune globulin
SOL, IM (PF,LATEX-FREE)
50 mcg, ea 00562-7806-01 60.34
5s ea 00562-7806-05 301.68
25s ea 00562-7806-25 1508.40

MICRO-K (Ther-RX)
potassium chloride
CER, PO, 8 meq, 100s ea .. 64011-0010-04 80.34 AB
(DIS-CO-PACKS)
8 meq, 100s ea UD ... 64011-0010-11 84.47 AB
500s ea .... 64011-0010-08 396.19 AB

(PD-Rx Pharm)
REPACK
CER, PO, 10 meq, 30s ea .. 55289-0899-30 27.38 AB

(Phys Total Care)
REPACK
CER, PO, 8 meq, 30s ea ... 54868-1851-01 10.14 AB

MICRO-K 10 (Ther-RX)
potassium chloride
CER, PO, 10 meq, 100s ea . 64011-0009-04 84.76 AB
(DIS-CO PACK)
10 meq, 100s ea UD .. 64011-0009-11 88.94 AB
500s ea .... 64011-0009-08 420.95 AB

MICROBORE PRIMARY PUMP W/OL (Abbott Hosp)
tubing, connecting
DEV, NA (60" DISTAL TUBING)
24s ea 00074-1169-02 533.09 533.04

MICROCRYSTALLINE CELLULOSE (Letco)
cellulose, microcrystalline
POW, NA (NF,AVICEL PH 105)
500 gm 62991-2007-01 63.00
2500 gm 62991-2007-02 222.00

(PCCA)
POW, NA (NF, (PH-105))
1 gm 51927-1130-00 0.15
(NF)
1 gm 51927-2460-00 1.20

MICROGESTIN 1.5/30 (Watson)
ethinyl estradiol/norethindrone acetate
TAB, PO (COMPACK,6X21)
30 mcg-1.5 mg,
126s ea .... 52544-0951-21 173.61 AB

MICROGESTIN 1/20 (Watson)
ethinyl estradiol/norethindrone acetate
TAB, PO (COMPACK,6X21)
20 mcg-1 mg,
126s ea .... 52544-0950-21 171.94 AB

MICROGESTIN FE 1.5/30 (Watson)
ethinyl estradiol/ferrous fum/norethindrone ace
TAB, PO (6X28)
30 mcg-75 mg-1.5 mg,
168s ea .... 52544-0631-28 173.61 AB

(Phys Total Care)
REPACK
TAB, PO (COMPACK)
30 mcg-75 mg-1.5 mg,
168s ea .... 54868-4745-00 78.45 AB

MICROGESTIN FE 1/20 (Watson)
ethinyl estradiol/ferrous fum/norethindrone ace
TAB, PO (6X28)
20 mcg-75 mg-1 mg,
168s ea .... 52544-0630-28 171.94 AB

(A-S Medication)
REPACK
TAB, PO, 20 mcg-75 mg-1 mg,
28s ea 54569-5797-00 28.66

(Physician Partner)
REPACK
TAB, PO, 20 mcg-75 mg-1 mg,
28s ea .... 21695-0856-01 57.31 AB

MICRONASE (Pfizer)
glyburide
TAB, PO, 2.5 mg,
100s ea UD .... 00009-0141-02 69.90 58.25 AB

(Pharma Pac)
REPACK
TAB, PO, 5 mg, 30s ea .... 52959-0177-30 24.20 AB

(Phys Total Care)
REPACK
TAB, PO, 1.25 mg, 60s ea .. 54868-1688-01 22.96 AB
2.5 mg, 20s ea .... 54868-1244-04 17.86 AB
30s ea .... 54868-1244-01 25.85 AB
60s ea .... 54868-1244-03 49.83 AB
100s ea .... 54868-1244-02 71.68 AB

MICRONIZED COLESTIPOL HYDROCHLORIDE
(Greenstone)
colestipol hydrochloride, micronized
TAB, PO, 1 gm, 120s ea ... 59762-0450-01 78.94

(Phys Total Care)
REPACK
TAB, PO (MICRONIZED)
1 gm, 30s ea 54868-0610-01 66.18

MICROPORE PLUS SURGICAL PAPER
(3M Health Care)
tape, adhesive
DEV, NA (3"X10 YDS W/DISPENSER)
4s ea 08333-1536-03 10.90
(3"X10 YDS)
4s ea 08333-1532-03 9.30
(2"X10 YDS W/DISPENSER)
6s ea 08333-1536-02 10.90
(2"X10 YDS)
6s ea 08333-1532-02 9.30
(1"X10 YDS W/DISPENSER)
12s ea 08333-1536-01 10.90
(1"X10 YDS)
12s ea 08333-1532-01 9.30
(1/2"X10 YDS W/DISPENSER)
24s ea 08333-1536-00 10.90
(1/2"X10 YDS)
24s ea 08333-1532-00 9.30

MICROTHENE FN50100 (PCCA)
polyethylene
POW, NA (1X1GM)
1 gm 51927-3218-00 0.20

MICROZIDE (Watson)
hydrochlorothiazide
CAP, PO (HARD GELATIN)
12.5 mg, 100s ea ..... 52544-0622-01 95.06 AB

MIDAMOR (Paddock)
amiloride hydrochloride
TAB, PO (COMPRESSED)
5 mg, 100s ea .... 00574-0291-01 150.50 EE

MIDAZOLAM (Gallipot)
POW, NA, 0.5 gm, C-IV 51552-1023-09 588.00 420.00

(PCCA)
POW, NA (CIV)
1 gm, C-IV 51927-3265-00 2010.00

(Spectrum Pharmacy)
CRY, NA (BP,EP)
0.5 gm, C-IV 49452-4722-03 1190.00
1 gm, C-IV 49452-4722-04 1837.50
5 gm, C-IV 49452-4722-01 7563.50

(Pharma Pac)
REPACK
midazolam hydrochloride
SYR, PO (1X118ML)
2 mg/ml,
118 ml, C-IV 52959-0915-01 131.10

(Phys Total Care)
REPACK
SOL, IJ (10X2ML)
1 mg/ml,
2 ml 10s, C-IV 54868-5711-00 61.15

MIDAZOLAM HCL (Baxter)
midazolam hydrochloride
SOL, IJ, 1 mg/ml,
2 ml, C-IV .... 10019-0028-36 0.72 AP
(1X2ML)
1 mg/ml,
2 ml, C-IV .... 10019-0028-59 0.78 AP
(10X2ML)
1 mg/ml,
2 ml 10s, C-IV ..... 10019-0028-01 7.80 AP
2 ml 10s, C-IV ..... 10019-0028-02 7.44 AP
(25X2ML)
1 mg/ml,
2 ml 25s, C-IV ..... 10019-0028-04 19.50 AP
(DOSETTE)
1 mg/ml,
2 ml 25s, C-IV ..... 10019-0028-03 18.00 AP
5 ml, C-IV .... 10019-0028-37 1.67 AP
(M.D.V.)
1 mg/ml,
5 ml 10s, C-IV ..... 10019-0028-05 16.68 AP
10 ml, C-IV .... 10019-0028-39 2.64 AP
(M.D.V.)
1 mg/ml,
10 ml 10s, C-IV .... 10019-0028-10 26.40 AP
5 mg/ml,
1 ml, C-IV .... 10019-0027-37 1.25 AP
(1X1ML)
5 mg/ml,
1 ml, C-IV .... 10019-0027-64 1.44 AP
(10X1ML)
5 mg/ml,
1 ml 10s, C-IV ..... 10019-0027-01 12.00 AP
1 ml 10s, C-IV ..... 10019-0027-06 14.40 AP
(25X1ML)
5 mg/ml,
1 ml 25s, C-IV ..... 10019-0027-09 36.00 AP

PROD/MFR	NDC	AWP	DP	OBC
(DOSETTE)				
5 mg/ml,				
1 ml 25s, C-IV	10019-0027-03	31.20		AP
2 ml, C-IV	10019-0027-36	1.58		AP
(1X2ML)				
5 mg/ml,				
2 ml, C-IV	10019-0027-59	1.50		AP
(10X2ML)				
5 mg/ml,				
2 ml 10s, C-IV	10019-0027-02	15.84		AP
2 ml 10s, C-IV	10019-0027-07	15.00		AP
(25X2ML)				
5 mg/ml,				
2 ml 25s, C-IV	10019-0027-08	37.50		AP
(DOSETTE)				
5 mg/ml,				
2 ml 25s, C-IV	10019-0027-04	33.90		AP
10 ml, C-IV	10019-0027-39	8.28		AP
(M.D.V.)				
5 mg/ml,				
10 ml 10s, C-IV	10019-0027-10	82.80		AP
(Bedford)				
SOL, IJ (SDV, W/O PRESERVATIVE)				
1 mg/ml,				
2 ml 10s, C-IV	55390-0137-02	10.14		AP
5 ml 10s, C-IV	55390-0137-05	18.00		AP
(VIAL,PF)				
1 mg/ml,				
10 ml 10s, C-IV	55390-0125-10	36.00		AP
(SDV, W/O PRESERVATIVE)				
5 mg/ml,				
1 ml 10s, C-IV	55390-0138-01	18.00		AP
2 ml 10s, C-IV	55390-0138-02	36.00		AP
(VIAL,PF)				
5 mg/ml,				
5 ml 10s, C-IV	55390-0126-05	90.00		AP
10 ml 10s, C-IV	55390-0126-10	180.00		AP
(Hospira)				
SOL, IJ (LUER LOCK,STERILE,PF)				
1 mg/ml,				
2 ml 10s, C-IV	00409-2306-62	14.76	12.90	AP
(VIAL, FLIPTOP,PF)				
1 mg/ml,				
2 ml 10s, C-IV	00409-2305-02	5.28	4.60	AP
(PF)				
1 mg/ml,				
5 ml 10s, C-IV	00409-2305-05	9.96	8.70	AP
(10X1ML,PF,CARPUJECT)				
5 mg/ml,				
1 ml 10s, C-IV	00409-2307-60	23.04	20.20	AP
(10X1ML,PF)				
5 mg/ml,				
1 ml 10s, C-IV	00409-2308-01	11.28	9.90	AP
(VIAL)				
5 mg/ml,				
1 ml 10s, C-IV	61703-0321-42	15.60	13.65	AP
(VIAL,FLIPTOP,PF)				
5 mg/ml,				
2 ml 10s, C-IV	00409-2308-02	19.32	16.90	AP
(VIAL)				
5 mg/ml,				
2 ml 10s, C-IV	61703-0321-07	30.00	26.25	AP
(VIAL,FLIPTOP,LATEX-FREE)				
5 mg/ml,				
5 ml 10s, C-IV	00074-2596-03	72.60	63.50	AP
5 ml 10s, C-IV	00409-2596-03	70.80	62.00	AP
(VIAL)				
5 mg/ml,				
5 ml 10s, C-IV	61703-0321-53	74.22	64.94	AP
(VIAL, FLIPTOP)				
5 mg/ml,				
10 ml 10s, C-IV	00409-2596-05	75.24	65.80	AP
(VIAL)				
5 mg/ml,				
10 ml 10s, C-IV	61703-0321-32	138.36	121.07	AP
(Paddock)				
SYR, PO (W/ORAL DISPENSERS)				
2 mg/ml,				
118 ml, C-IV	00574-0150-04	81.25		AA
(Parenta Pharma)				
SOL, IJ, 1 mg/ml,				
10 ml, C-IV	66758-0018-01	7.08	5.90	AP
10 ml 10s, C-IV	66758-0018-02	70.80	59.00	AP
5 mg/ml,				
10 ml, C-IV	66758-0019-01	31.12	25.93	EE
10 ml 10s, C-IV	66758-0019-02	311.20	259.30	EE

PROD/MFR	NDC	AWP	DP	OBC
(Ranbaxy Pharm)				
SYR, PO, 2 mg/ml,				
118 ml, C-IV	63304-0205-18	129.50	98.10	AA
(Roxane)				
SYR, PO (WITH ORAL DISPENSERS)				
2 mg/ml,				
118 ml, C-IV	00054-3566-99	127.15		AA
(Dispensing Solutions)				
REPACK				
SOL, IJ (10X2ML)				
1 mg/ml,				
2 ml 10s, C-IV	55045-2887-02	24.14		AP
(Phys Total Care)				
REPACK				
SOL, IJ (VIAL,PF)				
5 mg/ml,				
5 ml 10s, C-IV	54868-4580-00	309.18		EE
MIDAZOLAM HCL AMERINET CHOICE (Hospira)				
midazolam hydrochloride				
SOL, IJ (VIAL,FLIPTOP,PF)				
1 mg/ml,				
2 ml 10s, C-IV	00409-2305-61	4.68	4.10	AP
5 ml 10s, C-IV	00409-2305-62	9.72	8.50	AP
MIDAZOLAM HCL NOVATION (Hospira)				
midazolam hydrochloride				
SOL, IJ (10X2ML,PF)				
1 mg/ml,				
2 ml 10s, C-IV	00409-2305-49	5.04	4.40	AP
(FTV,10X5ML,PF)				
1 mg/ml,				
5 ml 10s, C-IV	00409-2305-50	9.36	8.20	AP
(FLIPTOP VIAL,PF)				
5 mg/ml,				
1 ml 10s, C-IV	00409-2308-49	8.40	7.40	AP
(VIAL,FLIPTOP,PF)				
5 mg/ml,				
2 ml 10s, C-IV	00409-2308-50	8.16	7.10	AP
(FTV,10X10ML,LATEX-FREE)				
5 mg/ml,				
10 ml 10s, C-IV	00409-2596-53	68.64	60.10	AP
MIDAZOLAM HYDROCHLORIDE				
FUL				
SYR, PO, 2 mg/ml, 118 ml		97.50		
(APP)				
SOL, IJ (M.D.V.)				
1 mg/ml,				
2 ml, C-IV	63323-0411-12	5.55		AP
(M.D.V,25X5ML)				
1 mg/ml,				
5 ml 25s, C-IV	63323-0411-25	305.00		AP
(M.D.V.)				
1 mg/ml,				
10 ml, C-IV	63323-0411-10	21.81		AP
((M.D.V.),25X1ML)				
5 mg/ml,				
1 ml 25s, C-IV	63323-0412-25	89.50		AP
(M.D.V.)				
5 mg/ml,				
2 ml, C-IV	63323-0412-02	21.81		AP
5 ml, C-IV	63323-0412-05	51.49		AP
10 ml, C-IV	63323-0412-10	95.90		AP
(Baxter) *See MIDAZOLAM HCL*				
(Bedford) *See MIDAZOLAM HCL*				
(Cura Pharm)				
SOL, IJ (10X2ML,SINGLE-DOSE,PF)				
1 mg/ml,				
2 ml 10s, C-IV	66860-0130-02	22.00		AP
(10X2ML)				
1 mg/ml,				
2 ml 10s, C-IV	66860-0140-02	22.00		AP
(10X5ML)				
1 mg/ml,				
5 ml 10s, C-IV	66860-0141-02	122.20		AP
(10X10ML)				
1 mg/ml,				
10 ml 10s, C-IV	66860-0142-02	38.40		AP
(10X1ML,SINGLE-DOSE,PF)				
5 mg/ml,				
1 ml 10s, C-IV	66860-0132-02	35.00		AP
(10X2ML,SINGLE-DOSE,PF)				
5 mg/ml,				
2 ml 10s, C-IV	66860-0133-02	35.00		AP
(10X5ML)				
5 mg/ml,				
5 ml 10s, C-IV	66860-0145-02	51.49		AP
(10X10ML)				
5 mg/ml,				
10 ml 10s, C-IV	66860-0146-02	95.50		AP
(Hospira) *See MIDAZOLAM HCL*				

PROD/MFR	NDC	AWP	DP	OBC
(Hospira) *See MIDAZOLAM HCL AMERINET CHOICE*				
(Hospira) *See MIDAZOLAM HCL NOVATION*				
(Hospira) *See NOVAPLUS MIDAZOLAM HCL*				
(Hospira) *See NOVAPLUS MIDAZOLAM HYDROCHLORIDE*				
(Hospira)				
SOL, IJ (10X2ML,PF)				
1 mg/ml,				
2 ml 10s, C-IV	00409-2306-22	14.16	12.40	AP
(10X10ML,FLIPTOPVIAL)				
1 mg/ml,				
10 ml 10s, C-IV	00409-2587-05	30.60	26.80	AP
(10X1ML,PF)				
5 mg/ml,				
1 ml 10s, C-IV	00409-2307-21	14.16	12.40	AP
(Paddock) *See MIDAZOLAM HCL*				
(Parenta Pharma) *See MIDAZOLAM HCL*				
(Ranbaxy Pharm) *See MIDAZOLAM HCL*				
(Roxane) *See MIDAZOLAM HCL*				
(Wockhardt USA)				
SOL, IJ (10X2ML)				
1 mg/ml,				
2 ml 10s, C-IV	64679-0762-01	7.38		AP
(10X5ML)				
1 mg/ml,				
5 ml 10s, C-IV	64679-0762-02	17.28		AP
(10X10ML)				
1 mg/ml,				
10 ml 10s, C-IV	64679-0762-03	36.05		AP
(10X1ML)				
5 mg/ml,				
1 ml 10s, C-IV	64679-0763-01	16.28		AP
(10X2ML)				
5 mg/ml,				
2 ml 10s, C-IV	64679-0763-02	31.28		AP
(10X5ML)				
5 mg/ml,				
5 ml 10s, C-IV	64679-0763-03	77.38		AP
(10X10ML)				
5 mg/ml,				
10 ml 10s, C-IV	64679-0763-04	144.08		AP
(Dispensing Solutions)				
REPACK				
SOL, IJ, 5 mg/ml,				
1 ml 10s, C-IV	55045-2857-01	42.50		
(Palmetto)				
REPACK				
SOL, IJ, 1 mg/ml,				
2 ml, C-IV	23490-5932-01	2.50		
5 mg/ml, 2 ml, C-IV	23490-5933-01	2.50		
(10X10ML)				
5 mg/ml,				
10 ml 10s, C-IV	23490-5933-02	48.50		
(Phys Total Care)				
REPACK				
SOL, IJ (1X2ML,MDV)				
1 mg/ml,				
2 ml, C-IV	54868-6092-01	7.42		AP
(25X2ML,MDV)				
1 mg/ml,				
2 ml 25s, C-IV	54868-6092-00	117.65		AP
(Quality Care Prod)				
REPACK				
SOL, IJ (1X10ML)				
1 mg/ml,				
10 ml, C-IV	35356-0482-10	13.00		AP
MIDODRINE HCL (Global Pharm)				
midodrine hydrochloride				
TAB, PO, 2.5 mg, 100s ea.	00115-4211-01	120.10		AB
5 mg, 100s ea.	00115-4222-01	241.80		AB
10 mg, 100s ea	00115-4233-01	483.64		AB
(Mylan)				
TAB, PO, 2.5 mg, 100s ea.	00378-1901-01	120.10		
5 mg, 100s ea.	00378-1902-01	241.80		
10 mg, 100s ea	00378-1903-01	483.60		
(Sandoz)				
TAB, PO, 2.5 mg, 100s ea.	00185-0040-01	120.22		AB
5 mg, 100s ea.	00185-0043-01	242.06		AB
500s ea.	00185-0043-05	1210.28		AB
10 mg, 100s ea	00185-0149-01	483.60		
(Upsher-Smith)				
TAB, PO, 2.5 mg, 100s ea.	00245-0211-11	120.82		AB

PROD/MFR	NDC	AWP	DP	OBC
5 mg, ea	00245-0212-89	2.62		AB
100s ea	00245-0212-11	243.01		AB
(10X10)				
5 mg, 100s ea UD	00245-0212-01	262.45		AB
10 mg, 100s ea	00245-0213-11	486.02		AB
(Phys Total Care)				
REPACK				
TAB, PO, 5 mg, 10s ea	54868-5435-01	42.21		AB
90s ea	54868-5435-00	249.66		AB
MIDODRINE HYDROCHLORIDE				
FUL				
TAB, PO, 2.5 mg, 100s ea		111.72		
5 mg, 100s ea		183.83		
10 mg, 100s ea		313.38		
(Apotex Corp.)				
TAB, PO, 2.5 mg, 100s ea	60505-1320-01	120.82		AB
1000s ea	60505-1320-08	1208.20		AB
5 mg, 100s ea	60505-1321-01	243.01		AB
1000s ea	60505-1321-08	2430.10		AB
10 mg, 100s ea	60505-1325-01	486.02		AB
1000s ea	60505-1325-08	4860.20		AB
(Global Pharm) *See MIDODRINE HCL*				
(Mylan) *See MIDODRINE HCL*				
(Sandoz) *See MIDODRINE HCL*				
(Shire US Inc.) *See PROAMATINE*				
(UDL)				
TAB, PO (10X10)				
5 mg, 100s ea UD	51079-0453-20	270.98		AB
(Upsher-Smith) *See MIDODRINE HCL*				
(American Health)				
REPACK				
TAB, PO (10X10)				
2.5 mg, 100s ea UD	68084-0240-01	143.13		AB
5 mg, 100s ea UD	68084-0241-01	205.23		AB
(Phys Total Care)				
REPACK				
TAB, PO, 2.5 mg, 90s ea	54868-5930-00	122.19		AB
(Physician Partner)				
REPACK				
TAB, PO, 10 mg, 100s ea	21695-0181-00	967.20		
MIDRIN (Caraco)				
apap/dichloralphenazone/isometheptene mucate				
CAP, PO, 325 mg-100 mg-65 mg,				
100s ea, C-IV	14508-0304-08	74.99		
(Phys Total Care)				
REPACK				
CAP, PO, 325 mg-100 mg-65 mg,				
30s ea, C-IV	54868-1435-03	23.94		
50s ea, C-IV	54868-1435-01	38.65		
60s ea, C-IV	54868-1435-00	46.00		
100s ea, C-IV	54868-1435-02	74.80		
(Quality Care Prod)				
REPACK				
CAP, PO, 325 mg-100 mg-65 mg,				
4s ea, C-IV	35356-0447-04	12.00		
30s ea, C-IV	35356-0447-30	90.08		
60s ea, C-IV	35356-0447-60	175.87		
90s ea, C-IV	35356-0447-90	261.67		
MIFEPREX (Danco Labs.)				
mifepristone				
TAB, PO (S.D. BLISTER PACK)				
200 mg, 3s ea	64875-0001-03	270.00	270.00	
MIFEPRISTONE				
(Danco Labs.) *See MIFEPREX*				
MIGERGOT (G&W)				
caffeine/ergotamine tartrate				
SUP, RC, 100 mg-2 mg,				
12s ea	00713-0166-12	77.05		
MIGLITOL				
(Pfizer) *See GLYSET*				
MIGLUSTAT				
(Actelion Pharm) *See ZAVESCA*				
MIGRANAL (Valeant Pharm Intl)				
dihydroergotamine mesylate				
SPR, NS (VIAL W/SPRAYER)				
4 mg/ml, 1 ml 8s	00187-0245-03	756.86		
MIGRATEN (Azur Pharma, Inc.)				
acetaminophen/caffeine/isometheptene mucate				
CAP, PO, 325 mg-100 mg-65 mg,				
100s ea	66663-0112-01	166.26		

PROD/MFR	NDC	AWP	DP	OBC
MIGRAZONE (Breckenridge Pharm)				
apap/dichloralphenazone/isometheptene mucate				
CAP, PO, 325 mg-100 mg-65 mg,				
100s ea, C-IV	51991-0395-01	53.00		
MILK THISTLE				
(Medisca) *See SILYMARIN*				
(PCCA)				
POW, NA (SILYBUM MARIANUM)				
1 gm	51927-2419-00	1.80		
MILK THISTLE SEED (PCCA)				
POW, NA, 1 gm	51927-3517-00	0.54		
MILLIPRED (Laser Pharma)				
prednisolone sodium phosphate				
SOL, PO (1X237ML,AF,DYE-FREE)				
10 mg/5 ml, 237 ml	16477-0510-08	77.50		
(Laser Pharma)				
prednisolone				
TAB, PO, 5 mg, 100s ea	16477-0505-01	39.50		
MILLIPRED DP (Laser Pharma)				
prednisolone				
TAB, PO (1X21)				
5 mg, 21s ea UD	16477-0505-21	22.50		EE
MILNACIPRAN HYDROCHLORIDE				
(Forest Pharm) *See SAVELLA*				
(Forest Pharm) *See SAVELLA TITRATION PACK*				
MILRINONE LACTATE (Apotex Corp.)				
SOL, IV (PF)				
1 mg/ml, 10 ml 10s	60505-0718-00	147.50		AP
20 ml 10s	60505-0718-01	295.00		AP
(APP)				
SOL, IV (S.D.V.)				
1 mg/ml, 10 ml	63323-0617-10	94.80		AP
20 ml	63323-0617-20	171.70		AP
50 ml	63323-0617-50	432.00		AP
(Baxter)				
SOL, IV (SDV,PF)				
1 mg/ml, 10 ml	10019-0070-10	7.50		AP
(S.D.V.,PF)				
1 mg/ml, 10 ml 10s	10019-0070-01	75.00		AP
(SDV,PF)				
1 mg/ml, 20 ml	10019-0070-20	11.72		AP
(S.D.V.,PF)				
1 mg/ml, 20 ml 10s	10019-0070-02	117.24		AP
(Bedford) *See MILRINONE LACTATE NOVAPLUS*				
(Bedford)				
SOL, IV (S.D.V.)				
1 mg/ml, 10 ml 10s	55390-0019-10	144.00		AP
20 ml 10s	55390-0020-10	288.00		AP
50 ml	55390-0021-01	78.00		AP
(Hospira)				
SOL, IV (VIAL,FLIPTOP,LATEX-FREE)				
1 mg/ml, 10 ml 25s	00074-2775-01	328.50	287.50	AP
(VIAL,FLIPTOP,PF)				
1 mg/ml, 20 ml 25s	00409-2775-02	655.50	573.50	AP
(Hospira)				
dextrose/milrinone lactate				
(10X100ML,LATEX-FREE)				
5%-20 mg/100 ml,				
100 ml 10s	00409-2776-23	202.20	176.90	AP
(IN 5% DEXTROSE,10X200ML)				
5%-20 mg/100 ml,				
200 ml 10s	00409-2776-02	481.56	421.40	AP
MILRINONE LACTATE (Mayne Pharma)				
SOL, IV (PF,LATEX-FREE)				
1 mg/ml, 10 ml 10s	61703-0242-32	118.56	103.74	
20 ml 10s	61703-0242-21	232.80	203.70	
50 ml	61703-0242-50	59.40	51.98	
(Teva)				
SOL, IV (S.D.V.)				
1 mg/ml, 50 ml	00703-8008-01	246.25		
MILRINONE LACTATE IN DEXTROSE (Bedford)				
dextrose/milrinone lactate				
SOL, IV (10X100ML,SINGLE DOSE)				
5%-20 mg/100 ml,				
100 ml 10s	55390-0078-01	240.00		AP
(10X200ML,SINGLE DOSE)				
5%-20 mg/100 ml,				
200 ml 10s	55390-0079-01	480.00		AP
MILRINONE LACTATE NOVAPLUS (Bedford)				
milrinone lactate				
SOL, IV (S.D.V.,PRIVATE LABEL)				
1 mg/ml, 10 ml 10s	55390-0074-10	67.20		AP
20 ml 10s	55390-0075-10	135.60		AP
50 ml	55390-0076-01	34.80		AP

PROD/MFR	NDC	AWP	DP	OBC
MIMYX (Stiefel Labs)				
cream, multi ingredient				
CRE, TP (PF,FRAGRANCE-FREE)				
140 gm	00145-4200-02	116.28		
(Quality Care Prod)				
REPACK				
CRE, TP (1X140GM,PF)				
140 gm	35356-0232-14	214.09		
MINERAL OIL				
(Amend) *See BENOL*				
(Amend) *See BLANDOL*				
(Amend) *See CARNATION LIGHT*				
(Amend) *See ERVOL LIGHT*				
(Amend) *See GLORIA*				
(Amend) *See KAYDOL*				
(Amend) *See KLEAROL LIGHT*				
(Amend) *See PROTOL HEAVY*				
(Amend) *See RUDOL LIGHT*				
(APP) *See MURI-LUBE*				
(Baker, J.T.) *See MINERAL OIL HEAVY*				
(Mallinckrodt Lab) *See MINERAL OIL WHITE*				
(Marlex) *See MINERAL OIL HEAVY*				
MINERAL OIL (Medisca)				
mineral oil, light				
OIL, NA (1X500ML,NF,LIGHT)				
500 ml	38779-0037-08	27.00		
MINERAL OIL (Medisca)				
(1X500ML,USP,HEAVY)				
500 ml	38779-0949-08	27.00		
(Medisca)				
mineral oil, light				
(1X1000ML,NF,LIGHT)				
1000 ml	38779-0037-09	45.00		
MINERAL OIL (Medisca)				
(1X1000ML,USP,HEAVY)				
1000 ml	38779-0949-09	45.00		
(Medisca)				
mineral oil, light				
(1X2000ML,NF,LIGHT)				
2000 ml	38779-0037-06	60.00		
MINERAL OIL (Medisca)				
(1X2000ML,USP,HEAVY)				
2000 ml	38779-0949-07	60.00		
(Medisca)				
mineral oil, light				
(1X4000ML,NF,LIGHT)				
4000 ml	38779-0037-01	108.00		
MINERAL OIL (Medisca)				
(1X4000ML,USP,HEAVY)				
4000 ml	38779-0949-01	108.00		
(PCCA)				
OIL, NA (LIGHT; NF)				
1 ml	51927-1291-00	0.08		
(USP; HEAVY)				
1 ml	51927-1074-00	0.08		
(Spectrum Pharmacy) *See MINERAL OIL EXTRA HEAVY*				
(Spectrum Pharmacy) *See MINERAL OIL HEAVY*				
(Spectrum Pharmacy) *See MINERAL OIL LIGHT*				
(Spectrum Pharmacy) *See MINERAL OIL MEDIUM*				
(Phys Total Care)				
REPACK				
OIL, NA, 480 ml	54868-2403-00	35.64		
960 ml	54868-2403-01	20.55		
MINERAL OIL EXTRA HEAVY (Spectrum Pharmacy)				
mineral oil				
OIL, NA (1X500ML)				
500 ml	49452-4750-01	58.45		
(1X1000ML)				
1000 ml	49452-4750-04	88.90		
(1X4000ML)				
4000 ml	49452-4750-02	158.55		
(1X20000ML)				
20000 ml	49452-4750-03	549.50		
MINERAL OIL HEAVY (Baker, J.T.)				
mineral oil				
OIL, NA (U.S.P.)				
500 ml	10106-2705-01	14.77		
(Marlex)				
OIL, NA (U.S.P.)				
120 ml	10135-0110-04	0.93		

PROD/MFR	NDC	AWP	DP	OBC
180 ml	10135-0110-06	0.94		
480 ml	10135-0110-08	1.96		
3785 ml	10135-0110-18	13.45		
(Spectrum Pharmacy)				
OIL, NA (U.S.P., N.F.)				
500 ml	49452-4740-01	58.45		
1000 ml	49452-4740-05	88.90		
(U.S.P.)				
4000 ml	49452-4740-02	158.55		
20000 ml	49452-4740-03	549.50		
MINERAL OIL LIGHT (Spectrum Pharmacy)				
mineral oil				
OIL, NA (U.S.P./N.F.)				
500 ml	49452-4720-01	56.70		
1000 ml	49452-4720-02	86.10		
(N.F.)				
4000 ml	49452-4720-03	156.10		
20000 ml	49452-4720-04	535.50		
MINERAL OIL MEDIUM (Spectrum Pharmacy)				
mineral oil				
OIL, NA (U.S.P./N.F.)				
500 ml	49452-4730-01	56.35		
1000 ml	49452-4730-02	85.40		
(N.F.)				
4000 ml	49452-4730-03	155.05		
20000 ml	49452-4730-04	535.50		
MINERAL OIL WHITE (Mallinckrodt Lab)				
mineral oil				
OIL, NA (U.S.P.)				
500 ml	00406-6357-04	11.07		
MINERAL OIL, LIGHT				
(Medisca) *See MINERAL OIL*				
MINI TRANSFER PIN (APP)				
transfer unit, iv fluid				
DEV, NA (VENTED)				
100s ea	63323-0905-90	182.44		
MINIBORE EXTENSION (Abbott Hosp)				
kit, intravenous extension tubing				
DEV, NA (60" W/SLIDE CLAMP,LTXFR)				
50s ea	00074-1739-02	255.00	255.00	
(36" W/SLIDE CLAMP,LTXFR)				
120s ea	00074-1738-02	486.72	487.20	
MINIMED PARADIGM CGM STARTER (Medtronic Minimed)				
device				
DEV, NA, ea	76300-0006-01	1248.75	999.00	
MINIMED PARADIGM REAL-TIME TRANSMITTER (Medtronic Minimed)				
device				
DEV, NA, ea	76300-0770-11	1198.80		
MINIMED SYRINGE RESERVOIR (Medtronic Minimed)				
infusion pump, parenteral				
DEV, NA, 10s ea	76300-0103-10	41.58		
MINIPRESS (Pfizer)				
prazosin hydrochloride				
CAP, PO, 1 mg, 250s ea	00069-4310-71	203.93	169.94	AB
2 mg, 250s ea	00069-4370-71	283.86	236.55	AB
5 mg, 250s ea	00069-4380-71	483.92	403.27	AB
(Phys Total Care)				
REPACK				
CAP, PO, 1 mg, 30s ea	54868-0704-01	17.85		AB
2 mg, 100s ea	54868-1290-01	74.15		AB
(Southwood)				
REPACK				
CAP, PO, 1 mg, 30s ea	58016-0549-30	21.38		AB
60s ea	58016-0549-60	42.76		AB
90s ea	58016-0549-90	64.14		AB
100s ea	58016-0549-00	71.27		AB
MINIRIN (Ferring)				
desmopressin acetate				
SPR, NS, 0.01 mg/actuation,				
5 ml	55566-5010-01	153.46		AB
MINITRAN (Graceway)				
nitroglycerin				
TDM, TD, 0.1 mg/hr,				
30s ea	29336-0301-02	85.26		AB1
0.2 mg/hr, 30s ea	29336-0302-02	86.64		AB1
0.4 mg/hr, 30s ea	29336-0303-02	97.08		AB1
0.6 mg/hr, 30s ea	29336-0304-02	105.24		AB1
(Phys Total Care)				
REPACK				
TDM, TD, 0.2 mg/hr,				
30s ea	54868-2716-01	74.70		AB1
MINK OIL (PCCA)				
OIL, NA, 1 ml	51927-2839-00	0.47		

PROD/MFR	NDC	AWP	DP	OBC
MINOCIN (Triax Pharm)				
minocycline hydrochloride				
CAP, PO, 50 mg, ea	14290-0551-98	335.06		AB
60s ea	14290-0571-98	335.06		AB
100s ea	14290-0501-88	579.31		AB
(COMBO PACK)				
100 mg, ea	14290-0550-98	668.75		AB
50s ea	14290-0500-86	579.31		AB
60s ea	14290-0570-98	668.75		AB
MINOCYCLINE (Bryant Ranch)				
REPACK				
minocycline hydrochloride				
CAP, PO, 100 mg, 20s ea	63629-2759-01	93.23		
(Quality Care Prod)				
REPACK				
CAP, PO, 100 mg, 20s ea	49999-0505-20	56.68		
MINOCYCLINE HCL (Global Pharm)				
minocycline hydrochloride				
CAP, PO, 50 mg, 100s ea	00115-7017-01	167.50		AB
75 mg, 100s ea	00115-7054-01	248.04		AB
100 mg, 50s ea	00115-7018-06	167.50		AB
60s ea	00115-7018-13	201.00		AB
(Par)				
TAB, PO (FILM-COATED)				
50 mg, 100s ea	49884-0511-01	343.47		
75 mg, 100s ea	49884-0512-01	504.25		
1000s ea	49884-0512-10	5039.94		
100 mg, 50s ea	49884-0513-03	300.99		
(PCCA)				
POW, NA (USP)				
1 gm	51927-2197-00	18.60		
(Ranbaxy Pharm)				
CAP, PO, 50 mg, 100s ea	63304-0694-01	169.87		AB
75 mg, 100s ea	63304-0695-01	197.96		AB
100 mg, 50s ea	63304-0696-50	169.87		AB
500s ea	63304-0696-05	1664.75		AB
(Teva)				
CAP, PO, 50 mg, 100s ea	00093-3165-01	169.87		AB
75 mg, 100s ea	00093-7300-01	197.96		AB
100 mg, 50s ea	00093-3167-53	169.87		AB
(Watson Labs)				
CAP, PO, 50 mg, 100s ea	00591-5694-01	45.26		AB
75 mg, 100s ea	00591-3153-01	95.66		AB
100 mg, 50s ea	00591-5695-50	45.26		AB
(A-S Medication)				
REPACK				
CAP, PO, 50 mg, 60s ea	54569-4712-00	101.92		EE
100 mg, 20s ea	54569-4713-02	67.95		AB
60s ea	54569-4713-00	203.84		EE
(American Health)				
REPACK				
CAP, PO (10X10)				
100 mg, 100s ea UD	68084-0289-01	167.50		AB
(PD-Rx Pharm)				
REPACK				
CAP, PO, 50 mg, 30s ea	55289-0202-30	60.73		AB
100 mg, 30s ea	55289-0201-30	110.43		AB
30s ea	58864-0848-30	110.43		AB
(Phys Total Care)				
REPACK				
CAP, PO, 50 mg, 30s ea	54868-2390-01	24.69		AB
60s ea	54868-2390-00	44.88		AB
75 mg, 10s ea	54868-5040-01	48.24		AB
30s ea	54868-5040-00	104.82		AB
100 mg, 10s ea	54868-2391-00	19.47		EE
30s ea	54868-2391-02	52.44		EE
50s ea	54868-2391-03	66.00		AB
60s ea	54868-2391-01	78.60		EE
(USP)				
100 mg, 100s ea	54868-2391-04	129.00		EE
(Physician Partner)				
REPACK				
CAP, PO, 50 mg, 30s ea	21695-0693-30	101.92		AB
(Quality Care Prod)				
REPACK				
CAP, PO, 50 mg, 7s ea	49999-0504-07	28.56		EE
100 mg, 28s ea	49999-0505-28	79.35		AB
(Southwood)				
REPACK				
CAP, PO, 50 mg, 15s ea	58016-0873-15	21.40		EE
20s ea	58016-0873-20	32.90		EE
30s ea	58016-0873-30	42.25		EE
100s ea	58016-0873-00	163.35		EE
100 mg, 15s ea	58016-0284-15	40.80		EE
20s ea	58016-0284-20	54.40		EE
30s ea	58016-0284-30	81.60		EE
50s ea	58016-0284-50	136.06		EE

PROD/MFR	NDC	AWP	DP	OBC
(Stat Rx)				
REPACK				
CAP, PO, 100 mg, 28s ea	16590-0560-28	20.00		AB
30s ea	16590-0560-30	24.00		AB
(Vibranta)				
REPACK				
CAP, PO, 100 mg, 30s ea	57866-4034-01	82.00		AB
MINOCYCLINE HYDROCHLORIDE				
FUL				
CAP, PO, 50 mg, 100s ea		90.00		
75 mg, 100s ea		195.75		
100 mg, 50s ea		90.00		
TAB, PO, 50 mg, 100s ea		300.00		
75 mg, 100s ea		444.00		
100 mg, 50s ea		262.50		
(Aurobindo Pharma)				
CAP, PO (USP,HARD GELATIN)				
50 mg, 100s ea	65862-0209-01	169.87		AB
75 mg, 100s ea	65862-0210-01	197.96		AB
100 mg, 50s ea	65862-0211-50	169.87		AB
(Dr Reddy's)				
TAB, PO (USP,FILM-COATED)				
50 mg, 100s ea	55111-0637-01	343.47		AB
75 mg, 100s ea	55111-0638-01	504.25		AB
100 mg, 60s ea	55111-0639-60	361.18		AB
(Global Pharm) *See MINOCYCLINE HCL*				
(Medicis) *See DYNACIN*				
(Medicis) *See SOLODYN*				
(Par) *See MINOCYCLINE HCL*				
(PCCA) *See MINOCYCLINE HCL*				
(Ranbaxy Pharm) *See MINOCYCLINE HCL*				
(Ranbaxy Pharm)				
TAB, PO (USP,FILM-COATED)				
50 mg, 100s ea	63304-0697-01	343.47		AB
75 mg, 100s ea	63304-0698-01	504.25		AB
100 mg, 50s ea	63304-0699-50	300.98		AB
(Sandoz)				
TER, PO (USP,FILM COATED)				
45 mg, 30s ea	00781-5385-31	605.01		AB
100s ea	00781-5385-01	2016.68		AB
90 mg, 30s ea	00781-5386-31	605.01		AB
100s ea	00781-5386-01	2016.68		AB
135 mg, 30s ea	00781-5387-31	605.01		AB
100s ea	00781-5387-01	2016.68		AB
(Teva) *See MINOCYCLINE HCL*				
(Teva)				
TER, PO (FILM-COATED)				
45 mg, 30s ea	00555-0178-01	554.02		AB
100s ea	00555-0178-02	1846.75		AB
90 mg, 30s ea	00555-0179-01	554.02		AB
100s ea	00555-0179-02	1846.75		AB
135 mg, 30s ea	00555-0180-01	554.02		AB
100s ea	00555-0180-02	1846.75		AB
(Triax Pharm) *See MINOCIN*				
(Watson Labs)				
CAP, PO (USP)				
50 mg, 60s ea	00591-5694-60	27.16		AB
(Watson Labs) *See MINOCYCLINE HCL*				
(Altura)				
REPACK				
CAP, PO, 100 mg, 15s ea	63874-0241-15	42.84		
20s ea	63874-0241-20	57.12		
30s ea	63874-0241-30	85.68		
50s ea	63874-0241-50	142.86		
60s ea	63874-0241-60	171.43		
(Phys Total Care)				
REPACK				
CAP, PO, 75 mg, 60s ea	54868-5040-02	205.14		
MINOXIDIL				
FUL				
TAB, PO, 2.5 mg, 100s ea		31.70		
10 mg, 100s ea		69.65		
(Gallipot)				
POW, NA (U.S.P.)				
5 gm	51552-0536-02	28.00		
25 gm	51552-0536-04	56.00		
100 gm	51552-0536-05	182.00		
(Hawkins)				
POW, NA (U.S.P.)				
5 gm	63370-0157-15	76.00		
25 gm	63370-0157-25	160.00		
100 gm	63370-0157-35	520.00		
1000 gm	63370-0157-50	1960.00		

PROD/MFR	NDC	AWP	DP	OBC
(Medisca)				
POW, NA (U.S.P.)				
25 gm	38779-0574-04	147.00		
100 gm	38779-0574-05	465.00		
500 gm	38779-0574-08	1485.00		
1000 gm	38779-0574-09	2385.00		
(Mutual)				
TAB, PO, 2.5 mg, 100s ea	53489-0386-01	58.78		AB
10 mg, 100s ea	53489-0387-01	129.09		AB
(Par)				
TAB, PO, 2.5 mg, 100s ea	49884-0256-01	78.17		AB
10 mg, 100s ea	49884-0257-01	168.75		AB
500s ea	49884-0257-05	816.15		AB
(PCCA)				
POW, NA (U.S.P.)				
1 gm	51927-2885-00	18.00		
(Spectrum Pharmacy)				
POW, NA (U.S.P.)				
5 gm	49452-4780-01	119.70		
25 gm	49452-4780-02	245.35		
100 gm	49452-4780-03	714.00		
(Watson Labs)				
TAB, PO, 2.5 mg, 100s ea	00591-5642-01	58.78		AB
500s ea	00591-5642-05	279.18		AB
10 mg, 100s ea	00591-5643-01	129.14		AB
500s ea	00591-5643-05	613.41		AB
(American Health) REPACK				
TAB, PO (USP,10X10)				
2.5 mg, 100s ea UD	68084-0204-01	169.52		
10 mg, 100s ea UD	68084-0205-01	211.74		
(Phys Total Care) REPACK				
TAB, PO, 2.5 mg, 30s ea	54868-3465-00	30.12		
10 mg, 30s ea	54868-3467-01	42.24		AB
100s ea	54868-3467-02	99.18		AB
(Southwood) REPACK				
TAB, PO, 10 mg, 30s ea	58016-0914-30	9.63		EE
MINT CHOCOLATE CHIP FLAVOR SOLN (PCCA)				
flavoring aid				
SOL, NA, 1 ml	51927-3311-00	0.70		
MINTUSS DR (Breckenridge Pharm)				
cpm/dm/phenyleph hcl				
SYR, PO (RED,STRAWBERRY,AF)				
473 ml	51991-0286-16	31.45		
MINTUSS G (Breckenridge Pharm)				
gg/hydrocod bit/phenyleph hcl				
SYR, PO (AF,GRAPE)				
473 ml, C-III	51991-0279-16	29.90		
MINTUSS HC (Breckenridge Pharm)				
cpm/hydrocod bit/phenyleph hcl				
SYR, PO (BLACK CHERRY)				
473 ml, C-III	51991-0287-16	31.15		
MINTUSS MR (Breckenridge Pharm)				
hydrocod bit/phenyleph hcl/pyril mal				
SYR, PO (AF,ORANGE-PINEAPPLE)				
473 ml, C-III	51991-0274-16	36.44		
MINTUSS MS (Breckenridge Pharm)				
cpm/hydrocod bit/phenyleph hcl				
SYR, PO (AF,ORANGE)				
473 ml, C-III	51991-0276-16	29.50		
MINTUSS NX (Breckenridge Pharm)				
hydrocodone bitartrate/potassium guaiacolsulfonate				
SOL, PO (AF,SF,DYE-FREE,CHERRY)				
3 mg/5 ml-150 mg/5 ml, 473 ml, C-III	51991-0273-16	35.88		
MIO-REL (Intl Ethical)				
orphenadrine citrate				
SOL, IJ (AMP)				
30 mg/ml, 2 ml 5s	11584-1016-05	29.89		EE
2 ml 25s	11584-1016-02	142.50		EE
MIOCHOL-E (Novartis Pharm)				
acetylcholine chloride				
PDS, IO (W/DILUENT)				
20 mg, ea	00078-0474-61	48.54		
MIOSTAT (Alcon Surgical)				
carbachol				
SOL, IO (12X1.5ML)				
0.01%, 1.5 ml 12s	00065-0023-15	388.80		AT
MIRALAX (Phys Total Care) REPACK				
polyethylene glycol 3350				
PDS, PO, 17 gm/dose, 527 gm	54868-4265-00	52.11		
(Quality Care Prod) REPACK				
PDS, PO, 17 gm/dose, 255 gm	49999-0612-55	67.00		
(Southwood) REPACK				
PDS, PO, 17 gm/dose, 527 gm	58016-4668-01	35.63		
MIRALUMA (Lantheus)				
technetium tc 99m sestamibi				
KIT, IV (SRN,PREFILLED)				
ea	11994-0001-99	128.10		
MIRAPEX (Boehr Ingelheim Cons)				
pramipexole dihydrochloride				
TAB, PO, 0.75 mg, 90s ea	00597-0101-90	294.97		EE
(Boehr Ingelheim Phar)				
TAB, PO, 0.125 mg, 90s ea	00597-0183-90	294.97		
0.25 mg, 90s ea (10X10)	00597-0184-90	294.97	94.58	
0.25 mg, 100s ea UD	00597-0184-61	344.08	106.22	
0.5 mg, 90s ea (10X10)	00597-0185-90	294.97	166.91	
0.5 mg, 100s ea UD	00597-0185-61	344.08	194.69	
1 mg, 90s ea (10X10)	00597-0190-90	294.97	166.91	
1 mg, 100s ea UD	00597-0190-61	344.08	194.69	
1.5 mg, 90s ea (10X10)	00597-0191-90	294.97	166.91	
1.5 mg, 100s ea UD	00597-0191-61	344.08	194.69	
(Phys Total Care) REPACK				
TAB, PO, 0.125 mg, 30s ea	54868-4912-01	63.16		
60s ea	54868-4912-02	124.46		
63s ea	54868-4912-00	130.59		
0.25 mg, 30s ea	54868-4211-01	125.85		
90s ea	54868-4211-00	351.14		
0.5 mg, 30s ea	54868-5412-01	125.85		
60s ea	54868-5412-00	235.40		
90s ea	54868-5412-02	351.79		
1 mg, 30s ea	54868-5746-00	89.22		
(Physician Partner) REPACK				
TAB, PO, 0.5 mg, 90s ea	21695-0867-90	589.94		
(Quality Care Prod) REPACK				
TAB, PO, 0.125 mg, 30s ea	35356-0392-30	147.36		
(Stat Rx) REPACK				
TAB, PO, 0.25 mg, 30s ea	16590-0751-30	96.84		
0.5 mg, 30s ea	16590-0752-30	116.90		
MIRAPEX ER (Boehr Ingelheim Phar)				
pramipexole dihydrochloride				
TER, PO, 0.375 mg, 30s ea	00597-0109-30	294.97		
0.75 mg, 30s ea	00597-0285-30	294.97		
1.5 mg, 30s ea	00597-0113-30	294.97		
3 mg, 30s ea	00597-0115-30	294.97		
4.5 mg, 30s ea	00597-0116-30	294.97		
MIRCETTE (Teva)				
desogestrel/ethinyl estradiol				
TAB, PO (6X28)				
168s ea	51285-0114-58	441.00		AB
(A-S Medication) REPACK				
TAB, PO, 28s ea	54569-4890-00	95.55		AB
(Palmetto) REPACK				
TAB, PO, 28s ea	23490-7670-01	42.63		
(Phys Total Care) REPACK				
TAB, PO, 28s ea	54868-4731-00	59.34		AB
MIRENA (Bayer)				
levonorgestrel				
ICR, IU, 52 mg, ea	50419-0421-01	562.45		
MIRTAZAPINE FUL				
ODT, PO, 30 mg, 30s ea		37.95		
TAB, PO, 15 mg, 30s ea		36.90		
30 mg, 30s ea		37.95		
45 mg, 30s ea		38.54		
(Apotex Corp.)				
TAB, PO (USP,FILM-COATED)				
15 mg, 30s ea	60505-0247-01	81.46		AB
1000s ea	60505-0247-08	2715.33		AB
30 mg, 30s ea	60505-0248-01	83.91		AB
1000s ea	60505-0248-08	2797.00		AB
45 mg, 30s ea	60505-0249-01	85.53		AB
1000s ea	60505-0249-08	2851.00		AB
(Aurobindo Pharma)				
ODT, PO (5X6)				
15 mg, 30s ea UD	65862-0021-06	70.65		AB
30 mg, 30s ea UD	65862-0022-06	72.79		AB
45 mg, 30s ea UD	65862-0023-06	77.56		AB
TAB, PO (FILM-COATED)				
15 mg, 30s ea	13107-0031-30	81.00		AB
30s ea	65862-0031-30	81.00		AB
30 mg, 30s ea	13107-0003-30	83.00		AB
30s ea	65862-0003-30	83.00		AB
45 mg, 30s ea	13107-0032-30	85.00		AB
30s ea	65862-0032-30	85.00		AB
(Caraco)				
TAB, PO (FILM-COATED)				
7.5 mg, 30s ea	57664-0510-83	77.00		AB
1000s ea	57664-0510-18	2561.43		AB
15 mg, 30s ea	57664-0499-83	81.46		AB
1000s ea	57664-0499-18	2709.85		AB
30 mg, 30s ea	57664-0500-83	83.91		AB
1000s ea	57664-0500-18	2791.30		AB
45 mg, 30s ea	57664-0501-83	85.52		AB
1000s ea	57664-0501-18	2845.10		AB
(Greenstone)				
ODT, PO (ONCE-A-DAY,5X6)				
15 mg, 30s ea UD	59762-1410-07	70.65		
30 mg, 30s ea UD	59762-1412-07	72.79		
45 mg, 30s ea UD	59762-1414-07	77.56		
TAB, PO (USP,FILM-COATED)				
7.5 mg, 30s ea	59762-1415-03	79.00		
60s ea	59762-1415-06	158.00		
90s ea	59762-1415-09	237.00		
500s ea	59762-1415-05	1316.67		
15 mg, 30s ea	59762-1416-03	81.40		
60s ea	59762-1416-06	162.80		
90s ea	59762-1416-09	244.20		
500s ea	59762-1416-05	1356.67		
30 mg, 30s ea	59762-1417-03	83.00		
60s ea	59762-1417-06	166.00		
90s ea	59762-1417-09	249.00		
500s ea	59762-1417-05	1383.33		
45 mg, 30s ea	59762-1418-03	85.00		
60s ea	59762-1418-06	170.00		
90s ea	59762-1418-09	255.00		
500s ea	59762-1418-05	1416.67		
(Mylan)				
TAB, PO, 15 mg, 30s ea	00378-3515-93	81.45		
1000s ea	00378-3515-10	2715.00		
30 mg, 30s ea	00378-3530-93	83.90		
500s ea	00378-3530-05	1398.33		
45 mg, 30s ea	00378-3545-93	85.50		
500s ea	00378-3545-05	1425.00		
(Organon) *See REMERON*				
(Organon) *See REMERON SOLTAB*				
(Prasco Labs)				
ODT, PO (5X6,ORANGE)				
15 mg, 30s ea UD (5X6)	66993-0709-30	77.90		
30 mg, 30s ea UD (5X6,ORANGE)	66993-0711-30	80.27		
45 mg, 30s ea UD	66993-0712-30	85.53		
(Sandoz)				
TAB, PO (FILM COATED)				
15 mg, 30s ea	00185-0020-30	81.46		AB
1000s ea	00185-0020-10	2709.87		AB
30 mg, 30s ea	00185-0212-30	83.91		AB
1000s ea	00185-0212-10	2791.31		AB
45 mg, 30s ea	00185-0222-30	85.53		AB
1000s ea	00185-0222-10	2845.20		AB
(Teva)				
ODT, PO (5X6)				
15 mg, 30s ea UD	00093-7303-65	77.90		AB
30 mg, 30s ea UD (10X3)	00093-7304-65	80.27		AB
45 mg, 30s ea UD	00093-7305-65	85.55		AB
TAB, PO, 15 mg, 30s ea (USP,10X10)	00093-7206-56	81.40		AB
15 mg, 100s ea UD	00093-7206-93	271.55		AB
30 mg, 30s ea	00093-7207-56	83.89		AB

PROD/MFR	NDC	AWP	DP	OBC
(USP,10X10)				
30 mg, 100s ea UD	00093-7207-93	279.65		AB
45 mg, 30s ea	00093-7208-56	85.49		AB
(USP,10X10)				
45 mg, 100s ea UD	00093-7208-93	285.05		AB
(UDL)				
TAB, PO (10X10)				
15 mg, 100s ea UD	51079-0086-20	271.50		AB
(10X30,PUNCH CARD,USP)				
15 mg, 300s ea UD	51079-0086-56	814.50		AB
(10X10)				
30 mg, 100s ea UD	51079-0087-20	279.60		AB
(10X30,PUNCH CARD,USP)				
30 mg, 300s ea UD	51079-0087-56	838.80		AB
(10X10)				
45 mg, 100s ea UD	51079-0088-20	285.00		AB
(10X30)				
45 mg, 300s ea UD	51079-0088-56	855.00		AB
(Watson Labs)				
ODT, PO (5X6)				
15 mg, 30s ea UD	00591-2230-15	67.32		AB
30 mg, 30s ea UD	00591-2231-15	69.36		AB
TAB, PO (FILM-COATED)				
15 mg, 30s ea	00591-1117-30	10.68		AB
(USP,FILM-COATED)				
15 mg, 1000s ea	00591-1117-10	320.40		AB
(FILM-COATED)				
30 mg, 30s ea	00591-1118-30	13.50		AB
(USP,FILM-COATED)				
30 mg, 1000s ea	00591-1118-10	405.00		AB
(FILM-COATED)				
45 mg, 30s ea	00591-1119-30	15.30		AB
(Wockhardt USA)				
TAB, PO (U.S.P.,FILM-COATED)				
15 mg, 30s ea	64679-0559-01	81.00		AB
30 mg, 30s ea	64679-0560-01	83.00		AB
45 mg, 30s ea	64679-0561-01	85.00		AB
(A-S Medication)				
REPACK				
TAB, PO, 15 mg, 30s ea	54569-5895-00	81.45		
30 mg, 30s ea	54569-5968-00	83.90		
60s ea	54569-5968-02	167.80		
(Aidarex)				
REPACK				
ODT, PO (ORANGE)				
30 mg, 7s ea	33261-0074-07	7.21		AB
10s ea	33261-0074-10	10.30		AB
14s ea	33261-0074-14	14.42		AB
20s ea	33261-0074-20	20.60		AB
30s ea	33261-0074-30	43.44		AB
40s ea	33261-0074-40	41.20		AB
60s ea	33261-0074-60	61.80		AB
TAB, PO, 15 mg, 7s ea	33261-0073-07	7.21		
14s ea	33261-0073-14	14.42		
20s ea	33261-0073-20	20.60		
21s ea	33261-0073-21	21.63		
28s ea	33261-0073-28	28.84		
30s ea	33261-0073-30	30.90		
60s ea	33261-0073-60	61.81		
90s ea	33261-0073-90	92.70		
(Altura)				
REPACK				
TAB, PO, 15 mg, 30s ea	63874-1098-03	81.46		AB
30 mg, 30s ea	63874-1097-03	83.91		AB
45 mg, 30s ea	63874-1155-03	89.99		
(American Health)				
REPACK				
TAB, PO (USP,10X10)				
15 mg, 100s ea UD	68084-0119-01	270.95		
30 mg, 100s ea UD	68084-0120-01	279.40		
45 mg, 100s ea UD	68084-0121-01	284.95		
(DHS, Inc.)				
REPACK				
TAB, PO, 15 mg, 30s ea	55887-0548-30	96.99		AB
30 mg, 30s ea	55887-0541-30	82.75		
(Dispensing Solutions)				
REPACK				
TAB, PO (FILM-COATED)				
15 mg, 30s ea	68258-7004-03	89.61		AB
30 mg, 30s ea	66258-7005-03	92.30		AB
45 mg, 30s ea	68258-7006-03	94.08		AB
(IPI)				
REPACK				
TAB, PO (FILM-COATED)				
15 mg, 30s ea	18837-0094-30	104.67		AB
60s ea	18837-0093-60	203.24		
(Keltman Pharma., Inc.)				
REPACK				
TAB, PO (FILM-COATED)				
15 mg, 60s ea	68387-0360-60	162.92		AB
30 mg, 7s ea	68387-0363-07	21.38		
15s ea	68387-0363-15	45.82		
30s ea	68387-0363-30	91.64		
(McKesson Packaging)				
REPACK				
TAB, PO, 15 mg, 100s ea UD	63739-0355-10	339.41		
(USP)				
30 mg, 100s ea UD	63739-0356-10	349.63		
(Medsource)				
REPACK				
TAB, PO (FILM-COATED)				
7.5 mg, 30s ea	45865-0372-30	75.00		AB
60s ea	45865-0372-60	150.00		AB
90s ea	45865-0372-90	225.00		AB
100s ea	45865-0372-00	250.00		AB
15 mg, 30s ea	45865-0382-30	59.70		AB
60s ea	45865-0382-60	119.40		AB
90s ea	45865-0382-90	179.10		AB
100s ea	45865-0382-00	199.00		AB
30 mg, 30s ea	45865-0361-30	59.70		AB
60s ea	45865-0361-60	119.40		AB
90s ea	45865-0361-90	179.10		AB
100s ea	45865-0361-00	199.00		AB
(Nucare Pharm)				
REPACK				
TAB, PO, 15 mg, 60s ea	68071-0486-60	209.34		AB
30 mg, 30s ea	66267-0724-30	74.79		AB
30s ea	68071-0685-30	109.90		AB
(Palmetto)				
REPACK				
TAB, PO, 15 mg, 30s ea	23490-6989-01	96.99		
60s ea	23490-6989-02	193.98		
30 mg, 30s ea	23490-6990-03	104.89		
45 mg, 30s ea	23490-7293-03	89.99		
(PD-Rx Pharm)				
REPACK				
TAB, PO (FILM COATED)				
30 mg, 15s ea	58864-0823-15	12.76		AB
30s ea	58864-0823-30	18.53		
(Pharma Pac)				
REPACK				
TAB, PO, 15 mg, 30s ea	52959-0774-30	94.50		
30s ea	52959-0901-30	94.50		
60s ea	52959-0774-60	188.98		
(Phys Total Care)				
REPACK				
TAB, PO, 30 mg, 30s ea	54868-5448-00	28.92		
45 mg, 30s ea	54868-5812-00	39.69		
(Physician Partner)				
REPACK				
TAB, PO, 15 mg, 30s ea	21695-0081-30	162.96		
60s ea	21695-0081-60	325.92		
100s ea	21695-0081-00	543.20		
30 mg, 30s ea	21695-0082-30	167.82		
60s ea	21695-0082-60	335.64		
100s ea	21695-0082-00	559.40		
45 mg, 30s ea	21695-0083-30	171.04		
(Quality Care Prod)				
REPACK				
TAB, PO, 15 mg, 30s ea	49999-0629-30	85.58		
30 mg, 30s ea	49999-0630-30	105.60		
45 mg, 30s ea	35356-0032-30	111.30		
(Southwood)				
REPACK				
ODT, PO, 15 mg, 30s ea	58016-4825-01	61.10		
30 mg, 30s ea	58016-4826-01	80.27		
TAB, PO (FILM-COATED)				
15 mg, 30s ea	58016-0894-30	77.80		AB
60s ea	58016-0894-60	155.60		AB
90s ea	58016-0894-90	233.40		AB
100s ea	58016-0894-00	259.33		AB
120s ea	58016-0894-02	311.20		AB
150s ea	58016-0894-03	389.00		AB
180s ea	58016-0894-99	466.80		AB
30 mg, 30s ea	58016-0986-30	80.15		AB
60s ea	58016-0986-60	160.30		AB
90s ea	58016-0986-90	240.45		AB
100s ea	58016-0986-00	267.17		AB
120s ea	58016-0986-02	320.60		AB
150s ea	58016-0986-03	400.75		AB
45 mg, 30s ea	58016-0282-30	85.53		
60s ea	58016-0282-60	171.06		
90s ea	58016-0282-90	256.59		
100s ea	58016-0282-00	285.10		
(Stat Rx)				
REPACK				
ODT, PO (ORANGE)				
30 mg, 30s ea	16590-0720-30	84.25		AB
TAB, PO, 15 mg, 30s ea	16590-0153-30	98.25		
60s ea	16590-0153-60	196.50		
30 mg, 30s ea	16590-0154-30	104.67		
(FILM-COATED)				
30 mg, 45s ea	16590-0154-45	126.00		AB
56s ea	16590-0154-56	184.80		AB
60s ea	16590-0154-60	198.00		
(FILM-COATED)				
30 mg, 90s ea	16590-0154-90	289.50		AB
45 mg, 30s ea	16590-0155-30	111.00		
60s ea	16590-0155-60	222.00		
(Vibranta)				
REPACK				
TAB, PO, 30 mg, 30s ea	57866-3061-02	104.89		
MISOPROST (Core)				
REPACK				
misoprostol				
TAB, PO, 100 mcg, 60s ea	33358-0247-60	54.48		
200 mcg, 20s ea	33358-0248-20	29.40		
30s ea	33358-0248-30	41.70		
60s ea	33358-0248-60	78.57		
100s ea	33358-0248-00	133.92		
MISOPROSTOL (Greenstone)				
TAB, PO, 100 mcg, 60s ea	59762-5007-01	49.45		EE
120s ea	59762-5007-02	98.86		EE
200 mcg, 60s ea	59762-5008-01	71.95		EE
100s ea	59762-5008-02	119.95		EE
(Hawkins)				
POW, NA (DISPERSION)				
1%, 2 gm	63370-0159-12	312.00		
10 gm	63370-0159-20	1440.00		
(Pfizer) *See CYTOTEC*				
(Teva)				
TAB, PO, 100 mcg, 60s ea	00172-4430-49	49.45		AB
120s ea	00172-4430-59	98.85		AB
200 mcg, 60s ea	00172-4431-49	71.95		AB
100s ea	00172-4431-60	119.95		AB
(Aidarex)				
REPACK				
TAB, PO, 200 mcg, 30s ea	33261-0076-30	55.50		AB
60s ea	33261-0076-60	111.00		AB
90s ea	33261-0076-90	166.50		AB
120s ea	33261-0076-02	222.00		AB
(Altura)				
REPACK				
TAB, PO, 200 mcg, 40s ea	63874-1076-04	51.80		
60s ea	63874-1076-06	77.70		
90s ea	63874-1076-09	129.54		
100s ea	63874-1076-01	129.50		
(Dispensing Solutions)				
REPACK				
TAB, PO, 100 mcg, 90s ea	55045-3375-09	74.70		
200 mcg, 30s ea	55045-3336-08	36.00		AB
60s ea	55045-3336-06	72.00		AB
(IPI)				
REPACK				
TAB, PO, 200 mcg, 60s ea	18837-0290-60	89.97		
(Nucare Pharm)				
REPACK				
TAB, PO, 200 mcg, 30s ea	68071-0461-30	94.47		AB
60s ea	68071-0461-60	91.97		AB
(PD-Rx Pharm)				
REPACK				
TAB, PO, 200 mcg, 2s ea	55289-0640-02	6.93		
4s ea	55289-0640-04	8.85		
6s ea	55289-0640-06	10.78		
8s ea	55289-0640-08	12.70		
13s ea	55289-0640-13	17.66		
(Pharma Pac)				
REPACK				
TAB, PO, 100 mcg, 12s ea	52959-0692-12	17.00		
28s ea	52959-0692-28	32.40		
30s ea	52959-0692-30	34.50		
40s ea	52959-0692-40	44.12		
60s ea	52959-0692-60	60.12		
200 mcg, 12s ea	52959-0693-12	19.25		
16s ea	52959-0693-16	24.35		
20s ea	52959-0693-20	30.25		

PROD/MFR	NDC	AWP	DP	OBC
28s ea	52959-0693-28	37.12		
30s ea	52959-0693-30	38.85		
40s ea	52959-0693-40	49.80		
60s ea	52959-0693-60	74.69		
(Phys Total Care)				
REPACK				
TAB, PO, 200 mcg, 30s ea	54868-4766-00	86.07		AB
60s ea	54868-4766-01	127.77		AB
(Quality Care Prod)				
REPACK				
TAB, PO, 200 mcg, 60s ea	49999-0589-60	86.09		AB
(Southwood)				
REPACK				
TAB, PO, 200 mcg, 30s ea	58016-0766-30	35.98		
60s ea	58016-0766-60	71.95		
90s ea	58016-0766-90	107.93		
100s ea	58016-0766-00	119.92		
120s ea	58016-0766-02	143.90		
150s ea	58016-0766-03	179.88		
200s ea	58016-0766-89	239.83		
300s ea	58016-0766-73	359.75		
(Vibranta)				
REPACK				
TAB, PO, 200 mcg, 60s ea	57866-3172-02	86.09		
MISTERNEB COMPRESSOR/NEBULIZER (Respironics)				
nebulizer, direct patient interface				
DEV, NA, ea	83730-0001-23	53.69		
MITOMYCIM (Accord)				
mitomycin				
PDS, IV (USP)				
20 mg, 20 ml	16729-0108-11	218.40		EE
MITOMYCIN				
(Accord) *See MITOMYCIM*				
(Accord)				
PDS, IV (USP)				
5 mg, ea	16729-0115-05	67.20		AP
(Bedford) *See MITOMYCIN NOVAPLUS*				
(Bedford)				
PDS, IV (S.D.V.,PF)				
5 mg, ea	55390-0251-01	67.20		AP
20 mg, ea	55390-0252-01	218.40		AP
40 mg, ea	55390-0253-01	300.00		AP
(Medisca)				
POW, NA (U.S.P.)				
0.01 gm	38779-0553-07	399.00		
0.1 gm	38779-0553-09	2907.00		
(PCCA)				
POW, NA (USP)				
0.001 gm	51927-3642-00	44.00		
(Spectrum Pharmacy)				
POW, NA (U.S.P.)				
0.1 gm	49452-4785-02	3475.50		
(Supergen)				
PDS, IV (VIAL)				
20 mg, ea	62701-0011-01	452.91		AP
MITOMYCIN NOVAPLUS (Bedford)				
mitomycin				
PDS, IV (S.D.V.,PF,PRIVATE LABEL)				
5 mg, ea	55390-0451-01	24.00		AP
20 mg, ea	55390-0452-01	87.60		AP
40 mg, ea	55390-0453-01	175.20		AP
MITOTANE				
(B/M Squibb Onc/Vir) *See LYSODREN*				
(Letco)				
POW, NA (1X5GM,USP)				
5 gm	62991-2604-01	240.00		
(1X25GM,USP)				
25 gm	62991-2604-02	585.00		
(1X100GM,USP)				
100 gm	62991-2604-03	1125.00		
(1X500GM,USP)				
500 gm	62991-2604-04	5250.00		
(Medisca)				
POW, NA (1X1GM,USP)				
1 gm	38779-2263-06	90.00		
(1X5GM,USP)				
5 gm	38779-2263-03	255.00		
(1X25GM,USP)				
25 gm	38779-2263-04	994.50		
(1X100GM,USP)				
100 gm	38779-2263-05	2295.00		
(1X500GM,USP)				
500 gm	38779-2263-08	8568.00		
(PCCA)				
POW, NA, 1 gm	51927-2807-00	111.00		

PROD/MFR	NDC	AWP	DP	OBC
(Spectrum Pharmacy)				
POW, NA (1X1GM, USP)				
1 gm	49452-4786-01	189.70		
(1X5GM, USP)				
5 gm	49452-4786-02	668.50		
(1X25GM, USP)				
25 gm	49452-4786-03	2107.00		
(B&B Pharm, Inc)				
REPACK				
POW, NA, 100 gm	63275-9956-05	755.00		
500 gm	63275-9956-08	3870.00		
1000 gm	63275-9956-09	7700.00		
MITOXANTRONE (APP)				
mitoxantrone hydrochloride				
SOL, IV (USP,PF,LATEX-FREE)				
2 mg/ml, 10 ml	63323-0132-10	456.25	365.00	
(MDV,USP,CONCENTRATE)				
2 mg/ml, 12.5 ml	10518-0105-11	568.75	455.00	AP
(USP,PF,LATEX-FREE)				
2 mg/ml, 12.5 ml	63323-0132-12	1857.50		
(MDV,USP,CONCENTRATE)				
2 mg/ml, 15 ml	10518-0105-12	687.50	550.00	AP
(USP,PF,LATEX-FREE)				
2 mg/ml, 15 ml	63323-0132-15	2676.00		
(Bedford)				
SOL, IV (USP,CONCENTRATE, MDV,PF)				
2 mg/ml, 10 ml	55390-0083-01	492.00		AP
(USP,CONCENTRATE,MDV,PF)				
2 mg/ml, 12.5 ml	55390-0084-01	540.00		AP
(USP,CONCENTRATE, MDV,PF)				
2 mg/ml, 15 ml	55390-0085-01	624.00		AP
(Hospira)				
SOL, IV (USP,CONCENTRATE,MDV,PF)				
2 mg/ml, 10 ml	61703-0343-18	217.32	190.16	AP
12.5 ml	61703-0343-65	303.98	265.99	AP
15 ml	61703-0343-66	369.92	323.68	AP
(Teva)				
SOL, IV (MDV,PF)				
2 mg/ml, 10 ml	00703-4685-01	600.00		AP
12.5 ml	00703-4680-01	603.60		AP
15 ml	00703-4686-01	606.00		AP
MITOXANTRONE HYDROCHLORIDE				
(APP) *See MITOXANTRONE*				
(Bedford) *See MITOXANTRONE*				
(EMD) *See NOVANTRONE*				
(Hospira) *See MITOXANTRONE*				
(Mayne Pharma) *See OTN MITOXANTRONE*				
(OTN) *See OTN MITOXANTRONE*				
(Teva) *See MITOXANTRONE*				
MIXED AMPHETAMINE SALT (Teva)				
amphetamine salt combination				
CER, PO, 5 mg,				
100s ea, C-II	00555-0790-02	613.15		AB
10 mg,				
100s ea, C-II	00555-0787-02	613.15		AB
15 mg,				
100s ea, C-II	00555-0791-02	613.15		AB
20 mg,				
100s ea, C-II	00555-0788-02	613.15		AB
25 mg,				
100s ea, C-II	00555-0792-02	613.15		AB
30 mg,				
100s ea, C-II	00555-0789-02	613.15		AB
(Phys Total Care)				
REPACK				
CER, PO, 10 mg,				
10s ea, C-II	54868-6033-00	162.70		AB
30s ea, C-II	54868-6033-01	430.42		AB
20 mg,				
10s ea, C-II	54868-6028-00	162.70		AB
30s ea, C-II	54868-6028-01	444.47		AB
60s ea, C-II	54868-6028-02	879.94		AB
25 mg,				
10s ea, C-II	54868-6029-00	162.70		AB
30s ea, C-II	54868-6029-01	444.47		AB
30 mg,				
10s ea, C-II	54868-6034-00	162.70		AB
30s ea, C-II	54868-6034-01	430.42		AB
MIXED AMPHETAMINE SALTS (Global Pharm)				
amphetamine salt combination				
CER, PO, 5 mg,				
100s ea, C-II	00115-1328-01	613.15		
10 mg,				
100s ea, C-II	00115-1329-01	613.15		
15 mg,				
100s ea, C-II	00115-1330-01	613.15		

PROD/MFR	NDC	AWP	DP	OBC
25 mg,				
100s ea, C-II	00115-1332-01	613.15		
30 mg,				
100s ea, C-II	00115-1333-01	613.15		
TAB, PO, 20 mg,				
100s ea, C-II	00115-1331-01	613.15		
MIXED VESPID TREATMENT (Alk-Abello)				
vespid venom, mixed				
PDS, IJ (KIT (6X1ML))				
0.3 mg, ea	52709-1201-01	259.44	196.10	
(M.D.V.)				
0.3 mg, ea	52709-1201-02	339.82	252.10	
(Hollister-Stier)				
PDS, IJ (M.D.V.)				
1.65 mg, ea	65044-9945-05	133.10		
3.9 mg, ea	65044-9945-06	275.15		
3ML FUTURA SAFETY SYRINGE (Arkray)				
syringe and needle				
DEV, NA (21G X 1.5",LATEX-FREE)				
50s ea	08317-1032-14	22.50	15.00	
(21G X 1",LATEX-FREE)				
50s ea	08317-1032-13	22.50	15.00	
(22G X 1.5",LATEX-FREE)				
50s ea	08317-1032-24	22.50	15.00	
(22G X 1",LATEX-FREE)				
50s ea	08317-1032-23	22.50	15.00	
(23G X 1",LATEX-FREE)				
50s ea	08317-1032-33	22.50	15.00	
(25G X 0.625",LATEX-FREE)				
50s ea	08317-1032-52	22.50	15.00	
(25G X 1",MICRODRAW)				
50s ea	08317-1032-53	22.50	15.00	
MMA/PA GEL (VITAFLO, LLC)				
amino acids, multivitamin, and minerals				
PDS, PO (UNFLAVORED)				
30s ea	50600-0543-55	148.68		
MOBAN (Endo Labs)				
molindone hydrochloride				
TAB, PO, 5 mg, 100s ea	63481-0072-70	178.61		
10 mg, 100s ea	63481-0073-70	256.80		
25 mg, 100s ea	63481-0074-70	301.62		
50 mg, 100s ea	63481-0076-70	511.61		
MOBIC (Boehr Ingelheim Phar)				
meloxicam				
SUS, PO (RASPBERRY)				
7.5 mg/5 ml,				
100 ml	00597-0034-01	125.78		
TAB, PO, 7.5 mg, 100s ea	00597-0029-01	472.34		
15 mg, 100s ea	00597-0030-01	722.24		
(A-S Medication)				
REPACK				
TAB, PO, 7.5 mg, 14s ea	54569-5121-00	56.93		
30s ea	54569-5121-01	121.99		
15 mg, 14s ea	54569-5179-00	87.05		
30s ea	54569-5179-01	186.53		
(Advanced Pharm Serv, Inc.)				
REPACK				
TAB, PO, 7.5 mg, 10s ea	13411-0116-01	67.00		
30s ea	13411-0116-03	201.00		
60s ea	13411-0116-06	402.00		
90s ea	13411-0116-09	603.00		
100s ea	13411-0116-10	404.89		
(Altura)				
REPACK				
TAB, PO, 7.5 mg, 14s ea	63874-1109-04	49.00		
15s ea	63874-1109-05	52.50		
20s ea	63874-1109-02	70.00		
30s ea	63874-1109-03	105.00		
60s ea	63874-1109-06	210.00		
90s ea	63874-1109-09	315.00		
100s ea	63874-1109-00	350.00		
120s ea	63874-1109-01	420.00		
15 mg, 14s ea	63874-1110-04	57.26		
15s ea	63874-1110-05	61.35		
20s ea	63874-1110-02	81.80		
30s ea	63874-1110-03	138.45		
60s ea	63874-1110-06	244.91		
90s ea	63874-1110-09	361.51		
100s ea	63874-1110-00	409.00		
120s ea	63874-1110-01	479.11		
(AQ)				
REPACK				
TAB, PO, 7.5 mg, 100s ea	66105-0551-10	452.30		
(DHS, Inc.)				
REPACK				
TAB, PO, 7.5 mg, 60s ea	55887-0454-60	325.95		
15 mg, 30s ea	55887-0455-30	156.03		

PROD/MFR	NDC	AWP	DP	OBC
(Dispensing Solutions)				
REPACK				
TAB, PO, 7.5 mg, 30s ea	**55045-3082-08**	121.50		
60s ea	**55045-3082-06**	243.00		
15 mg, 30s ea	**55045-2950-08**	184.50		
(Nucare Pharm)				
REPACK				
TAB, PO, 15 mg, 30s ea	**68071-0261-30**	159.99		
(PD-Rx Pharm)				
REPACK				
TAB, PO, 7.5 mg, 14s ea	**55289-0618-14**	89.34		
30s ea	**55289-0618-30**	191.48		
60s ea	**55289-0618-60**	382.92		
15 mg, 14s ea	**55289-0739-14**	136.64		
(Pharma Pac)				
REPACK				
TAB, PO, 7.5 mg, 15s ea	**52959-0623-15**	52.80		
20s ea	**52959-0623-20**	70.39		
30s ea	**52959-0623-30**	105.58		
60s ea	**52959-0623-60**	211.15		
100s ea	**52959-0623-00**	351.88		
15 mg, 14s ea	**52959-0663-14**	69.30		
15s ea	**52959-0663-15**	74.25		
30s ea	**52959-0663-30**	148.49		
60s ea	**52959-0663-60**	296.96		
90s ea	**52959-0663-90**	445.04		
(Phys Total Care)				
REPACK				
TAB, PO, 7.5 mg, 10s ea	**54868-4490-03**	56.44		
20s ea	**54868-4490-02**	110.26		
30s ea	**54868-4490-00**	155.11		
60s ea	**54868-4490-01**	307.60		
100s ea	**54868-4490-04**	510.27		
15 mg, 10s ea	**54868-5158-02**	64.59		
15s ea	**54868-5158-03**	96.88		
20s ea	**54868-5158-01**	128.54		
30s ea	**54868-5158-00**	181.31		
(Quality Care Prod)				
REPACK				
TAB, PO, 7.5 mg, 14s ea	**49999-0423-14**	46.34		
(Southwood)				
REPACK				
TAB, PO, 7.5 mg, 15s ea	**58016-0592-15**	52.81		
20s ea	**58016-0592-20**	70.41		
21s ea	**58016-0592-21**	81.97		
30s ea	**58016-0592-30**	117.11		
60s ea	**58016-0592-60**	234.22		
90s ea	**58016-0592-90**	351.33		
100s ea	**58016-0592-00**	390.37		
120s ea	**58016-0592-02**	422.48		
15 mg, 15s ea	**58016-0638-15**	89.53		
20s ea	**58016-0638-20**	119.38		
21s ea	**58016-0638-21**	125.34		
30s ea	**58016-0638-30**	179.07		
60s ea	**58016-0638-60**	358.13		
90s ea	**58016-0638-90**	537.20		
100s ea	**58016-0638-00**	596.89		
120s ea	**58016-0638-02**	716.27		
(St. Mary's MPP)				
REPACK				
TAB, PO, 7.5 mg, 30s ea	**60760-0028-30**	113.58		
15 mg, 30s ea	**60760-0030-30**	170.49		
(Stat Rx)				
REPACK				
TAB, PO, 7.5 mg, 30s ea	**16590-0156-30**	114.25		
60s ea	**16590-0156-60**	208.50		
15 mg, 30s ea	**16590-0157-30**	160.00		
60s ea	**16590-0157-60**	320.00		
MOBISYL (Keltman Pharma., Inc.)				
REPACK				
trolamine salicylate				
CRE, TP, 10%, 100 gm	**68387-0445-01**	18.85		
MODAFINIL				
(Cephalon) *See PROVIGIL*				
MODICON (Ortho-McNeil Pharm)				
ethinyl estradiol/norethindrone				
TAB, PO (DIALPAK, 6X28)				
35 mcg-0.5 mg,				
168s ea	**00062-1714-15**	347.59	289.66	AB
(Phys Total Care)				
REPACK				
TAB, PO, 35 mcg-0.5 mg,				
28s ea	**54868-0525-00**	47.21		AB
MOEXIPRIL HYDROCHLORIDE (Apotex Corp.)				
TAB, PO, 7.5 mg, 100s ea	**60505-0271-01**	138.91		AB
15 mg, 100s ea	**60505-0272-01**	145.52		AB
(Kremers Urban)				
TAB, PO (FILM-COATED)				
7.5 mg, 100s ea	**62175-0171-37**	138.15		
15 mg, 100s ea	**62175-0177-37**	144.73		
(Paddock)				
TAB, PO (FILM-COATED)				
7.5 mg, 100s ea	**00574-0110-01**	137.38		AB
15 mg, 100s ea	**00574-0112-15**	143.92		AB
(Teva)				
TAB, PO, 7.5 mg, 100s ea	**00093-0017-01**	138.92		AB
(FILM COATED,FILM-COATED)				
15 mg, 100s ea	**00093-5150-01**	145.54		AB
(UCB) *See UNIVASC*				
(Watson Labs)				
TAB, PO (FILM-COATED)				
7.5 mg, 100s ea	**16252-0610-01**	100.76		AB
15 mg, 100s ea	**16252-0611-01**	105.56		AB
(A-S Medication)				
REPACK				
TAB, PO (FILM-COATED)				
15 mg, 30s ea	**54569-5916-00**	43.48		AB
(Phys Total Care)				
REPACK				
TAB, PO, 7.5 mg, 90s ea	**54868-5928-00**	146.33		AB
(FILM-COATED)				
15 mg, 20s ea	**54868-4883-01**	79.23		AB
40s ea	**54868-4883-00**	153.99		AB
100s ea	**54868-4883-02**	288.78		AB
MOEXIPRIL HYDROCHLORIDE AND HYDROCHLOROTHIAZIDE (Kremers Urban)				
hydrochlorothiazide/moexipril hydrochloride				
TAB, PO (FILM-COATED)				
12.5 mg-7.5 mg,				
100s ea	**62175-0712-37**	132.83		
12.5 mg-15 mg,				
100s ea	**62175-0720-37**	132.83		
25 mg-15 mg,				
100s ea	**62175-0725-37**	132.83		
(Paddock)				
TAB, PO (FILM-COATED)				
12.5 mg-7.5 mg,				
100s ea	**00574-0133-01**	133.57		AB
12.5 mg-15 mg,				
100s ea	**00574-0134-01**	133.57		AB
25 mg-15 mg,				
100s ea	**00574-0135-01**	133.57		AB
(Teva)				
TAB, PO (FILM-COATED)				
12.5 mg-7.5 mg,				
100s ea	**00093-5213-01**	133.57		AB
12.5 mg-15 mg,				
100s ea	**00093-5214-01**	133.57		AB
25 mg-15 mg,				
100s ea	**00093-5215-01**	133.57		AB
(Phys Total Care)				
REPACK				
TAB, PO, 25 mg-15 mg,				
10s ea	**54868-3443-00**	56.52		
30s ea	**54868-3443-01**	123.84		
MOEXIPRIL HYDROCHLORIDE/ HYDROCHLOROTHIAZIDE (Watson Labs)				
hydrochlorothiazide/moexipril hydrochloride				
TAB, PO (FILM-COATED)				
12.5 mg-7.5 mg,				
100s ea	**16252-0612-01**	96.89		AB
12.5 mg-15 mg,				
100s ea	**16252-0613-01**	96.89		AB
25 mg-15 mg,				
100s ea	**16252-0614-01**	96.89		AB
MOLASSES FLAVOR (Spectrum Pharmacy)				
flavoring aid				
LIQ, NA (1X100ML)				
100 ml	**49452-4787-01**	59.50		
(1X500ML)				
500 ml	**49452-4787-02**	131.95		
MOLASSES-ADE FLAVOR (PCCA)				
flavoring aid				
POW, NA (DRY,MOLASSES-ADE)				
1 gm	**51927-3448-00**	0.08		
MOLD, SUPPOSITORY				
(Gallipot) *See MOLDS 1 GM*				
(Gallipot) *See MOLDS 2 GM*				
(Gallipot) *See MOLDS DS 3GM*				
(Gallipot) *See MOLDS DS 3ML*				
(Gallipot) *See MOLDS V-NOTCH 2 GM*				
MOLDS 1 GM (Gallipot)				
mold, suppository				
DEV, NA (WHITE)				
100s ea	**51552-0424-01**	11.20		
1000s ea	**51552-0424-02**	91.00		
MOLDS 2 GM (Gallipot)				
mold, suppository				
DEV, NA (AMBER)				
100s ea	**51552-0344-01**	11.20		
(WHITE)				
100s ea	**51552-0350-01**	9.80		
(AMBER)				
1000s ea	**51552-0344-02**	91.00		
(WHITE)				
1000s ea	**51552-0350-02**	81.20		
MOLDS DS 3GM (Gallipot)				
mold, suppository				
DEV, NA (BLUE)				
1000s ea	**51552-0389-02**	91.00		
MOLDS DS 3ML (Gallipot)				
mold, suppository				
DEV, NA (W/PEELAWAY)				
100s ea	**51552-0637-01**	12.53		
MOLDS V-NOTCH 2 GM (Gallipot)				
mold, suppository				
DEV, NA, 100s ea	**51552-0426-01**	11.76		
MOLINDONE HYDROCHLORIDE				
(Endo Labs) *See MOBAN*				
MOLYBDENUM (PCCA)				
POW, NA, 1 gm	**51927-2209-00**	4.08		
MOLYBDENUM TRIOXIDE (Baker, J.T.)				
POW, NA (A.C.S., REAGENT)				
500 gm	**10106-0208-01**	163.46		
MOLYBDIC ACID 85% (Amend)				
ammonium molybdate				
POW, NA, 500 gm	**17317-1907-01**	42.00		
(Baker, J.T.)				
POW, NA (A.C.S., REAGENT)				
500 gm	**10106-0206-01**	103.62		
2500 gm	**10106-0206-05**	465.51		
MOMETASONE FUROATE				
FUL				
CRE, TP, 0.1%, 45 gm		33.00		
OIN, TP, 0.1%, 45 gm		42.00		
(Fougera)				
CRE, TP, 0.1%, 15 gm	**00168-0270-15**	26.90		
45 gm	**00168-0270-46**	49.25		
LOT, TP (1X30ML,USP)				
0.1%, 30 ml	**00168-0272-30**	29.12		AB
(1X60ML,USP)				
0.1%, 60 ml	**00168-0272-60**	55.71		AB
OIN, TP (USP)				
0.1%, 15 gm	**00168-0271-15**	23.90		
45 gm	**00168-0271-46**	43.77		
(G&W)				
CRE, TP, 0.1%, 15 gm	**00713-0634-15**	27.00		AB
45 gm	**00713-0634-37**	49.00		AB
OIN, TP (USP)				
0.1%, 15 gm	**00713-0635-15**	24.00		AB
45 gm	**00713-0635-37**	47.50		AB
(Glenmark Pharmaceuticals)				
CRE, TP (1X15GM,USP)				
0.1%, 15 gm	**68462-0192-17**	27.00		AB
(1X45GM,USP)				
0.1%, 45 gm	**68462-0192-55**	49.00		AB
OIN, TP (1X15GM,USP)				
0.1%, 15 gm	**68462-0225-17**	24.46		AB
(1X45GM,USP)				
0.1%, 45 gm	**68462-0225-55**	47.50		AB
(Harris)				
CRE, TP (1X15GM)				
0.1%, 15 gm	**67405-0100-15**	9.22		AB
(1X45GM)				
0.1%, 45 gm	**67405-0100-45**	17.98		AB
LOT, TP (1X30ML,USP)				
0.1%, 30 ml	**67405-0275-30**	14.86		AB
(1X60ML,USP)				
0.1%, 60 ml	**67405-0275-60**	27.26		AB
OIN, TP (1X15GM,USP)				
0.1%, 15 gm	**67405-0300-15**	9.22		AB
(1X45GM,USP)				
0.1%, 45 gm	**67405-0300-45**	17.98		AB
(Medisca)				
POW, NA (1X1000GM)				
1000 gm	**38779-2413-09**	30000.00		
(Perrigo)				
CRE, TP, 0.1%, 15 gm	**45802-0257-35**	26.75		AB
45 gm	**45802-0257-42**	49.00		AB
OIN, TP, 0.1%, 15 gm	**45802-0119-37**	24.30		AB
45 gm	**45802-0119-42**	44.60		AB

PROD/MFR	NDC	AWP	DP	OBC
SOL, TP, 0.1%, 30 ml	45802-0118-59	29.85		AB
60 ml	45802-0118-46	57.04		AB
(Sandoz)				
CRE, TP (USP)				
0.1%, 15 gm	00781-7066-27	27.00		
45 gm	00781-7066-19	49.00		
LOT, TP (1X30ML)				
0.1%, 30 ml	00781-7067-30	29.85		AB
(1X60ML)				
0.1%, 60 ml	00781-7067-61	57.04		AB
OIN, TP (USP)				
0.1%, 15 gm	00781-7068-27	24.46		AB
45 gm	00781-7068-19	44.77		AB
(Schering) *See ASMANEX TWISTHALER*				
(Schering) *See ELOCON*				
(Schering) *See NASONEX*				
(Taro)				
LOT, TP (USP)				
0.1%, 30 ml	51672-1305-03	28.95		AB
60 ml	51672-1305-04	55.45		AB
(A-S Medication)				
REPACK				
CRE, TP, 0.1%, 45 gm	54569-5914-00	49.00		
OIN, TP, 0.1%, 15 gm	54569-5915-00	24.30		
(Dispensing Solutions)				
REPACK				
CRE, TP, 0.1%, 15 gm	55045-3430-05	27.00		
45 gm	55045-3430-06	49.00		
(Nucare Pharm)				
REPACK				
OIN, TP (1X15GM)				
0.1%, 15 gm	68071-1328-05	25.90		
(Palmetto)				
REPACK				
CRE, TP, 0.1%, 45 gm	23490-7095-04	62.30		
SPR, NS, 0.05 mg/actuation,				
17 gm	23490-7094-01	86.69		
(Pharma Pac)				
REPACK				
CRE, TP, 0.1%, 45 gm	52959-0859-45	50.97		
(Phys Total Care)				
REPACK				
CRE, TP, 0.1%, 15 gm	54868-5455-00	48.93		
45 gm	54868-5455-01	82.26		
SOL, TP, 0.1%, 60 ml	54868-3757-00	152.61		
(Physician Partner)				
REPACK				
CRE, TP (1X15GM)				
0.1%, 15 gm	21695-0786-15	54.00		AB
(Southwood)				
REPACK				
CRE, TP, 0.1%, 45 gm	58016-4738-01	46.58		
MONARC-M (Amer Red Cross-Blood)				
antihemophilic factor viii:c human				
PDS, IV (APPROX 220-2000 IU/VIAL)				
1 iu, ea	52769-0460-01	1.02		
(Baxter Bioscience)				
PDS, IV (1701IU-2000IU,PF)				
1 iu, ea	00944-1304-10	1.09		
(220IU-400IU,PF)				
1 iu, ea	00944-1301-10	1.09		
(401IU-800IU,PF)				
1 iu, ea	00944-1302-10	1.09		
(801IU-1700IU,PF)				
1 iu, ea	00944-1303-10	1.09		
MONISTAT 3 (Phys Total Care)				
REPACK				
miconazole nitrate				
SUP, VG (W/APPLICATOR)				
200 mg, 3s ea	54868-0436-00	17.92		AB
MONISTAT DERM (Southwood)				
REPACK				
miconazole nitrate				
CRE, TP, 2%, 15 gm	58016-3048-01	14.38		
MONOBENZONE				
(Spectrum Pharmacy) *See 4-BENZYLOXYPHENOL*				
MONOCHLOROACETIC ACID (Amend)				
chloroacetic acid				
POW, NA, 454 gm	17317-0891-01	21.70		
2270 gm	17317-0891-05	86.80		
MONOCLATE-P (CSL)				
antihemophilic factor viii:c human				
PDS, IV, 1 iu, ea	00053-7656-01	1.00		
ea	00053-7656-02	1.00		
ea	00053-7656-04	1.00		
ea	00053-7656-05	1.00		
MONODOX (Aqua Pharmaceuticals)				
doxycycline				
CAP, PO, 50 mg, 100s ea	16110-0260-06	600.00		AB
(GELATIN)				
75 mg, 100s ea	16110-0075-01	1080.00		AB
(GELATIN CAPSULE)				
100 mg, 50s ea	16110-0259-04	660.00		AB
250s ea	16110-0259-07	2340.00		AB
MONOETHANOLAMINE (Baker, J.T.)				
ethanolamine				
LIQ, NA (A.C.S., REAGENT)				
500 ml	10106-9314-01	92.80		
4000 ml	10106-9314-03	174.22		
(Medisca)				
LIQ, NA (U.S.P.)				
500 ml	38779-1262-08	1395.00		
1000 ml	38779-1262-09	2685.00		
(Spectrum Pharmacy)				
LIQ, NA (N.F.)				
500 ml	49452-4776-01	143.85		
4000 ml	49452-4776-02	434.00		
MONOJECT MAGELLAN (Covidien)				
syringe and needle				
DEV, NA (1ML,23GX1",LATEX-FREE)				
200s ea	08881-8113-10	137.98		
(1ML,25GX1",LATEX-FREE)				
200s ea	08881-8115-10	137.98		
(1ML,25GX5/8",LATEX-FREE)				
200s ea	08881-8115-58	137.98		
MONOJECT PREFILL ADVANCED (Covidien)				
sodium chloride				
SOL, IV (60X10ML,PF,LATEX-FREE)				
0.9%, 10 ml 60s	08881-5701-28	268.75		
(120X10ML,PF,LATEX-FREE)				
0.9%, 10 ml 120s	08881-5701-29	531.25		
MONOJECT PREFILL ADVANCED HEPARIN LOCK FLUSH (Covidien)				
heparin sodium				
SOL, IV (SRN,12ML,PF,LATEX-FREE)				
100 u/ml,				
3 ml 180s	08881-5901-23	548.10		
MONOJECT PREFILL HEPARIN LOCK FLUSH (Covidien)				
heparin sodium				
SOL, IV (SRN,12 ML,PF,LATEX-FREE)				
10 u/ml, 3 ml 180s	08881-5801-23	622.80		
5 ml 180s	08881-5801-25	622.80		
(SRN,12 ML,LATEX-FREE)				
10 u/ml,				
10 ml 180s	08881-5801-21	693.00		
(SRN,3 ML,LATEX-FREE)				
100 u/ml,				
2.5 ml 180s	08881-0125-02	533.40		
(SRN,12 ML,PF,LATEX-FREE)				
100 u/ml,				
5 ml 180s	08881-5901-25	637.20		
10 ml 180s	08881-5901-21	711.00		
MONOJECT PREFILL SODIUM CHLORIDE (Covidien)				
sodium chloride				
SOL, IV (SRN,3 ML,PF,LATEX-FREE)				
0.9%, 2.5 ml 180s	08881-5703-00	526.50		
(SRN,12 ML,PF,LATEX-FREE)				
0.9%, 3 ml 180s	08881-5701-23	587.40		
10 ml 180s	08881-5701-21	646.20		
(Tyco)				
SOL, IV (SRN,12 ML,PF,LATEX-FREE)				
0.9%, 5 ml 180s	08881-5701-25	587.40		
MONOKET (UCB)				
isosorbide mononitrate				
TAB, PO, 10 mg, 100s ea	00091-3610-01	171.66		AB
20 mg, 100s ea	00091-3620-01	251.82		AB
180s ea	00091-3620-18	334.53		AB
MONOLETTOR SAFETY LANCET (Kendall)				
lancet device				
DEV, NA (STERILE)				
50s ea	08881-6020-91	18.26		
MONONESSA (Watson)				
ethinyl estradiol/norgestimate				
TAB, PO (COATED)				
35 mcg-0.25 mg,				
28s ea	52544-0247-28	196.42		
(A-S Medication)				
REPACK				
TAB, PO, 35 mcg-0.25 mg,				
28s ea	54569-5816-00	34.10		
MONONINE (CSL)				
factor ix human, purified				
PDS, IV, 1 iu, ea	00053-7668-02	1.18		
ea	00053-7668-04	1.18		
MONOPRIL (Bristol-Myers)				
fosinopril sodium				
TAB, PO, 10 mg, 90s ea	00087-0158-46	148.20		
40 mg, 90s ea	00087-1202-13	148.20		
(AQ)				
REPACK				
TAB, PO, 10 mg, 90s ea	66105-0546-09	159.38		
(PD-Rx Pharm)				
REPACK				
TAB, PO (REDI-SCRIPT)				
10 mg, 30s ea	58864-0104-30	75.00		
20 mg, 30s ea	58864-0667-30	75.00		
40 mg, 15s ea	58864-0510-15	61.89		
(Phys Total Care)				
REPACK				
TAB, PO, 10 mg, 30s ea	54868-2368-01	51.09		
90s ea	54868-2368-02	148.88		
100s ea	54868-2368-00	165.90		
20 mg, 30s ea	54868-3279-03	51.04		
60s ea	54868-3279-00	100.20		
100s ea	54868-3279-02	165.14		
40 mg, 30s ea	54868-4209-00	48.54		
MONOSODIUM GLUTAMATE (PCCA)				
POW, NA (FCC)				
1 gm	51927-3022-00	0.12		
MONTE-G HC (Monte Sano)				
guaifenesin/hydrocodone bitartrate				
SOL, PO (AF,SF,DYE-FREE,CHERRY)				
100 mg/5 ml-4 mg/5 ml,				
473 ml, C-III	12162-0162-16	91.85		
MONTEFLU HC (Monte Sano)				
gg/hydrocod bit/phenyleph hcl				
SOL, PO (AF,SF,DYE-FREE)				
473 ml, C-III	12162-0161-16	91.85		
MONTELUKAST SODIUM				
(Merck) *See SINGULAIR*				
MONTEPHEN (Monte Sano)				
guaifenesin/phenylephrine hydrochloride				
TER, PO, 600 mg-25 mg,				
100s ea	12162-0701-01	91.85		
MONUROL (Forest Pharm)				
fosfomycin tromethamine				
PDS, PO (SINGLE DOSE SACHET)				
3 gm, 3s ea	00456-4300-08	141.20		
(Phys Total Care)				
REPACK				
PDS, PO (SINGLE DOSE SACHET)				
3 gm, ea	54868-4662-00	47.53		
8-MOP (Valeant Pharm Intl)				
methoxsalen				
CAP, PO, 10 mg, 50s ea	00187-0651-42	1843.80		
MORANTEL TARTRATE (PCCA)				
POW, NA (1X1GM)				
1 gm	51927-4337-00	45.00		
MORPHINE (Palmetto)				
REPACK				
morphine sulfate				
TAB, PO, 10 mg,				
30s ea, C-II	23490-9360-03	32.41		
60s ea, C-II	23490-9360-06	64.83		
90s ea, C-II	23490-9360-09	97.24		
MORPHINE SULF (Phys Total Care)				
REPACK				
morphine sulfate				
SOL, IJ (10X1ML)				
4 mg/ml,				
1 ml 10s, C-II	54868-5745-00	50.28		
MORPHINE SULFATE				
(Actavis) *See KADIAN*				
(Amphastar)				
SOL, IJ (SRN,PREFILLED,STICKGARD)				
1 mg/ml,				
10 ml 25s, C-II	00548-2901-25	203.16		EE
(SRN,PREFILL,PCA INJECT)				
1 mg/ml,				
30 ml 10s, C-II	00548-1931-10	159.60		EE
(SRN,PREFILLED,PUMP-JET)				
1 mg/ml,				
30 ml 25s, C-II	00548-1911-25	399.00		EE
(SRN,PREFIL,DILUTE-A-JET)				
25 mg/ml,				
4 ml 25s, C-II	00548-6045-25	251.04		
(APP) *See ASTRAMORPH/PF*				
(Baxter) *See DURAMORPH*				
(Baxter) *See INFUMORPH 200*				
(Baxter) *See INFUMORPH 500*				

PROD/MFR	NDC	AWP	DP	OBC
(Baxter)				
SOL, IJ (SRN,PREFILLED,GLASS)				
1 mg/ml,				
50 ml 10s, C-II	**00338-2689-75**	311.40	259.50	EE
(1X1ML,SDV,USP)				
5 mg/ml,				
1 ml, C-II	**10019-0176-39**	0.74		
(S.D.V.)				
5 mg/ml,				
1 ml 25s, C-II	**10019-0176-44**	18.60		
8 mg/ml, 1 ml, C-II	**10019-0177-37**	1.56		
(1X1ML,USP)				
8 mg/ml,				
1 ml, C-II	**10019-0177-39**	0.84		
(AMP)				
8 mg/ml,				
1 ml 25s, C-II	**10019-0177-68**	39.00		
(VIAL,DOSETTE)				
8 mg/ml,				
1 ml 25s, C-II	**10019-0177-44**	21.00		
10 mg/ml, 1 ml, C-II	**10019-0178-39**	0.76		
(1X1ML,USP)				
10 mg/ml,				
1 ml, C-II	**10019-0178-37**	0.71		
(AMP)				
10 mg/ml,				
1 ml 25s, C-II	**10019-0178-68**	17.70		
(S.D.V., 25X1ML)				
10 mg/ml,				
1 ml 25s, C-II	**10019-0178-44**	18.90		
(M.D.V.)				
10 mg/ml,				
10 ml, C-II	**10019-0178-62**	4.80		
(MDV)				
10 mg/ml,				
10 ml, C-II	**10019-0178-36**	4.80		
(S.D.V.)				
15 mg/ml,				
1 ml 25s, C-II	**10019-0179-44**	19.50		
(M.D.V.)				
15 mg/ml,				
20 ml, C-II	**10019-0179-63**	6.00		
(MDV)				
15 mg/ml,				
20 ml, C-II	**10019-0179-36**	6.00		
(Covidien)				
POW, NA, 5 gm, C-II	**00406-1521-53**	53.05		
25 gm, C-II	**00406-1521-55**	265.25		
50 gm, C-II	**00406-1521-56**	530.05		
100 gm, C-II	**00406-1521-57**	1061.00		
SOL, PO (RASPBERRY FLAVORED)				
20 mg/ml,				
15 ml, C-II	**00406-8003-15**	8.79		
30 ml, C-II	**00406-8003-30**	18.58		
120 ml, C-II	**00406-8003-12**	69.91		
240 ml, C-II	**00406-8003-24**	116.78		
TER, PO, 15 mg,				
100s ea, C-II	**00406-8315-01**	89.37		
100s ea UD, C-II	**00406-8315-62**	89.37		
30 mg, 100s ea, C-II	**00406-8330-01**	169.84		
100s ea UD, C-II	**00406-8330-62**	169.84		
60 mg, 100s ea, C-II	**00406-8380-01**	331.39		
100s ea UD, C-II	**00406-8380-62**	331.39		
100 mg,				
100s ea, C-II	**00406-8390-01**	490.65		
100s ea UD, C-II	**00406-8390-62**	490.65		
200 mg,				
100s ea, C-II	**00406-8320-01**	898.53		
(Elge, Inc.)				
POW, NA (USP)				
100 gm, C-II	**58298-0545-02**	500.00		
(Endo Generics)				
TER, PO, 15 mg,				
100s ea, C-II	**60951-0652-70**	89.17		AB
30 mg, 100s ea, C-II	**60951-0653-70**	169.46		AB
(CAPLET)				
60 mg,				
100s ea, C-II	**60951-0655-70**	330.61		AB
100 mg,				
100s ea, C-II	**60951-0658-70**	489.56		AB
200 mg,				
100s ea, C-II	**60951-0659-70**	896.53		AB
(Ethex)				
TER, PO (FILM-COATED)				
15 mg,				
100s ea, C-II	**58177-0310-04**	89.17		AB
(FILM COATED)				
30 mg,				
100s ea, C-II	**58177-0320-04**	169.46		AB
(FILM-COATED)				
60 mg,				
100s ea, C-II	**58177-0330-04**	330.61		AB
(FILM COATED)				
100 mg,				
100s ea, C-II	**58177-0340-04**	490.65		AB
200 mg,				
100s ea, C-II	**58177-0380-04**	898.53		AB
(Gallipot)				
POW, NA (1X5GM,USP)				
5 gm, C-II	**51552-0678-02**	39.90	28.50	
(1X25GM,USP)				
25 gm, C-II	**51552-0678-04**	107.80	77.00	
(1X100GM,USP)				
100 gm, C-II	**51552-0678-06**	399.00	285.00	
(Glenmark Pharmaceuticals)				
SOL, PO (1X30ML,BERRY)				
20 mg/ml,				
30 ml, C-II	**68462-0349-37**	19.60		
(1X120ML,BERRY)				
20 mg/ml,				
120 ml, C-II	**68462-0349-21**	73.63		
(1X240ML,BERRY)				
20 mg/ml,				
240 ml, C-II	**68462-0349-24**	131.22		
TAB, PO, 15 mg,				
100s ea, C-II	**68462-0202-01**	19.30		
500s ea, C-II	**68462-0202-05**	91.68		
30 mg, 100s ea, C-II	**68462-0203-01**	32.62		
500s ea, C-II	**68462-0203-05**	154.95		
(Hawkins)				
POW, NA (U.S.P.)				
25 gm, C-II	**63370-0950-25**	480.00		
100 gm, C-II	**63370-0950-35**	1689.60		
500 gm, C-II	**63370-0950-45**	7492.80		
1000 gm, C-II	**63370-0950-50**	14030.40		
(Hospira)				
SOL, IJ (5X10ML,PF,LATEX-FREE)				
0.5 mg/ml,				
10 ml 5s, C-II	**00409-3814-12**	28.38	24.85	AP
(PF,LATEX-FREE)				
0.5 mg/ml,				
10 ml 5s, C-II	**00409-4057-12**	11.70	10.25	AP
(5X10ML,LATEX-FREE)				
1 mg/ml,				
10 ml 5s, C-II	**00409-3815-12**	29.76	26.05	AP
(AMP,LATEX-FREE)				
1 mg/ml,				
10 ml 5s, C-II	**00409-4058-12**	15.36	13.45	AP
(LLK,SLIM PK,CARPUJECT)				
2 mg/ml,				
1 ml 10s, C-II	**00409-1762-30**	12.84	11.20	
(LUER LOCK,U.S.P.,10X1ML)				
4 mg/ml,				
1 ml 10s, C-II	**00409-1258-30**	13.20	11.60	
(CARPUJECT W/LUER LOCK)				
8 mg/ml,				
1 ml 10s, C-II	**00409-1260-69**	13.68	12.00	
(LLK,SLIM PK, 10X1ML)				
10 mg/ml,				
1 ml 10s, C-II	**00409-1261-30**	14.16	12.40	
(LUER LOCK,LATEX-FREE)				
15 mg/ml,				
1 ml 10s, C-II	**00409-1264-31**	13.32	11.70	
(ADD-VANTAGE, 10X4ML)				
25 mg/ml,				
4 ml 10s, C-II	**00409-6177-14**	120.00	105.00	
(HIGH CONCENTRATION,PF)				
25 mg/ml,				
10 ml, C-II	**00409-1135-02**	6.20	5.43	
(ADD-VANTAGE,LATEX-FREE)				
25 mg/ml,				
10 ml 10s, C-II	**00409-6179-14**	111.48	97.50	
(VIAL, FLIPTOP)				
50 mg/ml,				
20 ml, C-II	**00409-1134-03**	10.72	9.38	
(LATEX-FREE)				
50 mg/ml,				
50 ml, C-II	**00409-1134-05**	22.02	19.27	
IV (10X30ML,USP,S.D.V,PF)				
1 mg/ml,				
30 ml 10s, C-II	**00409-2029-02**	102.12	89.40	AP
(SDV,30MLX10,PF)				
5 mg/ml,				
30 ml 10s, C-II	**00409-6028-04**	119.40	104.50	EE
(King Pharm) *See AVINZA*				
(Lannett)				
SOL, PO, 20 mg/ml,				
30 ml, C-II	**00527-1425-36**	18.62		
120 ml, C-II	**00527-1425-62**	73.63		
240 ml, C-II	**00527-1425-63**	131.22		
(Letco)				
POW, NA (1X25GM,USP)				
25 gm, C-II	**62991-1403-03**	368.00	92.00	
(1X100GM,USP)				
100 gm, C-II	**62991-1403-05**	1320.00	330.00	
(1X500GM,USP)				
500 gm, C-II	**62991-1403-07**	6400.00	1600.00	
(Medisca)				
POW, NA (U.S.P.)				
5 gm, C-II	**38779-0673-03**	89.40		
25 gm, C-II	**38779-0673-04**	285.00		
100 gm, C-II	**38779-0673-05**	985.50		
250 gm, C-II	**38779-0673-07**	2295.00		
(1X500GM,USP)				
500 gm, C-II	**38779-0673-08**	3825.00		
(Paddock)				
POW, NA, 25 gm, C-II	**00574-2006-25**	265.25		
SOL, PO (1X30ML,CONCENTRATE)				
20 mg/ml,				
30 ml, C-II	**00574-0127-30**	22.50		
SUP, RC, 5 mg,				
12s ea UD, C-II	**00574-7110-12**	53.40		
10 mg,				
12s ea UD, C-II	**00574-7112-12**	66.15		
20 mg,				
12s ea UD, C-II	**00574-7114-12**	80.50		
30 mg,				
12s ea UD, C-II	**00574-7116-12**	101.25		
(PCCA)				
POW, NA (U.S.P.; CII)				
1 gm, C-II	**51927-1000-00**	90.00		
(PharMEDium Services)				
SOL, IJ (5X50ML,LATEX-FREE)				
50 mg/ml,				
50 ml 5s, C-II	**61553-0649-75**	33.00	27.50	
(Purdue Pharma) *See MS CONTIN*				
(Roxane)				
SOL, PO (40X5ML)				
10 mg/5 ml,				
5 ml 40s UD, C-II	**00054-0237-55**	30.67		EE
(1X100ML)				
10 mg/5 ml,				
100 ml, C-II	**00054-0237-49**	11.17		EE
(1X500ML)				
10 mg/5 ml,				
500 ml, C-II	**00054-0237-63**	38.56		EE
(1X100ML)				
20 mg/5 ml,				
100 ml, C-II	**00054-0238-49**	15.92		EE
(1X500ML)				
20 mg/5 ml,				
500 ml, C-II	**00054-0238-63**	65.03		EE
(1X30ML,AF,SF)				
20 mg/ml,				
30 ml, C-II	**00054-0352-44**	22.91		
(1X120ML,AF,SF)				
20 mg/ml,				
120 ml, C-II	**00054-0352-50**	87.61		
TAB, PO, 15 mg,				
100s ea, C-II	**00054-0235-25**	18.32		EE
(25X4)				
15 mg,				
100s ea UD, C-II	**00054-0235-24**	32.28		EE
30 mg, 100s ea, C-II	**00054-0236-25**	31.22		EE
(25X4)				
30 mg,				
100s ea UD, C-II	**00054-0236-24**	54.80		EE
(Spectrum Pharmacy)				
POW, NA (U.S.P.)				
5 gm, C-II	**49452-0028-01**	145.25		
25 gm, C-II	**49452-0028-02**	423.50		
100 gm, C-II	**49452-0028-03**	1473.50		
250 gm, C-II	**49452-0028-04**	2205.00		
(Teva)				
SOL, IJ (USP,5X10ML,PF)				
0.5 mg/ml,				
10 ml 5s, C-II	**00555-1129-10**	155.25		AP
1 mg/ml,				
10 ml 5s, C-II	**00555-1128-10**	75.25		AP
10 ml 5s, C-II	**00555-1130-10**	146.00		AP
(Watson Labs)				
TER, PO (USP)				
15 mg,				
100s ea, C-II	**00591-3511-01**	45.78		
30 mg, 100s ea, C-II	**00591-3512-01**	81.84		
60 mg, 100s ea, C-II	**00591-3513-01**	198.49		
100 mg,				
100s ea, C-II	**00591-3514-01**	335.30		AB
200 mg,				
100s ea, C-II	**00591-3515-01**	484.88		
(Xanodyne Pharma) *See ORAMORPH SR*				
(4u)				
REPACK				
TAB, PO, 15 mg,				
28s ea, C-II	**42549-0602-28**	48.86		
28s ea, C-II	**42549-0623-28**	48.86		
56s ea, C-II	**42549-0602-56**	97.72		
56s ea, C-II	**42549-0623-56**	97.72		
TER, PO, 15 mg,				
28s ea, C-II	**10544-0401-28**	86.92		
28s ea, C-II	**10544-0414-28**	86.92		

PROD/MFR	NDC	AWP	DP	OBC
28s ea, C-II	42549-0601-28	86.92		
28s ea, C-II	42549-0614-28	86.92		
56s ea, C-II	10544-0401-56	166.34		
56s ea, C-II	42549-0601-56	166.34		
56s ea, C-II	42549-0614-56	166.34		
60s ea, C-II	10544-0414-60	174.44		
60s ea, C-II	42549-0601-60	174.44		
60s ea, C-II	42549-0614-60	174.44		
30 mg, 28s ea, C-II	10544-0372-28	79.36		
28s ea, C-II	10544-0379-28	101.56		
28s ea, C-II	42549-0572-28	79.36		
28s ea, C-II	42549-0579-28	101.56		
30s ea, C-II	10544-0379-30	104.24		
30s ea, C-II	42549-0579-30	104.24		
56s ea, C-II	10544-0379-56	156.72		
56s ea, C-II	42549-0572-56	156.72		
56s ea, C-II	42549-0579-56	156.72		
60s ea, C-II	10544-0379-60	164.88		
60s ea, C-II	42549-0579-60	164.88		
60 mg, 60s ea, C-II	42549-0616-60	274.16		
(Altura)				
REPACK				
TER, PO (FILM-COATED)				
15 mg,				
30s ea, C-II	63874-1238-03	72.75		AB
60s ea, C-II	63874-1238-06	145.52		AB
(FILM COATED)				
30 mg,				
30s ea, C-II	63874-1234-03	80.53		AB
60s ea, C-II	63874-1234-06	161.08		AB
60 mg, 30s ea, C-II	63874-1235-03	141.19		
60s ea, C-II	63874-1235-06	282.40		
(B&B Pharm, Inc)				
REPACK				
POW, NA (U.S.P.)				
25 gm, C-II	63275-1025-04	525.00		
100 gm, C-II	63275-1100-05	2100.00		
(DHS, Inc.)				
REPACK				
TAB, PO, 15 mg,				
30s ea, C-II	55887-0887-30	46.96		
TER, PO, 30 mg,				
30s ea, C-II	55887-0092-30	71.20		
60 mg, 30s ea, C-II	55887-0093-30	120.00		
60s ea, C-II	55887-0093-60	240.00		
100 mg, 30s ea, C-II	55887-0094-30	180.00		
60s ea, C-II	55887-0094-60	360.00		AB
(Dispensing Solutions)				
REPACK				
TER, PO, 15 mg,				
60s ea, C-II	66336-0172-60	64.95		
30 mg, 30s ea, C-II	66336-0173-30	52.12		
60s ea, C-II	66336-0173-60	122.88		
60 mg, 60s ea, C-II	66336-0963-60	228.00		
(Palmetto)				
REPACK				
TAB, PO, 15 mg,				
4s ea, C-II	23490-5945-00	16.19		
6s ea, C-II	23490-5945-01	18.59		
60s ea, C-II	23490-5945-02	63.00		
30 mg, 60s ea, C-II	23490-5946-01	117.00		
TER, PO, 15 mg,				
15s ea, C-II	23490-7792-01	33.75		
30s ea, C-II	23490-7792-03	67.50		
60s ea, C-II	23490-7792-06	135.00		
90s ea, C-II	23490-7792-09	202.50		
30 mg, 15s ea, C-II	23490-7777-01	41.25		
30s ea, C-II	23490-7777-03	82.50		
60s ea, C-II	23490-7777-06	165.00		
90s ea, C-II	23490-7777-09	247.50		
60 mg, 30s ea, C-II	23490-7912-03	127.07		
60s ea, C-II	23490-7912-06	254.14		
90s ea, C-II	23490-7912-09	381.12		
100 mg, 30s ea, C-II	23490-7913-03	188.16		
60s ea, C-II	23490-7913-06	376.32		
90s ea, C-II	23490-7913-09	564.48		
200 mg, 30s ea, C-II	23490-7914-03	344.87		
60s ea, C-II	23490-7914-06	689.75		
90s ea, C-II	23490-7914-09	1034.62		
(Phys Total Care)				
REPACK				
POW, NA, 25 gm, C-II	54868-4050-00	560.40		
SOL, IJ, 10 mg/ml,				
1 ml, C-II	54868-4752-01	7.77		
(22G,SLIM PK,LATEX-FREE)				
10 mg/ml,				
1 ml 10s, C-II	54868-4804-00	44.43		
(TUBEX,22GX1 1/4")				
10 mg/ml,				
1 ml 10s, C-II	54868-0115-00	52.62		
1 ml 25s, C-II	54868-4752-00	87.75		

PROD/MFR	NDC	AWP	DP	OBC
(AMP,DOSETTE)				
10 mg/ml,				
1 ml 25s, C-II	54868-4189-00	84.06		
PO, 20 mg/ml,				
30 ml, C-II	54868-5508-01	44.68		
120 ml, C-II	54868-5508-00	124.47		
TAB, PO, 15 mg,				
30s ea, C-II	54868-3191-04	13.38		EE
60s ea, C-II	54868-3191-03	26.77		EE
30 mg, 30s ea, C-II	54868-4973-02	20.94		EE
60s ea, C-II	54868-4973-01	34.38		EE
100s ea, C-II	54868-4973-05	50.72		EE
150s ea, C-II	54868-4973-04	71.58		EE
TER, PO, 15 mg,				
10s ea, C-II	54868-5132-02	20.79		
30s ea, C-II	54868-5132-00	50.34		
60s ea, C-II	54868-5132-01	94.68		
90s ea, C-II	54868-5132-04	92.61		
120s ea, C-II	54868-5132-03	141.60		
30 mg, 20s ea, C-II	54868-4033-01	50.91		
30s ea, C-II	54868-4033-03	81.07		
60s ea, C-II	54868-4033-00	120.81		
90s ea, C-II	54868-4033-04	175.23		
100s ea, C-II	54868-4033-05	165.81		
120s ea, C-II	54868-4033-02	235.65		
60 mg, 20s ea, C-II	54868-5054-03	64.86		
30s ea, C-II	54868-5054-02	124.14		
60s ea, C-II	54868-5054-00	139.08		
90s ea, C-II	54868-5054-01	203.40		
100s ea, C-II	54868-5054-04	249.81		
100 mg, 20s ea, C-II	54868-5590-01	87.45		
30s ea, C-II	54868-5590-03	127.44		
60s ea, C-II	54868-5590-00	247.38		
90s ea, C-II	54868-5590-02	347.34		
100s ea, C-II	54868-5590-04	287.56		AB
(Quality Care Prod)				
REPACK				
SOL, PO, 20 mg/ml,				
240 ml, C-II	35356-0008-08	140.14		
TER, PO, 15 mg,				
90s ea, C-II	49999-0845-90	140.88		
30 mg, 90s ea, C-II	49999-0846-90	213.60		
(FILM COATED)				
100 mg,				
30s ea, C-II	35356-0521-30	189.00		AB
60s ea, C-II	35356-0521-60	378.00		AB
200 mg, 30s ea, C-II	35356-0528-30	497.30		AB
(Stat Rx)				
REPACK				
TAB, PO, 15 mg,				
30s ea, C-II	16590-0658-30	11.25		EE
56s ea, C-II	16590-0658-56	21.00		EE
60s ea, C-II	16590-0658-60	22.50		EE
90s ea, C-II	16590-0658-90	33.75		EE
30 mg, 30s ea, C-II	16590-0683-30	15.00		EE
60s ea, C-II	16590-0683-60	26.50		EE
90s ea, C-II	16590-0683-90	38.01		EE
TER, PO, 15 mg,				
30s ea, C-II	16590-0645-30	40.00		
45s ea, C-II	16590-0645-45	45.00		
56s ea, C-II	16590-0645-56	71.68		
60s ea, C-II	16590-0645-60	78.75		
75s ea, C-II	16590-0645-75	75.00		
84s ea, C-II	16590-0645-62	107.50		
90s ea, C-II	16590-0645-90	115.00		
120s ea, C-II	16590-0645-72	149.50		
30 mg, 30s ea, C-II	16590-0607-30	65.00		
56s ea, C-II	16590-0607-56	95.20		
60s ea, C-II	16590-0607-60	128.75		
84s ea, C-II	16590-0607-62	142.75		
90s ea, C-II	16590-0607-90	188.25		
120s ea, C-II	16590-0607-72	204.00		
60 mg, 30s ea, C-II	16590-0695-30	120.25		
60s ea, C-II	16590-0695-60	220.50		
90s ea, C-II	16590-0695-90	328.09		
120s ea, C-II	16590-0695-72	404.25		
100 mg, 30s ea, C-II	16590-0696-30	162.03		AB
60s ea, C-II	16590-0696-60	284.00		AB
90s ea, C-II	16590-0696-90	431.00		AB
120s ea, C-II	16590-0696-72	525.00		AB
MORPHINE SULFATE ER (Quality Care Prod)				
REPACK				
morphine sulfate				
TER, PO, 15 mg,				
30s ea, C-II	49999-0845-30	50.50		
60s ea, C-II	49999-0845-60	145.52		
120s ea, C-II	49999-0845-01	183.02		
30 mg,				
30s ea, C-II	49999-0846-30	80.54		
60s ea, C-II	49999-0846-60	161.08		
120s ea, C-II	49999-0846-01	291.11		

PROD/MFR	NDC	AWP	DP	OBC
60 mg,				
30s ea, C-II	49999-0847-30	141.20		
60s ea, C-II	49999-0847-60	282.40		
90s ea, C-II	49999-0847-90	343.44		
120s ea, C-II	49999-0847-01	461.50		
MORPHINE SULFATE IN 5% DEXTROSE (Hospira)				
dextrose/morphine sulfate				
SOL, IV (PREMIX)				
5%-100 mg/100 ml,				
250 ml, C-II	00409-6062-02	13.98	12.23	
MORPHINE SULFATE IR (Phys Total Care)				
REPACK				
morphine sulfate				
TAB, PO, 15 mg,				
4s ea, C-II	54868-3191-00	7.38		
10s ea, C-II	54868-3191-01	9.45		
90s ea, C-II	54868-3191-05	37.14		
100s ea, C-II	54868-3191-06	38.05		
120s ea, C-II	54868-3191-02	47.54		
30 mg,				
90s ea, C-II	54868-4973-03	47.82		
120s ea, C-II	54868-4973-00	61.29		
(Quality Care Prod)				
REPACK				
TAB, PO, 15 mg,				
30s ea, C-II	49999-0848-30	46.96		
60s ea, C-II	49999-0848-60	93.92		
30 mg,				
30s ea, C-II	49999-0849-30	71.20		
60s ea, C-II	49999-0849-60	142.40		
MORPHINE SULFATE LIPOSOME (EKR) *See DEPODUR*				
MORPHINE SULFATE-SODIUM CHLORIDE (PharMEDium Services)				
morphine sulfate/sodium chloride				
SOL, IV (5X55ML,LATEX-FREE)				
1 mg/ml-0.9%,				
55 ml 5s, C-II	61553-0651-76	17.62	14.68	
(5X100ML, CASSETTE)				
1 mg/ml-0.9%,				
100 ml 5s, C-II	61553-0821-48	131.40	109.50	
(5X50ML, CASSETTE)				
5 mg/ml-0.9%,				
50 ml 5s	61553-0822-41	141.30	117.75	
MORPHINE SULFATE/NALTREXONE HYDROCHLORIDE (King Pharm) *See EMBEDA*				
MORPHINE SULFATE/SODIUM CHLORIDE (PharMEDium Services) *See MORPHINE SULFATE-SODIUM CHLORIDE*				
(PharMEDium Services)				
SOL, IV (INTRAVIA)				
50 mg/50 ml-0.9%,				
50 ml, C-II	61553-0177-41	25.40	21.17	
(INTRAVIA,BAG SIZE 150ML)				
100 mg/100 ml-0.9%,				
100 ml, C-II	61553-0179-48	26.56	22.13	
(IPUMP BAG)				
100 mg/100 ml-0.9%,				
100 ml, C-II	61553-0178-48	40.51	33.76	
(INTRAVIA)				
250 mg/250 ml-0.9%,				
250 ml, C-II	61553-0181-02	32.04	26.70	
MORRHUATE SODIUM (Amer Regent)				
SOL, IV (M.D.V.)				
50 mg/ml, 30 ml	00517-3065-01	87.50		
(Consolidated Midland) *See SODIUM MORRHUATE*				
(Phys Total Care)				
REPACK				
SOL, IV (M.D.V.)				
50 mg/ml, 30 ml	54868-4596-00	76.24		
MOTOFEN (Valeant Pharm Intl)				
atropine sulfate/difenoxin hydrochloride				
TAB, PO (DYE-FREE)				
0.025 mg-1 mg,				
50s ea, C-IV	00187-0500-01	56.19		
100s ea, C-IV	00187-0500-02	98.33		
(Phys Total Care)				
REPACK				
TAB, PO, 0.025 mg-1 mg,				
20s ea, C-IV	54868-3510-00	21.31		
50s ea, C-IV	54868-3510-01	49.55		
MOTRIN (PD-Rx Pharm)				
REPACK				
ibuprofen				
TAB, PO, 800 mg, 21s ea	55289-0041-21	38.95		AB
30s ea	55289-0041-30	53.50		AB

PROD/MFR	NDC	AWP	DP	OBC
(REDI-SCRIPT)				
800 mg, 30s ea	58864-0026-30	53.51		AB
(Pharma Pac)				
REPACK				
SUS, PO, 100 mg/5 ml,				
120 ml	52959-0266-03	9.95		AB
(Phys Total Care)				
REPACK				
TAB, PO, 400 mg, 30s ea	54868-0438-00	7.66		AB
600 mg, 30s ea	54868-0439-03	8.87		AB
60s ea	54868-0439-04	15.88		AB
(USP)				
800 mg, 20s ea	54868-0437-01	8.41		AB
30s ea	54868-0437-03	11.68		AB
60s ea	54868-0437-04	21.48		AB
100s ea	54868-0437-00	34.55		AB
(Southwood)				
REPACK				
SUS, PO, 100 mg/5 ml,				
120 ml	58016-0270-04	6.18		AB
TAB, PO, 800 mg, 30s ea	58016-0313-30	8.06		AB
60s ea	58016-0313-60	16.12		AB
90s ea	58016-0313-90	24.17		AB
100s ea	58016-0313-00	26.86		AB
MOTRIN PEDIATRIC (Phys Total Care)				
REPACK				
ibuprofen				
SUS, PO (BERRY,DROPS)				
40 mg/ml, 120 ml	54868-1904-01	8.23		
MOUTHWASH				
(Carrington) *See SALICEPT ORAL RINSE*				
MOVIPREP (Salix Pharm)				
peg electrolyte lavage solution				
PDS, PO (W/CONTAINER,POUCH A & B)				
ea	65649-0201-75	57.34		
(Phys Total Care)				
REPACK				
PDS, PO (W/CONTAINER, POUCH A &B)				
ea	54868-5890-00	68.47		
MOXATAG (MiddleBrook)				
amoxicillin				
TER, PO (FILM-COATED)				
775 mg, 30s ea	11042-0142-03	294.30		
MOXIFLOXACIN HYDROCHLORIDE				
(Alcon Ophthalmic) *See VIGAMOX*				
(Schering) *See AVELOX*				
(Schering) *See AVELOX I.V.*				
MOXILIN (Intl Ethical)				
amoxicillin				
CAP, PO, 250 mg, 100s ea	11584-0391-00	9.15		EE
500 mg, 100s ea	11584-0401-00	17.08		EE
500s ea	11584-0401-05	81.60		EE
PDR, PO, 250 mg/5 ml,				
100 ml	11584-0381-00	2.50		EE
150 ml	11584-0381-05	2.87		EE
MOZOBIL (Genzyme)				
plerixafor				
SOL, SC (PF)				
20 mg/ml, 1.2 ml	58468-0140-01	7500.00	6250.00	
MPI DMSA (GE)				
technetium tc 99m succimer				
KIT, IV (5 VIALS)				
ea	17156-0525-01	823.66		
MPI DTPA (GE)				
technetium tc 99m pentetate				
KIT, IV (CHELATE, 10 VIALS)				
ea	17156-0439-04	242.30		AP
MPI MAA (GE)				
technetium tc 99m albumin aggregated				
KIT, IV (10 VIALS)				
ea	17156-0520-01	998.82		EE
MPI MDP (GE)				
technetium tc 99m medronate				
KIT, IV (10 MG, 10 VIALS)				
ea	17156-0438-04	257.29		AP
(30 MG, 10 VIALS)				
ea	17156-0438-05	644.88		AP
MPI PYROPHOSPHATE (GE)				
technetium tc 99m pyrophosphate				
KIT, IV (10 VIALS)				
ea	17156-0521-01	210.83		EE
MS CONTIN (Purdue Pharma)				
morphine sulfate				
TER, PO, 15 mg,				
100s ea, C-II	59011-0260-10	146.17		
30 mg,				
100s ea, C-II	59011-0261-25	277.76		
500s ea, C-II	59011-0261-05	1277.64		
60 mg,				
100s ea, C-II	59011-0262-10	542.00		
500s ea, C-II	59011-0262-05	2493.24		
100 mg,				
100s ea, C-II	59011-0263-10	802.48		
500s ea, C-II	59011-0263-05	3691.42		
200 mg,				
100s ea, C-II	59011-0264-10	1469.63		
(DHS, Inc.)				
REPACK				
TER, PO, 15 mg,				
60s ea, C-II	55887-0072-60	70.14		
30 mg,				
60s ea, C-II	55887-0068-60	133.28		
(Palmetto)				
REPACK				
TER, PO, 30 mg,				
30s ea, C-II	23490-9280-03	90.00		
60s ea, C-II	23490-9280-06	180.00		
90s ea, C-II	23490-9280-09	270.00		
100 mg,				
30s ea, C-II	23490-9281-03	210.00		
60s ea, C-II	23490-9281-06	420.00		
90s ea, C-II	23490-9281-09	630.00		
200 mg,				
30s ea, C-II	23490-9282-03	360.00		
60s ea, C-II	23490-9282-06	720.00		
(Phys Total Care)				
REPACK				
TER, PO, 15 mg,				
30s ea, C-II	54868-3081-00	38.11		AB
90s ea, C-II	54868-3081-01	108.08		AB
30 mg,				
60s ea, C-II	54868-2115-01	127.26		
90s ea, C-II	54868-2115-00	189.34		
(Quality Care Prod)				
REPACK				
TER, PO, 15 mg,				
30s ea, C-II	35356-0335-30	112.17		
60s ea, C-II	35356-0335-60	217.39		
90s ea, C-II	35356-0335-90	322.62		
100s ea, C-II	35356-0335-00	357.69		
30 mg,				
100s ea, C-II	35356-0338-00	409.37		
60 mg,				
100s ea, C-II	35356-0334-00	795.20		
100 mg,				
100s ea, C-II	35356-0336-00	1175.48		
200 mg,				
100s ea, C-II	35356-0337-00	2149.56		
(Stat Rx)				
REPACK				
TER, PO, 60 mg,				
56s ea, C-II	16590-0884-56	354.94		
MST 600 (Cypress Pharm)				
magnesium salicylate				
TAB, PO, 600 mg, 100s ea	60258-0106-01	55.93		
MUCINEX ER (PD-Rx Pharm)				
REPACK				
guaifenesin				
TER, PO, 600 mg, 40s ea	58864-0196-40	26.45		
(REDI-SCRIPT,USP)				
600 mg, 60s ea	58864-0196-60	29.68		
MUIRA PUAMA (PCCA)				
POW, NA, 1 gm	51927-3275-00	0.33		
MULTAQ (Sanofi-Aventis)				
dronedarone hydrochloride				
TAB, PO (FILM-COATED)				
400 mg, 60s ea	00024-4142-60	259.20		
(10X10,FILM-COATED)				
400 mg, 100s ea UD	00024-4142-10	432.00		
(FILM-COATED)				
400 mg, 180s ea	00024-4142-18	777.60		
MULTI B PLUS (Phys Total Care)				
REPACK				
multivitamin and minerals				
TAB, PO, 100s ea	54868-1815-01	39.55		
MULTI VITA-BETS W/FLUORIDE (Phys Total Care)				
multivitamin and fluoride				
CTB, PO, 100s ea	54868-4915-00	28.35		
MULTI-VIT WITH FLUORIDE (Qualitest)				
multivitamin and fluoride				
LIQ, PO (1X50ML,DROPS)				
50 ml	00603-1449-47	11.80		
50 ml	00603-1450-47	11.80		
MULTI-VIT WITH FLUORIDE AND IRON (Qualitest)				
multivitamin, iron, and fluoride				
LIQ, PO (1X50ML,DROPS)				
50 ml	00603-1452-47	12.00		
MULTI-VITAMIN W/FLUORIDE (Phys Total Care)				
REPACK				
multivitamin and fluoride				
LIQ, PO (DROPS)				
50 ml	54868-1942-00	10.38		
MULTI-VITAMIN WITH FLUORIDE (Qualitest)				
multivitamin and fluoride				
CTB, PO (GRAPE)				
100s ea	00603-4381-21	34.73		
100s ea	00603-4382-21	34.73		
100s ea	00603-4383-21	34.73		
MULTICHEW (Vertical)				
multivitamin and minerals				
CTB, PO (BERRY)				
100s ea	68025-0021-10	43.46		
MULTIFOL PLUS (Breckenridge Pharm)				
multivitamin, minerals, and iron				
TAB, PO (FILM-COATED)				
100s ea	51991-0254-01	47.96		
MULTIGEN (Breckenridge Pharm)				
vitamin b complex, iron, and vitamin c				
TAB, PO (FILM-COATED CAPLET)				
90s ea	51991-0543-90	112.30		
MULTIGEN FOLIC (Breckenridge Pharm)				
vitamin b complex, iron, and vitamin c				
TAB, PO (FILM-COATED CAPLET)				
90s ea	51991-0546-90	112.30		
MULTIGEN PLUS (Breckenridge Pharm)				
vitamin b complex, iron, and vitamin c				
TAB, PO (FILM-COATED CAPLET)				
90s ea	51991-0544-90	112.30		
MULTIHANCE (Bracco Diag)				
gadobenate dimeglumine				
SOL, IV, 529 mg/ml,				
5 ml 5s	00270-5164-12	189.06	151.25	
10 ml 5s	00270-5164-13	370.94	296.75	
15 ml 5s	00270-5164-14	542.81	434.25	
20 ml 5s	00270-5164-15	670.31	536.25	
(MULTIPACK,BULK PACKAGE)				
529 mg/ml,				
50 ml 5s	00270-5264-16	1762.50	1410.00	
100 ml 5s	00270-5264-17	3525.00	2820.00	
MULTILYTE-20 CONCENTRATE (APP)				
multimineral				
SOL, IV (S.D.V.,PF)				
25 ml	63323-0425-25	4.48		
MULTILYTE-40 CONCENTRATE (APP)				
multimineral				
SOL, IV (S.D.V.,PF)				
25 ml	63323-0420-25	4.83		
MULTIMINERAL				
(APP) *See MULTILYTE-20 CONCENTRATE*				
(APP) *See MULTILYTE-40 CONCENTRATE*				
MULTIMINERAL/MULTIVITAMIN				
(Everett) *See STROVITE PLUS*				
(Pharmics) *See O-CAL FA*				
(Trigen) *See ELITE-OB*				
MULTIPLE VITAMINS W/FLUORIDE (A-S Medication)				
REPACK				
multivitamin and fluoride				
CTB, PO, 100s ea	54569-4629-00	15.07		
30s ea	54569-3372-02	4.52		
100s ea	54569-3372-01	15.07		
30s ea	54569-2384-01	4.52		
100s ea	54569-2384-00	15.07		
LIQ, PO (DROPS)				
50 ml	54569-1270-00	11.80		
MULTITRACE-4 CONCENTRATED (Amer Regent)				
chromium/copper/manganese/zinc				
SOL, IV (S.D.V.,PF)				
1 ml 25s	00517-7201-25	93.75		
(M.D.V.)				
10 ml 25s	00517-7210-25	310.94		
MULTITRACE-4 NEONATAL (Amer Regent)				
chromium/copper/manganese/zinc				
SOL, IV (S.D.V.,PF)				
2 ml 25s	00517-6202-25	109.38		
MULTITRACE-4 PEDIATRIC (Amer Regent)				
chromium/copper/manganese/zinc				
SOL, IV (S.D.V.,PF)				
3 ml 25s	00517-9203-25	125.00		

PROD/MFR	NDC	AWP	DP	OBC

MULTITRACE-4 REGULAR (Amer Regent)
chromium/copper/manganese/zinc
SOL, IV (M.D.V.)
10 ml 25s........... 00517-7410-25 132.81

MULTITRACE-5 (Amer Regent)
chromium/copper/manganese/selenium/zinc
SOL, IV (M.D.V.)
10 ml 25s........... 00517-8510-25 132.81

MULTITRACE-5 CONCENTRATE (Amer Regent)
chromium/copper/manganese/selenium/zinc
SOL, IV (S.D.V.,PF)
1 ml 25s............ 00517-8201-25 164.06
(M.D.V.)
10 ml 25s........... 00517-8210-25 140.63

MULTIVITAMIN
(Baxter) *See INFUVITE*
(Baxter) *See INFUVITE PEDIATRIC*
(Hospira) *See M.V.I.-12 W/O VITAMIN K*
(Hospira) *See M.V.I.ADULT*
(Hospira) *See MVI PEDIATRIC*
(Llorens Pharma Int) *See NUTRIVIT*
(Nnodum) *See RENO CAPS*

MULTIVITAMIN AND FLUORIDE
(Breckenridge Pharm) *See MULTIVITAMIN WITH FLUORIDE*
(Hi-Tech) *See POLYVITAMIN W/FLUORIDE*
(Major) *See CHEWABLE MULTIVITAMIN WITH FLUORIDE*
(Propharma) *See MULTIVITAMIN W/FLUORIDE*
(Qualitest) *See MULTI-VIT WITH FLUORIDE*
(Qualitest) *See MULTI-VITAMIN WITH FLUORIDE*
(Sancilio) *See MVC FLUORIDE*
(Silarx) *See POLY-VITAMIN W/FLUORIDE*
(Teva) *See MULTIVITE PLUS FLUORIDE*
(Palmetto)
REPACK
CTB, PO, 100s ea......... 23490-7396-01 15.81
100s ea.......... 23490-7203-01 15.07

MULTIVITAMIN AND IRON
(Breckenridge Pharm) *See FERREX 28*
(Nephro-Tech) *See NEPHRON FA*
(Ther-RX) *See NIFEREX GOLD*
(U.S. Pharm) *See INTEGRA-F*

MULTIVITAMIN AND MINERALS
(A. G. Marin) *See SUPPORT*
(Acella) *See CALCIUM-FOLIC ACID PLUS D CHEWABLE WAFER*
(Alaven) *See CALAFOL RX*
(Azur Pharma, Inc.) *See FEMTABS*
(Breckenridge Pharm) *See FERROCITE PLUS*
(Breckenridge Pharm) *See V•C FORTE*
(Contract Pharmacal) *See B-PLEX PLUS*
(Contract Pharmacal) *See PRENATAL*
(Everett) *See CALCIFOL*
(Everett) *See CALCIFOLIC-D*
(Everett) *See RENAX*
(Everett) *See RENAX 5.5*
(Everett) *See STROVITE FORTE*
(Gil Pharmaceutical) *See PROTECT PLUS*
(Hawthorn Pharm) *See RENATABS*
(Hawthorn Pharm) *See RENATABS WITH IRON*
(Major) *See FORMULA B PLUS*
(Major) *See VICAP FORTE*
(Mayne Pharma) *See M.V.I-12*
(Nephro-Tech) *See VITAL-D*
(Nnodum) *See VITAROCA PLUS*
(PGD, Inc.) *See GENESUPP-500*
(PGD, Inc.) *See GENETECT PLUS*
(Qualitest) *See THEROBEC PLUS*
(Qualitest) *See VICA-FORTE*
(Rising) *See VITA S FORTE*
(Seyer Pharmatec) *See HEMATRON*
(Seyer Pharmatec) *See SUPERVITE*
(Ther-RX) *See PRECARE PREMIER*
(U.S. Pharm) *See HEMOCYTE PLUS*
(Vertical) *See CORVITE*
(Vertical) *See MULTICHEW*

MULTIVITAMIN AND MINERALS/NUTRICEUTICAL
(Ther-RX) *See ENCORA*

MULTIVITAMIN AND NUTRICEUTICALS
(Boca Pharmacal) *See FEROTRIN*
(Contract Pharmacal) *See FEROTRINSIC*
(SJ) *See CARDIOTEK-RX*

MULTIVITAMIN W/FLUORIDE (Propharma)
multivitamin and fluoride
LIQ, PO (DROPS)
50 ml............... 50313-0110-43 5.75
50 ml............... 50313-0113-43 6.00

(Phys Total Care)
REPACK
CTB, PO, 30s ea.......... 54868-4914-01 27.22
100s ea............ 54868-4914-00 78.74
30s ea.............. 54868-1313-01 12.09

MULTIVITAMIN W/FLUORIDE & IRON (Propharma)
multivitamin, iron, and fluoride
LIQ, PO, 50 ml........... 50313-0111-43 6.20
50 ml............... 50313-0112-43 6.50

MULTIVITAMIN WITH FLUORIDE (Breckenridge Pharm)
multivitamin and fluoride
CTB, PO (ORANGE)
100s ea............. 51991-0679-01 34.73
100s ea............. 51991-0680-01 34.73
100s ea............. 51991-0681-01 34.73

MULTIVITAMIN, IRON, AND FLUORIDE
(Hi-Tech) *See POLY-VITAMIN W/FLUORIDE/IRON*
(Propharma) *See MULTIVITAMIN W/FLUORIDE & IRON*
(Qualitest) *See MULTI-VIT WITH FLUORIDE AND IRON*
(Silarx) *See POLY-VITAMIN W/FLUORIDE/IRON*

MULTIVITAMIN, MINERALS, AND IRON
(Breckenridge Pharm) *See FERROCITE PLUS*
(Breckenridge Pharm) *See MULTIFOL PLUS*
(Breckenridge Pharm) *See MUTIFOL*
(Contract Pharmacal) *See HEMOPLEX PLUS*
(Cypress Pharm) *See HEMATINIC PLUS VITAMINS & MINERALS*
(Everett) *See VITAFOL*
(Everett) *See VITAFOL-OB*
(Kenwood) *See GLUTOFAC-MX*
(Kramer-Novis) *See LYSIPLEX PLUS*
(McNeil,R.A.) *See M-VIT*
(River's Edge) *See RE DUALVIT PLUS*
(Seton) *See SE-TAN PLUS*
(Seyer Pharmatec) *See HEMATRON-AF*
(U.S. Pharm) *See INTEGRA PLUS*
(U.S. Pharm) *See TANDEM PLUS*
(Vertical) *See OB COMPLETE*
(Vertical) *See OB COMPLETE WITH DHA*

MULTIVITAMIN, MINERALS, AND NUTRICEUTICALS
(A. G. Marin) *See SUPPORT 500*
(Breckenridge Pharm) *See VITATAB MV*
(Capellon) *See REQ49+*
(Everett) *See STROVITE ADVANCE*
(Everett) *See STROVITE ADVANCE+D*
(Everett) *See STROVITE ONE*
(Gil Pharmaceutical) *See BIOTECT PLUS*
(Gil Pharmaceutical) *See PROTECT CARDIO*
(Gil Pharmaceutical) *See PROTECT PLUS NR*
(Hillestad) *See DIALYVITE 5000*
(Kenwood) *See GLUTOFAC-ZX*
(Kowa) *See UDAMIN*
(Kowa) *See UDAMIN SP*
(PGD, Inc.) *See GENEVIT PLUS*
(Seyer Pharmatec) *See SUPERVITE*
(U.S. Pharm) *See DIVISTA*
(Vertical) *See CORVITE FREE*

MULTIVITAMIN, MINERALS, IRON, AND FLUORIDE
(Teva) *See MULTIVITE W/FLUORIDE & IRON*

MULTIVITAMIN, MINERALS, IRON, AND NUTRICEUTICALS
(A. G. Marin) *See SIDEROL*
(Breckenridge Pharm) *See MEGAVITE RX*
(Marnel) *See BACMIN*
(Trigen) *See CORVITA*

MULTIVITAMIN/IRON/FLUORIDE (Palmetto)
REPACK
multivitamin, iron, and fluoride
LIQ, PO (1X50ML)
50 ml............... 23490-7400-01 13.22

MULTIVITE PLUS FLUORIDE (Teva)
multivitamin and fluoride
CTB, PO, 1000s ea........ 00093-9158-10 143.17
1000s ea........... 00093-9166-10 143.17

(PD-Rx Pharm)
REPACK
CTB, PO (REDI-SCRIPT)
45s ea.............. 58864-0880-45 7.95

(Phys Total Care)
REPACK
CTB, PO, 100s ea......... 54868-1313-00 29.85

MULTIVITE W/FLUORIDE & IRON (Teva)
multivitamin, minerals, iron, and fluoride
CTB, PO, 100s ea......... 00093-9159-01 15.07

MULTIWAX 110-X (Amend)
yellow wax
WAX, NA, 25424 gm...... 17317-2414-00 156.80

MULTIWAX 180-M (Amend)
yellow wax
WAX, NA, 27240 gm...... 17317-1077-00 168.00

MULTIWAX 180-W (Amend)
yellow wax
WAX, NA, 27240 gm...... 17317-1078-00 168.00

MULTIWAX H.S. (Amend)
yellow wax
WAX, NA, 27240 gm...... 17317-1073-00 168.00

MULTIWAX ML-445 (Amend)
yellow wax
WAX, NA, 27240 gm...... 17317-1074-00 168.00
(W/2% BUTYL RUBBER)
27240 gm........... 17317-1079-00 168.00

MULTIWAX W-445 (Amend)
yellow wax
WAX, NA, 27240 gm...... 17317-1075-00 168.00

MULTIWAX W-835 (Amend)
yellow wax
WAX, NA, 27240 gm...... 17317-1076-00 168.00

MULTIWAX X-145A (Amend)
yellow wax
WAX, NA, 27240 gm...... 17317-1072-00 168.00

MUMPS VIRUS VACCINE, LIVE
(Merck) *See MUMPSVAX*

MUMPSVAX (Merck)
mumps virus vaccine, live
PDS, SC (SDV W/DILUENT,TAX INCL)
20000 tcid50,
10s ea............. 00006-4584-00 265.42

MUPIROCIN
FUL
OIN, TP, 2%, 22 gm.................................. 41.45

(Fougera)
OIN, TP, 2%, 22 gm....... 00168-0352-22 44.65 AB

(Glaxo) *See BACTROBAN*

(Hawkins)
POW, NA (USP)
1 gm............... 63370-0137-10 128.00
5 gm............... 63370-0137-15 520.00
25 gm.............. 63370-0137-25 2400.00

(Letco)
POW, NA (USP)
25 gm.............. 62991-2701-01 1245.00

(Medimetriks) *See CENTANY*

(PCCA)
POW, NA (USP,1X1GM)
1 gm............... 51927-3844-00 72.00

(Perrigo)
OIN, TP, 2%, 22 gm....... 45802-0112-22 44.85

PROD/MFR	NDC	AWP	DP	OBC
(Taro)				
OIN, TP, 2%, 22 gm	51672-1312-00	42.50		AB
(Teva)				
OIN, TP, 2%, 22 gm	00093-1010-42	42.75		
(A-S Medication) REPACK				
OIN, TP, 2%, 22 gm	54569-5644-00	44.85		
(Aidarex) REPACK				
OIN, TP (1X22GM)				
2%, 22 gm	33261-0380-01	70.95		
(Altura) REPACK				
OIN, TP, 2%, 15 gm	63874-0131-15	29.10		
22 gm	63874-0131-22	52.88		
30 gm	63874-0131-30	30.08		
(DHS, Inc.) REPACK				
OIN, TP, 2%, 22 gm	55887-0468-22	41.69		
(Dispensing Solutions) REPACK				
OIN, TP, 2%, 22 gm	55045-3202-07	44.50		
(IPI) REPACK				
OIN, TP (1X22GM)				
2%, 22 gm	18837-0320-22	56.06		AB
(Keltman Pharma., Inc.) REPACK				
OIN, TP, 2%, ea	68387-0550-01	46.59		
(Palmetto) REPACK				
OIN, TP, 2%, 22 gm	23490-0945-02	42.50		
22 gm	23490-5949-01	55.33		
(Pharma Pac) REPACK				
OIN, TP, 2%, 22 gm	52959-0743-22	71.95		
(Phys Total Care) REPACK				
OIN, TP, 2%, 22 gm	54868-4958-00	48.00		
(Physician Partner) REPACK				
OIN, TP, 2%, 22 gm	21695-0188-22	89.70		
(Quality Care Prod) REPACK				
OIN, TP, 2%, 22 gm	49999-0644-22	100.94		
(Southwood) REPACK				
OIN, TP, 2%, 22 gm	58016-4624-01	42.75		
(Stat Rx) REPACK				
OIN, TP, 2%, 22 gm	16590-0158-22	56.06		
(Vibranta) REPACK				
OIN, TP (USP)				
2%, 22 gm	57866-3093-06	100.94		
MUPIROCIN CALCIUM				
(Glaxo) *See BACTROBAN*				
MURI-LUBE (APP)				
mineral oil				
OIL, NA, 2 ml 25s	63323-0254-02	201.56		
10 ml 25s	63323-0254-10	232.81		
MUROMONAB-CD3				
(Centocor) *See ORTHOCLONE OKT 3*				
MUSE (Vivus)				
alprostadil				
SUP, UR, 125 mcg, ea UD	62541-0110-01	27.73		
6s ea	62541-0110-06	176.33		
250 mcg, ea UD	62541-0120-01	29.02		
6s ea	62541-0120-06	184.54		
500 mcg, ea UD	62541-0130-01	31.06		
6s ea	62541-0130-06	197.50		
1000 mcg, ea UD	62541-0140-01	33.54		
6s ea	62541-0140-06	213.26		
MUSK OIL (Medisca)				
muskseed oil				
OIL, NA (1X14ML)				
14 ml	38779-1446-03	12.00		
(1X25ML)				
25 ml	38779-1446-04	18.00		
(1X100ML)				
100 ml	38779-1446-05	52.50		
(1X500ML)				
500 ml	38779-1446-08	150.00		

PROD/MFR	NDC	AWP	DP	OBC
(PCCA)				
fragrance				
SOL, NA, 1 ml	51927-2429-00	0.45		
MUSKSEED OIL				
(Medisca) *See MUSK OIL*				
MUSTARD OIL (PCCA)				
OIL, NA, 1 ml	51927-1620-00	0.68		
(NATURAL)				
1 ml	51927-2291-00	11.70		
(Spectrum Pharmacy)				
OIL, NA (SYNTHETIC)				
100 ml	49452-4790-02	213.15		
500 ml	49452-4790-03	644.00		
2500 ml	49452-4790-04	1942.50		
MUSTARGEN (Lundbeck)				
mechlorethamine hydrochloride				
PDS, IV, 10 mg, 4s ea	67386-0911-51	714.82	50.55	
MUTIFOL (Breckenridge Pharm)				
multivitamin, minerals, and iron				
TAB, PO (10X10,FILM-COATED)				
100s ea UD	51991-0126-11	35.64		
MVC FLUORIDE (Sancilio)				
multivitamin and fluoride				
CTB, PO (SF,DYE-FREE,ORANGE)				
30s ea	44946-1012-04	13.00		
90s ea	44946-1012-05	18.00		
30s ea	44946-1013-04	13.00		
90s ea	44946-1013-05	18.00		
30s ea	44946-1014-04	13.00		
90s ea	44946-1014-05	18.00		
MVI PEDIATRIC (Hospira)				
multivitamin				
PDS, IV (SDV)				
10s ea	61703-0421-53	105.36	92.20	
MY-O-DEN (Legere)				
adenosine phosphate				
SOL, IM (M.D.V.)				
25 mg/ml, 10 ml	25332-0043-03	24.95		
MYAMBUTOL (X-Gen)				
ethambutol hydrochloride				
TAB, PO (FILM-COATED)				
100 mg, 100s ea	68850-0010-01	61.50		AB
(10X10 BLISTER PACK)				
400 mg, 100s ea	68850-0012-02	180.00		AB
(FILM-COATED)				
400 mg, 100s ea	68850-0012-01	180.00		AB
(A-S Medication) REPACK				
TAB, PO, 400 mg, 60s ea	54569-3070-00	108.00		AB
(Phys Total Care) REPACK				
TAB, PO, 400 mg, 30s ea	54868-2876-04	68.86		AB
60s ea	54868-2876-01	132.98		AB
100s ea	54868-2876-02	213.59		AB
MYCAMINE (Astellas)				
micafungin sodium				
PDS, IV (PF)				
50 mg, 10s ea	00469-3250-10	1122.00	935.00	
(W/RED FLIP-OFF CAP)				
100 mg, 10s ea	00469-3211-10	2244.00		EE
MYCELEX (Southwood) REPACK				
clotrimazole				
CRE, TP, 1%, 15 gm	58016-3192-01	13.50		BT
MYCELEX TROCHE (Phys Total Care) REPACK				
clotrimazole				
LOZ, MM, 10 mg, 70s ea	54868-2498-01	147.63		
140s ea	54868-2498-02	263.21		
MYCOBUTIN (Pfizer)				
rifabutin				
CAP, PO, 150 mg, 100s ea	00013-5301-17	1275.06	1062.55	
(Phys Total Care) REPACK				
CAP, PO, 150 mg, 50s ea	54868-2841-00	233.39		
60s ea	54868-2841-01	279.83		
100s ea	54868-2841-02	464.98		
MYCOLOG-II (Southwood) REPACK				
nystatin/triamcinolone acetonide				
CRE, TP, 100000 u/gm-0.1%,				
15 gm	58016-9411-01	19.50		AT
MYCOPHENOLATE MOFETIL				
FUL				
CAP, PO, 250 mg, 100s ea		52.91		
TAB, PO, 500 mg, 100s ea		105.80		

PROD/MFR	NDC	AWP	DP	OBC
(Accord)				
CAP, PO (HARD GELATIN)				
250 mg, 100s ea	16729-0094-01	392.32		AB
500s ea	16729-0094-16	1961.61		AB
TAB, PO (FILM COATED)				
500 mg, 100s ea	16729-0019-01	784.65		AB
500s ea	16729-0019-16	3923.24		AB
(Apotex Corp.)				
CAP, PO, 250 mg, 100s ea	60505-2968-01	396.72		AB
500s ea	60505-2968-05	1983.63		AB
TAB, PO (FILM-COATED)				
500 mg, 100s ea	60505-2967-01	793.46		AB
500s ea	60505-2967-05	3967.27		AB
(Mylan)				
CAP, PO (HARD GELATIN)				
250 mg, 100s ea	00378-2250-01	396.24		AB
500s ea	00378-2250-05	1981.20		AB
TAB, PO (FILM-COATED)				
500 mg, 100s ea	00378-4472-01	792.59		AB
500s ea	00378-4472-05	3962.93		AB
(Roche Labs) *See CELLCEPT*				
(Roxane)				
CAP, PO, 250 mg, 100s ea	00054-0163-25	396.73		AB
500s ea	00054-0163-29	1983.65		AB
TAB, PO, 500 mg, 100s ea	00054-0166-25	793.47		AB
500s ea	00054-0166-29	3967.32		AB
(Sandoz)				
CAP, PO (HARD GELATIN)				
250 mg, 100s ea	00781-2067-01	396.73		AB
500s ea	00781-2067-05	1983.65		AB
(12X120,HARD GELATIN)				
250 mg, 1440s ea	00781-2067-89	5712.98		AB
TAB, PO (FILM-COATED)				
500 mg, 100s ea	00781-5175-01	793.47		AB
500s ea	00781-5175-05	3967.32		AB
(Teva)				
CAP, PO (HARD GELATIN)				
250 mg, 100s ea	00093-7334-01	396.73		AB
100s ea UD	00093-7334-93	396.73		AB
500s ea	00093-7334-05	1983.65		AB
TAB, PO (FILM-COATED)				
500 mg, 100s ea	00093-7477-01	793.47		AB
500s ea	00093-7477-05	3967.32		AB
(UDL)				
CAP, PO (10 X 10,HARD GELATIN)				
250 mg, 100s ea UD	51079-0721-20	396.29		AB
TAB, PO (10X10,FILM-COATED)				
500 mg, 100s ea UD	51079-0379-20	792.59		AB
(Zydus Pharm.)				
CAP, PO (HARD GELATIN)				
250 mg, 100s ea	68382-0130-01	396.28		EE
500s ea	68382-0130-05	1981.40		EE
TAB, PO (FILM-COATED)				
500 mg, 100s ea	68382-0131-01	792.58		EE
500s ea	68382-0131-05	3962.90		EE
(American Health) REPACK				
TAB, PO (FILM-COATED)				
500 mg, 100s ea UD	68084-0178-01	156.25		EE
MYCOPHENOLATE MOFETIL HYDROCHLORIDE				
(Roche Labs) *See CELLCEPT*				
MYCOPHENOLATE SODIUM				
(Novartis Pharm) *See MYFORTIC*				
MYCOSTATIN (Southwood) REPACK				
nystatin				
POW, TP, 100000 u/gm,				
15 gm	58016-3155-01	26.58		AT
MYDFRIN (Alcon Ophthalmic)				
phenylephrine hydrochloride				
SOL, OP (UNIT OF USE)				
2.5%, 3 ml	00065-0342-03	15.84		
5 ml	00998-0342-05	29.64		
MYDOCS (Centurion)				
guaifenesin/phenylephrine hydrochloride				
TER, PO (DYE-FREE)				
600 mg-20 mg,				
100s ea	23359-0001-10	56.64		
MYDRAL (Ocusoft)				
tropicamide				
SOL, OP, 0.5%, 15 ml	54799-0529-15	12.81		AT
1%, 15 ml	54799-0528-12	13.12		AT
MYDRIACYL (Alcon Ophthalmic)				
tropicamide				
SOL, OP (UNIT OF USE)				
1%, 3 ml	00065-0355-03	16.62		AT
15 ml	00998-0355-15	56.58		AT

PROD/MFR NDC AWP DP OBC

MYFERON 150 (ME Pharm)
iron polysaccharide
CAP, PO, 150 mg, 100s ea . 58607-0111-85 13.74

MYFERON 150 FORTE (ME Pharm)
cyanocobalamin/folic acid/iron polysaccharide
CAP, PO, 25 mcg-1 mg-150 mg,
100s ea.......... 58607-1011-00 13.74

MYFORTIC (Novartis Pharm)
mycophenolate sodium
ECT, PO (K-30,FILM-COATED)
180 mg, 120s ea 00078-0385-66 461.50
360 mg, 120s ea 00078-0386-66 922.97

MYHIST-DM (Larken Labs, Inc.)
dm/phenyleph hcl/pyril mal
SOL, PO (AF,SF,DYE-FREE,GRAPE)
473 ml 68047-0230-16 51.58

MYHIST-PD (Larken Labs, Inc.)
cpm/phenyleph hcl/pyril mal
SOL, PO (AF,SF,DYE-FREE)
473 ml 68047-0233-16 50.47

MYKIDZ IRON FL (NextWave)
fe/na fluoride/vit a/vit c/vit d
SUS, PO (W/DISPENSER,AF,DYE-FREE)
118 ml 24478-0102-04 23.75

MYLERAN (Glaxo)
busulfan
TAB, PO, 2 mg, 25s ea 00173-0713-25 111.56

MYLOTARG (Wyeth)
gemtuzumab ozogamicin
PDS, IV (VIAL,PF)
5 mg, ea............ 00008-4510-01 3104.82 2587.35

MYNATAL (ME Pharm)
prenatal vitamins
SGL, PO (SOFTGEL)
100s ea............. 58607-0103-59 21.79

MYNATAL ADVANCE (ME Pharm)
prenatal vitamins
TAB, PO (9X10,DYE-FREE)
90s ea UD 58607-0326-00 16.95

MYNATAL FC (ME Pharm)
prenatal vitamins
TAB, PO, 100s ea 58607-0102-59 13.74

MYNATAL PLUS (ME Pharm)
prenatal vitamins
TAB, PO (CAPLET)
100s ea............. 58607-0811-20 13.74

MYNATAL PN (ME Pharm)
prenatal vitamins
TAB, PO (CAPLET)
100s ea............. 58607-0104-58 13.74

MYNATAL PN FORTE (ME Pharm)
prenatal vitamins
TAB, PO, 100s ea 58607-0104-59 13.74

MYNATAL RX (ME Pharm)
prenatal vitamins
TAB, PO, 100s ea 58607-0103-10 13.74

MYNATAL ULTRA (ME Pharm)
prenatal vitamins
TAB, PO (CAPLET)
100s ea............. 58607-0125-83 18.95

MYNATAL-Z (ME Pharm)
prenatal vitamins
TAB, PO (CAPLET)
100s ea............. 58607-0105-65 13.74

MYNATE 90 PLUS (ME Pharm)
prenatal vitamins
TAB, PO, 100s ea 58607-0103-90 13.74

MYOBLOC (Solstice)
rimabotulinumtoxinb
SOL, IM, 2500 u/0.5 ml,
0.5 ml............ 10454-0710-10 299.40
5000 u/ml, 1 ml...... 10454-0711-10 598.80
(10000U/2ML)
5000 u/ml, 2 ml...... 10454-0712-10 1197.60

MYOCHRYSINE (Akorn)
gold sodium thiomalate
SOL, IM (VIAL)
50 mg/ml, 1 ml 6s.... 11098-0533-01 204.84
10 ml............ 11098-0533-10 283.46

MYOFLEX (Palmetto)
REPACK
trolamine salicylate
CRE, TP (1X60GM)
10%, 60 gm 23490-8011-01 8.85

(Quality Care Prod)
REPACK
CRE, TP, 10%, 120 gm 49999-0424-04 20.12

MYOVIEW (GE)
technetium tc 99m tetrofosmin
KIT, IJ (5 VIALS)
0.23 mg, ea.......... 17156-0024-05 3640.68

MYOZYME (Genzyme)
alglucosidase alfa
PDS, IV (PF)
50 mg, ea........... 58468-0150-01 720.00 600.00

MYPHETANE DX COUGH (Morton Grove)
bpm/dm/pse hcl
SYR, PO (BUTTERSCOTCH)
473 ml .... 60432-0482-16 62.44 AA

MYRRH (Gallipot)
TIN, NA, 100 ml 51552-0206-05 13.65
500 ml 51552-0206-06 34.16

(Lorann Oil) *See MYRRH OIL*

(Medisca) *See MYRRH OIL*

(Medisca)
TIN, NA, 100 ml 38779-0859-05 33.00
500 ml 38779-0859-08 67.50

(PCCA) *See MYRRH GUM*

(PCCA) *See MYRRH OIL*

MYRRH GUM (PCCA)
myrrh
TIN, NA, 1 ml............ 51927-1245-00 0.38

MYRRH OIL (Lorann Oil)
myrrh
OIL, NA, 9.9 ml 23535-0151-45 15.00

(Medisca)
OIL, NA (1X14ML)
14 ml............... 38779-0901-03 37.50
(1X25ML)
25 ml............... 38779-0901-04 58.50
(1X100ML)
100 ml 38779-0901-05 223.50

(PCCA)
OIL, NA, 1 ml............ 51927-2585-00 2.80

MYSOLINE (Valeant Pharm Intl)
primidone
TAB, PO, 50 mg, 100s ea .. 66490-0690-10 169.51 15.92 AB
250 mg, 100s ea ..... 66490-0691-10 611.88 AB

(Phys Total Care)
REPACK
TAB, PO, 50 mg, 60s ea ... 54868-3689-01 38.10 AB
90s ea............ 54868-3689-03 56.20 AB
100s ea........... 54868-3689-02 62.24 AB
500s ea........... 54868-3689-00 286.33 AB

MYTELASE CHLORIDE (Sanofi-Aventis)
ambenonium chloride
TAB, PO (CAPLET)
10 mg, 100s ea 00024-1287-04 172.27

MYTUSSIN AC COUGH (Morton Grove)
codeine phosphate/guaifenesin
SOL, PO (SF)
10 mg/5 ml-100 mg/5 ml,
480 ml, C-V........ 60432-0045-16 8.45

MYTUSSIN DAC (Morton Grove)
codeine phos/gg/pse hcl
SOL, PO (SF)
120 ml, C-V.......... 60432-0541-04 11.00
473 ml, C-V.......... 60432-0541-16 39.66

N-ACETYL D-GLUCOSAMINE (Gallipot)
n-acetyl glucosamine
POW, NA, 5 gm 51552-0951-02 21.00 15.00
25 gm.............. 51552-0951-04 37.10 26.50
100 gm............. 51552-0951-05 91.00 65.00
500 gm............. 51552-0951-06 350.00 250.00

N-ACETYL GLUCOSAMINE
(Gallipot) *See N-ACETYL D-GLUCOSAMINE*

(Letco) *See ACETYL-D-GLUCOSAMINE*

(Medisca) *See ACETYL-D-GLUCOSAMINE*

(PCCA) *See ACETYL-D-GLUCOSAMINE*

(Spectrum Pharmacy) *See N-ACETYL-D-GLUCOSAMINE*

N-ACETYL-D-GLUCOSAMINE (Spectrum Pharmacy)
n-acetyl glucosamine
POW, NA (1X25GM)
25 gm.............. 49452-0102-01 131.60
(1X100GM)
100 gm............. 49452-0102-02 344.05
(1X500GM)
500 gm............. 49452-0102-03 955.50

N-ACETYL-L-CYSTEINE (Spectrum Pharmacy)
acetylcysteine
POW, NA (U.S.P.)
25 gm.............. 49452-0097-01 76.65
100 gm............. 49452-0097-02 176.40
500 gm............. 49452-0097-04 658.00
1000 gm............ 49452-0097-03 829.50

N-ACETYL-PENICILLAMINE
(PCCA) *See ACETYL-DL-PENICILLAMINE*

N-HEPTANE (Baker, J.T.)
heptane
LIQ, NA (ULTRA RESI-ANALYZED)
1000 ml 10106-9338-02 39.40
(HPLC)
4000 ml 10106-9177-03 122.78
(ULTRA RESI-ANALYZED)
4000 ml 10106-9338-03 110.55

N,N-DIMETHYLGLYCINE HCL (Spectrum Pharmacy)
dimethylglycine hydrochloride
POW, NA (20-60 MESH)
100 gm............. 49452-2622-01 166.95
500 gm............. 49452-2622-02 577.50

NA PHOS, DIBASIC/NA PHOS, MONOBASIC
(Rite Aid) *See RITE AID ENEMA*

(Salix Pharm) *See OSMOPREP*

(Salix Pharm) *See VISICOL*

NABI-HB (Biotest)
hepatitis b immune globulin
SOL, IM (S.D.V.,312 IU/ML)
1 ml............... 59730-4202-01 183.69
5 ml............... 59730-4203-01 804.44

(A-S Medication)
REPACK
SOL, IM, 5 ml 54569-4739-00 804.44

(Quality Care Prod)
REPACK
SOL, IM (S.D.V.,312 IU/ML)
5 ml............... 49999-0425-05 872.00

NABUMETONE (Dr Reddy's)
TAB, PO (USP,FILM-COATED)
500 mg, 100s ea ..... 55111-0486-01 129.70 AB
500s ea........... 55111-0486-05 629.05 AB
750 mg, 100s ea ..... 55111-0487-01 153.17 AB
500s ea........... 55111-0487-05 742.87 AB

(Glenmark Pharmaceuticals)
TAB, PO (USP,FILM-COATED)
500 mg, 100s ea ..... 68462-0358-01 137.59 AB
500s ea........... 68462-0358-05 687.96 AB
750 mg, 100s ea ..... 68462-0359-01 162.49 AB
500s ea........... 68462-0359-05 812.43 AB

(Major)
TAB, PO (10X10,FILM-COATED)
500 mg, 100s ea UD.. 00904-5939-61 123.02 AB
(USP,FILM COATED)
750 mg, 100s ea UD.. 00904-5940-61 147.39 AB

(Sandoz)
TAB, PO (FILM-COATED)
500 mg, 100s ea ..... 00185-0145-01 129.65 AB
500s ea........... 00185-0145-05 615.84 AB
750 mg, 100s ea ..... 00185-0146-01 153.15 AB
500s ea........... 00185-0146-05 727.46 AB

(Teva)
TAB, PO, 500 mg, 100s ea . 00093-1015-01 129.70 AB
1000s ea .... 00093-1015-10 1297.00 AB
750 mg, 100s ea ..... 00093-1016-01 153.17 AB
1000s ea .... 00093-1016-10 1531.70 AB

(UDL)
TAB, PO (10X10)
500 mg, 100s ea UD .. 51079-0989-20 129.49 AB

(4u)
REPACK
TAB, PO, 500 mg, 60s ea .. 10544-0323-60 98.92
(FILM-COATED)
500 mg, 60s ea ...... 42549-0523-60 98.92 AB
60s ea............ 42549-0552-60 98.92 AB

(A-S Medication)
REPACK
TAB, PO (FILM-COATED)
500 mg, 14s ea ...... 54569-5303-04 18.38 AB
15s ea............ 54569-5303-01 19.69 AB
20s ea............ 54569-5303-05 26.25 AB
28s ea............ 54569-5303-02 36.75 AB
30s ea............ 54569-5303-07 39.38 AB
60s ea............ 54569-5303-00 78.76 AB
750 mg, 14s ea ...... 54569-5429-02 21.70 AB
30s ea............ 54569-5429-00 46.51 AB
60s ea............ 54569-5429-03 93.02 AB

PROD/MFR	NDC	AWP	DP	OBC
(Aidarex)				
REPACK				
TAB, PO, 500 mg, 7s ea	33261-0077-07	14.35		AB
14s ea	33261-0077-14	28.70		AB
20s ea	33261-0077-20	41.00		AB
21s ea	33261-0077-21	43.05		AB
28s ea	33261-0077-28	57.40		AB
30s ea	33261-0077-30	61.50		AB
40s ea	33261-0077-40	82.00		AB
60s ea	33261-0077-60	123.00		AB
90s ea	33261-0077-90	184.50		AB
100s ea	33261-0077-00	205.00		AB
120s ea	33261-0077-02	246.00		AB
180s ea	33261-0077-03	369.00		AB
(FILM-COATED)				
750 mg, 7s ea	33261-0078-07	14.84		AB
14s ea	33261-0078-14	29.68		AB
20s ea	33261-0078-20	42.40		AB
21s ea	33261-0078-21	44.52		AB
28s ea	33261-0078-28	59.08		AB
30s ea	33261-0078-30	63.60		AB
40s ea	33261-0078-40	84.40		AB
60s ea	33261-0078-60	126.60		AB
90s ea	33261-0078-90	189.90		AB
100s ea	33261-0078-01	212.00		AB
120s ea	33261-0078-02	253.20		AB
180s ea	33261-0078-03	379.80		AB
(Altura)				
REPACK				
TAB, PO, 500 mg, 6s ea	63874-0607-06	9.79		
10s ea	63874-0607-10	16.31		
12s ea	63874-0607-12	19.58		
14s ea	63874-0607-14	22.84		
15s ea	63874-0607-15	24.47		
20s ea	63874-0607-20	32.63		
30s ea	63874-0607-30	48.94		
40s ea	63874-0607-40	65.25		
50s ea	63874-0607-50	81.57		
60s ea	63874-0607-60	97.88		
100s ea	63874-0607-01	163.13		
(FILM COATED)				
500 mg, 120s ea	63874-0607-04	195.76		
750 mg, 14s ea	63874-0687-14	26.97		AB
60s ea	63874-0687-60	115.58		AB
90s ea	63874-0687-90	173.37		AB
100s ea	63874-0687-01	198.69		AB
(American Health)				
REPACK				
TAB, PO (USP,10X10)				
500 mg, 100s ea UD	68084-0246-01	82.36		
(Bryant Ranch)				
REPACK				
TAB, PO, 500 mg, 20s ea	63629-1620-01	31.99		
30s ea	63629-1620-02	45.00		
60s ea	63629-1620-03	94.96		
(FILM-COATED)				
750 mg, 20s ea	63629-2682-04	49.25		AB
30s ea	63629-2682-03	55.87		AB
42s ea	63629-2682-05	69.54		AB
60s ea	63629-2682-01	107.32		
(FILM-COATED)				
750 mg, 90s ea	63629-2682-02	162.58		AB
(Core)				
REPACK				
TAB, PO, 500 mg, 6s ea	33358-0251-06	10.91		
14s ea	33358-0251-14	23.72		
20s ea	33358-0251-20	32.79		
24s ea	33358-0251-24	36.76		
28s ea	33358-0251-28	41.33		
30s ea	33358-0251-30	46.13		
60s ea	33358-0251-60	97.33		
90s ea	33358-0251-90	143.09		
120s ea	33358-0251-01	187.37		
750 mg, 28s ea	33358-0252-28	49.44		
30s ea	33358-0252-30	52.57		
60s ea	33358-0252-60	110.00		
90s ea	33358-0252-90	155.97		
120s ea	33358-0252-01	188.40		
(DHS, Inc.)				
REPACK				
TAB, PO, 500 mg, 14s ea	55887-0440-14	18.63		
(FILM-COATED)				
500 mg, 30s ea	55887-0440-30	39.92		AB
60s ea	55887-0440-60	79.89		AB
90s ea	55887-0440-90	119.83		AB
750 mg, 30s ea	55887-0683-30	74.44		AB
90s ea	55887-0683-90	223.30		AB
(Dispensing Solutions)				
REPACK				
TAB, PO, 500 mg, 14s ea	66336-0316-14	21.78		EE
15s ea	55045-3007-06	23.70		
20s ea	55045-3007-07	31.50		AB
30s ea	55045-3007-08	47.40		AB
30s ea	66336-0316-30	50.80		EE
60s ea	55045-3007-02	94.80		AB
60s ea	66336-0316-60	93.35		AB
90s ea	55045-3007-03	142.20		AB
90s ea	66336-0316-90	144.15		AB
100s ea	55045-3007-01	158.00		AB
120s ea	55045-3007-00	189.60		
135s ea	55045-3007-04	213.30		
750 mg, 14s ea	55045-3056-02	22.82		AB
30s ea	55045-3056-08	48.90		AB
30s ea	66336-0925-30	55.74		
40s ea	55045-3056-04	65.20		
60s ea	55045-3056-06	97.80		AB
(FILM-COATED)				
750 mg, 60s ea	66336-0925-60	110.88		AB
90s ea	55045-3056-00	146.70		AB
(FILM-COATED)				
750 mg, 90s ea	66336-0925-90	166.32		AB
100s ea	55045-3056-01	163.00		AB
120s ea	55045-3056-05	195.60		
135s ea	55045-3056-03	220.05		
(IPI)				
REPACK				
TAB, PO (FILM-COATED)				
500 mg, 90s ea	18837-0097-90	138.56		AB
750 mg, 30s ea	18837-0098-30	60.93		AB
60s ea	18837-0098-60	121.50		
(Keltman Pharma., Inc.)				
REPACK				
TAB, PO, 500 mg, 30s ea	68387-0272-30	47.23		
(FILM-COATED)				
500 mg, 60s ea	68387-0272-60	94.46		AB
750 mg, 20s ea	68387-0270-20	46.67		
30s ea	68387-0270-30	70.00		AB
60s ea	68387-0270-60	140.00		AB
(Medsource)				
REPACK				
TAB, PO (FILM-COATED)				
500 mg, 30s ea	45865-0464-30	55.50		AB
60s ea	45865-0464-60	135.00		AB
90s ea	45865-0464-90	202.50		AB
100s ea	45865-0464-00	225.00		AB
120s ea	45865-0464-01	270.00		AB
150s ea	45865-0464-02	337.50		AB
300s ea	45865-0464-05	675.00		AB
750 mg, 30s ea	45865-0351-30	105.00		AB
60s ea	45865-0351-60	210.00		AB
90s ea	45865-0351-90	315.00		AB
100s ea	45865-0351-00	350.00		AB
120s ea	45865-0351-01	420.00		AB
150s ea	45865-0351-02	525.00		AB
300s ea	45865-0351-05	1050.00		AB
(Nucare Pharm)				
REPACK				
TAB, PO, 500 mg, 20s ea	66267-0482-20	32.38		AB
30s ea	66267-0482-30	66.98		AB
40s ea	66267-0482-40	86.99		AB
(FILM-COATED)				
500 mg, 60s ea	66267-0482-60	162.53		AB
90s ea	66267-0482-90	229.98		AB
750 mg, 20s ea	66267-0529-20	42.89		AB
(FILM-COATED)				
750 mg, 30s ea	66267-0529-30	67.02		AB
40s ea	66267-0529-40	76.05		AB
60s ea	66267-0529-60	127.58		AB
(Palmetto)				
REPACK				
TAB, PO, 500 mg, 14s ea	23490-5950-01	33.05		
30s ea	23490-5950-02	70.83		
60s ea	23490-5950-03	141.66		
90s ea	23490-5950-04	212.49		
750 mg, 20s ea	23490-5951-00	43.00		
30s ea	23490-5951-01	64.50		
60s ea	23490-5951-02	129.00		
90s ea	23490-5951-03	193.50		
(PD-Rx Pharm)				
REPACK				
TAB, PO (FILM-COATED)				
500 mg, 20s ea	55289-0611-20	58.14		AB
30s ea	55289-0611-30	70.83		AB
(USP)				
500 mg, 60s ea	55289-0611-60	102.00		
750 mg, 20s ea	55289-0609-20	58.14		AB
30s ea	55289-0609-30	82.23		
(FILM-COATED)				
750 mg, 40s ea	55289-0609-40	89.97		AB
(USP)				
750 mg, 60s ea	55289-0609-60	106.32		
(Pharma Pac)				
REPACK				
TAB, PO, 500 mg, 14s ea	52959-0650-14	26.00		AB
20s ea	52959-0650-20	37.14		AB
28s ea	52959-0650-28	51.99		
30s ea	52959-0650-30	55.70		AB
40s ea	52959-0650-40	74.20		AB
(FILM-COATED)				
500 mg, 42s ea	52959-0650-42	77.90		AB
60s ea	52959-0650-60	111.21		AB
90s ea	52959-0650-90	166.81		
100s ea	52959-0650-00	185.21		
750 mg, 20s ea	52959-0656-20	37.88		EE
28s ea	52959-0656-28	53.04		
30s ea	52959-0656-30	56.81		EE
40s ea	52959-0656-40	75.73		EE
(FILM-COATED)				
750 mg, 42s ea	52959-0656-42	79.49		AB
60s ea	52959-0656-60	113.57		EE
90s ea	52959-0656-90	170.33		
100s ea	52959-0656-00	189.23		AB
(FILM-COATED)				
750 mg, 120s ea	52959-0656-02	227.04		AB
(Phys Total Care)				
REPACK				
TAB, PO (FILM-COATED)				
500 mg, 20s ea	54868-4556-01	35.19		AB
30s ea	54868-4556-03	51.30		AB
60s ea	54868-4556-00	76.86		AB
100s ea	54868-4556-02	124.62		AB
750 mg, 20s ea	54868-4558-01	41.85		
(FILM-COATED)				
750 mg, 30s ea	54868-4558-03	61.29		AB
60s ea	54868-4558-00	92.16		
(FILM-COATED)				
750 mg, 100s ea	54868-4558-02	150.09		AB
(Physician Partner)				
REPACK				
TAB, PO, 500 mg, 14s ea	21695-0230-14	45.57		
20s ea	21695-0230-20	65.53		
30s ea	21695-0230-30	83.55		
60s ea	21695-0230-60	167.10		
750 mg, 14s ea	21695-0231-14	54.07		
(FILM-COATED)				
750 mg, 20s ea	21695-0231-20	65.66		AB
30s ea	21695-0231-30	98.41		
60s ea	21695-0231-60	196.98		
(FILM-COATED)				
750 mg, 90s ea	21695-0231-90	295.47		AB
(Quality Care Prod)				
REPACK				
TAB, PO, 500 mg, 14s ea	49999-0102-14	36.82		AB
(FILM-COATED)				
500 mg, 15s ea	49999-0102-15	39.44		AB
20s ea	49999-0102-20	52.60		AB
30s ea	49999-0102-30	78.90		AB
60s ea	49999-0102-60	157.80		AB
100s ea	49999-0102-00	263.00		
750 mg, 14s ea	49999-0103-14	30.00		AB
(FILM-COATED)				
750 mg, 20s ea	49999-0103-20	34.27		AB
30s ea	49999-0103-30	61.30		AB
60s ea	49999-0103-60	117.36		AB
100s ea	49999-0103-00	192.66		
(Southwood)				
REPACK				
TAB, PO, 500 mg, 6s ea	58016-0619-06	8.64		EE
10s ea	58016-0619-10	14.40		EE
12s ea	58016-0619-12	17.28		EE
14s ea	58016-0619-14	20.16		EE
15s ea	58016-0619-15	21.60		EE
20s ea	58016-0619-20	28.80		EE
24s ea	58016-0619-24	34.56		EE
28s ea	58016-0619-28	40.32		EE
(FILM-COATED)				
500 mg, 30s ea	58016-0619-30	57.00		AB
40s ea	58016-0619-40	57.60		EE
50s ea	58016-0619-50	72.00		EE
(FILM-COATED)				
500 mg, 60s ea	58016-0619-60	114.00		AB
90s ea	58016-0619-90	171.00		AB
100s ea	58016-0619-00	190.00		AB
120s ea	58016-0619-02	228.00		AB
750 mg, 14s ea	58016-0628-14	22.13		AB
28s ea	58016-0628-28	44.23		EE
(FILM-COATED)				
750 mg, 30s ea	58016-0628-30	60.30		AB
60s ea	58016-0628-60	120.60		AB
90s ea	58016-0628-90	180.90		AB
100s ea	58016-0628-00	201.00		AB

PROD/MFR	NDC	AWP	DP	OBC
120s ea	58016-0628-02	241.20		AB
150s ea	58016-0628-03	236.95		AB
200s ea	58016-0628-89	315.93		AB
300s ea	58016-0628-73	473.90		AB
(St. Mary's MPP)				
REPACK				
TAB, PO, 500 mg, 60s ea	60760-0015-60	87.29		AB
(Stat Rx)				
REPACK				
TAB, PO, 500 mg, 14s ea	16590-0163-14	24.90		AB
(FILM-COATED)				
500 mg, 30s ea	16590-0159-30	51.61		AB
45s ea	16590-0159-45	73.58		AB
56s ea	16590-0159-56	111.81		AB
60s ea	16590-0159-60	103.21		AB
90s ea	16590-0159-90	154.82		AB
(FILM-COATED)				
500 mg, 100s ea	16590-0159-71	164.00		AB
750 mg, 20s ea	16590-0160-20	40.60		AB
30s ea	16590-0160-30	60.93		AB
56s ea	16590-0160-56	113.74		AB
60s ea	16590-0160-60	121.87		AB
(Vibranta)				
REPACK				
TAB, PO, 500 mg, 60s ea	57866-6333-05	117.36		
750 mg, 14s ea	57866-6334-01	39.45		
30s ea	57866-6334-02	70.42		
60s ea	57866-6334-03	117.36		

NADIDE
(Spectrum Pharmacy) *See BETA-NICOTINAMIDE ADENINE DINUCLEOTIDE*

NADOLOL

PROD/MFR	NDC	AWP	DP	OBC
FUL				
TAB, PO, 20 mg, 100s ea		46.50		
40 mg, 100s ea		42.89		
80 mg, 100s ea		80.25		
(King Pharm) *See CORGARD*				
(Mylan)				
TAB, PO, 20 mg, 100s ea	00378-0028-01	89.80		AB
40 mg, 100s ea	00378-1171-01	105.00		AB
1000s ea	00378-1171-10	1028.70		AB
80 mg, 100s ea	00378-1132-01	142.30		AB
1000s ea	00378-1132-10	1391.30		AB
(PCCA)				
POW, NA (U.S.P.)				
1 gm	51927-2776-00	31.20		
(Sandoz)				
TAB, PO (USP)				
20 mg, 90s ea	00781-1181-92	80.82		EE
100s ea	00781-1181-01	89.80		EE
(USP)				
20 mg, 1000s ea	00781-1181-10	898.00		EE
40 mg, 90s ea	00781-1182-92	94.50		EE
100s ea	00781-1182-01	105.00		EE
100s ea	59772-2462-01	103.75		AB
(USP)				
40 mg, 1000s ea	00781-1182-10	1050.00		EE
80 mg, 90s ea	00781-1183-92	128.07		EE
100s ea	00781-1183-01	142.30		EE
100s ea	59772-2463-01	141.70		AB
(USP)				
80 mg, 1000s ea	00781-1183-10	1423.00		EE
160 mg, 100s ea	59772-2465-01	206.27		AB
(Spectrum Pharmacy)				
POW, NA (U.S.P.)				
1 gm	49452-4806-01	226.10		
5 gm	49452-4806-02	945.00		
(Teva)				
TAB, PO (USP)				
20 mg, 100s ea	00093-4235-01	89.80		
40 mg, 100s ea	00093-4236-01	105.00		
80 mg, 100s ea	00093-4237-01	142.30		EE
(UDL)				
TAB, PO (10X10)				
20 mg, 100s ea UD	51079-0812-20	92.49		AB
40 mg, 100s ea UD	51079-0813-20	108.15		AB
(Phys Total Care)				
REPACK				
TAB, PO, 20 mg, 30s ea	54868-5295-01	19.29		AB
90s ea	54868-5295-00	48.90		AB
40 mg, 10s ea	54868-3257-04	12.34		AB
30s ea	54868-3257-02	28.01		EE
45s ea	54868-3257-03	31.47		AB
60s ea	54868-3257-05	51.52		EE
90s ea	54868-3257-06	76.53		AB
100s ea	54868-3257-01	62.93		EE
80 mg, 30s ea	54868-3721-01	42.74		AB
100s ea	54868-3721-02	102.79		AB
(USP)				
160 mg, 15s ea	54868-5588-00	45.81		
(Quality Care Prod)				
REPACK				
TAB, PO, 40 mg, 30s ea	49999-0201-30	37.80		
80 mg, 30s ea	49999-0202-30	42.99		
160 mg, 30s ea	49999-0203-30	70.72		
(Vibranta)				
REPACK				
TAB, PO, 20 mg, 30s ea	57866-6339-01	26.75		
40 mg, 30s ea	57866-6337-01	31.76		
80 mg, 30s ea	57866-6338-01	42.84		

NADOLOL AND BENDROFLUMETHIAZIDE (Global Pharm)
bendroflumethiazide/nadolol

PROD/MFR	NDC	AWP	DP	OBC
TAB, PO (USP)				
5 mg-40 mg, 100s ea	00115-5311-01	246.24		AB
5 mg-80 mg, 100s ea	00115-5322-01	324.90		AB
(Mylan)				
TAB, PO (USP)				
5 mg-40 mg, 100s ea	00378-0096-01	246.45		AB
5 mg-80 mg, 100s ea	00378-0099-01	325.20		AB

NAFARELIN ACETATE
(Pfizer) *See SYNAREL*

NAFCILLIN (Sandoz)
nafcillin sodium

PROD/MFR	NDC	AWP	DP	OBC
PDS, IV (ADD-VANTAGE VIAL)				
1 gm, ea	00781-3128-15	14.90		
(USP,ADD-VANTAGE VIAL)				
1 gm, 10s ea	00781-3128-92	148.99		

NAFCILLIN SODIUM (Baxter)

PROD/MFR	NDC	AWP	DP	OBC
SOL, IV (GALAXY,PREMIX)				
1 gm/50 ml, 50 ml	00338-1017-41	21.67	18.06	
2 gm/100 ml, 100 ml	00338-1019-48	31.19	25.99	
(Sandoz) *See NAFCILLIN*				
(Sandoz) *See NOVAPLUS NAFCILLIN*				
(Sandoz)				
PDS, IJ, 1 gm, ea	00781-3124-85	12.41		AP
(ADD-VANTAGE)				
1 gm, ea	00015-7225-18	10.36		AP
(VIAL)				
1 gm, 10s ea	00781-3124-95	124.14		AP
2 gm, ea	00781-3125-85	24.08		AP
(ADD-VANTAGE)				
2 gm, ea	00015-7226-18	20.11		AP
(ADD-VANTAGE VIAL)				
2 gm, 10s ea	00781-3125-92	201.03		AP
(VIAL)				
2 gm, 10s ea	00781-3125-95	240.83		AP
10 gm, ea	00781-3126-46	118.01		AP
(VIAL,PHARMACY BULK)				
10 gm, ea	00015-7101-28	74.63		AP
10s ea	00781-3126-95	1180.11		AP
IV (ADD-VANTAGE)				
2 gm, ea	00781-3129-15	28.90		AP
(2GMX10, ADD-VANTAGE)				
2 gm, 10s ea	00781-3129-92	289.01		AP

NAFTIFINE HYDROCHLORIDE
(Merz) *See NAFTIN*

NAFTIN (Merz)
naftifine hydrochloride

PROD/MFR	NDC	AWP	DP	OBC
CRE, TP, 1%, 30 gm	00259-4126-30	96.05		
(1X30GM)				
1%, 30 gm	00259-4126-03	96.05		
60 gm	00259-4126-60	176.52		
90 gm	00259-4126-90	238.72		
(1X90GM)				
1%, 90 gm	00259-4126-09	238.72		
GEL, TP, 1%, 40 gm	00259-4770-40	146.34		
60 gm	00259-4770-60	202.96		
90 gm	00259-4770-90	278.92		
(Phys Total Care)				
REPACK				
GEL, TP, 1%, 60 gm	54868-2185-01	97.68		
(Quality Care Prod)				
REPACK				
CRE, TP (1X30GM)				
1%, 30 gm	35356-0244-30	123.60		
GEL, TP (1X20GM)				
1%, 20 gm	35356-0244-20	116.40		
(Southwood)				
REPACK				
CRE, TP, 1%, 30 gm	58016-3288-01	77.86		

NAGLAZYME (Biomarin)
galsulfase

PROD/MFR	NDC	AWP	DP	OBC
SOL, IV (PF)				
1 mg/ml, 5 ml	68135-0020-01	1956.00		

NALBUPHINE HCL (Hospira)
nalbuphine hydrochloride

PROD/MFR	NDC	AWP	DP	OBC
SOL, IJ (AMP,LATEX-FREE)				
10 mg/ml, 1 ml 10s	00409-1463-01	14.88	13.00	AP
(25X10ML)				
10 mg/ml, 10 ml 25s	00409-1464-01	478.50	418.75	AP
(AMP,LATEX-FREE)				
20 mg/ml, 1 ml 10s	00409-1465-01	30.84	27.00	AP
(VIAL,FLIPTOP)				
20 mg/ml, 10 ml 25s	00409-1467-01	675.60	591.25	AP
(PCCA)				
POW, NA, 1 gm	51927-2140-00	144.00		
(Spectrum Pharmacy)				
POW, NA, 0.1 gm	49452-4800-01	133.70		
1 gm	49452-4800-02	270.20		
5 gm	49452-4800-03	889.00		
(A-S Medication)				
REPACK				
SOL, IJ (10X1ML)				
10 mg/ml, 1 ml 10s	54569-5795-00	20.00		EE
(Phys Total Care)				
REPACK				
SOL, IJ, 10 mg/ml, 1 ml	54868-3608-00	11.31		AP
(10X1ML)				
10 mg/ml, 1 ml 10s	54868-3608-01	86.04		AP
(Southwood)				
REPACK				
SOL, IJ (10X1ML AMPS)				
10 mg/ml, 1 ml 10s	58016-4770-01	20.10		EE
(M.D.V.)				
10 mg/ml, 10 ml	58016-9384-01	20.40		EE

NALBUPHINE HYDROCHLORIDE
(Hospira) *See AMERINET CHOICE NALBUPHINE HYDROCHLORIDE*
(Hospira) *See NALBUPHINE HCL*
(Hospira) *See NOVAPLUS NALBUPHINE HYDROCHLORIDE*

PROD/MFR	NDC	AWP	DP	OBC
(Medisca)				
POW, NA (1X100GM)				
100 gm	38779-0448-05	7200.00		
(PCCA) *See NALBUPHINE HCL*				
(Spectrum Pharmacy) *See NALBUPHINE HCL*				
(Teva)				
SOL, IJ (10X1ML)				
10 mg/ml, 1 ml 10s	00555-1121-05	20.00		AP
(25X10ML)				
10 mg/ml, 10 ml 25s	00555-1119-09	443.13		AP
(10X1ML)				
20 mg/ml, 1 ml 10s	00555-1122-05	36.10		AP
(A-S Medication)				
REPACK				
SOL, IJ (10X1ML)				
20 mg/ml, 1 ml 10s	54569-4112-00	36.10		
(Palmetto)				
REPACK				
SOL, IJ, 10 mg/ml, 10 ml	23490-5955-01	21.50		

NALEX A 12 (Blansett)
cpm tan/phenyleph tan/pyril tan

PROD/MFR	NDC	AWP	DP	OBC
SUS, PO (RASPBERRY)				
120 ml	51674-0027-04	31.95		

NALEX DH (Blansett)
hydrocodone bitartrate/phenylephrine hydrochloride

PROD/MFR	NDC	AWP	DP	OBC
LIQ, PO (AF,SF,CHERRY)				
2.5 mg/5 ml-5 mg/5 ml, 480 ml, C-III	51674-0025-07	40.69		

NALEX EXPECTORANT (Blansett)
gg/hydrocod bit/pse hcl

PROD/MFR	NDC	AWP	DP	OBC
LIQ, PO, 480 ml, C-III	51674-0002-07	44.13		

NALEX-A (Blansett)
cpm/phenyleph hcl/phenyltoloxamine cit

PROD/MFR	NDC	AWP	DP	OBC
LIQ, PO (AF,SF,COTTON CANDY)				
473 ml	51674-0007-07	45.97		
TER, PO, 4 mg-20 mg-40 mg, 100s ea	51674-0008-01	87.33		

NALFON (Pedinol)
fenoprofen calcium

PROD/MFR	NDC	AWP	DP	OBC
CAP, PO, 200 mg, 100s ea	00884-6600-10	81.25		AB
400 mg, 90s ea	00884-7308-09	122.50		EE

PROD/MFR NDC AWP DP OBC

NALIDIXIC ACID (Medisca)
CRY, NA (1X25GM,USP)
25 gm 38779-0241-04 129.00
(U.S.P.)
25 gm 38779-0241-01 64.50
100 gm..............38779-0241-05 459.00
500 gm..............38779-0241-02 184.50

(PCCA)
POW, NA (U.S.P.)
1 gm 51927-2647-00 5.16

NALOXONE HCL (Amphastar)
naloxone hydrochloride
SOL, IJ (SRN,PREFIL,LUERJET,PF)
1 mg/ml, 2 ml 10s....00548-3369-00 203.40 AP
(21GX1 1/2",MINIJET,PF)
1 mg/ml, 2 ml 25s....00548-1469-00 563.59 AP

(Covidien)
POW, NA (U.S.P.)
1 gm 00406-1492-52 70.90

(Hospira)
SOL, IJ (10X1ML AMP,LATEX-FREE)
0.4 mg/ml,
1 ml 10s...........00409-1212-01 40.80 35.70 AP
(10X1ML, CARPUJECT)
0.4 mg/ml,
1 ml 10s...........00409-1782-69 19.56 17.10 AP
(INTERLINK,CARPUJECT)
0.4 mg/ml,
1 ml 10s...........00074-1782-21 16.80 14.70 AP
(VIAL,FLIPTOP,10X1ML)
0.4 mg/ml,
1 ml 10s...........00409-1215-01 69.60 60.90 AP
(VIAL, FLIPTOP)
0.4 mg/ml,
10 ml 25s..........00074-1219-01 81.00 71.00 AP

(A-S Medication)
REPACK
SOL, IJ (VIAL, FLIPTOP)
0.4 mg/ml,
1 ml 10s...........54569-5247-00 23.38 EE

(Phys Total Care)
REPACK
SOL, IJ (AMP)
0.4 mg/ml,
1 ml 10s...........54868-2062-00 24.78 AP
(SRN,PREFILLED,MIN-I-JET)
0.4 mg/ml,
1 ml 25s...........54868-0748-00 152.40 AP

NALOXONE HCL DIHYDRATE (Medisca)
naloxone hydrochloride
POW, NA (U.S.P.)
0.5 gm 38779-0767-00 240.00
1 gm 38779-0767-06 375.00
5 gm 38779-0767-03 1125.00

(PCCA)
POW, NA (U.S.P.)
1 gm 51927-3335-00 444.00

(Spectrum Pharmacy)
POW, NA (U.S.P.)
0.25 gm 49452-4836-02 198.80
1 gm 49452-4836-03 591.50
5 gm 49452-4836-04 1704.50

NALOXONE HYDROCHLORIDE
(Amphastar) *See NALOXONE HCL*
(Covidien) *See NALOXONE HCL*
(Hospira) *See NALOXONE HCL*

(Hospira)
SOL, IJ, 0.4 mg/ml,
10 ml 25s..........00409-1219-01 876.30 766.75 AP

(Medisca) *See NALOXONE HCL DIHYDRATE*
(PCCA) *See NALOXONE HCL DIHYDRATE*
(Spectrum Pharmacy) *See NALOXONE HCL DIHYDRATE*

(Dispensing Solutions)
REPACK
SOL, IJ, 0.4 mg/ml,
1 ml 10s...........55045-3515-01 9.50

NALOXONE HYDROCHLORIDE/PENTAZOCINE HYDROCHLORIDE
(Sanofi-Aventis) *See TALWIN NX*
(Watson Labs) *See NALOXONE/PENTAZOCINE*

(Palmetto)
REPACK
TAB, PO, 0.5 mg-50 mg,
30s ea, C-IV.......23490-6073-03 40.50
60s ea, C-IV.......23490-6073-01 81.00
120s ea, C-IV......23490-6073-08 121.50

PROD/MFR NDC AWP DP OBC

NALOXONE/PENTAZOCINE (Watson Labs)
naloxone hydrochloride/pentazocine hydrochloride
TAB, PO, 0.5 mg-50 mg,
100s ea, C-IV......00591-0395-01 124.84 AB

(A-S Medication)
REPACK
TAB, PO, 0.5 mg-50 mg,
60s ea, C-IV........54569-5772-01 73.06 AB

(Altura)
REPACK
TAB, PO, 0.5 mg-50 mg,
10s ea, C-IV........63874-0220-10 16.64 AB
12s ea, C-IV........63874-0220-12 19.97 AB
15s ea, C-IV........63874-0220-15 24.96 AB
20s ea, C-IV........63874-0220-20 33.28 AB
30s ea, C-IV........63874-0220-30 49.92 AB
35s ea, C-IV........63874-0220-35 58.24 AB
40s ea, C-IV........63874-0220-40 66.56 AB
60s ea, C-IV........63874-0220-60 99.84 AB
90s ea, C-IV........63874-0220-90 149.76 AB
100s ea, C-IV.......63874-0220-01 166.40 AB
120s ea, C-IV.......63874-0220-04 199.68 AB
300s ea, C-IV.......63874-0220-03 499.20 AB

(Dispensing Solutions)
REPACK
TAB, PO, 0.5 mg-50 mg,
60s ea, C-IV........55045-3099-08 60.00 AB

(Keltman Pharma., Inc.)
REPACK
TAB, PO, 0.5 mg-50 mg,
30s ea, C-IV........68387-0531-30 49.74 AB

(Nucare Pharm)
REPACK
TAB, PO, 0.5 mg-50 mg,
30s ea, C-IV........66267-0487-30 39.99 EE

(PD-Rx Pharm)
REPACK
TAB, PO, 0.5 mg-50 mg,
20s ea, C-IV........43063-0142-20 36.15 AB

(Pharma Pac)
REPACK
TAB, PO, 0.5 mg-50 mg,
10s ea, C-IV........52959-0545-10 18.63 EE
12s ea, C-IV........52959-0545-12 22.35 EE
15s ea, C-IV........52959-0545-15 27.93 EE
20s ea, C-IV........52959-0545-20 37.23 EE
24s ea, C-IV........52959-0545-24 44.67 EE
30s ea, C-IV........52959-0545-30 55.83 EE
35s ea, C-IV........52959-0545-35 65.13 EE
40s ea, C-IV........52959-0545-40 74.43 EE
50s ea, C-IV........52959-0545-50 93.03 EE
60s ea, C-IV........52959-0545-60 111.62 AB
90s ea, C-IV........52959-0545-90 167.40 EE
120s ea, C-IV.......52959-0545-02 223.18 EE

(Phys Total Care)
REPACK
TAB, PO, 0.5 mg-50 mg,
30s ea, C-IV........54868-4788-00 59.10 AB

(Quality Care Prod)
REPACK
TAB, PO, 0.5 mg-50 mg,
30s ea, C-IV........35356-0176-30 78.90 AB

(Southwood)
REPACK
TAB, PO, 0.5 mg-50 mg,
10s ea, C-IV........58016-0392-10 10.41 EE
12s ea, C-IV........58016-0392-12 12.48 EE
20s ea, C-IV........58016-0392-20 20.82 EE
30s ea, C-IV........58016-0392-30 31.23 EE
40s ea, C-IV........58016-0392-40 41.64 EE
60s ea, C-IV........58016-0392-60 62.46 EE
100s ea, C-IV.......58016-0392-00 104.10 EE

(Stat Rx)
REPACK
TAB, PO, 0.5 mg-50 mg,
30s ea, C-IV........16590-0556-30 91.18 AB
40s ea, C-IV........16590-0556-40 121.57 AB
60s ea, C-IV........16590-0556-60 183.36 AB
90s ea, C-IV........16590-0556-90 275.04 AB
120s ea, C-IV.......16590-0556-72 366.72 AB

NALTREXONE
(Alkermes, Inc.) *See VIVITROL*
(Gallipot) *See NALTREXONE HYDROCHLORIDE*

(PCCA)
POW, NA, 1 gm...........51927-3548-00 63.00

PROD/MFR NDC AWP DP OBC

(Phys Total Care)
REPACK
naltrexone hydrochloride
TAB, PO, 50 mg, 30s ea ...54868-5574-00 138.12

NALTREXONE HCL (Covidien)
naltrexone hydrochloride
TAB, PO (CAPLET)
50 mg, 30s ea........00406-1170-03 128.25 AB
100s ea............00406-1170-01 427.51 AB

(Hawkins)
POW, NA, 1 gm...........63370-0158-10 163.20
5 gm 63370-0158-15 672.00
25 gm 63370-0158-25 3072.00
100 gm..............63370-0158-35 10080.00

(Medisca)
POW, NA, 1 gm...........38779-0887-06 126.00
5 gm 38779-0887-03 597.00
25 gm 38779-0887-04 2085.00
100 gm..............38779-0887-05 6615.00

(PCCA)
POW, NA, 1 gm...........51927-2753-00 177.00

(Sandoz)
TAB, PO (CAPLET)
50 mg, 30s ea........00185-0039-30 137.21 AB
100s ea............00185-0039-01 457.34 AB

(Spectrum Pharmacy)
POW, NA (U.S.P.)
1 gm 49452-4835-01 205.45
5 gm 49452-4835-02 892.50
25 gm 49452-4835-03 3041.50

(Teva)
TAB, PO (FILM-COATED)
50 mg, 30s ea........00555-0902-01 128.25 AB
100s ea............00555-0902-02 427.51 AB

NALTREXONE HYDROCHLORIDE
FUL
TAB, PO, 50 mg, 100s ea.......................... 404.00

(Covidien) *See NALTREXONE HCL*

NALTREXONE HYDROCHLORIDE (Gallipot)
naltrexone
POW, NA (1X1GM,USP)
1 gm 51552-0737-01 50.75 36.25
(1X5GM,USP)
5 gm 51552-0737-02 231.00 165.00

NALTREXONE HYDROCHLORIDE
(Hawkins) *See NALTREXONE HCL*

(Letco)
POW, NA (1X1GM,USP)
1 gm 62991-1243-01 87.00
(1X5GM,USP)
5 gm 62991-1243-02 360.00
(1X25GM,USP)
25 gm 62991-1243-03 1575.00
(1X100GM,USP)
100 gm..............62991-1243-04 5700.00

(Medisca) *See NALTREXONE HCL*
(PCCA) *See NALTREXONE HCL*

(PCCA)
POW, NA (ANHYDROUS)
1 gm 51927-3602-00 150.00

(Sandoz) *See NALTREXONE HCL*
(Spectrum Pharmacy) *See NALTREXONE HCL*
(Teva) *See NALTREXONE HCL*
(Teva) *See REVIA*

NAMENDA (Forest Pharm)
memantine hydrochloride
SOL, PO (AF,SF,PEPPERMINT)
2 mg/ml, 360 ml 00456-3202-12 417.80
TAB, PO (TITRATION PAK)
49s ea..............00456-3200-14 162.55
(FILM COATED)
5 mg, 60s ea........00456-3205-60 199.08
100s ea UD.........00456-3205-63 331.78
10 mg, 60s ea.......00456-3210-60 199.08
100s ea UD 00456-3210-63 331.78

(AQ)
REPACK
TAB, PO (FILM COATED)
5 mg, 30s ea........66105-0650-03 163.86
10 mg, 30s ea.......66105-0651-03 163.86

(Nucare Pharm)
REPACK
TAB, PO (FILM COATED)
5 mg, 30s ea........68071-0798-30 132.00
10 mg, 30s ea.......68071-0799-30 132.00

PROD/MFR	NDC	AWP	DP	OBC
(PD-Rx Pharm)				
REPACK				
TAB, PO, 10 mg, 30s ea	**58864-0887-30**	123.68		
(FILM COATED)				
10 mg, 30s ea	**55289-0937-30**	147.95		
60s ea	**55289-0937-60**	295.89		
(Phys Total Care)				
REPACK				
TAB, PO, 5 mg, 60s ea	**54868-5654-00**	190.42		
(FILM COATED)				
10 mg, 60s ea	**54868-5161-00**	237.62		
(Physician Partner)				
REPACK				
TAB, PO, 5 mg, 15s ea	**21695-0232-15**	115.08		
60s ea	**21695-0232-60**	391.28		
(FILM COATED)				
10 mg, 30s ea	**21695-0169-30**	195.64		
60s ea	**21695-0169-60**	391.28		
(Quality Care Prod)				
REPACK				
TAB, PO (FILM COATED)				
5 mg, 60s ea	**35356-0105-60**	267.40		
10 mg, 30s ea	**49999-0804-30**	133.70		
60s ea	**49999-0804-60**	267.40		
(Stat Rx)				
REPACK				
TAB, PO (FILM COATED)				
10 mg, 15s ea	**16590-0769-15**	60.78		
30s ea	**16590-0769-30**	118.31		
60s ea	**16590-0769-60**	233.37		
NANDROLONE DEC (Phys Total Care)				
REPACK				
nandrolone decanoate				
OIL, IM, 100 mg/ml,				
20 ml, C-III	**54868-5555-00**	187.45		
NANDROLONE DECANOATE (Gallipot)				
POW, NA (U.S.P.)				
5 gm, C-III	**51552-1043-02**	238.00	170.00	
(Hawkins)				
POW, NA (U.S.P.)				
1 gm, C-III	**63370-0955-10**	96.00		
5 gm, C-III	**63370-0955-15**	336.00		
25 gm, C-III	**63370-0955-25**	1200.00		
100 gm, C-III	**63370-0955-35**	3120.00		
500 gm, C-III	**63370-0955-45**	43200.00		
(Letco)				
POW, NA (USP)				
25 gm, C-III	**62991-2186-03**	570.00		
100 gm, C-III	**62991-2186-04**	1650.00		
500 gm, C-III	**62991-2186-05**	6600.00		
(USP, 1X1000GM)				
1000 gm, C-III	**62991-2186-02**	12250.00		
(Medisca)				
POW, NA (1X5GM)				
5 gm, C-III	**38779-2218-03**	450.00		
(1X25GM)				
25 gm, C-III	**38779-2218-04**	1485.00		
(1X100GM)				
100 gm, C-III	**38779-2218-05**	2925.00		
(PCCA)				
POW, NA (U.S.P.; CIII)				
1 gm, C-III	**51927-3514-00**	150.00		
(Spectrum Pharmacy)				
CRY, NA (U.S.P.)				
1 gm, C-III	**49452-4838-03**	188.30		
5 gm, C-III	**49452-4838-04**	626.50		
25 gm, C-III	**49452-4838-05**	1837.50		
NAPHAZOLINE (Palmetto)				
REPACK				
naphazoline hydrochloride				
SOL, OP (1X15ML)				
0.1%, 15 ml	**23490-6031-01**	19.60		
(Stat Rx)				
REPACK				
SOL, OP, 0.1%, 15 ml	**16590-0161-15**	16.50		
NAPHAZOLINE HCL (Amend)				
naphazoline hydrochloride				
POW, NA (U.S.P.)				
25 gm	**17317-0376-02**	28.00		
100 gm	**17317-0376-03**	105.00		
1000 gm	**17317-0376-06**	455.00		
(Gallipot)				
CRY, NA (U.S.P.)				
5 gm	**51552-0488-02**	21.28		

PROD/MFR	NDC	AWP	DP	OBC
(PCCA)				
POW, NA (U.S.P.)				
1 gm	**51927-2112-00**	6.60		
(Spectrum Pharmacy)				
POW, NA (U.S.P.)				
5 gm	**49452-4810-01**	118.30		
25 gm	**49452-4810-02**	329.35		
100 gm	**49452-4810-03**	752.60		
(A-S Medication)				
REPACK				
SOL, OP, 0.1%, 15 ml	**54569-2657-00**	7.13		EE
(DHS, Inc.)				
REPACK				
SOL, OP, 0.1%, 15 ml	**55887-0800-15**	13.80		AT
(Dispensing Solutions)				
REPACK				
SOL, OP, 0.1%, 15 ml	**55045-1354-00**	13.85		AT
(Nucare Pharm)				
REPACK				
SOL, OP, 0.1%, 15 ml	**66267-0959-15**	13.98		EE
(Phys Total Care)				
REPACK				
SOL, OP, 0.1%, 15 ml	**54868-1023-01**	19.95		AT
(Quality Care Prod)				
REPACK				
SOL, OP, 0.1%, 15 ml	**49999-0441-15**	16.56		AT
(Southwood)				
REPACK				
SOL, OP, 0.1%, 15 ml	**58016-6077-01**	13.80		EE
NAPHAZOLINE HYDROCHLORIDE				
FUL				
SOL, OP, 0.1%, 15 ml		4.71		
(Akorn) *See AK-CON*				
(Amend) *See NAPHAZOLINE HCL*				
(Gallipot) *See NAPHAZOLINE HCL*				
(PCCA) *See NAPHAZOLINE HCL*				
(Spectrum Pharmacy) *See NAPHAZOLINE HCL*				
NAPHCON A (Keltman Pharma., Inc.)				
REPACK				
naphazoline hydrochloride/pheniramine maleate				
SOL, OP (DROPS)				
0.025%-0.3%, 15 ml	**68387-0449-01**	18.84		
NAPHTHOL				
(Amend) *See BETA NAPHTHOL*				
(PCCA)				
POW, NA (BETA; 99%)				
1 gm	**51927-1215-00**	0.21		
2-NAPHTHOL (Spectrum Pharmacy)				
betanaphthol				
POW, NA (1X500GM)				
500 gm	**49452-4825-01**	103.25		
(1X2500GM)				
2500 gm	**49452-4825-02**	283.50		
NAPRELAN (Victory Pharma, Inc.)				
naproxen sodium				
TER, PO, 375 mg, 100s ea	**68453-0375-10**	374.55		AB
500 mg, 75s ea	**68453-0850-75**	318.72		
750 mg, 30s ea	**68453-0777-03**	229.81		EE
(Nucare Pharm)				
REPACK				
TER, PO, 375 mg, 60s ea	**68071-0705-60**	151.32		AB
(Pharma Pac)				
REPACK				
TER, PO, 500 mg, 14s ea	**52959-0485-14**	32.55		
15s ea	**52959-0485-15**	34.72		
20s ea	**52959-0485-20**	44.53		
21s ea	**52959-0485-21**	46.64		
30s ea	**52959-0485-30**	65.01		
40s ea	**52959-0485-40**	84.12		
60s ea	**52959-0485-60**	122.76		
(Phys Total Care)				
REPACK				
TER, PO (CAPLET)				
375 mg, 30s ea	**54868-3974-00**	112.71		
60s ea	**54868-3974-01**	223.45		
500 mg, 30s ea	**54868-3973-00**	59.41		
40s ea	**54868-3973-01**	78.59		
60s ea	**54868-3973-02**	116.94		
(Physician Partner)				
REPACK				
TER, PO, 375 mg, 60s ea	**21695-0905-60**	449.46		AB
500 mg, 60s ea	**21695-0906-60**	509.95		

PROD/MFR	NDC	AWP	DP	OBC
(Quality Care Prod)				
REPACK				
TER, PO, 375 mg, 30s ea	**35356-0529-30**	213.60		AB
500 mg, 30s ea	**35356-0530-30**	243.40		
750 mg, 30s ea	**35356-0531-30**	416.30		EE
(Southwood)				
REPACK				
TER, PO, 500 mg, 10s ea	**58016-0388-10**	27.29		
20s ea	**58016-0388-20**	54.59		
30s ea	**58016-0388-30**	81.88		
40s ea	**58016-0388-40**	109.17		
60s ea	**58016-0388-60**	163.76		
75s ea	**58016-0388-75**	204.70		
90s ea	**58016-0388-90**	245.64		
100s ea	**58016-0388-00**	272.93		
(Stat Rx)				
REPACK				
TER, PO, 375 mg, 30s ea	**16590-0551-30**	181.78		AB
56s ea	**16590-0551-56**	221.45		AB
60s ea	**16590-0551-60**	237.04		AB
90s ea	**16590-0551-90**	265.53		AB
500 mg, 30s ea	**16590-0794-30**	135.88		
750 mg, 30s ea	**16590-0242-30**	240.51		EE
NAPRELAN 500 (A-S Medication)				
REPACK				
naproxen sodium				
TER, PO, 500 mg, 30s ea	**54569-4364-00**	165.73		AB
NAPRELAN CR (IPI)				
REPACK				
naproxen sodium				
TER, PO, 375 mg, 60s ea	**18837-0270-60**	235.43		
90s ea	**18837-0270-90**	401.30		
180s ea	**18837-0270-96**	802.60		
NAPRELAN DOSE CARD (Victory Pharma, Inc.)				
naproxen sodium				
TER, PO, 20s ea	**68453-0900-02**	119.68		
NAPROSYN (Roche Labs)				
naproxen				
SUS, PO, 25 mg/ml,				
480 ml	**00004-0028-28**	74.80		AB
TAB, PO, 250 mg, 100s ea	**00004-6313-01**	147.38		AB
375 mg, 100s ea	**00004-6314-01**	189.43		AB
(CAPLET)				
500 mg, 100s ea	**00004-6316-01**	231.37		AB
(A-S Medication)				
REPACK				
TAB, PO (CAPLET)				
500 mg, 20s ea	**54569-0294-01**	41.92		AB
(PD-Rx Pharm)				
REPACK				
TAB, PO (CAPLET)				
500 mg, 10s ea	**55289-0420-10**	29.82		AB
14s ea	**55289-0420-14**	41.87		AB
15s ea	**55289-0420-15**	44.85		AB
20s ea	**55289-0420-20**	59.81		AB
30s ea	**55289-0420-30**	89.70		AB
40s ea	**55289-0420-40**	119.27		AB
(Pharma Pac)				
REPACK				
TAB, PO, 250 mg, 20s ea	**52959-0110-20**	22.50		AB
30s ea	**52959-0110-30**	28.90		AB
500 mg, 14s ea	**52959-0111-14**	26.70		AB
20s ea	**52959-0111-20**	38.00		AB
28s ea	**52959-0111-28**	53.00		AB
30s ea	**52959-0111-30**	56.00		AB
40s ea	**52959-0111-40**	74.00		AB
60s ea	**52959-0111-60**	90.00		AB
(Phys Total Care)				
REPACK				
TAB, PO, 500 mg, 10s ea	**54868-0300-06**	24.02		AB
20s ea	**54868-0300-04**	46.53		AB
30s ea	**54868-0300-00**	68.85		AB
NAPROXEN				
FUL				
TAB, PO, 250 mg, 100s ea		10.32		
375 mg, 100s ea		7.61		
500 mg, 100s ea		8.24		
(Amneal)				
TAB, PO, 250 mg, 100s ea	**53746-0188-01**	77.25		AB
500s ea	**53746-0188-05**	377.79		AB
375 mg, 100s ea	**53746-0189-01**	106.35		AB
500s ea	**53746-0189-05**	467.40		AB
500 mg, 100s ea	**53746-0190-01**	125.77		AB
500s ea	**53746-0190-05**	573.39		AB
(Dava Pharma)				
TAB, PO, 250 mg, 100s ea	**67253-0620-10**	77.65		AB
1000s ea	**67253-0620-11**	755.58		AB

PROD/MFR	NDC	AWP	DP	OBC
(CAPLET)				
375 mg, 30s ea	**67253-0621-03**	32.80		AB
50s ea	**67253-0621-05**	52.66		AB
100s ea	**67253-0621-10**	106.35		AB
1000s ea	**67253-0621-11**	869.08		AB
500 mg, 30s ea	**67253-0622-03**	34.04		AB
50s ea	**67253-0622-05**	58.82		AB
100s ea	**67253-0622-10**	129.85		AB
500s ea	**67253-0622-50**	596.35		AB
(Dr Reddy's)				
TAB, PO, 250 mg, 100s ea	**55111-0366-01**	77.60		AB
500s ea	**55111-0366-05**	380.00		AB
375 mg, 100s ea	**55111-0367-01**	106.30		AB
500s ea	**55111-0367-05**	488.00		AB
500 mg, 100s ea	**55111-0368-01**	129.80		AB
500s ea	**55111-0368-05**	596.30		AB
(Ethex) *See NAPROXEN EC*				
(Gallipot)				
POW, NA (U.S.P.)				
25 gm	**51552-0401-04**	31.50		
100 gm	**51552-0401-05**	116.55		
(Glenmark Pharmaceuticals)				
TAB, PO, 250 mg, 100s ea	**68462-0188-01**	77.50		AB
500s ea	**68462-0188-05**	379.50		AB
375 mg, 100s ea	**68462-0189-01**	106.00		AB
500s ea	**68462-0189-05**	488.25		AB
500 mg, 100s ea	**68462-0190-01**	129.50		AB
500s ea	**68462-0190-05**	596.25		AB
(Hawkins)				
POW, NA (USP)				
25 gm	**63370-0164-25**	64.00		
100 gm	**63370-0164-35**	240.00		
500 gm	**63370-0164-45**	1040.00		
1000 gm	**63370-0164-50**	1920.00		
(Letco)				
POW, NA (U.S.P.)				
100 gm	**62991-1354-02**	135.00		
(Major)				
TAB, PO (10X10)				
250 mg, 100s ea UD	**00904-5535-61**	87.60		AB
(USP, 10X10)				
250 mg, 100s ea UD	**00904-6069-61**	87.60		AB
375 mg, 100s ea	**00904-5590-60**	89.10		AB
(CAPLET)				
375 mg, 100s ea UD	**00904-5536-61**	111.50		
(USP, 10X10)				
375 mg, 100s ea UD	**00904-5590-61**	111.50		AB
500 mg, 100s ea	**00904-5591-60**	109.25		AB
(USP, 10X10)				
500 mg, 100s ea UD	**00904-5591-61**	135.50		AB
500s ea	**00904-5591-40**	517.00		AB
(Medisca)				
POW, NA (U.S.P.)				
ea	**38779-0548-09**	1485.00		
25 gm	**38779-0548-04**	55.50		
100 gm	**38779-0548-05**	202.50		
500 gm	**38779-0548-08**	885.00		
(Mylan)				
TAB, PO, 250 mg, 100s ea	**00378-0377-01**	77.70		AB
500s ea	**00378-0377-05**	380.10		AB
375 mg, 100s ea	**00378-0555-01**	106.40		AB
500s ea	**00378-0555-05**	488.30		AB
500 mg, 100s ea	**00378-0451-01**	129.90		AB
500s ea	**00378-0451-05**	596.40		AB
(PCCA)				
POW, NA (U.S.P.)				
1 gm	**51927-2715-00**	3.00		
(Roche Labs) *See EC NAPROSYN*				
(Roche Labs) *See NAPROSYN*				
(Roxane)				
SUS, PO (ORANGE PINEAPPLE)				
25 mg/ml, 500 ml	**00054-3630-63**	45.65		AB
(Sandoz) *See NAPROXEN DELAYED-RELEASE*				
(Sandoz)				
TAB, PO, 250 mg, 100s ea	**00781-1163-01**	73.96		AB
500s ea	**00781-1163-05**	360.40		AB
375 mg, 100s ea	**00781-1164-01**	94.99		AB
500s ea	**00781-1164-05**	461.28		AB
500 mg, 100s ea	**00781-1165-01**	115.99		AB
500s ea	**00781-1165-05**	562.99		AB
(Spectrum Pharmacy)				
POW, NA (U.S.P., N.F.)				
25 gm	**49452-4815-03**	89.25		
100 gm	**49452-4815-04**	312.20		
500 gm	**49452-4815-05**	1288.00		
1000 gm	**49452-4815-01**	1988.00		

PROD/MFR	NDC	AWP	DP	OBC
(Teva) *See NAPROXEN DELAYED-RELEASE*				
(Teva)				
TAB, PO, 250 mg, 100s ea	**00093-0147-01**	77.70		AB
(USP,10X10)				
250 mg, 100s ea UD	**00093-0147-93**	80.00		AB
500s ea	**00093-0147-05**	380.10		AB
375 mg, 100s ea	**00093-0148-01**	106.40		AB
500s ea	**00093-0148-05**	488.30		AB
500 mg, 100s ea	**00093-0149-01**	129.90		AB
(10X10)				
500 mg, 100s ea UD	**00093-0149-93**	133.75		AB
500s ea	**00093-0149-05**	596.40		AB
1000s ea	**00093-0149-10**	1126.00		AB
(UDL)				
TAB, PO (10X10)				
250 mg, 100s ea UD	**51079-0793-20**	80.03		AB
375 mg, 100s ea UD	**51079-0794-20**	109.59		AB
500 mg, 100s ea UD	**51079-0795-20**	133.80		AB
(West-Ward)				
TAB, PO, 250 mg, 100s ea	**00143-1346-01**	77.60		AB
500s ea	**00143-1346-05**	377.80		AB
375 mg, 100s ea	**00143-1347-01**	106.30		AB
500s ea	**00143-1347-05**	465.50		AB
500 mg, 100s ea	**00143-1348-01**	129.75		AB
500s ea	**00143-1348-05**	596.20		AB
(4u)				
REPACK				
TAB, PO, 375 mg, 60s ea	**10544-0325-60**	71.44		
60s ea	**42549-0525-60**	71.44		AB
500 mg, 30s ea	**10544-0392-30**	62.86		AB
30s ea	**42549-0540-30**	62.86		AB
30s ea	**42549-0592-30**	62.86		AB
60s ea	**10544-0392-60**	112.26		AB
60s ea	**42549-0540-60**	112.26		AB
60s ea	**42549-0592-60**	112.26		AB
(4u)				
naproxen sodium				
550 mg, 60s ea	**10544-0324-60**	106.64		
NAPROXEN (A-S Medication)				
REPACK				
TAB, PO, 250 mg, 20s ea	**54569-3758-00**	15.53		AB
28s ea	**54569-3758-02**	21.74		AB
30s ea	**54569-3758-04**	23.30		AB
60s ea	**54569-3758-01**	46.59		AB
375 mg, 14s ea	**54569-3759-03**	14.89		AB
20s ea	**54569-3759-04**	21.27		AB
21s ea	**54569-3759-01**	22.33		AB
30s ea	**54569-3759-02**	31.91		AB
45s ea	**54569-3759-06**	47.86		AB
100s ea	**54569-3759-08**	106.35		AB
500 mg, 10s ea	**54569-3760-03**	12.99		AB
14s ea	**54569-3760-04**	18.18		AB
15s ea	**54569-3760-00**	19.48		AB
20s ea	**54569-3760-01**	25.97		AB
21s ea	**54569-4255-00**	27.27		AB
30s ea	**54569-3760-02**	38.96		AB
40s ea	**54569-3760-05**	51.94		AB
60s ea	**54569-3760-07**	77.91		AB
100s ea	**54569-3760-06**	129.85		AB
(Aidarex)				
REPACK				
TAB, PO, 375 mg, 7s ea	**33261-0080-07**	10.43		AB
10s ea	**33261-0080-10**	14.90		AB
12s ea	**33261-0080-12**	17.88		AB
14s ea	**33261-0080-14**	20.86		AB
20s ea	**33261-0080-20**	29.80		AB
21s ea	**33261-0080-21**	31.29		AB
28s ea	**33261-0080-28**	41.72		AB
30s ea	**33261-0080-30**	44.70		AB
40s ea	**33261-0080-40**	59.60		AB
52s ea	**33261-0080-52**	77.48		AB
60s ea	**33261-0080-60**	89.40		AB
90s ea	**33261-0080-90**	134.10		AB
500 mg, 7s ea	**33261-0081-07**	12.60		AB
10s ea	**33261-0081-10**	18.00		AB
12s ea	**33261-0081-12**	21.60		AB
14s ea	**33261-0081-14**	25.20		AB
20s ea	**33261-0081-20**	36.00		AB
21s ea	**33261-0081-21**	37.80		AB
28s ea	**33261-0081-28**	50.40		AB
30s ea	**33261-0081-30**	54.00		AB
40s ea	**33261-0081-40**	72.00		AB
52s ea	**33261-0081-52**	93.60		AB
60s ea	**33261-0081-60**	108.00		AB
90s ea	**33261-0081-90**	162.00		AB
(Altura)				
REPACK				
TAB, PO, 250 mg, 20s ea	**63874-0301-20**	19.95		EE
21s ea	**63874-0301-21**	20.94		EE
100s ea	**63874-0301-01**	99.75		EE

PROD/MFR	NDC	AWP	DP	OBC
500s ea	**63874-0301-50**	498.75		EE
375 mg, 10s ea	**63874-0325-10**	13.68		EE
14s ea	**63874-0325-14**	19.15		EE
15s ea	**63874-0325-15**	20.52		EE
20s ea	**63874-0325-20**	27.36		EE
21s ea	**63874-0325-21**	28.73		EE
28s ea	**63874-0325-28**	38.30		EE
30s ea	**63874-0325-30**	41.04		EE
40s ea	**63874-0325-40**	54.72		EE
45s ea	**63874-0325-45**	61.56		EE
60s ea	**63874-0325-60**	82.08		EE
90s ea	**63874-0325-90**	123.12		EE
100s ea	**63874-0325-01**	136.80		EE
120s ea	**63874-0325-04**	164.16		EE
500s ea	**63874-0325-03**	684.00		EE
1000s ea	**63874-0325-02**	1368.00		EE
500 mg, 10s ea	**63874-0326-10**	15.43		AB
14s ea	**63874-0326-14**	21.60		EE
15s ea	**63874-0326-15**	23.14		EE
20s ea	**63874-0326-20**	30.85		EE
21s ea	**63874-0326-21**	32.40		AB
25s ea	**63874-0326-25**	38.57		AB
28s ea	**63874-0326-28**	43.19		AB
30s ea	**63874-0326-30**	46.28		EE
40s ea	**63874-0326-40**	61.71		EE
42s ea	**63874-0326-42**	64.79		AB
45s ea	**63874-0326-45**	69.42		AB
50s ea	**63874-0326-50**	77.13		AB
56s ea	**63874-0326-56**	86.39		AB
60s ea	**63874-0326-60**	92.56		AB
90s ea	**63874-0326-90**	138.84		AB
100s ea	**63874-0326-01**	154.27		EE
120s ea	**63874-0326-04**	185.12		AB
500s ea	**63874-0326-03**	824.50		AB
(Bryant Ranch)				
REPACK				
TAB, PO, 250 mg, 30s ea	**63629-3202-01**	32.99		
60s ea	**63629-3202-02**	72.39		
375 mg, 20s ea	**63629-1476-01**	33.33		
30s ea	**63629-1476-02**	56.50		
40s ea	**63629-1476-03**	62.67		
60s ea	**63629-1476-05**	93.99		
90s ea	**63629-1476-06**	153.51		
120s ea	**63629-1476-04**	169.99		
500 mg, 20s ea	**63629-1477-05**	36.65		
30s ea	**63629-1477-01**	55.08		
45s ea	**63629-1477-03**	82.53		
50s ea	**63629-1477-07**	98.52		
60s ea	**63629-1477-02**	152.00		
90s ea	**63629-1477-04**	166.00		
(Core)				
REPACK				
TAB, PO, 250 mg, 30s ea	**33358-0253-30**	33.81		
60s ea	**33358-0253-60**	74.20		
375 mg, 20s ea	**33358-0254-20**	34.16		
30s ea	**33358-0254-30**	57.91		
60s ea	**33358-0254-60**	96.34		
120s ea	**33358-0254-01**	174.24		
500 mg, 14s ea	**33358-0255-14**	28.95		
15s ea	**33358-0255-15**	31.00		
20s ea	**33358-0255-20**	43.45		
28s ea	**33358-0255-28**	48.54		
30s ea	**33358-0255-30**	56.47		
45s ea	**33358-0255-45**	84.59		
60s ea	**33358-0255-60**	112.92		
90s ea	**33358-0255-90**	170.15		
120s ea	**33358-0255-01**	198.50		
(DHS, Inc.)				
REPACK				
TAB, PO, 250 mg, 30s ea	**55887-0085-30**	26.75		
60s ea	**55887-0085-60**	53.50		
90s ea	**55887-0085-90**	80.25		
375 mg, 20s ea	**55887-0901-20**	25.99		AB
21s ea	**55887-0901-21**	27.19		
30s ea	**55887-0901-30**	38.84		AB
60s ea	**55887-0901-60**	75.96		AB
500 mg, 15s ea	**55887-0959-15**	26.75		AB
20s ea	**55887-0959-20**	35.58		AB
28s ea	**55887-0959-28**	49.80		AB
30s ea	**55887-0959-30**	53.35		AB
40s ea	**55887-0959-40**	70.00		AB
60s ea	**55887-0959-60**	99.00		AB
120s ea	**55887-0959-82**	198.00		AB
(Dispensing Solutions)				
REPACK				
TAB, PO, 250 mg, 20s ea	**55045-2281-07**	25.20		AB
30s ea	**55045-3764-08**	27.00		
30s ea	**66336-0816-30**	27.95		AB
60s ea	**55045-2281-09**	54.00		AB
60s ea	**55045-3764-06**	54.00		

PROD/MFR	NDC	AWP	DP	OBC
(CAPLET)				
375 mg, 15s ea	55045-2065-05	22.35		AB
20s ea	55045-2065-07	29.80		AB
20s ea	66336-0817-20	26.40		AB
30s ea	55045-2065-08	44.70		AB
30s ea	66336-0817-30	39.44		AB
40s ea	55045-2065-04	59.60		AB
60s ea	55045-2065-02	89.40		
(CAPLET)				
375 mg, 90s ea	55045-2065-09	134.10		AB
100s ea	55045-2065-00	149.00		AB
120s ea	55045-2065-01	178.80		AB
135s ea	55045-2065-03	201.15		AB
500 mg, 6s ea	55045-2066-06	9.48		AB
10s ea	66336-0815-10	16.50		AB
(CAPLET)				
500 mg, 10s ea	55045-2066-03	15.80		AB
14s ea	66336-0815-14	23.10		AB
15s ea	55045-2066-05	23.70		AB
15s ea	66336-0815-15	24.75		AB
20s ea	55045-2066-07	31.60		AB
20s ea	55045-3926-01	31.60		AB
20s ea	66336-0815-20	33.00		AB
30s ea	55045-2066-08	47.40		AB
30s ea	66336-0815-30	49.50		AB
40s ea	55045-2066-04	63.20		
(CAPLET)				
500 mg, 50s ea	55045-3269-05	79.00		AB
60s ea	55045-2066-02	94.80		AB
60s ea	66336-0815-60	99.00		AB
(CAPLET)				
500 mg, 80s ea	55045-2066-00	126.40		AB
84s ea	55045-3722-04	132.72		
90s ea	55045-2066-09	142.20		
90s ea	66336-0815-90	172.02		AB
(CAPLET)				
500 mg, 100s ea	55045-2066-01	158.00		AB
120s ea	55045-3269-01	189.60		
(CAPLET)				
500 mg, 135s ea	55045-3269-03	213.30		AB
180s ea	55045-3269-08	284.40		AB
(GSMS)				
REPACK				
TAB, PO (UNIT OF USE)				
250 mg, 20s ea	60429-0133-20	12.60	4.20	AB
30s ea	60429-0133-30	16.05	5.35	AB
60s ea	60429-0133-60	32.40	10.80	AB
120s ea	60429-0133-12	67.95	22.65	AB
180s ea	60429-0133-18	107.40	35.80	AB
375 mg, 60s ea	60429-0134-60	46.80	15.60	AB
180s ea	60429-0134-18	132.45	44.15	AB
500 mg, 20s ea	60429-0135-20	24.15	8.05	AB
60s ea	60429-0135-60	66.00	22.00	AB
180s ea	60429-0135-18	188.55	62.85	AB
(HomeMed)				
REPACK				
TAB, PO, 250 mg, 30s ea	51655-0685-24	22.64		EE
375 mg, 14s ea	51655-0625-84	19.70		EE
20s ea	51655-0625-52	36.89		EE
30s ea	51655-0625-24	54.89		EE
60s ea	51655-0625-25	56.35		EE
500 mg, 10s ea	51655-0626-53	12.26		EE
14s ea	51666-0268-84	32.99		
20s ea	51655-0626-52	45.89		
30s ea	51655-0626-24	58.99		
60s ea	51655-0626-25	108.94		
(IPI)				
REPACK				
ECT, PO, 500 mg, 60s ea	18837-0102-60	97.43		
TAB, PO, 500 mg, 14s ea	18837-0101-14	20.87		AB
20s ea	18837-0101-20	29.75		AB
30s ea	18837-0101-30	35.78		AB
60s ea	18837-0101-60	82.95		
90s ea	18837-0101-90	134.15		AB
180s ea	18837-0101-96	285.89		
(IPI)				
naproxen sodium				
550 mg, 30s ea	18837-0330-30	50.25		
NAPROXEN (Keltman Pharma., Inc.)				
REPACK				
TAB, PO, 250 mg, 30s ea	68387-0801-30	29.75		AB
375 mg, 60s ea	68387-0802-60	119.93		
500 mg, 14s ea	68387-0800-14	27.16		
30s ea	68387-0800-30	58.20		AB
60s ea	68387-0800-60	116.40		AB
90s ea	68387-0800-90	174.60		AB
(LWP)				
REPACK				
TAB, PO (CAPLET)				
500 mg, 60s ea	64038-0093-60	82.80		AB
100s ea	64038-0093-01	136.34		AB

PROD/MFR	NDC	AWP	DP	OBC
(Nucare Pharm)				
REPACK				
TAB, PO, 250 mg, 20s ea	66267-0151-20	23.74		EE
30s ea	66267-0151-30	32.69		EE
40s ea	66267-0151-40	47.48		EE
60s ea	66267-0151-60	72.36		EE
375 mg, 20s ea	66267-0152-20	33.61		EE
30s ea	66267-0152-30	47.36		EE
40s ea	66267-0152-40	62.49		EE
60s ea	66267-0152-60	88.73		EE
90s ea	66267-0152-90	129.86		EE
500 mg, 10s ea	66267-0153-10	20.31		EE
14s ea	66267-0153-14	28.24		EE
15s ea	66267-0153-15	30.24		EE
20s ea	66267-0153-20	42.39		EE
30s ea	66267-0153-30	53.36		EE
40s ea	66267-0153-40	71.15		EE
42s ea	66267-0153-42	69.61		EE
60s ea	66267-0153-60	96.83		EE
90s ea	66267-0153-90	149.86		EE
120s ea	66267-0153-91	193.66		AB
(Palmetto)				
REPACK				
SUS, PO (1X5ML)				
25 mg/ml, 5 ml	23490-7919-00	2.61		
TAB, PO, 250 mg, 20s ea	23490-5969-00	21.00		
28s ea	23490-5969-02	29.40		
30s ea	23490-5969-01	31.50		
60s ea	23490-5969-06	63.00		
375 mg, 14s ea	23490-5970-00	23.10		
20s ea	23490-5970-01	33.00		
21s ea	23490-5970-06	34.65		
28s ea	23490-5970-02	46.20		
30s ea	23490-5970-03	49.50		
60s ea	23490-5970-05	99.00		
90s ea	23490-5970-04	148.50		
500 mg, 6s ea	23490-5971-01	16.80		
10s ea	23490-5971-02	20.00		
14s ea	23490-5971-03	28.00		
15s ea	23490-5971-04	30.00		
20s ea	23490-5971-05	40.00		
30s ea	23490-0961-03	60.41		
30s ea	23490-5971-06	60.00		
40s ea	23490-5971-00	80.00		
60s ea	23490-0961-06	120.81		
60s ea	23490-5971-07	120.00		
90s ea	23490-0961-09	181.22		
90s ea	23490-5971-09	180.00		
100s ea	23490-5971-08	200.00		
120s ea	23490-0961-05	241.62		
120s ea	23490-7918-04	240.00		
(PD-Rx Pharm)				
REPACK				
TAB, PO, 250 mg, 6s ea	43063-0092-06	44.90		AB
12s ea	55289-0445-12	50.80		AB
15s ea	55289-0445-15	52.11		AB
20s ea	55289-0445-20	60.00		AB
21s ea	55289-0445-21	61.33		AB
28s ea	55289-0445-28	62.11		AB
30s ea	55289-0445-30	62.33		AB
60s ea	55289-0445-60	91.33		AB
(REDI-SCRIPT)				
250 mg, 90s ea	58864-0359-90	128.39		AB
375 mg, 10s ea	55289-0297-10	44.78		AB
14s ea	55289-0297-14	54.00		AB
15s ea	55289-0297-15	54.11		AB
20s ea	55289-0297-20	56.22		AB
(REDI-SCRIPT)				
375 mg, 20s ea	58864-0360-20	56.22		AB
21s ea	55289-0297-21	57.89		AB
24s ea	55289-0297-24	64.67		AB
30s ea	55289-0297-30	67.67		AB
42s ea	55289-0297-42	85.78		AB
60s ea	55289-0297-60	102.00		AB
(REDI-SCRIPT)				
375 mg, 90s ea	58864-0360-90	136.33		AB
500 mg, 6s ea	55289-0298-06	34.00		AB
7s ea	55289-0298-07	39.56		AB
10s ea	55289-0298-10	42.22		AB
14s ea	55289-0298-14	45.78		AB
15s ea	55289-0298-15	46.67		AB
20s ea	55289-0298-20	51.11		AB
(REDI-SCRIPT)				
500 mg, 20s ea	58864-0400-20	51.10		AB
24s ea	55289-0298-24	54.67		AB
28s ea	55289-0298-28	58.22		AB
30s ea	55289-0298-30	60.00		AB
(REDI-SCRIPT)				
500 mg, 30s ea	58864-0400-30	60.00		AB
40s ea	55289-0298-40	68.89		AB
60s ea	55289-0298-60	86.67		AB

PROD/MFR	NDC	AWP	DP	OBC
(REDI-SCRIPT)				
500 mg, 60s ea	58864-0400-60	86.70		AB
90s ea	55289-0298-90	146.70		AB
(USP)				
500 mg, 180s ea	55289-0298-93	193.30		AB
(Pharma Pac)				
REPACK				
TAB, PO, 250 mg, 20s ea	52959-0190-20	19.90		EE
28s ea	52959-0190-28	23.57		EE
30s ea	52959-0190-30	27.17		EE
40s ea	52959-0190-40	39.88		EE
60s ea	52959-0190-60	59.62		EE
90s ea	52959-0190-90	89.32		AB
375 mg, 10s ea	52959-0191-10	14.83		EE
14s ea	52959-0191-14	20.75		EE
15s ea	52959-0191-15	22.23		EE
20s ea	52959-0191-20	29.63		EE
28s ea	52959-0191-28	41.47		EE
30s ea	52959-0191-30	44.43		EE
40s ea	52959-0191-40	59.22		EE
42s ea	52959-0191-42	62.18		EE
60s ea	52959-0191-60	88.80		EE
100s ea	52959-0191-00	147.97		EE
(CAPLET)				
375 mg, 120s ea	52959-0191-02	177.52		AB
500 mg, 10s ea	52959-0193-10	19.99		EE
14s ea	52959-0193-14	27.98		EE
15s ea	52959-0193-15	29.97		EE
20s ea	52959-0193-20	39.95		EE
21s ea	52959-0193-21	41.94		EE
24s ea	52959-0193-24	47.93		EE
28s ea	52959-0193-28	55.91		EE
30s ea	52959-0193-30	59.90		EE
35s ea	52959-0193-35	69.87		EE
40s ea	52959-0193-40	79.83		EE
42s ea	52959-0193-42	83.81		AB
60s ea	52959-0193-60	118.85		EE
90s ea	52959-0193-90	178.20		EE
100s ea	52959-0193-00	198.20		EE
(CAPLET)				
500 mg, 120s ea	52959-0193-02	237.90		AB
(Phys Total Care)				
REPACK				
TAB, PO, 250 mg, 20s ea	54868-2964-03	7.35		EE
30s ea	54868-2964-01	9.51		EE
60s ea	54868-2964-02	16.02		EE
375 mg, 20s ea	54868-2965-06	7.14		EE
30s ea	54868-2965-02	9.21		EE
40s ea	54868-2965-03	11.28		EE
50s ea	54868-2965-01	13.35		EE
60s ea	54868-2965-04	15.42		EE
100s ea	54868-2965-05	22.23		EE
500 mg, 15s ea	54868-2966-07	7.89		EE
20s ea	54868-2966-06	9.00		EE
30s ea	54868-2966-04	13.77		EE
40s ea	54868-2966-03	13.53		EE
60s ea	54868-2966-02	18.03		EE
90s ea	54868-2966-09	23.36		AB
(CAPLET)				
500 mg, 100s ea	54868-2966-08	25.56		AB
500s ea	54868-2966-00	114.45		EE
(Physician Partner)				
REPACK				
ECT, PO, 500 mg, 20s ea	21695-0343-20	50.08		
30s ea	21695-0343-30	75.12		
60s ea	21695-0343-60	150.24		
TAB, PO, 250 mg, 60s ea	21695-0084-60	90.67		
(CAPLET)				
375 mg, 20s ea	21695-0085-20	50.05		AB
30s ea	21695-0085-30	63.81		
60s ea	21695-0085-60	127.62		
90s ea	21695-0085-90	191.43		
120s ea	21695-0085-72	255.24		
500 mg, 14s ea	21695-0086-14	39.84		
20s ea	21695-0086-20	56.91		
28s ea	21695-0086-28	67.72		
30s ea	21695-0086-30	72.56		
40s ea	21695-0086-40	113.79		AB
45s ea	21695-0086-45	128.01		
60s ea	21695-0086-60	145.12		
90s ea	21695-0086-90	217.68		
(Quality Care Prod)				
REPACK				
TAB, PO, 250 mg, 30s ea	49999-0473-30	30.90		EE
60s ea	49999-0473-60	61.80		EE
375 mg, 10s ea	49999-0049-10	13.77		AB
15s ea	49999-0049-15	40.65		AB
20s ea	49999-0049-20	27.60		EE
28s ea	49999-0049-28	38.54		EE
30s ea	49999-0049-30	41.30		EE
60s ea	49999-0049-60	91.36		EE

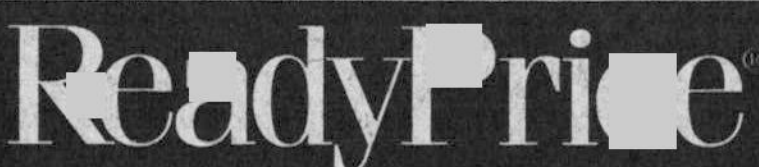

PROD/MFR	NDC	AWP	DP	OBC
120s ea	49999-0049-01	165.60		AB
500 mg, 10s ea	49999-0009-10	23.60		AB
14s ea	49999-0009-14	33.04		EE
15s ea	49999-0009-15	35.40		EE
20s ea	49999-0009-20	47.20		EE
30s ea	49999-0009-30	70.91		AB
42s ea	49999-0009-42	99.12		EE
45s ea	49999-0009-45	106.20		AB
60s ea	49999-0009-60	141.81		AB
90s ea	49999-0009-90	212.40		EE
100s ea	49999-0009-00	236.00		EE
(Southwood)				
REPACK				
TAB, PO, 250 mg, 10s ea	58016-0314-10	8.93		EE
12s ea	58016-0314-12	10.71		EE
14s ea	58016-0314-14	12.50		EE
15s ea	58016-0314-15	13.39		EE
20s ea	58016-0314-20	17.85		EE
21s ea	58016-0314-21	18.74		EE
24s ea	58016-0314-24	21.42		EE
28s ea	58016-0314-28	24.99		EE
30s ea	58016-0314-30	26.78		EE
40s ea	58016-0314-40	35.70		EE
60s ea	58016-0314-60	53.55		EE
100s ea	58016-0314-00	89.25		EE
120s ea	58016-0314-02	107.10		AB
150s ea	58016-0314-03	133.88		AB
200s ea	58016-0314-89	178.50		AB
300s ea	58016-0314-73	267.75		AB
375 mg, 10s ea	58016-0267-10	12.49		EE
12s ea	58016-0267-12	14.98		EE
14s ea	58016-0267-14	17.48		EE
15s ea	58016-0267-15	18.73		EE
20s ea	58016-0267-20	24.97		EE
21s ea	58016-0267-21	26.22		EE
24s ea	58016-0267-24	29.97		EE
28s ea	58016-0267-28	34.96		EE
30s ea	58016-0267-30	50.40		AB
40s ea	58016-0267-40	49.94		EE
42s ea	58016-0267-42	52.44		EE
60s ea	58016-0267-60	100.80		AB
90s ea	58016-0267-90	151.20		AB
100s ea	58016-0267-00	168.00		AB
120s ea	58016-0267-02	201.60		AB
(CAPLET)				
375 mg, 150s ea	58016-0267-03	187.29		AB
200s ea	58016-0267-89	249.72		AB
300s ea	58016-0267-73	374.58		AB
500 mg, 10s ea	58016-0289-10	15.26		EE
12s ea	58016-0289-12	18.31		EE
14s ea	58016-0289-14	21.36		EE
15s ea	58016-0289-15	22.89		EE
18s ea	58016-0289-18	27.46		EE
20s ea	58016-0289-20	30.51		EE
21s ea	58016-0289-21	32.04		EE
24s ea	58016-0289-24	36.62		EE
28s ea	58016-0289-28	42.72		EE
30s ea	58016-0289-30	54.60		AB
40s ea	58016-0289-40	61.03		EE
42s ea	58016-0289-42	64.08		EE
50s ea	58016-0289-50	76.29		EE
56s ea	58016-0289-56	85.44		EE
60s ea	58016-0289-60	109.20		AB
90s ea	58016-0289-90	163.80		AB
100s ea	58016-0289-00	182.00		AB
120s ea	58016-0289-02	218.40		AB
(CAPLET)				
500 mg, 135s ea	58016-0289-67	205.97		AB
150s ea	58016-0289-03	228.86		EE
(CAPLET)				
500 mg, 180s ea	58016-0289-99	274.63		AB
200s ea	58016-0289-89	305.14		AB
300s ea	58016-0289-73	457.71		AB
(St. Mary's MPP)				
REPACK				
TAB, PO (USP,CAPLET)				
375 mg, 15s ea	60760-0140-15	20.34		AB
20s ea	60760-0140-20	25.12		AB
60s ea	60760-0140-60	63.36		AB
500 mg, 30s ea	60760-0460-30	45.36		AB
60s ea	60760-0460-60	84.72		AB
90s ea	60760-0460-90	124.06		AB
(Stat Rx)				
REPACK				
TAB, PO, 375 mg, 30s ea	16590-0162-30	48.25		
(CAPLET)				
375 mg, 56s ea	16590-0162-56	113.74		AB
60s ea	16590-0162-60	96.50		
500 mg, 15s ea	16590-0163-15	24.25		AB
20s ea	16590-0163-20	35.57		
30s ea	16590-0163-30	55.10		
56s ea	16590-0163-56	90.55		AB

PROD/MFR	NDC	AWP	DP	OBC
60s ea	16590-0163-60	110.12		
90s ea	16590-0163-90	134.15		AB
120s ea	16590-0163-72	152.00		AB
(Vibranta)				
REPACK				
TAB, PO, 250 mg, 20s ea	57866-6607-02	19.32		
375 mg, 15s ea	57866-6608-04	19.70		
20s ea	57866-6608-03	27.80		
30s ea	57866-6608-01	76.65		
60s ea	57866-6608-02	91.36		
500 mg, 14s ea	57866-6609-02	23.20		
15s ea	57866-6609-07	25.24		
20s ea	57866-6609-06	27.07		
30s ea	57866-6609-01	58.90		
60s ea	57866-6609-03	125.65		
NAPROXEN COMFORT PAC (PD-Rx Pharm)				
REPACK				
naproxen				
KIT, MR, 500 mg, ea	55289-0466-92	74.75		
NAPROXEN D/R (Stat Rx)				
REPACK				
naproxen				
ECT, PO, 500 mg, 20s ea	16590-0164-20	52.00		
30s ea	16590-0164-30	78.00		
60s ea	16590-0164-60	156.00		
90s ea	16590-0164-90	170.00		
NAPROXEN DELAYED-RELEASE (Sandoz)				
naproxen				
ECT, PO, 375 mg, 100s ea	00781-1646-01	101.21		AB
500 mg, 100s ea	00781-1653-01	123.62		AB
(Teva)				
ECT, PO (CAPLET)				
375 mg, 100s ea	00093-1005-01	106.40		AB
500s ea	00093-1005-05	495.00		AB
500 mg, 100s ea	00093-1006-01	129.90		AB
500s ea	00093-1006-05	605.00		AB
(A-S Medication)				
REPACK				
ECT, PO (CAPLET)				
500 mg, 15s ea	54569-4520-00	19.48		EE
30s ea	54569-4520-01	38.96		EE
60s ea	54569-4520-03	77.91		EE
(Altura)				
REPACK				
ECT, PO (CAPLET)				
500 mg, 10s ea	63874-0984-10	15.74		AB
20s ea	63874-0984-20	31.47		AB
28s ea	63874-0984-28	44.06		AB
30s ea	63874-0984-30	47.21		AB
45s ea	63874-0984-45	70.81		AB
60s ea	63874-0984-60	94.42		AB
84s ea	63874-0984-84	132.19		AB
90s ea	63874-0984-90	141.63		AB
(DHS, Inc.)				
REPACK				
ECT, PO, 500 mg, 20s ea	55887-0705-20	34.20		AB
30s ea	55887-0705-30	51.30		AB
60s ea	55887-0705-60	98.00		AB
(Dispensing Solutions)				
REPACK				
ECT, PO (CAPLET)				
500 mg, 15s ea	55045-2516-07	28.65		AB
30s ea	55045-2516-08	57.30		AB
(Nucare Pharm)				
REPACK				
ECT, PO, 500 mg, 60s ea	66267-0373-60	105.53		AB
(PD-Rx Pharm)				
REPACK				
ECT, PO (CAPLET)				
500 mg, 60s ea	55289-0307-60	71.94		AB
(Pharma Pac)				
REPACK				
ECT, PO (CAPLET)				
500 mg, 15s ea	52959-0516-15	28.80		AB
42s ea	52959-0516-42	76.44		AB
NAPROXEN EC (Ethex)				
naproxen				
ECT, PO (CAPLET)				
375 mg, 100s ea	58177-0302-04	101.31		AB
500 mg, 100s ea	58177-0303-04	125.20		AB
(Aidarex)				
REPACK				
ECT, PO, 375 mg, 10s ea	33261-0082-10	16.00		
14s ea	33261-0082-14	22.40		
20s ea	33261-0082-20	32.00		
21s ea	33261-0082-21	33.60		
28s ea	33261-0082-28	44.80		

PROD/MFR	NDC	AWP	DP	OBC
30s ea	33261-0082-30	48.00		
40s ea	33261-0082-40	64.00		
60s ea	33261-0082-60	96.50		
90s ea	33261-0082-90	144.00		
120s ea	33261-0082-02	192.00		
500 mg, 10s ea	33261-0083-10	18.00		
14s ea	33261-0083-14	25.20		
20s ea	33261-0083-20	36.00		
21s ea	33261-0083-21	37.80		
28s ea	33261-0083-28	50.40		
30s ea	33261-0083-30	54.00		
40s ea	33261-0083-40	72.00		
60s ea	33261-0083-60	108.00		
90s ea	33261-0083-90	162.00		
120s ea	33261-0083-02	216.00		
(Core)				
REPACK				
ECT, PO, 500 mg, 60s ea	33358-0256-60	84.99		
(Dispensing Solutions)				
REPACK				
ECT, PO (CAPLET)				
500 mg, 20s ea	55045-2516-06	38.20		AB
60s ea	55045-2516-00	171.90		AB
60s ea	55045-2516-09	114.60		AB
100s ea	55045-2516-01	191.00		AB
120s ea	55045-2516-02	229.20		AB
(Keltman Pharma., Inc.)				
REPACK				
ECT, PO (CAPLET)				
500 mg, 60s ea	68387-0811-60	121.35		AB
(PD-Rx Pharm)				
REPACK				
ECT, PO (CAPLET)				
375 mg, 28s ea	55289-0921-28	75.00		AB
500 mg, 15s ea	55289-0307-15	27.12		AB
24s ea	55289-0307-24	38.64		AB
30s ea	55289-0307-30	47.70		AB
(Pharma Pac)				
REPACK				
ECT, PO, 375 mg, 30s ea	52959-0194-30	45.00		EE
(CAPLET)				
500 mg, 10s ea	52959-0516-10	19.50		EE
14s ea	52959-0516-14	27.02		EE
20s ea	52959-0516-20	37.15		EE
30s ea	52959-0516-30	55.19		EE
40s ea	52959-0516-40	72.80		EE
60s ea	52959-0516-60	107.99		EE
120s ea	52959-0516-02	148.08		EE
(Phys Total Care)				
REPACK				
ECT, PO, 500 mg, 30s ea	54868-4051-00	26.22		EE
40s ea	54868-4051-01	33.45		EE
(Quality Care Prod)				
REPACK				
ECT, PO, 500 mg, 30s ea	49999-0897-30	70.91		
60s ea	49999-0897-60	90.16		
(Southwood)				
REPACK				
ECT, PO, 500 mg, 20s ea	58016-0372-20	31.47		EE
30s ea	58016-0372-30	47.21		EE
40s ea	58016-0372-40	62.94		EE
60s ea	58016-0372-60	94.42		EE
84s ea	58016-0372-84	132.19		EE
90s ea	58016-0372-90	141.63		EE
100s ea	58016-0372-00	157.37		EE
(Vibranta)				
REPACK				
ECT, PO, 500 mg, 15s ea	57866-6602-02	78.21		
20s ea	57866-6602-03	83.58		
NAPROXEN SOD (Physician Partner)				
REPACK				
naproxen sodium				
TAB, PO, 550 mg, 14s ea	21695-0090-14	42.62		
30s ea	21695-0090-30	77.63		
60s ea	21695-0090-60	155.26		
90s ea	21695-0090-90	232.88		
NAPROXEN SOD. (Stat Rx)				
REPACK				
naproxen sodium				
TAB, PO, 550 mg, 20s ea	16590-0165-20	31.00		
90s ea	16590-0165-90	139.50		
NAPROXEN SODIUM (Amneal)				
TAB, PO (USP,FILM-COATED)				
275 mg, 100s ea	53746-0193-01	89.30		
500s ea	53746-0193-05	141.31		
550 mg, 100s ea	53746-0194-01	139.02		
500s ea	53746-0194-05	670.35		

PROD/MFR	NDC	AWP	DP	OBC
(Dr Reddy's)				
TAB, PO (USP,FILM COATED)				
275 mg, 100s ea	**55111-0107-01**	89.30		
550 mg, 100s ea	**55111-0108-01**	139.02		
500s ea	**55111-0108-05**	670.00		
(Gallipot)				
POW, NA (U.S.P.)				
25 gm	**51552-0450-04**	35.70		
(Glenmark Pharmaceuticals)				
TAB, PO (USP,FILM-COATED)				
275 mg, 100s ea	**68462-0178-01**	89.30		AB
500s ea	**68462-0178-05**	431.02		AB
550 mg, 100s ea	**68462-0179-01**	139.02		AB
500s ea	**68462-0179-05**	670.00		AB
(Intl Ethical) *See AFLAXEN*				
(Medisca)				
POW, NA (U.S.P.)				
25 gm	**38779-0484-04**	64.50		
100 gm	**38779-0484-05**	234.00		
500 gm	**38779-0484-08**	885.00		
(PCCA)				
POW, NA (U.S.P.)				
1 gm	**51927-2771-00**	2.67		
(Roche Labs) *See ANAPROX*				
(Roche Labs) *See ANAPROX DS*				
(Sandoz)				
TAB, PO, 275 mg, 100s ea	**00781-1187-01**	89.30		AB
1000s ea	**00781-1187-10**	893.00		AB
550 mg, 100s ea	**00781-1188-01**	139.02		AB
(Spectrum Pharmacy)				
POW, NA (U.S.P.)				
25 gm	**49452-4817-02**	98.00		
100 gm	**49452-4817-03**	353.50		
500 gm	**49452-4817-06**	1235.50		
1000 gm	**49452-4817-01**	1778.00		
(Teva)				
TAB, PO, 275 mg, 100s ea	**00093-0536-01**	84.55		AB
500s ea	**00093-0536-05**	414.31		AB
1000s ea	**00093-0536-10**	803.26		AB
550 mg, 100s ea	**00093-0537-01**	129.38		AB
500s ea	**00093-0537-05**	635.43		AB
1000s ea	**00093-0537-10**	1263.75		AB
(Victory Pharma, Inc.) *See NAPRELAN*				
(Victory Pharma, Inc.) *See NAPRELAN DOSE CARD*				
(West-Ward)				
TAB, PO, 275 mg, 100s ea	**00143-9916-01**	83.75		
550 mg, 100s ea	**00143-9908-01**	138.95		AB
500s ea	**00143-9908-05**	670.00		AB
(4u) REPACK				
TAB, PO (FILM-COATED)				
550 mg, 60s ea	**10544-0366-60**	106.64		
60s ea	**42549-0324-60**	106.64		AB
60s ea	**42549-0524-60**	106.64		AB
60s ea	**42549-0566-60**	106.64		
(A-S Medication) REPACK				
TAB, PO, 275 mg, 20s ea	**54569-3761-00**	17.52		AB
30s ea	**54569-3761-02**	26.27		AB
(FILM-COATED)				
550 mg, 14s ea	**54569-3762-07**	19.05		
16s ea	**54569-3762-02**	21.77		
20s ea	**54569-3762-03**	27.21		
21s ea	**54569-3762-04**	28.57		
30s ea	**54569-3762-05**	40.82		
60s ea	**54569-3762-06**	81.64		
(Aidarex) REPACK				
TAB, PO, 550 mg, 10s ea	**33261-0085-10**	2.92		
14s ea	**33261-0085-14**	40.88		
20s ea	**33261-0085-20**	58.40		
21s ea	**33261-0085-21**	61.32		
28s ea	**33261-0085-28**	81.76		
30s ea	**33261-0085-30**	87.60		
40s ea	**33261-0085-40**	116.80		
60s ea	**33261-0085-60**	175.20		
90s ea	**33261-0085-90**	262.80		
120s ea	**33261-0085-02**	350.40		
(Altura) REPACK				
TAB, PO (FILM-COATED)				
275 mg, 12s ea	**63874-0489-12**	10.32		
14s ea	**63874-0489-14**	12.04		
20s ea	**63874-0489-20**	17.20		
30s ea	**63874-0489-30**	25.80		
60s ea	**63874-0489-60**	51.60		
90s ea	**63874-0489-90**	77.40		
100s ea	**63874-0489-01**	86.00		
(CAPLET)				
550 mg, 10s ea	**63874-0339-10**	15.88		EE
12s ea	**63874-0339-12**	19.05		EE
14s ea	**63874-0339-14**	22.23		EE
15s ea	**63874-0339-15**	23.81		EE
20s ea	**63874-0339-20**	31.75		EE
21s ea	**63874-0339-21**	33.34		EE
24s ea	**63874-0339-24**	38.10		EE
26s ea	**63874-0339-26**	41.27		EE
28s ea	**63874-0339-28**	44.45		EE
30s ea	**63874-0339-30**	47.63		EE
40s ea	**63874-0339-40**	63.51		EE
42s ea	**63874-0339-42**	66.68		EE
50s ea	**63874-0339-50**	79.38		EE
56s ea	**63874-0339-56**	88.91		EE
60s ea	**63874-0339-60**	95.26		EE
90s ea	**63874-0339-90**	142.89		EE
100s ea	**63874-0339-01**	158.77		EE
(Bryant Ranch) REPACK				
TAB, PO, 220 mg, 30s ea	**63629-1793-01**	0.10		
550 mg, 20s ea	**63629-1260-01**	43.56		
30s ea	**63629-1260-03**	53.34		
(FILM-COATED)				
550 mg, 60s ea	**63629-1260-05**	119.82		
90s ea	**63629-1260-06**	176.58		
100s ea	**63629-1260-02**	209.80		
(Core) REPACK				
TAB, PO, 220 mg, 30s ea	**33358-0257-30**	26.64		
550 mg, 14s ea	**33358-0259-14**	36.13		
20s ea	**33358-0259-20**	44.65		
21s ea	**33358-0259-21**	48.54		
30s ea	**33358-0259-30**	54.67		
60s ea	**33358-0259-60**	147.32		
100s ea	**33358-0259-00**	215.05		
TER, PO, 500 mg, 75s ea	**33358-0258-75**	133.85		
(DHS, Inc.) REPACK				
TAB, PO (FILM-COATED)				
275 mg, 15s ea	**55887-0042-15**	12.89		AB
30s ea	**55887-0042-30**	25.78		AB
60s ea	**55887-0042-60**	51.55		AB
90s ea	**55887-0042-90**	77.33		AB
550 mg, 20s ea	**55887-0923-20**	28.01		AB
30s ea	**55887-0923-30**	42.00		AB
60s ea	**55887-0923-60**	79.00		AB
90s ea	**55887-0923-90**	126.00		
TER, PO, 500 mg, 30s ea	**55887-0410-30**	58.00		
(Dispensing Solutions) REPACK				
TAB, PO, 220 mg, 20s ea	**55045-2737-07**	5.00		
275 mg, 14s ea	**66336-0875-14**	14.20		AB
30s ea	**55045-2109-08**	24.45		AB
550 mg, 10s ea	**55045-2068-01**	16.20		AB
14s ea	**66336-0826-14**	18.11		AB
15s ea	**66336-0826-15**	23.29		AB
20s ea	**66336-0826-20**	31.05		AB
21s ea	**55045-2068-09**	34.02		AB
30s ea	**55045-2068-08**	48.60		AB
30s ea	**66336-0826-30**	46.58		AB
60s ea	**55045-2068-07**	97.20		AB
60s ea	**66336-0826-60**	94.17		AB
90s ea	**55045-2068-06**	145.80		AB
(FILM-COATED)				
550 mg, 90s ea	**66336-0826-90**	139.73		AB
100s ea	**55045-2068-02**	162.00		AB
120s ea	**55045-2068-00**	194.40		AB
(FILM-COATED)				
550 mg, 120s ea	**66336-0826-94**	186.31		AB
(HomeMed) REPACK				
TAB, PO, 275 mg, 20s ea	**51655-0629-52**	16.70		EE
550 mg, 20s ea	**51655-0627-52**	40.99		EE
30s ea	**51655-0627-24**	61.99		EE
(IPI) REPACK				
TAB, PO (FILM-COATED)				
550 mg, 60s ea	**18837-0330-60**	80.44		
(Keltman Pharma., Inc.) REPACK				
TAB, PO, 550 mg, 30s ea	**68387-0545-30**	48.26		
60s ea	**68387-0545-60**	96.52		
(Medsource) REPACK				
TAB, PO (FILM-COATED)				
550 mg, 30s ea	**45865-0349-30**	49.50		
60s ea	**45865-0349-60**	99.00		
90s ea	**45865-0349-90**	148.50		
100s ea	**45865-0349-00**	165.00		
120s ea	**45865-0349-01**	198.00		
150s ea	**45865-0349-02**	247.50		
300s ea	**45865-0349-05**	495.00		
(Nucare Pharm) REPACK				
TAB, PO, 550 mg, 14s ea	**66267-0154-14**	19.80		EE
20s ea	**66267-0154-20**	27.00		EE
30s ea	**66267-0154-30**	60.02		AB
60s ea	**66267-0154-60**	105.53		AB
(Palmetto) REPACK				
TAB, PO, 220 mg, 30s ea	**23490-6709-01**	18.99		
60s ea	**23490-6709-02**	37.98		
100s ea	**23490-6709-03**	63.30		
275 mg, 14s ea	**23490-5972-01**	15.87		
30s ea	**23490-5972-03**	34.00		
60s ea	**23490-5972-06**	68.00		
90s ea	**23490-5972-09**	102.00		
550 mg, 14s ea	**23490-5973-01**	24.50		
15s ea	**23490-5973-02**	26.25		
20s ea	**23490-5973-03**	35.00		
21s ea	**23490-5973-00**	36.75		
25s ea	**23490-5973-07**	43.75		
30s ea	**23490-5973-04**	52.50		
60s ea	**23490-5973-05**	105.00		
90s ea	**23490-5973-06**	157.50		
(PD-Rx Pharm) REPACK				
TAB, PO, 275 mg, 6s ea	**55289-0467-06**	16.23		AB
10s ea	**55289-0467-10**	18.00		AB
21s ea	**55289-0467-21**	28.80		AB
30s ea	**55289-0467-30**	34.00		AB
30s ea	**58864-0751-30**	33.99		AB
550 mg, 6s ea	**55289-0367-06**	19.87		AB
10s ea	**55289-0367-10**	21.50		AB
14s ea	**55289-0367-14**	29.80		AB
15s ea	**55289-0367-15**	29.83		AB
20s ea	**55289-0367-20**	30.00		AB
28s ea	**55289-0367-28**	39.93		AB
30s ea	**55289-0367-30**	43.00		AB
30s ea	**58864-0752-30**	42.99		AB
42s ea	**55289-0367-42**	59.73		AB
(USP,FILM-COATED)				
550 mg, 60s ea	**55289-0367-60**	76.23		
(Pharma Pac) REPACK				
TAB, PO, 275 mg, 21s ea	**52959-0357-21**	20.87		EE
30s ea	**52959-0357-30**	29.80		EE
(FILM-COATED)				
275 mg, 42s ea	**52959-0357-42**	41.71		
42s ea	**52959-0375-42**	41.71		AB
60s ea	**52959-0357-60**	59.59		EE
550 mg, 10s ea	**52959-0271-10**	29.38		EE
14s ea	**52959-0271-14**	41.15		EE
15s ea	**52959-0271-15**	43.95		EE
20s ea	**52959-0271-20**	58.62		EE
21s ea	**52959-0271-21**	61.42		EE
28s ea	**52959-0271-28**	81.84		EE
30s ea	**52959-0271-30**	87.70		EE
40s ea	**52959-0271-40**	116.76		EE
42s ea	**52959-0271-42**	122.54		AB
60s ea	**52959-0271-60**	174.96		EE
90s ea	**52959-0271-90**	261.90		EE
120s ea	**52959-0271-02**	349.08		EE
(Phys Total Care) REPACK				
TAB, PO, 275 mg, 30s ea	**54868-3359-00**	12.42		EE
550 mg, 15s ea	**54868-3043-01**	12.39		EE
20s ea	**54868-3043-03**	15.54		EE
30s ea	**54868-3043-02**	26.37		EE
60s ea	**54868-3043-05**	48.24		EE
(Physician Partner) REPACK				
TAB, PO (FILM COATED)				
550 mg, 20s ea	**21695-0090-20**	60.89		AB
56s ea	**21695-0090-56**	144.90		AB
(Quality Care Prod) REPACK				
TAB, PO, 275 mg, 60s ea	**49999-0200-60**	51.03		AB
550 mg, 14s ea	**49999-0058-14**	23.10		AB
15s ea	**49999-0058-15**	24.70		EE
20s ea	**49999-0058-20**	32.93		AB
28s ea	**49999-0058-28**	46.11		EE
30s ea	**49999-0058-30**	49.42		EE
60s ea	**49999-0058-60**	98.84		EE
90s ea	**49999-0058-90**	148.26		AB
TER, PO, 500 mg, 30s ea	**49999-0194-30**	129.60		

PROD/MFR	NDC	AWP	DP	OBC
(Southwood)				
REPACK				
TAB, PO, 275 mg, 12s ea	**58016-0694-12**	9.43		EE
14s ea	**58016-0694-14**	12.03		EE
20s ea	**58016-0694-20**	17.18		EE
30s ea	**58016-0694-30**	25.78		EE
60s ea	**58016-0694-60**	51.55		EE
90s ea	**58016-0694-90**	77.33		EE
100s ea	**58016-0694-00**	85.92		EE
120s ea	**58016-0694-02**	103.10		EE
150s ea	**58016-0694-03**	128.88		EE
200s ea	**58016-0694-89**	171.84		EE
300s ea	**58016-0694-73**	257.76		EE
550 mg, 10s ea	**58016-0321-10**	15.70		EE
12s ea	**58016-0321-12**	18.83		EE
14s ea	**58016-0321-14**	21.97		EE
15s ea	**58016-0321-15**	23.54		EE
20s ea	**58016-0321-20**	31.39		EE
24s ea	**58016-0321-24**	37.67		EE
28s ea	**58016-0321-28**	43.95		EE
30s ea	**58016-0321-30**	47.09		EE
40s ea	**58016-0321-40**	62.78		EE
42s ea	**58016-0321-42**	65.92		EE
56s ea	**58016-0321-56**	87.89		EE
60s ea	**58016-0321-60**	94.17		EE
90s ea	**58016-0321-90**	141.26		EE
100s ea	**58016-0321-00**	156.95		EE
120s ea	**58016-0321-02**	188.34		EE
150s ea	**58016-0321-03**	235.43		EE
200s ea	**58016-0321-89**	313.90		EE
300s ea	**58016-0321-73**	470.85		EE
(St. Mary's MPP)				
REPACK				
TAB, PO (USP)				
550 mg, 6s ea	**60760-0537-06**	17.90		
15s ea	**60760-0537-15**	28.11		AB
20s ea	**60760-0537-20**	35.48		AB
30s ea	**60760-0537-30**	50.22		AB
60s ea	**60760-0537-60**	94.44		AB
(Stat Rx)				
REPACK				
TAB, PO, 550 mg, 30s ea	**16590-0165-30**	50.25		AB
60s ea	**16590-0165-60**	100.50		AB
(Vibranta)				
REPACK				
TAB, PO, 275 mg, 21s ea	**57866-3612-02**	16.25		
30s ea	**57866-3612-03**	24.88		
550 mg, 10s ea	**57866-6613-03**	23.10		
14s ea	**57866-6613-04**	24.00		
15s ea	**57866-6613-02**	25.40		
16s ea	**57866-6613-05**	19.50		
20s ea	**57866-6613-00**	30.30		
21s ea	**57866-6613-06**	31.01		
30s ea	**57866-6613-01**	42.30		
60s ea	**57866-6613-07**	63.45		
NAPROXEN SODIUM/SUMATRIPTAN SUCCINATE				
(Glaxo) *See TREXIMET*				
NARATRIPTAN HYDROCHLORIDE				
(Glaxo) *See AMERGE*				
NARCAN (Phys Total Care)				
REPACK				
naloxone hydrochloride				
SOL, IJ (AMP)				
0.4 mg/ml,				
1 ml 10s	**54868-0114-00**	43.18		AP
NARDIL (Pfizer)				
phenelzine sulfate				
TAB, PO (FILM-COATED)				
15 mg, 60s ea	**00071-0350-60**	55.69	46.41	
NARIZ (Hawthorn Pharm)				
guaifenesin/phenylephrine hydrochloride				
SOL, PO (BUBBLE GUM,COTTON CANDY)				
200 mg/5 ml-7.5 mg/5 ml,				
473 ml	**63717-0262-16**	68.74		
NARIZ-HC (Hawthorn Pharm)				
gg/hydrocod bit/phenyleph hcl				
SOL, PO (BUBBLE GUM,COTTON CANDY)				
473 ml, C-III	**63717-0714-16**	82.49		
NAROPIN (APP)				
ropivacaine hydrochloride				
SOL, IJ (POLYAMPDUOFIT STERL-PAK)				
2 mg/ml, 10 ml 5s	**63323-0285-10**	22.14		EE
20 ml 5s	**63323-0285-20**	36.85		EE
(1X100ML, SINGLE DOSE,PF)				
2 mg/ml, 100 ml	**63323-0285-65**	26.08		EE
(S.D. INFUSION BOTTLE)				
2 mg/ml, 100 ml	**00186-0859-81**	27.16		
(1X200ML,SINGLE DOSE,PF)				
2 mg/ml, 200 ml	**63323-0285-64**	45.72		EE

PROD/MFR	NDC	AWP	DP	OBC
(POLYAMPDUOFIT STERL-PAK)				
5 mg/ml, 20 ml 5s	**63323-0286-20**	61.14		EE
(SDV,PF)				
5 mg/ml, 30 ml	**63323-0286-30**	17.51		EE
(5X30ML,SDV,PF)				
5 mg/ml, 30 ml 5s	**63323-0286-31**	99.24		EE
(POLYAMP DUOFIT,STER-PAK)				
7.5 mg/ml,				
20 ml 5s	**63323-0287-20**	86.40		
(5X10ML,POLYAMP DUOFIT)				
10 mg/ml, 10 ml 5s	**63323-0288-10**	51.90		
(5X20ML,PF)				
10 mg/ml, 20 ml 5s	**63323-0288-20**	97.20		
NASACORT AQ (Sanofi-Aventis)				
triamcinolone acetonide				
SPR, NS, 55 mcg/actuation,				
16.5 gm	**00075-1506-16**	111.83		
(A-S Medication)				
REPACK				
SPR, NS, 55 mcg/actuation,				
16.5 gm	**54569-4476-00**	139.79		
(Dispensing Solutions)				
REPACK				
SPR, NS, 55 mcg/actuation,				
16.5 gm	**55045-2920-01**	85.00		
(Palmetto)				
REPACK				
SPR, NS (1X16.5GM)				
55 mcg/actuation,				
16.5 gm	**23490-6987-01**	84.12		
(Phys Total Care)				
REPACK				
SPR, NS, 55 mcg/actuation,				
16.5 gm	**54868-4207-00**	134.34		
(Quality Care Prod)				
REPACK				
SPR, NS, 55 mcg/actuation,				
16.5 gm	**49999-0567-16**	154.18		
NASALIDE (Phys Total Care)				
REPACK				
flunisolide				
SPR, NS, 0.025 mg/actuation,				
25 ml	**54868-1015-01**	62.40		AB
NASAREL (Phys Total Care)				
flunisolide				
SPR, NS, 0.025 mg/actuation,				
25 ml	**54868-4162-00**	49.60		BX
NASCOBAL (Par)				
cyanocobalamin				
SPR, NS (8 DOSES)				
500 mcg/0.1 ml,				
2.3 ml	**49884-0270-14**	281.18		
NASOFED (Hawthorn Pharm)				
pseudoephedrine tannate				
SUS, PO (STRAWBERRY)				
50 mg/5 ml, 118 ml	**63717-0265-04**	31.24		
NASOHIST (Hawthorn Pharm)				
cpm/phenyleph hcl				
SOL, PO (PEDIATRIC)				
1 mg/ml-2 mg/ml,				
30 ml	**63717-0290-30**	19.99		
NASOHIST DM (Hawthorn Pharm)				
cpm/dm/phenyleph hcl				
SOL, PO (PEDIATRIC)				
1 mg/ml-3 mg/ml-2 mg/ml,				
30 ml	**63717-0291-30**	47.49		
NASONEX (Schering)				
mometasone furoate				
SPR, NS (SCENT-FREE MIST)				
0.05 mg/actuation,				
17 gm	**00085-1288-01**	108.37		
(A-S Medication)				
REPACK				
SPR, NS, 0.05 mg/actuation,				
17 gm	**54569-4601-00**	140.88		
(DHS, Inc.)				
REPACK				
SPR, NS, 0.05 mg/actuation,				
17 gm	**55887-0467-17**	133.72		
(Dispensing Solutions)				
REPACK				
SPR, NS, 0.05 mg/actuation,				
17 gm	**55045-2922-01**	93.00		

PROD/MFR	NDC	AWP	DP	OBC
(Pharma Pac)				
REPACK				
SPR, NS, 0.05 mg/actuation,				
17 gm	**52959-0798-00**	77.85		
(Phys Total Care)				
REPACK				
SPR, NS, 0.05 mg/actuation,				
17 gm	**54868-4174-00**	137.80		
(Quality Care Prod)				
REPACK				
SPR, NS, 0.05 mg/actuation,				
17 gm	**49999-0474-50**	147.97		
NASOP (Hawthorn Pharm)				
phenylephrine hydrochloride				
ODT, PO (BUBBLE GUM)				
10 mg, 100s ea	**63717-0260-01**	53.74		
(Hawthorn Pharm)				
phenylephrine tannate				
SUS, PO (AF,SF,GLUTEN-FREE)				
7.5 mg/5 ml,				
118 ml	**63717-0261-04**	21.99		
NASOP12 (Hawthorn Pharm)				
phenylephrine tannate				
CTB, PO (GRAPE)				
10 mg, 100s ea	**63717-0259-01**	112.49		
NATACHEW (Mission)				
prenatal vitamins				
CTB, PO, 90s ea	**00430-0223-23**	80.99		
NATACYN (Alcon Ophthalmic)				
natamycin				
SUS, OP, 5%, 15 ml	**00065-0645-15**	212.40		
NATAFORT (Mission)				
prenatal vitamins				
TAB, PO (FILM-COATED)				
90s ea	**00430-0224-23**	80.99	64.80	
NATAL (Contract Pharmacal)				
prenatal vitamins				
TAB, PO, 100s ea	**10267-1121-01**	19.70		
NATALCARE PLUS (PD-Rx Pharm)				
REPACK				
prenatal vitamins				
TAB, PO (REDI-SCRIPT)				
30s ea	**58864-0786-30**	9.25		
NATALIZUMAB				
(Elan Pharmaceuticals) *See TYSABRI*				
NATAMYCIN				
(Alcon Ophthalmic) *See NATACYN*				
NATATAB CFE (Ethex)				
prenatal vitamins				
TAB, PO, 100s ea	**58177-0328-04**	28.30		
NATEGLINIDE (Dr Reddy's)				
TAB, PO, 60 mg, 90s ea	**55111-0328-90**	149.59		AB
120 mg, 90s ea	**55111-0329-90**	155.42		AB
(Novartis Pharm) *See STARLIX*				
(Par)				
TAB, PO (COATED)				
60 mg, 100s ea	**49884-0984-01**	166.22		AB
120 mg, 100s ea	**49884-0985-01**	172.70		AB
NATELLE C (Azur Pharma, Inc.)				
prenatal vitamins				
TAB, PO (SUGAR-COATED)				
90s ea	**66663-0724-01**	65.34		
NATELLE ONE (Azur Pharma, Inc.)				
prenatal vitamins				
SGL, PO (SOFT GELATIN)				
30s ea	**18860-0852-01**	72.00		
NATELLE PLUS W/ DHA (Azur Pharma, Inc.)				
prenatal vitamins				
KIT, PO (6X(5+5),SOFTGEL)				
60s ea	**66663-0333-30**	58.69		
NATELLE-EZ (Azur Pharma, Inc.)				
prenatal vitamins				
TAB, PO (SUGAR-COATED)				
90s ea	**66663-0668-01**	71.88		
NATRECOR (Scios)				
nesiritide				
PDS, IV (S.D.V.)				
1.5 mg, ea	**65847-0205-25**	716.36	596.97	
NATURAL BITTERNESS MASKING (Gallipot)				
bitterness masking agent				
POW, NA, 454 gm	**51552-1033-06**	49.00	35.00	

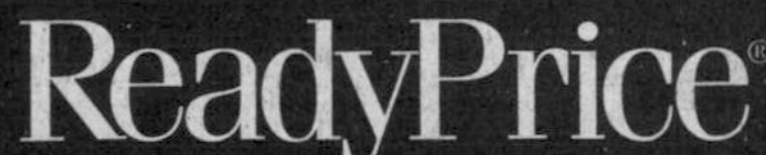

PROD/MFR	NDC	AWP	DP	OBC
NATURE-THROID (RLC)				
thyroid				
TAB, PO (MICRO-COATED)				
16.25 mg, 100s ea	64727-3298-01	6.89		
1000s ea	64727-3298-02	77.87		
32.5 mg, 100s ea	64727-3299-01	8.92		
1000s ea	64727-3299-02	83.33		
65 mg, 100s ea	64727-3300-01	9.91		
1000s ea	64727-3300-02	101.64		
130 mg, 100s ea	64727-3308-01	17.95		
1000s ea	64727-3308-02	131.56		
195 mg, 100s ea	64727-3312-01	27.48		
1000s ea	64727-3312-02	172.70		
NAVANE (Pfizer)				
thiothixene				
CAP, PO, 2 mg, 100s ea	00049-5720-66	102.11	85.09	AB
5 mg, 100s ea	00049-5730-66	159.66	133.05	AB
10 mg, 100s ea	00049-5740-66	220.15	183.46	AB
20 mg, 100s ea	00049-5770-66	308.88	257.40	AB
NAVELBINE (Pierre Fabre)				
vinorelbine tartrate				
SOL, IV (1X1ML,SINGLE USE,PF)				
10 mg/ml, 1 ml	64370-0532-01	114.74		
(1X5ML,SINGLE USE,PF)				
10 mg/ml, 5 ml	64370-0532-02	573.72		
NAVOGAN (Intl Ethical)				
benzocaine/trimethobenzamide hydrochloride				
SUP, RC, 2%-100 mg,				
10s ea	11584-0421-01	9.98		
NEATSFOOT OIL (Amend)				
OIL, NA, 480 ml	17317-0738-01	5.60		
3840 ml	17317-0738-06	28.00		
19200 ml	17317-0738-08	105.00		
(PCCA)				
OIL, NA, 1 ml	51927-1545-00	0.08		
NEBIVOLOL HYDROCHLORIDE				
(Forest Pharm) *See BYSTOLIC*				
NEBULIZER AEROSOL MASK ADULT (Pari)				
mask, face				
DEV, NA (FITS LC-PLUS NEB SET)				
ea	83490-0140-10	1.42		
NEBULIZER, DIRECT PATIENT INTERFACE				
(Monaghan Medical) *See AEROECLIPSE NEBULIZER*				
(Pari) *See PARI LC SPRINT REUSABLE NEBULIZER SET*				
(Pari) *See PARI LC-PLUS REUSABLE NEBULIZER SET*				
(Pari) *See PRONEB ULTRA II*				
(Pari) *See PRONEB ULTRA II PEDIATRIC*				
(Respironics) *See INSPIRATION COMPRESSOR/NEBULIZER*				
(Respironics) *See MISTERNEB COMPRESSOR/NEBULIZER*				
(Respironics) *See ZOEY INSPIRATION626 COMPRESSOR/NEBULIZER*				
(Sunrise Medical) *See PULMO-AIDE COMPACT COMPRESSOR/NEBULIZER*				
(Sunrise Medical) *See PULMO-AIDE COMPRESSOR/NEBULIZER*				
(Sunrise Medical) *See PULMOMATE COMPRESSOR/NEBULIZER*				
NEBUPENT (APP)				
pentamidine isethionate				
PDS, IH (S.D.V.,PF)				
300 mg, ea	63323-0877-15	98.75		
(Phys Total Care) REPACK				
PDS, IH (S.D.V.,PF)				
300 mg, ea	54868-2528-00	116.84		
NECON 0.5/35 (Watson)				
ethinyl estradiol/norethindrone				
TAB, PO (6 X 28)				
35 mcg-0.5 mg,				
168s ea	52544-0550-28	192.84		AB
(A-S Medication) REPACK				
TAB, PO, 35 mcg-0.5 mg,				
28s ea	54569-5358-00	41.86		AB
(Phys Total Care) REPACK				
TAB, PO, 35 mcg-0.5 mg,				
28s ea	54868-4538-00	81.00		AB
NECON 1/35 (Watson)				
ethinyl estradiol/norethindrone				
TAB, PO (6 X 28)				
35 mcg-1 mg,				
168s ea	52544-0552-28	176.81		AB
(A-S Medication) REPACK				
TAB, PO, 35 mcg-1 mg,				
28s ea	54569-4999-00	29.48		AB
(Phys Total Care) REPACK				
TAB, PO, 35 mcg-1 mg,				
28s ea	54868-4045-00	94.26		AB
(Physician Partner) REPACK				
TAB, PO (1X28)				
35 mcg-1 mg,				
28s ea	21695-0857-01	58.94		AB
(Quality Care Prod) REPACK				
TAB, PO, 35 mcg-1 mg,				
28s ea	35356-0365-28	93.22		AB
NECON 1/50 (Watson)				
mestranol/norethindrone				
TAB, PO (3X28)				
0.05 mg-1 mg,				
84s ea	52544-0245-31	79.57		
NECON 10/11 (Watson)				
ethinyl estradiol/norethindrone				
TAB, PO (6 X 28)				
168s ea	52544-0554-28	192.84		AB
NECON 7/7/7 (Watson)				
ethinyl estradiol/norethindrone				
TAB, PO (DIALPAK, 6X28)				
168s ea	52544-0936-28	193.18		AB
NEDOCROMIL SODIUM				
(Allergan Inc) *See ALOCRIL*				
NEEDLE				
(BD Dickinson Hosp Prod) *See B-D FILTER NEEDLES*				
(BD Dickinson Hosp Prod) *See B-D NOKOR ADMIX NEEDLES*				
(BD Dickinson Hosp Prod) *See B-D NOKOR VENTED NEEDLE*				
(Cardinal Health) *See LEADER NEEDLES*				
NEEDLE AND/OR SYRINGE SUPPLIES				
(APP) *See FLOW-EZE VENTED*				
(BD Dickinson Hosp Prod) *See B-D BLUNT FILL NEEDLE*				
(BD Dickinson Hosp Prod) *See B-D INTEGRA SYRINGE*				
(BD Dickinson Hosp Prod) *See B-D SYRINGE W/BLUNT FILL NEEDLE*				
(Terumo) *See TERUMO*				
NEEDLE, HYPODERMIC				
(BD Dickinson Hosp Prod) *See B-D BULK NEEDLES REGULAR BEVEL*				
(BD Dickinson Hosp Prod) *See B-D BULK NEEDLES SHORT BEVEL*				
(BD Dickinson Hosp Prod) *See B-D NEEDLES*				
(BD Dickinson Hosp Prod) *See B-D NEEDLES REGULAR BEVEL*				
(BD Dickinson Hosp Prod) *See B-D NEEDLES SHORT BEVEL*				
(BD Dickinson Hosp Prod) *See B-D SPECIALTY USE NEEDLES*				
(Portex) *See THORACENTESIS SET*				
(Terumo) *See NEOLUS HYPODERMIC NEEDLES*				
NEEVO (Pamlab)				
vitamin b complex, iron, and vitamin c				
TAB, PO (GLUTEN-FREE)				
90s ea	00525-2010-90	177.68		
NEEVODHA (Pamlab)				
medical food				
CAP, PO (GELCAP)				
30s ea	00525-2030-30	59.23		
NEFAZODONE (Southwood) REPACK				
nefazodone hydrochloride				
TAB, PO, 100 mg, 30s ea	58016-0100-30	46.17		
60s ea	58016-0100-60	92.35		
90s ea	58016-0100-90	138.52		
100s ea	58016-0100-00	153.91		
150 mg, 30s ea	58016-0546-30	47.04		
60s ea	58016-0546-60	94.08		
90s ea	58016-0546-90	141.12		
100s ea	58016-0546-00	156.80		
200 mg, 30s ea	58016-0336-30	47.93		
60s ea	58016-0336-60	95.85		
90s ea	58016-0336-90	143.78		
100s ea	58016-0336-00	159.75		
(Stat Rx) REPACK				
TAB, PO, 100 mg, 30s ea	16590-0166-30	48.00		
60s ea	16590-0166-60	96.00		
90s ea	16590-0166-90	144.00		
NEFAZODONE HCL (Mylan)				
nefazodone hydrochloride				
TAB, PO, 100 mg, 60s ea	00378-2052-91	92.25		
150 mg, 60s ea	00378-2053-91	94.00		
200 mg, 60s ea	00378-2054-91	95.75		
250 mg, 60s ea	00378-2055-91	97.55		
(Sandoz)				
TAB, PO, 50 mg, 60s ea	00185-0038-60	90.17		
100 mg, 60s ea	00185-0016-60	92.34		
150 mg, 60s ea	00185-0081-60	94.08		
200 mg, 60s ea	00185-0126-60	95.85		
250 mg, 60s ea	00185-0148-60	97.63		
(Teva)				
TAB, PO, 50 mg, 100s ea	00093-7178-01	150.28		AB
100 mg, 60s ea	00093-1024-06	92.34		
150 mg, 60s ea	00093-7113-06	94.08		
200 mg, 60s ea	00093-1025-06	95.85		
250 mg, 60s ea	00093-1026-06	97.63		
(Phys Total Care) REPACK				
TAB, PO, 200 mg, 60s ea	54868-4924-00	115.50		
NEFAZODONE HYDROCHLORIDE				
(Mylan) *See NEFAZODONE HCL*				
(Sandoz) *See NEFAZODONE HCL*				
(Teva) *See NEFAZODONE HCL*				
(Palmetto) REPACK				
TAB, PO, 100 mg, 30s ea	23490-6577-01	63.75		
200 mg, 30s ea	23490-6579-01	50.47		
60s ea	23490-6579-02	100.93		
90s ea	23490-6579-03	151.40		
(Phys Total Care) REPACK				
TAB, PO, 150 mg, 60s ea	54868-5562-00	85.11		
(Physician Partner) REPACK				
TAB, PO, 100 mg, 60s ea	21695-0174-60	184.68		
150 mg, 60s ea	21695-0175-60	188.16		
200 mg, 30s ea	21695-0176-30	95.85		
60s ea	21695-0176-60	191.70		
250 mg, 30s ea	21695-0177-30	97.62		
60s ea	21695-0177-60	195.26		
NELARABINE				
(Glaxo) *See ARRANON*				
NELFINAVIR MESYLATE				
(Pfizer) *See VIRACEPT*				
NEMBUTAL SODIUM (Lundbeck)				
pentobarbital sodium				
SOL, IJ, 50 mg/ml,				
20 ml, C-II	67386-0501-52	344.12		AP
(VIAL)				
50 mg/ml,				
50 ml, C-II	67386-0501-55	641.84		AP
NEO DM (Laser Pharma)				
brompheniramine tan/dm tan/phenyleph tan				
SUS, PO (AF,SF,CHERRY)				
473 ml	16477-0560-01	85.00		
(Laser Pharma)				
bpm/dm/pse hcl				
SYR, PO (1X473ML,BERRY-VANILLA)				
473 ml	16477-0562-01	49.75		
NEO DM DROPS (Laser Pharma)				
cpm/dm/phenyleph hcl				
SOL, PO (W/ DROPPER,AF,SF)				
30 ml	16477-0620-30	22.00		
NEO HC (Laser Pharma)				
cpm/hydrocod bit/phenyleph hcl				
SYR, PO (AF,SF,ORANGE-CREAM)				
473 ml, C-III	16477-0625-01	59.00		
NEO-FRADIN (X-Gen)				
neomycin sulfate				
SOL, PO, 125 mg/5 ml,				
480 ml	39822-0330-05	55.30		

PROD/MFR	NDC	AWP	DP	OBC

NEO-POLY-GRAM (Quality Care Prod)
REPACK
gramicidin/neomycin sulfate/polymyxin b sulfate
SOL, OP, 10 ml 49999-0591-10 32.92

NEO-RX (X-Gen)
neomycin sulfate
POW, NA (U.S.P.)
10 gm .... 39822-0300-02 6.00 AA
100 gm .... 39822-0300-01 19.75 AA

NEO-SYNEPHRINE HCL (Hospira)
phenylephrine hydrochloride
SOL, IJ (AMP,25X1ML)
10 mg/ml,
1 ml 25s UD 00409-1800-01 137.70 120.50
(AMP,LATEX-FREE)
10 mg/ml, 1 ml 25s ... 00074-1800-01 137.70 120.50

NEO/POLY B SUL & GRAMICIDIN (Altura)
REPACK
gramicidin/neomycin sulfate/polymyxin b sulfate
SOL, OP, 10 ml 63874-0168-10 32.24

NEO/POLY-B/BAC. (Stat Rx)
REPACK
bacitracin zinc/neomycin/polymyxin b sulfate
OIN, OP, 3.5 gm 16590-0170-35 35.00

NEO/POLY-B/DEX (Stat Rx)
dexamethasone/neomycin sulfate/polymyxin b sulfate
OIN, OP, 3.5 gm 16590-0168-35 27.00
SUS, OP, 5 ml 16590-0167-05 14.00

NEO/POLY-B/HC (Stat Rx)
hc/neomycin sulf/polymyxin b sulf
SOL, OT, 1%-0.35%-10000 u/ml,
10 ml.............. 16590-0169-10 51.00

NEOASMA (Tarmac)
guaifenesin/theophylline
TAB, PO, 100 mg-125 mg,
48s ea 11096-0216-01 7.26
200s ea 11096-0216-02 27.29

NEOBEE M-5 (Amend)
coconut oil
OIL, NA, 480 ml 17317-1367-01 14.00
3840 ml 17317-1367-06 70.00
20640 ml 17317-1367-08 240.80

NEOBENZ MICRO (Intendis, Inc.)
benzoyl peroxide
CRE, TP, 3.5%, 45 gm 67402-0020-45 123.75 99.00
5.5%, 45 gm 67402-0021-45 123.75 99.00
8.5%, 45 gm 67402-0022-45 123.75 99.00

NEOBENZ MICRO CREAM PLUS PACK (Intendis, Inc.)
benzoyl peroxide
CRE, TP, ea 67402-0021-23 135.06

NEOBENZ MICRO SD (Intendis, Inc.)
benzoyl peroxide
CRE, TP, 3.5%, 30s ea UD . 67402-0020-06 187.50 150.00
(PRE-FILLED SPONGE APP)
5.5%, 30s ea 67402-0023-30 208.46 150.00
8.5%, 30s ea UD 67402-0022-06 187.50 150.00

NEOBENZ MICRO WASH PLUS PACK (Intendis, Inc.)
benzoyl peroxide
KIT, TP, ea 67402-0029-23 146.63

NEOCIDIN (Major)
gramicidin/neomycin sulfate/polymyxin b sulfate
SOL, OP, 10 ml 00904-3016-10 28.81

NEOFRIN (Ocusoft)
phenylephrine hydrochloride
SOL, OP, 2.5%, 15 ml 54799-0530-15 8.68
10%, 5 ml 54799-0531-05 9.31

NEOLUS HYPODERMIC NEEDLES (Terumo)
needle, hypodermic
DEV, NA (18G X 1" T.W.)
100s ea............. 08970-6000-11 8.10
(18GX1-1/2" T.W.)
100s ea............. 08970-6000-21 8.10
(19G X 1" T.W.)
100s ea............. 08970-6000-31 8.10
(19GX1-1/2" T.W.)
100s ea............. 08970-6000-41 8.10
(20G X 1" U.T.W.)
100s ea............. 08970-6000-51 8.10
(20GX1-1/2" U.T.W.)
100s ea............. 08970-6000-61 8.10
(21G X 1" U.T.W.)
100s ea............. 08970-6000-70 8.10
(21GX1-1/2" U.T.W.)
100s ea............. 08970-6000-81 8.10
(22G X 1" U.T.W.)
100s ea............. 08970-6000-91 8.10
(22GX1-1/2" U.T.W.)
100s ea............. 08970-6001-01 8.10
(22GX3/4" U.T.W.)
100s ea............. 08970-6001-71 8.10
(23GX1-1/2" U.T.W.)
100s ea............. 08970-6001-21 8.10
(23GX1" U.T.W.)
100s ea............. 08970-6001-11 8.10
(25G X 1" T.W.)
100s ea............. 08970-6001-41 8.10
(25GX5/8" T.W.)
100s ea............. 08970-6001-31 8.10
(26GX1/2" R.W.)
100s ea............. 08970-6001-51 8.10
(27GX1/2" R.W.)
100s ea............. 08970-6001-61 8.10

NEOMYCIN AND POLYMYXIN B SULFATES
(Watson Labs)
neomycin sulfate/polymyxin b sulfate
SOL, IL (USP)
40 mg/ml-200000 u/ml,
1 ml 10s........... 00591-2190-45 159.39 AT
1 ml 50s........... 00591-2190-50 749.25 AT

(X-Gen)
SOL, IL (USP,1MLX10)
40 mg/ml-200000 u/ml,
1 ml 10s........... 39822-1201-02 128.50 AT
(USP)
40 mg/ml-200000 u/ml,
1 ml 50s........... 39822-1201-05 604.50 AT
(MDV)
40 mg/ml-200000 u/ml,
20 ml.............. 39822-1220-01 145.95 AT

NEOMYCIN AND POLYMYXIN B SULFATES AND GRAMICIDIN (Paddock)
gramicidin/neomycin sulfate/polymyxin b sulfate
SOL, OP (1X10ML,USP)
10 ml.............. 00574-4009-10 25.30 AT

NEOMYCIN SULF/POLYMYXIN B SULF/ PREDNISOLONE ACE
(Allergan Inc) *See POLY PRED*

(Palmetto)
REPACK
SUS, OP (1X5ML)
0.35%-10000 u/ml-0.5%,
5 ml.............. 23490-6562-00 28.55

NEOMYCIN SULFATE (Gallipot)
POW, NA (1X10GM,USP,MICRONIZED)
10 gm 51552-0969-03 13.30 9.50
(1X50GM,USP,MICRONIZED)
50 gm 51552-0969-09 37.10 26.50
(1X100GM,USP,MICRONIZED)
100 gm 51552-0969-05 67.20 48.00

(Major)
TAB, PO (5X10,USP)
500 mg, 50s ea UD ... 00904-5941-06 177.75 AA

(Medisca)
POW, NA (U.S.P.)
10 gm 38779-0348-01 31.50
50 gm 38779-0348-02 79.50
100 gm 38779-0348-05 147.00
(1X500GM,USP)
500 gm 38779-0348-08 612.00
(U.S.P.)
500 gm 38879-0348-08 612.00
(1X1000GM,USP)
1000 gm 38779-0348-09 1107.00

(Spectrum Pharmacy)
POW, NA (U.S.P.)
10 gm .... 49452-4830-01 62.30 EE
100 gm .... 49452-4830-04 218.05 EE

(Teva)
TAB, PO, 500 mg, 100s ea . 00093-1177-01 124.57 AA

(UDL)
TAB, PO (10X10)
500 mg, 100s ea UD .. 51079-0015-20 197.50 AA

(X-Gen) *See NEO-FRADIN*

(X-Gen) *See NEO-RX*

(Phys Total Care)
REPACK
TAB, PO, 500 mg, 100s ea . 54868-1560-00 290.94 AA

NEOMYCIN SULFATE MICRONIZED (PCCA)
neomycin sulfate, micronized
POW, NA (USP)
1 gm 51927-1167-00 2.16

NEOMYCIN SULFATE, MICRONIZED
(PCCA) *See NEOMYCIN SULFATE MICRONIZED*

NEOMYCIN SULFATE/POLYMYXIN B SULFATE
(Monarch) *See NEOSPORIN G.U. IRRIGANT*

(Watson Labs) *See NEOMYCIN AND POLYMYXIN B SULFATES*

(X-Gen) *See NEOMYCIN AND POLYMYXIN B SULFATES*

NEOMYCIN-POLYMYXIN-DEXAMETHASONE
(Quality Care Prod)
REPACK
dexamethasone/neomycin sulfate/polymyxin b sulfate
SUS, OP (DROPS)
5 ml 49999-0141-05 29.25

NEOMYCIN/BACITRACIN ZN/POLYMYXIN
(Physician Partner)
REPACK
bacitracin zinc/neomycin/polymyxin b sulfate
OIN, OP, 3.5 gm 21695-0192-35 31.54

NEOMYCIN/POLY B/BACITRACIN (Altura)
REPACK
bacitracin zinc/neomycin/polymyxin b sulfate
OIN, OP, 3.5 gm 63874-0167-04 11.55

NEOMYCIN/POLY B/DEXAMETHASONE (Physician Partner)
REPACK
dexamethasone/neomycin sulfate/polymyxin b sulfate
SUS, OP, 5 ml 21695-0595-05 16.00

(Quality Care Prod)
REPACK
OIN, OP, 3.5 gm 49999-0220-35 10.61

NEOMYCIN/POLY B/GRAMICIDIN (Physician Partner)
REPACK
gramicidin/neomycin sulfate/polymyxin b sulfate
SOL, OP, 10 ml 21695-0528-10 63.08

NEOMYCIN/POLY B/HYDROCORTISONE
(Physician Partner)
hc/neomycin sulf/polymyxin b sulf
SOL, OT, 1%-0.35%-10000 u/ml,
10 ml............. 21695-0437-10 61.60
SUS, OT, 1%-0.35%-10000 u/ml,
10 ml............. 21695-0438-10 61.60

(Quality Care Prod)
REPACK
SUS, OT, 1%-0.35%-10000 u/ml,
10 ml............. 49999-0439-10 36.96

NEOMYCIN/POLYMYXIN B SULFATES & HC
(Dispensing Solutions)
REPACK
hc/neomycin sulf/polymyxin b sulf
SUS, OP, 1%-0.35%-10000 u/ml,
7.5 ml 55045-1185-03 67.00

NEOMYCIN/POLYMYXIN B SULFATES/ DEXAMETHASONE (Keltman Pharma., Inc.)
REPACK
dexamethasone/neomycin sulfate/polymyxin b sulfate
SUS, OP, 5 ml 68387-0568-01 19.26

NEOMYCIN/POLYMYXIN B SULFATES/ HYDROCORTISONE (Paddock)
hc/neomycin sulf/polymyxin b sulf
SOL, OT (1X10ML,USP,W/DROPPER)
1%-0.35%-10000 u/ml,
10 ml............. 00574-4100-10 18.50 AT
SUS, OT (USP,1X10ML)
1%-0.35%-10000 u/ml,
10 ml............. 00574-4103-10 18.50 AT

NEOPROFEN (Lundbeck)
ibuprofen lysine
SOL, IV (3X2ML,PF)
10 mg/ml, 2 ml 3s 67386-0122-52 1827.00

NEORAL (Novartis Pharm)
cyclosporine, modified
SGL, PO (SOFTGEL)
25 mg, 30s ea UD 00078-0246-15 45.85 AB1
100 mg, 30s ea UD ... 00078-0248-15 183.21 AB1
SOL, PO, 100 mg/ml,
50 ml............. 00078-0274-22 332.83 AB

NEOSALUS (Quinnova)
foam, multi ingredient
FOA, TP (1X70GM,FRAGRANCE-FREE)
70 gm 23710-0000-70 143.75
(1X200GM,FRAGRANCE-FREE)
200 gm 23710-0000-02 231.25

NEOSPORIN (Monarch)
gramicidin/neomycin sulfate/polymyxin b sulfate
SOL, OP, 10 ml .... 61570-0045-10 53.52 AT

PROD/MFR | NDC | AWP | DP | OBC

(A-S Medication)
REPACK
SOL, OP, 10 ml .... 54569-0874-00 47.80 AT
(Phys Total Care)
REPACK
SOL, OP, 10 ml .... 54868-0593-00 49.66 AT
NEOSPORIN G.U. IRRIGANT (Monarch)
neomycin sulfate/polymyxin b sulfate
SOL, IL (AMP)
40 mg/ml-200000 u/ml,
1 ml 10s........... 61570-0047-10 231.23
1 ml 50s........... 61570-0047-50 1086.95
(M.D.V.)
40 mg/ml-200000 u/ml,
20 ml............. 61570-0048-20 262.34
NEOSTIGMINE BROMIDE (Medisca)
POW, NA (U.S.P.)
1 gm................ 38779-1450-06 31.50
5 gm................ 38779-1450-03 114.00
25 gm.............. 38779-1450-04 505.50
(PCCA)
POW, NA, 1 gm........... 51927-1980-00 77.40
(Spectrum Pharmacy)
POW, NA (U.S.P.)
1 gm................ 49452-4832-01 123.90
5 gm................ 49452-4832-02 416.50
25 gm.............. 49452-4832-03 1193.50
(Valeant Pharm Intl) *See PROSTIGMIN BROMIDE*
NEOSTIGMINE METHYLSULFATE (Amer Regent)
SOL, IJ (M.D.V.)
0.5 mg/ml,
10 ml 25s.......... 00517-0034-25 125.00
1 mg/ml, 10 ml 25s... 00517-0033-25 125.00
(APP)
SOL, IJ (M.D.V.,AMBER)
0.5 mg/ml, 10 ml..... 63323-0382-10 8.93
1 mg/ml, 10 ml....... 63323-0383-10 11.43
(Baxter)
SOL, IJ (1X10ML,USP,MDV)
0.5 mg/ml, 10 ml..... 10019-0271-37 4.08
((M.D.V.),USP)
0.5 mg/ml,
10 ml 10s.......... 10019-0271-10 40.80
(1X10ML,USP,MDV)
1 mg/ml, 10 ml....... 10019-0270-39 1.79
((M.D.V.),USP)
1 mg/ml, 10 ml 10s... 10019-0270-10 17.88
(Gallipot)
POW, NA, 5 gm........... 51552-0701-02 81.90 58.50
NEOTIC (Arbor)
antipyrine/benzocaine/glycerin/zinc acetate
SOL, OT (W/5 ALCOHOL PADS)
5.4%-1%-2%-1%,
10 ml 2s........... 24338-0810-20 55.00 44.00
NEOTRACE-4 (APP)
chromium/copper/manganese/zinc
SOL, IV (S.D.V.,PF)
2 ml................ 63323-0141-02 6.33
NEOTUSS-D (A. G. Marin)
cpm/dm/gg/phenyleph hcl
LIQ, PO (AF,SF,DYE-FREE)
473 ml 12539-0888-16 56.10
NEPAFENAC
(Alcon Ophthalmic) *See NEVANAC*
NEPHPLEX RX (Nephro-Tech)
vitamin b complex, mineral, and vitamin c
TAB, PO, 100s ea 59528-0317-01 34.50
NEPHRAMINE (B. Braun)
amino acids
SOL, IV (1X250ML)
5.4%, 250 ml .... 00264-1909-55 26.15 EE
NEPHRO-VITE RX (Watson)
vitamin b complex and vitamin c
TAB, PO (FILM-COATED)
100s ea............. 52544-0977-01 54.17
NEPHROCAPS (Fleming)
vitamin b complex and vitamin c
SGL, PO (SOFTGEL)
30s ea.............. 00256-0185-04 18.08
90s ea.............. 00256-0185-05 54.16
(American Health)
REPACK
SGL, PO (10X10,SOFTGEL)
100s ea UD 68084-0065-01 57.44
(15X30,SOFTGEL)
450s ea............. 68084-0065-85 193.73

PROD/MFR | NDC | AWP | DP | OBC

(Phys Total Care)
REPACK
SGL, PO (SOFTGEL)
100s ea.............. 54868-3008-01 37.09
NEPHRON FA (Nephro-Tech)
multivitamin and iron
TAB, PO, 100s ea 59528-4456-01 44.25
NEPHRONEX (Llorens Pharma Int)
vitamin b complex
TAB, PO (CAPLET)
100s ea............. 54859-0716-01 20.00
NESACAINE (APP)
chloroprocaine hydrochloride
SOL, IJ (M.D.V.)
1%, 30 ml 00186-0971-66 21.65
(1X30ML,MDV)
2%, 30 ml .... 63323-0476-30 22.19 AP
(Phys Total Care)
REPACK
SOL, IJ (M.D.V.)
2%, 30 ml .... 54868-4925-00 27.55 EE
NESACAINE-MPF (APP)
chloroprocaine hydrochloride
SOL, IJ (SDV, 1X20ML)
2%, 20 ml .... 63323-0477-20 26.63 AP
3%, 20 ml .... 63323-0478-20 27.97 AP
NESIRITIDE
(Scios) *See NATRECOR*
NESTABS CBF (Novavax)
prenatal vitamins
TAB, PO (9 BLISTER CARDS 5X2)
90s ea.............. 66500-0001-01 36.87
NESTABS FA (Novavax)
prenatal vitamins
TAB, PO (FILM-COATED)
100s ea............. 66500-0594-01 25.14
NESTABS RX (Novavax)
prenatal vitamins
TAB, PO (FILM-COATED)
90s ea.............. 66500-0317-01 38.62
NETTLE LEAF (PCCA)
POW, NA, 1 gm........... 51927-3482-00 0.45
NEULASTA (Amgen USA Inc.)
pegfilgrastim
SOL, SC (SRN,PREFILLED,PF)
6 mg/0.6 ml,
0.6 ml 55513-0190-01 3871.20
(Phys Total Care)
REPACK
SOL, SC (PF)
6 mg/0.6 ml,
0.6 ml 54868-5229-00 4102.37
NEUMEGA (Wyeth)
oprelvekin
PDS, SC (PF,LYOPHILIZED)
5 mg, ea............. 58394-0004-08 2937.60 2448.00 EE
(Phys Total Care)
REPACK
PDS, SC, 5 mg, ea 54868-5569-00 336.84
NEUPOGEN (Amgen USA Inc.)
filgrastim
SOL, IJ (S.D.V.,PF)
300 mcg/ml, 1 ml 55513-0530-01 275.04
((S.D.V.),1MLX10,PF)
300 mcg/ml,
1 ml 10s........... 55513-0530-10 2750.40
(S.D.V.,PF)
480 mcg/1.6 ml,
1.6 ml 55513-0546-01 437.94
((S.D.V.),1.6MLX10,PF)
480 mcg/1.6 ml,
1.6 ml 10s......... 55513-0546-10 4379.40
((26GX5/8"),SINGLE-USE)
300 mcg/0.5 ml,
0.5 ml 55513-0924-01 301.74
((26GX5/8"),0.5MLX10,PF)
300 mcg/0.5 ml,
0.5 ml 10s......... 55513-0924-10 3017.40
(26GX5/8",PF,SINGLEJECT)
480 mcg/0.8 ml,
0.8 ml 55513-0209-01 480.60
((26GX5/8"),0.8MLX10,PF)
480 mcg/0.8 ml,
0.8 ml 10s......... 55513-0209-10 4806.00

PROD/MFR | NDC | AWP | DP | OBC

(Phys Total Care)
REPACK
SOL, IJ (S.D.V.,PF)
300 mcg/ml, 1 ml 54868-2522-00 218.56
(PF,SINGLEJECT)
300 mcg/0.5 ml,
0.5 ml 10s......... 54868-5020-00 2768.75
480 mcg/0.8 ml,
0.8 ml 10s......... 54868-3050-00 4583.94
NEUPRO (UCB)
rotigotine
TDM, TD, 2 mg/24 hr,
7s ea............. 00091-6486-21 18.90
30s ea............ 00091-6486-01 81.00
4 mg/24 hr, 7s ea..... 00091-6487-21 64.68
30s ea............ 00091-6487-01 277.20
6 mg/24 hr, 7s ea..... 00091-6488-21 64.68
30s ea............ 00091-6488-01 277.20
NEURAGEN (Integra LifeSciences Corp)
collagen nerve encasement
DEV, NA (5MM IDX2CM)
ea.................. 08478-6109-02 1168.00
(5MM IDX3CM)
ea.................. 08478-6110-03 1390.00
(6MM IDX2CM)
ea.................. 08478-6111-02 1168.00
(6MM IDX3CM)
ea.................. 08478-6112-03 1390.00
(7MM IDX2CM)
ea.................. 08478-6113-02 1168.00
(7MM IDX3CM)
ea.................. 08478-6114-03 1390.00
(SINGLE USE,2MM IDX2CM)
ea UD 08478-6102-02 1168.00
(SINGLE USE,2MM IDX3CM)
ea UD 08478-6103-03 1390.00
(SINGLE USE,3MM IDX2CM)
ea UD 08478-6104-02 1168.00
(SINGLE USE,3MM IDX3CM)
ea.................. 08478-6105-03 1390.00
(SINGLE USE,4MM IDX2CM)
ea UD 08478-6106-02 1168.00
(SINGLE USE,4MM IDX3CM)
ea UD 08478-6107-03 1390.00
NEURAWRAP (Integra LifeSciences Corp)
collagen nerve encasement
DEV, NA (SINGLE USE,10MM IDX2CM)
ea.................. 08478-6210-02 1175.00
(SINGLE USE,10MM IDX4CM)
ea.................. 08478-6210-04 1510.00
(SINGLE USE,3MM IDX2CM)
ea UD 08478-6203-02 1175.00
(SINGLE USE,3MM IDX4CM)
ea UD 08478-6203-04 1510.00
(SINGLE USE,5MM IDX2CM)
ea.................. 08478-6205-02 1175.00
(SINGLE USE,5MM IDX4CM)
ea.................. 08478-6205-04 1510.00
(SINGLE USE,7MM IDX2CM)
ea UD 08478-6207-02 1175.00
(SINGLE USE,7MM IDX4CM)
ea UD 08478-6207-04 1510.00
NEUROFORTE-R (Intl Ethical)
cyanocobalamin
SOL, IM (VIAL)
1000 mcg/ml, 10 ml .. 11584-1025-01 12.51 EE
NEUROFORTE-SIX (Intl Ethical)
ascorbic acid/vitamin b complex
SOL, IJ (VIAL)
10 ml............... 11584-1018-06 17.69
NEUROKININ A (PCCA)
POW, NA, ea............. 51927-2567-00 1485.00
NEUROLITE (Lantheus)
technetium tc 99m bicisate
KIT, IV (SRN,PREFILLED)
ea.................. 11994-0006-00 446.51
NEUROMATRIX (Stryker)
collagen nerve encasement
DEV, NA (2.0MM IDX2.5CM)
ea.................. 08572-0020-25 1072.00
(2.5MM IDX2.5CM)
ea.................. 08572-0025-25 1072.00
(3.0MM IDX2.5CM)
ea.................. 08572-0030-25 1072.00
(4.0MM IDX2.5CM)
ea.................. 08572-0040-25 1072.00
(5.0MM IDX2.5CM)
ea.................. 08572-0050-25 1072.00
(6.0MM IDX2.5CM)
ea.................. 08572-0060-25 1072.00

PROD/MFR	NDC	AWP	DP	OBC
NEUROMEND COLLAGEN NERVE WRAP (Stryker)				
collagen nerve encasement				
DEV, NA (12MMX2.5CM,SINGLE USE)				
ea	**08572-0120-25**	1408.24		
(12MMX5CM,SINGLE USE)				
ea	**08572-0120-50**	1410.04		
(4MMX2.5CM,SINGLE USE)				
ea	**08572-0840-25**	1380.35		
(4MMX5CM,SINGLE USE)				
ea	**08572-0840-50**	1384.15		
(6MMX2.5CM,SINGLE USE)				
ea	**08572-0860-25**	1414.07		
(6MMX5CM,SINGLE USE)				
ea	**08572-0860-50**	1385.61		
NEURONTIN (Pfizer)				
gabapentin				
CAP, PO, 100 mg, 100s ea	**00071-0803-24**	81.36	67.80	AB
300 mg, 50s ea UD	**00071-0805-40**	111.24	92.70	AB
100s ea	**00071-0805-24**	203.44	169.53	AB
(5-2X5 BLISTER PACK)				
400 mg, 50s ea UD	**00071-0806-40**	129.18	107.65	AB
100s ea	**00071-0806-24**	244.07	203.39	AB
SOL, PO (ANISE-BERRY)				
250 mg/5 ml,				
470 ml	**00071-2012-23**	151.76	126.47	
TAB, PO (FILM-COATED)				
600 mg, 100s ea	**00071-0513-24**	386.48	322.07	
800 mg, 100s ea	**00071-0401-24**	463.72	386.43	
(A-S Medication)				
REPACK				
CAP, PO, 100 mg, 30s ea	**54569-4576-01**	22.84		
100s ea	**54569-4576-02**	76.14		AB
300 mg, 30s ea	**54569-4577-01**	57.12		
100s ea	**54569-4577-00**	190.39		
(Altura)				
REPACK				
CAP, PO, 100 mg, 10s ea	**63874-0706-10**	11.66		AB
14s ea	**63874-0706-14**	16.33		AB
20s ea	**63874-0706-20**	23.33		AB
21s ea	**63874-0706-21**	24.49		AB
28s ea	**63874-0706-28**	32.66		AB
30s ea	**63874-0706-30**	34.99		AB
40s ea	**63874-0706-40**	46.65		AB
60s ea	**63874-0706-60**	69.98		AB
90s ea	**63874-0706-90**	104.97		AB
100s ea	**63874-0706-01**	116.63		AB
120s ea	**63874-0706-04**	139.96		AB
180s ea	**63874-0706-18**	209.94		AB
300 mg, 10s ea	**63874-0629-10**	14.97		AB
14s ea	**63874-0629-14**	20.95		AB
21s ea	**63874-0629-21**	31.43		AB
28s ea	**63874-0629-28**	41.90		AB
30s ea	**63874-0629-30**	44.90		AB
40s ea	**63874-0629-40**	59.86		AB
50s ea	**63874-0629-50**	74.83		AB
60s ea	**63874-0629-60**	89.79		AB
90s ea	**63874-0629-90**	134.69		AB
100s ea	**63874-0629-01**	149.65		AB
120s ea	**63874-0629-04**	179.58		AB
180s ea	**63874-0629-18**	269.37		AB
TAB, PO (FILM-COATED)				
600 mg, 14s ea	**63874-1073-07**	45.31		
20s ea	**63874-1073-02**	64.73		
28s ea	**63874-1073-08**	90.63		
30s ea	**63874-1073-03**	97.10		
40s ea	**63874-1073-04**	129.47		
50s ea	**63874-1073-05**	161.83		
60s ea	**63874-1073-06**	194.20		
90s ea	**63874-1073-09**	291.30		
100s ea	**63874-1073-01**	323.67		
120s ea	**63874-1073-00**	388.40		
800 mg, 60s ea	**63874-1127-06**	212.41		
(AQ)				
REPACK				
CAP, PO, 100 mg, 100s ea	**66105-0539-10**	84.95		
300 mg, 100s ea	**66105-0540-10**	204.91		
400 mg, 100s ea	**66105-0541-10**	244.85		
TAB, PO, 600 mg, 100s ea	**66105-0542-10**	283.25		
800 mg, 10s ea	**66105-0543-01**	45.00		
30s ea	**66105-0543-03**	135.00		
60s ea	**66105-0543-06**	270.00		
90s ea	**66105-0543-09**	405.00		
100s ea	**66105-0543-10**	431.14		
(DHS, Inc.)				
REPACK				
TAB, PO, 600 mg, 30s ea	**55887-0539-30**	94.30		
60s ea	**55887-0539-60**	171.01		
(FILM-COATED)				
800 mg, 30s ea	**55887-0500-30**	101.02		
60s ea	**55887-0500-60**	199.99		
(Dispensing Solutions)				
REPACK				
CAP, PO, 100 mg, 30s ea	**55045-2696-08**	23.40		AB
45s ea	**55045-2696-09**	35.10		AB
60s ea	**55045-2696-06**	46.80		AB
100s ea	**55045-2696-00**	78.00		AB
300 mg, 30s ea	**55045-2616-08**	54.00		AB
45s ea	**55045-2616-09**	81.00		AB
60s ea	**55045-2616-06**	108.00		AB
90s ea	**55045-2616-05**	162.00		AB
100s ea	**55045-2616-00**	180.00		AB
400 mg, 30s ea	**55045-2545-08**	56.00		AB
100s ea	**55045-2545-00**	185.00		AB
(Nucare Pharm)				
REPACK				
CAP, PO, 100 mg, 30s ea	**66267-0339-30**	34.99		
45s ea	**66267-0339-45**	50.99		
90s ea	**66267-0339-90**	69.99		
300 mg, 30s ea	**66267-0155-30**	62.89		AB
45s ea	**66267-0155-45**	69.99		
60s ea	**66267-0155-60**	89.79		
90s ea	**66267-0155-90**	189.42		AB
180s ea	**66267-0155-92**	299.99		
(PD-Rx Pharm)				
REPACK				
CAP, PO, 100 mg, 30s ea	**55289-0843-30**	34.23		AB
(REDI-SCRIPT)				
100 mg, 60s ea	**58864-0712-60**	54.60		AB
300 mg, 10s ea	**55289-0570-10**	28.52		AB
30s ea	**55289-0570-30**	85.58		AB
60s ea	**55289-0570-60**	171.15		AB
TAB, PO (FILM-COATED)				
600 mg, 30s ea	**55289-0850-30**	127.14		
(Pharma Pac)				
REPACK				
CAP, PO, 100 mg, 20s ea	**52959-0506-20**	22.65		AB
21s ea	**52959-0506-21**	23.68		
30s ea	**52959-0506-30**	32.26		
45s ea	**52959-0506-45**	47.30		
60s ea	**52959-0506-60**	73.87		
90s ea	**52959-0506-90**	110.79		
100s ea	**52959-0506-00**	73.87		
120s ea	**52959-0506-02**	88.64		
300 mg, 20s ea	**52959-0434-20**	45.94		
30s ea	**52959-0434-30**	63.87		
35s ea	**52959-0434-35**	65.42		AB
45s ea	**52959-0434-45**	67.96		
60s ea	**52959-0434-60**	89.70		AB
90s ea	**52959-0434-90**	132.03		
100s ea	**52959-0434-00**	145.13		
120s ea	**52959-0434-02**	174.12		AB
TAB, PO, 600 mg, 30s ea	**52959-0640-30**	98.70		
60s ea	**52959-0640-60**	197.38		
90s ea	**52959-0640-90**	296.05		
120s ea	**52959-0640-02**	364.69		
(Phys Total Care)				
REPACK				
CAP, PO, 100 mg, 50s ea	**54868-3529-02**	35.88		AB
90s ea	**54868-3529-01**	64.20		
100s ea	**54868-3529-00**	70.50		
300 mg, 20s ea	**54868-3768-05**	39.45		AB
30s ea	**54868-3529-03**	22.65		
30s ea	**54868-3768-01**	58.54		
60s ea	**54868-3768-04**	115.84		AB
90s ea	**54868-3768-03**	163.58		
100s ea	**54868-3768-02**	181.61		
400 mg, 10s ea	**54868-3931-02**	22.65		
30s ea	**54868-3931-00**	64.19		
100s ea	**54868-3931-01**	197.43		
TAB, PO (FILM-COATED)				
600 mg, 10s ea	**54868-4491-01**	34.78		
30s ea	**54868-4491-03**	100.56		
60s ea	**54868-4491-02**	188.28		
90s ea	**54868-4491-00**	281.48		
100s ea	**54868-4491-04**	311.91		
800 mg, 10s ea	**54868-4600-02**	41.34		
30s ea	**54868-4600-01**	120.28		
100s ea	**54868-4600-00**	373.99		
(Quality Care Prod)				
REPACK				
CAP, PO, 300 mg, 100s ea	**49999-0257-00**	336.12		
TAB, PO, 800 mg, 30s ea	**35356-0061-30**	148.80		
(Southwood)				
REPACK				
CAP, PO, 100 mg, 10s ea	**58016-0427-10**	8.50		
14s ea	**58016-0427-14**	11.90		
15s ea	**58016-0427-15**	12.75		
20s ea	**58016-0427-20**	17.00		
21s ea	**58016-0427-21**	17.85		
28s ea	**58016-0427-28**	23.80		
30s ea	**58016-0427-30**	25.50		
40s ea	**58016-0427-40**	34.00		
50s ea	**58016-0427-50**	42.50		
60s ea	**58016-0427-60**	51.00		
90s ea	**58016-0427-90**	76.50		
100s ea	**58016-0427-00**	85.00		
300 mg, 10s ea	**58016-0481-10**	18.28		
14s ea	**58016-0481-14**	25.59		
15s ea	**58016-0481-15**	27.42		
20s ea	**58016-0481-20**	36.55		
21s ea	**58016-0481-21**	38.38		
28s ea	**58016-0481-28**	51.18		
30s ea	**58016-0481-30**	54.83		
40s ea	**58016-0481-40**	73.11		
50s ea	**58016-0481-50**	91.39		
60s ea	**58016-0481-60**	109.66		
90s ea	**58016-0481-90**	164.49		
100s ea	**58016-0481-00**	182.77		
400 mg, 10s ea	**58016-0433-10**	21.93		
14s ea	**58016-0433-14**	30.70		
15s ea	**58016-0433-15**	32.89		
20s ea	**58016-0433-20**	43.86		
21s ea	**58016-0433-21**	46.05		
28s ea	**58016-0433-28**	61.40		
30s ea	**58016-0433-30**	65.79		
40s ea	**58016-0433-40**	87.72		
50s ea	**58016-0433-50**	109.65		
60s ea	**58016-0433-60**	131.57		
90s ea	**58016-0433-90**	197.36		
100s ea	**58016-0433-00**	219.29		
TAB, PO, 600 mg, 10s ea	**58016-0482-10**	34.72		
14s ea	**58016-0482-14**	48.61		
15s ea	**58016-0482-15**	52.09		
20s ea	**58016-0482-20**	69.45		
21s ea	**58016-0482-21**	72.92		
28s ea	**58016-0482-28**	97.23		
30s ea	**58016-0482-30**	104.17		
40s ea	**58016-0482-40**	138.90		
50s ea	**58016-0482-50**	173.62		
60s ea	**58016-0482-60**	208.34		
90s ea	**58016-0482-90**	312.52		
100s ea	**58016-0482-00**	347.24		
800 mg, 10s ea	**58016-0483-10**	27.54		
10s ea	**58016-0483-20**	83.33		
30s ea	**58016-0483-30**	124.99		
40s ea	**58016-0483-40**	166.66		
50s ea	**58016-0483-50**	208.32		
60s ea	**58016-0483-60**	249.98		
90s ea	**58016-0483-90**	374.98		
100s ea	**58016-0483-00**	416.64		
(Stat Rx)				
REPACK				
CAP, PO, 400 mg, 84s ea	**16590-0870-62**	226.06		AB
TAB, PO (FILM-COATED)				
600 mg, 90s ea	**16590-0627-90**	382.55		
112s ea	**16590-0627-73**	475.27		
NEUT (Hospira)				
sodium bicarbonate				
SOL, IV (ADD-VANTAGE,FTV,25X5ML)				
4%, 5 ml 25s	**00409-6609-02**	119.70	104.75	
NEUTRAGARD ADVANCED (Pascal Co.)				
sodium fluoride				
GEL, DE (WINTERMINT)				
1.1%, 60 gm	**10866-0113-01**	4.60		
NEUTRAHIST (Cypress Pharm)				
cpm/pse hcl				
SOL, PO (W/DROPPER,CHERRY,DROPS)				
0.8 mg/ml-9 mg/ml,				
30 ml	**60258-0395-30**	46.79		
NEUTRAHIST PDX (Cypress Pharm)				
cpm/dm/pse hcl				
SOL, PO (W/DROPPER,AF,SF,GRAPE)				
30 ml	**60258-0396-30**	53.49		
NEUTRAL SODIUM FLUORIDE (Cypress Pharm)				
sodium fluoride				
SOL, PO (MINT)				
0.2%, 473 ml	**60258-0158-16**	9.19		
NEUTRASAL (Invado)				
saliva substitutes				
PDS, MM, 30s ea UD	**49939-1001-01**	181.25		
120s ea UD	**49939-1001-04**	725.00		
NEVANAC (Alcon Ophthalmic)				
nepafenac				
SUS, OP (3ML IN 4ML DROPTAINER)				
0.1%, 3 ml	**00065-0002-03**	109.20		
NEVIRAPINE				
(Boehr Ingelheim Phar) *See VIRAMUNE*				

PROD/MFR	NDC	AWP	DP	OBC
NEW AMI-TEX LA (Actavis)				
guaifenesin/phenylephrine hydrochloride				
TER, PO, 600 mg-30 mg,				
100s ea	52152-0253-02	114.10		
NEXAVAR (Bayer)				
sorafenib tosylate				
TAB, PO (FILM-COATED)				
200 mg, 120s ea	50419-0488-58	7993.14		
NEXIUM (AstraZeneca)				
esomeprazole magnesium				
ECC, PO (UNIT OF USE)				
20 mg, 30s ea	00186-5020-31	195.06		
90s ea	00186-5020-54	585.16		
100s ea UD	00186-5022-28	650.14		
1000s ea	00186-5020-82	6501.38		
(UNIT OF USE)				
40 mg, 30s ea	00186-5040-31	195.06		
90s ea	00186-5040-54	585.16		
100s ea UD	00186-5042-28	650.14		
1000s ea	00186-5040-82	6501.38		
PKT, PO, 10 mg/packet,				
30s ea UD	00186-4010-01	195.06		EE
20 mg/packet,				
30s ea UD	00186-4020-01	195.06		EE
40 mg/packet,				
30s ea UD	00186-4040-01	195.06		
(A-S Medication) REPACK				
ECC, PO, 20 mg, 30s ea	54569-5273-00	241.50		
40 mg, 30s ea	54569-5274-00	241.50		
90s ea	54569-5274-01	724.48		
(Altura) REPACK				
ECC, PO, 40 mg, 15s ea	63874-1060-05	111.29		
30s ea	63874-1060-03	269.88		
60s ea	63874-1060-06	335.00		
90s ea	63874-1060-09	437.52		
100s ea	63874-1060-00	494.61		
(AQ) REPACK				
ECC, PO, 40 mg, 30s ea	66105-0830-03	356.93		
(Core) REPACK				
ECC, PO, 40 mg, 30s ea	33358-0260-30	183.36		
60s ea	33358-0260-60	348.57		
(Dispensing Solutions) REPACK				
ECC, PO, 20 mg, 30s ea	55045-3450-08	181.50		
40 mg, 30s ea	55045-3432-08	199.15		
(IPI) REPACK				
ECC, PO, 40 mg, 90s ea	18837-0107-90	581.82		
(Nucare Pharm) REPACK				
ECC, PO, 40 mg, 10s ea	66267-0592-10	179.85		
30s ea	68071-1366-00	207.76		
60s ea	66267-0592-60	509.00		
(Palmetto) REPACK				
ECC, PO, 20 mg, 30s ea	23490-9020-03	155.42		
(PD-Rx Pharm) REPACK				
ECC, PO, 40 mg, 30s ea	58864-0763-30	276.09		
(Pharma Pac) REPACK				
ECC, PO, 20 mg, 10s ea	52959-0917-10	68.02		
40 mg, 30s ea	52959-0642-30	158.20		
90s ea	52959-0642-90	477.86		
(Phys Total Care) REPACK				
ECC, PO, 20 mg, 30s ea	54868-4635-00	206.59		
40 mg, 10s ea	54868-4510-01	84.11		
30s ea	54868-4510-00	232.87		
60s ea	54868-4510-03	449.53		
90s ea	54868-4510-02	672.33		
(Physician Partner) REPACK				
ECC, PO, 20 mg, 30s ea	21695-0091-30	390.12		
(HARD GELATIN)				
20 mg, 60s ea	21695-0091-60	780.17		
40 mg, 15s ea	21695-0092-15	227.66		
30s ea	21695-0092-30	390.12		
(Quality Care Prod) REPACK				
ECC, PO, 40 mg, 15s ea	49999-0307-15	135.69		
30s ea	49999-0307-30	371.00		
90s ea	49999-0307-90	1113.30		
(Southwood) REPACK				
ECC, PO, 20 mg, 30s ea	58016-0210-30	146.72		
30s ea	58016-0824-30	134.94		
60s ea	58016-0210-60	293.44		
60s ea	58016-0824-60	269.88		
90s ea	58016-0210-90	440.15		
90s ea	58016-0824-90	404.82		
100s ea	58016-0210-00	489.06		
100s ea	58016-0824-00	449.80		
120s ea	58016-0210-02	586.87		
40 mg, 30s ea	58016-0669-30	173.41		
60s ea	58016-0669-60	346.81		
90s ea	58016-0669-90	520.22		
100s ea	58016-0669-00	578.02		
120s ea	58016-0669-02	693.62		
(St. Mary's MPP) REPACK				
ECC, PO, 40 mg, 30s ea	60760-0504-30	287.79		
(Stat Rx) REPACK				
ECC, PO, 20 mg, 15s ea	16590-0625-15	106.38		
28s ea	16590-0625-28	203.67		
30s ea	16590-0625-30	217.99		
60s ea	16590-0625-60	432.72		
40 mg, 15s ea	16590-0509-15	110.62		
28s ea	16590-0509-28	203.67		
30s ea	16590-0509-30	217.98		
60s ea	16590-0509-60	432.72		
90s ea	16590-0509-90	647.45		
120s ea	16590-0509-72	567.25		
NEXIUM I.V. (AstraZeneca)				
esomeprazole sodium				
PDS, IV (2 TRAYSX5 S.D.V.)				
20 mg, 10s ea	00186-6020-01	339.10		
40 mg, 10s ea	00186-6040-01	339.10		
NEXT CHOICE (Watson)				
levonorgestrel				
TAB, PO, 0.75 mg, 2s ea	52544-0275-36	35.10		AB
(Pharma Pac) REPACK				
TAB, PO, 0.75 mg, 2s ea	52959-0450-02	35.18		AB
(Physician Partner) REPACK				
TAB, PO, 0.75 mg, 2s ea	21695-0443-02	73.12		AB
NIACIN FUL				
TAB, PO, 500 mg, 100s ea		3.90		
(Abbott Pharm) *See NIASPAN*				
(Baker, J.T.)				
POW, NA (F.C.C.)				
25 gm	10106-2745-03	32.55		
(Gallipot)				
POW, NA (U.S.P.)				
1000 gm	51552-0559-07	48.23		
(Medisca) *See NICOTINIC ACID*				
(PCCA)				
POW, NA (USP; NICOTINIC ACID)				
1 gm	51927-1105-00	0.36		
(Spectrum Pharmacy)				
POW, NA (U.S.P.)				
100 gm	49452-4840-01	76.13		
1000 gm	49452-4840-02	227.50		
(Upsher-Smith) *See NIACOR*				
(Bryant Ranch) REPACK				
TAB, PO, 50 mg, 100s ea	63629-1486-01	2.65		
NIACIN/SIMVASTATIN				
(Abbott Pharm) *See SIMCOR*				
NIACINAMIDE (Medisca)				
POW, NA (U.S.P.)				
100 gm	38779-0377-05	28.50		
500 gm	38779-0377-08	43.50		
1000 gm	38779-0377-09	267.00		
(PCCA) *See NICOTINAMIDE ADENINE DINUCLEOTIDE*				
(PCCA)				
POW, NA (U.S.P.)				
1 gm	51927-1689-00	0.36		
(Spectrum Pharmacy) *See NICOTINAMIDE*				
NIACINAMIDE ASCORBATE (Spectrum Pharmacy)				
POW, NA (F.C.C.)				
100 gm	49452-4848-01	100.10		
500 gm	49452-4848-02	247.80		
2500 gm	49452-4848-03	850.50		
NIACOR (Upsher-Smith)				
niacin				
TAB, PO, 500 mg, 100s ea	00245-0067-11	28.17		AA
NIASPAN (Abbott Pharm)				
niacin				
TER, PO (FILM-COATED)				
500 mg, 90s ea	00074-3074-90	228.35	200.31	
750 mg, 90s ea	00074-3079-90	325.70	285.70	
1000 mg, 90s ea	00074-3080-90	403.87	354.27	
(A-S Medication) REPACK				
TER, PO, 500 mg, 30s ea	54569-5267-01	67.98		
(CAPLET)				
1000 mg, 30s ea	54569-5261-01	120.23		
(Phys Total Care) REPACK				
TER, PO (CAPLET)				
500 mg, 10s ea	54868-4899-01	36.84		
30s ea	54868-4899-00	105.30		
60s ea	54868-4899-03	196.58		
90s ea	54868-4899-04	293.56		
(CAPLET)				
500 mg, 100s ea	54868-4899-02	325.23		
(FILM-COATED)				
500 mg, 120s ea	54868-4899-05	390.54		
(CAPLET)				
750 mg, 10s ea	54868-4867-01	51.43		
30s ea	54868-4867-00	140.93		
60s ea	54868-4867-02	279.25		
1000 mg, 10s ea	54868-0017-01	63.15		
15s ea	54868-0017-00	93.42		
30s ea	54868-0017-02	174.13		
45s ea	54868-0017-03	259.89		
60s ea	54868-0017-05	345.65		
90s ea	54868-0017-04	517.16		
(Quality Care Prod) REPACK				
TER, PO (FILM-COATED)				
500 mg, 90s ea	49999-0475-90	402.14		
750 mg, 90s ea	35356-0301-90	572.09		
1000 mg, 90s ea	35356-0302-90	708.54		
(Southwood) REPACK				
TER, PO (CAPLET)				
1000 mg, 30s ea	58016-0583-30	72.53		
60s ea	58016-0583-60	145.05		
90s ea	58016-0583-90	217.58		
100s ea	58016-0583-00	241.75		
NICARDIPINE HCL (Mylan)				
nicardipine hydrochloride				
CAP, PO, 20 mg, 90s ea	00378-1020-77	41.20		AB
500s ea	00378-1020-05	223.70		AB
30 mg, 90s ea	00378-1430-77	59.00		AB
500s ea	00378-1430-05	320.30		AB
NICARDIPINE HYDROCHLORIDE FUL				
CAP, PO, 20 mg, 100s ea		33.75		
30 mg, 100s ea		40.50		
(Amneal)				
CAP, PO, 20 mg, 100s ea	65162-0588-10	42.40		AB
30 mg, 100s ea	65162-0589-10	63.80		AB
(Caraco)				
SOL, IV (10X10ML)				
2.5 mg/ml,				
10 ml 10s	41616-0882-44	2501.25		AP
(EKR) *See CARDENE*				
(EKR) *See CARDENE I.V.*				
(EKR) *See CARDENE SR*				
(GeneraMedix)				
SOL, IV (1X10ML, SDV)				
2.5 mg/ml, 10 ml	10139-0700-10	99.20		AP
(10X10ML, SDV)				
2.5 mg/ml,				
10 ml 10s UD	10139-0700-11	992.04		AP
(Mylan) *See NICARDIPINE HCL*				
(PharmaForce)				
SOL, IV (10X10ML,SDV)				
2.5 mg/ml,				
10 ml 10s	40042-0047-10	308.00		AP
(Sandoz)				
SOL, IV (1X10ML,SINGLE DOSE)				
2.5 mg/ml, 10 ml	00781-3204-70	252.94		AP
(10X10ML,SINGLE DOSE)				
2.5 mg/ml,				
10 ml 10s	00781-3204-95	2529.36		AP

PROD/MFR	NDC	AWP	DP	OBC

(Teva)
SOL, IV (10X10ML)
2.5 mg/ml,
10 ml 10s.......... 00703-8315-03 1000.74 AP

(Wockhardt USA)
SOL, IV (1X10ML)
2.5 mg/ml, 10 ml..... 64679-0631-01 104.24 AP
(10X10ML,SDV)
2.5 mg/ml,
10 ml 10s.......... 64679-0631-02 1042.44 AP

NICARDIPINE HYDROCHLORIDE/SODIUM CHLORIDE
(EKR) *See CARDENE*

NICKEL ACETATE
(Baker, J.T.) *See NICKELOUS ACETATE TETRAHYDRATE*

NICKEL AMMONIUM SULFATE
(Baker, J.T.) *See NICKELOUS AMMONIUM SULFATE*

NICKEL CARBONATE
(Baker, J.T.) *See NICKELOUS CARBONATE*

NICKEL CHLORIDE
(Baker, J.T.) *See NICKELOUS CHLORIDE HEXAHYDRATE*

NICKEL NITRATE
(Baker, J.T.) *See NICKELOUS NITRATE HEXAHYDRATE*

NICKEL OXIDE
(Baker, J.T.) *See NICKEL OXIDE BLACK*
(Baker, J.T.) *See NICKELOUS OXIDE GREEN*

NICKEL OXIDE BLACK (Baker, J.T.)
nickel oxide
POW, NA (REAGENT)
125 gm............. 10106-2792-04 129.93
500 gm............. 10106-2792-01 229.54

NICKEL SULFATE
(Baker, J.T.) *See NICKELOUS SULFATE HEXAHYDRATE*
(Medisca) *See NICKLE SULFATE*

NICKELOUS ACETATE TETRAHYDRATE (Baker, J.T.)
nickel acetate
CRY, NA (REAGENT)
125 gm............. 10106-2756-04 138.59
500 gm............. 10106-2756-01 251.89

NICKELOUS AMMONIUM SULFATE (Baker, J.T.)
nickel ammonium sulfate
CRY, NA (REAGENT, HEXAHYDRATE)
125 gm............. 10106-2760-04 61.75
500 gm............. 10106-2760-01 111.03

NICKELOUS CARBONATE (Baker, J.T.)
nickel carbonate
POW, NA (REAGENT)
125 gm............. 10106-2764-04 125.09
500 gm............. 10106-2764-01 224.90

NICKELOUS CHLORIDE HEXAHYDRATE (Baker, J.T.)
nickel chloride
CRY, NA (REAGENT)
125 gm............. 10106-2768-04 49.08
500 gm............. 10106-2768-01 131.89

NICKELOUS NITRATE HEXAHYDRATE (Baker, J.T.)
nickel nitrate
CRY, NA (REAGENT)
125 gm............. 10106-2784-04 59.95
500 gm............. 10106-2784-01 108.77

NICKELOUS OXIDE GREEN (Baker, J.T.)
nickel oxide
POW, NA (REAGENT)
125 gm............. 10106-2796-04 154.60
500 gm............. 10106-2796-01 192.56

NICKELOUS SULFATE HEXAHYDRATE (Baker, J.T.)
nickel sulfate
CRY, NA (A.C.S., REAGENT)
125 gm............. 10106-2808-04 49.90
500 gm............. 10106-2808-01 141.78

NICKLE SULFATE (Medisca)
nickel sulfate
CRY, NA (PURIFIED)
25 gm.............. 38779-1455-04 61.50

NICLOSAMIDE (PCCA)
POW, NA (NP (ANHYDROUS))
1 gm............... 51927-3001-00 6.00

NICOTINAMIDE (Spectrum Pharmacy)
niacinamide
POW, NA (U.S.P.)
100 gm............. 49452-4850-01 69.13
(1X500GM,U.S.P.)
500 gm............. 49452-4850-03 129.33
(U.S.P.)
1000 gm............ 49452-4850-02 204.75
(1X5000GM,U.S.P.)
5000 gm............ 49452-4850-04 682.50

NICOTINAMIDE ADENINE DINUCLEOTIDE (PCCA)
niacinamide
POW, NA, 1 gm.......... 51927-3546-00 53.40
(REDUCED; BETA)
1 gm............... 51927-3174-00 390.00

NICOTINAMIDE W/ZINC AND CUPRIC OXIDES & FOLIC ACID (PruGen)
copper oxide/folic acid/niacinamide/zinc oxide
TER, PO (MULTIPHASIC RELEASE)
60s ea............. 42546-0917-60 85.01

NICOTINAMIDE/ZINC OXIDE/CUPRIC OXIDE/FOLIC ACID (Acella)
copper oxide/folic acid/niacinamide/zinc oxide
TAB, PO, 60s ea 42192-0308-60 84.95

NICOTINE
(Pfizer) *See NICOTROL*
(Pfizer) *See NICOTROL NS*
(Pharmacia Consumer) *See NICOTROL*
(Pharmacia Consumer) *See NICOTROL NS*

NICOTINE BITARTRATE
(PCCA) *See NICOTINE TARTRATE*

NICOTINE POLACRILEX (Gallipot)
POW, NA (U.S.P.)
15%, 5 gm.......... 51552-1009-02 63.00 45.00

(PCCA)
POW, NA (U.S.P.; 15% NICOTINE)
1 gm............... 51927-3406-00 27.00

(Spectrum Pharmacy)
POW, NA (1X1GM)
20%, 1 gm.......... 49452-1084-01 99.40
(1X5GM)
20%, 5 gm.......... 49452-1084-02 297.50
(1X25GM)
20%, 25 gm 49452-1084-03 910.00

NICOTINE TARTRATE (PCCA)
nicotine bitartrate
POW, NA, 1 gm.......... 51927-3465-00 75.00

NICOTINIC ACID (Medisca)
niacin
POW, NA (U.S.P.)
100 gm............. 38779-0378-05 22.50
500 gm............. 38779-0378-08 58.50
(1X1000GM,USP)
1000 gm............ 38779-0378-09 87.00

NICOTINIC ACID N-HEXYL ESTER (PCCA)
hexyl nicotinate
SOL, NA (1X1ML)
1 ml............... 51927-3167-00 21.00

NICOTROL (Pfizer)
nicotine
DEV, IH, 4 mg/actuation,
168s ea........... 00009-5400-01 214.90 179.08

(Pharmacia Consumer)
KIT, MR (MOUTHPIECE/PLASTIC CASE)
4 mg/actuation,
168s ea........... 00009-5195-08 133.20

(A-S Medication)
REPACK
DEV, IH, 4 mg/actuation,
ea................ 54569-6152-00 197.15

(Phys Total Care)
REPACK
DEV, IH, 4 mg/actuation,
168s ea........... 54868-5052-00 170.46

NICOTROL NS (Pfizer)
nicotine
SPR, NS (4X10ML)
10 mg/ml, 10 ml 4s... 00009-5401-01 214.90 179.08

(Pharmacia Consumer)
SPR, NS, 0.5 mg/actuation,
10 ml 4s.......... 00009-5194-02 133.20

(A-S Medication)
REPACK
SPR, NS (4X10ML)
10 mg/ml, 10 ml 4s... 54569-6153-00 197.15

NIFEDIAC CC (Teva)
nifedipine
TER, PO (FILM-COATED)
30 mg, 100s ea 00093-5272-01 115.35 AB1
(USP,10X10,FILM-COATED)
30 mg, 100s ea UD... 00093-5272-93 132.40
(FILM-COATED)
30 mg, 300s ea 00093-5272-55 339.13 AB1
(FILM COATED)
60 mg, 100s ea 00093-1022-01 216.79 AB1
(USP,10X10,FILM-COATED)
60 mg, 100s ea UD... 00093-1022-93 229.10
(FILM COATED)
60 mg, 300s ea 00093-1022-55 637.36 AB1
(10X10, USP,FILM-COATED)
90 mg, 100s ea UD... 00093-1023-93 256.10

NIFEDICAL XL (Teva)
nifedipine
TER, PO, 30 mg, 100s ea.. 00093-0819-01 136.46 AB2
300s ea........... 00093-0819-55 401.24 AB2
60 mg, 100s ea 00093-5173-01 236.17 AB2
300s ea........... 00093-5173-55 694.29 AB2

NIFEDIPINE (Actavis)
SGL, PO, 10 mg, 100s ea.. 00228-2497-10 92.90 AB
20 mg, 100s ea ...... 00228-2530-10 166.86 AB
TER, PO (FILM-COATED)
30 mg, 100s ea 67767-0153-01 139.40 AB1
500s ea........... 67767-0153-05 697.00 AB1
60 mg, 100s ea 67767-0151-01 248.31 AB1
500s ea........... 67767-0151-05 1241.55 AB1

(Gallipot)
POW, NA (1X5GM,USP)
5 gm............... 51552-0720-02 32.20 23.00
(1X25GM,USP)
25 gm.............. 51552-0720-04 80.50 57.50
(1X100GM,USP)
100 gm............. 51552-0720-05 273.00 195.00

(Hawkins)
POW, NA (U.S.P.)
5 gm............... 63370-0163-15 92.00
25 gm.............. 63370-0163-25 224.00
100 gm............. 63370-0163-35 760.00
500 gm............. 63370-0163-45 3400.00

(Kremers Urban)
TER, PO (USP,COATED)
30 mg, 90s ea........ 62175-0260-46 120.31 AB2
100s ea........... 62175-0260-37 133.69 AB2
300s ea........... 62175-0260-55 393.08 AB2
1000s ea.......... 62175-0260-43 2314.38 AB2
(USP,COATED)
60 mg, 90s ea........ 62175-0261-46 208.30 AB2
100s ea........... 62175-0261-37 231.44 AB2
300s ea........... 62175-0261-55 679.95 AB2
1000s ea.......... 62175-0261-43 2314.38 AB2
(COATED)
90 mg, 30s ea........ 62175-0262-32 79.87 AB2
(USP,COATED)
90 mg, 90s ea........ 62175-0262-46 239.63 AB2

(Letco)
POW, NA (U.S.P.)
5 gm............... 62991-1106-01 60.00
25 gm.............. 62991-1106-02 165.00

(Medisca)
POW, NA, 5 gm.......... 38779-0280-03 75.00
(U.S.P.)
25 gm.............. 38779-0280-04 201.00
100 gm............. 38779-0280-05 615.00
500 gm............. 38779-0280-08 2685.00

(Mylan) *See NIFEDIPINE ER*

(PCCA)
POW, NA, 1 gm.......... 51927-2311-00 17.40

(Pfizer) *See PROCARDIA*
(Pfizer) *See PROCARDIA XL*
(Schering) *See ADALAT CC*

(Spectrum Pharmacy)
POW, NA (U.S.P,MICRONIZED)
5 gm............... 49452-4852-01 119.00
(U.S.P.,MICRONIZED)
25 gm.............. 49452-4852-02 345.10
100 gm............. 49452-4852-03 822.50

(Teva) *See NIFEDIAC CC*
(Teva) *See NIFEDICAL XL*
(Teva) *See NIFENDIAC CC*

(UCB)
TER, PO (USP,COATED)
90 mg, 100s ea 62175-0262-37 267.00 AB2

(UDL) *See NIFEDIPINE ER*
(Watson Labs) *See AFEDITAB CR*

(A-S Medication)
REPACK
SGL, PO, 10 mg, 15s ea... 54569-3121-04 13.94 AB

PROD/MFR	NDC	AWP	DP	OBC
(Altura)				
REPACK				
SGL, PO, 10 mg, 8s ea	63874-0338-08	5.28		
10s ea	63874-0338-10	6.60		
12s ea	63874-0338-12	7.92		
15s ea	63874-0338-15	9.90		
20s ea	63874-0338-20	13.20		
30s ea	63874-0338-30	19.80		
50s ea	63874-0338-50	33.00		
60s ea	63874-0338-60	39.60		
90s ea	63874-0338-90	59.40		
100s ea	63874-0338-01	66.00		
300s ea	63874-0338-03	198.00		
TER, PO, 30 mg, 10s ea	63874-0582-10	26.70		AB1
14s ea	63874-0582-14	37.38		AB1
15s ea	63874-0582-15	40.05		AB1
20s ea	63874-0582-20	53.40		AB1
24s ea	63874-0582-24	64.08		AB1
30s ea	63874-0582-30	79.99		AB1
60s ea	63874-0582-60	160.20		AB1
100s ea	63874-0582-01	267.00		AB1
(American Health)				
REPACK				
TER, PO (10X10,FILM-COATED)				
30 mg, 100s ea UD	68084-0142-01	138.21		AB1
60 mg, 100s ea UD	68084-0143-01	209.09		AB1
(Bryant Ranch)				
REPACK				
SGL, PO, 10 mg, 20s ea	63629-1558-01	26.87		
30s ea	63629-1558-03	30.99		
90s ea	63629-1558-04	69.95		
100s ea	63629-1558-02	75.86		
TER, PO, 30 mg, 30s ea	63629-1559-01	57.31		
100s ea	63629-1559-02	191.04		
60 mg, 30s ea	63629-1560-01	97.20		
(Core)				
REPACK				
SGL, PO, 10 mg, 20s ea	33358-0261-20	27.54		
30s ea	33358-0261-30	31.76		
90s ea	33358-0261-90	71.70		
100s ea	33358-0261-00	77.76		
(DHS, Inc.)				
REPACK				
SGL, PO, 10 mg, 10s ea	55887-0668-10	7.50		
13s ea	55887-0668-13	9.75		
15s ea	55887-0668-15	11.25		
30s ea	55887-0668-30	22.50		
100s ea	55887-0668-01	60.00		
TER, PO, 30 mg, 15s ea	55887-0361-15	33.54		
60 mg, 90s ea	55887-0802-90	206.23		
(Nucare Pharm)				
REPACK				
SGL, PO, 10 mg, 10s ea	66267-0401-10	24.30		AB
(Palmetto)				
REPACK				
TER, PO, 30 mg, 30s ea	23490-5991-01	79.99		
60 mg, 30s ea	23490-5992-01	151.49		
(PD-Rx Pharm)				
REPACK				
SGL, PO (SOFTGEL)				
10 mg, ea	55289-0907-79	10.16		AB
8s ea	55289-0907-08	14.48		AB
(REDI-SCRIPT)				
10 mg, 20s ea	58864-0796-20	34.27		AB
(SOFTGEL)				
10 mg, 30s ea	55289-0907-30	46.82		AB
(REDI-SCRIPT)				
20 mg, 30s ea	58864-0797-30	29.07		AB
(Pharma Pac)				
REPACK				
SGL, PO, 10 mg, 8s ea	52959-0273-08	6.50		EE
10s ea	52959-0273-10	7.29		EE
30s ea	52959-0273-30	20.00		EE
20 mg, 30s ea	52959-0488-30	19.86		EE
TER, PO (FILM-COATED)				
30 mg, 60s ea	52959-0996-60	145.18		AB1
(Phys Total Care)				
REPACK				
SGL, PO (USP)				
10 mg, 15s ea	54868-1326-06	49.91		EE
20s ea	54868-1326-05	65.04		AB
30s ea	54868-1326-04	73.95		AB
60s ea	54868-1326-07	126.30		AB
100s ea	54868-1326-02	234.49		EE
20 mg, 30s ea	54868-1521-02	9.62		EE
60s ea	54868-1521-00	16.24		EE
TER, PO (FILM-COATED)				
60 mg, 60s ea	54868-4531-03	188.38		AB1
90s ea	54868-4531-04	262.66		AB1
(Physician Partner)				
REPACK				
TER, PO, 30 mg, 30s ea	21695-0776-30	80.21		AB2
(FILM-COATED)				
30 mg, 30s ea	21695-0908-30	83.64		AB1
60 mg, 30s ea	21695-0909-30	148.99		AB1
(Quality Care Prod)				
REPACK				
SGL, PO, 10 mg, 30s ea	49999-0161-28	56.20		AB
(Southwood)				
REPACK				
SGL, PO, 10 mg, 8s ea	58016-0622-08	5.03		EE
12s ea	58016-0622-12	7.27		EE
15s ea	58016-0622-15	9.09		EE
20s ea	58016-0622-20	12.12		EE
30s ea	58016-0622-30	18.17		EE
50s ea	58016-0622-50	30.29		EE
60s ea	58016-0622-60	36.35		EE
90s ea	58016-0622-90	54.52		EE
100s ea	58016-0622-00	60.58		EE
20 mg, 12s ea	58016-0620-12	13.08		EE
15s ea	58016-0620-15	16.35		EE
20s ea	58016-0620-20	21.80		EE
30s ea	58016-0620-30	32.70		EE
90s ea	58016-0620-90	98.10		EE
100s ea	58016-0620-00	109.01		EE
(Vibranta)				
REPACK				
TER, PO, 30 mg, 30s ea	57866-4068-01	57.36		
60 mg, 30s ea	57866-4069-01	111.13		
90 mg, 30s ea	57866-4070-01	132.33		
NIFEDIPINE ER (Mylan)				
nifedipine				
TER, PO, 30 mg, 100s ea	00378-3475-01	132.45		AB2
300s ea	00378-3475-30	389.40		AB2
60 mg, 100s ea	00378-3482-01	229.15		AB2
300s ea	00378-3482-30	674.00		AB2
90 mg, 100s ea	00378-3495-01	256.15		AB2
(UDL)				
TER, PO (10X10)				
30 mg, 100s ea UD	51079-0940-20	132.45		AB2
60 mg, 100s ea UD	51079-0968-20	229.15		AB2
90 mg, 100s ea UD	51079-0969-20	256.15		AB2
(A-S Medication)				
REPACK				
TER, PO, 30 mg, 30s ea	54569-5155-00	40.54		EE
60 mg, 30s ea	54569-5156-00	70.15		EE
90 mg, 30s ea	54569-5157-00	78.47		EE
(Core)				
REPACK				
TER, PO, 30 mg, 30s ea	33358-0262-30	58.74		
100s ea	33358-0262-00	195.82		
(Dispensing Solutions)				
REPACK				
TER, PO, 30 mg, 30s ea	66336-0683-30	50.23		AB2
60 mg, 30s ea	66336-0424-30	88.15		AB2
(PD-Rx Pharm)				
REPACK				
TER, PO, 30 mg, 7s ea	55289-0798-07	15.42		
14s ea	58864-0824-14	29.69		
30s ea	55289-0798-30	43.12		AB2
(REDI-SCRIPT)				
30 mg, 100s ea	58864-0824-01	152.82		
(Phys Total Care)				
REPACK				
TER, PO, 30 mg, 10s ea	54868-4532-01	28.82		AB1
30s ea	54868-4532-00	80.47		EE
60s ea	54868-4532-04	121.48		
90s ea	54868-4532-02	179.22		
100s ea	54868-4532-03	198.96		
60 mg, 10s ea	54868-4531-01	43.50		EE
30s ea	54868-4531-00	121.50		EE
100s ea	54868-4531-02	371.34		AB1
90 mg, 10s ea	54868-4875-01	81.00		AB2
30s ea	54868-4875-00	181.95		AB2
60s ea	54868-4875-02	341.01		AB2
(Quality Care Prod)				
REPACK				
TER, PO, 30 mg, 30s ea	49999-0357-30	95.05		AB2
60 mg, 30s ea	49999-0476-30	77.94		
NIFENDIAC CC (Teva)				
nifedipine				
TER, PO (FILM-COATED TABLET)				
90 mg, 100s ea UD	00093-1023-01	256.54		AB1
NIFEREX FORTE-150 (Phys Total Care)				
REPACK				
vitamin b complex, iron, and vitamin c				
CAP, PO, 10s ea	54868-2600-02	12.18		
30s ea	54868-2600-01	32.78		
NIFEREX GOLD (Ther-RX)				
multivitamin and iron				
TAB, PO (FILM-COATED)				
90s ea	64011-0162-26	94.79		
NIFEREX-150 (Ther-RX)				
ascorbic acid/iron/succinic acid				
CAP, PO, 50 mg-150 mg-50 mg,				
90s ea	64011-0163-26	123.34		
NIFEREX-150 FORTE (Ther-RX)				
fe/folic acid/succinic acid/vit b12/vit c				
CAP, PO, 90s ea	64011-0164-26	123.34		
(Phys Total Care)				
REPACK				
vitamin b complex, iron, and vitamin c				
CAP, PO, 60s ea	54868-2600-00	63.66		
NIFEREX-PN FORTE (Phys Total Care)				
prenatal vitamins				
TAB, PO, 30s ea	54868-4841-01	14.95		
100s ea	54868-4841-00	44.83		
NIKETHAMIDE				
(PCCA) *See DIETHYLNICOTINAMIDE (N,N)*				
NILANDRON (Sanofi-Aventis)				
nilutamide				
TAB, PO, 150 mg, 30s ea	00088-1111-14	490.97		
(Phys Total Care)				
REPACK				
TAB, PO, 150 mg, 30s ea	54868-5734-00	438.35		
NILOTINIB HYDROCHLORIDE				
(Novartis Pharm) *See TASIGNA*				
NILUTAMIDE				
(Sanofi-Aventis) *See NILANDRON*				
NIMBEX (Abbott Pharm)				
cisatracurium besylate				
SOL, IV (VIAL)				
2 mg/ml, 5 ml 10s (M.D.V.)	00074-4378-05	145.72	127.82	
2 mg/ml, 10 ml 10s (S.D.V.)	00074-4380-10	255.62	224.23	
10 mg/ml, 20 ml 10s	00074-4382-20	2760.32	2421.34	
NIMODIPINE				
(Bayer Corp.) *See NIMOTOP*				
(Caraco)				
SGL, PO (SOFTGEL)				
30 mg, 30s ea UD	57664-0135-64	287.43		AB
100s ea UD	57664-0135-65	915.45		AB
(Heritage)				
SGL, PO (SOFTGEL)				
30 mg, 30s ea UD	23155-0108-30	288.50		AB
100s ea UD	23155-0108-00	920.50		AB
(Teva)				
SGL, PO (SOFT GELATIN)				
30 mg, 30s ea UD	00555-0980-37	290.63		AB
100s ea UD	00555-0980-40	925.63		AB
NIMOTOP (Bayer Corp.)				
nimodipine				
SGL, PO, 30 mg,				
30s ea UD	00026-2855-70	310.04		
100s ea UD	00026-2855-48	987.44		
NIPENT (Hospira)				
pentostatin				
PDS, IV (SDV)				
10 mg, ea	00409-0801-01	2182.80	1909.95	
NIRAVAM (Azur Pharma, Inc.)				
alprazolam				
ODT, PO (ORANGE)				
0.25 mg, 100s ea, C-IV	00091-3321-01	242.78		
0.5 mg, 100s ea, C-IV	00091-3322-01	302.48		
1 mg, 100s ea, C-IV	00091-3323-01	403.57		
2 mg, 100s ea, C-IV	00091-3324-01	686.22		
(A-S Medication)				
REPACK				
ODT, PO (ORANGE)				
1 mg, ea, C-IV	54569-5787-00	2.80		

PROD/MFR	NDC	AWP	DP	OBC
(Core)				
REPACK				
ODT, PO, 0.25 mg,				
100s ea, C-IV	**33358-0263-00**	137.57		
0.5 mg,				
100s ea, C-IV	**33358-0264-00**	168.70		
NISOLDIPINE (Mylan)				
TER, PO (FILM-COATED)				
20 mg, 100s ea	**00378-2222-01**	255.86		
30 mg, 100s ea	**00378-2223-01**	278.84		
40 mg, 100s ea	**00378-2224-01**	278.84		
(Shionogi) *See SULAR*				
(Phys Total Care)				
REPACK				
TER, PO (FILM-COATED)				
40 mg, 10s ea	**54868-5931-00**	81.26		
30s ea	**54868-5931-01**	234.78		
NITAZOXANIDE				
(Romark) *See ALINIA*				
NITISINONE				
(Rare Disease) *See ORFADIN*				
NITRIC ACID				
(Baker, J.T.) *See NITRIC ACID 69%-70%*				
(Baker, J.T.) *See NITRIC ACID FUMING 90%*				
(Baker, J.T.) *See NITRIC ACID HUEY 65%*				
(Medisca)				
SOL, NA (1X500ML)				
500 ml	**38779-0580-08**	93.00		
(PCCA)				
LIQ, NA (A.C.S.)				
1 ml	**51927-3002-00**	0.48		
NITRIC ACID 69%-70% (Baker, J.T.)				
nitric acid				
LIQ, NA (N.F., A.C.S., GLASS)				
2500 ml	**10106-9607-04**	31.63		
NITRIC ACID FUMING 90% (Baker, J.T.)				
nitric acid				
LIQ, NA (A.C.S., REAGENT)				
500 ml	**10106-9624-02**	118.76		
2500 ml	**10106-9624-05**	210.48		
NITRIC ACID HUEY 65% (Baker, J.T.)				
nitric acid				
LIQ, NA (REAGENT)				
2500 ml	**10106-9597-04**	38.68		
NITRIC OXIDE				
(Ikaria / Ino) *See INOMAX*				
NITRO-BID (Savage)				
nitroglycerin				
OIN, TD (48X1GM)				
2%, 1 gm 48s	**00281-0326-08**	34.82		
(1X30GM)				
2%, 30 gm	**00281-0326-30**	8.48		
(1X60GM)				
2%, 60 gm	**00281-0326-60**	15.26		
(Phys Total Care)				
REPACK				
OIN, TP, 2%, 30 gm	**54868-2736-00**	5.58		
NITRO-DUR (Schering)				
nitroglycerin				
TDM, TD, 0.1 mg/hr,				
30s ea UD	**00085-3305-30**	102.01		AB1
0.2 mg/hr,				
30s ea UD	**00085-3310-30**	103.57		AB1
0.3 mg/hr,				
30s ea UD	**00085-3315-30**	116.04		
0.4 mg/hr,				
30s ea UD	**00085-3320-30**	116.04		AB1
0.6 mg/hr,				
30s ea UD	**00085-3330-30**	125.83		AB1
0.8 mg/hr,				
30s ea UD	**00085-0819-30**	125.83		BX
(Phys Total Care)				
REPACK				
TDM, TD, 0.1 mg/hr,				
30s ea	**54868-3633-00**	54.61		AB1
0.2 mg/hr, 30s ea	**54868-1289-01**	62.20		AB1
0.3 mg/hr, 30s ea	**54868-4426-00**	72.74		
0.8 mg/hr, 30s ea	**54868-5084-00**	103.89		BX
NITRO-TIME (Time-Cap)				
nitroglycerin				
CER, PO, 2.5 mg, 60s ea	**49483-0221-06**	11.35		
100s ea	**49483-0221-10**	13.62		
6.5 mg, 60s ea	**49483-0222-06**	13.68		
100s ea	**49483-0222-10**	18.24		
9 mg, 60s ea	**49483-0223-06**	15.18		
100s ea	**49483-0223-10**	21.42		

PROD/MFR	NDC	AWP	DP	OBC
NITROANILINE				
(Gallipot) *See 2-NITROANILINE*				
2-NITROANILINE (Gallipot)				
nitroaniline				
POW, NA (NON-STERILE)				
500 gm	**51552-0600-06**	219.94		
NITROFURANTOIN				
(Gallipot) *See NITROFURANTOIN ANHYDROUS*				
(Shionogi) *See FURADANTIN*				
(Spectrum Pharmacy) *See NITROFURANTOIN ANHYDROUS*				
NITROFURANTOIN (Teva)				
nitrofurantoin, macrocrystals				
CAP, PO (USP,MACROCRYSTAL)				
100 mg, 100s ea UD	**00093-2131-93**	186.37		AB
(Bryant Ranch)				
REPACK				
CAP, PO, 100 mg, 14s ea	**63629-1748-02**	25.90		
20s ea	**63629-1748-01**	37.00		
28s ea	**63629-1459-02**	98.32		
30s ea	**63629-1459-03**	98.32		
40s ea	**63629-1459-01**	109.32		
(Core)				
REPACK				
CAP, PO, 100 mg, 14s ea	**33358-0265-14**	36.50		
14s ea	**33358-0267-14**	47.69		
20s ea	**33358-0265-20**	37.93		
28s ea	**33358-0267-28**	90.27		
30s ea	**33358-0267-30**	96.35		
40s ea	**33358-0267-40**	126.76		
(Dispensing Solutions)				
REPACK				
CAP, PO, 100 mg, 14s ea	**66336-0008-14**	37.07		AB
28s ea	**66336-0008-28**	74.20		AB
NITROFURANTOIN (HomeMed)				
REPACK				
TAB, PO, 100 mg, 20s ea	**51655-0597-52**	52.04		
(Quality Care Prod)				
REPACK				
nitrofurantoin, macrocrystals				
CAP, PO, 100 mg, 20s ea	**49999-0210-20**	72.81		
28s ea	**49999-0210-28**	101.94		
NITROFURANTOIN ANHYDROUS (Gallipot)				
nitrofurantoin				
POW, NA (U.S.P.)				
25 gm	**51552-0566-04**	59.50		
(Spectrum Pharmacy)				
POW, NA (U.S.P.)				
25 gm	**49452-4856-04**	173.95		
100 gm	**49452-4856-01**	556.50	12.50	
NITROFURANTOIN MACROCRYSTALS (Medisca)				
nitrofurantoin, macrocrystals				
CRY, NA (ANHYDROUS, U.S.P.)				
5 gm	**38779-0539-03**	34.50		
25 gm	**38779-0539-04**	117.00		
100 gm	**38779-0539-05**	387.00		
POW, NA (U.S.P.)				
ea	**38779-0539-09**	1606.50		
(Mylan)				
CAP, PO, 50 mg, 100s ea	**00378-1650-01**	109.05		AB
500s ea	**00378-1650-05**	545.25		AB
100 mg, 100s ea	**00378-1700-01**	185.30		AB
500s ea	**00378-1700-05**	926.45		AB
(PCCA)				
CRY, NA (USP; ANHYDROUS)				
1 gm	**51927-2237-00**	6.60		
(Sandoz)				
CAP, PO (MONOHYDRATE)				
100 mg, 100s ea	**00185-0122-01**	203.75		AB
1000s ea	**00185-0122-10**	2037.50		AB
(Teva)				
CAP, PO (USP,GELCAP)				
50 mg, 100s ea	**00093-2130-01**	109.44		AB
(USP)				
50 mg, 100s ea UD	**00093-2130-93**	109.94		
(USP,GELCAP)				
50 mg, 1000s ea	**00093-2130-10**	1090.93		AB
100 mg, 100s ea	**00093-2131-01**	185.87		AB
1000s ea	**00093-2131-10**	1858.70		AB
(UDL)				
CAP, PO (10X10)				
50 mg, 100s ea UD	**51079-0584-20**	126.99	49.89	AB
100 mg, 100s ea UD	**51079-0585-20**	215.67	89.49	AB

PROD/MFR	NDC	AWP	DP	OBC
(A-S Medication)				
REPACK				
CAP, PO, 50 mg, 28s ea	**54569-0181-00**	30.64		EE
30s ea	**54569-0181-01**	32.83		EE
100 mg, 20s ea	**54569-1969-02**	37.17		EE
28s ea	**54569-1969-00**	52.04		EE
40s ea	**54569-1969-01**	74.35		EE
(PD-Rx Pharm)				
REPACK				
CAP, PO, 50 mg, 12s ea	**55289-0186-12**	31.95		AB
14s ea	**55289-0186-14**	36.00		AB
20s ea	**55289-0186-20**	48.00		AB
21s ea	**55289-0186-21**	50.13		AB
28s ea	**55289-0186-28**	64.47		AB
40s ea	**55289-0186-40**	89.61		AB
100 mg, 2s ea	**43063-0173-02**	17.43		AB
10s ea	**55289-0203-10**	36.78		AB
12s ea	**55289-0203-12**	48.87		AB
14s ea	**55289-0203-14**	94.17		AB
14s ea	**55289-0822-14**	70.77		AB
14s ea	**58864-0371-14**	87.80		AB
20s ea	**55289-0203-20**	102.24		AB
(REDI-SCRIPT)				
100 mg, 20s ea	**58864-0371-20**	102.24		AB
28s ea	**55289-0203-28**	135.30		AB
30s ea	**55289-0203-30**	143.58		AB
30s ea	**58864-0371-30**	143.58		AB
40s ea	**55289-0203-40**	184.89		AB
(Pharma Pac)				
REPACK				
CAP, PO, 50 mg, 30s ea	**52959-0406-30**	33.50		EE
100 mg, 8s ea	**52959-0405-08**	14.94		EE
10s ea	**52959-0405-10**	18.67		EE
10s ea	**52959-0783-10**	27.56		EE
14s ea	**52959-0405-14**	26.13		EE
14s ea	**52959-0783-14**	37.65		EE
15s ea	**52959-0405-15**	28.00		EE
16s ea	**52959-0405-16**	29.86		EE
20s ea	**52959-0405-20**	37.32		EE
21s ea	**52959-0405-21**	39.18		EE
28s ea	**52959-0405-28**	52.23		EE
30s ea	**52959-0405-30**	55.96		EE
40s ea	**52959-0405-40**	74.60		EE
100s ea	**52959-0405-00**	186.44		EE
(Phys Total Care)				
REPACK				
CAP, PO, 50 mg, 20s ea	**54868-0107-06**	53.49		EE
30s ea	**54868-0107-05**	53.49		AB
40s ea	**54868-0107-02**	80.22		EE
100s ea	**54868-0107-00**	187.98		AB
100 mg, 6s ea	**54868-0473-06**	27.93		EE
10s ea	**54868-0473-05**	44.55		AB
14s ea	**54868-0473-01**	61.14		EE
15s ea	**54868-0473-03**	65.31		EE
20s ea	**54868-0473-02**	86.07		EE
30s ea	**54868-0473-04**	98.28		AB
40s ea	**54868-0473-00**	130.05		EE
60s ea	**54868-0473-07**	213.09		EE
(Physician Partner)				
REPACK				
CAP, PO, 100 mg, 14s ea	**21695-0300-14**	67.07		
20s ea	**21695-0300-20**	95.88		
(Quality Care Prod)				
REPACK				
CAP, PO, 100 mg, 14s ea	**49999-0210-14**	50.97		AB
(Southwood)				
REPACK				
CAP, PO, 50 mg, 10s ea	**58016-0142-10**	7.15		EE
12s ea	**58016-0142-12**	8.58		EE
14s ea	**58016-0142-14**	10.01		EE
15s ea	**58016-0142-15**	10.73		EE
20s ea	**58016-0142-20**	14.31		EE
24s ea	**58016-0142-24**	17.17		EE
28s ea	**58016-0142-28**	20.03		EE
30s ea	**58016-0142-30**	21.46		EE
40s ea	**58016-0142-40**	29.76		EE
100s ea	**58016-0142-00**	71.53		EE
100 mg, 10s ea	**58016-0141-10**	12.14		EE
12s ea	**58016-0141-12**	14.57		EE
14s ea	**58016-0141-14**	17.00		EE
15s ea	**58016-0141-15**	18.21		EE
20s ea	**58016-0141-20**	24.28		EE
20s ea	**58016-0886-20**	36.54		AB
21s ea	**58016-0141-21**	25.50		EE
24s ea	**58016-0141-24**	29.14		EE
28s ea	**58016-0141-28**	34.00		EE
30s ea	**58016-0034-30**	55.76		EE
30s ea	**58016-0886-30**	54.81		AB
60s ea	**58016-0034-60**	111.52		EE
60s ea	**58016-0886-60**	109.63		AB

PROD/MFR	NDC	AWP	DP	OBC
90s ea	58016-0034-90	167.28		EE
90s ea	58016-0886-90	164.44		AB
100s ea	58016-0034-00	185.87		EE
100s ea	58016-0886-00	182.71		AB
(Vibranta)				
REPACK				
CAP, PO, 100 mg, 40s ea	57866-6590-03	68.43		
NITROFURANTOIN MONO/MACRO (HomeMed)				
REPACK				
nitrofurantoin monohydrate/nitrofurantoin, macro				
CAP, PO, 100 mg, 14s ea	51655-0593-84	87.80		
NITROFURANTOIN MONOHYDRATE (Dispensing Solutions)				
REPACK				
nitrofurantoin monohydrate/nitrofurantoin, macro				
CAP, PO (MACROCRYSTALS)				
100 mg, 14s ea	66336-0590-14	35.27		
20s ea	66336-0590-20	50.39		
NITROFURANTOIN MONOHYDRATE & MACROCRYSTALS (Dispensing Solutions)				
nitrofurantoin monohydrate/nitrofurantoin, macro				
CAP, PO, 100 mg, 14s ea	55045-3182-05	29.40		
NITROFURANTOIN MONOHYDRATE/ MACROCRYSTALS (Mylan)				
nitrofurantoin monohydrate/nitrofurantoin, macro				
CAP, PO, 100 mg, 100s ea	00378-3422-01	203.70		
(Ranbaxy Pharm)				
CAP, PO, 100 mg, 100s ea	63304-0518-01	203.70		AB
(UDL)				
CAP, PO (10X10,USP)				
100 mg, 100s ea UD	51079-0348-20	235.45		AB
(A-S Medication)				
REPACK				
CAP, PO, 100 mg, 10s ea	54569-5576-01	20.37		
14s ea	54569-5576-00	28.52		
(DHS, Inc.)				
REPACK				
CAP, PO, 100 mg, 6s ea	55887-0407-06	8.76		
14s ea	55887-0407-14	20.65		
(Palmetto)				
REPACK				
CAP, PO, 100 mg, 6s ea	23490-6840-01	15.96		
14s ea	23490-5994-01	26.60		
14s ea	23490-6840-02	26.60		
20s ea	23490-5994-00	38.00		
20s ea	23490-6840-03	38.00		
28s ea	23490-5994-02	53.20		
30s ea	23490-5994-03	57.00		
30s ea	23490-6840-04	57.00		
(PD-Rx Pharm)				
REPACK				
CAP, PO (REDI-SCRIPT)				
100 mg, 6s ea	55289-0822-06	40.38		
20s ea	55289-0822-20	93.66		AB
(Pharma Pac)				
REPACK				
CAP, PO, 100 mg, 20s ea	52959-0783-20	52.11		AB
(Stat Rx)				
REPACK				
CAP, PO, 100 mg, 14s ea	16590-0380-14	20.00		
NITROFURANTOIN MONOHYDRATE/ NITROFURANTOIN, MACRO				
(Mylan) *See NITROFURANTOIN MONOHYDRATE/MACROCRYSTALS*				
(P & G Pharm) *See MACROBID*				
(Ranbaxy Pharm) *See NITROFURANTOIN MONOHYDRATE/MACROCRYSTALS*				
(UDL) *See NITROFURANTOIN MONOHYDRATE/ MACROCRYSTALS*				
NITROFURANTOIN, MACROCRYSTALS				
(Medisca) *See NITROFURANTOIN MACROCRYSTALS*				
(Mylan) *See NITROFURANTOIN MACROCRYSTALS*				
(P & G Pharm) *See MACRODANTIN*				
(PCCA) *See NITROFURANTOIN MACROCRYSTALS*				
(Sandoz) *See NITROFURANTOIN MACROCRYSTALS*				
(Teva) *See NITROFURANTOIN*				
(Teva) *See NITROFURANTOIN MACROCRYSTALS*				
(UDL) *See NITROFURANTOIN MACROCRYSTALS*				
NITROFURAZONE (Consolidated Midland)				
OIN, TP, 0.2%, 30 gm	00223-4380-01	2.40		EE
454 gm	00223-4380-02	9.50		EE
(Gallipot)				
POW, NA (U.S.P.)				
25 gm	51552-0272-04	14.00		
100 gm	51552-0272-05	34.65		
(PCCA)				
POW, NA (U.S.P.)				
1 gm	51927-1638-00	1.20		
NITROGLYCERIN				
(3M Pharm) *See NITROGLYCERIN TRANSDERMAL SYSTEM*				
(Amer Regent)				
SOL, IV (S.D.V.,PF)				
5 mg/ml, 10 ml 25s	00517-4810-25	175.00		AP
(Glenmark Pharmaceuticals)				
TAB, SL, 0.3 mg, 100s ea	68462-0145-01	13.89		
0.4 mg, 25s ea	68462-0146-25	8.50		
100s ea	68462-0146-01	13.89		
(4X25)				
0.4 mg, 100s ea	68462-0146-45	30.30		
0.6 mg, 100s ea	68462-0147-01	13.89		
(Graceway) *See MINITRAN*				
(Graceway)				
TDM, TD (3.3 CM2)				
0.1 mg/hr, 30s ea	29336-0321-30	48.60		
(Hercon Labs) *See NITROGLYCERIN TRANSDERMAL SYSTEM*				
(Kremers Urban)				
TDM, TD (FILM)				
0.2 mg/hr,				
30s ea UD	62175-0123-01	25.44		AB1
0.4 mg/hr, 30s ea UD	62175-0124-01	30.63		AB1
(Major)				
CER, PO, 2.5 mg, 100s ea	00904-0643-60	14.23		
6.5 mg, 100s ea	00904-0644-60	19.75		
(Major) *See NITROGLYCERIN TRANSDERMAL SYSTEM*				
(Mylan) *See NITROGLYCERIN TRANSDERMAL SYSTEM*				
(Pfizer) *See NITROSTAT*				
(Sandoz) *See NITROGLYCERIN SLOCAPS*				
(Savage) *See NITRO-BID*				
(Schering) *See NITRO-DUR*				
(Sciele) *See NITROLINGUAL*				
(Shionogi) *See NITROLINGUAL*				
(Time-Cap) *See NITRO-TIME*				
(A-S Medication)				
REPACK				
TAB, SL, 0.4 mg, 25s ea	54569-5929-00	7.58		
100s ea	54569-4631-00	13.89		
(Altura)				
REPACK				
TAB, SL, 0.4 mg, 25s ea	63874-0466-25	1.77		
100s ea	63874-0466-01	7.10		
(Core)				
REPACK				
TAB, SL, 0.4 mg, 25s ea	33358-0268-25	8.57		
100s ea	33358-0268-00	12.87		
(DHS, Inc.)				
REPACK				
TDM, TD, 0.2 mg/hr, 30s ea	55887-0142-30	49.45		
(Dispensing Solutions)				
REPACK				
TAB, SL, 0.4 mg, 100s ea	55045-3504-01	10.00		
(Nucare Pharm)				
REPACK				
TAB, SL, 0.4 mg, 25s ea	68071-1330-05	10.57		
(Palmetto)				
REPACK				
TAB, SL, 0.4 mg, 25s ea	23490-6002-01	16.18		
100s ea	23490-6002-02	64.73		
(Phys Total Care)				
REPACK				
CER, PO, 2.5 mg, 100s ea	54868-1554-02	29.55		
6.5 mg, 60s ea	54868-0689-02	26.18		
100s ea	54868-0689-01	41.64		
TAB, SL, 0.4 mg, 100s ea	54868-6045-00	62.15		
TDM, TD, 0.1 mg/hr, 30s ea	54868-3115-00	68.31		
0.2 mg/hr, 30s ea	54868-2183-01	66.81		EE
0.4 mg/hr, 30s ea	54868-1992-01	72.57		EE
0.6 mg/hr, 30s ea	54868-2744-00	99.06		EE
(Physician Partner)				
REPACK				
TAB, SL, 0.4 mg, 100s ea	21695-0810-00	27.78		
(4X25)				
0.4 mg, 100s ea	21695-0697-25	36.48		
(Quality Care Prod)				
REPACK				
TAB, SL, 0.4 mg, 25s ea	49999-0384-25	19.42		
100s ea	49999-0384-00	77.68		
TDM, TD, 0.1 mg/hr, 30s ea	35356-0042-30	46.00		
(Southwood)				
REPACK				
TAB, SL, 0.4 mg, 25s ea	58016-0296-25	16.18		
25s ea	58016-0297-25	16.18		
30s ea	58016-0296-30	19.42		
60s ea	58016-0296-60	38.83		
90s ea	58016-0296-90	58.25		
100s ea	58016-0296-00	64.72		
120s ea	58016-0296-02	77.66		
NITROGLYCERIN DISTAL EXTENSION (Abbott Hosp)				
device				
DEV, NA (60",LOW ABSORPTION)				
48s ea	00074-1736-48	112.90	112.80	
NITROGLYCERIN PRIMARY PUMP (Abbott Hosp)				
kit, administration, intravenous				
DEV, NA (CONV PIN-OL)				
48s ea	00074-1772-78	624.38	624.48	
NITROGLYCERIN SLOCAPS (Sandoz)				
nitroglycerin				
CER, PO, 2.5 mg, 60s ea	00185-5174-60	16.60		
100s ea	00185-5174-01	27.66		
6.5 mg, 60s ea	00185-1235-60	43.16		
100s ea	00185-1235-01	71.93		
9 mg, 60s ea	00185-1217-60	59.75		
100s ea	00185-1217-01	99.59		
NITROGLYCERIN SR (Physician Partner)				
REPACK				
nitroglycerin				
CER, PO, 2.5 mg, 60s ea	21695-0635-60	25.64		
6.5 mg, 60s ea	21695-0636-60	27.82		
NITROGLYCERIN TRANSDERMAL SYSTEM (3M Pharm)				
nitroglycerin				
TDM, TD, 0.2 mg/hr,				
30s ea	00089-1302-30	50.40		AB1
0.4 mg/hr, 30s ea	00089-1303-30	55.80		AB1
0.6 mg/hr, 30s ea	00089-1304-30	59.40		AB1
(Hercon Labs)				
TDM, TD, 0.2 mg/hr,				
30s ea	49730-0111-30	49.45	18.70	AB2
0.4 mg/hr, 30s ea	49730-0112-30	56.30	20.16	AB2
0.6 mg/hr, 30s ea	49730-0113-30	61.90	29.40	AB2
(Major)				
TDM, TD, 0.2 mg/hr,				
30s ea	00904-5495-46	48.50		AB2
0.4 mg/hr, 30s ea	00904-5496-46	55.40		AB2
0.6 mg/hr, 30s ea	00904-5497-46	61.10		AB2
(Mylan)				
TDM, TD, 0.1 mg/hr,				
30s ea	00378-9102-93	47.40		AB2
0.2 mg/hr, 30s ea	00378-9104-93	48.50		AB2
0.4 mg/hr, 30s ea	00378-9112-93	55.40		AB2
0.6 mg/hr, 30s ea	00378-9116-93	61.10		AB2
NITROGLYCERINE (Phys Total Care)				
REPACK				
nitroglycerin				
SOL, IV (S.D.V.,25X10ML)				
5 mg/ml, 10 ml 25s	54868-5718-00	469.68		
NITROLINGUAL (Sciele)				
nitroglycerin				
SPR, SL (PUMPSPRAY,DUO PACK)				
0.4 mg/actuation,				
16.9 gm	59630-0300-26	260.75		
(Shionogi)				
SPR, SL (PUMP)				
0.4 mg/actuation,				
4.9 gm	59630-0300-65	135.99		
12 gm	59630-0300-20	233.49		
(A-S Medication)				
REPACK				
SPR, SL (PUMP)				
0.4 mg/actuation,				
12 ml	54569-4974-00	282.31		
(Dispensing Solutions)				
REPACK				
SPR, SL, 0.4 mg/actuation,				
12 ml	55045-3664-01	200.00		
(Phys Total Care)				
REPACK				
SPR, SL (PUMP)				
0.4 mg/actuation,				
12 ml	54868-2165-00	171.19		

PROD/MFR	NDC	AWP	DP	OBC
NITROPRESS (Hospira)				
sodium nitroprusside				
PDS, IV (MDV,FTV,LATEX-FREE)				
50 mg, ea	**00409-3024-01**	19.43	17.00	AP
(Phys Total Care)				
REPACK				
PDS, IV (VIAL, ADD-VANTAGE)				
50 mg, ea	**54868-3582-00**	5.11		AP
NITROQUICK (Phys Total Care)				
nitroglycerin				
TAB, SL (DYE-FREE)				
0.3 mg, 100s ea	**54868-4756-00**	16.02		
0.6 mg, 100s ea	**54868-4717-00**	20.55		
NITROSTAT (Pfizer)				
nitroglycerin				
TAB, SL, 0.3 mg, 100s ea	**00071-0417-24**	16.27	13.56	
0.4 mg, 100s ea	**00071-0418-24**	16.27	13.56	
(4X25)				
0.4 mg, 100s ea	**00071-0418-13**	35.48	29.57	
0.6 mg, 100s ea	**00071-0419-24**	16.27	13.56	
(A-S Medication)				
REPACK				
TAB, SL, 0.4 mg, 25s ea	**54569-2140-00**	9.24		
(Dispensing Solutions)				
REPACK				
TAB, SL, 0.4 mg, 100s ea	**55045-3510-01**	19.00		
(25X4)				
0.4 mg, 100s ea	**55045-3510-02**	33.00		
(PD-Rx Pharm)				
REPACK				
TAB, SL (USP,REDI-SCRIPT)				
0.4 mg, 100s ea	**58864-0967-01**	12.00		
(Phys Total Care)				
REPACK				
TAB, SL, 0.3 mg, 100s ea	**54868-1538-01**	11.31		
0.4 mg, 25s ea	**54868-0691-00**	13.08		
100s ea	**54868-0691-01**	46.44		
0.6 mg, 100s ea	**54868-1508-01**	11.64		
(Southwood)				
REPACK				
TAB, SL, 0.3 mg, 100s ea	**58016-5108-00**	6.76		
0.4 mg, 100s ea	**58016-5006-00**	8.69		
NIZATIDINE				
FUL				
CAP, PO, 150 mg, 60s ea		109.84		
300 mg, 30s ea		109.85		
(Amneal)				
SOL, PO (PEPPERMINT)				
15 mg/ml, 473 ml	**65162-0659-90**	347.65		AA
(Apotex Corp.)				
CAP, PO, 150 mg, 60s ea	**60505-0230-04**	142.99		AB
300 mg, 30s ea	**60505-0231-01**	142.98		AB
(Braintree) *See AXID*				
(Dr Reddy's)				
CAP, PO (HARD GELATIN)				
150 mg, 60s ea	**55111-0310-60**	143.28		AB
500s ea	**55111-0310-05**	1194.00		AB
300 mg, 30s ea	**55111-0311-30**	143.28		AB
(Glaxo) *See AXID*				
(Mylan)				
CAP, PO, 150 mg, 60s ea	**00378-5150-91**	143.65		AB
500s ea	**00378-5150-05**	1196.95		AB
300 mg, 30s ea	**00378-5300-93**	140.80		AB
(Sandoz)				
CAP, PO, 150 mg, 60s ea	**00185-0150-60**	143.79		AB
500s ea	**00185-0150-05**	1198.23		AB
300 mg, 30s ea	**00185-0300-30**	140.94		AB
100s ea	**00185-0300-01**	469.80		AB
(Teva)				
CAP, PO, 150 mg, 60s ea	**00093-1065-06**	142.98		AB
(10X10)				
150 mg, 100s ea UD	**00093-1065-93**	245.05		AB
500s ea	**00093-1065-05**	1191.55		AB
300 mg, 30s ea	**00093-1066-56**	142.98		
(Watson Labs)				
CAP, PO, 150 mg, 60s ea	**00591-3137-60**	142.99		AB
300 mg, 30s ea	**00591-3138-30**	142.99		AB
(A-S Medication)				
REPACK				
CAP, PO, 150 mg, 60s ea	**54569-5924-00**	143.79		AB
(Aidarex)				
REPACK				
CAP, PO, 150 mg, 10s ea	**33261-0086-10**	24.03		
14s ea	**33261-0086-14**	34.02		
20s ea	**33261-0086-20**	48.60		

PROD/MFR	NDC	AWP	DP	OBC
21s ea	**33261-0086-21**	51.03		
28s ea	**33261-0086-28**	68.04		
30s ea	**33261-0086-30**	72.90		
40s ea	**33261-0086-40**	97.20		
60s ea	**33261-0086-60**	146.00		
90s ea	**33261-0086-90**	218.99		
120s ea	**33261-0086-02**	291.99		
(Altura)				
REPACK				
CAP, PO, 150 mg, 60s ea	**63874-1216-06**	182.37		AB
(Bryant Ranch)				
REPACK				
CAP, PO, 150 mg, 60s ea	**63629-3639-01**	184.32		AB
(DHS, Inc.)				
REPACK				
CAP, PO, 150 mg, 15s ea	**55887-0153-15**	35.74		
30s ea	**55887-0153-30**	71.49		
60s ea	**55887-0153-60**	142.99		
90s ea	**55887-0153-90**	214.48		
100s ea	**55887-0153-01**	238.26		
120s ea	**55887-0153-82**	285.91		
150s ea	**55887-0153-86**	357.39		
300 mg, 30s ea	**55887-0154-30**	142.98		
60s ea	**55887-0154-60**	285.96		
90s ea	**55887-0154-90**	428.94		
100s ea	**55887-0154-01**	476.60		
120s ea	**55887-0154-82**	571.92		
150s ea	**55887-0154-86**	714.90		
(Dispensing Solutions)				
REPACK				
CAP, PO, 150 mg, 60s ea	**55045-3748-06**	144.60		
90s ea	**55045-3748-09**	216.90		
120s ea	**55045-3748-08**	289.20		
300 mg, 30s ea	**68258-3006-01**	142.15		AB
(Palmetto)				
REPACK				
CAP, PO, 150 mg, 60s ea	**23490-6010-06**	142.98		
300 mg, 60s ea	**23490-6011-06**	280.30		
(Pharma Pac)				
REPACK				
CAP, PO, 150 mg, 30s ea	**52959-0824-30**	91.06		
60s ea	**52959-0824-60**	182.37		
300 mg, 30s ea	**52959-0903-30**	143.70		
60s ea	**52959-0903-60**	281.20		AB
90s ea	**52959-0903-90**	388.80		
(Phys Total Care)				
REPACK				
CAP, PO, 150 mg, 60s ea	**54868-4643-00**	139.77		AB
100s ea	**54868-4643-01**	195.62		EE
(Physician Partner)				
REPACK				
CAP, PO, 150 mg, 14s ea	**21695-0375-14**	78.94		
28s ea	**21695-0375-28**	157.88		AB
60s ea	**21695-0375-60**	287.58		
(Southwood)				
REPACK				
CAP, PO, 150 mg, 30s ea	**58016-0726-30**	71.49		AB
60s ea	**58016-0726-60**	142.98		AB
90s ea	**58016-0726-90**	214.47		AB
100s ea	**58016-0726-00**	238.30		AB
120s ea	**58016-0726-02**	285.96		AB
150s ea	**58016-0726-03**	357.45		AB
300 mg, 30s ea	**58016-0660-30**	140.15		AB
60s ea	**58016-0660-60**	280.29		AB
90s ea	**58016-0660-90**	420.44		AB
100s ea	**58016-0660-00**	467.15		AB
120s ea	**58016-0660-02**	560.58		AB
150s ea	**58016-0660-03**	700.73		AB
(Stat Rx)				
REPACK				
CAP, PO, 150 mg, 30s ea	**16590-0741-30**	83.58		AB
56s ea	**16590-0741-56**	156.00		AB
NIZORAL (Janssen)				
ketoconazole				
SHA, TP, 2%, 120 ml	**50580-0380-08**	43.38	36.15	
(1X120ML)				
2%, 120 ml	**50458-0680-08**	43.38	36.15	AB
(A-S Medication)				
REPACK				
SHA, TP, 2%, 120 ml	**54569-3394-00**	42.04		
(Pharma Pac)				
REPACK				
TAB, PO, 200 mg, 14s ea	**52959-0197-14**	59.99		AB
20s ea	**52959-0197-20**	85.36		AB
30s ea	**52959-0197-30**	127.39		AB

PROD/MFR	NDC	AWP	DP	OBC
(Phys Total Care)				
REPACK				
CRE, TP, 2%, 15 gm	**54868-1879-01**	25.80		AB
30 gm	**54868-1879-02**	41.42		AB
60 gm	**54868-1879-03**	62.59		AB
SHA, TP, 2%, 120 ml	**54868-2239-00**	37.40		
(Southwood)				
REPACK				
CRE, TP, 2%, 15 gm	**58016-1051-01**	20.45		AB
30 gm	**58016-3181-01**	28.25		AB
TAB, PO, 200 mg, 20s ea	**58016-0168-20**	61.88		AB
30s ea	**58016-0168-30**	90.04		AB
NO DOLO (Clint)				
sodium thiosalicylate				
SOL, IM (VIAL)				
50 mg/ml, 30 ml	**55553-0009-30**	36.00		
NOCLOT-50 (Citra)				
citric acid/dextrose/sodium citrate				
SOL, NA (NOT FOR DIRECT IV INFUS)				
50 ml 12s	**23731-6051-05**	450.00	375.00	
NOHIST (Larken Labs, Inc.)				
cpm/phenyleph hcl				
TER, PO (CAPLET)				
8 mg-20 mg,				
100s ea	**68047-0160-01**	28.09		
NOHIST DMX (Larken Labs, Inc.)				
cpm/dm/phenyleph hcl				
TER, PO, 8 mg-30 mg-20 mg,				
100s ea	**68047-0167-01**	68.78		
NOHIST-EXT (Larken Labs, Inc.)				
chlorpheniramine maleate/methscopolamine nitrate				
TER, PO (CAPLET)				
8 mg-2.5 mg,				
100s ea	**68047-0161-01**	46.20		
NOHIST-PDX (Larken Labs, Inc.)				
cpm/dm/phenyleph hcl				
SOL, PO (1X30ML,AF,SF,CHERRY)				
30 ml	**68047-0015-30**	18.39		
NOHIST-PE (Larken Labs, Inc.)				
cpm/methscopolamine nitrate/phenyleph hcl				
SOL, PO (1X473ML,AF,SF,GRAPE)				
473 ml	**68047-0169-16**	42.73		
NOHIST-PLUS (Larken Labs, Inc.)				
cpm/methscopolamine nitrate/phenyleph hcl				
CTB, PO, 2 mg-1.25 mg-10 mg,				
100s ea	**68047-0166-01**	48.17		
TER, PO, 8 mg-2.5 mg-20 mg,				
100s ea	**68047-0163-01**	60.29		
NOHIST-PLUS JR (Larken Labs, Inc.)				
cpm/methscopolamine nitrate/phenyleph hcl				
TER, PO, 4 mg-1.25 mg-10 mg,				
100s ea	**68047-0165-01**	36.48		
NOLVADEX (AQ)				
REPACK				
tamoxifen citrate				
TAB, PO, 10 mg, 10s ea	**66105-0832-01**	40.60		
30s ea	**66105-0832-03**	121.80		
60s ea	**66105-0832-06**	243.60		
90s ea	**66105-0832-09**	365.40		
100s ea	**66105-0832-10**	406.00		
NOMUC-PE (Cypress Pharm)				
guaifenesin/pseudoephedrine hydrochloride				
CER, PO, 200 mg-60 mg,				
100s ea	**60258-0353-01**	44.44		
NONBAC (Truxton)				
acetaminophen/butalbital/caffeine				
TAB, PO, 325 mg-50 mg-40 mg,				
500s ea	**00463-6326-05**	35.40		EE
NONBREAKABLE CREAM BASE (Medisca)				
cream base				
CRE, NA (1X100GM)				
100 gm	**38779-2376-05**	28.50		
(1X500GM)				
500 gm	**38779-2376-08**	120.00		
(1X1000GM)				
1000 gm	**38779-2376-09**	210.00		
NONOXYNOL 9 (PCCA)				
SOL, NA, 1 ml	**51927-1894-00**	0.47		
(Spectrum Pharmacy)				
SOL, NA (1X100ML, USP)				
100 ml	**49452-4861-01**	123.90		
(1X500ML, USP)				
500 ml	**49452-4861-02**	237.65		

PROD/MFR	NDC	AWP	DP	OBC
NOR-QD (Watson)				
norethindrone				
TAB, PO (6X28)				
0.35 mg, 168s ea	52544-0235-28	375.67		
(Phys Total Care)				
REPACK				
TAB, PO (1X28)				
0.35 mg, ea	54868-4712-00	50.19		AB1
NORA-BE (Watson)				
norethindrone				
TAB, PO (6X28)				
0.35 mg, 168s ea	52544-0629-28	221.52		
NORCO (Watson)				
acetaminophen/hydrocodone bitartrate				
TAB, PO, 325 mg-5 mg,				
100s ea, C-III	52544-0913-01	119.16		AA
325 mg-7.5 mg,				
100s ea, C-III	52544-0729-01	138.06		AA
325 mg-10 mg,				
100s ea, C-III	52544-0539-01	191.11		AA
500s ea, C-III	52544-0539-05	910.18		AA
(A-S Medication)				
REPACK				
TAB, PO, 325 mg-7.5 mg,				
30s ea, C-III	54569-5305-00	41.09		AA
(PD-Rx Pharm)				
REPACK				
TAB, PO, 325 mg-5 mg,				
15s ea, C-III	55289-0894-15	33.00		AA
325 mg-10 mg,				
30s ea, C-III	55289-0651-30	59.53		AA
(Pharma Pac)				
REPACK				
TAB, PO, 325 mg-10 mg,				
24s ea, C-III	52959-0533-24	22.35		AA
30s ea, C-III	52959-0533-30	27.90		AA
40s ea, C-III	52959-0533-40	36.80		AA
(Phys Total Care)				
REPACK				
TAB, PO, 325 mg-7.5 mg,				
100s ea, C-III	54868-5321-00	110.94		AA
325 mg-10 mg,				
10s ea, C-III	54868-4034-02	19.00		AA
30s ea, C-III	54868-4034-00	53.26		AA
100s ea, C-III	54868-4034-01	163.03		AA
500s ea, C-III	54868-4034-03	638.41		AA
(Quality Care Prod)				
REPACK				
TAB, PO, 325 mg-7.5 mg,				
30s ea, C-III	35356-0451-30	83.10		AA
90s ea, C-III	35356-0451-90	249.30		AA
325 mg-10 mg,				
20s ea, C-III	49999-0019-20	55.20		AA
30s ea, C-III	49999-0019-30	182.80		AA
90s ea, C-III	49999-0019-90	365.60		AA
(Southwood)				
REPACK				
TAB, PO, 325 mg-5 mg,				
6s ea, C-III	58016-0662-06	6.48		AA
9s ea, C-III	58016-0662-09	9.73		AA
10s ea, C-III	58016-0662-10	10.81		AA
12s ea, C-III	58016-0662-12	12.97		AA
14s ea, C-III	58016-0662-14	15.13		AA
15s ea, C-III	58016-0662-15	16.21		AA
16s ea, C-III	58016-0662-16	17.29		AA
18s ea, C-III	58016-0662-18	19.45		AA
20s ea, C-III	58016-0662-20	21.62		AA
21s ea, C-III	58016-0662-21	22.70		AA
24s ea, C-III	58016-0662-24	25.94		AA
25s ea, C-III	58016-0662-25	27.02		AA
28s ea, C-III	58016-0662-28	30.26		AA
30s ea, C-III	58016-0662-30	32.42		AA
40s ea, C-III	58016-0662-40	43.23		AA
42s ea, C-III	58016-0662-42	45.39		AA
45s ea, C-III	58016-0662-45	48.64		AA
50s ea, C-III	58016-0662-50	54.04		AA
56s ea, C-III	58016-0662-56	60.52		AA
60s ea, C-III	58016-0662-60	64.85		AA
75s ea, C-III	58016-0662-75	81.06		AA
80s ea, C-III	58016-0662-80	86.46		AA
84s ea, C-III	58016-0662-84	90.79		AA
90s ea, C-III	58016-0662-90	97.27		AA
100s ea, C-III	58016-0662-00	108.08		AA
112s ea, C-III	58016-0662-92	121.05		AA
120s ea, C-III	58016-0662-02	129.70		AA
180s ea, C-III	58016-0662-99	194.54		AA
240s ea, C-III	58016-0662-04	259.39		AA
325 mg-7.5 mg,				
6s ea, C-III	58016-0632-06	7.51		AA
9s ea, C-III	58016-0632-09	11.27		AA
10s ea, C-III	58016-0632-10	12.52		AA
12s ea, C-III	58016-0632-12	15.03		AA
14s ea, C-III	58016-0632-14	17.53		AA
15s ea, C-III	58016-0632-15	18.78		AA
16s ea, C-III	58016-0632-16	20.04		AA
18s ea, C-III	58016-0632-18	22.54		AA
20s ea, C-III	58016-0632-20	25.04		AA
21s ea, C-III	58016-0632-21	26.30		AA
24s ea, C-III	58016-0632-24	30.05		AA
25s ea, C-III	58016-0632-25	31.31		AA
28s ea, C-III	58016-0632-28	35.06		AA
30s ea, C-III	58016-0632-30	37.57		AA
40s ea, C-III	58016-0632-40	50.09		AA
42s ea, C-III	58016-0632-42	52.59		AA
45s ea, C-III	58016-0632-45	56.35		AA
50s ea, C-III	58016-0632-50	62.61		AA
56s ea, C-III	58016-0632-56	70.12		AA
60s ea, C-III	58016-0632-60	75.13		AA
75s ea, C-III	58016-0632-75	93.92		AA
80s ea, C-III	58016-0632-80	100.18		AA
84s ea, C-III	58016-0632-84	105.18		AA
90s ea, C-III	58016-0632-90	112.70		AA
100s ea, C-III	58016-0632-00	125.22		AA
112s ea, C-III	58016-0632-92	140.25		AA
120s ea, C-III	58016-0632-02	150.26		AA
180s ea, C-III	58016-0632-99	225.40		AA
240s ea, C-III	58016-0632-04	300.53		AA
325 mg-10 mg,				
30s ea, C-III	58016-0845-30	51.98		AA
60s ea, C-III	58016-0845-60	103.95		AA
90s ea, C-III	58016-0845-90	155.93		AA
100s ea, C-III	58016-0845-00	173.25		AA
(Stat Rx)				
REPACK				
TAB, PO, 325 mg-10 mg,				
112s ea, C-III	16590-0880-73	237.04		AA
NORDETTE-28 (Teva)				
ethinyl estradiol/levonorgestrel				
TAB, PO (PILPAK,6X28)				
30 mcg-0.15 mg,				
168s ea	51285-0091-58	441.00		AB
(Phys Total Care)				
REPACK				
TAB, PO (PILPAK, 1X28)				
30 mcg-0.15 mg,				
28s ea	54868-0507-00	60.79		AB
NORDIPEN 15 DELIVERY SYSTEM (Novo Nordisk)				
injector, medication (inoculator)				
DEV, NA (GROWTH HORMONE)				
ea	00169-7764-13	60.00		
NORDIPEN 5 DELIVERY SYSTEM (Novo Nordisk)				
injector, medication (inoculator)				
DEV, NA (GROWTH HORMONE)				
ea	00169-7764-11	60.00		
NORDITROPIN (Novo Nordisk)				
somatropin, e-coli derived				
SOL, SC (CARTRIDGE)				
5 mg/1.5 ml,				
1.5 ml	00169-7768-11	374.46		
(CARTRIDGE,GREEN)				
15 mg/1.5 ml,				
1.5 ml	00169-7770-11	1123.38		
NORDITROPIN NORDIFLEX (Novo Nordisk)				
somatropin, e-coli derived				
SOL, SC (PEN, ORANGE)				
5 mg/1.5 ml,				
1.5 ml	00169-7704-11	374.46		
(PEN,BLUE)				
10 mg/1.5 ml,				
1.5 ml	00169-7705-11	748.92		
(PEN,GREEN)				
15 mg/1.5 ml,				
1.5 ml	00169-7708-11	1123.38		
(1X3ML)				
30 mg/3 ml, 3 ml	00169-7703-11	2246.76		EE
NOREL SR (U.S. Pharm)				
apap/cpm/phenyleph hcl/phenyltoloxamine cit				
TER, PO, 325 mg-8 mg-40 mg-50 mg,				
100s ea	52747-0420-70	94.01		
NOREPHEDRINE (PCCA)				
phenylpropanolamine, l-				
POW, NA (1R,2S)				
1 gm	51927-3183-00	54.00		
NOREPINEPHRINE (Phys Total Care)				
REPACK				
norepinephrine bitartrate				
SOL, IV (10X4ML)				
1 mg/ml, 4 ml 10s	54868-5721-00	174.60		
NOREPINEPHRINE BITARTRATE (Bedford)				
SOL, IV (VIAL)				
1 mg/ml, 4 ml 10s	55390-0002-10	55.20		AP
(Hospira) *See LEVOPHED*				
(Hospira) *See LEVOPHED BITARTRATE*				
(Teva)				
SOL, IV (U.S.P.)				
1 mg/ml, 4 ml 10s	00703-1153-03	38.40		AP
NORETHINDRONE				
(Ortho-McNeil Pharm) *See ORTHO MICRONOR*				
(PCCA)				
POW, NA (U.S.P.)				
1 gm	51927-3623-00	288.00		
(Teva) *See CAMILA*				
(Teva) *See ERRIN*				
(Watson) *See JOLIVETTE*				
(Watson) *See NOR-QD*				
(Watson) *See NORA-BE*				
NORETHINDRONE (Core)				
REPACK				
norethindrone acetate				
TAB, PO, 5 mg, 50s ea	33358-0269-50	123.77		
(DHS, Inc.)				
REPACK				
TAB, PO, 5 mg, 30s ea	55887-0782-30	133.32		
NORETHINDRONE (Southwood)				
REPACK				
TAB, PO, 0.35 mg, 6s ea	58016-4827-01	221.52		
NORETHINDRONE ACETATE (Gallipot)				
POW, NA (U.S.P.)				
100 gm	51552-1055-09	46.34	33.10	
(Teva) *See AYGESTIN*				
(Teva)				
TAB, PO, 5 mg, 50s ea	00555-0211-10	129.26		AB
(Phys Total Care)				
REPACK				
TAB, PO, 5 mg, 10s ea	54868-4829-00	69.96		AB
20s ea	54868-4829-01	104.58		AB
30s ea	54868-4829-02	154.65		AB
NORETHINDRONE ACETATE MICRONIZED (PCCA)				
norethindrone acetate, micronized				
POW, NA (USP)				
1 gm	51927-2832-00	252.00		
NORETHINDRONE ACETATE, MICRONIZED				
(PCCA) *See NORETHINDRONE ACETATE MICRONIZED*				
NORETHINDRONE MICRONIZED (PCCA)				
norethindrone, micronized				
POW, NA (USP)				
1 gm	51927-3118-00	276.00		
NORETHINDRONE, MICRONIZED				
(PCCA) *See NORETHINDRONE MICRONIZED*				
NORETHINDRONE/ETH ESTRADIOL (DHS, Inc.)				
REPACK				
ethinyl estradiol/norethindrone				
TAB, PO (6X28)				
35 mcg-1 mg,				
168s ea	55887-0286-28	170.00		
NORFLEX (Graceway)				
orphenadrine citrate				
SOL, IJ (AMP)				
30 mg/ml, 2 ml 6s	00089-0540-06	171.72		AP
(Nucare Pharm)				
REPACK				
TER, PO, 100 mg, 14s ea	66267-0157-14	36.95		AB
20s ea	66267-0157-20	54.47		AB
(Pharma Pac)				
REPACK				
SOL, IJ, 30 mg/ml, 2 ml	52959-0179-06	103.25		AP
TER, PO, 100 mg, 10s ea	52959-0178-10	26.66		AB
14s ea	52959-0178-14	36.39		AB
15s ea	52959-0178-15	38.89		AB
20s ea	52959-0178-20	55.09		AB
30s ea	52959-0178-30	75.75		AB
(Phys Total Care)				
REPACK				
TER, PO, 100 mg, 15s ea	54868-1056-03	44.12		AB
20s ea	54868-1056-01	58.21		AB
30s ea	54868-1056-04	81.69		AB
50s ea	54868-1056-05	134.89		AB
100s ea	54868-1056-00	267.28		AB

PROD/MFR	NDC	AWP	DP	OBC
NORFLOXACIN				
(Merck) *See NOROXIN*				
NORGESIC FORTE (PD-Rx Pharm)				
REPACK				
aspirin/caffeine/orphenadrine citrate				
TAB, PO (CAPLET)				
770 mg-60 mg-50 mg,				
20s ea	55289-0846-20	55.83		AB
(Phys Total Care)				
REPACK				
TAB, PO, 770 mg-60 mg-50 mg,				
10s ea	54868-1101-00	24.36		AB
(CAPLET)				
770 mg-60 mg-50 mg,				
20s ea	54868-1101-02	46.84		AB
30s ea	54868-1101-03	69.33		AB
100s ea	54868-1101-04	226.70		AB
NORGESTREL/ETHINYL ESTRADIOL (Rouses)				
ethinyl estradiol/norgestrel				
TAB, PO, 30 mcg-0.3 mg,				
168s ea	24090-0961-84	164.74		
(Bryant Ranch)				
REPACK				
TAB, PO, 50 mcg-0.5 mg,				
4s ea	63629-2666-01	43.96		
NORINYL 1/35 (Watson)				
ethinyl estradiol/norethindrone				
TAB, PO (WALLETTE, 6X28)				
35 mcg-1 mg,				
168s ea	52544-0259-28	290.02		AB
(Phys Total Care)				
REPACK				
TAB, PO, 35 mcg-1 mg,				
28s ea	54868-0442-00	47.72		AB
NORINYL 1/50 (Watson)				
mestranol/norethindrone				
TAB, PO (3X28)				
0.05 mg-1 mg,				
84s ea	52544-0265-31	145.01		AB
NORIT A (Amend)				
activated charcoal				
POW, NA (N.F.)				
454 gm	17317-1345-01	84.00		
NORITATE (Dermik)				
metronidazole				
CRE, TP, 1%, 60 gm	00066-9850-60	150.42		
(Phys Total Care)				
REPACK				
CRE, TP, 1%, 30 gm	54868-4449-00	62.69		
60 gm	54868-4449-01	165.32		
NORMAL SALINE FLUSH (BD Dickinson Hosp Prod)				
sodium chloride				
SOL, IV (2ML SRN, 30X2ML,PF)				
0.9%, 2 ml 30s	08290-0910-02	17.10		
(3ML SRN,30X2ML,PF)				
0.9%, 2 ml 30s	08290-0310-02	18.00		
(SRN, W/CANNULA,30X2ML)				
0.9%, 2 ml 30s	08290-0911-02	23.06		
(10ML SRN,30X3ML,PF)				
0.9%, 3 ml 30s	08290-0330-03	20.10		
(3ML SRN, 30X3ML,PF)				
0.9%, 3 ml 30s	08290-0910-03	17.70		
(3ML SRN,30X3ML,PF)				
0.9%, 3 ml 30s	08290-0310-03	18.00		
(5ML SRN, 30X3ML,PF)				
0.9%, 3 ml 30s	08290-0320-03	18.90		AP
(SRN,3ML W/CANNULA,PF)				
0.9%, 3 ml 30s	08290-0311-03	24.53		
(SRN,W/CANNULA,30X3ML,PF)				
0.9%, 3 ml 30s	08290-0911-03	23.42		
(10ML SRN, 30X5ML,PF)				
0.9%, 5 ml 30s	08290-0330-05	20.10		
(5ML SRN, 30X5ML,PF)				
0.9%, 5 ml 30s	08290-0920-05	18.00		
(5ML SRN,30X5ML,PF)				
0.9%, 5 ml 30s	08290-0320-05	18.90		
(SRN, 10ML W/ CANN,PF)				
0.9%, 5 ml 30s	08290-0331-05	26.70		
(SRN, W/CANNULA, 30X5ML)				
0.9%, 5 ml 30s	08290-0921-05	23.78		
(SRN,5ML W/CANNULA,PF)				
0.9%, 5 ml 30s	08290-0321-05	25.65		
(10ML SRN, 10MLX30,PF)				
0.9%, 10 ml 30s	08290-0930-10	18.30		
(10ML SRN,30X10ML,PF)				
0.9%, 10 ml 30s	08290-0330-10	20.10		
(REG LENGTH PLUNGER ROD)				
0.9%, 10 ml 30s	08290-0940-10	18.30		
(SRN, 10ML W/CANN,PF)				
0.9%, 10 ml 30s	08290-0331-10	26.70		
(SRN,W/CANNULA,30X10ML)				
0.9%, 10 ml 30s	08290-0941-10	24.15		
(Medefil)				
SOL, IV (SRN,6 ML W/LUER LOCK,PF)				
0.9%, 1 ml	64253-0111-21	2.41		
2 ml	64253-0111-22	2.65		
(SRN,12 ML W/LUER LOK,PF)				
0.9%, 3 ml	64253-0111-33	3.09		
(SRN,6 ML W/LUER LOCK,PF)				
0.9%, 3 ml	64253-0111-23	2.79		
(SRN,12 ML W/LUER LOK,PF)				
0.9%, 5 ml	64253-0111-35	3.41		
(SRN,6 ML W/LUER LOCK,PF)				
0.9%, 5 ml	64253-0111-25	3.19		
(SRN W/LUER LOCK,PF)				
0.9%, 10 ml	64253-0111-30	3.65		
NORMAL SALINE IV FLUSH SYRINGE (Sierra)				
sodium chloride				
SOL, IV (PF)				
0.9%, 2 ml UD	64054-0902-03	3.10	3.10	
3 ml UD	64054-0903-02	3.10	3.10	
3 ml UD	64054-0903-06	3.10	3.10	
5 ml UD	64054-0905-02	3.10	3.10	
5 ml UD	64054-0905-06	3.10	3.10	
10 ml UD	64054-0910-02	3.10	3.10	
NORMODYNE (Phys Total Care)				
REPACK				
labetalol hydrochloride				
TAB, PO, 200 mg, 60s ea	54868-1004-01	59.80		AB
NORMOSOL-M W/5% DEXTROSE (Hospira)				
dextrose/k ace/mg ace/na cl				
SOL, IV (LIFECARE,LATEX-FREE)				
500 ml 24s	00409-7965-03	102.24	89.52	EE
1000 ml 12s	00409-7965-09	36.58	32.04	EE
NORMOSOL-R (Hospira)				
k cl/mg cl/na ace/na cl/na gluconate				
SOL, IV (LIFECARE,LATEX-FREE)				
500 ml 24s	00409-7967-03	98.21	85.92	
1000 ml 12s	00409-7967-09	37.87	33.12	
NORMOSOL-R PH 7.4 (Hospira)				
k cl/mg cl/na ace/na cl/na gluconate				
SOL, IV (LIFECARE,24X500ML)				
500 ml 24s	00409-7670-03	120.38	105.36	
(12X1000ML,LIFECARE,USP)				
1000 ml 12s	00409-7670-09	49.10	42.96	EE
(LIFECARE,LATEX-FREE)				
1000 ml 12s	00074-7670-09	40.06	35.05	
NORMOSOL-R W/5% DEXTROSE (Hospira)				
dextrose/k cl/mg cl/na ace/na cl/na gluconate				
SOL, IV (LIFECARE,LATEX-FREE)				
1000 ml 12s	00409-7968-09	36.58	32.04	
NOROXIN (Merck)				
norfloxacin				
TAB, PO (UNIT OF USE)				
400 mg, 20s ea	00006-0705-20	83.17		
100s ea	00006-0705-68	409.82		
(Phys Total Care)				
REPACK				
TAB, PO, 400 mg, 10s ea	54868-0889-00	49.31		
15s ea	54868-0889-05	69.09		
20s ea	54868-0889-01	91.49		
40s ea	54868-0889-03	181.10		
NORPACE (Pfizer)				
disopyramide phosphate				
CAP, PO, 100 mg, 100s ea	00025-2752-31	158.40	132.00	AB
150 mg, 100s ea	00025-2762-31	187.15	155.96	AB
NORPACE CR (Pfizer)				
disopyramide phosphate				
CER, PO, 100 mg, 100s ea	00025-2732-31	190.81	159.01	AB
500s ea	00025-2732-51	954.07	795.06	AB
150 mg, 100s ea	00025-2742-31	225.53	187.94	AB
500s ea	00025-2742-51	1127.64	939.70	AB
(Phys Total Care)				
REPACK				
CER, PO, 150 mg, 100s ea	54868-0692-00	177.83		AB
NORPRAMIN (Sanofi-Aventis)				
desipramine hydrochloride				
TAB, PO, 10 mg, 100s ea	00068-0007-01	102.76		AB
25 mg, 100s ea	00068-0011-01	123.44		AB
50 mg, 100s ea	00068-0015-01	232.40		AB
75 mg, 100s ea	00068-0019-01	295.79		AB
100 mg, 100s ea	00068-0020-01	388.70		AB
150 mg, 50s ea	00068-0021-50	281.60		AB
NORTHYX (Centrix)				
methimazole				
TAB, PO, 5 mg, 100s ea	11528-0300-01	28.80		
10 mg, 100s ea	11528-0310-01	47.10		
15 mg, 100s ea	11528-0320-01	81.90		
20 mg, 100s ea	11528-0330-01	94.20		
NORTREL (Teva)				
ethinyl estradiol/norethindrone				
TAB, PO (3X28)				
35 mcg-0.5 mg,				
84s ea	00555-9008-67	96.52		AB
(3X21)				
35 mcg-1 mg,				
63s ea	00555-9009-42	88.50		AB
(6X28)				
35 mcg-1 mg,				
168s ea	00555-9010-58	176.99		AB
(Phys Total Care)				
REPACK				
TAB, PO, 35 mcg-1 mg,				
28s ea	54868-4776-00	62.73		AB
(Quality Care Prod)				
REPACK				
TAB, PO, 35 mcg-1 mg,				
168s ea	35356-0014-68	212.40		
NORTREL 7/7/7 (Teva)				
ethinyl estradiol/norethindrone				
TAB, PO (28 DAY REGIMEN)				
168s ea	00555-9012-58	193.38		AB
(Phys Total Care)				
REPACK				
TAB, PO, 28s ea	54868-5286-00	79.44		AB
NORTRIPTYLINE (Bryant Ranch)				
REPACK				
nortriptyline hydrochloride				
CAP, PO, 10 mg, 30s ea	63629-3204-01	15.32		
(Core)				
REPACK				
CAP, PO, 10 mg, 30s ea	33358-0270-30	15.70		
60s ea	33358-0270-60	28.89		
90s ea	33358-0270-90	56.62		
25 mg, 30s ea	33358-0271-30	37.72		
60s ea	33358-0271-60	76.47		
120s ea	33358-0271-01	108.04		
(IPI)				
REPACK				
CAP, PO, 25 mg, 30s ea	18837-0114-30	28.50		
60s ea	18837-0114-60	58.26		
(PD-Rx Pharm)				
REPACK				
CAP, PO (USP)				
10 mg, 30s ea	55289-0586-30	20.00		
(Stat Rx)				
REPACK				
CAP, PO, 75 mg, 30s ea	16590-0510-30	76.00		
60s ea	16590-0510-60	152.00		
90s ea	16590-0510-90	228.00		
120s ea	16590-0510-72	260.00		
TAB, PO, 25 mg, 30s ea	16590-0171-30	35.00		
60s ea	16590-0171-60	70.00		
90s ea	16590-0171-90	105.00		
NORTRIPTYLINE HCL (Mylan)				
nortriptyline hydrochloride				
CAP, PO, 75 mg, 100s ea	00378-4175-01	247.30		AB
(PCCA)				
POW, NA (U.S.P.)				
1 gm	51927-2175-00	19.80		
(Pharm Assoc Inc)				
SOL, PO (CHERRY)				
10 mg/5 ml, 473 ml	00121-0678-16	182.95		AA
(Ranbaxy Pharm)				
SOL, PO, 10 mg/5 ml,				
473 ml	63304-0202-01	55.50		AA
(Spectrum Pharmacy)				
CRY, NA (U.S.P.)				
5 gm	49452-4858-01	155.05		
25 gm	49452-4858-02	626.50		
(Taro)				
CAP, PO, 10 mg, 90s ea	51672-4001-05	34.70		AB
25 mg, 90s ea	51672-4002-05	70.58		AB
50 mg, 90s ea	51672-4003-05	128.11		AB
75 mg, 90s ea	51672-4004-05	194.20		AB
(Watson Labs)				
CAP, PO, 10 mg, 100s ea	00591-5786-01	40.50		AB
500s ea	00591-5786-05	173.00		AB
25 mg, 100s ea	00591-5787-01	80.31		AB

PROD/MFR	NDC	AWP	DP	OBC
500s ea	00591-5787-05	374.34		AB
1000s ea	00591-5787-10	643.43		AB
50 mg, 100s ea	00591-5788-01	151.80		AB
500s ea	00591-5788-05	645.18		AB
75 mg, 100s ea	00591-5789-01	221.36		AB
(A-S Medication)				
REPACK				
CAP, PO, 10 mg, 30s ea	54569-4146-01	12.15		EE
60s ea	54569-4146-00	24.30		EE
25 mg, 15s ea	54569-3849-01	12.05		AB
30s ea	54569-3849-00	24.09		AB
(Aidarex)				
REPACK				
CAP, PO, 10 mg, 30s ea	33261-0532-30	39.50		AB
60s ea	33261-0532-60	79.00		AB
90s ea	33261-0532-90	118.50		AB
120s ea	33261-0532-02	158.00		AB
25 mg, 7s ea	33261-0348-07	11.20		AB
14s ea	33261-0348-14	22.40		AB
20s ea	33261-0348-20	32.00		AB
28s ea	33261-0348-28	44.80		AB
30s ea	33261-0348-30	48.00		AB
60s ea	33261-0348-60	96.00		AB
90s ea	33261-0348-90	144.00		AB
120s ea	33261-0348-02	192.00		AB
(Altura)				
REPACK				
CAP, PO, 10 mg, 30s ea	63874-1033-03	14.10		AB
60s ea	63874-1033-06	28.20		AB
100s ea	63874-1033-01	47.00		AB
120s ea	63874-1033-04	56.40		AB
25 mg, 14s ea	63874-0580-14	16.24		AB
15s ea	63874-0580-15	17.40		AB
20s ea	63874-0580-20	23.20		AB
30s ea	63874-0580-30	34.80		AB
60s ea	63874-0580-60	69.60		AB
90s ea	63874-0580-90	104.40		AB
100s ea	63874-0580-01	116.00		AB
50 mg, 60s ea	63874-1079-06	104.02		AB
75 mg, 100s ea	63874-1081-01	260.99		AB
(American Health)				
REPACK				
CAP, PO (10X10)				
10 mg, 100s ea UD	68084-0031-01	44.12		AB
25 mg, 100s ea UD	68084-0032-01	88.24		AB
(DHS, Inc.)				
REPACK				
CAP, PO, 10 mg, 30s ea	55887-0439-30	14.01		AB
60s ea	55887-0439-60	25.08		AB
25 mg, 15s ea	55887-0518-15	12.05		AB
30s ea	55887-0518-30	36.01		AB
90s ea	55887-0518-90	108.03		AB
50 mg, 30s ea	55887-0498-30	16.00		AB
60s ea	55887-0498-60	32.00		AB
(Dispensing Solutions)				
REPACK				
CAP, PO, 10 mg, 30s ea	55045-1920-08	26.40		AB
45s ea	55045-1920-09	39.60		AB
60s ea	55045-1920-06	52.80		AB
90s ea	55045-1920-02	79.20		AB
100s ea	55045-1920-01	88.00		AB
25 mg, 30s ea	55045-1956-08	33.00		AB
45s ea	55045-1956-04	49.50		AB
60s ea	55045-1956-09	66.00		AB
60s ea	66336-0757-60	206.07		AB
90s ea	55045-1956-06	99.00		AB
100s ea	55045-1956-01	110.00		AB
120s ea	55045-1956-02	132.00		AB
50 mg, 30s ea	55045-1982-08	51.00		AB
30s ea	66336-0621-30	388.34		AB
60s ea	55045-1982-09	102.00		AB
60s ea	66336-0621-60	91.08		AB
90s ea	55045-1982-02	153.00		AB
75 mg, 30s ea	55045-2360-08	74.10		AB
(IPI)				
REPACK				
CAP, PO, 10 mg, 60s ea	18837-0310-60	50.92		AB
(Keltman Pharma., Inc.)				
REPACK				
CAP, PO, 25 mg, 30s ea	68387-0330-30	33.06		
60s ea	68387-0330-60	66.12		AB
(McKesson Packaging)				
REPACK				
CAP, PO (USP)				
25 mg, 100s ea UD	63739-0190-10	78.53		AB
(Nucare Pharm)				
REPACK				
CAP, PO, 10 mg, 45s ea	66267-0483-45	21.99		AB
25 mg, 30s ea	66267-0484-30	34.99		AB
45s ea	66267-0484-45	52.49		AB

PROD/MFR	NDC	AWP	DP	OBC
(PD-Rx Pharm)				
REPACK				
CAP, PO (USP)				
25 mg, 30s ea	55289-0099-30	35.00		AB
50s ea	55289-0099-50	45.83		AB
(Pharma Pac)				
REPACK				
CAP, PO, 10 mg, 20s ea	52959-0358-20	9.42		EE
30s ea	52959-0358-30	14.12		EE
60s ea	52959-0358-60	24.58		EE
90s ea	52959-0358-90	36.85		EE
120s ea	52959-0358-02	49.10		EE
25 mg, 20s ea	52959-0359-20	19.49		EE
30s ea	52959-0359-30	29.22		EE
50s ea	52959-0359-50	41.37		AB
60s ea	52959-0359-60	49.70		EE
90s ea	52959-0359-90	75.59		EE
120s ea	52959-0359-02	100.75		EE
50 mg, 15s ea	52959-0519-15	24.92		AB
30s ea	52959-0519-30	50.33		AB
60s ea	52959-0519-60	101.40		AB
75 mg, 30s ea	52959-0840-30	85.75		AB
(Phys Total Care)				
REPACK				
CAP, PO, 10 mg, 30s ea	54868-2835-02	7.14		EE
60s ea	54868-2835-01	11.31		EE
90s ea	54868-2835-04	18.46		AB
100s ea	54868-2835-03	16.86		EE
25 mg, 25s ea	54868-2480-04	7.17		EE
30s ea	54868-2480-02	8.01		EE
60s ea	54868-2480-01	13.02		EE
100s ea	54868-2480-00	19.71		EE
50 mg, 30s ea	54868-2481-02	10.35		EE
60s ea	54868-2481-03	14.70		AB
100s ea	54868-2481-01	22.47		EE
75 mg, 30s ea	54868-2482-02	13.44		AB
100s ea	54868-2482-00	35.91		EE
(Quality Care Prod)				
REPACK				
CAP, PO, 25 mg, 25s ea	49999-0215-25	34.80		EE
60s ea	49999-0215-60	125.10		AB
(Southwood)				
REPACK				
CAP, PO, 10 mg, 12s ea	58016-0519-12	5.40		EE
12s ea	58016-0934-12	5.40		EE
15s ea	58016-0519-15	6.75		EE
15s ea	58016-0934-15	6.75		EE
20s ea	58016-0519-20	9.00		EE
20s ea	58016-0934-20	9.00		EE
30s ea	58016-0519-30	13.50		EE
30s ea	58016-0934-30	13.50		EE
40s ea	58016-0519-40	18.22		AB
50s ea	58016-0519-50	22.77		AB
60s ea	58016-0519-60	27.32		EE
70s ea	58016-0519-70	31.88		EE
80s ea	58016-0519-80	5.40		AB
90s ea	58016-0519-90	40.99		AB
100s ea	58016-0519-00	45.54		EE
100s ea	58016-0934-00	45.54		EE
120s ea	58016-0519-02	54.65		AB
180s ea	58016-0519-99	208.80		AB
25 mg, 15s ea	58016-0491-15	17.40		EE
20s ea	58016-0491-20	23.20		EE
25s ea	58016-0491-25	29.00		EE
30s ea	58016-0491-30	34.80		EE
40s ea	58016-0491-40	46.40		EE
60s ea	58016-0491-60	69.60		EE
70s ea	58016-0491-70	81.20		EE
80s ea	58016-0491-80	92.80		EE
90s ea	58016-0491-90	104.40		EE
100s ea	58016-0491-00	116.00		EE
120s ea	58016-0491-02	139.20		EE
50 mg, 15s ea	58016-0508-15	25.72		EE
30s ea	58016-0508-30	51.30		EE
50s ea	58016-0491-50	58.00		EE
60s ea	58016-0508-60	102.89		EE
100s ea	58016-0508-00	171.48		EE
75 mg, 12s ea	58016-0875-12	31.32		EE
12s ea	58016-0945-12	31.32		EE
15s ea	58016-0875-15	39.15		EE
15s ea	58016-0945-15	39.15		EE
20s ea	58016-0875-20	52.20		EE
20s ea	58016-0945-20	52.20		EE
30s ea	58016-0875-30	78.30		EE
30s ea	58016-0945-30	78.30		EE
60s ea	58016-0875-60	156.60		EE
100s ea	58016-0875-00	261.42		EE
100s ea	58016-0945-00	261.42		EE

PROD/MFR	NDC	AWP	DP	OBC
(St. Mary's MPP)				
REPACK				
CAP, PO, 10 mg, 30s ea	60760-0508-30	17.29		AB
60s ea	60760-0508-60	28.57		AB
(Stat Rx)				
REPACK				
CAP, PO, 10 mg, 30s ea	16590-0435-30	25.47		AB
60s ea	16590-0435-60	50.94		AB
25 mg, 100s ea	16590-0171-71	94.20		AB
50 mg, 30s ea	16590-0590-30	48.00		AB
60s ea	16590-0590-60	74.00		AB
90s ea	16590-0590-90	101.00		AB
120s ea	16590-0590-72	132.00		AB
(Vibranta)				
REPACK				
CAP, PO, 25 mg, 30s ea	57866-6650-01	41.76		AB
60s ea	57866-6650-02	83.52		AB
90s ea	57866-6650-03	125.28		AB
NORTRIPTYLINE HYDROCHLORIDE				
FUL				
CAP, PO, 10 mg, 100s ea		10.19		
25 mg, 100s ea		14.06		
50 mg, 100s ea		17.22		
75 mg, 100s ea		22.03		
(Covidien) *See PAMELOR*				
(Mylan) *See NORTRIPTYLINE HCL*				
(PCCA) *See NORTRIPTYLINE HCL*				
(Pharm Assoc Inc) *See NORTRIPTYLINE HCL*				
(Ranbaxy Pharm) *See NORTRIPTYLINE HCL*				
(Spectrum Pharmacy) *See NORTRIPTYLINE HCL*				
(Taro) *See NORTRIPTYLINE HCL*				
(Teva)				
CAP, PO, 10 mg, 100s ea	00093-0810-01	38.65		AB
500s ea	00093-0810-05	171.00		AB
25 mg, 100s ea	00093-0811-01	77.20		AB
500s ea	00093-0811-05	377.85		AB
50 mg, 100s ea	00093-0812-01	145.55		AB
500s ea	00093-0812-05	645.20		AB
75 mg, 100s ea	00093-0813-01	221.95		AB
500s ea	00093-0813-05	1054.30		AB
(Watson Labs) *See NORTRIPTYLINE HCL*				
(Bryant Ranch)				
REPACK				
CAP, PO, 25 mg, 30s ea	63629-2833-04	36.80		
60s ea	63629-2833-02	74.60		
(DHS, Inc.)				
REPACK				
CAP, PO, 10 mg, 180s ea	55887-0439-92	75.24		
(Keltman Pharma., Inc.)				
REPACK				
TAB, PO, 25 mg, 15s ea	68387-0330-15	16.53		
(Nucare Pharm)				
REPACK				
CAP, PO, 10 mg, 30s ea	66267-0483-30	34.05		AB
60s ea	66267-0483-60	56.05		AB
25 mg, 60s ea	66267-0484-60	64.09		AB
(Palmetto)				
REPACK				
CAP, PO, 10 mg, 30s ea	23490-6019-02	22.50		
60s ea	23490-6019-01	45.00		
90s ea	23490-6019-03	67.50		
180s ea	23490-6019-04	101.25		
25 mg, 30s ea	23490-6020-02	35.40		
60s ea	23490-6020-01	70.80		
90s ea	23490-6020-03	106.20		
50 mg, 60s ea	23490-6021-06	118.40		
(Pharma Pac)				
REPACK				
CAP, PO, 75 mg, 60s ea	52959-0840-60	156.56		
(Physician Partner)				
REPACK				
CAP, PO, 10 mg, 30s ea	21695-0093-30	24.30		
60s ea	21695-0093-60	48.60		
90s ea	21695-0093-90	72.90		
25 mg, 30s ea	21695-0094-30	44.92		
60s ea	21695-0094-60	89.84		
90s ea	21695-0094-90	134.76		
(Quality Care Prod)				
REPACK				
CAP, PO, 10 mg, 30s ea	49999-0538-30	17.55		
25 mg, 30s ea	49999-0215-30	41.76		
50 mg, 30s ea	49999-0915-30	51.64		AB
60s ea	49999-0915-60	103.28		AB
90s ea	49999-0915-90	154.92		

PROD/MFR	NDC	AWP	DP	OBC
(St. Mary's MPP)				
REPACK				
CAP, PO (USP)				
25 mg, 30s ea	**60760-0811-30**	30.94		
60s ea	**60760-0811-60**	55.88		
NORVASC (Pfizer)				
amlodipine besylate				
TAB, PO, 2.5 mg, 90s ea	**00069-1520-68**	206.89	172.41	
5 mg, 90s ea	**00069-1530-68**	206.89	172.41	
100s ea UD	**00069-1530-41**	229.87	191.56	
300s ea	**00069-1530-72**	689.63	574.69	
10 mg, 90s ea	**00069-1540-68**	283.92	236.60	
100s ea UD	**00069-1540-41**	315.46	262.88	
(A-S Medication)				
REPACK				
TAB, PO, 5 mg, 30s ea	**54569-3866-01**	85.38		
10 mg, 30s ea	**54569-4472-00**	89.42		
(Advanced Pharm Serv, Inc.)				
REPACK				
TAB, PO, 2.5 mg, 10s ea	**13411-0157-01**	27.80		
30s ea	**13411-0157-03**	73.40		
60s ea	**13411-0157-06**	141.80		
90s ea	**13411-0157-09**	210.25		
100s ea	**13411-0157-10**	233.00		
5 mg, 10s ea	**13411-0148-01**	33.84		
30s ea	**13411-0148-03**	101.52		
60s ea	**13411-0148-06**	203.04		
90s ea	**13411-0148-09**	304.57		
100s ea	**13411-0148-10**	338.41		
10 mg, 10s ea	**13411-0158-01**	45.33		
30s ea	**13411-0158-03**	135.99		
60s ea	**13411-0158-06**	271.98		
90s ea	**13411-0158-09**	407.98		
100s ea	**13411-0158-10**	453.31		
(AQ)				
REPACK				
TAB, PO, 5 mg, 10s ea	**66105-0528-01**	33.84		
30s ea	**66105-0528-03**	101.52		
60s ea	**66105-0528-06**	203.04		
90s ea	**66105-0528-09**	304.57		
100s ea	**66105-0528-10**	338.41		
10 mg, 10s ea	**66105-0529-01**	45.33		
30s ea	**66105-0529-03**	135.99		
60s ea	**66105-0529-06**	271.98		
90s ea	**66105-0529-09**	407.98		
100s ea	**66105-0529-10**	453.31		
(Bryant Ranch)				
REPACK				
TAB, PO, 5 mg, 30s ea	**63629-1566-01**	58.99		
10 mg, 30s ea	**63629-1565-01**	149.99		
(Direct Pharmaceutical, Inc.)				
REPACK				
TAB, PO, 5 mg, 30s ea UD	**67801-0307-03**	61.75		
30s ea UD	**67801-0307-30**	110.97		
10 mg, 30s ea	**67801-0408-03**	84.88		
30s ea UD	**67801-0408-30**	105.68		
(Dispensing Solutions)				
REPACK				
TAB, PO, 5 mg, 90s ea	**55045-3344-01**	185.40		
10 mg, 30s ea	**66336-0255-30**	96.25		
90s ea	**55045-3499-01**	253.80		
(PD-Rx Pharm)				
REPACK				
TAB, PO (USP)				
2.5 mg, 30s ea	**55289-0602-30**	97.64		
(REDI-SCRIPT)				
5 mg, 14s ea	**58864-0620-14**	44.32		
30s ea	**55289-0103-30**	97.64		
(REDI-SCRIPT)				
5 mg, 30s ea	**58864-0620-30**	75.73		
60s ea	**55289-0103-60**	195.24		
10 mg, 30s ea	**55289-0549-30**	133.95		
(REDI-SCRIPT)				
10 mg, 30s ea	**58864-0657-30**	133.95		
60s ea	**55289-0549-60**	267.93		
(Phys Total Care)				
REPACK				
TAB, PO, 2.5 mg, 30s ea	**54868-3853-01**	77.54		
60s ea	**54868-3853-02**	144.79		
90s ea	**54868-3853-03**	215.63		
5 mg, 5s ea	**54868-2873-05**	15.03		
30s ea	**54868-2873-01**	80.36		
60s ea	**54868-2873-03**	150.05		
90s ea	**54868-2873-04**	223.44		
100s ea	**54868-2873-00**	248.77		
10 mg, 30s ea	**54868-3464-01**	109.55		
90s ea	**54868-3464-02**	306.14		
(Physician Partner)				
REPACK				
TAB, PO, 5 mg, 15s ea	**21695-0151-15**	76.66		
(Quality Care Prod)				
REPACK				
TAB, PO, 5 mg, 30s ea	**49999-0436-30**	109.17		
90s ea	**49999-0436-90**	320.60		
10 mg, 30s ea	**49999-0478-30**	147.18		
90s ea	**49999-0478-90**	429.45		
NORVIR (Abbott Pharm)				
ritonavir				
SGL, PO (SOFTGEL)				
100 mg, 30s ea	**00074-6633-30**	308.60	270.71	
SOL, PO (PEPPERMINT-CARAMEL)				
80 mg/ml, 240 ml	**00074-1940-63**	1728.24	1516.00	
TAB, PO (FILM-COATED)				
100 mg, 30s ea	**00074-3333-30**	308.60	270.71	
(A-S Medication)				
REPACK				
SGL, PO (SOFTGEL)				
100 mg, 30s ea	**54569-5656-00**	401.18		
(Phys Total Care)				
REPACK				
SGL, PO, 100 mg, 30s ea (SOFTGEL)	**54868-3782-03**	395.80		
100 mg, 60s ea	**54868-3782-01**	763.63		
(Quality Care Prod)				
REPACK				
SGL, PO (SOFTGEL)				
100 mg, 30s ea	**35356-0138-30**	581.01		
NOTRIPTYLINE (Dispensing Solutions)				
REPACK				
nortriptyline hydrochloride				
CAP, PO, 10 mg, 60s ea	**66336-0973-60**	28.92		
NOTUSS-AC (SJ)				
chlorpheniramine maleate/codeine phosphate				
SOL, PO (1X473ML,AF,SF,DYE-FREE)				
2 mg/5 ml-10 mg/5 ml, 473 ml, C-V	**24839-0338-16**	106.88		
NOTUSS-DC (SJ)				
codeine phosphate/pseudoephedrine hydrochloride				
SOL, PO (1X473ML,AF,SF,DYE-FREE)				
10 mg/5 ml-30 mg/5 ml, 473 ml, C-V	**24839-0339-16**	106.88		
NOTUSS-FORTE (SJ)				
cpm/hydrocod bit/pse hcl				
SYR, PO (AF,SF,DYE-FREE)				
473 ml, C-III	**24839-0228-16**	95.75		
NOTUSS-PE (SJ)				
codeine phosphate/phenylephrine hydrochloride				
SOL, PO (1X473ML,AF,SF,DYE-FREE)				
10 mg/5 ml-10 mg/5 ml, 473 ml, C-V	**24839-0343-16**	106.88		
NOV-ONXOL (Teva)				
paclitaxel				
SOL, IV (M.D.V.)				
6 mg/ml, 5 ml	**00172-3754-94**	172.72		AP
25 ml	**00172-3756-95**	863.60		AP
50 ml	**00172-3753-96**	1727.19		AP
NOVA SUREFLEX (Nova)				
lancet				
DEV, NA, 100s ea	**08548-0434-21**	7.50		
NOVACORT (Primus Pharma)				
aloe/hc ace/pramoxine hcl				
GEL, RC (DYE-FREE,FRAGRANCE-FREE)				
1%-2%-1%, 29 gm	**68040-0704-26**	77.65		
NOVADYNE EXPECTORANT (Pharma Pac)				
REPACK				
codeine phos/gg/pse hcl				
LIQ, PO (CHERRY)				
120 ml, C-V	**52959-0610-03**	9.10		
NOVAFED A (Southwood)				
REPACK				
cpm/pse hcl				
CER, PO, 8 mg-120 mg, 16s ea	**58016-0659-16**	10.80		
NOVAGESIC (A. G. Marin)				
acetaminophen/phenyltoloxamine citrate				
TAB, PO (CAPLET)				
500 mg-30 mg, 100s ea	**12539-0101-00**	11.95		
NOVAMINE (Hospira)				
amino acids				
SOL, IV (BULK PKG,10X500ML,GLASS)				
15%, 500 ml 10s	**00409-0468-05**	298.44	261.10	
NOVANTRONE (EMD)				
mitoxantrone hydrochloride				
SOL, IV (M.D.V.)				
2 mg/ml, 10 ml	**44087-1520-01**	1585.88		
NOVAPLUS ACETAZOLAMIDE (X-Gen)				
acetazolamide				
PDS, IV (USP,LATEX-FREE)				
500 mg, ea	**39822-0190-07**	51.75		AP
NOVAPLUS ALFENTANIL (Hospira)				
alfentanil hydrochloride				
SOL, IJ (USP,10X5ML,PF)				
0.5 mg/ml, 5 ml 10s, C-II	**00409-2266-51**	82.80	72.50	AP
NOVAPLUS AMIODARONE HYDROCHLORIDE (Hospira)				
amiodarone hydrochloride				
SOL, IV (10X3ML,SD,PRIVATE LABEL)				
50 mg/ml, 3 ml 10s	**00409-4348-49**	20.52	18.00	AP
NOVAPLUS AMPHOTERICIN B (X-Gen)				
amphotericin b				
PDS, IV (PRIVATE LABEL)				
50 mg, ea	**39822-1055-07**	24.50		AP
NOVAPLUS AMPICILLIN (Sandoz)				
ampicillin sodium				
PDS, IJ (ADD-VANTAGE)				
1 gm, ea	**00781-9412-15**	14.90		
(PRIVATE LABEL)				
1 gm, ea	**00781-9404-85**	8.64		
(ADD-VANTAGE)				
1 gm, 10s ea	**00781-9412-92**	148.99		
2 gm, ea	**00781-9408-92**	26.39		
ea	**00781-9413-15**	28.90		
(PRIVATE LABEL)				
2 gm, ea	**00781-9408-80**	16.75		
(ADD-VANTAGE)				
2 gm, 10s ea	**00781-9413-92**	289.01		
(PRIVATE LABEL)				
10 gm, ea	**00781-9409-96**	107.77		
125 mg, ea	**00781-9401-78**	5.22		
250 mg, ea	**00781-9402-78**	4.19		
500 mg, ea	**00781-9407-78**	4.41		
NOVAPLUS AMPICILLIN AND SULBACTAM (Baxter)				
ampicillin sodium/sulbactam sodium				
PDS, IJ (PRIVATE LABEL)				
1 gm-0.5 gm, ea	**10019-0636-31**	4.74		AP
(USP,10MLX10)				
1 gm-0.5 gm, 10s ea	**10019-0636-01**	47.40		AP
(PRIVATE LABEL)				
2 gm-1 gm, ea	**10019-0637-33**	8.06		AP
(USP,20MLX10)				
2 gm-1 gm, 10s ea	**10019-0637-02**	80.64		AP
IV (PHARMACYBULKPACKAGE,USP)				
10 gm-5 gm, ea	**10019-0638-15**	43.15		AP
(USP,PHARMACYBULK)				
10 gm-5 gm, ea	**10019-0638-03**	43.15		AP
(Hospira)				
PDS, IV (USP,ADD-VANTAGE)				
1 gm-0.5 gm, 10s ea	**00409-2689-11**	44.76	39.20	AP
2 gm-1 gm, 10s ea	**00409-2987-13**	73.92	64.70	AP
NOVAPLUS ARGATROBAN (Glaxo)				
argatroban				
SOL, IV (1X2.5ML,SINGLE-USE)				
100 mg/ml, 2.5 ml	**00007-4407-54**	1486.98		
NOVAPLUS AZITHROMYCIN (APP)				
azithromycin				
PDS, IV (10X10ML)				
500 mg, 10s ea	**63323-0398-12**	299.50		
NOVAPLUS BACIIM (X-Gen)				
bacitracin				
PDS, IM (STERILE,USP)				
50000 u, 10s ea	**39822-0277-07**	198.00		AP
NOVAPLUS BUMETANIDE (Hospira)				
bumetanide				
SOL, IJ (SDV,USP,10X4ML)				
0.25 mg/ml, 4 ml 10s	**00409-1412-49**	9.96	8.70	AP
(MDV,USP,10X10ML)				
0.25 mg/ml, 10 ml 10s	**00409-1412-50**	18.96	16.60	AP
NOVAPLUS BUTORPHANOL TARTRATE (Hospira)				
butorphanol tartrate				
SOL, IJ (VHA,10X1ML)				
2 mg/ml, 1 ml 10s, C-IV	**00409-1626-49**	51.36	44.90	AP

PROD/MFR	NDC	AWP	DP	OBC
NOVAPLUS CAFFEINE CITRATE (Paddock)				
caffeine citrate				
SOL, IV (USP,10X3ML,PF)				
20 mg/ml, 3 ml 10s	00574-0823-81	33.12		
PO (10X3ML,PF,PRIVATE LABEL)				
20 mg/ml, 3 ml 10s	00574-0152-80	456.25		
NOVAPLUS CARBOPLATIN (Hospira)				
carboplatin				
SOL, IV (MDV,PRIVATE LABEL)				
10 mg/ml, 5 ml	61703-0360-18	7.91	6.92	AP
15 ml	61703-0360-22	17.02	14.89	AP
45 ml	61703-0360-50	55.18	48.28	AP
NOVAPLUS CEFAZOLIN (Sandoz)				
cefazolin sodium				
PDS, IJ (PRIVATE LABEL)				
1 gm, ea	00781-9339-85	6.46		
(USP,PRIVATE LABEL)				
1 gm, 25s ea	00781-9339-96	161.43		
25s ea	00781-9451-96	161.43		AP
(PHARMACY BULK PACKAGE)				
10 gm, ea	00781-9337-46	36.53		
10s ea	00781-9337-95	365.34		
(PRIVATE LABEL)				
500 mg, ea	00781-9338-85	3.23		
(USP,PRIVATE LABEL)				
500 mg, 10s ea	00781-9338-95	32.26		
(Sandoz)				
cefazolin				
PDS, IV (USP,PHARMACY BULK)				
10 gm, 10s ea	00781-9452-95	365.34		AP
NOVAPLUS CEFOXITIN (Apotex Corp.)				
cefoxitin sodium				
PDS, IV (USP,PRIVATE LABEL)				
1 gm, 25s ea	60505-6025-05	280.63		AP
2 gm, 25s ea	60505-6026-05	562.50		AP
NOVAPLUS CIPROFLOXACIN (Hospira)				
ciprofloxacin				
SOL, IV (SINGLE-DOSE,24X100ML)				
200 mg/100 ml,				
100 ml 24s	00409-4777-49	53.57	46.80	AP
(SINGLE-DOSE,24X200ML)				
400 mg/200 ml,				
200 ml 24s	00409-4777-50	66.24	58.08	AP
NOVAPLUS CLAFORAN (Hospira)				
cefotaxime sodium				
PDS, IJ (PRIVATE LABEL)				
1 gm, 10s ea	00039-0018-49	29.52	25.80	AP
(ADD-VANTAGE SYSTEM)				
1 gm, 25s ea	00039-0023-49	98.70	86.25	AP
(PRIVATE LABEL)				
2 gm, 10s ea	00039-0019-49	58.56	51.20	AP
(ADD-VANTAGE SYSTEM)				
2 gm, 25s ea	00039-0024-49	167.70	146.75	AP
(PHARMACY BULK PACKAGE)				
10 gm, ea	00039-0020-49	44.40	38.85	AP
NOVAPLUS CORVERT (Pfizer)				
ibutilide fumarate				
SOL, IV (1X10ML,SINGLE-DOSE)				
0.1 mg/ml, 10 ml	00009-3794-22	542.72	452.27	
NOVAPLUS DEPO-MEDROL (Pfizer)				
methylprednisolone acetate				
SUS, IJ (1X1ML,SINGLE-DOSE)				
40 mg/ml, 1 ml	00009-3073-22	9.04	7.53	
(SINGLE-DOSE,25X1ML)				
40 mg/ml, 1 ml 25s	00009-3073-23	225.90	188.25	
(SINGLE-DOSE,1X1ML)				
80 mg/ml, 1 ml	00009-3475-22	15.67	13.06	
(SINGLE-DOSE,25X1ML)				
80 mg/ml, 1 ml 25s	00009-3475-23	391.80	326.50	
NOVAPLUS DIPRIVAN (APP)				
propofol				
EMU, IV (25X20ML,PRIVATE LABEL)				
10 mg/ml,				
20 ml 25s	63323-0269-27	187.50		AB
(20X50ML,PRIVATE LABEL)				
10 mg/ml,				
50 ml 20s	63323-0269-57	375.00		AB
(10X100ML, INFUSION)				
10 mg/ml,				
100 ml 10s	63323-0269-67	375.00		AB
NOVAPLUS EPIRUBICIN HYDROCHLORIDE (Hospira)				
epirubicin hydrochloride				
SOL, IV (1X25ML,SINGLE USE,PF)				
2 mg/ml, 25 ml	61703-0359-01	84.73	74.14	
(1X100ML,SINGLE USE,PF)				
2 mg/ml, 100 ml	61703-0359-02	201.95	176.70	
NOVAPLUS ESMOLOL HYDROCHLORIDE (Bedford)				
esmolol hydrochloride				
SOL, IV (S.D.V.,PF,PRIVATE LABEL)				
10 mg/ml,				
10 ml 10s	55390-0340-10	64.80		AP
NOVAPLUS FENTANYL (Watson Labs)				
fentanyl				
TDM, TD (TRANSDERMAL SYSTEM)				
25 mcg/hr,				
5s ea, C-II	00591-3600-72	64.96		AB
50 mcg/hr,				
5s ea, C-II	00591-3601-72	118.73		AB
75 mcg/hr,				
5s ea, C-II	00591-3602-72	181.10		AB
100 mcg/hr,				
5s ea, C-II	00591-3603-72	240.36		AB
NOVAPLUS FLUCONAZOLE (Hospira)				
fluconazole				
SOL, IV (6X100ML,LATEX-FREE)				
200 mg/100 ml,				
100 ml 6s	00409-4688-28	60.05	52.56	AP
(6X200ML,LATEX-FREE)				
200 mg/100 ml,				
200 ml 6s	00409-4688-34	65.09	56.94	AP
NOVAPLUS FLUDARABINE PHOSPHATE (Teva)				
fludarabine phosphate				
SOL, IV (PRIVATE LABEL)				
25 mg/ml, 2 ml	00703-4852-92	240.00		
NOVAPLUS FLUMAZENIL (Teva)				
flumazenil				
SOL, IV, 0.1 mg/ml, 5 ml	00703-2084-93	198.00		
(M.D.V.)				
0.1 mg/ml,				
5 ml 10s	00703-2084-03	198.00		
10 ml	00703-2085-93	360.00		
(M.D.V.)				
0.1 mg/ml,				
10 ml 10s	00703-2085-03	360.00		
NOVAPLUS FLUTICASONE PROPIONATE (Apotex Corp.)				
fluticasone propionate				
SPR, NS (1X16GM,PRIVATE LABEL)				
0.05 mg/actuation,				
16 gm	60505-0847-03	85.26		AB
NOVAPLUS FOSPHENYTOIN SODIUM (Hospira)				
fosphenytoin sodium				
SOL, IJ (25X2ML,USP)				
75 mg/ml, 2 ml 25s	00409-4857-49	40.50	35.50	
(10X10ML,USP)				
75 mg/ml,				
10 ml 10s	00409-4857-50	58.56	51.20	
NOVAPLUS HALOPERIDOL DECANOATE (Apotex Corp.)				
haloperidol decanoate				
OIL, IM (1X5ML,MDV)				
50 mg/ml, 5 ml	60505-6020-02	140.00		AO
(1X5ML,MDV,PRIVATE LABEL)				
100 mg/ml, 5 ml	60505-6021-02	247.25		AO
NOVAPLUS HEPAGAM B (Apotex Corp.)				
hepatitis b immune globulin				
SOL, IJ (>312IU/ML,PF)				
1 ml	60492-0052-02	182.80		
(1X1ML,>312IU/ML,PF)				
1 ml	60505-6071-00	182.80		
1 ml	60505-6073-00	182.80		
(>1560/5ML,PF)				
5 ml	60492-0051-02	800.00		
(1X5ML,>312IU/ML,PF)				
5 ml	60505-6072-00	800.00		
5 ml	60505-6074-00	800.00		
NOVAPLUS HEPARIN SODIUM (APP)				
heparin sodium				
SOL, IJ (25X10ML, M.D.V.)				
1000 u/ml,				
10 ml 25s	63323-0540-57	218.10		
(25X1ML, M.D.V.)				
5000 u/ml,				
1 ml 25s	63323-0262-55	124.80		
NOVAPLUS HYDRALAZINE HYDROCHLORIDE (APP)				
hydralazine hydrochloride				
SOL, IJ (USP,SDV,LATEX-FREE)				
20 mg/ml, 1 ml 25s	63323-0614-55	375.00		AP
NOVAPLUS IDARUBICIN HYDROCHLORIDE (Teva)				
idarubicin hydrochloride				
SOL, IV (SDV,PF,PRIVATE LABEL)				
1 mg/ml, 5 ml	00703-4154-91	144.00		
10 ml	00703-4155-91	288.00		
20 ml	00703-4156-91	480.00		
NOVAPLUS IRINOTECAN HYDROCHLORIDE (Teva)				
irinotecan hydrochloride				
SOL, IV (1X5ML,PRIVATE LABEL)				
20 mg/ml, 5 ml	00703-4434-91	121.73		AP
NOVAPLUS LORAZEPAM (Baxter)				
lorazepam				
SOL, IJ (USP,PRIVATE LABEL)				
2 mg/ml,				
1 ml, C-IV	10019-0105-44	0.90		EE
1 ml, C-IV	10019-0105-71	7.68		EE
(25X1ML,SDV)				
2 mg/ml,				
1 ml 25s, C-IV	10019-0105-01	22.50		EE
(10X10ML,MDV)				
2 mg/ml,				
10 ml 10s, C-IV	10019-0105-02	76.80		EE
(PRIVATE LABEL)				
4 mg/ml,				
1 ml, C-IV	10019-0106-44	2.16		EE
1 ml, C-IV	10019-0106-71	11.06		EE
(25X1ML,SDV)				
4 mg/ml,				
1 ml 25s, C-IV	10019-0106-01	54.00		EE
(10X10ML,MDV)				
4 mg/ml,				
10 ml 10s, C-IV	10019-0106-02	110.64		EE
NOVAPLUS LOVENOX (Sanofi-Aventis)				
enoxaparin sodium				
SOL, IJ (1X3ML,MULTIPLE-DOSE)				
100 mg/ml, 3 ml	00075-0626-04	270.64		EE
SC (10X0.3ML,SINGLE-DOSE,PF)				
30 mg/0.3 ml,				
0.3 ml 10s	00075-0624-31	270.64		EE
(10X0.4ML,SINGLE-DOSE,PF)				
40 mg/0.4 ml,				
0.4 ml 10s	00075-0620-41	360.83		EE
(10X0.6ML,SINGLE-DOSE,PF)				
60 mg/0.6 ml,				
0.6 ml 10s	00075-0621-61	541.88		EE
(10X0.8ML,SINGLE-DOSE,PF)				
80 mg/0.8 ml,				
0.8 ml 10s	00075-0622-81	722.52		EE
(10X1ML,SINGLE-DOSE,PF)				
100 mg/ml,				
1 ml 10s	00075-0623-01	903.13		
(10X0.8ML,SINGLE-DOSE,PF)				
120 mg/0.8 ml,				
0.8 ml 10s	00075-2912-02	1084.12		EE
(10X1ML,SINGLE-DOSE,PF)				
150 mg/ml,				
1 ml 10s	00075-2915-02	1355.16		EE
NOVAPLUS MERREM (AstraZeneca)				
meropenem				
PDS, IV (PRIVATE LABEL)				
1 gm, 10s ea	00310-0321-65	781.90		
500 mg, 10s ea	00310-0325-64	390.95		
NOVAPLUS MIDAZOLAM HCL (Hospira)				
midazolam hydrochloride				
SOL, IJ (10X10ML,FTV)				
1 mg/ml,				
10 ml 10s, C-IV	00409-2587-53	18.84	16.50	AP
NOVAPLUS MIDAZOLAM HYDROCHLORIDE (Hospira)				
midazolam hydrochloride				
SOL, IJ (10X5ML,PRIVATE LABEL)				
5 mg/ml,				
5 ml 10s, C-IV	00409-2596-52	36.72	32.10	AP
NOVAPLUS NAFCILLIN (Sandoz)				
nafcillin sodium				
PDS, IJ (PRIVATE LABEL)				
1 gm, ea	00781-9124-85	12.41		AP
10s ea	00781-9124-95	124.14		AP
(INNER PACK)				
2 gm, ea	00781-9125-15	26.39		AP
(PRIVATE LABEL)				
2 gm, ea	00781-9125-85	24.08		AP
10s ea	00781-9125-95	240.83		AP
10 gm, ea	00781-9126-46	118.01		AP
(BULK PACKAGE)				
10 gm, 10s ea	00781-9126-95	1180.11		AP
IV (ADD-VANTAGE)				
1 gm, ea	00781-9224-15	14.90		AP
(USP,ADD-VANTAGE)				
1 gm, 10s ea	00781-9224-92	148.99		AP
(ADD-VANTAGE)				
2 gm, ea	00781-9225-20	26.39		AP
(USP,ADD-VANTAGE)				
2 gm, 10s ea	00781-9225-92	289.01		AP

PROD/MFR	NDC	AWP	DP	OBC
NOVAPLUS NALBUPHINE HYDROCHLORIDE (Hospira)				
nalbuphine hydrochloride				
SOL, IJ (10X1ML,PRIVATE LABEL)				
10 mg/ml, 1 ml 10s	00409-1463-49	14.64	12.80	AP
20 mg/ml, 1 ml 10s	00409-1465-49	30.00	26.30	AP
NOVAPLUS NAROPIN (APP)				
ropivacaine hydrochloride				
SOL, IJ (1X100ML, SINGLE DOSE,PF)				
2 mg/ml, 100 ml	63323-0285-67	26.08		EE
(1X30ML,SDV,PF)				
5 mg/ml, 30 ml	63323-0286-37	17.51		EE
(5X20ML,POLYAMP,PF)				
10 mg/ml, 20 ml 5s	63323-0288-27	97.20		
NOVAPLUS OCTREOTIDE ACETATE (Teva)				
octreotide acetate				
SOL, IJ (SDV)				
500 mcg/ml, 1 ml	00703-3321-94	600.00		
NOVAPLUS OMNISCAN (GE)				
gadodiamide				
SOL, IV (10X15ML,SINGLE-DOSE)				
287 mg/ml, 15 ml 10s	00407-0691-64	1052.89		
(10X20ML,SINGLE-DOSE)				
287 mg/ml, 20 ml 10s	00407-0691-65	1288.19		
NOVAPLUS ONDANSETRON (Baxter)				
ondansetron hydrochloride				
SOL, IJ (USP,SDV,1X2ML)				
2 mg/ml, 2 ml	10019-0905-02	0.48		AP
(USP,SDV,25X2ML)				
2 mg/ml, 2 ml 25s	10019-0905-03	12.00		AP
(USP,MDV,1X20ML)				
2 mg/ml, 20 ml	10019-0906-04	3.23		AP
20 ml	10019-0906-05	3.23		AP
NOVAPLUS OXACILLIN (Sandoz)				
oxacillin sodium				
PDS, IJ (PRIVATE LABEL)				
1 gm, ea	00781-9109-85	12.41		AP
(USP,PRIVATE LABEL)				
1 gm, 10s ea	00781-9109-95	124.14		AP
(PRIVATE LABEL)				
2 gm, ea	00781-9111-80	24.08		AP
(USP,PRIVATE LABEL)				
2 gm, 10s ea	00781-9111-95	240.83		AP
(PRIVATE LABEL)				
10 gm, ea	00781-9113-46	118.01		AP
10s ea	00781-9113-95	1180.11		AP
IV (USP,ADD-VANTAGE VIAL)				
1 gm, ea	00781-9110-15	14.90		AP
(1X10,USP,ADD-VANTAGE)				
1 gm, 10s ea	00781-9110-92	148.99		AP
(ADD-VANTAGE)				
2 gm, ea	00781-9112-15	28.90		AP
(USP,ADD-VANTAGE VIAL)				
2 gm, ea	00781-9112-20	26.39		AP
(1X10,USP,ADD-VANTAGE)				
2 gm, 10s ea	00781-9112-92	289.01		AP
NOVAPLUS OXYTOCIN (APP)				
oxytocin				
SOL, IJ (25X1ML,USP)				
10 u/ml, 1 ml 25s	63323-0012-12	117.18		AP
NOVAPLUS PAMIDRONATE DISODIUM (Hospira)				
pamidronate disodium				
SOL, IV (SDV,PRIVATE LABEL)				
9 mg/ml, 10 ml	61703-0356-18	58.96	51.59	AP
NOVAPLUS PFIZERPEN (Pfizer)				
penicillin g potassium				
PDS, IJ (PRIVATE LABEL)				
5000000 u, 10s ea	00049-0520-22	79.86	66.55	
IV, 20 million u, ea	00049-0530-22	23.41	19.51	
NOVAPLUS POLYMYXIN B (X-Gen)				
polymyxin b sulfate				
PDS, IJ (PRIVATE LABEL)				
500000 u, ea	39822-0166-07	13.65		AP
NOVAPLUS PROTAMINE SULFATE (APP)				
protamine sulfate				
SOL, IV (25X5ML,SDV,FLIPTOP,USP)				
10 mg/ml, 5 ml 25s	63323-0229-15	225.00		
(1X25ML,SDV,FLIPTOP,USP)				
10 mg/ml, 25 ml	63323-0229-35	27.00		
NOVAPLUS ROCURONIUM BROMIDE (Hospira)				
rocuronium bromide				
SOL, IV (10X5ML,MDV)				
10 mg/ml, 5 ml 10s	00409-9558-49	47.76	41.80	AP
(10X10ML,MDV)				
10 mg/ml, 10 ml 10s	00409-9558-50	93.48	81.80	AP
NOVAPLUS SOLU-MEDROL (Pharmacia)				
methylprednisolone sodium succinate				
PDS, IJ (SDV,ACT-O-VIAL SYSTEM)				
40 mg, 25s ea	00009-0039-32	90.44	75.37	AP
125 mg, 25s ea	00009-0047-26	145.84	121.53	AP
NOVAPLUS TAZICEF (Hospira)				
ceftazidime				
PDS, IJ, 1 gm, 25s ea	00409-5092-52	196.50	172.00	AP
(PRIVATE LABEL)				
1 gm, 25s ea	00409-5082-52	120.90	105.75	AP
(ADD-VANTAGE)				
2 gm, 10s ea	00409-5093-51	149.64	130.90	AP
(PRIVATE LABEL)				
2 gm, 10s ea	00409-5084-51	138.84	121.50	AP
(BULK PACKAGE)				
6 gm, 10s ea	00409-5086-51	269.64	235.90	AP
NOVAPLUS VECURONIUM BROMIDE (Bedford)				
vecuronium bromide				
PDS, IV (PRIVATE LABEL)				
20 mg, 10s ea	55390-0182-10	63.60		AP
NOVAPLUS VENTOLIN HFA (Glaxo)				
albuterol sulfate				
ARO, IH (1X8GM,PRIVATE LABEL)				
0.09 mg/actuation, 8 gm	00173-0682-54	18.00		BX
NOVAREL (Ferring)				
chorionic gonadotropin				
PDS, IM (M.D.V.)				
10000 u, ea	55566-1501-01	113.99		AP
NOVASUS (SJ)				
chlorpheniramine tannate/hydrocodone tannate				
SUS, PO (AF,SF,TROPICAL FRUIT)				
4 mg/5 ml-5 mg/5 ml, 120 ml, C-III	24839-0222-04	57.60		
NOVOBIOCIN SODIUM (Medisca)				
POW, NA (U.S.P.)				
5 gm	38779-0149-03	138.00		
10 gm	38779-0149-01	261.00		
25 gm	38779-0149-04	597.00		
NOVOCAIN (Hospira)				
procaine hydrochloride				
SOL, IJ (25X2ML,AMP.,LATEX-FREE)				
1%, 2 ml 25s	00409-1808-02	89.40	78.25	AP
(UNI-AMP,USP)				
10%, 2 ml 25s UD	00409-1810-02	120.00	105.00	
NOVOFINE 30 (Novo Nordisk)				
insulin syringe/needle				
DEV, NA, 100s ea	00169-1852-50	34.20		
(Phys Total Care)				
REPACK				
DEV, NA, 100s ea	54868-1369-00	39.41		
NOVOLOG (Novo Nordisk)				
insulin aspart, recombinant				
SOL, SC (PENFILL CARTRIDGE)				
100 u/ml, 3 ml 5s	00169-3303-12	222.12		
(VIAL)				
100 u/ml, 10 ml	00169-7501-11	119.58		
(Phys Total Care)				
REPACK				
SOL, SC, 100 u/ml, 10 ml	54868-2777-00	112.40		
NOVOLOG FLEXPEN (Novo Nordisk)				
insulin aspart, recombinant				
SOL, SC (PREFILLED SYRINGE)				
100 u/ml, 3 ml 5s	00169-6339-10	230.94		
(Phys Total Care)				
REPACK				
SOL, SC (5X3ML,PREFILLED SYRINGE)				
100 u/ml, 3 ml 5s	54868-6054-00	256.24		
NOVOLOG MIX 70/30 (Novo Nordisk)				
insulin aspart/insulin aspart protamine				
SUS, SC (FLEXPEN,SRN PREFILLED)				
70 u/ml-30 u/ml, 3 ml 5s	00169-3696-19	230.94		
(VIAL)				
70 u/ml-30 u/ml, 10 ml	00169-3685-12	119.58		
(Phys Total Care)				
REPACK				
SUS, SC (PREFILLED SYRINGE)				
70 u/ml-30 u/ml, 3 ml 5s	54868-5327-00	55.81		
10 ml	54868-5201-00	143.51		
NOVOSEVEN (Novo Nordisk)				
coagulation factor viia				
PDS, IV (1200MCG/VIAL)				
1 mcg, ea	00169-7060-01	1.64		
(2400MCG/VIAL)				
1 mcg, ea	00169-7061-01	1.64		
(4800MCG/VIAL)				
1 mcg, ea	00169-7062-01	1.64		
NOVOSEVEN RT (Novo Nordisk)				
coagulation factor viia				
PDS, IV (1000MCG/VIAL,LATEX-FREE)				
1 mcg, ea	00169-7010-01	1.79		
(2000MCG/VIAL,LATEX-FREE)				
1 mcg, ea	00169-7020-01	1.79		
(5000MCG/VIAL,LATEX-FREE)				
1 mcg, ea	00169-7050-01	1.79		
NOXAFIL (Schering)				
posaconazole				
SUS, PO (CHERRY)				
40 mg/ml, 105 ml	00085-1328-01	743.84		
NPLATE (Amgen USA Inc.)				
romiplostim				
PDS, SC (PF,STERILE, LYOPHILIZED)				
250 mcg, ea	55513-0221-01	1300.50		
500 mcg, ea	55513-0222-01	2601.00		
NUBAIN (Phys Total Care)				
REPACK				
nalbuphine hydrochloride				
SOL, IJ (AMP,W/O SULFITE/PARABEN)				
10 mg/ml, 1 ml	54868-3686-01	3.21		AP
1 ml 10s	54868-3686-00	20.85		AP
(M.D.V.)				
10 mg/ml, 10 ml	54868-3471-00	31.25		AP
20 mg/ml, 10 ml	54868-3609-00	4.06		AP
NUCORT (Wraser Pharm)				
hydrocortisone acetate				
LOT, TP (1X60ML)				
2%, 60 ml	66992-0185-02	84.19		
NUCYNTA (Ortho-McNeil Pharm)				
tapentadol hydrochloride				
TAB, PO, 50 mg, 100s ea, C-II	50458-0820-04	217.26	181.05	
(10X10)				
50 mg, 100s ea UD, C-II	50458-0820-02	217.26	181.05	
75 mg, 100s ea, C-II	50458-0830-04	254.33	211.94	
(10X10)				
75 mg, 100s ea UD, C-II	50458-0830-02	254.33	211.94	
100 mg, 100s ea, C-II	50458-0840-04	338.68	282.23	
(10X10)				
100 mg, 100s ea UD, C-II	50458-0840-02	338.68	282.23	
(Quality Care Prod)				
REPACK				
TAB, PO, 50 mg, 100s ea, C-II	35356-0525-00	336.88		
(Stat Rx)				
REPACK				
TAB, PO, 50 mg,				
15s ea, C-II	16590-0863-15	44.27		
60s ea, C-II	16590-0863-60	144.73		
75s ea, C-II	16590-0863-75	180.11		
90s ea, C-II	16590-0863-30	191.70		
90s ea, C-II	16590-0863-90	215.48		
75 mg,				
30s ea, C-II	16590-0889-30	84.23		
60s ea, C-II	16590-0889-60	168.67		
100 mg,				
60s ea, C-II	16590-0289-60	223.55		
120s ea, C-II	16590-0289-72	445.07		
NUFOL (Rising)				
cyanocobalamin/folic acid/pyridoxine				
TAB, PO (SF,DYE-FREE)				
1 mg-2.5 mg-25 mg, 90s ea	64980-0127-09	39.61		
NULEV (Alaven)				
hyoscyamine sulfate				
CTB, PO (PEPPERMINT)				
0.125 mg, 100s ea	68220-0118-10	91.61		
NULYTELY (Braintree)				
k cl/na bicarb/na cl/polyethylene glycol 3350				
PDS, PO (CHERRY,LEMON-LIME)				
4000 ml	52268-0300-01	26.89		AA
4000 ml	52268-0301-01	26.89		AA
4000 ml	52268-0302-01	26.89		AA
4000 ml	52268-0303-01	26.89		AA
4000 ml	52268-0400-01	29.39		AA

PROD/MFR	NDC	AWP	DP	OBC
(Phys Total Care)				
REPACK				
PDS, PO (CHERRY)				
4000 ml	**54868-4233-00**	31.28		
NUMOISYN (Align)				
saliva substitutes				
LOZ, MM, 100s ea	**08514-0210-01**	14.40		
SOL, MM, 300 ml	**08514-0110-02**	60.00		
NUOX (Wraser Pharm)				
benzoyl peroxide/sulfur				
GEL, TP, 6%-3%, 43 gm	**66992-0170-43**	63.91		
(Phys Total Care)				
REPACK				
GEL, TP (1X43GM)				
6%-3%, 43 gm	**54868-5947-00**	50.59		
NUQUIN HP (Stratus)				
hydroquinone				
CRE, TP (W/SUNSCREENS)				
4%, 15 gm	**58980-0574-05**	18.00		
30 gm	**58980-0574-10**	35.50		
60 gm	**58980-0574-20**	46.00		
GEL, TP, 4%, 14.2 gm	**58980-0475-05**	18.00		
28.4 gm	**58980-0475-10**	35.50		
NUTMEG OIL (Medisca)				
OIL, NA (1X14ML,MYRISTICA OIL)				
14 ml	**38779-1464-03**	16.50		
(1X25ML,MYRISTICA OIL)				
25 ml	**38779-1464-04**	31.50		
(1X100ML,MYRISTICA OIL)				
100 ml	**38779-1464-05**	45.00		
(1X500ML,MYRISTICA OIL)				
500 ml	**38779-1464-08**	261.00		
(PCCA)				
OIL, NA (MYRISTICA OIL)				
1 ml	**51927-2474-00**	1.20		
NUTRACARE (Blansett)				
prenatal vitamins				
CTB, PO (6X10,ORANGE-PINEAPPLE)				
60s ea UD	**51674-5001-06**	25.63	20.50	
NUTRASWEET ASPARTAME APM (Gallipot)				
aspartame				
GRA, NA, 10 gm	**51552-0060-03**	14.00		
100 gm	**51552-0060-05**	49.00		
NUTRESTORE ()				
glutamine				
PDS, PO (84X5GM)				
5 gm/packet,				
5 gm 84s	**42457-0001-84**	336.00	268.80	
NUTRICEUTICAL				
(Acella) *See BP VIT 3*				
(Heel/BHI) *See TRAUMEEL*				
(Midlothian Labs) *See MI-OMEGA NF*				
NUTRICEUTICAL/PRENATAL VITAMINS				
(Marnel) *See MARNATAL-F PLUS*				
(Ther-RX) *See PRIMACARE ADVANTAGE*				
NUTRIDOX CONVENIENCE (Advanced Vision)				
doxycycline/flaxseed oil/omega-3 fatty acids/vit e				
KIT, PO (GLUTEN-FREE)				
131s ea	**58790-0216-87**	112.18	89.74	
NUTRILYTE (Amer Regent)				
ca ace/k ace/k cl/mg ace/na ace/na gluconate				
SOL, IV (S.D.V.)				
20 ml 25s	**00517-3120-25**	109.38		
100 ml 25s	**00517-3100-25**	562.50		
NUTRILYTE II (Amer Regent)				
ca cl/k cl/mg cl/na ace/na cl				
SOL, IV (S.D.V.,PF)				
20 ml 25s	**00517-2020-25**	93.75		
(PF)				
100 ml 25s	**00517-2000-25**	375.00		
NUTRIMIX (Hospira)				
kit, feeding (enteral)				
DEV, NA (MACRO VENTED ADAPTER)				
48s ea	**00074-1968-48**	93.31	81.60	
(Hospira)				
amino acids/dextrose				
SOL, IV (DUAL CHAMBER,LATEX-FREE)				
3.5%-25%,				
1000 ml 6s	**00409-7700-29**	218.74	191.40	
5%-25%, 1000 ml 6s	**00409-7744-29**	218.59	191.28	
NUTRIMIX W/ELECTROLYTES (Hospira)				
amino acids/dextrose/k cl/mg cl/na cl/na phos				
SOL, IV (DUAL CHAMBER,4.25%-10%)				
1000 ml 6s	**00409-7742-29**	188.78	165.18	

PROD/MFR	NDC	AWP	DP	OBC
NUTRIVIT (Llorens Pharma Int)				
multivitamin				
SOL, PO (AF,SF,DYE-FREE)				
237 ml	**54859-0501-08**	9.40		
NUTROPIN (Genentech)				
somatropin, e-coli derived				
PDS, SC (VIAL W/DILUENT)				
5 mg, ea	**50242-0072-03**	392.35		BX
(VIAL)				
5 mg, ea	**50242-0019-02**	348.81		BX
(VIAL W/DILUENT)				
10 mg, ea	**50242-0018-21**	784.70		
(VIAL)				
10 mg, ea	**50242-0020-20**	697.58		
NUTROPIN AQ (Genentech)				
somatropin, e-coli derived				
SOL, SC (VIAL CARTON)				
5 mg/ml, 2 ml	**50242-0022-20**	759.55		
NUTROPIN AQ NUSPIN 5 (Genentech)				
somatropin, e-coli derived				
SOL, SC (1X2ML)				
5 mg/2 ml, 2 ml	**50242-0075-01**	379.78		EE
NUTROPIN AQ PEN (Genentech)				
somatropin, e-coli derived				
SOL, SC (1X2ML)				
10 mg/ml, 2 ml	**50242-0073-01**	1519.10		
NUTROPIN AQ PEN CARTRIDGE (Genentech)				
somatropin, e-coli derived				
SOL, SC, 5 mg/ml, 2 ml	**50242-0043-14**	759.55		
NUVARING (Organon)				
ethinyl estradiol/etonogestrel				
ICR, VG, ea	**00052-0273-01**	66.88		
(LATEX-FREE)				
3s ea	**00052-0273-03**	200.62		
(A-S Medication)				
REPACK				
ICR, VG (LATEX-FREE)				
ea	**54569-5865-00**	69.66		
(DHS, Inc.)				
REPACK				
ICR, VG, ea	**55887-0754-01**	67.48		
(Phys Total Care)				
REPACK				
ICR, VG, 3s ea	**54868-4832-01**	239.45		
(Quality Care Prod)				
REPACK				
ICR, VG (LATEX-FREE)				
3s ea	**35356-0410-03**	117.09		
NUVIGIL (Cephalon)				
armodafinil				
TAB, PO, 50 mg,				
60s ea, C-IV	**63459-0205-60**	214.80		
150 mg,				
60s ea, C-IV	**63459-0215-60**	646.80		
250 mg,				
60s ea, C-IV	**63459-0225-60**	646.80		
NUX VOMICA EXTRACT (PCCA)				
POW, NA, 1 gm	**51927-1062-00**	0.96		
NUZON (Wraser Pharm)				
hydrocortisone acetate				
GEL, TP, 2%, 43 gm	**66992-0180-43**	49.18		
NY-TANNIC (Allegis)				
chlorpheniramine tannate/phenylephrine tannate				
TAB, PO, 9 mg-25 mg,				
100s ea	**28595-0610-01**	116.09		
NYAMYC (Upsher-Smith)				
nystatin				
POW, TP, 100000 u/gm,				
15 gm	**00832-0465-15**	27.75		AT
30 gm	**00832-0465-30**	54.30		AT
60 gm	**00832-0465-60**	96.83		AT
NYDRAZID (Sandoz)				
isoniazid				
SOL, IM (VIAL)				
100 mg/ml, 10 ml	**00003-0643-50**	249.00		
NYLIDRIN HYDROCHLORIDE (PCCA)				
POW, NA (U.S.P.)				
1 gm	**51927-2596-00**	23.40		
NYSTAT-RX (X-Gen)				
nystatin				
POW, NA (U.S.P., 1 BU)				
ea	**39822-0900-07**	246.25		EE
(U.S.P., 2 BU))				
ea	**39822-0900-04**	447.00		EE
(U.S.P., 50 MU)				
ea	**39822-0900-05**	19.75		EE

PROD/MFR	NDC	AWP	DP	OBC
(U.S.P., 500 MU)				
ea	**39822-0900-02**	130.75		EE
(U.S.P.,150 MU)				
ea	**39822-0900-03**	42.25		EE
NYSTATIN				
FUL				
CRE, TP, 100000 u/gm,				
30 gm		2.97		
OIN, TP, 100000 u/gm,				
15 gm		1.53		
POW, TP, 100000 u/gm,				
15 gm		26.22		
SUS, PO, 100000 u/ml,				
60 ml		12.37		
(Actavis)				
POW, TP (SQUEEZE BOTTLE)				
100000 u/gm, 15 gm	**67767-0112-15**	27.46		
30 gm	**67767-0112-16**	53.83		
60 gm	**67767-0112-17**	95.88		
(Actavis Mid Atlantic)				
SUS, PO (5X10)				
100000 u/ml,				
5 ml 50s UD	**00472-5003-60**	83.30		AA
60 ml	**00472-1320-02**	16.94		AA
(USP)				
100000 u/ml,				
237 ml	**00472-1320-98**	63.60		AA
473 ml	**00472-1320-16**	116.07		AA
(Bio-Tech Pharm) *See BIO-STATIN*				
(Ethex)				
POW, TP (USP)				
100000 u/gm, 15 gm	**58177-0839-45**	27.46		AT
30 gm	**58177-0839-46**	53.83		AT
60 gm	**58177-0839-61**	95.88		AT
(Fougera)				
CRE, TP, 100000 u/gm,				
15 gm	**00168-0054-15**	3.00		AT
30 gm	**00168-0054-30**	7.12		AT
OIN, TP, 100000 u/gm,				
15 gm	**00168-0007-15**	2.12		AT
30 gm	**00168-0007-30**	3.23		AT
SUS, PO, 100000 u/ml,				
60 ml	**00168-0037-60**	16.94		AA
(Glenmark Pharmaceuticals)				
SUS, PO (USP,1X60ML,W/DROPPER)				
100000 u/ml, 60 ml	**68462-0148-02**	16.94		
(USP,1X473ML,CHERRY)				
100000 u/ml,				
473 ml	**68462-0148-16**	116.00		
(Hawkins)				
POW, NA (U.S.P.)				
ea	**63370-0160-72**	62.40		
ea	**63370-0160-73**	96.00		
ea	**63370-0160-74**	384.00		
ea	**63370-0160-75**	703.20		
ea	**63370-0160-76**	1357.20		
ea	**63370-0160-80**	2688.00		
(Letco)				
POW, NA (U.S.P., DOMESTIC)				
ea	**62991-2044-02**	87.00		EE
ea	**62991-2044-03**	240.00		EE
(Medisca)				
POW, NA (U.S.P., FOREIGN)				
ea	**38779-0242-00**	2955.00		EE
ea	**38779-0242-01**	52.50		EE
ea	**38779-0242-05**	405.00		EE
ea	**38779-0242-06**	645.00		EE
ea	**38779-0242-08**	1095.00		EE
ea	**38779-0242-09**	2055.00		EE
(Midlothian Labs)				
POW, TP (1X15GM,USP)				
100000 u/gm, 15 gm	**68308-0152-15**	26.95		AT
(1X30GM,USP)				
100000 u/gm, 30 gm	**68308-0152-30**	52.33		AT
(1X60GM,USP)				
100000 u/gm, 60 gm	**68308-0152-60**	93.39		AT
(Morton Grove)				
SUS, PO, 100000 u/ml,				
60 ml	**60432-0537-60**	16.94		AA
473 ml	**60432-0537-16**	116.07		AA
(Mutual)				
TAB, PO, 500000 u, 100s ea	**53489-0400-01**	68.07		AA
(Paddock) *See NYSTOP*				
(Paddock) *See PADDOCK NYSTATIN*				

PROD/MFR	NDC	AWP	DP	OBC
(Par)				
POW, TP, 100000 u/gm,				
15 gm	49884-0989-18	27.45		
60 gm	49884-0989-60	95.86		
(PCCA)				
POW, NA (U.S.P.)				
ea	51927-1084-00	5.64		
(Pedinol) *See PEDI-DRI*				
(Perrigo)				
CRE, TP, 100000 u/gm,				
15 gm	45802-0059-35	2.95		AT
30 gm	45802-0059-11	7.10		AT
OIN, TP, 100000 u/gm,				
15 gm	45802-0048-35	2.95		AT
30 gm	45802-0048-11	7.10		AT
(Precision Dose)				
SUS, PO (1X5ML,USP,CHERRY-MINT)				
100000 u/ml,				
5 ml UD	68094-0599-59	0.83		AA
(UNIT DOSE CUP)				
100000 u/ml,				
5 ml 30s UD	68094-0599-62	26.28		AA
(CHERRY-MINT)				
100000 u/ml,				
5 ml 50s UD	68094-0599-58	60.48		AA
(UNIT DOSE CUP)				
100000 u/ml,				
5 ml 100s UD	68094-0599-61	82.80		AA
(Qualitest)				
CRE, TP (USP)				
100000 u/gm, 15 gm	00603-7818-74	2.99		EE
30 gm	00603-7818-78	7.11		EE
SUS, PO (W/DROPPER,CHERRY-MINT)				
100000 u/ml, 60 ml	00603-1481-49	16.93		AA
(CHERRY-MINT)				
100000 u/ml,				
473 ml	00603-1481-58	116.00		AA
(Spectrum Pharmacy)				
POW, NA (U.S.P.)				
ea	49452-4870-01	106.40		EE
ea	49452-4870-02	672.00		EE
ea	49452-4870-03	1813.00		EE
(Taro)				
CRE, TP, 100000 u/gm,				
15 gm	51672-1289-01	2.71		AT
30 gm	51672-1289-02	5.96		AT
SUS, PO (USP,W/DROPPER)				
100000 u/ml, 60 ml	51672-4117-04	16.94		AA
(USP,CHERRY/MINT)				
100000 u/ml,				
473 ml	51672-4117-09	115.99		AA
(Teva)				
TAB, PO, 500000 u, 100s ea	00093-0983-01	68.08		AA
VG (W/APPLICATOR)				
100000 u, 15s ea	51285-0534-22	71.65		
15s ea	65473-0705-09	46.45		AT
(Upsher-Smith) *See NYAMYC*				
(X-Gen) *See NYSTAT-RX*				
(A-S Medication) REPACK				
CRE, TP, 100000 u/gm,				
15 gm	54569-1125-00	2.91		AT
30 gm	54569-1155-00	7.10		AT
OIN, TP, 100000 u/gm,				
15 gm	54569-1104-00	2.75		EE
SUS, PO, 100000 u/ml,				
60 ml	54569-1018-00	16.94		EE
(Altura) REPACK				
CRE, TP, 100000 u/gm,				
15 gm	63874-0805-15	5.82		EE
30 gm	63874-0805-30	7.17		EE
OIN, TP, 100000 u/gm,				
15 gm	63874-0840-15	1.98		EE
30 gm	63874-0840-30	3.41		EE
SUS, PO, 100000 u/ml,				
60 ml	63874-0727-60	21.90		AA
(Bryant Ranch) REPACK				
SUS, PO, 100000 u/ml,				
60 ml	63629-2598-01	20.31		
(DHS, Inc.) REPACK				
CRE, TP, 100000 u/gm,				
15 gm	55887-0689-15	7.67		AT

PROD/MFR	NDC	AWP	DP	OBC
(Dispensing Solutions) REPACK				
CRE, TP, 100000 u/gm,				
15 gm	55045-1333-05	10.96		AT
SUS, PO (1X60ML,CHERRY-MINT)				
100000 u/ml, 60 ml	55045-1407-09	17.00		AA
(Nucare Pharm) REPACK				
CRE, TP, 100000 u/gm,				
15 gm	66267-0953-15	7.36		EE
30 gm	66267-0952-30	7.89		EE
SUS, PO, 100000 u/ml,				
60 ml	66267-0951-60	9.89		EE
(Palmetto) REPACK				
CRE, TP, 100000 u/gm,				
15 gm	23490-6025-01	7.73		
30 gm	23490-6025-02	9.26		
30 gm	23490-6026-03	5.50		
SUS, PO, 100000 u/ml,				
60 ml	23490-6028-01	22.02		
120 ml	23490-6028-02	44.04		
180 ml	23490-6028-04	66.05		
240 ml	23490-6028-05	88.07		
(PD-Rx Pharm) REPACK				
TAB, PO, 500000 u, 40s ea	55289-0130-40	25.16		EE
(Pharma Pac) REPACK				
CRE, TP, 100000 u/gm,				
15 gm	52959-0551-03	7.73		EE
30 gm	52959-0551-01	9.33		EE
SUS, PO, 100000 u/ml,				
60 ml	52959-0496-60	24.50		EE
TAB, PO, 500000 u, 20s ea	52959-0648-20	15.80		
(Phys Total Care) REPACK				
CRE, TP, 100000 u/gm,				
15 gm	54868-0242-01	5.88		EE
30 gm	54868-0242-00	8.91		EE
OIN, TP, 100000 u/gm,				
15 gm	54868-1425-00	11.01		EE
POW, TP, 100000 u/gm,				
15 gm	54868-5216-00	37.08		
60 gm	54868-5216-01	107.65		
SUS, PO, 100000 u/ml,				
60 ml	54868-0243-01	22.80		EE
473 ml	54868-0243-00	91.31		EE
TAB, PO, 500000 u, 100s ea	54868-3492-00	140.64		EE
VG, 100000 u, 15s ea	54868-1459-01	97.45		EE
(Physician Partner) REPACK				
CRE, TP (1X15GM)				
100000 u/gm, 15 gm	21695-0761-15	15.42		AT
30 gm	21695-0761-30	21.92		AT
(Quality Care Prod) REPACK				
CRE, TP, 100000 u/gm,				
15 gm	49999-0251-15	15.30		AT
30 gm	49999-0251-30	30.56		
POW, TP (1X15GM)				
100000 u/gm, 15 gm	35356-0539-15	41.30		
SUS, PO, 100000 u/ml,				
60 ml	49999-0773-02	20.33		
(1X60ML)				
100000 u/ml, 60 ml	35356-0196-60	41.50		AA
(Southwood) REPACK				
CRE, TP, 100000 u/gm,				
15 gm	58016-3056-01	5.60		EE
30 gm	58016-3057-01	6.83		EE
SUS, PO, 100000 u/ml,				
60 ml	58016-1022-01	9.65		EE
TAB, PO, 500000 u, 100s ea	58016-0143-00	55.31		EE
VG, 100000 u, 15s ea	58016-9005-01	7.59		EE
(Stat Rx) REPACK				
CRE, TP, 100000 u/gm,				
15 gm	16590-0172-15	12.50		
SUS, PO, 100000 u/ml,				
60 ml	16590-0174-60	24.25		
NYSTATIN AND TRIAMCINOLONE ACET				
(Physician Partner) REPACK				
nystatin/triamcinolone acetonide				
CRE, TP, 100000 u/gm-0.1%,				
30 gm	21695-0185-30	23.28		
60 gm	21695-0185-60	37.58		

PROD/MFR	NDC	AWP	DP	OBC
NYSTATIN AND TRIAMCINOLONE ACETONIDE				
(Quality Care Prod) REPACK				
nystatin/triamcinolone acetonide				
OIN, TP, 100000 u/gm-0.1%,				
30 gm	49999-0242-30	28.44		
NYSTATIN/TRIAMCINOLONE (DHS, Inc.) REPACK				
nystatin/triamcinolone acetonide				
CRE, TP, 100000 u/gm-0.1%,				
15 gm	55887-0326-15	14.67		
30 gm	55887-0326-30	24.21		
60 gm	55887-0326-60	12.06		
(Stat Rx) REPACK				
CRE, TP, 100000 u/gm-0.1%,				
15 gm	16590-0173-15	15.00		
NYSTATIN/TRIAMCINOLONE ACETONIDE				
FUL				
CRE, TP, 100000 u/gm-0.1%,				
30 gm		2.93		
OIN, TP, 100000 u/gm-0.1%,				
30 gm		2.93		
(Consolidated Midland)				
CRE, TP, 100000 u/gm-0.1%,				
15 gm	00223-4221-15	3.25		EE
30 gm	00223-4221-30	5.50		EE
60 gm	00223-4221-60	12.50		EE
120 gm	00223-4221-12	18.00		EE
454 gm	00223-4221-16	57.50		EE
OIN, TP, 100000 u/gm-0.1%,				
15 gm	00223-4224-15	3.25		EE
30 gm	00223-4224-30	5.50		EE
60 gm	00223-4224-60	12.50		EE
120 gm	00223-4224-12	19.50		EE
454 gm	00223-4224-16	57.50		EE
(Fougera)				
CRE, TP, 100000 u/gm-0.1%,				
15 gm	00168-0081-15	4.60		AT
30 gm	00168-0081-30	7.09		AT
60 gm	00168-0081-60	12.06		AT
OIN, TP, 100000 u/gm-0.1%,				
15 gm	00168-0089-15	4.60		AT
30 gm	00168-0089-30	7.09		AT
60 gm	00168-0089-60	12.06		AT
(Taro)				
CRE, TP, 100000 u/gm-0.1%,				
15 gm	51672-1263-01	4.31		AT
30 gm	51672-1263-02	6.64		AT
60 gm	51672-1263-03	11.29		AT
OIN, TP, 100000 u/gm-0.1%,				
15 gm	51672-1272-01	4.31		AT
30 gm	51672-1272-02	6.64		AT
60 gm	51672-1272-03	11.29		AT
(A-S Medication) REPACK				
CRE, TP, 100000 u/gm-0.1%,				
15 gm	54569-0774-00	4.46		AT
30 gm	54569-2148-00	6.87		AT
OIN, TP, 100000 u/gm-0.1%,				
30 gm	54569-1143-00	6.87		AT
(Altura) REPACK				
CRE, TP, 100000 u/gm-0.1%,				
15 gm	63874-0813-15	15.20		EE
30 gm	63874-0813-30	24.89		EE
60 gm	63874-0813-60	10.06		EE
(DHS, Inc.) REPACK				
OIN, TP, 100000 u/gm-0.1%,				
15 gm	55887-0451-15	15.72		AT
30 gm	55887-0451-30	24.30		AT
(Dispensing Solutions) REPACK				
CRE, TP, 100000 u/gm-0.1%,				
15 gm	55045-1138-05	18.99		AT
(1X30GM)				
100000 u/gm-0.1%,				
30 gm	55045-1138-06	28.90		AT
(Nucare Pharm) REPACK				
CRE, TP, 100000 u/gm-0.1%,				
15 gm	66267-0950-15	14.78		EE
30 gm	66267-0949-30	23.89		EE

PROD/MFR	NDC	AWP	DP	OBC
(Palmetto)				
REPACK				
CRE, TP, 100000 u/gm-0.1%,				
15 gm	**23490-6030-01**	14.99		
30 gm	**23490-6030-02**	29.98		
60 gm	**23490-6030-03**	59.96		
(Pharma Pac)				
REPACK				
CRE, TP, 100000 u/gm-0.1%,				
15 gm	**52959-0558-03**	15.77		EE
30 gm	**52959-0558-01**	24.36		EE
OIN, TP, 100000 u/gm-0.1%,				
15 gm	**52959-0559-03**	6.98		EE
30 gm	**52959-0559-07**	11.25		EE
(Phys Total Care)				
REPACK				
CRE, TP, 100000 u/gm-0.1%,				
15 gm	**54868-0295-01**	6.66		EE
30 gm	**54868-0295-02**	8.43		EE
60 gm	**54868-0295-03**	12.03		EE
OIN, TP, 100000 u/gm-0.1%,				
30 gm	**54868-2470-00**	8.01		AT
(Physician Partner)				
REPACK				
CRE, TP (1X15GM)				
100000 u/gm-0.1%,				
15 gm	**21695-0185-15**	18.62		AT
(Quality Care Prod)				
REPACK				
CRE, TP, 100000 u/gm-0.1%,				
15 gm	**49999-0337-15**	17.74		AT
60 gm	**49999-0337-60**	118.27		AT
(Southwood)				
REPACK				
CRE, TP, 100000 u/gm-0.1%,				
15 gm	**58016-3053-01**	14.48		EE
30 gm	**58016-3054-01**	23.70		EE
OIN, TP, 100000 u/gm-0.1%,				
15 gm	**58016-3055-01**	5.25		EE
(Stat Rx)				
REPACK				
CRE, TP (1X30GM)				
100000 u/gm-0.1%,				
30 gm	**16590-0173-30**	6.52		AT
NYSTOP (Paddock)				
nystatin				
POW, TP, 100000 u/gm,				
15 gm	**00574-2008-15**	27.46		AT
30 gm	**00574-2008-30**	53.82		AT
60 gm	**00574-2008-02**	95.88		AT
O-CAL FA (Pharmics)				
multimineral/multivitamin				
TAB, PO (SF,DYE-FREE,GLUTEN-FREE)				
100s ea	**00813-9316-01**	28.34		
O-CAL PRENATAL (Pharmics)				
prenatal vitamins				
TAB, PO, 100s ea	**00813-0202-01**	15.44		
O-DICHLOROBENZENE (Baker, J.T.)				
dichlorobenzene				
LIQ, NA (REAGENT)				
500 ml	**10106-9217-01**	75.81		
O-TOLUIDINE				
(PCCA) *See ORTHO-TOLUIDINE*				
OB COMPLETE (Vertical)				
multivitamin, minerals, and iron				
TAB, PO (10X10,SF,GLUTEN-FREE)				
100s ea UD	**68025-0010-10**	151.56		
OB COMPLETE 400 (Vertical)				
prenatal vitamins				
SGL, PO (SOFTGEL CAPLET)				
30s ea UD	**68025-0038-30**	61.71		
OB COMPLETE WITH DHA (Vertical)				
multivitamin, minerals, and iron				
SGL, PO (SOFTGEL)				
60s ea	**68025-0022-60**	123.09		
OB-NATAL ONE (Lannett)				
prenatal vitamins				
SGL, PO (SOFTGEL)				
30s ea	**00527-1760-30**	51.98		
(SOFT GELATIN)				
30s ea	**00527-1766-30**	51.98		
OBSTETRIX EC (Seyer Pharmatec)				
prenatal vitamins				
ECT, PO (CAPLET)				
60s ea	**11026-2626-06**	13.20		
OBSTETRIX-100 (Seyer Pharmatec)				
prenatal vitamins				
TAB, PO (BLISTER PACK,CAPLET)				
30s ea UD	**11026-2616-03**	12.90		
OBTREX (Pronova)				
prenatal vitamins				
TAB, PO (CAPLET)				
60s ea	**67555-0145-60**	23.75		
OBTREX DHA (Pronova)				
omega-3 fatty acids/prenatal vitamins				
KIT, PO (CAPLET,SOFTGEL)				
60s ea	**67555-0148-30**	31.25		
OCELLA (Teva)				
drospirenone/ethinyl estradiol				
TAB, PO (3X28,FILM-COATED)				
3 mg-0.03 mg,				
84s ea	**00555-9131-67**	201.55		
(A-S Medication)				
REPACK				
TAB, PO (FILM-COATED)				
3 mg-0.03 mg,				
28s ea	**54569-6128-00**	67.18		
(Phys Total Care)				
REPACK				
TAB, PO (FILM-COATED)				
3 mg-0.03 mg,				
28s ea	**54868-5922-00**	143.12		
OCTAGAM (Octapharma USA)				
immune globulin				
SOL, IV (1GM/1VIAL,S/D TREATED)				
50 mg/ml, 20 ml	**68209-0843-01**	128.77		
(1GM/VIAL,S/D TREATED)				
50 mg/ml, 20 ml	**67467-0843-01**	128.77		
(2.5GM/VIAL,S/D TREATED)				
50 mg/ml, 50 ml	**67467-0843-02**	321.94		
(PF,SUCROSE-FREE)				
50 mg/ml, 50 ml	**68209-0843-02**	321.94		
(5GM/VIAL,S/D TREATED)				
50 mg/ml, 100 ml	**67467-0843-03**	643.86		
(PF,SUCROSE-FREE)				
50 mg/ml, 100 ml	**68209-0843-03**	643.86		
(10GM/VIAL,S/D TREATED)				
50 mg/ml, 200 ml	**67467-0843-04**	1287.72		
(PF,SUCROSE-FREE)				
50 mg/ml, 200 ml	**68209-0843-04**	1287.72		
500 ml	**67467-0843-05**	3219.30		
OCTANOIC ACID (Medisca)				
SOL, NA (CAPRYLIC ACID 99%)				
100 ml	**38779-1467-05**	52.50		
500 ml	**38779-1467-08**	166.50		
(PCCA) *See CAPRYLIC ACID*				
OCTINOXATE				
(PCCA) *See OCTYL METHOXYCINNAMATE*				
(Spectrum Pharmacy)				
SOL, NA (1X100GM, USP)				
100 gm	**49452-4605-02**	89.60		
(1X500GM, USP)				
500 gm	**49452-4605-03**	310.80		
(1X2500GM, USP)				
2500 gm	**49452-4605-04**	1022.00		
OCTISALATE				
(Medisca) *See OCTYL SALICYLATE*				
(PCCA) *See OCTYL SALICYLATE*				
(Spectrum Pharmacy) *See OCTYL SALICYLATE*				
OCTOCRYLENE/OXYBENZONE				
(Rite Aid) *See RITE AID DARK TANNING*				
OCTOXYNOL 1				
(Amend) *See TRITON X-15*				
OCTOXYNOL 16				
(Amend) *See TRITON X-165*				
OCTOXYNOL 3				
(Amend) *See TRITON X-35*				
OCTOXYNOL 5				
(Amend) *See TRITON X-45*				
(PCCA) *See TRITON X-45*				
OCTOXYNOL 8				
(Amend) *See TRITON X-114*				
OCTOXYNOL 9				
(Amend) *See TRITON X-100*				
(PCCA) *See TRITON X-100*				
OCTREOSCAN (Mallinckrodt Inc.)				
indium in 111 pentetreotide				
KIT, IJ (VIAL)				
3 mci/ml, ea	**00019-9050-40**	3405.60	2838.00	
OCTREOTIDE ACETATE (APP)				
SOL, IJ (SDV,1MLX10,PF)				
50 mcg/ml,				
1 ml 10s	**63323-0365-01**	111.80		AP
100 mcg/ml, 1 ml 10s	**63323-0376-01**	216.60		AP
(MDV)				
200 mcg/ml, 5 ml	**63323-0378-05**	223.39		
(SDV,1MLX10,PF)				
500 mcg/ml,				
1 ml 10s	**63323-0377-01**	1045.10		AP
(MDV)				
1000 mcg/ml, 5 ml	**63323-0379-05**	1099.18		
(Bedford) *See AMERINET CHOICE OCTREOTIDE ACETATE*				
(Bedford)				
SOL, IJ (S.D.V.)				
50 mcg/ml,				
1 ml 10s	**55390-0160-10**	119.16		AP
(SDV)				
100 mcg/ml,				
1 ml 10s	**55390-0161-10**	231.12		AP
(MDV)				
200 mcg/ml, 5 ml	**55390-0163-01**	238.28		AP
(SDV)				
500 mcg/ml,				
1 ml 10s	**55390-0162-10**	1114.80		AP
(MDV)				
1000 mcg/ml, 5 ml	**55390-0164-01**	1172.46		AP
(Caraco)				
SOL, IJ (10X1ML)				
50 mcg/ml,				
1 ml 10s	**62756-0348-44**	110.50		AP
100 mcg/ml, 1 ml 10s	**62756-0349-44**	214.25		AP
(1X5ML,MDV)				
200 mcg/ml, 5 ml	**62756-0350-40**	220.90		AP
(10X1ML)				
500 mcg/ml,				
1 ml 10s	**62756-0351-44**	1033.50		AP
(1X5ML,MDV)				
1000 mcg/ml, 5 ml	**62756-0352-40**	1086.95		AP
(Novartis Pharm) *See SANDOSTATIN*				
(Novartis Pharm) *See SANDOSTATIN LAR DEPOT*				
(Sandoz) *See OCTREOTIDE ACETATE NOVAPLUS*				
(Sandoz)				
SOL, IJ (1X5ML,MDV)				
200 mcg/ml, 5 ml	**00781-3165-75**	156.25		
1000 mcg/ml, 5 ml	**00781-3164-75**	787.50		
(Teva) *See NOVAPLUS OCTREOTIDE ACETATE*				
(Teva)				
SOL, IJ (1MLX25 VIALS)				
50 mcg/ml,				
1 ml 25s	**00703-3301-04**	132.00		AP
100 mcg/ml, 1 ml 25s	**00703-3311-04**	252.00		AP
200 mcg/ml, 5 ml	**00703-3333-01**	108.00		AP
(1MLX25 VIALS)				
500 mcg/ml,				
1 ml 25s	**00703-3321-04**	696.00		AP
1000 mcg/ml, 5 ml	**00703-3343-01**	504.00		AP
OCTREOTIDE ACETATE NOVAPLUS (Sandoz)				
octreotide acetate				
SOL, IJ (1X1ML,INNER PACK)				
50 mcg/ml, 1 ml	**00781-9166-71**	11.17		
(M.D.V.,PRIVATE LABEL)				
50 mcg/ml,				
1 ml 10s	**00781-9166-95**	111.71		
(1X1ML,INNER PACK)				
100 mcg/ml, 1 ml	**00781-9167-71**	21.67		
(M.D.V.,PRIVATE LABEL)				
100 mcg/ml,				
1 ml 10s	**00781-9167-95**	216.69		
200 mcg/ml, 5 ml	**00781-9165-75**	223.39		
(1X1ML,INNER PACK)				
500 mcg/ml, 1 ml	**00781-9168-71**	49.98		
(M.D.V.,PRIVATE LABEL)				
500 mcg/ml,				
1 ml 10s	**00781-9168-95**	1045.11		
1000 mcg/ml, 5 ml	**00781-9164-75**	1099.18		
OCTYL DIMETHYL PABA (PCCA)				
padimate o				
SOL, NA (PADIMATE O)				
1 ml	**51927-3366-00**	0.30		
OCTYL METHOXYCINNAMATE (PCCA)				
octinoxate				
SOL, NA, 1 gm	**51927-1805-00**	0.54		

PROD/MFR	NDC	AWP	DP	OBC
OCTYL SALICYLATE (Medisca)				
octisalate				
SOL, NA (1X100ML)				
100 ml	**38779-1470-05**	30.00		
(1X500ML)				
500 ml	**38779-1470-08**	73.50		
(PCCA)				
SOL, NA, 1 ml	**51927-1600-00**	0.30		
(Spectrum Pharmacy)				
SOL, NA (U.S.P.)				
100 ml	**49452-4885-01**	75.95		
500 ml	**49452-4885-02**	148.40		
OCUFEN (Allergan Inc)				
flurbiprofen sodium				
SOL, OP, 0.03%, 2.5 ml	**11980-0801-03**	21.26		AT
(Phys Total Care)				
REPACK				
SOL, OP, 0.03%, 2.5 ml	**54868-1158-00**	25.03		AT
(Southwood)				
REPACK				
SOL, OP, 0.03%, 2.5 ml	**58016-1131-01**	16.64		AT
OCUFLOX (Allergan Inc)				
ofloxacin				
SOL, OP, 0.3%, 5 ml	**11980-0779-05**	56.75		
10 ml	**11980-0779-10**	102.01		
(A-S Medication)				
REPACK				
SOL, OP, 0.3%, 5 ml	**54569-4160-00**	54.65		
(Altura)				
REPACK				
SOL, OP (1X5ML)				
0.3%, 5 ml	**63874-0998-05**	41.46		
(Pharma Pac)				
REPACK				
SOL, OP, 0.3%, 5 ml	**52959-0607-05**	49.67		
(Phys Total Care)				
REPACK				
SOL, OP, 0.3%, 5 ml	**54868-3900-00**	60.56		
10 ml	**54868-3900-01**	103.65		
(Quality Care Prod)				
REPACK				
SOL, OP, 0.3%, 5 ml	**49999-0358-05**	76.31		
(Southwood)				
REPACK				
SOL, OP, 0.3%, 5 ml	**58016-6498-01**	34.55		
10 ml	**58016-8711-01**	69.08		
OCULAR (Allergan Medical)				
ca cl/k cl/na cl				
SOL, IR, 0.048%-0.03%-0.64%,				
18 ml	**54849-0301-18**	1.99		
150 ml	**54849-0301-15**	2.85		
250 ml	**54849-0301-25**	3.00		
500 ml	**54849-0301-50**	3.35		
OCUPRESS (Phys Total Care)				
REPACK				
carteolol hydrochloride				
SOL, OP, 1%, 10 ml	**54868-3028-00**	68.34		AT
OCUSURG (Allergan Medical)				
balanced salt solution				
PDR, IR (W/TRANSFER SPIKE,SF)				
515 ml	**54849-0501-04**	29.00		
OFATUMUMAB				
(Glaxo) *See ARZERRA*				
OFLOXACIN				
FUL				
SOL, OP, 0.3%, 5 ml		17.25		
(Akorn)				
SOL, OP, 0.3%, 5 ml	**17478-0713-10**	41.71		AT
10 ml	**17478-0713-11**	80.80		AT
(Allergan Inc) *See OCUFLOX*				
(Apotex Corp.)				
SOL, OP, 0.3%, 5 ml	**60505-0560-00**	42.13		
10 ml	**60505-0560-01**	84.14		
OT, 0.3%, 5 ml	**60505-0363-01**	74.24		AT
10 ml	**60505-0363-02**	127.11		AT
(Bausch & Lomb Inc.)				
SOL, OP, 0.3%, 5 ml	**24208-0434-05**	13.75		AT
10 ml	**24208-0434-10**	20.00		AT
OT (1X5ML)				
0.3%, 5 ml	**24208-0410-05**	18.44		AT
(1X10ML)				
0.3%, 10 ml	**24208-0410-10**	30.94		AT
(Daiichi Sankyo) *See FLOXIN OTIC SINGLES*				

PROD/MFR	NDC	AWP	DP	OBC
(Dr Reddy's)				
TAB, PO (FILM COATED)				
200 mg, 50s ea	**55111-0160-50**	239.20		AB
300 mg, 50s ea	**55111-0161-50**	284.66		AB
400 mg, 100s ea	**55111-0162-01**	600.36		AB
(Falcon Ophthalmics)				
SOL, OP, 0.3%, 5 ml	**61314-0012-05**	42.17		
10 ml	**61314-0012-10**	84.23		
OT, 0.3%, 5 ml	**61314-0015-05**	18.00		AT
10 ml	**61314-0015-10**	30.00		AT
(Hi-Tech)				
SOL, OP, 0.3%, 5 ml	**50383-0024-05**	41.71		
10 ml	**50383-0024-10**	83.30		
OT (1X5ML)				
0.3%, 5 ml	**50383-0025-05**	74.24		AT
(1X10ML)				
0.3%, 10 ml	**50383-0025-10**	127.11		AT
(Pacific Pharma) *See OFLOXACIN*				
OFLOXACIN (Pacific Pharma)				
ofloxacin				
SOL, OP (USP)				
0.3%, 5 ml	**60758-0929-05**	42.21		
10 ml	**60758-0929-10**	84.42		
OFLOXACIN (Pack)				
SOL, OP (1X5ML,USP)				
0.3%, 5 ml	**16571-0130-50**	41.71		AT
(1X10ML,USP)				
0.3%, 10 ml	**16571-0130-11**	80.80		AT
(PharmaForce)				
SOL, OP (1X5ML,USP)				
0.3%, 5 ml	**40042-0012-05**	38.50		AT
(1X10ML,USP)				
0.3%, 10 ml	**40042-0012-10**	77.50		AT
(Ranbaxy Pharm)				
TAB, PO (FILM COATED)				
200 mg, 50s ea	**63304-0716-50**	239.20	170.10	
300 mg, 50s ea	**63304-0715-50**	284.66	202.43	
400 mg, 100s ea	**63304-0717-01**	600.39	426.95	
(Teva)				
TAB, PO (FILM-COATED)				
200 mg, 100s ea	**00093-7180-01**	478.37		AB
300 mg, 100s ea	**00093-7181-01**	569.29		AB
400 mg, 100s ea	**00093-7182-01**	600.36		AB
(A-S Medication)				
REPACK				
SOL, OP, 0.3%, 5 ml	**54569-5624-00**	42.17		
OT, 0.3%, 5 ml	**54569-6045-00**	74.24		AT
(Core)				
REPACK				
TAB, PO, 200 mg, 6s ea	**33358-0272-06**	35.36		
(DHS, Inc.)				
REPACK				
SOL, OP, 0.3%, 5 ml	**55887-0406-05**	47.17		
(Dispensing Solutions)				
REPACK				
SOL, OP (1X5ML)				
0.3%, 5 ml	**55045-3230-05**	41.00		
OT, 0.3%, 5 ml	**55045-3910-01**	70.00		AT
(IPI)				
REPACK				
SOL, OP (1X5ML)				
0.3%, 5 ml	**18837-0321-05**	52.14		
(Keltman Pharma., Inc.)				
REPACK				
SOL, OP (1X5ML)				
0.3%, 5 ml	**68387-0106-01**	43.15		
(PD-Rx Pharm)				
REPACK				
TAB, PO (FILM-COATED)				
400 mg, ea	**55289-0904-79**	18.16		AB
14s ea	**55289-0904-14**	128.94		AB
(Pharma Pac)				
REPACK				
SOL, OP, 0.3%, 5 ml	**52959-0763-05**	42.35		
(1X10ML)				
0.3%, 10 ml	**52959-0763-10**	95.16		
OT (1X5ML)				
0.3%, 5 ml	**52959-0979-05**	73.18		AT
(Phys Total Care)				
REPACK				
SOL, OT (1X5ML)				
0.3%, 5 ml	**54868-6035-00**	31.59		AT

PROD/MFR	NDC	AWP	DP	OBC
(Physician Partner)				
REPACK				
SOL, OP (1X5ML)				
0.3%, 5 ml	**21695-0439-05**	148.34		
OT, 0.3%, 5 ml	**21695-0881-05**	148.48		AT
(Quality Care Prod)				
REPACK				
SOL, OP, 0.3%, 5 ml	**49999-0891-05**	50.05		
10 ml	**49999-0891-10**	101.08		
(Southwood)				
REPACK				
SOL, OP, 0.3%, 5 ml	**58016-4660-01**	42.17		
10 ml	**58016-4666-01**	84.23		
(Stat Rx)				
REPACK				
SOL, OP, 0.3%, 5 ml	**16590-0175-05**	52.14		
OFORTA (Sanofi-Aventis)				
fludarabine phosphate				
TAB, PO (4X5 STRIP,FILM COATED)				
10 mg, 20s ea	**00024-5820-20**	1851.43		
OGEN 0.625 (Phys Total Care)				
REPACK				
estropipate				
TAB, PO, 0.75 mg, 10s ea.	**54868-1262-02**	13.58		AB
30s ea	**54868-1262-01**	36.99		AB
100s ea	**54868-1262-00**	118.28		AB
OGEN 1.25 (Phys Total Care)				
estropipate				
TAB, PO, 1.5 mg, 100s ea.	**54868-1261-00**	143.45		AB
OGEN 2.5 (Phys Total Care)				
estropipate				
TAB, PO, 3 mg, 25s ea	**54868-3653-00**	50.42		AB
OGESTREL-28 (Watson)				
ethinyl estradiol/norgestrel				
TAB, PO (3X28)				
50 mcg-0.5 mg,				
84s ea	**52544-0848-28**	134.77		AB
OINTMENT BASE				
(Amend) *See AQUAPHOR*				
(Gallipot) *See FATTY ACID BASE*				
(Gallipot) *See LIP BALM BASE*				
(Gallipot)				
OIN, NA (ANHYDROUS)				
454 gm	**51552-0695-06**	16.80	12.00	
(Med-Derm) *See DELBASE*				
(Medisca)				
OIN, NA (1X450GM)				
450 gm	**38779-0937-08**	177.00		
(Medisca) *See SILK BASE*				
(Quintess Corp) *See AQUASATE-P*				
(Spectrum Pharmacy) *See BASE, OINTMENT*				
(Spectrum Pharmacy) *See BASE, PEG*				
(Spectrum Pharmacy) *See OINTMENT BASE 10% CARBAMIDE*				
(Spectrum Pharmacy) *See OINTMENT BASE 20% CARBAMIDE*				
(Spectrum Pharmacy) *See OINTMENT BASE WASHABLE COAL TAR*				
(Spectrum Pharmacy) *See OINTMENT BASE WATER IN OIL*				
(Spectrum Pharmacy) *See PLASTICIZED OINTMENT BASE*				
(Spectrum Pharmacy) *See TRANSDERMAL OINTMENT BASE*				
OINTMENT BASE 10% CARBAMIDE				
(Spectrum Pharmacy)				
ointment base				
OIN, NA, 480 gm	**49452-0842-01**	96.95		
OINTMENT BASE 20% CARBAMIDE				
(Spectrum Pharmacy)				
ointment base				
OIN, NA, 480 gm	**49452-0843-01**	120.75		
OINTMENT BASE WASHABLE COAL TAR				
(Spectrum Pharmacy)				
ointment base				
OIN, NA (1%,HYDRATED,HYDROPHILIC)				
480 gm	**49452-0839-01**	128.10		
OINTMENT BASE WATER IN OIL (Spectrum Pharmacy)				
ointment base				
OIN, NA (1X425.2GM)				
425.2 gm	**49452-0857-01**	89.95		

PROD/MFR	NDC	AWP	DP	OBC
OLANZAPINE				
(Lilly) *See ZYPREXA*				
(Lilly) *See ZYPREXA INTRAMUSCULAR*				
(Lilly) *See ZYPREXA ZYDIS*				
OLANZAPINE PAMOATE				
(Lilly) *See ZYPREXA RELPREVV*				
OLEIC ACID (Baker, J.T.)				
LIQ, NA (N.F., F.C.C)				
500 ml	10106-0224-01	14.06		
(N.F., F.C.C.)				
4000 ml	10106-0224-03	114.25		
(Gallipot)				
LIQ, NA (N.F.)				
473 ml	51552-0259-06	16.17		
(Mallinckrodt Lab)				
LIQ, NA (N.F.)				
500 ml	00406-2744-04	28.52		
4000 ml	00406-2744-08	173.87		
(Medisca)				
LIQ, NA (N.F.)				
500 ml	38779-0734-08	30.00		
(1X4000ML,NF)				
4000 ml	38779-0734-01	114.00		
(PCCA)				
LIQ, NA (N.F.)				
1 ml	51927-1299-00	0.09		
(Spectrum Pharmacy)				
LIQ, NA (N.F.)				
500 ml	49452-4880-01	83.30		
4000 ml	49452-4880-03	243.60		
20000 ml	49452-4880-04	871.50		
OLEYL ALCOHOL (PCCA)				
LIQ, NA (TECHNICAL)				
1 ml	51927-2037-00	0.62		
OLIVE OIL (Gallipot)				
OIL, NA (F.C.C.)				
29.57 ml	51552-0403-02	2.17		
473 ml	51552-0403-06	16.10		
(U.S.P.,N.F.)				
473 ml	51552-0250-06	15.33		
(Medisca)				
OIL, NA (NF 18)				
400 ml	38779-0347-08	45.00		
(1X1000ML,NF)				
1000 ml	38779-0347-09	75.00		
(NF 18)				
4000 ml	38779-0347-01	240.00		
(PCCA)				
OIL, NA (NF)				
1 ml	51927-3025-00	0.13		
(Spectrum Pharmacy)				
OIL, NA (N.F.)				
500 ml	49452-4890-01	79.80		
4000 ml	49452-4890-03	348.60		
20000 ml	49452-4890-04	1337.00		
OLMESARTAN MEDOXOMIL				
(Daiichi Sankyo) *See BENICAR*				
OLOPATADINE HYDROCHLORIDE				
(Alcon Ophthalmic) *See PATADAY*				
(Alcon Ophthalmic) *See PATANASE*				
(Alcon Ophthalmic) *See PATANOL*				
OLSALAZINE SODIUM				
(Alaven) *See DIPENTUM*				
OLUX (Stiefel Labs)				
clobetasol propionate				
FOA, TP, 0.05%, 50 gm	63032-0031-50	222.74		
100 gm	63032-0031-00	410.60		
(Quality Care Prod)				
REPACK				
FOA, TP (1X100GM)				
0.05%, 100 gm	35356-0233-00	677.00		
OLUX-E (Stiefel Labs)				
clobetasol propionate				
FOA, TP, 0.05%, 50 gm	63032-0101-50	185.62		
100 gm	63032-0101-00	342.17		
(Quality Care Prod)				
REPACK				
FOA, TP (1X100GM)				
0.05%, 100 gm	35356-0234-00	590.12		
OLUX/OLUX-E COMPLETE PACK (Stiefel Labs)				
clobetasol propionate				
FOA, TP, ea	00145-2300-03	342.17		
ea	00145-2300-50	342.17		
OMACOR (Phys Total Care)				
REPACK				
omega-3-acid ethyl esters				
SGL, PO, 1 gm, 60s ea	54868-5454-00	92.45		
OMALIZUMAB				
(Genentech) *See XOLAIR*				
OMEDIA (Athlon Pharm)				
benzocaine				
SOL, OT, 20%, 15 ml	62022-0168-15	10.80		
OMEGA-3 FATTY ACIDS/PRENATAL VITAMINS				
(Pronova) *See OBTREX DHA*				
OMEGA-3-ACID ETHYL ESTERS				
(Glaxo) *See LOVAZA*				
OMEPRAZOLE				
FUL				
ECC, PO, 10 mg, 100s ea		354.63		
20 mg, 100s ea		397.90		
40 mg, 100s ea		173.43		
(Apotex Corp.)				
ECC, PO (HARD-GELATIN)				
10 mg, 30s ea	60505-0145-00	111.00		AB
100s ea	60505-0145-02	369.99		AB
1000s ea	60505-0145-01	3699.90		AB
20 mg, 30s ea	60505-0065-00	124.55		AB
100s ea	60505-0065-02	415.14		AB
(USP,10X10,HARD-GELATIN)				
20 mg, 100s ea UD	60505-0065-07	417.14		AB
(HARD-GELATIN)				
20 mg, 1000s ea	60505-0065-01	4151.40		AB
5000s ea	60505-0065-08	20757.00		AB
(USP,ENTERIC-COATED)				
40 mg, 30s ea	60505-0146-00	221.88		AB
90s ea	60505-0146-09	665.68		AB
100s ea	60505-0146-02	739.64		AB
500s ea	60505-0146-01	3698.20		AB
(AstraZeneca) *See PRILOSEC*				
(Dr Reddy's)				
ECC, PO (USP,ENTERIC COATED)				
10 mg, 30s ea	55111-0157-30	111.00		AB
100s ea	55111-0157-01	370.00		AB
20 mg, 30s ea	55111-0158-30	124.55		AB
100s ea	55111-0158-01	415.15		AB
1000s ea	55111-0158-10	4151.50		AB
(USP,HARD GELATIN)				
40 mg, 30s ea	55111-0159-30	221.86		AB
100s ea	55111-0159-01	739.56		AB
500s ea	55111-0159-05	3697.77		AB
(Gallipot)				
POW, NA (1X5GM,USP)				
5 gm	51552-1050-02	27.30	19.50	
(1X25GM,USP)				
25 gm	51552-1050-04	81.20	58.00	
(1X100GM,USP)				
100 gm	51552-1050-05	224.00	160.00	
(Hawkins)				
POW, NA (USP)				
25 gm	63370-0214-25	120.00		
100 gm	63370-0214-35	360.00		
1000 gm	63370-0214-50	1920.00		
(Kremers Urban)				
ECC, PO, 10 mg, 30s ea	62175-0114-32	90.16		AB
20 mg, 30s ea	62175-0118-32	101.20		AB
100s ea	62175-0118-37	337.34		AB
500s ea	62175-0118-41	1686.69		AB
1000s ea	62175-0118-43	3373.38		AB
40 mg, 30s ea	62175-0136-32	200.63		AB
100s ea	62175-0136-37	669.04		AB
1000s ea	62175-0136-43	6690.26		AB
(Letco)				
POW, NA (U.S.P.)				
100 gm	62991-2400-02	180.00		
1000 gm	62991-2400-01	1185.00		
(Major)				
ECC, PO, 20 mg,				
100s ea UD	00904-5684-61	318.49		
(Medisca)				
POW, NA (1X25GM,USP)				
25 gm	38779-1935-04	247.50		
(U.S.P.)				
100 gm	38779-1935-05	495.00		
500 gm	38779-1935-08	1155.00		
1000 gm	38779-1935-09	2115.00		
(1X10000GM,USP)				
10000 gm	38779-1935-00	13770.00		
(Mylan)				
ECC, PO, 10 mg, 30s ea	00378-5211-93	111.00		AB
20 mg, 30s ea	00378-6150-93	124.55		AB
90s ea	00378-6150-77	373.64		AB
100s ea	00378-6150-01	415.15		AB
(USP)				
40 mg, 30s ea	00378-5222-93	221.80		AB
(PCCA)				
POW, NA (U.S.P.)				
1 gm	51927-3445-00	105.00		
(Ranbaxy Pharm)				
ECC, PO (HARD GELATIN)				
40 mg, 30s ea	63304-0445-30	221.86		
100s ea	63304-0445-01	739.53		
1000s ea	63304-0445-10	7396.36		
(Sandoz)				
ECC, PO, 10 mg, 30s ea	00781-2232-31	119.56		EE
30s ea	66685-0421-00	111.00		AB
100s ea	00781-2232-01	398.53		EE
100s ea	66685-0421-01	369.99		AB
20 mg, 30s ea	00781-2233-31	133.46		
30s ea	66685-0422-00	124.55		AB
(USP)				
20 mg, 90s ea	00781-2233-92	400.38		
100s ea	00781-2233-01	444.86		
100s ea	66685-0422-01	415.14		AB
1000s ea	00781-2233-10	4448.64		
1000s ea	66685-0422-03	4151.40		AB
(USP,ENTERIC-COATED)				
40 mg, 30s ea	00781-2234-31	221.86		AB
100s ea	00781-2234-01	739.53		AB
(Spectrum Pharmacy)				
POW, NA (U.S.P.)				
25 gm	49452-4891-05	364.00		
100 gm	49452-4891-01	864.50		
(Teva)				
ECC, PO, 20 mg, 1000s ea	00093-5211-10	4151.50		AB
(USP)				
40 mg, 1000s ea	00093-5212-10	7840.15		AB
(UDL)				
ECC, PO (10X10)				
20 mg, 100s ea UD	51079-0007-20	390.00		AB
(USP,10X30)				
20 mg, 300s ea UD	51079-0007-56	1170.00		AB
(Watson)				
ECC, PO (HARD GELATIN)				
40 mg, 30s ea	62037-0640-30	43.81		
100s ea	62037-0640-01	138.74		
1000s ea	62037-0640-10	1318.07		
(4u)				
REPACK				
ECC, PO, 20 mg, 30s ea	10544-0341-30	220.56		
(HARD-GELATIN)				
20 mg, 30s ea	42549-0541-30	220.56		AB
(A-S Medication)				
REPACK				
ECC, PO, 20 mg, 15s ea	54569-5482-02	62.91		AB
30s ea	54569-5482-00	125.83		AB
30s ea	54569-6165-00	124.55		AB
60s ea	54569-5482-03	251.66		
60s ea	54569-6165-01	249.09		AB
(Aidarex)				
REPACK				
ECC, PO, 20 mg, 7s ea	33261-0087-07	38.50		
14s ea	33261-0087-14	77.00		
21s ea	33261-0087-21	115.50		
28s ea	33261-0087-28	154.00		
30s ea	33261-0087-30	165.00		
40s ea	33261-0087-40	220.00		
60s ea	33261-0087-60	330.00		
90s ea	33261-0087-90	495.00		
(Altura)				
REPACK				
ECC, PO, 20 mg, 10s ea	63874-0553-10	49.78		AB
14s ea	63874-0553-14	63.74		AB
15s ea	63874-0553-15	74.67		AB
30s ea	63874-0553-30	136.59		AB
60s ea	63874-0553-60	273.18		AB
90s ea	63874-0553-90	415.32		AB
(HARD-GELATIN)				
20 mg, 120s ea	63874-0553-04	558.00		AB
(American Health)				
REPACK				
ECC, PO (10X10)				
20 mg, 100s ea UD	68084-0128-01	111.40		
(Bryant Ranch)				
REPACK				
ECC, PO, 20 mg, 30s ea	63629-2607-01	123.60		
56s ea	63629-2607-03	230.72		
60s ea	63629-2607-02	247.20		
90s ea	63629-2607-06	367.85		AB

PROD/MFR	NDC	AWP	DP	OBC
(Core)				
REPACK				
ECC, PO, 20 mg, 10s ea	**33358-0273-10**	42.23		
18s ea	**33358-0273-18**	77.27		
28s ea	**33358-0273-28**	115.31		
30s ea	**33358-0273-30**	126.69		
60s ea	**33358-0273-60**	253.38		
90s ea	**33358-0273-90**	383.05		
(DHS, Inc.)				
REPACK				
ECC, PO, 20 mg, 20s ea	**55887-0396-20**	89.31		AB
30s ea	**55887-0396-30**	133.97		AB
60s ea	**55887-0396-60**	240.00		AB
90s ea	**55887-0396-90**	360.00		AB
(Dispensing Solutions)				
REPACK				
ECC, PO, 20 mg, 15s ea	**55045-3071-03**	64.80		AB
30s ea	**55045-3071-08**	129.50		AB
45s ea	**55045-3071-04**	194.40		AB
60s ea	**55045-3071-06**	259.20		AB
(HARD-GELATIN)				
20 mg, 60s ea	**66336-0706-60**	268.12		AB
90s ea	**55045-3071-09**	388.80		AB
100s ea	**55045-3071-01**	432.00		AB
120s ea	**55045-3071-02**	518.40		AB
(GSMS)				
REPACK				
ECC, PO (HARD-GELATIN)				
20 mg, 30s ea	**60429-0157-30**	15.00	5.00	AB
60s ea	**60429-0157-60**	26.25	8.75	AB
90s ea	**60429-0157-90**	37.50	12.50	AB
100s ea	**60429-0157-01**	42.00	14.00	AB
180s ea	**60429-0157-18**	73.50	24.50	AB
360s ea	**60429-0157-36**	150.00	50.00	AB
500s ea	**60429-0157-05**	210.00	70.00	AB
1000s ea	**60429-0157-10**	420.00	140.00	AB
3000s ea	**60429-0157-03**	1275.00	425.00	AB
4000s ea	**60429-0157-04**	1650.00	550.00	AB
8000s ea	**60429-0157-08**	3150.00	1050.00	AB
(IPI)				
REPACK				
ECC, PO, 10 mg, 30s ea	**18837-0269-30**	138.75		
20 mg, 7s ea	**18837-0116-07**	51.34		AB
(HARD-GELATIN)				
20 mg, 15s ea	**18837-0116-15**	77.86		AB
30s ea	**18837-0116-30**	155.63		
(Keltman Pharma., Inc.)				
REPACK				
ECC, PO, 20 mg, 30s ea	**68387-0370-30**	140.28		AB
(HARD-GELATIN)				
20 mg, 60s ea	**68387-0370-60**	277.35		AB
(McKesson Packaging)				
REPACK				
ECC, PO, 20 mg,				
100s ea UD	**63739-0358-10**	292.16		
(20X5)				
40 mg, 100s ea UD	**63739-0445-10**	203.13		AB
(Medsource)				
REPACK				
ECC, PO (HARD-GELATIN)				
20 mg, 30s ea	**45865-0342-30**	124.50		AB
60s ea	**45865-0342-60**	249.00		AB
100s ea	**45865-0342-00**	415.00		AB
(Nucare Pharm)				
REPACK				
ECC, PO, 20 mg, 15s ea	**68071-0230-15**	85.65		AB
30s ea	**66267-1017-03**	163.41		AB
60s ea	**68071-0230-60**	269.39		AB
90s ea	**68071-0230-90**	476.23		AB
(Palmetto)				
REPACK				
ECC, PO, 10 mg, 30s ea	**23490-6897-03**	158.57		
60s ea	**23490-6897-06**	317.14		
90s ea	**23490-6897-09**	475.70		
20 mg, 28s ea	**23490-6036-01**	139.99		
30s ea	**23490-6036-03**	149.99		
30s ea	**23490-7611-03**	140.00		
60s ea	**23490-6036-06**	299.98		
90s ea	**23490-6036-09**	449.97		
(PD-Rx Pharm)				
REPACK				
ECC, PO, 20 mg, 14s ea	**55289-0971-14**	59.67		
30s ea	**55289-0971-30**	124.55		
(REDI-SCRIPT)				
20 mg, 30s ea	**58864-0832-30**	66.51		AB
60s ea	**55289-0971-60**	250.01		
(REDI-SCRIPT)				
20 mg, 60s ea	**58864-0832-60**	125.96		AB
90s ea	**55289-0971-90**	277.50		

PROD/MFR	NDC	AWP	DP	OBC
(USP,HARD-GELATIN)				
20 mg, 180s ea	**55289-0971-93**	345.27		AB
(Pharma Pac)				
REPACK				
ECC, PO, 20 mg, 10s ea	**52959-0722-10**	47.15		AB
(ENTERIC COATED)				
20 mg, 14s ea	**52959-0722-14**	65.15		AB
15s ea	**52959-0722-15**	69.80		AB
18s ea	**52959-0722-18**	83.75		AB
20s ea	**52959-0722-20**	93.05		
30s ea	**52959-0722-30**	139.56		AB
60s ea	**52959-0722-60**	277.53		
90s ea	**52959-0722-90**	416.26		
(Phys Total Care)				
REPACK				
ECC, PO, 10 mg, 60s ea	**54868-6085-00**	71.35		AB
20 mg, 30s ea	**54868-4714-00**	60.96		AB
60s ea	**54868-4714-01**	100.38		AB
90s ea	**54868-4714-03**	139.44		
100s ea	**54868-4714-02**	154.59		
(HARD GELATIN)				
40 mg, 30s ea	**54868-5987-00**	71.38		AB
90s ea	**54868-5987-01**	116.64		AB
(Physician Partner)				
REPACK				
ECC, PO (HARD-GELATIN)				
10 mg, 30s ea	**21695-0097-30**	222.00		AB
60s ea	**21695-0097-60**	443.99		
120s ea	**21695-0097-72**	887.98		
20 mg, 7s ea	**21695-0098-07**	68.35		
10s ea	**21695-0098-10**	97.64		
14s ea	**21695-0098-14**	136.70		
(HARD-GELATIN)				
20 mg, 15s ea	**21695-0098-15**	146.46		AB
30s ea	**21695-0098-30**	249.00		
60s ea	**21695-0098-60**	498.00		
90s ea	**21695-0098-90**	747.00		
120s ea	**21695-0098-72**	996.00		
(Quality Care Prod)				
REPACK				
ECC, PO, 10 mg, 30s ea	**49999-0611-30**	114.00		AB
60s ea	**49999-0611-60**	228.00		AB
100s ea	**49999-0611-00**	380.00		
20 mg, 90s ea	**49999-0265-90**	247.60		AB
(Southwood)				
REPACK				
ECC, PO, 10 mg, 30s ea	**58016-4614-03**	111.00		AB
60s ea	**58016-4614-06**	221.99		AB
90s ea	**58016-4614-09**	332.99		AB
100s ea	**58016-4614-00**	369.99		AB
(HARD-GELATIN)				
20 mg, 14s ea	**58016-0877-14**	64.61		AB
15s ea	**58016-0877-15**	69.22		AB
30s ea	**58016-0877-30**	138.44		
30s ea	**58016-0925-30**	138.44		AB
(HARD-GELATIN)				
20 mg, 42s ea	**58016-0877-42**	193.82		AB
60s ea	**58016-0877-60**	276.88		
60s ea	**58016-0925-60**	276.88		AB
90s ea	**58016-0877-90**	415.32		
90s ea	**58016-0925-90**	415.32		AB
100s ea	**58016-0877-00**	461.47		
100s ea	**58016-0925-00**	461.47		AB
120s ea	**58016-0877-02**	553.76		
120s ea	**58016-0925-02**	553.76		AB
180s ea	**58016-0877-99**	830.65		
180s ea	**58016-0925-99**	830.64		AB
(St. Mary's MPP)				
REPACK				
ECC, PO (HARD-GELATIN)				
20 mg, 5s ea	**60760-0521-05**	28.83		AB
10s ea	**60760-0521-10**	51.67		
30s ea	**60760-0521-30**	143.00		AB
(Stat Rx)				
REPACK				
ECC, PO (ENTERIC COATED)				
10 mg, 15s ea	**16590-0793-15**	77.81		AB
30s ea	**16590-0793-30**	155.63		AB
(HARD-GELATIN)				
20 mg, 14s ea	**16590-0176-14**	73.85		AB
15s ea	**16590-0176-15**	79.13		AB
28s ea	**16590-0176-28**	147.70		AB
(HARD GELATIN)				
40 mg, 30s ea	**16590-0773-30**	316.50		AB
90s ea	**16590-0773-90**	665.68		AB
(Vibranta)				
REPACK				
ECC, PO, 10 mg, 60s ea	**57866-3122-01**	228.00		

PROD/MFR	NDC	AWP	DP	OBC
OMEPRAZOLE D/R (DHS, Inc.)				
REPACK				
omeprazole				
ECC, PO, 20 mg, 14s ea	**55887-0396-14**	62.52		
40s ea	**55887-0396-40**	178.62		
(Stat Rx)				
REPACK				
ECC, PO, 20 mg, 30s ea	**16590-0176-10**	50.00		
30s ea	**16590-0176-30**	135.70		
60s ea	**16590-0176-60**	270.08		
90s ea	**16590-0176-90**	450.00		
OMEPRAZOLE DR (Dispensing Solutions)				
REPACK				
omeprazole				
ECC, PO, 20 mg, 15s ea	**66336-0706-15**	67.03		
30s ea	**66336-0706-30**	134.06		
(Quality Care Prod)				
REPACK				
ECC, PO, 20 mg, 15s ea	**49999-0265-15**	123.90		
28s ea	**49999-0265-28**	115.73		
60s ea	**49999-0265-60**	247.99		
100s ea	**49999-0265-00**	882.03		
(Vibranta)				
REPACK				
ECC, PO, 20 mg, 30s ea	**57866-3125-02**	124.00		
60s ea	**57866-3125-01**	247.99		
OMEPRAZOLE MAGNESIUM				
(AstraZeneca) *See PRILOSEC*				
OMEPRAZOLE SODIUM (Medisca)				
POW, NA (1X100GM,BP)				
100 gm	**38779-2251-05**	535.50		
(1X500GM,BP)				
500 gm	**38779-2251-08**	1147.50		
(1X1000GM,BP)				
1000 gm	**38779-2251-09**	1912.50		
(1X5000GM,BP)				
5000 gm	**38779-2251-03**	8874.00		
(1X25000GM,BP)				
25000 gm	**38779-2251-07**	36720.00		
OMEPRAZOLE/SODIUM BICARBONATE				
(Santarus, Inc.) *See ZEGERID*				
OMNARIS (Sepracor)				
ciclesonide				
SPR, NS (1X12.5GM)				
50 mcg/actuation,				
12.5 gm	**63402-0701-01**	103.80		
(Phys Total Care)				
REPACK				
SPR, NS, 50 mcg/actuation,				
12.5 gm	**54868-6020-00**	125.88		
OMNICEF (Abbott Pharm)				
cefdinir				
CAP, PO, 300 mg, 60s ea	**00074-3769-60**	370.99	325.43	
PDR, PO, 125 mg/5 ml,				
60 ml	**00074-3771-60**	61.68	54.10	
100 ml	**00074-3771-13**	97.68	85.68	
(STRAWBERRY)				
250 mg/5 ml, 60 ml	**00074-6151-60**	120.26	105.49	
100 ml	**00074-6151-13**	190.49	167.09	
(A-S Medication)				
REPACK				
CAP, PO, 300 mg, 10s ea	**54569-5214-00**	56.83		
20s ea	**54569-5214-01**	113.65		
PDR, PO, 125 mg/5 ml,				
60 ml	**54569-5215-00**	62.36		
100 ml	**54569-4877-00**	123.27		
(STRAWBERRY)				
250 mg/5 ml, 60 ml	**54569-5649-00**	151.79		
100 ml	**54569-5650-00**	240.41		
(IPI)				
REPACK				
CAP, PO, 300 mg, 20s ea	**18837-0244-20**	333.16		
(PD-Rx Pharm)				
REPACK				
CAP, PO, 300 mg, 20s ea	**55289-0831-20**	165.20		
(Phys Total Care)				
REPACK				
CAP, PO, 300 mg, 10s ea	**54868-4366-00**	68.34		
20s ea	**54868-4366-01**	128.59		
PDR, PO, 125 mg/5 ml,				
60 ml	**54868-4682-01**	62.28		
100 ml	**54868-4682-00**	98.24		
(STRAWBERRY)				
250 mg/5 ml, 60 ml	**54868-0737-00**	130.53		
100 ml	**54868-0737-01**	195.81		

PROD/MFR NDC AWP DP OBC

(Quality Care Prod)
REPACK
CAP, PO, 300 mg, 20s ea . . **35356-0038-20** 165.60

OMNIHIST L.A. (Dexo)
cpm/methscopolamine nitrate/phenyleph hcl
TER, PO, 8 mg-2.5 mg-20 mg,
100s ea. **59196-0002-01** 64.80

OMNIPAQUE 140 (GE)
iohexol
SOL, IJ (PLUSPAK,10X50ML,PF)
30.2%, 50 ml 10s **00407-1401-52** 409.12

OMNIPAQUE 180 (GE)
iohexol
SOL, IJ (VIAL)
38.8%, 10 ml 10s **00407-1411-10** 480.54
20 ml 10s. **00407-1411-20** 536.95

OMNIPAQUE 240 (GE)
iohexol
SOL, IJ (VIAL)
51.8%, 10 ml 10s **00407-1412-10** 522.47
20 ml 10s. **00407-1412-20** 552.19
50 ml 10s. **00407-1412-50** 456.46
(PLUSPAK,10X50ML,PF)
51.8%, 50 ml 10s **00407-1412-30** 479.57
100 ml 10s **00407-1412-33** 907.56
100 ml 10s **00407-1412-60** 881.38
(10X125ML, REDIFLO)
51.8%, 125 ml 10s . . . **00407-1412-91** 2212.92
150 ml 10s **00407-1412-34** 1242.84
(10X150ML, REDIFLO)
51.8%, 150 ml 10s . . . **00407-1412-90** 2322.12
(VIAL, 200 ML)
51.8%, 150 ml 10s . . . **00407-1412-49** 1206.96
200 ml 10s **00407-1412-35** 1695.12

OMNIPAQUE 300 (GE)
iohexol
SOL, IJ (VIAL)
64.7%, 10 ml 10s **00407-1413-10** 482.40
30 ml 10s. **00407-1413-30** 485.16
(SRN,PREFILLED HAND-HELD)
64.7%, 50 ml **00407-1413-25** 539.98
(BOTTLE)
64.7%, 50 ml 10s **00407-1413-51** 539.98
(PLUSPAK,10X50ML,PF)
64.7%, 50 ml 10s **00407-1413-61** 567.32
(VIAL)
64.7%, 50 ml 10s **00407-1413-50** 539.98
75 ml 10s. **00407-1413-62** 835.80
100 ml 10s **00407-1413-63** 1089.48
(10X100ML, REDIFLO)
64.7%, 100 ml 10s . . . **00407-1413-70** 2170.20
(BOTTLE)
64.7%, 100 ml 10s . . . **00407-1413-60** 1058.08
(REDIFLO,FLS-2,10X100ML)
64.7%, 100 ml 10s . . . **00407-1413-74** 2088.38
(10X125ML, REDIFLO)
64.7%, 125 ml 10s . . . **00407-1413-71** 2425.92
(BOTTLE, 200 ML)
64.7%, 125 ml 10s . . . **00407-1413-53** 1308.72
(REDIFLO,FLS-2,10X125ML)
64.7%, 125 ml 10s . . . **00407-1413-75** 2344.10
150 ml 10s **00407-1413-65** 1589.04
(10X150ML, REDIFLO)
64.7%, 150 ml 10s . . . **00407-1413-72** 2665.08
(BOTTLE, 200 ML)
64.7%, 150 ml 10s . . . **00407-1413-90** 1543.20
(REDIFLO,FLS-2,10X150ML)
64.7%, 150 ml 10s . . . **00407-1413-76** 2583.26
200 ml 10s **00407-1413-66** 1974.18
500 ml 10s **00407-1413-68** 4833.24

OMNIPAQUE 350 (GE)
iohexol
SOL, IJ (SRN,PREFILLED HAND-HELD)
75.5%, 50 ml **00407-1414-26** 588.10
(BOTTLE)
75.5%, 50 ml 10s **00407-1414-51** 588.10
(PLUSPAK,10X50ML)
75.5%, 50 ml 10s **00407-1414-89** 617.88
(VIAL)
75.5%, 50 ml 10s **00407-1414-50** 588.10
75 ml 10s. **00407-1414-90** 906.12
100 ml 10s **00407-1414-91** 1210.68
(10X100ML, REDIFLO)
75.5%, 100 ml 10s . . . **00407-1414-31** 2290.20
(BOTTLE)
75.5%, 100 ml 10s . . . **00407-1414-60** 1175.72
(PLUSPAK,10X100ML,PF)
75.5%, 100 ml 10s . . . **00407-1414-84** 1210.68
(REDIFLO,FLS-2,10X100ML)
75.5%, 100 ml 10s . . . **00407-1414-36** 2208.38

PROD/MFR NDC AWP DP OBC

(BOTTLE, 200 ML)
75.5%, 125 ml **00407-1414-76** 1389.60
(10X125ML, REDIFLO)
75.5%, 125 ml 10s . . . **00407-1414-32** 2508.36
(REDIFLO,FLS-2,10X125ML)
75.5%, 125 ml 10s . . . **00407-1414-37** 2426.54
150 ml 10s **00407-1414-93** 1671.24
(BOTTLE, 200 ML)
75.5%, 150 ml 10s . . . **00407-1414-03** 1623.12
(10X200ML,PF)
75.5%, 200 ml 10s . . . **00407-1414-42** 1999.44
(BOTTLE, 200 ML)
75.5%, 200 ml 10s . . . **00407-1414-04** 1999.44
(PLASTIC BOTTLE)
75.5%, 200 ml 10s . . . **00407-1414-94** 2058.84
(BOTTLE, 300 ML)
75.5%, 250 ml 10s . . . **00407-1414-80** 2411.64
500 ml 10s **00407-1414-98** 4905.94

OMNIPRED (Alcon Ophthalmic)
prednisolone acetate
SUS, OP, 1%, 5 ml . . . . **00065-0638-27** 44.88 AB
10 ml. . . . . **00065-0638-25** 67.80 AB

OMNISCAN (GE)
gadodiamide
SOL, IV (S.D.V.)
287 mg/ml,
5 ml 10s. **00407-0690-05** 356.04
(PREFILLED)
287 mg/ml, 10 ml **00407-0690-12** 707.68
(S.D.V.)
287 mg/ml,
10 ml 10s. **00407-0690-10** 696.00
(PREFILLED)
287 mg/ml, 15 ml **00407-0690-17** 1022.53
(S.D.V.)
287 mg/ml,
15 ml 10s. **00407-0690-15** 999.96
(PREFILLED)
287 mg/ml, 20 ml **00407-0690-22** 1257.73
(S.D.V.)
287 mg/ml,
20 ml 10s. **00407-0690-20** 1235.24
(10X50ML)
287 mg/ml,
50 ml 10s. **00407-0690-55** 2941.06

OMNISCAN PREFILL PLUS (GE)
gadodiamide/sodium chloride
SOL, IV (15ML FILL IN 20ML,PF)
287 mg/ml-0.9%,
15 ml 10s. **00407-0690-62** 1052.89
(20ML FILL IN 20ML,PF)
287 mg/ml-0.9%,
20 ml 10s. **00407-0690-63** 1288.19

OMNITROPE (Sandoz)
somatropin, e-coli derived
PDS, SC, 5.8 mg, ea . . . . . . **00781-4014-71** 238.25 BX
(W/ 8 VIALS OF DILUENT)
5.8 mg, 8s ea . . . . **00781-4004-36** 2077.56 BX
SOL, SC (1X1.5ML,W/DILUENT)
5 mg/1.5 ml,
1.5 ml . . . . **00781-3001-07** 299.30 BX
(5X1.5ML,W/DILUENT)
5 mg/1.5 ml,
1.5 ml 5s . . . . **00781-3001-26** 1496.52 BX
(10X1.5ML,W/DILUENT)
5 mg/1.5 ml,
1.5 ml 10s . . . . **00781-3001-44** 2993.04 BX
(1X1.5ML)
10 mg/1.5 ml,
1.5 ml . . . . **00781-3004-07** 598.63 BX
(5X1.5ML)
10 mg/1.5 ml,
1.5 ml 5s . . . . **00781-3004-26** 2993.16 BX
(10X1.5ML)
10 mg/1.5 ml,
1.5 ml 10s . . . . **00781-3004-44** 5986.32 BX

ONABOTULINUMTOXINA
(Allergan Inc) *See BOTOX*

(Allergan Inc) *See BOTOX COSMETIC*

ONCASPAR (Enzon Pharma, Inc.)
pegaspargase
SOL, IJ (S.D.V.,PF)
750 iu/ml, 5 ml. **57665-0002-02** 3280.00

ONDANSETRON (Akorn)
ondansetron hydrochloride
SOL, IJ (USP,SDV,5X2ML)
2 mg/ml, 2 ml 5s . . . . . **23360-0016-02** 9.30 AP
(USP,MDV,1X20ML)
2 mg/ml, 20 ml. . . . . . . **23360-0016-20** 18.56 AP

PROD/MFR NDC AWP DP OBC

(Apotex Corp.)
SOL, IJ (5X2ML,SDV,USP)
2 mg/ml, 2 ml 5s . . . . . **60505-0744-01** 120.22 AP
(MDV,USP)
2 mg/ml, 20 ml. . . . . . . **60505-0744-06** 240.35 AP
PO (USP,1X50ML)
4 mg/5 ml, 50 ml. . . . . **60505-0381-05** 239.81 AA

(APP)
SOL, IJ (SDV,25X2ML,PF)
2 mg/ml, 2 ml 25s. . . . **63323-0373-02** 70.31 AP
(MDV)
2 mg/ml, 20 ml. . . . . . . **63323-0374-20** 25.31 AP

(Baxter)
SOL, IJ (LATEX-FREE)
2 mg/ml, 1 ml. . . . . **10019-0905-17** 1.14 AP
1 ml. . . . . **10019-0906-63** 10.20 AP
(2MLX25,SDV,USP)
2 mg/ml, 2 ml 25s. . . . **10019-0905-01** 28.50 AP
(MDV,USP,LATEX-FREE)
2 mg/ml, 20 ml. . . . . . . **10019-0906-03** 10.20 AP
IV (50MLX10,SD,USP,PREMIX)
32 mg/50 ml,
50 ml 10s. . . . . **00338-1762-41** 432.00 EE

(Bedford)
SOL, IJ (SDV,USP,10X2ML)
2 mg/ml, 2 ml 10s. . . . **55390-0121-10** 18.00 AP
(MDV,USP)
2 mg/ml, 20 ml. . . . . . . **55390-0121-01** 18.00 AP

ONDANSETRON (Caraco)
ODT, PO, 4 mg, 30s ea UD . **62756-0240-64** 667.50 AB
8 mg, 10s ea UD . . . . . **62756-0356-66** 369.90 AB
30s ea UD . . . . **62756-0356-64** 1099.90 AB

(Caraco)
ondansetron hydrochloride
SOL, IJ (5X2ML,SDA,USP)
2 mg/ml, 2 ml 5s **62756-0181-01** 118.85
(MDV,USP)
2 mg/ml, 20 ml. **62756-0182-01** 237.65

(Cura Pharm)
SOL, IJ (SDV,5X2ML)
2 mg/ml, 2 ml 5s . . . . . **66860-0087-06** 116.18 AP
(MDV,1X20ML)
2 mg/ml, 20 ml. . . . . . . **66860-0088-01** 232.37 AP

ONDANSETRON
(Glaxo) *See ZOFRAN ODT*

(Glenmark Pharmaceuticals)
ODT, PO (STRAWBERRY)
4 mg, 30s ea UD . . . . . **68462-0157-13** 693.40 AB
8 mg, 10s ea UD . . . . . **68462-0158-13** 384.97 AB
30s ea UD . . . . **68462-0158-11** 1154.97 AB

(Hospira)
ondansetron hydrochloride
SOL, IJ (5X2ML,SDV,USP)
2 mg/ml, 2 ml 5s . . . . . **00409-4755-01** 5.88 5.15 AP
(10X2ML,SDPFS,USP)
2 mg/ml, 2 ml 10s. . . . **00409-1120-62** 13.44 11.80 AP
(2MLX10,SDV,USP)
2 mg/ml, 2 ml 10s. . . . **61703-0244-07** 21.96 19.20 AP
(SINGLEDOSE,USP,10X2ML)
2 mg/ml, 2 ml 10s. . . . **00409-4755-02** 8.64 7.60 AP
(25X2ML,SDV,USP)
2 mg/ml, 2 ml 25s. . . . **00409-4755-03** 18.60 16.25 AP
(M.D.V.,USP)
2 mg/ml, 20 ml. . . . . . . **61703-0245-22** 27.60 24.15 AP
(MDV,USP)
2 mg/ml, 20 ml. . . . . . . **00409-4759-01** 10.72 9.38 AP
IV (PF,LATEX-FREE)
32 mg/50 ml,
50 ml 6s. . . . . **00409-4760-13** 115.56 101.10 AP

ONDANSETRON (Mylan)
ODT, PO (USP)
4 mg, 30s ea. . . . . **00378-7732-93** 668.78 AB
8 mg, 10s ea. . . . . **00378-7734-97** 371.30 AB
30s ea. . . . . **00378-7734-93** 1113.95 AB

(Northstar)
ondansetron hydrochloride
SOL, PO (USP,1X60ML,STRAWBERRY)
4 mg/5 ml, 60 ml. . . . . **16714-0671-01** 239.82 AA

(Roxane)
SOL, PO (1X50ML,USP,STRAWBERRY)
4 mg/5 ml, 50 ml. . . . . **00054-0064-47** 239.83 AA

(Sagent)
SOL, IV (6X50ML, W/DEXTROSE,PF)
32 mg/50 ml,
50 ml 6s. . . . . **25021-0776-50** 118.13 AP

PROD/MFR	NDC	AWP	DP	OBC
ONDANSETRON (Sandoz)				
ODT, PO (3X10,STRAWBERRY)				
4 mg, 30s ea UD	00781-5265-64	668.78		
(USP,3X10,STRAWBERRY)				
4 mg, 30s ea UD	00781-5238-64	668.78		AB
(1X10,STRAWBERRY)				
8 mg, 10s ea UD	00781-5266-80	371.30		
(STRAWBERRY)				
8 mg, 10s ea UD	00781-5239-80	371.30		AB
(3X10,STRAWBERRY)				
8 mg, 30s ea UD	00781-5266-64	1113.95		
(USP,3X10,STRAWBERRY)				
8 mg, 30s ea UD	00781-5239-64	1113.95		AB
(Taro)				
ondansetron hydrochloride				
SOL, PO (1X50ML,USP)				
4 mg/5 ml, 50 ml	51672-4091-03	239.82		AA
ONDANSETRON (Teva)				
ODT, PO (USP,STRAWBERRY)				
4 mg, 30s ea UD	00093-7301-65	668.78		AB
8 mg, 10s ea UD	00093-7302-03	371.30		AB
30s ea UD	00093-7302-65	1113.95		AB
(Teva)				
ondansetron hydrochloride				
SOL, IJ (SDV,USP,5X2ML)				
2 mg/ml, 2 ml 5s	00703-7221-02	12.00		AP
(SDV,USP,25X2ML)				
2 mg/ml, 2 ml 25s	00703-7221-04	60.00		AP
(MDV,USP)				
2 mg/ml, 20 ml	00703-7226-01	24.00		AP
(MDV,USP,10X20ML)				
2 mg/ml, 20 ml 10s	00703-7226-03	240.00		AP
IV (SINGLE DOSE,6X50ML,PF)				
32 mg/50 ml,				
50 ml 6s	00703-7239-39	239.58		AP
(West-Ward)				
SOL, IJ (USP,SINGLE DOSE)				
2 mg/ml, 2 ml 5s	00143-9891-05	6.25		AP
(USP,MULTIDOSE)				
2 mg/ml, 20 ml	00143-9890-01	3.44		AP
IV (48X50ML,SINGLE-DOSE)				
32 mg/50 ml,				
50 ml 48s	00143-9771-06	112.50		
(Wockhardt USA)				
SOL, IJ (5X2ML,SDV,USP)				
2 mg/ml, 2 ml 5s	64679-0726-01	116.18		AP
(MDV,USP)				
2 mg/ml, 20 ml	64679-0727-01	232.37		AP
ONDANSETRON (A-S Medication)				
REPACK				
ODT, PO (STRAWBERRY)				
8 mg, 4s ea	54569-6124-00	150.47		AB
(A-S Medication)				
ondansetron hydrochloride				
SOL, IJ (5X2ML,SDV)				
2 mg/ml, 2 ml 5s	54569-5874-00	84.07		
ONDANSETRON (Core)				
REPACK				
ODT, PO, 4 mg, 20s ea	33358-0471-20	72.66		AB
(DHS, Inc.)				
REPACK				
ondansetron hydrochloride				
TAB, PO, 4 mg, 3s ea	55887-0078-03	74.33		
ONDANSETRON (Dispensing Solutions)				
REPACK				
ODT, PO, 4 mg, 30s ea	55045-3848-09	600.00		AB
(STRAWBERRY)				
4 mg, 30s ea	55045-3848-04	600.00		AB
8 mg, 10s ea	55045-3815-01	370.00		
(Nucare Pharm)				
REPACK				
ODT, PO (STRAWBERRY)				
4 mg, 2s ea	68071-0692-02	59.59		AB
8 mg, 3s ea	68071-0758-03	125.28		AB
(PD-Rx Pharm)				
REPACK				
ODT, PO, 4 mg, 2s ea	43063-0052-02	49.50		AB
(USP,STRAWBERRY)				
4 mg, 3s ea	55289-0559-03	58.40		AB
4s ea	43063-0052-04	68.50		AB
(STRAWBERRY)				
4 mg, 5s ea	55289-0559-05	63.90		AB
(USP,STRAWBERRY)				
4 mg, 6s ea	55289-0559-06	89.50		AB
(Phys Total Care)				
REPACK				
ODT, PO (STRAWBERRY)				
4 mg, 10s ea	54868-5887-00	26.42		AB
(Phys Total Care)				
ondansetron hydrochloride				
SOL, IJ (1X10ML)				
2 mg/ml, 10 ml	54868-5888-00	21.74		AP
TAB, PO, 4 mg, 15s ea	54868-5801-01	40.13		
30s ea	54868-5801-00	108.46		
ONDANSETRON (Physician Partner)				
REPACK				
ODT, PO (STRAWBERRY)				
4 mg, 10s ea	21695-0380-10	524.53		AB
30s ea	21695-0380-30	1337.56		AB
8 mg, 10s ea	21695-0479-10	742.60		AB
(Stat Rx)				
REPACK				
ODT, PO (STRAWBERRY)				
8 mg, 20s ea	16590-0465-20	760.88		
30s ea	16590-0465-30	1165.51		
ONDANSETRON AND DEXTROSE (Mayne Pharma)				
ondansetron hydrochloride				
SOL, IV (SINGLE-USE,6X50ML,PF)				
32 mg/50 ml,				
50 ml 6s	61703-0415-49	276.00	241.50	
ONDANSETRON HCL (B&B Pharm, Inc)				
ondansetron hydrochloride				
POW, NA, 0.1 gm	63275-9955-06	377.00		
0.5 gm	63275-9955-07	1885.00		
1 gm	63275-9955-01	3770.00		
5 gm	63275-9955-02	17110.00		
ONDANSETRON HYDROCHLORIDE				
FUL				
TAB, PO, 4 mg, 30s ea		33.00		
8 mg, 30s ea		57.00		
(Actavis)				
TAB, PO (FILM-COATED)				
4 mg, 30s ea	52152-0538-30	746.67		AB
8 mg, 30s ea	52152-0539-30	1243.70		AB
(Akorn) *See ONDANSETRON*				
(Apotex Corp.) *See ONDANSETRON*				
(Apotex Corp.)				
TAB, PO (FILM-COATED)				
4 mg, 30s ea	60505-1311-03	743.40		AB
8 mg, 30s ea	60505-1312-03	1237.80		AB
(APP) *See ONDANSETRON*				
(Aurobindo Pharma)				
TAB, PO (FILM-COATED)				
4 mg, 3s ea UD	65862-0187-03	72.60		AB
30s ea	65862-0187-30	726.00		AB
500s ea	65862-0187-05	12100.00		AB
8 mg, 3s ea UD	65862-0188-03	120.00		AB
30s ea	65862-0188-30	1209.00		AB
500s ea	65862-0188-05	20150.00		AB
(B&B Pharm, Inc) *See ONDANSETRON HCL*				
(Baxter) *See NOVAPLUS ONDANSETRON*				
(Baxter) *See ONDANSETRON*				
(Bedford) *See ONDANSETRON*				
(Bedford) *See ONDANSETRON NOVAPLUS*				
(Caraco) *See ONDANSETRON*				
(Caraco)				
TAB, PO (FILM-COATED)				
4 mg, 30s ea	62756-0130-01	708.90		AB
8 mg, 30s ea	62756-0131-01	1179.95		AB
(Cura Pharm) *See ONDANSETRON*				
(Dr Reddy's)				
TAB, PO (1X3,FILM-COATED)				
4 mg, 3s ea UD	55111-0153-13	74.33		AB
(FILM-COATED)				
4 mg, 30s ea	55111-0153-30	743.30		AB
(1X3,FILM-COATED)				
8 mg, 3s ea UD	55111-0154-13	123.79		AB
(FILM-COATED)				
8 mg, 30s ea	55111-0154-30	1237.80		AB
(1X1,FILM-COATED)				
24 mg, ea UD	55111-0156-11	106.51		AB
(Glaxo) *See ZOFRAN*				
(Glenmark Pharmaceuticals)				
TAB, PO (FILM-COATED)				
4 mg, 30s ea	68462-0105-30	735.05		AB
8 mg, 30s ea	68462-0106-30	1070.26		AB
(Greenstone)				
TAB, PO (FILM-COATED)				
4 mg, 30s ea	59762-2990-01	726.00		
500s ea	59762-2990-02	12100.00		
8 mg, 30s ea	59762-2993-01	1209.00		
500s ea	59762-2993-02	20150.00		
(Hospira) *See AMERINET CHOICE ONDANSETRON*				
(Hospira) *See ONDANSETRON*				
(Letco)				
POW, NA (1X100GM)				
100 gm	62991-2599-01	735.00		
(1X1000GM)				
1000 gm	62991-2599-02	5400.00		
(Mayne Pharma) *See ONDANSETRON AND DEXTROSE*				
(Medisca)				
POW, NA (1X5GM,USP,DIHYDRATE)				
5 gm	38779-2415-03	885.00		
(1X25GM,USP,DIHYDRATE)				
25 gm	38779-2415-04	2850.00		
(1X100GM,USP,DIHYDRATE)				
100 gm	38779-2415-05	8985.00		
(Mylan)				
TAB, PO (FILM-COATED)				
4 mg, 3s ea UD	00378-0315-53	74.33		AB
30s ea	00378-0315-93	743.40		AB
8 mg, 3s ea UD	00378-0344-53	123.79		AB
30s ea	00378-0344-93	1237.80		AB
(Northstar) *See ONDANSETRON*				
(PCCA) *See ONDANSETRON HYDROCHLORIDE DIHYDRATE*				
(Perrigo)				
TAB, PO (FILM-COATED)				
4 mg, 3s ea UD	45802-0127-14	71.76		
30s ea	45802-0127-65	717.61		
8 mg, 3s ea UD	45802-0205-14	119.50		
30s ea	45802-0205-65	1195.28		
(Pfizer) *See ONDANSETRON IN 5% DEXTROSE*				
(Ranbaxy Pharm)				
TAB, PO (FILM-COATED)				
4 mg, 30s ea	63304-0458-30	743.35		AB
8 mg, 30s ea	63304-0459-30	1238.17		AB
(Roxane) *See ONDANSETRON*				
(Sagent) *See ONDANSETRON*				
(Sandoz)				
SOL, IJ (SDV,10X2ML)				
2 mg/ml, 10s ea	00781-3010-95	240.46		
(S.D.V,5X2ML)				
2 mg/ml, 2 ml 5s	00781-3057-14	120.23		
(MULTIPLE DOSE VIAL)				
2 mg/ml, 20 ml	00781-3057-80	240.38		
TAB, PO (FILM COATED)				
4 mg, 3s ea UD	00781-5257-33	70.89		
(FILM-COATED)				
4 mg, 3s ea UD	00781-1679-33	70.89		AB
(FILM COATED)				
4 mg, 30s ea	00781-5257-31	708.94		
(FILM-COATED)				
4 mg, 30s ea	00781-1679-31	708.94		AB
(FILM COATED)				
4 mg, 100s ea UD	00781-5257-13	2362.72		
8 mg, 3s ea UD	00781-5258-33	118.06		
(UNIT OF USE,FILM-COATED)				
8 mg, 3s ea	00781-1681-33	118.06		AB
(FILM COATED)				
8 mg, 30s ea	00781-5258-31	1180.85		
(FILM-COATED)				
8 mg, 30s ea	00781-1681-31	1180.85		AB
(FILM COATED)				
8 mg, 100s ea UD	00781-5258-13	3936.05		
(Taro) *See ONDANSETRON*				
(Teva) *See ONDANSETRON*				
(Teva)				
SOL, PO, 4 mg/5 ml, 50 ml	50111-0819-42	239.81		
TAB, PO (FILM COATED)				
4 mg, 3s ea	00093-0233-33	73.08		AB
30s ea	00093-0233-56	730.89		AB
8 mg, 3s ea	00093-7236-33	121.71		AB
30s ea	00093-7236-56	1217.42		AB
(UDL)				
TAB, PO (USP,10X10,FILM-COATED)				
4 mg, 100s ea UD	51079-0524-20	2478.00		AB
8 mg, 100s ea UD	51079-0525-20	4126.00		AB
(West-Ward) *See ONDANSETRON*				
(Wockhardt USA) *See ONDANSETRON*				
(A-S Medication)				
REPACK				
TAB, PO, 8 mg, 4s ea	54569-5873-00	165.04		
(FILM-COATED)				
8 mg, 10s ea	54569-5873-01	412.60		AB

PROD/MFR	NDC	AWP	DP	OBC
(Aidarex)				
REPACK				
TAB, PO (FILM-COATED)				
4 mg, 3s ea	**33261-0417-03**	75.00		**AB**
6s ea	**33261-0417-06**	150.00		**AB**
12s ea	**33261-0417-12**	300.00		**AB**
30s ea	**33261-0417-30**	750.00		**AB**
(Dispensing Solutions)				
REPACK				
TAB, PO (FILM-COATED)				
4 mg, 3s ea	**66336-0793-03**	72.77		**AB**
6s ea	**66336-0793-06**	145.54		**AB**
30s ea	**55045-3729-03**	720.00		
(FILM-COATED)				
8 mg, 3s ea	**66336-0268-03**	121.19		**AB**
6s ea	**66336-0268-06**	242.38		**AB**
(Pharma Pac)				
REPACK				
TAB, PO (FILM COATED)				
8 mg, 3s ea	**52959-0980-03**	127.74		
(Phys Total Care)				
REPACK				
TAB, PO, 8 mg, 10s ea	**54868-5738-00**	79.74		
(FILM-COATED)				
8 mg, 30s ea	**54868-5738-01**	70.73		**AB**
(Physician Partner)				
REPACK				
TAB, PO (FILM-COATED)				
4 mg, 4s ea	**21695-0834-04**	222.40		**AB**
12s ea	**21695-0834-12**	667.20		**AB**
15s ea	**21695-0834-15**	834.00		**AB**
30s ea	**21695-0834-30**	1417.80		**AB**
8 mg, 30s ea	**21695-0835-30**	2359.90		**AB**
(Quality Care Prod)				
REPACK				
TAB, PO (FILM COATED)				
4 mg, 30s ea	**35356-0197-30**	136.20		
8 mg, 30s ea	**35356-0445-30**	246.60		**AB**
(Stat Rx)				
REPACK				
TAB, PO (FILM-COATED)				
4 mg, 10s ea	**16590-0464-10**	243.63		**AB**
20s ea	**16590-0464-20**	494.30		**AB**
30s ea	**16590-0464-30**	744.20		**AB**
ONDANSETRON HYDROCHLORIDE DIHYDRATE (PCCA)				
ondansetron hydrochloride				
POW, NA (USP,1X1GM)				
1 gm	**51927-4320-00**	177.00		
ONDANSETRON IN 5% DEXTROSE (Pfizer)				
ondansetron hydrochloride				
SOL, IV (6X50ML,SINGLE DOSE,PF)				
32 mg/50 ml,				
50 ml 6s	**00069-0700-12**	124.80		
ONDANSETRON NOVAPLUS (Bedford)				
ondansetron hydrochloride				
SOL, IJ (SDV,USP)				
2 mg/ml, 2 ml 10s	**55390-0307-10**	12.00		**AP**
(MDV,USP)				
2 mg/ml, 20 ml	**55390-0307-01**	7.20		**AP**
ONDANSETRON ODT (Phys Total Care)				
REPACK				
ondansetron				
ODT, PO, 8 mg, 10s ea	**54868-5749-00**	72.96		
15s ea	**54868-5749-01**	104.82		
(Southwood)				
REPACK				
ODT, PO, 4 mg, 30s ea	**00490-0075-30**	668.78		
60s ea	**00490-0075-60**	1337.56		
90s ea	**00490-0075-90**	2006.34		
100s ea	**00490-0075-00**	2229.27		
ONGLYZA (Bristol-Myers)				
saxagliptin hydrochloride				
TAB, PO (FILM-COATED)				
2.5 mg, 30s ea	**00003-4214-11**	205.92		
90s ea	**00003-4214-21**	617.76		
5 mg, 30s ea	**00003-4215-11**	205.92		
90s ea	**00003-4215-21**	617.76		
100s ea UD	**00003-4215-41**	686.40		
500s ea	**00003-4215-31**	3432.00		
ONION EXTRACT (Medisca)				
POW, NA (1X1000GM,WATER SOLUBLE)				
1000 gm	**38779-1473-09**	229.50		
(PCCA)				
POW, NA (WATER SOLUBLE)				
1 gm	**51927-2598-00**	0.38		
ONOPORDON COMPOUND (Weleda)				
homeopathic substance				
TAB, PO, 100s ea	**55946-0320-30**	5.85		
ONSOLIS (Meda)				
fentanyl citrate				
FIL, BC (BILAYER)				
200 mcg,				
30s ea, C-II	**00037-5200-30**	637.50	510.00	
400 mcg,				
30s ea, C-II	**00037-5400-30**	937.50	750.00	
600 mcg,				
30s ea, C-II	**00037-5600-30**	1237.50	990.00	
800 mcg,				
30s ea, C-II	**00037-5800-30**	1537.50	1230.00	
1200 mcg,				
30s ea, C-II	**00037-5120-30**	1837.50	1470.00	
ONTAK (Eisai)				
denileukin diftitox				
SOL, IV (2ML,SINGLE USE)				
150 mcg/ml, 2 ml	**62856-0603-01**	1756.80		
OPANA (Endo Pharm)				
oxymorphone hydrochloride				
SOL, IJ (1MLX10,PARABEN-FREE)				
1 mg/ml,				
1 ml 10s, C-II	**63481-0624-10**	31.26		
TAB, PO, 5 mg,				
100s ea, C-II	**63481-0612-70**	327.34		
10 mg,				
100s ea, C-II	**63481-0613-70**	594.37		
(Quality Care Prod)				
REPACK				
TAB, PO, 5 mg,				
30s ea, C-II	**35356-0214-30**	149.75		
60s ea, C-II	**35356-0214-60**	294.61		
10 mg,				
30s ea, C-II	**35356-0380-30**	271.08		
60s ea, C-II	**35356-0380-60**	537.25		
120s ea, C-II	**35356-0380-01**	757.84		
(Stat Rx)				
REPACK				
TAB, PO, 5 mg,				
56s ea, C-II	**16590-0819-56**	215.14		
60s ea, C-II	**16590-0819-60**	230.28		
120s ea, C-II	**16590-0819-72**	431.78		
10 mg,				
28s ea, C-II	**16590-0765-28**	195.62		
30s ea, C-II	**16590-0765-30**	376.38		
56s ea, C-II	**16590-0765-56**	388.00		
60s ea, C-II	**16590-0765-60**	415.48		
90s ea, C-II	**16590-0765-90**	621.59		
OPANA ER (Endo Pharm)				
oxymorphone hydrochloride				
TER, PO (FILM-COATED)				
5 mg,				
100s ea, C-II	**63481-0907-70**	205.70		**EE**
7.5 mg,				
100s ea, C-II	**63481-0522-70**	300.35		**EE**
10 mg,				
100s ea, C-II	**63481-0674-70**	395.00		**EE**
15 mg,				
100s ea, C-II	**63481-0553-70**	547.80		**EE**
20 mg,				
100s ea, C-II	**63481-0617-70**	700.58		**EE**
30 mg,				
100s ea, C-II	**63481-0571-70**	1008.38		**EE**
40 mg,				
100s ea, C-II	**63481-0693-70**	1316.20		
(Quality Care Prod)				
REPACK				
TER, PO (FILM-COATED)				
5 mg,				
120s ea, C-II	**35356-0214-01**	379.26		**EE**
10 mg,				
30s ea, C-II	**35356-0388-30**	207.11		**EE**
60s ea, C-II	**35356-0388-60**	409.31		**EE**
90s ea, C-II	**35356-0388-90**	621.00		**EE**
15 mg,				
30s ea, C-II	**35356-0390-30**	285.78		**EE**
60s ea, C-II	**35356-0390-60**	566.67		**EE**
20 mg,				
20s ea, C-II	**35356-0389-20**	242.48		**EE**
30s ea, C-II	**35356-0389-30**	363.73		**EE**
60s ea, C-II	**35356-0389-60**	722.55		**EE**
30 mg,				
30s ea, C-II	**35356-0403-30**	521.82		**EE**
60s ea, C-II	**35356-0403-60**	1038.73		**EE**
40 mg,				
30s ea, C-II	**35356-0381-30**	654.45		
30s ea, C-II	**35356-0391-30**	679.17		
60s ea, C-II	**35356-0391-60**	1353.43		
90s ea, C-II	**35356-0391-90**	2030.40		
(St. Mary's MPP)				
REPACK				
TER, PO (FILM-COATED)				
20 mg,				
60s ea, C-II	**60760-0617-60**	579.73		**EE**
(Stat Rx)				
REPACK				
TER, PO (FILM-COATED)				
5 mg, 56s ea, C-II	**16590-0767-56**	123.50		**EE**
60s ea, C-II	**16590-0767-60**	236.40		**EE**
10 mg,				
56s ea, C-II	**16590-0747-56**	236.07		**EE**
60s ea, C-II	**16590-0747-60**	252.82		**EE**
90s ea, C-II	**16590-0747-90**	379.24		**EE**
15 mg,				
60s ea, C-II	**16590-0862-60**	347.13		**EE**
20 mg,				
28s ea, C-II	**16590-0608-28**	210.42		**EE**
30s ea, C-II	**16590-0608-30**	226.20		**EE**
56s ea, C-II	**16590-0608-56**	414.09		**EE**
60s ea, C-II	**16590-0608-60**	450.89		**EE**
90s ea, C-II	**16590-0608-90**	675.60		**EE**
40 mg,				
30s ea, C-II	**16590-0609-30**	423.54		
40s ea, C-II	**16590-0609-40**	564.72		
60s ea, C-II	**16590-0609-60**	837.64		
90s ea, C-II	**16590-0609-90**	1255.75		
OPHTHETIC (A-S Medication)				
REPACK				
proparacaine hydrochloride				
SOL, OP, 0.5%, 15 ml	**54569-2244-00**	15.86		**AT**
(Phys Total Care)				
REPACK				
SOL, OP, 0.5%, 15 ml	**54868-1674-00**	15.46		**AT**
(Quality Care Prod)				
REPACK				
SOL, OP, 0.5%, 15 ml	**49999-0590-15**	22.93		**AT**
(Southwood)				
REPACK				
SOL, OP, 0.5%, 15 ml	**58016-6447-01**	19.11		**AT**
OPIUM (Marathon)				
TIN, PO (1X118ML,DEODORIZED,USP)				
10 mg/ml,				
118 ml, C-II	**42998-0203-01**	756.20		
(1X473ML,DEODORIZED,USP)				
10 mg/ml,				
473 ml, C-II	**42998-0203-02**	3024.79		
OPRELVEKIN				
(Wyeth) *See NEUMEGA*				
OPTASE (Onset)				
castor oil/peru balsam/trypsin				
GEL, TP (6GMX10)				
6 gm 10s	**16781-0116-06**	87.50	70.00	
95 gm	**16781-0116-95**	65.86		
OPTICHAMBER (Respironics)				
spacer, inhalation				
DEV, NA, ea	**83730-0800-10**	20.20		
OPTICHAMBER FACE MASK (Respironics)				
mask, face				
DEV, NA (LARGE)				
ea	**83730-0813-10**	11.00		
(MEDIUM)				
ea	**83730-0812-10**	10.00		
(SMALL)				
ea	**83730-0811-10**	10.00		
OPTICHAMBER W/MASK (Respironics)				
spacer, inhalation				
DEV, NA (LARGE)				
ea	**83730-0803-10**	31.20		
(MEDIUM)				
ea	**83730-0802-10**	30.20		
(SMALL)				
ea	**83730-0801-10**	30.20		
OPTIHALER (Respironics)				
spacer, inhalation				
DEV, NA (DRUG DELIVERY SYSTEM)				
ea	**08373-0765-00**	12.84		
OPTIMARK (Mallinckrodt Inc.)				
gadoversetamide				
INJ, IJ (SDV,GLASS,PF)				
330.9 mg/ml, 5 ml	**00019-1177-02**	33.72	28.10	
10 ml	**00019-1177-04**	44.88	37.40	
(SRN,HAND HELD,PF)				
330.9 mg/ml, 10 ml	**00019-1177-10**	48.84	40.70	
(SDV,GLASS,PF)				
330.9 mg/ml, 15 ml	**00019-1177-06**	67.32	56.10	
(SRN,HAND HELD,PF)				
330.9 mg/ml, 15 ml	**00019-1177-15**	71.28	59.40	

PROD/MFR	NDC	AWP	DP	OBC
(SDV,GLASS,PF)				
330.9 mg/ml, 20 ml	**00019-1177-08**	89.76	74.80	
(SRN,HAND HELD,PF)				
330.9 mg/ml, 20 ml	**00019-1177-20**	93.72	78.10	
30 ml	**00019-1177-30**	138.60	115.50	
(BULK VIAL,GLASS,PF)				
330.9 mg/ml, 50 ml	**00019-1177-50**	205.92	171.60	
OPTIPRANOLOL (Bausch & Lomb Inc.)				
metipranolol				
SOL, OP, 0.3%, 5 ml	**24208-0275-07**	25.38		
10 ml	**24208-0275-09**	42.98		
(Phys Total Care)				
REPACK				
SOL, OP, 0.3%, 10 ml	**54868-3027-00**	39.41		AT
OPTIRAY 160 (Mallinckrodt Inc.)				
ioversol				
SOL, IJ (BOTTLE)				
34%, 50 ml	**00019-1325-06**	39.60	33.00	
OPTIRAY 240 (Mallinckrodt Inc.)				
ioversol				
SOL, IJ (BOTTLE)				
51%, 50 ml	**00019-1324-06**	46.50	38.75	
(SRN,PREFILLED)				
51%, 50 ml	**00019-1324-75**	19.68		
100 ml	**00019-1324-11**	83.40	69.50	
(SRN,PREFILLED)				
51%, 125 ml	**00019-1324-81**	117.60	98.00	
OPTIRAY 300 (Mallinckrodt Inc.)				
ioversol				
SOL, IJ (BOTTLE)				
64%, 50 ml	**00019-1332-06**	47.40	39.50	
(SRN,PREFILLED)				
64%, 50 ml	**00019-1332-75**	20.88		
(BOTTLE)				
64%, 100 ml	**00019-1332-11**	93.90	78.25	
(SRN,PREFILLED,ULTRAJECT)				
64%, 100 ml	**00019-1332-83**	115.20	96.00	
(BOTTLE)				
64%, 150 ml	**00019-1332-16**	135.00	112.50	
OPTIRAY 320 (Mallinckrodt Inc.)				
ioversol				
SOL, IJ, 68%, 50 ml	**00019-1323-06**	52.50	43.75	
(SRN,PREFILLED)				
68%, 50 ml	**00019-1323-75**	23.04		
100 ml	**00019-1323-11**	104.40	87.00	
(SRN,PREFILLED,ULTRAJECT)				
68%, 100 ml	**00019-1323-83**	117.60	98.00	
(SRN,PREFILLED)				
68%, 125 ml	**00019-1323-81**	143.40	119.50	
150 ml	**00019-1323-16**	150.30	125.25	
OPTIRAY 350 (Mallinckrodt Inc.)				
ioversol				
SOL, IJ, 74%, 50 ml	**00019-1333-06**	57.00	47.50	
(SRN,PREFILLED)				
74%, 50 ml	**00019-1333-75**	24.48		
(SRN,PREFILLED,ULTRAJECT)				
74%, 75 ml	**00019-1333-91**	100.20	83.50	
(BOTTLE)				
74%, 100 ml	**00019-1333-11**	114.00	95.00	
(SRN,PREFILLED)				
74%, 100 ml	**00019-1333-83**	123.60	103.00	
125 ml	**00019-1333-81**	147.60	123.00	
150 ml	**00019-1333-16**	159.60	133.00	
OPTISON (GE)				
perflutren protein type a microsphere				
SUS, IV ((SDV,MICROSPHERE),5X3ML)				
3 ml 5s	**00407-2707-03**	842.40		
OPTIVA IV CATHETER/OCR (J&J Medical)				
catheter				
DEV, NA (RADIOPAQUE,14X1 1/4")				
ea	**56091-0050-48**	1.24		
(RADIOPAQUE,14X2 1/4")				
ea	**56091-0050-58**	1.24		
(RADIOPAQUE,16X1 1/4")				
ea	**56091-0050-42**	1.24		
(RADIOPAQUE,16X2 1/4")				
ea	**56091-0050-52**	1.24		
(RADIOPAQUE,18X1 1/4")				
ea	**56091-0050-55**	1.24		
(RADIOPAQUE,18X1 3/4")				
ea	**56091-0050-54**	1.24		
(RADIOPAQUE,20X1 1/4")				
ea	**56091-0050-56**	1.24		
(RADIOPAQUE,20X1 3/4")				
ea	**56091-0050-59**	1.24		
(RADIOPAQUE,20X1")				
ea	**56091-0050-57**	1.24		
(RADIOPAQUE,22X1")				
ea	**56091-0050-50**	1.30		
(RADIOPAQUE,24X3/4")				
ea	**56091-0050-53**	1.69		

PROD/MFR	NDC	AWP	DP	OBC
OPTIVAR (Meda)				
azelastine hydrochloride				
SOL, OP, 0.05%, 6 ml	**00037-7025-60**	115.63		
(Pharma Pac)				
REPACK				
SOL, OP, 0.05%, 6 ml	**52959-0710-06**	68.50		
(Phys Total Care)				
REPACK				
SOL, OP, 0.05%, 6 ml	**54868-4696-00**	101.23		
ORACEA (Galderma)				
doxycycline				
CER, PO (HARD GELATIN)				
40 mg, 30s ea	**00299-3822-30**	373.75		EE
(Phys Total Care)				
REPACK				
CER, PO, 40 mg, 30s ea	**54868-5676-00**	279.88		
ORACIT (Carolina)				
citric acid/sodium citrate				
SOL, PO (10X15ML)				
640 mg/5 ml-490 mg/5 ml,				
15 ml 10s UD	**46287-0014-15**	16.20	13.00	
(10X30ML)				
640 mg/5 ml-490 mg/5 ml,				
30 ml 10s UD	**46287-0014-30**	17.65	14.00	
500 ml	**46287-0014-01**	17.65	14.00	
3840 ml	**46287-0014-99**	67.20	56.00	
ORAL SALINE LAXATIVE (Southwood)				
REPACK				
na phos, dibasic/na phos, monobasic				
SOL, PO, 0.9 gm/5 ml-2.4 gm/5 ml,				
90 ml	**58016-4848-01**	2.60		
ORAL TRANSMUCOSAL FENTANYL CITRATE (Teva)				
fentanyl citrate				
LOZ, MM (BERRY)				
0.2 mg,				
30s ea, C-II	**00555-1080-01**	564.12		
0.4 mg,				
30s ea, C-II	**00555-1081-01**	714.71		
0.6 mg,				
30s ea, C-II	**00555-1082-01**	875.40		
0.8 mg,				
30s ea, C-II	**00555-1083-01**	1037.22		
1.2 mg,				
30s ea, C-II	**00555-1084-01**	1348.50		
1.6 mg,				
30s ea, C-II	**00555-1085-01**	1663.15		
(Watson Labs)				
LOZ, MM (BERRY)				
0.2 mg,				
30s ea, C-II	**55253-0070-30**	487.40		
0.4 mg,				
30s ea, C-II	**55253-0071-30**	617.51		
0.6 mg,				
30s ea, C-II	**55253-0072-30**	756.35		
0.8 mg,				
30s ea, C-II	**55253-0073-30**	896.16		
1.2 mg,				
30s ea, C-II	**55253-0074-30**	1165.10		
1.6 mg,				
30s ea, C-II	**55253-0075-30**	1436.96		
(DHS, Inc.)				
REPACK				
LOZ, MM (BERRY)				
0.2 mg,				
30s ea, C-II	**55887-0922-30**	1014.12		
0.4 mg,				
30s ea, C-II	**55887-0918-30**	1164.71		
0.6 mg,				
30s ea, C-II	**55887-0915-30**	1275.40		
0.8 mg,				
30s ea, C-II	**55887-0087-30**	1400.00		
1.2 mg,				
30s ea, C-II	**55887-0086-30**	1800.00		
1.6 mg,				
30s ea, C-II	**55887-0906-30**	2286.90		
(Phys Total Care)				
REPACK				
LOZ, MM (BERRY)				
0.2 mg,				
30s ea, C-II	**54868-6025-00**	995.43		
0.4 mg,				
30s ea, C-II	**54868-5975-00**	1167.71		
0.6 mg,				
30s ea, C-II	**54868-6026-00**	1427.25		
0.8 mg,				
30s ea, C-II	**54868-6027-00**	1689.29		
1.2 mg,				
30s ea, C-II	**54868-6037-00**	2111.87		

PROD/MFR	NDC	AWP	DP	OBC
(Quality Care Prod)				
REPACK				
LOZ, MM (BERRY)				
1.2 mg,				
30s ea, C-II	**35356-0377-30**	1323.32		
ORALONE (Taro)				
triamcinolone acetonide				
PAS, MM (USP,1X5GM)				
0.1%, 5 gm	**51672-1335-05**	67.83		EE
ORAMAGICRX (MPM Medical Inc.)				
aloe vera				
PDR, MM (AF,LEMON-LIME)				
7.1 gm	**66977-0222-02**	7.06	6.04	
37.5 gm	**66977-0222-12**	22.73	19.43	
ORAMORPH SR (Xanodyne Pharma)				
morphine sulfate				
TER, PO (4X25)				
15 mg,				
4s ea UD, C-II	**66479-0540-25**	117.97		BC
100s ea, C-II	**66479-0540-10**	135.34		BC
30 mg,				
100s ea, C-II	**66479-0541-10**	257.17		BC
100s ea UD, C-II	**66479-0541-25**	235.58		BC
60 mg,				
25s ea UD, C-II	**66479-0542-25**	117.73		BC
100s ea, C-II	**66479-0542-10**	501.82		BC
100 mg,				
25s ea UD, C-II	**66479-0543-25**	179.03		BC
100s ea, C-II	**66479-0543-10**	742.99		BC
(Quality Care Prod)				
REPACK				
TER, PO, 15 mg,				
10s ea, C-II	**35356-0347-10**	41.20		BC
30 mg,				
10s ea, C-II	**35356-0348-10**	68.30		BC
60 mg,				
10s ea, C-II	**35356-0349-10**	217.60		BC
100 mg,				
10s ea, C-II	**35356-0350-10**	171.60		BC
ORANGE CREAM FLAVOR (PCCA)				
flavoring aid				
SOL, NA (ORANGE CREAM)				
1 ml	**51927-3310-00**	0.70		
ORANGE EXTRACT NATURAL (Gallipot)				
orange oil				
LIQ, NA, 59.14 ml	**51552-0166-03**	6.02		
ORANGE FLAVOR (Medisca)				
flavoring aid				
SOL, NA (1X100ML,CONCENTRATE)				
100 ml	**38779-1474-05**	25.50		
(1X500ML,CONCENTRATE)				
500 ml	**38779-1474-08**	55.50		
(PCCA)				
SOL, NA (CONCENTRATE, NATURAL)				
1 ml	**51927-1280-00**	0.23		
(CONCENTRATE; NATURAL)				
1 ml	**51927-2269-00**	0.23		
(Spectrum Pharmacy)				
LIQ, NA (NATURAL)				
100 ml	**49452-4920-01**	56.70		
500 ml	**49452-4920-02**	114.10		
ORANGE FOOD COLOR (PCCA)				
color additive				
POW, NA, 1 gm	**51927-1649-00**	6.50		
ORANGE OIL				
(Gallipot) *See ORANGE EXTRACT NATURAL*				
(Lorann Oil)				
OIL, NA, 9.9 ml	**23535-0151-48**	2.50		
(Lorann Oil) *See ORANGE OIL NATURAL*				
(Medisca)				
OIL, NA (1X14ML,SWEET)				
14 ml	**38779-0828-03**	12.00		
(1X100ML,SWEET)				
100 ml	**38779-0828-05**	22.50		
(1X500ML,SWEET)				
500 ml	**38779-0828-08**	45.00		
(PCCA) *See ORANGE OIL CALIFORNIA*				
(PCCA) *See ORANGE OIL FLAVOR*				
(Spectrum Pharmacy) *See ORANGE OIL FLORIDA*				
ORANGE OIL CALIFORNIA (PCCA)				
orange oil				
OIL, NA, 1 ml	**51927-3184-00**	0.27		

PROD/MFR NDC AWP DP OBC

ORANGE OIL FLAVOR (PCCA)
orange oil
OIL, NA (FLORIDA TYPE)
1 ml................51927-1396-00 0.30

ORANGE OIL FLORIDA (Spectrum Pharmacy)
orange oil
OIL, NA (F.C.C., COLDPRESSED)
125 ml 49452-4916-01 72.45
(F.C.C.,COLDPRESSED)
500 ml 49452-4916-02 119.70

ORANGE OIL NATURAL (Lorann Oil)
orange oil
OIL, NA (U.S.P.)
3.75 ml..............23535-0060-01 0.57
30 ml...............23535-0060-05 2.25
480 ml 23535-0060-10 18.00
1920 ml 23535-0060-15 60.00
(N.F.)
3840 ml 23535-0060-11 110.00

ORANGE SYRUP (Gallipot)
SYR, NA, 480 ml..........51552-0808-06 13.58 9.70

ORAP (Gate)
pimozide
TAB, PO, 1 mg, 100s ea ...57844-0151-01 121.83
(CAPLET)
2 mg, 100s ea..........57844-0187-01 162.44

ORAPRED (Biomarin)
prednisolone sodium phosphate
SOL, PO (20MLX10,DYE-FREE,GRAPE)
15 mg/5 ml,
20 ml 10s..........68135-0455-03 147.38 AA
(DYE-FREE,GRAPE)
15 mg/5 ml, 237 ml ..68135-0455-02 176.27 AA

(Shionogi)
SOL, PO (20MLX10,DYE-FREE,GRAPE)
15 mg/5 ml,
20 ml 10s..........59630-0710-10 214.34 AA
(DYE-FREE,GRAPE)
15 mg/5 ml, 237 ml ..59630-0710-08 256.58 AA

(Dispensing Solutions)
REPACK
SOL, PO (10X20ML)
15 mg/5 ml,
20 ml 10s..........55045-2885-00 125.00
237 ml 55045-2885-08 160.00

(Phys Total Care)
REPACK
SOL, PO (DYE-FREE,GRAPE)
15 mg/5 ml, 237 ml ..54868-0954-00 165.08

ORAPRED ODT (Shionogi)
prednisolone sodium phosphate
ODT, PO (8X6,GRAPE)
10 mg, 48s ea........59630-0700-48 233.15
15 mg, 48s ea........59630-0701-48 350.60
30 mg, 48s ea........59630-0702-48 499.59

(Phys Total Care)
REPACK
ODT, PO, 15 mg, 48s ea ...54868-0821-00 230.60

ORAQIX (Dentsply)
lidocaine/prilocaine
GEL, SG (W/STERILE APPLICATOR)
2.5%-2.5%,
1.7 gm 20s UD 66312-0110-20 93.46

ORATUSS (Vindex Pharma Inc)
carbetapentane citrate/guaifenesin
SOL, PO (GRAPE)
20 mg/5 ml-75 mg/5 ml,
473 ml 67204-0210-16 81.76

ORAVERSE (Novalar)
phentolamine mesylate
SOL, IJ (10X1.7ML,PF)
0.4 mg/1.7 ml,
1.7 ml 10s.........45293-0101-01 175.00 EE
(50X1.7ML,PF)
0.4 mg/1.7 ml,
1.7 ml 50s.........45293-0101-02 650.00 EE

ORAXYL (E5)
doxycycline hyclate
CAP, PO (HARD GELATIN)
20 mg, 100s ea ......13517-0131-01 93.75 AB

ORCEL (Ortec Int'l)
graftskin
SHE, TP (36 SQUARE CM)
ea...................30170-0000-01 1250.00 1250.00

OREGANO
(PCCA) *See ORIGANUM OIL*

OREGON GRAPE ROOT (PCCA)
POW, NA (1X1GM)
1 gm 51927-3221-00 0.36

ORENCIA (Bristol-Myers)
abatacept
PDS, IV (W/SYRINGE,PF)
250 mg, ea 00003-2187-10 591.49

ORFADIN (Rare Disease)
nitisinone
CAP, PO, 2 mg, 60s ea 66607-1002-06 3527.72
5 mg, 60s ea.........66607-1005-06 8819.31
10 mg, 60s ea........66607-1010-06 17638.60

ORFRO (Truxton)
orphenadrine citrate
SOL, IJ (VIAL)
30 mg/ml, 10 ml .....00463-1092-10 9.30 EE

ORGAN-1 NR (Qualitest)
guaifenesin
TAB, PO, 200 mg, 100s ea .00603-4886-21 19.95

ORGANIDIN NR (Meda)
guaifenesin
TAB, PO (SF)
200 mg, 100s ea 00037-4312-01 85.51

ORGOTEIN (Medisca)
POW, NA (1X25GM)
25 gm 38779-1475-04 28.50
(1X100GM)
100 gm..............38779-1475-05 93.00

ORIGANUM OIL (PCCA)
oregano
OIL, NA, 1 ml............51927-1833-00 1.90

ORLISTAT
(Roche Labs) *See XENICAL*

ORNIDAZOLE (PCCA)
POW, NA, 1 gm...........51927-3397-00 45.00

ORNITHINE
(Amend) *See L-ORNITHINE MONOHYDROCHLORIDE*
(Gallipot) *See L-ORNITHINE MONOHYDROCHLORIDE*

ORNITHINE (L) HYDROCHLORIDE (PCCA)
ornithine hydrochloride
POW, NA (1X1GM)
1 gm 51927-2057-00 1.05

ORNITHINE HYDROCHLORIDE
(Medisca) *See L-ORNITHINE HYDROCHLORIDE*
(PCCA) *See ORNITHINE (L) HYDROCHLORIDE*

ORPHENADRINE (Aidarex)
REPACK
orphenadrine citrate
TER, PO, 100 mg, 10s ea ..33261-0088-10 27.10
14s ea............33261-0088-14 37.94
20s ea............33261-0088-20 54.20
21s ea............33261-0088-21 56.91
28s ea............33261-0088-28 75.88
30s ea............33261-0088-30 81.30
60s ea............33261-0088-60 162.77
90s ea............33261-0088-90 243.90

(Dispensing Solutions)
REPACK
TER, PO, 100 mg, 30s ea ..66336-0554-30 78.82

(IPI)
REPACK
TER, PO, 100 mg, 30s ea ..18837-0117-30 81.75

(PD-Rx Pharm)
REPACK
TER, PO, 100 mg, 20s ea ..55289-0877-20 32.42

ORPHENADRINE CITRATE
FUL
TER, PO, 100 mg, 100s ea 104.25

(Actavis)
TER, PO, 100 mg, 100s ea. 52152-0340-02 207.67 AB

(Akorn)
SOL, IJ (10X2ML)
30 mg/ml, 2 ml 10s...17478-0538-02 222.04 AP

(Bedford)
SOL, IJ, 30 mg/ml,
2 ml 10s...........55390-0059-10 196.80 AP

(Clint) *See ANTIFLEX*

(Consolidated Midland)
SOL, IJ (VIAL)
30 mg/ml, 10 ml .....00223-8200-10 8.00 EE

(Gallipot)
POW, NA (U.S.P.)
100 gm.............51552-0839-05 46.00

(GeneraMedix)
SOL, IJ (1X2ML,SINGLE DOSE,USP)
30 mg/ml, 2 ml.......10139-0230-02 19.20 AP
(10X2ML,SINGLE DOSE,USP)
30 mg/ml, 2 ml 10s...10139-0230-10 192.00 AP

(Global Pharm)
TER, PO, 100 mg, 100s ea.00115-2011-01 217.29 AB
500s ea..........00115-2011-02 880.50 AB

(Graceway) *See NORFLEX*

(Intl Ethical) *See MIO-REL*

(PCCA)
POW, NA (USP)
1 gm 51927-2118-00 2.40

(Sandoz)
TER, PO, 100 mg, 100s ea.00185-0022-01 218.42 AB
1000s ea..........00185-0022-10 2075.00 AB

(Spectrum Pharmacy)
POW, NA (U.S.P.)
25 gm 49452-4936-01 209.30
100 gm.............49452-4936-02 518.00

(Truxton) *See ORFRO*

(Watson Labs)
SOL, IJ, 30 mg/ml,
2 ml 10s...........00591-3222-47 225.00 AP

(4u)
REPACK
TER, PO, 100 mg, 30s ea ..10544-0359-30 86.18 AB
30s ea............42549-0559-30 86.18 AB
56s ea............10544-0359-56 179.88 AB
56s ea............42549-0559-56 179.88 AB
60s ea............42549-0559-60 186.46 AB

(A-S Medication)
REPACK
TER, PO, 100 mg, 14s ea ..54569-0838-02 30.58 EE
20s ea............54569-0838-00 43.68 EE
30s ea............54569-0838-01 65.53 EE
100s ea...........54569-0838-06 218.42 EE

(Altura)
REPACK
TER, PO, 100 mg, 10s ea ..63874-0531-10 23.05 AB
14s ea............63874-0531-14 32.27 AB
20s ea............63874-0531-20 46.10
30s ea............63874-0531-30 69.15 AB
40s ea............63874-0531-40 92.20 AB
60s ea............63874-0531-60 138.30
90s ea............63874-0531-90 207.45
100s ea...........63874-0531-01 230.50
120s ea...........63874-0531-04 276.60

(Bryant Ranch)
REPACK
TER, PO, 100 mg, 20s ea ..63629-1564-01 47.99
60s ea............63629-1564-02 139.89

(DHS, Inc.)
REPACK
TER, PO, 100 mg, 15s ea ..55887-0670-15 36.67 AB
20s ea............55887-0670-20 48.90 AB
30s ea............55887-0670-30 72.50 AB
60s ea............55887-0670-60 139.70 AB
90s ea............55887-0670-90 205.08 AB

(Dispensing Solutions)
REPACK
TER, PO, 100 mg, 10s ea ..55045-1325-01 23.00 AB
14s ea............55045-1325-05 32.20 AB
20s ea............55045-1325-07 46.00 AB
30s ea............55045-1325-08 69.00 AB
60s ea............55045-1325-09 138.00 AB
60s ea............66336-0554-60 157.64 AB
84s ea............55045-1325-04 193.20 AB
90s ea............55045-1325-02 207.00 AB
90s ea............66336-0554-90 225.95 AB
100s ea...........55045-1325-00 230.00 AB
120s ea...........55045-1325-03 276.00 AB

(IPI)
REPACK
TER, PO, 100 mg, 14s ea ..18837-0117-14 30.42 AB
60s ea............18837-0117-60 130.37 AB
90s ea............18837-0117-90 195.56 AB

(Keltman Pharma., Inc.)
REPACK
TER, PO, 100 mg, 14s ea ..68387-0575-14 32.58
60s ea............68387-0575-60 139.62

(Medsource)
REPACK
TER, PO, 100 mg, 30s ea ..45865-0363-30 82.50 AB
60s ea............45865-0363-60 165.00 AB
90s ea............45865-0363-90 247.50 AB

PROD/MFR	NDC	AWP	DP	OBC
100s ea	45865-0363-00	275.00		AB
120s ea	45865-0363-01	330.00		AB
150s ea	45865-0363-02	412.50		AB
300s ea	45865-0363-05	825.00		AB
(Nucare Pharm)				
REPACK				
TER, PO, 100 mg, 14s ea	66267-0158-14	44.90		AB
15s ea	66267-0158-15	34.95		EE
30s ea	66267-0158-30	85.55		AB
60s ea	66267-0158-60	171.68		AB
90s ea	66267-0158-90	252.61		AB
(Palmetto)				
REPACK				
TER, PO, 100 mg, 20s ea	23490-6039-01	48.33		
30s ea	23490-6039-02	72.50		
60s ea	23490-6039-03	145.00		
90s ea	23490-6039-09	217.50		
100s ea	23490-6039-04	241.67		
(PD-Rx Pharm)				
REPACK				
TER, PO, 100 mg, 14s ea	55289-0877-14	24.24		AB
30s ea	55289-0877-30	39.00		AB
(Pharma Pac)				
REPACK				
TER, PO, 100 mg, 10s ea	52959-0527-10	23.33		EE
14s ea	52959-0527-14	32.66		EE
15s ea	52959-0527-15	34.98		EE
20s ea	52959-0527-20	46.35		EE
28s ea	52959-0527-28	64.88		AB
30s ea	52959-0527-30	69.51		EE
42s ea	52959-0527-42	97.31		AB
45s ea	52959-0527-45	104.06		AB
60s ea	52959-0527-60	138.30		EE
90s ea	52959-0527-90	207.59		EE
100s ea	52959-0527-00	229.55		AB
(Phys Total Care)				
REPACK				
TER, PO, 100 mg, 10s ea	54868-4102-01	27.93		EE
15s ea	54868-4102-00	40.38		EE
30s ea	54868-4102-02	60.18		AB
50s ea	54868-4102-04	98.29		AB
60s ea	54868-4102-05	118.86		EE
100s ea	54868-4102-03	192.09		EE
(Physician Partner)				
REPACK				
TAB, PO, 100 mg, 14s ea	21695-0099-14	71.95		
30s ea	21695-0099-30	131.05		
60s ea	21695-0099-60	262.10		
TER, PO, 100 mg, 28s ea	21695-0099-28	122.32		AB
56s ea	21695-0099-56	262.10		AB
(Quality Care Prod)				
REPACK				
TER, PO, 100 mg, 14s ea	49999-0046-14	38.73		EE
20s ea	49999-0046-20	46.10		EE
30s ea	49999-0046-30	69.30		AB
(Southwood)				
REPACK				
TER, PO, 100 mg, 7s ea	58016-0248-07	16.14		EE
10s ea	58016-0248-10	23.05		EE
12s ea	58016-0248-12	27.66		EE
14s ea	58016-0248-14	32.27		EE
15s ea	58016-0248-15	34.58		EE
20s ea	58016-0248-20	46.10		EE
21s ea	58016-0248-21	48.41		EE
28s ea	58016-0248-28	64.54		EE
30s ea	58016-0248-30	78.00		AB
40s ea	58016-0248-40	92.20		EE
42s ea	58016-0248-42	96.81		EE
50s ea	58016-0248-50	115.25		EE
60s ea	58016-0248-60	156.00		AB
90s ea	58016-0248-90	234.00		AB
100s ea	58016-0248-00	260.00		AB
120s ea	58016-0248-02	312.00		AB
(St. Mary's MPP)				
REPACK				
TER, PO, 100 mg, 30s ea	60760-0810-30	64.11		EE
(Vibranta)				
REPACK				
TER, PO, 100 mg, 14s ea	57866-7601-04	33.71		AB
15s ea	57866-7601-02	34.91		AB
20s ea	57866-7601-03	47.17		AB
60s ea	57866-7601-05	138.40		AB
90s ea	57866-7601-06	227.50		AB
ORPHENADRINE CITRATE ER (Core)				
REPACK				
orphenadrine citrate				
TER, PO, 100 mg, 20s ea	33358-0274-20	49.19		
30s ea	33358-0274-30	92.15		
60s ea	33358-0274-60	143.39		
ORPHENADRINE COMPOUND (Dispensing Solutions)				
REPACK				
aspirin/caffeine/orphenadrine citrate				
TAB, PO, 770 mg-60 mg-50 mg,				
24s ea	55045-2777-06	26.40		
ORPHENADRINE E/R (Stat Rx)				
REPACK				
orphenadrine citrate				
TER, PO, 100 mg, 30s ea	16590-0177-20	46.70		
30s ea	16590-0177-30	70.00		
60s ea	16590-0177-60	140.00		
90s ea	16590-0177-90	210.00		
120s ea	16590-0177-72	280.00		
ORRIS ROOT (Humco)				
POW, NA, 90 gm	00395-2105-93	9.59		
ORTHO EVRA (Ortho-McNeil Pharm)				
ethinyl estradiol/norelgestromin				
TDM, TD, ea	00062-1920-01	25.01	20.84	
(6X3)				
18s ea	00062-1920-15	450.48	375.40	
(A-S Medication)				
REPACK				
TDM, TD, 3s ea	54569-5413-00	71.16		
(Phys Total Care)				
REPACK				
TDM, TD, 3s ea	54868-4670-00	63.83		
ORTHO MICRONOR (Ortho-McNeil Pharm)				
norethindrone				
TAB, PO (ORTHO DIALPAK)				
0.35 mg, 168s ea	00062-1411-16	206.87	172.39	
(Phys Total Care)				
REPACK				
TAB, PO, 0.35 mg, 28s ea	54868-4369-00	69.69		
ORTHO TRI-CYCLEN (Ortho-McNeil Pharm)				
ethinyl estradiol/norgestimate				
TAB, PO (DIALPAK,COATED)				
28s ea	00062-1910-15	189.06	157.55	
(A-S Medication)				
REPACK				
TAB, PO (DIALPAK)				
28s ea	54569-4269-00	32.82		
(Phys Total Care)				
REPACK				
TAB, PO (DIALPAK,6X28)				
168s ea	54868-4093-00	38.29		
(Quality Care Prod)				
REPACK				
TAB, PO (DIAL-PACK)				
28s ea	35356-0021-68	346.18		
ORTHO TRI-CYCLEN LO (Ortho-McNeil Pharm)				
ethinyl estradiol/norgestimate				
TAB, PO (DIALPAK, 6X28)				
168s ea	00062-1251-15	450.35	375.29	
(A-S Medication)				
REPACK				
TAB, PO, 28s ea	54569-5493-00	88.79		
(6X28)				
168s ea	54569-5493-02	363.33		
(Phys Total Care)				
REPACK				
TAB, PO, 28s ea	54868-4730-00	79.85		
(Quality Care Prod)				
REPACK				
TAB, PO, 28s ea	35356-0411-28	120.71		
ORTHO-CEPT (Ortho-McNeil Pharm)				
desogestrel/ethinyl estradiol				
TAB, PO (DIALPAK, 6X28)				
0.15 mg-0.03 mg,				
168s ea	00062-1796-15	318.68	265.57	AB
(Phys Total Care)				
REPACK				
TAB, PO, 0.15 mg-0.03 mg,				
28s ea	54868-2701-00	54.87		AB
ORTHO-CYCLEN (Ortho-McNeil Pharm)				
ethinyl estradiol/norgestimate				
TAB, PO (DIALPAK)				
35 mcg-0.25 mg,				
28s ea	00062-1907-15	189.06	157.55	
(A-S Medication)				
REPACK				
TAB, PO (DIALPAK)				
35 mcg-0.25 mg,				
168s ea	54569-4273-01	316.85		
(Phys Total Care)				
REPACK				
TAB, PO (DIALPAK)				
35 mcg-0.25 mg,				
28s ea	54868-2606-00	57.50		
ORTHO-EST (Phys Total Care)				
estropipate				
TAB, PO, 0.75 mg, 30s ea	54868-3672-01	54.03		AB
100s ea	54868-3672-00	169.56		AB
1.5 mg, 30s ea	54868-3673-01	77.25		AB
100s ea	54868-3673-00	226.56		AB
ORTHO-NOVUM 1/35 (Ortho-McNeil Pharm)				
ethinyl estradiol/norethindrone				
TAB, PO (DIALPAK, 6X28)				
35 mcg-1 mg,				
168s ea	00062-1761-15	318.68	265.57	AB
(A-S Medication)				
REPACK				
TAB, PO, 35 mcg-1 mg,				
168s ea	54569-0685-01	414.28		AB
(Phys Total Care)				
REPACK				
TAB, PO, 35 mcg-1 mg,				
28s ea	54868-0443-00	60.19		AB
ORTHO-NOVUM 7/7/7 (Ortho-McNeil Pharm)				
ethinyl estradiol/norethindrone				
TAB, PO (DIALPAK, 6X28)				
168s ea	00062-1781-15	171.43	142.86	
(A-S Medication)				
REPACK				
TAB, PO (DIALPAK, 6X28)				
168s ea	54569-0689-01	222.86		
(Phys Total Care)				
REPACK				
TAB, PO (DIALPAK)				
21s ea	54868-0508-00	29.33		
28s ea	54868-0508-01	34.83		
ORTHO-PHENYLPHENOL (PCCA)				
POW, NA, 1 gm	51927-1554-00	0.36		
ORTHO-TOLUIDINE (PCCA)				
o-toluidine				
SOL, NA, 1 ml	51927-3342-00	0.99		
ORTHO/CS (Merit)				
ascorbic acid				
SOL, IJ, 250 mg/ml,				
100 ml	30727-0399-95	25.90	12.95	
ORTHOCLONE OKT 3 (Centocor)				
muromonab-cd3				
SOL, IV (AMP)				
1 mg/ml, 5 ml	59676-0101-01	1308.77		
ORTHOVISC (DePuy)				
hyaluronic acid				
SOL, IJ (PREFILLED SYRINGE)				
15 mg/ml, 2 ml	59676-0360-01	270.00	225.00	
(Quality Care Prod)				
REPACK				
SOL, IJ (1X2ML)				
15 mg/ml, 2 ml	35356-0035-02	612.00		
ORTHOWASH (Omnii Intl)				
acidulated phosphate fluoride				
SOL, MM (APF DAILY RINSE)				
0.044%, 480 ml	48878-3214-05	8.50		
ORUDIS (Phys Total Care)				
REPACK				
ketoprofen				
CAP, PO, 75 mg, 18s ea	54868-1052-04	28.43		AB
ORUVAIL (Pharma Pac)				
REPACK				
ketoprofen				
CER, PO, 200 mg, 15s ea	52959-0347-15	54.91		AB
20s ea	52959-0347-20	70.58		AB
30s ea	52959-0347-30	98.05		AB
(Phys Total Care)				
REPACK				
CER, PO, 150 mg, 10s ea	54868-3831-00	37.11		AB
200 mg, 10s ea	54868-3380-03	41.66		AB
15s ea	54868-3380-02	61.56		AB
30s ea	54868-3380-01	121.25		AB
100s ea	54868-3380-00	377.04		AB
OSCION (Prasco Labs)				
benzoyl peroxide				
PAD, TP, 3%, 30s ea	66993-0916-30	83.95		
6%, 30s ea	66993-0917-30	83.95		
9%, 30s ea	66993-0918-30	83.95		

PROD/MFR NDC AWP DP OBC

OSCION CLEANSER (Prasco Labs)
benzoyl peroxide
SOA, TP, 3%, 170.3 gm.... **66993-0906-06** 46.02
340.2 gm **66993-0906-12** 82.40
6%, 170.3 gm........ **66993-0907-06** 47.39
340.2 gm **66993-0907-12** 85.16
9%, 170.3 gm........ **66993-0908-06** 49.16
340.2 gm **66993-0908-12** 88.26

OSELTAMIVIR PHOSPHATE
(Roche Labs) *See TAMIFLU*

OSMITROL (Baxter)
mannitol
SOL, IV (VIAFLEX,AF)
5%, 1000 ml 12s ..... **00338-0351-04** 463.03 **AP**
(VIAFLEX)
10%, 500 ml 24s ..... **00338-0353-03** 1011.49 **AP**
(VIAFLEX;12X1000ML)
10%, 1000 ml 12s .... **00338-0353-04** 504.72 **AP**
(VIAFLEX,AF)
15%, 500 ml 24s ..... **00338-0355-03** 1442.04 **AP**
(VIAFLEX)
20%, 250 ml 36s ..... **00338-0357-02** 2209.68 **AP**
500 ml 24s .... **00338-0357-03** 1686.82 **AP**

OSMOPREP (Salix Pharm)
na phos, dibasic/na phos, monobasic
TAB, PO (GLUTEN-FREE)
0.398 gm-1.102 gm,
100s ea............ **65649-0701-41** 243.44

(Phys Total Care)
REPACK
TAB, PO (GLUTEN-FREE)
0.398 gm-1.102 gm,
32s ea............. **54868-5889-00** 78.01

OTICOT HC (Truxton)
acetic acid/hydrocortisone
SOL, OT, 2%-1%, 10 ml ... **00463-8054-10** 6.00 **EE**

OTIRX (Breckenridge Pharm)
chloroxylenol/hc/pramoxine hcl
SOL, OT, 10 ml **51991-0671-71** 14.20

(Palmetto)
REPACK
SOL, OT (1X10ML)
10 ml................ **23490-9377-00** 24.00

(Phys Total Care)
REPACK
SOL, OT (1X10ML)
10 ml................ **54868-6046-00** 39.65

(Physician Partner)
REPACK
SOL, OT (1X10ML)
10 ml................ **21695-0727-10** 28.40

OTN FLUDARABINE PHOSPHATE (Teva)
fludarabine phosphate
SOL, IV (SDV,PRIVATE LABEL)
25 mg/ml, 2 ml....... **00703-4852-81** 330.32

OTN MITOXANTRONE (Mayne Pharma)
mitoxantrone hydrochloride
SOL, IV (MDV,USP,PF)
2 mg/ml, 12.5 ml..... **15210-0403-36** 1744.32 1526.28 **AP**

(OTN)
SOL, IV (USP,MDV,PF)
2 mg/ml, 10 ml....... **15210-0403-35** 1407.60 1231.65
15 ml................ **15210-0403-37** 2254.93 1973.07

OTN PAMIDRONATE DISODIUM (OTN)
pamidronate disodium
SOL, IV (PRIVATE LABEL)
3 mg/ml, 10 ml....... **15210-0401-11** 101.70 **AP**
9 mg/ml, 10 ml....... **15210-0402-11** 305.10 **AP**

OTO-END 10 (Larken Labs, Inc.)
chloroxylenol/hc/pramoxine hcl
SOL, OT (1X10ML,DROPS)
10 ml................ **68047-0051-10** 21.14

OTOMAR (Marnel)
chloroxylenol/hc/pramoxine hcl
SOL, OT (W/DROPPER,DROPS)
15 ml................ **00682-9090-15** 34.40

OTOMAR-HC (Marnel)
benzalkonium cl/chloroxylenol/hc/pramoxine hcl
SOL, OT, 15 ml **00682-9080-15** 27.90

OTOMAX HC (A. G. Marin)
benzalkonium cl/chloroxylenol/hc/pramoxine hcl
SOL, OT, 15 ml **12539-0226-15** 23.44

OVACE WASH (Valeant Pharm Intl)
sulfacetamide sodium
LOT, TP, 10%, 360 ml **13548-0040-12** 165.25

OVCON 35 (Warner Chilcott)
ethinyl estradiol/norethindrone
TAB, PO (5X28)
35 mcg-0.4 mg,
140s ea............ **00430-0580-14** 409.71 **AB**

(Phys Total Care)
REPACK
TAB, PO, 35 mcg-0.4 mg,
28s ea............. **54868-0509-01** 59.73

OVCON 50 (Warner Chilcott)
ethinyl estradiol/norethindrone
TAB, PO (3X28)
50 mcg-1 mg,
84s ea............. **00430-0585-45** 245.83

(Phys Total Care)
REPACK
TAB, PO, 50 mcg-1 mg,
28s ea............. **54868-3772-00** 58.19

OVIDE (Taro)
malathion
LOT, TP, 0.5%, 59 ml...... **51672-5276-04** 173.85

OVIDREL (EMD)
chorionic gonadotropin alfa, recombinant
SOL, SC (SRN,PREFILLED SYRINGE)
0.25 mg/0.5 ml,
0.5 ml **44087-1150-01** 90.13

OVRAL-21 (Pharma Pac)
REPACK
ethinyl estradiol/norgestrel
TAB, PO (PILPAK, 6X21)
50 mcg-0.5 mg,
126s ea............ **52959-0460-04** 11.45 **AB**

OVRAL-28 (Phys Total Care)
REPACK
ethinyl estradiol/norgestrel
TAB, PO, 50 mcg-0.5 mg,
28s ea............. **54868-1276-00** 65.16 **AB**

OXACILLIN (Sandoz)
oxacillin sodium
PDS, IJ (USP)
2 gm, ea............. **00781-3101-80** 24.08 **AP**
IV (USP,ADD-VANTAGE VIAL)
1 gm, ea............. **00781-3094-15** 14.90 **AP**
(1X10,USP,ADD-VANTAGE)
1 gm, 10s ea......... **00781-3094-92** 148.99 **AP**
(ADD-VANTAGE)
2 gm, ea............. **00781-3095-15** 28.90 **AP**
(USP,ADD-VANTAGE VIAL)
2 gm, ea............. **00781-3095-80** 26.39 **AP**
(1X10,USP,ADD-VANTAGE)
2 gm, 10s ea......... **00781-3095-92** 289.01 **AP**

OXACILLIN SODIUM (Baxter)
SOL, IV (PREMIXED)
1 gm/50 ml,
50 ml 24s.......... **00338-1013-41** 533.04
2 gm/50 ml,
50 ml 24s.......... **00338-1015-41** 767.28

(Sandoz) *See NOVAPLUS OXACILLIN*

(Sandoz) *See OXACILLIN*

(Sandoz)
PDS, IJ, 1 gm, ea .... **00781-3099-85** 12.41 **AP**
(ADD-VANTAGE)
1 gm, ea............. **00015-7981-18** 10.36 **AP**
10s ea............... **00781-3099-95** 124.14 **AP**
(ADD-VANTAGE)
1 gm, 10s ea......... **00015-7981-89** 103.62 **AP**
2 gm, ea............. **00015-7970-18** 20.11 **AP**
10s ea............... **00015-7970-89** 201.03 **AP**
(VIAL,PIGGYBACK)
2 gm, 10s ea......... **00781-3101-95** 240.83 **AP**
10 gm, ea............ **00781-3103-46** 118.01 **AP**
(PHARMACY BULK PACKAGE)
10 gm, 10s ea........ **00781-3103-95** 1180.11 **AP**

OXALIC ACID
(Baker, J.T.) *See OXALIC ACID DIHYDRATE*

(Gallipot)
CRY, NA (TECHNICAL)
28.35 gm............. **51552-0034-02** 2.73
113.4 gm............. **51552-0034-04** 6.37
454 gm............... **51552-0034-06** 14.56
2270 gm.............. **51552-0034-09** 55.65

(Humco)
CRY, NA (TECHNICAL)
120 gm............... **00395-2117-94** 5.75
454 gm............... **00395-2117-01** 12.89

(Medisca)
CRY, NA (TECHNICAL)
100 gm............... **38779-0611-05** 27.00
500 gm............... **38779-0611-08** 67.50

(PCCA)
POW, NA (ACS)
1 gm **51927-9094-00** 0.60

OXALIC ACID DIHYDRATE (Baker, J.T.)
oxalic acid
CRY, NA (A.C.S., REAGENT)
500 gm............... **10106-0230-01** 102.38
2500 gm.............. **10106-0230-05** 401.39

OXALIPLATIN (APP)
PDS, IV (SINGLE USE,PF)
50 mg, ea............ **63323-0175-30** 712.80
100 mg, ea **63323-0176-50** 1483.92

(Caraco)
PDS, IV (SINGLE-USE,PF)
50 mg, ea............ **41616-0176-40** 825.00 **AP**
100 mg, ea .... **41616-0178-40** 1650.00 **AP**

(Hospira)
SOL, IV (1X10ML,SINGLE USE,PF)
5 mg/ml, 10 ml....... **61703-0363-18** 941.28 823.62 **AP**
(1X20ML,SINGLE USE,PF)
5 mg/ml, 20 ml....... **61703-0363-22** 1882.52 1647.21 **AP**
(1X40ML,SINGLE USE,PF)
5 mg/ml, 40 ml....... **61703-0363-40** 3765.01 3294.39 **AP**

(Parenta Pharma)
SOL, IV (1X10ML,SINGLE USE,PF)
5 mg/ml, 10 ml....... **66758-0053-01** 825.00 **AP**
(1X20ML,SINGLE USE,PF)
5 mg/ml, 20 ml....... **66758-0053-02** 1650.00 **AP**

(Sanofi-Aventis) *See ELOXATIN*

(Teva)
SOL, IV (1X10ML,SINGLE-USE,PF)
5 mg/ml, 10 ml....... **00703-3985-01** 825.35 **EE**
(1X20ML,SINGLE-USE,PF)
5 mg/ml, 20 ml....... **00703-3986-01** 1649.06 **EE**

OXANDRIN (Savient Pharm. Inc.)
oxandrolone
TAB, PO, 2.5 mg,
100s ea, C-III **54396-0111-11** 785.04
10 mg,
60s ea, C-III **54396-0110-60** 1597.22

(A-S Medication)
REPACK
TAB, PO, 10 mg,
60s ea, C-III **54569-5697-00** 1375.03

(Phys Total Care)
REPACK
TAB, PO, 2.5 mg,
10s ea, C-III **54868-4664-00** 80.97
30s ea, C-III **54868-4664-01** 224.85
(USP)
2.5 mg,
60s ea, C-III **54868-4664-02** 445.95
10 mg,
15s ea, C-III **54868-5408-00** 315.87

OXANDROLONE (B&B Pharm, Inc)
POW, NA, 0.5 gm, C-III.... **63275-9962-07** 875.00
1 gm, C-III.......... **63275-9962-01** 1740.00
5 gm, C-III.......... **63275-9962-02** 8700.00
25 gm, C-III......... **63275-9962-04** 43000.00

(Letco)
POW, NA (USP)
100 gm, C-III **62991-2699-02** 3150.00
(USP, 1X1000GM)
1000 gm, C-III **62991-2699-01** 23850.00

(Medisca)
POW, NA (1X5GM,USP)
5 gm, C-III.......... **38779-2286-03** 802.50
(1X25GM,USP)
25 gm, C-III......... **38779-2286-04** 2625.00
(1X100GM,USP)
100 gm, C-III **38779-2286-05** 9600.00
(1X500GM,USP)
500 gm, C-III **38779-2286-08** 48000.00

(Par)
TAB, PO (USP)
2.5 mg,
100s ea, C-III **49884-0301-01** 552.95
10 mg, 60s ea, C-III .. **49884-0302-02** 1125.03

PROD/MFR	NDC	AWP	DP	OBC
(Sandoz)				
TAB, PO (USP)				
2.5 mg,				
100s ea, C-III	**00185-0271-01**	552.95		AB
10 mg, 60s ea, C-III	**00185-0272-60**	1125.03		AB
(Savient Pharm. Inc.) *See OXANDRIN*				
(Upsher-Smith)				
TAB, PO (USP)				
2.5 mg,				
100s ea UD, C-III	**00245-0271-01**	552.95		AB
100s ea, C-III	**00245-0271-11**	552.95		AB
(UNCOATED)				
10 mg,				
60s ea, C-III	**00245-0272-06**	1125.03		AB
(10X10,UNCOATED)				
10 mg,				
100s ea UD, C-III	**00245-0272-01**	1875.05		AB
(Watson Labs)				
TAB, PO (USP)				
2.5 mg,				
100s ea, C-III	**00591-3544-01**	524.93		
10 mg, 60s ea, C-III	**00591-3545-60**	1068.02		
(A-S Medication)				
REPACK				
TAB, PO, 10 mg,				
60s ea, C-III	**54569-5875-00**	1125.03		
OXAPROZIN				
FUL				
TAB, PO, 600 mg, 100s ea		67.58		
(Apotex Corp.)				
TAB, PO (FILM-COATED)				
600 mg, 100s ea	**60505-0176-00**	151.50		AB
500s ea	**60505-0176-01**	757.50		AB
(Caraco)				
TAB, PO, 600 mg, 100s ea	**57664-0391-08**	151.48		AB
500s ea	**57664-0391-13**	742.25		AB
(Dr Reddy's)				
TAB, PO (FILM COATED)				
600 mg, 100s ea	**55111-0170-01**	151.25		AB
500s ea	**55111-0170-05**	741.50		AB
(Greenstone)				
TAB, PO (CAPLET)				
600 mg, 100s ea	**59762-5002-01**	149.80		AB
500s ea	**59762-5002-02**	743.27		AB
(Pfizer) *See DAYPRO*				
(Sandoz)				
TAB, PO (FILM-COATED)				
600 mg, 100s ea	**00185-0141-01**	163.40		AB
500s ea	**00185-0141-05**	817.10		AB
(Teva)				
TAB, PO, 600 mg,				
100s ea UD	**00172-4348-10**	153.50		AB
(FILM-COATED)				
600 mg, 100s ea	**00093-0924-01**	151.00		AB
500s ea	**00093-0924-05**	742.35		AB
(4u)				
REPACK				
TAB, PO, 600 mg, 60s ea	**42549-0526-60**	184.44		AB
(FILM-COATED)				
600 mg, 60s ea	**10544-0396-60**	184.44		AB
60s ea	**42549-0596-60**	184.44		AB
(A-S Medication)				
REPACK				
TAB, PO (CAPLET)				
600 mg, 15s ea	**54569-5212-01**	22.93		EE
20s ea	**54569-5212-03**	30.57		EE
30s ea	**54569-5212-00**	45.86		EE
60s ea	**54569-5212-02**	91.71		EE
(Aidarex)				
REPACK				
TAB, PO (FILM-COATED)				
600 mg, 7s ea	**33261-0089-07**	17.15		AB
14s ea	**33261-0089-14**	34.30		AB
28s ea	**33261-0089-28**	68.60		AB
30s ea	**33261-0089-30**	73.50		AB
60s ea	**33261-0089-60**	147.00		AB
90s ea	**33261-0089-90**	220.50		AB
120s ea	**33261-0089-02**	294.00		AB
(Altura)				
REPACK				
TAB, PO (FILM COATED)				
600 mg, 10s ea	**63874-0353-10**	22.57		AB
12s ea	**63874-0353-12**	27.08		AB
14s ea	**63874-0353-14**	31.60		AB
15s ea	**63874-0353-15**	33.86		AB
20s ea	**63874-0353-20**	45.14		AB
30s ea	**63874-0353-30**	67.71		AB
40s ea	**63874-0353-40**	90.28		AB
50s ea	**63874-0353-50**	112.85		AB
60s ea	**63874-0353-60**	135.42		AB
90s ea	**63874-0353-90**	203.13		AB
100s ea	**63874-0353-01**	225.70		AB
120s ea	**63874-0353-04**	180.00		AB
(Bryant Ranch)				
REPACK				
TAB, PO, 600 mg, 14s ea	**63629-1345-03**	37.02		
20s ea	**63629-1345-02**	52.98		
30s ea	**63629-1345-01**	55.65		
60s ea	**63629-1345-04**	112.98		
(Core)				
REPACK				
TAB, PO, 600 mg, 14s ea	**33358-0275-14**	33.81		
20s ea	**33358-0275-20**	54.31		
30s ea	**33358-0275-30**	61.49		
60s ea	**33358-0275-60**	116.39		
(DHS, Inc.)				
REPACK				
TAB, PO, 600 mg, 14s ea	**55887-0698-14**	35.00		AB
15s ea	**55887-0698-15**	40.52		AB
20s ea	**55887-0698-20**	48.35		AB
30s ea	**55887-0698-30**	72.52		AB
60s ea	**55887-0698-60**	147.34		AB
(Dispensing Solutions)				
REPACK				
TAB, PO, 600 mg, 10s ea	**55045-2916-02**	16.80		AB
15s ea	**55045-2916-03**	25.20		AB
20s ea	**55045-2916-07**	33.60		AB
30s ea	**55045-2916-08**	50.40		AB
45s ea	**55045-2916-04**	75.60		AB
60s ea	**55045-2916-06**	100.80		AB
(FILM COATED)				
600 mg, 60s ea	**66336-0722-60**	109.08		AB
90s ea	**55045-2916-09**	151.20		AB
(FILM-COATED)				
600 mg, 90s ea	**66336-0722-90**	163.62		AB
(FILM COATED)				
600 mg, 100s ea	**55045-2916-01**	168.00		AB
120s ea	**55045-2916-00**	201.60		
(GSMS)				
REPACK				
TAB, PO (FILM-COATED)				
600 mg, 60s ea	**60429-0752-60**	26.40	8.80	AB
180s ea	**60429-0752-18**	67.59	22.53	AB
(IPI)				
REPACK				
TAB, PO (FILM COATED)				
600 mg, 30s ea	**18837-0118-30**	55.67		AB
60s ea	**18837-0118-60**	30.00		AB
(Keltman Pharma., Inc.)				
REPACK				
TAB, PO (FILM COATED)				
600 mg, 30s ea	**68387-0180-30**	68.10		AB
60s ea	**68387-0180-60**	136.20		AB
(Nucare Pharm)				
REPACK				
TAB, PO, 600 mg, 14s ea	**66267-0407-14**	32.99		EE
20s ea	**66267-0407-20**	42.99		EE
30s ea	**66267-0407-30**	51.99		EE
60s ea	**66267-0407-60**	113.55		EE
(Palmetto)				
REPACK				
TAB, PO, 600 mg, 15s ea	**23490-6047-03**	28.50		
20s ea	**23490-6047-00**	38.00		
30s ea	**23490-6047-01**	57.00		
60s ea	**23490-6047-02**	114.00		
90s ea	**23490-6047-09**	171.00		
(PD-Rx Pharm)				
REPACK				
TAB, PO, 600 mg, 20s ea	**55289-0601-20**	46.22		EE
30s ea	**55289-0601-30**	62.67		EE
(USP)				
600 mg, 60s ea	**55289-0601-60**	75.96		EE
(Pharma Pac)				
REPACK				
TAB, PO, 600 mg, 14s ea	**52959-0800-14**	26.60		AB
15s ea	**52959-0800-15**	28.50		AB
20s ea	**52959-0800-20**	37.99		AB
21s ea	**52959-0800-21**	39.89		AB
24s ea	**52959-0800-24**	45.58		AB
(FILM COATED)				
600 mg, 28s ea	**52959-0800-28**	53.17		AB
30s ea	**52959-0800-30**	56.97		AB
(FILM COATED)				
600 mg, 40s ea	**52959-0800-40**	75.95		AB
42s ea	**52959-0800-42**	79.74		AB
45s ea	**52959-0800-45**	85.43		AB
60s ea	**52959-0800-60**	113.88		AB
90s ea	**52959-0800-90**	170.75		AB
100s ea	**52959-0800-00**	189.77		AB
(Phys Total Care)				
REPACK				
TAB, PO, 600 mg, 30s ea	**54868-4548-01**	22.44		
60s ea	**54868-4548-00**	40.35		
(FILM COATED)				
600 mg, 100s ea	**54868-4548-02**	62.76		AB
(Physician Partner)				
REPACK				
TAB, PO, 600 mg, 14s ea	**21695-0100-14**	49.82		
28s ea	**21695-0100-28**	24.42		AB
30s ea	**21695-0100-30**	90.75		
60s ea	**21695-0100-60**	62.38		AB
(Quality Care Prod)				
REPACK				
TAB, PO (FILM-COATED)				
600 mg, 30s ea	**49999-0376-30**	105.44		AB
OXAPROZIN (Quality Care Prod)				
60s ea	**49999-0376-60**	210.88		
OXAPROZIN (Southwood)				
REPACK				
TAB, PO (CAPLET)				
600 mg, 10s ea	**58016-0574-10**	18.15		EE
12s ea	**58016-0574-12**	21.78		EE
14s ea	**58016-0574-14**	25.42		EE
15s ea	**58016-0574-15**	27.23		EE
20s ea	**58016-0574-20**	36.31		EE
28s ea	**58016-0574-28**	50.83		EE
(FILM-COATED)				
600 mg, 30s ea	**58016-0574-30**	67.80		AB
(CAPLET)				
600 mg, 40s ea	**58016-0574-40**	72.62		EE
(FILM-COATED)				
600 mg, 60s ea	**58016-0574-60**	135.60		AB
90s ea	**58016-0574-90**	203.40		AB
100s ea	**58016-0574-00**	226.00		AB
120s ea	**58016-0574-02**	271.20		AB
150s ea	**58016-0574-03**	272.31		AB
(CAPLET)				
600 mg, 180s ea	**58016-0574-99**	326.78		EE
200s ea	**58016-0574-89**	363.08		AB
300s ea	**58016-0574-73**	544.62		AB
(St. Mary's MPP)				
REPACK				
TAB, PO (FILM COATED)				
600 mg, 10s ea	**60760-0382-10**	22.31		AB
20s ea	**60760-0382-20**	39.22		EE
30s ea	**60760-0382-30**	54.94		EE
60s ea	**60760-0382-60**	105.66		EE
(Stat Rx)				
REPACK				
TAB, PO, 600 mg, 20s ea	**16590-0178-20**	56.65		
30s ea	**16590-0178-30**	82.00		
(FILM-COATED)				
600 mg, 56s ea	**16590-0178-56**	107.46		AB
60s ea	**16590-0178-60**	164.00		
90s ea	**16590-0178-90**	246.00		
(Vibranta)				
REPACK				
TAB, PO (FILM-COATED)				
600 mg, 30s ea	**57866-2899-01**	105.44		AB
60s ea	**57866-2899-02**	210.88		AB
90s ea	**57866-2899-03**	137.51		AB
120s ea	**57866-2899-04**	182.93		AB
OXAZEPAM				
FUL				
CAP, PO, 10 mg, 100s ea		53.63		
15 mg, 100s ea		57.09		
30 mg, 100s ea		123.37		
(Actavis)				
CAP, PO, 10 mg,				
100s ea, C-IV	**00228-2067-10**	86.21		AB
500s ea, C-IV	**00228-2067-50**	422.41		AB
15 mg, 100s ea, C-IV	**00228-2069-10**	108.85		AB
500s ea, C-IV	**00228-2069-50**	533.35		AB
30 mg, 100s ea, C-IV	**00228-2073-10**	157.43		AB
(Faulding Labs) *See SERAX*				
(Sandoz)				
CAP, PO, 10 mg,				
100s ea, C-IV	**00781-2809-01**	87.08		AB
15 mg, 100s ea, C-IV	**00781-2810-01**	109.95		AB
30 mg, 100s ea, C-IV	**00781-2811-01**	159.02		AB

PROD/MFR	NDC	AWP	DP	OBC
(Teva)				
CAP, PO, 10 mg,				
100s ea, C-IV	00172-4804-60	86.99		AB
500s ea, C-IV	00172-4804-70	434.95		AB
15 mg, 100s ea, C-IV	00172-4805-60	108.99		AB
500s ea, C-IV	00172-4805-70	544.95		AB
30 mg, 100s ea, C-IV	00172-4806-60	163.99		AB
(American Health) REPACK				
CAP, PO (10X10)				
10 mg,				
100s ea UD, C-IV	62584-0812-01	86.01		AB
15 mg,				
100s ea UD, C-IV	62584-0813-01	108.50		AB
30 mg,				
100s ea UD, C-IV	62584-0814-01	158.23		AB
(HomeMed) REPACK				
CAP, PO, 15 mg,				
30s ea, C-IV	51655-0854-24	28.12		EE
90s ea, C-IV	51655-0854-26	82.36		EE
30 mg, 30s ea, C-IV	51655-0855-24	42.40		EE
(Nucare Pharm) REPACK				
CAP, PO, 15 mg,				
90s ea, C-IV	68071-0460-90	117.78		AB
(Pharma Pac) REPACK				
CAP, PO, 15 mg,				
90s ea, C-IV	52959-0837-90	115.78		
(Phys Total Care) REPACK				
CAP, PO (USP)				
10 mg,				
20s ea, C-IV	54868-1341-02	24.00		EE
60s ea, C-IV	54868-1341-01	58.47		EE
100s ea, C-IV	54868-1341-00	74.79		EE
15 mg, 30s ea, C-IV	54868-2182-01	49.47		EE
90s ea, C-IV	54868-2182-00	104.22		AB
100s ea, C-IV	54868-2182-02	150.87		EE
30 mg, 10s ea, C-IV	54868-5851-00	38.56		
30s ea, C-IV	54868-5851-01	80.70		
(Quality Care Prod) REPACK				
CAP, PO, 10 mg,				
20s ea, C-IV	35356-0170-20	20.80		AB
(Stat Rx) REPACK				
CAP, PO, 15 mg,				
90s ea, C-IV	16590-0304-90	117.61		AB
OXCARBAZEPINE FUL				
TAB, PO, 150 mg, 100s ea		90.00		
300 mg, 100s ea		171.00		
600 mg, 100s ea		342.00		
(Apotex Corp.)				
TAB, PO (10X10,FILM-COATED)				
150 mg, 100s ea UD	60505-2534-00	152.63		AB
(FILM-COATED)				
150 mg, 100s ea	60505-2534-01	145.36		AB
500s ea	60505-2534-05	719.53		AB
(10X10,FILM-COATED)				
300 mg, 100s ea UD	60505-2535-00	278.73		AB
(FILM-COATED)				
300 mg, 100s ea	60505-2535-01	265.46		AB
1000s ea	60505-2535-08	2628.05		AB
(10X10,FILM-COATED)				
600 mg, 100s ea UD	60505-2536-00	512.32		AB
(FILM-COATED)				
600 mg, 100s ea	60505-2536-01	487.92		AB
500s ea	60505-2536-05	2415.20		AB
(Ascend)				
TAB, PO (FILM-COATED)				
150 mg, 100s ea	67877-0129-01	147.66		AB
500s ea	67877-0129-05	738.30		AB
300 mg, 100s ea	67877-0130-01	269.43		AB
500s ea	67877-0130-05	1347.15		AB
600 mg, 500s ea	67877-0131-05	2460.55		AB
(Breckenridge Pharm)				
TAB, PO (FILM-COATED)				
150 mg, 100s ea	51991-0292-01	143.74		AB
500s ea	51991-0292-05	718.70		AB
300 mg, 100s ea	51991-0293-01	262.51		AB
500s ea	51991-0293-05	1312.55		AB
600 mg, 100s ea	51991-0294-01	482.50		AB
500s ea	51991-0294-05	2412.50		AB

PROD/MFR	NDC	AWP	DP	OBC
(Caraco)				
TAB, PO (FILM-COATED)				
150 mg, 100s ea	62756-0183-88	144.55		AB
500s ea	62756-0183-13	722.76		AB
1000s ea	62756-0183-18	1445.51		AB
300 mg, 100s ea	62756-0184-88	263.98		AB
500s ea	62756-0184-13	1319.90		AB
1000s ea	62756-0184-18	2639.80		AB
600 mg, 100s ea	62756-0185-88	485.21		AB
500s ea	62756-0185-13	2426.03		AB
1000s ea	62756-0185-18	4852.06		AB
(Glenmark Pharmaceuticals)				
TAB, PO (FILM-COATED)				
150 mg, 100s ea	68462-0137-01	142.94		AB
300 mg, 100s ea	68462-0138-01	261.03		AB
600 mg, 100s ea	68462-0139-01	479.79		AB
(Novartis Pharm) *See TRILEPTAL*				
(Ranbaxy Pharm)				
SUS, PO (1X250ML)				
300 mg/5 ml,				
250 ml	63304-0653-25	155.79		AB
(Roxane)				
TAB, PO, 150 mg,				
100s ea UD	00054-0097-20	152.63		AB
100s ea	00054-0097-25	145.36		AB
300 mg, 100s ea UD	00054-0098-20	278.73		AB
100s ea	00054-0098-25	265.46		AB
500s ea	00054-0098-29	1327.28		AB
600 mg, 100s ea UD	00054-0099-20	512.31		AB
100s ea	00054-0099-25	487.92		AB
(Sandoz)				
SUS, PO (1X250ML)				
300 mg/5 ml,				
250 ml	00781-6270-43	155.96		
TAB, PO (10X10,FILM-COATED)				
150 mg, 100s ea UD	00781-5278-13	145.36		
(FILM-COATED)				
150 mg, 100s ea	00781-5278-01	145.36		
(10X10,FILM-COATED)				
300 mg, 100s ea UD	00781-5279-13	265.46		
(FILM-COATED)				
300 mg, 100s ea	00781-5279-01	265.46		
(10X10,FILM-COATED)				
600 mg, 100s ea UD	00781-5280-13	487.92		
(FILM-COATED)				
600 mg, 100s ea	00781-5280-01	487.92		
(Teva)				
TAB, PO (FILM-COATED)				
150 mg, 100s ea	00093-7281-01	145.36		AB
300 mg, 100s ea	00093-7282-01	265.46		AB
600 mg, 100s ea	00093-7283-01	487.92		AB
(American Health) REPACK				
TAB, PO (10X10,FILM-COATED)				
150 mg, 100s ea UD	62584-0142-01	150.85		
300 mg, 100s ea UD	62584-0143-01	275.48		
600 mg, 100s ea UD	62584-0145-01	506.33		
(Nucare Pharm) REPACK				
TAB, PO (FILM-COATED)				
300 mg, 60s ea	68071-0814-60	161.28		AB
(Phys Total Care) REPACK				
TAB, PO, 150 mg, 20s ea	54868-5830-00	80.45		
60s ea	54868-5830-01	232.36		
(FILM-COATED)				
300 mg, 60s ea	54868-6073-00	100.57		AB
(Physician Partner) REPACK				
TAB, PO (FILM-COATED)				
150 mg, 30s ea	21695-0862-30	86.73		AB
60s ea	21695-0862-60	174.43		AB
300 mg, 60s ea	21695-0863-60	159.28		AB
600 mg, 60s ea	21695-0864-60	585.50		AB
(Stat Rx) REPACK				
TAB, PO (FILM-COATED)				
150 mg, 30s ea	16590-0748-30	43.13		AB
60s ea	16590-0748-60	86.25		AB
90s ea	16590-0748-90	129.38		AB
300 mg, 30s ea	16590-0569-30	78.75		AB
60s ea	16590-0569-60	157.51		AB
90s ea	16590-0569-90	96.75		
100s ea	16590-0569-71	268.75		AB
OXICONAZOLE NITRATE				
(PharmaDerm) *See OXISTAT*				

PROD/MFR	NDC	AWP	DP	OBC
OXILAN-300 (Cook Inc)				
ioxilan				
SOL, IJ (S.D.V.)				
62%, 50 ml 10s	58707-0001-07	450.00		
100 ml 10s	58707-0001-11	900.00		
150 ml 10s	58707-0001-08	1350.00		
200 ml 10s	58707-0001-12	1800.00		
OXILAN-350 (Cook Inc)				
ioxilan				
SOL, IJ (S.D.V.)				
73%, 50 ml 10s	58707-0002-07	500.00		
100 ml 10s	58707-0002-11	1000.00		
150 ml 10s	58707-0002-18	1500.00		
200 ml 10s	58707-0002-19	2000.00		
OXISTAT (PharmaDerm)				
oxiconazole nitrate				
CRE, TP, 1%, 15 gm	00462-0358-15	47.74		
30 gm	00462-0358-30	86.84		
60 gm	00462-0358-60	173.58		
LOT, TP, 1%, 30 ml	00462-0359-30	91.19		
(1X60ML)				
1%, 60 ml	00462-0359-60	182.38		
(Dispensing Solutions) REPACK				
CRE, TP, 1%, 15 gm	55045-2483-05	35.00		
60 gm	55045-2180-09	90.00		
(Physician Partner) REPACK				
LOT, TP (1X30ML)				
1%, 30 ml	21695-0459-30	182.38		
(Quality Care Prod) REPACK				
CRE, TP (1X60GM)				
1%, 60 gm	35356-0357-60	186.60		
OXSORALEN (Valeant Pharm Intl)				
methoxsalen				
LOT, TP, 1%, 29.57 ml	00187-0402-31	569.81		
OXSORALEN-ULTRA (Valeant Pharm Intl)				
methoxsalen				
CAP, PO, 10 mg, 50s ea	00187-0650-42	1843.80		
OXTRIPHYLLINE (PCCA)				
POW, NA (USP)				
1 gm	51927-2468-00	0.72		
(Spectrum Pharmacy)				
CRY, NA (U.S.P.)				
100 gm	49452-4940-01	133.35		
500 gm	49452-4940-02	430.50		
OXY IR (Bryant Ranch) REPACK				
oxycodone hydrochloride				
CAP, PO, 5 mg,				
60s ea, C-II	63629-3763-01	25.12		
120s ea, C-II	63629-3763-02	48.65		
150s ea, C-II	63629-3763-03	59.33		
(Phys Total Care) REPACK				
CAP, PO, 5 mg,				
10s ea, C-II	54868-5700-01	9.10		
90s ea, C-II	54868-5700-00	43.60		
(Stat Rx) REPACK				
CAP, PO, 5 mg,				
56s ea, C-II	16590-0684-56	26.26		
120s ea, C-II	16590-0684-72	81.77		
OXYBENZONE (Medisca)				
POW, NA (U.S.P.)				
25 gm	38779-0718-04	25.50		
100 gm	38779-0718-05	58.50		
500 gm	38779-0718-08	214.50		
(PCCA)				
POW, NA, 1 gm	51927-1171-00	1.20		
(Spectrum Pharmacy)				
POW, NA (U.S.P.)				
25 gm	49452-1012-01	67.90		
500 gm	49452-1012-03	353.50		
OXYBUTYNIN				
(Watson) *See OXYTROL*				
OXYBUTYNIN (DHS, Inc.) REPACK				
oxybutynin chloride				
TAB, PO, 5 mg, 30s ea	55887-0529-30	16.07		
(PD-Rx Pharm) REPACK				
TAB, PO, 5 mg, 30s ea	58864-0874-30	8.13		

PROD/MFR	NDC	AWP	DP	OBC
(Phys Total Care)				
REPACK				
TER, PO, 10 mg, 10s ea	54868-5728-00	81.84		
30s ea	54868-5728-01	236.49		
OXYBUTYNIN CHLORIDE				
FUL				
SYR, PO, 5 mg/5 ml, 473 ml		13.15		
TAB, PO, 5 mg, 100s ea		16.50		
(Apotex Corp.)				
SYR, PO (BERRY)				
5 mg/5 ml, 473 ml	60505-6008-09	66.32		AA
(Kremers Urban)				
TER, PO (USP,COATED)				
5 mg, 100s ea	62175-0270-37	307.28		AB
500s ea	62175-0270-41	1459.56		AB
10 mg, 100s ea	62175-0271-37	307.60		AB
500s ea	62175-0271-41	1461.10		AB
15 mg, 100s ea	62175-0272-37	315.66		AB
500s ea	62175-0272-41	1499.40		AB
(Major)				
TAB, PO (10X10)				
5 mg, 100s ea UD	00904-2821-61	61.96		AB
(Medisca)				
POW, NA (U.S.P.)				
1 gm	38779-0384-06	63.00		
5 gm	38779-0384-03	267.00		
(Morton Grove)				
SYR, PO, 5 mg/5 ml, 473 ml	60432-0092-16	51.95		AA
(Mylan)				
TER, PO (FILM-COATED)				
5 mg, 100s ea	00378-6605-01	328.40		AB
500s ea	00378-6605-05	1642.00		AB
10 mg, 100s ea	00378-6610-01	328.75		AB
500s ea	00378-6610-05	1643.75		AB
15 mg, 100s ea	00378-6015-01	336.95		
(Ortho-McNeil Pharm) *See DITROPAN XL*				
(PCCA) *See OXYBUTYNIN CL*				
(Pharm Assoc Inc)				
SYR, PO (40X5ML,CHERRY)				
5 mg/5 ml, 5 ml 40s UD	00121-0671-05	104.00		AA
(CHERRY)				
5 mg/5 ml, 473 ml	00121-0671-16	66.25		AA
(Qualitest)				
SYR, PO (APPLE-WATERMELON)				
5 mg/5 ml, 473 ml	00603-1491-58	38.95		AA
TAB, PO, 5 mg, 60s ea	00603-4975-20	32.62		AB
90s ea	00603-4975-02	48.94		AB
100s ea	00603-4975-21	56.32		AB
180s ea	00603-4975-04	92.98		AB
500s ea	00603-4975-28	275.87		AB
1000s ea	00603-4975-32	535.07		AB
(Silarx)				
SYR, PO (RASPBERRY)				
5 mg/5 ml, 473 ml	54838-0510-80	52.00		AA
(Teva)				
TAB, PO, 5 mg, 100s ea	50111-0456-01	54.38		AB
500s ea	50111-0456-02	258.31		AB
1000s ea	50111-0456-03	527.49		AB
TER, PO (FILM-COATED)				
5 mg, 100s ea	00093-5206-01	328.82		AB
10 mg, 100s ea	00093-5207-01	329.16		AB
15 mg, 100s ea	00093-5208-01	337.40		AB
(UDL)				
TAB, PO (ROBOT READY 25X1)				
5 mg, 25s ea UD	51079-0628-19	11.15		AB
(10X10)				
5 mg, 100s ea UD	51079-0628-20	44.59		AB
TER, PO (FILM-COATED)				
5 mg, 30s ea UD	51079-0722-63	295.56		AB
(10X10,FILM-COATED)				
5 mg, 100s ea UD	51079-0722-20	328.40		AB
(FILM-COATED)				
10 mg, 30s ea UD	51079-0723-63	295.89		AB
(10X10,FILM-COATED)				
10 mg, 100s ea UD	51079-0723-20	328.75		AB
(Upsher-Smith)				
TAB, PO, 5 mg, 100s ea	00832-0038-00	47.67		AB
500s ea	00832-0038-50	233.30		AB
1000s ea	00832-0038-10	535.07		AB
(Watson) *See GELNIQUE*				
(A-S Medication)				
REPACK				
TAB, PO, 5 mg, 30s ea	54569-1990-00	16.31		EE
(Altura)				
REPACK				
TAB, PO, 5 mg, 12s ea	63874-0660-12	5.63		
15s ea	63874-0660-15	7.04		
30s ea	63874-0660-30	14.08		
42s ea	63874-0660-42	19.71		
60s ea	63874-0660-60	28.26		
100s ea	63874-0660-01	46.92		
(American Health)				
REPACK				
TAB, PO, 5 mg, 100s ea UD	68084-0400-01	10.00		AB
(Bryant Ranch)				
REPACK				
TAB, PO, 5 mg, 30s ea	63629-1354-01	16.38		
100s ea	63629-1354-02	52.03		
(Dispensing Solutions)				
REPACK				
TAB, PO, 5 mg, 30s ea	55045-2050-08	16.20		AB
100s ea	55045-2050-00	54.00		
(HomeMed)				
REPACK				
TAB, PO, 5 mg, 90s ea	51655-0665-26	35.56		EE
(McKesson Packaging)				
REPACK				
TAB, PO (USP)				
5 mg, 100s ea UD	63739-0195-10	44.22		AB
(Nucare Pharm)				
REPACK				
TAB, PO, 5 mg, 30s ea	66267-0642-30	16.99		AB
90s ea	66267-0642-90	41.99		AB
120s ea	66267-0642-91	53.99		AB
270s ea	66267-0642-93	92.99		AB
(Palmetto)				
REPACK				
TAB, PO, 5 mg, 100s ea	23490-6051-04	56.63		
(PD-Rx Pharm)				
REPACK				
TAB, PO, 5 mg, 30s ea	43063-0145-30	12.38		AB
(REDI-SCRIPT)				
5 mg, 90s ea	58864-0874-90	14.38		AB
(Phys Total Care)				
REPACK				
TAB, PO, 5 mg, 30s ea	54868-2157-01	7.51		EE
60s ea	54868-2157-03	12.03		EE
100s ea	54868-2157-02	18.05		EE
100s ea	54868-2157-04	45.62		EE
TER, PO (FILM-COATED)				
15 mg, 180s ea	54868-5743-03	855.00		AB
(Physician Partner)				
REPACK				
TAB, PO, 5 mg, 30s ea	21695-0406-30	33.79		AB
60s ea	21695-0406-60	67.58		AB
(Southwood)				
REPACK				
TAB, PO, 5 mg, 30s ea	58016-0623-30	16.31		EE
60s ea	58016-0623-60	32.62		EE
90s ea	58016-0623-90	48.93		EE
100s ea	58016-0623-00	54.37		EE
120s ea	58016-0623-02	65.24		EE
180s ea	58016-0623-99	97.86		EE
(Stat Rx)				
REPACK				
TER, PO, 5 mg, 30s ea	16590-0321-30	17.00		
60s ea	16590-0321-60	34.00		
90s ea	16590-0321-90	51.00		
120s ea	16590-0321-72	68.00		
OXYBUTYNIN CL (PCCA)				
oxybutynin chloride				
POW, NA (USP)				
1 gm	51927-2455-00	54.00		
OXYBUTYNIN ER (Phys Total Care)				
REPACK				
oxybutynin chloride				
TER, PO, 5 mg, 10s ea	54868-5742-00	81.75		
30s ea	54868-5742-01	236.28		
60s ea	54868-5742-02	442.29		
15 mg, 10s ea	54868-5743-01	78.30		
30s ea	54868-5743-00	228.90		
90s ea	54868-5743-02	644.55		
OXYCODONE (Core)				
REPACK				
oxycodone hydrochloride				
TAB, PO, 5 mg,				
30s ea, C-II	33358-0276-30	14.68		
60s ea, C-II	33358-0276-60	27.83		
(DHS, Inc.)				
REPACK				
TAB, PO, 15 mg,				
30s ea, C-II	55887-0133-30	20.90		
32s ea, C-II	55887-0133-32	18.66		
60s ea, C-II	55887-0133-60	66.27		
90s ea, C-II	55887-0133-90	99.41		
120s ea, C-II	55887-0133-82	132.55		
150s ea, C-II	55887-0133-86	165.69		
180s ea, C-II	55887-0133-92	198.82		
240s ea, C-II	55887-0133-91	265.10		
30 mg,				
28s ea, C-II	55887-0132-28	37.60		
32s ea, C-II	55887-0132-32	42.98		
60s ea, C-II	55887-0132-60	130.03		
90s ea, C-II	55887-0132-90	195.04		
120s ea, C-II	55887-0132-82	260.06		
150s ea, C-II	55887-0132-86	325.08		
180s ea, C-II	55887-0132-92	390.09		
240s ea, C-II	55887-0132-91	520.12		
TER, PO, 40 mg,				
60s ea, C-II	55887-0131-60	480.00		
90s ea, C-II	55887-0131-90	720.00		
120s ea, C-II	55887-0131-82	960.00		
180s ea, C-II	55887-0131-92	1440.00		
80 mg,				
90s ea, C-II	55887-0130-90	1080.00		
120s ea, C-II	55887-0130-82	1440.00		
150s ea, C-II	55887-0130-86	1800.00		
(Dispensing Solutions)				
REPACK				
TAB, PO, 5 mg,				
90s ea, C-II	66336-0174-90	39.42		
120s ea, C-II	66336-0174-94	52.38		
180s ea, C-II	66336-0174-62	78.29		
240s ea, C-II	66336-0174-98	104.20		
(Phys Total Care)				
REPACK				
CAP, PO, 5 mg,				
30s ea, C-II	54868-3932-00	28.99		
50s ea, C-II	54868-3932-01	42.32		
60s ea, C-II	54868-3932-02	48.99		
90s ea, C-II	54868-3932-03	68.98		
120s ea, C-II	54868-3932-04	88.98		
SOL, PO, 20 mg/ml,				
30 ml, C-II	54868-5507-00	69.93		
OXYCODONE AND ACETAMINOPHEN (Amneal)				
acetaminophen/oxycodone hydrochloride				
TAB, PO, 325 mg-5 mg,				
100s ea, C-II	53746-0203-01	51.23		AA
500s ea, C-II	53746-0203-05	230.98		AA
325 mg-10 mg,				
100s ea, C-II	53746-0204-01	177.72		AA
500 mg-7.5 mg,				
100s ea, C-II	53746-0205-01	106.05		AA
650 mg-10 mg,				
100s ea, C-II	53746-0206-01	145.65		AA
(Mylan)				
TAB, PO (USP)				
325 mg-2.5 mg,				
100s ea, C-II	00378-7103-01	204.91		
325 mg-5 mg,				
100s ea, C-II	00378-7104-01	57.67		
325 mg-7.5 mg,				
100s ea, C-II	00378-7105-01	136.07		
325 mg-10 mg,				
100s ea, C-II	00378-7106-01	177.92		
500 mg-7.5 mg,				
100s ea, C-II	00378-7107-01	145.30		
650 mg-10 mg,				
100s ea, C-II	00378-7108-01	190.02		
(Watson Labs)				
CAP, PO (HARD GELATIN)				
500 mg-5 mg,				
100s ea, C-II	00591-0737-01	11.83		AA
500s ea, C-II	00591-0737-05	56.21		AA
(4u)				
REPACK				
TAB, PO, 325 mg-5 mg,				
28s ea, C-II	42549-0618-28	64.22		AA
30s ea, C-II	10544-0418-30	66.94		AA
30s ea, C-II	42549-0618-30	66.94		AA
40s ea, C-II	42549-0618-40	88.48		AA
60s ea, C-II	10544-0418-60	120.22		AA
60s ea, C-II	42549-0618-60	120.22		AA
84s ea, C-II	42549-0618-84	162.42		AA
90s ea, C-II	42549-0618-90	169.46		AA
325 mg-10 mg,				
30s ea, C-II	42549-0640-30	104.44		AA
60s ea, C-II	42549-0640-60	188.99		AA
84s ea, C-II	42549-0640-84	278.14		AA
112s ea, C-II	42549-0640-02	326.86		AA

PROD/MFR	NDC	AWP	DP	OBC
(American Health)				
REPACK				
TAB, PO, 325 mg-5 mg,				
100s ea UD, C-II	**68084-0355-01**	27.50		AA
(Bryant Ranch)				
REPACK				
TAB, PO, 325 mg-10 mg,				
20s ea, C-II	**63629-3953-06**	38.40		AA
(Dispensing Solutions)				
REPACK				
TAB, PO, 650 mg-10 mg,				
28s ea, C-II	**66336-0465-28**	91.90		AA
32s ea, C-II	**66336-0465-32**	105.05		AA
(PD-Rx Pharm)				
REPACK				
TAB, PO, 325 mg-5 mg,				
2s ea, C-II	**43063-0025-02**	9.32		AA
4s ea, C-II	**43063-0025-04**	9.60		AA
6s ea, C-II	**43063-0025-06**	9.75		AA
(USP)				
325 mg-5 mg,				
10s ea, C-II	**55289-0951-10**	9.90		AA
12s ea, C-II	**43063-0025-12**	10.62		AA
(USP)				
325 mg-5 mg,				
12s ea, C-II	**55289-0951-12**	10.08		AA
20s ea, C-II	**55289-0951-20**	10.80		AA
24s ea, C-II	**55289-0951-24**	11.10		AA
(USP)				
325 mg-5 mg,				
30s ea, C-II	**55289-0951-30**	11.70		AA
40s ea, C-II	**55289-0951-40**	12.60		AA
(USP)				
325 mg-5 mg,				
60s ea, C-II	**55289-0951-60**	14.42		AA
90s ea, C-II	**55289-0951-90**	17.12		AA
120s ea, C-II	**55289-0951-98**	19.83		AA
180s ea, C-II	**55289-0951-93**	25.23		AA
240s ea, C-II	**55289-0951-99**	30.65		AA
360s ea, C-II	**55289-0951-86**	41.48		AA
(Phys Total Care)				
REPACK				
TAB, PO, 325 mg-10 mg,				
150s ea, C-II	**54868-5024-08**	217.89		AA
180s ea, C-II	**54868-5024-09**	284.15		AA
650 mg-10 mg,				
150s ea, C-II	**54868-5004-08**	233.72		AA
(Physician Partner)				
REPACK				
TAB, PO, 325 mg-10 mg,				
40s ea, C-II	**21695-0619-40**	227.70		AA
(St. Mary's MPP)				
REPACK				
TAB, PO, 325 mg-5 mg,				
30s ea, C-II	**60760-0200-30**	29.05		AA
60s ea, C-II	**60760-0200-60**	52.11		AA
90s ea, C-II	**60760-0200-90**	75.16		AA
120s ea, C-II	**60760-0200-92**	98.21		AA
325 mg-10 mg,				
30s ea, C-II	**60760-0204-30**	85.70		AA
60s ea, C-II	**60760-0204-60**	165.41		AA
90s ea, C-II	**60760-0204-90**	245.11		AA
120s ea, C-II	**60760-0204-92**	324.82		AA
OXYCODONE HCL (Actavis)				
oxycodone hydrochloride				
TAB, PO, 15 mg,				
100s ea, C-II	**52152-0214-02**	73.75		
30 mg,				
100s ea, C-II	**52152-0215-02**	142.15		
(Covidien)				
CAP, PO, 5 mg,				
100s ea, C-II	**00406-0554-01**	33.89		
POW, NA (U.S.P.)				
5 gm, C-II	**00406-8865-53**	268.20		
SOL, PO (RASPBERRY)				
5 mg/5 ml,				
500 ml, C-II	**00406-8555-50**	37.00		
(W/DROPPER)				
20 mg/ml,				
30 ml, C-II	**00406-8558-30**	35.00		
TAB, PO, 5 mg,				
100s ea, C-II	**00406-0552-01**	47.94		
(10X10)				
5 mg,				
100s ea UD, C-II	**00406-0552-62**	41.05		
15 mg,				
100s ea, C-II	**00406-8515-01**	75.79		
30 mg,				
100s ea, C-II	**00406-8530-01**	143.57		

PROD/MFR	NDC	AWP	DP	OBC
(Ethex)				
TAB, PO, 5 mg,				
100s ea, C-II	**58177-0315-04**	35.75		
100s ea UD, C-II	**58177-0315-11**	41.05		
(Hawkins)				
POW, NA (U.S.P.)				
1 gm, C-II	**63370-0960-10**	192.00		
5 gm, C-II	**63370-0960-15**	504.00		
25 gm, C-II	**63370-0960-25**	2160.00		
100 gm, C-II	**63370-0960-35**	6960.00		
500 gm, C-II	**63370-0960-45**	34080.00		
(Lannett)				
SOL, PO (CONCENTRATED,BERRY)				
20 mg/ml,				
30 ml, C-II	**00527-1426-36**	34.42		
(Medisca)				
POW, NA (U.S.P.)				
5 gm, C-II	**38779-0725-03**	331.50		
25 gm, C-II	**38779-0725-04**	1362.00		
100 gm, C-II	**38779-0725-05**	4590.00		
(1X1000GM,USP)				
1000 gm, C-II	**38779-0725-09**	34731.00		
(PCCA)				
POW, NA (U.S.P.; CII)				
1 gm, C-II	**51927-1008-00**	162.00		
(Qualitest)				
TAB, PO (USP)				
5 mg,				
100s ea, C-II	**00603-4990-21**	47.21		
(Spectrum Pharmacy)				
POW, NA (U.S.P.)				
1 gm, C-II	**49452-0034-02**	240.10		
5 gm, C-II	**49452-0034-01**	511.00		
25 gm, C-II	**49452-0034-03**	1610.00		
100 gm, C-II	**49452-0034-04**	4487.00		
(4u)				
REPACK				
CAP, PO, 5 mg,				
56s ea, C-II	**42549-0610-56**	84.22		
TAB, PO, 5 mg,				
30s ea, C-II	**42549-0610-30**	62.42		
56s ea, C-II	**42549-0626-56**	84.22		
60s ea, C-II	**42549-0610-60**	89.56		
90s ea, C-II	**42549-0610-90**	108.48		
(Altura)				
REPACK				
TAB, PO, 15 mg,				
20s ea, C-II	**63874-1267-02**	41.54		
30s ea, C-II	**63874-1267-03**	62.31		
60s ea, C-II	**63874-1267-06**	124.62		
30 mg,				
20s ea, C-II	**63874-1266-02**	76.35		
30s ea, C-II	**63874-1266-03**	114.52		
60s ea, C-II	**63874-1266-06**	229.06		
(American Health)				
REPACK				
TAB, PO, 15 mg,				
100s ea UD, C-II	**68084-0184-01**	48.75		
30 mg,				
100s ea UD, C-II	**68084-0185-01**	73.75		
(B&B Pharm, Inc)				
REPACK				
POW, NA (U.S.P.)				
5 gm, C-II	**63275-3005-02**	810.00		
25 gm, C-II	**63275-3025-04**	4050.00		
100 gm, C-II	**63275-3100-05**	16200.00		
(Bryant Ranch)				
REPACK				
TAB, PO, 5 mg,				
30s ea, C-II	**63629-3803-01**	12.89		
60s ea, C-II	**63629-3803-02**	23.12		
(DHS, Inc.)				
REPACK				
CAP, PO, 5 mg,				
30s ea, C-II	**55887-0050-30**	14.89		
(Nucare Pharm)				
REPACK				
TAB, PO, 30 mg,				
60s ea, C-II	**68071-0454-60**	170.72		
(Phys Total Care)				
REPACK				
CAP, PO, 5 mg,				
100s ea, C-II	**54868-3932-05**	75.65		
TAB, PO, 5 mg,				
50s ea, C-II	**54868-4983-01**	48.60		
60s ea, C-II	**54868-4983-00**	56.52		

PROD/MFR	NDC	AWP	DP	OBC
150s ea, C-II	**54868-4983-09**	96.23		
15 mg,				
60s ea, C-II	**54868-4980-00**	100.20		
30 mg,				
30s ea, C-II	**54868-5390-01**	77.94		
60s ea, C-II	**54868-5390-00**	116.01		
(Quality Care Prod)				
REPACK				
TAB, PO, 5 mg,				
30s ea, C-II	**35356-0453-30**	48.60		
90s ea, C-II	**35356-0453-90**	115.43		
120s ea, C-II	**49999-0899-01**	93.28		
30 mg,				
90s ea, C-II	**49999-0851-90**	341.25		
(St. Mary's MPP)				
REPACK				
TAB, PO (USP)				
15 mg,				
90s ea, C-II	**60760-0855-90**	105.56		
(Stat Rx)				
REPACK				
CAP, PO, 5 mg,				
30s ea, C-II	**16590-0854-30**	10.59		
60s ea, C-II	**16590-0854-60**	21.18		
TAB, PO, 5 mg,				
30s ea, C-II	**16590-0835-30**	14.40		
60s ea, C-II	**16590-0835-60**	65.52		
90s ea, C-II	**16590-0835-90**	98.28		
TER, PO, 20 mg,				
30s ea, C-II	**16590-0610-30**	107.19		
60s ea, C-II	**16590-0610-60**	212.16		
90s ea, C-II	**16590-0610-90**	317.51		
180s ea, C-II	**16590-0610-82**	635.02		
(FILM-COATED)				
40 mg,				
30s ea, C-II	**16590-0611-30**	231.30		AB
56s ea, C-II	**16590-0611-56**	433.60		AB
60s ea, C-II	**16590-0611-60**	464.46		AB
90s ea, C-II	**16590-0611-90**	695.97		AB
OXYCODONE HYDROCHLORIDE				
FUL				
CAP, PO, 5 mg, 100s ea		21.38		
SOL, PO, 20 mg/ml, 30 ml		28.50		
TAB, PO, 5 mg, 100s ea		23.99		
15 mg, 100s ea		66.95		
30 mg, 100s ea		130.94		
(Actavis) *See OXYCODONE HCL*				
(Actavis)				
TER, PO (CONTROLLED-RELEASE)				
10 mg,				
100s ea, C-II	**52152-0408-02**	183.28		
20 mg, 100s ea, C-II	**52152-0409-02**	350.69		
40 mg, 100s ea, C-II	**52152-0410-02**	622.25		
80 mg, 100s ea, C-II	**52152-0411-02**	1170.17		
(Caraco)				
TAB, PO (USP,UNCOATED)				
5 mg,				
100s ea, C-II	**57664-0223-88**	47.94		AB
15 mg, 100s ea, C-II	**57664-0187-88**	125.05		AB
30 mg, 100s ea, C-II	**57664-0224-88**	245.25		AB
(CorePharma)				
TAB, PO (USP,COMPRESSED)				
5 mg,				
100s ea, C-II	**64720-0224-10**	47.94		AB
15 mg, 100s ea, C-II	**64720-0225-10**	74.19		AB
30 mg, 100s ea, C-II	**64720-0226-10**	145.57		AB
(Covidien) *See OXYCODONE HCL*				
(Covidien)				
SOL, PO (1X30ML,RASPBERRY)				
20 mg/ml,				
30 ml, C-II	**00406-8668-30**	35.00		
(Ethex) *See OXYCODONE HCL*				
(Ethex)				
TAB, PO, 5 mg,				
100s ea, C-II	**58177-0625-04**	32.80		
(10X10)				
5 mg,				
100s ea UD, C-II	**58177-0625-11**	44.91		
(USP)				
10 mg,				
100s ea, C-II	**58177-0461-04**	55.17		EE
15 mg, 100s ea, C-II	**58177-0445-04**	69.70		AB
(USP)				
20 mg, 100s ea	**58177-0462-04**	91.26		EE
30 mg, 100s ea, C-II	**58177-0446-04**	134.34		AB
TER, PO, 10 mg,				
100s ea, C-II	**58177-0677-04**	183.28		
20 mg, 100s ea, C-II	**58177-0679-04**	350.69		

PROD/MFR	NDC	AWP	DP	OBC
40 mg, 100s ea, C-II	**58177-0681-04**	622.25		
80 mg, 100s ea, C-II	**58177-0683-04**	1170.17		
(Gallipot)				
POW, NA (1X1GM,USP)				
1 gm, C-II	**51552-0685-01**	54.60	39.00	
(1X5GM,USP)				
5 gm, C-II	**51552-0685-02**	147.00	105.00	
(1X25GM,USP)				
25 gm, C-II	**51552-0685-04**	595.00	425.00	
(Glenmark Pharmaceuticals)				
CAP, PO, 5 mg,				
100s ea, C-II	**68462-0204-01**	35.30		
SOL, PO (USP,1X100ML,W/DROPPER)				
5 mg/5 ml,				
100 ml, C-II	**68462-0348-19**	34.00		
(USP,1X500ML,BERRY)				
5 mg/5 ml,				
500 ml, C-II	**68462-0348-57**	37.00		
(1X30ML,W/DROPPER,BERRY)				
20 mg/ml,				
30 ml, C-II	**68462-0347-37**	34.42		
(Hawkins) *See OXYCODONE HCL*				
(KVK)				
TAB, PO (USP)				
5 mg,				
100s ea, C-II	**10702-0018-01**	48.10		**AB**
10 mg, 100s ea, C-II	**10702-0056-01**	62.50		**AB**
15 mg, 100s ea, C-II	**10702-0008-01**	75.90		**AB**
20 mg, 100s ea	**10702-0057-01**	110.30		**AB**
30 mg, 100s ea, C-II	**10702-0009-01**	143.90		**AB**
(Lannett) *See OXYCODONE HCL*				
(Letco)				
POW, NA (1X5GM,USP)				
5 gm, C-II	**62991-1410-01**	488.00	122.00	
(1X25GM,USP)				
25 gm, C-II	**62991-1410-02**	1732.00	433.00	
(1X100GM,USP)				
100 gm, C-II	**62991-1410-03**	4620.00	1155.00	
(1X500GM,USP)				
500 gm, C-II	**62991-1410-04**	23100.00	5775.00	
(Medisca) *See OXYCODONE HCL*				
(Midlothian Labs)				
CAP, PO, 5 mg,				
100s ea, C-II	**68308-0145-10**	34.98		
(PCCA) *See OXYCODONE HCL*				
(Purdue Pharma) *See OXYCONTIN*				
(Qualitest) *See OXYCODONE HCL*				
(Qualitest)				
TAB, PO (USP)				
15 mg,				
100s ea, C-II	**00603-4991-21**	73.75		**AB**
30 mg, 100s ea, C-II	**00603-4992-21**	142.14		**AB**
(Ranbaxy Pharm)				
TER, PO (CONTROLLED-RELEASE)				
10 mg,				
100s ea, C-II	**63304-0400-01**	183.28		
20 mg, 100s ea, C-II	**63304-0401-01**	350.69		
(Spectrum Pharmacy) *See OXYCODONE HCL*				
(Xanodyne Pharma) *See ROXICODONE*				
(4u)				
REPACK				
TAB, PO, 5 mg,				
56s ea, C-II	**42549-0581-56**	84.22		
10 mg, 28s ea, C-II	**42549-0580-28**	78.84		**EE**
30s ea, C-II	**42549-0580-30**	81.26		**EE**
60s ea, C-II	**42549-0580-60**	144.34		**EE**
84s ea, C-II	**42549-0580-84**	176.56		**EE**
15 mg, 30s ea, C-II	**42549-0643-30**	81.84		**AB**
60s ea, C-II	**42549-0643-60**	144.46		**AB**
30 mg, 30s ea, C-II	**42549-0644-30**	88.26		**AB**
TER, PO, 10 mg,				
28s ea, C-II	**42549-0611-28**	78.84		**AB**
30s ea, C-II	**42549-0611-30**	81.26		**AB**
60s ea, C-II	**42549-0611-60**	144.34		**AB**
84s ea, C-II	**42549-0611-84**	176.56		**AB**
(American Health)				
REPACK				
TAB, PO, 5 mg,				
100s ea UD, C-II	**68084-0354-01**	37.50		**AB**
(DHS, Inc.)				
REPACK				
TAB, PO, 30 mg,				
30s ea, C-II	**55887-0132-30**	65.61		**AB**
(Dispensing Solutions)				
REPACK				
TAB, PO, 5 mg,				
30s ea, C-II	**66336-0174-30**	13.14		
60s ea, C-II	**66336-0174-60**	26.28		
15 mg, 28s ea, C-II	**66336-0470-28**	22.72		**AB**
32s ea, C-II	**66336-0470-32**	25.96		**AB**
90s ea, C-II	**66336-0470-90**	73.02		**AB**
30 mg, 28s ea, C-II	**66336-0135-28**	43.78		**AB**
32s ea, C-II	**66336-0135-32**	50.04		**AB**
90s ea, C-II	**66336-0135-90**	140.73		**AB**
(Palmetto)				
REPACK				
TAB, PO, 5 mg,				
12s ea, C-II	**23490-7781-01**	18.92		
20s ea, C-II	**23490-7781-02**	31.54		
30s ea, C-II	**23490-7781-03**	47.31		
60s ea, C-II	**23490-7781-06**	94.62		
90s ea, C-II	**23490-7781-09**	141.93		
100s ea, C-II	**23490-7781-08**	157.70		
15 mg, 20s ea, C-II	**23490-7819-02**	41.54		
30s ea, C-II	**23490-7819-03**	62.31		
60s ea, C-II	**23490-7819-06**	124.62		
90s ea, C-II	**23490-7819-09**	186.93		
100s ea, C-II	**23490-7819-08**	415.40		
30 mg, 20s ea, C-II	**23490-7820-02**	76.35		
30s ea, C-II	**23490-7820-03**	114.53		
60s ea, C-II	**23490-7820-06**	229.06		
90s ea, C-II	**23490-7820-09**	343.59		
100s ea, C-II	**23490-7820-08**	381.00		
TER, PO, 10 mg,				
6s ea, C-II	**23490-7799-01**	11.10		
30s ea, C-II	**23490-7799-03**	55.50		
56s ea, C-II	**23490-7799-04**	103.60		
90s ea, C-II	**23490-7799-09**	166.50		
20 mg, 6s ea, C-II	**23490-7800-01**	25.50		
56s ea, C-II	**23490-7800-04**	238.00		
60s ea, C-II	**23490-7800-06**	255.00		
90s ea, C-II	**23490-7800-09**	382.50		
40 mg, 6s ea, C-II	**23490-7801-01**	35.70		
60s ea, C-II	**23490-7801-06**	357.00		
(PD-Rx Pharm)				
REPACK				
TAB, PO (USP)				
15 mg,				
60s ea, C-II	**43063-0219-60**	44.10		**AB**
90s ea, C-II	**43063-0219-90**	61.14		**AB**
120s ea, C-II	**43063-0219-98**	78.18		**AB**
180s ea, C-II	**43063-0219-93**	112.30		**AB**
30 mg, 60s ea, C-II	**43063-0220-60**	65.64		**AB**
90s ea, C-II	**43063-0220-90**	93.48		**AB**
120s ea, C-II	**43063-0220-98**	121.30		**AB**
180s ea, C-II	**43063-0220-93**	176.92		**AB**
(Phys Total Care)				
REPACK				
TAB, PO, 5 mg,				
30s ea, C-II	**54868-4983-04**	32.76		
90s ea, C-II	**54868-4983-03**	80.28		
100s ea, C-II	**54868-4983-05**	88.20		
120s ea, C-II	**54868-4983-08**	104.04		
10 mg, 12s ea, C-II	**54868-3137-00**	17.35		**EE**
60s ea, C-II	**54868-3137-01**	56.76		**EE**
90s ea, C-II	**54868-3137-02**	81.40		**EE**
120s ea, C-II	**54868-3137-03**	106.03		**EE**
(USP)				
15 mg,				
30s ea, C-II	**54868-4980-02**	42.37		
90s ea, C-II	**54868-4980-03**	91.73		
100s ea, C-II	**54868-4980-04**	92.64		
120s ea, C-II	**54868-4980-01**	92.82		
150s ea, C-II	**54868-4980-05**	116.03		
180s ea, C-II	**54868-4980-06**	177.81		**AB**
20 mg, 12s ea	**54868-5902-00**	27.21		**EE**
60s ea	**54868-5902-01**	82.87		**EE**
90s ea	**54868-5902-02**	120.55		**EE**
120s ea	**54868-5902-03**	158.23		**EE**
30 mg, 20s ea, C-II	**54868-5390-02**	53.94		
90s ea, C-II	**54868-5390-05**	107.71		
100s ea, C-II	**54868-5390-03**	146.28		
120s ea, C-II	**54868-5390-04**	174.35		
150s ea, C-II	**54868-5390-06**	194.33		
180s ea, C-II	**54868-5390-07**	286.31		**AB**
200s ea, C-II	**54868-5390-08**	317.28		**AB**
(Quality Care Prod)				
REPACK				
TAB, PO, 5 mg,				
30s ea, C-II	**49999-0899-30**	23.32		
60s ea, C-II	**49999-0899-60**	46.64		
90s ea, C-II	**49999-0899-90**	69.96		
10 mg, 60s ea, C-II	**35356-0211-60**	181.33		**EE**
90s ea, C-II	**35356-0211-90**	272.00		**EE**
15 mg, 30s ea, C-II	**49999-0850-30**	62.80		
60s ea, C-II	**49999-0850-60**	125.60		
120s ea, C-II	**49999-0850-01**	251.20		
150s ea, C-II	**49999-0850-05**	314.00		
20 mg, 30s ea	**35356-0212-30**	226.00		**EE**
60s ea	**35356-0212-60**	452.00		**EE**
90s ea	**35356-0212-90**	678.00		**EE**
30 mg, 30s ea, C-II	**49999-0851-30**	113.75		
60s ea, C-II	**49999-0851-60**	227.50		
120s ea, C-II	**49999-0851-01**	409.00		
150s ea, C-II	**49999-0851-05**	484.43		
(Stat Rx)				
REPACK				
TAB, PO, 10 mg,				
10s ea, C-II	**16590-0798-10**	5.52		**EE**
30s ea, C-II	**16590-0855-30**	16.55		**EE**
56s ea, C-II	**16590-0855-56**	30.90		**EE**
60s ea, C-II	**16590-0855-60**	33.10		**EE**
90s ea, C-II	**16590-0855-90**	49.65		**EE**
15 mg, 30s ea, C-II	**16590-0659-30**	38.75		**AB**
56s ea, C-II	**16590-0659-56**	72.33		**AB**
60s ea, C-II	**16590-0659-60**	75.50		**AB**
84s ea, C-II	**16590-0659-62**	90.25		**AB**
90s ea, C-II	**16590-0659-90**	95.00		**AB**
112s ea, C-II	**16590-0659-73**	118.50		**AB**
120s ea, C-II	**16590-0659-72**	100.80		**AB**
150s ea, C-II	**16590-0659-83**	126.00		**AB**
20 mg, 84s ea	**16590-0610-62**	296.45		**EE**
30 mg, 30s ea, C-II	**16590-0671-30**	43.07		**AB**
60s ea, C-II	**16590-0671-60**	86.14		**AB**
90s ea, C-II	**16590-0671-90**	145.80		**AB**
120s ea, C-II	**16590-0671-72**	172.28		**AB**
TER, PO, 10 mg,				
56s ea, C-II	**16590-0798-56**	106.15		**AB**
60s ea, C-II	**16590-0798-60**	114.41		**AB**
OXYCODONE HYDROCHLORIDE AND IBUPROFEN				
(Actavis)				
ibuprofen/oxycodone hydrochloride				
TAB, PO (FILM-COATED)				
400 mg-5 mg,				
100s ea, C-II	**00228-4029-11**	147.26		**AB**
(Teva)				
TAB, PO (FILM-COATED)				
400 mg-5 mg,				
100s ea, C-II	**00555-0778-02**	147.40		**AB**
(Watson Labs)				
TAB, PO (FILM COATED)				
400 mg-5 mg,				
100s ea, C-II	**00591-3494-01**	141.53		**AB**
(Quality Care Prod)				
REPACK				
TAB, PO (FILM COATED)				
400 mg-5 mg,				
30s ea, C-II	**35356-0561-30**	79.20		**AB**
OXYCODONE HYDROCHLORIDE/ACETAMINOPHEN				
(Quality Care Prod)				
acetaminophen/oxycodone hydrochloride				
TAB, PO, 325 mg-5 mg,				
30s ea, C-II	**49999-0852-30**	98.20		
60s ea, C-II	**49999-0852-60**	196.40		
90s ea, C-II	**49999-0852-90**	294.60		
120s ea, C-II	**49999-0852-01**	392.80		
325 mg-7.5 mg,				
30s ea, C-II	**49999-0853-30**	127.20		
60s ea, C-II	**49999-0853-60**	254.40		
90s ea, C-II	**49999-0853-90**	381.60		
120s ea, C-II	**49999-0853-01**	498.67		
325 mg-10 mg,				
30s ea, C-II	**49999-0854-30**	104.80		
60s ea, C-II	**49999-0854-60**	209.60		
90s ea, C-II	**49999-0854-90**	314.40		
120s ea, C-II	**49999-0854-01**	419.20		
150s ea, C-II	**49999-0854-05**	497.70		
500 mg-7.5 mg,				
30s ea, C-II	**35356-0063-30**	127.00		
60s ea, C-II	**35356-0063-60**	254.00		
90s ea, C-II	**35356-0063-90**	498.00		
650 mg-10 mg,				
30s ea, C-II	**49999-0855-30**	90.25		
60s ea, C-II	**49999-0855-60**	180.50		
OXYCODONE/ACETAMINOPHEN (DHS, Inc.)				
REPACK				
acetaminophen/oxycodone hydrochloride				
TAB, PO, 325 mg-10 mg,				
30s ea, C-II	**55887-0129-30**	120.08		
90s ea, C-II	**55887-0129-90**	360.24		
120s ea, C-II	**55887-0129-82**	480.32		
150s ea, C-II	**55887-0129-86**	600.40		

PROD/MFR	NDC	AWP	DP	OBC
(Phys Total Care)				
REPACK				
CAP, PO, 500 mg-5 mg,				
40s ea, C-II	**54868-2771-02**	40.38		
TAB, PO (USP)				
325 mg-7.5 mg,				
40s ea, C-II	**54868-5338-03**	73.29		
90s ea, C-II	**54868-5338-04**	120.72		
120s ea, C-II	**54868-5338-05**	158.45		
OXYCODONE/APAP (Bryant Ranch)				
REPACK				
acetaminophen/oxycodone hydrochloride				
TAB, PO, 325 mg-5 mg,				
10s ea, C-II	**63629-3066-01**	10.99		
120s ea, C-II	**63629-3066-02**	142.99		
650 mg-10 mg,				
120s ea, C-II	**63629-3184-01**	306.89		
(Core)				
REPACK				
CAP, PO, 500 mg-5 mg,				
40s ea, C-II	**33358-0280-40**	20.69		
TAB, PO, 325 mg-5 mg,				
10s ea, C-II	**33358-0279-10**	6.02		
30s ea, C-II	**33358-0279-30**	10.47		
60s ea, C-II	**33358-0279-60**	41.32		
325 mg-10 mg,				
20s ea, C-II	**33358-0281-20**	76.97		
30s ea, C-II	**33358-0281-30**	107.83		
60s ea, C-II	**33358-0281-60**	214.42		
90s ea, C-II	**33358-0281-90**	325.19		
(DHS, Inc.)				
REPACK				
CAP, PO, 500 mg-5 mg,				
20s ea, C-II	**55887-0084-20**	24.95		
30s ea, C-II	**55887-0084-30**	37.42		
60s ea, C-II	**55887-0084-60**	74.85		
90s ea, C-II	**55887-0084-90**	112.26		
TAB, PO, 325 mg-5 mg,				
15s ea, C-II	**55887-0141-15**	38.67		
20s ea, C-II	**55887-0141-20**	51.56		
30s ea, C-II	**55887-0141-30**	77.34		
40s ea, C-II	**55887-0141-40**	103.12		
50s ea, C-II	**55887-0141-50**	128.90		
60s ea, C-II	**55887-0141-60**	154.68		
90s ea, C-II	**55887-0141-90**	232.02		
120s ea, C-II	**55887-0141-82**	309.37		
650 mg-10 mg,				
30s ea, C-II	**55887-0128-30**	41.30		
32s ea, C-II	**55887-0128-32**	30.92		
60s ea, C-II	**55887-0128-60**	82.60		
120s ea, C-II	**55887-0128-82**	165.21		
(Dispensing Solutions)				
REPACK				
TAB, PO, 325 mg-5 mg,				
60s ea, C-II	**66336-0145-60**	87.12		
90s ea, C-II	**66336-0145-90**	109.29		
120s ea, C-II	**66336-0145-94**	145.72		
180s ea, C-II	**66336-0145-62**	218.58		
240s ea, C-II	**66336-0145-98**	291.44		
325 mg-10 mg,				
15s ea, C-II	**66336-0147-15**	38.25		
30s ea, C-II	**66336-0147-30**	58.71		
90s ea, C-II	**66336-0147-90**	176.13		
120s ea, C-II	**66336-0147-94**	213.05		
(Nucare Pharm)				
REPACK				
TAB, PO, 325 mg-5 mg,				
20s ea, C-II	**68071-0224-20**	4.78		
30s ea, C-II	**68071-0224-30**	7.16		
(Phys Total Care)				
REPACK				
TAB, PO, 325 mg-7.5 mg,				
100s ea, C-II	**54868-5338-06**	125.88		
OXYCONTIN (Purdue Pharma)				
oxycodone hydrochloride				
TER, PO (2X10 BLISTER CARDS)				
10 mg,				
20s ea, C-II	**59011-0100-20**	41.81		
100s ea, C-II	**59011-0100-10**	203.64		
15 mg,				
100s ea, C-II	**59011-0815-10**	304.96		AB
(2X10 BLISTER CARDS)				
20 mg,				
20s ea, C-II	**59011-0103-20**	79.93		
100s ea, C-II	**59011-0103-10**	389.66		
30 mg,				
100s ea, C-II	**59011-0830-10**	551.52		AB
(2X10 BLISTER CARDS)				
40 mg,				
20s ea, C-II	**59011-0105-20**	141.76		
100s ea, C-II	**59011-0105-10**	691.39		
60 mg,				
100s ea, C-II	**59011-0860-10**	1006.12		AB
(2X10 BLISTER CARDS)				
80 mg,				
20s ea, C-II	**59011-0107-20**	266.71		
100s ea, C-II	**59011-0107-10**	1300.19		
(4u)				
REPACK				
TER, PO, 20 mg,				
30s ea, C-II	**42549-0645-30**	236.92		
(Bryant Ranch)				
REPACK				
TER, PO, 10 mg,				
60s ea, C-II	**63629-3775-02**	109.65		
90s ea, C-II	**63629-3775-01**	161.32		
20 mg,				
60s ea, C-II	**63629-3772-01**	199.89		
90s ea, C-II	**63629-3772-02**	299.65		
120s ea, C-II	**63629-3772-03**	399.23		
40 mg,				
60s ea, C-II	**63629-3774-01**	356.23		
90s ea, C-II	**63629-3774-02**	536.52		
120s ea, C-II	**63629-3774-03**	712.29		
(DHS, Inc.)				
REPACK				
TER, PO, 80 mg,				
60s ea, C-II	**55887-0130-60**	778.33		
(Palmetto)				
REPACK				
TER, PO, 40 mg,				
30s ea, C-II	**23490-9290-03**	165.00		
60s ea, C-II	**23490-9290-06**	330.00		
90s ea, C-II	**23490-9290-09**	495.00		
80 mg,				
30s ea, C-II	**23490-9291-03**	330.00		
60s ea, C-II	**23490-9291-06**	660.00		
90s ea, C-II	**23490-9291-09**	990.00		
(Phys Total Care)				
REPACK				
TER, PO, 10 mg,				
10s ea, C-II	**54868-3813-03**	29.45		
20s ea, C-II	**54868-3813-02**	54.97		
20s ea, C-II	**54868-3813-05**	51.63		
30s ea, C-II	**54868-3813-00**	80.49		
60s ea, C-II	**54868-3813-01**	148.56		
120s ea, C-II	**54868-3813-04**	293.19		
20 mg,				
10s ea, C-II	**54868-3814-06**	52.76		
20s ea, C-II	**54868-3814-02**	101.60		
20s ea, C-II	**54868-3814-04**	104.11		
30s ea, C-II	**54868-3814-00**	142.30		
60s ea, C-II	**54868-3814-01**	280.68		
90s ea, C-II	**54868-3814-03**	419.06		
120s ea, C-II	**54868-3814-05**	539.58		
30 mg,				
10s ea, C-II	**54868-5966-00**	73.05		AB
30s ea, C-II	**54868-5966-01**	199.78		AB
60s ea, C-II	**54868-5966-02**	395.63		AB
40 mg,				
10s ea, C-II	**54868-3815-03**	90.58		
20s ea, C-II	**54868-3815-02**	167.61		
30s ea, C-II	**54868-3815-00**	249.45		
60s ea, C-II	**54868-3815-01**	494.98		
90s ea, C-II	**54868-3815-04**	716.75		
120s ea, C-II	**54868-3815-05**	954.36		
60 mg,				
10s ea, C-II	**54868-5970-00**	130.03		AB
60s ea, C-II	**54868-5970-01**	695.46		AB
80 mg,				
10s ea, C-II	**54868-3986-03**	157.83		
20s ea, C-II	**54868-3986-01**	311.74		
30s ea, C-II	**54868-3986-02**	450.75		
60s ea, C-II	**54868-3986-00**	897.58		
90s ea, C-II	**54868-3986-05**	1319.19		
120s ea, C-II	**54868-3986-04**	1753.62		
(Quality Care Prod)				
REPACK				
TER, PO, 20 mg,				
60s ea, C-II	**35356-0091-60**	712.00		
90s ea, C-II	**35356-0091-90**	1068.30		
40 mg,				
60s ea, C-II	**35356-0399-30**	566.88		
60 mg,				
30s ea, C-II	**35356-0444-30**	512.30		AB
80 mg,				
90s ea, C-II	**35356-0400-90**	1037.96		
(St. Mary's MPP)				
REPACK				
TER, PO, 20 mg,				
90s ea, C-II	**60760-0049-90**	532.04		
(Stat Rx)				
REPACK				
TER, PO, 10 mg,				
15s ea, C-II	**16590-0677-15**	36.74		
20s ea, C-II	**16590-0677-20**	48.53		
30s ea, C-II	**16590-0677-30**	72.79		
60s ea, C-II	**16590-0677-60**	142.66		
84s ea, C-II	**16590-0677-62**	200.98		
90s ea, C-II	**16590-0677-90**	213.28		
120s ea, C-II	**16590-0677-72**	283.89		
15 mg,				
60s ea, C-II	**16590-0690-60**	209.46		AB
20 mg,				
30s ea, C-II	**16590-0616-30**	138.37		
56s ea, C-II	**16590-0616-56**	242.48		
60s ea, C-II	**16590-0616-60**	273.51		
84s ea, C-II	**16590-0616-62**	381.60		
90s ea, C-II	**16590-0616-90**	408.63		
112s ea, C-II	**16590-0616-73**	507.72		
30 mg,				
30s ea, C-II	**16590-0653-30**	194.50		AB
60s ea, C-II	**16590-0653-60**	397.00		AB
90s ea, C-II	**16590-0653-90**	577.01		AB
120s ea, C-II	**16590-0653-72**	768.26		AB
40 mg,				
30s ea, C-II	**16590-0615-30**	241.19		
40s ea, C-II	**16590-0611-40**	306.41		
56s ea, C-II	**16590-0615-56**	450.22		
60s ea, C-II	**16590-0615-60**	481.05		
84s ea, C-II	**16590-0615-62**	674.58		
90s ea, C-II	**16590-0615-90**	722.53		
120s ea, C-II	**16590-0615-72**	962.29		
60 mg,				
30s ea, C-II	**16590-0717-30**	352.14		AB
60s ea, C-II	**16590-0717-60**	701.04		AB
90s ea, C-II	**16590-0717-90**	1049.93		AB
80 mg,				
30s ea, C-II	**16590-0617-30**	454.12		
30s ea, C-II	**16590-0617-86**	4061.12		
60s ea, C-II	**16590-0617-60**	905.00		
90s ea, C-II	**16590-0617-90**	1355.87		
OXYCONTIN CR (Quality Care Prod)				
REPACK				
oxycodone hydrochloride				
TER, PO, 10 mg,				
5s ea, C-II	**35356-0090-05**	44.45		
10s ea, C-II	**35356-0090-10**	88.90		
30s ea, C-II	**35356-0090-30**	206.80		
20 mg,				
30s ea, C-II	**35356-0091-30**	356.00		
OXYMETAZOLINE HCL (PCCA)				
oxymetazoline hydrochloride				
POW, NA (U.S.P.)				
1 gm	**51927-3205-00**	57.00		
(Spectrum Pharmacy)				
POW, NA (U.S.P.)				
5 gm	**49452-4954-01**	364.00		
25 gm	**49452-4954-02**	931.00		
100 gm	**49452-4954-03**	3038.00		
OXYMETAZOLINE HYDROCHLORIDE				
(PCCA) *See OXYMETAZOLINE HCL*				
(Spectrum Pharmacy) *See OXYMETAZOLINE HCL*				
(Palmetto)				
REPACK				
SPR, NS, 0.05%, 15 ml	**23490-6720-01**	5.75		
OXYMETHOLONE				
(Alaven) *See ANADROL-50*				
(Medisca)				
POW, NA (1X25GM,USP)				
25 gm, C-III	**38779-1946-04**	1650.00		
(1X100GM,USP)				
100 gm, C-III	**38779-1946-05**	3750.00		
(1X500GM,USP)				
500 gm, C-III	**38779-1946-08**	14400.00		
(1X1000GM,USP)				
1000 gm, C-III	**38779-1946-09**	21000.00		
OXYMORPHONE HYDROCHLORIDE				
(Endo Pharm) *See OPANA*				
(Endo Pharm) *See OPANA ER*				
OXYPHENCYCLIMINE HCL (Gallipot)				
oxyphencyclimine hydrochloride				
POW, NA, 25 gm	**51552-0524-04**	229.88		

PROD/MFR	NDC	AWP	DP	OBC
(Medisca)				
POW, NA (U.S.P.)				
5 gm	38779-1479-03	117.00		
25 gm	38779-1479-04	450.00		
100 gm	38779-1479-05	1402.50		
(PCCA)				
POW, NA (U.S.P. XXII)				
1 gm	51927-1948-00	23.40		
OXYPHENCYCLIMINE HYDROCHLORIDE				
(Gallipot) *See OXYPHENCYCLIMINE HCL*				
(Medisca) *See OXYPHENCYCLIMINE HCL*				
(PCCA) *See OXYPHENCYCLIMINE HCL*				
OXYPURINOL (PCCA)				
POW, NA, 1 gm	51927-3645-00	456.42		
OXYQUINOLINE				
(PCCA) *See HYDROXYQUINOLINE*				
(Spectrum Pharmacy) *See 8-QUINOLINOL*				
OXYQUINOLINE SULFATE (Amend)				
POW, NA (C.P.)				
125 gm	17317-0396-04	22.40		
454 gm	17317-0396-01	67.20		
2270 gm	17317-0396-05	266.00		
(PCCA) *See HYDROXYQUINOLINE SULFATE*				
OXYTETRACYCLINE (PCCA)				
POW, NA (DIHYDRATE,USP)				
1 gm	51927-1508-00	24.00		
OXYTETRACYCLINE HCL (Gallipot)				
oxytetracycline hydrochloride				
POW, NA (U.S.P.)				
5 gm	51552-1069-02	11.20	8.00	
(Medisca)				
POW, NA (1X25GM,USP)				
25 gm	38779-0042-04	88.05		
(U.S.P.)				
100 gm	38779-0042-05	306.00		
(PCCA)				
POW, NA (U.S.P.)				
1 gm	51927-3258-00	3.60		
OXYTETRACYCLINE HYDROCHLORIDE				
(Gallipot) *See OXYTETRACYCLINE HCL*				
(Medisca) *See OXYTETRACYCLINE HCL*				
(PCCA) *See OXYTETRACYCLINE HCL*				
OXYTOCIN				
(APP) *See NOVAPLUS OXYTOCIN*				
(APP)				
SOL, IV (VIAL,P.C.,1MLX25)				
10 u/ml, 1 ml 25s	63323-0012-01	117.19		AP
(M.D.V.,10MLX25)				
10 u/ml, 10 ml 25s	63323-0012-10	1171.88		AP
(10X30ML,MDV)				
10 u/ml, 30 ml 10s	63323-0012-30	1406.25		AP
(Baxter)				
SOL, IJ (SDV,USP)				
10 u/ml, 1 ml	10019-0291-12	1.26		
(1MLX25,SDV,USP)				
10 u/ml, 1 ml 25s	10019-0291-02	31.50		
(MDV,USP)				
10 u/ml, 10 ml	10019-0291-71	12.54		
(10MLX25,MDV,USP)				
10 u/ml, 10 ml 25s	10019-0291-04	313.50		
(Gallipot)				
POW, NA, 0.01 gm	51552-0631-09	168.00	120.00	
(Hawkins)				
POW, NA, 0.01 gm	63370-0162-04	480.00		
(JHP) *See PITOCIN*				
(PCCA)				
POW, NA (USP)				
0.001 gm	51927-2843-00	53.70		
(Teva)				
SOL, IJ (25X1ML)				
10 u/ml, 1 ml 25s	00703-6271-04	36.00		AP
10 ml 10s	00703-6275-03	120.00		AP
(PD-Rx Pharm)				
REPACK				
SOL, IJ (10X1ML)				
10 u/ml, 1 ml 10s	43063-0029-01	105.75		AP
OXYTOCIN-LACTATED RINGERS (PharMEDium Services)				
lactated ringer's solution/oxytocin				
SOL, IV (USP,6X1000ML,VIAFLEX)				
20 u, 1000 ml 6s	61553-0769-04	33.00	27.50	
OXYTOCIN-SODIUM CHLORIDE (PharMEDium Services)				
oxytocin/sodium chloride				
SOL, IV (12X500ML, VIAFLEX BAG)				
10 u-0.9%,				
500 ml 12s	61553-0732-03	16.38	13.65	
OXYTOCIN/SODIUM CHLORIDE				
(PharMEDium Services) *See OXYTOCIN-SODIUM CHLORIDE*				
OXYTROL (Watson)				
oxybutynin				
TDM, TD, 3.9 mg/24 hr,				
8s ea	52544-0920-08	160.50		
(Phys Total Care)				
REPACK				
TDM, TD, 3.9 mg/24 hr,				
8s ea	54868-4834-00	101.90		
OYSTER SHELL CALCIUM (PCCA)				
calcium carbonate				
GRA, NA, 1 gm	51927-2445-00	0.04		
OZURDEX (Allergan Inc)				
dexamethasone				
IMP, IO (SINGLE-USE APPLICATOR)				
0.7 mg, ea	00023-3348-07	1554.00		
P CHLOR GG (Boca Pharmacal)				
cpm/gg/phenyleph hcl				
SOL, PO (PEACH)				
1 mg/ml-20 mg/ml-2 mg/ml,				
30 ml	64376-0707-30	5.95		
P-(AMINOMETHYL) BENZENESULFONAMIDE HYDROCHLORIDE (Spectrum Pharmacy)				
mafenide hydrochloride				
CRY, NA, 25 gm	49452-0421-01	344.75		
100 gm	49452-0421-02	927.50		
1000 gm	49452-0421-03	4882.50		
P-CHLOROPHENOL				
(PCCA) *See PARACHLOROPHENOL*				
P-D HISTINE D (PD-Rx Pharm)				
REPACK				
cough/cold combination				
CER, PO, 16 mg-50 mg-16 mg-16 mg,				
30s ea	55289-0960-30	16.01		
P-D NATAL W/FOLIC ACID (PD-Rx Pharm)				
prenatal vitamins				
TAB, PO, 100s ea	55289-0741-01	8.30		
P-DICHLOROBENZENE (Amend)				
dichlorobenzene				
CRY, NA, 2270 gm	17317-0400-05	28.00		
11350 gm	17317-0400-08	105.00		
P-DIMETHYLAMINOBENZALDEHYDE				
(PCCA) *See DIMETHYLAMINOBENZALDEHYDE-P*				
P-PHENOLSULFONIC ACID				
(Medisca) *See PHENOLSULFONIC ACID*				
(PCCA) *See PHENOLSULFONIC ACID*				
P.E.G. 1000 (Amend)				
polyethylene glycol				
POW, NA (N.F., F.C.C.)				
20430 gm	17317-0722-03	220.50		
SOL, NA, 454 gm	17317-0772-01	9.80		
(U.S.P./F.C.C.)				
4086 gm	17317-0772-06	56.00		
P.E.G. 1450 (Amend)				
polyethylene glycol				
SOL, NA (N.F., F.C.C.)				
454 gm	17317-0740-01	14.00		
4086 gm	17317-0740-06	56.00		
P.E.G. 1500 (Amend)				
polyethylene glycol				
SOL, NA (N.F., F.C.C.)				
454 gm	17317-0427-01	14.00		
(N.F./F.C.C.)				
20430 gm	17317-0427-08	220.50		
P.E.G. 200 (Amend)				
polyethylene glycol				
SOL, NA, 480 ml	17317-0769-01	14.00		
3840 ml	17317-0769-06	56.00		
22700 gm	17317-0769-03	245.00		
P.E.G. 300 (Amend)				
polyethylene glycol				
SOL, NA (N.F., F.C.C.)				
480 ml	17317-0770-01	14.00		
3840 ml	17317-0770-06	56.00		
22700 gm	17317-0770-03	245.00		
P.E.G. 3350 (Amend)				
polyethylene glycol				
FLA, NA (N.F., F.C.C.)				
454 gm	17317-0428-01	8.40		
2270 gm	17317-0428-05	35.00		
11350 gm	17317-0428-08	105.00		
P.E.G. 400 (Amend)				
polyethylene glycol				
SOL, NA (N.F., F.C.C.)				
480 ml	17317-0426-01	8.75		
3840 ml	17317-0426-06	49.00		
22700 gm	17317-0426-08	245.00		
P.E.G. 600 (Amend)				
polyethylene glycol				
SOL, NA (N.F., F.C.C.)				
480 ml	17317-0771-01	14.00		
3840 ml	17317-0771-06	56.00		
22700 gm	17317-0771-03	245.00		
P.E.G. 8000 (Amend)				
polyethylene glycol				
FLA, NA (N.F., F.C.C.)				
454 gm	17317-0741-01	8.75		
454 gm	17317-0741-05	35.00		
11350 gm	17317-0741-08	105.00		
POW, NA, 454 gm	17317-1936-01	12.60		
2270 gm	17317-1936-05	49.00		
11350 gm	17317-1936-08	113.75		
P.T.E.-4 (APP)				
chromium/copper/manganese/zinc				
SOL, IV (S.D.V.,PF)				
3 ml	63323-0082-03	4.79		
P.T.E.-5 (APP)				
chromium/copper/manganese/selenium/zinc				
SOL, IV (S.D.V.,PF)				
3 ml	63323-0144-03	5.25		
PACAPS (Lunsco)				
acetaminophen/butalbital/caffeine				
CAP, PO, 325 mg-50 mg-40 mg,				
100s ea	10892-0116-10	29.88		EE
PACERONE (Upsher-Smith)				
amiodarone hydrochloride				
TAB, PO, 100 mg, ea	00245-0144-89	7.06		AB
30s ea	00245-0144-30	222.89		AB
(10X10)				
100 mg, 100s ea UD	00245-0144-01	742.96		AB
200 mg, ea	00245-0147-89	3.53		AB
60s ea	00245-0147-60	197.93		AB
90s ea	00245-0147-90	290.96		AB
100s ea UD	00245-0147-01	353.08		AB
500s ea	00245-0147-15	1566.95		AB
(10X10)				
300 mg, 10s ea UD	00245-0140-01	706.17		
400 mg, ea	00245-0145-89	7.06		
30s ea	00245-0145-30	199.49		
100s ea UD	00245-0145-01	742.96		
PACLITAXEL (APP)				
SOL, IV (1X5ML,MDV,USP)				
6 mg/ml, 5 ml	63323-0763-05	15.52	12.93	
(1X16.7ML,MDV,USP)				
6 mg/ml, 16.7 ml	63323-0763-16	51.83	43.19	
(1X50ML,MDV,USP)				
6 mg/ml, 50 ml	63323-0763-50	155.16	129.30	
(Bedford) *See PACLITAXEL AMERINET CHOICE*				
(Bedford) *See PACLITAXEL NOVAPLUS*				
(Bedford)				
SOL, IV (M.D.V.)				
6 mg/ml, 5 ml	55390-0114-05	20.40		AP
16.7 ml	55390-0114-20	68.40		AP
50 ml	55390-0114-50	205.20		AP
(Hospira)				
SOL, IV (M.D.V.)				
6 mg/ml, 5 ml	61703-0342-09	10.20	8.93	AP
16.7 ml	61703-0342-22	34.31	30.02	AP
50 ml	61703-0342-50	144.00	126.00	AP
(Parenta Pharma)				
SOL, IV (USP,1X5ML,MULTI-DOSE)				
6 mg/ml, 5 ml	66758-0043-01	56.58		AP
(USP,1X16.7ML,MULTI-DOSE)				
6 mg/ml, 16.7 ml	66758-0043-02	188.94		AP
(USP,1X50ML,MULTI-DOSE)				
6 mg/ml, 50 ml	66758-0043-03	565.69		AP
(Teva) *See NOV-ONXOL*				
(Teva)				
SOL, IV (1X5ML,MULTIDOSE)				
6 mg/ml, 5 ml	00703-4764-01	17.70		AP
(1X16.7ML,MDV)				
6 mg/ml, 16.7 ml	00703-4766-01	49.88		AP

PROD/MFR	NDC	AWP	DP	OBC
(M.D.V,1X25ML)				
6 mg/ml, 25 ml	00703-4767-01	84.00		AP
(1X50ML,MDV)				
6 mg/ml, 50 ml	00703-4768-01	162.00		AP
PACLITAXEL AMERINET CHOICE (Bedford)				
paclitaxel				
SOL, IV (M.D.V.,PRIVATE LABEL)				
6 mg/ml, 5 ml	55390-0314-05	42.00		AP
16.7 ml	55390-0314-20	150.00		AP
50 ml	55390-0314-50	420.00		AP
PACLITAXEL NOVAPLUS (Bedford)				
paclitaxel				
SOL, IV (MDV,USP,PRIVATE LABEL)				
6 mg/ml, 5 ml	55390-0304-05	42.00		AP
16.7 ml	55390-0304-20	150.00		AP
(M.D.V.,USP)				
6 mg/ml, 50 ml	55390-0304-50	420.00		AP
PACLITAXEL PROTEIN-BOUND				
(Abraxis) *See ABRAXANE*				
PACNEX (Medimetriks)				
benzoyl peroxide				
SOA, TP (1X480GM)				
7%, 480 gm	43538-0110-16	119.47		
PADDOCK NYSTATIN (Paddock)				
nystatin				
POW, NA (U.S.P.,50 MILLION UNITS)				
ea	00574-0404-05	35.45		AA
(USP 150M UNITS)				
ea	00574-0404-15	91.05		AA
(USP 500M UNITS)				
ea	00574-0404-50	264.05		AA
PADIMATE O				
(PCCA) *See OCTYL DIMETHYL PABA*				
PALCAPS 10 (Breckenridge Pharm)				
amylase/lipase/protease				
ECC, PO, 33200 u-10000 u-37500 u,				
100s ea	51991-0410-01	72.00		
PALCAPS 20 (Breckenridge Pharm)				
amylase/lipase/protease				
ECC, PO, 66400 u-20000 u-75000 u,				
100s ea	51991-0411-01	155.75		
PALGIC (Pamlab)				
carbinoxamine maleate				
SOL, PO (ARTIFICIAL BUBBLE GUM)				
4 mg/5 ml, 480 ml	00525-6752-16	87.47		
TAB, PO, 4 mg, 100s ea	00525-6748-01	87.47		
(Phys Total Care)				
REPACK				
TAB, PO, 4 mg, 20s ea	54868-5149-01	15.43		
60s ea	54868-5149-00	42.54		
PALIFERMIN				
(Biovitrum) *See KEPIVANCE*				
PALIPERIDONE				
(Janssen) *See INVEGA*				
PALIPERIDONE PALMITATE				
(Janssen) *See INVEGA SUSTENNA*				
PALIVIZUMAB				
(Medimmune) *See SYNAGIS*				
PALLADIUM CHLORIDE (PCCA)				
POW, NA (II)				
1 gm	51927-3315-00	165.00		
PALM OIL (Medisca)				
OIL, NA (1X500ML)				
500 ml	38779-2140-08	87.00		
(PCCA)				
OIL, NA, 1 ml	51927-3141-00	0.18		
PALMAROSA OIL (PCCA)				
OIL, NA, 1 gm	51927-3556-00	1.35		
(Spectrum Pharmacy)				
OIL, NA (F.C.C.)				
125 ml	49452-4955-01	128.45		
PALMITIC ACID (Amend)				
SOL, NA, 454 gm	17317-0878-01	9.80		
2270 gm	17317-0878-05	25.20		
11350 gm	17317-0878-08	87.50		
(Spectrum Pharmacy)				
CRY, NA (1X500GM)				
500 gm	49452-4960-01	165.90		
PALONOSETRON HYDROCHLORIDE				
(Eisai) *See ALOXI*				
PAMABROM (PCCA)				
POW, NA, 1 gm	51927-1432-00	3.60		

PROD/MFR	NDC	AWP	DP	OBC
PAMELOR (Covidien)				
nortriptyline hydrochloride				
CAP, PO, 10 mg, 30s ea	00406-9910-03	721.20		AB
25 mg, 30s ea	00406-9911-03	721.20		AB
50 mg, 30s ea	00406-9912-03	721.20		AB
(USP)				
75 mg, 30s ea	00406-9913-03	721.20		AB
(Pharma Pac)				
REPACK				
CAP, PO, 25 mg, 30s ea	52959-0163-30	38.60		AB
(Phys Total Care)				
REPACK				
CAP, PO, 10 mg, 10s ea	54868-2833-01	26.86		AB
(Quality Care Prod)				
REPACK				
CAP, PO, 50 mg, 60s ea	35356-0369-60	1841.23		AB
PAMIDRONATE DISODIUM (Akorn)				
SOL, IV (4X10ML,SINGLE USE)				
3 mg/ml, 10 ml 4s	23360-0023-10	134.99		AP
(1X10ML,SINGLE USE)				
9 mg/ml, 10 ml	23360-0024-10	116.94		AP
(APP) *See PAMIDRONATE DISODIUM OTN*				
(APP)				
SOL, IV (S.D.V.)				
3 mg/ml, 10 ml	63323-0734-10	290.00		AP
9 mg/ml, 10 ml	63323-0735-10	872.00		AP
(Bedford) *See PAMIDRONATE DISODIUM NOVAPLUS*				
(Bedford)				
PDS, IV (VIAL)				
30 mg, ea	55390-0127-01	48.00		AP
90 mg, ea	55390-0129-01	144.00		AP
SOL, IV, 3 mg/ml, 10 ml	55390-0204-01	48.00		AP
(Hospira) *See NOVAPLUS PAMIDRONATE DISODIUM*				
(Hospira)				
SOL, IV (SDV)				
3 mg/ml, 10 ml	61703-0324-18	18.00	15.75	AP
10 ml 4s	61703-0324-39	137.23	120.08	AP
(PF)				
6 mg/ml, 10 ml	61703-0325-18	61.94	54.20	AP
9 mg/ml, 10 ml	61703-0326-18	84.42	73.87	AP
(SINGLE-USE VIAL)				
9 mg/ml, 10 ml	00703-4085-91	122.47	107.16	AP
(Novartis Pharm) *See AREDIA*				
(OTN) *See OTN PAMIDRONATE DISODIUM*				
(PharmaForce)				
SOL, IV (1X10ML,USP)				
3 mg/ml, 10 ml	40042-0019-10	39.60		AP
9 mg/ml, 10 ml	40042-0017-10	117.22		AP
(Sagent)				
SOL, IV (1X10ML,SINGLE-DOSE VIAL)				
3 mg/ml, 10 ml	25021-0802-10	24.00		AP
(1X10ML,SDV,PF)				
9 mg/ml, 10 ml	25021-0803-10	72.00		AP
(Sandoz)				
PDS, IV, 30 mg, 4s ea	00781-3147-84	447.78		
90 mg, ea	00781-3148-70	755.64		
(Teva)				
SOL, IV (S.D.V)				
3 mg/ml, 10 ml 4s	00703-4075-59	192.00		AP
9 mg/ml, 10 ml	00703-4085-51	192.00		AP
PAMIDRONATE DISODIUM NOVAPLUS (Bedford)				
pamidronate disodium				
PDS, IV, 30 mg, ea	55390-0157-01	48.00		AP
90 mg, ea	55390-0159-01	144.00		AP
SOL, IV (S.D.V.,FLIPTOP)				
3 mg/ml, 10 ml	55390-0604-01	48.00		AP
PAMIDRONATE DISODIUM OTN (APP)				
pamidronate disodium				
SOL, IV (S.D.V.,LATEX-FREE)				
3 mg/ml, 10 ml	63323-0734-35	290.00		AP
(S.D.V.,PRIVATE LABEL)				
9 mg/ml, 10 ml	63323-0735-35	872.00		AP
PAMINE (Kenwood)				
methscopolamine bromide				
TAB, PO, 2.5 mg, 100s ea	00482-0061-01	266.26		
PAMINE FORTE (Kenwood)				
methscopolamine bromide				
TAB, PO (DOSE PACK,LACTOSE-FREE)				
5 mg, 60s ea	00482-0062-06	234.05		
PAMINE FQ (Kenwood)				
lactobacillus combination				
KIT, PO (PF,GLUTEN-FREE)				
5 mg, ea	00482-0072-01	249.49		

PROD/MFR	NDC	AWP	DP	OBC
PANAFIL (Healthpoint)				
chlorophyllin copper complex/papain/urea				
SPR, TP, 0.5%-10%, 33 ml	00064-3510-33	88.00		
(Phys Total Care)				
REPACK				
OIN, TP, 0.5%-10%-10%,				
72 gm	54868-5598-00	317.59		
PANATUSS DXP (Seyer Pharmatec)				
dm/dexbrompheniramine maleate/gg/phenyleph hcl				
SOL, PO (AF,DYE-FREE,RASPBERRY)				
118 ml	11026-2675-04	12.00		
PANATUSS DXP PEDIATRIC (Seyer Pharmatec)				
dm/dexbrompheniramine maleate/gg/phenyleph hcl				
SOL, PO (DROPS,AF)				
60 ml	11026-2662-02	13.20		
PANCREASE (Phys Total Care)				
REPACK				
amylase/lipase/protease				
ECC, PO, 20000 u-4500 u-25000 u,				
100s ea	54868-1557-01	70.47		
PANCREASE MT 10 (Ortho-McNeil Pharm)				
amylase/lipase/protease				
ECC, PO (30,000U-10,000U-30,000U)				
30000 u-10000 u-30000 u,				
100s ea	00045-0342-60	130.66		
PANCREASE MT 16 (Ortho-McNeil Pharm)				
amylase/lipase/protease				
ECC, PO (48,000U-16,000U-48,000U)				
48000 u-16000 u-48000 u,				
100s ea	00045-0343-60	209.76		
PANCREASE MT 20 (Ortho-McNeil Pharm)				
amylase/lipase/protease				
ECC, PO (56,000U-20,000U-44,000U)				
56000 u-20000 u-44000 u,				
100s ea	00045-0346-60	261.24		
PANCREASE MT 4 (Ortho-McNeil Pharm)				
amylase/lipase/protease				
CAP, PO, 12000 u-4000 u-12000 u,				
100s ea	00045-0341-60	52.26		
PANCREATIN (Baker, J.T.)				
POW, NA (U.S.P.)				
500 gm	10106-2840-01	37.86		
(Medisca)				
POW, NA (U.S.P.)				
100 gm	38779-2142-05	28.50		
500 gm	38779-2142-08	76.50		
(PCCA)				
POW, NA (U.S.P. 8X)				
1 gm	51927-3532-00	3.24		
(USP)				
1 gm	51927-1556-00	0.45		
(Spectrum Pharmacy)				
POW, NA (U.S.P.)				
100 gm	49452-4970-01	67.90		
500 gm	49452-4970-02	155.40		
PANCRECARB MS-16 (Digestive Care Inc)				
amylase/lipase/protease				
ECC, PO (ENTERIC-COATED)				
52000 u-16000 u-52000 u,				
100s ea	59767-0003-01	307.50		
250s ea	59767-0003-02	768.75		
PANCRECARB MS-4 (Digestive Care Inc)				
amylase/lipase/protease				
ECC, PO (MICROSPHERES)				
25000 u-4000 u-25000 u,				
100s ea	59767-0002-01	90.90		
PANCRECARB MS-8 (Digestive Care Inc)				
amylase/lipase/protease				
ECC, PO, 40000 u-8000 u-45000 u,				
100s ea	59767-0001-01	164.60		
250s ea	59767-0001-02	411.50		
PANCRELIPASE (X-Gen)				
amylase/lipase/protease				
ECC, PO (ENTERICCOATEDMICROSPHER)				
20000 u-4500 u-25000 u,				
100s ea	39822-9045-01	63.53		
27000 u-5000 u-17000 u,				
100s ea	39822-0205-01	46.19		
(ENTERICCOATEDMICROSPHER)				
30000 u-10000 u-30000 u,				
100s ea	39822-9100-01	132.77		
48000 u-16000 u-48000 u,				
100s ea	39822-9160-01	194.70		
56000 u-20000 u-44000 u,				
100s ea	39822-9200-01	228.53		

PROD/MFR	NDC	AWP	DP	OBC
PANCRELIPASE 8000 (Contract Pharmacal)				
amylase/lipase/protease				
TAB, PO (FILM COATED)				
30000 u-8000 u-30000 u,				
100s ea	**10267-2737-01**	31.09		
PANCRELIPASE MT 16 (Contract Pharmacal)				
amylase/lipase/protease				
ECC, PO, 48000 u-16000 u-48000 u,				
100s ea	**10267-0506-01**	115.00		
PANCURONIUM BROMIDE (Hospira)				
SOL, IV (VIAL, FLIPTOP)				
1 mg/ml, 10 ml 25s	**00074-4646-01**	49.80	43.50	**AP**
10 ml 25s	**00409-4646-01**	48.00	42.00	**AP**
(Teva)				
SOL, IV (M.D.V.)				
1 mg/ml, 10 ml 10s	**00703-2804-03**	24.98		**AP**
(S.D.V.)				
2 mg/ml, 2 ml 25s	**00703-2812-04**	57.00		**AP**
(M.D.V.)				
2 mg/ml, 5 ml 25s	**00703-2823-04**	60.90		**AP**
PANDEL (PharmaDerm)				
hydrocortisone probutate				
CRE, TP, 0.1%, 15 gm	**00462-0153-15**	65.12		
45 gm	**00462-0153-46**	155.16		
80 gm	**00462-0153-80**	260.64		
PANGAMIC ACID SODIUM (PCCA)				
sodium pangamate				
POW, NA, 1 gm	**51927-2202-00**	10.20		
PANGESTYME EC (Phys Total Care)				
REPACK				
amylase/lipase/protease				
ECC, PO, 20000 u-4500 u-25000 u,				
100s ea	**54868-5737-00**	58.53		
PANGLOBULIN NF (Amer Red Cross-Blood)				
immune globulin				
PDS, IV (S.D.V.,PF,NANOFILTERED)				
6 gm, ea	**52769-0417-06**	606.00		
12 gm, ea	**52769-0418-12**	1212.00		
PANHEMATIN (Lundbeck)				
hemin				
PDS, IV, 313 mg, ea	**67386-0701-54**	3070.48		
PANITUMUMAB				
(Amgen USA Inc.) *See VECTIBIX*				
PANLOR SS (Pamlab)				
acetaminophen/caffeine/dihydrocodeine bitartrate				
TAB, PO, 712.8 mg-60 mg-32 mg,				
100s ea, C-III	**00525-0032-01**	187.96		
(DHS, Inc.)				
REPACK				
TAB, PO, 712.8 mg-60 mg-32 mg,				
60s ea, C-III	**55887-0456-60**	103.10		
(Phys Total Care)				
REPACK				
TAB, PO, 712.8 mg-60 mg-32 mg,				
30s ea, C-III	**54868-5594-00**	44.81		
(Quality Care Prod)				
REPACK				
TAB, PO, 712.8 mg-60 mg-32 mg,				
30s ea, C-III	**35356-0327-30**	121.30		
PANLOR-DC (Stat Rx)				
REPACK				
acetaminophen/caffeine/dihydrocodeine bitartrate				
CAP, PO, 356.4 mg-30 mg-16 mg,				
30s ea, C-III	**16590-0180-30**	60.00		
40s ea, C-III	**16590-0180-40**	80.00		
60s ea, C-III	**16590-0180-60**	120.00		
90s ea, C-III	**16590-0180-90**	180.00		
PANLOR-SS (Stat Rx)				
acetaminophen/caffeine/dihydrocodeine bitartrate				
TAB, PO, 712.8 mg-60 mg-32 mg,				
30s ea, C-III	**16590-0179-30**	62.00		
40s ea, C-III	**16590-0179-40**	82.66		
60s ea, C-III	**16590-0179-60**	124.00		
90s ea, C-III	**16590-0179-90**	186.00		
PANMIST DM (Phys Total Care)				
REPACK				
dm/gg/pse hcl				
SYR, PO (BERRY)				
473 ml	**54868-4204-00**	39.85		
PANOCAPS (Breckenridge Pharm)				
amylase/lipase/protease				
ECC, PO, 20000 u-4500 u-25000 u,				
100s ea	**51991-0406-01**	43.25		
PANOCAPS MT 16 (Breckenridge Pharm)				
amylase/lipase/protease				
ECC, PO, 48000 u-16000 u-48000 u,				
100s ea	**51991-0407-01**	131.10		
PANOCAPS MT 20 (Breckenridge Pharm)				
amylase/lipase/protease				
ECC, PO, 56000 u-20000 u-44000 u,				
100s ea	**51991-0408-01**	163.35		
PANOKASE (Breckenridge Pharm)				
amylase/lipase/protease				
TAB, PO, 30000 u-8000 u-30000 u,				
100s ea	**51991-0655-01**	34.50		
500s ea	**51991-0655-05**	149.95		
PANOKASE 16 (Breckenridge Pharm)				
amylase/lipase/protease				
TAB, PO, 60000 u-16000 u-60000 u,				
100s ea	**51991-0654-01**	65.80		
PANRETIN (Eisai)				
alitretinoin				
GEL, TP, 0.1%, 60 gm	**62856-0601-22**	2460.00		
PANTHENOL (Medisca)				
dexpanthenol				
POW, NA (1X10GM,USP)				
10 gm	**38779-1481-01**	24.00		
(U.S.P.)				
25 gm	**38779-1481-04**	46.50		
100 gm	**38779-1481-05**	90.00		
500 gm	**38779-1481-08**	315.00		
(1X1000GM,USP)				
1000 gm	**38779-1481-09**	525.00		
PANTHENOL				
(PCCA) *See PANTHENOL (DL)*				
PANTHENOL (DL) (PCCA)				
panthenol				
POW, NA (USP,1X1GM)				
1 gm	**51927-1711-00**	2.16		
PANTOPRAZOLE (IPI)				
REPACK				
pantoprazole sodium				
TAB, PO, 40 mg, 30s ea	**18837-0296-30**	122.74		
PANTOPRAZOLE SODIUM (Caraco)				
ECT, PO (DELAYED-RELEASE)				
20 mg, 90s ea	**41616-0144-81**	367.80		**AB**
40 mg, 90s ea	**62756-0580-81**	367.80		
(Teva)				
ECT, PO, 20 mg, 90s ea	**00093-0011-98**	368.22		**AB**
40 mg, 90s ea	**00093-0012-98**	368.22		**AB**
(Wyeth)				
ECT, PO, 20 mg, 90s ea	**00008-0606-01**	353.48	294.57	
40 mg, 90s ea	**00008-0607-01**	353.48	294.57	
(Wyeth) *See PROTONIX*				
(A-S Medication)				
REPACK				
ECT, PO, 40 mg, 30s ea	**54569-6062-00**	122.67		
(Aidarex)				
REPACK				
ECT, PO, 40 mg, 30s ea	**33261-0629-30**	450.00		**AB**
60s ea	**33261-0629-60**	900.00		**AB**
90s ea	**33261-0629-90**	1350.00		**AB**
120s ea	**33261-0629-02**	1800.00		**AB**
(Dispensing Solutions)				
REPACK				
ECT, PO, 40 mg, 30s ea	**66336-0405-30**	141.15		**AB**
(Nucare Pharm)				
REPACK				
ECT, PO, 40 mg, 30s ea	**68071-0782-30**	247.20		**AB**
(Phys Total Care)				
REPACK				
ECT, PO, 20 mg, 30s ea	**54868-6038-00**	285.35		
40 mg, 30s ea	**54868-5846-00**	294.78		
60s ea	**54868-5846-02**	535.50		**AB**
90s ea	**54868-5846-01**	873.84		
(Physician Partner)				
REPACK				
ECT, PO, 40 mg, 30s ea	**21695-0771-30**	245.20		
(Stat Rx)				
REPACK				
ECT, PO, 20 mg, 30s ea	**16590-0635-30**	167.69		
40 mg, 28s ea	**16590-0599-28**	156.97		
30s ea	**16590-0599-30**	168.17		
60s ea	**16590-0599-60**	333.63		
90s ea	**16590-0599-90**	459.60		
PAPACON (Consolidated Midland)				
papaverine hydrochloride				
CER, PO, 150 mg, 60s ea	**00223-1358-60**	4.25		
100s ea	**00223-1358-01**	6.75		
1000s ea	**00223-1358-03**	49.50		
PAPAIN (Amend)				
POW, NA (PURIFIED)				
125 gm	**17317-0702-04**	16.10		
454 gm	**17317-0702-01**	49.00		
2270 gm	**17317-0702-05**	203.00		
(Gallipot)				
POW, NA (PURIFIED)				
100 gm	**51552-0584-05**	27.30		
(PCCA)				
POW, NA (PURIFIED)				
1 gm	**51927-1221-00**	1.44		
(U.S.P.)				
1 gm	**51927-3625-00**	1.44		
(Spectrum Pharmacy)				
POW, NA (1X100GM)				
100 gm	**49452-4995-02**	140.70		
(1X454GM)				
454 gm	**49452-4995-03**	392.00		
PAPAIN/UREA				
(Allan Pharmaceutical) *See ALLANZYME*				
(Allan Pharmaceutical) *See ALLANZYME 650 OINTMENT*				
(Ethex) *See ETHEZYME 650*				
(Healthpoint) *See ACCUZYME*				
(Stratus) *See KOVIA*				
PAPAVERINE HYDROCHLORIDE (Amend)				
POW, NA (U.S.P.)				
100 gm	**17317-0398-04**	70.00		
500 gm	**17317-0398-01**	273.00		
(Amer Regent)				
SOL, IJ (S.D.V.)				
30 mg/ml, 2 ml 25s	**00517-4002-25**	93.75		
(M.D.V.)				
30 mg/ml, 10 ml	**00517-4010-01**	6.25		
(Consolidated Midland) *See PAPACON*				
(Gallipot)				
POW, NA (U.S.P.)				
5 gm	**51552-0416-02**	14.35		
25 gm	**51552-0416-04**	29.40		
100 gm	**51552-0416-05**	103.60		
1000 gm	**51552-0416-07**	828.80		
(Hawkins)				
POW, NA (U.S.P.)				
5 gm	**63370-0165-15**	41.00		
25 gm	**63370-0165-25**	84.00		
100 gm	**63370-0165-35**	296.00		
(Medisca)				
POW, NA (U.S.P.)				
5 gm	**38779-0454-03**	36.00		
25 gm	**38779-0454-04**	76.50		
100 gm	**38779-0454-05**	267.00		
(1X500GM,USP)				
500 gm	**38779-0454-08**	1185.00		
(1X1000GM,USP)				
1000 gm	**38779-0454-09**	2025.00		
(Parenta Pharma)				
SOL, IJ (USP,S.D.V.)				
30 mg/ml, 2 ml	**66758-0014-01**	3.36	2.80	
2 ml 10s	**66758-0014-02**	33.60	28.00	
(USP, W/CHLOROBUTANOL)				
30 mg/ml, 10 ml	**66758-0015-01**	16.20	13.50	
(PCCA)				
POW, NA (U.S.P.)				
1 gm	**51927-1775-00**	8.40		
(Sandoz)				
CER, PO, 150 mg, 100s ea	**00185-5156-01**	186.37		
1000s ea	**00185-5156-10**	1863.73		
(Spectrum Pharmacy)				
POW, NA (U.S.P.)				
5 gm	**49452-5000-01**	67.90		
25 gm	**49452-5000-02**	124.95		
100 gm	**49452-5000-03**	434.00		
(Truxton) *See PAVACOT*				
(B&B Pharm, Inc)				
REPACK				
POW, NA (U.S.P.)				
5 gm	**63275-9990-02**	27.00		
25 gm	**63275-9990-04**	68.00		
100 gm	**63275-9990-05**	230.00		

PROD/MFR | NDC | AWP | DP | OBC

(Phys Total Care)
REPACK
CER, PO (USP)
150 mg, 60s ea 54868-3663-02 22.35
100s ea 54868-3663-01 32.76

PARA-AMINOBENZOIC ACID (Gallipot)
aminobenzoic acid
POW, NA (U.S.P.,N.F.)
113.4 gm 51552-0097-04 16.66
454 gm 51552-0097-06 41.30

(Medisca)
POW, NA (U.S.P.)
100 gm 38779-0087-05 28.50
500 gm 38779-0087-08 87.00
1000 gm 38779-0087-09 153.00
2500 gm 38779-0087-01 337.50

(PCCA)
POW, NA (USP)
1 gm 51927-1040-00 0.42

(Spectrum Pharmacy)
POW, NA (U.S.P.)
100 gm 49452-0410-01 64.75
500 gm 49452-0410-02 155.05
2500 gm 49452-0410-03 584.50

PARA-FORMALDEHYDE (Spectrum Pharmacy)
paraformaldehyde
POW, NA (PURIFIED)
500 gm 49452-5010-01 89.25
2500 gm 49452-5010-02 246.05
12000 gm 49452-5010-03 861.00

PARACENTESIS TRAY (Covidien)
lidocaine hydrochloride
KIT, IJ (8FR 2.7MM X 4.75")
1%, 5s ea 08888-5680-06 341.74

PARACHLOROPHENOL (PCCA)
p-chlorophenol
CRY, NA (1X1GM)
1 gm 51927-1366-00 2.16

PARADIGM 515 (Medtronic Minimed)
infusion pump, insulin
DEV, NA (BLUE W/LINK)
ea 76300-0515-12 7743.75 6195.00
(CLEAR W/LINK)
ea 76300-0515-11 7743.75 6195.00
(PURPLE W/LINK)
ea 76300-0515-14 7743.75 6195.00
(SMOKE W/LINK)
ea 76300-0515-13 7743.75 6195.00

PARADIGM 522 (Medtronic Minimed)
infusion pump, insulin
DEV, NA (BLUE W/LINK)
ea 76300-0522-12 7805.70
(CLEAR W/LINK)
ea 76300-0522-11 7805.70
(PINK W/LINK)
ea 76300-0522-19 7805.70
ea 76300-0522-20 7805.70
(PURPLE W/LINK)
ea 76300-0522-14 7805.70
(SMOKE W/LINK)
ea 76300-0522-13 7805.70

PARADIGM 712 (Medtronic Minimed)
infusion pump, insulin
DEV, NA (4 YEAR WARRANTY)
ea 76300-0712-11 7493.75 5995.00
ea 76300-0712-12 7493.75 5995.00
ea 76300-0712-13 7493.75 5995.00
ea 76300-0712-14 7493.75 5995.00

PARADIGM 715 (Medtronic Minimed)
infusion pump, insulin
DEV, NA (BLUE W/LINK)
ea 76300-0715-12 7743.75 6195.00
(CLEAR W/LINK)
ea 76300-0715-11 7743.75 6195.00
(PURPLE W/LINK)
ea 76300-0715-14 7743.75 6195.00
(SMOKE W/LINK)
ea 76300-0715-13 7743.75 6195.00

PARADIGM 722 (Medtronic Minimed)
infusion pump, insulin
DEV, NA (BLUE W/LINK)
ea 76300-0722-12 7805.70
(CLEAR W/LINK)
ea 76300-0722-11 7805.70
(PINK W/LINK)
ea 76300-0722-19 7805.70
ea 76300-0722-20 7805.70
(PURPLE W/LINK)
ea 76300-0722-14 7805.70
(SMOKE W/LINK)
ea 76300-0722-13 7805.70

PARADIGM INSULIN INFUSION PUMP (Medtronic Minimed)
pump, infusion
DEV, NA (BLUE)
ea 76300-0511-12 6868.75 5495.00
(CHARCOAL)
ea 76300-0511-13 6868.75 5495.00
(CLEAR)
ea 76300-0511-11 6868.75 5495.00

PARADIGM INSULIN PUMP PATHWAY PROGRAM (Medtronic Minimed)
infusion pump, insulin
DEV, NA (511 TO 522)
ea 76300-0122-01 998.75 799.00
(512 TO 522)
ea 76300-0222-01 498.75 399.00
(515 TO 522)
ea 76300-0522-01 373.75 299.00

PARADIGM POLYFIN QR WITH WINGS (Medtronic Minimed)
infusion pump, parenteral
DEV, NA (24")
20s ea 76300-0312-21 182.50 146.00
(42")
20s ea 76300-0312-22 182.50 146.00

PARADIGM QUICK-SET INFUSION (Medtronic Minimed)
kit, administration, intravenous
DEV, NA (23" TUBING,6MM CATHETER)
ea 76300-0399-10 146.16
(23" TUBING,9MM CATHETER)
ea 76300-0397-10 146.16
(43" TUBING,6MM CATHETER)
ea 76300-0398-10 146.16
(43" TUBING,9MM CATHETER)
ea 76300-0396-10 146.16

PARADIGM REAL-TIME TRANSMITTER (Medtronic Minimed)
device
DEV, NA, ea 76300-0701-01 1248.75 999.00

PARADIGM RESERVOIR (Medtronic Minimed)
infusion pump, parenteral
DEV, NA, 10s ea 76300-0326-10 41.58
10s ea 76300-0332-10 41.58

PARADIGM SURE-T INFUSION SET (Medtronic Minimed)
infusion pump, insulin
DEV, NA (23")
10s ea 76300-0840-10 93.24

PARAFFIN (PCCA)
paraffin wax
WAX, NA (N.F.)
1 gm 51927-3087-00 0.10

(Spectrum Pharmacy)
WAX, NA (N.F.)
500 gm 49452-5005-01 78.75

PARAFFIN WAX
(Amend) *See ARISTOWAX 143*
(Amend) *See ARISTOWAX 165*
(Lorann Oil) *See PARRAFIN*
(PCCA) *See PARAFFIN*
(Spectrum Pharmacy) *See PARAFFIN*

PARAFON FORTE DSC (Ortho-McNeil Pharm)
chlorzoxazone
TAB, PO (CAPLET)
500 mg, 100s ea .... 00045-0325-60 264.86 220.72 AA

(PD-Rx Pharm)
REPACK
TAB, PO (CAPLET)
500 mg, 24s ea ..... 55289-0888-24 76.98 AA

(Phys Total Care)
REPACK
TAB, PO (CAPLET)
500 mg, 100s ea .... 54868-1017-00 209.70 AA

PARAFORMALDEHYDE (Amend)
POW, NA, 454 gm 17317-0586-01 10.50
2270 gm 17317-0586-05 29.40
11350 gm 17317-0586-08 105.00

(PCCA)
POW, NA (95-97%)
1 gm 51927-1149-00 0.13

(Spectrum Pharmacy) *See PARA-FORMALDEHYDE*

PARAGARD T380A (FEI Products LLC)
intrauterine device, contraceptive & introducer
DEV, NA (COPPER IUD)
ea 50907-0380-06 475.00
5s ea 50907-0380-07 2158.00

(Teva)
DEV, NA, ea 51285-0204-01 494.00
5s ea 51285-0204-02 2244.32

PARALDEHYDE (PCCA)
POW, NA, 1 gm, C-IV 51927-3537-00 0.80

PARCAINE (Ocusoft)
proparacaine hydrochloride
SOL, OP, 0.5%, 15 ml ..... 54799-0500-12 11.18 AT

PARCOPA (Azur Pharma, Inc.)
carbidopa/levodopa
ODT, PO (MINT)
10 mg-100 mg,
100s ea 00091-3341-01 194.60
25 mg-100 mg,
100s ea 00091-3342-01 219.74
25 mg-250 mg,
100s ea 00091-3343-01 279.98

PAREGORIC (Actavis Mid Atlantic)
LIQ, PO, 2 mg/5 ml,
473 ml, C-III 00472-0802-16 142.86

(Hi-Tech)
LIQ, PO (USP)
2 mg/5 ml,
473 ml, C-III 50383-0855-16 142.86

(Phys Total Care)
REPACK
LIQ, PO (ANISE)
2 mg/5 ml,
473 ml, C-III 54868-5063-00 220.65

PAREMYD (Akorn)
hydroxyamphetamine hydrobromide/tropicamide
SOL, OP, 1%-0.25%, 15 ml 17478-0704-12 19.20

PARI BABY (Pari)
mask, face
DEV, NA (FITS LC-PLUS NEB,SIZE 1)
ea 83490-0440-03 15.53
(FITS LC-PLUS NEB,SIZE 2)
ea 83490-0440-04 15.53
(FITS LC-PLUS NEB,SIZE 3)
ea 83490-0440-06 15.53

PARI LC SPRINT REUSABLE NEBULIZER SET (Pari)
nebulizer, direct patient interface
DEV, NA, ea 83490-0230-01 23.94
12s ea 83490-0230-02 287.28
50s ea 83490-0230-03 1197.00

PARI LC-PLUS REUSABLE NEBULIZER SET (Pari)
nebulizer, direct patient interface
DEV, NA (W/TUBING,REUSABLE 6 MO.)
ea 83490-0220-28 17.94

PARI TREK S COMBO PACK (Pari)
device, inhalation
DEV, NA, ea 83490-0470-05 370.80

PARI TREK S COMPACT COMPRESSOR (Pari)
device, inhalation
DEV, NA, ea 83490-0470-03 288.00

PARI TREK S PORT POWER KIT (Pari)
device
DEV, NA, ea 83490-0470-04 264.00

PARI TREK S W/ DC ADAPTOR (Pari)
device, inhalation
DEV, NA, ea 83490-0470-06 336.00

PARICALCITOL
(Abbott Pharm) *See ZEMPLAR*

PARLODEL (Novartis Pharm)
bromocriptine mesylate
CAP, PO, 5 mg, 30s ea 00078-0102-15 266.77
100s ea 00078-0102-05 842.41
TAB, PO, 2.5 mg, 30s ea... 00078-0017-15 166.07 AB
100s ea .... 00078-0017-05 552.04 AB

(Southwood)
REPACK
TAB, PO, 2.5 mg, 30s ea... 58016-0921-30 54.98 AB

PARLODION (Mallinckrodt Lab)
pyroxylin
POW, NA (PURIFIED)
125 gm 00406-6552-01 300.41
500 gm 00406-6552-12 1176.18

PROD/MFR	NDC	AWP	DP	OBC
PARNATE (Glaxo)				
tranylcypromine sulfate				
TAB, PO, 10 mg, 100s ea	00007-4471-20	160.70		
PAROMOMYCIN SULFATE (Caraco)				
CAP, PO, 250 mg, 100s ea	57664-0175-08	272.90		AA
(Heritage)				
CAP, PO (USP)				
250 mg, 100s ea	23155-0038-01	567.00		AA
(A-S Medication)				
REPACK				
CAP, PO, 250 mg, 60s ea	54569-5611-00	163.74		AA
PAROXETINE (Aurobindo Pharma)				
paroxetine hydrochloride				
TAB, PO (FILM-COATED)				
10 mg, 30s ea	65862-0154-30	78.55		AB
20 mg, 30s ea	13107-0155-30	79.30		AB
30s ea	65862-0155-30	79.30		AB
500s ea	13107-0155-05	1321.40		AB
500s ea	65862-0155-05	1321.40		AB
1000s ea	13107-0155-99	3643.00		AB
1000s ea	65862-0155-99	2643.00		AB
30 mg, 30s ea	65862-0156-30	84.43		AB
(USP,FILM-COATED)				
30 mg, 1000s ea	65862-0156-99	2814.33		AB
(FILM-COATED)				
40 mg, 30s ea	65862-0157-30	89.19		AB
(USP,FILM-COATED)				
40 mg, 1000s ea	65862-0157-99	2973.00		AB
(Caraco)				
TAB, PO (USP,FILM-COATED)				
10 mg, 30s ea	57664-0421-83	78.50		AB
90s ea	57664-0421-99	235.50		AB
500s ea	57664-0421-13	1308.33		AB
20 mg, 30s ea	57664-0422-83	79.95		AB
90s ea	57664-0422-99	239.85		AB
500s ea	57664-0422-13	1332.50		AB
1000s ea	57664-0422-18	2665.00		AB
30 mg, 30s ea	57664-0424-83	82.50		AB
90s ea	57664-0424-99	247.50		AB
500s ea	57664-0424-13	1375.00		AB
40 mg, 30s ea	57664-0425-83	86.25		AB
90s ea	57664-0425-99	258.75		AB
500s ea	57664-0425-13	1437.50		AB
(Greenstone)				
TAB, PO (FILM-COATED)				
10 mg, 30s ea	59762-1808-01	78.55		
500s ea	59762-1808-02	1309.17		
1000s ea	59762-1808-03	2618.33		
20 mg, 30s ea	59762-1810-01	79.30		
100s ea	59762-1810-02	264.33		
500s ea	59762-1810-03	1321.40		
1000s ea	59762-1810-04	2643.00		
30 mg, 30s ea	59762-1812-01	84.43		
500s ea	59762-1812-02	1407.17		
1000s ea	59762-1812-03	2814.33		
40 mg, 30s ea	59762-1815-01	89.19		
500s ea	59762-1815-02	1486.50		
1000s ea	59762-1815-03	2973.00		
(Mylan)				
TAB, PO (USP,FILM-COATED)				
10 mg, 30s ea	00378-7001-93	78.56		AB
1000s ea	00378-7001-10	2618.67		AB
20 mg, 30s ea	00378-7002-93	81.99		AB
1000s ea	00378-7002-10	2733.00		AB
30 mg, 30s ea	00378-7003-93	84.45		AB
1000s ea	00378-7003-10	2815.00		AB
40 mg, 30s ea	00378-7004-93	89.21		AB
1000s ea	00378-7004-10	2973.67		AB
(Zydus Pharm.)				
TAB, PO (USP,FILM-COATED)				
10 mg, 30s ea	68382-0097-06	78.56		AB
90s ea	68382-0097-16	235.00		AB
500s ea	68382-0097-05	1309.00		AB
1000s ea	68382-0097-10	1218.00		AB
20 mg, 30s ea	68382-0098-06	81.99		AB
90s ea	68382-0098-16	245.97		AB
(FILM-COATED)				
20 mg, 100s ea	68382-0098-01	273.30		AB
(USP,FILM-COATED)				
20 mg, 500s ea	68382-0098-05	1366.50		AB
(FILM-COATED)				
20 mg, 1000s ea	68382-0098-10	2733.00		AB
(USP,FILM-COATED)				
30 mg, 30s ea	68382-0099-06	84.44		AB
90s ea	68382-0099-16	253.30		AB
500s ea	68382-0099-05	1407.50		AB
1000s ea	68382-0099-10	2815.00		AB
40 mg, 30s ea	68382-0001-06	86.28		AB
90s ea	68382-0001-16	258.84		AB
500s ea	68382-0001-05	1486.50		AB

PROD/MFR	NDC	AWP	DP	OBC
(Aidarex)				
REPACK				
TAB, PO, 20 mg, 10s ea	33261-0090-10	27.40		
10s ea	33261-0091-10	28.00		
14s ea	33261-0090-14	38.36		
14s ea	33261-0091-14	39.20		
20s ea	33261-0090-20	54.80		
21s ea	33261-0091-21	58.80		
28s ea	33261-0090-28	76.72		
28s ea	33261-0091-28	78.40		
30s ea	33261-0090-30	82.30		
30s ea	33261-0091-30	84.00		
40s ea	33261-0091-40	112.00		
60s ea	33261-0090-60	164.40		
60s ea	33261-0091-60	168.00		
90s ea	33261-0090-90	246.60		
90s ea	33261-0091-90	252.00		
(FILM-COATED)				
40 mg, 7s ea	33261-0093-07	21.00		AB
14s ea	33261-0093-14	42.00		AB
20s ea	33261-0093-20	60.00		AB
21s ea	33261-0093-21	63.00		AB
28s ea	33261-0093-28	84.00		AB
30s ea	33261-0093-30	90.00		AB
40s ea	33261-0093-40	120.00		AB
60s ea	33261-0093-60	180.00		AB
(Bryant Ranch)				
REPACK				
TAB, PO, 20 mg, 30s ea	63629-1840-01	102.00		
(Core)				
REPACK				
TAB, PO, 20 mg, 30s ea	33358-0283-30	109.25		
60s ea	33358-0283-60	218.50		
90s ea	33358-0283-90	327.75		
(Dispensing Solutions)				
REPACK				
TAB, PO, 10 mg, 30s ea	55045-3171-08	75.90		
(IPI)				
REPACK				
TAB, PO, 40 mg, 30s ea	18837-0278-30	111.51		
(PD-Rx Pharm)				
REPACK				
TAB, PO (FILM-COATED)				
20 mg, 30s ea	55289-0972-30	17.31		AB
60s ea	55289-0972-60	23.69		
(Pharma Pac)				
REPACK				
TAB, PO, 10 mg, 30s ea	52959-0775-30	82.46		
60s ea	52959-0775-60	164.90		
(Physician Partner)				
REPACK				
TAB, PO, 10 mg, 30s ea	21695-0101-30	157.12		
60s ea	21695-0101-60	314.24		
90s ea	21695-0101-90	471.36		
20 mg, 30s ea	21695-0102-30	163.98		
60s ea	21695-0102-60	317.15		
90s ea	21695-0102-90	491.94		
30 mg, 30s ea	21695-0103-30	163.34		
90s ea	21695-0103-90	506.70		
40 mg, 30s ea	21695-0104-30	178.42		
90s ea	21695-0104-90	535.26		
(Quality Care Prod)				
REPACK				
TAB, PO, 20 mg, 100s ea	49999-0632-00	399.97		
(Southwood)				
REPACK				
TAB, PO, 30 mg, 30s ea	58016-0749-30	84.45		
60s ea	58016-0749-60	168.90		
90s ea	58016-0749-90	253.35		
100s ea	58016-0749-00	281.50		
120s ea	58016-0749-02	337.80		
(Stat Rx)				
REPACK				
TAB, PO, 10 mg, 30s ea	16590-0322-30	55.00		
56s ea	16590-0322-56	102.66		
60s ea	16590-0322-60	110.00		
90s ea	16590-0322-90	165.00		
120s ea	16590-0322-72	220.00		
20 mg, 30s ea	16590-0181-30	120.00		
60s ea	16590-0181-60	240.00		
30 mg, 5s ea	16590-0512-06	13.66		
30s ea	16590-0512-30	82.00		
60s ea	16590-0512-60	120.00		
90s ea	16590-0512-90	160.00		
120s ea	16590-0512-72	180.00		
40 mg, 30s ea	16590-0513-30	150.50		
56s ea	16590-0513-56	280.94		
60s ea	16590-0513-60	301.00		
90s ea	16590-0513-90	400.00		
120s ea	16590-0513-72	533.33		

PROD/MFR	NDC	AWP	DP	OBC
PAROXETINE HCL (Apotex Corp.)				
paroxetine hydrochloride				
TAB, PO (FILM COATED)				
10 mg, 30s ea	60505-0097-01	78.56		AB
100s ea	60505-0097-02	261.80		AB
1000s ea	60505-0097-04	2618.67		AB
20 mg, 30s ea	60505-0083-01	81.99		AB
100s ea	60505-0083-02	273.30		AB
1000s ea	60505-0083-04	2733.00		AB
(USP,FILM COATED)				
20 mg, 12500s ea	60505-0083-00	34162.50		AB
(FILM COATED)				
30 mg, 30s ea	60505-0084-01	84.45		AB
100s ea	60505-0084-02	281.50		AB
1000s ea	60505-0084-04	2815.00		AB
40 mg, 30s ea	60505-0101-01	89.21		AB
100s ea	60505-0101-02	297.30		AB
1000s ea	60505-0101-04	2973.67		AB
(USP,FILM COATED)				
40 mg, 7000s ea	60505-0101-07	20815.69		AB
(Major)				
TAB, PO (FILM COATED)				
10 mg, 100s ea	00904-5676-61	281.44		AB
20 mg, 100s ea	00904-5677-61	293.66		AB
30 mg, 100s ea	00904-5678-61	272.90		AB
40 mg, 100s ea	00904-5679-61	288.25		AB
(Teva)				
TAB, PO (FILM-COATED)				
10 mg, 90s ea	00093-7114-98	227.97		AB
20 mg, 90s ea	00093-7115-98	237.84		AB
30 mg, 90s ea	00093-7116-98	245.01		AB
40 mg, 90s ea	00093-7121-98	258.84		AB
(UDL)				
TAB, PO (10X10,FILM-COATED)				
20 mg, 100s ea UD	51079-0774-20	272.70		AB
(A-S Medication)				
REPACK				
TAB, PO, 20 mg, 30s ea	54569-5541-00	81.99		
(FILM-COATED)				
20 mg, 60s ea	54569-5541-01	163.98		AB
40 mg, 30s ea	54569-5682-00	89.21		AB
(Altura)				
REPACK				
TAB, PO (FILM-COATED)				
10 mg, 60s ea	63874-1125-06	173.97		
(FILM COATED)				
20 mg, 10s ea	63874-0538-10	29.24		AB
14s ea	63874-0538-14	40.94		AB
15s ea	63874-0538-15	43.86		AB
20s ea	63874-0538-20	58.49		AB
30s ea	63874-0538-30	99.67		AB
60s ea	63874-0538-60	145.78		AB
100s ea	63874-0538-01	292.43		AB
30 mg, 30s ea	63874-1151-03	129.99		AB
(American Health)				
REPACK				
TAB, PO (10X10,FILM COATED)				
10 mg, 100s ea UD	68084-0044-01	267.21		AB
(15X30,FILM COATED)				
10 mg, 450s ea	68084-0044-85	1202.45		AB
(10X10,FILM COATED)				
20 mg, 100s ea UD	68084-0045-01	278.88		AB
(15X30,FILM COATED)				
20 mg, 450s ea	68084-0045-85	1254.95		AB
(10X10,FILM COATED)				
30 mg, 100s ea UD	68084-0046-01	287.24		AB
(15X30,FILM COATED)				
30 mg, 450s ea	68084-0046-85	1292.60		AB
(10X10,FILM COATED)				
40 mg, 100s ea UD	68084-0047-01	303.44		AB
(15X30,FILM COATED)				
40 mg, 450s ea	68084-0047-85	1365.46		AB
(DHS, Inc.)				
REPACK				
TAB, PO, 20 mg, 30s ea	55887-0394-30	78.05		
60s ea	55887-0394-60	156.09		
90s ea	55887-0394-90	229.00		
(FILM COATED)				
40 mg, 30s ea	55887-0346-30	107.50		AB
(Dispensing Solutions)				
REPACK				
TAB, PO (FILM COATED)				
10 mg, 30s ea	68258-7007-03	86.42		AB
(FILM-COATED)				
20 mg, 30s ea	55045-3172-08	82.50		AB
(FILM COATED)				
20 mg, 60s ea	55045-3172-09	165.00		AB
(FILM-COATED)				
20 mg, 60s ea	66336-0799-60	191.24		AB
(FILM COATED)				
30 mg, 30s ea	68258-7008-03	92.87		AB

PROD/MFR	NDC	AWP	DP	OBC
(GSMS)				
REPACK				
TAB, PO (FILM COATED)				
10 mg, 30s ea	60429-0734-30	10.50	3.50	AB
90s ea	60429-0734-90	27.60	9.20	AB
500s ea	60429-0734-05	151.35	50.45	AB
20 mg, 30s ea	60429-0735-30	16.05	5.35	AB
90s ea	60429-0735-90	52.05	17.35	AB
100s ea	60429-0735-01	63.45	21.15	AB
500s ea	60429-0735-05	298.35	99.45	AB
30 mg, 30s ea	60429-0736-30	15.00	5.00	AB
90s ea	60429-0736-90	44.10	14.70	AB
500s ea	60429-0736-05	237.45	79.15	AB
40 mg, 30s ea	60429-0737-30	22.80	7.60	AB
90s ea	60429-0737-90	58.80	19.60	AB
500s ea	60429-0737-05	325.05	108.35	AB
(IPI)				
REPACK				
TAB, PO (FILM-COATED)				
10 mg, 30s ea	18837-0306-30	98.20		AB
(FILM COATED)				
20 mg, 30s ea	18837-0222-30	81.90		AB
(Medsource)				
REPACK				
TAB, PO, 10 mg, 30s ea	45865-0442-30	90.00		
60s ea	45865-0442-60	180.00		
90s ea	45865-0442-90	270.00		
100s ea	45865-0442-00	300.00		
20 mg, 30s ea	45865-0463-30	97.50		
60s ea	45865-0463-60	195.00		
90s ea	45865-0463-90	292.50		
100s ea	45865-0463-00	325.00		
(Nucare Pharm)				
REPACK				
TAB, PO (FILM COATED)				
20 mg, 30s ea	66267-0721-30	107.61		AB
40 mg, 30s ea	68071-0034-30	117.09		AB
(PD-Rx Pharm)				
REPACK				
TAB, PO (FILM-COATED)				
10 mg, 90s ea	55289-0037-90	30.53		AB
(REDI-SCRIPT)				
20 mg, 15s ea	58864-0741-15	44.92		
30s ea	58864-0741-30	84.82		
(FILM-COATED)				
20 mg, 90s ea	55289-0972-90	30.06		AB
(REDI-SCRIPT)				
40 mg, 15s ea	58864-0716-15	55.00		
30s ea	58864-0716-30	90.00		
(FILM-COATED)				
40 mg, 45s ea	55289-0053-45	23.05		AB
90s ea	55289-0053-90	35.12		AB
(Phys Total Care)				
REPACK				
TAB, PO, 10 mg, 30s ea	54868-5080-00	55.11		
20 mg, 30s ea	54868-4937-00	49.95		
90s ea	54868-4937-01	132.51		
(FILM-COATED)				
20 mg, 100s ea	54868-4937-04	54.67		AB
30 mg, 30s ea	54868-4938-00	58.35		
40 mg, 30s ea	54868-4817-00	67.23		
(FILM COATED)				
40 mg, 90s ea	54868-4817-02	67.19		AB
(Physician Partner)				
REPACK				
TAB, PO (FILM-COATED)				
20 mg, 90s ea	21695-0465-90	491.94		AB
(FILM COATED)				
40 mg, 60s ea	21695-0104-60	356.84		AB
(Quality Care Prod)				
REPACK				
TAB, PO, 10 mg, 30s ea	49999-0631-30	104.39		
60s ea	49999-0631-60	208.78		
(FILM-COATED)				
20 mg, 30s ea	49999-0632-30	119.99		AB
60s ea	49999-0632-60	239.98		AB
30 mg, 30s ea	49999-0613-30	100.00		
(Southwood)				
REPACK				
TAB, PO (FILM COATED)				
10 mg, 30s ea	58016-0817-30	76.17		AB
60s ea	58016-0817-60	152.34		AB
90s ea	58016-0817-90	228.51		AB
100s ea	58016-0817-00	253.90		AB
120s ea	58016-0817-02	304.68		AB
150s ea	58016-0817-03	380.85		AB
20 mg, 30s ea	58016-0818-30	76.28		AB

PROD/MFR	NDC	AWP	DP	OBC
60s ea	58016-0818-60	152.56		AB
90s ea	58016-0818-90	228.84		AB
100s ea	58016-0818-00	254.27		AB
120s ea	58016-0818-02	305.12		AB
150s ea	58016-0818-03	381.40		AB
(FILM-COATED)				
20 mg, 180s ea	58016-0818-99	457.68		AB
(Stat Rx)				
REPACK				
TAB, PO, 10 mg, 15s ea	16590-0322-15	27.50		
(FILM COATED)				
20 mg, 15s ea	16590-0181-15	52.75		AB
28s ea	16590-0181-28	98.47		AB
90s ea	16590-0181-90	307.88		AB
180s ea	16590-0181-82	615.75		AB
PAROXETINE HYDROCHLORIDE				
FUL				
TAB, PO, 10 mg, 30s ea		10.28		
20 mg, 30s ea		10.73		
30 mg, 30s ea		12.60		
40 mg, 30s ea		14.63		
(Apotex Corp.) *See PAROXETINE HCL*				
(Apotex Corp.)				
SUS, PO (ORANGE)				
10 mg/5 ml, 250 ml	60505-0374-01	158.06		AB
(Aurobindo Pharma) *See PAROXETINE*				
(Caraco) *See PAROXETINE*				
(Glaxo) *See PAXIL*				
(Glaxo) *See PAXIL CR*				
(Greenstone) *See PAROXETINE*				
(Major) *See PAROXETINE HCL*				
(Mylan) *See PAROXETINE*				
(Mylan)				
TER, PO (ENTERIC FILM-COATED)				
12.5 mg, 30s ea	00378-2003-93	102.50		AB
500s ea	00378-2003-05	1708.33		AB
25 mg, 30s ea	00378-2004-93	106.95		AB
500s ea	00378-2004-05	1782.50		AB
37.5 mg, 30s ea	00378-2006-93	110.15		
(Teva) *See PAROXETINE HCL*				
(UDL) *See PAROXETINE HCL*				
(UDL)				
TER, PO (ENTERIC FILM-COATED)				
12.5 mg, 30s ea	51079-0824-63	93.65		AB
25 mg, 30s ea	51079-0825-63	97.75		AB
(Zydus Pharm.) *See PAROXETINE*				
(Dispensing Solutions)				
REPACK				
TAB, PO, 20 mg, 30s ea	66336-0799-30	95.62		
(GSMS)				
REPACK				
TAB, PO (FILM-COATED)				
40 mg, 15s ea	60429-0737-15	12.90	4.30	
45s ea	60429-0737-45	28.65	9.55	
(McKesson Packaging)				
REPACK				
TAB, PO, 10 mg, 100s ea UD	63739-0407-10	205.66		
40 mg, 100s ea UD	63739-0408-10	233.52		
(Palmetto)				
REPACK				
TAB, PO, 10 mg, 30s ea	23490-6947-01	86.99		
60s ea	23490-6947-02	173.98		
20 mg, 28s ea	23490-6059-01	99.48		
30s ea	23490-6059-02	106.59		
60s ea	23490-6059-03	213.18		
30 mg, 30s ea	23490-6060-01	129.99		
60s ea	23490-6060-02	259.98		
40 mg, 28s ea	23490-6948-01	88.66		
30s ea	23490-6948-02	94.99		
60s ea	23490-6948-03	189.98		
(Pharma Pac)				
REPACK				
TAB, PO, 10 mg, 50s ea	52959-0775-50	137.41		
20 mg, 30s ea	52959-0776-30	87.62		
60s ea	52959-0776-60	175.20		
(Phys Total Care)				
REPACK				
TAB, PO, 20 mg, 60s ea	54868-4937-03	75.64		
100s ea	54868-4937-02	513.96		
40 mg, 60s ea	54868-4817-01	72.54		
TER, PO (ENTERIC FILM-COATED)				
25 mg, 30s ea	54868-1819-00	276.53		AB

PROD/MFR	NDC	AWP	DP	OBC
(Quality Care Prod)				
REPACK				
TAB, PO, 40 mg, 30s ea	49999-0828-30	126.30		
(Stat Rx)				
REPACK				
TER, PO (ENTERIC FILM-COATED)				
37.5 mg, 30s ea	16590-0896-30	128.95		
PAROXETINE MESYLATE				
(Noven) *See PEXEVA*				
PARRAFIN (Lorann Oil)				
paraffin wax				
WAX, NA, 454 gm	23535-0610-51	2.75		
PARSLEY LEAF				
(PCCA) *See PARSLEY LEAVES*				
PARSLEY LEAVES (PCCA)				
parsley leaf				
POW, NA, 1 gm	51927-3088-00	0.12		
PASER (Jacobus)				
aminosalicylic acid				
GER, PO, 4 gm/packet,				
30s ea UD	49938-0107-04	112.13		
PASSION FLOWER (PCCA)				
passionflower				
POW, NA, 1 gm	51927-3488-00	0.60		
PASSIONFLOWER				
(PCCA) *See PASSION FLOWER*				
PASTE BASE				
(Gallipot) *See BHRTBASE*				
(Gallipot) *See LIPOVAN BASE*				
PATADAY (Alcon Ophthalmic)				
olopatadine hydrochloride				
SOL, OP (LD POLYETHYLN DRPTAINER)				
0.2%, 2.5 ml	00065-0272-25	105.96		
(Quality Care Prod)				
REPACK				
SOL, OP, 0.2%, 2.5 ml	35356-0477-25	174.04		
PATANASE (Alcon Ophthalmic)				
olopatadine hydrochloride				
SPR, NS, 0.6%, 30.5 gm	00065-0332-30	114.78		
(Phys Total Care)				
REPACK				
SPR, NS (1X30.5GM)				
0.6%, 30.5 gm	54868-6049-00	133.94		
PATANOL (Alcon Ophthalmic)				
olopatadine hydrochloride				
SOL, OP, 0.1%, 5 ml	00065-0271-05	106.92		
(A-S Medication)				
REPACK				
SOL, OP, 0.1%, 5 ml	54569-4470-00	102.19		
(DHS, Inc.)				
REPACK				
SOL, OP, 0.1%, 5 ml	55887-0609-05	91.25		
(Dispensing Solutions)				
REPACK				
SOL, OP, 0.1%, 5 ml	55045-2640-05	95.00		
(Pharma Pac)				
REPACK				
SOL, OP, 0.1%, 5 ml	52959-0762-05	78.50		
(Phys Total Care)				
REPACK				
SOL, OP, 0.1%, 5 ml	54868-4528-00	124.93		
(Quality Care Prod)				
REPACK				
SOL, OP (1X5ML)				
0.1%, 5 ml	35356-0164-05	153.14		
(Southwood)				
REPACK				
SOL, OP, 0.1%, 5 ml	58016-8719-01	73.44		
PATCHOULI (Amend)				
OIL, NA, 30 ml	17317-0403-02	7.00		
120 ml	17317-0403-04	12.60		
500 ml	17317-0403-01	35.00		
(Lorann Oil) *See PATCHOULI OIL*				
(Medisca) *See PATCHOULI OIL*				
PATCHOULI OIL (Lorann Oil)				
patchouli				
OIL, NA, 9.9 ml	23535-0151-51	2.75		
(Medisca)				
OIL, NA (1X14ML,NATURAL)				
14 ml	38779-0773-03	19.50		

PROD/MFR	NDC	AWP	DP	OBC
(1X25ML,NATURAL)				
25 ml	38779-0773-04	25.50		
(1X100ML,NATURAL)				
100 ml	38779-0773-05	54.00		
(1X500ML,NATURAL)				
500 ml	38779-0773-08	229.50		
PATCHOULY OIL FRAGRANCE (PCCA)				
fragrance				
SOL, NA, 1 ml	51927-2551-00	2.00		
PATROL EASY-FEED (Abbott)				
kit, feeding (enteral)				
DEV, NA (W/PREATTACHED PUMP SET)				
ea	70074-0568-44	13.64	11.37	
PATROL PUMP SET (Abbott)				
kit, feeding (enteral)				
DEV, NA (W/SCREW CAP,LATEX-FREE)				
ea	70074-0568-42	6.95	5.79	
PAVACOT (Truxton)				
papaverine hydrochloride				
CER, PO, 150 mg, 100s ea	00463-3011-01	8.40		
1000s ea	00463-3011-10	79.80		
PAXIL (Glaxo)				
paroxetine hydrochloride				
SUS, PO (ORANGE)				
10 mg/5 ml, 250 ml	00029-3215-48	203.44		
TAB, PO (UNIT OF USE)				
10 mg, 30s ea	00029-3210-13	117.18		
20 mg, 30s ea	00029-3211-13	122.27		
90s ea	00029-3211-59	366.85		
(UNIT OF USE)				
30 mg, 30s ea	00029-3212-13	125.96		
40 mg, 30s ea	00029-3213-13	133.07		
500s ea	00029-3213-25	1474.75		
(A-S Medication) REPACK				
TAB, PO, 20 mg, 30s ea	54569-3810-00	115.54		
(Altura) REPACK				
TAB, PO (FILM COATED)				
30 mg, 30s ea	63874-1003-03	102.67		
(DHS, Inc.) REPACK				
TAB, PO, 20 mg, 60s ea	55887-0549-60	238.08		
(Dispensing Solutions) REPACK				
TAB, PO, 20 mg, 30s ea	55045-2546-08	95.75		
(PD-Rx Pharm) REPACK				
TAB, PO, 20 mg, 30s ea	55289-0216-30	173.07		
30s ea	58864-0372-30	134.37		
40 mg, 15s ea	58864-0628-15	70.48		
(Pharma Pac) REPACK				
TAB, PO, 10 mg, 30s ea	52959-0639-30	80.50		
20 mg, 12s ea	52959-0360-12	40.32		
15s ea	52959-0360-15	50.25		
20s ea	52959-0360-20	66.40		
30s ea	52959-0360-30	99.30		
60s ea	52959-0360-60	192.00		
(Phys Total Care) REPACK				
TAB, PO, 10 mg, 30s ea	54868-4065-00	103.55		
20 mg, 30s ea	54868-2976-02	136.02		
60s ea	54868-2976-03	255.27		
100s ea	54868-2976-00	409.95		
30 mg, 30s ea	54868-3526-00	152.32		
60s ea	54868-3526-01	286.62		
40 mg, 30s ea	54868-3962-00	128.30		
(Quality Care Prod) REPACK				
TAB, PO, 10 mg, 30s ea	49999-0597-30	129.00		
40 mg, 30s ea	35356-0246-30	150.88		
(Southwood) REPACK				
TAB, PO, 10 mg, 30s ea	58016-0661-30	106.28		
60s ea	58016-0661-60	212.56		
90s ea	58016-0661-90	318.84		
100s ea	58016-0661-00	354.27		
20 mg, 10s ea	58016-0485-10	36.97		
12s ea	58016-0485-12	44.37		
15s ea	58016-0485-15	55.46		
20s ea	58016-0485-20	73.94		
25s ea	58016-0485-25	92.43		
30s ea	58016-0485-30	110.92		
40s ea	58016-0485-40	147.89		
50s ea	58016-0485-50	184.86		
60s ea	58016-0485-60	221.83		

PROD/MFR	NDC	AWP	DP	OBC
70s ea	58016-0485-70	258.81		
80s ea	58016-0485-80	295.78		
90s ea	58016-0485-90	332.75		
100s ea	58016-0485-00	369.72		
120s ea	58016-0485-02	443.67		
30 mg, 30s ea	58016-0806-30	114.25		
60s ea	58016-0806-60	174.26		
90s ea	58016-0806-90	342.75		
100s ea	58016-0806-00	380.83		
40 mg, 30s ea	58016-0731-30	120.70		
60s ea	58016-0731-60	362.10		
90s ea	58016-0731-90	362.10		
100s ea	58016-0731-00	402.33		
PAXIL CR (Glaxo)				
paroxetine hydrochloride				
TER, PO (FILM-COATED)				
12.5 mg, 30s ea	00029-3206-13	120.70		
25 mg, 30s ea	00029-3207-13	125.95		
37.5 mg, 30s ea	00029-3208-13	129.73		
(A-S Medication) REPACK				
TER, PO, 12.5 mg, 30s ea	54569-5898-00	114.04		
(FILM-COATED)				
25 mg, 30s ea	54569-5598-00	124.95		
(DHS, Inc.) REPACK				
TER, PO, 12.5 mg, 30s ea	55887-0213-30	110.00		
(FILM-COATED)				
25 mg, 20s ea	55887-0511-20	80.31		
30s ea	55887-0214-30	120.00		
(Pharma Pac) REPACK				
TER, PO (FILM-COATED)				
25 mg, 30s ea	52959-0792-30	97.50		
(Phys Total Care) REPACK				
TER, PO (FILM-COATED)				
12.5 mg, 30s ea	54868-5347-00	122.25		
25 mg, 30s ea	54868-4791-00	131.76		
37.5 mg, 30s ea	54868-5365-00	143.59		
(Physician Partner) REPACK				
TER, PO (FILM-COATED)				
12.5 mg, 15s ea	21695-0159-15	134.17		
30s ea	21695-0159-30	228.08		
25 mg, 30s ea	21695-0160-30	238.00		
(Quality Care Prod) REPACK				
TER, PO, 12.5 mg, 30s ea	49999-0780-30	97.27		
(FILM-COATED)				
25 mg, 15s ea	49999-0601-15	65.75		
30s ea	49999-0601-30	196.40		
(Southwood) REPACK				
TER, PO (FILM-COATED)				
12.5 mg, 30s ea	58016-0897-30	109.48		
60s ea	58016-0897-60	218.96		
90s ea	58016-0897-90	328.44		
100s ea	58016-0897-00	364.93		
25 mg, 30s ea	58016-0761-30	114.24		
60s ea	58016-0761-60	228.48		
90s ea	58016-0761-90	342.72		
100s ea	58016-0761-00	380.80		
37.5 mg, 30s ea	58016-0907-30	117.67		
60s ea	58016-0907-60	235.34		
90s ea	58016-0907-90	353.01		
100s ea	58016-0907-00	392.23		
(Stat Rx) REPACK				
TER, PO (FILM-COATED)				
12.5 mg, 30s ea	16590-0514-30	134.30		
60s ea	16590-0514-60	227.82		
90s ea	16590-0514-90	329.00		
120s ea	16590-0514-72	429.53		
PAZOPANIB HYDROCHLORIDE (Glaxo) *See VOTRIENT*				
PBM ALLERGY (Boca Pharmacal)				
bpm/dm/pse hcl				
SOL, PO (1X473ML,AF,SF)				
473 ml	64376-0738-16	31.36		
PCA CONTINUOUS INFUSION-OL (Abbott Hosp)				
kit, administration, intravenous				
DEV, NA (MINIBORE, ANTI-SIPN VLV)				
24s ea	00074-6517-03	164.45	267.00	
PCA EXTENSION (Abbott Hosp)				
kit, intravenous extension tubing				
DEV, NA (10" W/BACKCHECK VALVE)				
50s ea	00074-6514-01	304.20	304.00	

PROD/MFR	NDC	AWP	DP	OBC
PCA INJECTOR (Abbott Hosp)				
kit, administration, intravenous				
DEV, NA, 48s ea	00074-4831-48	104.31	87.84	
PCA LONG W/INJECTOR-OL (Abbott Hosp)				
kit, administration, intravenous				
DEV, NA (MINIBORE, ANTI-SIPN VLV)				
24s ea	00074-6516-03	139.39	139.44	
PCA MINIBORE (Abbott Hosp)				
kit, administration, intravenous				
DEV, NA (W/ANTI-SIPHON VALVE)				
50s ea	00074-3559-01	290.40	290.50	
PCA PLUS 2 (Abbott Hosp)				
pump, infusion, patient controlled analgesia (pca)				
DEV, NA (ENHANCED)				
ea	00074-1950-07	8114.07	6832.90	
PCA W/INJECTOR-OL (Abbott Hosp)				
kit, administration, intravenous				
DEV, NA (MINIBORE, ANTI-SIPN VLV)				
24s ea	00074-3559-03	149.18	149.28	
PCCA GELATIN (PCCA)				
gelatin				
POW, NA (BASE; TM)				
1 gm	51927-1520-00	0.12		
PCCA LECITHIN ISOPROPYL PALMITATE (PCCA)				
liquid base				
LIQ, NA, 1 ml	51927-3222-00	0.23		
PCCA SWEET-SF (PCCA)				
liquid base				
LIQ, NA (SYRUP VEHICLE,SF)				
1 ml	51927-3228-00	0.09		
PCCA SYRUP VEHICLE (PCCA)				
liquid base				
LIQ, NA, 1 ml	51927-3521-00	0.13		
PCCA-PLUS (PCCA)				
liquid base				
LIQ, NA (ORAL SUSPENDING VEHICLE)				
1 ml	51927-3227-00	0.08		
PCE DISPERTAB (Abbott Pharm)				
erythromycin				
TCP, PO, 333 mg, 60s ea	00074-6290-60	137.77	120.85	
500 mg, 100s ea	00074-3389-13	302.82	265.63	
(PD-Rx Pharm) REPACK				
TCP, PO, 333 mg, 21s ea	55289-0426-21	64.27		
500 mg, 20s ea	55289-0027-20	70.08		
(Phys Total Care) REPACK				
TCP, PO, 500 mg, 15s ea	54868-1774-00	33.00		
20s ea	54868-1774-02	43.59		
PCM ALLERGY (Boca Pharmacal)				
cpm/methscopolamine nitrate/phenyleph hcl				
TER, PO, 12 mg-2.5 mg-20 mg,				
100s ea	64376-0036-01	45.69		
PCM LA (Cypress Pharm)				
cpm/methscopolamine nitrate/pse hcl				
TER, PO, 8 mg-1.25 mg-60 mg,				
100s ea	60258-0280-01	57.25		
PDM GG (Boca Pharmacal)				
dm/gg/phenyleph hcl				
SYR, PO (AF,CHERRY)				
473 ml	64376-0710-16	52.10		
PE-GUAI (Laser Pharma)				
guaifenesin/phenylephrine hydrochloride				
SOL, PO (W/CALIBRATED DROPPER,AF)				
20 mg/ml-1.5 mg/ml,				
30 ml	68134-0102-30	23.75		
PE-HIST DM (Larken Labs, Inc.)				
cpm/dm/phenyleph hcl				
SYR, PO (AF,STRAWBERRY)				
473 ml	68047-0320-16	35.18		
PEACH FLAVOR (Medisca)				
flavoring aid				
SOL, NA (1X25ML,ARTIFICIAL)				
25 ml	38779-2143-04	22.50		
(1X100ML,ARTIFICIAL)				
100 ml	38779-2143-05	34.50		
(PCCA)				
SOL, NA (ARTIFICIAL)				
1 ml	51927-2154-00	0.90		
PEANUT BUTTER FLAVOR (Medisca)				
flavoring aid				
SOL, NA (1X25ML)				
25 ml	38779-1486-04	22.50		
(1X100ML)				
100 ml	38779-1486-05	34.50		

PROD/MFR	NDC	AWP	DP	OBC
(PCCA)				
SOL, NA (ARTIFICIAL)				
1 ml	**51927-2226-00**	0.90		
(Spectrum Pharmacy)				
LIQ, NA (ARTIFICIAL)				
100 ml	**49452-5035-01**	63.70		
500 ml	**49452-5035-02**	170.10		
PEANUT OIL (Gallipot)				
OIL; NA (U.S.P.,N.F.)				
473 ml	**51552-0257-06**	9.73		
(Lorann Oil) *See PEANUT OIL NATURAL*				
(PCCA)				
OIL, NA (N.F.)				
1 ml	**51927-1387-00**	0.08		
(Spectrum Pharmacy)				
OIL, NA (N.F.)				
500 ml	**49452-5040-01**	67.55		
4000 ml	**49452-5040-02**	163.80		
PEANUT OIL NATURAL (Lorann Oil)				
peanut oil				
OIL, NA (U.S.P.)				
30 ml	**23535-0237-05**	1.00		
120 ml	**23535-0237-08**	1.80		
480 ml	**23535-0237-01**	4.00		
3840 ml	**23535-0237-11**	24.00		
PECTIN (Gallipot)				
POW, NA (U.S.P.,N.F.)				
100 gm	**51552-0196-05**	12.81		
454 gm	**51552-0196-06**	36.05		
(PCCA)				
POW, NA (USP; CITRUS)				
1 gm	**51927-1185-00**	0.38		
(Spectrum Pharmacy)				
POW, NA (U.S.P.)				
125 gm	**49452-5050-01**	77.00		
500 gm	**49452-5050-02**	172.20		
2500 gm	**49452-5050-03**	728.00		
PEDI-DRI (Pedinol)				
nystatin				
POW, TP, 100000 u/gm,				
56.7 gm	**00884-0396-02**	101.80		EE
PEDIADERM HC KIT (Arbor)				
hydrocortisone				
KIT, MR, 2%, ea	**24338-0420-01**	106.80	89.00	
PEDIAHIST DM (Boca Pharmacal)				
bpm/dm/pse hcl				
SOL, PO (W/DROPPER,GRAPE,DROPS)				
1 mg/ml-4 mg/ml-15 mg/ml,				
30 ml	**64376-0722-30**	27.04		
(1X38ML,GRAPE,DROPS)				
1 mg/ml-4 mg/ml-15 mg/ml,				
38 ml	**64376-0722-38**	40.52		
(Boca Pharmacal)				
bpm/dm/gg/pse hcl				
SYR, PO (AF,GRAPE)				
473 ml	**64376-0723-16**	45.20		
PEDIAPRED (UCB)				
prednisolone sodium phosphate				
SOL, PO (SF,DYE-FREE,RASPBERRY)				
5 mg/5 ml, 120 ml	**53014-0250-01**	48.80		
(A-S Medication)				
REPACK				
SOL, PO (SF,DYE-FREE,RASPBERRY)				
5 mg/5 ml, 120 ml	**54569-1335-00**	45.61		
(Phys Total Care)				
REPACK				
SOL, PO, 5 mg/5 ml,				
120 ml	**54868-1720-00**	43.09		
(Quality Care Prod)				
REPACK				
SOL, PO (SF,DYE-FREE,RASPBERRY)				
5 mg/5 ml, 120 ml	**35356-0488-04**	91.32		
(Southwood)				
REPACK				
SOL, PO, 5 mg/5 ml,				
120 ml	**58016-4144-01**	19.79		
PEDIARIX (Glaxo)				
dpt, hepatitis b, and polio vaccine				
SUS, IM (0.5X5,SD,TIPLOK,TAXINCL)				
0.5 ml 5s	**58160-0811-46**	420.59		
(SDV,0.5MLX10,TAXINCL,PF)				
0.5 ml 10s	**58160-0811-11**	841.18		
(A-S Medication)				
REPACK				
SUS, IM (SYRINGE W/O NEEDLE)				
0.5 ml 5s	**54569-5486-00**	456.09		
PEDIATEX TD (Zyber)				
pse hcl/triprolidine hcl				
SOL, PO (1X30ML,COTTON CANDY)				
10 mg/ml-0.938 mg/ml,				
30 ml	**65224-0539-30**	74.64		
PEDIATRIC MASK OPTICHAMBER (Respironics)				
mask, face				
DEV, NA (SMALL)				
ea	**83730-0811-11**	12.00		
PEDIAZOLE (Phys Total Care)				
REPACK				
erythromycin ethylsuccinate/sulfisoxazole acetyl				
PDR, PO, 200 mg/5 ml-600 mg/5 ml,				
100 ml	**54868-0302-01**	44.14		AB
200 ml	**54868-0302-02**	41.75		AB
(Southwood)				
REPACK				
PDR, PO, 200 mg/5 ml-600 mg/5 ml,				
100 ml	**58016-4114-01**	16.06		AB
100 ml	**58016-4847-01**	17.75		AB
200 ml	**58016-4113-01**	27.46		AB
PEDTRACE-4 (APP)				
chromium/copper/manganese/zinc				
SOL, IV (S.D.V.)				
3 ml	**63323-0138-03**	4.79		
10 ml	**63323-0138-10**	17.24		
PEDVAXHIB (Merck)				
haemophilus b conjugate vaccine				
SOL, IM (S.D.V.,FED TAX INCL)				
7.5 mcg/0.5 ml,				
0.5 ml 10s	**00006-4897-00**	273.23		
(A-S Medication)				
REPACK				
SOL, IM (S.D.V., TAX INCL)				
7.5 mcg/0.5 ml,				
0.5 ml 10s	**54569-5269-00**	282.74		
PEG 3350 & ELECTROLYTES (Kremers Urban)				
k cl/na bicarb/na cl/na sulf/peg				
PDR, PO, 4000 ml	**62175-0446-01**	12.50		AA
(Stat Rx)				
REPACK				
PDR, PO (1X4000ML)				
4000 ml	**16590-0591-04**	27.22		AA
PEG ELECTROLYTE LAVAGE SOLUTION				
(Alaven) *See COLYTE*				
(Braintree) *See GOLYTELY*				
(Mylan) *See POLYETHYLENE GLYCOL 3350 AND ELECTROLYTES*				
(Salix Pharm) *See MOVIPREP*				
PEG INTRON RP (Phys Total Care)				
REPACK				
peginterferon alfa-2b				
KIT, MR, 150 mcg, 4s ea	**54868-5036-01**	1976.94		
PEG-100 STEARATE				
(Gallipot) *See BRIJ 700*				
PEG-120 METHYL GLUCOSE DIOLEATE (PCCA)				
POW, NA, 1 gm	**51927-2440-00**	0.13		
PEG-150				
(PCCA) *See BASE E*				
(PCCA) *See POLYETHYLENE GLYCOL 6000*				
PEG-4 (PCCA)				
SOL, NA, 1 ml	**51927-3464-00**	0.11		
PEG-40 (Medisca)				
polyoxyethylene (40)				
WAX, NA (1X500GM)				
500 gm	**38779-1490-08**	96.00		
PEG-40 CASTOR (PCCA)				
castor oil				
OIL, NA (1X1ML)				
1 ml	**51927-2128-00**	0.29		
PEG-6				
(Medisca) *See MEDIBASE C*				
(PCCA) *See POLYETHYLENE GLYCOL 300*				
PEG-7 GLYCERYL COCOATE (PCCA)				
SOL, NA, 1 ml	**51927-2507-00**	0.12		
PEG-8 DISTEARATE				
(PCCA) *See BASE L*				
PEGADEMASE BOVINE				
(Enzon Pharma, Inc.) *See ADAGEN*				
PEGANONE (Lundbeck)				
ethotoin				
TAB, PO, 250 mg, 100s ea	**67386-0601-01**	130.20		
PEGAPTANIB OCTASODIUM				
(Eyetech) *See MACUGEN*				
PEGASPARGASE				
(Enzon Pharma, Inc.) *See ONCASPAR*				
PEGASYS (Roche Labs)				
peginterferon alfa-2a				
KIT, MR (S.D.V.)				
180 mcg/ml, 1 ml	**00004-0350-09**	633.30		
(MONTHLY CONVENIENCE PK)				
180 mcg/0.5 ml, ea	**00004-0352-39**	2533.20		
PEGFILGRASTIM				
(Amgen USA Inc.) *See NEULASTA*				
PEGINTERFERON ALFA-2A				
(Roche Labs) *See PEGASYS*				
PEGINTERFERON ALFA-2B				
(Schering) *See PEGINTRON*				
PEGINTRON (Schering)				
peginterferon alfa-2b				
KIT, MR (PF,REDIPEN)				
50 mcg, ea	**00085-1323-01**	553.40		
(VIAL/SRN/DILUENT,PF)				
50 mcg, ea	**00085-1368-01**	553.40		
(PF,REDIPEN)				
50 mcg, 4s ea	**00085-1323-02**	2213.63		
80 mcg, ea	**00085-1316-01**	581.02		
(VIAL/SRN/DILUENT,PF)				
80 mcg, ea	**00085-1291-01**	581.02		
(PF,REDIPEN)				
80 mcg, 4s ea	**00085-1316-02**	2324.12		
120 mcg, ea	**00085-1297-01**	610.09		
(VIAL/SRN/DILUENT,PF)				
120 mcg, ea	**00085-1304-01**	610.09		
(PF,REDIPEN)				
120 mcg, 4s ea	**00085-1297-02**	2440.46		
150 mcg, ea	**00085-1370-01**	640.61		
(VIAL/SRN/DILUENT,PF)				
150 mcg, ea	**00085-1279-01**	640.61		
(PF,REDIPEN)				
150 mcg, 4s ea	**00085-1370-02**	2562.41		
(Phys Total Care)				
REPACK				
KIT, MR (PF,REDIPEN)				
150 mcg, ea	**54868-5036-00**	505.95		
PEGVISOMANT				
(Pfizer) *See SOMAVERT*				
PEMETREXED				
(Lilly) *See ALIMTA*				
PEMIROLAST POTASSIUM				
(Vistakon) *See ALAMAST*				
PEMOLINE (PCCA)				
POW, NA (CIV)				
1 gm, C-IV	**51927-2690-00**	57.00		
(Dispensing Solutions)				
REPACK				
CTB, PO, 37.5 mg,				
60s ea, C-IV	**55045-3433-06**	120.00		
(Southwood)				
REPACK				
TAB, PO, 37.5 mg,				
30s ea, C-IV	**58016-0868-30**	41.06		AB
60s ea, C-IV	**58016-0868-60**	82.13		AB
90s ea, C-IV	**58016-0868-90**	123.19		AB
PEN-VK (Bryant Ranch)				
REPACK				
penicillin v potassium				
TAB, PO, 500 mg, 20s ea	**63629-1615-04**	44.65		
28s ea	**63629-1615-03**	52.85		
30s ea	**63629-1615-01**	78.91		
40s ea	**63629-1615-02**	89.21		
100s ea	**63629-1615-05**	79.99		
PENBUTOLOL SULFATE				
(UCB) *See LEVATOL*				
PENCICLOVIR				
(Novartis Consumer) *See DENAVIR*				
PENDEX (Cypress Pharm)				
guaifenesin/phenylephrine hydrochloride				
TER, PO, 600 mg-10 mg,				
100s ea	**60258-0242-01**	55.79		
PENICILLAMINE				
(Aton) *See CUPRIMINE*				

PROD/MFR	NDC	AWP	DP	OBC
(Meda) *See DEPEN*				
(Medisca) *See D-PENICILLAMINE*				
(PCCA)				
POW, NA ((D) USP)				
1 gm	**51927-1786-00**	9.00		
PENICILLIN (Bryant Ranch)				
REPACK				
penicillin v potassium				
TAB, PO, 250 mg, 20s ea	**63629-1614-01**	6.24		
28s ea	**63629-1614-03**	8.74		
30s ea	**63629-2738-01**	9.36		
40s ea	**63629-1614-02**	12.48		
40s ea	**63629-2738-02**	12.48		
PENICILLIN G BENZATHINE				
(King Pharm) *See BICILLIN L-A*				
PENICILLIN G BENZATHINE/ PENICILLIN G PROCAINE				
(King Pharm) *See BICILLIN C-R*				
(King Pharm) *See BICILLIN C-R 900/300*				
PENICILLIN G POTASSIUM (APP)				
PDS, IJ, 5000000 u, 10s ea	**63323-0323-20**	480.00		AP
(Baxter)				
SOL, IV (GALAXY,PREMIX)				
1 million u/50 ml, 50 ml 24s	**00338-1021-41**	304.13	253.44	
2 million u/50 ml, 50 ml 24s	**00338-1023-41**	316.51	263.76	
3 million u/50 ml, 50 ml 24s	**00338-1025-41**	328.61	273.84	
(Pfizer) *See AMERINET CHOICE PFIZERPEN*				
(Pfizer) *See NOVAPLUS PFIZERPEN*				
(Pfizer) *See PFIZERPEN*				
(Sandoz)				
PDS, IV, 5 million u, 10s ea	**00781-6135-95**	421.75		AP
20 million u, ea	**00781-6136-94**	160.26		AP
(Phys Total Care)				
REPACK				
PDS, IV (VIAL,PHARMACY BOTTLE)				
20 million u, ea	**54868-4488-00**	12.57		AP
PENICILLIN G PROCAINE (King Pharm)				
SUS, IM (21GX1&1/2,1MLX10)				
600000 u/ml, 1 ml 10s	**60793-0130-10**	159.89		
(21GX1&1/4,2MLX10) 600000 u/ml, 2 ml 10s	**60793-0131-10**	266.22		
PENICILLIN G SODIUM (Sandoz)				
PDS, IV, 5 million u, ea	**00781-6135-94**	42.18		EE
(VIAL) 5 million u, 10s ea	**00781-6153-95**	479.06		EE
PENICILLIN V POTASSIUM				
FUL				
TAB, PO, 250 mg, 100s ea		21.12		
500 mg, 100s ea		35.90		
(Aurobindo Pharma)				
TAB, PO (USP,FILM-COATED)				
250 mg, 100s ea	**65862-0175-01**	23.46		AB
1000s ea	**65862-0175-99**	222.90		AB
500 mg, 100s ea	**65862-0176-01**	39.88		AB
500s ea	**65862-0176-05**	189.40		AB
1000s ea	**65862-0176-99**	378.90		AB
(Dava Pharma)				
PDS, PO (USP,FRUIT)				
125 mg/5 ml, 100 ml	**67253-0202-10**	4.40		AA
(FRUIT) 125 mg/5 ml, 200 ml	**67253-0202-20**	6.30		AA
250 mg/5 ml, 100 ml	**67253-0203-10**	4.90		AA
200 ml	**67253-0203-20**	7.00		AA
(Dava Pharma) *See PENICILLIN VK*				
(Greenstone)				
TAB, PO (USP,FILM-COATED)				
250 mg, 100s ea	**59762-1534-01**	23.48		
1000s ea	**59762-1534-02**	222.87		
500 mg, 100s ea	**59762-1537-01**	39.88		
500s ea	**59762-1537-02**	199.40		
1000s ea	**59762-1537-03**	378.86		
(Sandoz) *See PENICILLIN VK*				
(Sandoz) *See VEETIDS*				
(Teva) *See PENICILLIN VK*				
(Teva) *See PENICILLIN-VK*				
(Truxton) *See TRUXCILLIN VK*				
(Altura)				
REPACK				
PDR, PO, 250 mg/5 ml, 100 ml	**63874-0170-10**	5.51		
200 ml	**63874-0170-20**	4.26		
TAB, PO, 250 mg, 10s ea	**63874-0232-10**	1.28		
12s ea	**63874-0232-12**	1.54		
16s ea	**63874-0232-16**	2.05		
20s ea	**63874-0232-20**	2.57		
21s ea	**63874-0232-21**	2.70		
24s ea	**63874-0232-24**	3.09		
28s ea	**63874-0232-28**	3.60		
30s ea	**63874-0232-30**	3.85		
40s ea	**63874-0232-40**	7.18		
50s ea	**63874-0232-50**	8.97		
100s ea	**63874-0232-01**	12.86		
500s ea	**63874-0232-03**	89.75		
1000s ea	**63874-0232-02**	128.60		
500 mg, 6s ea	**63874-0233-06**	1.45		
10s ea	**63874-0233-10**	2.42		
12s ea	**63874-0233-12**	2.90		
15s ea	**63874-0233-15**	3.62		
16s ea	**63874-0233-16**	3.86		
20s ea	**63874-0233-20**	4.83		
24s ea	**63874-0233-24**	5.80		
28s ea	**63874-0233-28**	6.93		
30s ea	**63874-0233-30**	7.25		
36s ea	**63874-0233-36**	8.69		
40s ea	**63874-0233-40**	9.20		
50s ea	**63874-0233-50**	12.08		
60s ea	**63874-0233-60**	14.49		
100s ea	**63874-0233-01**	24.16		
1000s ea	**63874-0233-02**	128.60		
(Dispensing Solutions)				
REPACK				
PDS, PO (1X200ML,FRUIT)				
250 mg/5 ml, 200 ml	**55045-1179-02**	8.91		AA
(Palmetto)				
REPACK				
PDS, PO, 125 mg/5 ml, 200 ml	**23490-6067-07**	6.25		
250 mg/5 ml, 200 ml	**23490-6069-07**	9.25		
TAB, PO, 250 mg, 6s ea	**23490-6068-01**	8.71		
20s ea	**23490-6068-02**	20.40		
28s ea	**23490-6068-03**	28.56		
30s ea	**23490-6068-05**	30.60		
40s ea	**23490-6068-04**	40.80		
500 mg, 6s ea	**23490-6070-01**	8.99		
10s ea	**23490-6070-02**	10.73		
20s ea	**23490-6070-03**	21.47		
28s ea	**23490-6070-04**	30.05		
30s ea	**23490-6070-05**	32.20		
40s ea	**23490-6070-06**	42.93		
(Physician Partner)				
REPACK				
PDS, PO (1X100ML,FRUIT)				
125 mg/5 ml, 100 ml	**21695-0772-00**	14.40		AA
PENICILLIN VK (Dava Pharma)				
penicillin v potassium				
TAB, PO, 250 mg, 100s ea	**67253-0200-10**	23.48		AB
1000s ea	**67253-0200-11**	222.90		AB
(USP 800,000 UNITS)				
500 mg, 100s ea	**67253-0201-10**	39.90		AB
500s ea	**67253-0201-50**	189.40		AB
(Sandoz)				
PDR, PO, 125 mg/5 ml, 100 ml	**00781-6120-46**	5.91		
250 mg/5 ml, 100 ml	**00781-6121-46**	6.57		
200 ml	**00781-6121-48**	9.38		
TAB, PO, 250 mg, 100s ea	**00781-1205-01**	23.46		AB
1000s ea	**00781-1205-10**	222.87		AB
500 mg, 100s ea	**00781-1655-01**	39.88		AB
1000s ea	**00781-1655-10**	378.86		AB
(Teva)				
TAB, PO, 250 mg, 100s ea	**00093-1172-01**	23.46		AB
500 mg, 100s ea	**00093-1174-01**	39.88		AB
(A-S Medication)				
REPACK				
PDR, PO, 250 mg/5 ml, 100 ml	**54569-2933-00**	4.75		EE
200 ml	**54569-2935-00**	5.51		EE
TAB, PO, 250 mg, 12s ea	**54569-2702-06**	2.82		EE
20s ea	**54569-2702-00**	4.70		EE
28s ea	**54569-2702-02**	6.57		EE
30s ea	**54569-2702-03**	7.04		EE
40s ea	**54569-2702-04**	9.39		EE
500 mg, 12s ea	**54569-2710-01**	4.79		EE
20s ea	**54569-2710-02**	7.98		EE
28s ea	**54569-2710-04**	11.17		EE
30s ea	**54569-2710-05**	11.97		EE
40s ea	**54569-2710-06**	15.96		EE
(Core)				
REPACK				
TAB, PO, 250 mg, 20s ea	**33358-0284-20**	12.79		
30s ea	**33358-0284-30**	14.47		
40s ea	**33358-0284-40**	17.44		
60s ea	**33358-0284-60**	21.69		
500 mg, 20s ea	**33358-0285-20**	45.77		
30s ea	**33358-0285-30**	80.88		
40s ea	**33358-0285-40**	91.44		
60s ea	**33358-0285-60**	108.64		
(DHS, Inc.)				
REPACK				
PDS, PO, 125 mg/5 ml, 100 ml	**55887-0218-01**	6.96		
250 mg/5 ml, 100 ml	**55887-0215-01**	6.57		
TAB, PO, 250 mg, 28s ea	**55887-0930-28**	16.01		AB
30s ea	**55887-0930-30**	17.08		AB
40s ea	**55887-0930-40**	22.77		AB
500 mg, 30s ea	**55887-0980-30**	21.00		AB
40s ea	**55887-0980-40**	28.00		AB
(Dispensing Solutions)				
REPACK				
TAB, PO, 250 mg, 20s ea	**55045-1201-07**	6.85		AB
20s ea	**66336-0414-20**	21.80		AB
28s ea	**66336-0414-28**	30.52		AB
30s ea	**55045-1201-08**	10.20		AB
40s ea	**55045-1201-03**	13.60		AB
40s ea	**66336-0414-40**	43.69		EE
500 mg, 6s ea	**55045-1202-06**	3.48		AB
6s ea	**66336-0095-06**	6.54		AB
12s ea	**55045-1202-04**	6.90		AB
15s ea	**55045-1202-05**	8.70		AB
20s ea	**55045-1202-07**	11.60		AB
20s ea	**66336-0095-20**	21.80		AB
28s ea	**66336-0095-28**	30.52		AB
30s ea	**55045-1202-08**	17.40		AB
30s ea	**66336-0095-30**	31.73		AB
40s ea	**55045-1202-03**	23.20		AB
40s ea	**66336-0095-40**	42.36		AB
(USP 800,000 UNITS)				
500 mg, 40s ea	**55045-3928-01**	23.20		AB
60s ea	**55045-1202-02**	34.80		AB
90s ea	**55045-1202-09**	52.20		AB
100s ea	**55045-1202-01**	58.00		AB
120s ea	**55045-1202-00**	69.60		AB
(GSMS)				
REPACK				
TAB, PO (UNIT OF USE)				
250 mg, 40s ea	**60429-0147-40**	87.75	29.25	AB
500 mg, 40s ea	**60429-0148-40**	163.05	54.35	AB
(HomeMed)				
REPACK				
TAB, PO, 250 mg, 6s ea	**51655-0009-87**	6.54		EE
20s ea	**51655-0009-52**	21.80		EE
28s ea	**51655-0009-29**	30.52		EE
40s ea	**51655-0009-51**	3.85		EE
500 mg, 20s ea	**51655-0010-52**	21.80		EE
28s ea	**51655-0010-29**	30.52		EE
30s ea	**51655-0010-24**	13.67		EE
40s ea	**51655-0010-51**	15.48		EE
(Nucare Pharm)				
REPACK				
TAB, PO, 250 mg, 20s ea	**66267-0159-20**	22.85		EE
30s ea	**66267-0159-30**	34.27		EE
40s ea	**66267-0159-40**	45.69		EE
500 mg, 20s ea	**66267-0160-20**	44.89		EE
28s ea	**66267-0160-28**	62.85		EE
40s ea	**66267-0160-40**	89.78		EE
(PD-Rx Pharm)				
REPACK				
TAB, PO (USP)				
250 mg, 6s ea	**43063-0054-06**	11.91		AB
10s ea	**55289-0206-10**	13.87		AB
20s ea	**55289-0206-20**	17.73		AB
28s ea	**55289-0206-28**	21.57		AB
30s ea	**55289-0206-30**	21.93		AB
40s ea	**55289-0206-40**	25.47		AB
(REDI-SCRIPT)				
250 mg, 40s ea	**58864-0379-40**	25.47		AB
56s ea	**55289-0206-56**	29.64		AB
500 mg, 4s ea	**55289-0207-04**	12.87		AB
(USP 800,000 UNITS)				
500 mg, 6s ea	**43063-0096-06**	12.48		AB
15s ea	**55289-0207-15**	22.53		AB
20s ea	**55289-0207-20**	24.80		AB
28s ea	**58864-0612-28**	30.37		

PROD/MFR	NDC	AWP	DP	OBC
(USP)				
500 mg, 28s ea	55289-0207-28	30.72		AB
30s ea	55289-0207-30	32.20		AB
30s ea	58864-0612-30	32.19		
40s ea	55289-0207-40	39.60		AB
(Pharma Pac)				
REPACK				
PDR, PO, 125 mg/5 ml,				
100 ml	52959-0560-00	6.25		AA
TAB, PO, 250 mg, 20s ea	52959-0333-20	13.87		EE
24s ea	52959-0333-24	16.09		EE
28s ea	52959-0333-28	18.57		EE
30s ea	52959-0333-30	19.27		EE
40s ea	52959-0333-40	22.66		EE
500 mg, 10s ea	52959-0213-10	21.72		EE
20s ea	52959-0213-20	43.43		EE
24s ea	52959-0213-24	51.94		EE
28s ea	52959-0213-28	60.32		EE
30s ea	52959-0213-30	64.34		EE
40s ea	52959-0213-40	72.33		EE
(USP 800,000 UNITS)				
500 mg, 100s ea	52959-0213-01	179.20		AB
(Phys Total Care)				
REPACK				
PDR, PO, 125 mg/5 ml,				
100 ml	54868-4125-01	10.08		EE
200 ml	54868-4125-02	18.06		EE
250 mg/5 ml,				
100 ml	54868-1780-01	11.04		EE
200 ml	54868-1780-02	15.21		EE
TAB, PO, 250 mg, 20s ea	54868-1171-00	11.88		EE
30s ea	54868-1171-03	15.57		EE
40s ea	54868-1171-01	19.26		EE
100s ea	54868-1171-02	41.43		EE
500 mg, 20s ea	54868-1173-05	19.41		EE
30s ea	54868-1173-01	31.26		EE
40s ea	54868-1173-02	40.66		EE
100s ea	54868-1173-00	83.61		EE
500s ea	54868-1173-06	243.09		EE
1000s ea	54868-1173-04	506.55		EE
(Physician Partner)				
REPACK				
TAB, PO, 500 mg, 12s ea	21695-0318-12	26.19		
20s ea	21695-0318-20	37.83		
28s ea	21695-0318-28	44.96		
30s ea	21695-0318-30	55.65		
40s ea	21695-0318-40	74.20		
(Quality Care Prod)				
REPACK				
PDR, PO, 250 mg/5 ml,				
200 ml	49999-0332-20	16.20		AA
TAB, PO, 250 mg, 6s ea	49999-0002-06	7.76		EE
20s ea	49999-0002-20	9.60		AB
24s ea	49999-0002-24	10.92		EE
30s ea	49999-0002-30	12.15		AB
40s ea	49999-0002-40	16.20		AB
500 mg, 10s ea	49999-0050-10	12.50		AB
12s ea	49999-0050-12	15.00		AB
14s ea	49999-0050-14	17.50		AB
20s ea	49999-0050-20	30.00		AB
21s ea	49999-0050-21	26.25		AB
28s ea	49999-0050-28	35.00		AB
30s ea	49999-0050-30	37.60		AB
40s ea	49999-0050-40	50.00		AB
(Southwood)				
REPACK				
PDR, PO, 125 mg/5 ml,				
100 ml	58016-1026-01	4.70		EE
200 ml	58016-1027-06	6.22		EE
250 mg/5 ml,				
100 ml	58016-1028-01	5.25		EE
200 ml	58016-1029-01	7.70		EE
TAB, PO, 250 mg, 10s ea	58016-0146-10	2.35		EE
12s ea	58016-0146-12	2.82		EE
16s ea	58016-0146-16	3.75		EE
20s ea	58016-0146-20	4.69		EE
21s ea	58016-0146-21	4.93		EE
24s ea	58016-0146-24	5.63		EE
28s ea	58016-0146-28	6.57		EE
30s ea	58016-0146-30	7.04		EE
40s ea	58016-0146-40	9.38		EE
60s ea	58016-0146-60	14.08		EE
90s ea	58016-0146-90	21.11		EE
100s ea	58016-0146-00	23.46		EE
120s ea	58016-0146-02	28.15		EE
150s ea	58016-0146-03	35.19		EE
200s ea	58016-0146-89	46.92		EE
300s ea	58016-0146-73	70.38		EE
500 mg, 6s ea	58016-0147-06	2.39		EE
10s ea	58016-0147-10	3.99		EE
12s ea	58016-0147-12	4.79		EE
15s ea	58016-0147-15	5.98		EE
16s ea	58016-0147-16	6.38		EE
20s ea	58016-0147-20	7.98		EE
21s ea	58016-0147-21	8.37		EE
24s ea	58016-0147-24	9.57		EE
28s ea	58016-0147-28	11.17		EE
30s ea	58016-0147-30	11.96		EE
40s ea	58016-0147-40	15.95		EE
50s ea	58016-0147-50	19.94		EE
60s ea	58016-0147-60	23.93		EE
90s ea	58016-0147-90	35.89		EE
100s ea	58016-0147-00	39.88		EE
120s ea	58016-0147-02	47.86		EE
150s ea	58016-0147-03	59.82		EE
200s ea	58016-0147-89	79.76		EE
300s ea	58016-0147-73	119.64		EE
(Stat Rx)				
REPACK				
TAB, PO (USP 800,000 UNITS)				
500 mg, 40s ea	16590-0183-40	13.65		AB
(Vibranta)				
REPACK				
TAB, PO, 250 mg, 40s ea	57866-3613-02	5.10		
500 mg, 40s ea	57866-3614-01	9.48		AB
PENICILLIN-VK (Teva)				
penicillin v potassium				
PDS, PO (CHERRY)				
125 mg/5 ml,				
100 ml	00093-4125-73	2.48		AA
200 ml	00093-4125-74	3.64		AA
250 mg/5 ml,				
100 ml	00093-4127-73	2.78		AA
200 ml	00093-4127-74	4.02		AA
TAB, PO, 250 mg,				
1000s ea	00093-1172-10	222.87		AB
500 mg, 1000s ea	00093-1174-10	378.86		AB
(Stat Rx)				
REPACK				
PDR, PO, 250 mg/5 ml,				
200 ml	16590-0182-36	15.00		
TAB, PO, 500 mg, 20s ea	16590-0183-20	6.00		
30s ea	16590-0183-30	9.00		
PENLAC (Dermik)				
ciclopirox				
SOL, TP, 8%, 6.6 ml	00066-8008-02	235.45		
(A-S Medication)				
REPACK				
SOL, TP, 8%, 6.6 ml	54569-5597-00	225.01		
(Phys Total Care)				
REPACK				
SOL, TP, 8%, 7 ml	54868-4633-01	191.18		
PENNYROYAL				
(Medisca) *See PENNYROYAL OIL*				
(PCCA) *See PENNYROYAL OIL*				
PENNYROYAL OIL (Medisca)				
pennyroyal				
OIL, NA (1X14ML,NATURAL)				
14 ml	38779-1735-03	31.50		
(1X25ML,NATURAL)				
25 ml	38779-1735-04	52.50		
(1X100ML,NATURAL)				
100 ml	38779-1735-05	150.00		
(1X500ML,NATURAL)				
500 ml	38779-1735-08	352.50		
(PCCA)				
OIL, NA, 1 gm	51927-1654-00	1.35		
PENTACEL (Sanofi)				
KIT, IM (5 DOSE PACKAGE)				
5s ea	49281-0510-05	448.23	376.65	
PENTAERYTHRITOL TETRANITRATE (PCCA)				
POW, NA (USP 22)				
20%, 1 gm	51927-2680-00	0.66		
PENTAM (APP)				
pentamidine isethionate				
PDS, IJ (S.D.V.,PF)				
300 mg, ea	63323-0113-10	98.75		AP
PENTAMIDINE ISETHIONATE (Abbott Hosp)				
PDS, IJ, 300 mg, ea	00074-4548-01	53.44	45.00	AP
(APP) *See NEBUPENT*				
(APP) *See PENTAM*				
PENTASA (Shire US Inc.)				
mesalamine				
CER, PO, 250 mg, 240s ea	54092-0189-81	309.61	258.01	
500 mg, 120s ea	54092-0191-12	309.61	258.01	
(Phys Total Care)				
REPACK				
CER, PO, 500 mg, 120s ea	54868-5302-00	197.56		
180s ea	54868-5302-01	417.24		
PENTASPAN (B. Braun)				
pentastarch/sodium chloride				
SOL, IV (LATEX-FREE)				
500 ml	00264-1970-10	76.33		
PENTASTARCH/SODIUM CHLORIDE				
(B. Braun) *See PENTASPAN*				
PENTAZOCIN/NALOXONE (Bryant Ranch)				
REPACK				
naloxone hydrochloride/pentazocine hydrochloride				
TAB, PO, 0.5 mg-50 mg,				
60s ea, C-IV	63629-3206-01	99.89		
PENTAZOCINE AND NALOXONE HYDROCHLORIDES (Phys Total Care)				
REPACK				
naloxone hydrochloride/pentazocine hydrochloride				
TAB, PO (USP)				
0.5 mg-50 mg,				
30s ea, C-IV	54868-4788-01	77.31		
PENTAZOCINE HYDROCHLORIDE/NALOXONE HYDROCHLORIDE (Keltman Pharma., Inc.)				
REPACK				
naloxone hydrochloride/pentazocine hydrochloride				
TAB, PO, 0.5 mg-50 mg,				
60s ea, C-IV	68387-0531-60	99.48		
120s ea, C-IV	68387-0531-12	198.96		
PENTAZOCINE LACTATE				
(Hospira) *See TALWIN LACTATE*				
PENTAZOCINE/APAP (Physician Partner)				
REPACK				
acetaminophen/pentazocine hydrochloride				
TAB, PO, 650 mg-25 mg,				
60s ea, C-IV	21695-0634-60	101.64		
PENTAZOCINE/NALOXONE (DHS, Inc.)				
REPACK				
naloxone hydrochloride/pentazocine hydrochloride				
TAB, PO, 0.5 mg-50 mg,				
30s ea, C-IV	55887-0171-30	34.05		
60s ea, C-IV	55887-0171-60	68.10		
90s ea, C-IV	55887-0171-90	102.15		
100s ea, C-IV	55887-0171-01	113.50		
150s ea, C-IV	55887-0171-86	170.25		
200s ea, C-IV	55887-0171-83	227.00		
300s ea, C-IV	55887-0171-84	340.50		
(Dispensing Solutions)				
REPACK				
TAB, PO, 0.5 mg-50 mg,				
30s ea, C-IV	55045-3099-07	30.00		
40s ea, C-IV	55045-3099-04	40.00		
45s ea, C-IV	55045-3099-05	45.00		
90s ea, C-IV	55045-3099-09	90.00		
100s ea, C-IV	55045-3099-00	100.00		
120s ea, C-IV	55045-3099-01	120.00		
135s ea, C-IV	55045-3099-03	135.00		
(Physician Partner)				
REPACK				
TAB, PO, 0.5 mg-50 mg,				
28s ea, C-IV	21695-0364-28	63.56		
60s ea, C-IV	21695-0364-60	136.20		
120s ea, C-IV	21695-0364-72	272.40		
PENTETATE CALCIUM TRISODIUM				
(Akorn) *See PENTETATE CALCIUM TRISODIUM*				
PENTETATE CALCIUM TRISODIUM (Akorn)				
pentetate calcium trisodium				
SOL, IV (10X5ML SINGLE-USE AMPS)				
200 mg/ml,				
5 ml 10s	52919-0001-03	900.00		
PENTETATE ZINC TRISODIUM				
(Akorn) *See PENTETATE ZINC TRISODIUM*				
PENTETATE ZINC TRISODIUM (Akorn)				
pentetate zinc trisodium				
SOL, IV (10X5ML SINGLE-USE AMPS)				
200 mg/ml,				
5 ml 10s	52919-0002-03	900.00		
PENTOBARBITAL SODIUM				
(Lundbeck) *See NEMBUTAL SODIUM*				
(PCCA)				
POW, NA (U.S.P.)				
1 gm, C-II	51927-3613-00	27.00		
PENTOSAN POLYSULFATE SODIUM				
(Ortho-McNeil Pharm) *See ELMIRON*				
PENTOSTATIN (Bedford)				
PDS, IV (SDV)				
10 mg, ea	55390-0244-01	2280.00		AP
(Hospira) *See NIPENT*				
PENTOTHAL (Hospira)				
thiopental sodium				
PDS, IV (COMBO PAK)				
1 gm,				
25s ea, C-III	00409-6435-01	1413.60	1237.00	
(USP)				
1 gm,				
25s ea, C-III	00409-6431-02	747.90	654.50	

PROD/MFR	NDC	AWP	DP	OBC
(SRN, RTM LIFESHIELD)				
250 mg,				
25s ea, C-III	00074-3351-01	361.20	316.00	
(RTMLIFESHLD,NACL DLUENT)				
400 mg,				
25s ea, C-III	00409-3352-01	675.00	590.75	
(SRN, RTM LIFESHIELD)				
400 mg,				
25s ea, C-III	00074-3352-01	583.20	510.25	
(COMBOPK W/20ML DILUENT)				
500 mg,				
25s ea, C-III	00409-3329-01	783.90	686.00	
(LIFESHIELD READY-TO-MIX)				
500 mg,				
25s ea, C-III	00409-3353-01	650.40	569.00	
(SRN, RTM LIFESHIELD)				
500 mg,				
25s ea, C-III	00074-3353-01	613.50	536.75	
(STERILE WATER COMBO PAK)				
500 mg,				
25s ea, C-III	00074-3329-01	944.10	826.00	
PENTOTHAL DISPENSING PIN (Abbott Hosp)				
device				
DEV, NA, 100s ea	00074-6682-02	418.80	419.00	
PENTOXIFYL XR (Core)				
REPACK				
pentoxifylline				
TER, PO, 400 mg, 30s ea	33358-0286-30	26.19		
PENTOXIFYLLINE				
FUL				
TER, PO, 400 mg, 100s ea		31.47		
(Apotex Corp.)				
TER, PO, 400 mg, 100s ea	60505-0033-06	59.51		AB
500s ea	60505-0033-07	297.80		AB
5500s ea	60505-0033-08	3275.80		AB
(Gallipot)				
POW, NA, 100 gm	51552-1059-05	101.50	72.50	
(Hawkins)				
POW, NA (BP)				
100 gm	63370-0168-35	168.00		
500 gm	63370-0168-45	768.00		
(Letco)				
POW, NA (PH.EUR.2002)				
100 gm	62991-2521-03	88.50		
500 gm	62991-2521-02	405.00		
1000 gm	62991-2521-01	750.00		
(Major)				
TER, PO (10X10)				
400 mg, 100s ea UD	00904-5448-61	66.56		EE
(Medisca)				
POW, NA (BP)				
25 gm	38779-2145-04	75.00		
100 gm	38779-2145-05	147.00		
500 gm	38779-2145-08	645.00		
(1X1000GM,BP)				
1000 gm	38779-2145-09	1134.00		
(Mylan)				
TER, PO, 400 mg, 100s ea	00378-0357-01	64.05		AB
500s ea	00378-0357-05	285.85		AB
(PCCA)				
POW, NA, 1 gm	51927-3012-00	4.20		
(Sanofi-Aventis) *See TRENTAL*				
(Spectrum Pharmacy)				
POW, NA (B.P.)				
5 gm	49452-5080-01	117.25		
25 gm	49452-5080-02	153.48		
100 gm	49452-5080-03	290.15		
500 gm	49452-5080-04	1102.50		
(Teva)				
TER, PO, 400 mg, 100s ea	00093-5116-01	59.50		AB
500s ea	00093-5116-05	288.57		AB
(UDL)				
TER, PO (25X1 ROBOT READY)				
400 mg, 25s ea UD	51079-0889-19	41.79		AB
(10X10)				
400 mg, 100s ea UD	51079-0889-20	65.71		AB
(Upsher-Smith) *See PENTOXIL*				
(A-S Medication)				
REPACK				
TER, PO, 400 mg, 30s ea	54569-5972-00	18.39		
(Bryant Ranch)				
REPACK				
TER, PO, 400 mg, 30s ea	63629-2910-01	25.02		
60s ea	63629-2910-02	50.03		
(DHS, Inc.)				
REPACK				
TER, PO (FILM-COATED)				
400 mg, 30s ea	55887-0293-30	17.85		AB
90s ea	55887-0293-90	40.22		AB
(GSMS)				
REPACK				
TER, PO (UNIT OF USE)				
400 mg, 90s ea	60429-0703-90	6.00	18.00	EE
100s ea	60429-0703-01	19.80	6.60	EE
500s ea	60429-0703-05	85.20	28.40	EE
(PD-Rx Pharm)				
REPACK				
TER, PO, 400 mg, 30s ea	43063-0188-30	18.54		AB
(Phys Total Care)				
REPACK				
TER, PO, 400 mg, 30s ea	54868-4515-01	14.12		AB
60s ea	54868-4515-03	23.75		AB
PENTOXIFYLLINE (Phys Total Care)				
REPACK				
TER, PO, 400 mg, 90s ea	54868-4515-00	33.37		
100s ea	54868-4515-02	35.08		AB
(Quality Care Prod)				
REPACK				
TER, PO, 400 mg, 24s ea	49999-0542-24	20.70		
60s ea	49999-0542-60	51.76		AB
100s ea	49999-0542-00	51.76		
(Stat Rx)				
REPACK				
TER, PO, 400 mg, 90s ea	16590-0856-90	53.64		AB
(Vibranta)				
REPACK				
TER, PO, 400 mg, 90s ea	57866-6778-01	64.70		EE
PENTOXIL (Upsher-Smith)				
pentoxifylline				
TER, PO, 400 mg, ea	00245-0027-89	0.62		AB
PENTYLENETETRAZOL				
(PCCA) *See PENTYLENETETRAZOLE*				
PENTYLENETETRAZOLE (PCCA)				
pentylenetetrazol				
POW, NA, 1 gm	51927-1103-00	2.28		
PEPCID (Merck)				
famotidine				
TAB, PO (UNIT OF USE)				
20 mg, 30s ea	00006-0963-31	62.44		AB
100s ea	00006-0963-58	208.10		AB
40 mg, 30s ea	00006-0964-31	120.67		AB
100s ea	00006-0964-58	402.24		AB
(Salix Pharm)				
PDR, PO (1X50ML)				
40 mg/5 ml, 50 ml	65649-0211-24	196.61		
(A-S Medication)				
REPACK				
TAB, PO, 20 mg, 10s ea	54569-2352-05	20.28		AB
30s ea	54569-2352-00	60.84		AB
(PD-Rx Pharm)				
REPACK				
TAB, PO, 20 mg, 6s ea	55289-0473-06	24.98		AB
20s ea	55289-0473-20	68.24		AB
40 mg, 4s ea	55289-0146-04	31.23		AB
(Pharma Pac)				
REPACK				
TAB, PO, 20 mg, 30s ea	52959-0465-30	60.68		AB
(Phys Total Care)				
REPACK				
TAB, PO, 20 mg, 30s ea	54868-0303-02	72.47		AB
60s ea	54868-0303-01	136.40		AB
40 mg, 30s ea	54868-0304-01	131.25		AB
(Quality Care Prod)				
REPACK				
TAB, PO, 20 mg, 10s ea	49999-0427-10	27.50		AB
30s ea	49999-0427-30	69.25		AB
PEPPERMINT				
(Gallipot) *See PEPPERMINT SPIRIT*				
PEPPERMINT OIL (Lorann Oil)				
OIL, NA (U.S.P., NATURAL)				
3.75 ml	23535-0070-01	0.57		
9.9 ml	23535-0151-54	3.25		
(U.S.P., NATURAL)				
30 ml	23535-0070-05	4.75		
480 ml	23535-0070-10	55.00		
1920 ml	23535-0070-15	160.00		
3840 ml	23535-0070-11	295.00		
(Medisca)				
OIL, NA (1X14ML,NATURAL)				
14 ml	38779-0827-03	23.25		
(1X25ML,NATURAL)				
25 ml	38779-0827-04	37.50		
(1X100ML,NATURAL)				
100 ml	38779-0827-05	58.50		
(1X500ML,NATURAL)				
500 ml	38779-0827-08	180.00		
(PCCA)				
OIL, NA (NF)				
1 ml	51927-3462-00	1.65		
(Spectrum Pharmacy)				
OIL, NA (N.F.)				
100 ml	49452-5090-02	103.95		
500 ml	49452-5090-03	275.45		
PEPPERMINT SPIRIT (Gallipot)				
peppermint				
LIQ, NA, 29.57 ml	51552-0563-02	8.89		
118.28 ml	51552-0563-04	28.49		
PEPSIN (Baker, J.T.)				
POW, NA (PURIFIED)				
500 gm	10106-2844-01	150.23		
(PCCA)				
POW, NA, 1 gm	51927-1409-00	0.57		
(Spectrum Pharmacy) *See PEPSIN 1:3000*				
(Spectrum Pharmacy)				
POW, NA (1:10,000)				
25 gm	49452-5110-01	105.00		
100 gm	49452-5110-02	138.95		
500 gm	49452-5110-03	472.50		
PEPSIN 1:3000 (Spectrum Pharmacy)				
pepsin				
POW, NA (1X100GM)				
100 gm	49452-5105-01	104.65		
(1X500GM)				
500 gm	49452-5105-02	250.95		
PERANEX HC (Kenwood)				
hydrocortisone acetate/lidocaine hydrochloride				
KIT, TP, 2%-2%, ea	00482-4801-24	368.71		
PAD, TP, 1%-3%, 60s ea	00482-4808-60	275.42		
PERCOCET (Endo Labs)				
acetaminophen/oxycodone hydrochloride				
TAB, PO (25X4,BLISTER PACK)				
325 mg-5 mg,				
100s ea UD, C-II	63481-0623-75	134.34		
(Endo Pharm)				
TAB, PO, 325 mg-2.5 mg,				
100s ea, C-II	63481-0627-70	259.74		
325 mg-5 mg,				
100s ea, C-II	63481-0623-70	363.53		
500s ea, C-II	63481-0623-85	1771.94		
325 mg-7.5 mg,				
100s ea, C-II	63481-0628-70	392.75		AA
325 mg-10 mg,				
100s ea, C-II	63481-0629-70	513.55		AA
500 mg-7.5 mg,				
100s ea, C-II	63481-0621-70	419.26		AA
650 mg-10 mg,				
100s ea, C-II	63481-0622-70	548.36		AA
(DHS, Inc.)				
REPACK				
TAB, PO, 325 mg-7.5 mg,				
60s ea, C-II	55887-0884-60	76.26		AA
(Phys Total Care)				
REPACK				
TAB, PO, 325 mg-5 mg,				
10s ea, C-II	54868-0510-03	36.83		AA
20s ea, C-II	54868-0510-02	70.54		
60s ea, C-II	54868-0510-00	194.14		AA
100s ea, C-II	54868-0510-01	321.49		AA
325 mg-7.5 mg,				
60s ea, C-II	54868-4603-01	252.11		
100s ea, C-II	54868-4603-00	382.32		
325 mg-10 mg,				
60s ea, C-II	54868-4710-01	368.67		
100s ea, C-II	54868-4710-00	611.84		
(CAPLET)				
500 mg-7.5 mg,				
10s ea, C-II	54868-4574-02	35.31		AA
30s ea, C-II	54868-4574-01	94.32		AA
100s ea, C-II	54868-4574-00	307.12		AA
650 mg-10 mg,				
30s ea, C-II	54868-4604-01	90.40		AA
60s ea, C-II	54868-4604-03	167.96		AA
100s ea, C-II	54868-4604-00	277.86		AA
120s ea, C-II	54868-4604-02	332.81		AA

PROD/MFR	NDC	AWP	DP	OBC
(Quality Care Prod)				
REPACK				
TAB, PO, 325 mg-5 mg,				
30s ea, C-II	**35356-0331-30**	176.62		
90s ea, C-II	**35356-0331-90**	529.86		
325 mg-7.5 mg,				
30s ea, C-II	**35356-0454-30**	296.60		**AA**
90s ea, C-II	**35356-0454-90**	889.80		**AA**
325 mg-10 mg,				
30s ea, C-II	**35356-0455-30**	322.00		**AA**
90s ea, C-II	**35356-0455-90**	966.00		**AA**
(Stat Rx)				
REPACK				
TAB, PO, 325 mg-5 mg,				
30s ea, C-II	**16590-0619-30**	129.31		
60s ea, C-II	**16590-0619-60**	255.37		
60s ea, C-II	**16590-0619-62**	356.22		
90s ea, C-II	**16590-0619-90**	381.43		
120s ea, C-II	**16590-0619-72**	360.00		
325 mg-7.5 mg,				
90s ea, C-II	**16590-0762-90**	382.27		**AA**
325 mg-10 mg,				
30s ea, C-II	**16590-0618-30**	181.34		**AA**
56s ea, C-II	**16590-0618-56**	335.68		**AA**
60s ea, C-II	**16590-0618-60**	359.42		**AA**
84s ea, C-II	**16590-0618-62**	467.73		**AA**
90s ea, C-II	**16590-0618-90**	537.51		**AA**
112s ea, C-II	**16590-0618-73**	668.11		**AA**
120s ea, C-II	**16590-0618-72**	715.60		**AA**
180s ea, C-II	**16590-0618-82**	1071.77		**AA**
650 mg-10 mg,				
30s ea, C-II	**16590-0620-30**	193.41		**AA**
56s ea, C-II	**16590-0620-56**	358.21		**AA**
60s ea, C-II	**16590-0620-60**	383.57		**AA**
84s ea, C-II	**16590-0620-62**	535.69		**AA**
90s ea, C-II	**16590-0620-90**	573.73		**AA**
112s ea, C-II	**16590-0620-73**	713.18		**AA**
120s ea, C-II	**16590-0620-72**	763.88		**AA**
150s ea, C-II	**16590-0620-83**	954.04		**AA**
PERCODAN (Endo Pharm)				
aspirin/oxycodone hydrochloride				
TAB, PO (USP)				
325 mg-4.8355 mg,				
100s ea, C-II	**63481-0121-70**	162.48		**AA**
PERFECT CHOICE (Biotrol)				
stannous fluoride				
GEL, DE, 0.4%, 129 gm	**50467-0110-04**	8.15		
129 gm	**50467-0811-04**	8.15		
129 gm	**50467-0812-04**	8.15		
129 gm	**50467-0816-04**	8.15		
(CREME DE MENTHE)				
0.4%, 129 gm	**50467-0813-04**	8.15		
(NO FLAVOR)				
0.4%, 129 gm	**50467-0815-04**	8.15		
PERFECTA (Amend)				
petrolatum				
POW, NA (U.S.P.)				
454 gm	**17317-1047-01**	4.90		
3178 gm	**17317-1047-06**	21.00		
16344 gm	**17317-1047-08**	88.20		
PERFLUTREN LIPID MICROSPHERE (Lantheus) *See DEFINITY*				
PERFLUTREN PROTEIN TYPE A MICROSPHERE (GE) *See OPTISON*				
PERFOROMIST (Dey, L.P.)				
formoterol fumarate				
SOL, IH, 20 mcg/2 ml,				
2 ml 60s	**49502-0605-61**	406.31		
PERGOLIDE MESYLATE (Gallipot)				
POW, NA, 0.5 gm	**51552-1065-09**	441.00	315.00	
(Hawkins)				
POW, NA, 0.1 gm	**63370-0169-06**	600.00		
0.5 gm	**63370-0169-09**	1800.00		
1 gm	**63370-0169-10**	2640.00		
5 gm	**63370-0169-15**	9600.00		
(Letco)				
POW, NA, 0.5 gm	**62991-2528-01**	675.00		
1 gm	**62991-2528-02**	1305.00		
(Medisca)				
POW, NA, 1 gm	**38779-1952-06**	1425.00		
5 gm	**38779-1952-03**	4950.00		
10 gm	**38779-1952-01**	8415.00		
(1X25GM,USP)				
25 gm	**38779-1952-04**	13500.00		
(PCCA)				
POW, NA (USP)				
1 gm	**51927-3512-00**	1950.00		
(Spectrum Pharmacy)				
POW, NA (1X0.5GM, USP)				
0.5 gm	**49452-5115-03**	1463.00		
(1X5GM, USP)				
5 gm	**49452-5115-05**	6828.50		
PERIDEX (Zila)				
chlorhexidine gluconate				
LIQ, PO, 0.12%, 473 ml	**51284-0620-22**	12.25		**AT**
(Quality Care Prod)				
REPACK				
LIQ, PO, 0.12%, 473 ml	**49999-0331-16**	20.83		**AT**
(Southwood)				
REPACK				
LIQ, PO, 0.12%, 480 ml	**58016-9062-01**	17.36		**AT**
PERILLYL ALCOHOL (PCCA)				
SOL, NA, 85%, 1 gm	**51927-3510-00**	25.50		
PERINDOPRIL ERBUMINE (Aurobindo Pharma)				
TAB, PO, 2 mg, 100s ea	**65862-0286-01**	197.45		**EE**
4 mg, 100s ea	**65862-0287-01**	230.24		**EE**
8 mg, 100s ea	**65862-0288-01**	279.64		**EE**
(Roxane)				
TAB, PO, 2 mg, 100s ea	**00054-0110-25**	189.77		**EE**
4 mg, 100s ea	**00054-0111-25**	221.27		**EE**
8 mg, 100s ea	**00054-0112-25**	268.76		**EE**
(Solvay) *See ACEON*				
PERIO MED (Omnii Intl)				
stannous fluoride				
GEL, DE (CINNAMON)				
0.63%, 283.5 gm	**48878-3316-00**	9.55		
(FRUIT,TROPICAL)				
0.63%, 283.5 gm	**48878-3317-00**	9.55		
(MINT)				
0.63%, 283.5 gm	**48878-3315-00**	9.55		
PERIOGARD (Colgate Oral)				
chlorhexidine gluconate				
LIQ, PO, 0.12%, 473 ml	**00126-0271-16**	10.40		**AT**
(Phys Total Care)				
REPACK				
LIQ, PO, 0.12%, 480 ml	**54868-3313-00**	8.51		**AT**
PERIOSTAT (Galderma)				
doxycycline hyclate				
TAB, PO, 20 mg, 100s ea	**00299-5960-02**	587.50		**AB**
(Southwood)				
REPACK				
TAB, PO, 20 mg, 30s ea	**58016-0955-30**	98.90		
60s ea	**58016-0955-60**	197.81		
90s ea	**58016-0955-90**	296.71		
100s ea	**58016-0955-00**	329.68		
PERITONEAL LAVAGE TRAY (Portex)				
lidocaine hydrochloride				
KIT, IJ, 1%, 10s ea	**00074-4961-20**	415.03	349.50	
PERMACOL (Covidien)				
implant insertion device				
DEV, NA (10CM X 10CM, 1MM)				
ea	**04523-0001-08**	2000.00		
(10CM X 15CM, 1.5MM)				
ea	**04523-0001-60**	3000.00		
(10CM X 15CM, 1MM)				
ea	**04523-0001-15**	3000.00		
(10CM X 20CM, 1.5MM)				
ea	**04523-0001-77**	4000.00		
(15CM X 20CM, 1.5MM)				
ea	**04523-0001-84**	6000.00		
(15CM X 20CM, 1MM)				
ea	**04523-0001-22**	6000.00		
(18CM X 28CM, 1.5MM)				
ea	**04523-0001-91**	11088.00		
(18CM X 28CM, 1MM)				
ea	**04523-0001-39**	11088.00		
(20CM X 30CM, 1.5MM)				
ea	**04523-0002-07**	13200.00		
(20CM X 40CM, 1.5MM)				
ea	**04523-0002-14**	17600.00		
(20CM X 50CM, 1.5MM)				
ea	**04523-0002-21**	22000.00		
(28CM X 40CM, 1.5MM)				
ea	**04523-0002-45**	24640.00		
(5CM X 10CM, 1MM)				
ea	**04523-0000-92**	1000.00		
(5CM X 5CM, 1MM)				
ea	**04523-0000-47**	500.00		
PERMETHRIN (Actavis Mid Atlantic)				
CRE, TP, 5%, 60 gm	**00472-0242-60**	29.25		**AB**
(Mylan) *See ACTICIN*				
(PCCA)				
SOL, NA (TECHNICAL)				
1 gm	**51927-3037-00**	1.20		
(Perrigo)				
CRE, TP (VANISHING CREAM)				
5%, 60 gm	**45802-0269-37**	29.25		**AB**
(A-S Medication)				
REPACK				
CRE, TP, 5%, 60 gm	**54569-5743-00**	29.25		
(Altura)				
REPACK				
CRE, TP (VANISHING CREAM)				
5%, 60 gm	**63874-0839-60**	29.95		**AB**
(Dispensing Solutions)				
REPACK				
CRE, TP, 5%, 60 gm	**55045-2613-06**	29.15		
(Palmetto)				
REPACK				
CRE, TP, 5%, 60 gm	**23490-6075-01**	30.29		
(Pharma Pac)				
REPACK				
CRE, TP, 5%, 60 gm	**52959-0159-06**	29.55		**AB**
(Phys Total Care)				
REPACK				
CRE, TP (VANISHING CREAM)				
5%, 60 gm	**54868-5391-00**	30.66		**AB**
(Physician Partner)				
REPACK				
CRE, TP (1X60GM,VANISHING CREAM)				
5%, 60 gm	**21695-0907-60**	58.50		**AB**
PERODERM (Breckenridge Pharm)				
benzoyl peroxide/urea				
GEL, TP (1X125ML)				
4.5%-10%, 125 ml	**51991-0499-07**	70.50		
6.5%-10%, 125 ml	**51991-0500-07**	71.00		
8.5%-10%, 125 ml	**51991-0501-07**	71.50		
PERODERM CLEANSER (Breckenridge Pharm)				
benzoyl peroxide/urea				
SOA, TP (1X400ML)				
4.5%-10%, 400 ml	**51991-0502-46**	70.50		
6.5%-10%, 400 ml	**51991-0503-46**	71.00		
8.5%-10%, 400 ml	**51991-0504-46**	71.50		
PERPHENAZINE (PCCA)				
POW, NA (U.S.P.)				
1 gm	**51927-2351-00**	24.00		
(Qualitest)				
TAB, PO (SUGAR-COATED)				
2 mg, 100s ea	**00603-5090-21**	82.52		**AB**
500s ea	**00603-5090-28**	391.97		**AB**
4 mg, 100s ea	**00603-5091-21**	112.91		**AB**
500s ea	**00603-5091-28**	536.32		**AB**
8 mg, 100s ea	**00603-5092-21**	136.99		**AB**
500s ea	**00603-5092-28**	650.70		**AB**
16 mg, 100s ea	**00603-5093-21**	184.29		**AB**
(Sandoz)				
TAB, PO, 2 mg, 100s ea	**00781-1046-01**	82.52		**AB**
100s ea UD	**00781-1046-13**	92.83		**AB**
1000s ea	**00781-1046-10**	783.89		**AB**
4 mg, 100s ea	**00781-1047-01**	112.91		**AB**
100s ea UD	**00781-1047-13**	127.01		**AB**
1000s ea	**00781-1047-10**	1072.65		**AB**
8 mg, 100s ea	**00781-1048-01**	136.99		**AB**
100s ea UD	**00781-1048-13**	154.10		**AB**
1000s ea	**00781-1048-10**	1301.37		**AB**
16 mg, 100s ea	**00781-1049-01**	184.29		**AB**
100s ea UD	**00781-1049-13**	207.32		**AB**
(GSMS)				
REPACK				
TAB, PO (UNIT OF USE)				
4 mg, 60s ea	**60429-0153-60**	33.60	11.20	**AB**
8 mg, 60s ea	**60429-0154-60**	42.00	14.00	**AB**
(Pharma Pac)				
REPACK				
TAB, PO (SUGAR-COATED)				
8 mg, 60s ea	**52959-0940-60**	241.85		**AB**
(Phys Total Care)				
REPACK				
TAB, PO, 4 mg, 30s ea	**54868-2686-00**	18.02		**EE**
8 mg, 60s ea	**54868-2687-02**	76.83		**EE**
100s ea	**54868-2687-01**	98.58		**EE**
(Physician Partner)				
REPACK				
TAB, PO, 4 mg, 60s ea	**21695-0414-60**	113.00		
(FILM-COATED)				
8 mg, 60s ea	**21695-0415-60**	137.10		

PROD/MFR	NDC	AWP	DP	OBC
(Quality Care Prod)				
REPACK				
TAB, PO, 8 mg, 60s ea	35356-0096-60	146.30		
(Southwood)				
REPACK				
TAB, PO, 4 mg, 30s ea	00490-0091-30	28.30		
60s ea	00490-0091-60	56.59		
90s ea	00490-0091-90	84.89		
100s ea	00490-0091-00	94.32		
(Vibranta)				
REPACK				
TAB, PO, 4 mg, 30s ea	57866-4132-01	20.60		AB
60s ea	57866-4132-02	41.10		AB
90s ea	57866-4132-03	60.25		AB
8 mg, 30s ea	57866-4133-01	25.50		AB
60s ea	57866-4133-02	47.90		AB
90s ea	57866-4133-03	94.70		AB
PERPHENAZINE/AMITRIPTYLINE (Southwood)				
REPACK				
amitriptyline hydrochloride/perphenazine				
TAB, PO, 25 mg-2 mg,				
30s ea	58016-0073-30	9.12		
60s ea	58016-0073-60	18.24		
90s ea	58016-0073-90	27.36		
100s ea	58016-0073-00	30.40		
PERSANTINE (Boehr Ingelheim Phar)				
dipyridamole				
TAB, PO, 25 mg, 100s ea	00597-0017-01	87.17		AB
50 mg, 100s ea	00597-0018-01	140.44		AB
75 mg, 100s ea	00597-0019-01	187.88		AB
(Phys Total Care)				
REPACK				
TAB, PO, 25 mg, 100s ea	54868-1288-00	55.13		AB
PERSONAL BEST PEAK FLOW METER (Respironics)				
meter, peak flow, spirometry				
DEV, NA (FULL RANGE)				
ea	83730-0755-00	24.67		
(LOW RANGE)				
ea	83730-0756-00	24.67		
PERTUDORON 1 (Weleda)				
homeopathic substance				
LIQ, PO, 20 ml	55946-0330-10	4.65		
PERTUDORON 2 (CUPRUM ACETICUM) (Weleda)				
homeopathic substance				
LIQ, PO (3X)				
20 ml	55946-0340-10	4.65		
PERU BALSAM				
(Gallipot) *See PERUVIAN BALSAM*				
(Lorann Oil) *See BALSAM PERU*				
(PCCA) *See PERUVIAN BALSAM*				
(Spectrum Pharmacy) *See PERUVIAN BALSAM*				
PERUVIAN BALSAM (Gallipot)				
peru balsam				
POW, NA, 113.4 gm	51552-0317-04	24.36		
454 gm	51552-0317-06	83.72		
(PCCA)				
POW, NA, 1 gm	51927-1118-00	0.51		
(Spectrum Pharmacy)				
SOL, NA (1X125GM)				
125 gm	49452-5125-01	77.35		
(1X500GM)				
500 gm	49452-5125-02	258.65		
PETROLATUM				
(Amend) *See ALBA PROTOPET*				
(Amend) *See PERFECTA*				
(Gallipot) *See PETROLATUM WHITE*				
(Gallipot) *See PETROLATUM YELLOW*				
(Letco) *See PETROLATUM WHITE*				
(Medisca) *See PETROLATUM WHITE*				
(Medisca) *See PETROLATUM YELLOW*				
(PCCA) *See PETROLATUM YELLOW*				
(PCCA)				
POW, NA (USP, WHITE)				
1 gm	51927-1024-00	0.13		
PETROLATUM HYDROPHILIC (Gallipot)				
petrolatum, hydrophilic				
OIN, NA, 454 gm	51552-0753-06	17.85	12.75	
PETROLATUM WHITE (Gallipot)				
petrolatum				
OIN, NA (U.S.P.)				
454 gm	51552-0239-06	10.22		
2270 gm	51552-0239-08	26.11		
15890 gm	51552-0239-09	154.00		
(Letco)				
OIN, NA (U.S.P.)				
500 gm	62991-1250-02	27.00		
2500 gm	62991-1250-01	60.00		
(Medisca)				
OIN, NA (U.S.P.)				
454 gm	38779-0040-08	25.50		
(1X5000GM,USP)				
5000 gm	38779-0040-03	105.00		
PETROLATUM YELLOW (Gallipot)				
petrolatum				
OIN, NA (U.S.P.,N.F.)				
454 gm	51552-0309-06	11.06		
(Medisca)				
OIN, NA (U.S.P.)				
454 gm	38779-0041-08	21.00		
(1X5000GM,USP)				
5000 gm	38779-0041-03	99.00		
(PCCA)				
OIN, NA (USP)				
1 gm	51927-2880-00	0.07		
PETROLATUM, HYDROPHILIC				
(Gallipot) *See PETROLATUM HYDROPHILIC*				
(Medisca) *See HYDROPHYLLIC PETROLATUM*				
PEXEVA (Noven)				
paroxetine mesylate				
TAB, PO (FILM COATED)				
10 mg, 30s ea	68968-2010-01	168.04		EE
20 mg, 30s ea	68968-2020-01	174.67		EE
(FILM-COATED)				
30 mg, 30s ea	68968-2030-01	181.32		EE
(FILM COATED)				
40 mg, 30s ea	68968-2040-01	187.98		
PFIZERPEN (Pfizer)				
penicillin g potassium				
PDS, IV (VIAL, PHARMACY BOTTLE)				
5 million u,				
10s ea	00049-0520-83	87.05	72.54	AP
20 million u, ea	00049-0530-28	25.52	21.27	AP
PHANATUSS-HC DIABETIC CHOICE (Pharmakon)				
guaifenesin/hydrocodone bitartrate				
SOL, PO (AF,SF,SODIUM-FREE,MINT)				
100 mg/5 ml-5 mg/5 ml,				
473 ml, C-III	55422-0888-16	17.26	17.26	
PHEN/CLOR TAN PED (Phys Total Care)				
REPACK				
chlorpheniramine tannate/phenylephrine tannate				
SUS, PO, 4.5 mg/5 ml-5 mg/5 ml,				
473 ml	54868-4962-01	159.69		
PHENA-HC (GM Pharm)				
cpm/hydrocod bit/phenyleph hcl/pyril mal				
SOL, PO (AF,SF,DYE-FREE,GRAPE)				
473 ml, C-III	58809-0442-01	39.95	31.96	
PHENA-PLUS (GM Pharm)				
cpm/phenyleph hcl/pyril mal				
TAB, PO, 2 mg-10 mg-10 mg,				
100s ea	58809-0281-01	57.50	46.00	
PHENA-S (GM Pharm)				
cpm/phenyleph hcl/pyril mal				
LIQ, PO (AF,SF,GRAPE)				
473 ml	58809-0112-01	74.00	59.20	
PHENA-S 12 (GM Pharm)				
cpm/phenyleph hcl/phenyleph tan/pyril tan				
SUS, PO (AF,SF,ORANGE-PINEAPPLE)				
473 ml	58809-0912-01	89.25	69.80	
PHENABID (Gil Pharmaceutical)				
cpm/phenyleph hcl				
TER, PO (12HR,PF,SF,DYE-FREE)				
8 mg-20 mg,				
100s ea	58552-0305-01	161.65		
PHENABID DM (Gil Pharmaceutical)				
cpm/dm/phenyleph hcl				
TER, PO (PF,SF,DYE-FREE)				
8 mg-30 mg-20 mg,				
100s ea	58552-0306-01	190.22		
PHENACEMIDE				
(PCCA) *See PHENYLACETYLUREA*				
PHENACETIN (Amend)				
POW, NA (PURIFIED)				
125 gm	17317-0412-04	8.70		
500 gm	17317-0412-01	21.00		
2270 gm	17317-0412-05	98.00		
11350 gm	17317-0412-08	420.00		
(Baker, J.T.)				
POW, NA (PURIFIED)				
125 gm	10106-2848-04	43.26		
PHENADOZ (Paddock)				
promethazine hydrochloride				
SUP, RC, 12.5 mg,				
12s ea UD	00574-7236-12	46.72	46.72	AB
25 mg, 12s ea UD	00574-7234-12	53.36	53.56	AB
(Quality Care Prod)				
REPACK				
SUP, RC, 25 mg, 12s ea	35356-0039-12	53.20		
PHENAVENT D (Ethex)				
guaifenesin/phenylephrine hydrochloride				
TER, PO (FILM-COATED)				
1200 mg-40 mg,				
100s ea	58177-0444-04	72.25		
PHENAZO HCL (Contract Pharmacal)				
phenazopyridine hydrochloride				
TAB, PO, 100 mg, 100s ea	10267-0025-01	47.75		
1000s ea	10267-0025-10	405.81		
PHENAZOPYRIDINE (Bryant Ranch)				
REPACK				
phenazopyridine hydrochloride				
TAB, PO, 100 mg, 9s ea	63629-1616-03	6.02		
12s ea	63629-1616-02	8.02		
20s ea	63629-1616-01	13.37		
200 mg, 9s ea	63629-1595-01	8.91		
10s ea	63629-1595-04	9.90		
15s ea	63629-1595-05	14.85		
20s ea	63629-1595-02	19.80		
30s ea	63629-1595-03	29.70		
(Core)				
REPACK				
TAB, PO, 100 mg, 12s ea	33358-0288-12	8.22		
20s ea	33358-0288-20	13.70		
200 mg, 9s ea	33358-0289-09	8.00		
10s ea	33358-0289-10	10.15		
30s ea	33358-0289-30	30.44		
(Dispensing Solutions)				
REPACK				
TAB, PO, 200 mg, 9s ea	66336-0105-09	15.23		
(Stat Rx)				
REPACK				
TAB, PO, 200 mg, 6s ea	16590-0184-06	9.50		
10s ea	16590-0184-10	15.84		
12s ea	16590-0184-12	19.00		
20s ea	16590-0184-20	31.66		
PHENAZOPYRIDINE HCL (Breckenridge Pharm)				
phenazopyridine hydrochloride				
TAB, PO, 100 mg, 100s ea	51991-0520-01	44.75		
(FILM-COATED)				
200 mg, 100s ea	51991-0525-01	84.95		
(Consolidated Midland)				
TAB, PO, 100 mg, 100s ea	00223-1442-01	5.50		
1000s ea	00223-1442-02	27.50		
200 mg, 100s ea	00223-1443-01	7.50		
1000s ea	00223-1443-02	34.50		
(Contract Pharmacal)				
TAB, PO, 200 mg, 100s ea	10267-0860-01	86.95		
1000s ea	10267-0860-10	749.52		
(Medisca)				
POW, NA (U.S.P.)				
100 gm	38779-0122-05	46.50		
500 gm	38779-0122-08	193.50		
(PCCA)				
POW, NA (U.S.P.)				
1 gm	51927-1069-00	1.86		
(Spectrum Pharmacy)				
POW, NA (U.S.P.)				
100 gm	49452-5166-01	310.10		
500 gm	49452-5166-02	1344.00		
(Vintage)				
TAB, PO, 100 mg, 100s ea	00254-4971-28	45.08		
200 mg, 100s ea	00254-4972-28	83.25		
(A-S Medication)				
REPACK				
TAB, PO, 100 mg, 6s ea	54569-0199-08	2.85		
10s ea	54569-0199-00	4.75		
12s ea	54569-0199-05	5.69		
(Altura)				
REPACK				
TAB, PO, 100 mg, 15s ea	63874-0376-15	8.24		
30s ea	63874-0376-30	16.62		
100s ea	63874-0376-10	68.23		
1000s ea	63874-0376-01	301.25		
200 mg, 15s ea	63874-0375-15	15.86		

PROD/MFR	NDC	AWP	DP	OBC
30s ea	63874-0375-30	32.00		
100s ea	63874-0375-10	115.63		
1000s ea	63874-0375-01	589.63		
(DHS, Inc.)				
REPACK				
TAB, PO, 200 mg, 6s ea	55887-0827-06	6.45		
10s ea	55887-0827-10	10.70		
12s ea	55887-0827-12	12.84		
20s ea	55887-0827-20	21.40		
(Dispensing Solutions)				
REPACK				
TAB, PO, 100 mg, 6s ea	55045-1235-06	5.10		
15s ea	55045-1235-05	12.75		
200 mg, 6s ea	55045-1409-02	6.15		
6s ea	66336-0105-06	10.34		
9s ea	55045-1409-08	9.27		
10s ea	55045-1409-03	10.30		
10s ea	66336-0105-10	16.87		
15s ea	55045-1409-05	15.45		
15s ea	66336-0105-15	25.03		
20s ea	66336-0105-20	33.37		
(HomeMed)				
REPACK				
TAB, PO, 100 mg, 10s ea	51655-0153-53	9.99		
12s ea	51655-0153-27	5.87		
200 mg, 6s ea	51655-0175-87	9.99		
9s ea	51655-0175-85	11.99		
12s ea	51655-0175-27	14.99		
15s ea	51655-0175-54	6.30		
(PD-Rx Pharm)				
REPACK				
TAB, PO, 100 mg, 6s ea	55289-0713-06	8.98		
8s ea	55289-0713-08	9.73		
10s ea	55289-0713-10	10.51		
(REDI-SCRIPT)				
100 mg, 10s ea	58864-0397-10	10.51		
12s ea	55289-0713-12	11.29		
(REDI-SCRIPT)				
100 mg, 15s ea	58864-0397-15	12.33		
18s ea	55289-0713-18	13.60		
(REDI-SCRIPT,USP)				
100 mg, 20s ea	58864-0397-20	13.90		
30s ea	55289-0713-30	14.34		
200 mg, 6s ea	55289-0209-06	8.38		
8s ea	55289-0209-08	8.93		
9s ea	55289-0209-09	9.22		
10s ea	55289-0209-10	9.51		
12s ea	55289-0209-12	10.07		
15s ea	55289-0209-15	10.93		
20s ea	55289-0209-20	12.36		
30s ea	55289-0209-30	15.20		
100s ea	55289-0209-01	35.11		
100s ea UD	55289-0209-17	41.71		
(Pharma Pac)				
REPACK				
TAB, PO, 100 mg, 6s ea	52959-0202-06	4.83		
10s ea	52959-0202-10	7.51		
20s ea	52959-0202-20	14.48		
30s ea	52959-0202-30	20.13		
200 mg, 3s ea	52959-0122-03	1.05		
4s ea	52959-0122-04	1.34		
6s ea	52959-0122-06	7.79		
9s ea	52959-0122-09	11.55		
10s ea	52959-0122-10	12.65		
12s ea	52959-0122-12	14.91		
15s ea	52959-0122-15	18.15		
20s ea	52959-0122-20	23.50		
30s ea	52959-0122-30	34.89		
(Phys Total Care)				
REPACK				
TAB, PO, 100 mg, 6s ea	54868-0249-06	6.51		
10s ea	54868-0249-00	6.36		
20s ea	54868-0249-03	9.69		
30s ea	54868-0249-02	13.05		
40s ea	54868-0249-05	16.38		
100s ea	54868-0249-04	34.95		
200 mg, 5s ea	54868-0250-04	5.13		
6s ea	54868-0250-06	5.55		
10s ea	54868-0250-01	7.26		
15s ea	54868-0250-07	9.39		
20s ea	54868-0250-02	11.52		
30s ea	54868-0250-08	15.78		
100s ea	54868-0250-00	44.10		
(Physician Partner)				
REPACK				
TAB, PO, 200 mg, 30s ea	21695-0301-30	43.88		
(Quality Care Prod)				
REPACK				
TAB, PO, 100 mg, 8s ea	49999-0047-08	7.73		
10s ea	49999-0047-10	6.33		
12s ea	49999-0047-12	7.60		
15s ea	49999-0047-15	9.46		
200 mg, 6s ea	49999-0176-06	7.32		
9s ea	49999-0176-09	13.66		
10s ea	49999-0176-10	15.18		
15s ea	49999-0176-15	22.77		
(Southwood)				
REPACK				
TAB, PO, 200 mg, 6s ea	58016-0152-06	6.09		
8s ea	58016-0152-08	8.12		
9s ea	58016-0152-09	9.14		
10s ea	58016-0152-10	10.16		
12s ea	58016-0152-12	12.19		
14s ea	58016-0152-14	14.22		
15s ea	58016-0152-15	15.24		
20s ea	58016-0152-20	20.32		
21s ea	58016-0152-21	21.34		
24s ea	58016-0152-24	24.38		
28s ea	58016-0152-28	28.45		
30s ea	58016-0152-30	30.48		
50s ea	58016-0152-50	50.80		
100s ea	58016-0152-00	101.60		
(Stat Rx)				
REPACK				
TAB, PO, 100 mg, 6s ea	16590-0728-06	2.74		
(Vibranta)				
REPACK				
TAB, PO, 200 mg, 6s ea	57866-4392-03	6.26		
9s ea	57866-4392-06	9.85		
10s ea	57866-4392-04	10.60		
PHENAZOPYRIDINE HYDROCHLORIDE (Amneal)				
TAB, PO (USP,FILM-COATED)				
100 mg, 100s ea	65162-0517-10	44.50		
200 mg, 100s ea	65162-0520-10	85.25		
(Breckenridge Pharm) *See PHENAZOPYRIDINE HCL*				
(Consolidated Midland) *See PHENAZOPYRIDINE HCL*				
(Contract Pharmacal) *See PHENAZO HCL*				
(Contract Pharmacal) *See PHENAZOPYRIDINE HCL*				
(Medisca) *See PHENAZOPYRIDINE HCL*				
(PCCA) *See PHENAZOPYRIDINE HCL*				
(SDA)				
TAB, PO (SUGAR COATED)				
100 mg, 100s ea	66424-0043-01	47.50	4.00	
200 mg, 100s ea	66424-0045-01	83.00	5.00	
1000s ea	66424-0045-10	725.00	38.00	
(Spectrum Pharmacy) *See PHENAZOPYRIDINE HCL*				
(Teva)				
TAB, PO, 100 mg, 100s ea	00182-0138-01	45.09		
200 mg, 100s ea	00182-0904-01	83.25		
(Truxton) *See PYRIDIATE*				
(Vintage) *See PHENAZOPYRIDINE HCL*				
(Warner Chilcott) *See PYRIDIUM*				
(A-S Medication)				
REPACK				
TAB, PO (SUGAR COATED)				
200 mg, 6s ea	54569-0197-04	5.13		
9s ea	54569-0197-07	7.69		
10s ea	54569-0197-00	8.54		
12s ea	54569-0197-06	10.25		
15s ea	54569-0197-01	12.81		
20s ea	54569-0197-02	17.09		
(American Health)				
REPACK				
TAB, PO (10X10,FILM-COATED)				
100 mg, 100s ea UD	68084-0292-01	50.73		
200 mg, 100s ea UD	68084-0293-01	93.69		
(McKesson Packaging)				
REPACK				
TAB, PO (USP)				
100 mg, 100s ea UD	63739-0309-10	50.73		
(Palmetto)				
REPACK				
TAB, PO, 200 mg, 6s ea	23490-6080-01	9.24		
9s ea	23490-6080-04	9.90		
10s ea	23490-6080-05	11.00		
12s ea	23490-6080-03	13.20		
15s ea	23490-6080-07	16.50		
18s ea	23490-6080-00	19.79		
20s ea	23490-6080-02	21.99		
(PD-Rx Pharm)				
REPACK				
TAB, PO (USP,FILM-COATED)				
100 mg, 6s ea	43063-0058-06	8.00		
(FILM-COATED)				
200 mg, 6s ea	43063-0022-06	8.38		
(USP,FILM-COATED)				
200 mg, 18s ea	55289-0209-18	11.96		
(Physician Partner)				
REPACK				
TAB, PO (SUGAR COATED)				
100 mg, 10s ea	21695-0638-10	11.16		
30s ea	21695-0638-30	28.47		
200 mg, 6s ea	21695-0301-06	10.43		
9s ea	21695-0301-09	15.65		
10s ea	21695-0301-10	17.21		
12s ea	21695-0301-12	20.65		
15s ea	21695-0301-15	25.81		
PHENAZOPYRIDINE PLUS (Breckenridge Pharm)				
belladonna alkaloids and analgesics				
TAB, PO (FILM-COATED)				
15 mg-0.3 mg-150 mg,				
30s ea	51991-0251-33	37.55		
(Contract Pharmacal)				
TAB, PO (FILM-COATED)				
15 mg-0.3 mg-150 mg,				
30s ea	10267-2929-03	28.12		
90s ea	10267-2929-05	77.00		
PHENCARB GG (Boca Pharmacal)				
carbetapentane cit/gg/phenyleph hcl				
SYR, PO (SPEARMINT)				
473 ml	64376-0537-16	41.36		
PHENCLOR TANNATE PEDIATRIC (Phys Total Care)				
REPACK				
chlorpheniramine tannate/phenylephrine tannate				
SUS, PO, 4.5 mg/5 ml-5 mg/5 ml,				
120 ml	54868-4962-00	80.28		
PHENDIET (Truxton)				
phendimetrazine tartrate				
TAB, PO, 35 mg,				
1000s ea, C-III	00463-6247-10	36.00		EE
PHENDIET-105 (Truxton)				
phendimetrazine tartrate				
CER, PO, 105 mg,				
1000s ea, C-III	00463-3029-10	150.00		EE
PHENDIMETRAZINE (Bryant Ranch)				
REPACK				
phendimetrazine tartrate				
CER, PO, 105 mg,				
28s ea, C-III	63629-3051-01	33.60		
(DHS, Inc.)				
REPACK				
TAB, PO, 35 mg,				
21s ea, C-III	55887-0225-21	17.05		
30s ea, C-III	55887-0225-30	21.95		
PHENDIMETRAZINE TARTRATE (Sandoz)				
CER, PO, 105 mg,				
100s ea, C-III	00185-5254-01	128.73		BC
1000s ea, C-III	00185-5254-10	1222.90		BC
TAB, PO, 35 mg,				
100s ea, C-III	00185-4057-01	21.07		AA
1000s ea, C-III	00185-4057-10	189.64		AA
(Truxton) *See PHENDIET*				
(Truxton) *See PHENDIET-105*				
(Truxton)				
TAB, PO (WHITE)				
35 mg,				
100s ea, C-III	00463-8000-01	19.90		EE
(YELLOW)				
35 mg,				
100s ea, C-III	00463-7500-01	19.90		EE
(WHITE)				
35 mg,				
1000s ea, C-III	00463-8000-10	178.90		EE
(YELLOW)				
35 mg,				
1000s ea, C-III	00463-7500-10	178.90		EE
(Valeant Pharm Intl) *See BONTRIL PDM*				
(Valeant Pharm Intl) *See BONTRIL SLOW-RELEASE*				
(A-S Medication)				
REPACK				
CER, PO, 105 mg,				
14s ea, C-III	54569-2198-00	18.02		BC
30s ea, C-III	54569-2198-01	38.62		BC
TAB, PO, 35 mg,				
7s ea, C-III	54569-2668-04	1.47		EE
14s ea, C-III	54569-2668-05	2.95		EE
(YELLOW)				
35 mg,				
14s ea, C-III	54569-5233-02	2.95		EE

PROD/MFR	NDC	AWP	DP	OBC
21s ea, C-III	54569-2668-06	4.42		EE
28s ea, C-III	54569-4336-00	5.90		EE
(YELLOW)				
35 mg,				
28s ea, C-III	54569-5195-06	5.90		EE
30s ea, C-III	54569-2668-09	6.32		EE
(YELLOW)				
35 mg,				
30s ea, C-III	54569-5195-00	6.32		EE
42s ea, C-III	54569-2668-01	8.85		EE
(YELLOW)				
35 mg,				
42s ea, C-III	54569-5195-04	8.85		EE
56s ea, C-III	54569-2668-07	11.80		EE
(YELLOW)				
35 mg,				
56s ea, C-III	54569-5195-08	11.80		EE
60s ea, C-III	54569-5195-01	12.64		EE
84s ea, C-III	54569-5195-07	17.70		EE
90s ea, C-III	54569-5195-02	18.96		EE
100s ea, C-III	54569-2668-00	21.07		EE
(YELLOW)				
35 mg,				
114s ea, C-III	54569-5195-09	23.60		EE
140s ea, C-III	54569-5233-00	29.50		EE
168s ea, C-III	54569-5195-05	35.40		EE
180s ea, C-III	54569-5195-03	37.93		EE
1000s ea, C-III	54569-5233-01	210.70		EE
(Altura)				
REPACK				
TAB, PO, 35 mg,				
7s ea, C-III	63874-0269-07	4.89		AA
10s ea, C-III	63874-0269-10	6.99		AA
12s ea, C-III	63874-0269-12	8.39		AA
14s ea, C-III	63874-0269-14	9.78		AA
15s ea, C-III	63874-0269-15	10.48		AA
20s ea, C-III	63874-0269-20	13.99		AA
21s ea, C-III	63874-0269-21	14.68		AA
24s ea, C-III	63874-0269-24	16.77		AA
30s ea, C-III	63874-0269-30	20.97		AA
40s ea, C-III	63874-0269-40	27.95		AA
60s ea, C-III	63874-0269-60	41.93		AA
100s ea, C-III	63874-0269-01	69.88		AA
120s ea, C-III	63874-0269-03	83.85		AA
(Bryant Ranch)				
REPACK				
TAB, PO, 35 mg,				
15s ea, C-III	63629-1604-03	3.15		
30s ea, C-III	63629-1604-02	6.30		
60s ea, C-III	63629-1604-01	12.60		
100s ea, C-III	63629-1604-04	21.00		
(Core)				
REPACK				
TAB, PO, 35 mg,				
15s ea, C-III	33358-0287-15	3.23		
30s ea, C-III	33358-0287-30	6.46		
60s ea, C-III	33358-0287-60	12.92		
(Dispensing Solutions)				
REPACK				
CER, PO, 105 mg,				
7s ea, C-III	66336-0562-07	9.91		BC
14s ea, C-III	66336-0562-14	19.82		BC
28s ea, C-III	66336-0562-28	39.65		BC
30s ea, C-III	66336-0562-30	42.48		BC
TAB, PO, 35 mg,				
21s ea, C-III	66336-0191-21	9.95		AA
28s ea, C-III	66336-0191-28	10.86		AA
30s ea, C-III	55045-2954-08	12.60		
30s ea, C-III	66336-0191-30	11.47		AA
42s ea, C-III	66336-0191-42	12.70		AA
56s ea, C-III	66336-0191-56	16.93		AA
60s ea, C-III	66336-0191-60	18.14		AA
84s ea, C-III	55045-3817-08	35.88		
84s ea, C-III	66336-0191-84	25.39		AA
90s ea, C-III	66336-0191-90	27.20		AA
(Palmetto)				
REPACK				
CER, PO, 105 mg,				
7s ea, C-III	23490-6081-01	10.56		
14s ea, C-III	23490-6081-02	16.21		
28s ea, C-III	23490-6081-03	32.42		
30s ea, C-III	23490-6081-04	34.74		
TAB, PO, 35 mg,				
21s ea, C-III	23490-6082-07	9.45		
28s ea, C-III	23490-6082-01	12.60		
30s ea, C-III	23490-6082-02	13.50		
42s ea, C-III	23490-6082-03	18.90		
56s ea, C-III	23490-6082-04	25.20		
60s ea, C-III	23490-6082-05	27.00		
84s ea, C-III	23490-6082-06	37.80		
90s ea, C-III	23490-6082-08	40.50		

PROD/MFR	NDC	AWP	DP	OBC
(PD-Rx Pharm)				
REPACK				
CER, PO, 105 mg,				
7s ea, C-III	55289-0302-07	15.09		BC
14s ea, C-III	55289-0302-14	31.23		BC
(BROWN/CLEAR)				
105 mg,				
28s ea, C-III	55289-0302-28	41.64		BC
30s ea, C-III	55289-0302-30	43.59		BC
TAB, PO (YELLOW)				
35 mg,				
7s ea, C-III	55289-0834-07	9.89		AA
14s ea, C-III	55289-0834-14	10.94		AA
21s ea, C-III	55289-0834-21	11.79		AA
28s ea, C-III	55289-0834-28	15.60		AA
(USP)				
35 mg,				
30s ea, C-III	55289-0834-30	15.90		AA
(YELLOW)				
35 mg,				
56s ea, C-III	55289-0834-56	22.16		AA
60s ea, C-III	55289-0834-60	26.20		AA
84s ea, C-III	55289-0834-84	37.80		AA
90s ea, C-III	55289-0834-90	40.50		AA
112s ea, C-III	55289-0834-88	50.40		AA
120s ea, C-III	55289-0834-98	54.00		AA
(YELLOW)				
35 mg,				
140s ea, C-III	55289-0834-89	60.12		AA
180s ea, C-III	55289-0834-93	63.66		AA
(YELLOW)				
35 mg,				
240s ea, C-III	55289-0834-99	72.21		AA
360s ea, C-III	55289-0834-86	127.07		AA
(Pharma Pac)				
REPACK				
CER, PO, 105 mg,				
7s ea, C-III	52959-0886-07	10.60		
30s ea, C-III	52959-0886-30	32.76		
TAB, PO, 35 mg,				
21s ea, C-III	52959-0282-21	8.74		EE
28s ea, C-III	52959-0282-28	11.66		EE
30s ea, C-III	52959-0282-30	12.50		EE
42s ea, C-III	52959-0282-42	17.46		EE
90s ea, C-III	52959-0282-90	37.38		EE
100s ea, C-III	52959-0282-00	41.49		EE
(Phys Total Care)				
REPACK				
CER, PO, 105 mg,				
7s ea, C-III	54868-3071-01	29.51		BC
30s ea, C-III	54868-3071-00	66.92		BC
TAB, PO, 35 mg,				
30s ea, C-III	54868-0252-00	22.29		EE
90s ea, C-III	54868-0252-04	59.42		AA
100s ea, C-III	54868-0252-03	63.84		EE
1000s ea, C-III	54868-0252-01	459.87		EE
PHENDIMETRAZINE TARTRATE (Physician Partner)				
REPACK				
TAB, PO, 35 mg,				
7s ea, C-III	21695-0597-07	7.95		
PHENDIMETRAZINE TARTRATE (Physician Partner)				
21s ea, C-III	21695-0597-21	23.85		AA
PHENDIMETRAZINE TARTRATE (Physician Partner)				
60s ea, C-III	21695-0597-60	42.95		
PHENDIMETRAZINE TARTRATE (Quality Care Prod)				
REPACK				
CER, PO, 105 mg,				
28s ea, C-III	49999-0360-28	39.76		BC
30s ea, C-III	49999-0360-30	42.60		BC
TAB, PO, 35 mg,				
28s ea, C-III	35356-0003-28	15.20		
28s ea, C-III	49999-0003-28	7.00		
30s ea, C-III	35356-0003-30	16.00		
30s ea, C-III	35356-0003-90	48.00		AA
60s ea, C-III	35356-0003-60	32.00		
(Stat Rx)				
REPACK				
TAB, PO, 35 mg,				
30s ea, C-III	16590-0642-30	22.50		AA
60s ea, C-III	16590-0642-60	29.00		AA
PHENELZINE SULFATE (PCCA)				
POW, NA (U.S.P.)				
1 gm	51927-2404-00	51.00		
(Pfizer) *See NARDIL*				
PHENERGAN (Baxter)				
promethazine hydrochloride				
SOL, IJ, 25 mg/ml, 1 ml	60977-0001-43	2.66		
1 ml	60977-0001-44	2.66		

PROD/MFR	NDC	AWP	DP	OBC
(25X1ML,DOSETTE)				
25 mg/ml, 1 ml 25s	60977-0001-03	66.60		
(AMP)				
25 mg/ml, 1 ml 25s	60977-0001-01	66.60		
50 mg/ml, 1 ml	60977-0002-43	3.68		
1 ml	60977-0002-44	3.68		
(1X25ML,DOSETTE)				
50 mg/ml, 1 ml 25s	60977-0002-04	92.10		
(AMP)				
50 mg/ml, 1 ml 25s	60977-0002-02	92.10		
(Wyeth)				
TAB, PO, 50 mg, 100s ea	00008-0227-01	90.54	72.43	BP
(Dispensing Solutions)				
REPACK				
SUP, RC, 25 mg, 4s ea	55045-1749-02	26.65		AB
(Pharma Pac)				
REPACK				
SUP, RC, 12.5 mg, 4s ea	52959-0561-04	28.39		
12s ea	52959-0561-01	52.17		
25 mg, 6s ea	52959-0562-06	26.03		AB
12s ea	52959-0562-01	47.90		AB
TAB, PO, 25 mg, 2s ea	52959-0451-02	5.77		BP
30s ea	52959-0451-30	16.23		BP
(Phys Total Care)				
REPACK				
SOL, IJ (AMP)				
25 mg/ml, 1 ml 25s	54868-0597-00	91.24		AP
SUP, RC, 12.5 mg, ea	54868-1932-01	6.37		
6s ea	54868-1932-02	32.59		
12s ea	54868-1932-00	62.68		
25 mg, 2s ea	54868-1933-00	12.99		BR
6s ea	54868-1933-02	37.10		BR
12s ea	54868-1933-01	71.69		BR
50 mg, 6s ea	54868-1406-01	46.99		BR
TAB, PO, 12.5 mg, 12s ea	54868-0721-00	6.57		
25 mg, 30s ea	54868-1285-01	22.63		BP
60s ea	54868-1285-00	43.36		BP
(Quality Care Prod)				
REPACK				
TAB, PO, 12.5 mg, 6s ea	49999-0269-06	30.84		BP
25 mg, 5s ea	49999-0594-05	12.75		BP
30s ea	49999-0594-30	76.39		
90s ea	49999-0594-90	229.16		
(Southwood)				
REPACK				
SUP, RC, 12.5 mg, 12s ea	58016-3066-01	30.50		
25 mg, 12s ea	58016-3067-01	33.25		AB
50 mg, 12s ea	58016-3068-01	44.81		BR
PHENETHYLAMINE (Baker, J.T.)				
LIQ, NA (REAGENT)				
500 ml	10106-2857-07	260.49		
PHENFLU CD (MCR American)				
apap/codeine phos/gg/phenyleph hcl				
TAB, PO, 100s ea, C-III	58605-0433-01	117.99		
PHENFLU CDX (MCR American)				
apap/codeine phos/gg/phenyleph hcl				
TAB, PO, 100s ea, C-III	58605-0434-01	121.76		
PHENIRAMINE MALEATE (Amend)				
POW, NA (PURIFIED)				
25 gm	17317-0885-02	14.00		
100 gm	17317-0885-03	42.00		
500 gm	17317-0885-05	175.00		
(Gallipot)				
POW, NA (1X25GM,USP/NF)				
25 gm	51552-0751-04	29.40	21.00	
(1X100GM,USP/NF)				
100 gm	51552-0751-05	86.80	62.00	
(PCCA)				
POW, NA (USP)				
1 gm	51927-3148-00	2.88		
(Spectrum Pharmacy)				
POW, NA (B.P.)				
25 gm	49452-5170-01	133.70		
100 gm	49452-5170-02	476.00		
PHENOBARBITAL (Amend)				
POW, NA (U.S.P.)				
25 gm, C-IV	17317-0413-02	10.50		
125 gm, C-IV	17317-0413-04	24.50		
(Consolidated Midland)				
TAB, PO, 15 mg,				
100s ea, C-IV	00223-1430-01	2.50		
1000s ea, C-IV	00223-1430-02	21.00		
30 mg, 100s ea, C-IV	00223-1431-01	2.75		
1000s ea, C-IV	00223-1431-02	22.50		
60 mg, 100s ea, C-IV	00223-1432-01	3.25		
1000s ea, C-IV	00223-1432-02	29.50		

PROD/MFR	NDC	AWP	DP	OBC
100 mg,				
100s ea, C-IV	**00223-1433-01**	3.75		
1000s ea, C-IV	**00223-1433-02**	32.50		
(Excellium)				
TAB, PO, 15 mg,				
100s ea, C-IV	**64125-0915-01**	3.60		
1000s ea, C-IV	**64125-0915-10**	21.95		
30 mg, 100s ea, C-IV	**64125-0901-01**	3.90		
1000s ea, C-IV	**64125-0901-10**	23.95		
60 mg, 100s ea, C-IV	**64125-0902-01**	5.75		
1000s ea, C-IV	**64125-0902-10**	29.95		
100 mg,				
100s ea, C-IV	**64125-0903-01**	6.95		
1000s ea, C-IV	**64125-0903-10**	64.95		
(Gallipot)				
POW, NA (1X5GM,USP)				
5 gm, C-IV	**51552-0745-02**	6.93	4.95	
(1X25GM,USP)				
25 gm, C-IV	**51552-0745-04**	16.10	11.50	
(1X125GM,USP)				
125 gm, C-IV	**51552-0745-09**	48.72	34.80	
(1X500GM,USP)				
500 gm, C-IV	**51552-0745-06**	147.00	105.00	
(Medisca)				
POW, NA (U.S.P.)				
ea, C-IV	**38779-0852-09**	750.00		
25 gm, C-IV	**38779-0852-04**	52.50		
100 gm, C-IV	**38779-0852-05**	114.00		
500 gm, C-IV	**38779-0852-08**	450.00		
(Ohm)				
TAB, PO, 15 mg,				
100s ea, C-IV	**51660-0784-01**	3.81		
1000s ea, C-IV	**51660-0784-10**	19.43		
30 mg, 100s ea, C-IV	**51660-0785-01**	3.89		
1000s ea, C-IV	**51660-0785-10**	19.34		
60 mg, 100s ea, C-IV	**51660-0786-01**	5.76		
1000s ea, C-IV	**51660-0786-10**	30.73		
100 mg,				
100s ea, C-IV	**51660-0787-01**	7.30		
1000s ea, C-IV	**51660-0787-10**	37.23		
(PCCA)				
POW, NA (U.S.P.; CIV)				
1 gm, C-IV	**51927-1015-00**	2.04		
(Qualitest)				
ELI, PO, 20 mg/5 ml,				
473 ml, C-IV	**00603-1508-58**	25.61		
TAB, PO (CAPLET)				
16.2 mg,				
100s ea, C-IV	**00603-5165-21**	3.90		
1000s ea, C-IV	**00603-5165-32**	19.40		
32.4 mg,				
30s ea, C-IV	**00603-5166-16**	1.05		
60s ea, C-IV	**00603-5166-20**	2.10		
90s ea, C-IV	**00603-5166-02**	3.15		
100s ea, C-IV	**00603-5166-21**	3.60		
120s ea, C-IV	**00603-5166-22**	4.08		
1000s ea, C-IV	**00603-5166-32**	22.50		
60 mg, 100s ea, C-IV	**00603-5167-21**	5.75		
1000s ea, C-IV	**00603-5167-32**	30.73		
100 mg,				
100s ea, C-IV	**00603-5168-21**	6.95		
1000s ea, C-IV	**00603-5168-32**	62.55		
(Spectrum Pharmacy)				
POW, NA (U.S.P.)				
125 gm, C-IV	**49452-5190-01**	173.60		
500 gm, C-IV	**49452-5190-02**	549.50		
(Truxton)				
TAB, PO, 15 mg,				
1000s ea, C-IV	**00463-6160-10**	9.60		
30 mg,				
1000s ea, C-IV	**00463-6145-10**	10.70		
60 mg,				
1000s ea, C-IV	**00463-6151-10**	24.00		
100 mg,				
1000s ea, C-IV	**00463-6152-10**	30.00		
(UDL)				
TAB, PO (10X10)				
30 mg,				
100s ea UD, C-IV	**51079-0095-20**	6.56		
(Vintage)				
TAB, PO, 15 mg,				
100s ea, C-IV	**00254-5011-28**	3.34		
30 mg, 100s ea, C-IV	**00254-5012-28**	3.40		
1000s ea, C-IV	**00254-5012-38**	16.95		
100 mg,				
100s ea, C-IV	**00254-5014-28**	6.40		
(West-Ward)				
TAB, PO, 15 mg,				
1000s ea, C-IV	**00143-1445-10**	19.30		
30 mg,				
1000s ea, C-IV	**00143-1450-10**	21.80		
60 mg,				
1000s ea, C-IV	**00143-1455-10**	29.80		
100 mg,				
100s ea, C-IV	**00143-1458-01**	7.15		
1000s ea, C-IV	**00143-1458-10**	35.10		
(Altura)				
REPACK				
ELI, PO, 20 mg/5 ml,				
120 ml, C-IV	**63874-0223-12**	5.16		
480 ml, C-IV	**63874-0223-48**	5.30		
TAB, PO, 15 mg,				
20s ea, C-IV	**63874-0254-20**	4.63		
(DHS, Inc.)				
REPACK				
TAB, PO, 97.2 mg,				
30s ea, C-IV	**55887-0755-30**	8.00		
60s ea, C-IV	**55887-0755-60**	16.00		
90s ea, C-IV	**55887-0755-90**	24.00		
(HomeMed)				
REPACK				
TAB, PO, 30 mg,				
30s ea, C-IV	**51655-0848-24**	3.88		
90s ea, C-IV	**51655-0848-26**	6.64		
120s ea, C-IV	**51655-0848-82**	8.52		
180s ea, C-IV	**51655-0848-83**	10.00		
270s ea, C-IV	**51655-0848-92**	14.49		
360s ea, C-IV	**51655-0848-93**	17.40		
(McKesson Packaging)				
REPACK				
TAB, PO, 16.2 mg,				
100s ea UD, C-IV	**63739-0200-10**	7.67		
(USP)				
32.4 mg,				
100s ea UD, C-IV	**63739-0201-10**	7.85		
(PD-Rx Pharm)				
REPACK				
TAB, PO, 30 mg,				
100s ea, C-IV	**55289-0337-01**	26.33		
(CAPLET)				
32.4 mg,				
30s ea, C-IV	**55289-0535-30**	11.76		
100s ea, C-IV	**55289-0535-01**	18.33		
(Pharma Pac)				
REPACK				
TAB, PO, 15 mg,				
100s ea, C-IV	**52959-0124-00**	7.40		
(Phys Total Care)				
REPACK				
TAB, PO, 30 mg,				
30s ea, C-IV	**54868-1698-03**	8.49		
100s ea, C-IV	**54868-1698-02**	14.25		
1000s ea, C-IV	**54868-1698-00**	31.96		
(CAPLET)				
32.4 mg,				
100s ea, C-IV	**54868-1254-00**	9.69		
60 mg, 30s ea, C-IV	**54868-1219-02**	7.20		
60s ea, C-IV	**54868-1219-04**	9.90		
(USP)				
60 mg,				
90s ea, C-IV	**54868-1219-03**	12.60		
100s ea, C-IV	**54868-1219-01**	13.50		
100 mg,				
100s ea, C-IV	**54868-3381-00**	15.88		
(Quality Care Prod)				
REPACK				
TAB, PO, 30 mg,				
30s ea, C-IV	**49999-0394-30**	9.71		
60s ea, C-IV	**49999-0394-60**	19.42		
90s ea, C-IV	**49999-0394-90**	29.13		
60 mg, 100s ea, C-IV	**49999-0867-00**	32.01		
(Southwood)				
REPACK				
TAB, PO, 30 mg,				
6s ea, C-IV	**58016-0826-06**	2.44		
50s ea, C-IV	**58016-0826-50**	6.20		
PHENOBARBITAL SODIUM				
(Amend) *See SODIUM PHENOBARBITAL*				
(Baxter)				
SOL, IJ (VIAL, DOSETTE)				
65 mg/ml,				
1 ml, C-IV	**00641-0476-21**	1.63		
1 ml 25s, C-IV	**00641-0476-25**	40.80		
(DOSETTE VIAL)				
130 mg/ml,				
1 ml, C-IV	**00641-0477-21**	4.32		
1 ml 25s, C-IV	**00641-0477-25**	108.00		
(Hospira) *See LUMINAL SODIUM*				
(Medisca)				
POW, NA (U.S.P.)				
25 gm, C-IV	**38779-0853-04**	150.00		
100 gm, C-IV	**38779-0853-05**	552.00		
(1X500GM,USP)				
500 gm, C-IV	**38779-0853-08**	2448.00		
(Spectrum Pharmacy)				
POW, NA (U.S.P.)				
25 gm, C-IV	**49452-5200-03**	955.50		
(Phys Total Care)				
REPACK				
SOL, IJ (TUBEX)				
30 mg/ml,				
1 ml 10s, C-IV	**54868-3859-01**	97.06		
PHENOL (Amend)				
CRY, NA (U.S.P.)				
500 gm	**17317-0414-01**	21.55		
2270 gm	**17317-0414-05**	91.00		
(Amend) *See PHENOL 90%*				
(Baker, J.T.)				
CRY, NA (A.C.S., REAGENT)				
125 gm	**10106-2858-04**	53.46		
500 gm	**10106-2858-01**	63.50		
(U.S.P., FUSED)				
500 gm	**10106-2862-01**	61.22		
2000 gm	**10106-2862-05**	163.46		
LIQ, NA (U.S.P.)				
500 ml	**10106-2864-01**	28.71		
(Gallipot)				
CRY, NA (U.S.P.,N.F.)				
1 gm	**51552-0131-02**	7.77		
113.4 gm	**51552-0131-04**	14.63		
454 gm	**51552-0131-06**	27.58		
(Gallipot) *See PHENOL LIQUIFIED*				
(Mallinckrodt Lab)				
CRY, NA (U.S.P.)				
500 gm	**00406-0605-04**	14.42		
2500 gm	**00406-0605-06**	97.35		
LIQ, NA, 500 gm	**00406-0221-03**	57.08		
2500 ml	**00406-0610-04**	43.37		
(Mallinckrodt Lab) *See PHENOL LIQUEFIED*				
(Medisca)				
CRY, NA (U.S.P.)				
100 gm	**38779-0558-05**	46.50		
500 gm	**38779-0558-08**	93.00		
SOL, NA (1X100ML,USP)				
100 ml	**38779-1938-05**	31.50		
(1X500ML,USP)				
500 ml	**38779-1938-08**	87.00		
(PCCA)				
CRY, NA (USP)				
1 gm	**51927-1064-00**	0.22		
LIQ, NA (U.S.P.)				
1 ml	**51927-1657-00**	0.21		
(Spectrum Pharmacy)				
GRA, NA (FUSED CRYSTAL, U.S.P.)				
125 gm	**49452-5210-04**	95.20		
500 gm	**49452-5210-01**	158.90		
1000 gm	**49452-5210-03**	250.60		
2500 gm	**49452-5210-02**	493.50		
LIQ, NA (U.S.P.)				
500 ml	**49452-5220-02**	146.65		
2500 ml	**49452-5220-03**	476.00		
4000 ml	**49452-5220-04**	581.00		
PHENOL 90% (Amend)				
phenol				
LIQ, NA (U.S.P.)				
500 ml	**17317-0415-01**	21.55		
3840 ml	**17317-0415-06**	91.00		
PHENOL LIQUEFIED (Mallinckrodt Lab)				
phenol				
LIQ, NA, 500 gm	**00406-0276-01**	100.63		
PHENOL LIQUIFIED (Gallipot)				
phenol				
LIQ, NA (U.S.P.,N.F.)				
60 ml	**51552-0118-03**	11.76		
118.28 ml	**51552-0118-04**	22.05		
473 ml	**51552-0118-06**	29.19		
3785 ml	**51552-0118-08**	111.44		
PHENOL RED (PCCA)				
phenolsulfonphthalein				
POW, NA (ACS;WATER SOLUBLE)				
1 gm	**51927-2581-00**	10.20		

PROD/MFR	NDC	AWP	DP	OBC
PHENOLPHTHALEIN				
(Baker, J.T.) *See PHENOPHTHALEIN*				
(Gallipot)				
POW, NA (1X125GM)				
125 gm	**51552-0534-09**	23.52	16.80	
(PCCA)				
POW, NA, 1 gm	**51927-3348-00**	9.00		
(WHITE)				
1 gm	**51927-3317-00**	1.20		
PHENOLSULFONIC ACID (Medisca)				
p-phenolsulfonic acid				
SOL, NA, 100 ml	**38779-1500-05**	43.50		
500 ml	**38779-1500-08**	114.00		
(PCCA)				
SOL, NA (1X1ML)				
1 ml	**51927-1385-00**	0.38		
PHENOLSULFONPHTHALEIN				
(PCCA) *See PHENOL RED*				
PHENOPHTHALEIN (Baker, J.T.)				
phenolphthalein				
POW, NA (U.S.P.)				
500 gm	**10106-2872-01**	125.16		
PHENOXYBENZAMINE HCL (Gallipot)				
phenoxybenzamine hydrochloride				
POW, NA, 1 gm	**51552-0599-01**	42.35		
(Hawkins)				
POW, NA (U.S.P.)				
1 gm	**63370-0171-10**	112.80		
5 gm	**63370-0171-15**	489.60		
10 gm	**63370-0171-20**	840.00		
(Letco)				
POW, NA, 1 gm	**62991-2045-01**	65.50		
5 gm	**62991-2045-02**	225.00		
(Medisca)				
POW, NA (U.S.P.)				
1 gm	**38779-0456-06**	88.50		
5 gm	**38779-0456-03**	387.00		
25 gm	**38779-0456-04**	1497.00		
(PCCA)				
POW, NA (U.S.P.)				
1 gm	**51927-3119-00**	141.00		
(Spectrum Pharmacy)				
POW, NA (1X1GM, USP)				
1 gm	**49452-5214-01**	159.60		
(1X5GM, USP)				
5 gm	**49452-5214-02**	658.00		
(1X25GM, USP)				
25 gm	**49452-5214-03**	2334.50		
PHENOXYBENZAMINE HYDROCHLORIDE				
(Gallipot) *See PHENOXYBENZAMINE HCL*				
(Hawkins) *See PHENOXYBENZAMINE HCL*				
(Letco) *See PHENOXYBENZAMINE HCL*				
(Medisca) *See PHENOXYBENZAMINE HCL*				
(PCCA) *See PHENOXYBENZAMINE HCL*				
(Spectrum Pharmacy) *See PHENOXYBENZAMINE HCL*				
(Wellspring Pharm) *See DIBENZYLINE*				
PHENOXYETHANOL (PCCA)				
LIQ, NA (REAGENT)				
1 ml	**51927-2141-00**	0.31		
PHENTERCOT (Truxton)				
phentermine hydrochloride				
CAP, PO (GRAY & YELLOW)				
18.75 mg,				
1000s ea, C-IV	**00463-3036-10**	48.00		
30 mg,				
1000s ea, C-IV	**00463-3025-10**	120.00		EE
37.5 mg,				
1000s ea, C-IV	**00463-3032-10**	96.00		EE
TAB, PO, 8 mg,				
1000s ea, C-IV	**00463-6338-10**	36.00		EE
37.5 mg,				
1000s ea, C-IV	**00463-6308-10**	150.00		EE
PHENTERMINE (Altura)				
REPACK				
phentermine hydrochloride				
CAP, PO, 30 mg,				
7s ea, C-IV	**63874-0260-07**	11.50		
14s ea, C-IV	**63874-0260-14**	23.01		
20s ea, C-IV	**63874-0260-20**	32.87		
30s ea, C-IV	**63874-0260-30**	49.30		
100s ea, C-IV	**63874-0260-01**	164.33		
500s ea, C-IV	**63874-0260-50**	821.67		
1000s ea, C-IV	**63874-0260-02**	1643.33		
(Bryant Ranch)				
REPACK				
CAP, PO, 15 mg,				
7s ea, C-IV	**63629-2950-01**	12.18		
14s ea, C-IV	**63629-2950-02**	24.36		
30s ea, C-IV	**63629-2950-03**	52.20		
100s ea, C-IV	**63629-2950-04**	174.00		
30 mg, 7s ea, C-IV	**63629-2949-02**	9.62		
14s ea, C-IV	**63629-2949-03**	19.23		
30s ea, C-IV	**63629-2949-01**	41.22		
100s ea, C-IV	**63629-2949-04**	137.39		
TAB, PO, 37.5 mg,				
7s ea, C-IV	**63629-1584-04**	16.17		
14s ea, C-IV	**63629-1584-05**	21.61		
15s ea, C-IV	**63629-1584-02**	34.65		
28s ea, C-IV	**63629-1584-03**	64.68		
30s ea, C-IV	**63629-1584-01**	69.30		
(DHS, Inc.)				
REPACK				
CAP, PO, 15 mg,				
7s ea, C-IV	**55887-0762-07**	13.51		
14s ea, C-IV	**55887-0762-14**	27.02		
15s ea, C-IV	**55887-0762-15**	29.00		
30s ea, C-IV	**55887-0762-30**	58.00		
60s ea, C-IV	**55887-0762-60**	116.00		
(BLUE & WHITE)				
30 mg,				
60s ea, C-IV	**55887-0712-60**	79.99		
100s ea, C-IV	**55887-0891-01**	205.35		
37.5 mg,				
7s ea, C-IV	**55887-0080-07**	10.99		
30s ea, C-IV	**55887-0080-30**	47.10		
60s ea, C-IV	**55887-0080-60**	94.20		
TAB, PO, 37.5 mg,				
30s ea, C-IV	**55887-0840-30**	60.66		AA
45s ea, C-IV	**55887-0840-45**	90.09		AA
60s ea, C-IV	**55887-0840-60**	120.09		AA
90s ea, C-IV	**55887-0840-90**	141.76		AA
(Dispensing Solutions)				
REPACK				
TAB, PO, 37.5 mg,				
7s ea, C-IV	**66336-0344-07**	12.58		
14s ea, C-IV	**66336-0344-14**	25.16		
28s ea, C-IV	**66336-0344-28**	49.68		
30s ea, C-IV	**66336-0344-30**	53.23		
56s ea, C-IV	**66336-0344-56**	98.64		
84s ea, C-IV	**66336-0344-84**	147.97		
(HomeMed)				
REPACK				
TAB, PO, 30 mg,				
30s ea, C-IV	**51655-0310-24**	88.00		
(Pharma Pac)				
REPACK				
TAB, PO, 37.5 mg,				
7s ea, C-IV	**52959-0812-07**	12.66		
10s ea, C-IV	**52959-0812-10**	18.09		
14s ea, C-IV	**52959-0812-14**	25.32		
30s ea, C-IV	**52959-0812-30**	54.08		
90s ea, C-IV	**52959-0812-90**	162.23		
(Quality Care Prod)				
REPACK				
CAP, PO, 15 mg,				
28s ea, C-IV	**49999-0724-28**	52.08		
60s ea, C-IV	**49999-0724-60**	111.60		
30 mg,				
28s ea, C-IV	**49999-0405-28**	169.40		
(Southwood)				
REPACK				
TAB, PO, 37.5 mg,				
30s ea, C-IV	**58016-0310-30**	47.10		
60s ea, C-IV	**58016-0310-60**	94.20		
90s ea, C-IV	**58016-0310-90**	141.30		
100s ea, C-IV	**58016-0310-00**	157.00		
(Stat Rx)				
REPACK				
CAP, PO, 30 mg,				
30s ea, C-IV	**16590-0185-30**	65.00		
60s ea, C-IV	**16590-0185-60**	130.00		
PHENTERMINE HCL (Cody Labs)				
phentermine hydrochloride				
POW, NA (U.S.P.)				
25 gm, C-IV	**65893-0400-02**	21.50		
100 gm, C-IV	**65893-0400-10**	74.00		
500 gm, C-IV	**65893-0400-50**	355.00		
1000 gm, C-IV	**65893-0400-11**	685.00		
(Hawkins)				
POW, NA (U.S.P.)				
25 gm, C-IV	**63370-0965-25**	92.00		
100 gm, C-IV	**63370-0965-35**	296.00		
1000 gm, C-IV	**63370-0965-50**	2740.00		
(Lannett)				
CAP, PO (USP)				
30 mg,				
100s ea, C-IV	**00527-0597-01**	158.38		AA
1000s ea, C-IV	**00527-0597-10**	1504.52		AA
(Medisca)				
POW, NA, 100 gm, C-IV	**38779-0854-05**	1050.00		
(1X1000GM,USP)				
1000 gm, C-IV	**38779-0854-09**	4500.00		
(Mutual)				
CAP, PO, 30 mg,				
100s ea, C-IV	**53489-0433-01**	103.35		AA
1000s ea, C-IV	**53489-0433-10**	981.83		AA
TAB, PO, 37.5 mg,				
100s ea, C-IV	**53489-0406-01**	152.25		AA
1000s ea, C-IV	**53489-0406-10**	1450.00		AA
(PCCA)				
POW, NA (USP; CIV)				
1 gm, C-IV	**51927-2937-00**	5.88		
(Qualitest)				
TAB, PO, 37.5 mg,				
100s ea, C-IV	**00603-5192-21**	152.25		AA
1000s ea, C-IV	**00603-5192-32**	1446.38		AA
(Sandoz)				
CAP, PO, 15 mg,				
100s ea, C-IV	**00185-0644-01**	156.71		AA
1000s ea, C-IV	**00185-0644-10**	1488.86		AA
(BLUE/CLEAR)				
30 mg,				
100s ea, C-IV	**00185-5000-01**	164.98		AA
(YELLOW)				
30 mg,				
100s ea, C-IV	**00185-0647-01**	129.19		AA
(BLUE/CLEAR)				
30 mg,				
1000s ea, C-IV	**00185-5000-10**	1567.21		AA
(YELLOW)				
30 mg,				
1000s ea, C-IV	**00185-0647-10**	1227.29		AA
(A-S Medication)				
REPACK				
CAP, PO (BLUE/CLEAR)				
30 mg,				
14s ea, C-IV	**54569-3069-03**	17.55		EE
15s ea, C-IV	**54569-3069-02**	18.81		EE
28s ea, C-IV	**54569-3069-06**	35.11		EE
30s ea, C-IV	**54569-3069-00**	37.61		EE
60s ea, C-IV	**54569-3069-04**	75.23		EE
37.5 mg,				
28s ea, C-IV	**54569-4816-02**	43.96		EE
30s ea, C-IV	**54569-4816-01**	47.10		EE
TAB, PO, 37.5 mg,				
7s ea, C-IV	**54569-3203-02**	10.80		EE
14s ea, C-IV	**54569-3203-01**	21.60		EE
(WHITE WITH BLUE SPECKS)				
37.5 mg,				
28s ea, C-IV	**54569-3203-08**	43.19		EE
30s ea, C-IV	**54569-3203-00**	46.28		EE
30s ea, C-IV	**54569-6100-00**	43.50		AA
45s ea, C-IV	**54569-3203-04**	69.41		EE
60s ea, C-IV	**54569-3203-03**	92.55		EE
100s ea, C-IV	**54569-5224-02**	154.25		EE
(Aidarex)				
REPACK				
TAB, PO, 37.5 mg,				
7s ea, C-IV	**33261-0471-07**	13.09		AA
14s ea, C-IV	**33261-0471-14**	26.18		AA
21s ea, C-IV	**33261-0471-21**	39.27		AA
30s ea, C-IV	**33261-0471-30**	56.10		AA
40s ea, C-IV	**33261-0471-40**	74.80		AA
60s ea, C-IV	**33261-0471-60**	112.20		AA
90s ea, C-IV	**33261-0471-90**	168.30		AA
(Altura)				
REPACK				
CAP, PO, 15 mg,				
7s ea, C-IV	**63874-0271-07**	8.03		AA
14s ea, C-IV	**63874-0271-14**	16.05		AA
15s ea, C-IV	**63874-0271-15**	17.20		AA
30s ea, C-IV	**63874-0271-30**	34.40		AA
100s ea, C-IV	**63874-0271-01**	114.67		AA
37.5 mg,				
7s ea, C-IV	**63874-0270-07**	10.65		AA
30s ea, C-IV	**63874-0270-30**	45.68		AA
100s ea, C-IV	**63874-0270-01**	154.25		AA
TAB, PO, 37.5 mg,				
10s ea, C-IV	**63874-0282-10**	15.22		AA
14s ea, C-IV	**63874-0282-14**	21.60		AA
15s ea, C-IV	**63874-0282-15**	26.45		AA
30s ea, C-IV	**63874-0282-30**	45.68		AA
100s ea, C-IV	**63874-0282-01**	154.25		AA
1000s ea, C-IV	**63874-0282-02**	649.80		AA

PROD/MFR	NDC	AWP	DP	OBC
(B&B Pharm, Inc)				
REPACK				
POW, NA (1X100GM)				
100 gm, C-IV	63275-9959-05	405.00		
(1X1000GM)				
1000 gm, C-IV	63275-9959-09	3375.00		
(DHS, Inc.)				
REPACK				
CAP, PO, 30 mg,				
30s ea, C-IV	55887-0891-30	60.01		AA
60s ea, C-IV	55887-0891-60	120.01		AA
(Dispensing Solutions)				
REPACK				
CAP, PO, 15 mg,				
7s ea, C-IV	66336-0133-07	16.73		
14s ea, C-IV	66336-0133-14	32.87		
28s ea, C-IV	66336-0133-28	65.13		
30s ea, C-IV	66336-0133-30	45.73		
30 mg, 7s ea, C-IV	66336-0185-07	18.48		AA
7s ea, C-IV	66336-0763-07	19.08		AA
14s ea, C-IV	66336-0185-14	36.96		AA
14s ea, C-IV	66336-0763-14	37.56		AA
28s ea, C-IV	66336-0185-28	73.92		AA
28s ea, C-IV	66336-0763-28	74.47		AA
30s ea, C-IV	55045-1264-08	39.00		
30s ea, C-IV	66336-0185-30	79.20		AA
30s ea, C-IV	66336-0763-30	79.75		AA
42s ea, C-IV	66336-0185-42	110.88		AA
37.5 mg,				
30s ea, C-IV	66336-0426-30	47.10		AA
TAB, PO, 37.5 mg,				
30s ea, C-IV	55045-1689-08	43.00		
45s ea, C-IV	66336-0344-45	79.27		AA
60s ea, C-IV	66336-0344-60	105.69		AA
(Nucare Pharm)				
REPACK				
TAB, PO, 37.5 mg,				
7s ea, C-IV	66267-0166-07	18.17		AA
30s ea, C-IV	66267-0166-30	71.30		AA
45s ea, C-IV	66267-0166-45	92.09		AA
60s ea, C-IV	66267-0166-60	117.69		AA
90s ea, C-IV	66267-0166-90	154.54		AA
(PD-Rx Pharm)				
REPACK				
CAP, PO (GRAY/YELLOW)				
15 mg, 7s ea, C-IV	55289-0791-07	28.97		AA
14s ea, C-IV	55289-0791-14	45.54		AA
15s ea, C-IV	55289-0791-15	47.93		AA
(USP)				
15 mg,				
21s ea, C-IV	55289-0791-21	66.50		AA
(GRAY/YELLOW)				
15 mg,				
28s ea, C-IV	55289-0791-28	67.07		AA
30s ea, C-IV	55289-0791-30	68.00		AA
60s ea, C-IV	55289-0791-60	126.00		AA
(BLUE/CLEAR)				
30 mg, 7s ea, C-IV	55289-0624-07	31.57		AA
(YELLOW)				
30 mg, 7s ea, C-IV	55289-0313-07	28.97		AA
(BLUE/CLEAR)				
30 mg,				
14s ea, C-IV	55289-0624-14	53.17		AA
(YELLOW)				
30 mg,				
14s ea, C-IV	55289-0313-14	47.90		AA
16s ea, C-IV	55289-0313-16	51.37		AA
21s ea, C-IV	55289-0313-21	66.83		AA
28s ea, C-IV	55289-0313-28	67.98		AA
(BLUE/CLEAR)				
30 mg,				
28s ea, C-IV	55289-0624-28	74.97		AA
30s ea, C-IV	55289-0624-30	75.03		AA
(YELLOW)				
30 mg,				
30s ea, C-IV	55289-0313-30	68.51		AA
60s ea, C-IV	55289-0313-60	126.00		AA
TAB, PO (WHITE/BLUE)				
37.5 mg,				
7s ea, C-IV	55289-0701-07	33.47		AA
14s ea, C-IV	55289-0701-14	56.90		AA
15s ea, C-IV	55289-0701-15	56.93		AA
21s ea, C-IV	55289-0701-21	80.33		AA
28s ea, C-IV	55289-0701-28	80.58		AA
(WHITE/BLUE)				
37.5 mg,				
30s ea, C-IV	55289-0701-30	80.63		AA
45s ea, C-IV	55289-0701-45	120.17		AA
60s ea, C-IV	55289-0701-60	154.23		AA
90s ea, C-IV	55289-0701-90	220.47		AA
120s ea, C-IV	55289-0701-98	292.47		AA
(Pharma Pac)				
REPACK				
CAP, PO, 15 mg,				
6s ea, C-IV	52959-0426-06	17.10		EE
7s ea, C-IV	52959-0426-07	19.51		EE
14s ea, C-IV	52959-0426-14	24.91		EE
15s ea, C-IV	52959-0426-15	26.11		EE
24s ea, C-IV	52959-0426-24	30.31		EE
28s ea, C-IV	52959-0426-28	35.35		EE
30s ea, C-IV	52959-0426-30	38.11		EE
60s ea, C-IV	52959-0426-60	76.20		EE
30 mg, 7s ea, C-IV	52959-0432-07	8.47		EE
7s ea, C-IV	52959-0440-07	8.47		EE
14s ea, C-IV	52959-0440-14	16.95		EE
(YELLOW)				
30 mg,				
14s ea, C-IV	52959-0432-14	14.12		EE
15s ea, C-IV	52959-0440-15	18.15		EE
28s ea, C-IV	52959-0440-28	33.88		EE
30s ea, C-IV	52959-0440-30	36.30		EE
(YELLOW)				
30 mg,				
30s ea, C-IV	52959-0432-30	30.15		EE
TAB, PO, 37.5 mg,				
20s ea, C-IV	52959-0812-20	36.06		AA
60s ea, C-IV	52959-0812-60	108.15		AA
(Phys Total Care)				
REPACK				
CAP, PO, 15 mg,				
30s ea, C-IV	54868-0283-00	74.10		EE
100s ea, C-IV	54868-0283-01	179.61		EE
18.75 mg,				
1000s ea, C-IV	54868-1051-01	117.44		
(BLUE/CLEAR)				
30 mg,				
30s ea, C-IV	54868-0192-04	77.34		EE
(YELLOW)				
30 mg,				
30s ea, C-IV	54868-0253-01	37.77		EE
(BLUE/CLEAR)				
30 mg,				
60s ea, C-IV	54868-0192-00	115.11		EE
(YELLOW)				
30 mg,				
60s ea, C-IV	54868-0253-00	69.54		EE
(BLUE/CLEAR)				
30 mg,				
100s ea, C-IV	54868-0192-01	187.86		EE
TAB, PO, 37.5 mg,				
7s ea, C-IV	54868-0087-03	10.09		EE
(BLUE/WHITE)				
37.5 mg,				
15s ea, C-IV	54868-0087-00	17.64		EE
30s ea, C-IV	54868-0087-02	28.44		EE
60s ea, C-IV	54868-0087-04	47.68		AA
90s ea, C-IV	54868-0087-05	68.52		AA
100s ea, C-IV	54868-0087-01	71.55		AA
(Physician Partner)				
REPACK				
CAP, PO, 15 mg,				
30s ea, C-IV	21695-0509-30	75.22		AA
TAB, PO, 37.5 mg,				
100s ea, C-IV	21695-0513-00	304.50		AA
(Quality Care Prod)				
REPACK				
CAP, PO, 15 mg,				
30s ea, C-IV	49999-0724-30	55.73		AA
100s ea, C-IV	49999-0724-00	186.00		AA
30 mg, 7s ea, C-IV	49999-0405-07	42.34		AA
30s ea, C-IV	49999-0405-30	181.44		AA
37.5 mg,				
7s ea, C-IV	49999-0517-07	25.60		AA
14s ea, C-IV	49999-0517-14	41.84		AA
15s ea, C-IV	49999-0361-15	35.21		AA
28s ea, C-IV	49999-0517-28	83.68		AA
30s ea, C-IV	49999-0361-30	89.64		AA
TAB, PO, 37.5 mg,				
15s ea, C-IV	49999-0517-15	27.41		AA
45s ea, C-IV	49999-0517-45	82.23		AA
60s ea, C-IV	49999-0517-60	109.64		AA
(Southwood)				
REPACK				
CAP, PO, 30 mg,				
14s ea, C-IV	58016-0861-14	13.85		EE
PHENTERMINE HYDROCHLORIDE				
(Cody Labs) *See PHENTERMINE HCL*				
(Gate) *See ADIPEX-P*				
(Hawkins) *See PHENTERMINE HCL*				
(KVK)				
CAP, PO (USP)				
15 mg,				
100s ea, C-IV	10702-0026-01	125.37		AA
1000s ea, C-IV	10702-0026-10	1191.09		AA
30 mg, 100s ea, C-IV	10702-0027-01	103.00		AA
100s ea, C-IV	10702-0028-01	103.35		AA
1000s ea, C-IV	10702-0027-10	981.00		AA
1000s ea, C-IV	10702-0028-10	981.83		AA
37.5 mg,				
100s ea, C-IV	10702-0029-01	157.00		AA
1000s ea, C-IV	10702-0029-10	1392.61		AA
TAB, PO, 37.5 mg,				
30s ea, C-IV	10702-0025-03	50.00		AA
100s ea, C-IV	10702-0025-01	154.25		AA
1000s ea, C-IV	10702-0025-10	1369.00		AA
(Lannett)				
CAP, PO (USP)				
30 mg,				
100s ea, C-IV	00527-1308-01	158.38		AA
100s ea, C-IV	00527-1310-01	124.02		AA
1000s ea, C-IV	00527-1308-10	1504.52		AA
1000s ea, C-IV	00527-1310-10	1177.20		AA
(Lannett) *See PHENTERMINE HCL*				
(Lannett)				
TAB, PO, 37.5 mg,				
100s ea, C-IV	00527-1445-01	185.10		AA
1000s ea, C-IV	00527-1445-10	1740.00		AA
(Medisca) *See PHENTERMINE HCL*				
(Mutual) *See PHENTERMINE HCL*				
(PCCA) *See PHENTERMINE HCL*				
(Qualitest) *See PHENTERMINE HCL*				
(Sandoz) *See PHENTERMINE HCL*				
(Truxton) *See PHENTERCOT*				
(A-S Medication)				
REPACK				
CAP, PO, 15 mg,				
14s ea, C-IV	54569-4143-02	21.94		AA
(GRAY & YELLOW)				
15 mg,				
28s ea, C-IV	54569-4143-00	43.88		AA
30s ea, C-IV	54569-4143-04	47.01		AA
60s ea, C-IV	54569-4143-05	94.03		AA
(YELLOW)				
30 mg, 7s ea, C-IV	54569-0392-03	8.50		AA
14s ea, C-IV	54569-0392-02	17.00		AA
28s ea, C-IV	54569-0392-04	33.99		AA
30s ea, C-IV	54569-0392-00	36.42		AA
(Dispensing Solutions)				
REPACK				
CAP, PO, 30 mg,				
30s ea, C-IV	55045-2231-08	39.00		AA
TAB, PO, 37.5 mg,				
7s ea, C-IV	55045-1689-07	10.01		AA
15s ea, C-IV	55045-1689-03	21.45		AA
28s ea, C-IV	55045-1689-06	40.04		AA
(Keltman Pharma., Inc.)				
REPACK				
TAB, PO, 37.5 mg,				
30s ea, C-IV	68387-0690-30	48.25		
(Palmetto)				
REPACK				
CAP, PO, 15 mg,				
7s ea, C-IV	23490-6090-01	20.66		
14s ea, C-IV	23490-6090-02	31.73		
28s ea, C-IV	23490-6090-03	63.47		
30s ea, C-IV	23490-6090-04	68.00		
60s ea, C-IV	23490-6090-06	136.00		
30 mg, 7s ea, C-IV	23490-6092-01	24.02		
7s ea, C-IV	23490-7240-00	18.48		
7s ea, C-IV	23490-7921-01	18.48		
14s ea, C-IV	23490-6092-03	31.73		
14s ea, C-IV	23490-7240-01	36.96		
14s ea, C-IV	23490-7921-02	36.96		
28s ea, C-IV	23490-6092-06	63.47		
28s ea, C-IV	23490-7240-02	73.92		
28s ea, C-IV	23490-7921-04	73.92		
30s ea, C-IV	23490-6092-07	68.00		
30s ea, C-IV	23490-7240-03	79.20		
30s ea, C-IV	23490-7921-03	79.20		
40s ea, C-IV	23490-6092-08	105.60		
42s ea, C-IV	23490-6092-09	110.88		
42s ea, C-IV	23490-7240-04	110.88		
60s ea, C-IV	23490-6092-00	158.40		
TAB, PO, 37.5 mg,				
7s ea, C-IV	23490-6094-00	18.81		
14s ea, C-IV	23490-6094-01	37.63		
28s ea, C-IV	23490-6094-02	75.26		

PROD/MFR	NDC	AWP	DP	OBC
30s ea, C-IV	23490-6094-03	80.63		
56s ea, C-IV	23490-6094-04	150.51		
60s ea, C-IV	23490-6094-06	161.26		
84s ea, C-IV	23490-6094-05	225.77		
90s ea, C-IV	23490-6094-09	241.89		
(PD-Rx Pharm)				
REPACK				
CAP, PO (USP)				
37.5 mg,				
30s ea, C-IV	43063-0182-30	54.08		AA
(Pharma Pac)				
REPACK				
CAP, PO, 30 mg,				
60s ea, C-IV	52959-0440-60	71.01		AA
37.5 mg, 7s ea, C-IV	52959-0417-04	13.66		AA
(Physician Partner)				
REPACK				
CAP, PO, 15 mg,				
100s ea, C-IV	21695-0509-00	250.74		
30 mg, 30s ea, C-IV	21695-0510-30	79.19		
(Quality Care Prod)				
REPACK				
TAB, PO, 37.5 mg,				
30s ea, C-IV	49999-0517-30	54.82		
(Stat Rx)				
REPACK				
TAB, PO, 37.5 mg,				
30s ea, C-IV	16590-0186-30	78.00		
60s ea, C-IV	16590-0186-60	156.00		
PHENTOLAMINE MESYLATE (Bedford)				
PDS, IJ (USP)				
5 mg, ea	55390-0113-01	64.80		AP
(Gallipot)				
POW, NA (U.S.P.)				
0.1 gm	51552-0496-04	49.00		
0.2 gm	51552-0496-09	91.00		
0.5 gm	51552-0496-05	196.00		
1 gm	51552-0496-01	364.00		
5 gm	51552-0496-02	1302.00		
(Hawkins)				
POW, NA (U.S.P.)				
0.1 gm	63370-0170-06	168.00		
0.5 gm	63370-0170-09	672.00		
1 gm	63370-0170-10	1248.00		
5 gm	63370-0170-15	4080.00		
(Letco)				
POW, NA (U.S.P.)				
0.1 gm	62991-1108-01	90.00		
0.5 gm	62991-1108-02	270.00		
1 gm	62991-1108-03	495.00		
5 gm	62991-1108-04	2100.00		
(Medisca)				
POW, NA (U.S.P.)				
0.1 gm	38779-1502-09	126.00		
0.5 gm	38779-1502-00	477.00		
1 gm	38779-1502-06	897.00		
5 gm	38779-1502-03	2385.00		
(Novalar) *See ORAVERSE*				
(PCCA)				
POW, NA (U.S.P.)				
1 gm	51927-2669-00	4500.00		
(Spectrum Pharmacy)				
POW, NA (U.S.P.)				
0.1 gm	49452-5217-01	206.15		
0.5 gm	49452-5217-02	714.00		
1 gm	49452-5217-04	955.50		
5 gm	49452-5217-05	3241.00		
(B&B Pharm, Inc)				
REPACK				
POW, NA (U.S.P.)				
0.1 gm	63275-9989-06	122.00		
0.5 gm	63275-9989-07	500.00		
1 gm	63275-9989-01	975.00		
PHENYL ACETATE (PCCA)				
SOL, NA (1X1ML)				
1 ml	51927-3252-00	0.84		
PHENYL SALICYLATE (Gallipot)				
CRY, NA (PURIFIED)				
100 gm	51552-0199-05	19.25		
(PCCA)				
POW, NA (PURIFIED)				
1 gm	51927-9010-00	0.48		
(Spectrum Pharmacy)				
CRY, NA (1X125GM)				
125 gm	49452-5330-01	95.20		
(1X500GM)				
500 gm	49452-5330-02	230.30		
(1X2500GM)				
2500 gm	49452-5330-03	770.00		
PHENYL/GUAIFENESIN (Bryant Ranch)				
REPACK				
guaifenesin/phenylephrine hydrochloride				
TER, PO, 600 mg-30 mg,				
20s ea	63629-1367-01	22.80		
30s ea	63629-1367-03	34.20		
PHENYLACETYLUREA (PCCA)				
phenacemide				
POW, NA, 1 gm	51927-3150-00	2.85		
PHENYLALANINE				
(Gallipot) *See DL-PHENYLALANINE*				
(Medisca)				
CRY, NA (1X25GM,USP)				
25 gm	38779-1809-04	34.50		
(1X100GM,USP)				
100 gm	38779-1809-05	90.00		
(1X1000GM,USP)				
1000 gm	38779-1809-09	585.00		
(PCCA)				
POW, NA (D)				
1 gm	51927-2830-00	8.64		
(FCC)				
1 gm	51927-1472-00	1.80		
(USP;L)				
1 gm	51927-2212-00	1.80		
(Spectrum Pharmacy) *See DL-PHENYLALANINE*				
(Spectrum Pharmacy) *See L-PHENYLALANINE*				
PHENYLBUTAZONE (Gallipot)				
POW, NA (U.S.P.)				
100 gm	51552-0608-05	35.00		
(Letco)				
POW, NA (U.S.P., VET USE ONLY)				
100 gm	62991-2160-01	75.00		
(U.S.P.)				
500 gm	62991-2160-03	270.00		
(U.S.P., VET USE ONLY)				
5000 gm	62991-2160-04	1050.00		
(Medisca)				
POW, NA (U.S.P.)				
ea	38779-0497-07	3825.00		
25 gm	38779-0497-04	28.50		
100 gm	38779-0497-05	90.00		
500 gm	38779-0497-08	345.00		
1000 gm	38779-0497-09	495.00		
5000 gm	38779-0497-03	1077.00		
(PCCA)				
POW, NA (U.S.P.)				
1 gm	51927-1011-00	1.44		
(Spectrum Pharmacy)				
POW, NA (U.S.P.)				
100 gm	49452-5285-02	164.85		
500 gm	49452-5285-04	535.50		
1000 gm	49452-5285-03	686.00		
5000 gm	49452-5285-05	1403.50		
PHENYLEPH HCL/PROMETHAZINE HCL				
(Actavis Mid Atlantic) *See PROMETHAZINE VC*				
(Qualitest) *See PROMETHAZINE VC*				
PHENYLEPHRINE COMPLEX (Breckenridge Pharm)				
bpm/dm/phenyleph hcl				
SOL, PO (1X473ML,AF,SF,DYE-FREE)				
473 ml	51991-0660-16	66.17		
PHENYLEPHRINE HCL (Amend)				
phenylephrine hydrochloride				
POW, NA (U.S.P.)				
25 gm	17317-0417-02	29.40		
100 gm	17317-0417-03	86.80		
500 gm	17317-0417-05	364.00		
(Amer Regent)				
SOL, IJ (S.D.V.)				
10 mg/ml, 1 ml 25s	00517-0299-25	78.13		
(VIAL)				
10 mg/ml, 5 ml 25s	00517-0405-25	390.75		
(Bausch & Lomb Inc.)				
SOL, OP, 2.5%, 2 ml 12s	24208-0740-59	3.73		
5 ml	24208-0740-02	4.14		
15 ml	24208-0740-06	4.90		
(Baxter)				
SOL, IJ (S.D.V.)				
10 mg/ml, 1 ml 25s	10019-0163-12	20.40		
(1X2ML,SDV,USP)				
10 mg/ml, 2 ml	10019-0163-39	0.82		
(1X5ML,SDV,USP)				
10 mg/ml, 5 ml	10019-0163-05	5.51		
(S.D.V.)				
10 mg/ml, 5 ml 25s	10019-0163-01	137.70		
(Consolidated Midland)				
SOL, OP, 2.5%, 5 ml	00223-6695-05	3.50		
15 ml	00223-6695-15	3.90		
10%, 5 ml	00223-6696-05	4.00		
15 ml	00223-6696-15	4.95		
(Falcon Ophthalmics)				
SOL, OP, 2.5%, 3 ml	61314-0342-01	4.10		
5 ml	61314-0342-02	4.15		
(Gallipot)				
POW, NA (U.S.P.,N.F.)				
5 gm	51552-0232-02	20.30		
25 gm	51552-0232-04	35.28		
100 gm	51552-0232-05	123.48		
(Medisca)				
POW, NA (U.S.P.)				
25 gm	38779-0247-04	88.50		
100 gm	38779-0247-05	297.00		
(Parenta Pharma)				
SOL, IJ (USP,PF)				
10 mg/ml, 5 ml	66758-0016-03	15.60	13.00	
(USP,25X5ML,PF)				
10 mg/ml, 5 ml 25s	66758-0016-04	390.00	325.00	
(USP, BULK PACKAGE,PF)				
10 mg/ml, 10 ml	66758-0017-01	41.52	34.60	
(PCCA)				
POW, NA (U.S.P.)				
1 gm	51927-1225-00	4.50		
(Spectrum Pharmacy)				
POW, NA (U.S.P.)				
5 gm	49452-5290-01	73.15		
25 gm	49452-5290-02	147.35		
100 gm	49452-5290-03	511.00		
(Dispensing Solutions)				
REPACK				
SOL, OP, 2.5%, 5 ml	55045-3326-01	6.00		
(Phys Total Care)				
REPACK				
SOL, OP, 2.5%, 5 ml	54868-2812-01	14.47		
15 ml	54868-2812-00	21.00		
(Southwood)				
REPACK				
SOL, OP, 2.5%, 15 ml	58016-6097-01	11.60		
PHENYLEPHRINE HYDROCHLORIDE				
(Akorn) *See AK-DILATE*				
(Alcon Ophthalmic) *See MYDFRIN*				
(Altaire) *See ALTAFRIN*				
(Amend) *See PHENYLEPHRINE HCL*				
(Amer Regent) *See PHENYLEPHRINE HCL*				
(Bausch & Lomb Inc.) *See PHENYLEPHRINE HCL*				
(Baxter) *See PHENYLEPHRINE HCL*				
(Consolidated Midland) *See PHENYLEPHRINE HCL*				
(Dexo) *See AH-CHEW D*				
(Falcon Ophthalmics) *See PHENYLEPHRINE HCL*				
(Gallipot) *See PHENYLEPHRINE HCL*				
(Hawthorn Pharm) *See NASOP*				
(Hospira) *See NEO-SYNEPHRINE HCL*				
(HUB Pharma)				
SOL, OP (USP)				
10%, 5 ml	17238-0520-05	6.70		
(Intl Ethical) *See DESPEC-SF*				
(Medisca) *See PHENYLEPHRINE HCL*				
(Ocusoft) *See NEOFRIN*				
(Parenta Pharma) *See PHENYLEPHRINE HCL*				
(PCCA) *See PHENYLEPHRINE HCL*				
(Spectrum Pharmacy) *See PHENYLEPHRINE HCL*				
(Teva)				
SOL, IJ (S.D.V.)				
10 mg/ml, 1 ml 25s	00703-1631-04	26.60		
(SINGLE USE,25X5ML)				
10 mg/ml, 5 ml 25s	00703-1633-04	144.29		
(Wraser Pharm) *See LUSONAL*				
(Phys Total Care)				
REPACK				
SOL, IJ (SDV,25X1ML)				
10 mg/ml, 1 ml 25s	54868-5716-00	60.69		

PROD/MFR NDC AWP DP OBC

PHENYLEPHRINE HYDROCHLORIDE/GUAIFENESIN
(Acella)
guaifenesin/phenylephrine hydrochloride
SOL, PO (1X30ML,AF,SF,RASPBERRY)
20 mg/ml-1.5 mg/ml,
30 ml.............. **42192-0510-30** 31.37

PHENYLEPHRINE HYDROCHLORIDE/ PYRILAMINE MALEATE
(Cornerstone) *See DECONSAL CT*
(Zyber) *See ALDEX D*

PHENYLEPHRINE TANNATE
(Hawthorn Pharm) *See NASOP*
(Hawthorn Pharm) *See NASOP12*

PHENYLEPHRINE TANNATE/PYRILAMINE TANNATE
(Allan Pharmaceutical) *See ALLANVAN-S*
(Athlon Pharm) *See PYRLEX PD*
(Breckenridge Pharm) *See V-TANN*
(Meda) *See RYNA-12*
(Meda) *See RYNA-12 S*
(Prasco Labs) *See K-TAN*

PHENYLETHYL ALCOHOL (PCCA)
LIQ, NA (USP)
1 ml.................. **51927-1307-00** 0.75
(Spectrum Pharmacy) *See ALCOHOL PHENETHYL*

PHENYLETHYLAMINE HCL (PCCA)
phenylethylamine hydrochloride
POW, NA, 1 gm........... **51927-2201-00** 2.55

PHENYLETHYLAMINE HYDROCHLORIDE
(PCCA) *See PHENYLETHYLAMINE HCL*

PHENYLHISTINE (Quality Care Prod)
REPACK
codeine phos/gg/pse hcl
LIQ, PO, 120 ml, C-V...... **49999-0404-04** 6.81
(Stat Rx)
REPACK
LIQ, PO, 120 ml, C-V...... **16590-0359-04** 26.50

PHENYLHISTINE DH (Qualitest)
cpm/codeine phos/pse hcl
SYR, PO (1X118ML)
118 ml, C-V.......... **00603-1520-54** 10.43
(1X473ML)
473 ml, C-V.......... **00603-1520-58** 39.65

PHENYLHISTINE DH EXPECTORANT
(Quality Care Prod)
REPACK
cpm/codeine phos/pse hcl
ELI, PO, 120 ml, C-V...... **49999-0721-04** 7.71

PHENYLMERCURIC ACETATE (Medisca)
POW, NA (N.F.)
25 gm.............. **38779-1507-04** 163.50
100 gm.............. **38779-1507-05** 478.50
(PCCA)
POW, NA (NF)
1 gm................ **51927-1219-00** 9.60
(Spectrum Pharmacy)
POW, NA (N.F.)
25 gm.............. **49452-5300-01** 344.75
100 gm.............. **49452-5300-02** 889.00

PHENYLMERCURIC NITRATE (Medisca)
POW, NA (N.F.)
25 gm.............. **38779-1749-04** 81.00
(1X100GM,NF)
100 gm.............. **38779-1749-05** 285.00
(PCCA)
POW, NA (NF)
1 gm................ **51927-1223-00** 4.80
(Spectrum Pharmacy)
POW, NA (N.F.)
25 gm.............. **49452-5310-01** 175.70
100 gm.............. **49452-5310-02** 591.50

PHENYLPROPANOLAMINE HCL (PCCA)
phenylpropanolamine hydrochloride
POW, NA (U.S.P.)
1 gm................ **51927-1043-00** 3.00

PHENYLPROPANOLAMINE HYDROCHLORIDE
(Gallipot)
POW, NA (U.S.P.,N.F.)
25 gm.............. **51552-0142-04** 13.30
100 gm.............. **51552-0142-05** 25.90
(PCCA) *See PHENYLPROPANOLAMINE HCL*

PROD/MFR NDC AWP DP OBC

(Spectrum Pharmacy)
POW, NA (U.S.P.)
25 gm.............. **49452-5320-01** 67.90
100 gm.............. **49452-5320-02** 123.90
500 gm.............. **49452-5320-03** 455.00
1000 gm............ **49452-5320-04** 693.00

PHENYLPROPANOLAMINE, L-
(PCCA) *See NOREPHEDRINE*

PHENYLTOL/PHEN/CHLOR (Phys Total Care)
REPACK
cpm/phenyleph hcl/phenyltoloxamine cit
TER, PO, 4 mg-20 mg-40 mg,
100s ea............ **54868-5541-00** 101.16

PHENYLTOLOXAMINE CITRATE
(Medisca) *See PHENYLTOLOXAMINE DIHYDROGEN CITRATE*
(PCCA) *See PHENYLTOLOXAMINE DIHYDROGEN CITRATE*

PHENYLTOLOXAMINE DIHYDROGEN CITRATE
(Medisca)
phenyltoloxamine citrate
POW, NA, 25 gm.......... **38779-0248-04** 64.50
(PCCA)
POW, NA, 1 gm........... **51927-1462-00** 2.16

PHENYLTOLOXAMINE PE CPM (Boca Pharmacal)
cpm/phenyleph hcl/phenyltoloxamine cit
SOL, PO (AF,SF,SACCHARIN-FREE)
473 ml.............. **64376-0431-16** 30.05

PHENYTEK (Mylan)
phenytoin sodium, extended
CER, PO (HARD-SHELL GELATIN)
200 mg, 30s ea ...... **00378-2670-93** 26.81 AB
100s ea........... **00378-2670-01** 89.35 AB
300 mg, 30s ea ...... **00378-3750-93** 40.16 AB
100s ea........... **00378-3750-01** 133.87 AB
(Southwood)
REPACK
CER, PO, 300 mg, 30s ea.. **58016-4863-01** 29.75

PHENYTOIN
FUL
SUS, PO, 125 mg/5 ml,
237 ml.................................. 36.05
(Actavis Mid Atlantic)
SUS, PO (ORANGE)
100 mg/4 ml,
4 ml 50s UD .... **00472-5002-60** 96.73 AB
(1X237ML,USP)
125 mg/5 ml,
237 ml .... **00472-5002-08** 33.30 AB
(Gallipot)
POW, NA, 25 gm.......... **51552-0553-04** 20.30
100 gm............. **51552-0553-05** 30.45
(Hawkins) *See PHENYTOIN BASE*
(Morton Grove)
SUS, PO (ORANGE,VANILLA)
125 mg/5 ml,
237 ml .... **60432-0131-08** 34.10 AB
(PCCA)
POW, NA (USP)
1 gm................ **51927-1216-00** 3.60
(Pfizer) *See DILANTIN INFATABS*
(Pfizer) *See DILANTIN-125*
(Prasco Labs)
SUS, PO (1X237ML,USP)
125 mg/5 ml,
237 ml **66993-0232-08** 36.97
(Precision Dose)
SUS, PO (ORANGE-VANILLA)
100 mg/4 ml,
4 ml 50s UD **68094-0533-58** 63.18
(Spectrum Pharmacy)
POW, NA (U.S.P.)
25 gm.............. **49452-5340-02** 98.70
100 gm.............. **49452-5340-03** 144.90
500 gm.............. **49452-5340-04** 420.00
(Taro)
SUS, PO (ORANGE-VANILLA)
125 mg/5 ml,
237 ml .... **51672-4069-01** 36.97 AB
(Phys Total Care)
REPACK
phenytoin sodium, extended
CER, PO (USP)
100 mg, 90s ea **54868-5534-00** 62.70

PROD/MFR NDC AWP DP OBC

PHENYTOIN (Phys Total Care)
SUS, PO, 125 mg/5 ml,
237 ml **54868-2038-00** 88.44

PHENYTOIN BASE (Hawkins)
phenytoin
POW, NA (USP)
5 gm................ **63370-0173-15** 28.00
25 gm.............. **63370-0173-25** 56.00
100 gm.............. **63370-0173-35** 84.00

PHENYTOIN SODIUM (Baxter)
phenytoin sodium, prompt
SOL, IV (USP)
50 mg/ml, 1 ml....... **00641-2555-41** 3.36 AP
(DOSETTE,VIAL)
50 mg/ml, 2 ml....... **00641-0493-21** 3.68 AP
2 ml 25s.......... **00641-0493-25** 92.10 AP
(VIAL, DOSETTE)
50 mg/ml, 5 ml 25s... **00641-2555-45** 84.00 AP
(Gallipot)
POW, NA, 25 gm.......... **51552-0532-04** 12.60

PHENYTOIN SODIUM (Hawkins)
POW, NA (U.S.P.)
25 gm.............. **63370-0176-25** 36.00
100 gm.............. **63370-0176-35** 84.00
500 gm.............. **63370-0176-45** 332.00
2500 gm............ **63370-0176-53** 1440.00
(Hospira)
phenytoin sodium, prompt
SOL, IV (CARPUJECT,10X2ML)
50 mg/ml, 2 ml 10s... **00409-1844-32** 16.68 14.60
(AMP,25X2ML,LATEX-FREE)
50 mg/ml, 2 ml 25s... **00409-1317-01** 48.30 42.25 AP
(AMP,LATEX-FREE)
50 mg/ml, 5 ml 25s... **00409-1317-02** 69.00 60.50 AP
(Medisca)
POW, NA (U.S.P.)
25 gm.............. **38779-0216-04** 28.50
100 gm.............. **38779-0216-05** 67.50
500 gm.............. **38779-0216-08** 267.00

PHENYTOIN SODIUM (PCCA)
POW, NA (U.S.P.)
1 gm................ **51927-1838-00** 1.32
(Spectrum Pharmacy)
phenytoin sodium, prompt
POW, NA (U.S.P.)
25 gm.............. **49452-5344-01** 67.90
100 gm.............. **49452-5344-02** 122.85
500 gm.............. **49452-5344-03** 434.00
(West-Ward)
SOL, IV (USP,25X2ML)
50 mg/ml, 2 ml 25s... **00143-9882-25** 30.00 AP
(USP,25X5ML)
50 mg/ml, 5 ml 25s... **00143-9881-25** 49.00 AP
(Wockhardt USA)
phenytoin sodium, extended
CER, PO (HARD GELATIN)
100 mg, 100s ea ..... **64679-0720-01** 33.88 AB
(USP,HARD GELATIN)
100 mg, 1000s ea .... **64679-0720-02** 322.93 AB
(Dispensing Solutions)
REPACK
CER, PO, 100 mg, 30s ea.. **55045-2899-08** 9.00
90s ea............ **55045-2899-09** 27.00
(Palmetto)
REPACK
CER, PO, 100 mg, 30s ea.. **23490-6524-01** 21.04
100s ea........... **23490-6524-02** 70.13
(Southwood)
REPACK
CER, PO, 100 mg, 30s ea.. **58016-0319-30** 19.95
60s ea............ **58016-0319-60** 39.90
90s ea............ **58016-0319-90** 59.85
100s ea........... **58016-0319-00** 66.50
(Stat Rx)
REPACK
CER, PO (HARD GELATIN)
100 mg, 90s ea ...... **16590-0815-60** 30.49 AB

PHENYTOIN SODIUM EXTENDED (Mylan)
phenytoin sodium, extended
CER, PO, 100 mg, 100s ea. **00378-1560-01** 33.90 AB
1000s ea .... **00378-1560-10** 339.00 AB
(UDL)
CER, PO (ROBOT READY 25X1)
100 mg, 25s ea UD ... **51079-0905-19** 10.30 AB
(10X10)
100 mg, 100s ea UD.. **51079-0905-20** 34.60 AB
(10X30 PUNCH CARD)
100 mg, 300s ea UD.. **51079-0905-56** 101.88 AB

PROD/MFR	NDC	AWP	DP	OBC
(A-S Medication)				
REPACK				
CER, PO, 100 mg, 100s ea	**54569-5151-00**	33.90		EE
(DHS, Inc.)				
REPACK				
CER, PO, 100 mg, 30s ea	**55887-0508-30**	21.04		AB
60s ea	**55887-0508-60**	38.49		AB
90s ea	**55887-0508-90**	49.09		AB
(Dispensing Solutions)				
REPACK				
CER, PO, 100 mg, 30s ea	**66336-0732-30**	19.25		AB
100s ea	**55045-2899-00**	30.00		AB
120s ea	**66336-0732-94**	76.96		AB
(PD-Rx Pharm)				
REPACK				
CER, PO, 100 mg, 30s ea	**55289-0906-30**	20.00		AB
(REDI-SCRIPT)				
100 mg, 30s ea	**58864-0746-30**	20.00		AB
60s ea	**55289-0906-60**	35.98		AB
(Phys Total Care)				
REPACK				
CER, PO, 100 mg, 30s ea	**54868-0040-02**	30.51		AB
30s ea	**54868-5534-02**	29.02		AB
60s ea	**54868-0040-01**	56.52		AB
100s ea	**54868-0040-00**	91.32		AB
100s ea	**54868-5534-01**	67.83		AB
(Quality Care Prod)				
REPACK				
CER, PO, 100 mg, 15s ea	**49999-0574-15**	12.79		AB
100s ea	**49999-0574-00**	85.00		AB
(Stat Rx)				
REPACK				
CER, PO, 100 mg, 150s ea	**16590-0815-83**	81.20		AB
180s ea	**16590-0815-82**	97.45		AB
PHENYTOIN SODIUM PROMPT (Palmetto)				
REPACK				
phenytoin sodium, prompt				
CAP, PO, 100 mg, 30s ea	**23490-6109-03**	13.50		
100s ea	**23490-6109-00**	45.00		
(Phys Total Care)				
REPACK				
CAP, PO, 100 mg, 90s ea	**54868-0040-03**	82.56		
PHENYTOIN SODIUM, EXTENDED				
(Amneal) *See EXTENDED PHENYTOIN SODIUM*				
(Caraco) *See EXTENDED PHENYTOIN SODIUM*				
(Mylan) *See PHENYTEK*				
(Mylan) *See PHENYTOIN SODIUM EXTENDED*				
(Pfizer) *See DILANTIN*				
(Taro) *See EXTENDED PHENYTOIN SODIUM*				
(UDL) *See PHENYTOIN SODIUM EXTENDED*				
(Wockhardt USA) *See PHENYTOIN SODIUM*				
(Vibranta)				
REPACK				
CER, PO, 100 mg, 30s ea	**57866-9031-01**	16.05		
PHENYTOIN SODIUM, PROMPT				
(Apotex Corp.) *See FOSPHENYTOIN SODIUM*				
(Baxter) *See PHENYTOIN SODIUM*				
(Gallipot) *See PHENYTOIN SODIUM*				
(Hospira) *See PHENYTOIN SODIUM*				
(Medisca) *See PHENYTOIN SODIUM*				
(Spectrum Pharmacy) *See PHENYTOIN SODIUM*				
(Teva) *See FOSPHENYTOIN SODIUM*				
(Truxton) *See DIPHEN*				
(West-Ward) *See PHENYTOIN SODIUM*				
PHISOHEX (Sanofi-Aventis)				
hexachlorophene				
LIQ, TP, 3%, 148 ml	**00024-1535-02**	26.72		
473 ml	**00024-1535-06**	51.61		
(Phys Total Care)				
REPACK				
LIQ, TP, 3%, 150 ml	**54868-3340-00**	23.55		
PHLEMEX (Cypress Pharm)				
dm/gg/phenyleph hcl				
TER, PO (DYE-FREE)				
30 mg-1200 mg-30 mg,				
100s ea	**60258-0323-01**	100.57		
PHLEMEX-PE (Cypress Pharm)				
dm/gg/phenyleph hcl				
TER, PO, 20 mg-800 mg-20 mg,				
100s ea	**60258-0321-01**	117.54		

PROD/MFR	NDC	AWP	DP	OBC
PHOS LO (PD-Rx Pharm)				
REPACK				
calcium acetate				
CAP, PO, 667 mg, 30s ea	**55289-0128-30**	14.59		
PHOS-FLUR (Colgate Oral)				
sodium fluoride				
GEL, DE (CHERRY)				
1.1%, 51 gm	**00126-0130-66**	9.28		
(MINT)				
1.1%, 51 gm	**00126-0131-66**	9.28		
PHOSLO (Fresenius)				
calcium acetate				
TAB, PO (GELCAP)				
667 mg, 200s ea	**49230-0640-21**	168.43	140.36	
(Phys Total Care)				
REPACK				
TAB, PO, 667 mg, 100s ea	**54868-3460-01**	41.26		
(GELCAP)				
667 mg, 200s ea	**54868-5691-00**	200.70		
PHOSPHA 250 NEUTRAL (Rising)				
k phos/na phos, dibasic/na phos, monobasic				
TAB, PO, 155 mg-852 mg-130 mg,				
100s ea	**64980-0104-01**	15.73		
PHOSPHATIDYL CHOLINE (Gallipot)				
POW, NA, 35%, 1000 gm	**51552-0823-07**	56.56	40.40	
(Letco) *See PHOSPHATIDYLCHOLINE*				
(Medisca) *See PHOSPHATIDYLCHOLINE*				
(PCCA) *See PHOSPHATIDYLCHOLINE*				
(Spectrum Pharmacy) *See PHOSPHATIDYLCHOLINE*				
PHOSPHATIDYLCHOLINE (Letco)				
phosphatidyl choline				
POW, NA, 94%, 25 gm	**62991-2688-01**	120.00		
100 gm	**62991-2688-02**	375.00		
(1X1000GM)				
94%, 1000 gm	**62991-2688-03**	2385.00		
(Medisca)				
GRA, NA (1X25GM)				
25 gm	**38779-2375-04**	225.00		
(1X100GM)				
100 gm	**38779-2375-05**	585.00		
(1X1000GM)				
1000 gm	**38779-2375-09**	2385.00		
(PCCA)				
POW, NA, 1 gm	**51927-3307-00**	4.80		
(Spectrum Pharmacy)				
GRA, NA (1X25GM)				
25 gm	**49452-5348-02**	208.95		
(1X100GM)				
100 gm	**49452-5348-03**	518.00		
(1X1000GM)				
1000 gm	**49452-5348-04**	2639.00		
PHOSPHATIDYLSERINE (PCCA)				
POW, NA (LECITHIN SOYBEAN)				
40%, 1 gm	**51927-3212-00**	13.20		
PHOSPHOLINE IODIDE (Wyeth)				
echothiophate iodide				
PDR, OP, 0.125%, 5 ml	**00046-1065-05**	80.45	67.04	
PHOSPHORIC ACID (Baker, J.T.)				
LIQ, NA (F.C.C., N.F., GLASS S/S)				
500 ml	**10106-0262-02**	27.18		
2500 ml	**10106-0262-05**	46.46		
(Mallinckrodt Lab) *See PHOSPHORIC ACID 85%*				
(Medisca)				
SOL, NA (1X500ML)				
500 ml	**38779-1817-08**	76.50		
(1X1000ML)				
1000 ml	**38779-1817-09**	78.00		
(PCCA) *See PHOSPHORIC ACID 85%*				
(Spectrum Pharmacy)				
LIQ, NA (N.F.)				
500 ml	**49452-5350-01**	85.75		
1000 ml	**49452-5350-02**	113.75		
2500 ml	**49452-5350-03**	180.95		
4000 ml	**49452-5350-04**	259.00		
PHOSPHORIC ACID 85% (Mallinckrodt Lab)				
phosphoric acid				
SOL, NA (N.F.)				
500 ml	**00406-2788-14**	29.91		
2500 ml	**00406-2788-46**	59.85		
(PCCA)				
SOL, NA (NF)				
1 ml	**51927-1303-00**	0.25		

PROD/MFR	NDC	AWP	DP	OBC
PHOSPHORUS PENTACHLORIDE (PCCA)				
POW, NA, 1 gm	**51927-3333-00**	2.94		
PHOSPHORUS PENTOXIDE (Baker, J.T.)				
POW, NA (PURIFIED)				
500 gm	**10106-9378-01**	50.83		
PHOSPHOTEC (Bracco Diag)				
technetium tc 99m pyrophosphate				
KIT, IV, ea	**00270-0064-25**	420.01		AP
PHOSPHOTUNGSTIC ACID				
(Baker, J.T.) *See PHOSPHOTUNGSTIC ACID N-HYDRATE*				
PHOSPHOTUNGSTIC ACID N-HYDRATE (Baker, J.T.)				
phosphotungstic acid				
CRY, NA (REAGENT)				
125 gm	**10106-2891-04**	144.92		
500 gm	**10106-2891-01**	448.93		
PHOTOFRIN (Axcan)				
porfimer sodium				
PDS, IV (VIAL)				
75 mg, ea	**58914-0155-75**	3317.04		
PHRENILIN (Valeant Pharm Intl)				
acetaminophen/butalbital				
TAB, PO (CAFFEINE-FREE)				
325 mg-50 mg,				
100s ea	**00187-0842-01**	137.97		AB
500s ea	**00187-0842-02**	253.89		AB
(PD-Rx Pharm)				
REPACK				
TAB, PO, 325 mg-50 mg,				
15s ea	**55289-0127-15**	16.93		AB
25s ea	**55289-0127-25**	22.93		AB
PHRENILIN FORTE (Valeant Pharm Intl)				
acetaminophen/butalbital				
CAP, PO (USP)				
650 mg-50 mg,				
100s ea	**00187-0844-01**	464.39		AB
500s ea	**00187-0844-02**	404.05		AB
(Phys Total Care)				
REPACK				
CAP, PO, 650 mg-50 mg,				
100s ea	**54868-1109-00**	83.93		AB
PHTHALIC ANHYDRIDE (Baker, J.T.)				
POW, NA (A.C.S., REAGENT)				
500 gm	**10106-0272-01**	22.71		
2500 gm	**10106-0272-05**	39.50		
PHYSIOLYTE (B. Braun)				
k cl/mg cl/na ace/na cl/na gluconate				
SOL, IR (PIC CONTAINER)				
1000 ml	**00264-2205-00**	2.56		AT
PHYSIOSOL (Hospira)				
k cl/mg cl/na ace/na cl/na gluconate				
SOL, IR (250MLX24,STERILE)				
250 ml 24s	**00409-6141-22**	150.91	132.00	EE
IV (AQUALITE,24X500ML)				
500 ml 24s	**00409-6141-03**	136.80	119.76	AT
(12X1000ML,LATEX-FREE)				
1000 ml 12s	**00409-7012-05**	65.38	57.24	
(AQUALITE)				
1000 ml 12s	**00409-6141-09**	57.89	50.64	AT
PHYSOSTIGMINE				
(PCCA) *See PHYSOSTIGMINE SALICYLATE*				
(Spectrum Pharmacy) *See PHYSOSTIGMINE SALICYLATE*				
PHYSOSTIGMINE SALICYLATE (Akorn)				
SOL, IJ (AMP)				
1 mg/ml, 2 ml 10s	**11098-0510-02**	48.60		
(PCCA)				
physostigmine				
POW, NA (U.S.P.)				
1 gm	**51927-2019-00**	228.00		
(Spectrum Pharmacy)				
POW, NA (U.S.P.)				
1 gm	**49452-5370-01**	342.65		
5 gm	**49452-5370-02**	1172.50		
PHYTIC ACID				
(PCCA) *See PHYTIC ACID (50% IN WATER)*				
PHYTIC ACID (50% IN WATER) (PCCA)				
phytic acid				
SOL, NA (1X1ML)				
50%, 1 ml	**51927-3157-00**	4.80		
PHYTIC ACID SODIUM				
(PCCA) *See INOSITOL HEXAPHOSPHATE SODIUM SALT*				
PHYTONADIONE (Amphastar)				
SOL, IJ (S.D.V.,MINIJET,25GX5/8")				
1 mg/0.5 ml,				
0.5 ml 25s	**00548-1140-00**	133.00		BP

PROD/MFR	NDC	AWP	DP	OBC
(SAF-T-JET, SRN,27GX1/2")				
1 mg/0.5 ml,				
0.5 ml 25s	00548-1240-00	141.31		BP
(Aton) *See MEPHYTON*				
(Hospira) *See VITAMIN K1*				
(Medisca)				
SOL, NA (1X1ML,USP)				
1 ml	38779-1822-06	57.00		
(1X5ML,USP)				
5 ml	38779-1822-03	183.00		
(1X25ML,USP)				
25 ml	38779-1822-04	675.00		
(1X100ML,USP)				
100 ml	38779-1822-05	2025.00		
(PCCA)				
SOL, NA (USP; VITAMIN K1)				
1 gm	51927-1925-00	60.00		
(Spectrum Pharmacy)				
POW, NA (U.S.P.)				
1 gm	49452-5390-01	95.90		
5 gm	49452-5390-02	313.25		
25 gm	49452-5390-03	1011.50		
PICRIC ACID (Baker, J.T.)				
CRY, NA (A.C.S., REAGENT)				
500 gm	10106-0276-01	181.43		
3000 gm	10106-0276-09	725.74		
PICROTOXIN (PCCA)				
POW, NA (1X1GM)				
1 gm	51927-1896-00	90.00		
PILOCARPINE (Phys Total Care)				
REPACK				
pilocarpine hydrochloride				
TAB, PO, 5 mg, 15s ea	54868-5436-00	39.09		
90s ea	54868-5436-01	163.17		
PILOCARPINE HCL (Actavis)				
pilocarpine hydrochloride				
TAB, PO (FILM-COATED)				
5 mg, 100s ea	00228-2801-11	152.11		
(Alcon Surgical)				
SOL, OP, 1%, 2 ml 12s	00065-0728-12	69.12		
2%, 2 ml 12s	00065-0752-12	69.12		
4%, 2 ml 12s	00065-0756-12	69.12		
(Bausch & Lomb Inc.)				
SOL, OP, 1%, 15 ml	24208-0676-15	23.81		
2%, 15 ml	24208-0681-15	25.06		
4%, 15 ml	24208-0686-15	26.31		
(Consolidated Midland)				
SOL, OP, 1%, 15 ml	00223-6700-15	4.95		
2%, 15 ml	00223-6701-15	7.50		
4%, 15 ml	00223-6702-15	8.50		
(Falcon Ophthalmics)				
SOL, OP (DROP-TAINER)				
1%, 15 ml	61314-0203-15	22.80		
2%, 15 ml	61314-0204-15	24.00		
4%, 15 ml	61314-0206-15	25.20		
6%, 15 ml	61314-0208-15	13.20		
(Gallipot)				
CRY, NA (U.S.P.)				
1 gm	51552-0477-01	19.95		
5 gm	51552-0477-02	50.40		
25 gm	51552-0477-04	255.50		
(Mallinckrodt Lab)				
CRY, NA (U.S.P.)				
30 gm	00406-6656-34	260.08		
125 gm	00406-6656-01	1021.52		
(Medisca)				
POW, NA (U.S.P.)				
1 gm	38779-0182-06	57.00		
5 gm	38779-0182-03	117.00		
25 gm	38779-0182-04	597.00		
(PCCA)				
POW, NA (U.S.P.)				
1 gm	51927-1528-00	31.80		
(Roxane)				
TAB, PO (FILM-COATED)				
5 mg, 100s ea	00054-0056-25	152.28		AB
500s ea	00054-0056-29	761.40		AB
(Spectrum Pharmacy)				
CRY, NA (U.S.P.)				
1 gm	49452-5400-01	106.40		
5 gm	49452-5400-02	214.55		
25 gm	49452-5400-03	910.00		
(Phys Total Care)				
REPACK				
SOL, OP, 0.5%, 15 ml	54868-2110-00	21.53		
1%, 15 ml	54868-1200-00	18.75		
2%, 15 ml	54868-1167-01	14.55		
4%, 15 ml	54868-1168-01	10.55		
6%, 15 ml	54868-1203-00	21.14		
(Physician Partner)				
REPACK				
SOL, OP (1X15ML)				
1%, 15 ml	21695-0368-01	18.40		
(Southwood)				
REPACK				
SOL, OP, 1%, 15 ml	58016-6403-01	10.24		
2%, 15 ml	58016-6088-01	10.24		
4%, 15 ml	58016-6037-01	11.04		
6%, 15 ml	58016-6327-01	21.35		
PILOCARPINE HYDROCHLORIDE				
FUL				
TAB, PO, 7.5 mg, 100s ea		194.25		
(Actavis) *See PILOCARPINE HCL*				
(Actavis)				
TAB, PO (FILM-COATED)				
7.5 mg, 100s ea	00228-2837-11	199.60		
(Alcon Ophthalmic) *See ISOPTO CARPINE*				
(Alcon Ophthalmic) *See PILOPINE-HS*				
(Alcon Surgical) *See PILOCARPINE HCL*				
(Bausch & Lomb Inc.) *See PILOCARPINE HCL*				
(Consolidated Midland) *See PILOCARPINE HCL*				
(Eisai) *See SALAGEN*				
(Falcon Ophthalmics) *See PILOCARPINE HCL*				
(Gallipot) *See PILOCARPINE HCL*				
(Global Pharm)				
TAB, PO (FILM COATED)				
5 mg, 100s ea	00115-5922-01	161.64		AB
7.5 mg, 100s ea	00115-5911-01	199.36		AB
(Lannett)				
TAB, PO (FILM-COATED)				
5 mg, 100s ea	00527-1313-01	152.28		AB
(FILM COATED)				
7.5 mg, 100s ea	00527-1407-01	239.52		AB
(Mallinckrodt Lab) *See PILOCARPINE HCL*				
(Medisca) *See PILOCARPINE HCL*				
(PCCA) *See PILOCARPINE HCL*				
(Roxane) *See PILOCARPINE HCL*				
(Roxane)				
TAB, PO (FILM-COATED)				
7.5 mg, 100s ea	00054-0144-25	199.60		AB
(Spectrum Pharmacy) *See PILOCARPINE HCL*				
PILOCARPINE NITRATE (Gallipot)				
POW, NA (USP,1X1GM)				
1 gm	51552-0669-01	19.60	14.00	
(USP,1X5GM)				
5 gm	51552-0669-02	49.00	35.00	
(Mallinckrodt Lab)				
CRY, NA (U.S.P.)				
30 gm	00406-6662-03	246.75		
(Spectrum Pharmacy)				
CRY, NA (U.S.P.)				
1 gm	49452-5410-01	103.95		
5 gm	49452-5410-02	209.65		
25 gm	49452-5410-03	850.50		
PILOPINE-HS (Alcon Ophthalmic)				
pilocarpine hydrochloride				
GEL, OP, 4%, 4 gm	00065-0215-35	60.96		
(Phys Total Care)				
REPACK				
GEL, OP, 4%, 4 gm	54868-0631-00	51.18		
PIMECROLIMUS				
(Novartis Pharm) *See ELIDEL*				
PIMENTA BERRY OIL (Medisca)				
pimenta oil				
OIL, NA (1X14ML,NATURAL)				
14 ml	38779-1511-03	52.50		
(1X25ML,NATURAL)				
25 ml	38779-1511-04	120.00		
(1X100ML,NATURAL)				
100 ml	38779-1511-05	352.50		
PIMENTA OIL				
(Medisca) *See PIMENTA BERRY OIL*				
PIMOZIDE				
(Gate) *See ORAP*				
PINA COLADA FLAVOR (Medisca)				
flavoring aid				
SOL, NA (1X25ML,ANHYDROUS)				
25 ml	38779-1512-04	21.00		
(1X100ML,ANHYDROUS)				
100 ml	38779-1512-05	31.50		
(1X100ML,CONCENTRATE)				
100 ml	38779-1513-05	28.50		
(1X500ML,ANHYDROUS)				
500 ml	38779-1512-08	55.50		
(1X500ML,CONCENTRATE)				
500 ml	38779-1513-08	55.50		
(PCCA)				
SOL, NA (ANHYDROUS; ARTIFICIAL)				
1 ml	51927-2328-00	0.90		
(CONCENTRATE)				
1 ml	51927-1623-00	0.30		
PINDOLOL (Martec)				
TAB, PO, 5 mg, 100s ea	52555-0454-01	69.30		AB
10 mg, 100s ea	52555-0455-01	94.50		AB
(Mylan)				
TAB, PO, 5 mg, 100s ea	00378-0052-01	72.80		AB
10 mg, 100s ea	00378-0127-01	99.20		AB
PINE NEEDLE OIL				
(Medisca) *See PINE NEEDLES OIL*				
(PCCA)				
OIL, NA (PINE NEEDLE)				
1 ml	51927-2792-00	0.43		
(SIBERIAN, FIR NEEDLE)				
1 gm	51927-2025-00	0.69		
PINE NEEDLES OIL (Medisca)				
pine needle oil				
OIL, NA (1X14ML,NATURAL)				
14 ml	38779-0902-03	12.00		
(1X100ML,NATURAL)				
100 ml	38779-0902-05	43.50		
(1X500ML,NATURAL)				
500 ml	38779-0902-08	160.50		
PINE OIL (Lorann Oil)				
OIL, NA, 9.9 ml	23535-0151-57	3.00		
(Medisca)				
OIL, NA (1X25ML,STEAM DISTILLED)				
25 ml	38779-1514-04	165.00		
(1X100ML,STEAM DISTILLED)				
100 ml	38779-1514-05	31.50		
(1X500ML,STEAM DISTILLED)				
500 ml	38779-1514-08	52.50		
(PCCA)				
OIL, NA (STEAM DISTILLED)				
1 ml	51927-1290-00	0.35		
PINE TAR (Humco)				
LIQ, NA (TECHNICAL)				
420 ml	00395-2279-14	12.37		
(Medisca)				
SOL, NA (1X250ML)				
250 gm	38779-1515-07	25.50		
(1X500ML)				
500 gm	38779-1515-08	31.50		
(PCCA)				
POW, NA, 1 gm	51927-1947-00	0.17		
PINEAPPLE FLAVOR (Medisca)				
flavoring aid				
SOL, NA (1X100ML,CONCENTRATE)				
100 ml	38779-1516-05	22.50		
(1X500ML,CONCENTRATE)				
500 ml	38779-1516-08	46.50		
(PCCA)				
POW, NA (ARTIFICIAL)				
1 gm	51927-3565-00	0.15		
SOL, NA (CONCENTRATE,PINEAPPLE)				
1 ml	51927-2015-00	0.23		
(PINEAPPLE)				
1 ml	51927-3435-00	0.90		
(Spectrum Pharmacy)				
LIQ, NA (1X100ML)				
100 ml	49452-5425-01	53.20		
(1X500ML)				
500 ml	49452-5425-02	109.55		
PINENE (PCCA)				
SOL, NA (FCC; L-ALPHA)				
1 ml	51927-3612-00	0.95		
PINK FOOD COLOR (PCCA)				
color additive				
SOL, NA, 1 ml	51927-2674-00	2.79		

PROD/MFR	NDC	AWP	DP	OBC
PIOGLITAZONE HYDROCHLORIDE				
(Takeda) *See ACTOS*				
PIPERACILLIN (APP)				
piperacillin sodium				
PDS, IJ (VIAL)				
2 gm, 10s ea	63323-0380-20	83.52		
3 gm, 10s ea	63323-0381-20	125.28		
4 gm, 10s ea	63323-0390-50	167.04		
40 gm, ea	63323-0391-74	161.25		
PIPERACILLIN AND TAZOBACTAM (Apotex Corp.)				
piperacillin sodium/tazobactam sodium				
PDS, IV (SDV)				
2 gm-0.25 gm,				
10s ea	60505-0686-04	143.10		AP
3 gm-0.375 gm,				
10s ea	60505-0687-04	214.69		AP
4 gm-0.5 gm,				
10s ea	60505-0688-04	271.89		AP
(PHARMACY BULK PACKAGE)				
36 gm-4.5 gm, ea	60505-0773-00	257.70		AP
PIPERACILLIN SODIUM				
(APP) *See PIPERACILLIN*				
PIPERACILLIN SODIUM/TAZOBACTAM SODIUM				
(Apotex Corp.) *See PIPERACILLIN AND TAZOBACTAM*				
(Wyeth) *See ZOSYN*				
PIPERAZINE (PCCA)				
POW, NA (HEXAHYDRATE)				
1 gm	51927-1855-00	1.20		
PIPERAZINE CITRATE (Spectrum Pharmacy)				
POW, NA (U.S.P.)				
100 gm	49452-5470-01	95.20		
500 gm	49452-5470-02	157.85		
PIPERINE (PCCA)				
POW, NA, 1 gm	51927-3474-00	120.00		
PIPERONYL BUTOXIDE (PCCA)				
POW, NA, 1 gm	51927-1867-00	3.75		
PIRACETAM (Gallipot)				
POW, NA (1X25GM)				
25 gm	51552-0622-04	19.95	14.25	
(1X100GM)				
100 gm	51552-0622-05	41.30	29.50	
(1X500GM)				
500 gm	51552-0622-06	154.00	110.00	
1000 gm	51552-0622-07	273.00		
(1X20000GM)				
20000 gm	51552-0622-09	2520.00	1800.00	
(Hawkins)				
POW, NA, 100 gm	63370-0180-35	110.40		
500 gm	63370-0180-45	456.00		
1000 gm	63370-0180-50	840.00		
5000 gm	63370-0180-55	3504.00		
25000 gm	63370-0180-62	16320.00		
(Medisca)				
POW, NA, 25 gm	38779-0177-04	47.85		
(1X25GM,BP)				
25 gm	38779-2491-04	47.85		
100 gm	38779-0177-05	97.50		
(1X100GM,BP)				
100 gm	38779-2491-05	97.50		
500 gm	38779-0177-08	345.00		
(1X500GM,BP)				
500 gm	38779-2491-08	345.00		
1000 gm	38779-0177-09	585.00		
(1X1000GM,BP)				
1000 gm	38779-2491-09	585.00		
(PCCA)				
POW, NA, 1 gm	51927-2213-00	2.16		
(Spectrum Pharmacy)				
POW, NA (1X25GM)				
25 gm	49452-5472-02	79.80		
(1X100GM)				
100 gm	49452-5472-03	168.00		
(1X1000GM)				
1000 gm	49452-5472-05	983.50		
PIRBUTEROL ACETATE				
(Graceway) *See MAXAIR AUTOHALER*				
PIROXICAM				
FUL				
CAP, PO, 10 mg, 100s ea		8.91		
20 mg, 100s ea		11.31		
(Gallipot)				
POW, NA (U.S.P.)				
5 gm	51552-0457-02	25.20		
25 gm	51552-0457-04	89.60		
(Hawkins)				
POW, NA (U.S.P.)				
5 gm	63370-0185-15	72.00		
25 gm	63370-0185-25	256.00		
100 gm	63370-0185-35	540.00		
500 gm	63370-0185-45	2360.00		
(Letco)				
POW, NA (U.S.P.)				
5 gm	62991-1113-01	37.50		
25 gm	62991-1113-02	120.00		
100 gm	62991-1113-03	300.00		
(Martec)				
CAP, PO, 10 mg, 100s ea	52555-0972-01	134.10		AB
20 mg, 100s ea	52555-0973-01	251.35		AB
500s ea	52555-0973-05	1231.60		AB
(Medisca)				
POW, NA (1X5GM,USP)				
5 gm	38779-0302-03	64.50		
(U.S.P.)				
25 gm	38779-0302-04	208.50		
100 gm	38779-0302-05	471.00		
500 gm	38779-0302-08	1485.00		
(Mylan)				
CAP, PO, 20 mg, 100s ea	00378-2020-01	263.90		AB
500s ea	00378-2020-05	1293.20		AB
(PCCA)				
POW, NA (U.S.P.)				
1 gm	51927-1699-00	13.80		
(Pfizer) *See FELDENE*				
(Spectrum Pharmacy)				
POW, NA (U.S.P.)				
5 gm	49452-5476-01	114.45		
25 gm	49452-5476-02	353.50		
100 gm	49452-5476-03	714.00		
(Teva)				
CAP, PO, 10 mg, 100s ea	00093-0756-01	140.80		AB
20 mg, 100s ea	00093-0757-01	263.90		AB
500s ea	00093-0757-05	1293.20		AB
(4u)				
REPACK				
CAP, PO, 20 mg, 30s ea	10544-0342-30	104.56		
30s ea	42549-0542-30	104.56		AB
(A-S Medication)				
REPACK				
CAP, PO, 10 mg, 21s ea	54569-3974-00	29.57		EE
20 mg, 10s ea	54569-3693-01	26.39		EE
14s ea	54569-3693-00	36.95		EE
15s ea	54569-3693-05	39.59		EE
20s ea	54569-3693-03	52.78		EE
30s ea	54569-3693-04	79.17		EE
(Aidarex)				
REPACK				
CAP, PO, 20 mg, 7s ea	33261-0096-07	22.75		AB
14s ea	33261-0096-14	45.50		AB
20s ea	33261-0096-20	65.00		AB
21s ea	33261-0096-21	68.25		AB
28s ea	33261-0096-28	91.00		AB
30s ea	33261-0096-30	97.50		AB
40s ea	33261-0096-40	130.00		AB
60s ea	33261-0096-60	195.00		AB
90s ea	33261-0096-90	292.50		AB
100s ea	33261-0096-00	325.00		AB
120s ea	33261-0096-02	390.00		AB
180s ea	33261-0096-03	702.00		AB
(Altura)				
REPACK				
CAP, PO, 10 mg, 7s ea	63874-0614-07	10.70		
10s ea	63874-0614-10	15.29		
14s ea	63874-0614-14	21.40		
15s ea	63874-0614-15	22.93		
20s ea	63874-0614-20	30.57		
21s ea	63874-0614-21	32.10		
28s ea	63874-0614-28	42.80		
30s ea	63874-0614-30	45.86		
40s ea	63874-0614-40	61.15		
50s ea	63874-0614-50	76.43		
60s ea	63874-0614-60	91.72		
90s ea	63874-0614-90	137.58		
100s ea	63874-0614-01	152.87		
20 mg, 7s ea	63874-0362-07	21.00		EE
10s ea	63874-0362-10	30.00		EE
12s ea	63874-0362-12	36.00		EE
14s ea	63874-0362-14	42.00		EE
15s ea	63874-0362-15	45.00		EE
20s ea	63874-0362-20	60.00		EE
21s ea	63874-0362-21	63.00		EE
24s ea	63874-0362-24	72.00		EE
28s ea	63874-0362-28	84.00		EE
30s ea	63874-0362-30	90.00		EE
36s ea	63874-0362-36	108.00		EE
40s ea	63874-0362-40	120.00		EE
42s ea	63874-0362-42	126.00		EE
50s ea	63874-0362-50	150.00		EE
56s ea	63874-0362-56	168.00		EE
60s ea	63874-0362-60	180.00		EE
90s ea	63874-0362-90	270.00		EE
100s ea	63874-0362-01	300.00		EE
120s ea	63874-0362-04	360.00		EE
128s ea	63874-0362-08	384.00		EE
500s ea	63874-0362-03	1575.75		EE
(Bryant Ranch)				
REPACK				
CAP, PO, 20 mg, 7s ea	63629-1383-03	25.35		
10s ea	63629-1383-01	36.21		
30s ea	63629-1383-02	108.63		
60s ea	63629-1383-04	179.56		
(Core)				
REPACK				
CAP, PO, 20 mg, 10s ea	33358-0290-10	37.12		
30s ea	33358-0290-30	111.35		
60s ea	33358-0290-60	184.05		
90s ea	33358-0290-90	243.45		
120s ea	33358-0290-01	318.30		
(DHS, Inc.)				
REPACK				
CAP, PO, 10 mg, 20s ea	55887-0688-20	30.05		AB
30s ea	55887-0688-30	43.98		AB
60s ea	55887-0688-60	80.05		AB
20 mg, 20s ea	55887-0784-20	57.78		AB
30s ea	55887-0784-30	86.66		AB
60s ea	55887-0784-60	173.32		AB
(Dispensing Solutions)				
REPACK				
CAP, PO, 10 mg, 60s ea	55045-1926-09	93.00		AB
20 mg, 7s ea	55045-1924-06	21.49		AB
10s ea	55045-1924-03	30.65		AB
10s ea	66336-0676-10	29.39		AB
15s ea	55045-1924-05	46.05		AB
20s ea	55045-1924-07	61.40		AB
20s ea	55045-1926-06	31.00		AB
30s ea	55045-1924-08	92.10		AB
30s ea	55045-3758-08	92.10		
30s ea	66336-0676-30	88.17		AB
42s ea	55045-3719-04	128.94		
45s ea	55045-1924-02	138.15		AB
50s ea	55045-3311-05	153.50		
60s ea	55045-1924-09	184.20		AB
60s ea	66336-0676-60	176.34		AB
90s ea	55045-1924-01	276.30		AB
100s ea	55045-1924-00	307.00		AB
120s ea	55045-1924-04	368.40		AB
(HomeMed)				
REPACK				
CAP, PO, 20 mg, 14s ea	51655-0567-84	16.09		EE
30s ea	51655-0567-24	94.99		EE
(IPI)				
REPACK				
CAP, PO (USP)				
20 mg, 30s ea	18837-0124-30	96.98		
60s ea	18837-0124-60	194.25		
(Keltman Pharma., Inc.)				
REPACK				
CAP, PO, 20 mg, 15s ea	68387-0700-15	45.00		
30s ea	68387-0700-30	90.13		AB
60s ea	68387-0700-60	180.26		AB
90s ea	68387-0700-90	270.39		AB
(LWP)				
REPACK				
CAP, PO, 20 mg, 30s ea	64038-0105-30	84.17		AB
60s ea	64038-0105-60	166.25		AB
100s ea	64038-0105-01	277.09		AB
(Nucare Pharm)				
REPACK				
CAP, PO, 20 mg, 10s ea	66267-0168-10	32.56		EE
14s ea	66267-0168-14	42.12		EE
20s ea	66267-0168-20	60.89		EE
30s ea	66267-0168-30	110.43		AB
60s ea	66267-0168-60	203.96		AB
90s ea	66267-0168-90	305.80		AB
(Palmetto)				
REPACK				
CAP, PO, 20 mg, 10s ea	23490-6125-01	35.00		
20s ea	23490-6125-00	70.00		
30s ea	23490-6125-02	105.00		
60s ea	23490-6125-03	210.00		
90s ea	23490-6125-09	315.00		

PROD/MFR	NDC	AWP	DP	OBC
(PD-Rx Pharm)				
REPACK				
CAP, PO, 10 mg, 10s ea	**55289-0515-10**	81.40		AB
20 mg, 7s ea	**55289-0052-07**	80.67		AB
10s ea	**55289-0052-10**	84.44		AB
14s ea	**55289-0052-14**	94.44		AB
(REDI-SCRIPT)				
20 mg, 14s ea	**58864-0643-14**	94.40		AB
20s ea	**55289-0052-20**	102.22		AB
(REDI-SCRIPT)				
20 mg, 20s ea	**58864-0643-20**	102.22		AB
21s ea	**55289-0052-21**	108.44		AB
30s ea	**55289-0052-30**	120.00		AB
(REDI-SCRIPT)				
20 mg, 30s ea	**58864-0643-30**	120.00		AB
(Pharma Pac)				
REPACK				
CAP, PO, 10 mg, 10s ea	**52959-0398-10**	16.19		EE
20s ea	**52959-0398-20**	32.38		EE
21s ea	**52959-0398-21**	33.99		EE
30s ea	**52959-0398-30**	48.56		EE
60s ea	**52959-0398-60**	97.11		EE
100s ea	**52959-0398-00**	161.83		EE
20 mg, 7s ea	**52959-0232-07**	23.97		EE
9s ea	**52959-0232-09**	30.82		EE
10s ea	**52959-0232-10**	34.24		EE
14s ea	**52959-0232-14**	47.93		EE
15s ea	**52959-0232-15**	51.36		EE
18s ea	**52959-0232-18**	61.62		EE
20s ea	**52959-0232-20**	68.47		EE
21s ea	**52959-0232-21**	71.89		EE
30s ea	**52959-0232-30**	102.69		EE
60s ea	**52959-0232-60**	205.35		EE
90s ea	**52959-0232-90**	308.00		EE
(Phys Total Care)				
REPACK				
CAP, PO, 10 mg, 30s ea	**54868-2198-00**	12.72		AB
20 mg, 10s ea	**54868-2199-04**	6.42		EE
15s ea	**54868-2199-03**	9.46		AB
30s ea	**54868-2199-01**	13.23		EE
60s ea	**54868-2199-00**	23.46		EE
100s ea	**54868-2199-05**	35.61		EE
(Physician Partner)				
REPACK				
CAP, PO, 10 mg, 60s ea	**21695-0520-60**	168.96		AB
90s ea	**21695-0520-90**	253.44		AB
20 mg, 15s ea	**21695-0285-15**	91.28		AB
20s ea	**21695-0285-20**	121.71		
30s ea	**21695-0285-30**	155.18		
60s ea	**21695-0285-60**	310.36		
90s ea	**21695-0285-90**	465.55		
120s ea	**21695-0285-72**	620.74		
(Quality Care Prod)				
REPACK				
CAP, PO, 20 mg, 7s ea	**49999-0074-07**	22.05		AB
10s ea	**49999-0074-10**	35.73		AB
14s ea	**49999-0074-14**	46.45		AB
30s ea	**49999-0074-30**	107.21		EE
60s ea	**49999-0074-60**	189.00		EE
(Southwood)				
REPACK				
CAP, PO, 10 mg, 7s ea	**58016-0705-07**	10.67		EE
10s ea	**58016-0705-10**	15.25		EE
14s ea	**58016-0705-14**	21.35		EE
15s ea	**58016-0705-15**	22.87		EE
20s ea	**58016-0705-20**	30.49		EE
21s ea	**58016-0705-21**	32.02		EE
28s ea	**58016-0705-28**	42.69		EE
30s ea	**58016-0705-30**	45.74		EE
40s ea	**58016-0705-40**	60.99		EE
50s ea	**58016-0705-50**	76.23		EE
60s ea	**58016-0705-60**	91.48		EE
90s ea	**58016-0705-90**	137.22		EE
100s ea	**58016-0705-00**	152.47		EE
126s ea	**58016-0705-97**	192.11		EE
20 mg, 7s ea	**58016-0666-07**	20.83		EE
10s ea	**58016-0666-10**	29.75		EE
14s ea	**58016-0666-14**	41.65		EE
15s ea	**58016-0666-15**	44.63		EE
20s ea	**58016-0666-20**	59.50		EE
21s ea	**58016-0666-21**	62.48		EE
28s ea	**58016-0666-28**	83.30		EE
30s ea	**58016-0666-30**	98.70		AB
40s ea	**58016-0666-40**	119.00		EE
45s ea	**58016-0666-45**	133.88		AB
50s ea	**58016-0666-50**	148.75		EE
60s ea	**58016-0666-60**	197.40		AB
90s ea	**58016-0666-90**	296.10		AB
100s ea	**58016-0666-00**	329.00		AB
120s ea	**58016-0666-02**	394.80		AB
126s ea	**58016-0666-97**	374.85		AB
150s ea	**58016-0666-03**	446.25		AB
200s ea	**58016-0666-89**	595.00		AB
300s ea	**58016-0666-73**	892.50		AB
(St. Mary's MPP)				
REPACK				
CAP, PO, 20 mg, 20s ea	**60760-0020-20**	62.90		AB
30s ea	**60760-0020-30**	91.35		AB
(USP)				
20 mg, 60s ea	**60760-0020-60**	176.70		AB
(Stat Rx)				
REPACK				
CAP, PO, 10 mg, 30s ea	**16590-0187-30**	45.00		
60s ea	**16590-0187-60**	90.00		
90s ea	**16590-0187-90**	135.00		
120s ea	**16590-0187-72**	180.00		AB
180s ea	**16590-0187-82**	270.00		AB
20 mg, 15s ea	**16590-0188-15**	48.49		AB
30s ea	**16590-0188-30**	102.80		
60s ea	**16590-0188-60**	184.00		
90s ea	**16590-0188-90**	276.00		
180s ea	**16590-0188-82**	582.46		AB
(Vibranta)				
REPACK				
CAP, PO, 20 mg, 10s ea	**57866-5559-04**	35.73		
14s ea	**57866-5559-02**	46.45		
30s ea	**57866-5559-01**	107.21		
PITOCIN (JHP)				
oxytocin				
SOL, IJ (25X1ML)				
10 u/ml, 1 ml 25s	**42023-0116-25**	39.95		AP
(1X10ML,MDV)				
10 u/ml, 10 ml	**42023-0116-01**	15.98		AP
PITRESSIN (JHP)				
vasopressin				
SOL, IJ (25X1ML)				
20 u/ml, 1 ml 25s	**42023-0117-25**	192.00		
PLACEBO				
(Forest Pharm) *See CEBOCAP*				
PLAN B (Teva)				
levonorgestrel				
TAB, PO, 0.75 mg, 2s ea	**51285-0038-20**	36.86		
2s ea	**51285-0769-93**	40.62		
(DHS, Inc.)				
REPACK				
TAB, PO, 0.75 mg, 2s ea	**55887-0204-02**	36.00		
(Dispensing Solutions)				
REPACK				
TAB, PO, 0.75 mg, 2s ea	**55045-2839-02**	36.00		
2s ea	**55045-3783-02**	40.00		
(Phys Total Care)				
REPACK				
TAB, PO, 0.75 mg, 2s ea	**54868-4894-00**	50.20		
PLAN B ONE-STEP (Teva)				
levonorgestrel				
TAB, PO (UNIT OF USE)				
1.5 mg, ea	**51285-0942-88**	40.62		EE
(A-S Medication)				
REPACK				
TAB, PO, 1.5 mg, ea	**54569-6145-00**	40.62		EE
PLANTAIN LEAF (PCCA)				
common plantain				
POW, NA, 1 gm	**51927-3198-00**	0.20		
PLAQUENIL (Sanofi-Aventis)				
hydroxychloroquine sulfate				
TAB, PO, 200 mg, 100s ea	**00024-1562-10**	265.40		AB
PLASBUMIN-25 (Talecris)				
albumin human				
SOL, IV (S.D.V.,PF)				
25%, 20 ml	**13533-0692-16**	27.74		
(SINGLE-DOSE,PF)				
25%, 20 ml	**13533-0684-16**	27.74		
(S.D.V.,PF)				
25%, 50 ml	**13533-0692-20**	55.51		
(SINGLE-DOSE,PF)				
25%, 50 ml	**13533-0684-20**	55.51		
(S.D.V.,PF)				
25%, 100 ml	**13533-0692-71**	110.96		
(SINGLE-DOSE,PF)				
25%, 100 ml	**13533-0684-71**	110.96		
PLASBUMIN-5 (Talecris)				
albumin human				
SOL, IV (S.D.V.,PF)				
5%, 50 ml	**13533-0690-20**	29.63		
(SINGLE-DOSE,PF)				
5%, 50 ml	**13533-0685-20**	29.63		
(S.D.V.,PF)				
5%, 250 ml	**13533-0690-25**	59.29		
(SINGLE-DOSE,PF)				
5%, 250 ml	**13533-0685-25**	59.29		
PLASMA PROTEIN FRACTION				
(Talecris) *See PLASMANATE*				
PLASMA-LYTE 148 (Baxter)				
k cl/mg cl/na ace/na cl/na gluconate				
SOL, IV, 500 ml 24s	**00338-0179-03**	387.65		AP
1000 ml 12s	**00338-0179-04**	221.76		AP
PLASMA-LYTE 56 W/DEXTROSE (Baxter)				
dextrose/k ace/mg ace/na cl				
SOL, IV, 500 ml 24s	**00338-0147-03**	398.88		AP
1000 ml 12s	**00338-0147-04**	232.13		AP
PLASMA-LYTE A PH-7.4 (Baxter)				
k cl/mg cl/na ace/na cl/na gluconate				
SOL, IV, 500 ml 24s	**00338-0221-03**	498.82		AP
1000 ml 12s	**00338-0221-04**	301.10		AP
PLASMANATE (Talecris)				
plasma protein fraction				
SOL, IV (SDV,USP)				
5%, 50 ml	**13533-0613-20**	23.52		
(SDV)				
5%, 250 ml	**13533-0613-25**	43.38		
PLASTER OF PARIS (Gallipot)				
calcium sulfate, dried				
POW, NA (DENTAL)				
454 gm	**51552-0240-06**	5.53		
2270 gm	**51552-0240-08**	12.18		
(Humco)				
POW, NA (DENTAL)				
454 gm	**00395-2285-01**	3.66		
PLASTICIZED OINTMENT BASE (Spectrum Pharmacy)				
ointment base				
OIN, TP, 100 gm	**49452-0853-01**	59.50		
454 gm	**49452-0853-02**	159.95		
PLAVIX (Bristol-Myers)				
clopidogrel hydrogen sulfate				
TAB, PO (FILM-COATED)				
75 mg, 30s ea	**63653-1171-06**	186.46		
90s ea	**63653-1171-01**	559.45		
(BLISTER PACK)				
75 mg, 100s ea UD	**63653-1171-03**	621.62		
(FILM-COATED)				
75 mg, 500s ea	**63653-1171-05**	3108.11		
300 mg, 30s ea UD	**63653-1332-02**	745.93		EE
100s ea UD	**63653-1332-03**	2130.55		EE
(A-S Medication)				
REPACK				
TAB, PO (FILM-COATED)				
75 mg, 30s ea	**54569-4700-00**	224.64		
90s ea	**54569-4700-02**	674.05		
(Advanced Pharm Serv, Inc.)				
REPACK				
TAB, PO, 75 mg, 10s ea	**13411-0117-01**	62.70		
20s ea	**13411-0117-02**	120.40		
(FILM-COATED)				
75 mg, 30s ea	**13411-0117-03**	178.10		
60s ea	**13411-0117-06**	351.20		
90s ea	**13411-0117-09**	524.33		
(Altura)				
REPACK				
TAB, PO (FILM-COATED)				
75 mg, 10s ea	**63874-0564-10**	42.16		
30s ea	**63874-0564-30**	126.48		
90s ea	**63874-0564-90**	379.46		
(AQ)				
REPACK				
TAB, PO, 75 mg, 10s ea	**66105-0119-01**	62.70		
15s ea	**66105-0119-15**	87.38		
30s ea	**66105-0119-03**	173.09		
60s ea	**66105-0119-06**	351.20		
90s ea	**66105-0119-09**	524.33		
(Bryant Ranch)				
REPACK				
TAB, PO, 75 mg, 30s ea	**63629-1598-01**	126.48		
(Nucare Pharm)				
REPACK				
TAB, PO (FILM-COATED)				
75 mg, 15s ea	**66267-0696-15**	135.00		
30s ea	**66267-1299-03**	266.36		
60s ea	**66267-0696-60**	512.00		
(PD-Rx Pharm)				
REPACK				
TAB, PO (FILM-COATED)				
75 mg, 15s ea	**55289-0911-15**	128.43		

PROD/MFR NDC AWP DP OBC

30s ea............55289-0911-30 256.89
(REDI-SCRIPT,FILM-COATED)
75 mg, 30s ea.......58864-0748-30 209.49

(Phys Total Care)
REPACK
TAB, PO, 75 mg, 30s ea...54868-4070-00 206.52
(FILM-COATED)
75 mg, 90s ea.......54868-4070-01 595.85

(Physician Partner)
REPACK
TAB, PO (FILM-COATED)
75 mg, 30s ea........21695-0665-30 360.00

(Quality Care Prod)
REPACK
TAB, PO (FILM-COATED)
75 mg, 30s ea........49999-0402-30 265.80
90s ea............49999-0402-90 797.40

(Stat Rx)
REPACK
TAB, PO (FILM-COATED)
75 mg, 30s ea........16590-0288-30 244.68

PLEGISOL (Hospira)
ca cl/k cl/mg cl/na cl
SOL, IR (LIFECARE,12X1000ML)
1000 ml 12s.........00409-7969-05 691.92 605.40 AT

PLENAXIS (Praecis Pharma Inc)
abarelix/sodium chloride
KIT, MR (S.D.V.,PF)
100 mg-0.9%, ea.....68158-0149-51 776.83

PLENDIL (A-S Medication)
REPACK
felodipine
TER, PO, 10 mg, 30s ea...54569-3719-00 95.18

(Bryant Ranch)
REPACK
TER, PO, 5 mg, 30s ea....63629-1597-01 36.55
10 mg, 30s ea........63629-1596-01 78.23

(PD-Rx Pharm)
REPACK
TER, PO (REDI-SCRIPT)
2.5 mg, 30s ea.......58864-0723-30 88.25
10 mg, 30s ea........58864-0713-30 112.57

(Phys Total Care)
REPACK
TER, PO, 5 mg, 10s ea....54868-2167-00 18.21
30s ea............54868-2167-02 50.88
10 mg, 10s ea........54868-2168-03 29.11
30s ea............54868-2168-02 79.11

(Quality Care Prod)
REPACK
TER, PO, 5 mg, 30s ea....49999-0296-30 95.70

PLENDIL ER (PD-Rx Pharm)
REPACK
felodipine
TER, PO (REDI-SCRIPT)
5 mg, 20s ea.........58864-0102-20 49.00

PLERIXAFOR
(Genzyme) *See MOZOBIL*

PLETAL (Otsuka)
cilostazol
TAB, PO, 50 mg, 60s ea...59148-0003-16 133.81 107.05
100 mg, 60s ea......59148-0002-16 133.81 107.05

(Phys Total Care)
REPACK
TAB, PO, 50 mg, 30s ea...54868-5027-00 73.06
60s ea............54868-5027-01 136.34
100 mg, 30s ea......54868-4427-00 79.56
60s ea............54868-4427-01 148.63

PLEXION (Medicis)
sulfacetamide sodium/sulfur
LOT, TP, 10%-5%,
170.3 gm.........99207-0741-06 126.89
340.2 gm.........99207-0741-12 232.80
PAD, TP, 10%-5%, 30s ea.99207-0745-30 194.26
60s ea............99207-0745-60 369.16

PLEXION SCT (Medicis)
sulfacetamide sodium/sulfur
CRE, TP, 10%-5%,
113.4 gm.........99207-0744-04 145.25

PLUG, EAR
(McKeon) *See MACK'S SAFE SOUND FOAM EARPLUGS*

PROD/MFR NDC AWP DP OBC

PLUM LC 5000 (Abbott Hosp)
pump, infusion
DEV, NA (INFUSER SYS RECERTIFIED)
ea..................00074-2507-12 5710.44 4808.79
(INFUSER SYSTEM)
ea..................00074-2507-11 5710.44 4808.79

(Abbott Hosp)
kit, administration, intravenous
(MINIPOLE)
ea..................00074-9295-01 40.22 32.15
(SECONDARY CONTNR SUPPRT)
ea..................00074-9294-01 39.06 39.06
(40 MM SCREW ETERNAL/98")
24s ea..............00074-1479-02 372.96 372.96

(Abbott Hosp)
kit, feeding (enteral)
(ENTRL W/INTGRL CO/105)
24s ea..............00074-6492-02 294.91 294.96

(Abbott Hosp)
kit, administration, intravenous
(SOLUSET W/HP,CNTPP 130")
24s ea..............00074-6445-03 546.05 546.00
(IV SET-SL NONVENTED)
48s ea..............00074-3260-48 85.25 85.44

PLUM LC 5000 LATEX-FREE (Abbott Hosp)
kit, administration, intravenous
DEV, NA (MICRDRP SLST/150 ML BUR)
24s ea..............00074-6446-03 536.26 536.16

PLUMSET LIFESHIELD H-FLOW (Abbott Hosp)
kit, administration, intravenous
DEV, NA (114", CONV PIN, OL)
48s ea..............00074-9097-48 1445.52 1217.28

PLUMSET MACRO INTEGRAL HP FILTER-OL
(Abbott Hosp)
device
DEV, NA (CONV PIN, 2-Y INJ)
48s ea..............00074-1649-48 1203.24 896.16

(Abbott Hosp)
filter, intravenous tubing
(LS CONV PIN, 2-LAV-Y)
48s ea..............00074-1647-48 691.20 691.20
(LS CONV PIN, 2-PP-Y)
48s ea..............00074-1645-48 864.00 864.00
(LS CONV PIN,PP SEC PORT)
48s ea..............00074-1644-48 630.72 1051.20

PLUMSET MICRO SECONDARY MIDLENGTH
(Abbott Hosp)
kit, administration, intravenous
DEV, NA (CONV PIERCING PIN, 40";)
48s ea..............00074-1139-48 130.53 109.92

PLUMSET MICRODRIP NITROGLYCERIN-OL
(Abbott Hosp)
kit, administration, intravenous
DEV, NA (CNVT PIN,LS)
48s ea..............00074-2427-78 637.06 636.96

PLUMSET MICRODRIP PRIMARY IV W/OL
(Abbott Hosp)
kit, administration, intravenous
DEV, NA (104" W/PP SITE,LTXF,LS)
24s ea..............00074-1735-78 249.12 249.12

PLUMSET MICRODRIP VENTED (Abbott Hosp)
kit, administration, intravenous
DEV, NA (SINGLE CHANNEL, OL)
48s ea..............00074-6440-12 943.49 943.20

PLUMSET PRIMARY IV W/OL (Abbott Hosp)
kit, administration, intravenous
DEV, NA (CONV PIN, DUAL CH, 1-Y)
48s ea..............00074-1651-48 896.61 755.04

PLUMSET SPECIALTY MICROBORE PUMP-OL
(Abbott Hosp)
kit, administration, intravenous
DEV, NA (76")
48s ea..............00074-2422-22 409.54 682.56

PLURONIC 20% (Gallipot)
poloxamer
GEL, NA, 100 ml..........51552-0549-05 10.99

(Letco)
GEL, NA (F127)
480 ml 62991-1565-01 63.00
3840 ml..............62991-1565-02 210.00

PLURONIC 30% (Gallipot)
poloxamer
GEL, NA, 473 ml..........51552-0589-06 26.46

(Letco)
GEL, NA (F127)
480 ml 62991-1566-02 66.00

PROD/MFR NDC AWP DP OBC

PLURONIC F-127 (Gallipot)
poloxamer
POW, NA (N.F.)
454 gm..............51552-0355-06 25.20
11350 gm 51552-0355-09 400.54

(Letco)
POW, NA (N.F.)
500 gm..............62991-1297-01 66.00
1000 gm.............62991-1297-02 96.00
2500 gm.............62991-1297-03 210.00

PNEUMOCOCCAL 7-VALENT VACCINE, DIPHTHERIA CONJUG
(Wyeth) *See PREVNAR*

PNEUMOCOCCAL VACCINE POLYVALENT
(Merck) *See PNEUMOVAX 23*

PNEUMODORON 1 (Weleda)
homeopathic substance
LIQ, PO, 20 ml...........55946-0350-10 4.65

PNEUMODORON 2 (Weleda)
homeopathic substance
LIQ, PO, 20 ml...........55946-0360-10 4.65

PNEUMOVAX 23 (Merck)
pneumococcal vaccine polyvalent
SOL, IM (S.D.V.,LATEX-FREE)
0.5 ml 10s...........00006-4943-00 510.97
(M.D.V.)
2.5 ml...............00006-4739-00 227.62

(A-S Medication)
REPACK
SOL, IM (M.D.V.)
2.5 ml...............54569-1412-00 227.62

(Dispensing Solutions)
REPACK
SOL, IM (1X2.5ML)
2.5 ml...............55045-3542-02 210.00

(Phys Total Care)
REPACK
SOL, IM (0.5MLX10)
0.5 ml 10s...........54868-4320-00 527.93
(M.D.V., FED TAX INCL)
2.5 ml...............54868-3339-01 180.00

PNV-DHA (Acella)
prenatal vitamins
SGL, PO, 30s ea..........42192-0321-30 51.21

PNV-SELECT (Acella)
prenatal vitamins
TAB, PO (FILM-COATED)
90s ea...............42192-0320-90 168.73

PODOCON-25 (Paddock)
benzoin compound/podophyllum
LIQ, TP, 75%-25%, 15 ml..00574-0601-15 92.95

(Phys Total Care)
REPACK
LIQ, TP, 75%-25%, 15 ml..54868-3003-01 69.26

PODODERM (Phys Total Care)
benzoin compound/podophyllum
LIQ, TP, 10%-25%, 5 ml...54868-3404-00 43.92
15 ml..............54868-3404-01 76.22

PODOFILOX (Paddock)
SOL, TP (W/24 ACCUTIP WANDS)
0.5%, 3.5 ml.........00574-0611-05 108.15 AT

(PCCA)
POW, NA, 1 gm............51927-2420-00 45.00

(Watson) *See CONDYLOX*

(Watson Labs) *See CONDYLOX*

(Watson Labs)
SOL, TP, 0.5%, 3.5 ml.....00591-3204-13 99.48 AT

PODOPHYLLUM RESIN (Amend)
POW, NA (U.S.P.)
30 gm...............17317-0425-02 42.00
125 gm..............17317-0425-04 140.00
500 gm..............17317-0425-01 490.00

(Baker, J.T.)
POW, NA (U.S.P.)
30 gm...............10106-2898-00 76.74

(Gallipot)
POW, NA (U.S.P.)
25 gm...............51552-0016-04 46.90
(BLISTER PACK)
30 gm...............51552-0068-09 49.00

(Humco)
POW, NA, 30 gm..........00395-2281-91 39.59

PROD/MFR	NDC	AWP	DP	OBC
(Mallinckrodt Lab)				
POW, NA (U.S.P.)				
30 gm	**00406-7700-12**	76.11		
125 gm	**00406-7700-01**	304.41		
(Medisca)				
POW, NA (U.S.P.)				
25 gm	**38779-0046-04**	111.00		
100 gm	**38779-0046-05**	415.50		
(PCCA)				
POW, NA (BP)				
1 gm	**51927-1673-00**	6.00		
(U.S.P.)				
1 gm	**51927-1220-00**	6.30		
(Spectrum Pharmacy)				
POW, NA (U.S.P.)				
5 gm	**49452-5480-01**	123.90		
(BP80)				
25 gm	**49452-5490-02**	148.40		
(U.S.P.)				
25 gm	**49452-5480-02**	162.05		
(BP80)				
125 gm	**49452-5490-03**	553.00		
(U.S.P.)				
125 gm	**49452-5480-03**	591.50		
POLIDOCANOL (Gallipot)				
polyoxyethylene lauryl ether				
SOL, NA, 120 ml	**51552-1075-09**	130.20	93.00	
(PCCA)				
SOL, NA, 1 ml	**51927-2783-00**	3.00		
POLIHEXANIDE				
(Covidien) *See KENDALL AMD ANTIMICROBIAL FENESTRATED FOAMDRESSING*				
(Covidien) *See KENDALL AMD ANTIMICROBIAL FOAM DRESSING*				
(Covidien) *See KENDALL AMD ANTIMICROBIAL FOAM DRESSING W/TOPSHEET*				
POLIOVIRUS VACCINE, INACTIVATED				
(Sanofi) *See IPOL*				
POLOCAINE (APP)				
mepivacaine hydrochloride				
SOL, IJ (1X50ML, MDV, USP)				
1%, 50 ml	**63323-0283-50**	11.46		**AP**
(1X50ML,MDV)				
2%, 50 ml	**63323-0296-50**	12.28		**AP**
POLOCAINE DENTAL (Dentsply)				
mepivacaine hydrochloride				
SOL, IJ (1.8MLX100)				
2%, 1.8 ml 100s	**66312-0460-14**	44.86		**AP**
3%, 1.8 ml 100s	**66312-0440-14**	44.86		**AP**
POLOCAINE-MPF (APP)				
mepivacaine hydrochloride				
SOL, IJ (SDV)				
1%, 30 ml	**63323-0260-30**	8.16		**AP**
(S.D.V.)				
1.5%, 30 ml	**00186-0418-01**	11.06		**AP**
(1X20ML, S.D.V.)				
2%, 20 ml	**63323-0294-20**	9.06		**AP**
POLOX 407 20% (Gallipot)				
poloxamer				
GEL, NA, 473 ml	**51552-0549-06**	21.35		
3785 ml	**51552-0549-08**	110.25		
POLOXAMER				
(Gallipot) *See PLURONIC 20%*				
(Gallipot) *See PLURONIC 30%*				
(Gallipot) *See PLURONIC F-127*				
(Gallipot) *See POLOX 407 20%*				
(Letco) *See PLURONIC 20%*				
(Letco) *See PLURONIC 30%*				
(Letco) *See PLURONIC F-127*				
(Medisca) *See POLOXAMER 407*				
(PCCA) *See POLOXAMER 188*				
(PCCA) *See POLOXAMER 407*				
(Spectrum Pharmacy) *See POLOXAMER 188*				
POLOXAMER 188 (PCCA)				
poloxamer				
POW, NA (NF)				
1 gm	**51927-2560-00**	0.22		
(Spectrum Pharmacy)				
FLA, NA (N.F.)				
500 gm	**49452-5503-01**	237.65		
POLOXAMER 407 (Medisca)				
poloxamer				
POW, NA (N.F.,PLURONIC F-127)				
500 gm	**38779-0834-08**	75.00		
(1X1000GM,NF)				
1000 gm	**38779-0834-09**	135.00		
(1X2500GM,NF)				
2500 gm	**38779-0834-01**	267.00		
(1X5000GM,NF)				
5000 gm	**38779-0834-03**	435.00		
(PCCA)				
POW, NA (NF)				
1 gm	**51927-2637-00**	0.16		
POLOXAMER 407 (Spectrum Pharmacy)				
GRA, NA (N.F.)				
500 gm	**49452-5507-01**	123.90		
2500 gm	**49452-5507-02**	406.00		
POLY HIST DHC (Poly)				
dihydrocodeine bitartrate/phenyleph hcl/pyril mal				
SOL, PO (1X473ML,AF,SF,DYE-FREE)				
473 ml, C-III	**50991-0521-16**	156.24		
POLY HIST DM (Poly)				
dm/phenyleph hcl/pyril mal				
SOL, PO (AF,SF,DYE-FREE,GRAPE)				
473 ml	**50991-0126-16**	59.20	49.51	
POLY HIST FORTE (Poly)				
cpm/phenyleph hcl/pyril mal				
TER, PO, 4 mg-10 mg-25 mg,				
100s ea	**50991-0201-01**	53.74	42.99	
POLY HIST HC (Poly)				
hydrocod bit/phenyleph hcl/pyril mal				
SOL, PO (AF,SF,DYE-FREE)				
473 ml, C-III	**50991-0714-16**	59.20	49.51	
POLY HIST NC (Poly)				
codeine phos/pse hcl/triprolidine hcl				
SOL, PO (1X473ML,AF,SF,DYE-FREE)				
473 ml, C-V	**50991-0528-16**	86.46		
POLY HIST PD (Poly)				
cpm/phenyleph hcl/pyril mal				
SOL, PO (AF,SF,DYE-FREE)				
473 ml	**50991-0405-16**	59.20	49.51	
POLY IRON PN (Contract Pharmacal)				
prenatal vitamins				
TAB, PO, 100s ea	**10267-2102-01**	24.50		
POLY IRON PN FORTE (Contract Pharmacal)				
prenatal vitamins				
TAB, PO, 100s ea	**10267-2101-01**	27.30		
POLY PRED (Allergan Inc)				
neomycin sulf/polymyxin b sulf/prednisolone ace				
SUS, OP, 0.35%-10000 u/ml-0.5%,				
5 ml	**00023-0028-05**	29.64		
POLY TAN D (Poly)				
dexbrompheniramine tannate/phenyleph tan/pyril mal				
SUS, PO (AF,SF)				
473 ml	**50991-0817-16**	129.77	108.14	
POLY TAN DM (Poly)				
cough/cold combination				
SUS, PO (AF,SF,CANDY APPLE)				
473 ml	**50991-0710-16**	129.77	108.14	
POLY-DEX (Ocusoft)				
dexamethasone/neomycin sulfate/polymyxin b sulfate				
OIN, OP, 3.5 gm	**54799-0519-35**	7.81		**AT**
SUS, OP, 5 ml	**54799-0520-05**	7.81		**AT**
POLY-IRON 150 FORTE (Cypress Pharm)				
cyanocobalamin/folic acid/iron polysaccharide				
CAP, PO, 25 mcg-1 mg-150 mg,				
100s ea	**60258-0186-01**	29.05		
POLY-RX (X-Gen)				
polymyxin b sulfate				
POW, NA (USP,100 MMU,MICRONIZED)				
13 gm	**39822-0100-01**	520.00		
POLY-TUSSIN (Poly)				
hydrocod bit/phenyleph hcl/pyril mal				
SOL, PO (AF,SF)				
473 ml, C-III	**50991-0707-16**	64.05	53.14	
POLY-TUSSIN AC (Poly)				
bpm/codeine phos/phenyleph hcl				
SOL, PO (1X473ML)				
473 ml, C-V	**50991-0713-16**	86.46	69.17	
POLY-TUSSIN DHC (Poly)				
bpm/dihydrocodeine bitartrate/phenyleph hcl				
SOL, PO (1X473ML,GRAPE)				
473 ml, C-V	**50991-0790-16**	86.46	69.17	
POLY-TUSSIN DM (Poly)				
cpm/dm/phenyleph hcl				
SYR, PO (AF,SF,BERRY)				
473 ml	**50991-0320-16**	41.28	33.87	
POLY-TUSSIN EX (Poly)				
dihydrocodeine bitartrate/gg/phenyleph hcl				
SOL, PO (1X473ML,AF,SF,DYE-FREE)				
473 ml, C-III	**50991-0529-16**	156.24		
POLY-TUSSIN HD (Poly)				
cpm/hydrocod bit/phenyleph hcl				
SYR, PO (AF,SF)				
473 ml, C-III	**50991-0603-16**	64.05	53.14	
POLY-TUSSIN XP (Poly)				
gg/hydrocod bit/phenyleph hcl				
SOL, PO (AF,SF)				
473 ml, C-III	**50991-0322-16**	64.05	53.14	
POLY-VI-FLOR (Southwood)				
REPACK				
multivitamin and fluoride				
LIQ, PO, 50 ml	**58016-9049-01**	5.93		
(DROPS)				
50 ml	**58016-9008-01**	6.05		
POLY-VITAMIN W/FLUORIDE (Silarx)				
multivitamin and fluoride				
LIQ, PO (WITH 0.25MG FLUORIDE)				
50 ml	**54838-0518-50**	5.60		
(WITH 0.5MG FLUORIDE)				
50 ml	**54838-0519-50**	5.60		
(Phys Total Care)				
REPACK				
LIQ, PO (DROPS)				
50 ml	**54868-6240-00**	10.86		
POLY-VITAMIN W/FLUORIDE/IRON (Hi-Tech)				
multivitamin, iron, and fluoride				
LIQ, PO (DROPS)				
50 ml	**50383-0634-50**	12.00		
50 ml	**50383-0633-50**	12.00		
(Silarx)				
LIQ, PO (DROPS)				
50 ml	**54838-0520-50**	6.10		
(Phys Total Care)				
REPACK				
LIQ, PO (DROPS)				
50 ml	**54868-4383-00**	10.86		
50 ml	**54868-1924-00**	4.38		
POLYCARBOPHIL (PCCA)				
POW, NA (USP)				
1 gm	**51927-2353-00**	2.16		
POLYCIN-B (Ocusoft)				
bacitracin zinc/polymyxin b sulfate				
OIN, OP, 500 u/gm-10000 u/gm,				
3.5 gm	**54799-0515-35**	12.43		**EE**
POLYDEXTROSE (Spectrum Pharmacy)				
POW, NA (1X500GM, UNTREATED)				
500 gm	**49452-5520-01**	116.55		
(1X2500GM, UNTREATED)				
2500 gm	**49452-5520-02**	325.50		
POLYETHYLENE				
(PCCA) *See MICROTHENE FN50100*				
POLYETHYLENE GLYCOL				
(Amend) *See P.E.G. 1000*				
(Amend) *See P.E.G. 1450*				
(Amend) *See P.E.G. 1500*				
(Amend) *See P.E.G. 200*				
(Amend) *See P.E.G. 300*				
(Amend) *See P.E.G. 3350*				
(Amend) *See P.E.G. 400*				
(Amend) *See P.E.G. 600*				
(Amend) *See P.E.G. 8000*				
(Gallipot) *See POLYETHYLENE GLYCOL 1000*				
(Gallipot) *See POLYETHYLENE GLYCOL 1450*				
(Gallipot) *See POLYETHYLENE GLYCOL 300*				
(Gallipot) *See POLYETHYLENE GLYCOL 3350*				
(Gallipot) *See POLYETHYLENE GLYCOL 400*				
(Gallipot) *See POLYETHYLENE GLYCOL 8000*				
(Gallipot) *See POLYETHYLENE GLYCOL BASE*				
(Gallipot) *See POLYETHYLENE GLYCOL BLEND*				
(Letco) *See POLYGLYCOL 1450*				
(Letco) *See POLYGLYCOL 300*				

PROD/MFR | NDC | AWP | DP | OBC

(Letco) *See POLYGLYCOL 3350*
(Letco) *See POLYGLYCOL 4500*
(Medisca) *See POLYETHYLENE GLYCOL 1000*
(Medisca) *See POLYETHYLENE GLYCOL 1450*
(Medisca) *See POLYETHYLENE GLYCOL 3350*
(Medisca) *See POLYETHYLENE GLYCOL 400*
(Medisca) *See POLYETHYLENE GLYCOL 4500*
(Medisca) *See POLYETHYLENE GLYCOL 8000*
(PCCA) *See POLYETHYLENE GLYCOL 1000*

(PCCA)
POW, NA (MONOSTEARATE)
1 gm 51927-1782-00 0.10
(NF; 3350)
1 gm 51927-3300-00 0.09

(Spectrum Pharmacy) *See POLYETHYLENE GLYCOL 1000*
(Spectrum Pharmacy) *See POLYETHYLENE GLYCOL 1450*
(Spectrum Pharmacy) *See POLYETHYLENE GLYCOL 3350*
(Spectrum Pharmacy) *See POLYETHYLENE GLYCOL 400*
(Spectrum Pharmacy) *See POLYETHYLENE GLYCOL 4500*
(Spectrum Pharmacy) *See POLYETHYLENE GLYCOL 600*
(Spectrum Pharmacy) *See POLYETHYLENE GLYCOL 8000*

POLYETHYLENE GLYCOL (Phys Total Care)
REPACK
polyethylene glycol 3350
PDS, PO, 17 gm/dose,
255 gm 54868-5160-01 34.95
527 gm 54868-5160-00 54.12

(Southwood)
REPACK
PDS, PO, 17 gm/dose,
14s ea 58016-4899-01 22.78

POLYETHYLENE GLYCOL 1000 (Gallipot)
polyethylene glycol
POW, NA (N.F.)
454 gm 51552-0089-06 13.23

(Medisca)
POW, NA (N.F.)
500 gm 38779-0288-08 30.00
2200 gm 38779-0288-09 49.50
(1X2500GM,NF)
2500 gm 38779-0288-01 117.00

(PCCA)
POW, NA (NF (BASE J))
1 gm 51927-1181-00 0.11

(Spectrum Pharmacy)
POW, NA (N.F.)
500 gm 49452-5550-01 53.90
2500 gm 49452-5550-02 190.75

POLYETHYLENE GLYCOL 1450 (Gallipot)
polyethylene glycol
FLA, NA (N.F.)
28.35 gm 51552-0019-02 4.76
454 gm 51552-0019-06 11.76

(Medisca)
POW, NA (1X100GM)
100 gm 38779-0778-05 30.00
(N.F.)
500 gm 38779-0778-08 25.50
(1X2500GM)
2500 gm 38779-0778-01 105.00
(1X5000GM)
5000 gm 38779-0778-03 184.50
(1X10000GM,NF)
10000 gm 38779-0778-00 297.00
(1X25000GM)
25000 gm 38779-0778-07 628.50

POLYETHYLENE GLYCOL 1450 (PCCA)
POW, NA (BASE A; NF)
1 gm 51927-9013-00 0.07

(Spectrum Pharmacy)
polyethylene glycol
FLA, NA (N.F.)
500 gm 49452-5555-01 53.90
2500 gm 49452-5555-02 189.35

POLYETHYLENE GLYCOL 300 (Gallipot)
polyethylene glycol
POW, NA (N.F.)
454 gm 51552-0293-06 12.53

(PCCA)
peg-6
SOL, NA (BASE C; NF)
1 ml 51927-9012-00 0.08

(Spectrum Pharmacy)
propylene glycol
LIQ, NA (N.F.)
500 ml 49452-5525-01 53.90
2500 ml 49452-5525-02 189.35

POLYETHYLENE GLYCOL 3350 (Breckenridge Pharm)
PDS, PO (NF)
17 gm/dose, 255 gm .. 51991-0457-58 19.50 AA
527 gm .... 51991-0457-57 38.99 AA

(Gallipot)
polyethylene glycol
POW, NA (N.F.)
454 gm 51552-0088-06 11.20

POLYETHYLENE GLYCOL 3350
(Kremers Urban) *See GLYCOLAX*

POLYETHYLENE GLYCOL 3350 (Medisca)
polyethylene glycol
POW, NA (N.F.)
500 gm 38779-0289-08 37.50
2200 gm 38779-0289-09 58.80
(1X2500GM)
2500 gm 38779-0289-01 76.50

POLYETHYLENE GLYCOL 3350 (Paddock)
PDS, PO (NF)
17 gm/dose, 14s ea ... 00574-0412-07 39.06 AA
255 gm .... 00574-0412-02 19.54 AA
527 gm .... 00574-0412-05 39.06 AA

(PCCA)
POW, NA (BASE B;NF)
1 gm 51927-9014-00 0.07

(Spectrum Pharmacy)
polyethylene glycol
POW, NA (N.F.)
500 gm 49452-5570-01 53.90
2500 gm 49452-5570-02 190.75

POLYETHYLENE GLYCOL 3350 (Teva)
PDS, PO, 17 gm/dose,
12s ea .... 00093-5299-22 19.54 AA
255 gm .... 00093-5299-25 19.54 AA
527 gm .... 00093-5299-82 39.06 AA

(IPI)
REPACK
PDS, PO, 17 gm/dose, ea .. 18837-0260-08 38.99 AA

(Nucare Pharm)
REPACK
PDS, PO, 17 gm/dose,
527 gm .... 68071-1316-07 56.12 AA

(Palmetto)
REPACK
PDS, PO, 17 gm/dose,
225 gm 23490-5006-01 22.78
527 gm 23490-5006-02 53.29

(Pharma Pac)
REPACK
PDS, PO, 17 gm/dose,
14s ea 52959-0893-14 40.10
(1X527GM)
17 gm/dose, 527 gm .. 52959-0893-57 39.06 AA

(Southwood)
REPACK
PDS, PO, 17 gm/dose,
527 gm 58016-4759-01 39.06

POLYETHYLENE GLYCOL 3350 AND ELECTROLYTES (Mylan)
peg electrolyte lavage solution
PDS, PO, ea .... 00378-6669-40 18.94 AA

POLYETHYLENE GLYCOL 400 (Gallipot)
polyethylene glycol
LIQ, NA (N.F.)
473 ml 51552-0003-06 12.39
3785 ml 51552-0003-08 70.98

(Medisca)
LIQ, NA (N.F.)
500 ml 38779-0251-08 31.50
1008 ml 38779-0251-09 52.50
4000 ml 38779-0251-01 193.50

(Spectrum Pharmacy)
LIQ, NA (N.F.)
500 ml 49452-5530-01 53.90
2500 ml 49452-5530-02 190.75

POLYETHYLENE GLYCOL 4500 (Medisca)
polyethylene glycol
POW, NA (N.F.)
500 gm 38779-1520-08 43.50
(1X2500GM)
2500 gm 38779-1520-01 187.50

POLYETHYLENE GLYCOL 4500 (PCCA)
POW, NA (BASE D; NF)
1 gm 51927-9015-00 0.07

(Spectrum Pharmacy)
polyethylene glycol
POW, NA (N.F.)
500 gm 49452-5575-01 53.90
2500 gm 49452-5575-02 189.35

POLYETHYLENE GLYCOL 600 (Spectrum Pharmacy)
polyethylene glycol
LIQ, NA (N.F.)
500 ml 49452-5540-01 53.90
2500 ml 49452-5540-02 190.75

POLYETHYLENE GLYCOL 6000 (PCCA)
peg-150
POW, NA, 1 gm 51927-3152-00 0.35

POLYETHYLENE GLYCOL 8000 (Gallipot)
polyethylene glycol
FLA, NA (N.F.)
454 gm 51552-0004-06 12.46
2270 gm 51552-0004-08 59.08
POW, NA, 454 gm 51552-0440-06 11.20

(Medisca)
POW, NA (N.F.)
500 gm 38779-0290-08 31.50
2500 gm 38779-0290-01 132.00

(Spectrum Pharmacy)
POW, NA (N.F.)
500 gm 49452-5580-01 53.90
2500 gm 49452-5580-02 190.75

POLYETHYLENE GLYCOL BASE (Gallipot)
polyethylene glycol
OIN, NA, 454 gm 51552-0527-06 19.04

POLYETHYLENE GLYCOL BLEND (Gallipot)
polyethylene glycol
POW, NA, 90 gm 51552-0008-05 6.09
454 gm 51552-0008-06 15.96
2270 gm 51552-0008-09 71.54

POLYETHYLENE OXIDE
(PCCA) *See POLYOX*

POLYFIN NEEDLE INFUSION (Medtronic Minimed)
kit, administration, intravenous
DEV, NA (24" BENT NDL,W/WINGS)
24s ea 76300-0307-24 143.75 115.00
(42" BENT NDL,W/WINGS)
24s ea 76300-0306-24 143.75 115.00
(42" BENT NDL)
24s ea 76300-0106-24 143.75 115.00

POLYFIN QR NEEDLE INFUSION (Medtronic Minimed)
kit, administration, intravenous
DEV, NA (24"BENT NDL,W/QR&WINGS)
24s ea 76300-0366-24 220.50
(42" QR BENT NDL)
24s ea 76300-0165-24 218.75 175.00
(42"BENT NDL,W/QR&WINGS)
24s ea 76300-0365-24 220.50

POLYFIN TUBING EXTENSION (Medtronic Minimed)
kit, intravenous extension tubing
DEV, NA (60")
24s ea 76300-0128-24 131.25 105.00

POLYGLYCOL 1450 (Letco)
polyethylene glycol
POW, NA, 500 gm 62991-1313-01 33.00
2500 gm 62991-1313-02 102.00

POLYGLYCOL 300 (Letco)
polyethylene glycol
LIQ, NA, 500 ml 62991-1334-01 29.25
3840 ml 62991-1334-02 135.00

POLYGLYCOL 3350 (Letco)
polyethylene glycol
POW, NA, 500 gm 62991-2009-01 34.50
2500 gm 62991-2009-02 90.00

POLYGLYCOL 4500 (Letco)
polyethylene glycol
POW, NA, 500 gm 62991-2010-01 42.00
2500 gm 62991-2010-02 135.00

PROD/MFR NDC AWP DP OBC

POLYMYCIN B/TRIMETHOPRIM SULFATE (DHS, Inc.)
REPACK
polymyxin b sulfate/trimethoprim sulfate
SOL, OP, 10000 u/ml-1 mg/ml,
10 ml.............. **55887-0357-10** 34.09 AT

POLYMYXIN B (APP)
polymyxin b sulfate
PDS, IJ (USP)
500000 u, 10s ea..... **63323-0321-10** 158.75 AP

POLYMYXIN B SULFATE
(APP) *See POLYMYXIN B*

(Bedford)
PDS, IJ (VIAL)
500000 u, 10s ea..... **55390-0139-10** 152.40 AP

(Gallipot)
POW, NA (1X12.66GM,MICRONIZED)
12.66 gm............ **51552-0946-09** 336.00 240.00

(Hawkins)
POW, NA (U.S.P.)
ea.................. **63370-0188-73** 2048.00

(Letco)
POW, NA (U.S.P., MICRO)
1 gm................ **62991-1548-01** 180.00
5 gm................ **62991-1548-02** 735.00

(Medisca)
POW, NA (U.S.P.,MICRONIZED)
50 ml............... **38779-0045-01** 2475.00 EE
(USP,1X100MU,MICRONIZED)
100 ml.............. **38779-0045-03** 3960.00 EE

(Spectrum Pharmacy)
POW, NA (U.S.P.)
16 gm............... **49452-5600-01** 2957.50 EE

(X-Gen) *See NOVAPLUS POLYMYXIN B*

(X-Gen)
PDS, IJ, 500000 u, ea..... **39822-0166-05** 13.65 AP

(X-Gen) *See POLY-RX*

POLYMYXIN B SULFATE MICRONIZED (PCCA)
polymyxin b sulfate, micronized
POW, NA (USP; NON-STERILE)
1 gm................ **51927-1086-00** 78.00

POLYMYXIN B SULFATE, MICRONIZED
(PCCA) *See POLYMYXIN B SULFATE MICRONIZED*

POLYMYXIN B SULFATE/NEOMYCIN SULFATE/GRAMICIDIN (Palmetto)
REPACK
gramicidin/neomycin sulfate/polymyxin b sulfate
SOL, OP, 10 ml........... **23490-7136-01** 31.50

POLYMYXIN B SULFATE/TRIMETHOPRIM SULFATE
FUL
SOL, OP, 10000 u/ml-1 mg/ml,
10 ml.. 12.36

(Allergan Inc) *See POLYTRIM*

(Bausch & Lomb Inc.) *See POLYMYXIN B/ TRIMETHOPRIM SULFATE*

(Falcon Ophthalmics) *See POLYMYXIN B/ TRIMETHOPRIM SULFATE*

(Pacific Pharma) *See POLYMYXIN B/ TRIMETHOPRIM SULFATE*

POLYMYXIN B/TRIMETHOPRIM (A-S Medication)
REPACK
polymyxin b sulfate/trimethoprim sulfate
SOL, OP, 10000 u/ml-1 mg/ml,
10 ml.............. **54569-4487-00** 17.42

POLYMYXIN B/TRIMETHOPRIM SULFATE
(Bausch & Lomb Inc.)
polymyxin b sulfate/trimethoprim sulfate
SOL, OP, 10000 u/ml-1 mg/ml,
10 ml.............. **24208-0315-10** 17.42 AT

(Falcon Ophthalmics)
SOL, OP, 10000 u/ml-1 mg/ml,
10 ml.............. **61314-0628-10** 17.42 AT

(Pacific Pharma)
SOL, OP, 10000 u/ml-1 mg/ml,
10 ml.............. **60758-0908-10** 17.23 AT

(Pharma Pac)
REPACK
SOL, OP, 10000 u/ml-1 mg/ml,
10 ml.............. **52959-0609-10** 19.75 AT

(Phys Total Care)
REPACK
SOL, OP, 10000 u/ml-1 mg/ml,
10 ml.............. **54868-4335-00** 9.78 AT

PROD/MFR NDC AWP DP OBC

(Quality Care Prod)
REPACK
SOL, OP, 10000 u/ml-1 mg/ml,
10 ml.............. **49999-0378-10** 9.42 AT
(1X10ML)
10000 u/ml-1 mg/ml,
10 ml.............. **35356-0536-10** 9.42 AT

(Southwood)
REPACK
SOL, OP, 10000 u/ml-1 mg/ml,
10 ml.............. **58016-5561-01** 27.75 EE

POLYMYXIN-B/TRIMETHOPRIM (Stat Rx)
REPACK
polymyxin b sulfate/trimethoprim sulfate
SOL, OP, 10000 u/ml-1 mg/ml,
10 ml.............. **16590-0233-10** 27.25

POLYOX (PCCA)
polyethylene oxide
POW, NA (WSR-301)
95%, 1 gm.......... **51927-2173-00** 0.39

POLYOXY PROPYLENE (15) STEARYL ETHER
(Amend) *See ARLAMOL E*

POLYOXYETHYLENE (2) OLEYL ETHER
(Gallipot) *See BRIJ 93*

(PCCA) *See BRIJ 93*

(Spectrum Pharmacy) *See BRIJ 35*

POLYOXYETHYLENE (20) ISOHEXADECYL ETHER
(Amend) *See ARLASOLVE 200*

POLYOXYETHYLENE (20) OLEYL ETHER
(Spectrum Pharmacy) *See BRIJ 98*

POLYOXYETHYLENE (200) CETYL ETHER
(Amend) *See BRIJ 58*

POLYOXYETHYLENE (40)
(Medisca) *See PEG-40*

POLYOXYETHYLENE (40) SORBITOL SEPTAOLEATE
(Amend) *See ARLATONE T*

(PCCA) *See POLYOXYETHYLENE 40 SORB SEPTAOLEATE*

POLYOXYETHYLENE (40) STEARATE
(Gallipot) *See POLYOXYL 40 STEARATE*

(Letco) *See POLYOXYL 40 STEARATE*

(PCCA) *See POLYOXYL 40 STEARATE*

(Spectrum Pharmacy) *See POLYOXYL 40 STEARATE*

POLYOXYETHYLENE (50) STEARATE
(Spectrum Pharmacy) *See POLYOXYL 50 STEARATE*

POLYOXYETHYLENE 100 STEARYL ETHER (PCCA)
steareth-100
POW, NA (BRIJ 700)
1 gm................ **51927-2302-00** 0.12

POLYOXYETHYLENE 40 SORB SEPTAOLEATE (PCCA)
polyoxyethylene (40) sorbitol septaoleate
LIQ, NA, 1 ml............ **51927-2521-00** 0.13

POLYOXYETHYLENE FATTY GLYCERIDE
(Amend) *See ARLATONE G*

POLYOXYETHYLENE LAURYL ETHER
(Gallipot) *See POLIDOCANOL*

(PCCA) *See POLIDOCANOL*

(Spectrum Pharmacy) *See BRIJ 30*

POLYOXYL 40 STEARATE (Gallipot)
polyoxyethylene (40) stearate
LIQ, NA (N.F.)
480 ml.............. **51552-0279-06** 12.39

(Letco)
POW, NA (MYRJ 52)
500 gm.............. **62991-2050-01** 36.00
2500 gm............. **62991-2050-02** 105.00

(PCCA)
POW, NA, 1 gm.......... **51927-1629-00** 0.29

(Spectrum Pharmacy)
POW, NA (N.F.)
500 gm.............. **49452-5610-01** 74.20
2500 gm............. **49452-5610-02** 206.85

POLYOXYL 50 STEARATE (Spectrum Pharmacy)
polyoxyethylene (50) stearate
LIQ, NA (N.F.)
500 gm.............. **49452-5615-01** 112.35
2500 gm............. **49452-5615-02** 357.00

PROD/MFR NDC AWP DP OBC

POLYSACCHARIDE IRON COMPLEX (DHS, Inc.)
REPACK
iron polysaccharide
CAP, PO, 150 mg, 60s ea.. **55887-0914-60** 47.96

POLYSACCHARIDE IRON FORTE (Contract Pharmacal)
cyanocobalamin/folic acid/iron polysaccharide
CAP, PO, 25 mcg-1 mg-150 mg,
100s ea............ **10267-2103-01** 34.56

POLYSORBATE 20 (Gallipot)
LIQ, NA (N.F.)
473 ml.............. **51552-0452-06** 21.00
3785 ml............. **51552-0452-08** 88.20

(PCCA)
LIQ, NA (NF)
1 ml................ **51927-1054-00** 0.42

(Spectrum Pharmacy)
LIQ, NA (N.F.)
500 ml.............. **49452-5620-01** 93.45
4000 ml............. **49452-5620-02** 364.00

POLYSORBATE 40 (Medisca)
SOL, NA (1X500ML,NF,TWEEN 40)
500 ml.............. **38779-2157-08** 54.00
(1X4000ML,NF,TWEEN 40)
4000 ml............. **38779-2157-01** 193.50

(PCCA)
LIQ, NA (NF)
1 ml................ **51927-2754-00** 0.12

(Spectrum Pharmacy)
LIQ, NA (N.F.)
500 ml.............. **49452-5630-01** 93.45
4000 ml............. **49452-5630-02** 364.00

POLYSORBATE 60 (Gallipot)
LIQ, NA (U.S.P.,N.F.)
473 ml.............. **51552-0111-06** 15.40

(Medisca)
LIQ, NA (N.F.)
500 ml.............. **38779-0940-08** 34.50
(1X4000ML)
4000 ml............. **38779-0940-01** 178.50

(PCCA)
LIQ, NA (NF)
1 gm................ **51927-1359-00** 0.12

(Spectrum Pharmacy)
LIQ, NA (N.F.)
500 ml.............. **49452-5640-01** 93.45
4000 ml............. **49452-5640-02** 364.00

POLYSORBATE 80 (Baker, J.T.)
LIQ, NA (N.F.)
500 ml.............. **10106-2903-01** 15.05

(Gallipot)
LIQ, NA (U.S.P.,N.F.)
236.56 ml........... **51552-0092-05** 9.59
473 ml.............. **51552-0092-06** 13.30
3785 ml............. **51552-0092-08** 65.80

(Letco)
LIQ, NA (U.S.P./N.F.)
500 ml.............. **62991-1296-01** 37.50
3840 ml............. **62991-1296-02** 120.00

(Medisca)
LIQ, NA (N.F.)
100 ml.............. **38779-0526-05** 21.00
500 ml.............. **38779-0526-08** 31.50
1008 ml............. **38779-0526-09** 52.50
4000 ml............. **38779-0526-01** 147.00

(PCCA)
LIQ, NA (NF)
1 ml................ **51927-1075-00** 0.23

(Spectrum Pharmacy)
LIQ, NA (N.F.)
500 ml.............. **49452-5650-01** 63.70
4000 ml............. **49452-5650-02** 244.65

POLYSORBATE 81 (Gallipot)
LIQ, NA (F.C.C., KOSHER)
3785 ml............. **51552-0645-08** 101.85

POLYSPORIN (Pharma Pac)
REPACK
bacitracin zinc/polymyxin b sulfate
OIN, OP, 500 u/gm-10000 u/gm,
3.5 gm.............. **52959-0563-03** 28.41 AT

POLYTETRAFLUOROETHYLENE (PCCA)
POW, NA (1X1GM)
1 gm................ **51927-2943-00** 3.75

POLYTHIAZIDE
(Pfizer) *See RENESE*

PROD/MFR	NDC	AWP	DP	OBC
POLYTRIM (Allergan Inc)				
polymyxin b sulfate/trimethoprim sulfate				
SOL, OP, 10000 u/ml-1 mg/ml,				
10 ml	00023-7824-10	35.87		AT
(A-S Medication)				
REPACK				
SOL, OP, 10000 u/ml-1 mg/ml,				
10 ml	54569-2867-00	34.55		AT
(Phys Total Care)				
REPACK				
SOL, OP, 10000 u/ml-1 mg/ml,				
10 ml	54868-1148-00	41.69		AT
(Quality Care Prod)				
REPACK				
SOL, OP (DROPS)				
10000 u/ml-1 mg/ml,				
10 ml	49999-0157-10	85.02		
POLYVINYL ALCOHOL (PCCA)				
POW, NA (USP)				
1 gm	51927-3120-00	0.84		
(Spectrum Pharmacy) *See ALCOHOL POLYVINYL*				
POLYVINYL ALCOHOL/POVIDONE				
(Focus Labs, Inc.) *See FRESHKOTE*				
POLYVINYL CHLORIDE, RADIOPAQUE				
(Konsyl) *See SITZMARKS*				
POLYVINYLPYRROLIDONE K-30 (Spectrum Pharmacy)				
povidone				
POW, NA (U.S.P.)				
100 gm	49452-5965-01	86.10		
500 gm	49452-5965-02	197.75		
POLYVINYLPYRROLIDONE K-90 (Spectrum Pharmacy)				
povidone				
POW, NA (U.S.P.)				
100 gm	49452-5967-01	102.20		
500 gm	49452-5967-02	235.20		
POLYVITAMIN W/ FLUORIDE (Pharma Pac)				
REPACK				
multivitamin and fluoride				
CTB, PO, 100s ea	52959-0256-00	19.20		
POLYVITAMIN W/FLUORIDE (Hi-Tech)				
multivitamin and fluoride				
LIQ, PO (DROPS)				
50 ml	50383-0642-50	11.80		
50 ml	50383-0641-50	11.80		
(Pharma Pac)				
REPACK				
LIQ, PO (DROPS)				
50 ml	52959-0593-50	9.72		
(W/DROPPER,DROPS)				
50 ml	52959-0863-50	9.72		
POMEGRANATE				
(PCCA) *See POMEGRANATE POWDER EXTRACT*				
POMEGRANATE POWDER EXTRACT (PCCA)				
pomegranate				
POW, NA (1X1GM)				
1 gm	51927-3561-00	1.19		
PONSTEL (Shionogi)				
mefenamic acid				
CAP, PO, 250 mg, 30s ea	59630-0400-30	341.96		
(PD-Rx Pharm)				
REPACK				
CAP, PO, 250 mg, 8s ea	55289-0759-08	124.34		
30s ea	55289-0759-30	139.89		
36s ea	55289-0759-36	167.85		
(Phys Total Care)				
REPACK				
CAP, PO, 250 mg, 10s ea	54868-0449-02	69.84		
30s ea	54868-0449-01	205.76		
50s ea	54868-0449-00	341.69		
PONTOCAINE (Dispensing Solutions)				
REPACK				
tetracaine hydrochloride				
SOL, TP, 2%, 120 ml	55045-3814-04	56.00		
PONTOCAINE HCL (Hospira)				
tetracaine hydrochloride				
PDS, IJ (NIPHANOID AMP)				
20 mg, 100s ea	00074-1849-06	1500.00	1313.00	
SOL, IJ (AMP,25X2ML,LATEX-FREE)				
1%, 2 ml 25s	00409-1846-02	173.70	152.00	
TP (LATEX-FREE)				
2%, 30 ml	00409-1866-01	19.67	17.21	
118 ml	00409-1866-02	54.02	47.27	
(Dispensing Solutions)				
REPACK				
SOL, TP (LATEX-FREE)				
2%, 118 ml	55045-3420-01	50.00		
(Physician Partner)				
REPACK				
SOL, TP (1X30ML,LATEX-FREE)				
2%, 30 ml	21695-0886-01	38.00		
PONTOCAINE HYDROCHLORIDE (Hospira)				
tetracaine hydrochloride				
PDS, IJ (NIPHANOID AMP,PF)				
20 mg, 100s ea	00409-1849-06	1500.00	1313.00	
PORACTANT ALFA				
(Cornerstone) *See CUROSURF*				
PORFIMER SODIUM				
(Axcan) *See PHOTOFRIN*				
PORTIA-28 (Teva)				
ethinyl estradiol/levonorgestrel				
TAB, PO (BLISTER PACK,6X28)				
30 mcg-0.15 mg,				
168s ea	00555-9020-58	185.58		AB
POSACONAZOLE				
(Schering) *See NOXAFIL*				
POSIFLUSH HEPARIN (BD Dickinson Hosp Prod)				
heparin sodium				
SOL, IV (30X3ML,SINGLEUSE,PF)				
10 u/ml, 3 ml 30s	08290-3064-13	16.80		
(30X5ML,SINGLEUSE,PF)				
10 u/ml, 5 ml 30s	08290-3064-14	17.10		
(30X3ML,SINGLEUSE,PF)				
100 u/ml, 3 ml 30s	08290-3064-23	16.80		
(30X5ML,SINGLEUSE,PF)				
100 u/ml, 5 ml 30s	08290-3064-24	17.10		
POT CIT/CITRIC ACID (Phys Total Care)				
REPACK				
citric acid/potassium citrate				
PDR, PO, 100s ea	54868-5529-00	77.27		
POTABA (Glenwood)				
aminobenzoate potassium				
CAP, PO, 0.5 gm, 250s ea	00516-0051-25	160.39		
1000s ea	00516-0051-10	594.61		
PDR, PO (ENVULE,50X2GM)				
2 gm/packet,				
2 gm 50s	00516-0052-50	135.63		
TAB, PO, 0.5 gm, 100s ea	00516-0054-01	66.24		
1000s ea	00516-0054-10	556.65		
POTASH SULFURATED (Baker, J.T.)				
LUM, NA (U.S.P.)				
125 gm	10106-2908-04	14.86		
500 gm	10106-2908-01	35.02		
(Gallipot)				
LUM, NA (U.S.P.)				
10 gm	51552-0419-03	6.65		
28.35 gm	51552-0419-02	7.35		
113.4 gm	51552-0419-04	12.88		
454 gm	51552-0419-06	29.05		
(Mallinckrodt Lab)				
LUM, NA (U.S.P.)				
100 gm	00406-6684-01	11.89		
500 gm	00406-6684-04	31.00		
(PCCA) *See SULFURATED POTASH*				
(Spectrum Pharmacy)				
LUM, NA (U.S.P.)				
125 gm	49452-5710-02	77.00		
500 gm	49452-5710-03	165.55		
POTASS CHL (Phys Total Care)				
REPACK				
potassium chloride				
SOL, PO, 20 meq/15 ml,				
473 ml	54868-5554-00	8.82		
POTASSIUM ACETATE (Amend)				
POW, NA (U.S.P.)				
454 gm	17317-0432-01	15.40		
(A.C.S., REAGENT)				
500 gm	17317-1614-05	25.20		
(U.S.P.)				
2270 gm	17317-0432-05	44.80		
(A.C.S., REAGENT)				
2500 gm	17317-1614-06	98.00		
(U.S.P.)				
11350 gm	17317-0432-08	192.50		
(Amer Regent)				
SOL, IV (S.D.V.)				
2 meq/ml,				
20 ml 25s	00517-2053-25	59.69		
(BULK VIAL)				
2 meq/ml,				
100 ml 25s	00517-2400-25	171.88		
(S.D.V.)				
4 meq/ml,				
50 ml 25s	00517-5024-25	156.25		
(Baker, J.T.)				
GRA, NA (U.S.P., A.C.S.)				
500 gm	10106-2914-01	27.80		
2500 gm	10106-2914-05	186.22		
(Hospira)				
SOL, IV (25X20ML,LATEX-FREE)				
2 meq/ml,				
20 ml 25s	00409-8183-01	14.40	12.50	
(25X50ML,LATEX-FREE)				
2 meq/ml,				
50 ml 25s	00409-3294-51	52.50	46.00	
(VIAL,FLIPTOP,BULK)				
2 meq/ml,				
100 ml 25s	00409-3294-06	68.10	59.50	
(Mallinckrodt Lab)				
CRY, NA (U.S.P.)				
500 gm	00406-6696-04	52.56		
(Medisca)				
POW, NA (U.S.P.)				
500 gm	38779-1523-08	34.50		
2200 gm	38779-1523-09	84.00		
(1X2500GM,USP)				
2500 gm	38779-1523-01	117.00		
(PCCA)				
POW, NA (USP)				
1 gm	51927-1470-00	0.17		
(Spectrum Pharmacy)				
GRA, NA (U.S.P.)				
500 gm	49452-5720-01	93.10		
2500 gm	49452-5720-02	267.05		
12000 gm	49452-5720-03	973.00		
POTASSIUM ALGINATE (Spectrum Pharmacy)				
POW, NA (F.C.C.)				
125 gm	49452-5722-01	150.50	14.30	
500 gm	49452-5722-02	357.00	31.40	
2500 gm	49452-5722-03	1060.50	109.80	
POTASSIUM ALUM DODECAHYDRATE (Medisca)				
alum, potassium				
POW, NA (U.S.P.)				
500 gm	38779-0600-08	31.50		
1000 gm	38779-0600-09	126.00		
POTASSIUM ASCORBATE (PCCA)				
POW, NA (1X1GM)				
1 gm	51927-3669-00	0.99		
POTASSIUM ASPARTATE (PCCA)				
POW, NA, 1 gm	51927-2190-00	0.54		
POTASSIUM BENZOATE (PCCA)				
POW, NA (NF)				
1 gm	51927-2050-00	0.17		
(Spectrum Pharmacy)				
POW, NA (N.F.)				
500 gm	49452-5723-01	108.85		
2500 gm	49452-5723-02	395.50		
12000 gm	49452-5723-03	1011.50		
POTASSIUM BICARBONATE (Amend)				
GRA, NA (U.S.P., F.C.C.)				
500 gm	17317-2641-01	8.40		
(U.S.P./F.C.C.)				
2270 gm	17317-2641-05	35.00		
11350 gm	17317-2641-08	122.50		
(Baker, J.T.)				
GRA, NA (U.S.P., F.C.C.)				
500 gm	10106-2943-01	18.95		
POW, NA, 500 gm	10106-2945-01	20.26		
(Gallipot)				
GRA, NA (U.S.P.,N.F.)				
454 gm	51552-0207-06	20.65		
(Major) *See K-VESCENT*				
(Mallinckrodt Lab)				
POW, NA (U.S.P.)				
500 gm	00406-6736-04	29.32		
(Medisca)				
POW, NA (U.S.P.)				
500 gm	38779-0619-08	31.50		
2200 gm	38779-0619-09	54.00		
(PCCA)				
GRA, NA (USP)				
1 gm	51927-1305-00	0.10		
(Qualitest) *See K-EFFERVESCENT*				

PROD/MFR	NDC	AWP	DP	OBC
(Spectrum Pharmacy)				
GRA, NA (U.S.P.)				
500 gm	**49452-5730-01**	64.75		
2500 gm	**49452-5730-02**	244.65		
12000 gm	**49452-5730-03**	794.50		
(Phys Total Care)				
REPACK				
potassium bicarbonate/potassium citrate				
TEF, PO, 25 meq, 30s ea	**54868-0355-00**	25.92		
POTASSIUM BICARBONATE/POTASSIUM CHLORIDE				
(Qualitest) *See POTASSIUM CHLORIDE*				
(TOWER) *See EFFERVESCENT POTASSIUM/CHLORIDE*				
POTASSIUM BICARBONATE/POTASSIUM CITRATE				
(TOWER) *See EFFERVESCENT POTASSIUM*				
(Upsher-Smith) *See KLOR-CON/EF*				
POTASSIUM BICHROMATE				
(Amend) *See POTASSIUM DICHROMATE*				
(Baker, J.T.) *See POTASSIUM DICHROMATE*				
(PCCA) *See POTASSIUM DICHROMATE*				
POTASSIUM BIPHTHALATE (Baker, J.T.)				
CRY, NA (A.C.S., REAGENT)				
100 gm	**10106-2958-00**	57.73		
500 gm	**10106-2958-01**	120.56		
POTASSIUM BISULFATE (Baker, J.T.)				
CRY, NA (REAGENT)				
500 gm	**10106-2960-01**	82.61		
2500 gm	**10106-2960-05**	292.01		
POTASSIUM BITARTRATE (Amend)				
POW, NA (F.C.C.)				
454 gm	**17317-0434-01**	14.00		
(PURIFIED, F.C.C.)				
2270 gm	**17317-0434-05**	56.00		
11350 gm	**17317-0434-08**	175.00		
(Baker, J.T.)				
POW, NA (REAGENT)				
500 gm	**10106-2982-01**	45.78		
(Gallipot)				
POW, NA (F.C.C.)				
56.7 gm	**51552-0160-03**	6.23		
454 gm	**51552-0160-06**	23.10		
(Lorann Oil)				
POW, NA, 30 gm	**23535-0610-75**	1.25		
120 gm	**23535-0610-78**	2.95		
454 gm	**23535-0610-71**	8.00		
(Medisca)				
POW, NA (PURIFIED,U.S.P.)				
500 gm	**38779-1526-08**	34.50		
1000 gm	**38779-1526-09**	61.50		
(PCCA)				
POW, NA (F.C.C.)				
1 gm	**51927-1691-00**	0.36		
(Spectrum Pharmacy)				
POW, NA (F.C.C.)				
500 gm	**49452-5737-01**	95.20		
(U.S.P.)				
500 gm	**49452-5731-01**	95.20		
(F.C.C.)				
2500 gm	**49452-5737-02**	371.00		
(U.S.P.)				
2500 gm	**49452-5731-02**	371.00		
(F.C.C.)				
12000 gm	**49452-5737-03**	1253.00		
(U.S.P.)				
12000 gm	**49452-5731-03**	1253.00		
POTASSIUM BROMATE (Baker, J.T.)				
POW, NA (A.C.S., REAGENT)				
500 gm	**10106-2992-01**	53.82		
(Spectrum Pharmacy)				
POW, NA (1X125GM)				
125 gm	**49452-5740-01**	112.35		
(1X500GM)				
500 gm	**49452-5740-02**	247.45		
(1X2500GM)				
2500 gm	**49452-5740-03**	836.50		
POTASSIUM BROMIDE (Amend)				
POW, NA (PURIFIED)				
454 gm	**17317-0435-01**	10.50		
2270 gm	**17317-0435-05**	42.00		
11350 gm	**17317-0435-08**	122.50		
(Baker, J.T.)				
CRY, NA (A.C.S., REAGENT)				
500 gm	**10106-2998-01**	87.09		
2500 gm	**10106-2998-05**	345.62		
(Gallipot)				
CRY, NA (A.C.S.,REAGENT)				
113.4 gm	**51552-0144-04**	8.82		
454 gm	**51552-0144-06**	17.85		
(Letco)				
GRA, NA (PURIFIED)				
500 gm	**62991-1116-01**	34.50		
1000 gm	**62991-1116-02**	45.00		
2500 gm	**62991-1116-03**	96.00		
(Medisca)				
PEL, NA (1X500GM)				
500 gm	**38779-2341-08**	31.50		
(1X1000GM)				
1000 gm	**38779-2341-09**	51.00		
(1X2500GM)				
2500 gm	**38779-2341-01**	117.00		
(1X5000GM)				
5000 gm	**38779-2341-03**	195.00		
(1X25000GM)				
25000 gm	**38779-2341-07**	705.00		
POW, NA (PURIFIED)				
500 gm	**38779-0816-08**	31.50		
1000 gm	**38779-0816-09**	51.00		
2500 gm	**38779-0816-01**	117.00		
5000 gm	**38779-0816-03**	195.00		
(1X25000GM)				
25000 gm	**38779-0816-07**	705.00		
(PCCA)				
GRA, NA (PURIFIED)				
1 gm	**51927-1718-00**	0.09		
(Spectrum Pharmacy)				
CRY, NA (A.C.S./REAGENT)				
125 gm	**49452-5742-02**	81.20		
500 gm	**49452-5742-03**	122.85		
2500 gm	**49452-5742-04**	406.00		
12000 gm	**49452-5742-05**	892.50		
POTASSIUM CARBONATE				
(Amend) *See POTASSIUM CARBONATE ANHYDROUS*				
(Baker, J.T.) *See POTASSIUM CARBONATE 1.5-HYDRATE*				
(Baker, J.T.) *See POTASSIUM CARBONATE ANHYDROUS*				
(Gallipot) *See POTASSIUM CARBONATE ANHYDROUS*				
(PCCA)				
GRA, NA (USP; ANHYDROUS)				
1 gm	**51927-3112-00**	0.11		
(Spectrum Pharmacy) *See POTASSIUM CARBONATE ANHYDROUS*				
POTASSIUM CARBONATE 1.5-HYDRATE (Baker, J.T.)				
potassium carbonate				
CRY, NA (A.C.S., REAGENT)				
500 gm	**10106-3010-01**	52.32		
2500 gm	**10106-3010-05**	185.71		
POTASSIUM CARBONATE ANHYDROUS (Amend)				
potassium carbonate				
GRA, NA (F.C.C.)				
25 gm	**17317-0436-01**	8.40		
125 gm	**17317-0436-05**	28.00		
(Baker, J.T.)				
GRA, NA (F.C.C.)				
2500 gm	**10106-3014-05**	54.98		
(Gallipot)				
GRA, NA (F.C.C.)				
454 gm	**51552-0339-06**	16.45		
(Spectrum Pharmacy)				
GRA, NA (U.S.P.)				
500 gm	**49452-5755-01**	144.90		
2500 gm	**49452-5755-02**	434.00		
12000 gm	**49452-5755-03**	1092.00		
POTASSIUM CHLORATE (Baker, J.T.)				
CRY, NA (A.C.S., REAGENT)				
500 gm	**10106-3024-01**	77.20		
(PURIFIED)				
500 gm	**10106-3028-01**	60.36		
(A.C.S., REAGENT)				
2500 gm	**10106-3024-05**	293.04		
(PURIFIED)				
2500 gm	**10106-3028-05**	220.27		
(PCCA)				
GRA, NA (PURIFIED)				
1 gm	**51927-1525-00**	0.17		
POTASSIUM CHLORIDE				
FUL				
TER, PO, 8 meq, 100s ea		10.44		
10 meq, 100s ea		25.38		
20 meq, 100s ea		46.25		
(Abbott Pharm) *See K-TAB*				
(Amend)				
GRA, NA (U.S.P., F.C.C.)				
500 gm	**17317-0438-01**	8.40		
(U.S.P./F.C.C.)				
2270 gm	**17317-0438-05**	28.00		
11350 gm	**17317-0438-08**	87.50		
(APP) *See POTASSIUM CHLORIDE CONCENTRATE*				
(B. Braun)				
SOL, IV (CONCENTRATE)				
2 meq/ml, 250 ml	**00264-1940-20**	23.32		**AP**
500 ml	**00264-1940-10**	28.60		**AP**
(Baker, J.T.)				
CRY, NA (U.S.P., F.C.C.)				
500 gm	**10106-3046-01**	16.28		
2500 gm	**10106-3046-05**	69.50		
POW, NA, 500 gm	**10106-3052-01**	23.66		
2500 gm	**10106-3052-05**	116.32		
(Baxter)				
SOL, IV, 10 meq/100 ml,				
100 ml 24s	**00338-0709-48**	351.12		
10 meq/50 ml,				
50 ml 24s	**00338-0705-41**	351.12		
20 meq/100 ml,				
100 ml 24s	**00338-0705-48**	351.12		
20 meq/50 ml,				
50 ml 24s	**00338-0703-41**	351.12		**AP**
40 meq/100 ml,				
100 ml 24s	**00338-0703-48**	351.12		**AP**
(BULK PACKAGE)				
2 meq/ml, 250 ml	**00338-0318-02**	12.00	10.00	**AP**
(Consolidated Midland) *See POTASSIUM CHLORIDE SOLUTION*				
(Consolidated Midland)				
SOL, IV (AMP)				
2 meq/ml,				
10 ml 100s	**00223-8330-01**	120.00		**EE**
(VIALS)				
2 meq/ml,				
30 ml 25s	**00223-8322-30**	50.00		**EE**
PO, 20 meq/15 ml,				
480 ml	**00223-6589-01**	2.75		
3840 ml	**00223-6589-02**	13.95		
(Ethex)				
CER, PO (USP)				
8 meq, 100s ea	**58177-0667-04**	75.24		**AB**
500s ea	**58177-0667-08**	371.02		**AB**
10 meq, 100s ea	**58177-0001-04**	58.14		**AB**
(10X10)				
10 meq, 100s ea UD	**58177-0001-11**	57.20		**AB**
500s ea	**58177-0001-08**	279.76		**AB**
1000s ea	**58177-0001-09**	546.13		**AB**
5000s ea	**58177-0001-12**	2594.09		**AB**
TER, PO (10X10)				
20 meq, 100s ea UD	**58177-0202-11**	56.45		**AB**
(Gallipot)				
CRY, NA (U.S.P.,N.F.)				
454 gm	**51552-0061-06**	14.56		
GRA, NA (U.S.P.)				
454 gm	**51552-0324-06**	11.90		
2270 gm	**51552-0324-08**	33.32		
POW, NA, 11350 gm	**51552-0324-09**	168.00		
(Hospira)				
SOL, IV (P.C.,LATEX-FREE)				
10 meq/100 ml,				
100 ml 24s	**00409-7074-26**	70.56	61.68	
(24X50ML,LATEX-FREE)				
10 meq/50 ml,				
50 ml 24s	**00409-7075-14**	66.53	58.32	
(PC,24X100ML,LATEX-FREE)				
20 meq/100 ml,				
100 ml 24s	**00409-7075-26**	68.26	59.76	
(100MLX24,USE W/DEVICE)				
30 meq/100 ml,				
100 ml 24s	**00409-7076-26**	66.82	58.56	**AP**
(24X50ML,LATEX-FREE)				
20 meq/50 ml,				
50 ml 24s	**00409-7077-14**	68.54	60.00	**AP**
(HIGHLY CONC.,24X100ML)				
40 meq/100 ml,				
100 ml 24s	**00409-7077-26**	66.53	58.32	**AP**
(FTV,25X5ML,10ML VIAL)				
2 meq/ml, 5 ml 25s	**00409-6635-01**	19.80	17.25	**AP**
(AMP,LATEX-FREE)				
2 meq/ml,				
10 ml 25s	**00409-3907-03**	30.30	26.50	**AP**
(VIAL, FLIPTOP, 20 ML)				
2 meq/ml,				
10 ml 25s	**00074-6651-06**	15.60	13.75	**AP**

PROD/MFR	NDC	AWP	DP	OBC
(VIAL,FLIPTOP,20ML)				
2 meq/ml,				
10 ml 25s	00409-6651-06	16.80	14.75	AP
(FTV,30ML,LATEX-FREE)				
2 meq/ml,				
15 ml 25s	00409-6636-01	21.60	19.00	AP
(AMP,LATEX-FREE)				
2 meq/ml,				
20 ml 25s	00074-3934-02	31.80	27.75	AP
(FTV,30ML,LATEX-FREE)				
2 meq/ml,				
20 ml 25s	00409-6653-05	17.70	15.50	AP
(12X250ML,LATEX-FREE)				
2 meq/ml,				
250 ml 12s	00409-1513-02	114.91	100.56	AP
(Hospira)				
dextrose/potassium/sodium chloride				
(IN 5% DEXROSE/.45% NACL)				
5%-30 meq-0.45%,				
1000 ml 12s	00409-7903-09	31.68	27.72	AP
POTASSIUM CHLORIDE (Humco)				
LIQ, NA (CHERRY)				
473 ml	00395-2300-16	2.67		
(Major)				
CER, PO (USP)				
10 meq, 100s ea UD	00904-6068-61	528.75		EE
(Major) *See POTASSIUM CHLORIDE SOLUTION*				
(Mallinckrodt Lab)				
CRY, NA (U.S.P.)				
500 gm	00406-6845-04	15.45		
GRA, NA (A.C.S.)				
500 gm	00406-6858-04	9.94		
(U.S.P.)				
500 gm	00406-6838-04	25.84		
2500 gm	00406-6838-06	78.83		
(Medisca)				
POW, NA (U.S.P.)				
500 gm	38779-0587-08	28.50		
(1X1000GM,USP)				
1000 gm	38779-0587-09	46.50		
(PCCA)				
GRA, NA (USP; GRANULAR)				
1 gm	51927-1090-00	0.08		
(Pharm Assoc Inc) *See POTASSIUM CHLORIDE SOLUTION*				
(Pharm Assoc Inc)				
SOL, PO (SF,CITRUS)				
20 meq/15 ml,				
15 ml 100s UD	00121-1465-15	39.43		
30 ml 100s UD	00121-1465-30	42.50		
(Qualitest)				
SOL, PO, 20 meq/15 ml,				
473 ml	00603-1534-58	6.44		
473 ml	00603-1535-58	6.44		
(AF,SF,DYE-FREE)				
20 meq/15 ml,				
473 ml	00603-1532-58	6.44		
(SF)				
40 meq/15 ml,				
473 ml	00603-1536-58	7.21		
(Qualitest)				
potassium bicarbonate/potassium chloride				
TEF, PO, 25 meq, 30s ea	00603-3508-16	28.10		
POTASSIUM CHLORIDE (Sandoz)				
TER, PO, 8 meq, 100s ea	00781-1516-01	17.74		EE
1000s ea	00781-1516-10	168.53		EE
10 meq, 100s ea	00781-1526-01	27.75		BC
(USP,MICROENCAPSULATED)				
10 meq, 100s ea	00781-5710-01	29.05		
1000s ea	00781-1526-10	263.63		BC
(USP,MICROENCAPSULATED)				
10 meq, 1000s ea	00781-5710-10	278.99		
20 meq, 100s ea	00781-5720-01	52.91		
500s ea	00781-5720-05	262.49		
1000s ea	00781-5720-10	516.10		
(Savage) *See KAON-CL 10*				
(Schering)				
TER, PO (USP)				
10 meq, 100s ea	00085-1717-01	27.75		
20 meq, 100s ea	00085-1718-02	50.50		
1000s ea	00085-1718-01	492.50		
(Spectrum Pharmacy)				
CRY, NA (U.S.P.)				
500 gm	49452-5770-01	53.90		
2500 gm	49452-5770-02	161.00		
12000 gm	49452-5770-03	518.00		
GRA, NA, 500 gm	49452-5780-01	53.90		

PROD/MFR	NDC	AWP	DP	OBC
2500 gm	49452-5780-02	161.00		
12000 gm	49452-5780-03	518.00		
(Ther-RX) *See MICRO-K*				
(Ther-RX) *See MICRO-K 10*				
(Upsher-Smith) *See KLOR-CON*				
(Upsher-Smith) *See KLOR-CON 10*				
(Upsher-Smith) *See KLOR-CON 8*				
(Upsher-Smith) *See KLOR-CON M10*				
(Upsher-Smith) *See KLOR-CON M15*				
(Upsher-Smith) *See KLOR-CON M20*				
(Upsher-Smith) *See KLOR-CON/25*				
(Upsher-Smith)				
TER, PO, 8 meq, 100s ea	00245-0242-11	17.74		AB
1000s ea	00245-0242-10	169.80		AB
5000s ea	00245-0042-55	1299.03		AB
10000s ea	00245-0042-00	2598.07		AB
10 meq, 1000s ea	00245-0243-10	261.20		BC
5000s ea	00245-0043-55	1683.92		BC
10000s ea	00245-0043-00	3367.83		BC
15 meq, 100s ea UD	00245-0150-01	49.77		
100s ea UD	00245-0336-01	54.75		
100s ea	00245-0336-11	50.53		
(Vintage)				
SOL, PO (SF)				
40 meq/15 ml,				
480 ml	00254-9384-58	5.60		
(Watson)				
CER, PO (USP)				
8 meq, 100s ea	62037-0559-01	72.23		AB
500s ea	62037-0559-05	356.18		AB
10 meq, 90s ea	62037-0560-90	68.65		AB
100s ea	62037-0560-01	76.28		AB
500s ea	62037-0560-05	362.34		AB
TER, PO, 20 meq, 100s ea	62037-0999-01	31.38		AB
500s ea	62037-0999-05	155.52		AB
1000s ea	62037-0999-10	305.82		AB
(A-S Medication)				
REPACK				
CER, PO, 10 meq, 30s ea	54569-3388-00	17.44		AB
60s ea	54569-3388-01	34.88		AB
80s ea	54569-3388-05	46.51		AB
TER, PO, 8 meq, 30s ea	54569-1899-01	6.33		EE
100s ea	54569-1899-00	21.09		EE
10 meq, 30s ea	54569-4903-01	8.72		EE
100s ea	54569-4903-04	29.05		EE
(MICROENCAPSULATED)				
20 meq, 30s ea	54569-5414-00	15.68		
60s ea	54569-5414-01	31.35		
(American Health)				
REPACK				
TER, PO, 20 meq,				
100s ea UD	68084-0360-01	16.50		AB
(Bryant Ranch)				
REPACK				
TER, PO, 10 meq, 30s ea	63629-2937-01	11.66		
20 meq, 30s ea	63629-2703-01	37.32		
60s ea	63629-2703-02	74.64		
(DHS, Inc.)				
REPACK				
TER, PO, 10 meq, 30s ea	55887-0580-30	16.66		AB
60s ea	55887-0580-60	33.03		BC
90s ea	55887-0580-90	51.00		BC
20 meq, 10s ea	55887-0460-10	8.00		AB
30s ea	55887-0460-30	18.96		AB
60s ea	55887-0460-60	37.02		AB
90s ea	55887-0460-90	55.05		AB
(Dispensing Solutions)				
REPACK				
CER, PO, 10 meq, 100s ea	55045-1695-00	22.40		AB
TER, PO (FILM-COATED)				
8 meq, 30s ea	55045-1404-07	6.55		AB
10 meq, 30s ea	66336-0112-30	12.04		BC
60s ea	66336-0161-60	23.53		BC
(GSMS)				
REPACK				
TER, PO, 8 meq, 90s ea	60429-0158-90	16.80	5.60	AB
180s ea	60429-0158-18	27.00	9.00	AB
10 meq, 90s ea	60429-0215-90	45.51	15.17	EE
(HomeMed)				
REPACK				
CER, PO, 10 meq, 30s ea	51655-0583-24	6.30		EE
TER, PO, 8 meq, 30s ea	51655-0582-24	6.35		
10 meq, 30s ea	51655-0511-24	21.99		EE
60s ea	51655-0593-25	14.54		EE

PROD/MFR	NDC	AWP	DP	OBC
(McKesson Packaging)				
REPACK				
TER, PO (10X10,USP)				
10 meq, 100s ea UD	63739-0446-10	34.87		
(MICROENCAPSULATED)				
10 meq, 100s ea UD	63739-0305-10	33.33		AB
750s ea UD	63739-0305-01	255.00		AB
(10X10,USP)				
20 meq, 100s ea UD	63739-0447-10	64.51		
(MICROENCAPSULATED)				
20 meq, 100s ea UD	63739-0396-10	61.69		AB
(25X30,USP)				
20 meq, 750s ea UD	63739-0447-01	483.84		
(PC25X30,USP)				
20 meq, 750s ea UD	63739-0447-03	483.84		
(USP)				
20 meq, 750s ea UD	63739-0396-01	471.95		AB
(Palmetto)				
REPACK				
TER, PO, 8 meq, 30s ea	23490-6135-01	7.50		
100s ea	23490-6135-02	25.00		
10 meq, 4s ea	23490-6130-01	2.88		
20s ea	23490-6130-05	9.00		
30s ea	23490-6130-02	13.50		
60s ea	23490-6130-03	27.00		
90s ea	23490-6130-04	40.50		
20 meq, 30s ea	23490-6131-03	22.50		
60s ea	23490-6131-06	45.00		
90s ea	23490-6131-09	67.50		
(PD-Rx Pharm)				
REPACK				
CER, PO, 10 meq, 30s ea	55289-0218-30	63.90		EE
TER, PO, 8 meq, 30s ea	55289-0697-30	20.47		AB
(FILM-COATED)				
8 meq, 90s ea	55289-0697-90	48.09		AB
(REDI-SCRIPT)				
8 meq, 90s ea	58864-0408-90	48.09		AB
10 meq, 30s ea	58864-0871-30	21.27		BC
45s ea	55289-0359-45	21.04		AB
60s ea	55289-0359-60	24.70		BC
90s ea	55289-0359-90	32.10		AB
100s ea	55289-0359-01	34.52		BC
180s ea	55289-0359-93	54.16		BC
270s ea	55289-0218-94	131.56		AB
270s ea	55289-0359-94	76.24		AB
20 meq, 12s ea	55289-0738-12	13.58		AB
(REDI-SCRIPT)				
20 meq, 30s ea	58864-0684-30	37.33		AB
90s ea	55289-0738-90	77.96		
180s ea	55289-0738-93	146.76		AB
(Pharma Pac)				
REPACK				
TER, PO, 20 meq, 30s ea	52959-0681-30	26.75		
(Phys Total Care)				
REPACK				
CER, PO, 10 meq, 12s ea	54868-1317-03	16.66		EE
30s ea	54868-1317-01	63.21		EE
60s ea	54868-1317-05	121.92		EE
90s ea	54868-1317-06	180.62		EE
100s ea	54868-1317-02	200.19		EE
500s ea	54868-1317-00	371.29		EE
PDS, PO, 20 meq, 30s ea	54868-0356-03	21.90		
50s ea	54868-0356-01	33.51		
100s ea	54868-0356-02	61.02		
SOL, IV (VIAL)				
2 meq/ml, 10 ml	54868-0767-00	6.33		EE
250 ml	54868-0767-01	48.45		EE
TER, PO, 8 meq, 30s ea	54868-0097-02	7.80		EE
60s ea	54868-0097-01	11.10		AB
100s ea	54868-0097-04	19.02		EE
500s ea	54868-0097-00	99.35		EE
10 meq, 20s ea	54868-3671-03	14.13		BC
30s ea	54868-3671-01	18.96		BC
60s ea	54868-3671-00	33.42		BC
90s ea	54868-3671-04	49.37		BC
100s ea	54868-3671-02	51.18		BC
20 meq, 30s ea	54868-4617-01	17.76		AB
50s ea	54868-4617-00	27.57		EE
60s ea	54868-4617-03	32.49		AB
90s ea	54868-4617-05	48.41		AB
100s ea	54868-4617-02	50.64		AB
1000s ea	54868-4617-04	287.12		AB
(Physician Partner)				
REPACK				
TER, PO, 10 meq, 30s ea	21695-0711-30	16.85		AB
20 meq, 30s ea	21695-0712-30	31.22		AB
(Quality Care Prod)				
REPACK				
TER, PO, 10 meq, 28s ea	49999-0271-28	14.31		BC
30s ea	49999-0271-30	15.33		

PROD/MFR	NDC	AWP	DP	OBC
40s ea	**49999-0271-40**	16.27		
90s ea	**49999-0271-90**	46.00		
100s ea	**49999-0271-00**	40.69		**BC**
20 meq, 30s ea	**49999-0740-30**	29.80		
100s ea	**49999-0740-00**	99.33		
(Southwood) REPACK				
CER, PO, 10 meq, 30s ea	**58016-0989-30**	5.75		**EE**
100s ea	**58016-0989-00**	17.45		**EE**
SOL, PO, 20 meq/15 ml,				
480 ml	**58016-5001-01**	5.15		
TER, PO, 8 meq, 8s ea	**58016-0564-08**	4.68		**AB**
10 meq, 30s ea	**58016-0522-30**	8.64		**BC**
60s ea	**58016-0522-60**	17.28		**BC**
90s ea	**58016-0522-90**	25.92		**BC**
100s ea	**58016-0522-00**	28.80		**BC**
20 meq, 30s ea	**58016-0569-30**	14.70		
60s ea	**58016-0569-60**	29.40		
90s ea	**58016-0569-90**	44.10		
100s ea	**58016-0569-00**	49.00		
(Vibranta) REPACK				
CER, PO, 10 meq, 30s ea	**57866-4311-01**	21.70		**AB**
60s ea	**57866-4311-02**	20.00		**AB**
80s ea	**57866-6670-04**	53.60		**AB**
POTASSIUM CHLORIDE CONCENTRATE (APP)				
potassium chloride				
SOL, IV (S.D.V.,P.C.)				
2 meq/ml, 5 ml	**63323-0965-05**	1.18		**AP**
10 ml	**63323-0965-10**	1.42		**AP**
15 ml	**63323-0965-15**	1.56		**AP**
20 ml	**63323-0965-20**	1.65		**AP**
(M.D.V.,P.C.)				
2 meq/ml, 30 ml	**63323-0967-30**	1.73		**AP**
POTASSIUM CHLORIDE ER (Dispensing Solutions) REPACK				
potassium chloride				
TER, PO, 10 meq, 60s ea	**66336-0112-60**	23.53		
POTASSIUM CHLORIDE IN DEXTROSE AND SODIUM CHLORIDE (Baxter)				
dextrose/potassium chloride/sodium chloride				
SOL, IV (USP,1X1000ML)				
5%-0.15%-0.45%,				
1000 ml	**00338-6330-04**	14.21	11.84	**AP**
POTASSIUM CHLORIDE IN SODIUM CHLORIDE (Hospira)				
potassium chloride/sodium chloride				
SOL, IV (1X1000ML,USP)				
2 meq/100 ml-0.45%,				
1000 ml	**00409-9257-39**	42.05	36.84	
POTASSIUM CHLORIDE SOLUTION (Baxter)				
ca cl/dextrose/k cl/na cl/na lact				
SOL, IV (5%,DEXTROSE & LAC-RING)				
1000 ml 12s	**00338-0811-04**	232.22		**AP**
1000 ml 12s	**00338-0815-04**	232.22		**AP**
(Consolidated Midland)				
potassium chloride				
SOL, IV (AMP)				
2 meq/ml,				
10 ml 25s	**00223-8330-10**	35.00		**EE**
20 ml 25s	**00223-8331-20**	40.00		**EE**
30 ml 25s	**00223-8332-30**	50.00		**EE**
PO, 20 meq/15 ml,				
480 ml	**00223-6591-01**	3.00		
3840 ml	**00223-6591-02**	12.50		
40 meq/15 ml,				
480 ml	**00223-6592-01**	3.00		
3840 ml	**00223-6592-02**	15.50		
(Major)				
SOL, PO, 20 meq/15 ml,				
473 ml	**00904-1007-16**	4.80		
(Pharm Assoc Inc)				
SOL, PO (SF,DYE-FREE)				
40 meq/15 ml,				
15 ml 100s UD	**00121-0466-15**	49.72		
473 ml	**00121-0466-16**	9.35		
POTASSIUM CHLORIDE SR (Dispensing Solutions) REPACK				
potassium chloride				
TER, PO, 10 meq, 100s ea	**55045-3009-01**	32.00		
POTASSIUM CHLORIDE/SODIUM CHLORIDE (B. Braun)				
SOL, IV (EXCEL)				
2 meq/100 ml-0.9%,				
1000 ml	**00264-7865-00**	3.60		**AP**
(Baxter)				
SOL, IV (VIAFLEX BAG,USP,PF)				
2 meq/100 ml-0.45%,				
1000 ml 14s	**00338-0704-34**	174.72	145.60	
2 meq/100 ml-0.9%,				
1000 ml 12s	**00338-0691-04**	201.46		**AP**
4 meq/100 ml-0.9%,				
1000 ml 12s	**00338-0695-04**	201.46		
(Hospira) *See POTASSIUM CHLORIDE IN SODIUM CHLORIDE*				
(Hospira)				
SOL, IV (12X1000ML,LATEX-FREE)				
2 meq/100 ml-0.9%,				
1000 ml 12s	**00409-7115-09**	36.00	31.56	**AP**
4 meq/100 ml-0.9%,				
1000 ml 12s	**00409-7116-09**	36.00	31.56	**AP**
POTASSIUM CHROMATE (Baker, J.T.)				
CRY, NA (A.C.S., REAGENT)				
125 gm	**10106-3058-04**	42.13		
500 gm	**10106-3058-01**	74.93		
(PCCA)				
POW, NA (ACS REAGENT)				
1 gm	**51927-2411-00**	1.18		
POTASSIUM CITRATE (Amend)				
GRA, NA (U.S.P., F.C.C.)				
454 gm	**17317-0440-01**	10.50		
(U.S.P./F.C.C.)				
2270 gm	**17317-0440-05**	29.40		
11350 gm	**17317-0440-08**	122.50		
(Baker, J.T.) *See POTASSIUM CITRATE MONOHYDRATE*				
(Gallipot) *See POTASSIUM CITRATE MONOHYDRATE*				
(Mallinckrodt Lab)				
GRA, NA (U.S.P.)				
500 gm	**00406-0714-04**	33.88		
(Medisca)				
POW, NA (USP,1X100GM)				
100 gm	**38779-0623-05**	13.50		
(U.S.P.)				
500 gm	**38779-0623-08**	38.85		
(Mission) *See UROCIT-K*				
(Mission) *See UROCIT-K 10*				
(Mission) *See UROCIT-K 5*				
(PCCA)				
POW, NA (U.S.P.; MONOHYDRATE)				
1 gm	**51927-1406-00**	0.10		
(Rising)				
TER, PO (USP)				
5 meq, 100s ea	**64980-0137-01**	29.65		**AB**
10 meq, 100s ea	**64980-0138-01**	41.15		**AB**
(Spectrum Pharmacy) *See POTASSIUM CITRATE MONOHYDRATE*				
(Upsher-Smith)				
TER, PO (WAX MATRIX TABLET)				
5 meq, 100s ea	**00245-0070-11**	37.75		
10 meq, 100s ea	**00245-0071-11**	52.35		
(Pharma Pac) REPACK				
TER, PO, 10 meq, 120s ea	**52959-0001-01**	66.40		**AB**
POTASSIUM CITRATE MONOHYDRATE (Baker, J.T.)				
potassium citrate				
GRA, NA (U.S.P., F.C.C.)				
500 gm	**10106-3068-01**	14.86		
2500 gm	**10106-3068-05**	75.29		
(Gallipot)				
GRA, NA (U.S.P.)				
454 gm	**51552-0342-06**	11.90		
(Spectrum Pharmacy)				
GRA, NA (U.S.P.)				
500 gm	**49452-5790-01**	71.40		
2500 gm	**49452-5790-02**	211.40		
12000 gm	**49452-5790-03**	829.50		
POTASSIUM CYANATE (Baker, J.T.)				
CRY, NA (REAGENT)				
500 gm	**10106-3076-01**	48.26		
POTASSIUM CYANIDE (Baker, J.T.)				
GRA, NA (A.C.S., REAGENT)				
125 gm	**10106-3080-04**	48.36		
500 gm	**10106-3080-01**	58.45		
POTASSIUM DICHROMATE (Amend)				
potassium bichromate				
GRA, NA, 454 gm	**17317-1630-01**	11.20		
2270 gm	**17317-1630-05**	35.00		
11350 gm	**17317-1630-08**	140.00		
(Baker, J.T.)				
CRY, NA (A.C.S., REAGENT)				
125 gm	**10106-3090-04**	53.15		
500 gm	**10106-3090-01**	105.83		
(PCCA)				
GRA, NA (GRANULAR)				
1 gm	**51927-1809-00**	0.75		
POTASSIUM FERRICYANIDE (Baker, J.T.)				
CRY, NA (A.C.S., REAGENT)				
500 gm	**10106-3104-01**	156.61		
2500 gm	**10106-3104-05**	563.87		
(Baker, J.T.) *See POTASSIUM FERROCYANIDE TRIHYDRATE*				
(PCCA) *See POTASSIUM HEXACYANOFERRATE TRIHYDRATE REAGENT*				
POTASSIUM FERROCYANIDE TRIHYDRATE (Baker, J.T.)				
potassium ferricyanide				
CRY, NA (A.C.S., REAGENT)				
500 gm	**10106-3114-01**	84.82		
2500 gm	**10106-3114-05**	303.23		
POTASSIUM FLUORIDE				
(Baker, J.T.) *See POTASSIUM FLUORIDE ANHYDROUS*				
(PCCA)				
POW, NA (ACS;ANHYDROUS)				
1 gm	**51927-1482-00**	1.66		
POTASSIUM FLUORIDE ANHYDROUS (Baker, J.T.)				
potassium fluoride				
POW, NA (A.C.S., REAGENT)				
125 gm	**10106-3123-04**	56.19		
500 gm	**10106-3123-01**	101.51		
2500 gm	**10106-3123-05**	363.49		
POTASSIUM GLUCONATE				
(Amend) *See POTASSIUM GLUCONATE ANHYDROUS*				
(Consolidated Midland)				
ELI, PO, 20 meq/15 ml,				
480 ml	**00223-6295-01**	5.00		
3840 ml	**00223-6295-02**	32.50		
(Gallipot) *See POTASSIUM GLUCONATE ANHYDROUS*				
(PCCA) *See POTASSIUM GLUCONATE ANHYDROUS*				
(Spectrum Pharmacy) *See POTASSIUM GLUCONATE ANHYDROUS*				
POTASSIUM GLUCONATE ANHYDROUS (Amend)				
potassium gluconate				
POW, NA (U.S.P.)				
454 gm	**17317-0625-01**	9.10		
2270 gm	**17317-0625-05**	35.00		
11350 gm	**17317-0625-08**	131.25		
(Gallipot)				
POW, NA (U.S.P.)				
454 gm	**51552-0607-06**	15.40		
(PCCA)				
POW, NA (U.S.P.)				
1 gm	**51927-1356-00**	0.29		
(Spectrum Pharmacy)				
POW, NA (U.S.P.)				
500 gm	**49452-5830-01**	77.70		
2500 gm	**49452-5830-02**	215.25		
12000 gm	**49452-5830-03**	871.50		
POTASSIUM GUAIACOLSULFONATE (Amend)				
POW, NA (U.S.P.)				
125 gm	**17317-0441-04**	14.00		
500 gm	**17317-0441-01**	28.00		
2270 gm	**17317-0441-05**	126.00		
11350 gm	**17317-0441-08**	525.00		
(PCCA)				
POW, NA (USP; HEMIHYDRATE)				
1 gm	**51927-1694-00**	0.48		
(Spectrum Pharmacy)				
POW, NA (U.S.P.)				
100 gm	**49452-5840-01**	97.30		
500 gm	**49452-5840-02**	205.10		
POTASSIUM HEXACYANOFERRATE TRIHYDRATE REAGENT (PCCA)				
potassium ferricyanide				
POW, NA (1X1GM)				
1 gm	**51927-1688-00**	0.90		
POTASSIUM HYDROXIDE (Amend)				
PEL, NA (N.F., F.C.C.)				
454 gm	**17317-0442-01**	12.30		
11350 gm	**17317-0442-08**	115.00		
(Baker, J.T.)				
FLA, NA (TECHNICAL)				
2500 gm	**10106-3150-05**	52.53		
PEL, NA (N.F., F.C.C.)				
125 gm	**10106-3146-04**	13.69		
500 gm	**10106-3146-01**	16.04		

PROD/MFR NDC AWP DP OBC

(Baker, J.T.) *See POTASSIUM HYDROXIDE 45%*

(Gallipot)
FLA, NA (TECHNICAL)
454 gm.............. **51552-0292-06** 20.65
PEL, NA (N.F.)
454 gm.............. **51552-0067-06** 15.05

(Gallipot) *See POTASSIUM HYDROXIDE 10%*

(Gallipot) *See POTASSIUM HYDROXIDE 20%*

(Gallipot) *See POTASSIUM HYDROXIDE 30%*

(Gallipot) *See POTASSIUM HYDROXIDE 50%*

(Gordon) *See POTASSIUM HYDROXIDE 5%*

(Mallinckrodt Lab)
PEL, NA (N.F.)
500 gm.............. **00406-6976-09** 28.25

(Medisca)
PEL, NA (1X500GM)
500 gm.............. **38779-0909-08** 43.50
(1X2500GM)
2500 gm............. **38779-0909-01** 102.00
SOL, NA (1X500ML,45%)
500 ml **38779-1534-08** 48.00

(PCCA)
PEL, NA (NF)
1 gm UD............. **51927-1255-00** 0.13

(PCCA) *See POTASSIUM HYDROXIDE 45%*

(Spectrum Pharmacy)
PEL, NA (N.F.)
500 gm.............. **49452-5850-01** 78.75
(U.S.P.)
2500 gm............. **49452-5850-02** 232.40
(N.F.)
12000 gm **49452-5850-03** 766.50

(Spectrum Pharmacy) *See POTASSIUM HYDROXIDE 10%*

POTASSIUM HYDROXIDE 10% (Gallipot)
potassium hydroxide
SOL, NA, 473 ml.......... **51552-0071-06** 13.16

(Spectrum Pharmacy)
SOL, NA, 500 ml.......... **49452-5857-03** 73.50
1000 ml **49452-5857-01** 137.20
4000 ml **49452-5857-02** 252.70

POTASSIUM HYDROXIDE 20% (Gallipot)
potassium hydroxide
SOL, NA, 473 ml.......... **51552-0072-06** 14.35

POTASSIUM HYDROXIDE 30% (Gallipot)
potassium hydroxide
SOL, NA, 473 ml.......... **51552-0073-06** 17.71

POTASSIUM HYDROXIDE 45% (Baker, J.T.)
potassium hydroxide
SOL, NA (REAGENT)
500 ml **10106-3143-01** 33.37

(PCCA)
SOL, NA (REAGENT)
1 ml................. **51927-2671-00** 0.18

POTASSIUM HYDROXIDE 5% (Gordon)
potassium hydroxide
SOL, NA, 60 ml........... **10481-3012-01** 23.75

POTASSIUM HYDROXIDE 50% (Gallipot)
potassium hydroxide
SOL, NA, 473 ml.......... **51552-0511-06** 17.64

POTASSIUM IODATE (Baker, J.T.)
POW, NA (A.C.S., REAGENT)
125 gm.............. **10106-3156-04** 69.32
500 gm.............. **10106-3156-01** 215.53
2500 gm............. **10106-3156-05** 903.67

(Spectrum Pharmacy)
POW, NA (1X25GM)
25 gm............... **49452-5858-01** 105.70
(1X125GM)
125 gm.............. **49452-5858-02** 204.05

POTASSIUM IODIDE (Amend)
GRA, NA (U.S.P.)
500 gm.............. **17317-0443-01** 49.00
2270 gm............. **17317-0443-05** 196.00
11350 gm **17317-0443-08** 700.00
POW, NA (A.C.S., REAGENT)
500 gm.............. **17317-1497-05** 35.00
2500 gm............. **17317-1497-04** 140.00

(Baker, J.T.)
GRA, NA (U.S.P., F.C.C.)
125 gm.............. **10106-3168-04** 15.21
500 gm.............. **10106-3168-01** 47.82

(Baker, J.T.) *See POTASSIUM IODIDE COMPACTED*

(Gallipot)
GRA, NA (U.S.P.,N.F.)
113.4 gm............ **51552-0235-04** 15.33
454 gm.............. **51552-0235-06** 43.82

(Mallinckrodt Lab)
GRA, NA (U.S.P.)
125 gm.............. **00406-1112-02** 43.59
500 gm.............. **00406-1112-12** 114.48
POW, NA, 500 gm......... **00406-1115-04** 35.92

(PCCA)
GRA, NA (USP)
1 gm................ **51927-1393-00** 0.48

(Spectrum Pharmacy)
GRA, NA (U.S.P.)
125 gm.............. **49452-5860-01** 66.50
500 gm.............. **49452-5860-02** 213.85
(USP,1X2500GM)
2500 gm............. **49452-5860-04** 882.00

(Spectrum Pharmacy) *See POTASSIUM IODIDE 10%*

(Upsher-Smith) *See SSKI*

POTASSIUM IODIDE 10% (Spectrum Pharmacy)
potassium iodide
SOL, NA (1X500ML)
500 ml **49452-5859-01** 121.45
4000 ml **49452-5859-02** 399.00

POTASSIUM IODIDE COMPACTED (Baker, J.T.)
potassium iodide
CRY, NA (A.C.S., REAGENT)
500 gm.............. **10106-3165-01** 160.99
2500 gm............. **10106-3165-05** 605.49

POTASSIUM IODIDE/THEOPHYLLINE
(Consolidated Midland) *See THEOPHYLLINE-KI*

POTASSIUM METABISULFITE (Amend)
POW, NA (F.C.C.)
454 gm.............. **17317-0444-01** 9.45
2270 gm............. **17317-0444-05** 37.80
11350 gm **17317-0444-08** 131.25

(Baker, J.T.)
CRY, NA (REAGENT)
500 gm.............. **10106-2976-01** 87.24
2500 gm............. **10106-2976-05** 209.14

(PCCA)
POW, NA (FCC)
1 gm................ **51927-1886-00** 0.33

(Spectrum Pharmacy)
CRY, NA (F.C.C.)
500 gm.............. **49452-5870-01** 175.35
(N.F.)
500 gm.............. **49452-5867-01** 219.10
(F.C.C.)
2500 gm............. **49452-5870-02** 402.50
(N.F.)
2500 gm............. **49452-5867-02** 493.50

POTASSIUM METAPERIODATE (Baker, J.T.)
CRY, NA (A.C.S., REAGENT)
125 gm.............. **10106-3224-04** 86.47
500 gm.............. **10106-3224-01** 336.35

POTASSIUM NITRATE (Baker, J.T.)
GRA, NA (A.C.S., F.C.C.)
2500 gm............. **10106-3194-05** 65.57

(Gallipot)
GRA, NA (PURIFIED)
56.7 gm **51552-0082-03** 2.80
113.4 gm **51552-0082-04** 3.71
454 gm.............. **51552-0082-06** 10.22

(Humco)
GRA, NA, 120 gm......... **00395-2637-94** 2.46
454 gm.............. **00395-2637-01** 9.15

(Lorann Oil)
GRA, NA, 120 gm......... **23535-0611-08** 1.50
480 gm.............. **23535-0611-01** 3.95

(Mallinckrodt Lab)
CRY, NA, 500 gm **00406-6715-04** 25.91

(Medisca)
POW, NA (1X100GM,USP)
100 gm.............. **38779-0351-05** 25.50
500 gm.............. **38779-0351-08** 40.50

(PCCA)
POW, NA (USP)
1 gm................ **51927-1460-00** 0.09

(Spectrum Pharmacy)
CRY, NA (F.C.C.,B.P.)
500 gm.............. **49452-5890-02** 80.15
(U.S.P.)
500 gm.............. **49452-5880-02** 80.15
(F.C.C.,B.P.)
2500 gm............. **49452-5890-03** 236.25
(U.S.P.)
2500 gm............. **49452-5880-03** 236.25

POTASSIUM NITRATE/SILVER NITRATE
(Arzol) *See SILVER NITRATE*

POTASSIUM NITRATE/SODIUM FLUORIDE
(Discus Dental) *See FLUORIDEX DAILY DEFENSE SENSITIVITY RELIEF*

(Glaxo) *See AQUAFRESH SENSITIVE*

POTASSIUM OXALATE
(Baker, J.T.) *See POTASSIUM OXALATE MONOHYDRATE*

(PCCA)
CRY, NA (MONOHYDRATE; C.P.)
1 gm................ **51927-1656-00** 0.42

POTASSIUM OXALATE MONOHYDRATE (Baker, J.T.)
potassium oxalate
CRY, NA (A.C.S., REAGENT)
500 gm.............. **10106-3212-01** 86.37
2500 gm............. **10106-3212-05** 308.07

POTASSIUM PERCHLORATE (Baker, J.T.)
CRY, NA (A.C.S., REAGENT)
500 gm.............. **10106-3220-01** 77.46
2500 gm............. **10106-3220-05** 276.09

(Medisca)
CRY, NA (1X100GM)
100 gm.............. **38779-1538-05** 58.50
(1X500GM)
500 gm.............. **38779-1538-08** 150.00

(PCCA)
POW, NA (ACS REAENT)
1 gm................ **51927-2119-00** 1.32

(Spectrum Pharmacy)
CRY, NA (1X25GM)
25 gm............... **49452-5891-01** 105.00
125 gm.............. **49452-5891-02** 248.15

POTASSIUM PERMANGANATE (Baker, J.T.)
CRY, NA (U.S.P.)
500 gm.............. **10106-3232-01** 24.58
2500 gm............. **10106-3232-05** 127.93

(Gallipot)
CRY, NA (U.S.P.)
113.4 gm............ **51552-0040-04** 5.81
454 gm.............. **51552-0040-06** 16.52
2270 gm............. **51552-0040-09** 51.45

(Mallinckrodt Lab)
CRY, NA (U.S.P.)
500 gm.............. **00406-7056-12** 48.20
2500 gm............. **00406-7056-06** 148.03

(Medisca)
POW, NA (U.S.P.)
500 gm.............. **38779-0603-08** 49.50
1000 gm............. **38779-0603-09** 81.00

(PCCA)
POW, NA (U.S.P.)
1 gm................ **51927-1224-00** 0.17

(Spectrum Pharmacy)
CRY, NA (U.S.P.)
500 gm.............. **49452-5900-01** 91.70
2500 gm............. **49452-5900-02** 290.15
12000 gm **49452-5900-03** 913.50

POTASSIUM PERSULFATE (Baker, J.T.)
POW, NA (REAGENT)
500 gm.............. **10106-3238-01** 52.07
2500 gm............. **10106-3238-05** 210.69

POTASSIUM PHOSPHATE
(Amend) *See POTASSIUM PHOSPHATE DIBASIC*

(Amend) *See POTASSIUM PHOSPHATE MONOBASIC*

(Amer Regent) *See POTASSIUM PHOSPHATES*

(Baker, J.T.) *See POTASSIUM PHOSPHATE DIBASIC*

(Baker, J.T.) *See POTASSIUM PHOSPHATE MONOBASIC*

(Baker, J.T.) *See POTASSIUM PHOSPHATE TRIBASIC*

(Hospira)
SOL, IV (25X5ML,LATEX-FREE)
3 mmole/ml,
5 ml 25s........... **00409-7296-01** 15.00 13.25

PROD/MFR NDC AWP DP OBC

(25X15ML,LATEX-FREE)
3 mmole/ml,
15 ml 25s.......... **00409-7295-01** 17.10 15.00
(BULK ADD,LATEX-FREE)
3 mmole/ml,
50 ml 25s.......... **00409-4201-01** 74.70 65.25

(Mallinckrodt Lab) *See POTASSIUM PHOSPHATE DIBASIC*

(PCCA) *See POTASSIUM PHOSPHATE DIBASIC*

(PCCA)
POW, NA (NF; MONOBASIC)
1 gm................ **51927-1566-00** 0.09
(TRIBASIC)
1 gm................ **51927-2693-00** 0.36

(Spectrum Pharmacy) *See POTASSIUM PHOSPHATE DIBASIC*

(Spectrum Pharmacy) *See POTASSIUM PHOSPHATE MONOBASIC*

(Spectrum Pharmacy) *See POTASSIUM PHOSPHATE TRIBASIC*

POTASSIUM PHOSPHATE DIBASIC (Amend)
potassium phosphate
CRY, NA (REAGENT, DIHYDRATE)
500 gm.............. **17317-1374-01** 42.00
2500 gm............. **17317-1374-05** 140.00
POW, NA (F.C.C., ANHYDROUS)
454 gm.............. **17317-0448-01** 11.20
2270 gm............. **17317-0448-05** 46.20
11350 gm **17317-0448-08** 157.50

(Baker, J.T.)
POW, NA (F.C.C.)
500 gm.............. **10106-3254-01** 27.25
2500 gm............. **10106-3254-05** 171.56

(Mallinckrodt Lab)
GRA, NA, 500 gm......... **00406-7080-04** 39.37

(PCCA)
POW, NA (U.S.P.)
1 gm................ **51927-3114-00** 0.15

(Spectrum Pharmacy)
POW, NA (ANHYDROUS/U.S.P.)
500 gm.............. **49452-5921-01** 93.10
2500 gm............. **49452-5921-02** 296.80
12000 gm **49452-5921-03** 1067.50

POTASSIUM PHOSPHATE MONOBASIC (Amend)
potassium phosphate
CRY, NA (N.F., F.C.C.)
454 gm.............. **17317-0449-01** 9.80
2270 gm............. **17317-0449-05** 35.00
11350 gm **17317-0449-08** 113.75

(Baker, J.T.)
CRY, NA (A.C.S., F.C.C., N.F.)
2500 gm............. **10106-3247-05** 106.19

(Spectrum Pharmacy)
CRY, NA (N.F.)
500 gm.............. **49452-5910-01** 74.20
2500 gm............. **49452-5910-02** 231.70
12000 gm **49452-5910-03** 735.00

POTASSIUM PHOSPHATE TRIBASIC (Baker, J.T.)
potassium phosphate
POW, NA (REAGENT, N-HYDRATE)
500 gm.............. **10106-3256-01** 112.73
2500 gm............. **10106-3256-05** 300.25

(Spectrum Pharmacy)
CRY, NA (F.C.C.)
125 gm.............. **49452-5928-01** 94.85
500 gm.............. **49452-5928-02** 236.25

POTASSIUM PHOSPHATE, MONOBASIC
(Beach Pharm) *See K-PHOS ORIGINAL*

POTASSIUM PHOSPHATES (Amer Regent)
potassium phosphate
SOL, IV (S.D.V.,PF)
3 mmole/ml,
5 ml 25s........... **00517-2305-25** 20.94
15 ml 25s.......... **00517-2315-25** 32.19
50 ml 25s.......... **00517-2350-25** 85.94

POTASSIUM PYROPHOSPHATE (Spectrum Pharmacy)
POW, NA (F.C.C.)
500 gm.............. **49452-5929-01** 156.10

POTASSIUM PYROSULFATE (Baker, J.T.)
POW, NA (REAGENT)
500 gm.............. **10106-2964-01** 126.54
2500 gm............. **10106-2964-05** 485.59

PROD/MFR NDC AWP DP OBC

POTASSIUM SODIUM TARTRATE (Amend)
POW, NA (U.S.P.)
454 gm.............. **17317-0450-01** 14.00
2270 gm............. **17317-0450-05** 49.00
11350 gm **17317-0450-08** 175.00

(Baker, J.T.) *See POTASSIUM SODIUM TARTRATE 4-HYDRATE*

(Gallipot)
GRA, NA (U.S.P.)
454 gm.............. **51552-0479-06** 24.15

(Mallinckrodt Lab)
potassium tartrate
POW, NA (U.S.P.)
500 gm.............. **00406-2370-04** 77.73

POTASSIUM SODIUM TARTRATE (Medisca)
POW, NA (U.S.P.)
100 gm.............. **38779-1539-05** 28.50
500 gm.............. **38779-1539-08** 46.50
1000 gm............. **38779-1539-09** 87.00

(PCCA)
POW, NA (USP; TETRAHYDRATE)
1 gm................ **51927-1468-00** 0.36

(Spectrum Pharmacy)
GRA, NA (U.S.P.)
500 gm.............. **49452-5930-01** 93.10
2500 gm............. **49452-5930-02** 281.40
12000 gm **49452-5930-03** 973.00
POW, NA, 500 gm......... **49452-5940-01** 93.10
2500 gm............. **49452-5940-02** 281.40
12000 gm............ **49452-5940-03** 973.00

POTASSIUM SODIUM TARTRATE 4-HYDRATE
(Baker, J.T.)
potassium sodium tartrate
CRY, NA (A.C.S., REAGENT)
500 gm.............. **10106-3262-01** 109.80
2500 gm............. **10106-3262-05** 350.25

POTASSIUM SORBATE (Amend)
POW, NA (N.F., F.C.C.)
125 gm.............. **17317-0661-04** 8.40
454 gm.............. **17317-0661-01** 18.90
2270 gm............. **17317-0661-05** 52.50

(Baker, J.T.)
POW, NA (N.F., F.C.C.)
500 gm.............. **10106-3273-01** 43.42

(Gallipot)
POW, NA (U.S.P.,N.F.)
113.4 gm............ **51552-0214-04** 11.06
454 gm.............. **51552-0214-06** 21.00

(Letco)
POW, NA (N.F.)
500 gm.............. **62991-1293-02** 36.00
2500 gm............. **62991-1293-03** 120.00

(PCCA)
POW, NA (NF)
1 gm................ **51927-1107-00** 1.08

(Spectrum Pharmacy)
GRA, NA (N.F.)
125 gm.............. **49452-5951-01** 60.55
500 gm.............. **49452-5951-02** 89.60
(U.S.P., N.F.)
2500 gm............. **49452-5951-03** 241.50
POW, NA (N.F.)
125 gm.............. **49452-5950-01** 53.90
500 gm.............. **49452-5950-02** 81.90
2500 gm............. **49452-5950-03** 222.60

POTASSIUM STARCH (Amend)
starch
POW, NA (N.F., FOOD GRADE)
454 gm.............. **17317-1227-01** 8.40
11350 gm **17317-1227-08** 8.40

POTASSIUM SULFATE (Amend)
GRA, NA (A.C.S., REAGENT)
500 gm.............. **17317-1217-05** 19.90
2500 gm............. **17317-1217-06** 69.50
POW, NA (PURIFIED, F.C.C.)
454 gm.............. **17317-0451-01** 7.00
2270 gm............. **17317-0451-05** 26.60
11350 gm **17317-0451-08** 113.75

(Baker, J.T.)
CRY, NA (FINE, A.C.S., REAGENT)
500 gm.............. **10106-3278-01** 40.79
2500 gm............. **10106-3278-05** 150.28
POW, NA (A.C.S., REAGENT)
500 gm.............. **10106-3282-01** 78.13
2500 gm............. **10106-3282-05** 343.92

PROD/MFR NDC AWP DP OBC

(Mallinckrodt Lab)
GRA, NA (A.C.S.)
500 gm.............. **00406-7140-04** 31.94
POW, NA, 500 gm......... **00406-7144-04** 59.45

(PCCA)
POW, NA (FCC)
1 gm................ **51927-1417-00** 0.12

POTASSIUM TARTRATE
(Baker, J.T.) *See POTASSIUM TARTRATE HEMIHYDRATE*

(Mallinckrodt Lab) *See POTASSIUM SODIUM TARTRATE*

POTASSIUM TARTRATE HEMIHYDRATE (Baker, J.T.)
potassium tartrate
CRY, NA (REAGENT)
500 gm.............. **10106-3316-01** 73.23

POTASSIUM THIOCYANATE (Baker, J.T.)
CRY, NA (A.C.S., REAGENT)
500 gm.............. **10106-3326-01** 102.07
2500 gm............. **10106-3326-05** 412.98

(PCCA)
POW, NA (ACS REAGENT)
1 gm................ **51927-1851-00** 1.20

POVIDONE
(Amend) *See POVIDONE K2932*

(Amend) *See POVIDONE K30*

(Medisca)
POW, NA (1X100GM,USP)
100 gm.............. **38779-0252-05** 28.50

(PCCA)
POW, NA (USP;30)
1 gm................ **51927-1169-00** 0.54

(Spectrum Pharmacy) *See POLYVINYLPYRROLIDONE K-30*

(Spectrum Pharmacy) *See POLYVINYLPYRROLIDONE K-90*

POVIDONE IODINE
(Alcon Surgical) *See BETADINE*

(PCCA)
POW, NA (U.S.P.)
1 gm................ **51927-1076-00** 0.36

(Spectrum Pharmacy) *See POVIDONE-IODINE*

POVIDONE K2932 (Amend)
povidone
POW, NA (U.S.P.)
454 gm.............. **17317-0888-01** 54.60
2270 gm............. **17317-0888-05** 189.00

POVIDONE K30 (Amend)
povidone
POW, NA, 454 gm......... **17317-1289-01** 29.40
2270 gm............. **17317-1289-05** 105.00

POVIDONE-IODINE (Spectrum Pharmacy)
povidone iodine
POW, NA (U.S.P.)
100 gm.............. **49452-5970-01** 67.90
500 gm.............. **49452-5970-02** 207.20
2500 gm............. **49452-5970-03** 707.00

POWDER SCENT (Medisca)
fragrance
SOL, NA (1X25ML)
25 ml............... **38779-1544-04** 22.50
(1X100ML)
100 ml **38779-1544-05** 46.50

POWDER SCENT FRAGRANCE (PCCA)
fragrance
SOL, NA, 1 ml........... **51927-3225-00** 1.00

PPG-2 MYRISTYL ETHER PROPIONATE (PCCA)
SOL, NA, 1 ml........... **51927-2522-00** 0.14

PR BENZOYL PEROXIDE (PruGen)
benzoyl peroxide
SOA, TP (1X480ML)
7%, 480 ml.......... **42546-0145-16** 136.29

PR NATAL 400 (PruGen)
prenatal vitamins
KIT, PO (FILM-COATED,SOFTGEL)
60s ea.............. **42546-0811-30** 37.08

PR NATAL 400 EC (PruGen)
prenatal vitamins
KIT, PO (ENTERIC COATED SOFTGEL)
60s ea.............. **42546-0517-30** 42.52

PR NATAL 430 (PruGen)
prenatal vitamins
KIT, PO (FILM-COATED,SOFTGEL)
60s ea.............. **42546-0812-30** 37.08

PROD/MFR	NDC	AWP	DP	OBC
PR NATAL 430 EC (PruGen)				
prenatal vitamins				
KIT, PO (ENTERIC COATED SOFTGEL)				
60s ea	**42546-0518-30**	42.52		
PR NATAL 440 EC (PruGen)				
prenatal vitamins				
KIT, PO (ENTERIC COATED SOFTGEL)				
60s ea	**42546-0170-30**	43.68		
PR OTIC SOLUTION (PruGen)				
acetic acid/antipyrine/benzocaine/policosanol				
SOL, OT (1X14ML,DROPPERSCREWCAP)				
14 ml	**42546-0501-04**	160.65		
PRALATREXATE				
(Allos) *See FOLOTYN*				
PRALIDOXIME CHLORIDE				
(Baxter) *See PROTOPAM CHLORIDE*				
(PCCA)				
POW, NA, 1 gm	**51927-2300-00**	57.00		
(Spectrum Pharmacy)				
CRY, NA (U.S.P.)				
1 gm	**49452-5971-01**	89.60		
5 gm	**49452-5971-02**	312.90		
25 gm	**49452-5971-03**	1253.00		
PRALINES AND CREAM FLAVOR (PCCA)				
flavoring aid				
SOL, NA (PRALINES AND CREAM)				
1 ml	**51927-3309-00**	0.70		
PRAMIPEXOLE DIHYDROCHLORIDE				
(Boehr Ingelheim Cons) *See MIRAPEX*				
(Boehr Ingelheim Phar) *See MIRAPEX*				
(Boehr Ingelheim Phar) *See MIRAPEX ER*				
(Teva)				
TAB, PO, 0.125 mg, 63s ea	**00555-0617-62**	185.83		**AB**
0.25 mg, 90s ea	**00555-0612-14**	265.47		**AB**
0.5 mg, 90s ea	**00555-0613-14**	265.47		**AB**
1 mg, 90s ea	**00555-0614-14**	265.47		**AB**
1.5 mg, 90s ea	**00555-0615-14**	265.47		**AB**
PRAMLINTIDE ACETATE				
(Amylin) *See SYMLIN*				
(Amylin) *See SYMLINPEN*				
PRAMOSONE (Ferndale)				
hydrocortisone acetate/pramoxine hydrochloride				
CRE, TP, 1%-1%, 28.4 gm	**00496-0716-04**	78.08		
57 gm	**00496-0716-03**	106.97		
2.5%-1%, 28.4 gm	**00496-0717-04**	78.08		
57 gm	**00496-0717-03**	106.97		
LOT, TP, 1%-1%, 59 ml	**00496-0729-06**	97.63		
118 ml	**00496-0729-04**	152.90		
236 ml	**00496-0729-03**	228.59		
2.5%-1%, 59 ml	**00496-0726-06**	97.63		
118 ml	**00496-0726-04**	152.90		
OIN, TP, 1%-1%, 28.4 gm	**00496-0763-04**	76.52		
2.5%-1%, 28.4 gm	**00496-0777-04**	76.52		
PRAMOTIC (Hawthorn Pharm)				
chloroxylenol/pramoxine hydrochloride				
SOL, OT (DROPS)				
1 mg/ml-10 mg/ml,				
10 ml	**63717-0400-10**	20.89		
(Phys Total Care)				
REPACK				
SOL, OT (DROPS)				
1 mg/ml-10 mg/ml,				
10 ml	**54868-5091-00**	22.00		
PRAMOXGEL (Hawthorn Pharm)				
pramoxine hydrochloride				
GEL, TP (1X113GM)				
1%, 113 gm	**63717-0033-04**	14.37		
PRAMOXINE HYDROCHLORIDE				
(Alaven) *See PROCTOFOAM*				
(Hawthorn Pharm) *See PRAMOXGEL*				
(Medisca)				
POW, NA (U.S.P.)				
25 gm	**38779-0458-04**	87.00		
100 gm	**38779-0458-05**	297.00		
(1X1000GM,USP)				
1000 gm	**38779-0458-09**	1842.00		
(PCCA)				
POW, NA (U.S.P.)				
1 gm	**51927-1914-00**	5.10		
(Spectrum Pharmacy)				
POW, NA (U.S.P.)				
25 gm	**49452-5972-01**	147.70		
100 gm	**49452-5972-02**	465.50		
500 gm	**49452-5972-04**	1764.00		
1000 gm	**49452-5972-03**	2562.00		

PROD/MFR	NDC	AWP	DP	OBC
PRANDIMET (Novo Nordisk)				
metformin hydrochloride/repaglinide				
TAB, PO, 500 mg-1 mg,				
100s ea	**00169-0093-01**	194.14		
500 mg-2 mg,				
100s ea	**00169-0092-01**	194.14		
PRANDIN (Novo Nordisk)				
repaglinide				
TAB, PO, 0.5 mg, 100s ea	**00169-0081-81**	213.36		
1000s ea	**00169-0081-83**	2133.44		
1 mg, 100s ea	**00169-0082-81**	213.36		
1000s ea	**00169-0082-83**	2133.44		
2 mg, 100s ea	**00169-0084-81**	213.36		
1000s ea	**00169-0084-83**	2133.44		
(Phys Total Care)				
REPACK				
TAB, PO, 2 mg, 10s ea	**54868-5381-00**	16.96		
90s ea	**54868-5381-01**	130.16		
(Quality Care Prod)				
REPACK				
TAB, PO, 0.5 mg, 100s ea	**35356-0303-01**	350.32		
1 mg, 100s ea	**35356-0304-01**	350.32		
2 mg, 100s ea	**35356-0305-01**	350.32		
PRASCION (Prasco Labs)				
sulfacetamide sodium/sulfur				
SOA, TP (CLEANSER)				
10%-5%, 170.3 gm	**66993-0902-06**	45.15		
340.2 gm	**66993-0902-12**	82.80		
(Phys Total Care)				
REPACK				
SOA, TP, 10%-5%,				
170.3 gm	**54868-5509-00**	81.54		
PRASCION FC (Prasco Labs)				
sulfacetamide sodium/sulfur				
PAD, TP, 10%-5%, 30s ea	**66993-0905-30**	108.39		
60s ea	**66993-0905-60**	205.96		
PRASCION RA (Prasco Labs)				
sulfacetamide sodium/sulfur				
CRE, TP, 10%-5%, 45 gm	**66993-0904-45**	87.84		
(1X45GM,W/SUNSCREEN)				
10%-5%, 45 gm	**66993-0925-45**	87.84		
PRASCION TS (Prasco Labs)				
sulfacetamide sodium/sulfur				
SUS, TP, 10%-5%, 30 gm	**66993-0919-31**	67.90		
PRASUGREL HYDROCHLORIDE				
(Lilly) *See EFFIENT*				
PRAVACHOL (Bristol-Myers)				
pravastatin sodium				
TAB, PO, 10 mg, 90s ea	**00003-5154-05**	386.54		
20 mg, 90s ea	**00003-5178-05**	392.80		
40 mg, 90s ea	**00003-5194-10**	576.41		
80 mg, 90s ea	**00003-5195-10**	576.41		
(Advanced Pharm Serv, Inc.)				
REPACK				
TAB, PO, 20 mg, 10s ea	**13411-0118-01**	46.01		
20s ea	**13411-0118-02**	92.02		
30s ea	**13411-0118-03**	138.05		
60s ea	**13411-0118-06**	276.11		
90s ea	**13411-0118-09**	414.16		
40 mg, 10s ea	**13411-0119-01**	67.27		
20s ea	**13411-0119-02**	134.54		
30s ea	**13411-0119-03**	201.81		
60s ea	**13411-0119-06**	403.62		
90s ea	**13411-0119-09**	605.43		
(AQ)				
REPACK				
TAB, PO, 10 mg, 10s ea	**66105-0120-01**	45.30		
15s ea	**66105-0120-15**	67.95		
30s ea	**66105-0120-03**	135.89		
60s ea	**66105-0120-06**	271.77		
90s ea	**66105-0120-09**	407.65		
20 mg, 10s ea	**66105-0121-01**	46.02		
15s ea	**66105-0121-15**	69.03		
30s ea	**66105-0121-03**	138.06		
60s ea	**66105-0121-06**	276.11		
90s ea	**66105-0121-09**	414.16		
40 mg, 10s ea	**66105-0122-01**	67.27		
15s ea	**66105-0122-15**	100.91		
30s ea	**66105-0122-03**	201.81		
60s ea	**66105-0122-06**	403.62		
90s ea	**66105-0122-09**	605.43		
(Bryant Ranch)				
REPACK				
TAB, PO, 40 mg, 30s ea	**63629-1606-01**	153.99		
(PD-Rx Pharm)				
REPACK				
TAB, PO, 10 mg, 30s ea	**55289-0104-30**	191.51		

PROD/MFR	NDC	AWP	DP	OBC
(REDI-SCRIPT)				
10 mg, 30s ea	**58864-0653-30**	147.03		
20 mg, 30s ea	**55289-0871-30**	194.60		
(REDI-SCRIPT)				
40 mg, 15s ea	**58864-0743-15**	108.68		
30s ea	**55289-0873-30**	285.57		
(REDI-SCRIPT)				
40 mg, 30s ea	**58864-0743-30**	261.92		
(Phys Total Care)				
REPACK				
TAB, PO, 10 mg, 10s ea	**54868-2287-02**	42.09		
30s ea	**54868-2287-01**	122.50		
20 mg, 30s ea	**54868-2288-01**	128.34		
60s ea	**54868-2288-02**	240.74		
90s ea	**54868-2288-00**	359.55		
40 mg, 30s ea	**54868-3270-00**	230.06		
60s ea	**54868-3270-01**	456.85		
90s ea	**54868-3270-02**	683.63		
80 mg, 30s ea	**54868-4634-00**	188.53		
(Southwood)				
REPACK				
TAB, PO, 20 mg, 30s ea	**58016-0425-30**	130.93		
60s ea	**58016-0425-60**	261.87		
90s ea	**58016-0425-90**	392.80		
100s ea	**58016-0425-00**	436.44		
PRAVASTATIN (DHS, Inc.)				
REPACK				
pravastatin sodium				
TAB, PO, 20 mg, 30s ea	**55887-0203-30**	98.00		
90s ea	**55887-0203-90**	294.01		
40 mg, 90s ea	**55887-0192-90**	450.00		
(Southwood)				
REPACK				
TAB, PO, 20 mg, 30s ea	**58016-0013-30**	98.01		
60s ea	**58016-0013-60**	196.03		
90s ea	**58016-0013-90**	294.04		
100s ea	**58016-0013-00**	326.71		
40 mg, 30s ea	**58016-0012-30**	143.83		
60s ea	**58016-0012-60**	287.67		
90s ea	**58016-0012-90**	431.50		
100s ea	**58016-0012-00**	479.44		
(Vibranta)				
REPACK				
TAB, PO, 40 mg, 30s ea	**57866-3932-01**	51.54		
PRAVASTATIN SODIUM				
FUL				
TAB, PO, 10 mg, 90s ea		22.50		
20 mg, 90s ea		26.25		
40 mg, 90s ea		32.04		
80 mg, 90s ea		51.78		
(Apotex Corp.)				
TAB, PO, 10 mg, 90s ea	**60505-0168-09**	289.33		**AB**
500s ea	**60505-0168-05**	1607.39		**AB**
20 mg, 90s ea	**60505-0169-09**	294.01		**AB**
1000s ea	**60505-0169-07**	3267.26		**AB**
40 mg, 90s ea	**60505-0170-09**	431.45		**AB**
1000s ea	**60505-0170-07**	4793.89		**AB**
9000s ea	**60505-0170-08**	43145.01		**AB**
80 mg, 90s ea	**60505-1323-09**	431.50		**AB**
500s ea	**60505-1323-05**	2397.20		**AB**
(Bristol-Myers) *See PRAVACHOL*				
(Dr Reddy's)				
TAB, PO (COATED TABLET)				
10 mg, 90s ea	**55111-0229-90**	289.36		**AB**
500s ea	**55111-0229-05**	1607.55		**AB**
20 mg, 90s ea	**55111-0230-90**	294.04		**AB**
500s ea	**55111-0230-05**	1633.55		**AB**
40 mg, 90s ea	**55111-0231-90**	431.50		**AB**
500s ea	**55111-0231-05**	2397.20		**AB**
80 mg, 90s ea	**55111-0274-90**	431.50		**AB**
500s ea	**55111-0274-05**	2397.20		**AB**
(Glenmark Pharmaceuticals)				
TAB, PO, 10 mg, 90s ea	**68462-0195-90**	289.36		**AB**
500s ea	**68462-0195-05**	1607.55		**AB**
20 mg, 90s ea	**68462-0196-90**	294.04		**AB**
500s ea	**68462-0196-05**	1633.55		**AB**
40 mg, 90s ea	**68462-0197-90**	431.50		**AB**
500s ea	**68462-0197-05**	2397.20		**AB**
80 mg, 90s ea	**68462-0198-90**	431.50		**AB**
500s ea	**68462-0198-05**	2397.20		**AB**
(Lupin Pharma, Inc.)				
TAB, PO (FILM-COATED)				
10 mg, 90s ea	**68180-0485-09**	289.36		**AB**
500s ea	**68180-0485-02**	1607.55		**AB**
20 mg, 90s ea	**68180-0486-09**	294.04		**AB**
500s ea	**68180-0486-02**	1633.55		**AB**
40 mg, 90s ea	**68180-0487-09**	431.50		**AB**
500s ea	**68180-0487-02**	2397.20		**AB**

PROD/MFR	NDC	AWP	DP	OBC
80 mg, 90s ea	68180-0488-09	431.50		AB
500s ea	68180-0488-02	2397.22		AB
(Major)				
TAB, PO (10X10)				
10 mg, 100s ea UD	00904-5891-61	287.98		AB
20 mg, 100s ea UD	00904-5892-61	325.91		AB
40 mg, 100s ea UD	00904-5893-61	429.36		AB
(Mylan)				
TAB, PO, 10 mg, 90s ea	00378-8210-77	289.36		
1000s ea	00378-8210-10	3215.10		
20 mg, 90s ea	00378-8220-77	294.04		
1000s ea	00378-8220-10	3267.10		
40 mg, 90s ea	00378-8240-77	431.50		
1000s ea	00378-8240-10	4794.40		
80 mg, 90s ea	00378-8280-77	431.50		
500s ea	00378-8280-05	2397.00		
(Ranbaxy Pharm)				
TAB, PO, 10 mg, 90s ea	63304-0595-90	289.36		AB
20 mg, 90s ea	63304-0596-90	294.04		AB
40 mg, 90s ea	63304-0597-90	431.50		AB
(CAPLET)				
80 mg, 90s ea	63304-0598-90	431.50		AB
500s ea	63304-0598-05	2397.00		AB
(Sandoz)				
TAB, PO, 10 mg, 90s ea	00781-5231-92	289.36		AB
1000s ea	00781-5231-10	3215.10		AB
20 mg, 90s ea	00781-5232-92	294.04		AB
1000s ea	00781-5232-10	3267.10		AB
40 mg, 90s ea	00781-5234-92	431.50		AB
1000s ea	00781-5234-10	4794.40		AB
(Teva)				
TAB, PO, 10 mg, 90s ea	00093-0771-98	289.36		AB
90s ea	50111-0761-17	289.04		AB
(USP)				
10 mg, 1000s ea	00093-0771-10	3215.11		AB
20 mg, 90s ea	00093-7201-98	294.04		AB
90s ea	50111-0762-17	293.71		AB
1000s ea	00093-7201-10	3267.10		AB
1000s ea	50111-0762-03	3263.99		AB
40 mg, 90s ea	00093-7202-98	431.50		AB
90s ea	50111-0764-17	431.02		AB
1000s ea	00093-7202-10	4794.40		AB
1000s ea	50111-0764-03	4789.07		AB
(USP)				
80 mg, 90s ea	00093-7270-98	431.50		AB
1000s ea	00093-7270-10	4794.44		AB
(UDL)				
TAB, PO (10X10)				
20 mg, 100s ea UD	51079-0458-20	326.71		AB
40 mg, 100s ea UD	51079-0782-20	477.07		AB
(Watson Labs)				
TAB, PO, 10 mg, 90s ea	16252-0526-90	36.00		AB
20 mg, 90s ea	16252-0527-90	36.00		AB
500s ea	16252-0527-50	199.20		AB
40 mg, 90s ea	16252-0528-90	54.00		AB
500s ea	16252-0528-50	300.00		AB
80 mg, 90s ea	16252-0529-90	60.00		AB
(A-S Medication)				
REPACK				
TAB, PO, 20 mg, 30s ea	54569-5793-00	98.01		
40 mg, 30s ea	54569-5794-00	143.83		
(American Health)				
REPACK				
TAB, PO (10X10)				
10 mg, 100s ea UD	68084-0186-01	319.98		
20 mg, 100s ea UD	68084-0187-01	325.12		
40 mg, 100s ea UD	68084-0188-01	477.07		
(Dispensing Solutions)				
REPACK				
TAB, PO, 40 mg, 30s ea	66336-0813-30	143.83		AB
(Palmetto)				
REPACK				
TAB, PO, 10 mg, 30s ea	23490-9350-03	157.50		
60s ea	23490-9350-06	315.00		
90s ea	23490-9350-09	472.50		
20 mg, 30s ea	23490-9351-03	112.50		
60s ea	23490-9351-06	225.00		
90s ea	23490-9351-09	337.50		
40 mg, 30s ea	23490-9352-03	157.50		
60s ea	23490-9352-06	315.00		
90s ea	23490-9352-09	472.50		
(PD-Rx Pharm)				
REPACK				
TAB, PO (COATED TABLET)				
20 mg, 30s ea	43063-0143-30	158.38		AB
(USP,COATED TABLET)				
40 mg, 30s ea	43063-0195-30	23.38		AB
(Pharma Pac)				
REPACK				
TAB, PO, 20 mg, 30s ea	52959-0990-30	112.10		AB
(Phys Total Care)				
REPACK				
TAB, PO, 10 mg, 30s ea	54868-5576-00	58.26		
(COATED TABLET)				
10 mg, 90s ea	54868-5576-01	55.09		AB
20 mg, 30s ea	54868-5577-00	53.76		
90s ea	54868-5577-01	155.28		
40 mg, 30s ea	54868-5578-00	28.32		
60s ea	54868-5578-02	46.40		AB
90s ea	54868-5578-01	74.49		
80 mg, 30s ea	54868-5579-00	52.15		AB
90s ea	54868-5579-01	113.00		AB
(Physician Partner)				
REPACK				
TAB, PO, 10 mg, 30s ea	21695-0178-30	190.73		AB
(COATED TABLET)				
20 mg, 30s ea	21695-0179-30	194.15		AB
90s ea	21695-0179-90	588.08		
40 mg, 30s ea	21695-0180-30	287.66		AB
90s ea	21695-0180-90	862.98		AB
(Quality Care Prod)				
REPACK				
TAB, PO, 40 mg, 30s ea	35356-0125-30	248.00		AB
(Stat Rx)				
REPACK				
TAB, PO (COATED TABLET)				
40 mg, 30s ea	16590-0546-30	143.75		AB
60s ea	16590-0546-60	287.40		AB
90s ea	16590-0546-90	431.10		AB
PRAZIQUANTEL (Gallipot)				
POW, NA (USP,1X1000GM)				
1000 gm	51552-0911-07	1190.00	850.00	
(Hawkins)				
POW, NA (U.S.P.)				
5 gm	63370-0192-15	103.20		
25 gm	63370-0192-25	480.00		
100 gm	63370-0192-35	1824.00		
1000 gm	63370-0192-50	4800.00		
(Letco)				
POW, NA (U.S.P.)				
5 gm	62991-2053-01	57.00		
25 gm	62991-2053-02	225.00		
100 gm	62991-2053-03	865.00		
(Medisca)				
POW, NA (U.S.P.)				
5 gm	38779-0090-03	87.00		
25 gm	38779-0090-04	387.00		
100 gm	38779-0090-05	1155.00		
(PCCA)				
POW, NA (U.S.P.)				
1 gm	51927-2737-00	24.60		
(Schering) *See BILTRICIDE*				
(Spectrum Pharmacy)				
CRY, NA (U.S.P.)				
1 gm	49452-5976-01	105.00		
5 gm	49452-5976-02	169.05		
25 gm	49452-5976-03	626.50		
PRAZOSIN HCL (Medisca)				
prazosin hydrochloride				
POW, NA (1X10GM,USP)				
10 gm	38779-0307-01	87.00		
(U.S.P.)				
25 gm	38779-0307-04	229.50		
(1X50GM,USP)				
50 gm	38779-0307-02	435.00		
(U.S.P.)				
100 gm	38779-0307-05	765.00		
(Mylan)				
CAP, PO, 1 mg, 100s ea	00378-1101-01	32.00		AB
1000s ea	00378-1101-10	320.00		AB
2 mg, 100s ea	00378-2302-01	47.25		AB
1000s ea	00378-2302-10	472.50		AB
5 mg, 100s ea	00378-3205-01	78.00		AB
250s ea	00378-3205-25	195.00		AB
(UDL)				
CAP, PO (10X10)				
1 mg, 100s ea UD	51079-0630-20	29.36		AB
2 mg, 100s ea UD	51079-0631-20	38.21		AB
5 mg, 100s ea UD	51079-0632-20	65.41		AB
(A-S Medication)				
REPACK				
CAP, PO, 1 mg, 30s ea	54569-2582-01	11.88		AB
2 mg, 30s ea	54569-2583-01	16.55		EE
(PD-Rx Pharm)				
REPACK				
CAP, PO, 1 mg, 30s ea	58864-0415-30	14.87		AB
60s ea	55289-0536-60	23.07		AB
100s ea	55289-0536-01	34.00		AB
2 mg, 30s ea	58864-0416-30	23.33		EE
(Phys Total Care)				
REPACK				
CAP, PO, 1 mg, 30s ea	54868-0705-03	18.84		EE
60s ea	54868-0705-00	33.18		EE
100s ea	54868-0705-01	52.32		EE
2 mg, 100s ea	54868-1547-01	100.50		EE
5 mg, 30s ea	54868-2004-00	64.36		EE
100s ea	54868-2004-01	202.52		EE
(Southwood)				
REPACK				
CAP, PO, 1 mg, 30s ea	58016-0398-30	14.40		EE
60s ea	58016-0398-60	28.80		EE
90s ea	58016-0398-90	43.20		EE
100s ea	58016-0398-00	48.00		EE
PRAZOSIN HYDROCHLORIDE				
FUL				
CAP, PO, 5 mg, 250s ea		134.25		
(Medisca) *See PRAZOSIN HCL*				
(Mylan) *See PRAZOSIN HCL*				
(Pfizer) *See MINIPRESS*				
(Teva)				
CAP, PO (USP)				
1 mg, 100s ea	00093-4067-01	39.60		AB
250s ea	00093-4067-52	99.00		AB
(USP)				
1 mg, 1000s ea	00093-4067-10	396.00		AB
2 mg, 100s ea	00093-4068-01	55.15		
250s ea	00093-4068-52	137.85		
1000s ea	00093-4068-10	551.35		
5 mg, 100s ea	00093-4069-01	93.98		
250s ea	00093-4069-52	234.95		
500s ea	00093-4069-05	469.90		
(UDL) *See PRAZOSIN HCL*				
(Altura)				
REPACK				
CAP, PO, 1 mg, 10s ea	63874-0631-10	5.04		
12s ea	63874-0631-12	6.05		
15s ea	63874-0631-15	7.57		
20s ea	63874-0631-20	10.09		
30s ea	63874-0631-30	15.13		
90s ea	63874-0631-90	45.40		
100s ea	63874-0631-01	50.44		
(PD-Rx Pharm)				
REPACK				
CAP, PO (REDI-SCRIPT)				
1 mg, 90s ea	58864-0415-90	32.25		AB
(USP,REDI-SCRIPT)				
5 mg, 30s ea	58864-0826-30	39.68		
(REDI-SCRIPT)				
5 mg, 60s ea	58864-0826-60	72.68		AB
(Phys Total Care)				
REPACK				
CAP, PO, 2 mg, 30s ea	54868-1547-02	33.30		AB
PRE-PEN (Alk-Abello)				
benzylpenicilloyl polylysine				
SOL, ID, 0.25 ml 5s	49471-0001-05		345.00	
PRECARE (Ther-RX)				
prenatal vitamins				
CTB, PO (BERRY)				
30s ea	64011-0024-19	37.49		
PRECARE CONCEIVE (Ther-RX)				
prenatal vitamins				
TAB, PO, 30s ea	64011-0014-19	37.49		
PRECARE PREMIER (Ther-RX)				
multivitamin and minerals				
TAB, PO (DYE-FREE)				
30s ea	64011-0195-19	39.84		
PRECEDEX (Hospira)				
dexmedetomidine hydrochloride				
SOL, IV (VIAL,FLIPTOP,PF)				
100 mcg/ml,				
2 ml 25s	00409-1638-02	2065.80	1721.50	
PRECISION 200 URINE METER (Covidien)				
catheter supplies				
DEV, NA, 10s ea	08080-1000-04	129.89		

PROD/MFR	NDC	AWP	DP	OBC
PRECISION 200 URINE METER CATHETERIZATION TRAY (Covidien)				
collector, urine				
DEV, NA (16FR,5CC,LATEX-FREE)				
10s ea	08080-2601-04	234.72		
10s ea	08080-2601-22	181.50		
(18FR,5CC,LATEX-FREE)				
10s ea	08080-2801-04	234.72		
10s ea	08080-2801-22	181.50		
PRECISION 400 ADD-A-FOLEY CATHETER TRAY (Covidien)				
catheter supplies				
DEV, NA (LATEX-FREE)				
10s ea	08080-2000-05	212.43		
10s ea	08080-2000-06	196.63		
PRECISION 400 URINE METER (Covidien)				
collector, urine				
DEV, NA (LATEX-FREE)				
10s ea	08080-1000-05	134.85		
10s ea	08080-1000-06	153.07		
PRECISION 400 URINE METER CATHETERIZATION TRAY (Covidien)				
catheter supplies				
DEV, NA (14FR,5CC,LATEX-FREE)				
10s ea	08080-2401-05	257.93		
10s ea	08080-2401-06	266.73		
10s ea	08080-2401-07	257.93		
10s ea	08080-2401-08	266.73		
10s ea	08080-2411-06	317.78		
10s ea	08080-2412-05	223.62		
10s ea	08080-2412-06	231.26		
10s ea	08080-2412-07	223.62		
10s ea	08080-2412-08	231.26		
(16FR,5CC,LATEX-FREE)				
10s ea	08080-2601-05	257.93		
10s ea	08080-2601-06	266.73		
10s ea	08080-2601-07	257.93		
10s ea	08080-2601-08	266.73		
10s ea	08080-2605-08	285.42		
10s ea	08080-2611-06	317.78		
10s ea	08080-2612-05	223.62		
10s ea	08080-2612-06	231.26		
10s ea	08080-2612-07	223.62		
10s ea	08080-2612-08	231.26		
(18FR,5CC,LATEX-FREE)				
10s ea	08080-2801-05	257.93		
10s ea	08080-2801-06	266.73		
10s ea	08080-2801-07	257.93		
10s ea	08080-2801-08	266.73		
10s ea	08080-2811-06	317.78		
10s ea	08080-2812-05	223.62		
10s ea	08080-2812-06	231.26		
10s ea	08080-2812-07	223.62		
10s ea	08080-2812-08	231.26		
PRECISION 400 URINE METER CATHETERIZATION TRAY WITH TEMPERATURE SENSOR (Covidien)				
catheter supplies				
DEV, NA (14FR,5CC,LATEX-FREE)				
10s ea	08080-2401-10	270.18		
(16FR,5CC,LATEX-FREE)				
10s ea	08080-2605-06	270.18		
(18FR,5CC,LATEX-FREE)				
10s ea	08080-2805-06	270.18		
PRECISION ADD-A-FOLEY CATHETER TRAY (Covidien)				
catheter supplies				
DEV, NA (LATEX-FREE)				
10s ea	08080-2000-02	114.07		
PRECISION ADD-A-FOLEY DRAINAGE BAG TRAY (Covidien)				
foley catheter				
DEV, NA (LATEX-FREE)				
10s ea	08080-2000-03	107.99		
PRECISION DRAINAGE BAG (Covidien)				
bag, urinary collection				
DEV, NA (LATEX-FREE)				
20s ea	08080-1000-02	139.38		
20s ea	08080-1000-03	141.93		
20s ea	08080-1001-02	90.89		
PRECISION SURE-DOSE (Abbott)				
insulin syringe/needle				
DEV, NA (28GX1/2",0.5 CC)				
100s ea	57599-8547-01	17.42		
(28GX1/2",1 CC)				
100s ea	57599-8546-01	17.42		
(29GX1/2",0.3 CC)				
100s ea	57599-8550-01	21.19		
(29GX1/2",0.5 CC)				
100s ea	57599-8549-01	21.19		
(29GX1/2",1 CC)				
100s ea	57599-8548-01	21.19		
(30GX3/8",0.3 CC)				
100s ea	57599-8894-01	24.01		
(30GX3/8",0.5 CC)				
100s ea	57599-8895-01	24.01		
PRECOSE (Bayer Corp.)				
acarbose				
TAB, PO, 25 mg, 100s ea	00026-2863-51	97.02		
50 mg, 100s ea UD	00026-2861-48	109.74		
100s ea	00026-2861-51	104.46		
100 mg, 100s ea	00026-2862-51	125.10		
(A-S Medication) REPACK				
TAB, PO, 50 mg, 42s ea	54569-4501-00	42.32		
(Phys Total Care) REPACK				
TAB, PO, 25 mg, 10s ea	54868-5831-00	13.61		
90s ea	54868-5831-01	107.49		
50 mg, 20s ea	54868-3823-01	19.88		
PRED FORTE (Allergan Inc)				
prednisolone acetate				
SUS, OP, 1%, 1 ml	11980-0180-01	10.32		AB
5 ml	11980-0180-05	32.10		AB
10 ml	11980-0180-10	64.18		AB
15 ml	11980-0180-15	92.69		AB
(Phys Total Care) REPACK				
SUS, OP, 1%, 5 ml	54868-0636-01	31.00		AB
15 ml	54868-0636-00	86.94		AB
(Southwood) REPACK				
SUS, OP, 1%, 5 ml	58016-0637-01	17.48		AB
(Stat Rx) REPACK				
SUS, OP, 1%, 5 ml	16590-0189-05	28.75		
PRED MILD (Allergan Inc)				
prednisolone acetate				
SUS, OP, 0.12%, 5 ml	11980-0174-05	25.72		
10 ml	11980-0174-10	37.52		
(Pharma Pac) REPACK				
SUS, OP (1X5ML)				
0.12%, 5 ml	52959-0935-05	23.15		
(Southwood) REPACK				
SUS, OP, 0.12%, 5 ml	58016-6057-01	17.25		
PRED-G (Allergan Inc)				
gentamicin sulfate/prednisolone acetate				
SUS, OP, 0.3%-1%, 2 ml	00023-0106-02	10.23		
5 ml	00023-0106-05	30.72		
(Pharma Pac) REPACK				
SUS, OP, 0.3%-1%, 5 ml	52959-0565-03	26.25		
5 ml	52959-0629-03	26.25		
(Phys Total Care) REPACK				
SUS, OP, 0.3%-1%, 5 ml	54868-0640-01	35.89		
PRED-G S.O.P. (Allergan Inc)				
gentamicin sulfate/prednisolone acetate				
OIN, OP, 0.3%-0.6%,				
3.5 gm	00023-0066-04	29.88		
(Southwood) REPACK				
OIN, OP, 0.3%-0.6%,				
3.5 gm	58016-6445-01	23.73		
SUS, OP, 0.3%-1%, 5 ml	58016-0637-10	25.94		
PREDNICARBATE				
(Dermik) *See DERMATOP*				
(Fougera)				
OIN, TP (1X15GM)				
0.1%, 15 gm	00168-0410-15	30.00		
(1X60GM)				
0.1%, 60 gm	00168-0410-60	73.79		
(Medisca)				
POW, NA (1X50GM,USP)				
50 gm	38779-2486-02	4500.00		
(Prasco Labs)				
EMO, TP, 0.1%, 15 gm	66993-0880-15	23.08		
60 gm	66993-0880-61	56.76		
PREDNICOT (Truxton)				
prednisone				
TAB, PO, 5 mg, 1000s ea	00463-6155-10	18.00		EE
10 mg, 1000s ea	00463-6140-10	35.40		EE
20 mg, 1000s ea	00463-6141-10	54.00		EE
PREDNISOL (Ocusoft)				
prednisolone sodium phosphate				
SOL, OP, 1%, 5 ml	54799-0550-10	27.44		AT
PREDNISOLONE FUL				
SYR, PO, 15 mg/5 ml,				
480 ml		99.89		
(Adamis) *See PRELONE*				
(Amend) *See PREDNISOLONE ANHYDROUS*				
(Amneal)				
SYR, PO (GRAPE)				
15 mg/5 ml, 237 ml	65162-0667-88	118.70		AA
473 ml	65162-0667-90	225.53		AA
(Axiom Pharmaceutical)				
SYR, PO, 15 mg/5 ml,				
236 ml	67870-0103-08	74.00		AA
473 ml	67870-0103-16	119.05		AA
(Consolidated Midland)				
TAB, PO, 5 mg, 100s ea	00223-1512-01	3.95		EE
1000s ea	00223-1512-02	22.50		EE
(Dexo)				
SYR, PO, 15 mg/5 ml,				
240 ml	59196-0010-24	67.39		AA
480 ml	59196-0010-48	107.83		AA
(Ethex)				
SYR, PO, 5 mg/5 ml, 120 ml	58177-0912-03	17.35		AA
(Gallipot) *See PREDNISOLONE ANHYDROUS*				
(Hi-Tech)				
SOL, PO (USP,RED CHERRY)				
15 mg/5 ml, 240 ml	50383-0042-24	74.50		
480 ml	50383-0042-48	119.20		
(Laser Pharma) *See MILLIPRED*				
(Laser Pharma) *See MILLIPRED DP*				
(Letco) *See PREDNISOLONE ANHYDROUS*				
(Medisca) *See PREDNISOLONE ANHYDROUS*				
(PCCA) *See PREDNISOLONE MICRONIZED*				
(Spectrum Pharmacy)				
POW, NA (U.S.P.,MICRONIZED)				
5 gm	49452-5980-01	102.55		
25 gm	49452-5980-02	409.50		
100 gm	49452-5980-03	1130.50		
(Teva)				
SYR, PO, 15 mg/5 ml,				
240 ml	00093-6118-87	70.90		EE
480 ml	00093-6118-16	113.50		EE
(Truxton) *See COTOLONE*				
(A-S Medication) REPACK				
SOL, PO (4X60 ML,RED CHERRY)				
15 mg/5 ml,				
60 ml 4s	54569-4827-01	74.50		
(2X120 ML,RED CHERRY)				
15 mg/5 ml,				
120 ml 2s	54569-4827-00	74.50		
(Bryant Ranch) REPACK				
SYR, PO, 15 mg/5 ml,				
60 ml	63629-1862-01	20.86		
(Core) REPACK				
SYR, PO, 15 mg/5 ml,				
240 ml	33358-0291-08	77.49		
(DHS, Inc.) REPACK				
SYR, PO, 15 mg/5 ml, 8 ml	55887-0373-08	74.96		EE
(Palmetto) REPACK				
SYR, PO, 15 mg/5 ml,				
120 ml	23490-6144-03	74.99		
120 ml	23490-6145-03	74.99		
180 ml	23490-6144-02	111.60		
180 ml	23490-6145-02	111.60		
240 ml	23490-6144-01	148.80		
240 ml	23490-6145-01	148.80		
(Pharma Pac) REPACK				
SYR, PO (CHERRY)				
15 mg/5 ml, 480 ml	52959-0622-60	19.25		AA
(Phys Total Care) REPACK				
SYR, PO, 5 mg/5 ml,				
120 ml	54868-4748-00	52.38		AA

PROD/MFR	NDC	AWP	DP	OBC
15 mg/5 ml, 240 ml	**54868-4749-00**	37.98		
(CHERRY)				
15 mg/5 ml, 480 ml	**54868-4749-01**	54.48		**AA**
(Physician Partner)				
REPACK				
SYR, PO, 15 mg/5 ml,				
240 ml	**21695-0365-08**	150.00		
480 ml	**21695-0365-16**	240.00		
(Quality Care Prod)				
REPACK				
SYR, PO, 5 mg/5 ml,				
120 ml	**49999-0929-01**	24.38		
15 mg/5 ml, 240 ml	**49999-0335-08**	89.40		
(CHERRY)				
15 mg/5 ml, 240 ml	**49999-0335-24**	90.00		**AA**
(Southwood)				
REPACK				
prednisolone sodium phosphate				
SOL, OP, 0.125%, 5 ml	**58016-6031-01**	11.21		**EE**
1%, 5 ml	**58016-6029-01**	12.60		**EE**
PREDNISOLONE (Southwood)				
SYR, PO, 15 mg/5 ml,				
240 ml	**58016-4843-01**	5.71		
(Stat Rx)				
REPACK				
SOL, PO (1X240ML,RED CHERRY)				
15 mg/5 ml, 240 ml	**16590-0291-37**	88.86		
(Vibranta)				
REPACK				
TAB, PO, 5 mg, 90s ea	**57866-4327-01**	13.06		
PREDNISOLONE ACETATE				
FUL				
SUS, OP, 1%, 10 ml		16.95		
(Alcon Ophthalmic) *See OMNIPRED*				
(Allergan Inc) *See PRED FORTE*				
(Allergan Inc) *See PRED MILD*				
(Consolidated Midland)				
SUS, IJ (VIAL)				
25 mg/ml, 10 ml	**00223-8345-10**	5.50		
30 ml	**00223-8345-30**	6.50		
50 mg/ml, 10 ml	**00223-5346-10**	7.50		
10 ml	**00223-8346-10**	6.50		
30 ml	**00223-8341-30**	9.50		
30 ml	**00223-8346-30**	11.50		
(Falcon Ophthalmics)				
SUS, OP, 1%, 5 ml	**61314-0637-05**	12.60		**AB**
10 ml	**61314-0637-10**	23.10		**AB**
15 ml	**61314-0637-15**	34.10		**AB**
(Gallipot)				
POW, NA (U.S.P.)				
5 gm	**51552-0027-02**	18.90		
25 gm	**51552-0027-04**	76.30		
100 gm	**51552-0027-05**	268.80		
(Medisca)				
POW, NA (U.S.P.,MICRONIZED)				
10 gm	**38779-0152-01**	112.50		
25 gm	**38779-0152-04**	217.50		
100 gm	**38779-0152-05**	747.00		
500 gm	**38779-0152-08**	2655.00		
1000 gm	**38779-0152-09**	4155.00		
(Pacific Pharma)				
SUS, OP, 1%, 5 ml	**60758-0119-05**	12.60		**AB**
10 ml	**60758-0119-10**	23.10		**AB**
15 ml	**60758-0119-15**	34.06		**AB**
(Spectrum Pharmacy)				
POW, NA (U.S.P.,MICRONIZED)				
5 gm	**49452-5990-01**	99.75		
25 gm	**49452-5990-02**	402.50		
100 gm	**49452-5990-03**	1106.00		
(Truxton) *See COTOLONE*				
(Altura)				
REPACK				
SUS, OP, 1%, 5 ml	**63874-0875-05**	14.70		
(Pharma Pac)				
REPACK				
SUS, OP, 1%, 5 ml	**52959-0265-05**	22.60		**AB**
10 ml	**52959-0265-10**	33.10		**AB**
15 ml	**52959-0265-15**	44.06		**AB**
(Phys Total Care)				
REPACK				
SUS, OP (1X5ML)				
1%, 5 ml	**54868-4293-02**	40.82		**AB**
10 ml	**54868-4293-01**	64.02		**AB**
15 ml	**54868-4293-00**	57.48		**AB**
(Physician Partner)				
REPACK				
SUS, OP (1X5ML)				
1%, 5 ml	**21695-0409-05**	25.20		**AB**
(Southwood)				
REPACK				
SUS, OP, 1%, 5 ml	**58016-6557-01**	13.50		**AB**
15 ml	**58016-4633-01**	34.10		
PREDNISOLONE ACETATE MICRONIZED (Hawkins)				
prednisolone acetate, micronized				
POW, NA (U.S.P.)				
5 gm	**63370-0195-15**	54.00		
25 gm	**63370-0195-25**	196.00		
100 gm	**63370-0195-35**	768.00		
1000 gm	**63370-0195-50**	4800.00		
5000 gm	**63370-0195-55**	20000.00		
(Letco)				
POW, NA, 5 gm	**62991-1692-01**	39.00		
25 gm	**62991-1692-02**	144.00		
100 gm	**62991-1692-03**	495.00		
(PCCA)				
POW, NA (U.S.P.)				
1 gm	**51927-1325-00**	12.60		
PREDNISOLONE ACETATE, MICRONIZED				
(Hawkins) *See PREDNISOLONE ACETATE MICRONIZED*				
(Letco) *See PREDNISOLONE ACETATE MICRONIZED*				
(PCCA) *See PREDNISOLONE ACETATE MICRONIZED*				
PREDNISOLONE ACETATE/SULFACETAMIDE SODIUM				
(Allergan Inc) *See BLEPHAMIDE*				
(Allergan Inc) *See BLEPHAMIDE S.O.P.*				
PREDNISOLONE ANHYDROUS (Amend)				
prednisolone				
POW, NA (U.S.P.)				
5 gm	**17317-0477-08**	15.05		
25 gm	**17317-0447-02**	58.80		
100 gm	**17317-0447-03**	210.00		
(Gallipot)				
POW, NA (U.S.P.)				
5 gm	**51552-0026-02**	21.00		
25 gm	**51552-0026-04**	88.20		
100 gm	**51552-0026-05**	308.00		
(Letco)				
POW, NA (U.S.P.)				
5 gm	**62991-1257-01**	45.00		
(U.S.P., MICRO)				
25 gm	**62991-1257-02**	156.00		
(Medisca)				
POW, NA (U.S.P.,MICRONIZED)				
5 gm	**38779-0150-03**	49.50		
25 gm	**38779-0150-04**	202.50		
100 gm	**38779-0150-05**	795.00		
(ANHYDROUS,MICRONIZED)				
500 gm	**38779-0150-08**	2754.00		
(U.S.P.,MICRONIZED)				
1000 gm	**38779-0150-09**	6594.00		
PREDNISOLONE MICRONIZED (PCCA)				
prednisolone				
POW, NA (ANHYDROUS)				
1 gm	**51927-1148-00**	13.20		
PREDNISOLONE SOD PHOS/ SULFACETAMIDE SODIUM (Altura)				
REPACK				
prednisolone sodium phosphate/sulfacetamide sodium				
SOL, OP, 0.25%-10%, 5 ml	**63874-0197-05**	21.41		
10 ml	**63874-0197-10**	28.79		
PREDNISOLONE SOD PHOS/SULFACET SOD (Bausch & Lomb Inc.)				
prednisolone sodium phosphate/sulfacetamide sodium				
SOL, OP, 0.25%-10%, 5 ml	**24208-0317-05**	18.75		**AT**
10 ml	**24208-0317-10**	25.00		**AT**
(Falcon Ophthalmics)				
SOL, OP, 0.25%-10%, 5 ml	**61314-0297-05**	18.00		**AT**
10 ml	**61314-0297-10**	24.00		**AT**
(Pharma Pac)				
REPACK				
SOL, OP, 0.25%-10%, 5 ml	**52959-0567-03**	16.45		**EE**
(Quality Care Prod)				
REPACK				
SOL, OP, 0.25%-10%, 5 ml	**49999-0524-05**	24.23		**AT**
(Southwood)				
REPACK				
SOL, OP, 0.25%-10%, 5 ml	**58016-6571-01**	18.50		**EE**
10 ml	**58016-5566-01**	25.25		**AT**
PREDNISOLONE SOD. PHOS. (Stat Rx)				
REPACK				
prednisolone sodium phosphate				
SOL, OP, 1%, 10 ml	**16590-0190-10**	37.00		
15 ml	**16590-0190-15**	55.50		
PREDNISOLONE SODIUM PHOSPHATE				
FUL				
SOL, PO, 15 mg/5 ml,				
237 ml		49.51		
(Bausch & Lomb Inc.)				
SOL, OP, 1%, 10 ml	**24208-0715-10**	46.12		**AT**
(Biomarin) *See ORAPRED*				
(Ethex)				
SOL, PO (DYE-FREE,GRAPE)				
15 mg/5 ml, 237 ml	**58177-0932-05**	114.02		**AA**
(Gallipot)				
POW, NA (USP,1X5GM)				
5 gm	**51552-0735-02**	69.30	49.50	
(USP,1X100GM)				
100 gm	**51552-0735-05**	1043.00	745.00	
(Hawkins)				
POW, NA (U.S.P.)				
5 gm	**63370-0196-15**	184.00		
10 gm	**63370-0196-20**	344.00		
25 gm	**63370-0196-25**	832.00		
100 gm	**63370-0196-35**	2520.00		
(Hawthorn Pharm) *See VERIPRED 20*				
(Hi-Tech)				
SOL, PO (AF,SF,DYE-FREE)				
5 mg/5 ml, 120 ml	**50383-0040-04**	24.75		
(Laser Pharma) *See MILLIPRED*				
(Letco) *See PREGNENOLONE*				
(Medisca)				
POW, NA (U.S.P.)				
5 gm	**38779-0153-03**	177.00		
25 gm	**38779-0153-04**	696.00		
100 gm	**38779-0153-05**	2250.00		
(Morton Grove)				
SOL, PO (AF,SF,DYE-FREE)				
5 mg/5 ml, 118 ml	**60432-0089-04**	25.38		
(DYE-FREE,GRAPE)				
15 mg/5 ml, 237 ml	**60432-0212-08**	74.50		**AA**
(Novartis Pharm) *See INFLAMASE FORTE*				
(Ocusoft) *See PREDNISOL*				
(PCCA)				
POW, NA (U.S.P.)				
1 gm	**51927-1550-00**	60.00		
(Pharm Assoc Inc)				
SOL, PO (AF,DYE-FREE,GRAPE)				
15 mg/5 ml, 237 ml	**00121-0759-08**	121.95		
(Shionogi) *See ORAPRED*				
(Shionogi) *See ORAPRED ODT*				
(Spectrum Pharmacy)				
POW, NA (U.S.P.)				
5 gm	**49452-5995-01**	262.15		
25 gm	**49452-5995-02**	1099.00		
100 gm	**49452-5995-03**	3321.50		
(UCB) *See PEDIAPRED*				
(Upstate Pharma)				
SOL, PO (DYE-FREE,RASPBERRY)				
6.7 mg/5 ml,				
120 ml	**65580-0251-01**	25.38		
(A-S Medication)				
REPACK				
SOL, PO (DYE-FREE,GRAPE)				
15 mg/5 ml, 240 ml	**54569-5749-00**	108.65		**AA**
(Dispensing Solutions)				
REPACK				
SOL, PO (1X120ML,DYE-FREE)				
6.7 mg/5 ml,				
120 ml	**55045-3128-02**	25.00		
(Keltman Pharma., Inc.)				
REPACK				
SOL, OP (DROPS)				
1%, 5 ml	**68387-0640-01**	25.12		
(Phys Total Care)				
REPACK				
SOL, PO (DYE-FREE,GRAPE)				
15 mg/5 ml, 237 ml	**54868-5242-00**	179.46		**AA**

PROD/MFR	NDC	AWP	DP	OBC
(Physician Partner)				
REPACK				
SOL, PO (1X240ML,AF,DYE-FREE)				
15 mg/5 ml, 240 ml	21695-0405-08	243.90		
PREDNISOLONE SODIUM PHOSPHATE/SULFACETAMIDE SODIUM				
(Bausch & Lomb Inc.) *See PREDNISOLONE SOD PHOS/SULFACET SOD*				
(Falcon Ophthalmics) *See PREDNISOLONE SOD PHOS/SULFACET SOD*				
PREDNISONE				
FUL				
TAB, PO, 5 mg, 100s ea		2.03		
10 mg, 100s ea		6.15		
20 mg, 100s ea		8.04		
(4u)				
TAB, PO, 20 mg, 14s ea	42549-0647-14	16.88		AB
(Breckenridge Pharm)				
TAB, PO (U.S.P.)				
1 mg, 100s ea	51991-0458-01	19.42		AB
1000s ea	51991-0458-10	190.41		AB
(Cadista)				
TAB, PO, 1 mg, 100s ea	59746-0171-06	19.43		AB
1000s ea	59746-0171-10	190.41		AB
5 mg, 100s ea	59746-0007-06	3.40		AB
(USP)				
5 mg, 100s ea	59746-0172-06	8.25		
1000s ea	59746-0007-10	25.50		AB
(USP)				
5 mg, 1000s ea	59746-0172-10	37.75		
10 mg, 100s ea	59746-0008-06	4.27		AB
(USP)				
10 mg, 100s ea	59746-0173-06	8.95		
500s ea	59746-0173-09	43.63		
1000s ea	59746-0008-10	29.75		AB
(USP)				
10 mg, 1000s ea	59746-0173-10	85.00		
20 mg, 100s ea	59746-0175-06	18.00		
500s ea	59746-0175-09	76.00		
1000s ea	59746-0175-10	140.00		
(Consolidated Midland)				
TAB, PO, 5 mg, 100s ea	00223-1515-01	3.50		EE
1000s ea	00223-1515-02	22.50		EE
10 mg, 100s ea	00223-1516-01	6.00		EE
1000s ea	00223-1516-02	52.50		EE
20 mg, 100s ea	00223-1517-01	11.50		EE
1000s ea	00223-1517-02	99.50		EE
(Gallipot)				
POW, NA, 1 gm	51552-0028-01	13.23		
(U.S.P.)				
5 gm	51552-0028-02	20.51		
25 gm	51552-0028-04	94.08		
100 gm	51552-0028-05	301.00		
(Letco)				
POW, NA (U.S.P.,MICRONIZED)				
5 gm	62991-1206-01	43.50		
25 gm	62991-1206-02	150.00		
(Medisca)				
POW, NA (U.S.P.,MICRONIZED)				
5 gm	38779-0154-03	58.50		
25 gm	38779-0154-04	255.00		
100 gm	38779-0154-05	897.00		
(Medisca) *See PREDNISONE ANHYDROUS*				
(Mutual)				
TAB, PO, 5 mg, 100s ea	53489-0138-01	4.75		AB
1000s ea	53489-0138-10	28.50		AB
10 mg, 100s ea	53489-0139-01	7.93		AB
500s ea	53489-0139-05	26.30		AB
1000s ea	53489-0139-10	51.46		AB
20 mg, 100s ea	53489-0140-01	11.79		AB
500s ea	53489-0140-05	44.31		AB
1000s ea	53489-0140-10	86.54		AB
(Perrigo)				
TAB, PO (USP,BLISTER PACK)				
5 mg, 21s ea UD	45802-0733-21	5.40		AB
48s ea UD	45802-0733-67	11.71		AB
(USP)				
5 mg, 100s ea	10768-7733-03	8.40		
1000s ea	10768-7733-04	42.20		
(USP,BLISTER PACK)				
10 mg, 21s ea UD	45802-0303-21	9.45		AB
48s ea UD	45802-0303-67	13.28		AB
(USP)				
10 mg, 100s ea	10768-7283-03	9.90		
1000s ea	10768-7283-04	88.90		
20 mg, 100s ea	10768-7085-01	19.20		
(Qualitest)				
TAB, PO, 1 mg, 100s ea	00603-5335-21	19.42		AB
1000s ea	00603-5335-32	190.41		AB
2.5 mg, 100s ea	00603-5336-21	6.52		AB
(DOSE PACK)				
5 mg, 21s ea	00603-5337-15	5.40		AB
48s ea	00603-5337-31	11.70		AB
100s ea	00603-5337-21	8.46	1.35	AB
1000s ea	00603-5337-32	42.25	7.95	AB
(DOSE PACK)				
10 mg, 21s ea	00603-5338-15	9.45		AB
48s ea	00603-5338-31	13.28		AB
100s ea	00603-5338-21	9.96		AB
500s ea	00603-5338-28	47.31		AB
1000s ea	00603-5338-32	89.00		AB
20 mg, 100s ea	00603-5339-21	19.22		AB
500s ea	00603-5339-28	91.30		AB
1000s ea	00603-5339-32	173.47		AB
(Roxane) *See PREDNISONE INTENSOL*				
(Roxane)				
SOL, PO (PEPPERMINT-VANILLA)				
5 mg/5 ml,				
5 ml 40s UD	00054-8722-16	40.43		
120 ml	00054-3722-50	20.21		
500 ml	00054-3722-63	82.53		
TAB, PO, 1 mg, 100s ea	00054-4741-25	19.43		AB
(10X10)				
1 mg, 100s ea UD	00054-8739-25	23.32		AB
1000s ea	00054-4741-31	190.41		AB
2.5 mg, 100s ea	00054-4742-25	6.53		AB
(10X10)				
2.5 mg, 100s ea UD	00054-8740-25	10.66		AB
5 mg, 100s ea	00054-4728-25	4.23		AB
(10X10)				
5 mg, 100s ea UD	00054-8724-25	11.98		AB
1000s ea	00054-4728-31	25.99		AB
10 mg, 100s ea	00054-0017-25	6.09		AB
(10X10)				
10 mg, 100s ea UD	00054-0017-20	13.31		AB
500s ea	00054-0017-29	28.09		AB
20 mg, 100s ea	00054-0018-25	11.77		AB
(10X10)				
20 mg, 100s ea UD	00054-0018-20	17.41		AB
500s ea	00054-0018-29	57.72		AB
50 mg, 100s ea	00054-0019-25	30.76		AB
(10X10)				
50 mg, 100s ea UD	00054-0019-20	34.19		AB
(Spectrum Pharmacy)				
POW, NA (U.S.P.,ANH,MICRONIZED)				
5 gm	49452-6000-01	105.70		
25 gm	49452-6000-02	423.50		
100 gm	49452-6000-03	1263.50		
(Truxton) *See PREDNICOT*				
(UDL)				
TAB, PO (ROBOT READY 25X1)				
5 mg, 25s ea UD	51079-0032-19	4.26		AB
10 mg, 25s ea UD	51079-0033-19	4.96		AB
20 mg, 25s ea UD	51079-0022-19	6.40		AB
(Watson Labs)				
TAB, PO, 5 mg, 100s ea	00591-5052-01	8.22		AB
1000s ea	00591-5052-10	37.76		AB
10 mg, 100s ea	00591-5442-01	8.87		AB
500s ea	00591-5442-05	45.35		AB
1000s ea	00591-5442-10	84.00		AB
20 mg, 100s ea	00591-5443-01	17.94		AB
500s ea	00591-5443-05	75.95		AB
1000s ea	00591-5443-10	137.66		AB
(West-Ward)				
TAB, PO, 2.5 mg, 100s ea	00143-1425-01	6.45		AB
5 mg, 100s ea	00143-1475-01	6.50		AB
1000s ea	00143-1475-10	38.25		AB
10 mg, 100s ea	00143-1473-01	8.40		AB
1000s ea	00143-1473-10	63.00		AB
20 mg, 100s ea	00143-1477-01	14.25		AB
500s ea	00143-1477-05	41.80		AB
1000s ea	00143-1477-10	101.25		AB
(A-S Medication)				
REPACK				
TAB, PO, 5 mg, 21s ea	54569-0330-00	1.73		EE
21s ea	54569-3413-00	1.29		EE
30s ea	54569-0330-04	2.47		EE
(PACK)				
5 mg, 48s ea	54569-5911-00	11.71		EE
50s ea	54569-0330-01	4.11		EE
60s ea	54569-0330-07	4.93		EE
100s ea	54569-0330-03	8.22		EE
10 mg, 10s ea	54569-0331-00	0.86		EE
15s ea	54569-0331-01	1.29		EE
20s ea	54569-3302-01	1.72		EE
21s ea	54569-0331-02	1.80		EE
21s ea	54569-5840-00	9.45		EE
30s ea	54569-0331-05	2.58		EE
40s ea	54569-0331-08	3.44		EE
48s ea	54569-5841-00	13.28		EE
50s ea	54569-0331-04	4.30		EE
60s ea	54569-3302-00	5.15		EE
100s ea	54569-0331-07	8.59		EE
20 mg, 6s ea	54569-3043-02	0.93		AB
10s ea	54569-0332-01	1.55		AB
12s ea	54569-3043-01	1.86		AB
14s ea	54569-3043-05	2.17		AB
18s ea	54569-0332-09	2.79		AB
20s ea	54569-3043-00	3.10		AB
21s ea	54569-0332-02	3.26		AB
25s ea	54569-3043-06	3.88		AB
30s ea	54569-0332-03	4.65		AB
100s ea	54569-0332-05	15.50		AB
50 mg, 8s ea	54569-0333-00	2.46		EE
(Aidarex)				
REPACK				
TAB, PO, 5 mg, 7s ea	33261-0351-07	3.39		AB
14s ea	33261-0351-14	6.79		AB
20s ea	33261-0351-20	9.70		AB
21s ea	33261-0351-21	10.19		AB
28s ea	33261-0351-28	13.53		AB
30s ea	33261-0351-30	14.55		AB
40s ea	33261-0351-40	19.20		AB
60s ea	33261-0351-60	29.10		AB
10 mg, 12s ea	33261-0352-12	6.36		AB
14s ea	33261-0352-14	7.42		AB
20s ea	33261-0352-20	10.60		AB
21s ea	33261-0352-21	11.13		AB
28s ea	33261-0352-28	14.84		AB
30s ea	33261-0352-30	15.75		AB
60s ea	33261-0352-60	32.40		AB
90s ea	33261-0352-90	48.60		AB
20 mg, 12s ea	33261-0129-12	14.35		AB
30s ea	33261-0129-30	35.87		AB
60s ea	33261-0129-60	71.68		AB
90s ea	33261-0129-90	107.61		AB
(Altura)				
REPACK				
TAB, PO, 5 mg, 10s ea	63874-0373-10	1.97		
15s ea	63874-0373-15	2.95		
20s ea	63874-0373-20	3.33		
21s ea	63874-0373-21	3.50		
30s ea	63874-0373-30	5.92		
33s ea	63874-0373-33	6.51		
36s ea	63874-0373-36	7.10		
40s ea	63874-0373-40	7.89		
50s ea	63874-0373-50	9.87		
60s ea	63874-0373-60	11.83		
100s ea	63874-0373-01	19.73		
1000s ea	63874-0373-02	197.33		
10 mg, 10s ea	63874-0327-10	3.60		AB
12s ea	63874-0327-12	4.31		AB
14s ea	63874-0327-14	5.02		AB
15s ea	63874-0327-15	5.38		AB
18s ea	63874-0327-18	6.46		AB
19s ea	63874-0327-19	6.82		AB
20s ea	63874-0327-20	7.18		AB
21s ea	63874-0327-21	7.90		AB
24s ea	63874-0327-24	3.12		AB
25s ea	63874-0327-25	8.98		AB
28s ea	63874-0327-28	10.05		AB
30s ea	63874-0327-30	10.77		AB
32s ea	63874-0327-32	11.49		AB
40s ea	63874-0327-40	14.37		AB
42s ea	63874-0327-42	15.08		AB
50s ea	63874-0327-50	17.95		AB
60s ea	63874-0327-60	21.54		AB
100s ea	63874-0327-01	36.00		AB
1000s ea	63874-0327-02	359.17		AB
20 mg, 10s ea	63874-0392-10	2.55		
14s ea	63874-0392-14	3.57		
15s ea	63874-0392-15	3.82		
20s ea	63874-0392-20	5.10		
21s ea	63874-0392-21	5.35		
24s ea	63874-0392-24	6.12		
28s ea	63874-0392-28	7.14		
30s ea	63874-0392-30	7.65		
40s ea	63874-0392-40	10.20		
60s ea	63874-0392-06	15.30		
100s ea	63874-0392-01	25.50		
1000s ea	63874-0392-02	255.00		
(Bryant Ranch)				
REPACK				
TAB, PO, 5 mg, 15s ea	63629-1605-05	5.07		
21s ea	63629-1605-04	7.10		
30s ea	63629-1605-01	10.14		
36s ea	63629-1605-03	12.17		
78s ea	63629-1605-02	26.36		

PROD/MFR	NDC	AWP	DP	OBC
10 mg, 21s ea	**63629-1579-01**	9.85		
30s ea	**63629-1579-03**	10.65		
40s ea	**63629-1579-02**	13.53		
20 mg, 15s ea	**63629-1587-04**	7.99		
20s ea	**63629-1587-01**	11.84		
30s ea	**63629-1587-02**	15.25		
40s ea	**63629-1587-03**	19.67		
(Core)				
REPACK				
TAB, PO, 5 mg, 12s ea	**33358-0292-12**	3.21		
15s ea	**33358-0292-15**	5.20		
21s ea	**33358-0292-21**	7.28		
30s ea	**33358-0292-30**	10.39		
78s ea	**33358-0292-78**	27.02		
10 mg, 20s ea	**33358-0293-20**	10.08		
30s ea	**33358-0293-30**	10.92		
40s ea	**33358-0293-40**	13.87		
20 mg, 15s ea	**33358-0294-15**	8.19		
20s ea	**33358-0294-20**	12.14		
30s ea	**33358-0294-30**	15.63		
40s ea	**33358-0294-40**	20.16		
60s ea	**33358-0294-60**	28.03		
(DHS, Inc.)				
REPACK				
TAB, PO, 5 mg, 15s ea	**55887-0770-15**	5.50		
20s ea	**55887-0770-20**	6.46		
30s ea	**55887-0770-30**	9.69		
39s ea	**55887-0770-39**	12.59		
50s ea	**55887-0770-50**	16.14		
60s ea	**55887-0770-60**	19.37		
100s ea	**55887-0770-01**	30.00		
10 mg, 15s ea	**55887-0643-15**	5.99		AB
21s ea	**55887-0643-21**	6.99		AB
(DOSE PACK)				
10 mg, 21s ea	**55887-0696-21**	15.00		AB
30s ea	**55887-0643-30**	9.75		AB
40s ea	**55887-0643-40**	13.00		AB
42s ea	**55887-0643-42**	13.65		
50s ea	**55887-0643-50**	14.50		
60s ea	**55887-0643-60**	17.40		AB
90s ea	**55887-0643-90**	26.10		AB
20 mg, 15s ea	**55887-0796-15**	8.00		AB
18s ea	**55887-0796-18**	8.50		
20s ea	**55887-0796-20**	8.50		AB
21s ea	**55887-0796-21**	8.91		AB
30s ea	**55887-0796-30**	11.50		AB
90s ea	**55887-0796-90**	28.50		
(Dispensing Solutions)				
REPACK				
TAB, PO, 5 mg, 15s ea	**55045-1480-05**	4.20		
20s ea	**55045-1480-06**	5.60		
21s ea	**55045-1480-07**	5.85		AB
21s ea	**66336-0515-21**	8.02		AB
(DOSEPACK)				
5 mg, 21s ea UD	**55045-1260-09**	9.40		AB
30s ea	**55045-1480-08**	8.40		AB
30s ea	**66336-0515-30**	11.46		AB
40s ea	**55045-1480-09**	11.20		AB
40s ea	**66336-0515-40**	15.28		AB
48s ea	**68258-3013-01**	14.04		AB
(DOSEPACK)				
5 mg, 48s ea	**55045-1260-00**	11.50		
60s ea	**55045-1480-02**	16.80		
100s ea	**55045-1480-01**	28.00		AB
10 mg, 10s ea	**66336-0058-10**	5.42		AB
12s ea	**66336-0058-12**	6.50		EE
15s ea	**55045-3281-03**	4.50		AB
18s ea	**55045-3281-04**	5.40		AB
20s ea	**55045-1533-03**	6.00		AB
20s ea	**66336-0058-20**	8.54		AB
21s ea	**55045-1533-07**	6.25		AB
21s ea	**66336-0058-21**	8.80		AB
(DOSEPACK)				
10 mg, 21s ea	**55045-2963-01**	11.50		
30s ea	**55045-1533-08**	9.00		AB
30s ea	**66336-0058-30**	12.99		EE
40s ea	**55045-1533-09**	12.00		AB
40s ea	**66336-0058-40**	17.32		AB
42s ea	**55045-1533-06**	12.60		AB
(DOSEPACK)				
10 mg, 48s ea	**55045-2963-02**	14.99		
60s ea	**66336-0058-60**	25.98		AB
100s ea	**55045-1533-01**	30.00		AB
20 mg, 10s ea	**66336-0094-10**	5.92		
12s ea	**55045-1444-04**	6.00		AB
18s ea	**55045-1444-03**	9.00		AB
18s ea	**66336-0094-18**	10.65		
20s ea	**66336-0094-20**	11.84		
21s ea	**55045-1444-07**	10.50		AB
21s ea	**66336-0094-21**	12.43		AB
30s ea	**55045-1444-08**	15.00		AB
30s ea	**66336-0094-30**	17.76		
35s ea	**55045-1444-01**	17.50		
42s ea	**55045-1444-02**	21.00		AB
(HomeMed)				
REPACK				
TAB, PO, 5 mg, 12s ea	**51655-0086-27**	4.06		EE
30s ea	**51655-0086-24**	8.99		EE
40s ea	**51655-0086-51**	15.28		EE
10 mg, 21s ea	**51655-0087-28**	7.99		
30s ea	**51655-0087-24**	9.99		
42s ea	**51655-0087-49**	14.99		
20 mg, 8s ea	**51655-0020-80**	3.99		EE
10s ea	**51655-0020-53**	4.99		EE
20s ea	**51655-0020-52**	9.99		EE
30s ea	**51655-0020-24**	14.99		EE
(IPI)				
REPACK				
TAB, PO, 10 mg, 21s ea	**18837-0267-21**	11.65		
30s ea	**18837-0267-30**	12.52		
48s ea	**18837-0267-48**	23.78		
(Keltman Pharma., Inc.)				
REPACK				
TAB, PO, 10 mg, 15s ea	**68387-0241-15**	6.15		AB
20 mg, 10s ea	**68387-0240-10**	6.45		AB
25s ea	**68387-0240-25**	7.88		AB
(McKesson Packaging)				
REPACK				
TAB, PO (USP)				
5 mg, 100s ea UD	**63739-0207-10**	36.21		AB
10 mg, 100s ea UD	**63739-0208-10**	42.80		AB
20 mg, 100s ea UD	**63739-0209-10**	62.55		
(Nucare Pharm)				
REPACK				
TAB, PO, 5 mg, 20s ea	**66267-0173-20**	10.46		EE
(DOSEPACK)				
5 mg, 21s ea	**66267-0948-21**	10.99		EE
30s ea	**66267-0173-30**	15.70		EE
40s ea	**66267-0173-40**	20.73		EE
42s ea	**66267-0173-42**	21.77		EE
60s ea	**66267-0173-60**	31.10		EE
10 mg, 15s ea	**66267-0171-15**	9.16		EE
20s ea	**66267-0171-20**	12.20		EE
21s ea	**66267-0171-21**	12.82		AB
30s ea	**66267-0171-30**	17.05		AB
40s ea	**66267-0171-40**	21.80		EE
42s ea	**66267-0171-42**	22.89		EE
48s ea	**66267-0171-48**	26.16		AB
20 mg, 10s ea	**66267-0172-10**	7.59		EE
15s ea	**66267-0172-15**	10.99		EE
20s ea	**66267-0172-20**	13.58		EE
30s ea	**66267-0172-30**	20.38		EE
(Palmetto)				
REPACK				
SOL, PO (1X120ML)				
5 mg/5 ml, 120 ml	**23490-7854-00**	55.57		
TAB, PO, 5 mg, 10s ea	**23490-6159-01**	4.67		
20s ea	**23490-6159-02**	9.33		
21s ea	**23490-6159-03**	9.80		
28s ea	**23490-6159-05**	13.07		
30s ea	**23490-6159-06**	14.00		
40s ea	**23490-6159-04**	18.67		
10 mg, 10s ea	**23490-6157-01**	5.15		
20s ea	**23490-6157-02**	10.29		
PREDNISONE (Palmetto)				
REPACK				
TAB, PO, 10 mg, 21s ea	**23490-1113-02**	10.60		
21s ea	**23490-6157-05**	10.81		
30s ea	**23490-1113-03**	9.99		
30s ea	**23490-6157-06**	15.44		
37s ea	**23490-6157-04**	19.04		
40s ea	**23490-6157-03**	20.59		
60s ea	**23490-6157-07**	30.88		
100s ea	**23490-6157-08**	51.47		
20 mg, 6s ea	**23490-6158-00**	6.96		
10s ea	**23490-6158-01**	5.92		
15s ea	**23490-6158-08**	8.88		
18s ea	**23490-6158-02**	10.66		
20s ea	**23490-6158-03**	11.84		
21s ea	**23490-6158-05**	12.43		
25s ea	**23490-6158-07**	14.80		
30s ea	**23490-6158-04**	17.76		
90s ea	**23490-6158-09**	53.28		
(PD-Rx Pharm)				
REPACK				
TAB, PO (U.S.P.,REDI-SCRIPT)				
5 mg, 20s ea	**58864-0362-20**	13.33		AB
30s ea	**55289-0373-30**	14.00		AB
36s ea	**55289-0373-36**	15.20		AB
42s ea	**55289-0373-42**	16.40		AB
46s ea	**55289-0373-46**	16.53		AB
55s ea	**55289-0373-55**	17.83		AB
(U.S.P.,REDI-SCRIPT)				
5 mg, 56s ea	**58864-0362-56**	17.97		AB
60s ea	**55289-0373-60**	18.00		AB
72s ea	**55289-0373-72**	20.40		AB
100s ea	**55289-0373-01**	23.30		AB
(USP)				
10 mg, 10s ea	**43063-0109-10**	9.00		AB
15s ea	**58864-0423-15**	12.50		AB
20s ea	**55289-0438-20**	13.33		AB
20s ea	**58864-0423-20**	13.33		AB
21s ea	**55289-0438-21**	13.50		AB
30s ea	**55289-0438-30**	15.00		AB
(REDI-SCRIPT)				
10 mg, 30s ea	**58864-0423-30**	15.00		AB
36s ea	**55289-0438-36**	16.53		AB
38s ea	**55289-0438-38**	16.60		AB
40s ea	**55289-0438-40**	16.68		AB
(REDI-SCRIPT)				
10 mg, 40s ea	**58864-0423-40**	16.68		AB
(USP)				
10 mg, 42s ea	**55289-0438-42**	17.07		AB
50s ea	**55289-0438-50**	18.17		AB
60s ea	**55289-0438-60**	19.83		AB
(USP)				
20 mg, 5s ea	**55289-0352-05**	11.37		AB
6s ea	**43063-0097-06**	11.67		AB
7s ea	**55289-0352-07**	11.97		AB
9s ea	**55289-0352-09**	12.53		AB
10s ea	**55289-0352-10**	12.57		AB
(USP)				
20 mg, 12s ea	**55289-0352-12**	14.07		AB
14s ea	**55289-0352-14**	14.93		AB
(REDI-SCRIPT)				
20 mg, 14s ea	**58864-0424-14**	14.93		AB
15s ea	**55289-0352-15**	14.97		AB
20s ea	**55289-0352-20**	16.83		AB
(REDI-SCRIPT)				
20 mg, 20s ea	**58864-0424-20**	16.83		AB
21s ea	**55289-0352-21**	17.40		AB
30s ea	**55289-0352-30**	17.70		AB
30s ea	**58864-0424-30**	17.70		AB
(USP)				
50 mg, 5s ea	**55289-0330-05**	15.75		AB
7s ea	**55289-0330-07**	16.83		AB
10s ea	**55289-0330-10**	18.45		AB
(Pharma Pac)				
REPACK				
TAB, PO, 5 mg, 10s ea	**52959-0220-10**	3.38		EE
20s ea	**52959-0220-20**	5.73		EE
21s ea	**52959-0220-21**	5.95		EE
30s ea	**52959-0220-30**	8.06		EE
36s ea	**52959-0220-36**	9.41		EE
40s ea	**52959-0220-40**	10.35		EE
60s ea	**52959-0220-60**	12.59		EE
75s ea	**52959-0220-75**	13.11		EE
100s ea	**52959-0220-00**	15.52		EE
10 mg, 5s ea	**52959-0126-05**	3.75		EE
7s ea	**52959-0126-07**	4.75		EE
10s ea	**52959-0126-10**	4.20		EE
12s ea	**52959-0126-12**	5.43		EE
15s ea	**52959-0126-15**	6.54		EE
18s ea	**52959-0126-18**	6.78		EE
20s ea	**52959-0126-20**	7.13		EE
21s ea	**52959-0126-21**	7.49		EE
25s ea	**52959-0126-25**	8.57		EE
30s ea	**52959-0126-30**	9.50		EE
37s ea	**52959-0126-37**	11.47		EE
40s ea	**52959-0126-40**	12.47		EE
42s ea	**52959-0126-42**	13.36		EE
44s ea	**52959-0126-44**	13.99		EE
45s ea	**52959-0126-45**	14.01		EE
50s ea	**52959-0126-50**	15.44		EE
60s ea	**52959-0126-60**	17.81		EE
70s ea	**52959-0126-70**	18.59		AB
100s ea	**52959-0126-00**	21.00		EE
20 mg, 7s ea	**52959-0127-07**	3.64		EE
10s ea	**52959-0127-10**	5.10		EE
12s ea	**52959-0127-12**	6.01		EE
15s ea	**52959-0127-15**	7.07		EE
18s ea	**52959-0127-18**	8.67		AB
20s ea	**52959-0127-20**	9.36		EE
21s ea	**52959-0127-21**	9.84		EE
25s ea	**52959-0127-25**	11.46		EE
30s ea	**52959-0127-30**	12.57		EE
37s ea	**52959-0127-37**	14.35		EE
42s ea	**52959-0127-42**	15.80		EE
100s ea	**52959-0127-00**	21.84		EE
50 mg, 5s ea	**52959-0954-05**	12.98		AB
100s ea	**52959-0954-00**	14.35		AB
(Phys Total Care)				
REPACK				
TAB, PO, 1 mg, 15s ea	**54868-1119-04**	11.73		AB

PROD/MFR	NDC	AWP	DP	OBC
30s ea	**54868-1119-03**	17.22		EE
60s ea	**54868-1119-05**	33.39		AB
90s ea	**54868-1119-02**	45.66		EE
100s ea	**54868-1119-01**	52.65		EE
5 mg, 15s ea	**54868-0258-09**	4.26		EE
20s ea	**54868-0258-04**	4.71		EE
(6 DAY DOSEPAK)				
5 mg, 21s ea UD	**54868-4096-00**	14.97		AB
30s ea	**54868-0258-01**	5.55		EE
36s ea	**54868-0258-05**	6.06		EE
48s ea	**54868-5213-00**	26.25		AB
55s ea	**54868-0258-06**	7.68		EE
60s ea	**54868-0258-08**	8.10		EE
100s ea	**54868-0258-02**	11.49		EE
10 mg, 15s ea	**54868-0836-04**	4.80		EE
20s ea	**54868-0836-08**	5.40		EE
(DOSE PACK)				
10 mg, 21s ea	**54868-5230-00**	24.06		AB
30s ea	**54868-0836-07**	6.60		EE
40s ea	**54868-0836-00**	7.77		EE
(12 DAY DOSE PACK)				
10 mg, 48s ea	**54868-4095-00**	41.61		EE
50s ea	**54868-0836-03**	8.97		EE
60s ea	**54868-0836-05**	10.17		EE
100s ea	**54868-0836-02**	13.44		EE
20 mg, 10s ea	**54868-1183-08**	6.54		EE
15s ea	**54868-1183-01**	7.56		EE
20s ea	**54868-1183-07**	8.58		EE
25s ea	**54868-1183-09**	9.60		AB
30s ea	**54868-1183-03**	10.62		EE
60s ea	**54868-1183-02**	16.71		EE
100s ea	**54868-1183-00**	23.34		EE
50 mg, 3s ea	**54868-0908-02**	7.02		EE
5s ea	**54868-0908-05**	10.30		AB
10s ea	**54868-0908-01**	12.93		EE
30s ea	**54868-0908-00**	29.79		EE
(USP)				
50 mg, 50s ea	**54868-0908-03**	46.65		EE
60s ea	**54868-0908-04**	55.08		EE
(Physician Partner)				
REPACK				
TAB, PO, 5 mg, 30s ea	**21695-0305-30**	13.99		AB
10 mg, 20s ea	**21695-0306-20**	12.48		
21s ea	**21695-0306-21**	13.11		
28s ea	**21695-0306-28**	16.59		
30s ea	**21695-0306-30**	17.78		
39s ea	**21695-0306-39**	24.35		AB
42s ea	**21695-0306-42**	24.89		
48s ea	**21695-0765-48**	26.56		AB
20 mg, 10s ea	**21695-0307-10**	12.85		
12s ea	**21695-0307-12**	15.42		AB
14s ea	**21695-0307-14**	15.57		AB
15s ea	**21695-0307-15**	15.72		AB
18s ea	**21695-0307-18**	16.04		
20s ea	**21695-0307-20**	17.82		
21s ea	**21695-0307-21**	18.71		AB
30s ea	**21695-0307-30**	26.74		
50 mg, 5s ea	**21695-0580-05**	13.08		
(Quality Care Prod)				
REPACK				
TAB, PO, 5 mg, 5s ea	**49999-0008-05**	16.50		AB
20s ea	**49999-0008-20**	4.20		EE
30s ea	**49999-0008-30**	6.30		EE
40s ea	**49999-0008-40**	5.02		EE
42s ea	**49999-0008-42**	8.44		AB
55s ea	**49999-0008-55**	6.90		EE
100s ea	**49999-0008-00**	21.00		EE
10 mg, 5s ea	**49999-0028-05**	4.58		AB
12s ea	**49999-0028-12**	11.04		AB
14s ea	**49999-0028-14**	12.88		AB
15s ea	**49999-0028-15**	13.80		AB
20s ea	**49999-0028-20**	18.40		AB
21s ea	**49999-0028-21**	19.32		AB
28s ea	**49999-0028-28**	25.76		AB
30s ea	**49999-0028-30**	27.60		AB
40s ea	**49999-0028-40**	36.80		AB
48s ea	**49999-0028-48**	44.16		AB
50s ea	**49999-0028-50**	46.00		AB
60s ea	**49999-0028-60**	55.20		AB
90s ea	**49999-0028-90**	82.80		AB
20 mg, 6s ea	**49999-0110-06**	4.44		EE
7s ea	**49999-0110-07**	5.18		AB
10s ea	**49999-0110-10**	7.40		AB
12s ea	**49999-0110-12**	8.88		AB
14s ea	**49999-0110-14**	10.36		AB
15s ea	**49999-0110-15**	11.10		EE
18s ea	**49999-0110-18**	13.32		AB
20s ea	**49999-0110-20**	14.80		EE
21s ea	**49999-0110-21**	15.54		AB
30s ea	**49999-0110-30**	22.90		EE
100s ea	**49999-0110-00**	47.00		AB
50 mg, 3s ea	**49999-0437-03**	4.97		AB

PROD/MFR	NDC	AWP	DP	OBC
(Southwood)				
REPACK				
TAB, PO, 5 mg, 20s ea	**58016-0218-20**	1.44		EE
21s ea	**58016-0218-21**	1.51		EE
21s ea	**58016-4832-01**	5.40		EE
24s ea	**58016-0218-24**	1.73		EE
30s ea	**58016-0218-30**	4.20		EE
33s ea	**58016-0218-33**	2.38		EE
36s ea	**58016-0218-36**	2.59		EE
40s ea	**58016-0218-40**	2.88		EE
50s ea	**58016-0218-50**	3.60		EE
55s ea	**58016-0218-55**	3.96		EE
60s ea	**58016-0218-60**	8.40		EE
69s ea	**58016-0218-69**	9.66		EE
90s ea	**58016-0218-90**	12.60		AB
100s ea	**58016-0218-00**	14.00		EE
10 mg, 10s ea	**58016-0216-10**	1.30		EE
12s ea	**58016-0126-12**	1.12		EE
12s ea	**58016-0216-12**	1.56		EE
14s ea	**58016-0216-14**	1.82		EE
15s ea	**58016-0216-15**	1.95		EE
20s ea	**58016-0216-20**	2.60		EE
21s ea	**58016-0216-21**	2.73		EE
22s ea	**58016-0216-22**	2.86		EE
24s ea	**58016-0216-24**	3.12		EE
28s ea	**58016-0216-28**	3.64		EE
30s ea	**58016-0216-30**	3.90		EE
32s ea	**58016-0216-32**	4.16		EE
40s ea	**58016-0216-40**	5.20		EE
42s ea	**58016-0216-42**	5.46		EE
50s ea	**58016-0216-50**	6.50		EE
60s ea	**58016-0216-60**	7.80		EE
84s ea	**58016-0216-84**	10.92		EE
90s ea	**58016-0216-90**	11.70		EE
100s ea	**58016-0216-00**	13.00		EE
20 mg, 5s ea	**58016-0217-05**	0.83		EE
7s ea	**58016-0217-07**	1.16		EE
10s ea	**58016-0217-10**	1.65		EE
12s ea	**58016-0217-12**	1.98		EE
15s ea	**58016-0217-15**	2.48		EE
16s ea	**58016-0217-16**	2.64		EE
18s ea	**58016-0217-18**	2.98		EE
20s ea	**58016-0217-20**	3.31		EE
21s ea	**58016-0217-21**	3.47		EE
22s ea	**58016-0217-22**	3.64		EE
23s ea	**58016-0217-23**	3.80		EE
24s ea	**58016-0217-24**	3.97		EE
28s ea	**58016-0217-28**	4.63		EE
30s ea	**58016-0217-30**	4.96		EE
40s ea	**58016-0217-40**	6.61		EE
60s ea	**58016-0217-60**	9.92		EE
100s ea	**58016-0217-00**	16.53		EE
(St. Mary's MPP)				
REPACK				
TAB, PO, 20 mg, 21s ea	**60760-0002-21**	8.34		AB
(Stat Rx)				
REPACK				
TAB, PO, 5 mg, 21s ea	**16590-0365-21**	10.50		AB
21s ea	**16590-0373-21**	6.93		AB
28s ea	**16590-0373-28**	9.24		AB
30s ea	**16590-0373-30**	9.90		AB
40s ea	**16590-0373-40**	13.86		AB
42s ea	**16590-0373-42**	13.86		AB
44s ea	**16590-0373-44**	14.52		AB
48s ea	**16590-0365-48**	24.00		AB
10 mg, 3s ea	**16590-0404-03**	2.74		AB
10s ea	**16590-0404-10**	5.00		
20s ea	**16590-0404-20**	11.54		AB
21s ea	**16590-0404-21**	12.12		AB
21s ea	**16590-0624-21**	25.75		AB
30s ea	**16590-0404-30**	17.31		AB
36s ea	**16590-0404-31**	15.02		AB
45s ea	**16590-0404-45**	22.50		
48s ea	**16590-0624-48**	44.33		AB
20 mg, 10s ea	**16590-0326-10**	6.00		
13s ea	**16590-0326-13**	6.44		AB
16s ea	**16590-0326-16**	7.93		AB
20s ea	**16590-0326-20**	11.90		AB
21s ea	**16590-0326-21**	12.50		
30s ea	**16590-0326-30**	14.86		AB
45s ea	**16590-0326-45**	27.00		
48s ea	**16590-0326-48**	23.78		AB
60s ea	**16590-0326-60**	12.75		AB
(Vibranta)				
REPACK				
TAB, PO, 5 mg, 20s ea	**57866-4327-02**	3.14		
21s ea	**57866-4324-04**	5.96		
30s ea	**57866-4324-01**	41.22		
50s ea	**57866-4324-05**	1.93		
10 mg, 21s ea	**57866-4325-02**	6.46		AB
30s ea	**57866-4325-01**	15.44		AB
40s ea	**57866-4325-03**	9.50		AB

PROD/MFR	NDC	AWP	DP	OBC
60s ea	**57866-4325-08**	19.20		
90s ea	**57866-4325-07**	28.80		
20 mg, 5s ea	**57866-4326-07**	1.18		
15s ea	**57866-4326-05**	1.73		
18s ea	**57866-4326-08**	7.14		
20s ea	**57866-4326-01**	2.60		
21s ea	**57866-4326-04**	9.93		
30s ea	**57866-4326-02**	42.00		
PREDNISONE ANHYDROUS (Medisca)				
prednisone				
POW, NA (U.S.P.,MICRONIZED)				
500 gm	**38779-0154-08**	4155.00		
1000 gm	**38779-0154-09**	7350.00		
PREDNISONE INTENSOL (Roxane)				
prednisone				
SOL, PO, 5 mg/ml, 30 ml	**00054-3721-44**	34.97		
PREDNISONE MICRONIZED (Hawkins)				
prednisone, micronized				
POW, NA (U.S.P)				
5 gm	**63370-0194-15**	44.00		
25 gm	**63370-0194-25**	200.00		
100 gm	**63370-0194-35**	760.00		
500 gm	**63370-0194-45**	3600.00		
1000 gm	**63370-0194-50**	6400.00		
(PCCA)				
POW, NA (USP)				
1 gm	**51927-1435-00**	13.20		
PREDNISONE, MICRONIZED				
(Hawkins) *See PREDNISONE MICRONIZED*				
(PCCA) *See PREDNISONE MICRONIZED*				
PREFERAOB (Alaven)				
prenatal vitamins				
TAB, PO (FILM-COATED)				
90s ea	**68220-0088-90**	125.00		
PREFERAOB + DHA (Alaven)				
prenatal vitamins				
KIT, PO (30X30,FILM-COATED)				
60s ea	**68220-0089-30**	56.38		
PREFEST (Teva)				
estradiol/norgestimate				
TAB, PO (6X30)				
180s ea	**51285-0063-90**	396.73		AB
(Phys Total Care)				
REPACK				
TAB, PO, 30s ea	**54868-4269-00**	38.29		
PREGABALIN				
(Pfizer) *See LYRICA*				
PREGNENOLONE (Gallipot)				
POW, NA, 25 gm	**51552-0438-04**	58.80		
(1X25GM,MICRONIZED)				
25 gm	**51552-0757-04**	58.80	42.00	
100 gm	**51552-0438-05**	138.60		
(1X100GM,MICRONIZED)				
100 gm	**51552-0757-05**	138.60	99.00	
500 gm	**51552-0438-06**	658.00		
1000 gm	**51552-0438-07**	1120.00		
(1X5000GM,MICRONIZED)				
5000 gm	**51552-0757-08**	2555.00	1825.00	
(Letco)				
prednisolone sodium phosphate				
POW, NA, 25 gm	**62991-2052-02**	115.50		
100 gm	**62991-2052-03**	240.00		
500 gm	**62991-2052-04**	1125.00		
PREGNENOLONE (Medisca)				
POW, NA, 5 gm	**38779-0769-03**	46.50		
25 gm	**38779-0769-04**	177.00		
(1X25GM,MICRONIZED)				
25 gm	**38779-2233-04**	180.00		
100 gm	**38779-0769-05**	327.00		
(1X100GM,MICRONIZED)				
100 gm	**38779-2233-05**	405.00		
500 gm	**38779-0769-08**	1395.00		
(1X500GM,MICRONIZED)				
500 gm	**38779-2233-08**	1140.00		
(1X1000GM,MICRONIZED)				
1000 gm	**38779-2233-09**	2097.00		
(1X1000GM)				
1000 gm	**38779-0769-09**	2397.00		
(PCCA)				
POW, NA, 1 gm	**51927-2475-00**	10.80		
(Spectrum Pharmacy)				
POW, NA (1X5GM)				
5 gm	**49452-6065-02**	86.10		
(1X25GM)				
25 gm	**49452-6065-03**	285.60		

PROD/MFR	NDC	AWP	DP	OBC
(1X100GM)				
100 gm	49452-6065-04	626.50		
(1X1000GM)				
1000 gm	49452-6065-05	2880.50		
(B&B Pharm, Inc)				
REPACK				
POW, NA (1X100GM,MICRONIZED)				
100 gm	63275-9949-05	240.00		
(1X1000GM,MICRONIZED)				
1000 gm	63275-9949-09	1800.00		
PREGNYL (Organon)				
chorionic gonadotropin				
PDS, IM (W/DILUENT)				
10000 u, ea	00052-0315-10	57.23		AP
(Phys Total Care)				
REPACK				
PDS, IM (W/DILUENT)				
10000 u, ea	54868-4997-00	65.10		AP
PREHIST D (Marnel)				
cpm/methscopolamine nitrate/phenyleph hcl				
CER, PO, 8 mg-2.5 mg-20 mg,				
100s ea	00682-0100-01	81.80		
PRELONE (Adamis)				
prednisolone				
SYR, PO (CHERRY)				
15 mg/5 ml, 240 ml	38739-0150-08	128.64		
(Phys Total Care)				
REPACK				
SYR, PO (CHERRY)				
15 mg/5 ml, 240 ml	54868-3220-00	125.83		AA
(Southwood)				
REPACK				
SYR, PO, 15 mg/5 ml,				
60 ml	58016-0673-12	11.81		AA
120 ml	58016-0673-24	22.44		AA
240 ml	58016-0673-48	42.44		AA
PREMARIN (Wyeth)				
conjugated estrogens				
TAB, PO, 0.3 mg, 100s ea	00046-1100-81	194.02	161.68	
1000s ea	00046-1100-91	1940.23	1616.86	
0.45 mg, 100s ea	00046-1101-81	194.02	161.68	
0.625 mg, 100s ea	00046-1102-81	194.02	161.68	
1000s ea	00046-1102-91	1940.23	1616.86	
0.9 mg, 100s ea	00046-1103-81	194.02	161.68	
1.25 mg, 100s ea	00046-1104-81	194.02	161.68	
1000s ea	00046-1104-91	1940.23	1616.86	
(A-S Medication)				
REPACK				
TAB, PO, 0.625 mg,				
30s ea	54569-0812-05	72.06		
100s ea	54569-0812-00	240.21		
1.25 mg, 30s ea	54569-0813-01	72.06		
(Altura)				
REPACK				
TAB, PO, 0.3 mg, 10s ea	63874-0158-10	9.87		
14s ea	63874-0158-14	11.94		
15s ea	63874-0158-15	12.79		
20s ea	63874-0158-20	18.70		
30s ea	63874-0158-30	23.91		
100s ea	63874-0158-01	29.73		
(AQ)				
REPACK				
TAB, PO, 0.625 mg,				
100s ea	66105-0137-10	197.48		
1.25 mg, 100s ea	66105-0138-10	197.48		
(Core)				
REPACK				
TAB, PO, 0.9 mg, 30s ea	33358-0295-30	43.59		
(Direct Pharmaceutical, Inc.)				
REPACK				
TAB, PO, 0.625 mg,				
30s ea UD	67801-0326-03	85.48		
1.25 mg, 30s ea UD	67801-0327-03	85.48		
(Dispensing Solutions)				
REPACK				
TAB, PO, 0.625 mg,				
30s ea	66336-0599-30	65.69		
(HomeMed)				
REPACK				
TAB, PO, 0.625 mg,				
30s ea	51655-0452-24	25.34		
60s ea	51655-0452-25	31.68		
(PD-Rx Pharm)				
REPACK				
TAB, PO, 0.3 mg, 30s ea	55289-0123-30	109.76		
0.625 mg, 7s ea	55289-0943-07	27.22		
25s ea	55289-0943-25	91.46		
28s ea	55289-0943-28	102.44		
(REDI-SCRIPT)				
0.625 mg, 28s ea	58864-0422-28	102.44		
30s ea	55289-0943-30	109.76		
30s ea	58864-0422-30	109.76		
1.25 mg, 25s ea	55289-0047-25	91.46		
30s ea	55289-0047-30	109.76		
42s ea	55289-0047-42	153.66		
90s ea	55289-0047-90	329.26		
(Pharma Pac)				
REPACK				
TAB, PO, 0.625 mg,				
30s ea	52959-0223-30	29.88		
100s ea	52959-0223-00	55.76		
1.25 mg, 100s ea	52959-0222-00	128.35		
(Phys Total Care)				
REPACK				
TAB, PO, 0.3 mg, 10s ea	54868-2702-01	25.77		
30s ea	54868-2702-00	72.10		
60s ea	54868-2702-02	141.58		
90s ea	54868-2702-04	199.48		
100s ea	54868-2702-03	221.35		
0.45 mg, 10s ea	54868-4865-01	26.93		
30s ea	54868-4865-00	75.57		
60s ea	54868-4865-02	148.52		
90s ea	54868-4865-03	209.32		
0.625 mg, 10s ea	54868-0451-06	26.93		
25s ea	54868-0451-00	63.41		
30s ea	54868-0451-02	75.57		
50s ea	54868-0451-01	124.21		
90s ea	54868-0451-07	209.32		
100s ea	54868-0451-03	231.63		
0.9 mg, 10s ea	54868-0365-03	26.93		
30s ea	54868-0365-02	75.57		
100s ea	54868-0365-00	232.29		
1.25 mg, 10s ea	54868-0453-06	25.77		
25s ea	54868-0453-00	60.52		
30s ea	54868-0453-02	72.10		
90s ea	54868-0453-05	199.48		
100s ea	54868-0453-04	221.35		
2.5 mg, 100s ea	54868-0452-03	187.17		
(Quality Care Prod)				
REPACK				
TAB, PO, 0.3 mg, 100s ea	35356-0249-00	326.60		
0.45 mg, 100s ea	35356-0251-00	326.60		
0.625 mg, 30s ea	49999-0109-30	97.86		
90s ea	49999-0109-90	189.90		
100s ea	49999-0109-00	326.60		
0.9 mg, 100s ea	35356-0250-00	326.60		
1.25 mg, 30s ea	35356-0426-30	97.86		
(Southwood)				
REPACK				
TAB, PO, 0.3 mg, 10s ea	58016-0744-10	16.37		
12s ea	58016-0744-12	19.64		
14s ea	58016-0744-14	22.92		
15s ea	58016-0744-15	24.55		
20s ea	58016-0744-20	32.74		
30s ea	58016-0744-30	49.11		
60s ea	58016-0744-60	98.21		
90s ea	58016-0744-90	147.32		
100s ea	58016-0744-00	163.69		
0.625 mg, 10s ea	58016-0948-10	16.37		
12s ea	58016-0948-12	19.64		
14s ea	58016-0948-14	22.92		
15s ea	58016-0948-15	24.55		
20s ea	58016-0948-20	32.74		
30s ea	58016-0948-30	49.11		
50s ea	58016-0948-50	81.85		
60s ea	58016-0948-60	98.21		
90s ea	58016-0948-90	147.32		
100s ea	58016-0948-00	163.69		
1.25 mg, 10s ea	58016-0983-10	11.36		
12s ea	58016-0983-12	13.64		
14s ea	58016-0983-14	15.91		
15s ea	58016-0983-15	17.04		
20s ea	58016-0983-20	22.73		
PREMARIN INTRAVENOUS (Wyeth)				
conjugated estrogens				
PDS, IV (W/SECULE VIAL)				
25 mg, ea	00046-0749-05	107.54	89.62	
PREMARIN VAGINAL (Wyeth)				
conjugated estrogens				
CRE, VG (W/APPLICATOR)				
0.625 mg/gm,				
42.5 gm	00046-0872-93	128.90	107.42	
(A-S Medication)				
REPACK				
CRE, VG (W/APPLICATOR)				
0.625 mg/gm,				
42.5 gm	54569-0981-00	159.59		
(Phys Total Care)				
REPACK				
CRE, VG (REFILL)				
0.625 mg/gm, 43 gm	54868-3391-01	73.50		
(W/APPLICATOR)				
0.625 mg/gm, 45 gm	54868-0454-00	147.28		
(Quality Care Prod)				
REPACK				
CRE, VG, 0.625 mg/gm,				
42.5 gm	49999-0303-15	209.46		
PREMASOL (Baxter)				
amino acids				
SOL, IV (SULFITE-FREE,VIAFLEX)				
6%, 500 ml 24s	00338-1131-03	1497.60	1248.00	EE
(SULFITE-FREE)				
10%, 500 ml 24s	00338-1130-03	2059.20	1716.00	EE
(VIAFLEX,SULFITE-FREE)				
10%, 1000 ml 12s	00338-1130-04	1666.37	1388.64	EE
(SULFITE-FREE,VIAFLEX)				
10%, 2000 ml 6s	00338-1130-06	1286.64	1072.20	EE
PREMESIS RX (Ther-RX)				
calcium/cyanocobalamin/folic acid/pyridoxine				
TAB, PO (FILM-COATED)				
30s ea	64011-0019-19	37.49		
(Phys Total Care)				
REPACK				
TAB, PO (FILM-COATED)				
30s ea	54868-4839-01	29.58		
100s ea	54868-4839-00	53.97		
PREMPHASE (Wyeth)				
conjugated estrogens/medroxyprogesterone acetate				
TAB, PO, 28s ea	00046-2579-11	65.53	54.61	
(Phys Total Care)				
REPACK				
TAB, PO (EZ-DIAL DISPENSER)				
0.625 mg-5 mg,				
28s ea	54868-3800-00	31.78		
PREMPRO (Wyeth)				
conjugated estrogens/medroxyprogesterone acetate				
TAB, PO (1X28)				
0.3 mg-1.5 mg,				
28s ea	00046-1105-11	68.81	57.34	EE
0.45 mg-1.5 mg,				
28s ea	00046-1106-11	68.81	57.34	EE
0.625 mg-2.5 mg,				
28s ea	00046-0875-11	68.81	57.34	
0.625 mg-5 mg,				
28s ea	00046-0975-11	68.81	57.34	
(A-S Medication)				
REPACK				
TAB, PO, 0.625 mg-2.5 mg,				
28s ea	54569-4365-00	85.19		
(Phys Total Care)				
REPACK				
TAB, PO, 0.3 mg-1.5 mg,				
28s ea	54868-5047-00	88.21		
(EZ-DIAL)				
0.625 mg-2.5 mg,				
28s ea	54868-3799-00	74.46		
0.625 mg-5 mg,				
28s ea	54868-5540-00	53.65		
(Quality Care Prod)				
REPACK				
TAB, PO, 0.3 mg-1.5 mg,				
28s ea	35356-0276-28	121.41		
0.625 mg-2.5 mg,				
28s ea	35356-0277-28	121.41		
0.625 mg-5 mg,				
28s ea	35356-0278-28	121.41		
(Southwood)				
REPACK				
TAB, PO, 0.625 mg-2.5 mg,				
28s ea	58016-4074-01	124.77		
PREMPRO LOW DOSE (Phys Total Care)				
REPACK				
conjugated estrogens/medroxyprogesterone acetate				
TAB, PO, 0.45 mg-1.5 mg,				
28s ea	54868-4866-00	88.21		
(Quality Care Prod)				
REPACK				
TAB, PO, 0.45 mg-1.5 mg,				
28s ea	35356-0279-28	121.41		

PROD/MFR	NDC	AWP	DP	OBC
PRENACARE (Cypress Pharm)				
prenatal vitamins				
TAB, PO (DYE-FREE)				
100s ea	60258-0184-01	24.95		
PRENAFIRST (Cypress Pharm)				
prenatal vitamins				
TAB, PO (FILM-COATED)				
90s ea	60258-0178-09	34.96		
PRENAPLUS (Cypress Pharm)				
prenatal vitamins				
TAB, PO (FILM COATED)				
100s ea	60258-0183-01	27.94		
PRENATABS FA (Cypress Pharm)				
prenatal vitamins				
TAB, PO, 100s ea	60258-0190-01	20.05		
PRENATABS RX (Cypress Pharm)				
prenatal vitamins				
TAB, PO, 90s ea	60258-0193-09	30.77		
PRENATAL (Contract Pharmacal)				
multivitamin and minerals				
TAB, PO (CAPLET)				
200s ea	10267-2016-02	13.05		
PRENATAL 1 PLUS 1 (Dispensing Solutions)				
REPACK				
prenatal vitamins				
TAB, PO, 100s ea	55045-1504-01	28.15		
(Phys Total Care)				
REPACK				
TAB, PO, 100s ea	54868-0190-01	46.71		
(Southwood)				
REPACK				
TAB, PO, 30s ea	58016-0929-30	5.71		
100s ea	58016-0929-00	23.24		
PRENATAL 1 PLUS IRON (Phys Total Care)				
REPACK				
prenatal vitamins				
TAB, PO, 100s ea	54868-0330-01	60.75		
PRENATAL 19 (Cypress Pharm)				
prenatal vitamins				
CTB, PO (ORANGE)				
100s ea	60258-0197-01	44.25		
TAB, PO, 100s ea	60258-0196-01	38.16		
PRENATAL AD (Cypress Pharm)				
prenatal vitamins				
TAB, PO (9X10)				
90s ea UD	60258-0194-09	32.75		
PRENATAL ADVANTAGE (Contract Pharmacal)				
prenatal vitamins				
TAB, PO, 90s ea	10267-2926-05	27.45		
PRENATAL FA (Consolidated Midland)				
prenatal vitamins				
TAB, PO, 100s ea	00223-1412-01	5.50		
1000s ea	00223-1412-02	47.50		
PRENATAL FORTE (Contract Pharmacal)				
prenatal vitamins				
CAP, PO, 100s ea	10267-0737-01	20.00		
1000s ea	10267-0737-10	86.00		
TAB, PO (FILM COATED)				
90s ea	10267-2812-05	22.10		
PRENATAL LOW IRON (Contract Pharmacal)				
prenatal vitamins				
TAB, PO, 100s ea	10267-2069-01	18.00		
500s ea	10267-2069-05	84.90		
PRENATAL MULTITABS G (Contract Pharmacal)				
prenatal vitamins				
TAB, PO (BLISTER PACK)				
9s ea	10267-2813-05	27.45		
PRENATAL PLUS (Amneal)				
prenatal vitamins				
TAB, PO, 100s ea	65162-0668-10	31.05		
500s ea	65162-0668-50	147.77		
(A-S Medication)				
REPACK				
TAB, PO, 30s ea	54569-4552-01	5.55		
100s ea	54569-4552-00	18.49		
(PD-Rx Pharm)				
REPACK				
TAB, PO, 30s ea	58864-0736-30	12.10		
(Phys Total Care)				
REPACK				
TAB, PO, 30s ea	54868-0190-00	16.38		
(Physician Partner)				
REPACK				
TAB, PO, 30s ea	21695-0859-30	18.63		
100s ea	21695-0859-00	62.10		
(Quality Care Prod)				
REPACK				
TAB, PO, 30s ea	49999-0085-30	15.01		
PRENATAL PLUS IRON (Major)				
prenatal vitamins				
TAB, PO, 100s ea	00904-5339-60	21.39		
PRENATAL PLUS W/ IRON (Pharma Pac)				
REPACK				
prenatal vitamins				
TAB, PO, 100s ea	52959-0494-00	18.25		
PRENATAL RX (Contract Pharmacal)				
prenatal vitamins				
TAB, PO (FILM-COATED)				
100s ea	10267-0701-01	25.05		
(Phys Total Care)				
REPACK				
TAB, PO, 100s ea	54868-3828-00	65.16		
PRENATAL RX 1 (Phys Total Care)				
prenatal vitamins				
TAB, PO (FILM-COATED)				
30s ea	54868-5374-00	16.65		
PRENATAL RX W/BETA CAROTENE (Teva)				
prenatal vitamins				
TAB, PO, 200s ea	00093-9165-54	13.50		
PRENATAL VITAMIN 1PLUS 1 (PD-Rx Pharm)				
REPACK				
prenatal vitamins				
TAB, PO, 100s ea	55289-0365-01	7.73		

PRENATAL VITAMINS
(Acella) *See BP MULTINATAL PLUS*
(Acella) *See PNV-DHA*
(Acella) *See PNV-SELECT*
(Alaven) *See PREFERAOB*
(Alaven) *See PREFERAOB + DHA*
(Amneal) *See PRENATAL PLUS*
(Atley) *See PREQUE 10*
(Azur Pharma, Inc.) *See GESTICARE*
(Azur Pharma, Inc.) *See GESTICARE DHA*
(Azur Pharma, Inc.) *See NATELLE C*
(Azur Pharma, Inc.) *See NATELLE ONE*
(Azur Pharma, Inc.) *See NATELLE PLUS W/ DHA*
(Azur Pharma, Inc.) *See NATELLE-EZ*
(Blansett) *See NUTRACARE*
(Breckenridge Pharm) *See VINACAL*
(Breckenridge Pharm) *See VINATAL FORTE*
(Breckenridge Pharm) *See VINATE AZ*
(Breckenridge Pharm) *See VINATE AZ EXTRA*
(Breckenridge Pharm) *See VINATE C*
(Breckenridge Pharm) *See VINATE CALCIUM*
(Breckenridge Pharm) *See VINATE CARE*
(Breckenridge Pharm) *See VINATE GT*
(Breckenridge Pharm) *See VINATE IC*
(Breckenridge Pharm) *See VINATE II*
(Breckenridge Pharm) *See VINATE III*
(Breckenridge Pharm) *See VINATE M*
(Breckenridge Pharm) *See VINATE ONE*
(Breckenridge Pharm) *See VINATE PN CARE*
(Breckenridge Pharm) *See VINATE ULTRA*
(Consolidated Midland) *See PRENATAL FA*
(Contract Pharmacal) *See CO-NATAL CBF*
(Contract Pharmacal) *See CO-NATAL FA*
(Contract Pharmacal) *See MATERNITY VITAMIN LOW IRON*
(Contract Pharmacal) *See NATAL*
(Contract Pharmacal) *See POLY IRON PN*
(Contract Pharmacal) *See POLY IRON PN FORTE*
(Contract Pharmacal) *See PRENATAL ADVANTAGE*
(Contract Pharmacal) *See PRENATAL FORTE*
(Contract Pharmacal) *See PRENATAL LOW IRON*
(Contract Pharmacal) *See PRENATAL MULTITABS G*
(Contract Pharmacal) *See PRENATAL RX*
(Contract Pharmacal) *See PRENATAL-Z*
(Contract Pharmacal) *See ULTRA-NATAL VITAMIN*
(Cypress Pharm) *See PRENACARE*
(Cypress Pharm) *See PRENAFIRST*
(Cypress Pharm) *See PRENAPLUS*
(Cypress Pharm) *See PRENATABS FA*
(Cypress Pharm) *See PRENATABS RX*
(Cypress Pharm) *See PRENATAL 19*
(Cypress Pharm) *See PRENATAL AD*
(Cypress Pharm) *See PRENATAL-H*
(Cypress Pharm) *See PRENATAL-U*
(Cypress Pharm) *See TRINATE*
(Ethex) *See CAL-NATE*
(Ethex) *See NATATAB CFE*
(Everett) *See SELECT-OB*
(Everett) *See SELECT-OB+DHA*
(Everett) *See VITAFOL-OB+DHA*
(Everett) *See VITAFOL-PN*
(Gentex Pharma) *See GENTEX ADE*
(Hawthorn Pharm) *See ICAR PRENATAL*
(JayMac Pharma) *See VIVA DHA*
(Lannett) *See OB-NATAL ONE*
(Laser Pharma) *See LACTOCAL-F*
(Major) *See PRENATAL PLUS IRON*
(Marnel) *See MARNATAL-F*
(ME Pharm) *See MYNATAL*
(ME Pharm) *See MYNATAL ADVANCE*
(ME Pharm) *See MYNATAL FC*
(ME Pharm) *See MYNATAL PLUS*
(ME Pharm) *See MYNATAL PN*
(ME Pharm) *See MYNATAL PN FORTE*
(ME Pharm) *See MYNATAL RX*
(ME Pharm) *See MYNATAL ULTRA*
(ME Pharm) *See MYNATAL-Z*
(ME Pharm) *See MYNATE 90 PLUS*
(Midlothian Labs) *See FOLCAL DHA*
(Midlothian Labs) *See FOLCAPS CARE ONE*
(Midlothian Labs) *See FOLTABS 90 PLUS DHA*
(Midlothian Labs) *See FOLTABS PRENATAL*
(Midlothian Labs) *See FOLTABS PRENATAL PLUS DHA*
(Mission) *See CITRANATAL 90 DHA*
(Mission) *See CITRANATAL ASSURE*
(Mission) *See CITRANATAL DHA*
(Mission) *See CITRANATAL RX*
(Mission) *See NATACHEW*
(Mission) *See NATAFORT*
(Nnodum) *See INATAL ADVANCE*
(Nnodum) *See INATAL GT*
(Nnodum) *See INATAL ULTRA TAB*
(Novavax) *See NESTABS CBF*
(Novavax) *See NESTABS FA*
(Novavax) *See NESTABS RX*
(Pharmics) *See O-CAL PRENATAL*
(Pronova) *See OBTREX*
(PruGen) *See PR NATAL 400*
(PruGen) *See PR NATAL 400 EC*
(PruGen) *See PR NATAL 430*
(PruGen) *See PR NATAL 430 EC*
(PruGen) *See PR NATAL 440 EC*
(PruGen) *See PRUET DHA*
(PruGen) *See PRUET DHAEC*
(River's Edge) *See DOCOSAVIT*
(Seton) *See CAVAN ONE OMEGA*
(Seton) *See CAVAN PRENATAL TAB WITH EC CALCIUM*
(Seton) *See CAVAN-EC SOD DHA*
(Seton) *See SE-CARE CHEWABLE*

PROD/MFR | NDC | AWP | DP | OBC

(Seton) *See SE-CARE CONCEIVE*
(Seton) *See SE-NATAL 19*
(Seton) *See SE-NATAL 19 CHEWABLE*
(Seton) *See SE-NATAL 90*
(Seton) *See SE-NATAL ONE*
(Seton) *See SE-PLETE DHA*
(Seton) *See SE-TAN DHA*
(Seton) *See SETONET*
(Seton) *See SETONET-EC DHA*
(Seyer Pharmatec) *See OBSTETRIX EC*
(Seyer Pharmatec) *See OBSTETRIX-100*
(Shionogi) *See PRENATE DHA*
(Shionogi) *See PRENATE ELITE*
(Teva) *See PRENATAL RX W/BETA CAROTENE*
(Ther-RX) *See PRECARE*
(Ther-RX) *See PRECARE CONCEIVE*
(Ther-RX) *See PRIMACARE*
(Ther-RX) *See PRIMACARE ONE*
(Trigen) *See ELITE OB WITH DHA*
(U.S. Pharm) *See CONCEPT DHA*
(U.S. Pharm) *See CONCEPT OB*
(U.S. Pharm) *See TANDEM OB*
(Upsher-Smith) *See PRENEXA*
(Vertical) *See OB COMPLETE 400*
(Vertical) *See TRUST NATAL DHA*
(Xanodyne Pharma) *See DUET*
(Xanodyne Pharma) *See DUET DHA*
(Xanodyne Pharma) *See DUET DHA COMPLETE*
(Xanodyne Pharma) *See DUET STUARTNATAL*
(Xanodyne Pharma) *See DUETDHA STUARTNATAL*

(PD-Rx Pharm)
REPACK
TAB, PO (REDI-SCRIPT)
30s ea............... **58864-0609-30** 12.10

PRENATAL WITH FOLIC (Quality Care Prod)
REPACK
prenatal vitamins
TAB, PO, 100s ea......... **49999-0166-00** 25.56

PRENATAL-H (Cypress Pharm)
prenatal vitamins
CAP, PO, 100s ea UD...... **60258-0187-01** 30.39

PRENATAL-U (Cypress Pharm)
prenatal vitamins
CAP, PO, 100s ea **60258-0179-01** 34.70

PRENATAL-Z (Contract Pharmacal)
prenatal vitamins
TAB, PO (CAPLET)
100s ea............ **10267-1125-01** 23.20

PRENATE DHA (Shionogi)
prenatal vitamins
SGL, PO (WITH METAFOLIN,SOFTGEL)
30s ea UD **59630-0418-30** 76.01

PRENATE ELITE (Shionogi)
prenatal vitamins
TAB, PO (FILM-COATED)
90s ea............... **59630-0416-90** 187.48

(Phys Total Care)
REPACK
TAB, PO (FILM-COATED)
30s ea............... **54868-5069-01** 33.58
90s ea............... **54868-5069-00** 96.36

PRENEXA (Upsher-Smith)
prenatal vitamins
SGL, PO (WITH PLANT-BASED DHA)
30s ea............... **00245-0177-30** 59.98

PREPIDIL (Pfizer)
dinoprostone
GEL, VG (5X3GM)
0.5 mg/3 gm,
3 gm 5s **00009-3359-02** 1574.12 1311.77

PREQUE 10 (Atley)
prenatal vitamins
TAB, PO (COATED)
60s ea............... **59702-0710-60** 56.25

PREVACID (Takeda)
lansoprazole
ECC, PO (HARD GELATIN)
15 mg, 30s ea........ **64764-0541-30** 188.94 EE
100s ea UD .... **64764-0541-11** 629.80 EE
30 mg, 100s ea UD... **64764-0046-11** 629.80
100s ea............ **64764-0046-13** 629.80

(A-S Medication)
REPACK
ECC, PO (HARD GELATIN)
15 mg, 30s ea........ **54569-4450-00** 187.44 EE
30 mg, 7s ea......... **54569-4451-02** 39.67
30s ea............ **54569-4451-00** 187.44

(Advanced Pharm Serv, Inc.)
REPACK
ECC, PO, 15 mg, 15s ea... **13411-0120-15** 94.86
30s ea............ **13411-0120-03** 189.72
60s ea............ **13411-0120-06** 379.45
90s ea............ **13411-0120-09** 569.18
100s ea............ **13411-0120-10** 632.39
30 mg, 15s ea......... **13411-0121-15** 94.86
30s ea............ **13411-0121-03** 189.72
60s ea............ **13411-0121-06** 379.45
90s ea............ **13411-0121-09** 569.18
100s ea............ **13411-0121-10** 632.39

(AQ)
REPACK
ECC, PO, 15 mg, 10s ea... **66105-0134-01** 108.90
15s ea............ **66105-0134-15** 163.36
30s ea............ **66105-0134-03** 326.71
60s ea............ **66105-0134-06** 653.43
90s ea............ **66105-0134-09** 980.14
30 mg, 10s ea......... **66105-0135-01** 108.90
30s ea............ **66105-0135-03** 347.10
60s ea............ **66105-0135-06** 694.20
90s ea............ **66105-0135-09** 1041.30
100s ea............ **66105-0135-10** 1157.00

(Bryant Ranch)
REPACK
ECC, PO, 15 mg, 30s ea... **63629-3352-01** 163.17
30 mg, 30s ea......... **63629-1613-01** 236.99

(Core)
REPACK
ECC, PO, 30 mg, 30s ea... **33358-0298-30** 170.74

(Direct Pharmaceutical, Inc.)
REPACK
ECC, PO, 15 mg,
30s ea UD **67801-0318-03** 251.39
30 mg, 30s ea UD **67801-0313-30** 382.10

(Dispensing Solutions)
REPACK
ECC, PO, 15 mg, 30s ea... **55045-2740-08** 180.00
30 mg, 15s ea......... **55045-2560-02** 91.65
30s ea............ **55045-2560-08** 183.30
30s ea............ **66336-0869-30** 205.00
60s ea............ **66336-0869-60** 409.99
90s ea............ **66336-0869-90** 614.99

(Nucare Pharm)
REPACK
ECC, PO, 30 mg, 30s ea... **66267-0317-30** 285.00
60s ea............ **66267-0317-60** 387.00

(PD-Rx Pharm)
REPACK
ECC, PO (REDI-SCRIPT)
15 mg, 30s ea........ **58864-0679-30** 187.58
30 mg, 7s ea......... **55289-0704-07** 65.57
14s ea............ **55289-0704-14** 131.12
30s ea............ **55289-0704-30** 280.98
30s ea UD **58864-0614-30** 238.25
(REDI-SCRIPT)
30 mg, 60s ea UD **58864-0614-60** 382.10
90s ea............ **55289-0704-90** 768.06

(Pharma Pac)
REPACK
ECC, PO, 15 mg, 30s ea... **52959-0769-30** 154.50
60s ea............ **52959-0769-60** 308.99
30 mg, 20s ea......... **52959-0307-20** 113.54
30s ea............ **52959-0307-30** 163.95
60s ea............ **52959-0307-60** 327.99

(Phys Total Care)
REPACK
ECC, PO, 15 mg, 30s ea... **54868-3867-00** 197.03
30 mg, 10s ea......... **54868-4079-01** 77.79
30s ea............ **54868-4079-00** 215.62
60s ea............ **54868-4079-02** 414.89
90s ea............ **54868-4079-05** 621.02
100s ea............ **54868-4079-03** 689.08
1000s ea **54868-4079-04** 6589.79

(Physician Partner)
REPACK
ECC, PO, 30 mg, 15s ea... **21695-0106-15** 210.02

(Quality Care Prod)
REPACK
ECC, PO, 15 mg, 30s ea... **35356-0408-30** 343.91
30 mg, 30s ea......... **49999-0480-30** 306.80
100s ea............ **49999-0480-00** 892.54

(Southwood)
REPACK
ECC, PO, 30 mg, 30s ea... **58016-0683-30** 179.94
60s ea............ **58016-0683-60** 359.89
90s ea............ **58016-0683-90** 539.83
100s ea............ **58016-0683-00** 599.81

(Stat Rx)
REPACK
ECC, PO (HARD GELATIN)
15 mg, 30s ea........ **16590-0753-30** 221.65 EE
30 mg, 30s ea........ **16590-0515-30** 221.65
60s ea............ **16590-0515-60** 440.05
90s ea............ **16590-0515-90** 437.00
120s ea............ **16590-0515-72** 627.00

PREVACID DR (Quality Care Prod)
REPACK
lansoprazole
PKT, PO, 30 mg/packet,
30s ea............ **49999-0883-30** 213.37

PREVACID I.V. (Takeda)
lansoprazole
PDS, IV (SDV)
30 mg, ea............ **00300-3954-25** 27.31

PREVACID NAPRAPAC 375 (Takeda)
lansoprazole/naproxen
KIT, PO (WEEKLY)
15 mg-375 mg,
21s ea............ **00300-1545-07** 32.08

(Phys Total Care)
REPACK
KIT, PO, 15 mg-375 mg,
84s ea............ **54868-4659-00** 151.95

PREVACID NAPRAPAC 500 (Phys Total Care)
lansoprazole/naproxen
KIT, PO, 15 mg-500 mg,
84s ea............ **54868-5205-00** 161.39

PREVACID SOLUTAB (Takeda)
lansoprazole
TDR, PO (10X10)
15 mg, 100s ea UD... **64764-0543-11** 629.62 EE
(DELAYED RELEASE)
30 mg, 100s ea UD... **64764-0544-11** 629.62

(Phys Total Care)
REPACK
TDR, PO, 15 mg, 30s ea... **54868-5795-00** 135.22
(STRAWBERRY)
30 mg, 30s ea........ **54868-5303-00** 186.43

PREVALITE (Upsher-Smith)
cholestyramine
PDR, PO (PACKET)
4 gm/5.5 gm,
42s ea............ **00245-0036-42** 108.36 AB
60s ea............ **00245-0036-60** 154.99 AB
231 gm............ **00245-0036-23** 68.12 AB

PREVIDENT (Colgate Oral)
sodium fluoride
GEL, DE (CHERRY)
1.1%, 56 gm......... **00126-0088-02** 9.25
56 gm............ **00126-0288-02** 9.25
56 gm............ **00126-0290-02** 9.25

(Phys Total Care)
REPACK
GEL, DE, 1.1%, 60 gm..... **54868-3030-00** 11.30

PREVIDENT 5000 BOOSTER (Colgate Oral)
sodium fluoride
PAS, DE (SPEARMINT)
1.1%, 106 ml **00126-0075-34** 9.46

PREVIDENT 5000 PLUS (Colgate Oral)
sodium fluoride
CRE, DE (SPEARMINT)
1.1%, 51 gm......... **00126-0287-66** 9.46
51 gm............ **00126-0288-66** 9.38
51 gm 2s **00126-0287-33** 17.07

(Dispensing Solutions)
REPACK
CRE, DE (SPEARMINT)
1.1%, 51 gm......... **55045-3033-01** 13.75

PROD/MFR	NDC	AWP	DP	OBC

PREVIDENT DENTAL RINSE (Colgate Oral)
sodium fluoride
SOL, PO (MINT)
0.2%, 250 ml **00126-0179-99** 6.63

PREVIFEM (Qualitest)
ethinyl estradiol/norgestimate
TAB, PO (6X28)
35 mcg-0.25 mg,
168s ea........... **00603-7640-17** 193.38

PREVITE RX (Midlothian Labs)
calcium/cyanocobalamin/folic acid/pyridoxine
TAB, PO (FILM-COATED)
30s ea.............. **68308-0381-30** 32.75 22.92

PREVNAR (Wyeth)
pneumococcal 7-valent vaccine, diphtheria conjug
SUS, IM (PEDIATRIC USE,TAX INCLD)
16 mcg/0.5 ml,
0.5 ml 10s......... **00005-1970-50** 1005.06 838.80

PREVPAC (Takeda)
amoxicillin/clarithromycin/lansoprazole
KIT, PO (FILM-COATED)
500 mg-500 mg-30 mg,
ea................ **64764-0702-01** 414.82

(A-S Medication)
REPACK
KIT, PO (FILM-COATED)
500 mg-500 mg-30 mg,
14s ea............. **54569-4592-00** 539.27

(Phys Total Care)
REPACK
KIT, PO (FILMTAB)
500 mg-500 mg-30 mg,
14s ea............. **54868-4909-00** 469.62

PREZISTA (Tibotec Therapeutics)
darunavir ethanolate
TAB, PO (FILM-COATED)
75 mg, 480s ea ...... **59676-0563-01** 1102.20 EE
150 mg, 240s ea ..... **59676-0564-01** 1102.20 EE
400 mg, 60s ea **59676-0561-01** 1102.20
600 mg, 60s ea **59676-0562-01** 1102.20

(A-S Medication)
REPACK
TAB, PO (FILM-COATED)
400 mg, 60s ea **54569-6159-00** 1039.81
600 mg, 60s ea **54569-6086-00** 1351.75

(Phys Total Care)
REPACK
TAB, PO (FILM-COATED)
400 mg, 60s ea **54868-5969-00** 1108.31

(Quality Care Prod)
REPACK
TAB, PO (FILM-COATED)
600 mg, 60s ea **35356-0284-60** 1943.50

PRIALT (Elan Pharmaceuticals)
ziconotide
SOL, IN (PF)
25 mcg/ml, 20 ml **59075-0723-10** 3834.70
100 mcg/ml, 1 ml **59075-0720-10** 766.94
5 ml............. **59075-0722-10** 3834.70

PRIFTIN (Sanofi-Aventis)
rifapentine
TAB, PO, 150 mg, 32s ea .. **00088-2100-03** 113.78

PRILOCAINE (Letco)
POW, NA (USP)
100 gm............ **62991-2685-01** 315.00

PRILOCAINE HCL (Gallipot)
prilocaine hydrochloride
POW, NA (U.S.P.)
25 gm.............. **51552-0638-04** 39.90

(Letco)
POW, NA (U.S.P.)
25 gm.............. **62991-1693-02** 75.00
100 gm............ **62991-1693-03** 267.00

(Medisca)
POW, NA (U.S.P.)
25 gm.............. **38779-0155-04** 97.50
100 gm............ **38779-0155-05** 315.00
500 gm............ **38779-0155-08** 1245.00

(PCCA)
POW, NA (U.S.P.)
1 gm **51927-1720-00** 4.20

(Spectrum Pharmacy)
POW, NA (U.S.P.)
5 gm **49452-6010-04** 73.50
25 gm.............. **49452-6010-01** 145.60
100 gm............ **49452-6010-02** 497.00
500 gm............ **49452-6010-03** 1757.00

PRILOCAINE HYDROCHLORIDE
(Dentsply) *See CITANEST PLAIN DENTAL*
(Gallipot) *See PRILOCAINE HCL*
(Letco) *See PRILOCAINE HCL*
(Medisca) *See PRILOCAINE HCL*
(PCCA) *See PRILOCAINE HCL*
(Spectrum Pharmacy) *See PRILOCAINE HCL*

PRILOSEC (AstraZeneca)
omeprazole
ECC, PO (UNIT OF USE)
10 mg, 30s ea........ **00186-0606-31** 167.66 AB
1000s ea .... **00186-0606-82** 5588.29 AB
(UNIT OF USE)
20 mg, 30s ea........ **00186-0742-31** 187.15 AB
1000s ea .... **00186-0742-82** 6237.92 AB
40 mg, 30s ea........ **00186-0743-31** 276.59 AB
100s ea............ **00186-0743-68** 922.02 AB
1000s ea .... **00186-0743-82** 9220.01 AB

(AstraZeneca)
omeprazole magnesium
PKT, PO, 2.5 mg/packet,
30s ea UD .... **00186-0625-01** 167.66 EE
10 mg/packet,
30s ea UD **00186-0610-01** 167.66

(AQ)
REPACK
omeprazole
ECC, PO, 10 mg, 30s ea ... **66105-0556-03** 171.39
20 mg, 30s ea........ **66105-0557-03** 190.66
40 mg, 30s ea........ **66105-0558-03** 279.39

(Dispensing Solutions)
REPACK
ECC, PO, 40 mg, 30s ea ... **55045-3097-08** 232.50 AB

(Palmetto)
REPACK
ECC, PO, 20 mg, 30s ea ... **23490-7858-03** 135.00
60s ea............. **23490-7858-06** 270.00
90s ea............. **23490-7858-09** 405.00

(PD-Rx Pharm)
REPACK
ECC, PO, 20 mg, 10s ea ... **55289-0714-10** 79.00 AB
28s ea............. **55289-0714-28** 178.37 AB

(Pharma Pac)
REPACK
ECC, PO, 20 mg, 4s ea .... **52959-0536-04** 5.40 AB
10s ea............. **52959-0536-10** 57.01
14s ea............. **52959-0536-14** 74.48
15s ea............. **52959-0536-15** 79.75
28s ea............. **52959-0536-28** 138.35
30s ea............. **52959-0536-30** 146.23
60s ea............. **52959-0536-60** 277.45

(Phys Total Care)
REPACK
ECC, PO, 20 mg, 20s ea ... **54868-2169-03** 116.05 AB
30s ea............. **54868-2169-01** 163.88 AB
60s ea............. **54868-2169-04** 303.54 AB
100s ea............ **54868-2169-00** 514.18 AB
40 mg, 30s ea........ **54868-4495-00** 241.61 AB
90s ea............. **54868-4495-01** 699.07 AB

(Quality Care Prod)
REPACK
ECC, PO, 20 mg, 30s ea ... **49999-0265-30** 264.61

(Southwood)
REPACK
ECC, PO, 10 mg, 30s ea ... **58016-0776-30** 143.47 AB
60s ea............. **58016-0776-60** 286.94 AB
90s ea............. **58016-0776-90** 430.41 AB
100s ea............ **58016-0776-00** 478.23 AB
20 mg, 30s ea........ **58016-0327-30** 160.14
60s ea............. **58016-0327-60** 320.28
90s ea............. **58016-0327-90** 480.42
100s ea............ **58016-0327-00** 533.80
40 mg, 30s ea........ **58016-0384-30** 236.69 AB
60s ea............. **58016-0384-60** 473.37 AB
90s ea............. **58016-0384-90** 710.06 AB
100s ea............ **58016-0384-00** 788.95 AB
120s ea............ **58016-0384-02** 946.74 AB

(Stat Rx)
REPACK
ECC, PO, 20 mg, 30s ea ... **16590-0334-30** 196.50 AB
60s ea............. **16590-0334-60** 390.00 AB

PRIMABELLA (Alaven)
device
DEV, NA, ea **68220-0190-15** 212.50

PRIMACARE (Ther-RX)
prenatal vitamins
KIT, PO (DYE-FREE,FILM COATED)
60s ea UD **64011-0204-28** 92.42

(Phys Total Care)
REPACK
KIT, PO (DYE-FREE,FILM-COATED)
60s ea............... **54868-5191-00** 48.26

PRIMACARE ADVANTAGE (Ther-RX)
nutriceutical/prenatal vitamins
KIT, PO (DYE-FREE,FILM COATED)
60s ea............... **64011-0230-28** 53.75

PRIMACARE ONE (Ther-RX)
prenatal vitamins
SGL, PO (SOFT GELATIN)
30s ea............... **64011-0218-19** 52.87

PRIMACARE ONE PRENATAL VIT (Phys Total Care)
REPACK
prenatal vitamins
SGL, PO (SOFTGEL)
30s ea............... **54868-5535-00** 47.89

PRIMALEV (Atley)
acetaminophen/oxycodone hydrochloride
TAB, PO, 300 mg-2.5 mg,
100s ea, C-II **59702-0680-01** 287.50
300 mg-5 mg,
100s ea, C-II **59702-0681-01** 287.50
300 mg-7.5 mg,
100s ea, C-II **59702-0682-01** 287.50
300 mg-10 mg,
100s ea, C-II **59702-0683-01** 287.50

PRIMAQUINE PHOSPHATE (Gallipot)
POW, NA (B.P.)
25 gm............... **51552-0567-04** 116.06

(Sanofi-Aventis)
TAB, PO, 26.3 mg, 100s ea **00024-1596-01** 139.62

PRIMARY CONVERTABLE PIN LATEX FREE (Abbott Hosp)
kit, administration, intravenous
DEV, NA (P.B. MICRODRIP BKCK/INJ)
48s ea............... **00074-4968-78** 806.55 679.20

PRIMARY IV SET-SL W/IVEX-HP (Abbott Hosp)
kit, administration, intravenous
DEV, NA (112")
48s ea............... **00074-1769-78** 614.59 614.40

PRIMARY MACRO IV PUMP (Abbott Hosp)
kit, administration, intravenous
DEV, NA (105", VENTED)
48s ea............... **00074-3704-48** 856.14 720.96

PRIMARY NONVENTED IV SET-OL (Abbott Hosp)
kit, administration, intravenous
DEV, NA (BACKCHECK, 2-Y-INJ SITE)
48s ea............... **00074-1877-68** 660.63 556.32

PRIMATRIX DERMAL REPAIR SCAFFOLD (TEI Biosciences Inc.)
collagen, bovine
SHE, TP (10X12CM)
ea.................. **08533-6071-12** 4560.00
(10X25CM)
ea.................. **08533-6071-25** 6250.00
(20X25CM)
ea.................. **08533-6072-25** 10500.00
(4X4CM,FENESTRATED)
ea.................. **08533-6744-40** 672.00
(4X4CM)
ea.................. **08533-6074-40** 672.00
(6X6CM,FENESTRATED)
ea.................. **08533-6746-60** 1512.00
(6X6CM)
ea.................. **08533-6076-60** 1512.00
(8X12CM)
ea.................. **08533-6078-12** 4032.00
(8X8CM,FENESTRATED)
ea.................. **08533-6748-80** 2688.00
(8X8CM)
ea.................. **08533-6078-80** 2688.00
(0.2X26.5CM,SINGLE USE)
3s ea............... **08533-6070-09** 750.00

PRIMAXIN IM (Merck)
cilastatin sodium/imipenem
PDS, IM (VIAL)
500 mg-500 mg,
10s ea............. **00006-3582-75** 391.79

PRIMAXIN IV (Merck)
cilastatin sodium/imipenem
PDS, IV, 250 mg-250 mg,
25s ea............. **00006-3514-58** 520.39

PROD/MFR	NDC	AWP	DP	OBC
(ADD-VANTAGE)				
250 mg-250 mg,				
25s ea	00006-3551-58	550.68		
(P.B.)				
500 mg-500 mg,				
10s ea	00006-3517-75	412.58		
25s ea	00006-3516-59	979.54		
(ADD-VANTAGE)				
500 mg-500 mg,				
25s ea	00006-3552-59	1017.85		
(MONOVIAL)				
500 mg-500 mg,				
25s ea	00006-3666-59	1078.38		
PRIMIDONE				
FUL				
TAB, PO, 250 mg, 100s ea		80.55		
(Amneal)				
TAB, PO (USP)				
50 mg, 100s ea	65162-0544-10	49.50		AB
500s ea	65162-0544-50	232.25		AB
250 mg, 100s ea	65162-0545-10	99.60		AB
500s ea	65162-0545-50	489.15		AB
1000s ea	65162-0545-11	961.11		AB
(Consolidated Midland)				
TAB, PO, 250 mg, 100s ea	00223-1414-01	7.95		EE
1000s ea	00223-1414-02	67.50		EE
(Global Pharm)				
TAB, PO (USP)				
50 mg, 100s ea	00115-1030-01	49.75		
500s ea	00115-1030-02	232.50		
250 mg, 100s ea	00115-1031-01	99.60		AB
1000s ea	00115-1031-03	961.11		AB
(Hawkins)				
POW, NA (USP)				
25 gm	63370-0197-25	160.00		
100 gm	63370-0197-35	400.00		
500 gm	63370-0197-45	1600.00		
1000 gm	63370-0197-50	2800.00		
(Lannett)				
TAB, PO, 50 mg, 100s ea	00527-1301-01	50.25		AB
500s ea	00527-1301-05	242.00		AB
250 mg, 100s ea	00527-1231-01	99.60		AB
1000s ea	00527-1231-10	961.11		AB
(Major)				
TAB, PO, 50 mg, 100s ea	00904-5559-60	50.25		AB
500s ea	00904-5559-40	452.38		AB
250 mg, 100s ea	00904-0560-60	98.60		AB
(Marlex)				
TAB, PO (USP)				
250 mg, 500s ea	10135-0522-05	490.55		AB
(Medisca)				
POW, NA (U.S.P.)				
25 gm	38779-2164-04	201.00		
(1X100GM,USP)				
100 gm	38779-2164-05	510.00		
(1X500GM,USP)				
500 gm	38779-2164-08	1875.00		
(1X1000GM,USP)				
1000 gm	38779-2164-09	3285.00		
(Mutual)				
TAB, PO, 50 mg, 100s ea	53489-0602-01	46.52		AB
250 mg, 100s ea	53489-0603-01	98.65		AB
(PCCA)				
POW, NA (U.S.P.)				
1 gm	51927-2339-00	9.96		
(Qualitest)				
TAB, PO, 50 mg, 100s ea	00603-5371-21	46.49		AB
500s ea	00603-5371-28	224.00		AB
250 mg, 100s ea	00603-5372-21	99.60		AB
500s ea	00603-5372-28	961.11		AB
(Spectrum Pharmacy)				
POW, NA (1X25GM)				
25 gm	49452-6020-02	357.00		
100 gm	49452-6020-03	850.50		
(Valeant Pharm Intl) *See MYSOLINE*				
(Watson Labs)				
TAB, PO, 250 mg, 100s ea	00591-5321-01	43.42		AB
1000s ea	00591-5321-10	425.83		AB
(West-Ward)				
TAB, PO (USP)				
50 mg, 100s ea	00143-1482-01	49.75		AB
500s ea	00143-1482-05	232.50		AB
250 mg, 100s ea	00143-1484-01	99.60		AB

PROD/MFR	NDC	AWP	DP	OBC
(American Health)				
REPACK				
TAB, PO (USP,10X10)				
50 mg, 100s ea UD	68084-0202-01	79.39		
250 mg, 100s ea UD	68084-0203-01	94.90		
(HomeMed)				
REPACK				
TAB, PO, 250 mg, 30s ea	51655-0366-24	16.00		EE
(Phys Total Care)				
REPACK				
TAB, PO (USP)				
50 mg, 30s ea	54868-5067-01	46.41		
60s ea	54868-5067-03	46.49		AB
100s ea	54868-5067-00	109.83		EE
180s ea	54868-5067-02	127.46		AB
250 mg, 30s ea	54868-1691-02	50.76		EE
120s ea	54868-1691-00	119.15		AB
(Quality Care Prod)				
REPACK				
TAB, PO, 50 mg, 100s ea	49999-0559-00	49.32		AB
PRIMSOL (FSC Laboratories)				
trimethoprim hydrochloride				
SOL, PO (AF,DYE-FREE,BUBBLEGUM)				
50 mg/5 ml, 473 ml	13551-0501-05	186.12		
PRINIVIL (Merck)				
lisinopril				
TAB, PO (UNIT OF USE)				
5 mg, 90s ea	00006-0019-54	99.80		AB
(BULK PACKAGE)				
5 mg, 1000s ea	00006-0019-82	1097.24		AB
(UNIT OF USE)				
10 mg, 90s ea	00006-0106-54	103.06		AB
20 mg, 90s ea	00006-0207-54	110.33		AB
(AQ)				
REPACK				
TAB, PO, 5 mg, 100s ea	66105-0555-10	192.29		
20 mg, 30s ea	66105-0548-03	43.31		
(PD-Rx Pharm)				
REPACK				
TAB, PO, 10 mg, 8s ea	55289-0929-08	18.35		AB
30s ea	55289-0929-30	51.06		AB
(Phys Total Care)				
REPACK				
TAB, PO, 5 mg, 30s ea	54868-1960-00	39.83		AB
10 mg, 10s ea	54868-1970-03	14.94		AB
30s ea	54868-1970-02	41.06		AB
100s ea	54868-1970-01	124.61		AB
20 mg, 30s ea	54868-1502-00	43.81		AB
40 mg, 10s ea	54868-1501-01	22.33		AB
30s ea	54868-1501-00	63.21		AB
(Southwood)				
REPACK				
TAB, PO, 5 mg, 30s ea	58016-0564-30	31.12		AB
60s ea	58016-0564-60	62.24		AB
90s ea	58016-0564-90	93.36		AB
100s ea	58016-0564-00	103.73		AB
20 mg, 30s ea	58016-0760-30	34.40		AB
60s ea	58016-0760-60	68.81		AB
90s ea	58016-0760-90	103.21		AB
100s ea	58016-0760-00	114.68		AB
40 mg, 30s ea	58016-0646-30	50.31		AB
30s ea	58016-0646-90	150.92		AB
60s ea	58016-0646-60	100.61		AB
100s ea	58016-0646-00	150.92		AB
PRINZIDE (Merck)				
hydrochlorothiazide/lisinopril				
TAB, PO (UNIT OF USE)				
12.5 mg-10 mg,				
100s ea	00006-0145-58	127.75		AB
12.5 mg-20 mg,				
100s ea	00006-0140-58	138.30		AB
(PD-Rx Pharm)				
REPACK				
TAB, PO, 25 mg-20 mg,				
30s ea	55289-0573-30	59.30		AB
PRISTIQ (Wyeth)				
desvenlafaxine succinate				
TER, PO (FILM-COATED)				
50 mg, 14s ea	00008-1211-14	63.04	52.53	
30s ea	00008-1211-30	135.08	112.57	
90s ea	00008-1211-01	405.25	337.71	
(10X10,FILM-COATED)				
50 mg, 100s ea UD	00008-1211-50	450.29	375.24	
(FILM-COATED)				
100 mg, 14s ea	00008-1222-14	63.04	52.53	
30s ea	00008-1222-30	135.08	112.57	
90s ea	00008-1222-01	405.25	337.71	

PROD/MFR	NDC	AWP	DP	OBC
(10X10,FILM-COATED)				
100 mg, 100s ea UD	00008-1222-50	450.29	375.24	
(Phys Total Care)				
REPACK				
TER, PO (FILM-COATED)				
50 mg, 30s ea	54868-2932-00	146.62		
(Quality Care Prod)				
REPACK				
TER, PO (FILM-COATED)				
50 mg, 30s ea	35356-0491-30	207.88		
PRIVIGEN (CSL)				
immune globulin				
SOL, IV (PF,LATEX-FREE)				
10%, 50 ml	44206-0436-05	666.00		
100 ml	44206-0437-10	1332.00		
200 ml	44206-0438-20	2664.00		
PRO-CLEAR AC (Pro-Pharma LLC)				
codeine phosphate/pyrilamine maleate				
SOL, PO (1X473ML,AF,SF,DYE-FREE)				
9 mg/5 ml-8.33 mg/5 ml,				
473 ml, C-V	66594-0333-16	26.00		
PRO-RED AC (Pro-Pharma LLC)				
codeine phos/phenyleph hcl/pyril mal				
SOL, PO (1X473ML,AF,SF)				
473 ml, C-V	66594-0444-16	26.00		
PRO-TANNATE PEDIATRIC (Propharma)				
chlorpheniramine tannate/phenylephrine tannate				
SUS, PO, 4.5 mg/5 ml-5 mg/5 ml,				
473 ml	50313-0117-42	141.00		
PROAIR HFA (Teva)				
albuterol sulfate				
ARO, IH, 0.09 mg/actuation,				
8.5 gm	59310-0579-20	43.33		BX
(A-S Medication)				
REPACK				
ARO, IH, 0.09 mg/actuation,				
8.5 gm	54569-5777-00	42.69		BX
(Palmetto)				
REPACK				
ARO, IH (1X8.5GM)				
0.09 mg/actuation,				
8.5 gm	23490-7972-01	100.98		
(Pharma Pac)				
REPACK				
ARO, IH (1X8.5GM)				
0.09 mg/actuation,				
8.5 gm	52959-0978-01	65.20		BX
(Physician Partner)				
REPACK				
ARO, IH (1X8.5GM)				
0.09 mg/actuation,				
8.5 gm	21695-0851-85	73.44		BX
(Quality Care Prod)				
REPACK				
ARO, IH, 0.09 mg/actuation,				
8.5 gm	49999-0908-85	78.80		
PROAMATINE (Shire US Inc.)				
midodrine hydrochloride				
TAB, PO, 2.5 mg, 100s ea	54092-0003-01	152.93		
5 mg, 100s ea	54092-0004-01	307.93		
10 mg, 100s ea	54092-0007-01	615.84		
(Phys Total Care)				
REPACK				
TAB, PO, 5 mg, 10s ea	54868-5442-00	37.63		
60s ea	54868-5442-02	204.49		
90s ea	54868-5442-01	305.80		
PROBARIMIN QT (Fleming)				
medical food				
ODT, PO (SF,FRUIT PUNCH)				
60s ea	00256-0218-01	37.50		
PROBENECID				
FUL				
TAB, PO, 500 mg, 100s ea		70.59		
(Consolidated Midland)				
TAB, PO, 500 mg, 100s ea	00223-1472-01	17.50		EE
1000s ea	00223-1472-02	167.50		EE
(Lannett)				
TAB, PO (FILM COATED)				
500 mg, 100s ea	00527-1367-01	55.20		AB
1000s ea	00527-1367-10	486.00		AB
(Medisca)				
POW, NA (U.S.P.)				
100 gm	38779-0345-05	61.50		
500 gm	38779-0345-08	276.00		

PROD/MFR	NDC	AWP	DP	OBC
(Mylan)				
TAB, PO, 500 mg, 100s ea	**00378-0156-01**	98.25		**AB**
(Truxton)				
TAB, PO, 500 mg, 100s ea	**00463-6318-01**	9.00		**EE**
(Watson Labs)				
TAB, PO, 500 mg, 100s ea	**00591-5347-01**	98.33		**AB**
1000s ea	**00591-5347-10**	805.89		**AB**
(PD-Rx Pharm) REPACK				
TAB, PO, 500 mg, 2s ea	**55289-0715-02**	30.27		**AB**
15s ea	**55289-0715-15**	47.78		**AB**
100s ea UD	**55289-0715-17**	205.42		**AB**
(Phys Total Care) REPACK				
TAB, PO, 500 mg, 30s ea	**54868-0159-03**	51.00		**AB**
60s ea	**54868-0159-00**	75.63		**EE**
100s ea	**54868-0159-02**	121.56		**EE**
PROBENECID AND COLCHICINE (Rising) colchicine/probenecid				
TAB, PO (USP)				
0.5 mg-500 mg, 100s ea	**64980-0149-01**	59.75		**AB**
PROBUCOL (Gallipot)				
POW, NA (U.S.P.)				
100 gm	**51552-0666-05**	233.10		
(Medisca)				
POW, NA (U.S.P.)				
25 gm	**38779-0498-04**	150.00		
100 gm	**38779-0498-05**	459.00		
500 gm	**38779-0498-08**	1530.00		
(PCCA)				
POW, NA (U.S.P.)				
1 gm	**51927-2932-00**	0.75		
PROCAINAMIDE HCL (Gallipot) procainamide hydrochloride				
POW, NA, 25 gm	**51552-0397-04**	21.28		
100 gm	**51552-0397-05**	69.65		
(Hospira)				
SOL, IV, 500 mg/ml, 2 ml 25s	**00409-1903-01**	268.50	235.00	**AP**
(Medisca)				
POW, NA (U.S.P.)				
25 gm	**38779-0400-04**	43.50		
100 gm	**38779-0400-05**	120.00		
500 gm	**38779-0400-08**	435.00		
1000 gm	**38779-0400-09**	546.00		
(PCCA)				
POW, NA (U.S.P.)				
1 gm	**51927-3115-00**	2.28		
(Phys Total Care) REPACK				
CAP, PO, 250 mg, 100s ea	**54868-3468-00**	51.58		**EE**
500 mg, 100s ea	**54868-3469-00**	30.67		**EE**
SOL, IV (VIAL,FLIPTOP)				
100 mg/ml, 10 ml 25s	**54868-3136-00**	93.42		**AP**
PROCAINAMIDE HYDROCHLORIDE				
(Gallipot) *See PROCAINAMIDE HCL*				
(Hospira) *See PROCAINAMIDE HCL*				
(Hospira)				
SOL, IJ (25X10ML,FTV)				
100 mg/ml, 10 ml 25s	**00409-1902-01**	268.50	235.00	**AP**
(Medisca) *See PROCAINAMIDE HCL*				
(PCCA) *See PROCAINAMIDE HCL*				
PROCAINE				
(Spectrum Pharmacy) *See PROCAINE BASE*				
PROCAINE BASE (Spectrum Pharmacy) procaine				
POW, NA, 25 gm	**49452-6040-01**	215.25		
100 gm	**49452-6040-02**	570.50		
PROCAINE HCL (Amend) procaine hydrochloride				
CRY, NA (U.S.P.)				
125 gm	**17317-0452-01**	44.10		
125 gm	**17317-0452-04**	18.20		
2270 gm	**17317-0452-05**	182.00		
3632 gm	**17317-0452-08**	770.00		
(Consolidated Midland)				
SOL, IJ (VIAL)				
1%, 30 ml	**00223-8350-30**	3.50		**EE**
2%, 30 ml	**00223-8362-30**	4.00		**EE**
(Gallipot)				
CRY, NA (U.S.P.)				
100 gm	**51552-0505-05**	17.43		
454 gm	**51552-0505-06**	57.19		
(Medisca)				
CRY, NA (U.S.P.)				
100 gm	**38779-0156-05**	39.00		
500 gm	**38779-0156-08**	147.00		
1000 gm	**38779-0156-09**	240.00		
(PCCA)				
CRY, NA (U.S.P.)				
1 gm	**51927-1427-00**	0.63		
(Spectrum Pharmacy)				
CRY, NA (U.S.P.)				
100 gm	**49452-6050-01**	176.40		
500 gm	**49452-6050-02**	535.50		
5000 gm	**49452-6050-03**	2978.50		
PROCAINE HYDROCHLORIDE				
(Amend) *See PROCAINE HCL*				
(Consolidated Midland) *See PROCAINE HCL*				
(Gallipot) *See PROCAINE HCL*				
(Hospira) *See NOVOCAIN*				
(Medisca) *See PROCAINE HCL*				
(PCCA) *See PROCAINE HCL*				
(Spectrum Pharmacy) *See PROCAINE HCL*				
PROCALAMINE (B. Braun) amino acids and electrolytes				
SOL, IV (W/3% GLYCERIN)				
1000 ml	**00264-1915-00**	40.00		
(W/SOLID STOPPER) 1000 ml	**00264-1915-07**	30.52		
PROCARBAZINE HYDROCHLORIDE				
(Sigma-Tau) *See MATULANE*				
PROCARDIA (Pfizer) nifedipine				
SGL, PO, 10 mg, 100s ea	**00069-2600-66**	114.92	95.77	**AB**
(PD-Rx Pharm) REPACK				
SGL, PO, 10 mg, 30s ea	**55289-0290-30**	48.41		**AB**
50s ea	**55289-0290-50**	81.83		**AB**
PROCARDIA XL (Pfizer) nifedipine				
TER, PO (FILM-COATED)				
30 mg, 100s ea UD	**00069-2650-41**	255.82	213.18	**AB2**
100s ea	**00069-2650-66**	229.60	191.33	**AB2**
300s ea	**00069-2650-72**	688.79	573.99	**AB2**
60 mg, 100s ea UD	**00069-2660-41**	442.70	368.92	**AB2**
100s ea	**00069-2660-66**	397.31	331.09	**AB2**
300s ea	**00069-2660-72**	1191.91	993.26	**AB2**
90 mg, 100s ea	**00069-2670-66**	458.40	382.00	**BC**
(PD-Rx Pharm) REPACK				
TER, PO (FILM-COATED)				
30 mg, 30s ea	**55289-0323-30**	97.50		**AB2**
100s ea	**55289-0323-01**	324.99		**AB2**
60 mg, 30s ea	**55289-0357-30**	168.72		**AB2**
100s ea	**55289-0357-01**	568.40		**AB2**
(Phys Total Care) REPACK				
TER, PO, 30 mg, 30s ea	**54868-1006-02**	70.43		**AB2**
100s ea	**54868-1006-03**	217.04		**AB2**
60 mg, 10s ea	**54868-1008-00**	36.01		**AB2**
30s ea	**54868-1008-01**	104.29		**AB2**
100s ea	**54868-1008-02**	323.65		**AB2**
90 mg, 30s ea	**54868-1443-03**	125.94		**BC**
PROCHIEVE (Ascend) progesterone				
GEL, VG (PREFILLED APPLICATORS)				
4%, 1.45 gm 6s	**55056-0406-01**	51.34		
(Columbia Labs)				
GEL, VG (18X1.45GM,SINGLE-USE)				
8%, 1.45 gm 18s	**55056-1601-08**	256.68		
PROCHLORPERAZINE (G&W)				
SUP, RC, 25 mg, 12s ea	**00713-0135-12**	39.98		**AB**
(Paddock) *See COMPRO*				
(A-S Medication) REPACK				
SUP, RC, 25 mg, 3s ea	**54569-4720-02**	11.12		**AB**
12s ea	**54569-4720-00**	44.48		**AB**
(A-S Medication) prochlorperazine maleate				
TAB, PO, 10 mg, 30s ea	**54569-0355-00**	26.70		**EE**
PROCHLORPERAZINE (Altura) REPACK				
SUP, RC, 25 mg, 12s ea	**63874-0806-12**	35.70		
(Core) REPACK				
SUP, RC, 25 mg, 2s ea	**33358-0301-02**	12.57		
12s ea	**33358-0301-12**	46.84		
(Core) prochlorperazine maleate				
TAB, PO, 5 mg, 20s ea	**33358-0299-20**	12.10		
30s ea	**33358-0299-30**	23.37		
10 mg, 10s ea	**33358-0300-10**	13.53		
20s ea	**33358-0300-20**	27.00		
30s ea	**33358-0300-30**	40.39		
60s ea	**33358-0300-60**	75.65		
PROCHLORPERAZINE (DHS, Inc.) REPACK				
SUP, RC, 25 mg, 12s ea	**55887-0220-12**	38.63		
(Dispensing Solutions) REPACK				
SUP, RC, 25 mg, 3s ea	**66336-0150-03**	14.46		
6s ea	**66336-0150-06**	18.24		
12s ea	**55045-2400-02**	39.50		**AB**
(Dispensing Solutions) prochlorperazine maleate				
TAB, PO, 5 mg, 6s ea	**66336-0434-06**	10.74		
10s ea	**66336-0434-10**	17.90		
10 mg, 12s ea	**55045-1126-04**	13.80		**AB**
(HomeMed) REPACK				
TAB, PO, 5 mg, 6s ea	**51655-0093-87**	3.99		
10 mg, 4s ea	**51655-0294-89**	2.66		
PROCHLORPERAZINE (Palmetto) REPACK				
SUP, RC, 25 mg, 3s ea	**23490-6174-01**	10.00		
(PD-Rx Pharm) REPACK				
SUP, RC, 25 mg, 2s ea	**55289-0119-02**	11.82		**AB**
6s ea	**55289-0119-06**	25.18		**AB**
(Pharma Pac) REPACK				
SUP, RC, 25 mg, 6s ea	**52959-0355-06**	33.00		**EE**
12s ea	**52959-0355-12**	60.25		**EE**
(Phys Total Care) REPACK				
SUP, RC, 25 mg, 6s ea	**54868-3112-01**	27.57		**AB**
12s ea	**54868-3112-00**	49.14		**AB**
(Southwood) REPACK				
SUP, RC, 25 mg, 12s ea	**58016-6506-01**	34.00		**EE**
PROCHLORPERAZINE EDISYLATE (Baxter)				
SOL, IJ (VIAL, DOSETTE)				
5 mg/ml, 2 ml	**00641-0491-21**	3.00		**AP**
2 ml 25s	**00641-0491-25**	75.00		**AP**
(Bedford)				
SOL, IJ (USP)				
5 mg/ml, 2 ml 10s	**55390-0077-10**	36.00		**AP**
(U.S.P., M.D.V.) 5 mg/ml, 10 ml	**55390-0077-01**	24.00		**AP**
(Medisca)				
POW, NA (U.S.P.)				
1 gm	**38779-2165-06**	84.00		
5 gm (1X25GM)	**38779-2165-03**	324.00		
25 gm	**38779-2165-04**	1836.00		
(PCCA)				
POW, NA (USP)				
1 gm	**51927-2206-00**	87.00		
(Phys Total Care) REPACK				
SOL, IJ (CARPUJECT)				
5 mg/ml, 2 ml 10s	**54868-4137-00**	67.45		**EE**
(M.D.V.) 5 mg/ml, 10 ml	**54868-0261-00**	150.87		**EE**
PROCHLORPERAZINE MALEATE FUL				
TAB, PO, 5 mg, 100s ea		39.86		
10 mg, 100s ea		57.66		
(Breckenridge Pharm)				
TAB, PO, 5 mg, 100s ea	**51991-0196-01**	59.50		**AB**
10 mg, 100s ea	**51991-0197-01**	89.50		**AB**
(Cadista)				
TAB, PO, 5 mg, 100s ea	**59746-0113-06**	59.35		**AB**
10 mg, 100s ea	**59746-0115-06**	89.25		**AB**

PROD/MFR	NDC	AWP	DP	OBC
(Gallipot)				
POW, NA (U.S.P.)				
20 gm	**51552-0074-09**	30.80		
100 gm	**51552-0074-05**	147.00		
(Hawkins)				
POW, NA (USP)				
25 gm	**63370-0198-25**	104.00		
100 gm	**63370-0198-35**	402.00		
500 gm	**63370-0198-45**	1740.00		
(Letco)				
POW, NA (U.S.P.)				
25 gm	**62991-1122-04**	87.00		
100 gm	**62991-1122-02**	285.00		
(Medisca)				
POW, NA (U.S.P.)				
25 gm	**38779-0180-04**	117.00		
100 gm	**38779-0180-05**	447.00		
500 gm	**38779-0180-08**	1677.00		
(Mylan)				
TAB, PO, 5 mg, 100s ea	**00378-5105-01**	59.50		**AB**
10 mg, 100s ea	**00378-5110-01**	89.50		**AB**
(PCCA)				
POW, NA (U.S.P.)				
1 gm	**51927-2134-00**	6.90		
(Sandoz)				
TAB, PO (FILM-COATED)				
5 mg, 100s ea	**00781-5020-01**	59.25		**AB**
10 mg, 100s ea	**00781-5021-01**	89.00		**AB**
(Spectrum Pharmacy)				
POW, NA (U.S.P., N.F.)				
5 gm	**49452-6053-01**	107.45		
25 gm	**49452-6053-02**	191.10		
100 gm	**49452-6053-03**	700.00		
(U.S.P.)				
500 gm	**49452-6053-05**	2422.00		
(Teva)				
TAB, PO (10X10,FILM-COATED)				
5 mg, 100s ea UD	**00182-8210-89**	59.50		**AB**
(USP,FILM-COATED)				
5 mg, 100s ea	**00093-9643-01**	54.18		**AB**
(10X10,FILM-COATED)				
10 mg, 100s ea UD	**00182-8211-89**	89.50		**AB**
(FILM-COATED)				
10 mg, 100s ea	**00172-3691-60**	84.99		**AB**
(USP,FILM-COATED)				
10 mg, 100s ea	**00093-9652-01**	81.41		**AB**
(UDL)				
TAB, PO (10X10)				
5 mg, 100s ea UD	**51079-0541-20**	61.29		**AB**
10 mg, 100s ea UD	**51079-0542-20**	92.08		**AB**
(A-S Medication)				
REPACK				
TAB, PO (FILM-COATED)				
5 mg, 6s ea	**54569-0350-05**	3.58		**AB**
10 mg, 10s ea	**54569-0355-02**	8.90		**EE**
(Aidarex)				
REPACK				
TAB, PO (FILM-COATED)				
10 mg, 30s ea	**33261-0550-30**	40.52		**AB**
60s ea	**33261-0550-60**	81.03		**AB**
90s ea	**33261-0550-90**	121.55		**AB**
120s ea	**33261-0550-02**	162.08		**AB**
(Altura)				
REPACK				
TAB, PO (FILM-COATED)				
5 mg, 6s ea	**63874-0525-06**	10.74		**AB**
10s ea	**63874-0525-10**	26.16		**AB**
12s ea	**63874-0525-12**	31.40		**AB**
15s ea	**63874-0525-15**	39.24		**AB**
20s ea	**63874-0525-20**	52.32		**AB**
30s ea	**63874-0525-30**	78.48		**AB**
10 mg, 6s ea	**63874-0490-06**	7.37		**AB**
8s ea	**63874-0490-08**	9.83		**AB**
10s ea	**63874-0490-10**	13.12		**AB**
12s ea	**63874-0490-12**	10.74		**AB**
15s ea	**63874-0490-15**	19.86		**AB**
20s ea	**63874-0490-20**	26.24		**AB**
28s ea	**63874-0490-28**	36.73		**AB**
30s ea	**63874-0490-30**	39.36		**AB**
60s ea	**63874-0490-60**	73.72		**AB**
100s ea	**63874-0490-01**	131.20		**AB**
(Bryant Ranch)				
REPACK				
TAB, PO, 5 mg, 20s ea	**63629-1841-01**	11.80		
10 mg, 10s ea	**63629-1335-01**	11.90		
20s ea	**63629-1335-03**	23.80		
30s ea	**63629-1335-02**	35.70		

PROD/MFR	NDC	AWP	DP	OBC
(DHS, Inc.)				
REPACK				
TAB, PO (FILM-COATED)				
5 mg, 30s ea	**55887-0395-30**	16.50		**AB**
10 mg, 30s ea	**55887-0619-30**	21.20		**AB**
(Dispensing Solutions)				
REPACK				
TAB, PO (FILM-COATED)				
5 mg, 10s ea	**55045-1696-02**	7.85		**AB**
10 mg, 5s ea	**55045-1126-03**	5.75		**AB**
10s ea	**55045-1126-02**	11.50		**AB**
15s ea	**66336-0921-15**	13.43		**AB**
20s ea	**55045-1126-07**	23.00		**AB**
30s ea	**55045-1126-08**	34.50		**AB**
60s ea	**55045-1126-06**	69.00		
60s ea	**66336-0921-60**	53.70		**AB**
(Palmetto)				
REPACK				
TAB, PO, 5 mg, 6s ea	**23490-6512-01**	6.89		
10s ea	**23490-6512-02**	8.80		
10 mg, 30s ea	**23490-6509-03**	34.50		
(PD-Rx Pharm)				
REPACK				
TAB, PO, 5 mg, 10s ea	**55289-0568-10**	10.65		**AB**
12s ea	**55289-0568-12**	15.71		**AB**
15s ea	**58864-0702-01**	11.26		**AB**
20s ea	**55289-0568-20**	18.74		**AB**
30s ea	**55289-0568-30**	20.00		**AB**
10 mg, 4s ea	**55289-0224-04**	6.30		
(USP)				
10 mg, 4s ea	**43063-0160-04**	7.46		**AB**
6s ea	**43063-0160-06**	7.95		**AB**
10s ea	**55289-0224-06**	17.12		**AB**
12s ea	**55289-0224-12**	17.12		**AB**
(REDI-SCRIPT)				
10 mg, 42s ea	**58864-0644-42**	19.00		**AB**
(Pharma Pac)				
REPACK				
TAB, PO, 10 mg, 10s ea	**52959-0476-10**	9.87		**EE**
15s ea	**52959-0476-15**	13.65		**EE**
(FILM-COATED)				
10 mg, 20s ea	**52959-0476-20**	19.74		**AB**
24s ea	**52959-0476-24**	23.57		**EE**
30s ea	**52959-0476-30**	29.61		**EE**
60s ea	**52959-0476-60**	59.19		**EE**
120s ea	**52959-0476-02**	118.35		**EE**
(Phys Total Care)				
REPACK				
TAB, PO, 5 mg, 15s ea	**54868-4721-01**	8.91		
30s ea	**54868-4721-00**	13.35		
(FILM-COATED)				
5 mg, 60s ea	**54868-4721-02**	22.20		**AB**
100s ea	**54868-4721-03**	24.07		
10 mg, 10s ea	**54868-1082-01**	5.40		**EE**
15s ea	**54868-1082-00**	6.63		**EE**
20s ea	**54868-1082-02**	7.83		**AB**
30s ea	**54868-1082-04**	10.23		**AB**
60s ea	**54868-1082-05**	16.44		**AB**
90s ea	**54868-1082-06**	23.15		**EE**
100s ea	**54868-1082-03**	25.65		**EE**
100s ea	**54888-1082-03**	33.76		**AB**
(Physician Partner)				
REPACK				
TAB, PO, 5 mg, 30s ea	**21695-0571-30**	35.61		**AB**
(FILM-COATED)				
10 mg, 30s ea	**21695-0572-30**	51.00		
(Quality Care Prod)				
REPACK				
TAB, PO (FILM-COATED)				
10 mg, 5s ea	**35356-0325-05**	17.16		**AB**
60s ea	**35356-0564-60**	145.80		**AB**
(FILM-COATED)				
10 mg, 100s ea	**35356-0325-00**	115.00		**AB**
(Southwood)				
REPACK				
TAB, PO, 5 mg, 12s ea	**58016-0326-12**	31.40		**AB**
20s ea	**58016-0326-20**	21.00		**AB**
30s ea	**58016-0326-30**	31.49		
60s ea	**58016-0326-60**	62.98		
90s ea	**58016-0326-90**	94.46		
100s ea	**58016-0326-00**	104.96		
10 mg, 8s ea	**58016-0706-08**	5.32		
30s ea	**58016-0706-30**	19.95		**AB**
60s ea	**58016-0706-60**	39.90		**AB**
90s ea	**58016-0706-90**	59.85		**AB**
100s ea	**58016-0706-00**	66.50		**AB**
120s ea	**58016-0706-02**	79.80		**AB**
150s ea	**58016-0706-03**	99.75		**AB**

PROD/MFR	NDC	AWP	DP	OBC
(Stat Rx)				
REPACK				
TAB, PO (FILM-COATED)				
10 mg, 10s ea	**16590-0327-10**	8.95		**AB**
60s ea	**16590-0327-60**	53.70		**AB**
(Vibranta)				
REPACK				
TAB, PO, 5 mg, 10s ea	**57866-6299-02**	1.73		
30s ea	**57866-6299-01**	18.95		**AB**
10 mg, 30s ea	**57866-6298-01**	27.95		**AB**
PROCHLORPERAZINE MESYLATE (PCCA)				
POW, NA (BP)				
1 gm	**51927-3489-00**	71.40		
PROCRIT (Centocor)				
epoetin alfa				
SOL, IJ (VIAL)				
2000 u/ml, 1 ml 6s	**59676-0302-01**	218.16		
(VOLUME PACK VIAL)				
2000 u/ml, 1 ml 25s	**59676-0302-02**	909.00		
(VIAL)				
3000 u/ml, 1 ml 6s	**59676-0303-01**	327.24		
(VOLUME PACK VIAL)				
3000 u/ml, 1 ml 25s	**59676-0303-02**	1363.50		
(VIAL)				
4000 u/ml, 1 ml 6s	**59676-0304-01**	436.32		
(VOLUME PACK VIAL)				
4000 u/ml, 1 ml 25s	**59676-0304-02**	1818.00		
(VIAL)				
10000 u/ml, 1 ml 6s	**59676-0310-01**	1090.80		
(VOLUME PACK VIAL)				
10000 u/ml, 1 ml 25s	**59676-0310-02**	4545.00		
(4X2ML,MDV)				
10000 u/ml, 2 ml 4s	**59676-0312-04**	1454.40		**EE**
(MULTIDOSE)				
20000 u/ml, 1 ml 4s	**59676-0320-04**	1454.40		
(PF)				
40000 u/ml, 1 ml 4s	**59676-0340-01**	2908.80		
(Phys Total Care)				
REPACK				
SOL, IJ (S.D.V.)				
10000 u/ml, 1 ml	**54868-2523-00**	181.24		
1 ml 6s	**54868-2523-01**	1167.89		
(M.D.V,1X4ML)				
20000 u/ml, 4 ml	**54868-5673-01**	1556.54		
(MDV)				
20000 u/ml, 6 ml	**54868-5673-00**	2333.84		
(SDV,1MLX4)				
40000 u/ml, 1 ml 4s	**54868-5802-00**	3111.12		
PROCTO-KIT 1% (Ranbaxy Labs)				
hydrocortisone				
CRE, RC (W/APPLICATOR)				
1%, 28.35 gm	**10631-0405-01**	30.37		**AT**
PROCTO-KIT 2.5% (Ranbaxy Labs)				
hydrocortisone				
CRE, RC (W/APPLICATOR)				
2.5%, 28.35 gm	**10631-0406-01**	33.85		**AT**
PROCTO-PAK (Rising)				
hydrocortisone				
CRE, RC (W/APPLICATOR)				
1%, 30 gm	**64980-0302-30**	41.50		**AT**
PROCTOCARE-HC (Nucare Pharm)				
REPACK				
hydrocortisone				
CRE, RC, 2.5%, 30 gm	**66267-0947-30**	14.62		**AT**
PROCTOCORT (Salix Pharm)				
hydrocortisone				
CRE, RC, 1%, 28.35 gm	**65649-0501-30**	106.42		**AT**
(Salix Pharm)				
hydrocortisone acetate				
SUP, RC, 30 mg, 12s ea	**65649-0511-12**	118.30		
PROCTOCREAM-HC (Alaven)				
hydrocortisone				
CRE, TP, 2.5%, 30 gm	**00091-4640-24**	65.08		**AT**
(Phys Total Care)				
REPACK				
CRE, TP, 2.5%, 30 gm	**54868-4232-00**	20.34		**AT**

PROD/MFR NDC AWP DP OBC

PROCTOFOAM (Alaven)
pramoxine hydrochloride
FOA, TP (NON-STEROID)
1%, 15 gm........ **00091-4750-20** 43.33

PROCTOFOAM-HC (Alaven)
hydrocortisone acetate/pramoxine hydrochloride
FOA, TP (1X10GM)
1%-1%, 10 gm....... **68220-0142-10** 71.06

(Phys Total Care)
REPACK
FOA, RC, 1%-1%, 10 gm .. **54868-1225-00** 81.02 BX

PROCTOSOL-HC (Ranbaxy Labs)
hydrocortisone
CRE, RC, 2.5%, 28.35 gm . **10631-0407-01** 24.95 AT

(A-S Medication)
REPACK
CRE, RC, 2.5%, 30 gm .... **54569-4329-00** 29.40 AT

(DHS, Inc.)
REPACK
CRE, RC, 2.5%, 30 gm .... **55887-0252-01** 34.08 AT

PROCTOZONE-HC (Rising)
hydrocortisone
CRE, RC, 2.5%, 30 gm .... **64980-0301-30** 24.95 AT

(Physician Partner)
REPACK
CRE, RC (1X30GM)
2.5%, 30 gm......... **21695-0430-30** 49.90 AT

PRODRIN (Wraser Pharm)
acetaminophen/caffeine/isometheptene mucate
TAB, PO (CAPLET)
500 mg-20 mg-130 mg,
50s ea............ **66992-0165-50** 74.63

(Stat Rx)
REPACK
TAB, PO (CAPLET)
500 mg-20 mg-130 mg,
30s ea............ **16590-0844-30** 35.00
50s ea............ **16590-0844-50** 65.00
60s ea............ **16590-0844-60** 55.00
90s ea............ **16590-0844-90** 95.00
100s ea........... **16590-0844-71** 105.00

PRODROX (Legere)
hydroxyprogesterone caproate
OIL, IM (VIAL)
250 mg/ml, 5 ml ..... **25332-0088-05** 29.95 EE

PROFERRIN-FORTE (Colorado Biolabs)
folic acid/iron
TAB, PO, 1 mg-12 mg,
90s ea............ **67181-0216-90** 52.93

PROFILNINE SD (Grifols USA, Inc.)
factor ix complex human
PDS, IV (1000IU FIX/10ML SDV)
1 iu, ea............ **68516-3200-04** 0.90 0.75
(1500IU FIX/10ML SDV)
1 iu, ea............ **68516-3200-05** 0.90 0.75
(APPROX. 500 IU/VIAL)
1 iu, ea............ **68516-3200-02** 0.90 0.75

PROFLAVINE HEMISULFATE (PCCA)
proflavine sulfate
POW, NA, 1 gm......... **51927-1822-00** 5.76

PROFLAVINE SULFATE
(PCCA) *See PROFLAVINE HEMISULFATE*

PROGESTERONE (Amend)
POW, NA (U.S.P.)
5 gm.............. **17317-0626-08** 8.40
(WETTABLE)
5 gm.............. **17317-0934-08** 8.40
(U.S.P.)
10 gm............. **17317-0626-01** 14.00
(WETTABLE)
10 gm............. **17317-0934-01** 14.00
(U.S.P.)
25 gm............. **17317-0626-02** 28.00
(WETTABLE)
25 gm............. **17317-0934-02** 28.00
(U.S.P.)
100 gm............ **17317-0626-03** 105.00
(WETTABLE)
100 gm............ **17317-0934-03** 105.00

(APP) *See PROGESTERONE IN SESAME OIL*
(Ascend) *See PROCHIEVE*
(Columbia Labs) *See CRINONE*
(Columbia Labs) *See PROCHIEVE*
(Ferring) *See ENDOMETRIN*

PROGESTERONE (Gallipot)
progesterone, micronized
POW, NA (1X1GM,USP)
1 gm.............. **51552-0829-01** 5.46 3.90

PROGESTERONE (Gallipot)
(U.S.P.)
1 gm.............. **51552-0005-01** 5.46
(WETTABLE,U.S.P.)
1 gm.............. **51552-0006-01** 7.35

(Gallipot)
progesterone, micronized
(1X10GM,USP)
10 gm............. **51552-0829-03** 18.06 12.90

PROGESTERONE (Gallipot)
(U.S.P.)
10 gm............. **51552-0005-03** 18.06
(WETTABLE,U.S.P.)
10 gm............. **51552-0006-03** 24.50
(1X25GM,USP,MICRONIZED)
25 gm............. **51552-0738-04** 27.30 19.50

(Gallipot)
progesterone, micronized
(1X25GM,USP)
25 gm............. **51552-0829-04** 27.30 19.50

PROGESTERONE (Gallipot)
(U.S.P.)
25 gm............. **51552-0005-04** 30.10
(WETTABLE,U.S.P.)
25 gm............. **51552-0006-04** 36.75
(1X100GM,USP,MICRONIZED)
100 gm............ **51552-0738-05** 70.70 50.50

(Gallipot)
progesterone, micronized
(1X100GM,USP)
100 gm............ **51552-0829-05** 70.70 50.50

PROGESTERONE (Gallipot)
(U.S.P.)
100 gm............ **51552-0005-05** 78.40
(WETTABLE,U.S.P.)
100 gm............ **51552-0006-05** 102.90
(1X500GM,USP,MICRONIZED)
500 gm............ **51552-0738-06** 315.00 225.00

(Gallipot)
progesterone, micronized
(1X500GM,USP)
500 gm............ **51552-0829-06** 315.00 225.00

PROGESTERONE (Gallipot)
(1X1000GM,USP,MICRONIZED)
1000 gm........... **51552-0738-07** 518.00 370.00

(Gallipot)
progesterone, micronized
(1X1000GM,USP)
1000 gm........... **51552-0829-07** 518.00 370.00

PROGESTERONE (Gallipot)
(MILLED,U.S.P.)
1000 gm........... **51552-0643-07** 628.60
(U.S.P.,MICRONIZED)
1000 gm........... **51552-0005-07** 588.00
(WETTABLE,U.S.P.)
1000 gm........... **51552-0006-07** 805.00

(Gallipot)
progesterone, micronized
(1X5000GM,USP)
5000 gm........... **51552-0829-08** 2520.00 1800.00

PROGESTERONE (Hawkins)
POW, NA (USP,YAM)
100 gm............ **63370-0200-35** 196.00
500 gm............ **63370-0200-45** 900.00
5000 gm........... **63370-0200-55** 7200.00

(Hawkins) *See PROGESTERONE WETTABLE*

(Letco)
POW, NA (U.S.P.,MICRONIZED)
100 gm............ **62991-1124-02** 144.00

(Medisca)
POW, NA (U.S.P., WETTABLE)
10 gm............. **38779-0057-01** 45.00
(U.S.P.,MICRONIZED)
10 gm............. **38779-0043-01** 71.25 12.60
25 gm............. **38779-0043-04** 96.00
(USP, WETTABLE)
25 gm............. **38779-0057-04** 66.00
(U.S.P., WETTABLE)
100 gm............ **38779-0057-05** 237.00
(U.S.P.,MICRONIZED)
100 gm............ **38779-0043-05** 285.00
(MILLED, U.S.P.)
1000 gm........... **38779-0310-09** 1453.50
(U.S.P., WETTABLE)
1000 gm........... **38779-0057-09** 1515.00
(U.S.P.,MICRONIZED)
1000 gm........... **38779-0043-09** 1687.50

(Paddock) *See PROGESTERONE WETTABLE*

(PCCA)
POW, NA (U.S.P.; WETTABLE POWDER)
1 gm.............. **51927-9017-00** 7.80

(Solvay) *See PROMETRIUM*

(Spectrum Pharmacy)
POW, NA (MILLED/U.S.P.)
25 gm............. **49452-6070-02** 143.15
(USP, YAM,MICRONIZED)
25 gm............. **49452-6061-02** 91.70
(WETTABLE/U.S.P.)
25 gm............. **49452-6080-02** 143.15
(MILLED/U.S.P.)
100 gm............ **49452-6070-03** 430.50
(USP, YAM,MICRONIZED)
100 gm............ **49452-6061-03** 278.95
(WETTABLE/U.S.P.)
100 gm............ **49452-6080-03** 430.50
(MILLED/U.S.P.)
500 gm............ **49452-6070-06** 1722.00
(USP, YAM,MICRONIZED)
500 gm............ **49452-6061-04** 1134.00
(WETTABLE/U.S.P.)
500 gm............ **49452-6080-06** 1753.60
(MILLED/U.S.P.)
1000 gm........... **49452-6070-04** 2583.00
(USP, YAM,MICRONIZED)
1000 gm........... **49452-6061-05** 1767.50
(WETTABLE/U.S.P.)
1000 gm........... **49452-6080-04** 2810.50

(Watson Labs)
OIL, IM ((VIAL),USP)
50 mg/ml, 10 ml ..... **00591-3128-79** 38.75 2.50 AO

(X-Gen)
POW, NA (USP,WETTABLE)
10 gm............. **39822-6100-01** 14.00
25 gm............. **39822-6100-03** 32.50
100 gm............ **39822-6100-07** 89.50

PROGESTERONE IN SESAME OIL (APP)
progesterone
OIL, IM (M.D.V.)
50 mg/ml, 10 ml ..... **63323-0261-10** 38.75 AO

PROGESTERONE MICRONIZED (Hawkins)
progesterone, micronized
POW, NA (USP,SOY)
100 gm............ **63370-0199-35** 224.00
(YAM)
100 gm............ **63370-0204-35** 192.00
(USP,SOY)
500 gm............ **63370-0199-45** 992.00
(YAM)
500 gm............ **63370-0204-45** 868.80
(USP,SOY)
1000 gm........... **63370-0199-50** 1752.00
(YAM)
1000 gm........... **63370-0200-50** 1460.00
1000 gm........... **63370-0204-50** 1416.00
(USP,SOY)
5000 gm........... **63370-0199-55** 8300.00
(YAM)
5000 gm........... **63370-0204-55** 6600.00
(USP,SOY)
25000 gm **63370-0199-62** 41200.00
(YAM)
25000 gm **63370-0204-62** 40800.00

(Letco)
POW, NA, 100 gm........ **62991-2184-01** 210.00
100 gm............ **62991-2184-02** 825.00
(SOY, U.S.P. 23)
100 gm............ **62991-2504-02** 240.00
500 gm............ **62991-1124-03** 660.00
500 gm............ **62991-2184-03** 1470.00
(SOY, U.S.P. 23)
500 gm............ **62991-2504-03** 1125.00
1000 gm........... **62991-2184-04** 6450.00
(SOY, U.S.P.23, 1X1000GM)
1000 gm........... **62991-2504-04** 1920.00
5000 gm........... **62991-1124-05** 5550.00

(Medisca)
POW, NA (U.S.P.)
500 gm............ **38779-0043-08** 1200.00

PROD/MFR	NDC	AWP	DP	OBC
(PCCA)				
POW, NA (U.S.P.)				
1 gm	**51927-1046-00**	5.10		
1 gm	**51927-3530-00**	6.00		
(B&B Pharm, Inc)				
REPACK				
POW, NA, 100 gm	**63275-9981-05**	129.00		
500 gm	**63275-9981-08**	1000.00		
1000 gm	**63275-9981-09**	1690.00		
PROGESTERONE WETTABLE (Hawkins)				
progesterone				
POW, NA (U.S.P.,YAM)				
100 gm	**63370-0202-35**	200.00		
(Hawkins)				
progesterone, wettable				
(U.S.P.)				
100 gm	**63370-0201-35**	280.00		
(Hawkins)				
progesterone				
(U.S.P.,YAM)				
500 gm	**63370-0202-45**	1540.00		
1000 gm	**63370-0202-50**	7580.00		
(Hawkins)				
progesterone, wettable				
(U.S.P.)				
1000 gm	**63370-0201-50**	2300.00		
5000 gm	**63370-0201-55**	11000.00		
(Medisca)				
POW, NA, 500 gm	**38779-0057-08**	897.00		
(Paddock)				
progesterone				
POW, NA (USP)				
100 gm	**00574-0431-01**	170.00		
(Spectrum Pharmacy)				
progesterone, wettable				
POW, NA (1X25GM)				
25 gm	**49452-6081-01**	98.00		
(1X100GM)				
100 gm	**49452-6081-02**	347.90		
(1X500GM)				
500 gm	**49452-6081-03**	1403.50		
(1X1000GM)				
1000 gm	**49452-6081-04**	1967.00		
PROGESTERONE WETTABLE MICROCRYSTALLINE (Letco)				
progesterone, wettable microcrystalline				
POW, NA, 25 gm	**62991-1123-01**	75.00		
100 gm	**62991-1123-02**	225.00		
500 gm	**62991-1123-03**	900.00		
1000 gm	**62991-1123-04**	1560.00		
PROGESTERONE, MICRONIZED				
(Gallipot) *See PROGESTERONE*				
(Hawkins) *See PROGESTERONE MICRONIZED*				
(Letco) *See PROGESTERONE MICRONIZED*				
(Medisca) *See PROGESTERONE MICRONIZED*				
(PCCA) *See PROGESTERONE MICRONIZED*				
PROGESTERONE, WETTABLE				
(Cutispharma) *See FIRST-PROGESTERONE VGS 100*				
(Cutispharma) *See FIRST-PROGESTERONE VGS 200*				
(Cutispharma) *See FIRST-PROGESTERONE VGS 25*				
(Cutispharma) *See FIRST-PROGESTERONE VGS 400*				
(Cutispharma) *See FIRST-PROGESTERONE VGS 50*				
(Hawkins) *See PROGESTERONE WETTABLE*				
(Medisca) *See PROGESTERONE WETTABLE*				
(Spectrum Pharmacy) *See PROGESTERONE WETTABLE*				
PROGESTERONE, WETTABLE MICROCRYSTALLINE				
(Letco) *See PROGESTERONE WETTABLE MICROCRYSTALLINE*				
PROGLYCEM (Teva)				
diazoxide				
SUS, PO, 50 mg/ml, 30 ml	**00575-6200-30**	189.47		
PROGRAF (Astellas)				
tacrolimus				
CAP, PO, 0.5 mg, 100s ea	**00469-0607-73**	237.84		
1 mg, 100s ea	**00469-0617-73**	475.68		
(10X10,BLISTER PACK)				
1 mg, 100s ea UD	**00469-0617-11**	475.68		
5 mg, 100s ea	**00469-0657-73**	2378.40		
(10X10,BLISTER PACK)				
5 mg, 100s ea UD	**00469-0657-11**	2378.40		
SOL, IV (AMP,PF)				
5 mg/ml, 1 ml	**00469-3016-01**	163.94		

PROD/MFR	NDC	AWP	DP	OBC
(AQ)				
REPACK				
CAP, PO, 1 mg, 100s ea	**66105-0549-10**	500.50		
(Physician Partner)				
REPACK				
CAP, PO, 1 mg, 100s ea	**21695-0170-00**	952.88		
PROHANCE (Bracco Diag)				
gadoteridol				
SOL, IV (S.D.V.)				
279.3 mg/ml,				
5 ml 5s	**00270-1111-04**	189.06	151.25	
(S.D. SRN,PREFILLED)				
279.3 mg/ml,				
10 ml 5s	**00270-1111-16**	387.50	310.00	
(S.D.V.)				
279.3 mg/ml,				
10 ml 5s	**00270-1111-01**	370.94	296.75	
15 ml 5s	**00270-1111-02**	542.81	434.25	
(S.D. SRN,PREFILLED)				
279.3 mg/ml,				
17 ml 5s	**00270-1111-45**	587.50	470.00	
(S.D.V.)				
279.3 mg/ml,				
20 ml 5s	**00270-1111-03**	670.31	536.25	
(MDV, BULK PACKAGE)				
279.3 mg/ml,				
50 ml 5s	**00270-1111-70**	1762.50	1410.00	
PROLASTIN (Talecris)				
alpha-1 proteinase inhibitor human				
PDS, IV (W/20ML DILUENT,PF)				
1 mg, ea	**13533-0601-30**	0.46		
(W/40ML DILUENT,PF)				
1 mg, ea	**13533-0601-35**	0.46		
PROLASTIN-C (Talecris)				
alpha-1 proteinase inhibitor human				
PDS, IV (1000MG W/20ML DILUENT)				
1 mg, ea	**13533-0700-01**	0.46		
PROLEUKIN (Prometheus Labs)				
aldesleukin				
PDS, IV (PF,LYOPHILOZED)				
22 million iu, ea	**00078-0495-61**	1092.34		
(Phys Total Care)				
REPACK				
PDS, IV, 22 million iu, ea	**54868-5596-00**	950.44		
PROLEX DH (Blansett)				
hydrocodone bitartrate/potassium guaiacolsulfonate				
LIQ, PO, 4.5 mg/5 ml-300 mg/5 ml,				
480 ml, C-III	**51674-0212-07**	64.94		
PROLEX DM (Blansett)				
dm/k guai				
LIQ, PO (AF,SF)				
15 mg/5 ml-300 mg/5 ml,				
480 ml	**51674-0019-07**	53.25		
PROLEX PD (Blansett)				
guaifenesin/phenylephrine hydrochloride				
TER, PO, 600 mg-10 mg,				
100s ea	**51674-0126-01**	62.34		
PROLEX-D (Blansett)				
guaifenesin/phenylephrine hydrochloride				
TER, PO (DYE-FREE)				
600 mg-20 mg,				
100s ea	**51674-0124-01**	77.94		
PROLINE (PCCA)				
POW, NA (USP; (L))				
1 gm	**51927-2590-00**	1.92		
(Spectrum Pharmacy) *See L-PROLINE*				
PROMACET (MCR American)				
acetaminophen/butalbital				
TAB, PO, 650 mg-50 mg,				
100s ea	**58605-0524-01**	67.05		EE
PROMACOT (Truxton)				
promethazine hydrochloride				
TAB, PO, 25 mg, 1000s ea	**00463-6156-10**	15.00		EE
PROMACTA (Glaxo)				
eltrombopag olamine				
TAB, PO (FILM-COATED)				
25 mg, 30s ea	**00007-4640-13**	2158.20		
50 mg, 30s ea	**00007-4641-13**	4316.40		
PROMAR (Marlop)				
ferrous fum/folic acid/if/vit b12/vit c				
CAP, PO, 30s ea	**12939-0315-30**	25.45		

PROD/MFR	NDC	AWP	DP	OBC
PROMETH W/ DEXTROMETHORPHAN HYDROBROMIDE (Altura)				
REPACK				
dm/promethazine hcl				
SYR, PO, 15 mg/5 ml-6.25 mg/5 ml,				
120 ml	**63874-0707-12**	6.88		
480 ml	**63874-0707-48**	4.50		
PROMETH/CODEINE (Stat Rx)				
REPACK				
codeine phosphate/promethazine hydrochloride				
SYR, PO, 10 mg/5 ml-6.25 mg/5 ml,				
120 ml, C-V	**16590-0192-04**	15.00		
PROMETHAZINE (American Health)				
REPACK				
promethazine hydrochloride				
TAB, PO (USP,10X10)				
25 mg, 100s ea UD	**68084-0155-01**	54.15		BP
(Bryant Ranch)				
REPACK				
SYR, PO, 6.25 mg/5 ml,				
120 ml	**63629-1870-01**	7.71		
240 ml	**63629-1870-02**	15.43		
TAB, PO, 12.5 mg, 2s ea	**63629-1591-03**	1.37		
4s ea	**63629-1591-02**	2.74		
12s ea	**63629-1591-01**	8.23		
30s ea	**63629-1591-04**	20.54		
25 mg, 10s ea	**63629-1742-03**	6.99		
15s ea	**63629-1742-01**	7.59		
20s ea	**63629-1742-04**	12.32		
30s ea	**63629-1742-02**	14.99		
(Core)				
REPACK				
TAB, PO, 12.5 mg, 30s ea	**33358-0418-30**	25.99		
25 mg, 8s ea	**33358-0302-08**	14.20		
10s ea	**33358-0302-10**	17.75		
30s ea	**33358-0302-30**	53.25		
60s ea	**33358-0302-60**	106.50		
(DHS, Inc.)				
REPACK				
SUP, RC, 25 mg, 3s ea	**55887-0621-03**	15.47		
TAB, PO, 25 mg, 25s ea	**55887-0936-25**	33.33		
(Dispensing Solutions)				
REPACK				
TAB, PO, 25 mg, 10s ea	**66336-0085-10**	8.66		
12s ea	**66336-0085-12**	10.40		
30s ea	**66336-0085-30**	25.99		
(HomeMed)				
REPACK				
TAB, PO, 25 mg, 10s ea	**51655-0084-53**	16.89		EE
12s ea	**51655-0084-27**	4.20		EE
(IPI)				
REPACK				
TAB, PO, 25 mg, 10s ea	**18837-0127-10**	4.81		
60s ea	**18837-0127-60**	42.00		
(PD-Rx Pharm)				
REPACK				
SUP, RC, 25 mg, ea	**55289-0928-79**	8.08		
(USP)				
25 mg, 2s ea	**55289-0928-02**	10.04		
4s ea	**55289-0928-04**	45.28		
6s ea	**55289-0928-06**	15.13		
TAB, PO, 12.5 mg, 2s ea	**55289-0948-02**	5.52		
(Pharma Pac)				
REPACK				
SYR, PO, 6.25 mg/5 ml,				
120 ml	**52959-0804-04**	6.79		AA
240 ml	**52959-0804-08**	13.65		AA
TAB, PO, 12.5 mg, 30s ea	**52959-0914-30**	29.40		
(Phys Total Care)				
REPACK				
SUP, RC, 12.5 mg, 2s ea	**54868-4794-02**	8.83		
(USP)				
50 mg, 6s ea	**54868-1613-02**	155.28		
(Physician Partner)				
REPACK				
TAB, PO, 25 mg, 10s ea	**21695-0453-10**	21.92		
15s ea	**21695-0453-15**	38.68		
20s ea	**21695-0453-20**	43.84		
25s ea	**21695-0453-25**	54.80		
(Stat Rx)				
REPACK				
SUP, RC, 12.5 mg, 12s ea	**16590-0193-12**	45.00		
25 mg, 12s ea	**16590-0194-12**	51.00		
TAB, PO, 25 mg, 10s ea	**16590-0191-10**	13.20		
30s ea	**16590-0191-30**	39.50		
60s ea	**16590-0191-60**	79.00		

PROD/MFR	NDC	AWP	DP	OBC
(Vibranta) REPACK				
TAB, PO, 25 mg, 5s ea	**57866-4379-06**	15.80		
12s ea	**57866-0215-01**	7.29		
20s ea	**57866-4328-03**	11.76		
30s ea	**57866-4379-01**	94.80		
60s ea	**57866-4379-07**	189.60		
90s ea	**57866-4379-08**	284.40		
PROMETHAZINE DM (Qualitest)				
dm/promethazine hcl				
SYR, PO (ORANGE PINEAPPLE)				
15 mg/5 ml-6.25 mg/5 ml,				
118 ml	**00603-1586-54**	7.09		
473 ml	**00603-1586-58**	21.64		
(DHS, Inc.) REPACK				
SYR, PO, 15 mg/5 ml-6.25 mg/5 ml,				
118 ml	**55887-0247-04**	9.99		
(Pharma Pac) REPACK				
SYR, PO, 15 mg/5 ml-6.25 mg/5 ml,				
120 ml	**52959-0700-04**	5.89		
180 ml	**52959-0700-06**	8.84		
240 ml	**52959-0700-08**	11.79		
(Stat Rx) REPACK				
SYR, PO (1X120ML)				
15 mg/5 ml-6.25 mg/5 ml,				
120 ml	**16590-0292-04**	11.09		
PROMETHAZINE HCL ()				
promethazine hydrochloride				
SOL, IJ (1X25)				
25 mg/ml, 1 ml 25s	**66860-0098-03**	39.60		
50 mg/ml, 1 ml 25s	**66860-0099-03**	55.50		
(Baxter)				
SOL, IJ (DOSETTE,VIAL)				
25 mg/ml, 1 ml	**00641-0928-21**	1.13		**AP**
(USP)				
25 mg/ml, 1 ml	**00641-1495-31**	1.58		**AP**
(AMP, DOSETTE)				
25 mg/ml, 1 ml 25s	**00641-1495-35**	39.60		**AP**
(DOSETTE,VIAL)				
25 mg/ml, 1 ml 25s	**00641-0928-25**	28.20		**AP**
50 mg/ml, 1 ml	**00641-0929-21**	2.22		**AP**
(USP)				
50 mg/ml, 1 ml	**00641-1496-31**	2.22		**AP**
(AMP, DOSETTE)				
50 mg/ml, 1 ml 25s	**00641-1496-35**	55.50		**AP**
(DOSETTE,VIAL)				
50 mg/ml, 1 ml 25s	**00641-0929-25**	55.50		**AP**
(Consolidated Midland)				
SOL, IJ (VIAL)				
25 mg/ml, 1 ml 25s	**00223-8393-01**	20.00		**EE**
10 ml	**00223-8393-10**	4.00		**EE**
50 mg/ml, 1 ml 25s	**00223-8394-01**	25.00		**EE**
10 ml	**00223-8394-10**	4.25		**EE**
SYR, PO, 6.25 mg/5 ml,				
480 ml	**00223-6343-01**	4.50		**EE**
TAB, PO, 25 mg, 100s ea	**00223-1521-01**	4.25		**EE**
1000s ea	**00223-1521-02**	39.50		**EE**
(Gallipot)				
POW, NA (U.S.P.,N.F.)				
1 gm	**51552-0147-01**	8.82		
5 gm	**51552-0147-02**	11.76		
(U.S.P.,N.F)				
25 gm	**51552-0147-04**	17.22		
(U.S.P.,N.F.)				
100 gm	**51552-0147-05**	54.74		
(Hawkins)				
POW, NA (U.S.P.)				
25 gm	**63370-0203-25**	40.00		
100 gm	**63370-0203-35**	101.00		
500 gm	**63370-0203-45**	454.00		
1000 gm	**63370-0203-50**	780.00		
(Hi-Tech)				
SYR, PO (CHERRY)				
6.25 mg/5 ml,				
473 ml	**50383-0801-16**	22.20		**AA**
(Hospira)				
SOL, IJ (LUER LOCK,CARPUJECT)				
25 mg/ml, 1 ml 10s	**00409-2312-31**	17.64	15.40	**AP**
(Letco)				
POW, NA (U.S.P.)				
25 gm	**62991-1125-01**	30.00		
100 gm	**62991-1125-02**	75.00		
500 gm	**62991-1125-04**	330.00		
(Medisca)				
POW, NA (U.S.P.)				
25 gm	**38779-0253-04**	52.50		
100 gm	**38779-0253-05**	177.00		
500 gm	**38779-0253-08**	525.00		
1000 gm	**38779-0253-09**	945.00		
(Morton Grove)				
SYR, PO (TROPICAL FRUIT)				
6.25 mg/5 ml,				
118 ml	**60432-0608-04**	7.35		**AA**
473 ml	**60432-0608-16**	22.04		**AA**
(PCCA)				
POW, NA (U.S.P.)				
1 gm	**51927-9018-00**	3.24		
(Perrigo)				
SUP, RC, 12.5 mg, 12s ea	**45802-0758-30**	46.20		**AB**
25 mg, 12s ea	**45802-0759-30**	52.95		**AB**
(Sandoz)				
TAB, PO, 25 mg, 100s ea	**00781-1830-01**	50.64		**AB**
1000s ea	**00781-1830-10**	481.08		**AB**
50 mg, 100s ea	**00781-1832-01**	77.62		**AB**
(Spectrum Pharmacy)				
POW, NA (U.S.P.)				
25 gm	**49452-6087-01**	91.70		
100 gm	**49452-6087-02**	288.40		
500 gm	**49452-6087-04**	861.00		
(Teva)				
SOL, IJ, 25 mg/ml,				
1 ml 25s	**00703-2191-04**	33.00		**AP**
50 mg/ml, 1 ml 25s	**00703-2201-04**	75.00		**AP**
(Watson Labs)				
TAB, PO, 25 mg, 100s ea	**00591-5307-01**	50.64		**AB**
1000s ea	**00591-5307-10**	481.08		**AB**
50 mg, 100s ea	**00591-5319-01**	77.62		**AB**
(4u) REPACK				
TAB, PO, 25 mg, 10s ea	**42549-0543-10**	49.76		**AB**
20s ea	**42549-0543-20**	62.44		**AB**
30s ea	**10544-0343-30**	72.68		**AB**
30s ea	**42549-0543-30**	72.68		**AB**
(A-S Medication) REPACK				
SUP, RC, 25 mg, 12s ea	**54569-5745-00**	53.16		
SYR, PO, 6.25 mg/5 ml,				
120 ml	**54569-1046-00**	7.47		**EE**
TAB, PO, 25 mg, 5s ea	**54569-4168-00**	2.53		**EE**
10s ea	**54569-1754-01**	5.06		**EE**
12s ea	**54569-1754-00**	6.08		**EE**
20s ea	**54569-1754-06**	10.13		**EE**
30s ea	**54569-1754-09**	15.19		**EE**
60s ea	**54569-1754-05**	30.38		**EE**
(Altura) REPACK				
SYR, PO, 6.25 mg/5 ml,				
120 ml	**63874-0712-12**	5.46		**EE**
TAB, PO, 25 mg, 8s ea	**63874-0370-08**	6.57		**AB**
10s ea	**63874-0370-10**	8.21		**AB**
12s ea	**63874-0370-12**	9.85		**AB**
15s ea	**63874-0370-15**	12.31		**AB**
20s ea	**63874-0370-20**	16.42		**AB**
24s ea	**63874-0370-24**	19.70		**AB**
30s ea	**63874-0370-30**	24.63		**AB**
40s ea	**63874-0370-40**	32.84		**AB**
100s ea	**63874-0370-01**	82.10		**AB**
(DHS, Inc.) REPACK				
SUP, RC, 25 mg, 12s ea	**55887-0621-12**	61.89		**AB**
SYR, PO (TROPICAL FRUIT)				
6.25 mg/5 ml,				
120 ml	**55887-0675-04**	9.99		**AA**
TAB, PO, 25 mg, 10s ea	**55887-0936-10**	13.34		**AB**
12s ea	**55887-0936-12**	16.00		**AB**
15s ea	**55887-0936-15**	20.01		**AB**
20s ea	**55887-0936-20**	26.68		**AB**
30s ea	**55887-0936-30**	40.02		**AB**
60s ea	**55887-0936-60**	80.04		**AB**
90s ea	**55887-0936-90**	108.00		**AB**
(Dispensing Solutions) REPACK				
SUP, RC, 25 mg, 4s ea	**55045-3011-02**	19.50		
4s ea	**68258-3011-04**	19.50		**AB**
SYR, PO (TROPICAL FRUIT)				
6.25 mg/5 ml,				
118 ml	**55045-1643-09**	9.99		**AA**
TAB, PO, 25 mg, 10s ea	**55045-1596-03**	7.10		**AB**
12s ea	**55045-1596-02**	8.50		**AB**
15s ea	**55045-1596-05**	10.65		**AB**
20s ea	**55045-1596-06**	14.20		**AB**
30s ea	**55045-1596-08**	21.30		**AB**
60s ea	**55045-1596-04**	42.60		**AB**
90s ea	**55045-1596-09**	63.90		**AB**
100s ea	**55045-1596-00**	71.00		**AB**
120s ea	**55045-1596-01**	85.20		**AB**
(McKesson Packaging) REPACK				
TAB, PO (10X10,USP)				
50 mg, 100s ea UD	**63739-0389-10**	72.78		**AB**
(Nucare Pharm) REPACK				
TAB, PO, 25 mg, 10s ea	**66267-0177-10**	9.53		**AB**
30s ea	**66267-0177-30**	31.78		**AB**
60s ea	**66267-0177-60**	46.20		**AB**
90s ea	**66267-0177-90**	70.40		**AB**
(PD-Rx Pharm) REPACK				
SUP, RC (USP)				
25 mg, 2s ea	**43063-0060-02**	10.04		**AB**
TAB, PO, 25 mg, ea	**55289-0464-79**	10.68		**AB**
2s ea	**55289-0464-02**	11.38		**BP**
10s ea	**55289-0464-10**	16.88		**BP**
(REDI-SCRIPT)				
25 mg, 10s ea	**58864-0761-10**	18.56		**AB**
12s ea	**55289-0464-12**	18.26		**BP**
15s ea	**55289-0464-15**	20.32		**AB**
20s ea	**55289-0464-20**	23.76		**BP**
25s ea	**55289-0464-25**	27.20		**BP**
30s ea	**55289-0464-30**	30.62		**BP**
30s ea	**58864-0761-30**	30.66		**AB**
42s ea	**58864-0761-42**	40.27		**AB**
(USP)				
25 mg, 60s ea	**55289-0464-60**	51.26		**BP**
(Pharma Pac) REPACK				
TAB, PO, 25 mg, 2s ea	**52959-0534-02**	5.26		**BP**
10s ea	**52959-0534-10**	13.29		**BP**
12s ea	**52959-0534-12**	15.94		**BP**
15s ea	**52959-0534-15**	20.20		**BP**
20s ea	**52959-0534-20**	26.55		**BP**
28s ea	**52959-0534-28**	37.15		**BP**
30s ea	**52959-0534-30**	39.80		**BP**
45s ea	**52959-0534-45**	59.67		**BP**
60s ea	**52959-0534-60**	79.50		**BP**
90s ea	**52959-0534-90**	119.16		**BP**
120s ea	**52959-0534-01**	158.76		**BP**
(Phys Total Care) REPACK				
SOL, IJ (AMP)				
25 mg/ml, 1 ml 25s	**54868-4021-00**	115.14		**EE**
(M.D.V.)				
25 mg/ml, 10 ml	**54868-2695-00**	103.35		**EE**
50 mg/ml, 10 ml	**54868-0262-00**	116.88		**EE**
(10X25ML,MDV)				
50 mg/ml,				
10 ml 25s	**54868-0262-01**	89.73		**EE**
25 ml 25s	**54868-2088-00**	106.20		
SUP, RC, 25 mg, 2s ea	**54868-0601-01**	7.47		**AB**
12s ea	**54868-0601-02**	28.26		**AB**
SYR, PO, 6.25 mg/5 ml,				
120 ml	**54868-1867-00**	13.29		**EE**
TAB, PO, 25 mg, 10s ea	**54868-1323-01**	15.12		**EE**
12s ea	**54868-1323-02**	17.55		**EE**
15s ea	**54868-1323-04**	21.18		**EE**
20s ea	**54868-1323-05**	27.24		**EE**
30s ea	**54868-1323-06**	39.36		**EE**
50s ea	**54868-1323-08**	63.57		**AB**
60s ea	**54868-1323-07**	75.69		**AB**
100s ea	**54868-1323-00**	94.14		**EE**
50 mg, 30s ea	**54868-2844-01**	40.94		**AB**
60s ea	**54868-2844-00**	14.19		**EE**
(Physician Partner) REPACK				
SYR, PO (1X120ML,TROPICAL FRUIT)				
6.25 mg/5 ml,				
120 ml	**21695-0703-04**	14.70		**AA**
(Quality Care Prod) REPACK				
SUP, RC, 12.5 mg, 12s ea	**49999-0339-12**	54.72		**AB**
25 mg, 12s ea	**49999-0340-12**	98.42		**AB**
SYR, PO, 6.25 mg/5 ml,				
120 ml	**49999-0262-04**	14.73		**EE**
TAB, PO, 25 mg, 5s ea	**49999-0090-05**	15.80		**AB**
10s ea	**49999-0090-10**	31.60		**EE**
12s ea	**49999-0090-12**	37.92		**AB**
15s ea	**49999-0090-15**	47.40		**AB**
20s ea	**49999-0090-20**	63.20		**AB**
30s ea	**49999-0090-30**	94.80		**AB**
60s ea	**49999-0090-60**	189.60		**EE**
90s ea	**49999-0090-90**	284.40		**AB**

PROD/MFR	NDC	AWP	DP	OBC
(Southwood)				
REPACK				
SUP, RC, 25 mg, 12s ea	**58016-5009-01**	40.48		AB
SYR, PO, 6.25 mg/5 ml,				
120 ml	**58016-4008-01**	6.22		EE
TAB, PO, 25 mg, 10s ea	**58016-0424-10**	6.79		EE
12s ea	**58016-0424-12**	8.15		EE
15s ea	**58016-0424-15**	10.19		EE
20s ea	**58016-0424-20**	13.58		EE
30s ea	**58016-0424-30**	20.37		EE
40s ea	**58016-0424-40**	27.16		EE
48s ea	**58016-0424-48**	32.60		EE
50s ea	**58016-0424-50**	33.96		EE
60s ea	**58016-0424-60**	40.75		EE
90s ea	**58016-0424-90**	61.12		EE
100s ea	**58016-0424-00**	67.91		EE
120s ea	**58016-0424-02**	81.49		EE
150s ea	**58016-0424-03**	101.87		EE
200s ea	**58016-0424-89**	135.82		EE
300s ea	**58016-0424-73**	203.73		EE
(St. Mary's MPP)				
REPACK				
TAB, PO, 25 mg, 20s ea	**60760-0830-20**	16.58		AB
(Stat Rx)				
REPACK				
TAB, PO, 25 mg, 12s ea	**16590-0191-12**	9.35		AB
15s ea	**16590-0191-15**	11.69		AB
20s ea	**16590-0191-20**	19.70		AB
28s ea	**16590-0191-28**	27.58		AB
112s ea	**16590-0191-73**	87.26		AB
(Vibranta)				
REPACK				
TAB, PO, 25 mg, 10s ea	**57866-4379-04**	5.31		
12s ea	**57866-4379-02**	5.61		
PROMETHAZINE HCL AMERINET CHOICE (Baxter)				
promethazine hydrochloride				
SOL, IJ (PRIVATE LABEL)				
25 mg/ml, 1 ml	**10019-0097-44**	1.80		AP
1 ml 25s	**10019-0097-01**	45.00		AP
PROMETHAZINE HCL NOVAPLUS (Baxter)				
promethazine hydrochloride				
SOL, IJ (AMP,PRIVATE LABEL)				
25 mg/ml, 1 ml	**00641-0948-31**	1.01		AP
(PRIVATE LABEL,DOSETTE)				
25 mg/ml, 1 ml	**00641-0955-21**	1.03		AP
(AMP,PRIVATE LABEL)				
25 mg/ml, 1 ml 25s	**00641-0948-35**	25.20		AP
(VIAL,PRIVATE LABEL)				
25 mg/ml, 1 ml 25s	**00641-0955-25**	25.80		AP
(PRIVATE LABEL,DOSETTE)				
50 mg/ml, 1 ml	**00641-0949-31**	2.22		AP
1 ml	**00641-0956-21**	2.22		AP
(AMP,PRIVATE LABEL)				
50 mg/ml, 1 ml 25s	**00641-0949-35**	55.50		AP
(VIAL,PRIVATE LABEL)				
50 mg/ml, 1 ml 25s	**00641-0956-25**	55.50		AP
PROMETHAZINE HYDROCHLORIDE				
See PROMETHAZINE HCL				
PROMETHAZINE HYDROCHLORIDE				
FUL				
SUP, RC, 12.5 mg, 12s ea		11.53		
25 mg, 12s ea		12.43		
TAB, PO, 12,5 mg,				
100s ea		45.00		
(Baxter) *See PHENERGAN*				
(Baxter) *See PROMETHAZINE HCL*				
(Baxter) *See PROMETHAZINE HCL AMERINET CHOICE*				
(Baxter) *See PROMETHAZINE HCL NOVAPLUS*				
(Caraco)				
SYR, PO (1X118ML,USP)				
6.25 mg/5 ml,				
118 ml	**57664-0146-31**	7.35		AA
(1X473ML,USP)				
6.25 mg/5 ml,				
473 ml	**57664-0146-34**	22.20		AA
TAB, PO (USP)				
12.5 mg, 100s ea	**57664-0107-88**	49.00		AB
25 mg, 100s ea	**57664-0108-88**	50.64		AB
50 mg, 100s ea	**57664-0109-88**	77.62		AB
(Consolidated Midland) *See PROMETHAZINE HCL*				
(Consolidated Midland) *See PROMETHAZINE PEDIATRIC*				
(G&W) *See PROMETHEGAN*				
(Gallipot) *See PROMETHAZINE HCL*				
(Global Pharm)				
TAB, PO (USP)				
12.5 mg, 100s ea	**00115-1040-01**	49.00		EE
25 mg, 100s ea	**00115-1041-01**	50.64		AB
1000s ea	**00115-1041-03**	451.01		AB
50 mg, 100s ea	**00115-1042-01**	77.62		AB
(Hawkins) *See PROMETHAZINE HCL*				
(Hi-Tech) *See PROMETHAZINE HCL*				
(Hospira) *See PROMETHAZINE HCL*				
(Hospira)				
SOL, IJ (10X1ML,USP)				
25 mg/ml, 1 ml 10s	**00409-2312-02**	13.44	11.80	AP
(KVK)				
TAB, PO (USP)				
12.5 mg, 100s ea	**10702-0002-01**	46.05		AB
25 mg, 100s ea	**10702-0003-01**	47.48		AB
1000s ea	**10702-0003-10**	451.01		AB
50 mg, 100s ea	**10702-0004-01**	72.78		AB
(Letco) *See PROMETHAZINE HCL*				
(Major) *See PROMETHAZINE HYDROCHLORIDE*				
PROMETHAZINE HYDROCHLORIDE (Major)				
promethazine hydrochloride				
TAB, PO, 25 mg,				
100s ea UD	**00904-5840-61**	95.18		AB
PROMETHAZINE HYDROCHLORIDE				
(Medisca) *See PROMETHAZINE HCL*				
(Morton Grove) *See PROMETHAZINE HCL*				
(Paddock) *See PHENADOZ*				
(PCCA) *See PROMETHAZINE HCL*				
(Perrigo) *See PROMETHAZINE HCL*				
(Qualitest) *See PROMETHAZINE PLAIN*				
(Qualitest)				
TAB, PO (USP)				
12.5 mg, 100s ea	**00603-5437-21**	49.00		AB
25 mg, 100s ea	**00603-5438-21**	50.64		AB
1000s ea	**00603-5438-32**	481.08		AB
50 mg, 100s ea	**00603-5439-21**	77.62		AB
(Sandoz) *See PROMETHAZINE HCL*				
(Spectrum Pharmacy) *See PROMETHAZINE HCL*				
(Teva) *See PROMETHAZINE HCL*				
(Truxton) *See PROMACOT*				
(UDL)				
TAB, PO (10X10)				
25 mg, 100s ea UD	**51079-0895-20**	52.58		AB
(Watson Labs) *See PROMETHAZINE HCL*				
(West-Ward)				
SOL, IJ (25X1ML,USP)				
25 mg/ml, 1 ml 25s	**00143-9869-22**	27.50		AP
50 mg/ml, 1 ml 25s	**00143-9868-22**	56.25		AP
(Wyeth) *See PHENERGAN*				
(Zydus Pharm.)				
TAB, PO, 12.5 mg, 100s ea	**68382-0040-01**	49.00		
25 mg, 100s ea	**68382-0041-01**	50.64		AB
1000s ea	**68382-0041-10**	481.08		AB
50 mg, 100s ea	**68382-0042-01**	77.62		BP
(A-S Medication)				
REPACK				
SUP, RC, 12.5 mg, 6s ea	**54569-5744-01**	23.23		
12s ea	**54569-5744-00**	46.46		
25 mg, 4s ea	**54569-5745-01**	17.72		
6s ea	**54569-5745-02**	26.58		
(Aidarex)				
REPACK				
TAB, PO, 25 mg, 7s ea	**33261-0131-07**	9.80		AB
10s ea	**33261-0131-10**	14.00		AB
12s ea	**33261-0131-12**	16.80		AB
14s ea	**33261-0131-14**	19.60		AB
20s ea	**33261-0131-20**	28.00		AB
21s ea	**33261-0131-21**	29.40		AB
25s ea	**33261-0131-25**	35.00		AB
28s ea	**33261-0131-28**	39.20		AB
30s ea	**33261-0131-30**	42.00		AB
40s ea	**33261-0131-40**	56.00		AB
50s ea	**33261-0131-50**	70.00		AB
60s ea	**33261-0131-60**	84.00		AB
90s ea	**33261-0131-90**	126.00		AB
120s ea	**33261-0131-02**	168.00		AB
(Altura)				
REPACK				
TAB, PO, 25 mg, 60s ea	**63874-0370-60**	49.26		
(American Health)				
REPACK				
TAB, PO (10X10)				
12.5 mg,				
100s ea UD	**68084-0154-01**	56.18		
(Bryant Ranch)				
REPACK				
TAB, PO, 25 mg, 12s ea	**63629-1742-05**	7.59		AB
60s ea	**63629-1742-06**	36.65		AB
(Dispensing Solutions)				
REPACK				
SOL, IJ (25X1ML)				
25 mg/ml, 1 ml 25s	**55045-3514-01**	101.25		
SUP, RC, 25 mg, 12s ea	**55045-3011-03**	58.80		
TAB, PO, 25 mg, 20s ea	**55045-3929-01**	14.20		AB
20s ea	**66336-0085-20**	17.33		AB
25s ea	**66336-0085-25**	21.66		AB
60s ea	**66336-0085-60**	51.98		AB
(IPI)				
REPACK				
TAB, PO, 25 mg, 30s ea	**18837-0127-30**	15.19		AB
90s ea	**18837-0127-90**	45.58		AB
(Keltman Pharma., Inc.)				
REPACK				
TAB, PO, 25 mg, 12s ea	**68387-0536-12**	21.30		
30s ea	**68387-0536-30**	53.25		
60s ea	**68387-0536-60**	106.50		
90s ea	**68387-0536-90**	159.75		
(McKesson Packaging)				
REPACK				
TAB, PO (USP)				
25 mg, 100s ea UD	**63739-0213-10**	60.13		
(Palmetto)				
REPACK				
SUP, RC, 12.5 mg, 12s ea	**23490-6180-01**	46.20		
25 mg, 6s ea	**23490-6182-01**	26.63		
10s ea	**23490-6182-03**	44.40		
12s ea	**23490-6182-02**	53.28		
SYR, PO (1X120ML)				
6.25 mg/5 ml,				
120 ml	**23490-6187-01**	7.21		
TAB, PO, 25 mg, 10s ea	**23490-6183-01**	7.50		
12s ea	**23490-6183-02**	9.00		
20s ea	**23490-6183-04**	15.00		
30s ea	**23490-6183-03**	22.50		
60s ea	**23490-6183-06**	45.00		
90s ea	**23490-6183-07**	67.50		AB
100s ea	**23490-6183-08**	75.00		AB
(PD-Rx Pharm)				
REPACK				
SUP, RC (USP)				
12.5 mg, 2s ea	**55289-0940-02**	25.12		
6s ea	**55289-0940-06**	16.48		
TAB, PO (USP)				
25 mg, 2s ea	**43063-0049-02**	15.44		AB
4s ea	**43063-0049-04**	16.88		AB
(USP)				
25 mg, 6s ea	**43063-0049-06**	18.32		AB
50 mg, 4s ea	**55289-0531-04**	8.50		AB
(Pharma Pac)				
REPACK				
SUP, RC, 25 mg, 12s ea	**52959-0237-12**	53.78		
(Phys Total Care)				
REPACK				
TAB, PO, 12.5 mg, 20s ea	**54868-5121-04**	19.81		
30s ea	**54868-5121-02**	29.95		
100s ea	**54868-5121-03**	73.55		
25 mg, 90s ea	**54868-1323-09**	66.19		AB
(Physician Partner)				
REPACK				
SUP, RC, 25 mg, 12s ea	**21695-0649-12**	107.64		
TAB, PO, 12.5 mg, 15s ea	**21695-0589-15**	17.29		
25 mg, 60s ea	**21695-0453-60**	131.52		AB
50 mg, 10s ea	**21695-0885-10**	28.26		BP
(Quality Care Prod)				
REPACK				
TAB, PO, 12.5 mg, 20s ea	**49999-0902-20**	11.78		
(St. Mary's MPP)				
REPACK				
TAB, PO, 25 mg, 30s ea	**60760-0830-30**	20.88		AB
60s ea	**60760-0830-60**	35.77		AB
(Stat Rx)				
REPACK				
TAB, PO, 12.5 mg, 10s ea	**16590-0047-10**	7.36		AB
25 mg, 90s ea	**16590-0191-90**	64.00		AB

PROD/MFR	NDC	AWP	DP	OBC
PROMETHAZINE HYDROCHLORIDE/CODEINE (Altura)				
REPACK				
codeine phosphate/promethazine hydrochloride				
SYR, PO, 10 mg/5 ml-6.25 mg/5 ml,				
120 ml, C-V........	63874-0204-12	7.58		
180 ml, C-V........	63874-0204-18	8.60		
240 ml, C-V........	63874-0204-24	10.91		
PROMETHAZINE PEDIATRIC (Consolidated Midland)				
promethazine hydrochloride				
SYR, PO, 6.25 mg/5 ml,				
120 ml	00223-6347-01	3.25		EE
480 ml	00223-6347-02	8.00		EE
PROMETHAZINE PLAIN (Qualitest)				
promethazine hydrochloride				
SYR, PO (USP)				
6.25 mg/5 ml,				
118 ml	00603-1584-54	7.35		AA
473 ml	00603-1584-58	22.19		AA
PROMETHAZINE VC (Actavis Mid Atlantic)				
phenyleph hcl/promethazine hcl				
SYR, PO, 5 mg/5 ml-6.25 mg/5 ml,				
473 ml	00472-1628-16	40.55		AA
(Qualitest)				
SYR, PO (APRICOT PEACH)				
5 mg/5 ml-6.25 mg/5 ml,				
118 ml	00603-1587-54	11.26		
473 ml	00603-1587-58	40.55		
(A-S Medication)				
REPACK				
SYR, PO (APRICOT PEACH)				
5 mg/5 ml-6.25 mg/5 ml,				
120 ml	54569-1054-00	11.26		
(Altura)				
REPACK				
SYR, PO, 5 mg/5 ml-6.25 mg/5 ml,				
120 ml	63874-0711-12	9.36		EE
(Bryant Ranch)				
REPACK				
SYR, PO, 5 mg/5 ml-6.25 mg/5 ml,				
120 ml	63629-1868-01	12.90		
240 ml	63629-1868-02	25.80		
(Dispensing Solutions)				
REPACK				
SYR, PO, 5 mg/5 ml-6.25 mg/5 ml,				
118 ml	55045-1699-02	9.00		AA
(Pharma Pac)				
REPACK				
SYR, PO, 5 mg/5 ml-6.25 mg/5 ml,				
120 ml	52959-0568-04	7.75		EE
(Phys Total Care)				
REPACK				
SYR, PO, 5 mg/5 ml-6.25 mg/5 ml,				
120 ml	54868-3935-00	23.07		EE
473 ml	54868-3935-01	88.68		EE
(Quality Care Prod)				
REPACK				
SYR, PO, 5 mg/5 ml-6.25 mg/5 ml,				
120 ml	49999-0657-04	11.23		AA
(Southwood)				
REPACK				
SYR, PO, 5 mg/5 ml-6.25 mg/5 ml,				
120 ml	58016-4011-01	4.75		EE
PROMETHAZINE VC W/ CODEINE (Bryant Ranch)				
REPACK				
codeine phos/phenyleph hcl/promethazine hcl				
SYR, PO, 120 ml, C-V.....	63629-2959-01	17.58		
PROMETHAZINE VC W/CODEINE (Actavis Mid Atlantic)				
codeine phos/phenyleph hcl/promethazine hcl				
SYR, PO, 237 ml, C-V.....	00472-1629-08	12.22		AA
473 ml, C-V..........	00472-1629-16	55.26		AA
(Altura)				
REPACK				
SYR, PO, 120 ml, C-V.....	63874-0209-12	7.86		EE
(Dispensing Solutions)				
REPACK				
SYR, PO, 118 ml, C-V.....	55045-1266-08	10.75		AA
(Pharma Pac)				
REPACK				
SYR, PO, 120 ml, C-V.....	52959-0229-04	8.15		EE
(Phys Total Care)				
REPACK				
SYR, PO, 120 ml, C-V.....	54868-0263-00	31.23		EE
473 ml, C-V..........	54868-0263-01	96.54		EE
(Quality Care Prod)				
REPACK				
SYR, PO, 120 ml, C-V.....	49999-0326-04	35.78		AA
(Southwood)				
REPACK				
SYR, PO, 120 ml, C-V.....	58016-0491-24	7.39		EE
240 ml, C-V..........	58016-0491-48	10.88		EE
PROMETHAZINE VC WITH CODEINE (Qualitest)				
codeine phos/phenyleph hcl/promethazine hcl				
SYR, PO (STRAWBERRY MENTHOL)				
118 ml, C-V..........	00603-1588-54	15.35		
473 ml, C-V..........	00603-1588-58	55.26		
(A-S Medication)				
REPACK				
SYR, PO (STRAWBERRY MENTHOL)				
118 ml, C-V..........	54569-1047-00	15.35		
PROMETHAZINE VC/CODEINE (Physician Partner)				
REPACK				
codeine phosphate/promethazine hydrochloride				
SYR, PO, 10 mg/5 ml-6.25 mg/5 ml,				
120 ml, C-V........	21695-0336-04	18.10		
PROMETHAZINE W/ DM (Bryant Ranch)				
REPACK				
dm/promethazine hcl				
SYR, PO, 15 mg/5 ml-6.25 mg/5 ml,				
120 ml	63629-1588-01	3.60		
180 ml	63629-1588-02	5.40		
240 ml	63629-1588-03	7.20		
PROMETHAZINE W/CODEINE (Dispensing Solutions)				
REPACK				
codeine phosphate/promethazine hydrochloride				
SYR, PO, 10 mg/5 ml-6.25 mg/5 ml,				
118 ml, C-V........	55045-1687-02	11.50		AA
PROMETHAZINE WITH CODEINE (Qualitest)				
codeine phosphate/promethazine hydrochloride				
SYR, PO (GRAPE)				
10 mg/5 ml-6.25 mg/5 ml,				
118 ml, C-V........	00603-1585-54	9.05		
473 ml, C-V........	00603-1585-58	32.70		
PROMETHAZINE/CODEINE (Bryant Ranch)				
REPACK				
codeine phosphate/promethazine hydrochloride				
SYR, PO, 10 mg/5 ml-6.25 mg/5 ml,				
120 ml, C-V........	63629-1607-01	17.39		
180 ml, C-V........	63629-1607-02	26.09		
240 ml, C-V........	63629-1607-03	34.79		
PROMETHEGAN (G&W)				
promethazine hydrochloride				
SUP, RC, 12.5 mg, 12s ea .	00713-0536-12	46.82		
25 mg, 12s ea........	00713-0526-12	53.82		AB
50 mg, 12s ea........	00713-0132-12	82.50		BR
(Phys Total Care)				
REPACK				
SUP, RC, 25 mg, 6s ea	54868-4686-00	20.16		AB
12s ea............	54868-4686-01	34.35		AB
50 mg, 4s ea.........	54868-1613-01	106.02		BR
12s ea............	54868-1613-00	235.92		BR
PROMETRIUM (Solvay)				
progesterone				
SGL, PO (MICRONIZED)				
100 mg, 100s ea	00032-1708-01	197.94		
200 mg, 100s ea	00032-1711-01	376.04		
(Palmetto)				
REPACK				
SGL, PO, 200 mg, 30s ea ..	23490-9340-03	101.67		
(Phys Total Care)				
REPACK				
SGL, PO (MICRONIZED)				
100 mg, 10s ea	54868-4250-01	22.05		
30s ea............	54868-4250-00	62.39		
200 mg, 10s ea	54868-4230-01	46.26		
30s ea............	54868-4230-00	126.27		
PROMISEB (Promius)				
cream, multi ingredient				
CRE, TP (FRAGRANCE-FREE)				
30 gm..............	67857-0803-30	72.00		
PRONAP-100 (DHS, Inc.)				
REPACK				
acetaminophen/propoxyphene napsylate				
TAB, PO, 650 mg-100 mg,				
10s ea, C-IV........	55887-0943-10	9.90		EE
12s ea, C-IV........	55887-0943-12	11.80		EE
14s ea, C-IV........	55887-0943-14	13.85		EE
15s ea, C-IV........	55887-0943-15	14.75		EE
20s ea, C-IV........	55887-0943-20	17.95		EE
30s ea, C-IV........	55887-0943-30	26.91		EE
40s ea, C-IV........	55887-0943-40	36.05		EE
50s ea, C-IV........	55887-0943-50	45.00		EE
60s ea, C-IV........	55887-0943-60	54.50		EE
90s ea, C-IV........	55887-0943-90	80.73		EE
100s ea, C-IV	55887-0943-01	89.70		EE
120s ea, C-IV	55887-0943-82	107.64		EE
PRONEB ULTRA II (Pari)				
nebulizer, direct patient interface				
DEV, NA (LC SPRINT REUSABLE NEB)				
ea..................	83490-0860-19	87.00		
(W/LC PLUS REUSABLE NEB)				
ea..................	83490-0860-01	85.00		
PRONEB ULTRA II PEDIATRIC (Pari)				
nebulizer, direct patient interface				
DEV, NA (LC SPRINT REUSABLE NEB)				
ea..................	83490-0860-10	91.00		
(W/LC PLUS REUSABLE NEB)				
ea..................	83490-0860-06	89.00		
PRONESTYL (Phys Total Care)				
REPACK				
procainamide hydrochloride				
CAP, PO, 250 mg, 100s ea .	54868-3367-00	90.34		AB
PROPAFENONE (Southwood)				
REPACK				
propafenone hydrochloride				
TAB, PO, 150 mg, 30s ea ..	58016-0303-30	49.08		
60s ea............	58016-0303-60	98.16		
90s ea............	58016-0303-90	147.24		
100s ea............	58016-0303-00	163.60		
PROPAFENONE HCL (Ethex)				
propafenone hydrochloride				
TAB, PO, 150 mg, 100s ea .	58177-0331-04	163.60		AB
(10X10)				
150 mg, 100s ea UD ..	58177-0331-11	171.87		AB
5000s ea	58177-0331-12	7013.33		AB
225 mg, 100s ea	58177-0332-04	232.95		AB
300 mg, 100s ea	58177-0333-04	297.00		AB
(Mutual)				
TAB, PO, 150 mg, 100s ea .	53489-0551-01	163.58		AB
225 mg, 100s ea	53489-0552-01	232.93		AB
(FILM-COATED)				
300 mg, 100s ea	53489-0553-01	296.99		AB
(Qualitest)				
TAB, PO (FILM-COATED)				
150 mg, 100s ea	00603-5448-21	163.59		AB
300s ea............	00603-5448-25	480.95		AB
225 mg, 100s ea	00603-5449-21	232.95		AB
300 mg, 100s ea	00603-5450-21	297.00		AB
(Teva)				
TAB, PO (FILM COATED)				
150 mg, 100s ea	50111-0708-01	163.58		AB
225 mg, 100s ea	50111-0709-01	232.94		AB
300 mg, 100s ea	50111-0710-01	296.99		AB
(UDL)				
TAB, PO (10X10)				
150 mg, 100s ea UD ..	51079-0996-20	168.40		AB
(Watson Labs)				
TAB, PO, 150 mg, 100s ea .	00591-0582-01	88.39		AB
225 mg, 100s ea	00591-0583-01	124.99		AB
(A-S Medication)				
REPACK				
TAB, PO, 225 mg, 60s ea .	54569-6133-00	139.76		AB
(Phys Total Care)				
REPACK				
TAB, PO, 150 mg, 100s ea .	54868-4770-03	84.90		AB
250s ea............	54868-4770-00	198.42		AB
(FILM COATED)				
225 mg, 30s ea	54868-5950-01	40.68		AB
90s ea............	54868-5950-00	87.50		AB
PROPAFENONE HYDROCHLORIDE				
FUL				
TAB, PO, 150 mg, 100s ea..........................		110.49		
225 mg, 100s ea..........................		156.24		

(Ethex) *See PROPAFENONE HCL*
(Glaxo) *See RYTHMOL*
(Glaxo) *See RYTHMOL SR*
(Mutual) *See PROPAFENONE HCL*
(Qualitest) *See PROPAFENONE HCL*
(Teva) *See PROPAFENONE HCL*
(UDL) *See PROPAFENONE HCL*
(Watson Labs) *See PROPAFENONE HCL*

PROD/MFR	NDC	AWP	DP	OBC
(American Health)				
REPACK				
TAB, PO (10X10,FILM-COATED)				
150 mg, 100s ea UD ..	68084-0361-01	93.75		AB

PROD/MFR	NDC	AWP	DP	OBC
(Phys Total Care)				
REPACK				
TAB, PO, 150 mg, 20s ea	54868-4770-02	28.74		
30s ea	54868-4770-05	30.17		
60s ea	54868-4770-01	80.25		
90s ea	54868-4770-04	108.51		
PROPANTHELINE (Southwood)				
REPACK				
propantheline bromide				
TAB, PO, 15 mg, 30s ea	58016-0019-30	17.60		
60s ea	58016-0019-60	35.20		
90s ea	58016-0019-90	52.79		
100s ea	58016-0019-00	58.66		
PROPANTHELINE BROMIDE (Gallipot)				
POW, NA (U.S.P.)				
5 gm	51552-0922-02	34.86	24.90	
(Medisca)				
CRY, NA (1X5GM)				
5 gm	38779-2334-03	49.50		
(1X25GM)				
25 gm	38779-2334-04	135.00		
(1X100GM)				
100 gm	38779-2334-05	420.00		
POW, NA (U.S.P.)				
5 gm	38779-0304-03	37.50		
25 gm	38779-0304-04	102.00		
100 gm	38779-0304-05	373.50		
(PCCA)				
POW, NA (U.S.P.)				
1 gm	51927-1404-00	11.16		
(Roxane)				
TAB, PO, 15 mg, 100s ea	00054-4721-25	60.42		BP
(Spectrum Pharmacy)				
POW, NA, 5 gm	49452-6035-01	103.25		
25 gm	49452-6035-02	261.45		
(U.S.P.)				
100 gm	49452-6035-03	843.50		
PROPARACAINE (Stat Rx)				
REPACK				
proparacaine hydrochloride				
SOL, OP, 0.5%, 15 ml	16590-0195-15	19.00		
PROPARACAINE HCL (Akorn)				
proparacaine hydrochloride				
SOL, OP, 0.5%, 15 ml	17478-0263-12	11.25		AT
(Bausch & Lomb Inc.)				
SOL, OP, 0.5%, 15 ml	24208-0730-06	8.66		AT
(Falcon Ophthalmics)				
SOL, OP, 0.5%, 15 ml	61314-0016-01	11.25		AT
(PCCA)				
POW, NA (U.S.P.)				
1 gm	51927-2513-00	84.00		
(Spectrum Pharmacy)				
POW, NA (U.S.P.)				
1 gm	49452-6036-01	283.15		
5 gm	49452-6036-02	899.50		
(A-S Medication)				
REPACK				
SOL, OP, 0.5%, 15 ml	54569-1444-00	10.59		EE
(Altura)				
REPACK				
SOL, OP (1X15ML)				
0.5%, 15 ml	63874-0200-15	17.37		AT
(DHS, Inc.)				
REPACK				
SOL, OP, 0.5%, 15 ml	55887-0809-15	15.55		AT
(Dispensing Solutions)				
REPACK				
SOL, OP, 0.5%, 15 ml	55045-3153-01	15.99		AT
(Nucare Pharm)				
REPACK				
SOL, OP (1X15ML)				
0.5%, 15 ml	68071-1332-05	21.00		AT
(Phys Total Care)				
REPACK				
SOL, OP, 0.5%, 15 ml	54868-2079-00	16.50		EE
(Quality Care Prod)				
REPACK				
SOL, OP, 0.5%, 15 ml	49999-0442-15	19.85		AT
(Southwood)				
REPACK				
SOL, OP, 0.5%, 15 ml	58016-6052-01	16.54		EE
PROPARACAINE HYDROCHLORIDE				
(Akorn) *See PROPARACAINE HCL*				
(Alcon Ophthalmic) *See ALCAINE*				
(Bausch & Lomb Inc.) *See PROPARACAINE HCL*				
(Falcon Ophthalmics) *See PROPARACAINE HCL*				
(Ocusoft) *See PARCAINE*				
(PCCA) *See PROPARACAINE HCL*				
(Spectrum Pharmacy) *See PROPARACAINE HCL*				
(Pharma Pac)				
REPACK				
SOL, OP, 0.5%, 15 ml	52959-0705-01	18.50		
PROPECIA (Merck)				
finasteride				
TAB, PO (UNIT OF USE)				
1 mg, 30s ea	00006-0071-31	75.95		
(PROPAK)				
1 mg, 90s ea	00006-0071-54	212.06		
(A-S Medication)				
REPACK				
TAB, PO, 1 mg, 30s ea	54569-4544-00	79.11		
(PROPAK)				
1 mg, 90s ea	54569-5681-00	275.68		
(Core)				
REPACK				
TAB, PO, 1 mg, 30s ea	33358-0307-30	90.90		
(DHS, Inc.)				
REPACK				
TAB, PO, 1 mg, 30s ea	55887-0145-30	70.00		
60s ea	55887-0145-60	140.00		
90s ea	55887-0145-90	210.00		
(Phys Total Care)				
REPACK				
TAB, PO (UNIT OF USE)				
1 mg, 30s ea	54868-4120-00	97.15		
90s ea	54868-4120-01	271.67		
(Quality Care Prod)				
REPACK				
TAB, PO, 1 mg, 30s ea	49999-0276-30	67.58		
PROPINE (Phys Total Care)				
REPACK				
dipivefrin hydrochloride				
SOL, OP, 0.1%, 5 ml	54868-0624-01	28.26		AT
10 ml	54868-0624-02	50.82		AT
15 ml	54868-0624-03	79.20		AT
(Southwood)				
REPACK				
SOL, OP, 0.1%, 5 ml	58016-6058-01	18.56		AT
10 ml	58016-6438-01	33.44		AT
15 ml	58016-6464-01	48.63		AT
PROPIONIC ACID (PCCA)				
SOL, NA (NF)				
1 ml	51927-1564-00	0.24		
(Spectrum Pharmacy)				
SOL, NA (NF)				
500 ml	49452-6088-01	165.90		
1000 ml	49452-6088-02	236.25		
4000 ml	49452-6088-03	577.50		
PROPOFOL				
(APP) *See DIPRIVAN*				
(APP)				
EMU, IV (SDV,5X20ML)				
10 mg/ml, 20 ml 5s	63323-0270-20	24.00		
(20X50ML,SDV)				
10 mg/ml,				
50 ml 20s	63323-0270-50	240.00		
(10X100ML,SDV)				
10 mg/ml,				
100 ml 10s	63323-0270-65	240.00		
(APP) *See NOVAPLUS DIPRIVAN*				
(Hospira) *See AMERINET CHOICE PROPOFOL*				
(Hospira)				
EMU, IV (FLIPTOP VIAL)				
10 mg/ml,				
20 ml 25s	00409-4699-30	12.84	11.25	AB
50 ml 20s	00409-4699-33	128.40	112.40	AB
100 ml 10s	00409-4699-24	102.72	89.80	AB
(Teva)				
EMU, IV (SDV,25X20ML)				
10 mg/ml,				
20 ml 25s	00703-2856-04	66.00		AB
(SDV,20X50ML)				
10 mg/ml,				
50 ml 20s	00703-2858-09	132.00		AB
(SDV,10X100ML)				
10 mg/ml,				
100 ml 10s	00703-2859-03	132.00		AB
(A-S Medication)				
REPACK				
EMU, IV (SDV,5X20ML)				
10 mg/ml, 20 ml 5s	54569-5862-00	23.63		
(Phys Total Care)				
REPACK				
EMU, IV (S.D.V.)				
10 mg/ml,				
20 ml 25s	54868-4629-00	792.36		AB
PROPOLIS EXTRACT				
(Gallipot) *See BEE PROPOLIS EXTRACT*				
(PCCA)				
POW, NA, 1 gm	51927-3372-00	1.80		
PROPOXACET-N (Core)				
REPACK				
acetaminophen/propoxyphene napsylate				
TAB, PO, 650 mg-100 mg,				
60s ea, C-IV	33358-0308-60	60.99		
(Physician Partner)				
REPACK				
TAB, PO, 650 mg-100 mg,				
12s ea, C-IV	21695-0280-12	15.09		
(FILM-COATED)				
650 mg-100 mg,				
15s ea, C-IV	21695-0280-15	18.86		
20s ea, C-IV	21695-0280-20	26.89		
28s ea, C-IV	21695-0280-28	32.00		
30s ea, C-IV	21695-0280-30	34.29		
60s ea, C-IV	21695-0280-60	68.58		
90s ea, C-IV	21695-0280-90	102.87		
120s ea, C-IV	21695-0280-72	161.36		
(Quality Care Prod)				
REPACK				
TAB, PO, 650 mg-100 mg,				
6s ea, C-IV	49999-0767-06	4.06		
10s ea, C-IV	49999-0767-10	6.76		
12s ea, C-IV	49999-0767-12	8.72		
15s ea, C-IV	49999-0767-15	9.97		
20s ea, C-IV	49999-0767-20	20.75		
30s ea, C-IV	49999-0767-30	29.49		
50s ea, C-IV	49999-0767-50	31.73		
60s ea, C-IV	49999-0767-60	57.55		
90s ea, C-IV	49999-0767-90	72.10		
100s ea, C-IV	49999-0767-00	33.80		
120s ea, C-IV	49999-0767-01	115.10		
PROPOXACET-N 100 (Dispensing Solutions)				
REPACK				
acetaminophen/propoxyphene napsylate				
TAB, PO, 650 mg-100 mg,				
90s ea, C-IV	66336-0628-90	80.73		
120s ea, C-IV	66336-0628-94	107.64		
PROPOXY NAPS/APAP (Bryant Ranch)				
REPACK				
acetaminophen/propoxyphene napsylate				
TAB, PO, 650 mg-100 mg,				
20s ea, C-IV	63629-1344-01	21.02		
30s ea, C-IV	63629-1344-02	31.50		
40s ea, C-IV	63629-1344-06	42.32		
50s ea, C-IV	63629-1344-07	52.65		
60s ea, C-IV	63629-1344-03	60.99		
60s ea, C-IV	63629-1344-08	60.99		
90s ea, C-IV	63629-1344-09	80.65		
100s ea, C-IV	63629-1344-05	89.95		
120s ea, C-IV	63629-1344-04	108.09		
PROPOXY NAPS/APAP-100 (Stat Rx)				
REPACK				
acetaminophen/propoxyphene napsylate				
TAB, PO, 650 mg-100 mg,				
15s ea, C-IV	16590-0197-15	14.00		
30s ea, C-IV	16590-0197-30	28.00		
40s ea, C-IV	16590-0197-40	37.30		
45s ea, C-IV	16590-0197-45	42.00		
60s ea, C-IV	16590-0197-60	75.75		
75s ea, C-IV	16590-0197-75	70.00		
90s ea, C-IV	16590-0197-90	84.00		
120s ea, C-IV	16590-0197-72	112.00		
PROPOXY/APAP-65 (Stat Rx)				
acetaminophen/propoxyphene hydrochloride				
TAB, PO, 650 mg-65 mg,				
15s ea, C-IV	16590-0196-15	7.50		
20s ea, C-IV	16590-0196-20	10.00		
30s ea, C-IV	16590-0196-30	15.00		
PROPOXYPHENE (Core)				
REPACK				
propoxyphene hydrochloride				
CAP, PO, 65 mg,				
20s ea, C-IV	33358-0309-20	8.87		
30s ea, C-IV	33358-0309-30	12.98		
60s ea, C-IV	33358-0309-60	25.95		

PROD/MFR	NDC	AWP	DP	OBC
(DHS, Inc.)				
REPACK				
CAP, PO, 65 mg,				
40s ea, C-IV	**55887-0446-40**	25.17		
100s ea, C-IV	**55887-0446-01**	33.30		
(Quality Care Prod)				
REPACK				
CAP, PO, 65 mg,				
30s ea, C-IV	**49999-0798-30**	12.47		
60s ea, C-IV	**49999-0798-60**	24.94		
(Stat Rx)				
REPACK				
TAB, PO, 65 mg,				
30s ea, C-IV	**16590-0198-30**	22.00		
60s ea, C-IV	**16590-0198-60**	44.00		
90s ea, C-IV	**16590-0198-90**	66.00		
120s ea, C-IV	**16590-0198-72**	88.00		
PROPOXYPHENE COMPOUND (Pharma Pac)				
REPACK				
aspirin/caffeine/propoxyphene hydrochloride				
CAP, PO, 389 mg-32.4 mg-65 mg,				
20s ea, C-IV	**52959-0462-20**	9.15		AA
(Phys Total Care)				
REPACK				
CAP, PO, 389 mg-32.4 mg-65 mg,				
30s ea, C-IV	**54868-1467-01**	23.98		EE
100s ea, C-IV	**54868-1467-02**	71.42		EE
(Southwood)				
REPACK				
CAP, PO, 389 mg-32.4 mg-65 mg,				
15s ea, C-IV	**58016-0215-15**	5.40		EE
28s ea, C-IV	**58016-0215-28**	10.08		EE
30s ea, C-IV	**58016-0215-30**	10.80		EE
56s ea, C-IV	**58016-0215-56**	20.16		EE
60s ea, C-IV	**58016-0215-60**	21.60		EE
100s ea, C-IV	**58016-0215-00**	36.00		EE
120s ea, C-IV	**58016-0215-02**	43.20		EE
PROPOXYPHENE HCL (Mylan)				
propoxyphene hydrochloride				
CAP, PO, 65 mg,				
100s ea, C-IV	**00378-7065-01**	33.30		AA
500s ea, C-IV	**00378-7065-05**	161.20		AA
(Qualitest)				
CAP, PO, 65 mg,				
500s ea, C-IV	**00603-5459-28**	161.20	10.95	AA
(Teva)				
CAP, PO, 65 mg,				
100s ea, C-IV	**00093-0741-01**	33.30		AA
1000s ea, C-IV	**00093-0741-10**	303.50		AA
(A-S Medication)				
REPACK				
CAP, PO, 65 mg,				
12s ea, C-IV	**54569-0223-04**	4.09		AA
20s ea, C-IV	**54569-0223-00**	6.82		AA
30s ea, C-IV	**54569-0223-05**	10.23		AA
(Altura)				
REPACK				
CAP, PO, 65 mg,				
12s ea, C-IV	**63874-0215-12**	5.73		EE
30s ea, C-IV	**63874-0215-30**	22.13		EE
60s ea, C-IV	**63874-0215-60**	45.98		EE
500s ea, C-IV	**63874-0215-50**	368.83		EE
(DHS, Inc.)				
REPACK				
CAP, PO, 65 mg,				
30s ea, C-IV	**55887-0446-30**	20.00		AA
(Dispensing Solutions)				
REPACK				
CAP, PO, 65 mg,				
12s ea, C-IV	**55045-1599-04**	6.00		AA
15s ea, C-IV	**55045-1599-05**	7.50		AA
20s ea, C-IV	**55045-1599-07**	10.00		AA
30s ea, C-IV	**55045-1599-08**	15.00		AA
45s ea, C-IV	**55045-1599-03**	22.50		AA
60s ea, C-IV	**55045-1599-06**	30.00		AA
90s ea, C-IV	**55045-1599-09**	45.00		AA
100s ea, C-IV	**55045-2995-00**	50.00		AA
120s ea, C-IV	**55045-1599-00**	60.00		AA
135s ea, C-IV	**55045-1599-01**	67.50		AA
(HomeMed)				
REPACK				
CAP, PO, 65 mg,				
30s ea, C-IV	**51655-0849-24**	10.11		EE
60s ea, C-IV	**51655-0849-25**	19.21		EE
90s ea, C-IV	**51655-0849-26**	28.32		EE

PROD/MFR	NDC	AWP	DP	OBC
(Nucare Pharm)				
REPACK				
CAP, PO, 65 mg,				
20s ea, C-IV	**66267-0179-20**	16.66		EE
30s ea, C-IV	**66267-0179-30**	24.99		EE
(PD-Rx Pharm)				
REPACK				
CAP, PO, 65 mg,				
12s ea, C-IV	**55289-0324-12**	15.44		AA
16s ea, C-IV	**55289-0324-16**	17.76		AA
30s ea, C-IV	**55289-0324-20**	22.26		AA
60s ea, C-IV	**55289-0324-60**	39.98		AA
(Pharma Pac)				
REPACK				
CAP, PO, 65 mg,				
20s ea, C-IV	**52959-0334-20**	13.65		EE
30s ea, C-IV	**52959-0334-30**	20.47		EE
40s ea, C-IV	**52959-0334-40**	27.28		EE
45s ea, C-IV	**52959-0334-45**	30.70		EE
60s ea, C-IV	**52959-0334-60**	40.92		EE
(Phys Total Care)				
REPACK				
CAP, PO, 65 mg,				
20s ea, C-IV	**54868-1466-03**	23.88		EE
30s ea, C-IV	**54868-1466-00**	39.39		EE
60s ea, C-IV	**54868-1466-02**	62.65		EE
100s ea, C-IV	**54868-1466-01**	95.79		EE
(Southwood)				
REPACK				
CAP, PO, 65 mg,				
20s ea, C-IV	**58016-0214-20**	5.23		EE
30s ea, C-IV	**58016-0214-30**	18.88		EE
60s ea, C-IV	**58016-0214-60**	37.76		EE
90s ea, C-IV	**58016-0214-90**	56.64		EE
100s ea, C-IV	**58016-0214-00**	62.93		EE
120s ea, C-IV	**58016-0214-02**	75.52		EE
PROPOXYPHENE HYDROCHLORIDE (Heritage)				
CAP, PO (USP)				
65 mg,				
100s ea, C-IV	**23155-0012-01**	33.30		AA
500s ea, C-IV	**23155-0012-05**	161.20		AA
(Mylan) *See PROPOXYPHENE HCL*				
(Qualitest)				
CAP, PO (USP)				
65 mg,				
100s ea, C-IV	**00603-5110-21**	33.30	2.44	
(Qualitest) *See PROPOXYPHENE HCL*				
(Teva) *See PROPOXYPHENE HCL*				
(West-Ward)				
CAP, PO (USP)				
65 mg,				
100s ea, C-IV	**00143-3235-01**	18.00		AA
500s ea, C-IV	**00143-3235-05**	85.20		AA
1000s ea, C-IV	**00143-3235-10**	154.80	18.50	AA
(Xanodyne Pharma) *See DARVON*				
(Bryant Ranch)				
REPACK				
CAP, PO, 65 mg,				
20s ea, C-IV	**63629-1359-01**	8.65		
30s ea, C-IV	**63629-1359-02**	12.66		
60s ea, C-IV	**63629-1359-03**	25.32		
PROPOXYPHENE NAPSYLATE				
(Xanodyne Pharma) *See DARVON-N*				
PROPOXYPHENE NAPSYLATE & ACETAMINOPHEN				
(Keltman Pharma., Inc.)				
REPACK				
acetaminophen/propoxyphene napsylate				
TAB, PO, 650 mg-100 mg,				
15s ea, C-IV	**68387-0100-15**	18.75		
30s ea, C-IV	**68387-0100-30**	37.50		
40s ea, C-IV	**68387-0100-40**	50.00		
50s ea, C-IV	**68387-0100-50**	62.50		
60s ea, C-IV	**68387-0100-60**	75.00		
90s ea, C-IV	**68387-0100-90**	112.50		
100s ea, C-IV	**68387-0100-01**	125.00		
120s ea, C-IV	**68387-0100-12**	150.00		
PROPOXYPHENE NAPSYLATE AND ACETAMINOPHEN				
(Aristos)				
acetaminophen/propoxyphene napsylate				
TAB, PO (USP,FILM-COATED)				
325 mg-100 mg,				
100s ea, C-IV	**24486-0325-10**	266.23		EE
500 mg-100 mg,				
100s ea, C-IV	**24486-0326-10**	184.98		

PROD/MFR	NDC	AWP	DP	OBC
(Qualitest)				
TAB, PO (USP,FILM COATED)				
650 mg-100 mg,				
30s ea, C-IV	**00603-5467-16**	20.01		
(Teva)				
TAB, PO (FILM-COATED)				
500 mg-100 mg,				
100s ea, C-IV	**50111-0790-01**	137.83		
(FILM COATED)				
650 mg-100 mg,				
100s ea, C-IV	**00093-0890-01**	66.70		AB
(Aidarex)				
REPACK				
TAB, PO (FILM COATED)				
650 mg-100 mg,				
7s ea, C-IV	**33261-0097-07**	10.15		AB
14s ea, C-IV	**33261-0097-14**	20.30		AB
20s ea, C-IV	**33261-0097-20**	29.00		AB
21s ea, C-IV	**33261-0097-21**	30.45		AB
25s ea, C-IV	**33261-0097-25**	36.25		AB
28s ea, C-IV	**33261-0097-28**	40.60		AB
30s ea, C-IV	**33261-0097-30**	43.50		AB
36s ea, C-IV	**33261-0097-36**	52.20		AB
40s ea, C-IV	**33261-0097-40**	58.00		AB
50s ea, C-IV	**33261-0097-50**	72.50		AB
60s ea, C-IV	**33261-0097-60**	87.00		AB
90s ea, C-IV	**33261-0097-90**	130.50		AB
100s ea, C-IV	**33261-0097-00**	145.00		AB
120s ea, C-IV	**33261-0097-02**	174.00		AB
(IPI)				
REPACK				
TAB, PO, 650 mg-100 mg,				
15s ea, C-IV	**18837-0128-15**	22.00		
28s ea, C-IV	**18837-0128-28**	24.00		
30s ea, C-IV	**18837-0128-30**	26.00		
40s ea, C-IV	**18837-0128-40**	27.50		
50s ea, C-IV	**18837-0128-50**	34.38		
60s ea, C-IV	**18837-0128-60**	41.25		
120s ea, C-IV	**18837-0128-98**	82.50		
(Phys Total Care)				
REPACK				
TAB, PO (FILM COATED)				
650 mg-100 mg,				
16s ea, C-IV	**54868-0073-02**	18.77		AB
(Quality Care Prod)				
REPACK				
TAB, PO (FILM-COATED)				
325 mg-100 mg,				
30s ea, C-IV	**35356-0507-30**	196.82		EE
60s ea, C-IV	**35356-0507-60**	393.65		EE
90s ea, C-IV	**35356-0507-90**	590.47		EE
PROPOXYPHENE NAPSYLATE/ACETAMINOPHEN				
(Palmetto)				
REPACK				
acetaminophen/propoxyphene napsylate				
TAB, PO, 650 mg-100 mg,				
30s ea, C-IV	**23490-0120-03**	37.48		
60s ea, C-IV	**23490-0120-06**	74.95		
90s ea, C-IV	**23490-6197-00**	99.00		
(Phys Total Care)				
REPACK				
TAB, PO (USP)				
500 mg-100 mg,				
30s ea, C-IV	**54868-5517-00**	101.34		
PROPOXYPHENE NAPSYLATE/APAP (DHS, Inc.)				
REPACK				
acetaminophen/propoxyphene napsylate				
TAB, PO, 650 mg-100 mg,				
24s ea, C-IV	**55887-0943-24**	22.08		
PROPOXYPHENE-N W/ APAP (HomeMed)				
REPACK				
acetaminophen/propoxyphene napsylate				
TAB, PO, 650 mg-100 mg,				
10s ea, C-IV	**51655-0837-53**	5.84		
15s ea, C-IV	**51655-0837-54**	17.90		
20s ea, C-IV	**51655-0837-52**	23.87		
30s ea, C-IV	**51655-0837-24**	17.85		
40s ea, C-IV	**51655-0837-51**	20.36		
50s ea, C-IV	**51655-0837-77**	25.20		
60s ea, C-IV	**51655-0837-25**	30.04		
120s ea, C-IV	**51655-0837-82**	59.08		
(PCA, LLC)				
REPACK				
TAB, PO, 650 mg-100 mg,				
90s ea, C-IV	**51655-0837-26**	44.56		

PROD/MFR	NDC	AWP	DP	OBC
PROPRANOLOL (Phys Total Care)				
REPACK				
propranolol hydrochloride				
SOL, IV (S.D.V.,10X1ML)				
1 mg/ml, 1 ml 10s	54868-3873-00	310.68		
TAB, PO (USP)				
60 mg, 20s ea	54868-5564-01	43.38		
60s ea	54868-5564-00	93.72		
(Southwood)				
REPACK				
TAB, PO, 60 mg, 30s ea	58016-0001-30	30.69		
60s ea	58016-0001-60	61.39		
90s ea	58016-0001-90	92.08		
100s ea	58016-0001-00	102.31		
PROPRANOLOL ER (Phys Total Care)				
REPACK				
propranolol hydrochloride				
CER, PO, 80 mg, 10s ea	54868-5755-00	49.70		
30s ea	54868-5755-01	110.14		
PROPRANOLOL HCL (Bedford)				
propranolol hydrochloride				
SOL, IV (S.D.V.)				
1 mg/ml, 1 ml 10s	55390-0003-10	102.00		AP
(Consolidated Midland)				
TAB, PO, 10 mg, 100s ea	00223-2550-01	2.25		EE
1000s ea	00223-2550-02	12.50		EE
20 mg, 100s ea	00223-2551-01	2.50		EE
1000s ea	00223-2551-02	15.00		EE
40 mg, 100s ea	00223-2552-01	3.00		EE
1000s ea	00223-2552-02	22.50		EE
60 mg, 100s ea	00223-2553-01	4.25		EE
1000s ea	00223-2553-02	30.00		EE
80 mg, 100s ea	00223-2554-01	3.75		EE
1000s ea	00223-2554-02	37.50		EE
(Hawkins)				
POW, NA (U.S.P.)				
25 gm	63370-0205-25	80.00		
100 gm	63370-0205-35	240.00		
500 gm	63370-0205-45	880.00		
(Major)				
TAB, PO (10X10)				
10 mg, 100s ea UD	00904-0411-61	27.32		AB
(Medisca)				
POW, NA (U.S.P.)				
5 gm	38779-0183-03	57.00		
25 gm	38779-0183-04	87.00		
100 gm	38779-0183-05	246.00		
500 gm	38779-0183-08	643.50		
(Mylan)				
TAB, PO, 10 mg, 100s ea	00378-0182-01	24.75		AB
1000s ea	00378-0182-10	204.35		AB
20 mg, 100s ea	00378-0183-01	26.75		AB
1000s ea	00378-0183-10	277.85		AB
40 mg, 100s ea	00378-0184-01	50.95		AB
1000s ea	00378-0184-10	390.50		AB
80 mg, 100s ea	00378-0185-01	63.10		AB
500s ea	00378-0185-05	465.60		AB
(PCCA)				
POW, NA (U.S.P.)				
1 gm	51927-1606-00	18.00		
(Roxane)				
SOL, PO, 20 mg/5 ml,				
500 ml	00054-3727-63	40.17		
40 mg/5 ml, 500 ml	00054-3730-63	57.40		
(Spectrum Pharmacy)				
POW, NA (U.S.P.)				
5 gm	49452-6089-02	107.10		
25 gm	49452-6089-03	164.15		
100 gm	49452-6089-04	437.50		
(Teva)				
TAB, PO, 10 mg, 100s ea	50111-0467-01	33.55		AB
1000s ea	50111-0467-03	277.30		AB
20 mg, 100s ea	50111-0468-01	36.30		AB
1000s ea	50111-0468-03	344.80		AB
40 mg, 100s ea	50111-0469-01	69.15		AB
1000s ea	50111-0469-03	508.70		AB
60 mg, 100s ea	50111-0470-01	121.83		AB
80 mg, 100s ea	50111-0471-01	63.39		AB
500s ea	50111-0471-02	465.60		AB
(UDL)				
TAB, PO (10X10)				
10 mg, 100s ea UD	51079-0277-20	20.29		AB
20 mg, 100s ea UD	51079-0278-20	27.09		AB
40 mg, 100s ea UD	51079-0279-20	40.99		AB
(Watson Labs)				
TAB, PO, 10 mg, 100s ea	00591-5554-01	33.53		AB
1000s ea	00591-5554-10	277.25		AB
20 mg, 100s ea	00591-5555-01	36.29		AB
1000s ea	00591-5555-10	344.76		AB
40 mg, 100s ea	00591-5556-01	69.11		AB
1000s ea	00591-5556-10	508.64		AB
80 mg, 100s ea	00591-5557-01	85.58		AB
500s ea	00591-5557-05	374.13		AB
(A-S Medication)				
REPACK				
TAB, PO, 10 mg, 100s ea	54569-0557-01	33.55		EE
20 mg, 100s ea	54569-0559-01	36.30		EE
40 mg, 60s ea	54569-0561-01	41.49		EE
(American Health)				
REPACK				
TAB, PO (15X30)				
10 mg, 450s ea	62584-0842-85	111.78		AB
20 mg, 450s ea	62584-0843-85	155.14		AB
(DHS, Inc.)				
REPACK				
TAB, PO, 20 mg, 30s ea	55887-0559-30	9.03		AB
60s ea	55887-0559-60	18.00		AB
90s ea	55887-0559-90	27.00		AB
60 mg, 60s ea	55887-0453-60	66.05		AB
(Dispensing Solutions)				
REPACK				
TAB, PO, 20 mg, 20s ea	55045-1236-07	7.40		AB
60s ea	55045-1236-09	22.20		AB
100s ea	55045-1236-01	37.00		AB
40 mg, 100s ea	55045-1853-01	39.00		AB
60 mg, 30s ea	55045-3371-08	61.20		AB
80 mg, 100s ea	55045-1813-01	63.00		AB
(HomeMed)				
REPACK				
TAB, PO, 20 mg, 60s ea	51655-0350-24	12.94		EE
40 mg, 30s ea	51655-0349-24	9.49		EE
(PD-Rx Pharm)				
REPACK				
TAB, PO (REDI-SCRIPT)				
10 mg, 56s ea	58864-0645-56	38.60		AB
20 mg, 12s ea	55289-0233-12	24.00		AB
(REDI-SCRIPT)				
20 mg, 30s ea	58864-0363-30	23.27		AB
(USP)				
20 mg, 60s ea	55289-0233-60	35.94		AB
90s ea	55289-0233-90	49.40		AB
100s ea	55289-0233-01	52.68		AB
40 mg, 30s ea	55289-0234-30	32.07		AB
90s ea	55289-0234-90	56.07		AB
100s ea	55289-0234-01	60.07		AB
(REDI-SCRIPT)				
60 mg, 30s ea	58864-0680-30	81.83		AB
(Pharma Pac)				
REPACK				
TAB, PO, 10 mg, 30s ea	52959-0827-30	14.94		AB
20 mg, 10s ea	52959-0212-10	7.23		EE
20s ea	52959-0212-20	10.05		EE
45s ea	52959-0212-45	20.54		AB
50s ea	52959-0212-50	21.28		EE
60s ea	52959-0212-60	25.05		EE
100s ea	52959-0212-01	42.56		AB
(Phys Total Care)				
REPACK				
CER, PO, 60 mg, 10s ea	54868-1517-03	42.18		
30s ea	54868-1517-02	92.88		
60s ea	54868-1517-00	182.77		
100s ea	54868-1517-01	301.11		
120 mg, 10s ea	54868-1518-02	55.73		
30s ea	54868-1518-01	123.96		
100s ea	54868-1518-00	406.23		
160 mg, 10s ea	54868-0854-00	73.41		
30s ea	54868-0854-01	162.57		
TAB, PO, 10 mg, 30s ea	54868-0052-00	7.23		EE
60s ea	54868-0052-01	12.03		EE
100s ea	54868-0052-02	17.07		EE
20 mg, 30s ea	54868-0293-05	7.86		AB
60s ea	54868-0293-06	12.75		AB
90s ea	54868-0293-00	17.61		EE
100s ea	54868-0293-01	19.26		EE
40 mg, 30s ea	54868-0053-07	8.67		EE
60s ea	54868-0053-02	14.34		AB
100s ea	54868-0053-03	21.93		EE
80 mg, 30s ea	54868-0696-01	10.23		EE
60s ea	54868-0696-03	17.49		EE
100s ea	54868-0696-02	27.15		AB
(Physician Partner)				
REPACK				
TAB, PO, 40 mg, 30s ea	21695-0669-30	41.49		AB
(Quality Care Prod)				
REPACK				
TAB, PO, 20 mg, 90s ea	49999-0555-90	51.88		AB
40 mg, 60s ea	49999-0286-60	25.56		EE
(Southwood)				
REPACK				
CER, PO, 80 mg, 30s ea	58016-0604-30	25.67		
60s ea	58016-0604-60	51.35		
90s ea	58016-0604-90	77.02		
100s ea	58016-0604-00	85.58		
TAB, PO, 10 mg, 15s ea	58016-0528-15	4.69		EE
30s ea	58016-0528-30	9.39		EE
60s ea	58016-0528-60	18.77		EE
100s ea	58016-0528-00	31.29		EE
20 mg, 15s ea	58016-0529-15	7.21		EE
20s ea	58016-0529-20	9.61		EE
30s ea	58016-0529-30	14.41		EE
100s ea	58016-0529-00	48.04		EE
40 mg, 15s ea	58016-0531-15	8.55		EE
30s ea	58016-0531-30	17.10		EE
100s ea	58016-0531-00	56.99		EE
80 mg, 15s ea	58016-0532-15	13.13		EE
30s ea	58016-0532-30	26.25		EE
60s ea	58016-0532-60	52.50		EE
100s ea	58016-0532-00	87.50		EE
120s ea	58016-0532-02	105.00		EE
(Stat Rx)				
REPACK				
TAB, PO, 10 mg, 45s ea	16590-0808-45	12.48		AB
60s ea	16590-0808-60	16.64		AB
90s ea	16590-0808-90	24.96		AB
(Vibranta)				
REPACK				
CER, PO, 60 mg, 30s ea	57866-4911-01	57.64		
80 mg, 30s ea	57866-4912-01	67.28		
120 mg, 30s ea	57866-4913-01	83.20		
160 mg, 30s ea	57866-4914-01	99.96		
TAB, PO, 10 mg, 30s ea	57866-4309-01	9.90		AB
20 mg, 30s ea	57866-4313-01	16.02		AB
40 mg, 30s ea	57866-4314-01	19.80		AB
60 mg, 30s ea	57866-4315-01	19.90		AB
80 mg, 30s ea	57866-4316-01	29.04		AB
PROPRANOLOL HYDROCHLORIDE				
FUL				
CER, PO, 60 mg, 100s ea		132.24		
80 mg, 100s ea		154.47		
120 mg, 100s ea		191.60		
160 mg, 100s ea		250.88		
TAB, PO, 10 mg, 100s ea		5.85		
20 mg, 100s ea		7.05		
40 mg, 100s ea		8.48		
60 mg, 100s ea		127.92		
80 mg, 100s ea		11.40		
(Actavis)				
CER, PO, 60 mg, 100s ea	00228-2778-11	138.45		AB
(USP)				
60 mg, 500s ea	00228-2778-50	692.25		AB
80 mg, 100s ea	00228-2779-11	161.71		AB
(USP)				
80 mg, 500s ea	00228-2779-50	808.55		AB
120 mg, 100s ea	00228-2780-11	200.59		AB
(USP)				
120 mg, 500s ea	00228-2780-50	1002.95		AB
160 mg, 100s ea	00228-2781-11	262.62		AB
(USP)				
160 mg, 500s ea	00228-2781-50	1313.10		AB
(Akrimax) *See INDERAL LA*				
(APP)				
SOL, IV (S.D.V.)				
1 mg/ml, 1 ml	63323-0604-01	14.27		
(Bedford) *See PROPRANOLOL HCL*				
(Consolidated Midland) *See PROPRANOLOL HCL*				
(Gallipot)				
POW, NA (USP,1X25GM)				
25 gm	51552-0910-04	28.00	20.00	
(USP,1X100GM)				
100 gm	51552-0910-05	84.00	60.00	
(Glaxo) *See INNOPRAN XL*				
(Hawkins) *See PROPRANOLOL HCL*				
(Heritage)				
TAB, PO (USP)				
10 mg, 100s ea	23155-0110-01	33.55		AB
1000s ea	23155-0110-10	277.30		AB
20 mg, 100s ea	23155-0111-01	36.30		AB
1000s ea	23155-0111-10	344.80		AB
40 mg, 100s ea	23155-0112-01	69.15		AB
1000s ea	23155-0112-10	508.70		AB

PROD/MFR	NDC	AWP	DP	OBC
60 mg, 100s ea	**23155-0113-01**	121.83		AB
80 mg, 100s ea	**23155-0114-01**	63.39		AB
500s ea	**23155-0114-05**	465.60		AB
(Major)				
CER, PO (USP,10X10)				
60 mg, 100s ea UD	**00904-5947-61**	124.36		AB
80 mg, 100s ea UD	**00904-5948-61**	126.49		AB
120 mg, 100s ea UD	**00904-5949-61**	215.96		AB
160 mg, 100s ea UD	**00904-5950-61**	273.55		AB
(Major) *See PROPRANOLOL HCL*				
(Medisca) *See PROPRANOLOL HCL*				
(Mylan)				
CER, PO (USP)				
60 mg, 100s ea	**00378-6160-01**	132.59		AB
500s ea	**00378-6160-05**	662.94		AB
80 mg, 100s ea	**00378-6180-01**	154.89		AB
500s ea	**00378-6180-05**	774.45		AB
120 mg, 100s ea	**00378-6220-01**	192.09		AB
500s ea	**00378-6220-05**	960.43		AB
160 mg, 100s ea	**00378-6260-01**	251.47		AB
500s ea	**00378-6260-05**	1257.34		AB
(Mylan) *See PROPRANOLOL HCL*				
(Northstar)				
TAB, PO (USP)				
10 mg, 100s ea	**16714-0021-04**	33.55		AB
1000s ea	**16714-0021-06**	277.30		AB
20 mg, 100s ea	**16714-0022-04**	36.30		AB
1000s ea	**16714-0022-06**	344.80		AB
40 mg, 100s ea	**16714-0023-04**	69.15		AB
1000s ea	**16714-0023-06**	508.70		AB
60 mg, 100s ea	**16714-0024-04**	121.83		AB
80 mg, 100s ea	**16714-0025-04**	63.39		AB
500s ea	**16714-0025-05**	465.60		AB
(Par)				
CER, PO (USP)				
60 mg, 100s ea	**49884-0282-01**	132.74		AB
1000s ea	**49884-0282-10**	1327.38		AB
80 mg, 100s ea	**49884-0328-01**	155.07		AB
1000s ea	**49884-0328-10**	1550.66		AB
120 mg, 100s ea	**49884-0329-01**	192.31		AB
1000s ea	**49884-0329-10**	1923.06		AB
160 mg, 100s ea	**49884-0330-01**	251.76		AB
1000s ea	**49884-0330-10**	2517.57		AB
(PCCA) *See PROPRANOLOL HCL*				
(Rouses)				
CER, PO, 60 mg, 100s ea	**43478-0900-88**	109.20		
80 mg, 100s ea	**43478-0901-88**	127.20		
120 mg, 100s ea	**43478-0902-88**	158.40		
160 mg, 100s ea	**43478-0903-88**	207.60		
(Roxane) *See PROPRANOLOL HCL*				
(Sandoz)				
SOL, IV (USP,10X1ML)				
1 mg/ml, 1 ml 10s	**00781-3777-95**	98.50		AP
(Spectrum Pharmacy) *See PROPRANOLOL HCL*				
(Teva) *See PROPRANOLOL HCL*				
(Teva)				
TAB, PO (10X10)				
10 mg, 100s ea UD	**00182-1812-89**	22.29		AB
20 mg, 100s ea UD	**00182-1813-89**	32.54		AB
40 mg, 100s ea UD	**00182-1814-89**	45.27		AB
80 mg, 100s ea UD	**00182-1815-89**	57.62		AB
(UDL) *See PROPRANOLOL HCL*				
(Upsher-Smith)				
CER, PO, 60 mg, 100s ea	**00245-0084-11**	132.59		AB
1000s ea	**00245-0084-10**	1325.90		AB
80 mg, 100s ea	**00245-0085-11**	154.89		AB
1000s ea	**00245-0085-10**	1548.90		AB
120 mg, 100s ea	**00245-0086-11**	192.09		AB
1000s ea	**00245-0086-10**	1920.90		AB
160 mg, 100s ea	**00245-0087-11**	251.47		AB
1000s ea	**00245-0087-10**	2514.70		AB
(Watson Labs) *See PROPRANOLOL HCL*				
(West-Ward)				
SOL, IV (10X1ML)				
1 mg/ml, 1 ml 10s	**00143-9872-01**	100.00		AP
(A-S Medication)				
REPACK				
CER, PO, 80 mg, 30s ea	**54569-3097-00**	45.54		AB
(Altura)				
REPACK				
TAB, PO, 40 mg, 15s ea	**63874-0486-15**	8.98		
30s ea	**63874-0486-30**	17.96		
40s ea	**63874-0486-40**	23.95		

PROD/MFR	NDC	AWP	DP	OBC
60s ea	**63874-0486-60**	49.59		
100s ea	**63874-0486-01**	59.84		
1000s ea	**63874-0486-02**	598.67		
(American Health)				
REPACK				
CER, PO (10X10,USP)				
60 mg, 100s ea UD	**68084-0209-01**	166.55		
80 mg, 100s ea UD	**68084-0210-01**	189.36		
120 mg, 100s ea UD	**68084-0211-01**	227.33		
160 mg, 100s ea UD	**68084-0212-01**	287.95		
(Bryant Ranch)				
REPACK				
TAB, PO, 10 mg, 30s ea	**63629-1423-01**	11.65		
60s ea	**63629-1423-02**	23.29		
20 mg, 20s ea	**63629-2570-01**	9.65		
30s ea	**63629-2570-02**	14.48		
100s ea	**63629-2570-03**	48.27		
(Core)				
REPACK				
CER, PO, 60 mg, 30s ea	**33358-0194-30**	92.90		
TAB, PO, 10 mg, 30s ea	**33358-0192-30**	11.94		
20 mg, 30s ea	**33358-0193-30**	14.84		
(Dispensing Solutions)				
REPACK				
TAB, PO, 10 mg, 30s ea	**55045-2078-08**	10.50		
60s ea	**55045-2078-06**	21.00		
100s ea	**55045-2078-01**	35.00		
20 mg, 30s ea	**55045-1236-08**	11.10		
(Palmetto)				
REPACK				
TAB, PO, 40 mg, 30s ea	**23490-6203-03**	19.57		
60s ea	**23490-6203-06**	39.13		
90s ea	**23490-6203-09**	58.70		
(Pharma Pac)				
REPACK				
TAB, PO, 40 mg, 60s ea	**52959-0895-60**	42.20		
(Phys Total Care)				
REPACK				
CER, PO, 120 mg, 120s ea	**54868-1518-03**	333.56		AB
(Physician Partner)				
REPACK				
TAB, PO, 20 mg, 60s ea	**21695-0668-60**	43.56		AB
40 mg, 60s ea	**21695-0669-60**	82.98		
(Stat Rx)				
REPACK				
CER, PO, 120 mg, 30s ea	**16590-0328-30**	69.50		AB
PROPYL ALCOHOL (PCCA)				
SOL, NA (ACS REAGENT)				
1 ml	**51927-1832-00**	0.27		
PROPYL GALLATE (Amend)				
POW, NA, 100 gm	**17317-1777-03**	16.80		
454 gm	**17317-1777-05**	224.00		
2270 gm	**17317-1777-01**	56.00		
(PCCA)				
POW, NA (FOOD GRADE)				
1 gm	**51927-2121-00**	0.72		
(NF)				
1 gm	**51927-3621-00**	0.72		
(Spectrum Pharmacy)				
POW, NA (N.F.,F.C.C.)				
100 gm	**49452-6096-01**	123.20		
500 gm	**49452-6096-02**	413.00		
PROPYL-2-THIOURACIL (PCCA)				
propylthiouracil				
POW, NA (USP)				
1 gm	**51927-1183-00**	10.08		
PROPYLENE CARBONATE (PCCA)				
POW, NA (REAGENT)				
1 gm	**51927-3047-00**	0.21		
PROPYLENE GLYCOL (Baker, J.T.)				
LIQ, NA (U.S.P., F.C.C.)				
500 ml	**10106-9402-01**	11.74		
(Gallipot)				
LIQ, NA (U.S.P.,N.F.)				
473 ml	**51552-0103-06**	8.75		
3785 ml	**51552-0103-08**	29.40		
18925 ml	**51552-0103-09**	139.44		
(Letco)				
LIQ, NA (U.S.P.)				
500 ml	**62991-1292-01**	27.00		
3840 ml	**62991-1292-02**	69.00		
(Mallinckrodt Lab)				
LIQ, NA (U.S.P.)				
3000 gm	**00406-6263-06**	102.97		

PROD/MFR	NDC	AWP	DP	OBC
(Medisca)				
LIQ, NA (U.S.P.)				
500 ml	**38779-0510-08**	25.50		
1000 ml	**38779-0510-09**	43.50		
4000 ml	**38779-0510-01**	86.85		
(PCCA)				
LIQ, NA (USP)				
1 ml	**51927-1055-00**	0.07		
(Spectrum Pharmacy)				
LIQ, NA (U.S.P.)				
500 ml	**49452-6090-01**	46.20		
4000 ml	**49452-6090-02**	136.15		
20000 ml	**49452-6090-03**	602.00		
(Spectrum Pharmacy) *See POLYETHYLENE GLYCOL 300*				
PROPYLENE GLYCOL MONOSTEARATE (PCCA)				
POW, NA, 1 gm	**51927-2077-00**	0.75		
PROPYLPARABEN (Amend)				
POW, NA (N.F.)				
125 gm	**17317-0454-04**	6.30		
454 gm	**17317-0454-01**	14.70		
2270 gm	**17317-0454-05**	60.90		
3632 gm	**17317-0454-08**	210.00		
(Gallipot)				
POW, NA (U.S.P.,N.F.)				
113.4 gm	**51552-0102-04**	14.63		
454 gm	**51552-0102-06**	23.31		
(Letco)				
POW, NA (U.S.P./N.F.)				
100 gm	**62991-1270-01**	37.50		
(PCCA)				
POW, NA (NF)				
1 gm	**51927-1164-00**	1.02		
(Spectrum Pharmacy)				
POW, NA (B.P.,E.P.,J.P.,N.F.)				
100 gm	**49452-6100-05**	58.45		
500 gm	**49452-6100-01**	105.35		
2500 gm	**49452-6100-02**	364.00		
PROPYLPARABEN SODIUM (Spectrum Pharmacy)				
POW, NA (N.F.)				
500 gm	**49452-6106-02**	304.50		
2500 gm	**49452-6106-03**	822.50		
PROPYLTHIOURACIL (Actavis)				
TAB, PO, 50 mg, 100s ea	**00228-2348-10**	18.80		BD
(Consolidated Midland)				
TAB, PO, 50 mg, 100s ea	**00223-1540-01**	8.75		EE
1000s ea	**00223-1540-02**	77.50		EE
(Medisca)				
POW, NA (U.S.P.)				
25 gm	**38779-2169-04**	166.50		
100 gm	**38779-2169-05**	535.50		
(PCCA) *See PROPYL-2-THIOURACIL*				
(Spectrum Pharmacy)				
POW, NA (1X5GM)				
5 gm	**49452-6112-01**	115.50		
(1X25GM)				
25 gm	**49452-6112-02**	455.00		
(1X100GM)				
100 gm	**49452-6112-03**	1389.50		
(West-Ward)				
TAB, PO, 50 mg, 100s ea	**00143-1480-01**	15.75		BD
1000s ea	**00143-1480-10**	64.00		BD
(Phys Total Care)				
REPACK				
TAB, PO, 50 mg, 30s ea	**54868-1752-03**	14.13		BD
100s ea	**54868-1752-01**	36.57		BD
1000s ea	**54868-1752-02**	169.85		BD
(Southwood)				
REPACK				
TAB, PO, 50 mg, 30s ea	**58016-0157-30**	4.58		
60s ea	**58016-0157-60**	9.15		
90s ea	**58016-0157-90**	13.73		
100s ea	**58016-0157-00**	15.25		
PROQUAD (Merck)				
measles, mumps, rubella and varicella vaccine live				
PDS, SC (W/DILUENT,TAX INCL,PF)				
10s ea	**00006-4999-00**	1540.74		
PROQUIN XR (Depomed)				
ciprofloxacin/ciprofloxacin hydrochloride				
TER, PO (FILM-COATED)				
500 mg, 3s ea	**13913-0001-03**	36.54		
30s ea	**13913-0001-30**	328.18		

PROD/MFR NDC AWP DP OBC

PROSCAR (Merck)
finasteride
TAB, PO (UNIT OF USE,FILM-COATED)
5 mg, 30s ea **00006-0072-31** 107.09
(FILM-COATED)
5 mg, 100s ea UD **00006-0072-28** 333.88
(UNIT OF USE,FILM-COATED)
5 mg, 100s ea **00006-0072-58** 356.92
(BULK,FILM-COATED)
5 mg, 1000s ea **00006-0072-82** 3569.24
(Advanced Pharm Serv, Inc.)
REPACK
TAB, PO, 5 mg, 15s ea **13411-0122-15** 204.48
(FILM-COATED)
5 mg, 30s ea **13411-0122-03** 122.70
60s ea **13411-0122-06** 245.41
90s ea **13411-0122-09** 368.11
100s ea **13411-0122-10** 408.96
(Altura)
REPACK
TAB, PO (FILM-COATED)
5 mg, 10s ea **63874-0507-10** 19.55
30s ea **63874-0507-30** 58.65
40s ea **63874-0507-40** 78.20
60s ea **63874-0507-60** 117.30
100s ea **63874-0507-01** 195.46
(AQ)
REPACK
TAB, PO, 5 mg, 10s ea **66105-0547-01** 47.39
15s ea **66105-0547-15** 71.09
20s ea **66105-0547-02** 94.78
30s ea **66105-0547-03** 142.17
60s ea **66105-0547-06** 284.34
(Bryant Ranch)
REPACK
TAB, PO, 5 mg, 100s ea ... **63629-1585-01** 450.00
(PD-Rx Pharm)
REPACK
TAB, PO, 5 mg, 30s ea **55289-0936-30** 137.94
(REDI-SCRIPT,FILM-COATED)
5 mg, 30s ea **58864-0881-30** 137.94
(Phys Total Care)
REPACK
TAB, PO, 5 mg, 10s ea **54868-2719-03** 41.64
30s ea **54868-2719-01** 115.70
100s ea **54868-2719-02** 382.74
PROSED/DS (Ferring)
belladonna alkaloids and analgesics
TAB, PO (SUGAR COATED)
100s ea **55566-8101-01** 194.75
PROSOL (Baxter)
amino acids
SOL, IV (VIAFLEX,PC,SULFITE-FREE)
20%, 2000 ml **00338-0499-06** 470.40 392.00
PROSTAGLANDIN E1 (B&B Pharm, Inc)
alprostadil
POW, NA (U.S.P.)
0.01 gm **63275-9988-09** 285.00
(Gallipot)
POW, NA (1X1MG,USP)
0.001 gm **51552-0498-01** 37.73 26.95
(1X5MG,USP)
0.005 gm **51552-0498-09** 70.00 50.00
(U.S.P.)
0.01 gm **51552-0498-03** 105.00
(1X100MG,USP)
0.1 gm **51552-0498-05** 693.00 495.00
PROSTASCINT (EUSA)
indium in 111 capromab pendetide
KIT, IV, ea **57902-0817-01** 3756.61
PROSTIGMIN BROMIDE (Valeant Pharm Intl)
neostigmine bromide
TAB, PO, 15 mg, 100s ea .. **00187-3100-10** 156.10
PROSTIN E2 (Pfizer)
dinoprostone
SUP, VG, 20 mg, ea **00009-0827-01** 422.12 351.77
5s ea **00009-0827-03** 5885.21 4904.34
PROSTIN VR PEDIATRIC (Pfizer)
alprostadil
SOL, IV (AMP,5X1ML)
0.5 mg/ml, 1 ml 5s ... **00009-3169-06** 3103.12 2585.93 AP
PROTAMINE SULFATE
(APP) *See NOVAPLUS PROTAMINE SULFATE*
(APP)
SOL, IV (S.D.V.)
10 mg/ml, 5 ml 25s ... **63323-0229-05** 225.00 AP
25 ml .... **63323-0229-30** 27.00 AP

PROD/MFR NDC AWP DP OBC

(Gallipot)
POW, NA (USP,1X5GM)
5 gm **51552-0960-02** 55.30 39.50
(PCCA)
POW, NA (USP; SALMON SPERM)
1 gm **51927-3442-00** 37.20
(Spectrum Pharmacy)
CRY, NA (U.S.P.)
5 gm **49452-6109-01** 274.40
25 gm **49452-6109-02** 829.50
100 gm **49452-6109-03** 2226.00
PROTEASE (Spectrum Pharmacy)
CRY, NA, 300 mcu/mg,
100 gm **49452-6107-01** 195.30
500 gm **49452-6107-02** 535.50
2500 gm **49452-6107-03** 1904.00
PROTECT CARDIO (Gil Pharmaceutical)
multivitamin, minerals, and nutriceuticals
SGL, PO (SF,YEAST-FREE,SOFTGEL)
60s ea **58552-0311-60** 46.38
PROTECT PLUS (Gil Pharmaceutical)
multivitamin and minerals
LIQ, PO (AF,SF,DYE-FREE)
237 ml **58552-0109-08** 21.97
PROTECT PLUS NR (Gil Pharmaceutical)
multivitamin, minerals, and nutriceuticals
SGL, PO (SF,YEAST-FREE,SOFTGEL)
60s ea **58552-0309-60** 45.96
PROTECTIV IV CATHETER/SAFETY SYSTEM
(J&J Medical)
catheter
DEV, NA (PLASTIC HUB,RO,20X1")
ea **56091-0030-57** 2.34
(PLASTIC HUB,RO,22X1")
ea **56091-0030-50** 2.34
(PLASTIC HUB,RO,24X3/4")
ea **56091-0030-53** 2.34
(PLSTC HUB,RO,14X1 1/4")
ea **56091-0030-48** 2.34
(PLSTC HUB,RO,16X1 1/4")
ea **56091-0030-42** 2.34
(PLSTC HUB,RO,18X1 1/4")
ea **56091-0030-55** 2.34
(PLSTC HUB,RO,20X1 1/4")
ea **56091-0030-56** 2.34
PROTECTIV PLUS IV CATH SAFETY SYST
(J&J Medical)
catheter
DEV, NA (OCR POLY/R-0,14X1 1/4")
ea **56091-0030-68** 2.47
(OCR POLY/R-0,16X1 1/4")
ea **56091-0030-62** 2.47
(OCR POLY/R-0,18X1 1/4")
ea **56091-0030-65** 2.47
(OCR POLY/R-0,20X1 1/4")
ea **56091-0030-66** 2.47
(OCR POLY/R-0,20X1")
ea **56091-0030-67** 2.47
(OCR POLY/R-0,22X1")
ea **56091-0030-60** 2.47
(OCR POLY/R-0,24X3/4")
ea **56091-0030-63** 2.47
PROTECTIV PLUS-W IV CATH SAFETY SYS
(J&J Medical)
kit, catheterization, intravenous, winged
DEV, NA (WINGED,14X1 1/4")
ea **56091-0030-88** 2.60
(WINGED,16X1 1/4")
ea **56091-0030-72** 2.47
ea **56091-0030-82** 2.60
(WINGED,18X1 1/4")
ea **56091-0030-85** 2.60
(WINGED,20X1 1/4")
ea **56091-0030-86** 2.60
(WINGED,20X1")
ea **56091-0030-87** 2.60
(WINGED,22X1")
ea **56091-0030-70** 2.47
ea **56091-0030-80** 2.60
(WINGED,24X5/8")
ea **56091-0030-83** 2.60
PROTECTIV-W IV CATHETER SAFETY SYST
(J&J Medical)
kit, catheterization, intravenous, winged
DEV, NA (WINGED,14X1 1/4")
ea **56091-0030-78** 2.47
(WINGED,18X1 1/4")
ea **56091-0030-75** 2.47

PROD/MFR NDC AWP DP OBC

(WINGED,20X1 1/4")
ea **56091-0030-76** 2.47
(WINGED,20X1")
ea **56091-0030-77** 2.47
(WINGED,24X5/8")
ea **56091-0030-73** 2.47
PROTECTIVE SAFETY INTRODUCER SYSTEM
(J&J Medical)
catheter, central venous, peripheral insertion
DEV, NA (13G,SHEATH,15G NDL)
ea **56091-0979-99** 25.00
(15G,SHEATH,17G NDL)
ea **56091-0979-98** 25.00
(17G,SHEATH,19G NDL)
ea **56091-0979-97** 25.00
(20G,SHEATH,21G NDL)
ea **56091-0979-96** 25.00
PROTEIN C, HUMAN
(Baxter Bioscience) *See CEPROTIN*
PROTID (Lunsco)
apap/cpm/phenyleph hcl
TER, PO, 500 mg-8 mg-40 mg,
100s ea **10892-0127-10** 70.68
PROTIRELIN (PCCA)
POW, NA, 1 gm **51927-3484-00** 78.00
PROTOL HEAVY (Amend)
mineral oil
OIL, NA (U.S.P.)
480 ml **17317-1063-01** 4.90
3840 ml **17317-1063-06** 21.00
19200 ml **17317-1063-08** 70.00
PROTONIX (Wyeth)
pantoprazole sodium
ECT, PO, 20 mg, 90s ea ... **00008-0843-81** 470.18 391.82
40 mg, 90s ea **00008-0841-81** 470.18 391.82
(10X10)
40 mg, 100s ea UD ... **00008-0841-99** 522.49 435.41
PDS, IV, 40 mg, 10s ea **00008-0923-55** 144.00 120.00
PKT, PO (ENTERIC-COATED GRANULES)
40 mg/packet,
30s ea UD **00008-0844-02** 156.86 130.72
(A-S Medication)
REPACK
ECT, PO, 40 mg, 30s ea ... **54569-5118-00** 149.78
(AQ)
REPACK
ECT, PO, 20 mg, 30s ea ... **66105-0975-03** 235.60
40 mg, 30s ea **66105-0844-03** 280.04
(Direct Pharmaceutical, Inc.)
REPACK
ECT, PO, 20 mg,
30s ea UD **67801-0424-30** 248.75
40 mg, 30s ea UD **67801-0325-03** 248.75
(Dispensing Solutions)
REPACK
ECT, PO, 40 mg, 90s ea ... **55045-3077-09** 423.00
(IPI)
REPACK
ECT, PO, 40 mg, 30s ea ... **18837-0262-30** 160.13
(Keltman Pharma., Inc.)
REPACK
ECT, PO, 40 mg, 30s ea ... **68387-0293-30** 144.25
(Nucare Pharm)
REPACK
ECT, PO, 40 mg, 30s ea ... **66267-0479-30** 168.14
(PD-Rx Pharm)
REPACK
ECT, PO, 20 mg, 30s ea ... **58864-0892-30** 188.23
(REDI-SCRIPT)
40 mg, 30s ea **58864-0601-30** 188.23
(Pharma Pac)
REPACK
ECT, PO, 40 mg, 30s ea ... **52959-0819-30** 124.50
(Phys Total Care)
REPACK
ECT, PO, 20 mg, 30s ea ... **54868-4786-01** 132.89
90s ea **54868-4786-00** 382.23
40 mg, 30s ea **54868-4271-00** 188.14
60s ea **54868-4271-01** 373.66
90s ea **54868-4271-02** 540.58
(Physician Partner)
REPACK
ECT, PO, 40 mg, 15s ea ... **21695-0108-15** 160.44

PROD/MFR	NDC	AWP	DP	OBC
(Quality Care Prod) REPACK				
ECT, PO, 40 mg, 30s ea	49999-0481-30	248.75		
90s ea	49999-0481-90	746.10		
90s ea	49999-0756-90	746.10		
(Southwood) REPACK				
ECT, PO, 20 mg, 30s ea	58016-0072-30	137.20		
60s ea	58016-0072-60	274.41		
90s ea	58016-0072-90	411.61		
100s ea	58016-0072-00	457.34		
40 mg, 30s ea	58016-0525-30	137.22		
60s ea	58016-0525-60	274.43		
90s ea	58016-0525-90	411.65		
100s ea	58016-0525-00	457.39		
120s ea	58016-0525-02	548.87		
(Stat Rx) REPACK				
ECT, PO, 40 mg, 30s ea	16590-0516-30	169.32		
PROTONIX TR (Stat Rx) pantoprazole sodium				
ECT, PO, 40 mg, 60s ea	16590-0516-60	302.00		
90s ea	16590-0516-90	390.75		
120s ea	16590-0516-72	505.25		
PROTOPAM CHLORIDE (Baxter) pralidoxime chloride				
PDS, IJ, 1 gm, ea (S.D.V.)	60977-0141-27	104.04		
1 gm, 6s ea	60977-0141-01	624.24		
PROTOPIC (Astellas) tacrolimus				
OIN, TP, 0.03%, 30 gm	00469-5201-30	122.76		
60 gm	00469-5201-60	245.52		
100 gm	00469-5201-11	409.20		
0.1%, 30 gm	00469-5202-30	122.76		
60 gm	00469-5202-60	245.52		
100 gm	00469-5202-11	409.20		
(Phys Total Care) REPACK				
OIN, TP (1X30GM) 0.1%, 30 gm	54868-5233-01	130.81		
100 gm	54868-5233-00	251.61		
(Quality Care Prod) REPACK				
OIN, TP (1X100GM) 0.1%, 100 gm	35356-0235-00	645.62		
PROTRIPTYLINE HYDROCHLORIDE (Teva)				
TAB, PO (FILM-COATED) 5 mg, 100s ea	00555-0595-02	211.55		
10 mg, 100s ea	00555-0594-02	306.57		
(Teva) *See VIVACTIL*				
PROVENT SLEEP APNEA THERAPY, HR DEVICE (Ventus) device				
DEV, NA (SINGLE USE) ea	08592-0001-01	6.00		
30s ea	08592-0001-30	180.00		
PROVENT SLEEP APNEA THERAPY, SR DEVICE (Ventus) device				
DEV, NA (SINGLE USE) ea	08592-0002-01	6.00		
30s ea	08592-0002-30	180.00		
PROVENTIL (Schering) albuterol sulfate				
SOL, IH, 0.5%, 20 ml	00085-1336-01	25.06		AN
(Pharma Pac) REPACK albuterol				
ARO, IH, 0.09 mg/actuation, 17 gm	52959-0293-00	36.83		BN
(Phys Total Care) REPACK albuterol sulfate				
TAB, PO, 4 mg, 100s ea	54868-0308-01	92.47		AB
(Southwood) REPACK albuterol				
ARO, IH, 0.09 mg/actuation, 17 gm	58016-6059-01	28.60		BN
PROVENTIL HFA (Schering) albuterol sulfate				
ARO, IH (M.D.I.) 0.09 mg/actuation, 6.7 gm	00085-1132-01	48.44		BX
(A-S Medication) REPACK				
ARO, IH (M.D.I.) 0.09 mg/actuation, 6.7 gm	54569-4621-00	47.65		BX
(Pharma Pac) REPACK				
ARO, IH, 0.09 mg/actuation, 6.7 gm	52959-0569-01	34.65		BX
(Phys Total Care) REPACK				
ARO, IH (1X6.7GM) 0.09 mg/actuation, 6.7 gm	54868-6051-00	60.58		BX
(Quality Care Prod) REPACK				
ARO, IH, 0.09 mg/actuation, 6.7 gm	49999-0907-67	84.03		BX
PROVERA (Pfizer) medroxyprogesterone acetate				
TAB, PO, 2.5 mg, 100s ea	00009-0064-04	98.46	82.05	AB
5 mg, 100s ea	00009-0286-03	148.02	123.35	AB
10 mg, 100s ea	00009-0050-02	193.09	160.91	AB
500s ea	00009-0050-11	965.47	804.56	AB
(PD-Rx Pharm) REPACK				
TAB, PO, 2.5 mg, 30s ea	55289-0121-30	41.82		AB
10 mg, 10s ea	55289-0034-10	27.33		AB
(Phys Total Care) REPACK				
TAB, PO, 2.5 mg, 30s ea	54868-1010-01	27.26		AB
40s ea	54868-1010-03	35.72		AB
10 mg, 5s ea	54868-0290-02	10.18		AB
30s ea	54868-0290-03	51.64		AB
40s ea	54868-0290-04	68.22		AB
100s ea	54868-0290-00	167.76		AB
(Quality Care Prod) REPACK				
TAB, PO, 2.5 mg, ea	49999-0272-01	5.36		AB
30s ea	49999-0272-30	71.46		AB
(Southwood) REPACK				
TAB, PO, 2.5 mg, 30s ea	58016-0969-30	26.79		AB
60s ea	58016-0969-60	53.58		AB
90s ea	58016-0969-90	80.37		AB
100s ea	58016-0969-00	89.30		AB
PROVIDER PUMP (Abbott Hosp) kit, administration, intravenous				
DEV, NA (72", NON-VENTED) 24s ea	00074-4829-01	443.23	443.28	
(72") 24s ea	00074-4818-01	1378.26	1160.64	
PROVIGIL (Cephalon) modafinil				
TAB, PO, 100 mg, 100s ea, C-IV	63459-0101-01	1078.80		EE
200 mg, 100s ea, C-IV	63459-0201-01	1633.20		
(Altura) REPACK				
TAB, PO, 200 mg, 100s ea, C-IV	63874-1027-01	716.40		
(Bryant Ranch) REPACK				
TAB, PO, 200 mg, 100s ea, C-IV	63629-1611-01	861.99		
(Dispensing Solutions) REPACK				
TAB, PO, 100 mg, 60s ea, C-IV	55045-3086-06	420.00		
200 mg, 60s ea, C-IV	55045-3085-06	585.00		
(IPI) REPACK				
TAB, PO, 100 mg, 60s ea, C-IV	18837-0273-60	510.20		
200 mg, 90s ea, C-IV	18837-0130-90	1163.15		
(Nucare Pharm) REPACK				
TAB, PO, 100 mg, 60s ea, C-IV	68071-0665-60	572.44		
200 mg, 30s ea, C-IV	68071-0297-30	399.35		
60s ea, C-IV	68071-0297-60	790.94		
(PD-Rx Pharm) REPACK				
TAB, PO, 200 mg, 30s ea, C-IV	55289-0253-30	564.69		
(Phys Total Care) REPACK				
TAB, PO, 100 mg, 10s ea, C-IV	54868-4492-01	81.13		
30s ea, C-IV	54868-4492-00	227.05		
200 mg, 10s ea, C-IV	54868-4897-01	196.60		
30s ea, C-IV	54868-4897-00	564.54		
(Physician Partner) REPACK				
TAB, PO, 100 mg, 15s ea, C-IV	21695-0234-15	307.50		
30s ea, C-IV	21695-0234-30	522.75		
200 mg, 15s ea, C-IV	21695-0235-15	332.65		
30s ea, C-IV	21695-0235-30	979.92		
(Quality Care Prod) REPACK				
TAB, PO, 200 mg, 30s ea, C-IV	35356-0372-30	554.63		
(Southwood) REPACK				
TAB, PO, 100 mg, 30s ea, C-IV	58016-0909-30	250.92		
60s ea, C-IV	58016-0909-60	501.84		
90s ea, C-IV	58016-0909-90	752.76		
100s ea, C-IV	58016-0909-00	836.40		
200 mg, 30s ea, C-IV	58016-0976-30	346.68		
60s ea, C-IV	58016-0976-60	693.36		
90s ea, C-IV	58016-0976-90	1040.04		
100s ea, C-IV	58016-0976-00	1155.60		
(Stat Rx) REPACK				
TAB, PO, 200 mg, 7s ea, C-IV	16590-0199-07	135.62		
10s ea, C-IV	16590-0199-10	192.28		
14s ea, C-IV	16590-0199-14	267.85		
28s ea, C-IV	16590-0199-28	532.31		
30s ea, C-IV	16590-0199-30	570.09		
45s ea, C-IV	16590-0199-45	853.45		
60s ea, C-IV	16590-0199-60	1136.80		
90s ea, C-IV	16590-0199-90	1703.51		
PROVISC (Alcon Surgical) hyaluronate sodium				
SOL, IO (SRN) 10 mg/ml, 0.4 ml	08065-1830-04	105.78		
0.55 ml	08065-1830-55	134.28		
0.85 ml	08065-1830-85	176.28		
PROVOCHOLINE (Methapharm) methacholine chloride				
PDS, IH, 100 mg, 6s ea	64281-0100-06	264.00	264.00	
12s ea	64281-0100-12	528.00	528.00	
PROZAC (Dista) fluoxetine hydrochloride				
CAP, PO, 10 mg, 100s ea	00777-3104-02	651.06	542.55	AB
20 mg, 30s ea	00777-3105-30	200.34	166.95	AB
100s ea	00777-3105-02	667.80	556.50	AB
2000s ea	00777-3105-07	13356.00	11130.00	AB
40 mg, 30s ea	00777-3107-30	400.68	333.90	AB
(AQ) REPACK				
CAP, PO, 20 mg, 30s ea	66105-0564-03	201.88		
(Palmetto) REPACK				
CAP, PO, 20 mg, 60s ea	23490-9240-06	164.40		
(PD-Rx Pharm) REPACK				
CAP, PO, 10 mg, 14s ea	55289-0308-14	100.40		AB
30s ea	55289-0308-30	188.83		AB
20 mg, 22s ea	55289-0215-22	142.22		AB
30s ea	58864-0971-30	222.11		
(Pharma Pac) REPACK				
CAP, PO, 20 mg, 10s ea	52959-0233-10	40.20		AB
14s ea	52959-0233-14	54.32		AB
20s ea	52959-0233-20	73.00		AB
30s ea	52959-0233-30	103.94		AB
40s ea	52959-0233-40	133.60		AB
50s ea	52959-0233-50	162.50		AB
100s ea	52959-0233-00	259.10		AB

PROD/MFR	NDC	AWP	DP	OBC
(Phys Total Care) REPACK				
CAP, PO, 10 mg, 10s ea	54868-3033-02	49.55		AB
30s ea	54868-3033-00	135.56		AB
20 mg, 30s ea	54868-0511-01	158.61		AB
60s ea	54868-0511-05	307.03		AB
90s ea	54868-0511-02	510.79		AB
100s ea	54868-0511-00	527.27		AB
40 mg, 30s ea	54868-4394-00	371.38		AB
(Southwood) REPACK				
CAP, PO, 20 mg, 10s ea	58016-0828-10	57.78		AB
20s ea	58016-0828-20	115.56		AB
30s ea	58016-0828-30	173.34		AB
40s ea	58016-0828-40	231.12		AB
60s ea	58016-0828-60	346.68		AB
90s ea	58016-0828-90	520.02		AB
100s ea	58016-0828-00	577.80		AB
(Stat Rx) REPACK				
CAP, PO, 20 mg, 90s ea	16590-0843-90	657.80		AB
PROZAC WEEKLY (Lilly) fluoxetine hydrochloride				
ECC, PO (BLISTER PACK)				
90 mg, 4s ea	00002-3004-75	138.00	115.00	
(Pharma Pac) REPACK				
ECC, PO (BLISTER PACK)				
90 mg, 4s ea	52959-0638-04	87.75		
PRUCLAIR (PruGen) cream, multi ingredient				
CRE, TP (1X100GM)				
100 gm	42546-0412-11	105.83		
PRUDOXIN (Healthpoint) doxepin hydrochloride				
CRE, TP, 5%, 45 gm	00064-3600-45	137.03		
PRUET DHA (PruGen) prenatal vitamins				
KIT, PO (5X12,SOFTGEL)				
60s ea UD	42546-0809-30	37.08		
(SOFTGEL)				
60s ea UD	42546-0810-30	37.08		
PRUET DHAEC (PruGen) prenatal vitamins				
KIT, PO (5X12,SOFTGEL)				
60s ea UD	42546-0515-30	42.52		
(ENTERIC-COATED, SOFTGEL)				
60s ea UD	42546-0516-30	42.52		
PRUMYX (PruGen) cream, multi ingredient				
CRE, TP (1X140GM,PF)				
140 gm	42546-0710-05	108.89		
PRUSSIAN BLUE (Heyltex Corp) *See RADIOGARDASE*				
PRUTECT (PruGen) cream, multi ingredient				
CRE, TP (1X45GM)				
45 gm	42546-0130-45	30.24		
(1X90GM)				
90 gm	42546-0130-90	48.39		
PRUVEL (PruGen) cream, multi ingredient				
CRE, TP (1X100GM)				
100 gm	42546-0125-10	72.27		
PRYFLEX (Zylera) chondroitin/glucosamine/paba/thioctic acid/vit e				
TAB, PO (SF,DYE-FREE) 300 mg-400 mg,				
120s ea	23594-0500-10	195.56		
PSE BROM DM (Boca Pharmacal) bpm/dm/pse hcl				
SYR, PO (GRAPE,AF,SF,DYE-FREE)				
473 ml	64376-0706-16	38.88		
PSE HCL/TRIPROLIDINE HCL FUL				
TAB, PO, 60 mg-2.5 mg, 100s ea		3.36		
(Breckenridge Pharm) *See TRIPOHIST D*				
(Consolidated Midland) *See PSEUDOEPHEDRINE/TRIPROLIDINE*				
(Consolidated Midland) *See TRIACIN*				
(Ohm) *See TRISUDRINE*				
(Truxton) *See PSEUDOCOT-T*				
(Vindex Pharma Inc) *See ZYMINE-D*				

PROD/MFR	NDC	AWP	DP	OBC
(Vita-Rx) *See VI-SUDO*				
(Zyber) *See PEDIATEX TD*				
PSE-BPM (Boca Pharmacal) bpm/pse hcl				
SOL, PO (AF,SF,DYE-FREE,CHERRY) 4 mg/5 ml-60 mg/5 ml,				
480 ml	64376-0721-16	32.39		
PSEUBROM (Dispensing Solutions) REPACK bpm/pse hcl				
CER, PO, 12 mg-120 mg,				
30s ea	55045-1554-08	14.45		
PSEUDACARB (Breckenridge Pharm) carbetapentane tannate/pseudoephedrine tannate				
CTB, PO (DYE-FREE,GRAPE) 25 mg-75 mg,				
100s ea	51991-0108-01	162.50		
PSEUDATEX HC (Breckenridge Pharm) gg/hydrocod bit/pse hcl				
SOL, PO (AF,SF,GRAPE)				
473 ml, C-III	51991-0522-16	68.88		
PSEUDO COUGH (Boca Pharmacal) dm/gg/pse hcl				
SOL, PO (AF,GRAPE)				
118 ml	64376-0733-40	13.39		
473 ml	64376-0733-16	50.88		
PSEUDO DM GG (Boca Pharmacal) dm/gg/pse hcl				
SOL, PO (AF,SF,DYE-FREE)				
480 ml	64376-0712-16	36.85		
PSEUDO-CHLOR (Nucare Pharm) REPACK cpm/pse hcl				
CER, PO, 8 mg-120 mg,				
6s ea	66267-0184-06	6.07		
20s ea	66267-0184-20	8.49		
PSEUDO-G (Southwood) REPACK guaifenesin/pseudoephedrine hydrochloride				
CER, PO, 250 mg-120 mg,				
30s ea	58016-0790-30	27.35		
60s ea	58016-0790-60	52.65		
100s ea	58016-0790-00	84.92		
PSEUDO/BROMPHEN MALEATE (Phys Total Care) REPACK bpm/pse hcl				
TER, PO, 6 mg-45 mg,				
30s ea	54868-5491-00	39.42		
PSEUDO/GUAIFENESIN (Bryant Ranch) REPACK guaifenesin/pseudoephedrine hydrochloride				
TER, PO, 600 mg-120 mg,				
20s ea	63629-2872-01	12.16		
PSEUDOCOT-C (Truxton) cpm/pse hcl				
CER, PO, 8 mg-120 mg,				
100s ea	00463-3035-05	19.80		
PSEUDOCOT-G (Truxton) guaifenesin/pseudoephedrine hydrochloride				
TER, PO, 100 mg-60 mg,				
100s ea	00463-7014-01	10.80		
PSEUDOCOT-T (Truxton) pse hcl/triprolidine hcl				
TAB, PO, 60 mg-2.5 mg,				
1000s ea	00463-6277-10	24.00		EE
PSEUDOEPHEDRINE (Core) REPACK pseudoephedrine hydrochloride				
TAB, PO, 30 mg, 24s ea	33358-0311-24	9.21		
30s ea	33358-0311-30	13.34		
60 mg, 15s ea	33358-0312-15	5.14		
20s ea	33358-0312-20	5.70		
30s ea	33358-0312-30	7.24		
PSEUDOEPHEDRINE AND CODEINE (Breckenridge Pharm) codeine phosphate/pseudoephedrine hydrochloride				
SOL, PO (1X473ML,AF,SF,DYE-FREE) 10 mg/5 ml-30 mg/5 ml,				
473 ml, C-V	51991-0665-16	95.12		
PSEUDOEPHEDRINE GG (Boca Pharmacal) guaifenesin/pseudoephedrine hydrochloride				
SYR, PO (GRAPE) 200 mg/5 ml-40 mg/5 ml,				
473 ml	64376-0716-16	33.69		

PROD/MFR	NDC	AWP	DP	OBC
PSEUDOEPHEDRINE HCL (Gallipot) pseudoephedrine hydrochloride				
POW, NA (U.S.P.,N.F.)				
100 gm	51552-0125-05	43.75		
500 gm	51552-0125-06	150.71		
(Medisca)				
POW, NA (U.S.P.)				
10 gm	38779-0254-01	34.50		
25 gm	38779-0254-04	55.50		
100 gm	38779-0254-05	108.00		
500 gm	38779-0254-08	358.50		
(PCCA)				
POW, NA (U.S.P.)				
1 gm	51927-1159-00	3.60		
PSEUDOEPHEDRINE HYDROCHLORIDE				
(Amend) *See D-PSEUDOEPHEDRINE HYDROCHLORIDE*				
(Gallipot) *See PSEUDOEPHEDRINE HCL*				
(Medisca) *See PSEUDOEPHEDRINE HCL*				
(PCCA) *See PSEUDOEPHEDRINE HCL*				
(Bryant Ranch) REPACK				
TAB, PO, 30 mg, 24s ea	63629-2625-02	8.99		
30s ea	63629-2625-01	13.01		
60 mg, 15s ea	63629-1491-03	5.01		
20s ea	63629-1491-01	5.56		
30s ea	63629-1491-02	7.06		
(Palmetto) REPACK				
SYR, PO (1X120ML)				
30 mg/5 ml, 120 ml	23490-6751-01	6.29		
TAB, PO, 30 mg, 20s ea	23490-6749-01	8.66		
30s ea	23490-6749-02	12.99		
PSEUDOEPHEDRINE HYDROCHLORIDE/GUAIFENESIN (Pharma Pac) REPACK guaifenesin/pseudoephedrine hydrochloride				
CER, PO, 400 mg-120 mg,				
20s ea	52959-0867-20	28.60		
PSEUDOEPHEDRINE TANNATE				
(Athlon Pharm) *See ENTEX*				
(Hawthorn Pharm) *See NASOFED*				
PSEUDOEPHEDRINE TANNATE/ TRIPROLIDINE TANNATE (Vindex Pharma Inc) *See ZYMINE DXR*				
PSEUDOEPHEDRINE/CHLORPHENIRAM (DHS, Inc.) REPACK cpm/pse hcl				
CER, PO, 8 mg-120 mg,				
20s ea	55887-0354-20	9.60		
PSEUDOEPHEDRINE/GUAIFENESIN (Bryant Ranch) REPACK guaifenesin/pseudoephedrine hydrochloride				
TER, PO, 600 mg-120 mg,				
20s ea	63629-1755-01	15.20		
PSEUDOEPHEDRINE/TRIPROLIDINE (Consolidated Midland) pse hcl/triprolidine hcl				
TAB, PO, 60 mg-2.5 mg,				
100s ea	00223-2115-01	4.25		EE
1000s ea	00223-2115-02	29.50		EE
(A-S Medication) REPACK				
TAB, PO, 60 mg-2.5 mg,				
24s ea	54569-4606-02	2.14		EE
30s ea	54569-4606-01	2.67		EE
PSEUDOPHEDRINE HCL (Quality Care Prod) REPACK pseudoephedrine hydrochloride				
TAB, PO, 30 mg, 24s ea	49999-0652-24	3.22		
PSEUDOVENT DM (Ethex) dm/gg/pse hcl				
TER, PO (CAPLET) 32 mg-595 mg-48 mg,				
100s ea	58177-0438-04	49.20		
PSORCON (Phys Total Care) REPACK diflorasone diacetate				
CRE, TP, 0.05%, 15 gm	54868-2658-00	51.69		AB
30 gm	54868-2658-01	70.77		AB
OIN, TP, 0.05%, 60 gm	54868-2222-01	146.41		AB
(Southwood) REPACK				
OIN, TP, 0.05%, 30 gm	58016-3247-01	40.10		AB

PROD/MFR NDC AWP DP OBC

PSORCON E (Phys Total Care)
REPACK
diflorasone diacetate
OIN, TP, 0.05%, 60 gm **54868-4790-00** 118.16

PSORIZIDE FORTE (Loma Lux)
homeopathic
TAB, PO, 1 x-1 x-1 x,
90s ea **61480-0255-05** 85.00

PSORIZIDE ULTRA (Loma Lux)
kali bromatum/niccolum sulphuricum/zincum bromatum
TAB, PO, 1 x-1 x-4 x,
100s ea **61480-0124-05** 67.50

PSYLLIUM
(Gallipot) *See PSYLLIUM HUSK*

PSYLLIUM HUSK (Gallipot)
psyllium
POW, NA, 1000 gm **51552-1061-07** 24.50 17.50

PSYLLIUM HUSK (Medisca)
POW, NA (1X500GM,USP)
500 gm **38779-1552-08** 31.50
(1X1000GM,USP)
1000 gm **38779-1552-09** 55.50

(PCCA)
POW, NA, 1 gm **51927-1552-00** 0.09

PULMARI-GP (Cypress Pharm)
carbetapentane citrate/guaifenesin
SYR, PO (AF,GRAPE)
20 mg-100 mg,
472 ml **60258-0425-16** 48.41

PULMICORT FLEX (Phys Total Care)
REPACK
budesonide
POW, IH, 180 mcg/actuation,
ea **54868-5844-00** 179.03

PULMICORT FLEXHALER (AstraZeneca)
budesonide
POW, IH, 90 mcg/actuation,
ea **00186-0917-06** 117.29
180 mcg/actuation,
ea **00186-0916-12** 157.06

(A-S Medication)
REPACK
POW, IH (FLEXHALER)
180 mcg/actuation,
ea **54569-5928-00** 194.45

PULMICORT RESPULES (AstraZeneca)
budesonide
SUS, IH (5X6)
0.25 mg/2 ml,
2 ml 30s **00186-1988-04** 226.56
0.5 mg/2 ml,
2 ml 30s **00186-1989-04** 266.65
(30X2ML)
1 mg/2 ml,
2 ml 30s .... **00186-1990-04** 533.33 EE

(Phys Total Care)
REPACK
SUS, IH, 0.25 mg/2 ml,
60s ea **54868-5774-00** 234.18
0.5 mg/2 ml, 60 ml ... **54868-5621-00** 288.92

PULMO-AIDE COMPACT COMPRESSOR/NEBULIZER (Sunrise Medical)
nebulizer, direct patient interface
DEV, NA (MODEL #3655D)
ea **16958-0684-58** 134.00

PULMO-AIDE COMPRESSOR/NEBULIZER (Sunrise Medical)
nebulizer, direct patient interface
DEV, NA (AEROSOL COMPRESSOR)
ea **33413-0056-50** 170.00

PULMOLITE (Pharmlucence)
technetium tc 99m albumin aggregated
KIT, IV (5 VIALS,PF)
ea .... **45567-0415-01** 117.30 97.75 BS
(5 VLS/KIT,PF)
6s ea .... **45567-0415-02** 703.80 586.60 BS

PULMOMATE COMPRESSOR/NEBULIZER (Sunrise Medical)
nebulizer, direct patient interface
DEV, NA (METAL HEAD COMPRESSOR)
ea **33413-0046-50** 150.00

PULMONA (Physician Thera, LLC)
amino acids and nutriceuticals
CAP, PO (PF,SF,DYE-FREE)
90s ea **68405-1005-03** 164.74

(Altura)
REPACK
CAP, PO, 90s ea **63874-1181-09** 128.70

(Dispensing Solutions)
REPACK
CAP, PO (PF,SF,DYE-FREE)
90s ea **55045-3399-09** 128.70

PULMOZYME (Genentech)
dornase alfa
SOL, IH (AMP,INNER NDC)
2.5 mg/2.5 ml,
2.5 ml **50242-0100-39** 74.10
(AMP)
2.5 mg/2.5 ml,
2.5 ml 30s **50242-0100-40** 2222.93

PUMICE
(Gallipot) *See PUMICE STONE*

(Medisca)
POW, NA (1X500GM,USP)
500 gm **38779-1553-08** 37.50

(PCCA)
POW, NA (USP, FLOUR)
1 gm **51927-2049-00** 0.09

(Spectrum Pharmacy)
POW, NA (U.S.P.)
500 gm **49452-6130-01** 72.10
2500 gm **49452-6130-02** 219.10

PUMICE STONE (Gallipot)
pumice
POW, NA (EXTRA FINE,AF)
56.7 gm **51552-0486-03** 8.96

PUMP, INFUSION
(Abbott Hosp) *See CONTROLLER LIFECARE*

(Abbott Hosp) *See LIFECARE PUMP MODEL 4 PIGGYBACK*

(Abbott Hosp) *See PLUM LC 5000*

(Medtronic Minimed) *See PARADIGM INSULIN INFUSION PUMP*

PUMP, INFUSION, PATIENT CONTROLLED ANALGESIA (PCA)
(Abbott Hosp) *See PCA PLUS 2*

PUMPKIN FLAVOR (Medisca)
flavoring aid
SOL, NA (1X25ML)
25 ml **38779-1554-04** 22.50
(1X100ML)
100 ml **38779-1554-05** 34.50

(PCCA)
SOL, NA (ARTIFICIAL)
1 ml **51927-2659-00** 0.90

PUMPKIN SEED (PCCA)
POW, NA, 1 gm **51927-3487-00** 0.75

PURIFIED WATER (Medisca)
water, purified
SOL, NA (1X100ML,DISTILLED)
100 ml **38779-0946-05** 450.00
(1X4000ML,DISTILLED)
4000 ml **38779-0946-01** 40.50

PURINETHOL (Gate)
mercaptopurine
TAB, PO, 50 mg, 60s ea ... **57844-0522-06** 365.49

PYGEUM BARK (PCCA)
african pygeum bark
POW, NA, 1 gm **51927-3638-00** 0.46

PYLERA (Axcan)
bi subcitrate k/metronidazole/tetracycline hcl
CAP, PO, 140 mg-125 mg-125 mg,
120s ea **58914-0600-21** 416.74

PYRANTEL PAMOATE (Gallipot)
POW, NA (U.S.P.)
1000 gm **51552-0954-07** 595.00 425.00

(Hawkins)
POW, NA (U.S.P.)
25 gm **63370-0213-25** 56.00
100 gm **63370-0213-35** 187.00
1000 gm **63370-0213-50** 1560.00

(Medisca)
POW, NA (U.S.P.)
25 gm **38779-0059-04** 55.50
100 gm **38779-0059-05** 187.50
500 gm **38779-0059-08** 705.00
(1X1000GM,USP)
1000 gm **38779-0059-09** 1197.00

(PCCA)
POW, NA (USP)
1 gm **51927-2126-00** 2.40

(Spectrum Pharmacy)
POW, NA (U.S.P.)
25 gm **49452-8138-01** 89.60
100 gm **49452-8138-02** 292.25
1000 gm **49452-8138-04** 1704.50

PYRAZINAMIDE (Dava Pharma)
TAB, PO, 500 mg, 100s ea . **67253-0660-10** 120.55 AB
500s ea .... **67253-0660-50** 596.35 AB

(Spectrum Pharmacy)
CRY, NA (U.S.P.)
25 gm **49452-6135-01** 105.00
100 gm **49452-6135-02** 314.65
1000 gm **49452-6135-04** 1785.00

(VersaPharm)
TAB, PO, 500 mg, 60s ea .. **61748-0012-06** 69.75 AB
90s ea .... **61748-0012-09** 104.46 AB
100s ea .... **61748-0012-01** 113.38 AB
(10X10)
500 mg, 100s ea UD .. **61748-0012-11** 119.54 AB
500s ea .... **61748-0012-05** 559.75 AB

(A-S Medication)
REPACK
TAB, PO, 500 mg, 100s ea . **54569-3950-00** 120.55 EE

(Phys Total Care)
REPACK
TAB, PO, 500 mg, 120s ea . **54868-2487-01** 286.76 EE

PYRELLE HB (Azur Pharma, Inc.)
belladonna alkaloids and analgesics
TAB, PO, 15 mg-0.3 mg-150 mg,
30s ea **66663-0702-01** 46.21

PYRICHLOR PE (Breckenridge Pharm)
cpm/phenyleph hcl/pyril mal
SOL, PO (1X473ML,AF,SF,GRAPE)
473 ml **51991-0624-16** 65.86

PYRIDIATE (Truxton)
phenazopyridine hydrochloride
TAB, PO, 100 mg,
1000s ea **00463-6162-10** 31.20
200 mg, 1000s ea **00463-6163-10** 39.50

PYRIDIUM (Warner Chilcott)
phenazopyridine hydrochloride
TAB, PO (COATED)
100 mg, 100s ea **00430-0190-24** 108.75
(COATED,CAPLET)
200 mg, 100s ea **00430-0191-24** 209.54

(PD-Rx Pharm)
REPACK
TAB, PO, 200 mg, 6s ea ... **55289-0689-06** 23.60

(Phys Total Care)
REPACK
TAB, PO, 200 mg, 10s ea .. **54868-0456-02** 10.41

PYRIDOSTIGMINE BROMIDE
FUL
TAB, PO, 60 mg, 100s ea 58.32

(Global Pharm)
TAB, PO, 60 mg, 100s ea .. **00115-3511-01** 59.85 AB

(Oceanside)
TAB, PO (USP)
60 mg, 100s ea **68682-0302-10** 57.50

(PCCA)
POW, NA, 1 gm **51927-2798-00** 71.40

(Sandoz) *See REGONOL*

(Sandoz)
TAB, PO, 60 mg, 100s ea .. **00781-5015-01** 59.98

(Spectrum Pharmacy)
CRY, NA (1X5GM)
5 gm **49452-6138-02** 434.00
(1X25GM)
25 gm **49452-6138-03** 1172.50

(Valeant Pharm Intl) *See MESTINON*

(Valeant Pharm Intl) *See MESTINON TIMESPAN*

PYRIDOXAL PHOSPHATE
(Medisca) *See PYRIDOXAL-5-PHOSPHATE*

(PCCA) *See PYRIDOXAL-5-PHOSPHATE MONOHYDRATE*

(Spectrum Pharmacy) *See PYRIDOXAL-5-PHOSPHATE*

PYRIDOXAL-5-PHOSPHATE (Medisca)
pyridoxal phosphate
POW, NA (1X1GM)
1 gm **38779-1556-06** 24.00

PROD/MFR	NDC	AWP	DP	OBC
(1X5GM)				
5 gm	38779-1556-03	117.00		
(1X25GM)				
25 gm	38779-1556-04	447.00		
(1X100GM)				
100 gm	38779-1556-05	1362.00		
(Spectrum Pharmacy)				
POW, NA (1X5GM, MONOHYDRATE)				
5 gm	49452-6148-02	184.10		
(1X25GM, MONOHYDRATE)				
25 gm	49452-6148-03	675.50		
(1X100GM, MONOHYDRATE)				
100 gm	49452-6148-04	1921.50		
PYRIDOXAL-5-PHOSPHATE MONOHYDRATE (PCCA)				
pyridoxal phosphate				
POW, NA (1X1GM)				
1 gm	51927-2044-00	27.00		
PYRIDOXINE				
(APP) *See PYRIDOXINE HYDROCHLORIDE*				
(Baker, J.T.) *See PYRIDOXINE HCL*				
(Consolidated Midland) *See PYRIDOXINE HCL*				
(Consolidated Midland) *See VITABEE 6*				
(Gallipot) *See PYRIDOXINE HCL*				
(Legere) *See RODEX*				
(Letco) *See PYRIDOXINE HCL*				
(Medisca) *See PYRIDOXINE HCL*				
(PCCA) *See PYRIDOXINE HCL*				
(Spectrum Pharmacy) *See PYRIDOXINE HCL*				
(Core) REPACK				
SOL, IJ (SINGLE-DOSE)				
100 mg/ml, 1 ml	33358-0313-01	9.48		
(Pharma Pac) REPACK				
TAB, PO, 50 mg, 20s ea	52959-0218-20	2.18		
60s ea	52959-0218-60	6.16		
100s ea	52959-0218-00	10.22		
PYRIDOXINE HCL (Baker, J.T.)				
pyridoxine				
POW, NA (U.S.P., F.C.C.)				
5 gm	10106-3343-01	32.05		
(Consolidated Midland)				
SOL, IJ (VIAL)				
100 mg/ml, 10 ml	00223-8403-10	5.50		EE
30 ml	00223-8404-30	6.50		EE
(Gallipot)				
POW, NA (U.S.P.,N.F.)				
25 gm	51552-0149-04	9.80		
100 gm	51552-0149-05	18.20		
(Letco)				
POW, NA (U.S.P.)				
100 gm	62991-1130-02	37.50		
500 gm	62991-1130-03	120.00		
(Medisca)				
POW, NA (U.S.P.)				
25 gm	38779-0873-04	23.55		
100 gm	38779-0873-05	43.50		
500 gm	38779-0873-08	165.00		
1000 gm	38779-0873-09	297.00		
(PCCA)				
POW, NA (USP)				
1 gm	51927-1093-00	1.14		
(Spectrum Pharmacy)				
POW, NA (U.S.P.)				
25 gm	49452-6140-01	44.10		
100 gm	49452-6140-02	69.30		
1000 gm	49452-6140-03	511.00		
PYRIDOXINE HYDROCHLORIDE (APP)				
pyridoxine				
SOL, IJ (M.D.V.,AMBER,25X1ML)				
100 mg/ml,				
1 ml 25s	63323-0180-01	280.94		AP
PYRIL DM (Macoven)				
dm/phenyleph hcl/pyril mal				
SUS, PO (GRAPE)				
473 ml	44183-0210-16	262.15		
PYRILAMINE MALEATE (Gallipot)				
POW, NA, 10 gm	51552-0032-03	12.60		
25 gm	51552-0032-04	18.55		
100 gm	51552-0032-05	54.46		
500 gm	51552-0032-06	219.10		
(Medisca)				
POW, NA (U.S.P.)				
25 gm	38779-0255-04	40.50		
100 gm	38779-0255-05	117.00		
500 gm	38779-0255-08	469.50		
(Spectrum Pharmacy)				
POW, NA (U.S.P.)				
25 gm	49452-6150-01	89.95		
(U.S.P., N.F.)				
100 gm	49452-6150-02	249.90		
500 gm	49452-6150-03	850.50		
PYRILAMINE TANNATE				
(Athlon Pharm) *See PYRLEX*				
PYRIMETHAMINE (Gallipot)				
POW, NA (U.S.P.)				
100 gm	51552-0617-05	56.00		
1000 gm	51552-0617-07	308.00		
(Glaxo) *See DARAPRIM*				
(Medisca)				
POW, NA (U.S.P.)				
5 gm	38779-0884-03	43.50		
25 gm	38779-0884-04	70.50		
100 gm	38779-0884-05	126.00		
500 gm	38779-0884-08	465.00		
1000 gm	38779-0884-09	645.00		
(PCCA)				
POW, NA (U.S.P.)				
1 gm	51927-3122-00	7.20		
(Spectrum Pharmacy)				
POW, NA (U.S.P.)				
25 gm	49452-6151-02	108.90		
100 gm	49452-6151-03	194.25		
1000 gm	49452-6151-05	924.00		
PYRITHIONE ZINC				
(Gallipot) *See ZINC PYRITHIONE*				
(PCCA) *See ZINC PYRITHIONE*				
PYRLEX (Athlon Pharm)				
pyrilamine tannate				
SUS, PO (BUBBLE GUM)				
12 mg/5 ml, 473 ml	66813-0161-16	172.90		
PYRLEX CB (Athlon Pharm)				
carbetapentane tannate/pyrilamine tannate				
SUS, PO (1X473ML,SF)				
22.5 mg/5 ml-12 mg/5 ml,				
473 ml	66813-0162-16	196.48		
PYRLEX PD (Athlon Pharm)				
phenylephrine tannate/pyrilamine tannate				
SUS, PO (COTTON CANDY)				
9 mg/5 ml-12 mg/5 ml,				
473 ml	66813-0163-16	182.33		
PYROGALLIC ACID (Gordon)				
pyrogallol				
OIN, TP, 25%, 30 gm	10481-1028-01	37.50		
PYROGALLOL (Baker, J.T.)				
CRY, NA (PURIFIED)				
500 gm	10106-0290-01	123.70		
(Gordon) *See PYROGALLIC ACID*				
(PCCA)				
POW, NA (ACS)				
1 gm	51927-1506-00	4.20		
(Spectrum Pharmacy)				
CRY, NA (1X25GM)				
25 gm	49452-6157-01	131.95		
(1X125GM)				
125 gm	49452-6157-02	317.10		
(1X500GM)				
500 gm	49452-6157-03	707.00		
PYROXYLIN				
(Mallinckrodt Lab) *See PARLODION*				
PYRUVIC ACID				
(PCCA) *See PYRUVIC ACID SODIUM SALT*				
(PCCA)				
SOL, NA, 1 gm	51927-3374-00	2.76		
PYRUVIC ACID SODIUM SALT (PCCA)				
pyruvic acid				
POW, NA, 1 gm	51927-2916-00	6.00		
PYTEST (Kimberly-Clark Hc)				
14c urea				
CAP, PO, 1 uci, 10s ea	63584-0001-10	280.00		
100s ea	63584-0001-00	2408.00		
KIT, NA, 1 uci, ea	63584-0001-02	90.00		
Q-BID DM (Quality Care Prod) REPACK				
dextromethorphan hydrobromide/guaifenesin				
TER, PO, 30 mg-600 mg,				
30s ea	49999-0558-30	15.23		
QDALL (Phys Total Care) REPACK				
cpm/pse hcl				
C24, PO, 12 mg-100 mg,				
30s ea	54868-5094-01	43.03		
100s ea	54868-5094-00	10.63		
QUAD TANN (Breckenridge Pharm)				
cpm tan/carbetapentane tan/eph tan/phenyleph tan				
TAB, PO (CAPLET)				
60 mg-5 mg-10 mg-10 mg,				
100s ea	51991-0816-01	250.98		
QUAD TANN PEDIATRIC (Breckenridge Pharm)				
cpm tan/carbetapentane tan/eph tan/phenyleph tan				
SUS, PO (BERRY)				
473 ml	51991-0815-16	219.95		
QUADRAMET (EUSA)				
samarium sm 153 lexidronam pentasodium				
SOL, IV (1X3ML,SDV)				
50 mci/ml, 3 ml	57902-0860-01	6683.95		
QUADRATUSS PEDIATRIC (Unigen)				
cpm tan/carbetapentane tan/eph tan/phenyleph tan				
SUS, PO (GRAPE)				
473 ml	62305-0403-16	44.00	15.95	
QUALAQUIN (AR Scientific)				
quinine sulfate				
CAP, PO, 324 mg, 30s ea	13310-0153-07	183.42		
(Stat Rx) REPACK				
CAP, PO, 324 mg, 30s ea	16590-0595-30	199.56		
60s ea	16590-0595-60	291.00		
90s ea	16590-0595-90	428.50		
QUARTUSS (Breckenridge Pharm)				
cpm/dm/gg/phenyleph hcl				
SOL, PO (AF,SF,CHERRY)				
473 ml	51991-0513-16	31.15		
QUARTUSS DM (Breckenridge Pharm)				
cpm/dm/phenyleph hcl				
SOL, PO (1X30ML,W/DROPPER,AF,SF)				
30 ml	51991-0537-03	19.22		
QUASENSE (Watson)				
ethinyl estradiol/levonorgestrel				
TAB, PO (3X91)				
30 mcg-0.15 mg,				
273s ea	52544-0966-91	462.80		AB
QUATERNIUM-15 (PCCA)				
POW, NA, 1 gm	51927-2342-00	2.28		
QUAZEPAM				
(Questcor Pharm) *See DORAL*				
QUELICIN (Hospira)				
succinylcholine chloride				
SOL, IV, 20 mg/ml,				
5 ml 10s	00074-8065-15	96.12	84.10	AP
(VIAL, FLIPTOP)				
20 mg/ml,				
10 ml 25s	00074-6629-02	56.10	49.00	AP
(VIAL,FLIPTOP)				
20 mg/ml,				
10 ml 25s	00409-6629-02	56.10	49.00	AP
(FTV,25X10ML,20ML VIAL)				
100 mg/ml,				
10 ml 25s	00409-6970-10	290.10	253.75	
(VIAL, FLIPTOP, 20 ML)				
100 mg/ml,				
10 ml 25s	00074-6970-10	284.70	249.00	
QUERCETIN (PCCA)				
POW, NA (DIHYDRATE)				
1 gm	51927-2308-00	2.88		
QUESTRAN (Par)				
cholestyramine				
PDR, PO, 4 gm/9 gm,				
60s ea	49884-0936-65	253.86		
(USP,SCOOP ENCLOSED)				
4 gm/9 gm, 378 gm	49884-0936-66	111.18		
(Phys Total Care) REPACK				
PDR, PO, 4 gm/9 gm,				
60s ea	54868-2647-00	246.25		AB
(Southwood) REPACK				
PDR, PO (CAN)				
4 gm/9 gm, 378 gm	58016-9066-01	46.58		AB

PROD/MFR	NDC	AWP	DP	OBC
QUESTRAN LIGHT (Par)				
cholestyramine				
PDR, PO (W/SCOOP)				
4 gm/5 gm, 60s ea	**49884-0937-65**	255.24		
210 gm	**49884-0937-67**	111.82		
(Southwood)				
REPACK				
PDR, PO (PACKET)				
4 gm/5 gm, 60s ea	**58016-9111-01**	92.50		AB
(CAN)				
4 gm/5 gm, 210 gm	**58016-9967-01**	46.68		AB
QUETIAPINE FUMARATE				
(AstraZeneca) *See SEROQUEL*				
(AstraZeneca) *See SEROQUEL XR*				
(Palmetto)				
REPACK				
TAB, PO, 25 mg, 30s ea	**23490-7088-02**	65.57		
60s ea	**23490-7088-03**	119.43		
100 mg, 30s ea	**23490-7089-01**	99.31		
60s ea	**23490-7089-02**	223.30		
200 mg, 30s ea	**23490-7090-01**	200.83		
QUICK-SET INFUSION (Medtronic Minimed)				
kit, administration, intravenous				
DEV, NA (23"TUBING W/6MM CANNULA)				
10s ea	**76300-0393-10**	146.16		
(23"TUBING W/9MM CANNULA)				
10s ea	**76300-0392-10**	146.16		
(43"TUBING W/6MM CANNULA)				
10s ea	**76300-0391-10**	146.16		
(43"TUBING W/9MM CANNULA)				
10s ea	**76300-0390-10**	146.16		
QUICK-SET PARADIGM (Medtronic Minimed)				
diabetic supplies				
DEV, NA (6MM, 18")				
10s ea	**76300-0394-10**	146.16		
(6MM, 32")				
10s ea	**76300-0387-10**	146.16		
(9MM, 32")				
10s ea	**76300-0386-10**	146.16		
QUINACRINE HCL (Gallipot)				
quinacrine hydrochloride				
POW, NA (U.S.P.)				
25 gm	**51552-0358-04**	37.80		
100 gm	**51552-0358-05**	147.00		
(Hawkins)				
POW, NA, 25 gm	**63370-0215-25**	108.00		
100 gm	**63370-0215-35**	400.00		
500 gm	**63370-0215-45**	1840.00		
1000 gm	**63370-0215-50**	2920.00		
QUINACRINE HCL DIHYDRATE (Spectrum Pharmacy)				
quinacrine hydrochloride				
POW, NA (U.S.P.)				
5 gm	**49452-6168-01**	127.40	15.35	
25 gm	**49452-6168-02**	181.30	43.90	
100 gm	**49452-6168-03**	591.50	148.75	
(1X1000GM)				
1000 gm	**49452-6168-05**	3276.50		
QUINACRINE HYDROCHLORIDE				
(Gallipot) *See QUINACRINE HCL*				
(Hawkins) *See QUINACRINE HCL*				
(PCCA)				
POW, NA, 1 gm	**51927-2193-00**	5.16		
(Spectrum Pharmacy) *See QUINACRINE HCL DIHYDRATE*				
QUINAPRIL (Apotex Corp.)				
quinapril hydrochloride				
TAB, PO (USP,FILM COATED)				
5 mg, 90s ea	**60505-0172-00**	110.08		AB
1000s ea	**60505-0172-01**	1223.11		AB
10 mg, 90s ea	**60505-0173-00**	110.08		AB
1000s ea	**60505-0173-01**	1223.11		AB
20 mg, 90s ea	**60505-0174-00**	110.08		AB
1000s ea	**60505-0174-01**	1223.11		AB
40 mg, 90s ea	**60505-0175-00**	110.08		AB
1000s ea	**60505-0175-01**	1223.11		AB
(Dr Reddy's)				
TAB, PO (USP)				
5 mg, 90s ea	**55111-0621-90**	110.08		AB
10 mg, 90s ea	**55111-0622-90**	110.08		AB
20 mg, 90s ea	**55111-0623-90**	110.08		AB
40 mg, 90s ea	**55111-0624-90**	110.08		AB
(Lupin Pharma, Inc.)				
TAB, PO (USP,FILM COATED)				
5 mg, 90s ea	**68180-0556-09**	42.00		AB
10 mg, 90s ea	**68180-0557-09**	42.00		AB
20 mg, 90s ea	**68180-0558-09**	42.00		AB
40 mg, 90s ea	**68180-0559-09**	42.00		AB
(Mylan)				
TAB, PO (USP,FILM-COATED)				
5 mg, 90s ea	**00378-1117-77**	110.10		AB
(Ranbaxy Pharm)				
TAB, PO (USP,FILM-COATED)				
5 mg, 90s ea	**63304-0548-90**	110.10		AB
10 mg, 90s ea	**63304-0549-90**	110.10		AB
20 mg, 90s ea	**63304-0550-90**	110.10		AB
40 mg, 90s ea	**63304-0551-90**	110.10		AB
(Teva)				
TAB, PO (USP,FILM COATED)				
5 mg, 90s ea	**00093-1050-98**	141.37		AB
500s ea	**00093-1050-05**	785.40		AB
10 mg, 90s ea	**00093-1051-98**	141.37		AB
500s ea	**00093-1051-05**	785.40		AB
(USP,FILM COATED, CAPLET)				
20 mg, 90s ea	**00093-1045-98**	141.37		AB
500s ea	**00093-1045-05**	785.40		AB
(USP,FILM COATED)				
40 mg, 90s ea	**00093-1053-98**	141.37		AB
500s ea	**00093-1053-05**	785.40		AB
(A-S Medication)				
REPACK				
TAB, PO (FILM COATED, CAPLET)				
20 mg, 30s ea	**54569-5710-00**	38.18		AB
(FILM COATED)				
40 mg, 30s ea	**54569-5711-00**	38.18		AB
(Bryant Ranch)				
REPACK				
TAB, PO (FILM COATED, CAPLET)				
20 mg, 30s ea	**63629-1241-01**	35.92		AB
(Dispensing Solutions)				
REPACK				
TAB, PO (FILM COATED)				
5 mg, 90s ea	**55045-3641-09**	98.10		AB
10 mg, 90s ea	**55045-3642-09**	98.10		AB
(FILM COATED, CAPLET)				
20 mg, 90s ea	**55045-3643-09**	98.10		AB
(FILM COATED)				
40 mg, 90s ea	**55045-3644-09**	98.10		AB
(Phys Total Care)				
REPACK				
TAB, PO, 40 mg, 90s ea	**54868-5246-01**	68.66		
(Physician Partner)				
REPACK				
TAB, PO, 5 mg, 30s ea	**21695-0393-30**	73.38		
10 mg, 30s ea	**21695-0394-30**	73.38		
QUINAPRIL HCL (Greenstone)				
quinapril hydrochloride				
TAB, PO (FILM-COATED)				
5 mg, 90s ea	**59762-5019-01**	109.96		
10 mg, 90s ea	**59762-5020-01**	109.96		
20 mg, 90s ea	**59762-5021-01**	109.96		
40 mg, 90s ea	**59762-5022-01**	109.96		
(Mylan)				
TAB, PO (FILM-COATED)				
5 mg, 90s ea	**00378-0017-77**	110.05		AB
10 mg, 90s ea	**00378-0226-77**	110.10		AB
20 mg, 90s ea	**00378-0254-77**	110.10		AB
40 mg, 90s ea	**00378-0272-77**	110.10		AB
(Teva)				
TAB, PO (FILM-COATED)				
5 mg, 90s ea	**00093-5456-98**	110.08		AB
10 mg, 90s ea	**00093-5457-98**	110.08		AB
20 mg, 90s ea	**00093-5458-98**	110.08		AB
40 mg, 90s ea	**00093-5459-98**	110.08		AB
(A-S Medication)				
REPACK				
TAB, PO (FILM-COATED)				
10 mg, 30s ea	**54569-5709-00**	38.18		
(Phys Total Care)				
REPACK				
TAB, PO (FILM-COATED)				
5 mg, 30s ea	**54868-5279-00**	85.05		AB
10 mg, 30s ea	**54868-5245-00**	31.62		AB
60s ea	**54868-5245-01**	46.77		AB
90s ea	**54868-5245-02**	67.17		AB
20 mg, 30s ea	**54868-5241-00**	31.62		AB
60s ea	**54868-5241-01**	50.04		AB
90s ea	**54868-5241-02**	72.09		AB
40 mg, 30s ea	**54868-5246-00**	53.40		AB
QUINAPRIL HYDROCHLORIDE				
FUL				
TAB, PO, 5 mg, 90s ea		22.50		
10 mg, 90s ea		22.50		
20 mg, 90s ea		22.50		
40 mg, 90s ea		22.50		
(Apotex Corp.) *See QUINAPRIL*				
(Dr Reddy's) *See QUINAPRIL*				
(Greenstone) *See QUINAPRIL HCL*				
(Lupin Pharma, Inc.) *See QUINAPRIL*				
(Mylan) *See QUINAPRIL*				
(Mylan) *See QUINAPRIL HCL*				
(Pfizer) *See ACCUPRIL*				
(Ranbaxy Pharm) *See QUINAPRIL*				
(Teva) *See QUINAPRIL*				
(Teva) *See QUINAPRIL HCL*				
(Palmetto)				
REPACK				
TAB, PO, 40 mg, 30s ea	**23490-9364-03**	100.91		
QUINAPRIL HYDROCHLORIDE AND HYDROCHLOROTHIAZIDE (Aurobindo Pharma)				
hydrochlorothiazide/quinapril hydrochloride				
TAB, PO (FILM-COATED)				
12.5 mg-10 mg, 90s ea	**65862-0161-90**	110.10		AB
12.5 mg-20 mg, 30s ea	**65862-0162-30**	36.70		AB
90s ea	**65862-0162-90**	110.10		AB
25 mg-20 mg, 90s ea	**65862-0163-90**	110.10		AB
(Mylan)				
TAB, PO (FILM COATED)				
12.5 mg-10 mg, 90s ea	**00378-0542-77**	110.10		AB
12.5 mg-20 mg, 90s ea	**00378-0543-77**	110.10		AB
25 mg-20 mg, 90s ea	**00378-0544-77**	110.10		AB
QUINAPRIL HYDROCHLORIDE/ HYDROCHLOROTHIAZIDE (Greenstone)				
hydrochlorothiazide/quinapril hydrochloride				
TAB, PO (FILM-COATED)				
12.5 mg-10 mg, 90s ea	**59762-0222-01**	110.04		
12.5 mg-20 mg, 90s ea	**59762-0220-01**	110.04		
25 mg-20 mg, 90s ea	**59762-0223-01**	110.04		
QUINAPRIL/HCTZ (Phys Total Care)				
REPACK				
hydrochlorothiazide/quinapril hydrochloride				
TAB, PO, 12.5 mg-10 mg, 30s ea	**54868-1802-00**	90.36		
QUINIDEX EXTENTABS (Phys Total Care)				
quinidine sulfate				
TER, PO, 300 mg, 30s ea	**54868-2740-03**	36.16		AB
90s ea	**54868-2740-01**	106.08		AB
QUINIDINE GLUCONATE (Lilly)				
SOL, IJ (VIAL)				
80 mg/ml, 10 ml	**00002-1407-01**	21.56	17.97	
(Mutual)				
TER, PO (FILM-COATED)				
324 mg, 100s ea	**53489-0141-01**	93.50		
250s ea	**53489-0141-03**	225.74		
500s ea	**53489-0141-05**	428.94		
(UDL)				
TER, PO (10X10)				
324 mg, 100s ea UD	**51079-0027-20**	136.80		BX
(Watson Labs)				
TER, PO, 324 mg, 100s ea	**00591-5538-01**	93.37		BX
250s ea	**00591-5538-25**	225.51		BX
500s ea	**00591-5538-05**	428.76		BX
(Palmetto)				
REPACK				
TER, PO, 324 mg, 30s ea	**23490-9365-03**	35.06		
(Phys Total Care)				
REPACK				
TER, PO, 324 mg, 100s ea	**54868-0698-01**	113.05		EE
QUINIDINE SULFATE (Amend)				
POW, NA (U.S.P.)				
30 gm	**17317-0459-01**	35.00		
125 gm	**17317-0459-09**	114.80		
(Consolidated Midland)				
TAB, PO, 200 mg, 100s ea	**00223-1560-01**	11.95		EE
(Letco) *See QUINIDINE SULFATE DIHYDRATE*				
(Mutual)				
TAB, PO, 200 mg, 100s ea	**53489-0461-01**	20.10		AB
300 mg, 100s ea	**53489-0460-01**	38.68		AB

PROD/MFR	NDC	AWP	DP	OBC
(PCCA)				
POW, NA (USP; DIHYDRATE)				
1 gm	**51927-1804-00**	4.68		
(Sandoz)				
TAB, PO, 200 mg, 100s ea	**00185-4346-01**	21.00		AB
1000s ea	**00185-4346-10**	195.30		AB
300 mg, 100s ea	**00185-1047-01**	40.00		AB
1000s ea	**00185-1047-10**	372.00		AB
(Spectrum Pharmacy) *See QUINIDINE SULFATE DIHYDRATE*				
(Spectrum Pharmacy) *See QUININE SULFATE DIHYDRATE*				
(Teva)				
TER, PO, 300 mg, 100s ea	**00093-9175-01**	87.84		AB
250s ea	**00093-9175-52**	217.98		AB
(Watson Labs)				
TAB, PO, 200 mg, 100s ea	**00591-5438-01**	20.10		AB
300 mg, 100s ea	**00591-5454-01**	38.68		AB
(Phys Total Care)				
REPACK				
TAB, PO, 200 mg, 30s ea	**54868-0047-03**	21.81		EE
300 mg, 100s ea	**54868-0898-01**	44.86		EE
QUINIDINE SULFATE DIHYDRATE (Letco)				
quinidine sulfate				
POW, NA (USP)				
25 gm	**62991-2663-01**	90.00		
100 gm	**62991-2663-03**	324.00		
(Spectrum Pharmacy)				
POW, NA (U.S.P.)				
10 gm	**49452-6180-01**	79.10		
50 gm	**49452-6180-02**	321.65		
100 gm	**49452-6180-03**	584.50		
QUININE HCL (Amend)				
quinine hydrochloride				
POW, NA (N.F.)				
25 gm	**17317-0460-01**	23.10		
125 gm	**17317-0460-09**	72.80		
(PCCA)				
POW, NA (NF XI)				
1 gm	**51927-1529-00**	6.75		
QUININE HYDROCHLORIDE				
(Amend) *See QUININE HCL*				
(PCCA) *See QUININE HCL*				
QUININE SULFATE				
(Amend) *See QUININE SULFATE DIHYDRATE*				
(AR Scientific) *See QUALAQUIN*				
(Consolidated Midland)				
CAP, PO, 325 mg, 100s ea	**00223-1561-01**	14.50		
1000s ea	**00223-1561-02**	112.50		
TAB, PO, 260 mg, 500s ea	**00223-1560-05**	47.50		
(Contract Pharmacal)				
CAP, PO (5 GR.)				
325 mg, 100s ea	**10267-0231-01**	90.34		
500s ea	**10267-0231-05**	428.60		
1000s ea	**10267-0231-04**	844.06		
(Gallipot) *See QUININE SULFATE DIHYDRATE*				
(Letco) *See QUININE SULFATE DIHYDRATE*				
(PCCA)				
POW, NA (USP)				
1 gm	**51927-1588-00**	1.80		
(Altura)				
REPACK				
CAP, PO, 324 mg, 10s ea	**63874-0881-10**	3.09		
12s ea	**63874-0881-12**	3.71		
15s ea	**63874-0881-15**	4.64		
20s ea	**63874-0881-20**	6.18		
21s ea	**63874-0881-21**	32.05		
30s ea	**63874-0881-30**	9.27		
40s ea	**63874-0881-40**	12.36		
60s ea	**63874-0881-60**	18.55		
90s ea	**63874-0881-90**	27.82		
100s ea	**63874-0881-01**	30.91		
120s ea	**63874-0881-04**	37.09		
(Bryant Ranch)				
REPACK				
CAP, PO, 324 mg, 30s ea	**63629-1617-01**	29.99		
(Core)				
REPACK				
CAP, PO, 325 mg, 30s ea	**33358-0315-30**	36.70		
TAB, PO, 260 mg, 30s ea	**33358-0314-30**	30.20		
(Dispensing Solutions)				
REPACK				
CAP, PO, 325 mg, 30s ea	**55045-2296-08**	27.00		
180s ea	**55045-2296-09**	162.00		
(Pharma Pac)				
REPACK				
CAP, PO, 325 mg, 30s ea	**52959-0826-30**	27.31		
60s ea	**52959-0826-60**	54.60		
(Phys Total Care)				
REPACK				
CAP, PO, 324 mg, 30s ea	**54868-2858-01**	57.00		
325 mg, 100s ea	**54868-2858-00**	136.83		
TAB, PO, 260 mg, 30s ea	**54868-3652-01**	63.21		
100s ea	**54868-3652-00**	241.64		
(Quality Care Prod)				
REPACK				
CAP, PO, 325 mg, 60s ea	**49999-0801-60**	60.79		
(Southwood)				
REPACK				
CAP, PO, 325 mg, 10s ea	**58016-0651-10**	9.03		
20s ea	**58016-0651-20**	18.07		
30s ea	**58016-0651-30**	27.10		
40s ea	**58016-0651-40**	36.13		
60s ea	**58016-0651-60**	54.20		
90s ea	**58016-0651-90**	81.30		
100s ea	**58016-0651-00**	90.34		
120s ea	**58016-0651-02**	108.40		
180s ea	**58016-0651-99**	162.60		
240s ea	**58016-0651-04**	216.80		
TAB, PO, 260 mg, 10s ea	**58016-0832-10**	6.49		
20s ea	**58016-0832-20**	12.99		
30s ea	**58016-0832-30**	19.48		
40s ea	**58016-0832-40**	25.98		
60s ea	**58016-0832-60**	38.96		
90s ea	**58016-0832-90**	58.45		
100s ea	**58016-0832-00**	64.94		
120s ea	**58016-0832-02**	77.93		
180s ea	**58016-0832-99**	116.89		
240s ea	**58016-0832-04**	155.86		
(Vibranta)				
REPACK				
TAB, PO, 260 mg, 30s ea	**57866-4426-01**	10.66		
QUININE SULFATE DIHYDRATE (Amend)				
quinine sulfate				
POW, NA (U.S.P.)				
30 gm	**17317-0461-01**	23.10		
125 gm	**17317-0461-09**	84.00		
(Gallipot)				
POW, NA (U.S.P.)				
25 gm	**51552-0604-04**	44.10		
(Letco)				
POW, NA (USP)				
25 gm	**62991-2676-02**	90.00		
(1X100GM,USP)				
100 gm	**62991-2676-03**	267.00		
(1X500GM,USP)				
500 gm	**62991-2676-04**	1050.00		
(1X1000GM,USP)				
1000 gm	**62991-2676-01**	2250.00		
(Spectrum Pharmacy)				
quinidine sulfate				
POW, NA (U.S.P.)				
10 gm	**49452-6210-01**	97.30		
25 gm	**49452-6210-02**	156.10		
100 gm	**49452-6210-03**	406.00		
QUINNOSTIK (Quinnova)				
urea				
SOL, TP (RINNOVI NAIL SYSTEM)				
50%, 2.4 ml 6s	**23710-0050-02**	170.78		
8-QUINOLINOL (Spectrum Pharmacy)				
oxyquinoline				
CRY, NA, 125 gm	**49452-6175-02**	176.40		
500 gm	**49452-6175-03**	476.00		
QUINZYME (Zyber)				
medical food				
ODT, PO, 90s ea	**65224-0562-01**	46.46		
QUIXIN (Vistakon)				
levofloxacin				
SOL, OP, 0.5%, 5 ml	**68669-0135-05**	78.54		
(Phys Total Care)				
REPACK				
SOL, OP, 0.5%, 5 ml	**54868-4692-00**	57.74		
(Southwood)				
REPACK				
SOL, OP, 0.5%, 5 ml	**58016-1555-01**	42.85		
QVAR (Teva)				
beclomethasone dipropionate				
AER, IH, 0.04 mg/actuation,				
7.3 gm	**59310-0175-40**	82.86		
0.08 mg/actuation,				
7.3 gm	**59310-0177-80**	104.82		
(Dispensing Solutions)				
REPACK				
AER, IH, 0.04 mg/actuation,				
7.3 gm	**55045-3063-00**	83.00		
0.08 mg/actuation,				
7.3 gm	**55045-3695-08**	90.00		
(Nucare Pharm)				
REPACK				
AER, IH, 0.04 mg/actuation,				
100s ea	**66267-1300-00**	112.95		
(Phys Total Care)				
REPACK				
AER, IH (1X7.3ML)				
0.04 mg/actuation,				
7.3 ml	**54868-5857-00**	105.81		
0.08 mg/actuation,				
7.3 ml	**54868-5858-00**	126.33		
(Stat Rx)				
REPACK				
AER, IH, 0.04 mg/actuation,				
7.3 gm	**16590-0860-73**	92.44		
(1X7.3GM)				
0.04 mg/actuation,				
7.3 gm	**16590-0860-71**	92.44		
R-GENE 10 (Pfizer)				
arginine hydrochloride				
SOL, IV, 10%, 300 ml	**00009-0436-24**	12.71	10.59	
R-TANNA (Prasco Labs)				
chlorpheniramine tannate/phenylephrine tannate				
TAB, PO, 9 mg-25 mg,				
100s ea	**66993-0534-02**	135.53		
(PD-Rx Pharm)				
REPACK				
TAB, PO, 9 mg-25 mg,				
30s ea	**43063-0207-30**	57.00		
R-TANNA PEDIATRIC (Prasco Labs)				
chlorpheniramine tannate/phenylephrine tannate				
SUS, PO, 4.5 mg/5 ml-5 mg/5 ml,				
473 ml	**66993-0537-57**	199.94		
R-TANNAMINE (Phys Total Care)				
REPACK				
cpm tan/phenyleph tan/pyril tan				
TAB, PO, 8 mg-25 mg-25 mg,				
20s ea	**54868-2189-02**	91.05		
40s ea	**54868-2189-00**	177.60		
R-TANNAMINE PEDIATRIC (Phys Total Care)				
cpm tan/phenyleph tan/pyril tan				
SUS, PO, 480 ml	**54868-3897-00**	78.59		
R-TANNATE PEDIATRIC (Phys Total Care)				
cpm tan/phenyleph tan/pyril tan				
SUS, PO (RASPBERRY)				
118 ml	**54868-3897-01**	29.99		
RABAVERT (Novartis)				
rabies vaccine				
PDR, IM (TAX INCL)				
2.5 iu, ea	**63851-0501-01**	261.36	217.80	
(Phys Total Care)				
REPACK				
PDR, IM (SRN,NDL,W/DILUENT,PF)				
2.5 iu, ea	**54868-4340-00**	179.11		
RABEPRAZOLE SODIUM				
(Eisai) *See ACIPHEX*				
RABIES IMMUNE GLOBULIN				
(Sanofi) *See IMOGAM RABIES-HT*				
(Talecris) *See HYPERRAB S/D*				
RABIES VACCINE				
(Novartis) *See RABAVERT*				
(Sanofi) *See IMOVAX RABIES*				
RACEPINEPHRINE HYDROCHLORIDE				
(Spectrum Pharmacy)				
POW, NA (1X1GM)				
1 gm	**49452-6213-01**	234.85		
(1X5GM)				
5 gm	**49452-6213-02**	861.00		
RADIAFDG (Carrington)				
bandage				
DEV, NA (4" DIAMETER)				
ea	**53303-0003-04**	9.63		

PROD/MFR	NDC	AWP	DP	OBC
RADIAGEL (Carrington)				
bandage				
DEV, NA (HYDROGEL)				
14 gm	53303-0021-05	6.56		
85 gm	53303-0021-30	24.02		
RADIAPLEXRX (MPM Medical Inc.)				
dimethicone				
GEL, TP, 14 gm	66977-0101-05	4.25	3.64	
(MPM Medical Inc.)				
gel, multi ingredient				
170 gm	66977-0101-06	24.58	21.01	
RADIGEL (MCR American)				
gel, multi ingredient				
GEL, TP (1X85GM)				
85 gm	58605-0301-01	43.75		
RADIOGARDASE (Heyltex Corp)				
prussian blue				
CAP, PO, 0.5 gm, 30s ea	58060-0002-01	96.00	80.00	
RAIN FRAGRANCE (Medisca)				
fragrance				
OIL, NA, 14 ml	38779-1740-03	16.50		
25 ml	38779-1740-04	31.50		
100 ml	38779-1740-05	90.00		
500 ml	38779-1740-08	261.00		
RALIX (Cypress Pharm)				
cpm/methscopolamine nitrate/phenyleph hcl				
TER, PO, 8 mg-2.5 mg-40 mg, 100s ea	60258-0232-01	59.82		
RALOXIFENE HYDROCHLORIDE				
(Lilly) *See EVISTA*				
RALTEGRAVIR POTASSIUM				
(Merck) *See ISENTRESS*				
RAMELTEON				
(Takeda) *See ROZEREM*				
RAMIPRIL				
FUL				
CAP, PO, 1.25 mg, 100s ea		45.90		
2.5 mg, 100s ea		48.77		
5 mg, 100s ea		51.17		
10 mg, 100s ea		59.87		
(Actavis)				
CAP, PO (HARD GELATIN)				
2.5 mg, 100s ea	00228-2695-11	180.61		AB
500s ea	00228-2695-50	903.05		AB
5 mg, 100s ea	00228-2696-11	189.49		AB
500s ea	00228-2696-50	947.45		AB
10 mg, 100s ea	00228-2697-11	221.72		AB
500s ea	00228-2697-50	1108.60		AB
(Apotex Corp.)				
CAP, PO (HARD GELATIN)				
1.25 mg, 100s ea	60505-2875-01	152.99		AB
(10X10,HARD GELATIN)				
2.5 mg, 100s ea UD	60505-2876-00	180.59		AB
(HARD GELATIN)				
2.5 mg, 100s ea	60505-2876-01	180.59		AB
500s ea	60505-2876-05	902.88		AB
(10X10,HARD GELATIN)				
5 mg, 100s ea UD	60505-2877-00	189.46		AB
(HARD GELATIN)				
5 mg, 100s ea	60505-2877-01	189.46		AB
500s ea	60505-2877-05	947.11		AB
10 mg, 100s ea UD	60505-2878-00	221.70		AB
100s ea	60505-2878-01	221.70		AB
500s ea	60505-2878-05	1108.28		AB
(Camber)				
CAP, PO (HARD GELATIN)				
1.25 mg, 100s ea	31722-0271-01	145.50		AB
2.5 mg, 100s ea	31722-0272-01	171.46		AB
1000s ea	31722-0272-10	1530.00		AB
5 mg, 100s ea	31722-0273-01	179.89		AB
1000s ea	31722-0273-10	1619.00		AB
10 mg, 100s ea	31722-0274-01	210.49		AB
1000s ea	31722-0274-10	1894.41		AB
(Dava Pharma)				
CAP, PO (HARD GELATIN)				
1.25 mg, 100s ea	67253-0671-10	153.00		AB
2.5 mg, 100s ea	67253-0672-10	180.60		AB
1000s ea	67253-0672-11	1625.41		AB
5 mg, 100s ea	67253-0673-10	189.47		AB
1000s ea	67253-0673-11	1705.27		AB
10 mg, 100s ea	67253-0674-10	221.71		AB
1000s ea	67253-0674-11	1995.40		AB
(Dr Reddy's)				
CAP, PO (HARD GELATIN)				
1.25 mg, 90s ea	55111-0438-90	137.70		AB
2.5 mg, 90s ea	55111-0439-90	162.52		AB
500s ea	55111-0439-05	902.91		AB
5 mg, 90s ea	55111-0440-90	170.50		AB
500s ea	55111-0440-05	947.38		AB
10 mg, 90s ea	55111-0441-90	199.50		AB
500s ea	55111-0441-05	1108.60		AB
(King Pharm) *See ALTACE*				
(Lupin Pharma, Inc.)				
CAP, PO (HARD GELATIN)				
1.25 mg, 100s ea	68180-0588-01	153.01		AB
2.5 mg, 100s ea	68180-0589-01	180.61		AB
500s ea	68180-0589-02	902.97		AB
5 mg, 100s ea	68180-0590-01	189.48		AB
500s ea	68180-0590-02	947.43		AB
10 mg, 100s ea	68180-0591-01	221.72		AB
500s ea	68180-0591-02	1108.65		AB
(Monarch) *See ALTACE*				
(Roxane)				
CAP, PO (HARD GELATIN)				
1.25 mg, 100s ea	00054-0106-25	153.01		AB
(10X10,HARD GELATIN)				
2.5 mg, 100s ea UD	00054-0107-20	180.61		AB
(HARD GELATIN)				
2.5 mg, 100s ea	00054-0107-25	180.61		AB
500s ea	00054-0107-29	902.98		AB
(10X10,HARD GELATIN)				
5 mg, 100s ea UD	00054-0108-20	189.49		AB
(HARD GELATIN)				
5 mg, 100s ea	00054-0108-25	189.49		AB
500s ea	00054-0108-29	947.44		AB
10 mg, 100s ea	00054-0109-25	221.72		AB
500s ea	00054-0109-29	1108.67		AB
(Sandoz)				
CAP, PO (HARD GELATIN)				
1.25 mg, 100s ea	00781-2126-01	153.01		AB
2.5 mg, 100s ea	00781-2127-01	180.61		AB
500s ea	00781-2127-05	902.98		AB
5 mg, 100s ea	00781-2128-01	189.49		AB
500s ea	00781-2128-05	947.43		AB
10 mg, 100s ea	00781-2129-01	221.72		AB
500s ea	00781-2129-05	1108.62		AB
(Teva)				
CAP, PO (HARD GELATIN)				
2.5 mg, 100s ea	00093-7436-01	180.61		AB
5 mg, 100s ea	00093-7437-01	189.49		AB
10 mg, 100s ea	00093-7438-01	221.72		AB
(Watson Labs)				
CAP, PO (HARD GELATIN)				
1.25 mg, 30s ea	16252-0570-30	7.20		AB
2.5 mg, 100s ea	16252-0571-01	13.20		AB
500s ea	16252-0571-50	66.00		AB
5 mg, 100s ea	16252-0572-01	15.60		AB
500s ea	16252-0572-50	78.00		AB
10 mg, 100s ea	16252-0573-01	18.00		AB
500s ea	16252-0573-50	90.00		AB
(A-S Medication)				
REPACK				
CAP, PO, 5 mg, 30s ea	54569-6111-00	53.97		AB
90s ea	54569-6111-01	161.90		AB
10 mg, 30s ea	54569-6112-00	63.15		AB
90s ea	54569-6112-01	189.44		AB
(American Health)				
REPACK				
CAP, PO (3X10,HARD GELATIN)				
1.25 mg, 30s ea UD	68084-0294-21	56.92		AB
(10X10)				
2.5 mg, 100s ea UD	68084-0266-01	193.71		
5 mg, 100s ea UD	68084-0267-01	203.73		
10 mg, 100s ea UD	68084-0268-01	236.91		
(Bryant Ranch)				
REPACK				
CAP, PO, 5 mg, 20s ea	63629-1254-02	47.14		AB
(Phys Total Care)				
REPACK				
CAP, PO (HARD GELATIN)				
1.25 mg, 30s ea	54868-5896-00	18.76		AB
2.5 mg, 30s ea	54868-5856-00	141.76		
100s ea	54868-5856-01	435.10		AB
5 mg, 10s ea	54868-5842-02	64.68		AB
30s ea	54868-5842-00	148.49		
60s ea	54868-5842-01	280.62		
90s ea	54868-5842-03	34.83		AB
10 mg, 10s ea	54868-5843-02	77.94		AB
30s ea	54868-5843-00	172.99		
90s ea	54868-5843-01	481.89		
(Physician Partner)				
REPACK				
CAP, PO, 2.5 mg, 30s ea	21695-0821-30	102.88		AB
5 mg, 30s ea	21695-0822-30	107.93		AB
10 mg, 30s ea	21695-0823-30	52.41		AB
RANEXA (Gilead Sciences)				
ranolazine				
TER, PO (FILM-COATED)				
500 mg, 60s ea	61958-1001-01	242.12		EE
1000 mg, 60s ea	61958-1002-01	397.50		
RANIBIZUMAB				
(Genentech) *See LUCENTIS*				
RANITIDINE (Actavis Mid Atlantic)				
ranitidine hydrochloride				
SOL, PO (PEPPERMINT)				
15 mg/ml, 473 ml	00472-0383-16	350.14		AA
(Amneal)				
SYR, PO (1X473ML,PEPPERMINT)				
15 mg/ml, 473 ml	65162-0664-90	350.28		AA
TAB, PO (USP,FILM-COATED)				
150 mg, 60s ea	53746-0253-60	91.97		AB
100s ea	53746-0253-01	155.80		AB
180s ea	53746-0253-18	270.15		AB
500s ea	53746-0253-05	812.70		AB
1000s ea	53746-0253-10	1525.00		AB
300 mg, 30s ea	53746-0254-30	87.90		AB
100s ea	53746-0254-01	293.00		AB
250s ea	53746-0254-02	675.48		AB
(Apotex Corp.)				
SYR, PO (PEPPERMINT)				
15 mg/ml, 473 ml	60505-0351-01	350.49		AA
(Bedford)				
SOL, IJ (S.D.V.)				
25 mg/ml, 2 ml 10s	55390-0616-10	40.32		AP
(M.D.V.)				
25 mg/ml, 6 ml	55390-0616-01	9.26		AP
(PHARMACY BULK PACKAGE)				
25 mg/ml, 40 ml	55390-0618-01	48.00		AP
(Dr Reddy's)				
TAB, PO (FILM-COATED)				
150 mg, 60s ea	55111-0420-60	88.80		AB
100s ea	55111-0420-01	148.00		AB
500s ea	55111-0420-05	740.00		AB
1000s ea	55111-0420-10	1480.00		AB
300 mg, 30s ea	55111-0421-30	80.60		AB
100s ea	55111-0421-01	268.70		AB
250s ea	55111-0421-25	671.75		AB
(Major)				
TAB, PO (USP,FILM-COATED)				
150 mg, 60s ea	00904-6080-52	88.80		
100s ea	00904-6080-60	148.00		
500s ea	00904-6080-40	740.00		
(Pharm Assoc Inc)				
SYR, PO (10X10ML,AF,SPEARMINT)				
15 mg/ml, 10 ml 10s UD	00121-4727-10	276.75		AA
(AF,SPEARMINT)				
15 mg/ml, 473 ml	00121-0727-16	350.00		AA
(Ranbaxy Pharm)				
SYR, PO (1X480ML,PEPPERMINT)				
15 mg/ml, 480 ml	63304-0851-16	350.49		AA
(Wockhardt USA)				
SOL, PO (1X473ML,USP,PEPPERMINT)				
15 mg/ml, 473 ml	64679-0694-01	350.50		AA
(4u)				
REPACK				
TAB, PO, 150 mg, 60s ea	10544-0344-60	98.84		
(Advanced Pharm Serv, Inc.)				
REPACK				
TAB, PO, 300 mg, 15s ea	13411-0179-15	35.40		
30s ea	13411-0179-03	70.80		
60s ea	13411-0179-06	141.60		
90s ea	13411-0179-09	212.40		
100s ea	13411-0179-10	329.71		
(Aidarex)				
REPACK				
TAB, PO (FILM-COATED)				
150 mg, 7s ea	33261-0099-07	25.90		AB
14s ea	33261-0099-14	51.80		AB
20s ea	33261-0099-20	74.00		AB
21s ea	33261-0099-21	77.70		AB
28s ea	33261-0099-28	103.60		AB
30s ea	33261-0099-30	111.00		AB
60s ea	33261-0099-60	222.00		AB
90s ea	33261-0099-90	333.00		AB
100s ea	33261-0099-00	370.00		AB
120s ea	33261-0099-02	444.00		AB
300 mg, 15s ea	33261-0202-15	80.85		
30s ea	33261-0202-30	161.70		
60s ea	33261-0202-60	355.80		
90s ea	33261-0202-90	533.70		
100s ea	33261-0202-00	593.00		
120s ea	33261-0202-02	711.60		
180s ea	33261-0202-03	192.13		

PROD/MFR	NDC	AWP	DP	OBC
(Bryant Ranch) REPACK				
TAB, PO, 150 mg, 30s ea	63629-1671-01	48.00		
60s ea	63629-1671-03	192.99		
90s ea	63629-1671-05	281.20		
100s ea	63629-1671-02	312.99		
120s ea	63629-1671-04	375.25		
300 mg, 30s ea	63629-1672-01	112.85		
50s ea	63629-1672-04	188.52		
60s ea	63629-1672-03	225.71		
100s ea	63629-1672-02	376.18		
(Core) REPACK				
TAB, PO, 150 mg, 6s ea	33358-0316-06	11.34		
15s ea	33358-0316-15	99.11		
30s ea	33358-0316-30	102.30		
60s ea	33358-0316-60	197.81		
90s ea	33358-0316-90	288.23		
100s ea	33358-0316-00	320.81		
120s ea	33358-0316-01	384.63		
300 mg, 30s ea	33358-0317-30	115.67		
60s ea	33358-0317-60	231.35		
90s ea	33358-0317-90	297.97		
120s ea	33358-0317-01	398.32		
(DHS, Inc.) REPACK				
TAB, PO, 150 mg, 20s ea	55887-0667-20	66.63		
100s ea	55887-0667-01	333.16		
300 mg, 15s ea	55887-0415-15	49.97		
30s ea	55887-0415-30	99.95		
45s ea	55887-0415-45	149.92		
60s ea	55887-0415-60	199.89		
90s ea	55887-0415-90	240.00		
(Dispensing Solutions) REPACK				
TAB, PO, 150 mg, 30s ea	55045-3771-08	92.70		
84s ea	55045-3720-04	259.26		
300 mg, 90s ea	55045-2664-09	290.70		
(HomeMed) REPACK				
TAB, PO, 150 mg, 4s ea	51655-0881-89	8.93		EE
20s ea	51655-0881-52	44.60		EE
90s ea	51655-0881-26	134.20		EE
(IPI) REPACK				
TAB, PO, 150 mg, 30s ea	18837-0133-30	68.60		
40s ea	18837-0133-40	81.49		
60s ea	18837-0133-60	137.20		
90s ea	18837-0133-90	205.80		
300 mg, 30s ea	18837-0243-30	100.76		
60s ea	18837-0243-60	201.53		
(McKesson Packaging) REPACK				
TAB, PO (USP)				
150 mg, 100s ea UD	63739-0266-10	159.97		
(Palmetto) REPACK				
SYR, PO, 15 mg/ml,				
120 ml	23490-6251-01	115.00		
180 ml	23490-6251-02	172.49		
TAB, PO, 150 mg, 4s ea	23490-6249-01	20.80		
6s ea	23490-6249-02	27.30		
20s ea	23490-6249-07	65.00		
30s ea	23490-1192-03	95.69		
30s ea	23490-6249-03	97.50		
60s ea	23490-1192-06	181.81		
60s ea	23490-6249-04	195.00		
90s ea	23490-6249-06	292.50		
100s ea	23490-6249-05	325.00		
120s ea	23490-6249-08	331.50		
(Phys Total Care) REPACK				
SYR, PO, 15 mg/ml,				
473 ml	54868-5770-00	740.13		
TAB, PO, 300 mg, 100s ea	54868-4350-01	31.44		
(Physician Partner) REPACK				
TAB, PO, 150 mg, 30s ea	21695-0109-30	114.73		
60s ea	21695-0109-60	229.47		
90s ea	21695-0109-90	344.19		
100s ea	21695-0109-00	312.40		
120s ea	21695-0109-72	458.92		
(Southwood) REPACK				
TAB, PO (FILM-COATED)				
150 mg, 30s ea	58016-0345-30	88.80		AB
60s ea	58016-0345-60	177.60		AB
90s ea	58016-0345-90	266.40		AB
120s ea	58016-0345-02	355.20		AB
300 mg, 30s ea	58016-0570-30	105.60		AB
60s ea	58016-0570-60	211.20		AB
90s ea	58016-0570-90	316.80		AB
100s ea	58016-0570-00	352.00		AB
120s ea	58016-0570-02	422.40		AB
(St. Mary's MPP) REPACK				
TAB, PO (USP,FILM-COATED)				
150 mg, 10s ea	60760-0025-10	22.37		AB
(FILM-COATED)				
150 mg, 30s ea	60760-0025-30	57.06		AB
(USP)				
300 mg, 60s ea	60760-0026-60	183.34		
(Stat Rx) REPACK				
TAB, PO, 150 mg, 30s ea	16590-0200-30	99.25		
40s ea	16590-0200-40	132.34		
60s ea	16590-0200-60	160.35		
RANITIDINE HCL (Apotex Corp.) ranitidine hydrochloride				
TAB, PO, 150 mg, 60s ea	60505-0025-04	95.25		AB
100s ea	60505-0025-06	156.20		AB
500s ea	60505-0025-08	740.00		AB
300 mg, 30s ea	60505-0026-02	87.85		AB
100s ea	60505-0026-03	286.70		AB
250s ea	60505-0026-07	671.75		AB
(Dr Reddy's)				
CAP, PO, 150 mg, 60s ea	55111-0129-60	91.27		AB
500s ea	55111-0129-05	737.72		AB
300 mg, 30s ea	55111-0130-30	82.30		AB
100s ea	55111-0130-01	266.12		AB
(Gallipot)				
POW, NA (U.S.P.)				
5 gm	51552-0620-02	28.00		
25 gm	51552-0620-04	56.00		
100 gm	51552-0620-05	182.00		
(Hawkins)				
POW, NA (U.S.P.)				
25 gm	63370-0218-25	140.00		
100 gm	63370-0218-35	240.00		
500 gm	63370-0218-45	520.00		
1000 gm	63370-0218-50	880.00		
(Letco)				
POW, NA (U.S.P.)				
25 gm	62991-1132-03	84.00		
50 gm	62991-1132-01	120.00		
100 gm	62991-1132-02	165.00		
1000 gm	62991-1132-04	660.00		
(Major)				
TAB, PO (10X10)				
150 mg, 100s ea UD	00904-5261-61	156.22		AB
300 mg, 100s ea UD	00904-5262-61	329.57		AB
(Medisca)				
POW, NA (U.S.P.)				
25 gm	38779-0536-04	127.50		
100 gm	38779-0536-05	237.00		
500 gm	38779-0536-08	507.00		
1000 gm	38779-0536-09	795.00		
(Par)				
TAB, PO, 150 mg, 60s ea	49884-0544-02	95.30		AB
100s ea	49884-0544-01	156.20		AB
500s ea	49884-0544-05	780.00		AB
1000s ea	49884-0544-10	1528.00		AB
300 mg, 30s ea	49884-0545-11	87.90		AB
100s ea	49884-0545-01	286.70		AB
250s ea	49884-0545-04	697.00		AB
(PCCA)				
POW, NA (U.S.P.)				
1 gm	51927-3023-00	10.80		
(Precision Dose)				
SYR, PO (PEPPERMINT)				
15 mg/ml,				
5 ml 50s UD	68094-0205-58	180.60		
(1X10ML,PEPPERMINT)				
15 mg/ml, 10 ml UD	68094-0204-59	8.10		
(PEPPERMINT)				
15 mg/ml,				
10 ml 30s UD	68094-0204-62	243.90		
(10X10,PEPPERMINT)				
15 mg/ml,				
10 ml 100s UD	68094-0204-61	810.60		
(Sandoz)				
CAP, PO, 150 mg, 60s ea	00781-2855-60	91.27		AB
500s ea	00781-2855-05	737.74		AB
SGL, PO, 300 mg, 30s ea	00781-2865-31	82.30		AB
TAB, PO, 150 mg, 60s ea	00781-1883-60	88.80		AB
100s ea UD	00781-1883-13	150.85		AB
1000s ea	00781-1883-10	1480.00		AB
300 mg, 30s ea	00781-1884-31	80.60		AB
250s ea	00781-1884-25	671.75		AB
(Spectrum Pharmacy)				
POW, NA (1X5GM)				
5 gm	49452-6214-05	95.20		
(1X25GM)				
25 gm	49452-6214-06	227.50		
(1X100GM)				
100 gm	49452-6214-01	518.00		
(UDL)				
TAB, PO (10X10)				
150 mg, 100s ea UD	51079-0879-20	158.60		AB
(Wockhardt USA)				
TAB, PO (USP,FILM-COATED)				
150 mg, 60s ea	64679-0906-01	89.28		AB
100s ea	64679-0906-06	148.78		AB
500s ea	64679-0906-03	743.91		AB
(3X5000,USP,FILM-COATED)				
150 mg, 15000s ea	64679-0906-11	22317.30		AB
(USP,FILM-COATED)				
150 mg, 15000s ea	64679-0906-07	22317.30		AB
40000s ea	64679-0906-00	59512.80		AB
300 mg, 30s ea	64679-0907-01	81.04		AB
100s ea	64679-0907-04	270.13		AB
250s ea	64679-0907-02	671.75		AB
(2X3750,USP,FILM-COATED)				
300 mg, 7500s ea	64679-0907-08	20152.50		AB
(USP,FILM-COATED)				
300 mg, 7500s ea	64679-0907-05	20152.50		AB
20000s ea	64679-0907-00	53740.00		AB
(4u) REPACK				
TAB, PO, 150 mg, 60s ea	42549-0544-60	98.84		AB
(FILM-COATED)				
300 mg, 30s ea	10544-0360-30	132.28		AB
30s ea	42549-0560-30	132.28		AB
(A-S Medication) REPACK				
TAB, PO, 150 mg, 15s ea	54569-4507-06	23.82		AB
20s ea	54569-4507-02	31.77		EE
30s ea	54569-4507-00	47.65		EE
60s ea	54569-4507-01	95.30		EE
90s ea	54569-4507-05	142.95		
120s ea	54569-4507-07	190.60		EE
300 mg, 15s ea	54569-4508-00	43.01		AB
30s ea	54569-4508-01	86.01		AB
(Altura) REPACK				
TAB, PO, 150 mg, 90s ea	63874-0337-90	281.00		EE
300 mg, 10s ea	63874-0428-10	32.00		AB
14s ea	63874-0428-14	44.80		AB
15s ea	63874-0428-15	48.00		AB
20s ea	63874-0428-20	65.00		AB
21s ea	63874-0428-21	67.20		AB
28s ea	63874-0428-28	89.60		AB
30s ea	63874-0428-30	96.00		AB
40s ea	63874-0428-40	128.00		AB
50s ea	63874-0428-50	160.00		AB
56s ea	63874-0428-56	179.20		AB
60s ea	63874-0428-60	192.00		AB
90s ea	63874-0428-90	288.00		AB
100s ea	63874-0428-01	320.00		AB
120s ea	63874-0428-04	384.00		AB
(American Health) REPACK				
TAB, PO (10X10)				
150 mg, 100s ea UD	62584-0252-01	150.82		AB
(15X30)				
150 mg, 450s ea	62584-0252-85	702.00		AB
300 mg, 450s ea	62584-0253-85	1254.60		AB
(DHS, Inc.) REPACK				
TAB, PO, 150 mg, 30s ea	55887-0667-30	99.95		AB
60s ea	55887-0667-60	189.00		AB
90s ea	55887-0667-90	240.00		AB
(Dispensing Solutions) REPACK				
TAB, PO, 150 mg, 4s ea	66336-0009-44	10.58		AB
6s ea	55045-3280-01	18.54		AB
10s ea	55045-2511-03	30.90		AB
15s ea	55045-2511-05	46.35		AB
20s ea	55045-2511-07	61.80		AB
20s ea	66336-0009-20	52.92		AB
30s ea	55045-2511-08	92.70		AB
30s ea	66336-0009-30	79.38		EE
40s ea	55045-3280-04	123.60		
45s ea	55045-2511-00	139.05		AB
60s ea	55045-2511-09	185.40		AB
60s ea	66336-0009-60	158.76		EE

PROD/MFR	NDC	AWP	DP	OBC
80s ea	**55045-3280-08**	247.20		AB
90s ea	**55045-2511-01**	278.10		AB
(FILM-COATED)				
150 mg, 90s ea	**66336-0009-90**	238.14		AB
100s ea	**55045-2511-06**	309.00		AB
120s ea	**55045-2511-04**	370.80		AB
160s ea	**55045-3280-06**	494.40		AB
180s ea	**55045-2511-02**	556.20		AB
300 mg, 20s ea	**55045-2664-07**	64.60		AB
30s ea	**55045-2664-08**	96.90		AB
30s ea	**66336-0887-30**	92.98		AB
60s ea	**55045-2664-06**	193.80		AB
(FILM-COATED)				
300 mg, 60s ea	**66336-0887-60**	185.96		AB
100s ea	**55045-2664-00**	323.00		AB
(GSMS)				
REPACK				
TAB, PO, 150 mg, 60s ea	**60429-0704-60**	8.10	2.70	AB
100s ea	**60429-0704-01**	11.52	3.84	AB
(UNIT OF USE)				
150 mg, 180s ea	**60429-0704-18**	18.00	6.00	AB
500s ea	**60429-0704-05**	37.38	12.46	AB
10000s ea	**60429-0704-00**	704.10	234.70	AB
(FILM-COATED)				
300 mg, 30s ea	**60429-0705-30**	7.92	2.64	
250s ea	**60429-0705-25**	42.84	14.28	
5000s ea	**60429-0705-00**	859.50	286.50	
(IPI)				
REPACK				
TAB, PO, 150 mg, 14s ea	**18837-0133-14**	33.90		AB
28s ea	**18837-0133-28**	62.07		AB
(Keltman Pharma., Inc.)				
REPACK				
TAB, PO, 150 mg, 60s ea	**68387-0310-60**	188.12		AB
300 mg, 60s ea	**68387-0315-60**	190.03		AB
(LWP)				
REPACK				
TAB, PO, 150 mg, 60s ea	**64038-0118-60**	100.30		AB
(McKesson Packaging)				
REPACK				
TAB, PO, 150 mg,				
750s ea UD	**63739-0266-01**	1199.75		AB
(25X30)				
150 mg, 750s ea	**63739-0266-03**	1190.75		AB
(Nucare Pharm)				
REPACK				
TAB, PO, 150 mg, 15s ea	**66267-0188-15**	47.84		EE
30s ea	**66267-0188-30**	95.69		EE
40s ea	**66267-0188-40**	85.56		AB
60s ea	**66267-0188-60**	231.62		AB
60s ea	**68071-1321-00**	231.62		AB
90s ea	**66267-0188-90**	279.89		EE
120s ea	**66267-0188-91**	177.60		AB
300 mg, 30s ea	**66267-0452-30**	105.80		AB
60s ea	**66267-0452-60**	198.36		AB
(PD-Rx Pharm)				
REPACK				
TAB, PO, 150 mg, 6s ea	**55289-0319-06**	25.87		AB
(USP)				
150 mg, 10s ea	**55289-0319-10**	30.00		AB
14s ea	**55289-0319-14**	31.80		AB
(USP)				
150 mg, 15s ea	**55289-0319-15**	31.80		AB
20s ea	**55289-0319-20**	32.20		AB
28s ea	**55289-0319-28**	38.20		AB
(REDI-SCRIPT)				
150 mg, 28s ea	**58864-0364-28**	38.22		AB
30s ea	**55289-0319-30**	38.33		AB
(REDI-SCRIPT)				
150 mg, 30s ea	**58864-0364-30**	38.34		AB
60s ea	**55289-0319-60**	56.00		AB
(REDI-SCRIPT)				
150 mg, 60s ea	**58864-0364-60**	55.98		AB
100s ea	**58864-0364-01**	88.02		AB
(FILM-COATED)				
150 mg, 180s ea	**55289-0319-93**	128.00		AB
300 mg, 14s ea	**55289-0505-14**	37.07		AB
30s ea	**55289-0505-30**	59.60		AB
60s ea	**55289-0505-60**	98.67		AB
(Pharma Pac)				
REPACK				
TAB, PO, 150 mg, 6s ea	**52959-0502-06**	14.14		EE
10s ea	**52959-0502-10**	23.56		EE
12s ea	**52959-0502-12**	28.25		EE
14s ea	**52959-0502-14**	32.80		EE
15s ea	**52959-0502-15**	35.10		EE
20s ea	**52959-0502-20**	46.30		EE
21s ea	**52959-0502-21**	49.05		AB
28s ea	**52959-0502-28**	65.10		EE
30s ea	**52959-0502-30**	69.40		EE
40s ea	**52959-0502-40**	92.26		EE
50s ea	**52959-0502-50**	115.28		EE
60s ea	**52959-0502-60**	138.33		EE
90s ea	**52959-0502-90**	206.95		EE
120s ea	**52959-0502-02**	275.30		AB
300 mg, 15s ea	**52959-0526-15**	63.87		AB
30s ea	**52959-0526-30**	127.73		AB
60s ea	**52959-0526-60**	255.45		AB
90s ea	**52959-0526-90**	383.15		AB
120s ea	**52959-0526-02**	510.84		AB
(Phys Total Care)				
REPACK				
TAB, PO, 150 mg, 30s ea	**54868-4048-02**	8.19		EE
60s ea	**54868-4048-00**	11.88		EE
90s ea	**54868-4048-03**	15.80		EE
100s ea	**54868-4048-01**	22.14		EE
300 mg, 30s ea	**54868-4350-00**	9.57		AB
(Physician Partner)				
REPACK				
TAB, PO, 150 mg, 14s ea	**21695-0109-14**	53.54		AB
(CAPLET)				
300 mg, 15s ea	**21695-0110-15**	101.19		AB
30s ea	**21695-0110-30**	172.02		AB
(Quality Care Prod)				
REPACK				
TAB, PO, 150 mg, 2s ea	**49999-0043-02**	7.49		EE
14s ea	**49999-0043-14**	52.50		AB
15s ea	**49999-0043-15**	56.20		EE
20s ea	**49999-0043-20**	74.94		EE
30s ea	**49999-0043-30**	112.41		EE
60s ea	**49999-0043-60**	224.87		EE
90s ea	**49999-0043-90**	337.50		AB
180s ea	**49999-0043-80**	400.00		AB
300 mg, 15s ea	**49999-0428-15**	53.76		AB
30s ea	**49999-0428-30**	107.40		AB
60s ea	**49999-0428-60**	214.80		AB
(Southwood)				
REPACK				
TAB, PO, 150 mg, 15s ea	**58016-0345-15**	34.30		EE
20s ea	**58016-0345-20**	45.73		EE
21s ea	**58016-0345-21**	48.02		EE
28s ea	**58016-0345-28**	64.03		EE
40s ea	**58016-0345-40**	91.47		EE
50s ea	**58016-0345-50**	114.33		EE
56s ea	**58016-0345-56**	128.05		EE
80s ea	**58016-0345-80**	182.93		EE
100s ea	**58016-0345-00**	296.00		EE
(FILM-COATED)				
150 mg, 124s ea	**58016-0345-63**	283.54		AB
300 mg, 10s ea	**58016-0570-10**	32.00		EE
14s ea	**58016-0570-14**	44.80		EE
15s ea	**58016-0570-15**	48.00		EE
20s ea	**58016-0570-20**	65.00		EE
21s ea	**58016-0570-21**	67.20		EE
28s ea	**58016-0570-28**	89.60		EE
40s ea	**58016-0570-40**	128.00		EE
50s ea	**58016-0570-50**	160.00		EE
56s ea	**58016-0570-56**	179.20		EE
(St. Mary's MPP)				
REPACK				
TAB, PO, 150 mg, 20s ea	**60760-0025-20**	38.56		AB
(USP)				
150 mg, 60s ea	**60760-0025-60**	103.68		AB
300 mg, 30s ea	**60760-0026-30**	94.67		AB
(Stat Rx)				
REPACK				
SGL, PO, 300 mg, 20s ea	**16590-0381-20**	67.11		AB
30s ea	**16590-0381-30**	100.67		AB
90s ea	**16590-0381-90**	302.30		AB
(Vibranta)				
REPACK				
TAB, PO, 150 mg, 14s ea	**57866-6390-01**	41.50		
30s ea	**57866-6930-02**	125.25		
60s ea	**57866-6930-04**	224.87		
90s ea	**57866-6930-05**	110.90		
120s ea	**57866-6930-06**	184.61		
180s ea	**57866-6390-07**	268.91		
RANITIDINE HYDROCHLORIDE				
FUL				
SYR, PO, 15 mg/ml, 473 ml		112.48		
TAB, PO, 150 mg, 100s ea		6.00		
300 mg, 30s ea		3.75		
(Actavis Mid Atlantic) *See RANITIDINE*				
(Amneal) *See RANITIDINE*				
(Apotex Corp.)				
CAP, PO (USP,FILM-COATED)				
300 mg, 5000s ea	**60505-0026-08**	13435.00		AB
(Apotex Corp.) *See RANITIDINE*				
(Apotex Corp.) *See RANITIDINE HCL*				
(Bedford) *See RANITIDINE*				
(Dr Reddy's) *See RANITIDINE*				
(Dr Reddy's) *See RANITIDINE HCL*				
(Gallipot) *See RANITIDINE HCL*				
(Glaxo) *See ZANTAC*				
(Glaxo) *See ZANTAC 150*				
(Glaxo) *See ZANTAC 25*				
(Glaxo) *See ZANTAC 300*				
(Hawkins) *See RANITIDINE HCL*				
(Letco) *See RANITIDINE HCL*				
(Major) *See RANITIDINE*				
(Major) *See RANITIDINE HCL*				
(Medisca) *See RANITIDINE HCL*				
(Par) *See RANITIDINE HCL*				
(PCCA) *See RANITIDINE HCL*				
(Pharm Assoc Inc) *See RANITIDINE*				
(Precision Dose) *See RANITIDINE HCL*				
(PRX) *See TALADINE*				
(Ranbaxy Pharm) *See RANITIDINE*				
(Sandoz) *See RANITIDINE HCL*				
(Spectrum Pharmacy) *See RANITIDINE HCL*				
(Teva)				
TAB, PO (FILM COATED)				
150 mg, 60s ea	**00172-4357-49**	88.80		AB
500s ea	**00172-4357-70**	740.00		AB
300 mg, 30s ea	**00172-4358-46**	80.60		AB
100s ea	**00172-4358-60**	268.70		AB
(UDL) *See RANITIDINE HCL*				
(Wockhardt USA) *See RANITIDINE*				
(Wockhardt USA) *See RANITIDINE HCL*				
(Altura)				
REPACK				
TAB, PO (FILM-COATED)				
150 mg, 10s ea	**63874-0337-10**	31.20		AB
12s ea	**63874-0337-12**	37.46		AB
14s ea	**63874-0337-14**	43.68		AB
15s ea	**63874-0337-15**	46.83		AB
20s ea	**63874-0337-20**	62.45		AB
21s ea	**63874-0337-21**	65.56		AB
28s ea	**63874-0337-28**	87.42		AB
30s ea	**63874-0337-30**	93.67		AB
40s ea	**63874-0337-40**	124.89		AB
45s ea	**63874-0337-45**	140.40		AB
50s ea	**63874-0337-50**	156.11		AB
56s ea	**63874-0337-56**	175.00		AB
60s ea	**63874-0337-60**	187.39		AB
75s ea	**63874-0337-75**	234.24		AB
80s ea	**63874-0337-80**	249.78		AB
84s ea	**63874-0337-84**	262.35		AB
100s ea	**63874-0337-01**	312.23		AB
120s ea	**63874-0337-04**	374.40		AB
500s ea	**63874-0337-03**	1560.00		AB
(Palmetto)				
REPACK				
TAB, PO, 300 mg, 30s ea	**23490-6250-01**	111.81		
60s ea	**23490-6250-02**	223.62		
90s ea	**23490-6250-03**	335.43		
120s ea	**23490-6250-04**	447.24		
(Physician Partner)				
REPACK				
CAP, PO (GELCAP)				
150 mg, 60s ea	**21695-0337-60**	182.54		
300 mg, 30s ea	**21695-0338-30**	164.60		
TAB, PO, 300 mg, 60s ea	**21695-0110-60**	344.04		
(Quality Care Prod)				
REPACK				
TAB, PO, 300 mg, 100s ea	**49999-0428-00**	358.00		
(Stat Rx)				
REPACK				
TAB, PO (FILM COATED)				
150 mg, 20s ea	**16590-0200-20**	45.74		AB
56s ea	**16590-0200-56**	128.07		AB
90s ea	**16590-0200-90**	205.83		AB
180s ea	**16590-0200-82**	411.66		AB
RANOLAZINE				
(Gilead Sciences) *See RANEXA*				

PROD/MFR NDC AWP DP OBC

RAPAFLO (Watson)
silodosin
CAP, PO, 4 mg, 30s ea **52544-0151-30** 118.39
8 mg, 30s ea........ **52544-0152-30** 118.39
90s ea........ **52544-0152-19** 355.19

RAPAMUNE (Wyeth)
sirolimus
SOL, PO (M.D. BOTTLE)
1 mg/ml, 60 ml....... **00008-1030-06** 703.01 585.84
TAB, PO, 1 mg, 100s ea ... **00008-1041-05** 1171.21 976.01
(REDIPAK,10X10)
1 mg, 100s ea....... **00008-1041-10** 1171.21 976.01
2 mg, 100s ea....... **00008-1042-05** 2342.41 1952.01

(Quality Care Prod)
REPACK
TAB, PO, 1 mg, 100s ea ... **35356-0280-00** 1870.06

RAPESEED OIL (PCCA)
OIL, NA, 1 ml............ **51927-3428-00** 0.09

RAPIFLUX (PRX)
fluoxetine hydrochloride
TAB, PO, 20 mg, 100s ea .. **16241-0759-01** 311.21

RAPPORT RING LOADING SYSTEM (Owen Mumford)
device
DEV, NA, ea **08470-2210-01** 51.06

RAPPORT VACUUM THERAPY DEVICE (Owen Mumford)
device, impotence, mechanical
DEV, NA, ea **08470-2000-01** 134.38

RASAGILINE
(Teva Neuroscience) *See AZILECT*

RASBURICASE
(Sanofi-Aventis) *See ELITEK*

RASPBERRY ARTIFICIAL FLAVOR
(Spectrum Pharmacy)
flavoring aid
LIQ, NA (1X100ML, CONCENTRATE)
100 ml **49452-6217-02** 63.70
(1X500ML, CONCENTRATE)
500 ml **49452-6217-03** 146.65

RASPBERRY FLAVOR (Gallipot)
flavoring aid
LIQ, NA (ARTIFICIAL)
59.14 ml............ **51552-0236-03** 6.02

(Medisca)
SOL, NA (1X100ML,CONCENTRATE)
100 ml **38779-1559-05** 28.50
(1X500ML,CONCENTRATE)
500 ml **38779-1559-08** 54.00

(PCCA)
POW, NA (ARTIFICIAL)
1 gm **51927-3272-00** 0.69
SOL, NA (ARTIFICIAL,RASPBERRY)
1 ml............ **51927-2323-00** 0.90
(CONCENTRATE,RASPBERRY)
1 ml............ **51927-1519-00** 0.23

RAUWOLFEMMS (Truxton)
rauwolfia serpentina
TAB, PO, 50 mg, 1000s ea . **00463-6164-10** 16.80 EE
100 mg, 1000s ea .... **00463-6165-10** 19.80 EE

RAUWOLFIA (Weleda)
homeopathic substance
LIQ, PO (1X)
50 ml............ **55946-0373-15** 9.00

RAUWOLFIA SERPENTINA (PCCA)
POW, NA (USP)
1 gm **51927-3394-00** 12.00

(Truxton) *See RAUWOLFEMMS*

RAZADYNE (Ortho-McNeil Neuro)
galantamine hydrobromide
SOL, PO (W/CALIBRATED PIPETTE)
4 mg/ml, 100 ml **50458-0490-10** 244.31 203.59
TAB, PO (FILM-COATED)
4 mg, 60s ea......... **50458-0396-60** 219.89 183.24
8 mg, 60s ea......... **50458-0397-60** 219.89 183.24
(FILM-COATED)
12 mg, 60s ea........ **50458-0398-60** 219.89 183.24

(Physician Partner)
REPACK
TAB, PO (FILM-COATED)
4 mg, 30s ea........ **21695-0184-30** 204.21
12 mg, 30s ea........ **21695-0591-30** 248.98

RAZADYNE ER (Ortho-McNeil Neuro)
galantamine hydrobromide
CER, PO, 8 mg, 30s ea **50458-0387-30** 219.89 183.24
16 mg, 30s ea........ **50458-0388-30** 219.89 183.24
24 mg, 30s ea........ **50458-0389-30** 219.89 183.24

(Phys Total Care)
REPACK
CER, PO, 16 mg, 30s ea ... **54868-5453-00** 200.58

RE DUALVIT PLUS (River's Edge)
multivitamin, minerals, and iron
CAP, PO,............ **68032-0242-90** 50.97 37.24

RE KAR C PLUS SR (River's Edge)
ascorbic acid/cyanocobalamin/folic acid/iron
CAP, PO, 100s ea **68032-0188-10** 52.80

RE-PB HYOS (River's Edge)
atropine sulf/hyoscyamine sulf/pb/scop hydrobrom
ELI, PO (GRAPE)
473 ml **68032-0395-16** 61.00

READI-CAT (E-Z-EM)
barium sulfate
SUS, NA (24X450ML)
1.3%, 450 ml 24s **32909-0728-01** 147.40 122.83
(1X900ML)
1.3%, 900 ml **32909-0728-03** 156.85 130.71
(1X1900ML)
1.3%, 1900 ml **32909-0728-02** 87.58 72.98

READI-CAT 2 (E-Z-EM)
barium sulfate
SUS, NA (1X450ML)
2.1%, 450 ml **32909-0723-01** 162.14 135.12
(1X900ML)
2.1%, 900 ml **32909-0723-03** 156.85 130.71
(1X1900ML)
2.1%, 1900 ml **32909-0723-02** 87.58 72.98
PO (1X250ML,BANANA SMOOTHIE)
2.1%, 250 ml **32909-0725-07** 140.87 117.39
(1X450ML,APPLE SMOOTHIE)
2.1%, 450 ml **32909-0735-03** 150.94 125.78
(1X450ML,BANANA SMOOTHIE)
2.1%, 450 ml **32909-0725-03** 150.94 125.78
(1X450ML,BERRY SMOOTHIE)
2.1%, 450 ml **32909-0715-03** 150.94 125.78

REBETOL (Schering)
ribavirin
CAP, PO, 200 mg, 56s ea .. **00085-1351-05** 593.39
70s ea............ **00085-1385-07** 741.74
84s ea............ **00085-1194-03** 890.09
SOL, PO (BUBBLE GUM)
40 mg/ml, 100 ml **00085-1318-01** 232.80

(Phys Total Care)
REPACK
CAP, PO, 200 mg, 70s ea .. **54868-5035-00** 810.50

REBIF (EMD)
interferon beta-1a
SOL, SC (TITRATION PACK,PF)
4.2 ml............ **44087-8822-01** 2973.46
(SRN,PREFILLED,27G,PF)
22 mcg/0.5 ml,
0.5 ml 12s........ **44087-0022-03** 2973.46
44 mcg/0.5 ml,
0.5 ml 12s........ **44087-0044-03** 2973.46

RECLAST (Novartis Pharm)
zoledronic acid
SOL, IV, 5 mg/100 ml,
100 ml **00078-0435-61** 1287.72

(Quality Care Prod)
REPACK
SOL, IV (1X100ML)
5 mg/100 ml,
100 ml **35356-0351-01** 2132.30

RECLIPSEN (Watson)
desogestrel/ethinyl estradiol
TAB, PO (6X28)
0.15 mg-0.03 mg,
168s ea............ **52544-0954-28** 203.98

(A-S Medication)
REPACK
TAB, PO, 0.15 mg-0.03 mg,
28s ea............ **54569-6032-00** 35.41

RECOMBINATE (Baxter Bioscience)
antihemophilic factor viii (recombinant)
PDS, IV (APPROX. 1000 IU/VIAL)
1 iu, ea **00944-2938-03** 1.58
(APPROX. 250 IU/VIAL)
1 iu, ea **00944-2938-01** 1.58
(APPROX. 500 IU/VIAL)
1 iu, ea **00944-2938-02** 1.58
(SINGLE-DOSE,220-400 IU)
1 iu, ea **00944-2831-10** 1.63
(SINGLE-DOSE,401-800 IU)
1 iu, ea **00944-2832-10** 1.63
(SINGLE-DOSE,801-1240IU)
1 iu, ea **00944-2833-10** 1.63

RECOMBIVAX HB (Merck)
hepatitis b vaccine recombinant
SUS, IM (S.D.V.,TAX INCL.)
10 mcg/ml, 1 ml...... **00006-4995-00** 71.64
(TAX INCL,PF)
10 mcg/ml, 1 ml...... **00006-4094-31** 73.31
(6X1ML,TAX INCL,PF)
10 mcg/ml, 1 ml 6s... **00006-4094-09** 439.88
(S.D.V.,TAX INCL.)
10 mcg/ml,
1 ml 10s........ **00006-4995-41** 708.12
(S.D.V., TAX INCL.)
40 mcg/ml, 1 ml...... **00006-4992-00** 199.25

(A-S Medication)
REPACK
SUS, IM (S.D.V.,TAX INCL)
10 mcg/ml, 1 ml...... **54569-5630-00** 736.79

(Phys Total Care)
REPACK
SUS, IM (S.D.V.,TAX INCL)
10 mcg/ml, 1 ml...... **54868-2219-01** 83.10
(3 DOSE VIAL,TAX INCL)
10 mcg/ml, 3 ml...... **54868-2219-00** 214.51

RECOMBIVAX HB PEDIATRIC/ADOLESCENT (Merck)
hepatitis b vaccine recombinant
SUS, IM (S.D.V.,TAX INCL,PF)
5 mcg/0.5 ml,
0.5 ml 10s......... **00006-4981-00** 278.45

(A-S Medication)
REPACK
SUS, IM (S.D.V.,TAX INCL,PF)
5 mcg/0.5 ml,
0.5 ml 10s......... **54569-5629-00** 288.18

RECOTHROM (ZymoGenetics)
thrombin human, recombinant
PDS, TP (W/DILUENT)
5000 iu, ea.......... **28400-0105-41** 103.20
(W/DILUENT,PF,LATEX-FREE)
20000 iu, ea **28400-0120-41** 412.80
(W/SPRAY KIT,PF)
20000 iu, ea **28400-0120-50** 434.40

RECTAGEL HC (Azur Pharma, Inc.)
hydrocortisone acetate/lidocaine hydrochloride
GEL, RC (5X20GM)
0.55%-2.8%,
20 gm 5s **66663-0357-05** 136.30

RECTASOL-HC (Bio-Pharm)
hydrocortisone acetate
SUP, RC, 25 mg, 12s ea ... **59741-0301-12** 17.50
24s ea............ **59741-0301-24** 31.24

RED ALGAE
(PCCA) *See RED ALGAE (ALASKAN)*

RED ALGAE (ALASKAN) (PCCA)
red algae
POW, NA (1X1GM)
1 gm **51927-1523-00** 900.00

RED FOOD COLOR (PCCA)
color additive
POW, NA, 1 gm.......... **51927-1650-00** 6.50
SOL, NA (LIQUID)
1 ml............ **51927-1166-00** 3.86

RED RICE YEAST EXTRACT (Gallipot)
red yeast rice
POW, NA, 0.4%, 1000 gm . **51552-1004-07** 105.00 75.00

RED YEAST RICE
(Gallipot) *See RED RICE YEAST EXTRACT*

RED YEAST RICE EXTRACT (PCCA)
POW, NA, 1 gm.......... **51927-3392-00** 0.51

REFACTO (Wyeth)
antihemophilic factor viii (recombinant)
PDS, IV (1000IU,LYOPHILIZED)
1 iu, ea **58394-0005-04** 1.31 1.09
(2000IU,LYOPHILIZED)
1 iu, ea **58394-0011-04** 1.31 1.09
(250IU,LYOPHILIZED)
1 iu, ea **58394-0007-04** 1.31 1.09
(500IU,LYOPHILIZED)
1 iu, ea **58394-0006-04** 1.31 1.09
(APPROX 250 IU/VIAL)
1 iu, ea **58394-0007-02** 1.31 1.09
(APPROX 500 IU/VIAL)
1 iu, ea **58394-0006-02** 1.31 1.09

PROD/MFR	NDC	AWP	DP	OBC
REFISSA (Spear Dermatology)				
tretinoin				
CRE, TP (1X40GM)				
0.05%, 40 gm	**66530-0411-49**	150.00		
REFLUDAN (Bayer)				
lepirudin				
PDS, IV (VIAL)				
50 mg, 10s ea	**50419-0150-57**	2731.86		
REGADENOSON (Astellas) *See LEXISCAN*				
REGENECARE WOUND (MPM Medical Inc.)				
aloe/collagen/lidocaine hydrochloride				
GEL, TP, 2%, 14 gm	**66977-0100-05**	3.57	3.05	
85 gm	**66977-0100-03**	18.25	15.60	
REGLAN (Alaven)				
metoclopramide hydrochloride				
TAB, PO, 5 mg, 100s ea	**68220-0150-10**	175.39		AB
10 mg, 100s ea	**68220-0151-10**	175.39		AB
(Baxter)				
SOL, IV (PF)				
5 mg/ml, 2 ml	**60977-0451-17**	2.27		AP
(S.D.V.,PF)				
5 mg/ml, 2 ml 25s	**60977-0451-01**	56.70		AP
(PF)				
5 mg/ml, 10 ml	**60977-0451-71**	2.10		AP
(S.D.V.,PF)				
5 mg/ml, 10 ml 25s	**60977-0451-02**	52.50		AP
(PF)				
5 mg/ml, 30 ml	**60977-0451-82**	5.58		AP
(S.D.V.,PF)				
5 mg/ml, 30 ml 25s	**60977-0451-03**	139.50		AP
(Phys Total Care)				
REPACK				
TAB, PO, 10 mg, 30s ea	**54868-0513-00**	39.98		AB
100s ea	**54868-0513-01**	128.24		AB
(Southwood)				
REPACK				
SOL, IV (25X2ML)				
5 mg/ml, 2 ml 25s	**58016-4811-01**	56.70		
REGONOL (Sandoz)				
pyridostigmine bromide				
SOL, IJ (10X2ML)				
5 mg/ml, 2 ml 10s	**00781-3040-95**	272.83		AP
REGRANEX (Ortho-McNeil Pharm)				
becaplermin				
GEL, TP, 0.01%, 15 gm	**00045-0810-15**	695.98	579.98	
(Quality Care Prod)				
REPACK				
GEL, TP, 0.01%, 15 gm	**49999-0732-15**	641.68		
REJUVESOL (enCyte)				
electrolytes, adenine, and inosine				
INJ, IJ (NOT FOR DIRECT IV INFUS)				
50 ml 12s	**23731-7000-05**	594.60	495.50	
RELAFEN (Altura)				
REPACK				
nabumetone				
TAB, PO, 750 mg, 20s ea	**63874-0687-20**	38.53		AB
30s ea	**63874-0687-30**	57.79		AB
(DHS, Inc.)				
REPACK				
TAB, PO, 500 mg, 14s ea	**55887-0744-14**	25.42		AB
(Dispensing Solutions)				
REPACK				
TAB, PO, 500 mg, 15s ea	**55045-1908-05**	33.75		AB
20s ea	**55045-1908-07**	45.00		AB
30s ea	**55045-1908-08**	67.50		AB
750 mg, 30s ea	**55045-2440-08**	70.15		AB
(Nucare Pharm)				
REPACK				
TAB, PO, 500 mg, 14s ea	**66267-0189-14**	26.20		AB
20s ea	**66267-0189-20**	40.69		AB
28s ea	**66267-0189-28**	57.89		AB
750 mg, 30s ea	**66267-0190-30**	59.91		AB
(Pharma Pac)				
REPACK				
TAB, PO, 500 mg, 14s ea	**52959-0227-14**	27.49		AB
15s ea	**52959-0227-15**	29.45		AB
20s ea	**52959-0227-20**	38.90		AB
28s ea	**52959-0227-28**	56.43		AB
30s ea	**52959-0227-30**	59.70		AB
40s ea	**52959-0227-40**	73.45		AB
60s ea	**52959-0227-60**	103.67		AB
750 mg, 20s ea	**52959-0373-20**	38.90		AB
28s ea	**52959-0373-28**	54.41		AB
30s ea	**52959-0373-30**	57.50		AB
40s ea	**52959-0373-40**	76.13		AB
(Phys Total Care)				
REPACK				
TAB, PO, 500 mg, 20s ea	**54868-2014-00**	47.58		AB
30s ea	**54868-2014-02**	70.74		AB
40s ea	**54868-2014-04**	93.91		AB
60s ea	**54868-2014-03**	140.26		AB
750 mg, 20s ea	**54868-3208-02**	50.80		AB
30s ea	**54868-3208-01**	75.26		AB
60s ea	**54868-3208-00**	148.65		AB
(Quality Care Prod)				
REPACK				
TAB, PO, 500 mg, 14s ea	**49999-0124-14**	39.48		AB
30s ea	**49999-0124-30**	84.60		AB
40s ea	**49999-0124-40**	112.80		AB
750 mg, 14s ea	**49999-0125-14**	43.63		AB
30s ea	**49999-0125-30**	93.60		AB
RELAGARD (Blansett)				
acetic acid glacial/oxyquinoline sulfate				
GEL, VG (W/APPLICATOR)				
0.9%-0.025%, 50 gm	**51674-0130-05**	25.24		
RELAGESIC (Intl Ethical)				
acetaminophen/phenyltoloxamine citrate				
TAB, PO, 650 mg-50 mg,				
100s ea	**11584-0476-01**	39.65		
RELAHIST-DM (Cypress Pharm)				
cpm/dm/phenyleph hcl				
SOL, PO (1X30ML,PEDIATRIC DROPS)				
1 mg/ml-3 mg/ml-2 mg/ml,				
30 ml	**60258-0341-30**	38.65		
RELAMINE (Deston Therapeutics, LLC)				
chondroitin/glucosamine/paba/thioctic acid/vit e				
TAB, PO (SF,DYE-FREE)				
300 mg-400 mg,				
120s ea	**16881-0800-10**	176.00		
RELENZA (Glaxo)				
zanamivir				
DSK, IH (5X4,W/DISKHALER)				
5 mg/actuation,				
20s ea	**00173-0681-01**	70.80		
(Phys Total Care)				
REPACK				
DSK, IH (5X4,W/DISKHALER)				
5 mg/actuation,				
20s ea	**54868-4377-00**	90.71		
(Stat Rx)				
REPACK				
DSK, IH (5X4)				
5 mg/actuation,				
20s ea	**16590-0840-20**	76.00		
RELI ON INSULIN SYRINGE (Can-Am Care)				
insulin syringe/needle				
DEV, NA (29GX1/2",1 CC)				
ea	**81306-0526-13**	0.18		
(29GX1/2",1/2 CC)				
ea	**81306-0525-13**	0.18		
(29GX1/2",3/10 CC)				
ea	**81306-0524-13**	0.18		
(30GX5/16, 3/10 CC)				
ea	**81306-0524-23**	0.18		
(30GX5/16",1/2CC,SHT ND)				
ea	**81306-0525-23**	0.18		
(30GX5/16",1CC,SHT ND)				
ea	**81306-0526-23**	0.18		
RELIEFBAND (Abbott Hosp)				
transcutaneous nerve stimulator wristband				
DEV, NA (DISPOSABLE 150 HOUR)				
ea	**00074-2878-01**	52.80		
(REUSABLE)				
ea	**00074-2879-01**	102.00		
RELION VENTOLIN HFA (Glaxo)				
albuterol sulfate				
ARO, IH (1X8GM,60 ACTUATIONS)				
0.09 mg/actuation,				
8 gm	**00173-0682-81**	18.00		BX
RELISTOR (Wyeth)				
methylnaltrexone bromide				
SOL, SC, 12 mg/0.6 ml,				
7s ea	**00008-2513-02**	336.00	280.00	
(SINGLE USE VIAL)				
12 mg/0.6 ml,				
0.6 ml	**00008-1218-01**	48.00	40.00	
RELPAX (Pfizer)				
eletriptan hydrobromide				
TAB, PO (FILM COATED)				
20 mg, 6s ea	**00049-2330-45**	150.05	125.04	
40 mg, 6s ea	**00049-2340-45**	150.05	125.04	
12s ea	**00049-2340-05**	300.11	250.09	
(Phys Total Care)				
REPACK				
TAB, PO, 40 mg, 6s ea	**54868-5528-00**	171.13		
(Physician Partner)				
REPACK				
TAB, PO (FILM COATED)				
40 mg, 12s ea	**21695-0871-12**	600.22		
(Southwood)				
REPACK				
TAB, PO, 40 mg, 6s ea	**58016-4877-01**	114.48		
(Stat Rx)				
REPACK				
TAB, PO (6X2 DISPENSER PACK)				
40 mg, 2s ea	**16590-0201-12**	235.00		
RELURI (Cypress Pharm)				
guaifenesin/phenylephrine hydrochloride				
TER, PO (DYE-FREE,CAPLET)				
1200 mg-30 mg,				
100s ea	**60258-0355-01**	61.73		
REMERON (Organon)				
mirtazapine				
TAB, PO, 15 mg, 30s ea	**00052-0105-30**	129.90		
30 mg, 30s ea	**00052-0107-30**	133.80		
45 mg, 30s ea	**00052-0109-30**	136.34		
REMERON (Altura)				
REPACK				
mirtazapine				
TAB, PO, 30 mg, 30s ea	**63874-1020-03**	111.23		
(AQ)				
REPACK				
TAB, PO, 30 mg, 30s ea	**66105-0550-03**	136.61		
(Palmetto)				
REPACK				
ODT, PO, 15 mg, 15s ea	**23490-9210-00**	55,41		
30s ea	**23490-9210-03**	110.82		
TAB, PO, 15 mg, 15s ea	**23490-9220-00**	66.78		
30s ea	**23490-9220-03**	133.55		
(Phys Total Care)				
REPACK				
TAB, PO, 15 mg, 30s ea	**54868-4848-00**	127.51		
30 mg, 30s ea	**54868-4498-00**	115.93		
(Southwood)				
REPACK				
TAB, PO, 15 mg, 30s ea	**58016-0624-30**	122.66		
60s ea	**58016-0624-60**	245.32		
90s ea	**58016-0624-90**	367.98		
100s ea	**58016-0624-00**	408.87		
30 mg, 30s ea	**58016-0723-30**	126.35		
60s ea	**58016-0723-60**	252.70		
90s ea	**58016-0723-90**	379.05		
100s ea	**58016-0723-00**	421.17		
45 mg, 30s ea	**58016-0600-30**	128.75		
60s ea	**58016-0600-60**	257.50		
90s ea	**58016-0600-90**	386.25		
100s ea	**58016-0600-00**	429.17		
REMERON SOLTAB (Organon)				
mirtazapine				
ODT, PO (BLIST PK 5X6)				
15 mg, 30s ea UD	**00052-0106-30**	103.44		
30 mg, 30s ea UD	**00052-0108-30**	106.58		
(BLISTER PACK,5X6)				
45 mg, 30s ea UD	**00052-0110-30**	113.54		
(Phys Total Care)				
REPACK				
ODT, PO, 15 mg, 30s ea	**54868-4227-00**	102.60		
30 mg, 30s ea	**54868-4889-00**	105.68		
REMICADE (Centocor)				
infliximab				
PDS, IV (S.D.V.,PF)				
100 mg, ea	**57894-0030-01**	752.57		
REMIFENTANIL HYDROCHLORIDE (Bioniche Pharma) *See ULTIVA*				
REMODULIN (United Therapeutics)				
treprostinil sodium				
SOL, IJ (M.D.V.)				
1 mg/ml, 20 ml	**66302-0101-01**	1345.00		
2.5 mg/ml, 20 ml	**66302-0102-01**	3362.50		
5 mg/ml, 20 ml	**66302-0105-01**	6725.00		
10 mg/ml, 20 ml	**66302-0110-01**	13450.00		
REMULAR-S (Intl Ethical)				
chlorzoxazone				
TAB, PO, 250 mg, 100s ea	**11584-1033-01**	34.89		EE
RENA-VITE RX (Cypress Pharm)				
vitamin b complex and vitamin c				
TAB, PO, 100s ea	**60258-0161-01**	43.99		

PROD/MFR	NDC	AWP	DP	OBC
RENACIDIN (Guardian)				
citric acid/gluconolactone/magnesium carbonate				
SOL, IR, 500 ml	**00327-0011-05**	36.88	36.88	
RENAGEL (Genzyme)				
sevelamer hydrochloride				
TAB, PO, 400 mg, 360s ea	**58468-0020-01**	460.36	383.63	
800 mg, 180s ea	**58468-0021-01**	460.36	383.63	
(Altura)				
REPACK				
TAB, PO, 800 mg, 180s ea	**63874-1136-08**	333.85		
(Phys Total Care)				
REPACK				
TAB, PO, 800 mg, 180s ea	**54868-5615-00**	335.33		
(Southwood)				
REPACK				
TAB, PO, 800 mg, 30s ea	**58016-0778-30**	44.37		
60s ea	**58016-0778-60**	88.75		
90s ea	**58016-0778-90**	133.12		
100s ea	**58016-0778-00**	147.91		
RENAL CAPS (Cypress Pharm)				
vitamin b complex and vitamin c				
SGL, PO (SOFTGEL)				
100s ea	**60258-0162-01**	22.41		
RENAMIN (Baxter)				
amino acids				
SOL, IV, 6.5%,				
250 ml 12s	**00338-0471-02**	900.00		
500 ml 12s	**00338-0471-03**	1800.00		
RENATABS (Hawthorn Pharm)				
multivitamin and minerals				
TAB, PO, 100s ea	**63717-0160-01**	49.99		
RENATABS WITH IRON (Hawthorn Pharm)				
multivitamin and minerals				
TAB, PO (CAPLET)				
60s ea	**63717-0161-03**	22.49		
RENAX (Everett)				
multivitamin and minerals				
TAB, PO (CAPLET)				
90s ea	**00642-2746-90**	56.71		
RENAX 5.5 (Everett)				
multivitamin and minerals				
TAB, PO (CAPLET, FILM-COATED)				
90s ea	**00642-2755-90**	56.02		
RENESE (Pfizer)				
polythiazide				
TAB, PO, 2 mg, 100s ea	**00069-3760-66**	68.05	56.71	
RENO CAPS (Nnodum)				
multivitamin				
SGL, PO (SOFTGEL)				
100s ea	**63044-0622-01**	22.41		
RENO-30 (Bracco Diag)				
diatrizoate meglumine				
SOL, IV (VIAL)				
30%, 50 ml 25s	**00270-0804-45**	426.25	341.00	AT
RENO-60 (Bracco Diag)				
diatrizoate meglumine				
SOL, IV (10X50ML,SDV)				
60%, 50 ml 10s	**00270-0696-49**	176.50	141.20	AP
(VIAL)				
60%, 50 ml 25s	**00270-0696-50**	441.25	353.00	AP
RENO-DIP (Bracco Diag)				
diatrizoate meglumine				
SOL, IV, 30%, 300 ml 10s	**00270-0809-75**	540.00	432.00	AP
RENOCAL-76 (Bracco Diag)				
diatrizoate meglumine/diatrizoate sodium				
SOL, IV (S.D.V.)				
66%-10%, 50 ml 25s	**00270-0860-20**	606.25	485.00	AP
100 ml 10s	**00270-0860-30**	486.25	389.00	AP
(S.D. BOTTLE)				
66%-10%,				
150 ml 10s	**00270-0860-40**	647.50	518.00	AP
RENOGRAFIN-60 (Bracco Diag)				
diatrizoate meglumine/diatrizoate sodium				
SOL, IV (10X50ML,SDV)				
52%-8%, 50 ml 10s	**00270-0707-49**	441.25	353.00	
(BOTTLE)				
52%-8%, 100 ml 10s	**00270-0707-55**	353.75	283.00	
RENOVA (Ortho)				
tretinoin				
CRE, TP, 0.02%, 40 gm	**00062-0187-02**	178.22	148.52	
(1X44GM)				
0.02%, 44 gm	**00062-0187-15**	188.26	156.88	
(1X60GM)				
0.02%, 60 gm	**00062-0187-09**	216.62	180.52	
(Phys Total Care)				
REPACK				
CRE, TP, 0.02%, 40 gm	**54868-4641-00**	132.91		
0.05%, 40 gm	**54868-3710-00**	127.28		
60 gm	**54868-3710-01**	159.40		
RENVELA (Genzyme)				
sevelamer carbonate				
PDR, PO (CITRUS CREAM)				
0.8 gm/packet,				
90s ea	**58468-0132-02**	552.44	460.37	EE
2.4 gm/packet,				
90s ea	**58468-0131-02**	552.44	460.37	EE
TAB, PO (COMPRESSED TABLET)				
800 mg, 270s ea	**58468-0130-01**	552.44	460.37	
REOPRO (Lilly)				
abciximab				
SOL, IV (VIAL)				
2 mg/ml, 5 ml	**00002-7140-01**	778.86	649.05	
REPAGLINIDE				
(Novo Nordisk) *See PRANDIN*				
REPAN (Everett)				
acetaminophen/butalbital/caffeine				
TAB, PO, 325 mg-50 mg-40 mg,				
100s ea	**00642-0162-10**	114.67		AB
REPAN CF (Everett)				
acetaminophen/butalbital				
TAB, PO, 650 mg-50 mg,				
100s ea	**00642-0166-10**	61.70		AB
REPLACEMENT PEDIATRIC MONITOR				
(Medtronic Minimed)				
glucose meter				
DEV, NA, ea	**76300-0100-02**	660.00	550.00	
REPLIVA 21/7 (Ther-RX)				
fe/folic acid/succinic acid/vit b12/vit c				
TAB, PO (3X28,FILM-COATED)				
84s ea	**64011-0207-34**	93.67		
(Phys Total Care)				
REPACK				
TAB, PO (FILM-COATED)				
28s ea	**54868-5960-00**	40.44		
REPREXAIN (Centrix)				
hydrocodone bitartrate/ibuprofen				
TAB, PO (AQUEOUS FILM-COATED)				
5 mg-200 mg,				
100s ea, C-III	**11528-0410-01**	85.14		AB
7.5 mg-200 mg,				
100s ea, C-III	**11528-0420-01**	96.30		AB
(Hawthorn Pharm)				
TAB, PO (FILM-COATED)				
2.5 mg-200 mg,				
100s ea, C-III	**63717-0900-01**	75.00		EE
5 mg-200 mg,				
100s ea, C-III	**63717-0901-01**	82.50		
10 mg-200 mg,				
100s ea, C-III	**63717-0902-01**	108.75		EE
(Stat Rx)				
REPACK				
TAB, PO (FILM-COATED)				
2.5 mg-200 mg,				
30s ea, C-III	**16590-0877-30**	26.40		EE
40s ea, C-III	**16590-0877-40**	35.20		EE
5 mg-200 mg,				
30s ea, C-III	**16590-0878-30**	28.89		
40s ea, C-III	**16590-0878-40**	38.52		
10 mg-200 mg,				
30s ea, C-III	**16590-0276-30**	37.65		EE
40s ea, C-III	**16590-0276-40**	49.71		EE
REPRONEX (Ferring)				
follicle stimulating hormone/luteinizing hormone				
PDS, IM (SDV)				
75 iu-75 iu, 5s ea	**55566-7185-02**	469.27		BX
REQ49+ (Capellon)				
multivitamin, minerals, and nutriceuticals				
TAB, PO, 120s ea	**64543-0900-01**	62.49	47.49	
REQUIP (Glaxo)				
ropinirole hydrochloride				
TAB, PO, 0.25 mg,				
100s ea	**00007-4890-20**	322.42		
0.5 mg, 100s ea	**00007-4891-20**	322.42		
1 mg, 100s ea	**00007-4892-20**	322.42		
2 mg, 100s ea	**00007-4893-20**	322.42		
3 mg, 100s ea	**00007-4895-20**	334.43		
4 mg, 100s ea	**00007-4896-20**	334.43		
5 mg, 100s ea	**00007-4894-20**	334.43		
(IPI)				
REPACK				
TAB, PO, 1 mg, 30s ea	**18837-0136-30**	72.04		
(Keltman Pharma., Inc.)				
REPACK				
TAB, PO, 0.25 mg, 30s ea	**68387-0198-30**	77.89		
(PD-Rx Pharm)				
REPACK				
TAB, PO, 1 mg, 30s ea	**55289-0470-30**	119.76		
(Phys Total Care)				
REPACK				
TAB, PO, 0.25 mg, 10s ea	**54868-4213-00**	36.58		
30s ea	**54868-4213-01**	111.92		
0.5 mg, 10s ea	**54868-0607-01**	38.61		
30s ea	**54868-0607-02**	111.92		
100s ea	**54868-0607-00**	347.48		
1 mg, 10s ea	**54868-5373-01**	34.20		
30s ea	**54868-5373-00**	98.84		
60s ea	**54868-5373-03**	185.03		
100s ea	**54868-5373-02**	306.51		
2 mg, 10s ea	**54868-5433-00**	25.06		
30s ea	**54868-5433-01**	75.54		
3 mg, 10s ea	**54868-5613-00**	30.06		
30s ea	**54868-5613-01**	86.44		
4 mg, 10s ea	**54868-2830-00**	35.40		
30s ea	**54868-2830-01**	102.45		
(Quality Care Prod)				
REPACK				
TAB, PO, 0.25 mg, 30s ea	**35356-0522-30**	164.80		
0.5 mg, 30s ea	**35356-0523-30**	164.80		
2 mg, 30s ea	**49999-0950-30**	114.13		
(Stat Rx)				
REPACK				
TAB, PO, 1 mg, 20s ea	**16590-0537-20**	61.00		
30s ea	**16590-0537-30**	111.50		
60s ea	**16590-0537-60**	222.99		
90s ea	**16590-0537-90**	395.25		
120s ea	**16590-0537-72**	358.00		
REQUIP XL (Glaxo)				
ropinirole hydrochloride				
TER, PO (FILM-COATED)				
2 mg, 30s ea	**00007-4885-13**	86.10		
90s ea	**00007-4885-59**	258.31		
4 mg, 30s ea	**00007-4887-13**	172.21		
90s ea	**00007-4887-59**	516.64		
6 mg, 30s ea	**00007-4883-13**	258.31		
(FILM-COATED)				
8 mg, 30s ea	**00007-4888-13**	258.31		
90s ea	**00007-4888-59**	774.95		
12 mg, 30s ea	**00007-4882-13**	430.52		
(Phys Total Care)				
REPACK				
TER, PO (FILM-COATED)				
2 mg, 30s ea	**54868-6093-00**	104.74		
RESCON (Capellon)				
cpm/methscopolamine nitrate/phenyleph hcl				
TER, PO (BILAYERED)				
12 mg-2 mg-40 mg,				
90s ea	**64543-0095-90**	193.75		
RESCON-JR. (Capellon)				
cpm/phenyleph hcl				
TER, PO (IMPROVED FORMULA)				
4 mg-20 mg,				
100s ea	**64543-0085-01**	105.00		
RESCON-MX (Capellon)				
dexchlorpheniramine mal/phenyleph hcl				
TER, PO, 6 mg-40 mg,				
90s ea	**64543-0091-90**	251.88	201.50	
(Capellon)				
cpm/methscopolamine nitrate/phenyleph hcl				
8 mg-2.5 mg-40 mg,				
100s ea	**64543-0090-01**	193.75		
RESCRIPTOR (Pfizer)				
delavirdine mesylate				
TAB, PO, 100 mg, 360s ea	**63010-0020-36**	331.03	275.86	
200 mg, 180s ea	**63010-0021-18**	331.03	275.86	
(Phys Total Care)				
REPACK				
TAB, PO, 200 mg, 180s ea	**54868-4520-00**	336.99		
RESECTISOL (B. Braun)				
mannitol				
SOL, IL, 5%, 2000 ml	**00264-2303-50**	10.57		
RESERPINE (Medisca)				
POW, NA (U.S.P.)				
1 gm	**38779-0159-06**	525.00		
5 gm	**38779-0159-03**	1575.00		
10 gm	**38779-0159-01**	2685.00		
(1X25GM,USP)				
25 gm	**38779-0159-04**	5055.00		

PROD/MFR	NDC	AWP	DP	OBC
(PCCA)				
POW, NA, 1 gm	51927-1264-00	390.00		
(Sandoz)				
TAB, PO, 0.1 mg, 100s ea.	00185-0032-01	83.31		BP
1000s ea	00185-0032-10	833.07		BP
0.25 mg, 100s ea.	00185-0134-01	114.96		BP
1000s ea	00185-0134-10	1034.47		BP
RESORCINOL (Amend)				
acetone/fuchsin/resorcinol				
POW, NA (U.S.P.)				
125 gm	17317-0463-04	8.75		
500 gm	17317-0463-01	26.60		
2270 gm	17317-0463-05	112.00		
11350 gm	17317-0463-08	490.00		
RESORCINOL (Baker, J.T.)				
CRY, NA (U.S.P.)				
125 gm	10106-3368-04	13.52		
500 gm	10106-3368-01	39.44		
POW, NA, 125 gm	10106-3366-04	62.18		
500 gm	10106-3366-01	77.61		
(Gallipot)				
acetone/fuchsin/resorcinol				
POW, NA (U.S.P.,N.F.)				
100 gm	51552-0052-05	11.06		
480 gm	51552-0052-06	33.60		
RESORCINOL (Mallinckrodt Lab)				
CRY, NA (U.S.P.)				
125 gm	00406-7228-02	53.56		
500 gm	00406-7228-04	71.64		
POW, NA, 500 gm	00406-7232-03	92.33		
(Medisca)				
CRY, NA (U.S.P.)				
25 gm	38779-0494-04	28.50		
100 gm	38779-0494-05	54.00		
500 gm	38779-0494-08	117.00		
1000 gm	38779-0494-09	201.00		
(PCCA)				
POW, NA (U.S.P.)				
1 gm	51927-1298-00	1.14		
(Spectrum Pharmacy)				
POW, NA (U.S.P.)				
125 gm	49452-6230-01	62.65		
500 gm	49452-6230-02	167.65		
2500 gm	49452-6230-03	696.50		
RESPA C&C IR (Respa Pharm)				
apap/dm/diphenhydramine hcl/phenyleph hcl				
TAB, PO, 100s ea	60575-0513-19	110.33		
RESPA-A.R. (Respa Pharm)				
cough/cold combination				
TER, PO, 100s ea	60575-0177-19	106.79		
RESPA-BR (Respa Pharm)				
brompheniramine maleate				
TER, PO (DYE-FREE)				
11 mg, 100s ea	60575-0786-19	107.97		
RESPAHIST-II (Respa Pharm)				
bpm/phenyleph hcl				
TER, PO, 6 mg-18 mg,				
100s ea	60575-0619-19	128.91		
RESPAIRE-120 SR (Laser Pharma)				
guaifenesin/pseudoephedrine hydrochloride				
CER, PO, 250 mg-120 mg,				
100s ea	00277-0169-01	38.00		
RESPAIRE-30 (Laser Pharma)				
guaifenesin/pseudoephedrine hydrochloride				
CAP, PO, 150 mg-30 mg,				
100s ea	16477-0306-01	54.75		
RESPAIRE-60 SR (Laser Pharma)				
guaifenesin/pseudoephedrine hydrochloride				
CER, PO, 200 mg-60 mg,				
100s ea	00277-0174-01	59.33		
RESPERAL (Cypress Pharm)				
dm/dexchlorpheniramine mal/phenyleph hcl/pyril mal				
SOL, PO (AF,SF,DYE-FREE)				
473 ml	60258-0399-16	54.39		
RESPERAL-DM (Cypress Pharm)				
bpm/dm/pse hcl				
SYR, PO (AF,DYE-FREE,GLUTEN-FREE)				
1 mg/ml-5 mg/ml-12 mg/ml,				
30 ml	60258-0398-30	26.89		
RESPI-TANN (Accentia)				
carbetapentane tannate/pseudoephedrine tannate				
CTB, PO (DYE-FREE,CHERRY)				
25 mg-75 mg,				
100s ea	67336-0157-01	199.37		
SUS, PO, 25 mg/5 ml-75 mg/5 ml,				
473 ml	67336-0156-16	209.16		

PROD/MFR	NDC	AWP	DP	OBC
RESPI-TANN PD (Accentia)				
carbetapentane cit/pse hcl				
SUS, PO (BUBBLEGUM,GRAPE)				
7.5 mg/5 ml-30 mg/5 ml,				
473 ml	67336-0187-16	189.74		
RESPIVENT DOSEPACK DF (Aristos)				
chlorpheniramine maleate/methscopolamine nitrate				
TAB, PO, 20s ea	24486-0704-20	69.10		
60s ea	24486-0704-60	207.29		
RESPIVENT-D (Aristos)				
methscopolamine nitrate/pse hcl				
TER, PO, 2.5 mg-120 mg,				
60s ea	24486-0702-60	53.25		
RESTALL (Clint)				
hydroxyzine hydrochloride				
SOL, IM (VIAL)				
50 mg/ml, 10 ml	55553-0171-10	8.50		EE
RESTASIS (Allergan Inc)				
cyclosporine				
EMU, OP (30X0.4ML,PF,HOMOGENEOUS)				
0.05%, 30s ea	00023-9163-30	134.68		
(60X0.4ML,PF,HOMOGENEOUS)				
0.05%, 60s ea	00023-9163-60	269.35		
(Phys Total Care)				
REPACK				
EMU, OP (30X0.4ML,PF,HOMOGENEOUS)				
0.05%, 0.4 ml 30s	54868-4793-01	147.94		
(Quality Care Prod)				
REPACK				
EMU, OP (30X0.4ML,PF,HOMOGENEOUS)				
0.05%, 0.4 ml 30s	35356-0248-30	223.33		
(32X0.4ML,PF,HOMOGENEOUS)				
0.05%, 0.4 ml 32s	35356-0248-32	223.67		
RESTORIL (Covidien)				
temazepam				
CAP, PO (USP)				
7.5 mg,				
30s ea, C-IV	00406-9915-03	350.25		EE
100s ea, C-IV	00406-9915-01	1167.50		
15 mg,				
100s ea, C-IV	00406-9916-01	1167.50		AB
(USP)				
22.5 mg,				
30s ea, C-IV	00406-9914-03	350.25		
30 mg,				
100s ea, C-IV	00406-9917-01	1167.50		AB
(Dispensing Solutions)				
REPACK				
CAP, PO, 7.5 mg,				
30s ea, C-IV	55045-3303-08	90.00		
(Phys Total Care)				
REPACK				
CAP, PO, 7.5 mg,				
10s ea, C-IV	54868-3657-02	92.10		
30s ea, C-IV	54868-3657-01	256.17		
100s ea, C-IV	54868-3657-00	820.54		
15 mg,				
10s ea, C-IV	54868-0778-03	146.91		AB
15s ea, C-IV	54868-0778-02	218.72		AB
30s ea, C-IV	54868-0778-00	410.24		AB
60s ea, C-IV	54868-0778-01	817.21		AB
30 mg,				
15s ea, C-IV	54868-0779-01	66.57		AB
30s ea, C-IV	54868-0779-00	130.65		AB
RETAPAMULIN				
(Glaxo) *See ALTABAX*				
RETAVASE (EKR)				
reteplase, recombinant				
KIT, IV (1X18.1 MG VIALS,PF)				
10.4 u, ea.	24477-0040-01	2605.93		
(2X18.1 MG VIALS,PF)				
10.4 u, ea.	24477-0041-02	5211.86		
RETEPLASE, RECOMBINANT				
(EKR) *See RETAVASE*				
RETIN A MICRO (Phys Total Care)				
REPACK				
tretinoin				
GEL, TP, 0.04%, 20 gm	54868-5604-01	135.57		
45 gm	54868-5604-00	221.61		
(1X50GM)				
0.04%, 50 gm	54868-5854-00	243.04		
RETIN-A (Ortho)				
tretinoin				
CRE, TP, 0.025%, 20 gm	00062-0165-01	82.82	69.02	AB
45 gm	00062-0165-02	156.80	130.67	AB
0.05%, 20 gm	00062-0175-12	92.88	77.40	AB
45 gm	00062-0175-13	174.19	145.16	AB

PROD/MFR	NDC	AWP	DP	OBC
0.1%, 20 gm	00062-0275-23	108.41	90.34	AB
45 gm	00062-0275-01	202.98	169.15	AB
GEL, TP, 0.01%, 15 gm	00062-0575-44	65.77	54.81	
45 gm	00062-0575-46	155.27	129.39	
0.025%, 15 gm	00062-0475-42	66.36	55.30	AB
45 gm	00062-0475-45	156.53	130.44	AB
(A-S Medication)				
REPACK				
CRE, TP, 0.05%, 20 gm	54569-1152-00	113.91		AB
(Pharma Pac)				
REPACK				
CRE, TP, 0.025%, 20 gm	52959-0571-01	51.83		AB
GEL, TP, 0.025%, 15 gm	52959-0570-00	26.71		AB
45 gm	52959-0570-01	63.60		AB
(Phys Total Care)				
REPACK				
CRE, TP, 0.025%, 20 gm	54868-1760-01	57.41		AB
45 gm	54868-1760-02	87.80		AB
0.05%, 20 gm	54868-0267-01	64.22		AB
45 gm	54868-0267-02	110.77		AB
0.1%, 20 gm	54868-0268-01	55.40		AB
45 gm	54868-0268-02	99.67		AB
GEL, TP, 0.01%, 15 gm	54868-0269-02	37.13		
0.025%, 45 gm	54868-0270-01	93.56		AB
(Quality Care Prod)				
REPACK				
CRE, TP, 0.1%, 45 gm	49999-0163-45	243.40		
(Southwood)				
REPACK				
CRE, TP, 0.025%, 20 gm	58016-3072-01	67.72		AB
45 gm	58016-3299-01	57.94		AB
0.05%, 20 gm	58016-3073-01	75.94		AB
45 gm	58016-3142-01	59.56		AB
0.1%, 20 gm	58016-3074-01	88.63		AB
45 gm	58016-9039-01	68.44		AB
GEL, TP, 0.01%, 15 gm	58016-3075-01	53.77		
0.025%, 15 gm	58016-3076-01	54.25		AB
45 gm	58016-3173-01	127.97		AB
SOL, TP, 0.05%, 28 ml	58016-3277-01	41.58		AT
RETIN-A MICRO (Ortho)				
tretinoin				
GEL, TP, 0.04%, 20 gm	00062-0204-02	112.99	94.16	
45 gm	00062-0204-03	204.14	170.12	
50 gm	00062-0204-11	237.24	197.70	
0.1%, 20 gm	00062-0190-02	112.99	94.16	
45 gm	00062-0190-03	204.14	170.12	
50 gm	00062-0190-11	237.24	197.70	
(A-S Medication)				
REPACK				
GEL, TP, 0.1%, 20 gm	54569-4506-00	138.58		
45 gm	54569-5439-00	250.37		
(Phys Total Care)				
REPACK				
GEL, TP, 0.1%, 20 gm	54868-4497-00	135.57		
45 gm	54868-4497-01	167.00		
(1X50GM)				
0.1%, 50 gm	54868-5926-00	243.04		
(Quality Care Prod)				
REPACK				
GEL, TP (1X45GM)				
0.04%, 45 gm	35356-0236-45	299.52		
(1X50GM)				
0.04%, 50 gm	35356-0236-50	347.25		
50 gm	35356-0238-50	347.25		
(1X45GM)				
0.1%, 45 gm	35356-0237-45	299.52		
(1X50GM)				
0.1%, 50 gm	35356-0237-50	347.25		
50 gm	35356-0239-50	347.25		
(Southwood)				
REPACK				
GEL, TP, 0.1%, 20 gm	58016-4851-01	62.20		
RETINOIC ACID (Amend)				
tretinoin				
POW, NA (U.S.P.)				
1 gm	17317-1415-07	35.00		
(Gallipot)				
POW, NA, 1 gm	51552-0120-01	39.90		
100 gm	51552-0120-05	1890.00		
RETINOIC ACID ALL-TRANS (Letco)				
tretinoin				
POW, NA (VITAMIN A ACID)				
1 gm	62991-2057-01	45.00		
5 gm	62991-2057-02	180.00		
10 gm	62991-2057-03	330.00		

PROD/MFR | NDC | AWP | DP | OBC

RETINOL (PCCA)
vitamin a
POW, NA (ALL TRANS)
0.001 gm **51927-3175-00** 4.14

RETISERT (Bausch & Lomb Inc.)
fluocinolone acetonide
IMP, IO (DIRECT SHIP ONLY)
0.59 mg, ea.......... **24208-0416-01** 21900.00

RETROVIR (Glaxo)
zidovudine
CAP, PO, 100 mg, 100s ea . **00173-0108-55** 280.72
(2X5X10)
100 mg, 100s ea UD . **00173-0108-56** 280.72
SOL, IV (S.D.V.)
10 mg/ml,
20 ml 10s........... **00173-0107-93** 303.64
SYR, PO, 50 mg/5 ml,
240 ml **00173-0113-18** 67.37
TAB, PO, 300 mg, 60s ea .. **00173-0501-00** 505.31

(A-S Medication)
REPACK
TAB, PO, 300 mg, 60s ea .. **54569-4538-00** 656.90

(Pharma Pac)
REPACK
CAP, PO, 100 mg, 6s ea ... **52959-0509-06** 13.43
18s ea............ **52959-0509-18** 39.35
24s ea............ **52959-0509-24** 47.17
28s ea............ **52959-0509-28** 54.47
30s ea............ **52959-0509-30** 57.76
TAB, PO, 300 mg, 6s ea ... **52959-0387-06** 31.50

(Phys Total Care)
REPACK
CAP, PO, 100 mg, 10s ea .. **54868-1974-02** 28.25
15s ea............ **54868-1974-00** 41.44
100s ea........... **54868-1974-03** 250.35
SYR, PO, 50 mg/5 ml,
240 ml **54868-2504-01** 67.45

(Quality Care Prod)
REPACK
CAP, PO, 100 mg, 18s ea .. **49999-0386-18** 93.72

(Southwood)
REPACK
CAP, PO, 100 mg, 18s ea .. **58016-0690-18** 33.44
30s ea............ **58016-0690-30** 79.45
60s ea............ **58016-0690-60** 158.90
90s ea............ **58016-0690-90** 238.35
100s ea........... **58016-0690-00** 264.83
TAB, PO, 300 mg, 30s ea .. **58016-0864-30** 238.35
60s ea............ **58016-0864-60** 476.70
90s ea............ **58016-0864-90** 715.05
100s ea........... **58016-0864-00** 794.50

REVATIO (Pfizer)
sildenafil citrate
SOL, IV, 10 mg/12.5 ml,
12.5 ml........... **00069-0338-01** 112.00 93.33
TAB, PO (FILM-COATED)
20 mg, 90s ea........ **00069-4190-68** 1544.23 1286.86

REVIA (Teva)
naltrexone hydrochloride
TAB, PO (FILM-COATED)
50 mg, 30s ea........ **51285-0275-01** 268.08 **AB**
100s ea........... **51285-0275-02** 893.66 **AB**

REVINA (Prasco Labs)
castor oil/peru balsam/trypsin
OIN, TP, 60 gm **66993-0915-61** 55.53

REVITADERM 40 (Blaine)
urea
CRE, TP, 40%, 112 gm **65373-0102-01** 57.00

REVLIMID (Celgene Corp)
lenalidomide
CAP, PO, 5 mg, 28s ea **59572-0405-28** 10863.94
30s ea............ **59572-0405-30** 9722.32
100s ea........... **59572-0405-00** 38800.03
10 mg, 28s ea........ **59572-0410-28** 11369.38
30s ea............ **59572-0410-30** 10174.52
100s ea........... **59572-0410-00** 40604.68
15 mg, 21s ea........ **59572-0415-21** 8561.78
100s ea........... **59572-0415-00** 40770.41
25 mg, 21s ea........ **59572-0425-21** 8645.76
25s ea............ **59572-0425-25** 9811.92
100s ea........... **59572-0425-00** 41170.84

REYATAZ (Bristol-Myers)
atazanavir sulfate
CAP, PO, 100 mg, 60s ea .. **00003-3623-12** 1087.49
150 mg, 60s ea **00003-3624-12** 1087.49
200 mg, 60s ea **00003-3631-12** 1087.49
300 mg, 30s ea **00003-3622-12** 1077.22

(A-S Medication)
REPACK
CAP, PO, 150 mg, 60s ea .. **54569-5530-00** 1334.97
200 mg, 60s ea **54569-5532-00** 1334.97
300 mg, 30s ea **54569-5864-00** 1334.97

(Phys Total Care)
REPACK
CAP, PO, 150 mg, 60s ea .. **54868-4857-00** 1132.43
200 mg, 60s ea **54898-4854-00** 956.57
300 mg, 30s ea **54868-5838-00** 1132.44

(Quality Care Prod)
REPACK
CAP, PO, 150 mg, 6s ea ... **35356-0068-06** 345.60
60s ea............ **35356-0068-60** 3270.00
200 mg, 60s ea **35356-0207-60** 1980.99
300 mg, 6s ea........ **35356-0114-06** 397.75
30s ea............ **35356-0114-30** 1724.04

REZYST IM (Zyber)
medical food
TAB, PO, 60s ea **65224-0560-01** 35.49

RHEUMADORON 1 (Weleda)
homeopathic substance
LIQ, PO, 50 ml........... **55946-0380-15** 9.00

RHEUMADORON 102A (Weleda)
homeopathic substance
LIQ, PO, 50 ml........... **55946-0392-15** 9.00

RHEUMADORON 2 (Weleda)
homeopathic substance
LIQ, PO, 50 ml........... **55946-0390-15** 9.00

RHEUMATREX DOSE PACK (Dava Pharma)
methotrexate sodium
TAB, PO (4X2)
2.5 mg, 8s ea .... **67253-0580-42** 93.58 **AB**
(4X3)
2.5 mg, 12s ea .... **67253-0580-43** 140.16 41.85 **AB**
(4X4)
2.5 mg, 16s ea .... **67253-0580-44** 187.02 **AB**
(4X5)
2.5 mg, 20s ea .... **67253-0580-45** 233.90 **AB**
(4X6)
2.5 mg, 24s ea .... **67253-0580-46** 280.58 **AB**

RHINACON A (Breckenridge Pharm)
cpm/phenyleph hcl/phenyltoloxamine cit
TER, PO, 4 mg-20 mg-40 mg,
100s ea........... **51991-0138-01** 54.25

RHINOCORT (Phys Total Care)
REPACK
budesonide
ARO, NS, 0.032 mg/actuation,
7 gm **54868-3553-00** 55.55

(Quality Care Prod)
REPACK
SPR, NS, 0.032 mg/actuation,
8.6 gm **49999-0995-16** 110.16

RHINOCORT AQUA (AstraZeneca)
budesonide
SPR, NS (120 METERED SPRAYS)
0.032 mg/actuation,
8.6 gm **00186-1070-08** 111.41

(A-S Medication)
REPACK
SPR, NS (120 METERED SPRAYS)
0.032 mg/actuation,
8.4 ml **54569-5248-00** 110.53

(Phys Total Care)
REPACK
SPR, NS (120 METERED SPRAYS)
0.032 mg/actuation,
8.4 ml **54868-4411-01** 118.78

(Quality Care Prod)
REPACK
SPR, NS, 0.032 mg/actuation,
8.6 gm **49999-0995-32** 152.77

RHINOFLEX (Carwin)
acetaminophen/phenyltoloxamine citrate
TAB, PO, 500 mg-50 mg,
100s ea........... **15370-0007-10** 37.45

RHINOFLEX-650 (Carwin)
acetaminophen/phenyltoloxamine citrate
TAB, PO, 650 mg-50 mg,
100s ea........... **15370-0650-10** 51.98 41.58

RHO(D) IMMUNE GLOBULIN
(Baxter Bioscience) *See WINRHO SDF*
(CSL) *See RHOPHYLAC*
(Ortho-Clinical) *See MICRHOGAM ULTRA-FILTERED*
(Ortho-Clinical) *See MICRHOGAM ULTRA-FILTERED PLUS*
(Ortho-Clinical) *See RHOGAM*
(Ortho-Clinical) *See RHOGAM ULTRA-FILTERED PLUS*
(Talecris) *See HYPERRHO S/D*

RHODYMENIA PALMETTA
(PCCA) *See DULSE FLAKES*

RHOGAM (Ortho-Clinical)
rho(d) immune globulin
SOL, IM (ULTRA-FILTERED,SF)
ea.................. **00562-7807-01** 127.20
(SRN,SFTY~300 MCG ANTI-D)
5s ea............... **00562-7807-06** 636.00
25s ea.............. **00562-7807-26** 3180.00

RHOGAM ULTRA-FILTERED PLUS (Ortho-Clinical)
rho(d) immune globulin
SOL, IM (PF,LATEX-FREE)
300 mcg, ea **00562-7805-01** 141.60
5s ea............... **00562-7805-05** 708.00
25s ea.............. **00562-7805-25** 3540.00

RHOPHYLAC (CSL)
rho(d) immune globulin
SOL, IJ (SAFETY NEEDLE,FULL DOSE)
750 iu/ml, 2 ml....... **44206-0300-01** 192.46
2 ml 10s.......... **44206-0300-10** 1749.60

RHUBARB
(PCCA) *See RHUBARB FLUID EXTRACT*

RHUBARB FLUID EXTRACT (PCCA)
rhubarb
LIQ, NA (NF)
1 ml................ **51927-1756-00** 0.58

RIASTAP (CSL)
fibrinogen
PDS, IV, 1 mg, ea......... **63833-8915-01** 1.09

RIBASPHERE (Three Rivers Pharm)
ribavirin
CAP, PO (GELATIN CAPSULE)
200 mg, 42s ea ...... **66435-0101-42** 417.20 **AB**
56s ea............ **66435-0101-56** 556.26 **AB**
70s ea............ **66435-0101-70** 695.34 **AB**
84s ea............ **66435-0101-84** 834.41
180s ea........... **66435-0101-18** 1787.40 **AB**
TAB, PO (USP,FILM-COATED)
200 mg, 168s ea **66435-0102-16** 1393.43
400 mg, 56s ea **66435-0103-56** 928.95
600 mg, 56s ea **66435-0104-56** 1393.43

RIBASPHERE RIBAPAK (Three Rivers Pharm)
ribavirin
TAB, PO (1000 DOSEPACK)
56s ea UD **66435-0106-99** 1344.22
(800 DOSEPACK,14X4)
400 mg, 56s ea UD ... **66435-0105-99** 1071.90
(1200 DOSE PACK,4X14)
600 mg, 56s ea UD ... **66435-0107-99** 1613.07

RIBAVIRIN
FUL
CAP, PO, 200 mg, 84s ea......................... 636.42

(Aurobindo Pharma)
CAP, PO (HARD GELATIN)
200 mg, 42s ea ...... **65862-0290-42** 400.09 **AB**
56s ea............ **65862-0290-56** 533.46 **AB**
70s ea............ **65862-0290-70** 666.82 **AB**
84s ea............ **65862-0290-84** 800.19 **AB**
180s ea........... **65862-0290-18** 1715.40 **AB**

(Gallipot)
POW, NA (USP,1X25GM)
25 gm.............. **51552-0813-04** 73.50 52.50
(USP,1X100GM)
100 gm............. **51552-0813-05** 220.50 157.50

(Hawkins)
POW, NA, 100 gm......... **63370-0219-35** 640.00
500 gm............ **63370-0219-45** 2800.00
1000 gm........... **63370-0219-50** 4400.00
(U.S.P.)
5000 gm........... **63370-0219-55** 20400.00

(Letco)
POW, NA (U.S.P.)
100 gm............ **62991-2077-02** 300.00
1000 gm........... **62991-2077-03** 1800.00

(Medisca)
POW, NA (1X25GM,USP)
25 gm.............. **38779-0256-04** 144.00

PROD/MFR	NDC	AWP	DP	OBC
(USP)				
100 gm	38779-0256-05	465.00		
500 gm	38779-0256-08	2085.00		
1000 gm	38779-0256-09	3150.00		
(1X25000GM,USP)				
25000 gm	38779-0256-07	24480.00		
(PCCA)				
POW, NA (U.S.P.)				
1 gm	51927-1671-00	5.79		
(Roche Labs) *See COPEGUS*				
(Sandoz)				
CAP, PO, 200 mg, 42s ea	00781-2043-42	417.23		
56s ea	00781-2043-16	556.29		
70s ea	00781-2043-67	695.38		
84s ea	00781-2043-04	834.46		
TAB, PO (FILM COATED)				
200 mg, 168s ea	00781-5177-28	1514.46		AB
(Schering) *See REBETOL*				
(Spectrum Pharmacy)				
CRY, NA (U.S.P.)				
100 gm	49452-6221-03	700.00		
500 gm	49452-6221-04	1984.50		
1000 gm	49452-6221-01	2978.50		
(Teva)				
CAP, PO, 200 mg, 42s ea	00093-7227-72	417.23		AB
56s ea	00093-7227-63	556.30		AB
70s ea	00093-7227-77	695.37		AB
84s ea	00093-7227-58	834.46		AB
TAB, PO (COATED)				
200 mg, 168s ea	00093-7232-81	1393.52		AB
(Three Rivers Pharm) *See RIBASPHERE*				
(Three Rivers Pharm) *See RIBASPHERE RIBAPAK*				
(Valeant Pharm Intl) *See VIRAZOLE*				
(Zydus Pharm.)				
CAP, PO, 200 mg, 42s ea	68382-0260-04	417.23		AB
56s ea	68382-0260-07	556.29		AB
70s ea	68382-0260-09	695.37		AB
84s ea	68382-0260-12	834.46		AB
TAB, PO (FILM-COATED)				
200 mg, 168s ea	68382-0046-03	1390.00		AB
(American Health) REPACK				
CAP, PO (5X10)				
200 mg, 50s ea UD	68084-0179-65	496.02		
TAB, PO, 200 mg,				
50s ea UD	68084-0150-65	413.69		
(Phys Total Care) REPACK				
CAP, PO, 200 mg, 42s ea	54868-4521-01	383.01		
70s ea	54868-4521-00	634.84		
168s ea	54868-4521-02	1203.00		
180s ea	54868-4521-03	2601.86		
RIBOFLAVIN (Letco)				
POW, NA (U.S.P.)				
500 gm	62991-1695-03	315.00		
(Medisca)				
POW, NA (U.S.P.)				
25 gm	38779-0875-04	31.50		
100 gm	38779-0875-05	76.50		
500 gm	38779-0875-08	297.00		
1000 gm	38779-0875-09	450.00		
(PCCA)				
POW, NA (U.S.P.; VITAMIN B2)				
1 gm	51927-1532-00	0.87		
(Spectrum Pharmacy)				
POW, NA (ANHYDROUS/U.S.P.)				
25 gm	49452-6271-01	131.60		
(U.S.P.)				
25 gm	49452-6270-01	66.50		
(ANHYDROUS/U.S.P.)				
100 gm	49452-6271-02	342.30		
(U.S.P.)				
100 gm	49452-6270-05	126.70		
500 gm	49452-6270-02	609.00		
RIBOFLAVIN 5-PHOSPHATE SODIUM (Medisca) riboflavine sodium phosphate				
POW, NA, 25 gm	38779-1561-04	64.50		
100 gm	38779-1561-05	186.00		
500 gm	38779-1561-08	795.00		
RIBOFLAVIN-5-PHOSPHATE SODIUM (Gallipot) riboflavine sodium phosphate				
POW, NA (1X100GM,USP)				
100 gm	51552-0961-05	80.15	57.25	
(1X1000GM,USP)				
1000 gm	51552-0961-07	434.00	310.00	
RIBOFLAVINE SODIUM PHOSPHATE				
(Gallipot) *See RIBOFLAVIN-5-PHOSPHATE SODIUM*				
(Medisca) *See RIBOFLAVIN 5-PHOSPHATE SODIUM*				
(PCCA)				
POW, NA (USP)				
1 gm	51927-1598-00	3.00		
RIBONUCLEIC ACID (PCCA)				
POW, NA (RNA)				
1 gm	51927-1821-00	4.35		
RIBOSE (PCCA)				
POW, NA, 1 gm	51927-2640-00	3.00		
(Spectrum Pharmacy) *See D-RIBOSE*				
RICE BRAN OIL (Medisca)				
OIL, NA (1X500ML)				
500 ml	38779-1562-08	28.50		
(1X4000ML)				
4000 ml	38779-1562-01	184.50		
(PCCA)				
OIL, NA, 1 ml	51927-2503-00	0.09		
RICE PROTEIN (PCCA)				
POW, NA, 1 gm	51927-3495-00	0.30		
RID-A-PAIN W/CODEINE (Pfeiffer) apap/asa/caff/codeine phos/salicylamide				
TAB, PO, 24s ea, C-V	00927-0060-24	2.77		
RIDAURA (Prometheus Labs) auranofin				
CAP, PO, 3 mg, 60s ea	65483-0093-06	358.87		
RIFABUTIN				
(Pfizer) *See MYCOBUTIN*				
RIFADIN (Sanofi-Aventis) rifampin				
CAP, PO, 150 mg, 30s ea	00068-0510-30	71.34		AB
300 mg, 60s ea	00068-0508-60	202.09		AB
100s ea	00068-0508-61	336.97		AB
(A-S Medication) REPACK				
CAP, PO, 300 mg, 60s ea	54569-0295-02	262.72		AB
(Phys Total Care) REPACK				
CAP, PO, 300 mg, 30s ea	54868-2901-02	88.94		AB
60s ea	54868-2901-01	145.46		AB
RIFADIN IV (Sanofi-Aventis) rifampin				
PDS, IV, 600 mg, ea	00068-0597-01	130.46		AP
RIFAMATE (Sanofi-Aventis) isoniazid/rifampin				
CAP, PO, 150 mg-300 mg,				
60s ea	00068-0509-60	232.82		
RIFAMPIN FUL				
CAP, PO, 150 mg, 30s ea		44.34		
300 mg, 100s ea		188.60		
(Akorn)				
PDS, IV (USP)				
600 mg, ea	23360-0051-42	136.30		AP
(Bedford)				
PDS, IV (VIAL,30 ML)				
600 mg, ea	55390-0123-01	139.20		AP
(Gallipot)				
POW, NA (USP,1X25GM)				
25 gm	51552-0715-04	28.00	20.00	
(USP,1X100GM)				
100 gm	51552-0715-05	84.00	60.00	
(USP,1X500GM)				
500 gm	51552-0715-06	336.00	240.00	
(Hawkins)				
CRY, NA (U.S.P.)				
25 gm	63370-0217-25	68.00		
100 gm	63370-0217-35	220.00		
1000 gm	63370-0217-50	1560.00		
(Lannett)				
CAP, PO (USP)				
150 mg, 30s ea	00527-1393-30	47.40		AB
100s ea	00527-1393-01	133.14		AB
300 mg, 30s ea	00527-1315-30	69.60		AB
60s ea	00527-1315-06	130.50		AB
100s ea	00527-1315-01	213.60		AB
(Letco)				
POW, NA (U.S.P.)				
25 gm	62991-1133-01	51.00		
100 gm	62991-1133-02	150.00		
1000 gm	62991-1133-04	975.00		
(Major)				
CAP, PO (5X10,USP)				
300 mg, 50s ea UD	00904-5282-06	273.47		AB
(Medisca)				
POW, NA (U.S.P.)				
25 gm	38779-0123-04	97.50		
100 gm	38779-0123-05	297.00		
500 gm	38779-0123-08	594.00		
1000 gm	38779-0123-09	1035.00		
(PCCA)				
POW, NA (U.S.P.)				
1 gm	51927-1956-00	4.32		
(Sandoz)				
CAP, PO, 150 mg, 30s ea	00185-0801-30	68.18		AB
100s ea	00185-0801-01	227.27		AB
300 mg, 30s ea	00185-0799-30	77.29		AB
60s ea	00185-0799-60	154.57		AB
100s ea	00185-0799-01	257.62		AB
500s ea	00185-0799-05	1288.12		AB
(Sanofi-Aventis) *See RIFADIN*				
(Sanofi-Aventis) *See RIFADIN IV*				
(Spectrum Pharmacy)				
POW, NA (1X25GM)				
25 gm	49452-6222-03	81.55		
(U.S.P.)				
25 gm	49452-6222-05	168.00		
100 gm	49452-6222-04	469.00		
1000 gm	49452-6222-06	1428.00		
(UDL)				
CAP, PO (ROBOT READY 25X1)				
300 mg, 25s ea UD	51079-0890-19	71.65		AB
(10X10)				
300 mg, 100s ea UD	51079-0890-20	303.85		AB
(VersaPharm)				
CAP, PO, 150 mg, 30s ea	61748-0015-30	47.30		AB
100s ea UD	61748-0015-11	156.40		AB
300 mg, 30s ea	61748-0018-30	60.53		AB
60s ea	61748-0018-60	120.65		AB
100s ea	61748-0018-01	201.16		AB
(10X10)				
300 mg, 100s ea UD	61748-0018-11	207.04		AB
(A-S Medication) REPACK				
CAP, PO, 300 mg, 10s ea	54569-5770-01	25.76		AB
30s ea	54569-5770-00	77.29		AB
(Altura) REPACK				
CAP, PO, 300 mg, 10s ea	63874-0088-10	19.00		
30s ea	63874-0088-30	57.01		
60s ea	63874-0088-60	114.04		
(American Health) REPACK				
CAP, PO, 150 mg,				
30s ea UD	68084-0357-21	43.75		AB
300 mg, 100s ea UD	68084-0358-01	136.25		AB
(IPI) REPACK				
CAP, PO, 300 mg, 30s ea	18837-0329-30	96.61		AB
90s ea	18837-0329-90	289.82		AB
(Keltman Pharma., Inc.) REPACK				
CAP, PO, 300 mg, 20s ea	68387-0115-20	43.85		
(McKesson Packaging) REPACK				
CAP, PO (USP)				
300 mg, 100s ea UD	63739-0415-10	190.08		
(PD-Rx Pharm) REPACK				
CAP, PO, 300 mg, 8s ea	55289-0386-08	52.43		AB
(Pharma Pac) REPACK				
CAP, PO, 300 mg, 10s ea	52959-0653-10	19.89		
20s ea	52959-0653-20	39.76		
30s ea	52959-0653-30	59.61		
40s ea	52959-0653-40	79.50		
(Phys Total Care) REPACK				
CAP, PO, 150 mg, 30s ea	54868-5472-00	108.87		
300 mg, 15s ea	54868-4683-01	128.70		AB
20s ea	54868-4683-02	131.14		AB
30s ea	54868-4683-00	192.95		AB
(Physician Partner) REPACK				
CAP, PO, 300 mg, 15s ea	21695-0527-15	67.09		
20s ea	21695-0527-20	89.45		

PROD/MFR	NDC	AWP	DP	OBC
(Quality Care Prod) REPACK				
CAP, PO, 300 mg, 30s ea	**35356-0480-30**	121.54		AB
(Stat Rx) REPACK				
CAP, PO, 300 mg, 30s ea	**16590-0714-30**	85.27		AB
RIFAPENTINE				
(Sanofi-Aventis) *See PRIFTIN*				
RIFATER (Sanofi-Aventis)				
isoniazid/pyrazinamide/rifampin				
TAB, PO, 50 mg-300 mg-120 mg, 60s ea	**00088-0576-41**	172.31		
RIFAXIMIN				
(Salix Pharm) *See XIFAXAN*				
RILONACEPT				
(Regeneron) *See ARCALYST*				
RILUTEK (Sanofi-Aventis)				
riluzole				
TAB, PO (CAPLET)				
50 mg, 60s ea	**00075-7700-60**	1104.14		
RILUZOLE				
(Sanofi-Aventis) *See RILUTEK*				
RIMABOTULINUMTOXINB				
(Solstice) *See MYOBLOC*				
RIMACTANE (Phys Total Care) REPACK				
rifampin				
CAP, PO, 300 mg, 60s ea	**54868-2484-00**	140.95		AB
RIMANTADINE (Bryant Ranch) REPACK				
rimantadine hydrochloride				
TAB, PO, 100 mg, 30s ea	**63629-3552-01**	119.09		
(Stat Rx) REPACK				
TAB, PO, 100 mg, 10s ea	**16590-0202-10**	7.50		
20s ea	**16590-0202-20**	15.00		
RIMANTADINE HCL (Caraco)				
rimantadine hydrochloride				
TAB, PO, 100 mg, 100s ea	**00258-3711-01**	183.36		AB
(Global Pharm)				
TAB, PO, 100 mg, 100s ea	**00115-1911-01**	244.11		AB
(Sandoz)				
TAB, PO, 100 mg, 100s ea	**00781-5029-01**	183.16		AB
(DHS, Inc.) REPACK				
TAB, PO, 100 mg, 14s ea	**55887-0644-14**	36.07		AB
28s ea	**55887-0644-28**	72.00		AB
(Dispensing Solutions) REPACK				
TAB, PO, 100 mg, 14s ea	**55045-3339-04**	27.30		AB
(PD-Rx Pharm) REPACK				
TAB, PO, 100 mg, 14s ea	**55289-0832-14**	34.58		AB
(Stat Rx) REPACK				
TAB, PO, 100 mg, 14s ea	**16590-0202-14**	37.49		AB
RIMANTADINE HYDROCHLORIDE FUL				
TAB, PO, 100 mg, 100s ea		151.20		
(Caraco) *See RIMANTADINE HCL*				
(Forest Pharm) *See FLUMADINE*				
(Global Pharm) *See RIMANTADINE HCL*				
(Sandoz) *See RIMANTADINE HCL*				
(Dispensing Solutions) REPACK				
TAB, PO, 100 mg, 30s ea	**55045-3760-08**	58.50		
(Palmetto) REPACK				
TAB, PO, 100 mg, 10s ea	**23490-6500-01**	23.50		
(Quality Care Prod) REPACK				
TAB, PO, 100 mg, 30s ea	**49999-0920-30**	66.01		
RIMEXOLONE				
(Alcon Ophthalmic) *See VEXOL*				
RIMSO-50 (Bioniche Pharma)				
dimethyl sulfoxide				
SOL, IL (ODORLESS)				
50%, 50 ml	**67457-0177-50**	93.75	50.00	AT
RINDAL HD (Breckenridge Pharm)				
cpm/hydrocod bit/phenyleph hcl				
LIQ, PO (AF,SF,CHERRY)				
473 ml, C-III	**51991-0225-16**	39.95		
RINDAL HD PLUS (Breckenridge Pharm)				
cpm/hydrocod bit/phenyleph hcl				
SOL, PO (AF,SF,GLUTEN-FREE)				
473 ml, C-III	**51991-0299-16**	42.60		
RINGER'S INJECTION (B. Braun)				
ca cl/k cl/na cl				
SOL, IJ (EXCEL)				
1000 ml	**00264-7780-00**	2.21		AP
(Baxter)				
SOL, IJ, 500 ml 24s	**00338-0105-03**	260.06		AP
1000 ml 12s	**00338-0105-04**	148.32		AP
(Hospira)				
SOL, IJ (LIFECARE,LATEX-FREE)				
500 ml 24s	**00409-7982-24**	50.69	44.40	AP
(LIFECARE,12X1000ML)				
1000 ml 12s	**00409-7982-09**	23.76	20.76	AP
RINGER'S IRRIGATION (B. Braun)				
ca cl/k cl/na cl				
SOL, IR (PIC CONTAINER)				
1000 ml	**00264-2202-00**	4.36		AT
2000 ml	**00264-2202-50**	13.22		AT
(Baxter)				
SOL, IR, 1000 ml 12s	**00338-0104-04**	238.61		AT
(Hospira)				
SOL, IR (AQUALITE,12X1000ML,PF)				
1000 ml 12s	**00409-6140-09**	65.95	57.72	AT
RIOMET (Ranbaxy Labs)				
metformin hydrochloride				
SOL, PO (CHERRY)				
500 mg/5 ml,				
118 ml	**10631-0206-01**	32.11		
473 ml	**10631-0206-02**	128.77		
RISEDRONATE SODIUM				
(P & G Pharm) *See ACTONEL*				
RISPERDAL (Janssen)				
risperidone				
SOL, PO, 1 mg/ml, 30 ml	**50458-0305-03**	196.55	163.79	
TAB, PO, 0.25 mg, 60s ea	**50458-0301-04**	301.60	251.33	
100s ea UD	**50458-0301-01**	502.60	418.83	
500s ea	**50458-0301-50**	2512.97	2094.14	
0.5 mg, 60s ea	**50458-0302-06**	330.95	275.79	
100s ea UD	**50458-0302-01**	551.54	459.62	
500s ea	**50458-0302-50**	2757.78	2298.15	
1 mg, 60s ea	**50458-0300-06**	351.84	293.20	
(10X10,BLISTER PACK)				
1 mg, 100s ea UD	**50458-0300-01**	586.27	488.56	
500s ea	**50458-0300-50**	2931.67	2443.06	
2 mg, 60s ea	**50458-0320-06**	588.00	490.00	
(10X10,BLISTER PACK)				
2 mg, 100s ea UD	**50458-0320-01**	979.90	816.58	
500s ea	**50458-0320-50**	4899.89	4083.24	
3 mg, 60s ea	**50458-0330-06**	690.62	575.52	
(10X10,BLISTER PACK)				
3 mg, 100s ea UD	**50458-0330-01**	1151.04	959.20	
500s ea	**50458-0330-50**	5754.92	4795.77	
4 mg, 60s ea	**50458-0350-06**	927.61	773.01	
(10X10,BLISTER PACK)				
4 mg, 100s ea UD	**50458-0350-01**	1545.96	1288.30	
(A-S Medication) REPACK				
TAB, PO, 1 mg, 30s ea	**54569-4140-01**	151.73		
(Advanced Pharm Serv, Inc.) REPACK				
TAB, PO, 1 mg, 10s ea	**13411-0123-01**	61.13		
15s ea	**13411-0123-15**	91.70		
30s ea	**13411-0123-03**	183.41		
60s ea	**13411-0123-06**	366.83		
90s ea	**13411-0123-09**	550.24		
2 mg, 10s ea	**13411-0124-01**	102.17		
15s ea	**13411-0124-15**	153.29		
30s ea	**13411-0124-03**	306.53		
60s ea	**13411-0124-06**	613.06		
90s ea	**13411-0124-09**	919.58		
3 mg, 30s ea	**13411-0125-03**	360.03		
4 mg, 30s ea	**13411-0126-03**	483.57		
(AQ) REPACK				
TAB, PO, 0.5 mg, 60s ea	**66105-0126-06**	318.69		
1 mg, 60s ea	**66105-0472-06**	338.49		
2 mg, 10s ea	**66105-0123-01**	125.02		
15s ea	**66105-0123-15**	187.53		
30s ea	**66105-0123-03**	375.06		
60s ea	**66105-0123-06**	750.12		
90s ea	**66105-0123-09**	1125.18		
3 mg, 10s ea	**66105-0124-01**	155.90		
15s ea	**66105-0124-15**	233.85		
30s ea	**66105-0124-03**	467.69		
60s ea	**66105-0124-06**	935.37		
90s ea	**66105-0124-09**	1403.04		
4 mg, 10s ea	**66105-0125-01**	181.81		
15s ea	**66105-0125-15**	272.72		
30s ea	**66105-0125-03**	545.43		
60s ea	**66105-0125-06**	1090.87		
90s ea	**66105-0125-09**	1636.30		
(Core) REPACK				
TAB, PO, 0.5 mg, 30s ea	**33358-0318-30**	123.91		
60s ea	**33358-0318-60**	340.38		
(PD-Rx Pharm) REPACK				
TAB, PO, 0.5 mg, 30s ea	**55289-0463-30**	203.94		
1 mg, 30s ea	**55289-0491-30**	237.92		
(REDI-SCRIPT)				
1 mg, 30s ea	**58864-0038-30**	237.92		
2 mg, 30s ea	**55289-0465-30**	397.61		
4 mg, 30s ea	**55289-0519-30**	627.26		
(Pharma Pac) REPACK				
TAB, PO, 2 mg, 30s ea	**52959-0916-30**	280.58		
60s ea	**52959-0916-60**	482.01		
(Phys Total Care) REPACK				
SOL, PO, 1 mg/ml, 30 ml	**54868-5800-00**	163.31		
TAB, PO, 0.5 mg, 30s ea	**54868-4874-00**	148.28		
1 mg, 30s ea	**54868-3512-00**	174.38		
60s ea	**54868-3512-01**	346.14		
2 mg, 30s ea	**54868-3513-01**	290.76		
60s ea	**54868-3513-02**	559.67		
4 mg, 60s ea	**54868-3515-00**	471.59		
(Physician Partner) REPACK				
TAB, PO, 1 mg, 15s ea	**21695-0113-15**	178.50		
3 mg, 30s ea	**21695-0115-30**	557.19		
60s ea	**21695-0115-60**	1191.28		
(Quality Care Prod) REPACK				
TAB, PO, 0.25 mg, 60s ea	**49999-0775-60**	472.00		
0.5 mg, 15s ea	**49999-0911-15**	108.60		
1 mg, 15s ea	**49999-0633-15**	201.00		
2 mg, 30s ea	**49999-0634-30**	394.80		
60s ea	**49999-0634-60**	789.60		
3 mg, 60s ea	**35356-0106-60**	984.60		
(Southwood) REPACK				
TAB, PO, 0.25 mg, 30s ea	**58016-0050-30**	124.86		
60s ea	**58016-0050-60**	249.71		
90s ea	**58016-0050-90**	374.57		
100s ea	**58016-0050-00**	416.18		
0.5 mg, 30s ea	**58016-0049-30**	137.01		
60s ea	**58016-0049-60**	274.01		
90s ea	**58016-0049-90**	411.02		
100s ea	**58016-0049-00**	456.68		
(Stat Rx) REPACK				
TAB, PO, 1 mg, 30s ea	**16590-0572-30**	172.45		
60s ea	**16590-0572-60**	307.00		
2 mg, 30s ea	**16590-0575-30**	237.00		
60s ea	**16590-0575-60**	572.88		
RISPERDAL CONSTA (Janssen)				
risperidone				
GER, IM, 12.5 mg, ea	**50458-0309-11**	148.22	123.52	EE
25 mg, ea	**50458-0306-11**	296.46	247.05	EE
37.5 mg, ea	**50458-0307-11**	444.68	370.57	EE
50 mg, ea	**50458-0308-11**	592.93	494.11	
RISPERDAL M-TAB (Janssen)				
risperidone				
ODT, PO, 0.5 mg, 28s ea	**50458-0395-28**	161.36	134.47	
30s ea	**50458-0395-30**	172.91	144.09	
1 mg, 28s ea	**50458-0315-28**	188.54	157.12	
30s ea	**50458-0315-30**	202.06	168.38	
2 mg, 28s ea	**50458-0325-28**	306.55	255.46	
(28 INDIVIDUAL BLISTERS)				
3 mg, 28s ea UD	**50458-0335-28**	386.74	322.28	
4 mg, 28s ea UD	**50458-0355-28**	519.47	432.89	
RISPERIDONE FUL				
TAB, PO, 0.25 mg, 60s ea		78.03		
0.5 mg, 60s ea		85.64		
1 mg, 60s ea		91.04		
2 mg, 60s ea		152.15		
3 mg, 60s ea		178.70		
4 mg, 60s ea		240.01		

PROD/MFR	NDC	AWP	DP	OBC
(Apotex Corp.)				
SOL, PO (1X30ML)				
1 mg/ml, 30 ml	**60505-0380-01**	152.56		AA
TAB, PO (FILM-COATED)				
0.25 mg, 60s ea	**60505-2584-06**	234.07		AB
100s ea UD	**60505-2584-00**	390.07		AB
500s ea	**60505-2584-05**	1950.36		AB
0.5 mg, 60s ea	**60505-2585-06**	256.86		AB
100s ea UD	**60505-2585-00**	428.07		AB
500s ea	**60505-2585-05**	2140.37		AB
1 mg, 60s ea	**60505-2586-06**	273.07		AB
100s ea UD	**60505-2586-00**	455.02		AB
500s ea	**60505-2586-05**	2275.32		AB
2 mg, 60s ea	**60505-2587-06**	456.37		AB
100s ea UD	**60505-2587-00**	760.51		AB
500s ea	**60505-2587-05**	3802.89		AB
3 mg, 60s ea	**60505-2588-06**	536.02		AB
100s ea UD	**60505-2588-00**	893.34		AB
500s ea	**60505-2588-05**	4466.50		AB
4 mg, 60s ea	**60505-2589-06**	719.95		AB
100s ea UD	**60505-2589-00**	1199.85		AB
(Aurobindo Pharma)				
SOL, PO (1X30ML)				
1 mg/ml, 30 ml	**65862-0167-30**	152.56		AA
TAB, PO (USP,FILM-COATED)				
0.25 mg, 60s ea	**65862-0119-60**	233.58		AB
500s ea	**65862-0119-05**	1946.25		AB
(USP,FILM-COATED CAPLET)				
0.5 mg, 60s ea	**65862-0120-60**	256.31		AB
500s ea	**65862-0120-05**	2135.85		AB
1 mg, 60s ea	**65862-0121-60**	272.50		AB
500s ea	**65862-0121-05**	2270.51		AB
2 mg, 60s ea	**65862-0122-60**	455.40		AB
500s ea	**65862-0122-05**	3794.86		AB
3 mg, 60s ea	**65862-0123-60**	534.89		AB
500s ea	**65862-0123-05**	4457.06		AB
4 mg, 60s ea	**65862-0124-60**	718.43		AB
(Bio-Pharm)				
SOL, PO (1X30ML)				
1 mg/ml, 30 ml	**55111-0579-30**	152.56		
(Dr Reddy's)				
ODT, PO, 0.5 mg,				
30s ea UD	**55111-0207-81**	147.47		AB
1 mg, 30s ea UD	**55111-0208-81**	171.95		AB
2 mg, 30s ea UD	**55111-0209-81**	280.15		AB
(Dr Reddy's) *See RISPERIDONE ODT*				
(Dr Reddy's)				
TAB, PO (USP,FILM COATED)				
0.25 mg, 60s ea	**55111-0201-60**	234.10		AB
500s ea	**55111-0201-05**	1950.83		AB
0.5 mg, 60s ea	**55111-0202-60**	256.89		AB
500s ea	**55111-0202-05**	2140.75		AB
1 mg, 60s ea	**55111-0203-60**	273.11		AB
500s ea	**55111-0203-05**	2275.92		AB
2 mg, 60s ea	**55111-0204-60**	456.42		AB
500s ea	**55111-0204-05**	3803.50		AB
3 mg, 60s ea	**55111-0205-60**	536.08		AB
500s ea	**55111-0205-05**	4467.33		AB
4 mg, 60s ea	**55111-0206-60**	720.03		AB
(Janssen) *See RISPERDAL*				
(Janssen) *See RISPERDAL CONSTA*				
(Janssen) *See RISPERDAL M-TAB*				
(Major)				
TAB, PO (10X10,FILM-COATED)				
0.25 mg,				
100s ea UD	**00904-5973-61**	350.37		AB
0.5 mg, 100s ea UD	**00904-5974-61**	384.46		AB
1 mg, 100s ea UD	**00904-5975-61**	408.75		AB
2 mg, 100s ea UD	**00904-5976-61**	683.10		AB
3 mg, 100s ea UD	**00904-5977-61**	804.00		AB
4 mg, 100s ea UD	**00904-5978-61**	1077.64		AB
(Mylan)				
TAB, PO (USP,FILM-COATED)				
0.25 mg, 60s ea	**00378-3502-91**	233.58		AB
500s ea	**00378-3502-05**	1946.25		AB
0.5 mg, 60s ea	**00378-3505-91**	256.31		AB
500s ea	**00378-3505-05**	2135.85		AB
1 mg, 60s ea	**00378-3511-91**	272.50		AB
500s ea	**00378-3511-05**	2270.51		AB
2 mg, 60s ea	**00378-3512-91**	455.40		AB
500s ea	**00378-3512-05**	3794.86		AB
3 mg, 60s ea	**00378-3513-91**	534.89		AB
500s ea	**00378-3513-05**	4457.06		AB
4 mg, 60s ea	**00378-3514-91**	718.43		AB
(Par)				
ODT, PO (5X6)				
0.25 mg, 30s ea	**49884-0212-55**	134.41		
(7X4)				
0.5 mg, 28s ea UD	**49884-0311-91**	137.64		
(5X6)				
0.5 mg, 30s ea UD	**49884-0311-55**	147.49		
(7X4)				
1 mg, 28s ea	**49884-0315-91**	160.83		AB
(5X6)				
1 mg, 30s ea	**49884-0315-55**	172.34		AB
(7X4)				
2 mg, 28s ea	**49884-0401-91**	261.48		
3 mg, 28s ea	**49884-0402-91**	329.88		
4 mg, 28s ea	**49884-0403-91**	443.09		
(Patriot Pharmaceuticals) *See RISPERIDONE M-TAB*				
(Patriot Pharmaceuticals)				
SOL, PO (1X30ML)				
1 mg/ml, 30 ml	**50458-0596-01**	146.14		
TAB, PO, 0.25 mg, 60s ea	**50458-0590-60**	78.48		
500s ea	**50458-0590-50**	653.94		
0.5 mg, 60s ea	**50458-0591-60**	86.12		
500s ea	**50458-0591-50**	717.65		
1 mg, 60s ea	**50458-0592-60**	91.56		
100s ea UD	**50458-0592-10**	235.38		
500s ea	**50458-0592-50**	762.89		
2 mg, 60s ea	**50458-0593-60**	153.01		
100s ea UD	**50458-0593-10**	393.42		
500s ea	**50458-0593-50**	1275.07		
3 mg, 60s ea	**50458-0594-60**	179.72		
100s ea UD	**50458-0594-10**	462.13		
500s ea	**50458-0594-50**	1497.58		
4 mg, 60s ea	**50458-0595-60**	241.39		
100s ea UD	**50458-0595-10**	620.69		
(Qualitest)				
TAB, PO (FILM-COATED)				
0.25 mg, 60s ea	**00603-5683-20**	234.08		
500s ea	**00603-5683-28**	1950.35		
0.5 mg, 60s ea	**00603-5684-20**	256.87		
500s ea	**00603-5684-28**	2140.35		
1 mg, 60s ea	**00603-5685-20**	273.09		
500s ea	**00603-5685-28**	2275.30		
2 mg, 60s ea	**00603-5686-20**	456.41		
500s ea	**00603-5686-28**	3802.87		
3 mg, 60s ea	**00603-5689-20**	536.06		
500s ea	**00603-5689-28**	4466.08		
4 mg, 60s ea	**00603-5688-20**	720.01		
(Roxane)				
SOL, PO (1X30ML)				
1 mg/ml, 30 ml	**00054-0063-44**	167.67		AA
(Sandoz)				
ODT, PO (7X4)				
0.5 mg, 28s ea UD	**00781-5310-08**	131.86		AB
1 mg, 28s ea UD	**00781-5311-08**	154.07		AB
2 mg, 28s ea UD	**00781-5312-08**	250.49		AB
3 mg, 28s ea UD	**00781-5313-08**	316.12		AB
4 mg, 28s ea UD	**00781-5314-08**	424.45		AB
(Teva)				
SOL, PO (1X30ML)				
1 mg/ml, 30 ml	**00093-6169-31**	152.56		AA
TAB, PO (USP,FILM-COATED)				
0.25 mg, 60s ea	**00093-0221-06**	234.10		AB
500s ea	**00093-0221-05**	1902.06		AB
0.5 mg, 60s ea	**00093-0225-06**	256.89		AB
500s ea	**00093-0225-05**	2087.23		AB
(FILM-COATED)				
1 mg, 60s ea	**00555-1771-09**	273.08		AB
(USP,FILM-COATED)				
1 mg, 60s ea	**00093-7240-06**	273.11		AB
(FILM-COATED)				
1 mg, 500s ea	**00555-1771-04**	2275.32		AB
(USP,FILM-COATED)				
1 mg, 500s ea	**00093-7240-05**	2219.02		AB
(FILM-COATED)				
2 mg, 60s ea	**00555-1772-09**	456.37		AB
(USP,FILM-COATED)				
2 mg, 60s ea	**00093-7241-06**	456.42		AB
(FILM-COATED)				
2 mg, 500s ea	**00555-1772-04**	3802.89		AB
(USP,FILM-COATED)				
2 mg, 500s ea	**00093-7241-05**	3708.41		AB
(FILM-COATED)				
3 mg, 60s ea	**00555-1773-09**	536.02		AB
(USP,FILM-COATED)				
3 mg, 60s ea	**00093-7242-06**	536.08		AB
(FILM-COATED)				
3 mg, 500s ea	**00555-1773-04**	4466.50		AB
(USP,FILM-COATED)				
3 mg, 500s ea	**00093-7242-05**	4355.65		AB
(FILM-COATED)				
4 mg, 60s ea	**00555-1774-09**	719.95		AB
(USP,FILM-COATED)				
4 mg, 60s ea	**00093-7243-06**	720.03		AB
(Torrent)				
TAB, PO (USP,FILM COATED)				
0.25 mg, 60s ea	**13668-0035-60**	234.08		AB
100s ea	**13668-0035-01**	390.10		AB
100s ea UD	**13668-0035-74**	389.30		AB
500s ea	**13668-0035-05**	1950.35		AB
0.5 mg, 60s ea	**13668-0036-60**	256.87		AB
100s ea	**13668-0036-01**	428.11		AB
100s ea UD	**13668-0036-74**	427.18		AB
500s ea	**13668-0036-05**	2140.35		AB
1 mg, 60s ea	**13668-0037-60**	273.09		AB
100s ea	**13668-0037-01**	455.10		AB
100s ea UD	**13668-0037-74**	454.17		AB
500s ea	**13668-0037-05**	2275.30		AB
2 mg, 60s ea	**13668-0038-60**	456.41		AB
100s ea	**13668-0038-01**	760.68		AB
100s ea UD	**13668-0038-74**	759.00		AB
500s ea	**13668-0038-05**	3802.87		AB
3 mg, 60s ea	**13668-0039-60**	535.93		AB
100s ea	**13668-0039-01**	893.21		AB
100s ea UD	**13668-0039-74**	891.48		AB
500s ea	**13668-0039-05**	4466.00		AB
4 mg, 60s ea	**13668-0040-60**	720.01		AB
90s ea UD	**13668-0040-64**	1197.38		AB
100s ea	**13668-0040-01**	1200.01		AB
500s ea	**13668-0040-05**	5999.00		AB
(UDL)				
TAB, PO (10X10,USP,FILM-COATED)				
0.25 mg,				
100s ea UD	**51079-0460-20**	389.30		AB
0.5 mg, 100s ea UD	**51079-0461-20**	427.18		AB
1 mg, 100s ea UD	**51079-0462-20**	454.17		AB
2 mg, 100s ea UD	**51079-0463-20**	759.00		AB
3 mg, 100s ea UD	**51079-0464-20**	891.48		AB
4 mg, 100s ea UD	**51079-0465-20**	1197.38		AB
(Watson Labs)				
TAB, PO (USP,FILM-COATED)				
0.25 mg, 60s ea	**16252-0558-60**	43.20		AB
0.5 mg, 60s ea	**16252-0559-60**	48.00		AB
1 mg, 60s ea	**16252-0560-60**	50.40		AB
2 mg, 60s ea	**16252-0561-60**	84.00		AB
3 mg, 60s ea	**16252-0562-60**	98.40		AB
4 mg, 60s ea	**16252-0563-60**	133.20		AB
(Wockhardt USA)				
SOL, PO (1X30ML)				
1 mg/ml, 30 ml	**64679-0692-01**	152.56		AA
TAB, PO (FILM-COATED)				
0.25 mg, 60s ea	**64679-0553-04**	234.08		AB
500s ea	**64679-0553-02**	1950.47		AB
0.5 mg, 60s ea	**64679-0554-04**	256.87		AB
500s ea	**64679-0554-02**	2140.48		AB
1 mg, 60s ea	**64679-0555-04**	273.09		AB
500s ea	**64679-0555-02**	2275.44		AB
2 mg, 60s ea	**64679-0557-04**	456.39		AB
500s ea	**64679-0557-02**	3803.09		AB
3 mg, 60s ea	**64679-0571-04**	536.04		AB
500s ea	**64679-0571-02**	4466.74		AB
4 mg, 60s ea	**64679-0572-04**	719.98		AB
500s ea	**64679-0572-02**	5999.85		AB
(Zydus Pharm.)				
TAB, PO (USP,FILM-COATED)				
0.25 mg, 60s ea	**68382-0112-14**	234.08		AB
500s ea	**68382-0112-05**	1950.35		AB
0.5 mg, 60s ea	**68382-0113-14**	256.87		AB
500s ea	**68382-0113-05**	2140.35		AB
1 mg, 60s ea	**68382-0114-14**	273.09		AB
500s ea	**68382-0114-05**	2275.30		AB
2 mg, 60s ea	**68382-0115-14**	456.41		AB
500s ea	**68382-0115-05**	3802.87		AB
3 mg, 60s ea	**68382-0116-14**	536.06		AB
500s ea	**68382-0116-05**	4466.08		AB
4 mg, 60s ea	**68382-0117-14**	720.01		AB
500s ea	**68382-0117-05**	5999.00		AB
(American Health)				
REPACK				
TAB, PO (10X10,FILM-COATED)				
0.25 mg,				
100s ea UD	**68084-0270-01**	389.25		AB
0.5 mg, 100s ea UD	**68084-0271-01**	427.13		AB
1 mg, 100s ea UD	**68084-0272-01**	454.12		AB
2 mg, 100s ea UD	**68084-0273-01**	758.95		AB
3 mg, 100s ea UD	**68084-0274-01**	891.43		AB
4 mg, 100s ea UD	**68084-0277-01**	1197.33		AB
(Pharma Pac)				
REPACK				
TAB, PO (FILM-COATED)				
2 mg, 30s ea	**52959-0941-30**	333.85		AB
(FILM COATED)				
2 mg, 60s ea	**52959-0941-60**	560.56		AB

PROD/MFR NDC AWP DP OBC

(Phys Total Care)
REPACK
TAB, PO (FILM COATED)
0.5 mg, 30s ea .... **54868-6082-00** 27.16 **AB**
(FILM-COATED)
1 mg, 60s ea......... **54868-5918-00** 517.66 **AB**

(Physician Partner)
REPACK
TAB, PO (FILM COATED)
0.25 mg, 60s ea...... **21695-0072-60** 468.14 **AB**
(FILM-COATED)
1 mg, 60s ea......... **21695-0089-60** 273.08 **AB**
(FILM COATED)
2 mg, 60s ea......... **21695-0095-60** 912.74 **AB**
(FILM-COATED)
4 mg, 60s ea......... **21695-0141-60** 234.07 **AB**

(Stat Rx)
REPACK
TAB, PO (FILM-COATED)
2 mg, 30s ea......... **16590-0641-30** 284.57 **AB**
60s ea.............. **16590-0641-60** 567.71 **AB**
90s ea.............. **16590-0641-90** 679.00 **AB**

RISPERIDONE M-TAB (Patriot Pharmaceuticals)
risperidone
ODT, PO (7X4)
0.5 mg, 28s ea....... **50458-0601-28** 131.86
1 mg, 28s ea......... **50458-0602-28** 154.07
2 mg, 28s ea......... **50458-0603-28** 250.49
3 mg, 28s ea......... **50458-0604-28** 316.12
4 mg, 28s ea......... **50458-0605-28** 424.45

RISPERIDONE ODT (Dr Reddy's)
risperidone
ODT, PO (3X10)
3 mg, 30s ea UD ..... **55111-0470-81** 352.81 **AB**
4 mg, 30s ea UD ..... **55111-0471-81** 473.72 **AB**

RITALIN (Novartis Pharm)
methylphenidate hydrochloride
TAB, PO, 5 mg,
100s ea, C-II .... **00078-0439-05** 78.83 **AB**
10 mg,
100s ea, C-II .... **00078-0440-05** 112.38 **AB**
20 mg,
100s ea, C-II .... **00078-0441-05** 161.59 **AB**

(Phys Total Care)
REPACK
TAB, PO, 5 mg,
20s ea, C-II .... **54868-1706-02** 18.28 **AB**
60s ea, C-II .... **54868-1706-01** 48.59 **AB**
100s ea, C-II .... **54868-1706-00** 78.40 **AB**
(USP)
5 mg,
120s ea, C-II .... **54868-1706-03** 94.00 **AB**
20 mg,
60s ea, C-II .... **54868-2762-00** 90.21 **AB**

RITALIN LA (Novartis Pharm)
methylphenidate hydrochloride
CER, PO, 10 mg,
100s ea, C-II **00078-0424-05** 432.67
20 mg,
100s ea, C-II **00078-0370-05** 432.67
30 mg,
100s ea, C-II **00078-0371-05** 442.52
40 mg,
100s ea, C-II **00078-0372-05** 454.81

(Phys Total Care)
REPACK
CER, PO, 10 mg,
10s ea, C-II **54868-5367-00** 36.04
30s ea, C-II **54868-5367-01** 101.85
20 mg,
10s ea, C-II **54868-5720-00** 42.55
30s ea, C-II **54868-5720-01** 121.41
30 mg,
10s ea, C-II **54868-5544-01** 43.45
30s ea, C-II **54868-5544-02** 124.10
100s ea, C-II **54868-5544-00** 383.35
40 mg,
10s ea, C-II **54868-5407-00** 37.71
30s ea, C-II **54868-5407-01** 106.90

(Quality Care Prod)
REPACK
CER, PO, 20 mg,
30s ea, C-II **35356-0165-30** 197.74
90s ea, C-II **35356-0165-90** 585.20

RITALIN-SR (Novartis Pharm)
methylphenidate hydrochloride
TER, PO, 20 mg,
100s ea, C-II .... **00078-0442-05** 266.65 **AB**

PROD/MFR NDC AWP DP OBC

(Phys Total Care)
REPACK
TER, PO, 20 mg,
10s ea, C-II .... **54868-2418-02** 23.49 **AB**
30s ea, C-II .... **54868-2418-01** 64.21 **AB**
60s ea, C-II .... **54868-2418-00** 125.30 **AB**

RITE AID BRANDS (Rite Aid)
codeine phosphate/guaifenesin
SYR, PO (TUSSIN DM COUGH)
10 mg/5 ml-100 mg/5 ml,
120 ml, C-V **11822-3253-07** 3.59

RITE AID DARK TANNING (Rite Aid)
octocrylene/oxybenzone
LOT, TP (SPF4,PRIVATE LABEL)
1%-0.5%, 237 ml **11822-9049-04** 4.79

RITE AID ENEMA (Rite Aid)
na phos, dibasic/na phos, monobasic
NMA, RC (LATEX-FREE)
7 gm/118 ml-19 gm/118 ml,
133 ml 8s.......... **11822-0339-98** 3.99

RITONAVIR
(Abbott Pharm) *See NORVIR*

RITUXAN (Genentech)
rituximab
SOL, IV (S.D.V.,PF)
10 mg/ml, 10 ml **50242-0051-21** 664.32
50 ml.............. **50242-0053-06** 3321.60

RITUXIMAB
(Genentech) *See RITUXAN*

RIVASTIGMINE
(Novartis Pharm) *See EXELON*

RIVASTIGMINE TARTRATE
(Novartis Pharm) *See EXELON*

RIZATRIPTAN BENZOATE
(Merck) *See MAXALT*
(Merck) *See MAXALT-MLT*

ROBAFEN AC (Major)
codeine phosphate/guaifenesin
SYR, PO, 10 mg/5 ml-100 mg/5 ml,
473 ml, C-V **00904-5065-16** 8.05

ROBAFEN AC COUGH SYRUP (Major)
codeine phosphate/guaifenesin
SYR, PO (SF)
10 mg/5 ml-100 mg/5 ml,
120 ml, C-V **00904-5065-00** 3.11

ROBAXIN (Baxter)
methocarbamol
SOL, IJ (SDV)
100 mg/ml, 10 ml .... **60977-0150-71** 33.55 **AP**
(S.D.V.)
100 mg/ml,
10 ml 25s.......... **60977-0150-01** 838.80 **AP**

(UCB)
TAB, PO, 500 mg, 100s ea . **00091-7429-63** 139.10 **AA**

(Phys Total Care)
REPACK
TAB, PO, 500 mg, 100s ea . **54868-0604-00** 100.20 **AA**

ROBAXIN-750 (UCB)
methocarbamol
TAB, PO, 750 mg, 100s ea . **00091-7449-63** 198.83 77.21 **AA**
500s ea............ **00091-7449-70** 726.10 **AA**

(PD-Rx Pharm)
REPACK
TAB, PO, 750 mg, 20s ea .. **55289-0017-20** 55.25 **AA**
40s ea............. **55289-0017-40** 110.48 **AA**

ROBAXISAL (Southwood)
REPACK
aspirin/methocarbamol
TAB, PO, 325 mg-400 mg,
30s ea............. **58016-0281-30** 18.69 **AB**

ROBINUL (Baxter)
glycopyrrolate
SOL, IJ, 0.2 mg/ml, 1 ml .. **60977-0155-81** 0.77 **AP**
(S.D.V.)
0.2 mg/ml,
1 ml 25s........... **60977-0155-01** 19.20 19.56 **AP**
2 ml............... **60977-0155-17** 0.91 **AP**
(S.D.V)
0.2 mg/ml,
2 ml 25s........... **60977-0155-02** 22.80 35.50 **AP**
5 ml............... **60977-0155-54** 1.38 **AP**
(M.D.V.)
0.2 mg/ml,
5 ml 25s........... **60977-0155-03** 34.50 86.53 **AP**

PROD/MFR NDC AWP DP OBC

(MDV)
0.2 mg/ml, 20 ml..... **60977-0155-63** 5.46 **AP**
(10X20ML,MDV)
0.2 mg/ml,
20 ml 10s.......... **60977-0155-06** 54.60 **AP**

(Shionogi)
TAB, PO, 1 mg, 100s ea ... **59630-0200-10** 388.31

(Phys Total Care)
REPACK
SOL, IJ (VIAL)
0.2 mg/ml,
1 ml 25s........... **54868-3231-01** 31.45 **AP**

ROBINUL FORTE (Shionogi)
glycopyrrolate
TAB, PO, 2 mg, 100s ea ... **59630-0205-10** 621.04

ROCALTROL (Validus)
calcitriol
SGL, PO (SOFT GELATIN)
0.25 mcg, 30s ea..... **30698-0143-23** 51.18 **AB**
100s ea............ **30698-0143-01** 167.83 **AB**
0.5 mcg, 100s ea..... **30698-0144-01** 268.60 **AB**
SOL, PO (1X15ML)
1 mcg/ml, 15 ml...... **30698-0911-15** 214.80 **AA**

(Phys Total Care)
REPACK
SGL, PO, 0.25 mcg,
30s ea............. **54868-3461-00** 51.18 **AB**

ROCEPHIN (Roche Labs)
ceftriaxone sodium
PDS, IJ (S.D.V.)
1 gm, ea............ **00004-1964-04** 63.50
10s ea............. **00004-1964-01** 620.14
(VIAL, BULK)
10 gm, ea........... **00004-1971-01** 478.32
(S.D.V.)
500 mg, ea **00004-1963-02** 37.78
10s ea............. **00004-1963-01** 362.42

(A-S Medication)
REPACK
PDS, IJ (VIAL)
500 mg, 10s ea **54569-1377-00** 298.71

(Phys Total Care)
REPACK
PDS, IJ (S.D.V.)
1 gm, ea............ **54868-2488-01** 62.51
250 mg, ea **54868-0934-01** 22.00
(S.D.V.)
250 mg, 10s ea **54868-0934-00** 181.36
500 mg, ea **54868-3221-01** 37.69
10s ea............. **54868-3221-00** 328.25

(Quality Care Prod)
REPACK
PDS, IJ, 1 gm, ea **49999-0586-01** 64.76
10s ea............. **49999-0586-10** 647.60

(Southwood)
REPACK
PDS, IJ, 1 gm, ea **58016-9438-01** 50.24
250 mg, 10s ea **58016-9453-01** 157.00
500 mg, 10s ea **58016-9551-01** 285.00

ROCURONIUM BROMIDE (APP)
SOL, IV (MDV, 10X5ML)
10 mg/ml, 5 ml 10s... **63323-0426-05** 78.00 **AP**
(MDV, 10X10ML)
10 mg/ml,
10 ml 10s.......... **63323-0426-10** 156.00 **AP**

(GeneraMedix)
SOL, IV (1X5ML,MDV)
10 mg/ml, 5 ml...... **10139-0235-05** 13.87 **AP**
(10X5ML,MDV)
10 mg/ml, 5 ml 10s... **10139-0235-15** 138.72 **AP**
(1X10ML,MDV)
10 mg/ml, 10 ml ..... **10139-0235-10** 26.63 **AP**
(10X10ML,MDV)
10 mg/ml,
10 ml 10s.......... **10139-0235-11** 266.28 **AP**

(Hospira) *See NOVAPLUS ROCURONIUM BROMIDE*

(Hospira)
SOL, IV (10X5ML,MDV)
10 mg/ml, 5 ml 10s... **00409-9558-05** 55.08 48.20 **AP**
(10X10ML,MDV)
10 mg/ml,
10 ml 10s.......... **00409-9558-10** 102.72 89.90 **AP**

(Organon) *See ZEMURON*

(Sandoz) *See ROCURONIUM BROMIDE*

PROD/MFR	NDC	AWP	DP	OBC
ROCURONIUM BROMIDE (Sandoz)				
rocuronium bromide				
SOL, IV (MDV; 1X5ML)				
10 mg/ml, 5 ml	00781-3220-75	19.66		AP
(MDV; 10X5ML)				
10 mg/ml, 5 ml 10s	00781-3220-95	196.64		AP
(MDV; 1X10ML)				
10 mg/ml, 10 ml	00781-3220-70	37.76		AP
(MDV; 10X10ML)				
10 mg/ml, 10 ml 10s	00781-3220-92	377.55		AP
ROCURONIUM BROMIDE (Teva)				
SOL, IV (10X5ML,MDV)				
10 mg/ml, 5 ml 10s	00703-2394-03	52.46		AP
(10X10ML,MDV)				
10 mg/ml, 10 ml 10s	00703-2395-03	89.05		AP
RODEX (Legere)				
pyridoxine				
SOL, IJ (VIAL)				
100 mg/ml, 30 ml	25332-0073-30	17.95		EE
ROMAZICON (Roche Labs)				
flumazenil				
SOL, IV (VIAL)				
0.1 mg/ml, 5 ml 10s	00004-6911-06	1256.74		
10 ml 10s	00004-6912-06	1999.31		
ROMIPLOSTIM				
(Amgen USA Inc.) *See NPLATE*				
ROMYCIN (Ocusoft)				
erythromycin				
OIN, OP, 5 mg/gm, 3.5 gm	54799-0540-35	7.18		EE
RONDEC DM (Quality Care Prod)				
REPACK				
bpm/dm/pse hcl				
SYR, PO, 120 ml	49999-0379-04	88.27		
ROOT BEER FLAVOR (Medisca)				
flavoring aid				
SOL, NA (1X100ML,CONCENTRATE)				
100 ml	38779-1563-05	22.50		
(1X500ML,CONCENTRATE)				
500 ml	38779-1563-08	37.50		
(PCCA)				
SOL, NA, 1 ml	51927-2848-00	0.05		
ROOT BEER FLAVOR SOLN (PCCA)				
flavoring aid				
SOL, NA (ARTIFICIAL)				
1 ml	51927-2823-00	0.90		
(CONCENTRATE)				
1 ml	51927-1281-00	0.23		
ROOTBEER ARTIFICIAL FLAVOR (Spectrum Pharmacy)				
flavoring aid				
LIQ, NA (1X100ML)				
100 ml	49452-6290-01	57.40		
(1X500ML)				
500 ml	49452-6290-02	116.90		
ROPINIROLE HYDROCHLORIDE				
FUL				
TAB, PO, 0.25 mg, 100s ea		75.15		
0.5 mg, 100s ea		75.15		
1 mg, 100s ea		75.15		
2 mg, 100s ea		75.15		
3 mg, 100s ea		77.96		
4 mg, 100s ea		77.96		
5 mg, 100s ea		77.96		
(CorePharma)				
TAB, PO (COATED)				
0.25 mg, 100s ea	64720-0201-10	247.73		AB
0.5 mg, 100s ea	64720-0202-10	247.73		AB
1 mg, 100s ea	64720-0203-10	247.73		AB
2 mg, 100s ea	64720-0204-10	247.73		AB
3 mg, 100s ea	64720-0205-10	256.97		AB
4 mg, 100s ea	64720-0206-10	256.97		AB
5 mg, 100s ea	64720-0207-10	256.97		AB
(Glaxo) *See REQUIP*				
(Glaxo) *See REQUIP XL*				
(Major)				
TAB, PO (10X10,FILM-COATED)				
0.25 mg, 100s ea UD	00904-5994-61	73.13		AB
0.5 mg, 100s ea UD	00904-5995-61	80.34		AB
1 mg, 100s ea UD	00904-5996-61	88.26		AB
2 mg, 100s ea UD	00904-5997-61	96.96		AB
3 mg, 100s ea UD	00904-5998-61	106.52		AB
4 mg, 100s ea UD	00904-5999-61	117.02		AB
5 mg, 100s ea UD	00904-6000-61	128.56		AB

PROD/MFR	NDC	AWP	DP	OBC
(Mylan)				
TAB, PO, 0.25 mg, 100s ea.	00378-5525-01	250.21		AB
0.5 mg, 100s ea	00378-5550-01	250.21		AB
1 mg, 100s ea	00378-5501-01	250.21		AB
2 mg, 100s ea	00378-5502-01	250.21		AB
3 mg, 100s ea	00378-5503-01	259.54		AB
4 mg, 100s ea	00378-5504-01	259.54		AB
5 mg, 100s ea	00378-5505-01	259.54		AB
(Roxane)				
TAB, PO, 0.25 mg, 100s ea.	00054-0116-25	250.52		AB
0.5 mg, 100s ea	00054-0117-25	250.52		AB
1 mg, 100s ea	00054-0118-25	250.52		AB
2 mg, 100s ea	00054-0119-25	250.52		AB
3 mg, 100s ea	00054-0120-25	259.86		AB
4 mg, 100s ea	00054-0121-25	259.86		AB
5 mg, 100s ea	00054-0122-25	259.86		AB
(Teva)				
TAB, PO (FILM COATED)				
0.25 mg, 100s ea	00093-5282-01	250.52		AB
0.5 mg, 100s ea	00093-5283-01	250.52		AB
1 mg, 100s ea	00093-5284-01	250.52		AB
2 mg, 100s ea	00093-5285-01	250.52		AB
3 mg, 100s ea	00093-5286-01	259.86		AB
4 mg, 100s ea	00093-5287-01	259.86		AB
(FILM-COATED)				
5 mg, 100s ea	00093-5288-01	259.86		AB
(Wockhardt USA)				
TAB, PO (FILM-COATED)				
0.25 mg, 100s ea	64679-0154-02	250.21		AB
500s ea	64679-0154-03	1226.03		AB
0.5 mg, 100s ea	64679-0155-02	250.21		AB
500s ea	64679-0155-03	1226.03		AB
1 mg, 100s ea	64679-0171-02	250.21		AB
500s ea	64679-0171-03	1226.03		AB
2 mg, 100s ea	64679-0172-02	250.21		AB
500s ea	64679-0172-03	1226.03		AB
3 mg, 100s ea	64679-0174-02	259.54		AB
4 mg, 100s ea	64679-0175-02	259.54		AB
5 mg, 100s ea	64679-0177-02	259.54		AB
(Zydus Pharm.)				
TAB, PO (FILM-COATED)				
0.25 mg, 100s ea	68382-0338-01	250.51		AB
0.5 mg, 100s ea	68382-0339-01	250.51		AB
1 mg, 100s ea	68382-0340-01	250.51		AB
2 mg, 100s ea	68382-0341-01	250.51		AB
3 mg, 100s ea	68382-0342-01	259.85		AB
4 mg, 100s ea	68382-0343-01	259.85		AB
5 mg, 100s ea	68382-0344-01	259.85		AB
(A-S Medication)				
REPACK				
TAB, PO (COATED)				
4 mg, 30s ea	54569-6104-00	77.78		AB
(American Health)				
REPACK				
TAB, PO (10X10,FILM-COATED)				
0.25 mg, 100s ea UD	68084-0305-01	81.25		AB
(3X10,FILM-COATED)				
0.5 mg, 30s ea UD	68084-0306-21	24.38		AB
(10X10,FILM-COATED)				
1 mg, 100s ea UD	68084-0307-01	81.25		AB
(3X10,FILM-COATED)				
2 mg, 30s ea UD	68084-0308-21	24.38		AB
(Nucare Pharm)				
REPACK				
TAB, PO (COATED)				
0.25 mg, 30s ea	68071-0806-30	79.89		AB
(Phys Total Care)				
REPACK				
TAB, PO (COATED)				
0.25 mg, 90s ea	54868-5952-01	137.82		AB
0.5 mg, 60s ea	54868-5953-01	83.34		AB
(FILM COATED)				
1 mg, 30s ea	54868-5897-00	63.36		AB
60s ea	54868-5897-01	94.52		AB
(COATED)				
2 mg, 10s ea	54868-5912-01	21.65		AB
30s ea	54868-5912-00	55.94		AB
(FILM COATED)				
4 mg, 10s ea	54868-5914-00	28.19		AB
30s ea	54868-5914-01	75.57		AB
(COATED)				
4 mg, 60s ea	54868-5914-03	81.57		AB
90s ea	54868-5914-02	139.50		AB
(Physician Partner)				
REPACK				
TAB, PO (COATED)				
0.25 mg, 60s ea	21695-0792-60	297.28		AB
1 mg, 60s ea	21695-0794-60	297.28		AB
5 mg, 60s ea	21695-0798-60	311.83		AB

PROD/MFR	NDC	AWP	DP	OBC
(Stat Rx)				
REPACK				
TAB, PO, 0.25 mg, 30s ea	16590-0849-30	75.06		AB
0.5 mg, 30s ea	16590-0754-30	19.34		AB
60s ea	16590-0754-60	37.21		AB
90s ea	16590-0754-90	73.81		AB
1 mg, 30s ea	16590-0643-30	71.83		AB
60s ea	16590-0643-60	143.66		AB
90s ea	16590-0643-90	215.49		AB
2 mg, 30s ea	16590-0734-30	130.00		AB
ROPIVACAINE HYDROCHLORIDE				
(APP) *See NAROPIN*				
(APP) *See NOVAPLUS NAROPIN*				
(Medisca)				
POW, NA (1X25GM,USP)				
25 gm	38779-2431-04	525.00		
ROPIVACAINE HYDROCHLORIDE-SODIUM CHLORIDE				
(PharMEDium Services)				
ropivacaine hydrochloride/sodium chloride				
SOL, EP, 0.2%-0.9%, 250 ml 5s	61553-0228-02	156.96	130.80	
ROPIVACAINE HYDROCHLORIDE/SODIUM CHLORIDE				
(PharMEDium Services) *See ROPIVACAINE HYDROCHLORIDE-SODIUM CHLORIDE*				
ROSAC CREAM W/SUNSCREENS (Stiefel Labs)				
sulfacetamide sodium/sulfur				
CRE, TP, 10%-5%, 45 gm	00145-2617-05	127.20		
ROSAC WASH (Stiefel Labs)				
sulfacetamide sodium/sulfur				
SOA, TP, 10%-1%, 170.1 gm	00145-2681-05	95.50		
ROSANIL (Galderma)				
sulfacetamide sodium/sulfur				
SOA, TP, 10%-5%, ea	00299-3839-01	181.25		
ROSE BENGAL (Akorn)				
TES, OP (STRIP)				
1.3 mg, 100s ea	17478-0402-01	19.56		
(HUB Pharma) *See ROSE GLO*				
(PCCA)				
POW, NA (C.I. 45440)				
1 gm	51927-2229-00	9.60		
(Spectrum Pharmacy)				
POW, NA (1X10GM)				
10 gm	49452-6302-02	135.10		
(1X25GM)				
25 gm	49452-6302-03	234.50		
ROSE GLO (HUB Pharma)				
rose bengal				
TES, OP, 1.3 mg, 100s ea	64334-1123-01	19.50		
ROSE OIL (Gallipot)				
OIL, NA (ARTIFICIAL)				
100 ml	51552-0449-05	20.23		
(Medisca)				
OIL, NA (1X14ML)				
14 ml	38779-0903-03	16.50		
(1X25ML)				
25 ml	38779-0903-04	31.50		
(1X100ML)				
100 ml	38779-0903-05	50.40		
(1X500ML)				
500 ml	38779-0903-08	145.20		
(PCCA)				
OIL, NA, 1 ml	51927-1267-00	1.20		
1 ml	51927-1416-00	1.20		
ROSEMARY OIL (Lorann Oil)				
OIL, NA, 9.9 ml	23535-0151-60	2.50		
(Medisca)				
OIL, NA (1X14ML)				
14 ml	38779-1566-03	16.50		
(1X25ML)				
25 ml	38779-1566-04	27.60		
(1X100ML)				
100 ml	38779-1566-05	56.10		
(1X500ML)				
500 ml	38779-1566-08	139.20		
(PCCA)				
OIL, NA (FCC)				
ea	51927-1266-00	1.20		
(Spectrum Pharmacy)				
OIL, NA (TUNISIAN TYPE,FCC)				
100 ml	49452-6308-01	150.50		
500 ml	49452-6308-02	395.50		
ROSEWOOD OIL (Lorann Oil)				
OIL, NA, 9.9 ml	23535-0151-63	3.50		

PROD/MFR	NDC	AWP	DP	OBC
ROSIGLITAZONE MALEATE				
(Glaxo) *See AVANDIA*				
ROSIN (Amend)				
LUM, NA (PURIFIED, W/W)				
454 gm	**17317-0471-01**	8.75		
2270 gm	**17317-0471-05**	29.40		
11350 gm	**17317-0471-08**	105.00		
POW, NA (W/DILUENT)				
454 gm	**17317-0472-01**	21.00		
2270 gm	**17317-0472-05**	98.00		
11350 gm	**17317-0472-08**	210.00		
(Gallipot)				
LUM, NA (CLEAR,TECHNICAL)				
454 gm	**51552-0388-06**	25.20		
2270 gm	**51552-0388-09**	61.74		
(Humco)				
POW, NA (W/DILUTENT)				
454 gm	**00395-2531-12**	11.13		
(Medisca)				
POW, NA (1X500GM)				
500 gm	**38779-1567-08**	57.00		
(Medisca) *See ROSIN WHITE*				
(PCCA)				
LUM, NA (PURIFIED)				
1 gm	**51927-1474-00**	0.11		
POW, NA (W/DILUENT)				
1 gm	**51927-1226-00**	0.13		
ROSIN WHITE (Medisca)				
rosin				
LUM, NA (1X500GM)				
500 gm	**38779-1568-08**	42.00		
ROSULA (Doak)				
sulfacetamide sodium/sulfur				
SOA, TP (AQUEOUS,CLEANSER)				
10%-5%, 355 ml	**10337-0662-12**	245.00		
(Phys Total Care)				
REPACK				
SOA, TP (CLEANSER)				
10%-5%, 355 ml	**54868-5372-00**	129.61		
ROSULA AQUEOUS GEL (Doak)				
sulfacetamide sodium/sulfur				
GEL, TP, 10%-5%, 45 gm	**10337-0661-45**	216.01		
ROSULA CLARIFYING WASH (Doak)				
sulfacetamide sodium/sulfur				
SOA, TP, 10%-4%, 473 ml	**10337-0667-16**	254.04		
ROSULA CLK (Doak)				
KIT, MR, 5%-10%-4%-5%,				
ea	**10337-0668-01**	301.00		
ROSULA NS (Doak)				
sulfacetamide sodium				
PAD, TP (SINGLE-USE,MEDICATED)				
10%, 30s ea	**10337-0664-10**	165.41		
ROSUVASTATIN CALCIUM				
(AstraZeneca) *See CRESTOR*				
ROTARIX (Glaxo)				
rotavirus vaccine, live				
PDR, PO (TAX INCL,PF,LYOPHILIZED)				
10s ea	**58160-0805-11**	1228.50		
ROTATEQ (Merck)				
rotavirus vaccine, live, pentavalent				
SUS, PO (10X2ML, TAX INCL,PF)				
2 ml 10s	**00006-4047-41**	833.53		
ROTAVIRUS VACCINE, LIVE				
(Glaxo) *See ROTARIX*				
ROTAVIRUS VACCINE, LIVE, PENTAVALENT				
(Merck) *See ROTATEQ*				
ROTIGOTINE				
(UCB) *See NEUPRO*				
ROWASA (Alaven)				
mesalamine				
KIT, MR, 4 gm/60 ml,				
60 ml 7s	**68220-0066-05**	244.69		AB
(7X60ML)				
4 gm/60 ml,				
60 ml 7s	**68220-0066-07**	190.05		AB
60 ml 28s	**68220-0066-03**	929.69		AB
(28X60ML)				
4 gm/60 ml,				
60 ml 28s	**68220-0066-28**	722.22		AB
ROXANOL (Phys Total Care)				
REPACK				
morphine sulfate				
SOL, PO, 20 mg/ml,				
30 ml, C-II	**54868-3416-00**	20.06		
ROXICET (Roxane)				
acetaminophen/oxycodone hydrochloride				
SOL, PO (MINT)				
325 mg/5 ml-5 mg/5 ml,				
5 ml 40s UD, C-II	**00054-8648-16**	55.06		
500 ml, C-II	**00054-3686-63**	46.19		
TAB, PO, 325 mg-5 mg,				
100s ea, C-II	**00054-4650-25**	51.46		AA
(R.N.P., 4X25)				
325 mg-5 mg,				
100s ea UD, C-II	**00054-8650-24**	60.28		AA
500s ea, C-II	**00054-4650-29**	217.08		AA
(CAPLET)				
500 mg-5 mg,				
100s ea, C-II	**00054-4784-25**	115.20		
(Dispensing Solutions)				
REPACK				
TAB, PO, 325 mg-5 mg,				
10s ea, C-II	**66336-0736-10**	17.90		
ROXICODONE (Xanodyne Pharma)				
oxycodone hydrochloride				
SOL, PO, 5 mg/5 ml,				
5 ml 40s UD, C-II	**66479-0583-05**	93.52		
(W/UNIT DOSE CUP)				
5 mg/5 ml,				
500 ml, C-II	**66479-0583-50**	73.60		
(W/CALIBRATED DROPPER)				
20 mg/ml,				
30 ml, C-II	**66479-0584-03**	69.00		
TAB, PO, 5 mg,				
100s ea, C-II	**66479-0580-10**	55.58		
(4X25)				
5 mg,				
100s ea UD, C-II	**66479-0580-25**	61.30		
15 mg,				
100s ea, C-II	**66479-0581-10**	145.02		AB
30 mg,				
100s ea, C-II	**66479-0582-10**	284.52		AB
(Phys Total Care)				
REPACK				
TAB, PO, 15 mg,				
30s ea, C-II	**54868-4722-03**	38.96		
60s ea, C-II	**54868-4722-02**	74.81		
90s ea, C-II	**54868-4722-04**	110.65		
100s ea, C-II	**54868-4722-00**	122.60		
120s ea, C-II	**54868-4722-01**	138.53		
30 mg,				
30s ea, C-II	**54868-4783-03**	55.53		
60s ea, C-II	**54868-4783-02**	108.55		
90s ea, C-II	**54868-4783-04**	152.74		
100s ea, C-II	**54868-4783-00**	169.43		
120s ea, C-II	**54868-4783-01**	202.81		
(Quality Care Prod)				
REPACK				
TAB, PO, 15 mg,				
30s ea, C-II	**49999-0858-30**	114.75		
60s ea, C-II	**49999-0858-60**	229.50		
90s ea, C-II	**49999-0858-90**	344.25		
30 mg,				
30s ea, C-II	**49999-0859-30**	206.50		
60s ea, C-II	**49999-0859-60**	413.00		
ROYAL JELLY (Medisca)				
POW, NA (1X25GM)				
25 gm	**38779-1569-04**	46.50		
(1X100GM)				
100 gm	**38779-1569-05**	123.00		
(PCCA)				
POW, NA (3:1,1.6% HDA,40-100MS))				
1 gm	**51927-2454-00**	2.70		
ROZEREM (Takeda)				
ramelteon				
TAB, PO (FILM-COATED)				
8 mg, 30s ea	**64764-0805-30**	149.15		
100s ea	**64764-0805-10**	497.16		
(A-S Medication)				
REPACK				
TAB, PO (FILM-COATED)				
8 mg, 30s ea	**54569-5893-01**	143.19		
(IPI)				
REPACK				
TAB, PO (FILM-COATED)				
8 mg, 90s ea	**18837-0137-90**	425.07		
(Keltman Pharma., Inc.)				
REPACK				
TAB, PO, 8 mg, 30s ea	**68387-0194-30**	112.21		
(Nucare Pharm)				
REPACK				
TAB, PO (FILM-COATED)				
8 mg, 30s ea	**68071-0452-30**	148.77		
(Phys Total Care)				
REPACK				
TAB, PO, 8 mg, 30s ea	**54868-5649-00**	174.25		
(Physician Partner)				
REPACK				
TAB, PO, 8 mg, 30s ea	**21695-0183-30**	298.30		
(Quality Care Prod)				
REPACK				
TAB, PO (FILM-COATED)				
8 mg, 30s ea	**35356-0092-30**	184.36		
(Southwood)				
REPACK				
TAB, PO, 8 mg, 30s ea	**58016-0048-30**	126.70		
60s ea	**58016-0048-60**	253.39		
90s ea	**58016-0048-90**	380.09		
100s ea	**58016-0048-00**	422.32		
(Stat Rx)				
REPACK				
TAB, PO, 8 mg, 14s ea	**16590-0517-14**	46.20		
21s ea	**16590-0517-21**	69.30		
(FILM-COATED)				
8 mg, 30s ea	**16590-0517-30**	175.66		
60s ea	**16590-0517-60**	257.00		
90s ea	**16590-0517-90**	380.00		
120s ea	**16590-0517-72**	506.00		
RU-HIST FORTE (Carwin)				
cpm/phenyleph hcl/pyril mal				
TAB, PO (SF,DYE-FREE)				
4 mg-10 mg-25 mg,				
100s ea	**15370-0008-10**	65.20		
RU-TUSS (Carwin)				
bell alk/cpm/pse hcl				
TER, PO (DYE-FREE)				
0.24 mg-8 mg-90 mg,				
100s ea	**15370-0027-10**	49.61		
RU-TUSS DM (Carwin)				
dm/gg/pse hcl				
SOL, PO (AF,SF,DYE-FREE)				
480 ml	**15370-0006-16**	42.24		
RUBELLA VIRUS VACCINE, LIVE				
(Merck) *See MERUVAX II*				
RUBIDIUM CHLORIDE (Medisca)				
POW, NA (1X25GM,HIGH PURITY)				
25 gm	**38779-1570-04**	160.50		
(PCCA)				
POW, NA (HIGH PURITY)				
1 gm	**51927-2614-00**	7.80		
(Spectrum Pharmacy)				
POW, NA (1X5GM, HIGH PURITY)				
5 gm	**49452-6320-01**	121.80		
(1X25GM, HIGH PURITY)				
25 gm	**49452-6320-02**	283.15		
(1X100GM, HIGH PURITY)				
100 gm	**49452-6320-03**	777.00		
RUBIDIUM CHLORIDE RB 82				
(Bracco Diag) *See CARDIOGEN-82 GENERATOR*				
RUBRATOPE-57 (Bracco Diag)				
cyanocobalamin co 57				
CAP, PO, 5s ea	**00270-3866-10**	439.56		
10s ea	**00270-3866-20**	985.96		
(Bracco Diag)				
cobaltous cl co 57/cyanocobalamin co 57/if/vit b12				
KIT, NA, ea	**00270-3868-10**	496.48		
RUDOL LIGHT (Amend)				
mineral oil				
OIL, NA, 19200 ml	**17317-1083-02**	84.00		
RUFINAMIDE				
(Eisai) *See BANZEL*				
RUTIN (Medisca)				
CRY, NA (1X25GM)				
25 gm	**38779-2172-04**	34.50		
(1X100GM)				
100 gm	**38779-2172-05**	84.00		
(PCCA)				
POW, NA (NF)				
1 gm	**51927-2482-00**	1.44		

PROD/MFR NDC AWP DP OBC

(Spectrum Pharmacy)
POW, NA, 25 gm..........**49452-6340-01** 67.90
100 gm..............**49452-6340-02** 126.00
500 gm..............**49452-6340-03** 388.50 84.80

RX-OTIC DROPS (Taro)
antipyrine/benzocaine
SOL, OT, 54 mg/ml-14 mg/ml,
14.79 ml..........**51672-3006-05** 4.95

RYNA-12 (Meda)
phenylephrine tannate/pyrilamine tannate
TAB, PO (CAPLET)
25 mg-60 mg,
100s ea...........**00037-0673-10** 346.49

RYNA-12 S (Meda)
phenylephrine tannate/pyrilamine tannate
SUS, PO (STRAWBERRY-CURRANT)
5 mg/5 ml-30 mg/5 ml,
118 ml **00037-0655-04** 344.71

RYNA-12X (Meda)
gg/phenyleph tan/pyril tan
SUS, PO (GRAPE)
118 ml **00037-1809-04** 68.27
TAB, PO, 200 mg-25 mg-60 mg,
30s ea.............**00037-1708-03** 85.77

RYNATAN (Meda)
chlorpheniramine tannate/phenylephrine tannate
CTB, PO (GRAPE)
4.5 mg-5 mg,
30s ea.............**00037-0712-03** 85.77
TAB, PO, 9 mg-25 mg,
100s ea............**00037-0707-10** 360.76

RYNATUSS (Meda)
cpm tan/carbetapentane tan/eph tan/phenyleph tan
TAB, PO (CAPLET)
60 mg-5 mg-10 mg-10 mg,
100s ea............**00037-0717-92** 583.84

RYNEZE (SJ)
chlorpheniramine maleate/scopolamine methonitrate
SOL, PO (1X473ML,AF,SF,DYE-FREE)
4 mg/5 ml-1.25 mg/5 ml,
473 ml **24839-0346-16** 102.17

RYTHMOL (Glaxo)
propafenone hydrochloride
TAB, PO, 150 mg, 100s ea.**65726-0265-25** 462.37 AB
(FILM-COATED)
225 mg, 100s ea .....**65726-0266-25** 607.96 AB
300 mg, 100s ea .....**65726-0267-25** 607.96 AB

RYTHMOL SR (Glaxo)
propafenone hydrochloride
CER, PO (HARD-GELATIN)
225 mg, 60s ea ......**00173-0786-01** 405.26 EE
325 mg, 60s ea ......**00173-0788-01** 513.43 EE
425 mg, 60s ea **00173-0789-01** 513.43

RYZOLT (Purdue Pharma)
tramadol hydrochloride
TER, PO, 100 mg, 30s ea..**59011-0334-30** 121.30
200 mg, 30s ea **59011-0335-30** 200.60
300 mg, 30s ea **59011-0336-30** 279.90

(Quality Care Prod)
REPACK
TER, PO, 200 mg, 30s ea..**35356-0497-30** 291.07
300 mg, 30s ea **35356-0498-30** 405.18

(Stat Rx)
REPACK
TER, PO, 100 mg, 30s ea..**16590-0253-30** 141.65
200 mg, 30s ea **16590-0244-30** 288.14
300 mg, 30s ea **16590-0255-30** 329.33

S-CARBOXYMETHYL-L-CYSTEINE (PCCA)
carbocysteine
POW, NA, 1 gm..........**51927-2802-00** 5.85

S-ENTRY DRY MAT (J&J Medical)
device
DEV, NA (CONTAMINATION CONTROL)
20s ea...............**56091-0505-41** 46.19

SABRIL (Lundbeck)
vigabatrin
PDS, PO, 500 mg/packet,
50s ea............**67386-0211-65** 1618.14
TAB, PO (FILM-COATED)
500 mg, 100s ea **67386-0111-01** 3236.28

SACCHARIN (Gallipot)
POW, NA (U.S.P.,N.F.)
113.4 gm............**51552-0356-04** 10.22
454 gm..............**51552-0356-06** 21.63

(PCCA)
POW, NA (NF)
1 gm **51927-1661-00** 0.36

(Spectrum Pharmacy)
POW, NA (N.F.)
125 gm.............**49452-6360-01** 222.60
500 gm.............**49452-6360-02** 476.00
2500 gm............**49452-6360-03** 1830.50

SACCHARIN CALCIUM
(Amend) *See CALCIUM SACCHARIN*

(PCCA)
POW, NA (USP, HYDRATE)
1 gm **51927-2042-00** 0.38

SACCHARIN SODIUM (Baker, J.T.)
POW, NA (U.S.P., F.C.C.)
500 gm..............**10106-3875-01** 36.15

(Gallipot) *See SODIUM SACCHARIN*

(Letco) *See SODIUM SACCHARIN*

(Mallinckrodt Lab)
POW, NA (U.S.P.)
125 gm..............**00406-7260-01** 25.09

(PCCA)
POW, NA (USP; DIHYDRATE)
1 gm **51927-1466-00** 0.36

(Spectrum Pharmacy) *See SODIUM SACCHARIN DIHYDRATE*

SACROSIDASE
(QOL Medical) *See SUCRAID*

SAFFLOWER OIL (Gallipot)
OIL, NA, 473 ml **51552-0626-06** 11.06

(PCCA)
OIL, NA (USP)
1 ml................**51927-3153-00** 0.09

(Spectrum Pharmacy)
OIL, NA (U.S.P.)
500 ml **49452-6365-01** 72.10
4000 ml **49452-6365-02** 248.85
20000 ml **49452-6365-03** 815.50

SAFFLOWER OIL/SOYBEAN OIL
(Abbott Hosp) *See LIPOSYN II*

(Hospira) *See LIPOSYN II*

SAGE LEAF (PCCA)
POW, NA (1X1GM)
1 gm **51927-3575-00** 0.26

SAGE OIL (Lorann Oil)
OIL, NA, 9.9 ml..........**23535-0151-66** 3.50

(Spectrum Pharmacy) *See SAGE OIL SPANISH*

SAGE OIL SPANISH (Spectrum Pharmacy)
sage oil
OIL, NA (F.C.C.)
25 ml................**49452-6384-01** 144.90
100 ml **49452-6384-02** 371.00

SAIZEN (EMD)
somatropin, mammalian derived
PDS, IJ (VIAL W/DILUENT)
8.8 mg, ea..........**44087-1088-01** 602.02
SC (VIAL, W/DILUENT)
5 mg, ea.............**44087-1005-02** 376.26 BX

(A-S Medication)
REPACK
PDS, SC (VIAL, W/DILUENT)
5 mg, ea..............**54569-4930-00** 329.06 BX

SAIZEN CLICK EASY CARTRIDGE (EMD)
somatropin, mammalian derived
PDS, IJ (W/DILUENT)
8.8 mg, ea...........**44087-1080-01** 602.02

SAL-TROPINE (Hope)
atropine sulfate
TAB, PO, 0.4 mg, 100s ea..**60267-0742-30** 39.95

SALAGEN (Eisai)
pilocarpine hydrochloride
TAB, PO (FILM-COATED)
5 mg, 100s ea.......**62856-0705-10** 201.60 AB
(FILM COATED)
7.5 mg, 100s ea......**62856-0775-10** 247.20 AB

(Phys Total Care)
REPACK
TAB, PO, 5 mg, 100s ea ...**54868-3447-01** 208.54

SALEX (Valeant Pharm Intl)
salicylic acid
KIT, MR, 6%, ea **13548-0010-17** 306.17
597 ml **13548-0011-09** 163.30
SHA, TP, 6%, 177 ml......**13548-0012-06** 133.46

(Phys Total Care)
REPACK
LOT, TP, 6%, 414 ml **54868-5481-00** 119.05

SALICEPT (Carrington)
bandage
DEV, NA (ORAL PATCH)
12s ea...............**53303-0009-12** 9.75

SALICEPT FDG (Carrington)
hydrogel, aloe vera base
PAD, MM (PF)
ea...................**53303-0011-04** 2.95

SALICEPT ORAL RINSE (Carrington)
mouthwash
PDR, MM (VANILLA)
9.4 gm **53303-0011-08** 25.59

SALICYLAMIDE (Amend)
POW, NA (U.S.P.)
454 gm.............**17317-0475-01** 21.00
2270 gm............**17317-0475-05** 84.00

(PCCA)
POW, NA (U.S.P.)
1 gm **51927-1231-00** 0.30

SALICYLIC ACID (Acella)
FOA, TP (1X70GM)
6%, 70 gm...........**42192-0112-70** 129.37

(Auriga) *See AKURZA*

(Baker, J.T.)
CRY, NA (U.S.P., FINE)
125 gm.............**10106-0302-04** 21.28
500 gm.............**10106-0302-01** 43.57
POW, NA (U.S.P.)
125 gm.............**10106-0303-04** 27.14
500 gm.............**10106-0303-01** 51.52

(Breckenridge Pharm) *See SALITOP*

(Gallipot)
CRY, NA (U.S.P.)
454 gm..............**51552-0264-06** 12.11
POW, NA (U.S.P.,N.F.)
56.7 gm **51552-0053-03** 6.02
113.4 gm **51552-0053-04** 8.61
(U.S.P.)
454 gm..............**51552-0053-06** 12.11
(U.S.P.,N.F.)
2270 gm.............**51552-0053-09** 58.03

(Humco)
POW, NA, 454 gm.........**00395-2625-01** 20.36

(Letco)
POW, NA (U.S.P./N.F.)
500 gm..............**62991-2058-02** 33.00

(Mallinckrodt Lab)
CRY, NA (U.S.P.)
125 gm.............**00406-2016-01** 22.09
500 gm.............**00406-2016-03** 63.47
POW, NA, 125 gm.........**00406-2020-02** 9.95
500 gm.............**00406-2020-03** 64.67

(Medisca)
POW, NA (1X100GM,USP)
100 gm.............**38779-0091-05** 22.50
(U.S.P.)
500 gm.............**38779-0091-08** 31.50

(Onset) *See SALKERA*

(PCCA)
POW, NA (U.S.P.)
1 gm **51927-1555-00** 0.30

(Perrigo)
CRE, TP (1X400GM,MENTHOL)
6%, 400 gm **45802-0806-01** 120.25
LOT, TP, 6%, 414 ml **45802-0818-41** 120.05
SHA, TP (1X177ML)
6%, 177 ml..........**45802-0237-01** 68.65

(Prasco Labs) *See ALICLEN*

(PruGen) *See SALICYLIC ACID CREAM KIT*

(PruGen)
SHA, TP (1X177ML)
6%, 177 ml..........**00072-0279-06** 69.40

(Quinnova) *See SALVAX*

(Seton) *See SALICYLIC ACID CREAM*

(Seton) *See SALICYLIC ACID LOTION*

(Spectrum Pharmacy)
CRY, NA (U.S.P.)
500 gm.............**49452-6410-01** 59.15
2500 gm............**49452-6410-02** 229.60
POW, NA, 500 gm.........**49452-6420-01** 59.15
2500 gm............**49452-6420-02** 229.60

PROD/MFR	NDC	AWP	DP	OBC
(Summers) *See KERALYT GEL*				
(Summers) *See KERALYT SCALP*				
(Summers)				
SHA, TP, 6%, 177 ml	**11086-0041-06**	23.99		
(Valeant Pharm Intl) *See SALEX*				
SALICYLIC ACID CREAM (Seton)				
salicylic acid				
KIT, MR, 6%, ea	**13925-0040-10**	177.19		
SALICYLIC ACID CREAM KIT (PruGen)				
salicylic acid				
KIT, MR, 6%, ea	**42546-0270-01**	176.99		
SALICYLIC ACID LOTION (Seton)				
salicylic acid				
KIT, MR, 6%, ea	**13925-0050-10**	94.50		
SALICYLIC ACID/SODIUM THIOSULFATE				
(A. G. Marin) *See EXODERM*				
(Hope) *See VERSICLEAR*				
SALICYLIC ACID/UREA				
(Quinnova) *See SALVAX DUO*				
SALITOP (Breckenridge Pharm)				
salicylic acid				
CRE, TP, 6%, 400 gm	**51991-0476-46**	97.31		
LOT, TP, 6%, 414 ml	**51991-0477-47**	97.31		
SALIVA SUBSTITUTES				
(Align) *See NUMOISYN*				
(Auriga) *See AQUORAL*				
(EUSA) *See CAPHOSOL*				
(Invado) *See NEUTRASAL*				
SALKERA (Onset)				
salicylic acid				
FOA, TP (1X60GM)				
6%, 60 gm	**16781-0167-60**	122.50		
SALMETEROL XINAFOATE				
(Glaxo) *See SEREVENT DISKUS*				
SALSALATE (Amneal)				
TAB, PO (USP,FILM-COATED)				
500 mg, 100s ea	**65162-0512-10**	23.80		
500s ea	**65162-0512-50**	104.25		
1000s ea	**65162-0512-11**	190.00		
750 mg, 100s ea	**65162-0513-10**	28.65		
500s ea	**65162-0513-50**	134.00		
1000s ea	**65162-0513-11**	252.00		
(Caraco)				
TAB, PO, 500 mg, 100s ea	**57664-0353-08**	25.02		
(FILM-COATED)				
500 mg, 100s ea	**57664-0103-08**	25.02		
500s ea	**57664-0353-13**	102.73		
(FILM-COATED)				
500 mg, 500s ea	**57664-0103-13**	102.73		
1000s ea	**57664-0353-18**	179.78		
(FILM-COATED)				
500 mg, 1000s ea	**57664-0103-18**	179.78		
750 mg, 100s ea	**57664-0354-08**	31.65		
(FILM-COATED)				
750 mg, 100s ea	**57664-0105-08**	31.65		
500s ea	**57664-0354-13**	129.50		
(FILM-COATED)				
750 mg, 500s ea	**57664-0105-13**	129.50		
1000s ea	**57664-0354-18**	226.63		
(FILM-COATED)				
750 mg, 1000s ea	**57664-0105-18**	226.63		
(Major)				
TAB, PO (USP,FILM-COATED)				
500 mg, 100s ea UD	**00904-5628-61**	33.28		
750 mg, 100s ea UD	**00904-5629-61**	39.94		
(Marlex)				
TAB, PO (USP,FILM-COATED)				
500 mg, 100s ea	**10135-0492-01**	30.00		
(USP)				
500 mg, 100s ea	**10135-0403-01**	30.00		
(USP,FILM-COATED)				
500 mg, 500s ea	**10135-0492-05**	110.00		
(USP)				
500 mg, 500s ea	**10135-0403-05**	110.00		
(USP,FILM-COATED)				
500 mg, 1000s ea	**10135-0492-10**	220.00		
(USP)				
500 mg, 1000s ea	**10135-0403-10**	220.00		
(USP,CAPLET)				
750 mg, 100s ea	**10135-0404-01**	40.00		
(USP,FILM-COATED)				
750 mg, 100s ea	**10135-0493-01**	40.00		
(USP,CAPLET)				
750 mg, 500s ea	**10135-0404-05**	135.00		
(USP,FILM-COATED)				
750 mg, 500s ea	**10135-0493-05**	135.00		
(USP,CAPLET)				
750 mg, 1000s ea	**10135-0404-10**	270.00		
(USP,FILM-COATED)				
750 mg, 1000s ea	**10135-0493-10**	270.00		
(PCCA)				
POW, NA, 1 gm	**51927-3509-00**	16.80		
(Vintage)				
TAB, PO, 750 mg, 500s ea	**00254-5812-35**	170.75		
(A-S Medication)				
REPACK				
TAB, PO, 750 mg, 28s ea	**54569-1712-01**	10.30		
(FILM-COATED)				
750 mg, 30s ea	**54569-1712-04**	10.10		
40s ea	**54569-1712-00**	13.46		
60s ea	**54569-1712-03**	20.20		
100s ea	**54569-1712-02**	36.79		
(FILM-COATED)				
750 mg, 120s ea	**54569-1712-06**	40.39		
(Altura)				
REPACK				
TAB, PO, 500 mg, 28s ea	**63874-0479-28**	14.14		
30s ea	**63874-0479-30**	14.63		
40s ea	**63874-0479-40**	19.51		
500s ea	**63874-0479-50**	110.13		
750 mg, 28s ea	**63874-0308-28**	16.21		
30s ea	**63874-0308-30**	17.25		
40s ea	**63874-0308-40**	23.01		
100s ea	**63874-0308-10**	57.52		
500s ea	**63874-0308-50**	141.47		
(Core)				
REPACK				
TAB, PO, 500 mg, 120s ea	**33358-0319-01**	30.32		
(DHS, Inc.)				
REPACK				
TAB, PO (FILM-COATED)				
750 mg, 30s ea	**55887-0239-30**	18.00		
60s ea	**55887-0239-60**	33.13		
(Dispensing Solutions)				
REPACK				
TAB, PO, 750 mg, 20s ea	**66336-0034-20**	8.61		
(FILM-COATED)				
750 mg, 30s ea	**55045-1935-08**	24.30		
40s ea	**55045-1935-09**	32.40		
120s ea	**55045-1935-02**	97.20		
(GSMS)				
REPACK				
TAB, PO (UNIT OF USE)				
750 mg, 30s ea	**60429-0207-30**	11.10	3.70	
60s ea	**60429-0207-60**	19.50	6.50	
120s ea	**60429-0207-12**	36.54	12.18	
180s ea	**60429-0207-18**	54.75	18.25	
(HomeMed)				
REPACK				
TAB, PO, 750 mg, 20s ea	**51655-0592-52**	6.09		
60s ea	**51655-0592-25**	16.80		
(IPI)				
REPACK				
TAB, PO, 750 mg, 60s ea	**18837-0138-60**	21.00		
(Nucare Pharm)				
REPACK				
TAB, PO, 750 mg, 28s ea	**66267-0192-28**	26.89		
30s ea	**66267-0192-30**	27.99		
40s ea	**66267-0192-40**	33.89		
(Palmetto)				
REPACK				
TAB, PO, 750 mg, 20s ea	**23490-6259-01**	20.00		
40s ea	**23490-6259-02**	40.00		
(PD-Rx Pharm)				
REPACK				
TAB, PO, 500 mg, 28s ea	**55289-0275-28**	25.17		
30s ea	**55289-0275-30**	25.28		
(REDI-SCRIPT)				
500 mg, 56s ea	**58864-0672-56**	33.61		
60s ea	**55289-0275-60**	33.83		
(REDI-SCRIPT)				
500 mg, 90s ea	**58864-0672-90**	42.67		
750 mg, 20s ea	**55289-0844-20**	24.44		
30s ea	**55289-0844-30**	30.00		
40s ea	**55289-0844-40**	32.22		
(Pharma Pac)				
REPACK				
TAB, PO, 500 mg, 40s ea	**52959-0394-40**	10.83		
60s ea	**52959-0394-60**	15.21		
90s ea	**52959-0394-90**	22.79		
750 mg, 24s ea	**52959-0332-24**	24.95		
28s ea	**52959-0332-28**	27.93		
30s ea	**52959-0332-30**	29.16		
40s ea	**52959-0332-40**	35.42		
60s ea	**52959-0332-60**	45.78		
90s ea	**52959-0332-90**	49.77		
(Phys Total Care)				
REPACK				
TAB, PO (FILM-COATED)				
500 mg, 60s ea	**54868-0791-00**	11.25		
750 mg, 30s ea	**54868-0088-04**	9.45		
40s ea	**54868-0088-06**	11.10		
(FILM-COATED)				
750 mg, 60s ea	**54868-0088-02**	17.60		
100s ea	**54868-0088-01**	19.53		
(Physician Partner)				
REPACK				
TAB, PO (FILM-COATED)				
500 mg, 60s ea	**21695-0391-60**	30.02		
750 mg, 60s ea	**21695-0392-60**	30.54		
(Quality Care Prod)				
REPACK				
TAB, PO (FILM-COATED)				
750 mg, 28s ea	**49999-0367-28**	33.52		
60s ea	**49999-0367-60**	71.83		
(Southwood)				
REPACK				
TAB, PO, 500 mg, 10s ea	**58016-0219-10**	4.27		
12s ea	**58016-0219-12**	5.13		
15s ea	**58016-0219-15**	6.42		
20s ea	**58016-0219-20**	8.56		
28s ea	**58016-0219-28**	11.98		
30s ea	**58016-0219-30**	12.83		
100s ea	**58016-0219-00**	42.78		
120s ea	**58016-0219-02**	51.33		
750 mg, 10s ea	**58016-0221-10**	5.48		
12s ea	**58016-0221-12**	6.57		
14s ea	**58016-0221-14**	7.67		
15s ea	**58016-0221-15**	8.22		
20s ea	**58016-0221-20**	10.96		
21s ea	**58016-0221-21**	10.96		
24s ea	**58016-0221-24**	13.15		
28s ea	**58016-0221-28**	15.34		
30s ea	**58016-0221-30**	16.43		
40s ea	**58016-0221-40**	21.91		
60s ea	**58016-0221-60**	32.87		
100s ea	**58016-0221-00**	54.78		
(Stat Rx)				
REPACK				
TAB, PO, 750 mg, 30s ea	**16590-0204-30**	31.00		
60s ea	**16590-0204-60**	62.00		
90s ea	**16590-0204-90**	93.00		
SALVAX (Quinnova)				
salicylic acid				
FOA, TP (1X70GM)				
6%, 70 gm	**23710-0006-70**	143.75		
(1X200GM)				
6%, 200 gm	**23710-0006-02**	225.00		
SALVAX DUO (Quinnova)				
salicylic acid/urea				
FOA, TP, 6%-40%, ea	**23710-0006-03**	225.00		
SAMARIUM SM 153 LEXIDRONAM PENTASODIUM				
(EUSA) *See QUADRAMET*				
SAMSCA (Otsuka)				
tolvaptan				
TAB, PO, 15 mg, 10s ea	**59148-0020-50**	3000.00		
30 mg, 10s ea	**59148-0021-50**	3000.00		
SANCTURA (Allergan Inc)				
trospium chloride				
TAB, PO (GLOSSY COATED)				
20 mg, 60s ea	**00023-3513-60**	191.30		
SANCTURA XR (Allergan Inc)				
trospium chloride				
CER, PO, 60 mg, 30s ea	**00023-9350-30**	150.50		
SANCUSO (ProStrakan)				
granisetron				
TDM, TD, 3.1 mg/24 hr, ea	**42747-0726-01**	372.00		
(Phys Total Care)				
REPACK				
TDM, TD, 3.1 mg/24 hr, ea	**54868-5985-00**	393.74		
SANDALWOOD OIL (Lorann Oil)				
OIL, NA, 9.9 ml	**23535-0151-69**	9.50		
(Medisca)				
OIL, NA (1X14ML)				
14 ml	**38779-0774-03**	37.50		

PROD/MFR	NDC	AWP	DP	OBC
(1X25ML)				
25 ml	38779-0774-04	64.50		
(1X100ML)				
100 ml	38779-0774-05	199.50		
(1X500ML)				
500 ml	38779-0774-08	918.00		
(PCCA) *See SANDALWOOD OIL FRAGRANCE*				
SANDALWOOD OIL FRAGRANCE (PCCA)				
sandalwood oil				
OIL, NA (ARTIFICIAL)				
1 gm	51927-1927-00	3.00		
SANDIMMUNE (Novartis Pharm)				
cyclosporine				
SGL, PO (SANDOPAK,SOFTGEL)				
25 mg, 30s ea UD	00078-0240-15	74.35		AB2
(SOFTGEL)				
100 mg, 30s ea UD	00078-0241-15	296.81		AB2
SOL, IV (AMP)				
50 mg/ml, 5 ml 10s	00078-0109-01	385.62		AP
PO, 100 mg/ml,				
50 ml	00078-0110-22	480.40		BX
SANDOSTATIN (Novartis Pharm)				
octreotide acetate				
SOL, IJ (AMP)				
50 mcg/ml,				
1 ml 10s	00078-0180-01	119.17		
100 mcg/ml,				
1 ml 10s	00078-0181-01	231.13		
(M.D.V.)				
200 mcg/ml, 5 ml	00078-0183-25	238.28		
(AMP)				
500 mcg/ml,				
1 ml 10s	00078-0182-01	1114.79		
(M.D.V.)				
1000 mcg/ml, 5 ml	00078-0184-25	1172.46		
SANDOSTATIN LAR DEPOT (Novartis Pharm)				
octreotide acetate				
PDR, IM (1&1/2"X19G,PFS)				
10 mg, ea	00078-0340-61	1949.29		
(PFS)				
20 mg, ea	00078-0341-61	2553.92		
30 mg, ea	00078-0342-61	3824.28		
SANTYL (Healthpoint)				
collagenase				
OIN, TP (PF)				
250 u/gm, 15 gm	00064-5010-15	61.96		
(COLLAGENASE)				
250 u/gm, 30 gm	00074-2316-60	70.70		
(PF)				
250 u/gm, 30 gm	00064-5010-30	89.99		
(A-S Medication)				
REPACK				
OIN, TP (1X15GM,PF)				
250 u/gm, 15 gm	54569-6140-00	59.02		
(COLLAGENASE)				
250 u/gm, 30 gm	54569-3854-00	70.70		
(Dispensing Solutions)				
REPACK				
OIN, TP, 250 u/gm, 15 gm	55045-2134-05	52.00		
30 gm	55045-2134-06	72.00		
(Physician Partner)				
REPACK				
OIN, TP (1X15GM,PF)				
250 u/gm, 15 gm	21695-0852-15	111.36		
(Stat Rx)				
REPACK				
OIN, TP, 250 u/gm, 30 gm	16590-0203-30	64.00		
SAPHRIS (Schering)				
asenapine				
TAB, SL (6X10)				
5 mg, 60s ea	00052-0118-06	594.00		
(10X10)				
5 mg, 100s ea UD	00052-0118-90	990.00		
(6X10)				
10 mg, 60s ea	00052-0119-06	594.00		
(10X10)				
10 mg, 100s ea UD	00052-0119-90	990.00		
SAPONIN (Baker, J.T.)				
POW, NA (REAGENT)				
125 gm	10106-3388-04	142.96		
(PCCA)				
POW, NA (FOOD GRADE)				
1 gm	51927-2359-00	1.08		
SAPROPTERIN DIHYDROCHLORIDE				
(Biomarin) *See KUVAN*				
SAQUINAVIR MESYLATE				
(Roche Labs) *See INVIRASE*				
SARAFEM (Warner Chilcott)				
fluoxetine hydrochloride				
TAB, PO (4X7)				
10 mg, 28s ea	00430-0210-14	211.91		EE
15 mg, 28s ea	00430-0215-14	211.91		EE
(4X7)				
20 mg, 28s ea	00430-0220-14	211.91		EE
(Phys Total Care)				
REPACK				
CAP, PO (4X7 BLISTER CARD)				
10 mg, 28s ea	54868-4570-00	112.11		
SARAPIN (High)				
sarracenia purpura				
SOL, IJ (M.D.V.)				
50 ml	10541-0492-50	60.00	37.00	
SARDINE FLAVOR (Gallipot)				
flavoring aid				
LIQ, NA, 59.14 ml	51552-0639-09	10.22		
SARGRAMOSTIM				
(Genzyme) *See LEUKINE*				
SARRACENIA PURPURA				
(High) *See SARAPIN*				
SARSAPARILLA FLAVOR (PCCA)				
flavoring aid				
SOL, NA (FLUID EXTRACT)				
1 ml	51927-1757-00	0.26		
SASSAFRAS OIL (Gallipot)				
OIL, NA (BRAZILIAN)				
100 ml	51552-0598-05	15.05		
(Medisca)				
OIL, NA (1X14ML,NATURAL)				
14 ml	38779-1578-03	19.50		
(1X25ML,NATURAL)				
25 ml	38779-1578-04	31.50		
(1X100ML,NATURAL)				
100 ml	38779-1578-05	87.00		
(1X500ML,NATURAL)				
500 ml	38779-1578-08	138.00		
(PCCA) *See SASSAFRASS OIL FOOD GRADE*				
SASSAFRASS OIL FOOD GRADE (PCCA)				
sassafras oil				
OIL, NA (1X1ML)				
1 ml	51927-1619-00	0.36		
SAVELLA (Forest Pharm)				
milnacipran hydrochloride				
TAB, PO (FILM-COATED)				
12.5 mg, 60s ea	00456-1512-60	127.76		
25 mg, 60s ea	00456-1525-60	127.76		
50 mg, 60s ea	00456-1550-60	127.76		
100 mg, 60s ea	00456-1510-60	127.76		
(Phys Total Care)				
REPACK				
TAB, PO (FILM-COATED)				
50 mg, 60s ea	54868-6043-00	146.00		
180s ea	54868-6043-01	420.78		
100 mg, 60s ea	54868-6024-00	153.20		
(Quality Care Prod)				
REPACK				
TAB, PO (FILM-COATED)				
50 mg, 60s ea	35356-0545-60	200.91		
(Stat Rx)				
REPACK				
TAB, PO (FILM-COATED)				
25 mg, 60s ea	16590-0845-60	142.14		
50 mg, 60s ea	16590-0846-60	142.14		
100 mg, 60s ea	16590-0847-60	142.09		
SAVELLA TITRATION PACK (Forest Pharm)				
milnacipran hydrochloride				
TAB, PO (FILM-COATED)				
55s ea	00456-1500-55	117.12		
SAW PALMETTO BERRY (PCCA)				
POW, NA, 1 gm	51927-2942-00	0.54		
SAW PALMETTO EXTRACT				
(Medisca) *See SAW PALMETTO LIQUID EXTRACT*				
(Medisca) *See SAW PALMETTO POWDER EXTRACT*				
(PCCA)				
SOL, NA, 1 ml	51927-2073-00	1.25		
SAW PALMETTO LIQUID EXTRACT (Medisca)				
saw palmetto extract				
SOL, NA (1X50ML)				
50 ml	38779-1579-02	84.00		
SAW PALMETTO POWDER EXTRACT (Medisca)				
saw palmetto extract				
POW, NA (1X1000GM)				
1000 gm	38779-2422-09	420.00		
SAXAGLIPTIN HYDROCHLORIDE				
(Bristol-Myers) *See ONGLYZA*				
SCALACORT (Avidas)				
hydrocortisone				
LOT, TP (1X29.6ML)				
2%, 29.6 ml	43684-0100-10	97.20		
SCALACORT DK (Avidas)				
hydrocortisone/salicylic acid/sulfur				
KIT, TP, 2%-2%-2%,				
265.6 ml	43684-0100-11	97.20		
SCARLET RED (Medisca)				
POW, NA (1X25GM)				
25 gm	38779-1580-04	55.50		
(1X100GM)				
100 gm	38779-1580-05	163.50		
(PCCA)				
POW, NA (C.I.26105)				
1 gm	51927-1533-00	2.16		
SCLERON (Weleda)				
homeopathic substance				
TAB, PO, 100s ea	55946-0396-30	6.60		
SCLEROSOL INTRAPLEURAL (Bryan Corp.)				
talc				
SPR, PL, 4 gm	63256-0100-30	117.50	117.50	
SCOPACE (Hope)				
scopolamine hydrobromide				
TAB, PO, 0.4 mg, 100s ea	60267-0301-00	40.95		
(Dispensing Solutions)				
REPACK				
TAB, PO, 0.4 mg, 12s ea	55045-2962-02	8.40		
(PD-Rx Pharm)				
REPACK				
TAB, PO, 0.4 mg, 12s ea	55289-0235-12	12.95		
(Phys Total Care)				
REPACK				
TAB, PO (USP)				
0.4 mg, 20s ea	54868-5560-00	12.24		
100s ea	54868-5560-01	40.89		
(Southwood)				
REPACK				
TAB, PO, 0.4 mg, 30s ea	58016-0016-30	10.79		
60s ea	58016-0016-60	21.57		
90s ea	58016-0016-90	32.36		
100s ea	58016-0016-00	35.95		
SCOPOHIST (Larken Labs, Inc.)				
cpm/methscopolamine nitrate/phenyleph hcl				
SYR, PO (1X473ML,AF,GRAPE)				
473 ml	68047-0292-16	31.71		
(Larken Labs, Inc.)				
cpm/methscopolamine nitrate/pse hcl				
TER, PO, 8 mg-1.25 mg-60 mg,				
100s ea	68047-0290-01	50.35		
SCOPOHIST-PE (Larken Labs, Inc.)				
cpm/methscopolamine nitrate/phenyleph hcl				
TER, PO, 8 mg-1.25 mg-20 mg,				
100s ea	68047-0291-01	49.43		
SCOPOLAMINE				
(Baxter) *See TRANSDERM SCOP*				
(Novartis Consumer) *See TRANSDERM SCOP*				
SCOPOLAMINE HYDROBROMIDE				
(Alcon Ophthalmic) *See ISOPTO HYOSCINE*				
(APP)				
SOL, IJ (M.D.V.,AMBER)				
0.4 mg/ml, 1 ml	63323-0268-01	5.63		
(Gallipot) *See SCOPOLAMINE HYDROBROMIDE TRIHYDRATE*				
(Hawthorn Pharm) *See MALDEMAR*				
(Hope) *See SCOPACE*				
(Medisca)				
POW, NA (U.S.P.)				
1 gm	38779-0293-06	42.00		
5 gm	38779-0293-03	135.00		
(PCCA)				
POW, NA (U.S.P.; TRIHYDRATE)				
1 gm	51927-1372-00	54.00		
(Spectrum Pharmacy) *See SCOPOLAMINE HYDROBROMIDE TRIHYDRATE*				

PROD/MFR NDC AWP DP OBC

SCOPOLAMINE HYDROBROMIDE TRIHYDRATE (Gallipot)
scopolamine hydrobromide
POW, NA (U.S.P.)
0.025 gm **51552-0444-09** 7.00
1 gm **51552-0444-01** 16.31
5 gm **51552-0444-02** 58.52

(Spectrum Pharmacy)
POW, NA (U.S.P.)
1 gm **49452-6460-01** 88.55
5 gm **49452-6460-02** 246.75
25 gm **49452-6460-03** 815.50

SCOPOLAMINE METHYL BROMIDE (Spectrum Pharmacy)
methscopolamine bromide
POW, NA (1X1GM)
1 gm **49452-6480-01** 132.65
(1X5GM)
5 gm **49452-6480-02** 441.00
(1X25GM)
25 gm **49452-6480-03** 1235.50

SCOPOLAMINE METHYL NITRATE (PCCA)
methscopolamine nitrate
POW, NA, 1 gm **51927-2318-00** 72.00

SE BPO WASH (Seton)
benzoyl peroxide
SOA, TP (1X180GM)
7%, 180 gm **13925-0112-18** 129.23

SE-CARE CHEWABLE (Seton)
prenatal vitamins
CTB, PO, 30s ea **13925-0104-30** 31.47

SE-CARE CONCEIVE (Seton)
prenatal vitamins
TAB, PO (FILM-COATED CAPLET)
30s ea **13925-0105-30** 31.47

SE-NATAL 19 (Seton)
prenatal vitamins
TAB, PO, 100s ea **13925-0116-01** 38.16

SE-NATAL 19 CHEWABLE (Seton)
prenatal vitamins
CTB, PO, 100s ea **13925-0117-01** 44.24

SE-NATAL 90 (Seton)
prenatal vitamins
TAB, PO (FILM-COATED)
100s ea **13925-0102-01** 28.78

SE-NATAL ONE (Seton)
prenatal vitamins
TAB, PO (FILM-COATED)
100s ea **13925-0103-01** 28.78

SE-PLETE DHA (Seton)
prenatal vitamins
SGL, PO (SOFTGEL CAPLET)
60s ea **13925-0120-60** 99.29

SE-TAN DHA (Seton)
prenatal vitamins
SGL, PO (HARD CAPSULE)
90s ea **13925-0119-90** 80.10

SE-TAN PLUS (Seton)
multivitamin, minerals, and iron
CAP, PO, 90s ea **13925-0118-90** 50.46

SEASONALE (Duramed)
ethinyl estradiol/levonorgestrel
TAB, PO (EXTENDED-CYCLE, 3X91)
30 mcg-0.15 mg,
273s ea **51285-0058-66** 737.10

(Phys Total Care)
REPACK
TAB, PO (FILM-COATED)
30 mcg-0.15 mg,
91s ea **54868-2316-00** 197.05

SEASONIQUE (Duramed)
ethinyl estradiol/levonorgestrel
TAB, PO (2X91,FILM-COATED)
182s ea **51285-0087-87** 436.80

SEB-PREV (Perrigo)
sulfacetamide sodium
CRE, TP (1X30GM)
10%, 30 gm **45802-0954-94** 60.17
(1X60GM)
10%, 60 gm **45802-0954-96** 109.65
GEL, TP (1X30GM)
10%, 30 gm **45802-0960-94** 60.17
60 gm **45802-0960-96** 109.65

SEB-PREV WASH (Perrigo)
sulfacetamide sodium
SOA, TP (1X170ML)
10%, 170 ml **45802-0939-01** 70.80
(1X340ML)
10%, 340 ml **45802-0939-02** 123.95

SECOBARBITAL SODIUM
(Marathon) *See SECONAL SODIUM*

SECONAL SODIUM (Marathon)
secobarbital sodium
CAP, PO, 100 mg,
100s ea, C-II **42998-0679-01** 490.50

SECRETIN
(ChiRhoClin) *See CHIRHOSTIM*

SECRETIN, 99% MANNITOL (PCCA)
mannitol/secretin
POW, NA (1X0.001GM)
99%, 0.001 gm **51927-3186-00** 1.40

SECTRAL (Promius)
acebutolol hydrochloride
CAP, PO, 200 mg, 100s ea . **67857-0700-01** 335.46 AB
400 mg, 100s ea .... **67857-0701-01** 446.00 223.70 AB

SEDAPAP (Merz)
acetaminophen/butalbital
TAB, PO, 650 mg-50 mg,
100s ea .... **00259-0392-01** 88.11 AB

(PD-Rx Pharm)
REPACK
TAB, PO, 650 mg-50 mg,
18s ea .... **55289-0778-18** 22.57 AB

SELECT-OB (Everett)
prenatal vitamins
TAB, PO (SWALLOW OR CHEW,CAPLET)
90s ea **00642-0077-90** 74.99

SELECT-OB+DHA (Everett)
prenatal vitamins
KIT, PO (GLUTEN-FREE)
60s ea UD **00642-0075-30** 49.57

SELEGILINE
(Dey, L.P.) *See EMSAM*

SELEGILINE HCL (Apotex Corp.)
selegiline hydrochloride
CAP, PO, 5 mg, 60s ea .... **60505-0055-01** 138.10 AB
1000s ea .... **60505-0055-02** 2186.58 AB
TAB, PO, 5 mg, 60s ea .... **60505-3438-03** 126.10 AB
500s ea .... **60505-3438-08** 998.29 AB

(Boscogen)
TAB, PO, 5 mg, 60s ea .... **62033-0102-03** 122.45 AB
1000s ea .... **62033-0102-02** 209.00 AB

(Dava Pharma)
CAP, PO, 5 mg, 60s ea .... **67253-0700-06** 138.24 AB

(Hawkins)
POW, NA (U.S.P.)
1 gm **63370-0220-10** 100.00
5 gm **63370-0220-15** 316.00
25 gm **63370-0220-25** 1000.00

(Medisca)
POW, NA (U.S.P.)
1 gm **38779-0644-06** 177.00
5 gm **38779-0644-03** 624.00
25 gm **38779-0644-04** 1155.00

(Mylan)
CAP, PO, 5 mg, 60s ea .... **00378-2252-91** 138.25 AB
TAB, PO, 5 mg, 60s ea .... **00378-2011-91** 138.25 EE

(PCCA)
POW, NA (U.S.P.)
1 gm **51927-2911-00** 231.00

(Spectrum Pharmacy)
POW, NA (U.S.P.)
0.25 gm **49452-6496-02** 222.60
1 gm **49452-6496-03** 320.60
5 gm **49452-6496-04** 1288.00

(Stason Pharm)
TAB, PO, 5 mg, 60s ea .... **60763-0102-03** 122.45 AB
1000s ea .... **60763-0102-02** 209.00 AB

(Pharma Pac)
REPACK
TAB, PO, 5 mg, 4s ea .... **52959-0972-04** 10.69 AB

(Phys Total Care)
REPACK
TAB, PO, 5 mg, 60s ea .... **54868-4288-00** 49.32 EE

SELEGILINE HYDROCHLORIDE
FUL
TAB, PO, 5 mg, 60s ea 45.95

(Apotex Corp.) *See SELEGILINE HCL*
(Boscogen) *See SELEGILINE HCL*
(Dava Pharma) *See SELEGILINE HCL*

(Gallipot)
POW, NA (1X1GM)
1 gm **51552-0882-01** 56.00 40.00

(Hawkins) *See SELEGILINE HCL*
(Medisca) *See SELEGILINE HCL*
(Mylan) *See SELEGILINE HCL*
(PCCA) *See SELEGILINE HCL*
(Somerset) *See ELDEPRYL*
(Spectrum Pharmacy) *See SELEGILINE HCL*
(Stason Pharm) *See SELEGILINE HCL*
(Valeant Pharm Intl) *See ZELAPAR*

SELENIOUS ACID
(PCCA) *See SELENIOUS ACID REAGENT*

SELENIOUS ACID REAGENT (PCCA)
selenious acid
CRY, NA, 1 gm **51927-2954-00** 5.10

SELENIUM (Amer Regent)
SOL, IV (S.D.V.,PF)
40 mcg/ml,
10 ml 25s **00517-6510-25** 69.69

(Baker, J.T.)
POW, NA (REAGENT)
125 gm **10106-3395-04** 134.36
500 gm **10106-3395-01** 356.90

SELENIUM CHELATE (Gallipot)
selenium, chelated
POW, NA, 0.2%, 1000 gm . **51552-0973-07** 70.00 50.00

SELENIUM CHLORIDE
(PCCA) *See SELENIUM MONOCHLORIDE*

SELENIUM MONOCHLORIDE (PCCA)
selenium chloride
POW, NA, 1 gm **51927-2613-00** 57.00

SELENIUM SULFIDE
FUL
LOT, TP, 2.5%, 120 ml 9.00

(Breckenridge Pharm) *See SELENOS*

(Consolidated Midland)
LOT, TP, 2.5%, 120 ml .... **00223-6608-00** 2.75 EE

(Doak) *See SELSEB*

(Morton Grove)
LOT, TP, 2.5%, 118 ml .... **60432-0528-04** 11.40 AT

(PCCA)
POW, NA, 1 gm **51927-3571-00** 3.60

(Perrigo)
LOT, TP, 2.5%, 120 ml .... **45802-0040-64** 11.40 AT

(Quinnova) *See TERSI FOAM*

(Spectrum Pharmacy)
POW, NA (U.S.P.)
25 gm **49452-6493-04** 144.90
100 gm **49452-6493-05** 455.00
500 gm **49452-6493-06** 1501.50

(A-S Medication)
REPACK
LOT, TP, 2.5%, 120 ml .... **54569-1139-00** 11.40 EE

(Dispensing Solutions)
REPACK
LOT, TP, 2.5%, 120 ml **55045-1413-02** 12.00

(Palmetto)
REPACK
LOT, TP (1X120ML)
2.5%, 120 ml **23490-6262-00** 31.35

(Phys Total Care)
REPACK
LOT, TP, 2.5%, 120 ml .... **54868-1362-01** 22.38 EE

(Quality Care Prod)
REPACK
LOT, TP, 2.5%, 120 ml .... **49999-0747-04** 16.14 AT

SELENIUM YEAST
(PCCA) *See SELENIUM YEAST 1000*

SELENIUM YEAST 1000 (PCCA)
selenium yeast
POW, NA (1X1GM)
1 gm **51927-1492-00** 1.44

SELENIUM, CHELATED
(Gallipot) *See SELENIUM CHELATE*

PROD/MFR	NDC	AWP	DP	OBC
SELENOMETHIONINE (PCCA)				
POW, NA (L)				
1 gm	**51927-3494-00**	3.15		
SELENOS (Breckenridge Pharm)				
selenium sulfide				
SHA, TP, 2.25%, 180 ml	**51991-0472-68**	62.72		
SELF-CATH COUDE/OLIVE TIP (Mentor)				
foley catheter				
DEV, NA (10 FR, 16",GUIDE STRIPE)				
30s ea	**81317-0008-10**	83.40		
(12 FR, 16",GUIDE STRIPE)				
30s ea	**81317-0008-12**	83.40		
(14 FR, 16",GUIDE STRIPE)				
30s ea	**81317-0008-14**	83.40		
(16 FR, 16",GUIDE STRIPE)				
30s ea	**81317-0008-16**	83.40		
(18 FR, 16",GUIDE STRIPE)				
30s ea	**81317-0008-18**	83.40		
(6 FR, 16", GUIDE STRIPE)				
30s ea	**81317-0008-06**	83.40		
(8 FR, 16", GUIDE STRIPE)				
30s ea	**81317-0008-08**	83.40		
SELF-CATH COUDE/TAPERED TIP (Mentor)				
foley catheter				
DEV, NA (10 FR, 16")				
20s ea	**81317-0005-86**	63.80		
(12 FR, 16")				
20s ea	**81317-0005-82**	63.80		
(14 FR, 16")				
20s ea	**81317-0004-86**	63.80		
(8 FR, 16")				
20s ea	**81317-0005-88**	63.80		
(10 FR, 16",GUIDE STRIPE)				
30s ea	**81317-0006-10**	83.40		
(12 FR, 16",GUIDE STRIPE)				
30s ea	**81317-0006-12**	83.40		
(14 FR, 16",GUIDE STRIPE)				
30s ea	**81317-0006-14**	80.70		
(8 FR, 16", GUIDE STRIPE)				
30s ea	**81317-0006-08**	83.40		
SELF-CATH FEMALE SPECIMEN (Mentor)				
catheter				
DEV, NA, 25s ea	**81317-0006-25**	81.00		
SELF-CATH PEDIATRIC STRAIGHT TIP (Mentor)				
foley catheter				
DEV, NA (10 FR, 10", LUER END)				
30s ea	**81317-0003-10**	30.90		
(5 FR, 10", FUNNEL END)				
30s ea	**81317-0003-05**	30.90		
(6 FR, 10", FUNNEL END)				
30s ea	**81317-0003-06**	30.90		
(8 FR, 10", LUER END)				
30s ea	**81317-0003-08**	30.90		
SELF-CATH SOFT/STRAIGHT TIP (Mentor)				
catheter				
DEV, NA (10 FR, 16", FUNNEL END)				
30s ea	**81317-0001-10**	30.90		
(12 FR, 16", FUNNEL END)				
30s ea	**81317-0001-12**	30.90		
(14 FR, 16", FUNNEL END)				
30s ea	**81317-0001-14**	30.90		
(16 FR, 16", FUNNEL END)				
30s ea	**81317-0001-16**	30.90		
SELF-CATH STRAIGHT TIP/FEMALE (Mentor)				
catheter				
DEV, NA (10 FR, 6", FUNNEL END)				
30s ea	**81317-0002-10**	26.10		
(12 FR, 6", FUNNEL END)				
30s ea	**81317-0002-12**	26.10		
(14 FR, 6", FUNNEL END)				
30s ea	**81317-0002-14**	26.10		
(14 FR, 6")				
30s ea	**81317-0002-40**	23.10		
(8 FR, 6", FUNNEL END)				
30s ea	**81317-0002-08**	26.10		
SELF-CATH STRAIGHT TIP/FUNNEL END (Mentor)				
catheter				
DEV, NA (10 FR, 16")				
30s ea	**81317-0004-10**	30.90		
(12 FR, 16")				
30s ea	**81317-0004-12**	30.90		
(14 FR, 16")				
30s ea	**81317-0004-14**	30.90		
(16 FR, 16")				
30s ea	**81317-0004-16**	30.90		
(18 FR, 16")				
30s ea	**81317-0004-18**	30.90		
(8 FR, 16")				
30s ea	**81317-0004-08**	30.90		
(12 FR, 16", CURVED PAK)				
50s ea	**81317-0004-60**	52.50		
(14 FR, 16")				
50s ea	**81317-0004-50**	52.50		
SELFEMRA (Teva)				
fluoxetine hydrochloride				
CAP, PO (4X7,HARD GELATIN)				
10 mg, 28s ea	**00093-7225-28**	172.98		AB
20 mg, 28s ea	**00093-7226-28**	177.44		AB
SELSEB (Doak)				
selenium sulfide				
SHA, TP, 2.25%, 180 ml	**10337-0500-10**	146.08		
SELSUN SULFIDE (Southwood)				
REPACK				
selenium sulfide				
LOT, TP, 2.5%, 120 ml	**58016-3077-01**	6.73		EE
SELZENTRY (Pfizer)				
maraviroc				
TAB, PO (FILM-COATED)				
150 mg, 60s ea	**00069-0807-60**	1101.42	917.85	
300 mg, 60s ea	**00069-0808-60**	1101.42	917.85	
(A-S Medication)				
REPACK				
TAB, PO (FILM-COATED)				
150 mg, 60s ea	**54569-6143-00**	1431.85		
(Phys Total Care)				
REPACK				
TAB, PO, 300 mg, 60s ea	**54868-5809-00**	1155.40		
(Quality Care Prod)				
REPACK				
TAB, PO (FILM-COATED)				
150 mg, 60s ea	**35356-0208-60**	2099.14		
300 mg, 60s ea	**35356-0209-60**	2099.14		
SEMPREX-D (UCB)				
acrivastine/pseudoephedrine hydrochloride				
CAP, PO, 8 mg-60 mg,				
100s ea	**53014-0404-10**	177.50		
SEN-SERTER (Medtronic Minimed)				
device				
DEV, NA, ea	**76300-7500-01**	58.80	14.00	
SENATEC (Breckenridge Pharm)				
lidocaine hydrochloride				
LOT, TP, 3%, 177 ml	**51991-0296-63**	95.20		
SENILEZOL (Edwards)				
vitamin b complex, mineral, and vitamin c				
ELI, PO, 480 ml	**00485-0038-01**	20.00		
SENNA				
(Gallipot) *See SENNA LEAVES*				
(Medisca)				
POW, NA (1X250GM,USP)				
250 gm	**38779-1586-07**	31.50		
(1X500GM,USP)				
500 gm	**38779-1586-08**	49.50		
(PCCA)				
POW, NA (USP)				
1 gm	**51927-2029-00**	0.17		
(IPI)				
REPACK				
sennosides a and b				
TAB, PO, 8.6 mg, 60s ea	**18837-0139-60**	11.50		
120s ea	**18837-0139-98**	2.25		
SENNA CON/DOCUSATE SODIUM (Southwood)				
REPACK				
docusate sodium/senna				
TAB, PO, 50 mg-8.6 mg,				
30s ea	**58016-0915-30**	12.08		
60s ea	**58016-0915-60**	24.16		
90s ea	**58016-0915-90**	36.24		
100s ea	**58016-0915-00**	40.27		
120s ea	**58016-0915-02**	48.32		
SENNA DOCUSATE (Pharma Pac)				
REPACK				
docusate sodium/senna				
TAB, PO, 50 mg-8.6 mg,				
30s ea	**52959-0675-30**	5.52		
60s ea	**52959-0675-60**	10.99		
100s ea	**52959-0675-00**	18.28		
180s ea	**52959-0675-08**	32.81		
SENNA EXTRACT				
(PCCA) *See SENNA FLUID EXTRACT*				
SENNA FLUID EXTRACT (PCCA)				
senna extract				
SOL, NA (USP; LEAF)				
1 ml	**51927-2407-00**	0.53		
SENNA LEAVES (Gallipot)				
senna				
POW, NA (U.S.P.,N.F.)				
113.4 gm	**51552-0535-04**	8.33		
454 gm	**51552-0535-06**	36.05		
SENNOSIDES (Bryant Ranch)				
REPACK				
sennosides a and b				
TAB, PO, 8.6 mg, 100s ea	**63629-3207-01**	3.98		
SENOKOT NATURAL LAXATIVE (Palmetto)				
REPACK				
sennosides a and b				
TAB, PO, 8.6 mg, 120s ea	**23490-7863-00**	52.61		
SENSIPAR (Amgen USA Inc.)				
cinacalcet hydrochloride				
TAB, PO (FILM-COATED)				
30 mg, 30s ea	**55513-0073-30**	431.64		
60 mg, 30s ea	**55513-0074-30**	863.28		
90 mg, 30s ea	**55513-0075-30**	1294.92		
(Phys Total Care)				
REPACK				
TAB, PO, 30 mg, 30s ea	**54868-5616-00**	368.09		
SENSOR (Medtronic Minimed)				
device				
DEV, NA, 10s ea	**76300-0700-21**	420.00		
SENSORCAINE (APP)				
bupivacaine hydrochloride				
SOL, IJ (1X50ML,MULTIPLEDOSE)				
0.25%, 50 ml	**63323-0465-50**	10.07		AP
(1X50ML,MDV)				
0.5%, 50 ml	**63323-0467-50**	11.20		AP
SENSORCAINE WITH EPINEPHRINE (APP)				
bupivacaine hydrochloride/epinephrine bitartrate				
SOL, IJ (1X50ML,MDV)				
0.25%-1:200000,				
50 ml	**63323-0461-50**	12.35		AP
0.5%-1:200000,				
50 ml	**63323-0463-50**	13.21		AP
SENSORCAINE-MPF (APP)				
bupivacaine hydrochloride				
SOL, IJ (5X10ML,SINGLE DOSE)				
0.25%, 10 ml 5s	**63323-0464-10**	20.88		AP
(1X30ML,SINGLE DOSE)				
0.25%, 30 ml	**63323-0464-30**	5.80		AP
(5X30ML,SDV)				
0.25%, 30 ml 5s	**63323-0464-31**	41.44		AP
(S.D. AMP)				
0.25%, 30 ml 5s	**00186-1030-02**	30.44		AP
(5X10ML,SDV,E-Z OFF)				
0.5%, 10 ml 5s	**63323-0466-10**	22.80		AP
(1X30ML,SDV)				
0.5%, 30 ml	**63323-0466-30**	6.26		AP
(5X30ML,SDV)				
0.5%, 30 ml 5s	**63323-0466-31**	44.52		AP
(5X30ML)				
0.5%, 30 ml 5s	**63323-0466-33**	30.95		AP
(S.D.V.,STERILE-PAK)				
0.5%, 30 ml 5s	**00186-1033-91**	44.52		AP
(10X2ML)				
0.75%, 2 ml 10s	**63323-0473-02**	47.21		
(5X10ML,SDV,E-Z OFF)				
0.75%, 10 ml 5s	**63323-0472-10**	23.75		AP
(1X30ML,SDV)				
0.75%, 30 ml	**63323-0472-30**	6.55		AP
(S.D. AMP)				
0.75%, 30 ml 5s	**00186-1037-02**	39.54		AP
SENSORCAINE-MPF WITH EPINEPHRINE (APP)				
bupivacaine hydrochloride/epinephrine				
SOL, IJ (USP,SD E-Z OFF VIAL)				
0.25%-1:200000,				
10 ml 5s	**63323-0468-10**	24.36		AP
(1X30ML,SDV)				
0.25%-1:200000,				
30 ml	**63323-0468-30**	7.70		AP
(APP)				
bupivacaine hydrochloride/epinephrine bitartrate				
(5X10ML,SDV)				
0.5%-1:200000,				
10 ml 5s	**63323-0462-10**	24.98		AP
(1X30ML,SDV)				
0.5%-1:200000,				
30 ml	**63323-0462-30**	8.29		AP
(5X30ML,SDV)				
0.5%-1:200000,				
30 ml 5s	**63323-0462-31**	49.55		AP

PROD/MFR	NDC	AWP	DP	OBC
(APP)				
bupivacaine hydrochloride/epinephrine				
(1X30ML,SDV)				
0.75%-1:200000,				
30 ml	**63323-0460-30**	9.31		**AP**
SENTRA AM (Physician Thera, LLC)				
amino acids and nutriceuticals				
CAP, PO (PF,SF,DYE-FREE)				
40 mg-70 mg-35 mg,				
60s ea	**68405-1002-02**	203.52		
(Altura)				
REPACK				
CAP, PO, 40 mg-70 mg-35 mg,				
60s ea	**63874-1182-06**	192.50		
(PF,SF,DYE-FREE)				
40 mg-70 mg-35 mg,				
60s ea	**63874-1002-02**	192.50		
(Dispensing Solutions)				
REPACK				
CAP, PO (PF,SF,DYE-FREE)				
40 mg-70 mg-35 mg,				
60s ea	**55045-3395-06**	192.50		
SENTRA PM (Physician Thera, LLC)				
amino acids and nutriceuticals				
CAP, PO (PF,SF,DYE-FREE)				
40 mg-70 mg-15 mg,				
60s ea	**68405-1003-02**	184.32		
(Altura)				
REPACK				
CAP, PO, 40 mg-70 mg-15 mg,				
60s ea	**63874-1183-06**	130.35		
(Dispensing Solutions)				
REPACK				
CAP, PO (PF,SF,DYE-FREE)				
40 mg-70 mg-15 mg,				
60s ea	**55045-3396-06**	130.35		
SEPRAFILM (Genzyme)				
carboxymethylcellulose/hyaluronate sodium				
SHE, NA (ABSB ADHESION BAR,3X5)				
5s ea	**12664-0101-23**	570.00	475.00	
20s ea	**12664-0201-24**	2040.00	1700.00	
20s ea	**12664-0301-25**	1950.00	1625.00	
30s ea	**12508-0602-26**	2448.00	2040.00	
SEPTRA (Monarch)				
sulfamethoxazole/trimethoprim				
TAB, PO, 400 mg-80 mg,				
100s ea	**61570-0052-01**	149.15		**AB**
(Phys Total Care)				
REPACK				
SUS, PO, 200 mg/5 ml-40 mg/5 ml,				
100 ml	**54868-1420-01**	15.20		**AB**
SEPTRA DS (Monarch)				
sulfamethoxazole/trimethoprim				
TAB, PO, 800 mg-160 mg,				
20s ea	**61570-0053-20**	50.93		**AB**
100s ea	**61570-0053-01**	233.04		**AB**
500s ea	**61570-0053-05**	794.58		**AB**
SERADEX (Gentex Pharma)				
bpm/carbetapentane cit/phenyleph hcl				
SOL, PO (AF,SF,BUBBLE GUM)				
120 ml	**15014-0777-04**	37.40		
(Quality Care Prod)				
REPACK				
SOL, PO (1X120ML,AF,SF)				
120 ml	**35356-0434-04**	61.30		
SERAX (Faulding Labs)				
oxazepam				
CAP, PO, 10 mg,				
100s ea, C-IV	**63857-0327-10**	102.68	69.92	**AB**
15 mg,				
100s ea, C-IV	**63857-0328-10**	129.64	87.90	**AB**
30 mg,				
100s ea, C-IV	**63857-0329-10**	187.50	127.14	**AB**
TAB, PO, 15 mg,				
100s ea, C-IV	**63857-0332-10**	129.64	87.90	
SERENTIL (Phys Total Care)				
REPACK				
mesoridazine besylate				
TAB, PO, 100 mg, 30s ea	**54868-3311-00**	49.28		
SEREVENT DISKUS (Glaxo)				
salmeterol xinafoate				
DSK, IH, 0.046 mg/actuation,				
28s ea	**00173-0520-00**	103.76		
60s ea	**00173-0521-00**	175.78		
(A-S Medication)				
REPACK				
DSK, IH, 0.046 mg/actuation,				
60s ea	**54569-4867-00**	146.60		
(Phys Total Care)				
REPACK				
DSK, IH, 0.046 mg/actuation,				
60s ea	**54868-4481-00**	190.04		
(Quality Care Prod)				
REPACK				
DSK, IH (BLISTER)				
0.046 mg/actuation,				
28s ea UD	**49999-0300-28**	140.54		
SERINE (PCCA)				
POW, NA (USP; (L))				
1 gm	**51927-2589-00**	2.16		
(Spectrum Pharmacy) *See L-SERINE*				
SERINE, DL-				
(Spectrum Pharmacy) *See DL-SERINE*				
SEROMYCIN (The Chao Center)				
cycloserine				
CAP, PO, 250 mg, 40s ea	**00002-0604-40**	240.00	133.92	
SEROPHENE (EMD)				
clomiphene citrate				
TAB, PO, 50 mg, 10s ea	**44087-8090-06**	104.95		**AB**
30s ea	**44087-8090-01**	300.48		**AB**
SEROQUEL (AstraZeneca)				
quetiapine fumarate				
TAB, PO (FILM-COATED)				
25 mg, 100s ea	**00310-0275-10**	328.32		
100s ea UD	**00310-0275-39**	328.32		
1000s ea	**00310-0275-34**	3283.54		
50 mg, 100s ea	**00310-0278-10**	539.50		
1000s ea	**00310-0278-34**	5395.12		
100 mg, 100s ea	**00310-0271-10**	563.40		
100s ea UD	**00310-0271-39**	563.40		
200 mg, 100s ea	**00310-0272-10**	1062.88		
100s ea UD	**00310-0272-39**	1062.88		
300 mg, 60s ea	**00310-0274-60**	836.16		
100s ea UD	**00310-0274-39**	1393.60		
400 mg, 100s ea	**00310-0279-10**	1637.81		
(A-S Medication)				
REPACK				
TAB, PO (FILM-COATED)				
25 mg, 30s ea	**54569-5707-00**	114.33		
100 mg, 60s ea	**54569-5691-01**	392.37		
(Advanced Pharm Serv, Inc.)				
REPACK				
TAB, PO, 25 mg, 10s ea	**13411-0127-01**	31.68		
15s ea	**13411-0127-15**	47.52		
(FILM-COATED)				
25 mg, 30s ea	**13411-0127-03**	95.04		
60s ea	**13411-0127-06**	190.08		
90s ea	**13411-0127-09**	285.12		
100 mg, 10s ea	**13411-0128-01**	54.37		
15s ea	**13411-0128-15**	81.55		
(FILM-COATED)				
100 mg, 30s ea	**13411-0128-03**	163.11		
60s ea	**13411-0128-06**	319.63		
90s ea	**13411-0128-09**	489.35		
200 mg, 10s ea	**13411-0129-01**	102.57		
15s ea	**13411-0129-15**	153.85		
(FILM-COATED)				
200 mg, 30s ea	**13411-0129-03**	307.72		
60s ea	**13411-0129-06**	615.45		
90s ea	**13411-0129-09**	923.17		
300 mg, 10s ea	**13411-0130-01**	80.69		
15s ea	**13411-0130-15**	121.04		
(FILM-COATED)				
300 mg, 30s ea	**13411-0130-03**	242.08		
60s ea	**13411-0130-06**	484.17		
90s ea	**13411-0130-09**	726.26		
(AQ)				
REPACK				
TAB, PO, 25 mg, 10s ea	**66105-0140-01**	39.46		
30s ea	**66105-0140-03**	118.37		
60s ea	**66105-0140-06**	236.74		
90s ea	**66105-0140-09**	394.56		
100s ea	**66105-0140-10**	434.02		
100 mg, 10s ea	**66105-0141-01**	66.71		
30s ea	**66105-0141-03**	200.14		
60s ea	**66105-0141-06**	400.27		
90s ea	**66105-0141-09**	600.42		
100s ea	**66105-0141-10**	667.12		
200 mg, 10s ea	**66105-0142-01**	125.20		
30s ea	**66105-0142-03**	375.62		
60s ea	**66105-0142-06**	751.24		
90s ea	**66105-0142-09**	1126.86		
100s ea	**66105-0142-10**	1252.06		
(Core)				
REPACK				
TAB, PO, 25 mg, 30s ea	**33358-0320-30**	71.62		
60s ea	**33358-0320-60**	133.30		
(IPI)				
REPACK				
TAB, PO, 100 mg, 30s ea	**18837-0141-30**	124.78		
(Nucare Pharm)				
REPACK				
TAB, PO (FILM-COATED)				
25 mg, 30s ea	**68071-0329-30**	138.00		
60s ea	**68071-0329-60**	194.85		
100 mg, 30s ea	**68071-0413-30**	195.00		
200 mg, 30s ea	**68071-0428-30**	305.00		
(Palmetto)				
REPACK				
TAB, PO, 100 mg, 120s ea	**23490-7089-03**	467.56		
200 mg, 45s ea	**23490-7090-02**	301.25		
(PD-Rx Pharm)				
REPACK				
TAB, PO (FILM-COATED)				
25 mg, 30s ea	**55289-0872-30**	148.01		
(REDI-SCRIPT,FILM-COATED)				
25 mg, 30s ea	**58864-0738-30**	148.01		
(REDI-SCRIPT)				
25 mg, 60s ea	**58864-0738-60**	153.25		
(FILM-COATED)				
100 mg, 30s ea	**55289-0187-30**	248.61		
(REDI-SCRIPT)				
100 mg, 30s ea	**58864-0959-30**	131.49		
(FILM-COATED)				
200 mg, 30s ea	**55289-0447-30**	420.98		
(REDI-SCRIPT,FILM-COATED)				
200 mg, 30s ea	**58864-0961-30**	420.98		
300 mg, 30s ea	**58864-0888-30**	603.89		
(Phys Total Care)				
REPACK				
TAB, PO, 25 mg, 10s ea	**54868-4961-03**	56.43		
(FILM-COATED)				
25 mg, 20s ea	**54868-4961-01**	84.92		
30s ea	**54868-4961-02**	126.07		
(FILM-COATED)				
25 mg, 60s ea	**54868-4961-00**	235.80		
90s ea	**54868-4961-04**	352.39		
(FILM-COATED)				
50 mg, 10s ea	**54868-5581-03**	70.23		
20s ea	**54868-5581-01**	130.34		
30s ea	**54868-5581-02**	194.20		
60s ea	**54868-5581-00**	385.79		
100 mg, 10s ea	**54868-4257-04**	49.11		
30s ea	**54868-4257-02**	135.71		
60s ea	**54868-4257-03**	269.55		
100s ea	**54868-4257-01**	432.49		
150s ea	**54868-4257-00**	649.48		
(FILM-COATED)				
200 mg, 10s ea	**54868-4272-01**	81.94		
30s ea	**54868-4272-00**	228.73		
300 mg, 30s ea	**54868-5484-01**	317.16		
90s ea	**54868-5484-00**	947.10		
(Physician Partner)				
REPACK				
TAB, PO, 25 mg, 15s ea	**21695-0117-15**	91.03		
50 mg, 15s ea	**21695-0118-15**	149.59		
100 mg, 15s ea	**21695-0119-15**	184.94		
(FILM-COATED)				
100 mg, 30s ea	**21695-0119-30**	314.40		
200 mg, 15s ea	**21695-0120-15**	294.70		
(Quality Care Prod)				
REPACK				
TAB, PO (FILM-COATED)				
25 mg, 15s ea	**49999-0603-15**	62.30		
30s ea	**49999-0603-30**	124.60		
100s ea	**49999-0603-00**	415.33		
50 mg, 30s ea	**35356-0086-30**	431.00		
100s ea	**35356-0086-00**	1436.37		
100 mg, 15s ea	**49999-0602-15**	81.17		
30s ea	**49999-0602-30**	233.36		
(FILM-COATED)				
100 mg, 100s ea	**49999-0602-00**	541.00		
200 mg, 30s ea	**49999-0951-30**	415.50		
300 mg, 60s ea	**35356-0204-60**	1092.24		
(Southwood)				
REPACK				
TAB, PO, 200 mg, 30s ea	**58016-0046-30**	245.28		
60s ea	**58016-0046-60**	490.57		
90s ea	**58016-0046-90**	735.85		
100s ea	**58016-0046-00**	817.61		

PROD/MFR	NDC	AWP	DP	OBC
(Stat Rx)				
REPACK				
TAB, PO (FILM-COATED)				
25 mg, 30s ea	16590-0521-30	115.13		
60s ea	16590-0521-60	227.66		
90s ea	16590-0521-90	338.88		
120s ea	16590-0521-72	380.00		
(FILM-COATED)				
50 mg, 30s ea	16590-0519-30	170.30		
60s ea	16590-0519-60	337.35		
90s ea	16590-0519-90	553.00		
120s ea	16590-0519-72	415.00		
100 mg, 30s ea	16590-0520-30	177.69		
60s ea	16590-0520-60	352.13		
90s ea	16590-0520-90	526.57		
120s ea	16590-0520-72	447.00		
(FILM-COATED)				
200 mg, 30s ea	16590-0679-30	392.60		
60s ea	16590-0679-60	785.20		
90s ea	16590-0679-90	1177.80		
400 mg, 30s ea	16590-0782-30	483.04		
SEROQUEL XR (AstraZeneca)				
quetiapine fumarate				
TER, PO (FILM COATED)				
50 mg, 60s ea	00310-0280-60	291.91		EE
100s ea UD	00310-0280-39	486.53		EE
150 mg, 60s ea	00310-0281-60	524.16		EE
100s ea UD	00310-0281-39	873.60		EE
(FILM-COATED)				
200 mg, 60s ea	00310-0282-60	576.91		
100s ea UD	00310-0282-39	961.51		
300 mg, 60s ea	00310-0283-60	756.41		EE
100s ea UD	00310-0283-39	1260.68		EE
400 mg, 60s ea	00310-0284-60	888.96		EE
100s ea UD	00310-0284-39	1481.61		EE
(Quality Care Prod)				
REPACK				
TER, PO (FILM-COATED)				
200 mg, 30s ea	35356-0440-30	409.61		
300 mg, 30s ea	35356-0441-30	536.08		EE
400 mg, 30s ea	35356-0442-30	630.12		EE
SEROSTIM (EMD)				
somatropin, mammalian derived				
PDS, SC, 4 mg, 7s ea	44087-0004-07	1553.33		BX
(S.D.V., W/DILUENT)				
5 mg, 7s ea	44087-0005-07	1941.66		BX
6 mg, 7s ea	44087-0006-07	2329.99		BX
(W/DILUENT)				
8.8 mg, 4s ea	44087-0088-04	1674.62		
SEROTONIN HYDROCHLORIDE (PCCA)				
POW, NA (1X1GM)				
1 gm	51927-3229-00	75.00		
SERTACONAZOLE NITRATE				
(Ortho) *See ERTACZO*				
SERTRALINE (Bryant Ranch)				
REPACK				
sertraline hydrochloride				
TAB, PO, 25 mg, 30s ea	63629-3313-01	163.10		
60s ea	63629-3313-02	299.23		
90s ea	63629-3313-03	489.32		
50 mg, 30s ea	63629-3309-01	168.30		
60s ea	63629-3309-02	321.90		
90s ea	63629-3309-03	499.23		
(Core)				
REPACK				
TAB, PO, 25 mg, 30s ea	33358-0321-30	80.47		
60s ea	33358-0321-60	160.96		
90s ea	33358-0321-90	241.43		
50 mg, 30s ea	33358-0322-30	90.92		
60s ea	33358-0322-60	181.63		
90s ea	33358-0322-90	272.75		
100 mg, 30s ea	33358-0323-30	91.12		
60s ea	33358-0323-60	181.84		
90s ea	33358-0323-90	273.06		
(DHS, Inc.)				
REPACK				
TAB, PO, 25 mg, 15s ea	55887-0160-15	40.68		
30s ea	55887-0160-30	81.37		
60s ea	55887-0160-60	162.73		
90s ea	55887-0160-90	244.10		
50 mg, 30s ea	55887-0168-30	81.46		
100 mg, 30s ea	55887-0925-30	81.37		
60s ea	55887-0925-60	162.74		
90s ea	55887-0925-90	244.11		
120s ea	55887-0925-82	325.48		
(PD-Rx Pharm)				
REPACK				
TAB, PO, 25 mg, 30s ea	55289-0378-30	56.94		
50 mg, 14s ea	55289-0291-14	65.94		
30s ea	55289-0291-30	82.74		
(Pharma Pac)				
REPACK				
TAB, PO, 25 mg, 30s ea	52959-0872-30	82.60		
60s ea	52959-0872-60	165.18		
50 mg, 30s ea	52959-0875-30	82.60		
60s ea	52959-0875-60	165.18		
100 mg, 30s ea	52959-0876-30	82.60		
60s ea	52959-0876-60	165.18		
(Phys Total Care)				
REPACK				
TAB, PO, 25 mg, 30s ea	54868-5658-00	18.30		
(Physician Partner)				
REPACK				
TAB, PO, 50 mg, 30s ea	21695-0165-30	170.90		
60s ea	21695-0165-60	341.79		
90s ea	21695-0165-90	512.69		
100 mg, 30s ea	21695-0166-30	170.90		
(FILM COATED)				
100 mg, 60s ea	21695-0166-60	341.79		
90s ea	21695-0166-90	512.69		
(Quality Care Prod)				
REPACK				
TAB, PO, 25 mg, 30s ea	35356-0033-30	162.92		
50 mg, 30s ea	49999-0860-30	488.76		
60s ea	49999-0860-60	325.84		
100 mg, 30s ea	49999-0861-30	162.92		
60s ea	49999-0861-60	325.84		
90s ea	49999-0861-90	488.76		
(Southwood)				
REPACK				
TAB, PO, 25 mg, 30s ea	58016-0011-30	81.37		
60s ea	58016-0011-60	162.74		
90s ea	58016-0011-90	244.11		
100s ea	58016-0011-00	271.23		
50 mg, 30s ea	58016-0010-30	108.30		
60s ea	58016-0010-60	216.60		
90s ea	58016-0010-90	324.90		
100s ea	58016-0010-00	361.00		
120s ea	58016-0010-02	433.20		
100 mg, 30s ea	58016-0009-30	81.37		
60s ea	58016-0009-60	162.74		
90s ea	58016-0009-90	244.11		
100s ea	58016-0009-00	271.23		
(Stat Rx)				
REPACK				
TAB, PO, 50 mg, 90s ea	16590-0457-90	240.00		
120s ea	16590-0457-72	320.00		
100 mg, 120s ea	16590-0416-72	194.00		
SERTRALINE HCL (PD-Rx Pharm)				
REPACK				
sertraline hydrochloride				
TAB, PO, 100 mg, 30s ea	55289-0381-30	85.26		
SERTRALINE HYDROCHLORIDE				
FUL				
TAB, PO, 25 mg, 100s ea		12.83		
50 mg, 100s ea		12.83		
100 mg, 100s ea		12.83		
(Actavis)				
TAB, PO (FILM-COATED)				
25 mg, 30s ea	00228-2721-03	85.40		AB
90s ea	00228-2721-09	256.20		AB
500s ea	00228-2721-50	1423.33		AB
50 mg, 30s ea	00228-2722-03	85.40		AB
90s ea	00228-2722-09	256.20		AB
3000s ea	00228-2722-90	8540.00		AB
100 mg, 30s ea	00228-2723-03	85.40		AB
90s ea	00228-2723-09	256.20		AB
1000s ea	00228-2723-96	2846.67		AB
(Apotex Corp.)				
TAB, PO (FILM COATED)				
25 mg, 30s ea	60505-0180-03	85.53		AB
1000s ea	60505-0180-08	2850.00		AB
50 mg, 30s ea	60505-0181-03	85.53		AB
1000s ea	60505-0181-08	2850.00		AB
100 mg, 30s ea	60505-0182-03	85.53		AB
1000s ea	60505-0182-08	2850.00		AB
(Aurobindo Pharma)				
TAB, PO (FILM-COATED)				
25 mg, 30s ea	65862-0011-30	85.45		AB
500s ea	65862-0011-05	1424.15		AB
50 mg, 30s ea	65862-0012-30	85.45		AB
500s ea	65862-0012-05	1424.15		AB
100 mg, 30s ea	65862-0013-30	85.45		AB
500s ea	65862-0013-05	1424.15		AB
(Camber)				
TAB, PO (FILM-COATED)				
25 mg, 30s ea	31722-0212-30	85.30		AB
500s ea	31722-0212-05	1357.00		AB
50 mg, 30s ea	31722-0213-30	85.30		AB
500s ea	31722-0213-05	1357.00		AB
100 mg, 30s ea	31722-0214-30	85.30		AB
500s ea	31722-0214-05	1357.00		AB
(Greenstone)				
SOL, PO, 20 mg/ml, 60 ml	59762-4940-01	64.28		
TAB, PO, 25 mg, 30s ea	59762-4960-01	81.37		
50 mg, 30s ea	59762-4900-01	81.37		
100s ea UD	59762-4900-03	271.23		
100s ea	59762-4900-04	271.23		
500s ea	59762-4900-05	1356.14		
5000s ea	59762-4900-02	13561.42		
100 mg, 30s ea	59762-4910-01	81.37		
100s ea UD	59762-4910-03	271.23		
100s ea	59762-4910-04	271.23		
500s ea	59762-4910-05	1356.14		
5000s ea	59762-4910-02	13561.42		
(Lupin Pharma, Inc.)				
TAB, PO (FILM COATED)				
25 mg, 30s ea	68180-0351-06	85.54		AB
90s ea	68180-0351-09	256.61		AB
50 mg, 30s ea	68180-0352-06	85.54		AB
90s ea	68180-0352-09	256.61		AB
500s ea	68180-0352-02	1425.60		AB
5000s ea	68180-0352-05	14255.43		AB
100 mg, 30s ea	68180-0353-06	85.54		AB
90s ea	68180-0353-09	256.61		AB
500s ea	68180-0353-02	1425.60		AB
5000s ea	68180-0353-05	14255.43		AB
(Major)				
TAB, PO (10X10,FILM-COATED)				
25 mg, 100s ea UD	00904-6087-61	335.57		AB
(10X10,FILM COATED)				
50 mg, 100s ea UD	00904-6088-61	335.57		AB
(10X10,COATED)				
100 mg, 100s ea UD	00904-5868-61	335.57		AB
(10X10,FILM COATED)				
100 mg, 100s ea UD	00904-6089-61	335.57		AB
(Mylan)				
TAB, PO (FILM COATED)				
25 mg, 30s ea	00378-4186-93	85.43		AB
100s ea	00378-4186-01	284.75		AB
500s ea	00378-4186-05	1423.75		AB
50 mg, 30s ea	00378-4187-93	85.43		AB
100s ea	00378-4187-01	284.75		AB
500s ea	00378-4187-05	1423.75		AB
100 mg, 30s ea	00378-4188-93	85.43		AB
100s ea	00378-4188-01	284.75		AB
500s ea	00378-4188-05	1423.75		AB
(Northstar)				
SOL, PO (1X60ML,PEPPERMINT)				
20 mg/ml, 60 ml	16714-0601-01	65.93		AA
TAB, PO (FILM-COATED)				
25 mg, 30s ea	16714-0611-01	85.00		AB
100s ea	16714-0611-04	278.14		AB
500s ea	16714-0611-05	1423.54		AB
1000s ea	16714-0611-06	2715.33		AB
50 mg, 30s ea	16714-0612-01	85.00		AB
100s ea	16714-0612-04	284.75		AB
500s ea	16714-0612-05	1423.75		AB
1000s ea	16714-0612-06	2715.33		AB
100 mg, 30s ea	16714-0613-01	84.59		AB
100s ea	16714-0613-04	284.75		AB
500s ea	16714-0613-05	1424.15		AB
1000s ea	16714-0613-06	2715.33		AB
(Pfizer) *See ZOLOFT*				
(Ranbaxy Labs)				
SOL, PO (MULTIDOSE,W/DROPPER)				
20 mg/ml, 60 ml	63304-0840-05	67.57		AB
TAB, PO (COATED)				
25 mg, 30s ea	63304-0164-30	85.54		AB
50 mg, 30s ea	63304-0165-30	85.54		AB
100s ea	63304-0165-01	285.20		AB
500s ea	63304-0165-05	1426.00		AB
100 mg, 30s ea	63304-0166-30	85.54		AB
100s ea	63304-0166-01	285.20		AB
500s ea	63304-0166-05	1426.00		AB
(Sandoz)				
TAB, PO (FILM COATED)				
25 mg, 30s ea	00185-0057-30	85.45		AB
50 mg, 30s ea	00185-0153-30	85.45		AB
100 mg, 30s ea	00185-0265-30	85.45		AB

PROD/MFR	NDC	AWP	DP	OBC
(Teva)				
TAB, PO (FILM-COATED)				
25 mg, 30s ea	**50111-0930-10**	85.53		AB
50 mg, 30s ea	**50111-0931-10**	85.53		AB
100s ea	**50111-0931-01**	285.08		AB
500s ea	**50111-0931-02**	1357.50		AB
100 mg, 30s ea	**50111-0932-10**	85.53		AB
100s ea	**50111-0932-01**	285.08		AB
500s ea	**50111-0932-02**	1357.50		AB
(Torrent)				
TAB, PO (FILM-COATED)				
25 mg, 30s ea	**13668-0004-30**	82.50		AB
50s ea	**13668-0004-50**	136.50		AB
90s ea	**13668-0004-90**	243.90		AB
100s ea	**13668-0004-01**	271.00		AB
500s ea	**13668-0004-05**	1345.00		AB
1000s ea	**13668-0004-10**	2670.00		AB
50 mg, 30s ea	**13668-0005-30**	82.50		AB
50s ea	**13668-0005-50**	136.50		AB
90s ea	**13668-0005-90**	243.90		AB
100s ea	**13668-0005-01**	271.00		AB
500s ea	**13668-0005-05**	1345.00		AB
1000s ea	**13668-0005-10**	2670.00		AB
100 mg, 30s ea	**13668-0006-30**	82.50		AB
50s ea	**13668-0006-50**	136.50		AB
90s ea	**13668-0006-90**	243.90		AB
100s ea	**13668-0006-01**	271.00		AB
500s ea	**13668-0006-05**	1345.00		AB
1000s ea	**13668-0006-10**	2670.00		AB
(UDL)				
TAB, PO (10X10,FILM COATED)				
25 mg, 100s ea UD	**51079-0762-20**	284.75		AB
50 mg, 100s ea UD	**51079-0763-20**	284.75		AB
100 mg, 100s ea UD	**51079-0764-20**	284.75		AB
(Watson Labs)				
TAB, PO (FILM COATED)				
25 mg, 30s ea	**16252-0533-30**	4.80		AB
500s ea	**16252-0533-50**	79.98		AB
50 mg, 30s ea	**16252-0534-30**	4.80		AB
90s ea	**16252-0534-90**	14.40		AB
500s ea	**16252-0534-50**	79.98		AB
100 mg, 30s ea	**16252-0535-30**	4.80		AB
90s ea	**16252-0535-90**	14.40		AB
500s ea	**16252-0535-50**	79.98		AB
(West-Ward)				
TAB, PO (FILM-COATED)				
25 mg, 30s ea	**00143-9582-30**	79.95		AB
90s ea	**00143-9582-09**	233.87		AB
(FILM COATED)				
50 mg, 30s ea	**00143-9581-30**	79.95		
90s ea	**00143-9581-09**	233.87		
500s ea	**00143-9581-05**	1285.50		
100 mg, 30s ea	**00143-9580-30**	79.95		
90s ea	**00143-9580-09**	233.87		
500s ea	**00143-9580-05**	1285.50		
(Wockhardt USA)				
TAB, PO (FILM-COATED)				
50 mg, 100s ea	**64679-0752-01**	284.83		AB
500s ea	**64679-0752-04**	1424.15		AB
1000s ea	**64679-0752-07**	2848.30		AB
100 mg, 100s ea	**64679-0753-01**	284.83		AB
500s ea	**64679-0753-04**	1424.15		AB
1000s ea	**64679-0753-07**	2848.30		AB
(A-S Medication)				
REPACK				
TAB, PO, 50 mg, 30s ea	**54569-5818-00**	84.34		
60s ea	**54569-5818-01**	168.68		
100 mg, 30s ea	**54569-5819-00**	84.32		
60s ea	**54569-5819-01**	168.64		
(Aidarex)				
REPACK				
TAB, PO (FILM COATED)				
100 mg, 7s ea	**33261-0346-07**	22.75		AB
10s ea	**33261-0346-10**	32.50		AB
14s ea	**33261-0346-14**	45.50		AB
20s ea	**33261-0346-20**	65.00		AB
21s ea	**33261-0346-21**	68.25		AB
28s ea	**33261-0346-28**	91.00		AB
30s ea	**33261-0346-30**	97.50		AB
60s ea	**33261-0346-60**	195.00		AB
(American Health)				
REPACK				
TAB, PO (10X10)				
25 mg, 100s ea UD	**68084-0180-01**	40.21		
50 mg, 100s ea UD	**68084-0181-01**	40.21		
100 mg, 100s ea UD	**68084-0182-01**	40.21		
(Bryant Ranch)				
REPACK				
TAB, PO, 50 mg, 30s ea	**63629-3289-01**	166.33		
(Dispensing Solutions)				
REPACK				
TAB, PO, 25 mg, 30s ea	**55045-3568-01**	82.50		
(FILM-COATED)				
25 mg, 30s ea	**68258-7010-03**	85.50		AB
50 mg, 30s ea	**55045-3566-01**	82.50		
100 mg, 30s ea	**55045-3562-01**	110.30		
(IPI)				
REPACK				
TAB, PO (FILM-COATED)				
50 mg, 60s ea	**18837-0248-60**	213.62		AB
(FILM COATED)				
50 mg, 90s ea	**18837-0248-90**	256.28		AB
100 mg, 60s ea	**18837-0249-60**	213.62		
90s ea	**18837-0249-90**	256.28		AB
(Keltman Pharma., Inc.)				
REPACK				
TAB, PO, 50 mg, 30s ea	**68387-0119-30**	80.20		
(Nucare Pharm)				
REPACK				
TAB, PO (FILM COATED)				
50 mg, 30s ea	**68071-1317-00**	110.02		
(FILM-COATED)				
50 mg, 60s ea	**68071-0548-60**	220.03		AB
(FILM COATED)				
100 mg, 30s ea	**68071-1318-00**	110.02		
60s ea	**68071-0702-60**	220.03		
(Palmetto)				
REPACK				
TAB, PO, 25 mg, 30s ea	**23490-7050-01**	82.50		
60s ea	**23490-7050-02**	165.00		
50 mg, 28s ea	**23490-6264-01**	77.00		
30s ea	**23490-6264-02**	82.50		
60s ea	**23490-6264-03**	165.00		
100s ea	**23490-6264-04**	275.00		
100 mg, 28s ea	**23490-6263-01**	111.07		
30s ea	**23490-6263-02**	119.00		
60s ea	**23490-6263-03**	238.00		
(PD-Rx Pharm)				
REPACK				
TAB, PO (FILM COATED)				
50 mg, 30s ea	**55289-0291-60**	118.74		
90s ea	**43063-0033-01**	256.20		
100 mg, 60s ea	**55289-0381-60**	123.42		
(Pharma Pac)				
REPACK				
TAB, PO (COATED)				
50 mg, 90s ea	**52959-0875-90**	248.40		AB
(Phys Total Care)				
REPACK				
TAB, PO, 50 mg, 10s ea	**54868-5639-02**	8.64		
15s ea	**54868-5639-04**	9.89		
30s ea	**54868-5639-00**	18.93		
45s ea	**54868-5639-01**	26.88		
60s ea	**54868-5639-06**	29.37		
90s ea	**54868-5639-05**	45.83		
100s ea	**54868-5639-03**	46.00		
100 mg, 10s ea	**54868-5638-03**	8.31		
15s ea	**54868-5638-02**	10.95		
30s ea	**54868-5638-01**	18.93		
45s ea	**54868-5638-04**	26.88		
60s ea	**54868-5638-00**	34.86		
90s ea	**54868-5638-06**	45.83		
100s ea	**54868-5638-05**	54.57		
(FILM-COATED)				
100 mg, 180s ea	**54868-5638-07**	65.90		AB
(Physician Partner)				
REPACK				
TAB, PO (FILM-COATED)				
25 mg, 30s ea	**21695-0164-30**	170.90		
(Stat Rx)				
REPACK				
TAB, PO (FILM-COATED)				
25 mg, 30s ea	**16590-0700-30**	85.45		AB
180s ea	**16590-0700-82**	512.64		AB
50 mg, 15s ea	**16590-0457-15**	40.73		AB
28s ea	**16590-0457-28**	99.68		AB
30s ea	**16590-0457-30**	106.78		AB
(FILM-COATED)				
50 mg, 56s ea	**16590-0457-56**	152.06		AB
60s ea	**16590-0457-60**	213.56		AB
(FILM-COATED)				
100 mg, 15s ea	**16590-0416-15**	53.39		AB
30s ea	**16590-0416-30**	106.78		AB
60s ea	**16590-0416-60**	213.56		AB
90s ea	**16590-0416-90**	320.34		AB
SERZONE (AQ)				
REPACK				
nefazodone hydrochloride				
TAB, PO, 100 mg, 60s ea	**66105-0127-06**	85.80		
90s ea	**66105-0127-09**	158.36		
200 mg, 60s ea	**66105-0129-06**	68.03		
(Pharma Pac)				
REPACK				
TAB, PO, 100 mg, 90s ea	**52959-0645-90**	137.70		
(Phys Total Care)				
REPACK				
TAB, PO, 100 mg, 60s ea	**54868-3707-00**	127.35		
150 mg, 60s ea	**54868-3708-00**	129.73		
200 mg, 20s ea	**54868-4823-01**	43.43		
60s ea	**54868-4823-00**	125.91		
SESAME OIL (Gallipot)				
OIL, NA (U.S.P.,N.F.)				
473 ml	**51552-0442-06**	12.46		
3785 ml	**51552-0442-08**	58.80		
(Letco)				
OIL, NA, 500 ml	**62991-1353-01**	32.25		
(Medisca)				
OIL, NA (1X14ML)				
14 ml	**38779-1855-03**	12.00		
(1X25ML)				
25 ml	**38779-1855-04**	7.50		
(1X100ML)				
100 ml	**38779-1855-05**	13.50		
(1X500ML)				
500 ml	**38779-1855-08**	25.50		
(1X1000ML)				
1000 ml	**38779-1855-09**	46.50		
(1X4000ML)				
4000 ml	**38779-1855-01**	155.85		
(1X20000ML)				
20000 ml	**38779-1855-07**	582.00		
(Spectrum Pharmacy)				
OIL, NA (N.F.)				
500 ml	**49452-6510-01**	53.90		
4000 ml	**49452-6510-02**	252.00		
(U.S.P., N.F.)				
20000 ml	**49452-6510-03**	1004.50		
SET, ADMINISTRATION, INTRAVENOUS, NEEDLE-FREE				
(Medtronic Minimed) *See SILHOUETTE NON-NEEDLE INFUSION*				
(Medtronic Minimed) *See SOF-SET MICRO QR NON-NEEDLE*				
(Medtronic Minimed) *See SOF-SET NON-NEEDLE INFUSION*				
(Medtronic Minimed) *See SOF-SET QR NON-NEEDLE INFUSION*				
(Medtronic Minimed) *See SOF-SET ULTIMATE QR NON-NEEDLE*				
SETONET (Seton)				
prenatal vitamins				
KIT, PO (SOFTGEL)				
60s ea UD	**13925-0100-60**	37.08		
SETONET-EC DHA (Seton)				
prenatal vitamins				
KIT, PO (ENTERIC-COATED, SOFTGEL)				
30s ea UD	**13925-0101-60**	42.90		
SEVELAMER CARBONATE				
(Genzyme) *See RENVELA*				
SEVELAMER HYDROCHLORIDE				
(Genzyme) *See RENAGEL*				
SEVEN PLUS CONTINUOUS GLUCOSE MONITORING SYSTEM (DexCom)				
glucose data management				
DEV, NA (RECEIVER ONLY)				
ea	**08627-0731-01**	718.80		
(STARTER KIT: TRANS/REC)				
ea	**08627-0732-01**	1497.60		
(TRANSMITTER ONLY)				
ea	**08627-0730-01**	778.80		
SEVEN SYSTEM SENSOR PACK (DexCom)				
glucose data management				
DEV, NA, 4s ea	**08627-0741-04**	124.69		
SEVOFLURANE				
(Abbott Pharm) *See ULTANE*				
(Baxter) *See AMERINET CHOICE SEVOFLURANE*				
(Baxter)				
LIQ, IH, 100%, 250 ml 6s	**10019-0651-64**	1332.00		AN
(RxElite) *See SOJOURN*				

PROD/MFR	NDC	AWP	DP	OBC
SF 1.1% GEL (Cypress Pharm)				
sodium fluoride				
GEL, DE (FRESH MINT)				
1.1%, 56 gm	60258-0151-01	8.23		
SF 5000 PLUS (Cypress Pharm)				
sodium fluoride				
CRE, DE (SPEARMINT)				
1.1%, 51 gm	60258-0150-01	8.33		
SFROWASA (Alaven)				
mesalamine				
NMA, RC (7X60ML,W/APPLICATOR TIP)				
4 gm/60 ml, 60 ml 7s	68220-0022-07	195.75		AB
(28X60ML,W/APPLICATORTIP)				
4 gm/60 ml, 60 ml 28s	68220-0022-28	743.75		AB
SHARK CARTILAGE (Gallipot)				
POW, NA, 454 gm	51552-0650-06	161.56		
(Medisca)				
POW, NA (1X100GM)				
100 gm	38779-1791-05	90.00		
(1X500GM)				
500 gm	38779-1791-08	294.00		
(PCCA)				
POW, NA, 1 gm	51927-3610-00	0.90		
(DEODORIZED)				
1 gm	51927-2667-00	0.90		
SHAVEGRASS (PCCA)				
horsetail				
POW, NA, 1 gm	51927-3480-00	0.60		
SHEA BUTTER (PCCA)				
WAX, NA, 1 gm	51927-2401-00	0.23		
(Spectrum Pharmacy)				
WAX, NA (1X500GM)				
500 gm	49452-6512-01	169.05		
SHELLGEL (Cytosol Ophth)				
hyaluronate sodium				
SOL, IO (REFRIDGERATE)				
12 mg/ml, 0.8 ml	61534-1000-01	38.00	42.00	
SHIITAKE MUSHROOM MYCELIUM (PCCA)				
POW, NA (1X1GM)				
1 gm	51927-3233-00	0.53		
SHOHL'S SOLUTION (Humco)				
citric acid/sodium citrate				
SOL, PO, 334 mg/5 ml-500 mg/5 ml, 480 ml	00802-3962-16	6.91		
SIBUTRAMINE HYDROCHLORIDE				
(Abbott Pharm) *See MERIDIA*				
SIDEROL (A. G. Marin)				
multivitamin, minerals, iron, and nutriceuticals				
LIQ, PO, 237 ml	12539-0013-08	25.44		
TAB, PO, 60s ea	12539-0360-60	60.00		
SILDEC (Silarx)				
bpm/pse hcl				
SYR, PO (AF,SF,RASPBERRY)				
4 mg/5 ml-45 mg/5 ml, 473 ml	54838-0534-80	58.30		
SILDEC PE-DM (Silarx)				
cpm/dm/phenyleph hcl				
SOL, PO (SYRUP,AF,SF,GRAPE)				
473 ml	54838-0544-80	105.00		
SILDEC-DM (Silarx)				
bpm/dm/pse hcl				
SYR, PO (AF,SF,GRAPE)				
473 ml	54838-0536-80	80.99		
SILDEC-PE (Silarx)				
cpm/phenyleph hcl				
SOL, PO (SYRUP,AF,SF,RASPBERRY)				
4 mg/5 ml-12.5 mg/5 ml, 473 ml	54838-0542-80	61.00		
SILDENAFIL CITRATE				
(Pfizer) *See REVATIO*				
(Pfizer) *See VIAGRA*				
SILHOUETTE (Medtronic Minimed)				
device				
DEV, NA (13MM)				
10s ea	76300-0369-10	139.20		
(17MM)				
10s ea	76300-0370-10	139.20		
SILHOUETTE CATHETER/TUBING INFUSION (Medtronic Minimed)				
catheter				
DEV, NA (23"COMBO,10 SITE/5 TUBE)				
5s ea	76300-0380-10	125.00	100.00	
(43"COMBO,10 CATH/5 TBNG)				
5s ea	76300-0372-05	125.00	100.00	
(43"COMBO,10 SITE/5 TUBE)				
5s ea	76300-0379-10	125.00	100.00	
(23")				
10s ea	76300-0378-10	146.16		
SILHOUETTE NON-NEEDLE INFUSION (Medtronic Minimed)				
set, administration, intravenous, needle-free				
DEV, NA (23")				
10s ea	76300-0373-10	146.16		
(43")				
10s ea	76300-0371-10	146.16		
SILHOUETTE PARADIGM (Medtronic Minimed)				
diabetic supplies				
DEV, NA (13MM, 32")				
10s ea	76300-0383-10	146.16		
(17MM, 32")				
10s ea	76300-0384-10	146.16		
(18 IN.)				
10s ea	76300-0368-10	146.16		
SILHOUETTE PARADIGM INFUSION SET (Medtronic Minimed)				
infusion pump, insulin				
DEV, NA (13 MM, 23")				
10s ea	76300-0381-10	146.16		
(13MM, 43")				
10s ea	76300-0382-10	146.16		
(17 MM 43")				
10s ea	76300-0377-10	146.16		
SILICA (Gallipot)				
silicon dioxide				
GEL, NA, 0.072 gm	51552-0126-09	4.34		
100 gm	51552-0126-05	16.10		
(Letco)				
GEL, NA (MICRONIZED)				
100 gm	62991-1367-01	30.00		
400 gm	62991-1367-02	75.00		
SILICA GEL (Medisca)				
silica gel, micronized				
POW, NA (1X100GM)				
100 gm	38779-1933-05	52.50		
(1X500GM)				
500 gm	38779-1933-08	165.00		
(1X1000GM)				
1000 gm	38779-1933-09	285.00		
(Spectrum Pharmacy)				
POW, NA (ULTRAMICRONIZED)				
100 gm	49452-6517-01	86.10		
500 gm	49452-6517-02	236.60		
SILICA GEL MICRONIZED (PCCA)				
silica gel, micronized				
POW, NA (1X1GM)				
1 gm	51927-9009-00	1.50		
SILICA GEL, MICRONIZED				
(Medisca) *See SILICA GEL*				
(PCCA) *See SILICA GEL MICRONIZED*				
(Spectrum Pharmacy) *See SILICA GEL*				
SILICON (PCCA)				
POW, NA, 1 gm	51927-2210-00	1.32		
SILICON DIOXIDE				
(Amend) *See AEROSIL 200*				
(Amend) *See CABOSIL M-5*				
(Gallipot) *See SILICA*				
(Letco) *See SILICA*				
(PCCA)				
POW, NA (240 MESH)				
1 gm	51927-2138-00	0.17		
(FCC)				
1 gm	51927-3325-00	0.14		
(FINE GRANULAR)				
1 gm	51927-2107-00	0.05		
(Spectrum Pharmacy)				
POW, NA (F.C.C., MINUS 325 MESH)				
500 gm	49452-6515-01	99.75		
2500 gm	49452-6515-02	326.90		
12000 gm	49452-6515-03	955.50		
SILICONE				
(Amend) *See SILICONE FLUID*				
(Medisca) *See SILICONE ANTIFOAM*				
(PCCA) *See DOW CORNING 9040 SILICONE ELASTOMER BLEND*				
(PCCA) *See SILICONE FLUID*				
SILICONE ANTIFOAM (Medisca)				
silicone				
SOL, NA (1X100ML)				
100 ml	38779-1590-05	31.50		
(1X500ML)				
500 ml	38779-1590-08	61.50		
SILICONE FLUID (Amend)				
silicone				
LIQ, NA (350 C.P.S.)				
3840 ml	17317-0897-01	14.00		
3840 ml	17317-0897-06	67.20		
(PCCA)				
SOL, NA (556)				
1 gm	51927-1065-00	0.84		
SILK BASE (Medisca)				
ointment base				
OIN, NA (1X500GM)				
500 gm	38779-2302-08	58.50		
SILODOSIN				
(Watson) *See RAPAFLO*				
SILVADENE (Monarch)				
silver sulfadiazine				
CRE, TP, 1%, 20 gm	61570-0131-20	9.34		AB
50 gm	61570-0131-50	15.46		AB
85 gm	61570-0131-85	27.49		AB
400 gm	61570-0131-40	66.04		AB
1000 gm	61570-0131-98	129.18		AB
(A-S Medication)				
REPACK				
CRE, TP, 1%, 20 gm	54569-1086-00	9.09		AB
50 gm	54569-1088-00	15.05		AB
(Pharma Pac)				
REPACK				
CRE, TP, 1%, 20 gm	52959-0120-02	13.99		AB
25 gm	52959-0120-25	15.30		AB
50 gm	52959-0120-05	17.41		AB
(Phys Total Care)				
REPACK				
CRE, TP, 1%, 20 gm	54868-0272-00	9.06		AB
50 gm	54868-0272-02	14.56		AB
85 gm	54868-0272-01	30.85		AB
(Quality Care Prod)				
REPACK				
CRE, TP, 1%, 20 gm	49999-0143-20	18.58		AB
25 gm	49999-0185-25	24.36		AB
50 gm	49999-0143-50	46.45		AB
50 gm	49999-0185-50	21.36		AB
(Southwood)				
REPACK				
CRE, TP, 1%, 20 gm	58016-3078-01	14.45		AB
50 gm	58016-2018-01	7.95		AB
SILVER ACETATE (Baker, J.T.)				
POW, NA (PURIFIED)				
30 gm	10106-3410-00	193.95		
SILVER CYANIDE (Baker, J.T.)				
POW, NA (PURIFIED)				
125 gm	10106-3422-04	295.04		
SILVER NITRATE (Amend)				
CRY, NA (U.S.P.)				
25 gm	17317-0487-02	25.20		
125 gm	17317-0487-04	84.00		
(Arzol)				
potassium nitrate/silver nitrate				
SWA, TP, 25%-75%, 100s ea	12870-0001-01	30.96		
100s ea	12870-0001-02	29.52		
SILVER NITRATE (Baker, J.T.)				
CRY, NA (U.S.P.)				
30 gm	10106-3429-00	45.87		
125 gm	10106-3429-04	97.11		
500 gm	10106-3429-01	314.67		
(Gallipot)				
CRY, NA (U.S.P.,N.F.)				
25 gm	51552-0087-04	27.79		
100 gm	51552-0087-05	87.50		
(Gordon)				
OIN, TP, 10%, 30 gm	10481-3011-01	36.25		
SOL, TP, 10%, 30 ml	10481-1051-01	36.25		
25%, 30 ml	10481-1052-01	55.00		
50%, 30 ml	10481-1053-01	77.50		
(Mallinckrodt Lab)				
CRY, NA (U.S.P.)				
4 gm	00406-7992-01	244.23		
(A.C.S.)				
30 gm	00406-2169-34	47.36		

PROD/MFR	NDC	AWP	DP	OBC
(U.S.P.)				
30 gm	00406-7992-34	44.67		
(A.C.S.)				
120 gm	00406-2169-01	171.62		
(U.S.P.)				
480 gm	00406-7992-03	759.21		
(Medisca)				
CRY, NA (1X10GM,USP)				
10 gm	38779-0593-01	34.50		
(U.S.P.)				
25 gm	38779-0593-04	58.50		
100 gm	38779-0593-05	187.50		
(PCCA)				
POW, NA (USP)				
1 gm	51927-1293-00	4.80		
(Spectrum Pharmacy)				
CRY, NA (U.S.P.)				
25 gm	49452-6225-01	141.40		
100 gm	49452-6225-04	427.00		
125 gm	49452-6225-02	476.00		
500 gm	49452-6225-03	1501.50		
(Teva)				
SOL, TP, 0.5%, 960 ml	00093-9614-13	19.33		
(Phys Total Care)				
REPACK				
potassium nitrate/silver nitrate				
SWA, TP, 25%-75%,				
100s ea	54868-2916-00	18.53		
SILVER PROTEIN (Amend)				
POW, NA (N.F., MILD)				
25 gm	17317-0489-02	29.40		
125 gm	17317-0489-04	112.00		
(Baker, J.T.)				
POW, NA (PURIFIED, MILD)				
30 gm	10106-2704-00	88.77		
125 gm	10106-2704-04	239.91		
(PCCA)				
POW, NA (MILD)				
1 gm	51927-1263-00	6.00		
(Spectrum Pharmacy)				
GRA, NA (1X25GM)				
25 gm	49452-6530-01	192.85		
(1X100GM)				
100 gm	49452-6530-02	497.00		
(1X500GM)				
500 gm	49452-6530-04	1984.50		
SILVER SULFADIAZINE				
FUL				
CRE, TP, 1%, 400 gm		25.12		
(Ascend)				
CRE, TP (1X25GM,USP)				
1%, 25 gm	67877-0124-25	5.64		
(1X50GM,USP)				
1%, 50 gm	67877-0124-50	8.53		
(1X85GM,USP)				
1%, 85 gm	67877-0124-85	14.89		
(1X400GM,USP)				
1%, 400 gm	67877-0124-40	35.56		
(Covidien) *See THERMAZENE*				
(Hawkins)				
POW, NA (U.S.P.)				
5 gm	63370-0221-15	32.00		
25 gm	63370-0221-25	114.00		
100 gm	63370-0221-35	400.00		
(Monarch) *See SILVADENE*				
(Par) *See SSD*				
(Par) *See SSD AF*				
(PCCA)				
POW, NA (USP)				
1 gm	51927-1684-00	6.60		
(Spectrum Pharmacy)				
POW, NA (U.S.P,MICRONIZED)				
10 gm	49452-6545-01	138.25		
25 gm	49452-6545-04	200.38		
100 gm	49452-6545-02	647.50		
(Watson Labs)				
CRE, TP, 1%, 25 gm	00591-0810-83	4.95		AB
50 gm	00591-0810-55	8.22		AB
85 gm	00591-0810-85	14.63		AB
400 gm	00591-0810-46	35.09		AB
(A-S Medication)				
REPACK				
CRE, TP, 1%, 25 gm	54569-5348-00	5.20		EE
50 gm	54569-4519-00	8.68		AB
50 gm	54569-5202-00	9.18		EE
400 gm	54569-3417-00	35.07		EE
(Aidarex)				
REPACK				
CRE, TP (1X25GM)				
1%, 25 gm	33261-0400-25	13.45		AB
(1X50GM)				
1%, 50 gm	33261-0382-01	22.00		AB
(Altura)				
REPACK				
CRE, TP, 1%, 50 gm	63874-0807-20	7.60		EE
50 gm	63874-0807-50	9.81		EE
400 gm	63874-0807-40	44.00		EE
(DHS, Inc.)				
REPACK				
CRE, TP, 1%, 25 gm	55887-0934-25	7.00		
(Dispensing Solutions)				
REPACK				
CRE, TP, 1%, 25 gm	55045-1344-08	8.40		AB
50 gm	55045-1344-04	10.25		AB
400 gm	55045-1344-09	41.30		AB
(IPI)				
REPACK				
CRE, TP (1X50GM)				
1%, 50 gm	18837-0302-50	10.28		
(Keltman Pharma., Inc.)				
REPACK				
CRE, TP, 1%, 50 gm	68387-0450-01	19.87		AB
(Palmetto)				
REPACK				
CRE, TP, 1%, 20 gm	23490-6265-00	5.00		
25 gm	23490-6265-01	6.25		
50 gm	23490-6265-02	12.50		
400 gm	23490-6265-03	100.00		
(Pharma Pac)				
REPACK				
CRE, TP, 1%, 25 gm	52959-0635-25	9.35		EE
50 gm	52959-0635-50	10.45		EE
400 gm	52959-0635-00	44.75		EE
(Phys Total Care)				
REPACK				
CRE, TP, 1%, 20 gm	54868-0375-03	12.12		
30 gm	54868-0375-00	12.36		EE
50 gm	54868-0375-01	20.64		EE
400 gm	54868-0375-02	123.45		EE
(Physician Partner)				
REPACK				
CRE, TP, 1%, 25 gm	21695-0182-25	25.20		
50 gm	21695-0182-50	26.44		
85 gm	21695-0182-85	29.36		
(Quality Care Prod)				
REPACK				
CRE, TP, 1%, 400 gm	49999-0185-40	172.00		AB
(Southwood)				
REPACK				
CRE, TP, 1%, 20 gm	58016-3504-01	4.00		EE
25 gm	58016-1152-01	5.25		EE
50 gm	58016-3081-01	10.30		EE
400 gm	58016-3079-01	30.50		EE
(Stat Rx)				
REPACK				
CRE, TP, 1%, 50 gm	16590-0206-50	20.00		
85 gm	16590-0206-85	34.00		
400 gm	16590-0206-44	80.00		
SILVER SULFATE (Baker, J.T.)				
POW, NA (A.C.S., REAGENT)				
125 gm	10106-3436-04	421.94		
500 gm	10106-3436-01	1380.92		
SILYMARIN (Medisca)				
milk thistle				
POW, NA (1X25GM)				
25 gm	38779-1593-04	37.50		
(1X100GM)				
100 gm	38779-1593-05	123.00		
SIMCOR (Abbott Pharm)				
niacin/simvastatin				
TER, PO (FILM-COATED)				
500 mg-20 mg,				
90s ea	00074-3312-90	228.35	200.31	
750 mg-20 mg,				
90s ea	00074-3315-90	325.70	285.70	
1000 mg-20 mg,				
90s ea	00074-3316-90	403.87	354.27	
(Phys Total Care)				
REPACK				
TER, PO (FILM-COATED)				
500 mg-20 mg,				
30s ea	54868-5886-00	105.30		
60s ea	54868-5886-01	196.58		
750 mg-20 mg,				
30s ea	54868-5907-00	140.93		
60s ea	54868-5907-01	279.25		
1000 mg-20 mg,				
30s ea	54868-5904-00	174.13		
60s ea	54868-5904-01	345.65		
SIMETHICONE				
(Amend) *See SIMETHICONE 100%*				
(Gallipot)				
POW, NA (U.S.P.)				
0.004 gm	51552-0119-04	26.46		
480 gm	51552-0119-06	58.45		
(PCCA)				
SOL, NA (USP MED. ANTIFOAM A)				
1 ml	51927-1382-00	0.58		
(Spectrum Pharmacy)				
LIQ, NA (U.S.P.)				
500 ml	49452-6546-01	207.55		
4000 ml	49452-6546-02	1036.00		
(Phys Total Care)				
REPACK				
SUS, PO (DROPS)				
40 mg/0.6 ml,				
30 ml	54868-5620-00	15.46		
SIMETHICONE 100% (Amend)				
simethicone				
LIQ, NA, 3840 ml	17317-0924-06	224.00		
(U.S.P.)				
3840 ml	17317-0924-01	31.50		
SIMETYL (Kramer-Novis)				
belladonna alkaloids/simethicone				
ELI, PO, 120 ml	52083-0511-04	7.00		
SIMPONI (Centocor)				
golimumab				
SOL, SC (PREFILLED SYRINGE)				
50 mg/0.5 ml,				
0.5 ml	57894-0070-01	1982.62		
(SMARTJECT AUTOINJECTION)				
50 mg/0.5 ml,				
0.5 ml	57894-0070-02	1982.62		
SIMUC (Cypress Pharm)				
guaifenesin/phenylephrine hydrochloride				
TER, PO (CAPLET)				
900 mg-25 mg,				
100s ea	60258-0326-01	153.11		
SIMUC-DM (Cypress Pharm)				
dextromethorphan hydrobromide/guaifenesin				
SOL, PO (AF,SF,GRAPE)				
25 mg/5 ml-225 mg/5 ml,				
473 ml	60258-0426-16	139.99		
SIMULECT (Novartis Pharm)				
basiliximab				
PDS, IV (S.D.V.,PF)				
10 mg, ea	00078-0393-61	1883.11		
20 mg, ea	00078-0331-84	2471.60		
SIMVASTATIN				
FUL				
TAB, PO, 5 mg, 90s ea		15.75		
10 mg, 90s ea		15.75		
20 mg, 90s ea		18.90		
40 mg, 90s ea		23.00		
80 mg, 90s ea		23.00		
(Accord)				
TAB, PO (USP,FILM-COATED)				
10 mg, 30s ea	16729-0004-10	84.50		AB
90s ea	16729-0004-15	253.10		AB
1000s ea	16729-0004-17	2815.55		AB
20 mg, 30s ea	16729-0005-10	147.10		AB
90s ea	16729-0005-15	441.15		AB
1000s ea	16729-0005-17	4917.12		AB
40 mg, 30s ea	16729-0006-10	147.10		AB
90s ea	16729-0006-15	441.15		AB
1000s ea	16729-0006-17	4917.12		AB
80 mg, 30s ea	16729-0007-10	147.10		AB
90s ea	16729-0007-15	441.15		AB
1000s ea	16729-0007-17	4917.12		AB
(Aurobindo Pharma)				
TAB, PO (FILM COATED)				
5 mg, 30s ea	65862-0050-30	62.86		AB
90s ea	65862-0050-90	188.76		AB
(USP,FILM COATED)				
10 mg, 30s ea	65862-0051-30	84.25		AB
90s ea	65862-0051-90	252.96		AB
1000s ea	65862-0051-99	2810.73		AB
2500s ea	65862-0051-26	7026.83		AB
20 mg, 30s ea	65862-0052-30	147.12		AB

PROD/MFR	NDC	AWP	DP	OBC
90s ea	**65862-0052-90**	441.37		AB
1000s ea	**65862-0052-99**	4904.11		AB
2500s ea	**65862-0052-26**	12260.28		AB
40 mg, 30s ea	**65862-0053-30**	147.12		AB
90s ea	**65862-0053-90**	441.37		AB
1000s ea	**65862-0053-99**	4904.11		AB
2000s ea	**65862-0053-22**	9808.22		AB
80 mg, 30s ea	**65862-0054-30**	147.12		AB
90s ea	**65862-0054-90**	441.37		AB
1000s ea	**65862-0054-99**	4904.11		AB
(Blu)				
TAB, PO (USP,FILM-COATED)				
5 mg, 30s ea	**24658-0210-30**	1.59		
45s ea	**24658-0210-45**	2.21		
90s ea	**24658-0210-90**	3.59		
1000s ea	**24658-0210-10**	33.47		
10 mg, 30s ea	**24658-0211-30**	1.59		
45s ea	**24658-0211-45**	2.21		
90s ea	**24658-0211-90**	3.61		
1000s ea	**24658-0211-10**	33.63		
20 mg, 30s ea	**24658-0212-30**	2.57		
45s ea	**24658-0212-45**	2.97		
90s ea	**24658-0212-90**	5.39		
1000s ea	**24658-0212-10**	47.00		
40 mg, 30s ea	**24658-0213-30**	2.66		
45s ea	**24658-0213-45**	3.83		
90s ea	**24658-0213-90**	6.84		
1000s ea	**24658-0213-10**	69.62		
80 mg, 30s ea	**24658-0214-30**	4.06		
45s ea	**24658-0214-45**	5.96		
90s ea	**24658-0214-90**	11.10		
1000s ea	**24658-0214-10**	116.38		
(Dr Reddy's)				
TAB, PO (USP,FILM COATED)				
5 mg, 30s ea	**55111-0197-30**	62.78		AB
90s ea	**55111-0197-90**	188.33		AB
500s ea	**55111-0197-05**	1046.28		AB
10 mg, 30s ea	**55111-0735-30**	84.13		
(USP,FILM-COATED)				
10 mg, 30s ea	**55111-0198-30**	84.13		AB
(USP,FILM COATED)				
10 mg, 90s ea	**55111-0735-90**	252.40		
(USP,FILM-COATED)				
10 mg, 90s ea	**55111-0198-90**	252.40		AB
500s ea	**55111-0198-05**	1402.23		AB
(USP,FILM COATED)				
10 mg, 1000s ea	**55111-0735-10**	2804.46		
(USP,FILM-COATED)				
20 mg, 30s ea	**55111-0199-30**	146.79		AB
30s ea	**55111-0740-30**	146.79		
(FILM-COATED)				
20 mg, 90s ea	**55111-0199-90**	440.38		AB
(USP,FILM-COATED)				
20 mg, 90s ea	**55111-0740-90**	440.38		
(FILM-COATED)				
20 mg, 500s ea	**55111-0199-05**	2446.59		AB
(USP,FILM-COATED)				
20 mg, 1000s ea	**55111-0740-10**	4893.17		
40 mg, 30s ea	**55111-0200-30**	146.79		AB
30s ea	**55111-0749-30**	146.79		
90s ea	**55111-0200-90**	440.38		AB
90s ea	**55111-0749-90**	440.38		
500s ea	**55111-0200-05**	2446.59		AB
1000s ea	**55111-0749-10**	4893.17		
80 mg, 30s ea	**55111-0268-30**	146.79		AB
30s ea	**55111-0750-30**	146.79		
90s ea	**55111-0268-90**	440.38		AB
90s ea	**55111-0750-90**	440.38		
500s ea	**55111-0268-05**	2446.59		AB
1000s ea	**55111-0750-10**	4893.17		
(Lupin Pharma, Inc.)				
TAB, PO (USP,FILM-COATED)				
10 mg, 30s ea	**68180-0478-01**	84.60		AB
90s ea	**68180-0478-02**	253.81		AB
1000s ea	**68180-0478-03**	2820.13		AB
20 mg, 30s ea	**68180-0479-01**	147.61		AB
90s ea	**68180-0479-02**	442.85		AB
1000s ea	**68180-0479-03**	4920.51		AB
40 mg, 30s ea	**68180-0480-01**	147.61		AB
90s ea	**68180-0480-02**	442.85		AB
1000s ea	**68180-0480-03**	4920.51		AB
80 mg, 30s ea	**68180-0481-01**	147.61		AB
90s ea	**68180-0481-02**	442.85		AB
1000s ea	**68180-0481-03**	4920.51		AB
(Major)				
TAB, PO (10X10,USP,FILM-COATED)				
10 mg, 100s ea UD	**00904-5800-61**	252.40		AB
20 mg, 100s ea UD	**00904-5801-61**	440.39		AB
40 mg, 100s ea UD	**00904-5802-61**	440.39		AB
(Medisca)				
POW, NA (1X100GM,USP)				
100 gm	**38779-1785-05**	1650.00		
(1X1000GM,USP)				
1000 gm	**38779-1785-09**	10500.00		
(Merck) *See ZOCOR*				
(Northstar)				
TAB, PO (USP,FILM COATED)				
5 mg, 30s ea	**16714-0681-01**	62.78		AB
90s ea	**16714-0681-02**	189.01		AB
10 mg, 30s ea	**16714-0682-01**	84.19		AB
90s ea	**16714-0682-02**	253.60		AB
1000s ea	**16714-0682-03**	2820.00		AB
20 mg, 30s ea	**16714-0683-01**	147.12		AB
90s ea	**16714-0683-02**	442.60		AB
1000s ea	**16714-0683-03**	4920.00		AB
40 mg, 30s ea	**16714-0684-01**	146.96		AB
90s ea	**16714-0684-02**	442.60		AB
1000s ea	**16714-0684-03**	4920.00		AB
80 mg, 30s ea	**16714-0685-01**	146.96		AB
90s ea	**16714-0685-02**	442.70		AB
1000s ea	**16714-0685-03**	4912.31		AB
(Ranbaxy Pharm)				
TAB, PO (USP,FILM COATED)				
5 mg, 90s ea	**63304-0789-90**	189.39		AB
1000s ea	**63304-0789-10**	2105.00		AB
10 mg, 90s ea	**63304-0790-90**	253.81		AB
1000s ea	**63304-0790-10**	2821.00		AB
20 mg, 90s ea	**63304-0791-90**	442.85		AB
1000s ea	**63304-0791-10**	4921.00		AB
40 mg, 90s ea	**63304-0792-90**	442.85		AB
1000s ea	**63304-0792-10**	4921.00		AB
(FILM-COATED)				
80 mg, 90s ea	**63304-0793-90**	442.85		
1000s ea	**63304-0793-10**	4920.51		
(Sandoz)				
TAB, PO (USP)				
5 mg, 30s ea	**00781-5070-31**	63.13		AB
90s ea	**00781-5070-92**	189.39		AB
10 mg, 30s ea	**00781-5071-31**	84.60		AB
90s ea	**00781-5071-92**	253.81		AB
20 mg, 30s ea	**00781-5072-31**	147.61		AB
90s ea	**00781-5072-92**	442.85		AB
40 mg, 30s ea	**00781-5073-31**	147.61		AB
90s ea	**00781-5073-92**	442.85		AB
80 mg, 30s ea	**00781-5074-31**	147.61		AB
90s ea	**00781-5074-92**	442.85		AB
(Teva)				
TAB, PO (FILM-COATED)				
5 mg, 30s ea	**00093-7152-56**	63.13		
90s ea	**00093-7152-98**	189.39		
(10X10,USP,FILM-COATED)				
5 mg, 100s ea UD	**00093-7152-93**	210.44		
(FILM-COATED)				
10 mg, 30s ea	**00093-7153-56**	84.60		
90s ea	**00093-7153-98**	253.81		
(10X10,USP,FILM-COATED)				
10 mg, 100s ea UD	**00093-7153-93**	282.02		
(FILM-COATED)				
10 mg, 1000s ea	**00093-7153-10**	2820.13		
20 mg, 30s ea	**00093-7154-56**	147.61		
90s ea	**00093-7154-98**	442.85		
(10X10,USP,FILM-COATED)				
20 mg, 100s ea UD	**00093-7154-93**	492.06		
(FILM-COATED)				
20 mg, 1000s ea	**00093-7154-10**	4920.51		
40 mg, 30s ea	**00093-7155-56**	147.61		
90s ea	**00093-7155-98**	442.85		
(10X10,USP,FILM-COATED)				
40 mg, 100s ea UD	**00093-7155-93**	492.06		
(FILM-COATED)				
40 mg, 1000s ea	**00093-7155-10**	4920.51		
(USP,FILM-COATED)				
80 mg, 30s ea	**00093-7156-56**	147.61		EE
90s ea	**00093-7156-98**	442.85		EE
1000s ea	**00093-7156-10**	4920.51		EE
(UDL)				
TAB, PO (FILM-COATED)				
10 mg, 100s ea UD	**51079-0454-20**	278.88		AB
20 mg, 100s ea UD	**51079-0455-20**	492.06		AB
40 mg, 100s ea UD	**51079-0456-20**	492.06		AB
(Watson Labs)				
TAB, PO (USP)				
5 mg, 30s ea	**16252-0505-30**	1.92		EE
90s ea	**16252-0505-90**	6.00		EE
500s ea	**16252-0505-50**	33.30		EE
10 mg, 30s ea	**16252-0506-30**	2.40		EE
90s ea	**16252-0506-90**	7.20		EE
500s ea	**16252-0506-50**	39.60		EE
20 mg, 30s ea	**16252-0507-30**	2.76		EE
90s ea	**16252-0507-90**	8.40		EE
500s ea	**16252-0507-50**	46.68		EE
40 mg, 30s ea	**16252-0508-30**	3.60		EE
90s ea	**16252-0508-90**	10.80		EE
500s ea	**16252-0508-50**	60.00		EE
80 mg, 30s ea	**16252-0509-30**	3.96		EE
90s ea	**16252-0509-90**	12.00		EE
500s ea	**16252-0509-50**	66.60		EE
(Zydus Pharm.)				
TAB, PO (USP,FILM COATED)				
5 mg, 90s ea	**68382-0065-16**	189.38		AB
1000s ea	**68382-0065-10**	2104.22		AB
10 mg, 90s ea	**68382-0066-16**	253.80		AB
500s ea	**68382-0066-05**	1410.00		AB
1000s ea	**68382-0066-10**	2820.00		AB
20 mg, 90s ea	**68382-0067-16**	442.80		AB
500s ea	**68382-0067-05**	2460.00		AB
1000s ea	**68382-0067-10**	4920.00		AB
40 mg, 90s ea	**68382-0068-16**	442.80		AB
500s ea	**68382-0068-05**	2460.00		AB
1000s ea	**68382-0068-10**	4920.00		AB
80 mg, 90s ea	**68382-0069-16**	442.80		AB
500s ea	**68382-0069-05**	2460.00		AB
1000s ea	**68382-0069-10**	4920.00		AB
(A-S Medication)				
REPACK				
TAB, PO, 20 mg, 30s ea	**54569-5833-01**	146.79		
90s ea	**54569-5833-02**	440.37		
200s ea	**54569-5833-03**	978.60		
40 mg, 30s ea	**54569-5834-01**	146.79		
90s ea	**54569-5834-03**	440.37		
100s ea	**54569-5834-02**	489.30		
200s ea	**54569-5834-04**	978.60		
(FILM-COATED)				
80 mg, 30s ea	**54569-6113-00**	146.79		AB
(Aidarex)				
REPACK				
TAB, PO, 40 mg, 30s ea	**33261-0542-30**	166.00		
60s ea	**33261-0542-60**	332.00		
90s ea	**33261-0542-90**	498.00		
120s ea	**33261-0542-02**	664.00		
(American Health)				
REPACK				
TAB, PO (10X10,USP)				
5 mg, 100s ea UD	**68084-0161-01**	200.00		
10 mg, 100s ea UD	**68084-0162-01**	278.88		
20 mg, 100s ea UD	**68084-0163-01**	492.06		
40 mg, 100s ea UD	**68084-0164-01**	492.06		
80 mg, 100s ea UD	**68084-0165-01**	492.06		
(Bryant Ranch)				
REPACK				
TAB, PO (FILM COATED)				
20 mg, 30s ea	**63629-3393-01**	147.50		AB
60s ea	**63629-3393-02**	285.65		AB
(DHS, Inc.)				
REPACK				
TAB, PO, 10 mg, 30s ea	**55887-0861-30**	239.96		
60s ea	**55887-0861-60**	479.92		
90s ea	**55887-0861-90**	719.88		
20 mg, 30s ea	**55887-0327-30**	105.00		
60s ea	**55887-0327-60**	210.00		
90s ea	**55887-0327-90**	315.00		
(FILM-COATED)				
40 mg, 10s ea	**55887-0858-10**	48.98		
30s ea	**55887-0858-30**	146.95		
60s ea	**55887-0858-60**	293.90		
90s ea	**55887-0858-90**	440.85		
80 mg, 30s ea	**55887-0318-30**	120.00		
60s ea	**55887-0318-60**	240.00		
90s ea	**55887-0318-90**	360.00		
(Dispensing Solutions)				
REPACK				
TAB, PO, 20 mg, 30s ea	**66336-0954-30**	148.22		
90s ea	**66336-0954-90**	444.66		EE
(FILM-COATED)				
40 mg, 30s ea	**66336-0953-30**	147.53		
90s ea	**66336-0953-90**	442.59		
(FILM COATED)				
80 mg, 30s ea	**66336-0986-30**	148.22		AB
(McKesson Packaging)				
REPACK				
TAB, PO, 5 mg, 100s ea UD	**63739-0435-10**	263.03		
10 mg, 100s ea UD	**63739-0436-10**	352.50		
20 mg, 100s ea UD	**63739-0437-10**	615.00		
40 mg, 100s ea UD	**63739-0438-10**	615.00		
(Palmetto)				
REPACK				
TAB, PO, 5 mg, 30s ea	**23490-9356-03**	75.00		
60s ea	**23490-9356-06**	150.00		

PROD/MFR	NDC	AWP	DP	OBC
90s ea	23490-9356-09	225.00		
10 mg, 30s ea	23490-9353-03	142.50		
60s ea	23490-9353-06	285.00		
90s ea	23490-9353-09	427.50		
20 mg, 30s ea	23490-9354-03	150.00		
60s ea	23490-9354-06	300.00		
90s ea	23490-9354-09	450.00		
40 mg, 30s ea	23490-9355-03	154.50		
60s ea	23490-9355-06	309.00		
90s ea	23490-9355-09	463.50		
80 mg, 30s ea	23490-9357-03	159.00		
60s ea	23490-9357-06	318.00		
90s ea	23490-9357-09	477.00		
(PD-Rx Pharm)				
REPACK				
TAB, PO, 10 mg, 14s ea	55289-0338-14	58.89		
(USP)				
10 mg, 30s ea	55289-0338-30	84.60		
90s ea	55289-0338-90	105.20		EE
20 mg, 14s ea	55289-0293-14	102.75		
(USP)				
20 mg, 30s ea	55289-0293-30	147.62		
90s ea	43063-0008-01	440.38		EE
90s ea	55289-0293-90	179.00		EE
(USP)				
40 mg, 30s ea	55289-0395-30	155.00		
90s ea	55289-0395-90	226.29		EE
80 mg, 30s ea	43063-0080-30	156.05		EE
90s ea	43063-0080-90	231.85		EE
(Pharma Pac)				
REPACK				
TAB, PO, 10 mg, 30s ea	52959-0988-30	96.33		EE
(FILM-COATED)				
20 mg, 30s ea	52959-0989-30	147.09		AB
90s ea	52959-0989-90	441.09		AB
40 mg, 30s ea	52959-0944-30	147.89		EE
(Phys Total Care)				
REPACK				
TAB, PO, 5 mg, 90s ea	54868-6066-00	25.02		EE
10 mg, 30s ea	54868-5627-00	12.69		
90s ea	54868-5627-01	32.08		
20 mg, 30s ea	54868-5628-00	17.97		
(FILM-COATED)				
20 mg, 60s ea	54868-5628-02	20.06		AB
90s ea	54868-5628-01	44.88		
40 mg, 15s ea	54868-5629-03	10.68		
30s ea	54868-5629-00	19.26		
60s ea	54868-5629-02	34.05		
90s ea	54868-5629-01	48.81		
(FILM-COATED)				
40 mg, 150s ea	54868-5629-04	64.45		AB
80 mg, 30s ea	54868-5630-00	27.77		
90s ea	54868-5630-01	75.81		
(Physician Partner)				
REPACK				
TAB, PO (FILM COATED)				
5 mg, 90s ea	21695-0738-90	378.50		AB
10 mg, 30s ea	21695-0739-30	169.00		EE
90s ea	21695-0739-90	507.00		EE
20 mg, 30s ea	21695-0740-30	295.00		EE
90s ea	21695-0740-90	885.00		EE
40 mg, 30s ea	21695-0741-30	295.00		EE
90s ea	21695-0741-90	885.00		EE
80 mg, 30s ea	21695-0742-30	295.00		EE
(Quality Care Prod)				
REPACK				
TAB, PO, 5 mg, 90s ea	49999-0900-90	207.16		
20 mg, 30s ea	49999-0889-30	261.13		
60s ea	49999-0889-60	522.26		
90s ea	49999-0889-90	783.39		
40 mg, 15s ea	49999-0903-15	80.70		
30s ea	49999-0903-30	161.47		
90s ea	49999-0903-90	484.41		
(Southwood)				
REPACK				
TAB, PO, 10 mg, 30s ea	58016-0008-30	84.13		
60s ea	58016-0008-60	168.27		
90s ea	58016-0008-90	252.40		
100s ea	58016-0008-00	280.44		
20 mg, 30s ea	58016-0007-30	146.79		
60s ea	58016-0007-60	293.59		
90s ea	58016-0007-90	440.38		
100s ea	58016-0007-00	489.31		
40 mg, 30s ea	58016-0006-30	146.79		
60s ea	58016-0006-60	293.59		
90s ea	58016-0006-90	440.38		
100s ea	58016-0006-00	489.31		
(Stat Rx)				
REPACK				
TAB, PO (FILM-COATED)				
80 mg, 90s ea	16590-0726-90	442.00		AB
(Vibranta)				
REPACK				
TAB, PO, 20 mg, 30s ea	57866-3936-01	64.15		
40 mg, 30s ea	57866-3949-01	65.95		
SINA-12X (Meda)				
guaifenesin/phenylephrine tannate				
SUS, PO (GRAPE)				
100 mg/5 ml-5 mg/5 ml,				
118 ml	00037-6302-04	68.27		
TAB, PO, 200 mg-25 mg,				
30s ea	00037-6301-03	85.77		
SINCALIDE				
(Bracco Diag) *See KINEVAC*				
SINECATECHINS				
(Doak) *See VEREGEN*				
SINEMET 10-100 (Bristol-Myers)				
carbidopa/levodopa				
TAB, PO, 10 mg-100 mg,				
100s ea	00056-0647-68	103.39		AB
(Phys Total Care)				
REPACK				
TAB, PO, 10 mg-100 mg,				
100s ea	54868-1544-01	77.11		AB
SINEMET 25-100 (Bristol-Myers)				
carbidopa/levodopa				
TAB, PO, 25 mg-100 mg,				
100s ea	00056-0650-68	116.74		AB
(Phys Total Care)				
REPACK				
TAB, PO, 25 mg-100 mg,				
100s ea	54868-1270-01	91.06		AB
SINEMET 25-250 (Bristol-Myers)				
carbidopa/levodopa				
TAB, PO, 25 mg-250 mg,				
100s ea	00056-0654-68	148.75		AB
SINEMET CR (Bristol-Myers)				
carbidopa/levodopa				
TER, PO, 25 mg-100 mg,				
100s ea	00056-0601-68	130.56		AB
50 mg-200 mg,				
100s ea	00056-0521-68	251.53		AB
(Phys Total Care)				
REPACK				
TER, PO, 50 mg-200 mg,				
60s ea	54868-1882-01	143.16		AB
100s ea	54868-1882-00	204.54		AB
SINGULAIR (Merck)				
montelukast sodium				
CTB, PO (UNIT OF USE)				
4 mg, 30s ea	00006-0711-31	131.24		
90s ea	00006-0711-54	393.71		
(BLISTER PACK)				
4 mg, 100s ea UD	00006-0711-28	437.45		
(UNIT OF USE)				
5 mg, 30s ea	00006-0275-31	131.24		
90s ea	00006-0275-54	393.71		
100s ea UD	00006-0275-28	437.45		
1000s ea	00006-0275-82	4374.54		
PKT, PO, 4 mg/packet,				
30s ea UD	00006-3841-30	131.24		
TAB, PO (UNIT OF USE)				
10 mg, 30s ea	00006-0117-31	131.24		
90s ea	00006-0117-54	393.71		
100s ea UD	00006-0117-28	437.45		
(BULK PACKAGE)				
10 mg, 8000s ea	00006-0117-80	34996.08		
(A-S Medication)				
REPACK				
CTB, PO (UNIT OF USE)				
5 mg, 30s ea	54569-4736-00	170.61		
TAB, PO, 10 mg, 30s ea	54569-4605-00	170.61		
90s ea	54569-4605-01	511.82		
(Advanced Pharm Serv, Inc.)				
REPACK				
CTB, PO, 5 mg, 10s ea	13411-0160-01	47.74		
15s ea	13411-0160-15	71.61		
60s ea	13411-0160-06	286.44		
90s ea	13411-0160-09	429.64		
TAB, PO, 10 mg, 10s ea	13411-0151-01	47.74		
15s ea	13411-0151-15	56.76		
30s ea	13411-0151-03	143.22		
30s ea	13411-0160-03	143.22		
60s ea	13411-0151-06	286.44		
90s ea	13411-0151-09	429.66		
(AQ)				
REPACK				
TAB, PO, 10 mg, 20s ea	66105-0164-02	123.30		
30s ea	66105-0164-03	184.96		
60s ea	66105-0164-06	369.91		
90s ea	66105-0164-09	554.87		
100s ea	66105-0164-10	616.52		
(Bryant Ranch)				
REPACK				
TAB, PO, 10 mg, 30s ea	63629-1639-01	94.46		
(DHS, Inc.)				
REPACK				
CTB, PO, 5 mg, 90s ea	55887-0120-90	336.05		
(Direct Pharmaceutical, Inc.)				
REPACK				
TAB, PO, 10 mg,				
30s ea UD	67801-0305-03	155.43		
(Palmetto)				
REPACK				
TAB, PO, 10 mg, 30s ea	23490-8018-03	135.00		
(PD-Rx Pharm)				
REPACK				
CTB, PO, 4 mg, 21s ea	55289-0989-21	136.53		
30s ea	55289-0989-30	195.06		
5 mg, 21s ea	55289-0990-21	136.53		
30s ea	55289-0990-30	195.05		
(REDI-SCRIPT)				
5 mg, 30s ea	58864-0694-30	129.95		
TAB, PO, 10 mg, 15s ea	55289-0961-15	97.53		
30s ea	55289-0961-30	195.06		
(REDI-SCRIPT)				
10 mg, 30s ea	58864-0658-30	174.33		
(Phys Total Care)				
REPACK				
CTB, PO (UNIT OF USE)				
4 mg, 30s ea	54868-4630-00	157.33		
5 mg, 30s ea	54868-4847-00	157.33		
TAB, PO, 10 mg, 10s ea	54868-3283-00	57.45		
30s ea	54868-3283-01	157.33		
90s ea	54868-3283-02	468.07		
(Quality Care Prod)				
REPACK				
CTB, PO, 4 mg, 30s ea	49999-0952-30	182.60		
5 mg, 30s ea	49999-0884-30	184.30		
90s ea	49999-0884-90	565.56		
TAB, PO, 10 mg, 30s ea	49999-0533-30	182.40		
90s ea	49999-0533-90	551.30		
SINOGRAFIN (Bracco Diag)				
diatrizoate meglumine/iodipamide meglumine				
SOL, IV (VIAL)				
52.7%-26.8%,				
10 ml 10s	00270-0523-30	641.25	513.00	
SINUTUSS DM (Dexo)				
dm/gg/phenyleph hcl				
TER, PO, 30 mg-600 mg-15 mg,				
100s ea	59196-0045-01	62.40		
SINUVENT PE (Dexo)				
guaifenesin/phenylephrine hydrochloride				
TER, PO, 600 mg-15 mg,				
100s ea	59196-0035-01	48.50		
SIROLIMUS				
(Wyeth) *See RAPAMUNE*				
SITAGLIPTIN PHOSPHATE				
(Merck) *See JANUVIA*				
SITREX PD (Vindex Pharma Inc)				
guaifenesin/phenylephrine hydrochloride				
SOL, PO (AF,SF,DYE-FREE,PUNCH)				
75 mg/5 ml-7.5 mg/5 ml,				
473 ml	67204-0042-16	89.38		
SITZMARKS (Konsyl)				
polyvinyl chloride, radiopaque				
DEV, NA (GELCAP)				
10s ea	10858-0081-00	60.00		
SKELAXIN (King Pharm)				
metaxalone				
TAB, PO, 800 mg, 100s ea	60793-0136-01	415.34		
500s ea	60793-0136-05	2037.91		
(4u)				
REPACK				
TAB, PO, 800 mg, 30s ea	10544-0345-30	144.68		
30s ea	42549-0545-30	188.46		
(A-S Medication)				
REPACK				
TAB, PO, 800 mg, 7s ea	54569-5477-05	28.30		
10s ea	54569-5477-06	50.46		
15s ea	54569-5477-01	75.70		

PROD/MFR	NDC	AWP	DP	OBC
20s ea	**54569-5477-00**	100.93		
30s ea	**54569-5477-02**	151.39		
(Aidarex)				
REPACK				
TAB, PO, 800 mg, 14s ea	**33261-0531-14**	56.60		
30s ea	**33261-0531-30**	121.31		
60s ea	**33261-0531-60**	242.61		
90s ea	**33261-0531-90**	363.93		
(Altura)				
REPACK				
TAB, PO, 800 mg, 15s ea	**63874-1101-05**	56.40		
20s ea	**63874-1101-02**	75.20		
24s ea	**63874-1101-08**	90.24		
30s ea	**63874-1101-03**	133.44		
60s ea	**63874-1101-06**	266.87		
90s ea	**63874-1101-09**	400.31		
100s ea	**63874-1101-01**	307.27		
120s ea	**63874-1101-04**	451.20		
(Bryant Ranch)				
REPACK				
TAB, PO, 400 mg, 7s ea	**63629-1640-02**	9.65		
30s ea	**63629-1640-01**	27.79		
800 mg, 30s ea	**63629-2768-02**	175.10		
50s ea	**63629-2768-04**	292.13		
60s ea	**63629-2768-03**	348.20		
100s ea	**63629-2768-01**	570.00		
(Core)				
REPACK				
TAB, PO, 800 mg, 30s ea	**33358-0325-30**	94.48		
45s ea	**33358-0325-45**	182.60		
60s ea	**33358-0325-60**	193.90		
90s ea	**33358-0325-90**	283.87		
120s ea	**33358-0325-01**	377.96		
(DHS, Inc.)				
REPACK				
TAB, PO, 800 mg, 12s ea	**55887-0631-12**	43.20		
20s ea	**55887-0631-20**	72.00		
30s ea	**55887-0631-30**	84.67		
40s ea	**55887-0631-40**	124.76		
60s ea	**55887-0631-60**	169.34		
(Dispensing Solutions)				
REPACK				
TAB, PO, 800 mg, 16s ea	**55045-2972-05**	80.00		
20s ea	**55045-2972-07**	100.00		
20s ea	**66336-0709-20**	91.78		
24s ea	**55045-2972-06**	120.00		
30s ea	**55045-2972-08**	150.00		
30s ea	**66336-0709-30**	127.08		
60s ea	**55045-2972-04**	300.00		
60s ea	**66336-0709-60**	245.86		
90s ea	**66336-0709-90**	436.50		
100s ea	**55045-2972-00**	500.00		
(HomeMed)				
REPACK				
TAB, PO, 800 mg, 10s ea	**51655-0240-53**	24.66		
(IPI)				
REPACK				
TAB, PO, 800 mg, 30s ea	**18837-0144-30**	116.19		
60s ea	**18837-0144-60**	232.37		
270s ea	**18837-0144-94**	1055.21		
(Keltman Pharma., Inc.)				
REPACK				
TAB, PO, 800 mg, 60s ea	**68387-0108-60**	232.90		
(LWP)				
REPACK				
TAB, PO, 400 mg, 40s ea	**64038-0121-40**	66.34		
60s ea	**64038-0121-60**	97.01		
100s ea	**64038-0121-01**	158.35		
(Nucare Pharm)				
REPACK				
TAB, PO, 800 mg, 8s ea	**66267-0611-08**	63.36		
15s ea	**66267-0611-15**	118.96		
20s ea	**66267-0611-20**	152.96		
21s ea	**66267-0611-21**	161.39		
30s ea	**66267-0611-30**	230.40		
30s ea	**68071-0611-30**	175.00		
42s ea	**66267-0611-42**	332.64		
45s ea	**66267-0611-45**	356.40		
60s ea	**66267-0611-60**	475.20		
90s ea	**66267-0611-90**	691.20		
100s ea	**68071-1352-00**	791.39		
112s ea	**66267-0611-78**	866.66		
120s ea	**66267-0611-91**	915.60		
(PD-Rx Pharm)				
REPACK				
TAB, PO, 800 mg, 10s ea	**55289-0736-10**	76.92		
15s ea	**55289-0736-15**	115.40		
20s ea	**55289-0736-20**	153.86		

PROD/MFR	NDC	AWP	DP	OBC
(REDI-SCRIPT)				
800 mg, 20s ea	**58864-0846-20**	117.28		
21s ea	**55289-0736-21**	161.54		
30s ea	**55289-0736-30**	230.78		
40s ea	**58864-0846-40**	179.11		
(Pharma Pac)				
REPACK				
TAB, PO, 800 mg, 14s ea	**52959-0709-14**	84.10		
15s ea	**52959-0709-15**	90.00		
20s ea	**52959-0709-20**	119.90		
21s ea	**52959-0709-21**	125.85		
28s ea	**52959-0709-28**	167.75		
30s ea	**52959-0709-30**	179.70		
40s ea	**52959-0709-40**	239.40		
42s ea	**52959-0709-42**	251.25		
45s ea	**52959-0709-45**	269.15		
50s ea	**52959-0709-50**	299.00		
56s ea	**52959-0709-56**	334.85		
60s ea	**52959-0709-60**	349.90		
90s ea	**52959-0709-90**	519.90		
100s ea	**52959-0709-00**	567.95		
(Phys Total Care)				
REPACK				
TAB, PO, 400 mg, 30s ea	**54868-2956-03**	55.73		
40s ea	**54868-2956-00**	73.90		
60s ea	**54868-2956-04**	110.23		
90s ea	**54868-2956-01**	164.73		
100s ea	**54868-2956-05**	182.27		
800 mg, 10s ea	**54868-4733-01**	51.27		
15s ea	**54868-4733-00**	75.59		
30s ea	**54868-4733-04**	148.58		
40s ea	**54868-4733-07**	186.42		
50s ea	**54868-4733-03**	232.37		
60s ea	**54868-4733-06**	278.32		
90s ea	**54868-4733-02**	416.17		
100s ea	**54868-4733-05**	446.64		
120s ea	**54868-4733-08**	554.02		
(Physician Partner)				
REPACK				
TAB, PO, 800 mg, 15s ea	**21695-0123-15**	140.04		
16s ea	**21695-0123-16**	128.13		
30s ea	**21695-0123-30**	238.07		
60s ea	**21695-0123-60**	476.15		
90s ea	**21695-0123-90**	714.22		
(Quality Care Prod)				
REPACK				
TAB, PO, 400 mg, 20s ea	**49999-0070-20**	52.20		
30s ea	**49999-0070-30**	82.80		
40s ea	**49999-0070-40**	60.15		
42s ea	**49999-0070-42**	100.02		
60s ea	**49999-0070-60**	165.60		
800 mg, ea	**49999-0363-00**	480.00		
15s ea	**49999-0363-15**	120.00		
16s ea	**49999-0363-16**	121.07		
20s ea	**49999-0363-20**	154.00		
30s ea	**49999-0363-30**	227.00		
90s ea	**49999-0363-90**	720.00		
120s ea	**49999-0363-01**	960.00		
180s ea	**49999-0363-18**	1440.00		
(Southwood)				
REPACK				
TAB, PO, 400 mg, 10s ea	**58016-0682-10**	12.97		
12s ea	**58016-0682-12**	15.56		
14s ea	**58016-0682-14**	7.35		
15s ea	**58016-0682-15**	19.46		
20s ea	**58016-0682-20**	25.94		
28s ea	**58016-0682-28**	36.32		
30s ea	**58016-0682-30**	38.91		
40s ea	**58016-0682-40**	51.88		
42s ea	**58016-0682-42**	54.47		
50s ea	**58016-0682-50**	64.85		
60s ea	**58016-0682-60**	77.82		
90s ea	**58016-0682-90**	116.73		
100s ea	**58016-0682-00**	129.70		
800 mg, 30s ea	**58016-0927-30**	106.84		
60s ea	**58016-0927-60**	213.67		
90s ea	**58016-0927-90**	320.51		
100s ea	**58016-0927-00**	356.12		
120s ea	**58016-0927-02**	427.34		
150s ea	**58016-0927-03**	534.18		
200s ea	**58016-0927-89**	712.24		
300s ea	**58016-0927-73**	1068.36		
300s ea	**58016-0927-77**	651.75		
(St. Mary's MPP)				
REPACK				
TAB, PO, 800 mg, 6s ea	**60760-0136-06**	31.14		
20s ea	**60760-0136-20**	89.80		
30s ea	**60760-0136-30**	177.41		
60s ea	**60760-0136-60**	348.83		
90s ea	**60760-0136-90**	520.24		

PROD/MFR	NDC	AWP	DP	OBC
(Stat Rx)				
REPACK				
TAB, PO, 800 mg, 20s ea	**16590-0207-20**	91.18		
28s ea	**16590-0207-28**	127.65		
30s ea	**16590-0207-30**	179.01		
40s ea	**16590-0207-40**	183.47		
56s ea	**16590-0207-56**	256.85		
60s ea	**16590-0207-60**	275.20		
84s ea	**16590-0207-62**	385.28		
90s ea	**16590-0207-90**	439.56		
100s ea	**16590-0207-71**	451.95		
120s ea	**16590-0207-72**	550.40		
SKELID (Sanofi-Aventis)				
tiludronate disodium				
TAB, PO, 200 mg, 56s ea	**00024-1800-16**	642.17		
SKIN SOFT FRAGRANCE (PCCA)				
fragrance				
SOL, NA, 1 ml	**51927-2430-00**	1.20		
SKIN TEST ANTIGENS, MULTIPLE				
(Allerderm Labs.) *See T.R.U.E. TEST*				
SLIPPERY ELM BARK				
(PCCA) *See ELM BARK*				
SMZ-TMP (Amneal)				
sulfamethoxazole/trimethoprim				
TAB, PO, 400 mg-80 mg,				
100s ea	**53746-0271-01**	66.45		AB
500s ea	**53746-0271-05**	299.03		AB
(Hi-Tech)				
SUS, PO, 200 mg/5 ml-40 mg/5 ml,				
473 ml	**50383-0824-16**	58.10		AB
(CHERRY)				
200 mg/5 ml-40 mg/5 ml,				
473 ml	**50383-0823-16**	58.10		AB
(Mutual)				
TAB, PO, 400 mg-80 mg,				
100s ea	**53489-0145-01**	66.45		AB
500s ea	**53489-0145-05**	299.03		AB
800 mg-160 mg,				
100s ea	**53489-0146-01**	109.02		AB
500s ea	**53489-0146-05**	426.53		AB
(Teva)				
SOL, IV (M.D.V.)				
80 mg/ml-16 mg/ml,				
30 ml	**00703-9526-01**	10.98		AP
(A-S Medication)				
REPACK				
SUS, PO (CHERRY)				
200 mg/5 ml-40 mg/5 ml,				
480 ml	**54569-4003-00**	58.96		EE
(Altura)				
REPACK				
TAB, PO, 800 mg-160 mg,				
6s ea	**63874-0118-06**	7.49		EE
7s ea	**63874-0118-07**	9.71		EE
10s ea	**63874-0118-10**	12.48		EE
12s ea	**63874-0118-12**	16.14		EE
14s ea	**63874-0118-14**	17.68		EE
15s ea	**63874-0118-15**	20.18		EE
18s ea	**63874-0118-18**	24.22		EE
20s ea	**63874-0118-20**	26.92		EE
21s ea	**63874-0118-21**	28.26		EE
24s ea	**63874-0118-24**	32.30		EE
28s ea	**63874-0118-28**	37.69		EE
30s ea	**63874-0118-30**	40.38		EE
40s ea	**63874-0118-40**	53.85		EE
50s ea	**63874-0118-50**	67.30		EE
60s ea	**63874-0118-60**	80.79		EE
100s ea	**63874-0118-01**	134.66		EE
500s ea	**63874-0118-03**	250.90		EE
(American Health)				
REPACK				
TAB, PO (DOUBLE STRENGTH,10X10)				
800 mg-160 mg,				
100s ea UD	**68084-0230-01**	29.40		AB
(DHS, Inc.)				
REPACK				
TAB, PO, 400 mg-80 mg,				
20s ea	**55887-0263-20**	24.00		AB
30s ea	**55887-0263-30**	36.00		AB
800 mg-160 mg,				
15s ea	**55887-0983-15**	58.50		AB
(Dispensing Solutions)				
REPACK				
TAB, PO, 400 mg-80 mg,				
14s ea	**55045-1514-06**	10.78		
800 mg-160 mg,				
10s ea	**55045-1210-03**	15.00		AB
14s ea	**55045-1210-05**	21.00		AB

PROD/MFR	NDC	AWP	DP	OBC
15s ea	55045-3385-05	22.50		AB
20s ea	55045-1210-07	30.00		AB
20s ea	55045-3914-02	30.00		AB
28s ea	55045-1210-08	42.00		AB
30s ea	55045-1210-06	45.00		AB
42s ea	55045-1210-09	63.00		AB
50s ea	55045-3288-05	75.00		AB
80s ea	55045-3288-08	120.00		AB
90s ea	55045-1210-01	135.00		AB
100s ea	55045-1210-00	150.00		AB
120s ea	55045-3288-02	180.00		AB
(Keltman Pharma., Inc.) REPACK				
TAB, PO, 800 mg-160 mg,				
20s ea	68387-0385-20	40.06		AB
30s ea	68387-0385-30	60.09		AB
(McKesson Packaging) REPACK				
TAB, PO, 800 mg-160 mg,				
100s ea UD	63739-0228-10	37.08		AB
(Nucare Pharm) REPACK				
TAB, PO, 800 mg-160 mg,				
6s ea	66267-0196-06	21.83		AB
10s ea	66267-0196-10	36.38		AB
14s ea	66267-0196-14	50.94		AB
20s ea	66267-0196-20	77.06		AB
28s ea	66267-0196-28	101.86		AB
30s ea	66267-0196-30	109.14		AB
60s ea	66267-0196-60	218.30		AB
(PD-Rx Pharm) REPACK				
TAB, PO, 400 mg-80 mg,				
10s ea	55289-0457-10	14.67		AB
20s ea	55289-0457-20	16.74		AB
800 mg-160 mg,				
2s ea	43063-0024-02	14.10		AB
4s ea	43063-0024-04	14.85		AB
6s ea	43063-0024-06	16.05		AB
(REDI-SCRIPT) 800 mg-160 mg,				
6s ea	58864-0478-06	16.05		
30s ea	58864-0478-30	20.10		AB
(Phys Total Care) REPACK				
TAB, PO, 400 mg-80 mg,				
30s ea	54868-4711-00	12.24		AB
(Physician Partner) REPACK				
TAB, PO, 800 mg-160 mg,				
10s ea	21695-0125-10	25.65		AB
28s ea	21695-0125-28	71.82		AB
(Quality Care Prod) REPACK				
TAB, PO, 400 mg-80 mg,				
20s ea	49999-0503-20	7.46		AB
800 mg-160 mg,				
28s ea	49999-0077-28	49.80		AB
30s ea	49999-0077-30	53.36		AB
60s ea	49999-0077-60	106.72		AB
90s ea	49999-0077-90	160.08		AB
(Southwood) REPACK				
TAB, PO, 400 mg-80 mg,				
20s ea	58016-0171-20	6.22		EE
30s ea	58016-0171-30	7.12		EE
(Vibranta) REPACK				
TAB, PO, 800 mg-160 mg,				
14s ea	57866-4693-04	18.86		
20s ea	57866-4693-02	26.94		
28s ea	57866-4693-01	38.04		
SMZ-TMP CONCENTRATE (Teva)				
sulfamethoxazole/trimethoprim				
SOL, IV (S.D.V.) 80 mg/ml-16 mg/ml,				
5 ml 10s	00703-9503-03	42.16		AP
(M.D.V.) 80 mg/ml-16 mg/ml,				
10 ml 10s	00703-9514-03	53.56		AP
SMZ-TMP DS (Amneal)				
sulfamethoxazole/trimethoprim				
TAB, PO, 800 mg-160 mg,				
100s ea	53746-0272-01	115.40		AB
500s ea	53746-0272-05	454.60		AB
(Major)				
TAB, PO, 800 mg-160 mg,				
100s ea	00904-2725-60	108.49		AB
(10X10) 800 mg-160 mg,				
100s ea UD	00904-2725-61	114.20		AB
500s ea	00904-2725-40	424.39		AB
(Sandoz)				
TAB, PO, 800 mg-160 mg,				
100s ea	00185-0112-01	144.12		AB
500s ea	00185-0112-05	451.62		AB
(UDL)				
TAB, PO (10X10) 800 mg-160 mg,				
100s ea UD	51079-0128-20	146.40		AB
(A-S Medication) REPACK				
TAB, PO, 800 mg-160 mg,				
4s ea	54569-0075-09	5.03		AB
6s ea	54569-0075-07	7.55		AB
10s ea	54569-0075-00	12.58		AB
14s ea	54569-0075-01	17.61		AB
20s ea	54569-0075-02	25.16		AB
28s ea	54569-0075-03	35.23		AB
40s ea	54569-5813-00	50.32		AB
100s ea	54569-0075-05	125.81		AB
(DHS, Inc.) REPACK				
TAB, PO, 800 mg-160 mg,				
6s ea	55887-0983-06	25.44		AB
10s ea	55887-0983-10	41.70		AB
14s ea	55887-0983-14	55.50		AB
20s ea	55887-0983-20	81.36		AB
28s ea	55887-0983-28	91.00		AB
30s ea	55887-0983-30	114.21		AB
(Dispensing Solutions) REPACK				
TAB, PO, 800 mg-160 mg,				
6s ea	55045-1210-02	9.00		
6s ea	66336-0087-06	8.40		AB
10s ea	66336-0087-10	13.63		AB
14s ea	66336-0087-14	18.86		AB
20s ea	66336-0087-20	27.76		AB
40s ea	66336-0087-40	52.88		AB
60s ea	55045-1210-04	90.00		
(GSMS) REPACK				
TAB, PO (UNIT OF USE) 800 mg-160 mg,				
14s ea	60429-0170-14	15.00	5.00	AB
20s ea	60429-0170-20	18.00	6.00	AB
(HomeMed) REPACK				
TAB, PO, 800 mg-160 mg,				
2s ea	51655-0112-31	2.88		EE
6s ea	51655-0112-87	8.65		EE
10s ea	51655-0112-53	13.88		EE
14s ea	51655-0112-84	16.75		EE
20s ea	51655-0112-52	22.55		EE
28s ea	51655-0112-29	34.25		EE
30s ea	51655-0112-24	26.85		EE
40s ea	51655-0112-51	55.51		EE
60s ea	51655-0112-25	83.27		EE
(PD-Rx Pharm) REPACK				
TAB, PO, 800 mg-160 mg,				
2s ea	55289-0241-02	14.10		AB
4s ea	55289-0241-04	14.85		AB
6s ea	55289-0241-06	16.05		AB
10s ea	55289-0241-10	19.50		AB
(REDI-SCRIPT) 800 mg-160 mg,				
10s ea	58864-0478-10	19.50		AB
14s ea	55289-0241-14	22.14		AB
(REDI-SCRIPT) 800 mg-160 mg,				
14s ea	58864-0478-14	22.14		AB
15s ea	55289-0241-15	23.07		AB
20s ea	55289-0241-20	27.75		AB
(REDI-SCRIPT) 800 mg-160 mg,				
20s ea	58864-0478-20	27.75		AB
28s ea	55289-0241-28	37.08		AB
40s ea	55289-0241-40	46.68		AB
60s ea	55289-0241-60	71.85		AB
100s ea UD	55289-0241-17	41.77		AB
(Pharma Pac) REPACK				
TAB, PO, 800 mg-160 mg,				
6s ea	52959-0144-06	14.05		EE
10s ea	52959-0144-10	23.40		EE
14s ea	52959-0144-14	32.69		EE
15s ea	52959-0144-15	35.01		EE
20s ea	52959-0144-20	46.65		EE
21s ea	52959-0144-21	48.96		EE
28s ea	52959-0144-28	65.27		EE
30s ea	52959-0144-30	69.87		EE
40s ea	52959-0144-40	93.12		EE
60s ea	52959-0144-60	139.62		EE
100s ea	52959-0144-00	255.00		EE
(Phys Total Care) REPACK				
TAB, PO, 800 mg-160 mg,				
10s ea	54868-0021-06	7.86		EE
14s ea	54868-0021-02	18.60		EE
15s ea	54868-0021-05	19.71		EE
20s ea	54868-0021-01	25.29		EE
30s ea	54868-0021-07	36.44		EE
60s ea	54868-0021-04	69.87		EE
100s ea	54868-0021-00	86.73		EE
500s ea	54868-0021-09	406.32		EE
(Quality Care Prod) REPACK				
TAB, PO, 800 mg-160 mg,				
6s ea	49999-0077-06	8.28		AB
10s ea	49999-0077-10	17.78		EE
14s ea	49999-0077-14	19.31		EE
20s ea	49999-0077-20	35.57		EE
(Southwood) REPACK				
TAB, PO, 800 mg-160 mg,				
6s ea	58016-0109-06	8.33		EE
7s ea	58016-0109-07	9.71		EE
10s ea	58016-0109-10	13.88		EE
12s ea	58016-0109-12	16.16		EE
14s ea	58016-0109-14	19.43		EE
15s ea	58016-0109-15	20.20		EE
18s ea	58016-0109-18	24.98		EE
20s ea	58016-0109-20	27.76		EE
21s ea	58016-0109-21	29.14		EE
24s ea	58016-0109-24	33.31		EE
28s ea	58016-0109-28	38.86		EE
30s ea	58016-0109-30	41.63		EE
40s ea	58016-0109-40	55.51		EE
50s ea	58016-0109-50	69.39		EE
60s ea	58016-0109-60	83.27		EE
80s ea	58016-0109-80	111.02		EE
90s ea	58016-0109-90	124.90		EE
100s ea	58016-0109-00	138.78		EE
120s ea	58016-0109-02	166.54		EE
150s ea	58016-0109-03	208.17		EE
200s ea	58016-0109-89	277.56		EE
300s ea	58016-0109-73	416.34		EE
(Stat Rx) REPACK				
TAB, PO, 800 mg-160 mg,				
10s ea	16590-0210-10	11.30		AB
SMZ-TMP PEDIATRIC (Pharma Pac) REPACK				
sulfamethoxazole/trimethoprim				
SUS, PO, 200 mg/5 ml-40 mg/5 ml,				
100 ml	52959-0766-05	20.35		
120 ml	52959-0766-07	23.48		
200 ml	52959-0766-03	28.99		
(Phys Total Care) REPACK				
SUS, PO, 200 mg/5 ml-40 mg/5 ml,				
100 ml	54868-0276-01	76.50		EE
(Southwood) REPACK				
SUS, PO, 200 mg/5 ml-40 mg/5 ml,				
50 ml	58016-0164-10	3.35		EE
100 ml	58016-0164-20	5.60		EE
100 ml	58016-1035-01	15.75		EE
120 ml	58016-0164-24	6.73		EE
150 ml	58016-0164-30	7.59		EE
180 ml	58016-0164-36	8.37		EE
200 ml	58016-0164-40	8.74		EE
240 ml	58016-0164-48	9.44		EE
SODA LIME INDICATING TYPE (Baker, J.T.)				
calcium oxide/sodium hydroxide				
POW, NA (4-8 MESH,A.C.S.,REAGENT)				
500 gm	10106-3448-01	44.19		
2500 gm	10106-3448-05	137.76		
SODIUM (Baker, J.T.)				
LUM, NA (A.C.S., REAGENT)				
100 gm	10106-9410-04	89.61		
500 gm	10106-9410-01	98.62		
(PURIFIED)				
2300 gm	10106-9412-05	242.05		

PROD/MFR | NDC | AWP | DP | OBC

SODIUM ACETATE
(Amend) *See SODIUM ACETATE TRIHYDRATE*

(Amer Regent)
SOL, IV (S.D.V.)
2 meq/ml,
20 ml 25s.......... **00517-2096-25** 59.69
(BULK PACKAGE,PF)
2 meq/ml,
100 ml 25s **00517-2500-25** 156.25
(S.D.V.,PF)
4 meq/ml,
50 ml 25s.......... **00517-5023-25** 117.19

(APP)
SOL, IV (MAXIVIAL,BULK PACK,PF)
4 meq/ml, 100 ml **63323-0032-61** 14.63

(Baker, J.T.) *See SODIUM ACETATE ANHYDROUS*

(Baker, J.T.) *See SODIUM ACETATE TRIHYDRATE*

(Baxter)
SOL, IV ((BULK PACKAGE),USP)
2 meq/ml,
250 ml 12s **00338-0875-02** 144.00 120.00

(Gallipot)
POW, NA (U.S.P.,TRIHYDRATE)
500 gm............. **51552-0752-06** 14.56 10.40

(Gallipot) *See SODIUM ACETATE ANHYDROUS*

(Hospira)
SOL, IV (VIAL,FLIPTOP)
2 meq/ml,
20 ml 25s.......... **00409-7299-73** 18.30 16.00
(VIAL,FLIPTOP,BULK)
2 meq/ml,
50 ml 25s.......... **00409-3299-05** 45.90 40.25
(VIAL, FLIPTOP)
2 meq/ml,
100 ml 25s **00409-3299-06** 70.50 61.75

(Mallinckrodt Lab) *See SODIUM ACETATE TRIHYDRATE*

(PCCA)
POW, NA (USP;TRIHYDRATE)
1 gm............... **51927-1531-00** 0.10

(Spectrum Pharmacy) *See SODIUM ACETATE ANHYDROUS*

(Spectrum Pharmacy) *See SODIUM ACETATE TRIHYDRATE*

SODIUM ACETATE ANHYDROUS (Baker, J.T.)
sodium acetate
POW, NA (A.C.S., REAGENT)
500 gm............. **10106-3470-01** 73.23
(PURIFIED)
500 gm............. **10106-3472-01** 60.51
2000 gm............ **10106-3472-05** 182.26
(A.C.S., REAGENT)
2500 gm............ **10106-3470-05** 277.33
(U.S.P., F.C.C., A.C.S.)
2500 gm............ **10106-3473-05** 183.27

(Gallipot)
POW, NA (U.S.P.)
454 gm............. **51552-0633-06** 13.51

(Spectrum Pharmacy)
POW, NA (U.S.P.)
500 gm............. **49452-6550-01** 71.40

SODIUM ACETATE TRIHYDRATE (Amend)
sodium acetate
POW, NA (U.S.P.)
454 gm............. **17317-0492-01** 9.80
2270 gm............ **17317-0492-05** 39.20
11350 gm **17317-0492-08** 113.75

(Baker, J.T.)
CRY, NA (U.S.P., F.C.C., A.C.S.)
500 gm............. **10106-3462-01** 17.90
2500 gm............ **10106-3462-05** 89.13

(Mallinckrodt Lab)
GRA, NA (U.S.P.)
500 gm............. **00406-7356-01** 13.16

(Spectrum Pharmacy)
GRA, NA (U.S.P.)
500 gm............. **49452-6560-01** 71.40

SODIUM ACID PYROPHOSPHATE
(Spectrum Pharmacy)
sodium pyrophosphate
POW, NA (F.C.C.)
500 gm............. **49452-6568-01** 135.80
2500 gm............ **49452-6568-02** 271.25

SODIUM ALGINATE (Amend)
POW, NA (FOOD GRADE)
454 gm............. **17317-0493-01** 21.00
2270 gm............ **17317-0493-05** 84.00
11350 gm **17317-0493-08** 297.50

(Gallipot)
POW, NA, 454 gm........ **51552-0623-06** 24.85

(Medisca)
POW, NA (1X100GM)
100 gm............. **38779-1598-05** 31.50
(1X500GM)
500 gm............. **38779-1598-08** 67.50
(1X2500GM)
2500 gm............ **38779-1598-01** 211.50

(PCCA)
POW, NA (1X1GM)
1 gm............... **51927-3629-00** 1.17
(FOOD GRADE)
1 gm............... **51927-1102-00** 0.45

(Spectrum Pharmacy)
POW, NA (F.C.C.)
500 gm............. **49452-6570-01** 139.30
(N.F.)
500 gm............. **49452-6569-01** 139.30
(F.C.C.)
2500 gm............ **49452-6570-02** 539.00
(N.F.)
2500 gm............ **49452-6569-02** 539.00

SODIUM ALUMINUM PHOSPHATE
(Spectrum Pharmacy) *See SODIUM ALUMINUM PHOSPHATE ACIDIC*

(Spectrum Pharmacy) *See SODIUM ALUMINUM PHOSPHATE BASIC*

SODIUM ALUMINUM PHOSPHATE ACIDIC (Spectrum Pharmacy)
sodium aluminum phosphate
POW, NA (F.C.C.)
500 gm............. **49452-6572-01** 143.85
2500 gm............ **49452-6572-02** 353.50

SODIUM ALUMINUM PHOSPHATE BASIC (Spectrum Pharmacy)
sodium aluminum phosphate
POW, NA, 500 gm........ **49452-6571-01** 143.85
(F.C.C.)
2500 gm............ **49452-6571-02** 353.50

SODIUM AMMONIUM PHOSPHATE
(Baker, J.T.) *See SODIUM AMMONIUM PHOSPHATE 4-HYDRATE*

SODIUM AMMONIUM PHOSPHATE 4-HYDRATE
(Baker, J.T.)
sodium ammonium phosphate
CRY, NA (REAGENT)
500 gm............. **10106-3478-01** 48.56
2500 gm............ **10106-3478-05** 167.27

SODIUM ARSENATE
(Baker, J.T.) *See SODIUM ARSENATE DIBASIC 7-HYDRATE*

SODIUM ARSENATE DIBASIC 7-HYDRATE
(Baker, J.T.)
sodium arsenate
GRA, NA (A.C.S., REAGENT)
125 gm............. **10106-3486-04** 80.80
500 gm............. **10106-3486-01** 126.64

SODIUM ARSENITE
(Baker, J.T.) *See SODIUM META-ARSENITE*

SODIUM ASCORBATE (Amend)
POW, NA (U.S.P., FINE)
125 gm............. **17317-0494-04** 9.80
500 gm............. **17317-0494-05** 35.00
2000 gm............ **17317-0494-02** 117.60

(Gallipot)
POW, NA (U.S.P.)
100 gm............. **51552-0337-05** 13.02

(PCCA)
POW, NA (USP)
1 gm............... **51927-1238-00** 0.33

(Spectrum Pharmacy)
GRA, NA (U.S.P.)
100 gm............. **49452-6580-03** 69.13
500 gm............. **49452-6580-01** 183.75
5000 gm............ **49452-6580-02** 1172.50
POW, NA, 100 gm........ **49452-7398-01** 64.75
500 gm............. **49452-7398-02** 154.70
5000 gm............ **49452-7398-03** 1022.00

SODIUM ASCORBYL PHOSPHATE
(PCCA) *See SODIUM-L-ASCORBYL-2-PHOSPHATE*

SODIUM BENZOATE (Baker, J.T.)
POW, NA (N.F., F.C.C.)
500 gm............. **10106-3500-01** 22.26
2500 gm............ **10106-3500-05** 163.32

(Gallipot)
POW, NA (U.S.P.,N.F.)
454 gm............. **51552-0221-06** 11.62

(Letco)
POW, NA (U.S.P./N.F.)
500 gm............. **62991-1381-01** 29.25
1000 gm............ **62991-1381-04** 39.00
(U.S.P./N.F.)
2500 gm............ **62991-1381-02** 75.00

(Mallinckrodt Lab)
POW, NA (N.F.)
500 gm............. **00406-0168-04** 40.97
2500 gm............ **00406-0168-05** 189.94

(Medisca)
POW, NA (N.F.)
500 gm............. **38779-0551-08** 31.50
1000 gm............ **38779-0551-09** 55.95
(1X5000GM)
5000 gm............ **38779-0551-03** 251.85

(PCCA)
POW, NA (N.F.)
1 gm............... **51927-1234-00** 0.23

(Spectrum Pharmacy)
POW, NA (N.F.)
500 gm............. **49452-6595-01** 61.25
2500 gm............ **49452-6595-02** 232.05
12000 gm **49452-6595-03** 672.00

SODIUM BENZOATE/SODIUM PHENYLACETATE
(Ucyclyd) *See AMMONUL*

SODIUM BICARBONATE (Amer Regent)
SOL, IV (S.D.V.,PF)
7.5%, 50 ml 25s **00517-0639-25** 54.69
8.4%, 50 ml 25s **00517-1550-25** 57.19

(Amphastar)
SOL, IV (SRN,PREFILLED,LUER-JET)
4.2%, 10 ml 10s **00548-3331-00** 53.20
8.4%, 50 ml 10s **00548-3352-00** 53.20
(MIN-I-JET,18GX1 1/2")
8.4%, 50 ml 25s **00548-1052-00** 205.82
(SRN,PREFILLED,STICKGARD)
8.4%, 50 ml 25s **00548-2052-00** 215.79

(APP)
SOL, IV (S.D.V.,PF)
4.2%, 5 ml........... **63323-0026-05** 3.33

(Baker, J.T.)
POW, NA (A.C.S., REAGENT)
500 gm............. **10106-3506-01** 25.75
(U.S.P., F.C.C.)
500 gm............. **10106-3509-01** 24.01
(A.C.S., REAGENT)
2500 gm............ **10106-3506-05** 60.41
(U.S.P., F.C.C.)
2500 gm............ **10106-3509-05** 37.84
(A.C.S., REAGENT)
12000 gm **10106-3506-07** 128.34

(Baxter)
SOL, IV, 5%, 500 ml 12s .. **00338-0374-03** 470.74

(Claris)
SOL, IV (12X250ML,SINGLEDOSE,USP)
8.4%, 250 ml 12s **36000-0027-12** 105.00
(12X500ML,SINGLEDOSE,USP)
8.4%, 500 ml 12s **36000-0026-12** 180.00

(Cura Pharm)
SOL, IV, 8.4%, 500 ml 10s. **66860-0120-02** 400.00

(Gallipot)
POW, NA, 454 gm........ **51552-0059-06** 8.75
2270 gm............ **51552-0059-09** 21.77

(Hospira) *See NEUT*

(Hospira)
SOL, IV (INFANT LS,LATEX-FREE)
4.2%, 10 ml 10s **00074-5534-34** 30.00 26.30
10 ml 10s.......... **00409-5534-34** 30.00 26.30
(12X500ML)
5%, 500 ml 12s **00409-1594-03** 111.74 97.80
(10X50ML,SINGLE-DOSE)
7.5%, 50 ml 10s **00409-4916-34** 42.96 37.60
(LIFESHIELD,LATEX-FREE)
7.5%, 50 ml 10s **00074-4916-34** 41.52 36.30
(USP,10X50ML,SINGLE-DOSE)
7.5%, 50 ml 10s **00409-3486-16** 35.64 31.20
(10X10ML,ABBOJECT)
8.4%, 10 ml 10s **00409-4900-34** 53.04 46.40

PROD/MFR	NDC	AWP	DP	OBC
(INFANT LS,LATEX-FREE)				
8.4%, 10 ml 10s	00074-4900-34	53.04	46.40	
(LIFESHEILD,ABBOJECT)				
8.4%, 50 ml 10s	00409-6637-34	30.12	26.40	
(LIFESHIELD,LATEX-FREE)				
8.4%, 50 ml 10s	00074-6637-34	30.12	26.40	
(USP,10X50ML,SINGLE-DOSE)				
8.4%, 50 ml 10s	00409-3495-16	31.20	27.30	
(VIAL,FLIPTOP,LATEX-FREE)				
8.4%, 50 ml 25s	00409-6625-02	25.80	22.50	
(Mallinckrodt Lab)				
POW, NA (U.S.P.)				
500 gm	00406-7396-04	22.43		
(Medisca)				
POW, NA (U.S.P.)				
500 gm	38779-0640-08	28.50		
(1X1000GM,USP)				
1000 gm	38779-0640-09	51.00		
(U.S.P.)				
2500 gm	38779-0640-01	57.75		
(PCCA)				
POW, NA (USP)				
1 gm	51927-1088-00	0.06		
(Spectrum Pharmacy)				
POW, NA (U.S.P.,E.P.,B.P.,J.P.)				
500 gm	49452-6610-01	49.00		
2500 gm	49452-6610-02	92.75		
12000 gm	49452-6610-03	364.00		
(DHS, Inc.)				
REPACK				
TAB, PO, 650 mg, 15s ea	55887-0161-15	5.25		
30s ea	55887-0161-30	7.00		
45s ea	55887-0161-45	10.49		
60s ea	55887-0161-60	13.98		
(Phys Total Care)				
REPACK				
SOL, IV (S.D.V.,25X5ML)				
4.2%, 5 ml 25s	54868-5723-00	182.97		
(SDV,25X50ML)				
8.4%, 50 ml 25s	54868-2061-00	84.93		
SODIUM BIPHOSPHATE (Amend)				
sodium phosphate				
GRA, NA (U.S.P., F.C.C.)				
454 gm	17317-0498-01	14.00		
(U.S.P./F.C.C.)				
2270 gm	17317-0498-05	56.00		
11350 gm	17317-0498-08	253.75		
SODIUM BISULFATE				
(Baker, J.T.) *See SODIUM BISULFATE MONOHYDRATE*				
(Mallinckrodt Lab) *See SODIUM BISULFATE MONOHYDRATE*				
(PCCA)				
POW, NA (PURIFIED)				
1 gm	51927-1849-00	0.54		
SODIUM BISULFATE MONOHYDRATE (Baker, J.T.)				
sodium bisulfate				
CRY, NA (REAGENT)				
500 gm	10106-3534-01	74.78		
2500 gm	10106-3534-05	259.51		
(Mallinckrodt Lab)				
CRY, NA, 500 gm	00406-7432-12	65.01		
SODIUM BISULFITE (Amend)				
GRA, NA (F.C.C.)				
454 gm	17317-0499-01	8.40		
(A.C.S., REAGENT)				
500 gm	17317-1878-01	12.60		
(F.C.C.)				
2270 gm	17317-0499-05	33.60		
(A.C.S., REAGENT)				
2500 gm	17317-1878-05	50.40		
(F.C.C.)				
11350 gm	17317-0499-08	105.00		
(Baker, J.T.)				
GRA, NA (DRIED, PURIFIED)				
500 gm	10106-3557-01	23.18		
(Gallipot)				
GRA, NA (F.C.C.)				
454 gm	51552-0448-06	12.46		
(Mallinckrodt Lab)				
GRA, NA (PURIFIED)				
500 gm	00406-7444-03	22.03		
(PCCA)				
POW, NA (F.C.C.)				
1 gm	51927-1674-00	0.11		
(Spectrum Pharmacy)				
GRA, NA (F.C.C.)				
500 gm	49452-6620-01	64.75		
2500 gm	49452-6620-02	148.05		
12000 gm	49452-6620-03	574.00		
SODIUM BORATE (Amend)				
POW, NA (N.F.)				
500 gm	17317-0500-01	8.40		
2270 gm	17317-0500-05	33.60		
11350 gm	17317-0500-08	122.50		
(Baker, J.T.) *See SODIUM BORATE DECAHYDRATE*				
(Gallipot) *See BORAX*				
(Gallipot)				
POW, NA (REAGENT)				
454 gm	51552-0467-06	34.65		
(1X500GM)				
500 gm	51552-0908-06	9.94	7.10	
(1X1000GM)				
1000 gm	51552-0908-07	18.20	13.00	
(Medisca)				
POW, NA (N.F.)				
500 gm	38779-0617-08	37.50		
(1X1000GM,NF)				
1000 gm	38779-0617-09	46.50		
(N.F.)				
2500 gm	38779-0617-01	96.00		
(PCCA)				
POW, NA, 1 gm	51927-1233-00	0.14		
(Spectrum Pharmacy) *See SODIUM BORATE DECAHYDRATE*				
SODIUM BORATE DECAHYDRATE (Baker, J.T.)				
sodium borate				
POW, NA (N.F.)				
500 gm	10106-3574-01	16.30		
2500 gm	10106-3574-05	89.57		
(Spectrum Pharmacy)				
POW, NA (N.F.)				
500 gm	49452-6625-01	72.10		
2500 gm	49452-6625-02	204.40		
12000 gm	49452-6625-03	658.00		
SODIUM BROMIDE (Amend)				
GRA, NA (PURIFIED)				
454 gm	17317-0501-01	11.20		
2270 gm	17317-0501-05	44.80		
11350 gm	17317-0501-08	157.50		
(Baker, J.T.)				
CRY, NA (A.C.S., REAGENT)				
500 gm	10106-3588-01	55.72		
2500 gm	10106-3588-05	204.25		
(Gallipot)				
GRA, NA (PURIFIED)				
454 gm	51552-0408-06	15.19		
2270 gm	51552-0408-09	55.93		
(Medisca)				
GRA, NA (1X500GM)				
500 gm	38779-1913-08	82.50		
(1X1000GM)				
1000 gm	38779-1913-09	138.00		
(1X2500GM)				
2500 gm	38779-1913-01	345.00		
(PCCA)				
GRA, NA (PURIFIED)				
1 gm	51927-1518-00	0.30		
(Spectrum Pharmacy)				
GRA, NA (1X125GM)				
125 gm	49452-6637-01	87.85		
(1X500GM)				
500 gm	49452-6637-02	257.25		
(1X2500GM)				
2500 gm	49452-6637-03	570.50		
(1X12000GM)				
12000 gm	49452-6637-04	1753.50		
SODIUM BUTYRATE (Gallipot)				
POW, NA, 100 gm	51552-0254-05	49.00		
500 gm	51552-0254-06	224.00		
(Medisca)				
POW, NA (1X100GM)				
100 gm	38779-1936-05	229.50		
(PCCA)				
POW, NA, 1 gm	51927-1946-00	4.20		
SODIUM CACODYLATE (Medisca)				
POW, NA, 25 gm	38779-0357-04	138.00		
100 gm	38779-0357-05	337.50		
500 gm	38779-0357-08	1453.50		
(PCCA)				
POW, NA, 1 gm	51927-2505-00	6.00		
SODIUM CAPRATE (PCCA)				
POW, NA, 1 gm	51927-1509-00	9.00		
SODIUM CAPRYLATE (Letco)				
POW, NA (FOOD GRADE)				
100 gm	62991-2602-02	60.00		
(FOOD GRADE, 1X1000GM)				
1000 gm	62991-2602-01	300.00		
(PCCA)				
POW, NA (FOOD GRADE)				
1 gm	51927-3332-00	0.54		
SODIUM CARBONATE				
(Amend) *See SODIUM CARBONATE ANHYDROUS*				
(Amend) *See SODIUM CARBONATE MONOHYDRATE*				
(Baker, J.T.) *See SODIUM CARBONATE ANHYDROUS*				
(Baker, J.T.) *See SODIUM CARBONATE MONOHYDRATE*				
(Gallipot)				
GRA, NA (ANHYDROUS,REAGENT)				
454 gm	51552-0587-06	31.43	22.45	
(Gallipot) *See SODIUM CARBONATE MONOHYDRATE*				
(Mallinckrodt Lab) *See SODIUM CARBONATE ANHYDROUS*				
(PCCA)				
POW, NA (NF; ANHYDROUS)				
1 gm	51927-1375-00	0.42		
(Spectrum Pharmacy) *See SODIUM CARBONATE ANHYDROUS*				
(Spectrum Pharmacy) *See SODIUM CARBONATE MONOHYDRATE*				
SODIUM CARBONATE ANHYDROUS (Amend)				
sodium carbonate				
GRA, NA (REAGENT)				
500 gm	17317-1468-01	14.00		
POW, NA (N.F., F.C.C.)				
454 gm	17317-0502-01	9.80		
2270 gm	17317-0502-05	39.20		
11350 gm	17317-0502-08	105.00		
(Baker, J.T.)				
GRA, NA (N.F., F.C.C.)				
500 gm	10106-3605-01	18.18		
(Mallinckrodt Lab)				
GRA, NA (A.C.S.)				
500 gm	00406-7527-04	33.68		
2500 gm	00406-7527-06	100.43		
(Spectrum Pharmacy)				
POW, NA (N.F.)				
500 gm	49452-6665-01	97.30		
2500 gm	49452-6665-02	175.00		
12000 gm	49452-6665-03	553.00		
SODIUM CARBONATE MONOHYDRATE (Amend)				
sodium carbonate				
POW, NA (N.F.)				
454 gm	17317-0503-01	8.40		
2270 gm	17317-0503-05	33.60		
11350 gm	17317-0503-08	105.00		
(Baker, J.T.)				
CRY, NA (N.F., F.C.C.)				
500 gm	10106-3600-01	12.64		
2500 gm	10106-3600-05	99.84		
(Gallipot)				
POW, NA (U.S.P.,N.F.)				
454 gm	51552-0204-06	10.64		
(Spectrum Pharmacy)				
POW, NA (N.F.)				
500 gm	49452-6670-01	67.55		
2500 gm	49452-6670-02	169.75		
12000 gm	49452-6670-03	528.50		
SODIUM CHLORATE (Baker, J.T.)				
CRY, NA (A.C.S., REAGENT)				
500 gm	10106-3616-01	103.62		
2500 gm	10106-3616-05	427.97		
(PCCA)				
POW, NA, 1 gm	51927-2304-00	0.54		
SODIUM CHLORIDE				
(Amer Regent) *See SODIUM CHLORIDE BACTERIOSTATIC*				
(Amer Regent) *See SODIUM CHLORIDE CONCENTRATE*				
(Amer Regent)				
SOL, IV (S.D.V.,PF)				
0.9%, 2 ml 25s	00517-2802-25	31.25		EE
10 ml 25s	00517-2810-25	34.38		EE
(AMSINO) *See SODIUM CHLORIDE FLUSH*				

PROD/MFR	NDC	AWP	DP	OBC
(AMSINO)				
SOL, IV (IN 12ML SD SYRINGE,PF)				
0.9%, 3 ml 400s	**68883-0600-16**	110.00	184.00	
5 ml 400s	**68883-0600-05**	110.00	184.00	
10 ml 400s	**68883-0600-10**	110.00	184.00	
(APP) *See SODIUM CHLORIDE CONCENTRATE*				
(APP)				
SOL, IV (S.D.V.,P.C.)				
0.9%, 2 ml	**63323-0186-02**	1.40		AP
(M.D.V.,P.C.)				
0.9%, 10 ml	**63323-0924-10**	1.08		AP
(S.D.V.,P.C.)				
0.9%, 10 ml	**63323-0186-10**	1.44		AP
20 ml	**63323-0186-20**	1.76		AP
(M.D.V.,P.C.)				
0.9%, 30 ml	**63323-0924-30**	1.32		AP
(M.D.V.)				
0.9%, 30 ml	**63323-0259-30**	1.32		AP
(S.D.V.,TEAR TOP)				
0.9%, 100 ml	**63323-0186-00**	3.02		AP
(S.D.V.)				
14.6%, 20 ml	**63323-0139-20**	2.26		
40 ml	**63323-0139-40**	2.67		
(B. Braun)				
SOL, IR (PIC CONTAINER)				
0.9%, 500 ml	**00264-2201-10**	1.62		AT
1000 ml	**00264-2201-00**	4.87		AT
2000 ml	**00264-2201-50**	3.76		AT
4000 ml	**00264-2201-70**	11.70		AT
IV (EXCEL)				
0.45%, 500 ml	**00264-7802-10**	1.75		AP
(GLASS CONTAINER)				
0.45%, 500 ml	**00264-4021-55**	3.30		AP
(EXCEL)				
0.45%, 1000 ml	**00264-7802-00**	1.68		AP
(100 ML PAB)				
0.9%, 25 ml	**00264-1800-36**	1.99		AP
50 ml	**00264-1800-31**	1.60		AP
(150 ML PAB)				
0.9%, 100 ml	**00264-1800-32**	1.48		AP
(250 ML GLASS CONTAINER)				
0.9%, 150 ml	**00264-4002-55**	1.75		AP
(EXCEL)				
0.9%, 250 ml	**00264-7800-20**	1.66		AP
500 ml	**00264-7800-10**	1.80		AP
(GLASS CONTAINER)				
0.9%, 500 ml	**00264-4001-55**	1.97		AP
(EXCEL)				
0.9%, 1000 ml	**00264-7800-00**	1.74		AP
(GLASS CONTAINER)				
0.9%, 1000 ml	**00264-4000-55**	3.00		AP
(HYPERTONIC,EXCEL)				
3%, 500 ml	**00264-7805-10**	5.00		AP
5%, 500 ml	**00264-7806-10**	2.26		AP
(Baker, J.T.)				
GRA, NA (U.S.P., F.C.C.)				
500 gm	**10106-3628-01**	78.99		
2500 gm	**10106-3628-05**	48.69		
(Baxter)				
SOL, IR, 0.9%, 250 ml 24s	**00338-0048-02**	277.34		AT
500 ml 18s	**00338-0048-03**	208.01		AT
(P.C.)				
0.9%, 1000 ml 12s	**00338-0048-04**	169.92		AT
((ARTHROMATIC P.C.),USP)				
0.9%, 1000 ml 14s	**00338-0047-24**	61.32	51.10	AT
((UROMATIC P.C.),USP)				
0.9%, 1000 ml 14s	**00338-0047-44**	61.32	51.10	AT
1500 ml 9s	**00338-0048-05**	145.53		AT
2000 ml 6s	**00338-0047-46**	66.02		AT
3000 ml 4s	**00338-0047-27**	50.16		AT
3000 ml 4s	**00338-0047-47**	65.95		AT
(PROCESSING)				
0.9%, 3000 ml 4s	**00338-0050-47**	53.24		AT
5000 ml 2s	**00338-0047-29**	41.48		AT
IV, 0.45%, 500 ml 24s	**00338-0043-03**	232.13		AP
(USP,1X1000ML)				
0.45%, 1000 ml	**00338-6333-04**	14.21	11.84	AP
(USP,VIAFLEX)				
0.45%, 1000 ml 14s	**00338-0043-04**	111.72	93.10	AP
(QUAD PACK, MINI-BAG)				
0.9%, 25 ml 48s	**00338-0049-10**	542.88		AP
(MINI-BAG PLUS)				
0.9%, 50 ml 80s	**00338-0553-11**	1160.00		AP
(MULTI PACK, MINI-BAG)				
0.9%, 50 ml 96s	**00338-0049-31**	928.51		AP
(QUAD PACK, MINI-BAG)				
0.9%, 50 ml 96s	**00338-0049-11**	928.51		AP
(SINGLE PACK, MINI-BAG)				
0.9%, 50 ml 96s	**00338-0049-41**	928.51		AP
(MINI-BAG PLUS)				
0.9%, 100 ml 80s	**00338-0553-18**	1160.00		AP
(MULTI PACK, MINI-BAG)				
0.9%, 100 ml 96s	**00338-0049-38**	928.51		AP
(QUAD PACK, MINI-BAG)				
0.9%, 100 ml 96s	**00338-0049-18**	928.51		AP
(SINGLE PACK, MINI-BAG)				
0.9%, 100 ml 96s	**00338-0049-48**	928.51		AP
150 ml 36s	**00338-0049-01**	327.89		AP
250 ml 36s	**00338-0049-02**	327.89		AP
(USP,40X250ML)				
0.9%, 250 ml 40s	**00338-6304-02**	515.52	429.60	AP
(USP,1X500ML)				
0.9%, 500 ml	**00338-6304-03**	14.88	12.40	AP
500 ml 24s	**00338-0049-03**	218.59		AP
(USP,1X1000ML)				
0.9%, 1000 ml	**00338-6304-04**	14.21	11.84	AP
(USP,VIAFLEX)				
0.9%, 1000 ml 14s	**00338-0049-04**	97.61	81.34	AP
3%, 500 ml 24s	**00338-0054-03**	258.52		
5%, 500 ml 24s	**00338-0056-03**	285.12		
((BULK PACKAGE),USP)				
23.4%, 250 ml	**00338-0873-02**	12.00	10.00	
(BD Dickinson Hosp Prod) *See BD POSIFLUSH SF*				
(BD Dickinson Hosp Prod) *See NORMAL SALINE FLUSH*				
(Consolidated Midland)				
SOL, IV (AMP)				
0.9%, 5 ml 25s	**00223-8496-02**	22.50		EE
5 ml 25s	**00223-8496-05**	18.75		EE
10 ml 25s	**00223-8497-10**	18.75		EE
(VIAL)				
0.9%, 30 ml 25s	**00223-8500-30**	37.50		EE
(Covidien) *See MONOJECT PREFILL ADVANCED*				
(Covidien) *See MONOJECT PREFILL SODIUM CHLORIDE*				
(Deen Pre-Fld Syr LLC) *See SODIUM CHLORIDE FLUSH*				
(Dey, L.P.)				
SOL, IH, 3%, 15 ml 50s UD	**49502-0640-15**	40.00		
(PF)				
10%, 15 ml 50s UD	**49502-0641-15**	40.00		
(Excelsior) *See SYREX*				
(Gallipot)				
GRA, NA (U.S.P.)				
454 gm	**51552-0077-06**	6.65		
11350 gm	**51552-0077-09**	103.74		
POW, NA, 454 gm	**51552-0062-06**	11.20		
2270 gm	**51552-0077-08**	21.84		
(Hospira) *See SODIUM CHLORIDE BACTERIOSTATIC*				
(Hospira)				
SOL, IJ (SRN,PF,LATEX-FREE)				
0.9%, 2.5 ml 100s	**63807-0100-30**	48.00	42.00	
(USP,10X3ML SYRINGE,PF)				
0.9%, 3 ml 100s	**63807-0100-35**	48.00	42.00	
(100X5ML,PF,LATEX-FREE)				
0.9%, 5 ml 100s	**63807-0100-55**	48.00	42.00	
(SRN,PF,LATEX-FREE)				
0.9%, 5 ml 100s	**63807-0100-50**	50.40	44.00	
(30X10ML,PF,LATEX-FREE)				
0.9%, 10 ml 30s	**63807-0100-20**	70.56	61.80	
(PF,LATEX-FREE)				
0.9%, 10 ml 100s	**63807-0100-01**	48.00	42.00	
(SRN,PF,LATEX-FREE)				
0.9%, 10 ml 100s	**63807-0100-75**	48.00	42.00	
IR (AQUALITE,PF,LATEX-FREE)				
0.45%, 1500 ml 9s	**00074-6147-36**	36.07	31.59	AT
(USP,6X2000ML)				
0.45%, 2000 ml 6s	**00409-7975-07**	47.23	41.34	AP
(AQUALITE, 24X250ML,PF)				
0.9%, 250 ml 24s	**00409-6138-22**	44.06	38.64	AT
(USP,AQUALITE,PF)				
0.9%, 500 ml 24s	**00409-6138-03**	46.94	41.04	AT
(AQUALITE,12X1000ML,PF)				
0.9%, 1000 ml 12s	**00409-7138-09**	23.90	20.88	AT
(FLEXIBLE CONTAINER,PF)				
0.9%, 1000 ml 12s	**00409-7972-05**	51.55	45.12	AT
(AQUALITE,9X1500ML,PF)				
0.9%, 1500 ml 9s	**00409-7138-36**	27.22	23.85	AT
(FLEX CONTAINER,6X2000ML)				
0.9%, 2000 ml 6s	**00409-7972-07**	41.62	36.42	AT
(FLEX CONTAINER,4X3000ML)				
0.9%, 3000 ml 4s	**00409-7972-08**	37.58	32.88	AT
IV (QUAD-PK,48X25ML)				
0.45%, 25 ml 48s	**00409-7730-20**	123.26	108.00	AP
(ADD-VANTAGE,LATEX-FREE)				
0.45%, 50 ml 50s	**00409-7132-66**	109.80	96.00	AP
(80X50ML,LATEX-FREE)				
0.45%, 50 ml 80s	**00409-7730-36**	214.08	187.20	AP
(ADD-VANTAGE,LATEX-FREE)				
0.45%, 100 ml 50s	**00409-7132-67**	108.60	95.00	AP
(80X100ML,LATEX-FREE)				
0.45%, 100 ml 80s	**00409-7730-37**	205.44	180.00	AP
(24X250ML,LATEX-FREE)				
0.45%, 250 ml 24s	**00409-7985-02**	39.46	34.56	AP
(24X250ML,VISIVCONTAINER)				
0.45%, 250 ml 24s	**00409-7985-25**	48.96	42.84	AP
(USP,ADD-VANTAGE)				
0.45%, 250 ml 24s	**00409-7132-02**	69.41	60.72	AT
(LIFECARE,24X500ML)				
0.45%, 500 ml 24s	**00409-7985-03**	42.05	36.72	AP
(LIFECARE,12X1000ML)				
0.45%, 1000 ml 12s	**00409-7985-09**	23.90	20.88	AP
(25X2ML,PF)				
0.9%, 2 ml 25s	**00409-2102-02**	21.90	19.25	AP
(INTERLINK,50X2ML,PF)				
0.9%, 2 ml 50s	**00074-1812-22**	50.47	42.50	EE
(LUER LOCK,50X2ML,PF)				
0.9%, 2 ml 50s	**00409-1918-32**	46.80	41.00	EE
(25X5ML,PF)				
0.9%, 5 ml 25s	**00409-2102-05**	26.40	23.00	AP
(LUER LOCK,PF,LATEX-FREE)				
0.9%, 5 ml 25s	**00409-1918-33**	26.10	22.75	EE
5 ml 25s	**00409-1918-35**	23.40	20.50	EE
(VIAL,PF)				
0.9%, 5 ml 25s	**00074-2102-05**	13.80	12.25	AP
(ANSYR,FOR IV ,50X5ML,PF)				
0.9%, 5 ml 50s	**00074-5365-05**	71.25	60.00	AP
(25X10ML,PF,LATEX-FREE)				
0.9%, 10 ml 25s	**00409-4888-12**	27.00	23.75	AP
(ADDITIVE,25X10ML,PF)				
0.9%, 10 ml 25s	**00409-4888-10**	15.60	13.75	AP
(THERMOJECT, 25X10ML)				
0.9%, 10 ml 25s	**00409-1081-51**	214.20	187.50	AP
(ADDITIVE,25X20ML,PF)				
0.9%, 20 ml 25s	**00409-4888-20**	21.60	19.00	AP
(VIAL, FLIPTOP, ADDITIVE)				
0.9%, 20 ml 25s	**00074-4888-20**	21.60	19.00	AP
(LIFECARE,QUAD PACK,LF)				
0.9%, 25 ml 48s	**00409-7984-20**	119.23	104.16	AP
(150 ML CONTAINER,PF)				
0.9%, 50 ml 12s	**00074-1584-01**	105.12	92.04	AP
(ADDITIVE,25X50ML,PF)				
0.9%, 50 ml 25s	**00409-4888-50**	48.60	42.50	AP
(48X50ML,PF,LATEX-FREE)				
0.9%, 50 ml 48s	**00409-7984-13**	124.42	108.96	AT
(ADDVANT,50X50ML,PF)				
0.9%, 50 ml 50s	**00409-7101-66**	101.40	88.50	AP
(60X50ML,SINGLE-DOSE)				
0.9%, 50 ml 60s	**00409-7984-06**	160.56	141.00	AP
(LFCARE,QUAD,LF,80X50ML)				
0.9%, 50 ml 80s	**00409-7984-36**	180.48	157.60	AP
(12X100ML,150ML VIAL,PF)				
0.9%, 100 ml 12s	**00409-1584-11**	105.12	92.04	AP
(LIFECARE,P/F,48X100ML)				
0.9%, 100 ml 48s	**00409-7984-23**	109.44	96.00	AT
(50X100ML, ADD-VANTAGE)				
0.9%, 100 ml 50s	**00409-7101-67**	102.00	89.50	AP
(60X100ML,SINGLE-DOSE)				
0.9%, 100 ml 60s	**00409-7984-11**	160.56	141.00	AP
(LFCARE,QUAD,LF,80X100ML)				
0.9%, 100 ml 80s	**00409-7984-37**	177.60	155.20	AP
(12X150ML,PF)				
0.9%, 150 ml 12s	**00409-1583-01**	49.54	43.32	AP
(LIFECARE,P.C.,32X150ML)				
0.9%, 150 ml 32s	**00409-7983-61**	51.46	45.12	AP
(12X250ML,PF)				
0.9%, 250 ml 12s	**00409-1583-02**	66.67	58.32	AP
(24X250ML,VISIVCONTAINER)				
0.9%, 250 ml 24s	**00409-7983-25**	48.96	42.84	AP
(ADD-VANTAGE,24X250ML,PF)				
0.9%, 250 ml 24s	**00409-7101-02**	68.26	59.76	AP
(LIFECARE,2 PORTS,PC,LF)				
0.9%, 250 ml 24s	**00409-7983-53**	64.80	56.64	AP
(LIFECARE,24X250ML,PF)				
0.9%, 250 ml 24s	**00409-7983-02**	36.29	31.68	AP
(2PORTS,PC,LF,18X500ML)				
0.9%, 500 ml 18s	**00409-7983-55**	62.86	55.08	AP
(LIFECARE,P.C.,24X500ML)				
0.9%, 500 ml 24s	**00409-7983-03**	33.98	29.76	AP
(VISIV CONTAINER)				
0.9%, 500 ml 24s	**00409-7983-30**	35.14	30.72	AP
(LIFECARE,P.C.,12X1000ML)				
0.9%, 1000 ml 12s	**00409-7983-09**	19.58	17.16	AP
(VISIV CONTAINER)				
0.9%, 1000 ml 12s	**00409-7983-48**	19.15	16.80	AP
(BULK,ADDITIVE,14.6%)				
2.5%, 250 ml 12s	**00409-4219-02**	58.90	51.48	
(12X500ML)				
5%, 500 ml 12s	**00409-1586-03**	112.32	98.28	
(FTV,50MEQ,25X20ML)				
14.6%, 20 ml 25s	**00409-6657-73**	19.50	17.00	
(25X40ML,LATEX-FREE)				
14.6%, 40 ml 25s	**00409-6660-75**	21.00	18.50	
(VIAL,FLIPTOP,BULK PKG)				
23.4%, 100 ml 25s	**00409-1141-02**	48.90	42.75	
250 ml 12s	**00409-1130-02**	49.10	42.96	

PROD/MFR	NDC	AWP	DP	OBC
(Letco)				
GRA, NA (U.S.P./N.F.)				
1000 gm	62991-1372-02	33.00		
(Mallinckrodt Lab)				
GRA, NA (U.S.P.)				
500 gm	00406-7532-04	17.67		
2500 gm	00406-7532-06	52.62		
(Medefil) *See NORMAL SALINE FLUSH*				
(Medisca)				
POW, NA (USP)				
100 gm	38779-0629-05	22.50		
(U.S.P.)				
500 gm	38779-0629-08	31.50		
(USP)				
1000 gm	38779-0629-09	46.50		
2500 gm	38779-0629-01	87.00		
(Pari) *See HYPER-SAL*				
(PCCA)				
GRA, NA (USP)				
1 gm	51927-1087-00	0.07		
(Sierra) *See NORMAL SALINE IV FLUSH SYRINGE*				
(Spectrum Pharmacy)				
GRA, NA (U.S.P.)				
500 gm	49452-6690-01	46.55		
2500 gm	49452-6690-02	108.50		
12000 gm	49452-6690-03	331.80		
POW, NA, 500 gm	49452-6700-01	70.00		
2500 gm	49452-6700-02	191.45		
(Tyco) *See MONOJECT PREFILL SODIUM CHLORIDE*				
(Vital Signs) *See VASCEZE SODIUM CHLORIDE*				
(A-S Medication) REPACK				
SOL, IV (AMP)				
0.9%, 10 ml 25s	54569-1522-00	21.41		EE
(Dispensing Solutions) REPACK				
SOL, IJ (10MLX25)				
0.9%, 10 ml 25s	55045-3710-01	50.00		
(Phys Total Care) REPACK				
SOL, IH (AMP,PF)				
0.9%, 3 ml 100s	54868-5026-00	50.04		
IR (PF,LATEX-FREE)				
0.9%, 500 ml 24s	54868-0710-02	91.08		AT
IV (150X5ML)				
0.9%, 5 ml 150s	54868-2527-00	90.58		
(PF)				
0.9%, 10 ml 25s	54868-4464-00	15.95		EE
(20X25ML)				
0.9%, 20 ml 25s	54868-5714-00	53.76		
(NORMAL SALINE,48X50ML)				
0.9%, 50 ml 48s	54868-0710-05	333.12		
(NORMAL SALINE,48X100ML)				
0.9%, 100 ml 48s	54868-0710-03	323.59		EE
(NORMAL SALINE,24X250ML)				
0.9%, 250 ml 24s	54868-0710-06	133.96		
500 ml	54868-0710-01	91.08		EE
1000 ml	54868-0710-00	64.38		EE
(NORMAL SALINE,12X1000ML)				
0.9%, 1000 ml 12s	54868-0710-04	83.75		
(Southwood) REPACK				
SOL, IJ (10MLX100)				
0.9%, 10 ml 100s	58016-4995-01	69.34		
SODIUM CHLORIDE BACTERIOSTATIC (Amer Regent)				
sodium chloride				
SOL, IV (M.D.V.)				
0.9%, 30 ml 25s	00517-0648-25	35.94		EE
(Hospira)				
SOL, IV (25X10ML, LS-PLASTIC)				
0.9%, 10 ml 25s	00409-1966-12	28.80	25.25	AP
(25X10ML,LATEX-FREE)				
0.9%, 10 ml 25s	00409-1966-04	22.20	19.50	AP
(25X20ML,LATEX-FREE)				
0.9%, 20 ml 25s	00409-1966-05	25.20	22.00	AP
(FLIPTOP,LS-PLASTIC)				
0.9%, 30 ml 25s	00409-1966-14	51.00	44.75	AP
(VIAL,FLIPTOP PLASTIC)				
0.9%, 30 ml 25s	00409-1966-07	21.00	18.50	AP
(Phys Total Care) REPACK				
SOL, IV (1X750ML,LATEX-FREE)				
0.9%, 750 ml	54868-0116-01	74.31		AP
(Quality Care Prod) REPACK				
SOL, IV (1X30ML,LATEX-FREE)				
0.9%, 30 ml	35356-0181-30	6.32		AP
SODIUM CHLORIDE CONCENTRATE (Amer Regent)				
sodium chloride				
SOL, IV (S.D.V.)				
23.4%, 30 ml 25s	00517-2930-25	35.94		
(BULK PACKAGE)				
23.4%, 100 ml 25s	00517-2900-25	93.75		
(APP)				
SOL, IV (S.D.V.,PF)				
23.4%, 30 ml	63323-0187-30	2.39		
(MAXIVIAL,BULK PACK,PF)				
23.4%, 100 ml	63323-0088-61	9.30		
200 ml	63323-0088-63	17.10		
SODIUM CHLORIDE FLUSH (AMSINO)				
sodium chloride				
SOL, IV (IN 3ML SD SYRINGE,PF)				
0.9%, 2.5 ml 180s	68883-0900-01	570.60		
(IN 12ML SD SYRINGE,PF)				
0.9%, 3 ml 180s	68883-0900-16	556.20		
(IN 6ML SD SYRINGE,PF)				
0.9%, 3 ml 180s	68883-0900-03	576.00		
(IN 12ML SD SYRINGE,PF)				
0.9%, 5 ml 180s	68883-0900-05	649.80		
(IN 6ML SD SYRINGE,PF)				
0.9%, 5 ml 180s	68883-0900-04	586.80		
(IN 12ML SD SYRINGE,PF)				
0.9%, 10 ml 180s	68883-0900-10	729.00		
(Deen Pre-Fld Syr LLC)				
SOL, IV (3ML W/CANNULA)				
0.9%, 2 ml	08450-6011-02	3.70	3.08	
(3ML,PRE-FILLED SYRINGE)				
0.9%, 2 ml	08450-0901-02	2.90	2.42	
(6ML W/CANNULA)				
0.9%, 3 ml	08450-6012-03	3.84	3.20	
(6ML,PRE-FILLED SYRINGE)				
0.9%, 3 ml	08450-0903-03	3.05	2.54	
(12ML W/CANNULA)				
0.9%, 5 ml	08450-6013-05	4.10	3.42	
(12ML,PRE-FILLED SYRINGE)				
0.9%, 5 ml	08450-0905-05	3.30	2.75	
(12ML W/CANNULA)				
0.9%, 10 ml	08450-6014-10	4.50	3.75	
(12ML,PRE-FILLED SYRINGE)				
0.9%, 10 ml	08450-0906-10	3.70	3.08	
SODIUM CHLORIDE/TETRASTARCH				
(Hospira) *See VOLUVEN*				
SODIUM CHLORIDE/TOBRAMYCIN SULFATE				
(Hospira)				
SOL, IV (PREMIX,24X100ML)				
0.9%-80 mg/100 ml, 100 ml 24s	00409-3470-23	263.52	230.64	
(PREMIX,LATEX-FREE)				
0.9%-60 mg/50 ml, 50 ml 24s	00409-3469-13	229.54	200.88	
SODIUM CHLORIDE/VANCOMYCIN HYDROCHLORIDE				
(PharMEDium Services) *See VANCOMYCIN HYDROCHLORIDE-SODIUM CHLORIDE*				
SODIUM CHROMATE				
(Baker, J.T.) *See SODIUM CHROMATE TETRAHYDRATE*				
SODIUM CHROMATE CR 51				
(Bracco Diag) *See CHROMITOPE SODIUM*				
SODIUM CHROMATE TETRAHYDRATE (Baker, J.T.)				
sodium chromate				
CRY, NA (REAGENT)				
125 gm	10106-3640-04	55.26		
500 gm	10106-3640-01	100.37		
SODIUM CITRATE				
(Baker, J.T.) *See SODIUM CITRATE DIHYDRATE*				
(Citra) *See TRICITRASOL*				
(Gallipot) *See SODIUM CITRATE DIHYDRATE*				
(Humco)				
GRA, NA (U.S.P.)				
454 gm	00395-2691-01	12.59		
(Mallinckrodt Lab) *See SODIUM CITRATE DIHYDRATE*				
(Medisca) *See SODIUM CITRATE DIHYDRATE*				
(PCCA)				
POW, NA (USP, ANHYDROUS)				
1 gm	51927-1144-00	0.09		
(Spectrum Pharmacy) *See SODIUM CITRATE ANHYDROUS*				
(Spectrum Pharmacy) *See SODIUM CITRATE DIHYDRATE*				
SODIUM CITRATE ANHYDROUS (Spectrum Pharmacy)				
sodium citrate				
POW, NA (F.C.C.)				
500 gm	49452-6707-02	79.10		
(U.S.P.)				
500 gm	49452-6711-02	72.45		
(F.C.C.)				
2500 gm	49452-6707-03	248.85		
(U.S.P.)				
2500 gm	49452-6711-03	234.85		
SODIUM CITRATE DIHYDRATE (Baker, J.T.)				
sodium citrate				
GRA, NA (U.S.P., F.C.C., A.C.S.)				
500 gm	10106-3649-01	10.79		
2500 gm	10106-3649-05	82.09		
POW, NA (U.S.P., F.C.C.)				
500 gm	10106-3650-01	10.92		
2500 gm	10106-3650-05	91.20		
(Gallipot)				
GRA, NA (U.S.P.,N.F.)				
454 gm	51552-0191-06	10.08		
2270 gm	51552-0191-09	29.68		
(Mallinckrodt Lab)				
CRY, NA (U.S.P.)				
500 gm	00406-0734-04	29.53		
2500 gm	00406-0734-06	95.94		
(Medisca)				
POW, NA (U.S.P.)				
100 gm	38779-0543-05	22.50		
500 gm	38779-0543-08	34.50		
(USP)				
2500 gm	38779-0543-01	87.00		
(Spectrum Pharmacy)				
GRA, NA (U.S.P.)				
500 gm	49452-6710-01	57.40		
2500 gm	49452-6710-02	147.00		
12000 gm	49452-6710-03	651.00		
SODIUM COBALTINITRITE (Baker, J.T.)				
POW, NA (A.C.S., REAGENT)				
125 gm	10106-3656-04	69.78		
500 gm	10106-3656-01	209.55		
SODIUM CYANIDE (Baker, J.T.)				
GRA, NA (A.C.S., REAGENT)				
125 gm	10106-3662-04	23.90		
500 gm	10106-3662-01	42.02		
(Mallinckrodt Lab)				
GRA, NA (A.C.S.)				
500 gm	00406-7616-04	29.13		
SODIUM DEHYDROACETATE (PCCA)				
POW, NA, 1 gm	51927-3581-00	0.41		
SODIUM DEOXYCHOLATE (Medisca)				
sodium desoxycholate				
POW, NA, 1000 gm	38779-2329-09	765.00		
SODIUM DESOXYCHOLATE				
(Medisca) *See SODIUM DEOXYCHOLATE*				
(PCCA) *See DEOXYCHOLIC ACID*				
SODIUM DICHROMATE				
(Baker, J.T.) *See SODIUM DICHROMATE DIHYDRATE*				
SODIUM DICHROMATE DIHYDRATE (Baker, J.T.)				
sodium dichromate				
CRY, NA (A.C.S., REAGENT)				
125 gm	10106-3672-04	77.35		
500 gm	10106-3672-01	139.20		
SODIUM DITHIONITE (Baker, J.T.)				
POW, NA (PURIFIED)				
500 gm	10106-3712-01	31.83		
2500 gm	10106-3712-05	103.62		
SODIUM EDECRIN (Aton)				
ethacrynate sodium				
PDS, IV, 50 mg, ea	25010-0210-27	366.25		
SODIUM FERRIC GLUCONATE COMPLEX				
(Sanofi-Aventis) *See FERRLECIT*				
(Watson) *See FERRLECIT*				
SODIUM FERROCYANIDE (Spectrum Pharmacy)				
POW, NA (F.C.C.)				
125 gm	49452-6737-01	117.60		
500 gm	49452-6737-02	243.25		
SODIUM FLUORIDE (Amend)				
POW, NA (U.S.P.)				
125 gm	17317-0508-04	8.40		
500 gm	17317-0508-01	19.60		
2270 gm	17317-0508-05	84.00		

PROD/MFR	NDC	AWP	DP	OBC
(Baker, J.T.)				
POW, NA (U.S.P., A.C.S.)				
500 gm	**10106-3689-01**	33.10		
2000 gm	**10106-3689-05**	284.89		
(Breckenridge Pharm)				
CTB, PO (ORANGE)				
0.25 mg, 120s ea	**51991-0676-36**	17.60		
0.5 mg, 120s ea	**51991-0677-36**	17.60		
1 mg, 120s ea	**51991-0678-36**	17.60		
(Colgate Oral) *See LURIDE*				
(Colgate Oral) *See PHOS-FLUR*				
(Colgate Oral) *See PREVIDENT*				
(Colgate Oral) *See PREVIDENT 5000 BOOSTER*				
(Colgate Oral) *See PREVIDENT 5000 PLUS*				
(Colgate Oral) *See PREVIDENT DENTAL RINSE*				
(Colgate Oral) *See THERA-FLUR-N*				
(Consolidated Midland)				
CTB, PO, 1 mg, 100s ea	**00223-1773-01**	2.50		
1000s ea	**00223-1773-02**	15.75		
(Contract Pharmacal)				
CTB, PO (SF,GRAPE)				
1.1 mg, 100s ea	**10267-1640-01**	4.90		
1000s ea	**10267-1640-04**	54.10		
(SF,CHERRY)				
2.2 mg, 100s ea	**10267-1641-01**	5.10		EE
1000s ea	**10267-1641-04**	55.10		EE
(Cypress Pharm) *See FLUORIDE*				
(Cypress Pharm) *See NEUTRAL SODIUM FLUORIDE*				
(Cypress Pharm) *See SF 1.1% GEL*				
(Cypress Pharm) *See SF 5000 PLUS*				
(Discus Dental) *See FLUORIDEX DAILY DEFENSE*				
(Discus Dental) *See FLUORIDEX DAILY DEFENSE ENHANCED WHITENING*				
(Fluoritab) *See FLUORITAB*				
(Gallipot)				
POW, NA, 113.4 gm	**51552-0146-04**	10.99		
(U.S.P.)				
454 gm	**51552-0146-06**	28.91		
(Hi-Tech)				
LIQ, PO (SF,PEACH,DROPS)				
0.5 mg/ml, 50 ml	**50383-0656-50**	8.05		
(Humco)				
GEL, DE, 1%, 60 gm	**00802-3923-92**	10.93		
(Kirkman Labs) *See FLURA-DROPS*				
(Kirkman Labs) *See FLURA-LOZ*				
(Mallinckrodt Lab)				
POW, NA (A.C.S.)				
500 gm	**00406-7636-04**	81.55		
(Medisca)				
POW, NA (U.S.P.)				
100 gm	**38779-0094-05**	25.50		
500 gm	**38779-0094-08**	55.50		
2500 gm	**38779-0094-01**	255.00		
(Omnii Intl) *See CAVIRINSE*				
(Omnii Intl) *See CONTROL RX*				
(Oral B Lab) *See FLUORINSE*				
(Pascal Co.) *See NEUTRAGARD ADVANCED*				
(PCCA)				
POW, NA (USP)				
1 gm	**51927-1038-00**	0.48		
(Perry Med)				
CTB, PO (RASPBERRY)				
0.25 mg, 100s ea	**11763-0398-01**	2.52		
1000s ea	**11763-0398-04**	11.00		
0.5 mg, 100s ea	**11763-0217-01**	2.31		
1000s ea	**11763-0217-04**	11.00		
(SF,GRAPE)				
1 mg, 1000s ea	**11763-0318-04**	11.00		
(SF,RASPBERRY)				
1 mg, 1000s ea	**11763-0317-04**	11.00		
(Perry Med) *See FLUORABON*				
(Pharmascience Labs) *See FLUOR-A-DAY*				
(Rising) *See DENTA 5000 PLUS*				
(Rising) *See DENTAGEL*				
(Sancilio) *See LUDENT FLUORIDE*				
(Spectrum Pharmacy)				
POW, NA (U.S.P.)				
125 gm	**49452-6740-05**	79.45		
500 gm	**49452-6740-01**	163.10		
2500 gm	**49452-6740-02**	598.50		
(A-S Medication)				
REPACK				
CTB, PO, 0.5 mg, 100s ea	**54569-2870-01**	5.54		
LIQ, PO (SF,PEACH,DROPS)				
0.5 mg/ml, 50 ml	**54569-4607-00**	8.05		
(Dispensing Solutions)				
REPACK				
CTB, PO (SF,GRAPE)				
1.1 mg, 90s ea	**66336-0680-90**	12.98		
(SF,CHERRY)				
2.2 mg, 100s ea	**55045-3353-00**	9.00		EE
TAB, PO, 2.2 mg, 90s ea	**66336-0263-90**	8.01		
(Palmetto)				
REPACK				
CTB, PO, 2.2 mg, 90s ea	**23490-7679-01**	8.19		
100s ea	**23490-7679-00**	9.10		
(PD-Rx Pharm)				
REPACK				
CTB, PO, 1 mg, 120s ea	**55289-0676-98**	7.89		
(Phys Total Care)				
REPACK				
CTB, PO, 1 mg, 120s ea	**54868-5169-00**	21.45		
LIQ, PO (DROPS)				
0.125 mg/drp, 30 ml	**54868-1941-00**	13.68		
(SF,PEACH,DROPS)				
0.5 mg/ml, 50 ml	**54868-1941-01**	12.18		
(Southwood)				
REPACK				
CTB, PO, 1 mg, 100s ea	**58016-0978-00**	4.84		
LIQ, PO (DROPS)				
0.125 mg/drp, 30 ml	**58016-9077-01**	7.70		
SODIUM FORMALDEHYDE SULFOXYLATE (PCCA)				
sodium formaldehydesulfoxylate				
POW, NA, 1 gm	**51927-3421-00**	3.60		
SODIUM FORMALDEHYDESULFOXYLATE (PCCA) *See SODIUM FORMALDEHYDE SULFOXYLATE*				
SODIUM FORMATE (Baker, J.T.)				
CRY, NA (A.C.S., REAGENT)				
500 gm	**10106-3700-01**	48.26		
2500 gm	**10106-3700-05**	226.75		
12000 gm	**10106-3700-07**	769.00		
SODIUM GLUCONATE (Amend)				
POW, NA (F.C.C.)				
454 gm	**17317-0901-01**	8.40		
2270 gm	**17317-0901-05**	33.60		
11350 gm	**17317-0901-08**	105.00		
(PCCA)				
POW, NA (USP)				
1 gm	**51927-2377-00**	0.10		
(Spectrum Pharmacy)				
POW, NA (U.S.P.)				
500 gm	**49452-6745-01**	89.25		
2500 gm	**49452-6745-02**	246.40		
12000 gm	**49452-6745-03**	700.00		
SODIUM GLYCEROPHOSPHATE (Amend)				
POW, NA (N.F.)				
125 gm	**17317-0510-04**	18.20		
454 gm	**17317-0510-01**	44.80		
2270 gm	**17317-0510-05**	196.00		
SODIUM HEXAMETAPHOSPHATE (Amend)				
sodium polymetaphosphate				
POW, NA (FOOD GRADE)				
454 gm	**17317-1547-01**	8.40		
2270 gm	**17317-1547-05**	29.40		
11350 gm	**17317-1547-08**	87.50		
(Spectrum Pharmacy)				
GRA, NA (F.C.C.)				
500 gm	**49452-6770-01**	95.20		
2500 gm	**49452-6770-02**	175.70		
SODIUM HYALURONATE (Cypress Pharm)				
hyaluronate sodium				
GEL, TP (1X340GM)				
0.2%, 340 gm	**60258-0026-12**	101.12		
SODIUM HYALURONATE HYDRATING LOTION (Cypress Pharm)				
hyaluronate sodium				
LOT, TP (1X1000GM,VISCOELASTIC)				
0.1%, 1000 gm	**60258-0025-10**	140.47		
SODIUM HYDROXIDE (Amend)				
PEL, NA (A.C.S., REAGENT)				
500 gm	**17317-1357-01**	11.20		
2500 gm	**17317-1357-05**	38.50		
POW, NA (N.F., F.C.C.)				
454 gm	**17317-0511-01**	7.00		
2270 gm	**17317-0511-05**	23.10		
11350 gm	**17317-0511-08**	52.75		
(Baker, J.T.)				
FLA, NA (PURIFIED)				
500 gm	**10106-3734-01**	34.25		
2500 gm	**10106-3734-05**	88.84		
PEL, NA (F.C.C., N.F.)				
125 gm	**10106-3728-04**	25.88		
500 gm	**10106-3728-01**	20.85		
(Baker, J.T.) *See SODIUM HYDROXIDE 10N*				
(Baker, J.T.) *See SODIUM HYDROXIDE 25%*				
(Baker, J.T.) *See SODIUM HYDROXIDE 50%*				
(Baker, J.T.) *See SODIUM HYDROXIDE 6N*				
(Gallipot)				
FLA, NA (TECHNICAL)				
22700 gm	**51552-0624-09**	93.80		
PEL, NA (U.S.P.,N.F.)				
454 gm	**51552-0080-06**	14.42		
(Gallipot) *See SODIUM HYDROXIDE 0.1N*				
(Gallipot) *See SODIUM HYDROXIDE 10%*				
(Gallipot) *See SODIUM HYDROXIDE 20%*				
(Gordon) *See SODIUM HYDROXIDE 10%*				
(Letco)				
PEL, NA (N.F.)				
500 gm	**62991-2061-01**	32.25		
2500 gm	**62991-2061-02**	75.00		
(Mallinckrodt Lab)				
PEL, NA (N.F.)				
500 gm	**00406-7680-04**	29.26		
(PCCA)				
POW, NA (NF; (CAUSTIC SODA))				
1 gm	**51927-1237-00**	0.09		
(Spectrum Pharmacy)				
PEL, NA (N.F.)				
500 gm	**49452-6780-01**	61.60		
2500 gm	**49452-6780-02**	156.10		
12000 gm	**49452-6780-03**	546.00		
SODIUM HYDROXIDE 0.1N (Gallipot)				
sodium hydroxide				
SOL, NA, 473 ml	**51552-0556-06**	8.40		
SODIUM HYDROXIDE 10% (Gallipot)				
sodium hydroxide				
SOL, NA, 473 ml	**51552-0406-06**	14.49		
(Gordon)				
SOL, NA, 60 ml	**10481-3006-01**	32.50		
SODIUM HYDROXIDE 10N (Baker, J.T.)				
sodium hydroxide				
SOL, NA (REAGENT, VOLUMETRIC)				
1000 ml	**10106-5674-02**	30.39		
4000 ml	**10106-5674-03**	52.32		
4000 ml	**10106-5674-06**	52.32		
20000 ml	**10106-5674-07**	128.75		
SODIUM HYDROXIDE 20% (Gallipot)				
sodium hydroxide				
SOL, NA (W/V)				
473 ml	**51552-0616-06**	14.70		
SODIUM HYDROXIDE 25% (Baker, J.T.)				
sodium hydroxide				
SOL, NA (REAGENT)				
1000 ml	**10106-5661-02**	39.86		
4000 ml	**10106-5661-03**	68.60		
20000 ml	**10106-5661-07**	202.34		
SODIUM HYDROXIDE 50% (Baker, J.T.)				
sodium hydroxide				
SOL, NA (REAGENT)				
500 ml	**10106-3727-01**	46.66		
4000 ml	**10106-3727-03**	103.67		
19000 ml	**10106-3727-07**	288.06		
SODIUM HYDROXIDE 6N (Baker, J.T.)				
sodium hydroxide				
SOL, NA (REAGENT, VOLUMETRIC)				
1000 ml	**10106-5672-02**	28.63		
4000 ml	**10106-5672-03**	44.29		
20000 ml	**10106-5672-07**	105.94		
SODIUM HYPOCHLORITE (Baker, J.T.) *See SODIUM HYPOCHLORITE 5%*				
SODIUM HYPOCHLORITE 5% (Baker, J.T.)				
sodium hypochlorite				
SOL, NA (REAGENT)				
500 ml	**10106-9416-01**	38.93		
4000 ml	**10106-9416-03**	162.95		

PROD/MFR	NDC	AWP	DP	OBC
SODIUM HYPOPHOSPHITE				
(Baker, J.T.) *See SODIUM HYPOPHOSPHITE MONOHYDRATE*				
SODIUM HYPOPHOSPHITE MONOHYDRATE				
(Baker, J.T.)				
sodium hypophosphite				
CRY, NA (REAGENT)				
500 gm	**10106-3740-01**	75.71		
2500 gm	**10106-3740-05**	262.03		
SODIUM IODATE (Baker, J.T.)				
POW, NA (REAGENT)				
125 gm	**10106-3745-04**	46.35		
500 gm	**10106-3745-01**	125.04		
SODIUM IODIDE				
(APP) *See IODOPEN*				
(Baker, J.T.)				
CRY, NA (U.S.P.)				
125 gm	**10106-3750-04**	51.38		
(A.C.S., REAGENT)				
500 gm	**10106-3748-01**	199.25		
(U.S.P.)				
500 gm	**10106-3750-01**	144.85		
(A.C.S., REAGENT)				
2500 gm	**10106-3748-05**	801.34		
(Gallipot)				
POW, NA, 113.4 gm	**51552-0494-04**	24.43		
(Mallinckrodt Lab)				
GRA, NA (U.S.P.)				
500 gm	**00406-1136-12**	124.66		
(Medisca)				
POW, NA (U.S.P.)				
100 gm	**38779-0805-05**	54.00		
500 gm	**38779-0805-08**	159.00		
(USP)				
1000 gm	**38779-0805-09**	285.00		
(PCCA)				
POW, NA (U.S.P.)				
1 gm	**51927-1569-00**	0.66		
(Spectrum Pharmacy)				
GRA, NA (U.S.P.)				
125 gm	**49452-6820-01**	105.00		
500 gm	**49452-6820-02**	324.80		
2500 gm	**49452-6820-03**	1060.50		
SODIUM IODIDE I 123				
(GE) *See SODIUM IODIDE I-123*				
SODIUM IODIDE I 131				
(Bracco Diag) *See IODOTOPE*				
(Mallinckrodt Inc.)				
CAP, PO (GELATIN CAPSULE)				
10 mci, ea	**00019-N452-FA**	428.40	357.00	
SODIUM IODIDE I-123 (GE)				
sodium iodide i 123				
CAP, PO, 100 uci, ea	**17156-0201-05**	141.01		**AA**
200 uci, ea	**17156-0522-05**	241.43		**EE**
SODIUM LACTATE				
(Amend) *See SODIUM LACTATE 60%*				
(Baxter)				
SOL, IV (USP,VIAFLEX)				
167 meq/l,				
1000 ml 14s	**00338-0129-04**	186.65	155.54	**AP**
(Hospira)				
SOL, IV (USP,SDV,25X10ML)				
5 meq/ml,				
10 ml 25s	**00409-6664-02**	63.60	55.75	**EE**
(PCCA)				
SOL, NA (USP, 60%)				
1 ml	**51927-2095-00**	0.11		
(Spectrum Pharmacy) *See SODIUM-DL-LACTATE 60%*				
(Spectrum Pharmacy) *See SODIUM-L-LACTATE 60%*				
SODIUM LACTATE 60% (Amend)				
sodium lactate				
SOL, NA (U.S.P.)				
480 ml	**17317-0514-01**	9.80		
3840 ml	**17317-0514-06**	44.80		
20000 ml	**17317-0514-08**	154.00		
SODIUM LAURETH SULFATE (PCCA)				
POW, NA (STANDAPOL ES-2)				
1 gm	**51927-2703-00**	0.21		
SODIUM LAURYL SULFATE (Gallipot)				
POW, NA (U.S.P.,N.F.)				
113.4 gm	**51552-0263-04**	10.64		
454 gm	**51552-0263-06**	20.23		
2270 gm	**51552-0263-08**	91.84		

PROD/MFR	NDC	AWP	DP	OBC
(Medisca)				
CRY, NA (1X100GM)				
100 gm	**38779-0622-05**	28.50		
(1X500GM)				
500 gm	**38779-0622-08**	52.50		
(PCCA)				
POW, NA (NF)				
1 gm	**51927-1050-00**	0.30		
(Spectrum Pharmacy)				
POW, NA (N.F.,E.P.,B.P.,J.P.)				
125 gm	**49452-6840-01**	61.25		
500 gm	**49452-6840-02**	105.00		
2500 gm	**49452-6840-03**	346.50		
SODIUM META-ARSENITE (Baker, J.T.)				
sodium arsenite				
POW, NA (REAGENT)				
125 gm	**10106-3487-04**	83.79		
500 gm	**10106-3487-01**	393.51		
SODIUM META-PERIODATE (Baker, J.T.)				
sodium periodate				
POW, NA (A.C.S., REAGENT)				
125 gm	**10106-3756-04**	162.69		
500 gm	**10106-3756-01**	461.34		
SODIUM META-SILICATE 9-HYDRATE (Baker, J.T.)				
sodium silicate				
CRY, NA (REAGENT)				
500 gm	**10106-3868-01**	72.15		
2500 gm	**10106-3868-05**	299.06		
SODIUM METABISULFITE (Amend)				
GRA, NA (N.F., F.C.C.)				
500 gm	**17317-0677-01**	7.00		
2270 gm	**17317-0677-05**	28.00		
11350 gm	**17317-0677-08**	97.50		
(Baker, J.T.)				
GRA, NA (A.C.S., REAGENT)				
500 gm	**10106-3552-01**	26.06		
2500 gm	**10106-3552-05**	93.16		
(Gallipot) *See SODIUM METABISULFITE ANHYDROUS*				
(Letco)				
POW, NA (U.S.P./N.F.)				
500 gm	**62991-1374-01**	25.50		
(PCCA)				
GRA, NA (NF)				
1 gm	**51927-1349-00**	0.07		
(Spectrum Pharmacy)				
GRA, NA (N.F.,E.P.,B.P.,J.P.)				
500 gm	**49452-6865-01**	53.90		
2500 gm	**49452-6865-02**	158.90		
12000 gm	**49452-6865-03**	490.00		
SODIUM METABISULFITE ANHYDROUS (Gallipot)				
sodium metabisulfite				
GRA, NA (U.S.P.)				
0.075 gm	**51552-0069-09**	7.35		
454 gm	**51552-0069-06**	10.50		
2270 gm	**51552-0069-08**	35.98		
SODIUM METASILICATE (PCCA)				
POW, NA (1X1GM)				
1 gm	**51927-3250-00**	0.57		
SODIUM MOLYBDATE				
(Amend) *See SODIUM MOLYBDATE DIHYDRATE*				
(Baker, J.T.) *See SODIUM MOLYBDATE DIHYDRATE*				
(PCCA)				
POW, NA (DIHYDRATE)				
1 gm	**51927-2729-00**	1.08		
SODIUM MOLYBDATE DIHYDRATE (Amend)				
sodium molybdate				
POW, NA, 454 gm	**17317-0902-01**	57.40		
2270 gm	**17317-0902-05**	224.00		
(Baker, J.T.)				
POW, NA (A.C.S., REAGENT)				
500 gm	**10106-3764-01**	134.05		
2500 gm	**10106-3764-05**	441.05		
SODIUM MONOFLUOROPHOSPHATE (PCCA)				
POW, NA (USP)				
1 gm	**51927-1801-00**	2.04		
(Spectrum Pharmacy)				
POW, NA (U.S.P.)				
125 gm	**49452-6870-01**	194.25		
500 gm	**49452-6870-02**	416.50		
SODIUM MORRHUATE (Consolidated Midland)				
morrhuate sodium				
SOL, IV (M.D.V.)				
50 mg/ml, 30 ml	**00223-8541-30**	49.50		

PROD/MFR	NDC	AWP	DP	OBC
SODIUM NITRATE (Amend)				
GRA, NA (PURIFIED, F.C.C.)				
454 gm	**17317-0516-01**	8.40		
2270 gm	**17317-0516-05**	33.60		
11350 gm	**17317-0516-08**	105.00		
(Baker, J.T.)				
CRY, NA (U.S.P.)				
500 gm	**10106-3782-01**	36.19		
2500 gm	**10106-3782-05**	153.62		
(Gallipot)				
GRA, NA (F.C.C.)				
454 gm	**51552-0345-06**	11.41		
(U.S.P.,N.F.)				
454 gm	**51552-0169-06**	10.50		
(Medisca)				
CRY, NA (1X500GM)				
500 gm	**38779-1757-08**	27.00		
(PCCA)				
POW, NA (FCC)				
1 gm	**51927-1672-00**	0.11		
(Spectrum Pharmacy)				
GRA, NA (F.C.C.)				
500 gm	**49452-6880-01**	80.85		
2500 gm	**49452-6880-02**	219.80		
12000 gm	**49452-6880-03**	805.00		
SODIUM NITRITE (Amend)				
GRA, NA (U.S.P.)				
454 gm	**17317-0517-01**	7.70		
2270 gm	**17317-0517-05**	29.40		
11350 gm	**17317-0517-08**	96.25		
(Hope)				
SOL, IJ (STERILE VIAL)				
30 mg/ml, 10 ml 2s	**60267-0079-02**	108.00		
(Mallinckrodt Lab)				
GRA, NA (A.C.S.)				
500 gm	**00406-7824-04**	46.80		
2500 gm	**00406-7824-06**	203.66		
(Medisca)				
POW, NA (1X500GM,USP)				
500 gm	**38779-1607-08**	36.00		
(PCCA)				
POW, NA (USP)				
1 gm	**51927-1724-00**	0.11		
(Spectrum Pharmacy)				
GRA, NA (U.S.P.)				
500 gm	**49452-6890-01**	78.75		
2500 gm	**49452-6890-02**	186.20		
12000 gm	**49452-6890-03**	665.00		
SODIUM NITROFERRICYANIDE (Baker, J.T.)				
sodium nitroprusside				
CRY, NA (A.C.S,REAGENT,DIHYDRATE)				
125 gm	**10106-3792-04**	74.57		
500 gm	**10106-3792-01**	155.27		
SODIUM NITROPRUSSIDE				
(Baker, J.T.) *See SODIUM NITROFERRICYANIDE*				
(Hospira) *See NITROPRESS*				
SODIUM OLEATE (Baker, J.T.)				
POW, NA (PURIFIED)				
500 gm	**10106-3796-01**	64.07		
(Medisca)				
FLA, NA (1X25GM)				
25 gm	**38779-1610-04**	73.50		
(1X100GM)				
100 gm	**38779-1610-05**	102.00		
(1X500GM)				
500 gm	**38779-1610-08**	367.50		
(PCCA)				
POW, NA, 1 gm	**51927-2002-00**	3.36		
SODIUM ORTHOVANADATE (PCCA)				
POW, NA (1X1GM)				
1 gm	**51927-3282-00**	5.94		
SODIUM OXALATE (Baker, J.T.)				
POW, NA (A.C.S., REAGENT)				
500 gm	**10106-3800-01**	112.79		
2500 gm	**10106-3800-05**	397.63		
SODIUM OXYBATE				
(Jazz) *See XYREM*				
SODIUM PANGAMATE				
(PCCA) *See PANGAMIC ACID SODIUM*				
SODIUM PCA				
(PCCA) *See SODIUM PYRROLIDONE CARBOXYLATE*				
SODIUM PERBORATE (Amend)				
POW, NA (PURIFIED)				
125 gm	**17317-0518-04**	4.90		
454 gm	**17317-0518-01**	10.50		
2270 gm	**17317-0518-05**	35.00		
11350 gm	**17317-0518-08**	105.00		

PROD/MFR NDC AWP DP OBC

(Baker, J.T.) *See SODIUM PERBORATE TETRAHYDRATE*

(Gallipot)
GRA, NA (PURIFIED)
113.4 gm........... 51552-0105-04 8.75
454 gm............. 51552-0105-06 14.14

(PCCA)
POW, NA (PURIFIED; TETRAHYDRATE)
1 gm............... 51927-1334-00 0.11

(Spectrum Pharmacy)
GRA, NA (TETRAHYDRATE)
125 gm............. 49452-6905-01 58.80
500 gm............. 49452-6905-02 89.95
2500 gm............ 49452-6905-03 246.05
12000 gm........... 49452-6905-04 805.00

(Spectrum Pharmacy) *See SODIUM PERBORATE MONOHYDRATE*

SODIUM PERBORATE MONOHYDRATE
(Spectrum Pharmacy)
sodium perborate
POW, NA, 500 gm......... 49452-6900-01 99.75

SODIUM PERBORATE TETRAHYDRATE (Baker, J.T.)
sodium perborate
GRA, NA (PURIFIED)
500 gm............. 10106-3811-01 29.92
2500 gm............ 10106-3811-05 80.03

SODIUM PERIODATE
(Baker, J.T.) *See SODIUM META-PERIODATE*

SODIUM PEROXIDE (Baker, J.T.)
GRA, NA (A.C.S., REAGENT,20 MESH)
500 gm............. 10106-9418-01 407.88

SODIUM PHENOBARBITAL (Amend)
phenobarbital sodium
POW, NA (U.S.P.)
500 gm, C-IV......... 17317-0413-01 70.00

SODIUM PHENYLBUTYRATE (Medisca)
POW, NA, 100 gm......... 38779-1597-05 1020.00
500 gm............. 38779-1597-08 3960.00
1000 gm............ 38779-1597-09 6273.00

(Ucyclyd) *See BUPHENYL*

SODIUM PHOSPHATE
(Amend) *See SODIUM BIPHOSPHATE*

(Amend) *See SODIUM PHOSPHATE DIBASIC*

(Amend) *See SODIUM PHOSPHATE DIBASIC ANHYDROUS*

(Amend) *See SODIUM PHOSPHATE MONOBASIC*

(Amend) *See SODIUM PHOSPHATE TRIBASIC*

(Amer Regent)
SOL, IV (S.D.V.)
3 mmole/ml,
5 ml 25s........... 00517-3405-25 20.94
15 ml 25s.......... 00517-3415-25 32.19
50 ml 25s.......... 00517-3450-25 85.94

(Baker, J.T.) *See SODIUM PHOSPHATE DIBASIC*

(Baker, J.T.) *See SODIUM PHOSPHATE DIBASIC 12-HYDRATE*

(Baker, J.T.) *See SODIUM PHOSPHATE DIBASIC 7-HYDRATE*

(Baker, J.T.) *See SODIUM PHOSPHATE MONOBASIC*

(Baker, J.T.) *See SODIUM PHOSPHATE MONOBASIC DIHYDRATE*

(Baker, J.T.) *See SODIUM PHOSPHATE TRIBASIC 12-HYDRATE*

(Gallipot) *See SODIUM PHOSPHATE DIBASIC*

(Gallipot) *See SODIUM PHOSPHATE DIBASIC ANHYDROUS*

(Gallipot) *See SODIUM PHOSPHATE MONOBASIC*

(Gallipot) *See SODIUM PHOSPHATE TRIBASIC*

(Hospira)
SOL, IV (VIAL,FLIPTOP)
3 mmole/ml,
15 ml 25s.......... 00409-7391-72 19.50 17.00

(Letco) *See SODIUM PHOSPHATE DIBASIC*

(Letco) *See SODIUM PHOSPHATE MONOBASIC*

(Mallinckrodt Lab) *See SODIUM PHOSPHATE DIBASIC*

(Mallinckrodt Lab) *See SODIUM PHOSPHATE TRIBASIC*

SODIUM PHOSPHATE (Medisca)
POW, NA (1X500GM,DIBASIC)
500 gm............. 38779-0807-08 43.50
(1X2500GM,DIBASIC)
2500 gm............ 38779-0807-01 153.00

PROD/MFR NDC AWP DP OBC

(Medisca) *See SODIUM PHOSPHATE MONOBASIC*

(PCCA)
POW, NA, 1 gm.......... 51927-3095-00 0.10
(DIABASIC; USP; DRIED)
1 gm............... 51927-1329-00 0.07

(PCCA) *See SODIUM PHOSPHATE DIBASIC*

(PCCA) *See SODIUM PHOSPHATE TRIBASIC*

(Spectrum Pharmacy) *See SODIUM PHOSPHATE DIBASIC*

(Spectrum Pharmacy) *See SODIUM PHOSPHATE MONOBASIC*

SODIUM PHOSPHATE DIBASIC (Amend)
sodium phosphate
GRA, NA (HEPTAHYDRATE, U.S.P.)
454 gm............. 17317-0520-01 9.80
2270 gm............ 17317-0520-05 39.20
11350 gm........... 17317-0520-08 175.00
POW, NA (DRIED, U.S.P.)
454 gm............. 17317-1657-01 9.80
(A.C.S., REAGENT)
500 gm............. 17317-1465-05 14.00
(DRIED, U.S.P.)
2270 gm............ 17317-1657-05 35.00
(A.C.S., REAGENT)
2500 gm............ 17317-1465-06 56.00
(DRIED, U.S.P.)
11350 gm........... 17317-1657-08 140.00

(Baker, J.T.)
POW, NA (U.S.P., A.C.S.)
500 gm............. 10106-3827-01 22.91

(Gallipot)
CRY, NA (HEPTAHYDRATE,U.S.P.)
454 gm............. 51552-0503-06 16.24

(Letco)
CRY, NA (U.S.P./N.F.)
500 gm............. 62991-1376-02 37.50

(Mallinckrodt Lab)
GRA, NA (U.S.P.)
500 gm............. 00406-7896-04 38.16

(PCCA)
POW, NA (UPS;HEPTAHYDRATE)
1 gm............... 51927-2635-00 0.11

(Spectrum Pharmacy)
CRY, NA (HEPTAHYDRATE/U.S.P.)
500 gm............. 49452-6930-01 75.60
2500 gm............ 49452-6930-02 269.50
12000 gm........... 49452-6930-03 1036.00
POW, NA (ANHYDROUS, U.S.P.)
500 gm............. 49452-6925-01 57.40
(DIHYDRATE, F.C.C.)
500 gm............. 49452-6928-01 117.25
(ANHYDROUS, U.S.P.)
2500 gm............ 49452-6925-02 171.15
(DIHYDRATE, F.C.C.)
2500 gm............ 49452-6928-02 332.85
(ANHYDROUS, U.S.P.)
12000 gm........... 49452-6925-03 735.00
(DIHYDRATE, F.C.C.)
12000 gm........... 49452-6928-03 1113.00

SODIUM PHOSPHATE DIBASIC 12-HYDRATE
(Baker, J.T.)
sodium phosphate
CRY, NA (REAGENT)
500 gm............. 10106-3822-01 44.81
2500 gm............ 10106-3822-05 160.32

SODIUM PHOSPHATE DIBASIC 7-HYDRATE
(Baker, J.T.)
sodium phosphate
CRY, NA (U.S.P., A.C.S.)
500 gm............. 10106-3817-01 19.24
2500 gm............ 10106-3817-05 127.26

SODIUM PHOSPHATE DIBASIC ANHYDROUS (Amend)
sodium phosphate
POW, NA (F.C.C.)
454 gm............. 17317-0148-01 8.40
(A.C.S, REAGENT)
500 gm............. 17317-1212-05 21.00
(F.C.C.)
2270 gm............ 17317-0148-05 33.60
(A.C.S., REAGENT)
2500 gm............ 17317-1212-06 84.00
(F.C.C.)
11350 gm........... 17317-0148-08 122.50
(A.C.S., REAGENT)
12000 gm........... 17317-1212-08 235.20

PROD/MFR NDC AWP DP OBC

(Gallipot)
GRA, NA (U.S.P.,N.F.)
454 gm............. 51552-0477-06 11.06
POW, NA, 113.4 gm...... 51552-0447-04 7.35

SODIUM PHOSPHATE MONOBASIC (Amend)
sodium phosphate
POW, NA (ANHYDROUS, U.S.P.)
454 gm............. 17317-1658-01 9.10
2270 gm............ 17317-1658-05 36.40
11350 gm........... 17317-1658-08 122.50

(Baker, J.T.)
CRY, NA (USP,FCC,ACS,MONOHYDRATE)
500 gm............. 10106-3820-01 24.11

(Gallipot)
GRA, NA (U.S.P.)
454 gm............. 51552-0504-06 17.85

(Letco)
POW, NA (ANHYDROUS, U.S.P./N.F.)
500 gm............. 62991-1377-02 42.00

(Medisca)
POW, NA (U.S.P.)
500 gm............. 38779-0943-08 49.50
(USP)
2500 gm............ 38779-0943-01 214.50

(Spectrum Pharmacy)
GRA, NA (MONOHYDRATE,U.S.P.)
500 gm............. 49452-6910-01 99.75
(MONOHYDRATE, U.S.P.)
2500 gm............ 49452-6910-02 332.85
12000 gm........... 49452-6910-03 1403.50
POW, NA (ANHYDROUS, F.C.C.)
500 gm............. 49452-6920-01 87.85
(ANHYDROUS, U.S.P.)
500 gm............. 49452-6921-01 73.15
(ANHYDROUS, F.C.C.)
2500 gm............ 49452-6920-02 276.50
(ANHYDROUS, U.S.P.)
2500 gm............ 49452-6921-02 229.25
(ANHYDROUS, F.C.C.)
12000 gm........... 49452-6920-03 1022.00
(ANHYDROUS, U.S.P.)
12000 gm........... 49452-6921-03 843.50

SODIUM PHOSPHATE MONOBASIC DIHYDRATE
(Baker, J.T.)
sodium phosphate
CRY, NA (REAGENT)
500 gm............. 10106-3819-01 70.76
2500 gm............ 10106-3819-05 291.23

SODIUM PHOSPHATE TRIBASIC (Amend)
sodium phosphate
POW, NA (TECHNICAL)
454 gm............. 17317-0521-01 5.60
2270 gm............ 17317-0521-05 15.05
11350 gm........... 17317-0521-08 52.50

(Gallipot)
POW, NA (TECHNICAL)
454 gm............. 51552-0084-06 8.68

(Mallinckrodt Lab)
CRY, NA (A.C.S.)
500 gm............. 00406-7940-04 37.89

(PCCA)
POW, NA (FCC; ANHYDROUS)
1 gm............... 51927-3109-00 0.15

(Spectrum Pharmacy)
sodium phosphate, tribasic
CRY, NA (1X500GM)
500 gm............. 49452-6935-01 210.35

SODIUM PHOSPHATE TRIBASIC 12-HYDRATE
(Baker, J.T.)
sodium phosphate
CRY, NA (A.C.S., REAGENT)
500 gm............. 10106-3836-01 60.10
2500 gm............ 10106-3836-05 227.37

SODIUM PHOSPHATE, TRIBASIC
(Spectrum Pharmacy) *See SODIUM PHOSPHATE TRIBASIC*

SODIUM POLYMETAPHOSPHATE
(Amend) *See SODIUM HEXAMETAPHOSPHATE*

(Spectrum Pharmacy) *See SODIUM HEXAMETAPHOSPHATE*

SODIUM POLYSTYRENE SULFONATE (Carolina)
PDR, NA (FOR ORAL OR RECTAL USE)
ea................. 46287-0012-16 130.00 110.00 **AA**

(Carolina) *See SPS SUSPENSION*

(KVK) *See KALEXATE*

PROD/MFR	NDC	AWP	DP	OBC
(Major)				
PDR, NA (1X454GM,USP)				
454 gm	**00904-6041-27**	175.27		
(Marlex)				
POW, NA, 454 gm	**10135-0146-17**	35.66		
(Medisca)				
POW, NA (USP)				
50 gm	**38779-0258-02**	147.00		
(U.S.P.)				
500 gm	**38779-0258-08**	337.50		
(USP)				
1000 gm	**38779-0258-09**	535.50		
(Paddock) *See KIONEX*				
(PCCA)				
POW, NA (U.S.P.)				
1 gm	**51927-1901-00**	0.87		
(Sanofi-Aventis) *See KAYEXALATE*				
(Phys Total Care)				
REPACK				
SUS, PO (CARAMEL CHERRY)				
15 gm/60 ml, 60 ml	**54868-4439-00**	13.47		AA
SODIUM PROPIONATE (Amend)				
POW, NA (N.F., F.C.C.)				
454 gm	**17317-0522-01**	8.40		
2270 gm	**17317-0522-05**	35.00		
11350 gm	**17317-0522-08**	105.00		
(Gallipot)				
POW, NA (F.C.C.)				
454 gm	**51552-0501-06**	15.33		
(PCCA)				
POW, NA (NF)				
1 gm	**51927-1096-00**	0.27		
(Spectrum Pharmacy)				
POW, NA (F.C.C.)				
500 gm	**49452-6950-01**	84.35		
(N.F.)				
500 gm	**49452-0947-01**	84.35		
(F.C.C.)				
2500 gm	**49452-6950-02**	205.80		
(N.F.)				
2500 gm	**49452-0947-02**	205.80		
(F.C.C.)				
12000 gm	**49452-6950-03**	532.00		
(N.F.)				
12000 gm	**49452-0947-03**	532.00		
SODIUM PYROPHOSPHATE				
(Baker, J.T.) *See SODIUM PYROPHOSPHATE 10-HYDRATE*				
(Spectrum Pharmacy) *See SODIUM ACID PYROPHOSPHATE*				
(Spectrum Pharmacy) *See SODIUM PYROPHOSPHATE ANHYDROUS*				
SODIUM PYROPHOSPHATE 10-HYDRATE (Baker, J.T.)				
sodium pyrophosphate				
CRY, NA (A.C.S., REAGENT)				
500 gm	**10106-3850-01**	55.88		
2500 gm	**10106-3850-05**	196.37		
SODIUM PYROPHOSPHATE ANHYDROUS (Spectrum Pharmacy)				
sodium pyrophosphate				
POW, NA (F.C.C.)				
500 gm	**49452-6960-01**	99.75		
2500 gm	**49452-6960-02**	310.10		
12000 gm	**49452-6960-03**	1032.50		
SODIUM PYRROLIDONE CARBOXYLATE (PCCA)				
sodium pca				
SOL, NA, 1 ml	**51927-2577-00**	0.30		
SODIUM PYRUVATE (Baker, J.T.)				
POW, NA (REAGENT)				
100 gm	**10106-3354-04**	67.47		
1000 gm	**10106-3354-02**	385.43		
SODIUM SACCHARIN (Gallipot)				
saccharin sodium				
GRA, NA (U.S.P.,N.F.)				
25 gm	**51552-0174-04**	7.91		
454 gm	**51552-0174-06**	24.71		
POW, NA, 25 gm	**51552-0187-04**	7.91		
454 gm	**51552-0187-06**	24.71		
(Letco)				
POW, NA (U.S.P.)				
100 gm	**62991-1378-01**	27.00		
(U.S.P., FCC)				
500 gm	**62991-1378-02**	51.00		
1000 gm	**62991-1378-03**	66.00		

PROD/MFR	NDC	AWP	DP	OBC
SODIUM SACCHARIN DIHYDRATE (Spectrum Pharmacy)				
saccharin sodium				
GRA, NA (U.S.P.)				
500 gm	**49452-6970-01**	392.00		
2500 gm	**49452-6970-02**	1463.00		
POW, NA, 500 gm	**49452-6980-01**	392.00		
2500 gm	**49452-6980-02**	1463.00		
SODIUM SALICYLATE (Amend)				
POW, NA (U.S.P.)				
454 gm	**17317-0524-01**	18.20		
2270 gm	**17317-0524-05**	67.20		
11350 gm	**17317-0524-08**	210.00		
(Baker, J.T.)				
CRY, NA (U.S.P.)				
500 gm	**10106-3872-01**	20.93		
(Gallipot)				
POW, NA (U.S.P.)				
454 gm	**51552-0558-06**	24.99		
2270 gm	**51552-0558-09**	94.50		
(Hawkins)				
POW, NA (U.S.P.)				
500 gm	**63370-0223-45**	60.00		
2500 gm	**63370-0223-53**	240.00		
(Medisca)				
POW, NA (U.S.P.)				
500 gm	**38779-0259-08**	57.00		
1000 gm	**38779-0259-09**	112.50		
(PCCA)				
POW, NA (U.S.P.)				
1 gm	**51927-1679-00**	0.15		
(Spectrum Pharmacy)				
CRY, NA (U.S.P.)				
500 gm	**49452-6990-01**	110.60		
2500 gm	**49452-6990-02**	367.50		
SODIUM SELENATE (PCCA)				
POW, NA (DECAHYDRATE)				
1 gm	**51927-3280-00**	3.75		
SODIUM SELENITE (PCCA)				
POW, NA, 1 gm	**51927-2663-00**	1.05		
SODIUM SILICATE (Amend)				
SOL, NA, 500 ml	**17317-0525-01**	7.00		
3840 ml	**17317-0525-06**	16.80		
(AmerisourceBergen)				
SOL, NA (PRIVATE LABEL)				
900 ml	**87701-0396-14**	6.49		
(Baker, J.T.) *See SODIUM META-SILICATE 9-HYDRATE*				
(Baker, J.T.)				
SOL, NA, 500 ml	**10106-3877-01**	49.08		
(Gallipot)				
LIQ, NA (41 BE)				
473 ml	**51552-0172-06**	8.82		
3785 ml	**51552-0172-08**	21.84		
(Gallipot) *See SODIUM SILICATE PENTAHYDRATE*				
(Humco)				
SOL, NA, 900 ml	**00395-2727-30**	7.85		
3840 ml	**00395-2727-28**	34.22		
(Medisca)				
SOL, NA (1X500ML,40 BE SOLUTION)				
500 ml	**38779-0839-08**	25.50		
(1X1000ML,40 BE SOLUTION)				
1000 ml	**38779-0839-09**	47.25		
(1X4000ML,40 BE SOLUTION)				
4000 ml	**38779-0839-01**	75.00		
(PCCA)				
SOL, NA, 1 ml	**51927-1875-00**	0.09		
(Spectrum Pharmacy)				
SOL, NA, 500 ml	**49452-7000-02**	65.10		
4000 ml	**49452-7000-01**	122.50		
SODIUM SILICATE PENTAHYDRATE (Gallipot)				
sodium silicate				
GRA, NA, 454 gm	**51552-0516-06**	14.56		
SODIUM STANNATE				
(Baker, J.T.) *See SODIUM STANNATE TRIHYDRATE*				
SODIUM STANNATE TRIHYDRATE (Baker, J.T.)				
sodium stannate				
POW, NA (REAGENT)				
500 gm	**10106-3880-01**	218.51		
2500 gm	**10106-3880-05**	970.05		
SODIUM STARCH GLYCOLATE (Spectrum Pharmacy)				
POW, NA (1X500GM)				
500 gm	**49452-7001-01**	119.70		

PROD/MFR	NDC	AWP	DP	OBC
(1X2500GM)				
2500 gm	**49452-7001-02**	535.50		
SODIUM STEARATE (Amend)				
POW, NA (N.F.)				
454 gm	**17317-0745-01**	9.80		
2270 gm	**17317-0745-05**	36.40		
11350 gm	**17317-0745-08**	140.00		
(Medisca)				
POW, NA (1X100GM)				
100 gm	**38779-1614-05**	22.50		
(1X500GM)				
500 gm	**38779-1614-08**	34.50		
(PCCA)				
POW, NA (NF)				
1 gm	**51927-1229-00**	0.30		
(Spectrum Pharmacy)				
POW, NA (N.F.)				
500 gm	**49452-7010-01**	78.75		
2500 gm	**49452-7010-02**	252.35		
12000 gm	**49452-7010-03**	847.00		
SODIUM STEAROYL LACTYLATE (Spectrum Pharmacy)				
POW, NA, 500 gm	**49452-7011-01**	149.80		
SODIUM STEARYL FUMARATE (Spectrum Pharmacy)				
POW, NA (N.F.)				
25 gm	**49452-7012-01**	228.90		
125 gm	**49452-7012-02**	626.50		
(N.F.)				
500 gm	**49452-7012-03**	1823.50		
SODIUM SUCCINATE (PCCA)				
POW, NA, 1 gm	**51927-2518-00**	0.57		
(Spectrum Pharmacy) *See SODIUM SUCCINATE HEXAHYDRATE*				
SODIUM SUCCINATE HEXAHYDRATE (Spectrum Pharmacy)				
sodium succinate				
POW, NA (REAGENT)				
100 gm	**49452-7020-01**	97.30		
500 gm	**49452-7020-02**	225.75		
SODIUM SULFACETAMIDE (Fougera)				
sulfacetamide sodium				
PAD, TP, 10%, 30s ea	**18754-0664-10**	69.60		
(PCCA)				
POW, NA (USP,MONOHYDRATE)				
1 gm	**51927-1053-00**	1.20		
(Prasco Labs)				
LOT, TP, 10%, 118 ml	**66993-0875-55**	110.48		
SODIUM SULFACETAMIDE AND SULFUR (Actavis Mid Atlantic)				
sulfacetamide sodium/sulfur				
PAD, TP, 10%-5%, 30s ea	**00472-0460-30**	128.87		
60s ea	**00472-0460-60**	244.90		
SOA, TP (1X170.3GM)				
10%-5%, 170.3 gm	**00472-0461-06**	84.16		
(1X340.2GM)				
10%-5%, 340.2 gm	**00472-0461-12**	154.43		
(Perrigo)				
LOT, TP (1X25GM,TINT-FREE)				
10%-5%, 25 gm	**45802-0950-01**	69.20		
(1X25GM,W/COLOR TINTER)				
10%-5%, 25 gm	**45802-0978-01**	71.50		
(1X30GM)				
10%-5%, 30 gm	**45802-0946-94**	60.94		
(1X60GM)				
10%-5%, 60 gm	**45802-0946-96**	109.71		
SOA, TP (1X170.1GM)				
10%-5%, 170.1 gm	**45802-0942-01**	53.79		
(2X170.1GM)				
10%-5%, 170.1 gm 2s	**45802-0942-02**	98.83		
SUS, TP (1X30GM)				
10%-5%, 30 gm	**45802-0901-94**	67.86		
SODIUM SULFACETAMIDE/ SULFUR CLEANSING PADS (Acella)				
sulfacetamide sodium/sulfur				
PAD, TP, 10%-4%, 60s ea	**42192-0113-60**	198.33		
SODIUM SULFATE (Amend)				
GRA, NA, 454 gm	**17317-0529-01**	12.60		
2270 gm	**17317-0529-05**	49.00		
11350 gm	**17317-0529-08**	157.50		
(Amend) *See SODIUM SULFATE ANHYDROUS*				
(Baker, J.T.) *See SODIUM SULFATE 10-HYDRATE*				
(Baker, J.T.) *See SODIUM SULFATE ANHYDROUS*				
(Baker, J.T.) *See SODIUM SULFATE DRIED*				

PROD/MFR NDC AWP DP OBC

(Gallipot) *See SODIUM SULFATE ANHYDROUS*

(Mallinckrodt Lab)
GRA, NA (U.S.P.)
500 gm............**00406-8012-04** 24.04
POW, NA, 500 gm........**00406-8028-12** 22.90

(PCCA)
POW, NA (USP; ANHYDROUS)
1 gm................**51927-3103-00** 0.11
(USP; DECAHYDRATE)
1 gm................**51927-1459-00** 0.12

(Spectrum Pharmacy)
POW, NA (DECAHYDRATE,U.S.P.)
500 gm............**49452-7044-01** 121.80
2500 gm...........**49452-7044-02** 256.55

(Spectrum Pharmacy) *See SODIUM SULFATE ANHYDROUS*

SODIUM SULFATE 10-HYDRATE (Baker, J.T.)
sodium sulfate
CRY, NA (A.C.S., REAGENT)
500 gm............**10106-3890-01** 34.56
2500 gm...........**10106-3890-05** 112.73

SODIUM SULFATE ANHYDROUS (Amend)
sodium sulfate
GRA, NA (A.C.S., REAGENT)
500 gm............**17317-1244-05** 8.40
1200 gm...........**17317-1244-08** 134.40
2500 gm...........**17317-1244-04** 49.00
POW, NA (F.C.C.)
454 gm............**17317-1406-01** 9.80
2270 gm...........**17317-1406-05** 28.00
11350 gm..........**17317-1406-08** 87.50

(Baker, J.T.)
POW, NA (A.C.S., REAGENT)
500 gm............**10106-3898-01** 33.68
(GRANULAR, ACS, REAGENT)
500 gm............**10106-3891-01** 32.45
(A.C.S., REAGENT)
2500 gm...........**10106-3898-05** 103.05
(GRANULAR, ACS, REAGENT)
2500 gm...........**10106-3891-05** 99.29

(Gallipot)
GRA, NA (U.S.P.)
454 gm............**51552-0308-06** 13.30
2270 gm...........**51552-0308-09** 39.69

(Spectrum Pharmacy)
GRA, NA (U.S.P.)
500 gm............**49452-7030-01** 78.75
2500 gm...........**49452-7030-02** 208.25
12000 gm..........**49452-7030-03** 616.00

SODIUM SULFATE DRIED (Baker, J.T.)
sodium sulfate
POW, NA (PURIFIED)
500 gm............**10106-3887-01** 35.12

SODIUM SULFIDE
(Baker, J.T.) *See SODIUM SULFIDE 9-HYDRATE*

(PCCA)
POW, NA (HYDRATE; TECHNICAL)
1 gm................**51927-1540-00** 0.87

SODIUM SULFIDE 9-HYDRATE (Baker, J.T.)
sodium sulfide
CRY, NA (A.C.S., REAGENT)
500 gm............**10106-3910-01** 55.77
2500 gm...........**10106-3910-05** 220.73

SODIUM SULFITE
(Baker, J.T.) *See SODIUM SULFITE ANHYDROUS*

(Baker, J.T.) *See SODIUM SULFITE EXSICCATED*

(Gallipot) *See SODIUM SULFITE ANHYDROUS*

(PCCA) *See SODIUM SULFITE ANHYDROUS*

(Spectrum Pharmacy)
POW, NA (B.P.,E.P.,F.C.C.,J.P.)
500 gm............**49452-7055-01** 74.20
(F.C.C.)
2500 gm...........**49452-7055-02** 212.45
12000 gm..........**49452-7055-03** 637.00

SODIUM SULFITE ANHYDROUS (Baker, J.T.)
sodium sulfite
POW, NA (A.C.S., REAGENT)
500 gm............**10106-3922-01** 29.61
2500 gm...........**10106-3922-05** 91.62
12000 gm..........**10106-3922-07** 197.86

(Gallipot)
GRA, NA (F.C.C.)
454 gm............**51552-0193-06** 10.99
2270 gm...........**51552-0193-09** 38.64

(PCCA)
POW, NA (F.C.C.)
1 gm................**51927-1453-00** 0.10

SODIUM SULFITE EXSICCATED (Baker, J.T.)
sodium sulfite
POW, NA (PURIFIED)
500 gm............**10106-3888-01** 22.90

SODIUM TARTRATE
(Baker, J.T.) *See SODIUM TARTRATE DIHYDRATE*

(PCCA) *See SODIUM TARTRATE DIHYDRATE*

SODIUM TARTRATE DIHYDRATE (Baker, J.T.)
sodium tartrate
CRY, NA (A.C.S., REAGENT)
500 gm............**10106-3930-01** 88.79
2500 gm...........**10106-3930-05** 318.22

(PCCA)
POW, NA (ACS; REAGENT)
1 gm................**51927-3403-00** 6.00

SODIUM TETRADECYL SULFATE
(Bioniche Pharma) *See SOTRADECOL*

(Medisca) *See SODIUM TETRADECYL SULFATE 27%*

(PCCA)
POW, NA, 1 gm..........**51927-2466-00** 264.00
SOL, NA (AQUEOUS)
27%, 1 ml............**51927-3410-00** 4.00

SODIUM TETRADECYL SULFATE 27% (Medisca)
sodium tetradecyl sulfate
SOL, NA (1X1ML)
27%, 1 ml............**38779-2236-06** 19.50
(1X5ML)
27%, 5 ml............**38779-2236-03** 46.50
(1X25ML)
27%, 25 ml...........**38779-2236-04** 123.00
(1X100ML)
27%, 100 ml..........**38779-2236-05** 337.50
(1X1000ML)
27%, 1000 ml.........**38779-2236-09** 750.00
(1X4000ML)
27%, 4000 ml.........**38779-2236-01** 1350.00

SODIUM THIOCYANATE (Baker, J.T.)
CRY, NA (A.C.S., REAGENT)
500 gm............**10106-3938-01** 90.64
2500 gm...........**10106-3938-05** 315.13

SODIUM THIOGLYCOLATE
(PCCA) *See MERCAPTOACETIC ACID SODIUM SALT*

SODIUM THIOSALICYLATE
(Clint) *See NO DOLO*

(PCCA) *See THIOSALICYLIC ACID SODIUM SALT*

SODIUM THIOSULFATE (Amend)
CRY, NA (U.S.P.)
500 gm............**17317-0533-01** 9.80
2270 gm...........**17317-0533-05** 35.00
11350 gm..........**17317-0533-08** 131.25

(Amer Regent)
SOL, IV (S.D.V.,PF)
10%, 10 ml 5s.......**00517-1019-05** 93.75
25%, 50 ml..........**00517-5019-01** 22.50

(Baker, J.T.) *See SODIUM THIOSULFATE ANHYDROUS*

(Baker, J.T.) *See SODIUM THIOSULFATE PENTAHYDRATE*

(Consolidated Midland)
SOL, IV (VIAL)
10%, 10 ml 5s.......**00223-8573-05** 75.00
(AMPULES)
10%, 10 ml 25s......**00223-8573-10** 300.00
(VIAL)
25%, 30 ml..........**00223-8573-50** 8.00

(Gallipot)
CRY, NA (U.S.P.)
454 gm............**51552-0512-06** 14.00

(Humco)
GRA, NA, 454 gm.........**00395-2745-01** 9.21

(Mallinckrodt Lab)
CRY, NA (U.S.P.)
500 gm............**00406-7763-04** 26.11
2500 gm...........**00406-7763-06** 96.94

(PCCA)
POW, NA (USP; PENTAHYDRATE)
1 gm................**51927-1294-00** 0.11

(Spectrum Pharmacy) *See SODIUM THIOSULFATE PENTAHYDRATE*

SODIUM THIOSULFATE ANHYDROUS (Baker, J.T.)
sodium thiosulfate
GRA, NA (REAGENT)
500 gm............**10106-3954-01** 45.53
2500 gm...........**10106-3954-05** 157.13

SODIUM THIOSULFATE PENTAHYDRATE (Baker, J.T.)
sodium thiosulfate
CRY, NA (A.C.S., REAGENT)
500 gm............**10106-3946-01** 37.34
2500 gm...........**10106-3946-05** 122.16

(Spectrum Pharmacy)
CRY, NA (U.S.P.,E.P.,B.P.,J.P.)
500 gm............**49452-7070-01** 98.35

SODIUM TRIMETAPHOSPHATE (Spectrum Pharmacy)
POW, NA (F.C.C.)
500 gm............**49452-7078-01** 107.80

SODIUM TRIPOLYPHOSPHATE (Spectrum Pharmacy)
POW, NA (F.C.C.)
500 gm............**49452-7080-01** 118.30

SODIUM TUNGSTATE
(Baker, J.T.) *See SODIUM TUNGSTATE DIHYDRATE*

(PCCA) *See SODIUM TUNGSTATE DIHYDRATE*

SODIUM TUNGSTATE DIHYDRATE (Baker, J.T.)
sodium tungstate
POW, NA (C.P.)
113 gm............**10106-3964-04** 66.54
500 gm............**10106-3964-01** 136.94

(PCCA)
POW, NA, 1 gm..........**51927-3283-00** 1.65

SODIUM VALPROATE (Gallipot)
valproate sodium
POW, NA, 25 gm.........**51552-0967-04** 44.10 31.50

(Hawkins)
POW, NA (BP)
25 gm.............**63370-0226-25** 88.00
100 gm............**63370-0226-35** 268.00
500 gm............**63370-0226-45** 1200.00
1000 gm...........**63370-0226-50** 2200.00

(Medisca)
POW, NA, 25 gm.........**38779-1683-04** 75.00
100 gm............**38779-1683-05** 225.00
500 gm............**38779-1683-08** 930.00

(Spectrum Pharmacy)
POW, NA (1X25GM)
25 gm.............**49452-7085-01** 155.40
(1X100GM)
100 gm............**49452-7085-02** 459.38

SODIUM-DL-LACTATE 60% (Spectrum Pharmacy)
sodium lactate
SOL, NA (U.S.P.)
500 ml............**49452-6830-01** 76.30
4000 ml...........**49452-6830-02** 281.40
20000 ml..........**49452-6830-03** 892.50

SODIUM-L-ASCORBYL-2-PHOSPHATE (PCCA)
sodium ascorbyl phosphate
POW, NA (DIHYDRATE)
1 gm................**51927-3589-00** 1.65

SODIUM-L-LACTATE 60% (Spectrum Pharmacy)
sodium lactate
SOL, NA (U.S.P.)
500 ml............**49452-6821-01** 74.20
4000 ml...........**49452-6821-02** 269.15
20000 ml..........**49452-6821-03** 857.50

SOF-SENSOR (Medtronic Minimed)
device
DEV, NA, 4s ea..........**76300-0002-14** 174.00 145.00
10s ea..........**76300-0002-11** 420.00 350.00

SOF-SERTER INFUSION/INSERTION SYST (Medtronic Minimed)
kit, administration, intravenous
DEV, NA, ea............**76300-0300-01** 31.19 24.95

SOF-SET MICRO NON-NEEDLE INFUSION (Medtronic Minimed)
infusion pump, parenteral
DEV, NA (W/24" POLYFIN TUBING)
12s ea............**76300-0321-12** 173.88
(W/42" POLYFIN TUBING)
12s ea............**76300-0320-12** 173.88

SOF-SET MICRO QR NON-NEEDLE (Medtronic Minimed)
set, administration, intravenous, needle-free
DEV, NA (PLASTIC CANNULA,24"X6MM)
ea................**76300-0325-12** 173.88
(PLASTIC CANNULA,42"X6MM)
ea................**76300-0324-12** 173.88

PROD/MFR NDC AWP DP OBC

SOF-SET NON-NEEDLE INFUSION
(Medtronic Minimed)
set, administration, intravenous, needle-free
DEV, NA (CANNULA,24"POLYFIN TBNG)
24s ea............... **76300-0112-24** 270.00 216.00
(CANNULA,42"POLYFIN TBNG)
24s ea............... **76300-0111-24** 270.00 216.00

SOF-SET QR NON-NEEDLE INFUSION
(Medtronic Minimed)
set, administration, intravenous, needle-free
DEV, NA (TEFLON CANNULA,24"TUBNG)
12s ea............... **76300-0316-12** 173.88
(TEFLON CANNULA,42"TUBNG)
12s ea............... **76300-0315-12** 173.88

SOF-SET ULTIMATE QR NON-NEEDLE
(Medtronic Minimed)
set, administration, intravenous, needle-free
DEV, NA (PLASTIC CANNULA,24"X9MM)
ea................... **76300-0318-12** 173.88
(PLASTIC CANNULA,42"X9MM)
ea................... **76300-0317-12** 173.88

SOJOURN (RxElite)
sevoflurane
LIQ, IH, 100%, 250 ml .... **66794-0012-25** 248.00 **AN**

SOLAGE (Stiefel Labs)
mequinol/tretinoin
SOL, TP, 2%-0.01%, 30 ml **13478-0001-01** 148.84

SOLAQUIN FORTE (Southwood)
REPACK
hydroquinone
CRE, TP, 4%, 15 gm....... **58016-3189-01** 18.56

SOLARAZE (Doak)
diclofenac sodium
GEL, TP, 3%, 100 gm...... **10337-0803-01** 476.56

(Dispensing Solutions)
REPACK
GEL, TP, 3%, 50 gm....... **55045-3358-05** 225.00

SOLIA (Prasco Labs)
desogestrel/ethinyl estradiol
TAB, PO (6X28)
0.15 mg-0.03 mg,
168s ea........... **66993-0611-28** 183.12

SOLIFENACIN SUCCINATE
(Astellas) *See VESICARE*

SOLIRIS (Alexion Pharmaceuticals)
eculizumab
SOL, IV (PF)
10 mg/ml, 30 ml **25682-0001-01** 6300.00

SOLODYN (Medicis)
minocycline hydrochloride
TER, PO (FILM-COATED)
45 mg, 30s ea........ **99207-0460-30** 664.69
100s ea........... **99207-0460-10** 2215.67
65 mg, 30s ea........ **99207-0463-30** 664.69
90 mg, 30s ea........ **99207-0461-30** 664.69
100s ea........... **99207-0461-10** 2215.67
115 mg, 30s ea **99207-0464-30** 664.69
135 mg, 30s ea **99207-0462-30** 664.69
100s ea........... **99207-0462-10** 2215.67

SOLOTUSS (Hawthorn Pharm)
carbetapentane tannate
SUS, PO (GRAPE)
30 mg/5 ml, 118 ml .. **63717-0280-04** 31.24

SOLU MEDROL (Dispensing Solutions)
REPACK
methylprednisolone sodium succinate
PDS, IJ, 125 mg, 25s ea... **55045-3509-01** 175.00

SOLU-CORTEF (Pfizer)
hydrocortisone sodium succinate
PDS, IJ (ACT-O-VIAL)
1 gm, ea............ **00009-0920-03** 35.71 29.76 **AP**
100 mg, ea .... **00009-0825-01** 4.63 3.86 **AP**
(ACT-O-VIAL)
100 mg, ea .... **00009-0900-13** 4.85 4.04 **AP**
(ACT-O-VIAL,25 PACK)
100 mg, 25s ea ...... **00009-0900-20** 121.32 101.10 **AP**
(ACT-O-VIAL)
250 mg, ea .... **00009-0909-08** 8.58 7.15 **AP**
(ACT-O-VIAL,25 PACK)
250 mg, 25s ea ...... **00009-0909-16** 214.51 178.76 **AP**
(ACT-O-VIAL)
500 mg, ea .... **00009-0912-05** 19.04 15.87 **AP**

(Phys Total Care)
REPACK
PDS, IJ (ACT-O-VIAL)
1 gm, ea............ **54868-4508-00** 19.19 **AP**
(S.D.V.)
100 mg, 2s ea........ **54868-0605-00** 13.14 **AP**

SOLU-MEDROL (Pfizer)
methylprednisolone sodium succinate
PDS, IJ (VIAL)
1 gm, ea............ **00009-0698-01** 24.43 20.36 **AP**
(W/DILUENT)
2 gm, ea............ **00009-0796-01** 53.36 44.47 **AP**
(VIAL)
500 mg, ea .... **00009-0758-01** 12.90 10.75 **AP**

(Pharmacia)
PDS, IJ (SDV,ACT-O-VIAL SYSTEM)
1 gm, ea............ **00009-0018-20** 33.14 27.62 **AP**
40 mg, 25s ea........ **00009-0039-28** 90.44 75.37 **AP**
125 mg, 2 ml 25s .... **00009-0047-22** 145.84 121.53 **AP**
500 mg, ea .... **00009-0003-02** 20.90 17.42 **AP**

(A-S Medication)
REPACK
PDS, IJ (ACT-O-VIAL)
125 mg, ea .... **54569-1555-00** 3.41 **AP**
25s ea............ **54569-1555-01** 85.25 **AP**

(Phys Total Care)
REPACK
PDS, IJ (S.D.V.)
40 mg, ea............ **54868-0768-00** 4.96 **AP**
(ACT-O-VIAL)
125 mg, ea .... **54868-3637-00** 4.77 **AP**
25s ea............ **54868-3637-01** 110.24 **AP**
(W/DILUENT)
500 mg, ea .... **54868-3623-00** 15.99 **AP**

(Southwood)
REPACK
PDS, IJ (SDV)
40 mg, 25s ea........ **58016-4897-01** 64.22
125 mg, ea .... **58016-9452-01** 5.31 **AP**

SOLU-SILK PROTEIN 20 (PCCA)
hydrolyzed silk
SOL, NA, 1 ml **51927-3391-00** 0.70

SOLUTION ADMINISTRATION SET (Bracco Diag)
kit, administration, intravenous
DEV, NA (STER,NONPYRO FLUID PATH)
10s ea.............. **00270-0004-31** 85.00 68.00

SOLUTION TRANSFER DEVICE (Bracco Diag)
transfer unit, iv fluid
DEV, NA (W/5CAPS,MALE/MALE ADAPT)
10s ea.............. **00270-0051-10** 133.38 113.00

SOMA (Meda)
carisoprodol
TAB, PO, 250 mg, 30s ea .. **00037-2250-30** 95.21
100s ea........... **00037-2250-10** 317.39
350 mg, 100s ea ..... **00037-2001-01** 580.62 **AA**

(IPI)
REPACK
TAB, PO, 250 mg, 40s ea .. **18837-0294-40** 126.96

(Nucare Pharm)
REPACK
TAB, PO, 350 mg, 40s ea .. **68071-0610-40** 137.05 **AA**

(PD-Rx Pharm)
REPACK
TAB, PO, 350 mg, 20s ea .. **55289-0578-20** 172.59 **AA**
40s ea............ **55289-0578-40** 345.18 **AA**

(Phys Total Care)
REPACK
TAB, PO, 350 mg, 20s ea .. **54868-0020-02** 121.08 **AA**
60s ea............ **54868-0020-01** 338.45 **AA**
100s ea........... **54868-0020-00** 562.41 **AA**

(Quality Care Prod)
REPACK
TAB, PO, 250 mg, 30s ea .. **35356-0501-30** 222.21

(Southwood)
REPACK
TAB, PO, 350 mg, 30s ea .. **58016-0038-30** 162.79 **AA**
60s ea............ **58016-0038-60** 325.58 **AA**
90s ea............ **58016-0038-90** 488.38 **AA**
100s ea........... **58016-0038-00** 542.64 **AA**

(Stat Rx)
REPACK
TAB, PO, 250 mg, 30s ea .. **16590-0755-30** 107.09
40s ea............ **16590-0755-40** 142.79
60s ea............ **16590-0755-60** 212.76
120s ea........... **16590-0755-72** 424.09
350 mg, 30s ea ...... **16590-0568-30** 158.00 **AA**
60s ea............ **16590-0568-60** 382.17 **AA**

SOMA COMPOUND W/CODEINE (PD-Rx Pharm)
REPACK
aspirin/carisoprodol/codeine phosphate
TAB, PO, 325 mg-200 mg-16 mg,
20s ea, C-III .... **55289-0472-20** 112.52 **AB**

SOMATROPIN (Medisca)
POW, NA (1X1GM,FREEZE DRIED)
1 gm **38779-2305-06** 27000.00

(PCCA)
POW, NA (1X1GM)
1 gm **51927-3664-00** 24000.00

SOMATROPIN, E-COLI DERIVED
(Gate) *See TEV-TROPIN*
(Genentech) *See NUTROPIN*
(Genentech) *See NUTROPIN AQ*
(Genentech) *See NUTROPIN AQ NUSPIN 5*
(Genentech) *See NUTROPIN AQ PEN*
(Genentech) *See NUTROPIN AQ PEN CARTRIDGE*
(Lilly) *See HUMATROPE*
(Novo Nordisk) *See NORDITROPIN*
(Novo Nordisk) *See NORDITROPIN NORDIFLEX*
(Pfizer) *See GENOTROPIN*
(Pfizer) *See GENOTROPIN MINIQUICK*
(Sandoz) *See OMNITROPE*

SOMATROPIN, MAMMALIAN DERIVED
(EMD) *See SAIZEN*
(EMD) *See SAIZEN CLICK EASY CARTRIDGE*
(EMD) *See SEROSTIM*
(EMD) *See ZORBTIVE*

SOMATULINE DEPOT (Tercica)
lanreotide acetate
SOL, SC (1X0.5ML, SINGLE USE)
120 mg/0.5 ml,
0.5 ml **15054-0120-01** 4317.60
(1X0.2ML, SINGLE USE)
60 mg/0.2 ml,
0.2 ml **15054-0060-01** 2155.20
(1X0.3ML, SINGLE USE)
90 mg/0.3 ml,
0.3 ml **15054-0090-01** 2844.00

SOMAVERT (Pfizer)
pegvisomant
PDS, SC (SINGLE DOSE,LYOPHILIZED)
10 mg, ea............ **00009-5176-01** 104.18 86.82
15 mg, ea............ **00009-5178-01** 156.29 130.24
20 mg, ea............ **00009-5180-01** 208.38 173.65

SOMNOTE (Breckenridge Pharm)
chloral hydrate
SGL, PO (5X10,SOFTGEL)
500 mg,
50s ea UD, C-IV **51991-0080-51** 74.95
(SOFTGEL)
500 mg,
50s ea, C-IV........ **51991-0080-52** 64.95

SONATA (King Pharm)
zaleplon
CAP, PO, 5 mg,
100s ea, C-IV **60793-0145-01** 471.36
10 mg,
100s ea, C-IV **60793-0146-01** 484.20

(A-S Medication)
REPACK
CAP, PO, 10 mg,
10s ea, C-IV........ **54569-4837-00** 47.14

(Altura)
REPACK
CAP, PO, 5 mg,
100s ea, C-IV **63874-1070-01** 227.80

(Core)
REPACK
CAP, PO, 10 mg,
30s ea, C-IV........ **33358-0326-30** 135.40

(DHS, Inc.)
REPACK
CAP, PO, 5 mg,
20s ea, C-IV........ **55887-0515-20** 73.18
30s ea, C-IV........ **55887-0515-30** 109.69

(Dispensing Solutions)
REPACK
CAP, PO, 5 mg,
20s ea, C-IV........ **55045-3034-07** 86.40
10 mg,
30s ea, C-IV........ **55045-3302-08** 132.90

(IPI)
REPACK
CAP, PO, 10 mg,
30s ea, C-IV........ **18837-0147-30** 124.36

PROD/MFR	NDC	AWP	DP	OBC
(Nucare Pharm)				
REPACK				
CAP, PO, 5 mg,				
30s ea, C-IV	66267-0723-30	127.12		
10 mg,				
30s ea, C-IV	68071-0414-30	130.58		
(Pharma Pac)				
REPACK				
CAP, PO, 5 mg,				
30s ea, C-IV	52959-0881-30	114.75		
10 mg,				
10s ea, C-IV	52959-0727-10	34.32		
30s ea, C-IV	52959-0727-30	102.95		
100s ea, C-IV	52959-0727-00	343.12		
(Phys Total Care)				
REPACK				
CAP, PO, 5 mg,				
10s ea, C-IV	54868-5139-00	46.15		
30s ea, C-IV	54868-5139-01	126.17		
10 mg,				
10s ea, C-IV	54868-4431-01	46.71		
30s ea, C-IV	54868-4431-00	137.01		
50s ea, C-IV	54868-4431-03	213.60		
100s ea, C-IV	54868-4431-02	424.71		
(Quality Care Prod)				
REPACK				
CAP, PO, 10 mg,				
15s ea, C-IV	49999-0604-15	128.60		
30s ea, C-IV	49999-0604-30	257.60		
(Southwood)				
REPACK				
CAP, PO, 10 mg,				
30s ea, C-IV	58016-0596-30	135.76		
60s ea, C-IV	58016-0596-60	271.51		
90s ea, C-IV	58016-0596-90	407.27		
100s ea, C-IV	58016-0596-00	452.52		
(Stat Rx)				
REPACK				
CAP, PO, 10 mg,				
30s ea, C-IV	16590-0522-30	224.98		
60s ea, C-IV	16590-0522-60	236.00		
90s ea, C-IV	16590-0522-90	339.00		
120s ea, C-IV	16590-0522-72	441.00		
SORAFENIB TOSYLATE				
(Bayer) *See NEXAVAR*				
SORBIC ACID (Amend)				
POW, NA (N.F., F.C.C.)				
454 gm	17317-0755-01	13.30		
2270 gm	17317-0755-05	53.20		
11350 gm	17317-0755-08	192.50		
(Gallipot)				
POW, NA (N.F.)				
113.4 gm	51552-0441-04	9.17		
454 gm	51552-0441-06	20.09		
(Letco)				
POW, NA (N.F.)				
500 gm	62991-1380-02	45.00		
(Medisca)				
POW, NA (1X100GM,CRYSTALLINE)				
100 gm	38779-0771-05	25.50		
(1X500GM,CRYSTALLINE)				
500 gm	38779-0771-08	52.50		
(PCCA)				
POW, NA (NF)				
1 gm	51927-1544-00	0.29		
(Spectrum Pharmacy)				
POW, NA (N.F.)				
100 gm	49452-7090-01	45.50		
500 gm	49452-7090-02	82.25		
SORBITAN MONOLAURATE				
(Amend) *See ARLACEL 20*				
(Amend) *See SPAN 20*				
(PCCA)				
LIQ, NA (NF, SPAN<<20)				
1 ml	51927-2075-00	0.43		
SORBITAN MONOOLEATE				
(Amend) *See ARLACEL 80*				
(Amend) *See SPAN 80*				
(Gallipot) *See SPAN 80*				
(PCCA)				
LIQ, NA (NF, SPAN<<80)				
1 ml	51927-1355-00	0.16		
(Spectrum Pharmacy) *See SPAN 80*				
SORBITAN MONOPALMITATE				
(Amend) *See ARLACEL 40*				
(Amend) *See SPAN 40*				
(Gallipot) *See SPAN 40*				
(PCCA)				
POW, NA (NF; SPAN40; BASE I)				
1 gm	51927-1180-00	0.36		
(Spectrum Pharmacy) *See SPAN 40*				
SORBITAN MONOSTEARATE				
(Amend) *See ARLACEL 60*				
(Amend) *See SPAN 60*				
(Medisca) *See SPAN 60*				
(PCCA)				
POW, NA (NF; SPAN<<60)				
1 gm	51927-2076-00	0.13		
(Spectrum Pharmacy) *See SPAN 60*				
SORBITAN SESQUIOLEATE				
(Amend) *See ARLACEL 83*				
(Amend) *See ARLACEL C*				
(PCCA) *See ARLACEL 83*				
(Spectrum Pharmacy)				
LIQ, NA (N.F.)				
500 ml	49452-7155-01	121.80		
4000 ml	49452-7155-02	570.50		
SORBITAN TRIOLEATE				
(Amend) *See SPAN 85*				
(PCCA)				
LIQ, NA, 1 ml	51927-2716-00	0.40		
SORBITAN TRISTEARATE				
(Amend) *See SPAN 65*				
(Medisca)				
BEA, NA (1X500GM,SPAN 65)				
500 gm	38779-2184-08	55.50		
(1X2500GM,SPAN 65)				
2500 gm	38779-2184-01	223.50		
SORBITOL				
(Amend) *See ARLEX*				
(B. Braun)				
SOL, IL (PIC CONTAINER)				
3.3%, 2000 ml	00264-2301-50	6.30		
4000 ml	00264-2301-70	12.62		
(Baxter)				
SOL, IL (UROLOGIC)				
3%, 3000 ml 4s	00338-0295-47	81.36		
5000 ml 2s	00338-0295-49	65.75		
(Carolina) *See SORBITOL 70%*				
(Cypress Pharm) *See SORBITOL 70%*				
(Gallipot)				
POW, NA (N.F.)				
454 gm	51552-0216-06	13.30		
(Gallipot) *See SORIBITOL 70%*				
(Humco) *See SORBITOL 70%*				
(Letco) *See SORBITOL 70%*				
(Lorann Oil) *See SORBITOL 70%*				
(Medisca)				
POW, NA (N.F.)				
500 gm	38779-0527-08	31.50		
1000 gm	38779-0527-09	52.50		
(NF)				
2500 gm	38779-0527-01	99.00		
(Medisca) *See SORBITOL 70%*				
(PCCA)				
POW, NA (N.F.)				
1 gm	51927-1227-00	0.08		
(PCCA) *See SORBITOL 70% SOLUTION*				
(Pharm Assoc Inc) *See SORBITOL 70%*				
(Qualitest) *See SORBITOL 70%*				
(Spectrum Pharmacy)				
POW, NA (N.F.)				
500 gm	49452-7100-01	63.00		
2500 gm	49452-7100-02	193.90		
(Spectrum Pharmacy) *See SORBITOL 70%*				
SORBITOL 70% (Carolina)				
sorbitol				
SOL, NA (U.S.P.)				
30 ml 10s UD	46287-0500-30	10.80	8.50	
480 ml	46287-0500-01	5.40	4.25	
3840 ml	46287-0500-99	27.70	25.50	
(Cypress Pharm)				
SOL, NA (U.S.P.)				
473 ml	60258-0901-16	7.29		
(Humco)				
SOL, NA (U.S.P.)				
480 ml	00802-3913-16	7.57		
(Letco)				
SOL, NA (U.S.P.)				
500 ml	62991-1146-01	21.00		
3840 ml	62991-1146-02	60.00		
(Lorann Oil)				
SOL, NA (U.S.P.)				
3840 ml	23535-0611-91	22.00		
(Medisca)				
SOL, NA (U.S.P.)				
500 ml	38779-0525-08	23.85		
4000 ml	38779-0525-01	97.50		
(Pharm Assoc Inc)				
SOL, NA (U.S.P.)				
30 ml 40s UD	00121-0659-30	62.52		
473 ml	00121-0659-16	6.94		
(Qualitest)				
SOL, NA, 480 ml	00603-0900-58	25.00		
(Spectrum Pharmacy)				
SOL, NA (U.S.P.)				
500 ml	49452-7110-01	46.65		
4000 ml	49452-7110-02	164.85		
20000 ml	49452-7110-03	549.50		
SORBITOL 70% SOLUTION (PCCA)				
sorbitol				
SOL, NA (USP (W/W))				
1 ml	51927-1268-00	1.08		
SORBITOL-MANNITOL (Hospira)				
mannitol/sorbitol				
SOL, IR (4X3000ML,PF,LATEX-FREE)				
3000 ml 4s	00409-7981-08	56.11	49.08	AT
SORIATANE (Stiefel Labs)				
acitretin				
KIT, MR, 10 mg, ea	00145-3800-01	700.30		
25 mg, ea	00145-4300-01	863.20		
SORIBITOL 70% (Gallipot)				
sorbitol				
SOL, NA (U.S.P.)				
473 ml	51552-0096-06	7.70		
3785 ml	51552-0096-08	36.61		
SORINE (Upsher-Smith)				
sotalol hydrochloride				
TAB, PO (CAPLET)				
80 mg, ea	00245-0012-89	2.61		AB
100s ea UD	00245-0012-01	260.89		AB
120 mg, ea	00245-0013-89	3.46		AB
100s ea UD	00245-0013-01	346.39		AB
160 mg, ea	00245-0014-89	4.31		AB
100s ea UD	00245-0014-01	430.98		AB
240 mg, ea	00245-0015-89	5.60		AB
100s ea UD	00245-0015-01	559.97		AB
SOTALOL (Physician Partner)				
REPACK				
sotalol hydrochloride				
TAB, PO, 80 mg, 30s ea	21695-0397-30	153.76		
SOTALOL HCL (Apotex Corp.)				
sotalol hydrochloride				
TAB, PO, 80 mg, 100s ea	60505-0080-00	256.21		AB1
120 mg, 100s ea	60505-0159-00	341.84		AB1
160 mg, 100s ea	60505-0081-00	427.40		AB1
240 mg, 100s ea	60505-0082-00	555.59		AB1
(Mylan)				
TAB, PO, 80 mg, 100s ea	00378-0305-01	241.60		AB
120 mg, 100s ea	00378-0310-01	322.35		AB
160 mg, 100s ea	00378-0314-01	403.00		AB
(Qualitest)				
TAB, PO, 80 mg,				
100s ea UD	00603-5769-21	256.27		AB1
500s ea UD	00603-5769-28	1281.40		AB1
120 mg, 100s ea UD	00603-5770-21	341.88		AB1
160 mg, 100s ea UD	00603-5771-21	427.45		AB1
(Sandoz)				
TAB, PO, 80 mg, 100s ea	00185-0171-01	256.28		AB
500s ea	00185-0171-05	1281.40		AB
120 mg, 100s ea	00185-0170-01	341.89		AB
160 mg, 100s ea	00185-0177-01	427.45		AB
240 mg, 100s ea	00185-0174-01	555.64		AB
(Teva)				
TAB, PO (CAPLET)				
80 mg, 100s ea	00093-1061-01	234.72		AB

PROD/MFR	NDC	AWP	DP	OBC
120 mg, 100s ea	00093-1060-01	313.14		AB
160 mg, 100s ea	00093-1062-01	391.50		AB
240 mg, 100s ea	00093-1063-01	508.95		AB
(American Health) REPACK				
TAB, PO, 80 mg, 100s ea UD	68084-0387-01	31.25		AB1
(Dispensing Solutions) REPACK				
TAB, PO, 80 mg, 100s ea	55045-3160-00	250.00		AB
(GSMS) REPACK				
TAB, PO (CAPLET)				
80 mg, 100s ea	60429-0948-01	20.31	6.77	AB
120 mg, 100s ea	60429-0949-01	22.59	7.53	AB
160 mg, 100s ea	60429-0950-01	32.55	10.85	AB
240 mg, 100s ea	60429-0951-01	40.89	13.63	AB
(PD-Rx Pharm) REPACK				
TAB, PO (USP)				
80 mg, 30s ea	43063-0133-30	35.04		AB
(Phys Total Care) REPACK				
TAB, PO, 80 mg, 30s ea	54868-4435-00	15.51		EE
60s ea	54868-4435-01	28.02		AB
90s ea	54868-4435-03	40.43		EE
100s ea	54868-4435-02	43.17		AB
(Southwood) REPACK				
TAB, PO, 80 mg, 30s ea	58016-0188-30	63.81		
60s ea	58016-0188-60	127.63		
90s ea	58016-0188-90	191.44		
100s ea	58016-0188-00	212.71		
120s ea	58016-0188-02	255.25		
(Vibranta) REPACK				
TAB, PO, 80 mg, 30s ea	57866-9032-02	69.55		AB
60s ea	57866-9032-01	137.86		AB
90s ea	57866-9032-03	206.16		AB
120s ea	57866-9032-04	274.46		AB
120 mg, 30s ea	57866-9033-02	92.37		AB
60s ea	57866-9033-01	183.50		AB
90s ea	57866-9033-03	274.62		AB
120s ea	57866-9033-04	365.75		AB
160 mg, 30s ea	57866-9034-02	115.18		AB
60s ea	57866-9034-01	229.10		AB
90s ea	57866-9034-03	343.03		AB
120s ea	57866-9034-04	456.96		AB
SOTALOL HCL AF (Apotex Corp.) sotalol hydrochloride				
TAB, PO, 80 mg, 100s ea	60505-0222-01	256.28		AB2
120 mg, 100s ea	60505-0223-01	341.89		AB2
160 mg, 100s ea	60505-0224-01	427.45		AB2
(Phys Total Care) REPACK				
TAB, PO, 120 mg, 20s ea	54868-5614-01	21.74		AB2
SOTALOL HYDROCHLORIDE FUL				
TAB, PO, 80 mg, 100s ea		178.50		
120 mg, 100s ea		235.50		
160 mg, 100s ea		292.50		
240 mg, 100s ea		397.50		
(Amneal)				
TAB, PO (USP)				
80 mg, 100s ea	65162-0725-10	256.25		AB2
120 mg, 100s ea	65162-0727-10	341.85		AB2
160 mg, 100s ea	65162-0731-10	427.45		AB2
(Apotex Corp.) *See SOTALOL HCL*				
(Apotex Corp.) *See SOTALOL HCL AF*				
(Bayer) *See BETAPACE*				
(Bayer) *See BETAPACE AF*				
(Mylan) *See SOTALOL HCL*				
(Mylan)				
TAB, PO (USP)				
80 mg, 100s ea	00378-5123-01	256.25		AB2
120 mg, 100s ea	00378-5124-01	341.85		AB2
160 mg, 100s ea	00378-5125-01	427.45		AB2
(Qualitest) *See SOTALOL HCL*				
(Sandoz) *See SOTALOL HCL*				
(Teva) *See SOTALOL HCL*				
(Upsher-Smith) *See SORINE*				
(GSMS) REPACK				
TAB, PO, 80 mg, 100s ea	60429-0748-01	19.95	6.65	AB1
120 mg, 100s ea	60429-0749-01	22.20	7.40	AB1
160 mg, 100s ea	60429-0750-01	31.95	10.65	AB1
(Phys Total Care) REPACK				
TAB, PO, 120 mg, 60s ea	54868-5614-00	51.72		
160 mg, 20s ea	54868-5549-01	25.74		
60s ea	54868-5549-00	68.19		
SOTRADECOL (Bioniche Pharma) sodium tetradecyl sulfate				
SOL, IV, 1%, 2 ml 5s	67457-0162-02	186.25		
3%, 2 ml 5s	67457-0163-02	311.25		
SOTRET (Ranbaxy Labs) isotretinoin				
SGL, PO (U.S.P., 3X10 RX PAK)				
10 mg, 30s ea	10631-0584-31	219.43		AB
100s ea	10631-0584-77	703.31		AB
(U.S.P., 3X10 RX PAK)				
20 mg, 30s ea	10631-0585-31	260.21		AB
100s ea	10631-0585-77	834.01		AB
(U.S.P., 3X10 RX PAK)				
30 mg, 30s ea	10631-0447-31	253.05		
40 mg, 30s ea	10631-0586-31	302.31		AB
100s ea	10631-0586-77	968.95		AB
(Phys Total Care) REPACK				
SGL, PO, 30 mg, 30s ea	54868-5868-00	585.73		
SOYA LECITHIN (Letco) soybean lecithin				
GRA, NA, 2500 gm	62991-1275-03	105.00		
SOYABEAN CASEIN DIGEST MEDIUM (PCCA) casein				
POW, NA (1X1GM)				
1 gm	51927-3585-00	3.67		
SOYBEAN LECITHIN				
(Letco) *See SOYA LECITHIN*				
(PCCA) *See LECITHIN SOYA*				
SOYBEAN OIL				
(Baxter) *See INTRALIPID*				
(Gallipot)				
OIL, NA (U.S.P.,REFINED)				
473 ml	51552-0873-06	17.50	12.50	
(Hospira) *See LIPOSYN III*				
(Medisca)				
OIL, NA (1X500ML,USP)				
500 ml	38779-2185-08	28.50		
(1X4000ML)				
4000 ml	38779-2185-01	190.50		
(1X20000ML)				
20000 ml	38779-2185-07	765.00		
(PCCA)				
OIL, NA (U.S.P.; REFINED)				
1 ml	51927-2516-00	0.08		
(Spectrum Pharmacy)				
OIL, NA (U.S.P.)				
500 ml	49452-7120-01	70.00		
SPACER, INHALATION				
(Adamis) *See ACAPELLA*				
(Dexo) *See E-Z SPACER & MASK COMBO*				
(Dey, L.P.) *See ACE AEROSOL CLOUD ENHANCER*				
(Dey, L.P.) *See EASIVENT VALVED HOLDING CHAMBER*				
(Forest Pharm) *See AEROCHAMBER*				
(FSC Laboratories) *See E-Z SPACER*				
(FSC Laboratories) *See THE BODY GUARDS PACK WITH E-Z SPACER*				
(Monaghan Medical) *See AEROCHAMBER Z-STAT PLUS*				
(Monaghan Medical) *See AEROPEP PLUS*				
(Monaghan Medical) *See AEROTRACH PLUS*				
(Pari) *See VORTEX VALVED HOLDING CHAMBER*				
(Respironics) *See OPTICHAMBER*				
(Respironics) *See OPTICHAMBER W/MASK*				
(Respironics) *See OPTIHALER*				
(Respironics) *See ZOEY OPTICHAMBER*				
(Schering) *See INSPIREASE*				
SPAN 20 (Amend) sorbitan monolaurate				
LIQ, NA (N.F.)				
480 ml	17317-1025-01	15.00		
3840 ml	17317-1025-06	60.00		
22560 ml	17317-1025-03	214.32		
SPAN 40 (Amend) sorbitan monopalmitate				
POW, NA, 454 gm	17317-1026-01	15.00		
4540 gm	17317-1026-06	60.00		
22700 gm	17317-1026-03	215.00		
(Gallipot)				
POW, NA (N.F.)				
454 gm	51552-0595-06	28.49		
(Spectrum Pharmacy)				
LIQ, NA (N.F.)				
500 gm	49452-7135-01	128.45		
2500 gm	49452-7135-02	448.00		
SPAN 60 (Amend) sorbitan monostearate				
POW, NA (N.F.)				
454 gm	17317-1027-01	15.00		
4540 gm	17317-1027-06	60.00		
22700 gm	17317-1027-03	201.00		
(Medisca)				
POW, NA (N.F.)				
500 gm	38779-0907-08	46.50		
(NF)				
2500 gm	38779-0907-01	166.50		
(Spectrum Pharmacy)				
LIQ, NA (N.F.)				
500 gm	49452-7145-01	98.00		
2500 gm	49452-7145-02	319.55		
SPAN 65 (Amend) sorbitan tristearate				
POW, NA, 454 gm	17317-1029-01	15.00		
4540 gm	17317-1029-06	60.00		
22700 gm	17317-1029-03	204.50		
SPAN 80 (Amend) sorbitan monooleate				
LIQ, NA (N.F.)				
480 ml	17317-1030-01	15.00		
3840 ml	17317-1030-06	60.00		
21600 ml	17317-1030-02	182.25		
(Gallipot)				
LIQ, NA, 473 ml	51552-0321-06	23.10		
(Spectrum Pharmacy)				
LIQ, NA (N.F.)				
500 ml	49452-7165-01	98.00		
4000 ml	49452-7165-02	402.50		
SPAN 85 (Amend) sorbitan trioleate				
LIQ, NA, 480 ml	17317-1031-01	15.00		
3840 ml	17317-1031-06	60.00		
172800 ml	17317-1031-03	173.83		
SPEARMINT (Lorann Oil)				
OIL, NA (N.F., NATURAL)				
3.75 ml	23535-0090-01	0.57		
30 ml	23535-0090-05	3.75		
120 ml	23535-0090-08	11.75		
480 ml	23535-0090-10	40.00		
1920 ml	23535-0090-15	145.00		
3840 ml	23535-0090-11	265.00		
(Medisca) *See SPEARMINT OIL*				
(Spectrum Pharmacy)				
OIL, NA (F.C.C.)				
100 ml	49452-7205-01	95.20		
500 ml	49452-7205-02	270.90		
SPEARMINT OIL (Medisca) spearmint				
OIL, NA (1X14ML,NATURAL)				
14 ml	38779-1621-03	15.00		
(1X25ML,NATURAL)				
25 ml	38779-1621-04	22.50		
(1X100ML,NATURAL)				
100 ml	38779-1621-05	46.50		
(1X500ML,NATURAL)				
500 ml	38779-1621-08	163.50		
SPEARMINT OIL (PCCA)				
OIL, NA, 1 ml	51927-1178-00	0.90		
SPECTAZOLE (Phys Total Care) REPACK econazole nitrate				
CRE, TP, 1%, 15 gm	54868-2241-01	25.90		
30 gm	54868-2241-00	45.28		
85 gm	54868-2241-03	93.47		
SPECTINOMYCIN DIHYDROCHLORIDE PENTAHYDRATE (Medisca) spectinomycin hydrochloride				
POW, NA, 1000 gm	38779-2268-09	2754.00		

PROD/MFR	NDC	AWP	DP	OBC
SPECTINOMYCIN HYDROCHLORIDE				
(Medisca) *See SPECTINOMYCIN DIHYDROCHLORIDE PENTAHYDRATE*				
SPECTRACEF (Cornerstone)				
cefditoren pivoxil				
TAB, PO (DOSE PACK,FILM-COATED)				
200 mg, 20s ea	**10122-0801-20**	341.25	273.00	
(FILM-COATED)				
200 mg, 60s ea	**10122-0801-60**	375.38	300.30	
400 mg, 20s ea	**10122-0802-20**	341.25	273.00	
28s ea	**10122-0802-28**	477.25	382.20	
SPECTRAGEL (Spectrum Design Med.)				
device				
DEV, NA, 28.4 gm	**08176-0077-30**	22.00		
SPERMACETI (Gallipot)				
GRA, NA (SYNTHETIC,U.S.P.)				
454 gm	**51552-0471-06**	19.04		
(PCCA) *See CETYL ESTERS*				
(Spectrum Pharmacy)				
WAX, NA (N.F., SYNTHETIC)				
500 gm	**49452-7210-01**	95.20		
2500 gm	**49452-7210-02**	256.20		
SPIKE LAVENDER OIL				
(PCCA) *See SPIKE OIL*				
SPIKE OIL (PCCA)				
spike lavender oil				
OIL, NA (DARK TECHNICAL)				
1 ml	**51927-2307-00**	1.20		
SPINAL-22 ANESTHESIA TRAY (Portex)				
bupivacaine hcl/dextrose/epi hcl/lido hcl				
KIT, IJ (3-1/2" QUINCKE)				
0.75%-10%-1 mg/ml-1%, 10s ea	**00074-1224-20**	378.69	318.90	
(Portex)				
dextrose/lido hcl/tetracaine hcl				
10%-1%-1%, 10s ea	**00074-4733-20**	384.51	323.80	
(Portex)				
dextrose/epi hcl/lido hcl/tetracaine hcl				
10%-1 mg/ml-1%-1%, 10s ea	**00074-4773-20**	385.70	324.80	
(3-1/2" WHITACRE)				
10%-1 mg/ml-1%-1%, 10s ea	**00074-4805-20**	506.47	426.50	
SPINAL-25 ANESTHESIA TRAY (Portex)				
bupivacaine hcl/dextrose/epi hcl/lido hcl				
KIT, IJ (3-1/2" QUINCKE)				
0.75%-10%-1 mg/ml-1%, 10s ea	**00074-1225-20**	386.89	325.80	
(Portex)				
dextrose/lido hcl/tetracaine hcl				
(3-1/2" QUINCKE W/INTRO)				
10%-1%-1%, 10s ea	**00074-4735-20**	391.64	329.80	
(Portex)				
dextrose/epi hcl/lido hcl/tetracaine hcl				
(3 1/2" QUINCKE W/INTRO)				
10%-1 mg/ml-1%-1%, 10s ea	**00074-4774-21**	393.78	331.60	
SPINAL-26 ANESTHESIA TRAY (Portex)				
bupivacaine hcl/dextrose/epi hcl/lido hcl				
KIT, IJ (3 1/2" QUINCKE)				
0.75%-10%-1 mg/ml-1%, 10s ea	**00074-3099-20**	420.38	354.00	
(Portex)				
dextrose/epi hcl/lido hcl/tetracaine hcl				
10%-1 mg/ml-1%-1%, 10s ea	**00074-4796-20**	420.38	354.00	
SPIRIVA (Boehr Ingelheim Phar)				
tiotropium bromide				
CAP, IH (W/ HANDIHALER)				
18 mcg, 5s ea	**00597-0075-75**	61.09		
(W/HANDIHALER)				
18 mcg, 6s ea	**00597-0075-06**	37.85		
(W/ HANDIHALER)				
18 mcg, 30s ea	**00597-0075-41**	217.91		
(W/HANDIHALER)				
18 mcg, 30s ea	**00597-0075-37**	139.78		
(W/ HANDIHALER)				
18 mcg, 90s ea	**00597-0075-47**	653.81		
(Phys Total Care)				
REPACK				
CAP, IH (W/HANDIHALER)				
18 mcg, 30s ea	**54868-5109-00**	229.95		
(Quality Care Prod)				
REPACK				
CAP, IH (W/HANDIHALER)				
18 mcg, 30s ea	**35356-0215-30**	329.26		

PROD/MFR	NDC	AWP	DP	OBC
SPIRONOLACTONE				
FUL				
TAB, PO, 25 mg, 100s ea		30.00		
(Actavis)				
TAB, PO (FILM-COATED)				
25 mg, 100s ea	**00228-2803-11**	45.94		AB
500s ea	**00228-2803-50**	218.22		AB
50 mg, 100s ea	**00228-2672-11**	81.57		AB
500s ea	**00228-2672-50**	407.85		AB
100 mg, 100s ea	**00228-2673-11**	142.43		AB
500s ea	**00228-2673-50**	598.24		AB
(Consolidated Midland)				
TAB, PO, 25 mg, 100s ea	**00223-1724-01**	6.25		EE
1000s ea	**00223-1724-02**	55.00		EE
(Gallipot)				
POW, NA (U.S.P.)				
1 gm	**51552-0276-01**	14.70		
5 gm	**51552-0276-02**	48.93		
25 gm	**51552-0276-04**	169.40		
(Greenstone)				
TAB, PO, 25 mg, 100s ea	**59762-5011-01**	46.01		AB
500s ea	**59762-5011-02**	218.55		AB
(FILM-COATED)				
50 mg, 100s ea	**59762-5012-01**	81.72		AB
100 mg, 100s ea	**59762-5013-01**	142.49		AB
(Major)				
TAB, PO (10X10, USP,FILM-COATED)				
25 mg, 100s ea UD	**00904-5951-61**	49.08		AB
(5X10, USP,FILM-COATED)				
50 mg, 50s ea UD	**00904-5952-06**	143.63		AB
(5X10, USP)				
100 mg, 50s ea UD	**00904-5953-06**	132.74		AB
(Medisca)				
POW, NA (U.S.P.)				
5 gm	**38779-0096-03**	81.00		
10 gm	**38779-0096-01**	114.00		
25 gm	**38779-0096-04**	225.00		
100 gm	**38779-0096-05**	750.00		
(Mutual)				
TAB, PO, 25 mg, 100s ea	**53489-0143-01**	45.94		AB
500s ea	**53489-0143-05**	218.22		AB
1000s ea	**53489-0143-10**	414.62		AB
(USP,FILM COATED)				
50 mg, 30s ea	**53489-0328-07**	24.78		AB
60s ea	**53489-0328-06**	49.70		AB
100s ea	**53489-0328-01**	81.18		AB
500s ea	**53489-0328-05**	385.61		AB
(USP,FILM COATED)				
100 mg, 30s ea	**53489-0329-07**	43.58		AB
60s ea	**53489-0329-06**	87.66		AB
100s ea	**53489-0329-01**	141.57		AB
500s ea	**53489-0329-05**	646.55		AB
(Mylan)				
TAB, PO, 25 mg, 100s ea	**00378-2146-01**	45.90		AB
500s ea	**00378-2146-05**	218.20		AB
50 mg, 30s ea	**00378-0243-93**	24.47		AB
100s ea	**00378-0243-01**	81.55		AB
(USP,FILM-COATED)				
50 mg, 500s ea	**00378-0243-05**	407.75		AB
100 mg, 100s ea	**00378-0437-01**	142.40		AB
(Pfizer) *See ALDACTONE*				
(Qualitest)				
TAB, PO (USP,FILM COATED)				
25 mg, 100s ea	**00603-5763-21**	45.94		AB
500s ea	**00603-5763-28**	222.05		AB
1000s ea	**00603-5763-32**	435.94		AB
50 mg, 100s ea	**00603-5764-21**	81.45		AB
500s ea	**00603-5764-28**	407.25		AB
(USP,FILM-COATED)				
100 mg, 30s ea	**00603-5765-16**	42.75		
(USP,FILM COATED)				
100 mg, 100s ea	**00603-5765-21**	142.49		AB
(Sandoz)				
TAB, PO, 25 mg, 100s ea	**00781-1599-01**	45.92		AB
500s ea	**00781-1599-05**	223.86		AB
1000s ea	**00781-1599-10**	436.24		AB
(Spectrum Pharmacy)				
POW, NA (U.S.P.)				
5 gm	**49452-7220-02**	118.30		
25 gm	**49452-7220-03**	328.65		
(UDL)				
TAB, PO (ROBOT READY 25X1)				
25 mg, 25s ea UD	**51079-0103-19**	10.69		AB
(USP)				
25 mg, 30s ea	**51079-0103-63**	82.62		AB
(10X10)				
25 mg, 100s ea UD	**51079-0103-20**	42.75		AB
50 mg, 100s ea UD	**51079-0979-20**	88.12		AB
100 mg, 100s ea UD	**51079-0980-20**	147.74		AB

PROD/MFR	NDC	AWP	DP	OBC
(A-S Medication)				
REPACK				
TAB, PO, 25 mg, 30s ea	**54569-0505-01**	13.78		EE
60s ea	**54569-0505-03**	27.56		EE
100s ea	**54569-0505-00**	45.94		EE
(American Health)				
REPACK				
TAB, PO (10X10,USP)				
25 mg, 100s ea UD	**68084-0206-01**	40.07		
50 mg, 100s ea UD	**68084-0207-01**	86.07		
100 mg, 100s ea UD	**68084-0208-01**	140.41		
(DHS, Inc.)				
REPACK				
TAB, PO, 25 mg, 100s ea	**55887-0821-01**	110.00		
(Dispensing Solutions)				
REPACK				
TAB, PO, 25 mg, 14s ea	**66336-0916-14**	11.49		AB
28s ea	**66336-0916-28**	22.98		AB
30s ea	**55045-1330-08**	15.00		AB
100s ea	**55045-1330-01**	50.00		AB
100 mg, 100s ea	**55045-3493-01**	163.00		
(GSMS)				
REPACK				
TAB, PO (UNIT OF USE)				
25 mg, 60s ea	**60429-0229-60**	54.45	18.15	AB
120s ea	**60429-0229-12**	105.75	35.25	AB
180s ea	**60429-0229-18**	156.75	52.25	AB
360s ea	**60429-0229-36**	312.00	104.00	AB
(IPI)				
REPACK				
TAB, PO, 25 mg, 30s ea	**18837-0274-30**	15.55		
50 mg, 30s ea	**18837-0280-30**	30.59		
100 mg, 30s ea	**18837-0275-30**	53.43		
(McKesson Packaging)				
REPACK				
TAB, PO (USP)				
25 mg, 100s ea UD	**63739-0226-10**	54.53		AB
(10X10,USP,FILM COATED)				
50 mg, 100s ea UD	**63739-0416-10**	96.40		AB
(Palmetto)				
REPACK				
TAB, PO, 25 mg, 30s ea	**23490-6299-02**	37.30		
(PD-Rx Pharm)				
REPACK				
TAB, PO (REDI-SCRIPT)				
25 mg, 28s ea	**58864-0673-28**	37.07		AB
30s ea	**55289-0507-30**	24.36		AB
90s ea	**55289-0507-90**	50.61		AB
100s ea	**55289-0507-01**	56.52		AB
(Phys Total Care)				
REPACK				
TAB, PO, 25 mg, 30s ea	**54868-0700-01**	22.38		EE
60s ea	**54868-0700-05**	41.73		EE
90s ea	**54868-0700-06**	61.11		EE
100s ea	**54868-0700-00**	67.56		EE
50 mg, 30s ea	**54868-4477-02**	48.63		AB
60s ea	**54868-4477-01**	74.28		AB
100s ea	**54868-4477-00**	119.28		AB
100 mg, 30s ea	**54868-5015-00**	77.85		
60s ea	**54868-5015-02**	134.44		AB
100s ea	**54868-5015-01**	259.11		AB
(Physician Partner)				
REPACK				
TAB, PO, 25 mg, 30s ea	**21695-0766-30**	27.56		AB
(Quality Care Prod)				
REPACK				
TAB, PO (FILM COATED)				
25 mg, 30s ea	**49999-0811-30**	25.20		AB
100s ea	**49999-0811-00**	59.72		
(FILM COATED)				
100 mg, 100s ea	**35356-0419-00**	170.00		AB
(Southwood)				
REPACK				
TAB, PO, 25 mg, 30s ea	**58016-0842-30**	13.78		
60s ea	**58016-0842-60**	27.56		
90s ea	**58016-0842-90**	41.35		
100s ea	**58016-0842-00**	45.94		
(Vibranta)				
REPACK				
TAB, PO, 25 mg, 60s ea	**57866-4575-02**	24.79		AB
SPIRONOLACTONE MICRONIZED (Hawkins)				
spironolactone, micronized				
POW, NA (U.S.P.)				
5 gm	**63370-0224-15**	48.00		
25 gm	**63370-0224-25**	188.00		
100 gm	**63370-0224-35**	660.00		

PROD/MFR	NDC	AWP	DP	OBC
(PCCA)				
POW, NA (U.S.P.)				
1 gm	51927-1377-00	11.70		
SPIRONOLACTONE, MICRONIZED				
(Hawkins) *See SPIRONOLACTONE MICRONIZED*				
(PCCA) *See SPIRONOLACTONE MICRONIZED*				
SPIRONOLACTONE/HCTZ (Southwood)				
REPACK				
hydrochlorothiazide/spironolactone				
TAB, PO, 25 mg-25 mg,				
30s ea	58016-0357-30	15.12		
60s ea	58016-0357-60	30.24		
90s ea	58016-0357-90	45.36		
100s ea	58016-0357-00	50.40		
SPIRULINA (PCCA)				
POW, NA, 1 gm	51927-3496-00	0.45		
SPORANOX (Centocor)				
itraconazole				
SOL, PO, 10 mg/ml,				
150 ml	50458-0295-15	202.94		
(Janssen)				
CAP, PO (7X4,PULSE PAK)				
100 mg, 28s ea	50458-0290-28	406.61	338.84	
30s ea	50458-0290-04	434.46	362.05	
(3X10,BLISTER PACK)				
100 mg, 30s ea UD	50458-0290-01	434.46	362.05	
(Advanced Pharm Serv, Inc.)				
REPACK				
CAP, PO, 100 mg, 10s ea	13411-0155-01	154.36		
15s ea	13411-0155-15	231.54		
30s ea	13411-0155-03	463.08		
60s ea	13411-0155-06	926.17		
90s ea	13411-0155-09	1389.26		
(AQ)				
REPACK				
CAP, PO, 100 mg, 10s ea	66105-0148-01	141.99		
15s ea	66105-0148-15	212.90		
30s ea	66105-0148-03	425.99		
60s ea	66105-0148-06	851.98		
90s ea	66105-0148-09	1277.97		
(Bryant Ranch)				
REPACK				
CAP, PO, 100 mg, 30s ea	63629-1647-01	296.88		
(Phys Total Care)				
REPACK				
CAP, PO, 100 mg, 30s ea	54868-3706-00	343.14		
SPRAY AND STRETCH (Gebauer)				
1,1,1,3,3-pentafluoropropane/norflurane				
SPR, TP (FINE STREAM)				
103.5 ml	00386-0004-04	34.25		
SPRINTEC (Teva)				
ethinyl estradiol/norgestimate				
TAB, PO (BLISTER PACK, 6X28)				
35 mcg-0.25 mg,				
168s ea	00555-9016-58	193.38		AB
(Phys Total Care)				
REPACK				
TAB, PO, 35 mcg-0.25 mg,				
28s ea	54868-4828-00	66.18		AB
(Physician Partner)				
REPACK				
TAB, PO, 35 mcg-0.25 mg,				
28s ea	21695-0769-01	64.46		AB
28s ea	21695-0769-28	386.76		AB
SPRYCEL (Bristol-Myers)				
dasatinib				
TAB, PO (FILM-COATED)				
20 mg, 60s ea	00003-0527-11	4173.67		
50 mg, 60s ea	00003-0528-11	8347.33		
70 mg, 60s ea	00003-0524-11	8347.33		
100 mg, 30s ea	00003-0852-22	8347.33		
(Phys Total Care)				
REPACK				
TAB, PO, 70 mg, 60s ea	54868-5759-00	6572.99		
SPS SUSPENSION (Carolina)				
sodium polystyrene sulfonate				
SUS, NA (FOR ORAL OR RECTAL USE)				
15 gm/60 ml,				
60 ml 10s UD	46287-0006-60	67.20	50.00	AA
120 ml	46287-0006-04	30.80	25.30	AA
473 ml	46287-0006-01	35.35	27.75	AA
SQ CAT HAIR (Alk-Abello)				
cat hair extract				
INJ, ID (M.D.V.)				
5000 bau/ml, 5 ml	52709-0701-02	72.12	54.60	

PROD/MFR	NDC	AWP	DP	OBC
SQUALANE (Medisca)				
squalene				
OIL, NA (1X100ML)				
100 ml	38779-0260-05	135.00		
(1X500ML)				
500 ml	38779-0260-08	660.00		
(PCCA)				
SOL, NA (NF)				
1 gm	51927-3093-00	1.80		
SQUALENE				
(Medisca) *See SQUALANE*				
(PCCA) *See SQUALANE*				
(Spectrum Pharmacy)				
OIL, NA (NF)				
100 ml	49452-7024-01	198.45		
500 ml	49452-7024-02	598.50		
SQUARIC ACID DI-N-BUTYL ESTER (Spectrum Pharmacy)				
squaric acid dibutylester				
SOL, NA (1X1GM)				
1 gm	49452-7225-01	253.05		
(1X5GM)				
5 gm	49452-7225-02	637.00		
SQUARIC ACID DIBUTYLESTER				
(Letco) *See DIBUTYL SQUARATE*				
(Medisca) *See DIBUTYL SQUARATE*				
(Spectrum Pharmacy) *See SQUARIC ACID DI-N-BUTYL ESTER*				
SRONYX (Watson)				
ethinyl estradiol/levonorgestrel				
TAB, PO (6X28)				
0.02 mg-0.1 mg,				
168s ea	52544-0967-28	170.63		
SSD (Par)				
silver sulfadiazine				
CRE, TP, 1%, 25 gm	49884-0600-57	5.20		AB
50 gm	49884-0600-36	8.26		AB
50 gm	49884-0600-58	9.18		AB
85 gm	49884-0600-85	14.68		AB
400 gm	49884-0600-40	35.07		AB
(Altura)				
REPACK				
CRE, TP (1X25GM)				
1%, 25 gm	63874-0807-25	5.25		AB
(Core)				
REPACK				
CRE, TP, 1%, 25 gm	33358-0327-25	8.41		
50 gm	33358-0327-50	16.38		
400 gm	33358-0327-94	41.79		
(DHS, Inc.)				
REPACK				
CRE, TP, 1%, 20 gm	55887-0934-20	8.00		AB
50 gm	55887-0934-50	10.50		AB
85 gm	55887-0934-85	21.98		AB
400 gm	55887-0934-01	31.65		AB
(Nucare Pharm)				
REPACK				
CRE, TP (1X25GM)				
1%, 25 gm	68071-1333-05	10.41		AB
50 gm	66267-0943-50	12.98		AB
(1X400GM)				
1%, 400 gm	68071-1334-00	43.79		AB
(Phys Total Care)				
REPACK				
CRE, TP (1X25GM)				
1%, 25 gm	54868-0375-05	18.92		AB
85 gm	54868-0375-04	35.43		AB
(Physician Partner)				
REPACK				
CRE, TP (1X20GM)				
1%, 20 gm	21695-0182-20	20.82		AB
(1X400GM)				
1%, 400 gm	21695-0182-40	71.12		AB
(St. Mary's MPP)				
REPACK				
CRE, TP (1X50GM)				
1%, 50 gm	60760-0600-50	15.77		AB
SSD AF (Par)				
silver sulfadiazine				
CRE, TP, 1%, 50 gm	49884-0601-36	10.52		BX
400 gm	49884-0601-40	40.84		BX
SSKI (Upsher-Smith)				
potassium iodide				
SOL, PO, 1 gm/ml, 30 ml	00245-0003-31	15.20		
237 ml	00245-0003-08	70.75		

PROD/MFR	NDC	AWP	DP	OBC
ST JOHN'S WORT				
(PCCA) *See ST. JOHN'S WORT*				
ST. JOHN'S WORT (PCCA)				
st john's wort				
POW, NA (HYPERICUM PERFORATUM)				
1 gm	51927-3000-00	0.23		
STADOL (Sandoz)				
butorphanol tartrate				
SOL, IJ (VIAL)				
1 mg/ml,				
1 ml, C-IV	00015-5645-20	8.43		AP
2 mg/ml,				
1 ml, C-IV	00015-5646-20	8.78		AP
(Dispensing Solutions)				
REPACK				
SOL, IJ, 2 mg/ml,				
10 ml, C-IV	55045-2533-00	90.00		AP
(Phys Total Care)				
REPACK				
SOL, IJ (M.D.V.)				
2 mg/ml,				
10 ml, C-IV	54868-0186-00	96.01		AP
STAFLEX (MAGNA Pharm)				
acetaminophen/phenyltoloxamine citrate				
TAB, PO (CAPLET)				
500 mg-55 mg,				
100s ea	58407-0407-01	59.45	42.45	
STAGESIC (MAGNA Pharm)				
acetaminophen/hydrocodone bitartrate				
CAP, PO, 500 mg-5 mg,				
100s ea, C-III	58407-0091-01	43.72		EE
STAHIST (MAGNA Pharm)				
cough/cold combination				
TER, PO (NEW FORMULA (10/05))				
100s ea	58407-0527-01	104.43	82.95	
STALEVO 100 (Novartis Pharm)				
carbidopa/entacapone/levodopa				
TAB, PO, 25 mg-200 mg-100 mg,				
100s ea	00078-0408-05	345.07		
STALEVO 125 (Novartis Pharm)				
carbidopa/entacapone/levodopa				
TAB, PO (FILM-COATED)				
31.25 mg-200 mg-125 mg,				
100s ea	00078-0545-05	345.07		EE
STALEVO 150 (Novartis Pharm)				
carbidopa/entacapone/levodopa				
TAB, PO, 37.5 mg-200 mg-150 mg,				
100s ea	00078-0409-05	345.07		
STALEVO 200 (Novartis Pharm)				
carbidopa/entacapone/levodopa				
TAB, PO, 50 mg-200 mg-200 mg,				
100s ea	00078-0527-05	345.07		
STALEVO 50 (Novartis Pharm)				
carbidopa/entacapone/levodopa				
TAB, PO, 12.5 mg-200 mg-50 mg,				
100s ea	00078-0407-05	345.07		
STALEVO 75 (Novartis Pharm)				
carbidopa/entacapone/levodopa				
TAB, PO (FILM-COATED)				
18.75 mg-200 mg-75 mg,				
100s ea	00078-0544-05	345.07		EE
STANGARD PERIO RINSE (Pascal Co.)				
stannous fluoride				
SOL, DE (MINT)				
0.63%, 284 ml	10866-0105-01	7.65		
STANNIC CHLORIDE				
(Baker, J.T.) *See STANNIC CHLORIDE PENTAHYDRATE*				
(PCCA)				
POW, NA (PENTAHYDRATE)				
1 gm	51927-3281-00	0.78		
STANNIC CHLORIDE PENTAHYDRATE (Baker, J.T.)				
stannic chloride				
LUM, NA (REAGENT)				
500 gm	10106-3972-01	131.58		
2500 gm	10106-3972-05	563.26		
STANNIC OXIDE (Baker, J.T.)				
POW, NA (REAGENT)				
500 gm	10106-3975-01	188.44		
2500 gm	10106-3975-05	761.63		
STANNOUS CHLORIDE				
(Baker, J.T.) *See STANNOUS CHLORIDE DIHYDRATE*				
(PCCA)				
CRY, NA (DIHYDRATE)				
1 gm	51927-1810-00	1.44		

PROD/MFR | NDC | AWP | DP | OBC

STANNOUS CHLORIDE DIHYDRATE (Baker, J.T.)
stannous chloride
CRY, NA (A.C.S., REAGENT)
500 gm.............10106-3980-01 189.88
2500 gm............10106-3980-05 818.64

STANNOUS FLUORIDE (Amend)
POW, NA (U.S.P.)
125 gm.............17317-0540-04 26.60
454 gm.............17317-0540-01 71.40

(Biotrol) *See PERFECT CHOICE*

(Colgate Oral) *See GEL-KAM*

(Omnii Intl) *See PERIO MED*

(Oral B Lab) *See STOP*

(Pascal Co.) *See STANGARD PERIO RINSE*

(PCCA)
POW, NA (U.S.P.)
1 gm...............51927-9019-00 1.68

(Spectrum Pharmacy)
POW, NA (U.S.P.)
25 gm..............49452-7230-01 88.55
100 gm.............49452-7230-02 208.60
500 gm.............49452-7230-03 514.50

STANNOUS OXIDE (Baker, J.T.)
POW, NA (REAGENT)
500 gm.............10106-3990-01 167.99

STANOZOLOL (Gallipot)
POW, NA (U.S.P.)
25 gm, C-III.........51552-1049-04 308.00 220.00

(Hawkins)
POW, NA (U.S.P.)
5 gm, C-III..........63370-0231-15 220.00
25 gm, C-III.........63370-0231-25 900.00
100 gm, C-III........63370-0231-35 3100.00
500 gm, C-III........63370-0231-45 13100.00
1000 gm, C-III.......63370-0231-50 22800.00

(Letco)
POW, NA (USP)
100 gm, C-III........62991-2560-05 2250.00

(Medisca)
POW, NA, 5 gm, C-III.....38779-1986-03 169.50
25 gm, C-III.........38779-1986-04 688.50
100 gm, C-III........38779-1986-05 2371.50
500 gm, C-III........38779-1986-08 11628.00
1000 gm, C-III.......38779-1986-09 20196.00

(B&B Pharm, Inc)
REPACK
POW, NA, 5 gm, C-III.....63275-9969-02 350.00
25 gm, C-III.........63275-9969-04 1750.00
100 gm, C-III........63275-9969-05 7000.00
1000 gm, C-III.......63275-9969-09 39000.00

STANOZOLOL MICRONIZED (PCCA)
stanozolol, micronized
POW, NA (USP)
1 gm, C-III..........51927-3402-00 300.00

STANOZOLOL, MICRONIZED
(PCCA) *See STANOZOLOL MICRONIZED*

STARCH
(Amend) *See POTASSIUM STARCH*

(Baker, J.T.) *See STARCH LINTNER*

(Baker, J.T.) *See STARCH POTATO*

(Spectrum Pharmacy) *See STARCH ARROWROOT*

STARCH ARROWROOT (Spectrum Pharmacy)
starch
POW, NA (1X500GM)
500 gm.............49452-7255-01 121.80

STARCH LINTNER (Baker, J.T.)
starch
POW, NA (REAGENT, SOLUBLE)
500 gm.............10106-4010-01 149.71

STARCH POTATO (Baker, J.T.)
starch
POW, NA (A.C.S., REAGENT)
125 gm.............10106-4006-04 33.11
500 gm.............10106-4006-01 68.50

STARCH, CORN
(Gallipot) *See CORN STARCH*

(Medisca) *See CORN STARCH*

(PCCA) *See CORN STARCH*

(Spectrum Pharmacy) *See CORN STARCH*

STARLIX (Novartis Pharm)
nateglinide
TAB, PO, 60 mg, 100s ea..00078-0351-05 194.87
120 mg, 100s ea.....00078-0352-05 202.46

(Phys Total Care)
REPACK
TAB, PO, 60 mg, 10s ea...54868-5156-01 15.86
30s ea..............54868-5156-00 43.83
120 mg, 10s ea......54868-5380-00 17.55
90s ea..............54868-5380-01 135.14

STAVUDINE
FUL
CAP, PO, 15 mg, 60s ea.............................. 135.33
20 mg, 60s ea.............................. 140.74
30 mg, 60s ea.............................. 149.47
40 mg, 60s ea.............................. 161.25

(Aurobindo Pharma)
CAP, PO (HARD GELATIN)
15 mg, 60s ea........65862-0111-60 365.08 AB
20 mg, 60s ea........65862-0112-60 379.64 AB
30 mg, 60s ea........65862-0046-60 403.25 AB
40 mg, 60s ea........65862-0047-60 410.70 AB

(B/M Squibb Onc/Vir) *See ZERIT*

(Camber)
CAP, PO (USP)
15 mg, 60s ea........31722-0515-60 365.48 EE
20 mg, 60s ea........31722-0516-60 380.06 EE
30 mg, 60s ea........31722-0517-60 403.70 EE
40 mg, 60s ea........31722-0518-60 411.16 EE

(Dava Pharma)
PDS, PO (1X200ML,DYE-FREE,FRUIT)
1 mg/ml, 200 ml.....67253-0761-20 75.51 AA

(Greenstone)
CAP, PO (USP,HARD GELATIN)
15 mg, 60s ea........59762-1190-01 365.08
20 mg, 60s ea........59762-1191-01 379.64
30 mg, 60s ea........59762-1192-01 403.25
40 mg, 60s ea........59762-1193-01 410.70

(Mylan)
CAP, PO (USP)
15 mg, 60s ea........00378-5040-91 365.08 AB
20 mg, 60s ea........00378-5041-91 379.64 AB
30 mg, 60s ea........00378-5042-91 403.25 AB
40 mg, 60s ea........00378-5043-91 410.70 AB

(A-S Medication)
REPACK
CAP, PO, 20 mg, 60s ea...54569-6122-00 379.75 AB
40 mg, 60s ea........54569-6123-00 410.82 AB

STAVZOR (Noven)
valproic acid
ECC, PO, 125 mg, 100s ea.68968-3125-01 109.43
250 mg, 100s ea.....68968-3250-01 214.94
500 mg, 100s ea.....68968-3500-01 396.34

STAYBELITE ESTER 5 (PCCA)
glyceryl hydrogenated rosinate
POW, NA (1X1GM)
1 gm...............51927-1966-00 0.09

STEARAMIDOPROPYL DIMETHYLAMINE LACTATE (PCCA)
SOL, NA (1X1ML)
1 ml...............51927-2696-00 0.13

STEARETH-100
(PCCA) *See POLYOXYETHYLENE 100 STEARYL ETHER*

STEARETH-20
(Spectrum Pharmacy) *See BRIJ 78*

STEARIC ACID (Baker, J.T.)
POW, NA (N.F.)
500 gm.............10106-0340-01 14.06
1500 gm............10106-0340-05 55.94

(Gallipot)
POW, NA (NF, FCC)
454 gm.............51552-0215-06 17.85

(Humco)
POW, NA (N.F.)
420 gm.............00395-2769-14 14.77

(Letco)
POW, NA (1X454GM,FLAKES)
454 gm.............62991-2575-01 30.00
(1X1000GM,FLAKES)
1000 gm............62991-2575-02 51.00
(1X2500GM,FLAKES)
2500 gm............62991-2575-03 105.00

(Lorann Oil)
POW, NA (N.F.)
120 gm.............23535-0611-78 1.50
480 gm.............23535-0611-71 3.50

(Mallinckrodt Lab)
POW, NA, 500 gm.........00406-2216-04 30.47

(PCCA)
FLA, NA (NF; TRIPLE PRESSED)
1 gm...............51927-2204-00 0.10
POW, NA (NF)
1 gm...............51927-1230-00 0.10

(Spectrum Pharmacy)
POW, NA (N.F.)
500 gm.............49452-7296-01 80.85
2500 gm............49452-7296-02 277.90

STEARYL ALCOHOL
(Amend) *See ALCOHOL STEARYL*

(Gallipot) *See ALCOHOL STEARYL*

(Letco) *See ALCOHOL STEARYL*

(Medisca) *See ALCOHOL STEARYL*

(PCCA)
POW, NA (NF)
1 gm...............51927-1354-00 0.09

(Spectrum Pharmacy) *See ALCOHOL STEARYL*

STELARA (Centocor)
ustekinumab
SOL, SC, 45 mg/0.5 ml,
0.5 ml.............57894-0060-02 5595.60
(1X0.5ML,SINGLE DOSE)
45 mg/0.5 ml,
0.5 ml.............57894-0060-03 5595.60 EE
(1X1ML,SINGLE DOSE)
90 mg/ml, 1 ml.......57894-0061-03 11191.20 EE

STERAPRED (Quality Care Prod)
REPACK
prednisone
TAB, PO, 5 mg, 21s ea....49999-0390-21 12.60 AB

STERAPRED DS (Phys Total Care)
REPACK
prednisone
TAB, PO (12 DAY UNI-PAK)
10 mg, 48s ea........54868-3234-00 32.68 AB

STERILE 70% ISOPROPANOL (Medisca)
isopropyl alcohol
SOL, NA (12X240ML)
240 ml 12s..........38779-2409-06 327.45
(12X480ML)
480 ml 12s..........38779-2407-01 407.55
(1X3800ML)
3800 ml.............38779-2408-06 157.50
(4X3800ML)
3800 ml 4s..........38779-2408-00 543.30

STERILE VANCOMYCIN HYDROCHLORIDE (Akorn)
vancomycin hydrochloride
PDS, IV (USP,LYOPHILIZED)
1 gm, 10s ea.........23360-0152-50 77.80 AP
5 gm, 5 gm...........23360-0153-65 37.60 AP
500 mg, 10s ea......23360-0151-40 45.90 AP

(Physician Partner)
REPACK
PDS, IV (LYOPHILIZED)
500 mg, ea..........21695-0424-01 75.20 AP

STERILE WATER (Hospira)
water, sterile
SOL, IJ (5MLX25,USP)
5 ml 25s.............00409-4027-02 27.90 24.50
(USP)
1000 ml 6s..........00409-1590-05 18.22 15.96

STERILE WATER BACTERIOSTATIC (APP)
water, sterile
SOL, IV (M.D.V.)
30 ml...............63323-0249-30 1.32

STERILE WATER FOR INJECTION (Baxter)
water, sterile
SOL, IV (USP,1X1000ML)
1000 ml.............00338-6351-04 14.21 11.84 AP

STEVIA EXTRACT (Letco)
POW, NA, 25 gm..........62991-1261-01 31.50
100 gm.............62991-1261-02 90.00
500 gm.............62991-1261-03 240.00

(Medisca) *See STEVIA POWDER/STEVIOSIDE*

(PCCA) *See STEVIOSIDE 90%*

(PCCA) *See STEVIOSIDE EXTRACT 15%*

(Spectrum Pharmacy)
SOL, NA (1X25ML)
15%, 25 ml..........49452-7307-01 53.20
(1X100ML)
15%, 100 ml.........49452-7307-04 89.95

PROD/MFR NDC AWP DP OBC

(Spectrum Pharmacy) *See STEVIA LEAVES EXTRACT*

STEVIA LEAVES EXTRACT (Spectrum Pharmacy)
stevia extract
POW, NA (1X100GM, SWEET)
100 gm 49452-7306-01 199.50
(1X500GM, SWEET)
500 gm 49452-7306-02 605.50

STEVIA POWDER/STEVIOSIDE (Medisca)
stevia extract
POW, NA (1X25GM)
25 gm 38779-1930-04 46.50
(1X100GM)
100 gm 38779-1930-05 123.00
(1X500GM)
500 gm 38779-1930-08 555.00
(1X2500GM)
2500 gm 38779-1930-01 1497.00

STEVIOSIDE 90% (PCCA)
stevia extract
POW, NA, 1 gm 51927-2892-00 2.28

STEVIOSIDE EXTRACT 15% (PCCA)
stevia extract
SOL, NA, 15%, 1 ml 51927-3145-00 1.00

STIMATE (CSL)
desmopressin acetate
SPR, NS (1X2.5ML)
0.15 mg/actuation,
2.5 ml .... 00053-6871-00 668.40 EE

STIMATE DS (Phys Total Care)
REPACK
desmopressin acetate
SPR, NS, 0.15 mg/actuation,
2.5 ml 54868-5805-00 718.95

STINGING NETTLE
(PCCA) *See STINGING NETTLE 2%*

STINGING NETTLE 2% (PCCA)
stinging nettle
POW, NA, 2%, 1 gm 51927-3234-00 0.32

STOP (Oral B Lab)
stannous fluoride
GEL, DE (GRAPE)
0.4%, 120 gm 00041-0710-34 4.30
120 gm 00041-0711-34 4.30
120 gm 00041-0712-34 4.30

STORAX
(PCCA) *See STORAX GUM*

(Spectrum Pharmacy)
GUM, NA (U.S.P.)
100 gm 49452-7310-01 122.85
500 gm 49452-7310-02 347.90

STORAX GUM (PCCA)
storax
GUM, NA (USP; STYRAX)
1 gm 51927-1771-00 1.05

STRATTERA (Lilly)
atomoxetine hydrochloride
CAP, PO, 10 mg, 30s ea ... 00002-3227-30 162.11 135.09
18 mg, 30s ea 00002-3238-30 162.11 135.09
25 mg, 30s ea 00002-3228-30 162.11 135.09
40 mg, 30s ea 00002-3229-30 175.97 146.64
60 mg, 30s ea 00002-3239-30 175.97 146.64
80 mg, 30s ea 00002-3250-30 189.86 158.22
100 mg, 30s ea 00002-3251-30 189.86 158.22

(Phys Total Care)
REPACK
CAP, PO, 25 mg, 30s ea ... 54868-4740-00 152.39
40 mg, 30s ea 54868-4741-00 165.35
60s ea 54868-4741-01 330.07
60 mg, 30s ea 54868-4884-00 198.47
80 mg, 30s ea 54868-1911-00 213.30

(Quality Care Prod)
REPACK
CAP, PO, 18 mg, 30s ea ... 35356-0141-30 229.46
25 mg, 30s ea 49999-0636-30 218.65
90s ea 49999-0636-90 719.48
40 mg, 30s ea 35356-0142-30 252.63
90s ea 35356-0142-90 779.61
60 mg, 30s ea 49999-0637-30 252.63

STRAWBERRY (Medisca)
flavoring aid
SOL, NA (1X25ML,ARTIFICIAL)
25 ml 38779-1633-04 15.00
(1X100ML,ARTIFICIAL)
100 ml 38779-1633-05 24.00
(1X500ML,ARTIFICIAL)
500 ml 38779-1633-08 46.50

STRAWBERRY FLAVOR (Gallipot)
flavoring aid
LIQ, NA (ARTIFICIAL, CONCENTRATE)
59.14 ml 51552-0283-03 6.02

(PCCA)
SOL, NA (ANHYDROUS; ARTIFICIAL)
1 ml 51927-2245-00 0.90
(CONCENTRATE,STRAWBERRY)
1 ml 51927-1282-00 0.23
1 ml 51927-2117-00 0.23

(Spectrum Pharmacy)
LIQ, NA (1X100ML)
100 ml 49452-7330-01 67.90
(1X500ML)
500 ml 49452-7330-02 170.10

STREPTOCOCCUS
(PCCA) *See ENTEROCOCCUS FAECIUM*

STREPTOMYCIN SULFATE (Gallipot)
POW, NA (U.S.P.)
100 gm 51552-0978-05 92.19 65.85

(Hawkins)
POW, NA (U.S.P., NON-STERILE)
100 gm 63370-0233-35 128.00
1000 gm 63370-0233-50 560.00

(Medisca)
POW, NA (B.P.)
25 gm 38779-0813-04 55.50
100 gm 38779-0813-05 99.00
500 gm 38779-0813-08 214.50
1000 gm 38779-0813-09 414.00

(PCCA)
POW, NA, 1 gm 51927-1788-00 3.84

(X-Gen)
PDS, IM (STERILE)
1 gm, 10s ea 39822-0706-02 146.50

STREPTOZOCIN
(Teva) *See ZANOSAR*

STRIANT (Columbia Labs)
testosterone
TDM, BC (MUCOADHESIVE TABLET)
30 mg,
60s ea, C-III 55056-3060-01 258.30

STROMECTOL (Merck)
ivermectin
TAB, PO, 3 mg, 20s ea UD . 00006-0032-20 111.66

(Southwood)
REPACK
TAB, PO, 3 mg, 20s ea 00490-0057-20 108.80

STRONG IODINE TINCTURE (Spectrum Pharmacy)
iodine
TIN, NA (1X480ML)
7%, 480 ml 49452-3750-04 138.25

STRONTIUM BROMIDE (Amend)
POW, NA (PURIFIED)
454 gm 17317-0543-01 35.00

STRONTIUM CHLORIDE
(Baker, J.T.) *See STRONTIUM CHLORIDE HEXAHYDRATE*

(PCCA)
CRY, NA (ACS)
1 gm 51927-2616-00 0.75

(Spectrum Pharmacy)
CRY, NA (1X25GM)
25 gm 49452-7347-01 72.45
(1X125GM)
125 gm 49452-7347-02 119.35
(1X500GM)
500 gm 49452-7347-03 312.55
(1X2500GM)
2500 gm 49452-7347-04 962.50

STRONTIUM CHLORIDE HEXAHYDRATE (Baker, J.T.)
strontium chloride
CRY, NA (A.C.S., REAGENT)
125 gm 10106-4036-04 36.67
500 gm 10106-4036-01 108.61

STRONTIUM CHLORIDE SR 89
(GE) *See METASTRON*

STRONTIUM NITRATE (PCCA)
CRY, NA (1X1GM)
1 gm 51927-3417-00 6.00
1 gm 51927-4329-00 6.24

(Spectrum Pharmacy)
CRY, NA (REAGENT,ACS)
25 gm 49452-7345-01 90.65

STROVITE (Everett)
vitamin b complex and vitamin c
TAB, PO, 100s ea 00642-0200-10 63.62

STROVITE ADVANCE (Everett)
multivitamin, minerals, and nutriceuticals
TAB, PO (CAPLET)
100s ea 00642-0208-10 67.52

STROVITE ADVANCE+D (Everett)
multivitamin, minerals, and nutriceuticals
TAB, PO (SF,DYE-FREE,GLUTEN-FREE)
60s ea UD 00642-0209-30 34.35

STROVITE FORTE (Everett)
multivitamin and minerals
SYR, PO (AF,SF)
473 ml 00642-0203-16 48.84
TAB, PO (CAPLET)
100s ea 00642-0204-10 79.48

STROVITE ONE (Everett)
multivitamin, minerals, and nutriceuticals
TAB, PO (DYE-FREE,GLUTEN-FREE)
90s ea 00642-0207-90 56.12

STROVITE PLUS (Everett)
multimineral/multivitamin
TAB, PO (CAPLET)
100s ea 00642-0201-10 78.33

STRYCHNINE (Baker, J.T.)
POW, NA (PURIFIED)
5 gm 10106-4061-02 46.09
30 gm 10106-4061-00 96.56

STRYCHNINE SULFATE
(Amend) *See STRYCHNINE SULFATE PENTAHYDRATE*

(Baker, J.T.) *See STRYCHNINE SULFATE PENTAHYDRATE*

(PCCA)
POW, NA (PENTAHYDRATE, PURIFIED)
1 gm 51927-1358-00 18.00

STRYCHNINE SULFATE PENTAHYDRATE (Amend)
strychnine sulfate
POW, NA (PURIFIED)
3.75 gm 17317-0545-07 11.20
30 gm 17317-0545-02 28.00

(Baker, J.T.)
POW, NA (PURIFIED)
5 gm 10106-4060-02 42.75
30 gm 10106-4060-00 83.07

SU-TUSS DM (Cypress Pharm)
dextromethorphan hydrobromide/guaifenesin
ELI, PO (FRUIT)
20 mg/5 ml-200 mg/5 ml,
473 ml 60258-0245-16 33.99

SUBLIMAZE (Akorn)
fentanyl citrate
SOL, IJ (AMP)
0.05 mg/ml,
2 ml 10s, C-II .... 11098-0030-02 4.50 AP
5 ml 10s, C-II .... 11098-0030-05 5.22 AP
20 ml 5s, C-II .... 11098-0030-20 10.98 AP

SUBOXONE (Reckitt Benckiser)
buprenorphine hydrochloride/naloxone hydrochloride
TAB, SL (LEMON-LIME)
2 mg-0.5 mg,
30s ea, C-III 12496-1283-02 114.00
8 mg-2 mg,
30s ea, C-III 12496-1306-02 202.80

(A-S Medication)
REPACK
TAB, SL (LEMON-LIME)
8 mg-2 mg,
7s ea, C-III 54569-5739-01 49.29
15s ea, C-III 54569-5739-02 131.82
30s ea, C-III 54569-5739-00 263.64

(Altura)
REPACK
TAB, SL (LEMON-LIME)
2 mg-0.5 mg,
30s ea, C-III 63874-1085-03 78.00
8 mg-2 mg,
30s ea, C-III 63874-1084-03 138.00

(DHS, Inc.)
REPACK
TAB, SL, 8 mg-2 mg,
4s ea, C-III 55887-0312-04 31.00
15s ea, C-III 55887-0312-15 116.25

PROD/MFR	NDC	AWP	DP	OBC
(Dispensing Solutions)				
REPACK				
TAB, SL, 8 mg-2 mg,				
30s ea, C-III	**55045-3784-03**	180.90		
(Nucare Pharm)				
REPACK				
TAB, SL (LEMON-LIME)				
2 mg-0.5 mg,				
30s ea, C-III	**68071-1510-03**	142.89		
8 mg-2 mg,				
30s ea, C-III	**68071-1380-03**	249.89		
(Palmetto)				
REPACK				
TAB, SL, 8 mg-2 mg,				
30s ea, C-III	**23490-9270-03**	158.94		
60s ea, C-III	**23490-9270-06**	317.98		
90s ea, C-III	**23490-9270-09**	476.82		
(PD-Rx Pharm)				
REPACK				
TAB, SL (LEMON-LIME)				
8 mg-2 mg,				
30s ea, C-III	**43063-0184-30**	301.42		
(Pharma Pac)				
REPACK				
TAB, SL, 2 mg-0.5 mg,				
30s ea, C-III	**52959-0749-30**	90.20		
8 mg-2 mg,				
30s ea, C-III	**52959-0304-30**	168.02		
(Phys Total Care)				
REPACK				
TAB, SL, 2 mg-0.5 mg,				
30s ea, C-III	**54868-5750-00**	125.35		
(LEMON-LIME)				
8 mg-2 mg,				
7s ea, C-III	**54868-5707-04**	62.58		
14s ea, C-III	**54868-5707-02**	115.30		
21s ea, C-III	**54868-5707-01**	171.32		
28s ea, C-III	**54868-5707-03**	227.34		
30s ea, C-III	**54868-5707-00**	243.34		
(Quality Care Prod)				
REPACK				
TAB, SL (LEMON-LIME)				
2 mg-0.5 mg,				
15s ea, C-III	**49999-0395-15**	100.20		
30s ea, C-III	**49999-0395-30**	201.00		
8 mg-2 mg,				
30s ea, C-III	**35356-0004-30**	174.00		
(Southwood)				
REPACK				
TAB, SL, 2 mg-0.5 mg,				
30s ea, C-III	**00490-0051-30**	89.81		
60s ea, C-III	**00490-0051-60**	179.62		
90s ea, C-III	**00490-0051-90**	269.43		
100s ea, C-III	**00490-0051-00**	299.37		
(Stat Rx)				
REPACK				
TAB, SL (LEMON-LIME)				
2 mg-0.5 mg,				
5s ea, C-III	**16590-0666-05**	23.40		
30s ea, C-III	**16590-0666-30**	140.40		
8 mg-2 mg,				
5s ea, C-III	**16590-0667-05**	40.51		
30s ea, C-III	**16590-0667-30**	243.06		
SUBUTEX (Reckitt Benckiser)				
buprenorphine hydrochloride				
TAB, SL, 2 mg,				
30s ea, C-III	**12496-1278-02**	150.00		
8 mg,				
30s ea, C-III	**12496-1310-02**	282.00		
(Altura)				
REPACK				
TAB, SL, 8 mg,				
30s ea, C-III	**63874-1173-03**	152.58		
(Quality Care Prod)				
REPACK				
TAB, SL, 2 mg,				
30s ea, C-III	**49999-0638-30**	261.36		
8 mg,				
30s ea, C-III	**49999-0639-30**	483.28		

SUCCIMER
(Gallipot) *See 2,3 DIMERCAPTOSUCCINIC ACID*
(Hawkins) *See DIMERCAPTOSUCCINIC ACID*
(Letco) *See DIMERCAPTOSUCCINIC ACID*
(Lundbeck) *See CHEMET*
(Medisca) *See DIMERCAPTOSUCCINIC ACID*
(PCCA) *See DIMERCAPTOSUCCINIC ACID*

PROD/MFR	NDC	AWP	DP	OBC
(Spectrum Pharmacy) *See MESO-2,3-DIMERCAPTO-SUCCINIC ACID*				
SUCCINIC ACID (Baker, J.T.)				
POW, NA (A.C.S., REAGENT)				
500 gm	**10106-0346-01**	85.49		
2500 gm	**10106-0346-05**	198.28		
(PCCA)				
POW, NA, 1 gm	**51927-2930-00**	0.33		
(Spectrum Pharmacy)				
CRY, NA (F.C.C.)				
500 gm	**49452-7392-02**	243.60		
2500 gm	**49452-7392-03**	801.50		
SUCCINYLCHOLINE CHLORIDE				
(Hospira) *See AMERINET CHOICE SUCCINYLCHOLINE CHLORIDE*				
(Hospira) *See QUELICIN*				
(PCCA)				
POW, NA (DIHYDRATE; BP)				
1 gm	**51927-3536-00**	3.96		
(Sandoz) *See ANECTINE*				
(Spectrum Pharmacy) *See SUCCINYLCHOLINE CHLORIDE DIHYDRATE*				
SUCCINYLCHOLINE CHLORIDE DIHYDRATE				
(Spectrum Pharmacy)				
succinylcholine chloride				
POW, NA (1X25GM)				
25 gm	**49452-7394-01**	218.75		
(1X100GM)				
100 gm	**49452-7394-02**	490.00		
SUCCINYLSULFATHIAZOLE (PCCA)				
POW, NA, 1 gm	**51927-3028-00**	2.55		
SUCCUS CINERARIA MARITIMA (Walker Pharmacal)				
glycerin/witch hazel				
SOL, OP, 7 ml	**00619-4021-38**	10.00		
SUCRAID (QOL Medical)				
sacrosidase				
SOL, PO, 8500 iu/ml,				
118 ml 2s	**67871-0011-04**	6510.00	684.12	
(2X118ML)				
8500 iu/ml,				
118 ml 2s	**67871-0111-04**	6781.25		
SUCRALFATE				
FUL				
TAB, PO, 1 gm, 100s ea		36.90		
(Axcan) *See CARAFATE*				
(Gallipot)				
POW, NA, 100 gm	**51552-0039-05**	26.53		
500 gm	**51552-0039-06**	63.00		
1000 gm	**51552-0039-07**	105.00		
(Hawkins)				
POW, NA (U.S.P.)				
500 gm	**63370-0225-45**	180.00		
1000 gm	**63370-0225-50**	260.00		
(Letco)				
POW, NA (U.S.P.)				
100 gm	**62991-1148-01**	51.00		
500 gm	**62991-1148-02**	120.00		
1000 gm	**62991-1148-03**	207.00		
(Martec)				
TAB, PO, 1 gm, 100s ea	**52555-0057-01**	72.94		AB
500s ea	**52555-0057-05**	354.04		AB
(Medisca)				
POW, NA (U.S.P.)				
100 gm	**38779-0318-05**	58.50		
500 gm	**38779-0318-08**	160.50		
1000 gm	**38779-0318-09**	297.00		
(Nostrum)				
TAB, PO (USP)				
1 gm, 100s ea	**29033-0003-01**	72.95		
500s ea	**29033-0003-05**	354.05		
(Precision Dose)				
SUS, PO (1X10ML)				
1 gm/10 ml,				
10 ml UD	**68094-0171-59**	2.74		
10 ml 30s UD	**68094-0171-62**	90.88		
(10X10)				
1 gm/10 ml,				
10 ml 100s UD	**68094-0171-61**	298.52		
(Sandoz)				
TAB, PO, 1 gm, 100s ea	**00185-2100-01**	84.60		AB
500s ea	**00185-2100-05**	410.47		AB
(Spectrum Pharmacy)				
POW, NA (U.S.P.)				
100 gm	**49452-7401-01**	90.65		
1000 gm	**49452-7401-02**	479.50		

PROD/MFR	NDC	AWP	DP	OBC
(Teva)				
TAB, PO, 1 gm, 100s ea	**00093-2210-01**	72.95		AB
(10X10)				
1 gm, 100s ea UD	**00093-2210-93**	77.06		AB
500s ea	**00093-2210-05**	354.05		AB
(UDL)				
TAB, PO (ROBOT READY 25X1)				
1 gm, 25s ea UD	**51079-0871-19**	20.76		AB
(10X10)				
1 gm, 100s ea UD	**51079-0871-20**	77.06		AB
(VistaPharm, Inc.)				
SUS, PO (5X10)				
1 gm/10 ml,				
10 ml 50s UD	**66689-0790-50**	136.80		
(Watson Labs)				
TAB, PO, 1 gm, 90s ea	**00591-0780-19**	27.97		
100s ea	**00591-0780-01**	29.52		AB
360s ea	**00591-0780-36**	100.96		
500s ea	**00591-0780-05**	130.14		AB
(A-S Medication)				
REPACK				
TAB, PO, 1 gm, 60s ea	**54569-4446-00**	43.77		EE
(Altura)				
REPACK				
TAB, PO, 1 gm, 20s ea	**63874-0305-20**	18.77		EE
30s ea	**63874-0305-30**	28.81		EE
(Bryant Ranch)				
REPACK				
TAB, PO, 1 gm, 20s ea	**63629-1307-04**	15.87		
30s ea	**63629-1307-03**	22.50		
60s ea	**63629-1307-02**	45.00		
100s ea	**63629-1307-01**	75.00		
(Dispensing Solutions)				
REPACK				
TAB, PO, 1 gm, 30s ea	**55045-1659-08**	22.50		AB
60s ea	**55045-1659-06**	45.00		AB
90s ea	**55045-1659-09**	67.50		AB
100s ea	**55045-1659-00**	75.00		AB
120s ea	**55045-1659-02**	90.00		AB
(McKesson Packaging)				
REPACK				
TAB, PO (USP)				
1 gm, 100s ea UD	**63739-0261-10**	76.97		AB
(PD-Rx Pharm)				
REPACK				
TAB, PO, 1 gm, 40s ea	**55289-0292-40**	21.34		AB
(Phys Total Care)				
REPACK				
SUS, PO (1X1000ML)				
1 gm/10 ml,				
1000 ml	**54868-5299-01**	632.37		
TAB, PO, 1 gm, 30s ea	**54868-3933-00**	30.00		EE
60s ea	**54868-3933-01**	57.00		AB
120s ea	**54868-3933-02**	111.00		EE
(Quality Care Prod)				
REPACK				
TAB, PO, 1 gm, 100s ea	**49999-0914-00**	76.01		
(Stat Rx)				
REPACK				
TAB, PO, 1 gm, 30s ea	**16590-0523-30**	25.75		
60s ea	**16590-0523-60**	45.00		
90s ea	**16590-0523-90**	67.00		
120s ea	**16590-0523-72**	90.00		
(Vibranta)				
REPACK				
TAB, PO, 1 gm, 60s ea	**57866-6109-01**	45.58		AB
SUCROSE (Amend)				
CRY, NA (N.F.)				
500 gm	**17317-0705-01**	8.40		
(REAGENT)				
500 gm	**17317-1759-01**	9.80		
(N.F.)				
2270 gm	**17317-0705-05**	29.40		
(REAGENT)				
2500 gm	**17317-1759-05**	46.20		
(N.F.)				
11350 gm	**17317-0705-08**	105.00		
(Baker, J.T.)				
CRY, NA (A.C.S., REAGENT)				
500 gm	**10106-4072-01**	43.36		
(N.F.)				
12000 gm	**10106-4074-07**	245.12		
(Gallipot)				
CRY, NA (U.S.P.,N.F.)				
454 gm	**05152-0502-06**	12.53		
(Humco) *See SYRPALTA*				

PROD/MFR	NDC	AWP	DP	OBC
(Medisca)				
POW, NA (N.F.,BEET SUGAR)				
500 gm	38779-1637-08	39.00		
(NF,BEET SUGAR)				
1000 gm	38779-1637-09	70.50		
(PCCA)				
POW, NA (CONFECTIONERS)				
1 gm	51927-1039-00	0.07		
(Spectrum Pharmacy)				
CRY, NA (N.F.)				
500 gm	49452-7410-01	53.20		
2500 gm	49452-7410-02	118.30		
12000 gm	49452-7410-03	490.00		
(Spectrum Pharmacy) *See SYRUP*				
SUCROSE OCTAACETATE (Amend)				
POW, NA (N.F.)				
454 gm	17317-0546-01	24.00		
2270 gm	17317-0546-05	105.00		
(PCCA)				
POW, NA (NF)				
1 gm	51927-2246-00	0.51		
(Spectrum Pharmacy)				
POW, NA (N.F.)				
125 gm	49452-7420-02	88.55		
500 gm	49452-7420-03	203.00		
2500 gm	49452-7420-04	556.50		
SUDAHIST (Larken Labs, Inc.)				
cpm/pse hcl				
TER, PO, 12 mg-120 mg,				
100s ea	68047-0330-01	77.77		
SUDAL-12 (Atley)				
cpm/pse hcl				
CTB, PO (SF,CAFFEINE-FREE,GRAPE)				
4 mg-30 mg,				
100s ea	59702-0819-01	178.75		
(Atley)				
(UNIT SIZE)				
4 mg-30 mg,				
100s ea	59702-0809-01	120.31		
SUDATEX-DM (Larken Labs, Inc.)				
dm/gg/pse hcl				
TAB, PO, 20 mg-400 mg-40 mg,				
100s ea	68047-0242-01	81.88		
SUDATRATE (Larken Labs, Inc.)				
methscopolamine nitrate/pse hcl				
TER, PO, 2.5 mg-120 mg,				
100s ea	68047-0245-01	74.57		
SUDATUSS DM (PGD, Inc.)				
cpm/dm/pse hcl				
SYR, PO (AF,CHERRY)				
473 ml	65615-0404-16	8.75		
SUDATUSS-2 (PGD, Inc.)				
codeine phos/gg/pse hcl				
LIQ, PO (AF)				
473 ml, C-V	65615-0405-16	39.00		
SUDATUSS-SF (PGD, Inc.)				
codeine phos/gg/pse hcl				
LIQ, PO (AF,SF,CHERRY)				
473 ml, C-V	65615-0406-16	39.00		
SUFENTA (Akorn)				
sufentanil citrate				
SOL, IJ (AMP)				
50 mcg/ml,				
1 ml 10s, C-II	11098-0050-01	53.82		AP
2 ml 10s, C-II	11098-0050-02	90.90		AP
5 ml 10s, C-II	11098-0050-05	192.00		AP
SUFENTANIL CITRATE				
(Akorn) *See SUFENTA*				
(Baxter)				
SOL, IJ, 50 mcg/ml,				
1 ml, C-II	10019-0050-39	5.87		AP
(AMP)				
50 mcg/ml,				
1 ml, C-II	10019-0050-43	5.87		AP
2 ml, C-II	10019-0050-37	9.78		AP
(AMP)				
50 mcg/ml,				
2 ml, C-II	10019-0050-21	9.78		AP
5 ml, C-II	10019-0050-36	17.40		AP
(AMP)				
50 mcg/ml,				
5 ml, C-II	10019-0050-06	17.40		AP
(Covidien)				
POW, NA (U.S.P.)				
1 gm, C-II	00406-0672-52	18927.00		

PROD/MFR	NDC	AWP	DP	OBC
(Gallipot)				
POW, NA (1X10MG,USP)				
0.01 gm, C-II	51552-0889-02	420.00	300.00	
(1X50MG,USP)				
0.05 gm, C-II	51552-0889-03	2100.00	1500.00	
(1X100MG,USP)				
0.1 gm, C-II	51552-0889-04	3500.00	2500.00	
(1X500MG,USP)				
0.5 gm, C-II	51552-0889-09	15365.00	10975.00	
(GeneraMedix)				
SOL, IJ (1X1ML,IV/EPI,PF)				
50 mcg/ml,				
1 ml UD, C-II	10139-0075-01	5.34		AP
(1MLX10,USP,IV/EPI,PF)				
50 mcg/ml,				
1 ml 10s UD, C-II	10139-0075-10	53.40		AP
(1X2ML,IV/EPI,PF)				
50 mcg/ml,				
2 ml UD, C-II	10139-0075-02	9.00		AP
(2MLX10,USP,IV/EPI,PF)				
50 mcg/ml,				
2 ml 10s UD, C-II	10139-0075-12	90.00		AP
(1X5ML,IV/EPI,PF)				
50 mcg/ml,				
5 ml UD, C-II	10139-0075-05	19.14		AP
(5MLX10,USP,IV/EPI,PF)				
50 mcg/ml,				
5 ml 10s UD, C-II	10139-0075-15	191.40		AP
(Hawkins)				
POW, NA (U.S.P.)				
0.01 gm, C-II	63370-0968-04	1296.00		
0.1 gm, C-II	63370-0968-06	11040.00		
(Hospira)				
SOL, IJ (10X1ML,LATEX-FREE)				
50 mcg/ml,				
1 ml 10s, C-II	00409-3382-21	68.16	59.60	AP
(LATEX-FREE)				
50 mcg/ml,				
1 ml 10s, C-II	00409-3380-31	41.88	36.60	AP
(10X2ML,LATEX-FREE)				
50 mcg/ml,				
2 ml 10s, C-II	00409-3382-22	122.28	107.00	AP
(AMP,10X2ML,LATEX-FREE)				
50 mcg/ml,				
2 ml 10s, C-II	00409-3380-32	78.24	68.50	AP
(AMP,LATEX-FREE)				
50 mcg/ml,				
5 ml 10s, C-II	00409-3380-35	168.60	147.50	AP
(FTV,LATEX-FREE)				
50 mcg/ml,				
5 ml 10s, C-II	00049-3382-25	263.16	230.30	AP
(USP,10X5ML)				
50 mcg/ml,				
5 ml 10s, C-II	00409-3382-25	261.72	229.00	AP
(VIAL, FLIPTOP)				
50 mcg/ml,				
5 ml 10s, C-II	00074-3382-25	263.16	230.30	AP
(Hospira) *See SUFENTANIL CITRATE NOVAPLUS*				
(Medisca)				
POW, NA (USP)				
0.01 gm, C-II	38779-1968-07	957.00		
0.1 gm, C-II	38779-1968-09	4785.00		
(PCCA)				
POW, NA (U.S.P)				
0.001 gm, C-II	51927-3213-00	105.00		
(B&B Pharm, Inc)				
REPACK				
POW, NA (U.S.P.)				
0.01 gm, C-II	63275-6200-09	725.00		
0.1 gm, C-II	63275-6200-06	6210.00		
0.5 gm, C-II	63275-6200-07	26975.00		
1 gm, C-II	63275-6200-01	46240.00		
SUFENTANIL CITRATE NOVAPLUS (Hospira)				
sufentanil citrate				
SOL, IJ (AMP,PF,LATEX-FREE)				
50 mcg/ml,				
1 ml 10s, C-II	00409-3380-49	34.44	30.10	AP
(10X2ML,PF,LATEX-FREE)				
50 mcg/ml,				
2 ml 10s, C-II	00409-3380-50	64.44	56.40	AP
(AMP,10X5ML,PF)				
50 mcg/ml,				
5 ml 10s, C-II	00409-3380-51	149.28	130.60	AP
SULAR (Shionogi)				
nisoldipine				
TER, PO (FILM COATED)				
8.5 mg, 100s ea	59630-0500-10	412.55		
17 mg, 100s ea	59630-0501-10	517.06		
25.5 mg, 100s ea	59630-0502-10	563.88		EE
34 mg, 100s ea	59630-0503-10	563.88		

PROD/MFR	NDC	AWP	DP	OBC
(Phys Total Care)				
REPACK				
TER, PO (FILM-COATED)				
10 mg, 10s ea	54868-4011-01	25.43		
30s ea	54868-4011-00	72.51		
90s ea	54868-4011-03	202.03		
(FILM-COATED)				
10 mg, 100s ea	54868-4011-02	223.64		
20 mg, 10s ea	54868-4200-01	34.93		
30s ea	54868-4200-00	101.03		
90s ea	54868-4200-02	282.83		
(FILM COATED)				
25.5 mg, 10s ea	54868-5993-00	43.51		EE
30s ea	54868-5993-01	125.31		EE
(FILM-COATED)				
40 mg, 10s ea	54868-4202-01	27.85		
30s ea	54868-4202-00	79.80		
(Quality Care Prod)				
REPACK				
TER, PO, 10 mg, 14s ea	35356-0040-14	70.50		
SULCONAZOLE NITRATE				
(Ranbaxy Labs) *See EXELDERM*				
SULFACETAMIDE (Gallipot)				
POW, NA (U.S.P.,N.F.)				
100 gm	51552-0190-05	22.33		
500 gm	51552-0190-06	71.82		
(Medisca)				
POW, NA (U.S.P.)				
25 gm	38779-0050-04	22.50		
100 gm	38779-0050-05	43.50		
500 gm	38779-0050-08	141.00		
(PCCA)				
POW, NA (U.S.P.)				
1 gm	51927-1428-00	1.68		
(Spectrum Pharmacy)				
POW, NA (U.S.P.)				
100 gm	49452-7440-01	138.25		
500 gm	49452-7440-02	402.50		
SULFACETAMIDE SOD. (Stat Rx)				
REPACK				
sulfacetamide sodium				
OIN, OP, 10%, 3.5 gm	16590-0208-35	21.00		
SULFACETAMIDE SODIUM				
FUL				
SOL, OP, 10%, 15 ml		2.54		
(Allergan Inc) *See BLEPH-10*				
(Bausch & Lomb Inc.)				
SOL, OP, 10%, 15 ml	24208-0670-04	5.08		AT
(Consolidated Midland)				
OIN, OP, 10%, 3.5 gm	00223-4430-03	2.75		EE
SOL, OP, 10%, 15 ml	00223-6710-15	2.75		EE
30%, 15 ml	00223-0000-00	4.75		EE
15 ml	00223-6711-15	6.50		EE
(Dermik) *See KLARON*				
(Doak) *See CARMOL SCALP TREATMENT*				
(Doak) *See ROSULA NS*				
(Falcon Ophthalmics)				
SOL, OP, 10%, 15 ml	61314-0701-01	5.05		AT
(Fougera) *See SODIUM SULFACETAMIDE*				
(Fougera)				
SUS, TP (USP)				
10%, 118 ml	00168-0382-04	109.99		
(Gallipot)				
POW, NA (U.S.P.,N.F.)				
100 gm	51552-0244-05	19.60		
500 gm	51552-0244-06	71.82		
(Hawthorn Pharm) *See MEXAR*				
(Major)				
SOL, OP, 10%, 15 ml	00904-2728-35	3.30		AT
(PCCA) *See SODIUM SULFACETAMIDE*				
(Perrigo) *See SEB-PREV*				
(Perrigo) *See SEB-PREV WASH*				
(Prasco Labs) *See SODIUM SULFACETAMIDE*				
(Spectrum Pharmacy)				
POW, NA (U.S.P.)				
100 gm	49452-7450-01	87.85		
500 gm	49452-7450-02	263.20		
(Taro)				
LOT, TP (1X118ML,USP)				
10%, 118 ml	51672-1346-08	131.25		AB
(Valeant Pharm Intl) *See OVACE WASH*				

PROD/MFR	NDC	AWP	DP	OBC
(A-S Medication)				
REPACK				
SOL, OP, 10%, 15 ml......	**54569-1186-00**	5.05		EE
(Altura)				
REPACK				
OIN, OP, 10%, 4 gm.......	**63874-0157-04**	23.12		EE
SOL, OP, 10%, 15 ml......	**63874-0136-15**	31.79		EE
(DHS, Inc.)				
REPACK				
OIN, OP, 10%, 3.5 gm.....	**55887-0910-35**	15.04		AT
SOL, OP, 10%, 15 ml......	**55887-0886-15**	21.69		EE
(Dispensing Solutions)				
REPACK				
OIN, OP, 10%, 3.5 gm.....	**55045-1559-09**	15.25		AT
SOL, OP, 10%, 15 ml......	**55045-1310-05**	21.65		AT
(1X15ML)				
10%, 15 ml........	**55045-3937-01**	21.65		AT
(Keltman Pharma., Inc.)				
REPACK				
OIN, OP, 10%, 3.75 gm....	**68387-0498-01**	19.96		AT
SOL, OP (1X15ML)				
10%, 15 ml..........	**68387-0491-01**	19.96		AT
(Nucare Pharm)				
REPACK				
OIN, OP, 10%, 3.5 gm.....	**66267-0942-35**	16.89		EE
SOL, OP, 10%, 15 ml......	**66267-0941-15**	25.69		AT
(Palmetto)				
REPACK				
OIN, OP (1X3.5GM)				
10%, 3.5 gm.........	**23490-6290-01**	23.09		
SOL, OP, 10%, 15 ml......	**23490-6289-01**	31.79		
(Pharma Pac)				
REPACK				
OIN, OP, 10%, 3.5 gm.....	**52959-0572-03**	23.09		EE
SOL, OP, 10%, 15 ml......	**52959-0117-01**	22.03		EE
(Phys Total Care)				
REPACK				
OIN, OP, 10%, 4 gm.......	**54868-1955-00**	6.72		EE
SOL, OP, 10%, 15 ml......	**54868-0727-01**	13.92		EE
(Physician Partner)				
REPACK				
SOL, OP (1X15ML)				
10%, 15 ml..........	**21695-0525-15**	15.10		AT
(Quality Care Prod)				
REPACK				
OIN, OP, 10%, 3.5 gm.....	**49999-0173-35**	20.10		AT
SOL, OP, 10%, 15 ml......	**49999-0144-15**	26.40		AT
(Southwood)				
REPACK				
OIN, OP, 10%, 3.5 gm.....	**58016-6063-01**	14.86		EE
SOL, OP, 10%, 15 ml......	**58016-6064-01**	21.94		EE
(St. Mary's MPP)				
REPACK				
SOL, OP (1X15ML)				
10%, 15 ml..........	**60760-0272-15**	6.95		AT
(Stat Rx)				
REPACK				
SOL, OP, 10%, 15 ml......	**16590-0209-15**	233.51		
(Vibranta)				
REPACK				
OIN, OP, 10%, 3.5 gm.....	**57866-7320-01**	18.75		
SOL, OP, 10%, 15 ml......	**57866-7351-01**	21.33		
SULFACETAMIDE SODIUM/PREDNISOLONE ACETATE (Altura)				
REPACK				
prednisolone acetate/sulfacetamide sodium				
SUS, OP, 0.2%-10%, 5 ml.	**63874-0175-05**	43.85		
SULFACETAMIDE SODIUM/SULFUR				
(Acella) *See BP 10-1*				
(Acella) *See BP CLEANSING WASH*				
(Acella) *See SODIUM SULFACETAMIDE/SULFUR CLEANSING PADS*				
(Actavis Mid Atlantic) *See SODIUM SULFACETAMIDE AND SULFUR*				
(Breckenridge Pharm) *See SULFATOL C*				
(Breckenridge Pharm) *See SULFATOL CLEANSER*				
(Breckenridge Pharm) *See SULFATOL GEL*				
(Breckenridge Pharm) *See SULFATOL SS*				
(Breckenridge Pharm) *See SULFATOL-M*				
(Breckenridge Pharm) *See SULFATOL-M TINT FREE*				
(Doak) *See ROSULA*				
(Doak) *See ROSULA AQUEOUS GEL*				
(Doak) *See ROSULA CLARIFYING WASH*				
(Galderma) *See ROSANIL*				
(Hawthorn Pharm) *See SUPHERA*				
(Larken Labs, Inc.) *See SULZEE WASH*				
(Medicis) *See PLEXION*				
(Medicis) *See PLEXION SCT*				
(Medimetriks) *See SUMAXIN*				
(Onset) *See CLARIFOAM EF*				
(Perrigo) *See SODIUM SULFACETAMIDE AND SULFUR*				
(Prasco Labs) *See PRASCION*				
(Prasco Labs) *See PRASCION FC*				
(Prasco Labs) *See PRASCION RA*				
(Prasco Labs) *See PRASCION TS*				
(Stiefel Labs) *See ROSAC CREAM W/SUNSCREENS*				
(Stiefel Labs) *See ROSAC WASH*				
(Tiber) *See AVAR CLEANSER*				
(Tiber) *See AVAR GEL*				
(Tiber) *See AVAR-E*				
(Tiber) *See AVAR-E GREEN*				
(Upsher-Smith) *See CLENIA*				
SULFACETAMIDE SODIUM/UREA				
(Doak) *See CARMOL SCALP TREATMENT*				
SULFACETAMIDE/PREDNISOLONE (Dispensing Solutions)				
REPACK				
prednisolone sodium phosphate/sulfacetamide sodium				
SOL, OP, 0.25%-10%, 5 ml.	**55045-3023-02**	19.95		
SULFACETAMINE-PREDNISOLONE (Physician Partner)				
REPACK				
prednisolone sodium phosphate/sulfacetamide sodium				
SOL, OP, 0.25%-10%, 5 ml.	**21695-0186-05**	47.98		
10 ml.............	**21695-0186-10**	47.98		
SULFADIAZINE (Gallipot)				
POW, NA (U.S.P.)				
100 gm.............	**51552-0305-05**	22.40		
454 gm.............	**51552-0305-06**	45.50		
(Letco)				
POW, NA (U.S.P.)				
1000 gm............	**62991-1149-04**	135.00		
2500 gm............	**62991-1149-05**	315.00		
5000 gm............	**62991-1149-06**	555.00		
25000 gm	**62991-1149-07**	2400.00		
(Medisca)				
POW, NA (U.S.P.)				
100 gm.............	**38779-0550-05**	45.75		
500 gm.............	**38779-0550-08**	126.00		
1000 gm............	**38779-0550-09**	225.00		
2500 gm............	**38779-0550-01**	688.50		
5000 gm............	**38779-0550-03**	675.00		
25000 gm	**38779-0550-07**	2985.00		
(PCCA)				
POW, NA (U.S.P.)				
1 gm...............	**51927-1109-00**	0.96		
(Sandoz)				
TAB, PO (CAPLET)				
500 mg, 100s ea	**00185-0757-01**	249.56		
1000s ea	**00185-0757-10**	2395.77		
(Spectrum Pharmacy)				
POW, NA (U.S.P.)				
100 gm.............	**49452-7460-01**	80.85		
500 gm.............	**49452-7460-02**	218.75		
2500 gm............	**49452-7460-05**	612.50		
5000 gm............	**49452-7460-06**	875.00		
SULFADIAZINE SODIUM (Letco)				
POW, NA (U.S.P.)				
1000 gm............	**62991-1150-03**	177.00		
2500 gm............	**62991-1150-04**	387.00		
5000 gm............	**62991-1150-05**	750.00		
25000 gm	**62991-1150-06**	3300.00		
(Medisca)				
POW, NA (USP)				
100 gm.............	**38779-0705-05**	43.50		
500 gm.............	**38779-0705-08**	117.00		
(U.S.P.)				
1000 gm............	**38779-0705-09**	217.50		
(USP)				
2500 gm............	**38779-0705-01**	387.00		
(U.S.P.)				
5000 gm............	**38779-0705-03**	1035.00		
25000 gm	**38779-0705-07**	4665.00		
(PCCA)				
POW, NA (U.S.P.)				
1 gm...............	**51927-2332-00**	0.51		
(Spectrum Pharmacy)				
POW, NA (U.S.P.)				
100 gm.............	**49452-7463-01**	80.85		
500 gm.............	**49452-7463-02**	218.75		
2500 gm............	**49452-7463-03**	612.50		
SULFADIMETHOXINE (PCCA)				
sulfadimethoxine sodium				
POW, NA, 1 gm...........	**51927-2821-00**	10.44		
SULFADIMETHOXINE SODIUM				
(PCCA) *See SULFADIMETHOXINE*				
SULFADOXINE (PCCA)				
POW, NA (U.S.P.)				
1 gm...............	**51927-2908-00**	4.80		
SULFAGUANIDINE (PCCA)				
POW, NA, 1 gm...........	**51927-2340-00**	2.46		
SULFAMERAZINE (Gallipot)				
POW, NA (1X100GM)				
100 gm.............	**51552-0990-05**	31.50	22.50	
(1X500GM)				
500 gm.............	**51552-0990-06**	126.00	90.00	
(PCCA)				
POW, NA, 1 gm...........	**51927-2098-00**	0.57		
SULFAMETH/TRIMETH (Physician Partner)				
REPACK				
sulfamethoxazole/trimethoprim				
TAB, PO (DS)				
800 mg-160 mg,				
14s ea.............	**21695-0125-14**	35.91		
20s ea.............	**21695-0125-20**	51.29		
30s ea.............	**21695-0125-30**	65.41		
60s ea.............	**21695-0125-60**	130.82		
SULFAMETH/TRIMETH DS (Core)				
REPACK				
sulfamethoxazole/trimethoprim				
TAB, PO, 800 mg-160 mg,				
6s ea..............	**33358-0329-06**	14.34		
14s ea.............	**33358-0329-14**	25.61		
20s ea.............	**33358-0329-20**	31.76		
30s ea.............	**33358-0329-30**	39.96		
SULFAMETH/TRIMETH-DS (Stat Rx)				
REPACK				
sulfamethoxazole/trimethoprim				
TAB, PO, 800 mg-160 mg,				
20s ea.............	**16590-0210-20**	34.29		
28s ea.............	**16590-0210-28**	48.00		
SULFAMETHAZINE (PCCA)				
POW, NA (U.S.P.)				
1 gm...............	**51927-1501-00**	1.08		
(Spectrum Pharmacy)				
POW, NA (U.S.P.)				
100 gm.............	**49452-7500-01**	150.50		
500 gm.............	**49452-7500-02**	434.00		
SULFAMETHAZINE SODIUM (Medisca)				
POW, NA, 50 gm..........	**38779-1120-02**	55.50		
100 gm.............	**38779-1120-05**	82.50		
SULFAMETHOXAZOLE (Medisca)				
POW, NA (1X100GM,CRYSTALLINE)				
100 gm.............	**38779-2320-05**	40.50		
(U.S.P.)				
100 gm.............	**38779-0261-05**	40.50		
(1X500GM,CRYSTALLINE)				
500 gm.............	**38779-2320-08**	135.00		
(U.S.P.)				
500 gm.............	**38779-0261-08**	135.00		
(1X1000GM,CRYSTALLINE)				
1000 gm............	**38779-2320-09**	238.50		
(U.S.P.)				
1000 gm............	**38779-0261-09**	238.50		
SULFAMETHOXAZOLE AND TRIMETHOPRIM (Precision Dose)				
sulfamethoxazole/trimethoprim				
SUS, PO (1X20ML,USP,CHERRY)				
200 mg/5 ml-40 mg/5 ml,				
20 ml UD	**68094-0120-59**	3.40		AB
(30X20ML,USP,CHERRY)				
200 mg/5 ml-40 mg/5 ml,				
20 ml 30s UD	**68094-0120-62**	102.00		AB
(Qualitest)				
SUS, PO (USP,1X473ML,CHERRY)				
200 mg/5 ml-40 mg/5 ml,				
473 ml	**00603-1684-58**	57.95		

PROD/MFR | NDC | AWP | DP | OBC

(USP,1X473ML,GRAPE)
200 mg/5 ml-40 mg/5 ml,
473 ml 00603-1685-58 57.95
TAB, PO (USP)
400 mg-80 mg,
100s ea........... 00603-5780-21 66.45 AB
500s ea........... 00603-5780-28 299.03 AB

(IPI)
REPACK
TAB, PO, 800 mg-160 mg,
20s ea............ 18837-0145-20 27.26
30s ea............ 18837-0145-30 40.88
60s ea............ 18837-0145-60 81.77

SULFAMETHOXAZOLE AND TRIMETHOPRIM DS (Qualitest)
sulfamethoxazole/trimethoprim
TAB, PO (USP,DOUBLE STRENGTH)
800 mg-160 mg,
100s ea........... 00603-5781-21 144.11 AB
500s ea........... 00603-5781-28 451.60 AB

(Aidarex)
REPACK
TAB, PO, 800 mg-160 mg,
7s ea.............. 33261-0148-07 10.57 AB
10s ea............ 33261-0148-10 15.10 AB
14s ea............ 33261-0148-14 21.14 AB
20s ea............ 33261-0148-20 30.20 AB
21s ea............ 33261-0148-21 31.71 AB
28s ea............ 33261-0148-28 42.28 AB
30s ea............ 33261-0148-30 45.30 AB
60s ea............ 33261-0148-60 90.60 AB

(St. Mary's MPP)
REPACK
TAB, PO (USP)
800 mg-160 mg,
20s ea............ 60760-0069-20 25.87

SULFAMETHOXAZOLE MICRONIZED (PCCA)
sulfamethoxazole, micronized
POW, NA (USP)
1 gm 51927-1696-00 0.90

SULFAMETHOXAZOLE, MICRONIZED
(PCCA) *See SULFAMETHOXAZOLE MICRONIZED*

SULFAMETHOXAZOLE/TRIMETHO DS (Vibranta)
REPACK
sulfamethoxazole/trimethoprim
TAB, PO, 800 mg-160 mg,
10s ea............ 57866-4693-06 19.20

SULFAMETHOXAZOLE/TRIMETHOPRIM
FUL
TAB, PO, 400 mg-80 mg,
100s ea 13.25
800 mg-160 mg,
100s ea 37.88

(Actavis Mid Atlantic) *See SULFATRIM PEDIATRIC*
(Amneal) *See SMZ-TMP*
(Amneal) *See SMZ-TMP DS*
(AR Scientific) *See BACTRIM*
(AR Scientific) *See BACTRIM DS*
(Hi-Tech) *See SMZ-TMP*

(Lannett)
TAB, PO, 400 mg-80 mg,
100s ea........... 00527-1442-01 22.80 AB
800 mg-160 mg,
100s ea........... 00527-1443-01 30.30 AB
500s ea........... 00527-1443-05 144.00 AB

(Major) *See SMZ-TMP DS*
(Monarch) *See SEPTRA*
(Monarch) *See SEPTRA DS*
(Mutual) *See SMZ-TMP*
(Precision Dose) *See SULFAMETHOXAZOLE AND TRIMETHOPRIM*
(Qualitest) *See SULFAMETHOXAZOLE AND TRIMETHOPRIM*
(Qualitest) *See SULFAMETHOXAZOLE AND TRIMETHOPRIM DS*
(Sandoz) *See SMZ-TMP DS*
(Teva) *See SMZ-TMP*
(Teva) *See SMZ-TMP CONCENTRATE*

(Teva)
SUS, PO (USP,CHERRY)
200 mg/5 ml-40 mg/5 ml,
473 ml .... 00093-5476-16 57.95 AB

(UDL) *See SMZ-TMP DS*

(DHS, Inc.)
REPACK
TAB, PO, 800 mg-160 mg,
60s ea............ 55887-0983-60 228.42

(Keltman Pharma., Inc.)
REPACK
TAB, PO, 800 mg-160 mg,
60s ea............ 68387-0385-60 120.18

(Palmetto)
REPACK
SUS, PO, 200 mg/5 ml-40 mg/5 ml,
100 ml 23490-6449-01 18.50
120 ml 23490-6449-03 38.52
160 ml 23490-6449-02 51.36
180 ml 23490-6449-04 57.78
480 ml 23490-6449-05 154.00
TAB, PO, 400 mg-80 mg,
14s ea............ 23490-9367-01 23.24
20s ea............ 23490-9367-02 33.20

(Phys Total Care)
REPACK
SUS, PO, 200 mg/5 ml-40 mg/5 ml,
473 ml 54868-0276-00 76.50

(Stat Rx)
REPACK
TAB, PO, 800 mg-160 mg,
14s ea............ 16590-0210-14 25.72 AB
40s ea............ 16590-0210-40 68.57 AB

SULFAMETHOXAZOLE/TRIMETHOPRIM DS (Palmetto)
REPACK
sulfamethoxazole/trimethoprim
TAB, PO, 800 mg-160 mg,
6s ea.............. 23490-6448-01 12.60
10s ea............ 23490-6448-02 15.00
14s ea............ 23490-6448-03 21.00
20s ea............ 23490-1244-02 33.20
20s ea............ 23490-6448-04 30.00
28s ea............ 23490-6448-05 42.00
30s ea............ 23490-6448-09 45.00
40s ea............ 23490-6448-06 60.00
60s ea............ 23490-6448-07 90.00
90s ea............ 23490-6448-08 135.00
120s ea.......... 23490-6448-00 252.00

SULFAMYLON (Mylan Bertek)
mafenide acetate
PDS, TP (5% SOLUTION)
50 gm/packet, ea 62794-0111-17 122.50

(UDL)
CRE, TP, 85 mg/gm,
56.7 gm 51079-0623-81 32.66
113.4 gm 51079-0623-82 62.79
453.6 gm 51079-0623-83 225.04
PDS, TP, 50 gm/packet,
5s ea.............. 51079-0624-85 738.95

SULFANILAMIDE
(Azur Pharma, Inc.) *See AVC*

(Baker, J.T.)
POW, NA (PURIFIED,NOT STERILIZED)
500 gm............. 10106-4079-01 69.58

(Gallipot)
POW, NA (U.S.P.)
100 gm............. 51552-0294-05 16.10
454 gm............. 51552-0294-06 47.95

(Letco)
POW, NA (200 MESH)
100 gm............. 62991-1499-01 30.00
500 gm............. 62991-1499-02 93.00

(Mallinckrodt Lab)
POW, NA, 500 gm......... 00406-0267-03 316.75

(Medisca)
POW, NA (PURIFIED)
25 gm.............. 38779-0170-04 25.50
100 gm............. 38779-0170-05 37.50
500 gm............. 38779-0170-08 105.00
1000 gm........... 38779-0170-09 190.50

(PCCA)
POW, NA, 1 gm.......... 51927-1261-00 0.57

(Spectrum Pharmacy)
POW, NA, 100 gm......... 49452-7510-01 67.90
500 gm............. 49452-7510-02 205.80
2500 gm........... 49452-7510-03 794.50

(Southwood)
REPACK
CRE, VG, 15%, 120 gm.... 58016-3006-01 37.21 EE
120 gm............. 58016-9109-01 24.38 EE

SULFANILIC ACID
(Baker, J.T.) *See SULFANILIC ACID ANHYDROUS*

SULFANILIC ACID ANHYDROUS (Baker, J.T.)
sulfanilic acid
POW, NA (A.C.S., REAGENT)
125 gm............. 10106-0354-04 91.77
500 gm............. 10106-0354-01 169.95

SULFAPYRIDINE (Gallipot)
POW, NA (U.S.P.,N.F.)
100 gm............. 51552-0255-05 52.92
454 gm............. 51552-0255-06 168.00

(PCCA)
POW, NA (USP)
1 gm 51927-2071-00 0.66

(Spectrum Pharmacy)
POW, NA (U.S.P.)
100 gm............. 49452-7520-01 141.75
500 gm............. 49452-7520-02 493.50

SULFAQUINOXALINE (PCCA)
POW, NA (1X1GM)
98%, 1 gm.......... 51927-2114-00 37.50

SULFASALAZINE
FUL
TAB, PO, 500 mg, 100s ea........................ 15.65

(Consolidated Midland)
TAB, PO, 500 mg, 100s ea . 00223-1727-01 12.75 EE
500s ea........... 00223-1727-05 57.50 EE
1000s ea .... 00223-1727-02 97.50 EE

(Gallipot)
POW, NA (U.S.P.)
100 gm............. 51552-1044-05 94.85 67.75

(Greenstone)
ECT, PO, 500 mg, 100s ea . 59762-0104-01 38.42 AB
(ENTERIC COATED)
500 mg, 300s ea ..... 59762-0104-02 110.01 AB
TAB, PO, 500 mg, 100s ea . 59762-5000-01 24.25 AB
300s ea........... 59762-5000-02 65.60 AB

(Letco)
POW, NA (USP)
100 gm............. 62991-2704-01 120.00

(Major)
TAB, PO, 500 mg, 100s ea . 00904-1152-60 25.49
500s ea........... 00904-1152-40 121.00 AB

(Medisca)
POW, NA (U.S.P.)
25 gm.............. 38779-0176-04 52.50
100 gm............. 38779-0176-05 157.50
500 gm............. 38779-0176-08 555.00
1000 gm........... 38779-0176-09 705.00

(PCCA)
POW, NA (U.S.P.)
1 gm 51927-1045-00 2.04

(Pfizer) *See AZULFIDINE*
(Pfizer) *See AZULFIDINE ENTABS*
(Qualitest) *See SULFAZINE*
(Qualitest) *See SULFAZINE EC*

(Qualitest)
TAB, PO, 500 mg, 100s ea . 00603-5801-21 25.49 AB
500s ea........... 00603-5801-28 121.00 AB

(Spectrum Pharmacy)
POW, NA (U.S.P.)
25 gm.............. 49452-7523-01 84.35
100 gm............. 49452-7523-02 240.10

(Watson Labs)
TAB, PO, 500 mg, 100s ea . 00591-0796-01 25.50 AB
500s ea........... 00591-0796-05 121.01 AB
1000s ea .... 00591-0796-10 177.36 AB

(A-S Medication)
REPACK
TAB, PO, 500 mg, 30s ea .. 54569-0313-03 7.55 AB

(Dispensing Solutions)
REPACK
TAB, PO, 500 mg, 100s ea . 55045-3496-01 27.00

(Palmetto)
REPACK
TAB, PO, 500 mg, 100s ea . 23490-6313-00 32.63

(PD-Rx Pharm)
REPACK
TAB, PO, 500 mg, 40s ea .. 55289-0176-40 18.37 AB

(Phys Total Care)
REPACK
TAB, PO, 500 mg, 30s ea .. 54868-1138-03 12.18 EE

PROD/MFR	NDC	AWP	DP	OBC
50s ea	54868-1138-00	18.33		EE
60s ea	54868-1138-08	21.39		EE
90s ea	54868-1138-07	30.57		EE
100s ea	54868-1138-04	32.16		EE
120s ea	54868-1138-01	39.78		EE
120s ea	54868-1139-00	100.98		EE
180s ea	54868-1138-05	58.17		EE
500s ea	54868-1138-06	177.97		EE
(Quality Care Prod)				
REPACK				
TAB, PO, 500 mg, 100s ea	49999-0981-00	31.00		
(Southwood)				
REPACK				
TAB, PO, 500 mg, 30s ea	58016-0074-30	7.28		
60s ea	58016-0074-60	14.55		
90s ea	58016-0074-90	21.83		
100s ea	58016-0074-00	24.25		
SULFATED CASTOR OIL				
(Medisca) *See TURKEY RED OIL*				
SULFATHIAZOLE (Baker, J.T.)				
POW, NA (PURIFIED)				
125 gm	10106-4082-04	72.36		
(Gallipot)				
POW, NA, 100 gm	51552-0664-05	24.92		
(PCCA)				
POW, NA (BP)				
1 gm	51927-3441-00	0.54		
SULFATOL C (Breckenridge Pharm)				
sulfacetamide sodium/sulfur				
CRE, TP (1X28GM)				
10%-5%, 28 gm	51991-0559-41	51.51		
SULFATOL CLEANSER (Breckenridge Pharm)				
sulfacetamide sodium/sulfur				
SOA, TP, 10%-5%, 355 ml	51991-0173-26	86.15		
SULFATOL GEL (Breckenridge Pharm)				
sulfacetamide sodium/sulfur				
GEL, TP, 10%-5%, 45 ml	51991-0172-45	70.07		
SULFATOL SS (Breckenridge Pharm)				
sulfacetamide sodium/sulfur				
CRE, TP (1X45GM,WITH SUNSCREENS)				
10%-5%, 45 gm	51991-0302-45	117.93		
SULFATOL-M (Breckenridge Pharm)				
sulfacetamide sodium/sulfur				
LOT, TP, 10%-5%, 25 gm	51991-0447-65	45.37		
SULFATOL-M TINT FREE (Breckenridge Pharm)				
sulfacetamide sodium/sulfur				
LOT, TP (TINT-FREE)				
10%-5%, 25 gm	51991-0448-65	45.37		
SULFATRIM (Bryant Ranch)				
REPACK				
sulfamethoxazole/trimethoprim				
SUS, PO, 200 mg/5 ml-40 mg/5 ml,				
100 ml	63629-1490-03	16.90		
150 ml	63629-1490-01	25.35		
200 ml	63629-1490-02	33.80		
300 ml	63629-1490-04	50.71		
(Quality Care Prod)				
REPACK				
SUS, PO, 200 mg/5 ml-40 mg/5 ml,				
100 ml	49999-0164-00	36.64		
SULFATRIM PEDIATRIC (Actavis Mid Atlantic)				
sulfamethoxazole/trimethoprim				
SUS, PO, 200 mg/5 ml-40 mg/5 ml,				
100 ml	00472-1285-33	12.63		AB
473 ml	00472-1285-16	57.95		AB
(A-S Medication)				
REPACK				
SUS, PO, 200 mg/5 ml-40 mg/5 ml,				
100 ml	54569-1017-00	12.63		AB
(Altura)				
REPACK				
SUS, PO, 200 mg/5 ml-40 mg/5 ml,				
100 ml	63874-0150-10	10.05		AB
480 ml	63874-0150-20	13.51		AB
(Dispensing Solutions)				
REPACK				
SUS, PO, 200 mg/5 ml-40 mg/5 ml,				
100 ml	55045-1176-01	18.50		AB
(Nucare Pharm)				
REPACK				
SUS, PO, 200 mg/5 ml-40 mg/5 ml,				
100 ml	66267-0939-00	12.36		AB
(Physician Partner)				
REPACK				
SUS, PO (1X100ML)				
200 mg/5 ml-40 mg/5 ml,				
100 ml	21695-0701-00	25.26		AB
(Quality Care Prod)				
REPACK				
SUS, PO, 200 mg/5 ml-40 mg/5 ml,				
100 ml	49999-0164-10	36.64		AB
(Stat Rx)				
REPACK				
SUS, PO, 200 mg/5 ml-40 mg/5 ml,				
100 ml	16590-0212-32	22.43		AB
SULFAZINE (Qualitest)				
sulfasalazine				
TAB, PO, 500 mg, 180s ea	00603-5801-04	45.88		AB
1000s ea	00603-5801-32	234.74		AB
SULFAZINE EC (Qualitest)				
sulfasalazine				
ECT, PO, 500 mg, 100s ea	00603-5803-21	38.42		AB
300s ea	00603-5803-25	110.65		AB
SULFINPYRAZONE (Spectrum Pharmacy)				
POW, NA, 25 gm	49452-7524-03	714.00		
100 gm	49452-7524-04	2184.00		
SULFISOXAZOLE (Consolidated Midland)				
TAB, PO, 500 mg, 100s ea	00223-1980-01	8.50		EE
1000s ea	00223-1980-02	72.50		EE
(Medisca)				
POW, NA (U.S.P.)				
100 gm	38779-0661-05	120.00		
500 gm	38779-0661-08	597.00		
1000 gm	38779-0661-09	885.00		
(PCCA)				
CRY, NA (USP)				
1 gm	51927-1106-00	2.52		
(Spectrum Pharmacy)				
CRY, NA (U.S.P.)				
25 gm	49452-7550-01	101.85		
100 gm	49452-7550-02	241.50		
POW, NA, 1000 gm	49452-7550-03	1344.00		
SULFOSALICYLIC ACID				
(Baker, J.T.) *See SULFOSALICYLIC ACID DIHYDRATE*				
(PCCA)				
POW, NA (DIHYDRATE; ACS REAGENT)				
1 gm	51927-3385-00	0.98		
SULFOSALICYLIC ACID DIHYDRATE (Baker, J.T.)				
sulfosalicylic acid				
CRY, NA (A.C.S., REAGENT)				
500 gm	10106-0364-01	160.47		
2000 gm	10106-0364-05	571.80		
SULFUR				
(AmerisourceBergen) *See SULFUR SUBLIMED*				
(Baker, J.T.) *See SULFUR PRECIPITATED*				
(Baker, J.T.) *See SULFUR SUBLIMED*				
(Gallipot)				
LUM, NA (TECHNICAL)				
454 gm	51552-0288-06	7.35		
11350 gm	51552-0288-04	31.50		
22700 gm	51552-0288-09	51.45		
(Gallipot) *See SULFUR COMMERCIAL*				
(Gallipot) *See SULFUR PRECIPITATED*				
(Gallipot) *See SULFUR SUBLIMED*				
(Humco) *See SULFUR SUBLIMED*				
(Mallinckrodt Lab) *See SULFUR PRECIPITATED*				
(Mallinckrodt Lab) *See SULFUR SUBLIMED*				
(Medisca)				
POW, NA (1X100GM)				
100 gm	38779-1640-05	40.50		
(1X500GM)				
500 gm	38779-1640-08	105.00		
(Medisca) *See SULFUR PRECIPITATED*				
(Medisca) *See SULFUR SUBLIMED*				
(PCCA) *See SULFUR PRECIPITATED*				
(PCCA) *See SULFUR SUBLIMED*				
(Spectrum Pharmacy) *See SULFUR PRECIPITATED*				
(Spectrum Pharmacy) *See SULFUR SUBLIMED*				
SULFUR COLLOIDAL (PCCA)				
colloidal sulfur				
POW, NA, 1 gm	51927-1448-00	0.42		
SULFUR COMMERCIAL (Gallipot)				
sulfur				
POW, NA (TECHNICAL)				
454 gm	51552-0287-06	5.88		
2270 gm	51552-0287-09	17.22		
SULFUR PRECIPITATED (Baker, J.T.)				
sulfur				
POW, NA (U.S.P.)				
500 gm	10106-4084-01	17.50		
2500 gm	10106-4084-05	38.16		
(Gallipot)				
POW, NA (U.S.P.,N.F.)				
454 gm	51552-0208-06	9.94		
2270 gm	51552-0208-09	31.85		
(Mallinckrodt Lab)				
POW, NA (U.S.P.)				
500 gm	00406-8400-04	27.52		
2500 gm	00406-8400-05	92.20		
(Medisca)				
POW, NA (U.S.P.)				
500 gm	38779-0098-08	24.00		
(1X2500GM,USP)				
2500 gm	38779-0098-01	76.50		
(U.S.P.)				
2500 gm	38779-0098-09	79.50		
(1X12000GM,USP)				
12000 gm	38779-0098-07	313.50		
(PCCA)				
POW, NA (U.S.P.)				
1 gm	51927-1218-00	0.10		
(Spectrum Pharmacy)				
POW, NA (U.S.P.)				
500 gm	49452-7399-01	57.40		
2500 gm	49452-7399-02	172.90		
12000 gm	49452-7399-03	616.00		
SULFUR SUBLIMED (AmerisourceBergen)				
sulfur				
POW, NA (PRIVATE LABEL)				
120 gm	24385-0936-94	2.51		
360 gm	24385-0936-12	4.22		
(Baker, J.T.)				
POW, NA (U.S.P.)				
500 gm	10106-4088-01	15.34		
2000 gm	10106-4088-05	25.05		
(Gallipot)				
POW, NA (U.S.P.)				
113.4 gm	51552-0133-04	4.20		
454 gm	51552-0133-06	9.45		
2270 gm	51552-0133-09	29.12		
(Humco)				
POW, NA (U.S.P.)				
120 gm	00395-2799-94	1.92		
360 gm	00395-2799-12	4.44		
(Mallinckrodt Lab)				
POW, NA (U.S.P.)				
500 gm	00406-8420-04	11.52		
(Medisca)				
POW, NA (U.S.P.)				
500 gm	38779-0606-08	40.50		
(PCCA)				
POW, NA (U.S.P.)				
1 gm	51927-2447-00	0.08		
(Spectrum Pharmacy)				
POW, NA (B.P.,E.P.,J.P.,U.S.P.)				
500 gm	49452-7570-01	67.55		
2500 gm	49452-7570-02	162.75		
12000 gm	49452-7570-03	490.00		
SULFURATED LIME (Medisca)				
calcium sulfide				
SOL, TP (1X500ML)				
500 ml	38779-1641-08	73.50		
(1X1000ML)				
1000 ml	38779-1641-09	117.00		
(PCCA)				
SOL, NA (VLEMINCKX SOL)				
1 ml	51927-1383-00	0.15		
SULFURATED POTASH (PCCA)				
potash sulfurated				
LUM, NA, 1 gm	51927-1232-00	0.45		
SULFURIC ACID (Amend)				
LIQ, NA (A.C.S., REAGENT)				
500 ml	17317-0562-01	21.00		
2500 ml	17317-0562-09	28.00		

PROD/MFR	NDC	AWP	DP	OBC
(Baker, J.T.)				
LIQ, NA (A.C.S., REAGENT)				
500 ml	**10106-9681-02**	32.70		
2500 ml	**10106-9681-05**	54.54		
(Baker, J.T.) *See SULFURIC ACID 0.1N*				
(PCCA)				
LIQ, NA (ACS)				
1 ml	**51927-1721-00**	0.17		
(Spectrum Pharmacy)				
LIQ, NA (F.C.C., 66 DEGREE BE)				
500 ml	**49452-7580-01**	123.20		
(N.F.)				
500 ml	**49452-7575-01**	130.20		
(F.C.C., 66 DEGREE BE)				
2500 ml	**49452-7580-02**	205.10		
(N.F.)				
2500 ml	**49452-7575-02**	220.85		
(Spectrum Pharmacy) *See SULFURIC ACID 50%*				
SULFURIC ACID 0.1N (Baker, J.T.)				
sulfuric acid				
LIQ, NA (REAGENT, VOLUMETRIC)				
1000 ml	**10106-5641-02**	21.63		
4000 ml	**10106-5641-03**	40.58		
20000 ml	**10106-5641-07**	106.97		
SULFURIC ACID 50% (Spectrum Pharmacy)				
sulfuric acid				
LIQ, NA (F.C.C.)				
500 ml	**49452-7579-01**	117.60		
4000 ml	**49452-7579-02**	232.75		
SULFUROUS ACID (Baker, J.T.)				
SOL, NA (A.C.S., REAGENT)				
500 ml	**10106-0370-02**	107.27		
2500 ml	**10106-0370-05**	206.72		
SULINDAC				
FUL				
TAB, PO, 150 mg, 100s ea		33.17		
200 mg, 100s ea		42.89		
(Heritage)				
TAB, PO (USP)				
150 mg, 100s ea	**23155-0005-01**	98.20		EE
500s ea	**23155-0005-05**	470.00		EE
200 mg, 100s ea	**23155-0006-01**	120.69		EE
500s ea	**23155-0006-05**	575.00		EE
(Major)				
TAB, PO, 200 mg, 100s ea	**00904-3379-60**	126.48		AB
(Merck) *See CLINORIL*				
(Mutual)				
TAB, PO, 150 mg, 100s ea	**53489-0478-01**	98.21		AB
500s ea	**53489-0478-05**	466.50		AB
200 mg, 100s ea	**53489-0479-01**	120.69		AB
500s ea	**53489-0479-05**	573.28		AB
(Mylan)				
TAB, PO, 150 mg, 100s ea	**00378-0427-01**	98.20		AB
200 mg, 100s ea	**00378-0531-01**	120.60		AB
(PCCA)				
POW, NA (U.S.P.)				
1 gm	**51927-2125-00**	4.50		
(Spectrum Pharmacy)				
POW, NA (U.S.P.)				
5 gm	**49452-7583-01**	74.90		
25 gm	**49452-7583-02**	159.25		
100 gm	**49452-7583-03**	563.50		
(UDL)				
TAB, PO (10X10)				
200 mg, 100s ea UD	**51079-0667-20**	124.22		AB
(Watson Labs)				
TAB, PO, 150 mg, 100s ea	**00591-5661-01**	98.21		AB
500s ea	**00591-5660-05**	603.44		AB
500s ea	**00591-5661-05**	491.01		AB
200 mg, 100s ea	**00591-5660-01**	120.69		AB
(West Point)				
TAB, PO, 150 mg, 500s ea	**59591-0170-74**	359.90		AB
200 mg, 500s ea	**59591-0154-74**	430.87		AB
(A-S Medication)				
REPACK				
TAB, PO, 200 mg, 14s ea	**54569-4032-00**	17.06		EE
20s ea	**54569-4032-05**	24.37		EE
30s ea	**54569-4032-01**	36.55		EE
(Altura)				
REPACK				
TAB, PO, 150 mg, 12s ea	**63874-0450-12**	12.13		EE
15s ea	**63874-0450-15**	19.03		EE
20s ea	**63874-0450-20**	25.01		EE
30s ea	**63874-0450-30**	34.15		EE
100s ea	**63874-0450-01**	101.01		EE
500s ea	**63874-0450-03**	428.00		EE
200 mg, 10s ea	**63874-0350-10**	17.03		EE
12s ea	**63874-0350-12**	20.44		EE
14s ea	**63874-0350-14**	23.85		EE
15s ea	**63874-0350-15**	25.55		EE
20s ea	**63874-0350-20**	34.07		EE
28s ea	**63874-0350-28**	47.69		EE
30s ea	**63874-0350-30**	51.10		EE
50s ea	**63874-0350-50**	85.16		EE
60s ea	**63874-0350-60**	102.20		EE
90s ea	**63874-0350-90**	153.30		EE
100s ea	**63874-0350-01**	170.33		EE
500s ea	**63874-0350-03**	851.67		EE
(Bryant Ranch)				
REPACK				
TAB, PO, 200 mg, 30s ea	**63629-3208-01**	70.12		
(Core)				
REPACK				
TAB, PO, 150 mg, 60s ea	**33358-0330-60**	71.36		
200 mg, 30s ea	**33358-0331-30**	51.24		
60s ea	**33358-0331-60**	77.23		
(DHS, Inc.)				
REPACK				
TAB, PO, 200 mg, 30s ea	**55887-0857-30**	39.11		AB
60s ea	**55887-0857-60**	78.22		
(Dispensing Solutions)				
REPACK				
TAB, PO, 150 mg, 14s ea	**55045-1791-05**	14.00		
20s ea	**55045-1791-07**	20.00		
30s ea	**55045-1791-08**	30.00		
60s ea	**55045-1791-06**	60.00		AB
100s ea	**55045-1791-00**	100.00		
200 mg, 14s ea	**55045-1676-05**	16.52		
30s ea	**55045-1676-08**	35.40		
60s ea	**55045-1676-09**	70.80		AB
60s ea	**66336-0686-60**	81.93		AB
(GSMS)				
REPACK				
TAB, PO (UNIT OF USE)				
200 mg, 60s ea	**60429-0172-60**	126.00	42.00	AB
(IPI)				
REPACK				
TAB, PO, 200 mg, 60s ea	**18837-0211-60**	90.52		
(Keltman Pharma., Inc.)				
REPACK				
TAB, PO, 200 mg, 60s ea	**68387-0588-60**	81.02		
(Nucare Pharm)				
REPACK				
TAB, PO, 150 mg, 20s ea	**66267-0264-20**	22.64		EE
200 mg, 15s ea	**66267-0197-15**	21.00		EE
20s ea	**66267-0197-20**	29.50		EE
30s ea	**66267-0197-30**	43.99		EE
40s ea	**66267-0197-40**	58.99		EE
(Palmetto)				
REPACK				
TAB, PO, 200 mg, 15s ea	**23490-6318-01**	35.00		
30s ea	**23490-6318-02**	69.99		
60s ea	**23490-6318-03**	139.98		
(PD-Rx Pharm)				
REPACK				
TAB, PO, 150 mg, 10s ea	**55289-0930-10**	27.16		AB
20s ea	**55289-0930-20**	40.96		AB
30s ea	**55289-0541-30**	39.52		AB
(USP)				
200 mg, 30s ea	**55289-0930-30**	54.80		AB
(Pharma Pac)				
REPACK				
TAB, PO, 150 mg, 10s ea	**52959-0196-10**	12.18		EE
14s ea	**52959-0196-14**	17.04		EE
15s ea	**52959-0196-15**	18.26		EE
20s ea	**52959-0196-20**	24.33		EE
30s ea	**52959-0196-30**	36.49		EE
60s ea	**52959-0196-60**	72.97		EE
100s ea	**52959-0196-00**	121.57		EE
200 mg, 14s ea	**52959-0195-14**	29.25		EE
15s ea	**52959-0195-15**	30.71		EE
20s ea	**52959-0195-20**	38.85		EE
28s ea	**52959-0195-28**	52.63		EE
30s ea	**52959-0195-30**	55.13		EE
60s ea	**52959-0195-60**	94.82		EE
180s ea	**52959-0195-18**	284.40		EE
(Phys Total Care)				
REPACK				
TAB, PO, 150 mg, 20s ea	**54868-0879-01**	15.36		EE
30s ea	**54868-0879-03**	21.54		EE
60s ea	**54868-0879-00**	40.08		EE
200 mg, 30s ea	**54868-1118-00**	27.72		EE
60s ea	**54868-1118-01**	58.08		EE
90s ea	**54868-1118-02**	78.65		EE
100s ea	**54868-1118-03**	86.88		EE
(Quality Care Prod)				
REPACK				
TAB, PO, 150 mg, 30s ea	**49999-0656-30**	83.98		AB
60s ea	**49999-0656-60**	167.96		AB
(Southwood)				
REPACK				
TAB, PO, 150 mg, 12s ea	**58016-0743-12**	11.03		EE
15s ea	**58016-0743-15**	13.79		EE
20s ea	**58016-0743-20**	18.38		EE
30s ea	**58016-0743-30**	27.57		EE
60s ea	**58016-0743-60**	55.15		AB
90s ea	**58016-0743-90**	82.72		AB
100s ea	**58016-0743-00**	91.91		EE
120s ea	**58016-0743-02**	110.29		AB
150s ea	**58016-0743-03**	137.87		AB
200s ea	**58016-0743-89**	183.82		AB
300s ea	**58016-0743-73**	275.73		AB
200 mg, 12s ea	**58016-0294-12**	14.22		EE
15s ea	**58016-0294-15**	17.78		EE
20s ea	**58016-0294-20**	23.70		EE
28s ea	**58016-0294-28**	33.18		EE
30s ea	**58016-0294-30**	50.10		AB
40s ea	**58016-0294-40**	47.40		EE
60s ea	**58016-0294-60**	100.20		AB
90s ea	**58016-0294-90**	150.30		AB
100s ea	**58016-0294-00**	167.00		AB
120s ea	**58016-0294-02**	200.40		AB
150s ea	**58016-0294-03**	177.75		AB
200s ea	**58016-0294-89**	237.00		AB
300s ea	**58016-0294-73**	355.50		AB
(Stat Rx)				
REPACK				
TAB, PO, 150 mg, 60s ea	**16590-0211-60**	140.00		AB
60s ea	**16590-0775-60**	20.25		AB
200 mg, 30s ea	**16590-0211-30**	70.00		
(Vibranta)				
REPACK				
TAB, PO, 150 mg, 60s ea	**57866-4621-03**	72.60		AB
200 mg, 15s ea	**57866-4622-03**	42.10		
30s ea	**57866-4622-02**	69.50		
60s ea	**57866-4622-05**	92.60		
SULPHAN BLUE (PCCA)				
POW, NA (1X1GM)				
1 gm	**51927-2085-00**	18.00		
SULZEE WASH (Larken Labs, Inc.)				
sulfacetamide sodium/sulfur				
SOA, TP (1X170.1GM)				
10%-1%, 170.1 gm	**68047-0040-06**	50.72		
SUMA ROOT (PCCA)				
POW, NA (1X1GM)				
1 gm	**51927-3232-00**	0.38		
SUMATRIPTAN				
(Glaxo) *See IMITREX*				
SUMATRIPTAN (Par)				
sumatriptan succinate				
SOL, SC (2X0.5ML)				
4 mg/0.5 ml,				
0.5 ml 2s	**49884-0482-52**	184.44		
0.5 ml 2s	**49884-0482-99**	194.73		
6 mg/0.5 ml,				
0.5 ml 2s	**49884-0483-52**	184.44		
0.5 ml 2s	**49884-0483-99**	194.73		
SUMATRIPTAN (Sandoz)				
SPR, NS, 5 mg, ea	**00781-6524-06**	38.89		
6s ea	**00781-6524-86**	233.32		
20 mg, ea	**00781-6523-06**	38.89		
6s ea	**00781-6523-86**	233.32		
(Phys Total Care)				
REPACK				
SPR, NS, 20 mg, 6s ea	**54868-6052-00**	573.90		
SUMATRIPTAN SUCCINATE (APP)				
SOL, SC (1X0.5ML,SDV)				
6 mg/0.5 ml,				
0.5 ml	**63323-0273-01**	61.25		AP
(Aurobindo Pharma)				
TAB, PO, 25 mg, 9s ea UD	**65862-0146-36**	243.47		AB
50 mg, 9s ea UD	**65862-0147-36**	226.26		AB
100 mg, 9s ea UD	**65862-0148-36**	226.26		AB
(Bedford)				
SOL, SC (10X0.5ML,SDV)				
6 mg/0.5 ml,				
0.5 ml 10s	**55390-0315-10**	969.60		AP
(Caraco)				
TAB, PO (UNIT-OF-USE,FILM-COATED)				
25 mg, 9s ea	**62756-0520-69**	243.49		AB

PROD/MFR	NDC	AWP	DP	OBC
(FILM-COATED)				
25 mg, 100s ea	62756-0520-88	2705.44		AB
(UNIT-OF-USE,FILM-COATED)				
50 mg, 9s ea	62756-0521-69	226.27		AB
(FILM-COATED)				
50 mg, 100s ea	62756-0521-88	2514.11		AB
(UNIT-OF-USE,FILM-COATED)				
100 mg, 9s ea	62756-0522-69	226.27		AB
(FILM-COATED)				
100 mg, 100s ea	62756-0522-88	2514.11		AB
(Cura Pharm)				
SOL, SC (SDV,5X0.5ML)				
6 mg/0.5 ml,				
0.5 ml 5s	66860-0022-06	400.00		AP
(Dr Reddy's)				
TAB, PO (1X9,FILM-COATED)				
25 mg, 9s ea UD	55111-0291-09	243.47		AB
(FILM-COATED)				
25 mg, 9s ea	55111-0738-09	243.47		EE
36s ea	55111-0291-36	973.87		AB
90s ea	55111-0291-90	2434.68		AB
(1X9,FILM-COATED)				
50 mg, 9s ea UD	55111-0292-09	226.26		AB
(FILM-COATED)				
50 mg, 9s ea	55111-0736-09	226.26		EE
36s ea	55111-0292-36	905.03		AB
90s ea	55111-0292-90	2262.57		AB
(1X9,FILM-COATED)				
100 mg, 9s ea UD	55111-0293-09	226.26		AB
(FILM-COATED)				
100 mg, 9s ea	55111-0737-09	226.26		EE
36s ea	55111-0293-36	905.03		AB
90s ea	55111-0293-90	2262.57		AB
(Glaxo) *See IMITREX*				
(Glaxo) *See IMITREX STATDOSE*				
(Glaxo) *See IMITREX STATDOSE REFILL*				
(Glaxo) *See IMITREX STATDOSE SYSTEM*				
(Greenstone)				
TAB, PO, 25 mg, 9s ea UD	59762-1850-09	243.47		
50 mg, 9s ea UD	59762-1851-09	226.26		
100 mg, 9s ea UD	59762-1852-09	226.26		
(JHP)				
SOL, SC (5X0.5ML,SDV)				
6 mg/0.5 ml,				
0.5 ml 5s	42023-0121-05	372.00		AP
(Mylan)				
TAB, PO (FILM COATED)				
25 mg, 9s ea	00378-5630-59	243.50		AB
50 mg, 9s ea	00378-5631-59	226.29		AB
100 mg, 9s ea	00378-5632-59	226.29		AB
(Par) *See SUMATRIPTAN*				
(Ranbaxy Pharm)				
TAB, PO, 25 mg, 9s ea	63304-0097-19	254.25		AB
50 mg, 9s ea	63304-0098-19	226.26		AB
100 mg, 9s ea	63304-0099-19	226.26		AB
(Sandoz)				
SOL, SC (1X0.5ML,SINGLE DOSE)				
4 mg/0.5 ml,				
0.5 ml	00781-3231-47	60.56		AP
(2X0.5ML,SDV)				
6 mg/0.5 ml,				
0.5 ml	00781-3174-71	90.84		EE
(2X0.5ML,SINGLE DOSE)				
6 mg/0.5 ml,				
0.5 ml 2s	00781-3173-07	184.46		EE
(5X0.5ML,SINGLE DOSE)				
6 mg/0.5 ml,				
0.5 ml 5s	00781-3174-14	454.21		EE
(Teva)				
SOL, SC (SINGE DOSE)				
6 mg/0.5 ml,				
0.5 ml 5s	00703-7351-02	367.91		EE
TAB, PO (3X3,FILM-COATED)				
25 mg, 9s ea	00093-0222-90	243.50		AB
50 mg, 9s ea	00093-0223-90	226.29		AB
100 mg, 9s ea	00093-0224-90	226.29		AB
(Watson Labs)				
TAB, PO (1X9)				
25 mg, 9s ea UD	16252-0590-99	30.00		AB
50 mg, 9s ea UD	16252-0591-99	30.00		AB
100 mg, 9s ea UD	16252-0592-99	30.00		AB
(Wockhardt USA)				
SOL, SC (5X0.5ML,SINGLE-DOSE)				
6 mg/0.5 ml,				
0.5 ml 5s	64679-0728-01	406.67		AP
(Zogenix) *See SUMAVEL DOSEPRO*				

PROD/MFR	NDC	AWP	DP	OBC
(A-S Medication)				
REPACK				
TAB, PO (FILM-COATED)				
50 mg, 9s ea	54569-6126-00	226.29		AB
100 mg, 9s ea	54569-6127-00	226.29		EE
(Aidarex)				
REPACK				
TAB, PO, 25 mg, 9s ea	33261-0662-09	251.50		AB
50 mg, 9s ea	33261-0663-09	241.90		AB
100 mg, 9s ea	33261-0664-09	241.90		AB
(American Health)				
REPACK				
TAB, PO, 25 mg, 27s ea UD	68084-0339-97	68.75		AB
50 mg, 27s ea UD	68084-0340-97	68.75		AB
100 mg, 27s ea UD	68084-0341-97	68.75		AB
(Dispensing Solutions)				
REPACK				
TAB, PO (FILM-COATED)				
50 mg, 9s ea	68258-3008-01	248.89		EE
100 mg, 9s ea	68258-3009-01	248.89		EE
(Nucare Pharm)				
REPACK				
TAB, PO (FILM-COATED)				
25 mg, 9s ea	66267-1265-09	270.56		AB
50 mg, 9s ea	66267-1264-09	251.43		AB
100 mg, 9s ea	66267-1263-09	251.43		AB
(Phys Total Care)				
REPACK				
TAB, PO (FILM-COATED)				
50 mg, 9s ea	54868-6023-00	504.33		EE
100 mg, 9s ea	54868-5978-00	535.97		EE
(Physician Partner)				
REPACK				
TAB, PO (FILM-COATED)				
25 mg, 9s ea	21695-0872-09	486.95		EE
50 mg, 9s ea	21695-0873-09	452.52		EE
100 mg, 9s ea	21695-0874-09	452.52		EE
(Quality Care Prod)				
REPACK				
TAB, PO (FILM-COATED)				
50 mg, 9s ea	35356-0439-09	526.60		EE
100 mg, 9s ea	35356-0438-09	526.60		EE
(Stat Rx)				
REPACK				
TAB, PO (FILM-COATED)				
100 mg, 9s ea	16590-0247-09	226.26		EE
SUMAVEL DOSEPRO (Zogenix)				
sumatriptan succinate				
SOL, SC, 6 mg/0.5 ml,				
0.5 ml 6s	43376-0106-06	99.60		
SUMAXIN (Medimetriks)				
sulfacetamide sodium/sulfur				
PAD, TP (60X3.7GM)				
10%-4%, 3.7 gm 60s	43538-0100-60	213.92		
SUMYCIN (Phys Total Care)				
REPACK				
tetracycline hydrochloride				
CAP, PO, 250 mg, 30s ea	54868-1047-02	3.11		AB
40s ea	54868-1047-01	3.83		AB
60s ea	54868-1047-03	5.01		AB
90s ea	54868-1047-04	6.91		AB
100s ea	54868-1047-00	6.94		AB
500 mg, 30s ea	54868-1048-01	9.48		AB
40s ea	54868-1048-03	12.01		AB
60s ea	54868-1048-02	17.09		AB
SUS, PO, 125 mg/5 ml,				
480 ml	54868-3424-00	14.31		AB
SUNFLOWER OIL				
(Amend) *See SUNFLOWER SEED OIL*				
(PCCA) *See SUNFLOWER SEED OIL*				
SUNFLOWER SEED OIL (Amend)				
sunflower oil				
OIL, NA, 500 ml	17317-1951-01	14.00		
3840 ml	17317-1951-06	49.00		
(PCCA)				
OIL, NA, 1 ml	51927-2985-00	0.25		
SUNITINIB MALATE				
(Pfizer) *See SUTENT*				
SUPARTZ (Smith & Nephew)				
hyaluronate sodium				
SOL, IJ (SRN,PREFILLED)				
10 mg/ml, 2.5 ml	08363-7761-01	162.50	130.00	
2.5 ml 5s	08363-7765-01	797.00		

PROD/MFR	NDC	AWP	DP	OBC
(Quality Care Prod)				
REPACK				
SOL, IJ, 10 mg/ml, 2s ea	35356-0036-02	632.00		
SUPER SYNERSWEET FLAVOR (PCCA)				
flavoring aid				
POW, NA (SUPER SYNERSWEET)				
1 gm	51927-3520-00	0.23		
SUPER THIN COMFORT ASSURED (Walgreens)				
insulin syringe/needle				
DEV, NA (29GX1/2",0.3CC,U100)				
100s ea	11917-0014-92	18.00		
(29GX1/2",0.5CC,U100)				
100s ea	11917-0014-89	18.00		
(29GX1/2",1CC,U100)				
100s ea	11917-0014-87	18.00		
SUPER THIN II COMFORT ASSURED (Walgreens)				
insulin syringe/needle				
DEV, NA (30GX5/16",0.3CC,U100)				
100s ea	11917-0025-27	19.00		
(30GX5/16",0.5CC,U100)				
100s ea	11917-0025-28	19.00		
(30GX5/16",1CC,U100)				
100s ea	11917-0025-29	19.00		
SUPEROXIDE DISMUTASE (PCCA)				
POW, NA, 1 gm	51927-2557-00	1.80		
(WATER SOLUBLE)				
1 ml	51927-3347-00	0.01		
SUPERVITE (Seyer Pharmatec)				
multivitamin, minerals, and nutriceuticals				
LIQ, PO (AF,SF,DYE-FREE)				
237 ml	11026-2841-08	16.50		
(Seyer Pharmatec)				
multivitamin and minerals				
TAB, PO (CAPLET)				
30s ea	11026-3020-03	14.70		
SUPHERA (Hawthorn Pharm)				
sulfacetamide sodium/sulfur				
CRE, TP, 10%-5%,				
113.4 gm	63717-0037-04	58.99		
SUPPORT (A. G. Marin)				
multivitamin and minerals				
LIQ, PO, 240 ml	12539-0083-08	16.80		
SUPPORT 500 (A. G. Marin)				
multivitamin, minerals, and nutriceuticals				
SGL, PO (SOFTGEL)				
60s ea	12539-0011-01	27.90		
SUPPOSITORY BASE				
(PCCA) *See BASE, PCCA MBK*				
(Spectrum Pharmacy) *See BASE, SUPPOSIBASE*				
SUPPRELIN LA (Endo Pharm)				
histrelin acetate				
IMP, SC, 50 mg, ea	67979-0002-01	17388.00		
SUPRANE (Baxter)				
desflurane				
LIQ, IH, 99%, 240 ml 6s	10019-0641-24	1088.28	906.90	
SUPRAX (Lupin Pharma, Inc.)				
cefixime				
PDR, PO (STRAWBERRY)				
100 mg/5 ml, 50 ml	68180-0202-03	126.11		
75 ml	68180-0202-02	76.81		
100 ml	68180-0202-01	255.42		
200 mg/5 ml, 50 ml	27437-0206-03	241.96		
75 ml	27437-0206-02	344.88		
TAB, PO (FILM-COATED)				
400 mg, 50s ea	27437-0201-08	603.41		EE
(A-S Medication)				
REPACK				
TAB, PO, 400 mg, ea	54569-2861-02	12.57		
(PD-Rx Pharm)				
REPACK				
TAB, PO (FILM-COATED)				
400 mg, ea	55289-0954-79	24.35		EE
(Phys Total Care)				
REPACK				
PDR, PO, 100 mg/5 ml,				
50 ml	54868-1384-01	58.61		
100 ml	54868-1384-02	168.72		
TAB, PO, 400 mg, 10s ea	54868-1383-00	105.25		
(Southwood)				
REPACK				
PDR, PO, 100 mg/5 ml,				
100 ml	58016-4807-01	201.56		

PROD/MFR NDC AWP DP OBC

SURE-T PARADIGM (Medtronic Minimed)
diabetic supplies
DEV, NA (10MM, 32")
10s ea **76300-0886-10** 93.24
(6MM, 18")
10s ea **76300-0862-10** 93.24
(6MM, 23")
10s ea **76300-0864-10** 93.24
(6MM, 32")
10s ea **76300-0866-10** 93.24
(8MM, 23")
10s ea **76300-0874-10** 93.24
(8MM, 32")
10s ea **76300-0876-10** 93.24

SURGICAL INSTRUMENT, DISPOSABLE
(Arkray) *See FUTURA SAFETY SCALPEL*

SURGIMEND COLLAGEN MATRIX (TEI Biosciences Inc.)
collagen, bovine
SHE, TP (.3X25CM,STRIP,SINGLEUSE)
ea **08533-6030-01** 195.00
(.6X25CM,STRIP,SINGLEUSE)
ea **08533-6030-02** 390.00
(10CMX15CM,PRS)
ea **08533-6041-00** 3900.00
(10CMX15CM,SINGLE USE)
ea **08533-6200-06** 4050.00
ea **08533-6300-06** 4200.00
ea **08533-6400-06** 4350.00
(10X10CM,THICK,SINGLEUSE)
ea **08533-6010-05** 2600.00
(10X15CM,FENESTRATEDOVAL)
ea **08533-6050-02** 2700.00
(10X15CM,RECTANGLE)
ea **08533-6050-04** 2700.00
(10X15CM,THICK,SINGLEUSE)
ea **08533-6010-06** 3900.00
(10X20CM,THICK,SINGLEUSE)
ea **08533-6010-07** 5200.00
(13CMX25CM,SINGLE USE)
ea **08533-6200-09** 8775.00
ea **08533-6300-09** 9100.00
ea **08533-6400-09** 9425.00
(13X25CM,THICK,SINGLEUSE)
ea **08533-6010-09** 8450.00
(16X20CM,THICK,SINGLEUSE)
ea **08533-6010-08** 8320.00
(1X25CM,SINGLE USE)
ea **08533-6030-03** 650.00
(20CMX30CM,SINGLE USE)
ea **08533-6200-17** 16200.00
ea **08533-6300-17** 16800.00
ea **08533-6400-17** 17400.00
(25CMX40CM,SINGLE USE)
ea **08533-6200-16** 27000.00
ea **08533-6300-16** 28000.00
ea **08533-6400-16** 29000.00
(25X40CM,THICK)
ea **08533-6010-16** 26000.00
(3X3CM,THICK,SINGLE USE)
ea **08533-6010-12** 234.00
(3X3CM,THIN,SINGLE USE)
ea **08533-6020-05** 234.00
(4X12CM,THICK,SINGLE USE)
ea **08533-6010-14** 1248.00
(4X16CM,THICK,SINGLE USE)
ea **08533-6010-10** 1664.00
(4X7CM,THICK,SINGLE USE)
ea **08533-6010-13** 728.00
(4X7CM,THIN,SINGLE USE)
ea **08533-6020-02** 728.00
(5X6CM,THICK,SINGLE USE)
ea **08533-6010-02** 780.00
(5X6CM,THIN,SINGLE USE)
ea **08533-6020-03** 780.00
(6CMX12CM,SINGLE USE)
ea **08533-6200-04** 1944.00
ea **08533-6300-04** 2016.00
ea **08533-6400-04** 2088.00
(6X12CM,THICK,SINGLE USE)
ea **08533-6010-04** 1872.00
(6X16CM,THICK)
ea **08533-6010-15** 2496.00
(8CMX16CM)
ea **08533-6010-18** 3328.00
(8X12CM,FENESTRATED OVAL)
ea **08533-6050-01** 1728.00
(8X12CM,RECTANGLE)
ea **08533-6050-03** 1728.00
(10X15CM,FENESTRATEDOVAL)
3s ea **08533-6051-02** 8100.00
(10X15CM,RECTANGLE)
3s ea **08533-6051-04** 8100.00

PROD/MFR NDC AWP DP OBC

(8X12CM,FENESTRATEDOVAL)
3s ea **08533-6051-01** 5184.00
(8X12CM,RECTANGLE)
3s ea **08533-6051-03** 5184.00

SURMONTIL (Teva)
trimipramine maleate
CAP, PO, 25 mg, 100s ea .. **51285-0538-02** 237.86
100s ea **65473-0718-01** 136.95
50 mg, 100s ea **51285-0539-02** 389.10
100s ea **65473-0719-01** 224.24
100 mg, 100s ea **51285-0554-02** 565.67
100s ea **65473-0720-01** 325.71

SURVANTA (Abbott Pharm)
beractant
SUS, IT (VIAL)
25 mg/ml, 4 ml **00074-1040-04** 459.60 383.00
8 ml **00074-1040-08** 813.46 677.88

SUSTIVA (B/M Squibb Onc/Vir)
efavirenz
CAP, PO, 50 mg, 30s ea ... **00056-0470-30** 53.16
200 mg, 90s ea **00056-0474-92** 637.50
TAB, PO (FILM COATED)
600 mg, 30s ea **00056-0510-30** 637.50

(A-S Medication)
REPACK
CAP, PO, 200 mg, 90s ea .. **54569-4611-00** 602.95
TAB, PO (FILM COATED)
600 mg, 30s ea **54569-5374-00** 782.57

(Phys Total Care)
REPACK
TAB, PO, 600 mg, 30s ea .. **54868-4668-00** 588.31

(Quality Care Prod)
REPACK
CAP, PO, 200 mg, 90s ea .. **35356-0069-90** 712.00
TAB, PO (FILM COATED)
600 mg, 6s ea **35356-0115-06** 295.85
30s ea **35356-0115-30** 1446.30

SUTAN (Cypress Pharm)
dexchlorpheniramine tan/pse tan
SUS, PO (CANDY APPLE)
3 mg/5 ml-50 mg/5 ml,
473 ml **60258-0480-16** 105.72

SUTAN-DM (Cypress Pharm)
dm tan/dexchlorpheniramine tan/pse tan
SUS, PO (GRAPE)
473 ml **60258-0401-16** 133.13

SUTENT (Pfizer)
sunitinib malate
CAP, PO, 12.5 mg, 28s ea .. **00069-0550-38** 2570.53 2142.11
25 mg, 28s ea **00069-0770-38** 5141.06 4284.22
50 mg, 28s ea **00069-0980-38** 9151.86 7626.55

SUTTAR-2 (Gil Pharmaceutical)
codeine phos/gg/pse hcl
SYR, PO, 473 ml, C-V **58552-0112-16** 18.00

SUTTAR-SF (Gil Pharmaceutical)
codeine phos/gg/pse hcl
SYR, PO (SF)
473 ml, C-V **58552-0111-16** 18.72

SWEETNESS ENHANCE FLAVOR (PCCA)
flavoring aid
SOL, NA, 1 ml **51927-3437-00** 3.00

SYMAX DUOTAB (Capellon)
hyoscyamine sulfate
TER, PO (BIPHASIC,BILAYERED)
0.375 mg, 90s ea **64543-0118-90** 172.50

SYMAX FASTABS (Capellon)
hyoscyamine sulfate
ODT, PO (CHEWABLE MELT)
0.125 mg, 100s ea **64543-0114-01** 97.50

SYMAX-SL (Capellon)
hyoscyamine sulfate
TAB, SL, 0.125 mg,
100s ea **64543-0111-01** 93.75

SYMAX-SR (Capellon)
hyoscyamine sulfate
TER, PO, 0.375 mg,
100s ea **64543-0112-01** 112.50

SYMBICORT (AstraZeneca)
budesonide/formoterol fumarate
AER, IH, 10.2 gm **00186-0372-20** 199.07
10.2 gm **00186-0370-20** 227.53

(Phys Total Care)
REPACK
AER, IH (1X10.2ML)
10.2 ml **54868-5937-00** 220.92
10.2 ml **54868-5936-00** 271.30

PROD/MFR NDC AWP DP OBC

SYMBYAX (Lilly)
fluoxetine hydrochloride/olanzapine
CAP, PO, 25 mg-3 mg,
30s ea .... **00002-3230-30** 272.66 227.22 EE
25 mg-6 mg, 30s ea .. **00002-3231-30** 372.82 310.68
(IDENTI-DOSE)
25 mg-6 mg,
100s ea UD **00002-3231-33** 1242.72 1035.60
25 mg-12 mg,
30s ea **00002-3232-30** 561.60 468.00
(IDENTI-DOSE)
25 mg-12 mg,
100s ea UD **00002-3232-33** 1872.00 1560.00
50 mg-6 mg, 30s ea .. **00002-3233-30** 372.82 310.68
(IDENTI-DOSE)
50 mg-6 mg,
100s ea UD **00002-3233-33** 1242.72 1035.60
50 mg-12 mg,
30s ea **00002-3234-30** 561.60 468.00
(IDENTI-DOSE)
50 mg-12 mg,
100s ea UD **00002-3234-33** 1872.00 1560.00

SYMLIN (Amylin)
pramlintide acetate
SOL, SC, 0.6 mg/ml, 5 ml .. **66780-0110-01** 226.42

(Phys Total Care)
REPACK
SOL, SC, 0.6 mg/ml, 5 ml .. **54868-5382-00** 117.58

(Quality Care Prod)
REPACK
SOL, SC (MDV)
0.6 mg/ml, ea **35356-0308-01** 246.73

SYMLINPEN (Amylin)
pramlintide acetate
SOL, SC (2X1.5ML)
1000 mcg/ml,
1.5 ml 2s .... **66780-0115-02** 201.04 EE
(2X2.7ML)
1000 mcg/ml,
2.7 ml 2s .... **66780-0121-02** 324.71 EE

SYMTAN (Athlon Pharm)
hydrocodone tannate/pseudoephedrine tannate
SOL, PO, 10 mg/5 ml-45 mg/5 ml,
480 ml, C-III **66813-0980-16** 162.53

SYMTAN A (Athlon Pharm)
brompheniramine tan/hydrocodone tannate/pse tan
SOL, PO (BUBBLE GUM)
480 ml, C-III **66813-0982-16** 229.49

SYNAGIS (Medimmune)
palivizumab
SOL, IM (PF)
50 mg/0.5 ml,
0.5 ml **60574-4114-01** 1145.47
100 mg/ml, 1 ml **60574-4113-01** 2162.99

SYNALGOS-DC (Cáraco)
aspirin/caffeine/dihydrocodeine bitartrate
CAP, PO, 356.4 mg-30 mg-16 mg,
100s ea, C-III **10551-0419-10** 196.45

(PD-Rx Pharm)
REPACK
CAP, PO, 356.4 mg-30 mg-16 mg,
15s ea, C-III **55289-0339-15** 43.32

SYNAREL (Pfizer)
nafarelin acetate
SPR, NS, 0.2 mg/actuation,
8 ml **00025-0166-08** 1105.92 921.60

SYNERA (Zars)
lidocaine/tetracaine
TDM, TP, 70 mg-70 mg,
10s ea **43469-0864-10** 153.60

SYNERCID (Monarch)
dalfopristin/quinupristin
PDS, IV (PF)
350 mg-150 mg,
10s ea **61570-0260-10** 1910.82

SYNTEST DS (Phys Total Care)
REPACK
esterified estrogens/methyltestosterone
TAB, PO (FILM COATED)
1.25 mg-2.5 mg,
10s ea **54868-4771-01** 23.79
30s ea **54868-4771-00** 62.40
90s ea **54868-4771-02** 168.51

SYNTHETIC IRON OXIDE
(PCCA) *See IRON OXIDE*

PROD/MFR	NDC	AWP	DP	OBC
SYNTHROID (Abbott Pharm)				
levothyroxine sodium				
TAB, PO, 0.025 mg,				
100s ea	**00074-4341-13**	47.87	41.99	**BX**
1000s ea	**00074-4341-19**	415.22	364.23	**BX**
0.05 mg, 100s ea	**00074-4552-13**	54.40	47.72	**BX**
(10X10)				
0.05 mg,				
100s ea UD	**00074-4552-11**	57.41	47.84	**BX**
1000s ea	**00074-4552-19**	463.66	406.72	**BX**
0.075 mg, 100s ea	**00074-5182-13**	60.08	52.70	**BX**
(10X10)				
0.075 mg,				
100s ea UD	**00074-5182-11**	64.02	53.35	**BX**
1000s ea	**00074-5182-19**	517.10	453.60	**BX**
0.088 mg, 100s ea	**00074-6594-13**	61.14	53.63	**BX**
1000s ea	**00074-6594-19**	528.61	463.69	**BX**
0.1 mg, 100s ea	**00074-6624-13**	61.56	54.00	**BX**
(10X10)				
0.1 mg, 100s ea UD	**00074-6624-11**	66.41	55.34	**BX**
1000s ea	**00074-6624-19**	533.56	468.03	**BX**
0.112 mg, 100s ea	**00074-9296-13**	71.11	62.38	**BX**
1000s ea	**00074-9296-19**	618.74	542.76	**BX**
0.125 mg, 100s ea	**00074-7068-13**	72.10	63.24	**BX**
(10X10)				
0.125 mg,				
100s ea UD	**00074-7068-11**	77.21	64.34	**BX**
1000s ea	**00074-7068-19**	620.57	544.36	**BX**
0.137 mg, 100s ea	**00074-3727-13**	73.75	64.69	**BX**
0.15 mg, 100s ea	**00074-7069-13**	74.24	65.13	**BX**
(10X10)				
0.15 mg,				
100s ea UD	**00074-7069-11**	79.25	66.04	**BX**
1000s ea	**00074-7069-19**	640.52	561.86	**BX**
0.175 mg, 100s ea	**00074-7070-13**	88.31	77.46	**BX**
1000s ea	**00074-7070-19**	763.43	669.67	**BX**
0.2 mg, 100s ea	**00074-7148-13**	88.49	77.62	**BX**
(10X10)				
0.2 mg, 100s ea UD	**00074-7148-11**	95.17	79.31	**BX**
1000s ea	**00074-7148-19**	766.70	672.55	**BX**
0.3 mg, 100s ea	**00074-7149-13**	120.43	105.64	**AB1**
1000s ea	**00074-7149-19**	1035.96	908.74	**AB1**
(A-S Medication)				
REPACK				
TAB, PO, 0.05 mg, 30s ea	**54569-0908-02**	16.04		**BX**
0.075 mg, 30s ea	**54569-0907-01**	17.71		**BX**
0.1 mg, 30s ea	**54569-0909-00**	18.15		**BX**
0.125 mg, 30s ea	**54569-3369-01**	19.86		**BX**
0.15 mg, 30s ea	**54569-0910-02**	21.89		**BX**
(AQ)				
REPACK				
TAB, PO, 0.025 mg,				
100s ea	**66105-0508-10**	52.04		
0.05 mg, 100s ea	**66105-0509-10**	58.46		
0.075 mg, 100s ea	**66105-0510-10**	64.04		
0.088 mg, 100s ea	**66105-0511-10**	65.42		
0.1 mg, 100s ea	**66105-0512-10**	65.49		
0.112 mg, 100s ea	**66105-0513-10**	74.89		
0.125 mg, 100s ea	**66105-0514-10**	75.85		
0.175 mg, 100s ea	**66105-0515-10**	91.79		
0.2 mg, 100s ea	**66105-0516-10**	72.83		
0.3 mg, 100s ea	**66105-0517-10**	99.11		
(DHS, Inc.)				
REPACK				
TAB, PO, 0.025 mg,				
30s ea	**55887-0303-30**	22.50		
0.05 mg, 30s ea	**55887-0302-30**	24.00		
0.075 mg, 30s ea	**55887-0301-30**	27.00		
0.1 mg, 30s ea	**55887-0300-30**	27.00		
0.125 mg, 30s ea	**55887-0299-30**	31.50		
(Direct Pharmaceutical, Inc.)				
REPACK				
TAB, PO, 0.125 mg,				
30s ea UD	**67801-0446-30**	66.20		
(PD-Rx Pharm)				
REPACK				
TAB, PO (USP,REDI-SCRIPT)				
0.025 mg, 100s ea	**58864-0965-01**	45.21		
(REDI-SCRIPT)				
0.05 mg, 30s ea	**58864-0722-30**	20.71		**BX**
0.075 mg, 30s ea	**58864-0487-30**	22.94		**BX**
0.1 mg, 30s ea	**55289-0129-30**	23.50		
(REDI-SCRIPT)				
0.1 mg, 30s ea	**58864-0730-30**	26.30		**BX**
(USP,REDI-SCRIPT)				
0.1 mg, 100s ea	**58864-0730-01**	58.71		
0.125 mg, 30s ea	**58864-0779-30**	27.53		**BX**
90s ea	**43063-0178-90**	92.18		**BX**
0.15 mg, 90s ea	**43063-0177-90**	83.99		**BX**

PROD/MFR	NDC	AWP	DP	OBC
(Pharma Pac)				
REPACK				
TAB, PO, 0.15 mg,				
100s ea	**52959-0206-00**	40.18		**BX**
0.2 mg, 100s ea	**52959-0148-00**	41.60		**BX**
(Phys Total Care)				
REPACK				
TAB, PO (USP)				
0.025 mg, 10s ea	**54868-3389-02**	7.12		**BX**
30s ea	**54868-3389-01**	24.31		**BX**
100s ea	**54868-3389-00**	53.66		**BX**
0.05 mg, 10s ea	**54868-1011-03**	9.95		**BX**
30s ea	**54868-1011-02**	23.98		**BX**
60s ea	**54868-1011-00**	46.65		**BX**
90s ea	**54868-1011-04**	68.01		**BX**
100s ea	**54868-1011-01**	76.00		**BX**
0.075 mg, 10s ea	**54868-2005-03**	10.72		**BX**
30s ea	**54868-2005-00**	26.93		**BX**
(USP)				
0.075 mg, 90s ea	**54868-2005-02**	75.56		**BX**
100s ea	**54868-2005-01**	83.01		**BX**
0.088 mg, 10s ea	**54868-2705-02**	10.86		**BX**
30s ea	**54868-2705-01**	27.36		**BX**
60s ea	**54868-2705-03**	52.10		**BX**
100s ea	**54868-2705-00**	84.44		**BX**
0.1 mg, 30s ea	**54868-0376-03**	27.53		**BX**
90s ea	**54868-0376-00**	77.35		**BX**
100s ea	**54868-0376-01**	85.66		**BX**
0.112 mg, 10s ea	**54868-5105-01**	12.21		**BX**
20s ea	**54868-5105-02**	21.80		**BX**
30s ea	**54868-5105-00**	31.39		**BX**
90s ea	**54868-5105-03**	88.95		
0.125 mg, 10s ea	**54868-2638-03**	12.34		**BX**
30s ea	**54868-2638-00**	31.79		**BX**
(USP)				
0.125 mg, 60s ea	**54868-2638-04**	60.97		**BX**
90s ea	**54868-2638-02**	90.14		**BX**
100s ea	**54868-2638-01**	99.22		**BX**
0.137 mg, 30s ea	**54868-5671-00**	30.77		**BX**
90s ea	**54868-5671-01**	87.08		**BX**
0.15 mg, 10s ea	**54868-1092-03**	12.63		**BX**
30s ea	**54868-1092-01**	32.66		**BX**
90s ea	**54868-1092-02**	92.76		**BX**
100s ea	**54868-1092-00**	102.78		**BX**
0.175 mg, 10s ea	**54868-3069-02**	13.85		**BX**
30s ea	**54868-3069-01**	36.33		**BX**
90s ea	**54868-3069-03**	103.76		**BX**
100s ea	**54868-3069-00**	114.35		**BX**
0.2 mg, 10s ea	**54868-1012-04**	14.55		**BX**
30s ea	**54868-1012-03**	38.43		**BX**
90s ea	**54868-1012-02**	110.05		**BX**
100s ea	**54868-1012-00**	121.98		**BX**
0.3 mg, 10s ea	**54868-1506-03**	14.66		**BX**
30s ea	**54868-1506-00**	40.22		**BX**
(Quality Care Prod)				
REPACK				
TAB, PO, 0.025 mg,				
100s ea	**35356-0309-00**	94.66		**BX**
0.05 mg, 30s ea	**35356-0107-30**	36.60		**BX**
100s ea	**35356-0107-00**	96.14		**BX**
0.075 mg, 30s ea	**35356-0310-30**	36.00		**BX**
100s ea	**35356-0310-00**	114.16		**BX**
0.088 mg, 100s ea	**49999-0824-00**	119.51		**BX**
0.1 mg, 30s ea	**49999-0825-30**	36.30		**BX**
30s ea	**49999-0954-30**	25.50		
100s ea	**49999-0825-00**	103.40		**BX**
0.112 mg, 100s ea	**35356-0311-00**	134.22		**BX**
0.125 mg, 30s ea	**49999-0953-30**	28.50		
100s ea	**49999-0953-00**	114.16		**BX**
0.137 mg, 100s ea	**35356-0312-00**	138.52		**BX**
0.15 mg, 30s ea	**49999-0393-30**	21.19		**BX**
100s ea	**49999-0373-00**	121.23		**BX**
0.175 mg, 30s ea	**35356-0313-30**	53.40		**BX**
100s ea	**35356-0313-00**	170.45		**BX**
0.2 mg, 100s ea	**35356-0314-00**	170.82		**BX**
0.3 mg, 100s ea	**35356-0315-00**	230.67		**BX**
SYNVISC (Genzyme)				
hylan polymers a and b				
SOL, IJ (3X2 ML SRN,PREFILLED)				
8 mg/ml, 2 ml 3s	**58468-0090-01**	904.80	754.00	
(Nucare Pharm)				
REPACK				
SOL, IJ (3X2ML SRN,PREFILLED)				
8 mg/ml, 2 ml 3s	**66267-0921-03**	799.99		
(Phys Total Care)				
REPACK				
SOL, IJ, 8 mg/ml,				
2 ml 3s	**54868-4219-00**	1001.99		

PROD/MFR	NDC	AWP	DP	OBC
(Physician Partner)				
REPACK				
SOL, IJ (1X2ML)				
8 mg/ml, 2 ml	**21695-0313-01**	603.20		
SYNVISC HYLAN G-F (Physician Partner)				
hylan polymers a and b				
SOL, IJ (3X2ML SYRINGES)				
8 mg/ml, 2 ml 3s	**21695-0313-03**	1809.60		
SYNVISC HYLAN GF (Quality Care Prod)				
REPACK				
hylan polymers a and b				
SOL, IJ, 8 mg/ml, 2 ml	**35356-0034-01**	483.00		
SYNVISC ONE (Genzyme)				
hylan polymers a and b				
SOL, IJ (3X2ML DOSES)				
8 mg/ml, 6 ml	**58468-0090-03**	904.80	754.00	
SYPRINE (Aton)				
trientine hydrochloride				
CAP, PO, 250 mg, 100s ea	**25010-0710-15**	815.06		
SYREX (Excelsior)				
sodium chloride				
SOL, IJ (PF,LATEX-FREE)				
0.9%, 2.5 ml	**63807-0100-33**	2.68		
5 ml	**63807-0100-51**	3.34		
5 ml	**63807-0100-56**	3.30		
10 ml	**63807-0100-11**	3.59		
10 ml	**63807-0102-11**	3.59		
(2X10ML,PF,LATEX-FREE)				
0.9%, 10 ml 2s	**63807-0100-92**	8.20		
IV (1X3ML,PF,LATEX-FREE)				
0.9%, 3 ml	**63807-0160-31**	2.68		
(1X5ML,PF,LATEX-FREE)				
0.9%, 5 ml	**63807-0160-51**	3.34		
(1X10ML,PF,LATEX-FREE)				
0.9%, 10 ml	**63807-0160-11**	3.59		
SYRINGE				
(Terumo) *See TERUMO HYPODERMIC SYRINGES*				
SYRINGE AND NEEDLE				
(Arkray) *See 3ML FUTURA SAFETY SYRINGE*				
(BD Consumer) *See B-D SAFETY GLIDE*				
(BD Consumer) *See B-D SAFETY GLIDE TB*				
(BD Dickinson Hosp Prod) *See B-D BULK SYRINGES CATHETER TIP*				
(BD Dickinson Hosp Prod) *See B-D BULK SYRINGES LUER-LOK TIP*				
(BD Dickinson Hosp Prod) *See B-D BULK SYRINGES SLIP TIP*				
(BD Dickinson Hosp Prod) *See B-D CORNWALL FLUID DISPENSING*				
(BD Dickinson Hosp Prod) *See B-D LAB SYRINGE ECCENTRIC TIP*				
(BD Dickinson Hosp Prod) *See B-D SAFETY-LOK W/ATTACHED NEEDLE*				
(BD Dickinson Hosp Prod) *See B-D SYRINGE CONVENIENCE PAK TRAY*				
(BD Dickinson Hosp Prod) *See B-D SYRINGE LUER-LOK TIP*				
(BD Dickinson Hosp Prod) *See B-D SYRINGE SLIP TIP*				
(Covidien) *See MONOJECT MAGELLAN*				
SYRINGE FILTER 1.0 MICRON (Abbott Hosp)				
filter, syringe				
DEV, NA, 48s ea	**00074-1837-01**	120.38	120.48	
SYRINGE INSUL (Phys Total Care)				
REPACK				
insulin syringe/needle				
DEV, NA (100U,G28 1/2,1ML)				
100s ea	**54868-1311-00**	84.30		
SYRINGE, ALLERGY				
(BD Dickinson Hosp Prod) *See B-D ALLERGIST TRAY*				
(BD Dickinson Hosp Prod) *See B-D ALLERGY SYRINGE*				
SYRINGEAVITENE (Davol)				
collagen hemostat				
POW, NA (PRELOADED 1GM)				
6s ea	**03031-0103-40**	858.96	715.80	
SYRPALTA (Humco)				
sucrose				
SYR, NA, 480 ml	**00802-3927-16**	9.71		
(RED)				
480 ml	**00802-3920-16**	10.17		

PROD/MFR	NDC	AWP	DP	OBC
SYRUP (Spectrum Pharmacy)				
sucrose				
SYR, NA (N.F.)				
500 ml	49452-7590-01	54.90		
4000 ml	49452-7590-02	284.55		
SYSTANE (DHS, Inc.)				
REPACK				
peg-400/propylene glycol				
SOL, OP, 0.4%-0.3%,				
15 ml	55887-0735-15	19.48		
T.R.U.E. TEST (Allerderm Labs.)				
skin test antigens, multiple				
TES, TP, 5s ea	00173-0457-01	295.00		
TACLONEX (Warner Chilcott)				
betamethasone dipropionate/calcipotriene				
OIN, TP, 0.064%-0.005%,				
60 gm	00430-3230-15	505.22		
100 gm	00430-3230-16	842.04		
(Phys Total Care)				
REPACK				
OIN, TP, 0.064%-0.005%,				
60 gm	54868-5680-00	521.06		
TACLONEX SCALP (Warner Chilcott)				
betamethasone dipropionate/calcipotriene				
SUS, TP (1X60GM)				
0.064%-0.005%,				
60 gm	00430-3240-15	505.22		
(Phys Total Care)				
REPACK				
SUS, TP (1X60GM)				
0.064%-0.005%,				
60 gm	54868-6091-00	557.57		
TACROLIMUS				
(Astellas) *See PROGRAF*				
(Astellas) *See PROTOPIC*				
(Letco)				
POW, NA (1X1GM)				
1 gm	62991-2664-03	2175.00		
(1X5GM)				
5 gm	62991-2664-04	7800.00		
(1X100MG)				
100 ml	62991-2664-01	336.00		
(1X500MG)				
500 ml	62991-2664-02	1125.00		
(Medisca)				
POW, NA (1X1GM)				
1 gm	38779-2272-06	2625.00		
(1X5GM)				
5 gm	38779-2272-03	8850.00		
(1X25GM)				
25 gm	38779-2272-04	29985.00		
(1X250MG)				
250 ml	38779-2272-07	1047.15		
(1X500MG)				
500 ml	38779-2272-00	1650.00		
(PCCA)				
POW, NA, 0.001 gm	51927-3557-00	6.72		
(Sandoz)				
CAP, PO (HARD GELATIN)				
0.5 mg, 100s ea	00781-2102-01	222.98		AB
1 mg, 100s ea	00781-2103-01	445.95		AB
5 mg, 100s ea	00781-2104-01	2229.75		AB
(B&B Pharm, Inc)				
REPACK				
POW, NA, 0.1 gm	63275-9958-06	310.00		
0.5 gm	63275-9958-07	1450.00		
1 gm	63275-9958-01	2800.00		
5 gm	63275-9958-02	13500.00		
TADALAFIL				
(Lilly) *See ADCIRCA*				
(Lilly) *See CIALIS*				
TAGAMET (Glaxo)				
cimetidine				
TAB, PO (CAPLET)				
400 mg, 500s ea	00108-5026-25	1083.78		AB
(Pharma Pac)				
REPACK				
TAB, PO, 300 mg, 12s ea	52959-0270-12	13.83		AB
30s ea	52959-0270-30	33.47		AB
35s ea	52959-0270-35	38.87		AB
(Phys Total Care)				
REPACK				
TAB, PO, 400 mg, 30s ea	54868-0319-02	77.11		AB
40s ea	54868-0319-06	96.62		AB
60s ea	54868-0319-01	152.36		AB

PROD/MFR	NDC	AWP	DP	OBC
TALACEN (Sanofi-Aventis)				
acetaminophen/pentazocine hydrochloride				
TAB, PO (CAPLET)				
650 mg-25 mg,				
100s ea, C-IV	00024-1937-04	169.67		AB
(PD-Rx Pharm)				
REPACK				
TAB, PO (CAPLET)				
650 mg-25 mg,				
15s ea UD, C-IV	55289-0889-15	39.92		AB
(Pharma Pac)				
REPACK				
TAB, PO (CAPLET)				
650 mg-25 mg,				
100s ea, C-IV	52959-0523-00	121.90		AB
TALADINE (PRX)				
ranitidine hydrochloride				
CAP, PO (HARD GELATIN)				
150 mg, 60s ea	16241-0757-02	102.00		
300 mg, 30s ea	16241-0758-11	92.00		
TALC (Baker, J.T.)				
POW, NA (U.S.P.)				
500 gm	10106-4100-01	18.45		
2000 gm	10106-4100-05	33.29		
(Bryan Corp.)				
POW, PL (STERILE)				
5 gm 10s	63256-0200-05	900.00	900.00	
(Bryan Corp.) *See SCLEROSOL INTRAPLEURAL*				
(Gallipot)				
POW, NA, 454 gm	51552-0219-06	8.68		
2270 gm	51552-0219-08	28.00		
11350 gm	51552-0219-04	96.74		
22700 gm	51552-0219-09	154.70		
(Lorann Oil)				
POW, NA (U.S.P.)				
454 gm	23535-0613-01	2.00		
2270 gm	23535-0613-50	8.25		
11350 gm	23535-0613-25	41.25		
(Mallinckrodt Lab)				
POW, NA (U.S.P.,SF)				
500 gm	00406-8476-04	16.03		
(Medisca)				
POW, NA (1X500GM,USP)				
500 gm	38779-0519-08	25.50		
(1X1000GM,USP)				
1000 gm	38779-0519-09	40.50		
(1X2500GM,USP)				
2500 gm	38779-0519-01	75.00		
(PCCA)				
POW, NA, 1 gm	51927-3101-00	0.02		
(USP)				
1 gm	51927-1239-00	0.07		
(Spectrum Pharmacy)				
POW, NA (U.S.P.)				
500 gm	49452-7600-01	54.95		
2500 gm	49452-7600-02	120.75		
12000 gm	49452-7600-03	332.85		
TALWIN (Physician Partner)				
REPACK				
pentazocine lactate				
SOL, IJ, 30 mg/ml,				
1 ml, C-IV	21695-0241-01	34.91		
TALWIN LACTATE (Hospira)				
pentazocine lactate				
SOL, IJ (UNI-AMP,LATEX-FREE)				
30 mg/ml,				
1 ml 25s, C-IV	00409-1941-01	399.60	349.75	
(VIAL,LATEX-FREE)				
30 mg/ml,				
10 ml, C-IV	00409-1920-10	119.70	104.74	
(Phys Total Care)				
REPACK				
SOL, IJ (VIAL)				
30 mg/ml,				
10 ml, C-IV	54868-2530-00	46.21		
TALWIN NX (Sanofi-Aventis)				
naloxone hydrochloride/pentazocine hydrochloride				
TAB, PO (CAPLET)				
0.5 mg-50 mg,				
100s ea, C-IV	00024-1951-04	187.03		AB
(Dispensing Solutions)				
REPACK				
TAB, PO (CAPLET)				
0.5 mg-50 mg,				
40s ea, C-IV	55045-2038-03	65.20		AB

PROD/MFR	NDC	AWP	DP	OBC
(Pharma Pac)				
REPACK				
TAB, PO, 0.5 mg-50 mg,				
10s ea, C-IV	52959-0340-10	19.72		AB
12s ea, C-IV	52959-0340-12	23.37		AB
24s ea, C-IV	52959-0340-24	37.52		AB
30s ea, C-IV	52959-0340-30	46.20		AB
40s ea, C-IV	52959-0340-40	59.99		AB
(Phys Total Care)				
REPACK				
TAB, PO, 0.5 mg-50 mg,				
20s ea, C-IV	54868-1465-01	36.53		AB
(Quality Care Prod)				
REPACK				
TAB, PO (CAPLET)				
0.5 mg-50 mg,				
30s ea, C-IV	35356-0329-30	122.60		AB
TAMBOCOR (Graceway)				
flecainide acetate				
TAB, PO, 50 mg, 100s ea	29336-0305-10	261.18		AB
100 mg, 100s ea	29336-0307-10	409.68		AB
150 mg, 100s ea	00089-0314-10	563.76		AB
100s ea	29366-0314-10	563.76		AB
(AQ)				
REPACK				
TAB, PO, 50 mg, 20s ea	66105-0152-02	55.41		
30s ea	66105-0152-03	83.11		
60s ea	66105-0152-06	166.23		
90s ea	66105-0152-09	249.34		
100s ea	66105-0152-10	277.06		
(Phys Total Care)				
REPACK				
TAB, PO, 50 mg, 20s ea	54868-5065-01	52.83		AB
60s ea	54868-5065-00	146.24		AB
100 mg, 60s ea	54868-4407-00	185.80		AB
TAMIFLU (Roche Labs)				
oseltamivir phosphate				
CAP, PO (HARD GELATIN)				
30 mg, 10s ea	00004-0802-85	97.63		EE
45 mg, 10s ea	00004-0801-85	97.63		EE
(BLISTER PACK)				
75 mg, 10s ea	00004-0800-85	97.63		
PDR, PO (TUTTI FRUTTI)				
12 mg/ml, 25 ml	00004-0810-95	48.82		
(A-S Medication)				
REPACK				
CAP, PO (BLISTER PACK)				
75 mg, 10s ea	54569-4888-00	126.92		
PDR, PO (TUTTI FRUTTI)				
12 mg/ml, 25 ml	54569-5615-00	46.25		
(Altura)				
REPACK				
CAP, PO (BLISTER PACK)				
75 mg, 10s ea	63874-0098-10	84.19		
(DHS, Inc.)				
REPACK				
CAP, PO, 75 mg, 10s ea	55887-0755-10	93.00		
10s ea UD	55887-0851-10	93.00		
(Dispensing Solutions)				
REPACK				
CAP, PO, 75 mg, 10s ea	55045-2759-01	101.00		
PDR, PO, 12 mg/ml, 25 ml	55045-3198-02	47.00		
(Pharma Pac)				
REPACK				
CAP, PO, 75 mg, 10s ea	52959-0801-10	159.82		
PDR, PO, 12 mg/ml, 25 ml	52959-0832-00	39.25		
(Phys Total Care)				
REPACK				
CAP, PO (HARD GELATIN)				
45 mg, 10s ea	54868-6083-00	117.53		EE
75 mg, 10s ea	54868-4476-00	125.05		
PDR, PO (TUTTI FRUTTI)				
12 mg/ml, 25 ml	54868-4684-00	62.50		
(Quality Care Prod)				
REPACK				
CAP, PO, 75 mg, 10s ea	49999-0298-10	171.04		
PDR, PO (TUTTI FRUTTI)				
12 mg/ml, 25 ml	35356-0478-25	97.60		
(Southwood)				
REPACK				
CAP, PO, 75 mg, 10s ea	58016-4789-01	97.63		
(Stat Rx)				
REPACK				
CAP, PO, 75 mg, 10s ea	16590-0213-10	193.41		
20s ea	16590-0213-20	202.00		
30s ea	16590-0213-30	303.00		

PROD/MFR	NDC	AWP	DP	OBC
TAMOXIFEN CITRATE				
FUL				
TAB, PO, 10 mg, 60s ea		58.28		
20 mg, 30s ea		58.28		
(Gallipot)				
POW, NA (U.S.P.)				
5 gm	51552-0838-02	123.20	88.00	
(Hawkins)				
POW, NA (U.S.P.)				
1 gm	63370-0251-10	76.00		
5 gm	63370-0251-15	352.00		
25 gm	63370-0251-25	1520.00		
100 gm	63370-0251-35	5200.00		
(Medisca)				
POW, NA (U.S.P.)				
5 gm	38779-0341-03	270.00		
10 gm	38779-0341-01	490.50		
25 gm	38779-0341-04	1197.00		
100 gm	38779-0341-05	3975.00		
(Mylan)				
TAB, PO, 10 mg, 60s ea	00378-0144-91	113.65		AB
500s ea	00378-0144-05	947.10		AB
20 mg, 30s ea	00378-0274-93	113.65		AB
100s ea	00378-0274-01	378.85		AB
(PCCA)				
POW, NA (U.S.P.)				
1 gm	51927-2976-00	72.00		
(Spectrum Pharmacy)				
POW, NA (U.S.P.)				
1 gm	49452-7571-01	107.80		
5 gm	49452-7571-02	420.00		
25 gm	49452-7571-06	1659.00		
100 gm	49452-7571-03	5250.00		
(Teva)				
TAB, PO (FILM COATED)				
10 mg, 60s ea	00093-0784-06	113.77		AB
180s ea	00093-0784-86	341.31		AB
500s ea	00093-0784-05	942.80		AB
1000s ea	00093-0784-10	1885.60		AB
20 mg, 30s ea	00093-0782-56	113.77		AB
(USP)				
20 mg, 30s ea	00172-5657-46	116.30		AB
(FILM COATED)				
20 mg, 100s ea	00093-0782-01	379.24		AB
500s ea	00093-0782-05	1885.50		AB
1000s ea	00093-0782-10	3771.15		AB
(Watson Labs)				
TAB, PO (USP,UNIT-OF-USE)				
10 mg, 60s ea	00591-2232-60	27.42		AB
180s ea	00591-2232-18	82.26		AB
20 mg, 30s ea	00591-2233-30	27.42		AB
90s ea	00591-2233-19	82.26		AB
(A-S Medication)				
REPACK				
TAB, PO, 10 mg, 60s ea	54569-3765-01	113.77		
(FILM COATED)				
20 mg, 30s ea	54569-5857-00	114.57		AB
(McKesson Packaging)				
REPACK				
TAB, PO (USP)				
10 mg, 100s ea UD	63739-0269-10	236.81		
(Phys Total Care)				
REPACK				
TAB, PO (USP)				
10 mg, 30s ea	54868-3004-05	22.38		
60s ea	54868-3004-02	40.26		
(USP)				
10 mg, 100s ea	54868-3004-04	67.62		
120s ea	54868-3004-01	59.01		
(USP)				
10 mg, 180s ea	54868-3004-03	89.55		
(FILM COATED)				
20 mg, 10s ea	54868-4287-01	13.95		AB
30s ea	54868-4287-00	35.82		AB
60s ea	54868-4287-04	70.13		
90s ea	54868-4287-03	78.27		AB
100s ea	54868-4287-02	85.14		
TAMSULOSIN HYDROCHLORIDE				
(Boehr Ingelheim Phar) *See FLOMAX*				
TANAFED DMX (Health Care Products)				
dm tan/dexchlorpheniramine tan/pse tan				
SUS, PO (COTTON CANDY)				
118 ml	61787-0866-04	63.30	50.64	
473 ml	61787-0866-16	230.33	184.26	
TANAHIST-D (Larken Labs, Inc.)				
chlorpheniramine tannate/phenylephrine tannate				
SER, PO (1X60ML,W/DROPPER)				
2 mg/ml-6 mg/ml,				
60 ml	68047-0031-02	35.04		
TANAHIST-PD (Larken Labs, Inc.)				
chlorpheniramine tannate				
SUS, PO (COTTON CANDY,DROPS)				
2 mg/ml, 60 ml	68047-0030-02	18.29		
TANDEM F (U.S. Pharm)				
ferrous fumarate/folic acid/iron polysaccharide				
CAP, PO, 162 mg-1 mg-115.2 mg,				
90s ea	52747-0901-60	36.69		
TANDEM OB (U.S. Pharm)				
prenatal vitamins				
CAP, PO, 90s ea	52747-0903-60	53.02		
TANDEM OB PRENATAL VIT (Phys Total Care)				
REPACK				
prenatal vitamins				
CAP, PO, 90s ea	54868-5815-00	62.04		
TANDEM PLUS (U.S. Pharm)				
multivitamin, minerals, and iron				
CAP, PO, 90s ea	52747-0902-60	57.43		
(Phys Total Care)				
REPACK				
CAP, PO, 30s ea	54868-5785-00	26.61		
TANGERINE FLAVOR (PCCA)				
flavoring aid				
POW, NA, 1 gm	51927-3273-00	0.60		
TANGERINE OIL (Lorann Oil)				
OIL, NA, 9.9 ml	23535-0151-72	2.50		
(Medisca)				
OIL, NA (1X14ML,NATURAL)				
14 ml	38779-0776-03	12.00		
(1X25ML,NATURAL)				
25 ml	38779-0776-04	19.50		
(1X100ML,NATURAL)				
100 ml	38779-0776-05	28.50		
(1X500ML,NATURAL)				
500 ml	38779-0776-08	76.50		
(PCCA) *See TANGERINE OIL FLAVOR*				
TANGERINE OIL FLAVOR (PCCA)				
tangerine oil				
OIL, NA (NATURAL)				
1 ml	51927-2155-00	0.90		
TANNATE-V-DM (Palmetto)				
REPACK				
dm tan/phenyleph tan/pyril tan				
SUS, PO, 480 ml	23490-7970-04	167.50		
TANNIC ACID (Baker, J.T.)				
POW, NA (F.C.C.)				
125 gm	10106-0380-04	24.10		
500 gm	10106-0380-01	169.05		
(Gallipot)				
POW, NA (U.S.P.,N.F.)				
28.35 gm	51552-0127-02	8.82		
113.4 gm	51552-0127-04	13.23		
454 gm	51552-0127-06	32.90		
(Lorann Oil)				
POW, NA, 30 gm	23535-0614-02	2.25		
120 gm	23535-0614-08	5.95		
480 gm	23535-0614-01	19.95		
(Mallinckrodt Lab)				
POW, NA (F.C.C.)				
125 gm	00406-1674-02	19.14		
500 gm	00406-1674-03	39.38		
(Medisca) *See TANNIN*				
(PCCA)				
POW, NA (USP)				
1 gm	51927-1123-00	0.45		
(Spectrum Pharmacy)				
POW, NA (U.S.P.)				
500 gm	49452-7610-01	144.90		
2500 gm	49452-7610-02	563.50		
TANNIC-12 (Cypress Pharm)				
carbetapentane tannate/chlorpheniramine tannate				
TAB, PO (DYE-FREE,CAPLET)				
60 mg-5 mg,				
100s ea	60258-0303-01	129.99		
TANNIN (Medisca)				
tannic acid				
POW, NA, 100 gm	38779-0604-05	37.50		
500 gm	38779-0604-08	31.50		
TAPAZOLE (King Pharm)				
methimazole				
TAB, PO, 5 mg, 100s ea	60793-0104-01	84.44		AB
10 mg, 100s ea	60793-0105-01	145.90		AB
(Phys Total Care)				
REPACK				
TAB, PO, 10 mg, 100s ea	54868-4639-00	130.84		AB
TAPE, ADHESIVE				
(3M Health Care) *See MICROPORE PLUS SURGICAL PAPER*				
(J&J Medical) *See DERMIVIEW HYPOALLERGENIC ADHESIVE*				
TAPENTADOL HYDROCHLORIDE				
(Ortho-McNeil Pharm) *See NUCYNTA*				
TARAXACUM (STANNO CULTUM) (Weleda)				
homeopathic substance				
LIQ, PO, 50 ml	55946-0398-15	9.00		
TARCEVA (Genentech)				
erlotinib				
TAB, PO (FILM-COATED)				
25 mg, 30s ea	50242-0062-01	1552.43		
100 mg, 30s ea	50242-0063-01	4264.03		
150 mg, 30s ea	50242-0064-01	4822.91		
(A-S Medication)				
REPACK				
TAB, PO, 150 mg, 30s ea	54569-5848-00	3906.71		
(Phys Total Care)				
REPACK				
TAB, PO (FILM-COATED)				
25 mg, 30s ea	54868-5290-00	1583.02		
100 mg, 30s ea	54868-5474-00	4556.07		
(FILM-COATED)				
150 mg, 30s ea	54868-5447-00	5046.76		
TARGRETIN (Eisai)				
bexarotene				
CAP, PO (SOFT GELATIN)				
75 mg, 100s ea	62856-0602-10	3654.00		
GEL, TP, 1%, 60 gm	62856-0604-22	1804.80		
TARKA (Abbott Pharm)				
trandolapril/verapamil hydrochloride				
TER, PO (FILM-COATED)				
1 mg-240 mg,				
100s ea	00074-3288-13	332.87	291.99	
2 mg-180 mg,				
100s ea	00074-3287-13	332.87	291.99	
(FILM COATED)				
2 mg-240 mg,				
100s ea	00074-3289-13	332.87	291.99	
4 mg-240 mg,				
100s ea	00074-3290-13	332.87	291.99	
(Phys Total Care)				
REPACK				
TER, PO, 2 mg-180 mg,				
20s ea	54868-5548-01	67.40		
30s ea	54868-5548-02	100.15		
60s ea	54868-5548-00	187.51		
(FILM COATED)				
2 mg-240 mg,				
10s ea	54868-5311-01	44.98		
30s ea	54868-5311-00	129.70		
4 mg-240 mg,				
10s ea	54868-5320-04	47.52		
20s ea	54868-5320-01	92.42		
30s ea	54868-5320-03	137.33		
(FILM COATED)				
4 mg-240 mg,				
60s ea	54868-5320-00	257.07		
100s ea	54868-5320-02	426.06		
(Quality Care Prod)				
REPACK				
TER, PO, 2 mg-180 mg,				
30s ea	35356-0268-30	194.67		
TARTARIC ACID				
(Baker, J.T.) *See D-TARTARIC ACID*				
(Baker, J.T.)				
GRA, NA (N.F., F.C.C.)				
500 gm	10106-4104-01	38.13		
(Gallipot)				
GRA, NA (N.F.)				
113.4 gm	51552-0268-04	12.25		
454 gm	51552-0268-06	32.13		
2270 gm	51552-0268-09	97.30		

PROD/MFR	NDC	AWP	DP	OBC
(Letco)				
POW, NA (1X100GM,USP)				
100 gm	62991-2612-01	23.50		
(1X500GM,USP)				
500 gm	62991-2612-02	75.00		
(Lorann Oil)				
POW, NA, 30 gm	23535-0615-05	1.25		
120 gm	23535-0615-08	2.95		
480 gm	23535-0615-01	8.95		
(Mallinckrodt Lab)				
GRA, NA (N.F.)				
500 gm	00406-2307-04	94.80		
(PCCA)				
POW, NA (NF)				
1 gm	51927-1524-00	0.36		
(Spectrum Pharmacy)				
GRA, NA (N.F.)				
500 gm	49452-7620-01	133.35		
2500 gm	49452-7620-02	409.50		
TASIGNA (Novartis Pharm)				
nilotinib hydrochloride				
CAP, PO, 200 mg, 28s ea	00078-0526-51	2221.90		
(4X28)				
200 mg, 112s ea	00078-0526-87	8887.61		
TASMAR (Valeant Pharm Intl)				
tolcapone				
TAB, PO, 100 mg, 90s ea	00187-0938-01	723.91		
TAURINE (Medisca)				
POW, NA (1X100GM)				
100 gm	38779-1949-05	55.50		
(1X500GM)				
500 gm	38779-1949-08	204.00		
(1X1000GM)				
1000 gm	38779-1949-09	297.00		
(PCCA)				
POW, NA, 1 gm	51927-2320-00	0.60		
SOL, NA, 1 gm	51927-4364-00	0.69		
TAVIST (Phys Total Care)				
REPACK				
clemastine fumarate				
SYR, PO, 0.5 mg/5 ml,				
120 ml	54868-1210-01	32.20		AA
(Southwood)				
REPACK				
SYR, PO, 0.5 mg/5 ml,				
120 ml	58016-4062-01	29.06		AA
TAXOTERE (Sanofi-Aventis)				
docetaxel				
SOL, IV (S.D.V. W/DILUENT)				
20 mg/0.5 ml,				
0.5 ml	00075-8001-20	469.16		
2 ml	00075-8001-80	1876.63		
TAZAROTENE				
(Allergan Inc) *See AVAGE*				
(Allergan Inc) *See TAZORAC*				
TAZICEF (Abbott Hosp)				
ceftazidime				
PDS, IJ (VIAL,LATEX-FREE)				
1 gm, 25s ea	00074-5082-16	192.60	168.50	AP
(VIAL)				
2 gm, 10s ea	00074-5084-11	141.24	123.60	AP
(Hospira)				
PDS, IJ (ADD-VANTAGE,LATEX-FREE)				
1 gm, 25s ea	00074-5092-16	210.60	184.25	AP
(LATEX-FREE)				
1 gm, 25s ea	00409-5082-16	160.50	140.50	AP
(SINGLE-DOSE ADD-VANTAGE)				
1 gm, 25s ea	00409-5092-16	218.70	191.25	AP
2 gm, 10s ea	00409-5084-11	141.24	123.60	AP
(ADD-VANTAGE,USP)				
2 gm, 10s ea	00409-5093-11	157.44	137.80	AP
(VIAL, BULK)				
6 gm, 10s ea	00074-5086-11	441.00	385.90	AP
IV (BULK PHARMACY)				
6 gm, 10s ea	00409-5086-11	432.00	378.00	AP
TAZORAC (Allergan Inc)				
tazarotene				
CRE, TP, 0.05%, 30 gm	00023-9155-30	157.82		
60 gm	00023-9155-60	315.59		
0.1%, 30 gm	00023-9156-30	167.68		
60 gm	00023-9156-60	335.29		
GEL, TP, 0.05%, 30 gm	00023-8335-03	157.82		
100 gm	00023-8335-10	525.95		
0.1%, 30 gm	00023-0042-03	167.68		
100 gm	00023-0042-10	558.85		
(Phys Total Care)				
REPACK				
CRE, TP, 0.05%, 30 gm	54868-4649-00	116.33		
60 gm	54868-4649-01	239.89		
GEL, TP, 0.1%, 100 gm	54868-4456-00	424.34		
TAZTIA XT (Watson)				
diltiazem hydrochloride				
C24, PO, 120 mg, 30s ea	62037-0696-30	29.30		AB4
90s ea	62037-0696-90	79.62		AB4
500s ea	62037-0696-05	439.56		AB4
180 mg, 30s ea	62037-0697-30	35.39		AB4
90s ea	62037-0697-90	96.10		AB4
500s ea	62037-0697-05	530.82		AB4
240 mg, 30s ea	62037-0698-30	50.18		AB4
90s ea	62037-0698-90	136.36		AB4
500s ea	62037-0698-05	752.76		AB4
300 mg, 30s ea	62037-0699-30	65.04		AB4
90s ea	62037-0699-90	176.66		AB4
500s ea	62037-0699-05	975.60		AB4
360 mg, 30s ea	62037-0700-30	66.29		AB4
90s ea	62037-0700-90	180.06		AB4
500s ea	62037-0700-05	994.32		AB4
TBC (Delta Pharm)				
castor oil/peru balsam/trypsin				
SPR, TP, 113.4 gm	53706-1001-01	17.35		
56.7 gm	53706-1001-02	12.60		
TDAP VACCINE				
(Glaxo) *See BOOSTRIX*				
(Sanofi) *See ADACEL*				
TEA TREE OIL (Lorann Oil)				
OIL, NA, 9.9 ml	23535-0151-75	4.75		
(Medisca)				
OIL, NA (1X14ML,NATURAL)				
14 ml	38779-0945-03	33.00		
(1X25ML,NATURAL)				
25 ml	38779-0945-04	43.50		
(1X100ML,NATURALL)				
100 ml	38779-0945-05	142.50		
(1X500ML,NATURAL)				
500 ml	38779-0945-08	399.00		
(PCCA)				
OIL, NA (MELALEUCA ALTERNIFOLIA)				
1 ml	51927-2416-00	1.99		
TEABERRY OIL FLAVOR (PCCA)				
flavoring aid				
SOL, NA, 1 ml	51927-3308-00	0.70		
TEARS AGAIN HYDRATE (Ocusoft)				
bilberry extract/evening primrose oil/flaxseed oil				
SGL, PO (SOFTGEL)				
40 mg-500 mg-1000 mg,				
120s ea	54799-0918-17	50.00		
TEARS RENEWED (Dispensing Solutions)				
REPACK				
mineral oil/petrolatum				
OIN, OP, 3.5 gm	55045-1352-09	4.95		
TECHNESCAN HDP (Mallinckrodt Inc.)				
technetium tc 99m oxidronate				
KIT, IJ (5 VIALS)				
ea	00019-9091-20	264.00	220.00	
TECHNESCAN MAG3 (Mallinckrodt Inc.)				
technetium tc 99m mertiatide				
KIT, IJ (5 VIALS)				
ea	00019-N096-B0	3096.00	2580.00	
TECHNESCAN PYP (Mallinckrodt Inc.)				
technetium tc 99m pyrophosphate				
KIT, IV (5 VIALS)				
ea	00019-N094-B0	214.80	179.00	AP
TECHNETIUM TC 99M ALBUMIN AGGREGATED				
(Bracco Diag) *See MACROTEC*				
(GE) *See MPI MAA*				
(Pharmlucence) *See PULMOLITE*				
TECHNETIUM TC 99M BICISATE				
(Lantheus) *See NEUROLITE*				
TECHNETIUM TC 99M DISOFENIN				
(Pharmlucence) *See HEPATOLITE*				
TECHNETIUM TC 99M EXAMETAZIME				
(GE) *See CERETEC*				
TECHNETIUM TC 99M MEBROFENIN				
(Bracco Diag) *See CHOLETEC*				
(Pharmlucence) *See KIT PREPARATION OF TECHNETIUM TC 99M MEBROFENIN*				
TECHNETIUM TC 99M MEDRONATE				
(GE) *See MPI MDP*				
(Pharmlucence) *See KIT FOR PREPARATION OF TECHNETIUM TC 99M MEDRONATE*				
TECHNETIUM TC 99M MERTIATIDE				
(Mallinckrodt Inc.) *See TECHNESCAN MAG3*				
TECHNETIUM TC 99M OXIDRONATE				
(Mallinckrodt Inc.) *See TECHNESCAN HDP*				
TECHNETIUM TC 99M PENTETATE				
(GE) *See MPI DTPA*				
(Pharmlucence) *See KIT FOR PREPARATION OF TECHNETIUM TC 99M PENTETATE*				
TECHNETIUM TC 99M PYROPHOSPHATE				
(Bracco Diag) *See PHOSPHOTEC*				
(GE) *See MPI PYROPHOSPHATE*				
(Mallinckrodt Inc.) *See TECHNESCAN PYP*				
(Pharmlucence) *See KIT PREPARATION OF TECHNETIUM TC 99M PYROPHOSPHATE*				
TECHNETIUM TC 99M RED BLOOD CELLS				
(Mallinckrodt Inc.) *See ULTRATAG RBC*				
TECHNETIUM TC 99M SESTAMIBI				
(Lantheus) *See CARDIOLITE*				
(Lantheus) *See MIRALUMA*				
(Pharmlucence) *See KIT FOR PREPARATION OF TECHNETIUM TC 99M SESTAMIBI*				
TECHNETIUM TC 99M SUCCIMER				
(GE) *See MPI DMSA*				
TECHNETIUM TC 99M SULFURCOLLOID				
(GE) *See TECHNETIUM TC 99M TSC*				
(Pharmlucence) *See KIT PREPARATION OF TECHNETIUM 99M SULFUR COLLOID*				
TECHNETIUM TC 99M TETROFOSMIN				
(GE) *See MYOVIEW*				
TECHNETIUM TC 99M TSC (GE)				
technetium tc 99m sulfurcolloid				
KIT, NA (5 VIALS)				
ea	17156-0526-05	320.84		AP
TEGRETOL (Novartis Pharm)				
carbamazepine				
CTB, PO, 100 mg, 100s ea	00078-0492-05	56.62		AB
100s ea UD	00078-0492-35	63.62		AB
SUS, PO (1X450ML,CITRUS-VANILLA)				
100 mg/5 ml,				
450 ml	00078-0508-83	69.48		AB
TAB, PO, 200 mg, 100s ea	00078-0509-05	107.87		AB
(PD-Rx Pharm)				
REPACK				
TAB, PO (REDI-SCRIPT)				
200 mg, 28s ea	58864-0631-28	58.53		AB
(Phys Total Care)				
REPACK				
CTB, PO, 100 mg, 30s ea	54868-1235-01	13.98		AB
100s ea	54868-1235-03	42.20		AB
TAB, PO, 200 mg, 100s ea	54868-1975-00	84.61		AB
TEGRETOL XR (PD-Rx Pharm)				
REPACK				
carbamazepine				
TER, PO, 200 mg, 30s ea	58864-0788-30	35.45		
(Phys Total Care)				
REPACK				
TER, PO, 200 mg, 20s ea	54868-5610-01	23.86		
60s ea	54868-5610-00	67.83		
TEGRETOL-XR (Novartis Pharm)				
carbamazepine				
TER, PO (COATED)				
100 mg, 100s ea	00078-0510-05	54.98		EE
200 mg, 100s ea	00078-0511-05	109.76		EE
400 mg, 100s ea	00078-0512-05	219.36		EE
(Phys Total Care)				
REPACK				
TER, PO, 100 mg, 90s ea	54868-4067-01	51.43		
100s ea	54868-4067-00	56.31		
400 mg, 100s ea	54868-3862-00	101.17		
TEKRAL (Capellon)				
diphenhydramine hcl/pse hcl				
TAB, PO, 100 mg-120 mg,				
90s ea	64543-0025-90	156.00	125.00	
TEKTURNA (Novartis Pharm)				
aliskiren				
TAB, PO (FILM-COATED)				
150 mg, 30s ea	00078-0485-15	87.64		
100s ea UD	00078-0485-35	292.09		
300 mg, 30s ea	00078-0486-15	110.56		
100s ea UD	00078-0486-35	368.50		

PROD/MFR	NDC	AWP	DP	OBC
(Phys Total Care)				
REPACK				
TAB, PO, 150 mg, 30s ea	54868-5772-00	103.77		
(FILM-COATED)				
300 mg, 30s ea	54868-6042-00	130.39		
(Quality Care Prod)				
REPACK				
TAB, PO (FILM-COATED)				
150 mg, 30s ea	35356-0133-30	121.60		
TEKTURNA HCT (Novartis Pharm)				
aliskiren/hydrochlorothiazide				
TAB, PO (FILM-COATED)				
150 mg-12.5 mg,				
30s ea	00078-0521-15	87.64		
150 mg-25 mg,				
30s ea	00078-0522-15	87.64		
300 mg-12.5 mg,				
30s ea	00078-0523-15	110.56		
300 mg-25 mg,				
30s ea	00078-0524-15	110.56		
(Phys Total Care)				
REPACK				
TAB, PO (FILM-COATED)				
150 mg-12.5 mg,				
30s ea	54868-6041-00	103.77		
TELAVANCIN HYDROCHLORIDE				
(Astellas) *See VIBATIV*				
TELBIVUDINE				
(Novartis Pharm) *See TYZEKA*				
TELITHROMYCIN				
(Sanofi-Aventis) *See KETEK*				
TELMISARTAN				
(Boehr Ingelheim Phar) *See MICARDIS*				
TEMAZEPAM				
FUL				
CAP, PO, 15 mg, 100s ea		13.65		
30 mg, 100s ea		17.48		
(Actavis)				
CAP, PO, 15 mg,				
100s ea, C-IV	00228-2076-10	73.45		AB
500s ea, C-IV	00228-2076-50	353.05		AB
30 mg, 100s ea, C-IV	00228-2077-10	88.45		AB
500s ea, C-IV	00228-2077-50	427.20		AB
(Covidien)				
CAP, PO, 7.5 mg,				
100s ea, C-IV	00406-9960-01	994.01		
(USP)				
22.5 mg,				
30s ea, C-IV	00406-9959-03	298.21		
(Covidien) *See RESTORIL*				
(Major)				
CAP, PO (USP,10X10)				
15 mg,				
100s ea UD, C-IV	00904-5885-61	92.40		AB
30 mg,				
100s ea UD, C-IV	00904-5886-61	102.93		AB
(Mutual)				
CAP, PO (USP)				
7.5 mg,				
100s ea, C-IV	53489-0648-01	994.03		EE
22.5 mg,				
30s ea, C-IV	53489-0650-07	298.21		AB
(Mylan)				
CAP, PO (USP,HARD-SHELL GELATIN)				
15 mg,				
90s ea, C-IV	00378-4010-77	66.11		AB
100s ea, C-IV	00378-4010-01	73.45		AB
500s ea, C-IV	00378-4010-05	367.25		AB
(USP,HARD-SHELL GELATIN)				
22.5 mg,				
30s ea, C-IV	00378-3120-93	298.21		AB
30 mg, 90s ea, C-IV	00378-5050-77	79.61		AB
100s ea, C-IV	00378-5050-01	88.45		AB
500s ea, C-IV	00378-5050-05	442.25		AB
(Sandoz)				
CAP, PO, 15 mg,				
100s ea, C-IV	00781-2201-01	69.30		AB
500s ea, C-IV	00781-2201-05	336.00		AB
30 mg, 100s ea, C-IV	00781-2202-01	80.90		AB
500s ea, C-IV	00781-2202-05	391.70		AB
(UDL)				
CAP, PO (10X10)				
15 mg,				
100s ea UD, C-IV	51079-0418-20	71.38		AB
(R.N.P., 5X20)				
15 mg,				
100s ea UD, C-IV	51079-0418-21	71.38		AB
(10X10)				
30 mg,				
100s ea UD, C-IV	51079-0419-20	83.33		AB
(4u)				
REPACK				
CAP, PO, 30 mg,				
30s ea, C-IV	10544-0361-30	35.84		AB
30s ea, C-IV	42549-0561-30	35.84		AB
(A-S Medication)				
REPACK				
CAP, PO, 15 mg,				
8s ea, C-IV	54569-0905-01	5.77		EE
30s ea, C-IV	54569-0905-00	21.62		EE
30 mg, 10s ea, C-IV	54569-1726-04	8.59		AB
30s ea, C-IV	54569-1726-01	25.78		EE
(Aidarex)				
REPACK				
CAP, PO, 15 mg,				
7s ea, C-IV	33261-0101-07	22.05		AB
14s ea, C-IV	33261-0101-14	44.10		AB
20s ea, C-IV	33261-0101-20	63.00		AB
21s ea, C-IV	33261-0101-21	66.15		AB
28s ea, C-IV	33261-0101-28	88.20		AB
30s ea, C-IV	33261-0101-30	94.50		AB
60s ea, C-IV	33261-0101-60	189.00		AB
90s ea, C-IV	33261-0101-90	283.50		AB
30 mg, 7s ea, C-IV	33261-0102-07	22.96		AB
14s ea, C-IV	33261-0102-14	45.92		AB
20s ea, C-IV	33261-0102-20	65.60		AB
21s ea, C-IV	33261-0102-21	68.88		AB
28s ea, C-IV	33261-0102-28	91.84		AB
30s ea, C-IV	33261-0102-30	98.40		AB
40s ea, C-IV	33261-0102-40	131.20		AB
60s ea, C-IV	33261-0102-60	196.80		AB
82s ea, C-IV	33261-0102-82	268.96		AB
90s ea, C-IV	33261-0102-90	295.20		AB
120s ea, C-IV	33261-0102-02	393.60		AB
(Altura)				
REPACK				
CAP, PO, 15 mg,				
10s ea, C-IV	63874-0292-10	9.19		EE
12s ea, C-IV	63874-0292-12	11.03		EE
15s ea, C-IV	63874-0292-15	13.79		EE
20s ea, C-IV	63874-0292-20	18.38		EE
30s ea, C-IV	63874-0292-30	27.57		EE
60s ea, C-IV	63874-0292-60	55.14		EE
90s ea, C-IV	63874-0292-90	82.71		AB
100s ea, C-IV	63874-0292-01	91.90		EE
120s ea, C-IV	63874-0292-04	110.28		AB
200s ea, C-IV	63874-0292-74	183.80		AB
30 mg, 12s ea, C-IV	63874-0713-12	12.34		EE
15s ea, C-IV	63874-0713-15	15.42		AB
20s ea, C-IV	63874-0713-20	20.56		EE
30s ea, C-IV	63874-0713-30	30.84		EE
40s ea, C-IV	63874-0713-40	41.12		AB
60s ea, C-IV	63874-0713-60	61.68		AB
90s ea, C-IV	63874-0713-90	92.52		AB
100s ea, C-IV	63874-0713-01	102.80		EE
120s ea, C-IV	63874-0713-04	123.36		AB
200s ea, C-IV	63874-0713-74	205.60		AB
(Bryant Ranch)				
REPACK				
CAP, PO, 15 mg,				
20s ea, C-IV	63629-1619-01	39.99		
30s ea, C-IV	63629-1619-02	51.98		
60s ea, C-IV	63629-1619-03	149.65		
30 mg, 20s ea, C-IV	63629-1621-02	23.92		
30s ea, C-IV	63629-1621-01	35.88		
60s ea, C-IV	63629-1621-04	197.85		
90s ea, C-IV	63629-1621-05	225.32		
100s ea, C-IV	63629-1621-03	119.62		
(Core)				
REPACK				
CAP, PO, 15 mg,				
20s ea, C-IV	33358-0332-20	40.99		
30s ea, C-IV	33358-0332-30	53.28		
60s ea, C-IV	33358-0332-60	153.39		
30 mg, 60s ea, C-IV	33358-0333-60	202.59		
90s ea, C-IV	33358-0333-90	230.95		
(DHS, Inc.)				
REPACK				
CAP, PO, 15 mg,				
7s ea, C-IV	55887-0437-07	6.12		
15s ea, C-IV	55887-0437-15	13.12		
30s ea, C-IV	55887-0437-30	26.25		AB
60s ea, C-IV	55887-0437-60	69.50		AB
90s ea, C-IV	55887-0437-90	72.18		AB
30 mg, 7s ea, C-IV	55887-0436-07	6.91		
15s ea, C-IV	55887-0436-15	14.82		
30s ea, C-IV	55887-0436-30	29.65		AB
90s ea, C-IV	55887-0436-90	80.01		AB
(Dispensing Solutions)				
REPACK				
CAP, PO, 15 mg,				
10s ea, C-IV	66336-0668-10	8.75		AB
20s ea, C-IV	55045-2152-07	18.00		AB
30s ea, C-IV	55045-2152-08	27.00		AB
30s ea, C-IV	55045-3754-08	27.00		
30s ea, C-IV	66336-0668-30	26.25		AB
40s ea, C-IV	55045-2152-04	36.00		AB
45s ea, C-IV	55045-2152-03	40.50		AB
60s ea, C-IV	55045-2152-09	54.00		AB
90s ea, C-IV	55045-2152-06	81.00		AB
100s ea, C-IV	55045-2152-01	90.00		
120s ea, C-IV	55045-2152-00	108.00		AB
30 mg, 7s ea, C-IV	55045-1746-02	7.07		AB
30s ea, C-IV	55045-1746-08	30.30		AB
30s ea, C-IV	66336-0005-30	31.50		
40s ea, C-IV	55045-1746-03	40.40		AB
45s ea, C-IV	55045-1746-04	45.45		AB
60s ea, C-IV	55045-1746-09	60.60		
60s ea, C-IV	66336-0005-60	63.00		
90s ea, C-IV	55045-1746-06	90.90		AB
100s ea, C-IV	55045-1746-01	101.00		AB
120s ea, C-IV	55045-1746-00	121.20		AB
(HomeMed)				
REPACK				
CAP, PO, 15 mg,				
30s ea, C-IV	51655-0856-24	18.64		EE
30 mg, 30s ea, C-IV	51655-0845-24	20.58		EE
(IPI)				
REPACK				
CAP, PO, 15 mg,				
30s ea, C-IV	18837-0150-30	21.18		AB
30 mg, 30s ea, C-IV	18837-0151-30	25.63		AB
(Keltman Pharma., Inc.)				
REPACK				
CAP, PO, 15 mg,				
24s ea, C-IV	68387-0195-24	21.60		AB
30s ea, C-IV	68387-0195-30	27.00		
30 mg, 30s ea, C-IV	68387-0196-30	121.55		
(McKesson Packaging)				
REPACK				
CAP, PO (USP)				
15 mg,				
100s ea UD, C-IV	63739-0231-10	86.62		
(Nucare Pharm)				
REPACK				
CAP, PO, 15 mg,				
30s ea, C-IV	66267-0415-30	33.59		AB
60s ea, C-IV	66267-0415-60	49.60		AB
30 mg, 10s ea, C-IV	66267-0321-10	17.19		AB
30s ea, C-IV	66267-0321-30	39.79		AB
60s ea, C-IV	66267-0321-60	53.60		AB
(Palmetto)				
REPACK				
CAP, PO, 15 mg,				
10s ea, C-IV	23490-6322-01	17.33		
15s ea, C-IV	23490-6322-02	25.99		
30s ea, C-IV	23490-6322-03	51.98		
60s ea, C-IV	23490-6322-05	103.96		
100s ea, C-IV	23490-6322-04	173.27		
30 mg, 10s ea, C-IV	23490-6323-01	17.50		
30s ea, C-IV	23490-6323-02	52.50		
60s ea, C-IV	23490-6323-03	105.00		
100s ea, C-IV	23490-6323-04	175.00		
(PD-Rx Pharm)				
REPACK				
CAP, PO, 15 mg,				
14s ea, C-IV	55289-0196-14	17.90		AB
30s ea, C-IV	55289-0196-30	28.00		AB
30 mg, 30s ea, C-IV	55289-0660-30	23.40		AB
(Pharma Pac)				
REPACK				
CAP, PO, 15 mg,				
10s ea, C-IV	52959-0535-10	9.45		AB
12s ea, C-IV	52959-0535-12	11.34		AB
24s ea, C-IV	52959-0535-24	22.63		AB
28s ea, C-IV	52959-0535-28	26.46		AB
30s ea, C-IV	52959-0535-30	28.34		AB
40s ea, C-IV	52959-0535-40	37.78		AB
60s ea, C-IV	52959-0535-60	56.66		AB
30 mg, 10s ea, C-IV	52959-0459-10	11.30		EE
12s ea, C-IV	52959-0459-12	13.50		EE
15s ea, C-IV	52959-0459-15	16.75		EE
15s ea, C-IV	52959-0535-15	14.18		AB

PROD/MFR	NDC	AWP	DP	OBC
20s ea, C-IV	52959-0459-20	22.33		AB
30s ea, C-IV	52959-0459-30	31.50		AB
60s ea, C-IV	52959-0459-60	62.25		EE
100s ea, C-IV	52959-0459-00	103.50		AB
(Phys Total Care) REPACK				
CAP, PO, 15 mg,				
10s ea, C-IV	54868-0038-01	8.98		EE
15s ea, C-IV	54868-0038-00	7.47		EE
20s ea, C-IV	54868-0038-03	10.44		EE
30s ea, C-IV	54868-0038-02	13.44		EE
60s ea, C-IV	54868-0038-05	22.35		EE
100s ea, C-IV	54868-0038-04	34.26		EE
30 mg, 15s ea, C-IV	54868-0039-04	8.70		AB
20s ea, C-IV	54868-0039-03	10.62		EE
30s ea, C-IV	54868-0039-02	15.93		EE
60s ea, C-IV	54868-0039-05	27.36		AB
100s ea, C-IV	54868-0039-06	41.07		AB
(Physician Partner) REPACK				
CAP, PO, 15 mg,				
30s ea, C-IV	21695-0282-30	44.07		
60s ea, C-IV	21695-0282-60	88.14		
30 mg, 30s ea, C-IV	21695-0283-30	53.04		
(Quality Care Prod) REPACK				
CAP, PO, 15 mg,				
15s ea, C-IV	49999-0045-15	16.55		AB
30s ea, C-IV	49999-0045-30	33.09		EE
60s ea, C-IV	49999-0045-60	66.20		EE
90s ea, C-IV	49999-0045-90	99.27		EE
30 mg, 15s ea, C-IV	49999-0346-15	41.10		AB
30s ea, C-IV	49999-0346-30	82.20		AB
60s ea, C-IV	49999-0346-60	164.40		AB
90s ea, C-IV	49999-0346-90	246.60		EE
(Southwood) REPACK				
CAP, PO, 15 mg,				
12s ea, C-IV	58016-0829-12	11.03		EE
15s ea, C-IV	58016-0829-15	13.79		EE
20s ea, C-IV	58016-0829-20	18.38		EE
30s ea, C-IV	58016-0829-30	27.57		EE
60s ea, C-IV	58016-0829-60	55.14		EE
90s ea, C-IV	58016-0829-90	82.71		AB
100s ea, C-IV	58016-0829-00	91.90		EE
120s ea, C-IV	58016-0829-02	110.28		AB
150s ea, C-IV	58016-0829-03	137.85		AB
200s ea, C-IV	58016-0829-89	183.80		AB
300s ea, C-IV	58016-0829-73	275.70		AB
30 mg, 12s ea, C-IV	58016-0831-12	12.34		EE
15s ea, C-IV	58016-0831-15	15.42		EE
20s ea, C-IV	58016-0831-20	20.56		EE
28s ea, C-IV	58016-0831-28	28.78		EE
30s ea, C-IV	58016-0831-30	30.84		EE
30s ea, C-IV	58016-0831-45	46.26		EE
60s ea, C-IV	58016-0831-60	61.68		EE
90s ea, C-IV	58016-0831-90	92.52		AB
100s ea, C-IV	58016-0831-00	102.80		EE
120s ea, C-IV	58016-0831-02	123.36		AB
150s ea, C-IV	58016-0831-03	154.20		AB
200s ea, C-IV	58016-0831-89	205.60		AB
300s ea, C-IV	58016-0831-73	308.40		AB
(St. Mary's MPP) REPACK				
CAP, PO (USP)				
15 mg,				
30s ea, C-IV	60760-0206-30	29.30		
30 mg, 30s ea, C-IV	60760-0207-30	34.19		
(Stat Rx) REPACK				
CAP, PO, 7.5 mg,				
30s ea, C-IV	16590-0744-30	264.50		
15 mg, 15s ea, C-IV	16590-0214-15	17.75		AB
28s ea, C-IV	16590-0214-28	32.67		AB
30s ea, C-IV	16590-0214-30	35.00		
30s ea, C-IV	16590-0438-30	42.50		AB
60s ea, C-IV	16590-0214-60	70.00		
90s ea, C-IV	16590-0214-90	105.00		
30 mg, 28s ea, C-IV	16590-0438-28	33.77		AB
60s ea, C-IV	16590-0438-60	60.00		
90s ea, C-IV	16590-0438-90	90.00		
120s ea, C-IV	16590-0438-72	120.00		
TEMODAR (Schering)				
temozolomide				
CAP, PO, 5 mg, 5s ea	00085-3004-02	53.24		EE
14s ea	00085-1248-03	136.67		EE
14s ea	00085-3004-01	150.90		EE
20 mg, 5s ea	00085-1519-02	214.51		EE
14s ea	00085-1519-01	600.59		EE
100 mg, 5s ea	00085-1366-02	1072.46		EE
14s ea	00085-1366-01	3002.94		EE
140 mg, 5s ea	00085-1425-01	1501.46		EE
14s ea	00085-1425-02	4204.09		EE
180 mg, 5s ea	00085-1430-01	1930.44		EE
14s ea	00085-1430-02	5405.27		EE
250 mg, 5s ea	00085-1417-01	2681.92		
PDS, IV, 100 mg, 100 ml	00085-1381-01	565.94		
(Phys Total Care) REPACK				
CAP, PO, 5 mg, 5s ea	54868-5348-01	52.84		
25s ea	54868-5348-00	245.49		
20 mg, 5s ea	54868-4142-00	202.54		
10s ea	54868-4142-02	378.54		
20s ea	54868-4142-06	755.20		
25s ea	54868-4142-01	963.78		
30s ea	54868-4142-05	1109.28		
40s ea	54868-4142-04	1478.62		
60s ea	54868-4142-03	2217.30		
100 mg, 5s ea	54868-5350-02	1159.68		
10s ea	54868-5350-03	2269.31		
15s ea	54868-5350-00	3402.66		
25s ea	54868-5350-01	5553.82		
30s ea	54868-5350-04	6662.49		
180 mg, 14s ea	54868-5980-00	5486.51		EE
250 mg, 5s ea	54868-5354-00	2892.76		
TEMOVATE (PharmaDerm)				
clobetasol propionate				
CRE, TP, 0.05%, 30 gm	00462-0163-30	125.83		AB1
60 gm	00462-0163-60	225.18		AB1
GEL, TP, 0.05%, 60 gm	00462-0293-60	225.18		AB
OIN, TP, 0.05%, 15 gm	00462-0162-15	76.27		AB
30 gm	00462-0162-30	127.45		AB
(Phys Total Care) REPACK				
CRE, TP, 0.05%, 15 gm	54868-1807-03	44.93		AB1
30 gm	54868-1807-02	60.31		AB1
45 gm	54868-1807-01	63.32		AB1
OIN, TP, 0.05%, 15 gm	54868-1589-01	28.87		AB
30 gm	54868-1589-02	61.69		AB
60 gm	54868-1589-00	109.04		AB
SOL, TP, 0.05%, 25 ml	54868-2993-01	36.28		AT
(Southwood) REPACK				
CRE, TP, 0.05%, 30 gm	58016-1133-01	34.94		AB1
TEMOVATE E (PharmaDerm)				
clobetasol propionate				
EMO, TP, 0.05%, 60 gm	00462-0301-60	225.18		AB2
(Phys Total Care) REPACK				
EMO, TP, 0.05%, 30 gm	54868-3734-01	41.52		AB2
60 gm	54868-3734-00	104.23		AB2
TEMOVATE SCALP APPLICATION (PharmaDerm)				
clobetasol propionate				
SOL, TP, 0.05%, 50 ml	00462-0269-50	187.66		AT
TEMOZOLOMIDE				
(Schering) *See TEMODAR*				
TEMSIROLIMUS				
(Wyeth) *See TORISEL*				
TENCON (Intl Ethical)				
acetaminophen/butalbital				
CAP, PO, 650 mg-50 mg,				
100s ea	11584-1029-01	25.92		AB
TENDERWET CAVITY SYSTEM (Medline)				
dressing				
DEV, NA (W/1.6" PAD)				
ea	53329-0990-54	124.33		
(W/2.2" PAD)				
ea	53329-0990-24	154.78		
(W/3"X3" PAD)				
ea	53329-0990-50	142.85		
(W/4"X4" PAD)				
ea	53329-0994-40	274.20		
TENECTEPLASE				
(Genentech) *See TNKASE*				
TENEX (Promius)				
guanfacine hydrochloride				
TAB, PO, 1 mg, 100s ea	67857-0705-01	288.52		AB
500s ea	67857-0705-05	1221.19	612.49	AB
2 mg, 100s ea	67857-0706-01	428.54	214.93	AB
TENIPOSIDE				
(B/M Squibb Onc/Vir) *See VUMON*				
TENOFOVIR DISOPROXIL FUMARATE				
(Gilead Sciences) *See VIREAD*				
TENOGLIDE (Integra LifeSciences Corp)				
collagen tendon encasement				
DEV, NA (2"X2")				
ea	08478-4015-02	1447.00		
(4"X5")				
ea	08478-4015-05	2266.00		
TENORETIC 100 (AstraZeneca)				
atenolol/chlorthalidone				
TAB, PO, 100 mg-25 mg,				
100s ea	00310-0117-10	291.10		AB
TENORETIC 50 (AstraZeneca)				
atenolol/chlorthalidone				
TAB, PO, 50 mg-25 mg,				
100s ea	00310-0115-10	207.40		AB
(Phys Total Care) REPACK				
TAB, PO, 50 mg-25 mg,				
30s ea	54868-0321-00	49.40		AB
TENORMIN (AstraZeneca)				
atenolol				
TAB, PO, 25 mg, 100s ea	00310-0107-10	184.99		AB
50 mg, 100s ea	00310-0105-10	188.71		AB
100 mg, 100s ea	00310-0101-10	283.14		AB
(PD-Rx Pharm) REPACK				
TAB, PO, 50 mg, 30s ea	55289-0254-30	67.18		AB
100 mg, 30s ea	55289-0587-30	92.07		AB
(Pharma Pac) REPACK				
TAB, PO, 50 mg, 30s ea	52959-0280-30	41.06		AB
(Phys Total Care) REPACK				
TAB, PO, 50 mg, 100s ea	54868-0701-00	167.80		AB
TEQUILA SUNRISE FLAVOR (PCCA)				
flavoring aid				
SOL, NA (CONCENTRATE)				
1 ml	51927-2602-00	0.23		
TERAZOL (Dispensing Solutions) REPACK				
terconazole				
CRE, VG, 0.4%, 45 gm	55045-1538-08	56.00		
TERAZOL 3 (Ortho-McNeil Pharm)				
terconazole				
CRE, VG (W/APPLICATOR)				
0.8%, 20 gm	00062-5356-01	52.79	43.99	
SUP, VG, 80 mg, 3s ea	00062-5351-01	52.79	43.99	
(A-S Medication) REPACK				
CRE, VG (W/APPLICATOR)				
0.8%, 20 gm	54569-3195-00	54.99		
SUP, VG, 80 mg, 3s ea	54569-2012-00	54.99		
(Altura) REPACK				
CRE, VG (W/ APPLICATOR)				
0.8%, 20 gm	63874-0890-20	35.53		
SUP, VG, 80 mg, 3s ea	63874-0831-03	30.39		
(Pharma Pac) REPACK				
SUP, VG (W/APPLICATOR)				
80 mg, 3s ea	52959-0574-00	29.80		
(Phys Total Care) REPACK				
CRE, VG, 0.8%, 20 gm	54868-1687-01	65.10		
SUP, VG, 80 mg, 3s ea	54868-0515-01	65.10		
(Southwood) REPACK				
CRE, VG, 0.8%, 20 gm	58016-2021-01	33.84		
SUP, VG, 80 mg, 3s ea	58016-3149-01	28.94		
TERAZOL 7 (Ortho-McNeil Pharm)				
terconazole				
CRE, VG (W/APPLICATOR)				
0.4%, 45 gm	00062-5350-01	52.79	43.99	
(A-S Medication) REPACK				
CRE, VG, 0.4%, 45 gm	54569-2013-00	54.99		
(Altura) REPACK				
CRE, VG, 0.4%, 45 gm	63874-0850-45	35.53		
(Phys Total Care) REPACK				
CRE, VG (W/APPLICATOR)				
0.4%, 45 gm	54868-2862-00	59.83		

PROD/MFR	NDC	AWP	DP	OBC
(Southwood) REPACK				
CRE, VG, 0.4%, 45 gm	58016-3119-01	33.84		
TERAZOSIN (Dispensing Solutions) REPACK				
terazosin hydrochloride				
CAP, PO, 1 mg, 30s ea	55045-2834-08	48.30		
(Pharma Pac) REPACK				
CAP, PO, 5 mg, 60s ea	52959-0829-60	94.15		
(Phys Total Care) REPACK				
CAP, PO, 1 mg, 60s ea	54868-4803-01	26.61		
TERAZOSIN HCL (Apotex Corp.)				
terazosin hydrochloride				
CAP, PO, 1 mg, 100s ea	60505-0115-00	160.17		AB
500s ea	60505-0115-05	786.45		AB
2 mg, 100s ea	60505-0116-00	160.17		AB
500s ea	60505-0116-05	786.45		AB
7000s ea	60505-0116-07	11010.30		AB
5 mg, 100s ea	60505-0117-00	160.17		AB
500s ea	60505-0117-05	786.45		AB
7000s ea	60505-0117-07	11010.30		AB
10 mg, 100s ea	60505-0118-00	160.17		AB
500s ea	60505-0118-05	786.45		AB
(Cadista)				
CAP, PO, 1 mg, 100s ea	59746-0383-06	160.50		AB
500s ea	59746-0383-09	778.42		AB
1000s ea	59746-0383-10	1556.84		AB
2 mg, 100s ea	59746-0384-06	160.50		AB
500s ea	59746-0384-09	778.42		AB
1000s ea	59746-0384-10	1556.84		AB
5 mg, 100s ea	59746-0385-06	160.50		AB
500s ea	59746-0385-09	778.42		AB
10 mg, 100s ea	59746-0386-06	160.50		AB
500s ea	59746-0386-09	778.42		AB
1000s ea	59746-0386-10	1556.84		AB
(Major)				
CAP, PO, 1 mg,				
100s ea UD	00904-5650-61	144.50		AB
10 mg, 100s ea UD	00904-5653-61	144.50		AB
(Mylan)				
CAP, PO, 1 mg, 100s ea	00378-2260-01	160.50		AB
2 mg, 100s ea	00378-2264-01	160.50		AB
5 mg, 100s ea	00378-2268-01	160.50		AB
10 mg, 100s ea	00378-1570-01	160.50		AB
(PCCA)				
POW, NA (DIHYDRATE)				
1 gm	51927-3268-00	135.00		
(Sandoz)				
CAP, PO, 1 mg, 100s ea	00781-2051-01	160.38		AB
500s ea	00781-2051-05	777.84		AB
2 mg, 100s ea	00781-2052-01	160.38		AB
500s ea	00781-2052-05	777.84		AB
5 mg, 100s ea	00781-2053-01	160.38		AB
500s ea	00781-2053-05	777.84		AB
10 mg, 100s ea	00781-2054-01	160.38		AB
500s ea	00781-2054-05	777.84		AB
(UDL)				
CAP, PO (10X10)				
1 mg, 100s ea UD	51079-0936-20	160.56		AB
2 mg, 100s ea UD	51079-0937-20	160.56		AB
5 mg, 100s ea UD	51079-0938-20	160.56		AB
(A-S Medication) REPACK				
CAP, PO, 1 mg, 30s ea	54569-4873-00	48.12		EE
5 mg, 30s ea	54569-4875-00	48.12		EE
10 mg, 30s ea	54569-4876-00	48.12		EE
(DHS, Inc.) REPACK				
CAP, PO, 5 mg, 30s ea	55887-0481-30	45.81		AB
90s ea	55887-0481-90	119.19		AB
10 mg, 30s ea	55887-0482-30	48.99		AB
(GSMS) REPACK				
CAP, PO (UNIT OF USE)				
1 mg, 30s ea	60429-0707-30	28.65	9.55	AB
90s ea	60429-0707-90	420.00	140.00	AB
2 mg, 30s ea	60429-0708-30	28.65	9.55	AB
90s ea	60429-0708-90	420.00	140.00	AB
5 mg, 30s ea	60429-0709-30	28.65	9.55	AB
90s ea	60429-0709-90	420.00	140.00	AB
10 mg, 30s ea	60429-0710-30	28.65	9.55	AB
90s ea	60429-0710-90	420.00	140.00	AB
(PD-Rx Pharm) REPACK				
CAP, PO (REDI-SCRIPT)				
1 mg, 60s ea	58864-0648-60	20.00		AB
90s ea	58864-0648-90	22.53		AB
2 mg, 30s ea	58864-0463-30	12.47		AB
5 mg, 30s ea	58864-0719-30	12.47		AB
90s ea	58864-0719-90	27.40		AB
10 mg, 30s ea	58864-0878-30	34.55		AB
(Pharma Pac) REPACK				
CAP, PO, 1 mg, 150s ea	52959-0828-05	235.45		AB
(Phys Total Care) REPACK				
CAP, PO, 1 mg, 30s ea	54868-4803-00	14.04		AB
2 mg, 30s ea	54868-4247-00	13.41		EE
100s ea	54868-4247-01	36.15		AB
5 mg, 30s ea	54868-4248-00	13.44		EE
90s ea	54868-4248-02	34.32		EE
100s ea	54868-4248-01	36.30		EE
10 mg, 25s ea	54868-4249-02	13.41		AB
30s ea	54868-4249-00	15.51		EE
100s ea	54868-4249-01	43.17		EE
(Physician Partner) REPACK				
CAP, PO, 2 mg, 90s ea	21695-0812-90	288.90		AB
5 mg, 30s ea	21695-0813-30	96.30		AB
90s ea	21695-0813-90	288.90		AB
(Southwood) REPACK				
CAP, PO, 1 mg, 30s ea	58016-0431-30	59.23		AB
60s ea	58016-0431-60	118.45		AB
90s ea	58016-0431-90	177.68		AB
100s ea	58016-0431-00	197.42		AB
120s ea	58016-0431-02	236.90		AB
2 mg, 30s ea	58016-0736-30	59.23		AB
60s ea	58016-0736-60	118.45		AB
90s ea	58016-0736-90	177.68		AB
100s ea	58016-0736-00	197.42		AB
120s ea	58016-0736-02	236.90		AB
5 mg, 30s ea	58016-0673-30	46.65		EE
60s ea	58016-0673-60	93.30		EE
90s ea	58016-0673-90	139.95		EE
100s ea	58016-0673-00	155.50		EE
10 mg, 30s ea	58016-0674-30	59.23		AB
60s ea	58016-0674-60	118.45		AB
90s ea	58016-0674-90	177.68		AB
100s ea	58016-0674-00	197.42		AB
120s ea	58016-0674-02	236.90		AB
(Vibranta) REPACK				
CAP, PO, 1 mg, 30s ea	57866-6486-01	49.18		
2 mg, 30s ea	57866-6487-01	52.31		
90s ea	57866-6487-02	145.44		
5 mg, 30s ea	57866-6488-01	52.31		
90s ea	57866-6488-02	145.44		
10 mg, 30s ea	57866-6489-01	49.99		
TERAZOSIN HYDROCHLORIDE FUL				
CAP, PO, 1 mg, 100s ea		14.25		
2 mg, 100s ea		14.25		
5 mg, 100s ea		14.25		
10 mg, 100s ea		14.25		
(Apotex Corp.) *See TERAZOSIN HCL*				
(Cadista)				
CAP, PO, 5 mg, 1000s ea	59746-0385-10	1556.84		AB
(Cadista) *See TERAZOSIN HCL*				
(Major)				
CAP, PO (10X10)				
2 mg, 100s ea UD	00904-6127-61	144.50		EE
5 mg, 100s ea UD	00904-6128-61	144.50		EE
(Major) *See TERAZOSIN HCL*				
(Mylan) *See TERAZOSIN HCL*				
(PCCA) *See TERAZOSIN HCL*				
(Sandoz) *See TERAZOSIN HCL*				
(Teva)				
CAP, PO (HARD GELATIN)				
1 mg, 100s ea	00093-4336-01	160.50		
500s ea	00093-4336-05	786.45		
2 mg, 100s ea	00093-4337-01	160.50		
1000s ea	00093-4337-10	1556.85		
5 mg, 100s ea	00093-4338-01	160.50		
1000s ea	00093-4338-10	1556.85		
10 mg, 100s ea	00093-4339-01	160.50		
500s ea	00093-4339-05	786.45		
(UDL) *See TERAZOSIN HCL*				
(Bryant Ranch) REPACK				
CAP, PO, 5 mg, 30s ea	63629-1414-02	67.41		
100s ea	63629-1414-01	224.70		
(Dispensing Solutions) REPACK				
CAP, PO, 2 mg, 30s ea	55045-3104-08	54.30		
100s ea	55045-3104-00	181.00		
(Palmetto) REPACK				
CAP, PO, 5 mg, 30s ea	23490-6814-03	52.31		
10 mg, 30s ea	23490-6815-03	59.70		
(Quality Care Prod) REPACK				
CAP, PO, 5 mg, 30s ea	49999-0227-30	57.99		
100s ea	49999-0227-00	192.67		
TERBINAFINE (Phys Total Care) REPACK				
terbinafine hydrochloride				
TAB, PO, 250 mg, 30s ea	54868-5794-00	30.48		
TERBINAFINE HCL (B&B Pharm, Inc) REPACK				
terbinafine hydrochloride				
POW, NA, 100 gm	63275-9950-05	2350.00		
500 gm	63275-9950-08	11000.00		
1000 gm	63275-9950-09	19000.00		
TERBINAFINE HYDROCHLORIDE FUL				
TAB, PO, 250 mg, 100s ea		70.50		
(Actavis)				
TAB, PO, 250 mg, 30s ea	00228-2101-03	391.82		AB
100s ea	00228-2101-11	1306.07		AB
(Apotex Corp.)				
TAB, PO, 250 mg, 30s ea	60505-2572-03	392.21		AB
100s ea	60505-2572-01	1307.04		AB
(Aurobindo Pharma)				
TAB, PO, 250 mg, 30s ea	65862-0079-30	383.54		AB
(Camber)				
TAB, PO, 250 mg, 30s ea	31722-0209-30	390.70		AB
100s ea	31722-0209-01	1307.50		AB
(Dr Reddy's)				
TAB, PO, 250 mg, 30s ea	55111-0250-30	391.82		AB
90s ea	55111-0250-90	1175.46		AB
(Glenmark Pharmaceuticals)				
TAB, PO, 250 mg, 30s ea	68462-0136-30	385.72		AB
100s ea	68462-0136-01	1285.40		AB
(Harris)				
TAB, PO, 250 mg, 30s ea	67405-0543-03	20.88		AB
100s ea	67405-0543-10	69.60		AB
(Medisca)				
POW, NA (1X25GM)				
25 gm	38779-1824-04	1050.00		
(1X100GM)				
100 gm	38779-1824-05	2475.00		
(1X1000GM)				
1000 gm	38779-1824-09	13500.00		
(Mylan)				
TAB, PO, 250 mg, 30s ea	00378-5710-93	391.75		AB
100s ea	00378-5710-01	1305.55		AB
(Northstar)				
TAB, PO, 250 mg, 30s ea	16714-0501-01	391.82		AB
100s ea	16714-0501-02	1306.56		AB
(Novartis Pharm) *See LAMISIL*				
(Roxane)				
TAB, PO, 250 mg, 30s ea	00054-0065-13	392.26		AB
100s ea	00054-0065-25	1307.19		AB
(Sandoz)				
TAB, PO, 250 mg, 30s ea	00781-5417-31	392.26		
100s ea	00781-5417-01	1307.52		
(Teva)				
TAB, PO, 250 mg, 30s ea	00093-7294-56	392.26		AB
30s ea	00555-0544-01	392.21		AB
100s ea	00093-7294-01	1307.52		AB
100s ea	00555-0544-02	1307.04		AB
(Wockhardt USA)				
TAB, PO, 250 mg, 30s ea	64679-0209-01	392.26		AB
30s ea	64679-0743-01	392.26		AB
100s ea	64679-0209-02	1307.19		AB
100s ea	64679-0743-03	1307.19		AB
(A-S Medication) REPACK				
TAB, PO, 250 mg, 30s ea	54569-5944-00	391.82		

PROD/MFR	NDC	AWP	DP	OBC
(Aidarex) REPACK				
TAB, PO, 250 mg, 7s ea	33261-0414-07	105.00		AB
14s ea	33261-0414-14	210.00		AB
21s ea	33261-0414-21	315.00		AB
28s ea	33261-0414-28	420.00		AB
30s ea	33261-0414-30	415.00		AB
40s ea	33261-0414-40	600.00		AB
60s ea	33261-0414-60	900.00		AB
90s ea	33261-0414-90	1350.00		AB
(DHS, Inc.) REPACK				
TAB, PO, 250 mg, 30s ea	55887-0115-30	380.00		
60s ea	55887-0115-60	759.99		
90s ea	55887-0115-90	1139.99		
(Palmetto) REPACK				
TAB, PO, 250 mg, 10s ea	23490-6961-01	203.09		
14s ea	23490-6961-00	284.32		
30s ea	23490-6961-03	609.26		
(PD-Rx Pharm) REPACK				
TAB, PO, 250 mg, 42s ea	55289-0054-42	31.67		AB
(Pharma Pac) REPACK				
TAB, PO, 250 mg, 21s ea	52959-0999-21	305.18		AB
30s ea	52959-0999-30	388.10		AB
(Phys Total Care) REPACK				
TAB, PO, 250 mg, 90s ea	54868-5794-01	75.08		AB
(Physician Partner) REPACK				
TAB, PO, 250 mg, 30s ea	21695-0630-30	235.09		AB
45s ea	21695-0630-45	352.64		AB
90s ea	21695-0630-90	705.27		AB
(Quality Care Prod) REPACK				
TAB, PO, 250 mg, 30s ea	35356-0243-30	36.80		AB
TERBUTALINE SULFATE (APP)				
SOL, SC (25X1ML)				
1 mg/ml, 1 ml 25s	63323-0665-01	562.25		AP
(Bedford)				
SOL, SC (SDV, USP, 10X1ML)				
1 mg/ml, 1 ml 10s	55390-0101-10	48.00		AP
(Bedford) *See TERBUTALINE SULFATE NOVAPLUS*				
(Gallipot)				
POW, NA (U.S.P., NF)				
10 gm	51552-0446-03	84.00		
(U.S.P.)				
25 gm	51552-0446-04	238.00		
(Global Pharm)				
TAB, PO, 2.5 mg, 100s ea	00115-2611-01	43.24		AB
5 mg, 100s ea	00115-2622-01	62.21		AB
(Hawkins)				
POW, NA (U.S.P.)				
5 gm	63370-0250-15	132.00		
10 gm	63370-0250-20	240.00		
25 gm	63370-0250-25	460.00		
100 gm	63370-0250-35	1620.00		
(Lannett)				
TAB, PO (U.S.P.)				
2.5 mg, 100s ea	00527-1318-01	43.24		AB
1000s ea	00527-1318-10	419.43		AB
5 mg, 100s ea	00527-1311-01	62.21		AB
1000s ea	00527-1311-10	603.44		AB
(Letco)				
POW, NA (U.S.P.)				
10 gm	62991-1152-01	150.00		
25 gm	62991-1152-02	270.00		
(Medisca)				
POW, NA (U.S.P.)				
5 gm	38779-0381-03	102.00		
10 gm	38779-0381-01	184.50		
25 gm	38779-0381-04	367.50		
100 gm	38779-0381-05	1300.50		
(PCCA)				
POW, NA (U.S.P.)				
1 gm	51927-2765-00	81.00		
(Spectrum Pharmacy)				
POW, NA (U.S.P.)				
1 gm	49452-7631-01	86.10		
5 gm	49452-7631-02	212.10		
25 gm	49452-7631-05	668.50		
(Teva)				
SOL, SC, 1 mg/ml,				
1 ml 25s	00703-1271-04	539.70		AP
(American Health) REPACK				
TAB, PO (3X10, USP)				
2.5 mg, 30s ea UD	68084-0256-21	21.48		AB
5 mg, 30s ea UD	68084-0257-21	26.61		AB
(PD-Rx Pharm) REPACK				
TAB, PO, 5 mg, 4s ea	43063-0059-04	15.48		AB
(USP)				
5 mg, 8s ea	43063-0059-08	12.32		AB
(Phys Total Care) REPACK				
TAB, PO, 2.5 mg, 15s ea	54868-4557-00	25.23		AB
(Physician Partner) REPACK				
TAB, PO, 2.5 mg, 30s ea	21695-0122-30	25.94		AB
(Quality Care Prod) REPACK				
TAB, PO, 2.5 mg, 30s ea	35356-0367-30	51.46		AB
TERBUTALINE SULFATE NOVAPLUS (Bedford)				
terbutaline sulfate				
SOL, SC (S.D.V.,PRIVATE LABEL)				
1 mg/ml, 1 ml 10s	55390-0193-10	42.00		AP
TERCONAZOLE FUL				
CRE, VG, 0.4%, 45 gm		43.43		
0.8%, 20 gm		39.74		
(Fougera)				
CRE, VG (W/APPLICATOR, 1X45GM)				
0.4%, 45 gm	00168-0346-46	43.07		
(W/APPLICATOR, 1X20GM)				
0.8%, 20 gm	00168-0347-20	47.08		
(Ortho-McNeil Pharm) *See TERAZOL 3*				
(Ortho-McNeil Pharm) *See TERAZOL 7*				
(Perrigo)				
SUP, VG (W/APPLICATOR)				
80 mg, 3s ea	45802-0717-08	48.94		AB
(PharmaDerm) *See ZAZOLE*				
(Taro)				
CRE, VG (W/APPLICATOR)				
0.4%, 45 gm	51672-1304-06	44.54		AB
(W/ 3 APPLICATORS)				
0.8%, 20 gm	51672-1302-00	40.75		
(Watson Labs)				
CRE, VG (MEASURED-DOSE APP)				
0.4%, 45 gm	00591-3196-89	40.93		
(3 DAY,W/APPLICATOR)				
0.8%, 20 gm	00591-3197-52	40.93		
(A-S Medication) REPACK				
CRE, VG, 0.4%, 45 gm	54569-5675-00	42.83		AB
(DHS, Inc.) REPACK				
CRE, VG, 0.8%, 20 gm	55887-0921-20	40.84		
(Dispensing Solutions) REPACK				
CRE, VG, 0.4%, 45 gm	55045-3612-01	44.00		
(Palmetto) REPACK				
CRE, VG, 0.4%, 45 gm	23490-6334-01	44.00		
0.8%, 20 gm	23490-6335-01	40.84		
(Pharma Pac) REPACK				
CRE, VG, 0.4%, 45 gm	52959-0811-03	43.25		
(Phys Total Care) REPACK				
CRE, VG, 0.8%, 20 gm	54868-5183-00	66.66		
(Physician Partner) REPACK				
CRE, VG (1X45GM)				
0.4%, 45 gm	21695-0844-45	81.86		
(Quality Care Prod) REPACK				
CRE, VG, 0.4%, 45 gm	49999-0762-45	80.17		
TERFENADINE (Medisca)				
POW, NA (U.S.P.)				
100 gm	38779-0703-05	190.50		
TERIPARATIDE				
(Lilly) *See FORTEO*				
TERPIN HYDRATE (Amend)				
POW, NA (U.S.P.)				
2270 gm	17317-0566-05	175.00		
(Gallipot)				
POW, NA (U.S.P.,N.F.)				
113.4 gm	51552-0319-04	19.39		
454 gm	51552-0319-06	41.30		
(PCCA)				
POW, NA (U.S.P.)				
1 gm	51927-1860-00	0.51		
(Spectrum Pharmacy)				
POW, NA (U.S.P.)				
100 gm	49452-7640-03	99.75		
500 gm	49452-7640-01	232.05		
TERRAMYCIN W/POLYMYXIN B SULFATE (Southwood) REPACK				
oxytetracycline hydrochloride/polymyxin b sulfate				
OIN, OP, 5 mg/gm-10000 u/gm,				
3.5 gm	58016-6452-03	12.38		
TERRELL (RxElite)				
isoflurane				
SOL, IH (USP)				
99.9%, 100 ml	66794-0011-10	15.00		AN
250 ml	66794-0011-25	30.00		AN
TERSI FOAM (Quinnova)				
selenium sulfide				
FOA, TP (1X70GM)				
2.25%, 70 gm	23710-0225-70	138.51		
TERT-BUTYL ALCOHOL (Baker, J.T.)				
butyl alcohol				
LIQ, NA (A.C.S., REAGENT)				
500 ml	10106-9056-01	41.51		
4000 ml	10106-9056-05	125.56		
20000 ml	10106-9056-07	276.92		
TERUMO (Terumo)				
needle and/or syringe supplies				
DEV, NA (ALLERGY,27G,1 ML.-DISP)				
100s ea.	08970-5010-21	18.25		
TERUMO HYPODERMIC SYRINGES (Terumo)				
syringe				
DEV, NA (20 ML, ECCENTRIC TIP)				
25s ea	08970-7530-01	12.25		
(20 ML, LUER SLIP TIP)				
25s ea	08970-7520-01	12.25		
(20 ML,LUER LOCK TIP)				
25s ea	08970-7510-01	12.25		
(30 ML,ECCENTRIC TIP)				
25s ea	08970-7630-01	14.25		
(30 ML,LUER LOCK TIP)				
25s ea	08970-7610-01	14.25		
(30 ML,LUER SLIP LOCK)				
25s ea	08970-7620-01	14.25		
(60 ML,ECCENTRIC TIP)				
25s ea	08970-7730-01	22.00		
(60 ML,LUER LOCK TIP)				
25s ea	08970-7710-01	22.00		
(60 ML,LUER SLIP TIP)				
25s ea	08970-7720-01	22.00		
(1 ML, 22GX1")				
100s ea	08970-7210-91	13.00		
(1 ML, 22GX3/4")				
100s ea	08970-7211-71	13.00		
(1 ML, TB W/O NDL)				
100s ea	08970-7120-01	12.00		
(1 ML, TB, 25GX5/8", LDS)				
100s ea	08970-7121-31	17.00		
(1 ML, TB, 26GX3/8" ,LDS)				
100s ea	08970-7121-51	17.00		
(1 ML, TB, 27GX1/2" ,LDS)				
100s ea	08970-7121-61	17.00		
(10 ML,20GX1-1/2")				
100s ea	08970-7410-61	27.00		
(10 ML,20GX1")				
100s ea	08970-7410-51	27.00		
(10 ML,21GX1-1/2")				
100s ea	08970-7410-81	27.00		
(10 ML,21GX1")				
100s ea	08970-7410-71	27.00		
(10 ML,22GX1-1/2")				
100s ea	08970-7411-01	27.00		
(10 ML,ECCENTRIC TIP)				
100s ea	08970-7430-01	18.00		
(10 ML,LUER LOCK TIP)				
100s ea	08970-7410-01	18.00		
(10 ML,LUER SLIP LOCK)				
100s ea	08970-7420-01	18.00		
(3 ML,20GX1-1/2")				
100s ea	08970-7210-61	13.00		

PROD/MFR	NDC	AWP	DP	OBC
(3 ML,20GX1")				
100s ea	08970-7210-51	13.00		
(3 ML,21GX1-1/2")				
100s ea	08970-7210-81	13.00		
(3 ML,21GX1")				
100s ea	08970-7210-71	13.00		
(3 ML,22GX1-1/2")				
100s ea	08970-7211-01	13.00		
(3 ML,23GX1-1/2")				
100s ea	08970-7211-21	13.00		
(3 ML,23GX1")				
100s ea	08970-7211-11	13.00		
(3 ML,25GX1")				
100s ea	08970-7211-41	13.00		
(3 ML,25GX5/8")				
100s ea	08970-7211-31	13.00		
(3 ML,LUER LOCK TIP)				
100s ea	08970-7210-01	8.70		
(3 ML,LUER SLIP TIP)				
100s ea	08970-7220-01	8.70		
(5 ML,20GX1-1/2")				
100s ea	08970-7310-61	25.00		
(5 ML,20GX1")				
100s ea	08970-7310-51	25.00		
(5 ML,21GX1-1/2")				
100s ea	08970-7310-81	25.00		
(5 ML,21GX1")				
100s ea	08970-7310-71	25.00		
(5 ML,22GX1-1/2")				
100s ea	08970-7311-01	25.00		
(5 ML,22GX1")				
100s ea	08970-7310-91	25.00		
(5 ML,LUER LOCK TIP)				
100s ea	08970-7310-01	16.00		
(5 ML,LUER SLIP TIP)				
100s ea	08970-7320-01	16.00		
TERUMO INSULIN (Terumo)				
insulin syringe/needle				
DEV, NA (27G,1 ML -DISP)				
100s ea	08970-2010-21	18.25		
(27G,1/2 ML -DISP)				
100s ea	08970-2005-21	18.25		
(28G X 1/2", 1 ML)				
100s ea	08970-2010-41	18.25		
(28G X 1/2", 1/2 ML)				
100s ea	08970-2005-41	18.25		
(29G, 1/4ML)				
100s ea	08970-2025-31	19.50		
(29G,1 ML)				
100s ea	08970-2010-31	19.50		
(29G,1/2 ML)				
100s ea	08970-2005-31	19.50		
TERUMO SURE DOSE (Terumo)				
insulin syringe/needle				
DEV, NA (U100, 28GX1/2CC)				
100s ea	08970-2105-41	18.25		
(U100, 28GX1/2X1CC)				
100s ea	08970-2110-41	18.25		
TERUMO SURE DOSE PLUS (Terumo)				
insulin syringe/needle				
DEV, NA (U100, 29G X 1/2, 1CC)				
100s ea	08970-2110-31	19.50		
(U100, 29GX1/2, 0.3 CC)				
100s ea	08970-2130-31	19.50		
(U100, 29GX1/2, 0.5CC)				
100s ea	08970-2105-31	19.50		
TESSALON PERLES (Forest Pharm)				
benzonatate				
SGL, PO, 100 mg, 100s ea	00456-0688-01	140.38		AA
500s ea	00456-0688-02	698.92		AA
200 mg, 100s ea	00456-0698-01	275.51		
(PD-Rx Pharm)				
REPACK				
SGL, PO, 100 mg, 12s ea	55289-0750-12	23.61		AA
21s ea	55289-0750-21	41.34		AA
30s ea	55289-0750-30	59.06		AA
(Phys Total Care)				
REPACK				
SGL, PO, 100 mg, 20s ea	54868-0714-01	30.59		AA
(Quality Care Prod)				
REPACK				
SGL, PO, 100 mg, 30s ea	35356-0344-30	82.52		AA
TESTIM (Auxilium Pharm, Inc)				
testosterone				
GEL, TP (GEL)				
1%,				
5 gm 30s UD, C-III	66887-0001-05	225.91		BX

PROD/MFR	NDC	AWP	DP	OBC
(A-S Medication)				
REPACK				
GEL, TP (GEL)				
1%,				
5 gm 30s UD, C-III	54569-5595-00	370.40		BX
(Phys Total Care)				
REPACK				
GEL, TP (GEL)				
1%,				
5 gm 30s UD, C-III	54868-4989-00	273.59		BX
(Stat Rx)				
REPACK				
GEL, TP (30X5GM,GEL)				
1%,				
5 gm 30s, C-III	16590-0853-30	330.79		BX
TESTOPEL PELLETS (Slate)				
testosterone				
IMP, SC, 75 mg,				
10s ea, C-III	43773-1001-02	750.00	600.00	EE
24s ea, C-III	43773-1001-04	1800.00		EE
100s ea, C-III	43773-1001-03	7500.00	6000.00	EE
TESTOSTERONE (Amend)				
POW, NA (U.S.P.,MICRONIZED)				
5 gm, C-III	17317-0567-08	14.55		
25 gm, C-III	17317-0567-02	58.80		
100 gm, C-III	17317-0567-03	196.00		
(Auxilium Pharm, Inc) *See TESTIM*				
(Columbia Labs) *See STRIANT*				
(Gallipot)				
POW, NA (U.S.P.)				
1 gm, C-III	51552-0029-01	10.50		
5 gm, C-III	51552-0029-02	17.50		
25 gm, C-III	51552-0029-04	61.60		
25 gm, C-III	51552-0564-04	61.60		
(U.S.P.,MICRONIZED)				
100 gm, C-III	51552-0564-05	203.00		
1000 gm, C-III	51552-0029-07	1813.00		
(U.S.P.)				
1000 gm, C-III	51552-0564-07	1610.00		
(Medisca)				
POW, NA (U.S.P.,MICRONIZED)				
5 gm, C-III	38779-0163-03	112.50		
25 gm, C-III	38779-0163-04	262.50		
100 gm, C-III	38779-0163-05	731.25		
500 gm, C-III	38779-0163-08	2493.75		
1000 gm, C-III	38779-0163-09	4256.25		
(Paddock)				
POW, NA (U.S.P.,MICRONIZED)				
5 gm, C-III	00574-0460-05	31.25		
25 gm, C-III	00574-0460-25	125.95		
(PCCA)				
POW, NA (USP;NONMICRONIZED;SOY)				
1 gm, C-III	51927-1026-00	9.00		
(Slate) *See TESTOPEL PELLETS*				
(Spectrum Pharmacy)				
POW, NA (U.S.P.,MICRONIZED)				
5 gm, C-III	49452-7652-01	117.25		
(U.S.P.)				
5 gm, C-III	49452-7650-01	88.55		
(U.S.P.,MICRONIZED)				
25 gm, C-III	49452-7652-02	402.50		
(U.S.P.)				
25 gm, C-III	49452-7650-02	273.35		
(U.S.P.,MICRONIZED)				
100 gm, C-III	49452-7652-03	1015.00		
(U.S.P.)				
100 gm, C-III	49452-7650-03	815.50		
(Truxton) *See TESTRO AQ*				
(Unimed Pharm) *See ANDROGEL*				
(Watson) *See ANDRODERM*				
TESTOSTERONE CYPIONATE (Gallipot)				
POW, NA (U.S.P.,N.F.)				
5 gm, C-III	51552-0104-02	21.00		
(Hawkins)				
POW, NA (U.S.P.)				
25 gm, C-III	63370-0980-25	350.40		
100 gm, C-III	63370-0980-35	916.80		
1000 gm, C-III	63370-0980-50	8208.00		
(Letco)				
POW, NA (U.S.P.)				
5 gm, C-III	62991-1707-01	45.00		
25 gm, C-III	62991-1707-02	156.00		
100 gm, C-III	62991-1707-03	510.00		
1000 gm, C-III	62991-1707-05	4200.00		

PROD/MFR	NDC	AWP	DP	OBC
(Medisca)				
POW, NA (U.S.P.)				
5 gm, C-III	38779-0164-03	160.50		
25 gm, C-III	38779-0164-04	393.75		
100 gm, C-III	38779-0164-05	1106.25		
500 gm, C-III	38779-0164-08	3900.00		
1000 gm, C-III	38779-0164-09	6600.00		
(Paddock)				
OIL, IM (1X1ML,USP)				
200 mg/ml,				
1 ml, C-III	00574-0820-01	23.18		AO
(1X10ML,USP)				
200 mg/ml,				
10 ml, C-III	00574-0820-10	101.39		AO
(PCCA)				
POW, NA (U.S.P.; CIII)				
1 gm, C-III	51927-2706-00	18.00		
(Pfizer) *See DEPO-TESTOSTERONE*				
(Sandoz)				
OIL, IM (USP,MDV)				
100 mg/ml,				
10 ml, C-III	00781-3073-70	59.14		AO
200 mg/ml,				
1 ml, C-III	00781-3074-71	23.18		AO
10 ml, C-III	00781-3074-70	112.86		AO
(Spectrum Pharmacy)				
POW, NA (U.S.P.)				
5 gm, C-III	49452-7660-01	125.65		
25 gm, C-III	49452-7660-02	455.00		
100 gm, C-III	49452-7660-03	959.00		
(Teva)				
OIL, IM (USP,MDV)				
200 mg/ml,				
1 ml, C-III	00703-6121-01	19.80		AO
10 ml, C-III	00703-6125-01	84.00		AO
(Watson Labs)				
OIL, IM (M.D.V.)				
200 mg/ml,				
10 ml, C-III	00591-3223-79	101.39		AO
(B&B Pharm, Inc)				
REPACK				
POW, NA (U.S.P.)				
25 gm, C-III	63275-9982-04	162.00		
100 gm, C-III	63275-9982-05	540.00		
1000 gm, C-III	63275-9982-09	4590.00		
(Palmetto)				
REPACK				
OIL, IM, 200 mg/ml,				
10 ml, C-III	23490-6343-01	112.22		
(Phys Total Care)				
REPACK				
OIL, IM, 200 mg/ml,				
1 ml, C-III	54868-3618-01	63.83		EE
(M.D.V.)				
200 mg/ml,				
10 ml, C-III	54868-3618-00	276.00		EE
TESTOSTERONE DECANOATE (Spectrum Pharmacy)				
POW, NA (1X5GM)				
5 gm	49452-7662-03	111.65		
(1X25GM)				
25 gm	49452-7662-04	327.25		
(1X100GM)				
100 gm	49452-7662-05	910.00		
TESTOSTERONE ENANTHATE				
(Endo Pharm) *See DELATESTRYL*				
(Hawkins)				
POW, NA (U.S.P.)				
5 gm, C-III	63370-0983-15	100.00		
25 gm, C-III	63370-0983-25	460.00		
100 gm, C-III	63370-0983-35	1760.00		
1000 gm, C-III	63370-0983-50	16000.00		
(Letco)				
POW, NA (USP, 1X1000GM)				
1000 gm, C-III	62991-2700-01	4590.00		
(Medisca)				
POW, NA, 5 gm, C-III	38779-0855-03	99.00		
25 gm, C-III	38779-0855-04	429.00		
100 gm, C-III	38779-0855-05	1653.00		
1000 gm, C-III	38779-0855-09	9825.00		
(Paddock)				
OIL, IM (USP,MULTIPLE DOSE)				
200 mg/ml,				
5 ml, C-III	00574-0821-05	84.95		AO
(Watson Labs)				
OIL, IM, 200 mg/ml,				
5 ml, C-III	00591-3221-26	84.95		AO

PROD/MFR | NDC | AWP | DP | OBC

TESTOSTERONE MICRONIZED (Hawkins)
testosterone, micronized
POW, NA (U.S.P.)
25 gm, C-III.........**63370-0970-25** 192.00
(USP,YAM)
25 gm, C-III.........**63370-0971-25** 136.00
(U.S.P.)
100 gm, C-III........**63370-0970-35** 672.00
(USP,YAM)
100 gm, C-III........**63370-0971-35** 456.00
(U.S.P.)
500 gm, C-III........**63370-0970-45** 2640.00
(USP,YAM)
500 gm, C-III........**63370-0971-45** 1680.00
(U.S.P.)
1000 gm, C-III.......**63370-0970-50** 4800.00
(USP,YAM)
1000 gm, C-III.......**63370-0971-50** 3048.00

(Letco)
POW, NA (U.S.P.)
5 gm, C-III..........**62991-2150-01** 34.50
25 gm, C-III.........**62991-2150-02** 96.00
100 gm, C-III........**62991-2150-03** 315.00
500 gm, C-III........**62991-2150-04** 1800.00

(PCCA)
POW, NA (U.S.P.; SOY; CIII)
1 gm, C-III..........**51927-1027-00** 24.00

(Spectrum Pharmacy)
POW, NA (1X100GM,U.S.P.)
.....................**49452-7657-03** 1015.00
(1X5GM,E.P.)
5 gm, C-III..........**49452-7656-01** 90.30
(1X5GM,U.S.P.)
5 gm, C-III..........**49452-7657-01** 117.25
(1X25GM,E.P.)
25 gm, C-III.........**49452-7656-02** 305.20
(1X25GM,U.S.P.)
25 gm, C-III.........**49452-7657-02** 402.50
(1X100GM,E.P.)
100 gm, C-III........**49452-7656-03** 843.50
(U.S.P.)
500 gm, C-III........**49452-7652-07** 2432.50
(1X1000GM,E.P.)
1000 gm, C-III.......**49452-7656-04** 3773.00
(1X1000GM,U.S.P.)
1000 gm, C-III.......**49452-7652-04** 4532.50
1000 gm, C-III.......**49452-7657-04** 4532.50

(B&B Pharm, Inc)
REPACK
POW, NA, 25 gm, C-III....**63275-9983-04** 450.00
100 gm, C-III........**63275-9983-05** 1800.00
500 gm, C-III........**63275-9983-08** 9000.00
1000 gm, C-III.......**63275-9983-09** 18000.00

TESTOSTERONE PHENYLPROPIONATE (Medisca)
POW, NA (1X100GM)
100 gm...............**38779-2396-05** 705.00
(1X500GM)
500 gm...............**38779-2396-08** 2865.00
(1X1000GM)
1000 gm..............**38779-2396-09** 4995.00

TESTOSTERONE PROPIONATE (Amend)
POW, NA (U.S.P.)
5 gm, C-III..........**17317-0568-08** 14.55
25 gm, C-III.........**17317-0568-02** 58.80
100 gm, C-III........**17317-0568-03** 196.00

(Cutispharma) *See FIRST-TESTOSTERONE*

(Cutispharma) *See FIRST-TESTOSTERONE MC*

(Gallipot)
POW, NA (U.S.P.,MICRONIZED)
0.3 gm, C-III........**51552-0030-08** 3.15
0.6 gm, C-III........**51552-0030-09** 3.99
(U.S.P.)
1 gm, C-III..........**51552-0030-01** 9.10
5 gm, C-III..........**51552-0030-02** 16.66
25 gm, C-III.........**51552-0030-04** 57.40
100 gm, C-III........**51552-0030-05** 203.00

(Hawkins)
POW, NA (U.S.P.)
25 gm, C-III.........**63370-0985-25** 184.00
100 gm, C-III........**63370-0985-35** 652.00
500 gm, C-III........**63370-0985-45** 3152.00
1000 gm, C-III.......**63370-0985-50** 6100.00

(Medisca)
POW, NA (USP,MICRONIZED)
5 gm, C-III..........**38779-0165-03** 206.25
25 gm, C-III.........**38779-0165-04** 487.50
(U.S.P.,MICRONIZED)
100 gm, C-III........**38779-0165-05** 1556.25
500 gm, C-III........**38779-0165-08** 2756.25

(Paddock)
POW, NA, 5 gm, C-III......**00574-0461-05** 31.25
25 gm, C-III.........**00574-0461-25** 125.95

(Spectrum Pharmacy)
POW, NA (U.S.P.,MICRONIZED)
5 gm, C-III..........**49452-0011-01** 126.88
25 gm, C-III.........**49452-0011-02** 330.75
100 gm, C-III........**49452-0011-03** 1032.50

(Truxton)
OIL, IM (VIAL)
100 mg/ml,
10 ml, C-III.........**00463-1073-10** 8.40

TESTOSTERONE PROPIONATE MICRONIZED (Letco)
testosterone propionate, micronized
POW, NA (U.S.P.)
5 gm, C-III..........**62991-1412-01** 33.00
25 gm, C-III.........**62991-1412-02** 120.00
100 gm, C-III........**62991-1412-03** 375.00

(PCCA)
POW, NA (U.S.P., MICRONIZED)
1 gm, C-III..........**51927-1029-00** 11.40

TESTOSTERONE PROPIONATE, MICRONIZED
(Letco) *See TESTOSTERONE PROPIONATE MICRONIZED*

(PCCA) *See TESTOSTERONE PROPIONATE MICRONIZED*

TESTOSTERONE, MICRONIZED
(Hawkins) *See TESTOSTERONE MICRONIZED*

(Letco) *See TESTOSTERONE MICRONIZED*

(PCCA) *See TESTOSTERONE MICRONIZED*

(Spectrum Pharmacy) *See TESTOSTERONE MICRONIZED*

TESTRED (Valeant Pharm Intl)
methyltestosterone
CAP, PO, 10 mg,
100s ea, C-III.......**00187-0901-01** 1668.33 BP

(Southwood)
REPACK
CAP, PO, 10 mg,
30s ea, C-III........**58016-0967-30** 90.94 BP
60s ea, C-III........**58016-0967-60** 181.88 BP
90s ea, C-III........**58016-0967-90** 272.82 BP
100s ea, C-III.......**58016-0967-00** 303.13 BP

TESTRO AQ (Truxton)
testosterone
SUS, IM (VIAL)
100 mg/ml,
10 ml, C-III.........**00463-1069-10** 8.40

TETANUS AND DIPHTHERIA TOXOIDS ADSORBED (Akorn)
diphtheria toxoid, adsorbed/tetanus toxoid
SUS, IM (10X0.5ML,ADULT,SDV,PF)
0.5 ml 10s...........**17478-0131-01** 235.50

(Physician Partner)
REPACK
SUS, IM (1X0.5ML,PF,LATEX-FREE)
0.5 ml...............**21695-0413-01** 44.10

TETANUS IMMUNE GLOBULIN
(Talecris) *See HYPERTET S/D*

TETANUS TOXOID
(Sanofi) *See TETANUS TOXOID ADSORBED*

(Quality Care Prod)
REPACK
SOL, IJ (1X7.5ML)
4 lf u/0.5 ml,
7.5 ml...............**35356-0182-75** 416.00

TETANUS TOXOID AD (Phys Total Care)
REPACK
tetanus toxoid
SUS, IM (S.D.V.)
5 lf u/0.5 ml,
5 ml.................**54868-3597-00** 271.95

TETANUS TOXOID ADSORBED (Sanofi)
tetanus toxoid
SUS, IM (TAX INCL, 10EA)
5 lf u/0.5 ml,
0.5 ml 10s...........**49281-0820-10** 322.99

TETCAINE HCL (Ocusoft)
tetracaine hydrochloride
SOL, OP, 0.5%, 15 ml.....**54799-0502-15** 9.37

TETRA-MAG (Stat Rx)
REPACK
magnesium salicylate/phenyltoloxamine citrate
TAB, PO, 600 mg-25 mg,
28s ea...............**16590-0219-28** 12.75

TETRABENAZINE
(Lundbeck) *See XENAZINE*

TETRACAINE (Akorn)
tetracaine hydrochloride
SOL, IJ (PF)
1%, 2 ml 25s.........**11098-0045-32** 131.63

TETRACAINE (Gallipot)
POW, NA (U.S.P.)
5 gm.................**51552-0323-02** 16.10
25 gm................**51552-0323-04** 49.00
100 gm...............**51552-0323-05** 168.00

(Hawkins)
POW, NA (U.S.P.,BASE)
5 gm.................**63370-0255-15** 52.80
25 gm................**63370-0255-25** 144.00
100 gm...............**63370-0255-35** 518.40
1000 gm..............**63370-0255-50** 3720.00

(Letco)
POW, NA (U.S.P.,BASE)
25 gm................**62991-1708-02** 90.00
100 gm...............**62991-1708-03** 300.00

(Medisca)
POW, NA (U.S.P.)
5 gm.................**38779-0374-03** 40.50
25 gm................**38779-0374-04** 117.00
100 gm...............**38779-0374-05** 417.00
1000 gm..............**38779-0374-09** 2355.00

(PCCA)
POW, NA (U.S.P. (FREE BASE))
1 gm.................**51927-2652-00** 13.20

(Spectrum Pharmacy)
POW, NA (U.S.P.)
5 gm.................**49452-7675-01** 74.20
25 gm................**49452-7675-02** 190.75
100 gm...............**49452-7675-03** 654.50

(Stat Rx)
REPACK
tetracaine hydrochloride
SOL, OP, 0.5%, 15 ml.....**16590-0215-15** 30.00

TETRACAINE HCL (Alcon Surgical)
tetracaine hydrochloride
SOL, OP, 0.5%, 2 ml 12s..**00065-0741-12** 87.41

(Altaire)
SOL, OP (STERILE)
0.5%, 0.7 ml 12s.....**59390-0181-07** 28.00

(Bausch & Lomb Inc.)
SOL, OP, 0.5%, 15 ml.....**24208-0920-64** 8.11

(A-S Medication)
REPACK
SOL, OP, 0.5%, 15 ml.....**54569-4362-00** 7.38

(Altura)
REPACK
SOL, OP, 0.5%, 15 ml.....**63874-0909-15** 27.02

(DHS, Inc.)
REPACK
SOL, OP, 0.5%, 15 ml.....**55887-0743-15** 21.80

(Nucare Pharm)
REPACK
SOL, OP, 0.5%, 15 ml.....**66267-0924-15** 20.58

(Phys Total Care)
REPACK
SOL, OP, 0.5%, 15 ml.....**54868-0901-00** 19.65

(Quality Care Prod)
REPACK
SOL, OP, 0.5%, 15 ml.....**49999-0268-15** 32.42

(Southwood)
REPACK
SOL, OP, 0.5%, 15 ml.....**58016-6098-01** 23.11

TETRACAINE HYDROCHLORIDE
(Akorn) *See TETRACAINE*

(Alcon Surgical) *See TETRACAINE HCL*

(Altaire) *See ALTACAINE*

(Altaire) *See TETRACAINE HCL*

(Amend)
POW, NA (U.S.P.)
125 gm...............**17317-0570-04** 56.00
1000 gm..............**17317-0570-06** 350.00

(Bausch & Lomb Inc.) *See TETRACAINE HCL*

(Gallipot)
POW, NA (U.S.P.,N.F.)
25 gm................**51552-0269-04** 22.68

PROD/MFR	NDC	AWP	DP	OBC
(U.S.P.)				
100 gm	51552-0269-05	63.00		
(Hawkins)				
POW, NA, 0.5 gm	63370-0256-09	24.00		
25 gm	63370-0256-25	66.00		
100 gm	63370-0256-35	232.00		
(Hospira) *See PONTOCAINE HCL*				
(Hospira) *See PONTOCAINE HYDROCHLORIDE*				
(Letco)				
POW, NA (U.S.P.)				
25 gm	62991-2067-01	54.00		
100 gm	62991-2067-02	165.00		
(Medisca)				
POW, NA (USP)				
25 gm	38779-0566-04	50.55		
100 gm	38779-0566-05	168.45		
1000 gm	38779-0566-09	1259.25		
(Ocusoft) *See TETCAINE HCL*				
(Ocusoft) *See TETRAVISC*				
(Ocusoft) *See TETRAVISC FORTE*				
(PCCA)				
POW, NA (U.S.P.)				
1 gm	51927-1241-00	4.08		
(Spectrum Pharmacy)				
POW, NA (U.S.P.)				
25 gm	49452-7680-01	84.00		
100 gm	49452-7680-02	254.80		
1000 gm	49452-7680-03	1603.00		
(Physician Partner)				
REPACK				
SOL, OP (1X15ML)				
0.5%, 15 ml	21695-0682-15	19.10		
TETRACHLOROETHYLENE (Baker, J.T.)				
LIQ, NA, 150 ml	10106-9465-04	30.49		
500 ml	10106-9465-01	45.37		
4000 ml	10106-9465-03	184.32		
20000 ml	10106-9465-07	442.95		
TETRACON (Consolidated Midland)				
tetracycline hydrochloride				
CAP, PO, 250 mg, 100s ea	00223-1655-01	7.50		EE
1000s ea	00223-1655-02	57.50		EE
500 mg, 100s ea	00223-1656-01	12.50		EE
1000s ea	00223-1656-02	112.50		EE
TETRACYCLINE (PCCA)				
POW, NA (U.S.P.)				
1 gm	51927-2449-00	6.00		
(DHS, Inc.)				
REPACK				
tetracycline hydrochloride				
CAP, PO, 250 mg, 21s ea	55887-0889-21	7.50		
(Physician Partner)				
REPACK				
CAP, PO, 250 mg, 28s ea	21695-0302-28	23.80		
(Stat Rx)				
REPACK				
CAP, PO, 250 mg, 30s ea	16590-0216-30	8.50		
500 mg, 30s ea	16590-0217-30	11.00		
60s ea	16590-0217-60	22.00		
TETRACYCLINE HCL (Gallipot)				
tetracycline hydrochloride				
POW, NA, 25 gm	51552-0463-04	23.80		
100 gm	51552-0463-05	56.00		
100 gm	51552-1067-05	133.00	95.00	
(Medisca)				
POW, NA (USP)				
25 gm	38779-0053-04	52.50		
100 gm	38779-0053-05	172.50		
500 gm	38779-0053-08	777.00		
1000 gm	38779-0053-09	1305.00		
(PCCA)				
POW, NA (U.S.P.)				
1 gm	51927-1945-00	2.28		
(Spectrum Pharmacy)				
POW, NA (U.S.P.)				
25 gm	49452-7701-01	83.30		
100 gm	49452-7701-02	258.30		
500 gm	49452-7701-03	1081.50		
(A-S Medication)				
REPACK				
CAP, PO, 250 mg, 20s ea	54569-2279-01	1.37		EE
28s ea	54569-2279-00	1.92		EE
30s ea	54569-2279-08	2.05		EE
40s ea	54569-2279-02	2.74		EE
100s ea	54569-2279-06	6.84		EE

PROD/MFR	NDC	AWP	DP	OBC
500 mg, 20s ea	54569-2501-04	2.36		EE
28s ea	54569-2501-00	3.30		EE
40s ea	54569-2501-02	4.72		EE
60s ea	54569-2501-08	7.08		EE
100s ea	54569-2501-03	11.80		EE
(Altura)				
REPACK				
CAP, PO, 250 mg, 8s ea	63874-0125-80	1.31		AB
10s ea	63874-0125-10	1.58		AB
14s ea	63874-0125-14	1.84		AB
15s ea	63874-0125-15	2.10		AB
20s ea	63874-0125-20	5.39		AB
21s ea	63874-0125-21	5.66		AB
24s ea	63874-0125-24	6.47		AB
28s ea	63874-0125-28	7.54		AB
30s ea	63874-0125-30	8.09		AB
40s ea	63874-0125-40	10.78		AB
60s ea	63874-0125-60	16.17		AB
100s ea	63874-0125-01	26.95		AB
1000s ea	63874-0125-02	269.50		AB
500 mg, 10s ea	63874-0124-10	1.14		AB
12s ea	63874-0124-12	1.38		AB
14s ea	63874-0124-14	1.61		AB
15s ea	63874-0124-15	1.72		AB
20s ea	63874-0124-20	7.74		AB
21s ea	63874-0124-21	8.12		AB
24s ea	63874-0124-24	9.29		AB
28s ea	63874-0124-28	10.84		AB
30s ea	63874-0124-30	11.61		AB
40s ea	63874-0124-40	15.48		AB
50s ea	63874-0124-50	19.35		AB
56s ea	63874-0124-56	21.67		AB
60s ea	63874-0124-60	23.22		AB
100s ea	63874-0124-01	38.70		AB
1000s ea	63874-0124-02	387.00		AB
(DHS, Inc.)				
REPACK				
CAP, PO, 250 mg, 28s ea	55887-0889-28	8.95		AB
(Dispensing Solutions)				
REPACK				
CAP, PO, 250 mg, 6s ea	66336-0609-06	7.03		AB
12s ea	55045-1206-04	3.00		AB
12s ea	66336-0609-12	7.55		AB
20s ea	55045-1206-07	5.00		AB
28s ea	55045-1206-08	7.00		AB
28s ea	66336-0609-28	8.98		AB
30s ea	55045-1206-09	7.50		AB
40s ea	55045-1206-03	10.00		AB
100s ea	55045-1206-01	25.00		AB
500 mg, 12s ea	55045-1322-04	6.00		AB
14s ea	55045-1322-07	7.00		AB
15s ea	55045-3414-05	7.50		AB
20s ea	55045-1322-02	10.00		AB
28s ea	55045-1322-09	14.00		AB
28s ea	66336-0435-28	12.52		AB
30s ea	55045-1322-08	15.00		AB
40s ea	55045-1322-03	20.00		AB
40s ea	66336-0435-40	17.88		AB
60s ea	55045-1322-05	30.00		AB
90s ea	55045-1322-06	45.00		AB
100s ea	55045-1322-01	50.00		AB
120s ea	55045-1322-00	60.00		AB
(GSMS)				
REPACK				
CAP, PO (UNIT OF USE)				
250 mg, 40s ea	60429-0208-40	9.96	3.32	AB
500 mg, 40s ea	60429-0209-40	13.77	4.59	AB
(Nucare Pharm)				
REPACK				
CAP, PO, 250 mg, 12s ea	66267-0200-12	4.35		EE
28s ea	66267-0200-28	6.82		EE
40s ea	66267-0200-40	10.99		EE
500 mg, 14s ea	66267-0201-14	5.89		EE
20s ea	66267-0201-20	7.71		EE
28s ea	66267-0201-28	8.91		EE
40s ea	66267-0201-40	11.24		EE
(PD-Rx Pharm)				
REPACK				
CAP, PO, 250 mg, 10s ea	55289-0256-10	24.00		AB
12s ea	55289-0256-12	26.27		AB
20s ea	55289-0256-20	28.00		AB
28s ea	55289-0256-28	31.20		AB
40s ea	55289-0256-40	36.00		AB
60s ea	55289-0256-60	44.00		AB
90s ea	55289-0256-90	56.00		AB
100s ea	55289-0256-01	53.47		AB
500 mg, 10s ea	55289-0446-10	26.27		AB
12s ea	55289-0446-12	29.00		AB
16s ea	55289-0446-16	30.00		AB
20s ea	55289-0446-20	32.47		AB
28s ea	55289-0446-28	37.47		AB

PROD/MFR	NDC	AWP	DP	OBC
30s ea	55289-0446-30	38.73		AB
40s ea	55289-0446-40	45.00		AB
(USP)				
500 mg, 56s ea	55289-0446-56	50.70		AB
60s ea	55289-0446-60	57.40		AB
100s ea	55289-0446-01	82.33		AB
(Pharma Pac)				
REPACK				
CAP, PO, 250 mg, 12s ea	52959-0283-12	5.95		EE
20s ea	52959-0283-20	8.25		EE
28s ea	52959-0283-28	9.01		EE
30s ea	52959-0283-30	9.21		EE
40s ea	52959-0283-40	11.06		EE
100s ea	52959-0283-00	18.96		EE
500 mg, 14s ea	52959-0336-14	5.80		EE
20s ea	52959-0336-20	7.71		EE
28s ea	52959-0336-28	9.24		EE
30s ea	52959-0336-30	9.50		EE
40s ea	52959-0336-40	11.48		EE
56s ea	52959-0336-56	14.15		EE
90s ea	52959-0336-90	21.52		EE
(Phys Total Care)				
REPACK				
CAP, PO, 250 mg, 20s ea	54868-0024-07	7.44		EE
30s ea	54868-0024-03	8.94		EE
40s ea	54868-0024-01	10.41		EE
60s ea	54868-0024-04	13.35		EE
90s ea	54868-0024-08	17.79		EE
100s ea	54868-0024-05	19.26		EE
500 mg, 30s ea	54868-0025-01	16.08		EE
40s ea	54868-0025-03	19.92		EE
60s ea	54868-0025-04	27.66		EE
90s ea	54868-0025-07	39.24		EE
100s ea	54868-0025-05	43.08		EE
500s ea	54868-0025-08	115.68		EE
1000s ea	54868-0025-00	141.97		EE
(Quality Care Prod)				
REPACK				
CAP, PO, 250 mg, 28s ea	49999-0541-28	3.40		
(Southwood)				
REPACK				
CAP, PO, 250 mg, 8s ea	58016-0101-08	1.25		EE
10s ea	58016-0101-10	1.50		EE
12s ea	58016-0101-12	1.60		EE
14s ea	58016-0101-14	1.41		EE
15s ea	58016-0101-15	2.00		EE
20s ea	58016-0101-20	2.02		EE
21s ea	58016-0101-21	2.25		EE
24s ea	58016-0101-24	2.50		EE
28s ea	58016-0101-28	2.83		EE
30s ea	58016-0101-30	3.03		EE
40s ea	58016-0101-40	4.04		EE
50s ea	58016-0101-50	6.59		EE
60s ea	58016-0101-60	6.12		EE
90s ea	58016-0101-90	9.17		EE
100s ea	58016-0101-00	10.10		EE
500 mg, 10s ea	58016-0102-10	1.09		EE
12s ea	58016-0102-12	1.31		EE
14s ea	58016-0102-14	1.53		EE
15s ea	58016-0102-15	1.64		EE
20s ea	58016-0102-20	1.96		EE
21s ea	58016-0102-21	2.29		EE
24s ea	58016-0102-24	2.62		EE
28s ea	58016-0102-28	3.05		EE
30s ea	58016-0102-30	2.94		EE
40s ea	58016-0102-40	4.36		EE
50s ea	58016-0102-50	5.46		EE
60s ea	58016-0102-60	5.87		EE
100s ea	58016-0102-00	9.79		EE
TETRACYCLINE HYDROCHLORIDE				
FUL				
CAP, PO, 500 mg, 100s ea		9.75		
(Consolidated Midland) *See TETRACON*				
(Gallipot) *See TETRACYCLINE HCL*				
(Medisca) *See TETRACYCLINE HCL*				
(PCCA) *See TETRACYCLINE HCL*				
(Spectrum Pharmacy) *See TETRACYCLINE HCL*				
(Teva)				
CAP, PO, 250 mg, 100s ea	00172-2416-60	6.80		AB
(USP, 10X10)				
250 mg, 100s ea UD	00172-2416-10	8.24		AB
1000s ea	00172-2416-80	55.50		AB
500 mg, 100s ea	00172-2407-60	11.80		AB
(USP)				
500 mg, 100s ea UD	00172-2407-10	19.02		AB
1000s ea	00172-2407-80	89.30		AB

PROD/MFR	NDC	AWP	DP	OBC
(Watson Labs)				
CAP, PO (USP)				
250 mg, 100s ea	**00591-2234-01**	5.45		**AB**
1000s ea	**00591-2234-10**	38.10		**AB**
500 mg, 100s ea	**00591-2235-01**	7.80		**AB**
1000s ea	**00591-2235-10**	74.68		**AB**
(Wesley) *See WESMYCIN*				
(Aidarex)				
REPACK				
CAP, PO, 500 mg, 7s ea	**33261-0395-07**	3.71		**AB**
14s ea	**33261-0395-14**	7.42		**AB**
20s ea	**33261-0395-20**	10.60		**AB**
21s ea	**33261-0395-21**	11.13		**AB**
28s ea	**33261-0395-28**	14.84		**AB**
30s ea	**33261-0395-30**	15.90		**AB**
40s ea	**33261-0395-40**	21.20		**AB**
60s ea	**33261-0395-60**	31.80		**AB**
(Altura)				
REPACK				
CAP, PO, 250 mg, 8s ea	**63874-0125-08**	2.16		**AB**
70s ea	**63874-0125-70**	18.87		**AB**
(Bryant Ranch)				
REPACK				
CAP, PO, 250 mg, 20s ea	**63629-1501-01**	14.00		
30s ea	**63629-1501-04**	11.09		
40s ea	**63629-1501-02**	28.00		
60s ea	**63629-1501-03**	42.00		
500 mg, 30s ea	**63629-1502-03**	10.99		
40s ea	**63629-1502-02**	5.00		
56s ea	**63629-1502-04**	7.00		
60s ea	**63629-1502-01**	9.99		
(Core)				
REPACK				
CAP, PO, 250 mg, 20s ea	**33358-0334-20**	14.35		
40s ea	**33358-0334-40**	28.70		
60s ea	**33358-0334-60**	43.05		
500 mg, 40s ea	**33358-0335-40**	5.13		
56s ea	**33358-0335-56**	7.18		
(DHS, Inc.)				
REPACK				
CAP, PO, 250 mg, 40s ea	**55887-0889-40**	12.50		**AB**
(Dispensing Solutions)				
REPACK				
CAP, PO, 250 mg, 40s ea	**66336-0609-40**	10.99		**AB**
(HomeMed)				
REPACK				
CAP, PO, 250 mg, 12s ea	**51655-0097-27**	20.03		**EE**
28s ea	**51655-0097-29**	2.23		**EE**
40s ea	**51655-0097-51**	12.99		**EE**
500 mg, 28s ea	**51655-0194-29**	10.99		**EE**
(Palmetto)				
REPACK				
CAP, PO, 250 mg, 6s ea	**23490-6352-01**	2.44		
7s ea	**23490-6352-00**	2.01		
12s ea	**23490-6352-02**	3.44		
14s ea	**23490-6352-07**	4.01		
21s ea	**23490-6352-08**	6.02		
28s ea	**23490-6352-03**	8.03		
30s ea	**23490-6352-04**	8.60		
40s ea	**23490-6352-05**	11.47		
100s ea	**23490-6352-06**	28.67		
500 mg, 7s ea	**23490-6353-04**	3.50		
14s ea	**23490-6353-05**	7.00		
21s ea	**23490-6353-07**	10.50		
28s ea	**23490-6353-01**	14.00		
30s ea	**23490-6353-03**	15.00		
40s ea	**23490-6353-02**	20.00		
(Physician Partner)				
REPACK				
CAP, PO, 500 mg, 28s ea	**21695-0640-28**	27.77		
40s ea	**21695-0640-40**	39.67		**AB**
56s ea	**21695-0640-56**	55.54		**AB**
(Quality Care Prod)				
REPACK				
CAP, PO, 250 mg, 100s ea	**49999-0541-00**	12.12		**AB**
500 mg, 14s ea	**49999-0224-14**	5.01		**AB**
30s ea	**49999-0224-30**	10.73		**AB**
40s ea	**49999-0224-40**	8.64		**AB**
100s ea	**49999-0224-00**	21.60		
(Southwood)				
REPACK				
CAP, PO, 500 mg, 90s ea	**58016-0102-90**	8.81		**AB**
TETRAHYDROFURAN (Baker, J.T.)				
LIQ, NA (A.C.S., REAGENT)				
500 ml	**10106-9450-01**	61.13		
4000 ml	**10106-9450-03**	234.22		
4000 ml	**10106-9450-05**	243.60		
(Baker, J.T.) *See TETRAHYDROFURAN LOW WATER*				
(Baker, J.T.) *See TETRAHYDROFURAN STABILIZED*				
TETRAHYDROFURAN LOW WATER (Baker, J.T.)				
tetrahydrofuran				
LIQ, NA (HPLC)				
4000 ml	**10106-9439-03**	173.35		
TETRAHYDROFURAN STABILIZED (Baker, J.T.)				
tetrahydrofuran				
LIQ, NA (HPLC)				
4000 ml	**10106-9440-03**	144.41		
TETRAHYDROZOLINE HCL (PCCA)				
tetrahydrozoline hydrochloride				
POW, NA, 1 gm	**51927-1796-00**	93.00		
(Spectrum Pharmacy)				
POW, NA (U.S.P.)				
1 gm	**49452-7705-01**	185.15		
5 gm	**49452-7705-02**	518.00		
TETRAHYDROZOLINE HYDROCHLORIDE				
(Kenwood) *See TYZINE*				
(Kenwood) *See TYZINE PEDIATRIC*				
(PCCA) *See TETRAHYDROZOLINE HCL*				
(Spectrum Pharmacy) *See TETRAHYDROZOLINE HCL*				
TETRAVISC (Ocusoft)				
tetracaine hydrochloride				
SOL, OP (12X0.6ML SD)				
0.5%, 0.6 ml 12s	**54799-0505-01**	97.20		
(SINGLE DROP)				
0.5%, 5 ml	**54799-0505-05**	26.18		
TETRAVISC FORTE (Ocusoft)				
tetracaine hydrochloride				
SOL, OP (1X5ML)				
0.5%, 5 ml	**54799-0504-05**	26.20		
TETRIX CREAM (Valeant Pharm Intl)				
cream, multi ingredient				
CRE, TP (4X56.7GM)				
226.8 gm	**08569-0000-03**	82.50		
TEV-TROPIN (Gate)				
somatropin, e-coli derived				
PDS, SC (VIAL W/DILUENT)				
5 mg, ea	**57844-0713-19**	249.47		**BX**
TEVETEN (Abbott Pharm)				
eprosartan mesylate				
TAB, PO (AQUEOUS FILM-COATED)				
400 mg, 100s ea	**00074-3025-11**	282.17	247.52	
(CAPLET)				
600 mg, 100s ea	**00074-3040-11**	330.25	289.69	
(Phys Total Care)				
REPACK				
TAB, PO, 600 mg, 10s ea	**54868-5466-01**	25.00		
10s ea	**57868-5466-01**	24.08		
30s ea	**54868-5466-00**	71.26		
TEVETEN HCT (Abbott Pharm)				
eprosartan mesylate/hydrochlorothiazide				
TAB, PO (FILM-COATED)				
600 mg-12.5 mg,				
100s ea	**00074-3015-11**	350.24	307.23	**EE**
600 mg-25 mg,				
100s ea	**00074-3020-11**	350.24	307.23	
(Phys Total Care)				
REPACK				
TAB, PO (FILM-COATED)				
600 mg-12.5 mg,				
10s ea	**54868-5281-00**	36.62		
30s ea	**54868-5281-01**	106.11		
(FILM-COATED TABLET)				
600 mg-25 mg,				
10s ea	**54868-0009-01**	40.67		
30s ea	**54868-0009-00**	118.08		
TEXACORT (JSJ Pharma)				
hydrocortisone				
SOL, TP (W/ APPLICATOR TIP)				
2.5%, 30 ml	**68712-0011-01**	54.00		
THALIDOMIDE				
(Celgene Corp) *See THALOMID*				
THALITONE (Monarch)				
chlorthalidone				
TAB, PO, 15 mg, 100s ea	**61570-0024-01**	152.26		
THALLOUS CHLORIDE TL 201 (GE)				
SOL, IJ (VIAL)				
1 mci/ml, 6.6 ml	**17156-0299-16**	1091.81		**AP**
8.8 ml	**17156-0299-18**	1374.38		**AP**
(Lantheus) *See THALLOUS CHLORIDE TL-201*				
(Mallinckrodt Inc.)				
SOL, IJ (VIAL)				
1 mci/ml, 1 ml	**00019-N120-00**	36.00	30.00	**AP**
THALLOUS CHLORIDE TL-201 (Lantheus)				
thallous chloride tl 201				
SOL, IJ, 1 mci/0.5 ml,				
0.5 ml	**11994-0427-01**	34.98		
THALOMID (Celgene Corp)				
thalidomide				
CAP, PO (BLISTER PACK)				
50 mg, 28s ea UD	**59572-0205-14**	4204.30		
(10X28, BLISTER PACK)				
50 mg, 280s ea	**59572-0205-94**	42042.85		
100 mg, 28s ea UD	**59572-0210-15**	6824.56		
140s ea	**59572-0210-95**	34122.82		
150 mg, 28s ea	**59572-0215-13**	7297.13		**EE**
(4X28)				
150 mg, 112s ea	**59572-0215-93**	29188.50		**EE**
200 mg, 28s ea UD	**59572-0220-16**	7769.98		
84s ea	**59572-0220-96**	23309.93		
THAM (Hospira)				
tromethamine				
SOL, IV, 3.6 gm/100 ml,				
500 ml 6s	**00409-1593-04**	1442.95	1262.58	
THE BODY GUARDS PACK WITH E-Z SPACER (FSC Laboratories)				
spacer, inhalation				
DEV, NA, ea	**59196-0111-01**	42.00		
THEO-24 (UCB)				
theophylline				
C24, PO, 100 mg, 100s ea	**50474-0100-01**	76.36		**BC**
200 mg, 100s ea	**50474-0200-01**	113.77		**BC**
500s ea	**50474-0200-50**	512.03		**BC**
300 mg, 100s ea	**50474-0300-01**	140.35		**BC**
100s ea	**50474-0400-01**	196.54		**BC**
500s ea	**50474-0300-50**	631.63		**BC**
(Phys Total Care)				
REPACK				
C24, PO, 300 mg, 10s ea	**54868-2710-00**	12.08		**BC**
30s ea	**54868-2710-01**	32.48		**BC**
THEO-DUR (PD-Rx Pharm)				
REPACK				
theophylline				
T12, PO, 200 mg, 60s ea	**55289-0003-60**	19.52		**AB**
THEOBROMINE (PCCA)				
POW, NA, 1 gm	**51927-2632-00**	10.20		
THEOCHRON (Forest Pharm)				
theophylline				
T12, PO, 100 mg, 100s ea	**00456-4310-01**	23.05		**AB**
200 mg, 100s ea	**00456-4320-01**	36.94		**AB**
300 mg, 100s ea	**00456-4330-01**	60.48		**AB**
THEOCON (Consolidated Midland)				
guaifenesin/theophylline				
ELI, PO				
90 mg/15 ml-150 mg/15 ml,				
480 ml	**00223-6622-01**	5.50		
THEOPHYLLINE				
FUL				
TER, PO, 200 mg, 100s ea		21.60		
(Amend) *See THEOPHYLLINE ANHYDROUS*				
(Caraco)				
T12, PO, 100 mg, 100s ea	**00258-3584-01**	25.60		**AB**
500s ea	**00258-3584-05**	120.66		**AB**
200 mg, 100s ea	**00258-3583-01**	41.04		**AB**
500s ea	**00258-3583-05**	193.56		**AB**
1000s ea	**00258-3583-10**	365.50		**AB**
300 mg, 100s ea	**00258-3581-01**	48.73		**AB**
500s ea	**00258-3581-05**	229.89		**AB**
1000s ea	**00258-3581-10**	444.83		**AB**
(Consolidated Midland)				
ELI, PO, 80 mg/15 ml,				
480 ml	**00223-6308-01**	3.95		**EE**
THEOPHYLLINE (Consolidated Midland)				
3840 ml	**00223-6308-02**	19.50		**EE**
THEOPHYLLINE				
(Consolidated Midland) *See THEOPHYLLINE*				
(Forest Pharm) *See ELIXOPHYLLIN*				
(Forest Pharm) *See THEOCHRON*				
(Gallipot) *See THEOPHYLLINE ANHYDROUS*				
(Major)				
T12, PO, 100 mg,				
100s ea UD	**00904-5887-61**	23.02		**AB**
200 mg, 100s ea UD	**00904-5888-61**	36.50		**AB**
300 mg, 100s ea UD	**00904-5889-61**	31.10		**AB**

PROD/MFR	NDC	AWP	DP	OBC
(Medisca) *See THEOPHYLLINE ANHYDROUS*				
(Nostrum)				
TER, PO, 400 mg, 100s ea	**29033-0001-01**	122.38		AB
600 mg, 100s ea	**29033-0002-01**	176.83		AB
(PCCA)				
POW, NA (USP, ANHYDROUS)				
1 gm	**51927-1510-00**	0.36		
(Pharm Assoc Inc)				
SOL, PO (1X15ML,MIXED FRUIT)				
80 mg/15 ml,				
15 ml 40s UD	**00121-4794-15**	500.82		
(Purdue Pharmaceutical) *See UNIPHYL*				
(Spectrum Pharmacy) *See THEOPHYLLINE ANHYDROUS*				
(Teva)				
T12, PO, 100 mg, 100s ea	**50111-0483-01**	21.79		AB
(10X10)				
100 mg, 100s ea UD	**00182-1589-89**	54.85		AB
500s ea	**50111-0483-02**	103.49		AB
200 mg, 100s ea	**50111-0482-01**	39.31		AB
500s ea	**50111-0482-02**	185.37		AB
1000s ea	**50111-0482-03**	350.02		AB
300 mg, 100s ea	**50111-0459-01**	46.68		AB
500s ea	**50111-0459-02**	220.14		AB
1000s ea	**50111-0459-03**	425.98		AB
450 mg, 100s ea	**50111-0518-01**	62.35		AB
(UCB) *See THEO-24*				
(A-S Medication)				
REPACK				
T12, PO, 300 mg, 30s ea	**54569-2483-02**	15.84		AB
100s ea	**54569-2483-01**	52.80		AB
(Altura)				
REPACK				
C12, PO, 300 mg, 30s ea	**63874-0675-30**	10.21		EE
ELI, PO, 80 mg/15 ml,				
120 ml	**63874-0744-12**	5.10		EE
240 ml	**63874-0744-24**	7.37		EE
T12, PO, 100 mg, 15s ea	**63874-0443-15**	2.93		EE
20s ea	**63874-0443-20**	3.95		EE
30s ea	**63874-0443-30**	5.91		EE
100s ea	**63874-0443-01**	19.72		EE
200 mg, 15s ea	**63874-0447-15**	4.29		EE
20s ea	**63874-0447-20**	5.73		EE
30s ea	**63874-0447-30**	8.59		EE
60s ea	**63874-0447-60**	12.18		EE
100s ea	**63874-0447-01**	28.64		EE
300 mg, 15s ea	**63874-0675-15**	5.10		EE
20s ea	**63874-0675-20**	6.80		EE
100s ea	**63874-0675-01**	34.02		EE
(Bryant Ranch)				
REPACK				
T12, PO, 100 mg, 30s ea	**63629-3551-01**	6.99		
200 mg, 30s ea	**63629-2792-01**	13.01		
60s ea	**63629-2792-02**	26.01		
(Dispensing Solutions)				
REPACK				
T12, PO, 100 mg, 30s ea	**55045-3768-08**	7.50		
(Palmetto)				
REPACK				
T12, PO, 300 mg, 30s ea	**23490-7355-01**	23.91		
(PD-Rx Pharm)				
REPACK				
T12, PO, 200 mg, 60s ea	**55289-0259-60**	39.58		AB
100s ea	**55289-0259-01**	61.49		AB
300 mg, 20s ea	**55289-0260-20**	18.18		AB
30s ea	**55289-0260-30**	23.91		AB
60s ea	**55289-0260-60**	41.16		AB
100s ea	**55289-0260-01**	52.89		AB
(Phys Total Care)				
REPACK				
C12, PO (USP)				
300 mg, 20s ea	**54868-5531-01**	33.00		
60s ea	**54868-5531-00**	90.00		
T12, PO, 100 mg, 30s ea	**54868-1461-01**	15.89		
90s ea	**54868-1461-02**	43.17		
200 mg, 30s ea	**54868-0028-06**	17.88		AB
50s ea	**54868-0028-03**	27.78		EE
60s ea	**54868-0028-01**	32.73		EE
100s ea	**54868-0028-02**	40.92		EE
500s ea	**54868-0028-00**	340.73		EE
1000s ea	**54868-0028-05**	521.82		EE
300 mg, 30s ea	**54868-0029-06**	21.90		EE
50s ea	**54868-0029-03**	34.47		EE
60s ea	**54868-0029-05**	40.77		EE
90s ea	**54868-0029-07**	65.10		EE
100s ea	**54868-0029-02**	51.15		EE
1000s ea	**54868-0029-00**	631.05		EE

PROD/MFR	NDC	AWP	DP	OBC
(Quality Care Prod)				
REPACK				
T12, PO, 200 mg, 60s ea	**35356-0126-60**	48.30		AB
(Southwood)				
REPACK				
T12, PO, 100 mg, 30s ea	**00490-0080-30**	6.14		
60s ea	**00490-0080-60**	12.29		
90s ea	**00490-0080-90**	18.43		
100s ea	**00490-0080-00**	20.48		
(Vibranta)				
REPACK				
T12, PO, 300 mg, 60s ea	**57866-4652-02**	27.10		AB
TER, PO, 200 mg, 60s ea	**57866-4651-02**	22.99		
450 mg, 60s ea	**57866-4653-01**	35.63		
THEOPHYLLINE ACETIC ACID (PCCA)				
acefylline				
POW, NA (1X1GM)				
1 gm	**51927-3176-00**	4.20		
THEOPHYLLINE ANHYDROUS (Amend)				
theophylline				
POW, NA (ANHYDROUS, U.S.P.)				
125 gm	**17317-0571-04**	9.80		
454 gm	**17317-0571-01**	29.40		
2270 gm	**17317-0571-05**	126.00		
11350 gm	**17317-0571-08**	350.00		
(Gallipot)				
POW, NA (U.S.P.)				
100 gm	**51552-0487-05**	13.93		
(Medisca)				
POW, NA (USP)				
100 gm	**38779-1816-05**	40.50		
500 gm	**38779-1816-08**	127.50		
(Spectrum Pharmacy)				
POW, NA (U.S.P.)				
100 gm	**49452-7720-01**	64.75		
500 gm	**49452-7720-02**	194.60		
2500 gm	**49452-7720-03**	801.50		
THEOPHYLLINE ER (DHS, Inc.)				
REPACK				
theophylline				
T12, PO, 450 mg, 60s ea	**55887-0079-60**	48.55		
(Quality Care Prod)				
REPACK				
T12, PO, 100 mg, 30s ea	**49999-0921-30**	11.65		
THEOPHYLLINE IN DEXTROSE (Hospira)				
dextrose/theophylline				
SOL, IV (24X250ML,LATEX-FREE)				
5%-160 mg/100 ml,				
250 ml 24s	**00409-7666-62**	139.10	121.68	AP
(24X100ML,SINGLEDOSE,USP)				
5%-200 mg/100 ml,				
100 ml 24s	**00409-7668-23**	147.74	129.36	AP
(USP,250MLX24,SINGLEDOSE)				
5%-320 mg/100 ml,				
250 ml 24s	**00409-7705-62**	161.57	141.36	AP
THEOPHYLLINE-KI (Consolidated Midland)				
potassium iodide/theophylline				
ELI, PO				
130 mg/15 ml-80 mg/15 ml,				
480 ml	**00223-6623-01**	4.00		
THERA-FLUR-N (Colgate Oral)				
sodium fluoride				
GEL, DE, 1.1%, 24 ml	**00126-0196-54**	5.63		
THERA-GESIC (Physician Partner)				
REPACK				
menthol/methyl salicylate				
CRE, TP, 1%-15%, 90 gm	**21695-0312-03**	17.26		
THERACYS (Sanofi)				
bacillus of calmette and guerin vaccine, live				
PDR, IL (S.D.V. W/DILUENT,PF)				
81 mg, ea	**49281-0880-01**	189.36	157.80	
THERAMINE (Physician Thera, LLC)				
amino acids and nutriceuticals				
CAP, PO (PF,SF,STARCH-FREE)				
90s ea	**68405-1008-03**	284.80		
101.5 mg-72.5 mg,				
60s ea	**68405-1008-02**	189.44		
(Altura)				
REPACK				
CAP, PO, 101.5 mg-72.5 mg,				
60s ea	**63874-1184-06**	132.00		
(Dispensing Solutions)				
REPACK				
CAP, PO (PF,SF,STARCH-FREE)				
101.5 mg-72.5 mg,				
60s ea	**55045-3397-06**	132.00		

PROD/MFR	NDC	AWP	DP	OBC
THERAPEUTIC-M (Dispensing Solutions)				
multimineral/multivitamin				
TAB, PO, 130s ea	**55045-3417-01**	8.75		
THERMAZENE (Covidien)				
silver sulfadiazine				
CRE, TP (24X20GM)				
1%, 20 gm 24s	**08880-9505-02**	96.56		AB
(JAR)				
1%, 50 gm 6s	**08880-9505-05**	47.24		AB
(36X50GM)				
1%, 50 gm 36s	**08880-9505-50**	155.51		AB
(JAR)				
1%, 85 gm 12s	**08880-9505-85**	143.78		AB
(6X400GM)				
1%, 400 gm 6s	**08880-9505-40**	172.78		AB
(6X1000GM)				
1%, 1000 gm 6s	**08880-9505-10**	408.11		AB
(Palmetto)				
REPACK				
CRE, TP, 1%, 50 gm	**23490-1325-01**	2.75		
400 gm	**23490-1325-02**	19.69		
(Quality Care Prod)				
REPACK				
CRE, TP, 1%, 20 gm	**49999-0187-20**	181.15		AB
(1X50GM)				
1%, 50 gm	**49999-0187-50**	28.60		AB
THEROBEC (Qualitest)				
vitamin b complex and vitamin c				
TAB, PO, 100s ea	**00603-5969-21**	33.99		
THEROBEC PLUS (Qualitest)				
multivitamin and minerals				
TAB, PO, 100s ea	**00603-5970-21**	37.77		
THIABENDAZOLE (Gallipot)				
POW, NA (U.S.P.)				
100 gm	**51552-0481-05**	85.68		
(Medisca)				
POW, NA (USP)				
100 gm	**38779-0111-05**	127.50		
500 gm	**38779-0111-08**	567.00		
(U.S.P.)				
1000 gm	**38779-0111-09**	1095.00		
(PCCA)				
POW, NA (U.S.P.)				
1 gm	**51927-2278-00**	1.92		
(Spectrum Pharmacy)				
POW, NA (U.S.P.)				
100 gm	**49452-7723-01**	198.45		
500 gm	**49452-7723-02**	812.00		
THIACETAZONE (PCCA)				
amithiozone				
POW, NA (1X1GM)				
1 gm	**51927-2975-00**	4.05		
THIAMINE				
(Amend) *See THIAMINE HCL*				
(APP) *See THIAMINE HYDROCHLORIDE*				
(Baker, J.T.) *See THIAMINE HCL*				
(Consolidated Midland) *See THIAMINE HCL*				
(Gallipot) *See THIAMINE HCL*				
(Spectrum Pharmacy) *See THIAMINE HCL*				
(Truxton) *See THIAMINE HCL*				
THIAMINE HCL (Amend)				
thiamine				
POW, NA (U.S.P.)				
25 gm	**17317-0572-02**	4.90		
100 gm	**17317-0572-03**	14.70		
500 gm	**17317-0572-05**	58.80		
1000 gm	**17317-0572-06**	98.00		
(Baker, J.T.)				
POW, NA (U.S.P., F.C.C.)				
100 gm	**10106-4110-05**	31.02		
(Consolidated Midland)				
SOL, IJ (AMP)				
100 mg/ml,				
1 ml 25s	**00223-8709-01**	25.00		EE
(VIAL)				
100 mg/ml, 30 ml	**00223-8711-02**	8.50		EE
(Gallipot)				
POW, NA (U.S.P.,N.F.)				
25 gm	**51552-0143-04**	7.98		
100 gm	**51552-0143-05**	18.20		
(Spectrum Pharmacy)				
POW, NA (U.S.P.)				
25 gm	**49452-7730-01**	53.90		
100 gm	**49452-7730-02**	86.10		
1000 gm	**49452-7730-03**	518.00		

PROD/MFR	NDC	AWP	DP	OBC
(Truxton)				
SOL, IJ (VIAL)				
100 mg/ml, 30 ml	00463-1074-30	4.20		EE
(Phys Total Care) REPACK				
SOL, IJ, 100 mg/ml, 2 ml	54868-2489-01	407.73		EE
THIAMINE HYDROCHLORIDE (APP)				
thiamine				
SOL, IJ (M.D.V.,25X2ML)				
100 mg/ml,				
2 ml 25s	63323-0013-02	310.94		AP
THIAMINE HYDROCHLORIDE (Letco)				
POW, NA (1X100GM, USP)				
100 gm	62991-2068-02	40.50		
(1X500GM, USP)				
500 gm	62991-2068-03	120.00		
(1X1000GM,USP)				
1000 gm	62991-2068-04	180.00		
(PCCA)				
POW, NA (USP)				
1 gm	51927-1242-00	1.08		
(Phys Total Care) REPACK				
thiamine				
SOL, IJ (1X2ML)				
100 mg/ml, 2 ml	54868-2489-00	17.21		AP
THIAMINE MONONITRATE (PCCA)				
POW, NA (USP)				
1 gm	51927-2738-00	0.90		
(Spectrum Pharmacy)				
POW, NA (U.S.P.)				
100 gm	49452-7740-02	159.60		
1000 gm	49452-7740-03	728.00		
THIMEROSAL (Amend)				
POW, NA (U.S.P.)				
25 gm	17317-0574-02	58.80		
100 gm	17317-0574-04	210.00		
THIMEROSAL (PCCA)				
POW, NA (U.S.P.)				
1 gm	51927-1244-00	11.40		
(Spectrum Pharmacy)				
POW, NA (U.S.P.)				
5 gm	49452-7750-03	197.05		
25 gm	49452-7750-01	665.00		
100 gm	49452-7750-02	1732.50		
THIOACETAMIDE (Baker, J.T.)				
CRY, NA (A.C.S., REAGENT)				
125 gm	10106-8984-04	136.73		
500 gm	10106-8984-01	453.56		
THIOCTIC ACID				
(Medisca) *See LIPOIC ACID*				
(PCCA) *See LIPOIC ACID*				
(Spectrum Pharmacy) *See LIPOIC ACID*				
THIOGUANINE (Glaxo)				
TAB, PO, 40 mg, 25s ea	00173-0880-25	247.10		
(PCCA)				
POW, NA, 1 gm	51927-2803-00	276.00		
THIOLA (Mission)				
tiopronin				
TAB, PO, 100 mg, 100s ea	00178-0900-01	126.00	105.00	
THIONYL CHLORIDE (Baker, J.T.)				
LIQ, NA (PURIFIED)				
500 ml	10106-8660-01	174.02		
THIOPENTAL SODIUM				
(Hospira) *See PENTOTHAL*				
THIORIDAZINE HCL (Consolidated Midland)				
thioridazine hydrochloride				
TAB, PO, 10 mg, 100s ea	00223-2128-01	6.25		EE
1000s ea	00223-2128-02	55.00		EE
15 mg, 100s ea	00223-2129-01	7.75		EE
1000s ea	00223-2129-02	66.00		EE
25 mg, 100s ea	00223-2130-01	9.50		EE
1000s ea	00223-2130-02	87.50		EE
50 mg, 100s ea	00223-2131-01	12.50		EE
1000s ea	00223-2131-02	120.00		EE
100 mg, 100s ea	00223-2132-01	19.50		EE
1000s ea	00223-2132-02	165.00		EE
150 mg, 100s ea	00223-2133-01	30.00		EE
1000s ea	00223-2133-02	270.00		EE
200 mg, 100s ea	00223-2134-01	34.50		EE
1000s ea	00223-2134-02	335.00		EE
(Mutual)				
TAB, PO, 10 mg, 100s ea	53489-0148-01	33.20		AB
1000s ea	53489-0148-10	325.10		AB
(FILM-COATED)				
25 mg, 100s ea	53489-0149-01	46.70		AB
1000s ea	53489-0149-10	457.40		AB
50 mg, 100s ea	53489-0150-01	58.40		AB
1000s ea	53489-0150-10	562.30		AB
100 mg, 100s ea	53489-0500-01	66.50		AB
(Mylan)				
TAB, PO, 10 mg, 100s ea	00378-0612-01	33.20		AB
1000s ea	00378-0612-10	325.10		AB
25 mg, 100s ea	00378-0614-01	46.70		AB
1000s ea	00378-0614-10	457.40		AB
50 mg, 100s ea	00378-0616-01	58.40		AB
1000s ea	00378-0616-10	562.30		AB
100 mg, 100s ea	00378-0618-01	66.50		AB
1000s ea	00378-0618-10	645.20		AB
(PCCA)				
POW, NA, 1 gm	51927-1928-00	11.16		
(UDL)				
TAB, PO (10X10)				
10 mg, 100s ea UD	51079-0565-20	34.20		AB
25 mg, 100s ea UD	51079-0566-20	48.10		AB
50 mg, 100s ea UD	51079-0567-20	60.15		AB
100 mg, 100s ea UD	51079-0580-20	68.50		AB
(Phys Total Care) REPACK				
TAB, PO, 25 mg, 30s ea	54868-0067-04	24.57		EE
60s ea	54868-0067-05	44.64		EE
100s ea	54868-0067-00	69.93		AB
50 mg, 30s ea	54868-1832-02	15.49		EE
100s ea	54868-1832-03	43.13		EE
1000s ea	54868-1832-00	169.96		EE
100 mg, 100s ea	54868-1828-02	37.18		EE
1000s ea	54868-1828-00	251.74		EE
(Vibranta) REPACK				
TAB, PO, 10 mg, 90s ea	57866-1042-01	30.44		AB
25 mg, 90s ea	57866-4642-03	40.52		AB
50 mg, 90s ea	57866-4643-01	48.08		
100 mg, 90s ea	57866-4644-01	52.96		
THIORIDAZINE HYDROCHLORIDE				
(Consolidated Midland) *See THIORIDAZINE HCL*				
(Mutual) *See THIORIDAZINE HCL*				
(Mylan) *See THIORIDAZINE HCL*				
(PCCA) *See THIORIDAZINE HCL*				
(UDL) *See THIORIDAZINE HCL*				
THIOSALICYLIC ACID SODIUM SALT (PCCA)				
sodium thiosalicylate				
POW, NA, 1 gm	51927-2582-00	16.20		
THIOTEPA (Bedford)				
PDS, IJ (S.D.V.)				
15 mg, ea	55390-0030-10	138.00		AP
(PCCA) *See TRIETHYLENETHIOPHOSPHORAMIDE/T*				
(Teva)				
PDS, IJ (S.D.V.)				
30 mg, ea	00703-4303-01	296.88		
THIOTHIXENE FUL				
CAP, PO, 1 mg, 100s ea		13.88		
2 mg, 100s ea		18.60		
5 mg, 100s ea		29.63		
10 mg, 100s ea		40.65		
(Mylan)				
CAP, PO, 1 mg, 100s ea	00378-1001-01	23.00		AB
2 mg, 100s ea	00378-2002-01	30.40		AB
1000s ea	00378-2002-10	294.80		AB
5 mg, 100s ea	00378-3005-01	46.10		AB
1000s ea	00378-3005-10	447.60		AB
10 mg, 100s ea	00378-5010-01	65.00		AB
1000s ea	00378-5010-10	630.80		AB
(PCCA)				
POW, NA (U.S.P.)				
1 gm	51927-2294-00	900.00		
(Pfizer) *See NAVANE*				
(Sandoz)				
CAP, PO, 1 mg, 100s ea	00781-2226-01	23.00		AB
2 mg, 100s ea	00781-2227-01	30.40		AB
5 mg, 100s ea	00781-2228-01	46.10		AB
10 mg, 100s ea	00781-2229-01	65.00		AB
(UDL)				
CAP, PO (10X10)				
2 mg, 100s ea UD	51079-0587-20	31.31		AB
5 mg, 100s ea UD	51079-0588-20	47.48		AB
10 mg, 100s ea UD	51079-0589-20	66.95		AB
(Phys Total Care) REPACK				
CAP, PO, 2 mg, 100s ea	54868-2343-00	23.42		EE
5 mg, 100s ea	54868-2358-00	30.45		EE
(Physician Partner) REPACK				
CAP, PO, 5 mg, 30s ea	21695-0161-30	27.66		AB
(Vibranta) REPACK				
CAP, PO, 5 mg, 30s ea	57866-4437-01	14.51		
60s ea	57866-4437-02	27.92		
90s ea	57866-4437-03	41.33		
10 mg, 30s ea	57866-4438-01	20.00		
60s ea	57866-4438-02	38.90		
90s ea	57866-4438-03	57.80		
THIOUREA (Amend)				
POW, NA (PURIFIED)				
454 gm	17317-0749-01	7.00		
2270 gm	17317-0749-05	28.00		
(Baker, J.T.)				
POW, NA (A.C.S., REAGENT)				
125 gm	10106-4123-04	42.59		
500 gm	10106-4123-01	78.49		
2500 gm	10106-4123-05	295.66		
(PCCA)				
POW, NA (ACS)				
1 gm	51927-3423-00	0.60		
(Spectrum Pharmacy)				
POW, NA (A.C.S. REAGENT)				
125 gm	49452-7760-04	110.95		
THORACENTESIS SET (Portex)				
needle, hypodermic				
DEV, NA (30" W/15G NDL)				
48s ea	00074-4653-48	544.92	458.88	
THORAZINE (Glaxo)				
chlorpromazine				
SUP, RC, 100 mg, 12s ea	00007-5071-03	57.36		
THREONINE				
(Gallipot) *See L-THREONINE*				
(Medisca) *See L-THREONINE*				
(PCCA)				
POW, NA (USP)				
1 gm	51927-3564-00	1.44		
(Spectrum Pharmacy) *See L-THREONINE*				
THROMBATE III (Talecris)				
antithrombin iii human				
PDS, IV (W/DILUENT,~1000IU/VIAL)				
1 iu, ea	13533-0603-30	3.54		
(W/DILUENT,~500IU/VIAL)				
1 iu, ea	13533-0603-20	3.54		
THROMBI-GEL (King Pharm)				
dressing				
DEV, NA (100 SQ CM)				
5s ea	60793-0909-10	701.88		
(40 SQ CM)				
5s ea	60793-0908-04	386.40		
(10 SQ CM)				
10s ea	60793-0907-01	578.52		
THROMBIN HUMAN, RECOMBINANT				
(ZymoGenetics) *See RECOTHROM*				
THROMBIN-JMI (King Pharm)				
thrombin, bovine				
PDS, TP (EPISTAXIS,PF)				
5000 iu, ea	60793-0205-05	87.85		
(W/DILUENT,PF)				
5000 iu, ea	60793-0215-05	86.12		
(PUMP SPRAY KIT,USP)				
20000 iu, ea	60793-0217-21	356.64		
(USP)				
20000 iu, ea	60793-0217-20	339.65		
(W/SYRINGE SPRAY KIT)				
20000 iu, ea	60793-0217-22	356.64		
THROMBIN, BOVINE				
(King Pharm) *See THROMBIN-JMI*				
THUJA OIL				
(Amend) *See CEDARLEAF OIL*				
(PCCA) *See CEDAR LEAF*				
(Spectrum Pharmacy) *See CEDAR LEAF OIL*				
THYME OIL				
(Amend) *See THYME OIL WHITE*				
(Lorann Oil)				
OIL, NA, 9.9 ml	23535-0151-78	5.00		

PROD/MFR	NDC	AWP	DP	OBC
(Medisca)				
OIL, NA (RED,NATURAL)				
14 ml	38779-1644-03	16.50		
25 ml	38779-1644-04	31.50		
100 ml	38779-1644-05	84.00		
500 ml	38779-1644-08	300.00		
(Medisca) *See THYME OIL WHITE*				
(PCCA)				
OIL, NA (FCC)				
1 ml	51927-1628-00	1.40		
THYME OIL WHITE (Amend)				
thyme oil				
OIL, NA, 100 ml	17317-0576-04	21.00		
500 ml	17317-0576-01	84.00		
(Medisca)				
OIL, NA (WHITE,NATURAL)				
14 ml	38779-1650-03	16.50		
25 ml	38779-1650-04	31.50		
100 ml	38779-1650-05	84.00		
500 ml	38779-1650-08	300.00		
THYMOGLOBULIN (Genzyme)				
antithymocyte globulin rabbit				
PDS, IV (VIAL,DILUENT)				
25 mg, ea	58468-0080-01	636.48	530.40	
THYMOL (Amend)				
CRY, NA (N.F.)				
125 gm	17317-0577-04	14.00		
454 gm	17317-0577-01	36.40		
2270 gm	17317-0577-05	112.00		
11350 gm	17317-0577-08	323.75		
(Baker, J.T.)				
CRY, NA (N.F.)				
125 gm	10106-4128-04	28.55		
500 gm	10106-4128-01	63.27		
(Gallipot)				
CRY, NA (U.S.P.,N.F.)				
25 gm	51552-0173-04	8.82		
100 gm	51552-0173-05	16.59		
(Mallinckrodt Lab)				
CRY, NA (N.F.)				
125 gm	00406-8528-02	28.51		
500 gm	00406-8528-03	202.26		
(Medisca)				
CRY, NA (N.F.)				
25 gm	38779-0309-04	25.50		
100 gm	38779-0309-05	37.50		
500 gm	38779-0309-08	112.50		
(PCCA) *See THYMOL CRYSTALS*				
(Spectrum Pharmacy)				
CRY, NA (N.F.)				
100 gm	49452-7790-01	68.95		
500 gm	49452-7790-02	201.95		
2500 gm	49452-7790-03	756.00		
THYMOL CRYSTALS (PCCA)				
thymol				
CRY, NA (N.F.)				
1 gm	51927-1246-00	1.14		
THYMOL IODIDE (Amend)				
POW, NA (PURIFIED)				
25 gm	17317-0578-02	19.60		
125 gm	17317-0578-04	56.00		
500 gm	17317-0578-01	168.00		
2500 gm	17317-0578-05	672.00		
(Baker, J.T.)				
POW, NA (PURIFIED)				
30 gm	10106-4131-00	25.16		
125 gm	10106-4131-04	55.91		
(Gallipot)				
POW, NA (PURIFIED,U.S.P.,N.F.)				
25 gm	51552-0150-04	18.97		
100 gm	51552-0150-05	51.59		
(Mallinckrodt Lab)				
POW, NA (PURIFIED)				
30 gm	00406-1155-12	24.45		
125 gm	00406-1155-02	45.20		
500 gm	00406-1155-04	578.58		
(Medisca)				
POW, NA (1X25GM)				
25 gm	38779-1651-04	51.75		
(1X100GM)				
100 gm	38779-1651-05	205.50		
(1X500GM)				
500 gm	38779-1651-08	964.50		
(PCCA)				
POW, NA (PURIFIED)				
1 gm	51927-1240-00	2.37		
(Spectrum Pharmacy)				
POW, NA (PURIFIED)				
25 gm	49452-7800-01	99.40		
125 gm	49452-7800-03	248.15		
500 gm	49452-7800-04	742.00		
THYROGEN (Genzyme)				
thyrotropin alfa				
PDS, IJ (W/2 VIALS DILUENT)				
1.1 mg, 2s ea	58468-1849-04	2392.80	1994.00	
THYROID (Amend)				
POW, NA (U.S.P.)				
125 gm	17317-0579-04	23.80		
500 gm	17317-0579-01	84.00		
(Bio-Tech Pharm)				
CAP, PO, 15 mg, 100s ea	53191-0289-01	8.40		
30 mg, 100s ea	53191-0290-01	9.00		
1000s ea	53191-0290-10	66.00		
60 mg, 100s ea	53191-0291-01	9.60		
1000s ea	53191-0291-10	72.00		
90 mg, 100s ea	53191-0292-01	10.20		
1000s ea	53191-0292-10	78.00		
120 mg, 100s ea	53191-0293-01	14.25		
1000s ea	53191-0293-10	120.00		
180 mg, 100s ea	53191-0297-01	12.00		
1000s ea	53191-0297-10	96.00		
240 mg, 100s ea	53191-0294-01	13.20		
1000s ea	53191-0294-10	108.00		
(Consolidated Midland)				
TAB, PO, 30 mg, 100s ea	00223-2072-01	5.00		
1000s ea	00223-2072-02	17.50		
60 mg, 100s ea	00223-2074-01	5.50		
1000s ea	00223-2074-02	22.50		
(Forest Pharm) *See ARMOUR THYROID*				
(Major)				
TAB, PO, 120 mg, 100s ea	00904-0762-60	14.44		
(RLC) *See NATURE-THROID*				
(RLC) *See WESTHROID*				
(Spectrum Pharmacy) *See THYROID 0.23%*				
(Truxton)				
TAB, PO, 30 mg, 1000s ea	00463-6199-10	16.80		
60 mg, 1000s ea	00463-6201-10	12.90		
120 mg, 1000s ea	00463-6203-10	17.40		
(Bryant Ranch) REPACK				
TAB, PO, 60 mg, 30s ea	63629-2713-01	0.82		
100s ea	63629-2713-02	2.73		
(DHS, Inc.) REPACK				
TAB, PO, 65 mg, 30s ea	55887-0927-30	13.86		
(Dispensing Solutions) REPACK				
TAB, PO, 30 mg, 30s ea	55045-3774-03	5.40		
(Nucare Pharm) REPACK				
TAB, PO, 65 mg, 30s ea	66267-0203-30	15.86		
60s ea	66267-0203-60	24.24		
90s ea	66267-0203-90	37.86		
(Palmetto) REPACK				
TAB, PO, 30 mg, 60s ea	23490-6374-01	12.00		
90 mg, 60s ea	23490-6377-01	18.60		
90s ea	23490-6377-02	27.69		
(PD-Rx Pharm) REPACK				
TAB, PO, 65 mg, 30s ea	55289-0261-30	43.68		
90s ea	55289-0261-90	73.04		
130 mg, 90s ea	55289-0262-90	28.27		
(Phys Total Care) REPACK				
TAB, PO, 32.4 mg, 30s ea	54868-0794-01	20.07		
100s ea	54868-0794-00	56.43		
64.8 mg, 30s ea	54868-0084-01	5.67		
100s ea	54868-0084-00	11.85		
1000s ea	54868-0084-02	91.62		
130 mg, 100s ea	54868-0041-00	16.62		
180 mg, 100s ea	54868-0083-00	23.37		
(Quality Care Prod) REPACK				
TAB, PO, 30 mg, 28s ea	49999-0288-28	14.60		
30s ea	49999-0288-30	5.46		
60s ea	49999-0288-60	10.92		
32.5 mg, 100s ea	49999-0288-00	18.20		
65 mg, 28s ea	49999-0702-28	14.60		
30s ea	49999-0084-30	4.95		
60s ea	49999-0084-60	9.90		
120 mg, 28s ea	49999-0088-28	15.21		
130 mg, 60s ea	49999-0088-60	8.96		
180 mg, 60s ea	49999-0282-60	14.84		
195 mg, 100s ea	49999-0282-00	24.73		
THYROID 0.23% (Spectrum Pharmacy)				
thyroid				
POW, NA (U.S.P.)				
25 gm	49452-7811-01	81.90		
100 gm	49452-7811-02	172.20		
THYROID PORCINE (Medisca)				
POW, NA (U.S.P.)				
100 gm	38779-1654-05	101.25		
500 gm	38779-1654-08	345.00		
(PCCA)				
POW, NA (U.S.P.)				
1 gm	51927-1467-00	0.66		
THYROLAR (Forest Pharm)				
levothyroxine sodium/liothyronine sodium				
TAB, PO, 12.5 mcg-3.1 mcg,				
100s ea	00456-0040-01	54.83		
25 mcg-6.25 mcg,				
100s ea	00456-0045-01	60.85		
50 mcg-12.5 mcg,				
100s ea	00456-0050-01	76.06		
100 mcg-25 mcg,				
100s ea	00456-0055-01	89.44		
150 mcg-37.5 mcg,				
100s ea	00456-0060-01	109.33		
THYROTROPIN ALFA				
(Genzyme) *See THYROGEN*				
THYROXINE SODIUM PENTAHYDRATE (PCCA)				
levothyroxine sodium				
POW, NA (1X1GM)				
1 gm	51927-1877-00	492.00		
TIAGABINE HYDROCHLORIDE				
(Cephalon) *See GABITRIL*				
TIAZAC (Forest Pharm)				
diltiazem hydrochloride				
C24, PO, 120 mg, 30s ea	00456-2612-30	47.23		AB4
90s ea	00456-2612-90	128.35		AB4
(10X10)				
120 mg, 100s ea UD	00456-2612-63	157.46		AB4
1000s ea	00456-2612-00	1258.81		AB4
180 mg, 30s ea	00456-2613-30	57.02		AB4
90s ea	00456-2613-90	154.90		AB4
(10X10)				
180 mg, 100s ea UD	00456-2613-63	189.28		AB4
1000s ea	00456-2613-00	1519.12		AB4
240 mg, 30s ea	00456-2614-30	80.90		AB4
90s ea	00456-2614-90	219.83		AB4
(10X10)				
240 mg, 100s ea UD	00456-2614-63	221.58		AB4
1000s ea	00456-2614-00	2177.15		AB4
300 mg, 30s ea	00456-2615-30	104.86		AB4
90s ea	00456-2615-90	284.78		AB4
(10X10)				
300 mg, 100s ea UD	00456-2615-63	346.72		AB4
1000s ea	00456-2615-00	2834.52		AB4
360 mg, 30s ea	00456-2616-30	106.86		AB4
90s ea	00456-2616-90	290.26		AB4
(10X10)				
360 mg, 100s ea UD	00456-2616-63	353.40		AB4
1000s ea	00456-2616-00	2862.04		AB4
420 mg, 30s ea	00456-2617-30	112.02		
90s ea	00456-2617-90	304.21		
1000s ea	00456-2617-00	3028.32		
(PD-Rx Pharm) REPACK				
C24, PO (REDI-SCRIPT)				
120 mg, 30s ea	58864-0724-30	75.90		AB4
180 mg, 14s ea	58864-0635-14	84.27		AB4
240 mg, 30s ea	58864-0714-30	252.93		AB4
(Phys Total Care) REPACK				
C24, PO, 120 mg, 15s ea	54868-3774-00	21.03		BC
180 mg, 15s ea	54868-3956-02	29.20		BC
30s ea	54868-3956-01	56.54		BC
60s ea	54868-3956-00	111.20		BC
240 mg, 30s ea	54868-3958-00	72.39		BC
300 mg, 30s ea	54868-4418-00	104.54		AB4
360 mg, 30s ea	54868-4068-00	108.30		AB4
420 mg, 30s ea	54868-5053-00	119.44		
90s ea	54868-5053-01	336.12		

PROD/MFR	NDC	AWP	DP	OBC
TICAR (Abbott Hosp)				
ticarcillin disodium				
PDS, IJ (VIAL, BULK)				
20 gm, 10s ea	**00029-6558-21**	824.96	694.70	
TICARCILLIN DISODIUM				
(Abbott Hosp) *See TICAR*				
TICE BCG (Organon)				
bacillus of calmette and guerin vaccine, live				
PDR, IL (VIAL)				
800 million cfu,				
ea	**00052-0602-02**	169.10		
TICLID (Roche Labs)				
ticlopidine hydrochloride				
TAB, PO, 250 mg, 30s ea	**00004-0018-23**	80.64		AB
60s ea	**00004-0018-22**	156.50		AB
500s ea	**00004-0018-14**	1303.46		AB
(AQ)				
REPACK				
TAB, PO, 250 mg, 10s ea	**66105-0139-01**	31.24		
20s ea	**66105-0139-02**	62.48		
30s ea	**66105-0139-03**	93.74		
60s ea	**66105-0139-06**	187.48		
100s ea	**66105-0139-10**	312.46		
(Phys Total Care)				
REPACK				
TAB, PO, 250 mg, 30s ea	**54868-3783-01**	81.71		AB
TICLOPIDINE HCL (Apotex Corp.)				
ticlopidine hydrochloride				
TAB, PO, 250 mg, 30s ea	**60505-0027-02**	57.69		AB
60s ea	**60505-0027-04**	111.97		AB
500s ea	**60505-0027-07**	932.67		AB
(Caraco)				
TAB, PO (FILM COATED)				
250 mg, 30s ea	**57664-0327-83**	57.69		AB
60s ea	**57664-0327-06**	111.98		AB
500s ea	**57664-0327-13**	932.67		AB
(Major)				
TAB, PO (10X10)				
250 mg, 100s ea UD	**00904-5378-61**	198.72		EE
(Sandoz)				
TAB, PO, 250 mg, 30s ea	**00185-0115-30**	57.69		AB
60s ea	**00185-0115-60**	111.98		AB
500s ea	**00185-0115-05**	932.67		AB
(Teva)				
TAB, PO, 250 mg, 100s ea	**00093-0154-01**	186.00		AB
(GSMS)				
REPACK				
TAB, PO, 250 mg, 30s ea	**60429-0764-30**	12.06	4.02	AB
60s ea	**60429-0764-60**	21.96	7.32	AB
500s ea	**60429-0764-05**	158.40	52.80	AB
(Phys Total Care)				
REPACK				
TAB, PO, 250 mg, 60s ea	**54868-5062-00**	43.77		AB
TICLOPIDINE HYDROCHLORIDE				
FUL				
TAB, PO, 250 mg, 60s ea		16.39		
(Apotex Corp.) *See TICLOPIDINE HCL*				
(Caraco) *See TICLOPIDINE HCL*				
(Major) *See TICLOPIDINE HCL*				
(Roche Labs) *See TICLID*				
(Sandoz) *See TICLOPIDINE HCL*				
(Teva) *See TICLOPIDINE HCL*				
TIGAN (JHP)				
trimethobenzamide hydrochloride				
SOL, IM (SDV,25X2ML)				
100 mg/ml,				
2 ml 25s	**42023-0119-25**	197.74		AP
(MDV,1X20ML)				
100 mg/ml, 20 ml	**42023-0118-01**	67.80		AP
(Monarch)				
CAP, PO, 300 mg, 100s ea	**61570-0079-01**	187.33		
(Dispensing Solutions)				
REPACK				
SOL, IM, 100 mg/ml,				
20 ml	**55045-3565-01**	72.00		
(Phys Total Care)				
REPACK				
CAP, PO, 300 mg, 100s ea	**54868-5181-00**	145.13		
SOL, IM (VIAL)				
100 mg/ml, 20 ml	**54868-0756-00**	83.26		AP

PROD/MFR	NDC	AWP	DP	OBC
(Physician Partner)				
REPACK				
SOL, IM (1X20ML)				
100 mg/ml, 20 ml	**21695-0853-20**	141.26		AP
TIGECYCLINE				
(Wyeth) *See TYGACIL*				
TIKOSYN (Pfizer)				
dofetilide				
CAP, PO, 0.125 mg,				
40s ea UD	**00069-5800-43**	142.40	118.67	
60s ea	**00069-5800-60**	213.61	178.01	
0.25 mg, 40s ea UD	**00069-5810-43**	142.40	118.67	
60s ea	**00069-5810-60**	213.61	178.01	
0.5 mg, 40s ea UD	**00069-5820-43**	142.40	118.67	
60s ea	**00069-5820-60**	213.61	178.01	
TILIA FE (Watson)				
ethinyl estradiol/ferrous fum/norethindrone ace				
TAB, PO (5X28)				
140s ea UD	**52544-0175-72**	274.36		
TILUDRONATE DISODIUM				
(Sanofi-Aventis) *See SKELID*				
TIMENTIN (Glaxo)				
clavulanate potassium/ticarcillin disodium				
PDS, IV (BULK VIAL)				
1 gm-30 gm, ea	**00029-6579-21**	159.56		
(ADD-VANTAGE)				
100 mg-3 gm, ea	**00029-6571-40**	16.31		
(VIAL)				
100 mg-3 gm, ea	**00029-6571-26**	16.00		
SOL, IV (PREMIX)				
100 ml 12s	**00029-6571-31**	222.11		
TIMOLOL				
(Vistakon) *See BETIMOL*				
TIMOLOL (Phys Total Care)				
REPACK				
timolol maleate				
GFS, OP, 0.5%, 5 ml	**54868-4691-00**	92.19		AB
TIMOLOL MALEATE				
FUL				
SOL, OP, 0.25%, 10 ml		6.98		
0.5%, 15 ml		13.50		
(Apotex Corp.)				
SOL, OP, 0.25%, 5 ml	**60505-0552-02**	15.00		AT
10 ml	**60505-0552-03**	27.75		AT
15 ml	**60505-0552-04**	42.02		AT
0.5%, 5 ml	**60505-0551-02**	17.00		AT
10 ml	**60505-0551-03**	32.33		AT
15 ml	**60505-0551-04**	48.43		AT
(Aton)				
GFS, OP (1X5ML)				
0.25%, 5 ml	**25010-0816-56**	49.50		
0.5%, 5 ml	**25010-0817-56**	58.50		
(Aton) *See TIMOPTIC IN OCUDOSE*				
(Aton) *See TIMOPTIC OCUMETER PLUS*				
(Aton) *See TIMOPTIC-XE OCUMETER PLUS*				
(Falcon Ophthalmics)				
GFS, OP, 0.25%, 5 ml	**61314-0224-05**	36.96		AB
0.5%, 5 ml	**61314-0225-05**	43.68		AB
SOL, OP, 0.25%, 5 ml	**61314-0226-05**	15.00		AT
10 ml	**61314-0226-10**	27.75		AT
15 ml	**61314-0226-15**	42.00		AT
0.5%, 5 ml	**61314-0227-05**	17.00		AT
10 ml	**61314-0227-10**	32.35		AT
15 ml	**61314-0227-15**	48.75		AT
(Gallipot)				
POW, NA (U.S.P.)				
1 gm	**51552-0433-01**	77.00		
(ISTA Pharm.) *See ISTALOL*				
(Medisca)				
POW, NA (USP)				
1 gm	**38779-0366-06**	135.00		
(U.S.P.)				
5 gm	**38779-0366-03**	525.00		
10 gm	**38779-0366-01**	897.00		
(Mylan)				
TAB, PO, 5 mg, 100s ea	**00378-0055-01**	39.95		AB
10 mg, 100s ea	**00378-0221-01**	49.80		AB
20 mg, 100s ea	**00378-0715-01**	92.20		AB
(Pacific Pharma)				
SOL, OP, 0.25%, 5 ml	**60758-0802-05**	14.06		AT
10 ml	**60758-0802-10**	27.18		AT
15 ml	**60758-0802-15**	41.55		AT
0.5%, 5 ml	**60758-0801-05**	16.64		AT
10 ml	**60758-0801-10**	32.29		AT
15 ml	**60758-0801-15**	48.32		AT

PROD/MFR	NDC	AWP	DP	OBC
(Pack)				
SOL, OP (1X5ML,USP)				
0.25%, 5 ml	**16571-0140-50**	15.00		AT
(1X10ML,USP)				
0.25%, 10 ml	**16571-0140-10**	27.75		AT
(1X5ML,USP)				
0.5%, 5 ml	**16571-0141-50**	17.00		AT
(1X10ML,USP)				
0.5%, 10 ml	**16571-0141-10**	32.35		AT
(PCCA)				
POW, NA (U.S.P.)				
1 gm	**51927-2003-00**	147.00		
(Spectrum Pharmacy)				
POW, NA (U.S.P.)				
0.1 gm	**49452-7813-03**	44.80	82.50	
1 gm	**49452-7813-02**	214.20		
5 gm	**49452-7813-04**	843.50		
(A-S Medication)				
REPACK				
SOL, OP, 0.5%, 10 ml	**54569-4289-00**	32.35		AT
(Phys Total Care)				
REPACK				
SOL, OP, 0.25%, 5 ml	**54868-3713-01**	11.58		AT
10 ml	**54868-3713-00**	11.43		EE
0.5%, 5 ml	**54868-3714-02**	23.01		AT
10 ml	**54868-3714-01**	38.38		EE
15 ml	**54868-3714-00**	21.81		EE
TIMONACIC (PCCA)				
l-4-thiazolidinecarboxylic acid				
POW, NA (1X1GM)				
1 gm	**51927-3304-00**	6.51		
TIMOPTIC IN OCUDOSE (Aton)				
timolol maleate				
SOL, OP (60X0.2ML,PF,DROP)				
0.25%,				
0.2 ml 60s UD	**25010-0814-66**	237.29		
0.5%,				
0.2 ml 60s UD	**25010-0815-66**	285.69		
TIMOPTIC OCUDOSE (Phys Total Care)				
REPACK				
timolol maleate				
SOL, OP (PF)				
0.5%, 0.2 ml 60s	**54868-4707-00**	146.86		
TIMOPTIC OCUMETER (Pharma Pac)				
REPACK				
timolol maleate				
SOL, OP, 0.5%, 5 ml	**52959-0584-03**	39.65		AT
(Phys Total Care)				
REPACK				
SOL, OP, 0.25%, 5 ml	**54868-0621-01**	23.66		AT
10 ml	**54868-0621-02**	42.36		AT
15 ml	**54868-0621-00**	63.10		AT
0.5%, 5 ml	**54868-0664-01**	24.74		AT
10 ml	**54868-0664-02**	51.44		AT
15 ml	**54868-0664-03**	70.72		AT
(Southwood)				
REPACK				
SOL, OP, 0.25%, 2.5 ml	**58016-1126-01**	9.94		AT
0.5%, 2.5 ml	**58016-6331-01**	11.54		AT
5 ml	**58016-6216-01**	21.07		AT
10 ml	**58016-6069-01**	39.63		AT
TIMOPTIC OCUMETER PLUS (Aton)				
timolol maleate				
SOL, OP (1X5ML)				
0.25%, 5 ml	**25010-0812-56**	38.15		AT
0.5%, 5 ml	**25010-0813-56**	44.96		AT
(1X10ML)				
0.5%, 10 ml	**25010-0813-16**	87.20		AT
TIMOPTIC-XE OCUMETER (Phys Total Care)				
REPACK				
timolol maleate				
GFS, OP, 0.25%, 5 ml	**54868-3263-00**	35.43		AB
0.5%, 5 ml	**54868-3264-00**	41.90		AB
TIMOPTIC-XE OCUMETER PLUS (Aton)				
timolol maleate				
GFS, OP (1X5ML)				
0.25%, 5 ml	**25010-0810-56**	59.95		AB
0.5%, 5 ml	**25010-0811-56**	70.85		AB
TIN (Baker, J.T.)				
GRA, NA (A.C.S.,REAGENT,20 MESH)				
500 gm	**10106-4150-01**	223.05		
2500 gm	**10106-4150-05**	654.20		
TINDAMAX (Mission)				
tinidazole				
TAB, PO (FILM-COATED)				
250 mg, 40s ea	**00178-8250-40**	164.88	137.40	EE
500 mg, 20s ea	**00178-8500-20**	164.88	137.40	
60s ea	**00178-8500-60**	494.64	412.20	

PROD/MFR	NDC	AWP	DP	OBC
(A-S Medication)				
REPACK				
TAB, PO, 500 mg, 12s ea	**54569-5753-00**	54.72		
(PD-Rx Pharm)				
REPACK				
TAB, PO, 500 mg, 4s ea	**55289-0910-04**	30.58		
TINIDAZOLE (Gallipot)				
POW, NA, 100 gm	**51552-0683-05**	119.70	85.50	
(Medisca)				
POW, NA, 25 gm	**38779-0786-04**	76.50		
100 gm	**38779-0786-05**	246.00		
500 gm	**38779-0786-08**	945.00		
1000 gm	**38779-0786-09**	1425.00		
(Mission) *See TINDAMAX*				
(PCCA)				
POW, NA (USP)				
1 gm	**51927-2391-00**	3.36		
(Spectrum Pharmacy)				
POW, NA (U.S.P.)				
25 gm	**49452-0046-01**	93.98		
100 gm	**49452-0046-03**	381.50		
500 gm	**49452-0046-04**	1358.00		
TINZAPARIN SODIUM				
(Celgene Corp) *See INNOHEP*				
TIOPRONIN				
(Mission) *See THIOLA*				
TIOTROPIUM BROMIDE				
(Boehr Ingelheim Phar) *See SPIRIVA*				
TIPRANAVIR				
(Boehr Ingelheim Phar) *See APTIVUS*				
TIROFIBAN HYDROCHLORIDE				
(Medicure) *See AGGRASTAT*				
TIS-U-SOL (Baxter)				
k cl/k phos/mg sulf/na cl/na phos				
SOL, IR, 1000 ml 12s	**00338-0190-04**	272.74		AT
TISSEEL (Baxter Bioscience)				
aprotinin/calcium chloride/fibrinogen/thrombin				
KIT, NA (VHSD)				
3000 kiu/ml-40/ml, 2 ml,	**00944-4201-04**	171.20		
(6X2ML,VALUPAK,VHSD) 3000 kiu/ml-40/ml, 2 ml 6s	**00944-4201-03**	980.90		
(VHSD) 3000 kiu/ml-40/ml, 4 ml	**00944-4201-08**	293.68		
(6X4ML,VALUPAK,VHSD) 3000 kiu/ml-40/ml, 4 ml 6s	**00944-4201-07**	1703.52		
(VHSD) 3000 kiu/ml-40/ml, 10 ml	**00944-4201-12**	707.78		
(6X10ML,VALUPAK,VHSD) 3000 kiu/ml-40/ml, 10 ml 6s	**00944-4201-11**	4179.92		
SOL, NA (FROZEN)				
2 ml	**00944-8402-02**	170.12		
4 ml	**00944-8402-04**	283.92		
10 ml	**00944-8402-10**	696.66		
TISSUEMEND (TEI Biosciences Inc.)				
collagen, bovine				
SHE, IP (3X3CM,STERILE) ea	**08533-6495-06**	1200.00		
(4X4CM,STERILE) ea	**08533-6495-03**	2250.00		
(5X6CM,STERILE) ea	**08533-6495-01**	2595.00		
(6X10CM,STERILE) ea	**08533-6495-04**	3056.00		
TITANIUM DIOXIDE (Amend)				
POW, NA (U.S.P.)				
454 gm	**17317-0706-01**	9.80		
2270 gm	**17317-0706-05**	28.00		
11350 gm	**17317-0706-08**	112.50		
(Gallipot)				
POW, NA (U.S.P.)				
454 gm	**51552-0635-06**	14.21		
(Medisca)				
POW, NA (1X500GM,USP)				
500 gm	**38779-1658-08**	28.50		
(1X2500GM,USP) 2500 gm	**38779-1658-01**	117.00		
(1X12000GM,USP) 12000 gm	**38779-1658-07**	405.00		
(PCCA)				
PAS, NA (1X1GM)				
1 gm	**51927-3820-00**	1.62		
POW, NA (USP)				
1 gm	**51927-1150-00**	0.11		
(Spectrum Pharmacy)				
POW, NA (U.S.P.)				
500 gm	**49452-7820-01**	74.20		
2500 gm	**49452-7820-02**	246.05		
12000 gm	**49452-7820-03**	787.50		
TITANIUM TETRACHLORIDE (Baker, J.T.)				
LIQ, NA (PURIFIED)				
500 ml	**10106-4167-01**	124.84		
TIZANIDINE (4u)				
REPACK				
tizanidine hydrochloride				
TAB, PO, 2 mg, 60s ea	**10544-0349-60**	86.63		
4 mg, 90s ea	**10544-0350-90**	192.08		
(Aidarex)				
REPACK				
TAB, PO, 2 mg, 10s ea	**33261-0103-10**	15.20		
14s ea	**33261-0103-14**	21.28		
20s ea	**33261-0103-20**	30.40		
21s ea	**33261-0103-21**	31.92		
28s ea	**33261-0103-28**	42.56		
30s ea	**33261-0103-30**	45.60		
60s ea	**33261-0103-60**	91.20		
90s ea	**33261-0103-90**	136.80		
4 mg, 10s ea	**33261-0104-10**	18.30		
14s ea	**33261-0104-14**	25.62		
20s ea	**33261-0104-20**	36.60		
21s ea	**33261-0104-21**	38.43		
28s ea	**33261-0104-28**	51.24		
30s ea	**33261-0104-30**	54.90		
60s ea	**33261-0104-60**	110.00		
90s ea	**33261-0104-90**	165.00		
(Bryant Ranch)				
REPACK				
TAB, PO, 2 mg, 30s ea	**63629-3209-01**	46.85		
60s ea	**63629-3209-02**	91.32		
4 mg, 30s ea	**63629-1673-01**	65.52		
60s ea	**63629-1673-02**	101.32		
(Core)				
REPACK				
TAB, PO, 2 mg, 30s ea	**33358-0338-30**	48.02		
60s ea	**33358-0338-60**	93.60		
4 mg, 30s ea	**33358-0339-30**	67.16		
60s ea	**33358-0339-60**	103.85		
120s ea	**33358-0339-01**	182.98		
(DHS, Inc.)				
REPACK				
TAB, PO, 2 mg, 100s ea	**55887-0493-01**	122.19		
4 mg, 28s ea	**55887-0555-28**	60.44		
(IPI)				
REPACK				
TAB, PO, 2 mg, 30s ea	**18837-0152-30**	46.81		
60s ea	**18837-0152-60**	92.62		
100s ea	**18837-0152-99**	122.17		
120s ea	**18837-0152-98**	146.60		
4 mg, 30s ea	**18837-0153-30**	68.00		
60s ea	**18837-0153-60**	110.25		
90s ea	**18837-0153-90**	165.38		
120s ea	**18837-0153-98**	219.78		
270s ea	**18837-0153-94**	494.46		
360s ea	**18837-0153-96**	659.28		
(Phys Total Care)				
REPACK				
TAB, PO, 4 mg, 150s ea	**54868-4939-03**	45.58		
(Physician Partner)				
REPACK				
TAB, PO, 2 mg, 28s ea	**21695-0126-28**	68.41		
30s ea	**21695-0126-30**	73.30		
120s ea	**21695-0126-72**	344.94		
4 mg, 14s ea	**21695-0127-14**	48.26		
30s ea	**21695-0127-30**	87.90		
60s ea	**21695-0127-60**	175.60		
90s ea	**21695-0127-90**	263.70		
120s ea	**21695-0127-72**	351.60		
(Quality Care Prod)				
REPACK				
TAB, PO, 4 mg, 90s ea	**49999-0347-90**	232.59		
(Stat Rx)				
REPACK				
TAB, PO, 2 mg, 20s ea	**16590-0220-20**	30.17		
30s ea	**16590-0220-30**	45.25		
60s ea	**16590-0220-60**	91.50		
90s ea	**16590-0220-90**	137.46		
4 mg, 20s ea	**16590-0221-20**	48.00		
30s ea	**16590-0221-30**	72.00		
60s ea	**16590-0221-60**	144.00		
90s ea	**16590-0221-90**	216.00		
TIZANIDINE HCL (Apotex Corp.)				
tizanidine hydrochloride				
TAB, PO, 2 mg, 150s ea	**60505-0251-03**	183.28		AB
1000s ea	**60505-0251-02**	1221.90		AB
4 mg, 150s ea	**60505-0252-03**	219.76		AB
1000s ea	**60505-0252-02**	1465.24		AB
(Caraco)				
TAB, PO, 2 mg, 30s ea	**57664-0502-83**	36.65		AB
100s ea	**57664-0502-88**	122.17		AB
150s ea	**57664-0502-89**	183.25		AB
500s ea	**57664-0502-13**	610.83		AB
1000s ea	**57664-0502-18**	1221.66		AB
4 mg, 30s ea	**57664-0503-83**	43.95		AB
100s ea	**57664-0503-88**	146.50		AB
150s ea	**57664-0503-89**	219.75		AB
500s ea	**57664-0503-13**	732.50		AB
1000s ea	**57664-0503-18**	1465.00		AB
(Dr Reddy's)				
TAB, PO, 2 mg, 150s ea	**55111-0179-15**	183.28		AB
1000s ea	**55111-0179-10**	1221.87		AB
4 mg, 150s ea	**55111-0180-15**	219.76		AB
1000s ea	**55111-0180-10**	1465.07		AB
(Mylan)				
TAB, PO, 2 mg, 150s ea (USP)	**00378-0722-19**	183.25		AB
2 mg, 500s ea	**00378-0722-05**	610.83		AB
4 mg, 150s ea (USP)	**00378-0724-19**	219.75		AB
4 mg, 500s ea	**00378-0724-05**	732.50		AB
(Sandoz)				
TAB, PO, 2 mg, 150s ea	**00185-0034-51**	183.29		AB
1000s ea	**00185-0034-10**	1221.93		AB
4 mg, 150s ea	**00185-4400-51**	219.78		AB
300s ea	**00185-4400-23**	441.00		AB
1000s ea	**00185-4400-10**	1465.20		AB
(UDL)				
TAB, PO (10X10)				
4 mg, 100s ea UD	**51079-0998-20**	146.50		AB
(4u)				
REPACK				
TAB, PO, 2 mg, 28s ea	**10544-0349-28**	58.28		AB
28s ea	**42549-0549-28**	58.28		AB
60s ea	**42549-0549-60**	86.63		AB
4 mg, 28s ea	**42549-0550-28**	69.92		AB
60s ea	**42549-0350-60**	144.64		AB
60s ea	**42549-0550-60**	144.64		AB
90s ea	**42549-0550-90**	192.08		AB
140s ea	**10544-0350-04**	292.68		AB
140s ea	**42549-0550-04**	292.68		AB
(A-S Medication)				
REPACK				
TAB, PO, 2 mg, 30s ea	**54569-5443-00**	36.66		EE
60s ea	**54569-5443-01**	73.32		EE
4 mg, 14s ea	**54569-5500-07**	20.51		
15s ea	**54569-5500-03**	21.98		
30s ea	**54569-5500-04**	43.96		AB
60s ea	**54569-5500-02**	87.91		AB
90s ea	**54569-5500-06**	131.87		
120s ea	**54569-5500-00**	175.82		AB
(Aidarex)				
REPACK				
TAB, PO, 2 mg, 120s ea	**33261-0103-02**	182.40		AB
(Altura)				
REPACK				
TAB, PO, 2 mg, 16s ea	**63874-0087-16**	23.94		AB
20s ea	**63874-0087-20**	29.40		AB
24s ea	**63874-0087-24**	35.28		AB
25s ea	**63874-0087-25**	36.75		AB
30s ea	**63874-0087-30**	44.88		AB
40s ea	**63874-0087-40**	58.80		AB
45s ea	**63874-0087-45**	66.15		AB
60s ea	**63874-0087-60**	89.76		AB
90s ea	**63874-0087-90**	134.64		AB
100s ea	**63874-0087-01**	149.60		AB
120s ea	**63874-0087-04**	179.52		AB
150s ea	**63874-0087-05**	220.50		AB
4 mg, 20s ea	**63874-1075-02**	34.00		AB
30s ea	**63874-1075-03**	51.00		AB
40s ea	**63874-1075-07**	68.00		AB
45s ea	**63874-1075-08**	76.50		AB
60s ea	**63874-1075-06**	102.00		AB
84s ea	**63874-1075-00**	142.80		AB
90s ea	**63874-1075-09**	153.00		AB
100s ea	**63874-1075-01**	170.00		AB
120s ea	**63874-1075-04**	204.00		AB
150s ea	**63874-1075-05**	255.00		AB

PROD/MFR	NDC	AWP	DP	OBC
(American Health)				
REPACK				
TAB, PO (10X10)				
4 mg, 100s ea UD	68084-0013-01	151.40		AB
(15X30)				
4 mg, 450s ea	68084-0013-85	659.40		AB
(Bryant Ranch)				
REPACK				
TAB, PO, 2 mg, 90s ea	63629-3209-03	140.55		AB
4 mg, 90s ea	63629-1673-03	195.32		AB
120s ea	63629-1673-04	295.64		AB
(DHS, Inc.)				
REPACK				
TAB, PO, 2 mg, 30s ea	55887-0493-30	47.81		AB
60s ea	55887-0493-60	85.69		AB
90s ea	55887-0493-90	128.54		AB
4 mg, 15s ea	55887-0555-15	36.33		EE
30s ea	55887-0555-30	64.76		EE
60s ea	55887-0555-60	129.52		EE
120s ea	55887-0555-82	259.04		EE
(Dispensing Solutions)				
REPACK				
TAB, PO, 2 mg, 30s ea	55045-3219-08	46.50		AB
30s ea	66336-0842-30	47.81		AB
60s ea	55045-3219-06	93.00		EE
60s ea	66336-0842-60	95,62		
90s ea	55045-3219-09	139.50		EE
100s ea	55045-3219-01	155.00		EE
120s ea	55045-3219-02	186.00		EE
135s ea	55045-3219-00	209.25		EE
150s ea	55045-3219-03	232.50		EE
180s ea	55045-3219-04	279.00		EE
4 mg, 15s ea	55045-2926-01	24.50		EE
30s ea	55045-2926-08	48.90		AB
30s ea	66336-0843-30	50.62		AB
60s ea	55045-2926-06	97.80		EE
60s ea	66336-0843-60	100.92		
90s ea	55045-2926-09	146.70		EE
90s ea	66336-0843-90	151.38		AB
100s ea	55045-2926-00	163.00		EE
120s ea	55045-2926-02	195.60		EE
120s ea	66336-0843-94	201.84		AB
150s ea	55045-2926-03	244.50		EE
(IPI)				
REPACK				
TAB, PO, 2 mg, 90s ea	18837-0152-90	137.46		AB
(Keltman Pharma., Inc.)				
REPACK				
TAB, PO, 4 mg, 30s ea	68387-0140-30	64.68		AB
60s ea	68387-0140-60	129.36		AB
90s ea	68387-0140-90	194.04		AB
(Nucare Pharm)				
REPACK				
TAB, PO, 2 mg, 30s ea	66267-0749-30	51.49		AB
60s ea	66267-0749-60	97.25		AB
90s ea	66267-0749-90	144.33		AB
100s ea	66267-0749-00	160.37		AB
120s ea	66267-0749-91	192.44		AB
4 mg, 15s ea	66267-0598-15	30.22		AB
30s ea	66267-0598-30	74.80		AB
45s ea	66267-0598-45	95.68		AB
60s ea	66267-0598-60	115.76		AB
90s ea	66267-0598-90	189.36		AB
120s ea	66267-0598-91	319.43		AB
(PD-Rx Pharm)				
REPACK				
TAB, PO, 2 mg, 12s ea	55289-0809-12	13.55		AB
30s ea	55289-0809-30	17.45		
60s ea	55289-0809-60	34.98		
4 mg, 20s ea	55289-0784-20	19.70		AB
(Pharma Pac)				
REPACK				
TAB, PO, 2 mg, 20s ea	52959-0691-20	35.00		
24s ea	52959-0691-24	39.00		
25s ea	52959-0691-25	40.00		
30s ea	52959-0691-30	45.00		
45s ea	52959-0691-45	52.02		
60s ea	52959-0691-60	69.30		
63s ea	52959-0691-63	72.50		AB
90s ea	52959-0691-90	103.25		
100s ea	52959-0691-00	114.65		AB
120s ea	52959-0691-02	137.50		
150s ea	52959-0691-05	147.50		
4 mg, 15s ea	52959-0689-15	25.12		AB
20s ea	52959-0689-20	33.48		AB
21s ea	52959-0689-21	35.15		AB
30s ea	52959-0689-30	50.19		AB
42s ea	52959-0689-42	70.26		AB
45s ea	52959-0689-45	75.24		AB
60s ea	52959-0689-60	100.29		AB
90s ea	52959-0689-90	150.34		AB
120s ea	52959-0689-02	181.43		AB
150s ea	52959-0689-05	250.27		AB
180s ea	52959-0689-08	272.07		AB
(Phys Total Care)				
REPACK				
TAB, PO, 2 mg, 30s ea	54868-4964-01	12.48		AB
60s ea	54868-4964-02	35.76		EE
100s ea	54868-4964-00	57.60		EE
4 mg, 30s ea	54868-4939-02	14.43		AB
60s ea	54868-4939-00	25.86		AB
90s ea	54868-4939-01	37.32		AB
120s ea	54868-4939-04	40.05		AB
270s ea	54868-4939-05	84.51		AB
(Physician Partner)				
REPACK				
TAB, PO, 2 mg, 90s ea	21695-0126-90	219.91		AB
180s ea	21695-0126-78	517.41		AB
4 mg, 15s ea	21695-0127-15	51.71		AB
(Quality Care Prod)				
REPACK				
TAB, PO, 2 mg, 60s ea	49999-0584-60	128.40		AB
90s ea	49999-0584-90	192.60		AB
4 mg, 28s ea	49999-0347-28	72.36		AB
30s ea	49999-0347-30	65.50		AB
60s ea	49999-0347-60	155.06		AB
120s ea	49999-0347-01	310.13		AB
(Southwood)				
REPACK				
TAB, PO, 2 mg, 30s ea	58016-0737-30	34.36		EE
60s ea	58016-0737-60	68.72		EE
63s ea	58016-0737-88	72.15		AB
90s ea	58016-0737-90	103.08		EE
100s ea	58016-0737-00	114.53		EE
120s ea	58016-0737-02	137.44		EE
180s ea	58016-0737-99	206.16		AB
240s ea	58016-0737-04	274.88		AB
4 mg, 20s ea	58016-0730-20	29.52		EE
63s ea	58016-0730-88	92.99		AB
140s ea	58016-0730-81	206.64		EE
180s ea	58016-0730-99	265.68		AB
240s ea	58016-0730-04	354.24		AB
248s ea	58016-0730-61	366.05		AB
270s ea	58016-0730-79	398.52		AB
280s ea	58016-0730-77	413.28		AB
(St. Mary's MPP)				
REPACK				
TAB, PO (USP)				
2 mg, 15s ea	60760-0782-15	26.13		AB
20s ea	60760-0782-20	32.88		AB
30s ea	60760-0782-30	46.31		AB
60s ea	60760-0782-60	86.63		AB
(Stat Rx)				
REPACK				
TAB, PO, 2 mg, 28s ea	16590-0220-28	42.24		AB
56s ea	16590-0220-56	85.34		AB
75s ea	16590-0220-75	112.25		AB
84s ea	16590-0220-62	126.70		AB
240s ea	16590-0220-84	362.00		AB
270s ea	16590-0220-86	413.10		AB
4 mg, 28s ea	16590-0221-28	53.68		AB
45s ea	16590-0221-45	86.25		EE
84s ea	16590-0221-62	161.00		AB
100s ea	16590-0221-71	191.67		EE
112s ea	16590-0221-73	214.66		AB
150s ea	16590-0221-83	287.51		EE
180s ea	16590-0221-82	288.00		AB
240s ea	16590-0221-84	460.08		AB
270s ea	16590-0221-86	517.59		AB

TIZANIDINE HYDROCHLORIDE

PROD/MFR	NDC	AWP	DP	OBC
FUL				
TAB, PO, 2 mg, 150s ea		39.00		
4 mg, 150s ea		48.00		
(Acorda Therapeutics) *See ZANAFLEX*				
(Acorda Therapeutics) *See ZANAFLEX CAPSULE*				
(Apotex Corp.) *See TIZANIDINE HCL*				
(Caraco) *See TIZANIDINE HCL*				
(CorePharma)				
TAB, PO (COMPRESSED TABLET)				
2 mg, 150s ea	64720-0106-15	183.28		AB
500s ea	64720-0106-50	610.09		AB
1000s ea	64720-0106-11	1221.86		AB
4 mg, 150s ea	64720-0138-15	219.76		AB
500s ea	64720-0138-50	732.49		AB
1000s ea	64720-0138-11	1464.98		AB
(Dr Reddy's) *See TIZANIDINE HCL*				
(Major)				
TAB, PO (10X10)				
4 mg, 100s ea UD	00904-5703-61	143.83		AB
(Mylan) *See TIZANIDINE HCL*				
(Sandoz) *See TIZANIDINE HCL*				
(Teva)				
TAB, PO, 2 mg, 150s ea	00172-5735-29	183.25		AB
500s ea	00172-5735-70	580.29		AB
4 mg, 150s ea	00172-5736-29	219.75		AB
500s ea	00172-5736-70	695.88		AB
(UDL) *See TIZANIDINE HCL*				
(4u)				
REPACK				
TAB, PO (COMPRESSED TABLET)				
4 mg, 60s ea	10544-0397-60	144.64		AB
60s ea	42549-0597-60	144.64		AB
(Dispensing Solutions)				
REPACK				
TAB, PO (COMPRESSED TABLET)				
2 mg, 90s ea	66336-0842-90	139.25		AB
4 mg, 7s ea	55045-3775-07	11.41		
84s ea	55045-3721-04	136.92		
(Keltman Pharma., Inc.)				
REPACK				
TAB, PO (COMPRESSED TABLET)				
2 mg, 30s ea	68387-0130-30	46.16		AB
90s ea	68387-0130-90	138.48		
4 mg, 10s ea	68387-0140-10	21.56		
45s ea	68387-0140-45	97.02		
(Medsource)				
REPACK				
TAB, PO (COMPRESSED TABLET)				
2 mg, 30s ea	45865-0386-30	43.80		AB
60s ea	45865-0386-60	87.60		AB
90s ea	45865-0386-90	131.40		AB
100s ea	45865-0386-00	146.00		AB
120s ea	45865-0386-01	175.20		AB
150s ea	45865-0386-02	219.00		AB
300s ea	45865-0386-05	438.00		AB
4 mg, 30s ea	45865-0348-30	52.20		AB
60s ea	45865-0348-60	104.40		AB
90s ea	45865-0348-90	156.60		AB
100s ea	45865-0348-00	174.00		AB
120s ea	45865-0348-01	208.80		AB
150s ea	45865-0348-02	261.00		AB
300s ea	45865-0348-05	522.00		AB
(Palmetto)				
REPACK				
TAB, PO, 2 mg, 30s ea	23490-7388-02	47.81		
60s ea	23490-7388-01	95.62		
90s ea	23490-7388-09	143.43		
120s ea	23490-7388-04	191.24		
4 mg, 15s ea	23490-7040-04	26.25		
30s ea	23490-7040-01	52.50		
60s ea	23490-7040-02	105.00		
90s ea	23490-7040-03	157.50		
100s ea	23490-7040-05	175.00		
120s ea	23490-7040-06	178.50		
180s ea	23490-7040-07	252.00		
(PD-Rx Pharm)				
REPACK				
TAB, PO, 4 mg, 30s ea	55289-0784-30	29.38		
60s ea	55289-0784-60	41.18		
90s ea	55289-0784-90	53.75		
(Pharma Pac)				
REPACK				
TAB, PO (COMPRESSED TABLET)				
4 mg, 63s ea	52959-0689-63	105.26		AB
(Quality Care Prod)				
REPACK				
TAB, PO, 2 mg, 30s ea	49999-0584-30	64.21		
150s ea	49999-0584-15	321.00		
(Southwood)				
REPACK				
TAB, PO (COMPRESSED TABLET)				
4 mg, 30s ea	58016-0730-30	55.20		AB
60s ea	58016-0730-60	110.40		AB
90s ea	58016-0730-90	165.60		AB
100s ea	58016-0730-00	184.00		AB
120s ea	58016-0730-02	220.80		AB
(St. Mary's MPP)				
REPACK				
TAB, PO (USP,COMPRESSED TABLET)				
4 mg, 15s ea	60760-0503-15	30.17		AB
(USP)				
4 mg, 30s ea	60760-0503-30	54.35		
60s ea	60760-0503-60	102.58		
90s ea	60760-0503-90	153.87		

PROD/MFR NDC AWP DP OBC

(Vibranta)
REPACK
TAB, PO, 2 mg, 30s ea **57866-6755-01** 46.50
60s ea **57866-6755-02** 80.25
90s ea **57866-6755-03** 120.38
4 mg, 30s ea **57866-6756-01** 65.50
60s ea **57866-6756-02** 155.06
90s ea **57866-6756-03** 232.59

TNKASE (Genentech)
tenecteplase
KIT, IV (VIAL W/DILUENT,SRN,PADS)
50 mg, ea **50242-0038-61** 3238.76

TOBI (Novartis Pharm)
tobramycin sulfate
SOL, IH (56X5ML,SDA,PF)
300 mg/5 ml,
5 ml 56s **00078-0494-71** 4924.07

TOBRADEX (Alcon Ophthalmic)
dexamethasone/tobramycin
OIN, OP, 0.1%-0.3%,
3.5 gm **00065-0648-35** 121.80
SUS, OP, 0.1%-0.3%,
2.5 ml .... **00065-0647-25** 48.12 AB
5 ml .... **00065-0647-05** 96.36 AB
10 ml .... **00065-0647-10** 192.72 AB

(A-S Medication)
REPACK
OIN, OP, 0.1%-0.3%,
3.5 gm **54569-2590-00** 116.38
SUS, OP, 0.1%-0.3%,
2.5 ml .... **54569-4400-00** 46.00 AB
5 ml .... **54569-2285-00** 92.06 AB
10 ml .... **54569-4493-00** 178.75 AB

(DHS, Inc.)
REPACK
OIN, OP, 0.1%-0.3%,
3.5 gm **55887-0700-35** 93.25
SUS, OP, 0.1%-0.3%,
2.5 ml .... **55887-0732-25** 43.00 AB

(Dispensing Solutions)
REPACK
OIN, OP, 0.1%-0.3%,
3.5 gm **55045-2213-05** 100.00
SUS, OP, 0.1%-0.3%,
2.5 ml .... **55045-2187-02** 44.50 AB
5 ml .... **55045-2187-05** 89.00 AB

(IPI)
REPACK
SUS, OP, 0.1%-0.3%,
2.5 ml .... **18837-0326-67** 50.03 AB

(Nucare Pharm)
REPACK
SUS, OP, 0.1%-0.3%, 5 ml. **66267-0937-05** 42.56 AB

(PD-Rx Pharm)
REPACK
SUS, OP, 0.1%-0.3%,
2.5 ml .... **43063-0005-01** 44.69 AB

(Pharma Pac)
REPACK
OIN, OP, 0.1%-0.3%,
3.5 gm **52959-0592-03** 119.90
SUS, OP, 0.1%-0.3%, 5 ml. **52959-0092-00** 129.90 AB
10 ml .... **52959-0092-01** 193.83 AB

(Phys Total Care)
REPACK
OIN, OP, 0.1%-0.3%,
3.5 gm **54868-2788-00** 69.56
SUS, OP, 0.1%-0.3%,
2.5 ml .... **54868-2789-01** 55.74 AB
5 ml .... **54868-2789-00** 112.73 AB
10 ml .... **54868-2789-02** 132.06 AB

(Physician Partner)
REPACK
OIN, OP, 0.1%-0.3%,
3.5 gm **21695-0628-35** 232.76
SUS, OP, 0.1%-0.3%, 5 ml. **21695-0203-05** 178.76 AB

(Quality Care Prod)
REPACK
OIN, OP, 0.1%-0.3%,
3.5 gm **49999-0174-35** 184.82
SUS, OP, 0.1%-0.3%,
2.5 ml .... **49999-0147-25** 89.19 AB
5 ml .... **49999-0147-05** 168.59 AB
(1X10ML)
0.1%-0.3%, 10 ml .... **49999-0147-10** 327.71 AB

PROD/MFR NDC AWP DP OBC

(Southwood)
REPACK
OIN, OP, 0.1%-0.3%,
3.5 gm **58016-6073-01** 96.78
SUS, OP, 0.1%-0.3%,
2.5 ml .... **58016-6527-01** 42.90 AB
5 ml .... **58016-5014-01** 62.13 AB

(Stat Rx)
REPACK
SUS, OP, 0.1%-0.3%,
2.5 ml .... **16590-0223-25** 60.71 AB
5 ml .... **16590-0223-05** 102.15 AB

TOBRAMYCIN
FUL
SOL, OP, 0.3%, 5 ml 3.36

(Akorn) *See AKTOB*

TOBRAMYCIN (Akorn)
tobramycin sulfate
SOL, IJ (USP,MDV,25X2ML)
40 mg/ml, 2 ml 25s... **23360-0014-02** 62.00 AP
(USP,MDV,1X30ML)
40 mg/ml, 30 ml ..... **23360-0014-30** 27.23 AP

TOBRAMYCIN
(Alcon Ophthalmic) *See TOBREX*

(Apotex Corp.)
SOL, OP, 0.3%, 5 ml ...... **60505-0558-00** 15.50 AT

(Bausch & Lomb Inc.)
SOL, OP, 0.3%, 5 ml ...... **24208-0290-05** 15.00 AT

(Falcon Ophthalmics)
SOL, OP, 0.3%, 5 ml ...... **61314-0643-05** 15.00 AT

(Major)
SOL, OP, 0.3%, 5 ml ...... **00904-2970-05** 14.95 AT

(Ocusoft) *See TOBRASOL*

(PCCA)
POW, NA (USP)
1 gm **51927-2375-00** 174.00

(Spectrum Pharmacy)
POW, NA (U.S.P.)
1 gm **49452-7823-01** 184.45
(USP)
5 gm **49452-7823-02** 637.00

(A-S Medication)
REPACK
SOL, OP, 0.3%, 5 ml ...... **54569-3781-00** 15.00 EE

(Altura)
REPACK
SOL, OP, 0.3%, 5 ml ...... **63874-0733-05** 54.50 EE

(DHS, Inc.)
REPACK
SOL, OP, 0.3%, 5 ml ...... **55887-0728-05** 22.78 AT

(Dispensing Solutions)
REPACK
SOL, OP, 0.3%, 5 ml ...... **55045-2114-05** 22.25 AT

(IPI)
REPACK
OIN, OP (1X3.5GM)
0.3%, 3.5 gm **18837-0324-68** 75.66
SOL, OP (1X5ML)
0.3%, 5 ml .... **18837-0325-05** 20.75 AT

(Keltman Pharma., Inc.)
REPACK
SOL, OP, 0.3%, 5 ml **68387-0495-01** 19.89

(Nucare Pharm)
REPACK
SOL, OP, 0.3%, 5 ml ...... **66267-0936-05** 22.83 AT

(Palmetto)
REPACK
SOL, OP, 0.3%, 5 ml **23490-6395-01** 54.50

(Pharma Pac)
REPACK
SOL, OP, 0.3%, 5 ml ...... **52959-0108-03** 31.95 EE

(Phys Total Care)
REPACK
SOL, OP, 0.3%, 5 ml ...... **54868-3118-00** 14.79 EE

(Physician Partner)
REPACK
SOL, OP, 0.3%, 5 ml **21695-0204-05** 30.00

(Southwood)
REPACK
SOL, OP, 0.3%, 5 ml ...... **58016-6489-01** 28.95 EE

PROD/MFR NDC AWP DP OBC

(Stat Rx)
REPACK
SOL, OP, 0.3%, 5 ml **16590-0224-05** 36.25

TOBRAMYCIN AND DEXAMETHASONE
(Bausch & Lomb Inc.)
dexamethasone/tobramycin
SUS, OP (USP,1X2.5ML)
0.1%-0.3%, 2.5 ml ... **24208-0295-25** 40.25 AB
(USP,1X5ML)
0.1%-0.3%, 5 ml ..... **24208-0295-05** 80.49 AB
(USP,1X10ML)
0.1%-0.3%, 10 ml .... **24208-0295-10** 160.98 AB

(Falcon Ophthalmics)
SUS, OP (1X2.5ML,DROP TAINER)
0.1%-0.3%, 2.5 ml ... **61314-0647-25** 34.32 AB
(1X5ML,DROP-TAINER)
0.1%-0.3%, 5 ml ..... **61314-0647-05** 68.64 AB
(1X10ML,DROP-TAINER)
0.1%-0.3%, 10 ml .... **61314-0647-10** 137.28 AB

(A-S Medication)
REPACK
SUS, OP, 0.1%-0.3%,
2.5 ml .... **54569-6134-00** 40.57 AB
(1X5GM)
0.1%-0.3%, 5 ml ..... **54569-6135-00** 81.14 AB

(Aidarex)
REPACK
SUS, OP (1X2.5ML)
0.1%-0.3%, 2.5 ml ... **33261-0401-01** 44.05 AB

(Pharma Pac)
REPACK
SUS, OP (1X5ML)
0.1%-0.3%, 5 ml ..... **52959-0984-01** 88.51 AB

TOBRAMYCIN SULFATE
(Akorn) *See TOBRAMYCIN*

(APP)
PDS, IV (BULK VIAL,PF,LATEX-FREE)
1.2 gm, 6s ea **63323-0303-51** 1417.50
SOL, IJ (PEDIATRIC M.D.V.,25X2ML)
10 mg/ml, 2 ml 25s... **63323-0305-02** 91.88 AP
(M.D.V.,25X2ML)
40 mg/ml, 2 ml 25s... **63323-0306-02** 105.94 AP
(M.D.V.,10X30ML)
40 mg/ml,
30 ml 10s .... **63323-0306-30** 275.00 AP
(PHARMACY BULK PACKAGE)
40 mg/ml, 50 ml ..... **63323-0307-51** 40.00 AP

(APP) *See TOBRAMYCIN SULFATE NOVAPLUS*

(Gallipot)
POW, NA (1X1GM,USP)
1 gm **51552-0789-01** 35.00 25.00
(1X5GM,USP)
5 gm **51552-0789-02** 137.90 98.50
(1X25GM,USP)
25 gm **51552-0789-04** 564.20 403.00
(1X100GM,USP)
100 gm **51552-0789-05** 1757.00 1255.00

(Hawkins)
POW, NA (U.S.P.)
1 gm **63370-0275-10** 100.80
5 gm **63370-0275-15** 472.80
25 gm **63370-0275-25** 1934.40
100 gm **63370-0275-35** 5472.00

(Hospira)
SOL, IJ (VIAL,FLIPTOP,LATEX-FREE)
10 mg/ml, 2 ml 25s... **00409-3577-01** 80.70 70.50 AP
(VIAL,ADD-VANTAGE)
10 mg/ml, 8 ml 25s... **00409-3255-03** 137.70 120.50 AP
(VIAL, FLIPTOP)
40 mg/ml, 2 ml 25s... **00074-3578-01** 48.30 42.25 AP
(VIAL,FLIPTOP)
40 mg/ml, 2 ml 25s... **00409-3578-01** 48.30 42.25 AP
(BULK PACKAGE)
40 mg/ml, 50 ml ..... **00409-3590-02** 43.08 37.70 AP

(Letco)
POW, NA, 1 gm **62991-1351-01** 51.00
5 gm **62991-1351-02** 240.00
10 gm **62991-1351-03** 450.00
(U.S.P.)
25 gm **62991-1351-04** 1080.00
100 gm **62991-1351-05** 2700.00

(Medisca)
POW, NA (U.S.P.)
1 gm **38779-0319-06** 70.50
5 gm **38779-0319-03** 297.00
10 gm **38779-0319-01** 525.00
25 gm **38779-0319-04** 1245.00

PROD/MFR	NDC	AWP	DP	OBC
(Novartis Pharm) *See TOBI*				
(Teva)				
SOL, IJ (M.D.V.)				
40 mg/ml, 2 ml 25s	**00703-9402-04**	61.88		**AP**
30 ml	**00703-9416-01**	28.80		**AP**
(X-Gen)				
PDS, IV (BULK VIAL,PF)				
1.2 gm, ea	**39822-0412-01**	338.25		**AP**
6s ea	**39822-0412-06**	1919.88		**AP**
(Medisca) REPACK				
POW, NA (U.S.P.)				
100 gm	**38779-0319-05**	3285.00		
(Phys Total Care) REPACK				
SOL, IJ (M.D.V.)				
40 mg/ml, 2 ml 25s	**54868-4106-00**	148.35		**AP**
TOBRAMYCIN SULFATE NOVAPLUS (APP)				
tobramycin sulfate				
PDS, IV (BULK PKG,50ML VIAL X 6)				
1.2 gm, 6s ea	**63323-0303-55**	1417.50		**AP**
TOBRASOL (Ocusoft)				
tobramycin				
SOL, OP, 0.3%, 5 ml	**54799-0513-05**	8.43		**AT**
TOBREX (Alcon Ophthalmic)				
tobramycin				
OIN, OP, 0.3%, 3.5 gm	**00065-0644-35**	75.96		
SOL, OP, 0.3%, 5 ml	**00065-0643-05**	64.98		**AT**
(A-S Medication) REPACK				
OIN, OP, 0.3%, 3.5 gm	**54569-1182-00**	75.38		
SOL, OP, 0.3%, 5 ml	**54569-0878-00**	64.44		**AT**
(DHS, Inc.) REPACK				
OIN, OP, 0.3%, 3.5 gm	**55887-0725-35**	79.56		
(Dispensing Solutions) REPACK				
OIN, OP, 0.3%, 3.5 gm	**55045-1634-09**	85.00		
SOL, OP, 0.3%, 5 ml	**55045-1367-05**	60.00		
(Nucare Pharm) REPACK				
OIN, OP (1X3.5GM)				
0.3%, 3.5 gm	**68071-1335-05**	98.93		
(Pharma Pac) REPACK				
OIN, OP, 0.3%, 3.5 gm	**52959-0051-01**	85.50		
SOL, OP, 0.3%, 5 ml	**52959-0590-00**	44.79		**AT**
(Phys Total Care) REPACK				
OIN, OP, 0.3%, 4 gm	**54868-1682-00**	76.44		
SOL, OP, 0.3%, 5 ml	**54868-0638-00**	57.90		**AT**
(Physician Partner) REPACK				
OIN, OP, 0.3%, 3.5 gm	**21695-0458-35**	150.76		
(Quality Care Prod) REPACK				
OIN, OP, 0.3%, 3.5 gm	**49999-0259-35**	118.00		
SOL, OP, 0.3%, 5 ml	**49999-0148-05**	53.23		**AT**
(Southwood) REPACK				
OIN, OP, 0.3%, 3.5 gm	**58016-5013-01**	67.62		
3.5 gm	**58016-5013-03**	25.60		
SOL, OP, 0.3%, 5 ml	**58016-6074-05**	22.10		**AT**
(1X5ML)				
0.3%, 5 ml	**58016-6074-01**	58.92		**AT**
(Stat Rx) REPACK				
OIN, OP, 0.3%, 3.5 gm	**16590-0222-35**	87.39		
3.5 gm	**16590-0225-35**	80.86		
TOCILIZUMAB				
(Genentech) *See ACTEMRA*				
TOCOPHERSOLAN				
(PCCA) *See TOCOPHERYL PEG 1000 SUCCINATE (D-ALPHA)*				
TOCOPHERYL ACID SUCCINATE (PCCA)				
d-alpha tocopheryl acid succinate				
POW, NA (FCC)				
1 gm	**51927-1374-00**	1.71		
TOCOPHERYL PEG 1000 SUCCINATE (D-ALPHA) (PCCA)				
tocophersolan				
WAX, NA (NF)				
1 gm	**51927-2396-00**	3.54		
TOFRANIL (Covidien)				
imipramine hydrochloride				
TAB, PO (SUGAR-COATED)				
10 mg, 30s ea	**00406-9920-03**	179.96		**AB**
25 mg, 30s ea	**00406-9921-03**	179.96		**AB**
50 mg, 30s ea	**00406-9922-03**	179.96		**AB**
TOFRANIL-PM (Covidien)				
imipramine pamoate				
CAP, PO (USP)				
75 mg, 30s ea	**00406-9923-03**	565.70		
100 mg, 30s ea	**00406-9924-03**	565.70		
125 mg, 30s ea	**00406-9925-03**	565.70		
150 mg, 30s ea	**00406-9926-03**	565.70		
TOLAZAMIDE (Consolidated Midland)				
TAB, PO, 100 mg, 100s ea	**00223-2081-01**	12.50		**EE**
500s ea	**00223-2081-05**	67.50		**EE**
250 mg, 100s ea	**00223-2082-01**	21.00		**EE**
1000s ea	**00223-2082-02**	190.00		**EE**
500 mg, 100s ea	**00223-2083-01**	35.00		**EE**
500s ea	**00223-2083-05**	175.00		**EE**
(Mylan)				
TAB, PO, 250 mg, 100s ea	**00378-0217-01**	106.53		**AB**
500 mg, 100s ea	**00378-0551-01**	160.88		**AB**
(PD-Rx Pharm) REPACK				
TAB, PO, 250 mg, 90s ea	**55289-0265-90**	63.87		**AB**
(Phys Total Care) REPACK				
TAB, PO, 250 mg, 100s ea	**54868-1020-00**	120.33		**EE**
TOLAZOLINE HCL (PCCA)				
tolazoline hydrochloride				
POW, NA, 1 gm	**51927-2593-00**	10.20		
TOLAZOLINE HYDROCHLORIDE (Medisca)				
POW, NA (1X100GM)				
100 gm	**38779-2278-05**	375.00		
(1X1000GM)				
1000 gm	**38779-2278-09**	2550.00		
(PCCA) *See TOLAZOLINE HCL*				
(Spectrum Pharmacy)				
CRY, NA (1X25GM)				
25 gm	**49452-7831-02**	296.45		
(1X100GM)				
100 gm	**49452-7831-04**	868.00		
(1X1000GM)				
1000 gm	**49452-7831-05**	3892.00		
TOLBUTAMIDE (Consolidated Midland)				
TAB, PO, 500 mg, 100s ea	**00223-1076-01**	8.75		**EE**
1000s ea	**00223-1076-02**	52.50		**EE**
(Mylan)				
TAB, PO, 500 mg, 100s ea	**00378-0215-01**	37.16		**AB**
500s ea	**00378-0215-05**	185.80		**AB**
(Phys Total Care) REPACK				
TAB, PO, 500 mg, 100s ea	**54868-1361-01**	20.58		**EE**
TOLCAPONE				
(Valeant Pharm Intl) *See TASMAR*				
TOLMETIN SODIUM (Mutual)				
TAB, PO, 200 mg, 100s ea	**53489-0506-01**	75.00		**AB**
(Mylan)				
CAP, PO, 400 mg, 100s ea	**00378-5200-01**	170.05		**AB**
TAB, PO, 600 mg, 100s ea	**00378-0313-01**	180.10		**AB**
(Teva)				
CAP, PO, 400 mg, 100s ea	**00093-8815-01**	118.25		**AB**
(HomeMed) REPACK				
CAP, PO, 400 mg, 24s ea	**51655-0562-30**	19.24		**AB**
(Pharma Pac) REPACK				
CAP, PO, 400 mg, 21s ea	**52959-0342-21**	19.10		**EE**
30s ea	**52959-0342-30**	42.28		**EE**
50s ea	**52959-0342-50**	38.80		**EE**
60s ea	**52959-0342-60**	46.25		**EE**
90s ea	**52959-0342-90**	130.47		**EE**
100s ea	**52959-0342-00**	144.98		**EE**
(Phys Total Care) REPACK				
TAB, PO, 600 mg, 30s ea	**54868-2421-01**	150.98		**EE**
100s ea	**54868-2421-00**	460.93		**EE**
(Quality Care Prod) REPACK				
CAP, PO, 400 mg, 30s ea	**35356-0330-30**	94.64		**AB**
100s ea	**35356-0330-90**	315.00		**AB**
(Southwood) REPACK				
CAP, PO, 400 mg, 30s ea	**58016-0614-30**	42.00		**EE**
60s ea	**58016-0614-60**	84.00		**EE**
90s ea	**58016-0614-90**	126.00		**EE**
100s ea	**58016-0614-00**	140.00		**EE**
TAB, PO, 600 mg, 30s ea	**58016-0658-30**	40.35		**AB**
60s ea	**58016-0658-60**	80.70		**AB**
90s ea	**58016-0658-90**	121.05		**AB**
100s ea	**58016-0658-00**	134.50		**AB**
120s ea	**58016-0658-02**	161.40		**AB**
150s ea	**58016-0658-03**	201.75		**AB**
TOLNAFTATE (Gallipot)				
POW, NA (U.S.P.,N.F.)				
10 gm	**51552-0198-03**	25.13		
50 gm	**51552-0198-09**	95.90		
(Medisca)				
POW, NA (U.S.P.)				
25 gm	**38779-0052-04**	117.00		
100 gm	**38779-0052-05**	429.00		
(PCCA)				
POW, NA (U.S.P.)				
1 gm	**51927-1574-00**	6.30		
(Spectrum Pharmacy)				
POW, NA (U.S.P.)				
10 gm	**49452-7834-01**	118.30		
50 gm	**49452-7834-04**	395.50		
250 gm	**49452-7834-05**	1113.00		
(Keltman Pharma., Inc.) REPACK				
CRE, TP, 1%, 15 gm	**68387-0447-01**	48.00		
TOLONIUM CHLORIDE				
(PCCA) *See TOLUIDINE BLUE O*				
(Spectrum Pharmacy) *See TOLUIDINE BLUE O*				
TOLTERODINE TARTRATE				
(Pfizer) *See DETROL*				
(Pfizer) *See DETROL LA*				
TOLU BALSAM				
(Amend) *See BALSAM TOLU*				
(PCCA)				
POW, NA (USP)				
1 gm	**51927-1700-00**	2.11		
TIN, NA, 1 ml	**51927-2689-00**	0.28		
TOLUENE (Amend)				
LIQ, NA (PURE)				
480 ml	**17317-0581-01**	4.90		
(A.C.S., REAGENT)				
500 ml	**17317-1385-01**	7.00		
(PURE)				
3840 ml	**17317-0581-06**	13.30		
(A.C.S., REAGENT)				
4000 ml	**17317-1385-05**	28.00		
19200 ml	**17317-1385-08**	72.80		
(PURE)				
19200 ml	**17317-0581-08**	49.00		
(Baker, J.T.)				
LIQ, NA (A.C.S., REAGENT)				
500 ml	**10106-9460-01**	19.62		
4000 ml	**10106-9460-03**	86.31		
(Mallinckrodt Lab)				
LIQ, NA (A.C.S.)				
500 ml	**00406-8608-04**	12.79		
(PCCA)				
LIQ, NA (ACS REAGENT)				
1 ml	**51927-2296-00**	0.12		
TOLUIDINE BLUE O (PCCA)				
tolonium chloride				
POW, NA, 1 gm	**51927-1315-00**	9.00		
(Spectrum Pharmacy)				
POW, NA (C.I. 52040)				
10 gm	**49452-7840-01**	110.95		
25 gm	**49452-7840-02**	156.10		
100 gm	**49452-7840-04**	476.00		
TOLVAPTAN				
(Otsuka) *See SAMSCA*				
TOPAMAX (Ortho-McNeil Neuro)				
topiramate				
CAP, PO (HARD GELATIN)				
15 mg, 60s ea	**50458-0647-65**	176.77	147.31	**AB**
25 mg, 60s ea	**50458-0645-65**	213.70	178.08	**AB**
(Ortho-McNeil Pharm)				
TAB, PO (COATED)				
25 mg, 60s ea	**50458-0639-65**	186.91	155.76	
50 mg, 60s ea	**50458-0640-65**	373.03	310.86	**EE**
100 mg, 60s ea	**50458-0641-65**	509.44	424.53	**EE**
200 mg, 60s ea	**50458-0642-65**	596.39	496.99	**EE**

PROD/MFR	NDC	AWP	DP	OBC
(A-S Medication)				
REPACK				
TAB, PO (FILM-COATED)				
25 mg, 60s ea	54569-4831-00	212.80		
100 mg, 30s ea	54569-5473-00	290.00		
(Altura)				
REPACK				
TAB, PO (FILM COATED)				
25 mg, 60s ea	63874-1128-06	136.20		
(Core)				
REPACK				
TAB, PO, 25 mg, 56s ea	33358-0341-56	133.50		
(DHS, Inc.)				
REPACK				
TAB, PO (FILM-COATED)				
25 mg, 60s ea	55887-0517-60	151.71		
50 mg, 30s ea	55887-0186-30	125.98		
(FILM-COATED)				
100 mg, 30s ea	55887-0489-30	185.00		
60s ea	55887-0489-60	361.16		
90s ea	55887-0489-90	462.00		
(Dispensing Solutions)				
REPACK				
CAP, PO, 25 mg, 60s ea	55045-3076-06	150.00		
TAB, PO (FILM-COATED)				
25 mg, 120s ea	55045-3076-01	300.00		
100 mg, 30s ea	55045-3124-08	195.00		
60s ea	55045-3124-06	390.00		
(IPI)				
REPACK				
TAB, PO, 25 mg, 180s ea	18837-0155-96	499.72		
50 mg, 60s ea	18837-0156-60	332.44		
(Keltman Pharma., Inc.)				
REPACK				
TAB, PO (FILM-COATED)				
25 mg, 60s ea	68387-0555-60	132.25		
120s ea	68387-0555-12	289.45		
100 mg, 30s ea	68387-0556-30	184.63		
(Nucare Pharm)				
REPACK				
TAB, PO (FILM-COATED)				
100 mg, 30s ea	68071-0320-30	233.81		
(COATED)				
100 mg, 60s ea	66267-1301-06	512.21		EE
(FILM-COATED)				
200 mg, 60s ea	66267-1302-06	598.47		
(Palmetto)				
REPACK				
TAB, PO, 100 mg, 20s ea	23490-9000-00	103.60		
30s ea	23490-9000-03	155.40		
(PD-Rx Pharm)				
REPACK				
TAB, PO, 25 mg, 30s ea	55289-0901-30	121.65		
50 mg, 30s ea	55289-0433-30	242.78		
(FILM-COATED)				
100 mg, 30s ea	55289-0497-30	303.24		
(Pharma Pac)				
REPACK				
TAB, PO, 25 mg, 60s ea	52959-0780-60	164.40		
(Phys Total Care)				
REPACK				
TAB, PO (FILM-COATED)				
25 mg, 30s ea	54868-4672-01	105.20		
60s ea	54868-4672-00	195.73		
90s ea	54868-4672-03	292.61		
210s ea	54868-4672-02	599.81		
50 mg, 30s ea	54868-5343-01	195.97		
60s ea	54868-5343-00	388.67		
100 mg, 10s ea	54868-4674-00	94.90		
(FILM-COATED)				
100 mg, 30s ea	54868-4674-01	218.78		
60s ea	54868-4674-02	435.07		
(FILM-COATED)				
200 mg, 30s ea	54868-5190-01	265.09		
60s ea	54868-5190-00	527.56		
(Physician Partner)				
REPACK				
TAB, PO (FILM-COATED)				
25 mg, 15s ea	21695-0128-15	85.38		
(COATED,FILM-COATED)				
25 mg, 60s ea	21695-0128-60	341.02		
50 mg, 15s ea	21695-0129-15	170.39		
(FILM-COATED)				
100 mg, 15s ea	21695-0130-15	232.69		

PROD/MFR	NDC	AWP	DP	OBC
(Quality Care Prod)				
REPACK				
TAB, PO (FILM-COATED)				
25 mg, 15s ea	49999-0698-15	75.00		
30s ea	49999-0698-30	151.00		
60s ea	49999-0698-60	316.00		
(FILM-COATED)				
25 mg, 90s ea	49999-0698-90	452.70		
50 mg, 60s ea	49999-0955-60	393.33		
(FILM-COATED)				
100 mg, 15s ea	49999-0605-15	165.00		
30s ea	49999-0605-30	397.00		
60s ea	49999-0605-60	794.00		
(FILM-COATED)				
100 mg, 120s ea	49999-0605-01	1320.00		
120s ea	49999-0698-01	632.00		
200 mg, 30s ea	35356-0401-30	381.00		
(Southwood)				
REPACK				
CAP, PO, 15 mg, 30s ea	58016-0626-30	70.44		
60s ea	58016-0626-60	140.87		
90s ea	58016-0626-90	211.31		
100s ea	58016-0626-00	234.78		
TAB, PO, 25 mg, 10s ea	58016-0478-10	24.82		
30s ea	58016-0478-30	74.47		
40s ea	58016-0478-40	99.29		
60s ea	58016-0478-60	148.94		
90s ea	58016-0478-90	223.41		
100s ea	58016-0478-00	248.23		
(FILM-COATED)				
100 mg, 30s ea	58016-0961-30	202.98		
60s ea	58016-0961-60	405.96		
90s ea	58016-0961-90	608.94		
100s ea	58016-0961-00	676.60		
200 mg, 30s ea	58016-0047-30	237.63		
60s ea	58016-0047-60	475.25		
90s ea	58016-0047-90	712.88		
100s ea	58016-0047-00	792.08		
(St. Mary's MPP)				
REPACK				
TAB, PO (FILM-COATED)				
25 mg, 30s ea	60760-0639-30	133.88		
60s ea	60760-0639-60	261.77		
90s ea	60760-0639-90	389.65		
100 mg, 30s ea	60760-0641-30	354.56		
60s ea	60760-0641-60	703.11		
90s ea	60760-0641-90	1051.67		
(Stat Rx)				
REPACK				
TAB, PO (FILM-COATED)				
25 mg, 30s ea	16590-0226-30	96.67		
56s ea	16590-0226-56	179.12		
60s ea	16590-0226-60	191.91		
90s ea	16590-0226-90	287.14		
120s ea	16590-0226-72	382.38		
50 mg, 30s ea	16590-0227-30	191.53		
60s ea	16590-0227-60	381.62		
90s ea	16590-0227-90	474.00		
120s ea	16590-0227-72	761.79		
(FILM-COATED)				
100 mg, 30s ea	16590-0228-30	261.03		
45s ea	16590-0228-45	390.82		
60s ea	16590-0228-60	520.07		
90s ea	16590-0228-90	780.20		
200 mg, 30s ea	16590-0543-30	305.34		
60s ea	16590-0543-60	609.25		
90s ea	16590-0543-90	913.15		
TOPICORT (Taro)				
desoximetasone				
CRE, TP, 0.25%, 15 gm	51672-5204-01	64.76		AB
60 gm	51672-5204-03	221.38		AB
(1X100GM)				
0.25%, 100 gm	51672-5204-07	254.35		AB
(2X100GM)				
0.25%, 100 gm 2s	51672-5204-09	431.38		AB
GEL, TP, 0.05%, 15 gm	51672-5202-01	55.17		AB
60 gm	51672-5202-03	176.55		AB
OIN, TP, 0.25%, 15 gm	51672-5203-01	69.63		AB
60 gm	51672-5203-03	231.23		AB
(1X100GM)				
0.25%, 100 gm	51672-5203-07	265.25		AB
(Phys Total Care)				
REPACK				
CRE, TP, 0.25%, 15 gm	54868-0976-01	45.36		AB
60 gm	54868-0976-02	105.25		AB
OIN, TP, 0.25%, 15 gm	54868-2662-01	45.36		AB
60 gm	54868-2662-02	105.25		AB
(Southwood)				
REPACK				
CRE, TP, 0.25%, 15 gm	58016-3187-01	64.76		AB

PROD/MFR	NDC	AWP	DP	OBC
TOPICORT LP (Taro)				
desoximetasone				
CRE, TP, 0.05%, 15 gm	51672-5205-01	51.76		
60 gm	51672-5205-03	191.83		
(3X100GM)				
0.05%, 100 gm 3s	51672-5205-08	662.40		
TOPIRAGEN (Upsher-Smith)				
topiramate				
TAB, PO (COATED)				
25 mg, 60s ea	00245-0711-60	127.72		
50 mg, 60s ea	00245-0712-60	254.90		
100 mg, 60s ea	00245-0713-60	348.11		
200 mg, 60s ea	00245-0714-60	407.53		
TOPIRAMATE				
FUL				
TAB, PO, 25 mg, 60s ea		14.52		
50 mg, 60s ea		28.89		
100 mg, 60s ea		39.56		
200 mg, 60s ea		46.31		
(Apotex Corp.)				
TAB, PO (FILM-COATED)				
25 mg, 60s ea	60505-2760-06	153.46		EE
500s ea	60505-2760-05	1240.47		EE
50 mg, 60s ea	60505-2761-06	306.27		EE
500s ea	60505-2761-05	2475.68		EE
100 mg, 60s ea	60505-2762-06	418.26		EE
500s ea	60505-2762-05	3380.94		EE
200 mg, 60s ea	60505-2763-06	489.65		EE
500s ea	60505-2763-05	3958.00		EE
(Aurobindo Pharma)				
TAB, PO (FILM-COATED)				
25 mg, 60s ea	65862-0171-60	153.25		AB
50 mg, 60s ea	65862-0172-60	305.90		AB
100 mg, 60s ea	65862-0173-60	417.80		AB
200 mg, 60s ea	65862-0174-60	489.10		AB
(Camber)				
TAB, PO, 25 mg, 60s ea	31722-0278-60	151.57		
1000s ea	31722-0278-10	2273.55		
50 mg, 60s ea	31722-0279-60	302.53		
1000s ea	31722-0279-10	4537.95		
100 mg, 60s ea	31722-0280-60	413.15		
1000s ea	31722-0280-10	6197.25		
200 mg, 60s ea	31722-0281-60	483.68		AB
1000s ea	31722-0281-10	7255.20		AB
(Caraco)				
TAB, PO (FILM-COATED)				
25 mg, 60s ea	62756-0707-86	153.25		AB
500s ea	62756-0707-13	1277.00		AB
50 mg, 60s ea	62756-0710-86	305.90		AB
500s ea	62756-0710-13	2549.00		AB
100 mg, 60s ea	62756-0711-86	417.00		AB
500s ea	62756-0711-13	3475.00		AB
200 mg, 60s ea	62756-0712-86	489.00		AB
500s ea	62756-0712-13	4075.00		AB
(Dava Pharma)				
TAB, PO (FILM-COATED)				
25 mg, 100s ea	67253-0751-10	252.92		AB
1000s ea	67253-0751-11	2276.31		AB
50 mg, 100s ea	67253-0752-10	504.78		AB
1000s ea	67253-0752-11	4543.01		AB
100 mg, 100s ea	67253-0753-10	689.36		AB
1000s ea	67253-0753-11	6204.28		AB
200 mg, 100s ea	67253-0754-10	807.02		AB
(Glenmark Pharmaceuticals)				
TAB, PO (FILM-COATED)				
25 mg, 60s ea	68462-0108-60	132.99		AB
1000s ea	68462-0108-10	1994.94		AB
50 mg, 60s ea	68462-0153-60	265.43		AB
1000s ea	68462-0153-10	3981.46		AB
100 mg, 60s ea	68462-0109-60	362.47		AB
1000s ea	68462-0109-10	5437.06		AB
200 mg, 60s ea	68462-0110-60	424.37		AB
1000s ea	68462-0110-10	6365.46		AB
(Greenstone)				
TAB, PO (FILM-COATED)				
25 mg, 60s ea	59762-1030-01	153.29		AB
50 mg, 60s ea	59762-1031-01	305.93		AB
100 mg, 60s ea	59762-1032-01	417.80		AB
200 mg, 60s ea	59762-1033-01	489.11		AB
(Major)				
TAB, PO (3X10,FILM-COATED)				
25 mg, 30s ea UD	00904-6016-04	74.64		AB
50 mg, 30s ea UD	00904-6017-04	148.74		AB
100 mg, 30s ea UD	00904-6018-04	203.13		AB
(Medisca)				
POW, NA (1X100GM,USP)				
100 gm	38779-2443-05	1545.00		

PROD/MFR	NDC	AWP	DP	OBC
(1X500GM,USP)				
500 gm	**38779-2443-08**	4935.00		
(1X1000GM,USP)				
1000 gm	**38779-2443-09**	8550.00		
(1X1000GM)				
1000 gm	**38779-2333-09**	8550.00		
(Mylan)				
CAP, PO (SPRINKLE,SPRINKLE)				
15 mg, 500s ea	**00378-2035-05**	1196.00		**AB**
(SPRINKLE,HARD GELATIN)				
25 mg, 500s ea	**00378-2036-05**	1445.92		**AB**
TAB, PO (FILM-COATED)				
25 mg, 60s ea	**00378-6101-91**	153.27		**AB**
500s ea	**00378-6101-05**	1277.26		**AB**
50 mg, 60s ea	**00378-6102-91**	305.90		**AB**
500s ea	**00378-6102-05**	2549.13		**AB**
100 mg, 60s ea	**00378-6103-91**	417.75		**AB**
500s ea	**00378-6103-05**	3481.29		**AB**
200 mg, 60s ea	**00378-6105-91**	489.06		**AB**
500s ea	**00378-6105-05**	4075.46		**AB**
(Ortho-McNeil Neuro) *See TOPAMAX*				
(Ortho-McNeil Pharm) *See TOPAMAX*				
(Sandoz)				
CAP, PO (HARD GELATIN)				
15 mg, 60s ea	**00781-2275-60**	145.13		**AB**
25 mg, 60s ea	**00781-2276-60**	175.46		**AB**
(Teva)				
CAP, PO (SPRINKLE CAP)				
15 mg, 60s ea	**00093-7335-06**	145.13		**AB**
25 mg, 60s ea	**00093-7336-06**	175.46		**AB**
TAB, PO, 25 mg, 60s ea	**00093-0155-06**	153.46		**AB**
1000s ea	**00093-0155-10**	2429.77		**AB**
50 mg, 60s ea	**00093-7540-06**	306.54		**AB**
1000s ea	**00093-7540-10**	4853.55		**AB**
100 mg, 60s ea	**00093-7219-06**	418.27		**AB**
1000s ea	**00093-7219-10**	6622.54		**AB**
200 mg, 60s ea	**00093-7220-06**	489.65		**AB**
1000s ea	**00093-7220-10**	7752.85		**AB**
(Torrent)				
TAB, PO (FILM COATED)				
25 mg, 30s ea	**13668-0031-30**	74.34		
60s ea	**13668-0031-60**	148.68		
100s ea	**13668-0031-01**	247.80		
100s ea UD	**13668-0031-74**	247.80		
500s ea	**13668-0031-05**	1239.00		
50 mg, 30s ea	**13668-0032-30**	148.74		
60s ea	**13668-0032-60**	297.48		
100s ea	**13668-0032-01**	495.80		
100s ea UD	**13668-0032-74**	495.80		
500s ea	**13668-0032-05**	2479.00		
100 mg, 60s ea	**13668-0033-60**	406.26		
90s ea UD	**13668-0033-64**	609.39		
100s ea	**13668-0033-01**	677.10		
500s ea	**13668-0033-05**	3385.50		
200 mg, 60s ea	**13668-0034-60**	477.54		
80s ea UD	**13668-0034-77**	636.72		
100s ea	**13668-0034-01**	795.90		
500s ea	**13668-0034-05**	3979.50		
(UDL)				
TAB, PO (10X10,FILM-COATED)				
25 mg, 100s ea UD	**51079-0726-20**	255.48		**AB**
50 mg, 100s ea UD	**51079-0727-20**	509.88		**AB**
100 mg, 100s ea UD	**51079-0728-20**	696.34		**AB**
(Upsher-Smith) *See TOPIRAGEN*				
(Watson Labs)				
CAP, PO (ANISEED,HARD GELATIN)				
15 mg, 60s ea	**16252-0568-60**	139.32		**AB**
25 mg, 60s ea	**16252-0569-60**	168.42		**AB**
TAB, PO (FILM- COATED)				
25 mg, 60s ea	**16252-0564-60**	6.00		**AB**
500s ea	**16252-0564-50**	50.00		**AB**
50 mg, 60s ea	**16252-0565-60**	9.00		**AB**
500s ea	**16252-0565-50**	75.00		**AB**
100 mg, 60s ea	**16252-0566-60**	12.00		**AB**
200 mg, 60s ea	**16252-0567-60**	19.20		**AB**
(Zydus Pharm.)				
CAP, PO (HARD GELATIN)				
15 mg, 60s ea	**68382-0004-14**	144.97		**AB**
25 mg, 60s ea	**68382-0005-14**	175.26		**AB**
TAB, PO (FILM-COATED)				
25 mg, 60s ea	**68382-0138-14**	153.29		**EE**
500s ea	**68382-0138-05**	1277.42		**EE**
50 mg, 60s ea	**68382-0139-14**	305.93		**EE**
500s ea	**68382-0139-05**	2549.42		**EE**
100 mg, 60s ea	**68382-0140-14**	417.80		**EE**
500s ea	**68382-0140-05**	3481.67		**EE**
200 mg, 60s ea	**68382-0141-14**	489.11		**EE**
500s ea	**68382-0141-05**	4075.92		**EE**
(4u)				
REPACK				
TAB, PO (FILM-COATED)				
25 mg, 60s ea	**10544-0419-60**	162.86		**AB**
60s ea	**42549-0619-60**	162.86		**AB**
50 mg, 60s ea	**10544-0420-60**	186.44		**AB**
60s ea	**42549-0620-60**	186.44		**AB**
100 mg, 60s ea	**10544-0421-60**	286.16		**AB**
60s ea	**42549-0621-60**	286.16		**AB**
(A-S Medication)				
REPACK				
TAB, PO (FILM-COATED)				
25 mg, 60s ea	**54569-6137-00**	134.62		**AB**
50 mg, 60s ea	**54569-6138-00**	268.74		**AB**
100 mg, 60s ea	**54569-6139-00**	366.92		**AB**
(Aidarex)				
REPACK				
TAB, PO, 25 mg, 7s ea	**33261-0106-07**	17.36		
14s ea	**33261-0106-14**	34.72		
20s ea	**33261-0106-20**	49.60		
21s ea	**33261-0106-21**	52.08		
28s ea	**33261-0106-28**	68.44		
30s ea	**33261-0106-30**	74.40		
60s ea	**33261-0106-60**	148.80		
90s ea	**33261-0106-90**	223.20		
100s ea	**33261-0106-00**	248.00		
120s ea	**33261-0106-02**	297.60		
180s ea	**33261-0106-03**	446.40		
50 mg, 7s ea	**33261-0400-07**	34.58		
14s ea	**33261-0400-14**	69.16		
20s ea	**33261-0400-20**	98.80		
21s ea	**33261-0400-21**	103.74		
28s ea	**33261-0400-28**	138.32		
30s ea	**33261-0400-30**	148.20		
60s ea	**33261-0400-60**	296.40		
90s ea	**33261-0400-90**	444.60		
100s ea	**33261-0400-00**	494.00		
120s ea	**33261-0400-02**	592.80		
180s ea	**33261-0400-03**	889.20		
100 mg, 7s ea	**33261-0480-07**	47.25		
14s ea	**33261-0480-14**	94.50		
20s ea	**33261-0480-20**	135.00		
21s ea	**33261-0480-21**	141.75		
28s ea	**33261-0480-28**	189.00		
30s ea	**33261-0480-30**	202.50		
60s ea	**33261-0480-60**	405.00		
90s ea	**33261-0480-90**	607.50		
100s ea	**33261-0480-00**	675.00		
120s ea	**33261-0480-02**	810.00		
180s ea	**33261-0480-03**	1215.00		
200 mg, 7s ea	**33261-0481-07**	55.30		**AB**
14s ea	**33261-0481-14**	110.60		**AB**
20s ea	**33261-0481-20**	158.00		**AB**
21s ea	**33261-0481-21**	165.90		**AB**
28s ea	**33261-0481-28**	221.20		**AB**
30s ea	**33261-0481-30**	237.00		**AB**
60s ea	**33261-0481-60**	474.00		**AB**
90s ea	**33261-0481-90**	711.00		**AB**
100s ea	**33261-0481-00**	790.00		**AB**
120s ea	**33261-0481-02**	948.00		**AB**
180s ea	**33261-0481-03**	1422.00		**AB**
(American Health)				
REPACK				
TAB, PO (10X10,FILM- COATED)				
25 mg, 100s ea UD	**68084-0342-01**	210.00		**AB**
(3X10,FILM- COATED)				
50 mg, 30s ea UD	**68084-0343-21**	134.00		**AB**
(10X10,FILM- COATED)				
100 mg, 100s ea UD	**68084-0344-01**	620.00		**AB**
(3X10,FILM- COATED)				
200 mg, 30s ea UD	**68084-0345-21**	218.00		**AB**
(Dispensing Solutions)				
REPACK				
TAB, PO (FILM-COATED)				
25 mg, 60s ea	**68258-3000-01**	150.50		**AB**
50 mg, 60s ea	**55045-3964-01**	300.00		**AB**
(FILM-COATED)				
50 mg, 60s ea	**68258-3001-01**	297.88		**AB**
(GSMS)				
REPACK				
TAB, PO (FILM-COATED)				
25 mg, 60s ea	**60429-0769-60**	9.36	3.12	**EE**
500s ea	**60429-0769-05**	64.80	21.60	**EE**
1000s ea	**60429-0769-10**	127.80	42.60	**AB**
(FILM-COATED)				
50 mg, 60s ea	**60429-0770-60**	14.40	4.80	**EE**
500s ea	**60429-0770-05**	113.40	37.80	**EE**
1000s ea	**60429-0770-10**	225.00	75.00	**AB**
(FILM-COATED)				
100 mg, 60s ea	**60429-0771-60**	43.20	14.40	**EE**
500s ea	**60429-0771-05**	345.60	115.20	**EE**
1000s ea	**60429-0771-10**	689.40	229.80	**AB**
(FILM-COATED)				
200 mg, 60s ea	**60429-0772-60**	53.28	17.76	**EE**
500s ea	**60429-0772-05**	421.20	140.40	**EE**
1000s ea	**60429-0772-10**	840.60	280.20	**AB**
(Keltman Pharma., Inc.)				
REPACK				
TAB, PO (FILM COATED)				
25 mg, 30s ea	**68387-0558-90**	178.33		
100 mg, 90s ea	**68387-0559-90**	235.18		
(Nucare Pharm)				
REPACK				
TAB, PO, 100 mg, 30s ea	**68071-0813-30**	197.00		**AB**
200 mg, 30s ea	**68071-0181-30**	299.50		**AB**
(PD-Rx Pharm)				
REPACK				
TAB, PO (FILM COATED)				
25 mg, 30s ea	**43063-0094-30**	112.90		
50 mg, 30s ea	**43063-0114-30**	124.50		
100 mg, 60s ea	**43063-0189-60**	142.50		
(Pharma Pac)				
REPACK				
TAB, PO (FILM COATED)				
25 mg, 30s ea	**52959-0441-30**	83.06		
60s ea	**52959-0441-60**	165.09		
120s ea	**52959-0441-01**	329.82		
50 mg, 60s ea	**52959-0994-60**	311.47		
120s ea	**52959-0994-02**	615.42		
(Phys Total Care)				
REPACK				
TAB, PO (FILM-COATED)				
25 mg, 30s ea	**54868-6016-01**	12.20		**AB**
60s ea	**54868-6016-00**	16.91		**AB**
90s ea	**54868-6016-02**	24.61		**AB**
50 mg, 30s ea	**54868-6017-01**	15.37		**AB**
60s ea	**54868-6017-00**	23.25		**AB**
90s ea	**54868-6017-02**	30.22		**AB**
100 mg, 30s ea	**54868-6014-01**	17.70		**AB**
60s ea	**54868-6014-00**	30.59		**AB**
90s ea	**54868-6014-02**	45.13		**AB**
(Physician Partner)				
REPACK				
TAB, PO (FILM-COATED)				
25 mg, 30s ea	**21695-0162-30**	306.50		**AB**
60s ea	**21695-0162-60**	306.50		**AB**
50 mg, 30s ea	**21695-0205-30**	305.90		**AB**
60s ea	**21695-0205-60**	611.80		**AB**
90s ea	**21695-0205-90**	917.70		**AB**
100 mg, 30s ea	**21695-0348-30**	417.80		**AB**
60s ea	**21695-0348-60**	835.60		**AB**
200 mg, 30s ea	**21695-0349-30**	489.00		**AB**
(Quality Care Prod)				
REPACK				
TAB, PO (FILM-COATED)				
25 mg, 30s ea	**35356-0469-30**	75.50		**AB**
60s ea	**35356-0469-60**	151.00		**AB**
90s ea	**35356-0469-90**	226.50		**AB**
50 mg, 30s ea	**35356-0470-30**	92.00		**AB**
60s ea	**35356-0470-60**	184.00		**AB**
100 mg, 30s ea	**35356-0471-30**	128.00		**AB**
60s ea	**35356-0471-60**	256.00		**AB**
200 mg, 30s ea	**35356-0472-30**	153.00		**AB**
60s ea	**35356-0472-60**	206.00		**AB**
(St. Mary's MPP)				
REPACK				
TAB, PO (FILM COATED)				
25 mg, 90s ea	**60760-0278-90**	251.32		
50 mg, 90s ea	**60760-0279-90**	496.84		
(Stat Rx)				
REPACK				
TAB, PO (FILM COATED)				
25 mg, 30s ea	**16590-0824-30**	74.40		
56s ea	**16590-0824-56**	165.26		
60s ea	**16590-0824-60**	148.80		
84s ea	**16590-0824-62**	229.40		
90s ea	**16590-0824-90**	223.20		
100s ea	**16590-0824-71**	248.00		
120s ea	**16590-0824-72**	297.60		
180s ea	**16590-0824-82**	446.40		
50 mg, 30s ea	**16590-0825-30**	148.80		
60s ea	**16590-0825-60**	297.60		
90s ea	**16590-0825-90**	446.40		
120s ea	**16590-0825-72**	595.20		
180s ea	**16590-0825-82**	892.80		
100 mg, 30s ea	**16590-0817-30**	203.13		
45s ea	**16590-0817-45**	304.70		
60s ea	**16590-0817-60**	406.26		
90s ea	**16590-0817-90**	609.39		
120s ea	**16590-0817-72**	812.52		

PROD/MFR	NDC	AWP	DP	OBC
200 mg, 30s ea	16590-0823-30	74.34		
60s ea	16590-0823-60	148.68		
90s ea	16590-0823-90	223.02		
TOPOSAR (Teva)				
etoposide				
SOL, IV (M.D.V. POLYMER)				
20 mg/ml, 5 ml	00703-5653-01	11.24		AP
(M.D.V. POLYMER)				
20 mg/ml, 25 ml	00703-5656-01	26.40		AP
(M.D.V.)				
20 mg/ml, 50 ml	00703-5657-01	55.80		AP
TOPOTECAN HYDROCHLORIDE				
(Glaxo) *See HYCAMTIN*				
TOPROL XL (AstraZeneca)				
metoprolol succinate				
TER, PO, 25 mg, 100s ea	00186-1088-05	123.94		
(BLISTER PACK,10X10)				
25 mg, 100s ea UD	00186-1088-39	123.94		
50 mg, 100s ea UD	00186-1090-39	123.94		
(FILM-COATED)				
50 mg, 100s ea	00186-1090-05	123.94		
100 mg, 100s ea	00186-1092-05	186.24		
(BLISTER PACK,10X10)				
100 mg, 100s ea UD	00186-1092-39	186.24		
(FILM-COATED)				
200 mg, 100s ea	00186-1094-05	296.32		
(A-S Medication)				
REPACK				
TER, PO (FILM-COATED)				
50 mg, 30s ea	54569-4441-00	36.89		
100 mg, 30s ea	54569-4442-00	55.43		
(Direct Pharmaceutical, Inc.)				
REPACK				
TER, PO, 50 mg,				
30s ea UD	67801-0304-30	64.97		
100 mg, 30s ea UD	67801-0315-30	64.97		
200 mg, 30s ea UD	67801-0316-03	81.88		
(Dispensing Solutions)				
REPACK				
TER, PO, 25 mg, 30s ea	55045-3361-08	33.60		
100s ea	55045-3361-01	112.00		
50 mg, 30s ea	55045-2431-08	33.60		
100s ea	55045-2431-01	112.00		
(PD-Rx Pharm)				
REPACK				
TER, PO, 25 mg, 30s ea	55289-0902-30	52.64		
(FILM-COATED)				
50 mg, 30s ea	55289-0855-30	52.64		
30s ea	58864-0765-30	44.39		
(EXTENDED-RELEASE)				
100 mg, 30s ea	58864-0759-30	63.98		
(Phys Total Care)				
REPACK				
TER, PO, 25 mg, 10s ea	54868-4661-01	17.41		
15s ea	54868-4661-03	24.81		
30s ea	54868-4661-00	47.00		
60s ea	54868-4661-02	91.38		
(FILM-COATED)				
50 mg, 10s ea	54868-3587-02	14.74		
30s ea	54868-3587-01	39.65		
50s ea	54868-3587-00	65.87		
(FILM-COATED)				
50 mg, 60s ea	54868-3587-04	78.65		
90s ea	54868-3587-05	116.99		
100s ea	54868-3587-03	129.12		
100 mg, 10s ea	54868-4223-02	20.41		
30s ea	54868-4223-00	57.48		
60s ea	54868-4223-03	113.08		
90s ea	54868-4223-04	158.79		
100s ea	54868-4223-01	186.59		
(FILM-COATED)				
200 mg, 10s ea	54868-5068-01	29.70		
30s ea	54868-5068-00	85.34		
60s ea	54868-5068-02	159.51		
90s ea	54868-5068-03	238.34		
(Physician Partner)				
REPACK				
TER, PO, 50 mg, 30s ea	21695-0291-30	60.13		
(Quality Care Prod)				
REPACK				
TER, PO, 25 mg, 30s ea	49999-0482-30	85.86		
(FILM-COATED)				
50 mg, 30s ea	49999-0483-30	236.60		
100s ea	49999-0483-00	384.90		
100 mg, 30s ea	49999-0484-30	64.97		
100s ea	49999-0484-00	216.57		
200 mg, 100s ea	49999-0996-00	288.00		

PROD/MFR	NDC	AWP	DP	OBC
(Southwood)				
REPACK				
TER, PO, 25 mg, 30s ea	58016-0974-30	31.82		
60s ea	58016-0974-60	63.64		
90s ea	58016-0974-90	95.45		
100s ea	58016-0974-00	106.06		
(FILM-COATED)				
50 mg, 30s ea	58016-0373-30	31.82		
60s ea	58016-0373-60	63.64		
90s ea	58016-0373-90	95.45		
100s ea	58016-0373-00	106.06		
120s ea	58016-0373-02	83.77		
TOPROL-XL (DHS, Inc.)				
REPACK				
metoprolol succinate				
TER, PO, 50 mg, 30s ea	55887-0729-30	44.98		
(Southwood)				
REPACK				
TER, PO, 200 mg, 30s ea	58016-0045-30	76.07		
60s ea	58016-0045-60	152.13		
90s ea	58016-0045-90	228.20		
100s ea	58016-0045-00	253.55		
TORADOL (Nucare Pharm)				
REPACK				
ketorolac tromethamine				
TAB, PO, 10 mg, 8s ea	66267-0204-08	17.56		AB
21s ea	66267-0204-21	36.99		AB
(Pharma Pac)				
REPACK				
TAB, PO, 10 mg, 8s ea	52959-0224-08	16.10		AB
10s ea	52959-0224-10	20.01		AB
12s ea	52959-0224-12	23.81		AB
14s ea	52959-0224-14	27.69		AB
15s ea	52959-0224-15	29.62		AB
20s ea	52959-0224-20	38.68		AB
30s ea	52959-0224-30	57.13		AB
40s ea	52959-0224-40	73.88		AB
60s ea	52959-0224-60	109.26		AB
(Quality Care Prod)				
REPACK				
TAB, PO, 10 mg, 20s ea	49999-0429-20	38.50		AB
TORECAN (Phys Total Care)				
REPACK				
thiethylperazine maleate				
SOL, IM (AMP)				
5 mg/ml, 2 ml 20s	54868-4579-00	119.07		
TAB, PO, 10 mg, 10s ea	54868-1963-01	9.02		
15s ea	54868-1963-00	12.61		
TOREMIFENE CITRATE				
(GTX) *See FARESTON*				
TORISEL (Wyeth)				
temsirolimus				
SOL, IV (WITH DILUENT)				
25 mg/ml, 1 ml	00008-1179-01	1467.89	1223.24	
TORSEMIDE				
FUL				
TAB, PO, 5 mg, 100s ea		45.00		
10 mg, 100s ea		48.00		
20 mg, 100s ea		52.50		
100 mg, 100s ea		291.75		
(Apotex Corp.)				
TAB, PO, 5 mg, 100s ea	60505-0232-01	63.45		AB
10 mg, 100s ea	60505-0233-01	70.30		AB
20 mg, 100s ea	60505-0234-01	82.10		AB
100 mg, 100s ea	60505-0235-01	304.15		AB
(Aurobindo Pharma)				
TAB, PO, 5 mg, 100s ea	65862-0125-01	63.40		AB
10 mg, 100s ea	65862-0126-01	70.25		AB
20 mg, 100s ea	65862-0127-01	82.05		AB
100 mg, 100s ea	65862-0128-01	304.00		AB
(Camber)				
TAB, PO, 5 mg, 100s ea	31722-0529-01	63.42		AB
10 mg, 100s ea	31722-0530-01	70.27		AB
20 mg, 100s ea	31722-0531-01	82.05		AB
100 mg, 100s ea	31722-0532-01	304.00		AB
(Caraco)				
TAB, PO, 5 mg, 100s ea	62756-0761-88	63.40		AB
10 mg, 100s ea	62756-0762-88	70.25		AB
20 mg, 100s ea	62756-0763-88	82.10		AB
500s ea	62756-0763-13	410.40		AB
100 mg, 100s ea	62756-0764-88	304.10		AB
(Greenstone)				
TAB, PO (UNCOATED)				
5 mg, 100s ea	59762-1700-01	63.40		
10 mg, 100s ea	59762-1701-01	70.27		
20 mg, 100s ea	59762-1702-01	82.05		
100 mg, 100s ea	59762-1703-01	304.00		

PROD/MFR	NDC	AWP	DP	OBC
(Meda) *See DEMADEX*				
(Par)				
TAB, PO, 5 mg, 100s ea	49884-0106-01	63.40		AB
1000s ea	49884-0651-10	624.49		AB
10 mg, 100s ea	49884-0652-01	70.25		AB
20 mg, 100s ea	49884-0108-01	82.06		AB
500s ea	49884-0108-05	410.30		AB
100 mg, 100s ea	49884-0109-01	304.00		AB
1000s ea	49884-0654-10	2994.40		AB
(Roxane)				
TAB, PO, 20 mg, 100s ea	00054-0077-25	82.08		AB
500s ea	00054-0077-29	410.40		AB
(Teva)				
TAB, PO, 5 mg, 100s ea	00093-7127-01	63.41		AB
100s ea	50111-0915-01	63.45		AB
10 mg, 100s ea	00093-7128-01	70.27		AB
100s ea	50111-0916-01	70.30		AB
20 mg, 100s ea	50111-0917-01	82.10		AB
1000s ea	50111-0917-03	821.00		AB
100 mg, 100s ea	50111-0918-01	304.15		AB
(UDL)				
TAB, PO (10X10)				
10 mg, 100s ea UD	51079-0025-20	75.04		AB
20 mg, 100s ea UD	51079-0026-20	87.65		AB
(Bryant Ranch)				
REPACK				
TAB, PO, 10 mg, 100s ea	63629-1346-01	53.62		
(McKesson Packaging)				
REPACK				
TAB, PO, 10 mg,				
100s ea UD	63739-0330-10	87.83		
20 mg, 100s ea UD	63739-0331-10	130.27		
(Phys Total Care)				
REPACK				
TAB, PO, 10 mg, 30s ea	54868-6048-00	25.52		AB
20 mg, 15s ea	54868-5180-01	19.32		AB
30s ea	54868-5180-02	34.11		AB
100s ea	54868-5180-00	78.48		AB
100 mg, 10s ea	54868-1234-01	42.12		AB
15s ea	54868-1234-02	60.93		AB
30s ea	54868-1234-00	117.36		AB
100s ea	54868-1234-03	358.29		AB
TOSITUMOMAB				
(Glaxo) *See BEXXAR*				
TOTECT (TopoTarget)				
dexrazoxane hydrochloride				
PDS, IV (W/10 VIALS OF DILUENT)				
500 mg, 10s ea	38423-0110-01	8125.00	6500.00	
TOVIAZ (Pfizer)				
fesoterodine fumarate				
TER, PO (FILM-COATED)				
4 mg, 30s ea	00069-0242-30	144.49	120.41	
8 mg, 30s ea	00069-0244-30	144.49	120.41	
TPN ELECTROLYTES (Hospira)				
ca cl/k cl/mg cl/na ace/na cl				
SOL, IV (VIAL,FLIPTOP)				
20 ml 25s	00409-5779-01	67.50	59.00	
(VIAL,FLIPTOP,BULK)				
100 ml 25s	00409-3296-06	145.80	127.50	
TPN ELECTROLYTES II (Hospira)				
ca cl/k cl/mg cl/na ace/na cl				
SOL, IV (VIAL, FLIP TOP)				
20 ml 25s	00074-3236-01	106.80	93.50	
(25X100ML)				
100 ml 25s	00409-3297-06	144.00	126.00	
TPN ELECTROLYTES II MULTIPLE ELECTROLYTE ADDITIVE (Hospira)				
ca cl/k cl/mg cl/na ace/na cl				
SOL, IV (25X20ML,SDV)				
20 ml 25s	00409-3236-01	76.80	67.25	
TRACE ELEMENT PEDIATRIC (Amer Regent)				
chromium/copper/manganese/zinc				
SOL, IV (M.D.V.)				
10 ml 25s	00517-9310-25	132.81		
TRACE METALS (Hospira)				
chromium/copper/manganese/zinc				
SOL, IV (VIAL,FLIPTOP,LATEX-FREE)				
5 ml 25s	00409-4592-10	56.70	49.50	
(25X50ML,LATEX-FREE)				
50 ml 25s	00409-4592-50	283.20	247.75	
TRACLEER (Actelion Pharm)				
bosentan				
TAB, PO, 62.5 mg, 60s ea	66215-0101-06	6516.00		
125 mg, 60s ea	66215-0102-06	6516.00		

PROD/MFR	NDC	AWP	DP	OBC
TRAGACANTH (Gallipot)				
POW, NA (U.S.P.,N.F.)				
120 gm	51552-0352-04	16.10		
454 gm	51552-0352-06	50.96		
(Medisca)				
POW, NA (N.F.)				
100 gm	38779-0099-05	63.00		
(U.S.P.)				
500 gm	38779-0099-08	288.00		
(PCCA)				
POW, NA (NF, POWDERED)				
1 gm	51927-1100-00	0.45		
(Spectrum Pharmacy)				
POW, NA (N.F.)				
125 gm	49452-7870-01	79.45		
500 gm	49452-7870-02	224.35		
2500 gm	49452-7870-03	857.50		
(Spectrum Pharmacy) *See TRAGACANTH NO.1 RIBBON*				
TRAGACANTH NO.1 RIBBON (Spectrum Pharmacy)				
tragacanth				
FLA, NA (N.F.)				
125 gm	49452-7860-01	248.15		
500 gm	49452-7860-02	728.00		
TRAINER, INJECTION				
(Dey, L.P.) *See EPIPEN TRAINER*				
TRAMADOL (4u)				
REPACK				
tramadol hydrochloride				
TAB, PO, 50 mg, 30s ea	10544-0327-30	68.48		
60s ea	10544-0327-60	99.46		
90s ea	10544-0327-90	132.52		
(Aidarex)				
REPACK				
TAB, PO, 50 mg, 10s ea	33261-0105-10	16.20		
12s ea	33261-0105-12	19.44		
14s ea	33261-0105-14	22.68		
20s ea	33261-0105-20	32.40		
21s ea	33261-0105-21	34.02		
30s ea	33261-0105-30	48.60		
60s ea	33261-0105-60	97.20		
90s ea	33261-0105-90	145.80		
100s ea	33261-0105-00	162.00		
120s ea	33261-0105-02	194.40		
180s ea	33261-0105-03	291.60		
240s ea	33261-0105-04	388.80		
(Bryant Ranch)				
REPACK				
TAB, PO, 50 mg, 20s ea	63629-2868-07	44.32		
30s ea	63629-2868-01	47.08		
40s ea	63629-2868-09	62.78		
50s ea	63629-2868-00	74.32		
60s ea	63629-2868-02	86.39		
90s ea	63629-2868-03	129.59		
100s ea	63629-2868-04	162.87		
120s ea	63629-2868-05	171.32		
180s ea	63629-2868-06	272.35		
(Core)				
REPACK				
TAB, PO, 50 mg, 20s ea	33358-0342-20	33.33		
30s ea	33358-0342-30	49.80		
40s ea	33358-0342-40	66.40		
45s ea	33358-0342-45	74.70		
50s ea	33358-0342-50	83.00		
60s ea	33358-0342-60	100.00		
90s ea	33358-0342-90	149.40		
120s ea	33358-0342-01	155.67		
(Dispensing Solutions)				
REPACK				
TAB, PO, 50 mg, 15s ea	66336-0915-15	22.50		
90s ea	66336-0915-90	135.00		
120s ea	66336-0915-94	180.00		
(HomeMed)				
REPACK				
TAB, PO, 50 mg, 20s ea	51655-0633-52	43.69		
60s ea	51655-0633-25	98.99		
(IPI)				
REPACK				
TAB, PO, 50 mg, 20s ea	18837-0157-20	37.00		
30s ea	18837-0157-30	45.00		
40s ea	18837-0157-40	41.65		
45s ea	18837-0157-45	46.69		
50s ea	18837-0147-50	52.06		
60s ea	18837-0157-60	62.25		
90s ea	18837-0157-90	93.38		
100s ea	18837-0157-99	104.11		
180s ea	18837-0157-96	186.45		
240s ea	18837-0157-95	249.00		
(Palmetto)				
REPACK				
TAB, PO, 50 mg, 6s ea	23490-6832-01	14.70		
15s ea	23490-6832-02	26.25		
20s ea	23490-6832-00	35.00		
30s ea	23490-1347-03	56.80		
30s ea	23490-6832-03	52.50		
40s ea	23490-7846-02	87.19		
60s ea	23490-1347-06	113.60		
60s ea	23490-6832-04	105.00		
90s ea	23490-6832-05	157.50		
100s ea	23490-6832-08	175.00		
120s ea	23490-7846-03	209.26		
180s ea	23490-6832-06	236.25		
240s ea	23490-6832-07	315.00		
300s ea	23490-6832-09	393.75		
360s ea	23490-7846-01	392.40		
450s ea	23490-7846-00	590.63		
(Physician Partner)				
REPACK				
TAB, PO (FILM-COATED)				
50 mg, 10s ea	21695-0132-10	40.01		
20s ea	21695-0132-20	39.23		
(FILM-COATED)				
50 mg, 24s ea	21695-0132-24	40.01		
28s ea	21695-0132-28	46.68		
30s ea	21695-0132-30	50.02		
45s ea	21695-0132-45	75.02		
50s ea	21695-0132-50	83.37		
60s ea	21695-0132-60	100.04		
90s ea	21695-0132-90	150.06		
120s ea	21695-0132-72	200.08		
180s ea	21695-0132-78	300.15		
(FILM-COATED)				
50 mg, 240s ea	21695-0132-64	400.20		
(Stat Rx)				
REPACK				
TAB, PO, 50 mg, 24s ea	16590-0229-24	40.00		
30s ea	16590-0229-30	50.00		
40s ea	16590-0229-40	66.66		
45s ea	16590-0229-45	75.00		
60s ea	16590-0229-60	90.63		
90s ea	16590-0229-90	105.00		
120s ea	16590-0229-72	135.00		
TRAMADOL HCL (Apotex Corp.)				
tramadol hydrochloride				
TAB, PO (FILM COATED)				
50 mg, 100s ea	60505-0171-01	83.40		AB
500s ea	60505-0171-02	418.30		AB
28000s ea	60505-0171-07	23424.80		AB
(Caraco)				
TAB, PO (CAPLET)				
50 mg, 100s ea	57664-0377-08	83.81		AB
500s ea	57664-0377-13	419.11		AB
(FILM COATED)				
50 mg, 1000s ea	57664-0377-18	838.00		AB
(Covidien)				
TAB, PO (CAPLET)				
50 mg, 1000s ea	00406-7171-10	790.00		AB
(BULK,CAPLET)				
50 mg, 5000s ea	00406-7171-91	3950.00		AB
(Major)				
TAB, PO, 50 mg,				
100s ea UD	00904-5556-61	90.99		AB
(Mylan)				
TAB, PO, 50 mg, 100s ea	00378-4151-01	83.75		AB
500s ea	00378-4151-05	418.75		AB
(Sandoz)				
TAB, PO, 50 mg, 100s ea	00185-0311-01	83.84		AB
1000s ea	00185-0311-10	838.40		AB
(Teva)				
TAB, PO, 50 mg, 100s ea	00093-0058-01	82.90		AB
500s ea	00093-0058-05	414.55		AB
(UDL)				
TAB, PO (10X10)				
50 mg, 100s ea UD	51079-0991-20	79.60		AB
(A-S Medication)				
REPACK				
TAB, PO, 50 mg, 15s ea	54569-5436-04	12.51		EE
20s ea	54569-5436-01	16.68		EE
30s ea	54569-5436-00	25.02		EE
45s ea	54569-5436-07	37.53		EE
50s ea	54569-5436-02	41.70		EE
60s ea	54569-5436-05	50.04		EE
90s ea	54569-5967-01	75.06		EE
100s ea	54569-5436-03	83.40		EE
120s ea	54569-5436-09	100.08		EE
240s ea	54569-5967-00	200.16		EE
(Aidarex)				
REPACK				
TAB, PO, 50 mg, 25s ea	33261-0105-25	40.50		AB
45s ea	33261-0105-45	72.90		AB
50s ea	33261-0105-50	81.00		AB
140s ea	33261-0105-01	226.80		AB
200s ea	33261-0105-91	324.00		AB
(Altura)				
REPACK				
TAB, PO (CAPLET)				
50 mg, 7s ea	63874-0532-07	6.61		AB
10s ea	63874-0532-10	9.44		AB
15s ea	63874-0532-15	14.16		AB
20s ea	63874-0532-23	18.88		AB
25s ea	63874-0532-25	23.60		AB
28s ea	63874-0532-28	26.43		AB
30s ea	63874-0532-33	28.32		AB
35s ea	63874-0532-35	33.04		AB
50s ea	63874-0532-53	47.20		AB
60s ea	63874-0532-63	56.64		AB
84s ea	63874-0532-84	79.29		AB
90s ea	63874-0532-93	84.96		AB
100s ea	63874-0532-01	94.40		AB
120s ea	63874-0532-00	113.28		AB
(American Health)				
REPACK				
TAB, PO (10X10)				
50 mg, 100s ea UD	62584-0559-01	78.75		AB
(DHS, Inc.)				
REPACK				
TAB, PO, 50 mg, 20s ea	55887-0658-20	38.95		AB
30s ea	55887-0658-30	45.00		AB
(CAPLET)				
50 mg, 40s ea	55887-0658-40	49.75		AB
45s ea	55887-0658-45	52.00		AB
60s ea	55887-0658-60	75.00		AB
90s ea	55887-0658-90	99.00		AB
100s ea	55887-0658-01	95.00		AB
120s ea	55887-0658-82	135.95		AB
300s ea	55887-0658-03	285.00		AB
(Dispensing Solutions)				
REPACK				
TAB, PO, 50 mg, 15s ea	55045-2928-06	15.00		AB
20s ea	55045-2928-07	20.00		AB
20s ea	66336-0915-20	30.00		AB
(FILM-COATED TABLET)				
50 mg, 25s ea	55045-2928-05	25.00		AB
(FILM COATED)				
50 mg, 28s ea	55045-3262-05	28.00		AB
30s ea	66336-0915-30	45.00		AB
(FILM-COATED TABLET)				
50 mg, 30s ea	55045-2928-08	30.00		AB
(FILM COATED)				
50 mg, 40s ea	55045-3262-07	40.00		AB
50s ea	55045-2928-02	50.00		AB
56s ea	55045-2928-03	56.00		AB
60s ea	66336-0915-60	90.00		AB
(FILM-COATED TABLET)				
50 mg, 60s ea	55045-2928-09	60.00		AB
90s ea	55045-2928-04	90.00		AB
(FILM-COATED TABLET)				
50 mg, 100s ea	55045-2928-01	100.00		AB
(CAPLET)				
50 mg, 120s ea	55045-2928-00	120.00		AB
160s ea	55045-3262-04	160.00		AB
180s ea	55045-3262-01	180.00		AB
200s ea	55045-3262-02	200.00		AB
(FILM COATED)				
50 mg, 240s ea	55045-3262-06	240.00		AB
300s ea	55045-3262-03	300.00		AB
(Keltman Pharma., Inc.)				
REPACK				
TAB, PO (CAPLET)				
50 mg, 30s ea	68387-0900-30	50.70		AB
50s ea	68387-0900-50	84.50		AB
60s ea	68387-0900-60	101.40		AB
90s ea	68387-0900-90	152.10		AB
120s ea	68387-0900-12	202.80		AB
240s ea	68387-0900-24	405.60		AB
(Medsource)				
REPACK				
TAB, PO (FILM-COATED TABLET)				
50 mg, 30s ea	45865-0357-30	31.50		AB
60s ea	45865-0357-60	63.00		AB
90s ea	45865-0357-90	94.50		AB
100s ea	45865-0357-00	105.00		AB
120s ea	45865-0357-01	126.00		AB
150s ea	45865-0357-02	157.50		AB
300s ea	45865-0357-05	315.00		AB

PROD/MFR	NDC	AWP	DP	OBC
(Nucare Pharm)				
REPACK				
TAB, PO, 50 mg, 15s ea	**66267-0563-15**	22.49		EE
20s ea	**66267-0563-20**	30.00		EE
30s ea	**66267-0563-30**	44.99		EE
40s ea	**66267-0563-40**	59.98		EE
60s ea	**66267-0563-60**	75.99		EE
(FILM-COATED)				
50 mg, 100s ea	**68071-1351-00**	149.96		AB
120s ea	**66627-0563-91**	101.50		AB
(PD-Rx Pharm)				
REPACK				
TAB, PO, 50 mg, 15s ea	**55289-0719-15**	51.50		AB
20s ea	**55289-0719-20**	54.60		AB
(REDI-SCRIPT)				
50 mg, 20s ea	**58864-0678-20**	54.60		AB
30s ea	**55289-0719-30**	65.30		AB
(REDI-SCRIPT,CAPLET)				
50 mg, 30s ea	**58864-0678-30**	65.30		AB
50s ea	**55289-0719-50**	86.70		AB
(Pharma Pac)				
REPACK				
TAB, PO (FILM-COATED TABLET)				
50 mg, 10s ea	**52959-0688-10**	15.81		AB
15s ea	**52959-0688-15**	23.69		AB
20s ea	**52959-0688-20**	31.57		AB
21s ea	**52959-0688-21**	33.14		AB
24s ea	**52959-0688-24**	37.87		AB
28s ea	**52959-0688-28**	44.17		AB
30s ea	**52959-0688-30**	47.32		AB
40s ea	**52959-0688-40**	63.08		AB
(CAPLET)				
50 mg, 50s ea	**52959-0688-50**	78.84		AB
(FILM-COATED TABLET)				
50 mg, 56s ea	**52959-0688-56**	88.30		AB
60s ea	**52959-0688-60**	94.60		AB
90s ea	**52959-0688-90**	141.10		AB
100s ea	**52959-0688-00**	155.80		AB
120s ea	**52959-0688-02**	184.92		AB
(FILM COATED)				
50 mg, 180s ea	**52959-0688-18**	277.06		AB
(Phys Total Care)				
REPACK				
TAB, PO, 50 mg, 20s ea	**54868-4638-02**	7.41		EE
30s ea	**54868-4638-00**	8.85		EE
50s ea	**54868-4638-03**	11.76		EE
60s ea	**54868-4638-01**	13.20		EE
90s ea	**54868-4638-07**	17.55		AB
100s ea	**54868-4638-05**	18.99		AB
120s ea	**54868-4638-04**	21.95		AB
(Physician Partner)				
REPACK				
TAB, PO (FILM COATED)				
50 mg, 8s ea	**21695-0132-08**	15.69		AB
16s ea	**21695-0132-16**	31.38		AB
100s ea	**21695-0132-00**	166.80		AB
(Quality Care Prod)				
REPACK				
TAB, PO (FILM-COATED TABLET)				
50 mg, 15s ea	**49999-0125-15**	13.94		AB
20s ea	**49999-0129-20**	43.59		AB
30s ea	**49999-0129-30**	65.39		AB
(FILM COATED)				
50 mg, 60s ea	**49999-0129-60**	98.99		AB
90s ea	**49999-0129-90**	149.69		AB
100s ea	**49999-0129-00**	93.00		AB
(FILM COATED)				
50 mg, 120s ea	**49999-0129-01**	199.56		AB
(CAPLET)				
50 mg, 180s ea	**49999-0129-18**	299.34		AB
(Southwood)				
REPACK				
TAB, PO, 50 mg, 7s ea	**58016-0708-07**	6.51		EE
10s ea	**58016-0708-10**	9.30		EE
12s ea	**58016-0708-12**	11.15		EE
15s ea	**58016-0708-15**	13.94		EE
20s ea	**58016-0708-20**	18.59		EE
21s ea	**58016-0708-21**	19.52		EE
25s ea	**58016-0708-25**	23.24		EE
28s ea	**58016-0708-28**	26.03		EE
40s ea	**58016-0708-40**	37.18		EE
42s ea	**58016-0708-42**	39.04		EE
50s ea	**58016-0708-50**	46.48		EE
56s ea	**58016-0708-56**	52.05		EE
84s ea	**58016-0708-84**	78.07		EE
(FILM COATED)				
50 mg, 112s ea	**58016-0708-92**	104.11		AB
140s ea	**58016-0708-81**	130.13		EE
150s ea	**58016-0708-03**	139.43		EE
(FILM-COATED TABLET)				
50 mg, 180s ea	**58016-0708-99**	167.31		AB
200s ea	**58016-0708-89**	185.90		EE
(FILM COATED)				
50 mg, 240s ea	**58016-0708-04**	223.12		AB
(FILM-COATED TABLET)				
50 mg, 300s ea	**58016-0708-73**	278.85		AB
(St. Mary's MPP)				
REPACK				
TAB, PO, 50 mg, 20s ea	**60760-0377-20**	32.28		EE
30s ea	**60760-0377-30**	45.42		EE
(CAPLET)				
50 mg, 60s ea	**60760-0377-60**	84.84		AB
90s ea	**60760-0377-90**	124.26		AB
(FILM COATED)				
50 mg, 120s ea	**60760-0377-92**	163.68		AB
180s ea	**60760-0377-98**	242.52		AB
240s ea	**60760-0377-99**	321.26		AB
(Stat Rx)				
REPACK				
TAB, PO (CAPLET)				
50 mg, 2s ea	**16590-0229-02**	31.39		AB
20s ea	**16590-0229-20**	37.00		AB
(CAPLET)				
50 mg, 28s ea	**16590-0229-28**	51.80		AB
50s ea	**16590-0229-50**	63.06		AB
56s ea	**16590-0229-56**	103.60		AB
84s ea	**16590-0229-62**	92.63		AB
100s ea	**16590-0229-71**	185.00		AB
150s ea	**16590-0229-83**	175.00		AB
180s ea	**16590-0229-82**	198.38		AB
240s ea	**16590-0229-84**	264.51		AB
270s ea	**16590-0229-86**	226.34		AB
(Vibranta)				
REPACK				
TAB, PO, 50 mg, 30s ea	**57866-8787-02**	65.39		
60s ea	**57866-8787-03**	109.20		
90s ea	**57866-8787-07**	149.69		
120s ea	**57866-8787-06**	199.59		
180s ea	**57866-8787-08**	167.34		
240s ea	**57866-8787-09**	523.12		
TRAMADOL HYDROCHLORIDE				
FUL				
TAB, PO, 50 mg, 100s ea		9.00		
(Amneal)				
TAB, PO (FILM-COATED)				
50 mg, 100s ea	**65162-0627-10**	83.40		
500s ea	**65162-0627-50**	416.90		
1000s ea	**65162-0627-11**	832.90		
(Apotex Corp.)				
TAB, PO (FILM COATED)				
50 mg, 1000s ea	**60505-0171-08**	836.60		
27000s ea	**60505-0171-05**	22588.20		
(Apotex Corp.) *See TRAMADOL HCL*				
(Caraco) *See TRAMADOL HCL*				
(Covidien) *See TRAMADOL HCL*				
(Major) *See TRAMADOL HCL*				
(Marlex)				
TAB, PO (FILM-COATED)				
50 mg, 100s ea	**10135-0519-01**	83.40		AB
500s ea	**10135-0519-05**	416.90		AB
1000s ea	**10135-0519-10**	832.90		AB
(Medisca)				
POW, NA (1X25GM)				
25 gm	**38779-2374-04**	465.00		
(1X100GM)				
100 gm	**38779-2374-05**	1485.00		
(Mylan) *See TRAMADOL HCL*				
(Ortho-McNeil Pharm) *See ULTRAM ER*				
(Par)				
TER, PO, 100 mg, 30s ea	**49884-0821-11**	109.16		AB
200 mg, 30s ea	**49884-0822-11**	180.53		AB
(Patriot Pharmaceuticals)				
TER, PO, 100 mg, 30s ea	**10147-0901-03**	108.92		AB
200 mg, 30s ea	**10147-0902-03**	180.14		AB
(PCCA)				
POW, NA, 1 gm	**51927-3404-00**	18.00		
(PriCara) *See ULTRAM*				
(PriCara) *See ULTRAM ER*				
(Purdue Pharma) *See RYZOLT*				
(Sandoz) *See TRAMADOL HCL*				
(Spectrum Pharmacy)				
POW, NA (1X5GM,EP)				
5 gm	**49452-7861-01**	136.15		
(1X25GM,EP)				
25 gm	**49452-7861-02**	518.00		
(1X100GM,EP)				
100 gm	**49452-7861-03**	1722.00		
(Teva)				
TAB, PO (FILM COATED)				
50 mg, 100s ea UD	**00172-6515-10**	91.70		AB
100s ea	**00172-6515-60**	83.35		AB
500s ea	**00172-6515-70**	416.85		AB
(Teva) *See TRAMADOL HCL*				
TRAMADOL HYDROCHLORIDE (UDL)				
tramadol hydrochloride				
TAB, PO (PUNCH CARDS,10X30)				
50 mg, 300s ea UD	**51079-0991-56**	238.80		AB
TRAMADOL HYDROCHLORIDE				
(UDL) *See TRAMADOL HCL*				
(UDL) *See TRAMADOL HYDROCHLORIDE*				
(4u)				
REPACK				
TAB, PO (FILM-COATED)				
50 mg, 30s ea	**42549-0327-30**	68.48		
30s ea	**42549-0527-30**	68.48		
40s ea	**42549-0527-40**	78.12		
60s ea	**42549-0327-60**	99.46		
60s ea	**42549-0527-60**	99.46		
90s ea	**42549-0527-90**	132.52		
112s ea	**10544-0327-02**	154.06		
112s ea	**42549-0527-02**	154.06		
120s ea	**42549-0527-12**	144.18		
224s ea	**42549-0527-24**	278.92		
(A-S Medication)				
REPACK				
TAB, PO (FILM-COATED)				
50 mg, 10s ea	**54569-5967-02**	8.34		
(Altura)				
REPACK				
TAB, PO (FILM COATED)				
50 mg, 40s ea	**63874-0532-40**	37.76		
(Dispensing Solutions)				
REPACK				
TAB, PO (FILM-COATED)				
50 mg, 50s ea	**66336-0915-50**	77.73		
60s ea	**55045-3769-06**	60.00		
168s ea	**55045-3724-06**	168.00		
(FILM-COATED)				
50 mg, 180s ea	**66336-0915-62**	270.00		
(IPI)				
REPACK				
TAB, PO (FILM-COATED)				
50 mg, 28s ea	**18837-0157-28**	39.15		
50s ea	**18837-0157-50**	52.06		
120s ea	**18837-0157-98**	99.95		
(Keltman Pharma., Inc.)				
REPACK				
TAB, PO, 50 mg, 15s ea	**68387-0900-15**	25.35		
20s ea	**68387-0900-20**	33.80		
(FILM-COATED)				
50 mg, 40s ea	**68387-0900-40**	67.60		
(Nucare Pharm)				
REPACK				
TAB, PO (FILM COATED)				
50 mg, 28s ea	**66267-0563-28**	41.99		
45s ea	**66267-0563-45**	67.48		
50s ea	**66267-0563-50**	74.98		
90s ea	**66267-0563-90**	134.96		
(FILM-COATED)				
50 mg, 180s ea	**66267-0563-92**	269.94		
240s ea	**66267-0563-99**	359.92		
(PD-Rx Pharm)				
REPACK				
TAB, PO (FILM-COATED)				
50 mg, 6s ea	**43063-0055-06**	36.40		
12s ea	**55289-0719-12**	48.20		
40s ea	**55289-0719-40**	76.00		
60s ea	**55289-0719-60**	89.50		
90s ea	**55289-0719-90**	109.90		
(FILM-COATED)				
50 mg, 270s ea	**55289-0719-94**	329.70		
(Pharma Pac)				
REPACK				
TAB, PO (FILM-COATED)				
50 mg, 8s ea	**52959-0688-08**	13.50		
12s ea	**52959-0688-12**	18.96		
25s ea	**52959-0688-25**	39.44		
35s ea	**52959-0688-35**	55.20		
(FILM-COATED)				
50 mg, 84s ea	**52959-0688-84**	130.87		
150s ea	**52959-0688-05**	230.94		
240s ea	**52959-0688-03**	369.34		

PROD/MFR	NDC	AWP	DP	OBC
(Phys Total Care)				
REPACK				
TAB, PO (FILM-COATED)				
50 mg, 150s ea	54868-4638-09	27.74		
(Physician Partner)				
REPACK				
TER, PO, 100 mg, 30s ea	21695-0699-30	218.32		AB
200 mg, 30s ea	21695-0700-30	361.06		AB
(Quality Care Prod)				
REPACK				
TAB, PO, 50 mg, 240s ea	49999-0129-24	523.12		
TER, PO, 100 mg, 30s ea	35356-0546-30	168.30		AB
200 mg, 30s ea	35356-0547-30	316.20		AB
(Southwood)				
REPACK				
TAB, PO (FILM-COATED)				
50 mg, 30s ea	58016-0708-30	48.30		
60s ea	58016-0708-60	96.60		
90s ea	58016-0708-90	144.90		
100s ea	58016-0708-00	161.00		
120s ea	58016-0708-02	193.20		
(St. Mary's MPP)				
REPACK				
TAB, PO, 50 mg, 9s ea	60760-0377-09	17.83		
TRAMADOL HYDROCHLORIDE & APAP (Dispensing Solutions)				
REPACK				
acetaminophen/tramadol hydrochloride				
TAB, PO, 325 mg-37.5 mg,				
40s ea	55045-3350-03	40.80		
TRAMADOL HYDROCHLORIDE AND ACETAMINOPHEN (Amneal)				
acetaminophen/tramadol hydrochloride				
TAB, PO (FILM-COATED)				
325 mg-37.5 mg,				
100s ea	65162-0617-10	102.49		AB
500s ea	65162-0617-50	512.18		AB
1000s ea	65162-0617-11	1024.00		AB
(Mylan)				
TAB, PO (FILM-COATED)				
325 mg-37.5 mg,				
100s ea	00378-8088-01	102.49		AB
500s ea	00378-8088-05	512.18		AB
(Par)				
TAB, PO (FILM-COATED)				
325 mg-37.5 mg,				
100s ea	49884-0946-01	102.48		AB
500s ea	49884-0946-05	483.59		AB
(Aidarex)				
REPACK				
TAB, PO (FILM-COATED)				
325 mg-37.5 mg,				
7s ea	33261-0389-07	9.73		AB
10s ea	33261-0389-10	13.90		AB
14s ea	33261-0389-14	19.46		AB
20s ea	33261-0389-20	27.80		AB
21s ea	33261-0389-21	29.19		AB
28s ea	33261-0389-28	38.92		AB
30s ea	33261-0389-30	41.70		AB
60s ea	33261-0389-60	83.40		AB
90s ea	33261-0389-90	125.10		AB
100s ea	33261-0389-00	139.00		AB
120s ea	33261-0389-02	166.80		AB
180s ea	33261-0389-03	250.20		AB
(American Health)				
REPACK				
TAB, PO (10X10)				
325 mg-37.5 mg,				
100s ea UD	68084-0139-01	107.10		
(Bryant Ranch)				
REPACK				
TAB, PO (FILM-COATED)				
325 mg-37.5 mg,				
60s ea	63629-3406-02	124.20		AB
(Nucare Pharm)				
REPACK				
TAB, PO (FILM-COATED)				
325 mg-37.5 mg,				
20s ea	68071-0287-20	28.16		AB
100s ea	68071-1359-00	134.79		AB
(Pharma Pac)				
REPACK				
TAB, PO (FILM-COATED)				
325 mg-37.5 mg,				
120s ea	52959-0814-12	150.42		AB

PROD/MFR	NDC	AWP	DP	OBC
(Phys Total Care)				
REPACK				
TAB, PO, 325 mg-37.5 mg,				
50s ea	54868-5291-04	79.14		
100s ea	54868-5291-05	119.44		
TRAMADOL HYDROCHLORIDE-ACETAMINOPHEN (Quality Care Prod)				
REPACK				
acetaminophen/tramadol hydrochloride				
TAB, PO, 325 mg-37.5 mg,				
60s ea	49999-0693-60	136.80		
100s ea	49999-0693-00	228.00		
TRAMADOL HYDROCHLORIDE/ACETAMINOPHEN (Caraco)				
acetaminophen/tramadol hydrochloride				
TAB, PO (FILM-COATED)				
325 mg-37.5 mg,				
100s ea	57664-0537-88	102.47		AB
500s ea	57664-0537-13	512.00		AB
1000s ea	57664-0537-18	1024.00		AB
(Teva)				
TAB, PO (COATED)				
325 mg-37.5 mg,				
500s ea	00172-6359-70	512.18		
(4u)				
REPACK				
TAB, PO (FILM-COATED)				
325 mg-37.5 mg,				
30s ea	10544-0369-30	72.86		AB
30s ea	42549-0569-30	72.86		AB
112s ea	10544-0369-02	194.36		AB
112s ea	42549-0569-02	194.36		AB
(Altura)				
REPACK				
TAB, PO (FILM-COATED)				
325 mg-37.5 mg,				
20s ea	63874-1163-02	21.40		AB
30s ea	63874-1163-03	32.10		AB
40s ea	63874-1163-04	42.80		AB
60s ea	63874-1163-06	64.20		AB
90s ea	63874-1163-09	96.30		AB
100s ea	63874-1163-00	107.00		AB
120s ea	63874-1163-01	128.40		AB
180s ea	63874-1163-08	192.60		AB
(IPI)				
REPACK				
TAB, PO (FILM-COATED)				
325 mg-37.5 mg,				
30s ea	18837-0158-30	30.72		AB
40s ea	18837-0158-40	40.96		AB
60s ea	18837-0158-60	61.44		AB
100s ea	18837-0158-99	102.70		AB
180s ea	18837-0138-96	230.40		AB
(Nucare Pharm)				
REPACK				
TAB, PO (COATED)				
325 mg-37.5 mg,				
30s ea	68071-0287-30	44.92		
40s ea	68071-0287-40	56.32		
60s ea	68071-0287-60	84.48		
90s ea	68071-0287-90	120.96		
120s ea	68071-0287-91	161.28		
(PD-Rx Pharm)				
REPACK				
TAB, PO (FILM-COATED)				
325 mg-37.5 mg,				
15s ea	55289-0895-15	48.66		AB
60s ea	55289-0895-60	72.51		AB
(Pharma Pac)				
REPACK				
TAB, PO (FILM-COATED)				
325 mg-37.5 mg,				
180s ea	52959-0814-18	223.74		AB
(St. Mary's MPP)				
REPACK				
TAB, PO, 325 mg-37.5 mg,				
20s ea	60760-0053-20	28.53		
(FILM-COATED)				
325 mg-37.5 mg,				
30s ea	60760-0053-30	39.79		AB
60s ea	60760-0053-60	73.58		
90s ea	60760-0053-90	107.38		
TRAMADOL HYDROCHLORIDE/APAP (Keltman Pharma., Inc.)				
REPACK				
acetaminophen/tramadol hydrochloride				
TAB, PO, 325 mg-37.5 mg,				
20s ea	68387-0497-20	26.67		

PROD/MFR	NDC	AWP	DP	OBC
TRAMADOL/ACETAMINOPHEN (DHS, Inc.)				
REPACK				
acetaminophen/tramadol hydrochloride				
TAB, PO, 325 mg-37.5 mg,				
20s ea	55887-0211-20	31.48		
30s ea	55887-0211-30	47.22		
40s ea	55887-0211-40	62.96		
50s ea	55887-0211-50	78.70		
60s ea	55887-0211-60	94.44		
90s ea	55887-0211-90	119.41		
TRAMADOL/APAP (Bryant Ranch)				
REPACK				
acetaminophen/tramadol hydrochloride				
TAB, PO, 325 mg-37.5 mg,				
50s ea	63629-3406-03	102.30		
(Core)				
REPACK				
TAB, PO, 325 mg-37.5 mg,				
30s ea	33358-0343-30	42.48		
50s ea	33358-0343-50	58.95		
60s ea	33358-0343-60	69.91		
90s ea	33358-0343-90	102.43		
(Dispensing Solutions)				
REPACK				
TAB, PO, 325 mg-37.5 mg,				
30s ea	66336-0909-30	32.89		
60s ea	66336-0909-60	65.17		
(Physician Partner)				
REPACK				
TAB, PO, 325 mg-37.5 mg,				
30s ea	21695-0236-30	62.49		
50s ea	21695-0236-50	102.43		
60s ea	21695-0236-60	122.92		
120s ea	21695-0236-72	245.83		
(Southwood)				
REPACK				
TAB, PO, 325 mg-37.5 mg,				
180s ea	58016-0617-99	183.60		
240s ea	58016-0617-04	244.80		
300s ea	58016-0617-73	306.00		
360s ea	58016-0617-98	367.20		
(Stat Rx)				
REPACK				
TAB, PO, 325 mg-37.5 mg,				
30s ea	16590-0230-30	62.10		
40s ea	16590-0230-40	111.00		
45s ea	16590-0230-45	124.88		
60s ea	16590-0230-60	166.50		
90s ea	16590-0230-90	249.75		
100s ea	16590-0230-71	277.00		
120s ea	16590-0230-72	333.00		
(Vibranta)				
REPACK				
TAB, PO, 325 mg-37.5 mg,				
60s ea	57866-3159-01	75.82		
90s ea	57866-3159-02	112.44		
120s ea	57866-3159-03	142.12		
TRANCOT (Truxton)				
meprobamate				
TAB, PO, 200 mg,				
1000s ea, C-IV	00463-6176-10	21.00		EE
400 mg,				
1000s ea, C-IV	00463-6177-10	30.00		EE
TRANDATE (Prometheus Labs)				
labetalol hydrochloride				
TAB, PO, 100 mg, 100s ea	65483-0391-10	74.77		AB
200 mg, 100s ea	65483-0392-10	105.56		AB
300 mg, 100s ea	65483-0393-10	127.78		AB
(Phys Total Care)				
REPACK				
SOL, IV (MDV)				
5 mg/ml, 20 ml	54868-3920-00	23.31		AP
TAB, PO, 100 mg, 60s ea	54868-2864-01	39.76		AB
100s ea	54868-2864-00	64.87		AB
TRANDOLAPRIL				
FUL				
TAB, PO, 1 mg, 100s ea		66.66		
2 mg, 100s ea		66.66		
4 mg, 100s ea		66.66		
(Abbott Pharm) *See MAVIK*				
(Aurobindo Pharma)				
TAB, PO, 1 mg, 100s ea	65862-0164-01	121.18		AB
2 mg, 100s ea	65862-0165-01	121.18		AB
4 mg, 100s ea	65862-0166-01	121.18		AB
(Dava Pharma)				
TAB, PO, 1 mg, 100s ea	67253-0106-10	123.93		AB
2 mg, 100s ea	67253-0107-10	123.93		AB
4 mg, 100s ea	67253-0108-10	123.93		AB

PROD/MFR	NDC	AWP	DP	OBC
(Greenstone)				
TAB, PO, 1 mg, 100s ea	59762-2140-01	115.20		
1000s ea	59762-2140-06	1152.00		
2 mg, 100s ea	59762-2141-01	115.20		
1000s ea	59762-2141-06	1152.00		
4 mg, 100s ea	59762-2142-01	115.20		
1000s ea	59762-2142-06	1152.00		
(Lupin Pharma, Inc.)				
TAB, PO, 1 mg, 100s ea	68180-0566-01	123.93		AB
2 mg, 100s ea	68180-0567-01	123.93		AB
4 mg, 100s ea	68180-0568-01	123.93		AB
(Mylan)				
TAB, PO, 1 mg, 100s ea	00378-3241-01	123.93		AB
2 mg, 100s ea	00378-3242-01	123.93		AB
4 mg, 100s ea	00378-3243-01	123.93		AB
(Sandoz)				
TAB, PO (COMPRESSED)				
1 mg, 100s ea	00781-5320-01	123.93		AB
2 mg, 100s ea	00781-5321-01	123.93		AB
4 mg, 100s ea	00781-5322-01	123.93		AB
(Teva)				
TAB, PO, 1 mg, 100s ea	00093-7325-01	120.32		AB
2 mg, 100s ea	00093-7326-01	120.32		AB
4 mg, 100s ea	00093-7327-01	120.32		AB
(Watson Labs)				
TAB, PO, 1 mg, 30s ea	16252-0541-30	14.40		AB
2 mg, 90s ea	16252-0542-90	48.00		AB
4 mg, 90s ea	16252-0543-90	48.00		AB
(Phys Total Care) REPACK				
TAB, PO, 4 mg, 90s ea	54868-6061-01	105.48		AB
100s ea	54868-6061-00	115.04		AB
TRANDOLAPRIL/VERAPAMIL HYDROCHLORIDE				
(Abbott Pharm) *See TARKA*				
TRANEXAMIC ACID (Gallipot)				
POW, NA, 50 gm	51552-0513-09	118.30		
(Hawkins)				
POW, NA, 25 gm	63370-0280-25	178.00		
100 gm	63370-0280-35	660.00		
(Letco)				
POW, NA (BP2000)				
100 gm	62991-2581-02	465.00		
(PCCA)				
POW, NA, 1 gm	51927-2793-00	9.00		
(Pfizer) *See CYKLOKAPRON*				
(Spectrum Pharmacy)				
POW, NA (1X25GM)				
25 gm	49452-7877-02	324.10		
(1X100GM)				
100 gm	49452-7877-03	805.00		
TRANILAST (PCCA)				
POW, NA (1X1GM)				
1 gm	51927-3178-00	5.04		
TRANSCUTANEOUS NERVE STIMULATOR WRISTBAND				
(Abbott Hosp) *See RELIEFBAND*				
TRANSDERM SCOP (Baxter)				
scopolamine				
TDM, TD, 0.33 mg/24 hr,				
ea	10019-0553-88	11.90		
(Novartis Consumer)				
TDM, TD, 0.33 mg/24 hr,				
4s ea	00067-4345-04	43.67		
(PD-Rx Pharm) REPACK				
TDM, TD, 0.33 mg/24 hr,				
ea	43063-0003-01	108.86		
(Phys Total Care) REPACK				
TDM, TD, 0.33 mg/24 hr,				
4s ea	54868-2803-01	56.69		
10s ea	54868-2803-00	123.33		
TRANSDERMAL OINTMENT BASE (Spectrum Pharmacy)				
ointment base				
OIN, NA (1X454GM)				
454 gm	49452-7878-01	163.80		
TRANSDERMAL PAIN BASE (Medisca)				
cream base				
CRE, NA (1X500GM)				
500 gm	38779-2493-08	207.00		
(1X2500GM)				
2500 gm	38779-2493-01	897.00		
(1X5000GM)				
5000 gm	38779-2493-03	1647.00		
TRANSFER PIN (APP)				
transfer unit, iv fluid				
DEV, NA, 100s ea	63323-0907-90	183.00		
TRANSFER UNIT, IV FLUID				
(Abbott Hosp) *See DOUBLE-NEEDLE TRANSFER DEVICE*				
(APP) *See CHEMO TRANSFER PIN*				
(APP) *See IV TRANSFER SPIKE*				
(APP) *See MAXIFILL TRANSFER SET*				
(APP) *See MINI TRANSFER PIN*				
(APP) *See TRANSFER PIN*				
(Bracco Diag) *See SOLUTION TRANSFER DEVICE*				
TRANXENE T-TAB (Lundbeck)				
clorazepate dipotassium				
TAB, PO, 3.75 mg,				
100s ea, C-IV	67386-0301-01	320.68		AB
7.5 mg,				
100s ea, C-IV	67386-0302-01	398.96		AB
500s ea, C-IV	67386-0302-05	1954.87		AB
15 mg,				
100s ea, C-IV	67386-0303-01	541.27		AB
TRANXENE-SD (Lundbeck)				
clorazepate dipotassium				
TER, PO, 11.25 mg,				
100s ea, C-IV	67386-0404-01	777.44		
22.5 mg,				
100s ea, C-IV	67386-0405-01	995.69		
TRANYLCYPROMINE SULFATE				
(Glaxo) *See PARNATE*				
(Par)				
TAB, PO (FILM-COATED)				
10 mg, 100s ea	49884-0032-01	124.85		
TRANZGEL (Gensco)				
homeopathic				
GEL, TP (1X50ML)				
50 ml	35781-0194-05	26.87		
TRASTUZUMAB				
(Genentech) *See HERCEPTIN*				
TRASYLOL (Bayer Corp.)				
aprotinin				
SOL, IV, 10000 kiu/ml,				
100 ml	00026-8196-36	325.94		
200 ml	00026-8197-63	599.06		
TRAUMANIL (Gensco)				
homeopathic				
GEL, TP (1X50ML,ODOR-FREE)				
50 ml	35781-0192-05	97.80		
(Aidarex) REPACK				
GEL, TP (1X50ML,ODOR-FREE)				
50 ml	33261-0455-01	97.80		
(Dispensing Solutions) REPACK				
GEL, TP (1X50ML,ODOR-FREE)				
50 ml	68258-3022-01	97.80		
(Nucare Pharm) REPACK				
GEL, TP (1X50ML,ODOR-FREE)				
50 ml	66267-1262-01	129.80		
(Quality Care Prod) REPACK				
GEL, TP (1X50ML,ODOR-FREE)				
50 ml	35356-0137-50	97.80		
TRAUMEEL (Heel/BHI)				
nutriceutical				
OIN, TP, 50 gm	51885-3302-03	7.95	7.95	
100 gm	51885-3302-01	13.95	13.95	
(Keltman Pharma., Inc.) REPACK				
OIN, TP (1X50GM)				
50 gm	68387-0107-01	18.25		
(Stat Rx) REPACK				
OIN, TP (1X50GM)				
50 gm	16590-0664-50	19.00		
TRAVASOL (Baxter)				
amino acids				
SOL, IV (VIAFLEX,SULF. FREE,BULK)				
10%, 500 ml 6s	00338-0644-03	503.93		
(VIAFLEX,BULK,AF)				
10%, 1000 ml	00338-0644-04	93.37		
2000 ml 6s	00338-0644-06	2001.67		
TRAVATAN (Alcon Ophthalmic)				
travoprost				
SOL, OP, 0.004%, 2.5 ml	00065-0266-25	91.74		
5 ml	00065-0266-34	183.48		
(A-S Medication) REPACK				
SOL, OP, 0.004%, 2.5 ml	54569-5393-00	79.50		
(Phys Total Care) REPACK				
SOL, OP, 0.004%, 2.5 ml	54868-4688-00	74.05		
5 ml	54868-4688-01	163.49		
TRAVATAN Z (Alcon Ophthalmic)				
travoprost				
SOL, OP, 0.004%, 2.5 ml	00065-0260-25	91.74		
5 ml	00065-0260-05	183.48		
(Phys Total Care) REPACK				
SOL, OP (1X5ML)				
0.004%, 5 ml	54868-5968-00	193.45		
TRAVOPROST				
(Alcon Ophthalmic) *See TRAVATAN*				
(Alcon Ophthalmic) *See TRAVATAN Z*				
TRAZODO (Altura) REPACK				
trazodone hydrochloride				
TAB, PO, 50 mg, 40s ea	63874-0560-40	65.17		
TRAZODONE (4u) REPACK				
trazodone hydrochloride				
TAB, PO, 50 mg, 30s ea	10544-0346-30	84.82		
60s ea	10544-0346-60	118.78		
(Bryant Ranch) REPACK				
TAB, PO, 50 mg, 20s ea	63629-1513-01	43.59		
30s ea	63629-1513-02	63.38		
60s ea	63629-1513-03	121.67		
100 mg, 30s ea	63629-3210-01	99.87		
60s ea	63629-3210-02	199.99		
150 mg, 30s ea	63629-2867-01	55.54		
60s ea	63629-2867-02	111.07		
90s ea	63629-2867-03	166.61		
(Core) REPACK				
TAB, PO, 50 mg, 20s ea	33358-0344-20	44.68		
30s ea	33358-0344-30	64.96		
60s ea	33358-0344-60	124.71		
100 mg, 30s ea	33358-0345-30	64.96		
90s ea	33358-0345-90	204.99		
150 mg, 30s ea	33358-0346-30	56.93		
60s ea	33358-0346-60	113.85		
90s ea	33358-0346-90	170.78		
(DHS, Inc.) REPACK				
TAB, PO, 100 mg, 20s ea	55887-0256-20	47.96		
150 mg, 60s ea	55887-0871-60	117.00		
(HomeMed) REPACK				
TAB, PO, 50 mg, 30s ea	51655-0634-24	47.49		EE
(IPI) REPACK				
TAB, PO, 50 mg, 30s ea	18837-0162-30	15.52		
(Physician Partner) REPACK				
TAB, PO, 50 mg, 30s ea	21695-0133-30	33.91		
60s ea	21695-0133-60	67.82		
90s ea	21695-0133-90	101.73		
100 mg, 30s ea	21695-0134-30	92.00		
60s ea	21695-0134-60	184.00		
90s ea	21695-0134-90	275.99		
(Stat Rx) REPACK				
TAB, PO, 50 mg, 30s ea	16590-0231-30	47.48		
60s ea	16590-0231-60	74.20		
90s ea	16590-0231-90	142.44		
100 mg, 30s ea	16590-0232-30	60.00		
45s ea	16590-0232-45	60.00		
90s ea	16590-0232-90	180.00		
TRAZODONE HCL (Major)				
trazodone hydrochloride				
TAB, PO (10X10)				
50 mg, 100s ea UD	00904-3990-61	43.51		AB
100 mg, 100s ea UD	00904-3991-61	78.43		AB

PROD/MFR	NDC	AWP	DP	OBC
(Medisca)				
POW, NA (USP)				
5 gm	**38779-0559-03**	40.50		
(U.S.P.)				
25 gm	**38779-0559-04**	165.00		
100 gm	**38779-0559-05**	555.00		
(Mutual)				
TAB, PO, 50 mg, 100s ea	**53489-0510-01**	56.72		AB
100 mg, 100s ea	**53489-0511-01**	73.26		AB
150 mg, 100s ea	**53489-0517-01**	146.92		AB
(Qualitest)				
TAB, PO (USP,FILM-COATED)				
50 mg, 100s ea	**00603-6147-21**	56.50		AB
1000s ea	**00603-6147-32**	413.80		AB
100 mg, 100s ea	**00603-6148-21**	73.20		AB
1000s ea	**00603-6148-32**	576.85		AB
(Sandoz)				
TAB, PO (DIVIDOSE)				
150 mg, 500s ea	**59772-3171-02**	716.44		AB
(Spectrum Pharmacy)				
CRY, NA (U.S.P.)				
5 gm	**49452-7073-02**	72.45		
25 gm	**49452-7073-03**	285.60		
(Teva)				
TAB, PO, 50 mg, 100s ea	**50111-0433-01**	56.52		AB
500s ea	**50111-0433-02**	220.65		AB
1000s ea	**50111-0433-03**	413.82		AB
100 mg, 100s ea	**50111-0434-01**	73.25		AB
500s ea	**50111-0434-02**	347.95		AB
1000s ea	**50111-0434-03**	576.90		AB
150 mg, 100s ea	**50111-0441-01**	146.91		AB
500s ea	**50111-0441-02**	661.15		AB
(4u)				
REPACK				
TAB, PO, 50 mg, 30s ea	**42549-0546-30**	84.82		AB
60s ea	**42549-0546-60**	118.78		AB
(A-S Medication)				
REPACK				
TAB, PO, 50 mg, 30s ea	**54569-1470-00**	16.96		EE
(USP)				
50 mg, 45s ea	**54569-1470-08**	25.43		EE
60s ea	**54569-1470-06**	33.91		EE
90s ea	**54569-1470-09**	50.87		EE
100s ea	**54569-1470-01**	56.52		EE
100 mg, 30s ea	**54569-1999-00**	21.98		EE
90s ea	**54569-1999-03**	65.93		EE
150 mg, 15s ea	**54569-3732-03**	22.04		EE
30s ea	**54569-3732-02**	44.08		EE
(Aidarex)				
REPACK				
TAB, PO, 50 mg, 14s ea	**33261-0107-14**	32.60		AB
20s ea	**33261-0107-20**	46.60		AB
21s ea	**33261-0107-21**	48.93		AB
28s ea	**33261-0107-28**	65.24		AB
30s ea	**33261-0107-30**	69.90		AB
40s ea	**33261-0107-40**	93.20		AB
60s ea	**33261-0107-60**	139.80		AB
90s ea	**33261-0107-90**	209.70		AB
100 mg, 30s ea	**33261-0385-30**	89.50		AB
60s ea	**33261-0385-60**	179.00		AB
90s ea	**33261-0385-90**	268.50		AB
120s ea	**33261-0385-02**	358.00		AB
150 mg, 30s ea	**33261-0386-30**	117.00		AB
60s ea	**33261-0386-60**	234.00		AB
90s ea	**33261-0386-90**	351.00		AB
120s ea	**33261-0386-02**	468.00		AB
(Altura)				
REPACK				
TAB, PO, 50 mg, 10s ea	**63874-0560-10**	15.80		AB
12s ea	**63874-0560-12**	18.96		AB
14s ea	**63874-0560-14**	22.12		AB
15s ea	**63874-0560-15**	23.70		AB
20s ea	**63874-0560-20**	31.60		AB
28s ea	**63874-0560-28**	44.24		AB
30s ea	**63874-0560-30**	48.89		AB
60s ea	**63874-0560-60**	97.76		AB
90s ea	**63874-0560-90**	142.20		AB
100s ea	**63874-0560-01**	162.96		AB
120s ea	**63874-0560-04**	189.60		AB
100 mg, 10s ea	**63874-0537-10**	22.81		
12s ea	**63874-0537-12**	27.37		
14s ea	**63874-0537-14**	31.93		
15s ea	**63874-0537-15**	34.21		
20s ea	**63874-0537-20**	45.61		
30s ea	**63874-0537-30**	68.42		
40s ea	**63874-0537-40**	91.23		
60s ea	**63874-0537-60**	136.84		
90s ea	**63874-0537-90**	205.25		
100s ea	**63874-0537-01**	228.06		
120s ea	**63874-0537-04**	273.67		
150 mg, 12s ea	**63874-0775-12**	23.58		AB
15s ea	**63874-0775-15**	29.47		AB
20s ea	**63874-0775-20**	39.30		AB
30s ea	**63874-0775-30**	58.94		AB
100s ea	**63874-0775-01**	196.48		AB
(DHS, Inc.)				
REPACK				
TAB, PO, 50 mg, 30s ea	**55887-0524-30**	46.95		AB
60s ea	**55887-0524-60**	93.90		AB
90s ea	**55887-0524-90**	140.85		AB
120s ea	**55887-0524-82**	187.80		AB
100 mg, 30s ea	**55887-0256-30**	71.95		AB
60s ea	**55887-0256-60**	143.90		AB
90s ea	**55887-0256-90**	215.84		AB
(Dispensing Solutions)				
REPACK				
TAB, PO, 50 mg, 7s ea	**55045-1715-02**	10.50		AB
28s ea	**55045-1715-07**	42.00		AB
28s ea	**66336-0620-28**	43.82		AB
30s ea	**55045-1715-08**	45.00		AB
30s ea	**66336-0620-30**	46.95		AB
60s ea	**55045-1715-09**	90.00		AB
60s ea	**66336-0620-60**	93.90		AB
90s ea	**55045-1715-03**	135.00		AB
90s ea	**66336-0620-90**	140.85		AB
100s ea	**55045-1715-00**	150.00		AB
120s ea	**55045-1715-01**	180.00		AB
100 mg, 30s ea	**55045-1724-08**	62.50		AB
30s ea	**66336-0014-30**	80.40		AB
60s ea	**55045-1724-09**	125.00		AB
60s ea	**66336-0014-60**	160.80		AB
90s ea	**55045-1724-06**	187.50		AB
100s ea	**55045-1724-01**	208.00		AB
120s ea	**55045-1724-00**	249.60		AB
150 mg, 14s ea	**66336-0838-14**	45.60		AB
30s ea	**55045-2509-08**	68.10		AB
60s ea	**55045-2509-06**	136.20		AB
90s ea	**55045-2509-09**	204.30		AB
100s ea	**55045-2509-01**	227.00		AB
120s ea	**55045-2509-00**	272.40		AB
(GSMS)				
REPACK				
TAB, PO (UNIT OF USE)				
50 mg, 30s ea	**60429-0187-30**	4.11	1.37	AB
60s ea	**60429-0187-60**	6.39	2.13	AB
90s ea	**60429-0187-90**	8.79	2.93	AB
100 mg, 30s ea	**60429-0188-30**	5.79	1.93	AB
60s ea	**60429-0188-60**	9.87	3.29	AB
(HomeMed)				
REPACK				
TAB, PO, 100 mg, 30s ea	**51655-0666-24**	18.31		EE
(IPI)				
REPACK				
TAB, PO, 50 mg, 60s ea	**18837-0162-60**	12.41		AB
100 mg, 30s ea	**18837-0160-30**	17.31		AB
150 mg, 30s ea	**18837-0376-30**	39.67		AB
(Keltman Pharma., Inc.)				
REPACK				
TAB, PO, 50 mg, 30s ea	**68387-0165-30**	48.15		AB
(USP)				
50 mg, 60s ea	**68387-0165-60**	96.30		AB
100 mg, 30s ea	**68387-0166-30**	67.50		AB
60s ea	**68387-0166-60**	135.00		AB
(Nucare Pharm)				
REPACK				
TAB, PO, 50 mg, 30s ea	**66267-0205-30**	45.39		AB
100 mg, 30s ea	**66267-0392-30**	83.56		AB
60s ea	**66267-0392-60**	169.35		AB
(PD-Rx Pharm)				
REPACK				
TAB, PO, 50 mg, 7s ea	**55289-0064-07**	31.50		AB
14s ea	**55289-0064-14**	32.88		AB
(REDI-SCRIPT)				
50 mg, 14s ea	**58864-0025-14**	24.60		AB
30s ea	**55289-0064-30**	36.18		AB
(REDI-SCRIPT)				
50 mg, 30s ea	**58864-0025-30**	28.80		AB
60s ea	**55289-0064-60**	42.30		AB
90s ea	**55289-0064-90**	48.48		AB
(REDI-SCRIPT)				
50 mg, 100s ea	**58864-0025-01**	44.80		AB
100 mg, 30s ea	**55289-0223-30**	34.27		AB
30s ea	**58864-0783-30**	34.27		AB
90s ea	**55289-0223-90**	54.30		AB
150 mg, 14s ea	**55289-0060-14**	35.79		AB
(REDI-SCRIPT)				
150 mg, 30s ea	**58864-0708-30**	52.94		AB
(Pharma Pac)				
REPACK				
TAB, PO, 50 mg, 15s ea	**52959-0378-15**	28.90		EE
20s ea	**52959-0378-20**	33.19		EE
30s ea	**52959-0378-30**	49.78		EE
60s ea	**52959-0378-60**	99.54		AB
90s ea	**52959-0378-90**	149.30		EE
100 mg, 30s ea	**52959-0140-30**	88.73		EE
60s ea	**52959-0140-60**	177.45		EE
90s ea	**52959-0140-90**	266.15		EE
150 mg, 60s ea	**52959-0894-60**	202.80		AB
(Phys Total Care)				
REPACK				
TAB, PO, 50 mg, 15s ea	**54868-0122-04**	5.82		AB
20s ea	**54868-0122-07**	6.38		AB
30s ea	**54868-0122-02**	8.67		EE
60s ea	**54868-0122-03**	14.34		EE
90s ea	**54868-0122-05**	19.98		AB
100s ea	**54868-0122-00**	20.37		EE
100 mg, 30s ea	**54868-1223-01**	13.11		EE
60s ea	**54868-1223-04**	23.25		AB
90s ea	**54868-1223-03**	33.36		AB
100s ea	**54868-1223-00**	36.75		EE
150 mg, 15s ea	**54868-1959-02**	17.79		EE
30s ea	**54868-1959-01**	32.61		EE
(USP)				
150 mg, 60s ea	**54868-1959-04**	33.33		EE
100s ea	**54868-1959-03**	100.17		AB
(Physician Partner)				
REPACK				
TAB, PO, 50 mg, 120s ea	**21695-0133-72**	159.59		AB
(Quality Care Prod)				
REPACK				
TAB, PO, 50 mg, 15s ea	**49999-0343-15**	28.49		AB
30s ea	**49999-0343-30**	57.57		AB
60s ea	**49999-0343-60**	113.76		EE
100s ea	**49999-0343-00**	189.96		EE
100 mg, 14s ea	**49999-0156-14**	38.47		AB
30s ea	**49999-0156-30**	82.12		AB
60s ea	**49999-0156-60**	168.00		EE
100s ea	**49999-0156-00**	274.80		EE
(Southwood)				
REPACK				
TAB, PO, 50 mg, 10s ea	**58016-0263-10**	16.30		EE
12s ea	**58016-0263-12**	19.56		EE
15s ea	**58016-0263-15**	24.44		EE
20s ea	**58016-0263-20**	32.59		EE
28s ea	**58016-0263-28**	45.63		EE
30s ea	**58016-0263-30**	48.89		EE
40s ea	**58016-0263-40**	65.18		AB
60s ea	**58016-0263-60**	97.78		EE
90s ea	**58016-0263-90**	146.66		EE
100s ea	**58016-0263-00**	162.96		EE
120s ea	**58016-0263-02**	195.55		EE
150s ea	**58016-0263-03**	244.44		EE
200s ea	**58016-0263-89**	325.92		EE
300s ea	**58016-0263-73**	488.88		EE
100 mg, 12s ea	**58016-0862-12**	34.17		EE
15s ea	**58016-0862-15**	42.72		EE
20s ea	**58016-0862-20**	56.95		EE
30s ea	**58016-0862-30**	85.43		EE
50s ea	**58016-0862-50**	142.39		EE
60s ea	**58016-0862-60**	170.86		EE
90s ea	**58016-0862-90**	256.29		EE
100s ea	**58016-0862-00**	284.77		EE
120s ea	**58016-0862-02**	341.72		EE
150s ea	**58016-0862-03**	427.16		EE
200s ea	**58016-0862-89**	569.54		EE
300s ea	**58016-0862-73**	854.31		EE
150 mg, 12s ea	**58016-0880-12**	23.58		EE
15s ea	**58016-0880-15**	29.47		EE
20s ea	**58016-0880-20**	39.30		EE
30s ea	**58016-0880-30**	58.94		EE
100s ea	**58016-0880-00**	196.48		EE
(St. Mary's MPP)				
REPACK				
TAB, PO, 50 mg, 60s ea	**60760-0440-60**	35.13		AB
(Stat Rx)				
REPACK				
TAB, PO, 50 mg, 15s ea	**16590-0231-15**	23.74		AB
180s ea	**16590-0231-82**	222.60		AB
100 mg, 28s ea	**16590-0232-28**	26.09		AB
60s ea	**16590-0232-60**	75.00		AB
150 mg, 28s ea	**16590-0585-28**	51.88		AB
30s ea	**16590-0585-30**	55.59		AB
60s ea	**16590-0585-60**	134.00		AB
90s ea	**16590-0585-90**	195.00		AB
120s ea	**16590-0585-72**	250.00		AB
300 mg, 30s ea	**16590-0713-30**	163.00		AB
60s ea	**16590-0713-60**	325.80		AB
90s ea	**16590-0713-90**	488.75		AB

PROD/MFR	NDC	AWP	DP	OBC
(Vibranta) REPACK				
TAB, PO, 50 mg, 30s ea	57866-4715-01	46.10		AB
60s ea	57866-4715-02	93.05		AB
90s ea	57866-4715-03	129.39		AB
120s ea	57866-4715-04	34.70		AB
100 mg, 30s ea	57866-4688-01	69.00		
60s ea	57866-4688-02	139.15		
90s ea	57866-4688-03	188.56		
120s ea	57866-4688-04	55.10		
TRAZODONE HYDROCHLORIDE				
FUL				
TAB, PO, 50 mg, 100s ea		7.42		
100 mg, 100s ea		11.40		
150 mg, 100s ea		31.13		
(Apotex Corp.)				
TAB, PO (USP)				
50 mg, 100s ea UD	60505-2653-00	43.51		AB
100s ea	60505-2653-01	56.72		AB
500s ea	60505-2653-05	220.71		AB
17000s ea	60505-2653-07	7504.14		AB
100 mg, 100s ea UD	60505-2654-00	78.43		AB
100s ea	60505-2654-01	73.26		AB
500s ea	60505-2654-05	347.92		AB
9000s ea	60505-2654-07	6262.56		AB
150 mg, 100s ea	60505-2655-01	146.92		AB
500s ea	60505-2655-05	661.14		AB
5500s ea	60505-2655-07	7272.54		AB
300 mg, 100s ea	60505-2659-01	543.52		AB
(Gallipot)				
POW, NA (1X25GM)				
25 gm	51552-0778-04	86.45	61.75	
(Major) *See TRAZODONE HCL*				
(Medisca) *See TRAZODONE HCL*				
(Mutual) *See TRAZODONE HCL*				
(Mylan)				
TAB, PO, 50 mg, 100s ea	00378-3471-01	56.72		AB
100 mg, 100s ea	00378-3472-01	73.26		AB
150 mg, 100s ea	00378-3473-01	146.92		AB
300 mg, 100s ea	00378-3474-01	543.52		AB
(PCCA)				
POW, NA (USP)				
1 gm	51927-2148-00	7.20		
(Qualitest) *See TRAZODONE HCL*				
(Sandoz) *See TRAZODONE HCL*				
(Spectrum Pharmacy) *See TRAZODONE HCL*				
(Teva)				
TAB, PO, 50 mg,				
100s ea UD	00182-1259-89	42.42		AB
100 mg, 100s ea UD	00182-1260-89	73.59		AB
(Teva) *See TRAZODONE HCL*				
(Dispensing Solutions) REPACK				
TAB, PO, 50 mg, 30s ea	55045-3757-08	45.00		
(Keltman Pharma., Inc.) REPACK				
TAB, PO, 50 mg, 90s ea	68387-0165-90	144.45		
150 mg, 30s ea	68387-0160-30	59.03		
(Nucare Pharm) REPACK				
TAB, PO, 50 mg, 60s ea	66267-0205-60	117.17		AB
90s ea	66267-0205-90	136.17		AB
(Palmetto) REPACK				
TAB, PO, 50 mg, 28s ea	23490-6407-01	55.99		
30s ea	23490-6407-02	59.99		
60s ea	23490-6407-03	119.98		
90s ea	23490-6407-04	179.97		
100 mg, 30s ea	23490-6405-01	98.99		
60s ea	23490-6405-02	197.98		
90s ea	23490-6405-09	296.97		
150 mg, 14s ea	23490-6406-01	45.60		
30s ea	23490-6406-02	97.72		
60s ea	23490-6406-06	195.43		
90s ea	23490-6406-09	293.15		
(Pharma Pac) REPACK				
TAB, PO, 150 mg, 30s ea	52959-0894-30	101.40		
(Physician Partner) REPACK				
TAB, PO, 150 mg, 60s ea	21695-0135-60	176.29		
(Quality Care Prod) REPACK				
TAB; PO, 100 mg, 20s ea	49999-0156-20	54.96		
150 mg, 30s ea	49999-0913-30	52.89		

PROD/MFR	NDC	AWP	DP	OBC
(St. Mary's MPP) REPACK				
TAB, PO (USP)				
50 mg, 30s ea	60760-0044-30	20.56		
100 mg, 30s ea	60760-0434-30	28.96		
60s ea	60760-0434-60	51.93		
TREANDA (Cephalon)				
bendamustine hydrochloride				
PDS, IV (SINGLE-USE,LYOPHILIZED)				
25 mg, 8 ml	63459-0390-08	540.00		
100 mg, ea	63459-0391-20	2160.00		
TRECATOR (Wyeth)				
ethionamide				
TAB, PO (FILM-COATED)				
250 mg, 100s ea	00008-4117-01	422.09	351.74	
TREHALOSE (PCCA)				
POW, NA ((D) DIHYDRATE)				
1 gm	51927-3563-00	5.25		
TRELSTAR DEPOT (Watson)				
triptorelin pamoate				
PDR, IM (W/MIXJECT SYSTEM)				
3.75 mg, ea	52544-0189-76	870.00		
TRELSTAR LA (Watson)				
triptorelin pamoate				
PDR, IM (W/MIXJECT SYSTEM)				
11.25 mg, ea	52544-0188-76	2610.00		
TRENTAL (Sanofi-Aventis)				
pentoxifylline				
TER, PO (FILM-COATED)				
400 mg, 100s ea	00039-0078-10	117.34		AB
(Phys Total Care) REPACK				
TER, PO, 400 mg, 30s ea	54868-0374-03	31.25		AB
100s ea	54868-0374-01	99.16		AB
(Southwood) REPACK				
TER, PO, 400 mg, 30s ea	58016-0568-30	32.30		AB
60s ea	58016-0568-60	64.59		AB
90s ea	58016-0568-90	96.89		AB
100s ea	58016-0568-00	107.65		AB
TREPADONE (Physician Thera, LLC)				
medical food				
CAP, PO, 90s ea	68405-1016-03	274.43		
TREPROSTINIL				
(United Therapeutics) *See TYVASO*				
TREPROSTINIL SODIUM				
(United Therapeutics) *See REMODULIN*				
TRETIN-X (Triax Pharm)				
tretinoin				
CRE, TP, 0.025%, 35 gm	14290-0352-97	205.15		AB
0.05%, 35 gm	14290-0351-97	233.84		AB2
0.1%, 35 gm	14290-0350-97	248.43		AB
GEL, TP, 0.01%, 35 gm	14290-0354-97	194.23		AB
0.025%, 35 gm	14290-0353-97	205.15		AB
(Phys Total Care) REPACK				
CRE, TP (COMBO PK)				
0.05%, 35 gm	54868-5696-00	142.13		
0.1%, ea	54868-5758-00	150.90		
TRETINOIN				
FUL				
CRE, TP, 0.025%, 45 gm		70.62		
(Actavis Mid Atlantic)				
CRE, TP, 0.025%, 20 gm	00472-0117-20	43.33		AB
45 gm	00472-0117-45	82.04		AB
(Amend) *See RETINOIC ACID*				
(Gallipot) *See RETINOIC ACID*				
(Letco) *See RETINOIC ACID ALL-TRANS*				
(Medisca)				
POW, NA (U.S.P.)				
1 gm	38779-0000-16	96.00		
1 gm	38779-0001-06	90.00		
1 gm 10s	38779-0001-01	675.00		
(USP,25X5GM)				
1 gm 25s	38779-0001-04	1488.00		
(U.S.P.)				
5 gm	38779-0000-13	375.00		
(USP)				
.5 gm	38779-0001-03	366.00		
(U.S.P.)				
10 gm	38779-0000-11	705.00		
25 gm	38779-0000-14	1497.00		
(Mylan) *See AVITA*				
(Ortho) *See RENOVA*				

PROD/MFR	NDC	AWP	DP	OBC
(Ortho) *See RETIN-A*				
(Ortho) *See RETIN-A MICRO*				
(PCCA)				
POW, NA (USP, ALL TRANS-RET ACID)				
1 gm	51927-1270-00	105.00		
(Perrigo)				
CRE, TP, 0.025%, 20 gm	45802-0182-02	43.33		
45 gm	45802-0182-42	82.05		
0.05%, 20 gm	45802-0361-02	50.28		AB
45 gm	45802-0361-42	94.28		AB
0.1%, 20 gm	45802-0183-02	58.69		
45 gm	45802-0183-42	109.90		
GEL, TP, 0.01%, 15 gm	45802-0362-35	35.59		
45 gm	45802-0362-42	84.02		
0.025%, 15 gm	45802-0363-35	35.91		
45 gm	45802-0363-42	84.72		
(Roche Labs) *See VESANOID*				
(Rouses)				
CRE, TP (1X20GM)				
0.025%, 20 gm	43478-0243-20	29.83		
(1X45GM)				
0.025%, 45 gm	43478-0243-45	56.50		
(1X20GM)				
0.05%, 20 gm	43478-0242-20	40.39		
(1X45GM)				
0.05%, 45 gm	43478-0242-45	75.71		
(1X20GM)				
0.1%, 20 gm	43478-0241-20	47.12		
(1X45GM)				
0.1%, 45 gm	43478-0241-45	88.26		
GEL, TP (1X15GM)				
0.01%, 15 gm	43478-0245-15	38.65		
(1X45GM)				
0.01%, 45 gm	43478-0245-45	91.25		
(1X15GM)				
0.025%, 15 gm	43478-0244-15	39.00		
(1X45GM)				
0.025%, 45 gm	43478-0244-45	91.98		
(Spear Dermatology)				
CRE, TP, 0.05%, 40 gm	66530-0411-40	129.60		AB2
60 gm	66530-0411-60	184.68		AB2
(Spear Dermatology) *See REFISSA*				
(Spectrum Pharmacy)				
POW, NA (U.S.P.)				
1 gm	49452-6243-01	157.15		
5 gm	49452-6243-04	553.00		
25 gm	49452-6243-02	2065.00		
(Teva)				
SGL, PO (HARD GELATIN)				
10 mg, 100s ea	00555-0808-02	2248.98		AB
(Triax Pharm)				
CRE, TP, 0.025%, 20 gm	14290-0243-20	42.65		
45 gm	14290-0243-45	80.74		AB
0.05%, 20 gm	14290-0242-20	50.22		AB
(EMOLLIENT)				
0.05%, 40 gm	66530-0247-40	129.60		
45 gm	14290-0242-45	94.17		
(EMOLLIENT)				
0.05%, 60 gm	66530-0247-60	184.68		
0.1%, 20 gm	14290-0241-20	58.62		
45 gm	14290-0241-45	109.77		
GEL, TP, 0.01%, 15 gm	14290-0245-15	40.26		AB
45 gm	14290-0245-45	95.05		
0.025%, 15 gm	14290-0244-15	40.63		
45 gm	14290-0244-45	95.81		
(Triax Pharm) *See TRETIN-X*				
(Valeant Pharm Intl) *See ATRALIN*				
(A-S Medication) REPACK				
CRE, TP, 0.025%, 20 gm	54569-4808-00	46.84		
0.05%, 40 gm	54569-5788-00	135.00		
0.1%, 45 gm	54569-5457-00	109.90		AB
(Altura) REPACK				
CRE, TP, 0.05%, 20 gm	63874-0835-20	39.50		
45 gm	63874-0835-45	62.54		
0.1%, 20 gm	63874-0836-20	43.25		
45 gm	63874-0836-45	54.89		
GEL, TP, 0.01%, 15 gm	63874-0837-15	30.20		
45 gm	63874-0837-45	110.93		
(DHS, Inc.) REPACK				
CRE, TP, 0.1%, 45 gm	55887-0174-45	109.77		
(Dispensing Solutions) REPACK				
CRE, TP, 0.05%, ea	55045-2783-08	89.00		AB
0.1%, ea	05045-3191-14	104.00		AB
20 gm	55045-3691-01	60.00		

PROD/MFR	NDC	AWP	DP	OBC
(Palmetto)				
REPACK				
CRE, TP, 0.025%, 20 gm	23490-6409-01	43.48		
0.1%, 20 gm	23490-6412-01	74.26		
(Pharma Pac)				
REPACK				
CRE, TP, 0.05%, 20 gm	52959-0934-20	44.09		AB
0.1%, 20 gm	52959-0933-20	42.15		
(Phys Total Care)				
REPACK				
CRE, TP, 0.025%, 20 gm	54868-4126-00	82.74		AB
45 gm	54868-4126-01	103.02		AB
0.05%, 20 gm	54868-4378-00	116.55		EE
45 gm	54868-4378-01	167.04		EE
(1X20GM)				
0.1%, 20 gm	54868-4379-01	71.22		
(1X45GM)				
0.1%, 45 gm	54868-4379-00	154.76		
GEL, TP, 0.025%, 15 gm	54868-4444-01	62.34		
45 gm	54868-4444-00	121.32		
(Physician Partner)				
REPACK				
CRE, TP (1X20GM)				
0.1%, 20 gm	21695-0805-20	85.30		
(Southwood)				
REPACK				
CRE, TP, 0.025%, 20 gm	58016-5569-01	35.50		EE
0.05%, 20 gm	58016-5568-01	39.50		EE
TREXALL (Teva)				
methotrexate sodium				
TAB, PO (FILM-COATED)				
5 mg, 30s ea	51285-0366-01	248.31		
7.5 mg, 30s ea	51285-0367-01	372.47		
10 mg, 30s ea	51285-0368-01	496.62		
15 mg, 30s ea	51285-0369-01	744.93		
TREXBROM (Capellon)				
bpm/carbetapentane cit/phenyleph hcl				
SOL, PO (1X120ML,AF,SF)				
120 ml	64543-0500-04	37.20		
(1X473ML,AF,SF)				
473 ml	64543-0500-16	119.04		
TREXIMET (Glaxo)				
naproxen sodium/sumatriptan succinate				
TAB, PO (FILM-COATED)				
500 mg-85 mg,				
9s ea	00173-0750-00	208.31		
(Quality Care Prod)				
REPACK				
TAB, PO (FILM-COATED)				
500 mg-85 mg,				
12s ea	35356-0395-12	456.60		
TREZIX (Wraser Pharm)				
acetaminophen/caffeine/dihydrocodeine bitartrate				
CAP, PO, 356.4 mg-30 mg-16 mg,				
100s ea, C-III	66992-0340-10	128.38		
TRI-CHLOR (Gordon)				
trichloroacetic acid				
LIQ, TP, 80%, 15 ml	10481-3008-01	51.25		
TRI-LEGEST FE 28 (Teva)				
ethinyl estradiol/ferrous fum/norethindrone ace				
TAB, PO (5X28)				
140s ea	00555-9032-70	285.76		AB
TRI-LEVLEN (Phys Total Care)				
REPACK				
ethinyl estradiol/levonorgestrel				
TAB, PO (3X28)				
84s ea	54868-3328-00	43.44		AB
TRI-LO-SPRINTEC (Teva)				
ethinyl estradiol/norgestimate				
TAB, PO (28X6,FILM-COATED)				
168s ea	00555-9065-58	349.60		
TRI-LUMA (Galderma)				
fluocinolone acetonide/hydroquinone/tretinoin				
CRE, TP, 0.01%-4%-0.05%,				
30 gm	00299-5950-30	200.00		
(Phys Total Care)				
REPACK				
CRE, TP, 0.01%-4%-0.05%,				
30 gm	54868-4820-00	109.53		
TRI-NORINYL (Watson)				
ethinyl estradiol/norethindrone				
TAB, PO (WALLETTE,6X28,BLISTERPK)				
168s ea	52544-0274-28	338.27		AB

PROD/MFR	NDC	AWP	DP	OBC
TRI-PREVIFEM (Qualitest)				
ethinyl estradiol/norgestimate				
TAB, PO (6X28)				
168s ea	00603-7665-17	235.92		
(Quality Care Prod)				
REPACK				
TAB, PO, 168s ea	35356-0015-68	283.10		
TRI-SPRINTEC (Dispensing Solutions)				
REPACK				
ethinyl estradiol/norgestimate				
TAB, PO, 168s ea	55045-3781-06	240.00		
TRI-SPRINTEC 28 (Teva)				
ethinyl estradiol/norgestimate				
TAB, PO (BLISTER PACK, 6X28)				
168s ea	00555-9018-58	235.94		AB
(Physician Partner)				
REPACK				
TAB, PO, 28s ea	21695-0770-28	471.88		AB
TRI-VIT W/FLUORIDE (Qualitest)				
ascorbic acid/sodium fluoride/vitamin a/vitamin d				
SOL, PO (AF,DROPS)				
50 ml	00603-1786-47	11.80		
(Phys Total Care)				
REPACK				
SOL, PO (AF,DROPS)				
50 ml	54868-1928-00	4.18		
TRI-VIT WITH FLUORIDE (Qualitest)				
ascorbic acid/sodium fluoride/vitamin a/vitamin d				
SOL, PO (DROPS)				
50 ml	00603-1785-47	11.80		
TRI-VIT WITH FLUORIDE AND IRON (Qualitest)				
fe/na fluoride/vit a/vit c/vit d				
SOL, PO (DROPS)				
50 ml	00603-1787-47	12.00		
TRI-VITAMIN W/ FLUORIDE (Pharma Pac)				
REPACK				
ascorbic acid/sodium fluoride/vitamin a/vitamin d				
SOL, PO, 50 ml	52959-0242-50	10.37		
TRI-VITAMIN W/FLUORIDE (Hi-Tech)				
ascorbic acid/sodium fluoride/vitamin a/vitamin d				
SOL, PO (DROPS)				
50 ml	50383-0637-50	11.80		
50 ml	50383-0636-50	11.80		
TRI-VITAMIN W/FLUORIDE & IRON (Hi-Tech)				
fe/na fluoride/vit a/vit c/vit d				
SOL, PO (DROPS)				
50 ml	50383-0628-50	12.00		
TRI-VITAMIN WITH 0.25MG FLUORIDE (Silarx)				
ascorbic acid/sodium fluoride/vitamin a/vitamin d				
SOL, PO (DROPS)				
50 ml	54838-0515-50	8.70		
TRIACETIN (PCCA)				
LIQ, NA (U.S.P.)				
1 ml	51927-3104-00	0.10		
(Spectrum Pharmacy)				
LIQ, NA (U.S.P.)				
500 ml	49452-7880-01	72.10		
4000 ml	49452-7880-02	295.05		
TRIACIN (Consolidated Midland)				
pse hcl/triprolidine hcl				
SYR, PO, 30 mg/5 ml-1.25 mg/5 ml,				
120 ml	00223-6199-01	2.25		EE
480 ml	00223-6199-02	5.50		EE
TRIALL (Breckenridge Pharm)				
cpm/methscopolamine nitrate/phenyleph hcl				
SYR, PO (AF,SF,GRAPE)				
473 ml	51991-0524-16	28.84		
TRIAMCINOLONE (Gallipot)				
POW, NA (1X1GM,USP)				
1 gm	51552-0768-01	21.56	15.40	
(Medisca)				
POW, NA (U.S.P.)				
5 gm	38779-0051-03	156.00		
10 gm	38779-0051-01	267.00		
25 gm	38779-0051-04	507.00		
100 gm	38779-0051-05	1797.00		
(PCCA)				
POW, NA (USP, NON-MICRONIZED)				
1 gm	51927-2575-00	43.80		
(Spectrum Pharmacy)				
CRY, NA (U.S.P.)				
1 gm	49452-7890-02	116.55		
5 gm	49452-7890-03	252.35		

PROD/MFR	NDC	AWP	DP	OBC
(Stat Rx)				
REPACK				
triamcinolone acetonide				
CRE, TP, 0.1%, 15 gm	16590-0234-15	13.00		
30 gm	16590-0234-30	26.00		
OIN, TP, 0.1%, 15 gm	16590-0235-15	12.00		
TRIAMCINOLONE ACET (Physician Partner)				
REPACK				
triamcinolone acetonide				
CRE, TP, 0.1%, 15 gm	21695-0189-15	7.10		
80 gm	21695-0189-80	23.10		
TRIAMCINOLONE ACETONIDE				
FUL				
CRE, TP, 0.025%, 80 gm		3.00		
0.1%, 80 gm		3.75		
0.5%, 15 gm		3.56		
OIN, TP, 0.1%, 80 gm		4.02		
(Actavis Mid Atlantic)				
CRE, TP, 0.1%, 15 gm	00472-0301-15	4.25		AT
80 gm	00472-0301-80	5.75		AT
453.6 gm	00472-0301-16	22.14		AT
2268 gm	00472-0301-05	77.49		AT
OIN, TP, 0.1%, 15 gm	00472-0306-15	2.75		AT
80 gm	00472-0306-80	5.75		AT
(Alcon Ophthalmic) *See TRIESENCE*				
(Amend)				
POW, NA (U.S.P.)				
1 gm	17317-0719-07	15.40		
10 gm	17317-0719-01	114.00		
(Auriga) *See ZYTOPIC*				
(Bristol-Myers Squibb Mature Brands) *See KENALOG-10*				
(Bristol-Myers Squibb Mature Brands) *See KENALOG-40*				
(Carolina) *See TRIAMCINOLONE ACETONIDE IN ABSORBASE*				
(Del-Ray) *See TRIDERM*				
(Fougera)				
CRE, TP, 0.025%, 15 gm	00168-0003-15	3.00		AT
80 gm	00168-0003-80	5.25		AT
0.1%, 15 gm	00168-0004-15	3.60		AT
80 gm	00168-0004-80	6.25		AT
454 gm	00168-0004-16	23.14		AT
0.5%, 15 gm	00168-0002-15	5.14		AT
LOT, TP, 0.025%, 60 ml	00168-0336-60	37.80		AT
0.1%, 60 ml	00168-0337-60	42.44		AT
OIN, TP, 0.025%, 80 gm	00168-0005-80	5.25		AT
0.1%, 15 gm	00168-0006-15	3.60		AT
80 gm	00168-0006-80	6.25		AT
454 gm	00168-0006-16	23.14		AT
(Gallipot)				
POW, NA (U.S.P.)				
1 gm	51552-0033-01	19.88		
(U.S.P.,MICRONIZED)				
5 gm	51552-0033-02	52.92		
(U.S.P.)				
10 gm	51552-0033-03	98.00		
100 gm	51552-0033-05	693.00		
(Letco)				
POW, NA (U.S.P.,BP,EP,MICRONIZED)				
5 gm	62991-1156-01	102.00		
10 gm	62991-1156-02	177.00		
25 gm	62991-1156-03	375.00		
(Medisca)				
POW, NA (USP,MICRONIZED)				
1 gm	38779-0011-06	43.50		
(U.S.P.,MICRONIZED)				
5 gm	38779-0011-03	126.00		
10 gm	38779-0011-01	225.00		
25 gm	38779-0011-04	420.00		
100 gm	38779-0011-05	1497.00		
(Morton Grove)				
LOT, TP, 0.025%, 60 ml	60432-0560-60	37.79		AT
0.1%, 60 ml	60432-0561-60	42.42		AT
(PCCA)				
POW, NA (U.S.P.,MICRONIZED)				
1 gm	51927-1326-00	27.60		
(Perrigo)				
CRE, TP, 0.025%, 15 gm	45802-0063-35	3.55		AT
80 gm	45802-0063-36	6.10		AT
(USP)				
0.025%, 454 gm	45802-0063-05	17.50		AT
0.1%, 15 gm	45802-0064-35	3.55		AT
(USP,1X80GM)				
0.1%, 80 gm	45802-0064-36	6.55		AT
(USP)				
0.1%, 454 gm	45802-0064-05	26.35		AT
0.5%, 15 gm	45802-0065-35	5.80		AT

PROD/MFR	NDC	AWP	DP	OBC
OIN, TP, 0.025%, 15 gm	45802-0054-35	3.60		AT
80 gm	00414-0054-36	5.20		AT
(USP)				
0.025%, 454 gm	45802-0054-05	17.50		AT
0.1%, 15 gm	45802-0055-35	3.55		AT
80 gm	45802-0055-36	6.55		AT
(USP)				
0,1%, 454 gm	45802-0055-05	26.35		AT
0.5%, 15 gm	45802-0049-35	5.80		AT
(Qualitest)				
CRE, TP (USP)				
0.025%, 15 gm	00603-7861-74	3.53		AT
80 gm	00603-7861-90	6.09		AT
0.1%, 15 gm	00603-7862-74	4.24		AT
80 gm	00603-7862-90	6.57		AT
LOT, TP, 0.1%, 60 ml	00603-7864-49	42.43		AT
(Ranbaxy Labs) *See KENALOG*				
(Sandoz)				
SUS, IJ (MDV, USP, 1X5ML)				
10 mg/ml, 5 ml	00781-3243-75	10.88		AB
(MDV, USP, 1X1ML)				
40 mg/ml, 1 ml	00781-3245-72	8.42		AB
(Sanofi-Aventis) *See NASACORT AQ*				
(Spectrum Pharmacy)				
POW, NA (U.S.P.)				
1 gm	49452-7900-01	78.75		
5 gm	49452-7900-02	184.45		
10 gm	49452-7900-03	331.80		
100 gm	49452-7900-04	2107.00		
(Taro)				
CRE, TP, 0.1%, 15 gm	51672-1282-01	3.48		AT
30 gm	51672-1282-02	4.20		AT
(Taro) *See ORALONE*				
(Taro)				
PAS, MM, 0.1%, 5 gm	51672-1267-05	64.43		AT
(Teva)				
CRE, TP, 0.5%, 15 gm	00182-1218-51	4.55		AT
(Truxton) *See TRIAMCOT*				
(X-Gen)				
POW, NA (U.S.P.,MICRONIZED)				
5 gm	39822-5300-05	53.50		
(4u)				
REPACK				
OIN, TP (1X15GM)				
0.1%, 15 gm	10544-0367-15	14.88		AT
15 gm	42549-0567-15	14.88		AT
(A-S Medication)				
REPACK				
CRE, TP, 0.025%, 15 gm	54569-1121-00	3.55		EE
80 gm	54569-1774-01	6.10		EE
0.1%, 15 gm	54569-1084-00	4.25		EE
80 gm	54569-0765-00	6.28		EE
454 gm	54569-4781-00	22.64		AT
0.5%, 15 gm	54569-2025-00	5.80		EE
OIN, TP, 0.025%, 15 gm	54569-2452-00	3.60		EE
0.1%, 15 gm	54569-1124-00	3.30		EE
80 gm	54569-0767-00	6.18		EE
PAS, MM (DENTAL)				
0.1%, 5 gm	54569-3473-00	66.13		AT
(Altura)				
REPACK				
CRE, TP, 0.1%, 15 gm	63874-0820-15	12.19		EE
30 gm	63874-0820-30	13.25		EE
80 gm	63874-0820-80	8.79		EE
0.5%, 15 gm	63874-0802-15	11.55		
OIN, TP, 0.1%, 15 gm	63874-0822-15	11.65		
(DHS, Inc.)				
REPACK				
CRE, TP, 0.1%, 15 gm	55887-0944-15	11.51		AT
30 gm	55887-0944-01	16.75		
30 gm	55887-0944-30	16.75		AT
OIN, TP, 0.1%, 15 gm	55887-0459-15	11.09		AT
(Dispensing Solutions)				
REPACK				
CRE, TP, 0.1%, 15 gm	55045-1241-05	10.75		AT
(1X15GM)				
0.1%, 15 gm	55045-3935-01	10.75		AT
30 gm	55045-1241-06	12.55		AT
80 gm	55045-1241-09	15.10		AT
0.5%, 15 gm	55045-1772-05	10.75		AT
PAS, MM, 0.1%, 5 gm	55045-2397-05	32.00		
(IPI)				
REPACK				
CRE, TP (1X15GM)				
0.1%, 15 gm	18837-0323-15	12.31		
(Keltman Pharma., Inc.)				
REPACK				
CRE, TP, 0.1%, 15 gm	68387-0625-01	14.95		
(Nucare Pharm)				
REPACK				
CRE, TP, 0.1%, 15 gm	66267-0935-15	13.54		EE
30 gm	66267-0934-30	13.56		EE
80 gm	66267-0933-80	15.99		EE
0.5%, 15 gm	66267-0932-15	8.22		EE
(Palmetto)				
REPACK				
CRE, TP, 0.1%, 15 gm	23490-6416-01	11.89		
80 gm	23490-6416-02	16.99		
0.5%, 15 gm	23490-6420-01	10.75		
OIN, TP, 0.1%, 15 gm	23490-6418-01	8.37		
80 gm	23490-6418-02	12.19		
PAS, MM, 0.1%, 5 gm	23490-6419-01	32.00		
(Pharma Pac)				
REPACK				
CRE, TP, 0.025%, 15 gm	52959-0199-03	9.95		EE
80 gm	52959-0199-01	12.75		EE
0.1%, 15 gm	52959-0096-00	12.16		EE
30 gm	52959-0096-30	13.91		EE
45 gm	52959-0096-45	15.23		EE
80 gm	52959-0096-01	16.34		EE
0.5%, 15 gm	52959-0136-00	8.24		EE
OIN, TP, 0.1%, 15 gm	52959-0156-00	10.05		EE
30 gm	52959-0156-01	19.20		EE
80 gm	52959-0156-02	13.95		EE
(Phys Total Care)				
REPACK				
CRE, TP, 0.025%, 15 gm	54868-1060-01	6.42		EE
80 gm	54868-1060-00	7.92		EE
454 gm	54868-1060-02	50.45		EE
0.1%, 15 gm	54868-0843-01	5.94		EE
80 gm	54868-0843-02	7.59		AT
454 gm	54868-0843-03	35.76		EE
0.5%, 15 gm	54868-0844-01	9.85		EE
LOT, TP, 0.1%, 60 ml	54868-3097-00	82.41		EE
OIN, TP, 0.025%, 15 gm	54868-1590-01	8.91		EE
80 gm	54868-1590-02	7.96		EE
0.1%, 15 gm	54868-1591-01	5.04		EE
80 gm	54868-1591-02	8.64		EE
454 gm	54868-1591-03	5.04		EE
PAS, MM, 0.1%, 5 gm	54868-2742-00	163.64		AT
(Physician Partner)				
REPACK				
CRE, TP (1X80GM)				
0.025%, 80 gm	21695-0501-80	20.50		AT
(1X30GM)				
0.1%, 30 gm	21695-0189-30	18.40		AT
(1X15GM)				
0.5%, 15 gm	21695-0502-15	10.28		AT
OIN, TP, 0.1%, 15 gm	21695-0504-15	7.10		AT
(1X80GM)				
0.1%, 80 gm	21695-0504-80	13.10		AT
(Quality Care Prod)				
REPACK				
CRE, TP, 0.025%, 80 gm	49999-0149-80	31.20		AT
0.1%, 15 gm	49999-0150-15	13.18		AT
30 gm	49999-0150-30	26.34		AT
80 gm	49999-0150-80	42.40		AT
0.5%, 15 gm	49999-0285-15	9.84		AT
OIN, TP, 0.1%, 15 gm	49999-0216-15	13.82		
PAS, MM (1X5GM)				
0.1%, 5 gm	35356-0088-01	34.14		
(Southwood)				
REPACK				
CRE, TP, 0.025%, 15 gm	58016-3034-01	4.88		EE
0.1%, 15 gm	58016-3035-01	4.25		EE
30 gm	58016-3543-01	4.20		EE
80 gm	58016-3108-01	8.37		EE
453 gm	58016-4894-01	22.14		EE
0.5%, 15 gm	58016-3127-01	6.83		EE
OIN, TP, 0.025%, 30 gm	58016-3161-01	5.13		EE
0.1%, 15 gm	58016-3208-01	3.20		EE
80 gm	58016-3253-01	8.37		EE
(St. Mary's MPP)				
REPACK				
CRE, TP (1X15GM)				
0.1%, 15 gm	60760-0040-15	7.40		AT
(Stat Rx)				
REPACK				
CRE, TP, 0.1%, 80 gm	16590-0234-80	4.82		AT
TRIAMCINOLONE ACETONIDE IN ABSORBASE				
(Carolina)				
triamcinolone acetonide				
OIN, TP, 0.05%, 430 gm	46287-0010-16	28.35	23.00	
TRIAMCINOLONE ACETONIDE MICRONIZED				
(Hawkins)				
triamcinolone acetonide, micronized				
POW, NA, 5 gm	63370-0300-15	172.80		
10 gm	63370-0300-20	321.60		
25 gm	63370-0300-25	624.00		
100 gm	63370-0300-35	2304.00		
TRIAMCINOLONE ACETONIDE, MICRONIZED				
(Hawkins) *See TRIAMCINOLONE ACETONIDE MICRONIZED*				
TRIAMCINOLONE DIACETATE				
(Clint) *See CLINACORT*				
(Gallipot)				
POW, NA (U.S.P.,MICRONIZED)				
1 gm	51552-0278-01	19.88		
5 gm	51552-0278-02	55.65		
10 gm	51552-0278-03	100.10		
(Medisca)				
POW, NA (USP)				
5 gm	38779-0166-03	127.50		
25 gm	38779-0166-04	495.00		
100 gm	38779-0166-05	1497.00		
(PCCA)				
POW, NA (USP)				
1 gm	51927-3370-00	27.60		
(Spectrum Pharmacy)				
CRY, NA (U.S.P.,MICRONIZED)				
1 gm	49452-7910-01	88.55		
5 gm	49452-7910-02	201.25		
10 gm	49452-7910-03	360.50		
POW, NA, 100 gm	49452-7910-04	2282.00		
(Truxton) *See TRIAMCOT*				
TRIAMCINOLONE HEXACETONIDE				
(Sabex) *See ARISTOSPAN*				
(Sandoz) *See ARISTOSPAN*				
TRIAMCINOLONE MICRONIZED (PCCA)				
triamcinolone, micronized				
POW, NA (1X1GM)				
1 gm	51927-1049-00	41.40		
TRIAMCINOLONE, MICRONIZED				
(PCCA) *See TRIAMCINOLONE MICRONIZED*				
TRIAMCOT (Truxton)				
triamcinolone acetonide				
CRE, TP, 0.1%, 15 gm	00463-8052-15	2.40		EE
(Truxton)				
triamcinolone diacetate				
SUS, IJ (VIAL)				
40 mg/ml, 5 ml	00463-1091-05	8.40		EE
TRIAMTERENE (Gallipot)				
POW, NA (U.S.P.)				
100 gm	51552-1008-05	69.93	49.95	
(PCCA)				
POW, NA (U.S.P.)				
1 gm	51927-1615-00	2.04		
(Spectrum Pharmacy)				
POW, NA (U.S.P.)				
5 gm	49452-7912-04	106.05		
25 gm	49452-7912-01	160.65		
100 gm	49452-7912-02	511.00		
(Wellspring Pharm) *See DYRENIUM*				
TRIAMTERENE AND HYDROCHLOROTHIAZIDE				
(Apotex Corp.)				
hydrochlorothiazide/triamterene				
TAB, PO, 25 mg-37.5 mg,				
100s ea	60505-2656-01	33.95		AB
500s ea	60505-2656-05	161.20		AB
50 mg-75 mg,				
100s ea	60505-2657-01	88.70		AB
500s ea	60505-2657-05	430.20		AB
(DHS, Inc.)				
REPACK				
TAB, PO, 25 mg-37.5 mg,				
30s ea	55887-0588-30	22.00		AB
(Pharma Pac)				
REPACK				
TAB, PO, 25 mg-37.5 mg,				
30s ea	52959-0977-30	29.17		AB
(Physician Partner)				
REPACK				
TAB, PO, 50 mg-75 mg,				
30s ea	21695-0497-30	17.27		AB
90s ea	21695-0497-90	51.81		AB

PROD/MFR	NDC	AWP	DP	OBC
TRIAMTERENE/HCTZ (Altura)				
REPACK				
hydrochlorothiazide/triamterene				
CAP, PO, 25 mg-50 mg,				
10s ea	**63874-0310-10**	8.01		
12s ea	**63874-0310-12**	9.61		
14s ea	**63874-0310-14**	11.21		
15s ea	**63874-0310-15**	12.02		
20s ea	**63874-0310-20**	16.02		
30s ea	**63874-0310-30**	24.03		
60s ea	**63874-0310-60**	48.06		
90s ea	**63874-0310-90**	72.09		
100s ea	**63874-0310-01**	80.10		
120s ea	**63874-0310-04**	96.12		
TAB, PO (FILM COATED)				
25 mg-50 mg,				
1000s ea	**63874-0310-02**	538.11		
50 mg-75 mg,				
10s ea	**63874-0477-10**	8.25		
14s ea	**63874-0477-14**	11.55		
15s ea	**63874-0477-15**	12.50		
20s ea	**63874-0477-20**	16.50		
30s ea	**63874-0477-30**	24.75		
50s ea	**63874-0477-50**	41.25		
90s ea	**63874-0477-90**	74.25		
100s ea	**63874-0477-01**	82.50		
(Bryant Ranch)				
REPACK				
CAP, PO, 25 mg-37.5 mg,				
30s ea	**63629-1507-02**	15.15		
60s ea	**63629-1507-03**	30.30		
100s ea	**63629-1507-01**	50.50		
TAB, PO, 25 mg-37.5 mg,				
30s ea	**63629-2647-01**	13.57		
50 mg-75 mg,				
30s ea	**63629-2585-01**	39.39		
(Core)				
REPACK				
TAB, PO, 25 mg-37.5 mg,				
30s ea	**33358-0349-30**	19.90		
(DHS, Inc.)				
REPACK				
TAB, PO, 25 mg-37.5 mg,				
90s ea	**55887-0588-90**	38.09		
(Dispensing Solutions)				
REPACK				
TAB, PO, 25 mg-37.5 mg,				
90s ea	**55045-2958-09**	36.00		
120s ea	**55045-2958-02**	48.00		
(HomeMed)				
REPACK				
CAP, PO, 25 mg-50 mg,				
30s ea	**51655-0510-24**	30.00		EE
TAB, PO, 25 mg-37.5 mg,				
30s ea	**51655-0575-24**	20.26		
50 mg-75 mg,				
30s ea	**51655-0534-24**	33.14		
(Pharma Pac)				
REPACK				
CAP, PO, 25 mg-37.5 mg,				
15s ea	**52959-0712-15**	14.99		
30s ea	**52959-0712-30**	18.35		
90s ea	**52959-0712-90**	35.75		
100s ea	**52959-0712-00**	38.68		
TRIANT-HC (Hawthorn Pharm)				
cpm/hydrocod bit/phenyleph hcl				
SOL, PO (AF,SF,STRAWBERRY)				
473 ml, C-III	**63717-0703-16**	43.75		
TRIAZ (Medicis)				
benzoyl peroxide				
PAD, TP (FOIL-WRAPPED PADS)				
3%, 30s ea UD	**99207-0221-30**	153.78		
(FOIL-WRAPPED CLOTH)				
3%, 60s ea	**99207-0224-60**	277.84		
(FOIL-WRAPPED PADS)				
3%, 60s ea UD	**99207-0221-60**	292.13		
6%, 30s ea UD	**99207-0222-30**	153.78		
60s ea UD	**99207-0222-60**	292.13		
9%, 30s ea UD	**99207-0223-30**	153.78		
60s ea UD	**99207-0223-60**	292.13		
TRIAZ CLEANSER (Medicis)				
benzoyl peroxide				
GEL, TP, 3%, 170.3 gm	**99207-0206-12**	81.94		
340.2 gm	**99207-0206-09**	146.76		
6%, 170.3 gm	**99207-0116-12**	84.41		
340.2 gm	**99207-0116-09**	151.64		
9%, 170.3 gm	**99207-0208-12**	87.55		
340.2 gm	**99207-0208-09**	157.18		

PROD/MFR	NDC	AWP	DP	OBC
(Phys Total Care)				
REPACK				
GEL, TP, 6%, 170.3 gm	**54868-5133-00**	63.09		
TRIAZ FOAMING CLOTHS (Medicis)				
benzoyl peroxide				
PAD, TP, 6%, 3.2 gm 60s	**99207-0225-60**	277.84		
TRIAZOLAM				
FUL				
TAB, PO, 0.125 mg,				
10s ea		3.01		
0.25 mg, 10s ea		3.25		
(Greenstone)				
TAB, PO (10X10)				
0.125 mg,				
100s ea UD, C-IV	**59762-3717-04**	67.28		AB
0.25 mg,				
100s ea UD, C-IV	**59762-3718-04**	72.28		AB
500s ea, C-IV	**59762-3718-03**	337.43		AB
(Pfizer) *See HALCION*				
(Roxane)				
TAB, PO (USP)				
0.125 mg,				
10s ea, C-IV	**00054-4858-51**	6.49		AB
(10X10)				
0.125 mg,				
100s ea UD, C-IV	**00054-8858-25**	64.00		AB
(USP)				
0.25 mg,				
10s ea, C-IV	**00054-4859-51**	6.66		AB
(10X10)				
0.25 mg,				
100s ea UD, C-IV	**00054-8859-25**	69.00		AB
500s ea, C-IV	**00054-4859-29**	315.00		AB
(4u)				
REPACK				
TAB, PO, 0.25 mg,				
300s ea, C-IV	**42549-0547-30**	64.62		AB
(A-S Medication)				
REPACK				
TAB, PO, 0.25 mg,				
6s ea, C-IV	**54569-3966-03**	3.96		AB
(10 X 10)				
0.25 mg,				
30s ea, C-IV	**54569-3966-00**	19.80		EE
100s ea, C-IV	**54569-3966-01**	65.99		EE
(Aidarex)				
REPACK				
TAB, PO, 0.25 mg,				
14s ea, C-IV	**33261-0108-14**	27.58		AB
30s ea, C-IV	**33261-0108-30**	59.10		AB
60s ea, C-IV	**33261-0108-60**	118.20		AB
90s ea, C-IV	**33261-0108-90**	177.30		AB
(Altura)				
REPACK				
TAB, PO, 0.125 mg,				
12s ea, C-IV	**63874-0808-12**	9.33		AB
15s ea, C-IV	**63874-0808-15**	10.68		AB
20s ea, C-IV	**63874-0808-20**	14.20		AB
30s ea, C-IV	**63874-0808-30**	21.35		AB
0.25 mg, 5s ea, C-IV	**63874-0281-05**	6.45		AB
10s ea, C-IV	**63874-0281-10**	12.90		AB
15s ea, C-IV	**63874-0281-15**	19.35		AB
20s ea, C-IV	**63874-0281-20**	25.80		AB
30s ea, C-IV	**63874-0281-30**	38.70		AB
50s ea, C-IV	**63874-0281-50**	64.50		AB
60s ea, C-IV	**63874-0281-60**	77.40		AB
90s ea, C-IV	**63874-0281-90**	116.10		AB
100s ea, C-IV	**63874-0281-01**	129.00		AB
120s ea, C-IV	**63874-0281-04**	154.80		AB
150s ea, C-IV	**63874-0281-72**	193.50		AB
200s ea, C-IV	**63874-0281-74**	258.00		AB
300s ea, C-IV	**63874-0281-77**	387.00		AB
(Bryant Ranch)				
REPACK				
TAB, PO, 0.25 mg,				
10s ea, C-IV	**63629-2956-01**	9.45		
30s ea, C-IV	**63629-2956-02**	23.98		
60s ea, C-IV	**63629-2956-03**	42.32		
(Core)				
REPACK				
TAB, PO, 0.25 mg,				
10s ea, C-IV	**33358-0350-10**	9.69		
15s ea, C-IV	**33358-0350-15**	17.24		
30s ea, C-IV	**33358-0350-30**	24.58		
60s ea, C-IV	**33358-0350-60**	43.38		

PROD/MFR	NDC	AWP	DP	OBC
(DHS, Inc.)				
REPACK				
TAB, PO, 0.25 mg, ea, C-IV	**55887-0319-01**	106.66		
60s ea, C-IV	**55887-0319-60**	39.59		
90s ea, C-IV	**55887-0319-90**	59.39		
(Dispensing Solutions)				
REPACK				
TAB, PO, 0.125 mg,				
10s ea, C-IV	**55045-2550-01**	6.70		AB
30s ea, C-IV	**55045-2550-08**	20.10		AB
45s ea, C-IV	**55045-2550-04**	30.15		AB
0.25 mg, 3s ea, C-IV	**66336-0886-03**	5.20		
5s ea, C-IV	**55045-2086-02**	4.60		
10s ea, C-IV	**55045-2086-04**	9.20		AB
30s ea, C-IV	**55045-2086-08**	27.50		AB
45s ea, C-IV	**55045-2086-05**	41.40		AB
60s ea, C-IV	**55045-2086-06**	55.00		
90s ea, C-IV	**55045-2086-09**	82.80		
100s ea, C-IV	**55045-2086-00**	92.00		AB
(HomeMed)				
REPACK				
TAB, PO, 0.25 mg,				
4s ea, C-IV	**51655-0835-89**	5.79		
(Keltman Pharma., Inc.)				
REPACK				
TAB, PO, 0.25 mg,				
15s ea, C-IV	**68387-0530-15**	17.00		
30s ea, C-IV	**68387-0530-30**	34.00		AB
(Nucare Pharm)				
REPACK				
TAB, PO, 0.25 mg,				
30s ea, C-IV	**66267-0492-30**	42.40		AB
(Palmetto)				
REPACK				
TAB, PO, 0.25 mg,				
3s ea, C-IV	**23490-6432-01**	7.40		
4s ea, C-IV	**23490-6432-02**	9.28		
21s ea, C-IV	**23490-6432-03**	30.45		
30s ea, C-IV	**23490-6432-04**	43.50		
(PD-Rx Pharm)				
REPACK				
TAB, PO, 0.125 mg,				
2s ea, C-IV	**55289-0790-02**	5.68		
(USP)				
0.25 mg,				
2s ea, C-IV	**55289-0787-02**	8.55		
(Pharma Pac)				
REPACK				
TAB, PO, 0.25 mg,				
10s ea, C-IV	**52959-0402-10**	10.23		EE
20s ea, C-IV	**52959-0402-20**	20.45		AB
30s ea, C-IV	**52959-0402-30**	30.66		EE
50s ea, C-IV	**52959-0402-50**	51.15		EE
60s ea, C-IV	**52959-0402-60**	60.73		EE
100s ea, C-IV	**52959-0402-01**	101.10		EE
(Phys Total Care)				
REPACK				
TAB, PO, 0.125 mg,				
3s ea, C-IV	**54868-2931-03**	6.87		EE
30s ea, C-IV	**54868-2931-00**	29.58		EE
100s ea, C-IV	**54868-2931-01**	84.54		EE
0.25 mg, 6s ea, C-IV	**54868-2983-01**	9.93		EE
10s ea, C-IV	**54868-2983-02**	12.00		EE
15s ea, C-IV	**54868-2983-04**	15.81		AB
20s ea, C-IV	**54868-2983-03**	19.08		EE
30s ea, C-IV	**54868-2983-00**	24.12		EE
60s ea, C-IV	**54868-2983-06**	45.21		AB
100s ea, C-IV	**54868-2983-05**	69.84		AB
(Physician Partner)				
REPACK				
TAB, PO, 0.125 mg,				
30s ea, C-IV	**21695-0303-30**	37.00		
60s ea, C-IV	**21695-0303-60**	74.00		
0.25 mg,				
100s ea, C-IV	**21695-0284-00**	141.90		AB
(Quality Care Prod)				
REPACK				
TAB, PO, 0.25 mg, ea, C-IV	**49999-0055-01**	4.67		EE
2s ea, C-IV	**49999-0055-02**	4.00		AB
10s ea, C-IV	**49999-0055-10**	16.79		AB
30s ea, C-IV	**49999-0055-30**	49.90		EE
60s ea, C-IV	**49999-0055-60**	99.80		AB
100s ea UD, C-IV	**49999-0055-00**	167.94		AB
(Southwood)				
REPACK				
TAB, PO, 0.125 mg,				
12s ea, C-IV	**58016-0338-12**	8.89		EE
15s ea, C-IV	**58016-0338-15**	10.17		EE

PROD/MFR	NDC	AWP	DP	OBC
20s ea, C-IV	58016-0338-20	13.56		EE
30s ea, C-IV	58016-0338-30	20.33		EE
0.25 mg, 5s ea, C-IV	58016-0757-05	4.76		EE
10s ea, C-IV	58016-0757-10	9.51		EE
12s ea, C-IV	58016-0757-12	11.41		EE
15s ea, C-IV	58016-0757-15	14.27		EE
20s ea, C-IV	58016-0757-20	19.02		EE
30s ea, C-IV	58016-0757-30	28.53		EE
60s ea, C-IV	58016-0757-60	57.06		EE
90s ea, C-IV	58016-0757-90	85.59		AB
100s ea, C-IV	58016-0757-00	95.10		EE
120s ea, C-IV	58016-0757-02	114.12		AB
150s ea, C-IV	58016-0757-03	142.65		AB
200s ea, C-IV	58016-0757-89	190.20		AB
300s ea, C-IV	58016-0757-73	285.30		AB
(St. Mary's MPP)				
REPACK				
TAB, PO, 0.25 mg,				
30s ea, C-IV	60760-0454-30	28.27		AB
(Stat Rx)				
REPACK				
TAB, PO, 0.25 mg,				
20s ea, C-IV	16590-0236-20	20.00		
30s ea, C-IV	16590-0236-30	30.00		
40s ea, C-IV	16590-0236-40	40.00		
TRICHLORMETHIAZIDE (Letco)				
POW, NA (U.S.P.)				
25 gm	62991-2071-01	165.00		
(Medisca)				
POW, NA (U.S.P.)				
25 gm	38779-0268-04	201.00		
100 gm	38779-0268-05	645.00		
(USP)				
500 gm	38779-0268-08	2895.00		
1000 gm	38779-0268-09	4665.00		
(PCCA)				
POW, NA (U.S.P.)				
1 gm	51927-2477-00	12.60		
(Spectrum Pharmacy)				
CRY, NA (U.S.P.)				
5 gm	49452-7921-01	105.70		
25 gm	49452-7921-02	313.25		
100 gm	49452-7921-04	889.00		
(Truxton) *See AQUACOT*				
(Southwood)				
REPACK				
TAB, PO, 4 mg, 14s ea	58016-0588-14	4.68		EE
15s ea	58016-0588-15	5.01		EE
30s ea	58016-0588-30	5.36		EE
TRICHLOROACETIC ACID (Amend)				
POW, NA (PURIFIED)				
25 gm	17317-0584-02	10.15		
125 gm	17317-0584-04	16.80		
500 gm	17317-0584-01	42.00		
(Baker, J.T.)				
CRY, NA (PURIFIED)				
30 gm	10106-0417-00	18.93		
125 gm	10106-0417-04	19.77		
(Gallipot)				
CRY, NA (A.C.S.,REAGENT)				
28.35 gm	51552-0049-02	9.59		
(A.C.S.,REAGENT.)				
113.4 gm	51552-0049-04	17.22		
(A.C.S.,REAGENT)				
454 gm	51552-0049-06	52.01		
(Gallipot) *See TRICHLOROACETIC ACID 10%*				
(Gallipot) *See TRICHLOROACETIC ACID 100%*				
(Gallipot) *See TRICHLOROACETIC ACID 15%*				
(Gallipot) *See TRICHLOROACETIC ACID 20%*				
(Gallipot) *See TRICHLOROACETIC ACID 25%*				
(Gallipot) *See TRICHLOROACETIC ACID 3%*				
(Gallipot) *See TRICHLOROACETIC ACID 30%*				
(Gallipot) *See TRICHLOROACETIC ACID 35%*				
(Gallipot) *See TRICHLOROACETIC ACID 40%*				
(Gallipot) *See TRICHLOROACETIC ACID 50%*				
(Gallipot) *See TRICHLOROACETIC ACID 75%*				
(Gallipot) *See TRICHLOROACETIC ACID 80%*				
(Gallipot) *See TRICHLOROACETIC ACID 85%*				
(Gallipot) *See TRICHLOROACETIC ACID 90%*				
(Gordon) *See TRI-CHLOR*				
(Letco)				
CRY, NA (U.S.P.)				
100 gm	62991-2070-01	57.00		
500 gm	62991-2070-02	183.00		
(Mallinckrodt Lab)				
CRY, NA (PURIFIED)				
30 gm	00406-2924-34	18.31		
125 gm	00406-2924-08	35.35		
(Medisca)				
CRY, NA (U.S.P., REAGENT)				
100 gm	38779-0100-05	49.50		
500 gm	38779-0100-08	135.00		
(PCCA)				
CRY, NA (U.S.P., ACS REAGENT)				
1 gm	51927-1243-00	0.57		
(Spectrum Pharmacy)				
CRY, NA (REAGENT, A.C.S.)				
25 gm	49452-7915-01	71.40		
125 gm	49452-7915-02	101.50		
500 gm	49452-7915-03	247.80		
(Spectrum Pharmacy) *See TRICHLOROACETIC ACID 85%*				
TRICHLOROACETIC ACID 10% (Gallipot)				
trichloroacetic acid				
SOL, NA, 473 ml	51552-0275-06	28.70		
TRICHLOROACETIC ACID 100% (Gallipot)				
trichloroacetic acid				
SOL, NA, 473 ml	51552-0274-06	183.75		
TRICHLOROACETIC ACID 15% (Gallipot)				
trichloroacetic acid				
SOL, NA, 29.57 ml	51552-0365-02	16.94		
TRICHLOROACETIC ACID 20% (Gallipot)				
trichloroacetic acid				
SOL, NA, 29.57 ml	51552-0273-02	18.27		
473 ml	51552-0273-06	62.09		
TRICHLOROACETIC ACID 25% (Gallipot)				
trichloroacetic acid				
SOL, NA, 29.57 ml	51552-0469-02	20.93		
473 ml	51552-0469-06	67.20		
TRICHLOROACETIC ACID 3% (Gallipot)				
trichloroacetic acid				
SOL, NA, 473 ml	51552-0329-06	21.14		
TRICHLOROACETIC ACID 30% (Gallipot)				
trichloroacetic acid				
SOL, NA, 29.57 ml	51552-0311-02	22.75		
473 ml	51552-0311-06	73.15		
TRICHLOROACETIC ACID 35% (Gallipot)				
trichloroacetic acid				
SOL, NA, 29.57 ml	51552-0312-02	23.80		
TRICHLOROACETIC ACID 40% (Gallipot)				
trichloroacetic acid				
SOL, NA, 29.57 ml	51552-0434-02	25.69		
TRICHLOROACETIC ACID 50% (Gallipot)				
trichloroacetic acid				
SOL, NA, 29.57 ml	51552-0316-02	27.86		
59.14 ml	51552-0316-03	49.98		
473 ml	51552-0316-06	103.25		
TRICHLOROACETIC ACID 75% (Gallipot)				
trichloroacetic acid				
SOL, NA, 29.57 ml	51552-0493-02	29.75		
TRICHLOROACETIC ACID 80% (Gallipot)				
trichloroacetic acid				
SOL, NA, 59.14 ml	51552-0364-03	49.70		
473 ml	51552-0364-06	119.70		
TRICHLOROACETIC ACID 85% (Gallipot)				
trichloroacetic acid				
SOL, NA, 29.57 ml	51552-0261-02	30.80		
473 ml	51552-0261-06	133.00		
(Spectrum Pharmacy)				
SOL, NA (1X500ML)				
500 ml	49452-7916-01	609.00		
(1X1000ML)				
1000 ml	49452-7916-02	882.00		
TRICHLOROACETIC ACID 90% (Gallipot)				
trichloroacetic acid				
SOL, NA, 29.57 ml	51552-0478-02	31.15		
TRICHLOROETHANE				
(Gallipot) *See 1,1,1 TRICHLOROETHANE*				
1,1,1 TRICHLOROETHANE (Gallipot)				
trichloroethane				
LIQ, NA, 473 ml	51552-0252-06	27.93		
3785 ml	51552-0252-08	73.50		
TRICHLOROETHANE (Medisca)				
SOL, NA (1X500ML)				
500 ml	38779-1664-08	76.50		
TRICHLOROETHYLENE (Baker, J.T.)				
LIQ, NA (ACS,REAGENT,STABILIZED)				
150 ml	10106-9458-04	20.19		
500 ml	10106-9458-01	28.58		
(PCCA)				
LIQ, NA (ACS; REAGENT)				
1 ml	51927-3334-00	0.65		
TRICHLOROFON (PCCA)				
POW, NA (1X1GM)				
1 gm	51927-3217-00	1.52		
TRICHOPHYTON (Alk-Abello)				
trichophyton mentagrophytes				
SOL, IJ (MDV)				
1:200, 2 ml	00268-0432-02	56.88	41.00	
TRICHOPHYTON MENTAGROPHYTES				
(Alk-Abello) *See TRICHOPHYTON*				
TRICITRASOL (Citra)				
sodium citrate				
SOL, IJ (NOT FOR DIRECT IV INFUS)				
46.7%, 30 ml 50s	23731-6030-03	3780.00	3150.00	
TRICITRATES (Pharm Assoc Inc)				
citric acid/potassium citrate/sodium citrate				
SOL, PO (AF,SF,RASPBERRY)				
473 ml	00121-0677-16	35.60		
SYR, PO (AF,RASPBERRY)				
473 ml	00121-0779-16	35.60		
TRICLOSAN (PCCA)				
POW, NA (U.S.P.)				
1 gm	51927-3576-00	4.20		
TRICON (Nnodum)				
ferrous fum/folic acid/if/vit b12/vit c				
CAP, PO, 100s ea	63044-0635-10	50.99		
TRICOR (Abbott Pharm)				
fenofibrate				
TAB, PO, 48 mg, 90s ea	00074-6122-90	137.87	120.94	
145 mg, 90s ea	00074-6123-90	413.60	362.81	
(A-S Medication)				
REPACK				
TAB, PO, 145 mg, 30s ea	54569-5750-00	135.48		
90s ea	54569-5750-01	507.25		
(Bryant Ranch)				
REPACK				
TAB, PO, 160 mg, 30s ea	63629-1514-01	125.00		
(Dispensing Solutions)				
REPACK				
TAB, PO, 48 mg, 30s ea	68258-6004-03	50.55		
145 mg, 30s ea	68258-6005-03	151.65		
(Nucare Pharm)				
REPACK				
TAB, PO, 145 mg, 30s ea	68071-0800-30	183.00		
(PD-Rx Pharm)				
REPACK				
TAB, PO, 145 mg, 30s ea	55289-0973-30	203.85		
(Phys Total Care)				
REPACK				
TAB, PO, 48 mg, 30s ea	54868-5224-00	61.10		
90s ea	54868-5224-01	167.67		
145 mg, 30s ea	54868-5203-00	178.27		
90s ea	54868-5203-01	511.92		
(Quality Care Prod)				
REPACK				
TAB, PO, 145 mg, 30s ea	49999-0885-30	218.30		
90s ea	49999-0885-90	582.30		
(Southwood)				
REPACK				
TAB, PO, 145 mg, 30s ea	58016-0044-30	123.99		
60s ea	58016-0044-60	247.97		
90s ea	58016-0044-90	371.96		
100s ea	58016-0044-00	413.29		
TRIDERM (Del-Ray)				
triamcinolone acetonide				
CRE, TP, 0.1%, 30 gm	00316-0170-01	13.71		AT
90 gm	00316-0170-03	19.96		AT
TRIENTINE HYDROCHLORIDE				
(Aton) *See SYPRINE*				
TRIESENCE (Alcon Ophthalmic)				
triamcinolone acetonide				
SUS, IJ, 40 mg/ml, 1 ml	00065-0543-01	148.80		

PROD/MFR	NDC	AWP	DP	OBC
TRIETHANOLAMINE (Baker, J.T.)				
trolamine				
LIQ, NA (REAGENT)				
500 ml	**10106-9468-01**	65.92		
4000 ml	**10106-9468-03**	287.78		
TRIETHANOLAMINE 85% (Amend)				
trolamine				
LIQ, NA, 500 ml	**17317-0935-01**	9.80		
3840 ml	**17317-0093-06**	35.70		
20000 ml	**17317-0935-08**	140.00		
TRIETHANOLAMINE LAURYL SULFATE (Amend)				
LIQ, NA, 500 ml	**17317-0708-01**	11.20		
3840 ml	**17317-0708-06**	56.00		
(PCCA)				
LIQ, NA, 1 ml	**51927-1489-00**	0.09		
TRIETHANOLAMINE SALICYLATE (Spectrum Pharmacy)				
trolamine salicylate				
POW, NA, 25 gm	**49452-7918-01**	171.15		
100 gm	**49452-7918-02**	497.00		
TRIETHYL CITRATE (Spectrum Pharmacy)				
SOL, NA (1X100ML)				
100 ml	**49452-7922-01**	120.40		
(1X500ML)				
500 ml	**49452-7922-02**	326.90		
TRIETHYLENETHIOPHOSPHORAMIDE/T (PCCA)				
thiotepa				
POW, NA, 1 gm	**51927-2762-00**	486.00		
TRIFLUOPERAZINE HCL (Mylan)				
trifluoperazine hydrochloride				
TAB, PO, 1 mg, 100s ea	**00378-2401-01**	58.30		AB
2 mg, 100s ea	**00378-2402-01**	85.90		AB
5 mg, 100s ea	**00378-2405-01**	108.20		AB
10 mg, 100s ea	**00378-2410-01**	163.10		AB
(Sandoz)				
TAB, PO (FILM-COATED)				
1 mg, 100s ea	**00781-1030-01**	56.64		AB
2 mg, 100s ea	**00781-1032-01**	83.54		AB
100s ea UD	**00781-1032-13**	100.25		AB
5 mg, 100s ea	**00781-1034-01**	105.14		AB
10 mg, 100s ea	**00781-1036-01**	158.47		AB
(UDL)				
TAB, PO (10X10)				
1 mg, 100s ea UD	**51079-0572-20**	60.05		AB
2 mg, 100s ea UD	**51079-0573-20**	88.48		AB
5 mg, 100s ea UD	**51079-0574-20**	111.45		AB
10 mg, 100s ea UD	**51079-0575-20**	167.99		AB
(GSMS)				
REPACK				
TAB, PO (UNIT OF USE)				
2 mg, 30s ea	**60429-0192-30**	39.00	13.00	AB
60s ea	**60429-0192-60**	75.00	25.00	AB
90s ea	**60429-0192-90**	111.00	37.00	AB
180s ea	**60429-0192-18**	219.00	73.00	AB
5 mg, 30s ea	**60429-0193-30**	36.45	12.15	AB
60s ea	**60429-0193-60**	69.75	23.25	AB
90s ea	**60429-0193-90**	103.20	34.40	AB
180s ea	**60429-0193-18**	203.40	67.80	AB
10 mg, 30s ea	**60429-0194-30**	57.75	19.25	AB
(Nucare Pharm)				
REPACK				
TAB, PO, 2 mg, 30s ea	**68071-0807-30**	41.20		AB
(Phys Total Care)				
REPACK				
TAB, PO, 5 mg, 100s ea	**54868-1352-00**	219.18		EE
10 mg, 100s ea	**54868-2356-01**	98.33		EE
(Stat Rx)				
REPACK				
TAB, PO, 2 mg, 30s ea	**16590-0305-30**	30.06		AB
TRIFLUOPERAZINE HYDROCHLORIDE				
(Mylan) *See TRIFLUOPERAZINE HCL*				
(Sandoz) *See TRIFLUOPERAZINE HCL*				
(UDL) *See TRIFLUOPERAZINE HCL*				
TRIFLUORACETIC ACID				
(PCCA) *See TRIFLUOROACETIC ACID REAGENT*				
TRIFLUOROACETIC ACID REAGENT (PCCA)				
trifluoracetic acid				
SOL, NA (1X1ML)				
1 ml	**51927-2862-00**	1.20		
TRIFLURIDINE (Falcon Ophthalmics)				
SOL, OP, 1%, 7.5 ml	**61314-0044-75**	114.58		AT
(Monarch) *See VIROPTIC*				

PROD/MFR	NDC	AWP	DP	OBC
(PCCA)				
POW, NA (TRIFLUOROTHYMIDINE)				
1 gm	**51927-2875-00**	1470.00		
(Phys Total Care)				
REPACK				
SOL, OP, 1%, 7.5 ml	**54868-4757-00**	209.01		AT
TRIGLIDE (Shionogi)				
fenofibrate				
TAB, PO, 50 mg, 30s ea	**59630-0480-30**	62.63		
160 mg, 30s ea	**59630-0485-30**	187.85		BX
(Phys Total Care)				
REPACK				
TAB, PO, 50 mg, 30s ea	**54868-5784-00**	41.38		
TRIHEXYPHENIDYL HCL (Consolidated Midland)				
trihexyphenidyl hydrochloride				
TAB, PO, 2 mg, 100s ea	**00223-2126-01**	15.00		EE
1000s ea	**00223-2126-02**	135.00		EE
5 mg, 100s ea	**00223-2127-01**	27.50		EE
1000s ea	**00223-2127-02**	227.50		EE
(Pharm Assoc Inc)				
ELI, PO (SF,DYE-FREE,LIME-MINT)				
2 mg/5 ml, 473 ml	**00121-0658-16**	30.74		AA
(Qualitest)				
TAB, PO, 2 mg, 100s ea	**00603-6240-21**	18.28		AA
1000s ea	**00603-6240-32**	148.06		AA
5 mg, 100s ea	**00603-6241-21**	36.37		AA
1000s ea	**00603-6241-32**	342.71		AA
(VersaPharm)				
ELI, PO (LIME-PEPPERMINT)				
2 mg/5 ml, 473 ml	**61748-0054-16**	25.65		AA
(Vintage)				
TAB, PO, 2 mg, 100s ea	**00254-5971-28**	18.28		AA
(Watson Labs)				
TAB, PO, 2 mg, 100s ea	**00591-5335-01**	18.29		AA
1000s ea	**00591-5335-10**	148.06		AA
5 mg, 100s ea	**00591-5337-01**	36.38		AA
1000s ea	**00591-5337-10**	342.71		AA
(West-Ward)				
TAB, PO, 2 mg, 100s ea	**00143-1764-01**	18.28		AA
1000s ea	**00143-1764-10**	148.06		AA
5 mg, 100s ea	**00143-1763-01**	36.37		AA
1000s ea	**00143-1763-10**	342.71		AA
(American Health)				
REPACK				
TAB, PO, 2 mg,				
100s ea UD	**62584-0886-01**	15.00		AA
5 mg, 30s ea UD	**62584-0887-21**	20.00		AA
(Phys Total Care)				
REPACK				
TAB, PO, 2 mg, 30s ea	**54868-2340-02**	13.38		EE
60s ea	**54868-2340-03**	22.29		EE
TRIHEXYPHENIDYL HYDROCHLORIDE				
FUL				
TAB, PO, 2 mg, 100s ea		12.75		
5 mg, 100s ea		22.95		
(Consolidated Midland) *See TRIHEXYPHENIDYL HCL*				
(Pharm Assoc Inc) *See TRIHEXYPHENIDYL HCL*				
(Qualitest) *See TRIHEXYPHENIDYL HCL*				
(VersaPharm) *See TRIHEXYPHENIDYL HCL*				
(Vintage) *See TRIHEXYPHENIDYL HCL*				
(Watson Labs) *See TRIHEXYPHENIDYL HCL*				
(West-Ward) *See TRIHEXYPHENIDYL HCL*				
TRIHIBIT (Sanofi)				
dtap and haemophilus b vaccine				
KIT, IM (5 DOSE PKG,TAX INCL,PF)				
ea	**49281-0597-05**	275.08	231.73	
TRIIODO-L-THYRONINE SODIUM (PCCA)				
liothyronine sodium				
POW, NA (1X1GM, USP)				
1 gm	**51927-3090-00**	516.00		
TRILEPTAL (Novartis Pharm)				
oxcarbazepine				
SUS, PO, 300 mg/5 ml,				
250 ml	**00078-0357-52**	190.45		
TAB, PO (10X10,FILM-COATED)				
150 mg, 100s ea UD	**00078-0456-35**	216.30		
(FILM-COATED)				
150 mg, 100s ea	**00078-0456-05**	205.99		
300 mg, 100s ea	**00078-0337-05**	376.20		
100s ea UD	**00078-0337-06**	395.00		
(10X10,FILM-COATED)				
600 mg, 100s ea UD	**00078-0457-35**	726.01		
(FILM-COATED)				
600 mg, 100s ea	**00078-0457-05**	691.45		

PROD/MFR	NDC	AWP	DP	OBC
(DHS, Inc.)				
REPACK				
TAB, PO (FILM-COATED)				
150 mg, 30s ea	**55887-0190-30**	53.67		
60s ea	**55887-0190-60**	107.34		
300 mg, 30s ea	**55887-0189-30**	86.15		
(IPI)				
REPACK				
TAB, PO, 150 mg, 90s ea	**18837-0163-90**	156.06		
(Nucare Pharm)				
REPACK				
TAB, PO (FILM-COATED)				
300 mg, 100s ea	**68071-1319-00**	329.50		
(PD-Rx Pharm)				
REPACK				
TAB, PO (FILM-COATED)				
300 mg, 30s ea	**55289-0007-30**	139.59		
(Phys Total Care)				
REPACK				
TAB, PO, 150 mg, 10s ea	**54868-4836-03**	19.59		
(FILM-COATED)				
150 mg, 20s ea	**54868-4836-01**	39.39		
30s ea	**54868-4836-04**	58.14		
(FILM-COATED)				
150 mg, 60s ea	**54868-4836-00**	114.40		
90s ea	**54868-4836-02**	222.60		
(FILM-COATED)				
300 mg, 20s ea	**54868-4837-01**	70.37		
30s ea	**54868-4837-03**	104.63		
(FILM-COATED)				
300 mg, 60s ea	**54868-4837-00**	195.96		
210s ea	**54868-4837-02**	659.25		
(Quality Care Prod)				
REPACK				
TAB, PO, 150 mg, 30s ea	**49999-0640-30**	87.30		
(FILM-COATED)				
150 mg, 60s ea	**49999-0640-60**	174.60		
300 mg, 30s ea	**49999-0641-30**	161.70		
(Southwood)				
REPACK				
TAB, PO, 600 mg, 30s ea	**58016-0068-30**	171.74		
60s ea	**58016-0068-60**	343.49		
90s ea	**58016-0068-90**	515.23		
100s ea	**58016-0068-00**	572.48		
(Stat Rx)				
REPACK				
TAB, PO, 150 mg, 30s ea	**16590-0237-30**	42.50		
60s ea	**16590-0237-60**	85.00		
90s ea	**16590-0237-90**	125.00		
120s ea	**16590-0237-72**	160.00		
300 mg, 30s ea	**16590-0238-30**	120.00		
(FILM-COATED)				
300 mg, 60s ea	**16590-0238-60**	238.24		
90s ea	**16590-0238-90**	356.64		
120s ea	**16590-0238-72**	476.87		
TRILIPIX (Abbott Pharm)				
fenofibric acid				
ECC, PO (ENTERIC COATED)				
45 mg, 90s ea	**00074-9642-90**	131.44	115.29	
135 mg, 90s ea	**00074-9189-90**	394.28	345.86	
(Phys Total Care)				
REPACK				
ECC, PO (ENTERIC COATED)				
135 mg, 30s ea	**54868-5986-00**	160.58		
90s ea	**54868-5986-01**	460.57		
TRILOSTANE (Medisca)				
POW, NA (1X5GM)				
5 gm	**38779-2387-03**	637.50		
(1X25GM)				
25 gm	**38779-2387-04**	2606.25		
(1X100GM)				
100 gm	**38779-2387-05**	8812.50		
(1X500GM)				
500 gm	**38779-2387-08**	33750.00		
(1X1000GM)				
1000 gm	**38779-2387-09**	56250.00		
TRILYTE W/FLAVOR PACKS (Alaven)				
k cl/na bicarb/na cl/polyethylene glycol 3350				
PDS, PO (CHERRY,CITRUS BERRY)				
4000 ml	**68220-0131-04**	27.98		
TRIMEPRAZINE TARTRATE (Gallipot)				
POW, NA (USP)				
25 gm	**51552-0983-04**	157.50	112.50	
(Medisca)				
POW, NA (1X5GM,USP)				
5 gm	**38779-2339-03**	75.00		

PROD/MFR	NDC	AWP	DP	OBC
(1X25GM,USP)				
25 gm	38779-2339-04	285.00		
(1X100GM,USP)				
100 gm	38779-2339-05	1050.00		
(PCCA)				
POW, NA (USP)				
1 gm	51927-3191-00	13.20		
TRIMETHOBENZAMIDE (Core)				
REPACK				
trimethobenzamide hydrochloride				
CAP, PO, 250 mg, 10s ea	33358-0352-10	21.53		
20s ea	33358-0352-20	31.78		
SUP, RC, 100 mg, 10s ea	33358-0351-10	19.98		
(Phys Total Care)				
REPACK				
CAP, PO, 300 mg, 100s ea	54868-5741-00	170.97		
(Stat Rx)				
REPACK				
CAP, PO, 250 mg, 10s ea	16590-0240-10	11.00		
20s ea	16590-0240-20	22.00		
TRIMETHOBENZAMIDE HCL (Actavis)				
trimethobenzamide hydrochloride				
CAP, PO, 250 mg, 100s ea	52152-0166-02	45.75		
300 mg, 100s ea	52152-0185-02	112.30		
(Concord Labs)				
CAP, PO, 250 mg, 100s ea	20254-0018-01	27.00		
500s ea	20254-0018-03	121.50		
(Consolidated Midland)				
SOL, IM (VIAL)				
100 mg/ml, 20 ml	00223-8700-20	10.00		EE
(Consolidated Midland)				
benzocaine/trimethobenzamide hydrochloride				
SUP, RC, 2%-100 mg,				
10s ea	00223-5904-10	9.50		
2%-200 mg, 10s ea	00223-5905-10	7.25		
50s ea	00223-5905-50	34.50		
(Hospira)				
trimethobenzamide hydrochloride				
SOL, IM (LUER LOCK,CARPUJECT)				
100 mg/ml,				
2 ml 10s	00409-1952-32	27.00	23.60	AP
(Medisca)				
POW, NA (U.S.P.)				
5 gm	38779-2196-03	46.50		
25 gm	38779-2196-04	165.00		
100 gm	38779-2196-05	435.00		
(Mutual)				
CAP, PO, 300 mg, 100s ea	53489-0376-01	163.74		AB
(PCCA)				
POW, NA, 1 gm	51927-1981-00	24.00		
1 gm	51927-3572-00	24.00		
(Spectrum Pharmacy)				
CRY, NA (U.S.P.)				
5 gm	49452-7924-01	190.75		
25 gm	49452-7924-02	518.00		
100 gm	49452-7924-03	1274.00		
(A-S Medication)				
REPACK				
CAP, PO, 300 mg, 6s ea	54569-5589-01	8.24		AB
12s ea	54569-5589-00	16.48		AB
(Dispensing Solutions)				
REPACK				
CAP, PO, 250 mg, 10s ea	55045-1628-03	8.75		
300 mg, 10s ea	55045-3203-03	18.00		AB
(HomeMed)				
REPACK				
CAP, PO, 250 mg, 10s ea	51655-0523-53	9.40		
(Nucare Pharm)				
REPACK				
CAP, PO, 250 mg, 10s ea	66267-0208-10	9.88		
20s ea	66267-0208-20	15.39		
(PD-Rx Pharm)				
REPACK				
CAP, PO, 300 mg, 6s ea	55289-0953-06	18.65		
(Pharma Pac)				
REPACK				
CAP, PO, 250 mg, 10s ea	52959-0479-10	10.37		
12s ea	52959-0479-12	12.59		
20s ea	52959-0479-20	16.16		
30s ea	52959-0479-30	22.89		
300 mg, 10s ea	52959-0817-10	12.75		
(Phys Total Care)				
REPACK				
CAP, PO, 250 mg, 10s ea	54868-2973-04	29.43		
15s ea	54868-2973-00	41.88		
30s ea	54868-2973-03	79.26		
100s ea	54868-2973-02	193.59		
SOL, IM, 100 mg/ml,				
2 ml 25s	54868-0608-00	73.36		EE
(Phys Total Care)				
benzocaine/trimethobenzamide hydrochloride				
SUP, RC, 2%-200 mg,				
4s ea	54868-3487-05	16.70		
(Physician Partner)				
REPACK				
trimethobenzamide hydrochloride				
CAP, PO, 300 mg, 10s ea	21695-0448-10	38.19		AB
(Quality Care Prod)				
REPACK				
CAP, PO, 300 mg, 10s ea	35356-0473-00	38.12		AB
(Southwood)				
REPACK				
CAP, PO, 250 mg, 8s ea	58016-0973-08	5.21		
10s ea	58016-0973-10	6.52		
12s ea	58016-0973-12	7.82		
15s ea	58016-0973-15	9.77		
20s ea	58016-0973-20	13.03		
24s ea	58016-0973-24	15.64		
30s ea	58016-0973-30	19.55		
50s ea	58016-0973-50	32.58		
60s ea	58016-0973-60	39.10		
90s ea	58016-0973-90	58.64		
100s ea	58016-0973-00	65.16		
120s ea	58016-0973-02	78.19		
150s ea	58016-0973-03	97.74		
200s ea	58016-0973-89	130.32		
300s ea	58016-0973-73	195.48		
(Stat Rx)				
REPACK				
CAP, PO, 300 mg, 10s ea	16590-0570-10	18.45		AB
30s ea	16590-0570-30	47.00		
60s ea	16590-0570-60	70.00		
90s ea	16590-0570-90	120.00		
TRIMETHOBENZAMIDE HYDROCHLORIDE				
FUL				
CAP, PO, 300 mg, 100s ea		101.93		
(Actavis) *See TRIMETHOBENZAMIDE HCL*				
(Concord Labs) *See TRIMETHOBENZAMIDE HCL*				
(Consolidated Midland) *See TRIMETHOBENZAMIDE HCL*				
(Hospira) *See TRIMETHOBENZAMIDE HCL*				
(JHP) *See TIGAN*				
(Medisca) *See TRIMETHOBENZAMIDE HCL*				
(Monarch) *See TIGAN*				
(Mutual) *See TRIMETHOBENZAMIDE HCL*				
(PCCA) *See TRIMETHOBENZAMIDE HCL*				
(Spectrum Pharmacy) *See TRIMETHOBENZAMIDE HCL*				
(Truxton) *See BENZACOT*				
(DHS, Inc.)				
REPACK				
CAP, PO, 300 mg, 6s ea	55887-0081-06	9.00		
TRIMETHOPRIM (Gallipot)				
POW, NA (U.S.P.)				
25 gm	51552-0953-04	23.10	16.50	
(Medisca)				
POW, NA (U.S.P.,MICRONIZED)				
25 gm	38779-0770-04	52.50		
100 gm	38779-0770-05	135.00		
(U.S.P.)				
100 gm	38779-0270-05	175.50		
(U.S.P.,MICRONIZED)				
500 gm	38779-0770-08	435.00		
(U.S.P.)				
500 gm	38779-0270-08	688.50		
(USP,MICRONIZED)				
1000 gm	38779-0770-09	585.00		
(USP)				
1000 gm	38779-0270-09	994.50		
(USP,MICRONIZED)				
5000 gm	38779-0770-03	1606.50		
(USP)				
5000 gm	38779-0270-03	2983.50		
(USP,MICRONIZED)				
25000 gm	38779-0770-07	7950.00		
(USP)				
25000 gm	38779-0270-07	3978.00		
(Spectrum Pharmacy)				
POW, NA (U.S.P.,MICRONIZED)				
25 gm	49452-7925-01	103.25		
100 gm	49452-7925-02	257.25		
500 gm	49452-7925-03	728.00		
(Teva)				
TAB, PO, 100 mg, 100s ea	00093-2158-01	68.40		AB
(Watson Labs)				
TAB, PO, 100 mg, 100s ea	00591-5571-01	68.40		AB
(A-S Medication)				
REPACK				
TAB, PO, 100 mg, 30s ea	54569-3153-03	20.52		EE
(Dispensing Solutions)				
REPACK				
TAB, PO, 100 mg, 14s ea	55045-2302-03	11.20		AB
(PD-Rx Pharm)				
REPACK				
TAB, PO, 100 mg, 6s ea	55289-0746-06	10.12		AB
10s ea	55289-0746-10	11.34		AB
(Phys Total Care)				
REPACK				
TAB, PO, 100 mg, 30s ea	54868-1616-01	47.49		AB
60s ea	54868-1616-03	90.48		
90s ea	54868-1616-02	103.14		AB
TRIMETHOPRIM & POLYMYXIN (Dispensing Solutions)				
REPACK				
polymyxin b sulfate/trimethoprim sulfate				
SOL, OP, 10000 u/ml-1 mg/ml,				
10 ml	55045-2595-00	17.50		
TRIMETHOPRIM HYDROCHLORIDE				
(FSC Laboratories) *See PRIMSOL*				
TRIMETHOPRIM MICRONIZED (Hawkins)				
trimethoprim, micronized				
POW, NA (U.S.P.)				
25 gm	63370-0301-25	44.00		
100 gm	63370-0301-35	120.00		
500 gm	63370-0301-45	360.00		
1000 gm	63370-0301-50	640.00		
(Letco)				
POW, NA (U.S.P.)				
500 gm	62991-2072-02	225.00		
1000 gm	62991-2072-03	435.00		
(PCCA)				
POW, NA (USP)				
1 gm	51927-1693-00	1.92		
TRIMETHOPRIM SULFATE/POLYMYXIN B SULFATE				
(Palmetto)				
REPACK				
polymyxin b sulfate/trimethoprim sulfate				
SOL, OP, 10000 u/ml-1 mg/ml,				
10 ml	23490-6446-01	34.09		
TRIMETHOPRIM W/ SULFA DS (Bryant Ranch)				
REPACK				
sulfamethoxazole/trimethoprim				
TAB, PO, 800 mg-160 mg,				
6s ea	63629-1765-06	8.59		
10s ea	63629-1765-03	19.65		
14s ea	63629-1765-02	26.70		
20s ea	63629-1765-01	37.29		
28s ea	63629-1765-04	44.41		
40s ea	63629-1765-05	74.58		
TRIMETHOPRIM, MICRONIZED				
(Hawkins) *See TRIMETHOPRIM MICRONIZED*				
(Letco) *See TRIMETHOPRIM MICRONIZED*				
(PCCA) *See TRIMETHOPRIM MICRONIZED*				
TRIMETHOPRIM/POLYMYXIN B SULF				
(Physician Partner)				
REPACK				
polymyxin b sulfate/trimethoprim sulfate				
SOL, OP, 10000 u/ml-1 mg/ml,				
10 ml	21695-0335-10	34.84		
TRIMETHYLAMINE HYDROCHLORIDE (PCCA)				
CRY, NA (1X1GM)				
1 gm	51927-3263-00	0.51		
TRIMIPRAMINE MALEATE (PCCA)				
POW, NA, 1 gm	51927-2451-00	51.00		
(Teva) *See SURMONTIL*				
TRIMOX (Sandoz)				
amoxicillin				
CAP, PO, 500 mg,				
3000s ea	00003-0109-70	1141.88		AB
(PD-Rx Pharm)				
REPACK				
CAP, PO (REDI-SCRIPT)				
500 mg, 30s ea	58864-0611-30	8.43		AB
TRIMPEX (Southwood)				
REPACK				
trimethoprim				
TAB, PO, 100 mg, 20s ea	58016-0373-20	17.81		AB

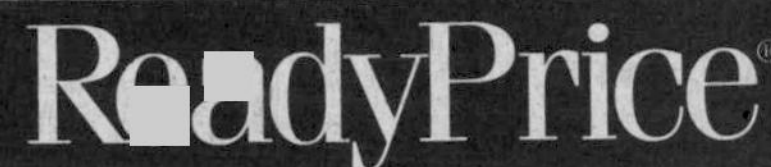

PROD/MFR	NDC	AWP	DP	OBC
TRINALIN REPETABS (Phys Total Care)				
REPACK				
azatadine maleate/pseudoephedrine sulfate				
TER, PO, 1 mg-120 mg,				
20s ea	**54868-1271-02**	30.28		
30s ea	**54868-1271-01**	44.82		
60s ea	**54868-1271-04**	88.43		
(Southwood)				
REPACK				
TER, PO, 1 mg-120 mg,				
40s ea	**58016-0446-40**	36.81		
TRINATE (Cypress Pharm)				
prenatal vitamins				
TAB, PO, 100s ea	**60258-0192-01**	31.27		
TRINESSA (Watson Labs)				
ethinyl estradiol/norgestimate				
TAB, PO (COATED)				
28s ea	**52544-0248-28**	226.51		
(A-S Medication)				
REPACK				
TAB, PO (6X28)				
28s ea	**54569-5796-00**	39.32		
(Quality Care Prod)				
REPACK				
TAB, PO, 28s ea	**35356-0368-28**	96.80		
TRINESSA 28 (Phys Total Care)				
REPACK				
ethinyl estradiol/norgestimate				
TAB, PO, 28s ea	**54868-5826-00**	73.89		
TRIONATE (Breckenridge Pharm)				
carbetapentane tannate/chlorpheniramine tannate				
SUS, PO (STRAWBERRY)				
30 mg/5 ml-4 mg/5 ml,				
480 ml	**51991-0071-16**	114.95		
TRIONATE NF (Breckenridge Pharm)				
carbetapentane tannate/chlorpheniramine tannate				
TAB, PO (CAPLET)				
60 mg-5 mg,				
100s ea	**51991-0072-01**	136.15		
TRIOSTAT (JHP)				
liothyronine sodium				
SOL, IV (6X1ML)				
0.01 mg/ml,				
1 ml 6s	**42023-0120-06**	3767.39		AP
TRIOXIN (Vertical)				
benzocaine/chloroxylenol/hydrocortisone acetate				
SUS, OT, 15 ml	**68025-0041-15**	92.50		
TRIOXSALEN (PCCA)				
POW, NA, 1 gm	**51927-3089-00**	852.00		
TRIPEDIA (Sanofi)				
dtap vaccine				
SUS, IM (S.D.V.,TAX INCL,PF)				
0.5 ml 10s	**49281-0298-10**	272.16	230.55	
TRIPELENNAMINE HCL (Gallipot)				
tripelennamine hydrochloride				
POW, NA, 25 gm	**51552-0186-04**	45.50		
100 gm	**51552-0186-05**	152.25		
(Medisca)				
POW, NA (U.S.P.)				
25 gm	**38779-2198-04**	99.00		
100 gm	**38779-2198-05**	343.50		
(USP)				
1000 gm	**38779-2198-09**	1989.00		
(PCCA)				
POW, NA (U.S.P.)				
1 gm	**51927-3355-00**	9.00		
(Spectrum Pharmacy)				
POW, NA (U.S.P.)				
25 gm	**49452-7941-01**	287.70		
100 gm	**49452-7941-02**	857.50		
TRIPELENNAMINE HYDROCHLORIDE				
(Gallipot) *See TRIPELENNAMINE HCL*				
(Medisca) *See TRIPELENNAMINE HCL*				
(PCCA) *See TRIPELENNAMINE HCL*				
(Spectrum Pharmacy) *See TRIPELENNAMINE HCL*				
TRIPHASIL-28 (Phys Total Care)				
REPACK				
ethinyl estradiol/levonorgestrel				
TAB, PO, 28s ea	**54868-0518-01**	42.01		AB
TRIPLE ANTIBIOTIC (Truxton)				
bacitracin zinc/neomycin/polymyxin b sulfate				
OIN, OP, 3.5 gm	**00463-8049-38**	2.52		EE
(Dispensing Solutions)				
REPACK				
OIN, TP, 30 gm	**55045-1436-06**	9.50		
(Keltman Pharma., Inc.)				
REPACK				
OIN, TP, 1 ml	**68387-0656-01**	33.45		
(Nucare Pharm)				
REPACK				
OIN, OP, 3.5 gm	**66267-0929-35**	8.71		EE
(Southwood)				
REPACK				
OIN, OP, 3.5 gm	**58016-6047-01**	6.22		EE
TRIPLE ANTIBIOTIC W/HYDROCORTISONE (Truxton)				
bacitracin zn/hc/neomycin sulf/polymyxin b sulf				
OIN, OP, 3.75 gm	**00463-8044-38**	2.70		EE
(Southwood)				
REPACK				
OIN, OP, 3.5 gm	**58016-6016-01**	8.37		EE
TRIPLE DYE (William Labs)				
brilliant green/gentian violet/proflavine sulfate				
SOL, TP (PIN-POINT APPL, AMP)				
0.5 ml 200s	**51101-2826-05**	57.15		
TRIPLE SULFA (Phys Total Care)				
REPACK				
sulfabenzamide/sulfacetamide/sulfathiazole				
CRE, VG, 3.7%-2.86%-3.42%,				
78 gm	**54868-0164-01**	13.96		EE
(Southwood)				
REPACK				
CRE, VG, 3.7%-2.86%-3.42%,				
78 gm	**58016-3082-01**	28.68		EE
TRIPLE VITAMIN W/FLUORIDE (Vintage)				
ascorbic acid/sodium fluoride/vitamin a/vitamin d				
SOL, PO (DROPS)				
50 ml	**00254-9451-48**	8.50		
50 ml	**00254-9452-48**	8.50		
(A-S Medication)				
REPACK				
SOL, PO (DROPS)				
50 ml	**54569-1280-00**	11.80		
TRIPLEX AD (Breckenridge Pharm)				
cpm/phenyleph hcl/pyril mal				
SOL, PO (1X473ML,AF,SF,DYE-FREE)				
473 ml	**51991-0549-16**	52.69		
TRIPLEX DM (Breckenridge Pharm)				
dm/phenyleph hcl/pyril mal				
SOL, PO (AF,SF,DYE-FREE,GRAPE)				
473 ml	**51991-0493-16**	51.50		
TRIPOHIST (Breckenridge Pharm)				
triprolidine hydrochloride				
SOL, PO (1X473ML,AF,SF,APPLE)				
1.25 mg/5 ml,				
473 ml	**51991-0531-16**	65.09		
TRIPOHIST D (Breckenridge Pharm)				
pse hcl/triprolidine hcl				
SOL, PO (1X473ML,AF,SF,BLUEBERRY)				
45 mg/5 ml-1.25 mg/5 ml,				
473 ml	**51991-0532-16**	63.14		
TRIPROLIDINE (Centurion)				
triprolidine hydrochloride				
SOL, PO (AF,SF,APPLE)				
1.25 mg/5 ml,				
473 ml	**23359-0002-16**	56.64		
TRIPROLIDINE HCL (Medisca)				
triprolidine hydrochloride				
POW, NA (U.S.P.)				
1 gm	**38779-0272-06**	31.50		
(PCCA)				
POW, NA (U.S.P.)				
1 gm	**51927-2038-00**	54.00		
TRIPROLIDINE HYDROCHLORIDE				
(Breckenridge Pharm) *See TRIPOHIST*				
(Centurion) *See TRIPROLIDINE*				
(Medisca) *See TRIPROLIDINE HCL*				
(PCCA) *See TRIPROLIDINE HCL*				
(Vindex Pharma Inc) *See ZYMINE*				
TRIPROLIDINE TANNATE				
(Vindex Pharma Inc) *See ZYMINE XR*				
TRIPTORELIN PAMOATE				
(Watson) *See TRELSTAR DEPOT*				
(Watson) *See TRELSTAR LA*				
TRIS (HYDROXYMETHYL) AMINOMETHANE (PCCA)				
tromethamine				
POW, NA, 1 gm	**51927-1283-00**	0.54		
TRISENOX (Cephalon)				
arsenic trioxide				
SOL, IV (10X10 AMP,PF)				
1 mg/ml, 10 ml 10s	**63459-0600-10**	4358.40		
TRISUDRINE (Ohm)				
pse hcl/triprolidine hcl				
TAB, PO, 60 mg-2.5 mg,				
24s ea	**51660-0160-24**	1.15		EE
100s ea	**51660-0160-01**	2.35		EE
1000s ea	**51660-0160-10**	14.00		EE
TRITAL DM (Breckenridge Pharm)				
cpm/dm/phenyleph hcl				
SOL, PO (AF,SF,DYE-FREE,GRAPE)				
473 ml	**51991-0131-16**	35.95		
TRITAL SR (Breckenridge Pharm)				
apap/cpm/phenyleph hcl/phenyltoloxamine cit				
TER, PO, 325 mg-8 mg-40 mg-50 mg,				
100s ea	**51991-0529-01**	82.61		
TRITON X-100 (Amend)				
octoxynol 9				
SOL, NA, 500 ml	**17317-0931-01**	10.85		
3840 ml	**17317-0931-06**	56.00		
22272 ml	**17317-0931-08**	218.40		
(PCCA)				
SOL, NA, 1 gm	**51927-1425-00**	0.11		
TRITON X-114 (Amend)				
octoxynol 8				
LIQ, NA, 500 ml	**17317-1779-01**	14.70		
3840 ml	**17317-1779-08**	56.00		
TRITON X-15 (Amend)				
octoxynol 1				
LIQ, NA, 500 ml	**17317-1452-01**	10.85		
3840 ml	**17317-1452-03**	56.00		
20812.8008 ml	**17317-1452-06**	204.75		
TRITON X-165 (Amend)				
octoxynol 16				
LIQ, NA, 500 ml	**17317-1311-01**	10.85		
500 ml	**17317-1311-06**	63.00		
TRITON X-35 (Amend)				
octoxynol 3				
LIQ, NA, 500 ml	**17317-1671-01**	10.85		
3840 ml	**17317-1671-06**	63.00		
TRITON X-45 (Amend)				
octoxynol 5				
LIQ, NA, 500 ml	**17317-0930-01**	10.85		
3840 ml	**17317-0930-06**	63.00		
19968 ml	**17317-0930-09**	195.65		
(PCCA)				
LIQ, NA, 1 ml	**51927-2708-00**	0.16		
TRITUSS (Everett)				
dm/gg/phenyleph hcl				
SOL, PO (AF,SF,STRAWBERRY)				
473 ml	**00642-0700-16**	154.22		
TRITUSS-ER (Everett)				
dm/gg/phenyleph hcl				
TER, PO (CAPLET)				
30 mg-600 mg-10 mg,				
100s ea	**00642-0661-10**	167.64		
TRIVORA-28 (Watson)				
ethinyl estradiol/levonorgestrel				
TAB, PO (6X28)				
168s ea	**52544-0291-28**	164.92		AB
(A-S Medication)				
REPACK				
TAB, PO, 28s ea	**54569-5115-00**	27.49		AB
(Phys Total Care)				
REPACK				
TAB, PO, 28s ea	**54868-4239-00**	35.36		AB
TRIZIVIR (Glaxo)				
abacavir sulfate/lamivudine/zidovudine				
TAB, PO (FILM-COATED)				
300 mg-150 mg-300 mg,				
60s ea	**00173-0691-00**	1518.76		
(A-S Medication)				
REPACK				
TAB, PO (FILM-COATED)				
300 mg-150 mg-300 mg,				
60s ea	**54569-5191-00**	1974.39		

PROD/MFR NDC AWP DP OBC

(Quality Care Prod)
REPACK
TAB, PO (FILM-COATED)
300 mg-150 mg-300 mg,
6s ea.............35356-0116-06 331.19
60s ea.............35356-0116-60 3111.06

TROCHE BASE (Medisca)
PEL, NA, 50 gm..........38779-2378-02 16.50
100 gm..............38779-2378-05 31.50
500 gm..............38779-2378-08 103.50
2500 gm..............38779-2378-01 435.00

TROLAMINE
(Amend) *See TRIETHANOLAMINE 85%*
(Amend) *See TROLAMINE 99%*
(Baker, J.T.)
LIQ, NA (N.F.)
500 ml.............10106-9467-01 68.86
4000 ml.............10106-9467-03 309.93
(Baker, J.T.) *See TRIETHANOLAMINE*
(Gallipot)
LIQ, NA (U.S.P.,N.F.)
60 ml..............51552-0132-03 7.42
473 ml.............51552-0132-06 16.80
3785 ml.............51552-0132-08 55.65
(Medisca) *See TROLAMINE 99%*
(PCCA)
LIQ, NA (NF)
1 ml..............51927-1097-00 0.23
(Spectrum Pharmacy)
LIQ, NA (1X500ML, N.F.)
500 ml.............49452-7930-00 64.75
(1X4000ML, N.F.)
4000 ml.............49452-7930-01 213.85
(1X20000ML, N.F.)
20000 ml............49452-7930-02 819.00

TROLAMINE 99% (Amend)
trolamine
LIQ, NA (N.F.)
500 ml.............17317-0585-01 9.80
3840 ml.............17317-0585-06 35.00
20000 ml............17317-0585-08 140.00
(Medisca)
SOL, NA (1X100ML)
100 ml.............38779-1671-05 22.50
(1X500ML)
500 ml.............38779-1671-08 28.50
(1X4000ML)
4000 ml.............38779-1671-01 105.00
(1X20000ML)
20000 ml............38779-1671-07 429.00

TROLAMINE SALICYLATE
(Spectrum Pharmacy) *See TRIETHANOLAMINE SALICYLATE*
(Altura)
REPACK
CRE, TP, 10%, 100 gm....63874-1115-01 6.31

TROMETHAMINE
(Hospira) *See THAM*
(Medisca)
POW, NA (1X100GM,USP)
100 gm..............38779-1672-05 49.50
(1X500GM,USP)
500 gm..............38779-1672-08 108.00
(1X1000GM,USP)
1000 gm.............38779-1672-09 205.50
(PCCA) *See TRIS (HYDROXYMETHYL) AMINOMETHANE*
(Spectrum Pharmacy)
POW, NA (U.S.P.)
500 gm..............49452-7955-01 236.25
2500 gm.............49452-7955-02 969.50

TROPAZONE (ECR)
lotion, multi ingredient
LOT, TP (1X140GM)
140 gm..............00095-0070-14 80.62

TROPHAMINE (B. Braun)
amino acids
SOL, IV, 6%, 500 ml......00264-9361-55 50.82
(GLASS)
10%, 500 ml.........00264-9341-55 67.68

TROPICACYL (Akorn)
tropicamide
SOL, OP, 0.5%, 15 ml.....17478-0101-12 10.00 AT
1%, 15 ml...........17478-0102-12 10.65 AT

TROPICAL PUNCH (Medisca)
flavoring aid
SOL, NA (1X25ML)
25 ml..............38779-1673-04 22.50
(1X100ML)
100 ml.............38779-1673-05 37.50
(1X500ML)
500 ml.............38779-1673-08 61.50
(Spectrum Pharmacy)
LIQ, NA (1X100ML)
100 ml.............49452-7985-01 53.20
(1X500ML)
500 ml.............49452-7985-02 118.30

TROPICAL PUNCH FLAVOR (PCCA)
flavoring aid
SOL, NA (ARTIFICIAL)
1 ml...............51927-2153-00 0.90

TROPICAMIDE
FUL
SOL, OP, 0.5%, 15 ml.............................. 9.83
1%, 15 ml.. 10.50
(Akorn) *See TROPICACYL*
(Alcon Ophthalmic) *See MYDRIACYL*
(Bausch & Lomb Inc.)
SOL, OP, 0.5%, 15 ml.....24208-0590-64 15.97 AT
1%, 2 ml 12s........24208-0585-59 5.03 AT
15 ml..............24208-0585-64 17.07 AT
(Falcon Ophthalmics)
SOL, OP, 0.5%, 15 ml.....61314-0354-01 15.95 AT
1%, 3 ml...........61314-0355-01 5.00 AT
15 ml..............61314-0355-02 17.00 AT
(Gallipot)
POW, NA (U.S.P.)
5 gm...............51552-1016-02 224.35 160.25
(Medisca)
POW, NA (USP)
1 gm...............38779-0273-06 88.50
(U.S.P.)
5 gm...............38779-0273-03 357.00
10 gm..............38779-0273-01 597.00
(USP)
100 gm.............38779-0273-05 3450.00
(Ocusoft) *See MYDRAL*
(PCCA)
POW, NA (U.S.P.)
1 gm...............51927-2670-00 105.00
(Spectrum Pharmacy)
POW, NA (U.S.P.)
1 gm...............49452-7988-01 133.00
5 gm...............49452-7988-02 535.50
(Nucare Pharm)
REPACK
SOL, OP (1X15ML)
0.5%, 15 ml........68071-1337-05 18.76 AT
(Phys Total Care)
REPACK
SOL, OP, 0.5%, 15 ml.....54868-3833-00 39.54 EE
1%, 15 ml..........54868-2108-00 38.85 AT
(Southwood)
REPACK
SOL, OP, 1%, 15 ml.......58016-6332-01 13.06 EE

TROSPIUM CHLORIDE
(Allergan Inc) *See SANCTURA*
(Allergan Inc) *See SANCTURA XR*

TRUSOPT OCUMETER (Phys Total Care)
REPACK
dorzolamide hydrochloride
SOL, OP, 2%, 5 ml........54868-3593-01 31.06
10 ml..............54868-3593-00 67.41

TRUSOPT OCUMETER PLUS (Merck)
dorzolamide hydrochloride
SOL, OP, 2%, 10 ml.......00006-3519-36 76.20

TRUST NATAL DHA (Vertical)
prenatal vitamins
KIT, PO (FILM-COATED,SOFTGEL)
60s ea UD..........68025-0901-30 34.89

TRUVADA (Gilead Sciences)
emtricitabine/tenofovir disoproxil fumarate
TAB, PO (GLUTEN-FREE,FILM-COATED)
200 mg-300 mg,
30s ea.............61958-0701-01 1118.00

(A-S Medication)
REPACK
TAB, PO (GLUTEN-FREE,FILM-COATED)
200 mg-300 mg,
30s ea.............54569-5588-00 1453.40
(Dispensing Solutions)
REPACK
TAB, PO, 200 mg-300 mg,
2s ea..............55045-3481-03 68.86
(Pharma Pac)
REPACK
TAB, PO (GLUTEN-FREE,FILM-COATED)
200 mg-300 mg,
3s ea..............52959-0969-03 198.69
(Phys Total Care)
REPACK
TAB, PO (GLUTEN-FREE,FILM-COATED)
200 mg-300 mg,
30s ea.............54868-5141-00 1034.35
(Quality Care Prod)
REPACK
TAB, PO (GLUTEN-FREE,FILM-COATED)
200 mg-300 mg,
6s ea..............35356-0070-06 462.40
30s ea.............35356-0070-30 2212.00

TRUXADRYL (Truxton)
diphenhydramine hydrochloride
SOL, IJ (VIAL)
10 mg/ml, 30 ml.....00463-1080-30 5.40
50 mg/ml, 10 ml.....00463-1089-10 5.40 EE

TRUXCILLIN VK (Truxton)
penicillin v potassium
TAB, PO, 250 mg,
1000s ea..........00463-5017-10 36.00 EE
500 mg, 1000s ea.....00463-5023-10 69.76 EE

TRUZONE PEAK FLOW METER (Monaghan Medical)
meter, peak flow, spirometry
DEV, NA, ea..............04351-0965-10 13.95

TRYPAN BLUE
(Dutch Ophthalmic USA) *See MEMBRANEBLUE*
(Dutch Ophthalmic USA) *See VISIONBLUE*
(PCCA)
POW, NA (1X1GM)
1 gm...............51927-3155-00 2.04
(Spectrum Pharmacy)
POW, NA (1X25GM)
25 gm..............49452-7992-01 159.25
(1X100GM)
100 gm.............49452-7992-02 455.00

TRYPSIN (PCCA)
POW, NA, 1 gm...........51927-1971-00 1.05
(Spectrum Pharmacy) *See TRYPSIN 1:100*

TRYPSIN 1:100 (Spectrum Pharmacy)
trypsin
POW, NA, 100 gm.........49452-7990-01 221.55
500 gm.............49452-7990-02 493.50

TRYPSIN COMPLEX (Breckenridge Pharm)
castor oil/peru balsam/trypsin
OIN, TP, 60 gm...........51991-0124-22 64.79

TRYPTOPHAN
(Gallipot) *See L-5-HYDROXYTRYPTOPHAN*
(Letco) *See 5-HYDROXY-L-TRYPTOPHAN*
(Letco) *See L-TRYPTOPHAN*
(PCCA)
POW, NA (USP)
1 gm...............51927-2873-00 2.40

TUBE, GASTROINTESTINAL
(Abbott) *See LAP J LAPAROSCOPIC JEJUNOSTOMY*
(Abbott) *See LAP J REPLACEMENT JEJUNOSTOMY TUBE*

TUBERCULIN
(JHP) *See APLISOL*
(Sanofi) *See TUBERSOL*

TUBERCULIN/PPD (Southwood)
REPACK
tuberculin
SOL, ID, 5 tu/0.1 ml,
5 ml...............58016-9474-01 404.40

TUBERSOL (Sanofi)
tuberculin
SOL, ID (VIAL, 10 TEST)
5 tu/0.1 ml, 1 ml.....49281-0752-21 36.46 30.38
(VIAL, 50 TEST)
5 tu/0.1 ml, 5 ml.....49281-0752-22 132.68 110.57

PROD/MFR	NDC	AWP	DP	OBC

(Dispensing Solutions)
REPACK
SOL, ID (1X1ML)
5 tu/0.1 ml, 1 ml **55045-3253-01** 32.00
(1X5ML)
5 tu/0.1 ml, 5 ml **55045-3253-02** 130.00

(Phys Total Care)
REPACK
SOL, ID (VIAL, 10 TEST)
5 tu/0.1 ml, 1 ml **54868-2972-01** 38.71
(VIAL, 50 TEST)
5 tu/0.1 ml, 5 ml **54868-3356-01** 152.13

(Quality Care Prod)
REPACK
SOL, ID (1X1ML)
5 tu/0.1 ml, 1 ml **35356-0183-01** 232.60
5 ml............... **49999-0430-05** 116.20

TUBING, CONNECTING
(Abbott Hosp) *See MICROBORE PRIMARY PUMP W/OL*

TUBING, FLUID DELIVERY
(Abbott Hosp) *See FAT EMULSION IV*

TUBING, IRRIGATION
(Alcon Surgical) *See BSS & BSS PLUS*

TUNA (Medisca)
flavoring aid
POW, NA (1X25GM)
25 gm............... **38779-1954-04** 22.50
(1X100GM)
100 gm............... **38779-1954-05** 43.50
(1X500GM)
500 gm............... **38779-1954-08** 114.00

TUNA FLAVOR (PCCA)
flavoring aid
POW, NA (ARTIFICIAL)
1 gm............... **51927-3239-00** 0.26

TUNGSTEN CHLORIDE (PCCA)
POW, NA, 1 gm........ **51927-9132-00** 37.50

TUNGSTIC ACID (Baker, J.T.)
POW, NA (REAGENT)
500 gm............... **10106-0422-01** 266.51

TURKEY RED OIL (Medisca)
sulfated castor oil
OIL, NA (1X500ML)
500 ml **38779-1675-08** 58.50

TURMERIC (PCCA)
POW, NA (CURCUMA LONGA)
1 gm............... **51927-3018-00** 0.11

TURPENTINE
(Lorann Oil) *See TURPENTINE RECTIFIED*
(Medisca) *See TURPENTINE STEAM DISTILLED*
(PCCA)
LIQ, NA (PURIFIED GUM SPIRITS)
1 ml............... **51927-1973-00** 0.09
(PCCA) *See TURPENTINE RECTIFIED*
(Spectrum Pharmacy)
LIQ, NA (PURIFIED)
500 ml **49452-8030-01** 76.30
4000 ml **49452-8030-02** 263.55

TURPENTINE RECTIFIED (Lorann Oil)
turpentine
OIL, NA (N.F.)
30 ml............... **23535-0248-05** 1.55
120 ml **23535-0248-08** 3.25
480 ml **23535-0248-01** 8.00
3840 ml **23535-0248-11** 38.00
(PCCA)
OIL, NA, 1 ml............... **51927-1437-00** 0.13

TURPENTINE STEAM DISTILLED (Medisca)
turpentine
SOL, NA (1X1000ML)
1000 ml **38779-2260-09** 123.00

TUSDEC-DM (Cypress Pharm)
bpm/dm/phenyleph hcl
SOL, PO (AF,SF,DYE-FREE)
473 ml **60258-0431-16** 43.35

TUSNEL (Llorens Pharma Int)
bpm/dm/gg
SOL, PO (AF,SF,DYE-FREE)
178 ml **54859-0502-06** 8.45

TUSNEL PEDIATRIC (Llorens Pharma Int)
dm/gg/pse hcl
SOL, PO (AF,GRAPE)
118 ml **54859-0544-04** 6.95

(Llorens Pharma Int)
guaifenesin/pseudoephedrine hydrochloride
(DROPS)
50 mg/ml-5 mg/ml,
60 ml............... **54859-0602-02** 8.95

TUSS-DA (Intl Ethical)
dm/pse hcl
LIQ, PO, 20 mg/5 ml-30 mg/5 ml,
120 ml **11584-1026-04** 9.15

TUSSAFED-EX (Everett)
dm/gg/phenyleph hcl
SYR, PO (AF,CHERRY,VANILLA)
473 ml **00642-0765-16** 41.00

TUSSAFED-EX PEDIATRIC (Everett)
dm/gg/phenyleph hcl
LIQ, PO (AF,SF,DROPS)
30 ml............... **00642-0769-30** 24.60

TUSSAFED-HC (Everett)
gg/hydrocod bit/phenyleph hcl
SYR, PO (AF,SF)
480 ml, C-III **00642-0460-16** 155.44

TUSSAFED-HCG (Everett)
gg/hydrocod bit/phenyleph hcl
SOL, PO (AF,SF,CHERRY)
473 ml, C-III **00642-0455-16** 171.98

TUSSAFED-LA (Everett)
dm/gg/pse hcl
TER, PO (DYE-FREE,CAPLET)
30 mg-600 mg-60 mg,
100s ea............ **00642-0650-10** 61.50

TUSSALL (Everett)
dm/dexbrompheniramine maleate/phenyleph hcl
SOL, PO (AF,SF,STRAWBERRY)
473 ml **00642-0470-16** 165.88

TUSSALL-ER (Everett)
dm/dexbrompheniramine maleate/phenyleph hcl
TER, PO, 6 mg-30 mg-20 mg,
100s ea............ **00642-0471-10** 166.77

TUSSCOUGH DHC (Breckenridge Pharm)
cpm/dihydrocodeine bitartrate/phenyleph hcl
SOL, PO (1X473ML,AF,SF,DYE-FREE)
473 ml, C-V.......... **51991-0608-16** 90.48

TUSSI-12 (Meda)
carbetapentane tannate/chlorpheniramine tannate
TAB, PO, 60 mg-5 mg,
100s ea............ **00037-0681-10** 360.76

TUSSI-12 S (Meda)
carbetapentane tannate/chlorpheniramine tannate
SUS, PO (STRAWBERRY-CURRANT)
30 mg/5 ml-4 mg/5 ml,
118 ml 4s.......... **00037-0682-04** 344.71

(Phys Total Care)
REPACK
cpm tan/carbetapentane tan/phenyleph tan
SUS, PO (STRAWBERRY-CURRANT)
118 ml **54868-4738-00** 58.19

TUSSI-12D (Meda)
carbetapentane tan/phenyleph tan/pyril tan
TAB, PO, 60 mg-10 mg-40 mg,
100s ea............ **00037-0692-10** 284.49

TUSSI-12D S (Meda)
carbetapentane tan/phenyleph tan/pyril tan
SUS, PO (UNIT/USE-CURRANT)
118 ml **00037-0693-04** 78.68

TUSSI-BID (Capellon)
dextromethorphan hydrobromide/guaifenesin
TER, PO (CAPLET)
60 mg-1200 mg,
100s ea............ **64543-0171-01** 101.95

TUSSI-PRES (Kramer-Novis)
dm/gg/phenyleph hcl
LIQ, PO (AF,SF,CHERRY)
120 ml **52083-0233-04** 4.50
3785 ml **52083-0233-10** 44.00

TUSSI-PRES PEDIATRIC (Kramer-Novis)
dm/gg/phenyleph hcl
SOL, PO (AF,SF,DYE-FREE)
120 ml **52083-0232-04** 5.65

TUSSICAPS (Covidien)
chlorpheniramine polistirex/hydrocodone polistirex
CER, PO, 4 mg-5 mg,
100s ea, C-III **23635-0054-01** 448.50
8 mg-10 mg,
20s ea, C-III **23635-0108-20** 89.70
100s ea, C-III **23635-0108-01** 448.50

(Phys Total Care)
REPACK
CER, PO, 8 mg-10 mg,
20s ea, C-III **54868-5957-00** 96.47

TUSSIGON (Monarch)
homatropine methylbromide/hydrocodone bitartrate
TAB, PO, 1.5 mg-5 mg,
100s ea, C-III ...... **61570-0081-01** 54.68 AA

TUSSIONEX PENNKINETIC (UCB)
chlorpheniramine polistirex/hydrocodone polistirex
SER, PO, 8 mg/5 ml-10 mg/5 ml,
473 ml, C-III **53014-0548-67** 332.42
(A-S Medication)
REPACK
SER, PO, 8 mg/5 ml-10 mg/5 ml,
480 ml, C-III **54569-4510-00** 403.88
(Phys Total Care)
REPACK
SER, PO, 8 mg/5 ml-10 mg/5 ml,
473 ml, C-III **54868-0534-02** 353.52
(Quality Care Prod)
REPACK
SER, PO (1X480ML)
8 mg/5 ml-10 mg/5 ml,
480 ml, C-III **35356-0127-16** 289.40
(Southwood)
REPACK
SER, PO, 8 mg/5 ml-10 mg/5 ml,
60 ml, C-III **58016-0490-12** 13.69
120 ml, C-III **58016-0490-24** 26.11
473 ml, C-III **58016-4852-01** 231.23

TUSSO-C (Everett)
codeine phosphate/guaifenesin
SOL, PO (AF,SF,DYE-FREE)
10 mg/5 ml-200 mg/5 ml,
473 ml, C-V........ **00642-0461-16** 185.28

TUSSO-DF (Everett)
guaifenesin/hydrocodone bitartrate
SYR, PO (CHERRY)
100 mg/5 ml-2.5 mg/5 ml,
473 ml, C-III **00642-0468-16** 165.60

TUSSO-DM (Everett)
dm/gg/phenyleph hcl
TER, PO (SF,GLUTEN-FREE)
23 mg-600 mg-9 mg,
100s ea............ **00642-0630-10** 129.45

TUSSO-DMR (Everett)
dm/gg/phenyleph hcl
CAP, PO (SF,GLUTEN-FREE)
14 mg-288 mg-7 mg,
100s ea............ **00642-0645-10** 105.29

TUSSO-HC (Everett)
guaifenesin/hydrocodone bitartrate
TER, PO (CAPLET)
1200 mg-10 mg,
100s ea, C-III **00642-0421-10** 133.24

TUSSO-XR (Everett)
dm/gg/phenyleph hcl
SUS, PO (AF,SF,GLUTEN-FREE)
473 ml **00642-0616-16** 191.08

TUSSO-ZMR (Everett)
carbetapentane citrate/guaifenesin
CAP, PO, 8 mg-200 mg,
100s ea............ **00642-0647-10** 104.96

TUSSO-ZR (Everett)
carbetapentane citrate/guaifenesin
SOL, PO (1X473ML,AF,SF)
7.5 mg/5 ml-150 mg/5 ml,
473 ml **00642-0649-16** 145.53

TUSSPLEX (Breckenridge Pharm)
hydrocod bit/phenyleph hcl/pyril mal
SOL, PO (AF,SF,BLACK CHERRY)
473 ml, C-III **51991-0523-16** 48.85

TUSSPLEX DM (Breckenridge Pharm)
cpm/dm/phenyleph hcl
SOL, PO (AF,SF)
473 ml **51991-0491-16** 36.94

TUTTI FRUTTI ARTIFICIAL FLAVOR (Spectrum Pharmacy)
flavoring aid
LIQ, NA (1X100ML,CONCENTRATE)
100 ml **49452-8035-02** 63.70
(1X500ML,CONCENTRATE)
500 ml **49452-8035-03** 146.65

PROD/MFR NDC AWP DP OBC

TUTTI FRUTTI FLAVOR (PCCA)
flavoring aid
SOL, NA (ARTIFICIAL)
1 ml................51927-2152-00 0.90

TUTTI-FRUTTI (Medisca)
flavoring aid
SOL, NA (1X25ML)
25 ml................38779-1677-04 22.50
(1X100ML)
100 ml 38779-1677-05 37.50
(1X500ML)
500 ml 38779-1677-08 82.50

TUTTI-FRUTTI CONCENTRATE (Gallipot)
flavoring aid
SOL, NA (ARTIFICIAL,TUTTI-FRUTTI)
60 ml................51552-0957-03 6.02 4.30

TWINJECT (Shionogi)
epinephrine
SOL, IJ (DELIVERS 0.15MG)
1 mg/ml, 0.15 ml.....59630-0801-01 100.13
(DELIVERS0.15MG,2X0.15ML)
1 mg/ml,
0.15 ml 2s.........59630-0801-02 192.72
(1X0.3ML,DELIVERS 0.3MG)
1 mg/ml, 0.3 ml......59630-0802-01 100.13
0.3 ml 2s..........59630-0802-02 192.72

(Verus)
SOL, IJ (0.15MG DELIVERY)
1 mg/ml, ea..........13436-0701-01 83.16
ea.................13436-0701-02 160.06
(0.3MG DELIVERY)
1 mg/ml, ea..........13436-0700-01 83.16
ea.................13436-0700-02 160.06

TWINRIX (Glaxo)
hep a vac, inactivated/hep b vac recombinant
SUS, IM (TPLOK,SNGLE DSE,TAXINCL)
720 el u/ml-20 mcg/ml,
1 ml 5s............58160-0815-46 537.60
(TAX INCLUDED,1MLX10,PF)
720 el u/ml-20 mcg/ml,
1 ml 10s...........58160-0815-11 1075.20

(A-S Medication)
REPACK
SUS, IM (TIP-LOK SYR)
720 el u/ml-20 mcg/ml,
1 ml 5s............54569-5578-00 510.03

TWYNSTA (Boehr Ingelheim Phar)
amlodipine besylate/telmisartan
TAB, PO (2X5X3)
5 mg-40 mg,
30s ea UD 00597-0124-37 126.00
5 mg-80 mg,
30s ea UD 00597-0126-37 126.00
10 mg-40 mg,
30s ea UD 00597-0125-37 126.00
10 mg-80 mg,
30s ea UD 00597-0127-37 126.00

TYGACIL (Wyeth)
tigecycline
PDS, IV (SDV,PF)
50 mg, 10s ea........00008-4990-02 734.94 612.45

TYKERB (Glaxo)
lapatinib ditosylate
TAB, PO (FILM-COATED)
250 mg, 150s ea 00173-0752-00 4259.65

TYLENOL W/CODEINE (Dispensing Solutions)
REPACK
acetaminophen/codeine phosphate
TAB, PO, 300 mg-30 mg,
18s ea, C-III 55045-2651-02 16.20

TYLENOL W/CODEINE #3 (Ortho-McNeil Pharm)
acetaminophen/codeine phosphate
TAB, PO, 300 mg-30 mg,
100s ea, C-III ......00045-0513-60 79.81 66.51 AA
1000s ea, C-III .....00045-0513-80 627.78 523.15 AA

(A-S Medication)
REPACK
TAB, PO, 300 mg-30 mg,
20s ea, C-III ....54569-0024-02 15.47 AA

(PD-Rx Pharm)
REPACK
TAB, PO, 300 mg-30 mg,
15s ea, C-III ....55289-0048-15 22.86 AA

(Phys Total Care)
REPACK
TAB, PO, 300 mg-30 mg,
20s ea, C-III ....54868-0285-02 15.33 AA
24s ea, C-III ....54868-0285-01 17.89 AA
30s ea, C-III ....54868-0285-03 21.74 AA
100s ea, C-III ......54868-0285-04 66.64 AA
120s ea, C-III ......54868-0285-00 79.46 AA

TYLENOL W/CODEINE #4 (Ortho-McNeil Pharm)
acetaminophen/codeine phosphate
TAB, PO, 300 mg-60 mg,
500s ea, C-III ......00045-0515-70 609.19 507.66 AA

(Phys Total Care)
REPACK
TAB, PO, 300 mg-60 mg,
100s ea, C-III ......54868-0519-00 113.56 AA

TYLENOL W/CODEINE NO 4 (Southwood)
REPACK
acetaminophen/codeine phosphate
TAB, PO, 300 mg-60 mg,
30s ea, C-III 58016-0062-30 35.81
60s ea, C-III 58016-0062-60 71.63
90s ea, C-III 58016-0062-90 107.44
100s ea, C-III 58016-0062-00 119.38

TYLENOL WITH CODEINE NO. 4 (PriCara)
acetaminophen/codeine phosphate
TAB, PO, 300 mg-60 mg,
100s ea, C-III ......50458-0515-60 141.04 117.53 AA

TYLOSIN TARTRATE (Medisca)
POW, NA (B.P.)
1 gm.................38779-0916-06 31.50
5 gm.................38779-0916-03 138.00
25 gm................38779-0916-04 612.00
100 gm...............38779-0916-05 1147.50
500 gm...............38779-0916-08 1530.00

(Spectrum Pharmacy)
POW, NA (B.P.)
1000 gm.............49452-8045-02 1802.50

TYLOX (Ortho-McNeil Pharm)
acetaminophen/oxycodone hydrochloride
CAP, PO, 500 mg-5 mg,
100s ea, C-II.......00045-0526-60 189.34 157.78 AA
100s ea UD, C-II....00045-0526-79 248.99 207.49 AA

(Phys Total Care)
REPACK
CAP, PO, 500 mg-5 mg,
10s ea, C-II........54868-0364-00 21.24 AA
20s ea, C-II........54868-0364-01 39.36 AA
90s ea, C-II........54868-0364-02 174.65 AA

TYPHIM VI (Sanofi)
typhoid vi polysaccharide vaccine
SOL, IM, 25 mcg/0.5 ml,
0.5 ml.............49281-0790-51 61.08 50.90
(20 DOSE VIAL)
25 mcg/0.5 ml,
10 ml..............49281-0790-20 1099.62 916.35

(Dispensing Solutions)
REPACK
SOL, IM, 25 mcg/0.5 ml,
0.5 ml.............55045-3786-05 55.00

TYPHOID VACCINE, LIVE
(Berna) *See VIVOTIF*

TYPHOID VI POLYSACCHARIDE (Physician Partner)
REPACK
typhoid vi polysaccharide vaccine
SOL, IM, 25 mcg/0.5 ml,
0.5 ml.............21695-0460-05 112.60

TYPHOID VI POLYSACCHARIDE VACCINE
(Sanofi) *See TYPHIM VI*

TYRAMINE HCL (PCCA)
tyramine hydrochloride
POW, NA (REAGENT)
1 gm...............51927-2103-00 33.00

TYRAMINE HYDROCHLORIDE
(PCCA) *See TYRAMINE HCL*

TYROSINE
(Gallipot) *See L-TYROSINE*
(Medisca) *See L-TYROSINE*

(PCCA)
POW, NA (USP)
1 gm...............51927-1560-00 1.08

(Spectrum Pharmacy)
POW, NA (U.S.P.)
100 gm.............49452-8052-01 80.85
1000 gm............49452-8052-03 595.00

TYSABRI (Elan Pharmaceuticals)
natalizumab
SOL, IV, 20 mg/ml, 15 ml..59075-0730-15 3109.72

TYVASO (United Therapeutics)
treprostinil
SOL, IH, 0.6 mg/ml,
2.9 ml 4s..........66302-0206-03 1920.00
2.9 ml 28s.........66302-0206-01 15050.00
2.9 ml 28s.........66302-0206-02 13420.00

TYZEKA (Novartis Pharm)
telbivudine
TAB, PO (FILM-COATED)
600 mg, 30s ea 00078-0538-15 801.68

TYZINE (Kenwood)
tetrahydrozoline hydrochloride
SOL, NS, 0.1%, 30 ml.....00482-4760-30 67.57
SPR, NS, 0.1%, 15 ml.....00482-4760-15 55.18

TYZINE PEDIATRIC (Kenwood)
tetrahydrozoline hydrochloride
SOL, NS, 0.05%, 15 ml....00482-4770-15 59.21

U-CORT (Taro)
hydrocortisone acetate
CRE, TP (PARABEN-FREE)
1%, 28.35 gm........51672-3009-02 29.65 AT

U-KERA (Taro)
urea
CRE, TP, 40%, 28.35 gm...51672-1329-02 49.34
85.05 gm..........51672-1329-08 77.40
198.45 gm.........51672-1329-07 142.40

UDAMIN (Kowa)
multivitamin, minerals, and nutriceuticals
TAB, PO (FILM-COATED CAPLET)
100s ea.............66869-0220-10 87.44 69.95

UDAMIN SP (Kowa)
multivitamin, minerals, and nutriceuticals
TAB, PO (CAPLET, FILM-COATED)
100s ea.............66869-0820-10 79.50 63.60

ULESFIA (Shionogi)
benzyl alcohol
LOT, TP, 5%, 227 gm......59630-0780-08 41.01

ULORIC (Takeda)
febuxostat
TAB, PO, 40 mg, 30s ea ...64764-0918-30 162.00
80 mg, 30s ea........64764-0677-30 162.00

ULTANE (Abbott Pharm)
sevoflurane
LIQ, IH (PLASTIC)
100%, 250 ml........00074-4456-04 225.60 197.89

ULTICARE (UltiMed)
insulin syringe/needle
DEV, NA (1/2CC,28GX1/2",U-100)
100s ea.............08222-0825-89 18.95
(1/2CC,29GX1/2",U-100)
100s ea.............08222-0925-95 18.95
(1/2CC,30GX5/16",U-100)
100s ea.............08222-0935-92 20.95
(1CC,28GX1/2",U-100)
100s ea.............08222-0821-83 18.95
(1CC,29GX1/2",U-100)
100s ea.............08222-0921-99 18.95
(1CC,30GX5/16",U-100)
100s ea.............08222-0931-96 20.95
(3/10 CC,29GX1/2",U-100)
100s ea.............08222-0923-97 18.95
(3/10 CC,30GX5/16",U-100)
100s ea.............08222-0933-94 20.95

ULTIGUARD (UltiMed)
insulin syringe/needle
DEV, NA (1/2ML,29G,1/2")
100s ea.............08222-0725-97 23.75
(1/2ML,30G,5/16")
100s ea.............08222-0735-94 25.70
(1ML,29G,1/2")
100s ea.............08222-0721-91 23.75
(1ML,30G,5/16")
100s ea.............08222-0731-98 25.70
(3/10ML,29G,1/2")
100s ea.............08222-0723-99 23.75
(3/10ML,30G,5/16")
100s ea.............08222-0733-96 25.70

ULTIVA (Bioniche Pharma)
remifentanil hydrochloride
PDS, IV (PF,LYOPHILIZED)
1 mg, 10s ea, C-II....67457-0198-03 314.50 EE
2 mg, 10s ea, C-II....67457-0198-05 595.80 EE
5 mg, 10s ea, C-II....67457-0198-10 1230.70

PROD/MFR	NDC	AWP	DP	OBC
ULTRA COMFORT (Cardinal Health)				
insulin syringe/needle				
DEV, NA (1/2CC,28GX1/2",U-100)				
100s ea	96295-0104-94	23.90		
(1/2CC,29GX1/2",U-100)				
100s ea	96295-0104-96	23.90		
(1/2CC,30GX1/2",U-100)				
100s ea	96295-0106-43	23.90		
(1CC,28GX1/2",U-100)				
100s ea	96295-0104-95	23.90		
(1CC,29GX1/2",U-100)				
100s ea	96295-0104-97	23.90		
(1CC,30GX1/2",U-100)				
100s ea	96295-0106-45	23.90		
(3/10CC,29GX1/2",U-100)				
100s ea	96295-0104-98	23.90		
(3/10CC,30GX1/2",U-100)				
100s ea	96295-0106-29	23.90		
ULTRA NATALCARE (Phys Total Care)				
REPACK				
prenatal vitamins				
TAB, PO, 100s ea	54868-4777-00	58.14		
ULTRA-NATAL VITAMIN (Contract Pharmacal)				
prenatal vitamins				
TAB, PO, 100s ea	10267-0043-01	26.90		
ULTRABROM (Dexo)				
bpm/pse hcl				
CER, PO, 12 mg-120 mg,				
100s ea	59196-0006-01	67.80		
ULTRABROM PD (Dexo)				
bpm/pse hcl				
CER, PO, 6 mg-60 mg,				
100s ea	59196-0004-01	64.20		
ULTRACAPS MT 20 (Breckenridge Pharm)				
amylase/lipase/protease				
ECC, PO, 65000 u-20000 u-65000 u,				
100s ea	51991-0409-01	147.75		
ULTRACET (Ortho-McNeil Pharm)				
acetaminophen/tramadol hydrochloride				
TAB, PO (10X10)				
325 mg-37.5 mg,				
100s ea UD	00045-0650-10	179.15	149.29	
(PriCara)				
TAB, PO (COATED)				
325 mg-37.5 mg,				
100s ea	50458-0650-60	162.88	135.73	AB
(A-S Medication)				
REPACK				
TAB, PO (FILM-COATED CAPLET)				
325 mg-37.5 mg,				
20s ea	54569-5308-00	31.57		
30s ea	54569-5308-01	47.35		
100s ea	54569-5308-02	143.61		
(DHS, Inc.)				
REPACK				
TAB, PO (FILM-COATED CAPLET)				
325 mg-37.5 mg,				
60s ea	55887-0521-60	96.00		
(Dispensing Solutions)				
REPACK				
TAB, PO (FILM-COATED CAPLET)				
325 mg-37.5 mg,				
20s ea	55045-2918-06	32.00		
25s ea	55045-2918-07	40.00		
30s ea	55045-2918-08	48.00		
50s ea	55045-2918-05	80.00		
60s ea	55045-2918-09	96.00		
90s ea	55045-2918-01	144.00		
100s ea	55045-2918-00	160.00		
160s ea	55045-2918-02	256.00		
180s ea	55045-2918-03	288.00		
(Nucare Pharm)				
REPACK				
TAB, PO, 325 mg-37.5 mg,				
20s ea	66267-0468-20	23.99		
40s ea	66267-0468-40	47.99		
60s ea	66267-0468-60	59.99		
(PD-Rx Pharm)				
REPACK				
TAB, PO (FILM-COATED CAPLET)				
325 mg-37.5 mg,				
20s ea	55289-0617-20	45.03		
(Pharma Pac)				
REPACK				
TAB, PO (FILM-COATED CAPLET)				
325 mg-37.5 mg,				
20s ea	52959-0666-20	25.85		
28s ea	52959-0666-28	34.75		
30s ea	52959-0666-30	36.75		
40s ea	52959-0666-40	48.99		
56s ea	52959-0666-56	64.32		
60s ea	52959-0666-60	68.35		
90s ea	52959-0666-90	99.75		
100s ea	52959-0666-00	108.75		
120s ea	52959-0666-02	128.30		
(Phys Total Care)				
REPACK				
TAB, PO (FILM-COATED CAPLET)				
325 mg-37.5 mg,				
10s ea	54868-4703-01	17.46		
30s ea	54868-4703-00	48.63		
40s ea	54868-4703-06	64.22		
60s ea	54868-4703-04	95.39		
90s ea	54868-4703-03	142.14		
(FILM-COATED CAPLET)				
325 mg-37.5 mg,				
100s ea	54868-4703-05	157.10		
120s ea	54868-4703-02	178.51		
(Physician Partner)				
REPACK				
TAB, PO (FILM-COATED CAPLET)				
325 mg-37.5 mg,				
120s ea	21695-0143-72	445.64		
(Quality Care Prod)				
REPACK				
TAB, PO (FILM-COATED CAPLET)				
325 mg-37.5 mg,				
30s ea	49999-0118-30	68.40		
(Southwood)				
REPACK				
TAB, PO (FILM-COATED CAPLET)				
325 mg-37.5 mg,				
24s ea	58016-0629-24	36.39		
30s ea	58016-0629-30	45.49		
60s ea	58016-0629-60	90.98		
90s ea	58016-0629-90	136.47		
100s ea	58016-0629-00	151.63		
ULTRAM (PriCara)				
tramadol hydrochloride				
TAB, PO (COATED)				
50 mg, 100s ea	50458-0659-60	175.92	146.60	AB
(A-S Medication)				
REPACK				
TAB, PO, 50 mg, 15s ea	54569-4089-05	25.57		
20s ea	54569-4089-00	34.09		
30s ea	54569-4089-01	63.82		
(Altura)				
REPACK				
TAB, PO, 50 mg, 20s ea	63874-5323-02	35.27		
30s ea	63874-5323-03	52.91		
40s ea	63874-5323-04	70.54		
50s ea	63874-5323-05	88.18		
60s ea	63874-5323-06	105.81		
(AQ)				
REPACK				
TAB, PO, 50 mg, 100s ea	66105-0500-10	175.46		
(Dispensing Solutions)				
REPACK				
TAB, PO, 50 mg, 15s ea	55045-2219-05	22.55		AB
20s ea	55045-2219-07	32.15		AB
25s ea	55045-2219-02	44.35		AB
30s ea	55045-2219-08	48.85		AB
56s ea	55045-2219-06	94.00		AB
(Nucare Pharm)				
REPACK				
TAB, PO, 50 mg, 12s ea	66267-0210-12	23.98		
20s ea	66267-0210-20	38.49		
25s ea	66267-0210-25	46.59		
30s ea	66267-0210-30	54.92		
40s ea	66267-0210-40	73.22		
56s ea	66267-0210-56	99.59		
(PD-Rx Pharm)				
REPACK				
TAB, PO, 50 mg, 15s ea	55289-0650-15	54.38		
20s ea	55289-0650-20	64.88		
24s ea	55289-0650-24	77.86		
30s ea	55289-0650-30	96.34		
(Pharma Pac)				
REPACK				
TAB, PO, 50 mg, 10s ea	52959-0414-10	22.23		
15s ea	52959-0414-15	30.31		
20s ea	52959-0414-20	38.64		
21s ea	52959-0414-21	40.57		
24s ea	52959-0414-24	44.69		
28s ea	52959-0414-28	50.18		
30s ea	52959-0414-30	52.92		
40s ea	52959-0414-40	63.84		
60s ea	52959-0414-60	101.21		
100s ea	52959-0414-00	135.10		
120s ea	52959-0414-02	159.60		
(Phys Total Care)				
REPACK				
TAB, PO, 50 mg, 15s ea	54868-3605-03	25.30		
20s ea	54868-3605-00	33.31		
30s ea	54868-3605-02	49.34		
60s ea	54868-3605-05	97.44		
100s ea	54868-3605-04	152.65		
(Quality Care Prod)				
REPACK				
TAB, PO, 50 mg, 15s ea	49999-0022-15	34.35		AB
20s ea	49999-0022-20	43.48		
21s ea	49999-0022-21	34.53		
25s ea	49999-0022-25	52.59		
30s ea	49999-0022-30	75.70		
56s ea	49999-0022-56	125.64		
60s ea	49999-0022-60	151.80		
(Southwood)				
REPACK				
TAB, PO, 50 mg, 7s ea	58016-0387-07	10.42		
10s ea	58016-0387-10	14.89		
15s ea	58016-0387-15	22.34		
20s ea	58016-0387-20	29.78		
21s ea	58016-0387-21	31.27		
25s ea	58016-0387-25	37.23		
28s ea	58016-0387-28	41.69		
30s ea	58016-0387-30	44.67		
40s ea	58016-0387-40	59.56		
42s ea	58016-0387-42	62.54		
50s ea	58016-0387-50	74.46		
60s ea	58016-0387-60	89.35		
90s ea	58016-0387-90	134.02		
100s ea	58016-0387-00	148.91		
ULTRAM ER (Ortho-McNeil Pharm)				
tramadol hydrochloride				
TER, PO, 100 mg, 30s ea	00062-0653-30	133.31	111.09	
200 mg, 30s ea	00062-0655-30	220.46	183.72	
(PriCara)				
TER, PO, 300 mg, 30s ea	50458-0657-30	307.61	256.34	BC
(Dispensing Solutions)				
REPACK				
TER, PO, 200 mg, 30s ea	55045-3806-03	210.00		
(IPI)				
REPACK				
TER, PO, 100 mg, 30s ea	18837-0169-30	123.32		
300 mg, 30s ea	18837-0259-30	284.57		
(Keltman Pharma., Inc.)				
REPACK				
TER, PO, 100 mg, 30s ea	68387-0910-30	111.74		
200 mg, 30s ea	68387-0920-30	187.04		
300 mg, 30s ea	68387-0930-30	235.70		
(Nucare Pharm)				
REPACK				
TER, PO, 100 mg, 30s ea	66267-1303-03	169.69		
200 mg, 30s ea	66267-1304-03	271.64		
300 mg, 30s ea	68071-1320-00	380.00		
(Pharma Pac)				
REPACK				
TER, PO, 200 mg, 30s ea	52959-0600-30	189.00		
(Phys Total Care)				
REPACK				
TER, PO, 100 mg, 30s ea	54868-5584-00	125.36		
200 mg, 30s ea	54868-5790-00	239.43		
300 mg, 30s ea	54868-5791-00	254.78		
(Physician Partner)				
REPACK				
TER, PO, 100 mg, 30s ea	21695-0292-30	252.70		
200 mg, 30s ea	21695-0563-30	417.92		
300 mg, 30s ea	21695-0913-30	583.12		
(Quality Care Prod)				
REPACK				
TER, PO, 100 mg, 30s ea	35356-0055-30	192.00		
200 mg, 10s ea	49999-0896-10	120.00		
30s ea	49999-0896-30	372.00		
300 mg, 30s ea	35356-0056-30	668.00		
90s ea	35356-0056-90	1994.00		
(Southwood)				
REPACK				
TER, PO, 100 mg, 30s ea	58016-0028-30	110.36		
60s ea	58016-0028-60	220.72		
90s ea	58016-0028-90	331.08		
100s ea	58016-0028-00	367.87		

PROD/MFR	NDC	AWP	DP	OBC
(St. Mary's MPP)				
REPACK				
TER, PO, 100 mg, 30s ea	60760-0653-30	195.53		
200 mg, 30s ea	60760-0655-30	319.44		
300 mg, 30s ea	60760-0657-30	443.34		
(Stat Rx)				
REPACK				
TER, PO, 100 mg, 30s ea	16590-0557-30	142.57		
40s ea	16590-0557-40	190.09		
60s ea	16590-0557-60	71.29		
200 mg, 30s ea	16590-0558-30	234.87		
60s ea	16590-0558-60	469.70		
90s ea	16590-0558-90	578.99		
300 mg, 30s ea	16590-0561-30	469.70		
60s ea	16590-0561-60	486.40		
90s ea	16590-0561-90	729.60		
ULTRASE (Axcan)				
amylase/lipase/protease				
ECC, PO, 20000 u-4500 u-25000 u,				
100s ea	58914-0045-10	72.90		
ULTRASE MT12 (Axcan)				
amylase/lipase/protease				
ECC, PO, 39000 u-12000 u-39000 u,				
100s ea	58914-0002-10	151.49		
ULTRASE MT18 (Axcan)				
amylase/lipase/protease				
ECC, PO, 58500 u-18000 u-58500 u,				
100s ea	58914-0018-10	250.79		
ULTRASE MT20 (Axcan)				
amylase/lipase/protease				
ECC, PO, 65000 u-20000 u-65000 u,				
100s ea	58914-0004-10	278.44		
500s ca	58914-0004-50	1356.16		
(Quality Care Prod)				
REPACK				
ECC, PO, 65000 u-20000 u-65000 u,				
30s ea	49999-0956-30	126.30		
ULTRATAG RBC (Mallinckrodt Inc.)				
technetium tc 99m red blood cells				
KIT, IV (5 TESTS)				
ea	00019-N068-B0	560.40	467.00	
ULTRAVATE (Ranbaxy Labs)				
halobetasol propionate				
CRE, TP, 0.05%, 15 gm	00072-1400-15	60.99		
(1X15GM)				
0.05%, 15 gm	10631-0103-15	64.04		AB
(1X50GM)				
0.05%, 50 gm	10631-0103-50	154.00		AB
OIN, TP (1X15GM)				
0.05%, 15 gm	10631-0102-15	64.04		AB
50 gm	00072-1450-50	154.00		
(Phys Total Care)				
REPACK				
CRE, TP, 0.05%, 50 gm	54868-2382-00	101.26		
OIN, TP, 0.05%, 15 gm	54868-4006-00	43.01		
50 gm	54868-4006-01	101.26		
ULTRAVATE PAC (Ranbaxy Labs)				
ammonium lactate/halobetasol propionate				
KIT, TP, 12%-0.05%,				
275 gm	10631-0110-01	162.47		
ULTRAVIST (Bayer)				
iopromide				
SOL, IJ (150 MG IODINE/ML)				
311.7 mg/ml,				
50 ml 10s	50419-0340-05	198.00		
(240 MG IODINE/ML)				
498.72 mg/ml,				
50 ml 10s	50419-0342-05	228.00		
100 ml 10s	50419-0342-10	456.00		
150 ml 10s	50419-0342-15	684.00		
200 ml 10s	50419-0342-20	912.00		
200 ml 10s	50419-0342-21	912.00		
(300 MG IODINE/ML)				
623.4 mg/ml,				
50 ml 10s	50419-0344-05	252.00		
75 ml 10s	50419-0344-07	360.00		
100 ml 10s	50419-0344-10	480.00		
125 ml 10s	50419-0344-12	600.00		
150 ml 10s	50419-0344-15	708.00	619.50	
200 ml 10s	50419-0344-21	960.00		
500 ml 8s	50419-0344-58	2016.00		
(370 MG IODINE/ML)				
768.86 mg/ml,				
50 ml 10s	50419-0346-05	288.00		
75 ml 10s	50419-0346-07	422.82		
100 ml 10s	50419-0346-10	938.13		
125 ml 10s	50419-0346-12	704.70		
150 ml 10s	50419-0346-15	840.00		
200 ml 10s	50419-0346-20	1104.00		
250 ml 10s	50419-0346-25	1409.40		
500 ml 10s	50419-0346-58	2304.00		
(Hospira)				
SOL, IJ (PROVIDES 300MGI/1ML)				
623.4 mg/ml,				
500 ml	50419-0344-50	252.00	220.50	
(PROVIDES 370MGI/1ML)				
768.86 mg/ml,				
500 ml	50419-0346-50	288.00	252.00	
UMECTA (JSJ Pharma)				
urea				
EMU, TP, 40%, 120 ml	68712-0004-03	59.88		
240 ml	68712-0004-01	95.88		
SUS, TP, 40%, 300 ml	68712-0005-01	95.88		
UNASYN (Pfizer)				
ampicillin sodium/sulbactam sodium				
PDS, IJ (VIAL)				
1 gm-0.5 gm,				
10s ea	00049-0013-83	91.18	75.98	AP
2 gm-1 gm, 10s ea	00049-0014-83	172.15	143.46	AP
IV (ADD-VANTAGE,ADD-VANTAGE)				
1 gm-0.5 gm,				
10s ea	00049-0031-83	96.74	80.62	AP
(P.B.,ADD-VANTAGE)				
1 gm-0.5 gm,				
10s ea	00049-0022-83	105.68	88.07	AP
(ADD-VANTAGE,ADD-VANTAGE)				
2 gm-1 gm, 10s ea	00049-0032-83	177.66	148.05	AP
(P.B.,ADD-VANTAGE)				
2 gm-1 gm, 10s ea	00049-0023-83	187.45	156.21	AP
(BULK PACKAGE)				
10 gm-5 gm, ea	00049-0024-28	86.08	71.73	AP
UNDECYLENIC ACID (Amend)				
LIQ, NA (U.S.P.)				
500 ml	17317-0592-01	18.20		
3840 ml	17317-0592-08	102.00		
18000 ml	17317-0592-06	459.38		
(Gallipot)				
LIQ, NA, 473 ml	51552-0366-06	25.69		
(PCCA)				
LIQ, NA (USP)				
1 ml	51927-1274-00	0.30		
(Spectrum Pharmacy)				
LIQ, NA (U.S.P.)				
500 ml	49452-8057-01	132.65		
4000 ml	49452-8057-02	598.50		
UNIFINE PENTIPS (Owen Mumford)				
insulin syringe/needle				
DEV, NA (29G,12MM)				
100s ea	08470-3529-01	22.31		
(29GX12MM)				
100s ea	08214-3529-01	19.88		
(30G,6MM)				
100s ea	08470-3590-01	22.31		
(30G,8MM)				
100s ea	08470-3530-01	22.31		
(31GX6MM)				
100s ea	08214-3590-01	19.88		
(31GX8MM)				
100s ea	08214-3530-01	19.88		
UNIPHYL (Purdue Pharmaceutical)				
theophylline				
T24, PO, 400 mg, 100s ea	67781-0251-01	151.69		
600 mg, 100s ea	67781-0252-01	219.18		
(PD-Rx Pharm)				
REPACK				
T24, PO, 400 mg, 30s ea	55289-0789-30	65.49		BC
(Phys Total Care)				
REPACK				
T24, PO, 400 mg, 30s ea	54868-1438-00	43.43		BC
60s ea	54868-1438-01	84.99		BC
UNIRETIC (UCB)				
hydrochlorothiazide/moexipril hydrochloride				
TAB, PO, 12.5 mg-7.5 mg,				
100s ea	00091-3712-01	201.05		
12.5 mg-15 mg,				
100s ea	00091-3720-01	201.05		
25 mg-15 mg,				
100s ea	00091-3725-01	201.05		
(PD-Rx Pharm)				
REPACK				
TAB, PO (REDI-SCRIPT)				
12.5 mg-15 mg,				
30s ea	58864-0661-30	51.00		
25 mg-15 mg,				
30s ea	58864-0838-30	51.00		
(Phys Total Care)				
REPACK				
TAB, PO, 25 mg-15 mg,				
10s ea	54868-4479-02	17.05		
30s ea	54868-4479-01	47.41		
100s ea	54868-4479-00	144.61		
UNITHIOL				
(Medisca) *See DIMERCAPTOPROPANE SULPHONATE*				
(Medisca)				
POW, NA, 1 gm	38779-0643-06	169.50		
5 gm	38779-0643-03	612.00		
25 gm	38779-0643-04	2601.00		
100 gm	38779-0643-05	6450.00		
(1X500GM)				
500 gm	38779-0643-08	20250.00		
(PCCA) *See DIMERCAPTO-PROPANESULFONIC ACID SODIUM SALT ANHYDROUS*				
(PCCA) *See DIMERCAPTOPROPANESULFONIC ACID*				
UNITHROID (Lannett)				
levothyroxine sodium				
TAB, PO, 0.025 mg,				
90s ea	00527-1370-90	40.80		AB1
100s ea	00527-1370-01	26.40		AB
1000s ea	00527-1370-10	241.80		AB1
0.05 mg, 90s ea	00527-1371-90	40.80		AB1
100s ea	00527-1371-01	29.98		AB
1000s ea	00527-1371-10	274.80		AB1
0.075 mg, 90s ea	00527-1372-90	40.80		AB1
100s ea	00527-1372-01	33.11		AB
1000s ea	00527-1372-10	303.48		AB1
0.088 mg, 90s ea	00527-1373-90	40.80		AB1
100s ea	00527-1373-01	33.70		AB
1000s ea	00527-1373-10	308.76		AB1
0.1 mg, 90s ea	00527-1374-90	40.80		AB1
100s ea	00527-1374-01	33.94		AB
1000s ea	00527-1374-10	311.16		AB1
0.112 mg, 90s ea	00527-1375-90	40.80		AB1
100s ea	00527-1375-01	39.24		AB
1000s ea	00527-1375-10	359.76		AB1
0.125 mg, 90s ea	00527-1376-90	40.80		AB1
100s ea	00527-1376-01	39.78		AB
1000s ea	00527-1376-10	364.56		AB1
0.137 mg, 90s ea	00527-1639-90	40.80		AB1
1000s ea	00527-1639-10	371.04		AB1
0.15 mg, 90s ea	00527-1377-90	40.80		AB1
100s ea	00527-1377-01	40.95		AB
1000s ea	00527-1377-10	375.36		AB1
0.175 mg, 90s ea	00527-1378-90	40.80		AB1
100s ea	00527-1378-01	48.67		AB
1000s ea	00527-1378-10	446.16		AB1
0.2 mg, 90s ea	00527-1379-90	40.80		AB1
100s ea	00527-1379-01	50.38		AB
1000s ea	00527-1379-10	447.12		AB1
0.3 mg, 90s ea	00527-1380-90	40.80		AB1
100s ea	00527-1380-01	68.59		AB
UNIVASC (UCB)				
moexipril hydrochloride				
TAB, PO, 7.5 mg, 100s ea	00091-3707-01	209.11		
15 mg, 100s ea	00091-3715-01	219.06		
(A-S Medication)				
REPACK				
TAB, PO, 15 mg, 30s ea	54569-4276-00	48.51		
(Phys Total Care)				
REPACK				
TAB, PO, 7.5 mg, 10s ea	54868-5423-00	18.26		
30s ea	54868-5423-01	51.05		
15 mg, 20s ea	54868-4088-02	33.04		
30s ea	54868-4088-00	48.61		
40s ea	54868-4088-01	64.19		
UNIVERSAL SYRINGE TIP ADAPTER (APP)				
adapter, syringe				
DEV, NA, 250s ea	63323-0908-90	258.75		
URAMAXIN (Medimetriks)				
urea				
CRE, TP (1X270GM)				
45%, 270 gm	43538-0210-09	141.82		
FOA, TP (1X100GM)				
20%, 100 gm	43538-0220-10	112.03		
GEL, TP (1X28ML)				
45%, 20 ml	43538-0200-28	138.90		
UREA				
(Acella) *See BP-50% UREA EMULSION*				
(Acella) *See UREA NAIL FILM*				
(Amend)				
POW, NA (A.C.S., REAGENT)				
500 gm	17317-1466-01	13.30		
(U.S.P.)				
500 gm	17317-0593-01	7.70		
2270 gm	17317-0593-05	30.80		
(A.C.S., REAGENT)				
2500 gm	17317-1466-05	50.40		
(U.S.P.)				
11350 gm	17317-0593-08	113.75		

PROD/MFR	NDC	AWP	DP	OBC
(Baker, J.T.)				
POW, NA (U.S.P.)				
500 gm	**10106-4206-01**	20.86		
2500 gm	**10106-4206-05**	72.54		
(Blaine) *See REVITADERM 40*				
(Breckenridge Pharm) *See KERATOL 40*				
(Breckenridge Pharm) *See KERATOL PLUS*				
(Doak) *See CARMOL 40*				
(Doak) *See KERALAC*				
(Doak) *See KEROL*				
(Doak) *See KEROL REDI-CLOTHS*				
(Doak) *See KEROL ZX*				
(Fougera)				
CRE, TP, 40%, 28.35 gm	**18754-0652-52**	46.05		
85 gm	**18754-0652-19**	70.88		
(1X198.6GM)				
40%, 198.6 gm	**00168-0485-07**	34.54		
EMU, TP (1X300GM)				
50%, 300 gm	**00168-0646-10**	155.10		
LOT, TP (1X207ML)				
35%, 207 ml	**00168-0488-07**	73.04		
325 ml	**18754-0663-11**	130.39		
OIN, TP (1X45GM)				
50%, 45 gm	**00168-0492-45**	46.70		
SOL, TP (1X12ML)				
50%, 12 ml	**00168-0644-12**	215.42		
SUS, TP (1X284GM)				
50%, 284 gm	**18754-0645-10**	96.32		
(Fougera) *See UREA NAIL*				
(Fougera) *See UREA NAILSTIK*				
(Gallipot)				
POW, NA (U.S.P.,N.F.)				
113.4 gm	**51552-0057-04**	6.23		
454 gm	**51552-0057-06**	9.10		
2270 gm	**51552-0057-08**	35.98		
(Gordon) *See GORDON'S UREA*				
(Hawthorn Pharm) *See CEROVEL*				
(Hi-Tech)				
CRE, TP, 40%, 28.35 gm	**50383-0664-30**	26.17		
85.05 gm	**50383-0664-03**	42.28		
198.6 gm	**50383-0664-07**	79.54		
(JSJ Pharma) *See UMECTA*				
(Letco)				
POW, NA (U.S.P./N.F.)				
500 gm	**62991-1382-01**	58.50		
(Mallinckrodt Lab)				
CRY, NA (U.S.P.)				
500 gm	**00406-8642-12**	20.38		
(Medimetriks) *See URAMAXIN*				
(Medisca)				
POW, NA (USP)				
100 gm	**38779-0101-05**	13.50		
(U.S.P.)				
500 gm	**38779-0101-08**	22.50		
1000 gm	**38779-0101-09**	40.50		
(Onset) *See KERAFOAM*				
(Onset) *See KERAFOAM 42*				
(PCCA)				
CRY, NA (USP)				
1 gm	**51927-1269-00**	0.06		
(Perrigo)				
CRE, TP, 40%, 28.35 gm	**45802-0170-03**	43.61		
85 gm	**45802-0170-53**	68.39		
198.6 gm	**45802-0170-77**	125.84		
GEL, TP, 40%, 15 ml	**45802-0171-56**	121.30		
LOT, TP, 40%, 236.6 ml	**45802-0176-55**	125.27		
(PharmaDerm) *See KEROL AD*				
(Quinnova) *See HYDRO 35*				
(Quinnova) *See HYDRO 40*				
(Quinnova) *See QUINNOSTIK*				
(River's Edge) *See UREA NAIL GEL*				
(Spectrum Pharmacy)				
GRA, NA (1X500GM,USP)				
500 gm	**49452-8065-01**	99.40		
POW, NA (U.S.P.,J.P.)				
500 gm	**49452-8070-01**	46.90		
2500 gm	**49452-8070-02**	136.50		
12000 gm	**49452-8070-03**	539.00		
(Stratus) *See X-VIATE*				
(Taro) *See U-KERA*				

PROD/MFR	NDC	AWP	DP	OBC
(Phys Total Care)				
REPACK				
CRE, TP (1X198.6GM)				
40%, 198.6 gm	**54868-5880-00**	83.96		
(Physician Partner)				
REPACK				
CRE, TP (1X30GM)				
40%, 30 gm	**21695-0683-30**	52.34		
UREA NAIL (Fougera)				
urea				
GEL, TP, 50%, 18 ml	**18754-0659-15**	108.61		
UREA NAIL FILM (Acella)				
urea				
SUS, TP (1X18ML)				
40%, 18 ml	**42192-0707-18**	158.95		
UREA NAIL GEL (River's Edge)				
urea				
GEL, TP (1X18ML)				
50%, 18 ml	**68032-0121-18**	103.21		
UREA NAILSTIK (Fougera)				
urea				
SOL, TP (14.4MLX6)				
50%, 14.4 ml 6s	**18754-0648-10**	96.17		
URECHOLINE (Teva)				
bethanechol chloride				
TAB, PO, 5 mg, 100s ea	**65473-0697-01**	91.64	32.59	
(USP)				
5 mg, 100s ea	**51285-0697-02**	129.58		
10 mg, 100s ea	**65473-0703-01**	149.53	61.14	
(USP)				
10 mg, 100s ea	**51285-0690-02**	211.44		
25 mg, 100s ea	**65473-0704-01**	229.24		
(USP)				
25 mg, 100s ea	**51285-0691-02**	324.17		
50 mg, 100s ea	**65473-0700-01**	318.95	130.43	
(USP)				
50 mg, 100s ea	**51285-0692-02**	451.02		
URELLE (Azur Pharma, Inc.)				
antibacterial/analgesic combination				
TAB, PO, 90s ea	**66663-0219-01**	220.07		
URETRON D/S (A. G. Marin)				
belladonna alkaloids and analgesics				
TAB, PO (SUGAR COATED)				
100s ea	**12539-0144-01**	126.30		
100s ea	**12539-0120-10**	105.25		
URIC ACID (PCCA)				
POW, NA (REAGENT)				
1 gm	**51927-2517-00**	6.00		
URIDINE				
(PCCA) *See URIDINE REAGENT*				
URIDINE REAGENT (PCCA)				
uridine				
POW, NA (1X1GM)				
1 gm	**51927-3179-00**	9.00		
URIMAR-T (Marnel)				
belladonna alkaloids and analgesics				
TAB, PO (SUGAR COATED)				
100s ea	**00682-0333-01**	65.85		
(2006 FORMULA)				
100s ea	**00682-0334-01**	65.85		
URINARY ANTISEPTIC (Pharma Pac)				
REPACK				
belladonna alkaloids and analgesics				
TAB, PO, 12s ea	**52959-0555-12**	6.25		
40s ea	**52959-0555-40**	19.20		
URISPAS (Phys. Total Care)				
REPACK				
flavoxate hydrochloride				
TAB, PO, 100 mg, 20s ea	**54868-0467-01**	42.28		
30s ea	**54868-0467-00**	62.47		
URO-SAN PLUS (Mentor)				
catheter				
DEV, NA (MALE, 2 PIECE, LARGE)				
100s ea	**81317-0078-00**	123.00		
(MALE, 2 PIECE, MEDIUM)				
100s ea	**81317-0078-50**	123.00		
(MALE, 2 PIECE, SMALL)				
100s ea	**81317-0078-75**	123.00		
UROCIT-K (Mission)				
potassium citrate				
TER, PO, 15 meq, 100s ea	**00178-0615-01**	180.00	150.00	
UROCIT-K 10 (Mission)				
potassium citrate				
TER, PO, 10 meq, 100s ea	**00178-0610-01**	111.00	92.50	

PROD/MFR	NDC	AWP	DP	OBC
(Phys Total Care)				
REPACK				
TER, PO, 10 meq, 20s ea	**54868-4779-01**	12.61		
60s ea	**54868-4779-00**	34.09		
90s ea	**54868-4779-02**	50.20		
UROCIT-K 5 (Mission)				
potassium citrate				
TER, PO, 5 meq, 100s ea	**00178-0600-01**	79.20	66.00	
UROFOLLITROPIN				
(Ferring) *See BRAVELLE*				
UROGESIC-BLUE (Edwards)				
belladonna alkaloids and analgesics				
TAB, PO, 100s ea	**00485-0051-01**	27.00		
UROKINASE				
(ImaRx) *See KINLYTIC*				
UROQID-ACID NO. 2 (Beach Pharm)				
methenamine mandelate/sodium phosphate, monobasic				
TAB, PO (CAPLET)				
500 mg-500 mg,				
100s ea	**00486-1114-01**	42.65		
UROXATRAL (Sanofi-Aventis)				
alfuzosin hydrochloride				
TER, PO, 10 mg, 100s ea	**00024-4200-10**	394.64		
(A-S Medication)				
REPACK				
TER, PO, 10 mg, 30s ea	**54569-5571-00**	113.15		
(Nucare Pharm)				
REPACK				
TER, PO, 10 mg, 30s ea	**68071-0805-30**	145.57		
(Phys Total Care)				
REPACK				
TER, PO, 10 mg, 10s ea	**54868-5046-01**	43.20		
30s ea	**54868-5046-00**	142.76		
90s ea	**54868-5046-02**	423.06		
(Quality Care Prod)				
REPACK				
TER, PO, 10 mg, 100s ea	**35356-0281-00**	601.59		
(Stat Rx)				
REPACK				
TER, PO, 10 mg, 30s ea	**16590-0279-30**	142.06		
URSO 250 (Axcan)				
ursodiol				
TAB, PO (FILM COATED)				
250 mg, 100s ea	**58914-0785-10**	354.78		
500s ea	**58914-0785-50**	1747.28		
URSO FORTE (Axcan)				
ursodiol				
TAB, PO (FILM-COATED)				
500 mg, 100s ea	**58914-0790-10**	628.70		
URSODIOL				
(Axcan) *See URSO 250*				
(Axcan) *See URSO FORTE*				
(Gallipot)				
POW, NA (1X25GM,USP)				
25 gm	**51552-0906-04**	105.00	75.00	
(1X100GM,USP)				
100 gm	**51552-0906-05**	336.00	240.00	
(1X500GM,USP)				
500 gm	**51552-0906-06**	1428.00	1020.00	
(Hawkins)				
POW, NA (U.S.P.)				
25 gm	**63370-0325-25**	360.00		
100 gm	**63370-0325-35**	1104.00		
500 gm	**63370-0325-45**	4560.00		
1000 gm	**63370-0325-50**	8160.00		
(Lannett)				
CAP, PO (USP)				
300 mg, 100s ea	**00527-1326-01**	309.30		AB
(Letco)				
POW, NA (U.S.P.)				
25 gm	**62991-2185-01**	180.00		
100 gm	**62991-2185-02**	585.00		
500 gm	**62991-2185-03**	2850.00		
(Medisca)				
POW, NA (U.S.P.)				
25 gm	**38779-1987-04**	255.00		
100 gm	**38779-1987-05**	897.00		
500 gm	**38779-1987-08**	3270.00		
(Mylan)				
CAP, PO (USP,HARD-SHELL GELATIN)				
300 mg, 100s ea	**00378-1730-01**	282.25		AB
(PCCA)				
POW, NA (U.S.P.)				
1 gm	**51927-2909-00**	11.40		

PROD/MFR	NDC	AWP	DP	OBC
(Prasco Labs)				
TAB, PO (USP,FILM-COATED)				
250 mg, 100s ea	66993-0405-02	268.24		
500 mg, 100s ea	66993-0406-02	475.34		
(Rising)				
CAP, PO, 300 mg, 100s ea	64980-0139-01	282.25		AB
(Spectrum Pharmacy)				
CRY, NA (U.S.P.)				
25 gm	49452-8085-01	367.50		
100 gm	49452-8085-02	1246.00		
(Teva)				
CAP, PO, 300 mg, 100s ea	00093-9380-01	257.75		AB
TAB, PO (USP,FILM-COATED)				
250 mg, 100s ea	00093-5360-01	268.24		AB
500 mg, 100s ea	00093-5361-01	475.34		AB
(Watson) *See ACTIGALL*				
(Watson Labs)				
CAP, PO, 300 mg, 100s ea	00591-3159-01	92.58		
(American Health)				
REPACK				
CAP, PO (10X10,USP)				
300 mg, 100s ea UD	68084-0213-01	231.55		
(Phys Total Care)				
REPACK				
CAP, PO, 300 mg, 30s ea	54868-5033-01	65.34		
100s ea	54868-5033-00	158.13		AB
URTICA DIOICA (FERRO CULTA) (Weleda)				
homeopathic substance				
LIQ, PO, 50 ml	55946-0400-15	9.00		
USNIC ACID (PCCA)				
d-usnic acid				
POW, NA (1X1GM)				
1 gm	51927-2536-00	39.60		
USTEKINUMAB				
(Centocor) *See STELARA*				
UTA (SJ)				
belladonna alkaloids and analgesics				
CAP, PO, 100s ea	45985-0646-01	166.80		
(Phys Total Care)				
REPACK				
CAP, PO, 15s ea	54868-5003-00	14.40		
30s ea	54868-5003-01	26.94		
UTAC (Breckenridge Pharm)				
methenamine mandelate/sodium phosphate, monobasic				
TAB, PO (FILM-COATED)				
500 mg-500 mg,				
100s ea	51991-0199-01	37.96		
UTICAP (Cypress Pharm)				
belladonna alkaloids and analgesics				
CAP, PO, 100s ea	60258-0519-01	112.23		
UTIRA (Hawthorn Pharm)				
belladonna alkaloids and analgesics				
TER, PO, 100s ea	63717-0512-01	106.24		
UTIRA-C (Hawthorn Pharm)				
belladonna alkaloids and analgesics				
TAB, PO, 100s ea	63717-0513-01	143.74		
UTRONA-C (Cypress Pharm)				
belladonna alkaloids and analgesics				
TAB, PO, 100s ea	60258-0518-01	128.69		
UVA URSI LEAF (PCCA)				
POW, NA, 1 gm	51927-3223-00	0.30		
UVA URSI LEAF EXTRACT (PCCA)				
SOL, NA (1X1ML)				
1 ml	51927-3491-00	0.50		
UVADEX (Therakos)				
methoxsalen				
SOL, IJ (VIAL)				
0.02 mg/ml,				
10 ml 12s	64067-0216-01	755.00		
V-C FORTE (Breckenridge Pharm)				
multivitamin and minerals				
CAP, PO, 100s ea	51991-0645-01	15.00		
V-COF (Macoven)				
bpm/carbetapentane cit/phenyleph hcl				
SUS, PO (12X118ML,BUBBLE GUM)				
118 ml	44183-0514-04	72.59		
V-HIST (Macoven)				
bpm/phenyleph hcl				
SUS, PO (12X118ML,BUBBLE GUM)				
6 mg/5 ml-10 mg/5 ml,				
118 ml	44183-0512-04	70.61		
V-TANN (Breckenridge Pharm)				
phenylephrine tannate/pyrilamine tannate				
CTB, PO (DYE-FREE,GRAPE)				
25 mg-30 mg,				
100s ea	51991-0267-01	168.90		
SUS, PO (SUSPENSION BID,AF,GRAPE)				
12.5 mg/5 ml-30 mg/5 ml,				
118 ml	51991-0266-04	31.70		
473 ml	51991-0266-16	126.81		
VAGIFEM (Novo Nordisk)				
estradiol				
TAB, VG (W/SINGLE-USE APPLICATOR)				
10 mcg, 8s ea	00169-5176-03	54.20		EE
18s ea	00169-5176-04	121.91		EE
(W/BLISTERED APPLICATORS)				
25 mcg, 8s ea	00169-5173-03	54.20	18.32	
18s ea	00169-5173-04	121.91	41.24	
(Phys Total Care)				
REPACK				
TAB, VG, 25 mcg, 8s ea	54868-4833-00	69.90		
18s ea	54868-4833-01	133.28		
(Quality Care Prod)				
REPACK				
TAB, VG (FILM-COATED)				
25 mcg, 8s ea	35356-0475-08	88.61		
VALACYCLOVIR HYDROCHLORIDE				
(Glaxo) *See VALTREX*				
(Ranbaxy Pharm)				
TAB, PO (FILM-COATED)				
1 gm, 30s ea	63304-0905-30	379.26		AB
500 mg, 30s ea	63304-0904-30	216.72		AB
(PD-Rx Pharm)				
REPACK				
TAB, PO (FILM-COATED)				
500 mg, 10s ea	43063-0200-10	150.48		AB
(Phys Total Care)				
REPACK				
TAB, PO (FILM-COATED)				
500 mg, 10s ea	54868-6090-01	187.62		AB
20s ea	54868-6090-00	349.07		AB
VALCYTE (Roche Labs)				
valganciclovir hydrochloride				
PDS, PO (TUTTI-FRUTTI)				
50 mg/ml, 88 ml	00004-0039-09	568.82		
TAB, PO, 450 mg, 60s ea	00004-0038-22	2685.02		
(A-S Medication)				
REPACK				
TAB, PO, 450 mg, 60s ea	54569-6101-00	3490.53		
VALERIAN ROOT (PCCA)				
POW, NA (VALERIANA OFFICINALIS)				
1 gm	51927-2915-00	0.20		
TIN, NA, 1 ml	51927-1768-00	0.16		
(PCCA) *See VALERIAN ROOT FLUID EXTRACT*				
VALERIAN ROOT EXTRACT (Amend)				
LIQ, NA, 120 ml	17317-0759-04	14.00		
500 ml	17317-0759-01	29.40		
(Medisca) *See VALERIAN ROOT FLUID EXTRACT*				
VALERIAN ROOT FLUID EXTRACT (Medisca)				
valerian root extract				
SOL, NA (1X500ML)				
500 ml	38779-1681-08	70.50		
(PCCA)				
valerian root				
LIQ, NA, 1 ml	51927-1753-00	0.22		
VALGANCICLOVIR HYDROCHLORIDE				
(Roche Labs) *See VALCYTE*				
VALINE				
(Gallipot) *See L-VALINE*				
(Medisca) *See L-VALINE*				
(PCCA)				
POW, NA (USP)				
1 gm	51927-3566-00	0.84		
(Spectrum Pharmacy) *See L-VALINE*				
VALIUM (Roche Labs)				
diazepam				
TAB, PO, 2 mg,				
100s ea, C-IV	00140-0004-01	231.70		AB
10000s ea, C-IV	00140-0004-32	21403.27		AB
5 mg,				
100s ea, C-IV	00140-0005-01	360.36		AB
500s ea, C-IV	00140-0005-14	1792.91		AB
15000s ea, C-IV	00140-0005-35	49687.39		AB
10 mg,				
100s ea, C-IV	00140-0006-01	606.61		AB
500s ea, C-IV	00140-0006-14	3025.06		AB
15000s ea, C-IV	00140-0006-35	83835.48		AB
(PD-Rx Pharm)				
REPACK				
TAB, PO, 5 mg,				
6s ea, C-IV	55289-0117-06	26.47		AB
12s ea, C-IV	55289-0117-12	47.92		AB
20s ea, C-IV	55289-0117-20	76.67		AB
(Phys Total Care)				
REPACK				
SOL, IJ, 5 mg/ml,				
2 ml, C-IV	54868-3670-00	8.22		AP
(VIAL)				
5 mg/ml,				
10 ml, C-IV	54868-0716-00	29.23		AP
TAB, PO, 5 mg,				
10s ea, C-IV	54868-0703-03	28.85		AB
30s ea, C-IV	54868-0703-00	83.43		AB
90s ea, C-IV	54868-0703-01	231.81		AB
100s ea, C-IV	54868-0703-02	257.29		AB
10 mg,				
30s ea, C-IV	54868-0987-01	97.41		AB
90s ea, C-IV	54868-0987-00	271.41		AB
(Quality Care Prod)				
REPACK				
TAB, PO, 5 mg,				
100s ea, C-IV	35356-0022-00	282.00		
10 mg,				
100s ea, C-IV	35356-0006-00	393.00		
(Southwood)				
REPACK				
TAB, PO, 5 mg,				
30s ea, C-IV	00490-0044-30	64.15		
60s ea, C-IV	00490-0044-60	128.30		
90s ea, C-IV	00490-0044-90	192.46		
100s ea, C-IV	00490-0044-00	213.84		
(Stat Rx)				
REPACK				
TAB, PO, 10 mg,				
56s ea, C-IV	16590-0742-56	264.00		AB
VALPROATE SODIUM				
(Abbott Pharm) *See DEPACON*				
(APP)				
SOL, IV (PF,LATEX-FREE)				
100 mg/ml,				
5 ml 10s	63323-0494-05	83.95		
(Bedford)				
SOL, IV (S.D.V.,PF)				
100 mg/ml,				
5 ml 10s	55390-0007-10	119.18		AP
(Gallipot) *See SODIUM VALPROATE*				
(Hawkins) *See SODIUM VALPROATE*				
(Medisca) *See SODIUM VALPROATE*				
(PCCA)				
POW, NA, 1 gm	51927-1929-00	3.72		
(Spectrum Pharmacy) *See SODIUM VALPROATE*				
VALPROIC ACID				
FUL				
SGL, PO, 250 mg, 100s ea		52.50		
SYR, PO, 250 mg/5 ml,				
480 ml		28.51		
(Abbott Pharm) *See DEPAKENE*				
(Hi-Tech)				
SYR, PO, 250 mg/5 ml,				
473 ml	50383-0792-16	50.00		AA
(Medisca)				
SOL, NA (1X25ML,USP)				
25 ml	38779-2245-04	126.00		
(1X100ML,USP)				
100 ml	38779-2245-05	450.00		
(1X500ML,USP)				
500 ml	38779-2245-08	1050.00		
(1X1000ML,USP)				
1000 ml	38779-2245-09	2754.00		
(Morton Grove)				
SYR, PO (CHERRY)				
250 mg/5 ml,				
473 ml	60432-0621-16	72.75		AA
(Noven) *See STAVZOR*				
(PCCA)				
SOL, NA, 1 ml	51927-3210-00	10.20		

PROD/MFR NDC AWP DP OBC

(Pharm Assoc Inc)
SYR, PO (5ML-4X10,AF,CHERRY)
250 mg/5 ml,
5 ml 40s UD .... **00121-4675-05** 86.43 **AA**
(AF,CHERRY)
250 mg/5 ml,
473 ml .... **00121-0675-16** 72.50 **AA**

(Precision Dose)
SYR, PO (1X5ML,USP,CHERRY)
250 mg/5 ml,
5 ml UD .... **68094-0193-59** 0.63 **AA**
(USP,CHERRY)
250 mg/5 ml,
5 ml 30s UD .... **68094-0193-62** 20.90 **AA**
(USP, ORAL SYRINGE)
250 mg/5 ml,
5 ml 50s UD .... **68094-0193-58** 41.76 **AA**
(10X10, USP,CHERRY)
250 mg/5 ml,
5 ml 100s UD ...... **68094-0193-61** 63.01 **AA**
(1X10ML,USP,CHERRY)
250 mg/5 ml,
10 ml UD .... **68094-0701-59** 1.09 **AA**
(USP,30X10ML,CHERRY)
250 mg/5 ml,
10 ml 30s UD ...... **68094-0701-62** 33.54 **AA**
(USP,100X10ML,CHERRY)
250 mg/5 ml,
10 ml 100s UD ..... **68094-0701-61** 109.42 **AA**

(Qualitest)
SYR, PO (USP,CHERRY)
250 mg/5 ml,
473 ml .... **00603-1841-58** 72.74 **AA**

(Teva)
SGL, PO (SOFTGEL)
250 mg, 100s ea ..... **50111-0852-01** 66.25 **AB**
SYR, PO (CHERRY-MINT)
250 mg/5 ml,
480 ml .... **00093-9633-16** 72.75 **AA**

(UDL)
SGL, PO (10X10)
250 mg, 100s ea UD .. **51079-0298-20** 79.40 **AB**
(USP,10X30)
250 mg, 300s ea UD .. **51079-0298-56** 238.20 **AB**

(Upsher-Smith)
SGL, PO, 250 mg, 100s ea . **00832-1008-00** 82.15 **AB**

(Watson Labs)
SGL, PO, 250 mg, 100s ea . **00591-4012-01** 79.40 **AB**
SYR, PO, 250 mg/5 ml,
473 ml .... **00591-0426-16** 72.75 **EE**

(McKesson Packaging)
REPACK
SGL, PO (USP)
250 mg, 100s ea UD .. **63739-0251-10** 100.57 **EE**
(BLISTER PACK)
250 mg, 750s ea UD .. **63739-0251-01** 754.30 **EE**

(PD-Rx Pharm)
REPACK
SGL, PO (REDI-SCRIPT,SOFTGEL)
250 mg, 60s ea ...... **58864-0829-60** 34.57 **AB**

(Phys Total Care)
REPACK
SGL, PO (USP)
250 mg, 30s ea ...... **54868-1689-02** 27.18 **EE**
60s ea .... **54868-1689-03** 49.83 **EE**
100s ea .... **54868-1689-01** 80.04 **EE**
SYR, PO, 250 mg/5 ml,
480 ml .... **54868-4285-00** 57.99 **AA**

(Physician Partner)
REPACK
SGL, PO, 250 mg, 30s ea .. **21695-0417-30** 52.93
60s ea **21695-0417-60** 105.86
100s ea **21695-0417-00** 176.44

(Quality Care Prod)
REPACK
SGL, PO (SOFTGEL)
250 mg, 30s ea ...... **49999-0322-30** 29.90 **AB**

(Southwood)
REPACK
SGL, PO, 250 mg, 30s ea .. **58016-0085-30** 23.82
60s ea **58016-0085-60** 47.64
90s ea **58016-0085-90** 71.46
100s ea **58016-0085-00** 79.40

(Vibranta)
REPACK
SGL, PO, 250 mg, 30s ea .. **57866-4477-01** 24.92

PROD/MFR NDC AWP DP OBC

VALRUBICIN
(Endo Pharm) *See VALSTAR*

VALSARTAN
(Novartis Pharm) *See DIOVAN*

(Palmetto)
REPACK
TAB, PO, 160 mg, 30s ea .. **23490-7591-01** 72.61

VALSTAR (Endo Pharm)
valrubicin
SOL, IL (4X5ML)
40 mg/ml, 5 ml 4s **67979-0001-01** 4399.20
(24X5ML)
40 mg/ml, 5 ml 24s ... **67979-0001-02** 26395.20

VALTREX (Glaxo)
valacyclovir hydrochloride
TAB, PO (FILM-COATED CAPLET)
1 gm, 30s ea **00173-0565-04** 421.87
90s ea .... **00173-0565-10** 1265.63 **AB**
(CAPLET; FILM-COATED)
500 mg, 30s ea **00173-0933-08** 241.07
(FILM-COATED CAPLET)
500 mg, 90s ea ...... **00173-0933-10** 723.14 **AB**
(CAPLET; FILM-COATED)
500 mg, 100s ea UD .. **00173-0933-56** 821.42

(A-S Medication)
REPACK
TAB, PO (FILM-COATED CAPLET)
1 gm, 15s ea **54569-5324-00** 274.22
21s ea **54569-5324-01** 383.90
30s ea **54569-5324-03** 548.43
(CAPLET; FILM-COATED)
500 mg, 8s ea **54569-4280-07** 66.96
10s ea **54569-4280-00** 83.70
14s ea **54569-4280-01** 146.25
30s ea **54569-4280-06** 313.39

(AQ)
REPACK
TAB, PO (CAPLET)
500 mg, 30s ea **66105-0479-03** 256.11
42s ea **66105-0479-42** 356.55

(Core)
REPACK
TAB, PO, 500 mg, 6s ea ... **33358-0353-06** 40.77
10s ea UD **33358-0353-10** 66.69
12s ea **33358-0353-12** 72.63
30s ea **33358-0353-30** 201.42

(DHS, Inc.)
REPACK
TAB, PO, 500 mg, 20s ea .. **55887-0734-20** 344.98

(Dispensing Solutions)
REPACK
TAB, PO, 1 gm, 20s ea **55045-2619-02** 220.00
42s ea **55045-3547-01** 462.00

(PD-Rx Pharm)
REPACK
TAB, PO (REDI-SCRIPT)
1 gm, 20s ea **58864-0683-20** 264.29
21s ea **58864-0683-21** 320.20
(CAPLET; FILM-COATED)
500 mg, 4s ea **55289-0926-04** 47.78
6s ea **55289-0926-06** 71.66
7s ea **55289-0926-07** 73.60
8s ea **55289-0926-08** 95.55
10s ea **55289-0926-10** 119.43
14s ea **55289-0926-14** 167.22

(Pharma Pac)
REPACK
TAB, PO (CAPLET)
1 gm, 21s ea **52959-0384-21** 184.20
500 mg, 10s ea **52959-0641-10** 66.25
14s ea **52959-0641-14** 90.18
30s ea **52959-0641-30** 198.30
42s ea **52959-0641-42** 291.90

(Phys Total Care)
REPACK
TAB, PO (CAPLET)
1 gm, 3s ea **54868-3993-08** 55.49
4s ea **54868-3993-07** 73.12
(FILM-COATED CAPLET)
1 gm, 7s ea **54868-3993-04** 125.99
10s ea **54868-3993-01** 178.87
14s ea **54868-3993-03** 235.66
15s ea **54868-3993-00** 252.31
(CAPLET)
1 gm, 20s ea **54868-3993-05** 335.54
(FILM-COATED CAPLET)
1 gm, 21s ea **54868-3993-02** 351.53

PROD/MFR NDC AWP DP OBC

(CAPLET)
1 gm, 30s ea **54868-3993-06** 501.35
500 mg, 6s ea **54868-3804-04** 63.04
10s ea **54868-3804-00** 103.33
15s ea **54868-3804-02** 145.29
(CAPLET; FILM-COATED)
500 mg, 20s ea **54868-3804-06** 192.85
(CAPLET)
500 mg, 30s ea **54868-3804-03** 287.32
(CAPLET; FILM-COATED)
500 mg, 90s ea **54868-3804-05** 831.08

(Quality Care Prod)
REPACK
TAB, PO (FILM-COATED CAPLET)
1 gm, 3s ea **49999-0865-03** 40.65
18s ea **49999-0865-18** 243.90
30s ea **49999-0865-30** 406.50
(CAPLET)
500 mg, 7s ea **49999-0486-07** 73.78
30s ea **49999-0486-30** 276.26

(Southwood)
REPACK
TAB, PO (FILM-COATED CAPLET)
1 gm, 21s ea **58016-0855-01** 183.43
(CAPLET)
1 gm, 30s ea **00490-0052-30** 77.84
60s ea **00490-0052-60** 155.67
90s ea **00490-0052-90** 233.51
100s ea **00490-0052-00** 259.45

VALTURNA (Novartis Pharm)
aliskiren/valsartan
TAB, PO (FILM-COATED)
150 mg-160 mg,
30s ea **00078-0572-15** 81.22
300 mg-320 mg,
30s ea **00078-0574-15** 102.46

VANACOF (GM Pharm)
chlophedianol hcl/dexchlorpheniramine mal/pse hcl
SOL, PO (1X473ML,AF,SF,DYE-FREE)
473 ml **58809-0999-01** 112.24 89.79

VANACOF CD (GM Pharm)
codeine phos/dexchlorpheniramine mal/phenyleph hcl
SOL, PO (1X473ML,AF,SF,DYE-FREE)
473 ml, C-V **58809-0817-01** 74.00 59.20

VANACOF DX (GM Pharm)
chlophedianol hcl/gg/pse hcl
SOL, PO (1X473ML,AF,SF,DYE-FREE)
473 ml **58809-0907-01** 112.24 89.79

VANACON (GM Pharm)
gg/hydrocod bit/pse hcl
SYR, PO (PEPPERMINT)
480 ml, C-III **58809-0929-01** 33.30 26.64

VANADIUM (PCCA)
POW, NA, 1 gm **51927-2286-00** 120.00

VANADIUM PENTOXIDE (Baker, J.T.)
POW, NA (REAGENT)
500 gm **10106-4207-01** 147.96

VANADYL SULFATE (Medisca)
POW, NA (1X25GM)
25 gm **38779-0790-04** 60.00
(1X100GM)
100 gm **38779-0790-05** 147.00
(1X500GM)
500 gm **38779-0790-08** 429.00

(PCCA)
CRY, NA (HYDRATE)
1 gm **51927-2181-00** 3.36

VANCENASE (Pharma Pac)
REPACK
beclomethasone dipropionate
ARO, NS, 0.042 mg/actuation,
7 gm .... **52959-0585-00** 40.15 **BN**

(Southwood)
REPACK
ARO, NS, 0.042 mg/actuation,
17 gm .... **58016-6075-01** 37.44 **BN**

(Stat Rx)
REPACK
ARO, NS, 0.042 mg/actuation,
7 gm **16590-0243-07** 59.00

VANCENASE AQ (Pharma Pac)
REPACK
beclomethasone dipropionate monohydrate
SPR, NS, 0.042 mg/actuation,
25 gm .... **52959-0586-00** 39.71 **BN**

PROD/MFR	NDC	AWP	DP	OBC
(Phys Total Care)				
REPACK				
SPR, NS, 0.042 mg/actuation,				
25 gm	54868-1282-01	70.34		BN
(Southwood)				
REPACK				
SPR, NS, 0.042 mg/actuation,				
25 gm	58016-6204-01	36.54		BN
VANCENASE AQ DOUBLE STRENGTH (Pharma Pac)				
REPACK				
beclomethasone dipropionate monohydrate				
SPR, NS, 0.084 mg/actuation,				
19 gm	52959-0264-01	60.26		
VANCOCIN HCL (Baxter)				
dextrose/vancomycin hydrochloride				
SOL, IV (S.D. GALAXY PLASTIC)				
5%-500 mg/100 ml,				
100 ml	00338-3551-48	17.53		
200 ml 6s	00338-3552-48	207.36		
VANCOCIN HCL PULVULES (ViroPharma, Inc.)				
vancomycin hydrochloride				
CAP, PO, 125 mg, 20s ea	66593-3125-02	486.20		
250 mg, 20s ea UD	66593-3126-02	896.38		
VANCOMYCIN HCL (Hawkins)				
vancomycin hydrochloride				
POW, NA (U.S.P.)				
1 gm	63370-0350-10	163.20		
5 gm	63370-0350-15	686.40		
25 gm	63370-0350-25	2736.00		
100 gm	63370-0350-35	8160.00		
(Hospira)				
PDS, IV (VIAL,FLIPTOP,LATEX-FREE)				
1 gm, 10s ea	00409-6533-01	77.52	67.80	AP
(BULK,LATEX-FREE)				
5 gm, ea	00409-6509-01	33.70	29.48	AP
(ADD-VANTAGE,LATEX-FREE)				
500 mg, 10s ea	00409-6534-01	46.44	40.60	AP
(VIAL, FLIPTOP)				
500 mg, 10s ea	00074-4332-01	38.16	33.40	AP
(VIAL,FLIPTOP)				
500 mg, 10s ea	00409-4332-01	38.16	33.40	AP
(Medisca)				
POW, NA (U.S.P.)				
1 gm	38779-0274-06	105.00		
5 gm	38779-0274-03	420.00		
25 gm	38779-0274-04	1650.00		
(PCCA)				
POW, NA (U.S.P.)				
1 gm	51927-1742-00	105.00		
VANCOMYCIN HCL NOVAPLUS (Hospira)				
vancomycin hydrochloride				
PDS, IV (BULK,PRIVATE LABEL)				
5 gm, ea	00409-6509-49	30.85	27.00	AP
VANCOMYCIN HYDROCHLORIDE				
(Akorn) *See STERILE VANCOMYCIN HYDROCHLORIDE*				
VANCOMYCIN HYDROCHLORIDE (APP)				
vancomycin hydrochloride				
PDS, IV (VIAL,PF)				
1 gm, ea	63323-0284-20	20.35		AP
(BULK PACKAGE,PF)				
5 gm, ea	63323-0295-61	136.32		AP
VANCOMYCIN HYDROCHLORIDE (APP)				
10 gm, ea	63323-0314-61	272.64		AP
VANCOMYCIN HYDROCHLORIDE (APP)				
(VIAL,PF)				
500 mg, ea	63323-0221-10	10.97		AP
VANCOMYCIN HYDROCHLORIDE				
(APP) *See VANCOMYCIN HYDROCHLORIDE*				
(Gallipot)				
POW, NA (1X250MG,USP)				
0.25 gm	51552-1036-09	34.30	24.50	
(1X1GM,USP)				
1 gm	51552-1036-01	52.01	37.15	
(GeneraMedix)				
PDS, IV (USP,STERILE,LYOPHILIZED)				
1 gm, 10s ea	10139-0501-12	74.28		AP
(Hawkins) *See VANCOMYCIN HCL*				
(Hospira) *See AMERINET CHOICE VANCOMYCIN HYDROCHLORIDE*				
(Hospira)				
PDS, IV (ADD-VANTAGE,LATEX-FREE)				
1 gm, 10s ea	00409-6535-01	83.88	73.40	AP
(PHARMACY BULK, USP,PF)				
10 gm, ea	00409-6510-01	57.78	50.56	AP
(ADD-V VIAL)				
750 mg, 10s ea	00409-6531-01	68.88	60.30	EE
(SINGLE-DOSE,FLIPTOP)				
750 mg, 10s ea	00409-6531-02	58.32	51.00	EE
(Hospira) *See VANCOMYCIN HCL*				
(Hospira) *See VANCOMYCIN HCL NOVAPLUS*				
(Medisca) *See VANCOMYCIN HCL*				
(PCCA) *See VANCOMYCIN HCL*				
(ViroPharma, Inc.) *See VANCOCIN HCL PULVULES*				
VANCOMYCIN HYDROCHLORIDE-SODIUM CHLORIDE (PharMEDium Services)				
sodium chloride/vancomycin hydrochloride				
SOL, IV (VIAFLEX BAG,PF)				
0.9%-1.5 gm,				
250 ml 24s	61553-0078-02	42.00	35.00	
VANDAZOLE (Upsher-Smith)				
metronidazole				
GEL, VG, 0.75%, 70 gm	00245-0860-70	33.71		
(Phys Total Care)				
REPACK				
GEL, VG, 0.75%, 70 gm	54868-5666-00	145.65		
VANILLA BUTTERNUT (Medisca)				
flavoring aid				
SOL, NA (1X25ML)				
25 ml	38779-1685-04	25.50		
(1X100ML)				
100 ml	38779-1685-05	41.25		
(1X500ML)				
500 ml	38779-1685-08	91.50		
VANILLA BUTTERNUT ARTIFICIAL FLAVOR (Spectrum Pharmacy)				
flavoring aid				
LIQ, NA (1X100ML,CONCENTRATE)				
100 ml	49452-8095-02	63.70		
(1X500ML,CONCENTRATE)				
500 ml	49452-8095-03	146.65		
VANILLA BUTTERNUT FLAVOR (PCCA)				
flavoring aid				
SOL, NA (ARTIFICIAL)				
1 ml	51927-2151-00	0.90		
VANILLA EXTRACT				
(PCCA) *See VANILLA EXTRACT FLAVOR*				
VANILLA EXTRACT FLAVOR (PCCA)				
vanilla extract				
SOL, NA (PURE VANILLA)				
1 ml	51927-2770-00	0.26		
(PCCA)				
flavoring aid				
(PURE)				
1 ml	51927-3624-00	0.41		
VANILLIN (Lorann Oil)				
POW, NA (U.S.P.)				
30 gm	23535-0616-05	2.00		
120 gm	23535-0616-08	5.50		
480 gm	23535-0616-01	19.00		
(PCCA)				
POW, NA (NF)				
1 gm	51927-1526-00	0.36		
(Spectrum Pharmacy)				
POW, NA (N.F.)				
125 gm	49452-8100-01	65.80		
500 gm	49452-8100-02	164.85		
VANIQA (SkinMedica)				
eflornithine hydrochloride				
CRE, TP, 13.9%, 30 gm	67402-0040-30	76.25		
(2X30GM,TWIN PACK)				
13.9%, 30 gm 2s	67402-0040-32	131.25		
(Phys Total Care)				
REPACK				
CRE, TP, 13.9%, 30 gm	54868-5124-00	79.53		
VANISHING CREAM (Medisca)				
cream, multi ingredient				
CRE, NA (1X500GM)				
500 gm	38779-0763-08	87.00		
(1X2500GM)				
2500 gm	38779-0763-01	390.00		
VANISHING CREAM BASE (Spectrum Pharmacy)				
cream base				
CRE, NA (1X453.6GM)				
453.6 gm	49452-0827-01	99.75		
VANOS (Medicis)				
fluocinonide				
CRE, TP, 0.1%, 30 gm	99207-0525-30	138.79		
60 gm	99207-0525-60	248.40		
120 gm	99207-0525-10	471.95		
VANOXIDE HC (Summers)				
benzoyl peroxide/hydrocortisone				
LOT, TP, 5%-0.5%, ea	11086-0045-01	58.46		
VANOXIDE-HC (Summers)				
benzoyl peroxide/hydrocortisone				
LOT, TP (DYE-FREE)				
5%-0.5%, 25 ml	11086-0032-01	30.00	25.00	
VANSPAR (PRX)				
buspirone hydrochloride				
TAB, PO (USP)				
7.5 mg, 100s ea	16241-0720-01	118.15		
500s ea	16241-0720-05	581.82		
VANTAS (Endo Pharm)				
histrelin acetate				
IMP, SC, 50 mg, ea	67979-0500-01	6000.00		
VANTIN (Pfizer)				
cefpodoxime proxetil				
TAB, PO (UNIT OF USE)				
200 mg, 20s ea	00009-3618-01	193.33	161.11	
(A-S Medication)				
REPACK				
TAB, PO, 200 mg, 20s ea	54569-4783-00	174.36		
(PD-Rx Pharm)				
REPACK				
TAB, PO, 200 mg, ea	55289-0390-79	13.68		
2s ea	55289-0390-02	27.36		
10s ea	55289-0390-10	136.83		
20s ea	55289-0390-20	273.66		
28s ea	55289-0390-28	383.12		
(Pharma Pac)				
REPACK				
TAB, PO, 100 mg, 10s ea	52959-0627-10	35.50		
20s ea	52959-0627-20	66.50		
VAPRISOL (Astellas)				
conivaptan hydrochloride				
SOL, IV (10X100ML,SINGLE USE)				
20 mg/100 ml,				
100 ml 10s	00469-1602-11	5730.00		
20 mg/4 ml,				
4 ml 10s	00469-1601-04	5196.00		
VAQTA (Merck)				
hepatitis a vaccine, inactivated				
SOL, IM (TAX INCL, S.D.V.)				
50 u/ml, 1 ml	00006-4841-00	76.21		
(TAX INCL)				
50 u/ml, 1 ml	00006-4096-31	77.89		
(S.D.V.,TAX INCL)				
50 u/ml, 1 ml 10s	00006-4841-41	719.86		
(A-S Medication)				
REPACK				
SOL, IM (S.D.V., TAX INCL)				
50 u/ml, 1 ml	54569-5632-00	78.45		
VAQTA PEDIATRIC (Merck)				
hepatitis a vaccine, inactivated				
SOL, IM ((S.D.V.,TAX INCL)				
25 u/0.5 ml,				
0.5 ml 10s	00006-4831-41	364.43		
VARDENAFIL HYDROCHLORIDE				
(Schering) *See LEVITRA*				
VARENICLINE				
(Pfizer) *See CHANTIX*				
VARICELLA VIRUS VACCINE				
(Merck) *See VARIVAX*				
(Merck) *See ZOSTAVAX*				
VARIVAX (Merck)				
varicella virus vaccine				
PDS, SC (SDV W/DILUENT,TAX INCL)				
1350 pfu, ea	00006-4826-00	101.27		
10s ea	00006-4827-00	965.47		
(Phys Total Care)				
REPACK				
PDS, SC, 1350 pfu, ea	54868-3624-00	112.30		
VASCEZE HEPARIN LOCK FLUSH (Vital Signs)				
heparin sodium				
SOL, IV (LUER SLIP NOZZLE,PF)				
10 u/ml, 3 ml	08166-1110-03	2.50		EE
5 ml	08166-1110-05	2.50		EE
(LUER SLIP NOZZLE)				
100 u/ml, 3 ml	08166-1100-03	2.50		EE
5 ml	08166-1100-05	2.50		EE
VASCEZE SODIUM CHLORIDE (Vital Signs)				
sodium chloride				
SOL, IV (LUER SLIP NOZZLE)				
0.9%, 3 ml	08166-1109-03	2.25		EE
5 ml	08166-1109-05	2.25		EE
10 ml	08166-1109-10	2.25		EE

PROD/MFR	NDC	AWP	DP	OBC
VASCULAR CATHETER SUPPLIES				
(J&J Medical) *See BIOVUE PROCEDURE TRAY*				
VASERETIC (BTA)				
enalapril maleate/hydrochlorothiazide				
TAB, PO, 10 mg-25 mg,				
100s ea	64455-0146-01	282.65	235.54	AB
(PD-Rx Pharm)				
REPACK				
TAB, PO, 10 mg-25 mg,				
30s ea	55289-0484-30	60.40		AB
VASOCIDIN (Pharma Pac)				
REPACK				
prednisolone sodium phosphate/sulfacetamide sodium				
SOL, OP, 0.25%-10%, 5 ml	52959-0587-01	21.05		AT
(Phys Total Care)				
REPACK				
SOL, OP, 0.25%-10%, 5 ml	54868-1840-01	24.84		AT
10 ml	54868-1840-02	31.79		AT
(Southwood)				
REPACK				
SOL, OP, 0.25%-10%,				
10 ml	58016-6222-01	24.63		AT
VASOPRESSIN (Amer Regent)				
SOL, IJ (M.D.V.)				
20 u/ml,				
0.5 ml 25s	00517-0510-25	75.00		
1 ml 25s	00517-1020-25	135.00		
10 ml 10s	00517-0410-10	193.80		
(APP)				
SOL, IJ (VIAL)				
20 u/ml, 1 ml	63323-0302-01	8.50		
(JHP) *See PITRESSIN*				
(Phys Total Care)				
REPACK				
SOL, IJ (25X1ML)				
20 u/ml, 1 ml 25s	54868-5740-00	61.73		
VASOTEC (BTA)				
enalapril maleate				
TAB, PO, 2.5 mg, 30s ea	64455-0140-30	65.65	54.71	AB
90s ea	64455-0140-90	196.94	164.12	AB
5 mg, 30s ea	64455-0141-30	76.15	63.46	AB
90s ea	64455-0141-90	228.41	190.34	AB
1000s ea	64455-0141-10	2537.93	2114.94	AB
10 mg, 30s ea	64455-0142-30	83.74	69.78	AB
90s ea	64455-0142-90	251.24	209.37	AB
1000s ea	64455-0142-10	2791.44	2326.20	AB
20 mg, 30s ea	64455-0143-30	119.16	99.30	AB
90s ea	64455-0143-90	357.48	297.90	AB
1000s ea	64455-0143-10	3971.83	3309.86	AB
(PD-Rx Pharm)				
REPACK				
TAB, PO, 5 mg, 3s ea	55289-0622-03	9.75		AB
30s ea	55289-0622-30	52.45		AB
10 mg, 30s ea	55289-0483-30	54.78		AB
(Phys Total Care)				
REPACK				
TAB, PO, 2.5 mg, 30s ea	54868-2280-00	31.22		AB
60s ea	54868-2280-02	59.73		AB
5 mg, 30s ea	54868-1090-05	39.33		AB
60s ea	54868-1090-06	75.57		AB
100s ea	54868-1090-01	124.55		AB
10 mg, 30s ea	54868-0620-01	59.96		AB
60s ea	54868-0620-05	118.05		AB
90s ea	54868-0620-02	165.84		AB
100s ea	54868-0620-03	184.13		AB
20 mg, 30s ea	54868-0541-01	75.51		AB
60s ea	54868-0541-03	149.16		AB
90s ea	54868-0541-00	222.18		AB
(Southwood)				
REPACK				
TAB, PO, 20 mg, 30s ea	58016-0571-30	108.25		AB
60s ea	58016-0571-60	216.50		AB
90s ea	58016-0571-90	324.75		AB
100s ea	58016-0571-00	360.83		AB
VAZOBID (Wraser Pharm)				
bpm/phenyleph hcl				
SUS, PO (BUBBLE GUM)				
6 mg/5 ml-10 mg/5 ml,				
118 ml	66992-0230-04	79.34		
VAZOL (Wraser Pharm)				
brompheniramine maleate				
SOL, PO (AF,SF,DYE-FREE)				
2 mg/5 ml, 472 ml	66992-0130-16	73.78		
VAZOL-D (Wraser Pharm)				
bpm/phenyleph hcl				
SOL, PO (BUBBLE GUM)				
4 mg/5 ml-7.5 mg/5 ml,				
474 ml	66992-0136-16	61.48		
VAZOTAB (Wraser Pharm)				
bpm/phenyleph hcl				
CTB, PO (TANNATE,GRAPE)				
6 mg-15 mg, 60s ea	66992-0235-60	163.98		
VAZOTAN (Wraser Pharm)				
bpm/carbetapentane cit/phenyleph hcl				
SUS, PO (BUBBLE GUM)				
118 ml	66992-0220-04	81.56		
VECTIBIX (Amgen USA Inc.)				
panitumumab				
SOL, IV, 20 mg/ml, 5 ml	55513-0954-01	1018.50		
20 ml	55513-0956-01	4074.00		
VECTICAL (Galderma)				
calcitriol				
OIN, TP, 3 mcg/gm,				
100 gm	00299-2012-10	463.75		
VECURONIUM BROMIDE				
(Bedford) *See NOVAPLUS VECURONIUM BROMIDE*				
(Bedford)				
PDS, IV, 10 mg, 10s ea	55390-0037-10	48.00		AP
20 mg, 10s ea	55390-0039-10	96.00		AP
(Bedford) *See VECURONIUM BROMIDE NOVAPLUS*				
(Caraco)				
PDS, IV (FREEZE-DRIED)				
10 mg, 10s ea	41616-0931-44	106.25		AP
20 mg, 10s ea	41616-0932-44	212.50		AP
(Hospira)				
PDS, IV (FLIPTOP VIAL)				
10 mg, 10s ea	00409-1632-01	35.40	31.00	AP
(VIAL,FLIPTOP)				
10 mg, 10s ea	00074-1632-01	24.36	21.30	AP
(FTV)				
20 mg, 10s ea	00409-1634-01	63.72	55.80	AP
(Hospira) *See VECURONIUM BROMIDE NOVAPLUS*				
(Teva)				
PDS, IV, 10 mg, 10s ea	00703-2914-03	36.25		AP
VECURONIUM BROMIDE NOVAPLUS (Bedford)				
vecuronium bromide				
PDS, IV, 10 mg, 10s ea	55390-0181-10	36.00		AP
(Hospira)				
PDS, IV (FLIPTOP VIAL)				
10 mg, 10s ea	00409-1632-49	24.36	21.30	AP
(25ML FTV)				
20 mg, 10s ea	00409-1634-49	69.72	61.00	AP
VEEGUM (Gallipot)				
magnesium aluminum silicate				
POW, NA, 454 gm	51552-0422-06	25.55		
VEETIDS (Sandoz)				
penicillin v potassium				
TAB, PO, 250 mg, 100s ea	00003-0115-50	23.46		AB
1000s ea	00003-0115-75	222.87		AB
VEGETABLE OIL				
(PCCA) *See HYDROGENATED VEGETABLE OIL*				
VELCADE (Millennium Pharm)				
bortezomib				
PDS, IV (10ML SDV,LYOPHILIZED)				
3.5 mg, ea	63020-0049-01	1590.00		
VELIVET (Teva)				
desogestrel/ethinyl estradiol				
TAB, PO (BLISTER PACK,3X28)				
84s ea	00555-9051-67	100.93		AB
VENLAFAXINE (Upstate Pharma)				
venlafaxine hydrochloride				
TER, PO (COATED)				
37.5 mg, 30s ea	65580-0301-03	113.83		EE
90s ea	65580-0301-09	341.48		EE
75 mg, 30s ea	65580-0302-03	127.45		EE
90s ea	65580-0302-09	382.36		EE
150 mg, 30s ea	65580-0303-03	138.88		
90s ea	65580-0303-09	416.64		
225 mg, 30s ea	65580-0304-03	266.33		EE
90s ea	65580-0304-09	798.98		EE
(IPI)				
REPACK				
TAB, PO, 75 mg, 30s ea	18837-0047-30	81.93		
60s ea	18837-0047-60	163.86		
(Phys Total Care)				
REPACK				
TAB, PO, 37.5 mg, 10s ea	54868-4055-01	79.40		
30s ea	54868-4055-00	181.71		
(Southwood)				
REPACK				
TAB, PO, 37.5 mg, 30s ea	58016-0004-30	60.01		
60s ea	58016-0004-60	120.02		
90s ea	58016-0004-90	180.04		
100s ea	58016-0004-00	200.04		
50 mg, 30s ea	00490-0034-30	61.83		
60s ea	00490-0034-60	123.66		
90s ea	00490-0034-90	185.49		
100s ea	00490-0034-00	206.10		
75 mg, 30s ea	00490-0114-30	65.55		
60s ea	00490-0114-60	131.09		
90s ea	00490-0114-90	196.64		
100s ea	00490-0114-00	218.49		
(Stat Rx)				
REPACK				
TAB, PO, 75 mg, 30s ea	16590-0535-30	104.00		
60s ea	16590-0535-60	208.00		
90s ea	16590-0535-90	312.00		
100s ea	16590-0535-71	330.00		
120s ea	16590-0535-72	416.00		
TER, PO (COATED)				
150 mg, 30s ea	16590-0848-30	138.98		
60s ea	16590-0848-60	276.46		
VENLAFAXINE HYDROCHLORIDE				
FUL				
TAB, PO, 25 mg, 100s ea		116.58		
37.5 mg, 100s ea		120.03		
50 mg, 100s ea		123.66		
75 mg, 100s ea		131.10		
100 mg, 100s ea		138.92		
(Dr Reddy's)				
TAB, PO (COMPRESSED TABLET)				
25 mg, 90s ea	55111-0545-90	174.86		AB
37.5 mg, 90s ea	55111-0546-90	180.04		AB
500s ea	55111-0546-05	1000.20		AB
50 mg, 90s ea	55111-0547-90	185.49		AB
75 mg, 90s ea	55111-0548-90	196.64		AB
500s ea	55111-0548-05	1092.45		AB
100 mg, 90s ea	55111-0549-90	208.38		AB
(Mylan)				
TAB, PO, 25 mg, 100s ea	00378-4881-01	194.29		AB
37.5 mg, 100s ea	00378-4882-01	200.04		AB
50 mg, 100s ea	00378-4883-01	206.10		AB
75 mg, 100s ea	00378-4884-01	218.49		AB
100 mg, 100s ea	00378-4885-01	231.53		AB
(Teva)				
TAB, PO, 25 mg, 100s ea	00093-0199-01	194.29		AB
37.5 mg, 100s ea	00093-7380-01	200.04		AB
50 mg, 100s ea	00093-7381-01	206.10		AB
75 mg, 100s ea	00093-7382-01	218.49		AB
100 mg, 100s ea	00093-7383-01	231.53		AB
(UDL)				
TAB, PO (10X10)				
37.5 mg,				
100s ea UD	51079-0480-20	200.04		AB
75 mg, 100s ea UD	51079-0482-20	218.49		AB
(10X30)				
75 mg, 300s ea UD	51079-0482-56	655.47		AB
(Upstate Pharma) *See VENLAFAXINE*				
(Wyeth) *See EFFEXOR*				
(Wyeth) *See EFFEXOR-XR*				
(Zydus Pharm.)				
TAB, PO, 25 mg, 100s ea	68382-0018-01	194.29		AB
37.5 mg, 100s ea	68382-0019-01	200.04		AB
50 mg, 100s ea	68382-0020-01	206.10		AB
75 mg, 100s ea	68382-0021-01	218.49		AB
100 mg, 100s ea	68382-0101-01	231.53		AB
(A-S Medication)				
REPACK				
TAB, PO, 75 mg, 30s ea	54569-5872-00	65.55		
(American Health)				
REPACK				
TAB, PO (10X10)				
37.5 mg, 100s ea	68084-0330-01	200.04		AB
75 mg, 100s ea	68084-0331-01	218.49		AB
(DHS, Inc.)				
REPACK				
TAB, PO, 75 mg, 30s ea	55887-0125-30	65.54		
60s ea	55887-0125-60	159.99		
(IPI)				
REPACK				
TAB, PO, 75 mg, 90s ea	18837-0047-90	245.80		AB
(Keltman Pharma., Inc.)				
REPACK				
TAB, PO, 75 mg, 30s ea	68387-0348-30	76.23		

PROD/MFR	NDC	AWP	DP	OBC
(Nucare Pharm)				
REPACK				
TAB, PO, 75 mg, 30s ea	**68071-0694-30**	86.03		**AB**
60s ea	**68071-0694-60**	172.06		**AB**
(Palmetto)				
REPACK				
TAB, PO, 75 mg, 60s ea	**23490-6530-06**	222.54		
(Pharma Pac)				
REPACK				
TAB, PO, 75 mg, 30s ea	**52959-0890-30**	133.20		**AB**
90s ea	**52959-0890-90**	198.75		**AB**
100 mg, 60s ea	**52959-0606-60**	141.60		**AB**
(Phys Total Care)				
REPACK				
TAB, PO, 75 mg, 10s ea	**54868-5754-00**	78.63		
30s ea	**54868-5754-01**	176.49		
60s ea	**54868-5754-02**	332.22		
(Physician Partner)				
REPACK				
TAB, PO, 25 mg, 60s ea	**21695-0715-60**	233.15		**AB**
37.5 mg, 30s ea	**21695-0716-30**	120.02		**AB**
75 mg, 30s ea	**21695-0719-30**	131.09		**AB**
100 mg, 60s ea	**21695-0720-60**	277.84		**AB**
(Quality Care Prod)				
REPACK				
TAB, PO, 75 mg, 30s ea	**35356-0375-30**	162.33		**AB**
(St. Mary's MPP)				
REPACK				
TAB, PO, 75 mg, 30s ea	**60760-0121-30**	78.10		**AB**
(Stat Rx)				
REPACK				
TAB, PO, 37.5 mg, 30s ea	**16590-0644-30**	65.00		**AB**
60s ea	**16590-0644-60**	120.00		**AB**
90s ea	**16590-0644-90**	165.00		**AB**
75 mg, 84s ea	**16590-0535-62**	191.60		**AB**
100 mg, 30s ea	**16590-0650-30**	70.00		**AB**
60s ea	**16590-0650-60**	138.50		**AB**
90s ea	**16590-0650-90**	200.00		**AB**
VENOFER (Amer Regent)				
iron sucrose				
SOL, IV (S.D.V.,PF)				
20 mg/ml, 5 ml 10s	**00517-2340-10**	688.00		
(25X5ML SDV,PF)				
20 mg/ml, 5 ml 25s	**00517-2340-25**	1720.00		
(5X10ML,SDV,USP,PF)				
20 mg/ml, 10 ml 5s	**00517-2310-05**	688.00		
(Fresenius)				
SOL, IV (SDV,10X5ML)				
20 mg/ml, 5 ml 10s	**49230-0534-10**	660.00		
(SDV,25X5ML)				
20 mg/ml, 5 ml 25s	**49230-0534-25**	1650.00		
VENOMIL (Hollister-Stier)				
bee venom				
PDS, IJ (VIAL)				
0.12 mg, 6s ea	**65044-9940-04**	71.90		
(Hollister-Stier)				
white faced hornet venom				
6s ea	**65044-9941-04**	92.40		
(Hollister-Stier)				
yellow hornet venom				
6s ea	**65044-9942-04**	92.40		
(Hollister-Stier)				
wasp venom				
6s ea	**65044-9943-04**	104.75		
(Hollister-Stier)				
yellow jacket venom				
6s ea	**65044-9944-04**	92.40		
(Hollister-Stier)				
vespid venom, mixed				
0.36 mg, 6s ea	**65044-9945-04**	182.90		
VENOSET (Abbott Hosp)				
kit, administration, intravenous				
DEV, NA (SOLUSET 150X60, VENTED)				
20s ea	**00074-6646-01**	372.00	250.60	
(100 W/2 INJ,HP-OL,LTXFR)				
48s ea	**00074-1734-78**	889.20	748.80	
(100-SL PGBK NV 100 INCH)				
48s ea	**00074-8082-48**	801.42	674.88	
(70" ,CNVT PIN)				
48s ea	**00074-1820-78**	449.73	378.72	
(72 W/CAIR CLAMP NV)				
48s ea	**00074-1857-48**	58.18	58.08	
(78 W/CONV PIN)				
48s ea	**00074-1881-58**	475.95	400.80	
(78 W/MB PRC PIN&CAIR NV)				
48s ea	**00074-3084-48**	475.95	400.80	
(78" W/CAIR CLAMP NV)				
48s ea	**00074-1859-48**	428.07	360.48	
(LTX FR 106" P.B.,MCRDRP)				
48s ea	**00074-8083-78**	299.25	252.00	
(LTX FR SECONDARY P.B.)				
48s ea	**00074-1832-68**	69.12	69.12	
(LTXF 100 MICRODRIP PIN)				
48s ea	**00074-1723-78**	515.85	434.40	
(LTXF,101"W/2 BKCK/2 INJ)				
48s ea	**00074-8961-78**	881.22	742.08	
(LTXF,80",P.B. 0.22 MIC)				
48s ea	**00074-4985-78**	1128.60	950.40	
(LTXF,80",P.B.W/0.22 MIC)				
48s ea	**00074-4258-78**	1161.09	977.76	
(LTXF,90",0.22 MIC-SL)				
48s ea	**00074-8958-78**	299.52	299.52	
(LTXF,P.B. W/DETACH 19G)				
48s ea	**00074-1889-58**	69.12	69.12	
(LTXF,PRIM P.B. W/BKCK)				
48s ea	**00074-4967-78**	773.49	651.36	
(LTXF,SEC. P.B. MICRODRP)				
48s ea	**00074-1992-78**	84.10	84.00	
(NV 100 W/CAIR CLAMP)				
48s ea	**00074-1728-58**	491.91	414.24	
(NV 78 W/IVEX-2 FILTER)				
48s ea	**00074-4293-48**	768.36	647.04	
(NV P.B. SURG W/IVEX-RF)				
48s ea	**00074-4800-48**	1027.71	865.44	
(NV PGBK ANESTH W/CAIR)				
48s ea	**00074-5742-48**	748.98	630.72	
(NV PIGYBCK W/CAIR CLAMP)				
48s ea	**00074-1818-48**	698.82	588.48	
(NV SEC. P.B. W/PRE NDL)				
48s ea	**00074-1889-48**	364.23	306.72	
(NV SECONDARY)				
48s ea	**00074-1861-58**	70.27	70.08	
48s ea	**00074-1926-48**	72.00	72.00	
(NV SURGICAL)				
48s ea	**00074-8965-48**	744.99	627.36	
(NV TWINSITE W/CAIR CLMP)				
48s ea	**00074-1819-48**	492.48	414.72	
(PRIM.P.B. W/CAIR CLP NV)				
48s ea	**00074-1860-48**	705.09	593.76	
(SEC.P.B. W/5MIC FLT+PIN)				
48s ea	**00074-1911-48**	105.41	105.12	
(SECONDARY, VENTED, 22")				
48s ea	**00074-1702-48**	100.80	100.80	
(Y-TYPE W/CAIR CLAMP NV)				
48s ea	**00074-1879-58**	116.35	116.64	
(EXTENSION 20-SL)				
50s ea	**00074-3903-02**	436.41	367.50	
(EXTENSION 30-SL)				
50s ea	**00074-3229-03**	95.40	95.50	
VENTAVIS (Actelion Pharm)				
iloprost				
SOL, IH (1X1ML,SINGLE-USE)				
10 mcg/ml, 1 ml	**66215-0302-00**	74.40		
(30X1ML,SINGLE-USE)				
10 mcg/ml,				
1 ml 30s	**66215-0302-30**	2232.00		
(1X1ML,SINGLE-USE)				
20 mcg/ml, 1 ml UD	**66215-0303-00**	74.40		
(30X1ML,SINGLE-USE)				
20 mcg/ml,				
1 ml 30s	**66215-0303-30**	2232.00		
(CoTherix, Inc)				
SOL, IH (UNIT-DOSE VIAL,PF)				
10 mcg/ml,				
2 ml 100s UD	**10148-0101-01**	3876.00		
VENTOLIN (Phys Total Care)				
REPACK				
albuterol sulfate				
SOL, IH, 0.5%, 20 ml	**54868-3479-00**	24.15		**AN**
VENTOLIN HFA (Glaxo)				
albuterol sulfate				
ARO, IH (60 ACTUATIONS)				
0.09 mg/actuation,				
8 gm	**00173-0682-21**	18.00		**BX**
(WITH DOSE COUNTER)				
0.09 mg/actuation,				
18 gm	**00173-0682-20**	36.12		**BX**
(Pharma Pac)				
REPACK				
ARO, IH (1X18GM)				
0.09 mg/actuation,				
18 gm	**52959-0983-18**	35.86		**BX**
(Phys Total Care)				
REPACK				
ARO, IH (1X8GM)				
0.09 mg/actuation,				
8 gm	**54868-6050-01**	24.52		**BX**
(1X18GM)				
0.09 mg/actuation,				
18 gm	**54868-6050-00**	47.24		**BX**
(Physician Partner)				
REPACK				
ARO, IH, 0.09 mg/actuation,				
8 gm	**21695-0423-08**	36.00		**BX**
(Quality Care Prod)				
REPACK				
ARO, IH, 0.09 mg/actuation,				
18 gm	**35356-0166-01**	60.52		**BX**
VERAMYST (Glaxo)				
fluticasone furoate				
SPR, NS, 27.5 mcg/actuation,				
10 gm	**00173-0753-00**	106.73		
(Quality Care Prod)				
REPACK				
SPR, NS (10GMX1)				
27.5 mcg/actuation,				
10 gm	**35356-0474-10**	180.25		
VERAPAMIL (Bryant Ranch)				
REPACK				
verapamil hydrochloride				
TER, PO, 240 mg, 30s ea	**63629-3052-01**	64.68		
(Southwood)				
REPACK				
TER, PO, 120 mg, 30s ea	**58016-0721-30**	32.19		
60s ea	**58016-0721-60**	64.38		
90s ea	**58016-0721-90**	96.57		
100s ea	**58016-0721-00**	107.30		
VERAPAMIL ER (DHS, Inc.)				
REPACK				
verapamil hydrochloride				
TER, PO, 240 mg, 30s ea	**55887-0418-30**	46.62		
VERAPAMIL HCL (Consolidated Midland)				
verapamil hydrochloride				
TAB, PO, 80 mg, 100s ea	**00223-1735-01**	22.50		**EE**
1000s ea	**00223-1735-02**	195.00		**EE**
120 mg, 100s ea	**00223-1736-01**	22.50		**EE**
1000s ea	**00223-1736-02**	210.00		**EE**
(Gallipot)				
POW, NA, 25 gm	**51552-0525-04**	29.40		
(1X100GM,USP)				
100 gm	**51552-0525-05**	97.30	69.50	
(1X500GM,USP)				
500 gm	**51552-0525-06**	408.80	292.00	
(1X1000GM,USP)				
1000 gm	**51552-0525-07**	726.60	519.00	
(Hawkins)				
POW, NA (U.S.P.)				
25 gm	**63370-0355-25**	72.00		
100 gm	**63370-0355-35**	224.00		
500 gm	**63370-0355-45**	1040.00		
(Hospira)				
SOL, IV (AMP,LATEX-FREE)				
2.5 mg/ml, 2 ml 5s	**00409-4011-01**	7.68	6.70	**AP**
(VIAL,FLIPTOP,ABBOJECT)				
2.5 mg/ml, 2 ml 5s	**00409-1144-01**	8.64	7.55	**AP**
(ANSYR,LATEX-FREE)				
2.5 mg/ml, 4 ml	**00409-9633-05**	73.08	63.90	**AP**
(VIAL,FLIPTOP,ABBOJECT)				
2.5 mg/ml, 4 ml 5s	**00409-1144-02**	15.96	13.95	**AP**
(Letco)				
POW, NA (U.S.P.)				
100 gm	**62991-1161-01**	207.00		
(Major)				
TAB, PO (10X10)				
80 mg, 100s ea UD	**00904-2920-61**	57.00		**AB**
120 mg, 100s ea UD	**00904-2924-61**	75.00		**AB**
(Medisca)				
POW, NA (USP)				
25 gm	**38779-0275-04**	79.50		
100 gm	**38779-0275-05**	247.50		
(U.S.P.)				
500 gm	**38779-0275-08**	1125.00		
1000 gm	**38779-0275-09**	2055.00		
(Mylan)				
CER, PO, 120 mg, 30s ea	**00378-6320-93**	41.13		**AB**
100s ea	**00378-6320-01**	137.10		**AB**
180 mg, 30s ea	**00378-6380-93**	43.17		**AB**
100s ea	**00378-6380-01**	143.90		**AB**
240 mg, 30s ea	**00378-6440-93**	48.84		**AB**
100s ea	**00378-6440-01**	162.80		**AB**
TAB, PO, 80 mg, 100s ea	**00378-0512-01**	30.75		**AB**
1000s ea	**00378-0512-10**	284.95		**AB**
120 mg, 100s ea	**00378-0772-01**	39.35		**AB**
500s ea	**00378-0772-05**	180.30		**AB**

PROD/MFR	NDC	AWP	DP	OBC
(PCCA)				
POW, NA (U.S.P.)				
1 gm	**51927-1921-00**	3.72		
(Spectrum Pharmacy)				
POW, NA (U.S.P.)				
25 gm	**49452-8113-02**	116.90		
100 gm	**49452-8113-03**	367.50		
(UDL)				
CER, PO (10X10)				
120 mg, 100s ea UD	**51079-0917-20**	130.25		AB
TER, PO, 120 mg,				
100s ea UD	**51079-0894-20**	93.73		AB
180 mg, 100s ea UD	**51079-0899-20**	120.10		AB
240 mg, 100s ea UD	**51079-0869-20**	121.87		AB
(Watson Labs)				
CER, PO, 120 mg, 100s ea	**00591-2880-01**	129.05		AB
180 mg, 100s ea	**00591-2882-01**	135.16		EE
240 mg, 100s ea	**00591-2884-01**	152.54		EE
360 mg, 100s ea	**00591-2886-01**	209.94		
TAB, PO, 40 mg, 100s ea	**00591-0404-01**	18.58		AB
(WHITE)				
80 mg, 100s ea	**00591-0343-01**	53.38		AB
500s ea	**00591-0343-05**	239.68		AB
1000s ea	**00591-0343-10**	498.23		AB
120 mg, 100s ea	**00591-0345-01**	68.43		AB
500s ea	**00591-0345-05**	315.53		AB
1000s ea	**00591-0345-10**	606.01		AB
(A-S Medication)				
REPACK				
TAB, PO, 120 mg, 30s ea	**54569-0646-02**	20.53		EE
100s ea	**54569-0646-00**	68.43		EE
TER, PO, 180 mg, 30s ea	**54569-4447-04**	41.99		EE
(DHS, Inc.)				
REPACK				
TAB, PO, 120 mg, 30s ea	**55887-0449-30**	33.82		AB
60s ea	**55887-0449-60**	59.00		AB
90s ea	**55887-0449-90**	84.00		AB
(Dispensing Solutions)				
REPACK				
TAB, PO, 120 mg, 30s ea	**66336-0296-30**	30.00		AB
30s ea	**66336-0300-30**	47.60		AB
TER, PO, 180 mg, 30s ea	**66336-0781-30**	60.17		AB
(FILM-COATED)				
180 mg, 60s ea	**55045-3043-09**	88.80		AB
240 mg, 30s ea	**55045-2321-08**	45.60		AB
30s ea	**66336-0959-30**	68.09		AB
60s ea	**55045-2321-09**	91.20		AB
(GSMS)				
REPACK				
TAB, PO (UNIT OF USE)				
120 mg, 60s ea	**60429-0197-60**	21.00	7.00	AB
TER, PO, 180 mg, 90s ea	**60429-0237-90**	69.90	23.30	AB
240 mg, 30s ea	**60429-0198-30**	38.85	12.95	AB
60s ea	**60429-0198-60**	75.30	25.10	AB
90s ea	**60429-0198-90**	111.45	37.15	AB
(HomeMed)				
REPACK				
TAB, PO, 120 mg, 120s ea	**51655-0586-82**	37.20		EE
(PD-Rx Pharm)				
REPACK				
CER, PO (REDI-SCRIPT)				
120 mg, 30s ea	**58864-0677-30**	94.85		AB
TAB, PO, 80 mg, 8s ea	**55289-0896-08**	20.39		AB
30s ea	**55289-0896-30**	28.06		AB
(REDI-SCRIPT)				
80 mg, 30s ea	**58864-0720-30**	28.05		AB
60s ea	**58864-0720-60**	39.44		AB
120 mg, 30s ea	**55289-0481-30**	32.61		AB
30s ea	**58864-0530-30**	32.60		AB
60s ea	**55289-0481-60**	48.56		AB
TER, PO, 180 mg, 30s ea	**55289-0607-30**	87.33		AB
60s ea	**58864-0706-60**	115.14		AB
240 mg, 30s ea	**55289-0723-30**	68.17		AB
90s ea	**55289-0723-90**	171.17		AB
(Pharma Pac)				
REPACK				
TER, PO, 240 mg, 30s ea	**52959-0050-30**	56.06		EE
(Phys Total Care)				
REPACK				
CER, PO, 360 mg, 10s ea	**54868-5984-01**	66.31		
30s ea	**54868-5984-00**	144.36		
SOL, IV, 2.5 mg/ml, 2 ml	**54868-3809-00**	6.87		EE
(2ML VIAL,LATEX-FREE)				
2.5 mg/ml, 2 ml 5s	**54868-3809-01**	23.85		AP
TAB, PO, 40 mg, 30s ea	**54868-2885-00**	14.49		EE
80 mg, 30s ea	**54868-0120-03**	11.28		EE
60s ea	**54868-0120-00**	18.03		EE
100s ea	**54868-0120-01**	27.06		EE
120 mg, 30s ea	**54868-0121-06**	11.10		EE
60s ea	**54868-0121-05**	19.23		EE
100s ea	**54868-0121-01**	30.06		EE
500s ea	**54868-0121-02**	116.42		EE
TER, PO, 120 mg, 30s ea	**54868-4432-00**	58.56		EE
180 mg, 30s ea	**54868-3300-02**	53.22		EE
60s ea	**54868-3300-03**	103.47		EE
90s ea	**54868-3300-04**	118.23		EE
100s ea	**54868-3300-01**	129.54		EE
240 mg, 10s ea	**54868-2207-06**	15.02		EE
30s ea	**54868-2207-02**	60.63		EE
60s ea	**54868-2207-00**	91.14		EE
(USP)				
240 mg, 90s ea	**54868-2207-05**	135.21		EE
100s ea	**54868-2207-03**	148.38		EE
(Quality Care Prod)				
REPACK				
CER, PO, 180 mg, 30s ea	**49999-0284-30**	51.83		EE
TAB, PO, 80 mg, 100s ea	**49999-0310-00**	67.38		AB
120 mg, 30s ea	**49999-0283-30**	38.34		AB
100s ea	**49999-0283-00**	127.80		AB
TER, PO, 240 mg, 30s ea	**49999-0075-30**	55.72		AB
(Southwood)				
REPACK				
TAB, PO, 80 mg, 8s ea	**58016-0511-08**	4.49		EE
30s ea	**58016-0511-30**	16.85		EE
100s ea	**58016-0511-00**	56.15		EE
120 mg, 12s ea	**58016-0509-12**	12.78		EE
15s ea	**58016-0509-15**	15.98		EE
20s ea	**58016-0509-20**	21.30		EE
30s ea	**58016-0509-30**	31.95		EE
60s ea	**58016-0509-60**	63.90		EE
100s ea	**58016-0509-00**	106.50		EE
120s ea	**58016-0509-02**	127.80		EE
TER, PO, 240 mg, 12s ea	**58016-0860-12**	18.58		EE
15s ea	**58016-0860-15**	23.22		EE
20s ea	**58016-0860-20**	30.96		EE
30s ea	**58016-0860-30**	46.44		EE
100s ea	**58016-0860-00**	154.80		EE
(Vibranta)				
REPACK				
TER, PO, 120 mg, 30s ea	**57866-6912-01**	42.84		
VERAPAMIL HCL ER (PD-Rx Pharm)				
REPACK				
verapamil hydrochloride				
TER, PO (REDI-SCRIPT)				
240 mg, 30s ea	**58864-0649-30**	68.15		AB
VERAPAMIL HYDROCHLORIDE				
FUL				
TAB, PO, 80 mg, 100s ea		7.73		
120 mg, 100s ea		11.48		
TER, PO, 120 mg, 100s ea		82.50		
180 mg, 100s ea		48.38		
240 mg, 100s ea		43.50		
(Consolidated Midland) *See VERAPAMIL HCL*				
(Gallipot) *See VERAPAMIL HCL*				
(Glenmark Pharmaceuticals)				
TER, PO (FILM-COATED)				
240 mg, 100s ea	**68462-0260-01**	163.55		AB
500s ea	**68462-0260-05**	770.55		AB
(Hawkins) *See VERAPAMIL HCL*				
(Hospira) *See VERAPAMIL HCL*				
(Kremers Urban)				
CER, PO (HARD GELATIN)				
100 mg, 100s ea	**62175-0485-37**	195.84		
200 mg, 100s ea	**62175-0486-37**	252.23		
300 mg, 100s ea	**62175-0487-37**	366.98		
(Letco) *See VERAPAMIL HCL*				
(Major) *See VERAPAMIL HCL*				
(Medisca) *See VERAPAMIL HCL*				
(Mylan)				
CER, PO (PM,HARD GELATIN)				
100 mg, 100s ea	**00378-6201-01**	196.10		AB
500s ea	**00378-6201-05**	980.50		AB
200 mg, 100s ea	**00378-6202-01**	252.55		AB
500s ea	**00378-6202-05**	1262.75		AB
300 mg, 100s ea	**00378-6203-01**	367.20		AB
500s ea	**00378-6203-05**	1836.00		AB
TER, PO (USP,FILM-COATED)				
120 mg, 30s ea	**00378-2120-93**	32.19		AB
100s ea	**00378-2120-01**	107.29		AB
180 mg, 100s ea	**00378-2180-01**	135.96		AB
500s ea	**00378-2180-05**	678.80		AB
(USP,FILM COATED)				
240 mg, 100s ea	**00378-1411-01**	155.85		AB
500s ea	**00378-1411-05**	770.55		AB
(Mylan) *See VERAPAMIL HCL*				
(PCCA) *See VERAPAMIL HCL*				
(Pfizer) *See CALAN*				
(Pfizer) *See CALAN SR*				
(Pfizer) *See COVERA-HS*				
(Ranbaxy Labs) *See ISOPTIN SR*				
(Ranbaxy Pharm)				
TER, PO (FILM-COATED)				
120 mg, 100s ea	**63304-0488-01**	107.29		
180 mg, 100s ea	**63304-0489-01**	143.96		
240 mg, 100s ea	**63304-0490-01**	163.55		
500s ea	**63304-0490-05**	770.55		
(Spectrum Pharmacy) *See VERAPAMIL HCL*				
(Teva)				
TAB, PO (10X10)				
120 mg, 100s ea UD	**00182-1301-89**	57.85		AB
TER, PO, 120 mg, 100s ea	**00172-4285-60**	107.29		AB
(10X10,CAPLET)				
120 mg, 100s ea UD	**00172-4285-10**	107.29		AB
180 mg, 100s ea	**00172-4286-60**	143.96		AB
(10X10,CAPLET)				
180 mg, 100s ea UD	**00172-4286-10**	143.96		AB
500s ea	**00172-4286-70**	678.00		AB
240 mg, 100s ea	**00172-4280-60**	163.55		AB
(10X10,CAPLET)				
240 mg, 100s ea UD	**00172-4280-10**	163.55		AB
(FILM-COATED)				
240 mg, 500s ea	**00172-4280-70**	770.00		AB
(UCB) *See VERELAN*				
(UCB) *See VERELAN PM*				
(UDL)				
TER, PO (USP,10X30,PUNCH CARD)				
180 mg, 300s ea UD	**51079-0899-56**	360.30		AB
240 mg, 300s ea UD	**51079-0869-56**	365.61		AB
(UDL) *See VERAPAMIL HCL*				
(Watson Labs) *See VERAPAMIL HCL*				
(A-S Medication)				
REPACK				
TER, PO (FILM-COATED)				
240 mg, 30s ea	**54569-3691-00**	48.49		AB
(Altura)				
REPACK				
TER, PO, 180 mg, 10s ea	**63874-0458-10**	14.00		
14s ea	**63874-0458-14**	19.60		
20s ea	**63874-0458-20**	28.00		
30s ea	**63874-0458-30**	42.00		
60s ea	**63874-0458-60**	84.00		
100s ea	**63874-0458-01**	139.96		
(DHS, Inc.)				
REPACK				
TER, PO (CAPLET)				
120 mg, 30s ea	**55887-0402-30**	45.50		AB
60s ea	**55887-0402-60**	91.00		AB
90s ea	**55887-0402-90**	136.50		AB
(Dispensing Solutions)				
REPACK				
TAB, PO, 120 mg, 30s ea	**55045-3017-08**	20.70		
60s ea	**55045-3017-06**	41.40		
100s ea	**55045-3017-01**	69.00		
(Palmetto)				
REPACK				
TAB, PO, 120 mg, 30s ea	**23490-6462-01**	46.96		
TER, PO, 120 mg, 30s ea	**23490-6463-01**	45.50		
180 mg, 30s ea	**23490-6464-01**	58.80		
90s ea	**23490-6464-09**	176.40		
240 mg, 30s ea	**23490-6466-01**	68.17		
60s ea	**23490-6466-06**	136.34		
90s ea	**23490-6466-09**	204.51		
(PD-Rx Pharm)				
REPACK				
TER, PO (REDI-SCRIPT,CAPLET)				
180 mg, 14s ea	**58864-0706-14**	49.61		AB
(REDI-SCRIPT)				
240 mg, 14s ea	**58864-0649-14**	50.17		AB
60s ea	**58864-0649-60**	103.75		
(FILM-COATED)				
240 mg, 100s ea	**43063-0011-01**	163.55		
(USP)				
240 mg, 180s ea	**55289-0723-93**	226.00		AB
(Phys Total Care)				
REPACK				
CER, PO (HARD GELATIN)				
100 mg, 30s ea	**54868-2211-00**	106.00		
300 mg, 20s ea	**54868-5841-00**	158.84		

PROD/MFR	NDC	AWP	DP	OBC
(HARD GELATIN)				
300 mg, 30s ea	**54868-5841-02**	194.52		
60s ea	**54868-5841-01**	441.80		
TER, PO, 120 mg, 100s ea	**54868-4432-01**	143.13		AB
(FILM-COATED)				
240 mg, 45s ea	**54868-2207-04**	89.43		AB
(Quality Care Prod)				
REPACK				
TAB, PO, 80 mg, 60s ea	**49999-0310-60**	40.43		
TER, PO, 180 mg, 100s ea	**49999-0284-00**	172.75		AB
240 mg, 100s ea	**49999-0075-00**	185.73		AB
(Vibranta)				
REPACK				
TER, PO, 240 mg, 30s ea	**57866-6914-01**	53.30		AB
60s ea	**57866-6914-02**	104.34		AB
VERAPAMIL HYDROCHLORIDE ER (HomeMed)				
REPACK				
verapamil hydrochloride				
TER, PO, 180 mg, 30s ea	**51655-0934-24**	54.99		
240 mg, 30s ea	**51655-0604-24**	68.17		
VERDESO (Stiefel Labs)				
desonide				
FOA, TP, 0.05%, 50 gm	**63032-0111-50**	157.66		
100 gm	**63032-0111-00**	294.61		
VEREGEN (Doak)				
sinecatechins				
OIN, TP (1X15GM, ALUMINUM TUBE)				
15%, 15 gm	**10337-0450-15**	297.92		
VERELAN (UCB)				
verapamil hydrochloride				
CER, PO, 120 mg, 100s ea	**00091-2490-23**	387.30		AB
180 mg, 100s ea	**00091-2489-23**	405.61		AB
240 mg, 100s ea	**00091-2491-23**	457.76		AB
360 mg, 100s ea	**00091-2495-23**	672.89		
VERELAN PM (UCB)				
verapamil hydrochloride				
CER, PO, 100 mg, 100s ea	**00091-4085-01**	313.28		
200 mg, 100s ea	**00091-4086-01**	403.50		
300 mg, 100s ea	**00091-4087-01**	586.62		
VERIPRED 20 (Hawthorn Pharm)				
prednisolone sodium phosphate				
SOL, PO (1X237ML,AF,DYE-FREE)				
20 mg/5 ml, 237 ml	**63717-0915-08**	156.25		EE
VERITAS COLLAGEN MATRIX (Synovis)				
collagen, bovine				
SHE, IP (10CMX16CM)				
ea	**03221-1016-11**	3648.00	3040.00	
(12CMX25CM)				
ea	**03221-1225-11**	6840.00	5700.00	
(2CMX8CM)				
ea	**03221-0208-11**	474.00	395.00	
(4CMX15CM)				
ea	**03221-0415-11**	1194.00	995.00	
(4CMX7CM)				
ea	**03221-0407-11**	714.00	595.00	
(6CMX8CM)				
ea	**03221-0608-11**	1194.00	995.00	
(8CMX14CM)				
ea	**03221-0814-11**	1554.00	1295.00	
VERMOX (PD-Rx Pharm)				
REPACK				
mebendazole				
CTB, PO, 100 mg, ea	**55289-0416-79**	13.23		
VERSABASE GEL (PCCA)				
gel, multi ingredient				
GEL, TP, 1 gm	**51927-3656-00**	0.33		
VERSABASE LOTION (PCCA)				
lotion, multi ingredient				
LOT, TP, 1 gm	**51927-3653-00**	0.33		
VERSICLEAR (Hope)				
salicylic acid/sodium thiosulfate				
LOT, TP, 1%-25%, 120 ml	**60267-0531-04**	26.50		
VERTEPORFIN				
(Novartis Pharm) *See VISUDYNE*				
VERTIGOHEEL (Heel/BHI)				
homeopathic substance				
LIQ, PO (DROPS)				
50 ml	**50114-1170-04**	21.93	21.93	
TAB, SL, 100s ea	**50114-6155-02**	11.86	11.86	
VESANOID (Roche Labs)				
tretinoin				
SGL, PO, 10 mg, 100s ea	**00004-0250-01**	2759.06		
VESICARE (Astellas)				
solifenacin succinate				
TAB, PO, 5 mg, 30s ea	**51248-0150-01**	155.16		
90s ea	**51248-0150-03**	465.48		
100s ea UD	**51248-0150-52**	517.20		
(FILM-COATED)				
10 mg, 30s ea	**51248-0151-01**	155.16		
90s ea	**51248-0151-03**	465.48		
100s ea UD	**51248-0151-52**	517.20		
(A-S Medication)				
REPACK				
TAB, PO, 5 mg, 30s ea	**54569-5790-00**	152.25		
(Phys Total Care)				
REPACK				
TAB, PO, 5 mg, 30s ea	**54868-5398-00**	174.98		
10 mg, 30s ea	**54868-4705-00**	174.98		
(FILM-COATED)				
10 mg, 60s ea	**54868-4705-01**	328.41		
(Quality Care Prod)				
REPACK				
TAB, PO, 5 mg, 30s ea	**35356-0282-30**	257.47		
(FILM-COATED)				
10 mg, 30s ea	**35356-0283-30**	257.47		
VESPID VENOM, MIXED				
(Alk-Abello) *See MIXED VESPID TREATMENT*				
(Hollister-Stier) *See MIXED VESPID TREATMENT*				
(Hollister-Stier) *See VENOMIL*				
VETIVER OIL (Lorann Oil)				
OIL, NA, 9.9 ml	**23535-0151-81**	6.00		
(Medisca)				
OIL, NA (1X14ML,FRAGRANCE)				
14 ml	**38779-1686-03**	19.50		
(1X25ML,FRAGRANCE)				
25 ml	**38779-1686-04**	28.50		
(1X100ML,FRAGRANCE)				
100 ml	**38779-1686-05**	114.00		
(1X500ML,FRAGRANCE)				
500 ml	**38779-1686-08**	276.00		
VEXOL (Alcon Ophthalmic)				
rimexolone				
SUS, OP, 1%, 5 ml	**00065-0627-07**	39.06		
10 ml	**00065-0627-03**	71.40		
(Phys Total Care)				
REPACK				
SUS, OP, 1%, 5 ml	**54868-3766-00**	37.83		
VFEND (Pfizer)				
voriconazole				
PDR, PO (W/ADAPTER AND DISPENSER)				
40 mg/ml, 75 ml	**00049-3160-44**	837.23	697.69	
TAB, PO, 50 mg, 30s ea	**00049-3170-30**	365.71	304.76	
(CAPLET)				
200 mg, 30s ea	**00049-3180-30**	1462.86	1219.05	
VFEND I.V. (Pfizer)				
voriconazole				
PDS, IV (S.D.V.)				
200 mg, ea	**00049-3190-28**	143.50	119.58	
VI-ATRO (Vita-Rx)				
atropine sulfate/diphenoxylate hydrochloride				
TAB, PO, 0.025 mg-2.5 mg,				
100s ea, C-V	**49727-0266-02**	3.44		EE
1000s ea, C-V	**49727-0266-05**	13.75		EE
VI-SUDO (Vita-Rx)				
pse hcl/triprolidine hcl				
TAB, PO, 60 mg-2.5 mg,				
100s ea	**49727-0004-02**	3.30		EE
1000s ea	**49727-0004-05**	17.07		EE
VIADUR (Bayer Corp.)				
leuprolide acetate				
KIT, ID, 65 mg, ea	**00026-9711-01**	5684.00		
VIAGRA (Pfizer)				
sildenafil citrate				
TAB, PO, 25 mg, 30s ea	**00069-4200-30**	571.97	476.64	
50 mg, 30s ea	**00069-4210-30**	571.97	476.64	
100s ea	**00069-4210-66**	1906.55	1588.79	
100 mg, 30s ea	**00069-4220-30**	571.97	476.64	
100s ea	**00069-4220-66**	1906.55	1588.79	
(A-S Medication)				
REPACK				
TAB, PO, 50 mg, 10s ea	**54569-4569-00**	227.39		
100 mg, 4s ea	**54569-4570-08**	72.88		
5s ea	**54569-4570-03**	91.10		
6s ea	**54569-4570-02**	136.43		
10s ea	**54569-4570-00**	227.39		
30s ea	**54569-4570-01**	682.16		
(Altura)				
REPACK				
TAB, PO, 100 mg, 6s ea	**63874-0481-06**	81.12		
10s ea	**63874-0481-10**	135.20		
30s ea	**63874-0481-30**	405.60		
100s ea	**63874-0481-01**	1352.00		
(AQ)				
REPACK				
TAB, PO, 50 mg, 30s ea	**66105-0535-03**	551.60		
100 mg, 30s ea	**66105-0536-03**	551.60		
(Bryant Ranch)				
REPACK				
TAB, PO, 50 mg, 5s ea	**63629-2640-03**	79.65		
10s ea	**63629-2640-02**	146.98		
30s ea	**63629-2640-01**	464.32		
100 mg, 2s ea	**63629-1792-04**	31.26		
5s ea	**63629-1792-02**	78.15		
6s ea	**63629-1792-05**	93.78		
10s ea	**63629-1792-01**	156.30		
30s ea	**63629-1792-03**	468.90		
(Core)				
REPACK				
TAB, PO, 50 mg, 5s ea	**33358-0355-05**	81.64		
10s ea	**33358-0355-10**	150.65		
30s ea	**33358-0355-30**	475.93		
100 mg, 2s ea	**33358-0356-02**	32.04		
5s ea	**33358-0356-05**	80.10		
6s ea	**33358-0356-06**	96.12		
10s ea	**33358-0356-10**	160.21		
30s ea	**33358-0356-30**	480.62		
60s ea	**33358-0356-60**	808.01		
(Dispensing Solutions)				
REPACK				
TAB, PO, 100 mg, 30s ea	**55045-2581-08**	550.00		
(Nucare Pharm)				
REPACK				
TAB, PO, 100 mg, 10s ea	**66267-0406-10**	120.00		
(Palmetto)				
REPACK				
TAB, PO, 25 mg, 3s ea	**23490-9380-00**	56.25		
6s ea	**23490-9380-01**	112.50		
10s ea	**23490-9380-02**	187.50		
12s ea	**23490-9380-03**	225.00		
15s ea	**23490-9380-04**	281.25		
20s ea	**23490-9380-05**	375.00		
50 mg, 3s ea	**23490-9381-00**	56.25		
6s ea	**23490-9381-01**	112.50		
10s ea	**23490-9381-02**	187.50		
12s ea	**23490-9381-03**	225.00		
15s ea	**23490-9381-04**	281.25		
20s ea	**23490-9381-05**	375.00		
100 mg, 3s ea	**23490-9382-00**	56.25		
6s ea	**23490-9382-01**	112.50		
10s ea	**23490-9382-02**	187.50		
12s ea	**23490-9382-03**	225.00		
15s ea	**23490-9382-04**	281.25		
20s ea	**23490-9382-05**	375.00		
(PD-Rx Pharm)				
REPACK				
TAB, PO, 50 mg, 10s ea	**58864-0862-10**	143.10		
20s ea	**55289-0577-20**	519.98		
100 mg, 10s ea	**55289-0524-10**	260.00		
(Phys Total Care)				
REPACK				
TAB, PO, 50 mg, 5s ea	**54868-4084-00**	112.23		
6s ea	**54868-4084-03**	134.15		
10s ea	**54868-4084-01**	209.66		
30s ea	**54868-4084-02**	603.07		
100 mg, 2s ea	**54868-4706-06**	50.41		
4s ea	**54868-4706-03**	98.20		
5s ea	**54868-4706-01**	122.10		
6s ea	**54868-4706-04**	145.99		
10s ea	**54868-4706-02**	228.30		
15s ea	**54868-4706-00**	341.15		
30s ea	**54868-4706-05**	657.19		
(Physician Partner)				
REPACK				
TAB, PO, 50 mg, 15s ea	**21695-0157-15**	506.19		
30s ea	**21695-0157-30**	1049.48		
100 mg, 30s ea	**21695-0158-30**	1049.48		
(Quality Care Prod)				
REPACK				
TAB, PO, 25 mg, 15s ea	**35356-0340-15**	489.14		
50 mg, 30s ea	**49999-0642-30**	576.32		
100 mg, 15s ea	**49999-0316-15**	250.20		
30s ea	**49999-0316-30**	576.32		
(Southwood)				
REPACK				
TAB, PO, 50 mg, 30s ea	**58016-0355-30**	450.23		
60s ea	**58016-0355-60**	900.46		
90s ea	**58016-0355-90**	1350.69		
100s ea	**58016-0355-00**	1500.77		
100 mg, 30s ea	**58016-0371-30**	450.23		
60s ea	**58016-0371-60**	900.46		
90s ea	**58016-0371-90**	1350.68		
100s ea	**58016-0371-00**	1500.76		

PROD/MFR	NDC	AWP	DP	OBC
(Stat Rx)				
REPACK				
TAB, PO, 50 mg, 5s ea	16590-0525-05	75.00		
8s ea	16590-0525-08	120.00		
10s ea	16590-0525-10	205.43		
20s ea	16590-0525-20	259.00		
30s ea	16590-0525-30	374.00		
60s ea	16590-0525-60	725.00		
100 mg, 8s ea	16590-0524-08	120.00		
10s ea	16590-0524-10	142.00		
20s ea	16590-0524-20	353.89		
30s ea	16590-0524-30	374.00		
60s ea	16590-0524-60	725.00		
VIAL, MEDICATION				
(APP) *See EMPTY STERILIZED VIAL*				
VIASPAN COLD STORAGE/FLUSHING (Teva)				
device				
DEV, NA (ORGAN BAG)				
1000 ml 10s	01000-0046-06	3882.95		
VIBATIV (Astellas)				
telavancin hydrochloride				
PDS, IV (PF)				
250 mg, 10s ea	00469-3525-30	600.00		
750 mg, 10s ea	00469-3575-50	1800.00		
VIBRA-TABS (Pfizer)				
doxycycline hyclate				
TAB, PO, 100 mg, 50s ea	00069-0990-50	328.20	273.50	AB
VIBRAMYCIN CALCIUM (Pfizer)				
doxycycline calcium				
SYR, PO, 50 mg/5 ml,				
480 ml	00069-0971-93	308.89	257.41	
VIBRAMYCIN HYCLATE (Pfizer)				
doxycycline hyclate				
CAP, PO, 100 mg, 50s ea	00069-0950-50	328.20	273.50	AB
(PD-Rx Pharm)				
REPACK				
CAP, PO, 100 mg, 14s ea	55289-0043-14	105.00		AB
VIBRAMYCIN MONOHYDRATE (Pfizer)				
doxycycline				
PDR, PO, 25 mg/5 ml,				
60 ml	00069-0970-65	25.30	21.08	
VICA-FORTE (Qualitest)				
multivitamin and minerals				
CAP, PO, 100s ea	00603-6381-21	12.87		
VICAP FORTE (Major)				
multivitamin and minerals				
CAP, PO, 100s ea	00904-0304-60	14.00		
(A-S Medication)				
REPACK				
CAP, PO, 100s ea	54569-6073-00	14.00		
VICODIN (Abbott Pharm)				
acetaminophen/hydrocodone bitartrate				
TAB, PO, 500 mg-5 mg,				
100s ea, C-III	00074-1949-14	130.94	114.86	AA
(R.N.P.,4X25)				
500 mg-5 mg,				
100s ea UD, C-III	00074-1949-12	155.80	129.83	AA
500s ea, C-III	00074-1949-54	609.12	534.32	AA
(A-S Medication)				
REPACK				
TAB, PO, 500 mg-5 mg,				
16s ea, C-III	54569-0032-02	20.59		AA
20s ea, C-III	54569-0032-05	25.74		AA
(Dispensing Solutions)				
REPACK				
TAB, PO, 500 mg-5 mg,				
15s ea, C-III	55045-2464-05	17.25		AA
(PD-Rx Pharm)				
REPACK				
TAB, PO, 500 mg-5 mg,				
12s ea, C-III	55289-0116-12	24.30		AA
(Phys Total Care)				
REPACK				
TAB, PO, 500 mg-5 mg,				
10s ea, C-III	54868-0982-02	16.55		AA
30s ea, C-III	54868-0982-01	44.42		AA
100s ea, C-III	54868-0982-00	134.22		AA
(Quality Care Prod)				
REPACK				
TAB, PO, 500 mg-5 mg,				
30s ea, C-III	49999-0051-30	41.70		AA
(Southwood)				
REPACK				
TAB, PO, 500 mg-5 mg,				
30s ea, C-III	58016-0063-30	42.03		AA
60s ea, C-III	58016-0063-60	84.07		AA
90s ea, C-III	58016-0063-90	126.10		AA
100s ea, C-III	58016-0063-00	140.11		AA
VICODIN ES (Abbott Pharm)				
acetaminophen/hydrocodone bitartrate				
TAB, PO (R.N.P.,4X25)				
750 mg-7.5 mg,				
100s ea UD, C-III	00074-1973-12	171.89	143.24	AA
100s ea UD, C-III	00074-1973-14	144.38	126.65	AA
500s ea, C-III	00074-1973-54	676.21	593.17	AA
(A-S Medication)				
REPACK				
TAB, PO, 750 mg-7.5 mg,				
15s ea, C-III	54569-2736-05	20.29		AA
20s ea, C-III	54569-2736-01	27.05		AA
30s ea, C-III	54569-2736-02	42.57		AA
(Phys Total Care)				
REPACK				
TAB, PO, 750 mg-7.5 mg,				
30s ea, C-III	54868-3031-00	48.71		AA
100s ea, C-III	54868-3031-01	147.73		AA
120s ea, C-III	54868-3031-02	176.75		AA
(Quality Care Prod)				
REPACK				
TAB, PO, 750 mg-7.5 mg,				
30s ea, C-III	35356-0553-30	102.20		AA
VICODIN HP (Abbott Pharm)				
acetaminophen/hydrocodone bitartrate				
TAB, PO, 660 mg-10 mg,				
100s ea, C-III	00074-2274-14	170.95	149.96	AA
500s ea, C-III	00074-2274-54	764.40	670.53	AA
(Pharma Pac)				
REPACK				
TAB, PO, 660 mg-10 mg,				
20s ea, C-III	52959-0513-20	22.75		AA
(Phys Total Care)				
REPACK				
TAB, PO, 660 mg-10 mg,				
100s ea, C-III	54868-4940-01	111.86		AA
120s ea, C-III	54868-4940-00	133.74		AA
(Quality Care Prod)				
REPACK				
TAB, PO, 660 mg-10 mg,				
60s ea, C-III	35356-0402-60	205.46		AA
(Southwood)				
REPACK				
TAB, PO, 660 mg-10 mg,				
30s ea, C-III	58016-0096-30	46.12		
60s ea, C-III	58016-0096-60	92.24		
90s ea, C-III	58016-0096-90	138.37		
100s ea, C-III	58016-0096-00	153.74		
VICOPROFEN (Abbott Pharm)				
hydrocodone bitartrate/ibuprofen				
TAB, PO, 7.5 mg-200 mg,				
100s ea, C-III	00074-2277-14	261.38	229.28	
(4X25)				
7.5 mg-200 mg,				
100s ea UD, C-III	00074-2277-12	300.61	250.51	
500s ea, C-III	00074-2277-54	1215.41	1066.15	
(A-S Medication)				
REPACK				
TAB, PO, 7.5 mg-200 mg,				
15s ea, C-III	54569-4806-00	38.53		
(Dispensing Solutions)				
REPACK				
TAB, PO, 7.5 mg-200 mg,				
12s ea, C-III	55045-2522-06	20.45		
20s ea, C-III	55045-2522-07	25.45		
100s ea, C-III	55045-2522-00	127.00		
(Nucare Pharm)				
REPACK				
TAB, PO, 7.5 mg-200 mg,				
12s ea, C-III	66267-0320-12	18.99		
30s ea, C-III	66267-0320-30	41.99		
(PD-Rx Pharm)				
REPACK				
TAB, PO, 7.5 mg-200 mg,				
15s ea, C-III	55289-0348-15	54.98		
(Pharma Pac)				
REPACK				
TAB, PO, 7.5 mg-200 mg,				
12s ea, C-III	52959-0522-12	24.08		
15s ea, C-III	52959-0522-15	29.90		
20s ea, C-III	52959-0522-20	36.34		
30s ea, C-III	52959-0522-30	48.29		
40s ea, C-III	52959-0522-40	62.73		
(Phys Total Care)				
REPACK				
TAB, PO, 7.5 mg-200 mg,				
15s ea, C-III	54868-4035-03	53.16		
20s ea, C-III	54868-4035-01	69.80		
30s ea, C-III	54868-4035-00	103.06		
60s ea, C-III	54868-4035-04	191.76		
100s ea, C-III	54868-4035-02	317.43		
(Southwood)				
REPACK				
TAB, PO, 7.5 mg-200 mg,				
2s ea, C-III	58016-0422-02	2.30		
15s ea, C-III	58016-0422-15	17.25		
20s ea, C-III	58016-0422-20	23.00		
30s ea, C-III	58016-0422-30	34.50		
40s ea, C-III	58016-0422-40	46.00		
60s ea, C-III	58016-0422-60	69.00		
VICTOZA (Novo Nordisk)				
liraglutide				
SOL, SC, 6 mg/ml,				
3 ml 2s	00169-4060-12	288.96		
3 ml 3s	00169-4060-13	433.44		
VIDARABINE (Medisca)				
POW, NA (1X1GM,USP)				
1 gm	38779-2206-06	555.00		
(1X5GM,USP)				
5 gm	38779-2206-03	1797.00		
(PCCA)				
POW, NA, 1 gm	51927-2961-00	645.00		
(USP)				
1 gm	51927-3632-00	687.00		
VIDAZA (Celgene Corp)				
azacitidine				
PDR, IJ, 100 mg, ea	59572-0102-01	573.88		
VIDEX (Phys Total Care)				
REPACK				
didanosine				
CTB, PO (MANDARIN ORANGE)				
100 mg, 60s ea	54868-2502-00	170.84		
VIDEX EC (B/M Squibb Onc/Vir)				
didanosine				
ECC, PO, 125 mg, 30s ea	00087-6671-17	133.61		
200 mg, 30s ea	00087-6672-17	213.74		
250 mg, 30s ea	00087-6673-17	272.39		
400 mg, 30s ea	00087-6674-17	425.42		
(A-S Medication)				
REPACK				
ECC, PO, 250 mg, 30s ea	54569-5504-00	340.48		
(Phys Total Care)				
REPACK				
ECC, PO, 250 mg, 30s ea	54868-5595-00	270.38		
400 mg, 30s ea	54868-4666-00	408.01		
(Quality Care Prod)				
REPACK				
ECC, PO, 400 mg, 30s ea	35356-0186-30	596.60		
VIDEX PEDIATRIC (B/M Squibb Onc/Vir)				
didanosine				
PDR, PO, 10 mg/ml,				
100 ml	00087-6632-41	54.84		
200 ml	00087-6633-41	119.72		
VIGABATRIN				
(Lundbeck) *See SABRIL*				
VIGAMOX (Alcon Ophthalmic)				
moxifloxacin hydrochloride				
SOL, OP (DROP-TAINER)				
0.5%, 3 ml	00065-4013-03	81.66		
(A-S Medication)				
REPACK				
SOL, OP, 0.5%, 3 ml	54569-5561-00	97.42		
(Dispensing Solutions)				
REPACK				
SOL, OP, 0.5%, 3 ml	55045-3267-03	69.00		
(Pharma Pac)				
REPACK				
SOL, OP, 0.5%, 3 ml	52959-0877-03	79.87		
(Phys Total Care)				
REPACK				
SOL, OP (DROP-TAINER)				
0.5%, 3 ml	54868-4798-00	104.32		
(Quality Care Prod)				
REPACK				
SOL, OP, 0.5%, 3 ml	49999-0712-03	112.61		
(Stat Rx)				
REPACK				
SOL, OP, 0.5%, 3 ml	16590-0355-03	87.00		

PROD/MFR	NDC	AWP	DP	OBC
VIMPAT (UCB)				
lacosamide				
SOL, IV, 10 mg/ml,				
20 ml 10s, C-V	00131-1810-67	420.00		
TAB, PO (FILM-COATED)				
50 mg, 60s ea, C-V	00131-2477-35	280.39		
100 mg, 60s ea, C-V	00131-2478-35	438.36		
150 mg, 60s ea, C-V	00131-2479-35	464.26		
200 mg, 60s ea, C-V	00131-2480-35	464.40		
(Phys Total Care)				
REPACK				
TAB, PO (FILM-COATED)				
50 mg, 60s ea, C-V	54868-6077-00	305.82		
(Quality Care Prod)				
REPACK				
TAB, PO (FILM-COATED)				
50 mg, 60s ea, C-V	35356-0532-60	421.32		
VINACAL (Breckenridge Pharm)				
prenatal vitamins				
TAB, PO (FILM-COATED)				
90s ea	51991-0617-90	96.92		
VINATAL FORTE (Breckenridge Pharm)				
prenatal vitamins				
TAB, PO (FILM COATED)				
90s ea	51991-0357-90	58.57		
VINATE AZ (Breckenridge Pharm)				
prenatal vitamins				
TAB, PO (FILM COATED)				
90s ea	51991-0466-90	55.07		
VINATE AZ EXTRA (Breckenridge Pharm)				
prenatal vitamins				
TAB, PO (FILM-COATED)				
90s ea	51991-0514-90	55.07		
VINATE C (Breckenridge Pharm)				
prenatal vitamins				
TAB, PO (FILM-COATED)				
30s ea	51991-0581-33	34.75		
VINATE CALCIUM (Breckenridge Pharm)				
prenatal vitamins				
TAB, PO (FILM-COATED)				
100s ea	51991-0469-01	42.26		
VINATE CARE (Breckenridge Pharm)				
prenatal vitamins				
CTB, PO, 30s ea	51991-0576-33	34.75		
VINATE GT (Breckenridge Pharm)				
prenatal vitamins				
TAB, PO, 90s ea	51991-0159-90	32.55		
(9X10) 90s ea	51991-0159-91	32.55		
VINATE IC (Breckenridge Pharm)				
prenatal vitamins				
CAP, PO, 90s ea	51991-0530-90	46.59		
VINATE II (Breckenridge Pharm)				
prenatal vitamins				
TAB, PO (DAIRY-FREE,GLUTEN-FREE)				
100s ea	51991-0178-01	36.67		
VINATE III (Breckenridge Pharm)				
prenatal vitamins				
TAB, PO (FILM-COATED)				
100s ea	51991-0378-01	52.38		
VINATE M (Breckenridge Pharm)				
prenatal vitamins				
TAB, PO, 100s ea	51991-0155-01	25.95		
VINATE ONE (Breckenridge Pharm)				
prenatal vitamins				
TAB, PO (FILM-COATED)				
100s ea	51991-0566-01	28.78		
VINATE PN CARE (Breckenridge Pharm)				
prenatal vitamins				
TAB, PO (FILM-COATED)				
30s ea	51991-0584-33	36.94		
VINATE ULTRA (Breckenridge Pharm)				
prenatal vitamins				
TAB, PO (10X10)				
100s ea UD	51991-0154-11	24.95		
(FILM-COATED) 100s ea	51991-0154-01	25.95		
VINBLASTINE SULFATE (APP)				
SOL, IV (M.D.V.)				
1 mg/ml, 10 ml	63323-0278-10	43.23		
(Bedford)				
PDS, IV (VIAL)				
10 mg, 10s ea	55390-0091-10	115.20		AP
VINCAMINE (PCCA)				
POW, NA, 1 gm	51927-2533-00	204.00		
VINCRISTINE SULFATE (Hospira)				
SOL, IV (S.D.V.,PF)				
1 mg/ml, 1 ml	61703-0309-06	9.50	8.32	AP
2 ml	61703-0309-16	13.48	11.79	AP
(Teva)				
SOL, IV (S.D.V.)				
1 mg/ml, 1 ml	00703-4402-11	18.06		AP
2 ml	00703-4412-11	36.12		AP
VINORELBINE (Parenta Pharma)				
vinorelbine tartrate				
SOL, IV (1X1ML,PF)				
10 mg/ml, 1 ml	66758-0045-01	57.89		AP
(1X5ML,PF) 10 mg/ml, 5 ml	66758-0045-02	289.41		AP
VINORELBINE TARTRATE (APP)				
SOL, IV (USP,PF)				
10 mg/ml, 1 ml	63323-0148-01	94.00		
5 ml	63323-0148-05	470.25		
(Bedford)				
SOL, IV (S.D.V.,PF)				
10 mg/ml, 1 ml	55390-0069-01	36.48		AP
5 ml	55390-0070-01	182.40		AP
(Bedford) *See VINORELBINE TARTRATE AMERINET CHOICE*				
(Hospira)				
SOL, IV (S.D.V.,PF)				
10 mg/ml, 1 ml	61703-0341-06	25.02	21.89	AP
5 ml	61703-0341-09	76.80	67.20	AP
(Parenta Pharma) *See VINORELBINE*				
(Pierre Fabre) *See AMERINET CHOICE VINORELBINE TARTRATE*				
(Pierre Fabre) *See NAVELBINE*				
(Teva)				
SOL, IV (PF)				
10 mg/ml, 1 ml	00703-4182-81	42.60		AP
1 ml	00703-4182-91	44.38		AP
(S.D.V.,PF) 10 mg/ml, 1 ml	00703-4182-01	44.38		AP
(PF) 10 mg/ml, 5 ml	00703-4183-81	208.20		AP
5 ml	00703-4183-91	138.00		AP
(S.D.V.,PF) 10 mg/ml, 5 ml	00703-4183-01	138.00		AP
VINORELBINE TARTRATE AMERINET CHOICE (Bedford)				
vinorelbine tartrate				
SOL, IV (S.D.V.,PF,PRIVATE LABEL)				
10 mg/ml, 1 ml	55390-0267-01	90.30		AP
5 ml	55390-0268-01	451.50		AP
VINPOCETINE (PCCA)				
POW, NA, 1 gm	51927-3226-00	52.80		
VIOKASE (Axcan)				
amylase/lipase/protease				
TAB, PO, 30000 u-8000 u-30000 u,				
100s ea	58914-0111-10	93.30		
VIOKASE 16 (Axcan)				
amylase/lipase/protease				
TAB, PO, 60000 u-16000 u-60000 u,				
100s ea	58914-0116-10	169.38		
VIOLET FOOD COLOR (PCCA)				
color additive				
POW, NA, 1 gm	51927-1735-00	6.50		
VIRACEPT (Pfizer)				
nelfinavir mesylate				
PDR, PO, 50 mg/gm,				
144 gm	63010-0011-90	70.02	58.35	
TAB, PO (FILM-COATED)				
250 mg, 300s ea	63010-0010-30	796.99	664.16	
625 mg, 120s ea	63010-0027-70	796.99	664.16	
(A-S Medication)				
REPACK				
TAB, PO (FILM-COATED)				
250 mg, 300s ea	54569-4543-03	1036.09		
625 mg, 120s ea	54569-5573-00	830.20		
(Dispensing Solutions)				
REPACK				
TAB, PO (FILM-COATED)				
250 mg, 30s ea	55045-2682-08	90.00		
63s ea	55045-2682-06	189.00		
(Nucare Pharm)				
REPACK				
TAB, PO (FILM-COATED)				
250 mg, 18s ea	66267-0514-18	57.37		
63s ea	66267-0514-63	189.39		
(PD-Rx Pharm)				
REPACK				
TAB, PO (FILM-COATED)				
250 mg, 27s ea	55289-0477-27	106.61		
(Pharma Pac)				
REPACK				
TAB, PO (FILM-COATED)				
250 mg, 30s ea	52959-0289-30	109.90		
(Phys Total Care)				
REPACK				
TAB, PO (CAPLET)				
250 mg, 270s ea	54868-3947-00	729.85		
(Quality Care Prod)				
REPACK				
TAB, PO (FILM-COATED)				
250 mg, 300s ea	49999-0431-03	1196.13		
625 mg, 120s ea	35356-0117-01	1348.42		
(Southwood)				
REPACK				
TAB, PO, 625 mg, 30s ea	58016-0455-30	188.86		
60s ea	58016-0455-60	377.73		
90s ea	58016-0455-90	566.59		
100s ea	58016-0455-00	629.54		
120s ea	58016-0455-02	755.45		
(St. Mary's MPP)				
REPACK				
TAB, PO (CAPLET)				
250 mg, 18s ea	60760-0010-18	55.94		
63s ea	60760-0010-63	180.79		
VIRAMUNE (Boehr Ingelheim Phar)				
nevirapine				
SUS, PO, 50 mg/5 ml,				
240 ml	00597-0047-24	118.50		
TAB, PO, 200 mg, 60s ea	00597-0046-60	547.20		
(A-S Medication)				
REPACK				
TAB, PO, 200 mg, 60s ea	54569-4561-00	711.36		
(PD-Rx Pharm)				
REPACK				
TAB, PO, 200 mg, 3s ea	55289-0392-03	33.97		
(Phys Total Care)				
REPACK				
TAB, PO, 200 mg, 60s ea	54868-3844-01	537.11		
100s ea	54868-3844-00	875.55		
(Quality Care Prod)				
REPACK				
TAB, PO, 200 mg, 6s ea	35356-0071-06	115.69		
60s ea	35356-0071-60	1193.40		
VIRAMUNE O/S (Quality Care Prod)				
nevirapine				
SUS, PO (1X240ML)				
50 mg/5 ml, 240 ml	35356-0072-24	121.00		
VIRAZOLE (Valeant Pharm Intl)				
ribavirin				
PDS, IH, 6 gm, 4s ea	00187-0007-14	18800.86		
VIREAD (Gilead Sciences)				
tenofovir disoproxil fumarate				
TAB, PO, 300 mg, 30s ea	61958-0401-01	771.54		
(A-S Medication)				
REPACK				
TAB, PO, 300 mg, 30s ea	54569-5334-00	929.58		
(Phys Total Care)				
REPACK				
TAB, PO, 300 mg, 30s ea	54868-4669-00	588.36		
(Quality Care Prod)				
REPACK				
TAB, PO, 300 mg, 6s ea	35356-0073-06	246.92		
30s ea	35356-0073-30	1234.60		
VIRILEX (Physician Thera, LLC)				
amino acids and nutriceuticals				
CAP, PO (PF,DYE-FREE,STARCH-FREE)				
60s ea	68405-1006-02	126.72		
(Altura)				
REPACK				
CAP, PO, 60s ea	63874-1185-06	104.50		
VIROPTIC (Monarch)				
trifluridine				
SOL, OP, 1%, 7.5 ml	61570-0037-75	153.91		AT

PROD/MFR	NDC	AWP	DP	OBC
(Phys Total Care)				
REPACK				
SOL, OP, 1%, 7.5 ml	**54868-1175-00**	124.10		**AT**
(Southwood)				
REPACK				
SOL, OP, 1%, 7.5 ml	**58016-6459-01**	143.84		**AT**
VISCOAT (Alcon Surgical)				
chondroitin sulfate/hyaluronate sodium				
SOL, OP (SRN)				
40 mg/ml-30 mg/ml,				
0.5 ml	**08065-1839-05**	142.44		
0.75 ml	**08065-1839-75**	187.14		
VISICOL (Salix Pharm)				
na phos, dibasic/na phos, monobasic				
TAB, PO (USP,GLUTEN-FREE)				
0.398 gm-1.102 gm,				
40s ea	**65649-0601-04**	181.96		
100s ea	**65649-0601-41**	454.85		
(Phys Total Care)				
REPACK				
TAB, PO, 0.398 gm-1.102 gm,				
40s ea	**54868-5396-00**	87.58		
VISIONBLUE (Dutch Ophthalmic USA)				
trypan blue				
SOL, IO, 0.06%,				
0.5 ml 10s	**68803-0612-01**	460.00		
VISIPAQUE (GE)				
iodixanol				
SOL, IJ (10X50ML,PF)				
55%, 50 ml 10s	**00407-2222-05**	733.75		
(PLUSPAK,10X50ML,PF)				
55%, 50 ml 10s	**00407-2222-16**	657.19		
(VIAL)				
55%, 50 ml 10s	**00407-2222-01**	566.83		
(BOTTLE)				
55%, 100 ml 10s	**00407-2222-02**	1110.61		
(SINGLE UNIT)				
55%, 100 ml 10s	**00407-2222-17**	1143.48		
(REDIFLO,FLS-1,10X125ML)				
55%, 125 ml 10s	**00407-2222-32**	2070.08		
(BOTTLE, 200 ML)				
55%, 150 ml 10s	**00407-2222-03**	1619.82		
(PLASTIC,SINGLEUNITDOSE)				
55%, 150 ml 10s	**00407-2222-19**	1668.48		
(REDIFLO,FLS-1,10X150ML)				
55%, 150 ml 10s	**00407-2222-31**	2356.67		
(PLASTIC,SINGLEUNITDOSE)				
55%, 200 ml 10s	**00407-2222-21**	2022.96		
(PHARMACY BULK PKG)				
55%, 500 ml 6s	**00407-2222-24**	3173.51		
(10X50ML,PF)				
65.2%, 50 ml 10s	**00407-2223-05**	799.06		
50 ml 10s	**00407-2223-06**	694.84		
(PLUSPAK,10X50ML,PF)				
65.2%, 50 ml 10s	**00407-2223-16**	635.80		
(VIAL)				
65.2%, 50 ml 10s	**00407-2223-01**	617.28		
(BOTTLE)				
65.2%, 100 ml 10s	**00407-2223-02**	1234.09		
(PLASTIC,SINGLEUNITDOSE)				
65.2%, 100 ml 10s	**00407-2223-17**	1271.16		
(REDIFLO,FLS-1,10X100ML)				
65.2%, 100 ml 10s	**00407-2223-30**	1922.47		
(REDIFLO,FLS-1,10X125ML)				
65.2%, 125 ml 10s	**00407-2223-32**	2186.76		
(BOTTLE, 200 ML)				
65.2%, 150 ml 10s	**00407-2223-03**	1703.68		
(PLASTIC,SINGLEUNITDOSE)				
65.2%, 150 ml 10s	**00407-2223-19**	1789.97		
(BOTTLE)				
65.2%, 200 ml 10s	**00407-2223-04**	2098.69		
(PLASTIC,SINGLEUNITDOSE)				
65.2%, 200 ml 10s	**00407-2223-21**	2161.68		
(PLUSPAK,PHARMACYBULK)				
65.2%, 500 ml 10s	**00407-2223-23**	5845.30		
VISTACOT (Truxton)				
hydroxyzine hydrochloride				
SOL, IM (VIAL)				
50 mg/ml, 10 ml	**00463-1101-10**	6.30		**EE**
VISTARIL (Pfizer)				
hydroxyzine pamoate				
CAP, PO, 25 mg, 100s ea	**00069-5410-66**	157.46	131.22	**AB**
50 mg, 100s ea	**00069-5420-66**	191.99	159.99	**AB**
(Phys Total Care)				
REPACK				
CAP, PO, 25 mg, 100s ea	**54868-0169-01**	115.18		**AB**
VISTIDE (Gilead Sciences)				
cidofovir				
SOL, IV (S.D.V.,PF)				
75 mg/ml, 5 ml	**61958-0101-01**	888.00		
(Phys Total Care)				
REPACK				
SOL, IV, 75 mg/ml, 5 ml	**54868-3979-00**	982.94		
VISTRA 650 (Vision)				
acetaminophen/phenyltoloxamine citrate				
TAB, PO, 650 mg-60 mg,				
100s ea	**68013-0010-01**	58.21		
VISUDYNE (Novartis Pharm)				
verteporfin				
PDS, IV, 15 mg, ea	**00078-0437-61**	1702.64	1350.00	
VITA #12 (Clint)				
cyanocobalamin				
SOL, IM (VIAL)				
1000 mcg/ml, 10 ml	**55553-0091-10**	4.50		**EE**
30 ml	**55553-0091-30**	5.95		**EE**
VITA S FORTE (Rising)				
multivitamin and minerals				
TAB, PO (CAPLET)				
100s ea	**64980-0102-01**	29.99		
VITA-RESPA (Respa Pharm)				
cyanocobalamin/folic acid/pyridoxine				
TAB, PO, 1.3 mg-2.2 mg-25 mg,				
90s ea	**60575-0913-90**	70.50		
VITABEE 12 (Consolidated Midland)				
cyanocobalamin				
SOL, IM (VIAL)				
1000 mcg/ml, 10 ml	**00223-8870-00**	2.75		**EE**
30 ml	**00223-8870-30**	5.50		**EE**
VITABEE 6 (Consolidated Midland)				
pyridoxine				
SOL, IJ (VIAL)				
100 mg/ml, 10 ml	**00223-8410-10**	7.50		**EE**
VITAFOL (Everett)				
vitamin b complex and iron				
SYR, PO (AF,RASPBERRY MINT)				
473 ml	**00642-0074-16**	57.18		
(Everett)				
multivitamin, minerals, and iron				
TAB, PO (S.F, 10X10,PF,SF,CAPLET)				
100s ea UD	**00642-0072-12**	79.67		
VITAFOL-OB (Everett)				
multivitamin, minerals, and iron				
TAB, PO (10X10,CAPLET)				
100s ea UD	**00642-0079-12**	70.27		
VITAFOL-OB+DHA (Everett)				
prenatal vitamins				
KIT, PO (SF,GLUTEN-FREE)				
ea UD	**00642-0076-30**	48.79		
VITAFOL-PN (Everett)				
prenatal vitamins				
TAB, PO (10X10,CAPLET)				
100s ea UD	**00642-0078-12**	70.35		
VITAL-D (Nephro-Tech)				
multivitamin and minerals				
TAB, PO, 100s ea	**59528-1988-01**	32.00		
VITAMIN A (Consolidated Midland)				
CAP, PO (SOLUBLE)				
50000 u, 100s ea	**00223-1790-01**	5.50		**EE**
1000s ea	**00223-1790-02**	32.50		**EE**
SGL, PO (NATURAL)				
25000 u, 100s ea	**00223-1751-01**	4.50		
(SOLUBLE)				
25000 u, 100s ea	**00223-1750-01**	3.75		
1000s ea	**00223-1751-02**	27.50		
(SOLUBLE)				
25000 u, 1000s ea	**00223-1750-02**	29.50		
(SYNTHETIC)				
25000 u, 1000s ea	**00223-1740-02**	16.75		
(PCCA) *See RETINOL*				
VITAMIN A ACETATE (PCCA)				
GRA, NA (USP; 500,000 U/GM)				
1 gm	**51927-1030-00**	1.17		
(Spectrum Pharmacy)				
GRA, NA (U.S.P.)				
100 gm	**49452-8119-01**	178.15		
(1X500GM)				
500 gm	**49452-8119-02**	598.50		
VITAMIN A PALMITATE				
(Gallipot) *See VITAMIN A PALMITATE IN OIL*				
(Hospira) *See AQUASOL A*				
(Letco) *See VITAMIN A PALMITATE IN OIL*				
(PCCA)				
SOL, NA, 1.7 million iu/gm,				
1 gm	**51927-3124-00**	3.00		
10000 u/ml, 1 ml	**51927-3172-00**	0.80		
18000 u/ml, 1 ml	**51927-1035-00**	0.80		
(Spectrum Pharmacy) *See VITAMIN A PALMITATE IN OIL*				
VITAMIN A PALMITATE IN OIL (Gallipot)				
vitamin a palmitate				
OIL, NA, 100 ml	**51552-0853-05**	196.00	140.00	
(Letco)				
OIL, NA, 100 gm	**62991-1162-01**	87.00		
500 gm	**62991-1162-02**	291.00		
(Spectrum Pharmacy)				
OIL, NA (U.S.P.)				
25 ml	**49452-8117-02**	108.15		
100 ml	**49452-8117-03**	183.05		
VITAMIN B COMPLEX				
(Llorens Pharma Int) *See NEPHRONEX*				
VITAMIN B COMPLEX 100 (Bioniche Pharma)				
dexpanthenol/niacinamide/vit b1/vit b2/vit b6				
SOL, IJ (M.D.V.)				
30 ml	**67457-0146-30**	29.88		
(Truxton)				
SOL, IJ (VIAL)				
30 ml	**00463-1007-30**	9.75		
VITAMIN B COMPLEX AND IRON				
(Clint) *See INFERROUS*				
(Everett) *See VITAFOL*				
VITAMIN B COMPLEX AND MINERAL				
(Consolidated Midland) *See IRON/LIVER EXTRACT/ VITAMINS*				
(Truxton) *See FERBEE*				
VITAMIN B COMPLEX AND VITAMIN C				
(Breckenridge Pharm) *See FOLBEE PLUS*				
(Contract Pharmacal) *See B-PLEX*				
(Cypress Pharm) *See RENA-VITE RX*				
(Cypress Pharm) *See RENAL CAPS*				
(Everett) *See STROVITE*				
(Fleming) *See NEPHROCAPS*				
(Hillestad) *See DIALYVITE*				
(Nnodum) *See VITAROCA*				
(Qualitest) *See THEROBEC*				
(Watson) *See NEPHRO-VITE RX*				
VITAMIN B COMPLEX W/VITAMIN C (Consolidated Midland)				
ascorbic acid/vitamin b complex				
SOL, IJ (VIAL)				
10 ml	**00223-7215-00**	5.50		
VITAMIN B COMPLEX, IRON, AND VITAMIN C				
(Breckenridge Pharm) *See FERREX 150 FORTE PLUS*				
(Breckenridge Pharm) *See MULTIGEN*				
(Breckenridge Pharm) *See MULTIGEN FOLIC*				
(Breckenridge Pharm) *See MULTIGEN PLUS*				
(Centrix) *See MAXARON FORTE*				
(Pamlab) *See NEEVO*				
(Ther-RX) *See CHROMAGEN*				
(Ther-RX) *See CHROMAGEN FA*				
(Ther-RX) *See CHROMAGEN FORTE*				
VITAMIN B COMPLEX, MINERAL, AND VITAMIN C				
(Breckenridge Pharm) *See IVITES RX*				
(Edwards) *See SENILEZOL*				
(Hillestad) *See DIALYVITE 3000*				
(Hillestad) *See DIALYVITE WITH ZINC*				
(Nephro-Tech) *See NEPHPLEX RX*				
(Pamlab) *See DIATX ZN*				
VITAMIN B12 (Truxton)				
cyanocobalamin				
SOL, IM (VIAL)				
100 mcg/ml, 30 ml	**00463-1021-30**	2.20		**EE**
1000 mcg/ml, 30 ml	**00463-1015-30**	2.40		**EE**
(Vita-Rx)				
SOL, IM (VIAL)				
1000 mcg/ml, 10 ml	**49727-0722-10**	1.50		**EE**
30 ml	**49727-0722-30**	2.00		**EE**

PROD/MFR	NDC	AWP	DP	OBC
(Phys Total Care)				
REPACK				
SOL, IM (VIAL)				
1000 mcg/ml, 30 ml	**54868-0762-00**	18.76		EE
VITAMIN B6 (Palmetto)				
REPACK				
pyridoxine				
TAB, PO, 50 mg, 100s ea	**23490-8017-00**	8.66		
VITAMIN C (Neurovites)				
ascorbic acid				
CRY, NA (U.S.P.)				
120 gm	**93595-2041-01**	9.75		
(Phys Total Care)				
REPACK				
SOL, IJ, 500 mg/ml,				
50 ml	**54868-4115-00**	48.58		
VITAMIN D (Breckenridge Pharm)				
ergocalciferol				
SGL, PO (USP,SOFTGEL)				
50000 iu, 100s ea	**51991-0604-01**	197.19		AA
(Consolidated Midland)				
CAP, PO, 25000 iu,				
100s ea	**00223-1970-01**	8.00		
SGL, PO, 50000 iu,				
100s ea	**00223-1971-01**	20.00		EE
(Teva)				
SGL, PO (SOFTGEL)				
50000 iu, 100s ea	**50111-0990-01**	168.57		AA
(DHS, Inc.)				
REPACK				
SGL, PO, 50000 iu,				
12s ea	**55887-0041-12**	18.47		
(Phys Total Care)				
REPACK				
SGL, PO, 50000 iu, 4s ea	**54868-5799-01**	22.58		
10s ea	**54868-5799-00**	51.96		
(SOFTGEL)				
50000 iu, 12s ea	**54868-5799-02**	70.10		AA
20s ea	**54868-5799-03**	87.70		AA
(Quality Care Prod)				
REPACK				
SGL, PO (SOFTGEL)				
50000 iu, 30s ea	**35356-0516-30**	90.60		AA
VITAMIN D3 (Letco)				
cholecalciferol				
LIQ, NA, 100 gm	**62991-1163-03**	118.50		
(PCCA)				
POW, NA (DRY)				
100000 iu/gm, 1 gm	**51927-1371-00**	0.75		
SOL, NA, 1 million iu/gm,				
1 gm	**51927-1033-00**	5.40		
2400 u/ml, 1 ml	**51927-1034-00**	0.80		
VITAMIN E (Amend)				
POW, NA (U.S.P./F.C.C.)				
100 gm	**17317-0628-03**	16.10		
(Spectrum Pharmacy)				
LIQ, NA (U.S.P.)				
100 ml	**49452-8120-01**	100.45		
1000 ml	**49452-8120-02**	570.50		
(Dispensing Solutions)				
REPACK				
vitamin e acetate				
OIL, TP, 28000 iu, 30 ml	**55045-3324-02**	7.50		
VITAMIN E ACETATE (Amend)				
POW, NA (U.S.P./F.C.C.)				
100 gm	**17317-0629-03**	11.50		
1000 gm	**17317-0628-06**	91.00		
1000 gm	**17317-0629-06**	84.00		
(Letco)				
LIQ, NA (U.S.P.)				
100 gm	**62991-1165-02**	43.50		
500 gm	**62991-1165-03**	150.00		
1000 gm	**62991-1165-04**	255.00		
(PCCA)				
LIQ, NA (125 U/ML)				
1 ml	**51927-1036-00**	0.34		
SOL, NA, 1 iu/mg, 1 gm	**51927-1032-00**	1.32		
(PCCA) *See VITAMIN E ACETATE 50% SD*				
(Spectrum Pharmacy)				
LIQ, NA (1X100ML,USP)				
100 ml	**49452-8130-04**	107.10		
(1X1000ML,USP)				
1000 ml	**49452-8130-05**	528.50		
VITAMIN E ACETATE 50% SD (PCCA)				
vitamin e acetate				
POW, NA (500 IU/GM)				
1 gm	**51927-1344-00**	1.20		
VITAMIN E SUCCINATE (Medisca)				
POW, NA (1X25GM,USP)				
25 gm	**38779-1693-04**	52.50		
(1X100GM,USP)				
100 gm	**38779-1693-05**	157.50		
(1X500GM,USP)				
500 gm	**38779-1693-08**	447.00		
VITAMIN K1 (Hospira)				
phytonadione				
SOL, IJ ((AMP)25X0.5ML)				
1 mg/0.5 ml,				
0.5 ml 25s	**00409-9157-01**	165.00	144.50	BP
(AMP, 25X1ML,LATEX-FREE)				
10 mg/ml, 1 ml 25s	**00409-9158-01**	429.60	376.00	BP
(AMP,LATEX-FREE)				
10 mg/ml, 1 ml 25s	**00074-9158-01**	343.80	300.75	BP
(Phys Total Care)				
REPACK				
SOL, IJ (AMP)				
1 mg/0.5 ml,				
0.5 ml 25s	**54868-4434-00**	120.69		BP
VITAROCA (Nnodum)				
vitamin b complex and vitamin c				
TAB, PO, 100s ea	**63044-0141-01**	10.99		
500s ea	**63044-0141-05**	40.99		
VITAROCA PLUS (Nnodum)				
multivitamin and minerals				
TAB, PO, 100s ea	**63044-0152-02**	11.99		
500s ea	**63044-0152-01**	45.99		
VITATAB MV (Breckenridge Pharm)				
multivitamin, minerals, and nutriceuticals				
TAB, PO (FILM-COATED, CAPLET)				
60s ea	**51991-0641-06**	75.76		
VITIS COMPOUND (Weleda)				
homeopathic substance				
TAB, PO, 100s ea	**55946-0405-30**	5.85		
VITRASE (ISTA Pharm.)				
hyaluronidase				
PDS, SC (PF)				
6200 u, ea	**67425-0001-01**	1007.50		
SOL, SC (LYOPHILIZED,OVINE,SDV)				
200 u/ml, 1.2 ml	**67425-0002-10**	49.94		
VITRASERT (Bausch & Lomb Inc.)				
ganciclovir				
IMP, IO, 4.5 mg, ea	**24208-0412-01**	19200.00		
VIVA DHA (JayMac Pharma)				
prenatal vitamins				
SGL, PO (SOFTGEL)				
30s ea	**64661-0080-30**	59.85	40.65	
VIVACTIL (Teva)				
protriptyline hydrochloride				
TAB, PO, 5 mg, 100s ea	**65473-0701-01**	119.55		AB
(USP,FILM-COATED)				
5 mg, 100s ea	**51285-0595-02**	261.64		
10 mg, 100s ea	**65473-0702-01**	173.28		AB
(USP,FILM-COATED)				
10 mg, 100s ea	**51285-0594-02**	379.17		
VIVAGLOBIN (CSL)				
immune globulin				
SOL, SC (1X3ML,SINGLE-USE)				
160 mg/ml, 3 ml	**00053-7596-01**	69.12		
(PF)				
160 mg/ml,				
3 ml 10s	**00053-7596-03**	576.00		
10 ml	**00053-7596-10**	192.00		
10 ml 10s	**00053-7596-15**	1920.00		
20 ml	**00053-7596-20**	384.00		
20 ml 10s	**00053-7596-25**	3840.00		
VIVELLE (Phys Total Care)				
REPACK				
estradiol				
TDM, TD, 0.05 mg/24 hr,				
8s ea	**54868-3795-00**	47.55		AB1
0.1 mg/24 hr,				
8s ea	**54868-3796-00**	38.84		AB1
VIVELLE-DOT (Novartis Pharm)				
estradiol				
TDM, TD (CALENDAR PACK)				
0.025 mg/24 hr,				
8s ea	**00078-0365-42**	60.22		
(3X8 CALENDAR PACK)				
0.025 mg/24 hr,				
24s ea	**00078-0365-45**	180.67		
0.0375 mg/24 hr,				
ea	**00078-0343-62**	7.54		AB1
(CALENDAR PACK)				
0.0375 mg/24 hr,				
8s ea	**00078-0343-42**	60.30		AB1
(3X8 CALENDAR PACK)				
0.0375 mg/24 hr,				
24s ea	**00078-0343-45**	180.89		AB1
0.05 mg/24 hr, ea	**00078-0344-62**	7.61		AB1
(CALENDAR PACK)				
0.05 mg/24 hr,				
8s ea	**00078-0344-42**	60.85		AB1
(3X8 CALENDAR PACK)				
0.05 mg/24 hr,				
24s ea	**00078-0344-45**	182.52		AB1
0.075 mg/24 hr, ea	**00078-0345-62**	7.82		AB1
(CALENDAR PACK)				
0.075 mg/24 hr,				
8s ea	**00078-0345-42**	62.53		AB1
(3X8 CALENDAR PACK)				
0.075 mg/24 hr,				
24s ea	**00078-0345-45**	187.60		AB1
0.1 mg/24 hr, ea	**00078-0346-62**	7.88		AB1
(CALENDAR PACK)				
0.1 mg/24 hr,				
8s ea	**00078-0346-42**	63.08		AB1
(3X8 CALENDAR PACK)				
0.1 mg/24 hr,				
24s ea	**00078-0346-45**	189.25		AB1
(Phys Total Care)				
REPACK				
TDM, TD, 0.0375 mg/24 hr,				
8s ea	**54868-4920-00**	61.63		AB1
0.05 mg/24 hr,				
8s ea	**54868-4242-00**	43.06		AB1
0.075 mg/24 hr,				
8s ea	**54868-4243-00**	73.28		AB1
0.1 mg/24 hr,				
8s ea	**54868-4244-00**	73.91		AB1
VIVITROL (Alkermes, Inc.)				
naltrexone				
GER, IM (W/DILUENT)				
380 mg, ea	**65757-0300-01**	1104.00		
VIVOTIF (Berna)				
typhoid vaccine, live				
CAP, PO (LIVE,ENTERIC-COATED)				
4s ea	**58337-0003-01**	48.25		
(Nucare Pharm)				
REPACK				
CAP, PO (ENTERIC-COATED)				
4s ea	**68071-1339-04**	50.25		
(Quality Care Prod)				
REPACK				
CAP, PO (ENTERIC-COATED)				
4s ea	**49999-0686-04**	38.16		
VIVOTIF BERNA (A-S Medication)				
REPACK				
typhoid vaccine, live				
ECC, PO (LIVE,BLISTER PACK)				
4s ea	**54569-3927-00**	48.25		
(Phys Total Care)				
REPACK				
ECC, PO (LIVE ORAL)				
4s ea	**54868-3954-00**	45.36		
VOLTAREN (Novartis Pharm)				
diclofenac sodium				
ECT, PO, 75 mg, 100s ea	**00028-0264-01**	385.33		AB
SOL, OP (1X5ML)				
0.1%, 5 ml	**00078-0478-61**	78.78		AT
(Dispensing Solutions)				
REPACK				
SOL, OP, 0.1%, 2.5 ml	**55045-2073-02**	50.00		AB
5 ml	**55045-2073-05**	82.00		AB
(PD-Rx Pharm)				
REPACK				
ECT, PO, 75 mg, 15s ea	**55289-0595-15**	51.75		AB
20s ea	**55289-0595-20**	67.13		AB
30s ea	**55289-0595-30**	98.20		AB
(Pharma Pac)				
REPACK				
ECT, PO, 25 mg, 30s ea	**52959-0416-30**	24.25		AB
50 mg, 30s ea	**52959-0161-30**	44.71		AB
42s ea	**52959-0161-42**	57.99		AB
75 mg, 14s ea	**52959-0318-14**	22.86		AB
20s ea	**52959-0318-20**	35.15		AB
30s ea	**52959-0318-30**	51.90		AB
SOL, OP, 0.1%, 2.5 ml	**52959-0594-03**	28.51		AB

PROD/MFR	NDC	AWP	DP	OBC
(Phys Total Care)				
REPACK				
ECT, PO, 50 mg, 30s ea	54868-0896-02	47.67		AB
60s ea	54868-0896-03	96.46		AB
100s ea	54868-0896-01	201.93		AB
75 mg, 30s ea	54868-0897-04	139.41		AB
40s ea	54868-0897-02	175.10		AB
100s ea	54868-0897-05	434.30		AB
SOL, OP, 0.1%, 2.5 ml	54868-2584-02	50.28		AB
5 ml	54868-2584-01	80.63		AB
(Quality Care Prod)				
REPACK				
ECT, PO, 75 mg, 60s ea	35356-0356-60	198.60		AB
SOL, OP, 0.1%, 2.5 ml	49999-0369-25	95.04		AB
(1X5ML)				
0.1%, 5 ml	49999-0369-05	98.47		AB
(Southwood)				
REPACK				
SOL, OP, 0.1%, 2.5 ml	58016-6462-01	48.29		AB
5 ml	58016-6449-01	78.78		AB
VOLTAREN GEL (Endo Pharm)				
diclofenac sodium				
GEL, TP (1X100GM,GEL)				
1%, 100 gm	00067-6215-97	31.51		
(GEL)				
1%, 100 gm	63481-0684-47	31.51		
(3X100GM,GEL)				
1%, 100 gm 3s	00067-6215-93	94.56		
100 gm 3s	63481-0684-03	95.46		
(5X100GM,GEL)				
1%, 100 gm 5s	00067-6215-05	157.60		
100 gm 5s	63481-0684-05	157.60		
(4u)				
REPACK				
GEL, TP (1X100GM,GEL)				
1%, 100 gm	42549-0607-01	46.24		
100 gm	42549-0627-01	46.24		
(A-S Medication)				
REPACK				
GEL, TP (1X100GM,GEL)				
1%, 100 gm	54569-6060-00	28.86		
(Dispensing Solutions)				
REPACK				
GEL, TP (1X100GM,GEL)				
1%, 100 gm	68258-2000-01	26.32		
100 gm	68258-3021-01	44.07		
(Keltman Pharma., Inc.)				
REPACK				
GEL, TP (1X100GM,GEL)				
1%, 100 gm	68387-0456-01	67.35		
(Nucare Pharm)				
REPACK				
GEL, TP (1X100GM,GEL)				
1%, 100 gm	66267-1258-01	49.39		
(3X100 GM,GEL)				
1%, 100 gm 3s	66267-1305-03	103.92		
(Pharma Pac)				
REPACK				
GEL, TP (1X100GM,GEL)				
1%, 100 gm	52959-0601-00	49.90		
(Phys Total Care)				
REPACK				
GEL, TP (1X100GM,GEL)				
1%, 100 gm	54868-5965-00	37.91		
(Physician Partner)				
REPACK				
GEL, TP (1X100GM,GEL)				
1%, 100 gm	21695-0791-00	67.28		
(Quality Care Prod)				
REPACK				
GEL, TP (1X100GM,GEL)				
1%, 100 gm	35356-0187-00	104.60		
(3X100GM,GEL)				
1%, 100 gm 3s	35356-0187-03	313.80		
(5X100GM,GEL)				
1%, 100 gm 5s	35356-0187-05	523.00		
(St. Mary's MPP)				
REPACK				
GEL, TP (GEL)				
1%, 100 gm	60760-0621-00	49.29		
(Stat Rx)				
REPACK				
GEL, TP (1X100GM,GEL)				
1%, 100 gm	16590-0592-01	38.75		

PROD/MFR	NDC	AWP	DP	OBC
VOLTAREN-XR (Novartis Pharm)				
diclofenac sodium				
TER, PO (FILM-COATED)				
100 mg, 100s ea	00078-0446-05	773.28		AB
(Pharma Pac)				
REPACK				
TER, PO, 100 mg, 20s ea	52959-0472-20	62.86		AB
VOLUMEX (Daxor Corp)				
albumin, iodinated i-131				
SOL, IV (S.D.SRN,PREFILLED)				
25 uci/ml, 1 ml	50914-7731-04	325.00	325.00	
VOLUVEN (Hospira)				
sodium chloride/tetrastarch				
SOL, IV (15X500ML,FREEFLEX)				
0.9%-6%,				
500 ml 15s	00409-1029-01	1059.30	926.85	
VOPAC (Athlon Pharm)				
acetaminophen/codeine phosphate				
TAB, PO, 650 mg-30 mg,				
100s ea, C-III	66813-0922-01	61.90		
VORICONAZOLE				
(Pfizer) *See VFEND*				
(Pfizer) *See VFEND I.V.*				
VORINOSTAT				
(Merck) *See ZOLINZA*				
VORTEX VALVED HOLDING CHAMBER (Pari)				
spacer, inhalation				
DEV, NA (NON ELECTROSTATIC)				
ea	83490-0510-01	19.77		
(WITH ADULT (LG) MASK)				
ea	83490-0510-04	27.89		
(WITH CHILD (MED) MASK)				
ea	83490-0510-03	27.89		
(WITH TODDLER (SM) MASK)				
ea	83490-0510-02	27.89		
VOSOL HC (ECR)				
acetic acid/hydrocortisone				
SOL, OT (USP,1X10ML)				
2%-1%, 10 ml	00095-0201-10	215.00		
VOSPIRE (Dava Pharma)				
albuterol sulfate				
TER, PO (COATED)				
4 mg, 100s ea	68774-0600-01	186.23		
8 mg, 100s ea UD	68774-0601-01	349.22		
VOSPIRE ER (Phys Total Care)				
REPACK				
albuterol sulfate				
TER, PO, 4 mg, 20s ea	54868-5542-01	40.51		
60s ea	54868-5542-00	90.51		
VOTRIENT (Glaxo)				
pazopanib hydrochloride				
TAB, PO (FILM-COATED)				
200 mg, 120s ea	00173-0804-09	6595.60		
VUMON (B/M Squibb Onc/Vir)				
teniposide				
SOL, IV (AMP)				
10 mg/ml, 5 ml	00015-3075-19	376.55		
VUSION (Stiefel Labs)				
miconazole nitrate/petrolatum, white/zinc oxide				
OIN, TP, 0.25%-81.35%-15%,				
50 gm	13478-0002-04	230.93		
VYTORIN (Merck/Schering-Plough)				
ezetimibe/simvastatin				
TAB, PO, 10 mg-10 mg,				
30s ea	66582-0311-31	124.16	103.47	
90s ea	66582-0311-54	372.49	310.41	
100s ea UD	66582-0311-28	413.90	344.92	
1000s ea	66582-0311-82	4138.87	3449.06	
10 mg-20 mg,				
30s ea	66582-0312-31	124.16	103.47	EE
90s ea	66582-0312-54	372.49	310.41	EE
100s ea UD	66582-0312-28	413.90	344.92	EE
1000s ea	66582-0312-82	4138.87	3449.06	EE
10000s ea	66582-0312-87	41388.73	34490.61	EE
10 mg-40 mg,				
30s ea	66582-0313-31	124.16	103.47	EE
50s ea UD	66582-0313-52	206.94	172.45	EE
90s ea	66582-0313-54	372.49	310.41	EE
500s ea	66582-0313-74	2069.44	1724.53	EE
5000s ea	66582-0313-86	20694.36	17245.30	EE
10 mg-80 mg,				
30s ea	66582-0315-31	124.16	103.47	
50s ea UD	66582-0315-52	206.94	172.45	
90s ea	66582-0315-54	372.49	310.41	
500s ea	66582-0315-74	2069.44	1724.53	
2500s ea	66582-0315-66	10347.17	8622.64	

PROD/MFR	NDC	AWP	DP	OBC
(A-S Medication)				
REPACK				
TAB, PO, 10 mg-10 mg,				
30s ea	54569-5768-00	153.01		
10 mg-20 mg,				
30s ea	54569-5766-00	153.01		EE
10 mg-40 mg,				
30s ea	54569-5648-00	153.01		EE
(DHS, Inc.)				
REPACK				
TAB, PO, 10 mg-20 mg,				
30s ea	55887-0882-30	189.60		
10 mg-40 mg,				
30s ea	55887-0333-30	149.95		
(PD-Rx Pharm)				
REPACK				
TAB, PO, 10 mg-20 mg,				
21s ea	55289-0980-21	108.51		EE
10 mg-40 mg,				
30s ea	55289-0280-30	174.93		EE
10 mg-80 mg,				
30s ea	55289-0520-30	155.01		
(Phys Total Care)				
REPACK				
TAB, PO, 10 mg-10 mg,				
30s ea	54868-5250-00	148.95		
10 mg-20 mg,				
15s ea	54868-5187-02	80.43		EE
30s ea	54868-5187-00	148.95		
90s ea	54868-5187-01	442.92		
10 mg-40 mg,				
30s ea	54868-5189-00	148.95		
90s ea	54868-5189-01	442.92		EE
10 mg-80 mg,				
30s ea	54868-5259-00	141.29		
90s ea	54868-5259-01	420.61		
(Quality Care Prod)				
REPACK				
TAB, PO, 10 mg-20 mg,				
30s ea	49999-0957-30	193.22		EE
10 mg-40 mg,				
30s ea	49999-0958-30	193.22		EE
VYVANSE (Shire US Inc.)				
lisdexamfetamine dimesylate				
CAP, PO, 20 mg,				
100s ea, C-II	59417-0102-10	501.79	418.16	EE
30 mg,				
100s ea, C-II	59417-0103-10	501.79	418.16	
40 mg,				
100s ea, C-II	59417-0104-10	501.79	418.16	EE
50 mg,				
100s ea, C-II	59417-0105-10	501.79	418.16	
60 mg,				
100s ea, C-II	59417-0106-10	501.79	418.16	EE
70 mg,				
100s ea, C-II	59417-0107-10	501.79	418.16	
(Phys Total Care)				
REPACK				
CAP, PO, 30 mg,				
10s ea, C-II	54868-5916-00	62.70		
30s ea, C-II	54868-5916-01	170.46		
40 mg,				
10s ea, C-II	54868-6009-00	62.70		EE
30s ea, C-II	54868-6009-01	170.46		EE
50 mg,				
10s ea, C-II	54868-5827-00	66.81		
30s ea, C-II	54868-5827-01	182.12		
(Quality Care Prod)				
REPACK				
CAP, PO, 30 mg,				
100s ea, C-II	35356-0134-00	696.40		
50 mg,				
100s ea, C-II	35356-0135-00	696.40		
WARFARIN (PD-Rx Pharm)				
REPACK				
warfarin sodium				
TAB, PO, 2 mg, 30s ea	58864-0879-30	11.57		AB
(Southwood)				
REPACK				
TAB, PO, 4 mg, 30s ea	58016-0083-30	19.70		
60s ea	58016-0083-60	39.41		
90s ea	58016-0083-90	59.11		
100s ea	58016-0083-00	65.68		
10 mg, 30s ea	58016-0697-30	27.91		
60s ea	58016-0697-60	55.82		
90s ea	58016-0697-90	83.74		
100s ea	58016-0697-00	93.04		

PROD/MFR	NDC	AWP	DP	OBC
WARFARIN SOD (Core)				
REPACK				
warfarin sodium				
TAB, PO, 2 mg, 100s ea	**33358-0360-00**	90.66		
5 mg, 30s ea	**33358-0361-30**	47.08		
(Physician Partner)				
REPACK				
TAB, PO, 2 mg, 30s ea	**21695-0673-30**	36.53		
WARFARIN SODIUM				
FUL				
TAB, PO, 1 mg, 100s ea		54.03		
2 mg, 100s ea		56.39		
2.5 mg, 100s ea		58.16		
3 mg, 100s ea		58.43		
4 mg, 100s ea		58.56		
5 mg, 100s ea		58.97		
6 mg, 100s ea		83.64		
7.5 mg, 100s ea		86.49		
10 mg, 100s ea		89.70		
(Bristol-Myers) *See COUMADIN*				
(PCCA)				
POW, NA (CLATHRATE FORM)				
1 gm	**51927-2471-00**	21.00		
(Taro)				
TAB, PO, 1 mg, 100s ea	**51672-4027-01**	60.81		AB
1000s ea	**51672-4027-03**	583.83		AB
(USP)				
1 mg, 5000s ea	**51672-4027-07**	2919.15		AB
2 mg, 100s ea	**51672-4028-01**	63.45		AB
1000s ea	**51672-4028-03**	609.23		AB
(USP)				
2 mg, 5000s ea	**51672-4028-07**	3046.15		AB
2.5 mg, 100s ea	**51672-4029-01**	65.41		AB
1000s ea	**51672-4029-03**	627.95		AB
(USP)				
2.5 mg, 5000s ea	**51672-4029-07**	3139.75		AB
3 mg, 100s ea	**51672-4030-01**	65.69		AB
1000s ea	**51672-4030-03**	630.72		AB
(USP)				
3 mg, 5000s ea	**51672-4030-07**	3153.60		AB
4 mg, 100s ea	**51672-4031-01**	65.86		AB
1000s ea	**51672-4031-03**	632.38		AB
(USP)				
4 mg, 5000s ea	**51672-4031-07**	3161.90		AB
5 mg, 100s ea	**51672-4032-01**	67.43		AB
1000s ea	**51672-4032-03**	640.59		AB
(USP)				
5 mg, 5000s ea	**51672-4032-07**	3202.95		AB
6 mg, 100s ea	**51672-4033-01**	92.33		AB
1000s ea	**51672-4033-03**	877.14		AB
7.5 mg, 100s ea	**51672-4034-01**	95.53		AB
1000s ea	**51672-4034-03**	907.54		AB
10 mg, 100s ea	**51672-4035-01**	99.74		AB
1000s ea	**51672-4035-03**	967.48		AB
(Teva)				
TAB, PO, 1 mg, 100s ea	**00555-0831-02**	58.34		AB
1000s ea	**00555-0831-05**	583.83		AB
2 mg, 100s ea	**00555-0869-02**	60.89		AB
1000s ea	**00555-0869-05**	609.23		AB
2.5 mg, 100s ea	**00555-0832-02**	62.84		AB
1000s ea	**00555-0832-05**	627.95		AB
3 mg, 100s ea	**00555-0925-02**	63.07		AB
4 mg, 100s ea	**00555-0874-02**	63.25		AB
1000s ea	**00555-0874-05**	632.38		AB
5 mg, 100s ea	**00555-0833-02**	63.68		AB
1000s ea	**00555-0833-05**	636.81		AB
6 mg, 100s ea	**00555-0926-02**	90.30		AB
7.5 mg, 100s ea	**00555-0834-02**	93.44		AB
10 mg, 100s ea	**00555-0835-02**	96.91		AB
(Upsher-Smith) *See JANTOVEN*				
(Zydus Pharm.)				
TAB, PO (USP)				
1 mg, 100s ea	**68382-0052-01**	58.88		AB
1000s ea	**68382-0052-10**	583.83		AB
2 mg, 100s ea	**68382-0053-01**	63.40		AB
1000s ea	**68382-0053-10**	609.23		AB
2.5 mg, 100s ea	**68382-0064-01**	64.50		AB
1000s ea	**68382-0064-10**	627.95		AB
3 mg, 100s ea	**68382-0054-01**	65.40		AB
1000s ea	**68382-0054-10**	630.72		AB
4 mg, 100s ea	**68382-0055-01**	65.50		AB
1000s ea	**68382-0055-10**	632.38		AB
5 mg, 100s ea	**68382-0056-01**	66.80		AB
1000s ea	**68382-0056-10**	640.58		AB
6 mg, 100s ea	**68382-0057-01**	92.30		AB
7.5 mg, 100s ea	**68382-0058-01**	94.69		AB
(USP,DYE-FREE)				
10 mg, 100s ea	**68382-0059-01**	98.56		AB

PROD/MFR	NDC	AWP	DP	OBC
(A-S Medication)				
REPACK				
TAB, PO, 2.5 mg, 30s ea	**54569-5868-00**	19.62		AB
4 mg, 30s ea	**54569-5869-00**	19.76		AB
5 mg, 30s ea	**54569-4934-00**	20.23		AB
60s ea	**54569-4934-01**	40.46		AB
(Aidarex)				
REPACK				
TAB, PO, 1 mg, 7s ea	**33261-0355-07**	7.00		AB
14s ea	**33261-0355-14**	14.00		AB
20s ea	**33261-0355-20**	20.00		AB
21s ea	**33261-0355-21**	21.00		AB
28s ea	**33261-0355-28**	28.00		AB
30s ea	**33261-0355-30**	30.00		AB
60s ea	**33261-0355-60**	60.00		AB
90s ea	**33261-0355-90**	90.00		AB
2 mg, 7s ea	**33261-0356-07**	7.35		AB
14s ea	**33261-0356-14**	14.70		AB
20s ea	**33261-0356-20**	21.00		AB
21s ea	**33261-0356-21**	22.05		AB
28s ea	**33261-0356-28**	29.40		AB
30s ea	**33261-0356-30**	31.50		AB
60s ea	**33261-0356-60**	63.00		AB
90s ea	**33261-0356-90**	94.50		AB
5 mg, 7s ea	**33261-0357-07**	7.98		AB
14s ea	**33261-0357-14**	15.96		AB
20s ea	**33261-0357-20**	22.80		AB
21s ea	**33261-0357-21**	23.94		AB
28s ea	**33261-0357-28**	31.92		AB
30s ea	**33261-0357-30**	34.20		AB
60s ea	**33261-0357-60**	68.40		AB
90s ea	**33261-0357-90**	102.60		AB
(American Health)				
REPACK				
TAB, PO (10X10)				
2 mg, 100s ea UD	**62584-0984-01**	61.51		AB
(USP,HIGHLY POTENT)				
2.5 mg, 30s ea	**68084-0027-77**	21.78		
(10X10)				
2.5 mg, 100s ea UD	**68084-0027-01**	63.47		AB
5 mg, 30s ea	**62584-0994-77**	21.50		AB
(10X10)				
5 mg, 100s ea UD	**62584-0994-01**	64.32		AB
(Bryant Ranch)				
REPACK				
TAB, PO, 2.5 mg, 30s ea	**63629-3177-01**	25.20		
60s ea	**63629-3177-02**	49.99		
5 mg, 30s ea	**63629-2548-02**	21.02		
100s ea	**63629-2548-01**	82.36		
7.5 mg, 100s ea	**63629-1336-01**	101.32		
(DHS, Inc.)				
REPACK				
TAB, PO, 1 mg, 90s ea	**55887-0264-90**	55.00		AB
2 mg, 90s ea	**55887-0926-90**	71.00		AB
2.5 mg, 10s ea	**55887-0577-10**	6.45		
30s ea	**55887-0577-30**	18.70		AB
60s ea	**55887-0577-60**	33.00		AB
90s ea	**55887-0577-90**	48.00		AB
4 mg, 60s ea	**55887-0464-60**	57.05		AB
90s ea	**55887-0464-90**	79.09		AB
5 mg, 10s ea	**55887-0578-10**	9.57		
30s ea	**55887-0578-30**	29.99		AB
60s ea	**55887-0578-60**	57.44		AB
90s ea	**55887-0578-90**	79.79		AB
150s ea	**55887-0578-86**	143.60		
10 mg, 60s ea	**55887-0567-60**	92.81		AB
(Dispensing Solutions)				
REPACK				
TAB, PO, 1 mg, 30s ea	**55045-2880-08**	18.00		AB
100s ea	**55045-2880-00**	60.00		AB
120s ea	**55045-2880-01**	72.00		
2 mg, 30s ea	**55045-2902-08**	18.90		AB
30s ea	**66336-0250-30**	24.61		AB
100s ea	**55045-2902-00**	63.00		AB
2.5 mg, 30s ea	**66336-0251-30**	25.37		AB
5 mg, 30s ea	**55045-2881-08**	20.10		AB
30s ea	**66336-0252-30**	26.41		AB
100s ea	**55045-2881-00**	67.00		AB
(GSMS)				
REPACK				
TAB, PO, 1 mg, 100s ea	**60429-0784-01**	10.14	3.38	AB
1000s ea	**60429-0784-10**	90.12	30.04	AB
2 mg, 100s ea	**60429-0785-01**	10.29	3.43	AB
1000s ea	**60429-0785-10**	91.59	30.53	AB
2.5 mg, 100s ea	**60429-0786-01**	10.44	3.48	AB
1000s ea	**60429-0786-10**	91.89	30.63	AB
3 mg, 100s ea	**60429-0787-01**	10.59	3.53	AB
1000s ea	**60429-0787-10**	92.34	30.78	AB
4 mg, 100s ea	**60429-0788-01**	10.74	3.58	AB
1000s ea	**60429-0788-10**	92.61	30.87	AB
5 mg, 100s ea	**60429-0789-01**	10.89	3.63	AB

PROD/MFR	NDC	AWP	DP	OBC
1000s ea	**60429-0789-10**	93.06	31.02	AB
6 mg, 100s ea	**60429-0790-01**	11.04	3.68	AB
1000s ea	**60429-0790-10**	95.28	31.76	AB
7.5 mg, 100s ea	**60429-0791-01**	11.49	3.83	AB
10 mg, 100s ea	**60429-0792-01**	11.61	3.87	AB
(HomeMed)				
REPACK				
TAB, PO, 5 mg, 30s ea	**51655-0283-24**	29.99		
(Palmetto)				
REPACK				
TAB, PO, 1 mg, 30s ea	**23490-6478-01**	24.00		
45s ea	**23490-6478-02**	36.00		
60s ea	**23490-6478-03**	48.00		
2 mg, 30s ea	**23490-6480-01**	27.00		
45s ea	**23490-6480-02**	40.50		
60s ea	**23490-6480-03**	54.00		
2.5 mg, 30s ea	**23490-6481-01**	28.50		
45s ea	**23490-6481-02**	42.75		
60s ea	**23490-6481-03**	57.00		
4 mg, 30s ea	**23490-6482-01**	45.05		
45s ea	**23490-6482-02**	67.57		
60s ea	**23490-6482-03**	90.10		
5 mg, 30s ea	**23490-6483-01**	30.00		
45s ea	**23490-6483-02**	45.00		
60s ea	**23490-6483-03**	60.00		
7.5 mg, 30s ea	**23490-6484-01**	34.86		
45s ea	**23490-6484-02**	52.29		
60s ea	**23490-6484-03**	69.72		
(PD-Rx Pharm)				
REPACK				
TAB, PO, 1 mg, 15s ea	**58864-0773-15**	11.35		AB
30s ea	**55289-0340-30**	43.00		
(REDI-SCRIPT)				
1 mg, 30s ea	**58864-0773-30**	17.70		AB
2.5 mg, 30s ea	**58864-0035-30**	11.79		AB
5 mg, 14s ea	**55289-0773-14**	28.92		AB
(U.S.P.)				
5 mg, 14s ea	**58864-0698-14**	11.82		
30s ea	**55289-0773-30**	49.54		
(REDI-SCRIPT)				
5 mg, 30s ea	**58864-0698-30**	19.58		AB
(USP)				
5 mg, 90s ea	**55289-0773-90**	77.46		AB
(Pharma Pac)				
REPACK				
TAB, PO, 1 mg, 30s ea	**52959-0924-30**	26.30		AB
2 mg, 30s ea	**52959-0925-30**	27.80		AB
5 mg, 30s ea	**52959-0926-30**	29.18		AB
(Phys Total Care)				
REPACK				
TAB, PO, 1 mg, 15s ea	**54868-4349-02**	13.38		AB
30s ea	**54868-4349-00**	23.76		EE
60s ea	**54868-4349-03**	44.52		AB
90s ea	**54868-4349-05**	50.61		EE
100s ea	**54868-4349-01**	70.68		EE
150s ea	**54868-4349-04**	82.35		AB
2 mg, 15s ea	**54868-4422-02**	13.23		EE
30s ea	**54868-4422-00**	23.46		EE
60s ea	**54868-4422-01**	43.92		EE
100s ea	**54868-4422-03**	71.22		AB
2.5 mg, 15s ea	**54868-4400-02**	13.59		AB
30s ea	**54868-4400-00**	24.15		EE
45s ea	**54868-4400-03**	34.74		EE
60s ea	**54868-4400-04**	34.21		AB
100s ea	**54868-4400-01**	72.03		EE
3 mg, 15s ea	**54868-4871-00**	15.99		AB
30s ea	**54868-4871-01**	28.95		AB
100s ea	**54868-4871-02**	88.05		
4 mg, 15s ea	**54868-4402-03**	11.13		EE
30s ea	**54868-4402-00**	19.26		EE
60s ea	**54868-4402-02**	35.55		EE
100s ea	**54868-4402-01**	35.55		EE
5 mg, 15s ea	**54868-4286-03**	13.77		AB
30s ea	**54868-4286-00**	24.51		EE
60s ea	**54868-4286-02**	39.14		EE
90s ea	**54868-4286-04**	67.56		EE
100s ea	**54868-4286-01**	73.23		EE
6 mg, 15s ea	**54868-4873-00**	20.13		AB
30s ea	**54868-4873-01**	35.73		AB
60s ea	**54868-4873-03**	66.96		
90s ea	**54868-4873-04**	59.79		AB
100s ea	**54868-4873-02**	82.62		AB
7.5 mg, 15s ea	**54868-4950-00**	17.13		AB
30s ea	**54868-4950-02**	31.23		AB
100s ea	**54868-4950-01**	73.47		AB
10 mg, 30s ea	**54868-5258-00**	34.83		AB
(Physician Partner)				
REPACK				
TAB, PO, 1 mg, 30s ea	**21695-0672-30**	35.33		AB
2 mg, 60s ea	**21695-0673-60**	73.06		AB
2.5 mg, 30s ea	**21695-0674-30**	38.70		AB
5 mg, 30s ea	**21695-0677-30**	40.08		AB

PROD/MFR	NDC	AWP	DP	OBC
(Quality Care Prod) REPACK				
TAB, PO, 2.5 mg, 30s ea	**35356-0397-30**	42.60		AB
4 mg, 10s ea	**49999-0923-10**	7.86		
5 mg, 10s ea	**49999-0576-10**	12.25		AB
20s ea	**49999-0576-20**	24.50		AB
30s ea	**49999-0576-30**	36.75		AB
100s ea	**49999-0576-00**	79.60		
7.5 mg, 100s ea	**49999-0829-00**	112.13		
WASP TREATMENT (Alk-Abello)				
wasp venom				
PDS, IJ (KIT (6X1ML))				
0.1 mg, ea	**52709-1301-01**	141.96	107.30	
(MDV)				
0.1 mg, ea	**52709-1301-02**	206.16	152.90	
WASP VENOM				
(Alk-Abello) *See WASP TREATMENT*				
(Hollister-Stier) *See VENOMIL*				
(Hollister-Stier) *See WASP VENOM PROTEIN*				
WASP VENOM PROTEIN (Hollister-Stier)				
wasp venom				
PDS, IJ (M.D.V.)				
0.55 mg, ea	**65044-9943-05**	76.30		
1.3 mg, ea	**65044-9943-06**	168.10		
WATCHHALER (U.S. Pharm)				
device, inhalation				
DEV, NA (SPACER)				
ea	**52747-0515-01**	42.00		
WATER FOR INJECTION (Amer Regent)				
water, sterile				
SOL, IV (S.D.V.)				
5 ml 25s	**00517-3005-25**	31.25		EE
10 ml 25s	**00517-3010-25**	34.38		EE
20 ml 25s	**00517-3020-25**	35.94		EE
50 ml 25s	**00517-3050-25**	43.75		EE
(APP)				
SOL, IV (S.D.V.)				
5 ml	**63323-0185-05**	1.40		AP
(S.D.V.,P.C.)				
10 ml	**63323-0185-10**	1.05		AP
20 ml	**63323-0185-20**	2.34		AP
50 ml	**63323-0185-50**	2.18		AP
(S.D.V.,TEAR TOP)				
100 ml	**63323-0185-00**	3.27		AP
(B. Braun)				
SOL, IV (EXCEL)				
250 ml	**00264-7850-20**	4.03		AP
500 ml	**00264-7850-10**	4.00		AP
(GLASS W/SOLID STOPPER)				
500 ml	**00264-9201-55**	2.20		AP
(EXCEL)				
1000 ml	**00264-7850-00**	3.00		AP
(GLASS W/SOLID STOPPER)				
1000 ml	**00264-9200-55**	2.40		AP
2000 ml	**00264-9205-55**	6.40		AP
(Baxter)				
SOL, IV, 1000 ml 12s	**00338-0013-04**	119.66		AP
2000 ml 6s	**00338-0013-06**	65.52	54.60	AP
3000 ml 4s	**00338-0013-08**	58.80	49.00	AP
5000 ml 2s	**00338-0013-29**	49.20	41.00	AP
(Consolidated Midland)				
SOL, IV (AMP)				
5 ml 25s	**00223-8979-05**	20.00		
(VIAL)				
10 ml 25s	**00223-8980-10**	22.50		
(Hospira)				
SOL, IV (AMP,PF,LATEX-FREE)				
5 ml 25s	**00074-4027-02**	27.60	24.25	AP
(25X10ML,PF,LATEX-FREE)				
10 ml 25s	**00409-4044-02**	33.60	29.50	AP
(FTV,25X10ML,PF)				
10 ml 25s	**00409-4887-10**	16.50	14.50	AP
(25X20ML,STERILE,PF)				
20 ml 25s	**00409-4887-20**	20.10	17.50	AP
(AMP,PF,LATEX-FREE)				
20 ml 25s	**00409-4029-03**	63.00	55.25	AP
(FTV,25X50ML,PF)				
50 ml 25s	**00409-4887-50**	40.50	35.50	AP
(VIAL, FLIPTOP,PF)				
50 ml 25s	**00074-4887-50**	36.30	31.75	AP
(FTV,25X100ML,PF)				
100 ml 25s	**00409-4887-99**	73.50	64.25	AP
(12X250ML,PF,LATEX-FREE)				
250 ml 12s	**00409-1590-02**	62.06	54.36	AP
(LIFECARE,PF,LATEX-FREE)				
1000 ml 12s	**00409-7990-09**	27.50	24.12	AP
(Phys Total Care) REPACK				
SOL, IV (S.D.V.)				
5 ml 25s	**54868-3975-00**	56.84		EE
(500X20ML,SDV,PF)				
20 ml 500s	**54868-3433-00**	46.75		AP
500 ml	**54868-4311-00**	63.19		EE
6000 ml	**54868-3905-00**	386.84		EE
(Southwood) REPACK				
SOL, IV, 50 ml	**58016-9464-01**	1.25		EE
WATER FOR INJECTION BACTERIOSTATIC				
(Amer Regent)				
water, sterile				
SOL, IV (M.D.V.)				
30 ml 25s	**00517-0662-25**	39.06		EE
(Consolidated Midland)				
SOL, IV (VIAL)				
10 ml	**00223-8884-10**	1.25		
30 ml	**00223-8883-30**	27.50		
(Hospira)				
SOL, IV (VIAL,FLIPTOP,LATEX-FREE)				
30 ml 25s	**00409-3977-03**	17.40	15.25	AP
(Phys Total Care) REPACK				
SOL, IV (VIAL)				
30 ml	**54868-0183-00**	52.38		
WATER FOR IRRIGATION (B. Braun)				
water, sterile				
SOL, IR (PIC CONTAINER)				
500 ml	**00264-2101-10**	1.61		AT
1000 ml	**00264-2101-00**	1.87		AT
2000 ml	**00264-2101-50**	3.46		AT
4000 ml	**00264-2101-70**	10.39		AT
(Baxter)				
SOL, IR, 250 ml 24s	**00338-0004-02**	268.42		AT
500 ml 18s	**00338-0004-03**	201.32		AT
1000 ml 12s	**00338-0003-44**	68.68		AT
1000 ml 12s	**00338-0004-04**	138.34		AT
1500 ml 9s	**00338-0004-05**	141.66		AT
2000 ml 6s	**00338-0003-46**	52.82		AT
3000 ml 4s	**00338-0003-47**	63.00		AT
5000 ml 2s	**00338-0003-49**	43.55		AT
(Hospira)				
SOL, IR (AQUALITE,USP,24X250ML)				
250 ml 24s	**00409-6139-22**	43.78	38.40	AT
(AQUALITE,U.S.P.24X500ML)				
500 ml 24s	**00409-6139-03**	48.10	42.00	AT
(AQUALITE W/HANGER,PF)				
1000 ml 12s	**00409-7139-09**	25.06	21.96	AT
(FLEXIBLE CONTAINER,PF)				
1000 ml 12s	**00409-7973-05**	51.55	45.12	AT
(AQUALITE,U.S.P.9X1500ML)				
1500 ml 9s	**00409-7139-36**	24.41	21.33	AT
(BULK PACKAGE,PF)				
2000 ml 6s	**00409-7118-07**	42.77	37.44	AT
(FLEXIBLE, CONTAINER,PF)				
2000 ml 6s	**00409-7973-07**	41.62	36.42	AT
(4X3000ML,PF,LATEX-FREE)				
3000 ml 4s	**00409-7973-08**	44.40	38.84	AT
(Phys Total Care) REPACK				
SOL, IR, 500 ml 24s	**54868-4296-00**	118.14		AT
WATER, PURIFIED				
(Medisca) *See PURIFIED WATER*				
WATER, STERILE				
(Amer Regent) *See WATER FOR INJECTION*				
(Amer Regent) *See WATER FOR INJECTION BACTERIOSTATIC*				
(APP) *See STERILE WATER BACTERIOSTATIC*				
(APP) *See WATER FOR INJECTION*				
(B. Braun) *See WATER FOR INJECTION*				
(B. Braun) *See WATER FOR IRRIGATION*				
(Baxter) *See STERILE WATER FOR INJECTION*				
(Baxter) *See WATER FOR INJECTION*				
(Baxter) *See WATER FOR IRRIGATION*				
(Consolidated Midland) *See WATER FOR INJECTION*				
(Consolidated Midland) *See WATER FOR INJECTION BACTERIOSTATIC*				
(Hospira) *See STERILE WATER*				
(Hospira) *See WATER FOR INJECTION*				
(Hospira) *See WATER FOR INJECTION BACTERIOSTATIC*				
(Hospira) *See WATER FOR IRRIGATION*				
WATERMELON (Medisca)				
flavoring aid				
SOL, NA (1X25ML)				
25 ml	**38779-1695-04**	25.50		
(1X100ML)				
100 ml	**38779-1695-05**	37.50		
(1X500ML)				
500 ml	**38779-1695-08**	76.50		
WATERMELON ARTIFICIAL FLAVOR				
(Spectrum Pharmacy)				
flavoring aid				
LIQ, NA (1X100ML,CONCENTRATE)				
100 ml	**49452-8133-02**	63.70		
(1X500ML,CONCENTRATE)				
500 ml	**49452-8133-03**	146.65		
WATERMELON FLAVOR (PCCA)				
flavoring aid				
SOL, NA (ARTIFICIAL)				
1 ml	**51927-2150-00**	0.90		
WE ALLERGY (Dexo)				
cpm/methscopolamine nitrate/phenyleph hcl				
SYR, PO (GRAPE)				
473 ml	**59196-0070-16**	20.30		
WE MIST II LA (Dexo)				
guaifenesin/pseudoephedrine hydrochloride				
TER, PO, 800 mg-80 mg,				
100s ea	**59196-0065-01**	38.40		
WE MIST LA (Dexo)				
guaifenesin/pseudoephedrine hydrochloride				
TER, PO, 600 mg-90 mg,				
100s ea	**59196-0060-01**	48.29		
WELCHOL (Daiichi Sankyo)				
colesevelam hydrochloride				
PDR, PO (CITRUS,GRANULES)				
3.75 gm/packet,				
30s ea	**65597-0902-30**	235.44		
TAB, PO, 625 mg, 180s ea	**65597-0701-18**	235.44		
(Phys Total Care) REPACK				
TAB, PO, 625 mg, 30s ea	**54868-4474-01**	43.24		
60s ea	**54868-4474-02**	84.61		
90s ea	**54868-4474-03**	141.39		
180s ea	**54868-4474-00**	235.68		
(Quality Care Prod) REPACK				
TAB, PO, 625 mg, 30s ea	**49999-0959-30**	68.34		
(Southwood) REPACK				
TAB, PO, 625 mg, 30s ea	**58016-0869-30**	37.08		
60s ea	**58016-0869-60**	74.16		
90s ea	**58016-0869-90**	111.24		
100s ea	**58016-0869-00**	123.60		
180s ea	**58016-0869-99**	222.48		
WELLBUTRIN (Glaxo)				
bupropion hydrochloride				
TAB, PO, 75 mg, 100s ea	**00173-0177-55**	266.08		AB
100 mg, 100s ea	**00173-0178-55**	354.85		AB
(Bryant Ranch) REPACK				
TAB, PO, 100 mg, 60s ea	**63629-2642-01**	111.65		
(Palmetto) REPACK				
TAB, PO, 75 mg, 30s ea	**23490-9232-03**	96.34		
(Phys Total Care) REPACK				
TAB, PO, 75 mg, 30s ea	**54868-1449-00**	39.91		AB
100 mg, 50s ea	**54868-1450-00**	128.49		AB
(Vibranta) REPACK				
TAB, PO, 75 mg, 60s ea	**57866-1035-01**	64.28		AB
WELLBUTRIN SR (Glaxo)				
bupropion hydrochloride				
T12, PO (FILM-COATED)				
100 mg, 60s ea	**00173-0947-55**	219.31		
150 mg, 60s ea	**00173-0135-55**	235.04		
200 mg, 60s ea	**00173-0722-00**	436.48		
(Altura) REPACK				
T12, PO, 150 mg, 20s ea	**63874-0780-20**	43.63		
(AQ) REPACK				
T12, PO, 100 mg, 10s ea	**66105-0480-01**	37.09		
15s ea	**66105-0480-15**	55.63		
20s ea	**66105-0480-02**	74.18		
30s ea	**66105-0480-03**	111.29		
60s ea	**66105-0480-06**	222.58		

PROD/MFR	NDC	AWP	DP	OBC
150 mg, 10s ea	66105-0481-01	48.48		
15s ea	66105-0481-15	72.72		
20s ea	66105-0481-02	96.96		
30s ea	66105-0481-03	145.46		
60s ea	66105-0481-06	290.92		
(DHS, Inc.) REPACK				
T12, PO (FILM-COATED)				
150 mg, 90s ea	55887-0663-90	207.99		
(Dispensing Solutions) REPACK				
T12, PO (FILM-COATED)				
150 mg, 60s ea	55045-2631-08	129.00		
(Palmetto) REPACK				
T12, PO, 100 mg, 30s ea	23490-9231-03	173.81		
150 mg, 60s ea	23490-9230-06	186.27		
(PD-Rx Pharm) REPACK				
T12, PO (REDI-SCRIPT,FILM-COATED)				
100 mg, 30s ea	58864-0715-30	110.56		
150 mg, 30s ea	58864-0625-30	118.50		
(FILM-COATED)				
150 mg, 30s ea	55289-0905-30	166.35		
(REDI-SCRIPT,FILM-COATED)				
150 mg, 60s ea	58864-0625-60	175.78		
(Pharma Pac) REPACK				
T12, PO, 150 mg, 30s ea	52959-0285-30	70.61		
60s ea	52959-0285-60	122.33		
(Phys Total Care) REPACK				
T12, PO (FILM-COATED)				
100 mg, 30s ea	54868-4505-01	81.44		
60s ea	54868-4505-00	151.53		
(FILM-COATED)				
150 mg, 30s ea	54868-3984-01	92.75		
60s ea	54868-3984-00	172.90		
60s ea	54868-5010-01	443.25		
(FILM-COATED)				
200 mg, 60s ea	54868-4763-00	249.03		
(Quality Care Prod) REPACK				
T12, PO (FILM-COATED)				
100 mg, 30s ea	35356-0353-30	206.60		
150 mg, 20s ea	35356-0354-20	158.00		
(Southwood) REPACK				
T12, PO (FILM-COATED)				
150 mg, 30s ea	58016-0599-30	106.60		
60s ea	58016-0599-60	213.19		
90s ea	58016-0599-90	319.79		
100s ea	58016-0599-00	355.32		
(Vibranta) REPACK				
T12, PO (FILM-COATED)				
100 mg, 60s ea	57866-3083-05	111.79		
150 mg, 60s ea	57866-0901-02	120.33		
WELLBUTRIN XL (BTA)				
bupropion hydrochloride				
T24, PO, 150 mg, 30s ea	00173-0730-01	197.29	164.41	
90s ea	00173-0730-02	591.88	493.23	
300 mg, 30s ea	00173-0731-01	260.42	217.02	
(A-S Medication) REPACK				
T24, PO, 300 mg, 30s ea	54569-5599-00	229.94		
(DHS, Inc.) REPACK				
T24, PO, 150 mg, 60s ea	55887-0284-60	225.00		
300 mg, 60s ea	55887-0283-60	291.00		
(Direct Pharmaceutical, Inc.) REPACK				
T24, PO, 150 mg, 30s ea UD	67801-0433-30	258.90		
(IPI) REPACK				
T24, PO, 150 mg, 30s ea	18837-0175-30	138.97		
300 mg, 30s ea	18837-0176-30	183.45		
(PD-Rx Pharm) REPACK				
T24, PO, 150 mg, 15s ea	55289-0922-15	83.18		
30s ea	55289-0922-30	166.35		
300 mg, 15s ea	55289-0900-15	182.58		
30s ea	55289-0900-30	365.16		
(Pharma Pac) REPACK				
T24, PO, 150 mg, 60s ea	52959-0820-60	206.98		
(Phys Total Care) REPACK				
T24, PO, 150 mg, 30s ea	54868-5010-00	222.28		
300 mg, 30s ea	54868-4935-00	262.61		
(Physician Partner) REPACK				
T24, PO, 150 mg, 15s ea	21695-0137-15	215.18		
30s ea	21695-0137-30	387.76		
45s ea	21695-0137-45	490.90		
300 mg, 15s ea	21695-0138-15	247.18		
30s ea	21695-0138-30	511.86		
(Quality Care Prod) REPACK				
T24, PO, 150 mg, 30s ea	49999-0774-30	237.02		
60s ea	49999-0774-60	343.17		
90s ea	49999-0774-90	514.80		
300 mg, 15s ea	49999-0443-15	85.79		
30s ea	49999-0443-30	305.60		
(Southwood) REPACK				
T24, PO, 150 mg, 30s ea	58016-0031-30	167.23		
60s ea	58016-0031-60	334.45		
90s ea	58016-0031-90	501.68		
100s ea	58016-0031-00	557.42		
300 mg, 30s ea	58016-0671-30	220.74		
60s ea	58016-0671-60	441.48		
90s ea	58016-0671-90	662.22		
100s ea	58016-0671-00	735.80		
120s ea	58016-0671-02	882.96		
150s ea	58016-0671-03	1103.70		
(Stat Rx) REPACK				
T24, PO, 150 mg, 30s ea	16590-0526-30	274.70		
60s ea	16590-0526-60	433.53		
90s ea	16590-0526-90	648.67		
300 mg, 30s ea	16590-0246-30	287.24		
60s ea	16590-0246-60	571.24		
90s ea	16590-0246-90	408.75		
WESMYCIN (Wesley)				
tetracycline hydrochloride				
CAP, PO, 250 mg, 100s ea	00917-0809-01	7.25		EE
WESTCORT (Ranbaxy Labs)				
hydrocortisone valerate				
OIN, TP (1X15GM)				
0.2%, 15 gm	10631-0105-15	50.22		AB
(1X45GM)				
0.2%, 45 gm	10631-0105-45	104.13		AB
(1X60GM)				
0.2%, 60 gm	10631-0105-60	125.25		AB
(Phys Total Care) REPACK				
CRE, TP, 0.2%, 15 gm	54868-2229-03	21.74		AB
45 gm	54868-2229-02	45.58		AB
60 gm	54868-2229-01	53.28		AB
OIN, TP, 0.2%, 15 gm	54868-2230-00	21.72		AB
(Southwood) REPACK				
CRE, TP, 0.2%, 15 gm	58016-3102-01	17.53		AB
(Stat Rx) REPACK				
CRE, TP, 0.2%, 15 gm	16590-0247-15	22.00		
WESTHROID (RLC)				
thyroid				
TAB, PO (MICRO-COATED)				
32.5 mg, 100s ea	64727-7070-01	8.92		
1000s ea	64727-7070-02	83.33		
65 mg, 100s ea	64727-7073-01	9.91		
1000s ea	64727-7073-02	101.64		
130 mg, 100s ea	64727-7080-01	17.95		
1000s ea	64727-7080-02	131.56		
WHEAT GERM (Spectrum Pharmacy)				
wheat germ oil				
OIL, NA, 500 ml	49452-8180-01	99.75		
4000 ml	49452-8180-02	427.00		
WHEAT GERM OIL (Medisca)				
OIL, NA (1X14ML)				
14 ml	38779-1696-03	15.00		
(1X500ML)				
500 ml	38779-1696-08	75.00		
(1X1000ML)				
1000 ml	38779-1696-09	135.00		
(1X4000ML)				
4000 ml	38779-1696-01	465.00		
(Spectrum Pharmacy) *See WHEAT GERM*				
WHEY PROTEIN (PCCA)				
PDR, NA (COCOA)				
1 gm	51927-3541-00	0.08		
WHEY PROTEIN ISOLATE (PCCA)				
POW, NA (INSTANIZED)				
1 gm	51927-3475-00	0.07		
WHITE FACED HORNET TREATMENT (Alk-Abello)				
white faced hornet venom				
PDS, IJ (KIT (6X1ML))				
0.1 mg, ea	52709-1101-01	125.40	94.80	
(MDV)				
0.1 mg, ea	52709-1101-02	210.84	156.40	
WHITE FACED HORNET VENOM				
(Alk-Abello) *See WHITE FACED HORNET TREATMENT*				
(Hollister-Stier) *See VENOMIL*				
(Hollister-Stier) *See WHITE FACED HORNET VENOM PROTEIN*				
WHITE FACED HORNET VENOM PROTEIN (Hollister-Stier)				
white faced hornet venom				
PDS, IJ (M.D.V.)				
0.55 mg, ea	65044-9941-05	72.20		
1.3 mg, ea	65044-9941-06	173.30		
WHITE FOOD COLOR (PCCA)				
color,additive				
SOL, NA, 1 ml	51927-2660-00	0.38		
WHITE WAX				
(PCCA) *See WHITE WAX BEADLETS (BEES WAX)*				
WHITE WAX (Spectrum Pharmacy)				
yellow wax				
WAX, NA (PASTILLES)				
500 gm	49452-8160-02	144.90		
WHITE WAX BEADLETS (BEES WAX) (PCCA)				
white wax				
BEA, NA (NF,1X1GM)				
1 gm	51927-1143-00	0.45		
WHITE WILLOW BARK				
(Gallipot) *See WHITE WILLOW BARK EXTRACT*				
WHITE WILLOW BARK EXTRACT (Gallipot)				
white willow bark				
POW, NA, 15%, 1000 gm	51552-0998-07	209.44	149.60	
WHITING GROUND CACO3 (Gallipot)				
calcium carbonate				
POW, NA (TECHNICAL)				
454 gm	51552-0286-06	5.46		
WILATE (Octapharma USA)				
ahf human/von willebrand factor				
PDS, IV (450IU,SDV W/5ML DILUENT)				
1 iu-1 iu, ea	67467-0181-01	1.38		
(900IU,SDVW/10ML DILUENT)				
1 iu-1 iu, ea	67467-0181-02	1.38		
WILD CHERRY (Medisca)				
flavoring aid				
SOL, NA (1X100ML,CONCENTRATE)				
100 ml	38779-1697-05	25.50		
(1X500ML,CONCENTRATE)				
500 ml	38779-1697-08	46.50		
WILD CHERRY BARK (PCCA)				
POW, NA, 1 gm	51927-3166-00	0.26		
WILD CHERRY FLAVOR (Gallipot)				
flavoring aid				
POW, NA (ARTIFICIAL)				
56.7 gm	51552-0222-03	5.74		
(PCCA)				
SOL, NA (CONCENTRATE,WILD CHERRY)				
1 ml	51927-1162-00	0.23		
WILD YAM EXTRACT (PCCA)				
SOL, NA, 1 ml	51927-2545-00	0.95		
WILLOW BARK (PCCA)				
POW, NA, 1 gm	51927-3485-00	0.57		
WINRHO SDF (Baxter Bioscience)				
rho(d) immune globulin				
SOL, IV (SDV,PF)				
1500 iu, 1.3 ml	00944-2967-03	403.01		
2500 iu, 2.2 ml	00944-2967-07	675.85		
5000 iu, 4.4 ml	00944-2967-05	1351.72		
15000 iu, 13 ml	00944-2967-09	4055.14		
WINTERGREEN OIL (Medisca)				
methyl salicylate				
OIL, NA (1X14ML,NATURAL)				
14 ml	38779-1753-03	46.50		
(1X25ML,NATURAL)				
25 ml	38779-1753-04	60.00		

PROD/MFR	NDC	AWP	DP	OBC
(1X100ML,NATURAL)				
100 ml	38779-1753-05	135.00		
(1X500ML,NATURAL)				
500 ml	38779-1753-08	285.00		
WITCH HAZEL EXTRACT (PCCA)				
LIQ, NA (USP)				
1 ml	51927-2355-00	0.09		
(Spectrum Pharmacy)				
LIQ, NA (U.S.P.,DOUBLE DISTILLED)				
500 ml	49452-8185-01	64.75		
4000 ml	49452-8185-02	200.20		
WITEPSOL H 15 (Gallipot)				
GRA, NA, 454 gm	51552-0858-06	18.90	13.50	
(PCCA) *See WITEPSOL H15*				
(Spectrum Pharmacy) *See WITEPSOL H-15*				
WITEPSOL H-15 (Spectrum Pharmacy)				
witepsol h 15				
POW, NA, 500 gm	49452-8190-01	74.65		
2500 gm	49452-8190-02	288.05		
WITEPSOL H15 (PCCA)				
witepsol h 15				
POW, NA (BASE F; TM)				
1 gm	51927-9026-00	0.09		
WORMWOOD OIL				
(PCCA) *See ABSINTHIUM OIL*				
WOUND AND/OR DRESSING SUPPLIES				
(ACell) *See MATRISTEM MICROMATRIX*				
(ACell) *See MATRISTEM WOUND SHEET*				
WOUND CARE PREPARATION				
(Coloplast) *See COMFEEL PURILON*				
X-VIATE (Stratus)				
urea				
CRE, TP (1X28.5GM)				
40%, 28.5 gm	58980-0625-10	19.20		
85 gm	58980-0625-30	38.50		
199 gm	58980-0625-70	70.50		
GEL, TP (1X15ML)				
40%, 15 ml	58980-0624-15	52.95		
LOT, TP (1X237ML)				
40%, 237 ml	58980-0623-80	52.95		
XALATAN (Pfizer)				
latanoprost				
SOL, OP, 0.005%, 2.5 ml	00013-8303-04	90.11	75.09	
2.5 ml 3s	00013-8303-01	270.32	225.27	
(Pharma Pac) REPACK				
SOL, OP, 0.005%, 2.5 ml	52959-0845-00	63.82		
(Phys Total Care) REPACK				
SOL, OP, 0.005%, 2.5 ml	54868-3881-00	114.90		
(Quality Care Prod) REPACK				
SOL, OP, 0.005%, 2.5 ml	49999-0997-01	113.36		
XANAX (Pfizer)				
alprazolam				
TAB, PO, 0.25 mg,				
100s ea, C-IV	00009-0029-01	138.76	115.63	AB
500s ea, C-IV	00009-0029-02	693.78	578.15	AB
0.5 mg,				
100s ea, C-IV	00009-0055-01	172.87	144.06	AB
500s ea, C-IV	00009-0055-03	864.36	720.30	AB
1 mg,				
100s ea, C-IV	00009-0090-01	230.66	192.22	AB
500s ea, C-IV	00009-0090-04	1153.32	961.10	AB
2 mg,				
100s ea, C-IV	00009-0094-01	392.20	326.83	AB
(PD-Rx Pharm) REPACK				
TAB, PO, 0.25 mg,				
10s ea, C-IV	55289-0346-10	26.00		EE
20s ea, C-IV	55289-0346-20	45.33		EE
30s ea, C-IV	55289-0346-30	64.67		AB
0.5 mg,				
30s ea, C-IV	55289-0011-30	89.24		AB
1 mg, 30s ea, C-IV	55289-0345-30	100.82		AB
(Pharma Pac) REPACK				
TAB, PO, 0.25 mg,				
30s ea, C-IV	52959-0322-30	28.51		AB
0.5 mg,				
20s ea, C-IV	52959-0162-20	22.78		AB
(Phys Total Care) REPACK				
TAB, PO, 0.25 mg,				
10s ea, C-IV	54868-0992-04	14.95		AB
15s ea, C-IV	54868-0992-03	21.19		AB
30s ea, C-IV	54868-0992-01	39.86		AB
50s ea, C-IV	54868-0992-02	64.77		AB
90s ea, C-IV	54868-0992-00	114.60		AB
0.5 mg,				
3s ea, C-IV	54868-0522-07	9.77		AB
20s ea, C-IV	54868-0522-01	46.60		AB
30s ea, C-IV	54868-0522-03	68.27		AB
50s ea, C-IV	54868-0522-02	111.60		AB
60s ea, C-IV	54868-0522-05	133.27		AB
90s ea, C-IV	54868-0522-06	187.44		AB
100s ea, C-IV	54868-0522-04	207.90		AB
1 mg, 10s ea, C-IV	54868-1251-02	23.20		AB
30s ea, C-IV	54868-1251-01	63.99		AB
90s ea, C-IV	54868-1251-00	178.50		AB
(Quality Care Prod) REPACK				
TAB, PO, 0.25 mg,				
100s ea, C-IV	35356-0013-00	157.00		
(Southwood) REPACK				
TAB, PO, 1 mg,				
30s ea, C-IV	58016-0099-30	65.90		
60s ea, C-IV	58016-0099-60	131.81		
90s ea, C-IV	58016-0099-90	197.71		
100s ea, C-IV	58016-0099-00	219.68		
2 mg, 30s ea, C-IV	58016-0033-30	112.06		
60s ea, C-IV	58016-0033-60	224.11		
90s ea, C-IV	58016-0033-90	336.17		
100s ea, C-IV	58016-0033-00	373.52		
XANAX XR (Pfizer)				
alprazolam				
TER, PO, 0.5 mg,				
60s ea, C-IV	00009-0057-07	175.74	146.45	
1 mg, 60s ea, C-IV	00009-0059-07	218.66	182.22	
2 mg, 60s ea, C-IV	00009-0066-07	290.22	241.85	
3 mg, 60s ea, C-IV	00009-0068-07	435.29	362.74	
(Nucare Pharm) REPACK				
TER, PO, 2 mg,				
60s ea, C-IV	66267-1306-06	345.49		
(Stat Rx) REPACK				
TER, PO, 2 mg,				
30s ea, C-IV	16590-0682-30	163.01		
XANTHAN GUM (Gallipot)				
POW, NA (U.S.P.,N.F.)				
7 gm	51552-0100-02	5.25		
60 gm	51552-0100-09	9.10		
100 gm	51552-0100-05	11.90		
(Letco)				
POW, NA (U.S.P./N.F.)				
100 gm	62991-1359-01	27.00		
(NF)				
2500 gm	62991-1359-04	180.00		
(Medisca)				
POW, NA (1X100GM)				
100 gm	38779-1700-05	28.50		
(1X500GM)				
500 gm	38779-1700-08	79.50		
(1X1000GM)				
1000 gm	38779-1700-09	130.50		
(1X2500GM)				
2500 gm	38779-1700-01	291.00		
(1X5000GM)				
5000 gm	38779-1700-03	555.00		
(PCCA)				
POW, NA, 1 gm	51927-1637-00	0.33		
(Spectrum Pharmacy)				
POW, NA (N.F.)				
100 gm	49452-8200-01	54.95		
500 gm	49452-8200-02	140.35		
2500 gm	49452-8200-03	500.50		
XCLAIR (Align)				
cream, multi ingredient				
CRE, TP, 75 ml	08514-0010-01	66.00		
XEDEC II (Cypress Pharm)				
guaifenesin/phenylephrine hydrochloride				
TER, PO (DYE-FREE)				
1100 mg-30 mg,				
100s ea	60258-0358-01	52.81		
XELODA (Roche Labs)				
capecitabine				
TAB, PO, 150 mg, 60s ea	00004-1100-20	511.38		
500 mg, 120s ea	00004-1101-50	3408.79		
(Phys Total Care) REPACK				
TAB, PO, 150 mg, 28s ea	54868-4143-03	166.58		
30s ea	54868-4143-02	178.39		
60s ea	54868-4143-00	343.46		
120s ea	54868-4143-01	686.30		
500 mg, 14s ea	54868-5260-04	473.38		
20s ea	54868-5260-09	653.44		
28s ea	54868-5260-05	913.77		
30s ea	54868-5260-00	978.85		
42s ea	54868-5260-06	1340.57		
60s ea	54868-5260-01	1913.98		
70s ea	54868-5260-07	2232.54		
80s ea	54868-5260-08	2551.10		
90s ea	54868-5260-03	2869.66		
120s ea	54868-5260-02	3824.69		
XENADERM (Healthpoint)				
castor oil/peru balsam/trypsin				
OIN, TP, 30 gm	00064-3900-30	59.05		
60 gm	00064-3900-60	69.48		
XENAZINE (Lundbeck)				
tetrabenazine				
TAB, PO, 12.5 mg,				
112s ea	67386-0421-01	4176.02		
25 mg, 112s ea	67386-0422-01	8352.05		
XENICAL (Roche Labs)				
orlistat				
CAP, PO, 120 mg, 90s ea	00004-0256-52	399.41		
(A-S Medication) REPACK				
CAP, PO, 120 mg, 30s ea	54569-4742-02	150.51		
60s ea	54569-4742-01	301.01		
90s ea	54569-4742-00	451.52		
(AQ) REPACK				
CAP, PO, 120 mg, 10s ea	66105-0750-01	49.45		
30s ea	66105-0750-03	148.37		
60s ea	66105-0750-06	296.74		
90s ea	66105-0750-09	445.11		
100s ea	66105-0750-10	494.56		
(Bryant Ranch) REPACK				
CAP, PO, 120 mg, 30s ea	63629-2643-01	64.99		
90s ea	63629-2643-02	132.32		
(Dispensing Solutions) REPACK				
CAP, PO, 120 mg, 30s ea	55045-2700-08	99.90		
90s ea	55045-2700-09	299.70		
(PD-Rx Pharm) REPACK				
CAP, PO, 120 mg, 30s ea	55289-0848-30	172.07		
(Pharma Pac) REPACK				
CAP, PO, 120 mg, 90s ea	52959-0931-90	339.81		
(Phys Total Care) REPACK				
CAP, PO, 120 mg, 30s ea	54868-4158-01	117.82		
60s ea	54868-4158-00	220.88		
90s ea	54868-4158-02	329.75		
(Quality Care Prod) REPACK				
CAP, PO, 120 mg, 15s ea	49999-0432-15	39.82		
90s ea	49999-0432-90	198.78		
(Southwood) REPACK				
CAP, PO, 120 mg, 30s ea	58016-0361-30	95.86		
60s ea	58016-0361-60	191.71		
90s ea	58016-0361-90	287.57		
100s ea	58016-0361-00	319.52		
XENON XE 133				
(Lantheus) *See XENON XE-133*				
XENON XE-133 (Lantheus)				
xenon xe 133				
GAS, IH, 10 mci, ea	11994-0127-11	41.01		AA
20 mci, ea	11994-0128-21	82.03		AA
30 mci, ea	11994-0129-31	123.05		
40 mci, ea	11994-0130-41	164.05		
50 mci, ea	11994-0131-51	205.07		
XERAC AC (Person & Covey)				
aluminum chloride				
SOL, TP, 6.25%, 35 ml	00096-0709-35	5.54		
60 ml	00096-0709-60	7.47		
XIAFLEX (Auxilium Pharm, Inc)				
collagenase, clostridium histolyticum				
PDS, IJ (SINGLE USE VIAL)				
0.9 mg, ea	66887-0003-01	3900.00		

PROD/MFR	NDC	AWP	DP	OBC
XIBROM (ISTA Pharm.)				
bromfenac				
SOL, OP, 0.09%, 2.5 ml	67425-0004-12	134.75		
(5ML IN 10ML CONTAINER)				
0.09%, 5 ml	67425-0004-50	262.70		
XIFAXAN (Salix Pharm)				
rifaximin				
TAB, PO, 200 mg, 30s ea	65649-0301-03	181.06		
100s ea UD	65649-0301-05	576.14		
100s ea	65649-0301-41	548.70		
(DHS, Inc.)				
REPACK				
TAB, PO, 200 mg, 20s ea	55887-0741-20	119.98		
40s ea	55887-0741-40	239.96		
60s ea	55887-0741-60	359.94		
(Phys Total Care)				
REPACK				
TAB, PO, 200 mg, 30s ea	54868-5972-00	184.05		
(Southwood)				
REPACK				
TAB, PO, 200 mg, 30s ea	58016-4824-01	118.30		
XIGRIS (Lilly)				
drotrecogin alfa				
PDS, IV (VIAL,PF)				
5 mg, ea	00002-7559-01	370.42	308.68	
20 mg, ea	00002-7561-01	1481.66	1234.72	
XIRAHIST PEDIATRIC DROPS (Hawthorn Pharm)				
carbinoxamine maleate/phenylephrine hydrochloride				
SOL, PO (AF,SF,DYE-FREE)				
2 mg/ml-2 mg/ml,				
30 ml	63717-0360-30	37.49		
XIRAHISTDM PEDIATRIC DROPS (Hawthorn Pharm)				
carbinoxamine mal/dm/phenyleph hcl				
SOL, PO (AF,SF,DYE-FREE,PEACH)				
2 mg/ml-3 mg/ml-2 mg/ml,				
30 ml	63717-0361-30	42.49		
XIRATUSS (Hawthorn Pharm)				
cpm tan/carbetapentane tan/phenyleph tan				
TAB, PO, 60 mg-5 mg-10 mg,				
60s ea	63717-0551-06	99.99		
(DHS, Inc.)				
REPACK				
TAB, PO, 60 mg-5 mg-10 mg,				
30s ea	55887-0371-30	87.45		
XODOL (Victory Pharma, Inc.)				
acetaminophen/hydrocodone bitartrate				
TAB, PO, 300 mg-10 mg,				
100s ea, C-III	68453-0911-10	245.29	68.50	
(Core)				
REPACK				
TAB, PO, 325 mg-10 mg,				
90s ea, C-III	33358-0366-90	129.46		
(Stat Rx)				
REPACK				
TAB, PO, 300 mg-10 mg,				
120s ea, C-III	16590-0806-72	309.47		
180s ea, C-III	16590-0806-82	425.63		
XODOL 5/300 (Victory Pharma, Inc.)				
acetaminophen/hydrocodone bitartrate				
TAB, PO, 300 mg-5 mg,				
100s ea, C-III	68453-0912-10	173.65		
(Stat Rx)				
REPACK				
TAB, PO, 300 mg-5 mg,				
30s ea, C-III	16590-0315-30	57.73		
60s ea, C-III	16590-0315-60	112.22		
XODOL 7.5/300 (Victory Pharma, Inc.)				
acetaminophen/hydrocodone bitartrate				
TAB, PO, 300 mg-7.5 mg,				
100s ea, C-III	68453-0913-10	190.13		
(Quality Care Prod)				
REPACK				
TAB, PO, 300 mg-7.5 mg,				
30s ea, C-III	35356-0384-30	89.48		
XOLAIR (Genentech)				
omalizumab				
PDS, SC, 150 mg, ea	50242-0040-62	694.58		
XOLEGEL (Stiefel Labs)				
ketoconazole				
GEL, TP, 2%, 15 gm	13478-0003-01	104.00		
XOLEGEL COREPAK (Stiefel Labs)				
hydrocortisone/ketoconazole				
GEL, MR, 1%-2%, ea	13478-0003-09	274.02		
XOLEGEL DUO (Stiefel Labs)				
ketoconazole/pyrithione zinc				
KIT, MR, 2%-1%, ea	13478-0003-04	105.23		
ea	13478-0003-07	274.02		
XOLOX (Wraser Pharm)				
acetaminophen/oxycodone hydrochloride				
TAB, PO, 500 mg-10 mg,				
100s ea, C-II	66992-0310-10	133.65		
XOPENEX (Sepracor)				
levalbuterol hydrochloride				
SOL, IH (PF)				
0.63 mg/3 ml,				
3 ml 24s	63402-0512-24	112.32		
1.25 mg/3 ml,				
3 ml 24s	63402-0513-24	112.32		
1.25 mg/0.5 ml,				
0.5 ml 30s	63402-0515-30	140.40		
(A-S Medication)				
REPACK				
SOL, IH (PF)				
0.63 mg/3 ml,				
3 ml 24s	54569-4748-00	106.50		
1.25 mg/3 ml,				
3 ml 24s	54569-5445-00	106.50		
(DHS, Inc.)				
REPACK				
SOL, IH (24X3ML)				
0.63 mg/3 ml,				
3 ml 24s UD	55887-0332-24	112.48		
(Phys Total Care)				
REPACK				
SOL, IH (PF)				
0.021%, 3 ml 24s	54868-4409-00	142.74		
0.042%, 3 ml 24s	54868-5459-00	118.99		
1.25 mg/0.5 ml,				
0.5 ml 30s	54868-6021-00	153.25		
(Physician Partner)				
REPACK				
SOL, IH (PF)				
1.25 mg/3 ml,				
3 ml 24s	21695-0153-24	213.12		
(Quality Care Prod)				
REPACK				
SOL, IH (1X3ML,PF)				
0.63 mg/3 ml, 3 ml	35356-0489-03	192.60		
XOPENEX HFA (Sepracor)				
levalbuterol tartrate				
ARO, IH (200 ACTUATIONS)				
0.045 mg/actuation,				
15 gm	63402-0510-01	52.49		
(A-S Medication)				
REPACK				
ARO, IH, 0.045 mg/actuation,				
15 gm	54569-5853-00	54.68		
(Quality Care Prod)				
REPACK				
ARO, IH, 0.045 mg/actuation,				
15 gm	49999-0922-15	62.19		
XOPENEX PEDIATRIC (Sepracor)				
levalbuterol hydrochloride				
SOL, IH, 0.31 mg/3 ml,				
3 ml 24s UD	63402-0511-24	112.32		
XPECT-AT (Hawthorn Pharm)				
carbetapentane citrate/guaifenesin				
TER, PO (CAPLET)				
60 mg-600 mg,				
100s ea	63717-0240-01	109.99		
XPECT-HC (Hawthorn Pharm)				
guaifenesin/hydrocodone bitartrate				
TER, PO, 600 mg-5 mg,				
100s ea, C-III	63717-0705-01	99.99		
XPECT-PE (Hawthorn Pharm)				
guaifenesin/phenylephrine hydrochloride				
TER, PO (CAPLET)				
1200 mg-25 mg,				
100s ea	63717-0241-01	159.99		
XYLAREX (Arbor)				
medical food				
SOL, PO (1X473ML,NATURAL BERRY)				
473 ml	24338-0620-16	90.00	72.00	
XYLAZINE HYDROCHLORIDE (Letco)				
POW, NA, 25 gm	62991-1624-02	150.00		
100 gm	62991-1624-03	525.00		
(PCCA)				
POW, NA (USP)				
1 gm	51927-3413-00	12.00		
(Spectrum Pharmacy)				
POW, NA (1X5GM)				
5 gm	49452-8220-02	213.15		
(1X25GM)				
25 gm	49452-8220-03	437.50		
(1X100GM)				
100 gm	49452-8220-04	1113.00		
XYLENE (Baker, J.T.)				
LIQ, NA (A.C.S., REAGENT)				
500 ml	10106-9490-01	26.73		
4000 ml	10106-9490-03	96.25		
(Mallinckrodt Lab) *See XYLENES*				
(PCCA) *See XYLENES PURE*				
XYLENES (Mallinckrodt Lab)				
xylene				
LIQ, NA (A.C.S.)				
500 ml	00406-8668-04	14.27		
XYLENES PURE (PCCA)				
xylene				
SOL, NA (1X1ML)				
1 ml	51927-1824-00	0.08		
XYLITOL (Gallipot)				
POW, NA (N.F.)				
100 gm	51552-0754-05	13.86	9.90	
(PCCA)				
POW, NA (NF)				
1 gm	51927-2413-00	0.42		
(Spectrum Pharmacy)				
POW, NA (N.F.)				
100 gm	49452-8235-01	172.55		
500 gm	49452-8235-02	179.90		
XYLOCAINE (APP)				
lidocaine hydrochloride				
GEL, TP (10X5ML)				
2%, 5 ml 10s	00186-0330-36	83.98		AT
(1X30ML)				
2%, 30 ml	63323-0479-30	20.40		AT
SOL, EP (M.D.V.)				
1%, 10 ml 5s	00186-0275-12	12.48		AP
20 ml	00186-0110-01	2.95		AP
IJ, 0.5%, 50 ml	00186-0135-01	5.53		AP
(1X50ML,MDV)				
1%, 50 ml	63323-0485-50	4.97		AP
(M.D.V.)				
2%, 10 ml 5s	00186-0243-12	14.95		AP
(1X20ML,MDV)				
2%, 20 ml	63323-0486-20	3.34		AP
(M.D.V.)				
2%, 50 ml	00186-0155-01	6.20		AP
IV (AMP,CARDIAC)				
2%, 5 ml 10s	00186-0232-03	46.36		AP
TP, 4%, 50 ml	00186-0320-01	21.64		AT
(Pharma Pac)				
REPACK				
lidocaine				
OIN, TP, 5%, 35 gm	52959-0708-35	28.80		
(Phys Total Care)				
REPACK				
lidocaine hydrochloride				
GEL, TP, 2%, 30 gm	54868-3503-00	19.79		AT
SOL, EP (M.D.V.)				
1%, 50 ml	54868-1795-00	7.26		AP
IJ (VIAL)				
0.5%, 50 ml	54868-3392-00	13.27		AP
(AMP)				
2%, 5 ml 10s	54868-3894-00	43.41		AP
(M.D.V.)				
2%, 10 ml 5s	54868-1798-01	8.76		AP
MM (VISCOUS)				
2%, 100 ml	54868-1825-00	26.76		AT
(Physician Partner)				
REPACK				
SOL, EP (1X20ML,SDV)				
1%, 20 ml	21695-0466-20	15.90		AP
(Southwood)				
REPACK				
GEL, TP, 2%, 30 gm	58016-3125-01	17.48		AT
(1X30GM)				
2%, 30 gm	58016-0321-01	20.40		AT
(Southwood)				
lidocaine				
OIN, TP, 5%, 35 gm	58016-3248-01	14.85		AT
(Southwood)				
lidocaine hydrochloride				
SOL, TP, 4%, 50 ml	58016-1127-01	21.64		AT

PROD/MFR NDC AWP DP OBC

XYLOCAINE DENTAL (Dentsply)
lidocaine hydrochloride
SOL, IJ (1.8MLX100)
2%, 1.8 ml 100s ..... 66312-0170-14 43.79 AP

XYLOCAINE DENTAL W/EPINEPHRINE (Dentsply)
epinephrine/lidocaine hydrochloride
SOL, IJ (1.8MLX100)
1:100000-2%,
1.8 ml 100s........ 66312-0175-14 43.79
1:50000-2%,
1.8 ml 100s........ 66312-0180-14 43.79

XYLOCAINE W/EPINEPHRINE (APP)
epinephrine/lidocaine hydrochloride
SOL, IJ (M.D.V.)
1:200000-0.5%,
50 ml............. 00186-0140-01 6.11 AP
1:100000-2%, 20 ml.. 00186-0125-01 3.80 AP
50 ml............. 00186-0160-01 7.09 AP

(Phys Total Care)
REPACK
SOL, IJ (M.D.V.)
1:100000-1%, 50 ml.. 54868-1796-00 8.80 AP
1:100000-2%, 20 ml.. 54868-1797-00 6.91 AP

XYLOCAINE WITH EPINEPHRINE (APP)
epinephrine/lidocaine hydrochloride
SOL, IJ (5X10ML,MDV)
1:100000-1%,
10 ml 5s........... 63323-0482-10 14.94 AP
(1X20ML,MDV)
1:100000-1%, 20 ml.. 63323-0482-20 3.74 AP
(1X50ML,MDV)
1:100000-1%, 50 ml.. 63323-0482-50 6.23 AP

XYLOCAINE-MPF (APP)
lidocaine hydrochloride
SOL, EP (10X2ML,SDV)
1%, 2 ml 10s .... 63323-0492-02 20.36 AP
(10X2ML)
1%, 2 ml 10s .... 63323-0492-80 21.48 AP
(10X5ML,SDV)
1%, 5 ml 10s .... 63323-0492-05 27.16 AP
(10X5ML)
1%, 5 ml 10s .... 63323-0492-89 29.04 AP
(POLYAMP DUOFIT PACK)
1%, 10 ml 5s .... 63323-0492-97 31.00 AP
(1X30ML,SDV)
1%, 30 ml .... 63323-0492-30 10.25 AP
(S.D. AMP)
1%, 30 ml 5s .... 00186-0255-02 57.86 AP
(S.D.V.,STERILE-PAK)
1%, 30 ml 5s .... 00186-0112-91 56.81 AP
IJ (S.D.V.)
0.5%, 50 ml .... 00186-0137-01 12.59 AP
(5X10ML,POLYAMP DUOFIT)
1.5%, 10 ml 5s....... 63323-0493-97 39.84 AP
(5X20ML,SINGLE DOSE)
1.5%, 20 ml 5s....... 63323-0493-91 71.52 AP
(10X2ML,SDV)
2%, 2 ml 10s 63323-0495-02 30.60
(S.D. AMP)
2%, 2 ml 10s .... 00186-0215-03 27.06 AP
(10X5ML,SDV)
2%, 5 ml 10s 63323-0495-05 28.44
(POLYAMP DUOFIT)
2%, 10 ml 5s 63323-0496-97 36.14
(S.D. AMP)
4%, 5 ml 10s .... 00186-0235-03 75.47 AP

XYLOCAINE-MPF W/EPINEPHRINE (APP)
epinephrine/lidocaine hydrochloride
SOL, EP (S.D. AMP,EPIDURAL TEST)
1:200000-1.5%,
5 ml 10s........... 00186-0265-03 29.06 EE
(S.D.V.,E-Z O CLOSURE)
1:200000-1.5%,
10 ml 5s........... 00186-0117-12 41.68 EE
(S.D. AMP)
1:200000-1.5%,
30 ml 5s........... 00186-0265-02 78.96 EE
(S.D.V.,STERILE-PAK)
1:200000-1.5%,
30 ml 5s........... 00186-0117-91 68.81 EE
IJ (S.D. AMP)
1:200000-1%,
30 ml 5s........... 00186-0260-02 66.35 AP
(S.D.V.,STERILE-PAK)
1:200000-1%,
30 ml 5s........... 00186-0114-91 61.10 AP
1:200000-2%,
20 ml 5s........... 00186-0122-91 76.88 AP

(Phys Total Care)
REPACK
SOL, IJ (S.D.V.)
1:200000-1%, 30 ml.. 54868-4043-00 12.08 AP

XYLOCAINE-MPF WITH EPINEPHRINE (APP)
epinephrine/lidocaine hydrochloride
SOL, EP (1X30ML,SDV)
1:200000-1.5%,
30 ml.............. 63323-0488-30 13.60 AP
IJ (SDV,5X10ML)
1:200000-1%,
10 ml 5s........... 63323-0487-10 36.90 AP
(1X30ML,SDV)
1:200000-1%, 30 ml.. 63323-0487-30 12.35 AP
(5X30ML,SDV)
1:200000-1%,
30 ml 5s........... 63323-0487-31 61.08 AP
(5X10ML,E-Z OFF VIAL,SDV)
1:200000-2%,
10 ml 5s........... 63323-0489-10 44.64 AP
(1X20ML,SDV)
1:200000-2%, 20 ml.. 63323-0489-20 15.72 AP
(5X20ML, USP)
1:200000-2%,
20 ml 5s........... 63323-0489-91 73.68 AP
(5X20ML,SDV)
1:200000-2%,
20 ml 5s........... 63323-0489-21 76.92 AP

XYLOMETAZOLINE HYDROCHLORIDE (PCCA)
POW, NA, 1 gm........... 51927-2487-00 75.60

XYLOSE (PCCA)
POW, NA (USP)
1 gm................ 51927-3558-00 1.80

(Spectrum Pharmacy) *See D+XYLOSE*

XYNTHA (Wyeth)
antihemophilic factor (recomb) plasma/albumin-free
PDS, IV (1000IU VIAL,PF)
1 iu, ea............. 58394-0014-01 1.66 1.38
(2000IU VIAL,PF)
1 iu, ea............. 58394-0015-01 1.66 1.38
(250IU VIAL,PF)
1 iu, ea............. 58394-0012-01 1.66 1.38
(500IU VIAL,PF)
1 iu, ea............. 58394-0013-01 1.66 1.38

XYRALID (Auriga)
hydrocortisone acetate/lidocaine hydrochloride
KIT, MR (FRAGRANCE-FREE)
1%-3%, ea........... 14629-0512-01 128.75

XYRALID LP (Auriga)
hydrocortisone acetate/lidocaine hydrochloride
KIT, TP (FRAGRANCE-FREE)
0.5%-3%, 414 ml 14629-0511-01 178.75

XYRALID RC (Auriga)
hc ace/lido hcl/psyllium
KIT, MR (SF)
1%-3%-6 gm/dose,
ea................. 14629-0510-01 160.00

XYREM (Jazz)
sodium oxybate
SOL, PO, 500 mg/ml,
180 ml, C-III 68727-0100-01 828.00

XYZAL (Sanofi-Aventis)
levocetirizine dihydrochloride
SOL, PO, 0.5 mg/ml,
148 ml 00024-5801-20 102.55
TAB, PO (FILM-COATED)
5 mg, 90s ea......... 00024-5800-90 307.67

(Phys Total Care)
REPACK
TAB, PO, 5 mg, 30s ea 54868-5829-00 115.08

(Quality Care Prod)
REPACK
TAB, PO (FILM-COATED)
5 mg, 90s ea......... 35356-0462-90 486.91

Y-COF DM (Larken Labs, Inc.)
dm/dexbrompheniramine maleate/phenyleph hcl
TER, PO, 6 mg-30 mg-20 mg,
100s ea........... 68047-0210-01 48.57 24.91

YASMIN (Bayer)
drospirenone/ethinyl estradiol
TAB, PO (3X28,BLISTER PACK)
3 mg-0.03 mg,
84s ea............ 50419-0402-03 236.04

(A-S Medication)
REPACK
TAB, PO (BLISTER PACK)
3 mg-0.03 mg,
28s ea............ 54569-5349-00 102.28

(Phys Total Care)
REPACK
TAB, PO (BLISTER PACK)
3 mg-0.03 mg,
28s ea............ 54868-4590-00 100.58

YAZ (Bayer)
drospirenone/ethinyl estradiol
TAB, PO (3X28,FILM-COATED)
3 mg-0.02 mg,
84s ea UD 50419-0405-03 236.04

(A-S Medication)
REPACK
TAB, PO (FILM-COATED)
3 mg-0.02 mg,
28s ea............ 54569-6144-00 102.28

(Quality Care Prod)
REPACK
TAB, PO (FILM-COATED)
3 mg-0.02 mg,
28s ea............ 35356-0255-28 114.30

YAZ 28 (Phys Total Care)
REPACK
drospirenone/ethinyl estradiol
TAB, PO, 3 mg-0.02 mg,
28s ea............ 54868-5828-00 100.58

YELLOW FEVER VACCINE
(Sanofi) *See YF-VAX*

YELLOW FOOD COLOR (PCCA)
color additive
POW, NA, 1 gm........... 51927-1277-00 115.00
SOL, NA, 1 ml........... 51927-1424-00 3.86

YELLOW HORNET TREATMENT (Alk-Abello)
yellow hornet venom
PDS, IJ (KIT (6X1ML))
0.1 mg, ea.......... 52709-1001-01 125.40 94.80
(MDV)
0.1 mg, ea.......... 52709-1001-02 192.24 149.70

YELLOW HORNET VENOM
(Alk-Abello) *See YELLOW HORNET TREATMENT*
(Hollister-Stier) *See VENOMIL*
(Hollister-Stier) *See YELLOW HORNET VENOM PROTEIN*

YELLOW HORNET VENOM PROTEIN (Hollister-Stier)
yellow hornet venom
PDS, IJ (M.D.V.)
0.55 mg, ea......... 65044-9942-05 68.55

YELLOW JACKET TREATMENT (Alk-Abello)
yellow jacket venom
PDS, IJ (KIT (6X1ML))
0.1 mg, ea.......... 52709-0901-01 125.40 94.80
(MDV)
0.1 mg, ea.......... 52709-0901-02 170.88 126.70

YELLOW JACKET VENOM
(Alk-Abello) *See YELLOW JACKET TREATMENT*
(Hollister-Stier) *See VENOMIL*
(Hollister-Stier) *See YELLOW JACKET VENOM PROTEIN*

YELLOW JACKET VENOM PROTEIN (Hollister-Stier)
yellow jacket venom
PDS, IJ (M.D.V.)
0.55 mg, ea......... 65044-9944-05 68.55
1.3 mg, ea.......... 65044-9944-06 139.90

YELLOW WAX
(Amend) *See MULTIWAX 110-X*
(Amend) *See MULTIWAX 180-M*
(Amend) *See MULTIWAX 180-W*
(Amend) *See MULTIWAX H.S.*
(Amend) *See MULTIWAX ML-445*
(Amend) *See MULTIWAX W-445*
(Amend) *See MULTIWAX W-835*
(Amend) *See MULTIWAX X-145A*
(Humco) *See BEESWAX WHITE*
(PCCA)
WAX, NA (NF; BEE'S WAX)
1 gm 51927-2434-00 0.15
(Spectrum Pharmacy) *See BEESWAX WHITE*
(Spectrum Pharmacy) *See BEESWAX YELLOW*

PROD/MFR | NDC | AWP | DP | OBC

(Spectrum Pharmacy) *See WHITE WAX*

YERBA SANTA EXTRACT (PCCA)
SOL, NA (1X1ML)
1 ml................. **51927-2710-00** 0.22

YF-VAX (Sanofi)
yellow fever vaccine
PDR, SC (5 DOSE VIAL W/DILUENT)
47400000000 pfu,
ea................. **49281-0915-05** 389.04 324.20
(S.D.V. W/DILUENT,PF)
47400000000 pfu,
5s ea............... **49281-0915-01** 486.30 405.25

YLANG-YLANG FRAGRANCE (PCCA)
ylang-ylang oil
OIL, NA (CANANGA OIL)
1 ml................. **51927-2373-00** 1.80

YLANG-YLANG OIL (Lorann Oil)
OIL, NA, 9.9 ml........... **23535-0151-84** 6.95

(Medisca)
OIL, NA (1X14ML,FRAGRANCE)
14 ml................ **38779-0904-03** 28.50
(1X25ML,FRAGRANCE)
25 ml................ **38779-0904-04** 52.50
(1X100ML,FRAGRANCE)
100 ml **38779-0904-05** 160.50
(1X500ML,FRAGRANCE)
500 ml **38779-0904-08** 291.00

(PCCA) *See YLANG-YLANG FRAGRANCE*

YODOXIN (Glenwood)
iodoquinol
TAB, PO, 210 mg, 100s ea . **00516-0092-01** 103.53
650 mg, 100s ea **00516-0093-01** 136.28

YOHIMBINE HCL (Concord Labs)
yohimbine hydrochloride
TAB, PO, 5.4 mg, 100s ea.. **20254-0017-01** 12.15
1000s ea **20254-0017-04** 108.00

(Contract Pharmacal)
TAB, PO (PEPPERMINT)
5.4 mg, 100s ea....... **10267-0715-01** 21.90

(Gallipot)
POW, NA, 5 gm........... **51552-0509-02** 34.72

(Medisca)
POW, NA, 25 gm.......... **38779-0278-04** 345.00
100 gm.............. **38779-0278-05** 1185.00

(PCCA)
POW, NA, 1 gm........... **51927-1068-00** 18.00

(Sandoz)
TAB, PO, 5.4 mg, 100s ea.. **00185-0998-01** 103.70
1000s ea **00185-0998-10** 1037.02

(Spectrum Pharmacy)
POW, NA (U.S.P.)
5 gm **49452-8265-01** 148.75
25 gm **49452-8265-02** 570.50
100 gm.............. **49452-8265-03** 1757.00

(Vintage)
TAB, PO, 5.4 mg, 100s ea.. **00254-6377-28** 19.71
1000s ea **00254-6377-38** 179.36

(Phys Total Care)
REPACK
TAB, PO, 5.4 mg, 90s ea... **54868-1884-01** 15.00
100s ea............ **54868-1884-02** 16.17

YOHIMBINE HYDROCHLORIDE
(Concord Labs) *See YOHIMBINE HCL*
(Contract Pharmacal) *See YOHIMBINE HCL*
(Gallipot) *See YOHIMBINE HCL*
(Medisca) *See YOHIMBINE HCL*
(PCCA) *See YOHIMBINE HCL*
(Sandoz) *See YOHIMBINE HCL*
(Spectrum Pharmacy) *See YOHIMBINE HCL*
(Vintage) *See YOHIMBINE HCL*

Z-COF 8DM (Zyber)
dm/gg/pse hcl
SUS, PO (12X473ML,AF,GRAPE)*
473 ml 144s **65224-0616-16** 3317.64

Z-TUSS AC (MAGNA Pharm)
chlorpheniramine maleate/codeine phosphate
SOL, PO (1X473ML,AF,SF,CHERRY)
2 mg/5 ml-9 mg/5 ml,
473 ml, C-V......... **58407-0755-16** 50.36 40.29

Z-TUSS DM (MAGNA Pharm)
dm/gg/phenyleph hcl
SYR, PO (AF,SF,RASPBERRY)
473 ml **58407-0810-16** 77.77 55.55

ZACARE 4% (Hawthorn Pharm)
benzoyl peroxide/hyaluronate sodium
KIT, MR, 4%-0.2%, 410 gm **63717-0042-11** 93.74

ZACARE 8% (Hawthorn Pharm)
benzoyl peroxide/hyaluronate sodium
KIT, MR, 8%-0.2%, 410 gm **63717-0043-11** 99.99

ZACLIR 4% (Hawthorn Pharm)
benzoyl peroxide
SOA, TP (CLEANSING LOTION)
4%, 297 gm **63717-0030-11** 59.49

ZACLIR 8% (Hawthorn Pharm)
benzoyl peroxide
SOA, TP (CLEANSING LOTION)
8%, 297 gm **63717-0031-11** 61.79

ZADITOR (A-S Medication)
REPACK
ketotifen fumarate
SOL, OP, 0.025%, 5 ml **54569-5931-00** 12.19

(Pharma Pac)
REPACK
SOL, OP, 0.025%, 5 ml **52959-0608-05** 47.85

(Phys Total Care)
REPACK
SOL, OP, 0.025%, 5 ml **54868-4132-00** 15.59

ZAFIRLUKAST
(AstraZeneca) *See ACCOLATE*

ZALEPLON
FUL
CAP, PO, 5 mg, 100s ea............................. 71.91
10 mg, 100s ea................................ 73.86

(Aurobindo Pharma)
CAP, PO (HARD GELATIN)
5 mg,
100s ea, C-IV ...... **65862-0214-01** 364.64 AB
10 mg, 100s ea, C-IV . **65862-0215-01** 374.58 AB

(CorePharma)
CAP, PO, 5 mg,
100s ea, C-IV **64720-0322-10** 364.64
10 mg, 100s ea, C-IV . **64720-0323-10** 374.58

(Dava Pharma)
CAP, PO, 5 mg,
100s ea, C-IV ...... **67253-0950-10** 368.71 AB
10 mg, 100s ea, C-IV . **67253-0951-10** 378.77 AB

(Greenstone)
CAP, PO (HARD GELATIN)
5 mg,
100s ea, C-IV **59762-2630-01** 364.64
500s ea, C-IV **59762-2630-04** 1823.20
10 mg, 100s ea, C-IV . **59762-2631-01** 374.58
500s ea, C-IV **59762-2631-04** 1872.90

(King Pharm) *See SONATA*

(Mylan)
CAP, PO, 5 mg,
100s ea, C-IV ...... **00378-6805-01** 364.64 AB
10 mg, 100s ea, C-IV . **00378-6810-01** 374.58 AB
1000s ea, C-IV ..... **00378-6810-10** 3745.80 AB

(Roxane)
CAP, PO, 5 mg,
100s ea, C-IV ...... **00054-0084-25** 368.74 AB
10 mg, 100s ea, C-IV . **00054-0085-25** 378.79 AB

(Teva)
CAP, PO, 5 mg,
100s ea, C-IV ...... **00093-5268-01** 368.74 AB
10 mg, 100s ea, C-IV . **00093-5269-01** 378.79 AB

(Unichem)
CAP, PO (HARD GELATIN)
5 mg,
100s ea, C-IV ...... **29300-0131-01** 368.74 AB
10 mg, 100s ea, C-IV . **29300-0132-01** 378.79 AB

(Upsher-Smith)
CAP, PO (HARD GELATIN)
5 mg,
1000s ea, C-IV ..... **00832-0400-10** 3374.90 AB
10 mg,
1000s ea, C-IV ..... **00832-0401-10** 3473.90 AB

(A-S Medication)
REPACK
CAP, PO (HARD GELATIN)
10 mg,
10s ea, C-IV........ **54569-6118-00** 37.49 AB

(Aidarex)
REPACK
CAP, PO, 10 mg,
30s ea, C-IV........ **33261-0454-30** 135.00
60s ea, C-IV........ **33261-0454-60** 270.00
90s ea, C-IV........ **33261-0454-90** 405.00
120s ea, C-IV **33261-0454-02** 540.00

(Dispensing Solutions)
REPACK
CAP, PO (HARD GELATIN)
5 mg, 30s ea, C-IV.... **66336-0056-30** 116.15 AB
10 mg, 30s ea, C-IV .. **66336-0102-30** 119.32 AB

(Nucare Pharm)
REPACK
CAP, PO, 5 mg,
30s ea, C-IV........ **68071-0788-30** 43.99 AB
10 mg, 30s ea, C-IV .. **68071-0789-30** 44.38 AB

(Pharma Pac)
REPACK
CAP, PO (HARD GELATIN)
5 mg, 30s ea, C-IV.... **52959-0971-30** 28.15 AB
10 mg, 30s ea, C-IV .. **52959-0957-30** 46.19 AB

(Phys Total Care)
REPACK
CAP, PO (HARD GELATIN)
5 mg, 10s ea, C-IV.... **54868-5909-00** 19.59 AB
30s ea, C-IV........ **54868-5909-01** 46.78 AB
10 mg, 10s ea, C-IV .. **54868-5908-00** 19.94 AB
30s ea, C-IV........ **54868-5908-01** 47.83 AB

(Physician Partner)
REPACK
CAP, PO, 5 mg,
60s ea, C-IV........ **21695-0376-60** 437.57
(HARD GELATIN)
10 mg,
14s ea, C-IV........ **21695-0105-14** 124.78 AB
30s ea, C-IV........ **21695-0105-30** 224.75 AB
60s ea, C-IV........ **21695-0105-60** 449.50 AB

(Stat Rx)
REPACK
CAP, PO, 5 mg,
30s ea, C-IV........ **16590-0661-30** 109.50 AB
60s ea, C-IV........ **16590-0661-60** 219.00 AB
90s ea, C-IV........ **16590-0661-90** 328.50 AB
10 mg, 28s ea, C-IV .. **16590-0629-28** 104.25 AB
30s ea, C-IV........ **16590-0629-30** 111.70 AB

ZAMICET (Hawthorn Pharm)
acetaminophen/hydrocodone bitartrate
SOL, PO (1X473ML,FRUIT)
325 mg/15 ml-10 mg/15 ml,
473 ml, C-III **63717-0895-16** 149.99

ZANAFLEX (Acorda Therapeutics)
tizanidine hydrochloride
TAB, PO, 2 mg, 150s ea ... **10144-0592-15** 215.06 AB
4 mg, 150s ea........ **10144-0594-15** 343.24 AB

(A-S Medication)
REPACK
TAB, PO, 4 mg, 30s ea .... **54569-4975-01** 104.22 AB

(IPI)
REPACK
CAP, PO, 6 mg, 60s ea **18837-0266-60** 244.51

(PD-Rx Pharm)
REPACK
TAB, PO, 2 mg, 12s ea .... **55289-0716-12** 37.41 AB
4 mg, 10s ea......... **55289-0612-10** 33.84 AB
20s ea.............. **55289-0612-20** 67.67 AB

(Pharma Pac)
REPACK
TAB, PO, 2 mg, 20s ea **52959-0636-20** 32.00
25s ea.............. **52959-0636-25** 38.75
30s ea.............. **52959-0636-30** 46.57
40s ea.............. **52959-0636-40** 46.57
45s ea.............. **52959-0636-45** 69.85
90s ea.............. **52959-0636-90** 116.42
4 mg, 15s ea......... **52959-0637-15** 26.25
30s ea.............. **52959-0637-30** 48.90
45s ea.............. **52959-0637-45** 73.20
90s ea.............. **52959-0637-90** 145.00

(Phys Total Care)
REPACK
CAP, PO, 2 mg, 50s ea **54868-5803-00** 117.79
100s ea............ **54868-5803-01** 220.83
TAB, PO, 2 mg, 90s ea **54868-4404-01** 198.31
100s ea............ **54868-4404-00** 220.21
4 mg, 30s ea......... **54868-4145-02** 77.36
60s ea.............. **54868-4145-01** 152.85
90s ea.............. **54868-4145-00** 215.75

PROD/MFR	NDC	AWP	DP	OBC
(Quality Care Prod)				
REPACK				
CAP, PO, 2 mg, 30s ea	**35356-0341-30**	108.47		
4 mg, 30s ea	**35356-0342-30**	136.60		
6 mg, 150s ea	**35356-0446-15**	1089.68		
(Southwood)				
REPACK				
TAB, PO, 2 mg, 30s ea	**58016-0521-30**	34.50		
60s ea	**58016-0521-60**	69.00		
100s ea	**58016-0521-00**	115.00		
4 mg, 2s ea	**58016-0513-02**	4.16		
8s ea	**58016-0513-08**	16.64		
10s ea	**58016-0513-10**	20.80		
20s ea	**58016-0513-20**	41.61		
30s ea	**58016-0513-30**	62.41		
40s ea	**58016-0513-40**	83.21		
45s ea	**58016-0513-45**	93.61		
60s ea	**58016-0513-60**	124.82		
90s ea	**58016-0513-90**	187.22		
100s ea	**58016-0513-00**	208.03		
150s ea	**58016-0513-03**	312.04		
ZANAFLEX CAPSULE (Acorda Therapeutics)				
tizanidine hydrochloride				
CAP, PO, 2 mg, 150s ea	**10144-0602-15**	363.68		
4 mg, 150s ea	**10144-0604-15**	460.98		
6 mg, 150s ea	**10144-0606-15**	691.42		
(Physician Partner)				
REPACK				
CAP, PO, 4 mg, 30s ea	**21695-0373-30**	167.02		
(Quality Care Prod)				
REPACK				
CAP, PO, 2 mg, 60s ea	**35356-0341-60**	216.94		
90s ea	**35356-0341-90**	325.41		
4 mg, 60s ea	**35356-0342-60**	273.20		
90s ea	**35356-0342-90**	409.80		
6 mg, 30s ea	**35356-0446-30**	259.54		
60s ea	**35356-0446-60**	519.08		
90s ea	**35356-0446-90**	778.62		
(Stat Rx)				
REPACK				
CAP, PO, 4 mg, 84s ea	**16590-0871-62**	260.90		
6 mg, 60s ea	**16590-0756-60**	281.31		
ZANAMIVIR				
(Glaxo) *See RELENZA*				
ZANOSAR (Teva)				
streptozocin				
PDS, IV, 1 gm, ea	**00703-4636-01**	335.26		
ZANTAC (Glaxo)				
ranitidine hydrochloride				
SOL, IJ (VIAL)				
25 mg/ml, 2 ml 10s	**00173-0362-38**	39.91		
(M.D.V.)				
25 mg/ml, 6 ml	**00173-0363-01**	9.26		
(VIAL)				
25 mg/ml, 40 ml	**00173-0363-00**	60.54		
IV (PREMIX)				
1 mg/ml, 50 ml 24s	**00173-0441-00**	141.86		
SYR, PO (PEPPERMINT)				
15 mg/ml, 480 ml	**00173-0383-54**	373.90		
(AQ)				
REPACK				
TAB, PO, 150 mg, 30s ea	**66105-0749-03**	130.44		
60s ea	**66105-0749-06**	260.88		
90s ea	**66105-0749-09**	391.32		
100s ea	**66105-0749-10**	434.80		
180s ea	**66105-0749-18**	782.64		
(Phys Total Care)				
REPACK				
SOL, IJ, 25 mg/ml, 40 ml	**54868-5775-00**	74.49		
ZANTAC 150 (Glaxo)				
ranitidine hydrochloride				
TAB, PO (FILM-COATED)				
150 mg, 60s ea	**00173-0344-42**	257.93		AB
180s ea	**00173-0344-17**	773.53		AB
500s ea	**00173-0344-14**	2148.78		AB
(PD-Rx Pharm)				
REPACK				
TAB, PO, 150 mg, 14s ea	**55289-0551-14**	64.72		AB
28s ea	**55289-0551-28**	104.52		AB
(Pharma Pac)				
REPACK				
TAB, PO, 150 mg, 6s ea	**52959-0325-06**	17.04		AB
14s ea	**52959-0325-14**	39.12		AB
15s ea	**52959-0325-15**	41.08		AB
28s ea	**52959-0325-28**	67.20		AB
30s ea	**52959-0325-30**	73.55		AB
60s ea	**52959-0325-60**	136.09		AB
(Phys Total Care)				
REPACK				
TAB, PO, 150 mg, 30s ea	**54868-0323-02**	120.00		AB
40s ea	**54868-0323-07**	159.38		AB
50s ea	**54868-0323-04**	198.75		AB
60s ea	**54868-0323-01**	225.00		AB
90s ea	**54868-0323-00**	336.56		AB
100s ea	**54868-0323-06**	373.13		AB
(Quality Care Prod)				
REPACK				
TAB, PO (FILM-COATED)				
150 mg, 30s ea	**49999-0056-30**	88.26		AB
ZANTAC 25 (Glaxo)				
ranitidine hydrochloride				
TEF, PO (EFFERDOSE)				
25 mg, 60s ea	**00173-0734-00**	241.40		
ZANTAC 300 (Glaxo)				
ranitidine hydrochloride				
TAB, PO (FILM-COATED)				
300 mg, 30s ea	**00173-0393-40**	234.10		AB
(Pharma Pac)				
REPACK				
TAB, PO, 300 mg, 10s ea	**52959-0201-10**	31.93		AB
15s ea	**52959-0201-15**	47.44		AB
(Phys Total Care)				
REPACK				
TAB, PO, 300 mg, 30s ea	**54868-0324-01**	189.75		AB
ZARONTIN (Pfizer)				
ethosuximide				
SGL, PO, 250 mg, 100s ea	**00071-0237-24**	156.16	130.13	
SYR, PO (AF)				
250 mg/5 ml,				
480 ml	**00071-2418-23**	164.28	136.90	AA
ZAROXOLYN (UCB)				
metolazone				
TAB, PO, 2.5 mg, 100s ea	**53014-0975-71**	222.79		
5 mg, 100s ea	**53014-0850-71**	253.20		
(Phys Total Care)				
REPACK				
TAB, PO, 2.5 mg, 30s ea	**54868-2707-00**	59.16		
100s ea	**54868-2707-01**	181.61		
5 mg, 30s ea	**54868-0476-00**	76.11		
60s ea	**54868-0476-01**	142.02		
100s ea	**54868-0476-02**	234.74		
ZAVESCA (Actelion Pharm)				
miglustat				
CAP, PO (K30)				
100 mg, 90s ea UD	**66215-0201-90**	14460.00		
ZAZOLE (PharmaDerm)				
terconazole				
CRE, VG (W/ APPLICATOR)				
0.4%, 45 gm	**00462-0346-46**	46.44		
(W/DOSE APPLICATOR)				
0.8%, 20 gm	**00462-0347-20**	50.84		
SUP, VG (W/ VAG APPLICATOR)				
80 mg, 3s ea	**00462-0348-03**	52.81		
ZEBETA (Teva)				
bisoprolol fumarate				
TAB, PO (FILM-COATED)				
5 mg, 30s ea	**51285-0060-01**	101.06	32.53	AB
10 mg, 30s ea	**51285-0061-01**	101.06	32.53	AB
(Phys Total Care)				
REPACK				
TAB, PO, 5 mg, 30s ea	**54868-4621-00**	117.12		AB
ZEBUTAL (Victory Pharma, Inc.)				
acetaminophen/butalbital/caffeine				
CAP, PO, 500 mg-50 mg-40 mg,				
100s ea	**68453-0170-10**	184.54		
ZEGERID (Santarus, Inc.)				
omeprazole/sodium bicarbonate				
CAP, PO, 20 mg-1100 mg,				
30s ea	**68012-0102-30**	192.60	160.50	
40 mg-1100 mg,				
30s ea	**68012-0104-30**	192.60	160.50	
PKT, PO (PEACH MINT)				
30s ea UD	**68012-0052-30**	205.56	171.30	
30s ea UD	**68012-0054-30**	205.56	171.30	
(Phys Total Care)				
REPACK				
CAP, PO, 40 mg-1100 mg,				
30s ea	**54868-5611-00**	193.08		
(Stat Rx)				
REPACK				
CAP, PO, 40 mg-1100 mg,				
30s ea	**16590-0314-30**	207.17		
ZELAPAR (Valeant Pharm Intl)				
selegiline hydrochloride				
ODT, PO (GRAPEFRUIT)				
1.25 mg, 60s ea	**00187-0453-02**	520.59		
ZEMA-PAK (Macoven)				
dexamethasone				
TAB, PO (6 DAY)				
1.5 mg, 21s ea	**44183-0509-21**	27.26		
(10-DAY)				
1.5 mg, 35s ea	**44183-0507-35**	38.94		
(13-DAY)				
1.5 mg, 51s ea	**44183-0508-51**	43.95		
ZEMAIRA (CSL)				
alpha-1 proteinase inhibitor human				
PDS, IV (APPRX 1000 MG VIAL,PF)				
1 mg, ea	**00053-7201-02**	0.43		
ZEMPLAR (Abbott Pharm)				
paricalcitol				
SGL, PO (SOFTGEL)				
1 mcg, 30s ea	**00074-4317-30**	276.31	242.38	
2 mcg, 30s ea	**00074-4314-30**	552.60	484.74	
4 mcg, 30s ea	**00074-4315-30**	1105.21	969.48	
SOL, IV (VIAL,FLIPTOP)				
0.002 mg/ml,				
1 ml 100s	**00074-4637-01**	1121.40	934.50	
(S.D.V.,FLIPTOP)				
0.005 mg/ml,				
1 ml 100s	**00074-1658-01**	2803.20	2336.00	
2 ml 100s	**00074-1658-02**	5605.20	4671.00	
ZEMURON (Organon)				
rocuronium bromide				
SOL, IV (VIAL)				
10 mg/ml, 5 ml 10s	**00052-0450-15**	244.33		
(M.D.V.)				
10 mg/ml,				
10 ml 10s	**00052-0450-16**	469.13		
ZENCHENT (Watson)				
ethinyl estradiol/norethindrone				
TAB, PO (28 DAY,5X28)				
35 mcg-0.4 mg,				
140s ea	**52544-0210-28**	193.69		
ZENPEP (Eurand)				
amylase/lipase/protease				
ECC, PO, 27000 u-5000 u-17000 u,				
100s ea	**42865-0100-02**	78.89		
55000 u-10000 u-34000 u,				
100s ea	**42865-0101-02**	147.28		
82000 u-15000 u-51000 u,				
100s ea	**42865-0102-02**	208.76		
109000 u-20000 u-68000 u,				
100s ea	**42865-0103-02**	300.28		
ZERIT (B/M Squibb Onc/Vir)				
stavudine				
CAP, PO, 15 mg, 60s ea	**00003-1964-01**	405.49		
20 mg, 60s ea	**00003-1965-01**	421.66		
30 mg, 60s ea	**00003-1966-01**	447.89		
40 mg, 60s ea	**00003-1967-01**	456.16		
PDS, PO (DYE-FREE,FRUIT)				
1 mg/ml, 200 ml	**00003-1968-01**	84.72		
(A-S Medication)				
REPACK				
CAP, PO, 20 mg, 60s ea	**54569-5480-00**	422.34		
40 mg, 60s ea	**54569-4054-00**	456.89		
(Phys Total Care)				
REPACK				
CAP, PO, 15 mg, 60s ea	**54868-3360-00**	293.36		
20 mg, 60s ea	**54868-3353-00**	305.05		
30 mg, 60s ea	**54868-3448-00**	419.44		
40 mg, 30s ea	**54868-3352-01**	221.93		
60s ea	**54868-3352-00**	427.16		
(Quality Care Prod)				
REPACK				
CAP, PO, 30 mg, 60s ea	**35356-0028-60**	810.00		
40 mg, 60s ea	**35356-0074-60**	814.03		
ZERLOR (Pamlab)				
acetaminophen/caffeine/dihydrocodeine bitartrate				
TAB, PO, 712.8 mg-60 mg-32 mg,				
100s ea, C-III	**18011-0032-01**	159.78		
ZERVALX (Pamlab)				
l-methylfolate				
TAB, PO (SF,GLUTEN-FREE)				
1 mg, 90s ea	**00525-1010-90**	74.75		
ZESTORETIC (AstraZeneca)				
hydrochlorothiazide/lisinopril				
TAB, PO, 12.5 mg-10 mg,				
100s ea	**00310-0141-10**	175.33		AB
12.5 mg-20 mg,				
100s ea	**00310-0142-10**	189.79		AB
25 mg-20 mg,				
100s ea	**00310-0145-10**	192.07		AB

PROD/MFR	NDC	AWP	DP	OBC
(Pharma Pac)				
REPACK				
TAB, PO, 12.5 mg-10 mg,				
100s ea	**52959-0498-00**	128.00		AB
(Phys Total Care)				
REPACK				
TAB, PO, 12.5 mg-20 mg,				
30s ea	**54868-4003-00**	50.84		AB
ZESTRIL (AstraZeneca)				
lisinopril				
TAB, PO, 2.5 mg, 100s ea	**00310-0135-10**	102.46		AB
(UNCOATED)				
5 mg, 100s ea	**00310-0130-11**	153.61		AB
10 mg, 100s ea	**00310-0131-11**	158.60		AB
20 mg, 100s ea	**00310-0132-11**	169.81		AB
30 mg, 100s ea	**00310-0133-10**	240.42		AB
40 mg, 100s ea	**00310-0134-10**	248.33		AB
(PD-Rx Pharm)				
REPACK				
TAB, PO, 10 mg, 30s ea	**55289-0509-30**	70.73		AB
(REDI-SCRIPT)				
10 mg, 30s ea	**58864-0654-30**	52.23		AB
20 mg, 30s ea	**55289-0106-30**	75.72		AB
(Phys Total Care)				
REPACK				
TAB, PO, 5 mg, 30s ea	**54868-1961-01**	42.16		AB
100s ea	**54868-1961-02**	135.53		AB
10 mg, 30s ea	**54868-1296-01**	42.13		AB
100s ea	**54868-1296-02**	127.96		AB
20 mg, 30s ea	**54868-1001-01**	44.96		AB
(Southwood)				
REPACK				
TAB, PO, 5 mg, 30s ea	**58016-0956-30**	43.47		AB
60s ea	**58016-0956-60**	86.95		AB
90s ea	**58016-0956-90**	130.42		AB
100s ea	**58016-0956-00**	144.91		AB
10 mg, 14s ea	**58016-0362-14**	15.92		AB
21s ea	**58016-0362-21**	23.88		AB
28s ea UD	**58016-0362-28**	31.84		AB
20 mg, 14s ea	**58016-0363-14**	22.43		AB
21s ea	**58016-0363-21**	33.64		AB
30s ea	**58016-0363-30**	48.06		AB
60s ea	**58016-0363-60**	96.12		AB
90s ea	**58016-0363-90**	144.18		AB
100s ea	**58016-0363-00**	160.20		AB
ZETIA (Merck/Schering-Plough)				
ezetimibe				
TAB, PO (UNIT OF USE)				
10 mg, 30s ea	**66582-0414-31**	122.54	102.12	
90s ea	**66582-0414-54**	367.64	306.37	
100s ea	**66582-0414-28**	408.49	340.41	
500s ea	**66582-0414-74**	2042.46	1702.05	
5000s ea	**66582-0414-76**	20424.50	1720.42	
(A-S Medication)				
REPACK				
TAB, PO, 10 mg, 30s ea	**54569-5489-00**	151.00		
90s ea	**54569-5489-02**	453.01		
(AQ)				
REPACK				
TAB, PO, 10 mg, 30s ea	**66105-0979-03**	184.18		
(DHS, Inc.)				
REPACK				
TAB, PO, 10 mg, 30s ea	**55887-0878-30**	144.00		
(PD-Rx Pharm)				
REPACK				
TAB, PO, 10 mg, 15s ea	**55289-0966-15**	86.43		
30s ea	**55289-0966-30**	172.86		
(REDI-SCRIPT)				
10 mg, 30s ea	**58864-0889-30**	146.87		
(Phys Total Care)				
REPACK				
TAB, PO, 10 mg, 30s ea	**54868-4719-01**	147.68		
90s ea	**54868-4719-00**	437.16		
(Quality Care Prod)				
REPACK				
TAB, PO, 10 mg, 30s ea	**49999-0487-30**	181.35		
90s ea	**49999-0487-90**	480.15		
(Southwood)				
REPACK				
TAB, PO, 10 mg, 30s ea	**58016-0572-30**	108.66		
60s ea	**58016-0572-60**	217.32		
90s ea	**58016-0572-90**	325.98		
100s ea	**58016-0572-00**	362.20		
ZEVALIN IN-111 (Spectrum)				
ibritumomab tiuxetan/sodium acetate				
SOL, MR (PF)				
ea	**68152-0104-04**	4515.00	3500.00	EE

PROD/MFR	NDC	AWP	DP	OBC
ZEVALIN Y-90 (Spectrum)				
ibritumomab tiuxetan/sodium acetate				
SOL, MR (PF)				
ea	**68152-0103-03**	40635.00	31500.00	EE
ZGESIC (Capellon)				
acetaminophen/phenyltoloxamine citrate				
TER, PO, 600 mg-66 mg,				
90s ea	**64543-0400-90**	106.25	85.00	
ZHIST (Huckaby)				
cpm/gg/hydrocod bit/pse hcl				
SOL, PO (CHERRY)				
473 ml, C-III	**35501-0037-16**	62.93	41.95	
ZIAC (Teva)				
bisoprolol fumarate/hydrochlorothiazide				
TAB, PO (FILM-COATED)				
2.5 mg-6.25 mg,				
100s ea	**51285-0047-02**	336.88	108.48	AB
5 mg-6.25 mg,				
100s ea	**51285-0050-02**	336.88	108.48	AB
10 mg-6.25 mg,				
30s ea	**51285-0040-01**	101.06	32.53	AB
(Phys Total Care)				
REPACK				
TAB, PO, 5 mg-6.25 mg,				
30s ea	**54868-4173-00**	54.38		AB
10 mg-6.25 mg,				
30s ea	**54868-4179-00**	47.84		AB
ZIAGEN (Glaxo)				
abacavir sulfate				
SOL, PO (BANANA-STRAWBERRY)				
20 mg/ml, 240 ml	**00173-0664-00**	152.77		
TAB, PO (BLISTER PACK,CAPLET)				
300 mg, 60s ea UD	**00173-0661-00**	581.10		
(CAPLET)				
300 mg, 60s ea	**00173-0661-01**	581.10		
(A-S Medication)				
REPACK				
SOL, PO (BANANA-STRAWBERRY)				
20 mg/ml, 240 ml	**54569-5390-00**	198.60		
TAB, PO (CAPLET)				
300 mg, 60s ea	**54569-4883-00**	755.43		
(Phys Total Care)				
REPACK				
TAB, PO, 300 mg, 30s ea	**54868-4522-01**	325.77		
(CAPLET)				
300 mg, 60s ea	**54868-4522-00**	629.31		
(Quality Care Prod)				
REPACK				
TAB, PO (CAPLET)				
300 mg, 6s ea	**35356-0075-06**	182.49		
60s ea	**35356-0075-60**	1825.20		
ZIANA (Medicis)				
clindamycin phosphate/tretinoin				
GEL, TP, 1.2%-0.025%,				
30 gm	**99207-0300-30**	191.10		
60 gm	**99207-0300-60**	382.20		
(Phys Total Care)				
REPACK				
GEL, TP (1X30GM)				
1.2%-0.025%, 30 gm	**54868-5946-00**	192.39		
ZICONOTIDE				
(Elan Pharmaceuticals) *See PRIALT*				
ZIDOVUDINE				
FUL				
TAB, PO, 300 mg, 60s ea		54.66		
(Aurobindo Pharma)				
CAP, PO, 100 mg, 100s ea	**65862-0107-01**	201.94		AB
SYR, PO (STRAWBERRY)				
50 mg/5 ml, 240 ml	**65862-0048-24**	56.42		AA
TAB, PO (FILM-COATED)				
300 mg, 60s ea	**65862-0024-60**	360.97		AB
(Camber)				
TAB, PO (USP,FILM COATED)				
300 mg, 60s ea	**31722-0509-60**	360.97		AB
(Dava Pharma)				
CAP, PO (USP,HARDGEL)				
100 mg, 100s ea	**67253-0109-10**	201.94		AB
SYR, PO (1X240ML,USP,STRAWBERRY)				
50 mg/5 ml, 240 ml	**67253-0961-24**	58.92		AA
(Glaxo) *See RETROVIR*				
(Greenstone)				
TAB, PO (FILM-COATED)				
300 mg, 60s ea	**59762-3650-01**	360.97		
(Mylan)				
TAB, PO (USP,FILM-COATED)				
300 mg, 60s ea	**00378-6106-91**	365.04		AB

PROD/MFR	NDC	AWP	DP	OBC
(Ranbaxy Pharm)				
TAB, PO (FILM-COATED)				
300 mg, 60s ea	**63304-0920-60**	365.04		AB
(Roxane)				
TAB, PO (FILM-COATED)				
300 mg, 60s ea	**00054-0052-21**	365.09		AB
(Dispensing Solutions)				
REPACK				
TAB, PO, 300 mg, 10s ea	**55045-3549-01**	69.50		
(Physician Partner)				
REPACK				
TAB, PO (FILM-COATED)				
300 mg, 18s ea	**21695-0369-18**	254.81		AB
(Southwood)				
REPACK				
TAB, PO, 300 mg, 30s ea	**00490-7026-30**	182.52		
60s ea	**00490-7026-60**	365.04		
90s ea	**00490-7026-90**	547.56		
100s ea	**00490-7026-00**	608.40		
ZIKS HEMATOGEN (Nnodum)				
ferrous fum/stomach, desiccated/vit b12/vit c				
SGL, PO (10X10)				
100s ea UD	**63044-0631-19**	30.99		
ZIKS HEMATOGEN FA (Nnodum)				
ferrous fum/folic acid/vit b12/vit c				
SGL, PO, 100s ea UD	**63044-0632-17**	35.99		
ZIKS HEMATOGEN FORTE (Nnodum)				
ferrous fum/folic acid/vit b12/vit c				
SGL, PO (GELCAP)				
100s ea UD	**63044-0633-21**	50.99		
ZILEUTON				
(Cornerstone) *See ZYFLO*				
(Cornerstone) *See ZYFLO CR*				
ZINACEF (Glaxo)				
cefuroxime sodium				
PDS, IJ, 1.5 gm, 10s ea	**00173-0354-10**	134.52		AP
(ADD-VANTAGE)				
1.5 gm, 10s ea	**00173-0437-00**	139.39		AP
7.5 gm, 6s ea	**00173-0400-00**	395.66		AP
750 mg, 10s ea	**00173-0352-10**	67.68		AB
(ADD-VANTAGE)				
750 mg, 25s ea	**00173-0436-00**	181.10		AB
SOL, IV (PREMIX)				
1.5 gm/50 ml,				
50 ml 24s	**00173-0425-00**	387.79		
750 mg/50 ml,				
50 ml 24s	**00173-0424-00**	227.12		
ZINC (Baker, J.T.)				
GRA, NA (A.C.S., REAGENT,10 MESH)				
500 gm	**10106-4240-01**	65.30		
(A.C.S., REAGENT,20 MESH)				
500 gm	**10106-4244-01**	79.52		
(A.C.S., REAGENT,30 MESH)				
500 gm	**10106-4248-01**	65.30		
(A.C.S., REAGENT,40 MESH)				
500 gm	**10106-4252-01**	72.72		
(A.C.S., REAGENT,10 MESH)				
2500 gm	**10106-4240-05**	228.25		
(A.C.S., REAGENT,20 MESH)				
2500 gm	**10106-4244-05**	284.38		
(A.C.S., REAGENT,30 MESH)				
2500 gm	**10106-4248-05**	228.66		
ZINC ACETATE				
(Baker, J.T.) *See ZINC ACETATE DIHYDRATE*				
(Gallipot)				
CRY, NA (U.S.P.)				
454 gm	**51552-0716-06**	22.33	15.95	
(Gate) *See GALZIN*				
(Medisca)				
POW, NA (USP)				
100 gm	**38779-1702-05**	31.50		
(U.S.P.)				
500 gm	**38779-1702-08**	58.50		
(PCCA)				
POW, NA (U.S.P.)				
1 gm	**51927-1412-00**	0.48		
(Spectrum Pharmacy)				
CRY, NA (U.S.P.)				
500 gm	**49452-8275-01**	99.40		
2500 gm	**49452-8275-02**	329.70		
ZINC ACETATE DIHYDRATE (Baker, J.T.)				
zinc acetate				
CRY, NA (A.C.S., REAGENT)				
500 gm	**10106-4296-01**	43.05		
2500 gm	**10106-4296-05**	95.89		

PROD/MFR	NDC	AWP	DP	OBC
ZINC ASCORBATE (PCCA)				
POW, NA (1X1GM)				
1 gm	**51927-3670-00**	0.95		
ZINC BROMIDE (Baker, J.T.)				
GRA, NA (REAGENT)				
500 gm	**10106-4308-01**	150.38		
ZINC CARBONATE (Baker, J.T.)				
POW, NA (REAGENT)				
500 gm	**10106-4312-01**	128.49		
ZINC CHELATE (Gallipot)				
zinc, chelated				
POW, NA (AMINO ACID)				
1000 gm	**51552-0975-07**	105.00	75.00	
ZINC CHLORIDE (Baker, J.T.)				
GRA, NA (U.S.P.)				
500 gm	**10106-4326-01**	26.58		
(Gallipot)				
GRA, NA (U.S.P.)				
454 gm	**51552-0596-06**	30.31		
(Hospira)				
SOL, IV (VIAL,FLIPTOP,LATEX-FREE)				
1 mg/ml, 10 ml 25s	**00409-4090-01**	25.80	22.50	
(Mallinckrodt Lab)				
GRA, NA (U.S.P.)				
500 gm	**00406-8772-04**	22.66		
(PCCA)				
POW, NA (U.S.P.)				
1 gm	**51927-1481-00**	0.17		
(Spectrum Pharmacy)				
GRA, NA (U.S.P.)				
500 gm	**49452-8290-01**	109.90		
2500 gm	**49452-8290-02**	420.00		
12000 gm	**49452-8290-03**	1291.50		
ZINC CITRATE (PCCA)				
POW, NA (PURIFIED DIHYDRATE)				
1 gm	**51927-2360-00**	1.32		
ZINC GLUCONATE (Gallipot)				
GRA, NA (U.S.P.)				
454 gm	**51552-0547-06**	31.08		
POW, NA (USP,1X454GM)				
454 gm	**51552-0903-06**	31.08	22.20	
(PCCA)				
POW, NA (USP)				
1 gm	**51927-1248-00**	0.36		
(Spectrum Pharmacy) *See ZINC GLUCONATE TRIHYDRATE*				
ZINC GLUCONATE TRIHYDRATE (Spectrum Pharmacy)				
zinc gluconate				
POW, NA (U.S.P.)				
500 gm	**49452-8298-01**	130.55		
2500 gm	**49452-8298-02**	472.50		
12000 gm	**49452-8298-03**	1291.50		
ZINC IODIDE (PCCA)				
POW, NA (PURIFIED)				
1 gm	**51927-3611-00**	2.28		
ZINC MONOMETHIONINE (PCCA)				
POW, NA, 1 gm	**51927-3050-00**	0.91		
ZINC NITRATE				
(Baker, J.T.) *See ZINC NITRATE HEXAHYDRATE*				
ZINC NITRATE HEXAHYDRATE (Baker, J.T.)				
zinc nitrate				
CRY, NA (REAGENT)				
500 gm	**10106-4344-01**	44.75		
2500 gm	**10106-4344-05**	145.38		
ZINC OXIDE (Baker, J.T.)				
POW, NA (U.S.P.)				
500 gm	**10106-4360-01**	17.35		
(Gallipot)				
POW, NA (U.S.P.)				
454 gm	**51552-0083-06**	10.85		
(Letco)				
POW, NA (U.S.P.)				
500 gm	**62991-1458-01**	37.50		
(Lorann Oil)				
POW, NA, 30 gm	**23535-0617-05**	1.35		
120 gm	**23535-0617-08**	2.50		
480 gm	**23535-0617-01**	4.95		
(Mallinckrodt Lab)				
POW, NA (U.S.P.)				
500 gm	**00406-8824-04**	12.08		
2500 gm	**00406-8824-05**	83.96		

PROD/MFR	NDC	AWP	DP	OBC
(Medisca)				
POW, NA (U.S.P.)				
500 gm	**38779-0055-08**	28.50		
1000 gm	**38779-0055-09**	49.50		
(PCCA)				
POW, NA (MICROFINE)				
1 gm	**51927-3473-00**	0.45		
(USP)				
1 gm	**51927-1063-00**	0.07		
(Spectrum Pharmacy)				
POW, NA (U.S.P.)				
500 gm	**49452-8320-01**	53.90		
12000 gm	**49452-8320-03**	626.50		
2500 gm	**49452-8320-02**	159.25		
ZINC PEROXIDE				
(PCCA) *See ZINC PEROXIDE 50%*				
ZINC PEROXIDE 50% (PCCA)				
zinc peroxide				
POW, NA, ea	**51927-3467-00**	2.11		
ZINC PHENOLSULFONATE (PCCA)				
POW, NA (PURIFIED)				
1 gm	**51927-1919-00**	0.45		
ZINC PICOLINATE (PCCA)				
POW, NA, 1 gm	**51927-2511-00**	0.75		
(Spectrum Pharmacy)				
POW, NA (200-400 MESH)				
25 gm	**49452-8345-02**	74.90		
100 gm	**49452-8345-03**	119.35		
500 gm	**49452-8345-04**	423.50		
ZINC PYRITHIONE (Gallipot)				
pyrithione zinc				
POW, NA, 10 gm	**51552-0539-03**	31.36		
25 gm	**51552-0539-04**	69.30		
(PCCA)				
POW, NA (48% MIN. AQ DISPERSION)				
1 gm	**51927-1885-00**	0.60		
ZINC STEARATE (Baker, J.T.)				
POW, NA (U.S.P.)				
500 gm	**10106-4375-01**	19.22		
2000 gm	**10106-4375-05**	81.85		
(Gallipot)				
POW, NA (U.S.P.)				
113.4 gm	**51552-0500-04**	6.93		
454 gm	**51552-0500-06**	15.33		
(PCCA)				
POW, NA (USP)				
1 gm	**51927-1285-00**	0.27		
(Spectrum Pharmacy)				
POW, NA (U.S.P.)				
500 gm	**49452-8350-01**	76.30		
2500 gm	**49452-8350-02**	207.55		
12000 gm	**49452-8350-03**	787.50		
ZINC SULFATE (Amer Regent)				
SOL, IV (S.D.V.,PF)				
1 mg/ml, 10 ml 25s	**00517-6110-25**	62.19		
(Amer Regent) *See ZINC SULFATE CONCENTRATED*				
(Baker, J.T.) *See ZINC SULFATE HEPTAHYDRATE*				
(Gallipot)				
GRA, NA (U.S.P.)				
10 gm	**51552-0220-03**	5.88		
(Gallipot) *See ZINC SULFATE HEPTAHYDRATE*				
(Mallinckrodt Lab)				
GRA, NA (U.S.P.)				
500 gm	**00406-8872-12**	44.53		
2500 gm	**00406-8872-07**	123.46		
POW, NA, 500 gm	**00406-8868-04**	48.34		
(Medisca)				
POW, NA (U.S.P., DRIED)				
454 gm	**38779-0102-08**	34.50		
(1X500GM,HEPTAHYDRATE)				
500 gm	**38779-0702-08**	28.50		
(1X1000GM,HEPTAHYDRATE)				
1000 gm	**38779-0702-09**	75.00		
(USP)				
1000 gm	**38779-0102-09**	88.50		
(Paddock) *See ZINCATE*				
(PCCA)				
POW, NA (U.S.P, MONOHYDRATE)				
1 gm	**51927-1364-00**	0.10		
(USP; HEPTAHYDRATE)				
1 gm	**51927-1247-00**	0.08		

PROD/MFR	NDC	AWP	DP	OBC
(Spectrum Pharmacy)				
POW, NA (F.C.C.,DRIED)				
500 gm	**49452-8375-01**	68.25		
(Spectrum Pharmacy) *See ZINC SULFATE HEPTAHYDRATE*				
(Upsher-Smith)				
CAP, PO, 220 mg, 100s ea	**00245-0080-11**	13.31		
ZINC SULFATE CONCENTRATED (Amer Regent)				
zinc sulfate				
SOL, IV (S.D.V.,PF)				
5 mg/ml, 5 ml 25s	**00517-8105-25**	124.69		
ZINC SULFATE HEPTAHYDRATE (Baker, J.T.)				
zinc sulfate				
GRA, NA (U.S.P., F.C.C.)				
500 gm	**10106-4384-01**	15.93		
(Gallipot)				
GRA, NA (U.S.P.)				
454 gm	**51552-0220-06**	20.30		
2270 gm	**51552-0220-09**	83.65		
(Spectrum Pharmacy)				
GRA, NA (U.S.P.)				
500 gm	**49452-8370-01**	64.75		
2500 gm	**49452-8370-02**	194.95		
POW, NA (F.C.C.,DRIED)				
2500 gm	**49452-8375-02**	194.95		
ZINC UNDECYLENATE (Amend)				
POW, NA (U.S.P.)				
500 gm	**17317-0619-01**	19.30		
2270 gm	**17317-0619-05**	58.80		
11350 gm	**17317-0619-08**	280.00		
(Medisca)				
POW, NA (U.S.P.)				
100 gm	**38779-0692-05**	27.00		
500 gm	**38779-0692-08**	72.00		
(USP)				
1000 gm	**38779-0692-09**	100.50		
(PCCA)				
POW, NA (U.S.P.)				
1 gm	**51927-1534-00**	0.45		
(Spectrum Pharmacy)				
POW, NA (U.S.P.)				
100 gm	**49452-8380-01**	110.95		
(U.S.P./N.F.)				
500 gm	**49452-8380-02**	208.25		
2500 gm	**49452-8380-03**	707.00		
ZINC, CHELATED				
(Gallipot) *See ZINC CHELATE*				
ZINCATE (Paddock)				
zinc sulfate				
CAP, PO, 220 mg, 100s ea	**00574-9167-01**	14.05		
ZINECARD (Pfizer)				
dexrazoxane hydrochloride				
PDS, IV (SDV,CRYSTALLINE)				
250 mg, ea	**00013-8717-62**	281.86	234.88	**AP**
500 mg, ea	**00013-8727-89**	563.72	469.77	**AP**
ZINOTIC (Arbor)				
chloroxylenol/glycerin/pramoxine hcl/zn ace				
SOL, OT (1X15ML,DROPS)				
0.1%-1%-0.5%-0.1%,				
15 ml	**24338-0711-15**	82.50	66.00	
ZINOTIC ES (Arbor)				
chloroxylenol/glycerin/pramoxine hcl/zn ace				
SOL, OT (1X15ML,EXTRA STRENGTH)				
0.1%-1%-1%-1%,				
15 ml	**24338-0722-15**	78.75	63.00	
ZINX ALLERGY (Auriga)				
cpm/pse hcl/zincum aceticum				
KIT, MR (PEPPERMINT,HARD GELATIN)				
8 mg-120 mg-2 x,				
ea	**14629-0474-01**	43.75		
ZINX COLD (Auriga)				
carbetapentane tan/phenyleph tan/zincum aceticum				
KIT, MR (STRAWBERRY)				
ea	**14629-0472-01**	43.75		
ZINX CONGESTION (Auriga)				
gg/phenyleph hcl/zincum aceticum				
KIT, MR (DYE-FREE,PEPPERMINT)				
1000 mg-30 mg-2 x,				
ea	**14629-0475-01**	43.75		
ZINX COUGH (Auriga)				
cough/cold combination				
KIT, MR (AF,STRAWBERRY)				
ea	**14629-0473-01**	43.75		

PROD/MFR	NDC	AWP	DP	OBC
ZINX KIDS SNEEZE (Auriga)				
KIT, MR (BERRY)				
ea	**14629-0477-01**	43.75		
ZIOX 405 (Stratus)				
chlorophyllin copper complex, sodium/papain/urea				
OIN, TP, 0.5%-405900 u/gm-10%,				
3.5 gm 100s	**58980-0776-35**	778.90		
30 gm	**58980-0776-11**	59.92		
ZIPRASIDONE HYDROCHLORIDE				
(Pfizer) *See GEODON*				
ZIPRASIDONE MESYLATE				
(Pfizer) *See GEODON*				
ZIPSOR (Xanodyne Pharma)				
diclofenac potassium				
SGL, PO, 25 mg, 100s ea	**66479-0592-10**	262.80		
(PD-Rx Pharm)				
REPACK				
SGL, PO, 25 mg, 40s ea	**43063-0205-40**	205.76		
(Quality Care Prod)				
REPACK				
SGL, PO, 25 mg, 60s ea	**35356-0537-60**	299.47		
ZIRCONIUM OXIDE (PCCA)				
POW, NA, 1 gm	**51927-1365-00**	0.57		
ZITHRANOL-RR (Elorac)				
anthralin				
CRE, TP (1X45GM,RAPID RELEASE)				
1.2%, 45 gm	**42783-0101-45**	146.21		
ZITHROMAX (Pfizer)				
azithromycin				
PDR, PO (SINGLE DOSE PACKETS)				
1 gm/packet, 3s ea	**00069-3051-75**	113.66	94.72	
10s ea	**00069-3051-07**	378.89	315.74	
100 mg/5 ml, 15 ml	**00069-3110-19**	47.08	39.23	
200 mg/5 ml, 15 ml	**00069-3120-19**	47.08	39.23	
22.5 ml	**00069-3130-19**	47.08	39.23	
30 ml	**00069-3140-19**	47.08	39.23	
PDS, IV (VIAL)				
500 mg, 10s ea	**00069-3150-83**	343.94	286.62	
(W/VIAL MATE)				
500 mg, 10s ea	**00069-3150-14**	343.94	286.62	
TAB, PO (FILM-COATED)				
250 mg, 30s ea	**00069-3060-30**	333.53	277.94	
50s ea UD	**00069-3060-86**	555.88	463.23	
500 mg, 30s ea	**00069-3070-30**	667.06	555.88	
(5 X 10)				
500 mg, 50s ea UD	**00069-3070-86**	1111.74	926.45	
600 mg, 30s ea	**00069-3080-30**	800.46	667.05	
(A-S Medication)				
REPACK				
PDR, PO (SINGLE DOSE PACKETS)				
1 gm/packet, ea	**54569-4567-00**	37.95		
100 mg/5 ml, 15 ml	**54569-4232-00**	47.15		
200 mg/5 ml, 15 ml	**54569-4230-00**	44.90		
22.5 ml	**54569-4231-00**	47.15		
30 ml	**54569-4417-00**	47.15		
TAB, PO, 250 mg, 2s ea	**54569-4522-01**	21.21		
(FILM-COATED)				
250 mg, 4s ea	**54569-4522-00**	44.54		
30s ea	**54569-4522-02**	334.07		
(Advanced Pharm Serv, Inc.)				
REPACK				
TAB, PO, 250 mg, 10s ea	**13411-0131-01**	113.02		
15s ea	**13411-0131-15**	169.53		
(FILM-COATED)				
250 mg, 30s ea	**13411-0131-03**	339.06		
60s ea	**13411-0131-06**	678.12		
90s ea	**13411-0131-09**	1017.18		
(Altura)				
REPACK				
TAB, PO, 250 mg, 4s ea	**63874-0246-04**	30.12		
6s ea	**63874-0246-06**	45.19		
(Z-PACK)				
250 mg, 6s ea	**63874-0246-00**	135.56		
10s ea	**63874-0246-10**	75.31		
15s ea	**63874-0246-15**	112.97		
(AQ)				
REPACK				
TAB, PO, 250 mg, 10s ea	**66105-0507-01**	113.02		
30s ea	**66105-0507-03**	339.06		
60s ea	**66105-0507-06**	678.12		
90s ea	**66105-0507-09**	1017.18		
100s ea	**66105-0507-10**	1130.20		
(Core)				
REPACK				
PDR, PO, 1 gm/packet, ea	**33358-0367-01**	36.17		
3s ea	**33358-0367-03**	93.57		
TAB, PO, 250 mg, 4s ea	**33358-0368-04**	46.43		
30s ea	**33358-0368-30**	297.31		
50s ea	**33358-0368-50**	474.71		
(DHS, Inc.)				
REPACK				
TAB, PO, 250 mg, 6s ea	**55887-0933-06**	60.08		
(Dispensing Solutions)				
REPACK				
PDR, PO, 100 mg/5 ml,				
15 ml	**55045-2372-05**	41.00		
200 mg/5 ml, 15 ml	**55045-2373-05**	41.00		
22.5 ml	**55045-2373-06**	41.00		
30 ml	**55045-2373-08**	41.00		
(Nucare Pharm)				
REPACK				
TAB, PO, 250 mg, 6s ea	**66267-0928-06**	60.89		
(PD-Rx Pharm)				
REPACK				
TAB, PO, 250 mg, 4s ea	**58864-0655-04**	64.97		
(FILM-COATED)				
250 mg, 4s ea	**55289-0310-04**	70.94		
6s ea	**58864-0655-30**	68.25		
(FILM-COATED)				
250 mg, 6s ea	**55289-0310-06**	102.66		
(REDI-SCRIPT,FILM-COATED)				
250 mg, 6s ea	**58864-0655-06**	68.25		
(FILM-COATED)				
250 mg, 14s ea	**55289-0310-14**	229.52		
14s ea	**58864-0655-14**	183.90		
(Pharma Pac)				
REPACK				
PDR, PO, 100 mg/5 ml,				
15 ml	**52959-0313-15**	39.25		
200 mg/5 ml, 15 ml	**52959-0657-03**	38.26		
22.5 ml	**52959-0657-06**	38.26		
(Phys Total Care)				
REPACK				
PDR, PO, 100 mg/5 ml,				
15 ml	**54868-4076-00**	46.30		
200 mg/5 ml, 15 ml	**54868-4078-01**	46.30		
22.5 ml	**54868-4078-00**	45.45		
30 ml	**54868-4078-02**	45.45		
PDS, IV (VIAL)				
500 mg, 10s ea	**54868-4527-00**	324.35		
TAB, PO, 250 mg, 4s ea	**54868-4644-00**	41.43		
(FILM-COATED)				
250 mg, 6s ea	**54868-4644-01**	61.51		
30s ea	**54868-4644-02**	301.96		
(Quality Care Prod)				
REPACK				
PDR, PO, 100 mg/5 ml,				
15 ml	**35356-0128-15**	156.00		
15 ml	**49999-0582-15**	40.12		
200 mg/5 ml, 15 ml	**49999-0260-15**	79.84		
TAB, PO, 250 mg, 4s ea	**49999-0096-04**	76.64		
6s ea	**49999-0096-06**	114.96		
(Southwood)				
REPACK				
TAB, PO, 250 mg, 6s ea	**58016-0391-06**	61.08		
10s ea	**58016-0391-10**	101.81		
15s ea	**58016-0391-15**	152.71		
18s ea	**58016-0391-18**	183.25		
20s ea	**58016-0391-20**	203.61		
28s ea	**58016-0391-28**	285.06		
30s ea	**58016-0391-30**	305.42		
60s ea	**58016-0391-60**	610.84		
90s ea	**58016-0391-90**	916.26		
100s ea	**58016-0391-00**	1018.07		
ZITHROMAX TRI-PAK (Pfizer)				
azithromycin				
TAB, PO (3X3)				
500 mg, 9s ea	**00069-3070-75**	200.11	166.76	
(A-S Medication)				
REPACK				
TAB, PO, 500 mg, 3s ea	**54569-5448-00**	66.81		
(Phys Total Care)				
REPACK				
TAB, PO, 500 mg, 3s ea	**54868-3244-00**	62.00		
ZITHROMAX Z PACK (Dispensing Solutions)				
REPACK				
azithromycin				
TAB, PO, 250 mg, 6s ea	**55045-2492-06**	61.98		
ZITHROMAX Z-PAK (Pfizer)				
azithromycin				
TAB, PO (3X6)				
250 mg, 18s ea	**00069-3060-75**	200.11	166.76	
(A-S Medication)				
REPACK				
TAB, PO, 250 mg, 6s ea	**54569-4497-00**	66.81		
(Pharma Pac)				
REPACK				
TAB, PO, 250 mg, 6s ea	**52959-0505-06**	63.78		
(Phys Total Care)				
REPACK				
CAP, PO, 250 mg, 6s ea	**54868-4183-00**	73.61		
(Southwood)				
REPACK				
TAB, PO, 250 mg, 18s ea	**58016-0391-01**	183.25		
(Stat Rx)				
REPACK				
TAB, PO, 250 mg, 6s ea	**16590-0248-06**	91.00		
6s ea	**16590-0362-06**	200.44		
ZMAX (Pfizer)				
azithromycin				
GER, PO (1X60ML,PEDIATRIC&ADULT)				
2 gm/60 ml, 60 ml	**00069-4170-34**	70.39	58.66	
(Phys Total Care)				
REPACK				
GER, PO (CHERRY-BANANA)				
2 gm/60 ml, ea	**54868-5404-00**	68.26		
(Physician Partner)				
REPACK				
GER, PO (1X60ML,CHERRY-BANANA)				
2 gm/60 ml, 60 ml	**21695-0444-60**	134.08		
ZOCOR (Merck)				
simvastatin				
TAB, PO (UNIT OF USE,FILM-COATED)				
5 mg, 30s ea	**00006-0726-31**	71.98		
90s ea	**00006-0726-54**	215.95		
(BULK PACKAGE)				
5 mg, 1000s ea	**00006-0726-82**	2399.40		
(UNIT OF USE)				
10 mg, 30s ea	**00006-0735-31**	96.47		
(UNIT OF USE,FILM-COATED)				
10 mg, 90s ea	**00006-0735-54**	289.42		
(BULK PACKAGE)				
10 mg, 1000s ea	**00006-0735-82**	3215.70		
(UNIT OF USE)				
20 mg, 30s ea	**00006-0740-31**	168.31		
90s ea	**00006-0740-54**	504.96		
(BULK PACKAGE)				
20 mg, 1000s ea	**00006-0740-82**	5610.68		
(UNIT OF USE,FILM-COATED)				
40 mg, 30s ea	**00006-0749-31**	168.31		
90s ea	**00006-0749-54**	504.96		
(BULK PACKAGE)				
40 mg, 1000s ea	**00006-0749-82**	5610.68		
(UNIT OF USE,FILM-COATED)				
80 mg, 30s ea	**00006-0543-31**	168.31		
90s ea	**00006-0543-54**	504.96		
(Advanced Pharm Serv, Inc.)				
REPACK				
TAB, PO, 5 mg, 10s ea	**13411-0161-01**	27.49		
15s ea	**13411-0161-15**	96.43		
(FILM-COATED)				
5 mg, 30s ea	**13411-0161-03**	82.47		
60s ea	**13411-0161-06**	135.12		
90s ea	**13411-0161-09**	247.44		
10 mg, 10s ea	**13411-0162-01**	44.36		
15s ea	**13411-0162-15**	55.26		
30s ea	**13411-0162-03**	110.53		
60s ea	**13411-0162-06**	181.10		
90s ea	**13411-0162-09**	399.28		
20 mg, 10s ea	**13411-0132-01**	64.28		
15s ea	**13411-0132-15**	96.43		
30s ea	**13411-0132-03**	192.86		
60s ea	**13411-0132-06**	315.93		
90s ea	**13411-0132-09**	578.60		
40 mg, 10s ea	**13411-0133-01**	64.28		
15s ea	**13411-0133-15**	96.43		
(FILM-COATED)				
40 mg, 30s ea	**13411-0133-03**	192.86		
60s ea	**13411-0133-06**	385.72		
90s ea	**13411-0133-09**	578.60		
(AQ)				
REPACK				
TAB, PO, 20 mg, 30s ea	**66105-0505-03**	180.33		
40 mg, 10s ea	**66105-0506-01**	64.00		
30s ea	**66105-0506-03**	192.00		
60s ea	**66105-0506-06**	384.00		
90s ea	**66105-0506-09**	576.00		
100s ea	**66105-0506-10**	640.00		
(Dispensing Solutions)				
REPACK				
TAB, PO, 40 mg, 30s ea	**55045-3100-08**	185.10		

PROD/MFR	NDC	AWP	DP	OBC
(PD-Rx Pharm)				
REPACK				
TAB, PO (REDI-SCRIPT,FILM-COATED)				
5 mg, 30s ea	58864-0739-30	86.27		
(REDI-SCRIPT)				
20 mg, 30s ea	58864-0760-30	235.23		
(FILM-COATED)				
40 mg, 30s ea	55289-0874-30	250.16		
(REDI-SCRIPT,FILM-COATED)				
40 mg, 30s ea	58864-0682-30	235.23		
(Pharma Pac)				
REPACK				
TAB, PO (FILM-COATED)				
40 mg, 30s ea	52959-0112-30	138.03		
(Phys Total Care)				
REPACK				
TAB, PO, 10 mg, 30s ea	54868-2639-01	104.34		
(FILM-COATED)				
10 mg, 90s ea	54868-2639-00	284.35		
20 mg, 30s ea	54868-3104-00	188.35		
90s ea	54868-3104-01	542.45		
40 mg, 15s ea	54868-4157-02	97.10		
30s ea	54868-4157-00	181.75		
90s ea	54868-4157-01	540.88		
80 mg, 15s ea	54868-4181-00	96.48		
30s ea	54868-4181-01	180.50		
(Quality Care Prod)				
REPACK				
TAB, PO, 20 mg, 30s ea	49999-0306-30	290.30		
40 mg, 30s ea	49999-0488-30	290.30		
(Southwood)				
REPACK				
TAB, PO, 10 mg, 30s ea	58016-0364-30	90.24		
60s ea	58016-0364-60	180.48		
90s ea	58016-0364-90	270.72		
100s ea	58016-0364-00	300.80		
20 mg, 30s ea	58016-0385-30	157.46		
60s ea	58016-0385-60	314.91		
90s ea	58016-0385-90	472.37		
100s ea	58016-0385-00	524.86		
40 mg, 30s ea	58016-0365-30	157.45		
60s ea	58016-0365-60	314.90		
90s ea	58016-0365-90	472.35		
100s ea	58016-0365-00	524.83		
ZODERM (Doak)				
benzoyl peroxide/urea				
CRE, TP, 4.5%-10%,				
125 ml	10337-0740-21	237.16		
6.5%-10%, 125 ml	10337-0748-21	238.73		
8.5%-10%, 125 ml	10337-0741-21	246.53		
GEL, TP, 4.5%-10%,				
125 ml	10337-0742-21	234.66		
6.5%-10%, 125 ml	10337-0749-21	237.64		
8.5%-10%, 125 ml	10337-0743-21	239.93		
(Doak)				
benzoyl peroxide				
PAD, TP, 4.5%, 30s ea	10337-0752-10	172.96		
6.5%, 30s ea	10337-0753-10	173.48		
(REDI-PADS)				
8.5%, 30s ea	10337-0754-10	178.79		
(Doak)				
benzoyl peroxide/urea				
SOA, TP, 4.5%-10%,				
400 ml	10337-0744-51	157.64		
(CLEANSER)				
6.5%-10%, 400 ml	10337-0751-51	159.42		
8.5%-10%, 400 ml	10337-0745-51	161.82		
ZODERM HYDRATING WASH (Doak)				
benzoyl peroxide				
SOL, TP (1X473ML)				
5.75%, 473 ml	10337-0758-51	209.39		
ZODRYL AC 25 (CodaDose)				
chlorpheniramine maleate/codeine phosphate				
SUS, PO (1X118ML,GRAPE)				
0.333 mg/ml-1 mg/ml,				
118 ml	43378-0100-04	34.38		
ZODRYL AC 30 (CodaDose)				
chlorpheniramine maleate/codeine phosphate				
SUS, PO (1X118ML,GRAPE)				
0.286 mg/ml-1 mg/ml,				
118 ml	43378-0101-04	34.38		
ZODRYL AC 35 (CodaDose)				
chlorpheniramine maleate/codeine phosphate				
SUS, PO (1X118ML,GRAPE)				
0.25 mg/ml-1 mg/ml,				
118 ml	43378-0102-04	34.38		

PROD/MFR	NDC	AWP	DP	OBC
ZODRYL AC 40 (CodaDose)				
chlorpheniramine maleate/codeine phosphate				
SUS, PO (1X118ML,GRAPE)				
0.222 mg/ml-1 mg/ml,				
118 ml	43378-0103-04	34.38		
ZODRYL AC 50 (CodaDose)				
chlorpheniramine maleate/codeine phosphate				
SUS, PO (1X236ML,GRAPE)				
0.4 mg/ml-1 mg/ml,				
236 ml	43378-0104-08	38.75		
ZODRYL AC 60 (CodaDose)				
chlorpheniramine maleate/codeine phosphate				
SUS, PO (1X236ML,GRAPE)				
0.267 mg/ml-1 mg/ml,				
236 ml	43378-0105-08	38.75		
ZODRYL AC 80 (CodaDose)				
chlorpheniramine maleate/codeine phosphate				
SUS, PO (1X236ML,GRAPE)				
0.2 mg/ml-1 mg/ml,				
236 ml	43378-0106-08	38.75		
ZODRYL DAC 25 (CodaDose)				
cpm/codeine phos/pse hcl				
SUS, PO (1X118ML,GRAPE)				
118 ml, C-V	43378-0110-04	35.00		
ZODRYL DAC 30 (CodaDose)				
cpm/codeine phos/pse hcl				
SUS, PO (1X118ML,GRAPE)				
118 ml, C-V	43378-0111-04	35.00		
ZODRYL DAC 35 (CodaDose)				
cpm/codeine phos/pse hcl				
SUS, PO (1X118ML,GRAPE)				
118 ml, C-V	43378-0112-04	35.00		
ZODRYL DAC 40 (CodaDose)				
cpm/codeine phos/pse hcl				
SUS, PO (1X118ML,GRAPE)				
118 ml, C-V	43378-0113-04	35.00		
ZODRYL DAC 50 (CodaDose)				
cpm/codeine phos/pse hcl				
SUS, PO (1X236ML,GRAPE)				
236 ml, C-V	43378-0114-08	39.38		
ZODRYL DAC 60 (CodaDose)				
cpm/codeine phos/pse hcl				
SUS, PO (1X236ML,GRAPE)				
236 ml, C-V	43378-0115-08	39.38		
ZODRYL DAC 80 (CodaDose)				
cpm/codeine phos/pse hcl				
SUS, PO (1X236ML,GRAPE)				
236 ml, C-V	43378-0116-08	39.38		
ZODRYL DEC 25 (CodaDose)				
codeine phos/gg/pse hcl				
SUS, PO (1X118ML,GRAPE)				
1 mg/ml-20 mg/ml-5 mg/ml,				
118 ml, C-V	43378-0120-04	35.00		
ZODRYL DEC 30 (CodaDose)				
codeine phos/gg/pse hcl				
SUS, PO (1X118ML,GRAPE)				
118 ml, C-V	43378-0121-04	35.00		
ZODRYL DEC 35 (CodaDose)				
codeine phos/gg/pse hcl				
SUS, PO (1X118ML,GRAPE)				
118 ml, C-V	43378-0122-04	35.00		
ZODRYL DEC 40 (CodaDose)				
codeine phos/gg/pse hcl				
SUS, PO (1X118ML,GRAPE)				
118 ml, C-V	43378-0123-04	35.00		
ZODRYL DEC 50 (CodaDose)				
codeine phos/gg/pse hcl				
SUS, PO (1X236ML,GRAPE)				
1 mg/ml-20 mg/ml-6 mg/ml,				
236 ml, C-V	43378-0124-08	39.38		
ZODRYL DEC 60 (CodaDose)				
codeine phos/gg/pse hcl				
SUS, PO (1X236ML,GRAPE)				
1 mg/ml-20 mg/ml-4 mg/ml,				
236 ml, C-V	43378-0125-08	39.38		
ZODRYL DEC 80 (CodaDose)				
codeine phos/gg/pse hcl				
SUS, PO (1X236ML,GRAPE)				
1 mg/ml-20 mg/ml-3 mg/ml,				
236 ml, C-V	43378-0126-08	39.38		
ZOEY INSPIRATION626 COMPRESSOR/NEBULIZER (Respironics)				
nebulizer, direct patient interface				
DEV, NA, ea	83730-0626-30	75.00		

PROD/MFR	NDC	AWP	DP	OBC
ZOEY OPTICHAMBER (Respironics)				
spacer, inhalation				
DEV, NA (ADVANTAGE)				
ea	83730-0800-30	22.20		
ZOFRAN (Glaxo)				
ondansetron hydrochloride				
SOL, IJ (S.D.V.)				
2 mg/ml, 2 ml 5s	00173-0442-02	128.24		
(M.D.V.)				
2 mg/ml, 20 ml	00173-0442-00	256.40		
PO (BERRY)				
4 mg/5 ml, 50 ml	00173-0489-00	269.74		
TAB, PO (1X3 DAILY PACK)				
4 mg, 3s ea UD	00173-0446-04	79.73		
30s ea	00173-0446-00	797.34		
100s ea UD	00173-0446-02	2657.33		
(1X3 DAILY PACK)				
8 mg, 3s ea UD	00173-0447-04	132.78		
30s ea	00173-0447-00	1328.09		
100s ea UD	00173-0447-02	4426.85		
(Core)				
REPACK				
ondansetron				
ODT, PO, 4 mg, 2s ea	33358-0369-02	57.59		
(Core)				
ondansetron hydrochloride				
TAB, PO, 4 mg, 2s ea	33358-0370-02	57.30		
(Phys Total Care)				
REPACK				
SOL, IJ (S.D.V.)				
2 mg/ml, 2 ml 5s	54868-4509-00	147.75		
TAB, PO (1X3 DAILY PACK)				
4 mg, 3s ea	54868-3508-00	92.70		
10s ea	54868-3508-02	264.39		
30s ea	54868-3508-01	819.54		
(1X3 DAILY PACK)				
8 mg, 3s ea	54868-3509-00	144.51		
10s ea	54868-3509-02	465.41		
15s ea	54868-3509-01	697.49		
20s ea	54868-3509-03	929.56		
(Quality Care Prod)				
REPACK				
TAB, PO, 4 mg, 30s ea	35356-0524-30	1083.92		
(CAPLET)				
8 mg, 30s ea	49999-0783-30	1387.75		
(Southwood)				
REPACK				
TAB, PO, 4 mg, 30s ea	58016-0826-30	797.20		
60s ea	58016-0826-60	1594.40		
90s ea	58016-0826-90	2391.60		
100s ea	58016-0826-00	2657.33		
8 mg, 10s ea	58016-0084-10	380.84		
30s ea	58016-0084-30	1328.09		
60s ea	58016-0084-60	2656.18		
90s ea	58016-0084-90	3984.27		
100s ea	58016-0084-00	4426.97		
ZOFRAN ODT (Glaxo)				
ondansetron				
ODT, PO, 4 mg, 30s ea UD	00173-0569-00	752.17		
8 mg, 10s ea	54868-5089-02	462.91		
(5X2)				
8 mg, 10s ea UD	00173-0570-04	417.60		
30s ea UD	00173-0570-00	1252.86		
(Phys Total Care)				
REPACK				
ODT, PO, 8 mg, 2s ea	54868-5089-00	102.28		
3s ea	54868-5089-03	144.99		
15s ea	54868-5089-01	679.80		
20s ea	54868-5089-04	925.21		
30s ea	54868-5089-05	1359.59		
ZOLADEX (AstraZeneca)				
goserelin acetate				
IMP, SC (SAFESYSTEM SRN)				
3.6 mg, ea	00310-0950-36	451.19		
10.8 mg, ea	00310-0951-30	1353.58		
ZOLEDRONIC ACID				
(Novartis Pharm) *See RECLAST*				
(Novartis Pharm) *See ZOMETA*				
ZOLINZA (Merck)				
vorinostat				
CAP, PO, 100 mg, 120s ea	00006-0568-40	9973.33		
ZOLMITRIPTAN				
(AstraZeneca) *See ZOMIG*				
(AstraZeneca) *See ZOMIG-ZMT*				
ZOLOFT (Pfizer)				
sertraline hydrochloride				
SOL, PO, 20 mg/ml, 60 ml	00049-4940-23	91.62	76.35	

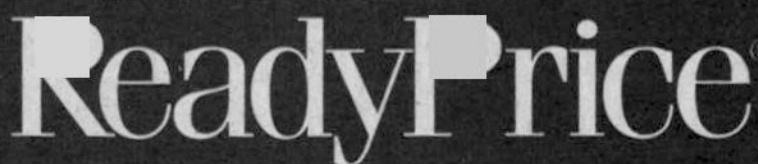

PROD/MFR	NDC	AWP	DP	OBC
TAB, PO (UNIT-OF-USE)				
25 mg, 30s ea	**00049-4960-30**	115.97	96.64	
50 mg, 30s ea	**00049-4900-30**	115.97	96.64	
100s ea UD	**00049-4900-41**	386.57	322.14	
(UNIT-OF-USE)				
100 mg, 30s ea	**00049-4910-30**	115.97	96.64	
100s ea UD	**00049-4910-41**	386.57	322.14	
(A-S Medication)				
REPACK				
TAB, PO, 50 mg, 30s ea	**54569-3724-00**	111.85		
(Advanced Pharm Serv, Inc.)				
REPACK				
TAB, PO, 50 mg, 10s ea	**13411-0152-01**	66.60		
15s ea	**13411-0152-15**	99.90		
30s ea	**13411-0152-03**	104.09		
60s ea	**13411-0152-06**	399.60		
90s ea	**13411-0152-09**	599.40		
100 mg, 10s ea	**13411-0153-01**	31.36		
15s ea	**13411-0153-15**	47.04		
30s ea	**13411-0153-03**	94.08		
60s ea	**13411-0153-06**	188.16		
90s ea	**13411-0153-09**	282.24		
(Altura)				
REPACK				
TAB, PO (FILM COATED)				
50 mg, 10s ea	**63874-0555-10**	33.20		
14s ea	**63874-0555-14**	46.48		
15s ea	**63874-0555-15**	49.80		
20s ea	**63874-0555-20**	66.40		
30s ea	**63874-0555-30**	99.60		
60s ea	**63874-0555-60**	199.20		
100s ea	**63874-0555-01**	332.00		
100 mg, 10s ea	**63874-0596-10**	30.40		
14s ea	**63874-0596-14**	42.56		
15s ea	**63874-0596-15**	45.60		
20s ea	**63874-0596-20**	60.80		
30s ea	**63874-0596-30**	91.20		
60s ea	**63874-0596-60**	182.40		
100s ea	**63874-0596-01**	225.76		
(AQ)				
REPACK				
TAB, PO, 50 mg, 100s ea	**66105-0560-10**	407.67		
100 mg, 100s ea	**66105-0561-10**	407.67		
(DHS, Inc.)				
REPACK				
TAB, PO, 25 mg, 30s ea	**55887-0519-30**	127.97		
60s ea	**55887-0519-60**	255.99		
100 mg, 30s ea	**55887-0967-30**	110.80		
60s ea	**55887-0967-60**	188.45		
(Direct Pharmaceutical, Inc.)				
REPACK				
TAB, PO, 50 mg,				
100s ea UD	**67801-0204-10**	347.56		
100 mg, 100s ea UD	**67801-0205-10**	347.56		
(Dispensing Solutions)				
REPACK				
TAB, PO, 25 mg, 30s ea	**55045-3386-08**	105.00		
50 mg, 7s ea	**55045-2224-02**	24.50		
20s ea	**55045-2224-07**	70.00		
30s ea	**55045-2224-08**	105.00		
100s ea	**55045-2224-00**	350.00		
100 mg, 15s ea	**55045-2208-03**	52.50		
20s ea	**55045-2208-07**	70.00		
30s ea	**55045-2208-08**	105.00		
100s ea	**55045-2208-01**	350.00		
(HomeMed)				
REPACK				
TAB, PO, 50 mg, 30s ea	**51655-0662-24**	99.99		
(PD-Rx Pharm)				
REPACK				
TAB, PO, 50 mg, 30s ea	**55289-0409-30**	148.86		
(REDI-SCRIPT)				
50 mg, 30s ea	**58864-0707-30**	107.90		
60s ea	**55289-0409-60**	297.73		
100 mg, 15s ea	**55289-0550-15**	75.60		
(REDI-SCRIPT)				
100 mg, 15s ea	**58864-0627-15**	75.61		
30s ea	**55289-0550-30**	146.87		
(REDI-SCRIPT)				
100 mg, 30s ea	**58864-0627-30**	146.87		
(Pharma Pac)				
REPACK				
TAB, PO, 25 mg, 30s ea	**52959-0787-30**	89.40		
50 mg, 14s ea	**52959-0361-14**	51.10		
30s ea	**52959-0361-30**	99.57		
60s ea	**52959-0361-60**	199.13		
100s ea	**52959-0361-00**	315.00		
100 mg, 30s ea	**52959-0781-30**	99.57		
60s ea	**52959-0781-60**	199.13		
(Phys Total Care)				
REPACK				
TAB, PO, 25 mg, 10s ea	**54868-4372-01**	37.19		
30s ea	**54868-4372-00**	107.83		
60s ea	**54868-4372-02**	202.01		
50 mg, 10s ea	**54868-2192-05**	36.91		
15s ea	**54868-2192-03**	54.43		
20s ea	**54868-2192-04**	71.94		
30s ea	**54868-2192-01**	106.98		
45s ea	**54868-2192-06**	150.76		
60s ea	**54868-2192-08**	200.40		
90s ea	**54868-2192-07**	299.66		
100s ea	**54868-2192-00**	332.12		
100 mg, 10s ea	**54868-2637-05**	38.04		
15s ea	**54868-2637-01**	56.43		
20s ea	**54868-2637-04**	74.82		
30s ea	**54868-2637-00**	111.61		
50s ea	**54868-2637-08**	174.96		
60s ea	**54868-2637-06**	209.70		
90s ea	**54868-2637-07**	313.93		
100s ea	**54868-2637-03**	348.04		
(Quality Care Prod)				
REPACK				
TAB, PO, 25 mg, 30s ea	**49999-0776-30**	117.74		
50s ea	**49999-0776-50**	196.23		
50 mg, 15s ea	**49999-0292-15**	67.73		
30s ea	**49999-0292-30**	202.78		
100 mg, 15s ea	**49999-0375-15**	134.27		
30s ea	**49999-0375-30**	202.78		
100s ea	**49999-0375-00**	357.94		
(Southwood)				
REPACK				
TAB, PO, 25 mg, 30s ea	**58016-0664-30**	107.38		
60s ea	**58016-0664-60**	214.76		
90s ea	**58016-0664-90**	322.14		
100s ea	**58016-0664-00**	357.93		
50 mg, 30s ea	**58016-0366-30**	107.38		
60s ea	**58016-0366-60**	214.76		
90s ea	**58016-0366-90**	322.14		
100s ea	**58016-0366-00**	357.93		
100 mg, 30s ea	**58016-0668-30**	107.38		
60s ea	**58016-0668-60**	214.76		
90s ea	**58016-0668-90**	322.15		
100s ea	**58016-0668-00**	357.94		
(Stat Rx)				
REPACK				
TAB, PO, 25 mg, 30s ea	**16590-0249-30**	110.75		
60s ea	**16590-0249-60**	221.50		
90s ea	**16590-0249-90**	332.25		
50 mg, 30s ea	**16590-0250-30**	135.71		
60s ea	**16590-0250-60**	234.00		
90s ea	**16590-0250-90**	351.00		
100 mg, 30s ea	**16590-0251-30**	136.38		
60s ea	**16590-0251-60**	244.50		
90s ea	**16590-0251-90**	366.75		
ZOLPIDEM (4u)				
REPACK				
zolpidem tartrate				
TAB, PO, 10 mg,				
30s ea, C-IV	**10544-0348-30**	172.82		
(Aidarex)				
REPACK				
TAB, PO, 10 mg,				
7s ea, C-IV	**33261-0173-07**	39.90		
14s ea, C-IV	**33261-0173-14**	79.80		
21s ea, C-IV	**33261-0173-21**	119.70		
28s ea, C-IV	**33261-0173-28**	159.60		
30s ea, C-IV	**33261-0173-30**	171.00		
60s ea, C-IV	**33261-0173-60**	342.00		
90s ea, C-IV	**33261-0173-90**	513.00		
(DHS, Inc.)				
REPACK				
TAB, PO, 5 mg,				
30s ea, C-IV	**55887-0124-30**	150.47		
60s ea, C-IV	**55887-0124-60**	277.20		
10 mg, 5s ea, C-IV	**55887-0123-05**	23.10		
7s ea, C-IV	**55887-0123-07**	35.11		
10s ea, C-IV	**55887-0123-10**	46.19		
15s ea, C-IV	**55887-0123-15**	69.30		
30s ea, C-IV	**55887-0123-30**	138.60		
60s ea, C-IV	**55887-0123-60**	277.20		
90s ea, C-IV	**55887-0123-90**	415.80		
(IPI)				
REPACK				
TAB, PO, 5 mg,				
30s ea, C-IV	**18837-0256-30**	174.23		
60s ea, C-IV	**18837-0256-60**	347.23		
(Nucare Pharm)				
REPACK				
TAB, PO, 5 mg,				
14s ea, C-IV	**68071-0703-14**	67.34		
60s ea, C-IV	**68071-0703-60**	274.20		
10 mg,				
14s ea, C-IV	**68071-0698-14**	67.34		
60s ea, C-IV	**68071-0698-60**	274.20		
(PD-Rx Pharm)				
REPACK				
TAB, PO, 5 mg,				
30s ea, C-IV	**55289-0399-30**	138.60		
10 mg,				
30s ea, C-IV	**55289-0419-30**	138.60		
(Phys Total Care)				
REPACK				
TAB, PO, 5 mg,				
30s ea, C-IV	**54868-0845-00**	12.02		
60s ea, C-IV	**54868-0845-02**	17.91		
100s ea, C-IV	**54868-0845-01**	25.85		
10 mg,				
10s ea, C-IV	**54868-0846-01**	7.98		
30s ea, C-IV	**54868-0846-00**	11.94		
100s ea, C-IV	**54868-0846-03**	22.38		
(Stat Rx)				
REPACK				
TAB, PO, 5 mg,				
10s ea, C-IV	**16590-0528-10**	20.00		
15s ea, C-IV	**16590-0528-15**	30.00		
30s ea, C-IV	**16590-0528-30**	169.38		
40s ea, C-IV	**16590-0528-40**	80.00		
90s ea, C-IV	**16590-0528-90**	180.00		
100s ea, C-IV	**16590-0528-71**	200.00		
10 mg,				
40s ea, C-IV	**16590-0527-40**	104.00		
100s ea, C-IV	**16590-0527-71**	244.00		
ZOLPIDEM TART (Physician Partner)				
REPACK				
zolpidem tartrate				
TAB, PO, 5 mg,				
7s ea, C-IV	**21695-0506-07**	75.34		
15s ea, C-IV	**21695-0506-15**	161.44		
30s ea, C-IV	**21695-0506-30**	274.44		
60s ea, C-IV	**21695-0506-60**	548.88		
10 mg, 7s ea, C-IV	**21695-0507-07**	75.34		
(FILM COATED)				
10 mg,				
10s ea, C-IV	**21695-0507-10**	107.63		
15s ea, C-IV	**21695-0507-15**	161.44		
30s ea, C-IV	**21695-0507-30**	274.44		
60s ea, C-IV	**21695-0507-60**	548.88		
ZOLPIDEM TARTRATE				
FUL				
TAB, PO, 5 mg, 100s ea		7.04		
10 mg, 100s ea		7.04		
(Actavis)				
TAB, PO (FILM-COATED)				
5 mg,				
100s ea, C-IV	**00228-2888-10**	462.02		
500s ea, C-IV	**00228-2888-50**	2310.06		
10 mg, 100s ea, C-IV	**00228-2889-10**	462.02		
500s ea, C-IV	**00228-2889-50**	2310.06		
(Apotex Corp.)				
TAB, PO (10X10,FILM-COATED)				
5 mg,				
100s ea UD, C-IV	**60505-2604-00**	464.49		AB
(FILM-COATED)				
5 mg,				
100s ea, C-IV	**60505-2604-01**	462.49		AB
1000s ea, C-IV	**60505-2604-08**	4624.90		AB
(10X10,FILM-COATED)				
10 mg,				
100s ea UD, C-IV	**60505-2605-00**	464.49		AB
(FILM-COATED)				
10 mg,				
100s ea, C-IV	**60505-2605-01**	462.49		AB
1000s ea, C-IV	**60505-2605-08**	4624.90		AB
(Aurobindo Pharma)				
TAB, PO (FILM-COATED)				
5 mg,				
100s ea, C-IV	**65862-0159-01**	513.93		AB
500s ea, C-IV	**65862-0159-05**	2569.65		AB
10 mg, 100s ea, C-IV	**65862-0160-01**	513.93		AB
500s ea, C-IV	**65862-0160-05**	2569.65		AB
(Caraco)				
TAB, PO (FILM-COATED)				
5 mg,				
100s ea, C-IV	**57664-0515-88**	457.40		AB
500s ea, C-IV	**57664-0515-13**	2286.99		AB
1000s ea, C-IV	**57664-0515-18**	4573.98		AB
10 mg, 100s ea, C-IV	**57664-0516-88**	457.40		AB
500s ea, C-IV	**57664-0516-13**	2286.99		AB
1000s ea, C-IV	**57664-0516-18**	4573.98		AB

PROD/MFR	NDC	AWP	DP	OBC
(Dr Reddy's)				
TAB, PO (FILM COATED)				
5 mg,				
100s ea, C-IV	**55111-0478-01**	462.02		**AB**
500s ea, C-IV	**55111-0478-05**	2310.06		**AB**
10 mg, 100s ea, C-IV	**55111-0479-01**	462.02		**AB**
500s ea, C-IV	**55111-0479-05**	2310.06		**AB**
(Glenmark Pharmaceuticals)				
TAB, PO (FILM COATED)				
5 mg,				
100s ea, C-IV	**68462-0279-01**	462.54		**AB**
500s ea, C-IV	**68462-0279-05**	2312.70		**AB**
10 mg, 100s ea, C-IV	**68462-0280-01**	462.54		**AB**
500s ea, C-IV	**68462-0280-05**	2312.70		**AB**
(Major)				
TAB, PO (10X10)				
5 mg, ea UD, C-IV	**00904-6082-61**	462.54		**AB**
10 mg, ea UD, C-IV	**00904-6083-61**	539.57		**AB**
(Meda) *See EDLUAR*				
(Mylan)				
TAB, PO (FILM-COATED)				
5 mg,				
100s ea, C-IV	**00378-5305-01**	461.95		**AB**
500s ea, C-IV	**00378-5305-05**	2309.80		**AB**
10 mg, 100s ea, C-IV	**00378-5310-01**	461.95		**AB**
500s ea, C-IV	**00378-5310-05**	2309.80		**AB**
(Northstar)				
TAB, PO (FILM-COATED)				
5 mg,				
100s ea, C-IV	**16714-0621-01**	462.02		**AB**
500s ea, C-IV	**16714-0621-02**	2309.80		**AB**
10 mg, 100s ea, C-IV	**16714-0622-01**	462.02		**AB**
500s ea, C-IV	**16714-0622-02**	2309.80		**AB**
(Prasco Labs)				
TAB, PO (FILM-COATED)				
5 mg,				
100s ea, C-IV	**66993-0715-02**	462.02		**AB**
500s ea, C-IV	**66993-0715-04**	2310.06		**AB**
10 mg, 100s ea, C-IV	**66993-0716-02**	462.02		**AB**
500s ea, C-IV	**66993-0716-04**	2310.06		**AB**
(Qualitest)				
TAB, PO (FILM-COATED)				
5 mg,				
100s ea, C-IV	**00603-6468-21**	462.54		**AB**
500s ea, C-IV	**00603-6468-28**	2312.70		**AB**
1000s ea, C-IV	**00603-6468-32**	4624.90		**AB**
10 mg, 100s ea, C-IV	**00603-6469-21**	462.54		**AB**
500s ea, C-IV	**00603-6469-28**	2312.70		**AB**
1000s ea, C-IV	**00603-6469-32**	4624.90		**AB**
(Ranbaxy Pharm)				
TAB, PO (FILM-COATED)				
5 mg,				
100s ea, C-IV	**63304-0159-01**	457.40		**AB**
500s ea, C-IV	**63304-0159-05**	2287.00		**AB**
10 mg, 100s ea, C-IV	**63304-0160-01**	457.40		**AB**
500s ea, C-IV	**63304-0160-05**	2287.00		**AB**
(Roxane)				
TAB, PO (FILM COATED)				
5 mg,				
100s ea UD, C-IV	**00054-0086-20**	485.69		**AB**
100s ea, C-IV	**00054-0086-25**	462.54		**AB**
500s ea, C-IV	**00054-0086-29**	2312.63		**AB**
10 mg,				
100s ea UD, C-IV	**00054-0087-20**	485.69		**AB**
100s ea, C-IV	**00054-0087-25**	462.54		**AB**
500s ea, C-IV	**00054-0087-29**	2312.63		**AB**
(Sandoz)				
TAB, PO (FILM-COATED)				
5 mg,				
100s ea, C-IV	**00781-5317-01**	462.54		**AB**
1000s ea, C-IV	**00781-5317-10**	4625.37		
10 mg, 100s ea, C-IV	**00781-5318-01**	462.54		**AB**
1000s ea, C-IV	**00781-5318-10**	4625.37		
(Sanofi-Aventis) *See AMBIEN*				
(Sanofi-Aventis) *See AMBIEN CR*				
(Synthon)				
TAB, PO (FILM-COATED)				
5 mg,				
100s ea, C-IV	**63672-3005-01**	462.27		**AB**
500s ea, C-IV	**63672-3005-02**	2311.38		**AB**
10 mg, 100s ea, C-IV	**63672-3010-01**	462.27		**AB**
500s ea, C-IV	**63672-3010-02**	2311.38		**AB**
(Teva)				
TAB, PO (FILM-COATED)				
5 mg,				
100s ea, C-IV	**00093-0073-01**	462.54		**AB**
10 mg, 100s ea, C-IV	**00093-0074-01**	462.54		**AB**
(Torrent)				
TAB, PO, 5 mg,				
30s ea, C-IV	**13668-0007-30**	145.70		**AB**
90s ea, C-IV	**13668-0007-90**	416.29		**AB**
100s ea, C-IV	**13668-0007-01**	462.54		**AB**
(10X10)				
5 mg,				
100s ea UD, C-IV	**13668-0007-74**	464.49		**AB**
500s ea, C-IV	**13668-0007-05**	2312.70		**AB**
1000s ea, C-IV	**13668-0007-10**	4625.10		**AB**
1500s ea, C-IV	**13668-0007-15**	6938.10		**AB**
10 mg, 30s ea, C-IV	**13668-0008-30**	145.70		**AB**
90s ea, C-IV	**13668-0008-90**	416.29		**AB**
100s ea, C-IV	**13668-0008-01**	462.54		**AB**
100s ea UD, C-IV	**13668-0008-74**	464.49		**AB**
500s ea, C-IV	**13668-0008-05**	2312.70		**AB**
1000s ea, C-IV	**13668-0008-10**	4625.10		**AB**
(UDL)				
TAB, PO (10X10,FILM-COATED)				
5 mg,				
100s ea UD, C-IV	**51079-0724-20**	461.95		**AB**
10 mg,				
100s ea UD, C-IV	**51079-0725-20**	461.95		**AB**
(Wockhardt USA)				
TAB, PO (FILM-COATED)				
5 mg,				
100s ea, C-IV	**64679-0714-01**	365.91		**AB**
500s ea, C-IV	**64679-0714-04**	1829.54		**AB**
10 mg, 100s ea, C-IV	**64679-0715-01**	365.91		**AB**
500s ea, C-IV	**64679-0715-04**	1829.54		**AB**
(4u)				
REPACK				
TAB, PO (FILM-COATED)				
10 mg,				
28s ea, C-IV	**10544-0348-28**	166.82		**AB**
28s ea, C-IV	**42549-0548-28**	166.82		**AB**
30s ea, C-IV	**42549-0548-30**	172.82		**AB**
30s ea, C-IV	**42549-0563-30**	172.82		**AB**
30s ea, C-IV	**42549-0593-30**	172.82		**AB**
(A-S Medication)				
REPACK				
TAB, PO, 5 mg,				
20s ea, C-IV	**54569-5906-00**	92.50		
30s ea, C-IV	**54569-5906-01**	138.75		
10 mg, 10s ea, C-IV	**54569-5907-00**	46.25		
30s ea, C-IV	**54569-5907-01**	138.75		
(Aidarex)				
REPACK				
TAB, PO (FILM COATED)				
5 mg, 7s ea, C-IV	**33261-0172-07**	39.00		**AB**
14s ea, C-IV	**33261-0172-14**	77.98		**AB**
21s ea, C-IV	**33261-0172-21**	116.97		**AB**
28s ea, C-IV	**33261-0172-28**	155.96		**AB**
30s ea, C-IV	**33261-0172-30**	167.10		**AB**
60s ea, C-IV	**33261-0172-60**	334.20		**AB**
90s ea, C-IV	**33261-0172-90**	501.30		**AB**
10 mg, 12s ea, C-IV	**33261-0173-12**	68.40		**AB**
(Altura)				
REPACK				
TAB, PO (FILM-COATED)				
5 mg, 10s ea, C-IV	**63874-1246-01**	46.90		**AB**
20s ea, C-IV	**63874-1246-02**	93.80		**AB**
30s ea, C-IV	**63874-1246-03**	140.77		**AB**
60s ea, C-IV	**63874-1246-06**	281.52		**AB**
(FILM COATED)				
10 mg,				
10s ea, C-IV	**63874-1247-09**	46.92		**AB**
30s ea, C-IV	**63874-1247-03**	140.77		**AB**
60s ea, C-IV	**63874-1247-06**	281.53		**AB**
100s ea, C-IV	**63874-1247-01**	469.21		**AB**
(American Health)				
REPACK				
TAB, PO (10X10,FILM-COATED)				
5 mg,				
100s ea UD, C-IV	**68084-0225-01**	331.40		**AB**
10 mg,				
100s ea UD, C-IV	**68084-0226-01**	331.40		**AB**
(Bryant Ranch)				
REPACK				
TAB, PO, 5 mg,				
30s ea, C-IV	**63629-3549-01**	148.66		
10 mg, 30s ea, C-IV	**63629-3548-01**	148.66		
60s ea, C-IV	**63629-3548-02**	297.32		
(DHS, Inc.)				
REPACK				
TAB, PO (FILM-COATED)				
5 mg, 5s ea, C-IV	**55887-0124-05**	25.07		**AB**
(Dispensing Solutions)				
REPACK				
TAB, PO, 5 mg,				
30s ea, C-IV	**55045-3812-03**	112.50		
30s ea, C-IV	**66336-0460-30**	150.47		
60s ea, C-IV	**66336-0460-60**	306.66		**AB**
100s ea, C-IV	**55045-3812-01**	375.00		
(FILM-COATED)				
10 mg, 2s ea, C-IV	**66336-0718-02**	11.03		**AB**
10s ea, C-IV	**55045-3811-02**	37.50		
30s ea, C-IV	**55045-3811-03**	112.50		
30s ea, C-IV	**66336-0718-30**	150.47		
60s ea, C-IV	**55045-3811-06**	225.00		
(FILM-COATED)				
10 mg,				
90s ea, C-IV	**66336-0718-90**	451.41		**AB**
100s ea, C-IV	**55045-3811-01**	375.00		
(IPI)				
REPACK				
TAB, PO (FILM-COATED)				
5 mg, 20s ea, C-IV	**18837-0256-20**	115.62		**AB**
10 mg, 15s ea, C-IV	**18837-0255-15**	86.72		**AB**
20s ea, C-IV	**18837-0255-20**	115.62		**AB**
30s ea, C-IV	**18837-0255-30**	138.75		**AB**
90s ea, C-IV	**18837-0255-90**	520.30		**AB**
(Medsource)				
REPACK				
TAB, PO (FILM-COATED)				
5 mg, 30s ea, C-IV	**45865-0409-30**	45.00		**AB**
60s ea, C-IV	**45865-0409-60**	90.00		**AB**
10 mg, 30s ea, C-IV	**45865-0413-30**	45.00		**AB**
60s ea, C-IV	**45865-0413-60**	90.00		**AB**
(Nucare Pharm)				
REPACK				
TAB, PO (FILM-COATED)				
5 mg, 30s ea, C-IV	**68071-0703-30**	182.94		**AB**
45s ea, C-IV	**68071-0703-45**	210.84		**AB**
10 mg, 20s ea, C-IV	**68071-0698-20**	121.40		**AB**
30s ea, C-IV	**68071-0698-30**	182.10		**AB**
(Palmetto)				
REPACK				
TAB, PO, 10 mg,				
30s ea, C-IV	**23490-6489-01**	113.88		
60s ea, C-IV	**23490-6489-06**	227.76		
90s ea, C-IV	**23490-6489-09**	341.64		
(PD-Rx Pharm)				
REPACK				
TAB, PO (FILM-COATED)				
5 mg, 10s ea, C-IV	**55289-0399-10**	65.94		**AB**
14s ea, C-IV	**55289-0399-14**	69.30		**AB**
60s ea, C-IV	**55289-0399-60**	253.20		**AB**
90s ea, C-IV	**55289-0399-90**	328.20		**AB**
10 mg, ea, C-IV	**43063-0068-79**	30.24		**AB**
6s ea, C-IV	**55289-0419-06**	35.28		**AB**
10s ea, C-IV	**55289-0419-10**	42.00		**AB**
14s ea, C-IV	**55289-0419-14**	59.34		**AB**
15s ea, C-IV	**55289-0419-15**	75.00		**AB**
60s ea, C-IV	**55289-0419-60**	277.20		**AB**
(Pharma Pac)				
REPACK				
TAB, PO, 5 mg,				
10s ea, C-IV	**52959-0879-10**	49.99		
14s ea, C-IV	**52959-0879-14**	69.98		
15s ea, C-IV	**52959-0879-15**	74.98		
20s ea, C-IV	**52959-0879-20**	99.97		
28s ea, C-IV	**52959-0879-28**	139.95		
30s ea, C-IV	**52959-0879-30**	149.95		
(FILM-COATED)				
5 mg, 42s ea, C-IV	**52959-0879-42**	209.92		**AB**
60s ea, C-IV	**52959-0879-60**	299.88		
90s ea, C-IV	**52959-0879-90**	449.73		
120s ea, C-IV	**52959-0879-02**	599.52		
10 mg, 2s ea, C-IV	**52959-0880-00**	15.20		
10s ea, C-IV	**52959-0880-10**	49.99		
14s ea, C-IV	**52959-0880-14**	69.98		
15s ea, C-IV	**52959-0880-15**	74.98		
20s ea, C-IV	**52959-0880-20**	99.97		
28s ea, C-IV	**52959-0880-28**	139.95		
30s ea, C-IV	**52959-0880-30**	149.95		
(FILM-COATED)				
10 mg,				
42s ea, C-IV	**52959-0880-42**	209.92		**AB**
45s ea, C-IV	**52959-0880-45**	224.91		**AB**
60s ea, C-IV	**52959-0880-60**	299.88		
90s ea, C-IV	**52959-0880-90**	449.73		
120s ea, C-IV	**52959-0880-02**	599.52		
(Phys Total Care)				
REPACK				
TAB, PO (FILM-COATED)				
10 mg,				
20s ea, C-IV	**54868-0846-05**	9.11		**AB**
(FILM COATED)				
10 mg,				
90s ea, C-IV	**54868-0846-04**	21.78		**AB**
(Quality Care Prod)				
REPACK				
TAB, PO, 5 mg,				
10s ea, C-IV	**49999-0932-00**	198.24		
30s ea, C-IV	**49999-0932-30**	660.80		
(FILM-COATED)				
10 mg, 2s ea, C-IV	**49999-0931-02**	13.22		**AB**
15s ea, C-IV	**49999-0931-15**	109.32		
30s ea, C-IV	**49999-0931-30**	198.24		

PROD/MFR	NDC	AWP	DP	OBC
(FILM-COATED)				
10 mg,				
60s ea, C-IV	49999-0931-60	396.48		AB
100s ea, C-IV	49999-0931-00	660.80		
(Southwood)				
REPACK				
TAB, PO (FILM-COATED)				
5 mg, 15s ea, C-IV	00490-7132-15	54.89		AB
20s ea, C-IV	00490-7132-20	73.19		AB
30s ea, C-IV	00490-7132-30	109.78		AB
40s ea, C-IV	00490-7132-40	146.37		AB
45s ea, C-IV	00490-7132-45	164.67		AB
50s ea, C-IV	00490-7132-50	182.97		AB
60s ea, C-IV	00490-7132-60	219.56		AB
90s ea, C-IV	00490-7132-90	329.34		AB
100s ea, C-IV	00490-7132-00	365.93		AB
10 mg, 15s ea, C-IV	00490-7131-15	54.89		AB
20s ea, C-IV	00490-7131-20	73.19		AB
30s ea, C-IV	00490-7131-30	109.78		AB
40s ea, C-IV	00490-7131-40	146.37		AB
45s ea, C-IV	00490-7131-45	164.67		AB
50s ea, C-IV	00490-7131-50	182.97		AB
60s ea, C-IV	00490-7131-60	219.56		AB
90s ea, C-IV	00490-7131-90	329.34		AB
100s ea, C-IV	00490-7131-00	365.93		AB
(St. Mary's MPP)				
REPACK				
TAB, PO, 5 mg,				
30s ea, C-IV	60760-0515-30	156.94		AB
10 mg, 30s ea, C-IV	60760-0288-30	158.46		
(Stat Rx)				
REPACK				
TAB, PO (FILM-COATED)				
5 mg, 20s ea, C-IV	16590-0528-20	112.92		AB
25s ea, C-IV	16590-0528-25	141.15		AB
56s ea, C-IV	16590-0528-56	112.00		AB
(FILM COATED)				
5 mg, 60s ea, C-IV	16590-0528-60	291.41		AB
10 mg, 10s ea, C-IV	16590-0527-10	46.25		AB
14s ea, C-IV	16590-0527-14	64.82		AB
15s ea, C-IV	16590-0527-15	69.38		AB
20s ea, C-IV	16590-0527-20	92.00		AB
25s ea, C-IV	16590-0527-25	115.63		AB
(FILM-COATED)				
10 mg,				
28s ea, C-IV	16590-0527-28	128.80		AB
(FILM COATED)				
10 mg,				
30s ea, C-IV	16590-0527-30	152.12		AB
45s ea, C-IV	16590-0527-45	208.14		AB
60s ea, C-IV	16590-0527-60	276.00		AB
90s ea, C-IV	16590-0527-90	454.57		AB
500s ea, C-IV	16590-0527-93	2312.63		AB
ZOMETA (Novartis Pharm)				
zoledronic acid				
SOL, IV (CONCENTRATE)				
4 mg/5 ml, 5 ml	00078-0387-25	1043.12		
ZOMIG (AstraZeneca)				
zolmitriptan				
SPR, NS, 5 mg, 6s ea	00310-0208-60	226.56		
TAB, PO (BLISTER PACK,1X6)				
2.5 mg, 6s ea	00310-0210-20	156.49		
(BLISTER PACK,1X3)				
5 mg, 3s ea	00310-0211-25	86.45		
(Phys Total Care)				
REPACK				
SPR, NS, 5 mg, 6s ea	54868-5361-00	181.29		
TAB, PO, 2.5 mg, 6s ea	54868-4215-00	169.99		
5 mg, 3s ea	54868-4086-00	100.25		
(Quality Care Prod)				
REPACK				
TAB, PO, 5 mg, 3s ea	35356-0412-03	152.26		
(Stat Rx)				
REPACK				
TAB, PO, 5 mg, 3s ea	16590-0760-03	98.42		
ZOMIG-ZMT (AstraZeneca)				
zolmitriptan				
ODT, PO (PACK,1X6)				
2.5 mg, 6s ea	00310-0209-20	153.52		
(BLISTER PACK,1X3)				
5 mg, 3s ea	00310-0213-21	84.82		
(Phys Total Care)				
REPACK				
ODT, PO, 2.5 mg, 6s ea	54868-5593-00	125.90		
5 mg, 3s ea	54868-0085-00	92.92		
6s ea	54868-0085-01	174.41		
ZONALON (Doak)				
doxepin hydrochloride				
CRE, TP, 5%, 30 gm	10337-0804-03	134.80		
45 gm	10337-0804-45	182.82		

PROD/MFR	NDC	AWP	DP	OBC
(Phys Total Care)				
REPACK				
CRE, TP, 5%, 30 gm	54868-3494-00	29.01		
(Quality Care Prod)				
REPACK				
CRE, TP, 5%, 30 gm	35356-0043-30	164.70		
ZONEGRAN (Eisai)				
zonisamide				
CAP, PO, 25 mg, 100s ea	62856-0681-10	88.27		
100 mg, 100s ea	62856-0680-10	353.10		
(Core)				
REPACK				
CAP, PO, 100 mg, 30s ea	33358-0371-30	96.20		
60s ea	33358-0371-60	160.91		
(Dispensing Solutions)				
REPACK				
CAP, PO, 100 mg, 30s ea	55045-3075-08	91.50		
60s ea	55045-3075-06	183.00		
(Pharma Pac)				
REPACK				
CAP, PO, 100 mg, 30s ea	52959-0899-30	95.20		
100s ea	52959-0899-00	301.98		
(Quality Care Prod)				
REPACK				
CAP, PO, 100 mg, 30s ea	35356-0140-30	207.40		
60s ea	35356-0140-60	386.53		
100s ea	35356-0140-00	543.34		
(Southwood)				
REPACK				
CAP, PO, 25 mg, 30s ea	58016-0636-30	21.69		
60s ea	58016-0636-60	43.39		
90s ea	58016-0636-90	65.08		
100s ea	58016-0636-00	72.31		
50 mg, 30s ea	58016-0650-30	36.57		
60s ea	58016-0650-60	73.14		
90s ea	58016-0650-90	109.71		
100s ea	58016-0650-00	121.90		
(Stat Rx)				
REPACK				
CAP, PO, 100 mg, 30s ea	16590-0252-30	90.50		
60s ea	16590-0252-60	181.00		
90s ea	16590-0252-90	271.00		
ZONISAMIDE				
FUL				
CAP, PO, 25 mg, 100s ea		19.31		
50 mg, 100s ea		21.12		
100 mg, 100s ea		49.98		
(Apotex Corp.)				
CAP, PO, 25 mg, 100s ea	60505-2545-01	54.80		AB
50 mg, 100s ea	60505-2546-01	109.60		AB
100 mg, 100s ea	60505-2547-01	219.60		AB
(Caraco)				
CAP, PO, 25 mg, 100s ea	62756-0258-02	54.75		AB
50 mg, 100s ea	62756-0259-02	109.52		AB
100 mg, 100s ea	62756-0260-02	219.17		AB
(CorePharma)				
CAP, PO (HARD GELATIN)				
25 mg, 100s ea	64720-0177-10	54.80		AB
50 mg, 100s ea	64720-0178-10	109.60		AB
100 mg, 100s ea	64720-0179-10	219.20		AB
500s ea	64720-0179-50	1096.00		AB
(Dr Reddy's)				
CAP, PO (HARD GELATIN)				
25 mg, 100s ea	55111-0402-01	54.83		AB
50 mg, 100s ea	55111-0403-01	109.60		AB
100 mg, 100s ea	55111-0288-01	219.20		AB
(Eisai) *See ZONEGRAN*				
(Glenmark Pharmaceuticals)				
CAP, PO, 25 mg, 100s ea	68462-0128-01	54.86		AB
500s ea	68462-0128-05	274.30		AB
50 mg, 100s ea	68462-0129-01	109.60		AB
500s ea	68462-0129-05	548.00		AB
100 mg, 100s ea	68462-0130-01	219.45		AB
500s ea	68462-0130-05	1097.25		AB
(Mylan)				
CAP, PO, 25 mg, 100s ea	00378-6725-01	54.80		AB
50 mg, 100s ea	00378-6726-01	109.60		AB
100 mg, 100s ea	00378-6727-01	219.20		AB
500s ea	00378-6727-05	1096.00		AB
(Ranbaxy Pharm)				
CAP, PO, 100 mg, 100s ea	63304-0992-01	219.45		AB
(Sandoz)				
CAP, PO, 25 mg, 100s ea	00185-0193-01	59.81		AB
50 mg, 100s ea	00185-0199-01	107.41		AB
100 mg, 100s ea	00185-0200-01	239.20		AB
(UDL)				
CAP, PO (10X10)				
100 mg, 100s ea UD	51079-0768-20	197.50		AB

PROD/MFR	NDC	AWP	DP	OBC
(Wockhardt USA)				
CAP, PO, 25 mg, 100s ea	64679-0945-01	54.80		AB
50 mg, 100s ea	64679-0946-01	109.60		AB
100 mg, 100s ea	64679-0990-01	207.15		AB
(American Health)				
REPACK				
CAP, PO (10X10)				
25 mg, 100s ea UD	68084-0190-01	52.45		
50 mg, 100s ea UD	68084-0191-01	63.90		
100 mg, 100s ea UD	68084-0183-01	123.13		
(IPI)				
REPACK				
CAP, PO (HARD GELATIN)				
25 mg, 60s ea	18837-0188-60	41.12		AB
(Keltman Pharma., Inc.)				
REPACK				
CAP, PO, 100 mg, 60s ea	68387-0650-60	103.45		
(Phys Total Care)				
REPACK				
CAP, PO, 100 mg, 30s ea	54868-5789-00	37.55		
(Physician Partner)				
REPACK				
CAP, PO, 100 mg, 60s ea	21695-0155-60	263.34		AB
(Quality Care Prod)				
REPACK				
CAP, PO, 25 mg, 30s ea	35356-0093-30	52.50		AB
60s ea	35356-0093-60	105.00		AB
90s ea	35356-0093-90	157.50		AB
120s ea	35356-0093-01	210.00		AB
50 mg, 30s ea	35356-0094-30	114.00		
100 mg, 30s ea	35356-0143-30	127.25		AB
60s ea	35356-0143-60	235.10		AB
(Southwood)				
REPACK				
CAP, PO, 100 mg, 30s ea	58016-0020-30	62.15		
60s ea	58016-0020-60	124.29		
90s ea	58016-0020-90	186.44		
100s ea	58016-0020-00	207.15		
(Stat Rx)				
REPACK				
CAP, PO, 25 mg, 30s ea	16590-0724-30	18.25		AB
60s ea	16590-0724-60	32.88		AB
90s ea	16590-0724-90	50.25		AB
50 mg, 60s ea	16590-0749-60	65.76		AB
100 mg, 30s ea	16590-0539-30	65.00		AB
60s ea	16590-0539-60	125.00		AB
90s ea	16590-0539-90	175.00		AB
120s ea	16590-0539-72	220.00		AB
ZORBTIVE (EMD)				
somatropin, mammalian derived				
PDS, SC (MDV, VIALS W/ DILUENT)				
8.8 mg, 7s ea	44087-3388-07	5983.49		
ZORPRIN (Par)				
aspirin				
TER, PO, 800 mg, 100s ea	49884-0657-01	138.85		
ZOSTAVAX (Merck)				
varicella virus vaccine				
PDS, SC (SDV,W/DILUENT,PF)				
19400 pfu, ea	00006-4963-00	193.80		
10s ea	00006-4963-41	1847.16		
ZOSYN (Wyeth)				
piperacillin sodium/tazobactam sodium				
PDS, IV, 2 gm-0.25 gm,				
10s ea	00206-8852-16	152.64	127.20	
(SDV,10X50ML)				
3 gm-0.375 gm,				
10s ea	00206-8854-16	229.00	190.83	
(SDV,10X100ML)				
4 gm-0.5 gm,				
10s ea	00206-8855-16	290.02	241.68	
(PHARMACY BULK VIAL)				
36 gm-4.5 gm, ea	00206-8859-10	274.87	229.06	
SOL, IV (24 PRE-MIX BAGS OF 50ML)				
2 gm/50 ml-0.25 gm/50 ml,				
50 ml 24s	00206-8860-02	439.38	366.15	
(12 PREMIX BAGS OF 100ML)				
100 ml 12s	00206-8862-02	417.72	348.10	
(24 PRE-MIX BAGS OF 50ML)				
50 ml 24s	00206-8861-02	659.22	549.35	
ZOTEX-12 (Vertical)				
dm tan/phenyleph tan/pyril tan				
SUS, PO (AF,SF,DYE-FREE,CHERRY)				
473 ml	68025-0024-16	169.81		
ZOTEX-12D (Vertical)				
cpm/dm/phenyleph hcl				
TER, PO, 8 mg-30 mg-20 mg,				
100s ea	68025-0033-10	242.76		

PROD/MFR	NDC	AWP	DP	OBC
ZOTEX-C (Vertical)				
codeine phos/phenyleph hcl/pyril mal				
SOL, PO (1X473ML,AF,SF,CHERRY)				
473 ml, C-V	68025-0037-16	153.13		
ZOTEX-D (Vertical)				
carbetapentane cit/pse hcl/pyril mal				
SOL, PO (1X473ML,AF,SF,DYE-FREE)				
473 ml	68025-0036-16	245.36		
ZOTEX-EX (Vertical)				
dm/gg/phenyleph hcl				
TAB, PO (CAPLET)				
15 mg-350 mg-12 mg,				
100s ea	68025-0035-10	206.39		
ZOTEX-PE (Vertical)				
bpm/phenyleph hcl				
TER, PO, 6 mg-30 mg,				
100s ea	68025-0034-10	215.51		
ZOTO-HC (Phys Total Care)				
REPACK				
chloroxylenol/hc/pramoxine hcl				
SOL, OT, 10 ml	54868-4364-00	19.53		
ZOVIA 1/35E (Watson)				
ethinyl estradiol/ethynodiol diacetate				
TAB, PO (6 X 28)				
35 mcg-1 mg,				
168s ea	52544-0383-28	179.27		AB
(A-S Medication)				
REPACK				
TAB, PO, 35 mcg-1 mg,				
28s ea	54569-4817-00	29.88		AB
(Phys Total Care)				
REPACK				
TAB, PO, 35 mcg-1 mg,				
28s ea	54868-4240-00	33.69		AB
ZOVIA 1/50E (Watson)				
ethinyl estradiol/ethynodiol diacetate				
TAB, PO (6 X 28)				
50 mcg-1 mg,				
168s ea	52544-0384-28	199.74		AB
(Phys Total Care)				
REPACK				
TAB, PO, 50 mcg-1 mg,				
28s ea	54868-4778-00	89.85		AB
ZOVIRAX (BTA)				
acyclovir				
CRE, TP, 5%, 2 gm	64455-0994-42	68.24	56.87	
5 gm	64455-0994-45	158.72	132.27	
OIN, TP, 5%, 15 gm	64455-0993-94	184.19	153.49	
(Glaxo)				
CAP, PO, 200 mg, 100s ea	00173-0991-55	307.46		AB
SUS, PO, 200 mg/5 ml,				
473 ml	00173-0953-96	254.74		AB
TAB, PO, 400 mg, 100s ea	00173-0949-55	596.71		AB
800 mg, 100s ea	00173-0945-55	1160.27		AB
(A-S Medication)				
REPACK				
OIN, TP, 5%, 15 gm	54569-0792-00	230.95		
(Altura)				
REPACK				
OIN, TP, 5%, 15 gm	63874-0882-15	39.48		
(PD-Rx Pharm)				
REPACK				
CAP, PO, 200 mg, 10s ea	55289-0006-10	28.25		AB
25s ea	55289-0006-25	70.75		AB
35s ea	55289-0006-35	97.88		AB
50s ea	55289-0006-50	121.20		AB
TAB, PO, 400 mg, 12s ea	55289-0691-12	94.75		AB
15s ea	55289-0691-15	94.80		AB
25s ea	55289-0691-25	139.75		AB
800 mg, 15s ea	55289-0564-15	179.38		AB
20s ea	55289-0564-20	180.33		AB
48s ea	55289-0564-48	424.20		AB
(Pharma Pac)				
REPACK				
CAP, PO, 200 mg, 25s ea	52959-0330-25	72.99		AB
50s ea	52959-0330-50	137.50		AB
100s ea	52959-0330-00	260.00		AB
(Phys Total Care)				
REPACK				
CAP, PO, 200 mg, 25s ea	54868-0163-02	56.00		AB
CRE, TP, 5%, 2 gm	54868-5410-01	66.79		
5 gm	54868-5410-00	145.19		
OIN, TP, 5%, 15 gm	54868-0165-01	175.03		
TAB, PO, 400 mg, 15s ea	54868-3025-00	61.68		AB
800 mg, 25s ea	54868-2184-03	195.68		AB
30s ea	54868-2184-02	221.51		AB
50s ea	54868-2184-04	367.93		AB
100s ea	54868-2184-00	709.75		AB

PROD/MFR	NDC	AWP	DP	OBC
(Quality Care Prod)				
REPACK				
OIN, TP (1X15GM)				
5%, 15 gm	35356-0241-15	301.78		
(Southwood)				
REPACK				
OIN, TP, 5%, 15 gm	58016-3103-01	152.30		
ZYBAN (Glaxo)				
bupropion hydrochloride				
TER, PO (ADVANTAGE PACK)				
150 mg, 60s ea	00173-0556-01	223.85		
(REFILL)				
150 mg, 60s ea	00173-0556-02	223.85		
(AQ)				
REPACK				
TER, PO, 150 mg, 60s ea	66105-0153-06	238.18		
(Pharma Pac)				
REPACK				
TER, PO (ADVANTAGE PACK)				
150 mg, 30s ea	52959-0487-30	49.47		
(Phys Total Care)				
REPACK				
TER, PO (ADVANTAGE PACK)				
150 mg, 60s ea	54868-4025-00	151.74		
ZYDONE (Endo Labs)				
acetaminophen/hydrocodone bitartrate				
TAB, PO, 400 mg-5 mg,				
100s ea, C-III	63481-0668-70	69.96		
400 mg-7.5 mg,				
100s ea, C-III	63481-0669-70	77.16		
400 mg-10 mg,				
100s ea, C-III	63481-0698-70	93.92		
(PD-Rx Pharm)				
REPACK				
TAB, PO, 400 mg-10 mg,				
30s ea, C-III	55289-0648-30	41.80		
(Phys Total Care)				
REPACK				
TAB, PO, 400 mg-5 mg,				
30s ea, C-III	54868-4099-00	23.50		
100s ea, C-III	54868-4099-01	72.51		
400 mg-7.5 mg,				
30s ea, C-III	54868-4097-00	27.28		
100s ea, C-III	54868-4097-01	85.10		
400 mg-10 mg,				
30s ea, C-III	54868-4098-00	33.73		
100s ea, C-III	54868-4098-01	106.60		
(Southwood)				
REPACK				
TAB, PO, 400 mg-5 mg,				
30s ea, C-III	58016-0090-30	19.08		
60s ea, C-III	58016-0090-60	38.16		
90s ea, C-III	58016-0090-90	57.24		
100s ea, C-III	58016-0090-00	63.60		
400 mg-10 mg,				
30s ea, C-III	58016-0067-30	25.61		
60s ea, C-III	58016-0067-60	51.23		
90s ea, C-III	58016-0067-90	76.84		
100s ea, C-III	58016-0067-00	85.38		
ZYFLO (Cornerstone)				
zileuton				
TAB, PO, 600 mg, 120s ea	68734-0700-10	749.09	599.27	
ZYFLO CR (Cornerstone)				
zileuton				
TER, PO (FILM-COATED)				
600 mg, 120s ea	68734-0710-10	749.09	599.27	
ZYLET (Bausch & Lomb Inc.)				
loteprednol etabonate/tobramycin				
SUS, OP, 0.5%-0.3%,				
2.5 ml	24208-0358-25	55.89		
5 ml	24208-0358-05	111.84		
10 ml	24208-0358-10	223.58		
ZYLOPRIM (Prometheus Labs)				
allopurinol				
TAB, PO, 100 mg, 100s ea	65483-0991-10	55.55		AB
300 mg, 100s ea	65483-0993-10	152.12		AB
500s ea	65483-0993-50	568.51		AB
(Phys Total Care)				
REPACK				
TAB, PO, 300 mg, 10s ea	54868-0678-00	15.96		AB
30s ea	54868-0678-02	54.66		AB
100s ea	54868-0678-01	166.46		AB
ZYMAR (Allergan Inc)				
gatifloxacin				
SOL, OP, 0.3%, 5 ml	00023-9218-05	83.75		
(Pharma Pac)				
REPACK				
SOL, OP, 0.3%, 5 ml	52959-0742-05	66.15		

PROD/MFR	NDC	AWP	DP	OBC
(Phys Total Care)				
REPACK				
SOL, OP, 0.3%, 5 ml	54868-4797-00	82.26		
ZYMECOT (Truxton)				
dehydrocholic acid/enzymes				
TAB, PO, 1000s ea	00463-0627-91	59.40		
ZYMINE (Vindex Pharma Inc)				
triprolidine hydrochloride				
SOL, PO (AF,SF,APPLE)				
1.25 mg/5 ml,				
473 ml	67204-0320-16	73.13		
ZYMINE DXR (Vindex Pharma Inc)				
pseudoephedrine tannate/triprolidine tannate				
SUS, PO (AF,SF,BERRY)				
45 mg/5 ml-2.5 mg/5 ml,				
473 ml	67204-0340-16	118.54		
ZYMINE XR (Vindex Pharma Inc)				
triprolidine tannate				
SUS, PO (AF,SF,APPLE)				
2.5 mg/5 ml,				
473 ml	67204-0325-16	106.55		
ZYMINE-D (Vindex Pharma Inc)				
pse hcl/triprolidine hcl				
SOL, PO (AF,SF,BERRY)				
45 mg/5 ml-1.25 mg/5 ml,				
473 ml	67204-0245-16	70.94		
ZYPRAM (Vertical)				
hydrocortisone acetate/pramoxine hydrochloride				
CRE, RC (1X30GM)				
2.35%-1%, 30 gm	68025-0040-30	76.05		
ZYPREXA (Lilly)				
olanzapine				
TAB, PO, 2.5 mg, 30s ea	00002-4112-30	263.16	219.30	
(IDENTI-DOSE)				
2.5 mg, 100s ea UD	00002-4112-33	877.20	731.00	
1000s ea	00002-4112-04	8772.00	7310.00	
5 mg, 30s ea	00002-4115-30	310.68	258.90	
100s ea UD	00002-4115-33	1035.60	863.00	
1000s ea	00002-4115-04	10356.00	8630.00	
7.5 mg, 30s ea	00002-4116-30	378.00	315.00	
100s ea UD	00002-4116-33	1260.00	1050.00	
1000s ea	00002-4116-04	12600.00	10500.00	
10 mg, 30s ea	00002-4117-30	468.00	390.00	
100s ea UD	00002-4117-33	1560.00	1300.00	
1000s ea	00002-4117-04	15600.00	13000.00	
15 mg, 30s ea	00002-4415-30	702.00	585.00	
(IDENTI-DOSE)				
15 mg, 100s ea UD	00002-4415-33	2340.00	1950.00	
1000s ea	00002-4415-04	23400.00	19500.00	
20 mg, 30s ea	00002-4420-30	936.00	780.00	
(IDENTI-DOSE)				
20 mg, 100s ea UD	00002-4420-33	3120.00	2600.00	
1000s ea	00002-4420-04	31200.00	26000.00	
(Advanced Pharm Serv, Inc.)				
REPACK				
TAB, PO, 2.5 mg, 10s ea	13411-0134-01	94.35		
15s ea	13411-0134-15	141.53		
30s ea	13411-0134-03	283.06		
60s ea	13411-0134-06	426.94		
90s ea	13411-0134-09	1280.82		
5 mg, 10s ea	13411-0135-01	111.37		
15s ea	13411-0135-15	167.06		
30s ea	13411-0135-03	334.12		
60s ea	13411-0135-06	504.07		
90s ea	13411-0135-09	1002.37		
7.5 mg, 10s ea	13411-0136-01	135.50		
15s ea	13411-0136-15	203.25		
30s ea	13411-0136-03	406.57		
60s ea	13411-0136-06	612.97		
90s ea	13411-0136-09	1219.54		
10 mg, 10s ea	13411-0137-01	181.22		
15s ea	13411-0137-15	167.75		
30s ea	13411-0137-03	543.67		
60s ea	13411-0137-06	1087.35		
90s ea	13411-0137-09	1509.75		
15 mg, 10s ea	13411-0138-01	251.62		
15s ea	13411-0138-15	377.43		
30s ea	13411-0138-03	754.87		
60s ea	13411-0138-06	1138.50		
90s ea	13411-0138-09	2264.62		
20 mg, 10s ea	13411-0139-01	335.43		
15s ea	13411-0139-15	503.14		
30s ea	13411-0139-03	1006.29		
60s ea	13411-0139-06	1516.35		
90s ea	13411-0139-09	3018.87		
(AQ)				
REPACK				
TAB, PO, 2.5 mg, 10s ea	66105-0133-01	146.10		
15s ea	66105-0133-15	219.15		
30s ea	66105-0133-03	438.30		
45s ea	66105-0133-45	657.45		
60s ea	66105-0133-06	876.60		
5 mg, 10s ea	66105-0132-03	179.10		
15s ea	66105-0132-15	268.65		

PROD/MFR	NDC	AWP	DP	OBC
45s ea	66105-0132-45	805.95		
60s ea	66105-0132-06	1074.60		
90s ea	66105-0132-09	1611.90		
7.5 mg, 10s ea	66105-0554-01	199.12		
15s ea	66105-0554-15	298.68		
30s ea	66105-0554-03	597.36		
60s ea	66105-0554-06	1194.72		
90s ea	66105-0554-09	1792.08		
10 mg, 15s ea	66105-0155-15	367.50		
30s ea	66105-0155-03	735.00		
45s ea	66105-0155-45	1102.50		
60s ea	66105-0155-06	1470.00		
90s ea	66105-0155-09	2205.00		
15 mg, 10s ea	66105-0562-01	248.75		
15s ea	66105-0562-15	365.63		
30s ea	66105-0562-03	736.25		
60s ea	66105-0562-06	1462.50		
90s ea	66105-0562-09	2193.75		
20 mg, 10s ea	66105-0563-01	330.00		
15s ea	66105-0563-15	489.17		
30s ea	66105-0563-03	975.00		
60s ea	66105-0563-06	1945.00		
90s ea	66105-0563-09	2910.00		
(Bryant Ranch)				
REPACK				
TAB, PO, 2.5 mg, 30s ea	63629-3633-01	208.35		
(Core)				
REPACK				
TAB, PO, 2.5 mg, 60s ea	33358-0372-60	384.51		
(DHS, Inc.)				
REPACK				
TAB, PO, 2.5 mg, 30s ea	55887-0272-30	188.99		
(PD-Rx Pharm)				
REPACK				
TAB, PO (REDI-SCRIPT)				
2.5 mg, 30s ea	58864-0704-30	391.14		
5 mg, 15s ea	58864-0768-15	230.91		
7.5 mg, 30s ea	58864-0896-30	561.83		
10 mg, 15s ea	58864-0968-15	347.81		
30s ea	55289-0213-30	695.58		
20 mg, 30s ea	55289-0499-30	1391.16		
(Pharma Pac)				
REPACK				
TAB, PO, 2.5 mg, 30s ea	52959-0579-30	540.30		
(Phys Total Care)				
REPACK				
TAB, PO, 2.5 mg, 15s ea	54868-4255-01	127.90		
30s ea	54868-4255-00	239.91		
5 mg, 30s ea	54868-4254-00	282.93		
60s ea	54868-4254-01	545.23		
7.5 mg, 30s ea	54868-5336-00	309.91		
10 mg, 30s ea	54868-3941-00	435.38		
(Physician Partner)				
REPACK				
TAB, PO, 5 mg, 30s ea	21695-0140-30	621.36		
10 mg, 15s ea	21695-0142-15	481.24		
20 mg, 30s ea	21695-0144-30	1872.00		
(Quality Care Prod)				
REPACK				
TAB, PO, 2.5 mg, 30s ea	35356-0316-30	473.90		
5 mg, 15s ea	49999-0739-15	270.19		
30s ea	49999-0739-30	559.02		
10 mg, 15s ea	49999-0606-15	192.60		
30s ea	49999-0606-30	840.70		
15 mg, 30s ea	35356-0317-30	1259.82		
20 mg, 30s ea	35356-0318-30	1677.86		
(Stat Rx)				
REPACK				
TAB, PO, 2.5 mg, 30s ea	16590-0511-30	307.44		
60s ea	16590-0511-60	611.64		
5 mg, 30s ea	16590-0621-30	362.37		
60s ea	16590-0621-60	561.00		
90s ea	16590-0621-90	840.00		
10 mg, 30s ea	16590-0818-30	457.50		
15 mg, 30s ea	16590-0529-30	544.00		
60s ea	16590-0529-60	1058.00		
90s ea	16590-0511-90	669.00		
90s ea	16590-0529-90	1570.00		
120s ea	16590-0511-72	890.00		
120s ea	16590-0529-72	2085.00		
ZYPREXA INTRAMUSCULAR (Lilly)				
olanzapine				
PDS, IM, 10 mg, ea	00002-7597-01	33.04	27.53	
ZYPREXA RELPREVV (Lilly)				
olanzapine pamoate				
GER, IM (W/3ML DILUENT VIAL)				
210 mg, ea	00002-7635-11	667.80	556.50	
300 mg, ea	00002-7636-11	954.00	795.00	
405 mg, ea	00002-7637-11	1287.90	1073.25	

PROD/MFR	NDC	AWP	DP	OBC
ZYPREXA ZYDIS (Lilly)				
olanzapine				
ODT, PO (DOSE PACK)				
5 mg, 30s ea	00002-4453-85	345.96	288.30	
10 mg, 30s ea	00002-4454-85	503.28		
15 mg, 30s ea	00002-4455-85	737.28	614.40	
20 mg, 30s ea	00002-4456-85	971.28	809.40	
(Quality Care Prod)				
REPACK				
ODT, PO, 5 mg, 30s ea	35356-0319-30	629.70		
10 mg, 30s ea	35356-0320-30	840.70		
15 mg, 30s ea	35356-0321-30	1371.59		
20 mg, 30s ea	35356-0322-30	1748.56		
ZYRTEC (Advanced Pharm Serv, Inc.)				
REPACK				
cetirizine hydrochloride				
TAB, PO, 5 mg, 10s ea	13411-0197-01	28.00		
30s ea	13411-0197-03	84.00		
60s ea	13411-0197-06	168.00		
90s ea	13411-0197-09	252.00		
100s ea	13411-0197-10	279.27		
10 mg, 10s ea	13411-0180-01	57.50		
30s ea	13411-0180-03	172.50		
60s ea	13411-0180-06	345.00		
90s ea	13411-0180-09	517.50		
100s ea	13411-0180-10	279.27		
(Altura)				
REPACK				
TAB, PO, 10 mg, 7s ea	63874-0554-07	21.50		
10s ea	63874-0554-10	30.71		
14s ea	63874-0554-14	43.00		
15s ea	63874-0554-15	46.07		
30s ea	63874-0554-30	73.20		
(Bryant Ranch)				
REPACK				
TAB, PO, 10 mg, 30s ea	63629-2798-01	99.21		
100s ea	63629-2798-02	300.88		
(DHS, Inc.)				
REPACK				
TAB, PO (FILM-COATED)				
10 mg, 30s ea	55887-0825-30	75.00		
(Direct Pharmaceutical, Inc.)				
REPACK				
TAB, PO, 5 mg, 30s ea	67801-0422-03	83.40		
10 mg, 30s ea UD	67801-0323-03	82.40		
(Dispensing Solutions)				
REPACK				
SYR, PO, 1 mg/ml, 120 ml	55045-2641-08	40.00		
480 ml	55045-2641-09	160.00		
TAB, PO, 10 mg, 7s ea	55045-2399-03	19.25		
(FILM-COATED)				
10 mg, 10s ea	55045-2399-01	27.50		
15s ea	55045-2399-05	41.25		
20s ea	55045-2399-02	55.00		
(FILM-COATED)				
10 mg, 30s ea	55045-2399-08	82.50		
30s ea	66336-0036-30	93.72		
(HomeMed)				
REPACK				
TAB, PO, 10 mg, 14s ea	51655-0143-84	39.50		
(Palmetto)				
REPACK				
TAB, PO, 10 mg, 14s ea	23490-6925-02	48.63		
30s ea	23490-6925-03	104.21		
(PD-Rx Pharm)				
REPACK				
TAB, PO (REDI-SCRIPT,FILM-COATED)				
5 mg, 30s ea	58864-0853-30	48.88		
10 mg, 7s ea	55289-0108-07	30.16		
14s ea	55289-0108-14	55.70		
15s ea	55289-0108-15	59.69		
25s ea	55289-0108-25	99.48		
30s ea	55289-0108-30	113.91		
(REDI-SCRIPT,FILM-COATED)				
10 mg, 30s ea	58864-0686-30	85.61		
(Pharma Pac)				
REPACK				
TAB, PO, 10 mg, 7s ea	52959-0482-07	21.47		
10s ea	52959-0482-10	29.86		
15s ea	52959-0482-15	41.50		
30s ea	52959-0482-30	77.15		
(FILM-COATED)				
10 mg, 100s ea	52959-0482-01	201.55		
(Phys Total Care)				
REPACK				
CTB, PO, 5 mg, 30s ea	54868-5763-00	97.93		
10 mg, 30s ea	54868-5278-00	97.30		
TAB, PO (FILM-COATED)				
5 mg, 10s ea	54868-4010-01	31.44		
30s ea	54868-4010-00	90.57		

PROD/MFR	NDC	AWP	DP	OBC
(Quality Care Prod)				
REPACK				
CTB, PO, 10 mg, 30s ea	35356-0168-30	148.96		
TAB, PO (FILM-COATED)				
10 mg, 6s ea	49999-0275-06	23.03		
7s ea	49999-0275-07	26.87		
(FILM-COATED)				
10 mg, 14s ea	49999-0275-14	53.76		
90s ea	49999-0275-90	494.90		
(Southwood)				
REPACK				
TAB, PO (FILM-COATED)				
5 mg, 30s ea	58016-0369-30	31.64		
60s ea	58016-0369-60	63.29		
90s ea	58016-0369-90	94.93		
100s ea	58016-0369-00	105.48		
10 mg, 20s ea	58016-0367-20	40.76		
30s ea	58016-0367-30	18.72		
60s ea	58016-0367-60	37.44		
90s ea	58016-0367-90	56.16		
100s ea	58016-0367-00	62.40		
(Stat Rx)				
REPACK				
CTB, PO, 10 mg, 15s ea	16590-0348-15	72.00		
30s ea	16590-0348-30	144.00		
60s ea	16590-0348-60	280.00		
90s ea	16590-0348-90	420.00		
120s ea	16590-0348-72	550.00		
ZYRTEC-D (AQ)				
REPACK				
cetirizine hcl/pse hcl				
TER, PO, 5 mg-120 mg,				
100s ea	66105-0567-10	113.59		
(DHS, Inc.)				
REPACK				
TER, PO, 5 mg-120 mg,				
20s ea	55887-0380-20	29.95		
(Pharma Pac)				
REPACK				
TER, PO, 5 mg-120 mg,				
20s ea	52959-0802-20	25.95		
(Phys Total Care)				
REPACK				
TER, PO, 5 mg-120 mg,				
20s ea	54868-4737-00	34.10		
30s ea	54868-4737-01	50.21		
(12HR)				
5 mg-120 mg,				
60s ea	54868-4737-02	98.55		
(Quality Care Prod)				
REPACK				
TER, PO, 5 mg-120 mg,				
8s ea	49999-0490-08	13.37		
12s ea	49999-0490-12	41.38		
24s ea	49999-0490-24	70.44		
60s ea	49999-0490-60	100.30		
ZYRTEC-D 12HR (Phys Total Care)				
REPACK				
cetirizine hcl/pse hcl				
TER, PO, 5 mg-120 mg,				
100s ea	54868-4737-03	153.42		
ZYTOPIC (Auriga)				
triamcinolone acetonide				
KIT, TP (FRAGRANCE-FREE)				
0.1%, ea	14629-0514-01	71.25		
ZYVOX (Pfizer)				
linezolid				
PDR, PO (ORANGE)				
100 mg/5 ml,				
150 ml	00009-5136-01	459.88	383.23	
SOL, IV (P.C.)				
2 mg/ml, 100 ml	00009-5137-01	60.05	50.04	
300 ml	00009-5140-01	120.11	100.09	
TAB, PO (CAPLET)				
600 mg, 20s ea	00009-5135-02	1839.48	1532.90	
(3X10,CAPLET)				
600 mg, 30s ea UD	00009-5135-03	2759.21	2299.34	
(Physician Partner)				
REPACK				
TAB, PO (CAPLET)				
600 mg, 20s ea	21695-0399-20	3649.76		
(Quality Care Prod)				
REPACK				
TAB, PO (CAPLET)				
600 mg, 20s ea	35356-0108-20	2687.64		

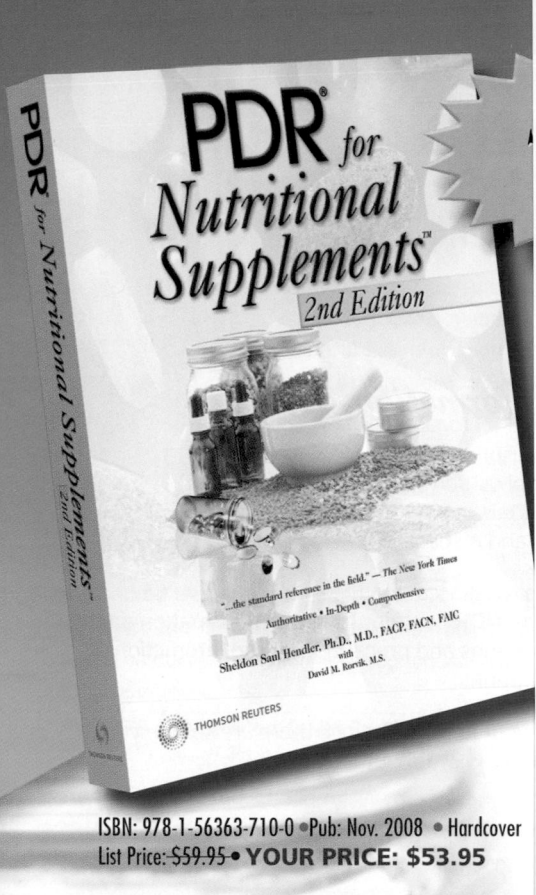

ODUCT LISTINGS

(AWP) and Suggested Retail Price
ach product form.

RI, or UPC		SRP (Suggested Retail Price)
53335-0080-11	12.70	25.40
53335-0080-11	12.70	25.40
53335-0080-11	12.70	25.40
ity	AWP (Average Wholesale Price)	

ook® are based on data *reported* by
as not performed any independent
d by wholesalers and providers in the
s paid by wholesalers and providers
contained in this publication and all
thout notice. Further, while care has
of the information contained herein,
its accuracy. For further explanation,
olicy" in the *Red Book* Foreword.
ed by subscribing to the monthly *Red*
Red Book for Windows™, *Red Book*
rices published in catalogs or other
by manufacturers or distributors.

ABBREVIATIONS

efers to the intake or application
ing abbreviations are used to indi-

OT..............Otic
PO..............Oral
RC..............Rectal
SC..............Subcutaneous
SL..............Sublingual
TD..............Transdermal
TP..............Topical
VG..............Vaginal

VIATIONS

used to provide additional descrip-

P.C.............Plastic container
P.F.............Preservative-free
R.N.P.........Reversed number package
S.D.............Single dose
S.D.V..........Single-dose vial
S.F.............Sugar-free
SRN...........Syringe
TAX INCL..Federal excise tax included
U.D............Unit dose
U.S.P..........U.S. Pharmacopeia

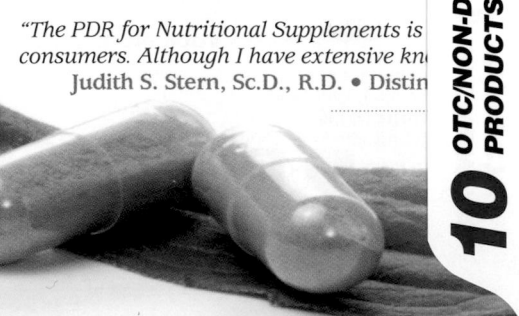

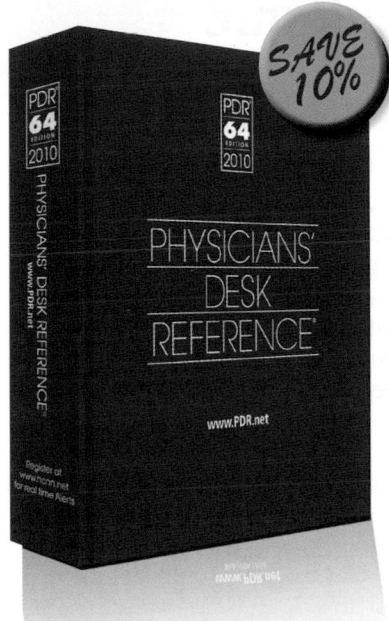

Continued on next page

STANDARD DOSAGE FORM DESCRIPTIONS

The following three-character abbreviations are used to indicate the form in which a product is available:

ACC	Accessory
AER	Aerosol liquid
BAN	Bandage
BAR	Bar
BEA	Beads
CAP	Capsule
CER	Capsule, extended release
CRE	Cream
CRY	Crystal
CTB	Tablet, chewable
DAP	Patch, device assisted
DEV	Device
DRE	Dressing
ECC	Capsule, delayed release
ECT	Tablet, enteric-coated
ELI	Elixir
EMO	Emollient cream
EMU	Emulsion
FDS	Food, solid
FIL	Film
FLA	Flake
FOA	Foam
GEF	Powder, effervescent
GEL	Gel/jelly
GRA	Granules
GUM	Gum
KIT	Kit
LIQ	Liquid
LOT	Lotion
LOZ	Lozenge/troche
NMA	Enema
ODT	Tablet, disintegrating
OIL	Oil
OIN	Ointment
PAD	Pad
PAS	Paste
PDR	Powder for suspension
PDS	Powder for solution
PEL	Pellet
PKT	Packet
POW	Powder
PRO	Prophylactic
PUD	Pudding
SER	Suspension, extended release
SGL	Capsule, liquid-filled
SHA	Shampoo
SHE	Sheet
SOA	Soap
SOL	Solution
SPE	Suppository, extended release
SPG	Sponge
SPR	Spray
STI	Stick
SUP	Suppository
SUS	Suspension
SWA	Swab
SYR	Syrup
T12	Tablet, extended release, 12-hr.
T24	Tablet, extended release, 24-hr.
TAB	Tablet
TAM	Tampon
TCP	Tablet, coated particles
TDM	Patch, extended release
TEF	Tablet, effervescent
TER	Tablet, extended release
TIN	Tincture
TSN	Tablet for solution
WAF	Wafer
WAX	Wax

ABBREVIATED INGREDIENT DESCRIPTIONS

Generic names are listed according to the following guidelines:

- Single-ingredient generic names will be spelled out in full (e.g., ACETAMINOPHEN)
- Multi-ingredient products (two or more) are listed in the alphabetical order of their ingredients using the following standard abbreviations:

ACE	ACETATE
AL	ALUMINUM
APAP	ACETAMINOPHEN
ASA	ASPIRIN
B	BORON
BI	BISMUTH
BICARB	BICARBONATE
BPM	BROMPHENIRAMINE
CA	CALCIUM
CAFF	CAFFEINE
CIT	CITRATE
CL	CHLORIDE
CPM	CHLORPHENIRAMINE
CR	CHROMIUM
CU	COPPER
DM	DEXTROMETHORPHAN
FE	IRON
FUM	FUMARATE
GG	GUAIFENESIN
HCL	HYDROCHLORIDE
K	POTASSIUM
LIDO	LIDOCAINE
MAL	MALEATE
MG	MAGNESIUM
MN	MANGANESE
PHOS	PHOSPHATE
PPA	PHENYLPROPANOLAMINE
PYRIL	PYRILAMINE
SAL	SALICYLATE
SE	SELENIUM
SI	SILICON
SULF	SULFATE
VIT	VITAMIN
ZN	ZINC

PROD/MFR	HRI, UPC,NDC	AWP	SRP
12-HOUR NASAL (A-S Medication)			
REPACK			
SPR,NS, 0.05%, 15 ml	54569-2154-00	3.46	
1ST TIER UNIFINE PENTIPS (Owen Mumford)			
DEV,NA (12MM,29G,ORIGINAL)			
100s ea	08571-3529-36	22.31	
(6MM,31G,MINI)			
100s ea	08571-3590-36	22.31	
(8MM,31G,SHORT)			
100s ea	08571-3530-36	22.31	
20/20 EYE DROPS (S.S.S.)			
SOL,OP, 0.4%-0.012%-0.25%,			
15 ml	12258-0215-05	1.99	2.99
20/20 LUBRICATING/REWETTING (S.S.S.)			
SOL,OP, 1.4%, 15 ml	12258-0116-02	2.80	
20/20 TEARS (S.S.S.)			
SOL,OP, 1.4%, 15 ml	12258-0121-05	2.80	
2ND SKIN BLISTER PAD (Spenco Medical)			
DEV,NA (60MMX45MM,STERILE)			
5s ea	38472-0504-10	3.30	7.89
2ND SKIN CUT CONTROL DRESSING (Spenco Medical)			
DEV,NA (2"X3",STERILE)			
4s ea	38472-0504-15	3.30	9.99
3M CLOTH ADHESIVE (3M Health Care)			
DEV,NA (3"X10 YDS)			
4s ea	08333-2950-03	13.20	
(2"X10 YDS)			
6s ea	08333-2950-02	13.20	
(1"X10 YDS)			
12s ea	08333-2950-01	13.20	
(1/2"X10 YDS)			
24s ea	08333-2950-00	13.20	
4 WAY FAST ACTING (Novartis Consumer)			
SPR,NS (1X14.8ML)			
1%, 14.8 ml	00067-2086-05	3.77	
(1X29.6ML)			
1%, 29.6 ml	00067-2086-01	6.05	
4 WEEK STOP SMOKING SYSTEM (Venturi)			
DEV,NA, ea	11120-0061-00	3.40	7.95
4-WAY FAST ACTING (B/M Squibb Cons Med)			
SPR,NS, 0.05%-0.5%-0.2%,			
15 ml	19810-0005-81	3.77	
(MENTHOLATED)			
0.05%-0.5%-0.2%,			
15 ml	19810-0005-61	3.77	
30 ml	19810-0005-82	6.05	
4-WAY LONG LASTING (B/M Squibb Cons Med)			
SPR,NS, 0.05%, 15 ml	19810-0057-51	3.77	
4-WAY NO DRIP (B/M Squibb Cons Med)			
SPR,NS (MAXSTRENGTH,FASTACTING)			
1%, 14.8 ml	19810-0301-19	4.48	
4-WAY SALINE MOISTURIZING MIST (B/M Squibb Cons Med)			
SPR,NS (AF)			
29.6 ml	19810-0002-65	2.81	
40+ MULTIPLE (ADH)			
TAB,PO, 60s ea	60142-0093-06	6.10	14.25
5-DAY DEODORANT (Numark)			
PAD,TP, 25%, 75s ea	38485-0110-42	4.62	
5-DAY ROLL-ON (Numark)			
SOL,TP, 44 ml	38485-0020-12	3.78	
74 ml	38485-0020-22	5.34	
5-HTP (Key Company)			
CAP,PO (PF,SF,CORN-FREE)			
50 mg, 60s ea	11694-0673-01	6.50	
666 COLD MAXIMUM STRENGTH (Monticello)			
TAB,PO (CAPLET)			
500 mg-30 mg,			
16s ea	11868-0237-16	1.85	
32s ea	11868-0237-32	2.48	
666 COLD PREPARATION (Monticello)			
LIQ,PO (MAXIMUM STRENGTH)			
118 ml	49580-1416-04	1.85	
177 ml	49580-1416-06	2.72	
666 COUGH & COLD FORMULA (Monticello)			
SYR,PO, 120 ml	11868-0044-04	2.60	4.68
666 PREPARATION W/QUININE (Monticello)			
LIQ,PO, 120 ml	11868-0001-04	2.33	4.20
A & D OINTMENT (Schering Plough)			
OIN,TP, 45 gm	00085-0096-01	2.34	
120 gm	00085-0096-02	3.86	
120 gm	00085-1410-02	3.86	
454 gm	00085-0096-04	8.94	
(Phys Total Care)			
REPACK			
OIN,TP, 120 gm	54868-2877-01	11.67	
454 gm	54868-2877-00	21.24	
A-25 (Bio-Tech Pharm)			
CAP,PO, 25000 iu,			
100s ea	53191-0218-01	4.44	
A-CARO-25 (Key Company)			
SGL,PO (SOFTGEL)			
25000 iu, 100s ea	11694-0853-01	6.00	
250s ea	11694-0853-04	12.00	
1000s ea	11694-0853-06	42.00	
A-FIL (Doak)			
CRE,TP (SPF 25)			
5%-5%, 42.5 gm	10337-0807-45	18.94	
A-FREE PRENATAL (Freeda)			
TAB,PO (PF,SF,DYE-FREE)			
100s ea	10432-0283-01	5.91	9.85
A-FREE ULTRA FREEDA (Freeda)			
TAB,PO (HIGH POTENCY)			
90s ea	10432-0339-01	13.05	21.75
A-SOY (PBM Pharmaceuticals)			
LIQ,PO (24X237ML)			
237 ml 24s	83744-0550-27	42.74	42.89
A-V IMPULSE SYSTEM IMPAD RIGID SOLE FOOT COVER (Covidien)			
DEV,NA (LEFT FOOT,STERILE)			
4s ea	08080-6067-01	299.25	
(RIGHT FOOT,STERILE)			
4s ea	08080-6066-01	299.25	
A-V IMPULSE SYSTEM IMPAD UNDER CAST INFLATION PADS (Covidien)			
DEV,NA (LEFT FOOT)			
12s ea	08080-5089-01	159.00	
(RIGHT FOOT)			
12s ea	08080-5087-01	159.00	
A-V IMPULSE SYSTEM TUBING ASSEMBLY (Covidien)			
DEV,NA (RIGHT)			
50s ea	08080-5007-01	25.00	
A.M.-75 MULTIVIT/MULTIMINERAL (ADH)			
TAB,PO, 100s ea	60142-0095-10	7.98	15.95
A/G PRO (Miller)			
TAB,PO, 180s ea	17204-0427-50	11.10	17.00
A+D (Schering Plough)			
CRE,TP, 1%-10%, 102 gm	41100-0895-43	4.68	
A200 LICE CONTROL (Hogil)			
SPR,NA, 0.5%, 170.1 gm	95814-0002-53	3.96	
A200 LICE TREATMENT (Hogil)			
KIT,NA (SHAMPOO, SPRAY, COMB)			
ea	95814-0000-05	10.29	
A200 MAXIMUM STRENGTH (Hogil)			
LIQ,TP (W/COMB)			
4%-0.33%, 120 ml	95814-0002-15	8.12	
A200 TIME-TESTED FORMULA (Hogil)			
SHA,TP (W/COMB)			
3%-0.3%, 60 ml	95814-0002-50	5.25	
ABLE EYES (Carlson,J.R.)			
SGL,PO (PF,SF,CORN-FREE)			
30s ea	88395-0048-44	9.95	19.90
90s ea	88395-0048-41	27.75	55.50
180s ea	88395-0048-42	49.50	99.00
ABLES FLATFOLD INCONTINENT BRIEFS (Covidien)			
DEV,NA (EXTRA LARGE,LATEX-FREE)			
60s ea	08080-6850-01	33.81	
(31"X50",LATEX-FREE)			
100s ea	08080-6400-00	61.69	
ABREVA (Glaxo)			
CRE,TP, 2 gm	00135-0200-01	15.14	
(1X2GM PUMP)			
2 gm	07660-0801-55	15.50	
(2GMX6)			
2 gm 6s	07660-0801-35	14.29	
(2GMX24)			
2 gm 24s	07660-0802-00	14.29	
ABSORBASE (Carolina)			
OIN,TP, 110 gm 12s	46287-0507-04	58.80	
454 gm	46287-0507-16	9.95	
ABSORBENT POUCH FOR MEN (Mentor)			
DEV,NA (250CC)			
10s ea	81317-0071-00	6.11	
ABSORBINE JR. (Young, W.F.)			
LIQ,TP, 1.27%, 59.2 ml	11444-0001-03	3.40	4.59
118 ml	11444-0001-04	4.70	6.49
473 ml	11444-0001-06	11.10	16.19
ABSORBINE JR. EXTRA STRENGTH (Young, W.F.)			
LIQ,TP, 4%, 59 ml	11444-0020-01	4.70	6.49
ABSORBINE JR. PAIN RELIEVING PATCH (Young, W.F.)			
PAD,TP, 6s ea	11444-0157-01	4.90	8.19
AC ADAPTER (Lumiscope)			
DEV,NA (3 VOLT)			
ea	38673-0006-05	6.25	12.95
ACCELWELL TRAVEL POUCH (Technological Investments)			
DEV,NA (8"X2 1/4"X6 3/4")			
ea	08605-0103-03	15.63	
ACCU-CHECK CMFT CURVE STRIP (Phys Total Care)			
REPACK			
DEV,NA, 50s ea	54868-5796-00	63.86	
ACCU-CHECK SOFT TOUCH LANCING (Roche Diag)			
DEV,NA (W/DIAL)			
ea	50924-0580-01	15.00	17.00
ACCU-CHEK ACTIVE (Roche Diag)			
DEV,NA (STRIP)			
50s ea	50924-0475-50	34.19	
(Phys Total Care)			
REPACK			
DEV,NA (STRIP)			
50s ea	54868-3590-00	64.49	
ACCU-CHEK ACTIVE GLUCOSE CONTROL (Roche Diag)			
DEV,NA (LOW/HIGH)			
2s ea	50924-0476-02	8.75	
ACCU-CHEK ACTIVE MONITORING (Roche Diag)			
DEV,NA (W/METER & LANCET DEV)			
ea	50924-0477-01	18.75	
ACCU-CHEK ADVANTAGE (Phys Total Care)			
REPACK			
DEV,NA, 100s ea	54868-0824-00	121.21	
ACCU-CHEK ADVANTAGE CARE (Roche Diag)			
DEV,NA, ea	50924-0860-01	68.75	
ACCU-CHEK AVIVA CONTROL SOLUTION (Roche Diag)			
DEV,NA (2X2.5ML,LEVELS 1 & 2)			
2s ea	65702-0107-10	8.75	
ACCU-CHEK AVIVA KIT (Roche Diag)			
DEV,NA, ea	65702-0101-10	19.94	
ACCU-CHEK AVIVA TEST STRIPS (Roche Diag)			
DEV,NA, 50s ea	65702-0103-10	60.06	
50s ea	65702-0212-10	60.06	
100s ea	65702-0104-10	120.13	
ACCU-CHEK COMFORT CURVE (Roche Diag)			
DEV,NA (NOT FOR RETAIL SALE)			
50s ea	50924-0882-50		
(STRIP)			
50s ea	50924-0373-50	63.13	
(2X50)			
100s ea	50924-0881-10	126.25	
(STRIP)			
100s ea	50924-0381-10	126.25	
ACCU-CHEK COMFORT CURVE CONTROL (Roche Diag)			
DEV,NA (LO/HI)			
2s ea	50924-0411-02	8.75	
ACCU-CHEK COMFORT CURVE TEST STRIPS (Roche Diag)			
DEV,NA, 50s ea	50924-0365-50	63.13	
50s ea	65702-0215-10	63.13	
ACCU-CHEK COMPACT DRUMS (Roche Diag)			
DEV,NA (STRIP,3X17)			
51s ea	50924-0988-50	60.06	
(STRIPS 6X17)			
102s ea	50924-0884-01	120.13	
ACCU-CHEK COMPACT GLUCOSE CONTROL (Roche Diag)			
DEV,NA (LOW/HIGH)			
2s ea	50924-0302-02	8.75	
ACCU-CHEK COMPACT PLUS (Roche Diag)			
DEV,NA, ea	50924-0019-01	19.94	
ACCU-CHEK COMPACT TEST STRIPS (Roche Diag)			
DEV,NA, 51s ea	65702-0223-10	60.06	
ACCU-CHEK INSTANT (Roche Diag)			
DEV,NA (STRIP)			
50s ea	50924-0913-50	43.31	

PROD/MFR	HRI, UPC,NDC	AWP	SRP
ACCU-CHEK INSTANT GLUCOSE CONTROL (Roche Diag)			
DEV,NA (LOW/HIGH)			
2s ea	50924-0919-01	11.88	
ACCU-CHEK MULTICLIX LANCET (Roche Diag)			
DEV,NA (W/12 LANCETS)			
ea	50924-0446-01	28.13	
ACCU-CHEK MULTICLIX LANCETS (Roche Diag)			
DEV,NA, 102s ea	50924-0450-01	12.50	
204s ea	50924-0981-01	19.69	
ACCU-CHEK SAFE-T-PRO PLUS (Roche Diag)			
DEV,NA (SINGLE-USE)			
200s ea	50924-0079-20	57.50	
ACCU-CHEK SOFT TOUCH (Roche Diag)			
DEV,NA, 100s ea	50924-0585-10	8.75	11.34
200s ea	50924-0937-20	11.88	
ACCU-CHEK SOFTCLIX (Roche Diag)			
DEV,NA, ea	50924-0957-01	28.13	
100s ea	50924-0971-10	10.94	
100s ea	65702-0156-10	10.94	
200s ea	65702-0124-10	16.56	
ACCU-CHEK VOICEMATE SYSTEM (Roche Diag)			
DEV,NA (W/LANCETS&CONTROL SOL.)			
ea	50924-0802-01	493.75	
ACCUTREND CHOLESTEROL (Roche Diag)			
DEV,NA, 25s ea	65702-0276-10	82.45	
ACCUTREND CHOLESTEROL CONTROL (Roche Diag)			
DEV,NA (2X2ML)			
ea	65702-0250-10	25.68	
ACCUTREND GLUCOSE (Roche Diag)			
DEV,NA, 50s ea	65702-0274-10	43.31	
ACCUTREND GLUCOSE CONTROL (Roche Diag)			
DEV,NA (2X4ML)			
4 ml 2s	65702-0275-10	10.11	
ACCUTREND PLUS (Roche Diag)			
DEV,NA, ea	65702-0284-10	187.90	
ACE + Z (Legere)			
TAB,PO, 100s ea	25332-1038-02	12.00	
ACEPHEN (G&W)			
SUP,RC, 120 mg, 6s ea	00713-0118-66	5.45	
12s ea	00713-0118-11	6.26	
12s ea UD	00713-0118-12	5.81	
50s ea UD	00713-0118-50	27.24	
100s ea UD	00713-0118-01	52.22	
325 mg, 6s ea	00713-0164-66	5.74	
12s ea	00713-0164-11	6.37	
12s ea	00713-0164-12	6.12	
50s ea	00713-0164-50	27.48	
100s ea	00713-0164-01	52.66	28.94
650 mg, 12s ea	00713-0165-12	6.34	
50s ea UD	00713-0165-50	27.69	
100s ea UD	00713-0165-01	53.14	
500s ea	00713-0165-05	233.23	
(A-S Medication)			
REPACK			
SUP,RC, 325 mg, 12s ea	54569-0004-00	6.87	
ACERFLEX (Nutricia)			
PDR,PO (MED. SUPV.,PINEAPPLE)			
454 gm 4s	49735-0100-26	210.60	
ACEROLA C500 (Mason Vit)			
CTB,PO (PF)			
500 mg, 60s ea	11845-0079-45	7.44	
ACES (Carlson,J.R.)			
SGL,PO (SOFTGEL)			
200s ea	88395-0044-32	21.00	42.00
360s ea	88395-0044-33	34.75	69.50
(PF,SF,CORN-FREE)			
50s ea	88395-0044-30	6.20	12.40
ACES GOLD (Carlson,J.R.)			
TAB,PO (PF,SF,SALT-FREE)			
60s ea	88395-0044-10	17.20	34.40
120s ea	88395-0044-11	32.20	64.40
180s ea	88395-0044-12	46.45	92.90
ACES PLUS ZINC (Carlson,J.R.)			
SGL,PO (SOFTGEL)			
60s ea	88395-0044-20	7.45	14.90
120s ea	88395-0044-21	13.25	26.50
180s ea	88395-0044-22	18.95	37.90
ACES+ZINC (Carlson,J.R.)			
PO (PF,SF,CORN-FREE)			
360s ea	88395-0044-24	36.00	72.00
ACETA-GESIC (Rugby)			
TAB,PO, 325 mg-30 mg,			
100s ea	00536-3014-01	5.10	
ACETADRINK (St. Paul)			
TEF,PO (EXTRA STRENGTH,FRUIT)			
500 mg, 30s ea	23110-0141-30	6.99	6.99
ACETAMINOPHEN (Actavis Mid Atlantic)			
SOL,PO (AF,DROPS)			
80 mg/0.8 ml, 15 ml	00472-1417-99	3.00	
(Advance)			
CAP,PO, 500 mg, 100s ea	17714-0037-01	3.50	
1000s ea	17714-0037-10	25.00	
TAB,PO, 325 mg, 100s ea	17714-0012-01	1.49	
1000s ea	17714-0012-10	9.99	
500 mg, 100s ea	17714-0013-01	2.49	
100s ea	17714-0014-01	2.80	
1000s ea	17714-0013-10	15.75	
1000s ea	17714-0014-10	18.99	
(Albertson's)			
SOL,PO (DROPS)			
80 mg/0.8 ml, 15 ml	41280-0220-51	2.37	
TAB,PO, 325 mg, 100s ea	12810-0453-78	2.16	
100s ea	41280-0220-40	2.16	
500 mg, 100s ea	12810-0484-78	2.88	
100s ea	41280-0220-48	2.88	
(Amneal)			
TAB,PO (REGULAR STRENGTH)			
325 mg, 50s ea	65162-0350-05	1.60	
100s ea	65162-0350-10	4.15	
1000s ea	65162-0350-11	14.85	
(EXTRA STRENGTH)			
500 mg, 100s ea	65162-0602-10	3.00	
100s ea	65162-0607-10	3.20	
1000s ea	65162-0602-11	22.20	
1000s ea	65162-0607-11	22.25	
(Concord Labs)			
TAB,PO, 325 mg, 100s ea	20254-0200-01	2.16	
1000s ea	20254-0200-04	13.50	
500 mg, 100s ea	20254-0201-01	2.70	
(COATED,CAPLET)			
500 mg, 100s ea	20254-0202-01	2.97	
(UN-COATED,CAPLET)			
500 mg, 100s ea	20254-0203-01	2.70	
1000s ea	20254-0201-04	18.90	
(COATED,CAPLET)			
500 mg, 1000s ea	20254-0202-04	21.60	
(UN-COATED,CAPLET)			
500 mg, 1000s ea	20254-0203-04	20.25	
(Consolidated Midland)			
SUP,RC, 120 mg, 12s ea	00223-5004-12	5.75	
100s ea	00223-5004-00	47.50	
325 mg, 12s ea	00223-5005-12	5.95	
100s ea	00223-5005-00	48.50	
650 mg, 12s ea	00223-5006-12	6.25	
100s ea	00223-5006-00	49.00	
(Family Phcy)			
TAB,PO (PRIVATE LABEL)			
325 mg, 100s ea	52735-0709-01	5.39	5.99
500 mg, 500s ea	52735-0710-70	8.99	9.99
(Geri-Care)			
TAB,PO, 325 mg, 50s ea	57896-0101-05	0.40	
100s ea	57896-0011-01	0.50	
100s ea	57896-0101-01	0.50	
1000s ea	57896-0100-10	4.15	
1000s ea	57896-0101-10	4.15	
500 mg, 100s ea	57896-0022-01	0.80	
(CAPLET)			
500 mg, 100s ea	57896-0221-01	0.90	
1000s ea	57896-0201-10	5.92	
(CAPLET)			
500 mg, 1000s ea	57896-0221-10	7.09	
(Marlex)			
TAB,PO, 325 mg, 24s ea	10135-0123-24	0.60	
30s ea	10135-0123-30	0.62	
50s ea	10135-0123-50	0.65	
60s ea	10135-0123-60	0.67	
90s ea	10135-0123-90	0.69	
100s ea	10135-0123-01	5.73	
(BLISTER PACK)			
325 mg, 100s ea UD	10135-0163-13	2.30	
(BOXED)			
325 mg, 100s ea	10135-0123-57	65.00	
120s ea	10135-0123-62	0.95	
(BLISTER PACK)			
325 mg, 200s ea UD	10135-0163-14	4.00	
240s ea	10135-0123-65	1.80	
700s ea	10135-0123-70	4.00	
1000s ea	10135-0123-10	4.10	
(Ohm)			
CAP,PO, 500 mg, 100s ea	51660-0600-01	1.95	
1000s ea	51660-0600-10	16.50	
TAB,PO, 325 mg, 100s ea	51660-0010-01	0.99	
1000s ea	51660-0010-10	5.95	
500 mg, 50s ea	51660-0311-51	0.99	
60s ea	51660-0011-60	0.99	
100s ea	51660-0011-01	1.45	
100s ea	51660-0311-01	1.60	
1000s ea	51660-0011-10	7.95	
1000s ea	51660-0311-10	9.00	
(Perrigo)			
SUP,RC, 120 mg, 12s ea	45802-0732-30	6.99	
100s ea	45802-0732-33	36.99	
(Pfeiffer)			
SUP,RC, 650 mg, 12s ea	00927-0678-12	3.11	5.59
(Pharm Assoc Inc)			
SOL,PO (AF,CHERRY)			
160 mg/5 ml,			
5 ml 100s UD	00121-0657-05	57.72	
(CHERRY)			
160 mg/5 ml,			
10.15 ml 100s UD	00121-0657-11	60.00	
20.3 ml 100s UD	00121-0657-21	85.47	
(Rugby)			
CTB,PO (ASPIRIN-FREE,FRUIT)			
80 mg, 30s ea	00536-3233-07	2.63	
SUP,RC, 120 mg, 12s ea	00536-1255-12	7.02	
325 mg, 12s ea	00536-1320-12	7.80	
650 mg, 12s ea	00536-1260-12	8.40	
(Teva)			
TAB,PO (10X10)			
325 mg, 100s ea UD	00182-8447-89	5.95	
1000s ea	00182-1000-10	14.85	
(10X10)			
500 mg, 100s ea UD	00182-8453-89	6.22	
(UDL)			
TAB,PO (ROBOT READY 25X1)			
325 mg, 25s ea UD	51079-0002-19	4.20	
(10X10)			
325 mg, 100s ea UD	51079-0002-20	6.35	
(10X10X2)			
325 mg, 200s ea UD	51079-0002-22	7.03	
(10X10,CAPLET)			
500 mg, 100s ea UD	51079-0396-20	8.36	
(Vita-Rx)			
CAP,PO, 500 mg, 100s ea	49727-0502-02	2.80	
1000s ea	49727-0502-05	19.30	
CTB,PO, 80 mg, 30s ea	49727-0499-33	1.43	
TAB,PO, 325 mg, 100s ea	49727-0500-02	2.10	
1000s ea	49727-0500-05	11.50	
500 mg, 100s ea	49727-0501-02	2.85	
(A-S Medication)			
REPACK			
CTB,PO, 80 mg, 30s ea	54569-3185-00	2.19	
ELI,PO, 160 mg/5 ml,			
120 ml	54569-2814-00	2.60	
SOL,PO (AF,DROPS)			
80 mg/0.8 ml,			
15 ml	54569-3178-00	2.70	
SUP,RC, 120 mg, 12s ea	54569-0003-00	6.13	
TAB,PO, 325 mg, 15s ea	54569-1533-01	0.22	
20s ea	54569-1533-04	0.30	
24s ea	54569-1533-08	0.36	
30s ea	54569-1533-03	0.45	
100s ea	54569-1533-02	1.49	
(ASPIRIN-FREE,CAPLET)			
500 mg, 15s ea	54569-2764-00	0.62	
20s ea	54569-2764-05	0.83	
24s ea	54569-2764-04	0.99	
30s ea	54569-2764-01	1.25	
50s ea	54569-2764-03	2.08	
60s ea	54569-2764-07	2.49	
100s ea	54569-2764-02	4.15	
(Altura)			
REPACK			
SOL,PO (DROPS)			
80 mg/0.8 ml,			
30 ml	63874-0064-30	7.60	
SUP,RC, 120 mg, 12s ea	63874-0060-12	10.54	
325 mg, 12s ea	63874-0059-12	13.24	
SYR,PO (CHERRY)			
160 mg/5 ml,			
120 ml	63874-0056-12	13.67	
TAB,PO, 325 mg, 15s ea	63874-0002-15	3.64	
16s ea	63874-0002-16	2.99	
20s ea	63874-0002-20	4.63	
24s ea	63874-0002-24	5.58	
25s ea	63874-0002-25	5.81	
30s ea	63874-0002-30	5.84	
40s ea	63874-0002-40	7.78	
50s ea	63874-0002-50	9.72	

PROD/MFR	HRI, UPC,NDC	AWP	SRP
60s ea	63874-0002-60	11.67	
100s ea	63874-0002-01	10.76	
1000s ea	63874-0002-02	34.64	
(CAPLET)			
500 mg, 10s ea	63874-0022-10	0.91	
12s ea	63874-0022-12	1.10	
14s ea	63874-0022-14	1.28	
15s ea	63874-0003-15	3.86	
(CAPLET)			
500 mg, 15s ea	63874-0022-15	1.38	
20s ea	63874-0003-20	5.18	
(GELCAPLET)			
500 mg, 20s ea	63874-0022-20	4.13	
(CAPLET)			
500 mg, 21s ea	63874-0022-21	1.93	
24s ea	63874-0003-24	5.73	
(CAPLET)			
500 mg, 24s ea	63874-0022-24	2.21	
25s ea	63874-0003-25	6.01	
(CAPLET)			
500 mg, 28s ea	63874-0022-28	2.57	
30s ea	63874-0003-30	7.94	
(GELCAPLET)			
500 mg, 30s ea	63874-0022-30	5.49	
40s ea	63874-0003-40	9.04	
(CAPLET)			
500 mg, 40s ea	63874-0022-40	3.68	
50s ea	63874-0003-50	10.14	
(GELCAPLET)			
500 mg, 50s ea	63874-0022-50	7.20	
60s ea	63874-0003-60	12.17	
(CAPLET)			
500 mg, 60s ea	63874-0022-60	8.64	
90s ea	63874-0003-90	18.25	
100s ea	63874-0003-01	20.20	
(GELCAPLET)			
500 mg, 100s ea	63874-0022-01	13.82	
500s ea	63874-0003-05	186.66	
(GELCAPLET)			
500 mg, 500s ea	63874-0022-05	36.26	
1000s ea	63874-0003-02	295.36	
(GELCAPLET)			
500 mg, 1000s ea	63874-0022-02	96.31	
(Bryant Ranch)			
REPACK			
TAB,PO, 500 mg, 15s ea	63629-1516-02	6.36	
20s ea	63629-1516-01	8.98	
30s ea	63629-1516-05	13.98	
40s ea	63629-1516-03	16.95	
45s ea	63629-1516-06	16.99	
100s ea	63629-1516-04	42.38	
(DHS, Inc.)			
REPACK			
SUP,RC, 120 mg, 12s ea	55887-0206-12	11.75	
TAB,PO, 500 mg, 20s ea	55887-0945-20	6.58	
40s ea	55887-0945-40	13.12	
45s ea	55887-0945-45	16.25	
50s ea	55887-0945-50	16.50	
60s ea	55887-0945-60	18.00	
90s ea	55887-0945-90	27.00	
(Dispensing Solutions)			
REPACK			
SUP,RC, 325 mg, 12s ea	55045-1499-04	7.80	
650 mg, 12s ea	55045-1196-04	8.40	
TAB,PO, 325 mg, 6s ea	66336-0107-06	3.38	
20s ea	55045-1376-07	4.00	
30s ea	55045-1376-08	6.05	
30s ea	66336-0107-30	10.11	
60s ea	55045-1376-02	12.00	
100s ea	55045-1376-01	20.00	
500 mg, 12s ea	55045-1864-01	3.24	
20s ea	55045-1864-07	5.40	
24s ea	55045-1864-04	6.48	
30s ea	55045-1864-08	8.10	
(CAPLET)			
500 mg, 30s ea	66336-0656-30	9.65	
40s ea	55045-1864-06	10.80	
50s ea	55045-1864-02	13.50	
(CAPLET)			
500 mg, 50s ea	66336-0656-50	11.22	
60s ea	55045-1864-09	16.20	
90s ea	55045-1864-03	24.30	
90s ea	66336-0656-90	14.36	
100s ea	55045-1864-00	27.00	
(CAPLET)			
500 mg, 120s ea	55045-1864-05	32.40	
500s ea	55045-3492-01	40.00	
(HomeMed)			
REPACK			
TAB,PO, 325 mg, 16s ea	51655-0130-74	2.78	
20s ea	51655-0130-52	3.01	

PROD/MFR	HRI, UPC,NDC	AWP	SRP
24s ea	51655-0130-30	3.25	
40s ea	51655-0130-51	4.00	
(McKesson Packaging)			
REPACK			
TAB,PO (25X30)			
325 mg, 750s ea UD	63739-0440-01	47.25	
750s ea	63739-0440-03	47.25	
(BLISTER PACK)			
325 mg, 750s ea UD	63739-0002-01	47.25	
(BLISTER PACK 25X30X2)			
325 mg,			
1500s ea UD	63739-0002-11	49.15	
(25X30,CAPLET)			
500 mg, 750s ea UD	63739-0439-01	60.90	
(Nucare Pharm)			
REPACK			
TAB,PO, 325 mg, 30s ea	66267-0003-30	5.89	
40s ea	66267-0003-40	7.89	
100s ea	66267-0999-00	10.86	
500 mg, 20s ea	66267-0005-20	5.68	
30s ea	66267-0005-30	7.98	
45s ea	66267-0005-45	11.97	
50s ea	66267-0005-50	10.89	
100s ea	66267-0998-00	20.36	
(Palmetto)			
REPACK			
CTB,PO, 80 mg, 30s ea	23490-6598-01	8.40	
ELI,PO (1X120ML)			
160 mg/5 ml,			
120 ml	23490-6590-01	6.13	
SOL,PO, 160 mg/5 ml,			
120 ml	23490-6591-02	6.13	
80 mg/0.8 ml,			
15 ml	23490-6599-01	6.29	
SUP,RC, 120 mg, 6s ea	23490-6589-01	7.06	
TAB,PO, 325 mg, 6s ea	23490-6593-01	3.11	
10s ea	23490-6593-02	3.66	
20s ea	23490-6593-03	7.33	
30s ea	23490-6593-04	10.99	
40s ea	23490-6593-05	14.65	
100s ea	23490-6593-06	36.63	
500 mg, 20s ea	23490-6595-01	7.33	
30s ea	23490-6595-02	10.99	
45s ea	23490-6595-03	16.48	
60s ea	23490-6595-05	21.98	
60s ea	23491-6595-05	10.32	
90s ea	23490-6595-06	32.97	
90s ea	23491-6595-06	14.48	
100s ea	23490-6595-04	36.63	
(PD-Rx Pharm)			
REPACK			
TAB,PO, 325 mg, 12s ea	55289-0563-12	5.39	
20s ea	55289-0563-20	5.80	
24s ea	55289-0563-24	6.20	
30s ea	55289-0563-30	6.20	
50s ea	55289-0563-50	8.67	
(REDI-SCRIPT)			
325 mg, 56s ea	58864-0002-56	9.77	
60s ea	55289-0563-60	10.50	
100s ea	55289-0563-01	15.25	
500 mg, 6s ea	55289-0880-06	5.35	
(USP,ASPIRIN-FREE,CAPLET)			
500 mg, 12s ea	55289-0880-12	5.48	
20s ea	55289-0880-20	6.00	
24s ea	55289-0880-24	6.20	
30s ea	55289-0880-30	6.50	
(REDI-SCRIPT)			
500 mg, 30s ea	58864-0061-30	6.50	
50s ea	55289-0880-50	8.25	
60s ea	55289-0880-60	8.66	
100s ea	55289-0880-01	9.12	
(Pharma Pac)			
REPACK			
CTB,PO (FRUIT)			
80 mg, 30s ea	52959-0170-03	7.15	
ELI,PO, 160 mg/5 ml,			
120 ml	52959-0309-04	4.75	
SOL,PO (DROPS)			
80 mg/0.8 ml,			
15 ml	52959-0097-00	6.10	
SUP,RC, 120 mg, 12s ea	52959-0101-00	9.35	
650 mg, 12s ea	52959-0109-03	11.75	
TAB,PO, 325 mg, 12s ea	52959-0302-12	4.74	
20s ea	52959-0302-20	5.70	
24s ea	52959-0302-24	5.95	
30s ea	52959-0302-30	6.63	
40s ea	52959-0302-40	8.82	
60s ea	52959-0302-60	9.88	
100s ea	52959-0302-00	10.88	
200s ea	52959-0302-95	20.45	
500 mg, 10s ea	52959-0002-10	4.09	

PROD/MFR	HRI, UPC,NDC	AWP	SRP
(CAPLET)			
500 mg, 10s ea	52959-0338-10	4.15	
12s ea	52959-0338-12	4.96	
15s ea	52959-0002-15	6.14	
20s ea	52959-0002-20	8.19	
(CAPLET)			
500 mg, 20s ea	52959-0338-20	8.19	
24s ea	52959-0002-24	8.55	
(CAPLET)			
500 mg, 24s ea	52959-0338-24	8.55	
25s ea	52959-0002-25	8.92	
30s ea	52959-0002-30	9.65	
(CAPLET)			
500 mg, 30s ea	52959-0338-30	9.65	
40s ea	52959-0002-40	10.47	
(CAPLET)			
500 mg, 40s ea	52959-0338-40	10.47	
(GELCAPLET)			
500 mg, 40s ea	52959-0412-40	4.85	
45s ea	52959-0002-45	11.36	
50s ea	52959-0002-50	11.22	
(CAPLET)			
500 mg, 50s ea	52959-0338-50	11.22	
(GELCAPLET)			
500 mg, 50s ea	52959-0412-50	7.20	
(CAPLET)			
500 mg, 60s ea	52959-0338-60	13.41	
90s ea	52959-0002-90	20.20	
100s ea	52959-0002-00	22.44	
(CAPLET)			
500 mg, 100s ea	52959-0338-00	22.44	
(Phys Total Care)			
REPACK			
ELI,PO, 160 mg/5 ml,			
120 ml	54868-1791-00	8.10	
SUP,RC, 120 mg, 12s ea	54868-1792-00	4.03	
325 mg, 12s ea	54868-2878-00	10.87	
650 mg, 12s ea	54868-4991-00	10.80	
TAB,PO, 325 mg, 50s ea	54868-0548-02	4.68	
100s ea	54868-0548-04	8.37	
500s ea	54868-0548-01	14.55	
1000s ea	54868-0548-03	26.42	
500 mg, 100s ea	54868-3832-02	7.94	
(Physician Partner)			
REPACK			
SOL,PO (1X30ML)			
80 mg/0.8 ml,			
30 ml	21695-0887-30	14.70	
TAB,PO, 325 mg, 30s ea	21695-0007-30	10.99	
60s ea	21695-0007-60	21.98	
500 mg, 14s ea	21695-0008-14	9.14	
15s ea	21695-0008-15	9.80	
20s ea	21695-0008-20	13.06	
30s ea	21695-0008-30	19.60	
50s ea	21695-0008-50	36.90	
60s ea	21695-0008-60	39.20	
100s ea	21695-0008-00	32.44	
(Quality Care Prod)			
REPACK			
SOL,PO (AF,ASPIRIN-FREE)			
160 mg/5 ml,			
120 ml	49999-0211-04	14.85	
TAB,PO, 325 mg, 30s ea	49999-0131-30	5.86	
500 mg, 20s ea	49999-0099-20	6.00	
30s ea	49999-0099-30	9.00	
60s ea	49999-0099-60	18.00	
100s ea	49999-0099-00	30.00	
(Southwood)			
REPACK			
CTB,PO, 80 mg, 20s ea	58016-0110-20	2.91	
30s ea	58016-0110-30	3.69	
ELI,PO, 160 mg/5 ml,			
118 ml	58016-2671-01	2.50	
SOL,PO (DROPS)			
80 mg/0.8 ml,			
15 ml	58016-2005-01	5.99	
SUP,RC, 120 mg, 12s ea	58016-2006-01	9.30	
TAB,PO, 325 mg, 16s ea	58016-0265-16	2.85	
20s ea	58016-0265-20	3.56	
24s ea	58016-0265-24	4.28	
30s ea	58016-0265-30	5.34	
40s ea	58016-0265-40	7.13	
50s ea	58016-0265-50	8.91	
100s ea	58016-0265-00	17.81	
(CAPLET)			
500 mg, 10s ea	58016-0287-10	0.87	
(GEL,CAPLET)			
500 mg, 10s ea	58016-0200-10	0.87	
(CAPLET)			
500 mg, 12s ea	58016-0287-12	1.04	

PROD/MFR	HRI, UPC,NDC	AWP	SRP
(GEL,CAPLET)			
500 mg, 12s ea	58016-0200-12	1.05	
(CAPLET)			
500 mg, 14s ea	58016-0287-14	1.22	
(GEL,CAPLET)			
500 mg, 14s ea	58016-0200-14	1.22	
(CAPLET)			
500 mg, 15s ea	58016-0287-15	1.31	
(GEL,CAPLET)			
500 mg, 15s ea	58016-0200-15	1.31	
(CAPLET)			
500 mg, 20s ea	58016-0287-20	1.74	
(GEL,CAPLET)			
500 mg, 20s ea	58016-0200-20	1.75	
(CAPLET)			
500 mg, 21s ea	58016-0287-21	1.83	
(GEL,CAPLET)			
500 mg, 21s ea	58016-0200-21	1.84	
(CAPLET)			
500 mg, 24s ea	58016-0287-24	2.09	
(GEL,CAPLET)			
500 mg, 24s ea	58016-0200-24	2.10	
25s ea	58016-0266-25	3.57	
(CAPLET)			
500 mg, 25s ea	58016-0287-25	2.18	
28s ea	58016-0287-28	2.44	
(GEL,CAPLET)			
500 mg, 28s ea	58016-0200-28	2.45	
(CAPLET)			
500 mg, 30s ea	58016-0287-30	2.61	
(GEL,CAPLET)			
500 mg, 30s ea	58016-0200-30	2.63	
(CAPLET)			
500 mg, 40s ea	58016-0287-40	3.48	
(GEL,CAPLET)			
500 mg, 40s ea	58016-0200-40	3.50	
(CAPLET)			
500 mg, 50s ea	58016-0287-50	4.35	
(GEL,CAPLET)			
500 mg, 50s ea	58016-0200-50	4.38	
60s ea	58016-0266-60	8.56	
(CAPLET)			
500 mg, 60s ea	58016-0287-60	5.22	
(GEL,CAPLET)			
500 mg, 60s ea	58016-0200-60	5.26	
(CAPLET)			
500 mg, 100s ea	58016-0287-00	8.70	
(GEL,CAPLET)			
500 mg, 100s ea	58016-0200-00	8.76	
120s ea	58016-0266-02	17.12	
(CAPLET)			
500 mg, 120s ea	58016-0287-02	10.44	
150s ea	58016-0266-03	21.40	
(CAPLET)			
500 mg, 150s ea	58016-0287-03	13.05	
(Stat Rx)			
REPACK			
TAB,PO, 500 mg, 60s ea	16590-0021-60	15.00	
ACETAMINOPHEN & DIPHENHYDRAMINE HYDROCHLORIDE (Dispensing Solutions)			
REPACK			
TAB,PO (CAPLET)			
500 mg-25 mg,			
24s ea	55045-3472-02	6.48	
ACETAMINOPHEN CHILDREN'S (Advance)			
CTB,PO, 80 mg, 30s ea	17714-0044-30	2.99	
(Geri-Care)			
CTB,PO, 80 mg, 30s ea	57896-0148-30	0.69	
(Dispensing Solutions)			
REPACK			
CTB,PO, 80 mg, 30s ea	55045-3042-03	5.10	
30s ea	55045-3042-08	5.10	
(Pharma Pac)			
REPACK			
ELI,PO, 160 mg/5 ml,			
120 ml	52959-0612-04	7.39	
480 ml	52959-0612-16	21.56	
ACETAMINOPHEN EXTRA STRENGTH (Marlex)			
TAB,PO, 500 mg, 24s ea	10135-0152-24	0.70	
(BOXED,CAPLET)			
500 mg, 24s ea	10135-0144-52	65.00	
(CAPLET)			
500 mg, 24s ea	10135-0144-24	0.70	
30s ea	10135-0152-30	0.74	
50s ea	10135-0152-50	0.76	
(BOXED,CAPLET)			
500 mg, 50s ea	10135-0144-55	65.00	
(CAPLET)			
500 mg, 50s ea	10135-0144-50	0.99	
60s ea	10135-0152-60	0.78	
(BOXED)			
500 mg, 60s ea	10135-0152-56	65.00	
(CAPLET)			
500 mg, 60s ea	10135-0144-60	1.00	
100s ea	10135-0152-01	0.84	
100s ea UD	10135-0152-13	2.40	
(BOXED,CAPLET)			
500 mg, 100s ea	10135-0144-57	65.00	
(BOXED)			
500 mg, 100s ea	10135-0152-57	65.00	
(CAPLET)			
500 mg, 100s ea	10135-0144-01	1.11	
100s ea UD	10135-0164-13	3.55	
175s ea	10135-0152-66	2.83	
(BOXED,CAPLET)			
500 mg, 175s ea	10135-0144-58	65.00	
(CAPLET)			
500 mg, 175s ea	10135-0144-66	2.81	
500s ea	10135-0144-05	5.51	
700s ea	10135-0152-70	5.00	
(CAPLET,CAPLET)			
500 mg, 700s ea	10135-0144-70	16.57	
1000s ea	10135-0152-10	5.80	
(CAPLET)			
500 mg, 1000s ea	10135-0144-10	8.19	
(Altura)			
REPACK			
TAB,PO, 500 mg, 6s ea	63874-0003-06	2.24	
(Dispensing Solutions)			
REPACK			
TAB,PO, 500 mg, 45s ea	66336-0656-45	10.10	
(McKesson Packaging)			
REPACK			
TAB,PO (EXTRA STRENGTH,CAPLET)			
500 mg, 100s ea UD	63739-0001-10	8.12	
(BLISTER PACK,CAPLET)			
500 mg, 750s ea UD	63739-0001-01	60.90	
ACETAMINOPHEN INFANT (Pharma Pac)			
REPACK			
SUS,PO (DROPS)			
80 mg/0.8 ml,			
15 ml	52959-0861-15	4.40	
ACETAMINOPHEN INFANTS (Dispensing Solutions)			
REPACK			
SOL,PO (DROPS)			
80 mg/0.8 ml,			
15 ml	55045-1289-04	3.75	
SUP,RC, 120 mg, 12s ea	55045-3002-04	7.00	
(Phys Total Care)			
REPACK			
SOL,PO (AF,FRUIT,DROPS)			
80 mg/0.8 ml,			
15 ml	54868-3267-00	10.14	
ACETAMINOPHEN JUNIOR (Family Phcy)			
CTB,PO (PRIVATE LABEL,FRUIT)			
160 mg, 30s ea	52735-0754-05	3.05	3.39
ACETAMINOPHEN PEDIATRIC (Family Phcy)			
SUP,RC (PRIVATE LABEL)			
120 mg, 12s ea	52735-0717-17	5.39	5.99
ACETEST (Bayer Diabetes Care)			
DEV,NA, 100s ea	00193-2381-21	31.14	
ACETYL-l-CARNITINE (Bio-Tech Pharm)			
ACETYL-L-CARNITINE			
CAP,PO, 500 mg, 100s ea	53191-0345-01	50.00	
ACID GONE (Major)			
SUS,PO, 355 ml	00904-7727-14	5.99	
ACID GONE EXTRA STRENGTH (Major)			
CTB,PO, 160 mg-105 mg,			
100s ea	00904-5365-60	5.23	
ACID REDUCER (AmerisourceBergen)			
TAB,PO (BLISTER PACK)			
10 mg, 30s ea	24385-0255-65	6.29	6.99
(Major)			
TAB,PO, 200 mg, 30s ea	00904-6047-29	6.44	
ACIDIL (Boiron)			
PEL,PO, 4 c-4 c-4 c-4 c,			
80s ea	06962-0002-03	3.87	6.49
TAB,PO, 4 c-4 c-4 c-4 c,			
60s ea	06962-0608-60	5.73	9.59
ACIDOLL (Key Company)			
CAP,PO (SF)			
260 mg-60 mg-230 mg,			
100s ea	11694-0925-01	7.00	
1000s ea	11694-0925-02	52.00	
ACIDOPHILUS (ADH)			
CAP,PO, 100s ea	60142-0103-10	2.98	5.95
(Basic Vitamins)			
CAP,PO (SF)			
100s ea	00761-0515-20	3.00	
(Major)			
CAP,PO, 100s ea	00904-4213-60	4.65	
(Marlex)			
CAP,PO, 100 mg-50 mg,			
100s ea	10135-0226-01	1.76	
(Nature's Bounty)			
CAP,PO (PF,SF,SOFTGEL)			
100 million u, 100s ea	74312-0026-10		6.09
(Rugby)			
TAB,PO, 25 million u-100 mg,			
100s ea	00536-7180-01	4.43	
(Torrance)			
CAP,PO, 2.5 billion u,			
100s ea	00389-0561-00	8.75	
LIQ,PO, 250 billion u/5 ml,			
180 ml	00389-0560-00	16.60	
(Freeda)			
MORE-DOPHILUS			
PDR,PO (PF,SF,DYE-FREE)			
12.4 billion u/5 ml,			
28 gm	10432-0276-00	6.87	11.45
112 gm	10432-0276-01	19.74	32.90
ACIDOPHILUS EXTRA STRENGTH (Rugby)			
TAB,PO (SOD FRE,PF,SF,DYE-FREE)			
100s ea	00536-7181-01	4.43	
(Phys Total Care)			
REPACK			
TAB,PO (PF,SF,DYE-FREE,CAPTAB)			
100s ea	54868-4891-00	18.51	
ACIDOPHILUS PROBIOTIC BLEND (21st Century)			
CAP,PO (HIGH POTENCY)			
150s ea	40985-0229-28		9.99
(Palmetto)			
REPACK			
CAP,PO, 30s ea	23490-1922-03	5.11	
ACIDOPHILUS W/BIFIDUS (Nature's Bounty)			
WAF,PO (PF,BERRY)			
100 mg, 100s ea	74312-0057-21		6.09
ACIDOPHILUS W/PECTIN (Health Products Corp)			
CAP,PO (PF,SF)			
100s ea	39686-0013-46	3.77	
(Mason Vit)			
CAP,PO, 100s ea	11845-0053-31	6.56	
100s ea	11845-0070-11	4.44	
(Nature's Bounty)			
CAP,PO (EX. STRENGTH,PF,SF)			
90 mg-100 mg, 100s ea	74312-0015-40		8.69
(Dispensing Solutions)			
REPACK			
CAP,PO, 100s ea	55045-3301-01	6.50	
ACIDOPHILUS/APPLE PECTIN COMPLEX (Rexall)			
CAP,PO (PF,SF)			
60s ea	30768-0001-56	2.01	3.05
ACIGEST (Key Company)			
TAB,PO, 120 mg-180 mg-60 mg,			
100s ea	11694-0998-02	5.50	
1000s ea	11694-0998-05	45.00	
ACIGEST II (Key Company)			
TAB,PO, 60s ea	11694-0997-91	5.75	
120s ea	11694-0997-92	9.50	
250s ea	11694-0997-25	17.50	
1000s ea	11694-0997-93	57.00	
ACIGEST IV (Key Company)			
CAP,PO, 100s ea	11694-0784-01	10.00	
250s ea	11694-0784-25	22.00	
ACIGEST-LPC (Key Company)			
TAB,PO, 17 mg-17 mg-8 mg,			
100s ea	11694-0916-01	8.00	
1000s ea	11694-0916-03	56.00	
ACNE (Nuage Labs)			
TAB,SL (TISSUE D)			
125s ea	00634-0904-68	3.05	5.09
ACNE 10 MAXIMUM STRENGTH (AmerisourceBergen)			
GEL,TP (PRIVATE LABEL)			
10%, 28 gm	24385-0423-49	3.50	3.89
ACNE CLEAR MAXIMUM STRENGTH (Altaire)			
GEL,TP, 10%, 45 gm	59390-0030-22	4.50	

PROD/MFR	HRI, UPC,NDC	AWP	SRP
ACNE MEDICATION 10 (Rugby)			
LOT,TP, 10%, 30 ml	00536-0815-95	3.45	
ACNE MEDICATION 5 (Rugby)			
TP, 5%, 30 ml	00536-0810-95	3.02	
ACNE PACK (Waltman)			
KIT,MR, ea	10768-0000-80	9.86	
ACNE-10 (A-S Medication)			
REPACK			
GEL,TP, 10%, 42.5 gm	54569-3405-00	16.35	
ACNE-5 (A-S Medication)			
GEL,TP, 5%, 42.5 gm	54569-3406-00	16.82	
ACNE-AID (Stiefel Consumer HealthCare)			
SOA,TP (3.5OZ)			
100 gm	73462-0101-23	2.64	3.99
ACNOMEL (Numark)			
CRE,TP, 2%-8%, 30 gm	38485-0911-61	7.14	
ACNOTEX (Genesis)			
LIQ,TP, 2%-8%, 60 ml	00398-0216-02	7.02	
ACONITE (Walker Pharmacal)			
TAB,SL (6X)			
250s ea	00619-0032-02	2.97	
ACONITE NAPELLUS (Luyties)			
TAB,SL (6X)			
6 x, 500s ea	00618-0032-03	3.99	
5500s ea	00618-0032-10	30.32	
12 x, 500s ea	00622-0032-03	4.19	
5500s ea	00622-0032-10	31.83	
30 x, 500s ea	00624-0032-03	4.19	
5500s ea	00624-0032-10	31.83	
ACTICAL (A. G. Marin)			
SGL,PO (SOFTGEL)			
60s ea	12539-0500-01	10.00	
ACTIDOSE W/SORBITOL (Paddock)			
SUS,PO (BOTTLE)			
25 gm/120 ml, 120 ml	00574-0120-04	16.28	
(TUBE) 25 gm/120 ml, 120 ml	00574-0120-74	16.28	
(BOTTLE) 25 gm/120 ml, 240 ml	00574-0120-08	23.05	
(TUBE) 25 gm/120 ml, 240 ml	00574-0120-76	23.05	
ACTIDOSE-AQUA (Paddock)			
SUS,PO (TUBE)			
15 gm/72 ml, 72 ml	00574-0121-25	10.65	
(BOTTLE) 25 gm/120 ml, 120 ml	00574-0121-04	16.28	
(TUBE) 25 gm/120 ml, 120 ml	00574-0121-74	16.28	
(BOTTLE) 25 gm/120 ml, 240 ml	00574-0121-08	23.05	
(TUBE) 25 gm/120 ml, 240 ml	00574-0121-76	23.05	
ACTIFED COLD & ALLERGY (McNeil Consumer Healthcare)			
TAB,PO, 4 mg-10 mg,			
12s ea	12547-0210-53	2.82	
24s ea	12547-0210-60	5.05	
ACTION FOR MEN (Action Labs)			
LIQ,PO, 120 ml	24675-0983-10	13.49	26.99
TAB,PO, 60s ea	24675-0983-60	10.49	20.99
ACTION-TABS MADE FOR MEN (Action Labs)			
TAB,PO (SF)			
42s ea	24675-0612-30	7.00	13.99
60s ea	24675-0612-60	10.99	21.99
ACTIPROTECT UF (Glaxo)			
DEV,NA (SINGLE USE, DISPOSABLE)			
1.8%, 240s ea	00135-0999-02	1025.28	
ACTIS (Vivus)			
DEV,NA, ea	62541-0210-01	11.25	
ACTIVATED CHARCOAL (Dispensing Solutions)			
REPACK			
CAP,PO, 260 mg, 60s ea	55045-3597-01	6.60	
ACTIVELIFE CONVEX ONE-PIECE (Convatec)			
DEV,NA (1 1/2",TRANS,DURAHESIVE)			
5s ea	68455-0102-57	51.35	66.84
5s ea	68455-0102-68	49.20	64.04
(1 1/4",TRANS,DURAHESIVE)			
5s ea	68455-0102-55	50.94	66.30
5s ea	68455-0102-66	48.29	62.85
(1 1/8",TRANS,DURAHESIVE)			
5s ea	68455-0102-54	50.94	66.30
5s ea	68455-0102-65	48.29	62.85
(1 3/4",TRANS,DURAHESIVE)			
5s ea	68455-0102-58	51.35	66.84
(1 3/8",TRANS,DURAHESIVE)			
5s ea	68455-0102-56	50.94	66.30
5s ea	68455-0102-67	48.29	62.85
(1",TRANS,DURAHESIVE)			
5s ea	68455-0102-53	50.94	66.30
5s ea	68455-0102-64	48.29	62.85
(1/2",TRANS,DURAHESIVE)			
5s ea	68455-0102-60	48.29	62.85
(2",TRANS,DURAHESIVE)			
5s ea	68455-0102-59	51.35	66.84
(3/4",TRANS,DURAHESIVE)			
5s ea	68455-0102-51	50.94	66.30
5s ea	68455-0102-62	48.29	62.85
(5/8",TRANS,DURAHESIVE)			
5s ea	68455-0102-61	48.29	62.85
(7/8",TRANS,DURAHESIVE)			
5s ea	68455-0102-52	50.94	66.30
5s ea	68455-0102-63	48.29	62.85
(1 1/2", TRANSPARENT)			
10s ea	68455-0102-22	88.94	115.77
(1 1/4", TRANSPARENT)			
10s ea	68455-0102-20	88.94	115.77
(1 1/8", TRANSPARENT)			
10s ea	68455-0102-19	88.94	115.77
(1 3/8", TRANSPARENT)			
10s ea	68455-0102-21	88.94	115.77
(1", TRANSPARENT)			
10s ea	68455-0102-18	88.94	115.77
(1/2", TRANSPARENT)			
10s ea	68455-0102-14	88.94	115.77
(12",TRANS,1 1/2",1-PC)			
10s ea	68455-0102-12	94.25	122.68
(12",TRANS,1 1/4",1-PC)			
10s ea	68455-0102-10	94.25	122.68
(12",TRANS,1 1/8",1-PC)			
10s ea	68455-0102-09	94.25	122.68
(12",TRANS,1 3/4",1-PC)			
10s ea	68455-0102-13	94.25	122.68
(12",TRANS,1 3/8",1-PC)			
10s ea	68455-0102-11	94.25	122.68
(12",TRANS,1",1-PC)			
10s ea	68455-0102-08	94.25	122.68
(12",TRANS,2",1-PC)			
10s ea	68455-0102-23	94.25	122.68
(12",TRANS,3/4",1-PC)			
10s ea	68455-0102-06	94.25	122.68
(12",TRANS,7/8",1-PC)			
10s ea	68455-0102-07	94.25	122.68
(3/4", TRANSPARENT)			
10s ea	68455-0102-16	88.94	115.77
(5/8", TRANSPARENT)			
10s ea	68455-0102-15	88.94	115.77
(7/8", TRANSPARENT)			
10s ea	68455-0102-17	88.94	115.77
ACTIVELIFE ONE-PIECE CLOSED-END POUCH (Convatec)			
DEV,NA (1 1/2", OPAQUE)			
15s ea	68455-0102-48	41.56	54.10
(1 1/2", TRANSPARENT)			
15s ea	68455-0102-40	41.56	54.10
(1 1/4", OPAQUE)			
15s ea	68455-0102-47	41.56	54.10
(1 1/4", TRANSPARENT)			
15s ea	68455-0102-39	41.56	54.10
(1 3/4", OPAQUE)			
15s ea	68455-0102-49	41.56	54.10
(1 3/4", TRANSPARENT)			
15s ea	68455-0102-41	41.56	54.10
(1", OPAQUE)			
15s ea	68455-0102-45	41.56	54.10
(1", TRANSPARENT)			
15s ea	68455-0102-38	41.56	54.10
(2", OPAQUE)			
15s ea	68455-0102-50	41.56	54.10
(2", TRANSPARENT)			
15s ea	68455-0102-42	41.56	54.10
(3/4", OPAQUE)			
15s ea	68455-0102-43	41.56	54.10
(3/4", TRANSPARENT)			
15s ea	68455-0102-37	41.56	54.10
ACTIVELIFE ONE-PIECE DRAINABLE POUCH (Convatec)			
DEV,NA (10",OPAQUE,1 1/2")			
10s ea	68455-0101-43	36.49	47.50
(10",OPAQUE,1 1/4")			
10s ea	68455-0101-42	36.49	47.50
(10",OPAQUE,1 3/4")			
10s ea	68455-0101-44	36.49	47.50
(10",OPAQUE,1")			
10s ea	68455-0101-41	36.49	47.50
(10",OPAQUE,2 1/2")			
10s ea	68455-0101-46	36.49	47.50
(10",OPAQUE,2")			
10s ea	68455-0101-45	36.49	47.50
(10",OPAQUE,3/4")			
10s ea	68455-0101-40	36.49	47.50
(12", TRANSPARENT, 1")			
10s ea	68455-0101-55	36.49	47.50
(12", TRANSPARENT, 2")			
10s ea	68455-0101-59	36.49	47.50
(12", TRANSPARENT, 3/4")			
10s ea	68455-0101-54	36.49	47.50
(12", TRANSPARENT)			
10s ea	68455-0101-56	36.49	47.50
10s ea	68455-0101-57	36.49	47.50
10s ea	68455-0101-58	36.49	47.50
10s ea	68455-0101-60	36.49	47.50
(12",OPAQUE,1 1/2")			
10s ea	68455-0101-50	36.49	47.50
(12",OPAQUE,1 1/4")			
10s ea	68455-0101-49	36.49	47.50
(12",OPAQUE,1 3/4")			
10s ea	68455-0101-51	36.49	47.50
(12",OPAQUE,1")			
10s ea	68455-0101-48	36.49	47.50
(12",OPAQUE,2 1/2")			
10s ea	68455-0101-53	36.49	47.50
(12",OPAQUE,2")			
10s ea	68455-0101-52	36.49	47.50
(12",OPAQUE,3/4")			
10s ea	68455-0101-47	36.49	47.50
(12",TRANS,3/4-2 1/2")			
10s ea	68455-0101-61	36.84	47.95
(10",OPAQUE,1 1/2",1-PC)			
20s ea	68455-0101-95	67.51	87.88
(10",OPAQUE,1 1/4",1-PC)			
20s ea	68455-0101-94	67.51	87.88
(10",OPAQUE,1 3/4",1-PC)			
20s ea	68455-0101-96	67.51	87.88
(10",OPAQUE,2 1/2",1-PC)			
20s ea	68455-0101-98	67.51	87.88
(10",OPAQUE,2",1-PC)			
20s ea	68455-0101-97	67.51	87.88
(10",OPAQUE,3/4",1-PC)			
20s ea	68455-0101-92	67.51	87.88
(12",OPAQUE,1 1/2",1-PC)			
20s ea	68455-0102-02	67.51	87.88
(12",OPAQUE,1 1/4",1-PC)			
20s ea	68455-0102-01	67.51	87.88
(12",OPAQUE,1 3/4",1-PC)			
20s ea	68455-0102-03	67.51	87.88
(12",OPAQUE,1",1-PC)			
20s ea	68455-0102-00	67.51	87.88
(12",OPAQUE,2 1/2",1-PC)			
20s ea	68455-0102-05	67.51	87.88
(12",OPAQUE,2",1-PC)			
20s ea	68455-0102-04	67.51	87.88
(12",OPAQUE,3/4",1-PC)			
20s ea	68455-0101-99	67.51	87.88
(12",TRANS,CUT-TO-FIT)			
20s ea	68455-0101-91	69.99	91.10
ACTIVELIFE ONE-PIECE STOMA CAP (Convatec)			
DEV,NA (WITH SKIN BARRIER)			
30s ea	68455-0102-36	73.44	95.59
ACTIVELIFE ONE-PIECE UROSTOMY POUCH (Convatec)			
DEV,NA (2",TRANSPARENT)			
10s ea	68455-0101-68	58.55	76.21
ACU-DYNE SKIN CLEANSER (Medical Action Ind.)			
LIQ,TP, 7.5%, 60 ml 48s	73577-0560-20	49.98	
240 ml 24s	73577-0560-19	59.76	
480 ml 12s	73577-0560-22	46.68	
960 ml 6s	73577-0560-24	36.18	
3840 ml 4s	73577-0560-16	73.44	
ACURA BLOOD GLUCOSE MONITORING SYSTEM (US DIAGNOSTICS, INC)			
DEV,NA (METER KIT)			
ea	08463-6103-01	44.28	
(STARTER KIT)			
ea	08463-6003-01	79.95	
ACURA BLOOD GLUCOSE TEST STRIPS (US DIAGNOSTICS, INC)			
DEV,NA, 50s ea	08463-6203-50	41.82	

PROD/MFR	HRI, UPC,NDC	AWP	SRP
ACURA CONTROL SOLUTION (US DIAGNOSTICS, INC)			
DEV,NA (NORMAL)			
ea	08463-6005-01	8.61	
ACYS-5 (Bio-Tech Pharm)			
CAP,PO, 500 mg, 100s ea	53191-0328-01	19.56	
ADAPTER PLUG MALE (Abbott Hosp)			
DEV,NA (PRN, 1")			
120s ea	00074-5877-01	289.28	
(REG, PRN, 1-1/2")			
120s ea	00074-5878-01	289.28	
(W/LUER LOCK, PRN, 1")			
120s ea	00074-5396-02	307.80	
(W/LUER LOCK,PRN,1-1/2")			
120s ea	00074-5395-01	307.80	
ADAPTIC NON-ADHERING PACKING STRIP (J&J Medical)			
DEV,NA (1/2"X4YD,STERILE)			
ea	56091-0020-01	5.03	
ADAPTIC NON-ADHERING STERILE (J&J Medical)			
DEV,NA (3"X60"/ROLL)			
ea	56091-0020-18	8.38	
(5"X9")			
12s ea	56091-0020-19	23.84	
(3"X8")			
24s ea	56091-0020-15	26.84	
(3"X16")			
36s ea	56091-0020-14	57.84	
(3"X3")			
50s ea	56091-0020-12	23.31	
(3"X8",3X36)			
108s ea	56091-0020-13	63.82	
ADAPTIC PG-PETROLATUM GAUZE (J&J Medical)			
DEV,NA (1"X36")			
12s ea	56091-0020-46	11.75	
(1/2"X72")			
12s ea	56091-0020-53	17.88	
(3"X18")			
12s ea	56091-0020-48	10.86	
(3"X36")			
12s ea	56091-0020-49	15.19	
(3"X9")			
12s ea	56091-0020-47	9.78	
(6"X36")			
12s ea	56091-0020-51	22.16	
(1"X8")			
50s ea	56091-0020-45	34.58	
ADAPTIC X-XEROFORM GAUZE (J&J Medical)			
DEV,NA (1"X8")			
50s ea	56091-0020-06	38.44	
(5"X9")			
50s ea	56091-0020-07	58.86	
ADAPTO-GEN (Bio-Tech Pharm)			
CAP,PO, 100s ea	53191-0360-01	22.50	
ADAPTOSODE FOR STRESS (HVS Labs)			
LIQ,PO (AF,SF)			
120 ml	52386-9601-04	9.00	
240 ml	52386-9626-04	14.00	
ADAPTOSODE R+R FOR ACUTE STRESS (HVS Labs)			
LIQ,PO (AF,SF)			
120 ml	52386-9602-04	9.00	
240 ml	52386-9627-04	14.00	
ADD-INS COMPLETE (Nutricia)			
POW,PO (60X18.2GM)			
18.2 gm 60s	49735-0126-41	382.20	
ADDAPRIN (Medique)			
TAB,PO (250X2)			
200 mg, 500s ea UD	51469-0314-01	12.61	15.30
ADDITIONS (Nestle)			
PDR,PO, 947 gm	00065-9270-91	29.40	
ADDITIVE CAP LIFECARE (Abbott Hosp)			
DEV,NA (SIDE-MOUNTED ADD. PORT)			
400s ea	00074-4929-01	187.20	
ADDITIVE HINGE CAP (Abbott Hosp)			
DEV,NA (DOWN PORT LIFECARE)			
1000s ea	00074-4858-01	444.00	
ADDITIVE PHARMACY TRANSFER (Abbott Hosp)			
DEV,NA (30 ", VENTED)			
10s ea	00074-3972-01	73.80	
ADE (Carlson,J.R.)			
CRE,TP, 120 gm	88395-0005-34	7.20	14.40
OIN,TP, 113 gm	88395-0005-44	7.20	14.40
ADE W/SELENIUM (Freeda)			
TAB,PO (PF,SF,DYE-FREE)			
100s ea	10432-0238-01	8.37	13.95
ADEKS (Axcan)			
TAB,PO (CAPLET)			
60s ea	58914-0010-06	21.35	
ADHESIVE PAD PLUS NEOSPORIN (Johnson & Johnson)			
BAN,TP (3"X3",ADHESIVE PADS)			
500 u/gm-10000 u/gm,			
5s ea	81370-0058-42	3.05	
ADHESIVE REMOVER (Mentor)			
OIL,TP, 240 ml	81317-0034-08	8.06	
PAD,TP (PACKET)			
50s ea	81317-0340-50	10.72	
ADRENAL (Bio-Tech Pharm)			
CAP,PO, 200 mg, 100s ea	53191-0340-01	7.95	
ADULT ACNE CLEARING (Waltman)			
GEL,TP (1X22ML)			
2%, 22 ml	10768-0000-90	4.20	
ADVACAL (Lane Labs)			
CAP,PO, 150 mg, 60s ea	02110-7706-06	7.63	16.95
150s ea	02110-7715-04	17.98	39.95
ADVANCE CONTROL SOLUTION (Arkray)			
DEV,NA, ea	08317-4105-01	7.20	
ADVANCE INTUITION (Arkray)			
DEV,NA, ea	08317-4200-01	45.00	
ADVANCE INTUITION BLOOD GLUCOSE MONITORING KIT (Arkray)			
DEV,NA (KIT)			
ea	08317-4211-00	52.50	
ADVANCE INTUITION BLOOD GLUCOSE TEST STRIPS (Arkray)			
DEV,NA, 50s ea	08317-4200-50	38.50	
ADVANCE INTUITION CONTROL (Arkray)			
DEV,NA (NORMAL)			
ea	08317-4200-05	7.20	
ADVANCE MICRO-DRAW CONTROL SOLUTION (Arkray)			
DEV,NA (LEVEL 1&2)			
2s ea	08317-4106-02	12.00	13.35
ADVANCE MICRO-DRAW TEST STRIPS (Arkray)			
DEV,NA, 50s ea	08317-4150-50	38.50	
(2X50)			
100s ea	08317-4100-00	77.00	
ADVANCE MICRODRAW BLOOD GLUCOSE METER (Arkray)			
DEV,NA, ea	08317-4100-01	45.00	
ADVANCE MICRODRAW BLOOD GLUCOSE MONITORING SYSTEM (Arkray)			
DEV,NA, ea	08317-4111-00	52.50	
ADVANCED EYE RELIEF (Bausch & Lomb Inc.)			
SOL,OP (1X118ML-STERILE EYE CUP)			
118 ml	10119-0002-52	3.46	
ADVANCED EYE RELIEF DRY EYE REJUVENATION (Bausch & Lomb Inc.)			
SOL,OP (1X15ML,DROPS)			
0.3%-1%, 15 ml	10119-0020-03	5.03	
ADVANCED EYE RELIEF NIGHT TIME (Bausch & Lomb Inc.)			
OIN,OP (1X3.5GM, DRY EYE,PF)			
20%-80%, 3.5 gm	10119-0020-13	8.18	
ADVANCED EYE RELIEF REDNESS INSTANT RELIEF (Bausch & Lomb Inc.)			
SOL,OP (1X15ML,DROPS)			
0.012%-0.2%, 15 ml	10119-0022-24	3.18	
ADVANCED EYE RELIEF REDNESS MAXIMUM RELIEF (Bausch & Lomb Inc.)			
SOL,OP (1X15ML,DROPS)			
0.5%-0.03%, 15 ml	10119-0022-25	3.18	
ADVANCED LANCING (Atlanta & Pacific)			
DEV,NA, ea	08214-0707-26	10.99	
ADVANCED LISTERINE ANTISEPTIC (Johnson & Johnson)			
SOL,MM (WITH TARTAR PROTECTION)			
95 ml	12547-0443-95	1.13	
250 ml	12547-0443-00	3.25	
500 ml	12547-0443-05	4.50	
1000 ml	12547-0443-15	5.95	
1500 ml	12547-0443-30	8.35	
ADVIL (Wyeth Consumer)			
TAB,PO (CAPLET)			
200 mg, 24s ea	00573-0150-20		3.49
24s ea	00573-0160-20		3.49
(GEL,CAPLET)			
200 mg, 24s ea	00573-0165-20		3.49
(CAPLET)			
200 mg, 50s ea	00573-0150-30		6.09
50s ea	00573-0160-30		9.09
(GEL,CAPLET)			
200 mg, 50s ea	00573-0165-30		6.09
(CAPLET)			
200 mg, 100s ea	00573-0150-40		9.99
100s ea	00573-0160-40		9.99
(GEL,CAPLET)			
200 mg, 100s ea	00573-0165-40		9.99
(CAPLET)			
200 mg, 150s ea	00573-0154-35		12.49
165s ea	00573-0150-43		12.49
165s ea	00573-0160-43		12.49
(GEL,CAPLET)			
200 mg, 165s ea	00573-0165-43		12.49
(CAPLET)			
200 mg, 200s ea	00573-0154-75		14.59
250s ea	00573-0150-46	13.86	
ADVIL CHILDREN'S (Wyeth Consumer)			
SUS,PO (AF,FRUIT)			
100 mg/5 ml,			
120 ml	00573-0170-30		5.89
ADVIL COLD & SINUS (Wyeth Consumer)			
SGL,PO (LIQUI-GELS,SOFTGEL)			
200 mg-30 mg,			
16s ea	00573-0184-16		6.29
(NON-DROWSY,LIQUI-GEL)			
200 mg-30 mg,			
32s ea	05730-0184-32		10.19
TAB,PO (CAPLET)			
200 mg-30 mg,			
20s ea	00573-0180-10		6.29
20s ea	00573-0185-10		4.99
(NON-DROWSY,CAPLET)			
200 mg-30 mg,			
40s ea	00573-0180-21		10.19
ADVIL JUNIOR (Wyeth Consumer)			
TAB,PO, 100 mg, 24s ea	00573-0175-10		4.19
ADVIL LIQUI-GELS (Wyeth Consumer)			
SGL,PO (SOFTGEL)			
200 mg, 20s ea	05730-0169-20		4.29
40s ea	05730-0169-30		7.19
(Southwood)			
REPACK			
SGL,PO, 200 mg, 30s ea	58016-0017-30	3.96	
60s ea	58016-0017-60	7.93	
80s ea	58016-0017-80	10.57	
90s ea	58016-0017-90	11.89	
100s ea	58016-0017-00	13.21	
ADVIL PM (Wyeth Consumer)			
TAB,PO (COATED CAPLET)			
38 mg-200 mg,			
20s ea	05730-0164-20		5.39
40s ea	05730-0164-30		8.49
AEROCHAMBER + MASK (Phys Total Care)			
REPACK			
DEV,NA, ea	54868-5852-00	44.71	
(SMALL)			
ea	54868-5131-00	59.16	
AEROSOL THERAPY NEBULIZER (Bestmed)			
DEV,NA (COMPRSSOR)			
ea	08466-0931-00	86.00	
AFRIN (Schering Plough)			
SPR,NS, 0.05%, 15 ml	00085-0756-12	5.64	
15 ml	11523-1167-06	5.02	
30 ml	00085-0756-08	7.98	
AFRIN SINUS (Schering Plough)			
SPR,NS, 0.05%, 15 ml	00085-4112-01	5.02	
AFRIN W/MENTHOL (Schering Plough)			
SPR,NS, 0.05%, 15 ml	00085-0474-05	5.02	
AFTER-TENS (Pharm Innov)			
CRE,TP, 10 gm	00036-3700-10	1.69	2.41
60 gm	00036-3700-60	5.09	7.28
AGIE-GRX (Geritrex)			
DEV,NA (4X4)			
10s ea	92771-0005-01	11.37	
AGRIMONY (Ellon)			
SOL,SL (DROPS)			
10.5 ml	51762-0001-10		9.25
AIMSCO ADJUSTABLE LANCET DEVICE (Delta Hi-Tech)			
DEV,NA (W/NEW ADJUSTABLE TIP)			
ea	51709-0007-60	8.95	

PROD/MFR	HRI, UPC,NDC	AWP	SRP
AIMSCO LANCETS (Delta Hi-Tech)			
DEV,NA (ULTRA THIN SAFTY AUTO)			
50s ea	51709-0007-29	11.00	
(ULTRA THIN,28 GAUGE)			
100s ea	51709-0007-26	6.00	
(ULTRA THIN,30 GAUGE)			
100s ea	51709-0007-28	6.00	
(ULTRA THIN,28 GAUGE)			
200s ea	51709-0007-27	11.00	
AIMSCO ULTRA-THIN II INSULIN PEN (Delta Hi-Tech)			
DEV,NA (29G,1/2",LATEX-FREE)			
100s ea	51709-0006-22	19.50	
AIMSCO ULTRA-THIN II SHORT INSULIN PEN (Delta Hi-Tech)			
DEV,NA (31G,5/16",LATEX-FREE)			
100s ea	51709-0006-30	21.60	
AIMSCO ULTRA-THIN II SHORT NEEDLE (Delta Hi-Tech)			
DEV,NA (31G,1/2CC,5/16"INSULIN)			
100s ea	51709-0007-42	24.55	
(31G,3/10CC,5/16",INSULN)			
100s ea	51709-0007-40	25.55	
AIR FILTER (Abbott Hosp)			
DEV,NA, 120s ea	00074-1830-03	102.24	
AIRGO NAVIGATOR ROLLING WALKER (Can-Am Care)			
DEV,NA (CRANBERRY RED)			
ea	38396-0118-99	307.50	
(PACIFIC BLUE)			
ea	38396-0116-99	307.50	
(TITANIUM SILVER)			
ea	38396-0117-99	307.50	
AKWA TEARS (Akorn)			
OIN,OP (PF)			
3.5 gm	17478-0062-35	3.88	
SOL,OP, 1.4%, 15 ml	17478-0060-12	3.69	
(A-S Medication)			
REPACK			
OIN,OP (1X3.5GM)			
3.5 gm	54569-6041-00	3.88	
AL-12 (JSJ Pharma)			
LOT,TP, 12%, 225 gm	58121-0000-21		12.58
ALA-BATH (Del-Ray)			
OIL,TP, 240 ml	00316-0110-08	10.31	
ALA-DERM (Del-Ray)			
LOT,TP, 240 ml	00316-0112-08	8.06	
360 ml	00316-0112-12	12.43	
ALA-SEB MEDICATED (Del-Ray)			
LIQ,TP, 120 ml	00316-0114-04	7.81	
360 ml	00316-0114-12	14.31	
ALA-SEB-T MEDICATED (Del-Ray)			
SHA,TP, 120 ml	00316-0116-04	7.81	
360 ml	00316-0116-12	14.31	
ALAMAG (Medique)			
CTB,PO (12X2)			
300 mg-150 mg,			
24s ea UD	47682-0103-64	2.60	
(50X2,SF,CHERRY)			
300 mg-150 mg,			
100s ea UD	47682-0103-33	8.15	
(250X2,SF,CHERRY)			
300 mg-150 mg,			
500s ea UD	47682-0103-13	33.34	
ALAMAG PLUS (Medique)			
CTB,PO (50X2, LACT-FREE)			
200 mg-200 mg-25 mg,			
100s ea UD	47682-0247-33	7.79	
(100X2, LACT-FREE)			
200 mg-200 mg-25 mg,			
200s ea UD	47682-0247-47	13.69	
(250X2, LACT-FREE)			
200 mg-200 mg-25 mg,			
500s ea UD	47682-0247-13	34.16	
ALAVERT (Wyeth Consumer)			
ODT,PO (ORIGINAL)			
10 mg, 6s ea	00573-2620-06		5.99
12s ea	00573-2620-12		10.99
24s ea	00573-2620-24		18.99
(ORIGINAL)			
10 mg, 30s ea	00573-2620-30		18.99
48s ea	00573-2620-48		26.99
TAB,PO, 10 mg, 15s ea	00573-2645-15		10.99
30s ea	00573-2645-30		18.99

PROD/MFR	HRI, UPC,NDC	AWP	SRP
(Palmetto)			
REPACK			
TAB,PO, 10 mg, 30s ea	23490-9358-03	36.69	
(Phys Total Care)			
REPACK			
ODT,PO, 10 mg, 30s ea	54868-5608-00	65.47	
(Quality Care Prod)			
REPACK			
ODT,PO, 10 mg, 6s ea	49999-0964-06	6.54	
ALAVERT D-12 HOUR (Wyeth Consumer)			
T12,PO, 5 mg-120 mg,			
12s ea	00573-2660-12		8.99
24s ea	00573-2660-24		9.99
(Phys Total Care)			
REPACK			
T12,PO, 5 mg-120 mg,			
24s ea	54868-3484-00	22.03	
ALAWAY (Bausch & Lomb Inc.)			
SOL,OP, 0.025%, 10 ml	24208-0601-10	9.99	
ALBERTSON'S GLUCOSE TABLETS (Can-Am Care)			
CTB,PO (SAVONOSCO BY ALBERTSONS)			
4 gm, 10s ea	41163-5022-03	1.99	
ALBOLENE (DSE Healthcare)			
GEL,TP (UNSCENTED)			
96 gm	38485-0016-30	3.90	
(SCENTED)			
180 gm	87900-0387-40	5.52	
(UNSCENTED)			
180 gm	38485-0016-40	5.52	
(SCENTED)			
360 gm	38485-0387-22	8.52	
(UNSCENTED)			
360 gm	38485-0016-22	8.52	
ALBUSTIX (Siemens)			
DEV,NA, 100s ea	08620-2191-21	45.60	45.60
ALC-FREE FOAM (Geritrex)			
FOA,TP (1X200ML,AF,FOAM)			
0.1%, 200 ml	54162-0575-07	3.78	3.70
ALCALAK (Medique)			
CTB,PO (50X2,SF)			
420 mg, 100s ea UD	47682-0101-33	5.40	
(100X2,SF)			
420 mg, 200s ea UD	47682-0101-47	10.24	
(250X2,SF)			
420 mg, 500s ea UD	47682-0101-13	24.18	
TAB,PO (3X2)			
420 mg, 6s ea UD	47682-0101-69	0.79	
(12X2)			
420 mg, 24s ea UD	47682-0101-64	1.59	
ALCO-GEL (Xttrium Labs)			
GEL,TP, 60%, 60 gm	00116-0600-01	0.60	1.30
120 gm	00116-0600-04	0.76	1.50
480 gm	00116-0600-16	2.17	3.10
ALCOHOL (Cardinal Health)			
DEV,NA (STERILE,PRIVATE LABEL)			
100s ea	37205-0155-78	1.68	
(Family Phcy)			
DEV,NA (PRIVATE LABEL)			
100s ea	52735-0910-01	1.79	1.99
ALCOHOL ETHYL (Denison)			
LIQ,TP, 70%, 480 ml	00295-1136-16	0.80	
(Cardinal Health)			
RUBBING ALCOHOL			
LIQ,TP (PRIVATE LABEL)			
70%, 480 ml 12s	37205-0012-43	9.36	
960 ml	37205-0012-45	1.37	
ALCOHOL ISOPROPYL (AmerisourceBergen)			
LIQ,TP (PRIVATE LABEL)			
70%, 480 ml	24385-0249-16	21.50	23.90
(Consolidated Midland)			
LIQ,TP, 70%, 480 ml 12s	00223-6350-00	17.50	
91%, 3840 ml	00223-6363-00	12.50	
(Denison)			
LIQ,TP, 70%, 480 ml	00295-1137-16	0.77	
3840 ml	00295-1137-28	7.43	
99%, 3840 ml	00295-1139-28	11.91	
(Major)			
DEV,NA, 100s ea	00904-4277-60	2.40	
(Lex)			
ALCOHOL MENTHOLATED			
SOL,TP, 60 ml	49523-0094-02	0.80	
ALCOHOL PREP (Rugby)			
PAD,TP, 70%, 100s ea	00536-9920-01	2.85	

PROD/MFR	HRI, UPC,NDC	AWP	SRP
(Specialty Medical)			
PAD,TP, 70%, 200s ea	68113-0996-02	31.18	
ALCOHOL PREP PADS WITH BENZOCAINE FOR PAIN RELIEF (Major)			
PAD,TP, 6%-70%, 80s ea	00904-5836-47	3.24	
ALCOHOL SALICYLIC (Lex)			
LIQ,TP, 5%, 60 ml	49523-0012-02	0.58	
ALCOLADO RELAMPAGO (Larkspur)			
SOL,TP, 180 ml	18864-0201-05	2.22	
480 ml	18864-0201-13	4.66	9.39
ALER-DRYL (Reese)			
TAB,PO, 50 mg, 24s ea	10956-0751-24	3.69	
48s ea	10956-0751-48	4.92	
ALERCAP (Magno-Humphries)			
CAP,PO, 25 mg, 100s ea	43292-0557-05	2.71	4.99
ALERTAB (Magno-Humphries)			
TAB,PO, 25 mg, 100s ea	43292-0556-31	2.33	4.99
ALERTNESS AID (Cardinal Health)			
TAB,PO (PRIVATE LABEL)			
200 mg, 16s ea	37205-0195-73	2.04	
ALEVE (Bayer HealthCare)			
TAB,PO (GELCAPLET)			
220 mg, 20s ea	25866-0054-20	2.86	
24s ea	25866-0105-01	2.98	
(CAPLET)			
220 mg, 24s ea	25866-0105-02	2.98	
(GELCAPLET)			
220 mg, 40s ea	25866-0054-40	5.13	
50s ea	25866-0105-03	5.13	
(CAPLET)			
220 mg, 50s ea	25866-0105-04	5.13	
(GELCAPLET)			
220 mg, 80s ea	25866-0054-80	8.05	
100s ea	25866-0105-05	8.05	
(CAPLET)			
220 mg, 100s ea	25866-0105-06	8.05	
150s ea	25866-0000-04	10.65	
(CAPLET)			
220 mg, 150s ea	25866-0000-03	10.65	
200s ea	25866-0001-02	12.32	
(A-S Medication)			
REPACK			
TAB,PO, 220 mg, 24s ea	54569-4490-00	3.35	
100s ea	54569-3853-04	9.11	
(Nucare Pharm)			
REPACK			
TAB,PO (CAPLET)			
220 mg, 30s ea	66267-0011-30	8.99	
(Phys Total Care)			
REPACK			
TAB,PO (CAPLET)			
220 mg, 100s ea	54868-3505-00	12.37	
(Southwood)			
REPACK			
TAB,PO (GELCAPLET)			
220 mg, 20s ea	58016-0128-20	2.86	
30s ea	58016-0128-30	2.72	
ALEVE ARTHRITIS (Bayer HealthCare)			
TAB,PO (CAPLET)			
220 mg, 100s ea	25866-0503-81	8.05	
ALEVE COLD & SINUS (Bayer HealthCare)			
TER,PO (CAPLET)			
220 mg-120 mg,			
10s ea	25866-0041-21	3.56	
20s ea	25866-0041-22	6.20	
ALEVE SINUS & HEADACHE (Bayer HealthCare)			
TER,PO (NON-DROWSY,CAPLET)			
220 mg-120 mg,			
10s ea	25866-0504-77	3.50	
ALFALFA (Basic Vitamins)			
TAB,PO, 650 mg, 100s ea	00761-0183-20	1.80	
(Botanical Labs.)			
SOL,PO, 30 ml	41954-0020-59	3.50	6.99
(Lex)			
TAB,PO, 650 mg, 100s ea	49523-0029-01	0.90	
(Marlex)			
TAB,PO, 520 mg, 500s ea	10135-0227-05	3.22	
(Mason Vit)			
TAB,PO, 650 mg, 100s ea	11845-0054-21	4.22	
250s ea	11845-0054-22	6.56	
(Nature's Bounty)			
TAB,PO (PF,SF)			
500 mg, 100s ea	74312-0023-70		2.99

PROD/MFR HRI, UPC,NDC AWP SRP

(Rexall)
TAB,PO (PF,SF)
650 mg, 100s ea **30768-0012-13** 1.30 1.97

(Dispensing Solutions)
REPACK
TAB,PO, 500 mg, 30s ea ... **66336-0025-30** 6.03

ALFALFA CONCENTRATE (Freeda)
TAB,PO (PF,SF,DYE-FREE)
600 mg, 100s ea **10432-0229-01** 4.50 7.50
250s ea **10432-0229-02** 9.00 15.00

ALFAMIN (Key Company)
TAB,PO, 520 mg, 100s ea .. **11694-0921-01** 4.25
500s ea **11694-0921-03** 19.00

ALGA (Bio-Tech Pharm)
CAP,PO, 225 mcg,
100s ea **53191-0020-01** 4.75

ALGA-K (Key Company)
CAP,PO, 500 mg-2000 iu,
100s ea **11694-0888-01** 6.50
250s ea **11694-0888-03** 13.00

ALGISITE M ALGINATE WOUND (Smith & Nephew)
DEV,NA (6"X8")
5s ea **40565-0118-31** 166.05 132.84
(12" ROPE)
10s ea **40565-0118-33** 82.13 65.70
(2"X2")
10s ea **40565-0118-27** 37.83 30.26
(4"X4")
10s ea **40565-0118-29** 59.95 47.96

ALIBOUR ASTRINGENT (Lex)
LIQ,TP, 120 ml **49523-0051-01** 0.80

ALICARE (Andersen)
LOT,TP, 60 ml **52145-0001-03** 2.07
240 ml **52145-0001-04** 3.91
473.6 ml **52145-0001-05** 5.88

ALITRAQ (Abbott)
POW,PO (W/GLUTAMINE.,PACKET)
76 gm 6s **70074-0506-31** 72.78

ALKA-GEST (Key Company)
TAB,PO (SF)
180 mg-190 mg-380 mg,
100s ea **11694-0802-01** 6.75
250s ea **11694-0802-03** 13.50

ALKA-MINTS (Bayer HealthCare)
CTB,PO (SPEARMINT)
850 mg, 75s ea **16500-0047-15** 1.49

ALKA-SELTZER (Bayer HealthCare)
TEF,PO, 325 mg, 12s ea ... **16500-0040-19** 1.93
12s ea **16500-0048-02** 2.64
24s ea **16500-0040-11** 2.72
24s ea **16500-0048-10** 2.72
36s ea **16500-0040-12** 3.67
36s ea **16500-0048-06** 3.67
72s ea **16500-0040-22** 6.94
100s ea **16500-0040-24** 10.22

ALKA-SELTZER EXTRA STRENGTH
(Bayer HealthCare)
TEF,PO, 500 mg, 12s ea ... **16500-0044-02** 2.48
24s ea **16500-0044-04** 3.67

ALKA-SELTZER GOLD (Bayer HealthCare)
TEF,PO, 832 mg-312 mg-958 mg,
36s ea **16500-0041-08** 3.67

ALKA-SELTZER HEARTBURN RELIEF
(Bayer HealthCare)
TEF,PO (LEMON,LIME)
1000 mg-1940 mg,
24s ea **16500-0500-55** 2.72
36s ea **16500-0500-56** 3.67

ALKA-SELTZER MORNING RELIEF
(Bayer HealthCare)
TEF,PO (CITRUS)
500 mg-65 mg,
24s ea **16500-0503-38** 3.67

ALKA-SELTZER PLUS COLD (Bayer HealthCare)
SGL,PO (LIQUIGEL)
325 mg-2 mg-30 mg,
12s ea **16500-0055-01** 3.56
20s ea **16500-0055-02** 4.51
TEF,PO, 250 mg-2 mg-5 mg,
12s ea **16500-0505-87** 2.96
20s ea **16500-0505-86** 3.56
(CHERRY)
250 mg-2 mg-5 mg,
20s ea **16500-0505-94** 3.56

PROD/MFR HRI, UPC,NDC AWP SRP

(ORANGE)
250 mg-2 mg-5 mg,
20s ea **16500-0505-93** 3.56
36s ea **16500-0505-88** 5.40
48s ea **16500-0505-89** 6.47

ALKA-SELTZER PLUS COLD & COUGH
(Bayer HealthCare)
SGL,PO (LIQUIGEL)
325 mg-2 mg-10 mg-30 mg,
12s ea **16500-0054-01** 3.56
20s ea **16500-0054-02** 4.51
TEF,PO, 2 mg-10 mg-5 mg,
20s ea **16500-0505-92** 4.51

ALKA-SELTZER PLUS COLD & SINUS
(Bayer HealthCare)
TEF,PO (NON-DROWSY)
250 mg-5 mg,
20s ea **16500-0505-95** 3.56

ALKA-SELTZER PLUS FLU & BODY ACHES
(Bayer HealthCare)
TEF,PO, 325 mg-2 mg-10 mg-20 mg,
20s ea **16500-0052-20** 3.56

ALKA-SELTZER PLUS NIGHT-TIME COLD
(Bayer HealthCare)
SGL,PO (LIQUIGEL)
12s ea **16500-0053-01** 3.56
20s ea **16500-0053-02** 4.51
TEF,PO, 10 mg-6.25 mg-5 mg,
20s ea **16500-0505-90** 4.51

ALKA-SELTZER PM (Bayer HealthCare)
TAB,PO, 325 mg-38 mg,
24s ea **16500-0040-30** 3.67

ALKALOL (Denison)
SOL,MM, 473 ml **10029-0189-60** 2.26

ALL DAY ALLERGY (Major)
TAB,PO, 10 mg, 14s ea **00904-5829-41** 7.20
30s ea **00904-5829-46** 10.80
45s ea **00904-5829-43** 34.49
90s ea **00904-5829-89** 23.97
(24 HOUR)
10 mg, 100s ea **00904-5829-60** 224.72

ALL DAY ALLERGY-D (Major)
TER,PO, 5 mg-120 mg,
12s ea **00904-5831-12** 38.23

ALL-NITE (Major)
SOL,PO (CHERRY)
177 ml **00904-5776-21** 2.70
(ORIGINAL)
177 ml **00904-5777-21** 2.70

ALL-PURPOSE FIRST AID KIT
(Johnson & Johnson)
DEV,NA, ea **81370-0081-23** 10.75

ALLBEE C-800 (Inverness)
TAB,PO, 60s ea **36652-0677-62** 8.75

ALLBEE C-800 W/IRON (Inverness)
TAB,PO, 60s ea **36652-0678-62** 9.36

ALLBEE W/C (Inverness)
TAB,PO (CAPLET)
130s ea **36652-0673-66** 8.32

ALLCLENZ (Healthpoint)
SPR,TP, 432 ml **08213-0200-12** 12.61

ALLER-CHLOR (Rugby)
SYR,PO (CHERRY)
2 mg/5 ml, 120 ml **00536-0370-97** 3.27
TAB,PO, 4 mg, 24s ea **00536-3467-35** 3.06
100s ea **00536-3467-01** 5.70
1000s ea **00536-3467-10** 17.17

(PD-Rx Pharm)
REPACK
TAB,PO (REDI-SCRIPT)
4 mg, 56s ea **58864-0664-56** 16.18

ALLER-G-TIME (Time-Cap)
TAB,PO (CAPLET)
25 mg, 100s ea **49483-0061-01** 3.60
1000s ea **49483-0061-10** 29.96

ALLEREST MAXIMUM STRENGTH
(Heritage/Insight)
TAB,PO, 2 mg-30 mg,
24s ea **63736-0585-01** 3.56

ALLEREST NO DROWSINESS (Heritage/Insight)
TAB,PO, 325 mg-30 mg,
20s ea **63736-0605-56** 3.56

PROD/MFR HRI, UPC,NDC AWP SRP

ALLERFRIM (Rugby)
SYR,PO (PINEAPPLE)
30 mg/5 ml-1.25 mg/5 ml,
120 ml **00536-0510-97** 2.80
480 ml **00536-0510-85** 9.21

ALLERGARD SYNTHETIC SURGICAL GLOVES
(J&J Medical)
DEV,NA (STERILE,50 PR,SZ 5.5)
100s ea **56091-0061-55** 168.48
(STERILE,50 PR,SZ 6.5)
100s ea **56091-0061-65** 168.48
(STERILE,50 PR,SZ 7.5)
100s ea **56091-0061-75** 168.48
(STERILE,50 PR,SZ 7)
100s ea **56091-0061-70** 168.48
(STERILE,50 PR,SZ 8.5)
100s ea **56091-0061-85** 168.48
(STERILE,50 PR,SZ 8)
100s ea **56091-0061-80** 168.48
(STERILE,50 PR,SZ 9)
100s ea **56091-0061-90** 168.48
(STERILE,50 PRSZ 6)
100s ea **56091-0061-60** 168.48

ALLERGY (AmerisourceBergen)
TAB,PO (PRIVATE LABEL)
4 mg, 24s ea **24385-0463-62** 3.50 3.89
100s ea **24385-0463-78** 5.39 5.99

(Basic Vitamins)
TAB,PO, 4 mg, 100s ea **00761-0913-20** 1.80

(Cardinal Health)
TAB,PO (PRIVATE LABEL)
4 mg, 24s ea **37205-0215-62** 3.07
100s ea **37205-0215-78** 6.42

(Family Phcy)
TAB,PO (PRIVATE LABEL)
4 mg, 100s ea **52735-0401-01** 5.39 5.99

(G&W)
CRE,TP, 2%-0.1%, 30 gm .. **00713-0295-31** 2.39

(Major)
ODT,PO (ORIG STRENGTH,FRUIT)
10 mg, 10s ea **00904-5806-15** 12.53
TAB,PO (12X1)
4 mg, 12s ea **00904-0012-05** 1.13
24s ea **00904-0012-24** 1.60
100s ea **00904-0012-59** 3.50
(10X10)
4 mg, 100s ea UD **00904-0012-61** 6.25
(NON-DROWSY 24HR)
10 mg, 10s ea **00904-5728-15** 4.50
30s ea **00904-5728-87** 8.25
90s ea **00904-5728-89** 16.50

ALLERGY CHILDREN'S (Chain Drug Marketing)
SOL,PO (AF,CHERRY)
12.5 mg/5 ml, 118 ml . **63868-0823-54** 1.38 4.99

ALLERGY EYE RELIEF (Similasan Corp.)
SOL,OP (DROPS)
6 x-6 x-6 x, 10 ml **59262-0346-11** 6.21 10.99

ALLERGY RELIEF INTENSE STRENGTH
(Chain Drug Marketing)
TAB,PO (CAPLET)
50 mg, 24s ea **63868-0751-24** 2.10 3.99

ALLERGY RELIEF MEDICINE (Mason Vit)
CAP,PO, 25 mg, 100s ea ... **11845-0896-01** 4.11

ALLERHIST-1 (Cardinal Health)
TAB,PO (PRIVATE LABEL)
1.34 mg, 16s ea **37205-0228-73** 5.19

(Family Phcy)
TAB,PO (PRIVATE LABEL)
1.34 mg, 8s ea **52735-0446-16** 3.05 3.39

ALLERMAX (Pfeiffer)
SOL,PO, 12.5 mg/5 ml,
120 ml **00927-0617-12** 1.76 3.17
TAB,PO, 50 mg, 24s ea ... **00927-0221-24** 2.33 4.19

ALLEVYN ADHESIVE (Smith & Nephew)
DEV,NA (3"X3")
10s ea **00223-0438-38** 59.01 47.21
(5"X5")
10s ea **00223-0438-39** 90.65 72.52
(7"X7")
10s ea **00223-0438-40** 169.93 135.94

ALLEVYN CAVITY (Smith & Nephew)
DEV,NA (4 3/4"X1 1/2" TUBULAR)
5s ea **00223-0438-48** 153.56 122.85
(4" CIRCULAR)
5s ea **00223-0438-47** 208.99 167.19

PROD/MFR	HRI, UPC,NDC	AWP	SRP
(2" CIRCULAR)			
10s ea	00223-0438-45	173.38	138.70
(3 1/2"X1" TUBULAR)			
10s ea	00223-0438-46	154.24	123.39
ALLEVYN HYDROCELLULAR FOAM (Smith & Nephew)			
DEV,NA (2"X2")			
10s ea	00223-0438-41	52.24	41.79
(4"X4")			
10s ea	00223-0438-42	80.03	64.02
(6"X6")			
10s ea	00223-0438-43	158.49	126.79
(8"X8")			
10s ea	00223-0438-44	266.95	213.56
(TRACHEOST,3 1/2"X3 1/2")			
10s ea	00223-0438-49	74.66	59.73
ALLFEN (MCR American)			
TAB,PO, 400 mg, 100s ea	58605-0400-01	22.46	
ALLFEN DM (MCR American)			
TAB,PO, 20 mg-400 mg,			
100s ea	58605-0401-01	27.71	
ALLI (Glaxo)			
CAP,PO (STARTER PACK)			
60 mg, 60s ea	00135-0461-01	40.20	
90s ea	00135-0461-02	51.52	
(REFILL PACK)			
60 mg, 120s ea	00135-0461-05	61.39	
(STARTER PACK)			
60 mg, 150s ea	53100-0471-00	97.44	
ALLIUM CEPA (Luyties)			
TAB,SL (6X)			
6 x, 500s ea	00618-0080-03	3.99	
5500s ea	00618-0080-10	30.32	
12 x, 500s ea	00622-0080-03	4.19	
5500s ea	00622-0080-10	31.83	
30 x, 500s ea	00624-0080-03	4.19	
(12X)			
30 x, 5500s ea	00624-0080-10	31.83	
ALLKARE ADHESIVE REMOVER WIPE (Convatec)			
DEV,NA, 100s ea	68455-0107-60	20.29	26.41
ALLKARE PROTECTIVE BARRIER WIPE (Convatec)			
DEV,NA, 50s ea	68455-0107-66	9.06	11.80
100s ea	68455-0107-61	17.33	22.55
ALMACONE (Rugby)			
CTB,PO (PEPPERMINT)			
200 mg-200 mg-20 mg,			
100s ea	00536-3035-01	3.78	
SUS,PO (MINT)			
360 ml	00536-0025-83	3.10	
ALMACONE DOUBLE STRENGTH (Rugby)			
SUS,PO (MINT)			
360 ml	00536-0015-83	4.45	
ALOE 99 (Lee Pharm)			
GEL,TP, 120 gm	23558-0684-60	2.15	
120 gm 12s	23558-0684-61	25.78	
ALOE GRANDE (Gordon)			
CRE,TP, 120 gm	10481-3013-03	14.40	
2270 gm	10481-3013-05	162.50	
ALOE GRANDE CREME (Gordon)			
TP, 75 gm	10481-3013-02	11.90	
480 gm	50217-0001-30	53.75	
ALOE VERA (ADH)			
CAP,PO (PF,SF)			
470 mg, 100s ea	60142-0901-21	5.48	10.95
(Coats Aloe Int'l)			
CRE,TP, 118 gm	58826-0703-04	12.00	18.00
473 gm	58826-0703-16	39.32	58.99
GEL,TP, 237 ml	58826-0705-08	12.00	18.00
1000 ml	58826-0705-33	39.32	58.99
LOT,TP, 60 ml	58826-0702-02	2.00	3.00
237 ml	58826-0702-08	12.00	18.00
240 ml	58826-0704-08	12.00	18.00
1000 ml	58826-0702-33	39.32	58.99
1000 ml	58826-0704-33	39.32	58.99
SOL,TP, 237 ml	58826-0701-08	12.00	18.00
(1X1000ML)			
1000 ml	58826-0701-33	19.32	29.00
(Nature's Bounty)			
CAP,PO (470MG)			
100s ea	74312-0051-01		7.99
ALOE VERA CONCENTRATE 5000 (Mason Vit)			
CAP,PO (PF,SF,SOFTGEL)			
60s ea	11845-0121-75	8.11	
SGL,PO, 25 mg, 60s ea	11845-0129-45	8.11	
ALOE VERA GEL (Carlson,J.R.)			
SGL,PO (PF,SF,CORN-FREE)			
25 mg, 100s ea	88395-0080-41	4.45	8.90
250s ea	88395-0080-42	10.38	20.75

PROD/MFR	HRI, UPC,NDC	AWP	SRP
ALOE VERA JUICE DRINK (Coats Aloe Int'l)			
SOL,PO (100%)			
1000 ml	58826-0707-33	8.00	12.00
ALOE VERA W/LIDOCAINE (AmerisourceBergen)			
GEL,TP (PRIVATE LABEL)			
0.5%, 227 gm	24385-0083-34	4.22	4.69
ALOE VESTA (Quality Care Prod)			
REPACK			
OIN,TP (2 IN 1)			
43.6%, 60 gm	49999-0864-02	7.13	
ALOPHEN (Numark)			
ECT,PO, 5 mg, 100s ea	38485-0140-01	5.70	
ALPH-E (Key Company)			
CRE,TP, 60 gm	11694-0126-08	5.00	
ALPHA BATH (Dermarite)			
OIL,TP, 60 ml	61924-0078-02	0.62	
240 ml	61924-0078-08	2.50	
ALPHA KERI (B/M Squibb Cons Med)			
OIL,TP, 240 ml	00723-0600-08	6.58	
480 ml	00723-0600-16	10.79	
(Phys Total Care)			
REPACK			
OIL,TP, 237 ml	54868-4995-00	9.50	
ALPHA LIPOIC (Carlson,J.R.)			
TAB,PO, 100 mg, 30s ea	88395-0080-60	4.45	8.90
90s ea	88395-0080-61	11.25	22.50
180s ea	88395-0080-62	19.95	39.90
300 mg, 30s ea	88395-0080-70	9.45	18.90
90s ea	88395-0080-71	24.95	49.90
ALPHA LIPOIC ACID (Freeda)			
TAB,PO (SF,GLUTEN-FREE)			
200 mg, 100s ea	10432-0365-01	13.17	21.95
ALPHA-E (Advanced Nutr)			
SGL,PO, 400 iu, 100s ea	62617-0505-06	20.25	27.00
ALPHA-LIPOIC ACID (Mason Vit)			
CAP,PO (PF,SF)			
100 mg, 60s ea	11845-0131-45	11.67	
(Nature's Bounty)			
CAP,PO (PF,SF,DAIRY-FREE)			
30 mg, 60s ea	74312-0003-60		6.99
(Rexall)			
TAB,PO (PF,SF)			
50 mg, 30s ea	30768-0001-30	3.93	5.95
ALPHA-LIPOIC-ACID-300 (Key Company)			
CAP,PO, 300 mg, 60s ea	11694-0654-01	12.50	
250s ea	11694-0654-02	44.00	
ALPHASOFT (Ameriderm Labs)			
OIL,TP (48X237ML)			
237 ml 48s	63921-0300-08	1.31	
ALPHIX (Topix)			
OIL,TP, 118 ml	58211-0360-04	3.58	
ALRA ONCOLOGY DEODORANT (Neue Medical)			
STI,TP, 67.5 gm	68374-0874-08	3.60	
ALTACHLORE (Altaire)			
OIN,OP (STERILE)			
5%, 3.5 gm	69390-0184-50	11.35	
SOL,OP, 5%, 15 ml	59390-0183-13	14.45	
30 ml	59390-0183-18	20.00	
ALTAFRIN (Altaire)			
SOL,OP, 0.12%, 15 ml	59390-0179-13	3.03	
ALTALUBE (Altaire)			
OIN,OP (STERILE)			
15%-85%, 3.5 gm	59390-0198-50	5.63	
ALTAMIST (Altaire)			
SPR,NS, 0.85%, 60 ml	59390-0035-26	2.75	
ALTAZINE (Altaire)			
SOL,OP (VASOCONSTRICTOR)			
0.05%, 15 ml	59390-0180-13	2.99	
ALTERNAGEL (J&J/Merck)			
SUS,PO, 600 mg/5 ml,			
355 ml	16837-0860-12	5.82	
ALUMINUM ACETATE (Amend)			
SOL,TP, 480 ml	17317-0213-01	10.15	
ALUMINUM HYDROXIDE (Pharm Assoc Inc)			
SUS,PO (100X30ML,SF,PEPPERMINT)			
320 mg/5 ml,			
30 ml 100s UD	00121-0733-30	68.94	
(SF,PEPPERMINT)			
320 mg/5 ml, 355 ml	00121-0733-12	6.55	
473 ml	00121-0733-16	7.20	
(SF,LEMON-MINT)			
600 mg/5 ml, 355 ml	00121-0601-12	7.20	

PROD/MFR	HRI, UPC,NDC	AWP	SRP
ALUMINUM HYDROXIDE GEL (Asafi Pharmaceutical)			
SUS,PO, 320 mg/5 ml,			
473 ml	65557-0772-16	5.95	
(R.I.J.)			
SUS,PO, 320 mg/5 ml,			
150 ml	53807-0132-02	2.54	
360 ml	53807-0132-01	3.64	
(Rugby)			
SUS,PO (SF,PEPPERMINT)			
320 mg/5 ml, 473 ml	00536-0091-85	5.60	
(Teva)			
SUS,PO, 320 mg/5 ml,			
480 ml	00182-0162-40	6.45	
ALUMINUM HYDROXIDE/MAGNESIUM HYDROXIDE/SIMETHICONE (Palmetto)			
REPACK			
SUS,PO, 360 ml	23490-7381-01	8.00	
ALUMINUM METALLICUM (Std Homeo)			
TAB,PO, 250s ea	54973-0094-01	4.37	7.29
ALUMINUM/MAGNESIUM (Pharma Pac)			
REPACK			
SUS,PO, 225 mg/5 ml-200 mg/5 ml,			
360 ml	52959-0235-03	7.65	
AMANTLE (Doak)			
CRE,TP, 30 gm	10337-0904-52	10.34	
120 gm	10337-0904-41	21.88	
480 gm	10337-0904-42	60.92	
AMBERDERM (Delta Pharm)			
SPR,TP, 113.4 gm	53706-1003-03	14.25	
AMBI 10PEH/400GFN (MCR American)			
TAB,PO, 400 mg-10 mg,			
100s ea	66870-0422-01	51.25	
AMBI 10PEH/400GFN/20DM (MCR American)			
TAB,PO, 20 mg-400 mg-10 mg,			
100s ea	66870-0423-01	53.75	
AMBI COCOA BUTTER (Johnson & Johnson)			
SOA,TP, 99 gm	81370-0022-33	1.18	
AMBI COMPLEXION (Johnson & Johnson)			
SOA,TP, 99 gm	81370-0022-32	1.18	
AMBI EVEN & CLEAR DAILY MOISTURIZER (Johnson & Johnson)			
LOT,TP (W/ SPF 30)			
3%-12%-5%-1.7%-3%,			
88 ml	81370-0022-27	8.48	
AMBI EVEN & CLEAR EXFOLIATING WASH (Johnson & Johnson)			
SOA,TP, 0.5%, 141 gm	81370-0022-26	5.09	
AMBI EVEN & CLEAR FOAMING CLEANSER (Johnson & Johnson)			
FOA,TP, 0.5%, 177 ml	81370-0022-19	5.09	
AMBI EVEN & CLEAR TARGETED MARK MINIMIZER (Johnson & Johnson)			
CRE,TP, 28 gm	81370-0022-55	8.48	
AMBI FADE CREAM (Johnson & Johnson)			
CRE,TP (FOR NORMAL SKIN)			
2%-2%, 56 gm	81370-0022-29	3.64	
(FOR OILY SKIN)			
2%-2%, 56 gm	81370-0022-30	3.64	
AMBI SOFT & EVEN CREAMY OIL LOTION (Johnson & Johnson)			
LOT,TP, 354 ml	81370-0019-78	5.94	
AMBI SOFT & EVEN SKIN TONE ENHANCING MOISTURE (Johnson & Johnson)			
CRE,TP, 113 gm	81370-0019-79	5.94	
AMBI SOFT & EVEN STRETCH MARK DIMINISHING BODY OIL (Johnson & Johnson)			
OIL,TP, 147 ml	81370-0019-80	5.94	
AMBIFED (MCR American)			
TAB,PO, 400 mg-30 mg,			
100s ea	58605-0414-01	82.46	
AMBIFED DM (MCR American)			
TAB,PO, 20 mg-400 mg-30 mg,			
100s ea	58605-0415-01	90.96	
AMBIFED-G (MCR American)			
TAB,PO, 400 mg-20 mg,			
100s ea	58605-0416-01	105.95	
AMBIFED-G DM (MCR American)			
TAB,PO, 20 mg-400 mg-20 mg,			
100s ea	58605-0417-01	112.36	

PROD/MFR	HRI, UPC,NDC	AWP	SRP
AMBULATORY FEEDING BAG (Abbott)			
DEV,NA (W/COMPANION PUMP SET)			
ea	70074-0005-07	15.23	
AMERICAINE (Heritage/Insight)			
OIN,TP, 0.1%-20%, 30 gm	63736-0037-51	3.63	
SPR,TP, 20%, 60 ml	63736-0378-82	3.63	
AMERICERIN (Ameriderm Labs)			
CRE,TP, 113 gm	63921-0130-04	3.13	
452 gm	63921-0130-16	6.50	
AMERIPHOR (Ameriderm Labs)			
OIN,TP, 113 gm	63921-0140-04	3.13	
452 gm	63921-0140-16	6.78	
AMERISTORE (Ameriderm Labs)			
LOT,TP, 118 ml	63921-0150-04	0.44	
237 ml	63921-0150-08	0.94	
AMERIWASH (Ameriderm Labs)			
LIQ,TP (4X3780ML)			
3780 ml 4s	63921-0200-01	11.86	
SOA,TP (24X473ML)			
473 ml 24s	63921-0209-16	2.60	
(12X800ML)			
800 ml 12s	63921-0200-80	3.85	
(12X1000ML)			
1000 ml 12s	63921-0200-10	4.28	
AMIELLE (Owen Mumford)			
DEV,NA (CARE VAGINAL TRAINER)			
ea	08470-2150-01	53.63	
(COMFORT VAG TRAINER)			
ea	08470-2100-01	53.63	60.00
AMINO 1500 (Nature's Bounty)			
TAB,PO, 150s ea	74312-0050-91		14.75
AMINO ACID #1 (Dispensing Solutions)			
REPACK			
CAP,PO, 350 mg-50 mg,			
30s ea	66336-0021-30	10.34	
AMINO ACID #2 (Dispensing Solutions)			
CAP,PO, 50 mg-350 mg,			
30s ea	66336-0023-30	10.34	
AMINO ACIDS (Mason Vit)			
CAP,PO (PF,SF)			
90s ea	11845-0054-89	7.44	
DAILY AMINO			
CTB,PO (PF,SF)			
60s ea	11845-0119-15	10.56	
TAB,PO, 60s ea	11845-0121-25	8.56	
SUPER AMINO ACIDS			
PO (PF,SF)			
90s ea	11845-0082-39	8.78	
AMINO BALANCE-NATURAL (Basic Vitamins)			
CAP,PO, 100s ea	00761-0742-20	4.00	
AMINO BLEND (Carlson,J.R.)			
POW,PO (PF,CORN-FREE,SOY-FREE)			
300 gm	88395-0067-06	31.65	63.30
AMINO-VIL (Carlson,J.R.)			
POW,PO, 370 gm	88395-0067-13	42.45	84.90
AMINOBRAIN (Med Prods Panamer)			
CAP,PO, 60s ea	00576-0103-60	10.60	
AMINOFEN (Medique)			
TAB,PO (250X2)			
325 mg, 500s ea UD	51469-0303-01	6.91	8.40
AMLACTIN (Upsher-Smith)			
CRE,TP (TUBE)			
12%, 140 gm	00245-0024-14	10.15	
LOT,TP, 12%, 225 gm	00245-0023-22	11.27	
400 gm	00245-0023-40	18.62	
AMLACTIN FOOT CREAM THERAPY (Upsher-Smith)			
CRE,TP (1X85GM,FRAGRANCE-FREE)			
85 gm	02450-0019-10	8.11	8.99
AMLACTIN XL (Upsher-Smith)			
LOT,TP (ULTRAPLEX FORMULATION)			
160 gm	00245-0022-16	27.98	
(Phys Total Care)			
REPACK			
LOT,TP (1X160GM,FRAGRANCE-FREE)			
160 gm	54868-5872-00	37.80	
AMMENS MEDICATED (Clairol, Inc.)			
POW,TP (ORIGINAL)			
187.5 gm	19810-0005-04	2.88	
(SHOWER FRESH)			
187.5 gm	19810-0008-21	2.88	
(ORIGINAL)			
330 gm	19810-0005-03	4.00	
(SHOWER FRESH)			
330 gm	19810-0071-02	4.00	

PROD/MFR	HRI, UPC,NDC	AWP	SRP
AMMONIA (Alexander, James)			
SOL,IH, 10s ea	46414-3333-03	1.58	2.82
100s ea	46414-3333-02	12.45	21.81
(Glenwood)			
SOL,IH (AMP)			
10s ea	00516-0121-01	12.48	
(X-Gen)			
SOL,IH (CRUSHABLE AMP)			
10s ea	39822-9900-01	3.10	
12s ea	39822-9900-02	3.75	
(A-S Medication)			
REPACK			
SOL,IH, 0.33 ml 12s	54569-2261-00	3.75	
(Phys Total Care)			
REPACK			
SOL,IH (10X0.33ML)			
0.33 ml 10s	54868-2525-00	10.15	
(Southwood)			
REPACK			
SOL,IH, 100s ea	58016-6317-01	11.60	
AMMONIUM LACTATE (Major)			
CRE,TP (FRAGRANCE-FREE)			
12%, 140 gm	00904-5983-48	20.49	
LOT,TP, 12%, 225 gm	00904-5984-26	38.12	
400 gm	00904-5984-63	42.49	
(Perrigo)			
LOT,TP (FRAGRANCE-FREE)			
12%, 225 gm	45802-0525-55	18.24	
400 gm	45802-0525-26	29.45	
(Phys Total Care)			
REPACK			
LOT,TP (FRAGRANCE-FREE)			
12%, 225 gm	54868-4599-00	23.76	
400 gm	54868-4599-01	40.04	
AMOSAN (Oral B Lab)			
PDS,PO, 20s ea	00041-0850-20	5.21	4.15
40s ea	00041-0850-40	8.46	7.57
AMYGDALUS (Std Homeo)			
TAB,PO, 250s ea	54973-0126-01	4.37	7.29
ANALGESIC (Dispensing Solutions)			
REPACK			
OIN,TP, 28.35 gm	55045-2663-08	3.55	
28.35 gm	55045-3352-08	3.55	
(Phys Total Care)			
REPACK			
OIN,TP, 480 gm	54868-2880-01	34.27	
(Southwood)			
REPACK			
OIN,TP, 30 gm	58016-3003-01	3.00	
ANALGESIC BALM (Geritrex)			
OIN,TP, 6%-14%, 454 gm	54162-0555-14	9.58	
(Altura)			
REPACK			
LOT,TP, 2%-1%-4.9%,			
60 ml	63874-0009-72	11.89	
OIN,TP, 30 gm	63874-0047-30	6.95	
ANALGESIC CREME RUB WITH ALOE (Major)			
CRE,TP (1X85GM)			
10%, 85 gm	00904-5857-56	3.95	
ANAMULEX (Lex)			
CAP,PO, 425 mg,			
1000s ea	49523-0044-01	6.00	
ANBESOL (Wyeth Consumer)			
GEL,MM, 6.3%, 7.5 gm	00573-0218-07	4.52	
9.35 gm	00573-0218-25		6.69
SOL,MM, 6.3%, 9.3 ml	00573-0221-10	4.52	
(MAXIMUM STRENGTH)			
20%, 12 ml	00573-0215-41		7.09
ANBESOL BABY (Wyeth Consumer)			
GEL,MM, 7.5%, 7.5 gm	00573-0219-07	3.95	
(GRAPE)			
7.5%, 7.5 gm	00573-0216-15	3.95	
(1X9.9GM,GRAPE)			
7.5%, 9.9 gm	00573-0216-26		5.79
ANBESOL MAXIMUM STRENGTH (Wyeth Consumer)			
GEL,MM, 20%, 7.5 gm	00573-0225-10	5.08	
(1X9.9GM)			
20%, 9.9 gm	00573-0225-67		7.09
SOL,MM, 20%, 9.3 ml	00573-0228-10	5.08	
ANDRODIM (Bio-Tech Pharm)			
CAP,PO, 90s ea	53191-0446-09	26.00	
ANDROVITE (Optimox)			
TAB,PO, 180s ea	50520-0004-01	13.00	

PROD/MFR	HRI, UPC,NDC	AWP	SRP
ANESTAFOAM (Onset)			
FOA,TP (1X30GM)			
4%, 30 gm	16781-0126-30	47.06	37.65
ANESTHESIA EXTENSION SET (Abbott Hosp)			
DEV,NA (32")			
120s ea	00074-1835-02	210.24	
ANGEL WING BLOOD COLLECTION SET (Covidien)			
DEV,NA (21G,.75",LUERADAPTER)			
50s ea	08080-2251-82	49.39	
(23G,0.75",W/HOLDER)			
50s ea	08080-2252-65	89.08	
(23G,0.75")			
50s ea	08080-2251-90	49.39	
(25G,3/4",TUBE HOLDER)			
50s ea	08080-2252-73	92.09	
ANGEL WING BLOOD COLLECTION/INFUSION SET (Covidien)			
DEV,NA (19G,3/4",FEMALE LUER)			
50s ea	08080-2251-74	49.39	
(19G,3/4",LUER ADAPTER)			
50s ea	08080-2252-81	62.13	
(21G,3/4",LUER ADAPTER)			
50s ea	08080-2252-99	60.32	
(25G,3/4",FEMALE LUER)			
50s ea	08080-2252-08	49.39	
(25G,3/4",LUER ADAPTER)			
50s ea	08080-2253-15	60.32	
(Tyco)			
DEV,NA (23G,3/4",LUER ADAPTER)			
50s ea	08080-2252-07	60.32	
ANGEL WING BLOOD TRANSFER (Covidien)			
DEV,NA, 50s ea	08080-2252-41	60.94	
ANGEL WING MULTI-SAMPLE LUER ADAPTER/ HOLDER SET (Covidien)			
DEV,NA (MALE)			
50s ea	08080-2252-24	58.44	
(TRANSFERSET,FEMALE)			
50s ea	08080-2252-40	58.47	
ANGEL WING TUBE HOLDER (Covidien)			
DEV,NA (FEMALE LUER ADAPTER)			
50s ea	08080-2252-32	42.22	
(W/ MALE LUER ADAPTER)			
50s ea	08080-2252-16	43.48	
ANIMAL SHAPES (Major)			
CTB,PO, 100s ea	00904-2621-60	3.53	
250s ea	00904-2621-70	6.54	
ANIMAL SHAPES + IRON (Major)			
CTB,PO, 100s ea	00904-0536-60	4.14	
250s ea	00904-0536-70	7.28	
ANIMAL SHAPES PLUS EXTRA C (Cardinal Health)			
CTB,PO (PRIVATE LABEL)			
100s ea	37205-0389-78	5.09	
ANIMAS PUMP CARTRIDGE (Animas Corp.)			
DEV,NA (STAMPED, STERILE)			
10s ea	65781-0310-10	47.09	
ANTACID (Albertson's)			
SUS,PO, 360 ml	41280-0200-41	2.37	
360 ml	41280-0200-75	3.24	
360 ml	41280-0230-19	2.19	
(AmerisourceBergen)			
SUS,PO (PRIVATE LABEL,MINT)			
225 mg/5 ml-200 mg/5 ml,			
360 ml	24385-0356-40	3.14	3.49
(Cardinal Health)			
CTB,PO (ASSORTED,PRIVATE LABEL)			
500 mg, 150s ea	37205-0200-47	3.52	
(PRIVATE LABEL)			
500 mg, 150s ea	37205-0210-47	3.52	
(Family Phcy)			
TAB,PO (ASSORTED,PRIVATE LABEL)			
150s ea	52735-0521-15	3.14	3.49
(PRIVATE LABEL)			
150s ea	52735-0519-15	3.05	3.39
(Major)			
CTB,PO (ASSORTED)			
200 mg, 150s ea	00904-1258-92	3.40	
(FRUIT)			
200 mg, 150s ea	00904-1257-92	3.40	
(FAST DISSOLVE,LEMON)			
600 mg, 85s ea	00904-5411-64	3.85	
(Teva)			
CTB,PO (ASSORTED)			
500 mg, 150s ea	00182-1139-20	3.59	

PROD/MFR	HRI, UPC, NDC	AWP	SRP
(Altura)			
REPACK			
SUS,PO, 225 mg/5 ml-200 mg/5 ml,			
355 ml	63874-0066-35	7.91	
(Phys Total Care)			
REPACK			
CTB,PO (UNFLAVORED)			
80 mg-20 mg,			
100s ea	54868-2410-03	8.25	
150s ea	54868-2410-04	10.89	
200 mg-200 mg,			
100s ea	54868-2326-00	8.91	
SUS,PO, 225 mg/5 ml-200 mg/5 ml,			
355 ml	54868-3054-00	9.36	
(Quality Care Prod)			
REPACK			
SUS,PO (MINT)			
225 mg/5 ml-200 mg/5 ml,			
360 ml	49999-0519-12	7.38	
ANTACID ANTI-GAS (Cardinal Health)			
SUS,PO, 360 ml	37205-0535-40	3.20	
(PRIVATE LABEL)			
360 ml	37205-0530-40	3.80	
ANTACID EFFERVESCENT (Albertson's)			
TEF,PO, 325 mg, 36s ea	41280-0220-75	3.57	
ANTACID EXTRA STRENGTH (Cardinal Health)			
CTB,PO (PRIVATE LABEL)			
160 mg-105 mg,			
100s ea	37205-0780-78	5.68	
(ASSORTED,PRIVATE LABEL)			
750 mg, 96s ea	37205-0205-80	3.52	
(PRIVATE LABEL,FRUIT)			
750 mg, 96s ea	37205-0706-80	3.52	
SUS,PO (PRIVATE LABEL,LEMON)			
355 ml	37205-0541-40	3.87	
ANTACID II W/SIMETHICONE (Southwood)			
REPACK			
SUS,PO, 360 ml	58016-7002-01	6.81	
ANTACID LIQUID (Cardinal Health)			
SUS,PO (PRIVATE LABEL,MINT)			
225 mg/5 ml-200 mg/5 ml,			
360 ml	37205-0540-40	2.16	
(Prime Marketing)			
SUS,PO (MINT)			
225 mg/5 ml-200 mg/5 ml,			
355 ml	62107-0020-11	2.90	
ANTACID LIQUID EXTRA STRENGTH (Prime Marketing)			
SUS,PO (LEMON)			
355 ml	62107-0021-11	3.75	
ANTACID M (Physician Partner)			
REPACK			
SUS,PO (1X360ML)			
360 ml	21695-0840-12	15.38	
ANTACID MULTI-SYMPTOM (Advance)			
CTB,PO (ASSORTED)			
500 mg, 150s ea	17714-0043-15	3.99	
ANTACID PLUS ANTI-GA (AmerisourceBergen)			
ANTACID PLUS ANTI-GAS			
SUS,PO (PRIVATE LABEL,CHERRY)			
360 ml	24385-0362-40	4.22	4.69
ANTACID ULTRA STRENGTH (AmerisourceBergen)			
CTB,PO (PRIVATE LABEL)			
1000 mg, 72s ea	24385-0595-23	3.14	3.49
ANTACID W/SIMETHICONE (Southwood)			
REPACK			
CTB,PO, 200 mg-200 mg-25 mg,			
100s ea	58016-0728-00	5.64	
SUS,PO, 360 ml	58016-7003-01	6.22	
ANTACID/ANTIGAS (A-S Medication)			
REPACK			
SUS,PO, 360 ml	54569-5201-00	3.73	
ANTI-ALLERGY FORMULA (Freeda)			
TAB,PO (PF,SF,DYE-FREE)			
100 mg-100 mg-50 mg,			
100s ea	10432-0307-01	6.57	10.95
250s ea	10432-0307-02	13.14	21.90
ANTI-DIARRHEAL (AmerisourceBergen)			
TAB,PO (PRIVATE LABEL,CAPLET)			
2 mg, 12s ea	24385-0554-53	3.23	3.59
24s ea	24385-0554-62	4.49	4.99
(Cardinal Health)			
LIQ,PO (PRIVATE LABEL,CHERRY)			
1 mg/5 ml, 120 ml	37205-0377-26	5.36	
TAB,PO (PRIVATE LABEL,CAPLET)			
2 mg, 12s ea	37205-0370-53	4.70	
18s ea	37205-0370-89	5.24	
(G&W)			
TAB,PO (CAPLET)			
2 mg, 6s ea	00713-0418-66	1.98	
12s ea	00713-0418-12	2.99	
18s ea	00713-0418-21	4.04	
24s ea	00713-0418-24	5.37	
(Major)			
LIQ,PO, 1 mg/5 ml,			
120 ml	00904-0036-20	5.65	
TAB,PO, 2 mg, 12s ea	00904-7725-12	3.99	
24s ea	00904-7725-24	6.37	
(Mason Vit)			
TAB,PO (BLISTER PACK,CAPLET)			
2 mg, 12s ea	11845-0984-20	5.00	
(Medicine Shoppe)			
TAB,PO (CAPLET)			
2 mg, 12s ea	49614-0554-53	3.99	3.99
ANTI-FUNGAL (AmerisourceBergen)			
SOL,TP (PRIVATE LABEL)			
10%, 30 ml	24385-0676-30		8.99
(MPM Medical Inc.)			
CRE,TP, 1%, 113 gm	66977-0023-04	8.00	8.89
ANTI-GAS 80 (Family Phcy)			
CTB,PO (PRIVATE LABEL)			
80 mg, 100s ea	52735-0531-01	5.39	5.99
ANTI-HIST (Basic Vitamins)			
CAP,PO, 25 mg, 100s ea	00761-0914-20	2.40	
ANTI-ITCH (AmerisourceBergen)			
SPR,TP (PRIVATE LABEL)			
2%, 60 ml	24385-0034-46	3.77	4.19
(Family Phcy)			
SPR,TP (PRIVATE LABEL)			
2%, 60 ml	52735-0742-36	3.77	4.19
(Taro)			
CRE,TP, 2%-0.1%,			
28.4 gm	51672-2066-02	2.43	
ANTI-ITCH MAXIMUM STRENGTH (AmerisourceBergen)			
CRE,TP (PRIVATE LABEL)			
1%-1%, 56 gm	24385-0240-46	4.13	4.59
GEL,TP, 2%-1%, 120 gm	24385-0023-16	3.77	4.19
(Cardinal Health)			
CRE,TP (PRIVATE LABEL)			
2%-0.1%, 28 gm	37205-0278-10	3.65	
(Teva)			
CRE,TP, 2%-0.1%, 30 gm	00182-5121-34	3.85	
ANTI-ITCH MEDICATED (McKesson)			
CRE,TP, 1%-1%, 30 gm	49348-0433-72	3.49	
ANTI-NAUSEA (Cardinal Health)			
SOL,PO (PRIVATE LABEL,CHERRY)			
120 ml	37205-0291-26	5.30	
ANTIBIOTIC PLUS (AmerisourceBergen)			
CRE,TP (MAX. STR.,PRIVATE LABEL)			
30 gm	24385-0144-03	4.76	5.29
ANTIHISTAMINE (Albertson's)			
ELI,PO, 12.5 mg/5 ml,			
120 ml	12810-0379-26	1.92	
TER,PO, 6 mg-120 mg,			
20s ea	12810-0475-60	5.37	
ANTIMONIUM TART (Luyties)			
TAB,SL (6X)			
6 x, 500s ea	00618-0177-03	3.99	
5500s ea	00618-0177-10	30.32	
12 x, 500s ea	00622-0177-03	4.19	
5500s ea	00622-0177-10	31.83	
30 x, 500s ea	00624-0177-03	4.19	
5500s ea	00624-0177-10	31.83	
ANTIOXIDANT (Major)			
TAB,PO (BOXED)			
60s ea	00904-5044-52	7.49	
(Miller)			
CAP,PO, 90s ea	17204-0363-85	12.60	21.00
(Nature's Bounty)			
SUPER ANTIOXIDANT FORMULA			
CAP,PO (PF,SF,SOFTGEL)			
50s ea	74312-0041-50		11.79
ANTIOXIDANT 4000 (Nature's Bounty)			
CAP,PO (PF,SF,SOFTGEL)			
60s ea	74312-0074-20		9.59
ANTIOXIDANT FORMULA (Rugby)			
SGL,PO (SOFTGEL)			
50s ea	00536-5588-06	5.40	
(Rx Vitamins)			
CAP,PO, 90s ea	08429-0140-90	14.48	28.95
ANTIOXIDANT PROTECTOR VITAMIN SUPER (Basic Vitamins)			
SGL,PO (SOFTGEL)			
60s ea	00761-0712-12	6.00	
ANTIOXIDANT PROTECTOR VITAMINS (Basic Vitamins)			
PO (SOFTGEL)			
60s ea	00761-0711-12	3.60	
100s ea	00761-0711-20	5.40	
ANTIOXIDANT ULTRA FORMULA (Rugby)			
SGL,PO (SOFTGEL)			
60s ea	00536-5589-08	13.43	
ANTIOXIDANT VISION VITAMINS (Mason Vit)			
TAB,PO (PF,SF)			
60s ea	11845-0122-95	6.11	
ANTIOXIDANT VITAMINS (Medicine Shoppe)			
TAB,PO, 60s ea	49614-0323-72	7.99	7.99
ANTIOXIDANT WITH CO Q-10 (Major)			
TAB,PO (PF,SF,GLUTEN-FREE)			
60s ea	00904-5907-52	5.49	
ANTISEPTIC CLEANSER (Family Phcy)			
SOL,MM (PRIVATE LABEL)			
10%, 60 ml	52735-0113-36	5.39	5.99
ANTISEPTIC CLEANSING (AmerisourceBergen)			
PAD,TP (PRIVATE LABEL)			
100s ea	24385-0200-33	4.49	4.99
ANTISEPTIC I.V. PREP (Animas Corp.)			
PAD,TP (WIPES)			
70%, 50s ea	65781-0610-50	16.77	
ANTISEPTIC MOUTH RINSE (Cardinal Health)			
SOL,MM (PRIVATE LABEL)			
1000 ml	37205-0318-45	2.02	
ANTISEPTIC MOUTHWASH BLUE MINT (Cardinal Health)			
SOL,MM (PRIVATE LABEL)			
1000 ml	37205-0664-45	2.02	
ANTISEPTIC WIPES (Family Phcy)			
PAD,TP (PRIVATE LABEL)			
100s ea	52735-0701-01	4.49	4.99
ANTISEPTIC WOUND & SKIN CLEANSER (MPM Medical Inc.)			
SPR,TP (1X60ML)			
0.1%, 60 ml	66977-0032-02	3.61	4.01
240 ml	66977-0032-08	9.34	10.37
ANTITUSSIN (Global Source)			
SYR,PO, 100 mg/5 ml,			
120 ml	59618-0061-33	2.00	
ANU-MED NF (Major)			
SUP,RC (NEW FORMULA)			
0.25%, 12s ea	00904-7688-22	2.95	
ANXIETY RELIEF (Similasan Corp.)			
PEL,PO (1X15GM)			
15 x-12 x, 15 gm	59262-0602-30	6.21	10.99
AODISC (Ciba Vision)			
TEF,NA (CATALYST)			
ea	47113-0687-01	3.80	
AOSEPT (Ciba Vision)			
DEV,NA (HOLDER/CUP)			
ea	47113-0605-20	4.20	
SOL,NA, 120 ml	47113-0605-04	2.50	
240 ml	47113-0605-00	4.70	
360 ml	47113-0605-12	5.80	
APAP (Bio-Pharm)			
ELI,PO (AF)			
160 mg/5 ml,			
120 ml	59741-0101-04	2.25	
240 ml	59741-0101-08	3.25	
480 ml	59741-0101-16	4.55	
(CHERRY)			
160 mg/5 ml,			
3840 ml	59741-0101-20	27.25	
SOL,PO (DROPS)			
80 mg/0.8 ml,			
15 ml	59741-0102-15	2.25	
(Consolidated Midland)			
ELI,PO, 160 mg/5 ml,			
325 ml	00223-6211-00	2.10	
480 ml	00223-6211-01	4.80	
TAB,PO, 325 mg, 100s ea	00223-6211-03	1.80	

PROD/MFR	HRI, UPC,NDC	AWP	SRP
1000s ea	00223-6404-01	14.50	
500 mg, 100s ea	00223-0053-01	2.00	
1000s ea	00223-0053-02	17.50	
(Medique)			
TAB,PO (12X2,SF)			
325 mg, 24s ea UD	47682-0145-64	1.34	
(75X2,SF)			
325 mg, 150s ea UD	47682-0145-36	5.89	
(125X2,SF)			
325 mg, 250s ea UD	47682-0145-48	9.35	
(250X2,SF)			
325 mg, 500s ea UD	47682-0145-13	15.86	
APAP 500 (Cypress Pharm)			
SOL,PO (AF,SF,CHERRY)			
500 mg/5 ml, 237 ml	60258-0050-08	12.77	
APAP EXTRA STRENGTH (Medique)			
TAB,PO (4X2, EXTRA STRENGTH)			
500 mg, 8s ea UD	47682-0175-30	0.81	
(12X2, EXTRA STRENGTH)			
500 mg, 24s ea UD	47682-0175-64	1.70	
(50X2)			
500 mg, 100s ea UD	47682-0175-33	5.69	
((125X2),EXTRA STRENGTH)			
500 mg, 250s ea UD	47682-0175-48	11.39	
(250X2)			
500 mg, 500s ea UD	47682-0175-13	21.40	
(Phys Total Care)			
REPACK			
TAB,PO, 500 mg, 50s ea	54868-3832-01	7.56	
100s ea	54868-2457-02	7.47	
1000s ea	54868-2457-01	57.35	
(CAPLET)			
500 mg, 1000s ea	54868-3832-00	37.05	
APATATE (Kenwood)			
LIQ,PO, 120 ml	00482-0130-13	34.07	
240 ml	00482-0130-14	60.98	
APETIGEN (Kramer-Novis)			
ELI,PO (AF,SF)			
120 ml	52083-0321-04	5.00	
(SF)			
240 ml	52083-0321-08	8.85	
APETIGEN PLUS (Kramer-Novis)			
LIQ,PO, 120 ml	52083-0329-04	6.85	
240 ml	52083-0329-08	12.10	
TAB,PO, 60s ea	52083-0352-60	16.00	
APETIMAR (Marlop)			
SOL,PO, 240 ml	12939-0998-31	7.40	
APHEDRID (Albertson's)			
TAB,PO, 60 mg-2.5 mg,			
24s ea	12810-0434-62	1.83	
100s ea	12810-0434-78	4.44	
APIS (Walker Pharmacal)			
TAB,SL (6X)			
250s ea	00619-0184-02	2.97	
APIS MEL (Luyties)			
TAB,SL (6X)			
6 x, 500s ea	00618-0184-03	3.99	
5500s ea	00618-0184-10	30.32	
(30X)			
12 x, 500s ea	00622-0184-03	4.19	
5500s ea	00622-0184-10	31.83	
(12X)			
30 x, 500s ea	00624-0184-03	4.19	
5500s ea	00624-0184-10	31.83	
APLICARE ANTIBACTERIAL (Aplicare)			
LOT,TP, 0.3%, 118 ml	52380-1865-04	1.75	
355 ml	52380-1865-03	4.68	
3785 ml	52380-1865-09	31.27	
APLICARE ANTISEPTIC CHLORHEXIDINE GLUCONATE (Aplicare)			
SOL,TP (SCRUB)			
2%, 118 ml	52380-1274-04	3.76	
4%, 118 ml	52380-1272-04	5.68	
237 ml	52380-1272-08	7.09	
473 ml	52380-1272-06	9.76	
946 ml	52380-1272-07	14.53	
3800 ml	52380-1272-09	50.72	
APLICARE ANTISEPTIC GEL HAND RINSE (Aplicare)			
GEL,TP (LATEX-FREE)			
62%, 118 ml	52380-1614-04	1.45	
(W/PUMP,LATEX-FREE)			
62%, 355 ml	52380-1614-03	5.04	
(LATEX-FREE)			
62%, 473 ml	52380-1614-06	4.51	
APLICARE ANTISEPTIC PERINEAL WASH (Aplicare)			
SPR,TP, 0.2%, 118 ml	52380-1617-04	1.87	
237 ml	52380-1617-08	3.17	
3785 ml	52380-1617-09	27.77	
APLICARE IODOPHOR PVP PREP (Aplicare)			
PAD,TP, 10%, 200s ea	52380-0001-05	13.40	
APLICARE ISOPROPYL ALCOHOL (Aplicare)			
GEL,TP (FRAGRANCE-FREE)			
70%, 118 ml	52380-1771-04	1.93	
APLICARE NINE CASTILE SOAP (Aplicare)			
LIQ,TP, 9 ml 125s	52380-9012-06	22.81	
APLICARE ONE HYDROGEN PEROXIDE (Aplicare)			
SOL,TP, 3%, 30 ml 20s	52380-0013-01	7.22	
APLICARE ONE IODOPHOR PVP (Aplicare)			
SOL,TP, 10%, 30 ml 20s	52380-0001-01	9.95	
SWA,TP, 10%, 50s ea	52380-1101-04	9.72	
APLICARE ONE IODOPHOR PVP SCRUB (Aplicare)			
SWA,TP, 7.5%, 50s ea	52380-1102-04	11.51	
APLICARE ONE ISOPROPYL ALCOHOL (Aplicare)			
LIQ,TP, 70%, 30 ml 20s	52380-0005-01	11.00	
APLICARE PHYSICIAN'S ANTIBACTERIAL (Aplicare)			
LOT,TP, 0.3%, 118 ml	52380-1845-04	1.61	
3785 ml	52380-1845-09	38.88	
APLICARE POVIDONE-IODINE (Aplicare)			
GEL,TP (LATEX-FREE)			
10%, 118 ml	52380-1738-04	2.71	
OIN,TP (200X1GM,LATEX-FREE)			
10%, 1 gm 200s	52380-0026-01	25.58	
SOL,TP (LATEX-FREE)			
10%, 59 ml	52380-1905-02	1.21	
118 ml	52380-1905-04	1.30	
237 ml	52380-1905-08	2.63	
473 ml	52380-1905-06	3.84	
946 ml	52380-1905-07	7.32	
3785 ml	52380-1905-09	24.68	
SPR,TP (USP)			
10%, 59 ml	52380-1905-00	5.74	
APLICARE POVIDONE-IODINE PREP (Aplicare)			
SWA,TP, 10%, 100s ea	52380-1721-01	28.60	
APLICARE POVIDONE-IODINE SCRUB (Aplicare)			
SOL,TP (LATEX-FREE)			
7.5%, 59 ml	52380-1855-02	1.42	
118 ml	52380-1855-04	1.54	
237 ml	52380-1855-08	2.59	
473 ml	52380-1855-06	4.32	
946 ml	52380-1855-07	7.82	
3785 ml	52380-1855-09	28.60	
APLICARE THREE IODOPHOR PVP (Aplicare)			
SWA,TP, 10%, 25s ea	52380-3101-05	9.44	
APLICARE THREE IODOPHOR PVP SCRUB (Aplicare)			
SWA,TP, 7.5%, 25s ea	52380-3102-05	10.48	
APPEAREX (Merz)			
TAB,PO, 2.5 mg, 28s ea	02590-0111-28	12.59	
84s ea	02590-0112-84	21.58	
APPLE BRAN (Freeda)			
CTB,PO (PF,SF,DYE-FREE)			
650 mg, 100s ea	10432-0259-01	5.85	9.75
APPLE CIDER VINEGAR DIET COMPLEX (Major)			
TAB,PO, 90s ea	00904-5595-89	7.50	
APRODINE (Major)			
TAB,PO, 60 mg-2.5 mg,			
24s ea	00904-0250-24	2.60	
100s ea	00904-0250-59	4.50	
AQUA CARE (Numark)			
CRE,TP, 10%, 75 gm	38485-0980-35	7.92	
LOT,TP, 10%, 240 ml	38485-0980-18	7.92	
AQUA DE AZAHAR FLAR (Flar Medicine)			
SOL,PO, 180 ml	53154-0020-21	1.25	
240 ml	53154-0020-08	1.95	
AQUA GEM-E (Carlson,J.R.)			
SGL,PO (SOFTGEL)			
400 iu, 60s ea	88395-0008-40	9.95	19.90
120s ea	88395-0008-41	17.75	35.50
AQUA GLYCOLIC FACE (Merz)			
CRE,TP, 60 gm	02590-0128-02	13.79	
AQUA GLYCOLIC FACIAL CLEANSER (Merz)			
SOL,TP, 180 ml	02596-0019-06	11.41	
AQUA GLYCOLIC HAND & BODY (Merz)			
LOT,TP, 180 ml	02596-0018-06	14.48	
AQUA GLYCOLIC SHAMPOO/BODY CLEANSER (Merz)			
SOL,TP, 240 ml	02596-0021-08	8.26	
AQUA GLYCOLIC TONER (Merz)			
SOL,TP, 177 ml	02596-0020-06	9.21	
AQUA LUBE (Mayer)			
GEL,TP (WATER BASED)			
60 gm	16169-0510-02	4.56	
120 gm	16169-0510-04	6.48	
AQUA LUBE ADVANCED FORMULA (Mayer)			
GEL,TP (WATER BASED)			
120 gm	16169-0520-04	7.80	
AQUA VELVA CLASSIC ICE BLUE (Combe)			
SOL,TP (FIRMS & TONES)			
103 ml	11509-0211-32	2.92	
206 ml	11509-0211-61	4.79	
AQUA VELVA ICE SPORT (Combe)			
SOL,TP (VITAMIN ENRICHED)			
103 ml	11509-0211-54	2.92	
AQUA VELVA MUSK (Combe)			
SOL,TP (AFTERSHAVE COLOGNE)			
103 ml	11509-0206-32	2.92	
AQUA-BAN (Blairex)			
TAB,PO, 50 mg, 30s ea	50486-0065-30	2.40	
AQUABALM (Quintess Corp)			
CRE,TP, 114 gm	53982-0301-12	4.49	
454 gm	53982-0301-08	8.98	
AQUACEL HYDROFIBER DRESSING (Convatec)			
DEV,NA (3/4"X18", ROPE)			
5s ea	68455-0107-43	57.55	75.64
(6"X6",STERILE)			
5s ea	68455-0107-22	93.44	122.81
(2"X2",STERILE)			
10s ea	68455-0107-20	50.33	66.15
(4"X4")			
10s ea	68455-0107-21	86.54	113.74
AQUADEKS (Axcan)			
SGL,PO (SOFTGEL)			
60s ea	58914-0011-06	36.23	
SUS,PO (W/GRADUATED DROPPER)			
60 ml	58914-0214-60	25.08	
AQUADERM (Teva)			
CRE,TP (FRAGRANCE-FREE)			
120 gm	00575-2002-04	11.69	
AQUAFILTER (Lee Pharm)			
DEV,NA, 3s ea	23558-0690-90	0.72	
10s ea	23558-0691-00	1.79	
(10X12)			
120s ea	23558-0691-08	21.46	
(3X48)			
144s ea	23558-0690-91	34.56	
(3X72)			
216s ea	23558-0690-92	51.84	
(10X24)			
240s ea	23558-0691-05	42.91	
(10X3X12)			
432s ea	23558-0691-07	64.37	
(12X36)			
432s ea	23558-0691-01	64.37	
(3X144)			
432s ea	23558-0690-93	103.68	
(10X72)			
720s ea	23558-0691-04	128.74	
(10X12X12)			
1440s ea	23558-0691-03	257.47	
(10X144)			
1440s ea	23558-0691-02	257.47	
AQUAFLEX (Parker)			
PAD,TP (2CM X 9CM, GEL)			
6s ea	00341-0004-02	25.68	42.80
AQUAFRESH (Glaxo)			
PAS,DE (CAVITY PROTECTION)			
0.15%, 70.5 gm	53100-0320-00	1.56	
(SENSITIVE)			
0.15%, 121.9 gm	53100-0324-20	2.28	
(FLUOR. PROTECTION,PUMP)			
0.15%, 130.4 gm	53100-0003-11	1.56	
(FLUORIDE PROTECTION)			
0.15%, 130.4 gm	53100-0321-00	1.56	
(SENSITIVE)			
0.15%, 168 gm	53100-0324-30	2.72	
170 gm	53100-0333-00	1.86	
(PUMP)			
0.15%, 170 gm	53100-0004-30	1.86	
(EXTRA FRESH,AF)			
0.15%, 181.4 gm	53100-0322-50	1.86	
(FLUOR. PROTECTION,PUMP)			
0.15%, 181.4 gm	53100-0003-18	1.86	

PROD/MFR	HRI, UPC,NDC	AWP	SRP
(FLUORIDE PROTECTION)			
0.15%, 181.4 gm	53100-0322-10	1.86	
(SENSITIVE)			
0.15%, 228 gm	53100-0324-35	3.22	
(EXTRA FRESH,AF)			
0.15%, 232.4 gm	53100-0325-50	2.23	
(FLUORIDE PROTECTION)			
0.15%, 232.4 gm	53100-0325-00	2.23	
AQUAFRESH ADVANCED (Glaxo)			
PAS,DE (1X158.8GM)			
0.14%, 158.8 gm	53100-0341-25	2.72	
AQUAFRESH CAVITY PROTECTION (Glaxo)			
PAS,DE (1X23GM)			
0.15%, 23 gm	53100-0005-97	0.38	
39.6 gm	53100-0003-24	0.43	
AQUAFRESH DEEP ACTION (Glaxo)			
DEV,NA (MEDIUM)			
ea	53100-0005-25	2.72	
(SOFT)			
ea	53100-0005-05	2.72	
AQUAFRESH DIRECT PLUS (Glaxo)			
DEV,NA (MEDIUM)			
ea	53100-0005-50	1.86	
(SOFT)			
ea	53100-0005-40	1.86	
AQUAFRESH DR SEUSS (Glaxo)			
DEV,NA (EXTRA SOFT)			
ea	53100-0001-33	1.86	
PAS,DE (SF,BUBBLE FRESH)			
0.15%, 130.4 gm	53100-0006-10	1.86	
AQUAFRESH EXTRA FRESH WHITENING (Glaxo)			
PAS,DE (WHITENING,TUBE)			
0.15%, 170 gm	53100-0336-51	2.72	
AQUAFRESH EXTREME CLEAN (Glaxo)			
PAS,DE (1X23GM,MINT)			
0.15%, 23 gm	53100-0005-79	0.65	
36.8 gm	53100-0005-61	0.73	
(WHITENING)			
0.15%, 36.8 gm	53100-0005-65	0.73	
121.9 gm	53100-0338-76	2.28	
(EMPOWERMINT)			
0.15%, 121.9 gm	53100-0338-96	2.28	
(WHITENING)			
0.15%, 121.9 gm	53100-0338-82	2.28	
158.7 gm	53100-0338-75	2.72	
(ARCTIC COOL)			
0.15%, 158.7 gm	53100-0339-81	2.72	
(EMPOWERMINT)			
0.15%, 158.7 gm	53100-0338-97	2.72	
(WHITENING)			
0.15%, 158.7 gm	53100-0338-83	2.72	
198.4 gm	53100-0338-99	3.22	
(EMPOWERMINT)			
0.15%, 198.4 gm	53100-0338-98	3.22	
(WHITENING)			
0.15%, 198.4 gm	53100-0338-84	3.22	
AQUAFRESH FOR KIDS (Glaxo)			
PAS,DE (PUMP,BUBBLEMINT)			
0.15%, 130.4 gm	53100-0003-03	1.56	
AQUAFRESH GEL FLEX (Glaxo)			
DEV,NA (MEDIUM)			
ea	53100-0002-65	2.72	
(SOFT)			
ea	53100-0002-55	2.72	
AQUAFRESH WHITE & SHINE (Glaxo)			
PAS,DE (BERRY FRESH)			
0.15%, 170 gm	53100-0361-75	2.72	
(DUAL ACTION)			
0.15%, 170 gm	53100-0361-00	2.72	
AQUAFRESH WHITE TRAYS (Glaxo)			
GEL,DE, 14s ea	53100-0442-00	32.28	
AQUAFRESH WHITENING (Glaxo)			
GEL,DE, 0.15%, 180 gm	53100-0335-50	2.72	
AQUAGEL (Parker)			
GEL,TP ((LUBRICATING),20X142GM)			
142 gm 20s	00341-0057-05	19.67	32.50
AQUALACTEN (Merz)			
LOT,TP, 473 ml	02596-0017-16	18.71	
AQUAMED (Merz)			
LOT,TP (1X473ML)			
473 ml	02596-0002-16	14.95	
AQUANIL (Person & Covey)			
LOT,TP, 240 ml	00096-0724-08	5.00	
480 ml	00096-0724-16	7.62	
AQUANIL HC (Person & Covey)			
LOT,TP, 1%, 120 ml	00096-0732-04	11.60	

PROD/MFR	HRI, UPC,NDC	AWP	SRP
AQUAPHILIC (Medco Lab)			
OIN,TP, 150 gm 12s	11940-0103-15	45.00	
180 gm	11940-0103-09	3.75	
454 gm	11940-0103-06	7.00	
AQUAPHILIC W/CARBAMIDE (Medco Lab)			
OIN,TP, 10%, 180 gm	11940-2113-09	4.25	
454 gm	11940-2113-06	8.00	
20%, 454 gm	11940-1118-06	8.50	
AQUAPHOR (Beiersdorf)			
OIN,TP, 50 gm	72140-0452-31		4.99
(Pharma Pac)			
REPACK			
OIN,TP, 50 gm	52959-0040-50	7.50	
(Phys Total Care)			
REPACK			
OIN,TP (1X50GM)			
50 gm	54868-6013-00	8.14	
396 gm	54868-5870-00	17.68	
AQUAPHOR BABY HEALING OINTMENT (Beiersdorf)			
OIN,TP (1X85GM)			
41%, 85 gm	72140-0633-77		7.99
AQUAPHOR HEALING OINTMENT (Beiersdorf)			
OIN,TP (1X99GM,FRAGRANCE-FREE)			
41%, 99 gm	72140-0032-63		8.49
(1X396GM,FRAGRANCE-FREE)			
41%, 396 gm	72140-0636-08		16.99
AQUASATE (Quintess Corp)			
OIN,TP (PF,FRAGRANCE-FREE)			
100 gm	53982-0303-12	5.91	
AQUASOL E (Hospira)			
SOL,PO (DROPS)			
15 iu/0.3 ml, 12 ml	61703-0419-77	36.20	
(W/DROPPER,DROPS)			
15 iu/0.3 ml, 12 ml	66591-0800-12	32.35	
(1X30ML,DROPS)			
15 iu/0.3 ml, 30 ml	61703-0419-78	68.68	
(W/DROPPER,DROPS)			
15 iu/0.3 ml, 30 ml	66591-0800-30	68.68	
AQUASONIC 100 (Parker)			
GEL,TP (48X20GM)			
20 gm 48s	00341-0001-01	44.11	73.15
(12X60GM)			
60 gm 12s	00341-0001-02	12.96	21.60
250 ml 12s	00341-0001-08	20.63	34.35
(DISPENSER BOTTLE)			
1000 ml 12s	00341-0001-34	64.80	108.00
(SONICPAC W/DISPENSER)			
5000 ml	00341-0001-50	16.04	25.85
AQUASONIC CLEAR (Parker)			
GEL,TP (12X60GM)			
60 gm 12s	00341-0003-02	12.96	21.60
(12X250ML)			
250 ml 12s	00341-0003-08	21.30	35.35
(SONICPAC-DISPENSER)			
1000 ml	00341-0003-34	33.05	110.20
(SONIC PAC)			
5000 ml	00341-0003-50	16.60	26.45
(ECONOPAC, 4X5000ML)			
5000 ml 4s	00341-0003-54	54.85	92.80
AQUAVIT-E (Cypress Pharm)			
SOL,PO (BUTTERSCOTCH,DROPS)			
15 iu/0.3 ml, 30 ml	60258-0111-30	64.00	
ARGINAID (Nestle)			
PDR,PO (4X14,PKT,CHERRY)			
4.5 gm/9.2 gm, 9.2 gm 56s	00212-5984-75	64.85	
(4X14,PKT,LEMON)			
4.5 gm/9.2 gm, 9.2 gm 56s	00212-5985-75	64.85	
(4X14,PKT,ORANGE)			
4.5 gm/9.2 gm, 9.2 gm 56s	00212-5983-75	64.85	
ARGININE (Bio-Tech Pharm)			
CAP,PO, 500 mg, 100s ea	53191-0210-01	7.35	
700 mg, 100s ea	53191-0365-01	9.00	
(VITAFLO, LLC)			
PDS,PO, 0.5 gm/4 gm, 30s ea	50600-0546-92	120.00	150.00
(Carlson,J.R.)			
L-ARGININE			
POW,PO, 1500 mg/dose, 100 gm	88395-0067-35	8.98	17.95

PROD/MFR	HRI, UPC,NDC	AWP	SRP
(Neurovites)			
TAB,PO, 500 mg, 100s ea	93595-2025-01	18.50	25.50
(Key Company)			
L-ARGININE-500			
TAB,PO (SF)			
500 mg, 60s ea	11694-0813-01	6.00	
250s ea	11694-0813-02	20.00	
500s ea	11694-0813-05	38.00	
ARGLAES FILM (Medline)			
DEV,NA (2 3/8"X3 1/3",STERILE)			
ea	53329-0300-34	28.75	
(4 3/4"X10",STERILE)			
ea	53329-0300-36	46.73	
(4"X4 3/4",STERILE)			
ea	53329-0300-35	35.59	
ARGLAES FILM POST-OP (Medline)			
DEV,NA (3 1/4"X14")			
10s ea	53329-0303-55	45.84	
ARGLAES ISLAND (Medline)			
DEV,NA (2-3/8X3-1/8,ALGINATEPAD)			
ea	53329-0301-34	31.48	
(4-3/4"X10",ALGINATEPAD)			
ea	53329-0301-36	66.40	
(4"X4 3/4",ALGINATE PAD)			
ea	53329-0301-35	39.30	
ARGLAES POWDER (Medline)			
POW,NA (ANTIMICROBIAL BARRIER)			
5 gm 20s	53329-0305-09	247.21	
(LATEX-FREE)			
10 gm 20s	53329-0304-09	529.95	
ARGYLE AUTOTRANSFUSION ACCESSORY UNIT (Covidien)			
DEV,NA, 5s ea	08080-7131-84	350.00	
ARGYLE CAROTID ARTERY SHUNT KIT (Covidien)			
DEV,NA (6",15CM)			
10s ea	08080-5777-75	289.33	
(8,10,12,14 FR,11IN)			
10s ea	08080-5777-00	312.50	
ARGYLE CLINICAL PRODUCTS EMERSON PUMP ADAPTER (Covidien)			
DEV,NA, 24s ea	08080-8472-30	100.65	
ARGYLE CLINICAL PRODUCTS TUBING SET (Covidien)			
DEV,NA, 6s ea	08080-8472-61	116.25	
(9/32")			
12s ea	08080-8472-96	167.64	
12s ea	88847-0261-00	115.10	
ARGYLE EZ-FLO (Covidien)			
DEV,NA (1-WAY W/PORT COVERS)			
50s ea	08080-1731-04	35.75	
(1WAYW/ADAPTR&PORT COVRS)			
50s ea	08080-1730-05	44.85	
(3-WAY W/PORT COVERS)			
50s ea	08080-1735-18	40.30	
(3-WAY)			
50s ea	08080-1735-00	36.40	
(3WAYW/20"EXT SET&COVERS)			
50s ea	08080-1735-26	77.99	
(3WAYW/33"EXT SET&COVERS)			
50s ea	08080-1735-34	87.35	
(3WAYW/INJ STE&20"EXTSET)			
50s ea	08080-1732-03	98.84	
(3WAYW/LOCK ADPTER&COVRS)			
50s ea	08080-1736-90	60.45	
(4WAYW/20"EXT SET&COVERS)			
50s ea	08080-1742-01	95.82	
(4WAYW/LOCKADAPTR&COVERS)			
50s ea	08080-1746-98	83.20	
(DOUBLE3WAYW/ADPTER&CVRS)			
50s ea	08080-1735-42	117.00	
ARGYLE FEEDING TUBE (Covidien)			
DEV,NA (1.7MMX41CM)			
50s ea	08888-2608-02	51.25	
ARGYLE FERGUSON LEFT VENTRICULAR VENT (Covidien)			
DEV,NA (X-RAY OPAQUE,SENTINEL)			
10s ea	08080-5900-18	300.00	
ARGYLE FERGUSON THORACIC CATHETER (Covidien)			
DEV,NA (28 FR)			
10s ea	08080-5720-40	245.00	
(32 FR)			
10s ea	08080-5720-57	245.00	
(36 FR)			
10s ea	08080-5720-65	322.50	
ARGYLE LEFT VENTRICULAR SUMP VENT (Covidien)			
DEV,NA (14 FR,20IN)			
10s ea	08080-5902-08	300.00	

PROD/MFR HRI, UPC,NDC AWP SRP

(18 FR,20IN)
10s ea 08080-5902-16 300.00
(20 FR,20IN)
10s ea 08080-5902-24 300.00

ARGYLE NEW AQUA-SEAL CHEST DRAINAGE
(Covidien)
DEV,NA, 5s ea 08080-5712-99 275.63
(AUTOTRANSFUSION CDU)
5s ea 08080-5713-15 236.32
(DUAL DRAIN CDU)
5s ea 08080-5714-06 343.25

ARGYLE PARALLEL "Y" CONNECTOR (Covidien)
DEV,NA, 5s ea 08080-5849-12 62.50

ARGYLE RIGHT ANGLE THORACIC CATHETER
(Covidien)
DEV,NA (16 FR,20")
10s ea 08080-5710-18 92.75
(20 FR,20")
10s ea 08080-5710-26 92.75
(24 FR,20")
10s ea 08080-5710-34 92.75
(28 FR,20")
10s ea 08080-5710-42 92.75
(32 FR,20")
10s ea 08080-5710-59 92.75
(36 FR,20")
10s ea 08080-5710-67 92.75
(40 FR,20")
10s ea 08080-5710-75 92.75

ARGYLE SARATOGA SUMP DRAIN (Covidien)
DEV,NA (16 FR,12")
10s ea 08080-5305-19 150.00
(20 FR,12")
10s ea 08080-5305-27 150.00
(20 FR,20")
10s ea 08080-5310-20 150.00
(24 FR,20")
10s ea 08080-5310-38 150.00
(28 FR,12")
10s ea 08080-5305-35 150.00
(28 FR,20")
10s ea 08080-5310-46 150.00

ARGYLE SENTINEL LOOPS (Covidien)
DEV,NA (BLUE/REGULAR)
100s ea 08080-5852-08 25.00
(BLUE/SMALL)
100s ea 08080-5852-40 25.00
(RED/REGULAR)
100s ea 08080-5852-16 25.00
(RED/SMALL)
100s ea 08080-5852-57 25.00
(WHITE/REGULAR)
100s ea 08080-5852-32 25.00
(WHITE/SMALL)
100s ea 08080-5852-73 25.00
(YELLOW/REGULAR)
100s ea 08080-5852-24 25.00
(YELLOW/SMALL)
100s ea 08080-5852-65 25.00

ARGYLE SENTINEL SEAL CHEST DRAINAGE
(Covidien)
DEV,NA, 5s ea 08080-5715-62 282.63
(AUTOTRANSFUSION CDU)
5s ea 08080-5714-89 300.00
(DUAL DRAIN CDU)
5s ea 08080-5715-13 399.44

ARGYLE SILICONE MEDIASTINAL CATHETER
(Covidien)
DEV,NA (28FR,20")
10s ea 08080-5735-50 171.88
(34FR,20")
10s ea 08080-5735-68 171.88

ARGYLE SILICONE RIGHT ANGLE THORACIC CATHETER (Covidien)
DEV,NA (28FR,20")
10s ea 08080-5730-48 147.50
(32FR,20")
10s ea 08080-5730-22 149.38
10s ea 08080-5730-55 147.50
(36FR,20")
10s ea 08080-5730-63 147.50

ARGYLE SILICONE STRAIGHT THORACIC CATHETER
(Covidien)
DEV,NA (28FR,20")
10s ea 08080-5725-52 106.88
(32FRX20",W/X-RAY LINE)
10s ea 08080-5725-60 106.88
(36FR,20")
10s ea 08080-5725-78 106.88
(40 FR,20")
10s ea 08080-5725-86 106.88

PROD/MFR HRI, UPC,NDC AWP SRP

ARGYLE STRAIGHT THORACIC CATHETER
(Covidien)
DEV,NA (12 FR,20")
10s ea 08080-5705-07 64.25
(16 FR,20")
10s ea 08080-5705-15 64.25
(20 FR,20")
10s ea 08080-5705-23 64.25
(24 FR,20")
10s ea 08080-5705-31 64.25
(28 FR,20")
10s ea 08080-5705-49 64.25
(32 FR,20")
10s ea 08080-5705-56 64.25
(36 FR,20")
10s ea 08080-5705-64 64.25
(40 FR,20")
10s ea 08080-5705-72 64.25

ARGYLE THI AORTIC PERFUSION CANNULA
(Covidien)
DEV,NA (ANGLED,3.3MM(10FR))
10s ea 08080-5910-08 262.50
(ANGLED,4.0MM(12FR))
10s ea 08080-5911-23 250.00
(ANGLED,4.7MM(14FR))
10s ea 08080-5910-24 262.50
(ANGLED,6.0MM(18FR))
10s ea 08080-5910-40 262.50
(ANGLED,7.0MM(21FR))
10s ea 08080-5910-65 250.00
(ANGLED,8.0MM(24FR))
10s ea 08080-5910-81 250.00
(STRAIGHT,6.0MM(18FR))
10s ea 08080-5910-57 262.50
(STRAIGHT,7.0MM(21FR))
10s ea 08080-5910-73 250.00
(STRAIGHT,8.0MM(24FR))
10s ea 08080-5910-99 250.00

ARGYLE THORA-SEAL ADAPTOR (Covidien)
DEV,NA (EMERSON PUMP ADAPTOR)
24s ea 08080-8472-35 175.00

ARGYLE THORA-SEAL III CHEST DRAINAGE
(Covidien)
DEV,NA (AUTOTRANSFUSION CDU)
3s ea 08080-7131-92 375.00
4s ea 08080-7133-08 220.50
(AUTOTRANSFUSION CDU)
4s ea 08080-7131-76 260.00
(REPLACEMENT CHAMBER)
6s ea 08080-8471-39 128.78

ARGYLE TROCAR THORACIC CATHETER (Covidien)
DEV,NA (10 FR,9")
10s ea 08080-5610-19 174.63
(12 FR,9")
10s ea 08080-5610-27 174.63
(16 FR,10")
10s ea 08080-5610-35 174.63
(20 FR,16")
10s ea 08080-5610-43 174.63
(24 FR,16")
10s ea 08080-5610-50 174.63
(28 FR,16")
10s ea 08080-5610-68 174.63
(32 FR,16")
10s ea 08080-5610-76 174.63
(8 FR,9")
10s ea 08080-5608-05 174.63

ARGYLE TUBING EXTENSION SET (Covidien)
DEV,NA (LATEX-FREE)
24s ea 08080-8471-42 206.54

ARGYLE VASCULAR TORNIQUET KIT (Covidien)
DEV,NA (5",13CM)
10s ea 08080-5850-00 64.15

ARNICA (Boiron)
CRE,TP (NON-GREASY,PERFUME-FREE)
1 x, 40 gm 00220-0513-60 3.71 6.19
GEL,TP, 7%, 45 gm 06960-0511-54 3.71 6.19
75 gm 06962-0035-59 5.86 9.79
(W/1 MULTIDOSE TUBE)
7%, 75 gm 06962-0747-24 7.44 12.39
OIN,TP, 4%, 30 gm 06960-0229-50 3.71 6.19

(Lex)
TIN,TP, 1.11%, 30 ml 49523-0039-01 0.92
60 ml 49523-0039-02 1.49

(Walker Pharmacal)
TAB,SL (6X)
250s ea 00619-0229-02 2.97

PROD/MFR HRI, UPC,NDC AWP SRP

(Weleda)
LIQ,PO (3X,DROPS)
50 ml 55946-0100-15 7.20
(6X)
50 ml 55946-0105-15 7.20

ARNICA ESSENCE (Weleda)
TP, 50 ml 55946-0110-15 7.20

ARNICA MONTANA (Luyties)
TAB,SL, 6 x, 500s ea 00618-0229-03 3.99
(6X)
6 x, 5500s ea 00618-0229-10 30.32
(30X)
12 x, 500s ea 00622-0229-03 4.19
5500s ea 00622-0229-10 31.83
30 x, 500s ea 00624-0229-03 4.19
(12X)
30 x, 5500s ea 00624-0229-10 31.83

ARNICALM ARTHRITIS (Boiron)
PEL,PO, 80s ea 06962-0005-03 3.87 6.49

ARNICALM TRAUMA (Boiron)
PEL,PO, 5 c-5 c-9 c,
80s ea 06962-0006-03 3.87 6.49

ARSENICUM (Walker Pharmacal)
TAB,SL (6X)
250s ea 00619-0230-02 2.97

ARSENICUM ALB (Luyties)
TAB,SL (6X)
6 x, 500s ea 00618-0230-03 3.99
5500s ea 00618-0230-10 30.32
(30X)
12 x, 500s ea 00622-0230-03 4.19
5500s ea 00622-0230-10 31.83
(12X)
30 x, 500s ea 00624-0230-03 4.19
5500s ea 00624-0230-10 31.83

ARTH-9 (Rx Vitamins)
CAP,PO, 120s ea 08429-0901-20 19.98 39.95

ARTHRICREAM (AmerisourceBergen)
CRE,TP (PRIVATE LABEL)
10%, 90 gm 24385-0165-53 3.86 4.29

(Cardinal Health)
CRE,TP (PRIVATE LABEL)
10%, 90 gm 37205-0198-21 3.76

(Family Phcy)
CRE,TP (PRIVATE LABEL)
10%, 90 gm 52735-0727-27 3.41 3.79

(Perrigo)
CRE,TP (STAINLESS)
10%, 85 gm 45802-0356-53 3.79

(Core)
REPACK
CRE,TP, 10%, 90 gm 33358-0034-03 5.63

ARTHRITIS PAIN FORMULA (Cardinal Health)
TER,PO (PRIVATE LABEL,CAPLET)
650 mg, 50s ea 37205-0034-71 5.36

(Medtech)
TAB,PO (CAPLET)
486 mg, 40s ea 75137-0271-10 4.53
100s ea 75137-0271-20 8.36

ARTHUR ITIS (Stellar Health)
CRE,TP, 0.025%-10%,
120 gm 89629-0019-40 16.00 24.98
LOT,TP (W/ALOE)
0.025%-10%, 105 ml 89629-0020-35 16.00 24.98

ARTIFICIAL TEARS (Cardinal Health)
SOL,OP (PRIVATE LABEL)
1.4%, 15 ml 37205-0137-05 2.40

(Chain Drug Marketing)
SOL,OP, 1.4%, 15 ml 63868-0223-05 1.26 5.99

(Consolidated Midland)
SOL,OP, 1.4%, 15 ml 00223-6009-15 2.75
30 ml 00223-6009-30 3.50

(Rugby)
OIN,OP (PF)
15%-83%, 3.5 gm 12s 00536-6550-91 44.39
SOL,OP, 1.4%, 15 ml 00536-1970-72 4.38

(A-S Medication)
REPACK
OIN,OP (PF)
3.5 gm 54569-1221-00 3.88
SOL,OP, 1.4%, 15 ml 54569-1231-00 3.69

(Altura)
REPACK
SOL,OP, 1.4%, 15 ml 63874-0054-15 5.58

PROD/MFR	HRI, UPC,NDC	AWP	SRP
(Nucare Pharm)			
REPACK			
SOL,OP, 15 ml	66267-0923-15	6.99	
(Palmetto)			
REPACK			
SOL,OP, 1.4%, 15 ml	23490-7857-00	6.95	
(Pharma Pac)			
REPACK			
SOL,OP, 15 ml	52959-0041-00	6.88	
(Phys Total Care)			
REPACK			
OIN,OP, 4 gm	54868-1650-00	15.00	
SOL,OP, 1.4%, 15 ml	54868-2496-01	18.18	
(Quality Care Prod)			
REPACK			
SOL,OP, 1.4%, 15 ml	49999-0133-15	13.60	
(Southwood)			
REPACK			
SOL,OP, 15 ml	58016-6201-01	5.31	
ARTIFICIAL TEARS PLUS			
(Consolidated Midland)			
SOL,OP, 15 ml	00223-6008-15	2.75	
30 ml	00223-6008-30	3.50	
ASC LOTIONIZED SKIN CLEANSER (Geritrex)			
LIQ,TP, 240 ml	92771-0251-08	1.82	
3840 ml	92771-0251-01	19.25	
ASCAREL (Pfeiffer)			
SUS,PO, 144 mg/ml,			
30 ml	00927-0726-31	5.28	9.49
ASCENSIA AUTODISC CONTROL			
(Bayer Diabetes Care)			
DEV,NA (NORMAL)			
ea	00193-3642-01	6.06	
(LOW & HIGH)			
2s ea	00193-3643-02	11.46	
ASCENSIA AUTODISC STRIPS (Phys Total Care)			
REPACK			
DEV,NA, 100s ea	54868-5797-00	115.33	
ASCENSIA AUTODISC TEST STRIPS			
(Bayer Diabetes Care)			
DEV,NA, 50s ea	00193-3610-50	60.48	
100s ea	00193-3627-21	110.82	
ASCO-CAPS-1000 (Key Company)			
CAP,PO (SF)			
1000 mg, 100s ea	11694-0722-01	10.50	
250s ea	11694-0722-25	25.00	
ASCO-CAPS-500 (Key Company)			
PO, 500 mg, 100s ea	11694-0984-01	8.50	
500s ea	11694-0984-03	39.00	
ASCOCID (Key Company)			
POW,PO (4300MG/5ML)			
240 gm	11694-0913-08	11.00	
(5000MG/5ML)			
240 gm	11694-0914-08	11.00	
(4300MG/5ML)			
480 gm	11694-0913-01	21.50	
(5000MG/5ML)			
480 gm	11694-0914-01	21.50	
4000 mg/5 ml,			
240 gm	11694-0845-06	12.00	
ASCOCID-1000 (Key Company)			
TER,PO, 1000 mg,			
100s ea	11694-0985-01	7.00	
250s ea	11694-0985-03	14.50	
1000s ea	11694-0985-02	55.00	
ASCOCID-500 (Key Company)			
TAB,PO, 500 mg, 100s ea	11694-0987-01	5.00	
ASCOCID-500-D (Key Company)			
TER,PO, 500 mg, 100s ea	11694-0986-01	5.50	
250s ea	11694-0986-03	11.00	
1000s ea	11694-0986-02	42.00	
ASCOCID-ISO-PH (Key Company)			
PDS,PO (BUFFERED,FRAGRANCE-FREE)			
150 gm	11694-0801-14	11.00	
480 gm	11694-0801-16	32.00	
ASCORBIC ACID (Palmetto)			
REPACK			
TAB,PO, 500 mg, 60s ea	23490-6888-06	4.90	
100s ea	23490-6888-01	5.36	
ASCRIPTIN (Novartis Consumer)			
TAB,PO (REGULAR STRENGTH)			
100s ea	00067-0149-10	7.62	
325 mg, 100s ea	00067-0145-68	7.19	
225s ea	00067-0145-77	13.85	
(Dispensing Solutions)			
REPACK			
TAB,PO, 60s ea	68258-2001-06	5.94	
(Phys Total Care)			
REPACK			
TAB,PO, 325 mg, 30s ea	54868-4094-00	3.60	
(Stat Rx)			
REPACK			
TAB,PO, 325 mg, 100s ea	16590-0783-71	10.34	
ASCRIPTIN MAXIMUM STRENGTH			
(Novartis Consumer)			
TAB,PO (CAPLET)			
500 mg, 85s ea	00067-0146-85	10.45	
ASPARATIC ACID (Carlson,J.R.)			
L-ASPARATIC ACID			
POW,PO, 1500 mg/dose,			
100 gm	88395-0067-55	3.75	7.50
ASPARTATE MG & K (Key Company)			
CAP,PO (SF)			
90 mg-90 mg, 100s ea	11694-0910-01	8.00	
250s ea	11694-0910-02	16.00	
ASPARTATE-700 (Key Company)			
PO (SF)			
40 mg-40 mg, 100s ea	11694-0824-01	9.00	
250s ea	11694-0824-04	20.00	
500s ea	11694-0824-05	37.00	
ASPEN (Ellon)			
SOL,SL (DROPS)			
10.5 ml	51762-0027-10		9.25
ASPER-FLEX (Geritrex)			
CRE,TP (24X85GM,ASPIRIN-FREE)			
10%, 85 gm 24s	54162-0010-03	66.00	
ASPERCREME (Phys Total Care)			
REPACK			
CRE,TP, 10%, 35 gm	54868-3617-00	5.21	
ASPERDRINK (St. Paul)			
TEF,PO (FRUIT)			
81 mg, 30s ea	23110-0144-30	6.49	6.49
ASPERGUM (Heritage/Insight)			
GUM,PO (CHERRY)			
227 mg, 12s ea	63736-0070-26	1.70	
(ORANGE)			
227 mg, 12s ea	63736-0070-28	1.70	
ASPI-COR (Health Products Corp)			
CTB,PO, 81 mg, 36s ea	39686-0014-91	1.60	
ECT,PO, 81 mg, 120s ea	39686-0014-92	4.50	
ASPIR 81 (Prime Marketing)			
ECT,PO, 81 mg, 120s ea	62107-0027-26	2.90	
1000s ea	62107-0027-32	17.50	
ASPIR-LOW (Major)			
TAB,PO, 81 mg, 120s ea	00904-7704-18	5.59	
250s ea	00904-7704-70	6.40	
1000s ea	00904-7704-80	20.99	
ASPIR-TRIN (Mason Vit)			
ECT,PO, 325 mg, 100s ea	11845-0706-01	2.78	
1000s ea	11845-0706-04	19.89	
650 mg, 100s ea	11845-0899-01	4.33	
ASPIRIN (Advance)			
CTB,PO, 81 mg, 36s ea	17714-0009-36	1.49	
ECT,PO, 325 mg, 100s ea	17714-0011-01	1.99	
1000s ea	17714-0011-10	10.99	
TAB,PO, 325 mg, 100s ea	17714-0010-01	1.19	
1000s ea	17714-0010-10	6.95	
(Albertson's)			
CTB,PO, 81 mg, 36s ea	41280-0000-24	1.29	
ECT,PO, 325 mg, 100s ea	04000-0001-06	3.09	
100s ea	12810-0429-78	3.08	
TAB,PO, 325 mg, 100s ea	04000-0003-26	1.71	
(AmerisourceBergen)			
ECT,PO (PRIVATE LABEL)			
325 mg, 500s ea	24385-0429-90	9.89	11.00
(Basic Vitamins)			
ECT,PO, 325 mg, 100s ea	00761-0218-20	2.00	
(Chain Drug Marketing)			
ECT,PO, 325 mg, 100s ea	63868-0914-10	1.68	4.99
(Consolidated Midland)			
ECT,PO, 325 mg, 100s ea	00223-0332-01	1.95	
1000s ea	00223-0332-02	12.00	
SUP,RC, 60 mg, 12s ea	00223-5030-12	3.25	
100s ea	00223-5030-00	22.50	
1000s ea	00223-5030-02	110.00	
120 mg, 12s ea	00223-5031-12	3.60	
100s ea	00223-5031-00	24.00	
1000s ea	00223-5031-02	110.00	
200 mg, 12s ea	00223-5033-00	1.85	
100s ea	00223-5033-01	14.00	
1000s ea	00223-5033-02	112.50	
300 mg, 12s ea	00223-5034-12	3.60	
100s ea	00223-5034-00	25.00	
1000s ea	00223-5034-02	115.00	
600 mg, 12s ea	00223-5035-12	3.75	
100s ea	00223-5035-00	26.00	
TAB,PO, 325 mg, 100s ea	00223-0331-01	1.50	
1000s ea	00223-0331-03	9.00	
650 mg, 100s ea	00223-0335-01	3.50	
1000s ea	00223-0335-02	27.50	
(Family Phcy)			
ECT,PO (PRIVATE LABEL)			
325 mg, 500s ea	52735-0703-70	8.99	9.99
TAB,PO, 325 mg, 300s ea	52735-0702-09	5.39	5.99
(Geri-Care)			
ECT,PO, 325 mg, 100s ea	57896-0921-01	0.80	
1000s ea	57896-0921-10	5.80	
TAB,PO, 325 mg, 100s ea	57896-0901-01	0.54	
1000s ea	57896-0901-10	3.25	
(Global Source)			
TAB,PO, 325 mg, 100s ea	59618-0099-15	1.50	
100s ea	59618-0101-15	1.80	
(Hart Health)			
TAB,PO (2X12)			
325 mg, 24s ea UD	50332-0102-05	0.96	
(2X25)			
325 mg, 50s ea UD	50332-0102-03	1.21	
(2X50)			
325 mg, 100s ea UD	50332-0102-04	2.26	
(2X125)			
325 mg, 250s ea UD	50332-0102-02	4.70	
(2X500)			
325 mg, 1000s ea UD	50332-0102-01	17.46	
(Humco)			
TAB,PO, 325 mg, 100s ea	00395-0134-10	1.17	
(Magno-Humphries)			
ECT,PO, 325 mg, 100s ea	43292-0555-95	1.81	3.69
250s ea	43292-0556-11	3.30	6.99
TAB,PO, 325 mg, 250s ea	43292-0555-90	1.85	3.29
(Major)			
ECT,PO, 325 mg, 100s ea	00904-2013-60	2.65	
(BOXED)			
325 mg, 100s ea	00904-2011-59	2.75	
300s ea	00904-2013-72	6.55	
1000s ea	00904-2013-80	20.99	
TAB,PO, 325 mg, 60s ea	00904-2019-59	2.20	
100s ea	00904-2009-60	1.55	
(TRI-BUFFERED, BOXED)			
325 mg, 100s ea	00904-2015-59	3.00	
250s ea	00904-2009-70	2.90	
500s ea	00904-2009-40	5.12	
1000s ea	00904-2009-80	7.90	
1000s ea	00904-2019-80	11.49	
(Marlex)			
ECT,PO, 81 mg, 36s ea	10135-0173-36	0.70	
100s ea	10135-0173-01	0.90	
120s ea	10135-0173-62	0.95	
250s ea	10135-0173-69	1.65	
500s ea	10135-0173-05	2.65	
1000s ea	10135-0173-10	4.95	
325 mg, 16s ea	10135-0126-75	0.67	
20s ea	10135-0126-20	0.74	
30s ea	10135-0126-30	0.78	
50s ea	10135-0126-50	0.80	
60s ea	10135-0126-60	0.82	
90s ea	10135-0126-90	0.84	
100s ea	10135-0126-01	0.91	
(BLISTER PACK)			
325 mg, 100s ea UD	10135-0126-13	2.50	
(BOXED)			
325 mg, 100s ea	10135-0126-57	65.00	
250s ea	10135-0126-69	3.20	
300s ea	10135-0126-03	2.99	
1000s ea	10135-0126-10	5.76	
TAB,PO, 325 mg, 20s ea	10135-0150-20	0.65	
24s ea	10135-0150-24	0.66	
30s ea	10135-0150-30	0.68	
100s ea	10135-0150-01	0.74	
(BLISTER PACK)			
325 mg, 100s ea UD	10135-0150-13	2.35	
250s ea	10135-0150-69	1.56	
500s ea	10135-0150-05	2.55	
1000s ea	10135-0150-10	4.27	
(Mason Vit)			
TAB,PO, 325 mg, 100s ea	11845-0930-01	2.20	
(Medicine Shoppe)			
ECT,PO, 325 mg, 100s ea	49614-0113-78	4.49	4.49
250s ea	49614-0429-85	6.99	6.99

PROD/MFR	HRI, UPC,NDC	AWP	SRP
(Medique)			
TAB,PO (2X12)			
325 mg, 24s ea UD	**47682-0116-64**	1.30	
(100X2)			
325 mg, 200s ea UD	**47682-0116-47**	5.55	
(250X2)			
325 mg, 500s ea UD	**47682-0116-13**	11.95	
(Paddock)			
SUP,RC, 300 mg,			
12s ea UD	**00574-7034-12**	13.75	
600 mg, 12s ea UD	**00574-7036-12**	14.05	
(Perrigo)			
TAB,PO (LOW DOSE)			
81 mg, 300s ea	**45802-0642-87**	8.10	
(Pfeiffer)			
TAB,PO, 325 mg, 100s ea	**00927-0058-01**	1.11	1.99
(Prime Marketing)			
TAB,PO, 325 mg, 100s ea	**62107-0025-07**	2.90	
1000s ea	**62107-0025-32**	15.50	
(Qualitest)			
ECT,PO (REGULAR STRENGTH)			
325 mg, 90s ea	**00603-0169-02**	2.85	
100s ea	**00603-0169-21**	3.10	
(REGULAR STRENGTH)			
325 mg, 100s ea	**00603-0168-21**	3.10	
1000s ea	**00603-0169-32**	39.20	
TAB,PO, 325 mg, 100s ea	**00603-0031-21**	2.47	
300s ea	**00603-0031-25**	5.69	
(Rugby)			
ECT,PO, 81 mg, 120s ea	**00536-3086-41**	5.48	
1000s ea	**00536-3086-10**	45.66	
325 mg, 100s ea	**00536-3313-01**	4.20	
1000s ea	**00536-3313-10**	26.55	
TAB,PO, 325 mg, 100s ea	**00536-3305-01**	3.45	
1000s ea	**00536-3305-10**	20.25	
(Teva)			
ECT,PO, 325 mg, 100s ea	**00182-0448-01**	2.79	
1000s ea	**00182-0448-10**	18.50	
TAB,PO, 325 mg,			
1000s ea	**00182-0444-10**	12.08	
(Time-Cap)			
ECT,PO, 325 mg, 100s ea	**49483-0052-01**	4.20	
1000s ea	**49483-0052-10**	22.48	
TAB,PO, 325 mg, 100s ea	**49483-0011-01**	3.52	
1000s ea	**49483-0011-10**	15.76	
(A-S Medication)			
REPACK			
CTB,PO, 81 mg, 36s ea	**54569-5659-00**	2.78	
ECT,PO, 81 mg, 120s ea	**54569-4233-01**	5.75	
325 mg, 30s ea	**54569-0014-01**	0.93	
100s ea	**54569-0014-03**	3.10	
TAB,PO, 325 mg, 14s ea	**54569-0005-06**	0.31	
20s ea	**54569-0005-04**	0.44	
(250X2,UNIT OF USE)			
325 mg, 500s ea	**54569-5676-00**	11.59	
(Altura)			
REPACK			
ECT,PO, 325 mg, 7s ea	**63874-0997-07**	1.83	
10s ea	**63874-0997-10**	2.62	
14s ea	**63874-0997-14**	3.67	
15s ea	**63874-0997-15**	3.93	
20s ea	**63874-0997-02**	5.24	
30s ea	**63874-0997-30**	7.02	
40s ea	**63874-0997-40**	8.83	
60s ea	**63874-0997-60**	13.25	
90s ea	**63874-0997-90**	12.80	
100s ea	**63874-0997-01**	14.23	
TAB,PO, 325 mg, 15s ea	**63874-0001-15**	3.96	
20s ea	**63874-0001-20**	5.61	
30s ea	**63874-0001-30**	8.70	
100s ea	**63874-0001-01**	14.74	
250s ea	**63874-0001-25**	14.79	
500s ea	**63874-0001-50**	16.87	
(Bryant Ranch)			
REPACK			
ECT,PO, 81 mg, 120s ea	**63629-2825-01**	1.73	
(Core)			
REPACK			
ECT,PO, 81 mg, 30s ea	**33358-0035-30**	6.14	
120s ea	**33358-0035-01**	11.49	
325 mg, 30s ea	**33358-0036-30**	2.56	
100s ea	**33358-0036-00**	6.87	
(DHS, Inc.)			
REPACK			
TAB,PO, 325 mg, 30s ea	**55887-0690-30**	6.69	
(Dispensing Solutions)			
REPACK			
ECT,PO, 81 mg, 30s ea	**55045-2823-08**	2.40	
100s ea	**55045-2875-00**	6.00	
(HomeMed)			
REPACK			
ECT,PO, 325 mg, 16s ea	**51655-0377-74**	2.37	
20s ea	**51655-0377-52**	2.45	
30s ea	**51655-0377-24**	22.00	
60s ea	**51655-0377-25**	4.06	
90s ea	**51655-0377-26**	4.97	
TAB,PO, 325 mg, 20s ea	**51655-0068-52**	2.50	
24s ea	**51655-0068-30**	2.53	
(McKesson Packaging)			
REPACK			
CTB,PO, 81 mg,			
750s ea UD	**63739-0434-01**	71.40	
750s ea	**63739-0434-03**	71.40	
ECT,PO, 81 mg,			
100s ea UD	**63739-0272-10**	9.95	
(BLISTER PACK)			
81 mg, 750s ea UD	**63739-0272-01**	74.66	
(PUNCH CARD 25X30)			
81 mg, 750s ea	**63739-0272-03**	74.66	
(BLISTER PACK)			
325 mg, 750s ea UD	**63739-0023-01**	46.05	
(PUNCH CARD 25X30)			
325 mg, 750s ea	**63739-0023-03**	46.05	
TAB,PO (FILM-COATED)			
325 mg, 100s ea UD	**63739-0433-10**	5.00	
750s ea UD	**63739-0433-01**	31.88	
(Palmetto)			
REPACK			
ECT,PO, 81 mg, 30s ea	**23490-6612-01**	9.80	
120s ea	**23490-6612-02**	39.20	
325 mg, 30s ea	**23490-6607-01**	8.89	
100s ea	**23490-6607-02**	29.63	
(PD-Rx Pharm)			
REPACK			
ECT,PO, 81 mg, 35s ea	**55289-0886-35**	6.51	
90s ea	**55289-0886-90**	7.57	
100s ea	**55289-0886-01**	7.72	
325 mg, 35s ea	**55289-0191-30**	6.91	
90s ea UD	**55289-0191-90**	9.05	
100s ea	**55289-0191-01**	9.47	
650 mg, 100s ea	**55289-0356-01**	12.27	
TAB,PO, 325 mg, 24s ea	**55289-0743-24**	5.80	
50s ea	**55289-0474-50**	6.47	
(Pharma Pac)			
REPACK			
ECT,PO, 81 mg, 30s ea	**52959-0770-30**	2.49	
325 mg, 14s ea	**52959-0018-14**	3.60	
20s ea	**52959-0018-20**	5.05	
24s ea	**52959-0018-24**	5.41	
30s ea	**52959-0018-30**	6.74	
40s ea	**52959-0018-40**	8.80	
60s ea	**52959-0018-60**	12.68	
80s ea	**52959-0018-80**	16.23	
100s ea	**52959-0018-00**	13.60	
TAB,PO, 325 mg, 10s ea	**52959-0724-10**	4.75	
14s ea	**52959-0724-14**	6.32	
15s ea	**52959-0724-15**	6.65	
20s ea	**52959-0724-20**	8.25	
24s ea	**52959-0724-24**	9.21	
30s ea	**52959-0724-30**	10.50	
100s ea	**52959-0724-00**	15.79	
(Phys Total Care)			
REPACK			
ECT,PO, 325 mg, 30s ea	**54868-2405-02**	3.38	
100s ea	**54868-2405-03**	7.77	
1000s ea	**54868-2405-01**	148.26	
650 mg, 100s ea	**54868-1996-01**	10.02	
TAB,PO, 325 mg, 100s ea	**54868-1198-00**	7.53	
250s ea	**54868-1198-03**	28.62	
1000s ea	**54868-1198-02**	39.36	
(Quality Care Prod)			
REPACK			
TAB,PO, 325 mg, 30s ea	**49999-0813-30**	6.67	
100s ea	**49999-0813-00**	3.94	
(Southwood)			
REPACK			
ECT,PO, 325 mg, 20s ea	**58016-0225-20**	4.46	
30s ea	**58016-0225-30**	6.69	
60s ea	**58016-0225-60**	13.38	
100s ea	**58016-0225-00**	22.30	
SUP,RC, 120 mg, 12s ea	**58016-2013-01**	4.39	
TAB,PO, 325 mg, 100s ea	**58016-0207-00**	14.04	
(Stat Rx)			
REPACK			
ECT,PO, 325 mg, 7s ea	**16590-0826-07**	0.60	
30s ea	**16590-0826-30**	2.55	
TAB,PO, 81 mg, 7s ea	**16590-0420-07**	2.52	
21s ea	**16590-0420-21**	2.73	
30s ea	**16590-0420-30**	2.96	
(Cardinal Health)			
BUFFERED ASPIRIN			
TAB,PO (PRIVATE LABEL)			
325 mg, 100s ea	**37205-0150-78**	3.99	
(Geri-Care)			
TAB,PO, 325 mg, 100s ea	**57896-0931-01**	0.95	
1000s ea	**57896-0931-10**	5.95	
(Hart Health)			
TAB,PO (2X50)			
325 mg, 100s ea UD	**50332-0111-04**	3.05	
(2X125)			
325 mg, 250s ea UD	**50332-0111-02**	6.80	
(Ohm)			
TAB,PO, 325 mg, 100s ea	**51660-0021-01**	1.25	
200s ea	**51660-0021-02**	1.80	
1000s ea	**51660-0021-10**	6.95	
(Medique)			
TRI-BUFFERED ASPIRIN			
TAB,PO (125X2,SF)			
325 mg, 250s ea UD	**47682-0119-48**	10.35	
(250X2,SF)			
325 mg, 500s ea UD	**47682-0119-13**	19.25	
(Ohm)			
TAB,PO, 325 mg, 100s ea	**51660-0320-01**	2.25	
200s ea	**51660-0320-02**	2.95	
1000s ea	**51660-0320-10**	7.95	
ASPIRIN ADULT LOW STRENGTH			
(AmerisourceBergen)			
ECT,PO (PRIVATE LABEL)			
81 mg, 120s ea	**24385-0535-76**	4.13	4.59
180s ea	**24385-0535-48**	6.29	6.99
300s ea	**24385-0535-87**	7.19	7.99
(Geri-Care)			
TAB,PO, 81 mg, 100s ea	**57896-0981-01**	1.00	
(Teva)			
ECT,PO, 81 mg, 500s ea	**00182-1061-05**	7.75	
ASPIRIN CHILDREN'S (AmerisourceBergen)			
CTB,PO (PRIVATE LABEL,CHERRY)			
81 mg, 36s ea	**24385-0278-68**	1.79	1.99
(PRIVATE LABEL,ORANGE)			
81 mg, 36s ea	**24385-0028-68**	1.79	1.99
(Cardinal Health)			
CTB,PO (PRIVATE LABEL,CHERRY)			
81 mg, 36s ea	**37205-0708-68**	1.79	
(PRIVATE LABEL,ORANGE)			
81 mg, 36s ea	**37205-0467-68**	1.54	
(Chain Drug Marketing)			
CTB,PO (ORANGE)			
81 mg, 36s ea	**63868-0241-36**	0.83	1.79
(Major)			
CTB,PO, 81 mg, 36s ea	**00904-4040-73**	1.45	
(Prime Marketing)			
CTB,PO, 81 mg, 36s ea	**62107-0026-36**	1.75	
(Qualitest)			
CTB,PO (ORANGE)			
81 mg, 36s ea	**00603-0024-36**	2.78	
(Rugby)			
CTB,PO (ORANGE)			
81 mg, 36s ea	**00536-3297-36**	2.25	
(Teva)			
CTB,PO (ORANGE)			
81 mg, 36s ea	**00182-1420-95**	1.39	
(Phys Total Care)			
REPACK			
CTB,PO (ORANGE)			
81 mg, 36s ea	**54868-4530-00**	4.31	
36s ea	**54868-4864-00**	6.63	
ASPIRIN E.C. (Phys Total Care)			
ECT,PO, 81 mg, 36s ea	**54868-2440-01**	6.60	
120s ea	**54868-2440-00**	7.86	
1000s ea	**54868-2440-02**	23.96	
ASPIRIN EC (Bryant Ranch)			
REPACK			
ECT,PO, 325 mg, 30s ea	**63629-1762-01**	0.76	
60s ea	**63629-1762-02**	1.52	
90s ea	**63629-1762-04**	2.28	
100s ea	**63629-1762-03**	2.54	

PROD/MFR	HRI. UPC.NDC	AWP	SRP
(Phys Total Care)			
REPACK			
ECT,PO, 500 mg, 60s ea	**54868-1412-00**	10.14	
(Physician Partner)			
REPACK			
ECT,PO, 81 mg, 30s ea	**21695-0684-30**	7.50	
(Vibranta)			
REPACK			
ECT,PO, 81 mg, 30s ea	**57866-0127-01**	9.80	
ASPIRIN ENTERIC COATED (Advance)			
ECT,PO, 81 mg, 120s ea	**17714-0121-12**	0.91	
ASPIRIN EXTRA STRENGTH (Medicine Shoppe)			
ECT,PO, 500 mg, 60s ea	**49614-0113-72**	3.49	3.49
ASPIRIN FOR ARTHRITIS (Cardinal Health)			
ECT,PO (PRIVATE LABEL)			
325 mg, 500s ea	**37205-0429-90**	9.76	
ASPIRIN FOR CHILDREN (Geri-Care)			
CTB,PO (ORANGE)			
81 mg, 36s ea	**57896-0911-36**	0.60	
(Nucare Pharm)			
REPACK			
CTB,PO (ORANGE)			
81 mg, 36s ea	**68071-1322-06**	4.78	
ASPIRIN LITE COATED (AmerisourceBergen)			
TAB,PO (PRIVATE LABEL)			
325 mg, 100s ea	**24385-0416-78**	2.69	2.99
300s ea	**24385-0416-87**	5.39	5.99
ASPIRIN LOW DOSE (Basic Vitamins)			
TAB,PO, 81 mg, 120s ea	**00761-0033-24**	2.00	
(Dispensing Solutions)			
REPACK			
ECT,PO, 81 mg, 30s ea	**66336-0323-30**	3.07	
(Quality Care Prod)			
REPACK			
ECT,PO, 81 mg, 30s ea	**49999-0359-30**	5.10	
ASPIRIN MICROTHIN COATING (Cardinal Health)			
TAB,PO (PRIVATE LABEL)			
325 mg, 100s ea	**37205-0145-78**	3.45	
300s ea	**37205-0145-87**	6.27	
ASPIRIN REGIMEN LOW STRENGTH (Cardinal Health)			
ECT,PO (PRIVATE LABEL)			
81 mg, 120s ea	**37205-0510-76**	5.37	
500s ea	**37205-0510-90**	6.18	
ASSESS PEAK FLOW METER (Respironics)			
DEV,NA (FULL RANGE)			
ea	**83730-0710-00**	20.60	
(LOW RANGE)			
ea	**83730-0750-00**	22.74	
ASSURA AC CONVEX LIGHT WITH STANDARD WEAR BASEPLATE (Coloplast)			
DEV,NA (1 1/2",RED,2-PIECE)			
5s ea	**11701-0904-87**	41.95	43.90
(1 1/4",RED,2-PIECE)			
5s ea	**11701-0904-85**	41.95	43.90
(1 1/8",RED,2-PIECE)			
5s ea	**11701-0904-84**	41.95	43.90
(1 3/8",RED,2-PIECE)			
5s ea	**11701-0904-86**	41.95	43.90
(1 5/8",RED,2-PIECE)			
5s ea	**11701-0904-88**	41.95	43.90
(1",RED,2-PIECE)			
5s ea	**11701-0904-83**	41.95	43.90
(3/4",GREEN,2-PIECE)			
5s ea	**11701-0904-81**	41.95	43.92
(5/8"-1 11/16",RED,2-PC)			
5s ea	**11701-0904-73**	40.85	42.75
(5/8"-15/16",GREN,2PIECE)			
5s ea	**11701-0904-71**	40.85	42.75
(7/8",GREEN,2-PIECE)			
5s ea	**11701-0904-82**	41.95	43.90
ASSURA AC EASICLOSE NON-CONVEX DRAINABLE POUCH (Coloplast)			
DEV,NA (2-PC,3/8"-2 3/4")			
5s ea	**11701-0907-03**	72.65	76.05
ASSURA BASEPLATE EXTRA EXTENDED WEAR (Coloplast)			
DEV,NA (3/8"-1 5/16")			
10s ea	**11701-0904-04**	83.10	86.90
(3/8"-1 7/8")			
10s ea	**11701-0904-05**	83.10	86.90
(3/8"-2 3/4")			
10s ea	**11701-0904-06**	92.50	96.80
ASSURA BASEPLATE STANDARD WEAR (Coloplast)			
DEV,NA (3/8"-1 5/16")			
10s ea	**11701-0904-01**	59.30	62.10
(3/8"-1 7/8")			
10s ea	**11701-0904-02**	59.30	62.10
(3/8"-2 3/4")			
10s ea	**11701-0904-03**	64.80	67.90
ASSURA CLOSED POUCH COUPLING (Coloplast)			
DEV,NA (OPAQUE,MAXI,1 3/8")			
30s ea	**11701-0904-31**	68.70	71.70
(OPAQUE,MAXI,2 3/4")			
30s ea	**11701-0904-34**	68.70	71.70
(OPAQUE,MAXI,2",CUSTOM)			
30s ea	**11701-0904-33**	68.70	71.70
(OPAQUE,MAXI,2")			
30s ea	**11701-0904-32**	68.70	71.70
(OPAQUE,MIDI,1 3/8")			
30s ea	**11701-0904-16**	68.70	71.70
30s ea	**11701-0904-18**	68.70	71.70
(OPAQUE,MIDI,2 3/4")			
30s ea	**11701-0904-19**	68.70	71.70
(OPAQUE,MIDI,2")			
30s ea	**11701-0904-17**	68.70	71.70
(TRANSP,MAXI,1 3/8")			
30s ea	**11701-0904-26**	68.70	71.70
(TRANSP,MAXI,2 3/4")			
30s ea	**11701-0904-29**	68.70	71.70
(TRANSP,MAXI,2",CUSTOM)			
30s ea	**11701-0904-28**	68.70	71.70
(TRANSP,MAXI,2")			
30s ea	**11701-0904-27**	68.70	71.70
(TRANSP,MIDI,1 3/8")			
30s ea	**11701-0904-11**	68.70	71.70
(TRANSP,MIDI,2 3/4")			
30s ea	**11701-0904-14**	68.70	71.70
(TRANSP,MIDI,2")			
30s ea	**11701-0904-12**	68.70	71.70
ASSURA CLOSED POUCH ONE PIECE (Coloplast)			
DEV,NA (5", 13/16"-2 1/8")			
30s ea	**11701-0838-16**	96.00	100.50
(5",OPAQUE,13/16"-2 1/8")			
30s ea	**11701-0838-11**	96.00	100.50
(7", 13/16"-2 1/8")			
30s ea	**11701-0853-56**	96.00	100.50
(7",OPAQUE,1 3/16")			
30s ea	**11701-0853-21**	98.10	102.60
(7",OPAQUE,1 3/8")			
30s ea	**11701-0853-31**	98.10	102.60
(7",OPAQUE,1 9/16")			
30s ea	**11701-0853-41**	98.10	102.60
(7",OPAQUE,1")			
30s ea	**11701-0853-11**	98.10	102.60
(7",OPAQUE,13/16"-2 1/8")			
30s ea	**11701-0838-75**	96.00	100.50
(7",OPAQUE,2")			
30s ea	**11701-0853-61**	98.10	102.60
(7",TRANSP,1 3/8")			
30s ea	**11701-0853-36**	98.10	102.60
(7",TRANSP,1 9/16")			
30s ea	**11701-0853-46**	98.10	102.60
(7",TRANSPARENT,1 3/16")			
30s ea	**11701-0852-26**	98.10	102.60
(7",TRANSPARENT,1")			
30s ea	**11701-0852-16**	98.10	102.60
(8",OPAQUE,1 3/16")			
30s ea	**11701-0838-81**	99.60	104.10
(8",OPAQUE,1 3/8")			
30s ea	**11701-0838-82**	99.60	104.10
(8",OPAQUE,1 9/16")			
30s ea	**11701-0838-83**	99.60	104.10
(8",OPAQUE,1")			
30s ea	**11701-0838-80**	99.60	104.10
(8"TRNSPAR,13/16"-2 3/4")			
30s ea	**11701-0838-76**	96.00	100.50
ASSURA CLOSED POUCH TWO PIECE (Coloplast)			
DEV,NA (7",OPAQUE,1/2"-1 9/16")			
30s ea	**11701-0848-11**	60.90	63.60
(7",OPAQUE,1/2"-2 3/8")			
30s ea	**11701-0848-21**	60.90	63.60
(7",OPAQUE,1/2"-2")			
30s ea	**11701-0848-16**	60.90	63.60
(7",TRANSPAR,1/2"-2 3/8")			
30s ea	**11701-0848-41**	60.90	63.60
(7",TRANSPAR,1/2"-2")			
30s ea	**11701-0848-36**	60.90	63.60
(7",TRNSPAR,1/2"-1 9/16")			
30s ea	**11701-0848-31**	60.90	63.60
(8 1/2", 1/2"-1 9/16")			
30s ea	**11701-0848-51**	56.70	59.40
30s ea	**11701-0848-71**	62.40	65.40
(8 1/2", 1/2"-2 3/8")			
30s ea	**11701-0848-61**	56.70	59.40
(8 1/2",OPAQ,1/2"-2 3/8")			
30s ea	**11701-0848-81**	62.40	65.40
(8 1/2",OPAQ,1/2"-2")			
30s ea	**11701-0848-76**	62.40	65.40
(8 1/2",TRANS,1/2"-2")			
30s ea	**11701-0848-56**	56.70	59.40
ASSURA CONVEX DRAINABLE POUCH (Coloplast)			
DEV,NA (12",OPAQUE,1 1/2")			
10s ea	**11701-0849-40**	78.40	82.10
(12",OPAQUE,1 1/4")			
10s ea	**11701-0849-30**	78.40	82.10
(12",OPAQUE,1 1/8")			
10s ea	**11701-0849-25**	78.40	82.10
(12",OPAQUE,1 3/8")			
10s ea	**11701-0849-35**	78.40	82.10
(12",OPAQUE,1 5/8")			
10s ea	**11701-0849-45**	78.40	82.10
(12",OPAQUE,1")			
10s ea	**11701-0849-20**	78.40	82.10
(12",OPAQUE,3/4")			
10s ea	**11701-0849-10**	78.40	82.10
(12",OPAQUE,7/8")			
10s ea	**11701-0849-15**	78.40	82.10
(12",STD, OPAQUE, 5/8")			
10s ea	**11701-0849-05**	78.40	82.10
ASSURA CONVEX FLANGE W/BELT LOOPS (Coloplast)			
DEV,NA (CUSTOM CUT,5/8"-1 5/16")			
5s ea	**11701-0844-10**	39.15	40.95
(CUSTOM CUT5/8"-1 11/16")			
5s ea	**11701-0844-15**	39.15	40.95
(PRE-CUT,1 1/2")			
5s ea	**11701-0834-45**	41.55	43.45
(PRE-CUT,1 1/4")			
5s ea	**11701-0834-35**	41.55	43.45
(PRE-CUT,1 1/8")			
5s ea	**11701-0834-30**	41.55	43.45
(PRE-CUT,1 3/8")			
5s ea	**11701-0834-40**	41.55	43.45
(PRE-CUT,1 5/8")			
5s ea	**11701-0834-50**	41.55	43.45
(PRE-CUT,1")			
5s ea	**11701-0834-25**	41.55	43.45
(PRE-CUT,3/4")			
5s ea	**11701-0834-15**	41.55	43.45
(PRE-CUT,5/8")			
5s ea	**11701-0834-10**	41.55	43.45
(PRE-CUT,7/8")			
5s ea	**11701-0834-20**	41.55	43.45
ASSURA CONVEX LIGHT CLOSED POUCH (Coloplast)			
DEV,NA (MAXI, 5/8"-1 11/16")			
10s ea	**11701-0889-42**	57.30	59.90
10s ea	**11701-0889-45**	57.30	59.90
(MAXI,5/8"-1 5/16")			
10s ea	**11701-0889-41**	57.30	59.90
10s ea	**11701-0889-44**	57.30	59.90
(MIDI, 5/8"-1 11/16")			
10s ea	**11701-0889-32**	57.30	59.90
(MIDI,5/8"-1 11/16")			
10s ea	**11701-0889-35**	57.30	59.90
(MIDI,5/8"-1 5/16")			
10s ea	**11701-0889-31**	57.30	59.90
(OPAQU,MIDI,5/8"-1 5/16")			
10s ea	**11701-0889-34**	57.30	59.90
(OPAQUE,MIDI,1 1/4")			
10s ea	**11701-0889-54**	57.30	59.90
(OPAQUE,MIDI,1 1/8")			
10s ea	**11701-0889-53**	57.30	59.90
(OPAQUE,MIDI,1")			
10s ea	**11701-0889-52**	57.30	59.90
(OPAQUE,MIDI,7/8")			
10s ea	**11701-0889-51**	57.30	59.90
ASSURA CONVEX LIGHT FLANGE W/BELT LOOPS (Coloplast)			
DEV,NA (CUSTOM CUT,5/8"-1 5/16")			
5s ea	**11701-0886-62**	39.15	40.95
(CUSTOM CUT,5/8"-15/16")			
5s ea	**11701-0886-61**	39.15	40.95
(CUSTOM CUT5/8"-1 11/16")			
5s ea	**11701-0886-63**	39.15	40.95
(PRE-CUT,1 1/2")			
5s ea	**11701-0886-77**	41.55	43.45
(PRE-CUT,1 1/4")			
5s ea	**11701-0886-75**	41.55	43.45
(PRE-CUT,1 1/8")			
5s ea	**11701-0886-74**	41.55	43.45
(PRE-CUT,1 3/8")			
5s ea	**11701-0886-76**	41.55	43.45
(PRE-CUT,1 5/8")			
5s ea	**11701-0886-78**	41.55	43.45

PROD/MFR HRI, UPC,NDC AWP

(PRE-CUT,1")
5s ea................11701-0886-73 41.55 43.45
(PRE-CUT,3/4")
5s ea................11701-0886-71 41.55 43.45
(PRE-CUT,7/8")
5s ea................11701-0886-72 41.55 43.45

ASSURA CONVEX POUCH ONE PIECE (Coloplast)
DEV,NA (12",DRAIN,5/8"-1 11/16")
10s ea................11701-0827-15 77.20 80.80
(12",DRAIN,5/8"-1 5/16")
10s ea................11701-0827-10 77.20 80.80

ASSURA CONVEX UROPOUCH 1 PIECE (Coloplast)
DEV,NA (10 3/4",TRANSPAR, 5/8")
10s ea................11701-0833-10 92.40 96.70
(10 3/4",TRANSPAR,1 1/4")
10s ea................11701-0833-35 92.40 96.70
(10 3/4",TRANSPAR,1 1/8")
10s ea................11701-0833-30 92.40 96.70
(10 3/4",TRANSPAR,1 3/8")
10s ea................11701-0833-40 92.40 96.70
(10 3/4",TRANSPAR,3/4")
10s ea................11701-0833-15 92.40 96.70
(10 3/4",TRANSPAR,7/8")
10s ea................11701-0833-20 92.40 96.70
(10 3/4",TRANSPARENT,1")
10s ea................11701-0833-25 92.40 96.70

ASSURA CONVEX UROPOUCH ONE PIECE (Coloplast)
DEV,NA (10 3/4", 5/8"-1 11/16")
10s ea................11701-0828-15 96.60 104.20
(10 3/4", 5/8"-1 5/16")
10s ea................11701-0828-10 96.60 104.20

ASSURA DRAINABLE POUCH 2 PIECE (Coloplast)
DEV,NA (10",OPAQUE,1/2"-1 1/2")
10s ea................11701-0847-10 28.70 30.10
(10",OPAQUE,1/2"-1 3/4")
10s ea................11701-0847-15 28.70 30.10
(10",OPAQUE,1/2"-2 1/4")
10s ea................11701-0847-20 28.70 30.10

ASSURA DRAINABLE POUCH TWO PIECE (Coloplast)
DEV,NA (12",OPAQUE,1/2"-1 1/2")
10s ea................11701-0846-10 28.70 30.10
(12",OPAQUE,1/2"-2 3/8")
10s ea................11701-0846-20 28.70 30.10
(12",OPAQUE,1/2"-2")
10s ea................11701-0846-15 28.70 30.10
(12",TRANSP,1/2"-1 9/16")
10s ea................11701-0846-25 28.70 30.10
(12",TRANSP,1/2"-2 3/8")
10s ea................11701-0846-35 28.70 30.10
(12",TRANSP,1/2"-2")
10s ea................11701-0846-30 28.70 30.10

ASSURA EASICLOSE CONVEX DRAINABLE POUCH (Coloplast)
DEV,NA (MAXI, 5/8"-1 11/16")
10s ea................11701-0887-30 101.00 105.70
(MIDI,5/8"-1 11/16")
10s ea................11701-0887-10 101.00 105.70
(OPAQUE,MAXI,1 1/4")
10s ea................11701-0887-34 101.00 105.70
(OPAQUE,MAXI,1 1/8")
10s ea................11701-0887-33 101.00 105.70
(OPAQUE,MAXI,1")
10s ea................11701-0887-32 101.00 105.70
(OPAQUE,MAXI,7/8")
10s ea................11701-0887-31 101.00 105.70
(TRANS,MAXI,1 1/4")
10s ea................11701-0887-24 101.00 105.70
(TRANS,MAXI,1 1/8")
10s ea................11701-0887-23 101.00 105.70
(TRANS,MAXI,1")
10s ea................11701-0887-22 101.00 105.70
(TRANS,MAXI,7/8")
10s ea................11701-0887-21 101.00 105.70
(TRANSMAXI,5/8"-1 11/16")
10s ea................11701-0887-20 101.00 105.70

ASSURA EASICLOSE CONVEX LIGHT DRAINABLE POUCH (Coloplast)
DEV,NA (2-PC,5/8"-1 11/16")
5s ea................11701-0907-01 85.15 92.25
(MIDI,5/8"-1 11/16")
10s ea................11701-0889-05 101.00 105.70
(MIDI,5/8"-1 5/16")
10s ea................11701-0889-04 101.00 105.70
(OPAQUE,MAXI, CUT-TO-FIT)
10s ea................11701-0889-14 101.00 105.70
10s ea................11701-0889-15 101.00 105.70
(OPAQUE,MAXI,1 1/4")
10s ea................11701-0889-24 101.00 105.70
(OPAQUE,MAXI,1 1/8")
10s ea................11701-0889-23 101.00 105.70
(OPAQUE,MAXI,1")
10s ea................11701-0889-22 101.00 105.70
(OPAQUE,MAXI,7/8")
10s ea................11701-0889-21 101.00 105.70
(TRANS,MAXI,5/8"-1 5/16")
10s ea................11701-0889-11 101.00 105.70
(TRANS,MAXI,CUT-TO-FIT)
10s ea................11701-0889-12 101.00 105.70

ASSURA EASICLOSE DRAINABLE POUCH (Coloplast)
DEV,NA (OPAQUE,MAXI,40MM)
10s ea................11701-0875-84 31.10 32.60
(OPAQUE,MAXI,50MM)
10s ea................11701-0875-85 31.10 32.60
(OPAQUE,MAXI,60MM)
10s ea................11701-0875-86 31.10 32.60
(OPAQUE,MIDI,40MM)
10s ea................11701-0875-64 32.50 34.00
(OPAQUE,MIDI,50MM)
10s ea................11701-0875-65 32.50 34.00
(OPAQUE,MIDI,60MM)
10s ea................11701-0875-66 32.50 34.00
(OPAQUE,MINI,40MM)
10s ea................11701-0875-24 31.10 32.60
(OPAQUE,MINI,50MM)
10s ea................11701-0875-25 31.10 32.60
(OPAQUE,MINI,60MM)
10s ea................11701-0875-26 31.10 32.60
(TRANSPARENT,MAXI,40MM)
10s ea................11701-0875-74 32.20 33.70
(TRANSPARENT,MAXI,50MM)
10s ea................11701-0875-75 32.20 33.70
(TRANSPARENT,MAXI,60MM)
10s ea................11701-0875-76 32.20 33.70

ASSURA EASICLOSE DRAINABLE POUCH COUPLING (Coloplast)
DEV,NA (OPAQ,MAXI,2",CUST PEEL)
20s ea................11701-0904-63 76.80 80.20
(OPAQ,MIDI,2",CUST PEEL)
20s ea................11701-0904-48 76.80 80.20
(OPAQUE,MAXI,1 3/8")
20s ea................11701-0904-61 76.80 80.20
(OPAQUE,MAXI,2 3/4")
20s ea................11701-0904-64 76.80 80.20
(OPAQUE,MAXI,2")
20s ea................11701-0904-62 76.80 80.20
(OPAQUE,MIDI,1 3/8")
20s ea................11701-0904-46 76.80 80.20
(OPAQUE,MIDI,2 3/4")
20s ea................11701-0904-49 76.80 80.20
(OPAQUE,MIDI,2")
20s ea................11701-0904-47 76.80 80.20
(TRANS,MAXI,2",CUST PEEL)
20s ea................11701-0904-58 78.00 81.80
(TRANSP,MAXI,1 3/8")
20s ea................11701-0904-56 78.00 81.80
(TRANSP,MAXI,2 3/4")
20s ea................11701-0904-59 78.00 81.80
(TRANSP,MAXI,2")
20s ea................11701-0904-57 78.00 81.80
(TRANSP,MIDI,1 3/8")
20s ea................11701-0904-41 78.00 81.80
(TRANSP,MIDI,2 3/4")
20s ea................11701-0904-44 78.00 81.80
(TRANSP,MIDI,2")
20s ea................11701-0904-42 78.00 81.80

ASSURA EASICLOSE NON-CONVEX DRAINABLE POUCH (Coloplast)
DEV,NA (1-PC,3/8"-2 3/4")
5s ea................11701-0907-05 50.30 52.65
(2-PC,3/8"-2 1/8")
5s ea................11701-0907-02 64.25 67.25
(GRAPHC,MIDI,3/8"-2 1/8")
10s ea................11701-0876-40 46.30 48.40
(GRAPHIC,MIDI,1 3/16")
10s ea................11701-0876-45 46.30 48.40
(GRAPHIC,MIDI,1 3/8")
10s ea................11701-0876-46 46.30 48.40
(GRAPHIC,MIDI,1")
10s ea................11701-0876-44 46.30 48.40
(OPAQUE,MAXI,1 3/16")
10s ea................11701-0876-82 46.30 48.40
(OPAQUE,MAXI,1 3/8")
10s ea................11701-0876-83 46.30 48.40
(OPAQUE,MAXI,1")
10s ea................11701-0876-81 46.30 48.40
(OPAQUE,MAXI,3/8"-2 3/4")
10s ea................11701-0876-70 46.30 48.40
(TRANSP,MAXI,3/8"-2 3/4")
10s ea................11701-0876-60 46.30 48.40

ASSURA EXTRA CONVEX DRAINABLE POUCH (Coloplast)
DEV,NA (11",OPAQU,5/8"-1 11/16")
10s ea................11701-0884-12 105.80 110.70
(11",OPAQUE,5/8"-1 5/16")
10s ea................11701-0884-11 105.80 110.70
(11",TRANS,5/8"-1 11/16")
10s ea................11701-0884-02 105.80 110.70
(11",TRANSP,5/8"-1 5/16")
10s ea................11701-0884-01 105.80 110.70

ASSURA EXTRA CONVEX FLANGE W/BELT LOOPS (Coloplast)
DEV,NA (CUSTOM CUT,5/8"-1 5/16")
5s ea................11701-0886-01 54.80 57.35
(CUSTOM CUT,5/8"-15/16")
5s ea................11701-0886-03 54.80 57.35
(CUSTOM CUT5/8"-1 11/16")
5s ea................11701-0886-02 54.80 57.35
(PRE-CUT,1 1/2")
5s ea................11701-0886-96 54.20 56.70
(PRE-CUT,1 1/4")
5s ea................11701-0886-94 54.20 56.70
(PRE-CUT,1 1/8")
5s ea................11701-0886-93 54.20 56.70
(PRE-CUT,1 3/8")
5s ea................11701-0886-95 54.20 56.70
(PRE-CUT,1 5/8")
5s ea................11701-0886-97 54.20 56.70
(PRE-CUT,1")
5s ea................11701-0886-92 54.20 56.70
(PRE-CUT,3/4")
5s ea................11701-0886-90 54.20 56.70
(PRE-CUT,7/8")
5s ea................11701-0886-91 54.20 56.70

ASSURA EXTRA CONVEX UROPOUCH 1 PIECE (Coloplast)
DEV,NA (375ML, 5/8"-1 11/16")
10s ea................11701-0885-02 105.80 110.70
(375ML, 5/8"-1 5/16")
10s ea................11701-0885-01 105.80 110.70

ASSURA EXTRA NON-CONVEX DRAINABLE POUCH (Coloplast)
DEV,NA (11",OPAQUE,3/8"-2 3/4")
10s ea................11701-0884-51 55.90 58.50
(11",TRANSP,3/8"-2 3/4")
10s ea................11701-0884-61 55.90 58.50

ASSURA EXTRA NON-CONVEX FLANGE W/BELT LOOPS (Coloplast)
DEV,NA (CUSTOM CUT,3/8"-1 3/4")
5s ea................11701-0886-52 37.75 39.50
(CUSTOM CUT,3/8"-1 3/8")
5s ea................11701-0886-51 37.75 39.50
(CUSTOM CUT,3/8"-2 1/8")
5s ea................11701-0886-53 37.75 39.50
(PRE-CUT,1 3/16")
5s ea................11701-0886-83 37.00 38.70
(PRE-CUT,1 3/4")
5s ea................11701-0886-86 37.00 38.70
(PRE-CUT,1 3/8")
5s ea................11701-0886-84 37.00 38.70
(PRE-CUT,1 9/16")
5s ea................11701-0886-85 37.00 38.70
(PRE-CUT,1")
5s ea................11701-0886-82 37.00 38.70
(PRE-CUT,13/16")
5s ea................11701-0886-81 37.00 38.70
(PRE-CUT,5/8")
5s ea................11701-0886-80 37.00 38.70

ASSURA EXTRA NON-CONVEX UROPOUCH 1 PIECE (Coloplast)
DEV,NA (150ML,OPAQ,3/8"-2 1/8")
10s ea................11701-0885-51 88.10 92.20
(150ML,TRANS,3/8"-2 1/8")
10s ea................11701-0885-61 88.10 92.20
(375ML,TRANS,3/8"-2 1/8")
10s ea................11701-0885-62 88.10 92.20

ASSURA EXTRA NON-CONVEX UROSTOMY POUCH (Coloplast)
DEV,NA (2-PC,3/8"-2 1/8")
5s ea................11701-0907-04 77.65 81.25

ASSURA FLANGE PEDIATRIC (Coloplast)
DEV,NA (OPAQUE 3/8"-1 3/8")
5s ea................11701-0830-10 27.95 29.25

ASSURA FLANGE W/BELT LOOPS (Coloplast)
DEV,NA (CUSTOM CUT,3/8"-1 3/4")
5s ea................11701-0843-15 27.60 28.90
(CUSTOM CUT,3/8"-2 1/8")
5s ea................11701-0843-20 27.60 28.90
(CUSTOM CUT,3/82"-1 3/8")
5s ea................11701-0843-10 27.60 28.90

PROD/MFR	HRI, UPC,NDC	AWP	SRP
(PRE-CUT,1 3/16")			
5s ea	**11701-0845-25**	28.45	29.80
(PRE-CUT,1 3/4")			
5s ea	**11701-0845-40**	28.45	29.80
(PRE-CUT,1 3/8")			
5s ea	**11701-0845-30**	28.45	29.80
(PRE-CUT,1")			
5s ea	**11701-0845-20**	28.45	29.80
(PRE-CUT,3/16")			
5s ea	**11701-0845-15**	28.45	29.80
(PRE-CUT,5/8")			
5s ea	**11701-0845-10**	28.45	29.80
(PRE-CUT,9/16")			
5s ea	**11701-0845-35**	28.45	29.80
ASSURA HIGH OUTPUT 2 PIECE SYSTEM (Coloplast)			
DEV,NA (ILEO NITE POUCH,1/2"-2")			
5s ea	**11701-0874-10**	87.70	91.80
(ILEO, 1/2"-2 3/8")			
5s ea	**11701-0874-15**	87.70	91.80
(HIGH OUTPUT POUCH,50 MM)			
10s ea	**11701-0874-50**	68.80	72.00
(HIGH OUTPUT POUCH,60 MM)			
10s ea	**11701-0874-55**	68.80	72.00
ASSURA IRRIGATION FACE PLATE (Coloplast)			
DEV,NA (1/2"-2")			
ea	**11701-0821-20**	12.95	13.55
ASSURA IRRIGATION SLEEVES (Coloplast)			
DEV,NA (FLANGE #2883, 1/2"- 2")			
5s ea	**11701-0822-40**	32.75	34.30
(FLANGE 2881,1/2"-1 1/2")			
5s ea	**11701-0822-30**	32.75	34.30
(FLANGE#2882,1/2"-1 3/4")			
5s ea	**11701-0822-35**	32.75	34.30
ASSURA NON-CONVEX 12" POUCH 1 PIECE (Coloplast)			
DEV,NA (OPAQUE,1 3/16")			
10s ea	**11701-0850-30**	43.90	45.90
(OPAQUE,1 3/8")			
10s ea	**11701-0850-40**	43.90	45.90
(OPAQUE,1 9/16")			
10s ea	**11701-0850-50**	43.90	45.90
(OPAQUE,1")			
10s ea	**11701-0850-20**	43.90	45.90
(OPAQUE,3/8"-2 3/4")			
10s ea	**11701-0850-10**	43.90	45.90
(TRANSPARENT,1 3/16")			
10s ea	**11701-0850-35**	43.90	45.90
(TRANSPARENT,1 3/8")			
10s ea	**11701-0850-45**	43.90	45.90
(TRANSPARENT,1")			
10s ea	**11701-0850-25**	43.90	45.90
(TRANSPARENT,19/16")			
10s ea	**11701-0850-55**	43.90	45.90
(TRANSPARENT,3/8"-2 3/4")			
10s ea	**11701-0850-15**	43.90	45.90
ASSURA NON-CONVEX POUCH 1 PIECE (Coloplast)			
DEV,NA (10",OPAQUE,1 3/16")			
10s ea	**11701-0851-30**	43.90	45.90
(10",OPAQUE,1 3/8")			
10s ea	**11701-0851-40**	43.90	45.90
(10",OPAQUE,1 9/16")			
10s ea	**11701-0851-50**	43.90	45.90
(10",OPAQUE,1")			
10s ea	**11701-0851-20**	43.90	45.90
(10",OPAQUE,3/8"-2 1/8")			
10s ea	**11701-0851-10**	43.90	45.90
(10",TRANSPAR,3/8-2 1/8")			
10s ea	**11701-0851-15**	43.90	45.90
(10",TRANSPARENT,1 3/16")			
10s ea	**11701-0851-35**	43.90	45.90
(10",TRANSPARENT,1 3/4")			
10s ea	**11701-0851-60**	43.90	45.90
(10",TRANSPARENT,1 3/8")			
10s ea	**11701-0851-45**	43.90	45.90
(10",TRANSPARENT,1 9/16")			
10s ea	**11701-0851-55**	43.90	45.90
(10",TRANSPARENT,1")			
10s ea	**11701-0851-25**	43.90	45.90
(10",TRANSPARENT,2")			
10s ea	**11701-0851-65**	43.90	45.90
ASSURA OSTOMY BELT (Coloplast)			
DEV,NA (ADJUSTABLE)			
10s ea	**11701-0835-10**	93.70	98.10
ASSURA PED. UROPOUCH ONE PIECE (Coloplast)			
DEV,NA (6",TRANSP,3/8"-1 3/8")			
10s ea	**11701-0837-21**	46.80	49.00
ASSURA PED. UROPOUCH TWO PIECE (Coloplast)			
DEV,NA (6",TRANSPARENT,150 ML)			
10s ea	**11701-0854-21**	38.00	39.80

PROD/MFR	HRI, UPC,NDC	AWP	SRP
ASSURA PEDIATRIC POUCH ONE PIECE (Coloplast)			
DEV,NA (6",DRAINABLE,TRANSPAREN)			
10s ea	**11701-0837-10**	38.70	40.50
(5",TRANSP,3/8"-1 3/8")			
30s ea	**11701-0837-11**	77.40	81.00
(5"OPAQ,CLSD,2/5"-1 2/5")			
30s ea	**11701-0837-15**	77.40	81.00
ASSURA PEDIATRIC POUCH TWO PIECE (Coloplast)			
DEV,NA (6",TRANS,DRANBLE,8 1/2")			
10s ea	**11701-0854-10**	24.80	25.90
(5",OPAQUE,CLOSED,5 3/4")			
30s ea	**11701-0854-15**	48.60	50.70
ASSURA POST-OP DRAINABLE POUCH (Coloplast)			
DEV,NA (W/O WINDOW,1/2"-2 3/4")			
5s ea	**11701-0831-20**	69.55	72.80
(W/WINDOW,1/2"-2 3/4")			
5s ea	**11701-0831-10**	77.25	80.80
(W/WINDOW,1/2"-4")			
5s ea	**11701-0831-15**	80.50	84.25
ASSURA POST-OP DRAINABLE STERILE (Coloplast)			
DEV,NA (W/O WINDOW,1/2"-2 3/4")			
5s ea	**11701-0831-35**	62.20	65.05
(W/WINDOW,1/2"-2 3/4")			
5s ea	**11701-0831-25**	79.65	83.35
(W/WINDOW,1/2"-4")			
5s ea	**11701-0831-30**	84.35	80.30
ASSURA STOMA CAP W/FILTER ONE PIECE (Coloplast)			
DEV,NA (OPAQUE,13/16"-2 1/8")			
30s ea	**11701-0839-10**	83.70	87.60
ASSURA STOMA CAP W/FILTER TWO PIECE (Coloplast)			
DEV,NA (OPAQUE,1/2"-1 1/2")			
30s ea	**11701-0841-10**	75.30	78.90
(OPAQUE,1/2"-1 3/4")			
30s ea	**11701-0841-15**	75.30	78.90
ASSURA URO MINICAP TWO PIECE (Coloplast)			
DEV,NA (OPAQ,CLOSE,1/2"-1 9/16")			
30s ea	**11701-0888-11**	90.90	95.10
(OPAQUE,CLOSED,1/2"-2")			
30s ea	**11701-0888-12**	90.90	95.10
ASSURA UROPOUCH ONE PIECE (Coloplast)			
DEV,NA (10 3/4",OPAQUE,180ML)			
10s ea	**11701-0840-11**	70.50	73.80
(10 3/4",OPAQUE,375ML)			
10s ea	**11701-0840-21**	70.50	73.80
(10 3/4",TRANSP,250ML)			
10s ea	**11701-0840-16**	70.50	73.80
(10 3/4",TRANSP,375ML)			
10s ea	**11701-0840-31**	70.50	73.80
ASSURA UROPOUCH TWO PIECE (Coloplast)			
DEV,NA (10",OPAQUE,1/2"-1 9/16")			
10s ea	**11701-0842-26**	41.10	43.00
(10",OPAQUE,1/2"-2 3/8")			
10s ea	**11701-0842-36**	41.10	43.00
(10",OPAQUE,1/2"-2")			
10s ea	**11701-0842-31**	41.10	43.00
(10",TRANSP,1/2"-1 9/16")			
10s ea	**11701-0842-11**	41.10	43.00
(10",TRANSP,1/2"-2 3/8")			
10s ea	**11701-0842-21**	41.10	43.00
(10",TRANSP,1/2"-2")			
10s ea	**11701-0842-16**	41.10	43.00
(7",TRANS,1/2"-1 9/16")			
10s ea	**11701-0842-41**	41.10	43.00
(7",TRANSPAR,1/2"-2")			
10s ea	**11701-0842-46**	41.10	43.00
ASSURA UROSTOMY MICRO-POUCH TWO-PIECE (Coloplast)			
DEV,NA (TRANSP,MATCHES RED SIZE)			
10s ea	**11701-0905-50**	40.90	42.80
(TRANSP,MATCHS BLUE SIZE)			
10s ea	**11701-0905-60**	40.90	42.80
(TRASP,MATCHES GRN SIZE)			
10s ea	**11701-0905-40**	40.90	42.80
ASSURA UROSTOMY MULTI-CHAMBER POUCH TWO-PIECE (Coloplast)			
DEV,NA (MAXI,OPAQUE,BLUE SIZES)			
10s ea	**11701-0905-26**	43.20	45.20
(MAXI,OPAQUE,GREEN SIZES)			
10s ea	**11701-0905-24**	43.20	45.20
(MAXI,OPAQUE,RED SIZES)			
10s ea	**11701-0905-25**	43.20	45.20
(MAXI,TRANSP,BLUE SIZES)			
10s ea	**11701-0905-29**	43.20	45.20

PROD/MFR	HRI, UPC,NDC	AWP	SRP
(MAXI,TRANSP,GREEN SIZES)			
10s ea	**11701-0905-27**	43.20	45.20
(MAXI,TRANSP,RED SIZES)			
10s ea	**11701-0905-28**	43.20	45.20
ASSURE (Arkray)			
DEV,NA (TEST STRIP)			
50s ea	**08317-7750-50**	35.40	
(TEST STRIPS)			
100s ea	**08317-7710-00**	63.15	
(Specialty Medical)			
DEV,NA (ULTRA THIN,G29)			
100s ea	**38415-0100-29**	10.20	
ASSURE 3 BLOOD GLUCOSE METER (Arkray)			
DEV,NA, ea	**08317-5501-01**	22.50	
ASSURE 3 BLOOD GLUCOSE TEST STRIPS (Arkray)			
DEV,NA, 50s ea	**08317-5550-50**	38.50	
(2X50)			
100s ea	**08317-5510-00**	77.00	
ASSURE 3 CONTROL SOLUTION (Arkray)			
DEV,NA (LEVEL 1&2)			
2s ea	**08317-5506-02**	10.35	
ASSURE 4 (Arkray)			
DEV,NA, ea	**08317-5600-01**	45.00	
ea	**08317-5600-06**	12.00	
50s ea	**08317-5600-50**	38.50	
100s ea	**08317-5601-00**	77.00	
ASSURE CONTROL (Arkray)			
DEV,NA (LEVELS 1 & 2)			
2s ea	**08317-7705-02**	12.60	
ASSURE DOSE NORMAL CONTROL SOLUTION (Arkray)			
DEV,NA, ea	**08317-5000-05**	7.50	
ASSURE DOSE NORMAL/HIGH CONTROL SOLUTION (Arkray)			
DEV,NA, ea	**08317-5000-06**	12.00	
ASSURE II (Arkray)			
DEV,NA, ea	**08317-2211-01**	22.50	
(CHECK STRIP)			
ea	**08317-2208-01**	7.50	
(GLUCOSE METER)			
ea	**08317-2200-01**	22.50	
(LEVEL 1 & 2)			
ea	**08317-2206-02**	12.00	
(LEVEL 1)			
ea	**08317-2205-01**	7.20	
(STRIP)			
50s ea	**08317-2250-50**	33.75	
(TEST STRIPS)			
100s ea	**08317-2210-00**	61.50	
ASSURE LANCE (Arkray)			
DEV,NA (1MM,28 GAUGE,MICROFLOW)			
100s ea	**08317-9801-28**	16.50	
(25G,LOW FLOW)			
100s ea	**08317-9801-25**	16.50	
(1MM,28 GAUGE,MICROFLOW)			
200s ea	**08317-9802-28**	30.00	
(25G,LOW FLOW)			
200s ea	**08317-9802-25**	30.00	
ASSURE PRO BLOOD GLUCOSE METER (Arkray)			
DEV,NA, ea	**08317-4600-01**	52.50	
ASSURE PRO BLOOD GLUCOSE TEST STRIPS (Arkray)			
DEV,NA, 50s ea	**08317-4600-50**	40.93	
100s ea	**08317-4601-00**	81.86	
ASSURE PRO LEVEL 1&2 CONTROL SOLUTION (Arkray)			
DEV,NA (2X3ML)			
2s ea	**08317-4600-06**	12.00	
ASSURE SORE THROAT (Dihoma Inc.)			
SPR,MM (CHERRY)			
1.4%, 15 ml	**62294-1004-02**	1.35	2.00
ASTHMA CHECK PEAK FLOW METER (Respironics)			
DEV,NA, ea	**83730-0740-00**	20.00	
ASTHMA MENTOR PEAK FLOW METER (Respironics)			
DEV,NA (UNIVERSAL RANGE)			
ea	**83730-0742-00**	24.67	
ASTRAGALUS (Botanical Labs.)			
LIQ,PO, 30 ml	**41954-0020-03**	4.00	7.99
60 ml	**41954-0020-04**	6.50	12.99
ASTRING-O-SOL (Oakhurst)			
SOL,MM (CONCENTRAT,.ALCOHOL38B)			
236 ml	**11969-0686-70**	7.84	11.77
ASTROGLIDE (Phys Total Care)			
REPACK			
GEL,TP, 66.5 gm	**54868-4818-00**	7.28	
71 gm	**54868-4818-01**	7.28	

PROD/MFR	HRI. UPC.NDC	AWP	SRP
ATHENA PELVIC MUSCLE TRAINER (Athena Feminine Tech)			
DEV,NA (WIRELESS)			
ea	38488-0001-01	522.75	
ATHLETE'S FOOT (Perrigo)			
CRE,TP (1X15GM)			
1%, 15 gm	45802-0434-01	5.99	
(1X28GM)			
1%, 28 gm	45802-0434-11	8.59	
ATHLETES FORMULA (Nature's Bounty)			
TER,PO (PF,SF,CAPLET)			
60s ea	74312-0075-90		7.49
ATRAC-TAIN (Coloplast)			
CRE,TP (PACKET)			
5%-10%, 2 gm 300s	11701-0022-21	108.00	114.00
57 gm 12s	11701-0022-23	87.72	91.80
142 gm 12s	11701-0022-14	140.52	147.12
LOT,TP, 2.5%-5%,			
118 ml 36s	11701-0024-04	213.48	223.56
237 ml 12s	11701-0024-05	136.20	142.56
ATTENDS BELTED UNDERGARMENT (Attends)			
DEV,NA (SUPER ABSORBANCY)			
120s ea	86679-0249-76	12.49	
ATTENDS BRIEF (Attends)			
DEV,NA (LARGE WAISTBAND)			
36s ea	37000-0684-53	12.36	
(MEDIUM WAISTBAND)			
88s ea	37000-0067-07	43.38	
(LARGE,BULK,CLASSIC)			
96s ea	86679-0248-86	43.77	
(MEDIUM,CLASSIC)			
96s ea	86679-0248-85	33.00	
(SMALL,CLASSIC)			
96s ea	86679-0248-84	8.50	
(YOUTH,BULK,CLASSIC)			
96s ea	86679-0250-17	31.39	
ATTENDS INSERTS (Attends)			
DEV,NA (BULK)			
144s ea	86679-0250-18	42.76	
ATTENDS PADS/PANTS (Attends)			
DEV,NA (EXTRA,SHAPED PAD 7)			
96s ea	86679-0249-73	34.49	
(SUPER,SHAPED PAD 8)			
96s ea	86679-0249-74	43.32	
(SHAPED PAD 5, MODERATE)			
120s ea	86679-0251-00	30.85	
ATTENDS UNDERPADS (Attends)			
DEV,NA (LG,CLASSIC EXTRA)			
80s ea	86679-0245-01	27.13	
(LRG,REG ABSORB,CLASSIC)			
100s ea	86679-0245-00	29.88	
(SUPER ABSORBENCY)			
120s ea	86679-0250-99	49.83	
AUDIOLOGIST'S CHOICE (Oaktree)			
SOL,OT, 6.5%, 15 ml	59256-0001-01	2.35	
(W/BULB SYRINGE)			
6.5%, 15 ml	59256-0001-02	3.50	
AURAPHENE-B (Reese)			
SOL,OT, 6.5%, 15 ml	10956-0616-53	3.69	
AURO EARACHE RELIEF (Del)			
SOL,OT (DROPS)			
12 x-6 x-4 x-4 x-12 x,			
29.6 ml	10310-0324-30	4.35	6.53
AURO-DRI (Del)			
SOL,OT, 5%-95%, 30 ml	10310-0221-02	2.29	3.44
AUTODROP EYEDROPPER AID (Owen Mumford)			
DEV,NA, ea	08470-6000-01	2.81	4.99
AUTOJECT 2 FIXED NEEDLE (Owen Mumford)			
DEV,NA (SELF INJEC DELIV SYSTEM)			
ea	08470-1310-01	32.19	
(FIXED NEEDLE,DELIV SYS)			
2s ea	08470-1300-01	32.19	40.00
AUTOJECT 2 REMOVABLE NEEDLE (Owen Mumford)			
DEV,NA (DRUG DELIVERY SYSTEM)			
ea	08470-1311-01	32.19	
AUTOLET II CLINISAFE (Owen Mumford)			
DEV,NA, ea	08470-0900-01	14.38	22.00
AUTOLET IMPRESSION (Owen Mumford)			
DEV,NA (BAG)			
ea	08470-0271-01	8.50	
(BOX)			
ea	08470-0270-01	11.25	
(WITHOUT HANGER TAB)			
ea	08470-0274-01	11.25	

PROD/MFR	HRI. UPC.NDC	AWP	SRP
AUTOLET LITE (Owen Mumford)			
DEV,NA (STARTER PACK)			
ea	08470-0569-01	10.63	20.00
AUTOLET LITE CLINISAFE (Owen Mumford)			
DEV,NA, ea	08740-0576-01	14.38	20.00
AUTOLET MINI (Owen Mumford)			
DEV,NA (SINGLE BOX)			
ea	08470-0265-01	4.69	5.99
2s ea	08470-0260-01	5.31	6.99
AUTOLET PLATFORMS (Owen Mumford)			
DEV,NA (ORANGE,3.0MM,DISPOSABLE)			
200s ea	08470-0301-01	5.31	7.25
(WHITE,1.8MM,DISPOSABLE)			
200s ea	08470-0302-01	5.31	7.25
(YELLOW,2.4MM,DISPOSABLE)			
200s ea	08470-0300-01	5.31	7.25
AUTOPEN (Owen Mumford)			
DEV,NA (1.5ML CART,1 UNIT INC)			
ea	08470-3100-01	35.63	35.00
(1.5ML CART,2 UNIT INC)			
ea	08470-3000-01	35.63	35.00
(3ML CART,1 UNIT INC)			
ea	08470-3810-01	36.88	35.00
(3ML CART,2 UNIT INC)			
ea	08470-3800-01	36.88	35.00
AUTOSENSOR (Sankyo Pharma)			
DEV,NA, 16s ea	08197-1001-16	144.00	
AUTOSQUEEZE EYEDROP BOTTLE AID (Owen Mumford)			
DEV,NA, ea	08470-6100-01	2.81	4.99
AVEENO 1% HYDROCORTISONE ANTI-ITCH CREAM (Johnson & Johnson)			
CRE,TP (MAX STRENGTH)			
1%, 28 gm	81370-0036-58	4.22	
AVEENO ACTIVE NATURALS ESSENTIAL MOISTURE (Johnson & Johnson)			
STI,TP (SPF15)			
1%-7.5%-5%, 4.2 gm	81370-0014-57	2.52	
AVEENO ACTIVE NATURALS POSITIVELY RADIANT (Johnson & Johnson)			
LOT,TP (SPF 30,OIL-FREE)			
3%-7.5%-2%, 75 ml	81370-0015-84	13.18	
(SPF 15,OIL-FREE)			
3%-7.5%-2%, 120 ml	81370-0036-95	13.18	
AVEENO ADVANCED CARE BODY WASH (Johnson & Johnson)			
SOA,TP (FRAGRANCE-FREE)			
295 ml	81370-0010-75	7.60	
AVEENO ADVANCED CARE MOISTURIZING CREAM (Johnson & Johnson)			
CRE,TP (FRAGRANCE-FREE)			
170 gm	81370-0010-74	7.60	
AVEENO ANTI-ITCH (Johnson & Johnson)			
LOT,TP (CONCENTRATED)			
3%-1%, 118 ml	81370-0036-90	5.20	
AVEENO ANTI-ITCH CREAM (Johnson & Johnson)			
CRE,TP, 3%-1%, 28 gm	81370-0036-80	2.59	
AVEENO BABY CALMING COMFORT BATH (Johnson & Johnson)			
SOL,TP (SOAP-FREE)			
236 ml	81370-0038-02	4.12	
AVEENO BABY CALMING COMFORT LOTION (Johnson & Johnson)			
LOT,TP, 1.2%, 227 gm	81370-0036-45	4.12	
AVEENO BABY CONTINUOUS PROTECTION SUNBLOCK LOTION (Johnson & Johnson)			
LOT,TP (SPF55,FRAGRANCE-FREE)			
3%-10%-5%-2.8%-6%,			
112 gm	81370-0012-74	8.14	
AVEENO BABY DAILY MOISTURE LOTION (Johnson & Johnson)			
LOT,TP (FRAGRANCE-FREE)			
1.2%, 227 gm	81370-0036-64	4.12	
354 gm	81370-0042-29	5.60	
AVEENO BABY ESSENTIAL MOISTURE (Johnson & Johnson)			
SHA,TP (1X236ML)			
236 ml	81370-0011-59	4.12	
AVEENO BABY SOOTHING BATH TREATMENT (Johnson & Johnson)			
PDR,TP (TEAR-FREE)			
43%, 5s ea	81370-0036-62	4.12	

PROD/MFR	HRI. UPC.NDC	AWP	SRP
AVEENO BABY SOOTHING RELIEF CREAMY WASH (Johnson & Johnson)			
SOA,TP (TEAR-FREE)			
236 ml	81370-0042-49	4.12	
AVEENO BABY SOOTHING RELIEF DIAPER RASH CREAM (Johnson & Johnson)			
CRE,TP (FRAGRANCE-FREE)			
13%, 51 gm	81370-0042-70	3.64	
105 gm	81370-0012-98	5.23	
AVEENO BABY SOOTHING RELIEF MOISTURE CREAM (Johnson & Johnson)			
CRE,TP (FRAGRANCE-FREE)			
140 gm	81370-0039-13	4.12	
227 gm	81370-0011-75	5.60	
AVEENO BABY WASH & SHAMPOO (Johnson & Johnson)			
SHA,TP (TEAR-FREE)			
236 ml	81370-0036-65	4.12	
354 ml	81370-0042-30	5.60	
AVEENO BATH TREATMENT (Johnson & Johnson)			
PDR,TP (SOOTHING, 8X42GM)			
100%, 42 gm 8s	81370-0036-40	5.50	
AVEENO CLEAR COMPLEXION CLEANSING BAR (Johnson & Johnson)			
SOA,TP (ACTIVE NATURALS)			
0.5%, 100 gm	81370-0036-22	2.23	
AVEENO CLEAR COMPLEXION CREAM CLEANSER (Johnson & Johnson)			
SOA,TP (OIL-FREE)			
2%, 141 gm	81370-0011-19	5.92	
AVEENO CLEAR COMPLEXION DAILY CLEANSING PADS (Johnson & Johnson)			
PAD,TP (AF,OIL-FREE,SOAP-FREE)			
0.5%, 28s ea	81370-0013-69	5.92	
AVEENO CLEAR COMPLEXION DAILY MOISTURIZER (Johnson & Johnson)			
LOT,TP (OIL-FREE)			
0.5%, 120 ml	81370-0038-11	13.18	
AVEENO CLEAR COMPLEXION FOAMING CLEANSER (Johnson & Johnson)			
FOA,TP (OIL-FREE,SOAP-FREE)			
0.5%, 180 ml	81370-0036-91	5.92	
AVEENO CONTINUOUS PROTECTION SUNBLOCK LOTION (Johnson & Johnson)			
LOT,TP (SPF30,FOR FACE,OIL-FREE)			
3%-10%-5%-2.4%-5%,			
84 gm	81370-0014-60	8.14	
(SPF55,OIL-FREE)			
3%-10%-5%-2.8%-6%,			
112 gm	81371-0010-33	8.14	
(ACTIVE,SPF 50,FOR FACE)			
3%-10%-5%-4%-6%,			
84 gm	81371-0010-65	8.14	
(SPF70,FOR FACE,OIL-FREE)			
3%-15%-5%-2.8%-6%,			
84 gm	81370-0011-27	8.90	
AVEENO CONTINUOUS PROTECTION SUNBLOCK SPRAY (Johnson & Johnson)			
SPR,TP (ACTIVE,SPF30,OIL-FREE)			
3%-8%-4%-2.4%-5%,			
141.5 gm	81371-0010-38	8.14	
(ACTIVE,SPF70,OIL-FREE)			
3%-15%-5%-4%-6%,			
141.5 gm	81371-0010-34	8.90	
(SPF50,OIL-FREE)			
3%-15%-5%-4%-6%,			
141.5 gm	81371-0010-31	8.14	
(SPF70,OIL-FREE)			
3%-15%-5%-4%-6%,			
141.5 gm	81370-0011-21	8.90	
AVEENO CONTINUOUS RADIANCE MOISTURIZING LOTION (Johnson & Johnson)			
LOT,TP (ALL SKIN TONES)			
212 gm	81370-0012-70	11.86	
(MEDIUM SKIN TONES)			
227 gm	81370-0015-87	7.13	
AVEENO CREAMY MOISTURIZING OIL (Johnson & Johnson)			
OIL,TP, 354 ml	81370-0039-21	7.13	
AVEENO DAILY MOISTURIZING (Johnson & Johnson)			
LOT,TP, 1.25%, 227 gm	81370-0036-01	5.50	
354 ml	81370-0036-00	7.13	
532 ml	81370-0038-44	8.93	
AVEENO DAILY MOISTURIZING FOAM BATH (Johnson & Johnson)			
FOA,TP, 295 ml	81371-0010-48	5.23	

PROD/MFR	HRI, UPC,NDC	AWP	SRP
AVEENO DAILY MOISTURIZING LOTION (Johnson & Johnson)			
LOT,TP (ACTIVE NATURALS)			
1.3%, 29 ml	81370-0013-82	0.79	
(FRAGRANCE-FREE)			
1.3%, 71 gm	81370-0036-02	2.42	
AVEENO DAILY MOISTURIZING LOTION WITH SUNSCREEN (Johnson & Johnson)			
LOT,TP (SPF 15)			
3%-5%-1.7%-3%,			
227 gm	81370-0011-74	7.13	
354 ml	81370-0011-73	8.93	
AVEENO INTENSE RELIEF (Johnson & Johnson)			
STI,TP, 1%-31%, 4.2 gm	81370-0014-76	2.52	
AVEENO INTENSE RELIEF HAND CREAM (Johnson & Johnson)			
CRE,TP, 100 gm	81370-0036-57	5.50	
AVEENO INTENSE RELIEF OVERNIGHT CREAM (Johnson & Johnson)			
CRE,TP (FRAGRANCE-FREE)			
1.3%, 207 gm	81370-0011-37	7.13	
AVEENO INTENSE RELIEF REPAIR CREAM (Johnson & Johnson)			
CRE,TP, 454 gm	81370-0015-59	11.86	
AVEENO MOISTURIZING BAR (Johnson & Johnson)			
BAR,TP (ACTIVE NATURALS)			
100 gm	81370-0036-23	2.23	
AVEENO OVERNIGHT ITCH RELIEF CREAM (Johnson & Johnson)			
CRE,TP (W/TRIPLE OAT COMPLEX)			
100 gm	81370-0042-69	5.20	
AVEENO POSITIVELY AGELESS DAILY CLEANSING PADS (Johnson & Johnson)			
PAD,TP (OIL-FREE,SOAP-FREE)			
28s ea	81371-0010-53	7.25	
AVEENO POSITIVELY AGELESS DAILY MOISTURIZER (Johnson & Johnson)			
LOT,TP (SPF 30)			
3%-12%-5%-1.7%-3%,			
75 ml	81370-0042-60	15.68	
(SPF 42)			
3%-12%-5%-2.35%-6%,			
47 ml	81371-0010-76	15.68	
AVEENO POSITIVELY AGELESS EXFOLIATING CLEANSER (Johnson & Johnson)			
SOA,TP, 150 ml	81370-0042-61	7.48	
AVEENO POSITIVELY AGELESS EYE SERUM (Johnson & Johnson)			
LOT,TP (FRAGRANCE-FREE,OIL-FREE)			
15 ml	81370-0011-18	15.68	
AVEENO POSITIVELY AGELESS FIRMING BODY LOTION (Johnson & Johnson)			
LOT,TP, 227 gm	81371-0010-77	7.25	
AVEENO POSITIVELY AGELESS LIFT & FIRM EYE CREAM (Johnson & Johnson)			
CRE,TP, 15 ml	81370-0011-78	15.68	
AVEENO POSITIVELY AGELESS LIFT & FIRM MOISTURIZER (Johnson & Johnson)			
LOT,TP (SPF30)			
3%-12%-5%-1.7%-3%,			
75 ml	81370-0011-77	15.68	
AVEENO POSITIVELY AGELESS LIFT & FIRM NIGHT (Johnson & Johnson)			
CRE,TP, 50 ml	81370-0011-76	15.68	
AVEENO POSITIVELY AGELESS NIGHT CREAM (Johnson & Johnson)			
CRE,TP, 50 ml	81370-0042-62	15.68	
AVEENO POSITIVELY AGELESS REJUVENATING SERUM (Johnson & Johnson)			
LOT,TP (OIL-FREE)			
50 ml	81370-0042-59	15.68	
AVEENO POSITIVELY AGELESS SUNBLOCK LOTION (Johnson & Johnson)			
LOT,TP (SPF70,FOR FACE,OIL-FREE)			
3%-15%-5%-2.8%-6%,			
84 gm	81371-0010-32	8.90	
AVEENO POSITIVELY AGELESS SUNBLOCK SPRAY (Johnson & Johnson)			
SPR,TP (SPF50,OIL-FREE)			
3%-15%-5%-4%-6%,			
141.5 gm	81371-0010-36	8.90	
AVEENO POSITIVELY AGELESS WARMING SCRUB (Johnson & Johnson)			
SOA,TP, 113 gm	81370-0022-66	7.25	
AVEENO POSITIVELY RADIANT CLEANSER (Johnson & Johnson)			
SOL,TP (ACTIVE NATURALS)			
200 ml	81370-0036-72	5.92	
AVEENO POSITIVELY RADIANT DAILY CLEANSING PADS (Johnson & Johnson)			
PAD,TP (ACTIVE NATURALS)			
28s ea	81370-0013-10	5.92	
AVEENO POSITIVELY RADIANT EXFOLIATING BODY WASH (Johnson & Johnson)			
SOL,TP (SOAP-FREE)			
354 ml	81370-0014-47	5.23	
AVEENO POSITIVELY RADIANT MAKEUP REMOVING CLEANSER (Johnson & Johnson)			
FOA,TP (1X163ML)			
163 ml	81371-0016-94	5.92	
AVEENO POSITIVELY RADIANT MOISTURIZING LOTION (Johnson & Johnson)			
LOT,TP, 305 ml	81370-0013-63	7.13	
AVEENO POSITIVELY RADIANT TRIPLE BOOSTING SERUM (Johnson & Johnson)			
LOT,TP (OIL-FREE)			
50 ml	81370-0022-67	13.18	
AVEENO POSITIVELY SMOOTH SHAVE GEL (Johnson & Johnson)			
GEL,TP, 198 gm	81370-0038-59	3.43	
AVEENO SKIN BRIGHTENING DAILY SCRUB (Johnson & Johnson)			
SOL,TP (ACTIVE NATURALS)			
140 gm	81370-0036-76	5.92	
AVEENO SKIN RELIEF BATH TREATMENT (Johnson & Johnson)			
PDR,TP (3 X 42GM,FRAGRANCE-FREE)			
100%, 42 gm 3s	81370-0036-89	2.59	
AVEENO SKIN RELIEF BODY WASH (Johnson & Johnson)			
SOL,TP (DYE-FREE,FRAGRANCE-FREE)			
354 ml	81370-0036-46	5.23	
(DYE-FREE,SOAP-FREE)			
354 ml	81370-0036-48	5.23	
(DYE-FREE,FRAGRANCE-FREE)			
532 ml	81370-0013-26	6.79	
(DYE-FREE,SOAP-FREE)			
532 ml	81370-0039-99	6.79	
AVEENO SKIN RELIEF MOISTURIZING CREAM (Johnson & Johnson)			
CRE,TP, 2.5%, 312 gm	81370-0013-65	8.93	
AVEENO SKIN RELIEF MOISTURIZING LOTION (Johnson & Johnson)			
LOT,TP (FRAGRANCE-FREE)			
1.3%, 227 gm	81370-0015-80	5.50	
354 ml	81370-0015-79	7.13	
532 ml	81370-0042-67	8.93	
(ACTIVE NATURALS)			
2.5%, 227 gm	81370-0036-84	5.50	
354 ml	81370-0036-85	7.13	
AVEENO SKIN RELIEF SHOWER & BATH OIL (Johnson & Johnson)			
OIL,TP, 295 ml	81371-0010-50	6.79	
AVEENO STRESS RELIEF BODY WASH (Johnson & Johnson)			
SOL,TP (DYE-FREE,SOAP-FREE)			
354 ml	81370-0039-55	5.23	
532 ml	81370-0013-27	6.79	
AVEENO STRESS RELIEF FOAMING BATH (Johnson & Johnson)			
FOA,TP, 295 ml	81371-0010-51	5.23	
AVEENO STRESS RELIEF MOISTURIZING LOTION (Johnson & Johnson)			
LOT,TP, 354 ml	81370-0039-16	7.13	
532 ml	81370-0015-31	8.93	
AVEENO THERAPEUTIC SHAVE GEL (Johnson & Johnson)			
GEL,TP, 198 gm	81370-0036-70	3.43	
AVEENO ULTRA-CALMING DAILY MOISTURIZER (Johnson & Johnson)			
LOT,TP (SPF 15,OIL-FREE)			
3%-7.5%-2%, 120 ml	81370-0014-23	13.18	
(SPF 30,FRAGRANCE-FREE)			
5%-7.5%-5%-2.3%,			
75 ml	81371-0016-23	13.18	
AVEENO ULTRA-CALMING FOAMING CLEANSER (Johnson & Johnson)			
FOA,TP (ACTIVE NATURALS)			
180 ml	81370-0014-24	5.92	
AVEENO ULTRA-CALMING SHAVE GEL (Johnson & Johnson)			
GEL,TP, 198 gm	81370-0012-60	3.43	
AVENA SATIVA (Luyties)			
TAB,SL (6X)			
6 x, 500s ea	00618-0288-03	3.99	
5500s ea	00618-0288-10	30.32	
12 x, 500s ea	00622-0288-03	4.19	
5500s ea	00622-0288-10	31.83	
30 x, 500s ea	00624-0288-03	4.19	
5500s ea	00624-0288-10	31.83	
AVENA SATIVA COMPOUND (Weleda)			
LIQ,PO, 50 ml	55946-0136-15	7.20	
AVENOC (Boiron)			
TAB,PO, 3 x-3 x-3 x-3 x,			
60s ea	06962-0603-60	5.73	9.59
AVITENE NON-WOVEN WEB (Davol)			
SHE,NA (35MMX35MM)			
6s ea	03031-0100-80	466.20	
(70MMX35MM)			
6s ea	03031-0100-90	858.96	
(70MMX70MM)			
6s ea	03031-0101-10	1097.46	
AVOGEL (Avocet Polymer Tech.)			
DEV,NA (6"X48",WOUND CARE)			
ea	76170-0106-48	75.00	
(8"X8", SCAR MGNT.)			
ea	76170-0108-81	30.00	
(4"X4", SCAR MGNT.)			
3s ea	76170-0104-43	26.75	
(6"X48",WOUND CARE)			
3s ea	76170-0164-83	225.00	
(8"X8", SCAR MGNT.)			
3s ea	76170-0108-83	85.50	
AVOSIL (Avocet Polymer Tech.)			
OIN,TP (FRAGRANCE-FREE)			
113.4 gm	76170-0400-01	30.00	
113.4 gm 20s	76170-0400-02	590.00	
AXID AR (Wyeth Consumer)			
TAB,PO, 75 mg, 30s ea	00573-2400-40	8.99	
50s ea	00573-2400-45		14.99
(Pharma Pac) REPACK			
TAB,PO, 75 mg, 20s ea	52959-0532-20	15.55	
AXSAIN (Rodlen Labs)			
CRE,TP (IN LIDOCARE VEHICLE)			
0.25%, 60 gm	66358-0100-60		37.50
AYR ALLERGY AND SINUS (Ascher)			
SPR,NS (HYPERTONIC SALINE MIST)			
2.65%, 50 ml	02250-0381-80	3.41	
AYR BABY SALINE (Ascher)			
SPR,NS (AF)			
0.65%, 30 ml	00225-0550-50	2.39	
AYR NO-DRIP SINUS SPRAY (Ascher)			
GEL,NS, 22 ml	02250-0528-48	5.24	
AYR SALINE (Ascher)			
SOL,NS (DROPS)			
0.65%, 50 ml	00225-0382-80	2.39	
SWA,NS (W/ALOE,INDWRPPD,MOIST)			
20s ea	02250-0526-86	6.91	
AYR SALINE MIST (Ascher)			
SPR,NS, 0.65%, 50 ml	00225-0380-80	2.39	
(A-S Medication) REPACK			
SPR,NS, 0.65%, 50 ml	54569-3425-00	2.39	
AYR SALINE NASAL (Ascher)			
GEL,TP, 14.1 gm	00225-0525-47	3.08	
AYR SALINE NASAL NETI RINSE KIT (Ascher)			
PKT,NS, 40s ea	02250-0710-19	7.45	
AYR SALINE NASAL RINSE KIT (Ascher)			
PKT,NS (W/APPLICATORT,SNUSWASH)			
1.6 gm 50s	02250-0700-10	7.45	
(SINUS WASH,PF)			
1.6 gm 100s	02250-0700-15	8.58	12.87
AYR SALINE NASAL RINSE KIT REFILL (Ascher)			
PKT,NS (PF,LATEX-FREE)			
51s ea	02250-0705-91	3.90	
(SINUS WASH,PF)			
1.6 gm 100s	02250-0705-15	7.74	
AYR SNORE RELIEVING THROAT SPRAY (Ascher)			
SPR,MM, 59 ml	02250-0680-51	8.10	
AYR VAPOR INHALER (Ascher)			
SOL,NS, 0.5 ml	00225-0655-23	3.30	

PROD/MFR	HRI, UPC,NDC	AWP	SRP
AZEC (Bio-Tech Pharm)			
CAP,PO, 100s ea..........	53191-0057-01	10.00	
AZO CRANBERRY (Amerifit)			
TAB,PO (PF,DYE-FREE,GLUTEN-FREE)			
450 mg, 50s ea	87651-0420-67	5.12	6.99
AZO STANDARD (Amerifit)			
TAB,PO, 95 mg, 30s ea	87651-0301-52	6.43	8.99
(MAXIMUM STRENGTH)			
97.5 mg, 12s ea	87651-0122-53	4.21	6.49
24s ea	87651-0241-53	7.15	9.99
AZO TEST STRIPS (Amerifit)			
DEV,NA, 3s ea	87651-0326-72	8.29	10.99
AZO YEAST (Amerifit)			
TAB,PO, 6 x-6 x, 60s ea ...	87651-0606-67	5.28	7.99
AZO-DINE (Cardinal Health)			
TAB,PO (PRIVATE LABEL)			
97.2 mg, 32s ea........	37205-0146-64	3.52	
AZO-GESIC (Alphagen)			
TAB,PO, 95 mg, 30s ea	59743-0115-30	3.95	
(Major)			
TAB,PO, 95 mg, 30s ea	00904-5025-46	6.45	
AZOSTIX (Siemens)			
DEV,NA, 25s ea	08620-2830-25	32.25	32.25
B-12 (Mason Vit)			
TER,PO (PF,SF)			
155 mg-1 mg, 60s ea .	11845-0080-55	7.22	
B-12 TIME (Carlson,J.R.)			
TER,PO (PF,SF,CORN-FREE)			
1000 mcg, 90s ea	88395-0024-21	5.95	11.90
B-12-SL (Carlson,J.R.)			
ODT,SL (PF,CORN-FREE,SALT FREE)			
1000 mcg, 180s ea ...	88395-0024-32	9.20	18.40
B-50 GEL (Carlson,J.R.)			
SGL,PO (SOFTGEL)			
50s ea..............	88395-0020-60	4.70	9.40
100s ea.............	88395-0020-61	8.95	17.90
200s ea.............	88395-0020-62	16.00	32.00
B-CARO-T (Bio-Tech Pharm)			
SGL,PO (SOFTGEL)			
25000 iu, 100s ea	53191-0011-01	4.20	
250s ea...........	53191-0011-25	8.80	
B-COMPLEET (Carlson,J.R.)			
TAB,PO (PF,SF,SALT-FREE)			
90s ea.............	88395-0020-10	6.45	12.90
180s ea............	88395-0020-14	11.15	22.30
B-COMPLEET-100 (Carlson,J.R.)			
TAB,PO, 30s ea	88395-0020-70	5.95	11.90
100s ea............	88395-0020-71	16.25	32.50
250s ea............	88395-0020-72	37.45	74.90
B-COMPLEET-50 (Carlson,J.R.)			
PO, 100s ea	88395-0020-21	8.70	17.40
250s ea............	88395-0020-22	19.45	38.90
B-COMPLEX (Nature's Bounty)			
SOL,SL (W/VITAMIN C,AF,SF)			
59 ml..............	74312-0028-71		5.99
B-COMPLEX 100 (Basic Vitamins)			
TER,PO, 60s ea........	00761-0225-20	3.50	
B-COMPLEX VIT PLUS (Bryant Ranch)			
REPACK			
TAB,PO, 30s ea	63629-1727-01	14.83	
100s ea	63629-1727-02	49.42	
B-COMPLEX WITH B-12 (Major)			
TER,PO (PF,SF,LACTOSE-FREE)			
100s ea............	00904-4220-60	5.10	
B-D ACE ADULT ATHLETIC SUPPORTER (BD Consumer)			
DEV,NA (LARGE)			
ea..................	08290-2073-42	5.48	
(MEDIUM)			
ea..................	08290-2073-41	5.48	
(SMALL)			
ea..................	08290-2073-40	5.48	
B-D ACE ANKLE BRACE (BD Consumer)			
DEV,NA (LARGE)			
ea..................	08290-2073-02	4.57	
(MEDIUM)			
ea..................	08290-2073-01	4.57	
(SMALL)			
ea..................	08290-2073-00	4.57	
B-D ACE ATHLETIC (BD Consumer)			
DEV,NA (2")			
ea..................	08290-2074-60	2.59	
(3")			
ea..................	08290-2074-61	3.24	
(4")			
ea..................	08290-2074-62	4.06	
B-D ACE BANDAGE CLIPS (BD Consumer)			
DEV,NA, 12s ea	08290-2074-07	2.10	
B-D ACE ELASTIC (BD Consumer)			
DEV,NA (2 1/2")			
ea..................	08290-2073-11	2.86	
(2")			
ea..................	08290-2073-10	2.46	
(3")			
ea..................	08290-2073-14	3.02	
(4")			
ea..................	08290-2073-13	3.76	
(6")			
ea..................	08290-2073-15	6.41	
B-D ACE ELBOW BRACE (BD Consumer)			
DEV,NA (LARGE)			
ea..................	08290-2073-19	5.08	
(MEDIUM)			
ea..................	08290-2073-18	5.08	
(SMALL)			
ea..................	08290-2073-17	5.08	
B-D ACE HOT/COLD COMPRESSION WRAP (BD Consumer)			
DEV,NA, ea	08290-2075-19	6.61	
B-D ACE INSTANT COLD COMPRESS (BD Consumer)			
DEV,NA, 6s ea	08290-2075-13	1.26	
B-D ACE KNEE BRACE (BD Consumer)			
DEV,NA (LARGE)			
ea..................	08290-2073-05	5.08	
(MEDIUM)			
ea..................	08290-2073-04	5.08	
(SMALL)			
ea..................	08290-2073-03	5.08	
B-D ACE NEOPRENE ANKLE BRACE (BD Consumer)			
DEV,NA (LARGE)			
ea..................	08290-2072-31	7.49	
(MEDIUM)			
ea..................	08290-2072-30	7.49	
(SMALL)			
ea..................	08290-2072-29	7.49	
B-D ACE NEOPRENE ANKLE WRAP (BD Consumer)			
DEV,NA (ONE SIZE FITS ALL)			
ea..................	08290-2072-48	6.61	
B-D ACE NEOPRENE ELBOW BRACE (BD Consumer)			
DEV,NA (LARGE)			
ea..................	08290-2072-27	7.60	
(MEDIUM)			
ea..................	08290-2072-26	7.60	
(ONE SIZE FITS ALL)			
ea..................	08290-2072-49	7.06	
(SMALL)			
ea..................	08290-2072-25	7.60	
(X-LARGE)			
ea..................	08290-2072-28	7.23	
B-D ACE NEOPRENE KNEE BRACE (BD Consumer)			
DEV,NA (ONE SIZE FITS ALL, OPEN)			
ea..................	08290-2072-47	8.11	
(ONE SIZE FITS ALL,CLOSE)			
ea..................	08290-2072-46	7.06	
B-D ACE NEOPRENE KNEE BRACE OPEN (BD Consumer)			
DEV,NA (LARGE)			
ea..................	08290-2072-39	8.51	
(MEDIUM)			
ea..................	08290-2072-38	8.51	
(SMALL)			
ea..................	08290-2072-37	8.51	
B-D ACE NEOPRENE KNEE BRACE REGULAR (BD Consumer)			
DEV,NA (LARGE)			
ea..................	08290-2072-35	7.97	
(MEDIUM)			
ea..................	08290-2072-34	7.97	
(SMALL)			
ea..................	08290-2072-33	7.97	
B-D ACE NEOPRENE PLUS KNEE BRACE (BD Consumer)			
DEV,NA (LARGE)			
ea..................	08290-2072-43	10.88	
(MEDIUM)			
ea..................	08290-2072-42	10.88	
(SMALL)			
ea..................	08290-2072-41	10.88	
B-D ACE NEOPRENE WRIST BRACE (BD Consumer)			
DEV,NA (ONE SIZE)			
ea..................	08290-2072-20	6.26	
B-D ACE PLUS KNEE BRACE (BD Consumer)			
DEV,NA (SIDE STABILIZER, LARGE)			
ea..................	08290-2073-55	7.86	
(SIDE STABILIZER, MEDIUM)			
ea..................	08290-2073-54	7.86	
(SIDE STABILIZER, SMALL)			
ea..................	08290-2073-53	7.86	
B-D ACE PLUS RIGID WRIST BRACE (BD Consumer)			
DEV,NA (LARGE)			
ea..................	08290-2073-22	10.88	
(MEDIUM)			
ea..................	08290-2073-21	10.80	
(SMALL)			
ea..................	08290-2073-20	10.80	
B-D ACE REUSABLE COLD COMPRESS (BD Consumer)			
DEV,NA, ea	08290-2075-16	3.82	
B-D ACE SPORTS TAPE (BD Consumer)			
DEV,NA (4 PACK)			
ea..................	08290-2074-64	7.37	
(SINGLE)			
ea..................	08290-2074-65	2.34	
B-D ACE VELCRO (BD Consumer)			
DEV,NA (3")			
ea..................	08290-2076-03	3.38	
(4")			
ea..................	08290-2076-04	4.22	
(2")			
10s ea..............	08290-8465-02	2.73	
B-D ACE WRIST BRACE (BD Consumer)			
DEV,NA, ea	08290-2073-06	2.87	
B-D AUTOMATIC INJECTOR (BD Consumer)			
DEV,NA, ea	08290-3282-45	20.40	
B-D BASAL DIGITAL THERMOMETER (BD Consumer)			
DEV,NA, ea	08290-5245-60	9.60	
B-D BAUER & BLACK (BD Consumer)			
ABOVE KNEE STOCKING			
DEV,NA (CLOSED TOE, LARGE,BEIGE)			
ea..................	08290-2060-12	12.17	
(CLOSED TOE,LARGE,BEIGE)			
ea..................	08290-2065-08	7.27	
(CLOSED TOE,MEDIUM,BEIGE)			
ea..................	08290-2050-31	12.17	
ea..................	08290-2064-97	7.27	
(CLOSED TOE,SMALL,BEIGE)			
ea..................	08290-2040-04	18.45	
ea..................	08290-2064-81	7.27	
(OPEN TOE,LARGE,BEIGE)			
ea..................	08290-2065-11	6.60	
(OPEN TOE,MEDIUM,BEIGE)			
ea..................	08290-2065-10	6.60	
(OPEN TOE,SMALL,BEIGE)			
ea..................	08290-2065-09	6.60	
ANKLE BRACE			
DEV,NA (ELASTIC, WHITE, LARGE)			
ea..................	08290-2032-24	4.66	
(ELASTIC, WHITE, MEDIUM)			
ea..................	08290-2030-31	4.66	
(ELASTIC, WHITE, SMALL)			
ea..................	08290-2028-38	4.66	
(NYLON, FLESH, LARGE)			
ea..................	08290-2063-38	5.65	
(NYLON, FLESH, MEDIUM)			
ea..................	08290-2061-61	5.65	
(NYLON, FLESH, SMALL)			
ea..................	08290-2060-06	5.65	
ARM SLING POUCH			
DEV,NA (ADULT)			
ea..................	08290-2039-51	10.69	
(YOUTH)			
ea..................	08290-2039-50	9.51	
ARTHRITIS RELIEF GLOVES			
DEV,NA (LARGE)			
ea..................	08290-2030-52	8.27	
(MEDIUM)			
ea..................	08290-2030-51	8.27	
(SMALL)			
ea..................	08290-2030-50	8.27	
ATHLETIC SUPPORTER A-3			
DEV,NA (ADULT, LARGE)			
ea..................	08290-2026-36	8.04	
(ADULT, MEDIUM)			
ea..................	08290-2025-49	8.04	
(ADULT, SMALL)			
ea..................	08290-2024-60	8.04	
ATHLETIC SUPPORTER S-10			
NA (SWIMMER, LARGE)			
ea..................	08290-2069-72	7.09	
(SWIMMER, MEDIUM)			
ea..................	08290-2069-31	7.09	
(SWIMMER, SMALL)			
ea..................	08290-2068-32	7.09	
BACK SUPPORT			
DEV,NA (WHITE, LARGE)			
ea..................	08290-2030-73	27.60	

PROD/MFR	HRI, UPC,NDC	AWP	SRP
(WHITE, MEDIUM)			
ea..................	08290-2030-72	27.60	
(WHITE, SMALL)			
ea..................	08290-2030-71	27.60	
BELOW KNEE STOCKING			
DEV,NA (CLOSED TOE,LARGE,BEIGE)			
ea..................	08290-2030-95	11.47	
(CLOSED TOE,MEDIUM,BEIGE)			
ea..................	08290-2037-75	11.47	
(CLOSED TOE,SMALL,BEIGE)			
ea..................	08290-2020-99	11.47	
(OPEN TOE,LARGE,BEIGE)			
ea..................	08290-2066-08	6.71	
(OPEN TOE,MEDIUM,BEIGE)			
ea..................	08290-2065-59	6.71	
(OPEN TOE,SMALL,BEIGE)			
ea..................	08290-2065-21	6.71	
ELBOW BRACE			
DEV,NA (NYLON, LARGE)			
ea..................	08290-2052-02	5.50	
(NYLON, MEDIUM)			
ea..................	08290-2052-01	5.50	
(NYLON, SMALL)			
ea..................	08290-2052-00	5.50	
(WHITE, LARGE)			
ea..................	08290-2032-57	4.91	
(WHITE, MEDIUM)			
ea..................	08290-2028-24	4.91	
(WHITE, SMALL)			
ea..................	08290-2063-90	4.91	
HERNIA BELT			
DEV,NA (X-LARGE)			
ea..................	08290-2023-87	26.60	
KNEE BRACE			
DEV,NA (ELASTIC, WHITE, LARGE)			
ea..................	08290-2026-57	4.91	
(ELASTIC, WHITE, MEDIUM)			
ea..................	08290-2024-95	4.91	
(ELASTIC, WHITE, SMALL)			
ea..................	08290-2023-28	4.91	
(NYLON, FLESH, LARGE)			
ea..................	08290-2014-93	5.50	
(NYLON, FLESH, MEDIUM)			
ea..................	08290-2012-12	5.50	
(NYLON, FLESH, SMALL)			
ea..................	08290-2010-90	8.71	
KNEE HIGH STOCKING			
DEV,NA (ULTRA SHEER,LARGE,BEIGE)			
ea..................	08290-2010-53	5.56	
(ULTRA SHEER,LARGE,BLACK)			
ea..................	08290-2010-56	5.56	
(ULTRA SHEER,MED.,BEIGE)			
ea..................	08290-2010-52	5.56	
(ULTRA SHEER,MED.,BLACK)			
ea..................	08290-2010-55	5.56	
(ULTRA SHEER,SMALL,BEIGE)			
ea..................	08290-2010-51	5.56	
(ULTRA SHEER,SMALL,BLACK)			
ea..................	08290-2010-54	5.56	
MATERNITY PANTY HOSE			
NA (ULTRA SHEER,MED.,BEIGE)			
ea..................	08290-2010-43	15.69	
(ULTRA SHEER,TALL,BEIGE)			
ea..................	08290-2010-44	15.69	
MEN'S ELASTIC HOSE			
NA (FIRM SUPPORT, LARGE)			
ea..................	08290-2062-31	11.47	
ea..................	08290-2062-57	11.47	
(FIRM SUPPORT, REGULAR)			
ea..................	08290-2062-28	11.47	
ea..................	08290-2062-44	11.47	
(FIRM SUPPORT, X-LARGE)			
ea..................	08290-2062-35	11.47	
ea..................	08290-2062-67	11.47	
(LIGHT SUPPORT, LARGE)			
ea..................	08290-2040-42	4.69	
ea..................	08290-2040-46	4.69	
(LIGHT SUPPORT, REGULAR)			
ea..................	08290-2040-41	4.69	
ea..................	08290-2040-45	4.69	
(LIGHT SUPPORT, X-LARGE)			
ea..................	08290-2040-43	4.69	
ea..................	08290-2040-47	4.69	
(MED. SUPPORT, LARGE)			
ea..................	08290-2019-69	7.07	
ea..................	08290-2077-25	7.07	
(MED. SUPPORT, REGULAR)			
ea..................	08290-2033-73	7.07	
ea..................	08290-2061-47	7.07	
(MED. SUPPORT, X-LARGE)			
ea..................	08290-2065-55	7.07	
ea..................	08290-2074-57	7.07	

PROD/MFR	HRI, UPC,NDC	AWP	SRP
PANTY HOSE			
NA (EXTRA-TALL, BEIGE)			
ea..................	08290-2040-18	19.20	
(MEDIUM, BEIGE)			
ea..................	08290-2040-16	19.20	
(PETITE, BEIGE)			
ea..................	08290-2040-15	19.20	
(SHEER, MEDIUM, BEIGE)			
ea..................	08290-2019-93	11.56	
(SHEER, MEDIUM, BLACK)			
ea..................	08290-2019-94	11.56	
(SHEER, PETITE, BEIGE)			
ea..................	08290-2017-91	11.56	
(SHEER, PETITE, BLACK)			
ea..................	08290-2017-92	11.56	
(SHEER, QUEEN, BEIGE)			
ea..................	08290-2024-68	11.56	
(SHEER, QUEEN, BLACK)			
ea..................	08290-2024-69	11.56	
(SHEER, TALL, BEIGE)			
ea..................	08290-2021-69	11.56	
(SHEER, TALL, BLACK)			
ea..................	08290-2021-70	11.56	
(SHEER, X-TALL, BEIGE)			
ea..................	08290-2024-66	11.56	
(SHEER,EXTRA-TALL, BLACK)			
ea..................	08290-2024-67	11.56	
(TALL, BEIGE)			
ea..................	08290-2040-17	19.20	
(ULTRA SHEER, MED.,BEIGE)			
ea..................	08290-2010-31	8.69	
(ULTRA SHEER, MED.,BLACK)			
ea..................	08290-2010-36	8.69	
(ULTRA SHEER, TALL,BEIGE)			
ea..................	08290-2010-32	8.69	
(ULTRA SHEER, TALL,BLACK)			
ea..................	08290-2010-37	8.69	
(ULTRA SHEER,PETIT,BEIGE)			
ea..................	08290-2010-30	8.69	
(ULTRA SHEER,PETIT,BLACK)			
ea..................	08290-2010-35	8.69	
(ULTRA SHEER,QUEEN,BEIGE)			
ea..................	08290-2010-34	8.69	
(ULTRA SHEER,QUEEN,BLACK)			
ea..................	08290-2010-39	8.69	
(ULTRA SHEER,XTALL,BEIGE)			
ea..................	08290-2010-33	8.69	
(ULTRA SHEER,XTALL,BLACK)			
ea..................	08290-2010-38	8.69	
RIB BELT FEMALE			
DEV,NA (LARGE)			
ea..................	08290-2039-54	12.94	
(MEDIUM)			
ea..................	08290-2039-53	12.94	
(SMALL)			
ea..................	08290-2039-52	12.99	
RIB BELT MALE			
NA (LARGE)			
ea..................	08290-2039-57	12.94	
(MEDIUM)			
ea..................	08290-2039-56	12.94	
(SMALL)			
ea..................	08290-2039-55	12.99	
RIGID KNEE BRACE			
DEV,NA (SIDE SUPPORTS, LARGE)			
ea..................	08290-2012-08	8.21	
(SIDE SUPPORTS, MEDIUM)			
ea..................	08290-2012-07	8.21	
(SIDE SUPPORTS, SMALL)			
ea..................	08290-2012-06	8.21	
RIGID WRIST BRACE			
DEV,NA (LARGE)			
ea..................	08290-2012-11	11.56	
(MEDIUM)			
ea..................	08290-2012-10	11.56	
(SMALL)			
ea..................	08290-2012-09	11.56	
SACROILLIAC BELT			
DEV,NA (LARGE)			
ea..................	08290-2062-54	26.60	
(SMALL)			
ea..................	08290-2022-54	26.60	
SUSPENSORY			
DEV,NA (EXTRA LARGE)			
ea..................	08290-2026-12	7.11	
(LARGE)			
ea..................	08290-2024-30	6.49	
(MEDIUM)			
ea..................	08290-2022-62	6.49	
(SMALL)			
ea..................	08290-2021-10	6.49	

PROD/MFR	HRI, UPC,NDC	AWP	SRP
SUSPENSORY/LEG STRAP			
NA (EXTRA LARGE)			
ea..................	08290-2013-52	12.94	
(LARGE)			
ea..................	08290-2012-55	11.46	
(MEDIUM)			
ea..................	08290-2011-61	11.46	
(SMALL)			
ea..................	08290-2010-70	11.46	
WRISTLET			
DEV,NA (DELUXE)			
ea..................	08290-2073-12	4.82	
B-D BAUER/BLACK CARPAL TUNNEL BRACE			
(BD Consumer)			
DEV,NA (LARGE, LEFT)			
ea..................	08290-2070-05	15.47	
(LARGE, RIGHT)			
ea..................	08290-2070-07	15.47	
(REGULAR, LEFT)			
ea..................	08290-2070-04	15.47	
(REGULAR, RIGHT)			
ea..................	08290-2070-06	15.47	
B-D DIGITAL FEVER THERMOMETER (BD Consumer)			
DEV,NA (FLEXIBLE)			
ea..................	08290-5240-34	9.09	
(STANDARD)			
ea..................	08290-5240-30	7.56	
B-D LANCETS (BD Consumer)			
DEV,NA (DME 33G)			
100s ea..............	08290-3220-65	8.81	
B-D ORAL MEDICATION CONTAINERS			
(BD Dickinson Hosp Prod)			
DEV,NA (15CC, ASSEMBLED)			
250s ea..............	08290-3052-03	42.00	
(15CC, UNASSEMBLED)			
250s ea..............	08290-3052-05	40.90	
(30CC, ASSEMBLED)			
250s ea..............	08290-3052-04	53.90	
(30CC, UNASSEMBLED)			
250s ea..............	08290-3052-06	52.80	
B-D ORAL SYRINGE FILLING DEVICES			
(BD Dickinson Hosp Prod)			
DEV,NA (BOTTLE ADAPTER)			
50s ea..............	08290-3052-22	21.80	
(FILLING CONNECTOR)			
50s ea..............	08290-3052-23	13.75	
B-D ORAL SYRINGE W/TIP CAP			
(BD Dickinson Hosp Prod)			
DEV,NA (10ML, AMBER)			
100s ea..............	82903-0052-09	20.95	
(10ML, CLEAR)			
100s ea..............	82903-0052-19	15.40	
(1ML, AMBER)			
100s ea..............	82903-0052-07	17.57	
(1ML, CLEAR)			
100s ea..............	82903-0052-17	12.75	
(3ML, AMBER)			
100s ea..............	82903-0052-10	15.75	
(3ML, CLEAR)			
100s ea..............	82903-0052-20	11.30	
(5ML, AMBER)			
100s ea..............	82903-0052-08	16.59	
(5ML, CLEAR)			
100s ea..............	82903-0052-18	11.90	
(5ML, AMBER)			
500s ea..............	08290-3052-08	80.80	
B-D SENSICARE MEDICAL GLOVES (BD Consumer)			
DEV,NA (SINGLE USE,LARGE)			
50s ea..............	08290-4870-53	5.52	
(SINGLE USE,MEDIUM)			
50s ea..............	08290-4870-52	5.52	
(SINGLE USE,SMALL)			
50s ea..............	08290-4870-51	5.52	
B-D SYRINGE LUER TIP CAP			
(BD Dickinson Hosp Prod)			
DEV,NA, 10s ea...........	82903-0083-41	0.71	
B-D SYRINGE TIP CONNECTOR			
(BD Dickinson Hosp Prod)			
DEV,NA, 50s ea...........	08290-3052-25	29.00	
B-D TRU-TOUCH VINYL GLOVES (BD Consumer)			
DEV,NA (SINGLE USE,MEDIUM)			
10s ea..............	08290-4870-82	15.55	
B-D YALE REUSABLE NEEDLE			
(BD Dickinson Hosp Prod)			
DEV,NA (27GX1"W/LUER LOCK)			
12s ea..............	08290-5110-05	59.79	
B-STRESS (Bio-Tech Pharm)			
CAP,PO, 100s ea...........	53191-0301-01	6.30	

PROD/MFR	HRI, UPC,NDC	AWP	SRP
B.F.I. (Numark)			
POW,TP, 16%, 37.5 gm	38485-0862-14	7.56	
B1-50 (Bio-Tech Pharm)			
CAP,PO, 50 mg, 100s ea	53191-0261-01	5.85	
B1-500 (Bio-Tech Pharm)			
CAP,PO, 500 mg, 100s ea	53191-0357-01	11.00	
B12-METHYL (Bio-Tech Pharm)			
CAP,PO, 1000 mcg,			
100s ea	53191-0455-01	8.40	
250s ea	53191-0455-25	15.75	
B2-50 (Bio-Tech Pharm)			
CAP,PO, 50 mg, 100s ea	53191-0262-01	5.85	
B3-250 (Bio-Tech Pharm)			
CAP,PO, 250 mg, 100s ea	53191-0368-01	4.25	
B3-50 (Bio-Tech Pharm)			
CAP,PO, 50 mg, 100s ea	53191-0356-01	3.15	
B3-500 (Bio-Tech Pharm)			
CAP,PO, 152 mg-500 mg,			
100s ea	53191-0369-01	12.00	
B5-250 (Bio-Tech Pharm)			
CAP,PO, 23 mg-250 mg,			
100s ea	53191-0247-01	3.65	
B6-50 (Bio-Tech Pharm)			
CAP,PO, 50 mg, 100s ea	53191-0348-01	3.15	
B6-FOLIC ACID (Bio-Tech Pharm)			
CAP,PO, 100s ea	53191-0248-01	6.00	
BABEE COF SYRUP (Pfeiffer)			
SYR,PO, 7.5 mg/5 ml,			
120 ml	00927-0513-12	1.76	3.17
BABEE TEETHING (Pfeiffer)			
LOT,MM, 2.5%, 15 ml	00927-0452-23	1.76	3.17
BABY GAS-X (Novartis Consumer)			
SOL,PO (1X30ML,DROPS)			
20 mg/0.3 ml,			
30 ml	00043-6243-01	8.38	
BABY LIZARD (Del-Ray)			
CRE,TP (1X89ML,SPF30+)			
5%-10%, 89 ml	00027-0000-39	7.80	9.99
BABY VITAMIN (Phys Total Care)			
REPACK			
SOL,PO (DROPS)			
50 ml	54868-5735-00	15.53	
BABYFRIDGE (Technological Investments)			
DEV,NA (PORTABLE,BF-7L)			
ea	08605-0104-04	93.75	
BABYTHERM PACIFIER DIGITAL (Lumiscope)			
DEV,NA (PEAK TEMP BEEPER)			
ea	38673-0020-19	5.99	11.99
BACID PROBIOTIC (Heritage/Insight)			
TAB,PO (PF,DYE-FREE,CAPLET)			
5%-80%-10%-5%,			
50s ea	63736-0105-04	16.28	
100s ea	63736-0105-06	29.90	
BACIGUENT (Lee Pharm)			
OIN,TP, 500 u/gm,			
15 gm 48s	23558-0520-13	345.60	
30 gm	23558-0520-12	7.20	
BACITRACIN (Albertson's)			
OIN,TP, 500 u/gm,			
30 gm 30s	41280-0200-78	2.04	
(Altaire)			
OIN,TP, 500 u/gm, 30 gm	59390-0026-17	1.75	
(AmerisourceBergen)			
OIN,TP (PRIVATE LABEL)			
500 u/gm, 30 gm	24385-0060-03	4.49	4.99
(Cardinal Health)			
OIN,TP (PRIVATE LABEL)			
500 u/gm, 30 gm	37205-0275-10	3.44	
(Consolidated Midland)			
OIN,TP, 500 u/gm,			
1 gm 144s	00223-4245-09	17.50	
15 gm	00223-4106-15	1.40	
30 gm	00223-4106-30	1.80	
120 gm	00223-4106-11	4.95	
454 gm	00223-4106-13	14.75	
(Denison)			
OIN,TP, 500 u/gm, 30 gm	00295-1223-95	1.55	
(Fougera)			
OIN,TP, 500 u/gm, 15 gm	00168-0011-35	2.90	
30 gm	00168-0011-31	4.24	
120 gm	00168-0011-04	16.80	
454 gm	00168-0011-16	57.10	
(G&W)			
OIN,TP, 500 u/gm, 30 gm	00713-0280-31	3.12	
(Hart Health)			
OIN,TP (FIRST AID ANTIBIOTIC)			
500 u/gm,			
0.9 gm 144s UD	50332-0030-04	13.47	
(Perrigo)			
OIN,TP, 500 u/gm,			
0.9 gm 144s UD	45802-0060-70	28.75	
15 gm	45802-0060-01	3.60	
30 gm	45802-0060-03	5.25	
(Pfeiffer)			
OIN,TP, 500 u/gm, 30 gm	00927-0094-30	1.09	1.96
(Qualitest)			
OIN,TP, 500 u/gm, 30 gm	00603-0441-50	5.88	
(Taro)			
OIN,TP, 500 u/gm, 15 gm	51672-2005-01	2.88	
(A-S Medication)			
REPACK			
OIN,TP, 500 u/gm,			
0.9 gm 144s UD	54569-5536-00	28.75	
30 gm	54569-5539-00	5.25	
(Altura)			
REPACK			
OIN,TP, 500 u/gm, 15 gm	63874-0033-15	5.98	
30 gm	63874-0033-30	9.04	
454 gm	63874-0149-45	20.37	
(DHS, Inc.)			
REPACK			
OIN,TP (1X3.5GM)			
500 u/gm, 3.5 gm	55887-0424-35	10.50	
15 gm	55887-0424-15	8.04	
30 gm	55887-0424-30	12.00	
(Dispensing Solutions)			
REPACK			
OIN,TP, 500 u/gm,			
0.9 gm 144s UD	55045-1422-01	28.00	
14 gm	55045-1422-05	6.45	
30 gm	55045-1422-06	11.42	
(Keltman Pharma., Inc.)			
REPACK			
OIN,TP (1X500GM)			
500 u/gm, 500 gm	68387-0546-01	6.15	
(Nucare Pharm)			
REPACK			
OIN,TP, 500 u/gm, 15 gm	66267-0989-15	6.47	
30 gm	66267-0988-30	6.79	
(1X30GM)			
500 u/gm, 30 gm	68071-1324-00	13.54	
(Palmetto)			
REPACK			
OIN,TP, 500 u/gm,			
144s ea	23490-6616-01	29.94	
(Phys Total Care)			
REPACK			
OIN,TP, 500 u/gm, 15 gm	54868-3269-00	8.91	
30 gm	54868-3269-01	8.76	
(Quality Care Prod)			
REPACK			
OIN,TP, 500 u/gm, 15 gm	49999-0142-15	12.34	
30 gm	49999-0142-30	20.60	
144 gm	49999-0142-44	23.00	
(Southwood)			
REPACK			
OIN,TP, 500 u/gm, 15 gm	58016-3009-01	4.13	
30 gm	58016-3011-01	5.11	
454 gm	58016-3008-01	19.40	
(Stat Rx)			
REPACK			
OIN,TP, 500 u/gm, 30 gm	16590-0363-30	5.99	
(Fougera)			
BACITRACIN ZINC			
OIN,TP (UNIT OF USE)			
500 u/gm,			
9.6 gm 144s	00168-0111-09	28.80	
(Actavis Mid Atlantic)			
OIN,TP (5 PANEL)			
500 u/gm, 15 gm	00472-1105-34	4.69	
30 gm	00472-1105-56	8.48	
(Taro)			
OIN,TP (U.S.P.)			
500 u/gm, 28.4 gm	51672-0207-52	4.21	
(Palmetto)			
REPACK			
OIN,TP (1X30GM)			
500 u/gm, 30 gm	23490-6817-03	11.54	
(Pharma Pac)			
REPACK			
OIN,TP, 500 u/gm,			
0.9 gm 144s	52959-0113-44	24.65	
15 gm	52959-0113-15	5.95	
30 gm	52959-0113-03	14.04	
BACITRACIN ZINC/POLY B SULFATE (DHS, Inc.)			
REPACK			
OIN,OP, 500 u/gm-10000 u/gm,			
15 gm	55887-0606-15	12.15	
BACITRACIN ZINC/POLYMYXIN B SULFATE (Southwood)			
REPACK			
OIN,TP, 500 u/gm-10000 u/gm,			
15 gm	58016-3153-01	12.15	
30 gm	58016-3239-01	18.16	
BACITRACIN ZN/NEOMYCIN/POLYMYXIN B SULFATE (Consolidated Midland)			
OIN,TP, 15 gm	00223-4108-01	1.95	
30 gm	00223-4108-02	2.50	
BACITRACIN ZN/POLYMYXIN B SULFATE (Fougera)			
OIN,TP (UNIT OF USE)			
500 u/gm-10000 u/gm,			
9.6 gm 144s	00168-0021-09	56.36	
15 gm	00168-0021-35	5.80	
30 gm	00168-0021-31	8.60	
(A-S Medication)			
REPACK			
OIN,TP, 500 u/gm-10000 u/gm,			
15 gm	54569-2034-00	5.80	
(Pharma Pac)			
REPACK			
OIN,TP, 500 u/gm-10000 u/gm,			
0.9 gm	52959-0054-04	5.95	
15 gm	52959-0054-03	14.15	
30 gm	52959-0054-07	23.35	
144 gm	52959-0054-44	48.78	
(Physician Partner)			
REPACK			
OIN,TP (1X30GM)			
500 u/gm-10000 u/gm,			
30 gm	21695-0400-30	21.08	
BACITRACIN-NEO-POLY (Consolidated Midland)			
CRE,TP, 1 gm 144s	00223-4247-01	17.50	
(Fougera)			
OIN,TP (UNIT OF USE)			
0.9 gm 144s	00168-0012-09	37.88	
15 gm	00168-0012-35	3.74	
30 gm	00168-0012-31	5.68	
(Quality Care Prod)			
REPACK			
OIN,TP, 3.34 gm	49999-0154-18	11.04	
BACITRACIN-POLYMYXIN (Consolidated Midland)			
OIN,TP, 500 u/gm-10000 u/gm,			
15 gm	00223-4255-01	2.25	
30 gm	00223-4255-02	2.75	
BACK PAIN-OFF (Medique)			
TAB,PO (50X2)			
250 mg-50 mg-290 mg,			
100s ea UD	47682-0073-33	9.41	
(100X2)			
250 mg-50 mg-290 mg,			
200s ea UD	47682-0073-47	18.14	
(250X2)			
250 mg-50 mg-290 mg,			
500s ea UD	47682-0073-13	40.09	
BACK-QUELL (Medique)			
TAB,PO (2X150,SF,LACTOSE-FREE)			
300s ea UD	47682-0155-87	41.89	33.51
BACKCHECK EXTENSION (Abbott Hosp)			
DEV,NA (32",STERILE PACK)			
120s ea	00074-1850-02	411.84	
BACTERICIN (Prime Marketing)			
OIN,TP, 500 u/gm, 15 gm	62107-0011-15	3.95	
30 gm	62107-0011-03	5.20	
BACTINE (Bayer HealthCare)			
SOL,TP, 0.13%-2.5%,			
60 ml	16500-0020-05	2.05	
120 ml	16500-0020-07	3.05	
BACTIVEX ATHLETE'S FOOT & CRACKED HEELS (BioRx)			
SOL,TP (1X30ML,AF)			
22%, 30 ml	63132-0014-01	11.98	

PROD/MFR	HRI, UPC,NDC	AWP	SRP
BAIN DE SOLEIL ORANGE GELEE (Schering Plough)			
OIN,TP (SPF 4,AF,SF)			
93.6 gm	74300-0770-93	7.51	
BAKER'S BEST (Scherer Labs)			
LOT,TP, 180 ml	00274-7500-08	2.35	
BALMEX (Johnson & Johnson)			
CRE,TP, 11.3%, 57 gm	81370-0024-23		3.49
113 gm	81370-0026-70		4.99
BALNEOL (Alaven)			
LOT,TP (20X2GM,CONVENIENCEPACK)			
2 gm 20s	68220-0077-10	6.88	
89 ml	68220-0077-03	11.98	
BALNEOL FOR HER (Alaven)			
LOT,TP (20X2GM,CONVENIENCEPACK)			
0.25%, 2 gm 20s	68220-0078-10	6.88	
(1X89ML)			
0.25%, 89 ml	68220-0078-03	11.98	
BALNETAR (Ranbaxy Labs)			
SOL,TP (1X221ML)			
2.5%, 221 ml	10631-0106-08	24.64	
(Phys Total Care) REPACK			
LIQ,TP, 2.5%, 240 ml	54868-3737-00	16.93	
BANALG (Forest Pharm)			
LOT,TP, 2%-1%-4.9%,			
60 ml 48s	00456-0523-21	2.94	
480 ml	00456-0523-16	18.26	
(A-S Medication) REPACK			
LOT,TP, 2%-1%-4.9%,			
60 ml	54569-2149-00	3.06	
(Altura) REPACK			
LOT,TP, 2%-1%-4.9%,			
60 ml	63874-0971-60	15.99	
(Core) REPACK			
LOT,TP, 2%-1%-4.9%,			
60 ml	33358-0044-02	5.60	
(DHS, Inc.) REPACK			
LOT,TP, 2%-1%-4.9%,			
60 ml	55887-0737-02	22.95	
(Dispensing Solutions) REPACK			
LOT,TP, 2%-1%-4.9%,			
60 ml	55045-3273-02	15.15	
(Nucare Pharm) REPACK			
LOT,TP, 2%-1%-4.9%,			
60 ml	66267-0985-02	17.55	
(Pharma Pac) REPACK			
LOT,TP, 2%-1%-4.9%,			
60 ml	52959-0255-03	17.18	
480 ml	52959-0255-01	30.41	
(Quality Care Prod) REPACK			
LOT,TP, 2%-1%-4.9%,			
60 ml	49999-0198-02	18.90	
(Stat Rx) REPACK			
LOT,TP, 2%-1%-4.9%,			
60 ml	16590-0342-02	16.00	
BANALG HOSPITAL STRENGTH (Forest Pharm)			
LOT,TP, 3%-14%,			
60 ml 48s	00456-0525-21	3.53	
(Dispensing Solutions) REPACK			
LOT,TP, 3%-14%, 60 ml	55045-3149-06	15.20	
(Pharma Pac) REPACK			
LOT,TP, 3%-14%, 60 ml	52959-0121-03	17.18	
(Southwood) REPACK			
LOT,TP, 3%-14%, 60 ml	58016-5613-01	13.95	
BANALG LOTION HOSPITAL STRENGTH (Palmetto) REPACK			
LOT,TP (1X60ML)			
3%-14%, 60 ml	23490-7839-00	3.53	
BAND-AID (Johnson & Johnson)			
DEV,NA (BUTTERFLY CLOSURES,MED)			
10s ea	81370-0055-41	0.86	
(GO DIEGO GO/ALL 1 SIZE)			
10s ea	81371-0040-15	0.91	
(HELLO KITTY/ALL 1 SIZE)			
10s ea	81370-0057-75	0.91	
(SPONGEBOB/ALL 1 SIZE)			
10s ea	81370-0057-74	0.91	
(SPONGEBOB/XL)			
10s ea	81370-0058-19	2.54	
(BATMAN,WATERPROOF,ASST)			
20s ea	81370-0058-18	2.54	
(BREAST CANCER AWARENESS)			
20s ea	81370-0051-95	1.99	
(GO DIEGO GO/ASST)			
20s ea	81370-0059-87	1.99	
(HELLO KITTY/ASST)			
20s ea	81370-0056-16	1.99	
(LITTLEST PET SHOP/ASST)			
20s ea	81371-0040-18	1.99	
(NASCAR,WATERPROOF,ASST)			
20s ea	81370-0057-54	2.54	
(SPIDERMAN/ASST)			
20s ea	81370-0045-22	1.99	
(SPONGEBOB/ASST)			
20s ea	81370-0044-73	1.99	
(STRAWBERRY SHORTCAKE)			
20s ea	81370-0057-55	2.54	
(TRANSFORMERS/ASST)			
20s ea	81371-0040-19	1.99	
(BARBIE,ASSORTED)			
25s ea	81370-0044-16	1.99	
(DORA THE EXPLORER/ASST)			
25s ea	81370-0044-84	1.99	
(SCOOBY DOO/ASST)			
25s ea	81370-0044-58	1.99	
BAND-AID ACTIV FLEX (Johnson & Johnson)			
DEV,NA (LARGE,LATEX-FREE)			
6s ea	81370-0044-13	3.31	
(REGULAR,LATEX-FREE)			
10s ea	81370-0044-14	3.31	
BAND-AID ADHESIVE PADS COMFORT-FLEX (Johnson & Johnson)			
DEV,NA (LARGE,2-7/8"X4")			
10s ea	81370-0047-68	2.71	
(MED,2-1/4"X3")			
10s ea	81370-0047-64	2.42	
BAND-AID ADVANCED HEALING BLISTER (Johnson & Johnson)			
DEV,NA, 6s ea	81370-0044-88	3.31	
BAND-AID ADVANCED HEALING BLISTER/ FINGERS & TOES (Johnson & Johnson)			
DEV,NA, 8s ea	81370-0045-82	3.32	
BAND-AID ARTHUR ADHESIVE STRIPS (J&J Medical)			
DEV,NA (3/4"X3",STERILE)			
100s ea	56091-0047-55	4.44	
BAND-AID BUTTERFLY CLOSURES STERILE (J&J Medical)			
DEV,NA (1 3/4"X3/8",MEDIUM)			
100s ea	56091-0043-31	6.15	
(2 3/4"X1/2",LARGE)			
100s ea	56091-0043-32	7.85	
BAND-AID CALAMINE SPRAY (Johnson & Johnson)			
SPR,TP, 5.25%-14.5%-0.77%,			
113 gm	81370-0039-41	4.58	
BAND-AID CLEAR COMFORT-FLEX (Johnson & Johnson)			
DEV,NA (ALL 1 SIZE)			
30s ea	81370-0046-70	1.81	
BAND-AID FLEXIBLE FABRIC (Johnson & Johnson)			
DEV,NA (TRAVEL SIZE)			
8s ea	81370-0047-54	0.59	
(XL,1 SIZE,1-3/4"X4")			
10s ea	81370-0056-85	2.54	
(ALL 1 SIZE)			
30s ea	81370-0044-31	2.54	
(ASSORTED)			
30s ea	81370-0044-30	2.54	
(ALL 1 SIZE)			
100s ea	81370-0044-44	5.33	
BAND-AID FLEXIBLE FABRIC STERILE (J&J Medical)			
DEV,NA (1"X3")			
100s ea	56091-0044-44	4.41	
(3/4"X3")			
100s ea	56091-0044-34	3.89	
(FINGERTIP)			
100s ea	56091-0044-36	6.58	
(KNUCKLE)			
100s ea	56091-0044-38	6.90	
BAND-AID FRICTION BLOCK (Johnson & Johnson)			
STI,TP, 9.6 gm	81370-0057-63	4.51	
BAND-AID HURT-FREE ANTISEPTIC WASH (Johnson & Johnson)			
SOL,TP, 0.13%-2%,			
177 ml	81370-0044-59	2.99	
BAND-AID ISLAND SURGICAL STERILE (J&J Medical)			
DEV,NA (4"X10")			
25s ea	56091-0043-18	37.22	
(4"X14")			
25s ea	56091-0043-19	45.50	
(4"X7")			
25s ea	56091-0043-17	26.90	
BAND-AID KNUCKLE & FINGERTIP (Johnson & Johnson)			
DEV,NA, 20s ea	81370-0044-52	2.54	
BAND-AID LIQUID BANDAGE (Johnson & Johnson)			
SOL,TP (W/APPLICATOR)			
10s ea	81370-0039-37	4.51	
BAND-AID MOLESKIN ADHESIVE (J&J Medical)			
DEV,NA (9"X4YD,UNCUT)			
ea	56091-0051-47	30.24	
BAND-AID NON-STICK STERILE (J&J Medical)			
DEV,NA (2"X4 1/2",X-LARGE)			
50s ea	56091-0057-16	6.01	
BAND-AID PERFECT BLEND CLEAR BANDAGES (Johnson & Johnson)			
DEV,NA (ASSORTED)			
45s ea	81370-0057-01	2.54	
(SPOTS,LIGHT,ALL 1 SIZE)			
50s ea	81370-0047-08	1.81	
BAND-AID PLASTIC COMFORT-FLEX (Johnson & Johnson)			
DEV,NA (ALL 1 SIZE)			
60s ea	81370-0056-35	1.81	
BAND-AID PLASTIC STRIPS STERILE (J&J Medical)			
DEV,NA (1"X3")			
100s ea	56091-0056-44	3.71	
(3/4"X3")			
100s ea	56091-0056-34	3.29	
BAND-AID PLUS ANTIBIOTIC (Johnson & Johnson)			
BAN,TP (XL/ALL 1 SIZE)			
500 u/gm-10000 u/gm,			
8s ea	81370-0055-67	3.01	
(WATERPROOF,ALL 1 SIZE)			
500 u/gm-10000 u/gm,			
15s ea	81371-0040-13	3.01	
(ALL 1 SIZE)			
500 u/gm-10000 u/gm,			
20s ea	81370-0055-69	3.01	
(ASSORTED)			
500 u/gm-10000 u/gm,			
20s ea	81370-0055-70	3.01	
(NEON COLORS)			
500 u/gm-10000 u/gm,			
20s ea	81370-0055-68	3.01	
BAND-AID SESAME STREET STRIPS (J&J Medical)			
DEV,NA (STERILE,3/4"X3")			
100s ea	56091-0047-53	4.94	
BAND-AID SHEER COMFORT-FLEX (Johnson & Johnson)			
DEV,NA (XL,1 3/4"X4")			
10s ea	81370-0057-05	2.54	
(ALL 1 SIZE)			
40s ea	81370-0046-66	1.81	
(ASSORTED)			
40s ea	81370-0046-67	1.81	
60s ea	81370-0046-68	2.12	
80s ea	81370-0046-69	2.54	
(ALL 1 SIZE,3/4")			
100s ea	81370-0046-34	3.80	
BAND-AID SHEER SPOTS STERILE (J&J Medical)			
DEV,NA (7/8")			
100s ea	56091-0049-30	3.99	
BAND-AID SHEER STRIPS STERILE (J&J Medical)			
DEV,NA (1"X3")			
100s ea	56091-0046-44	3.71	
(3/4"X3")			
100s ea	56091-0046-34	3.29	

PROD/MFR	HRI, UPC,NDC	AWP	SRP
(3/8"X1 1/2",JR)			
100s ea	56091-0046-33	2.20	
(1"X3")			
150s ea	56091-0046-51	4.96	
(3/4"X3")			
150s ea	56091-0046-50	4.30	
BAND-AID SPORT STRIP (Johnson & Johnson)			
DEV,NA (EXTRA WIDE,1")			
30s ea	81370-0047-23	2.54	
(ASSORTED)			
45s ea	81370-0056-93	2.54	
BAND-AID SURGICAL STERILE (J&J Medical)			
DEV,NA (4"X6")			
25s ea	56091-0043-11	21.76	
(8"X6")			
25s ea	56091-0043-13	33.38	
BAND-AID TOUGH-STRIPS (J&J/Merck)			
DEV,NA (XL,1-3/4"X4")			
10s ea	81370-0044-24	2.54	
(XL,WATERPROOF)			
10s ea	81370-0055-66	2.54	
(FINGER-CARE/ASST)			
15s ea	81370-0044-21	2.54	
(ALL 1 SIZE)			
20s ea	81370-0044-08	2.54	
(WATERPROOF,ASST)			
20s ea	81370-0048-34	2.54	
(WATERPROOF/ALL 1SIZE)			
20s ea	81370-0048-33	2.54	
BAND-AID ULTRA-STRIPS (Johnson & Johnson)			
DEV,NA (1 SIZE ADHESIVE PAD)			
8s ea	81370-0058-50	3.01	
(ALL 1 SIZE)			
20s ea	81370-0058-49	3.01	
(ASSORTED)			
20s ea	81370-0051-96	3.01	
BAND-AID VARIETY PACK (Johnson & Johnson)			
DEV,NA (ASST SIZES)			
30s ea	81370-0048-48	2.54	
280s ea	81370-0047-11	9.04	
BAND-AID WATER BLOCK PLUS (Johnson & Johnson)			
DEV,NA (LARGE,1 SIZE)			
10s ea	81370-0056-58	2.54	
(FINGER-CARE,ASST)			
20s ea	81370-0044-46	2.54	
(CLEAR,ALL 1 SIZE)			
30s ea	81370-0045-35	2.54	
(CLEAR,ASSORTED)			
30s ea	81370-0056-59	2.54	
BANISH II (Smith & Nephew)			
DEV,NA (DEODORANT)			
37.5 ml	40565-0112-47	10.09	8.07
(DEODORANT, ECONOMY SIZE)			
240 ml	40565-0115-00	33.71	26.97
BANOPHEN (Major)			
CAP,PO, 25 mg, 24s ea	00904-2035-24	2.20	
100s ea	00904-2035-59	4.45	
ELI,PO (AF)			
12.5 mg/5 ml, 120 ml	00904-1228-00	2.70	
(BOXED)			
12.5 mg/5 ml, 120 ml	00904-1228-20	2.70	
480 ml	00904-5174-16	5.50	
TAB,PO (MINITAB)			
25 mg, 24s ea	00904-5551-24	1.95	
(MINI TABS,MINI TAB)			
25 mg, 100s ea	00904-5551-59	5.95	
BANOPHEN MAXIMUM STRENGTH (Major)			
CRE,TP, 2%-0.1%,			
28.4 gm	00904-5354-31	4.35	
BARIDIUM (Pfeiffer)			
TAB,PO, 97.2 mg, 32s ea	00927-0031-93	3.10	5.57
BARLEY GRAIN (ADH)			
CAP,PO, 450 mg, 100s ea	60142-0104-10	5.48	10.95
BARNES HIND GP CLEANER (Allergan Inc)			
SOL,NA, 30 ml	00077-0664-30	2.91	
BARRIER FACE MASK (J&J Medical)			
DEV,NA (EXTRA PROTECTION PLUS)			
25s ea	56091-0042-32	25.35	
(EXTRA PROTECTION)			
50s ea	56091-0042-34	19.14	
(LASER PLUME)			
50s ea	56091-0042-36	58.50	
BARRIER FIELD STERILE (J&J Medical)			
DEV,NA (16"X29")			
35s ea	56091-0009-05	16.06	
(FENESTRATED,16"X29")			
35s ea	56091-0009-06	17.20	
BARRIER PARTICULATE RESPIRATOR MASK (J&J Medical)			
DEV,NA (TYPE N-95 TB,SMALL)			
20s ea	56091-0042-71	20.48	
(TYPE N-95 TB)			
20s ea	56091-0042-70	20.48	
BARRIER SURGICAL CAP (J&J Medical)			
DEV,NA (BLUE)			
100s ea	56091-0042-40	19.29	
(W/FABRIC 450)			
100s ea	56091-0042-41	32.88	
(W/TIRE STRINGS)			
100s ea	56091-0042-45	23.23	
BARRIER SURGICAL HOOD (J&J Medical)			
DEV,NA (BLUE)			
50s ea	56091-0042-42	18.26	
BASIC ONE (Advanced Nutr)			
SGL,PO (SOFTGEL)			
60s ea	62617-0005-02	15.75	21.00
BASIS SOAP (Beiersdorf)			
SOA,TP, ea	72140-0000-33	24.72	
12s ea	72140-0000-34	35.76	
12s ea	72140-0000-36	24.72	
12s ea	72140-0000-37	35.76	
12s ea	72140-0000-38	24.72	
12s ea	72140-0000-39	35.76	
12s ea	72140-0414-58	24.72	
12s ea	72140-0414-59	35.76	
(Phys Total Care)			
REPACK			
SOA,TP (NORMAL/DRY)			
ea	54868-2769-00	3.96	
BASLE (Del-Ray)			
CRE,TP, 60 gm	00316-0174-02	14.06	
BAY RUM (Humco)			
LIQ,TP, 480 ml	00395-0201-16	6.62	
BAYER ASPIRIN CHILDREN'S (Bayer HealthCare)			
CTB,PO (CHERRY)			
81 mg, 36s ea	12843-0132-31	1.79	
(ORANGE)			
81 mg, 36s ea	12843-0131-05	1.79	
(3X36,ORANGE)			
81 mg, 108s ea	12843-0101-05	5.02	
BAYER ASPIRIN REGIMEN (Bayer HealthCare)			
ECT,PO (LOW STRENGTH)			
81 mg, 32s ea	12843-0061-32	1.79	
120s ea	12843-0106-05	5.49	
325 mg, 100s ea	12843-0103-49	5.49	
BAYER BREEZE 2 CONTROL SOLUTION (Bayer Healthcare)			
DEV,NA (HIGH)			
2.5 ml	00193-1491-01	11.46	
(LOW)			
2.5 ml	00193-1490-01	11.46	
(NORMAL)			
2.5 ml	00193-1489-01	6.06	
BAYER BREEZE2 BLOOD GLUCOSE MONITORING SYSTEM (Bayer Healthcare)			
DEV,NA (10-TEST DISC)			
ea	00193-1440-01	24.00	
BAYER BREEZE2 BLOOD GLUCOSE TEST STRIPS (Bayer Healthcare)			
DEV,NA (5 DISCS)			
50s ea	00193-1465-50	58.26	
(10-TEST DISC)			
100s ea	00193-1466-21	106.80	
BAYER CONTOUR BLOOD GLUCOSE MONITORING SYSTEM (Bayer Diabetes Care)			
DEV,NA (GREEN)			
ea	00193-7184-01	18.00	
(Bayer Healthcare)			
DEV,NA (BLUE)			
ea	00193-7151-01	18.00	
(GRAY)			
ea	00193-7182-01	72.00	
(PURPLE)			
ea	00193-7183-01	18.00	
BAYER CONTOUR BLOOD GLUCOSE TEST STRIPS (Bayer Healthcare)			
DEV,NA, 25s ea	00193-7070-25	29.40	
50s ea	00193-7080-50	59.58	
100s ea	00193-7090-21	110.40	
BAYER CONTOUR CONTROL SOLUTION (Bayer Healthcare)			
DEV,NA (HIGH)			
ea	00193-7111-01	8.40	
(LOW)			
ea	00193-7110-01	8.40	
(NORMAL)			
ea	00193-7109-01	8.40	
BAYER EXTRA STRENGTH (Bayer HealthCare)			
TAB,PO (GELCAPLET)			
500 mg, 40s ea	12843-0363-66	3.83	
(CAPLET)			
500 mg, 50s ea	12843-0202-34	4.06	
BAYER MICROLET 2 LANCING (Bayer Healthcare)			
DEV,NA, ea	00193-6606-01	15.30	
BAYER PLUS EXTRA STRENGTH (Bayer HealthCare)			
TAB,PO (CAPLET)			
500 mg, 50s ea	12843-0124-22	4.06	
BAYER PM EXTRA STRENGTH (Bayer HealthCare)			
TAB,PO (CAPLET)			
500 mg-38.3 mg,			
40s ea	12843-0076-40	4.06	
BAZA ANTFUNGAL SKIN CARE PACK (Coloplast)			
CRE,TP (W/4 OZ PERI-WASH II)			
2%, 57 gm 12s	11701-0133-96	121.32	126.96
BAZA ANTIFUNGAL (Coloplast)			
CRE,TP (PACKET)			
2%, 4 gm 300s	11701-0045-22	159.00	168.00
57 gm 12s	11701-0045-23	87.36	91.32
142 gm 12s	11701-0045-14	157.68	165.00
BAZA CLEANSE & PROTECT (Coloplast)			
LOT,TP (PACKET)			
2%, 4 gm 300s	11701-0047-22	135.00	141.00
(ODOR CONTROL)			
2%, 237 ml 12s	11701-0062-05	129.60	135.60
(SPRAY)			
2%, 237 ml 12s	11701-0047-05	127.56	133.44
PAD,TP (3 X 100,CLOTH)			
2%, 300s ea	11701-0065-91	224.00	234.00
BAZA CLEAR (Coloplast)			
OIN,TP, 50 gm 12s	11701-0048-24	44.16	46.20
142 gm 12s	11701-0048-14	87.36	91.32
227 gm 12s	11701-0048-05	127.56	133.44
(SWEEN,4GM X 300)			
96%, 4 gm 300s	11701-0048-22	123.00	129.00
BAZA PROTECT (Coloplast)			
CRE,TP, 1%-12%,			
4 gm 300s UD	11701-0046-22	135.00	141.00
57 gm 12s	11701-0046-23	78.24	81.84
142 gm 12s	11701-0046-14	148.20	155.04
BC ALLERGY/SINUS/HEADACHE (Glaxo)			
PDR,PO, 6s ea	10158-0007-11	1.73	
12s ea	10158-0007-12	3.10	
BC HEADACHE POWDER (Glaxo)			
PDR,PO, 650 mg-33.3 mg-195 mg,			
1.165 gm 2s	10158-0009-08	0.39	
1.165 gm 6s	10158-0009-10	1.06	
1.165 gm 24s	10158-0009-12	3.01	
1.165 gm 50s	10158-0009-16	4.70	
BC POWDER ARTHRITIS STRENGTH (Glaxo)			
PDR,PO, 742 mg-36 mg-222 mg,			
1.165 gm 6s	10158-0008-04	1.20	
1.165 gm 24s	10158-0008-05	3.47	
1.165 gm 50s	10158-0008-06	5.41	
BCAD 1 (Mead Johnson & Co)			
PDR,PO, 454 gm	00087-4060-42	39.60	
BCAD 2 (Mead Johnson & Co)			
PDR,PO, 454 gm	00087-0083-41	68.99	
BD ALCOHOL (BD Consumer)			
DEV,NA (REGULAR)			
100s ea	08290-3268-95	1.76	2.69
BD AUTOSHIELD PEN (BD Consumer)			
DEV,NA (29G,1/2")			
50s ea	82903-0293-00	27.60	
(29G,3/16")			
200s ea	08290-3293-05	110.38	
(29G,5/16")			
200s ea	08290-3293-08	110.38	
BD GLUCOSE (BD Consumer)			
CTB,PO, 5 gm, 6s ea	08290-8230-00	1.08	
BD HOME SHARPS CONTAINER (BD Consumer)			
DEV,NA (DIABETES ACCESSORIES)			
ea	08290-3234-87	2.44	
BD INSULIN PEN (BD Consumer)			
DEV,NA (1.5 ML)			
ea	08290-3282-04	40.00	
BD LACTINEX (BD Consumer)			
CTB,PO, 1.4 mg, 50s ea	08290-2368-50	8.45	
GRA,PO (1GMX12)			
1 gm 12s	08290-2367-12	8.10	9.25

PROD/MFR	HRI, UPC,NDC	AWP	SRP

BD MAGNI-GUIDE INSULIN MAGNIFIER
(BD Consumer)
DEV,NA, ea 08290-3282-33 4.76

BD MICROTAINER CONTACT-ACTIVATED LANCET
(BD Consumer)
BD MICROTAINER CONTACT-ACTIVATED LANCET
DEV,NA (1.5MMX2MM,BLUE)
200s ea.............. 82903-0665-94 73.72
(21GX1.8MM,PINK)
200s ea.............. 82903-0665-93 73.72
(30GX1.5MM,PURPLE)
200s ea.............. 82903-0665-92 50.90

BD SAFE-CLIP **(BD Consumer)**
DEV,NA (NEEDLE CLIPPER)
ea.............. 08290-3282-35 3.10

BD SAFETY-LOK **(BD Dickinson Hosp Prod)**
DEV,NA (TUBERCULIN,27GX1/2")
100s ea.............. 08290-3055-53 38.41

BD SAFETYGLIDE **(BD Consumer)**
DEV,NA (23G,1")
50s ea.............. 08290-3059-02 18.92

BD SHARPS BY MAIL **(BD Consumer)**
DEV,NA, ea 08290-3234-88 20.64

BD SHARPS COLLECTOR **(Becton Dickinson)**
DEV,NA (3.3 QTS (3.1L))
24s ea.............. 82903-0054-88 112.56

BD TEST STRIPS **(Phys Total Care)**
REPACK
DEV,NA, 50s ea.......... 54868-5806-00 57.13

BD ULTRA FINE III **(Phys Total Care)**
DEV,NA (LATEX-FREE)
100s ea.............. 54868-6060-00 42.75

BD ULTRA-FINE **(BD Consumer)**
DEV,NA (3/10CC,30G,5/16")
10s ea.............. 08290-8440-01 2.73
(31GX5/16",1/2CC)
90s ea.............. 08290-3282-90 23.76
(31GX5/16",1CC)
90s ea.............. 08290-3282-89 23.76
(31GX5/16",3/10CC)
90s ea.............. 08290-3282-91 23.76

BD ULTRA-FINE II LANCETS **(BD Consumer)**
DEV,NA, 100s ea.......... 08290-3257-73 7.31
200s ea 08290-3257-72 13.26
(Phys Total Care)
REPACK
DEV,NA, 100s ea.......... 54868-5807-00 10.31

BD ULTRA-FINE MINI PEN NEEDLE **(BD Consumer)**
DEV,NA (31GX3/16")
90s ea.............. 08290-3208-82 29.30

BD ULTRA-FINE ORIGINAL PEN **(BD Consumer)**
DEV,NA (29GX1/2")
90s ea.............. 08290-3208-80 29.30

BD ULTRA-FINE PEN **(BD Consumer)**
DEV,NA (MINI,31GX3/16")
100s ea.............. 08290-3201-19 32.56
(SHORT,31GX5/16")
100s ea.............. 08290-3201-09 32.56

BD ULTRA-FINE SHORT **(BD Consumer)**
DEV,NA (31GX5/16",1 CC)
10s ea.............. 08290-8418-01 2.73
(31GX5/16",1/2CC)
10s ea.............. 08290-8468-01 2.73
(31GX5/16",3/10CC)
10s ea.............. 08290-8438-01 2.73
(31GX5/16",1/2CC,100X5)
100s ea.............. 08290-3284-68 27.30
(31GX5/16",1CC,100X5)
100s ea.............. 08290-3284-18 27.30
(31GX5/16",3/10CC,100X5)
100s ea.............. 08290-3284-38 27.30
100s ea 08290-3284-40 27.30

BD ULTRA-FINE SHORT PEN NEEDLE
(BD Consumer)
DEV,NA (31GX5/16")
90s ea.............. 08290-3208-81 29.30

BEANO **(Glaxo)**
CTB,PO, 150 u, 30s ea 41383-0062-00 3.91
60s ea 41383-0064-00 7.21
100s ea 41383-0063-00 11.14
LIQ,PO (DROPS)
30 u/drp, 15 ml 41383-0095-10 6.55
TAB,PO, 150 u, 12s ea..... 41383-0427-20 1.70

BEANO TO GO **(Glaxo)**
TAB,PO, 150 u, 12s ea..... 41383-0437-00 2.20

BEDSIDE-CARE **(Coloplast)**
LIQ,TP (BODY WASH/SHAMPOO)
0.1%, 118 ml 36s 11701-0020-04 72.36 75.96
237 ml 12s 11701-0020-05 42.36 44.28
3785 ml 4s 11701-0020-09 119.72 125.28

BEDSIDE-CARE FOAM **(Coloplast)**
FOA,TP (SWEEN BODY SHAMPOO,AF)
0.1%, 237 ml 12s 11701-0052-05 102.96 107.76

BEDSIDE-CARE PERINEAL WASH **(Coloplast)**
SPR,TP (36X118ML)
0.1%, 118 ml 36s 11701-0059-04 87.48 91.44
(12X237ML)
0.1%, 237 ml 12s 11701-0059-05 45.24 47.28
(4X3840ML)
0.1%, 3840 ml 4s 11701-0059-09 132.84 139.04

BEDSIDE-CARE UNSCENTED FOAM **(Coloplast)**
FOA,TP (SWEEN BODY SHAMPOO,AF)
0.1%, 237 ml 12s 11701-0053-05 102.96 107.76

BEE POLLEN **(Basic Vitamins)**
TAB,PO, 500 mg, 100s ea.. 00761-0007-10 3.00
(Health Products Corp)
TAB,PO (PF,SF)
500 mg, 100s ea 39686-0013-58 3.57
(Major)
TAB,PO, 500 mg, 100s ea.. 00904-3155-60 9.98
(Mason Vit)
TAB,PO, 500 mg, 100s ea.. 11845-0067-91 5.22
(PF,SF)
1000 mg, 90s ea 11845-0124-19 6.67
100s ea........... 11845-0079-51 6.11
(Nature's Bounty)
CTB,PO (PF,SF)
500 mg, 100s ea 74312-0008-20 6.25

BEE PROPOLIS **(ADH)**
CAP,PO (PF)
500 mg, 100s ea 60142-0454-01 5.98 11.95

BEE-ZEE **(Rugby)**
TAB,PO, 60s ea 00536-3357-08 4.85

BEECH **(Ellon)**
SOL,SL (DROPS)
10.5 ml.............. 51762-0013-10 9.25

BEEF,IRON & WINE **(Lex)**
LIQ,PO, 480 ml 49523-0071-16 1.75

BEELITH **(Beach Pharm)**
TAB,PO, 600 mg-25 mg,
100s ea........... 00486-1132-01 21.90

BELLADONNA **(Luyties)**
TAB,SL (6X)
6 x, 500s ea......... 00618-1033-03 3.99
5500s ea 00618-1033-10 30.32
(30X)
12 x, 500s ea 00622-1033-03 4.19
5500s ea 00622-1033-10 31.83
(12X)
30 x, 500s ea 00624-1033-03 4.19
5500s ea 00624-1033-10 31.83
(Walker Pharmacal)
TAB,SL (6X)
250s ea.............. 00619-1033-02 2.97
250s ea.............. 00619-1080-02 2.97

BELT RETAINER RING **(Coloplast)**
DEV,NA (1-1/2"-2 3/8")
ea.................. 11701-0826-20 4.64 4.86
(1-1/8"-2")
ea.................. 11701-0826-15 4.64 4.86
(3/4"-1")
ea.................. 11701-0826-10 4.64 4.86

BENADRYL **(Johnson & Johnson)**
CAP,PO, 25 mg, 24s ea.... 00071-0840-13 4.19
48s ea 00071-0840-18 6.89
CRE,TP (ORIGINAL STRENGTH)
1%-0.1%, 28.3 gm 12547-0171-62 3.74
(Dispensing Solutions)
REPACK
CRE,TP (ORIGINAL STRENGTH)
1%-0.1%, 28.3 gm ... 55045-3461-01 6.50
(Quality Care Prod)
REPACK
CRE,TP, 1%-0.1%, 30 gm.. 49999-0738-01 7.84

BENADRYL ALLERGY
(McNeil Consumer Healthcare)
SGL,PO (DYE-FREE,SOFTGEL)
25 mg, 24s ea........ 12547-0170-21 4.46
SOL,PO (AF,CHERRY)
12.5 mg/5 ml,
118 ml 00071-2333-17 4.87
TAB,PO (KAPGEL,CAPLET)
25 mg, 24s ea........ 00450-0108-25 4.46
(ULTRATAB)
25 mg, 24s ea........ 12547-0170-31 4.46
(KAPGEL,CAPLET)
25 mg, 48s ea........ 00450-0108-49 7.16
(ULTRATAB)
25 mg, 48s ea........ 12547-0171-36 7.16
100s ea 12547-0170-33 11.94

BENADRYL ALLERGY PLUS COLD
(McNeil Consumer Healthcare)
TAB,PO (KAPGEL,CAPLET)
325 mg-12.5 mg-5 mg,
24s ea............ 00450-0105-24 4.46

BENADRYL ALLERGY PLUS SINUS HEADACHE
(McNeil Consumer Healthcare)
TAB,PO (KAPGEL,CAPLET)
325 mg-12.5 mg-5 mg,
24s ea............ 00450-0107-24 4.46
48s ea 00450-0107-48 7.46

BENADRYL ALLERGY QUICK DISSOLVE STRIPS
(McNeil Consumer Healthcare)
FIL,PO (INDIVIDUALLY WRAPPED)
25 mg, 10s ea........ 12547-0170-41 4.46

BENADRYL EXTRA STRENGTH ITCH RELIEF SPRAY
(Johnson & Johnson)
SPR,TP, 2%-0.1%, 59 ml .. 12547-0170-04 5.02

BENADRYL EXTRA STRENGTH ITCH STOPPING CREAM **(Johnson & Johnson)**
CRE,TP, 2%-0.1%,
28.3 gm 12547-0171-67 4.02

BENADRYL ITCH RELIEF STICK
(Johnson & Johnson)
STI,TP (EXTRA STRENGTH)
2%-0.1%, 14 ml...... 12547-0171-40 2.20

BENADRYL ITCH STOPPING GEL
(Johnson & Johnson)
GEL,TP (EXTRA STRENGTH)
2%, 118 ml 12547-0171-60 5.02

BENADRYL SEVERE ALLERGY PLUS SINUS HEADACHE **(McNeil Consumer Healthcare)**
TAB,PO (MAX STRENGTH,CAPLET)
325 mg-25 mg-5 mg,
20s ea............ 12547-0175-84 4.46

BENADRYL-D ALLERGY PLUS SINUS
(McNeil Consumer Healthcare)
TAB,PO (ULTRATAB)
25 mg-10 mg,
24s ea............ 12547-0175-87 4.46

BENEFIBER **(Novartis Consumer)**
CTB,PO (SF,GLUTEN-FREE)
100s ea.............. 00067-0048-91 9.86
PDR,PO (FLAVOR FREE,SF)
4 gm/dose, 96 gm.... 00067-0042-96 6.18
POW,PO (1X80GM,SF,GLUTEN-FREE)
80 gm.............. 00670-0044-20 5.16
(1X155GM,SF,GLUTEN-FREE)
155 gm............. 00670-0044-38 7.02
(1X245GM,SF,GLUTEN-FREE)
245 gm............. 00670-0044-62 9.86
(1X350GM,SF,GLUTEN-FREE)
350 gm............. 00670-0044-90 13.50
(1X477GM,SF,GLUTEN-FREE)
477 gm............. 00670-0044-83 16.50

BENEFIBER FIBER DRINK MIX
(Novartis Consumer)
PKT,PO (SF,CHERRY POMEGRANATE)
8s ea............... 00067-0025-08 2.82
(SF,RASPBERRY TEA)
8s ea............... 00067-0021-08 2.82
(SF,CITRUS PUNCH)
16s ea.............. 00067-0024-16 5.64
(SF,KIWI STRAWBERRY)
16s ea.............. 00067-0023-16 5.64

BENEFIBER FOR CHILDREN **(Novartis Consumer)**
POW,PO (1X155GM,SF,GLUTEN-FREE)
155 gm............. 00067-0039-38 7.02

BENEFIN **(Lane Labs)**
PDR,PO, 454 gm.......... 02110-0007-16 62.98 139.00
TAB,PO (CAPLET)
750 mg, 60s ea 02110-0000-60 9.60 17.99
180s ea 02110-0001-80 29.25 65.00
270s ea 02110-0007-27 39.13 86.95

PROD/MFR	HRI, UPC,NDC	AWP	SRP
BENEFIT BAR (Health Management)			
BAR,PO (BLUEBERRY)			
24s ea	09355-0236-22	18.72	30.00
(HONEY GRAHAM)			
24s ea	09355-0236-24	18.72	30.00
(OATMEAL RAISIN)			
24s ea	09355-0236-23	18.72	30.00
(PEANUT BUTTER)			
24s ea	09355-0236-25	18.72	30.00
BENGAY ARTHRITIS FORMULA (Johnson & Johnson)			
CRE,TP, 8%-30%, 57 gm	74300-0005-37	4.72	
BENGAY GREASELESS (Johnson & Johnson)			
CRE,TP (GREASELESS)			
10%-15%, 57 gm	74300-0005-30	3.90	
113 gm	74300-0005-31	5.84	
BENGAY MOIST HEAT THERAPY (Johnson & Johnson)			
DEV,NA (LARGE,ODOR-FREE)			
3s ea	74300-0492-48	6.34	
(REGULAR,ODOR-FREE)			
4s ea	74300-0492-47	6.34	
BENGAY PM (Johnson & Johnson)			
CRE,TP, 10%, 57 gm	74300-0492-44	4.72	
BENGAY ULTRA STRENGTH (Johnson & Johnson)			
CRE,TP, 4%-10%-30%,			
57 gm	74300-0005-35	4.72	
113 gm	74300-0005-36	6.86	
TDM,TP (LARGE)			
5%, 4s ea	74300-0081-49	6.34	
(REGULAR)			
5%, 5s ea	74300-0081-50	6.34	
(Dispensing Solutions)			
REPACK			
CRE,TP, 4%-10%-30%,			
60 ml	55045-3312-01	7.50	
BENGAY VANISHING SCENT GEL (Johnson & Johnson)			
GEL,TP (GREASELESS)			
2.5%, 57 gm	74300-0005-39	3.90	
113 gm	74300-0005-45	5.84	
BENZ-O-STHETIC (Geritrex)			
GEL,MM (36X15GM,CHERRY)			
20%, 15 gm 36s	54162-0926-15	3.20	
(1X29GM,BUBBLE GUM)			
20%, 29 gm	54162-0926-01	7.00	
SPR,MM (1X56GM,W/200APPLICATORS)			
20%, 56 gm	54162-0925-03	30.73	
BENZ-PROTECT (Geritrex)			
SWA,TP (NON-STERILE)			
3 ml	54162-0100-10	2.14	
BENZALKONIUM CHLORIDE (Consolidated Midland)			
LIQ,TP, 480 ml	00223-6223-01	7.50	
3840 ml	00223-6223-00	39.50	
BENZEDREX (Ascher)			
LIQ,NS, 250 mg/actuation,			
0.42 ml	00225-0610-23	3.89	2.90
BENZOCAINE (Consolidated Midland)			
CRE,TP, 5%, 30 gm	00223-4112-30	1.60	
454 gm	00223-4112-13	7.50	
(Cypress Pharm)			
SPR,MM (1X59.7GM,WILD CHERRY)			
20%, 59.7 gm	60258-0034-02	27.50	
BENZOCAINE BURN SPRAY (Hart Health)			
SPR,TP, 20%-0.5%, 15 ml	50332-0033-01	2.17	
BENZODENT (Chattem)			
OIN,MM, 20%, 7.5 gm	41167-0005-32	2.18	2.17
30 gm	41167-0005-34	5.44	5.71
(A-S Medication)			
REPACK			
OIN,MM, 20%, 7.5 gm	54569-4973-00	2.62	
BENZOIN (Marlex)			
TIN,TP (N.F.)			
120 ml	10135-0103-04	3.10	
BENZOIN COMPOUND (Alexander, James)			
TIN,TP, 0.6 ml 100s	46414-8888-02	15.30	41.24
(AmerisourceBergen)			
TIN,TP (PRIVATE LABEL)			
60 ml	24385-0244-92	2.69	3.79
(Consolidated Midland)			
TIN,TP, 30 ml	00223-6225-01	2.75	
60 ml	00223-6225-02	3.00	
60 ml	00223-6225-03	3.95	
480 ml	00223-6225-04	12.50	

PROD/MFR	HRI, UPC,NDC	AWP	SRP
(Denison)			
TIN,TP, 30 ml	00295-1149-31	0.88	
60 ml	00295-1149-02	1.39	
(Geritrex)			
TIN,TP, 30 ml	54162-0100-01	3.24	
60 ml	54162-0100-02	4.46	
120 ml	54162-0100-04	8.79	
(Marlex)			
TIN,TP, 120 ml	10135-0101-04	2.53	
BENZOIN TINCTURE (Smith & Nephew)			
SPR,TP, 118 ml	40565-0111-82	25.06	20.05
BENZOYL PEROXIDE (Perrigo)			
GEL,TP (1X60GM)			
10%, 60 gm	45802-0915-96	20.77	
(1X90GM)			
10%, 90 gm	45802-0915-01	25.06	
(Rugby)			
GEL,TP, 5%, 45 gm	00536-4089-56	5.68	
10%, 45 gm	00536-4092-56	6.91	
(Altura)			
REPACK			
GEL,TP, 5%, 45 gm	63874-0827-45	9.22	
(Phys Total Care)			
REPACK			
GEL,TP, 5%, 43 gm	54868-2058-00	6.76	
(Quality Care Prod)			
REPACK			
GEL,TP, 5%, 45 gm	49999-0750-45	19.07	
(Southwood)			
REPACK			
GEL,TP, 5%, 45 gm	58016-3065-01	8.78	
LOT,TP, 10%, 30 ml	58016-3147-01	4.41	
BERBERIS VULG (Luyties)			
TAB,SL (6X)			
6 x, 500s ea	00618-1042-03	3.99	
5500s ea	00618-1042-10	30.32	
12 x, 500s ea	00622-1042-03	4.19	
5500s ea	00622-1042-10	31.83	
(12X)			
30 x, 500s ea	00624-1042-03	4.19	
5500s ea	00624-1042-10	31.83	
BERRYCONTENT (Ellon)			
ODT,PO (BERRY)			
30s ea	64723-0300-40		3.99
BESURE (Wakunaga)			
TAB,PO (CAPLET)			
30s ea	23542-0560-43	5.85	8.99
BETA CARE (Beta)			
CRE,TP, 240 gm	53062-0002-08	5.09	
LOT,TP, 480 ml	53062-0001-16	7.44	
BETA CAROTENE (ADH)			
TAB,PO (SF)			
25000 iu, 100s ea	60142-0490-51	5.25	10.50
(Basic Vitamins)			
SGL,PO, 25000 iu,			
100s ea	00761-0010-20	2.80	
(Freeda)			
TAB,PO (PF,SF,DYE-FREE)			
10000 iu, 100s ea	10432-0260-01	7.77	12.95
250s ea	10432-0260-02	15.54	25.90
500s ea	10432-0260-03	27.21	45.35
(Health Products Corp)			
TAB,PO (PF,SF,SOFTGEL)			
10000 iu, 100s ea	39686-0013-52	3.05	
25000 iu, 100s ea	39686-0013-53	4.80	
(Major)			
SGL,PO, 10000 iu,			
100s ea	00904-4222-60	3.25	
25000 iu, 100s ea	00904-4315-60	4.75	
(Mason Vit)			
SGL,PO (PF,SF,SOFTGEL)			
25000 iu, 100s ea	11845-0122-81	8.78	
TAB,PO, 10000 iu,			
100s ea	11845-0095-71	7.11	
25000 iu, 100s ea	11845-0078-01	8.78	
(Miller)			
SGL,PO, 25000 iu,			
100s ea	17204-0453-40	6.30	7.90
(Nature's Bounty)			
SGL,PO (PF,SF,SOFTGEL)			
10000 iu, 100s ea	74312-0015-20		5.99
25000 iu, 100s ea	74312-0012-20		7.69

PROD/MFR	HRI, UPC,NDC	AWP	SRP
(Pharmavite)			
SGL,PO (SOFTGEL)			
10000 iu, 100s ea	31604-0016-73	3.49	
25000 iu, 100s ea	31604-0013-14	4.72	
(Rexall)			
SGL,PO (PF,SF,SOFTGEL)			
10000 iu, 60s ea	30768-0010-93	2.12	3.22
25000 iu, 60s ea	30768-0001-42	2.90	4.40
(Rugby)			
SGL,PO (PF,SF,DYE-FREE,SOFTGEL)			
25000 iu, 100s ea	00536-4902-01	6.00	
(Phys Total Care)			
REPACK			
SGL,PO, 25000 iu,			
100s ea	54868-1025-01	16.27	
BETA HC (Beta)			
LOT,TP, 1%, 60 ml	53062-0012-02	8.16	
BETA MED (Beta)			
SHA,TP, 2%, 480 ml	53062-0013-16	10.80	
BETA-CARO PLUS (Bio-Tech Pharm)			
CAP,PO, 100s ea	53191-0315-01	31.50	
BETA-MIX (Key Company)			
SGL,PO (SOFTGEL)			
10 mg-15 mg-3 mg,			
60s ea	11694-0680-01	7.00	
BETADINE (Purdue Products L.P.)			
SOL,TP, 10%, 14.8 ml	67618-0150-05	1.16	
237 ml	67618-0150-08	11.99	
473 ml	67618-0150-16	18.46	
948 ml	67618-0150-32	7.43	
SPR,TP, 5%, 88.7 ml	67618-0148-03	9.67	
SWA,TP, 10%, 50s ea	67618-0153-03	16.87	
BETADINE SKIN CLEANSER (Purdue Products L.P.)			
SOL,TP, 7.5%, 118 ml	67618-0149-04	9.99	
BETAINE (Torrance)			
TAB,PO, 100s ea	00389-0260-00	5.00	
BETAINE HCL (Key Company)			
TAB,PO (SF)			
325 mg, 100s ea	11694-0800-01	5.00	
BETAINE HYDROCHLORIDE (Freeda)			
TAB,PO (PF,SF,DYE-FREE)			
300 mg, 100s ea	10432-0233-01	5.37	
250s ea	10432-0233-02	10.74	17.90
BETAMIDE (Beta)			
LOT,TP, 120 ml	53062-0005-04	7.08	
(SOOTHES CRACKED HEELS)			
120 ml	53062-0005-03	7.08	
480 ml	53062-0005-16	17.76	
BETASAL (Beta)			
LIQ,TP, 3%, 480 ml	53062-0014-16	10.80	
BETASEPT (Purdue Products L.P.)			
LIQ,TP (SURGICAL SCRUB)			
4%, 118 ml	67618-0200-04	5.47	
237 ml	67618-0200-08	6.90	
473 ml	67618-0200-16	9.20	
(SURGICAL SCRUB W/PUMP)			
4%, 946 ml	67618-0200-32	14.75	
(SURGICAL SCRUB)			
4%, 946 ml	67618-0200-30	13.82	
3785 ml	67618-0200-01	47.29	
BETATAR GEL (Beta)			
SHA,TP, 12.5%, 480 ml	53062-0023-16	10.80	
BEVITAMEL (Westlake Labs.)			
TAB,SL (PF,SF)			
1 mg-0.4 mg-3 mg,			
60s ea	10539-0832-01	10.50	15.00
BEYOND BODIHEAT BODIWRAP (Okamoto)			
DEV,NA (W/4 HEAT PADS)			
2s ea	28373-0779-84	2.99	3.99
BEYOND BODIHEAT KNEEWRAP (Okamoto)			
DEV,NA (W/HEAT PADS)			
2s ea	28373-0779-02	2.99	4.99
BEYOND BODIHEAT NECK AND SHOULDER (Okamoto)			
DEV,NA (W/HEAT PADS)			
4s ea	28373-0769-86	2.39	3.99
BEYOND BODY HEAT (Okamoto)			
DEV,NA, 4s ea	28373-0749-84	2.20	3.99
BEYOND SEVEN (Okamoto)			
DEV,NA (LIGHTLY LUBRICATED)			
3s ea	28373-0700-03	1.00	2.00
12s ea	28373-0700-12	3.80	6.99
(STUDDED)			
15s ea	28373-0510-12	4.10	5.95
(LIGHTLY LUBRICATED)			
1008s ea	28373-0710-00	88.00	125.00

PROD/MFR	HRI, UPC,NDC	AWP	SRP
BEYOND SEVEN PLUS (Okamoto)			
DEV,NA (W/SPERMICIDE)			
12s ea	28373-0900-12	3.80	10.00
(LUBRICATED W/SPERMICIDE)			
1008s ea	28373-0910-00	96.00	135.00
BEYOND SEVEN RIBS & DOTS (Okamoto)			
DEV,NA (LUBRICATED,TEXTURED)			
1008s ea	28373-0510-00	108.00	160.00
BI-ZETS (Reese)			
LOZ,MM (INTENSE STRENGTH)			
15 mg, 10s ea	10956-0713-10	3.38	
BIATAIN 3-D POLYMER FOAM (Coloplast)			
DEV,NA (ADHESIVE,7"X7")			
5s ea	11701-0880-89	82.05	85.85
(NON-ADHESIVE,6"X6")			
5s ea	11701-0881-90	80.75	84.50
(NON-ADHESIVE,8"X8")			
5s ea	11701-0881-70	136.40	142.75
(ADHESIVE,5"X5")			
10s ea	11701-0880-85	90.30	94.50
(NON-ADHESIVE,2" ROUND)			
10s ea	11701-0881-71	40.90	42.80
(NON-ADHESIVE,3" ROUND)			
10s ea	11701-0881-91	67.90	71.10
(NON-ADHESIVE,4"X4")			
10s ea	11701-0881-80	82.00	85.90
BIATAIN ADHESIVE FOAM DRESSING (Coloplast)			
DEV,NA (7 1/2"X8",HEEL)			
5s ea	11701-0880-50	76.45	80.00
(9"X9",SACRAL)			
5s ea	11701-0880-20	85.15	89.10
(4"X4")			
10s ea	11701-0880-80	68.10	71.30
BICARSIM (Kramer-Novis)			
TAB,PO, 250 mg-80 mg,			
60s ea	52083-0260-60	14.30	
BICARSIM FORTE (Kramer-Novis)			
PO (DUEL COATED)			
250 mg-125 mg, 60s ea	52083-0261-60	16.80	
BIDEX 400 (SJ)			
TAB,PO (CAPLET)			
400 mg, 100s ea	45985-0654-01	36.00	
BIFERA (Alaven)			
TAB,PO, 6 mg-22 mg,			
30s ea	68220-0087-30	14.88	
BIFIDONATE (Natren)			
CAP,PO (PF)			
60s ea	53983-0700-30	13.20	22.00
POW,PO, 2 billion org/gm,			
52.5 gm	53983-0700-15	12.60	21.00
(DAIRY,PF)			
2 billion org/gm,			
75 gm	53983-0200-25	13.20	22.00
(PF)			
2 billion org/gm,			
90 gm	53983-0700-25	18.60	31.00
(DAIRY,PF)			
2 billion org/gm,			
135 gm	53983-0200-45	18.60	31.00
BILBERRY (Cardinal Health)			
SGL,PO (PRIVATE LABEL)			
60 mg, 40s ea	37205-0051-58	7.15	
(Mason Vit)			
CAP,PO (PF,SF)			
60s ea	11845-1132-05	6.56	
(Nature's Bounty)			
CAP,PO, 100s ea	74312-0034-51		12.99
(Rexall)			
CAP,PO (PF,SF)			
40 mg, 50s ea	30768-0000-91	2.71	4.10
BILBERRY EXTRA STRENGTH (Yerba)			
CAP,PO, 160 mg, 50s ea	46352-0004-56	14.97	24.95
BILBERRY EXTRACT (ADH)			
CAP,PO (PF,SF)			
60 mg, 100s ea	60142-0903-61	16.48	32.95
(Mason Vit)			
CAP,PO (PF,SF)			
80 mg, 45s ea	11845-0129-57	13.22	
BIO-C-COMPLEX (Key Company)			
TAB,PO, 333 mg-667 mg,			
100s ea	11694-0778-01	7.00	
250s ea	11694-0778-02	14.00	
BIO-FLAV (Bio-Tech Pharm)			
CAP,PO, 100s ea	53191-0260-01	19.50	
BIO-IMMUNEX (Kramer-Novis)			
CAP,PO, 60s ea	52083-0992-60	20.00	
BIO-SPORT PHOSPHATE PLUS (Bio-Tech Pharm)			
CAP,PO, 100s ea	05105-0111-80	4.50	
500s ea	05105-0111-90	15.00	
1000s ea	05105-0112-00	27.50	
BIO-SPORT VIGOR (Bio-Tech Pharm)			
CAP,PO, 100s ea	05105-0112-10	11.00	
BIOBRANE (UDL)			
DEV,NA (15"X20")			
ea	08459-0095-79	394.94	
(10"X15")			
5s ea	08459-0095-77	1027.06	
(5"X15")			
5s ea	08459-0095-76	480.38	
(5"X5")			
5s ea	08459-0095-25	229.25	
BIOBRANE GLOVES (UDL)			
DEV,NA (LARGE)			
2s ea	08459-0099-68	762.63	
(MEDIUM)			
2s ea	08459-0099-67	666.00	
(PEDIATRIC)			
2s ea	08459-0099-65	343.19	
(SMALL)			
2s ea	08459-0099-66	622.44	
BIOBRANE-L (UDL)			
DEV,NA (10"X15")			
5s ea	08459-0096-77	1068.19	
(SHEET 5"X15")			
5s ea	08459-0096-76	538.00	
(SHEETS 5"X5")			
5s ea	08459-0096-25	291.00	
BIOCHEMIC PHOSPHATES (Hyland's)			
TAB,PO, 3 x-3 x-3 x-3 x-3 x,			
500s ea	54973-1069-01	6.77	11.29
1000s ea	54973-1069-02	9.89	16.49
BIOCLUSIVE MVP SELECT TRANSPARENT (J&J Medical)			
DEV,NA (1 3/4"X 2 3/4")			
25s ea	56091-0024-76	11.80	
(3"X4")			
25s ea	56091-0024-77	23.24	
(4"X5")			
25s ea	56091-0024-78	41.12	
(5"X7")			
25s ea	56091-0024-79	57.20	
BIOCLUSIVE SELECT TRANSPARENT (J&J Medical)			
DEV,NA (4"X10")			
20s ea	56091-0024-59	50.49	
(5"X7")			
20s ea	56091-0024-58	51.22	
(2 3/4"X2 3/8)			
50s ea	56091-0024-55	22.62	
(3"X4")			
50s ea	56091-0024-75	65.65	
(4"X5")			
50s ea	56091-0024-57	65.65	
(1 3/4"X2 3/4")			
100s ea	56091-0024-74	39.00	
BIOCLUSIVE TRANSPARENT STERILE (J&J Medical)			
DEV,NA (8"X10")			
10s ea	56091-0024-69	36.73	
(4"X10")			
20s ea	56091-0024-67	50.49	
(5"X7")			
20s ea	56091-0024-65	51.22	
(4"X5")			
50s ea	56091-0024-63	65.65	
(1 1/2"X1 1/2",MINI)			
100s ea	56091-0024-60	40.30	
(2"X3")			
100s ea	56091-0024-61	39.00	
BIOFED (Bio-Pharm)			
LIQ,PO, 30 mg/5 ml,			
120 ml	59741-0138-04	2.40	
240 ml	59741-0138-08	2.00	
480 ml	59741-0138-16	5.00	
3840 ml	59741-0138-20	13.44	
BIOFLAVON/VIT C (Nature's Bounty)			
C500 W/BIOFLAVONOIDS			
TAB,PO (PF,SF)			
100s ea	74312-0006-00		7.25
BIOFLAVONOID-1000 (Key Company)			
TAB,PO, 1000 mg,			
100s ea	11694-0856-01	6.00	
BIOFLAVONOIDS (Carlson,J.R.)			
TAB,PO (PF,SF,CORN-FREE)			
500 mg-5 mg, 100s ea	88395-0081-11	4.40	8.80
250s ea	88395-0081-12	9.95	19.90
BIOFLAVONOIDS/SELENIUM/VITAMIN C (Rexall)			
TAB,PO (PF,SF)			
60 mg-398 mg-0.2 mg,			
60s ea	30768-0001-06	3.30	5.00
BIOFLEXOR (Health Care Labs Inc)			
GEL,TP, 3%, 67.5 gm	62391-0001-02	8.10	
135 gm	62391-0001-04	13.62	
270 gm	62391-0001-08	36.70	
BIOFREEZE (Aidarex)			
REPACK			
GEL,TP (1X120GM)			
0.2%-3.5%, 120 gm	33261-0347-01	17.59	
(Altura)			
REPACK			
GEL,TP, 0.2%-3.5%,			
90 gm	63874-1067-03	6.89	
120 gm	63874-1067-04	8.63	
(Dispensing Solutions)			
REPACK			
GEL,TP, 0.2%-3.5%,			
120 gm	55045-9800-01	18.95	
(Nucare Pharm)			
REPACK			
GEL,TP, 0.2%-3.5%,			
113 gm	66267-1004-04	19.35	
(Palmetto)			
REPACK			
GEL,TP, 0.2%-3.5%,			
90 gm	23490-7840-00	11.50	
(Quality Care Prod)			
REPACK			
GEL,TP, 0.2%-3.5%,			
120 ml	49999-0530-04	25.80	
(Southwood)			
REPACK			
GEL,TP (ROLL-ON)			
0.2%-3.5%, 90 ml	58016-4732-01	7.28	
113.4 gm	58016-4593-01	5.81	
BIOFREEZE PAIN RELIEVING GEL (Hygenic Performance)			
GEL,TP (100X5GM)			
3.5%, 5 gm 100s	59316-0101-10		53.34
(1X118ML)			
3.5%, 118 ml	59316-0101-20		14.99
(1X473ML)			
3.5%, 473 ml	59316-0101-30		43.18
(1X946ML)			
3.5%, 946 ml	59316-0101-40		64.78
(1X3785ML)			
3.5%, 3785 ml	59316-0101-50		194.38
(Southwood)			
REPACK			
GEL,TP (W/PUMP)			
0.2%-3.5%, 3784 gm	58016-4772-01	111.69	
(Stat Rx)			
REPACK			
GEL,TP, 3.5%, 120 ml	16590-0098-04	11.44	
BIOFREEZE PAIN RELIEVING ROLL-ON (Hygenic Performance)			
GEL,TP (1X82GM)			
3.5%, 82 gm	59316-0101-15		14.99
BIOFREEZE PAIN RELIEVING SPRAY (Hygenic Performance)			
SPR,TP (1X60ML)			
10%, 60 ml	59316-0104-10		9.99
(1X118ML)			
10%, 118 ml	59316-0104-20		15.43
(1X473ML)			
10%, 473 ml	59316-0104-30		49.66
BION TEARS (Alcon Labs Cons Prod)			
SOL,OP (PF)			
0.1%-0.3%, 28s ea	00650-0419-28	11.88	
BIOPATCH W/CHLORHEXIDINE GLUCONATE (J&J Medical)			
DRE,TP (ANTIMICROBIAL,1.5MM)			
10s ea	56091-0021-51	52.24	
(ANTIMICROBIAL,7MM)			
10s ea	56091-0021-52	52.24	
(ANTIMICROBIAL)			
10s ea	56091-0021-50	52.24	

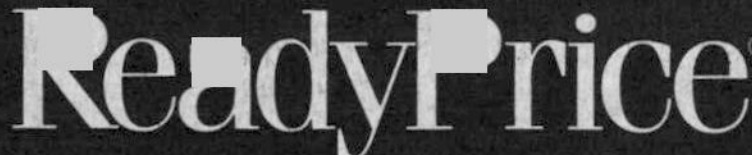

PROD/MFR	HRI, UPC,NDC	AWP	SRP
BIOPLASMA (Hyland's)			
TAB,PO, 1000s ea	54973-1068-02	9.89	16.49
4000s ea	54973-1068-07	49.43	82.39
(Nuage Labs)			
TAB,SL, 125s ea	00634-1212-68	3.05	5.09
BIOSODE (HVS Labs)			
LIQ,PO (AF,SF)			
120 ml	52386-9603-04	9.00	
240 ml	52386-9625-04	14.00	
BIOTENE DRY MOUTH (Glaxo)			
GEL,DE (1X127.6GM,GENTLEMINT)			
0.14%, 127.6 gm	48582-0003-20	5.28	
PAS,DE (1X21GM)			
0.14%, 21 gm	48582-0002-25	0.83	
(1X127.6GM)			
0.14%, 127.6 gm	48582-0002-20	5.28	
BIOTENE DRY MOUTH GUM WITH XYLITOL (Glaxo)			
GUM,DE (SF,MINT)			
16s ea	48582-0000-07	1.30	
BIOTENE DRY MOUTH MOUTHWASH (Glaxo)			
SOL,MM (1X59ML,AF)			
59 ml	48582-0005-92	0.77	
(1X473ML,AF)			
473 ml	48582-0003-30	5.28	
(1X1000ML,AF)			
1000 ml	48582-0004-40	8.28	
BIOTENE DRY MOUTH TOOTHPASTE (Southwood)			
REPACK			
PAS,DE, 135 gm	58016-4615-01	12.95	
BIOTENE MOISTURIZING MOUTH SPRAY (Glaxo)			
SPR,PO (1X44.3ML,AF,SF)			
44.3 ml	48582-0001-55	5.00	
BIOTENE MOUTHWASH W/ CALCIUM (Southwood)			
REPACK			
SOL,MM, 480 ml	58016-4602-01	12.95	
BIOTENE ORAL BALANCE (Glaxo)			
GEL,DE, 42 gm	48582-0512-01	5.28	
SOL,MM (1X44.3ML)			
44.3 ml	48582-0511-12	5.28	
BIOTENE PBF DRY MOUTH (Glaxo)			
PAS,DE (1X127.6GM)			
0.14%, 127.6 gm	48582-0005-20	6.24	
BIOTENE PBF DRY MOUTH CHEWING GUM WITH XYLITOL (Glaxo)			
GUM,DE (SF,APPLE MINT)			
20s ea	48582-0000-08	2.51	
BIOTENE PBF DRY MOUTH MOUTHWASH (Glaxo)			
SOL,MM (1X473ML,AF)			
473 ml	48582-0003-36	6.24	
(1X1000ML,AF)			
1000 ml	48582-0003-39	10.07	
BIOTENE SENSITIVE (Glaxo)			
PAS,DE (1X99.2GM)			
5%-0.14%, 99.2 gm	48582-0004-20	4.76	
BIOTIN (Basic Vitamins)			
TAB,PO, 300 mcg,			
100s ea	00761-0149-20	2.00	
(Carlson,J.R.)			
TAB,PO (PF,SF,CORN-FREE)			
1000 mcg, 100s ea	88395-0024-81	4.45	8.90
250s ea	88395-0024-82	9.95	19.90
(Freeda)			
TAB,PO (PF,SF,DYE-FREE)			
300 mcg, 100s ea	10432-0162-01	3.57	5.95
(Hillestad)			
TAB,PO, 5 mg, 120s ea	10542-0095-12	14.69	
(Major)			
TAB,PO, 0.3 mg-27 mg,			
100s ea	00904-5433-60	3.10	
(Mason Vit)			
TAB,PO (PF,SF)			
800 mcg-62 mg, 60s ea	11845-0073-65	5.22	
(Nature's Bounty)			
TAB,PO (PF,SF)			
300 mcg, 100s ea	74312-0027-60		4.59
(Rugby)			
TAB,PO, 300 mcg,			
100s ea	00536-6659-01	3.74	
(Freeda)			
D-BIOTIN			
TAB,PO (PF,SF,DYE-FREE)			
2.5 mg, 100s ea	10432-0296-01	7.17	11.95
10 mg, 100s ea	10432-0293-01	20.97	34.95
250s ea	10432-0293-02	41.94	69.90

PROD/MFR	HRI, UPC,NDC	AWP	SRP
BIOTUSS DM (Bio-Pharm)			
LIQ,PO, 15 mg/5 ml-100 mg/5 ml,			
120 ml	59741-0116-04	2.60	
240 ml	59741-0116-08	3.10	
480 ml	59741-0116-16	4.70	
3840 ml	59741-0116-20	29.50	
BIOVUE SECURING WINGS (J&J Medical)			
DEV,NA, ea	56091-0979-95	2.08	
(24G)			
ea	56091-0979-92	2.08	
BISA-LAX (AmerisourceBergen)			
ECT,PO (PRIVATE LABEL)			
5 mg, 100s ea	24385-0903-78	7.19	7.99
BISAC-EVAC (G&W)			
ECT,PO, 5 mg, 25s ea	00713-0416-25	3.30	
SUP,RC, 10 mg, 8s ea UD	00713-0109-08	3.09	
12s ea UD	00713-0109-12	2.93	
50s ea	00713-0109-50	10.14	
100s ea UD	00713-0109-01	17.80	
500s ea	00713-0109-05	84.43	
1000s ea	00713-0109-10	159.74	
BISACODYL (Bio-Pharm)			
SUP,RC, 10 mg, 12s ea	59741-0306-12	2.95	
50s ea	59741-0306-50	10.54	
100s ea	59741-0306-49	23.50	
(Consolidated Midland)			
ECT,PO, 5 mg, 12s ea	00223-5161-12	2.00	
50s ea	00223-5161-50	7.25	
100s ea	00223-0275-01	2.75	
100s ea	00223-5161-00	13.50	
1000s ea	00223-0275-02	21.50	
SUP,RC, 10 mg,			
12s ea UD	00223-5160-12	2.40	
50s ea	00223-5160-50	7.50	
100s ea	00223-5160-00	16.50	
(Family Phcy)			
ECT,PO (PRIVATE LABEL)			
5 mg, 25s ea	52735-0525-06	4.04	4.49
SUP,RC, 10 mg, 8s ea	52735-0516-16	4.49	4.99
(Major)			
ECT,PO, 5 mg, 25s ea	00904-7927-17	2.50	
100s ea	00904-7927-60	5.90	
(10X10)			
5 mg, 100s ea UD	00904-7927-61	8.86	
1000s ea	00904-7927-80	21.50	
(Marlex)			
ECT,PO, 5 mg, 10s ea	10135-0154-61	0.58	
25s ea	10135-0154-25	0.65	
50s ea	10135-0154-50	0.85	
100s ea	10135-0154-01	0.98	
(4X25 PUNCH CARD)			
5 mg, 100s ea UD	10135-0154-13	2.18	
1000s ea	10135-0154-10	5.75	
(Ohm)			
ECT,PO, 5 mg, 100s ea	51660-0230-01	1.35	
1000s ea	51660-0230-10	6.25	
(Paddock)			
ECT,PO (U.S.P.)			
5 mg, 100s ea	00574-0004-01	5.95	
(USP)			
5 mg, 100s ea UD	00574-0004-11	11.40	
SUP,RC (U.S.P.)			
10 mg, 12s ea UD	00574-7050-12	2.65	
50s ea UD	00574-7050-50	8.20	
(Qualitest)			
ECT,PO (USP,DELAYED RELEASE)			
5 mg, 100s ea	00603-2483-21	2.88	
1000s ea	00603-2483-32	21.30	
(Suppositoria)			
SUP,RC, 10 mg,			
12s ea UD	45802-0710-30	2.99	
50s ea	45802-0710-32	10.49	
100s ea UD	45802-0710-33	23.99	
(Time-Cap)			
ECT,PO, 5 mg, 100s ea	49483-0003-01	3.60	
1000s ea	49483-0003-10	20.30	
(Vintage)			
ECT,PO, 5 mg, 100s ea	00254-0060-28	2.88	
(A-S Medication)			
REPACK			
ECT,PO, 5 mg, 25s ea	54569-5699-00	2.95	
SUP,RC, 10 mg, 6s ea	54569-1895-02	2.21	
(Palmetto)			
REPACK			
SUP,RC, 10 mg, 12s ea	23490-6624-01	7.45	

PROD/MFR	HRI, UPC,NDC	AWP	SRP
(PD-Rx Pharm)			
REPACK			
ECT,PO (USP)			
5 mg, 10s ea	55289-0918-10	5.45	
25s ea	55289-0918-25	6.05	
(Pharma Pac)			
REPACK			
SUP,RC, 10 mg, 12s ea	52959-0672-12	9.31	
(Phys Total Care)			
REPACK			
ECT,PO, 5 mg, 100s ea	54868-2497-00	8.82	
SUP,RC, 10 mg, 12s ea	54868-2039-00	7.38	
(Quality Care Prod)			
REPACK			
ECT,PO, 5 mg, 10s ea	49999-0664-10	3.96	
(Southwood)			
REPACK			
ECT,PO, 5 mg, 25s ea	58016-0920-01	2.50	
30s ea	58016-0042-30	2.50	
60s ea	58016-0042-60	5.00	
90s ea	58016-0042-90	7.50	
100s ea	58016-0042-00	8.33	
SUP,RC, 10 mg, 12s ea	58016-3124-01	7.45	
(Stat Rx)			
REPACK			
ECT,PO, 5 mg, 30s ea	16590-0743-30	8.75	
BISACODYL LAXATIVE (Magno-Humphries)			
ECT,PO, 5 mg, 100s ea	43292-0556-86	1.80	3.99
BISCOLAX (Global Source)			
ECT,PO, 5 mg, 50s ea	59618-0125-11	2.95	
SUP,RC, 10 mg, 16s ea	59618-0126-77	2.95	
100s ea	59618-0126-76	16.50	
(Major)			
SUP,RC, 10 mg, 12s ea	00904-5058-12	3.25	
100s ea	00904-5058-60	17.99	
BISMATROL (Major)			
CTB,PO, 262 mg, 30s ea	00904-1315-46	3.75	
SUS,PO, 262 mg/15 ml,			
240 ml	00904-1313-09	2.50	
(1X236ML,MAXIMUMSTRENGTH)			
525 mg/15 ml, 236 ml	00904-1314-09	3.15	
TAB,PO (15X2)			
262 mg, 30s ea	00904-1315-03	2.55	
BISMUTH (Albertson's)			
PINK BISMUTH			
SUS,PO, 262 mg/15 ml,			
240 ml	12810-0302-34	2.40	
(AmerisourceBergen)			
CTB,PO (PRIVATE LABEL)			
262 mg, 30s ea	24385-0024-65	2.51	2.79
(PRIVATE LABEL,CAPLET)			
262 mg, 40s ea	24385-0017-58	3.59	3.99
SUS,PO (PRIVATE LABEL)			
262 mg/15 ml,			
240 ml	24385-0302-34	2.42	2.69
(Cardinal Health)			
CTB,PO (PRIVATE LABEL)			
262 mg, 30s ea	37205-0720-65	2.92	
SUS,PO (SF,PRIVATE LABEL)			
262 mg/15 ml,			
240 ml	37205-0302-34	2.85	
360 ml	37205-0302-40	3.28	
(Family Phcy)			
CTB,PO (PRIVATE LABEL)			
262 mg, 30s ea	52735-0511-08	2.51	2.79
(Qualitest)			
CTB,PO, 262 mg, 30s ea	00603-0235-16	3.51	
(Cardinal Health)			
PINK BISMUTH MAXIMUM STRENGTH			
SUS,PO (SF,PRIVATE LABEL)			
525 mg/15 ml,			
240 ml	37205-0337-34	3.20	
BISMUTH MAXIMUM STRENGTH (Chain Drug Marketing)			
SUS,PO, 525 mg/15 ml,			
237 ml	63868-0337-34	2.10	3.99
BISMUTH SUBSALICYLATE (Dispensing Solutions)			
REPACK			
CTB,PO, 262 mg, 30s ea	55045-3457-08	4.20	
SUS,PO, 262 mg/15 ml,			
240 ml	68258-3007-01	5.72	

PROD/MFR	HRI, UPC,NDC	AWP	SRP
BL (AmerisourceBergen)			
ABSORBENT SHIELDS			
DEV,NA (EXTRA ABSORBENCY)			
25s ea	87701-0555-55	23.35	25.95
(REGULAR ABSORBENCY)			
25s ea	87701-0555-53	22.45	29.99
ARM SLING			
DEV,NA (POUCH STYLE,ADULT)			
ea	87701-0706-15	9.29	
(POUCH STYLE,YOUTH)			
ea	87701-0706-12	11.69	14.69
BELTED UNDERGARMENT			
DEV,NA (REGULAR ABSORBENCY)			
10s ea	87701-0555-02	37.75	41.94
(EXTRA ABSORBENCY)			
60s ea	87701-0628-99	22.94	25.49
BETA CAROTENE NATURAL			
SGL,PO (PRIVATE LABEL,SOFTGEL)			
25000 iu, 100s ea	24385-0280-78	5.39	5.99
BLADDER CONTROL PADS			
DEV,NA (ULTRA PLUS)			
42s ea	87701-0702-55	46.76	39.24
(ULTRA,PRIVATE LABEL)			
52s ea	87701-0708-73	44.24	49.16
BLOOD GLUCOSE			
DEV,NA (STRIP,PRIVATE LABEL)			
50s ea	24385-0310-50	26.12	24.99
100s ea	24385-0310-01	50.00	45.95
BLOOD PRESSURE MONITOR SEMI-AUTO			
DEV,NA (PRIVATE LABEL)			
ea	87701-0173-23	35.99	44.89
CALCIUM/MAGNESIUM/ZINC NATURAL			
TAB,PO (PRIVATE LABEL)			
100s ea	24385-0277-78	3.77	4.19
COOL MIST HUMIDIFIER			
DEV,NA (#BL4100,1 GAL)			
ea	87701-0658-59	20.69	22.99
ELASTIC BANDAGE			
DEV,NA (2",PRIVATE LABEL)			
ea	87701-0706-07	3.59	3.99
(3",PRIVATE LABEL)			
ea	87701-0706-09	4.49	4.99
(4",PRIVATE LABEL)			
ea	87701-0706-11	4.49	4.99
ELBOW BRACE ELASTIC			
DEV,NA (PULL-ON,MEDIUM)			
ea	87701-0709-55	6.29	6.99
ELBOW BRACE NEOPRENE			
NA (HOOK/LOOP CLOSURE,OSFA)			
ea	87701-0709-69	10.25	11.39
EVAPORATIVE HUMIDIFIER			
DEV,NA (#BL3020,1 GAL)			
ea	87701-0670-99	26.99	29.99
EXAM GLOVES			
DEV,NA (LATEX,OSFA)			
50s ea	87701-0211-12	5.39	5.99
(OSFA,PRIVATE LABEL)			
50s ea	87701-0205-99	6.29	6.99
50s ea	87701-0213-22	5.39	5.99
(LARGE,PRIVATE LABEL)			
100s ea	87701-0104-21	8.09	8.99
(LATEX,LARGE)			
100s ea	87701-0104-23	8.99	8.99
(LATEX,MED,PRIVATE LABEL)			
100s ea	87701-0104-24	8.99	9.99
(LATEX,MEDIUM)			
100s ea	87701-0104-22	8.09	8.99
(LATEX,SMALL)			
100s ea	87701-0104-49	4.40	8.99
(MEDIUM,PRIVATE LABEL)			
100s ea	87701-0104-20	8.09	8.99
FEMININE PAD			
DEV,NA (SUPER,PRIVATE LABEL)			
20s ea	87701-0957-68	22.62	25.14
(PRIVATE LABEL)			
22s ea	87701-0957-67	22.62	25.14
(SUPER,BULK PACK)			
120s ea	87701-0629-41	35.09	38.99
(REGULAR,BULK PACK)			
132s ea	87701-0629-39	35.09	38.99
FITTED CONTOURED BRIEF			
NA (LARGE,PRIVATE LABEL)			
18s ea	87701-0563-44	22.12	24.58
(LARGE,BULK PACK)			
72s ea	87701-0558-00	45.89	50.99
(MEDIUM,BULK PACK)			
96s ea	87701-0558-43	45.89	50.99
GARLIC OIL NATURAL			
SGL,PO (PRIVATE LABEL,SOFTGEL)			
3 mg, 100s ea	24385-0336-78	3.32	3.69
LUBRICATING LOTION			
LOT,TP (W/PUMP,PRIVATE LABEL)			
480 ml	87701-0951-02	5.39	5.99
ONE STEP PREGNANCY			
DEV,NA (PRIVATE LABEL)			
ea	87701-0543-96	7.19	7.99
2s ea	87701-0894-74	9.89	10.99
ORAL SYRINGE			
DEV,NA (1 TSP,PRIVATE LABEL)			
ea	87701-0970-48	1.61	2.29
OVERNIGHT BRIEF SUPREME			
DEV,NA (LARGE,PRIVATE LABEL)			
16s ea	87701-0018-30	44.60	59.96
(MEDIUM,PRIVATE LABEL)			
20s ea	87701-0942-76	44.60	59.59
PILL BOX			
DEV,NA (1 DAY ADULT LOCK)			
ea	87701-0899-65	1.79	2.49
(7 DAY, 7 SIDED)			
ea	87701-0970-67	1.34	1.89
(VITAMIN,PRIVATE LABEL)			
ea	87701-0899-62	1.79	1.99
(WEEKLY MED. ORGANIZER)			
ea	87701-0970-56	6.53	8.29
PILL CRUSHER			
DEV,NA (DELUXE,PRIVATE LABEL)			
ea	87701-0899-61	3.58	4.69
PILL REMINDER			
DEV,NA (1 DAY,PRIVATE LABEL)			
ea	87701-0970-53	1.07	1.59
(7 DAY,MEDIUM)			
ea	87701-0970-51	1.34	1.49
(7 DAY,SMALL)			
ea	87701-0970-66	1.16	1.69
(WEEKLY ADULT LOCK,LARGE)			
ea	87701-0894-42	2.68	3.59
(WEEKLY,JUMBO)			
ea	87701-0894-43	2.51	2.79
PLASTIC FINGER GUARD			
DEV,NA (ASSORTED,PRIVATE LABEL)			
ea	87701-0970-95	1.70	2.39
POTASSIUM GLUCONATE NATURAL			
TAB,PO (PRIVATE LABEL)			
550 mg, 100s ea	24385-0345-78	3.59	3.99
PROTECTIVE UNDERWEAR			
DEV,NA (DISPOSABLE,SLIP-ON,LRG)			
18s ea	87701-0893-21	38.12	42.36
(DISPOSABLE,SLIP-ON,MED)			
20s ea	87701-0893-12	38.12	42.36
RIB BELT UNIVERSAL			
DEV,NA (FEMALE,PRIVATE LABEL)			
ea	87701-0652-16	13.49	14.99
(MALE,PRIVATE LABEL)			
ea	87701-0709-58	11.69	12.99
SENSITIVE SKIN MOISTURIZING			
CRE,TP (FRAGRANCE-FREE)			
480 gm	87701-0893-20	5.39	5.99
LOT,TP, 480 ml	87701-0893-18	5.39	5.99
SLIP-ON UNDERGARMENT			
DEV,NA (SUPER ABSORBENCY)			
16s ea	87701-0884-27	17.99	10.99
26s ea	87701-0742-25	29.31	14.99
STRETCH BANDAGE			
DEV,NA (2"X4 YDS,PRIVATE LABEL)			
ea	87701-0430-54	1.43	1.59
(3"X4 YDS,PRIVATE LABEL)			
ea	87701-0430-55	1.70	1.99
TABLET CRUSHER			
DEV,NA (PRIVATE LABEL)			
ea	87701-0970-55	5.84	7.49
TABLET CUTTER			
DEV,NA (DELUXE,PRIVATE LABEL)			
ea	87701-0899-60	1.69	2.19
(PRIVATE LABEL)			
ea	87701-0970-54	3.50	4.59
TALKING DIGITAL THERMOMETER			
DEV,NA (PRIVATE LABEL)			
ea	87701-0905-63	13.49	13.79
THERMOMETER PROBE COVERS			
DEV,NA (PRIVATE LABEL)			
25s ea	87701-0565-09	1.23	1.59
TUBULAR GAUZE			
DEV,NA (PRIVATE LABEL)			
ea	87701-0966-76	1.88	2.59
UNDERPADS			
DEV,NA (SUPER LARGE)			
10s ea	87701-0124-06	25.16	32.89
(LARGE,PRIVATE LABEL)			
18s ea	87701-0124-08	25.16	32.89
(LARGE,BULK PACK)			
150s ea	87701-0558-35	39.05	49.69
UNIVERSAL FINGER SPLINT			
DEV,NA (PRIVATE LABEL)			
ea	87701-0970-93	4.04	5.29
VAPORIZER			
DEV,NA (#BL2100,1 GAL)			
ea	87701-0665-63	10.79	17.19
VITAMIN A			
SGL,PO (PRIVATE LABEL,SOFTGEL)			
8000 iu, 100s ea	24385-0281-78	4.49	4.99
VITAMIN E			
OIL,TP (PRIVATE LABEL)			
30 ml	87701-0247-92	5.39	5.99
VITAMIN E MOISTURIZER			
CRE,TP (PRIVATE LABEL)			
120 gm	87701-0247-90	4.49	4.99
WRIST BRACE AMBIDEXTROUS			
DEV,NA (RESHAPABLE SPOON,XLRG)			
ea	87701-0709-53	13.29	15.99
WRIST BRACE ELASTIC			
NA (PULL-ON,EXTRA LARGE)			
ea	87701-0602-35	4.49	4.99
(PULL-ON,LARGE)			
ea	87701-0587-96	4.49	4.99
(PULL-ON,MEDIUM)			
ea	87701-0552-74	4.49	4.99
(PULL-ON,SMALL)			
ea	87701-0709-44	4.76	5.89
(WRAP,OSFA,PRIVATE LABEL)			
ea	87701-0709-43	4.76	5.89
WRIST SPLINT NEOPRENE			
DEV,NA (REMOV. STAYS,OSFA,LEFT)			
ea	87701-0061-41	10.79	21.99
(REMOV. STAYS,OSFA,RIGHT)			
ea	87701-0709-70	13.29	15.99
BL ANTACID EXTRA STRENGTH (AmerisourceBergen)			
ANTACID EXTRA STRENGTH			
CTB,PO (ASSORTED BERRY)			
750 mg, 96s ea	24385-0106-80	3.14	3.49
BL GARLIC (AmerisourceBergen)			
GARLIC			
ECT,PO (PF,DAIRY-FREE,ODOR-FREE)			
400 mg, 30s ea	24385-0957-65	5.39	5.99
BL IBUPROFEN CHILDREN'S (AmerisourceBergen)			
IBUPROFEN CHILDREN'S			
SUS,PO (AF,BUBBLE GUM)			
100 mg/5 ml,			
118 ml	24385-0361-26	4.49	4.99
BL MIGRAINE FORMULA (AmerisourceBergen)			
MIGRAINE FORMULA			
TAB,PO (COATED,CAPLET)			
250 mg-250 mg-65 mg,			
100s ea	24385-0365-78	7.19	7.99
BL OIL FREE SUNSCREEN (AmerisourceBergen)			
OIL FREE SUNSCREEN			
LOT,TP (SPF 15,OIL-FREE)			
7.5%-2.5%, 118 ml	24385-0228-26	4.49	5.79
BL SPORT SUNSCREEN (AmerisourceBergen)			
SPORT SUNSCREEN			
LOT,TP (SPF 30)			
7.5%-5.0%-5.0%,			
118 ml	24385-0230-26	4.49	5.79
BL SUNSCREEN (AmerisourceBergen)			
SUNSCREEN			
LOT,TP (MOISTURIZING)			
4.0%-2.0%, 118 ml	24385-0909-26	3.59	4.69
BL TIOCONAZOLE 1 (AmerisourceBergen)			
TIOCONAZOLE 1			
OIN,VG (W/APPLICATOR)			
6.5%, 8 gm	24385-0374-82	12.60	14.00
BL WART REMOVER (AmerisourceBergen)			
WART REMOVER			
SOL,TP, 17%, 15 ml	24385-0236-63	4.49	4.99
BLACK COHOSH (Mason Vit)			
SGL,PO (PF,SF)			
40 mg, 60s ea	11845-0130-45	8.33	
(Rexall)			
CAP,PO (PF,SF)			
540 mg, 75s ea	30768-0012-05	2.60	3.93
BLACK COHOSH EXTRACT (A-S Medication)			
REPACK			
CAP,PO, 200 mg, 60s ea	54569-4965-00	9.78	
BLACK CURRANT OIL (Neurovites)			
CAP,PO, 625 mg-15 mg,			
100s ea	93595-2020-01	22.95	
BLACK WALNUT (Botanical Labs.)			
LIQ,PO, 30 ml	41954-0020-61	3.50	6.99
BLACK-DRAUGHT (Lee Pharm)			
SYR,PO, 30 mg/5 ml,			
180 ml	23558-0510-90	3.60	
TAB,PO, 6 mg, 30s ea	23558-0510-80	2.52	2.19

PROD/MFR	HRI, UPC,NDC	AWP	SRP
BLACKSTONE CALLOUS & CORN REMOVER (Williams)			
DEV,NA (PUMICE STONE,JUMBO)			
ea	63922-0621-52	1.82	3.99
(PUMICE STONE,REGULAR)			
ea	63922-0621-51	0.90	1.99
BLAINE SCARCARE (Blaine)			
DEV,NA (W/E-SIL SCAR THERAPY)			
ea	65373-0200-01	37.00	65.00
BLAIREX STERILE SALINE SOLUTION (Blairex)			
SPR,NA, 360 ml	50486-0017-17	2.63	
BLENDERM SURGICAL (3M Health Care)			
DEV,NA (2"X5 YDS)			
6s ea	08333-1525-02	16.80	
(1"X5 YDS)			
12s ea	08333-1525-01	16.80	
(1/2"X5 YDS)			
24s ea	08333-1525-00	16.80	
BLIS-TO-SOL (Oakhurst)			
POW,TP, 12%, 60 gm	41167-0200-51	4.20	6.30
SOL,TP, 1%, 30 ml	41167-0200-11	2.85	4.28
55.5 ml	41167-0200-12	4.00	6.00
BLISTERFILM (Covidien)			
DEV,NA (TRANS PATCH,2"X3")			
100s ea	08080-4740-01	101.07	
(TRANS PATCH,3-1/2"X4")			
100s ea	08080-4740-19	139.90	
(TRANS PATCH,4"X5")			
100s ea	08080-4740-35	166.04	
(TRANS PATCH,5-1/2"X6")			
100s ea	08080-4740-27	238.57	
BLISTEX (Phys Total Care)			
REPACK			
OIN,TP (OINTMENT)			
1%-0.5%-0.6%-0.5%,			
100s ea	54868-3539-00	7.55	
500s ea	54868-3539-01	35.33	
BLOOD CLOTTING SPRAY (Hart Health)			
SPR,TP, 0.2%-4%, 85 gm	50332-0217-01	5.33	
BLOOD GLUCOSE (Albertson's)			
DEV,NA (STRIP)			
50s ea	56151-0321-50	28.60	
BLOOD GLUCOSE VALUE PACK (Albertson's)			
DEV,NA (STRIPS W/FREE METER)			
ea	56151-0221-01	22.18	
BLOOD NUTRIENTS (Carlson,J.R.)			
CAP,PO, 40s ea	88395-0044-66	4.75	9.50
90s ea	88395-0044-64	9.75	19.50
180s ea	88395-0044-61	17.45	34.90
BLOOD PRESSURE MONITOR (Cardinal Health)			
DEV,NA (DIGITAL,PRIVATE LABEL)			
ea	37205-0006-03	51.09	
(MANUAL,PRIVATE LABEL)			
ea	37205-0005-03	25.59	
(Lumiscope)			
DEV,NA (UPPER ARM,FUZZY LOGIC)			
ea	38673-0010-94	59.99	119.99
(WRIST,FUZZY LOGIC)			
ea	38673-0010-91	74.99	149.99
BLOOD PRESSURE MONITOR MANUAL (Lumiscope)			
DEV,NA (ANEROID SPHYGMOMANOMTR)			
ea	38673-0010-01	10.99	21.99
(MERCURY SPHYGMOMANOMTR)			
ea	38673-0000-10	24.99	49.99
(W/ATTACHED STETHOSCOPE)			
ea	38673-0000-21	12.99	25.99
(W/NURSE STETHOPSCOPE)			
ea	38673-0000-19	11.99	23.99
BLOOD PRESSURE/PULSE MONITOR (Lumiscope)			
DEV,NA (AUTO-INFL,DIGITAL,FING)			
ea	38673-0010-83	45.99	89.99
(AUTO-INFL,DIGITAL,WATCH)			
ea	38673-0050-20	84.99	179.99
(AUTO-INFL,DIGITAL)			
ea	38673-0010-85	49.99	99.99
(DIGITAL)			
ea	38673-0010-60	29.99	59.99
(UPPER ARM,SMART INFLATE)			
ea	38673-0010-95	74.99	149.99
ea	38673-0010-97	64.99	129.99
(WRIST TYPE, FUZZY LOGIC)			
ea	38673-0040-21	49.99	99.99
BLOOD SET 80 (Abbott Hosp)			
DEV,NA (W/CAIR CLAMP,Y-INJ)			
48s ea	00074-1845-68	210.24	
BLOOD SET W/PUMP (Abbott Hosp)			
DEV,NA (80")			
48s ea	00074-8954-68	279.36	
BLOOD WARMING COIL (Abbott Hosp)			
DEV,NA (24')			
20s ea	00074-4663-01	179.52	
BLOOD Y-TYPE SET 80 (Abbott Hosp)			
DEV,NA (W/CAIR CLAMP,NV,Y-INJ)			
48s ea	00074-1871-68	134.21	
BLOOD Y-TYPE SET W/PUMP (Abbott Hosp)			
DEV,NA (NV,82",CAIR CLAMP,Y-INJ)			
48s ea	00074-1873-68	155.52	
BLUE COHOSH (Botanical Labs.)			
LIQ,PO, 30 ml	41954-0020-05	3.50	6.99
BLUE GEL EXTERNAL ANALGESIC (Rugby)			
GEL,TP, 2%, 240 gm	00536-2302-59	3.97	
BLUE GREEN ALGAE (Rexall)			
CAP,PO, 50s ea	30768-0001-01	5.96	9.03
BLUE LIZARD (Del-Ray)			
CRE,TP (1X37ML,BABY,SPF30)			
5%-10%, 37 ml	00027-0000-14	3.11	3.99
(1X37ML,SENSITIVE,SPF30+)			
5%-10%, 37 ml	00027-0000-18	3.11	3.99
(1X89ML,SENSITIVE,SPF30+)			
5%-10%, 89 ml	00027-0000-35	7.80	9.99
(1X150ML,BABY,SPF30+)			
5%-10%, 148 ml	00027-0000-09	11.70	14.99
(1X266ML,BABY,SPF30+)			
5%-10%, 266 ml	00027-0000-04	18.00	24.99
(1X266ML,SENSITIVE,SPF30)			
5%-10%, 266 ml	00027-0000-20	18.00	24.99
(1X35.4GM,FACE,SPF30+)			
5.5%-8%, 35.4 gm	00027-0000-21	3.11	3.99
(1X89ML,FACE,SPF30+)			
5.5%-8%, 89 ml	00027-0000-38	7.80	9.99
(1X89ML,REGULAR,SPF30+)			
7.5%-2%-3%-6%,			
89 ml	00027-0000-30	7.80	9.99
(1X89ML,SPORT,SPF30+)			
7.5%-2%-3%-6%,			
89 ml	00027-0000-37	7.80	9.99
(SPF 30,REGULAR)			
8%-2%-3%-5.7%,			
30 gm	00027-0000-11	3.24	
(SPF 30,FACE,PABA-FREE)			
8%-2%-3%-5.7%,			
150 gm	00027-0000-08	12.19	
(SPF 30,REGULAR)			
8%-2%-3%-5.7%,			
150 gm	00027-0000-10	12.19	
(SPF 30,SPORT,PABA-FREE)			
8%-2%-3%-5.7%,			
150 gm	00027-0000-78	12.19	
(SPF 30,REGULAR)			
8%-2%-3%-5.7%,			
270 gm	00027-0000-03	18.75	
BLUE STAR (Quaker House)			
OIN,TP, 60 gm	70895-0054-32	3.37	
BODI BATH (Geritrex)			
SHA,TP (1X240ML)			
240 ml	92771-0767-08	1.05	1.03
3785 ml	92771-0767-01	11.84	11.59
BODI HEAT (Okamoto)			
DEV,NA, ea	28373-0749-82	0.60	0.99
3s ea	28373-0749-81	1.65	2.99
(POLYBAG)			
3s ea	28373-0749-83	1.65	2.99
BODI KLEEN (Geritrex)			
SPR,TP (48X240ML,DYE-FREE)			
240 ml 48s	92771-0772-08	1.21	
BODY BUILDER PROTEIN (Health Products Corp)			
TAB,PO, 60s ea	39686-0012-44	5.00	
BODY/HAIR/SKIN/NAILS BEAUTY FORMULA (Mason Vit)			
CAP,PO (PF,SF)			
60s ea	11845-0120-65	9.44	
BOIL-EASE (Del)			
OIN,TP, 5%-1.86%-0.44%,			
30 gm	10310-0004-13	5.82	8.73
BONA-BACILLUS (Westlake Labs.)			
CAP,PO (PF)			
100s ea	10539-0814-33	21.00	30.00
BONE DENSITY FORMULA (Rx Vitamins)			
CAP,PO (PF)			
180s ea	08429-0061-80	13.98	27.95
BONE MEAL (Marlex)			
TAB,PO, 214 mg-102 mg,			
250s ea	10135-0249-69	2.32	
BONE MEAL W/A & D (Mason Vit)			
TAB,PO, 100s ea	11845-0054-11	3.22	
BOOST (Nestle)			
LIQ,PO (LACTOSE-FREE,CHOCOLATE)			
237 ml 24s	43900-0675-30	31.68	
(LACTOSE-FREE,STRAWBERRY)			
237 ml 24s	43900-0676-30	31.68	
(LACTOSE-FREE,VANILLA)			
237 ml 24s	43900-0674-30	31.68	
(6X240ML,BUTTER PECAN)			
240 ml 6s	41679-0987-66	35.52	
(6X240ML,CHOCOLATE MALT)			
240 ml 6s	41679-0670-66	9.59	
(6X240ML,GLUTEN-FREE)			
240 ml 6s	41679-0674-66	35.52	
240 ml 6s	41679-0675-66	35.52	
240 ml 6s	41679-0676-66	35.52	
240 ml 6s	41679-0677-66	35.52	
BOOST HIGH PROTEIN (Nestle)			
LIQ,PO (LACTOSE-FREE,VANILLA)			
237 ml 24s	43900-0941-30	33.12	
(6X240ML,GLUTEN-FREE)			
240 ml 6s	41679-0940-66	37.73	
240 ml 6s	41679-0941-66	37.73	
240 ml 6s	41679-0944-66	37.73	
BOOST KID ESSENTIALS (Nestle)			
LIQ,PO (1X244ML,TETRA PAK)			
244 ml	41679-0332-51	2.09	
244 ml	41679-0332-61	2.09	
244 ml	41679-0332-81	2.09	
(24X244ML,TETRA PAK)			
244 ml 24s	41679-0332-50	50.16	
244 ml 24s	41679-0332-60	50.16	
244 ml 24s	41679-0332-80	50.16	
BOOST KID ESSENTIALS 1.0 CAL (Nestle)			
LIQ,PO (1X237ML,TETRA BRIK)			
237 ml	43900-0335-20	1.76	
237 ml	43900-0335-30	1.76	
(27X237ML,LACTOSE-FREE)			
237 ml 27s	00212-3352-13	47.63	
(27X237ML,TETRA BRIK)			
237 ml 27s	00212-3353-13	47.63	
SOL,PO (LACTOSE-FREE,VANILLA)			
237 ml	43900-0335-11	1.76	
237 ml 27s	00212-3351-13	47.63	
BOOST KID ESSENTIALS 1.5 CAL (Nestle)			
SOL,NA (1X237ML,TETRA BRIK)			
237 ml	43900-0335-40	2.36	
237 ml	43900-0335-88	2.36	
237 ml	43900-0335-90	2.36	
(27X237ML,TETRA BRIK)			
237 ml 27s	00212-3354-13	63.83	
237 ml 27s	00212-3358-13	63.83	
237 ml 27s	43900-0335-99	63.83	
BOOST KID ESSENTIALS 1.5 CAL W/FIBER (Nestle)			
SOL,PO (LACTOSE-FREE,VANILLA)			
237 ml	43900-0335-00	2.46	
237 ml 27s	00212-3350-13	66.42	
BOOST PLUS (Nestle)			
LIQ,PO (LACTOSE-FREE,CHOCOLATE)			
237 ml 24s	43900-0932-30	33.41	
(LACTOSE-FREE,STRAWBERRY)			
237 ml 24s	43900-0933-30	33.41	
(LACTOSE-FREE,VANILLA)			
237 ml 24s	43900-0931-30	33.41	
(6X240ML,GLUTEN-FREE)			
240 ml 6s	41679-0931-66	43.39	
240 ml 6s	41679-0932-66	43.39	
240 ml 6s	41679-0933-66	43.39	
BOOST PUDDING (Nestle)			
PUD,PO (48X150ML,VANILLA)			
150 ml 48s	41679-0945-03	65.95	
BOOST WITH BENEFIBER (Nestle)			
LIQ,PO (6X240ML,CHOCOLATE)			
240 ml 6s	41679-0158-01	11.32	
(6X240ML,ORANGE CREAM)			
240 ml 6s	41679-0157-61	11.32	
(6X240ML,VANILLA)			
240 ml 6s	41679-0157-21	11.32	
BORAGE (Bio-Tech Pharm)			
SGL,PO, 1000 mg-200 mg,			
30s ea	53191-0183-30	7.90	

PROD/MFR	HRI, UPC,NDC	AWP	SRP
BORAGE OIL (ADH)			
SGL,PO (PF,SF,SOFTGEL)			
1000 mg, 60s ea	60142-0755-56	10.48	20.95
BORDERED GAUZE (Dermarite)			
DEV,NA (2X2PAD;ABSORBENT ISLAND)			
100s ea	61924-0255-44	165.00	
(4X4PAD;ABSORBENT ISLAND)			
100s ea	61924-0256-66	195.00	
(Medline)			
DEV,NA (4"X4")			
ea	53329-0564-40	1.12	
(6"X6")			
ea	53329-0564-42	1.37	
(4"X10",STERILE)			
150s ea	08327-0510-09	206.05	
(4"X14",STERILE)			
150s ea	08327-0511-09	213.79	
(4"X4",STERILE)			
150s ea	08327-0510-40	71.25	
(6"X6",STERILE)			
150s ea	08327-0510-42	94.95	
BOROLEUM (Sinclair)			
OIN,TP, 6 gm	12350-0123-50	2.90	
BORON (Bio-Tech Pharm)			
CAP,PO, 3 mg, 100s ea	53191-0114-01	6.30	
BOSTON (Bausch & Lomb Inc.)			
SOL,NA (1 STEP ENZYME CLEANER)			
2.4 ml	47144-0056-02	8.83	
(REWETTING)			
10 ml	47144-0055-09	5.24	
(CLEANER)			
30 ml	47144-0061-01	9.53	
(CONDITIONING)			
105 ml	47144-0051-04	9.53	
BOSTON ADVANCE (Bausch & Lomb Inc.)			
KIT,NA (TRAVEL PACK)			
ea	47144-0074-20	5.50	
SOL,NA (CLEANER)			
30 ml	47144-0060-15	9.53	
BOSTON ADVANCE COMFORT FORMULA (Bausch & Lomb Inc.)			
SOL,NA (1X105ML,CONDITIONING)			
105 ml	10119-0056-09	9.53	
120 ml	47144-0050-12	9.53	
BOSTON LENS CASE (Bausch & Lomb Inc.)			
DEV,NA, ea	47144-0073-14	3.16	
BOSTON SIMPLUS (Bausch & Lomb Inc.)			
SOL,NA (MULTI-ACTION)			
105 ml	47144-0054-24	9.53	
BOUDREAUX'S BUTT PASTE (Boudreaux's)			
PAS,TP (16% ZINC OXIDE)			
10 gm	62103-3330-03	1.00	1.49
30 gm	62103-3330-00	2.25	3.99
60 gm	62103-3330-02	4.00	6.99
120 gm	62103-3330-04	6.50	10.99
480 gm	62103-3330-06	15.00	24.99
BOULES QUIES (Glenwood)			
DEV,NA (EAR PLUGS, 14X10)			
140s ea	00516-0013-12	125.84	
BOUNTY BUDDIES (Nature's Bounty)			
CTB,PO (ANIMAL SHAPES)			
100s ea	74312-0030-50		5.35
BOUNTY BUDDIES PLUS EXTRA C (Nature's Bounty)			
PO (ANIMAL SHAPES)			
100s ea	74312-0068-20		6.29
BOUNTY BUDDIES PLUS IRON (Nature's Bounty)			
CTB,PO, 100s ea	74312-0032-70		5.65
BRACELET (American)			
DEV,NA (10KT,PREMIER EMBOSSED)			
ea	08590-0103-00		279.95
(10KT.,CLASSIC)			
ea	08590-0048-00		229.95
(10KT.,HEART EMBOSSED)			
ea	08590-0001-00		199.95
(10KT.,HEART RED)			
ea	08590-0002-00		199.95
(14KT,PREMIER EMBOSSED)			
ea	08590-0112-00		349.95
(14KT.,CLASSIC)			
ea	08590-0051-00		229.95
(14KT.,HEART EMBOSSED)			
ea	08590-0005-00		271.95
(14KT.,HEART RED)			
ea	08590-0006-00		271.95
(GOLD-FILLED CLASSIC)			
ea	08590-0054-00		59.95
(GOLD-FILLED HEART RED)			
ea	08590-0010-00		51.95
(GOLD,HEART EMBOSSED)			
ea	08590-0009-00		51.95
(GOLD,PREMIER EMBOSSED)			
ea	08590-0118-00		69.95
(SILVER CLASSIC)			
ea	08590-0057-00		49.95
(SILVER,HEART EMBOSSED)			
ea	08590-0013-00		44.95
(SILVER,HEART,RED)			
ea	08590-0014-00		44.95
(SILVER,PREMIER EMBOSED)			
ea	08590-0124-00		59.95
(STAINLES,CLASIC,LRGE,RE)			
ea	08590-0061-00		29.95
(STAINLES,CLASIC,SMLL,OE)			
ea	08590-0062-00		24.95
(STAINLESS LYNX)			
ea	08590-0085-00		125.95
(TITANIUM LYNX)			
ea	08590-0091-00		195.95
BRASIVOL (Stiefel Consumer HealthCare)			
PAS,TP (FACIAL CLEANSER)			
70.9 gm	00145-0201-05	6.48	9.99
BREATHE FREE (Blairex)			
SPR,NS, 0.65%, 44.3 ml	50486-0641-15	2.32	
BREATHE RIGHT NASAL STRIPS (Glaxo)			
DEV,NA (ADULT -SM/MED,MENTHOL)			
10s ea	57145-0002-82	4.24	4.99
(ADULT, MENTHOLATED-LG)			
10s ea	57145-0002-85	4.24	4.99
(CLEAR,MED/LG)			
12s ea	57145-0002-38	4.24	4.99
(CLEAR,SM/MED)			
12s ea	57145-0002-34	4.24	4.99
(MED/LG,TAN)			
12s ea	57145-0002-30	4.24	4.99
(SM/MED,TAN)			
12s ea	57145-0002-26	4.24	4.99
(SM/MED,MENTHOLATED)			
28s ea	57145-0003-64	10.20	
(MED/LG,CLEAR)			
30s ea	57145-0002-46	10.20	11.99
(MED/LG,TAN)			
30s ea	57145-0001-32	10.20	11.99
(SM/MED,CLEAR)			
30s ea	57145-0002-42	10.20	11.99
(SM/MED,TAN)			
30s ea	57145-0001-22	10.20	11.99
BREATHE RIGHT SNORE RELIEF (Glaxo)			
SOL,MM (COOL MINT)			
300 ml	57145-0003-72	9.00	
SPR,MM, 60 ml	57145-0003-32	9.00	
BREEZE 2 BLOOD GLUCOSE MONITORING SYSTEM (Bayer Diabetes Care)			
DEV,NA (PURPLE FUSION)			
ea	00193-1461-01	56.40	
(TICKLED PINK)			
ea	00193-1460-01	56.40	
BREEZEE MIST FOOT POWDER (Pedinol)			
SPR,TP, 113 gm	00884-0659-04		13.00
BREWER'S YEAST (Basic Vitamins)			
TAB,PO, 500 mg, 250s ea	00761-0415-50	2.10	
(Major)			
TAB,PO, 486 mg, 250s ea	00904-3175-70	3.35	
(Marlex)			
TAB,PO, 486 mg, 250s ea	10135-0250-69	1.66	
1000s ea	10135-0250-10	4.48	
(Mason Vit)			
TAB,PO, 0.2 mg-0.02 mg-0.06 mg,			
100s ea	11845-0073-81	4.00	
250s ea	11845-0073-82	6.56	
(Modern Prod)			
PDR,PO, 198 gm	75820-0300-00	2.85	4.79
392 gm	75820-0300-01	5.33	8.99
(Nature's Bounty)			
TAB,PO (PF,SF)			
0.2 mg-0.02 mg-0.06 mg,			
250s ea	74312-0007-43		4.99
BRIGHT BEGINNINGS SOY (PBM Pharmaceuticals)			
LIQ,PO (PEDIATRIC,237MLX24)			
237 ml 24s	83744-0350-09	42.78	42.93
BRIOSCHI (Brioschi)			
GRA,PO (PACKET)			
6 gm 12s	10007-0123-50	2.15	
120 gm 12s	10007-0123-20	2.15	
240 gm 12s	10007-0123-10	3.50	
BRITE LIFE INSULIN SYRINGES (Can-Am Care)			
DEV,NA (31G,1/2CC,5/16")			
100s ea	38396-0430-90	17.50	
(31G,1CC,5/16")			
100s ea	38396-0431-90	17.50	
(31G,3/10CC,5/16")			
100s ea	38396-0429-90	17.50	
(ULTRA COMFORT, 28G)			
100s ea	38396-0421-90	15.50	
(ULTRA COMFORT, 29G)			
100s ea	38396-0423-90	17.50	
(ULTRA COMFORT,28G,1CC)			
100s ea	38396-0422-90	15.50	
(ULTRA COMFORT,29G,1CC)			
100s ea	38396-0424-90	17.50	
(ULTRA COMFORT,29G)			
100s ea	38396-0425-90	17.50	
(ULTRA COMFORT,30G,1/2CC)			
100s ea	38396-0426-90	17.50	
(ULTRA COMFORT,30G,1CC)			
100s ea	38396-0427-90	17.50	
(ULTRA COMFORT,30G)			
100s ea	38396-0428-90	17.50	
BRITE LIFE LANCETS (Can-Am Care)			
DEV,NA, 100s ea	38396-0323-90	5.85	
200s ea	38396-0324-90	9.50	
BRITE LIFE PSS STARTER (Home Diag)			
DEV,NA (MTR,STRP,LANCET,DEV,SOL)			
ea	56151-0210-01	22.18	
BRITE LIFE SUPER THIN LANCETS (Can-Am Care)			
DEV,NA, 100s ea	38396-0326-90	5.85	
BRITE LIFE THIN LANCETS (Can-Am Care)			
DEV,NA, 100s ea	38396-0327-90	5.85	
200s ea	38396-0325-90	9.50	
BRITE-LIFE ALLERGY RELIEF (AmerisourceBergen)			
ODT,PO (PRIVATE LABEL)			
10 mg, 10s ea	24385-0518-52	8.09	8.99
BRITE-LIFE ANKLE BRACE (AmerisourceBergen)			
DEV,NA (MEDIUM,ELASTIC)			
ea	87701-0709-40	7.19	7.99
BRITE-LIFE ANTIFUNGAL SPRAY LIQUID (AmerisourceBergen)			
SOL,TP (PRIVATE LABEL)			
1%, 151 gm	87701-0399-25	4.13	4.59
BRITE-LIFE ANTIFUNGAL SPRAY POWDER (AmerisourceBergen)			
POW,TP (PRIVATE LABEL)			
1%, 131 gm	87701-0399-26	4.13	4.59
BRITE-LIFE ANTISEPTIC (AmerisourceBergen)			
SOL,MM (MOUTH RINSE)			
1014 ml	87701-0649-31	2.87	3.19
BRITE-LIFE CALLUS CUSHIONS (AmerisourceBergen)			
DEV,NA (NON-MEDICATED)			
6s ea	87701-0399-42	1.79	1.99
BRITE-LIFE CALLUS REMOVERS (AmerisourceBergen)			
PAD,TP (W/6 PADS,MEDICATED)			
40%, 4s ea	87701-0399-43	1.88	2.09
BRITE-LIFE CARE SOX PLUS (AmerisourceBergen)			
DEV,NA (CREW,WHITE,LARGE)			
ea	87701-0752-81	7.25	8.39
(CREW,WHITE,X-LARGE)			
ea	87701-0752-84	7.25	8.39
BRITE-LIFE CORN & CALLUS REMOVER LIQUID (AmerisourceBergen)			
SOL,TP (W/3 CUSHIONS)			
12.6%, 15 ml	87701-0399-23	2.87	3.19

PROD/MFR HRI, UPC,NDC AWP SRP

BRITE-LIFE CORN CUSHIONS
(AmerisourceBergen)
DEV,NA (NON-MEDICATED)
9s ea 87701-0399-40 1.43 1.59

BRITE-LIFE CORN REMOVERS
(AmerisourceBergen)
PAD,TP (PAD W/PATCHES,MEDICATED)
40%, 9s ea 87701-0399-44 1.88 2.09

BRITE-LIFE DENTURE CLEANSER
(AmerisourceBergen)
TEF,NA (PRIVATE LABEL)
40s ea 87701-0910-36 2.24 2.49

BRITE-LIFE DOUBLE SOCK SYSTEM
(AmerisourceBergen)
DEV,NA (CREW,BLACK,LARGE)
ea 87701-0753-23 10.90 12.50
(CREW,BLACK,MEDIUM)
ea 87701-0753-21 10.90 12.50
(CREW,BLACK,SMALL)
ea 87701-0753-20 10.90 12.50
(CREW,BLACK,X-LARGE)
ea 87701-0753-24 10.90 12.50
(CREW,WHITE,LARGE)
ea 87701-0753-01 10.90 12.50
(CREW,WHITE,MEDIUM)
ea 87701-0752-98 10.90 12.50
(CREW,WHITE,SMALL)
ea 87701-0752-91 10.90 12.50
(CREW,WHITE,X-LARGE)
ea 87701-0753-10 10.90 12.50
(MINI-CREW,WHITE,LARGE)
ea 87701-0752-88 10.90 12.50
(MINI-CREW,WHITE,MEDIUM)
ea 87701-0752-86 10.90 12.50
(MINI-CREW,WHITE,SMALL)
ea 87701-0752-74 10.90 12.50
(MINI-CREW,WHITE,X-LARGE)
ea 87701-0752-90 10.90 12.50

BRITE-LIFE FIBER POWDER (AmerisourceBergen)
PDR,PO (NATURAL,REG FLAVOR)
3.4 gm/dose, 369 gm . 87701-0400-07 6.29 6.99
539 gm 24385-0301-37 6.29 8.29

BRITE-LIFE FIRM SUPPORT PANTYHOSE
(AmerisourceBergen)
DEV,NA (15-20MMHGCOMP,MED,FAWN)
ea 87701-0753-22 19.90 23.00
(15-20MMHGCOMP,MED,NUDE)
ea 87701-0753-48 19.90 23.00
(15-20MMHGCOMP,MED.BLK)
ea 87701-0753-39 19.90 23.00
(15-20MMHGCOMP,QUEEN,BLK)
ea 87701-0753-43 19.90 23.00
(15-20MMHGCOMP,TALL,BLK)
ea 87701-0753-41 19.90 23.00
(15-20MMHGCOMP,TALL,FAWN)
ea 87701-0753-27 19.90 23.00
(15-20MMHGCOMP,TALL,NUDE)
ea 87701-0753-49 19.90 23.00
(15-20MMHGCOMP,XTALL,BLK)
ea 87701-0753-42 19.90 23.00
(15-20MMHGCOMPPETITE,BLK)
ea 87701-0753-38 19.90 23.00
(15-20MMHGCOMPPETITEFAWN)
ea 87701-0753-11 19.90 23.00
(15-20MMHGCOMPPETITENUDE)
ea 87701-0753-44 19.90 23.00
(15-20MMHGCOMPQUEEN,FAWN)
ea 87701-0753-36 19.90 23.00
(15-20MMHGCOMPQUEEN,NUDE)
ea 87701-0753-86 19.90 23.00
(15-20MMHGCOMPX-TALLFAWN)
ea 87701-0753-32 19.90 23.00
(15-20MMHGCOMPX-TALLNUDE)
ea 87701-0753-78 19.90 23.00

BRITE-LIFE FIRM SUPPORT THIGH HIGH STOCKINGS (AmerisourceBergen)
DEV,NA (15-20MMHGL,FWNGRTRBLTRQ)
ea 87701-0753-94 15.40 17.70
(15-20MMHGM,FWNGRTRBLTRQ)
ea 87701-0753-88 15.40 17.70
(15-20MMHGXLFWN,GRTRBTRQ)
ea 87701-0753-95 15.40 17.70

BRITE-LIFE GLUCOSAMINE SULFATE
(AmerisourceBergen)
TAB,PO (PRIVATE LABEL,CAPLET)
750 mg, 120s ea 87701-0926-95 11.69 12.99

BRITE-LIFE HEMORRHOIDAL SUPPOSITORIES
(AmerisourceBergen)
SUP,RC (PRIVATE LABEL)
85.5%-0.25%-3%,
12s ea 87701-0537-68 4.31 5.79

BRITE-LIFE K-PEC (AmerisourceBergen)
SUS,PO (AF,PRIVATE LABEL)
262 mg/15 ml, 355 ml. 87701-0399-66 4.40 4.89

BRITE-LIFE KNEE BRACE (AmerisourceBergen)
DEV,NA (1-SIZE,NEOPRENE)
ea 87701-0709-73 10.49 12.59

BRITE-LIFE KNEE HIGH SHEER STOCKINGS
(AmerisourceBergen)
DEV,NA (15-20MMHGCOMP,LARGE,BLK)
ea 87701-0754-19 11.30 13.00
(15-20MMHGCOMP,MDIUM,BLK)
ea 87701-0754-18 11.30 13.00
(15-20MMHGCOMP,MED,FAWN)
ea 87701-0754-15 11.30 13.00
(15-20MMHGCOMP,MED,TAUPE)
ea 87701-0754-23 11.30 13.00
(15-20MMHGCOMP,XL,BLK)
ea 87701-0754-21 11.30 13.00
(15-20MMHGCOMPLARGE,FAWN)
ea 87701-0754-16 11.30 13.00
(15-20MMHGCOMPLARGETAUPE)
ea 87701-0754-28 11.30 13.00
(15-20MMHGCOMPX-LRGEFAWN)
ea 87701-0754-17 11.30 13.00

BRITE-LIFE LADIES' TROUSER SOCK
(AmerisourceBergen)
DEV,NA (15-20MMHGCOMP,LARGE,BLK)
ea 87701-0752-49 12.70 14.60
(15-20MMHGCOMP,LARGE,TAN)
ea 87701-0753-79 12.70 14.60
(15-20MMHGCOMP,MED,BLACK)
ea 87701-0752-48 12.70 14.60
(15-20MMHGCOMP,MED,NAVY)
ea 87701-0753-73 12.70 14.60
(15-20MMHGCOMP,MED,TAN)
ea 87701-0753-77 12.70 14.60
(15-20MMHGCOMP,SMALL,BLK)
ea 87701-0754-29 12.70 14.60
(15-20MMHGCOMP,XL,BLK)
ea 87701-0753-72 12.70 14.60
(15-20MMHGCOMP,XL,NAVY)
ea 87701-0753-74 12.70 14.60
(15-20MMHGCOMP,XL,TAN)
ea 87701-0753-80 12.70 14.60
(15-20MMHGCOMPLARGE,NAVY)
ea 87701-0753-76 12.70 14.60

BRITE-LIFE LICE BEDDING SPRAY
(AmerisourceBergen)
SPR,NA (PRIVATE LABEL)
0.5%, 124 gm 87701-0399-59 4.22 4.69

BRITE-LIFE MEDICATED WIPES
(AmerisourceBergen)
PAD,TP (PRE-MOISTENED)
50%, 48s ea 87701-0698-14 3.36 4.49

BRITE-LIFE MEN'S EXTRA FIRM SUPPORT SOCKS
(AmerisourceBergen)
DEV,NA (20-30MMHGCOMP,LARGE,BLK)
ea 87701-0751-59 13.10 15.00
(20-30MMHGCOMP,MED,BLK)
ea 87701-0751-57 13.10 15.00
(20-30MMHGCOMP,MED,BRWN)
ea 87701-0751-69 13.10 15.00
(20-30MMHGCOMP,MED,NAVY)
ea 87701-0751-65 13.10 15.00
(20-30MMHGCOMP,SMALL,BLK)
ea 87701-0751-55 13.10 15.00
(20-30MMHGCOMP,XL,BROWN)
ea 87701-0751-71 13.10 15.00
(20-30MMHGCOMP,XL,NAVY)
ea 87701-0751-68 13.10 15.00
(20-30MMHGCOMP,XLARG,BLK)
ea 87701-0751-63 13.10 15.00
(20-30MMHGCOMPLARGE,BRWN)
ea 87701-0751-70 13.10 15.00
(20-30MMHGCOMPLARGE,NAVY)
ea 87701-0751-67 13.10 15.00
(20-30MMHGCOMPSMALL,NAVY)
ea 87701-0751-64 13.10 15.00

BRITE-LIFE MEN'S FIRM SUPPORT SOCKS
(AmerisourceBergen)
DEV,NA (15-20MMHGCOMP,LARGE,BLK)
ea 87701-0753-83 12.70 14.60
(15-20MMHGCOMP,MED,BLK)
ea 87701-0753-82 12.70 14.60
(15-20MMHGCOMP,MED,BROWN)
ea 87701-0753-91 12.70 14.60
(15-20MMHGCOMP,MED,NAVY)
ea 87701-0753-87 12.70 14.60
(15-20MMHGCOMP,SMALL,BLK)
ea 87701-0753-81 12.70 14.60
(15-20MMHGCOMP,SMALLNAVY)
ea 87701-0753-85 12.70 14.60
(15-20MMHGCOMP,XL,BLK)
ea 87701-0753-84 12.70 14.60
(15-20MMHGCOMP,XL,NAVY)
ea 87701-0753-90 12.70 14.60
(15-20MMHGCOMP,XLRGE,BWN)
ea 87701-0753-93 12.70 14.60
(15-20MMHGCOMPLARGE,BRWN)
ea 87701-0753-92 12.70 14.60
(15-20MMHGCOMPLARGE,NAVY)
ea 87701-0753-89 12.70 14.60

BRITE-LIFE MICONAZOLE 3 (AmerisourceBergen)
CRE,MR (3 PREFILLED APPS/CREAM)
ea 87701-0962-87 9.90 11.99

BRITE-LIFE MOTION SICKNESS RELIEF
(AmerisourceBergen)
TAB,PO (PRIVATE LABEL)
25 mg, 8s ea 87701-0347-44 0.92 3.59

BRITE-LIFE ONE DAILY DIET SUPPORT
(AmerisourceBergen)
TAB,PO (PRIVATE LABEL)
50s ea 87701-0926-96 5.39 5.99

BRITE-LIFE OPTI-VITAMINS
(AmerisourceBergen)
TAB,PO (PRIVATE LABEL)
120s ea 87701-0926-92 10.79 11.99

BRITE-LIFE OVULATION PREDICTOR
(AmerisourceBergen)
DEV,NA (7-DAY KIT,PRIVATE LABEL)
ea 87701-0738-30 17.09 17.99

BRITE-LIFE PAIN RELIEF CREAM
(AmerisourceBergen)
CRE,TP (ULTRA STRENGTH)
4%-10%-30%, 57 gm . 87701-0399-52 3.50 3.99

BRITE-LIFE PAIN RELIEVING OINTMENT
(AmerisourceBergen)
OIN,TP (PRIVATE LABEL)
70 gm 87701-0399-58 3.77 4.19

BRITE-LIFE PLANTAR WART REMOVER
(AmerisourceBergen)
PAD,TP (FOR FEET,W/24 CVR PADS)
40%, 24s ea 87701-0399-37 4.75 5.99

BRITE-LIFE SENNA (AmerisourceBergen)
SGL,PO (NATURAL VEG LAXATIVE)
8.6 mg, 80s ea 87701-0964-65 8.99 9.99

BRITE-LIFE SINUS DAY (AmerisourceBergen)
TAB,PO (ASPIRIN-FREE)
500 mg-30 mg, 24s ea. 87701-0435-66 3.32 3.69
48s ea 87701-0868-37 5.21 5.79

BRITE-LIFE SLEEP SOCKS (AmerisourceBergen)
DEV,NA (ONE SIZE FITS ALL,BLUE)
ea 87701-0753-09 7.16 7.99

BRITE-LIFE SMARTKNIT SEAMLESS SOCKS
(AmerisourceBergen)
DEV,NA (CREW,LARGE,WHITE)
ea 87701-0752-96 10.90 12.50
(CREW,MEDIUM,WHITE)
ea 87701-0752-87 10.90 12.50
(CREW,SMALL,WHITE)
ea 87701-0752-85 10.90 12.50
(CREW,X-LARGE,WHITE)
ea 87701-0753-00 10.90 12.50

BRITE-LIFE SURGI-WEIGHT KNEE HIGH STOCKINGS
(AmerisourceBergen)
DEV,NA (20-30MMHGCLSETOEL,BEIGE)
ea 87701-0752-70 22.70 26.00
(20-30MMHGCLSETOEM,BEIGE)
ea 87701-0752-69 22.70 26.00
(20-30MMHGCLSETOES,BEIGE)
ea 87701-0752-67 22.70 26.00
(20-30MMHGCLSETOEXL,BEIG)
ea 87701-0752-72 22.70 26.00
(30-40MMHG,OPENTOESBEIGE)
ea 87701-0753-57 32.60 37.50
(30-40MMHG,OPENTOEXLBEIG)
ea 87701-0753-60 32.60 37.50
(30-40MMHGCLSETOE,S,BEIG)
ea 87701-0753-50 32.60 37.50
(30-40MMHGCLSETOEL,BEIGE)
ea 87701-0753-52 32.60 37.50
(30-40MMHGCLSETOEM,BEIGE)
ea 87701-0753-51 32.60 37.50

PROD/MFR	HRI, UPC,NDC	AWP	SRP
(30-40MMHGCLSETOEXL,BEIG) ea	87701-0753-53	32.60	37.50
(30-40MMHGOPENTOEL,BEIGE) ea	87701-0753-59	32.60	37.50
(30-40MMHGOPENTOEM,BEIGE) ea	87701-0753-58	32.60	37.50
BRITE-LIFE SURGI-WEIGHT PANTYHOSE (AmerisourceBergen)			
DEV,NA (20-30MMHGCLSETOEL,BEIGE) ea	87701-0753-40	33.50	38.50
(20-30MMHGCLSETOEM,BEIGE) ea	87701-0752-73	33.50	38.50
(20-30MMHGCLSETOEXL,BEIG) ea	87701-0753-46	33.50	38.50
BRITE-LIFE SURGI-WEIGHT THIGH HIGH STOCKINGS (AmerisourceBergen)			
DEV,NA (20-30MMHGCLSETOEL,BEIGE) ea	87701-0752-19	31.70	36.50
(20-30MMHGCLSETOEM,BEIGE) ea	87701-0752-15	31.70	36.50
(20-30MMHGCLSETOES,BEIGE) ea	87701-0751-24	31.70	36.50
(20-30MMHGCLSETOEXL,BEIG) ea	87701-0752-66	31.70	36.50
BRITE-LIFE THIGH HIGH STOCKINGS WITH LACE (AmerisourceBergen)			
DEV,NA (15-20MMHGCOMP,LARGE,BLK) ea	87701-0754-06	19.90	23.00
(15-20MMHGCOMP,MED,BLK) ea	87701-0754-05	19.90	23.00
(15-20MMHGCOMP,MED,FAWN) ea	87701-0753-96	19.90	23.00
(15-20MMHGCOMP,XL,BLK) ea	87701-0754-07	19.90	23.00
(15-20MMHGCOMP,XL,FAWN) ea	87701-0754-02	19.90	23.00
(15-20MMHGCOMPLARGE,FAWN) ea	87701-0753-98	19.90	23.00
BRITE-LIFE WART REMOVER (AmerisourceBergen)			
PAD,TP (FOR HANDS,W/20 CVR PADS) 40%, 18s ea	87701-0399-38	4.75	4.99
BRITE-LIFE WART REMOVER LIQUID (AmerisourceBergen)			
SOL,TP (MAX STRENGTH) 17%, 15 ml	87701-0399-50	2.18	4.29
BRITE-LIFE WIDE SOCK SYSTEM (AmerisourceBergen)			
DEV,NA (50% WIDER,CREW,LRGE,BLK) ea	87701-0753-34	10.90	12.50
(50% WIDER,CREW,MED,BLK) ea	87701-0753-31	10.90	12.50
(50% WIDER,CREW,XL,BLK) ea	87701-0753-35	10.90	12.50
(50% WIDER,CREW,XL,WHITE) ea	87701-0753-30	10.90	12.50
(50% WIDER,CREWMED,WHITE) ea	87701-0753-25	10.90	12.50
(50% WIDERCREWLARGEWHITE) ea	87701-0753-26	10.90	12.50
BRITE-LIFE WRIST BRACE (AmerisourceBergen)			
DEV,NA (1-SIZE,NEOPRENE,SPLINT) ea	87701-0709-71	13.29	15.99
(ELASTIC,MEDIUM) ea	87701-0709-46	4.76	5.89
BROCCOLI (Freeda)			
TAB,PO (PF,SF,DYE-FREE) 500 mg, 100s ea	10432-0308-01	5.37	8.95
250s ea	10432-0308-02	10.47	17.45
BROKOLI (Health Products Corp)			
TAB,PO (PF,SF) 60s ea	39686-0014-84	3.00	
BROM/PSEUD/DM (Phys Total Care) REPACK			
ELI,PO, 118 ml	54868-1936-00	14.13	
BROMAGEST (Key Company)			
CAP,PO, 500 mg-25 mg, 25s ea	11694-0750-25	6.00	
60s ea	11694-0750-60	12.50	
120s ea	11694-0750-12	21.50	
BROMALINE (Rugby)			
SYR,PO (AF,GRAPE) 1 mg/5 ml-15 mg/5 ml, 118 ml	00536-0880-97	2.70	
473 ml	00536-0880-85	6.37	
BROMALINE DM (Rugby)			
ELI,PO (AF,GRAPE) 120 ml	00536-1360-97	4.01	
480 ml	00536-1360-85	8.94	
BROMASE (Bio-Tech Pharm)			
CAP,PO, 15 mg-500 mg, 60s ea	53191-0151-60	11.50	
100s ea	53191-0151-01	18.25	
250s ea	53191-0151-25	40.00	
BROMELAIN (Freeda)			
TAB,PO (PF,SF,DYE-FREE) 500 mg, 100s ea	10432-0298-01	7.08	
250s ea	10432-0298-02	14.16	
BROMFED (Phys Total Care) REPACK			
SYR,PO (LEMON-ORANGE) 2 mg/5 ml-30 mg/5 ml, 120 ml	54868-4623-00	14.85	
BROMI-LOTION (Gordon)			
LOT,TP, 120 ml	10481-1006-02	13.25	
BROMI-TALC (Gordon)			
POW,TP (FOOT) 105 gm	10481-1011-01	9.30	
BROMI-TALC PLUS (Gordon)			
POW,TP, 120 gm	10481-6001-04	13.25	
BROMPHENEX DM (Breckenridge Pharm)			
SOL,PO (AF,SF,DYE-FREE,FRUIT) 473 ml	51991-0347-16	38.45	
BROMPHENIRAMINE MALEATE (Consolidated Midland)			
ELI,PO, 2 mg/5 ml, 480 ml	00223-6100-01	5.50	
3840 ml	00223-6100-02	29.00	
TAB,PO, 4 mg, 100s ea	00223-0550-01	2.95	
1000s ea	00223-0550-02	22.50	
BROMPHENIRAMINE/PHENYLEPHRINE DM (Macoven)			
SOL,PO (AF,BUBBLE GUM) 473 ml	44183-0313-16	98.66	
BROMPHENIRAMINE/PSE/DM (Southwood) REPACK			
ELI,PO, 120 ml	58016-4830-01	3.75	
BROMPHENIRAMINE/PSEUDOEPHEDRINE DM (Macoven)			
SOL,PO (AF,COTTON CANDY) 473 ml	44183-0311-16	94.13	
BRONCHO SALINE (Blairex)			
SOL,IH, 0.9%, 90 ml	50486-0078-22	5.48	
240 ml	50486-0078-23	7.12	
BRONCOTRON (Seyer Pharmatec)			
LIQ,PO (AF,SF,DYE-FREE,CHERRY) 10 mg/5 ml-100 mg/5 ml, 118 ml	11026-2640-04	9.90	
BRONKAID DUAL ACTION FORMULA (Bayer HealthCare)			
TAB,PO (CAPLET) 25 mg-400 mg, 24s ea	00024-4081-02	3.45	
60s ea	00024-4081-06	6.45	
BROTAPP (Silarx)			
LIQ,PO (AF,SF,GRAPE) 1 mg/5 ml-15 mg/5 ml, 118 ml	54838-0125-40	4.55	
237 ml	54838-0125-70	7.72	
473 ml	54838-0125-80	13.50	
BROTAPP PE (Silarx)			
SOL,PO (AF,SF,GRAPE) 1 mg/5 ml-2.5 mg/5 ml, 118 ml	54838-0143-40	4.55	
237 ml	54838-0143-70	7.72	
473 ml	54838-0143-80	13.50	
BROTAPP PE-DM (Silarx)			
SOL,PO (AF,SF,GRAPE) 118 ml	54838-0147-40	4.55	
237 ml	54838-0147-70	7.72	
BROTAPP-DM (Silarx)			
LIQ,PO (COLD & COUGH,AF,SF) 118 ml	54838-0136-40	4.55	
237 ml	54838-0136-70	7.72	
BROVEX PB (MCR American)			
TAB,PO, 4 mg-10 mg, 100s ea	42819-0101-01	105.24	
BROVEX PB DM (MCR American)			
TAB,PO, 4 mg-20 mg-10 mg, 100s ea	42819-0102-01	109.85	
BROVEX PSE (MCR American)			
TAB,PO, 4 mg-40 mg, 100s ea	58605-0440-01	114.99	
BROVEX PSE DM (MCR American)			
TAB,PO, 4 mg-20 mg-40 mg, 100s ea	58605-0441-01	119.99	
BRUSH'N FLOSS (Lee Pharm)			
DEV,NA, ea	23558-0683-40	1.43	
12s ea	23558-0683-41	102.82	
BRYONIA ALBA (Luyties)			
TAB,SL (6X) 6 x, 500s ea	00618-1080-03	3.99	
5500s ea	00618-1080-10	30.32	
12 x, 500s ea	00622-1080-03	4.19	
(30X) 12 x, 5500s ea	00622-1080-10	31.83	
30 x, 500s ea	00624-1080-03	4.19	
5500s ea	00624-1080-10	31.83	
BUF-PUF (3M Consumer)			
DEV,NA (BACK SCRUB) ea	51131-0916-01	5.24	
(BODY MATE) ea	51131-0908-01	3.84	
(EXTRA GENTLE) ea	51131-0587-88	3.18	
(GENTLE) ea	51131-0185-03	3.18	
(REGULAR) ea	51131-0910-01	3.18	
BUF-PUF SINGLES (3M Consumer)			
SPG,TP (W/ CLEANSER) 40s ea	51131-0083-62	3.68	
(W/CONDITIONING CLEANSER) 40s ea	51131-0002-15	3.68	
BUFEN (Lunsco)			
TAB,PO (250X2) 200 mg, 500s ea	10892-0138-02	26.28	
BUFFALO LIVER (Carlson,J.R.)			
CAP,PO (SF,CORN-FREE,SALT-FREE) 60s ea	88395-0070-50	6.45	12.90
(HYPOALLERGENIC,SF) 180s ea	88395-0070-51	17.75	35.50
BUFFERED SALT (Lannett)			
TAB,PO (BUFFERED TABLET) 287 mg-15 mg-180 mg, 100s ea	00527-1417-01	4.50	
BUFFERED VITAMIN C (Freeda)			
TAB,PO, 75 mg-500 mg, 100s ea	10432-0100-01	7.77	12.95
250s ea	10432-0100-02	15.30	25.50
500s ea	10432-0100-03	25.32	42.20
BUFFERIN (B/M Squibb Cons Med)			
TAB,PO, 325 mg, 39s ea	19810-0005-25	3.30	
65s ea	19810-0005-26	4.57	
130s ea	19810-0005-27	6.95	
(Novartis Consumer)			
TAB,PO (REGULAR STRENGTH,COATED) 325 mg, 39s ea	00067-2063-39	3.50	
(EXTRA STRENGTH,COATED) 500 mg, 65s ea	00067-2065-65	6.65	
130s ea	00067-2065-13	9.30	
BUFFERIN ARTHRITIS STRENGTH (B/M Squibb Cons Med)			
TAB,PO (CAPLET) 500 mg, 130s ea	19810-0059-56	8.77	
BUFFERIN EXTRA STRENGTH (B/M Squibb Cons Med)			
TAB,PO, 500 mg, 39s ea	19810-0071-71	3.86	
65s ea	19810-0071-72	6.28	
130s ea	19810-0071-73	8.77	
BUGS BEGONE (Amrita)			
SPR,TP (ALL NATURAL,AF) 120 ml	44037-0010-14	7.90	
BUGS BEGONE FOR KIDS (Amrita)			
SPR,TP (ALL NATURAL,AF) 120 ml	44037-0012-14	7.90	
BUGS BEGONE FOR PETS (Amrita)			
SPR,TP (ALL NATURAL,AF) 120 ml	44037-0011-14	7.90	
BUGS BUNNY COMPLETE (Bayer HealthCare)			
CTB,PO (SF) 60s ea	16500-0076-30	4.31	
BULGARICUM I.B. (Natren)			
POW,PO, 2 billion org/gm, 75 gm	53983-0300-50	13.20	22.00
135 gm	53983-0300-55	18.60	31.00

PROD/MFR	HRI, UPC,NDC	AWP	SRP
BULK-K (Key Company)			
PDR,PO, 3.4 gm/dose,			
392 gm	11694-0844-14	6.00	
BULLFROG AMPHIBIOUS FORMULA (Chattem)			
GEL,TP (SPF 36,AF,SF)			
118.2 ml	41167-0330-17	7.64	
(SPF36,SF,QUICKGEL)			
118.2 ml	41167-0330-52	7.64	
141 ml	41167-0330-58	7.20	
LOT,TP (S30,AF,SF)			
120 ml	41167-0330-44	7.20	
BULLFROG FOR KIDS (Chattem)			
LOT,TP (SPF36,PABA-FREE)			
120 ml	41167-0330-32	6.66	
BULLFROG MOISTURIZING FORMULA (Chattem)			
LOT,TP (SPF 30,SF)			
120 ml	41167-0330-45	7.20	
BULLSEYE SAFETY (Specialty Medical)			
DEV,NA (HIGH FLOW,SINGLE USE)			
100s ea	38415-0623-21	33.60	
BUNION CUSHION (Schering Plough)			
DEV,NA (FELT)			
ea	11017-0122-88	2.50	
(FOAM)			
ea	11017-0118-50	1.96	
BURDOCK (Botanical Labs.)			
LIQ,PO, 30 ml	41954-0020-07	3.75	7.49
BURN 'N BITE (Stanmar Labs)			
GEL,TP, 2%-1%, 22.5 gm	50263-0900-34	2.00	
150 gm	50263-0900-05	4.75	
BURN SPRAY (Hart Health)			
SPR,TP (W/ALOE VERA)			
0.13%-2.5%, 60 ml	50332-0214-01	2.27	
BURN-CARE (Weleda)			
GEL,TP, 34 gm	55946-0002-60	4.35	
BURN-O-JEL (S.S.S.)			
GEL,TP, 0.5%, 90 ml	12258-0128-03	2.33	3.49
BURNAMYCIN (Pfeiffer)			
SPR,TP, 0.5%, 60 ml	00927-0563-20	1.94	3.49
BUROW'S SOLUTION (Humco)			
SOL,TP, 480 ml	00395-0055-16	5.68	
BUTCHER'S BROOM (ADH)			
CAP,PO (PF,SF)			
470 mg, 100s ea	60142-0904-71	4.98	9.95
C & M CAPS-375 (Key Company)			
CAP,PO (SF)			
250 mg-125 mg,			
100s ea	11694-0808-01	5.00	
250s ea	11694-0808-02	10.50	
C-500 (Nature's Bounty)			
TER,PO, 500 mg, 200s ea	74312-0047-52		16.39
C-BUFF (Bio-Tech Pharm)			
POW,PO (1X227GM)			
227 gm	53191-0100-08	12.60	
C-GEL (Carlson,J.R.)			
CAP,PO (SOFTGEL)			
1000 mg, 60s ea	88395-0030-00	4.95	9.90
100s ea	88395-0030-01	7.75	15.50
250s ea	88395-0030-02	19.40	38.80
C-MAX (Bio-Tech Pharm)			
CAP,PO, 100s ea	53191-0374-01	6.85	
250s ea	53191-0374-25	15.40	
C-PLEX (Bio-Tech Pharm)			
CAP,PO, 750 mg-94 mg,			
100s ea	53191-0049-01	7.90	
C-TIME (Time-Cap)			
CER,PO, 500 mg, 100s ea	49483-0007-01	8.50	
1000s ea	49483-0007-10	87.85	
C-TIME W/ROSE HIPS (Nature's Bounty)			
TER,PO (PF,SF,DAIRY-FREE)			
1500 mg, 60s ea	74312-0028-01		9.59
C.P.M. TABLETS (Advance)			
TAB,PO, 4 mg, 100s ea	17714-0016-01	1.25	
1000s ea	17714-0016-10	4.99	
C1000 ASCORBIC ACID (Mason Vit)			
TAB,PO (PF,SF)			
1000 mg, 300s ea	11845-0071-60	22.11	
CA PLUS PROTEIN (Miller)			
TAB,PO, 100s ea	17204-0428-40	5.04	8.40
CAFFEINE (Marlex)			
TAB,PO, 200 mg, 16s ea	10135-0175-75	0.70	
1000s ea	10135-0175-10	9.28	

PROD/MFR	HRI, UPC,NDC	AWP	SRP
(Truxton)			
CAP,PO, 250 mg,			
1000s ea	00463-3034-10	39.00	
CAL CARB/VIT D (Key Company)			
LIQUA-CAL			
SGL,PO (PF,SOFTGEL)			
600 mg-200 iu,			
100s ea	11694-0770-01	7.25	
(Mason Vit)			
LIQUID CALCIUM PLUS VITAMIN D			
SGL,PO (PF,SF,SOFTGEL)			
600 mg-200 iu,			
60s ea	11845-0123-85	8.33	
SUPER CALCIUM W/VITAMIN D			
TAB,PO, 600 mg-125 iu,			
100s ea	11845-0088-91	7.56	
200s ea	11845-0088-92	14.11	
(PF,SF)			
600 mg-200 iu,			
60s ea	11845-0088-95	4.67	
CAL-AEP (Bio-Tech Pharm)			
CAP,PO, 42 mg-64 mg,			
100s ea	53191-0220-01	16.30	
CAL-C-CAPS (Key Company)			
CAP,PO, 800 mg, 100s ea	11694-0765-11	6.50	
500s ea	11694-0765-06	28.00	
CAL-CEE (Key Company)			
TAB,PO (SF)			
1150 mg, 100s ea	11694-0765-01	5.50	
250s ea	11694-0765-25	12.50	
500s ea	11694-0765-05	24.00	
CAL-CITRATE (Bio-Tech Pharm)			
CAP,PO, 225 mg, 100s ea	53191-0124-01	6.30	
250s ea	53191-0124-25	12.40	
CAL-CITRATE PLUS VITAMIN D (Freeda)			
TAB,PO (PURE,SF,GLUTEN-FREE)			
250 mg-100 iu,			
100s ea	10432-0351-01	6.57	10.95
250s ea	10432-0351-02	13.14	21.90
CAL-CO3S (Bio-Tech Pharm)			
CAP,PO, 200 mg, 100s ea	53191-0061-01	3.70	
CAL-G (Key Company)			
CAP,PO, 700 mg, 100s ea	11694-0864-01	4.50	
250s ea	11694-0864-25	9.50	
CAL-GEST (Rugby)			
CTB,PO (ASSORTED FLAVORS)			
500 mg, 150s ea	00536-4742-97	4.13	
CAL-GLU (Bio-Tech Pharm)			
CAP,PO, 50 mg, 100s ea	53191-0081-01	4.20	
CAL-K (Key Company)			
TAB,PO, 220 mg-5 mg-40 iu,			
100s ea	11694-0980-01	4.50	
250s ea	11694-0980-02	9.00	
CAL-LAC (Key Company)			
CAP,PO, 100 mg, 100s ea	11694-0919-01	6.25	
250s ea	11694-0919-25	12.50	
CAL-MINT (Freeda)			
CTB,PO (SF,GLUTEN-FREE)			
260 mg, 100s ea	10432-0300-01	5.97	9.95
250s ea	10432-0300-02	11.94	19.90
CAL-O.D.C. (Key Company)			
CAP,PO, 230 mg, 100s ea	11694-0873-01	5.00	
CAL-Y (Key Company)			
CAP,PO, 500 mg, 100s ea	11694-0918-01	7.00	
CAL/MAG (Freeda)			
CTB,PO (PF,SF,DYE-FREE)			
200 mg-100 mg,			
100s ea	10432-0326-01	5.67	9.45
(NATURAL)			
200 mg-100 mg,			
250s ea	10432-0326-02	11.34	18.90
CAL/MAG SUPER (Freeda)			
SUPER CAL MAG			
TAB,PO (PF,SF,DYE-FREE)			
333.3 mg-166.7 mg,			
100s ea	10432-0269-01	5.55	9.25
250s ea	10432-0269-02	11.10	18.50
500s ea	10432-0269-03	17.37	28.95
CAL/MG (Freeda)			
CAL/MAG CHELATED			
TAB,PO (PF,SF,DYE-FREE)			
100 mg-50 mg,			
100s ea	10432-0249-01	5.97	9.95
250s ea	10432-0249-02	11.94	19.90

PROD/MFR	HRI, UPC,NDC	AWP	SRP
MAG-CAL MEGA			
PO (PF,SF,DYE-FREE)			
133.3 mg-266.7 mg,			
100s ea	10432-0289-01	6.30	10.50
CALACLEAR (Humco)			
LOT,TP, 1%-0.1%, 177 ml	00395-0400-96	1.91	
CALADRYL (Johnson & Johnson)			
LOT,TP, 8%-1%, 177 ml	00713-0181-19	4.66	
CALADRYL CLEAR (Johnson & Johnson)			
LOT,TP, 1%-0.1%, 177 ml	12547-0311-80	4.66	
CALAGEL (Tec)			
LOT,TP, 0.15%-2%-0.215%,			
180 ml	83926-0860-00	3.40	5.99
CALAGESIC (Humco)			
LOT,TP (1X177ML)			
8%-1%, 177 ml	00395-0420-96	1.91	3.17
CALALGIN-GRX (Geritrex)			
DRE,TP (4"X4")			
30s ea	92771-0830-44	5.51	
(2"X2")			
50s ea	92771-0830-22	2.92	
CALALGIN-GRX ROPE (Geritrex)			
DRE,TP (3/4"X12")			
20s ea	92771-0831-12	7.65	
CALAMINE (Chain Drug Marketing)			
LOT,TP, 177 ml	63868-0317-06	1.07	3.99
(Consolidated Midland)			
LOT,TP, 480 ml	00223-6231-03	3.50	
(Humco)			
LOT,TP, 180 ml	00395-0413-96	1.43	
(Major)			
LOT,TP, 120 ml	00904-2533-00	1.29	
(Vi-Jon)			
LOT,TP (U.S.P.)			
8%-8%, 118 ml	00869-0063-26	0.84	
177 ml	00869-0063-30	1.15	
237 ml	00869-0063-34	1.37	
(A-S Medication)			
REPACK			
LOT,TP, 120 ml	54569-0752-00	1.31	
(Altura)			
REPACK			
LOT,TP, 120 ml	63874-0035-12	3.99	
(Phys Total Care)			
REPACK			
LOT,TP, 118 ml	54868-2056-00	6.18	
(Quality Care Prod)			
REPACK			
LOT,TP, 180 ml	49999-0350-06	8.37	
(Southwood)			
REPACK			
LOT,TP, 120 ml	58016-3112-01	4.65	
CALAMINE PHENOLATED (AmerisourceBergen)			
LOT,TP (PRIVATE LABEL)			
8%-1%, 180 ml	24385-0407-96	3.14	3.49
CALAMINE PLAIN (AmerisourceBergen)			
LOT,TP (PRIVATE LABEL)			
180 ml	24385-0413-96	2.42	2.69
CALAMINE W/PHENOL (Humco)			
LOT,TP (U.S.P.)			
8%-1%, 180 ml	00395-0407-96	1.92	
CALAMYCIN COOL & CLEAR (Pfeiffer)			
SPR,TP, 1%-0.1%, 60 ml	00927-0625-60	1.39	2.49
CALC FLUOR (Nuage Labs)			
TAB,SL (6X)			
125s ea	00634-2033-68	3.05	5.09
CALC PHOS (Nuage Labs)			
SL (6X)			
125s ea	00634-2043-68	3.05	5.09
CALC SULPH (Nuage Labs)			
SL (6X)			
125s ea	00634-2049-68	3.05	5.09
CALCARB 600 (Teva)			
TAB,PO, 600 mg, 60s ea	00182-4140-26	3.45	
500s ea	00182-4140-05	10.99	
CALCARB 600 WITH VITAMIN D (Teva)			
TAB,PO (PF,SF,SODIUM-FREE)			
600 mg-400 iu, 60s ea	00182-4141-26	3.59	
CALCAREA CARBONICA (Luyties)			
TAB,SL (6X)			
6 x, 500s ea	00618-2030-03	3.99	

PROD/MFR	HRI, UPC,NDC	AWP	SRP
5500s ea	00618-2030-10	30.32	
(30X)			
12 x, 500s ea	00622-2030-03	4.19	
5500s ea	00622-2030-10	31.83	
30 x, 500s ea	00624-2030-03	4.19	
5500s ea	00624-2030-10	31.83	
CALCAREA FLUOR (Hyland's)			
TAB,PO, 500s ea	54973-1002-01	5.87	9.79
1000s ea	54973-1002-02	10.49	17.49
CALCAREA PHOS (Hyland's)			
TAB,PO, 500s ea	54973-1008-01	5.87	9.79
1000s ea	54973-1008-02	10.49	17.49
CALCAREA SULPH (Hyland's)			
TAB,PO, 500s ea	54973-1014-01	5.87	9.79
1000s ea	54973-1014-02	10.49	17.49
CALCET (Mission)			
TAB,PO, 150 mg-100 iu,			
100s ea	01780-0251-01	6.87	
CALCET CITRATE CREAMY BITES (Mission)			
CTB,PO (LEMON CREAM)			
500 mg-400 iu,			
30s ea	01780-0277-30	16.24	
CALCET PLUS (Mission)			
TAB,PO (STRESS FORMULA)			
60s ea	00178-0252-60	8.00	
CALCI-CHEW (Rugby)			
CTB,PO (CHERRY)			
1250 mg, 100s ea	00536-3792-01	10.00	
CALCI-MIX (Rugby)			
CAP,PO, 1250 mg,			
100s ea	00536-3791-01	11.75	
CALCIBON (Kramer-Novis)			
SUS,PO, 180 ml	52083-0682-06	8.00	
CALCIFEROL (UCB)			
LIQ,PO (DROPS)			
8000 iu/ml, 60 ml	00091-4150-60	114.35	
CALCILO XD (Abbott)			
PDR,PO (1X375GM)			
375 gm	70074-0533-29	19.25	
400 gm	70074-0003-78	17.80	
423 gm	70074-0603-78	18.50	
CALCIMIN-300 (Key Company)			
TAB,PO (SF)			
300 mg, 100s ea	11694-0855-01	4.75	
250s ea	11694-0855-04	9.50	
CALCIO DEL MAR (Marlop)			
TAB,PO, 500 mg, 60s ea	12939-0517-60	5.32	
CALCIONATE (Rugby)			
SYR,PO (FRUIT)			
1.8 gm/5 ml, 473 ml	00536-2770-85	19.73	
CALCITRATE (Major)			
TAB,PO (COATED CAPLET)			
315 mg-200 iu,			
100s ea	00904-5272-60	5.05	
950 mg, 100s ea	00904-5062-60	6.14	
(Marlex)			
TAB,PO, 950 mg, 100s ea	10135-0252-01	2.22	
CALCIUM (AmerisourceBergen)			
TAB,PO (PRIVATE LABEL)			
600 mg, 60s ea	24385-0269-72	4.58	5.09
(Basic Vitamins)			
TAB,PO, 500 mg, 100s ea	00761-0930-20	2.40	
(Cardinal Health)			
TAB,PO (PF,PRIVATE LABEL)			
600 mg, 60s ea	37205-0391-72	4.14	
(Marlex)			
TAB,PO (CAPLET)			
600 mg, 60s ea	10135-0256-60	0.97	
150s ea	10135-0256-64	1.88	
(Rexall)			
TAB,PO (VITAMIN D,OYSTER SHELL)			
333.33 mg-133.33 iu,			
60s ea	30768-0001-51	1.73	2.63
(Nature's Bounty)			
LIQUID CALCIUM			
CAP,PO (PF,SF,SOFTGEL)			
200 mg-275 iu-200 iu,			
100s ea	74312-0076-80		4.99
(Mason Vit)			
SUPER CALCIUM			
TAB,PO (PF,SF)			
100s ea	11845-0130-21	8.56	
CALCIUM & MAGNESIUM CHELATE (Key Company)			
CAP,PO (SF)			
180 mg-90 mg, 100s ea	11694-0804-01	7.50	
250s ea	11694-0804-25	15.00	
CALCIUM + D (Rexall)			
TAB,PO (PROMOTES BONE HEALTH)			
500 mg-125 iu, 200s ea	30768-0070-86	6.59	8.99
CALCIUM 1200 W/VITAMIN D (Rexall)			
SGL,PO (SOFTGEL)			
600 mg-100 iu, 60s ea	30768-0001-08	4.39	6.65
CALCIUM 500 (Mason Vit)			
CTB,PO (PF,VANILLA)			
500 mg, 100s ea	11845-0124-41	6.33	
CALCIUM 500 + D (21st Century)			
TAB,PO, 500 mg-400 iu,			
200s ea	40985-0227-25	4.20	6.99
CALCIUM 500 W/VITAMIN D (Basic Vitamins)			
TAB,PO, 500 mg-125 iu,			
100s ea	00761-0129-20	2.40	
(Mason Vit)			
TAB,PO (PF,SF)			
500 mg-125 iu, 60s ea	11845-0075-55	4.11	
100s ea	11845-0075-51	6.56	
(Rexall)			
TAB,PO (PF,SF)			
500 mg-125 iu, 60s ea	30768-0001-34	3.63	5.50
CALCIUM 600 (Basic Vitamins)			
TAB,PO, 600 mg, 60s ea	00761-0811-12	1.90	
(Nature's Bounty)			
TAB,PO (PF)			
600 mg, 60s ea	74312-0042-20		3.89
250s ea	74312-0042-23		10.99
(Prime Marketing)			
TAB,PO (PF,SF)			
600 mg, 60s ea	62107-0042-06	4.62	
(Rugby)			
TAB,PO (SF)			
600 mg, 60s ea	00536-3426-08	4.79	
CALCIUM 600 PLUS VITAMIN D			
(Nature's Bounty)			
TAB,PO (PF)			
600 mg-125 iu, 60s ea	74312-0042-30		4.29
250s ea	74312-0042-33		11.99
CALCIUM 600-D (Rugby)			
TAB,PO (REFORMULATION)			
600 mg-400 iu, 60s ea	00536-3424-08	3.64	
CALCIUM 600/VITAMIN D (Basic Vitamins)			
TAB,PO, 600 mg-125 iu,			
60s ea	00761-0812-12	2.15	
CALCIUM 600MG+D (Major)			
TAB,PO (PF,SF,LACTOSE-FREE)			
600 mg-200 iu, 60s ea	00904-5856-52	3.45	
150s ea	00904-5856-92	3.45	
CALCIUM ACETATE (Hillestad)			
TAB,PO, 169 mg, 200s ea	10542-0045-20	19.86	
500s ea	10542-0045-50	47.94	
CALCIUM ANTACID (Chain Drug Marketing)			
CTB,PO (PEPPERMINT)			
500 mg, 150s ea	63868-0053-15	1.98	3.49
(Major)			
CTB,PO (EXTRA STRENGTH)			
750 mg, 96s ea	00904-5513-79	3.90	
(Qualitest)			
CTB,PO (PEPPERMINT)			
500 mg, 150s ea	00603-0095-26	4.03	
CALCIUM ANTACID EXTRA STRENGTH (Major)			
CTB,PO, 750 mg, 96s ea	00904-7695-91	3.90	
(Qualitest)			
CTB,PO (ASSORTED)			
750 mg, 96s ea	00603-0096-27	4.03	
CALCIUM ANTACID ULTRA			
(Chain Drug Marketing)			
CTB,PO (ASSORTED FRUIT)			
1000 mg, 72s ea	63868-0055-72	1.98	3.49
CALCIUM ASCORBATE (Freeda)			
PDR,PO (PF,SF,DYE-FREE)			
3256 mg/5 ml-400 mg/5 ml,			
120 gm	10432-0106-01	9.78	16.30
480 gm	10432-0106-03	28.74	47.90
CALCIUM ASPARTATE (Miller)			
TAB,PO, 625 mg, 100s ea	17204-0355-40	8.52	14.20
CALCIUM CARB (PD-Rx Pharm)			
REPACK			
TAB,PO, 500 mg, 180s ea	55289-0576-93	10.38	
CALCIUM CARB W/ VIT D (Core)			
REPACK			
TAB,PO, 600 mg-125 iu,			
60s ea	33358-0062-60	7.33	
(PD-Rx Pharm)			
REPACK			
TAB,PO, 600 mg-200 iu,			
180s ea	55289-0913-93	26.00	
CALCIUM CARB/W VIT D (Phys Total Care)			
REPACK			
TAB,PO, 600 mg-125 iu,			
60s ea	54868-3320-01	13.47	
300s ea	54868-3320-02	29.47	
CALCIUM CARBONATE (Advance)			
TAB,PO, 10 mg, 100s ea	17714-0025-01	1.30	
1000s ea	17714-0025-10	9.25	
(Freeda)			
CTB,PO, 260 mg, 100s ea	10432-0272-01	5.37	8.95
250s ea	10432-0272-02	10.74	17.90
500s ea	10432-0272-03	17.97	29.95
PDR,PO (PF,SF,DYE-FREE)			
1600 mg/5 ml, 16 ml	10432-0103-03	5.97	9.95
(Health Products Corp)			
TAB,PO (PF,SF)			
600 mg, 60s ea	39686-0012-86	2.60	
(Major)			
CTB,PO (REGULAR STRENGTH)			
500 mg, 100s ea	00904-5985-61	14.45	
600 mg, 60s ea	00904-3232-52	3.00	
150s ea	00904-3232-92	4.60	
(10X10)			
650 mg, 100s ea UD	00904-3232-61	10.95	
(Marlex)			
CTB,PO, 500 mg, 16s ea	10135-0254-16	1.20	
30s ea	10135-0254-30	1.40	
60s ea	10135-0254-60	1.60	
150s ea	10135-0254-64	2.13	
TAB,PO, 500 mg, 100s ea	10135-0362-01	5.90	
(Roxane)			
SUS,PO (SODIUM-FREE,MINT)			
1250 mg/5 ml,			
5 ml 40s UD	00054-8116-16	23.75	
500 ml	00054-3117-63	12.37	
TAB,PO (10X10,BLISTER PK,USP)			
1250 mg,			
100s ea UD	00054-8120-25	16.51	
(USP)			
1250 mg, 100s ea	00054-4120-25	9.19	
(Rugby)			
TAB,PO, 650 mg,			
1000s ea	00536-3414-10	15.75	
(PD-Rx Pharm)			
REPACK			
TAB,PO, 650 mg, 30s ea	55289-0442-30	10.38	
180s ea	55289-0442-93	16.24	
(Phys Total Care)			
REPACK			
CTB,PO, 500 mg, 150s ea	54868-3594-00	10.36	
TAB,PO, 500 mg, 60s ea	54868-2399-01	4.14	
120s ea	54868-2399-00	6.75	
150s ea	54868-2399-02	8.07	
901s ea	54868-2399-03	41.01	
(Quality Care Prod)			
REPACK			
CTB,PO, 600 mg, 60s ea	49999-0351-60	8.64	
CALCIUM CARBONATE WITH VITAMIN D			
(A-S Medication)			
REPACK			
TAB,PO, 600 mg-200 iu,			
60s ea	54569-5955-00	3.68	
CALCIUM CARBONATE/VITAMIN D (Major)			
TAB,PO, 600 mg-400 iu,			
60s ea	00904-3233-52	3.45	
150s ea	00904-3233-92	5.80	
(TriMarc Labs)			
TAB,PO (SF,GLUTEN-FREE)			
600 mg-400 iu, 60s ea	68752-0640-60	3.40	
120s ea	68752-0640-98	5.46	
180s ea	68752-0640-93	8.20	

PROD/MFR	HRI, UPC,NDC	AWP	SRP
(Palmetto)			
REPACK			
TAB,PO, 600 mg-125 iu,			
60s ea	23490-6631-01	6.00	
150s ea	23490-6631-00	9.54	
(PD-Rx Pharm)			
REPACK			
TAB,PO, 600 mg-125 iu,			
60s ea	55289-0763-60	6.00	
(Phys Total Care)			
REPACK			
TAB,PO, 600 mg-125 iu,			
150s ea	54868-3320-00	13.27	
CALCIUM CHELATED (Freeda)			
TAB,PO (PF,SF,DYE-FREE)			
200 mg, 100s ea	10432-0209-01	6.87	11.45
CALCIUM CITRATE (Freeda)			
TAB,PO (PF,SF,DYE-FREE)			
250 mg, 100s ea	10432-0284-01	6.27	10.45
250s ea	10432-0284-02	12.54	20.90
500s ea	10432-0284-03	21.57	35.95
(Marlex)			
TAB,PO, 950 mg,			
1000s ea	10135-0252-10	44.60	
(Nature's Bounty)			
TAB,PO (PF,SF)			
950 mg, 100s ea	74312-0075-10		5.99
(Teva)			
TAB,PO, 200 mg, 100s ea	00182-4151-01	5.99	
CALCIUM CITRATE + D (Cardinal Health)			
TAB,PO (PRIVATE LABEL,CAPLET)			
315 mg-200 iu, 60s ea	37205-0068-72	4.84	
(Family Phcy)			
TAB,PO (PRIVATE LABEL,CAPLET)			
315 mg-200 iu, 60s ea	52735-0130-13	4.58	5.09
(Physician Partner)			
REPACK			
TAB,PO (CAPLET)			
315 mg-200 iu,			
60s ea	21695-0784-60	23.98	
CALCIUM CITRATE 950 (Basic Vitamins)			
TAB,PO, 950 mg, 100s ea	00761-0195-20	3.00	
CALCIUM CITRATE FINE GRANULAR (Freeda)			
GRA,PO (760MG/3.5GM)			
760 mg/3.5 gm,			
480 gm	10432-0338-03	9.30	15.50
CALCIUM CITRATE W/VITAMIN D (Mason Vit)			
TAB,PO (PF,SF,CAPLET)			
1500 mg-200 iu, 60s ea	11845-0123-75	6.33	
CALCIUM FORMULA (Medicine Shoppe)			
TAB,PO (CAPLET)			
600 mg, 60s ea	59614-0629-72	4.79	4.79
CALCIUM GLUCONATE (Consolidated Midland)			
TAB,PO, 650 mg, 100s ea	00223-0592-01	3.25	
1000s ea	00223-0592-02	27.50	
975 mg, 100s ea UD	00223-0593-00	9.00	
(Freeda)			
POW,PO, 1040 mg/11.7 gm,			
448 gm	10432-0190-03	13.74	22.90
TAB,PO (PF,SF,DYE-FREE)			
50 mg, 100s ea	10432-0173-01	4.47	7.45
500s ea	10432-0173-03	15.57	25.95
(Global Source)			
TAB,PO, 650 mg, 100s ea	59618-0135-15	7.65	
(Marlex)			
TAB,PO, 500 mg, 100s ea	10135-0222-01	4.97	
1000s ea	10135-0222-10	10.82	
(Mason Vit)			
CTB,PO (PF,SF)			
650 mg, 100s ea	11845-0066-21	3.56	
(Pharmascience Labs)			
GEL,TP, 2.5%, 25 gm	57606-0303-34	28.00	39.20
(Roxane)			
TAB,PO (10X10, NOT USP)			
500 mg, 100s ea UD	00054-0262-20	24.67	
(Rugby)			
TAB,PO, 650 mg,			
1000s ea	00536-3416-10	17.32	
975 mg, 1000s ea	00536-3417-10	26.70	
(Southwood)			
REPACK			
CTB,PO (VANILLA)			
650 mg, 30s ea	58016-0140-30	0.52	
60s ea	58016-0140-60	1.04	
90s ea	58016-0140-90	1.57	
100s ea	58016-0140-00	1.74	
120s ea	58016-0140-02	2.09	
CALCIUM LACTATE (Consolidated Midland)			
TAB,PO, 325 mg, 100s ea	00223-0600-01	2.25	
1000s ea	00223-0600-02	19.50	
650 mg, 100s ea	00223-0601-01	2.75	
1000s ea	00223-0601-02	22.50	
(Freeda)			
TAB,PO (PF,SF,DYE-FREE)			
100 mg, 100s ea	10432-0232-01	4.77	7.95
(Major)			
TAB,PO, 650 mg, 100s ea	00904-2636-60	2.87	
(Mason Vit)			
TAB,PO (PF,SF)			
650 mg, 100s ea	11845-0055-91	3.89	
(Ohm)			
TAB,PO, 650 mg, 100s ea	51660-0031-01	1.95	
1000s ea	51660-0031-10	8.95	
(Rugby)			
TAB,PO, 650 mg, 100s ea	00536-3422-01	3.46	
1000s ea	00536-3422-10	18.15	
CALCIUM PANTOTHENATE (Freeda)			
TAB,PO (PF,SF,DYE-FREE)			
100 mg, 100s ea	10432-0002-01	3.57	5.95
200 mg, 100s ea	10432-0007-01	4.23	7.05
250s ea	10432-0007-02	8.46	14.10
500 mg, 100s ea	10432-0151-01	6.54	10.90
250s ea	10432-0151-02	13.08	21.80
CALCIUM PHOSPHATE (Freeda)			
POW,PO, 448 gm	10432-0189-03	10.95	18.25
CALCIUM PYRUVATE (Major)			
CAP,PO, 750 mg-5 mg,			
90s ea	09046-0040-89	5.94	
CALCIUM WITH D (Major)			
CTB,PO, 500 mg-400 iu,			
60s ea	09046-0036-52	4.89	
CALCIUM-500 (Rugby)			
CTB,PO (VANILLA)			
500 mg-100 iu, 60s ea	00536-6889-08	4.35	
CALCIUM-600 (Key Company)			
TAB,PO, 600 mg, 100s ea	11694-0723-01	3.50	
1000s ea	11694-0723-05	26.00	
CALCIUM/MAGNESIUM (ADH)			
TAB,PO (CHELATED)			
200 mg-200 mg,			
100s ea	60142-0114-10	2.48	4.95
(Family Phcy)			
TAB,PO (PRIVATE LABEL)			
100s ea	52735-0008-01	3.59	3.99
(Health Products Corp)			
TAB,PO (PF,SF)			
100s ea	39686-0013-74	3.91	
(Mason Vit)			
TAB,PO, 300 mg-300 mg,			
100s ea	11845-0075-01	5.89	
CALCIUM/MAGNESIUM CHELATED (Nature's Bounty)			
TAB,PO (PF,SF)			
500 mg-250 mg,			
100s ea	74312-0040-82		6.79
CALCIUM/MAGNESIUM CHELATED ZINC (ADH)			
TAB,PO (SF)			
1000 mg-400 mg-15 mg,			
100s ea	60142-0113-10	3.25	6.50
CALCIUM/MAGNESIUM W/VITAMIN D (Basic Organics, Inc.)			
TAB,PO, 1200 mg-500 mg-400 iu,			
100s ea	54458-0584-10	2.25	
CALCIUM/MAGNESIUM/ZINC (Basic Vitamins)			
TAB,PO, 333 mg-133 mg-5 mg,			
100s ea	00761-0019-20	2.00	
(Cardinal Health)			
TAB,PO (PF,PRIVATE LABEL)			
333 mg-133 mg-5 mg,			
100s ea	37205-0071-78	3.91	
(Health Products Corp)			
TAB,PO (PF,SF)			
100s ea	39686-0013-75	3.50	
(Major)			
TAB,PO, 100s ea	00904-5437-60	3.74	
(Mason Vit)			
TAB,PO, 334 mg-134 mg-5 mg,			
100s ea	11845-0096-81	5.89	
(Nature's Bounty)			
TAB,PO (PF,SF)			
333 mg-133 mg-8.3 mg,			
100s ea	74312-0042-90		4.99
(Pharmavite)			
TAB,PO, 333 mg-133 mg-5 mg,			
300s ea	31604-0018-93	5.65	
(Rexall)			
TAB,PO (PF,SF)			
1000 mg-500 mg-50 mg,			
100s ea	30768-0001-31	2.90	4.40
(Dispensing Solutions)			
REPACK			
TAB,PO (CAPLET)			
334 mg-134 mg-5 mg,			
100s ea	55045-3418-00	5.99	
CALCIUM/VITAMIN D (Rexall)			
CALCIUM 900 W/VITAMIN D			
SGL,PO (SOFTGEL,PF,SF,SOFTGEL)			
300 mg-100 iu,			
90s ea	30768-0000-31	4.09	6.20
CALCIUM/VITAMIN D (Cypress Pharm)			
TAB,PO (CAPLET)			
600 mg-200 iu, 60s ea	60258-0121-06	9.99	
(Lex)			
TAB,PO (SF,CAPLET)			
600 mg-125 iu, 60s ea	49523-0025-06	1.43	
(Marlex)			
TAB,PO, 600 mg-200 iu,			
60s ea	10135-0257-60	1.30	
150s ea	10135-0257-64	1.99	
(PD-Rx Pharm)			
REPACK			
TAB,PO, 500 mg-200 iu,			
90s ea	55289-0347-90	6.23	
100s ea	55289-0347-01	6.67	
CALDECORT (Heritage/Insight)			
CRE,TP, 1%, 15 gm	00235-0646-51	2.18	
CALDESENE (Heritage/Insight)			
OIN,TP, 37.5 gm	00235-1190-02	2.91	
POW,TP, 10%, 60 gm	00235-0363-01	1.82	
120 gm	00235-0363-04	2.91	
CALDYPHEN (AmerisourceBergen)			
LOT,TP (PRIVATE LABEL)			
7.5%-0.93%, 180 ml	24385-0072-82	3.59	3.99
(Cardinal Health)			
LOT,TP (PRIVATE LABEL)			
8%-1%, 180 ml	37205-0130-30	3.32	
CALDYPHEN CLEAR (Cardinal Health)			
LOT,TP (PRIVATE LABEL)			
1%-0.1%, 177 ml	37205-0281-30	3.87	
CALENDULA (Boiron)			
GEL,TP, 7%, 45 gm	06961-0105-54	3.71	6.19
(1X)			
7%, 75 gm	06962-0046-59	5.86	9.79
LOT,TP, 10%, 201 ml	06962-0714-70	6.54	10.89
OIN,TP, 4%, 30 gm	06962-0052-50	3.71	6.19
CALENDULA ESSENCE (Weleda)			
LIQ,TP, 50 ml	55946-0150-15	7.20	
CALENDULA OFFICINALIS (Luyties)			
TAB,SL (6X)			
6 x, 500s ea	00618-2052-03	3.99	
5500s ea	00618-2052-10	30.32	
(30X)			
12 x, 500s ea	00622-2052-03	4.19	
5500s ea	00622-2052-10	31.83	
(12X)			
30 x, 500s ea	00624-2052-03	4.19	
5500s ea	00624-2052-10	31.83	
(Std Homeo)			
OIN,TP, 1 x, 30 gm	05497-3205-21	3.77	6.29
105 gm	05497-3205-23	8.39	13.99
405 gm	05497-3115-29	23.99	39.99
CALIBRATED MEDICINE DROPPER (Apothecary)			
DEV,NA (GLASS,STRAIGHT TIP)			
ea	25715-0693-49	1.60	2.69
(PLASTIC)			
ea	25715-0693-47	1.19	1.99
CALICYLIC (Gordon)			
CRE,TP, 5%-10%, 60 gm	10481-1012-02	15.55	

PROD/MFR	HRI, UPC,NDC	AWP	SRP
CALLERGY CLEAR (Major)			
LOT,TP, 1%-0.1%, 177 ml	00904-7760-21	2.95	
(Pharma Pac) REPACK			
LOT,TP (1X60ML)			
1%-0.1%, 60 ml	52959-0960-02	2.80	
CALLUS CUSHIONS (Schering Plough)			
DEV,NA (ROUND)			
ea	11017-0103-90	1.96	
CALLUS REDUCER (Schering Plough)			
DEV,NA, ea	11017-0136-00	3.05	
CALLUS REMOVER (Schering Plough)			
DEV,NA, ea	11017-0100-42	2.50	
(EXTRA THICK PADS)			
ea	11017-0100-44	2.94	
CALMING ESSENCE (Ellon)			
CRE,TP, 37.5 gm	51762-0039-44	5.37	8.95
240 gm	51762-0040-27	17.40	29.00
SOL,SL (DROPS)			
10.5 ml	51762-0000-10		10.25
21 ml	51762-0000-21	7.17	11.95
CALMME (Mason Vit)			
TAB,PO (PF,SF)			
90s ea	11845-0078-69	7.22	
CALMOSEPTINE (Calmoseptine)			
OIN,TP (JAR)			
71 gm	00799-0001-03	4.00	6.00
(TUBE)			
71 gm	00799-0001-02	4.00	6.00
113 gm	00799-0001-04	5.00	7.50
(Phys Total Care) REPACK			
OIN,TP, 71 gm	54868-5287-00	7.05	
CALNA (Key Company)			
TAB,PO, 100s ea	11694-0979-01	8.50	
CALPHRON (Nephro-Tech)			
TAB,PO, 667 mg, 200s ea	59528-0331-02	25.00	
CALTRATE 600 (Wyeth Consumer)			
TAB,PO, 600 mg, 150s ea	00055-0510-20		12.69
(Phys Total Care) REPACK			
TAB,PO, 600 mg, 60s ea	54868-4845-00	8.55	
CALTRATE 600 + D (Wyeth Consumer)			
TAB,PO, 600 mg-200 iu,			
60s ea	00005-5509-19		7.69
120s ea	00055-0509-24		12.69
200s ea	00055-0509-25		15.99
CALTRATE PLUS (Wyeth Consumer)			
TAB,PO, 60s ea	00005-5556-19		7.69
(FRUIT)			
60s ea	00005-5567-19	5.78	
120s ea	00055-0556-23		12.69
CALVITE P&D (Cypress Pharm)			
TAB,PO, 105 mg-81 mg-120 iu,			
100s ea	60258-0128-01	16.94	
CAM LOTION (Merz)			
LOT,TP (SOAP-FREE)			
480 ml	02596-0014-16	14.95	
CAMEO OIL (Medco Lab)			
OIL,TP, 240 ml	11940-0315-02	4.00	
480 ml	11940-0315-03	6.00	
960 ml	11940-0315-04	10.00	
CAMILIA (Boiron)			
LIQ,PO (BABY TEETHING,AF,SF)			
1 ml 30s UD	06969-0020-09	6.07	10.19
CAMINO PRO 10 (Cambrooke)			
SUS,PO (11.4%,SORBET STIX,12X92)			
92 ml 12s	24359-0620-01	91.20	
92 ml 12s	24359-0620-02	91.20	
(11.9%,SORBET STIX,12X92)			
92 ml 12s	24359-0320-01	67.20	
92 ml 12s	24359-0320-02	67.20	
CAMINO PRO 15 (Cambrooke)			
LIQ,PO (11.1%,MSUD,28X140ML)			
140 ml 28s	24359-0610-01	320.20	
140 ml 28s	24359-0610-02	320.20	
(11.6%,PKU,28X140ML)			
140 ml,28s	24359-0310-01	237.20	
140 ml 28s	24359-0310-02	237.20	
PDS,PO (28X49GM,BETTERMILK)			
49 gm 28s	24359-0350-01	306.60	
CAMINO PRO 5 (Cambrooke)			
LIQ,PO (18.4%,MSUD,28X30ML)			
30 ml 28s	24359-0630-04	106.40	

PROD/MFR	HRI, UPC,NDC	AWP	SRP
(18.7%,MSUD,28X30ML)			
30 ml 28s	24359-0630-03	106.40	
(18.9%,PKU,28X30ML)			
30 ml 28s	24359-0330-04	78.40	
(19.4%,MSUD,28X30ML)			
30 ml 28s	24359-0630-02	106.40	
(19.4%,PKU,28X30ML)			
30 ml 28s	24359-0330-03	78.40	
(20%,PKU,28X30ML)			
30 ml 28s	24359-0330-02	78.40	
CAMPHO-PHENIQUE (Bayer HealthCare)			
GEL,TP, 10.8%-4.7%,			
6.9 gm	00024-0212-01	2.89	
15 gm	00024-0212-02	3.79	
LIQ,TP, 10.8%-4.7%,			
22.5 ml	00024-5150-05	2.53	
45 ml	00024-5150-06	4.40	
CAMPHOR & PHENOL (Major)			
LIQ,TP, 10.8%-4.7%,			
45 ml	00904-7851-75	4.75	
CANKAID (Dickinson Brands)			
SOL,MM (BLISTER PACK)			
10%, 22.2 ml	02590-0395-22	4.10	
CANTHARIS (Luyties)			
TAB,SL (6X)			
6 x, 500s ea	00618-2068-03	3.99	
5500s ea	00618-2068-10	30.32	
(30X)			
12 x, 500s ea	00622-2068-03	4.19	
5500s ea	00622-2068-10	31.83	
(12X)			
30 x, 500s ea	00624-2068-03	4.19	
5500s ea	00624-2068-10	31.83	
CAPSAICIN (Rugby)			
CRE,TP, 0.025%, 60 gm	00536-2525-25	9.95	
(A-S Medication) REPACK			
CRE,TP, 0.025%, 60 gm	54569-4332-00	16.50	
(Altura) REPACK			
CRE,TP, 0.025%, 60 gm	63874-0862-60	20.30	
(Nucare Pharm) REPACK			
CRE,TP, 0.025%, 60 gm	68071-1344-02	23.99	
(Pharma Pac) REPACK			
CRE,TP, 0.025%, 60 gm	52959-0257-02	21.20	
0.075%, 30 gm	52959-0275-03	8.79	
60 gm	52959-0275-07	28.00	
(Phys Total Care) REPACK			
CRE,TP (1X60GM)			
0.025%, 60 gm	54868-3760-00	33.19	
(Quality Care Prod) REPACK			
CRE,TP, 0.025%, 60 gm	49999-0409-60	11.94	
CAPSICUM OLEORESIN (Physician Partner) REPACK			
CRE,TP (1X60GM)			
0.025%, 60 gm	21695-0706-60	20.90	
(Stat Rx) REPACK			
CRE,TP, 0.025%, 60 gm	16590-0757-60	10.49	
CAPSIN (Pryde Pharmaceutical Corp)			
LOT,TP, 0.025%, 59 ml	59263-0025-02	10.20	
0.075%, 59 ml	59263-0075-02	11.40	
CARB-VANTAGE (Medicine Shoppe)			
TAB,PO (PRIVATE LABEL)			
50s ea	49614-0455-71	5.99	
CARBAMIDE PEROXIDE (Major)			
SOL,OT, 6.5%, 15 ml	00904-3220-35	2.48	
(A-S Medication) REPACK			
SOL,OT, 6.5%, 15 ml	54569-2494-00	4.99	
(Pharma Pac) REPACK			
SOL,OT, 6.5%, 15 ml	52959-0183-00	6.99	
(Phys Total Care) REPACK			
SOL,OT, 6.5%, 15 ml	54868-2850-01	12.27	
(Southwood) REPACK			
SOL,OT, 6.5%, 15 ml	58016-6094-01	8.68	

PROD/MFR	HRI, UPC,NDC	AWP	SRP
CARBAMOXIDE (R.I.J.)			
SOL,OT, 6.5%, 15 ml	53807-0133-01	1.70	
30 ml	53807-0133-02	2.60	
CARBO VEGETABILIS (Luyties)			
TAB,SL (6X)			
6 x, 500s ea	00618-2075-03	3.99	
5500s ea	00618-2075-10	30.32	
12 x, 500s ea	00622-2075-03	4.19	
5500s ea	00622-2075-10	31.83	
30 x, 500s ea	00624-2075-03	4.19	
(12X)			
30 x, 5500s ea	00624-2075-10	31.83	
(Walker Pharmacal)			
TAB,SL (6X)			
250s ea	00619-2075-02	2.97	
CARDENZ (Miller)			
TAB,PO, 100s ea	17204-0429-40	8.04	13.40
CARDI-RITE (Carlson,J.R.)			
TAB,PO (PF,SF,CORN-FREE)			
180s ea	88395-0042-22	24.95	49.90
360s ea	88395-0042-24	44.95	89.90
CARDIAC CATHETER (Abbott Hosp)			
DEV,NA (NON-VENTED, 67", Y-TYPE)			
48s ea	00074-6414-58	533.38	
CARDIOGEN-82 ACCESSORY PACK (Bracco Diag)			
DEV,NA, ea	00270-0151-00	94.38	
CARDIOTEK (SJ)			
TAB,PO, 100s ea	45985-0639-01	66.47	
(Phys Total Care) REPACK			
TAB,PO, 100s ea	54868-5090-00	46.50	
CARDIOVID PLUS (A. G. Marin)			
SGL,PO, 60s ea	12539-0865-60	26.10	
CAREFREE ULTRA PROTECTION (Johnson & Johnson)			
DEV,NA (UNSCENTED)			
16s ea	80041-0421-00	3.23	
(FRESH SCENT)			
32s ea	80041-0416-00	3.23	
32s ea	80041-0417-00	6.11	
(UNSCENTED)			
32s ea	80041-0439-00	6.11	
CAREONE ADVANCED LANCING DEVICE (Ahold)			
DEV,NA (PRIVATE LABEL)			
ea	08214-0707-21	10.99	
CAREONE THIN LANCET (Ahold)			
DEV,NA (SINGLE USE,23G)			
100s ea	08214-0157-21	4.56	
CAREONE ULTIGUARD HOME SYRINGE DISPENSER & SHARPS (UltiMed)			
DEV,NA (1/2CC,G29X1/2")			
100s ea	08474-7259-01	23.75	
(1/2CC,G30X5/16")			
100s ea	08474-7359-01	25.70	
(1CC,G29X1/2",LATEX-FREE)			
100s ea	08474-7219-01	23.75	
(1CC,G30X5/16")			
100s ea	08474-7319-01	25.70	
(3/10CC,G29X1/2")			
100s ea	08474-7239-01	23.75	
(3/10CC,G30X5/16")			
100s ea	08474-7339-01	25.70	
CAREONE ULTRA THIN LANCET (Ahold)			
DEV,NA (SINGLE USE,28G)			
100s ea	08214-0357-21	4.56	
CARLESTA (G&W)			
OIN,TP, 2%-26%, 60 gm	00713-0623-32	5.49	
120 gm	00713-0623-04	8.49	
CARLSON ABLE EYES (Carlson,J.R.)			
SGL,PO (PF,SF,CORN-FREE)			
60s ea	88395-0048-46	18.95	37.90
CARLSON ACES (Carlson,J.R.)			
SGL,PO (PF,SF,CORN-FREE)			
90s ea	88395-0044-39	10.95	21.90
CARLSON B-12 TIME (Carlson,J.R.)			
TER,PO, 1000 mcg,			
30s ea	88395-0024-20	2.45	4.90
CARLSON BABY DDROPS (Carlson,J.R.)			
SOL,PO (1X11ML,PF,SF,CORN-FREE)			
400 iu/0.03 ml,			
11 ml	88395-0019-00	13.25	26.50
CARLSON CHELATED MANGANESE (Carlson,J.R.)			
TAB,PO (PF,SF,GLUTEN-FREE)			
20 mg, 100s ea	88395-0056-31	3.85	7.70
250s ea	88395-0056-32	8.45	16.90

PROD/MFR	HRI, UPC, NDC	AWP	SRP
CARLSON CHEWABLE CALCIUM (Carlson,J.R.)			
CTB,PO (PF,SOY-FREE,STARCH-FREE)			
250 mg, 60s ea	88395-0050-80	4.45	8.90
120s ea	88395-0050-81	7.75	15.50
CARLSON COD LIVER OIL (Carlson,J.R.)			
SGL,PO (PF,SOFTGEL)			
150s ea	88395-0013-91	7.20	14.40
CARLSON DDROPS (Carlson,J.R.)			
SOL,PO (1X11ML,PF,SF,CORN-FREE)			
1000 iu/0.03 ml, 11 ml	88395-0019-10	12.25	24.50
2000 iu/0.03 ml, 11 ml	88395-0019-20	12.75	25.50
CARLSON E-GEMS ELITE (Carlson,J.R.)			
SGL,PO (SOFTGEL)			
20 mg-1000 iu-100 mg, 60s ea	88395-0007-96	17.25	34.50
120s ea	88395-0007-91	31.95	63.90
CARLSON EPA GEMS (Carlson,J.R.)			
SGL,PO (PF,CHOLESTEROL-FREE)			
580 mg-10 iu, 60s ea	88395-0016-86	9.95	19.90
120s ea	88395-0016-81	18.85	37.70
CARLSON FISH OIL MULTI (Carlson,J.R.)			
SGL,PO (PF,SF,CORN-FREE)			
60s ea	88395-0015-80	9.44	18.88
120s ea	88395-0015-81	17.95	35.90
180s ea	88395-0015-82	24.95	49.90
CARLSON FISH OIL Q (Carlson,J.R.)			
SGL,PO (PF,SOFTGEL)			
30s ea	88395-0016-63	7.40	14.80
60s ea	88395-0016-66	13.95	27.90
30s ea	88395-0016-73	11.45	22.90
60s ea	88395-0016-76	21.00	42.00
CARLSON FOR KIDS CHEWABLE CALCIUM (Carlson,J.R.)			
CTB,PO (PF,SOY-FREE,STARCH-FREE)			
250 mg, 60s ea	88395-0050-83	4.45	8.90
CARLSON FOR KIDS CHEWABLE DHA (Carlson,J.R.)			
SGL,PO (ORANGE,SOFTGEL)			
640 mg-10 iu, 60s ea	88395-0015-70	6.44	12.88
120s ea	88395-0015-71	11.95	23.90
CARLSON FOR KIDS CHEWABLE VITAMIN C (Carlson,J.R.)			
CTB,PO (PF,SUCROSE-FREE)			
250 mg-28 mg, 60s ea	88395-0031-00	3.95	7.90
120s ea	88395-0031-01	7.25	14.50
CARLSON FOR KIDS CHEWABLE VITAMINS AND MINERALS (Carlson,J.R.)			
CTB,PO (PF,WHEAT-FREE)			
60s ea	88395-0042-40	6.25	12.50
180s ea	88395-0042-42	14.95	29.90
CARLSON FOR KIDS DDROPS (Carlson,J.R.)			
SOL,PO (1X11ML,PF,SF,CORN-FREE)			
400 iu/0.028 ml, 11 ml	88395-0019-50	13.25	26.50
CARLSON FOR KIDS FISH OIL (Carlson,J.R.)			
SOL,PO (LEMON)			
200 ml	88395-0015-43	12.45	24.90
(ORANGE)			
200 ml	88395-0016-53	12.45	24.90
CARLSON FOR KIDS NORWEGIAN COD LIVER OIL (Carlson,J.R.)			
SOL,PO (LEMON)			
250 ml	88395-0013-53	13.45	26.90
CARLSON HOMOCYSTEINE GUARD (Carlson,J.R.)			
TAB,PO, 400 mcg-800 mcg-25 mg,			
120s ea	88395-0043-31	3.88	7.75
360s ea	88395-0043-33	9.95	19.90
CARLSON L-ARGININE (Carlson,J.R.)			
CAP,PO (PF,SF,CORN-FREE)			
675 mg, 90s ea	88395-0067-31	7.20	14.40
CARLSON MELLOW MOOD (Carlson,J.R.)			
TAB,PO (COATED)			
60s ea	88395-0044-80	13.85	27.70
120s ea	88395-0044-81	24.95	49.90
CARLSON MOLY-B (Carlson,J.R.)			
TAB,PO (PF,SF,CORN-FREE)			
500 mcg, 100s ea	88395-0056-41	3.95	7.90
CARLSON MOTHER'S DHA (Carlson,J.R.)			
SGL,PO (ORANGE,SOFTGEL)			
0.6 gm-10 iu, 60s ea	88395-0015-60	6.44	12.88
120s ea	88395-0015-61	11.95	23.90
CARLSON NORWEGIAN COD LIVER OIL (Carlson,J.R.)			
SGL,PO (PF,GLUTEN-FREE)			
230 mg-150 iu-80 iu-2 iu, 150s ea	88395-0013-81	9.40	18.80
(PF,LIGHT LEMON,SOFTGEL)			
230 mg-150 iu-80 iu-2 iu, 300s ea	88395-0013-83	16.45	32.90
CARLSON NORWEGIAN MEDOMEGA FISH OIL 2800 (Carlson,J.R.)			
SOL,PO (1X100ML,ORANGE)			
2.8 gm/5 ml-10 iu/5 ml, 100 ml	88395-0017-01	19.95	39.90
CARLSON NORWEGIAN SALMON OIL (Carlson,J.R.)			
SGL,PO (PF,SOFTGEL)			
375 mg-10 iu, 60s ea	88395-0015-00	4.25	8.50
180s ea	88395-0015-01	12.45	24.90
360s ea	88395-0015-03	22.20	44.40
CARLSON NUTRA-SUPPORT DIABETES (Carlson,J.R.)			
SGL,PO (PF,SF,CORN-FREE)			
60s ea	88395-0045-70	12.75	25.50
120s ea	88395-0045-71	24.45	48.90
180s ea	88395-0045-72	34.95	69.90
CARLSON PSYLLIUM (Carlson,J.R.)			
CAP,PO, 500 mg, 300s ea	88395-0085-35	9.95	19.90
CARLSON RIBOSE (Carlson,J.R.)			
PDS,PO (30X3GM,PF,CORN-FREE)			
3 gm/tsp, 3 gm 30s	88395-0088-24	14.95	29.90
(1X100GM,PF,CORN-FREE)			
3 gm/tsp, 100 gm	88395-0088-25	9.99	19.98
(1X500GM,PF,CORN-FREE)			
3 gm/tsp, 500 gm	88395-0088-23	44.95	89.90
CARLSON RIGHT FOR THE LIVER (Carlson,J.R.)			
CAP,PO (PF,SF,CORN-FREE)			
60s ea	88395-0047-30	9.99	19.98
CARLSON SOLAR D GEMS (Carlson,J.R.)			
SGL,PO (PF,LIGHT LEMON,SOFTGEL)			
120s ea	88395-0014-71	6.45	12.90
(PF,GLUTEN-FREE)			
360s ea	88395-0014-73	17.95	35.90
(PF,LIGHT LEMON,SOFTGEL)			
120s ea	88395-0014-81	8.45	16.90
(PF,GLUTEN-FREE)			
360s ea	88395-0014-83	22.45	44.90
CARLSON SUPER 2 DAILY (Carlson,J.R.)			
SGL,PO (PF,SF,CORN-FREE)			
180s ea	88395-0040-52	24.95	
CARLSON SUPER DAILY AMINO BLEND (Carlson,J.R.)			
CAP,PO, 30s ea	88395-0067-00	4.40	8.80
(PF,SF,CORN-FREE)			
100s ea	88395-0067-01	11.95	23.90
300s ea	88395-0067-03	29.95	59.90
CARLSON SUPER DHA GEMS (Carlson,J.R.)			
SGL,PO (SOFTGEL)			
1000 mg-10 iu, 60s ea	88395-0015-50	11.95	23.90
180s ea	88395-0015-52	32.95	65.90
CARLSON SUPER OMEGA-3 GEMS FISH OIL (Carlson,J.R.)			
SGL,PO (PF,CHOLESTEROL-FREE)			
600 mg-10 iu, 360s ea	88395-0015-23	39.95	79.90
CARLSON VITAMIN D (Carlson,J.R.)			
SGL,PO (PF,SF,CORN-FREE)			
2000 iu, 360s ea	88395-0014-63	10.75	21.50
10000 iu, 120s ea	88395-0014-21	9.45	18.90
CARLSON VITAMIN K2 (Carlson,J.R.)			
CAP,PO (PF,SF,CORN-FREE)			
5 mg, 60s ea	88395-0010-00	12.45	24.90
180s ea	88395-0010-01	34.50	69.00
CARMEX (Carma Labs)			
OIN,TP, 7.5 gm	83078-0113-11	0.72	1.59
(BLISTER PACK)			
7.5 gm	83078-0113-15	0.72	1.59
(BULK BLISTER PACK)			
7.5 gm 12s	83078-0123-15	8.64	17.88
(BULK PACK)			
7.5 gm 12s	83078-0123-11	8.64	17.88
10 gm	83078-0113-13	0.72	1.59
(BLISTER PACK)			
10 gm	83078-0113-14	0.72	1.59
(BULK BLISTER PACK)			
10 gm	83078-0123-14	8.64	17.88
(BULK PACK)			
10 gm 12s	83078-0123-13	8.64	17.88
15 gm 12s	83078-0112-12	13.32	2.39
(ORIGINAL)			
1.7%-0.7%-0.4%, 10 gm 3s	83078-0003-14		3.99
15 gm	83078-0112-16	1.11	2.39
(SPF 15,CHERRY)			
6.4%-5.4%, 7.5 gm	83078-0015-30	0.72	1.59
(SPF15,CHERRY)			
6.4%-5.4%, 7.5 gm	83078-0011-30		1.59
(SPF 15,CHERRY)			
6.4%-5.4%, 10 gm	83078-0014-30	0.72	1.59
(SPF15,CHERRY)			
6.4%-5.4%, 10 gm	83078-0013-30		1.59
(SPF15,STRAWBERRY)			
6.4%-5.4%, 10 gm	83078-0013-31		1.59
10 gm	83078-0014-31		1.59
(SPF15,CHERRY)			
6.4%-5.4%, 10 gm 3s	83078-0314-30		3.99
CARMEX CLICK STICK (Carma Labs)			
STI,TP (SPF 15,CHERRY)			
6.4%-5.4%, 4.25 gm	83078-0000-30	0.72	1.59
(SPF 15,STRAWBERRY)			
6.4%-5.4%, 4.25 gm	83078-0000-31	0.72	1.59
(SPF15,CHERRY)			
6.4%-5.4%, 4.25 gm	83078-0000-32		1.59
(SPF15,MINT)			
6.4%-5.4%, 4.25 gm	83078-0000-10		1.59
(SPF15,STRAWBERRY)			
6.4%-5.4%, 4.25 gm	83078-0000-33		1.59
CARMEX CLICK-STICK (Carma Labs)			
STI,TP, 4.25 gm	83078-0000-17		1.59
(BLISTER PACK)			
4.25 gm	83078-0113-17	0.72	1.59
4.25 gm 3s	83078-0003-17		3.99
(BULK BLISTER PACK)			
4.25 gm 12s	83078-0123-17	8.64	17.88
CARMOL (Doak)			
SHA,TP (DEEP CLEANSING)			
10%, 240 ml	10337-0654-51	33.52	
CARMOL 10 (Doak)			
LOT,TP, 10%, 180 ml	10337-0650-10	18.89	
CARMOL 20 (Doak)			
CRE,TP, 20%, 90 gm	10337-0651-19	17.38	
CARNATION INSTANT BREAKFAST (Nestle)			
LIQ,PO (163MLX24,LACTOSE-FREE)			
163 ml 24s	00065-9050-77	30.53	
163 ml 24s	00065-9050-78	30.53	
(250MLX24,CHOC SPLASH)			
250 ml 24s	00065-9050-71	28.51	
(250MLX24,LACTOSE-FREE)			
250 ml 24s	00065-9050-70	28.51	
(250MLX24,STRAW BURST)			
250 ml 24s	00065-9050-72	28.51	
CARNATION INSTANT BREAKFAST JUNIOR (Nestle)			
LIQ,PO (250MLX24,W/FIBER)			
250 ml 24s	00065-9050-79	61.20	
250 ml 24s	00065-9050-80	61.20	
CARNATION INSTANT BREAKFAST PLUS (Nestle)			
LIQ,PO (250MLX24, CHOC SPLASH)			
250 ml 24s	00065-9050-74	30.24	
(250MLX24,LACTOSE-FREE)			
250 ml 24s	00065-9050-73	30.24	
(250MLX24,STRAW BURST)			
250 ml 24s	00065-9050-75	30.24	
CARNATION INSTANT BREAKFAST VHC (Nestle)			
LIQ,PO (250MLX24,LACTOSE-FREE)			
250 ml 24s	00065-9050-76	42.62	
CARNITINE (Bio-Tech Pharm)			
CAP,PO, 400 mg, 30s ea	53191-0401-30	11.25	
100s ea	53191-0401-01	32.00	
(Miller)			
CAP,PO, 250 mg, 60s ea	17204-0572-20	17.64	25.20
(Carlson,J.R.)			
L-CARNITINE			
CAP,PO, 300 mg, 30s ea	88395-0067-60	8.25	16.50
90s ea	88395-0067-61	22.00	44.00
CAROZYME (Miller)			
CAP,PO, 200s ea	17204-0806-41	17.64	29.40
CARRADERM (Carrington)			
CRE,TP (MOISTURIZING)			
113 gm	53303-0030-40	6.50	
CARRADRES HYDROGEL (Carrington)			
DEV,NA (4"X4")			
ea	53303-0141-40	6.08	

PROD/MFR	HRI, UPC,NDC	AWP	SRP
CARRAFILM (Carrington)			
DEV,NA (2 3/4"X2 3/8")			
ea	53303-0000-21	0.52	
(4"X5 1/2")			
ea	53303-0000-18	1.98	
CARRAFOAM (Carrington)			
FOA,TP, 114 gm	53303-0022-40	6.63	
227 gm	53303-0022-80	10.10	
CARRAFOAM SKIN CARE (Carrington)			
KIT,TP, ea	53303-0102-04	12.75	
ea	53303-0102-05	16.83	
CARRAFREE (Carrington)			
SPR,NA (PUMP,UNSCENTED)			
29 ml	53303-0006-01	3.70	
236 ml	53303-0006-80	13.50	
CARRAFRESH (Carrington)			
SPR,NA (PUMP,CITRUS SCENT)			
59 ml	53303-0158-20	4.30	
236 ml	53303-0158-80	13.50	
CARRAGAUZE (Carrington)			
PAD,TP (2"X2")			
ea	53303-0011-17	4.59	
(4"X4")			
ea	53303-0011-15	6.63	
CARRAGINATE (Carrington)			
DEV,NA (14",ALGINATE,HYDROGEL)			
ea	53303-0144-14	8.04	
(2"X2",ALGINATE,HYDROGEL)			
ea	53303-0144-20	4.05	
(4"X4",ALGINATE,HYDROGEL)			
ea	53303-0144-40	7.82	
(4"X8",ALGINATE,HYDROGEL)			
ea	53303-0144-80	15.15	
CARRAKLENZ (Carrington)			
SPR,TP (PUMP)			
177 ml	53303-0020-60	8.66	
236 ml	53303-0020-62	11.22	
473 ml	53303-0020-16	18.87	
CARRASCENT (Carrington)			
SPR,TP (PUMP,SCENTED)			
29 ml	53303-0070-10	3.70	
236 ml	53303-0070-80	13.50	
CARRASMART FILM (Carrington)			
DEV,NA (4"X5",WATER RESISTANT)			
ea	53303-0140-40	3.90	
(6"X7",WATER RESISTANT)			
ea	53303-0140-60	7.90	
CARRASMART FOAM (Carrington)			
DEV,NA (2"X3",WATER RESISTANT)			
ea	53303-0142-20	3.41	
(4"X4",WATER RESISTANT)			
ea	53303-0142-40	5.40	
(6"X8",WATER RESISTANT)			
ea	53303-0142-60	17.04	
CARRASMART GEL (Carrington)			
DEV,NA (HYDROGEL)			
28 gm	53303-0118-01	8.44	
85 gm	53303-0118-03	19.47	
CARRASMART HYDROCOLLOID WOUND (Carrington)			
DEV,NA (4"X4")			
ea	53303-0143-40	7.50	
(6"X6")			
ea	53303-0143-60	15.00	
CARRASORB H (Carrington)			
DEV,NA (12" ROPE,ALGINATE)			
ea	53303-0000-10	6.10	
(2"X2",ALGINATE)			
ea	53303-0000-08	2.94	
(4"X4",ALGINATE)			
ea	53303-0000-09	6.32	
CARRASORB M (Carrington)			
DEV,NA (4",FDG,MED EXUDATE)			
ea	53303-0000-16	6.00	
CARRASYN (Carrington)			
DEV,NA, 28 gm	53303-0010-10	8.06	
85 gm	53303-0010-30	18.26	
(SPRAY BOTTLE)			
226 ml	53303-0010-80	46.82	
CARRASYN V (Carrington)			
GEL,TP, 85 gm	53303-0012-30	18.62	
CARRAWASH (Carrington)			
SPR,TP (PUMP,NO RINSE)			
236 ml	53303-0022-81	3.58	
CARRINGTON ANTIFUNGAL (Carrington)			
CRE,TP, 2%, 141 gm	53303-0050-50	12.75	
CARRINGTON BORDERED GAUZE (Carrington)			
DEV,NA (NON-STERILE,4"X4")			
15s ea	53303-0145-40	16.80	
(NON-STERILE,6"X6")			
15s ea	53303-0145-60	32.10	
(NON-STERILE,6"X9")			
15s ea	53303-0145-69	43.95	
CARRINGTON MOISTURE BARRIER (Carrington)			
CRE,TP, 99 gm	53303-0040-40	7.14	
CARRINGTON MOISTURE BARRIER W/ZINC (Carrington)			
CRE,TP, 99 gm	53303-0040-41	7.34	
CARRINGTON MOISTURE GUARD (Carrington)			
CRE,TP, 5%, 85 gm	53303-0025-30	8.30	
CARRINGTON ORAL WOUND RINSE (Carrington)			
PDR,MM, ea	53303-0011-01	25.59	
CARRINGTON SHAMPOO & BODY WASH (Carrington)			
SHA,TP, 236 ml	53303-0111-08	3.90	
CASANTHRANOL/DOCUSATE SODIUM (Family Phcy)			
SGL,PO (PRIVATE LABEL)			
30 mg-100 mg, 100s ea	52735-0515-01	6.29	6.99
(Marlex)			
SGL,PO (SOFTGEL)			
30 mg-100 mg, 60s ea	10135-0114-60	1.04	
(BOXED,SOFTGEL)			
30 mg-100 mg, 100s ea	10135-0114-57	65.00	
(SOFTGEL)			
30 mg-100 mg, 100s ea	10135-0114-01	1.56	
1000s ea	10135-0114-10	12.96	
(PD-Rx Pharm)			
REPACK			
SGL,PO, 30 mg-100 mg, 21s ea	55289-0621-21	6.60	
28s ea	55289-0621-28	7.13	
(Phys Total Care)			
REPACK			
SGL,PO, 30 mg-100 mg, 30s ea	54868-3463-00	5.82	
CASCARA SAGRADA (Consolidated Midland)			
SOL,PO, 120 ml	00223-6237-01	3.75	
480 ml	00223-6237-02	12.50	
TAB,PO, 325 mg, 100s ea	00223-0670-01	4.50	
1000s ea	00223-0670-02	39.50	
(Cypress Pharm)			
LIQ,PO (BERRY)			
50 mg/15 ml, 473 ml	60258-0959-16	10.68	
CASCARA SAGRADA FLUID EXTRACT (PCCA)			
SOL,PO (USP,PRIVATE LABEL)			
1 ml	51927-1543-00	0.35	
CASCARA-SAGRADA (Nature's Bounty)			
CAP,PO, 450 mg, 100s ea	74312-0035-51		5.99
CASTELLANI PAINT MODIFIED (Pedinol)			
LIQ,TP, 1.5%, 30 ml	00884-2893-01		25.00
(COLORLESS)			
1.5%, 30 ml	00884-2993-01		25.00
(Phys Total Care)			
REPACK			
LIQ,TP (1X29.57ML)			
1.5%, 29.57 ml	54868-0127-00	31.90	
CASTOR OIL (Albertson's)			
OIL,PO, 120 ml	04000-0003-22	8.35	
(AmerisourceBergen)			
OIL,PO (PRIVATE LABEL)			
60 ml	24385-0515-92	2.42	2.69
(Consolidated Midland)			
OIL,PO, 60 ml	00223-6238-02	2.00	
120 ml	00223-6238-03	2.50	
CAT'S CLAW (ADH)			
CAP,PO (PF,SF)			
500 mg, 100s ea	60142-0905-01	7.98	15.95
(Botanical Labs.)			
CAP,PO, 30s ea	41954-0032-74	7.50	14.99
60s ea	41954-0032-75	13.00	25.99
(Marlex)			
CAP,PO, 350 mg, 100s ea	10135-0262-01	2.50	
(Mason Vit)			
CAP,PO (PF,SF)			
350 mg, 60s ea	11845-0128-25	15.44	
500 mg, 60s ea	11845-0113-35	7.22	
(Rexall)			
CAP,PO (PF,SF)			
350 mg, 75s ea	30768-0000-85	8.05	12.20
CATARACT CARE (Similasan Corp.)			
SOL,OP, 6 x-6 x-12 x, 10 ml	59262-0349-11	6.21	10.99
CATHETER IRRIGATION SET (Abbott Hosp)			
DEV,NA (W/CAIR CLAMP, 70")			
20s ea	00074-6536-01	74.64	
CAULOPHYLLUM (Luyties)			
TAB,SL (6X)			
6 x, 500s ea	00618-2105-03	3.99	
5500s ea	00618-2105-10	30.32	
12 x, 500s ea	00622-2105-03	4.19	
(30X)			
12 x, 5500s ea	00622-2105-10	31.83	
30 x, 500s ea	00624-2105-03	4.19	
5500s ea	00624-2105-10	31.83	
CAUSTICUM (Luyties)			
TAB,SL (12X)			
500s ea	00624-2107-03	4.19	
(30X)			
500s ea	00622-2107-03	4.19	
(6X)			
500s ea	00618-2107-03	3.99	
(12X)			
5500s ea	00624-2107-10	31.83	
(30X)			
5500s ea	00622-2107-10	31.83	
(6X)			
5500s ea	00618-2107-10	30.32	
CAVILON ANTISEPTIC SKIN CLEANSER (3M Health Care)			
SPR,TP, 0.11%, 236 ml	17518-0020-01	7.00	
CAVILON DURABLE BARRIER (3M Health Care)			
CRE,TP, 1.3%, 97.5 gm	17518-0026-01	6.24	
CAVILON EMOLLIENT (3M Health Care)			
CRE,TP, 1.5%, 120 gm 12s	17518-0022-01	70.00	
CAVILON FOOT EMOLLIENT (3M Health Care)			
CRE,TP, 1.5%, 120 gm 12s	17518-0023-01	64.50	
CAVILON NO STING BARRIER FILM (3M Health Care)			
LIQ,TP (W/SMALL FOAM APPLICATOR)			
1 ml 25s	08333-3343-01	31.50	
(WIPE)			
1 ml 25s	08333-3344-01	15.75	
(W/LARGE FOAM APPLICATOR)			
3 ml 25s	08333-3345-01	64.75	
SPR,TP, 28 ml 12s	08333-3346-01	130.20	
CAVILON ONE-STEP SKIN CARE (3M Health Care)			
LOT,TP, 1.5%, 360 ml 12s	17518-0021-02	184.60	
CAYENNE (Botanical Labs.)			
CAP,PO, 100s ea	41954-0030-04	4.98	9.95
(Mason Vit)			
CAP,PO (PF,SF)			
500 mg, 60s ea	11845-0113-45	4.33	
(Nature's Bounty)			
CAP,PO (450MG)			
100s ea	74312-0032-90		6.49
CAYENNE PEPPER (ADH)			
CAP,PO (PF,SF)			
450 mg, 100s ea	60142-0905-11	4.98	9.95
(Major)			
CAP,PO, 450 mg, 100s ea	00904-5082-60	4.49	
CCP (Medique)			
TAB,PO (2X50,CAFFEINE-FREE)			
325 mg-200 mg-10 mg, 100s ea UD	47682-0105-33	9.76	
(2X250,CAFFEINE-FREE)			
325 mg-200 mg-10 mg, 500s ea UD	47682-0105-13	40.75	
CDA-21 (Rx Vitamins)			
CAP,PO, 90s ea	08429-0210-90	12.48	24.95
CEANOTHUS (Botanical Labs.)			
LIQ,PO, 30 ml	41954-0020-63	3.75	7.49
CEFINAL II (Alto)			
TAB,PO, 250 mg-25 mg-150 mg, 100s ea	00731-0135-01	12.00	
CELLERATERX (Wound Care Innov, LLC)			
GEL,TP, 60%, 6 gm	83779-8004-00	11.30	18.08
28.6 gm	83779-8004-01	45.25	72.40
POW,TP, 96%, 1 gm	83779-8005-00	21.44	34.30

PROD/MFR HRI, UPC,NDC AWP SRP

5 gm.............83779-8005-01 107.76 171.48
20 gm............83779-8005-02 428.68 685.88
40 gm............83779-8005-03 857.361371.96

CEMILL 1000 (Miller)
TER,PO, 1000 mg,
100s ea...........17204-0405-40 7.56 12.60

CEMILL 500 (Miller)
TER,PO, 500 mg, 100s ea .17204-0408-40 5.70 9.50

CENTAMIN (Silarx)
LIQ,PO, 237 ml..........54838-0010-70 5.05

CENTAURY (Ellon)
SOL,SL (DROPS)
10.5 ml...............51762-0009-10 9.25

CENTAVITE A-Z (Marlex)
TAB,PO, 30s ea..........10135-0224-30 1.29
100s ea...............10135-0224-01 1.99
130s ea...............10135-0224-63 2.38
300s ea...............10135-0224-03 6.75
1000s ea..............10135-0224-10 14.00

CENTERPOINTLOCK DRAINABLE POUCH (Hollister)
DEV,NA (1 1/2",OPAQUE FILM)
10s ea...............08380-0038-17 22.89
(1 1/2",TRANSPARENT FILM)
10s ea...............08380-0038-07 22.89
(1 3/4",OPAQUE FILM)
10s ea...............08380-0038-12 22.89
(1 3/4",TRANSPARENT FILM)
10s ea...............08380-0038-02 22.89
(2 1/4",OPAQUE FILM)
10s ea...............08380-0038-13 22.89
(2 3/4",OPAQUE FILM)
10s ea...............08380-0038-14 22.89
(2 3/4",TRANSPARENT FILM)
10s ea...............08380-0038-04 22.89
(2- 1/4")
10s ea...............08380-0038-03 22.89
(4",TRANSPARENT FILM)
10s ea...............08380-0038-06 27.66

CENTERPOINTLOCK FLEXWEAR BARRIER (Hollister)
DEV,NA (1 1/2",FLAT,W/TAPE)
5s ea................08380-0037-43 23.21
(1 1/4",FLAT,W/TAPE)
5s ea................08380-0037-48 23.21
(1",FLAT,W/TAPE)
5s ea................08380-0037-42 23.21
(13/4",FLAT,W/TAPE)
5s ea................08380-0037-49 23.21
(3/4",FLAT,W/TAPE)
5s ea................08380-0037-47 23.21

CENTERPOINTLOCK IRRIGATOR DRAIN (Hollister)
DEV,NA (1 1/2", FLANGE)
5s ea................08380-0038-27 25.44
(1 3/4", FLANGE)
5s ea................08380-0038-22 25.44
(2 1/4", FLANGE)
5s ea................08380-0038-23 25.44
(2 3/4", FLANGE)
5s ea................08380-0038-24 25.44
(4", FLANGE)
5s ea................08380-0038-26 25.44
(1 1/2",OPAQUE FILM)
10s ea...............08380-0038-37 33.26
(1 3/4",OPAQUE FILM)
10s ea...............08380-0038-32 33.26
(2 1/4",OPAQUE FILM)
10s ea...............08380-0038-33 33.26
(2 3/4",OPAQUE FILM)
10s ea...............08380-0038-34 33.26

CENTERPOINTLOCK MINIDRAINABLE POUCH (Hollister)
DEV,NA (1 1/2")
10s ea...............08380-0038-47 22.89
(1 3/4")
10s ea...............08380-0038-42 22.89
(2 1/4")
10s ea...............08380-0038-43 22.89
(2 3/4")
10s ea...............08380-0038-44 22.89

CENTERPOINTLOCK SOFTFLEX BARRIER (Hollister)
DEV,NA (1-1/2",FLAT,W/TAPE)
5s ea................08380-0037-07 22.68
(1-3/4",FLAT,W/TAPE)
5s ea................08380-0037-02 22.68
(2-1/4",FLAT,W/TAPE)
5s ea................08380-0037-03 22.68
(2-3/4",FLAT,W/TAPE)
5s ea................08380-0037-04 22.68
(4",FLAT,W/TAPE)
5s ea................08380-0037-06 22.68
(TO 1 1/4",FLAT,W/O TAPE)
5s ea................08380-0037-62 21.99
(TO 1 3/4",FLAT,W/O TAPE)
5s ea................08380-0037-63 21.99
(TO 1",FLAT,W/O TAPE)
5s ea................08380-0037-67 21.99
(TO 2 1/4",FLAT,W/O TAPE)
5s ea................08380-0037-64 21.99
(TO 3 1/2",FLAT,W/O TAPE)
5s ea................08380-0037-66 31.37

CENTRA-VIT (ADH)
TAB,PO, 100s ea.........60142-0077-10 2.95 5.50

CENTRAL-VITE SELECT (Cardinal Health)
TAB,PO (PRIVATE LABEL)
60s ea...............37205-0073-72 4.92

CENTRUM (Wyeth Consumer)
LIQ,PO, 240 ml..........00005-4343-61 8.99
TAB,PO (PERSONAL SIZE,CAPLET)
15s ea...............00054-0239-16 1.99
(CAPLET)
50s ea...............00054-0239-18 6.49
130s ea..............00005-4239-30 10.59
180s ea..............00054-0239-36 13.99
250s ea..............00054-0239-26 17.99

CENTRUM JR. + IRON (Wyeth Consumer)
CTB,PO, 60s ea..........00005-4234-19 5.39 4.99

CENTRUM PERFORMANCE (Wyeth Consumer)
TAB,PO, 45s ea..........00054-0430-45 9.49
75s ea...............00054-0430-19 14.99
120s ea..............00054-0430-13 20.99

CENTRUM SILVER (Wyeth Consumer)
CTB,PO (CITRUS BERRY)
60s ea...............00054-0461-19 11.19
TAB,PO, 60s ea..........00005-4177-19 7.99
100s ea..............00005-4177-23 11.19
150s ea..............00054-0177-58 15.99
220s ea..............00005-4177-90 20.99

(Phys Total Care)
REPACK
TAB,PO (CAPLET)
150s ea..............54868-5318-00 19.25

CENTURY ADVANTAGE (AmerisourceBergen)
TAB,PO (PRIVATE LABEL)
75s ea...............24385-0260-98 8.72 9.69

CEO-TWO (Beutlich)
SUP,RC, 12s ea..........00283-0808-12 13.50 18.00

CEPACOL (A-S Medication)
REPACK
LOZ,MM, 0.07%, 648s ea..54569-2807-00 31.96

CEPACOL ANTIBACTERIAL (Combe)
SOL,MM (1X710ML,GOLD)
710 ml...............00068-0210-24 3.59

CEPACOL DUAL RELIEF SORE THROAT (Combe)
SPR,MM (CHERRY,SF,CHERRY)
5%-33%, 22.5 ml.....11509-0230-17 3.28

CEPACOL FIZZLERS (Combe)
ODT,PO (CHERRY,GRAPE)
6 mg, 12s ea.........11509-0209-19 4.73

CEPACOL SORE THROAT (Combe)
LOZ,MM (9X72, REGULAR STRENGTH)
3 mg, 648s ea........01150-0900-01 34.20
(POST NASAL DRIP,CHERRY)
4.5 mg, 18s ea.......11509-0205-18 2.83
(MAXIMUM NUMBING,CITRUS)
15 mg-2.1 mg,
18s ea...............11509-0204-40 2.83
(MAX NUMBING,HONEY LEMON)
15 mg-2.5 mg,
18s ea...............11509-0208-18 2.36
(MAXIMUM NUMBING,SF)
15 mg-4 mg, 16s ea..11509-0215-16 2.36

CEPACOL SORE THROAT + COATING RELIEF (Combe)
LOZ,MM (MAXIMUM NUMBING,SF)
15 mg-5 mg, 18s ea..11509-0216-16 2.83

CEPACOL SORE THROAT+COUGH RELIEF (Combe)
LOZ,MM (MAXIMUM NUMBING)
7.5 mg-5 mg,
18s ea...............11509-0224-18 2.83

CEPASTAT (Heritage/Insight)
LOZ,MM (EXT. STR.,CHERRY)
18s ea...............63736-0219-18 2.56

(Insight)
LOZ,MM (CHERRY)
14.5 mg, 18s ea......63736-0204-18 2.75

CERALYTE (Cera Products)
SOL,PO (12X1000ML,GLUTEN-FREE)
1000 ml 12s..........00851-0500-31 25.53 43.40

CERALYTE 50 (Cera Products)
PKT,PO (100X10GM, MIXED BERRY)
300 mg-240 mg-580 mg,
100s ea..............00851-0000-09 108.00 199.00
(100X10GM,GLUTEN-FREE)
300 mg-240 mg-580 mg,
100s ea..............00851-0000-13 108.00 199.00

CERALYTE 70 (Cera Products)
PDS,PO (100X50GM, NATURAL)
100s ea..............00851-0000-01 240.00 480.00
(100X50GM,CHICKEN BROTH)
50 gm 100s...........00851-0000-03 240.00 480.00
(LEMON, 100X10GM)
100s ea..............00851-0000-12 108.00 199.00
(NATURAL, 100X10GM)
100s ea..............00851-0000-10 108.00 199.00
(100X10GM,CHICKEN BROTH)
10 gm 100s...........00851-0000-16 108.00 199.00
PKT,PO (100X50GM,GLUTEN-FREE)
1.5 gm-2.3 gm-2.9 gm,
100s ea..............00851-0000-05 240.00 480.00

CERALYTE 90 (Cera Products)
PKT,PO (100X50GM,GLUTEN-FREE)
1.3 gm-3.4 gm-2.9 gm,
100s ea..............00851-0000-02 240.00 480.00
1.5 gm-3.5 gm-2.9 gm,
100s ea..............00851-0000-06 240.00 480.00

CERASPORT (Cera Products)
SOL,PO (12X500ML,GLUTEN-FREE)
500 ml 12s...........00851-0500-55 20.71 30.00
(12X1000ML,CITRUS CONCEN)
1000 ml 12s..........00851-0230-04 79.88 135.80

CERASPORT ELECTROLYTE DRINK MIX (Cera Products)
PDS,PO (100X20GM, CHERRY BERRY)
75 mg/20 gm-200 mg/20 gm,
100s ea..............00851-0200-04 124.59 211.80
(100X20GM,GLUTEN-FREE)
75 mg/20 gm-200 mg/20 gm,
100s ea..............00851-0200-01 124.59 211.80
100s ea..............00851-0200-03 124.59 211.80

CERASPORT ELECTROLYTE HYDRATION DRINK MIX (Cera Products)
PDS,PO (6X402GM,GLUTEN-FREE)
6s ea................00851-0220-03 40.14 68.24

CERASPORT EX1 (Cera Products)
PDS,PO (100X12.5GM,GLUTEN-FREE)
12.5 gm 100s.........00851-0200-09 124.58 211.80
12.5 gm 100s.........00851-0200-10 124.58 211.80
12.5 gm 100s.........00851-0200-15 124.58 211.80
(100X12.5GMPOMACAIBLUBRY)
12.5 gm 100s.........00851-0200-12 124.58 211.80
SOL,PO (27X250ML, LIME RTD)
250 ml 27s...........00851-0500-13 19.06 32.39
(27X250ML, ORANGE RTD)
250 ml 27s...........00851-0500-14 19.06 32.39

CERATO (Ellon)
SOL,SL (DROPS)
10.5 ml..............51762-0010-10 9.25

CERAVE (Valeant Pharm Intl)
CRE,TP, 453 gm.........00644-0022-16 13.29
LIQ,TP, 360 ml.........00644-0020-12 10.20
LOT,TP, 360 ml.........00644-0021-12 10.88

CERAVE FACIAL MOISTURIZING LOTION PM (Valeant Pharm Intl)
LOT,TP (1X89ML)
89 ml................00187-1367-03 11.25

CEROVITE (Rugby)
LIQ,PO, 240 ml.........00536-2790-59 5.40

CEROVITE ADVANCED FORMULA (Rugby)
TAB,PO, 130s ea........00536-3442-38 6.45

CEROVITE JR. (Rugby)
CTB,PO, 60s ea.........00536-3443-08 3.82

(A-S Medication)
REPACK
CTB,PO, 60s ea.........54569-3800-00 3.82

CEROVITE SENIOR (Rugby)
TAB,PO, 60s ea.........00536-3445-08 4.65

CERTA VITE WITH LUTEIN (Major)
TAB,PO, 130s ea........00904-2641-13 9.10
300s ea..............00904-2641-72 18.03

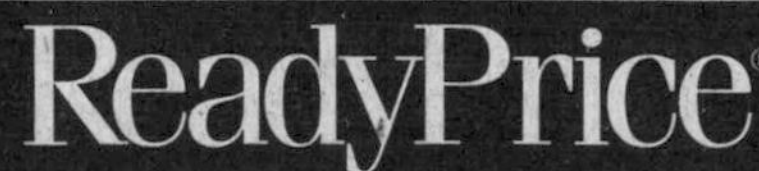

PROD/MFR	HRI, UPC,NDC	AWP	SRP
CERTAGEN (Teva)			
TAB,PO, 100s ea	00182-4162-01	5.80	
1000s ea	00182-4162-10	50.39	
CERTAIN DRI (DSE Healthcare)			
SOL,TP, 12%, 35.5 ml	89411-0011-40	4.26	
CERTAVITE (Major)			
LIQ,PO, 240 ml	00904-5023-09	6.30	
CERTAVITE SENIOR WITH LUTEIN (Major)			
TAB,PO, 60s ea	09045-0486-52	5.03	
CERTAVITE W/LUTEIN (Major)			
TAB,PO, 30s ea	00904-2641-46	2.03	
CERTAVITE WITH LUTEIN (Major)			
TAB,PO, 180s ea	00904-2641-93	7.62	
(PF,SF,LACTOSE-FREE)			
1000s ea	00904-2641-80	42.33	
CESIUM 1000 (Bio-Tech Pharm)			
CAP,PO, 1000 mg,			
100s ea	53191-0252-01	55.00	
CESIUM 500 (Bio-Tech Pharm)			
PO, 500 mg, 100s ea	53191-0225-01	34.00	
CETA-KLENZ (Major)			
SOL,TP (1X473ML,FRAGRANCE-FREE)			
473 ml	00904-5844-16	5.27	
CETAFEN (Hart Health)			
TAB,PO (2X12)			
325 mg, 24s ea UD	50332-0103-05	1.14	
(2X25)			
325 mg, 50s ea UD	50332-0103-03	1.47	
(2X50)			
325 mg, 100s ea UD	50332-0103-04	2.69	
(2X125)			
325 mg, 250s ea UD	50332-0103-02	5.92	
(2X500)			
325 mg,			
1000s ea UD	50332-0103-01	21.83	
CETAFEN COLD (Hart Health)			
TAB,PO (50 PACKETSX2,SF)			
500 mg-5 mg,			
100s ea UD	50332-0128-04	4.29	
(125 PACKETSX2,SF)			
500 mg-5 mg,			
250s ea UD	50332-0128-07	9.99	
CETAFEN COUGH & COLD (Hart Health)			
TAB,PO (50 PACKETSX2,SF)			
325 mg-15 mg-200 mg-5 mg,			
100s ea UD	50332-0129-04	5.88	
(125 PACKETSX2,SF)			
325 mg-15 mg-200 mg-5 mg,			
250s ea UD	50332-0129-07	13.94	
CETAFEN EXTRA (Hart Health)			
TAB,PO (2X50,CAPLET)			
500 mg, 100s ea UD	50332-0108-04	3.72	
(125X2,SF)			
500 mg, 250s ea UD	50332-0108-07	8.23	
(2X400,CAPLET)			
500 mg, 800s ea UD	50332-0108-01	24.64	
CETAKLENZ (Geritrex)			
SOL,TP, 480 ml	54162-0750-01	5.06	
(PUMP)			
480 ml	54162-0750-16	5.79	
CETAPHIL (Galderma)			
CRE,TP (THERAPEUTIC HAND,2X3OZ)			
85 gm 2s	00299-3915-06	11.25	
LOT,TP (SOAP-FREE)			
120 ml	00299-3921-40	3.62	
240 ml	00299-3921-08	6.31	
480 ml	00299-3921-16	10.12	
SOA,TP (4.5 OZ.)			
ea	00299-3923-04	3.50	
(Palmetto)			
REPACK			
LOT,TP, 480 ml	23490-9368-01	13.97	
(Phys Total Care)			
REPACK			
CRE,TP (FRAGRANCE-FREE)			
170 gm	54868-5988-00	16.91	
LOT,TP (1X240ML,SOAP-FREE)			
240 ml	54868-0177-00	9.06	
CETAPHIL ANTIBACTERIAL CLEANSING (Galderma)			
SOA,TP (4.5 OZ.)			
ea	00299-3925-04	3.50	
CETAPHIL COMPOUNDING VEHICLE (Galderma)			
LOT,TP, 480 ml	00299-3920-01	15.13	
CETAPHIL DAILY FACIAL CLEANSER (Galderma)			
SOL,TP (NON-COMEDOGENIC)			
240 ml	00299-3927-08	6.31	
480 ml	00299-3927-16	10.12	
CETAPHIL DAILY FACIAL MOISTURIZER (Galderma)			
LOT,TP (SPF 15,FRAGRANCE-FREE)			
3%-10%, 120 ml	00299-3928-04	10.12	
CETAPHIL MOISTURIZER (Galderma)			
CRE,TP, 90 gm	00299-3917-02	6.31	
480 gm	00299-3917-16	12.63	
LOT,TP, 240 ml	00299-3918-08	6.31	
480 ml	00299-3918-16	10.12	
(Phys Total Care)			
REPACK			
CRE,TP (1X90GM)			
90 gm	54868-0129-00	9.13	
LOT,TP (1X473ML)			
473 ml	54868-5873-00	13.87	
CETIRIZINE (Actavis)			
TAB,PO, 10 mg, 100s ea	00228-1198-55	249.47	
(PD-Rx Pharm)			
REPACK			
TAB,PO, 10 mg, 30s ea	55289-0995-30	72.00	
(Pharma Pac)			
REPACK			
TAB,PO, 10 mg, 15s ea	52959-0923-15	39.26	
(Phys Total Care)			
REPACK			
TAB,PO, 5 mg, 100s ea	54868-5855-00	33.46	
10 mg, 30s ea	54868-5845-02	13.74	
100s ea	54868-5845-00	33.46	
(Quality Care Prod)			
REPACK			
TAB,PO, 10 mg, 6s ea	35356-0085-06	14.94	
30s ea	35356-0085-30	74.70	
CETIRIZINE HCL AND PSEUDOEPHEDRINE HCL (Sandoz)			
TER,PO, 5 mg-120 mg,			
30s ea	00781-5285-31	37.46	
(Phys Total Care)			
REPACK			
TER,PO, 5 mg-120 mg,			
60s ea	54868-5884-00	140.01	
CETIRIZINE HYDROCHLORIDE (Actavis)			
TAB,PO, 5 mg, 100s ea	00228-1196-55	249.47	
(Apotex Corp.)			
TAB,PO (FILM-COATED)			
5 mg, 100s ea	60505-2632-01	249.72	
10 mg, 100s ea	60505-2633-01	249.72	
(Caraco)			
TAB,PO, 5 mg, 100s ea	57664-0540-88	246.98	
10 mg, 100s ea	57664-0541-88	246.98	
(Dr Reddy's)			
TAB,PO (FILM-COATED)			
10 mg, 90s ea	55111-0351-90	224.10	
(Major)			
TAB,PO (10X10)			
10 mg, 100s ea UD	00904-5852-61	248.55	
(Mylan)			
TAB,PO, 5 mg, 100s ea	00378-3635-01	249.40	
10 mg, 100s ea	00378-3637-01	249.40	
500s ea	00378-3637-05	1247.00	
(Northstar)			
TAB,PO (ALLERGY)			
10 mg, 100s ea	16714-0271-02	249.40	
300s ea	16714-0271-03	749.25	
(Perrigo)			
TAB,PO, 10 mg, 30s ea	45802-0919-39	11.73	
300s ea	45802-0919-87	749.25	
(Pharm Assoc Inc)			
SYR,PO (40X5ML,BANANA-GRAPE)			
5 mg/5 ml,			
5 ml 40s UD	00121-4780-05	62.50	
(Sandoz)			
CTB,PO (TUTTI FRUTTI)			
5 mg, 30s ea	00781-5283-64	112.40	
10 mg, 30s ea	00781-5284-64	112.40	
TAB,PO, 5 mg, 100s ea	00781-1683-01	249.75	
10 mg, 100s ea	00781-1684-01	249.75	
(TriMarc Labs)			
TAB,PO, 10 mg, 90s ea	68752-0005-90	11.70	
(UDL)			
TAB,PO (10X10,FILM-COATED)			
10 mg, 100s ea UD	51079-0597-20	249.40	
(A-S Medication)			
REPACK			
SYR,PO (1X120ML)			
5 mg/5 ml, 120 ml	54569-6068-00	9.78	
TAB,PO (FILM-COATED)			
10 mg, 14s ea	54569-6042-00	34.96	
30s ea	54569-6042-01	74.92	
(American Health)			
REPACK			
TAB,PO (10X10)			
10 mg, 100s ea UD	68084-0265-01	247.69	
(PD-Rx Pharm)			
REPACK			
TAB,PO, 10 mg, 7s ea	55289-0995-07	62.64	
10s ea	55289-0995-10	63.90	
90s ea	55289-0995-90	96.66	
(Pharma Pac)			
REPACK			
TAB,PO (FILM-COATED)			
10 mg, 7s ea	52959-0923-07	18.38	
10s ea	52959-0923-10	24.59	
20s ea	52959-0923-20	48.79	
30s ea	52959-0923-30	73.18	
(Physician Partner)			
REPACK			
TAB,PO (FILM-COATED)			
5 mg, 30s ea	21695-0708-30	149.83	
10 mg, 30s ea	21695-0709-30	149.83	
(Stat Rx)			
REPACK			
TAB,PO, 10 mg, 20s ea	16590-0538-20	49.88	
CETIRIZINE HYDROCHLORIDE AND PSEUDOEPHEDRINE HYDROCHLORIDE (Perrigo)			
TER,PO, 5 mg-120 mg,			
24s ea	45802-0721-62	17.55	
CETRA VITE SENIOR (Major)			
TAB,PO, 90s ea	00904-5486-89	6.56	
CGMS BELT CLIP (Medtronic Minimed)			
DEV,NA, ea	76300-0742-01	16.80	
CGMS CABLE (Medtronic Minimed)			
DEV,NA, ea	76300-0723-01	90.00	
(REPLACEMENT CABLE)			
ea	76300-0731-01	90.00	
CGMS TEST PLUG (Medtronic Minimed)			
DEV,NA, ea	76300-0400-01	62.50	
CHAMOMILE (Botanical Labs.)			
LIQ,PO, 30 ml	41954-0020-65	4.00	7.99
CHAMOMILLA (Luyties)			
TAB,SL, 6 x, 500s ea	00618-2127-03	3.99	
5500s ea	00618-2127-10	30.32	
12 x, 500s ea	00624-2127-03	4.19	
5500s ea	00624-2127-10	31.83	
30 x, 500s ea	00622-2127-03	4.19	
5500s ea	00622-2127-10	31.83	
(Walker Pharmacal)			
TAB,SL (6X)			
250s ea	00619-2127-02	2.97	
CHANTAL (Natl Vitamin)			
ALOE VERA			
CRE,TP, 480 gm	54629-0958-00	4.19	6.99
ELASTIN W/RETICULIN			
TP, 120 gm	54629-4601-04	2.81	4.69
FACIAL MOISTURIZER			
TP, 120 gm 120s	54629-4001-04	1.79	2.99
GENTLE CLEANSING			
CRE,TP, 120 gm	54629-4901-04	1.79	2.99
VITAMIN A PALMITATE/VITAMIN E			
GEL,TP, ea	54629-4442-08	2.03	3.39
VITAMIN E W/A & D			
CRE,TP, 120 gm	54629-4301-04	1.79	2.99
VITAMIN E W/ESTER C			
CRE,TP, 114 gm	54629-0461-10	2.09	3.49
LOT,TP, 278 ml	54629-0461-15	1.79	2.99
CHAP STICK (Wyeth Consumer)			
STI,TP (BLISTER PACK)			
4.5 gm 24s	36600-0813-31		1.39
4.5 gm 24s	36600-0814-01		1.39
4.5 gm 24s	36600-0814-61		1.39
(REFILL)			
4.5 gm 24s	36600-0810-45	22.46	
4.5 gm 24s	36600-0810-55	22.46	
4.5 gm 24s	36600-0810-75	22.46	
4.5 gm 24s	36600-0810-85	22.46	

PROD/MFR	HRI, UPC,NDC	AWP	SRP
CHAP STICK LIP MOISTURIZER (Wyeth Consumer)			
OIN,TP (SPF 15,TUBE,SF)			
10.5 gm 12s	36600-0827-01		1.79
STI,TP (SPF 15, BLISTER PACK,SF)			
4.5 gm 24s	36600-0828-03	26.50	
(SPF 15,SF)			
4.5 gm 24s	36600-0828-01		1.59
CHAP STICK ULTRA (Wyeth Consumer)			
STI,TP (SPF 30, REFILL,SF)			
4.5 gm 24s	36600-0813-05	35.42	
(SPF30, BLISTER PACK,SF)			
4.5 gm 24s	36600-0813-01		1.79
CHAP-ET (Glaxo)			
STI,TP (CHERRY)			
61.93%, 4.5 gm	11530-0007-01	0.48	
CHAP-ET MEDICATED (Glaxo)			
STI,TP, 0.5%-61.93%,			
4.5 gm	11530-0004-01	0.48	
CHAPSTICK (Wyeth Consumer)			
STI,TP (SPF 4,CLASSIC,1X4GM)			
1.5%-44%, 4 gm	00573-1900-24		1.59
4 gm	00573-1905-50		1.59
CHAPSTICK CLASSIC (Wyeth Consumer)			
STI,TP (1X4GM,SPF 4,STRAWBERRY)			
1.5%-44%, 4 gm	00573-1915-50		1.59
(SPF4,SPEARMINT)			
1.5%-44%, 4 gm	05731-0910-50		1.59
CHAPSTICK CLASSIC ORIGINAL (Wyeth Consumer)			
STI,TP (SPF4)			
1.5%-44%, 4 gm	36600-0814-81		1.59
CHAPSTICK FLAVA-CRAZE (Wyeth Consumer)			
STI,TP (1X4GM,BLUE CRAZEBERRY)			
44%, 4 gm	36600-0812-40		1.59
(3X4GM)			
44%, 4 gm 3s	00573-1945-12		3.99
CHAPSTICK MEDICATED (Wyeth Consumer)			
STI,TP (BLISTER CARD)			
1%-0.6%-41%-0.5%,			
4.5 gm 24s	36600-0833-31		1.59
CHAPSTICK PEPPERMINT (Wyeth Consumer)			
STI,TP (1X4GM,PEPPERMINT)			
4 gm	00573-1960-12		1.59
(1X4GM,REFILL,PEPPERMINT)			
4 gm	00573-1960-50		1.59
CHAR-CAPS (Key Company)			
CAP,PO, 260 mg, 100s ea	11694-0674-01	6.00	
CHARCOAL (Mason Vit)			
CAP,PO, 260 mg, 60s ea	11845-0078-75	6.33	
(Nature's Bounty)			
CAP,PO (ACTIVATED,PF,SF)			
260 mg, 50s ea	74312-0036-81	4.69	
CHARCOAL PLUS DS (Kramer Labs)			
ECT,PO, 250 mg, 36s ea	53076-0102-11	6.36	7.43
120s ea	53076-0105-16	12.77	15.96
CHARCOCAPS (Young, W.F.)			
CAP,PO, 12 x-12 x-12 x-12 x,			
36s ea	10961-0020-03	4.95	7.09
(PF,SF,CORN-FREE)			
260 mg, 36s ea	10961-0000-74	4.95	7.09
100s ea	10961-0010-03	9.30	13.49
CHECK VALVE EXTENSION (Abbott Hosp)			
DEV,NA (32" W/T-CONNECTOR)			
120s ea	00074-4730-02	444.96	
CHECKMATE PLUS (Quest Star Medical)			
DEV,NA (VALUE)			
ea	08312-3700-07	56.19	
(STRIP)			
50s ea	08312-3710-05	20.31	
CHEK-STIX (Siemens)			
DEV,NA, 25s ea	00193-1360-25	62.15	62.15
CHEK-STIX COMBO PAK (Siemens)			
DEV,NA, 50s ea	00193-1364-02	86.45	86.45
CHELATED CAL-MAG (Carlson,J.R.)			
TAB,PO (PF,SF,CORN-FREE)			
200 mg-100 mg,			
60s ea	88395-0054-70	6.45	12.90
180s ea	88395-0054-72	16.95	33.90
CHELATED CALCIUM (Carlson,J.R.)			
TAB,PO (PF,SF,CORN-FREE)			
250 mg, 60s ea	88395-0054-60	5.45	10.90
180s ea	88395-0054-62	14.45	28.90
CHELATED COPPER (Carlson,J.R.)			
TAB,PO (PF,CORN-FREE,SALT-FREE)			
5 mg, 100s ea	88395-0055-41	4.40	8.80
250s ea	88395-0055-42	9.95	19.90
CHELATED IRON (Carlson,J.R.)			
TAB,PO (PF,SF,SALT-FREE)			
27 mg, 100s ea	88395-0055-71	3.85	7.70
250s ea	88395-0055-72	8.45	16.90
CHELATED MAGNESIUM (Carlson,J.R.)			
TAB,PO (PF,SF,SALT-FREE)			
200 mg, 90s ea	88395-0056-11	9.95	19.90
180s ea	88395-0056-12	16.70	33.40
CHELATED ZINC (Carlson,J.R.)			
TAB,PO (PF,SF,CORN-FREE)			
30 mg, 100s ea	88395-0057-71	3.95	7.90
250s ea	88395-0057-72	8.95	17.90
CHELIDONIUM MAJUS (Luyties)			
TAB,SL (6X)			
6 x, 500s ea	00618-2133-03	3.99	
5500s ea	00618-2133-10	30.32	
12 x, 500s ea	00622-2133-03	4.19	
5500s ea	00622-2133-10	31.83	
(12X)			
30 x, 500s ea	00624-2133-03	4.19	
5500s ea	00624-2133-10	31.83	
CHEMSTRIP 10 MD (Roche Diag)			
DEV,NA, 100s ea	50924-0828-10	73.13	
CHEMSTRIP 10 WITH SG (Roche Diag)			
DEV,NA (STRIP)			
100s ea	50924-0145-10	73.13	
CHEMSTRIP 5 OB (Roche Diag)			
DEV,NA, 100s ea	50924-0467-06	42.86	
CHEMSTRIP 7 (Roche Diag)			
DEV,NA, 100s ea	50924-0218-07	66.08	
CHEMSTRIP 9 (Phys Total Care)			
DEV,NA (STRIP)			
100s ea	54868-2420-00	77.01	
(Roche Diag)			
DEV,NA (STRIP)			
100s ea	50924-0109-10	67.86	
CHEMSTRIP BG (Roche Diag)			
DEV,NA (SELF-TEST DIARY)			
25s ea	50924-0504-01	27.00	1.73
CHEMSTRIP GP (Roche Diag)			
DEV,NA (STRIP)			
100s ea	50924-0743-10	35.71	
CHEMSTRIP MICRAL (Roche Diag)			
DEV,NA (STRIP)			
30s ea	50924-0146-30	149.90	
CHERACOL D (Lee Pharm)			
SYR,PO, 10 mg/5 ml-100 mg/5 ml,			
120 ml	23558-0550-40	7.32	
120 ml 12s	23558-0550-41	87.84	
120 ml 12s	23558-0550-43	126.72	
180 ml	23558-0550-42	10.56	
CHERACOL PLUS (Lee Pharm)			
SYR,PO, 10 mg/5 ml-100 mg/5 ml,			
120 ml	23558-0550-70	6.12	
120 ml 12s	23558-0550-71	73.44	
CHERACOL SORE THROAT (Lee Pharm)			
SPR,MM (AF,SF)			
1.4%, 180 ml	23558-0550-50	5.52	
180 ml 12s	23558-0550-51	66.24	
CHERATUSSIN DAC (Qualitest)			
SOL,PO (SF)			
473 ml	00603-1078-58	39.66	
CHERRY FLAVORED (Covidien)			
SOL,PO (FOR METHADOSE)			
1000 ml	00406-0525-10	54.27	
CHERRY PLUM (Ellon)			
SOL,SL (DROPS)			
10.5 ml	51762-0028-10		9.25
CHEST RUB MEDICATED (Cardinal Health)			
OIN,TP (PRIVATE LABEL)			
4.2%-1.2%-2.6%,			
99 gm	37205-0360-25	3.68	
CHESTAL (Boiron)			
SYR,PO, 126 ml	06969-0032-15	4.04	6.79
253.5 ml	06969-0032-16	6.74	11.29
CHESTAL FOR CHILDREN (Boiron)			
SYR,PO, 126 ml	06969-0033-15	4.04	6.79
253.5 ml	06969-0033-16	6.74	11.29
CHESTNUT BUD (Ellon)			
SOL,SL (DROPS)			
10.5 ml	51762-0004-10		9.25
CHEW-12 (Key Company)			
CTB,PO (SF)			
100s ea	11694-0846-01	5.00	
CHEW-CAL (Key Company)			
WAF,PO, 333 mg-40 iu,			
100s ea	11694-0752-01	4.25	
250s ea	11694-0752-25	8.50	
CHEW-IRON (Carlson,J.R.)			
CTB,PO (PF,SALT-FREE,SOY-FREE)			
27 mg, 30s ea	88395-0055-80	2.20	4.40
CHEWABLE ASPIRIN (Major)			
CTB,PO (ORANGE)			
81 mg, 100s ea	00904-4040-61	10.93	
CHEWABLE VITE (Rugby)			
CTB,PO (FRUIT)			
100s ea	00536-3448-01	5.25	
CHEWABLE VITE W/IRON (Rugby)			
CTB,PO (FRUIT)			
100s ea	00536-3449-01	5.47	
CHICKEN SOUP (Health Products Corp)			
TAB,PO (PF,SF)			
60s ea	39686-0012-45	6.47	
CHICORY (Ellon)			
SOL,SL (DROPS)			
10.5 ml	51762-0011-10		9.25
CHIGGEREX (Scherer Labs)			
OIN,TP, 2%, 52.5 gm	00274-3870-01	1.73	
CHIGGERTOX (Scherer Labs)			
LIQ,TP, 2%, 30 ml	00274-3875-31	1.73	
CHILDREN'S ACETAMINOPHEN (Precision Dose)			
SUS,PO (1X5ML,GRAPE)			
160 mg/5 ml, 5 ml UD	68094-0593-59	0.60	
CHILDREN'S ALL DAY ALLERGY (Major)			
CTB,PO (TUTTI FRUTTI)			
5 mg, 5s ea	00904-5878-33	5.54	
10 mg, 12s ea	00904-5879-12	7.19	
SYR,PO (1X118ML,GRAPE)			
1 mg/ml, 118 ml	00904-5828-20	8.48	
CHILDREN'S BENADRYL ALLERGY (McNeil Consumer Healthcare)			
ODT,PO (FAST MELT,CHERRY)			
12.5 mg, 18s ea	00450-0180-18	5.20	
(FAST MELT,GRAPE)			
12.5 mg, 18s ea	00450-0190-18	5.20	
SYR,PO (PERFECT MEASURE,AF)			
12.5 mg/5 ml,			
5 ml 10s	12547-0175-40	5.20	
CHILDREN'S BENADRYL ANTI-ITCH GEL (Johnson & Johnson)			
GEL,TP (AGES 2 & UP)			
0.45%, 85 gm	12547-0171-03	4.02	
CHILDREN'S BENADRYL-D ALLERGY & SINUS (McNeil Consumer Healthcare)			
SOL,PO (AF,SF,GRAPE)			
12.5 mg/5 ml-5 mg/5 ml,			
118 ml	00450-0170-05	5.20	
CHILDREN'S CETIRIZINE (Actavis Mid Atlantic)			
SYR,PO (1X120ML,W/ DOSING CUP)			
1 mg/ml, 120 ml	00472-1180-94	10.11	
CHILDREN'S CETIRIZINE HYDROCHLORIDE (Ohm)			
SYR,PO (1X118ML,W/DOSING CUP)			
1 mg/ml, 118 ml	51660-0936-04	4.54	
(Perrigo)			
SOL,PO (W/DOSING CUP,1X118ML)			
1 mg/ml, 118 ml	45802-0974-26	10.13	
(Precision Dose)			
SOL,PO (1X5ML, INNER PACK NDC)			
1 mg/ml, 5 ml UD	68094-0720-59	1.21	
(30X5ML,GRAPE)			
1 mg/ml, 5 ml 30s UD	68094-0720-62	36.36	
(Taro)			
SOL,PO (W/DOSING CUP,1X120ML)			
1 mg/ml, 120 ml	51672-2088-08	9.95	
(Physician Partner)			
REPACK			
SYR,PO (GRAPE)			
1 mg/ml, 120 ml	21695-0878-04	72.98	
CHILDREN'S CHEWABLE VITALETS (Freeda)			
CTB,PO (SF,GLUTEN-FREE)			
100s ea	10432-0331-01	6.57	10.95
100s ea	10432-0332-01	6.57	10.95
100s ea	10432-0333-01	6.57	10.95
100s ea	10432-0334-01	6.57	10.95
250s ea	10432-0333-02	13.14	21.90
250s ea	10432-0334-02	13.14	21.90

PROD/MFR	HRI, UPC,NDC	AWP	SRP
CHILDREN'S CLARITIN (Schering Plough)			
CTB,PO (AGES 2YR +,GRAPE)			
5 mg, 10s ea	41100-0820-67	10.19	
40s ea	11523-7198-07	31.19	
SOL,PO (2-6YRS +,DYE-FREE,GRAPE)			
5 mg/5 ml, 60 ml	41100-0804-63	5.59	
120 ml	41100-0804-65	10.19	
CHILDREN'S DIMAPHEN (Major)			
SOL,PO (AF,GRAPE)			
1 mg/5 ml-2.5 mg/5 ml,			
118 ml	00904-5781-20	2.52	
237 ml	00904-5781-09	3.56	
CHILDREN'S DIMAPHEN DM (Major)			
SOL,PO (AF,RED GRAPE)			
118 ml	00904-5782-20	4.26	
CHILDREN'S DIMETAPP COLD & ALLERGY (Wyeth Consumer)			
CTB,PO (GRAPE)			
1 mg-2.5 mg,			
20s ea	00031-2293-20		5.49
SOL,PO (AF,GRAPE)			
1 mg/5 ml-2.5 mg/5 ml,			
118 ml	00031-2235-12		5.79
237 ml	00031-2235-18		9.49
355 ml	00031-2235-24		11.99
CHILDREN'S DIMETAPP DM COLD & COUGH (Wyeth Consumer)			
SOL,PO (AF,GRAPE)			
118 ml	00031-2234-12		5.79
(COLD & COUGH,AF,GRAPE)			
237 ml	00031-2234-18		9.49
CHILDREN'S DIMETAPP LONG ACTING COUGH PLUS COLD (Wyeth Consumer)			
SOL,PO (W/DOSAGE CUP,AF,GRAPE)			
1 mg/5 ml-7.5/5 ml,			
118 ml	00031-2238-12		5.79
CHILDREN'S DIMETAPP ND ALLERGY (Wyeth Consumer)			
ODT,PO (NON-DROWSY,COOL BLAST)			
10 mg, 12s ea	00031-2288-10		10.99
CHILDREN'S DIMETAPP NIGHTTIME FLU (Wyeth Consumer)			
SYR,PO (AF,RED GRAPE)			
118 ml	00031-2237-12		5.79
CHILDREN'S EARACHE RELIEF (Similasan Corp.)			
SOL,OT (DROPS)			
10 x-15 x-12 x-12 x,			
10 ml	59262-0274-11	6.21	10.99
CHILDREN'S IBUPROFEN (Actavis Mid Atlantic)			
SUS,PO (1X118ML,AF,BUBBLE GUM)			
100 mg/5 ml, 118 ml	00472-1263-94	2.94	
(1X118ML,AF,DYE-FREE)			
100 mg/5 ml, 118 ml	00472-1261-94	2.94	
(AF,BERRY)			
100 mg/5 ml, 118 ml	00472-1255-94	2.94	
(Precision Dose)			
SUS,PO (1X10ML,AF,BERRY)			
100 mg/5 ml, 10 ml UD	68094-0503-59	1.37	
CHILDREN'S LORATADINE (Taro)			
SYR,PO (W/DOSAGE CUP,AF,FRUIT)			
5 mg/5 ml, 120 ml	51672-0207-38	9.39	
(W/DOSAGE CUP,AF)			
5 mg/5 ml, 120 ml	51672-0208-58	9.39	
CHILDREN'S MAALOX (Novartis Consumer)			
CTB,PO (WILD BERRY)			
400 mg, 32s ea	00067-6241-32	4.19	
CHILDREN'S MAPAP (Major)			
ODT,PO (AGES 2-6,ASPIRIN-FREE)			
80 mg, 30s ea	00904-5791-46	2.95	
CHILDREN'S MAPAP COUGH & SINUS FORMULA (Major)			
SUS,PO (1X118ML,CHERRY)			
118 ml	00904-5874-20	3.17	
CHILDREN'S MOTRIN (McNeil Consumer Healthcare)			
SUS,PO (AF,BERRY)			
100 mg/5 ml, 60 ml	00450-0192-02	3.86	
120 ml	00450-0192-04	5.96	
(AF,BUBBLEGUM)			
100 mg/5 ml,			
120 ml	00450-0604-04	5.96	
(AF,DYE-FREE,BERRY)			
100 mg/5 ml,			
120 ml	00450-0184-04	5.96	
(AF,GRAPE)			
100 mg/5 ml,			
120 ml	00450-0603-04	5.96	
(AF,TROPICAL PUNCH)			
100 mg/5 ml,			
120 ml	00450-0215-04	5.96	
(Physician Partner) REPACK			
SUS,PO (1X120ML,AF,BERRY)			
100 mg/5 ml,			
120 ml	21695-0431-04	16.38	
CHILDREN'S MOTRIN COLD (McNeil Consumer Healthcare)			
SUS,PO (AF,BERRY)			
100 mg/5 ml-15 mg/5 ml,			
120 ml	00450-0902-04	5.50	
CHILDREN'S MUCINEX (Reckitt Benckiser)			
SYR,PO (W/ DOSAGE CUP,1X118ML)			
100 mg/5 ml,			
118 ml	63824-0273-64	6.41	
CHILDREN'S MUCINEX COLD (Reckitt Benckiser)			
SOL,PO (1X120ML,AF,MIXED BERRY)			
100 mg/5 ml-2.5 mg/5 ml,			
120 ml	63824-0277-64	6.83	
CHILDREN'S MUCINEX COUGH (Reckitt Benckiser)			
SYR,PO (W/ DOSAGE CUP,1X118ML)			
5 mg/5 ml-100 mg/5 ml,			
118 ml	63824-0274-64	6.83	
CHILDREN'S MUCINEX MINI-MELTS (Reckitt Benckiser)			
PKT,PO (ORANGE CREAM)			
5 mg-100 mg,			
12s ea	63824-0256-12	6.83	
(GRAPE)			
50 mg, 12s ea	63824-0253-12	6.41	
CHILDREN'S MYLANTA UPSET STOMACH RELIEF (J&J/Merck)			
CTB,PO (BUBBLEGUM)			
400 mg, 24s ea	16837-0810-24	3.56	
CHILDREN'S NORTEMP (Ballay Pharm., Inc)			
SUS,PO (AF,ASPIRIN-FREE)			
160 mg/5 ml, 118 ml	63162-0510-12	5.88	
CHILDREN'S PEDIA CARE (Johnson & Johnson)			
SOL,PO (LONG-ACTING,NON-DROWSY)			
7.5 mg/5 ml,			
120 ml	00501-2422-04	4.87	
SYR,PO (NIGHTTIME COUGH,AF)			
12.5 mg/5 ml,			
120 ml	00501-2431-04	4.87	
CHILDREN'S Q-PAP (Qualitest)			
SYR,PO (UNBOXED,W/MEASURING CUP)			
160 mg/5 ml, 118 ml	00603-0839-94	2.48	
118 ml	00603-0840-94	2.50	
(W/ MEASURING CUP,AF)			
160 mg/5 ml, 118 ml	00603-0839-54	2.48	
473 ml	00603-0839-58	7.94	
(Dispensing Solutions) REPACK			
SYR,PO (1X120ML,AF,ASPIRIN-FREE)			
160 mg/5 ml,			
120 ml	68258-3003-01	5.45	
CHILDREN'S SUDAFED (McNeil Consumer Healthcare)			
SOL,PO (NON-DROWSY,AF,SF,GRAPE)			
15 mg/5 ml, 118 ml	50580-0536-04	5.51	
CHILDREN'S SUDAFED PE COLD & COUGH (McNeil Consumer Healthcare)			
SOL,PO (NON-DROWSY,AF,SF,GRAPE)			
5 mg/5 ml-2.5 mg/5 ml,			
118 ml	00450-0538-04	5.51	
CHILDREN'S SUDAFED PE NASAL DECONGESTANT (McNeil Consumer Healthcare)			
SOL,PO (NON-DROWSY,AF,SF)			
2.5 mg/5 ml,			
118 ml	00450-0537-04	5.51	
CHILDREN'S TRIAMINIC ALLERGY (Novartis Consumer)			
FIL,MM (THIN STRIPS,GRAPE)			
12.5 mg, 14s ea	00067-6383-14	4.85	
CHILDREN'S TRIAMINIC CHEST & NASAL CONGESTION (Novartis Consumer)			
SOL,PO (1X118ML,W/DOSAGE CUP,AF)			
50 mg/5 ml-2.5 mg/5 ml,			
118 ml	00067-6347-04	4.85	
CHILDREN'S TRIAMINIC COLD & ALLERGY (Novartis Consumer)			
SOL,PO (1X118ML,W/DOSAGE CUP,AF)			
1 mg/5 ml-2.5 mg/5 ml,			
118 ml	00067-6346-04	4.85	
CHILDREN'S TRIAMINIC COUGH & RUNNY NOSE (Novartis Consumer)			
CTB,PO (SOFTCHEWS,CHERRY)			
1 mg-5 mg, 18s ea	00067-6357-18	4.85	
FIL,MM (THIN STRIPS,GRAPE)			
12.5 mg, 14s ea	00067-6354-14	4.85	
CHILDREN'S TRIAMINIC COUGH & SORE THROAT (Novartis Consumer)			
CTB,PO (SOFTCHEWS,GRAPE)			
160 mg-5 mg,			
18s ea	00067-6358-18	4.85	
SYR,PO (1X118ML,W/DOSAGE CUP,AF)			
160 mg/5 ml-5 mg/5 ml,			
118 ml	00067-6348-04	4.85	
CHILDREN'S TRIAMINIC DAY TIME COLD & COUGH (Novartis Consumer)			
FIL,PO (THIN STRIPS,WILD BERRY)			
5 mg-2.5 mg,			
14s ea	00067-6355-14	4.85	
SOL,PO (1X118ML,W/DOSAGE CUP,AF)			
5 mg/5 ml-2.5 mg/5 ml,			
118 ml	00067-6345-04	4.85	
(1X236ML,W/DOSAGE CUP,AF)			
5 mg/5 ml-2.5 mg/5 ml,			
236 ml	00067-6345-08	8.00	
CHILDREN'S TRIAMINIC FLU COUGH & FEVER (Novartis Consumer)			
SYR,PO (1X118ML,W/DOSAGE CUP,AF)			
118 ml	00067-6349-04	4.85	
CHILDREN'S TRIAMINIC LONG ACTING COUGH (Novartis Consumer)			
FIL,MM (THIN STRIP,CHERRY)			
7.5 mg, 14s ea	00067-6353-14	4.85	
SYR,PO (1X118ML,W/DOSAGE CUP,AF)			
7.5 mg/5 ml,			
118 ml	00067-6350-04	4.85	
CHILDREN'S TRIAMINIC NIGHT TIME COLD & COUGH (Novartis Consumer)			
FIL,MM (GRAPE)			
12.5 mg-5 mg,			
14s ea	00067-6356-14	4.85	
SOL,PO (1X118ML,W/DOSAGE CUP,AF)			
6.25 mg/5 ml-2.5 mg/5 ml,			
118 ml	00067-6344-04	4.85	
(1X236ML,W/DOSAGE CUP,AF)			
6.25 mg/5 ml-2.5 mg/5 ml,			
236 ml	00067-6344-08	8.00	
CHILDREN'S TYLENOL (McNeil Consumer Healthcare)			
ODT,PO (MELTAWAYS, AGES 2-6)			
80 mg, 30s ea	00450-0518-30	3.61	
30s ea	00450-0519-30	3.61	
SUS,PO (AGES 2-11,AF)			
160 mg/5 ml, 60 ml	00450-0123-02	3.85	
120 ml	00450-0123-04	5.95	
120 ml	00450-0296-04	5.95	
120 ml	00450-0407-04	5.95	
120 ml	00450-0493-04	5.95	
(NON-STAINING,AF)			
160 mg/5 ml,			
120 ml	00450-0166-04	5.95	
(Physician Partner) REPACK			
SUS,PO (1X120ML,AF,ASPIRIN-FREE)			
160 mg/5 ml,			
120 ml	21695-0435-04	16.90	
CHILDREN'S TYLENOL MELTAWAYS (Southwood) REPACK			
CTB,PO, 80 mg, 30s ea	00490-0070-30	5.02	
CHILDREN'S TYLENOL PLUS COLD (McNeil Consumer Healthcare)			
SUS,PO (GRAPE)			
120 ml	00450-0387-04	4.97	
120 ml	00450-0387-05	5.50	
CHILDREN'S TYLENOL PLUS COLD & ALLERGY (McNeil Consumer Healthcare)			
SUS,PO (BUBBLE GUM)			
120 ml	00045-0390-04	4.97	
120 ml	00450-0390-05	5.50	
CHILDREN'S TYLENOL PLUS COLD & COUGH (McNeil Consumer Healthcare)			
SUS,PO (NON-STAINING,DYE-FREE)			
120 ml	00450-0254-04	5.50	
CHILDREN'S TYLENOL PLUS COLD & STUFFY NOSE (McNeil Consumer Healthcare)			
SUS,PO (NON-STAINING,DYE-FREE)			
160 mg/5 ml-2.5 mg/5 ml,			
120 ml	00450-0253-04	5.50	

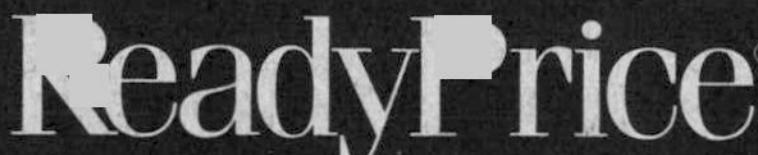

PROD/MFR	HRI, UPC,NDC	AWP	SRP
CHILDREN'S TYLENOL PLUS COUGH & RUNNY NOSE (McNeil Consumer Healthcare)			
SUS,PO (CHERRY)			
120 ml	00450-0249-04	4.97	
120 ml	00450-0249-05	5.50	
CHILDREN'S TYLENOL PLUS COUGH & SORE THROAT (McNeil Consumer Healthcare)			
SUS,PO (CHERRY)			
160 mg/5 ml-5 mg/5 ml,			
120 ml	00450-0247-04	4.97	
120 ml	00450-0247-05	5.50	
CHILDREN'S TYLENOL PLUS FLU (McNeil Consumer Healthcare)			
SUS,PO (BUBBLE GUM)			
120 ml	00045-0386-04	4.97	
120 ml	00450-0386-05	5.50	
CHILDREN'S TYLENOL PLUS MULTI-SYMPTOM COLD (McNeil Consumer Healthcare)			
PO (DYE-FREE,GRAPE)			
120 ml	00450-0255-04	5.50	
(GRAPE)			
120 ml	00450-0391-04	4.97	
120 ml	00450-0391-05	5.50	
CHILDREN'S ZYRTEC (McNeil Consumer Healthcare)			
CTB,PO (ALLERGY,GRAPE)			
5 mg, 15s ea	50580-0720-15	10.80	
10 mg, 12s ea	12547-0204-19	10.84	
SOL,PO (W/DOSING CUP,SF)			
5 mg/5 ml, 118 ml	00450-0205-04	10.84	
CHILDREN'S ZYRTEC ALLERGY (McNeil Consumer Healthcare)			
SOL,PO (10X5ML,24 HOUR,GRAPE)			
5 mg/5 ml,			
5 ml 10s	00450-0209-10	10.85	
(1X118ML,24 HOUR,SF)			
5 mg/5 ml, 118 ml	00450-0209-04	10.87	
CHILDRENS TRIAMINIC THIN STRIPS (Novartis Consumer)			
FIL,MM (RASPBERRY)			
2.5 mg, 14s ea	00067-6352-14	4.85	
CHIX CLEANERS (J&J Medical)			
DEV,NA (MEDIUM)			
40s ea	56091-0041-02	1.50	
(SMALL)			
40s ea	56091-0041-03	1.38	
(LARGE,BULK)			
250s ea	56091-0041-12	12.19	
(MEDIUM,BULK)			
250s ea	56091-0041-11	7.05	
CHLOR-PHEN (Truxton)			
TAB,PO, 4 mg, 1000s ea	00463-6065-10	7.20	
CHLOR-PHENIRAMINE (Chain Drug Marketing)			
TAB,PO, 4 mg, 24s ea	63868-0826-24	0.83	2.49
CHLOR-PHENITON (Global Source)			
TAB,PO, 4 mg-60 mg,			
24s ea	59618-0165-06	1.70	
CHLOR-TRIMETON ALLERGY (Schering Plough)			
TAB,PO, 4 mg, 24s ea	00085-0080-01	4.62	
TER,PO, 12 mg, 10s ea	00085-0009-09	4.62	
24s ea	00085-0009-03	10.19	
CHLOR-TRIPOLON (PGD, Inc.)			
SYR,PO (AF,CHERRY)			
2 mg/5 ml, 118 ml	65615-0429-04	4.75	
CHLORASEPTIC (Medtech)			
SPR,MM (1X177ML,MENTHOL)			
1.4%, 177 ml	78112-0011-04	4.31	
(Prestige Brands)			
LOZ,MM (CHERRY)			
6 mg-10 mg, 18s ea	78112-0011-06	2.75	
SPR,MM (AF,SF,ASPIRIN-FREE)			
1.4%, 177 ml	78112-0011-03	4.18	
(Phys Total Care)			
REPACK			
SPR,MM, 1.4%, 177 ml	54868-5810-00	6.62	
CHLORELLA (Bio-Tech Pharm)			
CAP,PO, 500 mg, 100s ea	53191-0229-01	11.25	
CHLORHIST (Magno-Humphries)			
TAB,PO, 4 mg, 100s ea	43292-0556-28	1.76	3.59
CHLORODEX GP (Palmetto)			
REPACK			
SYR,PO, 120 ml	23490-8031-01	15.63	
180 ml	23490-8031-02	23.46	
240 ml	23490-8031-03	31.27	
CHLOROPHYLL (Freeda)			
TAB,PO (PF,SF,DYE-FREE)			
20 mg, 100s ea	10432-0262-01	5.64	9.40
250s ea	10432-0262-02	11.28	18.80
(Rugby)			
TAB,PO (PF,SF,DYE-FREE)			
3 mg-0.6 mg, 100s ea	00536-3451-01	2.78	
CHLORPHEN (Medique)			
TAB,PO, 4 mg, 24s ea UD	47682-0241-64	1.59	
100s ea	47682-0241-33	2.84	
(250X1)			
4 mg, 250s ea UD	47682-0241-48	11.65	
CHLORPHENIRAMINE MALEATE (Consolidated Midland)			
SYR,PO, 2 mg/5 ml,			
480 ml	00223-6244-01	4.60	
TAB,PO, 4 mg, 100s ea	00223-0692-01	1.95	
1000s ea	00223-0692-02	9.75	
(Major)			
TAB,PO, 4 mg, 1000s ea	00904-0012-80	10.25	
(Marlex)			
TAB,PO, 4 mg, 24s ea	10135-0133-24	0.47	
(BOXED)			
4 mg, 24s ea	10135-0133-52	65.00	
30s ea	10135-0133-30	0.50	
100s ea	10135-0133-01	0.85	
(BOXED)			
4 mg, 100s ea	10135-0133-57	65.00	
120s ea	10135-0133-62	0.95	
250s ea	10135-0133-69	6.87	
1000s ea	10135-0133-10	10.00	
(Mason Vit)			
TAB,PO, 4 mg, 100s ea	11845-0860-01	2.33	
(Teva)			
TAB,PO, 4 mg, 100s ea	00182-0471-01	2.35	
1000s ea	00182-0471-10	8.99	
(UDL)			
TAB,PO (10X10)			
4 mg, 100s ea UD	51079-0163-20	6.19	
(A-S Medication)			
REPACK			
TAB,PO, 4 mg, 20s ea	54569-0243-06	0.80	
60s ea	54569-0243-07	2.39	
(HomeMed)			
REPACK			
TAB,PO, 4 mg, 24s ea	51655-0006-30	4.42	
TER,PO, 8 mg, 30s ea	51655-0007-24	8.12	
(PD-Rx Pharm)			
REPACK			
TAB,PO, 4 mg, 12s ea	55289-0560-12	7.47	
24s ea	55289-0560-24	8.27	
30s ea	55289-0560-30	8.67	
56s ea	58864-0093-56	5.39	
100s ea	55289-0560-01	13.33	
(Phys Total Care)			
REPACK			
TAB,PO, 4 mg, 100s ea	54868-2047-00	10.11	
1000s ea	54868-2047-02	74.07	
(Southwood)			
REPACK			
TAB,PO, 4 mg, 20s ea	58016-0484-20	2.63	
24s ea	58016-0484-24	3.47	
28s ea	58016-0484-28	3.69	
30s ea	58016-0484-30	3.94	
CHLORPHENIRAMINE MALEATE/PSEUDOEPHEDRINE HCL (Quality Care Prod)			
REPACK			
CER,PO, 8 mg-120 mg,			
20s ea	49999-0768-20	10.02	
30s ea	49999-0768-30	15.03	
CHOICE DM DIABETES RISK IN-HOME TEST KIT (Health Care Products)			
DEV,NA, ea	61787-0484-01	15.75	24.99
CHOLESTEROL MANAGEMENT (Major)			
TAB,PO (PF,SF,GLUTEN-FREE)			
90s ea	00904-5906-89	6.39	
CHOLINE (Bio-Tech Pharm)			
CAP,PO, 648 mg, 100s ea	53191-0233-01	4.20	
(Freeda)			
TAB,PO (PF,SF,DYE-FREE)			
650 mg, 100s ea	10432-0218-01	5.97	9.95
(Nature's Bounty)			
TAB,PO (PF,SF)			
650 mg, 100s ea	74312-0007-00		7.99
(Phys Total Care)			
REPACK			
TAB,PO, 250 mg, 100s ea	54868-3928-00	4.44	
CHOLINE & INOSITOL (Key Company)			
CAP,PO, 350 mg-350 mg,			
100s ea	11694-0683-01	7.00	
500s ea	11694-0683-05	30.00	
CHOLINE BITARTRATE (Marlex)			
TAB,PO (CAPLET)			
648 mg, 100s ea	10135-0265-01	2.91	
CHOLINE-10 (Key Company)			
TAB,PO, 648 mg, 100s ea	11694-0876-01	6.00	
250s ea	11694-0876-02	12.00	
CHOLINOID (Teva)			
CAP,PO, 100s ea	00182-4166-01	7.90	
CHONDROITIN COMPLEX/GLUCOSAMINE (Lex)			
CAP,PO, 200 mg-500 mg,			
50s ea	58537-0032-05	6.80	
CHONDROITIN SULFATE/GLUCOSAMINE HYDROCHLORIDE (Palmetto)			
REPACK			
CAP,PO, 400 mg-500 mg,			
120s ea	23490-7102-00	119.96	
CHONDROITIN/GLUCOSAMINE (AmerisourceBergen)			
TAB,PO (PRIVATE LABEL,CAPLET)			
200 mg-250 mg, 120s ea	24385-0258-76	15.29	16.99
(MAX. STR.,PRIVATE LABEL)			
400 mg-500 mg,			
110s ea	24385-0956-25	20.69	22.99
150s ea	24385-0956-47	22.49	24.99
(Breckenridge Pharm)			
CAP,PO (PF,SF)			
400 mg-500 mg,			
60s ea	51991-0031-06	17.44	
(Cardinal Health)			
TAB,PO (PRIVATE LABEL,CAPLET)			
200 mg-250 mg,			
48s ea	37205-0066-67	10.72	
(Major)			
CAP,PO (MAX. STR.)			
400 mg-500 mg,			
60s ea	00904-5481-52	19.35	
120s ea	00904-5481-18	38.20	
(Marlex)			
CAP,PO, 400 mg-500 mg,			
60s ea	10135-0284-60	7.27	
120s ea	10135-0284-62	14.26	
(Reese)			
CAP,PO, 250 mg-500 mg,			
60s ea	23513-0716-60	15.50	
(Teva)			
TAB,PO, 400 mg-500 mg,			
120s ea	00182-4095-07	32.99	
(United Research)			
CAP,PO, 400 mg-500 mg,			
60s ea	00677-1652-06	42.71	
120s ea	00677-1652-67	76.88	
(Altura)			
REPACK			
CAP,PO, 400 mg-500 mg,			
20s ea	63874-0871-20	29.99	
30s ea	63874-0871-30	44.99	
60s ea	63874-0871-60	89.98	
80s ea	63874-0871-80	119.97	
90s ea	63874-0871-90	134.97	
120s ea	63874-0871-04	179.96	
CHONDROITIN/GLUCOSAMINE COMPLEX (Southwood)			
REPACK			
CAP,PO, 30s ea	58016-0179-30	27.75	
60s ea	58016-0179-60	55.50	
80s ea	58016-0179-80	74.00	
90s ea	58016-0179-90	83.25	
100s ea	58016-0179-00	92.50	
120s ea	58016-0179-02	111.00	
CHOOZ (Heritage/Insight)			
CTB,PO, 500 mg, 16s ea	63736-0176-85	1.58	
CHROMA GUM (Health Products Corp)			
GUM,PO (SF,WINTERMINT)			
30s ea	39686-0013-68	7.50	
CHROMACAPS (Key Company)			
TAB,PO (SF)			
1 mg, 100s ea	11694-0836-01	6.25	
CHROMELIN (Summers)			
LOT,TP, 5%, 30 ml	11086-0014-01	12.84	

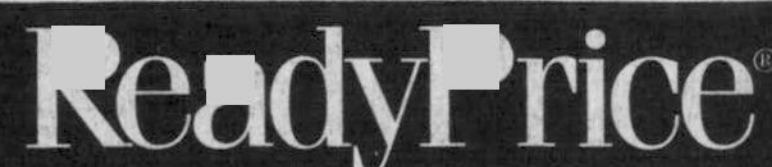

PROD/MFR	HRI, UPC, NDC	AWP	SRP
CHROMIMIN (Key Company)			
TAB,PO, 1 mg, 100s ea	11694-0936-01	5.50	
CHROMIUM (Basic Vitamins)			
TAB,PO, 200 mcg,			
100s ea	00761-0790-20	2.15	
(Carlson,J.R.)			
TAB,PO (PF,SF,CORN-FREE)			
200 mcg-474 mcg,			
100s ea	88395-0055-11	3.13	6.25
300s ea	88395-0055-13	8.20	16.40
(Major)			
TAB,PO, 200 mcg,			
130s ea	00904-4192-13	6.67	
(Mason Vit)			
TAB,PO, 100 mcg,			
100s ea	11845-0073-51	3.44	
200 mcg, 100s ea	11845-0077-41	7.78	
CHROMIUM ASPARTATE (Miller)			
TAB,PO, 1 mg, 100s ea	17204-0356-40	5.04	8.40
CHROMIUM CHELATED (Freeda)			
TAB,PO (PF,SF,DYE-FREE)			
200 mcg, 100s ea	10432-0247-01	3.87	6.45
400 mcg, 100s ea	10432-0278-01	5.28	8.80
CHROMIUM K6 (Rexall)			
TAB,PO (PF,SF)			
60s ea	30768-0000-81	3.69	5.58
CHROMIUM PICOLINATE (ADH)			
CAP,PO, 200 mcg,			
100s ea	60142-0111-10	5.48	10.95
(Basic Vitamins)			
TAB,PO, 200 mcg,			
100s ea	00761-0460-20	3.00	
(Health Products Corp)			
TAB,PO (PF,SF)			
200 mcg, 100s ea	39686-0013-67	4.25	
(Key Company)			
TAB,PO (CORN-FREE,RYE-FREE)			
192 mg-200 mcg,			
100s ea	11694-0672-01	5.00	
(Major)			
TAB,PO, 200 mcg,			
100s ea	00904-4314-60	6.95	
(Marlex)			
TAB,PO, 200 mcg, 50s ea	10135-0176-50	1.63	
100s ea	10135-0176-01	3.68	
130s ea	10135-0176-63	2.16	
1000s ea	10135-0176-10	19.62	
(Mason Vit)			
TAB,PO (PF,SF,DYE-FREE)			
51 mg-0.2 mg,			
200s ea	11845-0122-42	11.00	
(PF,SF)			
61 mg-500 mcg,			
60s ea	11845-0119-25	10.00	
200 mcg, 100s ea	11845-0098-11	7.22	
(PF,SF)			
200 mcg, 100s ea	11845-0122-41	7.22	
(Nature's Bounty)			
TAB,PO (PF,SF)			
200 mcg, 100s ea	74312-0063-90		6.59
(Rexall)			
TAB,PO (PF,SF)			
200 mcg, 50s ea	30768-0000-63	2.02	3.07
(Rugby)			
SGL,PO (PF,SF,DYE-FREE,SOFTGEL)			
200 mcg, 60s ea	00536-6668-08	7.43	
(PD-Rx Pharm)			
REPACK			
TAB,PO, 200 mcg, 21s ea	55289-0796-21	7.13	
28s ea	55289-0796-28	8.99	
CHROMIUM PICOLINATE FORTIFIED (Rexall)			
TAB,PO (PF,SF)			
0.4 mg-1 mg-400 mg,			
50s ea	30768-0001-07	5.52	8.37
CHROMIUM PICOLINATE KLB6 (Mason Vit)			
TAB,PO (PF,SF)			
100s ea	11845-0118-41	8.11	
CHROMIUM PICOLINATE W/ENHANCERS (Rexall)			
TAB,PO (PF,SF)			
0.2 mg-1 mg-400 mg,			
50s ea	30768-0000-71	4.17	6.32
CHROMIUN PICOLINATE (Cardinal Health)			
TAB,PO (PF,PRIVATE LABEL)			
200 mcg, 100s ea	37205-0168-78	5.77	

PROD/MFR	HRI, UPC, NDC	AWP	SRP
CHRONDROITIN GLUCOSAMINE COMPLEX (Alphagen)			
CAP,PO, 400 mg-500 mg,			
60s ea	59743-0911-60	18.15	
120s ea	59743-0911-12	33.15	
CIBA VISION SALINE (Ciba Vision)			
SOL,NA, 240 ml	47113-0606-20	2.90	
360 ml	47113-0606-27	3.60	
CICA-CARE SILICONE GEL SHEET (Smith & Nephew)			
DEV,NA (4 3/4"X6", 10 SHEETS)			
ea	00223-0410-79	600.54	480.43
CIDAFLEX (Pharmaceutica North)			
TAB,PO, 400 mg-500 mg,			
90s ea	45861-0000-00	89.10	
CIMETIDINE (AmerisourceBergen)			
TAB,PO (PRIVATE LABEL)			
200 mg, 30s ea	24385-0111-65	6.29	6.99
(Cardinal Health)			
TAB,PO (PRIVATE LABEL)			
200 mg, 30s ea	37205-0528-65	6.51	
(200X1 PACKETS)			
200 mg, 200s ea UD	37205-0528-93	27.30	
(Teva)			
TAB,PO, 200 mg, 30s ea	00182-2660-17	4.99	
CIMICIFUGA (Luyties)			
TAB,SL (6X)			
6 x, 500s ea	00618-2175-03	3.99	
(12X)			
6 x, 5500s ea	00624-2175-10	31.83	
(6X)			
6 x, 5500s ea	00618-2175-10	30.32	
12 x, 500s ea	00622-2175-03	4.19	
5500s ea	00622-2175-10	31.83	
30 x, 500s ea	00624-2175-03	4.19	
CINA (Luyties)			
TAB,SL (6X)			
6 x, 500s ea	00618-2176-03	3.99	
5500s ea	00618-2176-10	30.32	
(30X)			
12 x, 500s ea	00622-2176-03	4.19	
5500s ea	00622-2176-10	31.83	
30 x, 500s ea	00624-2176-03	4.19	
(12X)			
30 x, 5500s ea	00624-2176-10	31.83	
CINCHONA OFFICINALIS (Luyties)			
TAB,SL (6X)			
6 x, 500s ea	00618-2144-03	3.99	
5500s ea	00618-2144-10	30.32	
12 x, 500s ea	00622-2144-03	4.19	
5500s ea	00622-2144-10	31.83	
30 x, 500s ea	00624-2144-03	4.19	
5500s ea	00624-2144-10	31.83	
CINIS PREEMIE HALO (Lionhearted)			
DEV,NA (LARGE,LATEX-FREE)			
ea	85661-0236-01	43.74	
(MEDIUM,LATEX-FREE)			
ea	85661-0235-01	43.74	
(SMALL,LATEX-FREE)			
ea	85661-0234-01	43.74	
CINNABAR COMPOUND (Weleda)			
POW,TP, 30 gm	55946-0190-30	7.20	
CINNAMON (Key Company)			
CAP,PO, 500 mg, 100s ea	11694-0648-01	5.00	
(Major)			
CAP,PO (PF,SF,LACTOSE-FREE)			
500 mg, 100s ea	00904-5825-60	7.38	
CIRCUS CHEWS CHILDREN'S (Rexall)			
CTB,PO (PF,FRUIT)			
60s ea	30768-0000-34	1.64	2.48
CITRA PH (ValMed)			
SOL,PO, 450 mg/5 ml,			
30 ml 100s UD	54627-0502-30	94.00	
CITRACAL + D (Phys Total Care)			
REPACK			
TAB,PO (CAPLET)			
315 mg-200 iu,			
60s ea	54868-4849-00	8.66	
CITRACAL CALCIUM CITRATE PETITES WITH VITAMIN D (Bayer HealthCare)			
TAB,PO, 200 mg-200 iu,			
200s ea	00178-0800-20	8.58	
CITRACAL ULTRADENSE CALCIUM CITRATE (Bayer HealthCare)			
TAB,PO (W/VIT D,CAPLET)			
315 mg-200 iu,			
60s ea	01780-0815-60	5.04	

PROD/MFR	HRI, UPC, NDC	AWP	SRP
(ECONOMY,CAPLET)			
315 mg-200 iu,			
120s ea	01780-0815-12	8.58	
CITRACAL ULTRADENSE CALCIUM CITRATE PETITE W/VIT D (Bayer HealthCare)			
TAB,PO (SMALLER SIZE)			
200 mg-200 iu,			
100s ea	00178-0800-01	5.04	
CITRACAL ULTRADENSE CALCIUM CITRATE PLUS VIT D MAG (Bayer HealthCare)			
TAB,PO (MULTI-MINERAL SUPPLMNT)			
150s ea	01780-0825-15	8.58	
CITRATE OF MAGNES (Phys Total Care)			
REPACK			
SOL,PO (1X3552ML)			
1.75 gm/30 ml,			
3552 ml	54868-0010-01	63.26	
CITRATE OF MAGNESIA (Consolidated Midland)			
SOL,PO, 1.75 gm/30 ml,			
300 ml 24s	00223-6470-00	36.00	
(Humco)			
SOL,PO (LOW SODIUM,SF,CHERRY)			
300 ml	00395-4211-10	1.25	
(LOW SODIUM,SF,LEMON)			
1.75 gm/30 ml, 300 ml	00395-4210-10	1.25	
(Southwood)			
REPACK			
SOL,PO, 1.75 gm/30 ml,			
300 ml	58016-7032-01	4.86	
CITRATE OF MAGNESIUM (Cardinal Health)			
SOL,PO (PRIVATE LABEL)			
1.75 gm/30 ml, 300 ml	37205-0110-38	1.18	
CITRIMAX 250 (Mason Vit)			
TAB,PO (PF,SF)			
250 mg, 60s ea	11845-0115-45	7.44	
CITRIMAX 500 PLUS (Mason Vit)			
TAB,PO (PF,SF)			
75 mg-0.2 mg-500 mg,			
60s ea	11845-0118-55	13.00	
CITROCARBONATE (Lee Pharm)			
GEF,PO, 150 gm	23558-0510-20	9.00	
150 gm 12s	23558-0510-21	108.00	
300 gm	23558-0510-22	14.04	
300 gm 12s	23558-0510-23	168.48	
CITRUCEL (Glaxo)			
PDR,PO (ORANGE)			
2 gm/dose, 20s ea	00068-0418-25	7.63	
(PACKET,SF,ORANGE)			
2 gm/dose, 20s ea	00068-0420-25	7.63	
(SF,ORANGE)			
2 gm/dose, 245 gm	00068-0420-08	7.63	
(ORANGE)			
2 gm/dose, 454 gm	00068-0418-16	7.63	
(SF,ORANGE)			
2 gm/dose, 479 gm	00068-0420-17	12.91	
(CLEAR-MIX,ORANGE)			
2 gm/dose, 539 gm	07660-0421-00	13.05	
(ORANGE)			
2 gm/dose, 850 gm	00068-0418-30	12.91	
(SF,GLUTEN-FREE,ORANGE)			
2 gm/dose, 907 gm	07660-0420-50	20.53	
(CLEAR-MIX,ORANGE)			
2 gm/dose, 1021 gm	07660-0421-10	20.76	
(GLUTEN-FREE,ORANGE)			
2 gm/dose, 1418 gm	07660-0418-50	20.53	
TAB,PO (CAPLET)			
500 mg, 100s ea	00766-0425-20	12.91	
164s ea	07660-0419-40	20.53	
180s ea	07660-0419-70	20.53	
(Dispensing Solutions)			
REPACK			
TAB,PO (CAPLET)			
500 mg, 100s ea	55045-3110-00	14.99	
CITRUCEL FIBER SHAKE (Glaxo)			
PDR,PO (STARTER KIT + CUP)			
2 gm/dose, 5s ea	07660-0440-89	3.41	
(CHOCOLATE)			
2 gm/dose, 205 gm	07660-0442-00	7.63	
413 gm	07660-0443-00	12.91	
CITRULLINE 1000 (VITAFLO, LLC)			
POW,NA (30X4GM)			
4 gm 30s	50600-0550-95	120.00	150.00
CITRUS BIOFLAVONOIDS (Freeda)			
POW,PO, 700 mg/0.7 gm,			
120 gm	10432-0127-01	6.57	10.95

PROD/MFR	HRI, UPC,NDC	AWP	SRP
(Nature's Bounty)			
TAB,PO (PF,SF)			
1000 mg, 100s ea	74312-0020-30		8.65
CITRUS CALCIUM + D (Rugby)			
TAB,PO (LACTOSE-FREE,COATED)			
315 mg-250 iu, 60s ea	00536-3224-08	3.88	
CITRUS CALCIUM WITH VITAMIN D (Rugby)			
PO (LACTOSE-FREE,COATED)			
200 mg-250 iu, 100s ea	00536-3223-01	4.02	
CITRUS MAGIC (Beaumont Prod)			
SPR,NA (ODOR ELIMINATE,MANDARIN)			
90 ml	87052-0127-50	3.83	5.95
(ODOR ELIMINATOR)			
90 ml	87052-0127-47	3.83	5.95
90 ml	87052-0127-48	3.83	5.95
90 ml	87052-0127-49	3.83	5.95
90 ml	87052-0127-51	3.83	5.95
90 ml	87052-0127-95	3.83	5.95
180 ml	87052-0127-52	5.97	9.95
CITRUS MAGIC HAND SOAP (Beaumont Prod)			
LIQ,TP, 240 ml	87052-0129-20	1.80	2.95
240 ml	87052-0129-21	1.80	2.95
240 ml	87052-0129-22	1.80	2.95
CLARITIN (Schering Plough)			
TAB,PO, 10 mg, 5s ea	41100-0080-18	18.35	
5s ea	41100-0080-22	5.59	
(24 HOUR)			
10 mg, 5s ea	41100-0803-17	5.59	
10s ea	41100-0080-16	10.19	
30s ea	11523-7160-05	22.36	
(24HOUR)			
10 mg, 45s ea	11523-7237-01	29.16	
(24HOUR,NON-DROWSY)			
10 mg, 90s ea	11523-7237-05	39.77	
(A-S Medication)			
REPACK			
TAB,PO, 10 mg, 10s ea	54569-5495-00	10.19	
(Quality Care Prod)			
REPACK			
TAB,PO, 10 mg, 10s ea	49999-0123-10	61.74	
(Southwood)			
REPACK			
TAB,PO, 10 mg, 10s ea	58016-0560-10	10.19	
12s ea	58016-0560-12	12.23	
14s ea	58016-0560-14	14.27	
15s ea	58016-0560-15	15.29	
20s ea	58016-0560-20	20.38	
24s ea	58016-0560-24	24.46	
30s ea	58016-0560-30	30.57	
CLARITIN EYE (Schering Plough)			
SOL,OP (1X5ML,DROPS)			
0.025%, 5 ml	11523-7235-01	11.70	
CLARITIN LIQUI-GELS (Schering Plough)			
SGL,PO (NON-DROWSY)			
10 mg, 10s ea	11523-7200-01	10.96	
24s ea	11523-7200-02	23.16	
40s ea	11523-7200-03	31.15	
70s ea	11523-7200-04	41.39	
CLARITIN REDITABS (Schering Plough)			
ODT,PO (MINT)			
10 mg, 10s ea	41100-0806-02	10.19	
30s ea	41100-0806-04	22.36	
CLARITIN-D (Schering Plough)			
T24,PO, 10 mg-240 mg,			
5s ea	11523-7161-01	7.15	
5s ea	41100-0080-49	7.15	
10s ea	11523-7161-02	12.80	
CLARITIN-D 12HR (Schering Plough)			
T12,PO (NON-DROWSY)			
5 mg-120 mg,			
10s ea	11523-7162-01	11.12	
20s ea	41100-0802-17	18.86	
30s ea	41100-0803-19	23.26	
CLARITIN-D 24 HOUR (Schering Plough)			
T24,PO (NON-DROWSY)			
10 mg-240 mg,			
15s ea	11523-7161-03	17.70	
CLEAN & CLEAR ADVANTAGE 3 IN 1 EXFOLIATING CLEANSER (Johnson & Johnson)			
SOA,TP (1X141GM)			
5%, 141 gm	81371-0025-17	5.45	
CLEAN & CLEAR ADVANTAGE 3 IN 1 FOAMING ACNE WASH (Johnson & Johnson)			
SOA,TP (1X240ML,OIL-FREE)			
2%, 240 ml	81371-0025-80	5.45	
CLEAN & CLEAR ADVANTAGE ACNE CONTROL KIT (Johnson & Johnson)			
KIT,TP, ea	81370-0023-42	16.34	
CLEAN & CLEAR ADVANTAGE ACNE MOISTURIZER (Johnson & Johnson)			
LOT,TP (OIL-FREE)			
0.5%, 120 ml	81370-0023-40	5.45	
CLEAN & CLEAR ADVANTAGE ACNE SPOT TREATMENT (Johnson & Johnson)			
GEL,TP, 2%, 22 ml	81370-0039-91	5.45	
CLEAN & CLEAR ADVANTAGE BLACKHEAD ERASER (Johnson & Johnson)			
KIT,MR, 1%, ea	81370-0014-75	16.34	
CLEAN & CLEAR BLACKHEAD CLEARING SCRUB (Johnson & Johnson)			
SOA,TP, 2%, 226 gm	81370-0023-99	5.93	
CLEAN & CLEAR BLACKHEAD ERASER CLEANSING MASK (Johnson & Johnson)			
SOA,TP (1X113GM)			
0.5%, 113 gm	81371-0025-81	4.24	
CLEAN & CLEAR BLACKHEAD ERASER REFILL PACK (Johnson & Johnson)			
PAD,TP (+1ATTACHMENT HEAD)			
1%, 20s ea	81370-0015-60	4.97	
CLEAN & CLEAR BLACKHEAD ERASER SCRUB (Johnson & Johnson)			
SOA,TP, 2%, 141 gm	81370-0035-93	4.24	
CLEAN & CLEAR CONTINUOUS CONTROL ACNE CLEANSER (Johnson & Johnson)			
SOA,TP, 10%, 141 gm	81370-0032-89	4.97	
CLEAN & CLEAR CONTINUOUS CONTROL ACNE WASH (Johnson & Johnson)			
SOA,TP (OIL-FREE)			
2%, 177 ml	81370-0033-65	4.97	
CLEAN & CLEAR DAILY PORE CLEANSER (Johnson & Johnson)			
SOA,TP (OIL-FREE)			
156 gm	81370-0033-42	4.24	
CLEAN & CLEAR DEEP ACTION CREAM CLEANSER (Johnson & Johnson)			
CRE,TP (OIL-FREE)			
28 gm	81370-0016-42	0.78	
184 gm	81370-0033-61	4.24	
(SENSITIVE SKIN,OIL-FREE)			
184 gm	81370-0016-68	4.24	
(OIL-FREE)			
255 gm	81370-0023-98	4.97	
CLEAN & CLEAR DEEP ACTION EXFOLIATING SCRUB (Johnson & Johnson)			
SOA,TP (OIL-FREE)			
141 gm	81370-0019-36	4.24	
CLEAN & CLEAR DEEP CLEANING ASTRINGENT (Johnson & Johnson)			
SOL,TP (OIL-FIGHTING FORMULA)			
2%, 240 ml	81370-0033-67	3.38	
(Johnson Labs)			
SOL,TP (SENSITIVE SKIN)			
0.5%, 240 ml	81370-0033-77	3.38	
CLEAN & CLEAR DUAL ACTION MOISTURIZER (Johnson & Johnson)			
LOT,TP (OIL-FREE)			
0.5%, 120 ml	81370-0035-72	4.97	
CLEAN & CLEAR FOAMING FACIAL CLEANSER (Johnson & Johnson)			
SOA,TP (SENSITIVE SKIN,OIL-FREE)			
240 ml	81370-0033-87	3.76	
(OIL-FREE)			
0.25%, 240 ml	81370-0033-53	3.76	
CLEAN & CLEAR MAKEUP DISSOLVING FACIAL CLEANSING WIPES (Johnson & Johnson)			
PAD,TP (OIL-FREE)			
25s ea	81371-0015-03	4.97	
CLEAN & CLEAR MAKEUP DISSOLVING FOAMING CLEANSER (Johnson & Johnson)			
SOA,TP (OIL-FREE)			
177 ml	81371-0015-01	4.97	
CLEAN & CLEAR MORNING BURST DETOXIFYING CLEANSER (Johnson & Johnson)			
SOA,TP, 240 ml	81370-0027-86	4.97	
CLEAN & CLEAR MORNING BURST FACIAL CLEANSER (Johnson & Johnson)			
SOA,TP, 29 ml	81370-0016-38	0.78	
240 ml	81370-0016-17	4.97	
CLEAN & CLEAR MORNING BURST FACIAL SCRUB (Johnson & Johnson)			
SOA,TP, 141 gm	81370-0016-19	4.97	
CLEAN & CLEAR MORNING BURST IN-SHOWER FACIAL (Johnson & Johnson)			
SOA,TP (1X114GM)			
114 gm	81371-0025-53	4.97	
CLEAN & CLEAR MORNING BURST MOISTURIZER (Johnson & Johnson)			
LOT,TP (SHINE CONTROL,OIL-FREE)			
118 ml	81370-0023-97	4.97	
CLEAN & CLEAR MORNING BURST SHINE CONTROL CLEANSER (Johnson & Johnson)			
SOA,TP (OIL-FREE)			
240 ml	81370-0023-30	4.97	
CLEAN & CLEAR MORNING BURST SHINE CONTROL SCRUB (Johnson & Johnson)			
SOA,TP (OIL-FREE)			
141 gm	81370-0023-34	4.97	
CLEAN & CLEAR MORNING GLOW MOISTURIZER (Johnson & Johnson)			
LOT,TP (SPF15,OIL-FREE)			
3%-7.425%-2%,			
118 ml	81370-0016-20	4.97	
CLEAN & CLEAR OIL ABSORBING SHEETS (Johnson & Johnson)			
PAD,TP, 50s ea	81370-0035-66	4.24	
CLEAN & CLEAR OXYGENATING FIZZING CLEANSER (Johnson & Johnson)			
GEL,TP, 26 ml	81370-0021-39	0.78	
CLEAN & CLEAR PERSA-GEL 10 (Johnson & Johnson)			
GEL,TP, 10%, 28 gm	81370-0034-05	4.97	
CLEAN & CLEAR SOFT DAILY MOISTURIZER (Johnson & Johnson)			
LOT,TP (SPF15,OIL-FREE)			
118 ml	81370-0019-19	6.78	
CLEAN & CLEAR SOOTHING EYE MAKEUP REMOVER (Johnson & Johnson)			
SOL,TP (1X162ML,FRAGRANCE-FREE)			
162 ml	81371-0015-02	4.97	
CLEAN ZING! (Geritrex)			
SOL,MM (1X480ML,AF)			
0.06%, 480 ml	54162-0375-16	2.11	
CLEAN&CLEAR MORNING BURST DETOXIFYING FACIAL SCRUB (Johnson & Johnson)			
SOA,TP (1X141GM)			
141 gm	81370-0027-92	4.97	
CLEAR EYES (A-S Medication)			
REPACK			
SOL,OP, 0.012%, 15 ml	54569-2946-00	3.14	
CLEAR NASAL STRIPS (Major)			
DEV,NA (LATEX-FREE)			
30s ea	00904-5971-46	9.75	
(SMALL/MEDIUM STRIPS)			
30s ea	00904-5970-46	9.75	
CLEARBLUE EASY (Unipath)			
DEV,NA, ea	33472-0002-58	11.23	
2s ea	33472-0002-78	14.98	
CLEARPLAN EASY OVULATION (Unipath)			
DEV,NA (6 TESTS)			
ea	00573-0574-05	21.60	
CLEARSKIN MAXIMUM STRENGTH (Altaire)			
CRE,TP, 10%, 30 gm	59390-0079-17	3.75	
CLEMATIS (Ellon)			
SOL,SL (DROPS)			
10.5 ml	51762-0012-10		9.25
CLERZ 2 (Alcon Labs Cons Prod)			
SOL,OP, 15 ml	00580-0152-15	6.84	
CLERZ PLUS LENS DROPS (Alcon Labs Cons Prod)			
SOL,OP (THIMEROSAL-FREE)			
5 ml	00650-0192-05	3.06	
8 ml	00650-0192-10	4.46	
CLICKFINE UNIVERSAL PEN NEEDLE (Can-Am Care)			
DEV,NA (31G,6MM,1/4")			
100s ea	38396-0706-93	24.12	
(31G,8MM,5/16")			
100s ea	38396-0702-93	24.12	
CLINISTIX (Bayer Diabetes Care)			
DEV,NA, 50s ea	00193-2844-50	10.02	
CLINITEST (Bayer Diabetes Care)			
DEV,NA, 36s ea	00193-2127-36	7.56	
100s ea	00193-2126-21	17.28	
100s ea	00193-2159-21	22.92	

PROD/MFR	HRI, UPC,NDC	AWP	SRP
CLOFERA (Centrix)			
SOL,PO (1X473ML,AF,SF,DYE-FREE)			
12.5 mg/5 ml-30 mg/5 ml,			
473 ml	11528-0140-16	98.40	
CLORPACTIN WCS-90 (Guardian)			
PDR,TP, 2 gm, 2 gm 5s	00327-0001-10	25.25	
CLOSED POUCH ONE PIECE (Coloplast)			
DEV,NA (OPAQUE, 1 1/8")			
30s ea	11701-0809-22	96.90	101.40
(OPAQUE, 1 3/8")			
30s ea	11701-0809-23	96.90	101.40
(OPAQUE, 1 5/8")			
30s ea	11701-0809-24	96.90	101.40
(OPAQUE, 1 7/8")			
30s ea	11701-0809-25	96.90	101.40
(OPAQUE, 1")			
30s ea	11701-0809-21	96.90	101.40
(OPAQUE, 1/2"-2 1/4")			
30s ea	11701-0809-19	96.90	101.40
30s ea	11701-0809-20	96.90	101.40
(OPAQUE, 2 3/8")			
30s ea	11701-0809-27	96.90	101.40
(OPAQUE, 2")			
30s ea	11701-0809-26	96.90	101.40
(TRANSPARENT, 1 1/8")			
30s ea	11701-0809-13	96.90	101.40
(TRANSPARENT, 1 3/8")			
30s ea	11701-0809-14	96.90	101.40
(TRANSPARENT, 1 5/8")			
30s ea	11701-0809-15	96.90	101.40
(TRANSPARENT, 1 7/8")			
30s ea	11701-0809-16	96.90	101.40
(TRANSPARENT, 1")			
30s ea	11701-0809-12	96.90	101.40
(TRANSPARENT, 2 3/8")			
30s ea	11701-0809-18	96.90	101.40
(TRANSPARENT, 2")			
30s ea	11701-0809-17	96.90	101.40
(TRANSPARENT,1/2"-2 1/4")			
30s ea	11701-0809-10	96.90	101.40
30s ea	11701-0809-11	96.90	101.40
CLOSED POUCH TWO PIECE (Coloplast)			
DEV,NA (OPAQUE, UP TO 1 1/4")			
30s ea	11701-0814-25	59.40	62.10
(OPAQUE, UP TO 1 3/4")			
30s ea	11701-0814-30	59.40	62.10
(OPAQUE, UP TO 2")			
30s ea	11701-0814-35	59.40	62.10
(TRANSPARENT, UP TO 2")			
30s ea	11701-0814-20	59.40	62.10
(TRANSPARENT,TO 1 1/4")			
30s ea	11701-0814-10	59.40	62.10
(TRANSPARENT,TO 1 3/4")			
30s ea	11701-0814-15	59.40	62.10
CLOTRIM ANTIFUNGAL (Major)			
CRE,TP, 1%, 15 gm	00904-7822-36	5.29	
30 gm	00904-7822-31	8.29	
CLOTRIMAZOLE (Actavis Mid Atlantic)			
CRE,VG (W/1 APPLICATOR)			
1%, 45 gm	00472-0220-63	12.00	
(W/7 APPLICATORS)			
1%, 45 gm	00472-0220-41	12.00	
(AmerisourceBergen)			
CRE,TP (PRIVATE LABEL)			
1%, 15 gm	24385-0205-01	5.39	5.99
30 gm	24385-0205-03	7.19	7.99
(Taro)			
CRE,TP, 1%, 15 gm	51672-2002-01	4.25	
30 gm	51672-2002-02	5.50	
VG (W/APPLICATOR)			
1%, 45 gm	51672-2003-06	8.00	
(A-S Medication)			
REPACK			
CRE,VG, 1%, 15 gm	54569-3979-00	19.92	
30 gm	54569-4328-00	34.83	
(W/7 APPLICATORS)			
1%, 45 gm	54569-4546-00	12.00	
(Altura)			
REPACK			
CRE,TP, 1%, 15 gm	63874-0057-15	23.71	
30 gm	63874-0057-30	24.08	
(DHS, Inc.)			
REPACK			
CRE,TP, 1%, 15 gm	55887-0908-15	12.45	
30 gm	55887-0908-01	24.09	
45 gm	55887-0908-45	36.98	
(Dispensing Solutions)			
REPACK			
CRE,TP (1X15GM)			
1%, 15 gm	55045-3916-05	7.00	
(1X30GM)			
1%, 30 gm	55045-3916-03	10.00	
CRE,VG, 1%, 45 gm	55045-2174-07	10.99	
(PD-Rx Pharm)			
REPACK			
LOZ,MM, 10 mg, 35s ea	58864-0814-35	31.83	
(Pharma Pac)			
REPACK			
CRE,VG, 1%, 45 gm	52959-0621-01	25.64	
(Phys Total Care)			
REPACK			
CRE,TP, 1%, 15 gm	54868-3068-01	37.96	
TAB,VG, 100 mg, 7s ea	54868-3357-00	35.15	
(Physician Partner)			
REPACK			
CRE,TP (1X15GM)			
1%, 15 gm	21695-0035-15	24.32	
(Quality Care Prod)			
REPACK			
CRE,TP, 1%, 30 gm	49999-0170-30	26.76	
CRE,VG, 1%, 45 gm	49999-0302-45	40.14	
CLOTRIMAZOLE 3 (Taro)			
CRE,VG (W/APPLICATORS)			
2%, 21 gm	51672-6708-00	10.60	
CLOTRIMAZOLE 7 (Phys Total Care)			
REPACK			
CRE,VG, 1%, 45 gm	54868-3763-00	20.93	
CLOTRIMAZOLE A/F (Pharma Pac)			
REPACK			
CRE,TP, 1%, 15 gm	52959-0088-03	9.95	
30 gm	52959-0088-05	15.90	
CLOTRIMAZOLE ANTIFUNGAL (Cardinal Health)			
CRE,TP (PRIVATE LABEL)			
1%, 30 gm	37205-0160-10	6.42	
CLOVERINE SALVE (Medtech)			
OIN,TP (WHITE)			
30 gm	75137-0303-63	2.42	
CLUSIMAR (Marlop)			
LIQ,PO, 240 ml	12939-0160-08	7.50	
CLUSINEX (PGD, Inc.)			
SYR,PO, 480 ml	65615-0402-16	20.00	
(Pharmakon)			
SYR,PO (FRUIT)			
240 ml	55422-0402-08	5.24	10.91
CO Q-10 (Rexall)			
CAP,PO (SOFTGEL)			
50 mg, 30s ea	30768-0000-98	11.21	16.98
SGL,PO, 30 mg, 30s ea	30768-0000-27	8.25	12.50
100 mg-5 iu,			
30s ea	30768-0040-53	13.80	19.99
CO-APAP (Phys Total Care)			
REPACK			
TAB,PO, 325 mg-2 mg-15 mg-30 mg,			
1000s ea	54868-3643-00	99.90	
CO-Q-10 (Carlson,J.R.)			
SGL,PO (PF,CORN-FREE,WHEAT-FREE)			
30 mg-1 iu, 30s ea	88395-0082-10	3.75	7.50
60s ea	88395-0082-14	6.45	12.90
120s ea	88395-0082-11	11.95	23.90
240s ea	88395-0082-12	22.45	44.90
360s ea	88395-0082-13	32.50	65.00
50 mg-1 iu, 30s ea	88395-0082-20	5.45	10.90
60s ea	88395-0082-24	9.45	18.90
120s ea	88395-0082-21	17.95	35.90
100 mg-1 iu,			
30s ea	88395-0082-40	7.45	14.90
90s ea	88395-0082-41	19.95	39.90
200 mg-1 iu,			
30s ea	88395-0082-50	12.45	24.90
90s ea	88395-0082-51	34.95	69.90
CO-Q10 (ADH)			
SGL,PO, 30 mg, 60s ea	60142-0097-06	11.98	23.95
TAB,PO (AF,PF)			
60 mg, 60s ea	60142-0495-36	19.98	39.95
180s ea	60142-0495-38	55.48	110.95
(Carlson,J.R.)			
SGL,PO (SOFTGEL)			
300 mg-3 iu, 30s ea	88395-0082-60	17.45	34.90
90s ea	88395-0082-61	48.50	97.00
COACH ELASTIC BANDAGE (Johnson & Johnson)			
DEV,NA (2IN X 80IN)			
ea	81370-0079-28	2.62	
(3IN X 80IN)			
ea	81370-0079-29	3.28	
COACH SPORTS TAPE (Johnson & Johnson)			
DEV,NA (1 1/2INX10YDS)			
ea	81370-0079-02	2.48	
4s ea	81370-0079-49	8.16	
COAL TAR (Amend)			
SOL,TP (U.S.P.)			
20%, 3840 ml	17317-0123-06	56.00	
COATS ALOE VERA JUICE DRINK (Coats Aloe Int'l)			
SOL,PO (96%,KIWI-BERRY)			
1000 ml	32295-0708-33	8.00	12.00
(96%,LEMON,LIME)			
1000 ml	58826-0706-33	8.00	12.00
(96%,ORANGE-PAPAYA)			
1000 ml	32295-0709-33	8.00	12.00
COBAL COMPLEX (Merit)			
TAB,SL, 100s ea	30727-0445-07	17.95	
COBAN LATEX FREE SELF-ADHERENT WRAP (3M Health Care)			
DEV,NA (6"X5 YDS,NON-STERILE)			
12s ea	08333-2086-01	56.55	
(6"X5 YDS,STERILE)			
12s ea	08333-2086-10	95.75	
(4"X5 YDS,NON-STERILE)			
18s ea	08333-2084-01	60.40	
(4"X5 YDS,STERILE)			
18s ea	08333-2084-10	89.95	
(4"X6 1/2 YD,NON-STERILE)			
18s ea	08333-2084-30	72.50	
(3"X5 YDS,NON-STERILE)			
24s ea	08333-2083-01	64.35	
(3"X5 YDS,STERILE)			
24s ea	08333-2083-10	95.75	
(1"X5 YDS,NON-STERILE)			
30s ea	08333-2081-01	35.15	
(2"X5 YDS,NON-STERILE)			
36s ea	08333-2082-01	76.90	
COBAN SELF-ADHERENT WRAP (3M Health Care)			
DEV,NA (3"X5 YDS,ASSORTED)			
12s ea	08333-1583-26	28.00	
(3"X5 YDS,NEON ASSORTED)			
12s ea	08333-1583-14	28.00	
(6"X5 YDS,STERILE,TAN)			
12s ea	08333-1586-10	83.20	
(6"X5 YDS,TAN)			
12s ea	08333-1586-01	48.20	
(4"X5 YDS,BLUE)			
18s ea	08333-1584-02	52.50	
(4"X5 YDS,STERILE,TAN)			
18s ea	08333-1584-10	78.20	
(4"X5 YDS,TAN)			
18s ea	08333-1584-01	52.50	
(4"X6.5 YDS,TAN)			
18s ea	08333-1584-30	63.05	
(3"X5 YDS,BLUE)			
24s ea	08333-1583-02	55.90	
(3"X5 YDS,GREEN)			
24s ea	08333-1583-07	55.90	
(3"X5 YDS,RED)			
24s ea	08333-1583-18	55.90	
(3"X5 YDS,STERILE,TAN)			
24s ea	08333-1583-10	83.20	
(3"X5 YDS,TAN)			
24s ea	08333-1583-01	55.90	
(3"X5 YDS,WHITE)			
24s ea	08333-1583-23	55.90	
(3"X5 YDS,YELLOW)			
24s ea	08333-1583-25	55.90	
(1"X5 YDS,BLUE)			
30s ea	08333-1581-02	30.55	
(1"X5 YDS,TAN)			
30s ea	08333-1581-01	30.55	
(2"X5 YDS,BLUE)			
36s ea	08333-1582-02	62.80	
(2"X5 YDS,TAN)			
36s ea	08333-1582-01	66.85	
COCYNTAL (Boiron)			
LIQ,PO (BABY COLIC,AF,SF)			
1 ml 30s UD	06969-0045-09	6.07	10.19
COD LIVER OIL (Basic Vitamins)			
CAP,PO, 1250 iu-133 iu,			
90s ea	00761-0610-18	2.15	
(Carlson,J.R.)			
OIL,PO, 250 ml	88395-0013-21	13.45	26.90

PROD/MFR	HRI. UPC.NDC	AWP	SRP
(LEMON,LEMON)			
250 ml	88395-0013-51	13.45	26.90
500 ml	88395-0013-22	23.45	46.90
(LEMON,LEMON)			
500 ml	88395-0013-52	23.45	46.90
SGL,PO (PF,SOFT GEL)			
300s ea	88395-0013-93	12.45	24.90
(SOFTGEL)			
1250 iu-135 iu,			
100s ea	88395-0013-11	3.70	7.40
250s ea	88395-0013-12	7.30	14.60
(Chain Drug Marketing)			
OIL,PO, 118 ml	63868-0325-04	3.54	4.99
(Family Phcy)			
SGL,PO (PRIVATE LABEL)			
1250 iu-135 iu,			
100s ea	52735-0013-01	2.96	3.39
(Health Products Corp)			
SGL,PO (PF,SF,SOFTGEL)			
100s ea	39686-0013-76	2.80	
(Key Company)			
SGL,PO (SOFTGEL)			
1250 iu-135 iu,			
100s ea	11694-0828-01	3.75	
(Lex)			
SGL,PO (SF)			
1250 iu-135 iu,			
100s ea	58537-0721-05	0.90	
500s ea	58537-0072-10	1.80	
(Major)			
CAP,PO, 100s ea	00904-4225-60	3.72	
(Mason Vit)			
CAP,PO (PF,SF,SOFTGEL)			
2500 iu-270 iu, 60s ea	11845-0059-75	5.00	
(20 MIN)			
2500 iu-270 iu,			
100s ea	11845-0059-71	6.56	
SGL,PO (10 MIN)			
1250 iu-135 iu,			
100s ea	11845-0053-41	5.11	
(Nature's Bounty)			
SGL,PO (HIGH STRENGTH,PF,SF)			
1000 mg, 60s ea	74312-0077-41		4.89
(PF,SF,SOFTGEL)			
1250 iu-135 iu,			
100s ea	74312-0011-50		4.89
(Pharmavite)			
SGL,PO (SOFTGEL)			
1250 iu-130 iu,			
100s ea	31604-0013-25	2.93	
(Rexall)			
SGL,PO (SOFTGEL)			
100s ea	30768-0001-61	1.53	2.32
(Rugby)			
SGL,PO (SOFT GEL, SOD FREE,PF)			
1250 iu-130 iu,			
100s ea	00536-6384-01	3.30	
COD LIVER OIL EXTRACT/MINERAL (McCoy's)			
KIT,PO, 103s ea	31088-0791-03	3.80	5.70
COD LIVER OIL NATURAL (AmerisourceBergen)			
SGL,PO (PRIVATE LABEL,SOFTGEL)			
100s ea	24385-0284-78	3.32	3.69
CODAL-DM (Cypress Pharm)			
SYR,PO (AF,SF,DYE-FREE,CHERRY)			
473 ml	60258-0771-16	17.95	
CODIMAL DM (Phys Total Care)			
REPACK			
SYR,PO, 120 ml	54868-1612-01	17.84	
CODITUSS DM (Qualitest)			
SYR,PO (AF,SF,DYE-FREE,CHERRY)			
120 ml	00603-0728-54	5.92	
COENZYME Q-10 (Freeda)			
TAB,PO (SF,DYE-FREE)			
50 mg, 50s ea	10432-0323-00	17.37	28.95
(PURE,SF,GLUTEN-FREE)			
50 mg, 100s ea	10432-0323-01	31.74	
(SF,GLUTEN-FREE)			
100 mg, 50s ea	10432-0366-00	29.94	49.90
(Major)			
SGL,PO (PF,SF,GLUTEN-FREE)			
10 mg, 30s ea	00904-5615-46	4.50	
50 mg, 30s ea	00904-5616-46	19.50	
(SOFTGEL)			
100 mg, 30s ea	00904-5882-46	14.69	
200 mg, 30s ea	00904-5883-46	22.74	
400 mg, 30s ea	00904-5884-46	43.54	
(Westlake Labs.)			
CTB,PO (PF)			
100 mg, 60s ea	10539-0671-00	54.60	78.00
200 mg, 60s ea	10539-0672-00	100.80	144.00
COENZYME Q10 (Advanced Nutr)			
SGL,PO (SOFTGEL)			
30 mg-1 iu, 60s ea	62617-0405-02	22.13	29.50
(Basic Vitamins)			
SGL,PO, 30 mg, 30s ea	00761-0210-06	5.40	
(Bio-Tech Pharm)			
CAP,PO, 150 mg, 60s ea	53191-0230-06	49.00	
(Key Company)			
CAP,PO (PF,SF,STARCH-FREE)			
30 mg, 60s ea	11694-0689-01	15.50	
60 mg, 60s ea	11694-0685-01	23.50	
(Major)			
SGL,PO (SOFTGEL)			
30 mg, 30s ea	00904-5015-46	11.50	
(Mason Vit)			
CAP,PO (PF,SF,SOFTGEL)			
60 mg, 30s ea	11845-0131-88	24.33	
(BONUSPAK,PF,SF,SOFTGEL)			
60 mg, 60s ea	11845-0131-85	42.11	
(PF,SF,SOFTGEL)			
150 mg, 30s ea	11845-0132-38	48.78	
SGL,PO, 10 mg, 60s ea	11845-0123-15	12.78	
30 mg, 30s ea	11845-0123-28	15.44	
(BONUSPAK,PF,SF,SOFTGEL)			
30 mg, 60s ea	11845-0123-25	26.56	
(PF,SF,SOFTGEL)			
100 mg, 30s ea	11845-0131-98	33.22	
(Miller)			
CAP,PO, 10 mg, 60s ea	17204-0446-20	6.96	11.60
60 mg, 60s ea	17204-0449-20	24.60	
LIQ,PO, 30 mg/5 ml,			
480 ml	17204-0445-95	65.00	
SGL,PO, 30 mg, 30s ea	17204-0447-36	10.68	15.00
(SOFTGEL)			
100 mg-100 iu, 30s ea	17204-0583-36	45.00	
60s ea	17204-0463-20	81.00	
(Nature's Bounty)			
CAP,PO (PF,SF,SOFTGEL)			
10 mg, 50s ea	74312-0047-10		8.29
SGL,PO, 30 mg, 50s ea	74312-0072-70		15.50
(Rugby)			
SGL,PO (NATURAL,SOFTGEL)			
100 mg-10 iu, 30s ea	00536-1938-07	13.02	
200 mg-20 iu,			
30s ea	00536-2030-07	16.76	
COHERE-WRAP (Hart Health)			
DEV,NA (BLUE,2"X5 YD)			
ea	50332-0156-31	1.29	
(BLUE,3"X5 YD)			
ea	50332-0156-21	1.69	
ea	50332-0156-41	1.69	
(TAN,1"X5 YD)			
ea	50332-0156-01	1.49	
(TAN,2"X5 YD)			
ea	50332-0156-11	1.29	
COL-RITE (Rite Aid)			
SGL,PO (PRIVATE LABEL)			
100 mg, 100s ea	11822-0017-08	6.39	7.99
250s ea	11822-0003-96	8.79	10.99
COLACE (Purdue Products L.P.)			
LIQ,PO (W/DROPPER)			
100 mg/10 ml,			
30 ml	67618-0102-30	7.90	
SGL,PO, 50 mg, 30s ea	67618-0100-30	8.22	
60s ea	67618-0100-60	14.79	
100 mg, 10s ea UD	67618-0101-10	3.60	
30s ea	67618-0101-30	9.96	
60s ea	67618-0101-60	18.07	
250s ea	67618-0101-52	73.57	
SOL,PO (SYRUP,AF,SF)			
20 mg/5 ml, 473 ml	67618-0103-16	21.66	
SUP,RC, 2.1 gm, 24s ea	67618-0104-24	2.04	
(Phys Total Care)			
REPACK			
LIQ,PO, 150 mg/15 ml,			
30 ml	54868-3839-00	10.93	
SGL,PO, 100 mg, 60s ea	54868-2337-00	21.98	
(Quality Care Prod)			
REPACK			
SGL,PO, 100 mg, 30s ea	49999-0587-30	41.20	
60s ea	49999-0587-60	82.40	
(Southwood)			
REPACK			
LIQ,PO (1X30ML)			
100 mg/10 ml,			
30 ml	58016-4815-01	7.90	
COLACE INFANT/CHILD (Purdue Products L.P.)			
SUP,RC, 1.2 gm, ea	67618-0105-12	1.36	
COLAMINE (Bio-Tech Pharm)			
CAP,PO			
37 mg-23 mg-109 mg-29 mg,			
100s ea	53191-0353-01	13.50	
COLD & COUGH MEDICINE PLUS (Teva)			
SGL,PO (SOFTGEL)			
325 mg-2 mg-10 mg-30 mg,			
24s ea	00182-1177-16	6.99	
COLD & HOT PAIN RELIEF PATCH (Major)			
TDM,TP (EXTRA STRENGTH)			
5%, 5s ea	00904-5694-01	5.25	
COLD CONTROL PE (Reese)			
TAB,PO (CAPLET)			
650 mg-25 mg-10 mg,			
30s ea	10956-0792-30	4.92	7.49
COLD EEZE CHERRY (Dispensing Solutions)			
REPACK			
LOZ,MM, 13.3 mg, 18s ea	55045-3521-01	5.25	
COLD EEZE CITRUS (Dispensing Solutions)			
LOZ,MM, 13.3 mg, 18s ea	55045-3520-01	5.25	
COLD MEDICINE PLUS (Teva)			
SGL,PO (SOFTGEL)			
325 mg-2 mg-30 mg,			
24s ea	00182-1183-16	6.99	
COLD RELIEF-MULTI SYMPTOM (Basic Vitamins)			
TAB,PO, 500 mg-2 mg-15 mg-30 mg,			
50s ea	00761-0241-10	2.40	
COLD REMEDY (Major)			
ODT,PO (CHERRY)			
2 x-1 x, 25s ea	00904-5876-17	8.43	
COLD SORE (Pfeiffer)			
LOT,TP, 15 ml	00927-0435-23	1.68	3.02
COLD SPRAY (Hart Health)			
SPR,TP, 113 gm	50332-0216-01	2.44	
COLD-EEZE (Quigley)			
LOZ,MM (BAG,CHERRY)			
13.3 mg, 18s ea	91108-0100-01	3.50	5.95
(BAG,CITRUS)			
13.3 mg, 18s ea	91108-0100-00	3.50	5.95
(BAG,FRUIT,TROPICAL)			
13.3 mg, 18s ea	91108-0100-02	3.50	5.95
(BOX,CHERRY)			
13.3 mg, 18s ea	91108-0100-13	3.50	5.95
(BOX,CITRUS)			
13.3 mg, 18s ea	91108-0100-12	3.50	5.95
(A-S Medication)			
REPACK			
LOZ,MM, 13.3 mg, 18s ea	54569-5849-00	4.38	
COLDCALM (Boiron)			
TAB,PO, 60s ea	06962-0607-60	5.73	9.59
COLDONYL (Medique)			
TAB,PO (250X2,SF,CAFFEINE-FREE)			
325 mg-100 mg-5 mg,			
500s ea UD	47682-0253-07	24.41	
COLDS (Nuage Labs)			
TAB,SL (TISSUE J)			
125s ea	00634-0910-68	3.05	5.09
COLGATE TOTAL (Colgate-Palmolive)			
PAS,TP, 126 gm	35000-0740-02	2.05	
180 gm	35000-0740-03	2.45	
234 gm	35000-0740-04	2.86	
COLLADERM (Genesis)			
GEL,TP, 60 gm	00398-0112-02	8.46	
LOT,TP, 57 ml	00398-0094-23	8.46	
COLLOIDAL SILVER (Nature's Bounty)			
LIQ,PO (PF,DAIRY-FREE,DYE-FREE)			
118.3 ml	74312-0040-10		12.99
COLLYRIUM FOR FRESH EYES (Bausch & Lomb Inc.)			
SOL,OP (EYE WASH)			
5%, 120 ml	10119-0007-38	4.00	
COLOCYNTHIS (Luyties)			
TAB,SL (6X)			
6 x, 500s ea	00618-2212-03	3.99	
5500s ea	00618-2212-10	30.32	
(30X)			
12 x, 500s ea	00622-2212-03	4.19	

PROD/MFR	HRI, UPC,NDC	AWP	SRP
5500s ea	00622-2212-10	31.83	
30 x, 500s ea	00624-2212-03	4.19	
5500s ea	00624-2212-10	31.83	
COLON HERBAL CLEANSER (Mason Vit)			
CAP,PO (PF,SF)			
100s ea	11845-0122-21	7.33	
COLOPLAST PREP (Coloplast)			
LOT,TP (SECOND SKIN)			
59 ml 12s	11701-0007-03	45.36	47.52
SWA,TP (SECOND SKIN,54X12)			
648s ea	11701-0007-20	142.56	149.04
COLOR LANCETS (Cardinal Health)			
DEV,NA (PRIVATE LABEL)			
200s ea	37205-0118-82	9.79	
COLUMBIA ANTISEPTIC (Sturtevant,F.C.)			
POW,TP, 28.3 gm	17642-0010-01	2.55	3.99
170.1 gm	57464-0613-47	5.50	8.99
396.9 gm	57464-0226-72	9.00	13.99
COMBISTIX (Siemens)			
DEV,NA, 100s ea	08620-2183-21	61.30	
COMFEEL ALGINATE (Coloplast)			
DEV,NA (4"X4")			
10s ea	11701-0836-15	63.50	66.40
COMFEEL ALGINATE FILLER (Coloplast)			
DEV,NA (6"X6")			
10s ea	11701-0836-20	123.20	128.90
COMFEEL FILM TRANSPARENT (Coloplast)			
DEV,NA (ADHESIVE,11 1/2X15 3/4")			
10s ea	11701-0420-95	120.40	126.00
(ADHESIVE,8"X11 1/2")			
10s ea	11701-0420-92	62.10	65.00
(ADHESIVE,9"X5 1/2")			
10s ea	11701-0420-93	47.30	49.50
(ADHESIVE,4"X4 3/4")			
50s ea	11701-0420-82	87.00	91.00
(ADHESIVE,2 3/8"X2 3/4")			
100s ea	11701-0420-81	57.00	59.00
COMFEEL HYDROCOLLOID FILLER (Coloplast)			
DEV,NA (STERILE)			
6 gm 6s	11701-0411-41	69.96	73.20
12 gm 10s	11701-0410-40	46.30	48.40
50 gm 6s	11701-0410-24	105.18	110.04
COMFEEL PLUS CLEAR HYDROCOLLOID (Coloplast)			
DEV,NA (THIN, 6"X6")			
5s ea	11701-0406-90	49.30	51.55
(THIN, 6"X8")			
5s ea	11701-0406-85	60.80	63.65
(THIN, 8"X8")			
5s ea	11701-0406-91	72.50	75.85
(THIN, 2"X2-3/4")			
10s ea	11701-0406-74	35.80	37.40
(THIN, 3-1/2"X5-1/2")			
10s ea	11701-0406-75	66.90	70.00
(THIN, 4"X4")			
10s ea	11701-0406-80	53.80	56.30
COMFEEL PLUS CONTOUR HYDROCOLLOID (Coloplast)			
DEV,NA (BUTTERFLY, 24 SUBQ)			
5s ea	11701-0407-77	39.75	41.60
(BUTTERFLY, 42 SUBQ)			
5s ea	11701-0407-78	59.00	61.75
COMFEEL PLUS PRD HYDROCOLLOID (Coloplast)			
DEV,NA (4" ROUND)			
5s ea	11701-0408-61	50.20	52.55
(6" ROUND)			
5s ea	11701-0408-62	106.10	52.55
(BUTTERFLY, 3")			
5s ea	11701-0408-60	42.90	44.90
COMFEEL PLUS TRIANGLE (Coloplast)			
DEV,NA (7"X8")			
5s ea	11701-0407-72	87.70	91.90
COMFEEL PLUS ULCER DRESSING (Coloplast)			
DEV,NA (STERILE,1-1/2"X2-1/2")			
30s ea	11701-0406-73	125.40	131.10
COMFEEL PLUS ULCER HYDROCOLLOID (Coloplast)			
DEV,NA (4"X4")			
5s ea	11701-0405-80	36.05	37.70
(6"X6")			
5s ea	11701-0405-90	75.25	78.75
(8"X8")			
5s ea	11701-0405-91	128.55	134.55
COMFEEL ULCER CARE HYDROCOLLOID (Coloplast)			
DEV,NA (STERILE,4"X4")			
5s ea	11701-0409-80	31.30	32.75
(STERILE,6"X6")			
5s ea	11701-0409-90	67.35	70.45
(STERILE,8"X8")			
5s ea	11701-0409-91	113.10	118.35
(STERILE,1-1/2"X2-1/2")			
30s ea	11701-0409-73	85.20	89.10
COMFORT POINT INSULIN PEN NEEDLES (Exelint)			
DEV,NA (29GX 1/2",LATEX-FREE)			
100s ea	08287-1260-03	21.25	
(31GX 1/3",LATEX-FREE)			
100s ea	08287-1260-05	21.25	
(31GX 1/4",LATEX-FREE)			
100s ea	08287-1260-04	21.25	
COMFORT POINT INSULIN SYRINGE (Exelint)			
DEV,NA (28G,LATEX-FREE)			
100s ea	08287-1260-26	12.50	
100s ea	08287-1260-27	12.50	
(29G,LATEX-FREE)			
100s ea	08287-1260-21	12.50	
100s ea	08287-1260-28	12.50	
100s ea	08287-1260-29	12.50	
(30G,LATEX-FREE)			
100s ea	08287-1260-14	12.50	
100s ea	08287-1260-15	12.50	
100s ea	08287-1260-16	12.50	
COMFORTLANCETS (Diabetic Supplies)			
DEV,NA (STERILE,SINGLE-USE)			
100s ea	08214-0657-11	4.75	
COMLINK DOWNLOAD CABLE (Medtronic Minimed)			
DEV,NA, ea	76300-0734-01	124.94	
COMMIT (Glaxo)			
LOZ,MM (3X24,POPPAC,MINT)			
2 mg, 72s ea	00135-0208-01	39.37	
4 mg, 72s ea	00135-0209-01	39.37	
LOZ,PO (CHERRY)			
2 mg, 48s ea	07661-0551-00	28.03	
72s ea	07661-0551-30	28.03	
108s ea	07661-0400-15	54.56	
(CHERRY)			
2 mg, 108s ea	07661-0551-40	54.56	
(MINT)			
2 mg, 192s ea	07661-0500-56	78.10	
(CHERRY)			
4 mg, 48s ea	07661-0551-50	28.03	
72s ea	07661-0551-70	39.37	
108s ea	07661-0551-80	54.56	
(MINT)			
4 mg, 192s ea	07661-0500-66	78.10	
(A-S Medication)			
REPACK			
LOZ,MM (MINT)			
2 mg, 72s ea	54569-6158-00	39.37	
4 mg, 72s ea	54569-6157-00	39.37	
COMPANION AMBULATORY TRANSPORTER (Abbott)			
DEV,NA, ea	70074-0005-04	122.48	
COMPANION CLEARSTAR PUMP (Abbott)			
DEV,NA, ea	70074-0552-38	1318.80	
COMPANION ENTERAL NUTRITION PUMP (Abbott)			
DEV,NA (REFURBISHED)			
ea	70074-0547-48	940.50	
30s ea	70074-0000-86	7.76	
COMPAT BAGGLE CONTAINER (Nestle)			
DEV,NA (SEMI-RIGID, 1000 ML)			
30s ea	00212-9313-94	149.40	
(SEMI-RIGID, 500 ML)			
30s ea	00212-9312-94	142.20	
COMPAT CONTAINER GRAVITY DELIVERY (Nestle)			
DEV,NA (1000 ML)			
30s ea	00212-9211-94	136.44	
(500 ML)			
30s ea	00212-9210-94	122.04	
COMPAT DUALFLO ENTERAL FEEDING PUMP (Nestle)			
DEV,NA, 30s ea	00212-9255-94	612.00	
COMPAT DUALFLO PUMP (Nestle)			
DEV,NA (FORMULA & WATER BAGS)			
30s ea	00212-9447-94	336.24	
COMPAT DUALFLO PUMP PIERCING SPIKE (Nestle)			
DEV,NA (W/WATER BAG)			
30s ea	00212-9407-94	209.52	
COMPAT ENTERAL DELIVERY PUMP (Nestle)			
DEV,NA (W/DOSE LIMIT/MEMORY)			
ea	00212-9235-94	480.00	
COMPAT GASTROSTOMY/JEJUNOSTOMY TUBE (Nestle)			
DEV,NA (28/12 FR, SURGICAL)			
ea	00212-8800-93	239.40	
COMPAT JEJUNOSTOMY FEEDING TUBE (Nestle)			
DEV,NA (5 FR)			
10s ea	00212-7284-90	985.62	
(7 FR)			
10s ea	00212-7287-90	996.12	
COMPAT NASOGASTRIC TUBE W/STYLET (Nestle)			
DEV,NA (10 FR, W/WTD BOLUS)			
10s ea	00212-8316-91	274.44	
(12 FR, W/WTD BOLUS)			
10s ea	00212-8315-91	271.92	
(8 FR, W/WTD BOLUS)			
10s ea	00212-8314-91	269.40	
COMPAT NASOJEJUNAL/G-TUBE COMBO (Nestle)			
DEV,NA (9/18 FR,G-DECOMPRESSION)			
ea	00212-8231-91	236.04	
COMPAT REPLACEMENT G-TUBE (Nestle)			
DEV,NA (14 FR, 5CC BALLOON)			
5s ea	00212-8744-91	169.92	
(16 FR, 15CC BALLOON)			
5s ea	00212-8746-91	169.92	
(18 FR, 15CC BALLOON)			
5s ea	00212-8748-91	169.92	
(20 FR, 15CC BALLOON)			
5s ea	00212-8740-91	169.92	
(22 FR, 15CC BALLOON)			
5s ea	00212-8742-91	169.92	
(24 FR, 15CC BALLOON)			
5s ea	00212-8744-95	169.92	
COMPAT SELECTFLO FEEDING PUMP (Nestle)			
DEV,NA (ENTERAL)			
ea	00212-9245-94	480.00	
COMPAT VINYL BAG/GRAVITY (Nestle)			
DEV,NA (1000 ML)			
30s ea	00212-9216-94	96.84	
COMPAT Y SET (Nestle)			
DEV,NA (W/PIERCING SPIKE)			
30s ea	00212-9507-94	86.40	
(W/VINYL BAG,LATEX-FREE)			
30s ea	00212-9547-94	92.88	
COMPAT Y-ADAPTER LUER TIP (Nestle)			
DEV,NA (LARGE)			
5s ea	00212-8803-93	32.34	
(MEDIUM)			
5s ea	00212-8753-93	32.34	
(SMALL)			
5s ea	00212-8713-93	32.70	
COMPETE (Mission)			
TAB,PO, 100s ea	00178-0221-01	8.31	
COMPLEAT (Nestle)			
SUS,PO (6X1000ML)			
1000 ml 6s	43900-0141-80	89.50	
(6X1500ML)			
1500 ml 6s	43900-0141-82	127.87	
COMPLEAT PEDIATRIC (Nestle)			
LIQ,PO (BLENDERIZED TUBE FDG.)			
250 ml 24s	00212-1424-51	73.15	
COMPLEAT-MODIFIED (Nestle)			
LIQ,PO (BLENDERIZED TUBE FDG.)			
250 ml 24s	00212-1401-51	78.05	
(CLOSED SYSTEM TUBE FDG)			
1000 ml 6s	00212-1414-42	89.50	
1500 ml 6s	00212-1414-44	127.87	
COMPLERE (Miller)			
TAB,PO, 100s ea	17204-0807-40	6.96	11.60
COMPLETE (Major)			
CTB,PO (DUAL ACTION,BERRY)			
800 mg-10 mg-165 mg,			
25s ea	00904-5835-17	11.18	
(Prime Marketing)			
TAB,PO, 130s ea	62107-0041-13	8.24	
COMPLETE ALLERGY (Cardinal Health)			
ELI,PO (AF,PRIVATE LABEL,CHERRY)			
12.5 mg/5 ml,			
118 ml	37205-0565-26	3.59	
240 ml	37205-0565-34	3.12	
COMPLETE ALLERGY MEDICATION (Advance)			
TAB,PO (CAPLET)			
25 mg, 24s ea	17714-0042-24	1.99	
COMPLETE ALLERGY MEDICINE (Cardinal Health)			
CAP,PO (PRIVATE LABEL)			
25 mg, 24s ea	37205-0277-62	2.07	
100s ea	37205-0277-78	7.04	
TAB,PO, 25 mg, 24s ea	37205-0270-62	3.28	
100s ea	37205-0270-78	5.14	

PROD/MFR | HRI, UPC,NDC | AWP | SRP

COMPLETE AMINO ACID MIX (Nutricia)
PDR,PO (USE W/MED SUPV)
200 gm 2s........... 49735-0101-24 204.10

COMPLETE BRAND (Allergan Inc)
SOL,NA (LUBRICATING & REWETTING)
15 ml................ 00023-5363-15 4.49

COMPLETE BRAND MULTI-PURPOSE (Allergan Inc)
SOL,NA, 120 ml 00023-4343-04 3.24
360 ml 00023-4343-12 7.69

COMPLETE MAXIMUM STRENGTH (Family Phcy)
TAB,PO (COLD & COUGH RELIEF)
500 mg-2 mg-15 mg-30 mg,
24s ea............ 52735-0456-05 3.32 3.69

COMPLETE READY-TO-USE ENEMA (Cardinal Health)
NMA,RC (PRIVATE LABEL)
135 ml 37205-0030-11 1.00
(TWIN PACK,PRIVATE LABEL)
135 ml 2s............ 37205-0030-36 1.76

(Chain Drug Marketing)
NMA,RC (TWIN PACK - LATEX FREE)
133 ml 2s............ 63868-0380-90 1.18 1.79

COMPLETE READY-TO-USE ENEMA MINERAL OIL (Major)
NMA,RC (1X133ML,LATEX-FREE)
133 ml 00904-5895-78 2.50

COMPLETE SENIOR (Prime Marketing)
TAB,PO, 60s ea 62107-0045-06 5.52

COMPLETE WEEKLY ENZYMATIC CLEANER (Allergan Inc)
TEF,NA (W/2 ENZYME VIALS)
8s ea................ 11980-0151-08 4.24

COMPLEX 15 (Schering Plough)
CRE,TP (FACE)
75 gm............... 00085-4100-25 4.82
LOT,TP (HAND& BODY)
240 ml 00085-4115-08 6.48

COMPLEX ESSENTIAL MSD DRINK MIX (Applied Nutr. Corp.)
POW,PO (4X454GM,VANILLA)
454 gm 4s........... 00847-0597-22 285.00

COMPLEX MSUD AMINO ACID (Applied Nutr. Corp.)
BAR,PO (CHOCOLATE)
47 gm 12s........... 00847-0598-06 112.50

COMPLEX MSUD AMINO ACID BLEND (Applied Nutr. Corp.)
POW,PO (USE W/MED SUPV)
454 gm 4s........... 00847-0590-00 817.50

COMPLEX MSUD DRINK MIX (Applied Nutr. Corp.)
POW,PO (MED. SUPERV.,VANILLA)
454 gm 4s........... 00847-0598-22 285.00

COMPLEXED POTASSIUM (Carlson,J.R.)
TAB,PO (PF,SF,CORN-FREE)
99 mg, 100s ea 88395-0057-01 4.95 9.90
250s ea............ 88395-0057-02 11.45 22.90

COMPOUND W (Medtech)
GEL,TP, 17%, 7.5 gm...... 75137-0585-07 5.26
LIQ,TP, 17%, 9.3 ml...... 75137-0591-10 5.26

COMPOUND W ONE STEP WART REMOVER (Medtech)
PAD,TP (FOR KIDS)
40%, 12s ea 75137-0595-30 5.83
14s ea 75137-0595-10 5.83

COMPOZ NIGHTTIME SLEEP AID (Medtech)
TAB,PO, 50 mg, 12s ea.... 75137-0212-03 2.74
(GELCAPLET)
50 mg, 16s ea........ 75137-0212-15 2.63

COMTREX ACUTE HEAD COLD (B/M Squibb Cons Med)
TAB,PO (MAX STRENGTH)
500 mg-2 mg-30 mg,
20s ea.............. 19810-0300-78 4.40

COMTREX COLD & COUGH (B/M Squibb Cons Med)
TAB,PO (10 DAY+10 NIGHT,CAPLET)
20s ea.............. 19810-0300-82 4.40
(NON-DROWSY,MAX STRENGTH)
500 mg-15 mg-30 mg,
20s ea.............. 19810-0300-83 4.40

(Novartis Consumer)
TAB,PO (MAXIMUM STRENGTH)
ea.................. 00067-2082-30 4.40
(MAX STRENGTH,NON-DROWSY)
325 mg-10 mg-5 mg,
20s ea............ 00067-2077-20 4.40

PROD/MFR | HRI, UPC,NDC | AWP | SRP

COMTREX COLD & COUGH NIGHTTIME (B/M Squibb Cons Med)
TAB,PO (MAX STRENGTH,CAPLET)
500 mg-2 mg-15 mg-30 mg,
20s ea............ 19810-0300-84 4.40

COMTREX DEEP CHEST COLD (B/M Squibb Cons Med)
SGL,PO (MUTI-SYMP,NON-DROWSY)
20s ea.............. 19810-0300-79 4.40

(Novartis Consumer)
TAB,PO (NON-DROWSY,CAPLET)
325 mg-200 mg,
24s ea............ 00067-6227-24 4.40

COMTREX FLU THERAPY (B/M Squibb Cons Med)
TAB,PO (10 DAY+10 NIGHT,CAPLET)
20s ea.............. 19810-0300-80 4.40

COMTREX NIGHTIME COLD & COUGH (Novartis Consumer)
TAB,PO (MAXIMUM STRENGTH)
325 mg-2 mg-10 mg-5 mg,
20s ea............ 00067-2081-20 4.40

COMTREX SEVERE COLD & SINUS (Novartis Consumer)
TAB,PO (MAXIMUM STRENGTH)
ea.................. 00067-2083-30 4.40

COMTREX SINUS & NASAL DECONGESTANT (B/M Squibb Cons Med)
TAB,PO (MAX STRENGTH,CAPLET)
500 mg-2 mg-30 mg,
20s ea............ 19810-0300-81 4.40

COMTREX SORE THROAT RELIEF (B/M Squibb Cons Med)
SOL,PO, 500 mg/15 ml,
240 ml 19810-0300-12 4.40

CONCENTRATED MOTRIN INFANTS' DROPS (McNeil Consumer Healthcare)
SUS,PO (AF,BERRY,DROPS)
50 mg/1.25 ml,
15 ml............. 00450-0524-15 5.08
(AF,DYE-FREE,BERRY,DROPS)
50 mg/1.25 ml,
15 ml............. 00450-0198-15 5.08
30 ml 00450-0198-01 8.00
(DUAL PLACEMENT,AF)
50 mg/1.25 ml,
30 ml............. 00450-0198-11 8.00

CONCENTRATED TYLENOL INFANTS' DROPS (McNeil Consumer Healthcare)
SOL,PO (AF,ASPIRIN-FREE,CHERRY)
80 mg/0.8 ml,
15 ml............. 00450-0186-15 5.08
(AF,ASPIRIN-FREE,GRAPE)
80 mg/0.8 ml,
15 ml............. 00450-0122-15 5.08
(AF,ASPIRIN-FREE,CHERRY)
80 mg/0.8 ml,
30 ml............. 00450-0186-30 8.00
(AF,ASPIRIN-FREE,GRAPE)
80 mg/0.8 ml,
30 ml............. 00450-0122-01 8.00
(AF,ASPIRIN-FREE)
80 mg/0.8 ml,
30 ml............. 00450-0167-01 8.00
(DUAL PLACEMENT,AF)
80 mg/0.8 ml,
30 ml............. 00450-0122-10 8.00
30 ml 00450-0167-11 8.00

CONDOM (Rugby)
DEV,NA (PREM LUBRICATED)
12s ea.............. 00536-9995-12 3.78

CONFIRM HOME PREGNANCY (Durex)
DEV,NA, ea................ 02340-0891-00 5.02 10.04
2s ea.............. 02340-0892-00 7.62 15.24

CONFORM STRETCH (Covidien)
DEV,NA (6"X4.5YDS,NON-STERILE)
48s ea.............. 08080-2249-00 47.33
(6"X4.5YDS,STERILE)
48s ea.............. 08080-2238-00 69.10
(1"X4.1YDS,NON-STERILE)
96s ea.............. 08080-2239-00 24.38
(1"X4.1YDS,STERILE)
96s ea.............. 08080-2230-00 62.89
(2"X4.1YDS,NON-STERILE)
96s ea.............. 08080-2242-00 32.60
(2"X4.1YDS,STERILE)
96s ea.............. 08080-2231-00 60.03
(3"X4.1YDS,NON-STERILE)
96s ea.............. 08080-2244-00 40.92

PROD/MFR | HRI, UPC,NDC | AWP | SRP

(3"X4.1YDS,STERILE)
96s ea.............. 08080-2232-00 77.70
(4"X4.1YDS,NON-STERILE)
96s ea.............. 08080-2247-00 63.60
(4"X4.1YDS,STERILE)
96s ea.............. 08080-2236-00 93.24

CONGESTA DM (TriMarc Labs)
TAB,PO, 20 mg-400 mg,
90s ea............ 68752-0012-90 9.00

CONGESTAC (Ascher)
TAB,PO (CAPLET)
400 mg-60 mg,
12s ea............ 00225-0580-06 4.78
24s ea 00225-0580-08 8.26

CONIUM MACULATUM (Luyties)
TAB,SL (6X)
6 x, 500s ea.......... 00618-2219-03 3.99
5500s ea 00618-2219-10 30.32
12 x, 500s ea 00622-2219-03 4.19
5500s ea 00622-2219-10 31.83
30 x, 500s ea 00624-2219-03 4.19
5500s ea 00624-2219-10 31.83

CONSTANT CARE VASELINE (Covidien)
LOT,TP (MOISTURE BARRIER)
60 gm 12s.......... 08080-7375-00 31.87
((CONDITIONING),12X240GM)
240 gm 12s......... 08080-7374-00 47.50
(MOISTURE BARRIER)
240 gm 12s......... 08080-7376-00 55.69

CONSTANT CLENS (Covidien)
LIQ,TP (DERMAL WOUND W/SPRY NOZ)
60 ml 12s........... 08080-7389-08 69.07
480 ml 6s 08080-7389-16 50.13

CONTAC COLD+FLU (Glaxo)
TAB,PO (DUAL FORMULA PACK)
28s ea.............. 45800-0235-24 5.47
(MAXIMUM STRENGTH,CAPLET)
500 mg-2 mg-5 mg,
24s ea............ 45800-0234-25 4.40
36s ea 45800-0234-33 7.16
(MAX STRENGTH,NON-DROWSY)
500 mg-5 mg,
24s ea............ 45800-0238-17 4.40

CONTAC D COLD (Glaxo)
TAB,PO, 10 mg, 24s ea.... 45800-0239-15 4.40
36s ea 45800-0239-20 7.16

CONTAC DAY/NIGHT ALLERGY SINUS (Glaxo)
TAB,PO (CAPLET)
650 mg-50 mg-60 mg,
20s ea............ 45800-0235-30 5.47

CONTAC DAY/NIGHT COLD & FLU (Glaxo)
TAB,PO (CAPLET)
650 mg-30 mg-50 mg-60 mg,
20s ea............ 45800-0235-20 5.47

CONTAC SEVERE COLD & FLU (Glaxo)
TAB,PO (MAX. STR.,CAPLET)
500 mg-2 mg-15 mg-30 mg,
16s ea............ 45800-0234-16 4.40
30s ea 45800-0234-31 7.16

CONTAC SEVERE COLD & FLU/NON-DROWSY (Glaxo)
TAB,PO (CAPLET)
325 mg-15 mg-30 mg,
16s ea............ 45800-0238-16 4.40

CONTENTMINTS (Ellon)
ODT,PO (WINTERGREEN)
30s ea.............. 64723-0300-30 3.99

CONTI (Numark)
SOA,TP (3 OZ.,W/OLIVE OIL)
ea.................. 38485-0321-53 2.76

CONTOUR BLOOD GLUCOSE MONITORING SYSTEM (Bayer Diabetes Care)
DEV,NA, ea 00193-7190-01 78.00
ea 00193-7191-01 72.00

CONTOUR USB BLOOD GLUCOSE MONITORING SYSTEM (Bayer Diabetes Care)
DEV,NA, ea 00193-7393-01 70.68

CONTRAGESIC (Contract Pharmacal)
TAB,PO, 325 mg-30 mg,
90s ea............ 10267-1000-09 6.00
100s ea........... 10267-1000-01 7.00

(Southwood)
REPACK
TAB,PO, 325 mg-30 mg,
30s ea............ 58016-0718-30 18.95

PROD/MFR	HRI, UPC,NDC	AWP	SRP
CONTREET AG FOAM DRESSING (Coloplast)			
DRE,TP (2"X3" ADHESIVE)			
5s ea	11701-0422-52	47.30	49.50
(7.5"X7.75" ADHESIVE)			
5s ea	11701-0422-51	159.10	166.50
(9"X9" ADHESIVE)			
5s ea	11701-0422-50	210.70	220.50
(ADHESIVE,5"X5")			
5s ea	11701-0422-32	135.45	141.75
(ADHESIVE,7"X7")			
5s ea	11701-0422-35	264.10	276.40
(NON-ADHESIVE,4"X4")			
5s ea	11701-0422-22	118.25	123.75
(NON-ADHESIVE,6"X6")			
5s ea	11701-0422-25	230.90	241.65
CONTREET AG HYDROCOLLOID DRESSING (Coloplast)			
DRE,TP (STERILE,4"X4")			
5s ea	11701-0421-10	94.50	98.90
(STERILE,6"X6")			
5s ea	11701-0421-13	196.95	206.10
CONTROL BLOOD GLUCOSE MONITORING SYSTEM (US DIAGNOSTICS, INC)			
DEV,NA (STARTER KIT)			
ea	08463-3003-01	55.00	
(VALUE KIT)			
ea	08463-3104-01	50.00	
CONTROL METER KIT (US DIAGNOSTICS, INC)			
DEV,NA (METER,CONTROL SOLN,CASE)			
ea	08463-3103-01	45.00	
CONTROL SOLUTION (US DIAGNOSTICS, INC)			
DEV,NA (HIGH)			
ea	08463-3105-01	10.00	
(LOW)			
ea	08463-3205-01	10.00	
(NORMAL)			
ea	08463-3005-01	10.00	
CONTROL TEST STRIPS (US DIAGNOSTICS, INC)			
DEV,NA (2X25 STRIPS)			
50s ea	08463-3203-50	42.00	
CONVATEC NIGHT DRAINAGE CONTAINER TUBING (Convatec)			
DEV,NA, ea	68455-0107-09	8.71	11.34
CONVATEC OSTOMY APPLIANCE BELT (Convatec)			
DEV,NA, ea	68455-0107-18	7.36	9.58
CONVATEC STRAIGHT TAIL CLOSURES (Convatec)			
DEV,NA, 10s ea	68455-0107-19	18.46	24.03
CONVEEN BAG HANGER (Coloplast)			
DEV,NA, ea	11701-0866-10	5.52	5.78
CONVEEN CONTOURED URINE LEG BAG (Coloplast)			
DEV,NA (LARGE W/18" TUBING)			
10s ea	11701-0862-20	83.10	86.90
(MEDIUM W/18" TUBING)			
10s ea	11701-0862-10	81.90	85.70
(STERILE MED.W/18"TUBING)			
10s ea	11701-0862-15	88.10	92.20
CONVEEN DELUXE LEG BAG STRAPS (Coloplast)			
DEV,NA (25", 1 PAIR)			
10s ea	11701-0864-10	60.00	62.80
CONVEEN DRIP COLLECTOR (Coloplast)			
DEV,NA (EXTRA 4 OZ./100 ML)			
100s ea	11701-0868-15	129.00	135.00
(NORMAL 3 OZ./80 ML)			
100s ea	11701-0868-10	117.00	122.00
CONVEEN LEG/BEDSIDE DRAINAGE BAG (Coloplast)			
DEV,NA (EXTRA LARGE)			
10s ea	11701-0863-10	51.30	53.60
CONVEEN NET PANTS (Coloplast)			
DEV,NA (LARGE 150-200 LBS)			
10s ea	11701-0869-15	26.80	28.10
(MEDIUM 90-150 LBS)			
10s ea	11701-0869-10	26.80	28.10
(LARGE, 150-200 LBS)			
100s ea	11701-0869-25	122.00	128.00
(MEDIUM, 90-150 LBS)			
100s ea	11701-0869-20	122.00	128.00
(X-LARGE, OVER 200 LBS)			
100s ea	11701-0869-30	122.00	128.00
CONVEX 10" DRAINABLE POUCH (Coloplast)			
DEV,NA (1 1/2")			
10s ea	11701-0920-34	78.40	82.10
(1 1/4")			
10s ea	11701-0920-30	78.40	82.10
(1 1/8")			
10s ea	11701-0920-28	78.40	82.10
(1 3/8")			
10s ea	11701-0920-32	78.40	82.10
(1 5/8")			
10s ea	11701-0920-36	78.40	82.10
(1")			
10s ea	11701-0920-26	78.40	82.10
(3/4")			
10s ea	11701-0920-22	78.40	82.10
(5/8"-1 11/16")			
10s ea	11701-0920-12	77.20	80.80
(5/8"-1 5/16")			
10s ea	11701-0920-10	77.20	80.80
(5/8")			
10s ea	11701-0920-20	78.40	82.10
(7/8")			
10s ea	11701-0920-24	78.40	82.10
CONVEX 12" DRAINABLE POUCH (Coloplast)			
DEV,NA (1 1/2")			
10s ea	11701-0920-74	78.40	82.10
(1 1/4")			
10s ea	11701-0920-70	78.40	82.10
(1 1/8")			
10s ea	11701-0920-68	78.40	82.10
(1 3/8")			
10s ea	11701-0920-72	78.40	82.10
(1 5/8")			
10s ea	11701-0920-76	78.40	82.10
(1")			
10s ea	11701-0920-66	78.40	82.10
(3/4")			
10s ea	11701-0920-62	78.40	82.10
(5/8"-1 11/16")			
10s ea	11701-0920-52	77.20	80.80
(5/8"-1 5/16")			
10s ea	11701-0920-50	77.20	80.80
(5/8")			
10s ea	11701-0920-60	78.40	82.10
(7/8")			
10s ea	11701-0920-64	78.40	82.10
COOL 'N' HOT (Global Source)			
GEL,TP, 2%, 240 gm	59618-0175-57	2.95	
COOL MAGIC (MPM Medical Inc.)			
DEV,NA (1 3/4")			
ea	66977-0206-13	2.56	2.84
(8"X12")			
ea	66977-0206-12	15.78	17.53
COOL MINT LISTERINE ANTISEPTIC (Johnson & Johnson)			
SOL,MM (1X95ML)			
95 ml	12547-0427-95	1.13	
(1X250ML)			
250 ml	12547-0427-20	2.83	
(1X500ML)			
500 ml	12547-0427-25	3.91	
(1X1000ML)			
1000 ml	12547-0427-35	5.40	
(1X1500ML)			
1500 ml	12547-0427-55	7.60	
COOLING RELIEF PADS (Johnson & Johnson)			
DEV,NA (ASSORTED PADS)			
5s ea	81371-0040-24	4.22	
COOLMAGIC GEL SHEET (MPM Medical Inc.)			
DEV,NA (3 3/4"X3 3/4")			
ea	66977-0206-33	4.49	4.99
(6"X8")			
ea	66977-0206-68	10.25	11.39
COPA (Covidien)			
DEV,NA (SINGLE-USE,4"X4")			
50s ea	08080-5554-40	73.23	
(SINGLE-USE,4"X8")			
50s ea	08080-5554-80	130.00	
COPE (Lee Pharm)			
TAB,PO, 421 mg-32 mg,			
60s ea	23558-0570-10	6.96	
(60X36)			
421 mg-32 mg,			
2160s ea	23558-0570-11	250.56	
COPPER (Freeda)			
TAB,PO (PF,SF,DYE-FREE)			
2 mg, 100s ea	10432-0280-01	4.17	6.95
COPPERMIN (Key Company)			
TAB,PO, 5 mg, 100s ea	11694-0215-02	5.00	
COQ10 (Bio-Tech Pharm)			
CAP,PO, 30 mg, 100s ea	53191-0182-01	36.64	
60 mg, 60s ea	53191-0266-60	31.45	
150 mg, 60s ea	53191-0230-60	65.17	
100s ea	53191-0230-01	93.10	
250 mg, 100s ea	53191-0397-01	150.00	
POW,PO, 400 mg/scoopful,			
50 gm	53191-0254-50	250.00	
COQ10 IN OIL (Key Company)			
SGL,PO (PF,SF,DAIRY-FREE)			
100 mg-30 iu,			
60s ea	11694-0660-01	28.00	
CORAL CALCIUM (Key Company)			
CAP,PO (FROM OKINAWA,PF)			
500 mg-250 mg-400 iu,			
100s ea	11694-0662-01	10.00	
(Rexall)			
CAP,PO, 185 mg, 60s ea	30768-0038-80	5.50	7.99
CORBAN MAGNESIUM OXIDE (Blaine)			
TAB,PO (SF,GLUTEN-FREE)			
400 mg, 120s ea	68549-0100-12	7.50	
CORICIDIN HBP COLD & FLU (Schering Plough)			
TAB,PO, 325 mg-2 mg,			
12s ea	00085-0522-01	3.02	
24s ea	00085-0522-02	4.85	
48s ea	00085-0522-03	9.56	
CORN HUSKERS LOTION (Johnson & Johnson)			
LOT,TP, 210 ml	12547-0481-27	2.75	
CORN SILK (ADH)			
CAP,PO (PF,SF)			
450 mg, 100s ea	60142-0907-51	4.63	9.25
COROMEGA (The Coromega Company)			
EMU,PO (ORANGE)			
14s ea	89269-0001-00	7.25	11.49
30s ea	89269-0001-01	12.65	19.95
90s ea	89269-0001-06	20.99	39.95
COROMEGA CHILD BRAIN & BODY HIGH DHA OMEGA-3 (The Coromega Company)			
PKT,PO (LEMON LIME)			
850 mg-10 mg, 10s ea	89269-0454-01		9.99
30s ea	89269-0454-02		24.99
60s ea	89269-0454-03		36.99
COROMEGA OMEGA-3 (The Coromega Company)			
EMU,PO (SF,DAIRY-FREE)			
12 mg-650 mg-10 mg-3 iu,			
14s ea	89269-0452-00	7.25	11.49
30s ea	89269-0452-02	13.60	21.49
90s ea	89269-0452-06	20.99	39.95
PKT,PO (LEMON-LIME)			
14s ea	89269-0454-20		11.49
30s ea	89269-0454-22		19.95
90s ea	89269-0454-26		39.95
CORRECT-TABS (Time-Cap)			
ECT,PO, 5 mg, 100s ea	49483-0057-01	5.72	
1000s ea	49483-0057-10	39.25	
CORRECTIVE LAXATIVE (Qualitest)			
ECT,PO, 5 mg, 30s ea	00603-0129-16	2.61	
CORRECTOL (Schering Plough)			
ECT,PO, 5 mg, 10s ea	41100-0005-51	2.05	
30s ea	41100-0072-96	4.49	
30s ea	41100-0179-30	4.49	
90s ea	41100-0072-99	10.21	
CORTA-CAP (Dihoma Inc.)			
SPR,TP, 1%, 57 gm	62294-0690-04	4.09	5.73
142 gm	62294-0690-03	9.08	12.72
CORTA-CAP NEEDLE EASE (Dihoma Inc.)			
SPR,TP, 35%, 15 ml	62294-0409-02	20.46	30.69
CORTAID ADVANCED (Johnson & Johnson)			
CRE,TP (12HR ANTI-ITCH)			
1%, 42 gm	81371-0040-38	5.65	
CORTAID INTENSIVE THERAPY (Pharmacia Consumer)			
CRE,TP, 1%, 60 gm	00009-3991-08	5.63	
CORTAID INTENSIVE THERAPY COOLING SPRAY (Johnson & Johnson)			
SPR,TP (1X59ML)			
1%, 59 ml	81370-0050-06	5.65	
CORTAID INTENSIVE THERAPY MOISTURIZING CREAM (Johnson & Johnson)			
CRE,TP, 1%, 56 gm	81370-0050-25	5.65	
CORTAID MAXIMUM STRENGTH (Johnson & Johnson)			
CRE,TP (1X14GM)			
1%, 14 gm	81370-0050-09	2.89	
(1X28GM)			
1%, 28 gm	81370-0050-10	3.92	
56 gm	81370-0050-12	5.65	
OIN,TP, 1%, 28 gm	81370-0050-13	3.92	
(Pharmacia Consumer)			
CRE,TP, 1%, 15 gm	00009-3991-01	2.88	
30 gm	00009-3991-02	3.91	
39.9 gm	00009-3991-22	3.91	
60 gm	00009-3991-13	5.63	

PROD/MFR	HRI, UPC,NDC	AWP	SRP
60 gm 72s	00009-3991-99	6.20	
OIN,TP, 1%, 15 gm	00009-3486-01	2.88	
30 gm	00009-3486-02	3.91	
39.9 gm	00009-3486-16	3.91	
STI,TP (FASTSTICK)			
1%, 6.9 gm	00009-3990-08	1.67	
CORTAID POISON IVY CARE REMOVAL SCRUB (Johnson & Johnson)			
SOA,TP, 113 gm	81370-0050-57	10.84	
CORTAID POISON IVY CARE TOXIN REMOVAL CLOTHS (Johnson & Johnson)			
PAD,TP (PRE-MOISTENED CLOTH)			
6s ea	81370-0050-74	6.85	
CORTAID SENSITIVE SKIN W/ALOE (Pharmacia Consumer)			
CRE,TP, 0.5%, 15 gm	00009-3373-01	2.30	
CORTICOOL MAXIMUM STRENGTH (Tec)			
GEL,TP, 1%, 45 gm	83926-0110-00	3.40	5.99
CORVAC PLASMA SEPARATOR TUBES (Covidien)			
DEV,NA (6ML,RED/GREENSTOPPER)			
500s ea	08080-3021-30	162.52	
(9ML,RED/GREEN STOPPER)			
500s ea	08080-3020-64	168.34	
CORVAC PLASTIC TRANSPORT SERUM SEPARATOR TUBES (Covidien)			
DEV,NA (8ML,RED/GRAY STOPPER)			
500s ea	08080-3021-71	235.00	
CORVAC SERUM SEPARATOR TUBES (Covidien)			
DEV,NA (RED/GRAY STOPPER,9ML)			
500s ea	08080-3020-15	148.23	
(RED/GRAY,12.5ML)			
500s ea	08080-3021-14	175.63	
(THROMBIN,6ML,REDYELLOW)			
500s ea	08080-3023-12	262.35	
CORVAC TRANSPORT SERUM SEPARATOR TUBES (Covidien)			
DEV,NA (8.5ML,RED/GRAYSTOPPER)			
500s ea	08080-3020-31	169.64	
COSAMIN ASU (Nutramax Labs)			
CAP,PO, 200 mg-375 mg,			
90s ea	55970-0820-02	40.00	
COSAMIN DS (Nutramax Labs)			
TAB,PO (PF,SF,DAIRY-FREE)			
400 mg-500 mg, 75s ea	55970-0807-60	35.00	
150s ea	55970-0807-20	70.00	
(Phys Total Care) REPACK			
CAP,PO, 10 mg-5%-400 mg,			
180s ea	54868-3944-00	96.49	
(Southwood) REPACK			
CAP,PO			
66 mg-400 mg-500 mg-5 mg,			
30s ea	58016-0999-30	27.75	
60s ea	58016-0999-60	55.50	
80s ea	58016-0999-80	61.67	
90s ea	58016-0999-90	83.25	
100s ea	58016-0999-00	77.08	
120s ea	58016-0999-02	92.50	
COSAMINDS (Nutramax Labs)			
CAP,PO			
16 mg-400 mg-500 mg-3 mg,			
72s ea	55970-0808-72	30.00	
108s ea	55970-0808-25	45.00	
210s ea	55970-0808-41	87.50	
COTACORT (Truxton)			
LOT,TP, 0.5%, 120 ml	00463-8010-04	7.20	
COTTON GLOVES (Allerderm Labs.)			
DEV,NA (1 PAIR,LARGE)			
ea	34674-0111-30	1.00	
(1 PAIR,MEDIUM)			
ea	34674-0111-20	1.00	
(1 PAIR,SMALL)			
ea	34674-0111-10	1.00	
(1 PAIR,X-LARGE)			
ea	34674-0111-40	1.00	
COTTON SWAB (Medicine Shoppe)			
DEV,NA, 300s ea	49614-0506-87	2.19	2.19
COUGH & COLD (Major)			
TAB,PO, 4 mg-30 mg,			
16s ea	00904-5817-44	1.51	
COUGH & COLD PEDIATRIC (Silarx)			
LIQ,PO (MEDICINE,AF,CHERRY)			
120 ml	54838-0115-40	2.95	
COUGH DROPS (AmerisourceBergen)			
LOZ,MM (PRIVATE LABEL,CHERRY)			
30s ea	24385-0041-65	0.89	0.99
(PRIVATE LABEL,MENTHOL)			
30s ea	24385-0043-65	0.89	0.99
(PRIVATE LABEL)			
30s ea	24385-0042-65	0.89	0.99
COUGH RELIEVER INTENSE DOUBLE STRENGTH (Chain Drug Marketing)			
SOL,PO (NON-DROWSY,AF,SF)			
30 mg/5 ml-200 mg/5 ml,			
120 ml	63868-0674-04	3.59	5.99
COUGH/CONGESTION PEDIATRIC (Reese)			
LIQ,PO (AF,SF,DYE-FREE)			
10 mg/5 ml-100 mg/5 ml,			
120 ml	10956-0776-04	3.81	
COVRSITE (Smith & Nephew)			
DEV,NA (4"X4")			
10s ea	40565-0117-70	12.49	9.99
(6"X6")			
10s ea	40565-0117-74	20.80	16.64
(4"X4")			
30s ea	40565-0117-72	33.48	26.78
(6"X6")			
30s ea	40565-0117-76	53.90	43.12
CR PLUS PROTEIN (Miller)			
TAB,PO, 100s ea	17204-0423-40	4.08	6.80
CRAB APPLE (Ellon)			
SOL,SL (DROPS)			
10.5 ml	51762-0022-10		9.25
CRAMPLEX (Med Prods Panamer)			
CAP,PO, 90s ea	00576-1600-90	10.50	
CRAN-PLUS (Key Company)			
CAP,PO (SF,CORN-FREE,DAIRY-FREE)			
30s ea	11694-0663-30	5.00	
90s ea	11694-0663-90	12.00	
CRANBERRY (Cardinal Health)			
CAP,PO (PRIVATE LABEL)			
400 mg, 60s ea	37205-0053-72	8.33	
(Freeda)			
TAB,PO, 400 mg, 100s ea	10432-0368-01	7.17	11.95
CRANBERRY CONCENTRATE (Carlson,J.R.)			
SGL,PO (SOFTGEL)			
10 mg-1000 mg, 50s ea	88395-0081-80	9.40	18.80
100s ea	88395-0081-81	17.20	34.40
(Mason Vit)			
SGL,PO (PF,SF,SOFTGEL)			
100 mg-140 mg-3 iu,			
90s ea	11845-0129-69	7.33	
CRANBERRY FRUIT (Major)			
CAP,PO, 405 mg, 60s ea	00904-5527-52	6.81	
(Rexall)			
CAP,PO (PF,SF)			
425 mg, 50s ea	30768-0001-29	2.59	3.92
CRANGEL (Advanced Nutr)			
CAP,PO, 90s ea	62617-0410-03	18.00	24.00
CREAM BASE (Medco Lab)			
CRE,TP, 454 gm	11940-3313-06	7.00	
CREATINE (Bio-Tech Pharm)			
CAP,PO, 800 mg, 105s ea	53191-0231-01	9.50	
POW,PO, 2400 mg/tsp,			
500 gm	53191-0380-01	30.00	
(Carlson,J.R.)			
PDR,PO (PF,SF,CORN-FREE)			
3200 mg, 100 gm	88395-0068-05	4.95	9.90
1000 gm	88395-0068-06	34.00	68.00
CREO-TERPIN (Lee Pharm)			
LIQ,PO, 3.5 mg/5 ml,			
120 ml	23558-0681-10	6.96	
120 ml 36s	23558-0681-11	250.56	
CREOMULSION COUGH (Summit Industries)			
SYR,PO (AF,DYE-FREE)			
20 mg/15 ml,			
120 ml	12090-0001-41	3.25	3.99
CREOMULSION FOR CHILDREN (Summit Industries)			
SYR,PO (AF,CHERRY)			
5 mg/5 ml, 120 ml	12090-0001-51	3.25	3.99
CRITIC-AID (Coloplast)			
PAS,TP, 51%-20%,			
71 gm 12s	11701-0050-33	105.84	110.76
170 gm 12s	11701-0050-32	175.80	184.08
CRITIC-AID CLEAR (Coloplast)			
OIN,TP (4GM X 300)			
71.5%, 4 gm 300s	11701-0066-22	186.00	195.00
(71GM X 12)			
71.5%, 71 gm 12s	11701-0066-33	117.60	123.12
(170GM X 12)			
71.5%, 170 gm 12s	11701-0066-32	195.48	204.60
CRITIC-AID CLEAR AF (Coloplast)			
OIN,TP (300X4GM)			
2%, 4 gm 300s	11701-0067-22	192.00	201.00
(12X57GM)			
2%, 57 gm 12s	11701-0067-23	101.52	106.32
(12X142GM)			
2%, 142 gm 12s	11701-0067-14	183.12	191.64
CRM (Bio-Tech Pharm)			
CAP,PO, 200 mcg,			
100s ea	53191-0106-01	6.80	
CRO-MAN-ZIN (Freeda)			
TAB,PO (PF,SF,DYE-FREE)			
0.2 mg-5 mg-25 mg,			
100s ea	10432-0199-01	5.97	9.95
CROMOLYN SODIUM (Bausch & Lomb Inc.)			
SPR,NS, 5.2 mg/actuation,			
26 ml	57782-0397-26	12.90	
(Major)			
SPR,NS, 5.2 mg/actuation,			
26 ml	00904-5532-67	12.75	
CROWN (Okamoto)			
DEV,NA (LIGHTLY LUBRICATED)			
15s ea	28373-0200-12	2.05	4.75
(LUBRICATED)			
1008s ea	28373-0210-00	75.00	135.00
CRUCIAL (Nestle)			
LIQ,PO (250MLX24,UNFLAVORED)			
250 ml 24s	00065-9124-70	221.76	
CRUCIAL ULTRAPAK (Nestle)			
LIQ,PO (1000MLX6)			
1000 ml 6s	00065-9128-72	228.89	
CRUEX PRESCRIPTION STRENGTH (Novartis Consumer)			
CRE,TP, 1%, 15 gm	00067-9506-01	5.12	
SPR,TP, 2%, 85 gm	00235-9507-01	5.44	
CRUNCH AMINOS (Freeda)			
CTB,PO (SF,GLUTEN-FREE)			
100s ea	10432-0329-01	7.17	11.95
CRYOSERV (Bioniche Pharma)			
DEV,NA (12X10ML)			
10 ml 12s	67457-0178-10	17.50	
(6X50ML)			
50 ml 6s	67457-0178-50	68.75	
CU PLUS PROTEIN (Miller)			
TAB,PO, 100s ea	17204-0451-40	5.04	8.00
CU-5 (Bio-Tech Pharm)			
CAP,PO, 5 mg, 100s ea	53191-0211-01	4.20	
CULTURELLE (Amerifit)			
CAP,PO, 10 billion org,			
30s ea	49100-0363-74	13.44	21.99
CURAFIL GEL WOUND DRESSING (Covidien)			
DEV,NA (12X85GM)			
85 gm 12s	08080-9252-00	129.29	
CURAGEL HYDROGEL WOUND (Covidien)			
DEV,NA (4"X4")			
50s ea	08080-9901-00	177.05	
CURASILK HYPOALLERGENIC CLOTH (Covidien)			
DEV,NA (3"X10YDS)			
48s ea	08080-7140-00	134.71	
(2"X10YDS)			
72s ea	08080-7139-00	136.22	
(1"X10YDS)			
144s ea	08080-7138-00	135.85	
(1/2"X10YDS)			
288s ea	08080-7137-00	157.06	
CURASOL HYDROGEL SATURATED (Healthpoint)			
DEV,NA (4"X4")			
10s ea	08213-0060-44	48.10	
CURASOL WOUND DRESSING (Healthpoint)			
DEV,NA, 30 gm	08213-0050-01	8.03	
90 gm	08213-0050-03	14.29	
CURASORB CALCIUM ALGINATE (Covidien)			
DEV,NA (12" ROPE)			
20s ea	08080-9231-00	88.20	
CURASORE (S.S.S.)			
LIQ,TP, 1%, 15 ml	12258-0223-05	2.66	3.99

PROD/MFR	HRI, UPC,NDC	AWP	SRP
CURCUMIN (Bio-Tech Pharm)			
CAP,PO, 500 mg, 100s ea	53191-0422-01	14.00	
CURI-STRIP ADHESIVE WOUND CLOSURE (Covidien)			
DEV,NA (1/8"X3")			
1000s ea	08080-9890-00	196.85	
(1/4"X4")			
2000s ea	08080-9893-00	309.98	
CURITY 8000 URINE ME (Covidien)			
CURITY 8000 URINE METER FOLEY TRAY			
DEV,NA (16FR,5CC,SILICONE CATH)			
10s ea	08080-8122-00	249.77	
(W/PRE-FILLED SRN,10CC)			
10s ea	08080-8324-00	202.78	
CURITY ABSORBENT GAUZE (Covidien)			
DEV,NA (36"X100YDS,NON-STERILE)			
10s ea	08080-1473-00	675.00	
CURITY ABSORBENT WADDING ROLL (Covidien)			
DEV,NA (24" WIDE,8 LBS)			
4s ea	08080-7067-00	160.28	
CURITY ADHESIVE SURGICAL DRESSING (Covidien)			
DEV,NA (8"X6",STERILE)			
100s ea	08080-5113-00	137.50	
(4"X6",STERILE)			
200s ea	08080-5112-00	174.92	
(4"X8",PEEL-BACK)			
200s ea	08080-5111-00	139.53	
CURITY ALCOHOL PREP (Covidien)			
PAD,TP (MED,2 PLY,NON-STERILE)			
70%, 4000s ea	08080-5150-00	32.48	
CURITY ALCOHOL PREPS (Covidien)			
SWA,TP (MED,2 PLY)			
70%, 4000s ea	08080-5750-00	43.97	
CURITY AMD ANTIMICROBIAL PACKING STRIP (Covidien)			
DEV,NA (1"X5YDS)			
50s ea	08080-7833-10	55.02	
(1/2"X5YDS)			
50s ea	08080-7832-10	48.74	
(1/4"X5YDS)			
50s ea	08080-7831-10	46.89	
CURITY AMNIOCENTESIS TRAY (Covidien)			
CURITY AMNIOCENTESIS TRAY			
KIT,IJ, 1%, 10s ea	08080-9705-10	163.60	
CURITY APPLICATOR NON-STERILE (Covidien)			
DEV,NA (COTTON-TIPPED)			
10000s ea	08080-6553-00	178.67	
CURITY BANDAGE ROLL (Covidien)			
DEV,NA (4"X10YDS,READY-CUT)			
225s ea	08080-1824-00	330.90	
235s ea	08080-6021-00	533.02	
(3"X10YDS,READY-CUT)			
300s ea	08080-1522-00	330.90	
315s ea	08080-3250-00	533.02	
(2"X10YDS,READY-CUT)			
450s ea	08080-1334-00	330.90	
(1"X10 YDS)			
900s ea	08080-1143-00	330.90	
CURITY BURN DRESSING (Covidien)			
DEV,NA (18"X18",50PLY)			
24s ea	08080-7960-00	248.02	
(18"X18",10PLY)			
70s ea	08080-7911-00	153.00	
CURITY CLEAN CATCH (Covidien)			
DEV,NA (W/BZK TOWELETTES)			
48s ea	08080-5204-00	66.57	
CURITY COVER SPONGES (Covidien)			
DEV,NA (3"X4",STERILE)			
1200s ea	08080-3157-00	74.75	
(4"X4",STERILE)			
1200s ea	08080-2913-00	93.30	
(3"X4",NON-STERILE)			
2000s ea	08080-1713-00	89.62	
(4"X4",NON-STERILE)			
2000s ea	08080-1792-00	123.60	
(3"X3",NON-STERILE)			
4000s ea	08080-1700-00	141.95	
CURITY CRIB LINERS (Covidien)			
DEV,NA (10"X14")			
600s ea	08080-7209-00	73.84	
CURITY DISPOSABLE CLEANERS (Covidien)			
DEV,NA (LARGE)			
250s ea	08080-1913-00	86.52	
(MEDIUM,40X40)			
1600s ea	08080-2057-00	55.13	
(MEDIUM,12X250)			
3000s ea	08080-1429-00	72.92	
CURITY DISPOSABLE MESH BRIEFS (Covidien)			
DEV,NA (LARGE)			
100s ea	08080-7093-01	72.65	
(X-LARGE)			
100s ea	08080-7095-01	76.43	
CURITY DISPOSABLE NURSING (Covidien)			
DEV,NA, 288s ea	08080-2630-00	33.42	
CURITY DRAINAGE BAG (Covidien)			
DEV,NA (ANTREFLUXSPLSHGRD2000ML)			
20s ea	08080-6206-00	104.44	
CURITY DRESSING ROLL NON-STERILE (Covidien)			
DEV,NA (4 1/2"X100YDS,8 PLY)			
10s ea	08080-6474-00	816.04	
CURITY ELASTIC BANDAGE ROLLS (Covidien)			
DEV,NA (2"X5YDS,NON-STERILE)			
144s ea	08080-4422-00	107.82	
(3"X5YDS,NON-STERILE)			
144s ea	08080-4423-00	128.70	
(4"X5YDS,NON-STERILE)			
144s ea	08080-4424-00	172.69	
(6"X5YDS,NON-STERILE)			
144s ea	08080-4426-00	121.98	
CURITY EXTENSION SET (Tyco)			
DEV,NA (2.5MLX20")			
50s ea	08080-1559-22	49.28	
CURITY EYE PAD (Covidien)			
DEV,NA (1 5/8"X2 5/8",OVAL)			
600s ea	08080-2841-00	122.49	
CURITY FLEXIBLE ADHESIVE (Covidien)			
DEV,NA (1",FABRIC)			
50s ea	08080-6135-01	2.31	
(3/4",FABRIC)			
50s ea	08080-5024-10	2.04	
CURITY FOLEY CATHETER TRAY (Covidien)			
DEV,NA, 10s ea	08080-8944-00	136.80	
CURITY GAUZE BOLT NON-STERILE (Covidien)			
DEV,NA (20"X10YDS,FLAT FOLD)			
10s ea	08080-1267-00	675.00	
CURITY GAUZE PADS (Covidien)			
DEV,NA (4"X4",12 PLY,STERILE)			
1200s ea	08080-6309-00	256.22	
(2"X2",12 PLY,STERILE)			
2400s ea	08080-3381-00	232.48	
(3"X3",12 PLY,STERILE)			
2400s ea	08080-6132-00	303.65	
CURITY GAUZE SPONGES (Covidien)			
DEV,NA (4"X4",12PLY,STERILE)			
800s ea	08080-3967-00	92.83	
(3.5"X4",32PLY,NONSTERIL)			
1000s ea	08080-2438-00	167.07	
(4"X8",12 PLY,STERILE)			
1000s ea	08080-2259-00	225.45	
(3"X4",12 PLY,STERILE)			
1200s ea	08080-2029-00	88.78	
(4"X4",12 PLY,STERILE)			
1200s ea	08080-3033-00	81.95	
(4"X4",8 PLY,STERILE)			
1200s ea	08080-2187-00	81.98	
(12PLY,4"X4",USP TYPEVII)			
1280s ea	08080-6939-00	144.05	
(4"X4",12 PLY,STERILE)			
1600s ea	08080-3971-00	131.64	
(4"X4",16PLY,USP TYPEVII)			
1600s ea	08080-3973-00	176.43	
(4"X4",8 PLY,STERILE)			
1600s ea	08080-3968-00	106.35	
(3"X4",16 PLY)			
2000s ea	08080-7267-00	96.77	
(4"X4",12PLY,NON-STERILE)			
2000s ea	08080-2634-00	110.22	
(4"X4",16PLY,NON-STERILE)			
2000s ea	08080-2733-00	127.35	
(4"X8",12PLY,NON-STERILE)			
2000s ea	08080-2835-00	204.49	
(3"X3",12 PLY,STERILE)			
2400s ea	08080-1903-00	118.54	
(2"X2",8 PLY,STERILE)			
3000s ea	08080-1806-00	91.44	
(3"X3",12PLY,NON-STERILE)			
4000s ea	08080-2346-00	132.65	
(4"X4",8 PLY,NON-STERILE)			
4000s ea	08080-2556-00	129.72	
(2"X2",8 PLY,NON-STERILE)			
5000s ea	08080-2146-00	72.95	
(2"X2",12PLY,NON-STERILE)			
8000s ea	08080-2252-00	151.50	
CURITY GAUZE STERILE (Covidien)			
DEV,NA (4"X4",16 PLY,PLSTC TRAY)			
1280s ea	08080-7605-00	145.34	
(4"X4",8 PLY,PLSTC TRAY)			
1280s ea	08080-6318-00	150.98	
CURITY HEAVY DRAINAGE PACK (Covidien)			
DEV,NA (10"X12",SPONGE/PAD)			
48s ea	08080-3913-00	136.88	
CURITY HYPOALLERGENIC CLEAR (Covidien)			
DEV,NA (7.5CM X 9.1M)			
40s ea	08080-8536-10	173.70	
(5CM X 9.1M)			
60s ea	08080-8535-10	192.60	
(2.5CM X 9.1M)			
120s ea	08080-8534-10	161.30	
(1.25CM X 9.1M)			
240s ea	08080-8533-10	159.34	
(5CM X 1.3M)			
250s ea	08080-8538-00	141.38	
(2.5CM X 1.3M)			
500s ea	08080-8537-01	147.88	
CURITY INSERTION TRA (Covidien)			
CURITY INSERTION TRAY			
DEV,NA (BZK SWABSTICK PREP)			
20s ea	08080-7100-00	104.92	
(W/10CC PREFILLED SRN)			
20s ea	08080-5029-00	94.07	
(W/30CC PREFILLED SRN)			
20s ea	08080-5027-00	105.54	
CURITY IODOFORM PACKING STRIP (Covidien)			
DEV,NA (1"X5YD)			
12s ea	08080-7833-00	54.05	
(1/2"X5YD)			
12s ea	08080-7832-00	48.22	
(1/4"X5YD)			
12s ea	08080-7831-00	46.24	
(2"X5YD)			
12s ea	08080-7834-00	77.98	
CURITY IRRIGATION TR (Covidien)			
CURITY IRRIGATION TRAY			
DEV,NA (60CC,PISTON SRN)			
20s ea	08080-3685-00	40.92	
CURITY LUMBAR PUNCTU (Covidien)			
CURITY LUMBAR PUNCTURE TRAY			
DEV,NA (INF,22GX1/2",MANOMETER)			
10s ea	08080-7500-00	200.33	
(INFANT,22GX1/2" SPINAL)			
10s ea	08080-7039-00	161.19	
(PED,22GX2 1/2" SPINAL)			
10s ea	08080-1048-00	222.93	
(ADULT,18GX3.5" SPINAL)			
20s ea	08080-1017-00	386.57	
CURITY MATERNITY PADS (Covidien)			
DEV,NA (MATERNITY LENGTH)			
288s ea	08080-2022-00	34.62	
CURITY MULTI-TRAUMA (Covidien)			
DEV,NA (10"X30")			
50s ea	08080-1967-00	170.00	
CURITY NON-ADHERING DRESSING (Covidien)			
DEV,NA (1/2"X4YDS,STERILE)			
12s ea	08080-6111-00	57.83	
(5"X9",STERILE)			
72s ea	08080-6116-00	132.53	
(9"X16",STERILE)			
100s ea	08080-6121-00	312.02	
(3"X8",STERILE)			
144s ea	08080-6113-00	159.05	
(3"X16",STERILE)			
216s ea	08080-6114-00	331.25	
(3"X3")			
600s ea	08080-6112-00	276.33	
(3"X8",STERILE)			
648s ea	08080-6115-00	378.27	
CURITY O-B SPONGE (Covidien)			
DEV,NA (2 PLY,4"X4",100X20)			
2000s ea	08080-7420-00	149.53	
(2 PLY,4"X4",20X100)			
2000s ea	08080-7053-00	127.74	
(2 PLY,4"X4",50X40)			
2000s ea	08080-2818-00	165.37	
CURITY PLAIN PACKING STRIP (Covidien)			
DEV,NA (1"X5YD)			
12s ea	08080-7633-00	48.22	
(1/2"X5YD)			
12s ea	08080-7632-00	42.04	
(1/4"X5YD)			
12s ea	08080-7631-00	43.47	
(2"X5YD)			
12s ea	08080-7634-00	66.02	

PROD/MFR HRI, UPC,NDC AWP SRP

CURITY PLASTIC SPOT BANDAGES (Covidien)
DEV,NA (1"X3",PLASTIC)
50s ea............08080-7893-01 1.95
(7/8",SHEER SPOTS)
3600s ea..........08080-6403-01 145.29
(Kendall)
DEV,NA (3/4"X3",PLASTIC)
50s ea............08080-6193-01 1.72

CURITY PREPPING BALL (Covidien)
DEV,NA (LARGE)
2000s ea..........08080-2601-00 21.73
4000s ea..........08080-2602-00 85.82
(MEDIUM)
4000s ea..........08080-2600-00 16.10

CURITY READY-CUT GAUZE (Covidien)
DEV,NA (36"X36",NON-STERILE)
1000s ea..........08080-2798-00 782.28
(18"X18",NON-STERILE)
4000s ea..........08080-3195-00 714.57
(12"X12",NON-STERILE)
9000s ea..........08080-6122-00 695.50

CURITY RUNAROUNDS TRAINING PANTS (Covidien)
DEV,NA (X-LARGE,BIGBOYS,JUMBOPK)
84s ea............08080-7006-05 67.50
(X-LARGEBIGGIRLS,JUMBOPK)
84s ea............08080-7006-50 67.50
(LARGE,BIG BOYS,JUMBO PK)
96s ea............08080-7006-04 67.50
(LARGE,BIG GIRLS,JUMBOPK)
96s ea............08080-7006-40 67.50
(MEDIUM,BIG BOYS,JUMBOPK)
108s ea...........08080-7006-30 67.50
(MEDIUM,BIGGIRLS,JUMBOPK)
108s ea...........08080-7006-03 67.50

CURITY SLEEPPANTS (Covidien)
DEV,NA (XL)
52s ea............08080-7007-50 67.50
(LARGE)
56s ea............08080-7007-40 67.50
(MEDIUM)
68s ea............08080-7007-30 67.50

CURITY SPECIPAN COLL (Covidien)
CURITY SPECIPAN COLLECTION UNIT
DEV,NA, 100s ea.......08080-4014-00 114.25

CURITY STANDARD POROUS (Covidien)
DEV,NA (4"X10YDS)
36s ea............08080-3615-00 168.53
(3"X10YDS)
48s ea............08080-7046-00 147.64
(2"X10YDS, TAN)
72s ea............08080-5808-00 151.85
(2"X10YDS)
72s ea............08080-6613-00 144.84
(1 1/2"X10YDS, TAN)
96s ea............08080-5807-00 157.35
(1 1/2"X10YDS)
96s ea............08080-3027-00 147.65
(1"X10YDS, TAN)
144s ea...........08080-5806-00 156.46
(1"X10YDS)
144s ea...........08080-2531-00 170.14
(1/2"X10YDS,WHITE)
288s ea...........08080-2304-00 169.36

CURITY STERILE SALINE (Covidien)
SOL,IR (100MLX48)
0.9%, 100 ml 48s....08080-1020-00 39.74
100 ml 48s........08080-1022-00 39.14

CURITY STERILE WATER (Covidien)
SOL,IR, 100 ml 48s......08080-1000-00 39.74

CURITY SUTURE REMOVAL KIT (Covidien)
DEV,NA, 50s ea.........08080-6600-40 170.30

CURITY THORACENTESIS (Covidien)
CURITY THORACENTESIS TRAY
DEV,NA (W/CATHETER,14GX6")
10s ea............08080-5016-00 400.94
(W/NEEDLE,16GX3 1/2")
10s ea............08080-5014-00 279.75

CURITY TRACHEOSTOMY CARE TRAY (Covidien)
DEV,NA (W/ GLOVES)
20s ea............08080-4780-00 45.02
(W/LATEX GLOVES)
20s ea............08080-4220-10 70.28
(W/VINYL GLOVES)
20s ea............08080-4788-50 63.35
24s ea............08080-4780-20 91.94

CURITY TRIANGULAR BANDAGE (Covidien)
DEV,NA (40"X40"X56",NON-STERILE)
72s ea............08080-6286-00 121.25

CURITY ULTRA FITS DIAPERS (Covidien)
DEV,NA (FOR BOYS & GIRLS,6)
144s ea...........08080-8005-80 53.75
(FOR BOYS & GIRLS,5)
176s ea...........08080-8004-80 57.92
(FOR BOYS & GIRLS,4)
192s ea...........08080-8003-80 57.92
(FOR BOYS & GIRLS,3)
224s ea...........08080-8002-80 55.32
(FOR BOYS & GIRLS,2)
272s ea...........08080-8001-80 54.14
(FOR BOYS & GIRLS,1)
320s ea...........08080-8000-80 56.45

CURITY ULTRAMER CATH (Covidien)
CURITY ULTRAMER CATHETER
DEV,NA (16FR,30CC,2 WAY)
12s ea............08080-1416-00 107.83

CURITY ULTRAMER IRRIGATION (Covidien)
DEV,NA (18FR,30CC,3 WAY)
12s ea............08080-2819-00 157.58

CURITY UNIVERSAL FOL (Covidien)
CURITY UNIVERSAL FOLEY TRAY
NA (16FR,5CC,S.E.C.)
20s ea............08080-2101-00 206.02

CURITY URETHRAL CATH (Covidien)
CURITY URETHRAL CATHETER TRAY
NA (14FR,RUBBER,W/PVP,CSR)
20s ea............08080-3410-00 113.40
(14FR,VINYL,W/BZK SWABS)
20s ea............08080-2480-00 115.52
(14FR,VINYL,W/PVP,CSR)
20s ea............08080-3450-00 113.79
(14FR,VINYL INTERMITTENT)
50s ea............08080-3170-00 180.82

CURITY URINE METER (Covidien)
DEV,NA (200ML CAPACITY)
10s ea............08080-6500-00 136.93

CURITY VINYL URETHRAL (Covidien)
DEV,NA (14FR,FEMALE)
100s ea...........08080-2552-00 88.20
(14FR,REGULAR)
100s ea...........08080-2540-00 111.47

CURITY WET DRESSINGS SALINE (Covidien)
DEV,NA (8"X4",12PLY,STERILE)
192s ea...........08080-3606-00 188.98

CURITY WET DRESSINGS WATER (Covidien)
DEV,NA (8"X4",12PLY,STERILE)
192s ea...........08080-3337-00 131.20

CUTAR EMULSION (Summers)
EMU,TP, 1.5%, 180 ml....11086-0005-01 13.57
3840 ml...........11086-0005-02 117.90

CUTEMOL EMOLLIENT (Summers)
CRE,TP, 60 gm.........11086-0006-01 7.27
240 gm............11086-0006-02 17.68

CV-10 (Rx Vitamins)
CAP,PO, 150s ea........08429-0101-50 22.98 45.95

CVP UNIVERSAL MICRODRIP (Abbott Hosp)
DEV,NA (VENTED,Y-INJ)
20s ea............00074-1839-68 223.92

CVS GLUCOSE (Can-Am Care)
GEL,PO (3X38GM,PRIVATE LABEL)
15 gm, 38 gm 3s.....38396-0663-75 8.11
(CVS Corporation)
CTB,PO (CAFFEINE-FREE)
4 gm, 50s ea.......38396-0544-75 8.99
GEL,PO (3X38GM,PRIVATE LABEL)
15 gm, 38 gm 3s.....38396-0550-75 8.11

CVS GLUCOSE BITS (Can-Am Care)
CTB,PO (GLUTEN-FREE,SOUR BERRY)
60s ea............38396-0595-75 2.99

CVS GLUCOSE LIQUID SHOT (Can-Am Care)
SOL,PO (1X59ML,BERRY BLAST)
59 ml.............38396-0591-75 2.59

CVS LANCETS (Can-Am Care)
DEV,NA (PRIVATE LABEL)
200s ea...........38396-0502-75 9.50

CVS LANCING DEVICE (CVS Corporation)
DEV,NA (PRIVATE LABEL)
ea................38396-0510-75 6.49

CVS PRESTIGE SMART SYSTEM (Home Diag)
DEV,NA (STRIP)
50s ea............56151-0307-50 28.60

CVS PRESTIGE SMART SYSTEM STARTER (Home Diag)
DEV,NA (MTR,STRP,LANCET,DEV,SOL)
ea................56151-0207-01 22.18

CVS THIN LANCETS (Can-Am Care)
DEV,NA (PRIVATE LABEL)
100s ea...........38396-0501-75 5.85
200s ea...........38396-0503-75 9.50

CVS TRUETRACK BLOOD GLUCOSE TEST STRIPS (Home Diag)
DEV,NA, 25s ea........56151-0825-25 18.62

CVS ULTRA THIN LANCETS (Can-Am Care)
DEV,NA (PRIVATE LABEL)
100s ea...........38396-0521-75 5.85
200s ea...........38396-0522-75 9.50

CYCLEASE (Boiron)
PEL,SL (2X75)
150s ea...........06962-0431-42 5.27 8.49
TAB,SL, 60s ea........06969-0078-04 5.73 9.59

CYCLEASE PMS (Boiron)
ODT,PO, 15 c-12 c-12 c,
60s ea............00220-9081-04 5.73 9.59

CYCLINEX-1 (Abbott)
PDR,PO, 400 gm........70074-0511-45 20.34

CYCLINEX-2 (Abbott)
PDR,PO, 400 gm........70074-0511-47 44.56

CYDONOL (Gordon)
LOT,TP, 3840 ml.......10481-1016-01 53.75

CYLEX (Pharmakon)
LOZ,MM (SF,CHERRY) -
15 mg-5 mg, 12s ea..55422-0801-12 1.32 2.75

CYSTEINE-500 (Key Company)
CAP,PO (SF)
500 mg, 60s ea......11694-0912-01 8.50

CYSTEX (DSE Healthcare)
TAB,PO, 162 mg-162.5 mg,
40s ea............89411-0545-04 5.70
100s ea...........89411-0545-10 10.80

CYSTINE (VITAFLO, LLC)
PDS,PO, 0.5 gm/4 gm,
30s ea............50600-0547-77 120.00 150.00

CYSTOMANOMETER (Abbott Hosp)
DEV,NA (88")
20s ea............00074-6538-01 223.68

CYSTOSCOPY/IRRIGATION (Abbott Hosp)
DEV,NA (77")
20s ea............00074-6544-01 168.24
(LATEX)
20s ea............00074-6544-02 140.16

CYTO B2 (Solace)
POW,PO (1X100GM)
100 gm............57771-0007-03 42.00 70.00

CYTO-Q (Solace)
SOL,PO (30X10ML)
10 ml 30s.........57771-0007-01 78.00 130.00

CYTO-Q MAX (Solace)
SOL,PO (1X170ML)
170 ml............57771-0007-02 270.00 450.00

CYTOSE (Solace)
POW,PO (1X250GM)
250 gm............57771-0001-20 48.00 80.00

CYTOTINE (Solace)
SOL,PO (1X480ML)
480 ml............57771-0001-91 36.00 60.00

D-1000 (21st Century)
TAB,PO (MAXIMUM STRENGTH)
185 mg-1000 iu,
110s ea...........40985-0270-62 3.60 5.99

D-3 (Bio-Tech Pharm)
CAP,PO, 1000 iu,
100s ea...........53191-0454-01 3.50
250s ea...........53191-0454-25 7.25

D-MANNOSE (Bio-Tech Pharm)
CAP,PO, 300 mg, 50s ea...53191-0407-05 9.00
100s ea...........53191-0407-01 17.50
POW,PO (1X50GM)
0.9 gm/0.5 tsp, 50 gm.53191-0342-50 16.00
(1X100GM)
0.9 gm/0.5 tsp,
100 gm............53191-0342-10 25.00

PROD/MFR	HRI, UPC,NDC	AWP	SRP
D-NATURAL-5 (Key Company)			
SGL,PO (SOFTGEL)			
5000 u-10000 u,			
100s ea	11694-0915-01	4.50	
250s ea	11694-0915-25	9.00	
1000s ea	11694-0915-03	32.00	
D-R-C PERI-RECTAL CREME (Xttrium Labs)			
CRE,TP, 120 gm	00116-0851-03	4.38	4.90
D-RIBOSE (Bio-Tech Pharm)			
POW,PO (1X150GM)			
3 gm/tsp, 150 gm	53191-0467-15	22.10	
D-TRON ADAPTER (Disetronic)			
DEV,NA, 10s ea	08173-1062-01	71.40	
D-TRON POWER PACK (Disetronic)			
DEV,NA, ea	08173-1064-01	21.60	
D.O.C.'S EMERGENCY DENTURE REPAIR (Majestic Drug)			
DEV,NA (3 USES)			
ea	10705-0400-91	3.00	5.99
DAILY CALCIUM + VITAMIN D (Nature's Bounty)			
TAB,PO (PF)			
600 mg-125 iu, 60s ea.	74312-0042-36		4.49
DAILY HERBS BLOOD SUGAR BALANCE (Mason Vit)			
TAB,PO, 30s ea	11845-0134-38	19.98	
DAILY HERBS BREAST HEALTH (Mason Vit)			
TAB,PO (PF,SF)			
30s ea	11845-0134-28	19.98	
DAILY HERBS ENERGY (Mason Vit)			
TAB,PO (PF,SF)			
30s ea	11845-0133-88	19.98	
DAILY HERBS IMMUNE DEFENSE (Mason Vit)			
TAB,PO, 30s ea	11845-0133-68	19.98	
DAILY HERBS LEG VEIN & CIRCULATION (Mason Vit)			
TAB,PO (PF,SF)			
30s ea	11845-0133-78	19.98	
DAILY HERBS MEMORY (Mason Vit)			
TAB,PO (PF,SF)			
30s ea	11845-0133-58	19.98	
DAILY HERBS PROSTATE (Mason Vit)			
SGL,PO (PF,SF,SOFTGEL)			
30s ea	11845-0133-48	19.98	
DAILY HERBS RELAX & EASE TENSION (Mason Vit)			
TAB,PO (PF,SF)			
30s ea	11845-0134-18	19.98	
DAILY HERBS VISION HEALTH (Mason Vit)			
TAB,PO (PF,SF)			
30s ea	11845-0134-08	19.98	
DAILY MULTIPLE (ADH)			
TAB,PO, 100s ea	60142-0042-10	1.05	
(Mason Vit)			
TAB,PO (SF)			
100s ea	11845-0008-81	4.44	
DAILY MULTIPLE VITAMINS (Marlex)			
TAB,PO, 30s ea	10135-0115-30	0.99	
60s ea	10135-0115-60	1.11	
100s ea	10135-0115-01	1.28	
(BLISTER PACK)			
100s ea UD	10135-0160-13	2.60	
1000s ea	10135-0115-10	8.57	
(Rexall)			
TAB,PO (MULTIPLE CHOICE,PF,SF)			
90s ea	30768-0000-53	2.00	3.03
(Truxton)			
TAB,PO, 100s ea	00463-6133-01	3.00	
1000s ea	00463-6133-10	18.00	
(A-S Medication)			
REPACK			
TAB,PO, 100s ea	54569-2823-00	3.25	
DAILY MULTIPLE VITAMINS W/IRON (Marlex)			
TAB,PO, 100s ea	10135-0347-01	1.40	
250s ea	10135-0347-69	2.97	
1000s ea	10135-0347-10	9.75	
(Rexall)			
TAB,PO (PF,SF)			
90s ea	30768-0000-54	2.11	3.20
DAILY MULTIPLE VITAMINS/MINERALS (Rexall)			
PO (PF,SF)			
90s ea	30768-0000-60	3.84	5.82
DAILY MULTIPLE W/IRON (Mason Vit)			
TAB,PO (SF)			
365s ea	11845-0000-03	12.44	
DAILY MULTIPLE W/MINERALS (Mason Vit)			
TAB,PO, 60s ea	11845-0095-55	6.33	
DAILY VALUE MULTIVITAMIN (Freeda)			
TAB,PO (MODERATE,SF,GLUTEN-FREE)			
100s ea	10432-0314-01	5.07	8.45
250s ea	10432-0314-02	10.14	16.90
DAILY VITAMIN (Major)			
LIQ,PO (AF,SF)			
473 ml	00904-0985-16	13.93	
DAILY VITAMINS W/CALCIUM/IRON (Basic Vitamins)			
TAB,PO (FOR WOMEN)			
60s ea	00761-0334-12	2.15	
DAILY VITE (Rugby)			
TAB,PO, 100s ea	00536-3547-01	4.19	
1000s ea	00536-3547-10	20.92	
(Dispensing Solutions)			
REPACK			
TAB,PO, 100s ea	55045-3282-01	6.00	
DAILY VITE W/IRON (Rugby)			
TAB,PO, 100s ea	00536-3546-01	3.52	
1000s ea	00536-3546-10	20.92	
DAIRY DIGESTIVE SUPPLEMENT (Cardinal Health)			
TAB,PO (PRIVATE LABEL,CAPLET)			
60s ea	37205-0113-72	6.40	
DAIRY DIGESTIVE SUPPLEMENT ULTRA (Cardinal Health)			
CTB,PO (PRIVATE LABEL,CAPLET)			
9000 u, 32s ea	37205-0114-72	7.60	
DAIRYCARE (Plainview LLC)			
ECC,PO, 15 mg-190 mg,			
10s ea	44733-0480-10	2.14	2.99
30s ea	44733-0480-30	5.52	7.99
60s ea	44733-0480-60	9.84	12.99
DAKIN'S (Century)			
SOL,TP, 0.125%, 473 ml	00436-0672-16	8.58	9.50
DAKINS SOLUTION (Century)			
SOL,TP, 0.25%, 480 ml	00436-0936-16	8.58	9.50
0.5%, 480 ml	00436-0946-16	8.58	9.50
DAMIANA LEAVES (ADH)			
CAP,PO (PF,SF)			
450 mg, 100s ea	60142-0909-01	4.98	9.95
DANDELION (Botanical Labs.)			
LIQ,PO, 30 ml	41954-0020-11	4.00	7.99
DANDELION ROOT (ADH)			
CAP,PO (PF,SF)			
520 mg, 100s ea	60142-0907-71	4.98	9.95
DANDREX (Altaire)			
SHA,TP, 1%, 240 ml	59390-0045-41	3.75	
DARA (Valeant Pharm Intl)			
SHA,TP, 480 ml	00064-2010-16	17.71	
DARAGEN (Valeant Pharm Intl)			
SHA,TP, 240 ml	00064-2020-08	13.56	
DAY TIME MULTI-SYMPTOM COLD/FLU RELIEF (Major)			
SGL,PO, 325 mg-10 mg-5 mg,			
12s ea	00904-5763-12	4.15	
DAY-LEE DISPOSABLE WASHCLOTHS (J&J Medical)			
DEV,NA (REGULAR,13 1/2"X10 1/2")			
50s ea	56091-0041-35	3.21	
DAYHIST-1 (AmerisourceBergen)			
TAB,PO (PRIVATE LABEL)			
1.34 mg, 8s ea	24385-0183-51	3.14	3.49
DAYTIME COLD (Teva)			
SGL,PO (NON-DROWSY,AF,SOFTGEL)			
250 mg-10 mg-30 mg,			
12s ea	00182-1115-11	3.49	
DB-7 (Rx Vitamins)			
CAP,PO, 60s ea	08429-0700-60	10.98	21.95
DE WITT PILLS (Monticello)			
TAB,PO, 20s ea	11868-0010-12	1.11	
40s ea	11868-0010-11	1.66	
80s ea	11868-0010-13	2.47	
DEBROX (Glaxo)			
SOL,OT (W/ DROPPER)			
15 ml	07661-0021-09	5.89	
6.5%, 15 ml	00088-1021-05	4.39	
30 ml	00088-1021-01	6.98	
DECANTING SET (Abbott Hosp)			
DEV,NA (14")			
48s ea	00074-1721-48	315.65	
DECAVITAMIN (Consolidated Midland)			
TAB,PO, 100s ea	00223-0714-01	5.50	
1000s ea	00223-0714-02	52.50	
DECOLATE (Wesley)			
TAB,PO, 2 mg-100 mg-5 mg,			
100s ea	00917-0832-01	4.95	
DECONEX DMX (Poly)			
TAB,PO, 15 mg-380 mg-10 mg,			
60s ea	50991-0730-60	40.41	
DECONEX IR (Poly)			
TAB,PO, 380 mg-10 mg,			
60s ea	50991-0716-60	40.41	
DECONGESTANT (Albertson's)			
TAB,PO, 48s ea	41280-0201-75	3.06	
DECONGESTANT TABLETS (Basic Vitamins)			
TAB,PO, 30 mg, 60s ea	00761-0604-12	2.15	
DECONGESTANT/ANTIHISTAMINE (Basic Vitamins)			
TAB,PO, 60 mg-2.5 mg,			
100s ea	00761-0912-20	2.60	
DECOREL FORTE PLUS (Medique)			
TAB,PO (50X2)			
325 mg-15 mg-200 mg-5 mg,			
100s ea UD	47682-0425-33	7.71	
(250X2)			
325 mg-15 mg-200 mg-5 mg,			
500s ea UD	47682-0425-13	36.53	
DEEP SEA (Major)			
SPR,NS, 0.65%, 45 ml	00904-3865-75	2.10	
DEFENDER HOLDER CADDY (Covidien)			
DEV,NA, 10s ea	08080-2283-18	288.75	
DEFENSE SUN PADS (Topix)			
PAD,TP (SPF 30)			
6%-7.5%-5%, 60s ea	58211-0607-60	6.60	
DEL-CLENS (Del-Ray)			
SOL,TP, 240 ml	00316-0148-08	8.73	
DEL-RAY (Del-Ray)			
SHA,TP, 240 ml	00316-0146-08	7.43	
DELAZINC (Mericon)			
OIN,TP, 25%, 480 gm	00394-0014-41	11.75	
DELFEN FOAM (Phys Total Care)			
REPACK			
FOA,VG, 12.5%, 17 gm	54868-4196-00	13.04	
DELSYM (Reckitt Benckiser)			
SER,PO (1X89ML,ADULT,AF,ORANGE)			
30 mg/5 ml, 89 ml	63824-0175-63	7.86	
(1X89ML,AF,GRAPE)			
30 mg/5 ml, 89 ml	63824-0172-63	7.86	
(1X89ML,AF,ORANGE)			
30 mg/5 ml, 89 ml	63824-0176-63	7.86	
(AF,ORANGE)			
30 mg/5 ml, 89 ml	53014-0463-43	7.86	
89 ml	53014-0463-61	7.86	
(ADULT,GRAPE)			
30 mg/5 ml, 90 ml	63824-0171-63	7.86	
(1X148ML,12 HOUR,AF)			
30 mg/5 ml, 148 ml	63824-0171-65	10.69	
148 ml	63824-0172-65	10.69	
(1X148ML,ADULT,AF,ORANGE)			
30 mg/5 ml, 148 ml	63824-0175-65	10.69	
(1X148ML,AF,ORANGE)			
30 mg/5 ml, 148 ml	63824-0176-65	10.69	
(A-S Medication)			
REPACK			
SER,PO, 30 mg/5 ml,			
90 ml	54569-1051-00	7.72	
(Phys Total Care)			
REPACK			
SER,PO (1X89ML,AF,ORANGE)			
30 mg/5 ml, 89 ml	54868-6003-00	11.86	
(1X148ML,AF,ORANGE)			
30 mg/5 ml, 148 ml	54868-6003-01	15.43	
DELTA D3 (Freeda)			
TAB,PO (PF,SF,DYE-FREE)			
400 iu, 250s ea	10432-0170-02	6.57	10.95
500s ea	10432-0170-03	11.91	19.85
DELUXE FIRST AID KIT (Johnson & Johnson)			
DEV,NA, ea	81370-0059-98	17.70	

PROD/MFR	HRI, UPC, NDC	AWP	SRP
DENDRACIN NEURODENDRAXCIN (Physicians Science)			
LOT,TP (1X60ML)			
0.0375%-10%-30%, 60 ml	27495-0006-02	122.46	
(1X120ML)			
0.0375%-10%-30%, 120 ml	27495-0006-04	244.92	
(Aidarex) REPACK			
LOT,TP (1X60ML)			
15%-5%-30%, 60 ml	33261-0409-01	122.46	
(1X120ML)			
15%-5%-30%, 120 ml	33261-0410-01	244.92	
(Altura) REPACK			
LOT,TP (1X60ML)			
15%-5%-30%, 60 ml	63874-1269-06	146.95	
(1X120ML)			
15%-5%-30%, 120 ml	63874-1269-04	293.90	
(Pharma Pac) REPACK			
LOT,TP (1X60ML)			
15%-5%-30%, 60 ml	52959-0930-60	120.08	
DENT-O-KAIN/20 (Geritrex)			
SOL,MM (MAXIMUM STRENGTH)			
20%, 9 ml	54162-0950-09	4.90	
DENT'S EXTRA STRENGTH TOOTHACHE GUM (Dent,C.S.)			
WAX,DE, 20%, 1 gm 12s	10486-0001-00	31.68	
DENTAPAINE (Reese)			
GEL,MM, 20%, 11 gm	10956-0608-11	3.87	
DENTEMP (Majestic Drug)			
KIT,TP, ea	10705-0400-81	2.15	4.85
DENTEMP O.S. (Majestic Drug)			
PAS,TP, 2 gm	10705-0400-85	2.15	4.85
DENTEMP'S ORAL PAIN RELIEF (Majestic Drug)			
SWA,MM (GEL,CHERRY)			
20%, 8s ea	10705-0400-95	4.00	7.99
DENTIVA (Nuvora)			
LOZ,MM (AF,SF)			
12s ea	91124-0002-01	8.00	
120s ea	91124-0002-03	80.00	
DENTOOL (Majestic Drug)			
DEV,NA (4 IN 1)			
ea	10705-0400-93	3.00	6.99
DENTOOL JR (Majestic Drug)			
DEV,NA (2 IN 1,PIK & SCALER)			
ea	10705-0400-92	1.75	2.75
DENTUR-FIT (Regent Labs)			
CRE,NA (ORIGINAL,EXTRA HOLD)			
68 gm	83272-0881-02	2.78	
DENTURE CLEANSER (Major)			
TEF,NA, 40s ea	00904-7744-39	2.40	
DERM-APPLY SCENTED (Snuva)			
LOT,TP (HYPO-ALLERGENIC)			
59 ml	58291-0001-02	3.00	4.50
177 ml	58291-0001-01	5.00	8.75
DERM-APPLY UNSCENTED (Snuva)			
LOT,TP (HYPO-ALLERGENIC)			
59 ml	58291-0002-02	3.00	4.50
177 ml	58291-0002-01	5.00	8.75
DERMA CERIN (Dermarite)			
CRE,TP, 120 gm	61924-0178-04	4.57	
480 gm	61924-0178-16	5.05	
DERMA GRAN (Derma Sciences)			
OIN,TP (PACKET)			
0.275%, 5 gm UD	25382-0126-05	0.78	
120 gm	25382-0126-34	17.64	
120 gm	25382-0126-36	17.64	
SPR,TP, 120 ml	25382-0127-52	8.26	5.92
DERMA GRAN AF (Derma Sciences)			
OIN,TP, 2%, 113 gm	25382-0302-04	9.63	
DERMA PHOR (Dermarite)			
OIN,TP, 120 gm	61924-0184-04	5.18	
480 gm	61924-0184-16	11.02	
DERMA VANTAGE (Dermarite)			
LOT,TP, 60 ml	61924-0142-02	0.75	
240 ml	61924-0142-08	2.43	
DERMA-GEL SEMI-OCCLUSIVE (Medline)			
DEV,NA (4"X4", STERILE)			
100s ea	53329-0550-40	340.65	
DERMA-PAX (Recsei)			
LOT,TP, 0.5%, 120 ml	10952-0008-16	6.15	
DERMACLOUD (Carolina)			
OIN,TP (FANNY CREAM)			
430 gm	46287-0502-16	22.40	
DERMADAILY (Dermarite)			
LOT,TP, 118 ml	61924-0124-04	0.67	
240 ml	61924-0128-08	0.73	
DERMADRESS (Dermarite)			
DEV,NA (6"X6")			
10s ea	61924-0277-66	31.30	
(STERILE DRESSING)			
10s ea	61924-0276-44	25.50	
DERMADROX (Geritrex)			
OIN,TP (JAR)			
120 gm	54162-0221-04	10.56	
(TUBE)			
120 gm	54162-0221-01	10.67	
SPR,TP (12X118ML,FRAGRANCE-FREE)			
0.45%, 118 ml 12s	54162-0220-14	6.84	
DERMAFILM (Dermarite)			
DEV,NA (4"X4",EXTRA THIN)			
ea	61924-0259-44	7.20	
DERMAFIX (Ameriderm Labs)			
OIN,TP (PH BALANCED,JAR)			
113 gm	63921-0405-04	7.81	
(PH BALANCED,TUBE)			
113 gm	63921-0400-04	7.50	
(24X113GM)			
113 gm 24s	63921-0400-04	7.81	
SPR,TP (PH BALANCED)			
118 ml	63921-0410-04	5.00	
DERMAFUNGAL (Dermarite)			
OIN,TP, 2%, 113 gm	61924-0234-04	10.75	
DERMAGAUZE HYDROGEL (Dermarite)			
DEV,NA (2"X2")			
ea UD	61924-0248-22	3.61	
(4"X4")			
ea	61924-0248-99	3.95	
(2"X2")			
15s ea	61924-0240-02	36.75	
DERMAGINATE (Dermarite)			
DEV,NA (12" ROPE)			
ea	61924-0275-12	6.98	
(4"X4")			
ea	61924-0270-44	4.23	
DERMAGRAN HYDROGEL (Derma Sciences)			
DRE,TP, ea	25382-0250-03	7.21	
DERMAGRAN HYDROPHILIC WOUND (Derma Sciences)			
DEV,NA (2"X2")			
ea	25382-0200-20	2.16	
(4"X4")			
ea	25382-0200-21	3.79	
(8"X4")			
ea	25382-0200-24	4.23	
DERMAGRAN SALINE (Derma Sciences)			
DRE,TP, 32s ea	25382-0192-20	1.73	
DERMAGRAN TRI-ZINC (Derma Sciences)			
SPR,TP, 240 ml	25382-0300-08	2.61	
DERMAGRAN WOUND CLEANSER W/ZINC (Derma Sciences)			
LIQ,TP, 120 ml	25382-0128-04	1.79	
DERMAGRAN ZINC-SALINE (Derma Sciences)			
DRE,TP, 32s ea	25382-0195-10	1.77	
DERMAGRAN-B WOUND DRESSING (Derma Sciences)			
DEV,NA (HYDROPHILIC)			
90 gm	25382-0201-03	15.57	
DERMAKLENZ WOUND CLEANSER (Dermarite)			
SPR,TP, 473 ml	61924-0246-16	11.25	
DERMAL THERAPY (Bayer Diabetes Care)			
CRE,TP (HEEL CARE)			
18 gm	00193-5134-01	6.50	
(FINGER CARE)			
60 gm	00193-5170-01	5.35	
(FOOT MASSAGE)			
120 gm	00193-5171-01	6.50	
(HAND, ELBOW, KNEE)			
120 gm	00193-5169-01	6.90	
LOT,TP (EXT. STR. BODY)			
240 ml	00193-5168-01	8.00	
(FACE CARE)			
240 ml	00193-5167-01	9.25	
DERMAL WOUND CLEANSER (Smith & Nephew)			
LIQ,TP, 240 ml	50484-0492-00	10.61	8.49
480 ml	50484-0490-00	16.83	13.46
DERMALAB BATH & BODY OIL (Dermalab)			
OIL,TP, 240 ml	10641-0003-48	7.22	
DERMALAB CLEANSING BAR (Dermalab)			
SOA,TP (UNSCENTED)			
ea	10641-0003-02	2.71	
DERMALAB CONDITIONING SHAMPOO (Dermalab)			
SHA,TP, 240 ml	10641-0003-28	5.80	
DERMALAB LUBRICATING LOTION (Dermalab)			
LOT,TP (UNSCENTED)			
240 ml	10641-0003-08	7.22	
DERMALAB SKIN CLEANSER (Dermalab)			
SOL,TP, 240 ml	10641-0003-30	7.22	
DERMALAB SKIN CREAM (Dermalab)			
CRE,TP (UNSCENTED)			
120 gm	10641-0003-04	7.22	
DERMALAB SUNBLOCK (Dermalab)			
LIQ,TP (SPF 15,SF)			
120 ml	10641-0004-15	7.22	
DERMALAB SUPER FATTED SOAP (Dermalab)			
SOA,TP (UNSCENTED)			
ea	10641-0003-00	2.71	
DERMALEVIN (Dermarite)			
DEV,NA (ADHESIVE FOAM DRESSING)			
10s ea	61924-0285-66	60.90	
DERMALEVIN FOAM (Dermarite)			
DEV,NA (ADHESIVE FOAM DRESSING)			
10s ea	61924-0280-44	38.90	
DERMAMED (Dermarite)			
OIN,TP (JAR)			
120 gm	61924-0214-44	15.95	
(TUBE)			
120 gm	61924-0214-04	15.95	
SPR,TP, 118 ml	61924-0224-04	6.91	
DERMAMYCIN (Pfeiffer)			
CRE,TP, 2%, 28 gm	00927-0561-30	2.35	4.23
SPR,TP, 2%-1%, 60 ml	00927-0564-20	2.35	4.23
DERMANAIL (Summers)			
LIQ,TP, 30 ml	11086-0026-01	18.43	
DERMAPAIN (Pfeiffer)			
OIN,TP, 28.35 gm	00927-0194-30	3.05	5.49
DERMAPLEX (MPM Medical Inc.)			
GEL,TP (1X170GM)			
170 gm	66977-0306-06	24.58	27.32
DERMAREST ECZEMA BODY WASH (Del)			
SOL,TP, 177 ml	10310-0073-78	5.75	8.62
DERMAREST ECZEMA MEDICATED (Del)			
LOT,TP (FRAGRANCE-FREE)			
1%, 118 ml	10310-0339-42	7.16	10.75
DERMAREST ECZEMA MEDICATED MOISTURIZER (Del)			
CRE,TP, 1%, 56.6 gm	10310-0325-02	5.04	7.56
DERMAREST MOISTURIZING SCAR REDUCER (Del)			
GEL,TP, 28 gm	10310-0322-51	5.75	8.62
DERMAREST PSORIASIS MEDICATED MOISTURIZER (Del)			
LOT,TP (FRAGRANCE-FREE)			
2%, 118 ml	10310-0073-03	5.75	8.62
DERMAREST PSORIASIS OVERNIGHT TREATMENT (Del)			
CRE,TP (MAXIMUM STRENGTH)			
3%, 56.7 gm	10310-0328-18	5.04	7.56
DERMAREST PSORIASIS SCALP TREATMENT (Del)			
GEL,TP, 3%, 118 ml	10310-0073-12	5.87	8.80
DERMAREST PSORIASIS SHAMPOO (Del)			
SHA,TP (W/CONDITIONER,PF)			
3%, 236 ml	10310-0073-02	5.87	8.80
DERMAREST PSORIASIS SKIN TREATMENT (Del)			
GEL,TP (FRAGRANCE-FREE)			
3%, 118 ml	10310-0073-01	5.87	8.80
DERMAREST ROSACEA ADVANCED REDNESS TREATMENT (Del)			
CRE,TP, 56.7 gm	10310-0324-31	7.20	10.80
DERMAREST STRETCH MARK REPAIR (Del)			
CRE,TP, 85 gm	10310-0323-51	4.50	6.75
DERMASARRA (Dermarite)			
LOT,TP (ANTI-ITCH LOTION)			
0.5%-0.5%, 222 ml	61924-0188-08	7.11	

PROD/MFR	HRI, UPC,NDC	AWP	SRP
DERMASEPT ANTIFUNGAL (Pharmakon)			
SPR,TP, 1%, 30 ml	55422-0701-30	3.82	7.97
DERMASOFT (Ameriderm Labs)			
LOT,TP (W/ALOE)			
118 ml	63921-0110-04	0.39	
237 ml	63921-0110-08	0.65	
3780 ml	63921-0110-01	7.81	
DERMASORB (Med-Derm)			
GEL,TP, 114 gm	55747-0011-14	7.00	
DERMASYN GEL (Dermarite)			
SPR,TP, 228 gm	61924-0248-08	38.88	
DERMASYN HYDROGEL (Dermarite)			
DEV,NA, ea	61924-0248-03	15.95	
DERMATONE CAMPHOR ICE (Dermatone)			
STI,TP, 22.5 gm	20908-0023-11	1.84	
DERMATONE LIPS N FACE PROTECTOR (Dermatone)			
OIN,TP (SPF 23,AF,SF)			
12 gm	20908-0022-34	1.25	
DERMATONE MEDICATED LIP (Dermatone)			
STI,TP (SPF 23,SF)			
4.5 gm	20908-0022-73	1.10	
DERMATONE MEDICATED LIP BALM (Dermatone)			
STI,TP (SPF 23,SF)			
9 gm	20908-0022-70	1.20	
9 gm	20908-0022-72	1.40	
DERMATONE MOISTURIZING SUNBLOCK (Dermatone)			
CRE,TP (SPF 23,AF,SF)			
30 gm	20908-0022-66	2.10	
30 gm	20908-0022-67	1.95	
30 gm	20908-0422-66	1.95	
(SPF 33, KIDS,AF,SF)			
30 gm	20908-0022-69	2.25	
(SPF 33,AF,SF)			
30 gm	20908-0022-68	2.25	
(SPF 33, KIDS,AF,SF)			
120 gm	20908-0022-77	5.30	
DERMATONE SKIN PROTECTION STICK (Dermatone)			
STI,TP (SPF 23,SF)			
22.5 gm	20908-0022-56	2.90	
DERMATONE SKIN PROTECTOR (Dermatone)			
CRE,TP (SPF 15,AF,SF)			
15 gm	20908-0022-45	2.25	
OIN,TP (SPF 23,SF)			
4%-4.5%-8%, 14 gm	20908-0022-46	2.40	
31 gm	20908-0022-85	3.75	
STI,TP, 4.5%-4%-7%,			
14 gm	20908-0022-08	2.25	
DERMATONE TOPCOAT SUNBLOCK (Dermatone)			
SPR,TP (FOR SCALP/SKIN, SPF 20+)			
118 ml	20908-0022-96	3.95	
DERMATONE UVA/UVB SUNBLOCK (Dermatone)			
CRE,TP (SPF 15,SF)			
15 gm	20908-0022-05	2.25	
DERMATOX (Reese)			
LOT,TP (1X120ML, PAIN & ITCH)			
2%-1%, 120 ml	10956-0742-04	6.64	9.69
DERMAVIEW (Dermarite)			
DEV,NA (4"X5")			
50s ea	61924-0251-44	109.00	
(TRANSPARENT FILM;4X4.5)			
50s ea	61924-0253-44	76.50	
(2.2"X2.6")			
100s ea	61924-0241-23	185.00	
(TRANSPARENT;2.375X2.75)			
100s ea	61924-0252-23	42.00	
DERMAVITE (Stiefel Consumer HealthCare)			
TAB,PO, 60s ea	73462-0268-66	12.60	18.99
DERMICEL HYPO-ALLERGENIC CLOTH (J&J Medical)			
DEV,NA (3"X10 YD/ROLL)			
4s ea	56091-0051-46	9.95	
(2"X10YD/ROLL)			
6s ea	56091-0051-45	9.95	
(1"X10 YD/ROLL)			
12s ea	56091-0051-44	9.95	
(1/2"X10YD/ROLL)			
24s ea	56091-0051-43	9.95	
(2"X1YD/SINGLE USE ROLL)			
48s ea	56091-0051-40	21.52	
(1"X1YD/SINGLE USE ROLL)			
96s ea	56091-0051-39	21.52	
DERMICEL MONTGOMERY STRAPS (J&J Medical)			
DEV,NA (7 1/4"X11 1/8")			
24s ea	56091-0051-29	38.54	
DERMIFORM HYPO-ALLERGENIC KNITTED (J&J Medical)			
DEV,NA (3"X10YD/ROLL)			
4s ea	56091-0051-83	10.57	
(2"X10YD/ROLL)			
6s ea	56091-0051-82	10.57	
(1"X10YD/ROLL)			
12s ea	56091-0051-81	10.57	
(1/2"X10YD/ROLL)			
24s ea	56091-0051-80	10.57	
(2"X1YD/SINGLE USE ROLL)			
48s ea	56091-0051-79	29.76	
(1"X1YD/SINGLE USE ROLL)			
96s ea	56091-0051-78	29.76	
DERMOPLAST (Medtech)			
SPR,TP (W/ALOE& LANOLIN)			
20%-0.5%, 60 ml	63029-8504-01	3.26	
(W/ALOE & LANOLIN)			
20%-0.5%, 78 gm	75137-0855-20	5.78	7.57
DERMOPLAST ANTIBACTERIAL (Medtech)			
SPR,TP (HOSPITAL STRENGTH)			
0.2%-20%, 78 gm	75173-0857-00	4.82	
DERMTEX-HC (Pfeiffer)			
CRE,TP, 1%, 30 gm	00927-0041-30	2.47	4.44
SPR,TP, 1%, 52.5 ml	00927-0641-20	2.94	5.29
DESENEX (Novartis Consumer)			
CRE,TP (1X15GM)			
1%, 15 gm	00067-6190-05	5.17	
DESITIN (Johnson & Johnson)			
OIN,TP (OVERNIGHT RELIEF)			
40%, 90 gm	74300-0000-19	4.10	
DESITIN MAXIMUM STRENGTH ORIGINAL (Johnson & Johnson)			
OIN,TP, 40%, 56 gm	74300-0000-70	3.16	
113 gm	74300-0000-71	4.66	
DESITIN MULTI-PURPOSE (Johnson & Johnson)			
OIN,TP, 60.4%, 49 gm	58232-0071-31	3.60	
99 gm	74300-0495-21	5.41	
DESITIN ORIGINAL (Johnson & Johnson)			
OIN,TP (OVERNIGHT RELIEF)			
40%, 28 gm	74300-0000-68	2.28	
454 gm	74300-0000-65	11.75	
DESITIN RAPID RELIEF CREAMY (Johnson & Johnson)			
CRE,TP, 13%, 56 gm	74300-0003-00	3.16	
113 gm	74300-0003-01	4.66	
454 gm	74300-0495-16	11.75	
DETACHOL (Ferndale)			
LIQ,TP, 0.666 ml 48s	00496-0513-48	118.31	
15 ml UD	00496-0513-15	3.76	
60 ml	00496-0513-06	8.44	
120 ml	00496-0513-04	12.29	
DETANE (Del)			
GEL,MM, 7.5%, 15 gm	10310-0094-11	3.32	
DETOX (Reese)			
CAP,PO, 15s ea	23513-0696-15	4.55	
DETOXOSODE ALCOHOL (HVS Labs)			
LIQ,PO (AF,SF)			
120 ml	52386-9605-04	9.00	
DETOXOSODE ALLERGENS-ANTIGENS (HVS Labs)			
LIQ,PO (AF,SF)			
120 ml	52386-9606-04	9.00	
DETOXOSODE BACTERIA (HVS Labs)			
LIQ,PO (AF,SF)			
120 ml	52386-9607-04	9.00	
DETOXOSODE CHEMICALS (HVS Labs)			
LIQ,PO (AF,SF)			
120 ml	52386-9608-04	9.00	
DETOXOSODE DENTALS (HVS Labs)			
LIQ,PO (AF,SF)			
120 ml	52386-9609-04	9.00	
DETOXOSODE FOOD ADDITIVES I (HVS Labs)			
LIQ,PO (AF)			
120 ml	52386-9610-04	9.00	
DETOXOSODE FOOD ADDITIVES II (HVS Labs)			
LIQ,PO, 120 ml	52386-9611-04	9.00	
DETOXOSODE FREE RADICALS (HVS Labs)			
LIQ,PO (AF,SF)			
120 ml	52386-9614-04	9.00	
DETOXOSODE FUNGI-YEASTS (HVS Labs)			
LIQ,PO (AF,SF)			
120 ml	52386-9613-04	9.00	
DETOXOSODE METALS (HVS Labs)			
LIQ,PO (AF,SF)			
120 ml	52386-9615-04	9.00	
DETOXOSODE NEMATODES (HVS Labs)			
LIQ,PO (AF,SF)			
120 ml	52386-9616-04	9.00	
DETOXOSODE O-S (HVS Labs)			
LIQ,PO (AF,SF)			
120 ml	52386-9604-04	9.00	
DETOXOSODE PARASITES (HVS Labs)			
LIQ,PO (AF,SF)			
120 ml	52386-9617-04	9.00	
DETOXOSODE POLLUTION-AIR (HVS Labs)			
LIQ,PO (AF,SF)			
120 ml	52386-9618-04	9.00	
DETOXOSODE POLLUTION-ENVIRONS (HVS Labs)			
LIQ,PO (AF,SF)			
120 ml	52386-9619-04	9.00	
DETOXOSODE RADIATION (HVS Labs)			
LIQ,PO (AF,SF)			
120 ml	52386-9620-04	9.00	
DETOXOSODE RICKETTSIA (HVS Labs)			
LIQ,PO (AF,SF)			
120 ml	52386-9621-04	9.00	
DETOXOSODE TOBACCO (HVS Labs)			
LIQ,PO (AF,SF)			
120 ml	52386-9622-04	9.00	
DETOXOSODE VIRUSES (HVS Labs)			
LIQ,PO (AF,SF)			
120 ml	52386-9623-04	9.00	
DEVIL'S CLAW (ADH)			
CAP,PO (PF,SF)			
510 mg, 100s ea	60142-0908-51	5.95	11.95
DEVON ANDREWS FRAME KIT (Covidien)			
DEV,NA (SINGLE PATIENT USE)			
3s ea	08080-1510-40	70.05	
DEVON ANDREWS TABLE KIT (Covidien)			
DEV,NA (SINGLE PATIENT USE)			
6s ea	08080-1510-30	240.00	
DEVON JACKSON TABLE KIT (Covidien)			
DEV,NA (SINGLE PATIENT USE)			
6s ea	08080-1510-10	247.50	
DEVON JACKSON TABLE KIT, NO HEADREST (Covidien)			
DEV,NA (SINGLE PATIENT USE)			
6s ea	08080-1510-20	195.00	
DEVON SCHLEIN BEACH CHAIR KIT (Covidien)			
DEV,NA (SINGLE PATIENT USE)			
3s ea	08080-1510-50	90.90	
DEVON WILSON FRAME KIT (Covidien)			
DEV,NA (SINGLE PATIENT USE)			
6s ea	08080-1510-60	255.00	
DEWEE'S CARMINATIVE (Humco)			
LIQ,PO, 230 mg/5 ml,			
60 ml	00395-0713-92	3.88	
DEX 4 (Can-Am Care)			
CTB,PO (QUICK DISSOLVE)			
4 gm, 40s ea	38396-0560-63	5.18	
(CAFFEINE-FREE)			
4 gm, 50s ea	38396-0555-63	5.18	
50s ea	38396-0558-63	5.18	
DEX4 (Can-Am Care)			
CTB,PO (BITS,CAFFEINE-FREE)			
1.18 gm, 60s ea	38396-0595-63	3.49	
(GRAPE)			
4 gm, 10s ea	38396-0503-63	1.99	
(ORANGE)			
4 gm, 10s ea	38396-0501-63	1.99	
(RASPBERRY)			
4 gm, 10s ea	38396-0502-63	1.99	
10s ea	38396-0522-63	1.99	
(WATERMELON)			
4 gm, 10s ea	38396-0507-63	1.99	
(GRAPE)			
4 gm, 50s ea	38396-0543-63	7.99	
(ORANGE)			
4 gm, 50s ea	38396-0541-63	7.99	
(RASPBERRY)			
4 gm, 50s ea	38396-0542-63	7.99	
(WATERMELON)			
4 gm, 50s ea	38396-0547-63	7.99	
SOL,PO (6X59ML,CAFFEINE-FREE)			
59 ml 6s	38396-0592-63	17.92	
59 ml 6s	38396-0593-63	17.92	

PROD/MFR	HRI, UPC,NDC	AWP	SRP
DEX4 GLUCOSE (Can-Am Care)			
GEL,PO (3X38GM,TROPICAL BLAST)			
15 gm, 38 gm 3s	38396-0580-63	8.11	
DEXALONE (Dexgen)			
CAP,PO (BLISTER PACK,GELCAP)			
30 mg, 100s ea	65430-0105-01	33.75	
DEXTROMETHORPHAN HYDROBROMIDE/ GUAIFENESIN (Palmetto)			
REPACK			
SYR,PO, 10 mg/5 ml-100 mg/5 ml,			
120 ml	23490-6677-00	7.80	
(1X120ML)			
10 mg/5 ml-100 mg/5 ml,			
120 ml	23490-5655-01	5.76	
DEXTROMETHORPHAN/GUAIFENESIN (Rugby)			
SYR,PO (FRUIT)			
10 mg/5 ml-100 mg/5 ml,			
120 ml	00536-0970-97	3.27	
480 ml	00536-0970-85	8.09	
(A-S Medication)			
REPACK			
SYR,PO (10ML UD,FRUIT)			
10 mg/5 ml-100 mg/5 ml,			
10 ml UD	54569-3676-01	4.83	
DHEA (ADH)			
CAP,PO (PF,SF)			
25 mg, 60s ea	60142-0484-76	5.98	11.95
(Bio-Tech Pharm)			
CAP,PO (MICRONIZED)			
25 mg, 100s ea	53191-0419-01	10.00	
50 mg, 100s ea	53191-0253-01	17.50	
(Breckenridge Pharm)			
TAB,PO, 25 mg, 60s ea	51991-0022-06	5.95	
(Marlex)			
TAB,PO, 25 mg, 60s ea	10135-0273-60	1.50	
(Mason Vit)			
CAP,PO (PF,SF)			
25 mg, 30s ea	11845-0112-98	4.67	
60s ea	11845-0112-95	8.33	
50 mg, 30s ea	11845-0113-08	7.78	
(Rexall)			
TAB,PO, 25 mg, 100s ea	30768-0040-62	3.85	5.79
DHEA MAX (Nutraceutics)			
TER,PO (CAPLET)			
25 mg, 60s ea	02359-0710-07	25.00	
DHEA PLUS (Nutraceutics)			
TAB,PO (CAPLET)			
25 mg-700 mg-25 mg-6 mg,			
60s ea	02359-0110-01	28.00	
DHEA/GINKGO BILOBA (Applied Nutr. Inc.)			
CAP,PO, 25 mg-400 mg,			
30s ea	10363-0253-34	2.75	
60s ea	10363-0253-35	4.25	
DHS CLEAR (Person & Covey)			
SHA,TP, 240 ml	00096-0725-08	4.50	
480 ml	00096-0725-16	7.53	
DHS CONDITIONING RINSE (Person & Covey)			
LIQ,TP (W/PANTHENOL)			
240 ml	00096-0726-08	4.65	
DHS REGULAR (Person & Covey)			
SHA,TP, 240 ml	00096-0727-08	4.60	
480 ml	00096-0727-16	7.57	
DHS SAL (Person & Covey)			
LIQ,TP, 3%, 120 ml	00096-0731-04	4.50	
DHS TAR (Person & Covey)			
SHA,TP, 0.5%, 120 ml	00096-0728-04	4.22	
240 ml	00096-0728-08	6.39	
480 ml	00096-0728-16	9.62	
DHS TARGEL (Person & Covey)			
SHA,TP, 0.5%, 240 ml	00096-0730-08	6.75	
DHS ZINC (Person & Covey)			
SHA,TP, 2%, 240 ml	00096-0729-08	6.01	
360 ml	00096-0729-12	7.85	
(Phys Total Care)			
REPACK			
SHA,TP (1X360ML)			
2%, 360 ml	54868-5871-00	17.58	
DI-DAK-SOL (Century)			
SOL,TP, 0.0125%, 473 ml	00436-0669-16	8.58	9.50
DIAB CREAM (Carrington)			
CRE,TP, 85 gm	53303-0030-30	7.35	
DIAB DAILY CARE HYDROGEL (Carrington)			
DEV,NA, 14.1 gm	53303-0021-11	5.90	
DIAB KLENZ (Carrington)			
SPR,TP, 236 ml	53303-0080-81	11.55	
DIABETAID GINGIVITIS MOUTH RINSE (Del)			
SOL,MM, 0.1%, 473.6 ml	10310-0340-42	4.32	6.48
DIABETAID HAND & BODY LOTION (Del)			
LOT,TP (DEEP MOISTURIZING)			
113.2 gm	10310-0340-46	6.60	9.90
DIABETES TRIO (Mason Vit)			
TER,PO (CAPLET)			
60s ea	11845-0142-75	17.67	
DIABETI DERM HEEL & TOE (Health Care Products)			
CRE,TP (MAXIMUM RELIEF)			
120 gm	60569-0473-04	8.21	12.99
DIABETIC CARRY-ALL (Apothecary)			
DEV,NA, ea	25715-0669-62	6.25	10.49
DIABETIC DAILY LOG (Apothecary)			
DEV,NA, ea	25715-0669-67	2.77	4.69
DIABETIC I.D. CARD W/BRACELET (Apothecary)			
DEV,NA, ea	25715-0669-64	5.14	8.59
DIABETIC I.D. CARD W/NECKLACE (Apothecary)			
DEV,NA, ea	25715-0669-54	5.14	8.59
DIABETIC SILTUSSIN DAS-NA (Silarx)			
SOL,PO (AF,SF,SODIUM-FREE)			
100 mg/5 ml, 118 ml	54838-0138-40	4.46	
DIABETIC SILTUSSIN-DM (Silarx)			
SOL,PO (AF,SF,SODIUM-FREE)			
10 mg/5 ml-100 mg/5 ml,			
118 ml	54838-0139-40	4.46	
10 mg/5 ml-200 mg/5 ml,			
118 ml	54838-0140-40	4.48	
DIABETIC TUSSIN (Health Care Products)			
SOL,PO (1X118ML,AF,SF)			
100 mg/5 ml,			
118 ml	60569-0063-04	4.20	6.49
(1X118ML,AF,SF,DYE-FREE)			
200 mg/5 ml,			
118 ml	61787-0446-04	4.46	6.99
DIABETIC TUSSIN COLD & FLU (Health Care Products)			
SOL,PO (1X118ML,AF,SF,DYE-FREE)			
118 ml	61787-0452-04	4.46	6.99
(1X177ML,AF,SF,DYE-FREE)			
177 ml	61787-0452-06	5.70	8.49
(1X237ML,AF,SF,DYE-FREE)			
237 ml	61787-0452-08	6.93	9.99
DIABETIC TUSSIN COUGH DROPS (Health Care Products)			
LOZ,MM (EUCALYPTUS,SF,DYE-FREE)			
25s ea	60569-0058-25	1.75	2.39
DIABETIC TUSSIN DM (Health Care Products)			
SOL,PO (REGULAR STRENGTH,AF,SF)			
10 mg/5 ml-100 mg/5 ml,			
118 ml	61787-0062-04	4.20	6.49
DIABETIC TUSSIN DM MAXIMUM STRENGTH (Health Care Products)			
LIQ,PO (AF,SF,DYE-FREE)			
10 mg/5 ml-200 mg/5 ml,			
118 ml	60569-0064-04	4.46	6.99
237 ml	60569-0064-08	6.93	9.99
DIABETIC TUSSIN MUCUS RELIEF (Health Care Products)			
TAB,PO (SF,DYE-FREE,SODIUM-FREE)			
400 mg, 50s ea	61787-0445-50	6.30	9.99
DIABETIC TUSSIN NIGHT TIME FORMULA (Health Care Products)			
SOL,PO (AF,SF,DYE-FREE)			
118 ml	60569-0471-04	4.46	6.99
DIABETIC.COM PRESTIGE SMART SYSTEM (Home Diag)			
DEV,NA (STRIP)			
50s ea	56151-0316-50	26.12	
DIABETIC.COM PSS STARTER (Home Diag)			
DEV,NA (MTR,STRP,LANCET,DEV,SOL)			
ea	56151-0216-01	22.18	
DIABETIC'S FOOTCREAM (Stanmar Labs)			
CRE,TP, 141 gm	50263-0610-05	5.50	
DIABETIC'S HANDCREAM (Stanmar Labs)			
CRE,TP, 141 gm	50263-0600-05	5.00	
DIABETIDERM FOOT REJUVENATING (Health Care Products)			
CRE,TP, 113.4 gm	60569-0680-49	8.21	12.99
DIABETIDERM TOENAIL & FOOT FUNGUS (Health Care Products)			
CRE,TP (1X42GM)			
10%, 42 gm	60569-0481-15	10.50	15.99
DIABETIKS (Green Turtle)			
TAB,PO (PF,SF,DYE-FREE)			
60s ea	59074-0300-02	12.00	19.99
120s ea	59074-0300-01	20.40	33.99
DIABETISOURCE AC (Nestle)			
SUS,PO (6X1000ML)			
1000 ml 6s	43900-0365-08	80.14	
(6X1500ML)			
1500 ml 6s	43900-0365-82	120.17	
DIABETISWEET (Health Care Products)			
POW,PO (1X454GM)			
454 gm	60569-0464-16	5.78	7.99
480 gm	61787-0056-16	5.78	7.99
DIALYVITE 800 (Hillestad)			
TAB,PO, 100s ea	10542-0070-10	10.40	
DIALYVITE 800 W/ZINC (Hillestad)			
TAB,PO, 100s ea	10542-0050-10	11.80	
DIALYVITE 800 WITH IRON (Hillestad)			
TAB,PO, 100s ea	10542-0075-10	11.76	
DIALYVITE 800 WITH ZINC 15 (Hillestad)			
TAB,PO, 100s ea	10542-0015-10	11.09	
DIALYVITE 800/ULTRA D (Hillestad)			
TAB,PO, 90s ea	10542-0025-09	15.87	
DIAMODE (Medique)			
TAB,PO (50X1,CAPLET)			
2 mg, 50s ea UD	47682-0200-50	13.10	
(100X1,CAPLET)			
2 mg, 100s ea UD	47682-0200-33	28.70	
DIAPER RASH (Actavis Mid Atlantic)			
OIN,TP, 120 gm	00472-1802-04	3.10	
(G&W)			
OIN,TP, 120 gm	00713-0258-04	3.76	
DIAPER-CARE (Weleda)			
OIN,TP (PF)			
12%, 42 gm	55946-0003-57	3.84	
DIASCREEN 10 REAGENT STRIPS (Arkray)			
DEV,NA, 100s ea	08317-1100-00	33.00	
DIASCREEN 1B (Arkray)			
DIASCREEN 1B			
NA, 50s ea	08317-1315-50	7.35	
DIASCREEN 1G REAGENT STRIPS (Arkray)			
DEV,NA, 100s ea	08317-1110-00	6.98	
DIASCREEN 1K REAGENT STRIPS (Arkray)			
DEV,NA, 50s ea	08317-1215-50	6.08	
100s ea	08317-1215-00	6.98	
DIASCREEN 2GK REAGENT STRIPS (Arkray)			
DEV,NA, 100s ea	08317-1220-00	9.00	
DIASCREEN 2GP REAGENT STRIPS (Arkray)			
DEV,NA, 100s ea	08317-1120-00	15.83	
DIASCREEN 3 REAGENT STRIPS (Arkray)			
DEV,NA, 100s ea	08317-1130-00	27.23	
DIASCREEN 4NL REAGENT STRIPS (Arkray)			
DEV,NA, 100s ea	08317-1340-00	19.95	
DIASCREEN 4OBL REAGENT STRIPS (Arkray)			
DEV,NA, 100s ea	08317-1240-00	19.95	
DIASCREEN 4PH REAGENT STRIPS (Arkray)			
DEV,NA, 100s ea	08317-1140-00	20.85	
DIASCREEN 5 REAGENT STRIPS (Arkray)			
DEV,NA, 100s ea	08317-1150-00	24.53	
DIASCREEN 6 REAGENT STRIPS (Arkray)			
DEV,NA, 100s ea	08317-1160-00	32.55	
DIASCREEN 7 REAGENT STRIPS (Arkray)			
DEV,NA, 100s ea	08317-1170-00	33.75	
DIASCREEN 8 REAGENT STRIPS (Arkray)			
DEV,NA, 100s ea	08317-1180-00	36.98	
DIASCREEN 9 REAGENT STRIPS (Arkray)			
DEV,NA, 100s ea	08317-1190-00	37.05	
DIASCREEN URINE CONTROLS (Arkray)			
DEV,NA (2 EA POSITIVE/NEGATIVE)			
10 ml 4s	08317-7600-04	44.25	
DIASENSE CHROMIUM (Blaine)			
CAP,PO (SF,GLUTEN-FREE)			
200 mcg-60 mg,			
60s ea	01650-0088-60	9.30	

PROD/MFR	HRI, UPC,NDC	AWP	SRP
DIASENSE MAGNESIUM (Blaine)			
TAB,PO (SF,GLUTEN-FREE)			
241.3 mg, 60s ea	**01650-0077-60**	8.70	
DIASENSE MULTIVITAMIN (Blaine)			
TAB,PO (SF,GLUTEN-FREE,CINNAMON)			
30s ea	**01650-0099-30**	9.30	
DIASTIX (Bayer Diabetes Care)			
DEV,NA, 50s ea	**00193-2802-50**	7.32	
100s ea	**00193-2802-21**	12.48	
DIBUCAINE (Consolidated Midland)			
OIN,TP, 1%, 30 gm	**00223-4121-30**	1.80	
454 gm	**00223-4121-13**	12.95	
(Fougera)			
OIN,TP, 1%, 30 gm	**00168-0046-31**	3.65	
(Perrigo)			
OIN,TP (W/APPLICATOR)			
1%, 30 gm	**45802-0050-03**	3.49	
DICAL-D (Abbott Pharm)			
TAB,PO, 117 mg-133 iu,			
100s ea	**00074-3741-13**	22.84	
DICKINSON'S CLEANSING W/ALOE (Dickinson Brands)			
SOA,TP, 3s ea	**10331-0006-03**	3.43	
DICKINSON'S WITCH HAZEL ASTRINGENT (Dickinson Brands)			
LOT,TP (BLUE LABEL)			
60 ml	**05265-1000-07**	0.46	
240 ml	**05265-1000-05**	1.75	
480 ml	**05265-1000-06**	2.57	
DICKINSON'S WITCH HAZEL FORMULA (Dickinson Brands)			
LIQ,TP (YELLOW LABEL)			
60 ml	**10331-0000-07**	0.46	
240 ml	**10331-0000-08**	2.02	
480 ml	**10331-0000-16**	2.75	
960 ml	**10331-0000-32**	4.70	
3840 ml	**10331-0001-28**	15.13	
PAD,TP (TOWELETTES)			
20s ea	**10331-0000-20**	2.26	
50s ea	**10331-0000-09**	2.26	
DIET SYSTEM 6 (Applied Nutr. Inc.)			
CAP,PO, 60s ea	**10363-0253-37**	7.77	
100s ea	**10363-0253-59**	10.77	
GUM,PO (SF,COOL MINT)			
24s ea	**10363-0253-46**	2.99	
DIET SYSTEM 6 FOR MEN (Applied Nutr. Inc.)			
CAP,PO, 60s ea	**10363-0253-36**	7.77	
DIETEX FORTE (Kramer-Novis)			
CAP,PO, 60s ea	**52083-0470-60**	17.20	
DIFF-STAT (Medical Nutrition USA)			
CTB,PO (ORANGE,PINEAPPLE)			
30s ea	**26974-0410-80**	115.78	
PDR,PO (1X2GM)			
2 gm	**26974-0410-81**	129.64	
DIGESPLEN-PLUS (Med Prods Panamer)			
CAP,PO, 50s ea	**00576-0160-50**	12.60	
DIGEST I (Bio-Tech Pharm)			
CAP,PO, 130 mg-195 mg-65 mg,			
100s ea	**53191-0338-01**	5.75	
DIGESTIVE AID #34 (Carlson,J.R.)			
TAB,PO, 34 mg-340 mg,			
50s ea	**88395-0066-40**	4.30	8.60
100s ea	**88395-0066-41**	7.75	15.50
250s ea	**88395-0066-42**	17.75	35.50
500s ea	**88395-0066-45**	32.95	65.90
DIGESTIVE ENZYMES (Mason Vit)			
TAB,PO (PF,SF)			
90s ea	**11845-0118-69**	7.78	
DIGITAL EAR THERMOMETER (Lumiscope)			
DEV,NA (INSTANT READ,DUAL SCALE)			
ea	**38673-0022-15**	29.99	59.99
DIGITAL THERMOMETER (Lumiscope)			
DEV,NA (FAST READ,DUAL SCALE)			
ea	**38673-0022-10**	4.99	9.99
(SOFT TIP,FAST)			
ea	**38673-0022-14**	5.99	11.99
DIGITAL THERMOMETER PROBE COVERS (BD Consumer)			
DEV,NA (30 COUNT)			
ea	**08290-5240-35**	1.19	
DIMACID (Medique)			
CTB,PO (150X2,SF)			
265 mg-95 mg-20 mg,			
300s ea	**10244-0530-63**	30.71	
DIME (Med Prods Panamer)			
CAP,PO, 30s ea	**00576-0599-30**	12.60	
DIMENHYDRINATE (Albertson's)			
TAB,PO, 50 mg, 12s ea	**41280-0210-50**	1.32	
(Consolidated Midland)			
LIQ,PO, 12.5 mg/4 ml,			
480 ml	**00223-6250-01**	12.50	
TAB,PO, 50 mg, 100s ea	**00223-0860-01**	3.25	
1000s ea	**00223-0860-02**	27.00	
(Contract Pharmacal)			
TAB,PO, 50 mg, 100s ea	**10267-1006-01**	2.90	
1000s ea	**10267-1006-04**	22.90	
(Marlex)			
TAB,PO, 50 mg, 12s ea	**10135-0177-12**	0.78	
36s ea	**10135-0177-36**	0.85	
100s ea	**10135-0177-01**	1.35	
1000s ea	**10135-0177-10**	8.90	
(Qualitest)			
TAB,PO, 50 mg, 100s ea	**00603-3327-21**	3.70	
1000s ea	**00603-3327-32**	16.50	
(Truxton)			
TAB,PO, 50 mg, 1000s ea	**00463-6221-10**	12.00	
(A-S Medication) REPACK			
TAB,PO, 50 mg, 12s ea	**54569-2864-01**	0.44	
(HomeMed) REPACK			
TAB,PO, 50 mg, 20s ea	**51655-0681-52**	2.88	
(Phys Total Care) REPACK			
TAB,PO, 50 mg, 12s ea	**54868-1862-00**	7.26	
100s ea	**54868-1862-01**	7.27	
(Southwood) REPACK			
TAB,PO, 50 mg, 30s ea	**58016-0475-30**	1.02	
40s ea	**58016-0992-40**	4.27	
60s ea	**58016-0475-60**	2.04	
90s ea	**58016-0475-90**	3.06	
100s ea	**58016-0475-00**	3.40	
120s ea	**58016-0475-02**	4.08	
DIMETAPP DECONGESTANT PEDIATRIC (Wyeth Consumer)			
LIQ,PO (AF,DROPS),			
7.5 mg/0.8 ml,			
15 ml	**00031-2283-78**		5.49
DIMETAPP DM (Phys Total Care) REPACK			
ELI,PO (GRAPE)			
120 ml	**54868-1892-00**	7.51	
DIOCTO (Major)			
LIQ,PO, 150 mg/15 ml,			
480 ml	**00904-0936-16**	15.99	
(Rugby)			
LIQ,PO (VANILLA)			
150 mg/15 ml, 480 ml	**00536-0590-85**	12.00	
SYR,PO (PEPPERMINT)			
60 mg/15 ml, 480 ml	**00536-0600-85**	5.70	
(Teva)			
LIQ,PO, 150 mg/15 ml,			
480 ml	**00182-1774-40**	7.39	
DIOCTYL (R.I.J.)			
SYR,PO, 60 mg/15 ml,			
480 ml	**53807-0193-03**	3.64	
DIOSUCCIN (Consolidated Midland)			
SGL,PO, 100 mg, 100s ea	**00223-0854-01**	3.25	
1000s ea	**00223-0854-02**	32.50	
250 mg, 100s ea	**00223-0855-01**	5.25	
1000s ea	**00223-0855-02**	47.50	
DIOSUCCIN C (Consolidated Midland)			
SYR,PO, 30 mg/15 ml-60 mg/15 ml,			
480 ml	**00223-6341-01**	5.50	
DIOTAME (Medique)			
CTB,PO (50X2)			
262 mg, 100s ea UD	**47682-0220-33**	10.60	
(250X2)			
262 mg, 500s ea UD	**47682-0220-13**	47.39	
DIOTAME STOMACH RELIEF (Medique)			
PO (12X2)			
262 mg, 24s ea UD	**47682-0220-64**	2.84	
(15X2)			
262 mg, 30s ea UD	**47682-0220-83**	3.29	
DIPHEDRYL (AmerisourceBergen)			
TAB,PO (PRIVATE LABEL)			
25 mg, 24s ea	**24385-0479-62**	3.05	3.39
100s ea	**24385-0479-78**	8.09	8.99
DIPHEN (Medique)			
CAP,PO (SF)			
25 mg, 12s ea UD	**47682-0182-32**	1.34	
24s ea UD	**47682-0182-64**	1.75	
200s ea UD	**47682-0182-47**	11.69	
DIPHENHIST (Rugby)			
CAP,PO, 25 mg, 100s ea	**00536-3594-01**	6.38	
CRE,TP, 2%-0.1%, 30 gm	**00536-4180-95**	3.29	
SOL,PO, 12.5 mg/5 ml,			
120 ml	**00536-0770-97**	3.78	
480 ml	**00536-0770-85**	7.42	
TAB,PO (CAPTAB)			
25 mg, 100s ea	**00536-3597-01**	6.38	
DIPHENHYDRAMINE (Core) REPACK			
CAP,PO, 25 mg, 30s ea	**33358-0110-30**	24.60	
(Phys Total Care) REPACK			
ELI,PO (AF)			
12.5 mg/5 ml,			
473 ml	**54868-1227-00**	11.01	
SOL,PO, 12.5 mg/5 ml,			
120 ml	**54868-1227-02**	8.49	
(Physician Partner) REPACK			
CAP,PO, 25 mg, 30s ea	**21695-0304-30**	17.70	
90s ea	**21695-0304-90**	53.10	
(Quality Care Prod) REPACK			
CAP,PO, 25 mg, 20s ea	**49999-0003-20**	10.79	
(Stat Rx) REPACK			
CAP,PO, 25 mg, 20s ea	**16590-0078-20**	4.00	
30s ea	**16590-0078-30**	16.50	
50 mg, 20s ea	**16590-0079-20**	11.00	
DIPHENHYDRAMINE HCL (Advance)			
CAP,PO, 25 mg, 100s ea	**17714-0020-01**	3.50	
1000s ea	**17714-0020-10**	16.25	
TAB,PO (CAPLET)			
25 mg, 100s ea	**17714-0042-01**	3.99	
(Bio-Pharm)			
ELI,PO, 12.5 mg/5 ml,			
120 ml	**59741-0119-04**	2.20	
240 ml	**59741-0119-08**	3.05	
480 ml	**59741-0119-16**	4.70	
3840 ml	**59741-0119-20**	22.00	
(Concord Labs)			
TAB,PO (CAPLET)			
25 mg, 10s ea	**20254-0207-10**	1.49	
60s ea	**20254-0207-06**	5.27	
50 mg, 10s ea	**20254-0208-10**	1.76	
60s ea	**20254-0208-06**	6.62	
(Contract Pharmacal)			
CAP,PO, 25 mg, 100s ea	**10267-0835-01**	6.75	
1000s ea	**10267-0835-04**	53.75	
50 mg, 100s ea	**10267-0836-01**	8.25	
1000s ea	**10267-0836-04**	59.75	
(Magno-Humphries)			
TAB,PO (MAX. STR.)			
50 mg, 50s ea	**43292-0557-65**	1.50	3.19
(Major)			
CAP,PO, 25 mg, 100s ea	**00904-5306-60**	4.10	
(10X10)			
25 mg, 100s ea UD	**00904-5306-61**	12.50	
1000s ea	**00904-5306-80**	18.50	
50 mg, 100s ea	**00904-5307-60**	4.75	
(10X10)			
50 mg, 100s ea UD	**00904-2056-61**	13.45	
1000s ea	**00904-5307-80**	26.95	
(Marlex)			
CAP,PO, 25 mg, 10s ea	**10135-0149-61**	5.28	
24s ea	**10135-0149-24**	0.70	
100s ea	**10135-0149-01**	1.22	
1000s ea	**10135-0149-10**	8.70	
50 mg, 100s ea	**10135-0156-01**	5.94	
1000s ea	**10135-0156-10**	35.41	
TAB,PO (BOXED,CAPLET)			
25 mg, 24s ea	**10135-0151-52**	65.00	
(CAPLET)			
25 mg, 24s ea	**10135-0151-24**	0.72	
50s ea	**10135-0151-50**	0.94	
(BLISTER PACK,CAPLET)			
25 mg, 100s ea UD	**10135-0166-13**	4.00	

PROD/MFR	HRI, UPC,NDC	AWP	SRP
(BOXED,CAPLET)			
25 mg, 100s ea	10135-0151-57	65.00	
(CAPLET)			
25 mg, 100s ea	10135-0151-01	1.08	
1000s ea	10135-0151-10	7.90	
50 mg, 100s ea UD	10135-0156-13	3.26	
(Perrigo)			
CRE,TP, 2%, 30 gm	45802-0358-03	3.99	
(Rugby)			
TAB,PO, 50 mg, 50s ea	00536-3772-06	4.43	
(Sandoz)			
CAP,PO, 25 mg, 100s ea	00185-0648-01	8.26	
1000s ea	00185-0648-10	45.50	
50 mg, 100s ea	00185-0649-01	9.04	
1000s ea	00185-0649-10	58.24	
(UDL)			
TAB,PO (10X10)			
25 mg, 100s ea UD	51079-0967-20	11.15	
(A-S Medication)			
REPACK			
CAP,PO, 25 mg, 6s ea	54569-0239-08	0.50	
8s ea	54569-3504-00	0.66	
10s ea	54569-3504-01	0.83	
15s ea	54569-0239-02	1.24	
20s ea	54569-0239-03	1.65	
24s ea	54569-0239-01	1.98	
30s ea	54569-0239-00	2.48	
50 mg, 30s ea	54569-0241-00	2.51	
ELI,PO (AF)			
12.5 mg/5 ml,			
120 ml	54569-4197-00	2.18	
(Aidarex)			
REPACK			
CAP,PO, 25 mg, 7s ea	33261-0225-07	1.19	
10s ea	33261-0225-10	1.70	
14s ea	33261-0225-14	2.34	
20s ea	33261-0225-20	3.40	
25s ea	33261-0225-25	4.25	
28s ea	33261-0225-28	4.76	
30s ea	33261-0225-30	5.10	
60s ea	33261-0225-60	10.20	
50 mg, 14s ea	33261-0383-14	13.14	
28s ea	33261-0383-28	26.27	
30s ea	33261-0383-30	28.15	
60s ea	33261-0383-60	56.30	
(Altura)			
REPACK			
CAP,PO, 25 mg, 6s ea	63874-0005-06	4.51	
9s ea	63874-0005-09	6.76	
10s ea	63874-0005-10	7.51	
12s ea	63874-0005-12	9.01	
14s ea	63874-0005-14	10.51	
15s ea	63874-0005-15	11.27	
20s ea	63874-0005-20	15.02	
21s ea	63874-0005-21	15.77	
24s ea	63874-0005-24	18.02	
25s ea	63874-0005-25	18.78	
28s ea	63874-0005-28	21.03	
30s ea	63874-0005-30	22.53	
40s ea	63874-0005-40	30.04	
45s ea	63874-0005-45	33.80	
60s ea	63874-0005-60	45.06	
90s ea	63874-0005-90	67.59	
100s ea	63874-0005-01	75.10	
1000s ea	63874-0005-02	43.61	
50 mg, 15s ea	63874-0006-15	9.11	
20s ea	63874-0006-20	12.15	
30s ea	63874-0006-30	18.22	
1000s ea	63874-0006-02	190.27	
(DHS, Inc.)			
REPACK			
CAP,PO, 25 mg, 30s ea	55887-0973-30	14.52	
(Dispensing Solutions)			
REPACK			
CAP,PO, 25 mg, 12s ea	55045-1125-04	4.92	
15s ea	55045-1125-05	6.15	
20s ea	55045-1125-06	8.20	
30s ea	55045-1125-08	12.30	
50 mg, 30s ea	55045-1124-08	18.30	
CRE,TP, 2%, 30 gm	55045-3402-01	3.99	
ELI,PO (AF)			
12.5 mg/5 ml,			
118 ml	55045-1252-02	8.10	
(Nucare Pharm)			
REPACK			
CAP,PO, 25 mg, 15s ea	66267-0080-15	10.21	
20s ea	66267-0080-20	11.38	
30s ea	66267-0080-30	18.94	
60s ea	66267-0080-60	23.95	
50 mg, 15s ea	66267-0081-15	7.31	
20s ea	66267-0081-20	7.24	
30s ea	66267-0081-30	10.86	
60s ea	66267-0081-60	21.72	
(Pharma Pac)			
REPACK			
ELI,PO, 12.5 mg/5 ml,			
180 ml	52959-0123-06	12.53	
(Physician Partner)			
REPACK			
CAP,PO, 50 mg, 15s ea	21695-0500-15	12.71	
30s ea	21695-0500-30	18.17	
ELI,PO, 12.5 mg/5 ml,			
120 ml	21695-0689-04	7.56	
(Quality Care Prod)			
REPACK			
CAP,PO, 25 mg, 21s ea	49999-0003-21	11.33	
100s ea	49999-0003-00	47.38	
(Southwood)			
REPACK			
CAP,PO, 25 mg, 6s ea	58016-0408-06	1.30	
9s ea	58016-0408-09	1.95	
10s ea	58016-0408-10	2.17	
12s ea	58016-0408-12	2.60	
14s ea	58016-0408-14	3.04	
15s ea	58016-0408-15	3.25	
20s ea	58016-0408-20	4.34	
21s ea	58016-0408-21	4.55	
24s ea	58016-0408-24	5.21	
25s ea	58016-0408-25	5.42	
28s ea	58016-0408-28	6.07	
30s ea	58016-0408-30	6.51	
40s ea	58016-0408-40	8.68	
60s ea	58016-0408-60	13.01	
100s ea	58016-0408-00	21.69	
(Vibranta)			
REPACK			
CAP,PO, 25 mg, 12s ea	57866-3594-02	2.00	
20s ea	57866-3594-06	2.25	
30s ea	57866-3594-01	6.83	
90s ea	57866-3594-05	7.19	
DIPHENHYDRAMINE HYDROCHLORIDE (Advent)			
CAP,PO, 50 mg, 100s ea	60242-0202-01	1.35	
1000s ea	60242-0202-10	11.75	
(Amneal)			
CAP,PO (MAXIMUM STRENGTH)			
50 mg, 100s ea	65162-0518-10	8.45	
1000s ea	65162-0518-11	45.95	
(Qualitest)			
CAP,PO (USP)			
25 mg, 100s ea	00603-3339-21	8.26	
1000s ea	00603-3339-32	45.50	
(SDA)			
CAP,PO, 25 mg, 1000s ea	66424-0020-10	45.00	
(Palmetto)			
REPACK			
SOL,PO (1X120ML)			
12.5 mg/5 ml,			
120 ml	23490-5455-01	7.43	
(PD-Rx Pharm)			
REPACK			
CAP,PO (USP)			
25 mg, 6s ea	43063-0185-06	7.16	
(Physician Partner)			
REPACK			
CAP,PO, 25 mg, 15s ea	21695-0304-15	8.85	
DIPHENYL (Global Source)			
CAP,PO, 25 mg, 24s ea	59618-0200-06	2.70	
DIPHENYL ELIXIR (Global Source)			
ELI,PO, 12.5 mg/5 ml,			
120 ml	59618-0199-33	2.45	
DISCOUNT DRUG MART GLUCOSE (Can-Am Care)			
TAB,PO (GLUTEN-FREE)			
4 gm, 50s ea	38396-0541-57	6.49	
50s ea	38396-0542-57	6.49	
(Inverness)			
CTB,PO (RASPBERRY)			
4 gm, 50s ea	36652-5424-03	5.99	
DISCOUNT DRUG MART THIN LANCETS (Can-Am Care)			
DEV,NA (26G,SINGLE USE)			
100s ea	38396-0301-57	5.85	
DISCOUNT DRUG MART ULTRA THIN LANCETS (Can-Am Care)			
DEV,NA (30G,SINGLE USE)			
100s ea	38396-0305-57	5.85	
DISETRONIC GLASS CARTRIDGE (Disetronic)			
DEV,NA (EMPTY, 3.15 ML)			
25s ea	08173-0004-25	98.40	
DISETRONIC TENDER 1 INFUSION (Disetronic)			
DEV,NA (31", SET)			
ea	08173-0015-10	124.80	
DISETRONIC TENDER 2 INFUSION (Disetronic)			
DEV,NA (24", SET)			
ea	08173-9050-20	206.40	
(31", SET)			
ea	08173-0017-20	206.40	
DIUCAPS (Legere)			
CAP,PO (SF,DYE-FREE)			
1000s ea	25332-7200-01	89.95	
DIUREX WATER PILL (Alva-Amco)			
TAB,PO, 22s ea	72959-0060-22	1.99	2.98
42s ea	72959-0060-42	2.79	4.19
84s ea	72959-0060-84	4.92	7.36
DL-ALPHA TOCOPHERYL E400 (Mason Vit)			
SGL,PO (SOFT GEL,PF,SF,SOFTGEL)			
400 iu, 300s ea	11845-0050-50	22.78	
DL-PA-500 (Bio-Tech Pharm)			
CAP,PO, 500 mg, 100s ea	53191-0026-01	11.55	
DL-PHEN-500 (Key Company)			
CAP,PO (SF)			
500 mg, 60s ea	11694-0820-01	7.50	
DM/GG/PSEUDOEPH (Phys Total Care)			
REPACK			
LIQ,PO (AF)			
118 ml	54868-4493-00	8.94	
DMG (Miller)			
TAB,PO, 60s ea	17204-0550-20	4.08	6.80
DML (Person & Covey)			
LOT,TP, 240 ml	00096-0722-08	5.95	
480 ml	00096-0722-16	9.50	
DML FORTE (Person & Covey)			
CRE,TP, 120 gm	00096-0720-04	6.00	
DNZ-2 (Bio-Tech Pharm)			
CAP,PO, 100 mg, 100s ea	53191-0121-01	14.00	
250 mg, 100s ea	53191-0123-01	22.00	
DOAK TAR OIL 2% (Doak)			
OIL,TP, 0.8%, 240 ml	10337-0690-81	34.30	
DOAN'S (Novartis Consumer)			
SPR,TP, 8.4%-15%-0.6%,			
120 ml	00083-7550-87	4.76	
DOAN'S EXTRA STRENGTH (Novartis Consumer)			
TAB,PO, 500 mg, 24s ea	00083-0235-88	5.54	
DOAN'S PM (Novartis Consumer)			
TAB,PO, 25 mg-500 mg,			
20s ea	00083-0245-17	5.54	
DOAN'S REGULAR (Novartis Consumer)			
TAB,PO, 325 mg, 24s ea	00083-0230-88	4.36	
DOBELL'S SOLUTION (Lex)			
SOL,TP, 240 ml	49523-0098-08	0.90	
480 ml	49523-0099-16	1.12	
DOC DENTURE WIPES (Majestic Drug)			
DEV,NA, 40s ea	10705-0400-30	1.50	2.79
DOC-Q-LACE (Qualitest)			
LIQ,PO (VANILLA)			
150 mg/15 ml,			
480 ml	00603-0746-58	6.70	
SGL,PO (SOFTGEL)			
100 mg, 100s ea	00603-0145-21	3.11	
1000s ea	00603-0145-32	29.55	
SYR,PO, 60 mg/15 ml,			
480 ml	00603-0747-58	8.43	
DOC-Q-LAX (Qualitest)			
TAB,PO, 50 mg-8.6 mg,			
100s ea	00603-0149-21	23.98	
1000s ea	00603-0149-32	227.81	
(Quality Care Prod)			
REPACK			
TAB,PO, 50 mg-8.6 mg,			
60s ea	49999-0912-60	15.68	
DOCOMEGA (VITAFLO, LLC)			
POW,NA (30X4GM)			
30s ea	50600-0505-40	75.00	93.75

PROD/MFR | HRI, UPC,NDC | AWP | SRP

(30X)
12 x, 500s ea 00622-3053-03 4.19
5500s ea 00622-3053-10 31.83
(12X)
30 x, 500s ea 00624-3053-03 4.19
5500s ea 00624-3053-10 31.83

DULCOLAX (Boehr Ingelheim Cons)
ECT,PO (BLISTER PACK)
5 mg, 10s ea......... 00067-6200-48 2.02 3.52
25s ea 81421-0020-02 6.77
(BLISTER PACK)
5 mg, 25s ea......... 00067-6200-53 4.26 6.15
50s ea 00067-6200-55 7.24 10.40
100s ea 81421-0020-04 21.50
(BLISTER PACK)
5 mg, 100s ea........ 00067-6200-32 13.46 19.94
SGL,PO (STOOL SOFTENER)
100 mg, 10s ea 81421-0022-01 2.11
25s ea 81421-0220-26 6.19
50s ea 81421-0220-33 10.99
100s ea 81421-0220-40 19.99
SUP,RC, 10 mg, 4s ea 81421-0210-10 3.47 5.62
8s ea............. 00067-6100-08 6.66 10.06
16s ea 00067-6100-51 11.56 17.65
(COMFORT SHAPED)
10 mg, 16s ea........ 81421-0021-03 20.69
28s ea 81421-0021-05 19.02
50s ea 00067-6100-50 31.68 47.68

(Nucare Pharm)
REPACK
SUP,RC, 10 mg, 8s ea 68071-1345-00 13.60

(Palmetto)
REPACK
ECT,PO, 5 mg, 30s ea 23490-7880-03 12.69

(Phys Total Care)
REPACK
SUP,RC, 10 mg, 8s ea 54868-3155-00 8.37

DULCOLAX BOWEL CLEANSING KIT (Boehr Ingelheim Cons)
KIT,MR (LEMON)
ea.................. 81421-0024-01 6.50

DULCOLAX BOWEL PREP KIT (Boehr Ingelheim Cons)
KIT,MR, ea 81421-0023-01 2.50

DULCOLAX MILK OF MAGNESIA (Boehr Ingelheim Cons)
SUS,PO (SF,MINT)
400 mg/5 ml,
355 ml 81421-0026-02 3.53
(SF,ORIGINAL)
400 mg/5 ml,
355 ml 81421-0026-01 3.53
(SF,MINT)
400 mg/5 ml,
769 ml 81421-0026-04 5.50
(SF,ORIGINAL)
400 mg/5 ml,
769 ml 81421-0026-03 5.50

DUO-CARE (Forecare, Inc.)
DEV,NA, ea 08536-0100-00 52.50

DUO-CARE CONTROL SOLUTION (Forecare, Inc.)
DEV,NA (2X4ML)
2s ea.............. 08536-0120-00 9.94

DUO-CARE TEST STRIPS (Forecare, Inc.)
DEV,NA, 50s ea 08536-0115-00 26.25
100s ea 08536-0110-00 50.00

DUOCAL (Nutricia)
PDR,PO (USE W/MED SUPV)
400 gm 4s........... 49735-0102-80 100.10

DUODENUM (Key Company)
TAB,PO, 650 mg, 100s ea.. 11694-0898-01 9.25
500s ea............ 11694-0898-03 45.00

DUODERM CGF (Convatec)
DEV,NA (6"X8",STERILE)
5s ea............... 68455-0102-69 85.41 112.27
5s ea............... 68455-0102-72 70.60 92.80
(STERILE 4X4)
5s ea............... 68455-0106-97 32.84 43.16
(4"X4",STERILE)
20s ea.............. 68455-0102-70 127.16 167.14
(6"X6",STERILE)
20s ea.............. 68455-0102-71 268.14 353.75

ODERM HYDROACTIVE (Convatec)
,NA (4"X4",STERILE)
20s ea.............. 68455-0106-93 204.16 268.35

PROD/MFR | HRI, UPC,NDC | AWP | SRP

DUOFILM (Schering Plough)
SOL,TP (W/20 COVER-UP DISCS)
17%, 9.8 ml 11017-0252-20 6.07

(Quality Care Prod)
REPACK
LIQ,TP, 17%, 0.33 ml...... 49999-0716-13 12.08

DUOLOCK CURVED TAIL CLOSURE (Convatec)
DEV,NA, 10s ea 68455-0108-67 18.46 24.03

DUPLEX T (Genesis)
SHA,TP, 10%, 480 ml 00398-0096-16 11.46
3840 ml 00398-0096-28 71.94

DURAFLEX (TriMarc Labs)
TAB,PO, 60s ea 68752-0706-60 6.25
120s ea 68752-0706-98 11.95

DURAFLEX COMFORT GEL (TriMarc Labs)
GEL,TP (1X60ML)
60 ml................ 68752-0016-02 4.50

DURAMIST PLUS (Pfeiffer)
SPR,NS, 0.05%, 15 ml 00927-0889-23 1.86 3.34

DURAPORE SILK LIKE SURGICAL (3M Health Care)
DEV,NA (3"X10 YDS)
4s ea................ 08333-1538-03 12.20
(2"X10 YDS)
6s ea................ 08333-1538-02 12.20
(1"X10 YDS)
12s ea............... 08333-1538-01 12.20
(1/2"X10 YDS)
24s ea............... 08333-1538-00 12.20
(2"X1 1/2 YDS)
50s ea............... 08333-1538-12 48.10
(1"X1 1/2 YDS)
100s ea.............. 08333-1538-11 48.10

DURAPREP (3M Health Care)
SOL,TP (SURGICAL)
0.7%-74%, 6 ml...... 17518-0011-07 3.38
26 ml 17518-0011-08 6.70

DURASORB DISPOSABLE UNDERPADS (Covidien)
DEV,NA (30"X30")
100s ea.............. 08080-9490-10 34.80
(23"X36",10X15)
150s ea.............. 08080-1093-00 41.77
(23"X24",4X50)
200s ea.............. 08080-1038-00 36.70
(23"X24")
200s ea.............. 08080-6349-01 47.87
(17"X24")
300s ea.............. 08080-9490-00 42.73

DURASORB PLUS DISPOSABLE UNDERPADS (Covidien)
DEV,NA (23"X36",15X5)
75s ea............... 08080-7194-01 28.54
(23"X36")
75s ea............... 08080-7193-00 26.38

DUREX AVANTI (Durex)
DEV,NA (LUBRICATED,POLYURETHANE)
3s ea................ 02340-0560-00 2.88 5.76
6s ea................ 02340-0580-00 4.99 9.98

DUREX COLORS & SCENTS (Durex)
DEV,NA (LUBRICATED)
3s ea................ 02340-0090-00 1.38 2.76
12s ea 02340-0083-00 4.73 9.46

DUREX ENHANCED PLEASURE (Durex)
DEV,NA (LUBRICATED)
12s ea............... 02340-0038-00 4.73 9.46

DUREX EXTRA SENSITIVE (Durex)
DEV,NA (LUBRICATED)
3s ea................ 02340-0129-00 1.20 2.40
12s ea 02340-0130-00 3.99 7.98
24s ea 02340-0241-00 6.53 13.06

DUREX HIGH SENSATION (Durex)
DEV,NA (LUBRICATED)
3s ea................ 02340-0245-00 1.20 2.40
12s ea 02340-0246-00 3.99 7.98

DUREX NATURAL FEELING (Durex)
DEV,NA (LUBRICATED)
3s ea................ 02340-0054-00 1.20 2.40
12s ea 02340-0055-00 3.99 7.98
24s ea 02340-0067-00 6.53 13.06

DY-O-DERM (Galderma)
LIQ,TP, 120 ml............ 00299-1450-02 37.50

DYNA-FLEX COHESIVE COMPRESSION (J&J Medical)
DEV,NA (NON-STERILE,1 1/2"X5YD)
ea................... 56091-0070-32 1.33

PROD/MFR | HRI, UPC,NDC | AWP

(NON-STERILE,1"X5YD)
ea................... 56091-0070-31 0.94
(NON-STERILE,2"X5YD)
ea................... 56091-0070-33 1.71
(NON-STERILE,3"X5YD)
ea................... 56091-0070-34 2.14
(NON-STERILE,4"X5YD)
ea................... 56091-0070-35 2.68
(NON-STERILE,6"X5YD)
ea................... 56091-0070-36 3.77

DYNA-FLEX COMPRESSION SYSTEM (J&J Medical)
DEV,NA (MULTI-LAYER)
ea................... 56091-0070-25 18.85

DYNA-FLEX ELASTIC (J&J Medical)
DEV,NA (6"X5YD)
6s ea................ 56091-0070-06 18.44
(3"X5YD)
12s ea............... 56091-0070-03 21.32
(4"X5YD)
12s ea............... 56091-0070-04 27.20

DYNA-HEX (Xttrium Labs)
LIQ,TP, 4%, 120 ml 17187-1061-01 1.35 4.00
960 ml 17187-1061-04 3.60 25.00
3840 ml 17187-1061-05 12.60 40.00

DYNA-HEX2 (Xttrium Labs)
LIQ,TP, 2%, 120 ml 17187-1021-01 1.05 3.50
960 ml 17187-1021-04 2.90 20.00
3840 ml 17187-1021-05 9.80 35.00

E-400 (Nature's Bounty)
SGL,PO (SOFTGEL)
400 iu, 50s ea........ 74312-0005-42 5.99

E-400-CLEAR (Bio-Tech Pharm)
CAP,PO, 400 iu, 100s ea... 53191-0043-01 10.00

E-400-MIXED (Bio-Tech Pharm)
SGL,PO (SOFTGEL)
400 iu, 100s ea....... 53191-0053-01 8.90

E-600 (Nature's Bounty)
SGL,PO, 600 iu, 50s ea.... 74312-0026-21 7.99

E-GEMS (Carlson,J.R.)
SGL,PO (SOFTGEL)
100 iu, 100s ea....... 88395-0003-11 3.89 7.77
250s ea 88395-0003-12 8.95 17.90
200 iu, 90s ea 88395-0003-20 4.94 9.88
250s ea 88395-0003-22 12.45 24.90
500s ea 88395-0003-25 23.45 46.90
400 iu, 60s ea 88395-0003-41 6.25 12.50
90s ea 88395-0003-44 9.95 19.90
(PF,SF,CORN-FREE)
400 iu, 200s ea....... 88395-0003-42 14.95 29.90
(SOFTGEL)
400 iu, 500s ea....... 88395-0003-45 33.50 67.00
1000s ea 88395-0003-46 60.00 120.00
600 iu, 50s ea 88395-0003-60 6.45 12.90
100s ea 88395-0003-61 12.22 24.44
800 iu, 50s ea 88395-0003-80 7.95 15.90
100s ea 88395-0003-81 14.95 29.90
250s ea 88395-0003-82 34.95 69.90
1000 iu, 30s ea 88395-0003-90 6.48 12.95
90s ea 88395-0003-91 17.75 35.50
250s ea 88395-0003-92 46.45 92.90

E-GEMS ELITE (Carlson,J.R.)
PO (PF,SOFTGEL)
400 iu, 60s ea........ 88395-0007-70 14.75 29.50
120s ea........... 88395-0007-71 27.40 54.80
240s ea........... 88395-0007-72 47.50 95.00

E-GEMS PLUS (Carlson,J.R.)
SGL,PO (SOFTGEL)
200 iu, 100s ea....... 88395-0004-21 5.95 11.90
250s ea 88395-0004-22 13.95 27.90
400 iu, 50s ea 88395-0004-40 7.45 14.90
100s ea 88395-0004-41 14.75 29.50
250s ea 88395-0004-42 27.50 55.00
500s ea 88395-0004-45 50.00 100.00

E-MAX-1000 (Bio-Tech Pharm)
SGL,PO (SOFTGEL)
1000 iu, 100s ea 53191-0063-01 14.15

E-R-O (Scherer Labs)
SOL,OT (EAR WAX REMOVAL SYSTEM)
6.5%, 15 ml 00274-2300-15 3.20

E-R-O EAR DROPS (Scherer Labs)
SOL,OT, 6.5%, 15 ml...... 00274-2180-15 2.49

E-SEL (Carlson,J.R.)
SGL,PO (SOFTGEL)
0.1 mg-400 iu,
50s ea............. 88395-0008-00 5.45 10.90
100s ea 88395-0008-01 9.95 19.90
250s ea 88395-0008-02 23.75 47.50

PROD/MFR | HRI, UPC,NDC | AWP | SRP

DOCTOR'S CHOICE ADVANCED WOUND CARE BLISTER CARE (SciVolutions)
DEV,NA (ASSORTED SIZES)
12s ea.............. 08589-0506-12 5.63

DOCTOR'S CHOICE ADVANCED WOUND CARE BURNS, SCALDS, ABRASIONS (SciVolutions)
DEV,NA (LATEX-FREE)
5s ea............... 08589-0502-05 5.63

DOCTOR'S CHOICE ADVANCED WOUND CARE CORN & CALLUS REMOVER (SciVolutions)
PAD,TP (NIGHT TIME,LATEX-FREE)
40%, 12s ea 08589-0507-24 5.63

DOCTOR'S CHOICE ADVANCED WOUND CARE SKIN CLOSURE (SciVolutions)
DEV,NA (LATEX-FREE)
5s ea............... 08589-0504-05 5.63

DOCTOR'S CHOICE ADVANCED WOUND CARE ULTRA-FLEX FOR CUTS, SCRAPES & BLISTERS (SciVolutions)
DEV,NA (LATEX-FREE)
18s ea.............. 08589-0501-18 5.63

DOCTOR'S CHOICE DIABETIC CUSHIONED WOUND PADS (SciVolutions)
DEV,NA (W/ALOE SPRAY,ULTRAFLEX)
8s ea............... 08589-0519-08 9.38
(W/ALOE SPRAY)
10s ea.............. 08589-0509-10 9.38

DOCTOR'S CHOICE WITH DISSOLV AWAY ADHESIVE (SciVolutions)
DEV,NA (W/ALOE SPRAY,ULTRAFLEX)
8s ea............... 08589-0518-08 9.38
(W/ALOE SPRAY)
10s ea.............. 08589-0508-10 9.38

DOCU-LIQUID (Hi-Tech)
LIQ,PO, 150 mg/15 ml,
480 ml 50383-0771-16 6.70

DOCU-SOFT (Reese)
SGL,PO (SOFTGEL)
100 mg, 60s ea 10956-0643-60 3.38
100s ea 10956-0643-09 4.61

DOCUCAL (Global Source)
SGL,PO, 240 mg, 100s ea . 59618-0206-15 8.60

DOCULAX (Global Source)
SGL,PO, 100 mg, 100s ea . 59618-0210-15 3.55

DOCULAX PLUS (Global Source)
SGL,PO, 30 mg-100 mg,
100s ea............ 59618-0211-15 4.95

DOCUSATE CALCIUM (Consolidated Midland)
SGL,PO, 240 mg, 100s ea . 00223-0857-01 7.50
1000s ea 00223-0857-02 70.00

(Geri-Care)
SGL,PO (SOFTGEL)
240 mg, 100s ea 57896-0424-01 3.38
500s ea 57896-0424-05 17.99

(Marlex)
SGL,PO (SOFTGEL)
240 mg, 10s ea 10135-0138-61 2.20
30s ea............ 10135-0138-30 2.15
60s ea............ 10135-0138-60 2.87
100s ea........... 10135-0138-01 3.39
100s ea UD 10135-0138-13 4.99
300s ea........... 10135-0138-03 10.54
500s ea........... 10135-0138-05 17.00
1000s ea 10135-0138-10 35.00

(Rugby)
SGL,PO, 240 mg, 100s ea . 00536-3755-01 9.14
500s ea........... 00536-3755-05 40.91
1000s ea 00536-3755-10 77.48

(Vita-Rx)
SGL,PO, 240 mg, 100s ea . 49727-0079-02 8.30

(HomeMed)
REPACK
SGL,PO, 240 mg, 60s ea... 51655-0315-25 6.75

(McKesson Packaging)
REPACK
SGL,PO (BLISTER PACK)
240 mg, 750s ea UD.. 63739-0088-01 84.08

(PD-Rx Pharm)
REPACK
SGL,PO, 240 mg, 60s ea... 55289-0860-60 12.38

(Phys Total Care)
REPACK
SGL,PO, 240 mg, 100s ea . 54868-0035-00 35.76

PROD/MFR | HRI, UPC,NDC | AWP | SRP

DOCUSATE NA (PD-Rx Pharm)
REPACK
SGL,PO, 250 mg, 60s ea... 55289-0994-60 12.00

DOCUSATE SOD (Stat Rx)
REPACK
SGL,PO, 100 mg, 20s ea... 16590-0459-20 6.00
30s ea 16590-0459-30 9.00
60s ea 16590-0459-60 18.00
90s ea 16590-0459-90 27.00

DOCUSATE SODIUM (Amneal)
SGL,PO (STIMULANT-FREE,SOFTGEL)
100 mg, 100s ea 65162-0013-10 3.90
1000s ea 65162-0013-11 29.25

(Consolidated Midland)
LIQ,PO, 150 mg/15 ml,
480 ml 00223-6339-01 17.50
3840 ml 00223-6339-02 99.50
TAB,PO, 100 mg, 100s ea.. 00223-0852-01 3.50
1000s ea 00223-0852-02 22.50

(Cypress Pharm)
SGL,PO (SOFTGEL)
100 mg, 100s ea 60258-0955-01 25.27

(Geri-Care)
SGL,PO (SOFTGEL)
100 mg, 100s ea 57896-0401-01 1.00
1000s ea 57896-0401-10 8.75
250 mg, 100s ea 57896-0425-01 3.00
1000s ea 57896-0425-10 20.00

(Major)
SGL,PO (10X10)
100 mg, 100s ea UD.. 00904-2244-61 17.32

(Marlex)
SGL,PO (SOFTGEL)
100 mg, 30s ea 10135-0111-30 0.83
60s ea............ 10135-0111-60 0.96
90s ea............ 10135-0111-90 1.67
(BLISTER PACK,SOFTGEL)
100 mg, 100s ea UD.. 10135-0111-13 3.01
(BOXED,SOFTGEL)
100 mg, 100s ea 10135-0111-57 65.00
(SOFTGEL)
100 mg, 100s ea 10135-0111-01 1.36
120s ea........... 10135-0111-62 2.30
180s ea........... 10135-0111-67 2.92
300s ea........... 10135-0111-03 7.62
1000s ea 10135-0111-10 9.45
250 mg, 30s ea 10135-0136-30 1.34
60s ea............ 10135-0136-60 2.41
(BLISTER PACK,SOFTGEL)
250 mg, 100s ea UD.. 10135-0136-13 6.00
(BOXED,SOFTGEL)
250 mg, 100s ea 10135-0136-57 65.00
(SOFTGEL)
250 mg, 100s ea 10135-0136-01 3.04
500s ea........... 10135-0136-05 11.99
1000s ea 10135-0136-10 25.37
SYR,PO, 60 mg/15 ml,
480 ml 10135-0121-16 1.78

(Mason Vit)
SGL,PO, 250 mg, 100s ea . 11845-0059-41 8.78

(Perrigo)
SGL;PO (STIMULANT-FREE,SOFTGEL)
100 mg, 100s ea 45802-0486-78 5.47

(Pharm Assoc Inc)
LIQ,PO (SF,CHERRY)
100 mg/10 ml,
10 ml 100s UD 00121-0544-10 48.44
150 mg/15 ml,
25 ml 100s UD 00121-0544-25 71.10
473 ml 00121-0544-16 13.96
SOL,PO (U.S.P.,AF,SF,ANISE)
20 mg/5 ml, 473 ml .. 00121-0743-16 4.80

(Rugby)
SGL,PO (SOFTGEL)
100 mg, 100s ea 00536-3756-01 5.92
1000s ea 00536-3756-10 32.40
250 mg, 100s ea 00536-3757-01 6.57
1000s ea 00536-3757-10 40.83

(Vita-Rx)
SGL,PO, 100 mg, 100s ea . 49727-0077-02 3.03
1000s ea 49727-0077-05 18.70

(4u)
REPACK
SGL,PO (SOFTGEL)
100 mg, 60s ea 10544-0417-60 23.46
60s ea 42549-0617-60 23.46

PROD/MFR | HRI, UPC,NDC | AWP | SRP

(A-S Medication)
REPACK
SGL,PO, 100 mg, 20s ea... 54569-2385-00 1.09
30s ea 54569-2385-04 1.64
60s ea 54569-2385-02 3.28
100s ea 54569-2385-01 5.47

(Aidarex)
REPACK
SGL,PO (SOFTGEL)
100 mg, 30s ea 33261-0039-30 37.20
60s ea 33261-0039-60 74.40
90s ea 33261-0039-90 111.60
120s ea 33261-0039-02 148.80

(Altura)
REPACK
SGL,PO, 100 mg, 10s ea... 63874-0007-10 1.05
14s ea 63874-0007-14 1.47
20s ea 63874-0007-20 2.10
28s ea 63874-0007-28 2.94
30s ea 63874-0007-30 3.15
40s ea 63874-0007-40 4.20
60s ea 63874-0007-60 6.30
90s ea 63874-0007-90 9.45
100s ea 63874-0007-01 10.50
120s ea 63874-0007-04 12.60
1000s ea 63874-0007-02 158.34
(SOFT GEL)
250 mg, 10s ea 63874-0681-10 6.09
20s ea 63874-0681-20 12.18
30s ea 63874-0681-30 18.27
60s ea 63874-0681-60 36.54
90s ea 63874-0681-90 54.81
100s ea 63874-0681-01 60.90
120s ea 63874-0681-04 73.08

(American Health)
REPACK
SGL,PO (10X10)
100 mg, 100s ea UD.. 62584-0683-01 11.95
(15X30)
100 mg, 450s ea UD.. 62584-0683-85 20.93

(DHS, Inc.)
REPACK
SGL,PO, 100 mg, 30s ea... 55887-0981-30 9.00
60s ea 55887-0981-60 12.00

(Dispensing Solutions)
REPACK
SGL,PO, 100 mg, 6s ea.... 66336-0792-06 3.37
(SOFTGEL)
100 mg, 25s ea 55045-1403-07 4.25
30s ea 55045-1403-08 5.10
30s ea 66336-0792-30 39.14
(GEL CAP)
100 mg, 40s ea 55045-1403-04 6.80
(SOFTGEL)
100 mg, 60s ea 55045-1403-06 10.20
60s ea 66336-0792-60 17.17
90s ea 55045-1403-09 15.30
100s ea 55045-1403-01 17.00
120s ea 55045-1403-02 20.40
250 mg, 60s ea 66336-0010-60 11.02
(SOFTGEL)
250 mg, 60s ea 55045-1890-06 10.80
100s ea 55045-1890-01 18.00

(HomeMed)
REPACK
SGL,PO, 100 mg, 20s ea... 51655-0342-52 4.34
120s ea 51655-0342-82 5.75
180s ea 51655-0342-83 7.02

(IPI)
REPACK
SGL,PO (SOFTGEL)
100 mg, 60s ea 18837-0247-60 0.76

(McKesson Packaging)
REPACK
SGL,PO, 100 mg,
100s ea UD 63739-0089-10 11.41
(BLISTER PACK)
100 mg, 750s ea UD.. 63739-0089-01 85.58
(PUNCH CARD 25X30)
100 mg, 750s ea 63739-0089-03 85.58

(Nucare Pharm)
REPACK
SGL,PO (SOFTGEL)
100 mg, 30s ea 66267-0083-30 8.79
60s ea 66267-0083-60 12.84
90s ea 66267-0083-90 19.25
120s ea 66267-0083-91 25.66

PROD/MFR HRI, UPC,NDC AWP SRP

(Palmetto)
REPACK
LIQ,PO (1X120ML)
150 mg/15 ml,
120 ml 23490-6655-00 14.97
(PD-Rx Pharm)
REPACK
SGL,PO, 100 mg, 14s ea...55289-0493-14 5.63
20s ea 55289-0493-20 6.00
30s ea 55289-0493-30 6.50
60s ea 55289-0493-60 8.00
90s ea 55289-0493-90 9.50
(USP)
100 mg, 120s ea 55289-0493-98 11.39
180s ea 55289-0493-93 12.36
(Pharma Pac)
REPACK
SGL,PO, 100 mg, 20s ea...52959-0045-20 6.35
30s ea 52959-0045-30 9.52
60s ea 52959-0045-60 18.95
90s ea 52959-0045-90 24.46
100s ea 52959-0045-00 25.77
120s ea 52959-0045-02 27.58
(Phys Total Care)
REPACK
SGL,PO (SOFTGEL)
100 mg, 60s ea 54868-0096-01 10.02
100s ea 54868-0096-04 11.94
1000s ea 54868-0096-00 105.81
(Physician Partner)
REPACK
SGL,PO (SOFT GELATIN)
100 mg, 30s ea 21695-0590-30 11.72
90s ea 21695-0590-90 15.83
(Quality Care Prod)
REPACK
SGL,PO, 100 mg, 30s ea...49999-0725-30 4.60
(SOFTGEL)
100 mg, 30s ea 49999-0583-30 4.60
60s ea 49999-0725-60 9.20
90s ea 49999-0725-90 13.80
250 mg, 60s ea 49999-0790-60 2.70
(Southwood)
REPACK
SGL,PO, 100 mg, 20s ea...58016-0902-20 2.00
30s ea 58016-0902-30 3.00
60s ea 58016-0902-60 6.00
90s ea 58016-0902-90 9.00
100s ea 58016-0902-00 10.00
120s ea 58016-0902-02 12.00
150s ea 58016-0902-03 15.00
250 mg, 10s ea 58016-0903-10 2.75
15s ea 58016-0903-15 3.12
20s ea 58016-0903-20 3.50
30s ea 58016-0903-30 4.25
60s ea 58016-0903-60 6.50
90s ea 58016-0903-90 8.75
100s ea 58016-0903-00 9.50
120s ea 58016-0903-02 11.00
SYR,PO, 60 mg/15 ml,
120 ml 58016-0360-24 6.83
(Stat Rx)
REPACK
SGL,PO, 100 mg, 14s ea...16590-0459-14 4.20
56s ea 16590-0459-56 16.50
100s ea 16590-0459-71 30.00
120s ea 16590-0459-72 36.00

DOCUSATE SODIUM & SENNA (Rugby)
TAB,PO, 50 mg-8.6 mg,
100s ea............00536-0355-01 4.95
1000s ea............00536-0355-10 31.95
(Dispensing Solutions)
REPACK
TAB,PO, 50 mg-8.6 mg,
30s ea............66336-0003-30 9.31

DOCUSATE SODIUM AND SENNA (Pharma Pac)
REPACK
TAB,PO, 50 mg-8.6 mg,
120s ea............52959-0675-02 21.89

DOCUSATE SODIUM WITH SENNA (Phys Total Care)
REPACK
TAB,PO, 50 mg-8.6 mg,
60s ea............54868-4917-01 14.28
(Quality Care Prod)
REPACK
TAB,PO, 50 mg-8.6 mg,
30s ea............49999-0659-30 7.79

DOCUSATE SODIUM/SENNOSIDE (Phys Total Care)
REPACK
TAB,PO, 50 mg-8.6 mg,
100s ea............54868-4917-00 31.74

DOCUSIL (Prime Marketing)
SGL,PO (SOFTGEL)
100 mg, 100s ea 62107-0033-01 4.75
1000s ea 62107-0033-10 44.25

DOCUSOFT S (G&W)
SGL,PO, 100 mg, 60s ea...00713-0405-60 3.61
100s ea 00713-0405-99 4.72

DOCUSOL (Alliance)
NMA,RC, 283 mg, 5s ea...17433-9878-05 10.25 11.99

DOFUS (Miller)
CAP,PO, 1 billion u,
60s ea............17204-0412-20 6.30 10.50

DOK (Major)
SGL,PO, 100 mg, 100s ea ..00904-7889-59 4.79
100s ea 00904-7889-60 4.29
250 mg, 100s ea 00904-7891-59 11.50
TAB,PO, 100 mg, 100s ea..00904-5869-60 6.91

DOK COLACE (Major)
SGL,PO, 100 mg,
1000s ea 00904-7889-80 24.59

DOK PLUS (Major)
TAB,PO, 50 mg-8.6 mg,
100s ea............00904-5643-60 38.18
100s ea UD 00904-5643-61 18.65

DOLOGEN (Kramer-Novis)
TAB,PO (CAPLET)
500 mg-30 mg,
150s ea............52083-0480-10 18.00

DOLOMITE (Lex)
TAB,PO, 100s ea............49523-0031-01 0.70
(Mason Vit)
TAB,PO, 100s ea............11845-0055-41 2.78
250s ea............11845-0055-42 4.44
(Nature's Bounty)
TAB,PO (PF,SF)
130 mg-78 mg, 250s ea74312-0003-13 5.55

DOME-PASTE (Schering)
DEV,NA (3"X10 YD)
ea............00085-1808-02 18.16
(4"X10 YD)
ea............00085-1811-02 19.91

DOMEBORO (Bayer HealthCare)
PDR,TP, 12s ea 16500-0023-24 7.63
100s ea 00026-0232-20 50.41
TEF,TP, 12s ea 00026-0231-10 8.97
100s ea 00026-0231-20 60.49
(Phys Total Care)
REPACK
PDR,TP, 12s ea 54868-2091-00 14.21
(Physician Partner)
REPACK
PDR,TP, 12s ea 21695-0884-12 27.48

DONG QUAI (ADH)
CAP,PO (PF,SF)
500 mg, 100s ea 60142-0909-51 5.98 11.95
(Botanical Labs.)
LIQ,PO, 30 ml 41954-0020-13 4.00 7.99
60 ml............41954-0020-06 6.50 12.99
(Nature's Bounty)
CAP,PO (530MG)
100s ea............74312-0051-55 7.99

DONNAGEL (Phys Total Care)
REPACK
SUS,PO, 600 mg/15 ml,
240 ml 54868-3161-00 7.29

DORMIN SLEEP AID (Randob)
CAP,PO, 25 mg, 32s ea 30103-0322-54 4.05 6.75
72s ea 30103-0722-54 6.30 10.50

DOSER (Meditrack)
DEV,NA, ea 84665-0104-15 21.00 29.99

DOUBLE TUSSIN DM (Reese)
SOL,PO (1X120ML,DOUBLE STRENGTH)
20 mg/5 ml-300 mg/5 ml,
120 ml 10956-0674-04 4.61
(1X240ML,DOUBLE STRENGTH)
20 mg/5 ml-300 mg/5 ml,
240 ml 10956-0674-08 7.32 10.49

DOVER (Covidien)
DEV,NA (CATHETER LEG STRAP,30")
10s ea............08080-6001-49 33.62
(URETHRAL CATH TRAY 14FR)
20s ea............08080-6000-57 91.42
20s ea............08080-6000-73 91.65
(EXTEN TUBE W/CONN 18")
24s ea............08080-7319-01 48.62
(ELASTIC FOAM TAPE 1")
500s ea............08080-7306-00 49.32
(PED. URINE COLLECTOR)
500s ea............08080-6689-06 62.50
(TWO SIDE ADHESIVE STRAP)
500s ea............08080-7311-00 190.68
GEL,MM (LUBR JEL/PREFIL SYR10CC)
2.56 gm 50s 08080-6360-02 99.57

DOVER DRAINAGE BAG (Covidien)
DEV,NA (4000 ML,TURP)
20s ea............08080-6009-09 147.58
(URININARY, 2000 ML)
40s ea............08080-6016-01 292.10

DOVER FOLEY (Covidien)
DEV,NA (SILIC 3WAY FOL 18FR30CC)
10s ea............08080-6651-83 131.82
(SILIC 3WAY FOL 20FR30CC)
10s ea............08080-6652-09 131.82
(SILIC 3WAY FOL 22FR30CC)
10s ea............08080-6652-25 131.82
(SILIC 3WAY FOL 24FR30CC)
10s ea............08080-6652-41 131.82
(SILIC FOL CATH 18FR30CC)
10s ea............08080-6301-87 100.59
(SILICONE 10FR 3CC)
10s ea............08080-6031-01 107.99
(SILICONE 12FR 5CC)
10s ea............08080-6051-22 84.49
(SILICONE 14FR 5CC)
10s ea............08080-6051-48 84.49
(SILICONE 16FR 5CC)
10s ea............08080-7605-16 84.49
(SILICONE 18FR 5CC)
10s ea............08080-6051-89 84.49
(SILICONE 20FR 30CC)
10s ea............08080-7632-03 100.59
(SILICONE 20FR 5CC)
10s ea............08080-6052-05 84.49
(SILICONE 22FR 30CC)
10s ea............08080-7632-29 100.59
(SILICONE 24FR 30CC)
10s ea............08080-6302-45 100.59
(SILICONE 24FR 5CC)
10s ea............08080-6052-47 84.49
(SILICONE 26FR 30CC)
10s ea............08080-6302-60 100.59
(SILICONE 26FR 5CC)
10s ea............08080-6052-62 84.49
(SILICONE 8FR 3CC)
10s ea............08080-6030-85 107.99
(SILIC 16FR 5CC)
20s ea............08080-6061-61 215.65
(SILICONE 14FR 5CC)
20s ea............08080-6061-46 215.65
(SILICONE 18FR 5CC)
20s ea............08080-6061-87 215.65
(SILICONE 20FR 5CC)
20s ea............08080-6062-03 215.65

DOVER FOLEY 3WAY SILICONE ELASTOMER (Covidien)
DEV,NA (16FR,30CC)
10s ea............08080-6891-67 81.04
(16FR,5CC)
10s ea............08080-6881-69 75.93
(18FR,30CC)
10s ea............08080-6891-83 81.04
(18FR,5CC)
10s ea............08080-6881-85 75.93
(20FR,30CC)
10s ea............08080-6892-09 81.04
(20FR,5CC)
10s ea............08080-6882-01 75.93
(22FR,30CC)
10s ea............08080-6892-25 81.04
(22FR,5CC)
10s ea............08080-6882-27 75.93
(24FR,30CC)
10s ea............08080-6892-41 81.04
(24FR,5CC)
10s ea............08080-6882-43 75.93
(26FR,30CC)
10s ea............08080-6892-66 81.04
(26FR,5CC)
10s ea............08080-6882-68 75.93

PROD/MFR HRI, UPC,NDC AWP SRP

DOVER FOLEY CATHETER INSERTION TRAY (Covidien)
DEV,NA (PREP SOL/10CC INFL SRN)
20s ea............08080-6012-20 93.03

DOVER FOLEY TRAY (Covidien)
DEV,NA (W/UR MTR 16FR)
10s ea............08080-6408-63 276.82
10s ea............08080-6708-60 193.13

DOVER LEG BAG (Covidien)
DEV,NA (URINARY, MED 19 OZ)
20s ea............08080-6011-21 61.15
(URINARY,LG 32 OZ)
20s ea............08080-6011-39 61.15
(DELUXE LG 32 OZ)
24s ea............08080-7339-01 133.24
(LEG BAG-DELUXE MED 19OZ)
24s ea............08080-7332-00 130.48
(LEG BAG-DELUXE SM 9 OZ)
24s ea............08080-7331-00 121.05

DOVER MEC (Covidien)
DEV,NA (MALE EXTERNAL CATH-STND)
144s ea............08080-7323-00 129.90
(MALE EXTRNAL CATH-MED)
144s ea............08080-7320-01 152.50
144s ea............08080-7346-00 122.58
(MALE EXTRNAL CATH-STND)
144s ea............08080-7325-01 160.94
(TEXAS CATH W/FOAM TAPE)
144s ea............08080-7313-00 104.08
(TEXAS CATH W/STRAP STND)
144s ea............08080-7303-00 99.17

DOVER SILICONE FOLEY CATHETER TRAY (Covidien)
DEV,NA (16FR)
20s ea............08080-6007-76 244.63
(18FR)
20s ea............08080-6007-84 244.63

DOVER SILVER 400 URINE METER (Covidien)
DEV,NA (14FR,5CC,LATEX-FREE)
10s ea............08080-2431-08 294.94
(16FR,5CC,LATEX-FREE)
10s ea............08080-2631-08 294.94
(18FR,5CC,LATEX-FREE)
10s ea............08080-2831-08 294.94

DOVER SILVER CATHETERIZATION TRAY WITH URINE METER (Covidien)
DEV,NA (14FR, 5CC)
10s ea............08080-2431-06 294.94
(16FR, 5CC)
10s ea............08080-2631-06 294.94
(18FR, 5CC)
10s ea............08080-2831-06 294.94

DOVER URETHRAL CATHETER (Covidien)
DEV,NA (INTERMIT CATH TRAY 14FR)
20s ea............08080-6000-16 115.88
20s ea............08080-7600-32 121.27
(INTERMIT FEM CATH 14FR)
50s ea............08080-6609-03 26.82
(RED RUBBER ROBINSON 8FR)
100s ea............08080-6600-85 78.27
(RED RUBBER ROBINSON10FR)
100s ea............08080-6601-01 78.27
(RED RUBBER ROBINSON12FR)
100s ea............08080-6601-27 78.27
(RED RUBBER ROBINSON14FR)
100s ea............08080-6601-43 78.27
(REDRUBBER ROBINSON16FR)
100s ea............08080-6601-68 78.27
(REDRUBBER ROBINSON18FR)
100s ea............08080-6601-84 78.27
(REDRUBBER ROBINSON20FR)
100s ea............08080-6602-18 78.27
(ROB-NEL CATH 10FR)
100s ea............08888-4920-25 59.60
(ROB-NEL CATH 12FR)
100s ea............08888-4920-33 59.60
(ROB-NEL CATH 14FR)
100s ea............08888-4920-41 59.60
(ROB-NEL CATH 16FR)
100s ea............08888-4920-58 59.60
(ROB-NEL CATH 18FR)
100s ea............08888-4920-66 59.60
(ROB-NEL CATH 8FR)
100s ea............08888-4920-17 59.60

DOVER URINE COLLECTOR PEDIATRIC (Covidien)
DEV,NA (5 OZ)
500s ea............08080-6689-14 62.50

DOVER URINE METER (Covidien)
DEV,NA (400ML)
10s ea............08080-6008-91 149.68
(CLS DRAINAGE BAG 1800)
10s ea............08080-6008-00 147.27

DOXIDAN (Pharmacia Consumer)
SGL,PO, 30 mg-100 mg,
10s ea............00009-7572-01 2.08
30s ea............00009-7572-02 5.27
100s ea 00009-7572-03 11.94
100s ea UD............00009-7572-04 14.83

DR. BAKER'S CHILDREN'S ASPIRIN (Health Products Corp)
CTB,PO (ORANGE)
81 mg, 36s ea............39686-0015-03 1.97

DR. BLAINE'S ORTHO-NESIC (Blaine)
GEL,TP, 0.2%-3.5%,
170 gm............65373-0400-01 17.00 31.00

DR. CALDWELL SENNA LAXATIVE (Denison)
LIQ,PO, 33.3 mg/ml,
354 ml 00295-0008-12 5.48

DR. EDWARD'S OLIVE LAXATIVE (Oakhurst)
TAB,PO, 75s ea............11169-0075-12 4.98 5.97

DR. GREENFIELD'S RID-A-PAIN (Stanmar Labs)
GEL,TP (1X57GM,GREASELESS)
1.25%, 57 gm............50263-0100-02 19.95
(1X114GM,GREASELESS)
1.25%, 114 gm............50263-0100-04 32.95

DR. SMITH'S (Mission)
OIN,TP (DIAPER)
60 gm 53062-0010-02 6.88
90 gm............53062-0010-03 10.00

DR. SMITH'S RASH-N-ALL (Mission)
OIN,TP, 16%-57%-10%,
85 gm............53062-0022-03 10.00
18%-47%-10%,
56.6 gm 53062-0022-02 6.88

DRAINABLE POUCH CLAMP (Coloplast)
DEV,NA, 20s ea............11701-0824-10 47.40 49.60

DRAMAMINE (McNeil Consumer Healthcare)
CTB,PO (ORANGE)
50 mg, 8s ea............00450-0643-08 2.83
TAB,PO (LESS DROWSY)
25 mg, 8s ea............00450-0648-08 3.61
50 mg, 36s ea............00450-0642-36 9.06
(Pharmacia Consumer)
CTB,PO (PACKET OF 2)
50 mg, 2500s ea 00009-3643-03 826.80
TAB,PO, 50 mg, 100s ea....00009-3642-03 20.28
(Phys Total Care)
REPACK
CTB,PO, 50 mg, 12s ea....54868-1861-00 4.50
24s ea 54868-1861-02 8.57
100s ea 54868-1861-01 34.34

DRANOCHOL (A. G. Marin)
SGL,PO (CAFFEINE-FREE,SOFTGEL)
375 mg-84 mg,
30s ea............12539-0375-30 13.32

DRI-EAR (Pfeiffer)
SOL,OT, 5%-95%, 30 ml....00927-0086-31 1.58 2.85

DRIMINATE (Major)
TAB,PO, 50 mg, 12s ea....00904-2051-12 1.50
(BOXED)
50 mg, 100s ea 00904-2051-59 5.25

DRINEX (Breckenridge Pharm)
TAB,PO, 650 mg-4 mg-60 mg,
60s ea............51991-0595-06 44.65

DRISDOL (Sanofi-Aventis)
LIQ,PO (DROPS)
8000 iu/ml, 60 ml 00024-0391-02 143.16

DRISTAN 12-HR (Wyeth Consumer)
SPR,NS, 0.05%, 15 ml 00573-1191-20 4.99

DRISTAN COLD (Wyeth Consumer)
TAB,PO (ORIGINAL FORMULA,COATED)
325 mg-2 mg-5 mg,
20s ea............00573-1238-21 4.99

DRISTAN COLD MAXIMUM STRENGTH (Wyeth Consumer)
TAB,PO (NON-DROWSY,CAPLET)
500 mg-30 mg,
20s ea............00573-1120-21 4.99

DRISTAN SINUS (Wyeth Consumer)
TAB,PO (CAPLET)
200 mg-30 mg,
20s ea............00573-1265-10 4.99

DROSERA ROTUNDIFOLIA (Luyties)
TAB,SL (6X)
6 x, 500s ea............00618-3048-03 3.99
5500s ea 00618-3048-10 30.32
(30X)
12 x, 500s ea 00622-3048-03 4.19
5500s ea 00622-3048-10 31.83
(12X)
30 x, 500s ea 00624-3048-03 4.19
5500s ea 00624-3048-10 31.83

DROXY (Stratus)
CRE,TP, 56.7 gm............58980-0621-20 14.50

DRUG EMPORIUM PRESTIGE SMART SYSTEM (Home Diag)
DEV,NA (STRIP)
50s ea............56151-0318-50 26.12

DRUG EMPORIUM PSS STARTER (Home Diag)
DEV,NA (MTR,STRP,LANCET,DEV,SOL)
ea............56151-0218-01 22.18

DRUG MART ULTRA COMFORT INSULIN SYRINGE (Can-Am Care)
DEV,NA (29G,1ML,1/2",LATEX-FREE)
100s ea............38396-0413-57 17.50
(29G,3/10ML,1/2")
100s ea............38396-0411-57 17.50
(30G,1/2ML,5/16")
100s ea............38396-0415-57 17.50
(30G,1ML,5/16")
100s ea............38396-0416-57 17.50
(30G,3/10ML,5/16")
100s ea............38396-0414-57 17.50
(31G,1/2ML,5/16")
100s ea............38396-0420-57 17.50
(31G,3/10ML,5/16")
100s ea............38396-0419-57 17.50

DRY EYE RELIEF (Similasan Corp.)
SOL,OP (DROPS)
6 x-6 x-6 x, 10 ml 59262-0345-11 6.21 10.99

DRY EYES (Cardinal Health)
OIN,OP (PF,PRIVATE LABEL)
3.5 gm 37205-0134-79 2.60

DRY SKIN (Major)
CRE,TP, 480 gm 00904-7751-27 7.55
LOT,TP, 480 ml 00904-7752-16 7.99

DRYTERGENT (Genesis)
SOL,TP, 240 ml............00398-0010-08 5.34
480 ml 00398-0010-16 9.06
3840 ml 00398-0010-28 56.94

DRYTEX (Genesis)
LIQ,TP, 2%, 240 ml 00398-0011-08 7.62

DSS (Magno-Humphries)
SGL,PO (SOFTGEL)
100 mg, 100s ea 43292-0556-03 2.75 4.89
250 mg, 100s ea 43292-0556-04 5.00 7.99

DUAL INJECTION SITE (Abbott Hosp)
DEV,NA (W/LOCKING SPIN COLLAR)
120s ea............00074-5830-02 384.75

DUANE READE ALTERNATE SITE (Duane Reade)
DEV,NA (26G,SINGLE USE)
100s ea............08214-0435-14 4.75

DUANE READE PSS STARTER (Home Diag)
DEV,NA (MTR,STRP,LANCET,DEV,SOL)
ea............56151-0206-01 22.18

DUANE READE SUPER THIN (Duane Reade)
DEV,NA (30G,SINGLE USE)
100s ea............08214-0657-14 4.75

DUANE READE SUPER THIN LANCETS (Duane Reade)
DEV,NA (30G,RECAPPABLE)
100s ea............08214-4657-14 4

DUANE READE ULTRA THIN (Duane Reade)
DEV,NA (28G,SINGLE USE)
100s ea............08214-0257-14

DUCODYL (Prime Marketing)
ECT,PO, 5 mg, 100s ea 62107-0030-01
1000s ea 62107-0030-10

DULCAMARA (Luyties)
TAB,SL (6X)
6 x, 500s ea............00618-3053-0
5500s ea 00618-3053-

DU
DE

PROD/MFR	HRI, UPC,NDC	AWP	SRP
E-Z JECT LANCETS (Can-Am Care)			
DEV,NA (21 GAUGE)			
100s ea	38396-0303-00	5.85	
(COLOR,21 GAUGE)			
100s ea	38396-0305-00	5.85	
(21 GAUGE)			
200s ea	38396-0304-00	9.50	
(COLOR,21 GAUGE)			
200s ea	38396-0306-00	9.50	
E-Z JECT THIN LANCETS (Can-Am Care)			
DEV,NA, 100s ea	38396-0301-00	5.85	
200s ea	38396-0302-00	9.50	
E-ZJECT SUPER THIN (Can-Am Care)			
E-Z JECT SUPER THIN			
NA, 100s ea	38396-0308-00	5.85	
EAA (VITAFLO, LLC)			
PDR,PO (12.5GM)			
50s ea	50600-0549-06	147.50	199.95
EAKIN COHESIVE (Convatec)			
DEV,NA (4X8,LARGE)			
5s ea	00003-8390-03	62.20	80.96
EAR DROPS (Medicine Shoppe)			
SOL,OT, 6.5%, 15 ml	49614-0204-05	3.59	3.59
(Teva)			
SOL,OT, 6.5%, 15 ml	00182-6024-64	2.99	
EAR SYRINGE (Major)			
DEV,NA, ea	09046-0020-01	1.45	
EAR WAX DROPS (Quality Care Prod)			
REPACK			
SOL,OT (DROPS)			
6.5%, 15 ml	49999-0219-15	14.73	
(Southwood)			
REPACK			
SOL,OT, 6.5%, 15 ml	58016-6021-01	4.63	
EAR WAX RELIEF (Similasan Corp.)			
SOL,OT, 12 x-12 x-15 x-12 x,			
10 ml	59262-0272-11	6.21	10.99
EAR WAX REMOVAL (Cardinal Health)			
SOL,OT (PRIVATE LABEL)			
6.5%, 15 ml	37205-0457-05	3.99	
(W/BULB SYRINGE)			
6.5%, 15 ml	37205-0458-03	3.99	
(DHS, Inc.)			
REPACK			
SOL,OT (DROPS)			
6.5%, 15 ml	55887-0828-15	7.95	
EAR WAX REMOVER (Major)			
SOL,OT (1X15ML,WITH IRRIGATOR)			
6.5%, 15 ml	00904-6004-35	3.48	
EAR-DRY (Scherer Labs)			
SOL,OT, 5%-95%, 30 ml	00274-3495-31	1.54	
EARPOPPER MIDDLE EAR INFLATION (Micromedics)			
DEV,NA, ea	08564-0000-00	199.38	
EARSOL-HC (Parnell)			
SOL,OT, 1%, 30 ml	50930-0272-03	11.40	15.25
EARWAX (Nucare Pharm)			
REPACK			
SOL,OT, 6.5%, 15 ml	66267-0976-15	8.64	
EARWAX REMOVAL (Chain Drug Marketing)			
SOL,OT (DROPS)			
6.5%, 15 ml	63868-0051-15	1.92	5.99
EARWAX TREATMENT (Rugby)			
SOL,OT, 6.5%, 15 ml	00536-3000-94	2.54	
EASICLEANSE BATH (Coloplast)			
PAD,TP (NO RINSE,SELF-FOAMING)			
900s ea	11701-0100-91	270.90	283.50
EASY PRO PLUS BLOOD GLUCOSE MONITORING SYSTEM (Arkray)			
DEV,NA, ea	08480-4921-01	8.99	
EASY PRO PLUS BLOOD GLUCOSE TEST STRIPS (Arkray)			
DEV,NA, 50s ea	08480-4920-50	21.99	
EASY-FEED 500 (Abbott)			
DEV,NA (W/GRAVITY FEEDING SET)			
ea	70074-0515-85	10.31	
EASY-FEED ENTERAL NUTRITION BAG (Abbott)			
DEV,NA (W/GRAVITY FEEDING SET)			
ea	70074-0000-56	10.31	
(W/PATROL PUMP SET)			
ea	70074-0520-49	13.64	
EASY-FEED GASTROSTOMY TUBE (Abbott)			
DEV,NA (16 FRENCH)			
ea	70074-0501-13	35.93	
(18 FRENCH)			
ea	70074-0501-15	35.93	
(20 FRENCH)			
ea	70074-0501-17	35.93	
(22 FRENCH)			
ea	70074-0501-19	35.93	
EASYGLUCO BLOOD GLUCOSE MONITORING SYSTEM (US DIAGNOSTICS, INC)			
DEV,NA (METER KIT)			
ea	08463-0103-01	45.00	
(STARTER KIT)			
ea	08463-0003-01	65.00	
(VALUE KIT)			
ea	08463-0104-01	50.00	
EASYGLUCO BLOOD GLUCOSE TEST STRIPS (US DIAGNOSTICS, INC)			
DEV,NA, 50s ea	08463-0203-50	41.50	
EASYGLUCO CONTROL SOLUTION (US DIAGNOSTICS, INC)			
DEV,NA (HIGH)			
ea	08463-0105-01	10.00	
(LOW)			
ea	08463-0205-01	10.00	
(NORMAL)			
ea	08463-0005-01	10.00	
EASYPRO (Arkray)			
DEV,NA (W/LANCING DEV,LANCETS)			
ea	08480-4911-00	68.00	
(PRIVATE LABEL)			
50s ea	08480-4900-50	38.50	
EASYSOY (Carlson,J.R.)			
CAP,PO, 500 mg, 90s ea	88395-0083-21	6.48	12.95
180s ea	88395-0083-22	11.95	23.90
360s ea	88395-0083-23	22.44	44.88
POW,PO, 2.5 gm, 100 gm	88395-0083-25	7.45	14.90
300 gm	88395-0083-26	18.45	36.90
ECEE PLUS (Edwards)			
TAB,PO, 100s ea	00485-0023-01	17.00	
ECHINACE EXTRA STRENGTH (Yerba)			
CAP,PO, 305 mg, 30s ea	46352-0004-05	5.97	9.95
ECHINACEA (ADH)			
CAP,PO (PF,SF)			
450 mg, 100s ea	60142-0910-51	4.98	9.95
(AmerisourceBergen)			
TAB,PO (PF,PRIVATE LABEL,CAPLET)			
167 mg, 90s ea	24385-0662-75	8.09	8.99
(Botanical Labs.)			
LIQ,PO, 30 ml	41954-0032-00	5.00	9.99
60 ml	41954-0032-30	8.00	15.99
(Cardinal Health)			
CAP,PO (PRIVATE LABEL)			
380 mg, 100s ea	37205-0092-78	5.84	
(Contract Pharmacal)			
CAP,PO, 400 mg, 100s ea	10267-0841-01	8.00	
(Lex)			
CAP,PO, 400 mg, 100s ea	58537-0247-10	3.98	
(Mason Vit)			
CAP,PO (PF,SF)			
500 mg, 60s ea	11845-0113-65	7.22	
90s ea	11845-0113-69	8.11	
300s ea	11845-0113-60	18.33	
(Nature's Bounty)			
CAP,PO, 400 mg, 100s ea	74312-0056-32		6.99
(PF,SF)			
400 mg, 100s ea	74312-0056-33		6.99
(Rexall)			
CAP,PO (WHOLE HERB,PF,SF)			
400 mg, 75s ea	30768-0000-73	2.93	4.43
ECHINACEA ANGUSTIFOLIA (Luyties)			
TAB,SL (6X)			
6 x, 500s ea	00618-3212-03	3.99	
(30X)			
12 x, 500s ea	00622-3212-03	4.19	
(12X)			
12 x, 5500s ea	00624-3212-10	31.83	
(30X)			
12 x, 5500s ea	00622-3212-10	31.83	
(6X)			
12 x, 5500s ea	00618-3212-10	30.32	
(12X)			
30 x, 500s ea	00624-3212-03	4.19	
ECHINACEA COMPOUND (Weleda)			
LIQ,TP, 50 ml	55946-0228-15	7.20	
ECHINACEA PURPUREA (Mason Vit)			
CAP,PO (PF,SF)			
80 mg, 60s ea	11845-0128-15	8.33	
ECHINACEA ROOT (Key Company)			
CAP,PO (PF,SF)			
400 mg, 60s ea	11694-0697-01	6.00	
(Major)			
CAP,PO, 400 mg, 100s ea	00904-5085-60	5.99	
ECHINACEA STANDARDIZED (Rexall)			
CAP,PO (PF,SF)			
400 mg, 45s ea	30768-0001-23	2.06	3.12
ECHINACEA/GOLDEN SEAL (ADH)			
CAP,PO (PF,SF)			
450 mg, 100s ea	60142-0911-01	7.98	15.95
(Nature's Bounty)			
CAP,PO, 100s ea	74312-0009-22		9.59
ECHINACEA/GOLDEN SEAL ROOT (Cardinal Health)			
CAP,PO (PRIVATE LABEL)			
350 mg-50 mg, 50s ea	37205-0048-71	5.40	
ECHINACEA/GOLDENSEAL (AmerisourceBergen)			
TAB,PO (PF,PRIVATE LABEL,CAPLET)			
112.5 mg-25 mg, 90s ea	24385-0657-75	8.45	9.39
(Botanical Labs.)			
CAP,PO, 50s ea	41954-0032-62	6.00	11.99
90s ea	41954-0032-63	10.00	19.99
LIQ,PO, 30 ml	41954-0032-05	6.25	12.49
60 ml	41954-0032-35	10.00	19.99
(Mason Vit)			
CAP,PO (PF,SF)			
100 mg-100 mg, 60s ea	11845-0131-15	13.22	
ECHINACEA/GOLDENSEAL COMPLEX (Rexall)			
CAP,PO (PF,SF)			
50s ea	30768-0001-10	3.16	4.78
ECHINACEA/VITAMIN C (Cardinal Health)			
TAB,PO (PRIVATE LABEL)			
500 mg-100 mg, 60s ea	37205-0088-72	2.80	
ECLIPSE PROBE COVER (Parker)			
DEV,NA (PRE-GELLED)			
100s ea	00341-0038-01	43.66	64.25
ECOTRIN (Glaxo)			
ECT,PO, 81 mg, 45s ea	49692-0903-75	1.93	
150s ea	49692-0903-76	6.13	
365s ea	49692-0903-67	12.02	
(ENTERIC COATED)			
325 mg, 100s ea	49692-0901-20	5.95	
125s ea	00135-0014-27	6.50	
300s ea	49692-0903-79	12.02	
500 mg, 75s ea	49692-0903-78	6.13	
180s ea	49692-0903-80	12.02	
(Quality Care Prod)			
REPACK			
ECT,PO (ENTERIC COATED)			
325 mg, 30s ea	35356-0396-30	14.60	
ECPIRIN (Prime Marketing)			
ECT,PO, 325 mg, 100s ea	62107-0028-01	2.90	
1000s ea	62107-0028-32	17.50	
ED APAP (Edwards)			
LIQ,PO, 160 mg/5 ml,			
240 ml	00485-0057-08	7.80	
EFFERCLEANSE 1 LAYER (Global Source)			
TEF,NA, 40s ea	59618-0330-09	3.27	
90s ea	59618-0330-13	6.87	
EFFERCLEANSE 2 LAYER (Global Source)			
TEF,NA, 40s ea	59618-0331-09	3.60	
90s ea	59618-0331-13	7.50	
EFFERDENT (Johnson & Johnson)			
TEF,NA, 40s ea	12547-0636-34	2.51	
90s ea	12547-0636-39	4.07	
120s ea	12547-0636-32	6.11	
EFFERDENT PLUS (Johnson & Johnson)			
TEF,NA, 36s ea	12547-0639-37	2.51	
78s ea	12547-0639-38	4.88	
(W/Y LISTERINE,MINT)			
78s ea	12547-0636-22	4.88	
108s ea	12547-0636-33	6.11	
(W/Y LISTERINE,MINT)			
108s ea	12547-0636-26	6.11	
EFFERGRIP CREAM (Johnson & Johnson)			
CRE,NA, 45 gm	12547-0639-66	2.62	
75 gm	12547-0639-65	3.94	
EGG PRO (Nutra/Balance)			
POW,NA (6X283GM,SF)			
283 gm 6s	07249-0911-01		184.25
EGSENTIALS (Bio-Tech Pharm)			
CAP,PO, 9 mg, 235s ea	53191-0379-23	39.00	
ELA-MAX (Phys Total Care)			
REPACK			
CRE,TP, 4%, 30 gm	54868-4616-00	53.22	
ELASTIKON ELASTIC (J&J Medical)			
DEV,NA (3"X5YD/ROLL STRETCHED)			
4s ea	56091-0051-75	17.68	

PROD/MFR	HRI, UPC,NDC	AWP	SRP
(2"X5YD/ROLL STRETCHED)			
6s ea	56091-0051-74	17.68	
(4"X5YD/ROLL STRETCHED)			
6s ea	56091-0051-77	35.35	
(1"X5YD/ROLL STRETCHED)			
12s ea	56091-0051-72	17.68	
ELASTO-GEL (Southwest)			
DEV,NA (OCCLUSIVE WOUND, 4"X4")			
25s ea	61118-8000-01	332.05	116.25
ELASTO-GEL CAST & SPLINT PADDING (Southwest)			
DEV,NA (12"X12")			
5s ea	45713-0557-00	103.21	144.50
(6"X8")			
5s ea	45713-0556-00	43.13	60.40
(12"X12")			
25s ea	45713-0457-00	516.05	722.50
(6"X8")			
25s ea	45713-0456-00	215.65	302.00
(4"X4")			
100s ea	45713-0955-00	266.00	
ELASTO-GEL CERVICAL COLLAR (Southwest)			
DEV,NA (HOT/COLD PACK)			
10s ea	45713-0601-02	259.50	403.50
ELASTO-GEL COMFORT AID DRESSING (Southwest)			
DEV,NA (3"X4", GEL, DRESSING)			
3s ea	45713-0318-75	7.12	10.00
(1.5"X2.5",GEL,NON-DRYIN)			
144s ea	45713-0481-75	342.15	480.00
ELASTO-GEL CRANIAL CAP (Southwest)			
DEV,NA (LG/XL,HOT/COLD PACK)			
10s ea	45713-0606-02	397.00	618.00
(SM/MED,HOT/COLD PACK)			
10s ea	45713-0606-00	327.50	509.00
ELASTO-GEL CRANIAL HELMET (Southwest)			
DEV,NA (WATER RESIST PACK)			
6s ea	45713-0606-10	450.00	630.00
ELASTO-GEL FOOT/ANKLE WRAP (Southwest)			
DEV,NA (HOT/COLD PACK)			
10s ea	45713-0660-80	259.50	403.50
ELASTO-GEL HAND EXERCISER (Southwest)			
DEV,NA (LARGE,HOT/COLD PACK)			
10s ea	45713-0650-05	104.00	162.00
(SMALL,HOT/COLD PACK)			
10s ea	45713-0650-01	70.00	107.00
ELASTO-GEL HOT/COLD PACK (Southwest)			
DEV,NA (12"X12")			
10s ea	45713-0608-04	328.00	510.00
(6"X8")			
10s ea	45713-0608-01	173.00	269.00
(8"X16")			
10s ea	45713-0608-05	293.00	456.00
(3"X3")			
25s ea	45713-0407-50	140.00	218.75
ELASTO-GEL HOT/COLD WRIST WRAP (Southwest)			
DEV,NA, 10s ea	45713-0602-00	173.00	269.00
ELASTO-GEL KNEE WRAP (Southwest)			
DEV,NA (LG/XL, W/PATELLA HOLE)			
10s ea	45713-0660-04	328.00	510.00
(S/M, W/PATELLA HOLE)			
10s ea	45713-0660-03	259.50	403.50
ELASTO-GEL LUMBAR WRAP (Southwest)			
DEV,NA (LARGE,HOT/COLD WRAP)			
10s ea	45713-0602-03	415.00	646.00
ELASTO-GEL NECK/BACK COMBO WRAP (Southwest)			
DEV,NA (HOT/COLD PACK)			
10s ea	45713-0601-06	515.50	802.00
ELASTO-GEL PLUS WOUND DRESSING (Southwest)			
DEV,NA (2"X3",W/TAPE)			
5s ea	45713-0582-50	12.65	88.50
(4"X4",W/TAPE)			
5s ea	45713-0580-50	20.55	144.00
(2"X3",W/TAPE)			
100s ea	45713-0982-50	253.00	354.00
(4"X4",W/TAPE)			
100s ea	45713-0980-50	411.15	576.00
ELASTO-GEL SHOULDER SLEEVE (Southwest)			
DEV,NA (LG/XL,HOT/COLD PACK)			
10s ea	45713-0690-05	515.50	802.00
(SM/MED,HOT/COLD PACK)			
10s ea	45713-0690-04	483.00	751.50
(WRAP,HOT/COLD PACK)			
10s ea	45713-0690-01	587.00	913.00
ELASTO-GEL SINUS MASK (Southwest)			
DEV,NA (HOT/COLD PACK)			
10s ea	45713-0603-01	120.00	187.50
ELASTO-GEL SUPPORT ROLL (Southwest)			
DEV,NA (3"X10", SMALL)			
10s ea	45713-0640-01	225.00	350.00
(4"X10", LARGE)			
10s ea	45713-0640-05	293.00	456.00
ELASTO-GEL THERAPY MITT (Southwest)			
DEV,NA (HOT/COLD PACK)			
10s ea	45713-0670-01	293.00	456.00
ELASTO-GEL THERAPY WRAP (Southwest)			
DEV,NA (4"X24",HOT/COLD PACK)			
10s ea	45713-0660-01	190.00	296.00
(6"X16",HOT/COLD PACK)			
10s ea	45713-0660-02	190.00	296.00
(6"X24",HOT/COLD PACK)			
10s ea	45713-0660-05	259.50	403.50
(6"X30",HOT/COLD PACK)			
10s ea	45713-0660-30	328.00	510.00
(9"X24",HOT/COLD PACK)			
10s ea	45713-0660-10	328.00	510.00
(9"X30",HOT/COLD PACK)			
10s ea	45713-0660-40	414.50	645.00
ELASTO-GEL TOE AID DRESSING (Southwest)			
DEV,NA (T-SHAPED)			
3s ea	45713-0184-50	7.12	10.00
144s ea	45713-0484-50	342.10	480.00
ELASTO-GEL WOUND DRESSING (Southwest)			
DEV,NA (12"X12",THIN)			
5s ea	45713-0587-02	103.20	144.50
(12"X12")			
5s ea	45713-0587-00	103.20	144.50
(2"X3")			
5s ea	45713-0082-00	11.90	16.65
(4"X4",THIN)			
5s ea	45713-0580-02	16.60	23.25
(4"X4")			
5s ea	45713-0580-00	16.60	23.25
(6"X8",THIN)			
5s ea	45713-0586-02	43.15	60.40
(6"X8")			
5s ea	45713-0586-00	43.15	60.40
(8"X16",THIN)			
5s ea	45713-0588-02	91.45	128.00
(8"X16")			
5s ea	45713-0588-00	91.45	128.00
(8"X8",HORSESHOE SHAPED)			
5s ea	45713-0590-51	64.69	90.55
(12"X12",THIN)			
25s ea	45713-0487-02	516.05	722.50
(6"X8",THIN)			
25s ea	45713-0486-02	215.65	302.00
(6"X8")			
25s ea	45713-0486-00	215.65	302.00
(8"X16")			
25s ea	45713-0488-00	457.10	643.00
(8"X8",HORSESHOE SHAPED)			
25s ea	45713-0490-51	323.45	452.75
(4"X4",THIN)			
100s ea	45713-0980-02	332.05	465.00
(5"X5")			
100s ea	45713-0985-00	416.90	584.00
(2"X3")			
200s ea	45713-0282-00	475.80	666.00
ELDERTONIC (Merz)			
SYR,PO, 480 ml	02590-0351-16	26.34	
ELDOPAQUE (Valeant Pharm Intl)			
CRE,TP, 2%, 28.35 gm	00187-0518-31	30.10	
ELDOQUIN (Valeant Pharm Intl)			
CRE,TP, 2%, 28.35 gm	00187-0382-31	30.10	
ELECARE (Abbott)			
PDR,PO (PEDIATRIC)			
400 gm	70074-0546-66	34.32	
PDS,PO (VANILLA)			
400 gm	70074-0594-06	34.32	
ELECTRO-MIST (Pharm Innov)			
LIQ,TP, 60 ml	00036-3310-60	1.87	2.68
250 ml	00036-3310-25	4.46	6.37
4000 ml	00036-3310-04	44.90	64.15
ELECTROL PLUS (Medique)			
TAB,PO (250X2,SF)			
17 mg-9 mg-40 mg,			
500s ea	10244-0591-65	31.29	
ELECTROLYTE PEDIATRIC (AmerisourceBergen)			
SOL,PO (PRIVATE LABEL,BUBBLEGUM)			
1014 ml	24385-0101-47	28.70	31.90
(PRIVATE LABEL,FRUIT)			
1014 ml	24385-0096-47	28.70	31.90
(PRIVATE LABEL,GRAPE)			
1014 ml	24385-0103-47	28.70	31.90
(UNFLAVORED)			
1014 ml	24385-0100-47	28.70	31.90
(Family Phcy)			
SOL,PO (FLAVORED,PRIVATE LABEL)			
960 ml	52735-0621-40	3.59	3.99
(PRIVATE LABEL)			
960 ml	52735-0620-40	3.59	3.99
(Major)			
SOL,PO (FRUIT)			
1014 ml	00904-5118-69	39.20	
(Phys Total Care)			
REPACK			
SOL,PO (1X1000ML,FRUIT)			
1000 ml	54868-5999-00	8.91	
ELECTROTAB (Hart Health)			
TAB,PO (50X2,SF,SODIUM-FREE)			
18 mg-9 mg-40 mg,			
100s ea	50332-0125-04	2.96	
(125X2,SF,SODIUM-FREE)			
18 mg-9 mg-40 mg,			
250s ea	50332-0125-07	6.69	
ELITE CA/MG (Miller)			
TAB,PO, 100s ea	17204-0351-40	10.08	16.80
ELITE IRON (Miller)			
TAB,PO, 15 mg, 100s ea	17204-0349-40	6.96	
ELITE MAGNESIUM (Miller)			
TAB,PO, 100s ea	17204-0352-40	7.56	12.60
ELITE ZINC (Miller)			
TAB,PO, 100s ea	17204-0353-40	6.00	8.40
ELLIMAN'S LINIMENT (Consolidated Midland)			
OIN,TP, 75 gm	00223-6336-00	5.00	
ELLIS TONIC (Breckenridge Pharm)			
ELI,PO, 480 ml	51991-0215-16	20.26	
ELM (Ellon)			
SOL,SL (DROPS)			
10.5 ml	51762-0035-10		9.25
ELON BARRIER PROTECTANT (Dartmouth)			
LOT,TP (FRAGRANCE-FREE)			
60 ml	58869-0161-20	12.00	14.99
ELON DUAL DEFENSE (Dartmouth)			
TIN,TP, 25%, 15 ml	58869-0176-05	22.50	27.99
ELON HERBAL FOOT CREAM (Dartmouth)			
CRE,TP, 60 ml	58869-0131-01	9.60	11.99
180 ml	58869-0131-06	24.00	29.99
ELON MATRIX 5000 (Dartmouth)			
TAB,PO (PF,SF,CORN-FREE)			
5000 mcg-50 mg-100 mg,			
60s ea	58869-0125-01	22.50	27.99
ELON MATRIX 5000 COMPLETE (Dartmouth)			
TAB,PO (PF,SF,CORN-FREE)			
60s ea	58869-0126-01	26.50	32.99
ELON MATRIX MULTI-VITAMIN (Dartmouth)			
PO (PF,SF)			
60s ea	58869-0122-01	20.10	24.99
ELON MATRIX PLUS (Dartmouth)			
TAB,PO (PF,SF,CORN-FREE)			
3 mg-50 mg-100 mg,			
60s ea	58869-0121-01	16.08	19.99
ELON NAIL CARE SYSTEM (Dartmouth)			
DEV,NA (4 NAIL FILES)			
ea	58869-0111-05	12.00	14.99
ELON NAIL CONDITIONER (Dartmouth)			
CRE,TP (JAR)			
7.5 gm	58869-0101-01	9.60	11.99
(TUBE)			
10 gm	58869-0101-03	9.60	11.99
ELON NAIL REVITALIZING HAND SOAP (Dartmouth)			
SOL,TP, 180 ml	58869-0141-06	8.10	9.99
ELON SKIN REPAIR SYSTEM (Dartmouth)			
LOT,TP, 60 ml	58869-0151-02	9.60	11.99
180 ml	58869-0151-06	24.00	29.99
EMAGRIN (Medique)			
TAB,PO (2X150,SF,LACTOSE-FREE)			
410 mg-60 mg-30 mg,			
300s ea	47682-0155-70	24.99	23.80
EMAGRIN FORTE (Medique)			
TAB,PO (150X2,SF)			
260 mg-32 mg-100 mg-5 mg,			
300s ea	10244-0560-63	24.99	
EMBRACE BLOOD GLUCOSE METER (Omnis)			
DEV,NA, ea	94030-2010-01	29.99	29.99
EMBRACE BLOOD GLUCOSE TEST STRIPS (Omnis)			
DEV,NA, 25s ea	94030-2010-04	20.99	20.99
50s ea	94030-2010-03	39.99	39.99
100s ea	94030-2010-02	79.99	79.99

PROD/MFR	HRI, UPC,NDC	AWP	SRP
EMERGENCY FIRST AID KIT (Johnson & Johnson)			
DEV,NA, ea	**81370-0049-95**	26.75	
EMETROL (Johnson & Johnson)			
SOL,PO (CHERRY)			
118 ml	**00501-5005-04**	6.36	
(LEMON-MINT)			
118 ml	**00501-5006-04**	6.36	
(CHERRY)			
240 ml	**00501-5005-08**	9.76	
(Pharmacia Consumer)			
SOL,PO (LEMON-MINT)			
240 ml	**00009-7573-02**	9.56	
(Phys Total Care)			
REPACK			
SOL,PO (AF,CHERRY)			
120 ml	**54868-0574-00**	8.10	
EMOLLIA-CREME (Gordon)			
CRE,TP, 120 gm	**10481-2005-04**	11.05	
454 gm	**10481-2005-06**	47.50	
2270 gm	**10481-2005-05**	123.75	
EMOLLIA-LOTION (Gordon)			
LOT,TP, 120 ml	**10481-2004-04**	7.95	
240 ml	**10481-2004-08**	11.60	
3840 ml	**50217-0001-41**	72.50	
EMPTY 3-IN-1 MIXING CONTAINER (Abbott Hosp)			
DEV,NA (2000 ML, NON-DEHP)			
20s ea	**00074-7222-17**	959.03	
(3000 ML, NON-DEHP)			
20s ea	**00074-7222-18**	498.75	
EMPTY CONTAINER (Abbott Hosp)			
DEV,NA (W/ATCHD Y-TRANF,3000ML)			
24s ea	**00074-7927-08**	128.16	
(W/ATTCHD Y-TRNSF/1000ML)			
24s ea	**00074-7927-09**	928.82	
(LIFECARE,FLEXIBLE,500ML)			
48s ea	**00074-7951-13**	786.60	
(LIFECARE,FLEXIBLE,50ML)			
48s ea	**00074-7951-12**	296.40	
(LIFECARE,FLXIBLE,1000ML)			
48s ea	**00074-7951-19**	853.29	
(LIFECARE,FLEXIBLE,100ML)			
200s ea	**00074-7951-23**	2921.25	
EMPTY CONTAINER STERILE (Abbott Hosp)			
DEV,NA (VIAL & INJECTOR)			
25s ea	**00074-6021-03**	217.87	
(VIAL, FLIPTOP, 30 ML)			
25s ea	**00074-5816-31**	24.64	
(VIAL, TEARDROP, 10 ML)			
25s ea	**00074-5829-10**	18.41	
(VIAL, TEARDROP, 30 ML)			
25s ea	**00074-5829-30**	21.38	
(Hospira)			
DEV,NA (VIAL, FLIPTOP, 10 ML)			
25s ea	**00074-5816-11**	17.10	
EMPTY EVACUATED CONTAINER (Abbott Hosp)			
DEV,NA (1000 ML)			
6s ea	**00074-1614-05**	130.03	
(150 ML)			
12s ea	**00074-1614-01**	227.86	
(250 ML)			
12s ea	**00074-1614-02**	234.98	
(500 ML)			
12s ea	**00074-1614-03**	236.12	
ENCARE (Blairex)			
SUP,VG, 100 mg, 12s ea	**50486-0221-12**	9.20	
18s ea	**50486-0221-18**	13.06	
ENEMA (Albertson's)			
NMA,RC, 135 ml	**41280-0230-79**	2.55	
(AmerisourceBergen)			
NMA,RC (TWIN PACK,PRIVATE LABEL)			
135 ml 2s	**24385-0039-36**	1.43	1.59
(Family Phcy)			
NMA,RC (TWIN,PRIVATE LABEL)			
135 ml	**52735-0210-46**	1.34	1.49
(Major)			
NMA,RC, 135 ml	**00904-3535-78**	1.25	
(Qualitest)			
NMA,RC, 135 ml	**00603-0752-91**	1.78	
(Rugby)			
NMA,RC			
7 gm/118 ml-19 gm/118 ml,			
133 ml	**00536-7415-51**	1.03	
ENEMEEZ MINI ENEMA (Alliance)			
NMA,RC (SINGLE USE,5X30)			
283 mg, 30s ea	**17433-9876-03**	69.93	76.95
ENEMEEZ PLUS MINI ENEMA (Alliance)			
NMA,RC (SINGLE USE,30X5)			
20 mg-283 mg,			
30s ea	**17433-9877-03**	69.93	76.95
ENFACARE LIPIL (Mead Johnson & Co)			
PDR,PO (MILK-BASED)			
363 gm	**00087-0019-44**	16.96	
ENFAGROW GENTLEASE NEXT STEP LIPIL (Mead Johnson & Co)			
PDR,PO (1X680GM)			
680 gm	**00087-1461-42**	22.38	
ENFAGROW PREMIUM LIPIL (Mead Johnson & Co)			
PDR,PO (1X680GM,VANILLA)			
680 gm	**00087-8692-47**	22.38	
ENFAGROW PREMIUM NEXT STEP LIPIL (Mead Johnson & Co)			
LIQ,PO (1X946ML,READY TO USE)			
946 ml	**00087-1288-41**	7.03	
PDR,PO (MILK BASED)			
680 gm	**00087-1401-51**	22.38	
ENFAGROW SOY NEXT STEP LIPIL (Mead Johnson & Co)			
PDR,PO (MILK FREE,SOY BASED)			
680 gm	**00087-1409-44**	22.38	
ENFALYTE (Mead Johnson & Co)			
SOL,PO (R.T.U,NURSETTE)			
177 ml	**00087-0265-24**	2.11	
ENFAMIL 5% GLUCOSE IN WATER (Mead Johnson & Co)			
SOL,PO (6X59ML)			
5%, 59 ml 6s	**00087-1346-41**	65.28	
ENFAMIL A.R. LIPIL (Mead Johnson & Co)			
LIQ,PO (6X59ML,NURSETTE,20CAL)			
59 ml 6s	**00087-1453-41**	9.79	
(READY TO USE)			
946 ml	**00087-0203-73**	7.99	
PDR,PO, 366 gm	**00087-0201-42**	16.56	
(FREQUENTSPITUP)			
681 gm	**00087-0201-59**	30.49	
ENFAMIL D-VI-SOL (Mead Johnson & Co)			
SOL,PO (1X50ML,SF,GLUTEN-FREE)			
400 iu/ml, 50 ml	**00087-0866-44**	7.73	
ENFAMIL ENFACARE LIPIL (Mead Johnson & Co)			
LIQ,PO (6X59ML,NURSETTE)			
59 ml 6s	**00087-1390-41**	9.79	
946 ml	**00087-1287-41**	8.78	
ENFAMIL FER-IN-SOL (Mead Johnson & Co)			
SYR,PO (1X50ML,W/DROPPER,DROPS)			
15 mg/ml, 50 ml	**00087-0740-02**	9.65	
ENFAMIL GENTLEASE LIPIL (Mead Johnson & Co)			
LIQ,PO (6X59ML,READY TO USE)			
59 ml 6s	**00087-1464-41**	9.79	
PDR,PO, 341 gm	**00087-8693-42**	16.46	
680 gm	**00087-8693-43**	31.16	
ENFAMIL HUMAN MILK FORTIFIER (Mead Johnson & Co)			
PDR,PO (SACHET)			
0.71 gm	**00087-2014-48**	1.28	
ENFAMIL LACTOFREE LIPIL (Mead Johnson & Co)			
LIQ,PO (6X59ML,NURSETTE)			
59 ml 6s	**00087-1444-41**	9.79	
ENFAMIL LIPIL W/IRON (Mead Johnson & Co)			
LIQ,PO (CONCENTRATE)			
384 ml	**00087-1272-41**	5.39	
PDR,PO (MILK-BASED)			
366 gm	**00087-1273-41**	16.18	
729 gm	**00087-1273-52**	30.62	
ENFAMIL LIPIL WITH IRON (Mead Johnson & Co)			
LIQ,PO (6X59ML,NURSETTE)			
59 ml 6s	**00087-1388-41**	9.79	
946 ml	**00087-1271-43**	8.18	
ENFAMIL PREMATURE LIPIL (Mead Johnson & Co)			
LIQ,PO (6X59ML,NURSETTE)			
59 ml 6s	**00087-1392-41**	9.79	
59 ml 6s	**00087-1393-41**	9.79	
ENFAMIL PREMATURE LIPIL LOW IRON (Mead Johnson & Co)			
LIQ,PO (6X59ML,NURSETTE,20CAL)			
59 ml 6s	**00087-1394-41**	9.79	
(6X59ML,NURSETTE,24CAL)			
59 ml 6s	**00087-1391-41**	9.79	
ENFAMIL PREMIUM LIPIL (Mead Johnson & Co)			
LIQ,PO (6X59ML,READY TO USE)			
59 ml 6s	**00087-1366-41**	88.13	
(8X177ML,READY TO USE)			
177 ml 8s	**00087-1458-41**	19.67	
(4X237ML,READY TO USE)			
237 ml 4s	**00087-1459-41**	10.34	
(1X384ML,CONCENTRATED)			
384 ml	**00087-1367-41**	66.53	
(1X946ML,READY TO USE)			
946 ml	**00087-1459-42**	47.66	
PDR,PO (16X17.4GM,SINGLE-SERVE)			
17.4 gm 16s	**00087-1365-45**	12.08	
(1X354GM)			
354 gm	**00087-1365-42**	101.45	
(1X663GM)			
663 gm	**00087-1365-41**	180.36	
ENFAMIL PROSOBEE LIPIL (Mead Johnson & Co)			
LIQ,PO (6X59ML,NURSETTE,20CAL)			
59 ml 6s	**00087-1449-41**	9.79	
ENFAMIL RESTFULL LIPIL (Mead Johnson & Co)			
PDR,PO (1X354GM)			
354 gm	**00087-0201-63**	17.51	
ENFAMIL WATER (Mead Johnson & Co)			
LIQ,PO (6X59ML)			
59 ml 6s	**00087-1345-41**	65.28	
ENFAPORT LIPIL (Mead Johnson & Co)			
LIQ,PO (1X237ML)			
237 ml	**00087-1289-41**	3.28	
ENGYSTOL N (Heel/BHI)			
TAB,SL, 100s ea	**50114-6065-02**	5.85	10.80
ENNDS (Oakhurst)			
TAB,PO, 100s ea	**11169-0100-77**	7.54	9.05
ENSURE (Abbott)			
LIQ,PO (GLUTEN-FREE)			
237 ml	**70074-0582-94**	2.03	
237 ml	**70074-0582-96**	2.03	
237 ml	**70074-0582-98**	2.03	
237 ml 6s	**70074-0407-11**	11.84	
(CHOCOLATE)			
237 ml 6s	**70074-0407-01**	11.84	
(PECAN)			
237 ml 6s	**70074-0517-85**	12.22	
(STRAWBERRY)			
237 ml 6s	**70074-0407-05**	11.84	
(VANILLA)			
960 ml	**70074-0526-37**	6.90	
PDR,PO, 420 gm	**70074-0060-75**	10.54	
ENSURE ENLIVE (Abbott)			
LIQ,PO (BRIK PACK,APPLE)			
240 ml	**70074-0547-77**	1.02	
(BRIK PACK,PEACH)			
240 ml	**70074-0547-80**	1.02	
ENSURE FIBER W/FOS (Abbott)			
LIQ,PO, 240 ml 6s	**70074-0407-59**	11.84	
(CHOCOLATE)			
240 ml 6s	**70074-0407-56**	11.84	
ENSURE GLUCERNA SHAKE (Abbott)			
LIQ,PO (BERRY)			
237 ml	**70074-0559-05**	1.97	
(CHOCOLATE)			
237 ml 6s	**70074-0545-56**	11.84	
(PECAN)			
237 ml 6s	**70074-0545-70**	11.84	
(VANILLA)			
237 ml 6s	**70074-0545-69**	11.84	
ENSURE HEALTHY MOM (Abbott)			
BAR,PO (20GMX10,CHOCOLATE)			
20 gm 10s	**70074-0582-44**	4.44	
(20GMX10,FUDGE GRAHAM)			
20 gm 10s	**70074-0582-46**	4.44	
LIQ,PO (237MLX4,GLUTEN-FREE)			
237 ml 4s	**70074-0582-35**	7.62	
237 ml 4s	**70074-0582-38**	7.62	
ENSURE HIGH CALCIUM (Abbott)			
LIQ,PO (6X240ML,CHOCOLATE)			
240 ml 6s	**70074-0548-26**	12.22	
(6X240ML,VANILLA)			
240 ml 6s	**70074-0548-23**	12.22	
ENSURE HIGH PROTEIN (Abbott)			
LIQ,PO (BANANA)			
237 ml 6s	**70074-0520-65**	12.22	
(CHOCOLATE)			
237 ml 6s	**70074-0520-69**	12.22	
(VANILLA)			
237 ml 6s	**70074-0520-71**	12.22	
(WILD BERRY)			
237 ml 6s	**70074-0520-73**	12.22	
ENSURE NUTRA SHAKE HI-CAL (Abbott)			
LIQ,PO (USE W/ MED SUPV,VANILLA)			
946 ml	**70074-0553-06**	9.79	
ENSURE PLUS (Abbott)			
LIQ,PO (GLUTEN-FREE)			
237 ml	**70074-0583-00**	2.26	
237 ml	**70074-0583-02**	2.26	
237 ml	**70074-0583-04**	2.26	
(CHOCOLATE)			
240 ml 6s	**70074-0407-02**	13.13	
(PECAN)			
240 ml 6s	**70074-0517-87**	13.13	

PROD/MFR	HRI, UPC,NDC	AWP	SRP
(VANILLA)			
240 ml 6s	70074-0407-07	13.13	
240 ml 6s	70074-0407-18	13.13	
(RTF ASEPTIC BTL,VANILLA)			
960 ml	70074-0532-05	7.08	
ENSURE PLUS HN (Abbott)			
LIQ,PO, 240 ml	70074-0407-21	2.35	
ENTERAL FEEDING TUBE (Abbott)			
DEV,NA (10 FR 45" W/STYLET)			
ea	70074-0004-76	32.05	
(10FR 45" NON-BOLUS,STYL)			
ea	70074-0550-42	31.03	
(12 FR 36" W/STRIPE)			
ea	70074-0501-25	24.94	
(12 FR 36")			
ea	70074-0004-74	24.94	
(12 FR 45" W/STYLET)			
ea	70074-0004-75	33.20	
(14 FR 36")			
ea	70074-0004-77	25.67	
(16 FR 36" W/STRIPE)			
ea	70074-0501-39	26.44	
(8 FR 36" W/STYLET)			
ea	70074-0004-71	31.03	
(8 FR 45" W/STYLET)			
ea	70074-0004-73	31.03	
(8 FR 45")			
ea	70074-0004-72	26.74	
ENTERCOTE (Global Source)			
ECT,PO, 325 mg, 100s ea	59618-0100-15	2.70	
ENTEREX (Victus, Inc.)			
LIQ,PO (BANANA)			
237 ml	12197-0200-40	1.95	
(BERRY)			
237 ml	12197-0200-20	1.95	
ENTEREX (Victus, Inc.)			
LIQ,PO (CHOCOLATE)			
237 ml	12197-0200-60	1.95	
(VANILLA)			
237 ml	12197-0200-00	1.95	
PDR,PO (TUBE FEED,BANANA)			
400 gm	12197-0120-40	11.95	
(TUBE FEED,BERRY)			
400 gm	12197-0120-20	11.95	
(TUBE FEED,VANILLA)			
400 gm	12197-0120-00	11.95	
(TUBE FEED,BERRY)			
1000 gm	12197-0420-20	29.49	
(TUBE FEED,VANILLA)			
1000 gm	12197-0420-00	29.49	
ENTEREX DIABETIC (Victus, Inc.)			
LIQ,PO (SF,LACTOSE-FREE)			
237 ml	12197-0611-60	3.33	
(SF,VANILLA)			
237 ml	12197-0611-11	3.33	
ENTEREX GLUTAPAK-10 (Victus, Inc.)			
PDS,PO (PACKET)			
10 gm/15 gm, 15 gm 50s	12197-0700-10	150.00	
ENTSOL (Kenwood)			
GEL,NS (PF,HYPERTONIC)			
20 gm	00482-3300-20	9.97	
PDS,NS (HYPERTONIC,PACKET)			
3%, 10.5 gm 10s	00482-3200-10	11.30	
SPR,NS (HYPERTONIC,PF)			
3%, 100 ml	00482-3110-10	26.12	
ENTSOL ADAPTER NASAL WASH TIP (Kenwood)			
DEV,NA, ea	00482-3000-01	45.83	
ENTSOL MIST (Kenwood)			
SOL,NS (HYPERTONIC)			
3%, 30 ml	00482-3100-01	8.03	
ENTSOL REFILLABLE NASAL WASH BOTTLE (Kenwood)			
DEV,NA, ea	00482-3000-02	40.64	
ENTSOL SINGLE USE (Kenwood)			
SOL,NS (HYPERTONIC,PF)			
3%, 240 ml	00482-3120-08	8.04	
ENUCLENE (Alcon Surgical)			
SOL,OP, 0.02%-0.25%, 15 ml 12s	00065-0083-15	123.98	
EO28 SPLASH (Nutricia)			
LIQ,PO (27X237ML,GRAPE)			
237 ml 27s	49735-0126-70	135.20	
(27X237ML,TROPICAL FRUIT)			
237 ml 27s	49735-0126-66	135.20	
(27X237ML)			
237 ml 27s	49735-0110-50	135.20	
EPA/GARLIC (Miller)			
CAP,PO, 100s ea	17204-0562-40	11.22	18.70
EPHEDRINE SULFATE (Consolidated Midland)			
CAP,PO, 25 mg, 100s ea	00223-0620-01	4.95	
1000s ea	00223-0620-02	42.50	
(Truxton)			
CAP,PO, 25 mg, 1000s ea	00463-2010-10	22.00	
(West-Ward)			
CAP,PO, 25 mg, 100s ea	00143-3145-01	30.25	
EPHEDRINE-PHENOBARBITAL-THEOPHYLLINE (Consolidated Midland)			
TAB,PO, 100s ea	00223-2050-00	8.75	
EPI-CLENZ (Medline)			
FOA,TP (HAND CLEANSER)			
62%, 240 gm 24s	53329-0970-08	114.60	
GEL,TP, 70%, 120 gm 24s	53329-0970-44	27.10	
480 gm 12s	53329-0970-06	56.70	
EPIDERM BALM (Pharma Pac)			
REPACK			
LIQ,TP, 120 ml	52959-0578-04	15.65	
(Southwood)			
REPACK			
LIQ,TP, 60 ml	58016-3514-01	6.00	
120 ml	58016-3526-04	12.00	
EPILYT (Stiefel Consumer HealthCare)			
LOT,TP, 118 ml	00145-0624-04	9.12	13.79
(Phys Total Care)			
REPACK			
LOT,TP (1X118ML)			
118 ml	54868-0126-00	14.63	
EPINEPHRINE (Consolidated Midland)			
AER,IH, 0.22 mg/actuation, 15 ml	00223-6548-15	6.10	
EPINEPHRINE MIST (Cardinal Health)			
AER,IH (PRIVATE LABEL)			
0.22 mg/actuation, 15 ml	37205-0106-05	10.92	
(Phys Total Care)			
REPACK			
AER,IH, 0.22 mg/actuation, 15 ml	54868-3015-00	28.59	
EPSAL (Press)			
OIN,TP, 80%, 15 gm 12s	11649-0001-01	60.00	
60 gm 12s	11649-0001-03	119.40	
EQUALACTIN (Numark)			
CTB,PO, 625 mg, 24s ea	38485-0000-26	3.30	
48s ea	38485-0000-27	6.30	
EQUALINE COLOR LANCETS (Can-Am Care)			
DEV,NA, 100s ea	38396-0307-40	5.85	
EQUALINE INSULIN SYRINGE (Can-Am Care)			
DEV,NA (29GX1/2",1/2ML)			
100s ea	38396-0412-40	17.50	
(29GX1/2",1ML,SINGLE USE)			
100s ea	38396-0413-40	17.50	
(29GX1/2",3/10ML)			
100s ea	38396-0411-40	17.50	
(30GX5/16",1/2ML)			
100s ea	38396-0415-40	17.50	
(30GX5/16",1ML)			
100s ea	38396-0416-40	17.50	
(30GX5/16",3/10ML)			
100s ea	38396-0414-40	17.50	
(31GX5/16",1/2ML)			
100s ea	38396-0420-40	17.50	
(31GX5/16",1ML)			
100s ea	38396-0421-40	17.50	
(31GX5/16",3/10ML)			
100s ea	38396-0419-40	17.50	
EQUALINE SUPER THIN LANCETS (Can-Am Care)			
DEV,NA, 100s ea	38396-0305-40	5.85	
200s ea	38396-0306-40	9.50	
EQUALINE THIN LANCETS (Can-Am Care)			
DEV,NA, 100s ea	38396-0301-40	5.85	
200s ea	38396-0302-40	9.50	
EQUILIZER GAS RELIEF (Hi-Tech)			
SUS,PO (DROPS)			
40 mg/0.6 ml, 30 ml	50383-0785-30	5.00	
ERASE (Geritrex)			
SPR,NA (ODOR ELIMINATOR)			
240 ml	92771-0260-08	3.39	
ERASE RAS-POURI (Geritrex)			
SPR,NA (ODOR ELIMINATOR)			
240 ml	92771-0260-09	3.52	
ERGOCALCIFEROL (County Line)			
SOL,PO (1X60ML,USP)			
8000 iu/ml, 60 ml	43199-0015-60	100.19	
ESOTERICA FACIAL (Medicis)			
CRE,TP, 85 gm	00766-1121-14	6.49	
ESOTERICA REGULAR (Medicis)			
CRE,TP, 2%, 85 gm	00766-1101-14	6.49	
ESOTERICA SUNSCREEN (Medicis)			
CRE,TP, 85 gm	00766-1131-14	6.49	
ESPECOL (Pfeiffer)			
SOL,PO (CHERRY)			
120 ml	00927-0051-12	2.86	5.14
(LEMON-LIME)			
120 ml	00927-0052-12	2.86	5.14
ESSENTIAL AMINO ACID MIX (Nutricia)			
PDR,PO (USE W/MED SUPV)			
200 gm 2s	49735-0114-90	204.10	
ESSENTIAL NUTRIENTS PLUS SILICA (Action Labs)			
TAB,PO (SF)			
60s ea	24675-0710-61	5.99	11.99
ESTEEM SYNERGY CLOSED POUCH (Convatec)			
DEV,NA (LG,STD 9")			
30s ea	00034-0054-32	46.99	61.16
ESTER C (Nature's Bounty)			
TAB,PO (PF,SF)			
500 mg-200 mg-50 mg, 90s ea	74312-0069-90		9.99
ESTER-C 500 (Mason Vit)			
TAB,PO (PF,SF)			
60s ea	11845-0118-05	8.78	
ESTER-C W/BIOFLAVONOID COMPLEX (Linus)			
TAB,PO (CAPLET)			
700 mg-200 mg-64 mg, 90s ea	10363-0253-21	5.37	9.95
ESTER-C W/ROSE HIPS (Rexall)			
TAB,PO (NON-ACIDIC,PF,SF)			
500 mg-100 mg, 50s ea	30768-0000-92	3.51	5.32
EUCALYPTAMINT (Heritage/Insight)			
GEL,TP (POWDER FRESH)			
8%, 67.5 gm	63736-0342-59	3.63	
OIN,TP, 16%, 60 gm	63736-0340-98	3.74	
EUCERIN (Beiersdorf)			
CRE,TP (FRAGRANCE-FREE)			
57 gm	10356-0090-07	3.29	
57 gm	72140-0038-68		4.89
(1X113GM,ORIGINAL)			
113 gm	72140-0000-22		7.99
(FRAGRANCE-FREE)			
240 gm	10356-0090-05	7.37	
454 gm	10356-0090-01	9.45	9.30
LOT,TP, 120 ml	72140-0037-71	3.75	
240 ml	10356-0793-01	5.10	4.88
480 ml	10356-0793-04	7.37	7.54
SOA,TP (SOAP-FREE)			
ea	72140-0000-29	2.55	2.63
(A-S Medication)			
REPACK			
CRE,TP, 120 gm	54569-1936-00	6.78	
(Phys Total Care)			
REPACK			
CRE,TP, 120 gm	54868-2852-00	7.97	
EUCERIN CALMING CREME (Beiersdorf)			
CRE,TP (1X226GM,FRAGRANCE-FREE)			
226 gm	72140-0633-78		7.99
EUCERIN DAILY REPLENISHING LOTION (Beiersdorf)			
LOT,TP (1X400ML,FRAGRANCE-FREE)			
400 ml	72140-0110-18		7.99
EUCERIN EVERYDAY PROTECTION BODY LOTION (Beiersdorf)			
LOT,TP (1X400ML,SPF 15)			
400 ml	72140-0635-97		6.29
EUCERIN FACIAL (Beiersdorf)			
LOT,TP (SPF 25,AF)			
120 ml	10356-0972-01	5.49	
EUCERIN LIGHT (Beiersdorf)			
CRE,TP (FRAGRANCE-FREE)			
113 gm	10356-0282-01	5.10	
LOT,TP, 226 ml	10356-0032-01	5.10	
EUCERIN ORIGINAL MOISTURIZING LOTION (Beiersdorf)			
LOT,TP (1X250ML,FRAGRANCE-FREE)			
250 ml	72140-0110-19		7.99
(1X500ML,FRAGRANCE-FREE)			
500 ml	72140-0110-20		11.99

PROD/MFR	HRI, UPC,NDC	AWP	SRP
EUCERIN PLUS (Beiersdorf)			
LOT,TP (FRAGRANCE-FREE)			
177 ml	10356-0967-01	5.49	
354 ml	10356-0967-03	7.37	
EUCERIN SHOWER THERAPY (Beiersdorf)			
LOT,TP (FRAGRANCE-FREE)			
203 ml	72140-0032-41	5.10	
EUPATORIUM PERF (Luyties)			
TAB,SL (6X)			
6 x, 500s ea	00618-3270-03	3.99	
5500s ea	00618-3270-10	30.32	
(30X)			
12 x, 500s ea	00622-3270-03	4.19	
5500s ea	00622-3270-10	31.83	
(12X)			
30 x, 500s ea	00624-3270-03	4.19	
5500s ea	00624-3270-10	31.83	
EUPHORBIUM (Heel/BHI)			
SPR,NS, 20 ml	51885-3011-09	7.25	13.50
EUPHRASIA (Luyties)			
TAB,SL (6X)			
6 x, 500s ea	00618-3286-03	3.99	
5500s ea	00618-3286-10	30.32	
(30X)			
12 x, 500s ea	00622-3286-03	4.19	
5500s ea	00622-3286-10	31.83	
(12X)			
30 x, 500s ea	00624-3286-03	4.19	
5500s ea	00624-3286-10	31.83	
EVAC (Bio-Tech Pharm)			
PDR,PO, 3.4 gm/dose,			
480 gm	53191-0021-16	6.85	
EVAC-U-GEN (Lee Pharm)			
CTB,PO, 10 mg, 35s ea	23558-0510-40	3.96	3.28
80s ea	23558-0510-43	6.72	
(35X12)			
10 mg, 420s ea	23558-0510-41	47.52	
(80X12)			
10 mg, 960s ea	23558-0510-44	80.64	
EVENING PRIMROSE (Bio-Tech Pharm)			
SGL,PO, 500 mg-48 mg,			
100s ea	53191-0034-01	11.80	
180s ea	53191-0034-18	18.90	
(Major)			
SGL,PO (SOFTGEL)			
500 mg, 60s ea	00904-5317-52	7.49	
EVENING PRIMROSE OIL (ADH)			
SGL,PO (PF,SF,SOFTGEL)			
500 mg, 500s ea	60142-0755-01	8.48	16.95
(Mason Vit)			
SGL,PO (PF,SF,SOFTGEL)			
500 mg, 60s ea	11845-0122-15	9.11	
60s ea	11845-0128-45	9.11	
(Nature's Bounty)			
CAP,PO (PF,SF,SOFTGEL)			
365 mg-45 mg, 30s ea	74312-0036-30		4.99
EVOLVE (Bionutrics Health)			
SGL,PO (PF,SF,SOFTGEL)			
25 mg, 30s ea	10187-0125-30	10.28	12.99
90s ea	10187-0125-90	15.00	25.00
EX-L (Key Company)			
TAB,PO (SF)			
90s ea	11694-0973-01	9.00	
250s ea	11694-0973-02	23.00	
EX-LAX (Novartis Consumer)			
TAB,PO, 15 mg, 8s ea	00067-0003-08	1.88	
(CHOCOLATE)			
15 mg, 18s ea	00067-0005-18	3.17	
30s ea	00067-0003-30	5.17	
(CHOCOLATE)			
15 mg, 48s ea	00067-0005-48	7.10	
(MAXIMUM STRENGTH,PILL)			
25 mg, 90s ea	00067-0016-90	13.10	
EX-LAX MAXIMUM STRENGTH (Novartis Consumer)			
TAB,PO, 25 mg, 24s ea	00067-0016-24	5.17	
48s ea	00067-0016-48	8.70	
EX-LAX REGULAR STRENGTH (Novartis Consumer)			
CTB,PO (CHOCOLATE)			
15 mg, 24s ea	00067-0005-24	3.88	
EXAPRIN (Hart Health)			
TAB,PO (2X50)			
100s ea UD	50332-0105-04	3.08	
(2X125)			
250s ea UD	50332-0105-07	6.95	

PROD/MFR	HRI, UPC,NDC	AWP	SRP
EXCEDRIN (Novartis Consumer)			
TAB,PO (EXTRA STRENGTH)			
250 mg-250 mg-65 mg,			
10s ea	00067-2030-10	1.74	
24s ea	00067-2030-24	3.37	
(EXTRA STRENGTH,GELTAB)			
250 mg-250 mg-65 mg,			
50s ea	00067-2021-50	5.96	
100s ea	00067-2021-91	9.95	
(EXTRA STRENGTH)			
250 mg-250 mg-65 mg,			
200s ea	00067-2030-92	13.19	
250s ea	00067-2030-77	14.18	
EXCEDRIN BACK & BODY (Novartis Consumer)			
TAB,PO (EXTRA STRENGTH)			
250 mg-250 mg,			
6s ea	00067-6238-06	0.60	
(EXTRA STRENGTH,CAPLET)			
250 mg-250 mg,			
24s ea	00676-0238-24	3.37	
50s ea	00676-0238-50	5.75	
100s ea	00676-0238-91	9.59	
EXCEDRIN EXTRA STRENGTH (B/M Squibb Cons Med)			
TAB,PO, 250 mg-250 mg-65 mg,			
10s ea	19810-0300-89	2.12	
24s ea	19810-0077-29	3.18	
(CAPLET)			
250 mg-250 mg-65 mg,			
24s ea	19810-0000-21	3.18	
(GELTAB)			
250 mg-250 mg-65 mg,			
24s ea	19810-0002-96	3.18	
50s ea	19810-0001-65	5.42	
(CAPLET)			
250 mg-250 mg-65 mg,			
50s ea	19810-0000-22	5.42	
(GELTAB)			
250 mg-250 mg-65 mg,			
50s ea	19810-0002-97	5.42	
100s ea	19810-0001-66	9.05	
(CAPLET)			
250 mg-250 mg-65 mg,			
100s ea	19810-0000-23	9.05	
(GELTAB)			
250 mg-250 mg-65 mg,			
100s ea	19810-0002-98	9.05	
(CAPLET)			
250 mg-250 mg-65 mg,			
175s ea	19810-0006-19	12.29	
250s ea	19810-0300-87	13.38	
(Novartis Consumer)			
SGL,PO (EXPRESS GELS)			
250 mg-250 mg-65 mg,			
20s ea	00067-6270-20	3.85	
40s ea	00067-6270-40	6.56	
80s ea	00067-6270-80	10.94	
160s ea	00067-6270-16	16.20	
EXCEDRIN MIGRAINE (B/M Squibb Cons Med)			
TAB,PO, 250 mg-250 mg-65 mg,			
24s ea	19810-0007-90	3.18	
(CAPLET)			
250 mg-250 mg-65 mg,			
24s ea	19810-0008-63	3.18	
(GELTAB)			
250 mg-250 mg-65 mg,			
24s ea	19810-0054-06	3.18	
50s ea	19810-0008-08	5.42	
(CAPLET)			
250 mg-250 mg-65 mg,			
50s ea	19810-0008-65	5.42	
(GELTAB)			
250 mg-250 mg-65 mg,			
50s ea	19810-0057-02	5.42	
100s ea	19810-0008-09	9.05	
(CAPLET)			
250 mg-250 mg-65 mg,			
100s ea	19810-0008-66	9.05	
(GELTAB)			
250 mg-250 mg-65 mg,			
100s ea	19810-0057-03	9.05	
175s ea	19810-0052-06	12.29	
250s ea	19810-0300-88	13.38	
(Novartis Consumer)			
TAB,PO, 250 mg-250 mg-65 mg,			
24s ea	00067-2037-24	3.37	
(CAPLET)			
250 mg-250 mg-65 mg,			
50s ea	00067-2039-50	5.75	
100s ea	00067-2039-91	9.59	
200s ea	00067-2039-92	13.19	
250s ea	00067-2039-77	14.18	

PROD/MFR	HRI, UPC,NDC	AWP	SRP
EXCEDRIN PM (B/M Squibb Cons Med)			
TAB,PO, 500 mg-38 mg,			
24s ea	19810-0001-82	3.76	
(CAPLET)			
500 mg-38 mg,			
24s ea	19810-0003-22	3.76	
(GELTAB)			
500 mg-38 mg,			
24s ea	19810-0070-67	3.76	
50s ea	19810-0001-83	6.97	
(CAPLET)			
500 mg-38 mg,			
50s ea	19810-0003-23	6.97	
(GELTAB)			
500 mg-38 mg,			
50s ea	19810-0070-68	6.97	
100s ea	19810-0001-56	9.61	
(CAPLET)			
500 mg-38 mg,			
100s ea	19810-0003-26	9.61	
(GELTAB)			
500 mg-38 mg,			
100s ea	19810-0002-40	9.61	
(Novartis Consumer)			
TAB,PO (ASPIRIN-FREE,CAPLET)			
500 mg-38 mg,			
24s ea	00067-2055-24	3.98	
EXCEDRIN SINUS HEADACHE (Novartis Consumer)			
TAB,PO, 325 mg-5 mg,			
50s ea	00067-2060-50	5.75	
(CAPLET)			
325 mg-5 mg,			
50s ea	00067-2062-50	5.75	
100s ea	00067-2060-91	9.59	
EXCEDRIN TENSION HEADACHE (Novartis Consumer)			
CAP,PO (EXPRESS GELS)			
500 mg-65 mg,			
20s ea	00067-6272-20	3.85	
SGL,PO, 500 mg-65 mg,			
40s ea	00067-6272-40	6.56	
80s ea	00067-6272-80	10.94	
TAB,PO (ASPIRIN-FREE,CAPLET)			
500 mg-65 mg,			
24s ea	00067-2045-24	3.37	
(ASPIRIN-FREE,GELTAB)			
500 mg-65 mg,			
24s ea	00067-2050-24	3.50	
(ASPIRIN-FREE,CAPLET)			
500 mg-65 mg,			
50s ea	00067-2045-50	5.75	
100s ea	00067-2045-91	9.59	
(ASPIRIN-FREE,GELTAB)			
500 mg-65 mg,			
100s ea	00067-2050-91	9.95	
EXCEL AP (Aplicare)			
SWA,TP (1X25UD)			
72%-7.5%,			
25s ea UD	52380-0039-09	34.00	
EXCEL AP APLICARE (Aplicare)			
SWA,TP, 72%-7.5%,			
50s ea	52380-0039-04	46.97	
EXCEL-GEL (MPM Medical Inc.)			
GEL,TP, 28 gm	66977-0006-01	3.16	3.51
85 gm	66977-0006-03	11.51	12.79
EXCELGINATE AG (MPM Medical Inc.)			
DRE,TP (12" ROPE)			
ea	66977-0830-12	9.83	10.93
(2X2)			
ea	66977-0830-22	3.86	4.29
(4X4.75")			
ea	66977-0830-45	9.48	10.53
(6X6")			
ea	66977-0830-66	25.27	28.08
EXCILON I.V. STERILE (Covidien)			
DEV,NA (4"X4",6 PLY,PEEL-BACK)			
600s ea	08080-7086-00	135.90	
EXCILON NON-WOVEN ALL-PURPOSE (Covidien)			
DEV,NA (3"X4",6 PLY,PEEL-BACK)			
600s ea	08080-7083-00	83.19	
(4"X4",6 PLY,PEEL-BACK)			
600s ea	08080-7084-00	94.78	
(4"X4",6 PLY,PLSTIC TRAY)			
800s ea	08080-7085-00	127.02	
EXCILON WASHCLOTHS (Covidien)			
DEV,NA (12X50)			
600s ea	08080-6040-01	59.90	

PROD/MFR	HRI, UPC,NDC	AWP	SRP
EXEFEN DMX (Larken Labs, Inc.)			
TAB,PO, 20 mg-400 mg-60 mg,			
100s ea	68047-0155-01	76.88	
EXPANDOVER (Covidien)			
DEV,NA (ELASTIC ADHES,4"X5 YDS)			
24s ea	08080-6620-35	108.28	
(ELASTIC ADHES,2"X5YDS)			
48s ea	08080-6620-19	117.74	
(ELASTIC ADHES,3"X5 YDS)			
48s ea	08080-6620-27	159.25	
(ELASTIC ADHES,1"X5 YDS)			
96s ea	08080-6620-02	112.13	
EXPECTA (Mead Johnson & Co)			
SGL,PO (SOFTGEL)			
200 mg, 30s ea	00087-8695-42	9.60	
EXPRESS MED PRESTIGE SMART SYSTEM (Home Diag)			
DEV,NA (STRIP)			
50s ea	56151-0309-50	26.12	
EXPRESS MED PSS STARTER (Home Diag)			
DEV,NA (MTR,STRP,LANCET,DEV,SOL)			
ea	56151-0209-01	22.18	
EXTENSION SET (Abbott Hosp)			
DEV,NA (20")			
48s ea	00074-4429-48	72.00	
(30" W/SLIDE CLAMP)			
48s ea	00074-4481-48	78.91	
(32" W/STOPCOCK)			
48s ea	00074-1834-48	137.66	
(7" W/OPTION-LOK)			
50s ea	00074-4438-02	363.38	
(20", STERILE PACK)			
120s ea	00074-4620-02	188.64	
(30", STERILE PACK)			
120s ea	00074-4610-02	241.92	
EXTENSION SET INT-SL (Abbott Hosp)			
DEV,NA (6")			
50s ea	00074-4116-01	180.00	
EXTENSION WITH SLIDE CLAMP (Abbott Hosp)			
DEV,NA (71",IRRIGATION/DRAINAGE)			
20s ea	00074-4693-01	88.32	
(LATEX,71")			
20s ea	00074-4693-02	88.32	
EXTERNAL ITCH RELIEF (Johnson & Johnson)			
SPR,TP (SOOTHE & RELIEVE PACK)			
1%, 14.8 ml	80045-0506-00	7.24	
EXTRAPRIN (Magno-Humphries)			
TAB,PO, 250 mg-250 mg-65 mg,			
100s ea	43292-0556-34	2.14	4.89
250s ea	43292-0556-35	4.01	8.99
EXTRESS (Key Company)			
TAB,PO (SF,CAPLET)			
100s ea	11694-0974-01	5.25	
EXTRESS SUPER (Key Company)			
TAB,PO (SF)			
100s ea	11694-0112-05	6.50	
250s ea	11694-0112-25	14.00	
1000s ea	11694-0112-06	48.00	
EXTRESS-30 (Key Company)			
CER,PO (SF)			
100s ea	11694-0664-01	12.50	
250s ea	11694-0664-25	25.00	
1000s ea	11694-0664-05	89.00	
EXTRESS-60 (Key Company)			
CER,PO (SF)			
100s ea	11694-0831-01	16.00	
EXUDERM HYDROCOLLOID (Medline)			
DEV,NA (4"X4")			
5s ea	53329-0518-40	25.18	
(8"X8")			
5s ea	53329-0518-43	110.76	
EXUDERM LP HYDROCOLLOID (Medline)			
DEV,NA (6"X6")			
5s ea	53329-0519-42	61.05	
(4"X4")			
10s ea	53329-0519-40	27.50	
EXUDERM RCD HYDROCOLLOID (Medline)			
DEV,NA (4"X4")			
5s ea	53329-0517-40	14.89	
(6"X6")			
5s ea	53329-0517-42	40.24	
(8"X8")			
5s ea	53329-0517-43	55.11	
EXUDERM SACRUM HYDROCOLLOID (Medline)			
DEV,NA (4"X3.6")			
5s ea	53329-0523-40	40.20	
(6"X6.5")			
5s ea	53329-0522-49	96.18	
EXUDERM SATIN HYDROCOLLOID (Medline)			
DEV,NA (6"X6",STERILE)			
5s ea	08327-0513-42	32.54	
(8"X8",STERILE)			
5s ea	08327-0513-43	75.00	
(4"X4",STERILE)			
10s ea	08327-0513-40	58.49	
(2"X2",STERILE)			
20s ea	80196-0735-66	33.55	
EXUDERM ULTRA HYDROCOLLOID (Medline)			
DEV,NA (4"X4")			
10s ea	53329-0521-40	43.75	
EYE AREA REPLENISHER (Neurovites)			
CRE,TP, 60 gm	93595-2034-01	19.50	32.50
EYE BRIGHT (Advanced Nutr)			
CAP,PO, 50s ea	62617-0415-05	10.13	19.50
EYE CLEAN (Hart Health)			
SOL,OP (EYE WASH)			
15 ml	50332-0201-02	1.52	
(SQUEEZE BOTTLE)			
30 ml	50332-0201-03	1.56	
(EYE WASH)			
120 ml	50332-0201-01	1.78	
(EYE & SKIN WASH)			
480 ml	50332-0201-06	4.73	
960 ml	50332-0201-08	9.39	
EYE DROPS (AmerisourceBergen)			
SOL,OP (PRIVATE LABEL)			
0.05%, 15 ml	24385-0075-01	2.60	3.69
(Chain Drug Marketing)			
SOL,OP, 0.05%-0.25%,			
15 ml	63868-0377-05	1.20	2.99
EYE DROPS ALLERGY RELIEF (Cardinal Health)			
SOL,OP (PRIVATE LABEL)			
0.05%-0.25%, 15 ml	37205-0138-05	2.13	
EYE DROPS EXTRA (AmerisourceBergen)			
SOL,OP (PRIVATE LABEL)			
1%-0.05%, 15 ml	24385-0077-01	1.27	2.89
EYE DROPS MOISTURIZING RELIEF (Chain Drug Marketing)			
SOL,OP (STERILE)			
1%-0.05%, 15 ml	63868-0376-05	1.20	2.99
EYE DROPS REDNESS RELIEF (Cardinal Health)			
SOL,OP (PRIVATE LABEL)			
0.05%, 15 ml	37205-0139-05	2.00	
EYE IRRIGATING SOLUTION (Rugby)			
SOL,OP, 120 ml	00536-0901-97	4.12	
(A-S Medication)			
REPACK			
SOL,OP, 120 ml	54569-2594-00	3.81	
EYE ITCH RELIEF DROPS (Major)			
SOL,OP (1X5ML)			
0.025%, 5 ml	00904-5837-05	10.09	
EYE LUBE (Stat Rx)			
REPACK			
OIN,OP, 3.5 gm	16590-0094-35	6.25	
EYE SCRUB (Novartis Pharm)			
PAD,TP, 30s ea	00780-0520-30	10.14	
EYE WASH (Altaire)			
SOL,OP, 118 ml	59390-0195-35	6.91	
(STERILE BUFFERED SOLN)			
237 ml	59390-0175-41	2.25	
473 ml	59390-0175-46	3.00	
960 ml	59390-0175-48	3.75	
(AmerisourceBergen)			
SOL,OP (W/CUP,PRIVATE LABEL)			
120 ml	24385-0252-26	2.96	3.29
(Cardinal Health)			
SOL,OP (PRIVATE LABEL)			
118 ml	37205-0023-26	3.17	
(Major)			
SOL,OP, 118 ml	00904-5377-20	3.40	
(Altura)			
REPACK			
SOL,OP, 15 ml	63874-0051-15	5.88	
120 ml	63874-0051-12	10.54	
(Pharma Pac)			
REPACK			
SOL,OP, 118 ml	52959-0711-04	7.25	
(Phys Total Care)			
REPACK			
SOL,OP, 120 ml	54868-0226-01	14.97	
(Quality Care Prod)			
REPACK			
SOL,OP, 120 ml	49999-0241-04	6.82	
EYE WASH IRRIGATING SOLUTION (Southwood)			
REPACK			
SOL,OP, 120 ml	58016-6019-01	6.81	
EYE-CEPT REWETTING DROPS (Optics)			
SOL,OP (20X0.5ML,PF)			
0.5 ml 20s	64108-0411-12		5.95
EYE-RITE (Carlson,J.R.)			
CAP,PO, 60s ea	88395-0048-00	22.45	44.90
120s ea	88395-0048-01	42.45	84.90
180s ea	88395-0048-02	59.95	119.90
EYE-STREAM (Alcon Ophthalmic)			
SOL,OP, 30 ml	00065-0530-01	15.42	
120 ml	00065-0530-04	23.64	
EYE-VITES (Nature's Bounty)			
TAB,PO (SF)			
60s ea	74312-0074-30		6.65
EYETAMINS (Rexall)			
TAB,PO (WITH LUTEIN,PF,SF)			
50s ea	30768-0001-77	2.79	4.23
EZ DETECT (Biomerica)			
DEV,NA (STOOL BLOOD TEST)			
ea	83059-0100-01	4.50	
EZ-CHAR (Paddock)			
PDR,PO (PELLETS)			
25 gm/29.4 gm, ea	00574-0122-25	17.65	
(A-S Medication)			
REPACK			
PDR,PO (PELLETS)			
25 gm/29.4 gm,			
25 gm	54569-5677-00	17.65	
EZO DENTURE CUSHIONS (Medtech)			
DEV,NA (UPPER HEAVY)			
12s ea	75137-0286-98	2.12	
(LOWER HEAVY)			
15s ea	75137-0286-93	2.12	
EZY-DOSE 7-COMPARTMENT VITAMIN ORGANIZER (Apothecary)			
DEV,NA (W/ID PLATE)			
ea	25715-0671-50	2.36	3.99
EZY-DOSE 7-DAY AM/PM DUETS PILL REMINDER (Apothecary)			
DEV,NA, ea	25715-0675-97	4.14	6.99
EZY-DOSE ADULT-LOCK LOCKING TABLET CUTTER (Apothecary)			
DEV,NA, ea	25715-0678-30	4.76	7.99
EZY-DOSE ADULT-LOCK PILL REMINDER (Apothecary)			
DEV,NA (LOCKABLE, LARGE)			
ea	25715-0679-32	2.36	3.99
EZY-DOSE ALCOHOL APPLICATOR BOTTLE (Apothecary)			
DEV,NA (2OZ FOAM TIPPED DAUBER)			
ea	25715-0669-58	1.88	3.19
EZY-DOSE FOUR-A-DAY WEEKLY MEDTIME PLANNER (Apothecary)			
DEV,NA, ea	25715-0671-69	6.95	11.59
EZY-DOSE FOUR-A-DAY WEEKLY PHARMADOSE MEDICATION ORGANIZER (Apothecary)			
EZY-DOSE FOUR-A-DAY WEEKLY PHARMADOSE MEDICATION ORGANIZER			
NA, ea	25715-0913-40	6.94	11.59
EZY-DOSE LIQUID MEDICATION (Apothecary)			
DEV,NA, ea	25715-0671-91	2.13	3.59
EZY-DOSE UNIVERSAL PUSH 'N POP PILL REMINDER (Apothecary)			
DEV,NA (2XL)			
ea	25715-0675-64	2.71	4.59
F-A-A (Nestle)			
LIQ,PO (250MLX24,GLUTEN-FREE)			
250 ml 24s	00065-9092-70	166.75	
FA-8 (Bio-Tech Pharm)			
CAP,PO, 800 mcg,			
100s ea	53191-0265-01	3.15	
FABRIC STRIPS (AmerisourceBergen)			
DEV,NA (ASSORTED,PRIVATE LABEL)			
20s ea	24385-0158-60	1.26	1.79
FAMILY PHARMACY ALLERGY (AmerisourceBergen)			
TAB,PO (PRIVATE LABEL)			
25 mg, 24s ea	82468-0113-16	2.96	3.29
100s ea	52735-0404-01	8.09	8.99

PROD/MFR	HRI, UPC,NDC	AWP	SRP
FAMILY PHARMACY ALLERGY RELIEF (AmerisourceBergen)			
ODT,PO (PRIVATE LABEL)			
10 mg, 10s ea	82468-0620-46	8.81	9.79
(NON-DROWSY)			
10 mg, 12s ea	82468-0621-03	8.09	8.99
SYR,PO (PRIVATE LABEL,FRUIT)			
5 mg/5 ml, 120 ml	82468-0620-47	7.46	8.29
FAMILY PHARMACY ANIMAL SHAPES W/VITAMIN C (AmerisourceBergen)			
CTB,PO (PRIVATE LABEL)			
100s ea	82468-0615-76	4.67	5.19
FAMILY PHARMACY ANUSERT (AmerisourceBergen)			
SUP,RC (PRIVATE LABEL)			
51%, 12s ea	82468-0117-79	3.95	4.39
FAMILY PHARMACY ARTHRITIS PAIN RELIEF (AmerisourceBergen)			
TER,PO (ASPIRIN-FREE)			
650 mg, 100s ea	82468-0615-59	6.74	7.49
FAMILY PHARMACY ASPIRIN (AmerisourceBergen)			
ECT,PO (PRIVATE LABEL)			
81 mg, 180s ea	82468-0621-05	3.80	7.99
FAMILY PHARMACY B100 (AmerisourceBergen)			
TAB,PO (NATURAL,B-COMPLEX)			
60s ea	82468-0615-82	8.00	8.89
FAMILY PHARMACY CALCIUM 500 (AmerisourceBergen)			
TAB,PO (PRIVATE LABEL)			
500 mg, 75s ea	82468-0615-72	5.12	4.59
160s ea	82468-0620-62	8.99	18.99
FAMILY PHARMACY CALCIUM CITRATE + D (AmerisourceBergen)			
TAB,PO (PRIVATE LABEL)			
315 mg-200 iu, 120s ea	82468-0620-61	7.82	8.69
FAMILY PHARMACY CENTURY (AmerisourceBergen)			
TAB,PO (PRIVATE LABEL)			
300s ea	82468-0615-68	12.59	13.99
FAMILY PHARMACY CENTURY ADVANTAGE (AmerisourceBergen)			
TAB,PO (PRIVATE LABEL)			
75s ea	82468-0615-69	8.72	9.69
FAMILY PHARMACY CENTURY SENIOR (AmerisourceBergen)			
PO (IRON-FREE,PRIVATE LABEL)			
100s ea	82468-0615-70	6.74	7.49
300s ea	82468-0620-68	13.94	15.49
FAMILY PHARMACY CHROMIUM PICOLINATE (AmerisourceBergen)			
TAB,PO (PRIVATE LABEL)			
200 mcg, 100s ea	82468-0118-38	4.31	4.79
FAMILY PHARMACY COENZYME Q-10 (AmerisourceBergen)			
SGL,PO (PRIVATE LABEL,SOFTGEL)			
100 mg, 30s ea	82468-0622-08	13.49	14.99
FAMILY PHARMACY COLD RELIEF (AmerisourceBergen)			
TEF,PO (PRIVATE LABEL)			
250 mg-2 mg-5 mg, 20s ea	82468-0620-15	3.50	3.89
FAMILY PHARMACY CORAL CALCIUM (AmerisourceBergen)			
TAB,PO (PRIVATE LABEL,CAPLET)			
185 mg-20 mg, 60s ea	82468-0620-09	5.39	5.99
FAMILY PHARMACY ECHINACEA (AmerisourceBergen)			
TAB,PO (PRIVATE LABEL,CAPLET)			
167 mg, 90s ea	82468-0615-86	7.10	7.89
FAMILY PHARMACY ECHINACEA GOLDENSEAL (AmerisourceBergen)			
TAB,PO (PF,GLUTEN-FREE)			
112.5 mg-25 mg, 90s ea	82468-0615-87	8.18	9.09
FAMILY PHARMACY ESTROPLUS TAB (AmerisourceBergen)			
TAB,PO (PF,DYE-FREE,GLUTEN-FREE)			
30s ea	82468-0615-97	8.09	8.99
FAMILY PHARMACY EVENING PRIMROSE OIL (AmerisourceBergen)			
SGL,PO (PRIVATE LABEL,SOFTGEL)			
500 mg, 75s ea	82468-0620-52	5.39	5.99
FAMILY PHARMACY EYE HEALTH (AmerisourceBergen)			
TAB,PO (PRIVATE LABEL)			
120s ea	82468-0620-45	10.79	11.99
FAMILY PHARMACY FIBER (AmerisourceBergen)			
CAP,PO (PRIVATE LABEL)			
0.52 gm, 160s ea	82468-0621-18	8.09	8.99
FAMILY PHARMACY FISH OIL (AmerisourceBergen)			
SGL,PO (NATURAL,CONCENTRATE)			
120 mg-180 mg, 60s ea	82468-0615-93	5.39	5.99
(NATURAL,PRIVATE LABEL)			
175 mg-260 mg-880 mg, 60s ea	82468-0620-11	6.29	6.99
(PRIVATE LABEL)			
175 mg-260 mg-880 mg, 60s ea	82468-0621-16	8.09	8.99
FAMILY PHARMACY FLAX SEED OIL (AmerisourceBergen)			
SGL,PO (NATURAL,PRIVATE LABEL)			
1000 mg, 100s ea	82468-0615-94	7.19	7.99
FAMILY PHARMACY FOLIC ACID (AmerisourceBergen)			
TAB,PO (PRIVATE LABEL)			
0.4 mg, 250s ea	82468-0129-07	3.23	3.59
FAMILY PHARMACY GARLIC (AmerisourceBergen)			
ECT,PO (PF,SF,CAFFEINE-FREE)			
400 mg, 30s ea	82468-0620-67	5.39	5.99
FAMILY PHARMACY GINKO BILOBA (AmerisourceBergen)			
TAB,PO (CAFFEINE-FREE)			
40 mg, 36s ea	82468-0620-66	4.22	4.69
(PRIVATE LABEL,CAPLET)			
120 mg, 50s ea	82468-0615-88	5.39	5.99
FAMILY PHARMACY GINSENG (AmerisourceBergen)			
SGL,PO (PRIVATE LABEL,SOFTGEL)			
100 mg, 30s ea	82468-0620-65	2.60	2.89
FAMILY PHARMACY GLUCOSAMINE & CHONDROITIN (AmerisourceBergen)			
TAB,PO (REGULAR STRENGTH)			
200 mg-250 mg, 120s ea	82468-0620-60	14.39	16.99
(DOUBLE STRENGTH)			
400 mg-500 mg, 110s ea	82468-0615-78	26.99	29.99
150s ea	82468-0620-59	29.60	32.89
FAMILY PHARMACY GLUCOSAMINE COMPLEX (AmerisourceBergen)			
TAB,PO (NATURAL,PRIVATE LABEL)			
200 mg-300 mg, 60s ea	82468-0615-80	8.09	8.99
FAMILY PHARMACY GLUCOSAMINE SULFATE (AmerisourceBergen)			
TAB,PO (PRIVATE LABEL,CAPLET)			
750 mg, 120s ea	82468-0619-05	11.69	12.99
FAMILY PHARMACY HEMORRHOIDAL SUPPOSITORIES (AmerisourceBergen)			
SUP,RC (PRIVATE LABEL)			
85.5%-0.25%-3%, 12s ea	82468-0620-13	1.62	4.79
FAMILY PHARMACY IBUPROFEN COLD CHILDRENS (AmerisourceBergen)			
SUS,PO (AF,PRIVATE LABEL,BERRY)			
100 mg/5 ml-15 mg/5 ml, 120 ml	82468-0621-08	4.13	5.09
FAMILY PHARMACY IBUPROFEN INFANTS' (AmerisourceBergen)			
SUS,PO (CONCENTRATED DROPS,AF)			
50 mg/1.25 ml, 30 ml	82468-0621-07	6.81	8.39
FAMILY PHARMACY IBUPROFEN JUNIOR (AmerisourceBergen)			
CTB,PO (PRIVATE LABEL,ORANGE)			
100 mg, 24s ea	82468-0621-06	3.23	3.59
FAMILY PHARMACY INSULIN SYRINGES (Can-Am Care)			
DEV,NA (31G,1/2CC,5/16")			
100s ea	38396-0440-77	17.50	
(31G,1CC,5/16")			
100s ea	38396-0441-77	17.50	
(31G,3/10CC,5/16")			
100s ea	38396-0439-77	17.50	
(ULTRA COMFORT, 28G,1CC)			
100s ea	38396-0432-77	15.50	
(ULTRA COMFORT,28G,1/2CC)			
100s ea	38396-0431-77	15.50	
(ULTRA COMFORT,29G,1/2CC)			
100s ea	38396-0434-77	17.50	
(ULTRA COMFORT,29G,1CC)			
100s ea	38396-0433-77	17.50	
(ULTRA COMFORT,29G)			
100s ea	38396-0435-77	17.50	
(ULTRA COMFORT,30G,1/2CC)			
100s ea	38396-0436-77	17.50	
(ULTRA COMFORT,30G,1CC)			
100s ea	38396-0437-77	17.50	
(ULTRA COMFORT,30G)			
100s ea	38396-0438-77	17.50	
FAMILY PHARMACY IRON SLOW RELEASE (AmerisourceBergen)			
TER,PO (PRIVATE LABEL)			
160 mg, 30s ea	82468-0620-44	4.36	6.99
FAMILY PHARMACY IRON TABLETS (AmerisourceBergen)			
TAB,PO (PRIVATE LABEL)			
325 mg, 100s ea	82468-0135-03	6.11	6.79
FAMILY PHARMACY LANCETS (Can-Am Care)			
DEV,NA, 100s ea	38396-0331-77	5.85	
200s ea	38396-0332-77	9.50	
FAMILY PHARMACY MAGNESIUM (AmerisourceBergen)			
TAB,PO (NATURAL,PRIVATE LABEL)			
250 mg, 100s ea	82468-0620-48	2.78	3.09
FAMILY PHARMACY MOTION SICKNESS RELIEF (AmerisourceBergen)			
TAB,PO (PRIVATE LABEL)			
25 mg, 8s ea	82468-0621-19	2.51	2.79
FAMILY PHARMACY MSM GLUCOSAMINE COMPLEX (AmerisourceBergen)			
TAB,PO (NATURAL,PRIVATE LABEL)			
60s ea	82468-0620-58	8.36	9.29
FAMILY PHARMACY NIACIN (AmerisourceBergen)			
TER,PO (NATURAL,PRIVATE LABEL)			
250 mg, 100s ea	82468-0620-56	4.76	5.29
FAMILY PHARMACY ONE DAILY DIET SUPPORT (AmerisourceBergen)			
TAB,PO (PRIVATE LABEL)			
50s ea	82468-0620-10	5.39	5.99
FAMILY PHARMACY ONE DAILY ESSENTIAL (AmerisourceBergen)			
TAB,PO (PRIVATE LABEL)			
250s ea	82468-0620-63	7.19	7.99
FAMILY PHARMACY OPTI-VITAMINS (AmerisourceBergen)			
TAB,PO (PRIVATE LABEL)			
60s ea	52735-0391-13	5.03	5.59
FAMILY PHARMACY OYSTER SHELL CALCIUM (AmerisourceBergen)			
TAB,PO (NATURAL,PRIVATE LABEL)			
500 mg, 100s ea	82468-0620-57	2.96	3.29
FAMILY PHARMACY PAIN RELIEVER (AmerisourceBergen)			
TAB,PO (EXTRA STRENGTH)			
500 mg, 24s ea	82468-0118-84	2.42	2.69
FAMILY PHARMACY POTASSIUM (AmerisourceBergen)			
TAB,PO (NATURAL,PRIVATE LABEL)			
99 mg, 100s ea	82468-0615-96	2.69	2.99
FAMILY PHARMACY PRENATAL VITAMINS (AmerisourceBergen)			
TAB,PO (PRIVATE LABEL)			
200s ea	82468-0620-64	7.82	8.69
FAMILY PHARMACY SAW PALMETTO (AmerisourceBergen)			
SGL,PO (PF,CORN-FREE,DYE-FREE)			
160 mg, 50s ea	82468-0615-91	6.47	7.19
FAMILY PHARMACY SENNA (AmerisourceBergen)			
SGL,PO (PRIVATE LABEL,SOFTGEL)			
8.6 mg, 80s ea	82468-0621-09	5.82	10.99
FAMILY PHARMACY SINUS DAY (AmerisourceBergen)			
TAB,PO (ASPIRIN-FREE)			
500 mg-30 mg, 24s ea	82468-0620-69	3.32	4.29
48s ea	82468-0620-70	5.21	6.99
FAMILY PHARMACY ST. JOHN'S WORT (AmerisourceBergen)			
TAB,PO (PF,CORN-FREE,DYE-FREE)			
300 mg, 50s ea	82468-0615-92	5.57	6.19
FAMILY PHARMACY STARCH BLOCKER (AmerisourceBergen)			
TAB,PO (STIMULANT-FREE)			
500 mg, 80s ea	82468-0620-12	13.60	18.99
FAMILY PHARMACY SUPER THIN (Can-Am Care)			
DEV,NA, 100s ea	38396-0333-77	5.85	

PROD/MFR	HRI, UPC,NDC	AWP	SRP
FAMILY PHARMACY THIN (Can-Am Care)			
DEV,NA, 100s ea	38396-0335-77	5.85	
200s ea	38396-0334-77	9.50	
FAMILY PHARMACY VITAMIN A (AmerisourceBergen)			
SGL,PO (NATURAL,USP)			
8000 iu, 100s ea	82468-0615-81	2.96	3.29
FAMILY PHARMACY VITAMIN B12 (AmerisourceBergen)			
TAB,PO (PRIVATE LABEL)			
500 mcg, 100s ea	82468-0620-54	4.13	4.59
FAMILY PHARMACY VITAMIN B6 (AmerisourceBergen)			
TAB,PO (PRIVATE LABEL)			
50 mg, 100s ea	82468-0620-55	2.69	2.99
FAMILY PHARMACY VITAMIN C (AmerisourceBergen)			
CTB,PO (PRIVATE LABEL)			
500 mg, 100s ea	82468-0615-83	4.49	4.99
TAB,PO (NATURAL,W/ROSE HIPS)			
500 mg, 100s ea	82468-0615-85	3.68	4.09
(USP,PRIVATE LABEL)			
500 mg, 500s ea	82468-0620-53	11.87	13.19
FAMILY PHARMACY VITAMIN E (AmerisourceBergen)			
SGL,PO (NATURAL BLEND)			
400 iu, 100s ea	82468-0620-51	7.19	7.99
(NATURAL,PRIVATE LABEL)			
1000 iu, 50s ea	82468-0620-49	14.39	15.99
(PRIVATE LABEL,SOFTGEL)			
1000 iu, 100s ea	82468-0620-50	12.59	13.99
FAMOTIDINE (Teva)			
TAB,PO, 10 mg, 18s ea	00182-2662-14	3.59	
30s ea	00182-2662-17	4.69	
(USP)			
10 mg, 50s ea	00172-2662-48	7.49	
70s ea	00182-2662-22	9.49	
(DHS, Inc.)			
REPACK			
TAB,PO, 10 mg, 30s ea	55887-0968-30	9.95	
(Quality Care Prod)			
REPACK			
TAB,PO, 10 mg, 30s ea	49999-0546-30	9.38	
FANTASY (Line One Labs)			
DEV,NA (LUBRICATED W/SPERMICIDE)			
3s ea	05632-0868-10	1.20	
3s ea	05632-0868-30	1.20	
(LUBRICATED)			
3s ea	05632-0868-00	1.20	
3s ea	05632-0868-20	1.20	
(LUBRICATED W/SPERMICIDE)			
12s ea	05632-0868-15	4.50	
12s ea	05632-0868-35	4.75	
(LUBRICATED)			
12s ea	05632-0868-05	4.50	
12s ea	05632-0868-25	4.75	
FAST TAKE (Lifescan)			
DEV,NA (STRIP,2X25)			
50s ea	53885-0444-50	55.80	
(STRIP,4X25)			
100s ea	53885-0048-10	111.60	
FAT BURNERS (ADH)			
TAB,PO, 100s ea	60142-0102-10	9.48	18.95
FATHER JOHN'S MEDICINE (Oakhurst)			
SYR,PO, 10 mg/5 ml,			
120 ml	11169-0049-04	3.86	4.63
240 ml	11169-0049-08	5.15	7.73
FATHER JOHN'S MEDICINE PLUS (Oakhurst)			
LIQ,PO (AF,DROPS)			
120 ml	11169-0050-40	4.03	6.05
FAULTLESS (Abbott Ashland)			
HOT/COLD GELPACK			
DEV,NA, ea	00744-0321-01	3.13	
(W/COMPRESSION WRAP)			
ea	00744-3260-10	5.94	
ICE BAG			
DEV,NA (LARGE)			
ea	00074-2753-00	6.65	
(MEDIUM)			
ea	00074-2752-00	5.50	
(SMALL)			
ea	00074-2751-00	4.59	
INFANT EAR SYRINGE			
DEV,NA (1 OZ)			
ea	00074-2838-00	2.01	
(2 OZ)			
ea	00074-2839-00	2.30	
INFANT NASAL ASPIRATOR			
DEV,NA, ea	00074-2841-00	2.28	
INSTANT COLD PACK			
DEV,NA, ea	00074-2774-00	1.40	
INSTANT COLD PACK PLUS			
NA, ea	00074-1226-40	2.01	
INSTANT HOT PACK PLUS			
NA, ea	00074-1226-50	2.40	
SONATA REUSABLE DOUCHE			
DEV,NA (CONTROLLED-FLOW)			
ea	00074-2756-00	5.88	
TENDERCOOL PADS			
DEV,NA, ea	00074-1226-30	12.07	
TINYKIT REUSABLE DOUCHE			
DEV,NA, ea	00074-2700-00	4.48	
FE C TAB (Boca Pharmacal)			
TAB,PO, 250 mg-100 mg,			
100s ea	64376-0803-01	20.17	
FE PLUS PROTEIN (Miller)			
TAB,PO, 25 mg, 120s ea	17204-0431-55	5.04	
FE-20 (Bio-Tech Pharm)			
CAP,PO, 20 mg, 100s ea	53191-0326-01	4.20	
FEARN LECITHIN (Modern Prod)			
LIQ,PO, 473 ml	41178-0380-30	3.60	5.99
(MINT)			
473 ml	41178-0393-30	3.60	5.99
946 ml	41178-0382-40	6.75	10.99
(MINT)			
946 ml	41178-0394-40	6.75	10.99
FEARN SOYA PROTEIN ISOLATE (Modern Prod)			
PDR,PO, 283.5 gm	41178-0744-30	5.40	8.99
454 gm	41178-0744-35	7.80	12.99
FEM-CAL (Freeda)			
TAB,PO, 100s ea	10432-0292-01	5.55	9.25
250s ea	10432-0292-02	11.10	18.50
FEM-CAL CITRATE (Freeda)			
TAB,PO (DF,PF,SF)			
100s ea	10432-0342-01	6.30	10.50
250s ea	10432-0342-02	12.57	20.95
FEM-CAL PLUS (Freeda)			
TAB,PO (SF,DYE-FREE)			
100s ea	10432-0341-01	6.18	10.30
250s ea	10432-0341-02	12.36	20.60
FEM-PRIN (Hart Health)			
TAB,PO (50X2,SF)			
325 mg-25 mg-1 mg,			
100s ea UD	50332-0131-04	3.49	
(125X2,SF)			
325 mg-25 mg-1 mg,			
250s ea UD	50332-0131-07	8.07	
FEMATROL (Major)			
ECT,PO, 5 mg, 30s ea	00904-5312-46	2.40	
FEMCAPS (Medique)			
TAB,PO (2X150)			
325 mg-25 mg,			
300s ea UD	47682-0155-78	41.56	
FEMILAX (G&W)			
ECT,PO, 5 mg, 30s ea	00713-0422-30	1.85	
60s ea	00713-0422-60	3.32	
FEMINEASE (Parnell)			
CRE,VG, 60 gm	50930-0060-02	10.50	15.95
FEMININE SUPPORT FOR SKIN/HAIR/NAIL (Nature's Bounty)			
TAB,PO (PF,SF)			
60s ea	74312-0075-80		5.69
FEMINTROL (Global Source)			
TAB,PO, 100 mg-65 mg,			
30s ea	59618-0341-07	2.15	
60s ea	59618-0341-12	3.65	
FEMIRON (Lee Pharm)			
TAB,PO, 20 mg, 40s ea	23558-0530-50	9.00	
120s ea	23558-0530-51	13.44	
(40X12)			
20 mg, 480s ea	23558-0530-55	108.00	
(120X12)			
20 mg, 1440s ea	23558-0530-56	161.28	
FEMIRON MULTIVITAMINS W/IRON (Lee Pharm)			
TAB,PO, 35s ea	23558-0530-52	9.00	
60s ea	23558-0530-53	11.52	
90s ea	23558-0530-54	14.40	
(35X12)			
420s ea	23558-0530-57	108.00	
(60X12)			
720s ea	23558-0530-58	138.24	
(90X12)			
1080s ea	23558-0530-59	172.80	
FEMPAIN (S.S.S.)			
TAB,PO, 30s ea	12258-0117-12	2.17	3.25
FEMYSTIQUE (Majestic Drug)			
GEL,TP, 25 gm	10705-0800-87	2.25	5.99
FENUGREEK (Nature's Bounty)			
CAP,PO (PF)			
610 mg, 100s ea	74312-0060-20	7.99	9.99
FEOSOL (Glaxo)			
TAB,PO (CAPLET)			
45 mg, 40s ea	49692-0941-30	7.67	
75s ea	49692-0941-75	11.69	
65 mg, 125s ea	49692-0942-25	7.67	
(Stat Rx)			
REPACK			
TAB,PO (CAPLET)			
45 mg, 90s ea	16590-0831-90	22.02	
FER US PIC 150 (McNeil,R.A.)			
CAP,PO, 150 mg, 100s ea	12830-0811-01	17.64	
FER-GEN-SOL (Teva)			
LIQ,PO (DROPS)			
75 mg/0.6 ml,			
50 ml	00182-1381-67	4.59	
FER-IRON (Rugby)			
LIQ,PO (LEMON,DROPS)			
75 mg/0.6 ml, 50 ml	00536-0710-80	5.24	
FERATAB (Upsher-Smith)			
TAB,PO, 300 mg, ea	00245-0053-89	0.05	
FERATE (Major)			
TAB,PO (BOXED)			
27 mg, 100s ea	00904-5477-60	3.79	
FERGON (Bayer HealthCare)			
TAB,PO, 240 mg, 100s ea	00024-1015-10	5.54	
FEROSUL (Major)			
TAB,PO (GREEN, BLISTER PACK)			
325 mg, 100s ea	00904-7591-82	10.99	
(PF,SF)			
325 mg, 100s ea	00904-7591-60	2.45	
FERRETTS (Pharmics)			
TAB,PO, 325 mg,			
60s ea UD	00813-0012-06	8.53	13.95
FERRETTS IPS (Pharmics)			
SOL,PO (STRAWBERRY)			
40 mg/15 ml,			
237 ml	00813-2004-08	12.09	21.95
FERREX 150 (Breckenridge Pharm)			
CAP,PO (10X10,BLISTER PACK)			
150 mg, 100s ea UD	51991-0203-11	27.50	
(Major)			
CAP,PO (10X10)			
150 mg, 100s ea UD	00904-5395-61	25.00	
FERREX 150 PLUS (Breckenridge Pharm)			
CAP,PO, 50 mg-150 mg-50 mg,			
90s ea	51991-0703-90	114.35	
FERRIMIN 150 (Hillestad)			
TAB,PO, 150 mg, 120s ea	10542-0080-12	15.55	
FERRO-SEQUELS (Phys Total Care)			
REPACK			
TER,PO, 100 mg-150 mg,			
30s ea	54868-4075-00	8.72	
100s ea	54868-4075-01	22.01	
FERRO-TIME (Time-Cap)			
TAB,PO (FILM-COATED)			
325 mg, 100s ea	49483-0063-01	2.67	
100s ea	49483-0064-01	2.67	
1000s ea	49483-0063-10	11.07	
1000s ea	49483-0064-10	11.07	
FERROCITE (Breckenridge Pharm)			
TAB,PO (FILM-COATED)			
324 mg, 100s ea	51991-0181-42	22.25	
FERROMIN (Key Company)			
TAB,PO, 25 mg, 100s ea	11694-0140-22	5.75	
FERROTATE JUNIOR (Key Company)			
CAP,PO, 100s ea	11694-0825-01	8.50	
250s ea	11694-0825-02	17.00	
FERROTRIN (Bio-Tech Pharm)			
CAP,PO, 100s ea	53191-0327-01	6.30	
FERROUS FUMARATE (Consolidated Midland)			
TAB,PO, 300 mg, 100s ea	00223-0950-01	3.00	
1000s ea	00223-0950-02	27.00	
325 mg, 100s ea	00223-0949-01	3.25	
1000s ea	00223-0949-02	27.50	

PROD/MFR	HRI, UPC,NDC	AWP	SRP
(Freeda)			
TAB,PO (SF)			
29 mg, 100s ea	10432-0316-01	3.51	5.85
250s ea	10432-0316-02	7.02	11.70
(Phys Total Care)			
REPACK			
TAB,PO, 325 mg, 60s ea	54868-5514-00	29.49	
FERROUS FUMARATE DS (Vita-Rx)			
CER,PO, 100 mg-150 mg,			
100s ea	49727-0192-02	3.60	
FERROUS GLUCONATE (Consolidated Midland)			
ECT,PO, 325 mg, 100s ea	00223-0951-01	3.50	
1000s ea	00223-0951-02	27.50	
(Major)			
TAB,PO, 325 mg,			
100s ea UD	00904-2137-61	7.21	
(Mason Vit)			
TAB,PO (PF,SF)			
240 mg, 100s ea	11845-0137-51	5.00	
(Paddock)			
TAB,PO, 324 mg, 100s ea	00574-0508-01	5.15	
100s ea UD	00574-0508-11	9.45	
1000s ea	00574-0508-10	46.55	
(Vita-Rx)			
TAB,PO, 300 mg,			
1000s ea	49727-0188-05	12.25	
(Dispensing Solutions)			
REPACK			
TAB,PO, 325 mg, 100s ea	55045-3285-01	8.00	
FERROUS SULFATE (ADH)			
TAB,PO, 324 mg, 100s ea	60142-0001-10	0.85	
(Advance)			
TAB,PO, 325 mg, 100s ea	17714-0024-01	3.99	
1000s ea	17714-0024-10	8.25	
(Albertson's)			
TAB,PO, 325 mg, 100s ea	04000-0002-16	2.55	
(Cardinal Health)			
TAB,PO (PRIVATE LABEL)			
27 mg, 100s ea	37205-0414-78	2.32	
(Consolidated Midland)			
TAB,PO, 325 mg, 100s ea	00223-0960-01	1.95	
1000s ea	00223-0960-02	17.50	
(Geri-Care)			
TAB,PO, 325 mg, 100s ea	57896-0702-01	0.70	
1000s ea	57896-0702-10	3.50	
(Hi-Tech)			
ELI,PO, 220 mg/5 ml,			
480 ml	50383-0778-16	6.85	
(Major)			
ELI,PO, 220 mg/5 ml,			
480 ml	00904-1465-16	5.95	
SOL,PO (1X50ML,PEPPERMINT,DROPS)			
15 mg/ml, 50 ml	00904-6060-50	7.50	
TAB,PO, 325 mg, 100s ea	00904-7590-60	2.45	
(10X10, GREEN)			
325 mg, 100s ea UD	00904-7591-61	8.71	
(F.C., RED, BLISTER PACK)			
325 mg, 100s ea	00904-7590-82	10.99	
1000s ea	00904-7590-80	15.95	
(GREEN)			
325 mg, 1000s ea	00904-7591-80	15.95	
(Marlex)			
TAB,PO (BLISTER PACK,RED)			
324 mg, 100s ea UD	10135-0242-13	1.32	
(BLISTER PACK,S.C.,RED)			
324 mg, 100s ea UD	10135-0161-13	1.99	
(RED)			
324 mg, 1000s ea UD	10135-0242-19	6.05	
(BLISTER PACK,GREEN)			
325 mg, 100s ea UD	10135-0243-13	1.20	
(GREEN, BLISTER PACK)			
325 mg, 1000s ea UD	10135-0243-19	6.05	
(Mason Vit)			
TAB,PO (PF,SF,FRAGRANCE-FREE)			
325 mg, 100s ea	11845-0127-31	5.00	
(Nature's Bounty)			
TAB,PO (PF,SF)			
324 mg, 100s ea	74312-0017-90		4.25
(Nnodum)			
TAB,PO (FILM-COATED, RED)			
325 mg, 100s ea UD	63044-0165-66	2.90	
1000s ea UD	63044-0165-67	19.99	
(Paddock)			
ECT,PO, 324 mg, 100s ea	00574-0608-01	5.15	
100s ea UD	00574-0608-11	9.45	
1000s ea	00574-0608-10	46.55	
(Pharm Assoc Inc)			
LIQ,PO, 300 mg/5 ml,			
5 ml 100s UD	00121-0530-05	49.33	
(Propharma)			
LIQ,PO (DROPS)			
15 mg/0.6 ml, 50 ml	50313-0007-43	4.75	
(Qualitest)			
ELI,PO, 220 mg/5 ml,			
480 ml	00603-0763-58	7.19	
LIQ,PO (DROPS)			
75 mg/0.6 ml, 50 ml	00603-0762-47	4.71	
TAB,PO (4X25)			
325 mg, 100s ea UD	00603-0179-29	16.80	
1000s ea	00603-0179-32	194.23	
(Rugby)			
ELI,PO, 220 mg/5 ml,			
480 ml	00536-0650-85	5.93	
TAB,PO, 325 mg, 100s ea	00536-5890-01	4.04	
TER,PO (BLISTER PACK,PF,SF)			
160 mg, 30s ea	00536-3478-07	5.81	
60s ea	00536-3478-08	9.90	
(Silarx)			
ELI,PO, 220 mg/5 ml,			
473 ml	54838-0001-80	6.90	
LIQ,PO (DROPS)			
75 mg/0.6 ml, 50 ml	54838-0002-50	5.75	
(Teva)			
ELI,PO, 220 mg/5 ml,			
480 ml	00182-1201-40	7.19	
TAB,PO (GREEN,FILM-COATED)			
325 mg, 100s ea	00182-4028-01	3.39	
(RED,FILM-COATED)			
325 mg, 100s ea	00182-4029-01	3.39	
(Time-Cap)			
TAB,PO, 324 mg, 100s ea	49483-0008-04	3.45	
1000s ea	49483-0027-40	19.95	
(United Research)			
TAB,PO (GREEN,FILM-COATED)			
325 mg, 100s ea	00677-0070-01	2.80	
(RED,FILM-COATED)			
325 mg, 100s ea	00677-0071-01	2.80	
(GREEN,FILM-COATED)			
325 mg, 1000s ea	00677-0070-10	19.43	
(RED,FILM-COATED)			
325 mg, 1000s ea	00677-0071-10	19.43	
(Upsher-Smith)			
ECT,PO, 325 mg, ea	00245-0108-89	0.28	
100s ea	00245-0108-11	14.67	
(10X10)			
325 mg, 100s ea UD	00245-0108-01	27.60	
1000s ea	00245-0108-10	131.79	
(Vita-Rx)			
CER,PO, 159 mg, 100s ea	49727-0186-02	2.36	
1000s ea	49727-0186-05	17.36	
ECT,PO, 200 mg,			
1000s ea	49727-0184-05	7.86	
TAB,PO, 200 mg,			
1000s ea	49727-0183-05	5.64	
1000s ea	49727-0185-05	5.64	
(A-S Medication)			
REPACK			
ELI,PO, 220 mg/5 ml,			
480 ml	54569-3528-00	6.77	
LIQ,PO, 75 mg/0.6 ml,			
50 ml	54569-2393-00	5.57	
TAB,PO, 325 mg, 100s ea	54569-4537-00	4.15	
(Altura)			
REPACK			
TAB,PO (FILM-COATED)			
325 mg, 100s ea	63874-0008-01	5.51	
300s ea	63874-0008-30	13.41	
(Bryant Ranch)			
REPACK			
ELI,PO, 220 mg/5 ml,			
120 ml	63629-1808-01	1.77	
240 ml	63629-1808-02	3.54	
480 ml	63629-1808-03	7.07	
(DHS, Inc.)			
REPACK			
TAB,PO (FILM-COATED)			
325 mg, 100s ea	55887-0417-01	8.08	
(Dispensing Solutions)			
REPACK			
TAB,PO, 325 mg, 100s ea	55045-3939-01	5.50	
(FILM-COATED)			
325 mg, 100s ea UD	55045-1246-00	5.50	
(Palmetto)			
REPACK			
ELI,PO (1X480ML)			
220 mg/5 ml,			
480 ml	23490-6665-01	12.48	
LIQ,PO, 75 mg/0.6 ml,			
50 ml	23490-6669-01	6.40	
TAB,PO, 325 mg, 100s ea	23490-6668-01	8.00	
(PD-Rx Pharm)			
REPACK			
TAB,PO, 325 mg, 60s ea	55289-0013-60	7.78	
(FILM-COATED)			
325 mg, 90s ea	55289-0013-90	10.90	
(REDI-SCRIPT)			
325 mg, 100s ea	58864-0836-01	2.80	
(Pharma Pac)			
REPACK			
ECT,PO, 325 mg, 100s ea	52959-0976-00	9.75	
ELI,PO, 220 mg/5 ml,			
240 ml	52959-0862-08	3.60	
LIQ,PO (DROPS)			
75 mg/0.6 ml,			
50 ml	52959-0139-50	5.25	
(Phys Total Care)			
REPACK			
TAB,PO (FILM-COATED)			
325 mg, 25s ea	54868-0189-00	5.64	
(GREEN)			
325 mg, 100s ea	54868-0189-01	13.53	
(RED)			
325 mg, 100s ea	54868-3498-00	7.96	
(Physician Partner)			
REPACK			
TAB,PO, 325 mg, 30s ea	21695-0152-30	5.42	
90s ea	21695-0152-90	16.27	
100s ea	21695-0152-00	18.08	
(Quality Care Prod)			
REPACK			
TAB,PO, 325 mg, 100s ea	49999-0197-00	8.28	
(Southwood)			
REPACK			
ELI,PO, 220 mg/5 ml,			
120 ml	58016-4171-01	2.40	
480 ml	58016-4856-01	6.90	
LIQ,PO (DROPS)			
25 mg/ml, 50 ml	58016-9004-01	6.96	
FERROUSAL (Prime Marketing)			
TAB,PO (PF)			
325 mg, 100s ea	62107-0044-01	5.75	
FERRULE (Abbott Hosp)			
DEV,NA (12MM, FITS LIFECARE)			
ea	00074-7909-03	99.35	
(8MM,FITS NUTRIMIX MACRO)			
200s ea	00074-7909-02	51.07	
(5MM,FITS EMPTY LIFECARE)			
500s ea	00074-7909-01	42.00	
FERRUM PHOSPHORICUM (Hyland's)			
TAB,PO, 500s ea	54973-1020-01	5.87	9.79
1000s ea	54973-1020-02	10.49	17.49
(Nuage Labs)			
TAB,SL (6X)			
125s ea	00634-3431-68	3.05	5.09
(Walker Pharmacal)			
TAB,SL (6X)			
250s ea	00619-3431-02	2.97	
(Weleda)			
TAB,PO (6X)			
100s ea	55946-0250-30	6.60	
FEVER REDUCER (Perrigo)			
SUP,RC, 650 mg, 12s ea	45802-0730-30	7.99	
50s ea	45802-0730-32	29.70	
100s ea	45802-0730-33	42.99	
FEVERALL (Actavis Mid Atlantic)			
SUP,RC, 80 mg, 6s ea	00472-1200-06	4.81	
50s ea	00472-1200-50	37.06	
120 mg, 6s ea	00472-1201-06	4.81	
(CHILDREN'S)			
120 mg, 50s ea	00472-1201-50	26.61	
325 mg, 6s ea	00472-1202-06	4.81	
(UNISERTS)			
650 mg, 50s ea	00472-1203-50	33.08	
500s ea	00472-1203-05	216.29	
FEVERFEW (Botanical Labs.)			
CAP,PO, 100s ea	41954-0030-07	4.98	9.95
LIQ,PO, 30 ml	41954-0020-17	4.50	8.99

PROD/MFR	HRI, UPC,NDC	AWP	SRP
(Mason Vit)			
CAP,PO (PF,SF)			
500 mg, 60s ea	**11845-0113-85**	5.89	
SGL,PO, 100 mg, 60s ea	**11845-0129-75**	6.56	
(Nature's Bounty)			
CAP,PO, 100s ea	**74312-0052-11**		7.39
(Rexall)			
CAP,PO (PF,SF)			
400 mg, 75s ea	**30768-0012-00**	3.63	5.50
FEVERSCAN FOREHEAD (Hallcrest Products)			
DEV,NA, 12s ea	**74024-0004-45**	12.60	
FEVERSCAN MONITOR FOREHEAD (Hallcrest Products)			
DEV,NA (3 DISPOSABLE UNITS/PKG)			
12s ea	**75522-0000-35**	12.20	
FIBER (Cardinal Health)			
PDR,PO (SF,PRIVATE LABEL)			
3.4 gm/dose, 283 gm	**37205-0366-38**	6.40	
(ORIGINAL,PRIVATE LABEL)			
3.4 gm/dose, 369 gm	**37205-0303-27**	4.96	
(PRIVATE LABEL)			
3.4 gm/dose, 369 gm	**37205-0347-27**	4.89	
(REGULAR ORIGINAL)			
3.4 gm/dose, 369 gm	**37205-0301-27**	4.89	
(Major)			
TAB,PO, 625 mg, 90s ea	**00904-2500-91**	10.50	
FIBER CHOICE (Glaxo)			
CTB,PO (REGULAR,ORANGE)			
10s ea	**57145-0005-30**	1.80	2.49
90s ea	**57145-0005-36**	10.27	11.49
(SF,ASSORTED FRUIT)			
90s ea	**57145-0005-63**	10.27	11.99
(SF,ORANGE)			
90s ea	**57145-0005-38**	10.27	11.49
FIBER CHOICE PLUS CALCIUM (Glaxo)			
CTB,PO (SF,CHERRY,STRAWBERRY)			
90s ea	**57145-0005-69**	12.18	
FIBER CHOICE WEIGHT MANAGEMENT (Glaxo)			
CTB,PO (SF,STRAWBERRY)			
90s ea	**57145-0005-74**	12.18	
FIBER EASE (Plainview LLC)			
LIQ,PO (APPLE,RASPBERRY)			
420 ml	**44733-0003-16**	3.76	5.49
(ORANGE)			
420 ml	**44733-0001-16**	3.76	5.49
(SF,APPLE,RASPBERRY)			
420 ml	**44733-0004-16**	3.76	5.49
(SF,ORANGE)			
420 ml	**44733-0002-16**	3.76	5.49
FIBER HEALTH (Health Products Corp)			
TAB,PO, 105s ea	**39686-0013-04**	5.00	
FIBER LAXATIVE (Basic Vitamins)			
CTB,PO, 500 mg, 90s ea	**00761-0132-18**	4.20	
(Cardinal Health)			
TAB,PO (PRIVATE LABEL)			
625 mg, 90s ea	**37205-0213-75**	9.08	
FIBER OFF (Mason Vit)			
TAB,PO (PF,SF)			
8.88%-200 mg, 90s ea	**11845-0090-89**	3.89	
FIBER TABLETS (AmerisourceBergen)			
TAB,PO (PRIVATE LABEL)			
625 mg, 90s ea	**24385-0125-76**	7.64	8.49
FIBER THERAPY (Major)			
CAP,PO, 0.52 gm,			
160s ea	**00904-5716-91**	6.79	
PDR,PO (SF,ORANGE)			
3.4 gm/dose,			
283 gm	**00904-5788-77**	5.34	
TAB,PO (CAPLET)			
500 mg, 100s ea	**00904-5674-60**	7.00	
FIBER-LAX (Rugby)			
TAB,PO (CAPTAB)			
625 mg, 60s ea	**00536-4306-08**	6.59	
90s ea	**00536-4306-11**	11.24	
500s ea	**00536-4306-05**	44.62	
FIBER-STAT (Medical Nutrition USA)			
LIQ,PO (30MLX96,GLUTEN-FREE)			
30 ml 96s	**26974-0410-71**	105.55	
SOL,NA (887MLX6,GLUTEN-FREE)			
887 ml 6s	**26974-0410-70**	110.04	
FIBER-SURE (P & G Company)			
POW,PO (1X330.6GM,SF)			
330.6 gm	**37000-0077-45**	10.57	
FIBERALL (Heritage/Insight)			
PDR,PO (ORANGE)			
3.4 gm/dose,			
300 gm	**63736-0270-69**	6.76	
300 gm	**63736-0290-69**	6.76	
FIBERCON (Wyeth Consumer)			
TAB,PO (BLISTER PACK)			
625 mg, 36s ea	**00005-2500-02**		6.22
90s ea	**00005-2500-33**		11.62
(CAPLET)			
625 mg, 140s ea	**00005-2500-23**		14.99
FIBERLAX (Chain Drug Marketing)			
TAB,PO (CAPLET)			
625 mg, 90s ea	**63868-0530-90**	3.96	9.99
(PD-Rx Pharm)			
REPACK			
CTB,PO, 500 mg, 30s ea	**55289-0949-30**	6.75	
FIBERSOURCE (Nestle)			
LIQ,PO (TUBE FEEDING)			
250 ml 24s	**00212-1835-51**	29.38	
(CLOSED SYSTEM TUBE FDG)			
1000 ml 6s	**00212-1831-42**	36.58	
1500 ml 6s	**00212-1831-44**	54.86	
FIBERSOURCE HN (Nestle)			
LIQ,PO (TUBE FEEDING)			
250 ml 24s	**00212-1855-51**	30.24	
(CLOSED SYSTEM TUBE FDG)			
1000 ml 6s	**00212-1852-42**	37.51	
1500 ml 6s	**00212-1852-44**	56.23	
SUS,PO (6X1000ML)			
1000 ml 6s	**43900-0185-88**	37.51	
(6X1500ML)			
1500 ml 6s	**43900-0185-82**	56.23	
FIBERSOURCE HN WITH NUTRISHIELD (Nestle)			
SOL,PO (LACTOSE-FREE)			
250 ml	**43900-0185-56**	1.26	
250 ml 24s	**00212-1855-11**	30.24	
FIBERTAB (Qualitest)			
TAB,PO, 625 mg, 90s ea	**00603-0181-02**	11.41	
FIBRACOL COLLAGEN W/ALGINATE (J&J Medical)			
DEV,NA (4"X8 3/4")			
6s ea	**56091-0024-95**	72.31	
(PACKING)			
6s ea	**56091-0024-96**	56.24	
(2"X2")			
12s ea	**56091-0024-81**	36.33	
(4"X4 3/8")			
12s ea	**56091-0024-94**	96.41	
FIBRACOL PLUS COLLAGEN W/ALGINATE (J&J Medical)			
DEV,NA (4"X8 3/4")			
6s ea	**56091-0029-83**	72.31	
(PACKING ROPE)			
6s ea	**56091-0029-84**	56.24	
(2"X2")			
12s ea	**56091-0029-81**	36.33	
(4"X4 3/8")			
12s ea	**56091-0029-82**	96.41	
FIBRO MALIC (Trask)			
TAB,PO, 50 mg-200 mg,			
90s ea	**61339-0988-90**	11.97	19.95
180s ea	**61339-0967-18**	17.95	
FIBRO-TABS (Key Company)			
TAB,PO, 200s ea	**11694-0746-02**	4.00	
FIBRO-XL (Key Company)			
CAP,PO (SF)			
210s ea	**11694-0740-21**	8.75	
FILTRODOR POUCH FILTERS (Coloplast)			
DEV,NA, 50s ea	**11701-0823-10**	30.00	31.50
FINE TIP TRANSFER PIPETS (Lifescan)			
DEV,NA, 500s ea	**53885-0316-50**	15.63	
FING-R-FLEX (Nortech)			
DEV,NA (HAND/FINGER EXERCISER)			
ea	**10824-0003-13**	5.00	
FINGER (Family Phcy)			
CRE,TP (PRIVATE LABEL)			
113.4 gm	**52735-0353-41**	6.29	8.29
FINGERSTIX LANCETS (Bayer Diabetes Care)			
DEV,NA, 200s ea	**00193-5965-31**	37.14	
FIRM THIGHS (Health Products Corp)			
LOT,TP, 236 ml	**39686-0013-48**	12.00	
FIRST AID & BURN CREAM (Hart Health)			
CRE,TP, 0.13%-0.5%,			
0.9 gm 144s UD	**50332-0035-04**	10.09	
FIRST AID ALL PURPOSE CLEAR TAPE (Johnson & Johnson)			
DEV,NA (1"X10YDS)			
ea	**81370-0048-15**	2.17	
FIRST AID CLOTH TAPE (Johnson & Johnson)			
DEV,NA (1" X 10YDS,LATEX-FREE)			
ea	**81370-0048-71**	2.17	
(1/2"X5YDS,LATEX-FREE)			
ea	**81370-0048-31**	1.46	
(2" X 10YDS,LATEX-FREE)			
ea	**81370-0048-72**	3.62	
FIRST AID COLD PACK (Apothecary)			
DEV,NA, ea	**25715-0696-10**	1.97	2.59
FIRST AID COTTON BALLS (Johnson & Johnson)			
DEV,NA, 130s ea	**81370-0061-05**	2.24	
FIRST AID FINGER GUARD (Apothecary)			
DEV,NA (PLASTIC)			
ea	**25715-0696-03**	1.45	2.49
FIRST AID GAUZE PADS (Johnson & Johnson)			
DEV,NA (2"X2",SMALL)			
10s ea	**81370-0085-20**	1.21	
(3"X3",MEDIUM)			
10s ea	**81370-0085-22**	1.63	
(4"X4",LARGE)			
10s ea	**81370-0085-24**	2.66	
(2"X2",SMALL)			
25s ea	**81370-0085-21**	2.66	
(3"X3",MEDIUM)			
25s ea	**81370-0085-23**	3.92	
(4"X4",LARGE)			
25s ea	**81370-0085-25**	5.75	
FIRST AID HURT-FREE TAPE (Johnson & Johnson)			
DEV,NA (2"X2.3YDS,LATEX-FREE)			
ea	**81370-0049-02**	3.62	
FIRST AID HURT-FREE WRAP (Johnson & Johnson)			
DEV,NA (1"X2.3YDS,LATEX-FREE)			
ea	**81370-0049-00**	2.47	
FIRST AID PAPER TAPE (Johnson & Johnson)			
DEV,NA (1"X10YDS,LATEX-FREE)			
ea	**81370-0048-81**	2.17	
(1"X5YDS,LATEX-FREE)			
ea	**81370-0048-11**	2.47	
FIRST AID PLUS (Medicine Shoppe)			
OIN,TP, 30 gm	**49614-0416-10**	5.99	5.99
FIRST AID ROLLED GAUZE (Johnson & Johnson)			
DEV,NA (2"X90",2.5YDS)			
ea	**81370-0088-07**	1.63	
(3"X90",2.5YDS)			
ea	**81370-0088-08**	2.06	
(4"X90",2.5YDS)			
ea	**81370-0088-09**	2.66	
FIRST AID SECURE-COMFORT TAPE (Johnson & Johnson)			
DEV,NA (1"X5YDS,LATEX-FREE)			
ea	**81370-0051-62**	2.47	
FIRST AID SECURE-FLEX WRAP (Johnson & Johnson)			
DEV,NA (2"X2.5YDS)			
ea	**81370-0049-47**	3.62	
(3"X2.5YDS)			
ea	**81370-0049-46**	4.84	
FIRST AID SLIVER EXTRACTOR (Apothecary)			
DEV,NA (W/MAGNIFIER)			
ea	**25715-0696-08**	2.07	3.49
FIRST AID SPRAY (Hart Health)			
SPR,TP (PUMP)			
0.13%-2.5%, 60 ml	**50332-0211-01**	2.27	
FIRST AID TO GO (Johnson & Johnson)			
DEV,NA, ea	**81370-0082-95**	0.91	
FIRST AID TRIPLE LAYER NON-STICK PADS (Johnson & Johnson)			
DEV,NA (2"X3",MEDIUM)			
10s ea	**81370-0047-24**	1.63	
(3"X4",LARGE)			
10s ea	**81370-0047-28**	2.66	
FIRST AID WATERPROOF PAD (Johnson & Johnson)			
DEV,NA (2 7/8"X4",LARGE)			
6s ea	**81370-0049-84**	2.66	
FIRST AID WATERPROOF TAPE (Johnson & Johnson)			
DEV,NA (1"X10YDS)			
ea	**81370-0050-51**	3.62	
(1/2"X10YDS)			
ea	**81370-0050-50**	2.17	
(1/2"X5YDS)			
ea	**81370-0050-40**	1.46	

PROD/MFR	HRI, UPC,NDC	AWP	SRP
FIRST CHOICE COLORED LANCETS (Can-Am Care)			
DEV,NA, 100s ea	38396-0305-13	5.85	
FIRST CHOICE SUPER THIN LANCETS (Owen Mumford)			
DEV,NA (30G)			
100s ea	08517-0657-22	5.50	
FIRST CHOICE THIN LANCETS (Can-Am Care)			
DEV,NA, 100s ea	38396-0301-13	5.85	
200s ea	38396-0302-13	9.50	
(Owen Mumford)			
DEV,NA (23G)			
100s ea	08517-0157-22	4.60	
FIRST CHOICE ULTRA THIN LANCETS (Owen Mumford)			
DEV,NA (28G)			
100s ea	08517-0357-22	4.60	
200s ea	08517-0307-22	8.21	
FIRST CHOICE ULTRACOMFORT INSULIN SYRINGE (UltiMed)			
DEV,NA (1/2ML,29GX1/2")			
100s ea	08474-0108-78	18.95	
(1/2ML,30GX1/2")			
100s ea	08474-0110-78	20.95	
(1/2ML,31GX5/16")			
100s ea	08474-0112-78	21.95	
(1ML,29GX1/2")			
100s ea	08474-0109-78	18.95	
(1ML,30GX1/2")			
100s ea	08474-0111-78	20.95	
(1ML,31GX5/16")			
100s ea	08474-0113-78	21.95	
FIRST CHOICE ULTRACOMFORT MINI PEN (UltiMed)			
DEV,NA (6MM,31GX1/4")			
100s ea	08474-0100-78	28.75	
FIRST CHOICE ULTRACOMFORT SHORT PEN (UltiMed)			
NA (8MM,31GX5/16")			
100s ea	08474-0101-78	27.01	
FIRST CHOICE ULTRACOMFORT ULTIGUARD AND INSULIN (UltiMed)			
DEV,NA (1/2ML,29GX1/2")			
100s ea	08474-0102-78	23.75	
(1/2ML,30GX1/2")			
100s ea	08474-0104-78	25.70	
(1/2ML,31GX5/16")			
100s ea	08474-0106-78	26.35	
(1ML,29GX1/2")			
100s ea	08474-0103-78	23.75	
(1ML,30GX1/2")			
100s ea	08474-0105-78	25.70	
(1ML,31GX5/16")			
100s ea	08474-0107-78	26.35	
FISH OIL (21st Century)			
SGL,PO (ENTERIC COATED SOFTGEL)			
1000 mg, 90s ea	40985-0227-31		7.99
(SOFTGEL)			
1000 mg, 120s ea	40985-0228-72		8.49
300s ea	40985-0229-21	9.60	15.99
(Major)			
CAP,PO, 500 mg, 130s ea	00904-5604-13	5.50	
SGL,PO, 1000 mg,			
100s ea	00904-4043-60	7.05	
(Nature's Bounty)			
CAP,PO (SOFTGEL)			
120 mg-180 mg-5 iu,			
50s ea	74312-0038-30		5.99
100s ea	74312-0038-32		9.89
(Rexall)			
SGL,PO (SOFTGEL)			
1000 mg, 60s ea	30768-0036-60	4.32	6.55
(A-S Medication)			
REPACK			
SGL,PO, 1000 mg,			
100s ea	54569-5979-00	7.05	
(Keltman Pharma., Inc.)			
REPACK			
SGL,PO (SOFTGEL)			
1000 mg, 60s ea	68387-0432-60	14.25	
(Palmetto)			
REPACK			
SGL,PO (ENTERIC COATED SOFTGEL)			
1000 mg, 90s ea	23490-9407-00	20.00	
(SOFTGEL)			
1000 mg, 120s ea	23490-9408-00	20.00	
(Phys Total Care)			
REPACK			
SGL,PO, 1000 mg,			
100s ea	54868-5174-00	19.62	
FISH OIL CONCENTRATE (AmerisourceBergen)			
SGL,PO (PRIVATE LABEL,SOFTGEL)			
1000 mg, 60s ea	24385-0335-72	3.86	4.29
(Mason Vit)			
SGL,PO (AF,SF,DYE-FREE,SOFTGEL)			
1000 mg-3 iu, 120s ea	11845-1223-02	11.67	
FISHERMAN'S FRIEND (Phys Total Care)			
REPACK			
LOZ,MM, 19s ea	54868-3506-01	2.56	
30s ea	54868-3506-00	2.22	
FLANDERLACTIGLIDE (Neurovites)			
CRE,TP, 12%-6%, 60 gm	93595-2035-01	19.50	32.50
FLANDERS BUTTOCKS OINTMENT (Flanders)			
OIN,TP (FLIP TOP)			
120 gm	54323-0215-02	5.76	
FLAV-EIN (3 B's Limited)			
CAP,PO, 100 mg-560 mg,			
60s ea	30371-0000-32	9.75	15.95
FLAVONS-500 (Freeda)			
TAB,PO (PF,SF,DYE-FREE)			
500 mg, 100s ea	10432-0268-01	6.27	10.45
250s ea	10432-0268-02	12.54	20.90
FLAVOR PACKET (Nutricia)			
PDR,PO (CHERRY,VANILLA)			
5 gm 20s	49735-0102-49	15.60	
(FRUIT,GRAPE)			
5 gm 20s	49735-0101-33	15.60	
(LEMON,LIME)			
5 gm 20s	49735-0101-58	15.60	
FLAVOUR PAC (VITAFLO, LLC)			
PDR,PO (30X4GM,BLACKCURRANT)			
4 gm 30s	50600-0541-73	23.35	29.65
(4GMX30,BLACKCURRANT)			
4 gm 30s	50600-0541-59	23.35	29.65
(4GMX30,LEMON)			
4 gm 30s	50600-0540-98	23.35	29.65
(4GMX30,ORANGE)			
4 gm 30s	50600-0541-11	23.35	29.65
(4GMX30,RASPBERRY)			
4 gm 30s	50600-0541-35	23.35	29.65
FLAX OIL (Rexall)			
SGL,PO (SOFTGEL)			
1000 mg, 60s ea	30768-0036-57	4.00	6.07
FLAX SEED OIL (Mason Vit)			
SGL,PO (SOFT GEL,PF,SF,SOFTGEL)			
1000 mg, 100s ea	11845-0131-31	11.00	
FLAX SEED OIL NATURAL (AmerisourceBergen)			
SGL,PO (PRIVATE LABEL,SOFTGEL)			
1000 mg, 100s ea	24385-0933-78	6.74	7.99
FLAXSEED OIL (Major)			
SGL,PO (SOFTGEL)			
1000 mg, 60s ea	00904-5597-52	3.46	
(Rx Vitamins)			
SGL,PO (PF,SF,SOFTGEL)			
1300 mg, 60s ea	08429-0030-03	5.48	10.95
FLEET BABYLAX (Fleet,C.B.)			
NMA,RC (APPLICATORS)			
2.3 gm/2.3 ml,			
4 ml 6s	00132-0180-01	3.50	
FLEET BAGENEMA (Fleet,C.B.)			
DEV,NA (LARGE VOLUME)			
ea	00132-0901-10	2.80	
FLEET BISACODYL (Fleet,C.B.)			
ECT,PO, 5 mg, 25s ea	00132-0704-02	2.90	
SUP,RC, 10 mg, 4s ea	00132-0705-04	1.95	
FLEET BISACODYL ENEMA (Fleet,C.B.)			
NMA,RC, 10 mg/1.25 oz,			
37.5 ml	00132-0703-36	1.19	
FLEET ENEMA (Fleet,C.B.)			
NMA,RC, 135 ml	00132-0201-40	0.80	
(TWIN PACK)			
135 ml 2s	00132-0201-42	1.40	
(A-S Medication)			
REPACK			
NMA,RC, 135 ml	54569-0826-00	1.00	
(Phys Total Care)			
REPACK			
NMA,RC, 135 ml	54868-0022-00	2.51	
FLEET ENEMA CHILDREN (Fleet,C.B.)			
NMA,RC, 67.5 ml	00132-0202-20	1.09	
FLEET ENEMA EXTRA (Fleet,C.B.)			
NMA,RC (EASY SQUEEZE,LATEX-FREE)			
7 gm/197 ml-19 gm/197 ml,			
230 ml	01320-0020-11	1.27	
FLEET GLYCERIN LAXATIVE (Fleet,C.B.)			
NMA,RC (APPLICATORS)			
7.5 ml 4s	00132-0185-82	3.03	
FLEET GLYCERIN MAXIMUM STRENGTH (Fleet,C.B.)			
SUP,RC (FOIL WRAPPED)			
18s ea	00132-0084-18	1.68	
FLEET GLYCERIN SUPPOSITORIES (Fleet,C.B.)			
SUP,RC (ADULT,FOIL-WRAPPED)			
12s ea	00132-0080-12	1.14	
(ADULT)			
12s ea	00132-0791-12	0.99	
(CHILD)			
12s ea	00132-0081-12	0.99	
(ADULT)			
24s ea	00132-0079-24	1.68	
50s ea	00132-0079-50	2.49	
FLEET MINERAL OIL ENEMA (Fleet,C.B.)			
NMA,RC, 135 ml	00132-0301-40	1.53	
(Phys Total Care)			
REPACK			
NMA,RC, 135 ml	54868-3333-00	3.50	
FLEET PAIN RELIEF (Fleet,C.B.)			
PAD,TP (AF)			
12%-1%, 100s ea	00132-0487-00	4.04	
FLEET PHOSPHO-SODA EZ-PREP (Fleet,C.B.)			
LIQ,PO (SYSTEM W/45ML&30ML)			
75 ml	01320-0001-02	12.19	
FLEET PREP KIT 1 (Fleet,C.B.)			
KIT,NA (W/SUPPOSITORY)			
ea	00132-0101-01	4.36	
(Phys Total Care)			
REPACK			
KIT,NA, ea	54868-3177-00	7.66	
FLEET PREP KIT 2 (Fleet,C.B.)			
KIT,NA (W/LARGE-VOLUME ENEMA)			
ea	00132-0210-01	8.48	
FLEET PREP KIT 3 (Fleet,C.B.)			
KIT,NA (W/SMALL-VOLUME ENEMA)			
ea	00132-0103-01	5.96	
FLEET SOF-LAX (Fleet,C.B.)			
TAB,PO (GELCAPLET)			
100 mg, 60s ea	00132-0751-60	5.60	
FLETCHER'S CASTORIA (Mentholatum)			
LIQ,PO, 6.5%, 75 ml	10742-0003-21	3.59	
FLEX-WRAP SELF-ADHERENT WRAP (Covidien)			
DEV,NA (4"X5YD)			
18s ea	08080-4584-00	49.55	
FLEXALL 454 (Chattem)			
GEL,TP, 7%, 60 gm	41167-0160-11	3.24	
120 gm	41167-0160-13	4.86	
240 gm	41167-0160-15	7.60	
FLEXALL 454 MAXIMUM STRENGTH (Chattem)			
GEL,TP, 16%, 45 gm	41167-0160-21	3.24	
90 gm	41167-0160-22	4.86	
180 gm	41167-0160-24	7.68	
FLEXALL ULTRA PLUS (Chattem)			
GEL,TP, 3.1%-16%-10%,			
60 gm	41167-0160-31	4.06	
120 gm	41167-0160-33	5.88	
FLEXI-SEAL FECAL MANAGEMENT SYSTEM COLLECTION BAGS (Convatec)			
DEV,NA (WITH FILTERS)			
ea	68455-0108-62	126.98	166.90
FLEXI-TRAK ANCHORING DEVICE (Convatec)			
DEV,NA (4"X1 1/2", LARGE)			
50s ea	68455-0107-62	73.96	96.28
FLEXIFLO QUANTUM ENTERAL PUMP (Abbott)			
DEV,NA, ea	70074-0505-97	1380.00	
(40MM)			
ea	70074-0506-03	7.85	
FLEXIFLO QUANTUM PUMP (Abbott)			
DEV,NA (W/PIERC PIN& FLUSH BAG)			
ea	70074-0506-05	13.74	
(W/PIERCING PIN)			
ea	70074-0506-01	8.84	
FLEXISEAL FECAL MANAGEMENT SYSTEM (Convatec)			
DEV,NA (ADVANCED ODOR CONTROL)			
ea	68455-0101-37	672.95	884.53

PROD/MFR	HRI, UPC,NDC	AWP	SRP
FLEXITAINER 500 CONTAINER (Abbott)			
DEV,NA (ENTERAL NUTRITION)			
ea	70074-0000-68	5.23	
FLEXITAINER NUTRITION CONTAINER (Abbott)			
DEV,NA, ea	70074-0000-69	6.26	
FLEXPOWER (Flex-Power Inc)			
CRE,TP (CITRUS LIGHT SCENT)			
10%, 113 gm	55379-0464-04	38.00	
(CLEAN SCENT)			
10%, 113 gm	55379-0465-04	38.00	
FLEXZAN (UDL)			
DEV,NA (4"X8" SHEETS)			
5s ea	62794-0085-32	39.21	
(8"X8" SHEETS)			
5s ea	62794-0085-64	76.25	
(2"X3" SHEETS)			
10s ea	62794-0085-06	25.96	
(4"X4" SHEETS)			
10s ea	62794-0085-18	34.61	
FLINTSTONES (Bayer HealthCare)			
CTB,PO, 60s ea	16500-0078-18	3.94	
100s ea	16500-0078-14	5.56	
FLINTSTONES COMPLETE (Bayer HealthCare)			
CTB,PO, 60s ea	16500-0088-06	5.56	
150s ea	16500-0097-13	9.99	
FLINTSTONES PLUS CALCIUM (Bayer HealthCare)			
CTB,PO, 60s ea	16500-0077-06	5.01	
FLINTSTONES PLUS EXTRA C (Bayer HealthCare)			
CTB,PO, 60s ea	16500-0086-19	5.01	
FLINTSTONES W/IRON (Bayer HealthCare)			
CTB,PO, 60s ea	16500-0079-09	5.01	
FLORA Q 2 (Kenwood)			
CAP,PO (DOUBLE STRENGTH,PF)			
30s ea	04824-0001-30	50.29	
FLORA-Q (Kenwood)			
CAP,PO, 30s ea	00482-4000-30	40.66	
FLORANEX (Rising)			
CTB,PO, 0.2 mg-0.2 mg,			
50s ea	64980-0129-50	7.69	
(Phys Total Care)			
REPACK			
CTB,PO, 50s ea	54868-4905-00	7.16	
FLORANEX GRANULES (Rising)			
GRA,PO (12X1GM)			
5 mg, 1 gm 12s	64980-0146-12	9.07	
FLORASTOR (Biocodex)			
CAP,PO (EXTRA STRENGTH)			
250 mg, 10s ea	04142-0000-08	10.99	10.95
20s ea	04142-0000-24		21.95
50s ea	04142-0000-07	45.83	43.95
(Phys Total Care)			
REPACK			
CAP,PO, 250 mg, 20s ea	54868-6006-00	21.34	
FLORASTOR KIDS (Biocodex)			
PDR,PO (TUTTI-FRUTTI,SACHETS)			
250 mg/packet, 10s ea	04120-0000-16	9.24	12.95
20s ea	04142-0000-23		21.95
FLORICAL (Mericon)			
CAP,PO, 364 mg-8.3 mg,			
100s ea	00394-0102-02	12.36	
500s ea	00394-0102-05	58.52	
TAB,PO, 364 mg-8.3 mg,			
100s ea	00394-0100-02	11.39	
500s ea	00394-0100-05	53.57	
FLOW DETECTOR (Abbott Hosp)			
DEV,NA (54")			
ea	00074-1907-25	163.65	
FLU COLD & COUGH NIGHTTIME (Cardinal Health)			
PKT,PO (MAX. STR.,PRIVATE LABEL)			
6s ea	37205-0331-91	3.52	
FLU-RELIEF (Pfeiffer)			
TAB,PO, 325 mg-2 mg-30 mg,			
36s ea	00927-0324-63	2.94	5.29
FLU/COLD/COUGH MEDICINE (AmerisourceBergen)			
PDS,PO (PACKET,PRIVATE LABEL)			
6s ea	24385-0536-91	2.69	2.99
FLUORIGARD (Colgate Oral)			
SOL,PO, 0.05%, 473 ml	00126-0220-16	3.65	
FO-TI (Botanical Labs.)			
LIQ,PO, 30 ml	41954-0020-19	4.50	8.99
FOAM DRESSING (Geritrex)			
DEV,NA, ea	92771-0925-45	3.04	
(MPM Medical Inc.)			
DEV,NA (BORDERED, 2"X2")			
ea	66977-0500-44	3.09	3.43
(BORDERED, 4"X4")			
ea	66977-0500-66	5.69	6.32
(CIRCULAR BORD,2.5X2.5)			
ea	66977-0500-25	3.09	3.43
(NON-BORDERED, 2"X2")			
ea	66977-0500-22	1.76	1.95
(NON-BORDERED, 4"X4")			
ea	66977-0500-24	3.65	4.06
FOAM STRIPS (AmerisourceBergen)			
DEV,NA (ASSORTED,PRIVATE LABEL)			
45s ea	24385-0159-66	2.44	2.69
FOAMING ANTACID (AmerisourceBergen)			
CTB,PO (PRIVATE LABEL)			
80 mg-20 mg, 100s ea	24385-0126-78	4.94	5.49
SUS,PO			
95 mg/15 ml-358 mg/15 ml,			
360 ml	24385-0397-40	4.49	4.99
(Qualitest)			
CTB,PO, 80 mg-20 mg,			
100s ea	00603-0186-21	6.03	
(Dispensing Solutions)			
REPACK			
CTB,PO, 80 mg-20 mg,			
100s ea	55045-3475-01	7.00	
FOLACIN-800 (Key Company)			
TAB,PO (SF)			
0.8 mg, 100s ea	11694-0809-01	3.00	
250s ea	11694-0809-25	5.00	
FOLGARD (Upsher-Smith)			
TAB,PO, 0.115 mg-0.8 mg-10 mg,			
60s ea	00245-0017-60	16.44	
FOLIC & B12 & B6 (Key Company)			
TAB,PO (SF)			
1 mg-0.8 mg-20 mg,			
60s ea	11694-0696-01	6.00	
250s ea	11694-0696-02	20.00	
FOLIC + B12 (Key Company)			
TAB,PO (SF)			
1 mg-0.8 mg, 60s ea	11694-0712-01	5.25	
250s ea	11694-0712-02	18.00	
FOLIC ACID (ADH)			
TAB,PO (PF,SF)			
0.8 mg, 100s ea	60142-0241-01	2.48	4.95
(AmerisourceBergen)			
TAB,PO (PRIVATE LABEL)			
0.4 mg, 250s ea	24385-0286-85	3.32	3.69
(Basic Vitamins)			
TAB,PO, 0.4 mg, 200s ea	00761-0878-40	2.40	
(Cardinal Health)			
TAB,PO (PRIVATE LABEL)			
0.4 mg, 250s ea	37205-0188-85	3.56	
(Carlson,J.R.)			
TAB,PO (PF,SF,CORN-FREE)			
0.4 mg, 300s ea	88395-0026-53	3.25	6.50
(VEGETARIAN,PF,SF)			
0.8 mg, 300s ea	88395-0026-63	4.75	9.50
1000s ea	88395-0026-66	12.95	25.90
(Freeda)			
TAB,PO (PF,SF,DYE-FREE)			
0.4 mg, 100s ea	10432-0163-01	3.30	5.50
500s ea	10432-0163-03	11.37	18.95
0.8 mg, 100s ea	10432-0147-01	4.17	6.95
250s ea	10432-0147-02	8.34	13.90
(Major)			
TAB,PO, 0.4 mg, 100s ea	00904-3197-60	2.15	
250s ea	00904-3197-70	2.99	
800 mcg, 100s ea	09046-0037-60	3.96	
(Marlex)			
TAB,PO, 0.4 mg, 100s ea	10135-0180-01	0.93	
1000s ea	10135-0180-10	5.02	
0.8 mg, 100s ea	10135-0181-01	1.77	
1000s ea	10135-0181-10	4.75	
(Mason Vit)			
TAB,PO, 0.4 mg, 100s ea	11845-0065-31	3.00	
0.8 mg, 100s ea	11845-0067-61	3.67	
(Nature's Bounty)			
TAB,PO (PF,SF)			
0.4 mg, 100s ea	74312-0014-00		2.99
250s ea	74312-0014-03		4.29
0.8 mg, 250s ea	74312-0028-43		4.99
(Pharmavite)			
TAB,PO, 0.4 mg, 250s ea	31604-0012-74	2.51	
(Rexall)			
TAB,PO (PF,SF)			
0.8 mg, 75s ea	30768-0001-74	1.32	2.00
(Rugby)			
TAB,PO (PF,SF,DYE-FREE)			
0.4 mg, 100s ea	00536-3844-01	2.10	
0.8 mg, 100s ea	00536-3843-01	2.40	
FOLIC ACID B6 & B12 (Mason Vit)			
TAB,PO (PF,SF)			
90s ea	11845-0116-99	5.89	
FOLIC ACID XTRA (Rexall)			
TAB,PO, 60s ea	30768-0000-08	4.35	6.58
FOLIC ACID/VITAMIN B12 (Freeda)			
TAB,PO (PF,SF,DYE-FREE)			
0.5 mg-0.4 mg,			
100s ea	10432-0198-01	6.87	11.45
250s ea	10432-0198-02	13.74	22.90
FOLTABS 800 (Midlothian Labs)			
TAB,PO (FILM-COATED)			
0.115 mg-0.8 mg-10 mg,			
60s ea	68308-0325-60	14.63	
FOR PLAY (Pharm Innov)			
GEL,TP (MASSAGE/LUBRICATING)			
120 ml	00036-9690-20	5.21	7.44
150 ml	00036-9690-15	5.21	7.44
FOR STY RELIEF (Altaire)			
OIN,OP (STERILE)			
31.9%-57.7%, 3.5 gm	59390-0189-50	5.63	
FORA D10 BLOOD GLUCOSE PLUS BLOOD PRESSURE (Fora)			
DEV,NA, ea	98939-0002-00	43.00	
FORA D10 GLUCOSE TEST STRIPS (Fora)			
DEV,NA, 50s ea	98939-0002-01	16.50	
FORA G20 BLOOD GLUCOSE MONITORING SYSTEM (Fora)			
DEV,NA, ea	98939-0002-33	50.00	
FORA G20 BLOOD GLUCOSE TEST STRIPS (Fora)			
DEV,NA, 50s ea	98939-0002-34	40.00	
FORA V10 BLOOD GLUCOSE MONITORING SYSTEM (Fora)			
DEV,NA, ea	98939-0002-09	21.00	
ea	98939-0002-35	55.00	
FORA V10 BLOOD GLUCOSE TEST STRIP (Fora)			
DEV,NA, 50s ea	98939-0002-10	40.00	
FORMULA 3/6/9 (Advanced Nutr)			
CAP,PO, 60s ea	62617-0010-02	18.60	34.80
FORMULA 405 AHA FACE/BODY CLEANSER (Doak)			
LOT,TP (SOAP-FREE)			
240 ml	10337-0666-86	14.66	
FORMULA 405 AHA FACIAL NIGHT (Doak)			
CRE,TP, 60 gm	10337-0666-84	27.86	
FORMULA 405 BODY SMOOTHING (Doak)			
LOT,TP, 240 ml	10337-0666-72	13.51	
FORMULA 405 ENRICHED EYE CREAM (Doak)			
CRE,TP, 15 gm	10337-0666-64	17.65	
FORMULA 405 ENRICHED FACE CREAM (Doak)			
CRE,TP, 60 gm	10337-0666-63	21.13	
FORMULA 405 FACIAL & BODY CLEANSING (Doak)			
LOT,TP (W/BUFFING MITT)			
240 ml	10337-0666-69	15.53	
(SOAP-FREE)			
480 ml	10337-0666-70	21.37	
FORMULA 405 LE PONT NAIL TREATMENT (Doak)			
OIL,TP, 7.5 ml	10337-0666-71	12.62	
FORMULA 50 (Marlyn)			
CAP,PO, 252 mg-1 mg-320 mg,			
100s ea	10712-0601-00	5.75	11.49
250s ea	10712-0602-50	12.47	24.99
FORMULA 500 (Mason Vit)			
TAB,PO (PF,SF)			
75 mg-250 mg-250 mg,			
60s ea	11845-0116-75	7.44	
FORMULA E 400 (Miller)			
SGL,PO, 400 iu, 100s ea	17204-0937-40	8.82	10.00
FORMULA EM (Global Source)			
SOL,PO (CHERRY)			
120 ml	59618-0342-33	5.55	
(Major)			
SOL,PO, 120 ml	00904-0049-20	4.65	
FORMULATED FOR FINGERS (AmerisourceBergen)			
CRE,TP (FOR DIABETICS)			
113.4 gm	24385-0664-26	6.29	8.29

PROD/MFR	HRI, UPC,NDC	AWP	SRP
(Medicine Shoppe)			
CRE,TP, 120 gm	49614-0425-26	10.99	10.99
FORMULATION R (G&W)			
CRE,RC, 0.25%, 54 gm	00713-0604-35	4.81	
OIN,TP, 0.25%, 30 gm	00713-0298-31	3.79	
60 gm	00713-0298-32	4.68	
SUP,RC, 12s ea	00713-0535-12	4.17	
24s ea	00713-0535-24	7.55	
48s ea	00713-0535-48	13.64	
FORTEL ONE STEP PREGNANCY (Biomerica)			
DEV,NA, ea	83059-0001-44	5.99	
FOSFREE (Mission)			
TAB,PO, 60s ea	00178-0031-60	6.94	
120s ea	00178-0031-12	10.13	
FOSTEUM (Primus Pharma)			
CAP,PO (GLUTEN-FREE)			
60s ea	68040-0603-16	51.25	
FREE & CLEAR (Pharm Spec)			
SHA,TP, 240 ml	45334-0200-08	5.69	8.60
FREE & CLEAR CLEANSER (Pharm Spec)			
LIQ,TP (NORMAL & SENSITIVE SKIN)			
237 ml	45334-0220-08	5.69	8.60
FREE & CLEAR HAIR SPRAY (Pharm Spec)			
SPR,TP (FIRM HOLD,DYE-FREE)			
237 ml	45334-0231-08	7.65	11.55
(SOFT HOLD,DYE-FREE)			
237 ml	45334-0230-08	7.65	11.55
FREE & CLEAR HAIR STYLING (Pharm Spec)			
GEL,TP (AF,PF,DYE-FREE)			
198 gm	45334-0240-07	6.58	9.95
FREEDAVITE (Freeda)			
TAB,PO (PF,SF,DYE-FREE)			
100s ea	10432-0014-01	4.77	7.95
250s ea	10432-0014-02	9.54	15.90
FREEDOM LEG BAG STRAPS (Mentor)			
DEV,NA (1",PR,COMFORT,ADJUST)			
ea	81317-0070-90	7.37	
(2",PR,DELUXE,VELSTRETCH)			
ea	81317-0070-80	13.97	
FREEDOM LEG BAG W/CONNECTOR (Mentor)			
DEV,NA (18" CLR NON-LTX,1000ML)			
ea	81317-0070-82	10.93	
(18" CLR NON-LTX,500ML)			
ea	81317-0070-92	10.93	
FREEDOM LEG BAG W/STANDARD PORT (Mentor)			
DEV,NA (1000 ML)			
ea	81317-0070-85	4.39	
(1000ML,CLEAR 18" TUBING)			
ea	81317-0070-86	6.35	
(500 ML,CLEAR 18" TUBING)			
ea	81317-0070-76	6.35	
(500 ML)			
ea	81317-0070-75	4.54	
FREEDOM LEG BAG W/T-TAP PORT (Mentor)			
DEV,NA (1000 ML, COMFORT STRAPS)			
ea	81317-0070-89	11.29	
(1000 ML, VELCRO STRAPS)			
ea	81317-0070-88	11.29	
(1000 ML)			
ea	81317-0070-87	5.27	
(500 ML, COMFORT STRAPS)			
ea	81317-0070-79	11.29	
(500 ML, ELASTIC STRAPS)			
ea	81317-0070-78	7.11	
(500 ML)			
ea	81317-0070-77	5.27	
FREEDOM LEG BAG W/TWIST PORT (Mentor)			
DEV,NA (1000 ML)			
ea	81317-0070-97	4.54	
(1000ML,KIT)			
ea	81317-0070-96	4.39	
(500 ML)			
ea	81317-0070-93	4.54	
ea	81317-0070-94	6.35	
FREEDOM PAK SEVEN (Mentor)			
DEV,NA (INTERMEDIATE)			
ea	81317-0082-52	13.24	
(LARGE)			
ea	81317-0084-02	13.24	
(MEDIUM)			
ea	81317-0082-02	13.24	
(SMALL)			
ea	81317-0080-02	13.24	
FREESTYLE (Abbott)			
DEV,NA (STRIP,2X25)			
50s ea	99073-0120-50	63.89	
(STRIP,2X50)			
100s ea	99073-0121-01	114.02	

PROD/MFR	HRI, UPC,NDC	AWP	SRP
(Phys Total Care)			
REPACK			
DEV,NA, 100s ea	54868-5330-00	102.60	
FREESTYLE BLOOD GLUCOSE SYSTEM (Abbott)			
DEV,NA (10 LANCETS/TEST STRIPS)			
ea	99073-0110-01	75.00	
(100 STRIPS,FREE MONITOR)			
ea	99073-0120-51	92.76	
FREESTYLE CONTROL (Abbott)			
DEV,NA (HIGH/LOW)			
2s ea	99073-0140-03	7.50	
FREESTYLE FLASH (Abbott)			
DEV,NA, ea	99073-0170-01	73.75	
FREESTYLE FREEDOM BLOOD GLUCOSE MONITORING SYSTEM (Abbott)			
DEV,NA (VALUE PACK)			
ea	99073-0708-47	58.06	
FREESTYLE FREEDOM LITE (Abbott)			
DEV,NA, ea	99073-0709-14	18.00	
ea	99073-0709-20	30.00	
FREESTYLE LANCETS (Abbott)			
DEV,NA, 100s ea	99073-0130-01	8.98	
FREESTYLE LITE (Abbott)			
DEV,NA, 50s ea	99073-0708-19	65.82	
50s ea	99073-0708-22	65.82	
100s ea	99073-0708-23	113.04	
100s ea	99073-0708-27	117.44	
FREESTYLE LITE BLOOD GLUCOSE MONITORING SYSTEM (Abbott)			
DEV,NA, ea	99073-0708-04	30.00	
ea	99073-0708-05	18.00	
FREESTYLE UNISTIK 2 (Abbott)			
DEV,NA (LANCETS)			
200s ea	99073-0130-22	33.34	
FREEZONE MAXIMUM STRENGTH (Medtech)			
LIQ,TP, 17.6%, 9.3 ml	75137-0520-10	3.29	
FRESH 'N BRITE DENTURE (Johnson & Johnson)			
PAS,NA, 114 gm	12547-0639-21	2.29	
FRESH & PURE DOUCHE (Unico)			
SOL,VG (EXTRA MILD,AF)			
177 ml 2s	37513-0000-31	0.65	
FRESH N FREE (Geritrex)			
SOL,MM (AF)			
120 ml	54162-0350-04	0.51	
FRUIT PUNCH WITH FIBRE (Nutra/Balance)			
LIQ,PO (27X236ML)			
236 ml 27s	07249-0501-02		49.28
FRUITY CHEWS (Teva)			
CTB,PO, 100s ea	00182-4314-01	4.79	
FRUITY CHEWS W/IRON (Teva)			
CTB,PO, 100s ea	00182-4315-01	5.19	
FUNG-O (S.S.S.)			
LIQ,TP, 17%, 15 ml	12258-0326-05	2.10	
FUNGI NAIL (Kramer Labs)			
SOL,TP (1X1.7ML)			
25%, 1.7 ml	55505-0167-20	7.80	9.10
FUNGI-GUARD (Altaire)			
CRE,TP, 1%, 15 gm	59390-0024-14	2.00	
SOL,TP, 1%, 30 ml	59390-0062-18	5.75	
FUNGI-NAIL (Kramer Labs)			
SOL,TP, 25%, 30 ml	53076-0103-26	11.06	12.91
FUNGOID (Pedinol)			
KIT,TP (TINCTURE KIT)			
2%, ea	00884-5493-01		26.99
TIN,TP, 2%, 29.57 ml	00884-0293-01		20.00
(Phys Total Care)			
REPACK			
KIT,TP (TINCTURE NAIL KIT)			
2%, ea	54868-5878-00	42.61	
G-A-P (Freeda)			
CTB,PO (PF,SF,DYE-FREE)			
300 mg-300 mg,			
100s ea	10432-0309-01	7.53	12.55
G.F.S.-2000 (Westlake Labs.)			
CAP,PO (PF,SF)			
270s ea	10539-0770-42	41.30	59.00
G/C 1000 (Progressive Labs.)			
CAP,PO, 60s ea	51821-0723-60	11.00	22.00
GA (Mead Johnson & Co)			
PDR,PO (LYSINE/TRYPTOPHAN FREE)			
454 gm	00087-0198-41	52.80	

PROD/MFR	HRI, UPC,NDC	AWP	SRP
GA GEL (VITAFLO, LLC)			
PDS,PO (UNFLAVORED)			
30s ea	50600-0536-02	148.68	239.00
GALIUM-HEEL (Heel/BHI)			
LIQ,PO (DROPS)			
48 ml	50114-1063-04	5.95	10.95
GAMMA E PLUS (Key Company)			
SGL,PO (SOFTGEL)			
200 iu, 100s ea	11694-0667-01	12.00	
GAMMA E-GEMS (Carlson,J.R.)			
SGL,PO (W/500MG GAMMATOCOPHEROL)			
90 iu, 60s ea	88395-0008-66	10.95	21.90
120s ea	88395-0008-61	19.25	38.50
GAMMA GEL (Pharm Innov)			
GEL,TP, 90 ml	00036-1150-90	1.84	2.62
250 ml	00036-1150-25	2.06	2.94
4000 ml	00036-1150-04	15.17	21.67
GAMMA-LINIC 500 (Key Company)			
CAP,PO (SF,SOFTGEL)			
350 mg-40 mg,			
60s ea	11694-0868-01	7.00	
180s ea	11694-0868-03	18.00	
GARLIC (ADH)			
TAB,PO, 300 mg, 100s ea	60142-0101-10	4.48	8.95
(Basic Vitamins)			
TAB,PO, 500 mg, 100s ea	00761-0502-20	3.00	
(Bio-Tech Pharm)			
CAP,PO, 500 mg, 100s ea	53191-0223-01	6.30	
(Cardinal Health)			
SGL,PO (PRIVATE LABEL)			
500 mg, 100s ea	37205-0093-78	7.42	
(Contract Pharmacal)			
TAB,PO (DEODORIZED)			
300 mg, 100s ea	10267-0452-01	5.00	
(Freeda)			
TAB,PO (PF,SF,DYE-FREE)			
200 mg, 100s ea	10432-0181-01	3.42	5.70
500s ea	10432-0181-03	11.37	18.95
(Key Company)			
SGL,PO (SOFTGEL)			
345 mg, 100s ea	11694-0806-01	4.50	
250s ea	11694-0806-02	9.00	
(Major)			
SGL,PO, 500 mg, 100s ea	00904-3156-60	5.50	
(Mason Vit)			
CAP,PO (PF,SF)			
300 mg, 100s ea	11845-0123-41	8.33	
TAB,PO (PF)			
100 mg, 100s ea	11845-0098-51	5.56	
100s ea	11845-0123-61	5.22	
(Miller)			
SGL,PO, 345 mg, 100s ea	17204-0563-40	5.70	9.50
(Nature's Bounty)			
TAB,PO (DEODORIZED,PF,SF)			
300 mg, 100s ea	74312-0042-01		6.29
(Rexall)			
ECT,PO (PF,SF)			
400 mg, 60s ea	30768-0000-72	1.98	3.00
GARLIC & PARSLEY (Nature's Bounty)			
CAP,PO (PF,SF,SOFTGEL)			
2 mg-0.2 mg, 100s ea	74312-0028-50		4.99
(Rexall)			
TAB,PO (PF,SF,SOFTGEL)			
60s ea	30768-0001-65	1.20	1.82
GARLIC OIL (Basic Vitamins)			
CAP,PO, 2 mg, 100s ea	00761-0292-20	2.00	
(Health Products Corp)			
SGL,PO (PF,SF,SOFTGEL)			
1000 mg, 100s ea	39686-0014-06	2.75	
(Mason Vit)			
SGL,PO, 500 mg, 100s ea	11845-0053-21	3.44	
1000 mg, 100s ea	11845-0069-91	4.11	
300s ea	11845-0069-90	6.64	
1500 mg, 100s ea	11845-0072-31	5.89	
(Nature's Bounty)			
SGL,PO (PF,SF,SOFTGEL)			
1000 mg, 100s ea	74312-0029-70		4.15
5000 mg, 100s ea	74312-0029-80		5.59
GARLIC OIL NATURAL (Cardinal Health)			
SGL,PO (PRIVATE LABEL,SOFTGEL)			
3 mg, 100s ea	37205-0077-78	2.93	

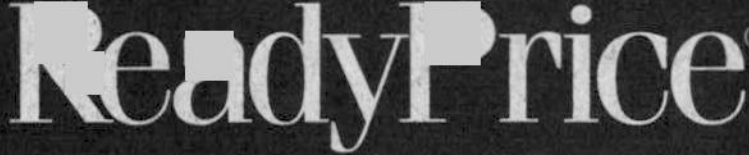

PROD/MFR	HRI, UPC,NDC	AWP	SRP
(Rexall)			
SGL,PO (PF,SF,SOFTGEL)			
1000 mg, 60s ea	30768-0000-59	1.33	2.02
1500 mg, 60s ea	30768-0001-76	1.80	2.73
GARLIC SUPPLEMENT (Mason Vit)			
CAP,PO (PF,SF)			
300 mg, 60s ea	11845-0131-55	8.78	
GARLIC-600 (Carlson,J.R.)			
TAB,PO (ODORLESS)			
600 mg, 100s ea	88395-0084-11	5.95	11.90
250s ea	88395-0084-12	13.85	27.70
GARLIC-PARSLEY (Freeda)			
TAB,PO (PF,SF,DYE-FREE)			
100 mg-200 mg,			
100s ea	10432-0239-01	3.75	6.25
500s ea	10432-0239-03	11.85	19.75
GARLIC-X (Mason Vit)			
TAB,PO, 400 mg, 100s ea	11845-0100-11	6.89	
(PF,SF)			
400 mg, 100s ea	11845-0123-51	6.67	
GARLIC/LECITHIN (Key Company)			
CAP,PO, 500 mg-500 mg,			
100s ea	11694-0805-01	9.00	
(Miller)			
CAP,PO, 500 mg-650 mg,			
100s ea	17204-0564-40	11.34	18.90
GARLIC/PARSLEY (Mason Vit)			
SGL,PO, 100s ea	11845-0072-51	5.56	
100s ea	11845-0074-01	3.67	
GAS FREE EXTRA STRENGTH (Major)			
SGL,PO (SOFTGEL)			
125 mg, 30s ea	00904-5458-46	3.86	
GAS RELIEF (AmerisourceBergen)			
SUS,PO (PRIVATE LABEL,DROPS)			
40 mg/0.6 ml, 30 ml	24385-0785-30	8.09	8.99
(Cardinal Health)			
CTB,PO (PRIVATE LABEL)			
80 mg, 100s ea	37205-0112-78	2.32	
(Family Phcy)			
SUS,PO (PRIVATE LABEL,DROPS)			
40 mg/0.6 ml, 30 ml	52735-0538-26	7.19	7.99
(Major)			
SGL,PO (ULTRA STRENGTH,SOFTGEL)			
180 mg, 60s ea	00904-5572-52	6.59	
(Perrigo)			
SOL,PO (W/DROPPER,1X30ML,AF)			
20 mg/0.3 ml,			
30 ml	45802-0406-49	6.99	
(Phys Total Care)			
REPACK			
CTB,PO, 80 mg, 100s ea	54868-2860-00	10.80	
GAS RELIEF 125 MAXIMUM STRENGTH (AmerisourceBergen)			
CTB,PO (PRIVATE LABEL)			
125 mg, 60s ea	24385-0123-72	3.95	4.39
GAS RELIEF 80 (AmerisourceBergen)			
PO (PRIVATE LABEL)			
80 mg, 100s ea	24385-0118-78	5.39	5.99
GAS RELIEF EXTRA STRENGTH (AmerisourceBergen)			
SGL,PO (PRIVATE LABEL,SOFTGEL)			
125 mg, 30s ea	24385-0428-65	4.13	4.59
(Cardinal Health)			
SGL,PO (PRIVATE LABEL,SOFTGEL)			
125 mg, 30s ea	37205-0295-65	3.28	
GAS RELIEF INFANTS (Global Source)			
SUS,PO (DROPS)			
40 mg/0.6 ml, 30 ml	59618-0355-29	8.25	
(Major)			
SUS,PO (W/DROPPER,DROPS)			
40 mg/0.6 ml, 30 ml	00904-5067-30	7.00	
GAS RELIEF INFANTS' (Chain Drug Marketing)			
SUS,PO (AF,DROPS)			
40 mg/0.6 ml, 30 ml	63868-0052-30	1.92	8.99
GAS-X (Novartis Consumer)			
CTB,PO, 80 mg, 12s ea	00043-0016-12	1.88	
36s ea	00043-0016-36	5.10	
(CHERRY)			
80 mg, 36s ea	00043-0113-36	5.10	
GAS-X EXTRA STRENGTH (Novartis Consumer)			
CTB,PO, 125 mg, 18s ea	00043-0129-18	3.88	
(CHERRY)			
125 mg, 18s ea	00043-0117-18	3.88	
48s ea	00043-0117-48	7.74	
SGL,PO (SOFTGEL)			
125 mg, 10s ea	00043-0134-10	2.00	
(SOFTGELS)			
125 mg, 20s ea	00067-6275-20	3.88	
(SOFTGEL)			
125 mg, 30s ea	00043-0134-30	5.38	
50s ea	00043-0134-50	8.38	
(SOFTGELS)			
125 mg, 50s ea	00067-6275-50	8.80	
GAS-X ULTRA STRENGTH (Novartis Consumer)			
SGL,PO (SOFTGELS)			
180 mg, 18s ea	00067-6274-18	4.79	
GAS-X WITH MAALOX (Novartis Consumer)			
CTB,PO (EXTRA STRENGTH)			
500 mg-125 mg,			
24s ea	00067-0130-24	5.59	
GASALIA (Boiron)			
TAB,PO, 6 c-6 c-6 c-6 c,			
60s ea	06962-0609-60	5.73	9.59
GASTROSTOMY TUBE (Abbott)			
DEV,NA (14 FR)			
ea	70074-0001-52	46.10	
(16 FR)			
ea	70074-0001-53	46.10	
(18 FR)			
ea	70074-0001-54	46.10	
(20 FR)			
ea	70074-0001-55	46.10	
(22 FR)			
ea	70074-0001-56	46.10	
(24 FR)			
ea	70074-0001-59	46.10	
(26 FRENCH)			
ea	70074-0501-59	46.10	
GAVISCON (Glaxo)			
CTB,PO, 80 mg-20 mg,			
30s ea	00088-1175-30	2.62	
100s ea	00088-1175-47	6.42	
(STRAWBERRY SMOOTHIE)			
500 mg, 25s ea	07661-0182-25	3.18	
75s ea	07661-0182-75	11.48	
SUS,PO			
95 mg/15 ml-358 mg/15 ml,			
360 ml	00088-1171-12	6.04	
GAVISCON ESRF (Glaxo)			
CTB,PO, 160 mg-105 mg,			
30s ea	00088-1174-30	3.02	
(CHERRY)			
160 mg-105 mg,			
30s ea	07661-0173-24	3.02	
100s ea	00088-1174-47	7.30	
(CHERRY)			
160 mg-105 mg,			
100s ea	07661-0173-25	7.30	
SUS,PO, 360 ml	00088-1173-12	7.30	
GE-150 (Bio-Tech Pharm)			
CAP,PO, 150 mg, 30s ea	53191-0142-30	29.35	
100s ea	53191-0142-01	89.20	
GEE WHIZ (Merlin Tech)			
DEV,NA (BEDSIDE DRAIN BAG)			
ea	08374-1040-01	11.50	
(CONDOM SHEATH)			
ea	34999-1020-01	5.82	
(EXTENSION TUBING)			
ea	34999-1080-01	3.95	
(LEG BAG 1000ML)			
ea	34999-0103-01	7.21	
(LEG BAG 500ML)			
ea	34999-1030-05	5.36	
(STARTER PAK)			
ea	34999-1000-01	84.63	
(CONNECTOR-FEMALE-MALE)			
5s ea	34999-1080-02	3.27	
(DISPOS. CONDOM SHEATHS)			
35s ea	34999-1020-05	72.80	
GEEWHIZ SILICONE MALE EXTERNAL CATHETER (Leading Edge)			
DEV,NA (29MM,SINGLE USE)			
35s ea	34999-0124-91	234.25	
(32MM,SINGLE USE)			
35s ea	34999-0212-49	234.25	
(36MM,SINGLE USE)			
35s ea	34999-0346-87	234.25	
(41MM,SINGLE USE)			
35s ea	34999-0429-81	234.25	
GEL-KAM (Colgate Oral)			
GEL,DE (BUBBLEGUM)			
0.4%, 122 gm	00126-0192-93	8.28	
129 gm	00126-0165-93	8.28	
129 gm	00126-0193-93	8.28	
GEL-STAT (Geritrex)			
GEL,TP (1X118ML)			
62%, 118 ml	54162-0254-04	1.86	1.82
120 gm	54162-0255-04	1.93	
(1X473ML)			
62%, 473 ml	92771-0254-16	6.27	6.14
480 gm	92771-0255-16	6.52	
GELATIN (Basic Vitamins)			
CAP,PO, 650 mg, 80s ea	00761-0615-16	2.40	
(Health Products Corp)			
CAP,PO (PF,SF)			
650 mg, 100s ea	39686-0013-97	3.65	
(Major)			
CAP,PO, 650 mg, 100s ea	00904-0078-60	5.48	
(Mason Vit)			
CAP,PO, 650 mg, 100s ea	11845-0053-61	6.33	
(Nature's Bounty)			
CAP,PO (PF,SF)			
650 mg, 100s ea	74312-0007-80		5.69
(Rexall)			
CAP,PO (PF,SF)			
650 mg, 50s ea	30768-0000-48	1.63	2.47
GELRITE (Dermarite)			
GEL,TP, 62%, 118 ml	61924-0106-04	1.87	
473 ml	61924-0100-27	4.75	
(LATEX-FREE)			
65%, 473 ml	61924-0106-16	5.52	
GELSEMIUM (Luyties)			
TAB,SL (6X)			
6 x, 500s ea	00618-4024-03	3.99	
5500s ea	00618-4024-10	30.32	
(30X)			
12 x, 500s ea	00622-4024-03	4.19	
5500s ea	00622-4024-10	31.83	
(12X)			
30 x, 500s ea	00624-4024-03	4.19	
5500s ea	00624-4024-10	31.83	
(Walker Pharmacal)			
TAB,SL (6X)			
250s ea	00619-4024-02	2.97	
GELUSIL (Johnson & Johnson)			
CTB,PO, 200 mg-200 mg-25 mg,			
100s ea	00071-0034-24	6.67	
GENAC (Teva)			
TAB,PO, 60 mg-2.5 mg,			
24s ea	00182-1605-16	2.39	
GENACOTE (Teva)			
ECT,PO, 325 mg, 100s ea	00182-1415-01	3.25	
GENAHIST (Teva)			
CAP,PO, 25 mg, 24s ea	00182-2092-16	2.39	
GENAPAP CHILDREN (Teva)			
CTB,PO (FRUIT)			
80 mg, 30s ea	00182-1585-17	1.90	
(GRAPE)			
80 mg, 30s ea	00182-2147-17	1.90	
ELI,PO (AF,CHERRY)			
160 mg/5 ml,			
120 ml	00182-1472-37	2.50	
(AF,GRAPE)			
160 mg/5 ml,			
120 ml	00182-2146-37	2.50	
GENAPHED (Teva)			
TAB,PO, 30 mg, 24s ea	00182-1459-16	1.59	
48s ea	00182-1459-98	3.59	
GENAPHED PLUS (Teva)			
TAB,PO, 4 mg-60 mg,			
24s ea	00182-1471-16	2.15	
GENASYME (Teva)			
CTB,PO, 80 mg, 100s ea	00182-1460-01	3.79	
(Phys Total Care)			
REPACK			
SUS,PO (DROPS)			
40 mg/0.6 ml,			
30 ml	54868-4347-00	8.98	
GENATON (Teva)			
CTB,PO, 80 mg-20 mg,			
100s ea	00182-2220-01	5.59	
SUS,PO (COOL MINT)			
95 mg/15 ml-358 mg/15 ml,			
360 ml	00182-1466-39	5.05	
GENEBS EXTRA STRENGTH (Teva)			
TAB,PO (CAPLET)			
500 mg, 100s ea	00182-1832-01	3.19	
1000s ea	00182-1832-10	23.39	

PROD/MFR	HRI, UPC,NDC	AWP	SRP
GENERATIONS (Health Products Corp)			
TAB,PO, 60s ea	39686-0012-51	7.63	
GENPRIL (Teva)			
TAB,PO (FILM COATED)			
200 mg, 50s ea	00182-2401-19	3.10	
100s ea	00182-2401-01	4.99	
GENTEAL (Novartis Pharm)			
GEL,OP (PF)			
0.25%-0.3%, 15 ml	00078-0425-24	8.08	
15 ml 8s	00078-0425-11	64.58	
25 ml	00078-0425-16	11.28	
(1X3.5ML,SEVERE)			
0.3%, 3.5 gm	00078-0429-97	4.14	
(SEVERE)			
0.3%, 10 gm	00078-0429-47	8.08	
(TWIN PACK)			
0.3%, 10 ml 2s	00078-0429-57	14.40	
SOL,OP (PF)			
0.3%, ea	58768-0789-15	8.13	
(1X15ML,MILD TO MODERATE)			
0.3%, 15 ml	00078-0518-24	8.08	
(MILD TO MODERATE,PF)			
0.3%, 25 ml	00078-0518-16	11.28	
(1X15ML,MILD,PF,DROPS)			
2%, 15 ml	00078-0517-24	8.08	
(MILD,PF)			
2%, 25 ml	00078-0517-16	11.28	
GENTEAL PM (Novartis Pharm)			
OIN,OP, 15%-85%, 3.5 gm	00078-0473-97	8.08	
GENTIAN (Ellon)			
SOL,SL (DROPS)			
10.5 ml	51762-0014-10		9.25
GENTIAN VIOLET (AmerisourceBergen)			
SOL,TP (PRIVATE LABEL)			
1%, 30 ml	24385-0003-91	3.14	3.49
(USP,1X59ML)			
1%, 59 ml	24385-0003-46	3.14	3.49
(Consolidated Midland)			
SOL,TP, 1%, 30 ml 12s	00223-6258-00	2.50	
2%, 30 ml 12s	00223-6259-00	36.00	
(Humco)			
SOL,TP (U.S.P.)			
1%, 30 ml	00395-1003-91	2.44	
2%, 30 ml	00395-1005-91	4.73	
(Lex)			
SOL,TP, 1%, 30 ml	49523-0083-01	0.67	
GENTLE CREAM (Geritrex)			
CRE,TP, 120 gm	54162-0850-04	3.85	
GENTLE DRAW (Home Diag)			
DEV,NA, ea	56151-0142-01	7.50	
GENTLE EXPRESSIONS BREAST PUMP (Lumiscope)			
DEV,NA (AC ADAPTABLE)			
ea	38673-0006-04	22.50	44.95
GENTLE EXPRESSIONS BREAST SHELLS (Lumiscope)			
DEV,NA (PLASTIC)			
ea	38673-0006-85	3.50	7.95
GENTLE EXPRESSIONS DELUXE PUMP (Lumiscope)			
DEV,NA (AC ADAPTER INCLUDED)			
ea	38673-0006-06	27.50	59.95
GENTLE EXPRESSIONS LACTO-STIM (Lumiscope)			
DEV,NA (BREAST PUMP INSERT)			
ea	38673-0060-15	4.50	9.99
GENTLE EXPRESSIONS NIPPLE SHIELD (Lumiscope)			
DEV,NA (SILICONE)			
ea	38673-0006-80	2.50	5.95
GENTLE EXPRESSIONS NURSING (Lumiscope)			
DEV,NA (WASHABLE)			
6s ea	38673-0006-32	2.49	4.99
GENTLE EXPRESSIONS TRAVEL PACK (Lumiscope)			
DEV,NA (PUMP,PADS,CRM,BOTT,BOOK)			
ea	38673-0006-60	39.90	79.95
GENTLE EXPRESSIONS ULTRA PUMP (Lumiscope)			
DEV,NA (W/LACTO-STIM)			
ea	38673-0006-07	25.00	49.99
GENTLE GEL (Pharm Innov)			
GEL,VG, 20 ml	00036-1500-20	0.90	1.28
90 ml	00036-1500-90	1.84	2.62
150 ml	00036-1500-15	2.43	3.48
GENTLE LAXATIVE (Chain Drug Marketing)			
ECT,PO, 5 mg, 25s ea	63868-0328-25	1.14	3.79

PROD/MFR	HRI, UPC,NDC	AWP	SRP
(Medicine Shoppe)			
ECT,PO, 5 mg, 25s ea	49614-0131-63	4.19	4.19
SUP,RC, 10 mg, 8s ea	49614-0133-35	3.59	3.59
GENTLE NATURALS BABY ECZEMA (Del)			
CRE,TP, 113 gm	10310-0340-16	5.70	8.55
GENTLE NATURALS CRADLE CAP TREATMENT (Del)			
LOT,TP, 113 gm	10310-0340-18	5.70	8.55
GENTLE NATURALS EARACHE DROPS (Del)			
SOL,OT (DROPS)			
30 ml	10310-0324-93	5.48	8.23
GENTLE NATURALS ECZEMA BABY WASH (Del)			
SOA,TP, 163 ml	10310-0340-17	3.96	5.94
GENTLE NATURALS WARM PACK (Del)			
DEV,NA (TEDDY BEAR W/GEL PACK)			
ea	10310-0340-20	7.20	10.80
GENTLE RAIN (Coloplast)			
SHA,TP (PACKET)			
5 ml 300s UD	11701-0102-22	30.00	33.00
59 ml 36s	11701-0102-03	32.04	33.84
(EXTRA MILD)			
59 ml 36s	11701-0041-03	29.16	30.60
118 ml 36s	11701-0102-04	59.40	62.28
(EXTRA MILD)			
237 ml 36s	11701-0041-05	89.64	93.96
473 ml 12s	11701-0102-06	55.68	58.32
621 ml 12s	11701-0102-26	66.48	69.60
(EXTRA MILD)			
621 ml 12s	11701-0041-26	59.88	62.64
1000 ml 12s	11701-0041-46	81.96	85.80
(REFILL)			
1000 ml 12s	11701-0102-46	92.88	97.20
3800 ml 4s	11701-0102-09	115.04	120.40
(EXTRA MILD)			
3840 ml 4s	11701-0041-09	110.76	115.92
GENTLE RAIN ANTIBACTERIAL (Coloplast)			
LIQ,TP (DYE-FREE)			
0.3%, 621 ml 12s	11701-0018-26	64.56	67.56
(REFILL,DYE-FREE)			
0.3%, 1000 ml 12s	11701-0622-46	94.08	98.52
GENTLE SENSITIVE EYES PLUS SALINE (Bausch & Lomb Inc.)			
SOL,NA (2X355ML,THIMEROSAL-FREE)			
355 ml 2s	10119-0028-03	4.54	
GENUINE SENSITIVE EYES REWETTING DROPS (Bausch & Lomb Inc.)			
SOL,NA (THIMEROSAL-FREE)			
15 ml	10119-0073-65	3.70	
GERAVIM (Major)			
LIQ,PO (SHERRY WINE)			
473 ml	00904-5414-16	9.98	
GERI RINSE-FREE (Geritrex)			
SHA,TP (W/ALOE VERA)			
60 ml	92771-0135-02	0.89	
240 ml	92771-0135-08	2.50	
GERI-FREEDA (Freeda)			
TAB,PO (PF,SF,DYE-FREE)			
100s ea	10432-0018-01	7.17	11.95
250s ea	10432-0018-02	14.34	23.90
GERI-HYDROLAC (Geritrex)			
CRE,TP (1X140GM,FRAGRANCE-FREE)			
12%, 140 gm	92771-0613-05	9.50	9.30
LOT,TP (FRAGRANCE-FREE)			
5%, 240 ml	92771-0610-08	5.24	
GERI-HYDROLAC 12 (Geritrex)			
TP, 12%, 240 ml	92771-0612-08	7.67	
420 ml	92771-0612-14	12.74	
GERI-KOT (Geri-Care)			
TAB,PO, 8.6 mg, 100s ea	57896-0451-01	1.10	
GERI-LAV RINSE FREE (Geritrex)			
SOL,TP (PF,DYE-FREE)			
240 ml	92771-0765-03	2.56	
GERI-PROTECT (Geritrex)			
OIN,TP (W/ALOE VERA,TUBE)			
120 gm	54162-0650-02	5.70	
GERI-SHAMPOO W/SHEA BUTTER (Geritrex)			
SOL,TP (SHAMPOO/BODY WASH)			
480 ml	92771-0130-16	3.57	
3840 ml	92771-0130-01	22.14	
GERI-SILK BATH (Geritrex)			
OIL,TP, 60 ml	54162-0300-02	0.81	
240 ml	54162-0300-08	2.28	
GERI-SOFT (Geritrex)			
LOT,TP, 60 ml	54162-0800-02	0.64	
240 ml	54162-0800-08	1.91	

PROD/MFR	HRI, UPC,NDC	AWP	SRP
GERI-VITE (Teva)			
LIQ,PO, 480 ml	00182-6054-40	9.00	
GERI-WASH (Geritrex)			
SOL,TP (BODY WASH/SHAMPOO)			
240 ml	92771-0125-08	1.42	
GERIATON (Silarx)			
LIQ,PO (SHERRY WINE)			
473 ml	54838-0007-80	7.95	
GERIDRYL (Geri-Care)			
TAB,PO, 25 mg, 100s ea	57896-0781-01	1.00	
(CAPLET)			
25 mg, 100s ea	57896-0782-01	1.00	
GERITABS W/BETA CAROTENE (Mason Vit)			
TAB,PO, 100s ea	11845-0099-61	8.11	
GERITOL (Glaxo)			
LIQ,PO, 120 ml	53100-0111-21	2.39	
360 ml	53100-0111-31	5.38	
GERITOL COMPLETE (Glaxo)			
TAB,PO, 40s ea	53100-0112-32	3.98	
100s ea	53100-0112-66	7.64	
180s ea	53100-0112-76	12.30	
GERITOL EXTEND (Glaxo)			
TAB,PO, 100s ea	53100-0002-95	7.64	
GERMANIUM FORTE (Key Company)			
TAB,SL (PF)			
150 mg, 30s ea	11694-0745-01	32.00	
GETS-IT CORN/CALLUS REMOVER (Oakhurst)			
LIQ,TP, 12%, 15 ml	11169-0012-06	3.98	5.97
GHOST SCENT (Monticello)			
TAB,PO, 33.3 mg, 60s ea	10327-0009-61	5.30	
GINGER (Botanical Labs.)			
LIQ,PO, 30 ml	41954-0020-21	4.00	7.99
(Key Company)			
CAP,PO, 250 mg, 100s ea	11694-0647-01	5.25	
(Mason Vit)			
CAP,PO (PF,SF)			
500 mg, 60s ea	11845-1139-05	4.33	
GINGER ROOT (Nature's Bounty)			
CAP,PO, 100s ea	74312-0051-45		5.99
(Rexall)			
CAP,PO (PF,SF)			
550 mg, 75s ea	30768-0012-09	2.27	3.43
GINGKO-GO (Wakunaga)			
TAB,PO (3X,CAPLET)			
120 mg, 20s ea	23542-0540-61	5.85	8.99
GINKGO (Botanical Labs.)			
CAP,PO, 50s ea	41954-0032-64	8.25	16.49
LIQ,PO, 30 ml	41954-0020-23	4.00	7.99
60 ml	41954-0020-10	6.50	12.99
(Mericon)			
TAB,PO, 60 mg, 60s ea	00394-0217-60	11.06	
GINKGO BILOBA (ADH)			
CAP,PO (PF,SF)			
60 mg, 50s ea	60142-0915-55	6.98	13.95
(AmerisourceBergen)			
TAB,PO (PF,PRIVATE LABEL,CAPLET)			
240 mg-120 mg,			
50s ea	24385-0641-71	6.29	6.99
(Cardinal Health)			
CAP,PO (PRIVATE LABEL)			
40 mg, 40s ea	37205-0094-58	7.20	
(Freeda)			
TAB,PO (SF)			
60 mg, 50s ea	10432-0349-00	5.97	9.95
100s ea	10432-0349-01	11.94	19.90
(Lex)			
CAP,PO, 400 mg, 60s ea	49523-0010-06	2.00	
(Major)			
CAP,PO, 60 mg, 50s ea	00904-5088-51	7.13	
(Mason Vit)			
CAP,PO (PF,SF,FRAGRANCE-FREE)			
60 mg, 60s ea	11845-0128-05	12.78	
(PF,SF)			
500 mg, 60s ea	11845-0114-05	5.89	
90s ea	11845-0114-09	7.22	
(Rexall)			
CAP,PO (WHOLE HERB,PF,SF)			
400 mg, 75s ea	30768-0000-74	2.93	4.43
GINKGO BILOBA COMPLEX (Rexall)			
CAP,PO (PF,SF)			
50s ea	30768-0001-11	3.39	5.13

PROD/MFR	HRI, UPC,NDC	AWP	SRP
GINKGO BILOBA EXTRACT (Nature's Bounty)			
TAB,PO (PF,SF)			
30 mg, 60s ea	74312-0056-31		4.99
120s ea	74312-0356-44		8.49
(Neurovites)			
CAP,PO, 40 mg, 100s ea	93595-2022-01	21.95	25.95
GINKGO BILOBA STANDARDIZED (Rexall)			
CAP,PO (PF,SF)			
450 mg, 45s ea	30768-0001-25	4.58	6.93
GINKGO EXTRA STRENGTH (Yerba)			
CAP,PO, 120 mg, 50s ea	46352-0004-55	14.97	24.95
GINKO BILOBA (Key Company)			
CAP,PO, 60 mg, 60s ea	11694-0679-01	6.00	
120 mg, 60s ea	11694-0678-01	8.00	
GINKOBA (Pharmaton)			
TAB,PO, 40 mg, 36s ea	93190-0020-03	6.50	8.21
72s ea	93190-0020-04	11.97	14.98
GINSANA (Pharmaton)			
SGL,PO, 100 mg, 30s ea	93190-0010-01	6.50	9.98
60s ea	93190-0010-02	11.97	14.86
GINSANA GOLD BLEND (Pharmaton)			
TAB,PO (GELCAPLET)			
50s ea	93190-0190-01	7.20	9.99
(CAPLET)			
80s ea	93190-0190-02	10.80	15.78
GINSENG (Basic Vitamins)			
SGL,PO, 250 mg, 50s ea	00761-0992-10	2.40	
(Contract Pharmacal)			
CAP,PO, 518 mg, 100s ea	10267-0158-01	8.00	
(Mason Vit)			
PANAX GINSENG			
SGL,PO (PF,SF)			
100 mg, 60s ea	11845-0128-75	7.22	
GINSENG AMERICAN (ADH)			
CAP,PO, 648 mg, 100s ea	60142-0916-51	8.48	16.95
SGL,PO (PF,SF)			
250 mg, 100s ea	60142-0916-01	6.48	12.95
(Botanical Labs.)			
LIQ,PO, 15 ml	41954-0022-01	3.00	5.99
30 ml	41954-0020-01	5.00	9.99
60 ml	41954-0020-02	8.00	15.99
GINSENG CHINESE (ADH)			
CAP,PO (PF,SF)			
648 mg, 100s ea	60142-0916-61	5.98	11.95
(Botanical Labs.)			
LIQ,PO, 30 ml	41954-0032-04	8.50	16.99
60 ml	41954-0032-34	13.50	26.99
GINSENG COMPLEX (Nature's Bounty)			
CAP,PO, 50s ea	74312-0376-40		9.99
(Rexall)			
CAP,PO, 0.3 mg-750 mg,			
50s ea	30768-0001-12	2.50	3.78
(PF,SF)			
518 mg, 50s ea	30768-0001-73	3.36	5.08
GINSENG CONCENTRATE (Cardinal Health)			
SGL,PO (PF,PRIVATE LABEL)			
100 mg, 30s ea	37205-0177-65	7.39	
GINSENG KOREAN (Health Products Corp)			
CAP,PO (PF,SF)			
518 mg, 50s ea	39686-0014-00	4.50	
(Mason Vit)			
CAP,PO (PF,SF)			
518 mg, 50s ea	11845-0064-29	6.33	
100s ea	11845-0064-21	8.78	
TAB,PO, 1000 mg, 60s ea	11845-0114-15	8.33	
GINSENG KOREAN STANDARDIZED (Rexall)			
CAP,PO (PF,SF)			
560 mg, 45s ea	30768-0001-26	4.00	6.07
GINSENG MANCHURIAN (Nature's Bounty)			
SGL,PO (SOFTGEL)			
250 mg, 50s ea	74312-0012-70		5.95
GINSENG POWER MAX 4X (Action Labs)			
CAP,PO, 500 mg, 50s ea	24675-0333-50	7.49	14.99
100s ea	24675-0333-00	13.49	26.99
LIQ,PO, 60 ml	24675-0333-20	7.99	15.99
GINSENG ROOT (Rexall)			
TAB,PO (PF)			
500 mg, 50s ea	30768-0001-72	3.77	5.72
GINSENG SIBERIAN (Botanical Labs.)			
LIQ,PO, 15 ml	41954-0022-09	2.50	4.99
(GOLD LABEL BOTANICAL)			
30 ml	41954-0020-47	4.00	7.99
(STANDARDIZED)			
30 ml	41954-0032-03	5.00	9.99
(GOLD LABEL BOTANICAL)			
60 ml	41954-0020-22	6.50	12.99
(STANDARDIZED)			
60 ml	41954-0032-33	8.00	15.99
(Cardinal Health)			
CAP,PO (PRIVATE LABEL)			
410 mg, 100s ea	37205-0095-78	3.84	
(Lex)			
CAP,PO, 500 mg, 60s ea	58537-0026-06	2.00	
(Nature's Bounty)			
TAB,PO, 100s ea	74312-0031-71		5.99
(Rexall)			
CAP,PO (PF,SF)			
450 mg, 75s ea	30768-0000-77	2.43	3.63
GLA (Carlson,J.R.)			
SGL,PO (PF,SF,CORN-FREE)			
500 mg, 30s ea	88395-0084-40	4.95	9.90
90s ea	88395-0084-44	12.45	24.90
GLEN-SLEEVE II ARM PROTECTOR (Western Medical)			
DEV,NA (HAND-WRIST-ARM, WHITE)			
12s ea	16926-0100-12	206.00	
(HAND-WRIST-THUMB, WHITE)			
12s ea	16926-0200-12	247.01	
GLEN-SLEEVE II LEG PROTECTOR (Western Medical)			
DEV,NA (BELOW KNEE, WHITE)			
12s ea	16926-0300-12	215.13	
GLUCERNA (Abbott)			
LIQ,PO (W/FIBER,RTU,VANILLA)			
240 ml 6s	70074-0502-41	19.87	
GLUCERNA 1.2 CAL (Abbott)			
LIQ,PO (1X240ML,READY-TO-HANG)			
240 ml	70074-0509-05	4.86	
(1X1000ML,READY-TO-HANG)			
1000 ml	70074-0509-07	25.55	
(1X1500ML,READY-TO-HANG)			
1500 ml	70074-0509-03	38.32	
GLUCERNA 1.5 CAL (Abbott)			
SOL,PO (GLUTEN-FREE)			
237 ml	70074-0535-35	5.46	
GLUCERNA MEAL (Abbott)			
BAR,PO (FOR PEOPLE W/DIABETES)			
58 gm 24s	70074-0576-04	42.05	
58 gm 24s	70074-0576-07	42.05	
58 gm 24s	70074-0576-17	42.05	
58 gm 24s	70074-0577-19	42.05	
GLUCERNA MEAL REPLACEMENT (Abbott)			
BAR,PO (CHOC PEANUT,MED SUPV)			
58 gm	70074-0569-68	1.75	
(CHOCOLATE PEANUT)			
58 gm 24s	70074-0569-67	42.05	
GLUCERNA ROSS READY-TO-HANG (Abbott)			
LIQ,PO, 1000 ml	70074-0512-07	16.80	
1500 ml	70074-0526-02	25.20	
GLUCERNA SELECT (Abbott)			
LIQ,PO (HIGH PROTEIN,VANILLA)			
237 ml	70074-0577-02	3.65	
(RTH,ENTERAL,HP,VANILLA)			
1000 ml	70074-0577-04	18.48	
1500 ml	70074-0577-06	27.72	
GLUCERNA SNACK (Abbott)			
BAR,PO (CHEWY,LEMON CRUNCH)			
4s ea	70074-0546-16	5.14	
(VANILLA,CARAMEL NUT)			
38 gm 4s	70074-0576-10	5.14	
(MED SUPV,CARAMEL)			
40 gm	70074-0569-59	1.28	
(STRAWBERRY YOGURT)			
40 gm 4s	70074-0579-73	5.14	
(CHOCOLATE CARAMEL)			
40 gm 24s	70074-0569-58	30.82	
GLUCERNA SNACK BAR (Abbott)			
BAR,PO (FUDGE GRAHAM)			
40 gm 4s	70074-0579-70	5.14	
GLUCERNA WEIGHT LOSS SHAKE (Abbott)			
LIQ,PO (BANANA,BANANA)			
325 ml 4s	70074-0576-49	11.87	
(CHOCOLATE,CHOCOLATE)			
325 ml 4s	70074-0576-46	11.84	
(DULCE DE LECHE)			
325 ml 4s	70074-0576-55	11.84	
(PEACH,PEACH)			
325 ml 4s	70074-0576-68	11.84	
(VANILLA,VANILLA)			
325 ml 4s	70074-0576-43	11.84	
GLUCOCARD 01 BLOOD GLUCOSE METER (Arkray)			
DEV,NA, ea	08317-7200-01	45.00	
GLUCOCARD 01 BLOOD GLUCOSE MONITORING SYSTEM (Arkray)			
DEV,NA, ea	08317-7211-00	50.00	
ea	08317-7411-00	20.25	
GLUCOCARD 01 CONTROL SOLUTION (Arkray)			
DEV,NA (2X2.5ML)			
2s ea	08317-7400-06	12.00	
2.5 ml	08317-7200-05	7.50	
GLUCOCARD 01 SENSOR BLOOD GLUCOSE TEST STRIPS (Arkray)			
DEV,NA, 50s ea	08317-7200-50	36.00	
50s ea	08317-7400-50	21.81	
GLUCOCARD 01-MINI (Arkray)			
DEV,NA, ea	08317-7311-00	15.75	
GLUCOCARD VITAL BLOOD GLUCOSE MONITORING SYSTEM (Arkray)			
DEV,NA, ea	08317-7611-00	22.50	
GLUCOCARD VITAL SENSOR BLOOD GLUCOSE TEST STRIPS (Arkray)			
DEV,NA, 50s ea	08317-7600-50	47.00	
GLUCOCARD X-METER BLOOD GLUCOSE MONITORING SYSTEM (Arkray)			
DEV,NA, ea	08317-7511-00	24.75	
GLUCOCARD X-METER CONTROL (Arkray)			
DEV,NA, 2.5 ml	08317-7500-05	9.00	
GLUCOCARD X-SENSOR BLOOD GLUCOSE TEST STRIPS (Arkray)			
DEV,NA, 50s ea	08317-7500-50	59.47	
GLUCOLET 2 (Bayer Diabetes Care)			
DEV,NA, 10s ea	00193-5976-10	106.44	
GLUCOS-AMINE (Bio-Tech Pharm)			
CAP,PO, 500 mg, 100s ea	53191-0199-01	15.25	
GLUCOSAMINE (Freeda)			
TAB,PO (100%VEGETARIAN,SF)			
500 mg, 100s ea	10432-0362-01	12.57	20.95
250s ea	10432-0362-02	25.14	41.90
GLUCOSAMINE & CHONDROITIN (Major)			
CAP,PO (DOUBLE STRENGTH)			
400 mg-500 mg,			
180s ea	00904-5481-93	26.20	
TAB,PO (DOUBLE STRENGTH,CAPLET)			
400 mg-500 mg,			
60s ea	00904-5592-52	17.25	
(CAPLET,PF,SF,DYE-FREE)			
400 mg-500 mg,			
180s ea	00904-5592-93	24.00	
(TRIPLE STRENGTH,CAPLET)			
600 mg-750 mg,			
90s ea	00904-5594-89	18.75	
TER,PO (CAPLET,PF,SF,DYE-FREE)			
600 mg-750 mg,			
150s ea	00904-5594-92	28.50	
(Aidarex)			
REPACK			
TER,PO (PF,SF,DYE-FREE,CAPLET)			
600 mg-750 mg,			
14s ea	33261-0350-14	15.50	
30s ea	33261-0350-30	33.30	
60s ea	33261-0350-60	66.60	
90s ea	33261-0350-90	99.90	
100s ea	33261-0350-00	111.00	
120s ea	33261-0350-02	133.20	
180s ea	33261-0350-03	199.80	
(Altura)			
REPACK			
TAB,PO, 400 mg-500 mg,			
100s ea	63874-0871-01	149.96	
(DHS, Inc.)			
REPACK			
CAP,PO (PF,SF,DYE-FREE)			
400 mg-500 mg,			
60s ea	55887-0520-60	24.00	
90s ea	55887-0520-90	36.00	
120s ea	55887-0520-82	51.00	
(Nucare Pharm)			
REPACK			
TAB,PO, 400 mg-500 mg,			
60s ea	68071-0313-60	37.75	
120s ea	68071-0313-91	33.98	

PROD/MFR	HRI, UPC,NDC	AWP	SRP
(Pharma Pac)			
REPACK			
CAP,PO (DOUBLE STRENGTH,PF,SF)			
400 mg-500 mg,			
30s ea	52959-0809-30	19.18	
60s ea	52959-0809-60	38.34	
120s ea	52959-0809-02	69.60	
TAB,PO (PF,SF,DYE-FREE,CAPLET)			
400 mg-500 mg,			
30s ea	52959-0768-30	19.18	
60s ea	52959-0768-60	38.34	
120s ea	52959-0768-02	69.60	
(Southwood)			
REPACK			
CAP,PO (PF,SF,DYE-FREE)			
400 mg-500 mg,			
40s ea	58016-0179-40	37.00	
56s ea	58016-0179-56	51.80	
GLUCOSAMINE & CHONDROITIN WITH MSM (Major)			
TAB,PO (PF,SF,STARCH-FREE)			
400 mg-250 mg-500 mg,			
90s ea	00904-5830-89	15.72	
GLUCOSAMINE CHONDROITIN 1500 COMPLX (Mason Vit)			
CAP,PO (PF,SF)			
60s ea	11845-0130-35	19.89	
100s ea	11845-0130-31	28.78	
(Dispensing Solutions)			
REPACK			
CAP,PO (PF,SF)			
60s ea	55045-3294-02	28.78	
100s ea	55045-3294-01	37.67	
GLUCOSAMINE CHONDROITIN 500 COMPLEX (Mason Vit)			
CAP,PO (PF,SF)			
200 mg-250 mg-5 mg-33 mg,			
30s ea	11845-0124-88	8.78	
100s ea	11845-0124-81	19.89	
GLUCOSAMINE COMPLEX (Rexall)			
TAB,PO (PF,SF)			
60s ea	30768-0000-29	8.79	13.32
GLUCOSAMINE FORTE (Miller)			
CAP,PO (SF)			
90s ea	17204-0938-85	33.55	
GLUCOSAMINE MSM COMPLEX (Major)			
TAB,PO, 60s ea	00904-5473-52	6.95	
GLUCOSAMINE SULFATE (ADH)			
CAP,PO (PF,SF)			
500 mg, 60s ea	60142-0482-96	10.98	21.95
(Breckenridge Pharm)			
CAP,PO (PF)			
500 mg, 30s ea	51991-0109-33	5.40	
60s ea	51991-0109-06	9.50	
(Carlson,J.R.)			
CAP,PO (PF,CORN-FREE,SALT-FREE)			
124 mg-750 mg-80 mg,			
60s ea	88395-0084-76	9.95	19.90
180s ea	88395-0084-72	27.50	55.00
(Key Company)			
CAP,PO (SF)			
750 mg, 60s ea	11694-0691-01	8.00	
120s ea	11694-0691-02	16.00	
(Major)			
CAP,PO, 500 mg, 60s ea	00904-5293-52	12.75	
(Mason Vit)			
TAB,PO (PF,SF)			
115 mg-500 mg-90 mg,			
30s ea	11845-0120-98	6.56	
90s ea	11845-0120-99	15.44	
(Mericon)			
TAB,PO (CAPLET)			
500 mg, 90s ea	00394-0250-09	10.74	
(Nature's Bounty)			
CAP,PO (PF,SF)			
500 mg, 80s ea	74312-0077-10		10.99
(Progressive Labs.)			
CAP,PO, 500 mg, 60s ea	51821-0812-60	8.00	16.00
(Teva)			
CAP,PO, 500 mg, 60s ea	00182-4048-26	11.99	
(A-S Medication)			
REPACK			
CAP,PO, 500 mg-62.5 mg,			
120s ea	54569-4977-00	25.27	
(Altura)			
REPACK			
CAP,PO, 500 mg, 30s ea	63874-1090-03	7.62	
60s ea	63874-1090-06	15.25	
90s ea	63874-1090-09	22.87	
120s ea	63874-1090-02	30.49	
GLUCOSAMINE, CHONDROITIN AND MSM (Rugby)			
TAB,PO (CAPLET)			
60s ea	00536-3111-08	10.56	
GLUCOSAMINE/CHONDRO (Physician Partner)			
REPACK			
CAP,PO, 400 mg-500 mg,			
30s ea	21695-0064-30	33.30	
60s ea	21695-0064-60	66.60	
90s ea	21695-0064-90	99.90	
GLUCOSAMINE/CHONDROITIN (21st Century)			
CAP,PO (DOUBLE STRENGTH)			
400 mg-500 mg-30 mg,			
400s ea	40985-0222-91	42.00	69.99
TAB,PO (TRIPLE STRENGTH)			
600 mg-750 mg,			
60s ea	40985-0224-76	12.00	19.99
(Basic Organics, Inc.)			
CAP,PO, 400 mg-500 mg,			
60s ea	54458-0100-22	11.49	
120s ea	54458-0200-22	21.49	
(A-S Medication)			
REPACK			
CAP,PO, 400 mg-500 mg,			
120s ea	54569-5250-00	31.04	
(Bryant Ranch)			
REPACK			
CAP,PO (DOUBLE STRENGTH)			
400 mg-500 mg-30 mg,			
90s ea	63629-3143-03	99.32	
100s ea	63629-3143-04	102.52	
(Keltman Pharma., Inc.)			
REPACK			
CAP,PO (DOUBLE STRENGTH)			
400 mg-500 mg-30 mg,			
60s ea	68387-0431-60	46.35	
(Nucare Pharm)			
REPACK			
CAP,PO, 400 mg-500 mg,			
60s ea	66267-1011-06	48.85	
(Quality Care Prod)			
REPACK			
CAP,PO, 400 mg-500 mg,			
60s ea	49999-0710-60	48.00	
90s ea	49999-0647-12	72.00	
90s ea	49999-0710-90	72.00	
120s ea	49999-0710-12	96.00	
240s ea	49999-0710-24	192.00	
(Stat Rx)			
REPACK			
CAP,PO, 400 mg-500 mg-30 mg,			
84s ea	16590-0668-62	59.79	
TAB,PO, 600 mg-750 mg,			
84s ea	16590-0686-62	59.81	
GLUCOSAMINE/CHONDROITIN 500 COMPLEX (Pharma Pac)			
REPACK			
CAP,PO (PF,SF)			
90s ea	52959-0486-90	46.35	
GLUCOSAMINE/CHONDROITIN DS (Phys Total Care)			
REPACK			
TAB,PO (PF)			
400 mg-500 mg-100 mg,			
120s ea	54868-4762-00	28.65	
160s ea	54868-4762-01	27.69	
GLUCOSAMINE/CHONDROITIN/MSM (Quality Care Prod)			
REPACK			
TAB,PO, 240s ea	49999-0648-24	175.00	
GLUCOSAMINE/MSM COMPLEX (Nature's Bounty)			
TAB,PO (MAXIMUM STRENGTH,PF,SF)			
60s ea	74312-0061-31		12.99
(Altura)			
REPACK			
TAB,PO (PF,SF,DAIRY-FREE)			
30s ea	63874-1021-03	28.00	
60s ea	63874-1021-06	56.00	
80s ea	63874-1021-08	74.67	
90s ea	63874-1021-09	84.00	
100s ea	63874-1021-01	93.33	
120s ea	63874-1021-04	112.00	
GLUCOSE (Major)			
TAB,PO (ORANGE)			
4 gm, 10s ea	00904-5896-15	1.89	
(Medicine Shoppe)			
CTB,PO (ORANGE)			
4 gm, 10s ea	49614-0620-52	1.59	1.59
(RASPBERRY)			
4 gm, 10s ea	49614-0621-52	1.59	1.59
(ORANGE)			
4 gm, 50s ea	49614-0620-71	5.99	5.99
(RASPBERRY)			
4 gm, 50s ea	49614-0621-71	5.99	5.99
(Medtronic Minimed)			
CTB,PO (CAFF FREE,AF,DYE-FREE)			
4 gm, 50s ea	63706-0031-50	11.94	
50s ea	63706-0032-50	11.94	
50s ea	63706-0033-50	11.94	
GLUCOSE/KETONE CONTROL SOLUTION (Abbott)			
DEV,NA (MID,1-NORMAL)			
ea	57599-0312-01	7.08	
(1-LOW,1-HIGH)			
2s ea	57599-0139-01	8.28	
(1-LOW,1-MED,1-HIGH)			
3s ea	57599-0138-01	10.50	
GLUCOSTIX (Phys Total Care)			
REPACK			
DEV,NA, 50s ea	54868-0863-00	54.19	
GLUTAMIC ACID (Carlson,J.R.)			
L-GLUTAMIC ACID			
POW,PO, 100 gm	88395-0068-15	2.95	5.90
(Mason Vit)			
TAB,PO, 500 mg, 100s ea	11845-0054-91	4.44	
(Neurovites)			
TAB,PO, 500 mg, 100s ea	93595-2026-01	10.95	
L-GLUTAMIC ACID HCL			
CAP,PO, 340 mg, 100s ea	93595-2027-01	32.95	
GLUTAMIC-500 (Key Company)			
TAB,PO (SF)			
500 mg, 100s ea	11694-0866-01	5.50	
250s ea	11694-0866-25	11.50	
GLUTAMINE (Baxter)			
PDS,PO, 10 gm/dose,			
450 gm	00338-9170-91	56.40	
(Bio-Tech Pharm)			
CAP,PO, 500 mg, 100s ea	53191-0236-01	7.50	
(Carlson,J.R.)			
L-GLUTAMINE			
CAP,PO, 750 mg, 90s ea	88395-0068-21	8.30	16.60
300s ea	88395-0068-23	24.50	49.00
POW,PO, 100 gm	88395-0068-25	7.45	14.90
1000 gm	88395-0068-26	49.95	99.90
(Freeda)			
PDR,PO (SF)			
4000 mg/5 ml,			
240 gm	10432-0340-02	17.37	28.95
480 gm	10432-0340-03	32.40	54.00
TAB,PO (PF,SF,DYE-FREE)			
500 mg, 100s ea	10432-0246-01	11.97	19.95
(Mason Vit)			
TAB,PO, 500 mg, 60s ea	11845-0077-05	6.89	
GLUTAMINE-500 (Key Company)			
CAP,PO, 500 mg, 100s ea	11694-0687-01	10.00	
250s ea	11694-0687-02	22.00	
GLUTANAC (Westlake Labs.)			
CAP,PO (PF,SF)			
42.3%-38.2%-19.5%,			
90s ea	10539-0806-77	14.00	20.00
GLUTAPAK R (Victus, Inc.)			
PDS,PO, 15 gm	12197-0700-22	170.00	
GLUTAREX-1 (Abbott)			
PDR,PO, 400 gm	70074-0511-41	40.46	
GLUTAREX-2 (Abbott)			
PDR,PO, 400 gm	70074-0511-43	81.12	
GLUTASOLVE (Nestle)			
PKT,PO (TUBE FEEDING)			
15 gm/packet,			
56s ea	00212-2833-78	109.20	
GLUTATHIONE BOOSTER (Carlson,J.R.)			
CAP,PO (PF,SF,CORN-FREE)			
60s ea	88395-0048-50	9.94	19.88
180s ea	88395-0048-52	27.75	55.50

PROD/MFR	HRI, UPC,NDC	AWP	SRP
GLUTOFAC (Kenwood)			
TAB,PO (CAPLET)			
90s ea	00482-0154-90	68.84	
GLUTOL (Paddock)			
SOL,PO, 100 gm/180 ml,			
180 ml	00574-1959-06	8.25	
GLUTOSE (Phys Total Care)			
REPACK			
CTB,PO, 5 gm, 12s ea	54868-3741-00	12.26	
GEL,PO, 40%, 15 gm 3s	54868-3981-00	10.20	
GLUTOSE 15 (Paddock)			
GEL,PO (DYE-FREE,GRAPE)			
15 gm, 15 gm	00574-0070-15	3.75	
(3X15GM,DYE-FREE,GRAPE)			
15 gm, 15 gm 3s	00574-0070-30	11.20	
40%, 15 gm	00574-0069-15	3.75	
15 gm 3s UD	00574-0069-30	11.20	
GLUTOSE 45 (Paddock)			
GEL,PO, 40%, 45 gm	00574-0069-45	11.20	
GLY-OXIDE (Glaxo)			
SOL,MM (AF)			
10%, 15 ml	00088-1010-05	4.58	
60 ml	00088-1010-02	8.27	
GLYCERIN PHENOLATE (Lex)			
SOL,OT, 95%-5%, 15 ml	49523-0073-05	0.65	
GLYCERIN SUPPOSITORIES (Albertson's)			
SUP,RC, 25s ea	12810-0320-63	1.29	
(AmerisourceBergen)			
SUP,RC (INFANT,PRIVATE LABEL)			
25s ea	24385-0317-63	1.43	1.59
(PRIVATE LABEL)			
25s ea	24385-0320-63	1.70	1.89
50s ea	24385-0320-71	2.42	2.69
(Cardinal Health)			
SUP,RC (PRIVATE LABEL)			
25s ea	37205-0320-63	5.42	
(Consolidated Midland)			
SUP,RC, 12s ea	00223-5500-12	1.75	
(PEDIATRIC)			
12s ea	00223-5501-12	1.75	
25s ea	00223-5500-25	2.10	
(PEDIATRIC)			
25s ea	00223-5501-25	2.10	
50s ea	00223-5500-50	3.25	
100s ea	00223-5500-00	4.80	
(Family Phcy)			
SUP,RC (PRIVATE LABEL)			
12s ea	52735-0506-02	1.79	1.99
25s ea	52735-0505-06	1.70	1.89
(G&W)			
SUP,RC, 12s ea	00713-0101-13	1.92	
12s ea	00713-0102-13	2.07	
25s ea	00713-0101-26	2.59	
25s ea	00713-0102-26	2.59	
50s ea	00713-0101-51	3.86	
100s ea	00713-0101-02	6.27	
(Major)			
SUP,RC, 12s ea	00904-2666-12	1.80	
25s ea	00904-2666-17	2.40	
25s ea	00904-2667-17	2.40	
100s ea	00904-2667-60	5.99	
(Qualitest)			
SUP,RC, 25s ea	00603-0511-35	2.62	
50s ea	00603-0511-19	3.53	
(Rose)			
SUP,RC, 12s ea	42037-0109-12	1.85	
(INFANT)			
12s ea	42037-0110-12	1.85	
25s ea	42037-0109-25	2.45	
(INFANT)			
25s ea	42037-0110-25	2.45	
50s ea	42037-0109-50	3.95	
100s ea	42037-0109-99	4.95	
(Southwood)			
REPACK			
SUP,RC, 12s ea	58016-7023-01	4.82	
GLYCERIN SUPPOSITORIES INFANT (Cardinal Health)			
SUP,RC (PRIVATE LABEL)			
25s ea	37205-0317-63	1.68	
GLYCERIN SUPPOSITORIES PEDIATRIC (Southwood)			
REPACK			
SUP,RC, 12s ea	58016-1053-01	4.82	
GLYCINE (Carlson,J.R.)			
PDR,PO (PF,CORN-FREE,SALT-FREE)			
2300 mg, 100 gm	88395-0068-35	4.45	8.90
(Freeda)			
POW,PO (PURE,FREE FORM,SF)			
2250 mg/2.25 gm,			
480 gm	10432-0185-03	16.17	26.95
GLYCO GEL (Topix)			
GEL,TP (OFFICE USE ONLY)			
120 gm	51326-0033-04	20.00	
120 gm	51326-0034-04	25.00	
120 gm	51326-0036-04	35.00	
GLYCOLIC ACID (Neurovites)			
CRE,TP, 12%, 60 gm	93595-2023-01	26.50	
120 gm	93595-2023-02	32.50	
GLYCOLIC ACID/PYRUVIC ACID (Neurovites)			
CRE,TP, 12%-1%, 60 gm	93595-2024-01	32.50	
120 gm	93595-2024-02	40.00	
GLYTROL ULTRAPAK (Nestle)			
LIQ,PO (1000MLX6)			
1000 ml 6s	00065-9086-72	63.50	
(1500MLX4)			
1500 ml 4s	00065-9086-73	63.50	
GNC CALCIUM/MAGNESIUM WITH VITAMIN D (Rite Aid)			
CAP,PO (SODIUM-FREE,YEAST-FREE)			
200 mg-100 mg-33.33 iu,			
180s ea	48107-0038-49	9.59	11.99
GNC L-ARGININE 500 (Rite Aid)			
CAP,PO (SODIUM-FREE,YEAST-FREE)			
500 mg, 90s ea	48107-0001-92	7.99	9.99
GNC NAC 600 (Rite Aid)			
CAP,PO (SODIUM-FREE,YEAST-FREE)			
600 mg, 60s ea	48107-0031-50	10.39	12.99
GNC NIACIN 250 (Rite Aid)			
TAB,PO (SODIUM-FREE,YEAST-FREE)			
250 mg, 100s ea	48107-0024-89	3.99	4.99
GNC NIACINAMIDE 100 (Rite Aid)			
PO (SODIUM-FREE,YEAST-FREE)			
100 mg, 250s ea	48107-0005-89	3.99	4.99
GNP (AmerisourceBergen)			
BLOOD GLUCOSE			
DEV,NA (STRIP,PRIVATE LABEL)			
50s ea	24385-0311-50	17.09	18.99
BLOOD GLUCOSE VALUE PACK			
DEV,NA (110 STRIPS/FREE METER)			
ea	87701-0523-73	44.99	49.99
CENTURY			
CTB,PO (PRIVATE LABEL,CHERRY)			
50s ea	24385-0261-71	7.19	7.99
COTTON BALLS			
DEV,NA (PRIVATE LABEL)			
300s ea	87701-0247-27	1.61	1.79
COTTON BALLS TRIPLE SIZE			
NA (PRIVATE LABEL)			
100s ea	87701-0247-25	1.16	1.29
COTTON ROUNDS			
NA (PRIVATE LABEL)			
80s ea	87701-0896-90	1.25	1.39
COTTON SQUARES			
NA (PRIVATE LABEL)			
200s ea	87701-0247-48	3.32	3.69
COTTON SWABS			
DEV,NA (PRIVATE LABEL)			
300s ea	87701-0485-70	1.79	1.99
DIGITAL FLEXIBLE-TIP THERMOMETER			
DEV,NA (PRIVATE LABEL)			
ea	87701-0892-49	8.99	9.99
DIGITAL THERMOMETER			
NA (PRIVATE LABEL)			
ea	87701-0391-30	7.19	7.99
FOREHEAD THERMOMETER			
NA (PRIVATE LABEL)			
ea	87701-0565-86	1.79	1.99
ONE STEP PREGNANCY			
DEV,NA (PRIVATE LABEL)			
ea	87701-0552-62	7.19	7.99
2s ea	87701-0894-80	9.89	10.99
PUMICE STONE SMOOTHING			
DEV,NA (PRIVATE LABEL)			
ea	87701-0838-25	1.34	1.89
SENSITIVE SKIN MOISTURIZING			
CRE,TP (FRAGRANCE-FREE)			
480 gm	87701-0893-01	5.39	5.99
LOT,TP, 480 ml	87701-0892-98	6.29	6.99
STRETCH BANDAGE			
DEV,NA (2"X4 YDS,PRIVATE LABEL)			
ea	87701-0486-12	1.16	1.29
(3"X4 YDS,PRIVATE LABEL)			
ea	87701-0486-13	1.70	2.59
TALKING DIGITAL THERMOMETER			
DEV,NA (PRIVATE LABEL)			
ea	87701-0905-62	13.49	17.19
THERMOMETER PROBE COVERS			
DEV,NA (PRIVATE LABEL)			
25s ea	87701-0565-80	1.25	1.39
GNP 12 HOUR COLD MAXIMUM STRENGTH (AmerisourceBergen)			
12 HOUR COLD MAXIMUM STRENGTH			
TER,PO (NON-DROWSY,CAPLET)			
120 mg, 10s ea	24385-0363-52	3.41	3.79
GNP 2 IN 1 DANDRUFF (AmerisourceBergen)			
2 IN 1 DANDRUFF			
SHA,TP (NORMAL OR DRY)			
1%, 400 ml	24385-0455-48	3.05	3.99
GNP 3 DAY VAGINAL CREAM (AmerisourceBergen)			
3 DAY VAGINAL CREAM			
CRE,VG (3 DISPOSABLE APPLICATRS)			
2%, 25 gm	24385-0110-09	8.99	9.99
GNP ANTI-GAS ULTRA STRENGTH (AmerisourceBergen)			
ANTI-GAS ULTRA STRENGTH			
SGL,PO (PRIVATE LABEL,SOFTGEL)			
180 mg, 60s ea	24385-0460-72	6.29	6.99
GNP ANTI-ITCH (AmerisourceBergen)			
ANTI-ITCH			
CRE,TP, 2%-0.1%, 28 gm	24385-0025-03	2.69	2.99
GNP ASPIRIN ADULT LOW STRENGTH (AmerisourceBergen)			
ASPIRIN ADULT LOW STRENGTH			
CTB,PO (ORANGE,LOW STRENGTH)			
81 mg, 36s ea	24385-0364-68	1.61	1.79
GNP COUGH DROPS (AmerisourceBergen)			
COUGH DROPS			
LOZ,MM (SF,SALT-FREE,MENTHOL)			
6.1 mg, 25s ea	24385-0057-63	1.16	1.29
GNP CROMOLYN SODIUM (AmerisourceBergen)			
CROMOLYN SODIUM			
SPR,NS, 5.2 mg/actuation,			
26 ml	24385-0224-36	11.69	12.99
GNP GLUCOSAMINE & CHONDROITIN (AmerisourceBergen)			
GLUCOSAMINE & CHONDROITIN			
TER,PO (PRIVATE LABEL)			
600 mg-750 mg,			
80s ea	24385-0381-41	19.79	21.99
GNP GLUCOSAMINE COMPLEX (AmerisourceBergen)			
GLUCOSAMINE COMPLEX			
TAB,PO (CAPLET)			
200 mg-300 mg,			
60s ea	24385-0950-72	8.99	9.99
GNP LAXATIVE MAXIMUM STRENGTH (AmerisourceBergen)			
LAXATIVE MAXIMUM STRENGTH			
TAB,PO (PILL)			
25 mg, 24s ea	24385-0369-62	3.95	4.39
GNP MOTION SICKNESS RELIEF (AmerisourceBergen)			
MOTION SICKNESS RELIEF			
TAB,PO (LESS DROWSY)			
25 mg, 8s ea	24385-0388-51	2.69	2.99
GNP MSM GLUCOSAMINE COMPLEX (AmerisourceBergen)			
MSM GLUCOSAMINE COMPLEX			
TAB,PO (PRIVATE LABEL,CAPLET)			
60s ea	24385-0672-72	8.99	9.99
GNP OIL FREE (AmerisourceBergen)			
OIL FREE			
LOT,TP (SPF 30 WATERPROOF)			
118 ml	24385-0229-26	4.49	5.79
GNP ORAL ANESTHETIC (AmerisourceBergen)			
ORAL ANESTHETIC			
GEL,MM (MAXIMUM STRENGTH)			
20%, 7 gm	24385-0631-67	4.49	4.99
GNP ORAL SALINE LAXATIVE (AmerisourceBergen)			
ORAL SALINE LAXATIVE			
SOL,PO (SF,LEMON)			
0.9 gm/5 ml-2.4 gm/5 ml,			
90 ml	24385-0358-21	2.96	2.99
GNP OYSTER SHELL CALCIUM (AmerisourceBergen)			
OYSTER SHELL CALCIUM			
TAB,PO (PRIVATE LABEL)			
500 mg, 100s ea	24385-0644-78	3.59	3.99

PROD/MFR	HRI, UPC,NDC	AWP	SRP
GNP URINARY PAIN RELIEF (AmerisourceBergen)			
URINARY PAIN RELIEF			
TAB,PO, 95 mg, 30s ea	24385-0013-65	4.49	4.99
GOLD BOND ANTI-ITCH (Chattem)			
CRE,TP, 1%-1%, 30 gm	41167-0050-10	3.30	
GOLD BOND MEDICATED BABY POWDER (Chattem)			
POW,TP, 120 gm	41167-0020-50	3.00	
120 gm	41167-0023-04	3.30	
300 gm	41167-0021-00	6.00	
300 gm	41167-0023-10	6.60	
GOLD BOND MEDICATED BODY POWDER (Chattem)			
POW,TP (TRIPLE ACTION)			
60 gm	41167-0012-40	12.00	
(EXT. STR.)			
120 gm	41167-0040-40	3.60	
(TRIPLE ACTION)			
120 gm	41167-0010-40	3.00	
(EXT. STR.)			
300 gm	41167-0041-00	7.20	
(TRIPLE ACTION)			
300 gm	41167-0011-00	6.00	
GOLD BOND MEDICATED FOOT POWDER (Chattem)			
POW,TP (TRIPLE ACTION,MAX. STR.)			
120 gm	41167-0017-04	3.00	
3000 gm	41167-0017-10	6.00	
GOLD DUST (Southwest)			
POW,TP (3GMX10X10)			
10s ea	45713-0993-00	420.00	85.70
(3GMX10)			
3 gm 10s UD	45713-0693-00	42.00	85.70
GOLDEN AGE (Hi-Tech)			
LIQ,PO, 240 ml	50383-0786-08	5.00	
GOLDEN ALOE (Carlson,J.R.)			
SGL,PO (PF,SF,SALT-FREE,SOFTGEL)			
100 mg, 60s ea	88395-0080-50	4.95	9.90
180s ea	88395-0080-52	13.85	27.70
GOLDEN PRIMROSE (Carlson,J.R.)			
SGL,PO (SOFTGEL)			
1300 mg, 50s ea	88395-0088-00	7.95	15.90
90s ea	88395-0088-01	13.45	26.90
GOLDEN SEAL (Key Company)			
CAP,PO, 300 mg, 60s ea	11694-0669-01	4.25	
GOLDEN SUNSHINE FAR INFRARED HERBAL (Golden Sunshine)			
TDM,TP (11CMX15CM,PRIVATE LABEL)			
3s ea	67475-0112-01	5.95	5.95
3s ea	67475-0112-03	5.95	5.95
GOLDEN SUNSHINE HERBAL (Golden Sunshine)			
CRE,TP (PRIVATE LABEL)			
50 gm	67475-0103-02	12.00	12.00
50 gm	67475-0113-02	12.00	12.00
450 gm	67475-0113-01	90.00	90.00
500 gm	67475-0103-01	96.00	96.00
PAS,TP, 300 gm	67475-0101-02	25.00	25.00
1200 gm	67475-0101-01	90.00	90.00
1200 gm	67475-0211-01	90.00	90.00
SPR,TP, 120 ml	67475-0104-01	12.50	12.50
120 ml	67475-0114-01	12.50	12.50
TDM,TP (11CMX15CM,PRIVATE LABEL)			
3s ea	67475-0102-01	4.95	4.95
3s ea	67475-0202-01	4.95	4.95
(36CMX15CM,PRIVATE LABEL)			
10s ea	67475-0102-03	60.00	60.00
GOLDEN SUNSHINE NATURAL HERBAL PAIN TERMINATOR (Golden Sunshine)			
CRE,TP (PRIVATE LABEL)			
2%-0.5%, 50 gm	67475-0313-02	12.00	12.00
450 gm	67475-0313-01	90.00	90.00
GOLDENSEAL (ADH)			
CAP,PO (PF,SF)			
500 mg, 100s ea	60142-0917-01	17.75	35.50
(Botanical Labs.)			
LIQ,PO, 15 ml	41954-0022-07	4.50	8.99
30 ml	41954-0020-25	7.00	13.99
30 ml	41954-0032-01	7.50	14.99
60 ml	41954-0020-12	11.00	21.99
60 ml	41954-0032-31	12.00	23.99
(Mason Vit)			
CAP,PO (PF,SF)			
500 mg, 60s ea	11845-0114-55	11.00	
GOLDENSEAL ROOT (Mason Vit)			
PO (PF,SF)			
100 mg, 60s ea	11845-0128-85	12.78	
(Rexall)			
CAP,PO (PF,SF)			
400 mg, 50s ea	30768-0000-78	5.46	8.27

PROD/MFR	HRI, UPC,NDC	AWP	SRP
GONAK (Akorn)			
SOL,OP, 2.5%, 15 ml	17478-0064-12	11.19	
GONIOSOFT (Ocusoft)			
SOL,OP, 2.5%, 15 ml	54799-0503-15	12.43	
GONIOVISC (HUB Pharma)			
SOL,OP, 2%, 15 ml	17238-0615-15	8.13	
2.5%, 15 ml	17238-0610-15	8.13	
GOOD BREATH (Scandinavian)			
SGL,PO (PF,SF,CORN-FREE)			
60s ea	51137-0011-10	2.99	4.99
GOOD NEIGHBOR ALCOHOL SWABS (AmerisourceBergen)			
PAD,TP (PRIVATE LABEL)			
70%, 100s ea	87701-0698-17	1.79	1.99
GOOD NEIGHBOR ALLERGY & CONGESTION RELIEF 24 HOUR (AmerisourceBergen)			
T24,PO (NON-DROWSY)			
10 mg-240 mg, 10s ea	24385-0351-52	8.99	9.99
GOOD NEIGHBOR ALLERGY RELIEF (AmerisourceBergen)			
ODT,PO (NON-DROWSY)			
10 mg, 12s ea	24385-0540-53	8.09	8.99
GOOD NEIGHBOR ANUSERT (AmerisourceBergen)			
SUP,RC (PRIVATE LABEL)			
51%, 12s ea	87701-0910-57	3.95	4.39
GOOD NEIGHBOR CALDYPHEN (AmerisourceBergen)			
LOT,TP (MEDICATED,PRIVATE LABEL)			
1%-0.1%, 177 ml	24385-0076-82	3.59	3.99
GOOD NEIGHBOR CAP-PROFEN (AmerisourceBergen)			
TAB,PO (PRIVATE LABEL,CAPLET)			
200 mg, 100s ea	24385-0483-78	6.29	6.99
GOOD NEIGHBOR CENTURY SENIOR (AmerisourceBergen)			
TAB,PO (IRON-FREE,PRIVATE LABEL)			
300s ea	24385-0127-87	14.39	15.99
GOOD NEIGHBOR CLOTRIMAZOLE (AmerisourceBergen)			
CRE,TP (ATHLETE'S FOOT)			
1%, 15 gm	87701-0800-42	5.39	5.99
GOOD NEIGHBOR COENZYME Q-10 (AmerisourceBergen)			
SGL,PO (PRIVATE LABEL,SOFTGEL)			
100 mg, 30s ea	24385-0508-65	14.40	16.00
GOOD NEIGHBOR FISH OIL (AmerisourceBergen)			
SGL,PO (EXTRA STRENGTH)			
175 mg-260 mg-880 mg,			
60s ea	24385-0584-72	8.09	8.99
(NATURAL,PRIVATE LABEL)			
175 mg-260 mg-880 mg,			
60s ea	24385-0513-72	7.19	7.99
GOOD NEIGHBOR HAIR, SKIN & NAILS (AmerisourceBergen)			
TAB,PO (PRIVATE LABEL,CAPLET)			
60s ea	24385-0583-72	8.09	8.99
GOOD NEIGHBOR IBUPROFEN (AmerisourceBergen)			
SGL,PO (PRIVATE LABEL,SOFTGEL)			
200 mg, 40s ea	24385-0499-58	4.04	4.49
80s ea	24385-0499-41	6.29	6.99
GOOD NEIGHBOR IBUPROFEN COLD CHILDREN'S (AmerisourceBergen)			
SUS,PO (AF,PRIVATE LABEL,BERRY)			
100 mg/5 ml-15 mg/5 ml,			
120 ml	24385-0549-26	4.49	4.99
GOOD NEIGHBOR IBUPROFEN INFANTS' (AmerisourceBergen)			
SUS,PO (CONCENTRATED DROPS,AF)			
50 mg/1.25 ml, 30 ml	24385-0550-10	7.19	7.99
GOOD NEIGHBOR IBUPROFEN JUNIOR STRENGTH (AmerisourceBergen)			
CTB,PO (PRIVATE LABEL,ORANGE)			
100 mg, 24s ea	24385-0546-62	3.59	3.99
GOOD NEIGHBOR INSULIN SYRINGES (Can-Am Care)			
DEV,NA (31G,1/2CC,5/16")			
100s ea	38396-0450-64	17.50	
(31G,1CC,5/16")			
100s ea	38396-0451-64	17.50	
(31G,3/10CC,5/16")			
100s ea	38396-0449-64	17.50	
(ULTRA COMFORT,28G,1/2CC)			
100s ea	38396-0441-64	15.50	
(ULTRA COMFORT,28G,1CC)			
100s ea	38396-0442-64	15.50	

PROD/MFR	HRI, UPC,NDC	AWP	SRP
(ULTRA COMFORT,29G,1/2CC)			
100s ea	38396-0443-64	17.50	
(ULTRA COMFORT,29G,1CC)			
100s ea	38396-0444-64	17.50	
(ULTRA COMFORT,29G)			
100s ea	38396-0445-64	17.50	
(ULTRA COMFORT,30G,1/2CC)			
100s ea	38396-0446-64	17.50	
(ULTRA COMFORT,30G,1CC)			
100s ea	38396-0447-64	17.50	
(ULTRA COMFORT,30G)			
100s ea	38396-0448-64	17.50	
GOOD NEIGHBOR IRON SLOW RELEASE (AmerisourceBergen)			
TER,PO (PRIVATE LABEL)			
160 mg, 30s ea	24385-0528-65	3.84	6.49
GOOD NEIGHBOR K-PEC (AmerisourceBergen)			
SUS,PO (AF,PRIVATE LABEL)			
262 mg/15 ml, 355 ml	87701-0399-67	4.31	4.79
GOOD NEIGHBOR LANCETS (Can-Am Care)			
DEV,NA, 100s ea	38396-0342-64	5.85	
200s ea	38396-0343-64	9.50	
GOOD NEIGHBOR LICE SOLUTION KIT (AmerisourceBergen)			
KIT,MR (SHAMPOO,GEL,COMB,SPRAY)			
0.5%-4%-0.33%, ea	24385-0634-23	13.49	14.99
GOOD NEIGHBOR MEDICATED WIPES (AmerisourceBergen)			
PAD,TP (PRE-MOISTENED)			
50%, 48s ea	87701-0698-00	3.59	3.99
GOOD NEIGHBOR MOTION SICKNESS RELIEF (AmerisourceBergen)			
TAB,PO (PRIVATE LABEL)			
25 mg, 8s ea	87701-0347-42	2.69	2.99
GOOD NEIGHBOR NASAL SPRAY PUMP (AmerisourceBergen)			
SPR,NS (ORIGINAL FORMULA)			
0.05%, 30 ml	24385-0498-10	3.95	4.39
GOOD NEIGHBOR PAIN RELIEVER (AmerisourceBergen)			
TAB,PO (EXTRA SRENGTH)			
500 mg, 24s ea	24385-0187-62	2.42	2.69
GOOD NEIGHBOR PHARMACY ACNE TREATMENT (AmerisourceBergen)			
CRE,TP (1X28GM,MAXIMUMSTRENGTH)			
10%, 28 gm	87701-0405-92	3.59	3.99
GOOD NEIGHBOR PHARMACY ADVANCED RECOVERY LOTION (AmerisourceBergen)			
LOT,TP (1X295ML,FRAGRANCE-FREE)			
295 ml	87701-0405-89	1.79	1.99
GOOD NEIGHBOR PHARMACY AIRWISE (AmerisourceBergen)			
TEF,PO (PRIVATE LABEL)			
10s ea	87701-0406-04	5.39	5.99
GOOD NEIGHBOR PHARMACY ALL DAY ALLERGY (AmerisourceBergen)			
TAB,PO (ORIGPRESCRIPTIONSTRNGTH)			
10 mg, 14s ea	24385-0175-74	8.99	9.99
14s ea	24385-0998-74	8.99	9.99
(24 HOUR,PRIVATE LABEL)			
10 mg, 90s ea	24385-0175-75	18.00	20.00
(Phys Total Care)			
REPACK			
TAB,PO, 10 mg, 14s ea	54868-5845-01	20.63	
GOOD NEIGHBOR PHARMACY ALLERGY (AmerisourceBergen)			
CAP,PO (PRIVATE LABEL)			
25 mg, 24s ea	24385-0462-62	2.96	3.29
100s ea	24385-0462-78	8.09	8.99
GOOD NEIGHBOR PHARMACY ANIMAL SHAPES (AmerisourceBergen)			
CTB,PO (PRIVATE LABEL)			
60s ea	24385-0275-72	4.13	5.99
GOOD NEIGHBOR PHARMACY ANIMAL SHAPES WITH IRON (AmerisourceBergen)			
CTB,PO (PRIVATE LABEL)			
60s ea	24385-0084-72	5.39	5.99
GOOD NEIGHBOR PHARMACY ANIMAL SHAPES WITH VIT C (AmerisourceBergen)			
CTB,PO (PRIVATE LABEL)			
60s ea	24385-0089-72	5.39	5.99
GOOD NEIGHBOR PHARMACY ANTACID (AmerisourceBergen)			
CTB,PO ((ASSORTED),REG STRENGTH)			
500 mg, 150s ea	24385-0478-47	3.14	3.49

PROD/MFR | HRI, UPC,NDC | AWP | SRP

(REGULAR STRENGTH)
500 mg, 150s ea 24385-0485-47 3.14 3.49
(EXTRA STRENGTH,SF)
750 mg, 80s ea 46122-0007-41 3.14 3.49

GOOD NEIGHBOR PHARMACY ANTI-DIARRHEAL (AmerisourceBergen)
SOL,PO (PRIVATE LABEL)
1 mg/5 ml, 120 ml.... 24385-0377-26 4.49 4.99

GOOD NEIGHBOR PHARMACY ANTI-NAUSEA (AmerisourceBergen)
SOL,PO (1X118ML,PRIVATE LABEL)
118 ml 24385-0291-26 4.85 5.39

GOOD NEIGHBOR PHARMACY BLOOD GLUCOSE TEST STRIPS (AmerisourceBergen)
DEV,NA, 100s ea.......... 87701-0335-86 31.94 45.95

GOOD NEIGHBOR PHARMACY CALCIUM 500 WITH D (AmerisourceBergen)
TAB,PO (PRIVATE LABEL)
500 mg-200 iu, 75s ea. 24385-0266-98 5.12 5.69
160s ea........... 24385-0266-06 8.99 9.99

GOOD NEIGHBOR PHARMACY CASTOR OIL (AmerisourceBergen)
OIL,PO (1X117ML,USP)
117 ml 24385-0515-30 3.95 4.39

GOOD NEIGHBOR PHARMACY CHEST RUB (AmerisourceBergen)
OIN,TP (1X100GM,PRIVATE LABEL)
4.8%-1.2%-2.6%,
100 gm.............. 87701-0405-90 4.40 4.89

GOOD NEIGHBOR PHARMACY CHILDREN'S ALLERGY (AmerisourceBergen)
SOL,PO (1X118ML,AF)
12.5 mg/5 ml, 118 ml. 24385-0379-26 3.23 3.59

GOOD NEIGHBOR PHARMACY CHILDREN'S IBUPROFEN (AmerisourceBergen)
SUS,PO (1X120ML,PRIVATE LABEL)
100 mg/5 ml, 120 ml . 24385-0372-26 4.49 4.99

GOOD NEIGHBOR PHARMACY CHILDREN'S MUCUS RELIEF (AmerisourceBergen)
SOL,PO (1X118ML,AF)
100 mg/5 ml, 118 ml . 24385-0982-26 5.39 5.99

GOOD NEIGHBOR PHARMACY CHILDREN'S TRIACTING (AmerisourceBergen)
SOL,PO (1X118ML,DAY TIME)
5 mg/5 ml-2.5 mg/5 ml,
118 ml 24385-0981-26 3.50 3.89
(1X118ML,NIGHT TIME)
6.25 mg/5 ml-2.5 mg/5 ml,
118 ml 24385-0121-26 3.50 3.89

GOOD NEIGHBOR PHARMACY CHILDRENS MUCUS RELIEF (AmerisourceBergen)
GOOD NEIGHBOR PHARMACY CHILDREN'S MUCUS RELIEF
SOL,PO (1X118ML,COUGH,AF)
5 mg/5 ml-100 mg/5 ml,
118 ml 24385-0985-26 5.39 5.99

GOOD NEIGHBOR PHARMACY CLEAR LAX (AmerisourceBergen)
PDS,PO (1X119GM,PRIVATE LABEL)
17 gm/dose, 119 gm.. 46122-0014-31 5.39 5.99
(1X238GM,PRIVATE LABEL)
17 gm/dose, 238 gm.. 46122-0014-33 8.54 9.49
(1X510GM,PRIVATE LABEL)
17 gm/dose, 510 gm.. 46122-0014-71 16.19 17.99

GOOD NEIGHBOR PHARMACY CLICKFINE (Can-Am Care)
DEV,NA (6MM)
100s ea............. 38396-0706-64 19.98
(8MM)
100s ea............. 38396-0702-64 19.98

GOOD NEIGHBOR PHARMACY COMPLETE (AmerisourceBergen)
CTB,PO (DUAL ACTION,25+15 FREE)
800 mg-10 mg-165 mg,
40s ea............. 24385-0201-58 8.99 9.99

GOOD NEIGHBOR PHARMACY COMPLETE ENEMA (AmerisourceBergen)
NMA,RC (READY-TO-USE,1X133ML)
7 gm/118 ml-19 gm/118 ml,
133 ml 24385-0039-28 0.89 0.99

GOOD NEIGHBOR PHARMACY COMPLETE READY-TO-USE ENEMA (AmerisourceBergen)
NMA,RC (1X133ML,LATEX-FREE)
133 ml 24385-0360-28 1.79 1.99

GOOD NEIGHBOR PHARMACY COUGH DROPS (AmerisourceBergen)
LOZ,MM (SF,PRIVATE LABEL)
5.8 mg, 25s ea 46122-0002-63 1.16 1.29
(PRIVATE LABEL)
9.1 mg, 30s ea 46122-0001-65 0.89 0.99

GOOD NEIGHBOR PHARMACY CRANBERRY (AmerisourceBergen)
TAB,PO (PRIVATE LABEL,CAPLET)
160 mg-400 mg, 90s ea 24385-0663-75 5.39 5.99

GOOD NEIGHBOR PHARMACY DAILY MOISTURIZING LOTION (AmerisourceBergen)
LOT,TP (1X354ML,FRAGRANCE-FREE)
1.25%, 354 ml 87701-0405-88 4.49 4.99

GOOD NEIGHBOR PHARMACY DAILY PRENATAL (AmerisourceBergen)
KIT,PO (COMBO PACK,GLUTEN-FREE)
ea.................. 46122-0009-25 12.60 14.00

GOOD NEIGHBOR PHARMACY DAIRY RELIEF (AmerisourceBergen)
CTB,PO (ORIGINAL STRENGTH)
3000 u, 120s ea...... 24385-0149-76 8.99 9.99

GOOD NEIGHBOR PHARMACY DAY TIME SINUS (AmerisourceBergen)
SGL,PO (NON-DROWSY,AF)
325 mg-5 mg, 20s ea . 46122-0004-60 3.86 4.29

GOOD NEIGHBOR PHARMACY DENTURE CLEANSER (AmerisourceBergen)
TEF,NA (DUAL ACTION)
42s ea.............. 46122-0011-04 2.42 2.69
(PRIVATE LABEL)
42s ea.............. 46122-0012-04 2.69 2.99

GOOD NEIGHBOR PHARMACY DIAPER RASH CREAMY (AmerisourceBergen)
OIN,TP (1X57GM,PRIVATE LABEL)
10%, 57 gm 46122-0013-46 2.06 2.29

GOOD NEIGHBOR PHARMACY DL-ALPHA VITAMIN E (AmerisourceBergen)
SGL,PO (PRIVATE LABEL,SOFTGEL)
400 iu, 100s ea....... 24385-0318-78 7.19 7.99

GOOD NEIGHBOR PHARMACY DOCUSATE CALCIUM (AmerisourceBergen)
SGL,PO (PRIVATE LABEL,SOFTGEL)
240 mg, 100s ea 24385-0435-78 10.80 12.00

GOOD NEIGHBOR PHARMACY EAR DROPS (AmerisourceBergen)
GOOD NEIGHBOR PHARMACY EAR DROPS
SOL,OT (PRIVATE LABEL)
6.5%, 15 ml 24385-0955-01 3.41 3.79

GOOD NEIGHBOR PHARMACY EYE DROPS (AmerisourceBergen)
SOL,OP (1X15ML,PRIVATE LABEL)
0.05%, 15 ml 24385-0075-05 2.60 3.69

GOOD NEIGHBOR PHARMACY EYE ITCH (AmerisourceBergen)
SOL,OP (PRESCRIPTION STRENGTH)
0.025%, 5 ml 24385-0494-64 9.89 11.00

GOOD NEIGHBOR PHARMACY FLU RELIEF THERAPY (AmerisourceBergen)
SOL,PO (1X245ML,PRIVATE LABEL)
245 ml 46122-0015-33 4.49 4.99
(1X245ML,NIGHTTIME)
245 ml 46122-0016-33 4.49 4.99

GOOD NEIGHBOR PHARMACY GINSENG (AmerisourceBergen)
SGL,PO (PRIVATE LABEL,SOFTGEL)
100 mg, 50s ea 24385-0948-71 5.84 6.49

GOOD NEIGHBOR PHARMACY GLUCOSE (AmerisourceBergen)
GEL,PO (3X38GM,PRIVATE LABEL)
15 gm, 38 gm 3s 87701-0402-05 8.99 9.99
(Can-Am Care)
CTB,PO (QUICK DISSOLVE)
4 gm, 40s ea......... 38396-0560-64 4.33
GEL,PO (PRIVATE LABEL)
15 gm, 38 gm 3s..... 38396-0550-64 8.11

GOOD NEIGHBOR PHARMACY GLYCERIN (AmerisourceBergen)
SOL,TP, 99.5%, 177 ml.... 24385-0033-30 4.49 4.99

GOOD NEIGHBOR PHARMACY HEADACHE RELIEF (AmerisourceBergen)
TAB,PO (ADDED STRENGTH)
500 mg-65 mg, 100s ea 24385-0544-78 7.19 7.99

GOOD NEIGHBOR PHARMACY HEATWRAPS (AmerisourceBergen)
DEV,NA (NECK,SHOULDER & WRIST)
3s ea................ 87701-0405-74 5.84 6.49

GOOD NEIGHBOR PHARMACY HEMORRHOIDAL OINTMENT (AmerisourceBergen)
OIN,TP (1X56.8GM)
14.0%-71.9%-0.25%-3.0%,
56.8 gm 24385-0387-46 5.39 5.99

GOOD NEIGHBOR PHARMACY HIGH POTENCY VITAMIN D (AmerisourceBergen)
TAB,PO (GLUTEN-FREE)
115 mg-2000 iu,
100s ea............ 87701-0405-77 7.19 7.99

GOOD NEIGHBOR PHARMACY IBUPROFEN (AmerisourceBergen)
TAB,PO (PRIVATE LABEL,COATED)
200 mg, 500s ea 24385-0604-90 12.30 13.70

GOOD NEIGHBOR PHARMACY IBUPROFEN COLD & SINUS (AmerisourceBergen)
TAB,PO (NON DROWSY)
200 mg-30 mg, 20s ea 24385-0465-60 4.40 4.89

GOOD NEIGHBOR PHARMACY IBUPROFEN JUNIOR STRENGTH (AmerisourceBergen)
CTB,PO (PRIVATE LABEL,GRAPE)
100 mg, 24s ea 46122-0010-62 3.59 3.99

GOOD NEIGHBOR PHARMACY IBUPROFEN PM (AmerisourceBergen)
TAB,PO (PRIVATE LABEL)
38 mg-200 mg, 20s ea. 24385-0937-60 3.59 3.99
40s ea............. 24385-0937-58 5.39 5.99

GOOD NEIGHBOR PHARMACY INSTANT HAND SANITIZER (AmerisourceBergen)
GEL,TP (1X59ML,PRIVATE LABEL)
62%, 59 ml 87701-0405-91 5.94

GOOD NEIGHBOR PHARMACY LORATADINE (AmerisourceBergen)
GOOD NEIGHBOR PHARMACY LORATADINE
TAB,PO (NON-DROWSY,90+30 FREE)
10 mg, 120s ea 24385-0471-76 14.40 16.00

GOOD NEIGHBOR PHARMACY MAGNESIUM CITRATE (AmerisourceBergen)
SOL,PO (1X296ML,SUCROSE-FREE)
1.75 gm/30 ml, 296 ml. 24385-0675-10 24.70 27.50
296 ml 24385-0910-10 24.70 27.50
(LOW SODIUM,1X296ML)
1.75 gm/30 ml, 296 ml 24385-0600-10 24.70 27.50

GOOD NEIGHBOR PHARMACY MARVEL HEROES BANDAGES (AmerisourceBergen)
DEV,NA (3/4"X3",LATEX-FREE)
25s ea.............. 87701-0405-93 1.79 1.99

GOOD NEIGHBOR PHARMACY MASANTI (AmerisourceBergen)
SUS,PO (ORIGINAL, REGULAR STR)
355 ml 24385-0357-40 3.59 3.99
(ORIGINAL, MAX STRENGTH)
355 ml 24385-0340-40 4.13 4.59

GOOD NEIGHBOR PHARMACY MICONAZOLE 3 (AmerisourceBergen)
KIT,MR (COMBINATION PACK)
ea.................. 24385-0606-02 12.00 13.30

GOOD NEIGHBOR PHARMACY MILK OF MAGNESIA (AmerisourceBergen)
SUS,PO (1X355ML,PRIVATE LABEL)
1200 mg/15 ml, 355 ml 24385-0608-40 3.23 3.59

GOOD NEIGHBOR PHARMACY MINI FIRST AID KIT (AmerisourceBergen)
DEV,NA (LATEX-FREE)
ea.................. 87701-0405-84 5.94

GOOD NEIGHBOR PHARMACY MUSCLE RUB (AmerisourceBergen)
CRE,TP (1X85GM,PRIVATE LABEL)
10%-15%, 85 gm 24385-0011-21 2.87 3.19

GOOD NEIGHBOR PHARMACY NASAL DECONGESTANT (AmerisourceBergen)
TAB,PO (NON-DROWSY,MAX STRENGTH)
30 mg, 24s ea........ 24385-0432-62 3.14 3.49

GOOD NEIGHBOR PHARMACY NATURAL NIACIN (AmerisourceBergen)
TER,PO (TIME RELEASE)
250 mg, 100s ea 24385-0969-78 5.39 5.99

GOOD NEIGHBOR PHARMACY NICOTINE (AmerisourceBergen)
GUM,PO (PRIVATE LABEL,MINT)
2 mg, 50s ea......... 24385-0594-71 18.00 20.00

GOOD NEIGHBOR PHARMACY NICOTINE GUM (AmerisourceBergen)
PO (PRIVATE LABEL,ORIGINAL)
2 mg, 50s ea......... 24385-0597-71 18.00 20.00

PROD/MFR	HRI, UPC,NDC	AWP	SRP
GOOD NEIGHBOR PHARMACY NIGHT TIME (AmerisourceBergen)			
SOL,PO (1X296ML,COLD & FLU)			
296 ml	46122-0008-38	4.40	4.89
GOOD NEIGHBOR PHARMACY NIGHT TIME SINUS (AmerisourceBergen)			
SGL,PO (AF,PRIVATE LABEL)			
325 mg-6.25 mg-5 mg, 20s ea	46122-0006-60	3.86	4.29
GOOD NEIGHBOR PHARMACY PAIN RELIEF (AmerisourceBergen)			
CAP,PO (EXTRA STRENGTH)			
500 mg, 24s ea	46122-0003-62	2.87	3.19
50s ea	46122-0003-71	5.39	5.99
100s ea	46122-0003-78	8.09	8.99
GOOD NEIGHBOR PHARMACY PAIN RELIEVER (AmerisourceBergen)			
TAB,PO (PRIVATE LABEL,CAPLET)			
500 mg, 10s ea	24385-0484-52	21.50	1.99
GOOD NEIGHBOR PHARMACY PEPPERMINT SPIRIT (AmerisourceBergen)			
LIQ,NA (1X30ML,PRIVATE LABEL)			
30 ml	24385-0932-91	3.86	4.29
GOOD NEIGHBOR PHARMACY PHOSPHATE LAXATIVE (AmerisourceBergen)			
SOL,PO (ORAL SALINE LAXATIVE)			
45 ml	24385-0370-21	2.69	2.99
GOOD NEIGHBOR PHARMACY PURIFIED NATURAL WATER (AmerisourceBergen)			
SOL,NA (1X591ML,PRIVATE LABEL)			
591 ml	87701-0399-95	8.91	9.90
GOOD NEIGHBOR PHARMACY SALINE NASAL SPRAY (AmerisourceBergen)			
SPR,NS (1X44ML,MOISTURIZING)			
0.65%, 44 ml	24385-0325-58	2.06	2.29
GOOD NEIGHBOR PHARMACY STOMACH RELIEF (AmerisourceBergen)			
SUS,PO (1X355ML,REGULARSTRENGTH)			
262 mg/15 ml, 355 ml	24385-0302-40	2.42	2.69
(MAXIMUM STRENGTH)			
525 mg/15 ml, 240 ml	24385-0337-34	3.23	3.59
GOOD NEIGHBOR PHARMACY STOOL SOFTENER (AmerisourceBergen)			
SOL,PO (1X473ML,PRIVATE LABEL)			
50 mg/5 ml, 473 ml	24385-0468-43	5.39	5.99
GOOD NEIGHBOR PHARMACY STOOL SOFTNER (AmerisourceBergen)			
SGL,PO (PRIVATE LABEL,SOFTGEL)			
100 mg, 100s ea	24385-0436-78	8.54	9.49
GOOD NEIGHBOR PHARMACY TERBINAFINE HYDROCHLORIDE (AmerisourceBergen)			
CRE,TP (1X12GM,PRIVATE LABEL)			
1%, 12 gm	24385-0524-40	7.19	7.99
(1X24GM,PRIVATE LABEL)			
1%, 24 gm	24385-0524-44	8.99	9.99
GOOD NEIGHBOR PHARMACY TRUERESULT (AmerisourceBergen)			
DEV,NA (FREE METER)			
ea	87701-0405-56	0.03	0.04
(PRIVATE LABEL)			
ea	56151-0124-01	17.10	19.00
GOOD NEIGHBOR PHARMACY TRUETEST TEST STRIPS (AmerisourceBergen)			
DEV,NA (PRIVATE LABEL)			
50s ea	56151-1030-05	34.00	34.00
GOOD NEIGHBOR PHARMACY TRUETRACK (AmerisourceBergen)			
DEV,NA (FREE METER)			
ea	87701-0405-57	0.03	0.04
GOOD NEIGHBOR PHARMACY TUSSIN (AmerisourceBergen)			
SOL,PO (NON-DROWSY,AF)			
100 mg/5 ml, 237 ml	24385-0310-34	4.49	4.99
GOOD NEIGHBOR PHARMACY TUSSIN CF COUGH & COLD (AmerisourceBergen)			
SOL,PO (1X118ML,NON-DROWSY,AF)			
118 ml	24385-0904-26	3.23	3.59
GOOD NEIGHBOR PHARMACY TUSSIN CHEST CONGESTION (AmerisourceBergen)			
SOL,PO (1X118ML,NON-DROWSY,AF)			
100 mg/5 ml, 118 ml	24385-0310-26	3.23	3.59
GOOD NEIGHBOR PHARMACY TUSSIN DM COUGH (AmerisourceBergen)			
SOL,PO (1X118ML,NON-DROWSY,AF)			
10 mg/5 ml-100 mg/5 ml, 118 ml	24385-0359-26	3.23	3.59
118 ml	24385-0578-26	3.23	3.59
GOOD NEIGHBOR PHARMACY TUSSIN DM MAX (AmerisourceBergen)			
PO (1X118ML,NON-DROWSY,AF)			
10 mg/5 ml-200 mg/5 ml, 118 ml	46122-0017-26	3.59	3.99
GOOD NEIGHBOR PHARMACY URINARY HEALTH (AmerisourceBergen)			
TAB,PO (PRIVATE LABEL)			
50s ea	87701-0405-34	4.94	5.49
GOOD NEIGHBOR PHARMACY VIT B50 BALANCED B-COMPLEX (AmerisourceBergen)			
TAB,PO (PRIVATE LABEL)			
100s ea	24385-0288-78	5.39	5.99
GOOD NEIGHBOR PHARMACY VITAMIN B1 (AmerisourceBergen)			
TAB,PO (PRIVATE LABEL)			
100 mg, 100s ea	24385-0108-78	3.14	3.49
GOOD NEIGHBOR PHARMACY VITAMIN B12 (AmerisourceBergen)			
TER,PO (PRIVATE LABEL)			
1000 mcg, 60s ea	24385-0999-72	5.39	5.99
GOOD NEIGHBOR PHARMACY ZINC OXIDE (AmerisourceBergen)			
OIN,TP (1X56.7GM,PRIVATE LABEL)			
20%, 56.7 gm	24385-0086-46	2.69	2.99
GOOD NEIGHBOR PRESTIGE SMART SYSTEM (Home Diag)			
DEV,NA (STRIP)			
50s ea	56151-0311-50	28.60	
100s ea	56151-0311-01	45.99	
GOOD NEIGHBOR PSS STARTER (Home Diag)			
DEV,NA (MTR,STRP,LANCET,DEV,SOL)			
ea	56151-0211-01	22.18	
GOOD NEIGHBOR SENNA (AmerisourceBergen)			
SGL,PO (NATURAL VEG LAXATIVE)			
8.6 mg, 80s ea	24385-0551-27	5.82	10.99
GOOD NEIGHBOR SINUS (AmerisourceBergen)			
TAB,PO (MAXIMUM STRENGTH)			
500 mg-30 mg, 24s ea	24385-0488-62	3.41	3.79
GOOD NEIGHBOR SINUS DAY (AmerisourceBergen)			
PO (ASPIRIN-FREE)			
500 mg-30 mg, 48s ea	87701-0944-32	5.39	5.99
GOOD NEIGHBOR STOOL SOFTENER (AmerisourceBergen)			
SGL,PO (PRIVATE LABEL,SOFTGEL)			
100 mg, 60s ea	24385-0436-72	6.29	6.99
GOOD NEIGHBOR STOOL SOFTENER EXTRA STRENGTH (AmerisourceBergen)			
PO (PRIVATE LABEL,SOFTGEL)			
250 mg, 100s ea	24385-0443-78	6.29	6.99
GOOD NEIGHBOR SUPER THIN LANCETS (Can-Am Care)			
DEV,NA, 100s ea	38396-0547-64	5.85	
GOOD NEIGHBOR SUPHEDRINE CHILDREN'S (AmerisourceBergen)			
SOL,PO (NON-DROWSY,AF,SF)			
15 mg/5 ml, 118 ml	24385-0489-26	3.41	3.79
GOOD NEIGHBOR TAB-PROFEN (AmerisourceBergen)			
TAB,PO (PRIVATE LABEL)			
200 mg, 100s ea	87701-0756-06	6.29	6.99
GOOD NEIGHBOR THERAPEUTIC BLUE GEL (AmerisourceBergen)			
GEL,TP (PRIVATE LABEL)			
2%, 227 gm	24385-0225-40	5.03	5.59
GOOD NEIGHBOR THIN LANCETS (Can-Am Care)			
DEV,NA, 100s ea	38396-0344-64	5.85	
200s ea	38396-0345-64	9.50	
GOOD NEIGHBOR TUSSIN (AmerisourceBergen)			
SYR,PO (MAX STRENGTH)			
15 mg/5 ml, 118 ml	24385-0493-26	3.59	3.99
GOOD SAMARITAN HEALING OINTMENT (Good Samaritan)			
OIN,TP, 37.5 gm	55251-0001-02	5.34	6.95
GOOD SENSE 12 HOUR DECONGESTANT (Perrigo)			
TER,PO (NON-DROWSY,MAXIMUM)			
120 mg, 10s ea	00113-0054-52	3.75	
GOOD SENSE ACID REDUCER (L. Perrigo)			
TAB,PO (SF,PRIVATE LABEL)			
75 mg, 30s ea	00113-0271-39	3.48	
(Perrigo)			
TAB,PO (ORIGINAL STRENGTH)			
10 mg, 30s ea	00113-0141-65	4.78	
(MAXIMUM STRENGTH)			
20 mg, 25s ea	00113-0194-02	5.73	7.49
(PRIVATE LABEL)			
75 mg, 60s ea	00113-0271-72	6.11	
(MAXIMUM STRENGTH,SF)			
150 mg, 24s ea	00113-0047-62	4.82	
50s ea	00113-0047-71	6.79	
GOOD SENSE ALL DAY ALLERGY (Perrigo)			
TAB,PO (PRIVATE LABEL)			
10 mg, 5s ea	00113-9458-13	5.46	
14s ea	00113-9458-66	7.98	
30s ea	00113-9458-39	11.73	
GOOD SENSE ALL DAY ALLERGY-D (Perrigo)			
TER,PO (PRIVATE LABEL)			
5 mg-120 mg, 12s ea	00113-0176-53	9.75	
24s ea	00113-0176-62	17.55	
GOOD SENSE ALL DAY PAIN RELIEF (Perrigo)			
TAB,PO (8-12 HOUR RELIEF)			
220 mg, 24s ea	00113-0368-62	2.52	
50s ea	00113-9490-71	4.02	
(PRIVATE LABEL,CAPLET)			
220 mg, 50s ea	00113-0368-71	4.02	
100s ea	00113-9490-78	6.95	
(PRIVATE LABEL,CAPLET)			
220 mg, 100s ea	00113-0368-78	6.95	
GOOD SENSE ALLERGY (Perrigo)			
TAB,PO (4 HOUR)			
4 mg, 24s ea	00113-0463-62	1.10	
100s ea	00113-0463-78	2.37	
GOOD SENSE ALLERGY MULTI-SYMPTOM (Perrigo)			
TAB,PO (PRIVATE LABEL,COOL ICE)			
325 mg-2 mg-5 mg, 24s ea	00113-0476-62	2.02	
GOOD SENSE ALLERGY RELIEF (Perrigo)			
ODT,PO (NON-DROWSY,MELTEEZ)			
10 mg, 10s ea	00113-0311-52	5.36	8.09
12s ea	00113-0824-53	6.32	7.69
TAB,PO (24 HOUR,PRIVATE LABEL)			
10 mg, 10s ea	00113-0612-46	3.52	7.49
(24 HOUR, NON-DROWSY)			
10 mg, 20s ea	00113-0612-60	6.33	13.29
30s ea	00113-0612-39	9.02	16.79
(24 HOUR,PRIVATE LABEL)			
10 mg, 30s ea	00113-0612-65	9.02	16.79
(EASY TO SWALLOW)			
25 mg, 24s ea	00113-0479-62	1.52	
100s ea	00113-0479-78	3.18	
GOOD SENSE ANTACID (L. Perrigo)			
SUS,PO (ANTI-GAS, REG STRENGTH)			
355 ml	00113-0851-40	3.14	
GOOD SENSE ANTACID PLUS ANTI-GAS RELIEF (Perrigo)			
SUS,PO (FAST ACTING)			
355 ml	00113-0357-40	3.03	
(MAXIMUM STRENGTH)			
355 ml	00113-0340-40	3.55	
GOOD SENSE ANTACID TABLETS (Perrigo)			
CTB,PO (REGULAR STRENGTH)			
500 mg, 150s ea	00113-0478-47	3.11	
150s ea	00113-0485-47	3.18	
(EXTRA STRENGTH)			
750 mg, 96s ea	00113-0468-80	2.95	
96s ea	00113-0489-80	3.27	
(ULTRA STRENGTH)			
1000 mg, 72s ea	00113-0595-23	2.86	
GOOD SENSE ANTACID W/ SIMETHICONE (Pharma Pac)			
REPACK			
SUS,PO (1X12ML)			
12 ml	52959-0938-12	12.36	
GOOD SENSE ANTI-DIARRHEAL (Perrigo)			
SOL,PO (PRIVATE LABEL)			
1 mg/5 ml, 120 ml	00113-0377-26	3.73	
TAB,PO (CAPLET)			
2 mg, 6s ea	00113-0224-91	1.64	
(PRIVATE LABEL,CAPLET)			
2 mg, 12s ea	00113-0224-53	2.25	
18s ea	00113-0224-89	2.59	
GOOD SENSE ANTI-ITCH (Perrigo)			
CRE,TP (MAXIMUM STRENGTH)			
1%, 28 gm	00113-0541-64	3.99	3.79
GOOD SENSE ANTI-NAUSEA (Perrigo)			
SOL,PO (ASPIRIN-FREE)			
118 ml	00113-0291-26	2.35	

PROD/MFR	HRI, UPC,NDC	AWP	SRP
GOOD SENSE ANTIHISTAMINE ALLERGY RELIEF (Perrigo)			
CAP,PO (EASY TO SWALLOW)			
25 mg, 24s ea	00113-0462-62	1.76	
GOOD SENSE ASPIRIN (Perrigo)			
CTB,PO (PRIVATE LABEL,CHERRY)			
81 mg, 36s ea	00113-0274-68	1.25	
ECT,PO, 81 mg, 120s ea	00113-0535-76	3.79	
(ADULT LOW STRENGTH)			
81 mg, 180s ea	00113-0277-48	5.40	6.49
(REGULAR STRENGTH)			
325 mg, 125s ea	00113-0429-02	2.59	5.19
TAB,PO (ORIGINAL STRENGTH)			
325 mg, 100s ea	00113-0416-78	1.21	
300s ea	00113-0416-87	2.80	
GOOD SENSE ATHLETE'S FOOT (Perrigo)			
SPR,TP (PRIVATE LABEL)			
1%, 150 gm	00113-0154-73	3.93	
GOOD SENSE BEDDING LICE TREATMENT (Perrigo)			
SPR,NA (STEP 3,1X142GM,INHOME)			
0.5%, 142 gm	70030-0148-61	4.45	7.99
GOOD SENSE CALCIUM ANTACID (Perrigo)			
CTB,PO (EXTRA STRENGTH)			
750 mg, 96s ea	00113-0179-80	2.95	
GOOD SENSE CHILDREN'S ALL DAY ALLERGY (Perrigo)			
SOL,PO (1X118ML,W/DOSAGE CUP)			
1 mg/ml, 118 ml	00113-0974-26	10.13	
GOOD SENSE CHILDREN'S ALLERGY RELIEF (Perrigo)			
SOL,PO (AF,PRIVATE LABEL,CHERRY)			
12.5 mg/5 ml, 118 ml	00113-0379-26	1.80	
GOOD SENSE CHILDREN'S ASPIRIN (Perrigo)			
CTB,PO (ORANGE)			
81 mg, 36s ea	00113-0467-68	1.25	
GOOD SENSE CHILDREN'S COLD & ALLERGY (Perrigo)			
SOL,PO (AF,PRIVATE LABEL,GRAPE)			
1 mg/5 ml-2.5 mg/5 ml, 118 ml	00113-0906-26	2.37	4.79
GOOD SENSE CHILDREN'S COLD & COUGH (Perrigo)			
SOL,PO (AF,PRIVATE LABEL)			
118 ml	00113-0987-26	2.64	4.79
GOOD SENSE CHILDREN'S IBUPROFEN (Perrigo)			
SUS,PO (AF,BERRY)			
100 mg/5 ml, 120 ml	00113-0897-26	4.86	
(AF,FRUIT)			
100 mg/5 ml, 120 ml	00113-0623-26	4.86	
(AF,PRIVATE LABEL)			
100 mg/5 ml, 120 ml	00113-0166-26	4.86	
(GRAPE,AF,GRAPE)			
100 mg/5 ml, 120 ml	00113-0660-26	4.68	
(AF,BERRY)			
100 mg/5 ml, 240 ml	00113-0897-34	7.60	
GOOD SENSE CHILDREN'S MUCUS RELIEF (Perrigo)			
SOL,PO (1X118ML,W/DOSAGE CUP,AF)			
100 mg/5 ml, 118 ml	00113-0288-26	2.81	
GOOD SENSE CHILDREN'S MUCUS RELIEF COUGH (Perrigo)			
SOL,PO (1X118ML,W/ DOSAGE CUP)			
5 mg/5 ml-100 mg/5 ml, 118 ml	00113-0419-26	2.81	
GOOD SENSE CHILDREN'S PAIN RELIEF (Perrigo)			
SUS,PO (AF,ASPIRIN-FREE)			
160 mg/5 ml, 118 ml	00113-0105-26	3.02	
118 ml	00113-0130-26	3.02	
118 ml	00113-0175-26	3.02	
GOOD SENSE CHILDREN'S TRIACTING COLD & COUGH SOLN (Perrigo)			
SOL,PO (NIGHT TIME)			
6.25 mg/5 ml-2.5 mg/5 ml, 118 ml	00113-0913-26	2.70	4.89
GOOD SENSE CLEARLAX (Perrigo)			
PDS,PO (ONCE-DAILY DOSES)			
17 gm/dose, 10s ea	00113-0306-52	9.07	
(1X119GM,PRIVATE LABEL)			
17 gm/dose, 119 gm	00113-0306-01	5.13	
(1X238GM,PRIVATE LABEL)			
17 gm/dose, 238 gm	00113-0306-02	9.07	
(1X510GM,PRIVATE LABEL)			
17 gm/dose, 510 gm	00113-0306-03	17.71	
GOOD SENSE COLD & ALLERGY (Perrigo)			
TAB,PO (PRIVATE LABEL)			
4 mg-10 mg, 24s ea	00113-0139-62	1.32	4.89
GOOD SENSE COLD DAYTIME MULTI-SYMPTOM (L. Perrigo)			
TAB,PO (PRIVATE LABEL,COOL ICE)			
325 mg-10 mg-200 mg-5 mg, 24s ea	00113-0308-62	3.02	
(Perrigo)			
TAB,PO (NON-DROWSY,COOL ICE)			
325 mg-10 mg-5 mg, 24s ea	00113-0371-62	2.26	
GOOD SENSE COLD HEAD CONGESTION DAYTIME (Perrigo)			
PO (NON-DROWSY)			
325 mg-10 mg-5 mg, 24s ea	00113-0402-62	2.26	4.49
GOOD SENSE COLD HEAD CONGESTION DAYTIME SEVERE (Perrigo)			
TAB,PO (NON-DROWSY)			
325 mg-10 mg-200 mg-5 mg, 24s ea	00113-0234-62	3.02	
GOOD SENSE COLD HEAD CONGESTION NIGHTTIME (Perrigo)			
GOOD SENSE COLD HEAD CONGESTION NIGHTTIME			
TAB,PO (PRIVATE LABEL,COOL ICE)			
325 mg-2 mg-10 mg-5 mg, 24s ea	00113-0393-62	2.58	4.49
GOOD SENSE COLD NIGHTTIME MULTI-SYMPTOM (Perrigo)			
PO (PRIVATE LABEL,COOL ICE)			
325 mg-2 mg-10 mg-5 mg, 24s ea	00113-0014-62	2.56	
GOOD SENSE COLD REMEDY (L. Perrigo)			
ODT,PO (PRIVATE LABEL,CHERRY)			
2 x-1 x, 25s ea	00113-0807-01	9.41	
GOOD SENSE COMPLETE (Perrigo)			
CTB,PO (DUAL ACTION)			
800 mg-10 mg-165 mg, 25s ea	00113-0546-63	10.00	
(PRIVATE LABEL,BERRY)			
800 mg-10 mg-165 mg, 25s ea	00113-0321-63	10.00	
GOOD SENSE COMPLETE LICE TREATMENT (L. Perrigo)			
KIT,MR (PRIVATE LABEL)			
0.5%-4%-0.33%, ea	00113-0173-24	12.35	
GOOD SENSE COUGH & SORE THROAT (Perrigo)			
SYR,PO (DAY, NON-DROWSY)			
500 mg/15 ml-15 mg/15 ml, 237 ml	00113-0698-34	4.18	4.99
(NIGHT TIME)			
237 ml	00113-0666-34	4.18	4.99
GOOD SENSE DAIRY DIGESTIVE (Perrigo)			
TAB,PO (CAPLET)			
3000 u, 60s ea	70030-0135-63	5.88	10.29
GOOD SENSE DAY TIME COLD & FLU (Perrigo)			
SOL,PO (NON-DROWSY,AF)			
177 ml	00113-0656-30	2.89	3.49
(MULTI-SYMPTOM,NONDROWSY)			
296 ml	00113-0656-38	3.79	
GOOD SENSE DAYHIST ALLERGY (Perrigo)			
TAB,PO (12 HOUR,PRIVATE LABEL)			
1.34 mg, 16s ea	00113-0282-73	5.13	
GOOD SENSE DAYTIME FLU & SEVERE COLD (Perrigo)			
PKT,PO (PRIVATE LABEL)			
6s ea	00113-0552-01	4.44	
GOOD SENSE DAYTIME PE COLD & FLU RELIEF (L. Perrigo)			
SGL,PO (NON-DROWSY,MULTISYMPTOM)			
325 mg-10 mg-5 mg, 12s ea	00113-0215-53	2.64	
20s ea	00113-0215-60	3.30	
GOOD SENSE FIBER LAXATIVE (Perrigo)			
TAB,PO (CAPLETS)			
625 mg, 90s ea	00113-0477-75	6.09	
GOOD SENSE GAS RELIEF (Perrigo)			
SGL,PO (EXTRA STRENGTH)			
125 mg, 30s ea	00113-0428-65	2.75	
(ULTRA STRENGTH,SOFTGEL)			
180 mg, 60s ea	00113-0657-72	3.50	
GOOD SENSE GOOD SENSE NIGHT TIME COLD & FLU RELIEF (Perrigo)			
SOL,PO (PRIVATE LABEL,ORIGINAL)			
177 ml	00113-0908-30	2.58	3.49
296 ml	00113-0908-38	3.66	4.49
GOOD SENSE HAIR REGROWTH TREATMENT (L. Perrigo)			
SOL,TP (3X60ML,USP)			
2%, 60 ml 3s	00113-0856-30	19.52	
GOOD SENSE HAIR REGROWTH TREATMENT FOR MEN (Perrigo)			
SOL,TP (3X60ML,UNSCENTED)			
5%, 60 ml 3s	00113-0798-30	25.97	
GOOD SENSE HEADACHE FORMULA (Perrigo)			
TAB,PO (ADDED STRENGTH)			
250 mg-250 mg-65 mg, 100s ea	00113-0430-78	3.93	
GOOD SENSE HEADACHE PM (Perrigo)			
TAB,PO (ASPIRIN-FREE)			
500 mg-25 mg, 50s ea	00113-0355-71	3.21	5.59
GOOD SENSE HEARTBURN RELIEF (Perrigo)			
TAB,PO (PRIVATE LABEL)			
200 mg, 30s ea	00113-0022-39	2.63	
GOOD SENSE HEMORRHOIDAL (Perrigo)			
CRE,RC (1X51GM,PRIVATE LABEL)			
14.4%-15%-0.25%-1%, 51 gm	00113-0944-24	3.32	
OIN,TP (PRIVATE LABEL)			
14.0%-71.9%-0.25%-3.0%, 57 gm	00113-0400-16	4.99	
SUP,RC, 85.5%-0.25%-3%, 12s ea	00113-0394-53	3.99	
24s ea	00113-0394-62	5.99	
GOOD SENSE IBUPROFEN (Perrigo)			
TAB,PO, 200 mg, 24s ea	00113-0604-62	1.48	
(COATED CAPLET)			
200 mg, 24s ea	00113-0647-62	1.48	
50s ea	00113-0604-71	1.74	
(COATED CAPLET)			
200 mg, 50s ea	00113-0647-71	1.74	
(PRIVATE LABEL,COATED)			
200 mg, 50s ea	00113-0074-71	1.74	
50s ea	00113-0517-71	1.74	
100s ea	00113-0604-78	2.86	
(COATED CAPLET)			
200 mg, 100s ea	00113-0647-78	2.86	
(PRIVATE LABEL,COATED)			
200 mg, 100s ea	00113-0074-78	2.86	
500s ea	00113-0604-90	10.18	
(PRIVATE LABEL,COATED)			
200 mg, 1000s ea	00113-0604-93	18.73	
GOOD SENSE IBUPROFEN COLD & SINUS (Perrigo)			
TAB,PO (NON-DROWSY,COATED)			
200 mg-30 mg, 20s ea	00113-0083-60	4.14	
GOOD SENSE IBUPROFEN JUNIOR STRENGTH (Perrigo)			
CTB,PO (PRIVATE LABEL,ORANGE)			
100 mg, 24s ea	00113-0461-62	3.97	
GOOD SENSE IBUPROFEN PM (L. Perrigo)			
TAB,PO (PRIVATE LABEL)			
38 mg-200 mg, 40s ea	00113-0050-58	6.96	
GOOD SENSE INFANTS IBUPROFEN (Perrigo)			
SUS,PO (AF,PRIVATE LABEL,BERRY)			
50 mg/1.25 ml, 15 ml	00113-0057-05	4.55	
GOOD SENSE INFANTS PAIN RELIEF (Perrigo)			
SUS,PO (AF,ASPIRIN-FREE,CHERRY)			
80 mg/0.8 ml, 15 ml	00113-0008-05	3.34	
(W/ DROPPER,AF)			
80 mg/0.8 ml, 15 ml	00113-0289-05	3.34	
(AF,ASPIRIN-FREE,CHERRY)			
80 mg/0.8 ml, 30 ml	00113-0008-10	4.18	
GOOD SENSE INFANTS' SIMETHICONE DROPS (Perrigo)			
SUS,PO (NON-STAINING,AF)			
20 mg/0.3 ml, 30 ml	00113-0882-10	6.99	
GOOD SENSE ITCH RELIEF (Perrigo)			
CRE,TP (EXTRA STRENGTH)			
2%-0.1%, 28 gm	00113-0622-64	3.99	3.79
GOOD SENSE JOCKITCH SPRAY (Perrigo)			
POW,TP (PRIVATE LABEL)			
1%, 130 gm	00113-0695-90	3.66	5.89
GOOD SENSE LAXATIVE (Perrigo)			
ECT,PO (COMFORT COATED)			
5 mg, 25s ea	00113-0086-63	1.48	5.09
GOOD SENSE LICE KILLING (Perrigo)			
SHA,TP (STEP 1,MAXIMUM STRENGTH)			
4%-0.33%, 118 ml	00113-0866-26	4.82	

PROD/MFR	HRI, UPC,NDC	AWP	SRP
GOOD SENSE MICONAZOLE 3 (Perrigo)			
KIT,MR (3 SUPPOSITORIES;APPL)			
ea	**00113-0605-00**	9.55	
(3 VAG SUPP-3 DISP APPS)			
ea	**00113-0081-00**	9.55	
GOOD SENSE MICONAZOLE 7 (Perrigo)			
CRE,VG (DISPOSABLE APPLICATORS)			
2%, 45 gm	**00113-0825-29**	7.01	
(REUSABLE APPLICATOR)			
2%, 45 gm	**00113-0214-29**	7.01	
GOOD SENSE MIGRAINE FORMULA (Perrigo)			
TAB,PO (PRIVATE LABEL)			
250 mg-250 mg-65 mg,			
24s ea	**00113-0374-62**	3.23	
GOOD SENSE MILK OF MAGNESIA (Perrigo)			
SUS,PO (ORIGINAL,SF)			
400 mg/5 ml, 355 ml	**00113-0396-40**	2.74	
(SF,STIMULANT-FREE)			
400 mg/5 ml, 355 ml	**00113-0332-40**	3.09	
(STIMULANT-FREE)			
400 mg/5 ml, 355 ml	**00113-0949-40**	3.56	4.09
GOOD SENSE MUSCLERUB (L. Perrigo)			
CRE,TP (1X113GM, ULTRA STRENGTH)			
4%-10%-30%, 113 gm	**00113-0049-26**	3.23	
GOOD SENSE NASAL DECONGESTANT (Perrigo)			
TAB,PO, 30 mg, 24s ea	**00113-0432-62**	2.45	
GOOD SENSE NASAL DECONGESTANT PE (Perrigo)			
TAB,PO (NON-DROWSY,MAX STRENGTH)			
10 mg, 18s ea	**00113-0094-89**	1.04	3.99
36s ea	**00113-0094-68**	1.68	5.59
72s ea	**00113-0094-23**	2.71	9.69
GOOD SENSE NASAL FOUR (Perrigo)			
SPR,NS, 1%, 29.6 ml	**00113-0648-10**	3.13	
GOOD SENSE NASAL MOISTURIZING (Perrigo)			
SPR,NS (PRIVATE LABEL)			
0.65%, 44 ml	**70030-0131-73**	3.99	2.99
GOOD SENSE NASAL SPRAY (Perrigo)			
SPR,NS (12 HOUR, MOISTURIZING)			
0.05%, 30 ml	**00113-0065-10**	1.78	
(12 HOUR, NO DRIP)			
0.05%, 30 ml	**00113-0388-10**	4.21	
(12 HOUR, SINUS)			
0.05%, 30 ml	**00113-0817-10**	1.78	
(ORIGINAL, 12 HOUR)			
0.05%, 30 ml	**00113-0304-10**	3.99	
GOOD SENSE NICOTINE POLACRILEX (Perrigo)			
GUM,PO (PRIVATE LABEL,COOL MINT)			
2 mg, 100s ea	**00113-0456-78**	36.61	41.99
(PRIVATE LABEL,MINT)			
2 mg, 110s ea	**00113-0206-25**	28.93	28.99
(PRIVATE LABEL,COOL MINT)			
4 mg, 100s ea	**00113-0532-78**	39.29	41.99
(PRIVATE LABEL,MINT)			
4 mg, 110s ea	**00113-0422-25**	34.91	41.99
LOZ,PO (3X24,PRIVATE LABEL,MINT)			
2 mg, 72s ea	**00113-0344-05**	35.43	
4 mg, 72s ea	**00113-0873-05**	35.43	
GOOD SENSE NIGHT TIME COLD & FLU RELIEF (Perrigo)			
SGL,PO (MULTI-SYMPTOM)			
325 mg-15 mg-6.25 mg,			
12s ea	**00113-0977-53**	2.64	3.99
20s ea	**00113-0977-60**	3.28	5.19
SOL,PO, 177 ml	**00113-0041-30**	2.58	3.49
296 ml	**00113-0041-38**	3.54	4.49
GOOD SENSE NIGHT TIME COUGH (Perrigo)			
SYR,PO (ASPIRIN-FREE)			
177 ml	**00113-0668-30**	2.63	3.49
GOOD SENSE NIGHTTIME SLEEP AID (Perrigo)			
TAB,PO (PRIVATE LABEL,CAPLETS)			
25 mg, 24s ea	**00113-0431-62**	1.80	
GOOD SENSE OMEPRAZOLE (Perrigo)			
TCP,PO (PRIVATE LABEL)			
20 mg, 14s ea	**00113-0915-74**	13.21	
28s ea	**00113-0915-30**	19.21	
42s ea	**00113-0915-55**	26.06	
GOOD SENSE PAIN RELIEF (Perrigo)			
TAB,PO (REGULAR STRENGTH)			
325 mg, 100s ea	**00113-0403-78**	2.13	
(EXTRA STRENGTH,CAPLET)			
500 mg, 24s ea	**00113-0484-62**	1.61	
(EXTRA STRENGTH)			
500 mg, 24s ea	**00113-0227-62**	1.59	3.19
(EXTRA STRENGTH,CAPLET)			
500 mg, 50s ea	**00113-0484-71**	2.05	
(EXTRA STRENGTH,COOL ICE)			
500 mg, 50s ea	**00113-0010-71**	2.04	
(EXTRA STRENGTH)			
500 mg, 50s ea	**00113-0227-71**	2.29	4.49
60s ea	**00113-0405-72**	2.14	
(EXTRA STRENGTH,CAPLET)			
500 mg, 100s ea	**00113-0484-78**	2.84	
(PRIVATE LABEL)			
500 mg, 100s ea	**00113-0405-78**	3.10	
(EXTRA STRENGTH,CAPLET)			
500 mg, 500s ea	**00113-0484-90**	9.77	
TER,PO (PRIVATE LABEL,CAPLET)			
650 mg, 24s ea	**00113-0544-62**	3.45	3.79
(8 HOUR,PRIVATE LABEL)			
650 mg, 50s ea	**00113-0217-71**	5.68	5.29
(PRIVATE LABEL,CAPLET)			
650 mg, 50s ea	**00113-0544-71**	4.82	5.29
GOOD SENSE PAIN RELIEF PM (Perrigo)			
TAB,PO (EXTRA STRENGTH)			
500 mg-25 mg, 50s ea	**00113-0437-71**	2.14	
GOOD SENSE PAIN RELIEVER (St. Mary's MPP)			
REPACK			
TAB,PO (EXTRA STRENGTH)			
500 mg, 24s ea	**60760-0048-24**	5.35	
GOOD SENSE PERSONAL LUBRICANT (Perrigo)			
GEL,VG (1X113GM,AF)			
113 gm	**70030-0147-65**	2.45	3.69
GOOD SENSE PREGNANCY TEST (Perrigo)			
DEV,NA, ea	**70030-0134-88**	3.04	9.79
2s ea	**70030-0134-89**	5.44	13.79
GOOD SENSE SINUS & ALLERGY PE (Perrigo)			
TAB,PO (MAXIMUM STRENGTH)			
4 mg-10 mg, 24s ea	**00113-0358-62**	2.09	4.19
GOOD SENSE SINUS CONGESTION & PAIN (Perrigo)			
TAB,PO (NON-DROWSY,DAYTIME)			
325 mg-5 mg, 24s ea	**00113-0272-62**	2.14	4.89
GOOD SENSE SLEEP AID (Perrigo)			
TAB,PO (PRIVATE LABEL)			
25 mg, 16s ea	**00113-0441-73**	3.36	
32s ea	**00113-0441-64**	4.90	
GOOD SENSE SORE THROAT (Perrigo)			
SPR,MM (FAST RELIEF/ACTING,AF)			
1.4%, 177 ml	**00113-0328-30**	3.10	
177 ml	**00113-0343-30**	3.10	
GOOD SENSE STAY AWAKE (Perrigo)			
TAB,PO (MAXIMUM STRENGTH)			
200 mg, 16s ea	**00113-0409-73**	1.70	
40s ea	**00113-0409-58**	3.45	
GOOD SENSE STOMACH RELIEF (L. Perrigo)			
SUS,PO (MAXIMUM STRENGTH)			
262 mg/15 ml, 237 ml	**00113-0337-34**	3.33	
(Perrigo)			
CTB,PO (REGULAR STRENGTH)			
262 mg, 30s ea	**00113-0469-65**	3.13	
SUS,PO (ORIGINAL STRENGTH)			
262 mg/15 ml, 237 ml	**00113-0302-34**	2.79	
(PRIVATE LABEL)			
262 mg/15 ml, 355 ml	**00113-0302-40**	3.72	
(REGULAR STRENGTH)			
262 mg/15 ml, 473 ml	**00113-0302-43**	4.46	
GOOD SENSE STOOL SOFTENER (Perrigo)			
SGL,PO, 100 mg, 60s ea	**00113-0486-72**	3.45	
GOOD SENSE TIOCONAZOLE 1 (L. Perrigo)			
OIN,VG (W/PREFILLED APPLICATOR)			
6.5%, 4.6 gm	**00113-0426-54**	14.12	
GOOD SENSE TRIPLE ANTIBIOTIC (Perrigo)			
OIN,TP (ORIGINAL STRENGTH)			
28 gm	**00113-0067-64**	6.15	5.89
GOOD SENSE TUSSIN CF (Perrigo)			
SOL,PO (NON-DROWSY,W/DOSAGE CUP)			
118 ml	**00113-0516-26**	2.36	
237 ml	**00113-0516-34**	3.39	
GOOD SENSE TUSSIN CHEST CONGESTION (Perrigo)			
SOL,PO (ALCOHOL FREE/COUGH,AF)			
100 mg/5 ml, 118 ml	**00113-0310-26**	1.96	
(AF,PRIVATE LABEL)			
100 mg/5 ml, 237 ml	**00113-0310-34**	3.21	
GOOD SENSE TUSSIN DM (Physician Partner)			
REPACK			
SYR,PO (1X120ML)			
10 mg/5 ml-100 mg/5 ml,			
120 ml	**21695-0737-04**	15.78	
GOOD SENSE TUSSIN DM COUGH (Perrigo)			
SOL,PO (ALCOHOL FREE, COUGH,AF)			
10 mg/5 ml-100 mg/5 ml,			
118 ml	**00113-0359-26**	2.04	
(SF)			
10 mg/5 ml-100 mg/5 ml,			
118 ml	**00113-0578-26**	2.75	
(COUGH FORMULA,W/DOSGCUP)			
10 mg/5 ml-100 mg/5 ml,			
237 ml	**00113-0359-34**	2.89	
GOOD SENSE WOMEN'S LAXATIVE (Perrigo)			
ECT,PO (COMFORT COATED)			
5 mg, 30s ea	**00113-0174-65**	1.92	
GOODHEALTH (Abbott Ashland)			
BULB DOUCHE			
DEV,NA, ea	**00742-0812-01**	4.98	
COMBINATION			
DEV,NA (DOUCHE/ENEMA/WATER BTL)			
ea	**00074-2808-01**	5.96	
EAR SYRINGE			
DEV,NA (ADULT,3 OZ.)			
ea	**00074-2840-00**	2.91	
FOAM CUSHION			
DEV,NA (MEDIUM)			
ea	**00074-2829-01**	12.48	
FOLDING DOUCHE			
DEV,NA, ea	**00074-2803-01**	5.44	
FOUNTAIN DOUCHE			
NA (ENEMA)			
ea	**00074-2812-01**	5.21	
PREMIUM COMBINATION			
NA (DOUCHE/ENEMA/WATER BTL)			
ea	**00074-2806-01**	8.35	
PREMIUM FOUNTAIN DOUCHE			
NA (ENEMA)			
ea	**00074-2810-01**	7.44	
PREMIUM WATER BOTTLE			
DEV,NA, ea	**00074-2814-01**	6.96	
RECTAL SYRINGE			
DEV,NA (ADULT,8 OZ.)			
ea	**00074-2843-01**	4.73	
VINYL INFLATABLE CUSHION			
DEV,NA (16")			
ea	**00074-2852-01**	6.75	
WATER BOTTLE			
DEV,NA, ea	**00074-2816-01**	4.81	
GOODSENSE ALLERGY & CONGESTION RELIEF (Perrigo)			
T24,PO (24 HOUR)			
10 mg-240 mg, 10s ea	**00113-0165-52**	5.74	
(NON-DROWSY)			
10 mg-240 mg, 15s ea	**00113-0165-22**	8.95	
GOODSENSE BABY SHAMPOO (Vi-Jon)			
SHA,TP (1X89ML,PRIVATE LABEL)			
89 ml	**79068-0006-65**	2.23	5.89
GOODY'S FAST PAIN RELIEF (Glaxo)			
PKT,PO (EXTRA STRENGTH)			
325 -500 mg-65 mg,			
4s ea	**74684-0021-00**	1.12	
24s ea	**74684-0021-50**	4.75	
TAB,PO (EXT STR)			
130 mg-260 mg-16.25 mg,			
4s ea	**74684-0007-08**	0.43	
60s ea	**74604-0007-07**	3.40	
GOODY'S HEADACHE POWDERS (Glaxo)			
PKT,PO (EXT. STR.)			
2s ea	**74684-0001-01**	0.39	
(EXT STR)			
6s ea	**74684-0001-02**	1.06	
24s ea	**74684-0001-03**	3.01	
50s ea	**74684-0001-04**	4.70	
GOODY'S PM ANALGESIC/SLEEP POWDERS (Glaxo)			
PKT,PO, 6s ea	**74684-0003-08**	1.10	
16s ea	**74684-0003-09**	2.68	
GORDOBALM (Gordon)			
LIQ,TP (GREEN OR PINK)			
0.075%-0.075%-2.5%,			
120 ml	**10481-1046-02**	7.40	
3840 ml	**10481-1046-03**	68.75	
GORDOCHOM (Gordon)			
SOL,TP, 3%-25%, 6 ml	**10481-8010-06**	10.00	
30 ml	**10481-8010-02**	17.10	
480 ml	**10481-8010-03**	178.75	
GORDOFILM (Gordon)			
LIQ,TP (BRUSH APPLICATOR)			
16.7%, 15 ml	**10481-3009-01**	12.85	
GORDOGESIC (Gordon)			
CRE,TP, 10%, 75 gm	**10481-3003-01**	5.95	
GORDOMATIC (Gordon)			
POW,TP (FOOT)			
105 gm	**10481-1009-01**	9.30	

PROD/MFR	HRI, UPC,NDC	AWP	SRP
GORDOMATIC CRYSTALS (Gordon)			
PDS,TP, 240 gm	10481-1008-01	7.35	
3360 gm	10481-1008-02	81.25	
GORDOMATIC LOTION (Gordon)			
SPR,TP (FOOT)			
92%, 120 ml	10481-1007-01	4.65	
GORDON'S BORO-PACKS (Gordon)			
PDR,TP (ASTRINGENT WET DRSG)			
49%-51%,			
2.7 gm 100s	10481-3018-01	55.00	
GORDON'S NO. FIVE (Gordon)			
SPR,TP (FOOT POWDER)			
120 ml	10481-1017-04	9.30	
GORDON'S VITE A (Gordon)			
CRE,TP, 75 gm	10481-1042-01	9.50	
120 gm	10481-1042-03	12.60	
2270 gm	10481-1042-05	148.75	
LOT,TP, 120 ml	10481-1043-01	7.40	
3840 ml	10481-1043-02	78.75	
GORDON'S VITE A CREME (Gordon)			
CRE,TP, 100000 u/30 gm,			
454 gm	50217-0001-19	51.25	
GORDON'S VITE E (Gordon)			
CRE,TP, 50 mg/gm, 15 gm	10481-3000-01	4.00	
75 gm	10481-3000-03	9.50	
2270 gm	10481-3000-05	142.50	
GORDON'S VITE E CREME (Gordon)			
TP, 1500 Iu/30 gm,			
454 gm	50217-0001-26	48.75	
GORDOPOOL (Gordon)			
LIQ,TP, 480 ml	50217-0001-65	36.25	
3840 ml	50217-0001-66	111.25	
GORMEL (Gordon)			
CRE,TP, 20%, 75 gm	10481-3001-01	10.65	
120 gm	10481-3001-05	13.95	
GORMEL CREME (Gordon)			
TP, 20%, 454 gm	50217-0001-14	56.25	
2270 gm	10481-3001-06	168.75	
GORMEL TEN (Gordon)			
LOT,TP, 10%, 228 gm	10481-6000-08	10.65	
GORSE (Ellon)			
SOL,SL (DROPS)			
10.5 ml	51762-0034-10		9.25
GOTU KOLA (ADH)			
GOTU KOLA			
CAP,PO (PF,SF)			
440 mg, 100s ea	60142-0917-51	5.48	10.95
(Botanical Labs.)			
LIQ,PO, 30 ml	41954-0020-67	4.00	7.99
(Mason Vit)			
CAP,PO (PF,SF)			
500 mg, 60s ea	11845-0114-65	5.67	
(Rexall)			
CAP,PO (PF,SF)			
450 mg, 75s ea	30768-0010-99	2.77	4.20
GRAM-O-LECI (Freeda)			
CTB,PO (PF,SF,DYE-FREE)			
1000 mg, 100s ea	10432-0020-01	5.97	9.95
250s ea	10432-0020-02	11.85	19.75
GRANDPA'S BAKING SODA SOAP (Grandpa Soap)			
SOA,TP (3.25OZ,UNSCENTED)			
24s ea	10486-0007-08	53.76	
GRANDPA'S INDIAN CORN SOAP (Grandpa Soap)			
TP (3.25 OZ)			
24s ea	10486-0007-18	53.76	
GRANDPA'S LOVE-MY-LOOFAH (Grandpa Soap)			
SOA,TP (3.25OZ)			
24s ea	10486-0007-20	53.76	
GRANDPA'S OATMEAL SOAP (Grandpa Soap)			
TP (3.25OZ)			
24s ea	10486-0007-07	53.76	
GRANDPA'S PATCHOULI SOAP (Grandpa Soap)			
SOA,TP (3.25OZ,W/ALOE VERA)			
24s ea	10486-0007-14	53.76	
GRANDPA'S PINE TAR (Grandpa Soap)			
SHA,TP, 240 ml 12s	10486-0007-10	71.76	
GRANDPA'S PINE TAR BATH & SHOWER (Grandpa Soap)			
GEL,TP, 237 ml 12s	10486-0007-24	71.76	
GRANDPA'S PINE TAR SOAP (Grandpa Soap)			
SOA,TP (3.25 OZ)			
25s ea	10486-0007-00	52.00	
(4.25 OZ)			
25s ea	10486-0007-01	68.00	
(1.25 OZ)			
48s ea	10486-0007-02	33.12	
GRANDPA'S SHEA BUTTER SOAP (Grandpa Soap)			
SOA,TP (3.25OZ)			
24s ea	10486-0007-25	53.76	
GRANDPA'S WITCH-HAZEL SOAP (Grandpa Soap)			
TP (3.25 OZ)			
24s ea	10486-0007-03	53.76	
GRAPE SEED EXTRACT (Cardinal Health)			
CAP,PO (PRIVATE LABEL)			
50 mg, 30s ea	37205-0054-65	3.97	
(Marlex)			
CAP,PO, 60 mg, 60s ea	10135-0287-60	2.99	
(Mason Vit)			
CAP,PO (YEAST FREE,PF,SF)			
146 mg-50 mg, 60s ea	11845-0128-65	12.89	
(PF,SF)			
146 mg-60 mg, 60s ea	11845-0115-85	6.89	
(Rexall)			
CAP,PO (PF,SF)			
30 mg, 30s ea	30768-0000-83	3.84	5.82
GRAPE-OPC (Key Company)			
CAP,PO, 400 mg-50 mg-65 mg,			
60s ea	11694-0646-01	11.50	
GRAPESEED EXTRACT (Nature's Bounty)			
CAP,PO (PF,SF)			
500 mg-50 mg, 50s ea	74312-0000-10		9.99
GRAPHITES (Luyties)			
TAB,SL (6X)			
6 x, 500s ea	00618-4044-03	3.99	
5500s ea	00618-4044-10	30.32	
12 x, 500s ea	00622-4044-03	4.19	
(30X)			
12 x, 5500s ea	00622-4044-10	31.83	
30 x, 500s ea	00624-4044-03	4.19	
(12X)			
30 x, 5500s ea	00624-4044-10	31.83	
GRAVITY FEEDING (Abbott)			
DEV,NA (USED W/FLEXITAINER)			
ea	70074-0000-61	4.27	
(W/PIERCING PIN)			
ea	70074-0059-01	4.85	
ea	70074-0553-80	4.85	
GREAT PLAINS BENTONITE DETOX (Yerba)			
SUS,PO, 480 ml	46352-0005-19	5.37	8.95
GREEN SOAP (Consolidated Midland)			
TIN,TP, 120 ml 125s	00223-6262-01	21.00	
480 ml	00223-6262-02	3.50	
3840 ml	00223-6262-03	22.50	
(Denison)			
TIN,TP, 480 ml	00295-1178-16	2.54	
GREEN SOURCE (Nature's Bounty)			
TAB,PO, 60s ea	74312-0062-20		14.65
GREEN TEA (Mason Vit)			
CAP,PO (PF,SF)			
150 mg, 60s ea	11845-0128-35	6.56	
GREEN TEA EXTRACT (Rexall)			
CAP,PO (STANDARDIZED)			
250 mg-150 mg, 60s ea	30768-0036-61	2.43	3.68
GRIPP-HEEL (Heel/BHI)			
TAB,SL, 100s ea	50114-6075-02	5.85	10.80
GROOM MATE (PHR)			
DEV,NA (LADY NASAL HAIR TRIMMER)			
ea	44582-0150-00	3.98	7.95
(NOSE HAIR TRIMMER)			
ea	44582-0100-00	3.98	7.95
GRX ANALGESIC BALM (Geritrex)			
OIN,TP, 30 gm	54162-0555-01	1.74	
(Quality Care Prod)			
REPACK			
OIN,TP, 30 gm	49999-0535-01	12.30	
GRX HYDROGEL GAUZE DRESSING (Geritrex)			
DEV,NA (4"X4",8PLY)			
30s ea	92771-0865-44	2.05	
(2"X2",8PLY)			
50s ea	92771-0865-22	1.45	
GRX HYDROPHOR GAUZE (Geritrex)			
DEV,NA (3"X3")			
ea	54162-0510-02	0.52	
(3"X8")			
ea	54162-0510-01	1.05	
GRX WOUND GEL DRESSING (Geritrex)			
DRE,TP (SRN)			
30 gm	54162-0222-01	5.39	
(100X30ML)			
30 ml 100s	54162-0222-10	0.95	
(TUBE)			
90 gm	54162-0222-03	4.34	
GTF CHROMIUM (ADH)			
TAB,PO, 200 mcg,			
100s ea	60142-0112-10	3.98	7.95
GUADALUPANO DE CAPSICO (McLean, Dr.)			
PAD,TP, 1.3%, ea	11169-0214-46	1.93	2.89
GUAIFENESIN (Bio-Pharm)			
SYR,PO, 100 mg/5 ml,			
120 ml	59741-0112-04	2.50	
240 ml	59741-0112-08	2.80	
480 ml	59741-0112-16	3.25	
3840 ml	59741-0112-20	16.75	
(Breckenridge Pharm)			
TAB,PO, 400 mg, 100s ea	51991-0606-01	28.98	
(Major)			
TAB,PO, 200 mg, 100s ea	00904-5154-60	23.95	
(Pharm Assoc Inc)			
SOL,PO (100X5ML,AF,SF)			
100 mg/5 ml,			
5 ml 100s UD	00121-1744-05	48.76	
(CUPS;10X10,AF,SF)			
100 mg/5 ml,			
10 ml 100s UD	00121-1744-10	51.46	
(100X15ML,AF,SF)			
100 mg/5 ml,			
15 ml 100s UD	00121-1744-15	58.80	
(AF,SF)			
100 mg/5 ml, 237 ml	00121-0744-08	4.21	
473 ml	00121-0744-16	6.35	
SYR,PO, 100 mg/5 ml,			
118 ml	00121-0744-04	1.93	
(Rugby)			
SYR,PO (AF,FRUIT)			
100 mg/5 ml, 120 ml	00536-0825-97	2.79	
480 ml	00536-0825-85	4.94	
(A-S Medication)			
REPACK			
SYR,PO (AF)			
100 mg/5 ml,			
120 ml	54569-4381-00	1.97	
(Pharma Pac)			
REPACK			
SOL,PO, 100 mg/5 ml,			
120 ml	52959-0851-04	2.89	
(Phys Total Care)			
REPACK			
SYR,PO, 100 mg/5 ml,			
3840 ml	54868-3883-00	93.48	
TAB,PO, 200 mg, 100s ea	54868-5847-00	24.23	
(Quality Care Prod)			
REPACK			
TAB,PO (DYE-FREE)			
400 mg, 20s ea	49999-0658-20	59.63	
GUAIFENESIN DM (Altura)			
REPACK			
SYR,PO, 10 mg/5 ml-100 mg/5 ml,			
120 ml	63874-0067-12	6.89	
240 ml	63874-0067-24	13.78	
480 ml	63874-0067-48	27.56	
(Phys Total Care)			
REPACK			
SYR,PO, 10 mg/5 ml-100 mg/5 ml,			
120 ml	54868-1986-01	11.24	
480 ml	54868-1986-00	28.44	
GUAIFENESIN EXPECTORANT (Dispensing Solutions)			
REPACK			
SYR,PO, 100 mg/5 ml,			
118 ml	55045-1254-02	3.65	
GUAIFENESIN-DM (Pharm Assoc Inc)			
SYR,PO (10X10X5ML,AF)			
10 mg/5 ml-100 mg/5 ml,			
5 ml 100s UD	00121-0638-05	42.19	
(10X10X10ML,AF)			
10 mg/5 ml-100 mg/5 ml,			
10 ml 100s UD	00121-0638-10	45.32	
(AF,PRIVATE LABEL)			
10 mg/5 ml-100 mg/5 ml,			
120 ml	00121-0638-04	2.40	
237 ml	00121-0638-08	5.89	
473 ml	00121-0638-16	8.05	

PROD/MFR	HRI, UPC,NDC	AWP	SRP
GUAIFENESIN/PSEUDOEPHEDRINE (Phys Total Care)			
REPACK			
SYR,PO (AF)			
100 mg/5 ml-30 mg/5 ml,			
118 ml	54868-4772-00	9.15	
GUAR GUM (Freeda)			
PDS,PO, 1800 mg/1.8 gm,			
480 gm	10432-0282-03	9.57	15.95
GUARANA (Mason Vit)			
CAP,PO (PF,SF)			
60s ea	11845-0114-75	7.22	
GUARDAL (Morton)			
TAB,PO, 100s ea	01277-0108-10	12.50	
GUIATUSCON (Consolidated Midland)			
LIQ,PO, 100 mg/5 ml,			
120 ml	00223-6263-01	1.95	
480 ml	00223-6263-02	3.95	
GUIATUSCON DM (Consolidated Midland)			
SYR,PO, 10 mg/5 ml-100 mg/5 ml,			
480 ml	00223-6516-02	6.50	
GUIATUSS (Teva)			
SYR,PO, 100 mg/5 ml,			
480 ml	00182-0259-40	4.45	
(A-S Medication)			
REPACK			
SYR,PO, 100 mg/5 ml,			
473 ml	54569-5474-00	6.65	
(Quality Care Prod)			
REPACK			
SYR,PO, 100 mg/5 ml,			
120 ml	49999-0192-04	6.43	
(Stat Rx)			
REPACK			
SYR,PO, 100 mg/5 ml,			
120 ml	16590-0111-04	7.00	
GUIATUSS DM (Dispensing Solutions)			
REPACK			
SYR,PO, 10 mg/5 ml-100 mg/5 ml,			
118 ml	55045-1603-02	6.85	
(Phys Total Care)			
REPACK			
LIQ,PO, 10 mg/5 ml-100 mg/5 ml,			
120 ml	54868-1934-01	8.97	
480 ml	54868-1934-00	22.98	
(Quality Care Prod)			
REPACK			
SYR,PO, 10 mg/5 ml-100 mg/5 ml,			
120 ml	49999-0188-04	9.24	
(Southwood)			
REPACK			
SYR,PO, 10 mg/5 ml-100 mg/5 ml,			
120 ml	58016-4018-01	7.70	
GUIATUSS PE (Consolidated Midland)			
SYR,PO, 100 mg/5 ml-30 mg/5 ml,			
120 ml	00223-6517-04	2.40	
480 ml	00223-6517-01	6.75	
(A-S Medication)			
REPACK			
SYR,PO, 100 mg/5 ml-30 mg/5 ml,			
118 ml	54569-2620-00	2.63	
GUMSOL (Kramer-Novis)			
SPR,MM, 2%, 30 ml	52083-0704-01	6.60	
GUMSOL SOLUTION (Kramer-Novis)			
LIQ,MM, 2%, 30 ml	52083-0703-01	5.50	
GY-NA-TREN (Natren)			
KIT,NA (VAGINAL/ORAL)			
ea	53983-0555-28	18.00	30.00
GYNE-LOTRIMIN (Phys Total Care)			
REPACK			
CRE,VG, 1%, 45 gm	54868-0418-01	10.03	
TAB,VG, 100 mg, 7s ea	54868-0417-02	9.51	
(Southwood)			
REPACK			
CRE,VG, 1%, 45 gm	58016-3028-01	23.69	
GYNE-LOTRIMIN 7 (Schering Plough)			
CRE,VG (1X45GM,W/APPLICATOR)			
1%, 45 gm	00085-0887-09	7.20	
GYNOVITE PLUS (Optimox)			
TAB,PO, 180s ea	50520-0008-02	13.00	18.00
H.E.A.R. (Prime Marketing)			
SOL,OT, 6.5%, 15 ml	62107-0009-84	3.70	
H&H THINLET LANCETS (Can-Am Care)			
DEV,NA (PRIVATE LABEL)			
100s ea	38396-0303-16	5.85	
(SUPER,PRIVATE LABEL)			
100s ea	38396-0304-16	5.85	
HAEMOLANCE LANCETS (Arkray)			
DEV,NA (LOW FLOW,RETRACTABLE)			
50s ea	08317-9550-00	11.10	
(RETRACTABLE,21G)			
50s ea	08317-0350-50	11.10	
(LOW FLOW,RETRACTABLE)			
150s ea	08317-9500-00	28.70	
(RETRACTABLE,21G)			
150s ea	08317-0150-01	28.70	
HAEMOLANCE PLUS (Arkray)			
DEV,NA (HIGH FLOW)			
150s ea	15482-0990-80	29.75	
HAEMOLANCE PLUS LANCETS (Arkray)			
DEV,NA (1.6MM,28GUAGE,MICROFLOW)			
50s ea	08317-9902-50	12.98	
(21G)			
50s ea	08317-9907-50	12.98	
(25G)			
50s ea	08317-9909-50	12.98	
(1.2MM,PEDIATRIC)			
150s ea	08317-9904-00	33.53	
(1.6MM,28GAUGE,MICROFLOW)			
150s ea	08317-9902-00	33.53	
(1.6MM,MAX FLOW)			
150s ea	08317-9906-00	33.53	
(21G)			
150s ea	08317-9907-00	33.53	
(25G)			
150s ea	08317-9909-00	33.53	
HAIR FORMULA EXTRA STRENGTH (Mason Vit)			
TAB,PO (PF,SF)			
60s ea	11845-0122-75	7.78	
HAIR VITAMINS EXTRA STRENGTH (Mason Vit)			
PO (PF,SF)			
60s ea	11845-0072-25	7.78	
90s ea	11845-0072-29	10.67	
HAIRVITE MEGA-POTENCY (Major)			
TAB,PO, 50s ea	00904-5043-51	5.38	
HALFPRIN (Kramer Labs)			
ECT,PO, 81 mg, 90s ea	53076-0109-14	4.40	5.15
162 mg, 60s ea	53076-0102-13	3.96	4.62
(Phys Total Care)			
REPACK			
ECT,PO, 162 mg, 60s ea	54868-4955-00	5.89	
HALLS (Cadbury)			
LOZ,MM (FAST RELIEF,SF)			
5 mg, 25s ea	12546-0625-42	1.67	
(ADVANCEDVAPORACTION)			
7 mg, 30s ea	12546-0627-49	1.45	
HAMAMELIS VIRGINIANA (Luyties)			
TAB,SL (6X)			
6 x, 500s ea	00618-4214-03	3.99	
5500s ea	00618-4214-10	30.32	
(30X)			
12 x, 500s ea	00622-4214-03	4.19	
5500s ea	00622-4214-10	31.83	
(12X)			
30 x, 500s ea	00624-4214-03	4.19	
5500s ea	00624-4214-10	31.83	
HAND AND SKIN LOTION (Mann)			
LOT,TP (TWIN PACK)			
473 ml 2s	99714-0032-29	7.80	12.00
HANDCLENS (Woodward Labs)			
SOL,TP (AF)			
120 ml	60193-0130-04	4.25	
480 ml	60193-0130-16	8.14	
800 ml	60193-0130-08	8.65	
HANDEZE THERAPEUTIC GLOVES (Dome)			
DEV,NA (BEIGE, SIZE 3, SMALL)			
ea	78509-0135-03	5.85	9.75
(BEIGE, SIZE 4, MEDIUM)			
ea	78509-0135-04	5.85	9.75
(BEIGE, SIZE 5, LARGE)			
ea	78509-0135-05	5.85	9.75
(BEIGE,SIZE 6)			
ea	78509-0135-06	5.85	9.75
(BEIGE,SIZE2,EXTRA SMALL)			
ea	78509-0135-02	5.85	9.75
HANDICARE GARMENT LINERS (Covidien)			
DEV,NA (4 1/2"X14",LATEX-FREE)			
125s ea	08080-1530-00	24.52	
(10"X24",LARGE)			
144s ea	08080-9310-24	57.54	
(7"X17",LATEX-FREE)			
200s ea	08080-6350-00	49.93	
200s ea	08080-9652-00	37.97	
HANDSHIELD (Stanmar Labs)			
CRE,TP, 22.5 gm	50263-0703-34	1.25	
150 gm	50263-0703-05	4.00	
480 gm	50263-0703-16	7.75	
960 gm	50263-0703-32	12.00	
HARD NAILS (Mericon)			
CAP,PO, 2.5 mg-57.5 mg-44.5 mg,			
42s ea	00394-0131-42	6.26	
HAWTHORN (Botanical Labs.)			
CAP,PO, 50s ea	41954-0032-65	4.00	7.99
LIQ,PO, 30 ml	41954-0020-27	3.75	7.49
HAWTHORN BERRY (Mason Vit)			
CAP,PO (PF,SF)			
500 mg, 60s ea	11845-0114-85	7.22	
HAWTHORNE (ADH)			
CAP,PO, 565 mg, 100s ea	60142-0105-10	4.98	9.95
(Mason Vit)			
CAP,PO (PF,SF)			
250 mg, 60s ea	11845-0129-25	8.33	
HAZELETES (Dickinson Brands)			
PAD,TP (W/ALOE)			
50s ea	52651-0000-11	3.50	
60s ea	52651-0000-10	2.21	
HC DERMA-PAX (Recsei)			
LOT,TP, 0.5%-0.5%,			
60 ml	10952-0050-12	6.15	
120 ml	10952-0050-16	9.95	
HCL AND PEPSIN (Carlson,J.R.)			
TAB,PO (PF,SF,LACTOSE-FREE)			
500 mg-150 mg, 100s ea	88395-0066-01	8.45	16.90
250s ea	88395-0066-02	18.50	37.00
HCU COOLER (VITAFLO, LLC)			
LIQ,PO (15GM PROTEIN EQUIVALENT)			
130 ml 30s	50600-0535-27	265.50	349.75
HCU EXPRESS (VITAFLO, LLC)			
PDR,PO (ENTERAL,UNFLAVORED)			
25 gm 30s	50600-0535-58	265.50	349.75
HCU GEL (VITAFLO, LLC)			
PO (ENTERAL,UNFLAVORED)			
20 gm 30s	50600-0535-03	148.68	239.00
HCY 1 (Mead Johnson & Co)			
PDR,PO, 454 gm	00087-0095-41	39.60	
HCY 2 (Mead Johnson & Co)			
PDR,PO, 454 gm	00087-0199-41	68.99	
HDA TOOTHACHE (S.S.S.)			
GEL,MM, 6.5%, 15 ml	12258-0124-05	2.53	3.79
HEADACHE FORMULA (Cardinal Health)			
TAB,PO (ADDED STRENGTH)			
100s ea	37205-0703-78	4.77	
HEALTH ALLIANCE PSS (Home Diag)			
DEV,NA (STRIP)			
50s ea	56151-0303-50	28.60	
HEALTH ALLIANCE PSS STARTER (Home Diag)			
DEV,NA (MTR,STRP,LANCET,DEV,SOL)			
ea	56151-0203-01	22.18	
HEALTH EPA (Health Products Corp)			
SGL,PO (PF,SF,SOFTGEL)			
60s ea	39686-0013-22	4.00	
HEALTH HAIR (Health Products Corp)			
TAB,PO, 60s ea	39686-0012-56	9.96	
HEALTH MART (McKesson)			
ADHESIVE STRIPS			
DEV,NA (EXTRA LARGE)			
10s ea	52297-0694-52	1.99	
ADHESIVE STRIPS CLEAR			
NA, 40s ea	52297-0693-58	1.99	
ASPIRIN			
ECT,PO, 325 mg, 100s ea	52297-0429-78	5.19	
500s ea	52297-0980-14	10.79	
BANDAGES FLEXIBLE			
DEV,NA (ASSORTED)			
30s ea	52297-0691-65	1.99	
BANDAGES SHEER			
NA (1")			
40s ea	52297-0692-58	1.99	
CLOTRIMAZOLE			
CRE,TP, 1%, 30 gm	52297-0499-10	7.49	
COTTON BALLS			
DEV,NA, 300s ea	52297-0685-87	1.09	

PROD/MFR	HRI, UPC,NDC	AWP	SRP
COTTON BALLS TRIPLE SIZE			
NA, 100s ea	**52297-0686-78**	1.09	
DAYHIST-1			
TAB,PO, 1.34 mg, 16s ea	**52297-0257-73**	5.79	
DIGITAL PROBE COVERS			
DEV,NA, 25s ea	**52297-0751-63**	1.39	
DIPHEDRYL			
CAP,PO, 25 mg, 24s ea	**52297-0462-62**	3.09	
48s ea	**52297-0268-67**	4.79	
TAB,PO, 25 mg, 24s ea	**52297-0521-62**	3.19	
DIPHEDRYL CHILDREN'S			
ELI,PO (AF,CHERRY)			
12.5 mg/5 ml,			
118 ml	**52297-0379-26**	3.79	
GAUZE BANDAGE			
DEV,NA (2"X2 YDS)			
ea	**52297-0695-00**	1.99	
HYDROCORTISONE			
CRE,TP, 1%, 30 gm	**52297-0105-10**	3.19	
OIN,TP, 1%, 30 gm	**52297-0104-10**	3.19	
HYDROGEN PEROXIDE			
SOL,TP, 3%, 240 ml	**52297-0722-34**	0.57	
480 ml	**52297-0722-43**	0.69	
IBUPROFEN			
TAB,PO (CAPLET)			
200 mg, 50s ea	**52297-0647-71**	4.19	
(COATED)			
200 mg, 50s ea	**52297-0604-71**	3.99	
100s ea	**52297-0497-78**	5.69	
(CAPLET)			
200 mg, 100s ea	**52297-0647-78**	5.69	
(COATED)			
200 mg, 100s ea	**52297-0604-78**	5.69	
250s ea	**52297-0604-19**	10.99	
(CAPLET)			
200 mg, 500s ea	**52297-0647-35**	14.29	
(COATED)			
200 mg, 500s ea	**52297-0979-14**	14.29	
L-LYSINE			
TAB,PO, 500 mg, 100s ea	**52297-0535-78**	5.99	
LANCETS			
DEV,NA, 100s ea	**52297-0956-10**	5.99	
(MONOLET)			
200s ea	**52297-0290-82**	9.59	
(THIN MONOLET)			
200s ea	**52297-0811-82**	9.59	
LAXATIVE			
ECT,PO, 5 mg, 25s ea	**52297-0235-63**	4.29	
SUP,RC, 10 mg, 8s ea	**52297-0109-51**	5.79	
MICONAZOLE 7			
CRE,VG, 2%, 47.7 gm	**52297-0248-29**	7.99	
MILK OF MAGNESIA			
SUS,PO, 400 mg/5 ml,			
360 ml	**52297-0396-40**	3.99	
(MINT)			
400 mg/5 ml,			
360 ml	**52297-0332-40**	3.99	
780 ml	**52297-0396-44**	6.69	
MULTIPLE VITAMINS ESSENTIAL			
TAB,PO, 100s ea	**52297-0648-78**	4.99	
250s ea	**52297-0650-65**	7.89	
MULTIPLE VITAMINS PLUS IRON			
TAB,PO, 250s ea	**52297-0654-85**	7.99	
MULTIPLE VITAMINS WOMEN'S			
TAB,PO, 100s ea	**52297-0656-78**	6.19	
MULTIVITAMIN & MULTIMINERAL			
TAB,PO, 100s ea	**52297-0426-78**	7.19	
NAPROXEN SODIUM			
TAB,PO, 220 mg, 50s ea	**52297-0843-71**	4.09	
(CAPLET)			
220 mg, 50s ea	**52297-0845-71**	4.09	
NASAL DECONGESTANT 12 HR			
SPR,NS, 0.05%, 30 ml	**52297-0304-10**	4.09	
NATURAL B-COMPLEX W/VITAMIN C			
TAB,PO, 100s ea	**52297-0237-78**	5.89	
NIACIN			
TAB,PO, 100 mg, 100s ea	**52297-0522-78**	2.99	
NIGHTTIME			
SGL,PO (LIQUICAP)			
12s ea	**52297-0530-53**	2.99	
NIGHTTIME COLD/FLU MEDICINE			
SOL,PO, 296 ml	**52297-0305-38**	3.99	
(CHERRY)			
296 ml	**52297-0322-38**	3.99	
NON-ASPIRIN ALLERGY/SINUS			
TAB,PO (MAX. STR.,GELCAP)			
325 mg-2 mg-30 mg,			
24s ea	**52297-0607-60**	3.39	
OCUMIN			
TAB,PO, 60s ea	**52297-0389-72**	6.19	
OYSTER SHELL CALCIUM			
TAB,PO (PF,SF)			
500 mg, 60s ea	**52297-0634-72**	5.59	
OYSTER SHELL CALCIUM/VITAMIN D			
TAB,PO, 250 mg-125 iu,			
100s ea	**52297-0546-78**	4.09	
(PF,SF)			
500 mg-200 iu,			
100s ea	**52297-0519-78**	6.69	
PAIN RELIEVER EXTRA STRENGTH			
TAB,PO (GELTAB)			
500 mg, 24s ea	**52297-0563-62**	2.09	
(CAPLET)			
500 mg, 50s ea	**52297-0484-71**	4.19	
(GELCAPLET)			
500 mg, 50s ea	**52297-0470-71**	4.19	
(GELTAB)			
500 mg, 50s ea	**52297-0563-71**	4.09	
100s ea	**52297-0405-78**	5.49	
(CAPLET)			
500 mg, 100s ea	**52297-0484-78**	5.59	
(GELCAPLET)			
500 mg, 100s ea	**52297-0470-78**	6.19	
PAIN RELIEVER W/SLEEP AID PM			
TAB,PO (EXT. STR.,GELTAB)			
500 mg-25 mg,			
50s ea	**52297-0983-09**	5.39	
(EXT.STR.,CAPLET)			
500 mg-25 mg,			
50s ea	**52297-0437-71**	5.19	
POTASSIUM GLUCONATE			
TAB,PO (PF,SF)			
550 mg, 100s ea	**52297-0558-78**	3.49	
POVIDONE-IODINE			
SOL,TP, 10%, 237 ml	**52297-0217-34**	5.39	
PREGNANCY TEST STRIP			
DEV,NA, ea	**52297-0790-00**	7.99	
PRENATAL			
TAB,PO, 100s ea	**52297-0259-78**	10.19	
SALINE MIST			
SPR,NS, 0.65%, 44 ml	**52297-0312-13**	2.09	
SENNA			
TAB,PO, 8.6 mg, 100s ea	**52297-0557-78**	10.69	
SINUS PAIN RELIEF MAXIMUM STRENGTH			
TAB,PO (NON-DROWSY,CAPLET)			
500 mg-30 mg,			
24s ea	**52297-0438-62**	3.69	
SORE THROAT			
LOZ,MM (CHERRY)			
18s ea	**52297-0194-73**	2.29	
SPR,MM (AF,SF,CHERRY)			
1.4%, 177 ml	**52297-0328-30**	3.79	
STOOL SOFTENER W/LAXATIVE			
SGL,PO, 30 mg-100 mg,			
60s ea	**52297-0270-72**	5.99	
STRESS B-COMPLEX			
TAB,PO, 60s ea	**52297-0624-72**	6.19	
STRESS B-COMPLEX W/ZINC			
TAB,PO, 60s ea	**52297-0628-72**	6.19	
THERAPEUTIC M			
TAB,PO, 130s ea	**52297-0644-97**	7.09	
THERMOMETER DIGITAL			
DEV,NA, ea	**52297-0759-00**	7.99	
TRIPLE ANTIBIOTIC			
OIN,TP, 15 gm	**52297-0114-05**	2.69	
30 gm	**52297-0106-10**	3.79	
TUSSIN			
SYR,PO (AF)			
100 mg/5 ml,			
118 ml	**52297-0310-26**	2.59	
237 ml	**52297-0310-34**	4.39	
TUSSIN COLD/COUGH			
CAP,PO (LIQUIGEL)			
10 mg-100 mg-30 mg,			
12s ea	**52297-0510-53**	3.49	
TUSSIN DM			
SYR,PO, 10 mg/5 ml-100 mg/5 ml,			
118 ml	**52297-0359-26**	3.39	
237 ml	**52297-0359-34**	5.19	
TUSSIN DM CLEAR			
LIQ,PO (NON-DROWSY,AF,SF)			
10 mg/5 ml-100 mg/5 ml,			
118 ml	**52297-0552-26**	4.19	
VITAMIN A			
SGL,PO (PF,SF,SOFTGEL)			
8000 iu, 100s ea	**52297-0502-78**	3.09	
VITAMIN B1 NATURAL			
TAB,PO, 100 mg, 100s ea	**52297-0580-78**	3.99	
VITAMIN B12			
TAB,PO, 100 mcg,			
100s ea	**52297-0586-78**	3.49	
500 mcg, 100s ea	**52297-0588-78**	5.79	
TER,PO (PF,SF)			
1000 mcg, 60s ea	**52297-0518-72**	6.39	
VITAMIN B6 NATURAL			
TAB,PO, 50 mg, 100s ea	**52297-0582-78**	3.79	
VITAMIN C			
CTB,PO, 500 mg, 100s ea	**52297-0606-78**	5.59	
TAB,PO, 250 mg, 100s ea	**52297-0594-78**	2.99	
500 mg, 100s ea	**52297-0596-78**	3.29	
250s ea	**52297-0598-85**	7.19	
500s ea	**52297-0435-90**	12.19	
1000 mg, 100s ea	**52297-0602-78**	5.79	
TER,PO, 500 mg, 100s ea	**52297-0600-78**	5.59	
VITAMIN C W/ROSE HIPS			
TAB,PO (PF,SF)			
500 mg, 100s ea	**52297-0534-78**	4.99	
1000 mg, 100s ea	**52297-0424-78**	7.19	
TER,PO, 1000 mg, 60s ea	**52297-0238-72**	6.19	
VITAMIN E			
SGL,PO (SOFTGEL)			
200 iu, 100s ea	**52297-0610-78**	4.49	
400 iu, 100s ea	**52297-0525-78**	7.69	
100s ea	**52297-0612-78**	5.69	
300s ea	**52569-0130-59**	14.09	
1000 iu, 50s ea	**52297-0616-71**	9.99	
VITAMIN E NATURAL			
PO (SOFTGEL)			
400 iu, 100s ea	**52297-0542-78**	10.19	
(PF,SF,SOFTGEL)			
1000 iu, 50s ea	**52297-0544-71**	14.69	
(SOFTGEL)			
1000 iu, 50s ea	**52569-0130-54**	8.19	
WITCH HAZEL			
LIQ,TP, 480 ml	**52297-0723-43**	2.57	
ZINC NATURAL			
TAB,PO, 50 mg, 100s ea	**52297-0562-78**	5.09	
HEALTH-A-DAY (Health Products Corp)			
TAB,PO (PF,SF)			
100s ea	**39686-0013-10**	2.35	
100s ea	**39686-0013-16**	2.45	
250s ea	**39686-0013-11**	5.00	
250s ea	**39686-0013-17**	5.10	
HEALTHMART (McKesson)			
ALCOHOL ETHYL			
LIQ,TP (RUBBING)			
70%, 480 ml	**52297-0717-43**	1.59	
ALCOHOL ISOPROPYL			
LIQ,TP, 70%, 480 ml	**52297-0718-43**	0.69	
480 ml	**52297-0719-43**	1.33	
ALCOHOL PREP			
DEV,NA, 110s ea	**52297-0707-00**	1.69	
ALLERGY			
TAB,PO, 4 mg, 24s ea	**52297-0463-62**	4.19	
ANIMAL SHAPES CHILDREN'S			
CTB,PO, 100s ea	**52297-0638-78**	5.59	
ANIMAL SHAPES PLUS EXTRA C			
PO, 100s ea	**52297-0239-72**	5.69	
ANIMAL SHAPES PLUS IRON CHILDREN'S			
CTB,PO (ASSORTED)			
100s ea	**52297-0640-78**	5.59	
ANTACID			
SUS,PO (MINT)			
225 mg/5 ml-200 mg/5 ml,			
355 ml	**52297-0356-40**	2.99	
780 ml	**52297-0356-35**	5.49	
ANTI-DIARRHEAL			
TAB,PO (CAPLET)			
2 mg, 12s ea	**52297-0288-53**	4.29	
(CAPELT,E-Z OPEN)			
2 mg, 18s ea	**52297-0288-89**	4.59	
ANTI-NAUSEA			
SOL,PO (CHERRY)			
118 ml	**52297-0455-26**	5.49	
ASPIRIN			
TAB,PO (MICRO-THIN COATED)			
325 mg, 100s ea	**52297-0416-78**	1.89	
ASPIRIN ADULT LOW STRENGTH			
ECT,PO, 81 mg, 120s ea	**52297-0507-76**	4.99	
ASPIRIN CHILDREN'S			
CTB,PO (CHERRY)			
81 mg, 36s ea	**52297-0820-68**	1.89	
ASPIRIN MAXIMUM STRENGTH			
ECT,PO, 500 mg, 60s ea	**52297-0266-72**	5.19	
BACITRACIN			
OIN,TP, 500 u/gm, 30 gm	**52297-0108-10**	2.99	
BETA CAROTENE			
SGL,PO (SOFTGEL)			
25000 iu, 100s ea	**52297-0514-78**	6.59	
CALCIUM			
TAB,PO (PF,SF)			
600 mg, 60s ea	**52297-0555-72**	5.09	
CALCIUM 500 + D			
TAB,PO, 500 mg-125 iu,			
60s ea	**52297-0988-12**	5.59	
250s ea	**52569-0130-53**	8.99	

PROD/MFR	HRI, UPC,NDC	AWP	SRP
CALCIUM ANTACID			
CTB,PO (PEPPERMINT)			
250 mg, 150s ea	**52297-0443-47**	3.29	
CALCIUM/VITAMIN D			
TAB,PO (PF,SF)			
600 mg-125 iu,			
60s ea	**52297-0540-72**	5.09	
CASTOR OIL			
OIL,PO, 60 ml	**52297-0712-16**	1.99	
CENTRAL-VITE ADVANCED FORMULA			
TAB,PO, 130s ea	**52297-0383-97**	7.19	
CHROMIUM PICOLINATE			
TAB,PO, 200 mcg,			
100s ea	**52297-0427-78**	6.19	
COD LIVER OIL			
SGL,PO (SOFTGEL)			
100s ea	**52297-0506-78**	4.59	
COMPLETE MAXIMUM STRENGTH			
TAB,PO, 500 mg-2 mg-15 mg-30 mg,			
24s ea	**52297-0888-62**	4.19	
COUGH SUPPRESSANT DROPS			
LOZ,MM (CHERRY)			
30s ea	**52297-0192-65**	1.09	
(HONEY,LEMON)			
30s ea	**52297-0750-65**	1.09	
(MENTHOL-EUCALYPTUS)			
30s ea	**52297-0193-65**	1.09	
DAILY VITAMINS W/IRON			
TAB,PO, 100s ea	**52297-0652-78**	4.99	
DAY TIME			
SGL,PO (LIQUICAP,NON-DROWSY)			
12s ea	**52297-0527-53**	2.99	
DIPHEDRYL ALLERGY			
CAP,PO, 25 mg, 100s ea	**52297-0948-10**	7.59	
ELECTROLYTE PEDIATRIC			
SOL,PO (FRUIT)			
1014 ml	**52297-0336-45**	4.29	
FIBER NATURAL			
PDR,PO (REGULAR)			
3.4 gm/dose,			
369 gm	**52297-0301-27**	4.79	
(ORANGE)			
3.4 gm/dose,			
539 gm	**52297-0303-37**	5.49	
FISH OIL CONCENTRATE			
SGL,PO (SOFTGEL)			
1000 mg, 60s ea	**52297-0431-20**	6.69	
FOLIC ACID			
TAB,PO, 0.4 mg, 250s ea	**52297-0879-85**	4.29	
GARLIC			
TAB,PO (PF,SF,DYE-FREE)			
400 mg, 30s ea	**52297-0985-44**	7.09	
GARLIC OIL NATURAL			
SGL,PO (SOFTGEL)			
1 mg, 100s ea	**52297-0995-10**	4.09	
GELATIN			
TAB,PO, 650 mg, 100s ea	**52297-0572-78**	4.79	
GINKGO BILOBA			
TAB,PO, 40 mg, 36s ea	**52569-0130-56**	7.49	
(CAPLET)			
120 mg, 50s ea	**52297-0897-71**	9.49	
GINSENG EXTRACT			
SGL,PO (SF,SOFTGEL)			
100 mg, 30s ea	**52297-0566-65**	7.79	
GLUCOSAMINE COMPLEX			
TAB,PO (CAPLET)			
200 mg-300 mg,			
60s ea	**52297-0990-12**	13.89	
GOLDENSEAL ROOT			
TAB,PO (CAPLET)			
250 mg, 50s ea	**52569-0130-57**	10.99	
HEARTBURN RELIEF 200			
TAB,PO, 200 mg, 30s ea	**52297-0961-44**	7.19	
IBUPROFEN CHILDREN'S			
SUS,PO (AF,BERRY)			
100 mg/5 ml,			
120 ml	**52297-0947-85**	4.19	
(AF,FRUIT)			
100 mg/5 ml,			
120 ml	**52297-0946-85**	4.19	
NASAL EXTRA MOISTURIZING 12 HOUR			
SPR,NS, 0.05%, 30 ml	**52297-0975-10**	4.09	
NASAL SINUS 12 HOUR			
NS, 0.05%, 30 ml	**52297-0976-10**	4.09	
PANAX GINSENG			
TAB,PO (SF,CAPLET)			
300 mg, 50s ea	**52569-0130-51**	9.19	
SAW PALMETTO STANDARDIZED EXTRACT			
SGL,PO (SF,SOFTGEL)			
160 mg, 50s ea	**52297-0905-71**	11.39	

PROD/MFR	HRI, UPC,NDC	AWP	SRP
VALERIAN ROOT			
TAB,PO (CAPLET)			
100 mg, 90s ea	**52569-0130-50**	6.19	
VITAL ADVANTAGE SUPER MEGA			
TAB,PO (CAPLET)			
100s ea	**52297-0989-45**	8.19	
HEALTHSENSE ANTACID (Prime Marketing)			
SUS,PO (SODIUM-FREE,MINT CREME)			
355 ml	**62107-0081-11**	2.90	4.90
(EXTRA STRENGTH)			
355 ml	**62107-0082-11**	3.75	5.95
HEALTHWISE PEN NEEDLES (Owen Mumford)			
DEV,NA (12MMX29G,ORIGINAL)			
100s ea	**08214-0297-37**	21.50	
(6MMX31G,MINI)			
100s ea	**08214-0907-37**	21.50	
(8MMX31G,SHORT)			
100s ea	**08214-0307-37**	21.50	
HEALTHY COLON (Major)			
CAP,PO, 240 mg, 30s ea	**00904-6035-46**	11.98	
HEALTHY LIVING COMPRESSOR NEBULIZER (Samsung America)			
DEV,NA (DESKTOP,CND-501S)			
ea	**81747-0911-92**	33.50	
HEALTHY LIVING REPLACEMENT FILTER (Samsung America)			
DEV,NA (CNF-520S)			
10s ea	**81747-0912-01**	1.30	
HEALTHY LIVING REPLACEMENT MASK (Samsung America)			
DEV,NA, 2s ea	**08495-1237-01**	2.50	
HEALTHY LIVING REPLACEMENT NEBULIZER (Samsung America)			
DEV,NA (W/OXYGEN TUBE,CNK-510S)			
ea	**81747-0912-00**	3.25	
HEALTHY MOOD 5-HTP ELITE (Carlson,J.R.)			
ODT,PO, 50 mg-1 mg,			
60s ea	**88395-0085-50**	7.75	15.50
120s ea	**88395-0085-51**	14.40	28.80
HEART (Miller)			
TAB,PO, 140 mg, 100s ea	**17204-0504-40**	5.70	9.00
HEART SMART (Health Products Corp)			
SGL,PO (PF,SF,SOFTGEL)			
60s ea	**39686-0014-85**	5.50	
HEARTBEAT ELITE (Carlson,J.R.)			
TAB,PO (PF,SF,CORN-FREE)			
180s ea	**88395-0041-52**	29.95	59.90
HEARTBURN 200 (Chain Drug Marketing)			
TAB,PO, 200 mg, 12s ea	**63868-0519-12**	1.22	4.49
30s ea	**63868-0519-30**	2.40	4.99
HEARTBURN 75 (Chain Drug Marketing)			
TAB,PO (SF,SODIUM-FREE)			
75 mg, 10s ea UD	**63868-0711-10**	1.32	3.19
30s ea UD	**63868-0711-30**	2.51	6.99
60s ea UD	**63868-0711-60**	4.08	11.99
HEARTBURN RELIEF (Major)			
TAB,PO, 10 mg, 30s ea	**00904-5529-87**	8.99	
60s ea	**00904-5529-52**	15.99	
(MAXIMUM STRENGTH)			
20 mg, 25s ea	**00904-5780-17**	5.99	
50s ea	**00904-5780-51**	7.49	
HEATHER (Ellon)			
SOL,SL (DROPS)			
10.5 ml	**51762-0006-10**		9.25
HEATHMART (McKesson)			
ECHINACEA			
TAB,PO (PF,SF,CAPLET)			
167 mg, 90s ea	**52569-0130-60**	6.69	
HEET (Medtech)			
LIQ,TP, 3.6%-0.25%-15%,			
69.9 ml	**75137-0701-10**	5.11	
HELIOCARE (Biopelle)			
CAP,PO, 240 mg, 60s ea	**42485-0200-01**	37.73	
HEM-PREP (Major)			
CRE,RC, 0.25%-3%,			
51.03 gm	**00904-5124-37**	3.55	
OIN,TP, 0.25%-3%, 60 gm	**00904-5184-02**	4.29	
SUP,RC, 24s ea	**00904-5304-24**	6.05	
HEMA ACCESS PORT (Abbott Hosp)			
DEV,NA, 48s ea	**00074-3129-48**	111.74	
HEMA II BLOOD SET W/SECURE LOCK (Abbott Hosp)			
DEV,NA (80")			
48s ea	**00074-9143-68**	778.62	

PROD/MFR	HRI, UPC,NDC	AWP	SRP
HEMA II NONVENTED SECONDARY BLOOD (Abbott Hosp)			
DEV,NA (36")			
24s ea	**00074-1783-02**	87.84	
HEMA II Y-TYPE W/SECURE LOCK NV (Abbott Hosp)			
DEV,NA (100", W/INLINE PUMP)			
48s ea	**00074-9165-58**	1092.69	
(100",DRIP CHAMBER PUMP)			
48s ea	**00074-9153-58**	1024.86	
(102",DRIP CHAMBER PUMP)			
48s ea	**00074-9149-58**	955.32	
(80",DRIP CHAMBER PUMP)			
48s ea	**00074-9155-68**	934.23	
HEMA TRANSFUSION FILTER PEDIATRIC (Abbott Hosp)			
DEV,NA (20 MICRON FILTER)			
48s ea	**00074-9136-48**	123.84	
HEMA-CHEK (Siemens)			
DEV,NA, 100s ea	**00193-2592-21**	102.20	102.20
25 ml 10s	**00193-2596-10**	94.10	94.10
HEMA-COMBISTIX (Siemens)			
DEV,NA, 100s ea	**08620-2182-21**	77.40	77.40
HEMASTIX (Siemens)			
DEV,NA (STRIP)			
50s ea	**00193-2190-50**	29.60	29.60
HEMATEST (Siemens)			
DEV,NA, 100s ea	**08620-2427-21**	65.00	65.00
HEMOCYTE (U.S. Pharm)			
TAB,PO (CHILD PROOF PACKAGING)			
324 mg, 30s ea	**52747-0307-30**	9.85	
(CHILD PROOF PKG)			
324 mg, 100s ea	**52747-0307-70**	32.80	
HEMORRHOID (Boiron)			
SUP,RC, 1 x-1 x-1 x,			
12s ea	**06960-0094-61**	7.66	11.99
HEMORRHOIDAL (Albertson's)			
OIN,TP, 60 gm 60s	**41280-0200-52**	3.36	
SUP,RC, 24s ea	**41280-0200-51**	3.60	
(AmerisourceBergen)			
OIN,TP (PRIVATE LABEL)			
60 gm	**24385-0387-16**	6.07	6.99
(Bio-Pharm)			
SUP,RC, 12s ea	**59741-0321-12**	2.25	
24s ea	**59741-0321-24**	4.05	
(Cardinal Health)			
CRE,RC (PRIVATE LABEL)			
51 gm	**37205-0572-24**	3.20	
OIN,TP, 0.25%-3%, 60 gm	**37205-0405-16**	3.20	
SUP,RC, 85.5%-0.25%-3%,			
12s ea	**37205-0715-16**	2.88	
(Consolidated Midland)			
SUP,RC, 12s ea	**00223-5174-12**	3.85	
24s ea	**00223-5174-24**	5.25	
(Dickinson Brands)			
PAD,TP, 100s ea	**52651-0000-30**	4.48	
(Family Phcy)			
OIN,TP (PRIVATE LABEL)			
60 gm	**52735-0714-36**	5.39	5.99
(Medicine Shoppe)			
OIN,TP, 0.25%-3%, 60 gm	**49614-0387-16**	4.19	4.19
(Qualitest)			
OIN,TP, 60 gm	**00603-0520-52**	4.21	
SUP,RC, 85.5%-0.25%-3%,			
12s ea	**00603-0524-11**	5.60	
(Rugby)			
SUP,RC, 0.25%, 12s ea	**00536-1389-12**	3.30	
(Phys Total Care)			
REPACK			
OIN,TP, 57 gm	**54868-2311-00**	16.78	
(Quality Care Prod)			
REPACK			
SUP,RC, 85.5%-0.25%-3%,			
12s ea	**35356-0192-12**	19.80	
HEMORRHOIDAL HC (Southwood)			
REPACK			
CRE,RC, 1%, 30 gm	**58016-3005-01**	27.96	
HEMORRHOIDAL OINTMENT (Reese)			
OIN,TP, 14.0%-71.9%-0.25%-3.0%,			
58 gm	**10956-0779-01**	5.66	
HEMORRHOIDAL PREP (Global Source)			
OIN,TP, 60 gm	**59618-0372-54**	4.15	
SUP,RC, 12s ea	**59618-0373-70**	3.35	

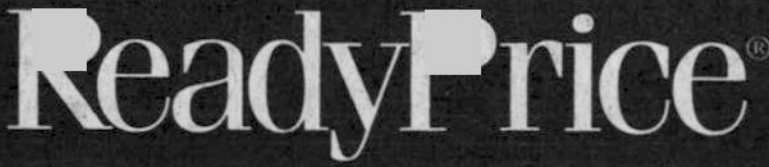

PROD/MFR	HRI, UPC,NDC	AWP	SRP
24s ea	59618-0373-72	4.95	
48s ea	59618-0373-74	8.95	
HEMORRODIL (Tarmac)			
OIN,TP, 30 gm	11096-0140-01	3.60	
1%, 15 gm	11096-0141-01	2.75	
SUP,RC, 12s ea	11096-0154-01	4.50	
HEMOSET (Abbott Hosp)			
DEV,NA (72", 100X10)			
20s ea	00074-8948-62	432.00	
HEP-FORTE (Marlyn)			
CAP,PO (SOFTGEL)			
300s ea	10712-0613-01	11.99	23.99
HEPAR SULPH (Luyties)			
TAB,SL (6X)			
6 x, 500s ea	00618-4232-03	3.99	
5500s ea	00618-4232-10	30.32	
(30X)			
12 x, 500s ea	00622-4232-03	4.19	
5500s ea	00622-4232-10	31.83	
(12X)			
30 x, 500s ea	00624-4232-03	4.19	
5500s ea	00624-4232-10	31.83	
(Walker Pharmacal)			
TAB,SL (6X)			
250s ea	00619-4232-02	2.97	
HEPATIC-AID II (Hormel Healthlabs)			
PDR,PO (GLUTEN-FREE)			
90 gm 24s	99429-0142-46	529.00	
90 gm 24s	99429-0148-53	529.00	
HERBAL ENERGY COMPLEX (Mason Vit)			
TAB,PO (PF,SF)			
60s ea	11845-0119-55	11.00	
(Rexall)			
CAP,PO (PF,SF)			
75s ea	30768-0011-97	2.73	4.13
HERBAL LAXATIVE (Health Products Corp)			
TAB,PO, 8.6 mg, 100s ea	39686-0015-04	2.75	
HERBAL SLEEP (Health Products Corp)			
TAB,PO (PF,SF)			
30s ea	39686-0015-00	3.50	
HERBAL SLIM COMPLEX (ADH)			
CAP,PO (PF,SF)			
470 mg, 100s ea	60142-0979-51	6.48	12.95
HERBAL WATER (Rexall)			
TAB,PO (PF,SF)			
30s ea	30768-0011-12	2.75	4.17
HERBALPAD (Zayco, Inc.)			
TDM,TD (SELF-ADHERING PAD)			
150 mg/24 hr,			
30s ea	77987-0210-00	7.80	12.95
30s ea	77987-0890-00	7.80	12.95
30s ea	77987-0790-00	7.80	12.95
30s ea	77987-0200-00	7.80	12.95
HERBCALM (Health Products Corp)			
TAB,PO (PF,SF)			
30s ea	39686-0014-86	3.50	
HERPALIEVE (Phyto Pharmica)			
CRE,TP, 1%, 5 gm	63948-0202-92	5.25	10.50
HERPECIN-L (Chattem)			
STI,TP (SPF 15,SF)			
2.8 gm	41167-0777-31	3.56	
HEX-ON (Coloplast)			
SPR,NA (FRESH LINEN)			
60 ml 12s	11701-0123-03	46.68	48.84
(LEMON)			
60 ml 12s	11701-0125-03	46.68	48.84
(FRESH LINEN)			
120 ml 12s	11701-0123-04	86.64	90.72
(LEMON)			
120 ml 12s	11701-0125-04	86.64	90.72
(FRESH LINEN)			
237 ml 12s	11701-0123-05	162.24	169.80
(LEMON)			
237 ml 12s	11701-0125-05	162.24	169.80
HEXAVITAMIN (Consolidated Midland)			
TAB,PO, 100s ea	00223-1052-01	3.25	
1000s ea	00223-1052-02	24.50	
(Upsher-Smith)			
TAB,PO, ea	00245-0082-89	0.06	
HI PRO-CAL (Hormel Healthlabs)			
POW,PO, 21.5 gm 50s	99429-0495-51	29.90	
HI-FIBER (Carlson,J.R.)			
PDR,PO, 6 gm/dose,			
448 gm	88395-0085-33	8.30	16.60
(PF,CORN-FREE,SALT-FREE)			
11 mg-1 mg-6 gm,			
35 gm	88395-0085-31	5.95	11.90
HI-KOVITE (Freeda)			
TAB,PO (2 TAB COMBO,PF,SF)			
200s ea	10432-0021-01	8.88	14.80
HI-PROTEIN (Mason Vit)			
CTB,PO, 500 mg, 100s ea	11845-0054-51	4.22	
HI-VEGI-LIP (Freeda)			
TAB,PO (PF,SF,DYE-FREE)			
60000 u-4800 u-60000 u,			
100s ea	10432-0277-01	14.97	24.95
250s ea	10432-0277-02	29.37	48.95
HIBICLENS (Molnlycke Healthcare)			
LIQ,TP (PACKETTE)			
4%, 15 ml 50s	00234-0575-17	49.81	
120 ml	00234-0575-04	4.48	
240 ml	00234-0575-08	6.34	
(PREFILLED GLOBE)			
4%, 480 ml	00234-0575-16	10.51	
(W/HAND WALL DISPENSER)			
4%, 480 ml	00234-0599-96	24.95	
960 ml	00234-0575-32	12.46	
(W/FOOT WALL DISPENSER)			
4%, 960 ml	00234-0599-94	74.94	
3840 ml	00234-0575-91	45.61	
(A-S Medication)			
REPACK			
LIQ,TP, 4%, 120 ml	54569-2996-00	4.07	
(Dispensing Solutions)			
REPACK			
SOL,TP, 4%, 480 ml	55045-3689-01	11.50	
(Phys Total Care)			
REPACK			
LIQ,TP, 4%, 120 ml	54868-3046-00	6.74	
240 ml	54868-3046-01	8.35	
HIBICLENS EMPTY GLOBE (Molnlycke Healthcare)			
DEV,NA, ea	00234-0599-95	2.84	
HIBICLENS FOOT PEDAL (Molnlycke Healthcare)			
DEV,NA, ea	00234-0599-05	24.95	
HIBICLENS HAND PUMP (Molnlycke Healthcare)			
DEV,NA (16 OZ GLOBE)			
ea	00234-0599-01	0.95	
(32 OZ BOTTLE)			
ea	00234-0599-02	1.50	
(GAL BOTTLE)			
ea	00234-0599-03	1.89	
HIBICLENS PUMP ASSEMBLY (Molnlycke Healthcare)			
DEV,NA, ea	00234-0599-04	37.43	
HIBISTAT (Molnlycke Healthcare)			
PAD,TP, 0.5%, 50s ea	00234-0587-17	22.50	
HIDE-A-PORT GASTROSTOMY BALLOON (Abbott)			
DEV,NA (LOW PROFILE,16FR,1.7CM)			
ea	70074-0541-54	102.00	
HIGH POTENCY FISH OIL (Major)			
SGL,PO (SOFTGEL)			
200 mg-300 mg-2 iu,			
100s ea	00904-5902-60	17.15	
HISTACOT (Truxton)			
CAP,PO, 1000s ea	00463-2045-10	35.40	
HISTAFED (AmerisourceBergen)			
SYR,PO (PRIVATE LABEL)			
30 mg/5 ml-1.25 mg/5 ml,			
118 ml	24385-0383-26	3.68	4.09
TAB,PO, 60 mg-2.5 mg,			
24s ea	24385-0434-62	3.68	4.09
HISTAPRIN (Hart Health)			
TAB,PO (SF,CAPLET)			
25 mg, 50s ea UD	50332-0132-04	3.16	
(CAPLET)			
25 mg, 200s ea UD	50332-0132-08	9.05	
HOLD DM (Ascher)			
LOZ,MM (CHERRY,CHERRY)			
5 mg, 10s ea	00225-0630-76	2.39	
(ORIGINAL)			
5 mg, 10s ea	00225-0620-76	2.39	
HOLLY (Ellon)			
SOL,SL (DROPS)			
10.5 ml	51762-0017-10		9.25
HOM 1 (Milupa North America)			
PDR,PO (2X500GM)			
500 gm 2s	81361-9356-01	181.25	
HOM 2 (Nutricia)			
PDR,PO (2X500GM)			
500 gm 2s	81361-9357-01	358.80	
HOME ACCESS (Home Access Health)			
DEV,NA, ea	83170-0448-55	31.68	
HOME ACCESS EXPRESS (Home Access Health)			
DEV,NA, ea	83170-0240-00	43.16	
HOME ACCESS HEPATITIS C CHECK (Home Access Health)			
DEV,NA, ea	83170-0510-00	40.00	69.95
HOME ACCESS INSTANT CHOLESTEROL TEST (Home Access Health)			
DEV,NA, ea	83170-0610-00	8.75	15.99
HOMEODENT (Boiron)			
PAS,TP (ANISE)			
99 gm	06969-0424-74	3.57	5.99
HOMEODENT 2 (Boiron)			
TP (LEMON)			
99 gm	06969-0384-74	3.57	5.99
HOMINEX-1 (Abbott)			
PDR,PO, 400 gm	70074-0511-17	40.46	
HOMINEX-2 (Abbott)			
PDR,PO, 400 gm	70074-0511-19	81.12	
HOMOCYSTEINE FORMULA (Mason Vit)			
TAB,PO (PF,SF,FRAGRANCE-FREE)			
0.1 mg-0.8 mg-50 mg,			
120s ea	11845-0125-52	6.56	
HONEYSUCKLE (Ellon)			
SOL,SL (DROPS)			
10.5 ml	51762-0021-10		9.25
HORNBEAM (Ellon)			
SL (DROPS)			
10.5 ml	51762-0007-10		9.25
HORSE CHESTNUT (Mason Vit)			
CAP,PO (PF,SF)			
300 mg, 60s ea	11845-0130-75	9.44	
HORSE CHESTNUT STANDARDIZED (Rexall)			
CAP,PO (PF,SF)			
300 mg, 60s ea	30768-0011-63	4.90	7.42
HORSETAIL (Botanical Labs.)			
LIQ,PO, 30 ml	41954-0020-29	3.75	7.49
HOSPITAL ANTISEPTIC (Chain Drug Marketing)			
SOL,TP, 10%, 236 ml	63868-0230-08	2.64	12.99
HOT AND COOL (Rose)			
CRE,TP, 10%-30%, 120 gm	42037-0425-40	3.25	
LOT,TP, 10%-30%, 210 ml	42037-0324-08	1.90	
OIN,TP, 7.6%-29%,			
210 gm	42037-0435-07	4.45	
HUGO BLUE FOLDING WALKER (Can-Am Care)			
DEV,NA, ea	38396-0075-95	46.74	
(WHEELS/GLIDERS INCLUDED)			
ea	38396-0097-95	60.27	
HUGO ROLLING WALKER (Can-Am Care)			
DEV,NA (CRANBERRY RED)			
ea	38396-0124-92	307.50	
(PACIFIC BLUE)			
ea	38396-0126-92	307.50	
(TITANIUM SILVER)			
ea	38396-0125-92	307.50	
HUGO ROLLING WALKER ELITE (Can-Am Care)			
DEV,NA (BLUE(COSTCO))			
ea	38396-0113-98	112.50	
(BLUE(SAM'S CLUB))			
ea	38396-0112-98	112.50	
HUMATRIX MICROCLYSMIC (Care-Tech Labs)			
GEL,TP, 255 gm	46706-0440-04	17.33	
HUMIST (Scherer Labs)			
SPR,NS, 0.65%, 45 ml	00274-2680-45	1.65	
HUMULIN 50/50 (Lilly)			
SUS,SC (VIAL)			
50 u/ml-50 u/ml,			
10 ml	00002-9515-01	53.16	
HUMULIN 70/30 (Lilly)			
SUS,SC (VIAL)			
70 u/ml-30 u/ml,			
10 ml	00002-8715-01	53.16	
(A-S Medication)			
REPACK			
SUS,SC, 70 u/ml-30 u/ml,			
10 ml	54569-3467-00	50.81	

PROD/MFR	HRI, UPC,NDC	AWP	SRP
(Phys Total Care)			
REPACK			
SUS,SC, 70 u/ml-30 u/ml,			
10 ml	54868-2746-00	52.78	
HUMULIN 70/30 PEN (Lilly)			
SUS,SC (PREFILLED DISPOSABLE)			
70 u/ml-30 u/ml,			
3 ml 5s	00002-8770-59	168.48	
HUMULIN N (Lilly)			
SUS,SC (VIAL)			
100 u/ml, 10 ml	00002-8315-01	53.16	
(A-S Medication)			
REPACK			
SUS,SC (VIAL)			
100 u/ml, 10 ml	54569-2318-00	50.81	
(Phys Total Care)			
REPACK			
SUS,SC, 100 u/ml, 10 ml	54868-1429-01	35.43	
HUMULIN N PEN (Lilly)			
SUS,SC (PREFILLED DISPOSABLE)			
100 u/ml, 3 ml 5s	00002-8730-59	168.48	
HUMULIN R (Lilly)			
SOL,IJ (1X3ML)			
100 u/ml, 3 ml	00002-8215-17	15.95	
(VIAL)			
100 u/ml, 10 ml	00002-8215-01	53.16	
(A-S Medication)			
REPACK			
SOL,IJ (VIAL)			
100 u/ml, 10 ml	54569-2319-00	50.81	
(Phys Total Care)			
REPACK			
SOL,IJ, 100 u/ml, 10 ml	54868-3619-00	52.78	
HURRICAINE (Beutlich)			
GEL,MM, 20%,			
5.25 gm 12s	00283-0871-12	66.06	101.64
(FRESH MINT)			
20%, 30 gm	00283-0998-31	7.92	12.18
(ORIGINAL WILD CHERRY)			
20%, 30 gm	00283-0871-31	7.92	12.18
(PINA COLADA)			
20%, 30 gm	00283-0886-31	7.92	12.18
(WATERMELON)			
20%, 30 gm	00283-0293-31	7.92	12.18
SOL,MM (CHERRY)			
20%, 30 ml	00283-0569-31	7.92	12.18
(PINA COLADA)			
20%, 30 ml	00283-1886-31	7.92	12.18
SPR,MM (CHERRY)			
20%, 60 gm	00283-0679-02	25.74	39.59
SWA,MM (ORIGINAL WILD CHERRY)			
20%, 0.15 ml 8s	00283-0569-08	4.83	8.06
0.15 ml 72s	00283-0569-72	26.71	44.52
(Southwood)			
REPACK			
GEL,TP, 20%, 30 gm	58016-4993-01	7.57	
HURRICAINE SPRAY KIT (Beutlich)			
SPR,MM (W/DISPOSABLE EXT TUBE)			
20%, 59.7 gm	00283-0679-60	35.50	54.62
HURRISEPT (Beutlich)			
GEL,TP (1X473ML)			
70%, 473 ml	00283-0304-16	13.78	21.20
HURRIVIEW II TWO-TONE PLAQUE INDICATING SNAP-N-GO (Beutlich)			
SWA,DE (0.15ML)			
8s ea	00283-1105-08	5.53	9.22
72s ea	00283-1105-72	30.72	51.20
HURRIVIEW PLAQUE INDICATING SNAP-N-GO (Beutlich)			
SWA,DE (0.15ML)			
8s ea	00283-0104-08	4.83	8.06
72s ea	00283-0104-72	26.71	44.52
HYALEX (Miller)			
TAB,PO, 100s ea	17204-0432-40	8.52	13.70
HYCOLOID-GRX (Geritrex)			
DEV,NA (4"X4")			
30s ea	92771-0826-44	3.71	
HYDRALIFE (Fleet,C.B.)			
PDR,PO (4X9GM,ORANGE TANGERINE)			
4s ea	01320-0002-22	6.34	
HYDRAMINE (Quality Care Prod)			
REPACK			
ELI,PO, 12.5 mg/5 ml,			
120 ml	49999-0247-04	6.65	
HYDRASTIS CAN (Luyties)			
TAB,SL (6X)			
6 x, 500s ea	00618-4253-03	3.99	
5500s ea	00618-4253-10	30.32	
(30X)			
12 x, 500s ea	00622-4253-03	4.19	
5500s ea	00622-4253-10	31.83	
(12X)			
30 x, 500s ea	00624-4253-03	4.19	
5500s ea	00624-4253-10	31.83	
HYDRISALIC (Pedinol)			
GEL,TP, 5%, 28.35 gm	00884-2296-01		12.00
HYDRISINOL (Pedinol)			
CRE,TP, 113.4 gm	00884-0142-04		12.00
480 gm	00884-0142-16		38.40
LOT,TP, 240 ml	00884-3042-08		10.50
HYDROCERIN (Geritrex)			
CRE,TP, 120 gm	54162-0600-02	4.20	
454 gm	54162-0600-01	8.81	8.81
LOT,TP, 240 ml	54162-0620-08	3.22	
(FRAGRANCE-FREE)			
480 ml	54162-0620-16	6.26	
HYDROCERIN PLUS (Geritrex)			
CRE,TP (24X140GM)			
140 gm 24s	54162-0601-05	102.96	
HYDROCIL INSTANT (Numark)			
PDR,PO (PACKET)			
3.5 gm/dose,			
3.7 gm 30s UD	55499-0808-57	12.60	
3.7 gm 500s UD	55499-0808-55	124.56	
(SF)			
3.5 gm/dose,			
300 gm	38485-0808-68	13.02	
HYDROCOL (Mylan Bertek)			
DEV,NA (STERILE,6"X8")			
5s ea	62794-0086-48	67.28	
HYDROCOL II (UDL)			
DEV,NA (STERILE,SACRAL)			
5s ea	62794-0088-75	76.04	
(STERILE,4"X4" THIN)			
10s ea	62794-0089-18	33.12	
(STERILE,4"X4")			
10s ea	62794-0088-18	43.93	
HYDROCORTISONE (Actavis Mid Atlantic)			
CRE,TP, 1%, 30 gm	00472-0343-56	3.48	
OIN,TP (5 PANEL)			
1%, 30 gm	00472-0345-56	3.48	
(Altaire)			
CRE,TP, 1%, 30 gm	59390-0023-17	2.30	
(AmerisourceBergen)			
CRE,TP (PRIVATE LABEL)			
0.5%, 30 gm	24385-0190-03	2.69	2.99
(W/ALOE,PRIVATE LABEL)			
1%, 30 gm	24385-0274-03	3.05	3.39
LOT,TP (PRIVATE LABEL)			
1%, 120 ml	24385-0283-06	7.19	7.99
OIN,TP (W/ALOE,PRIVATE LABEL)			
1%, 30 gm	24385-0276-03	3.05	3.39
(Consolidated Midland)			
CRE,TP, 0.5%, 1 gm	00223-4243-01	16.75	
15 gm	00223-4160-01	1.60	
15 gm	00223-4162-12	1.50	
30 gm	00223-4160-02	1.80	
30 gm	00223-4162-30	1.90	
120 gm	00223-4160-03	6.25	
120 gm	00223-4162-11	6.50	
454 gm	00223-4160-04	16.75	
454 gm	00223-4162-13	15.75	
LOT,TP, 0.5%, 60 ml	00223-6518-60	3.25	
(Fougera)			
CRE,TP, 0.5%, 30 gm	00168-0014-31	2.64	
(UNIT OF USE)			
1%, 1.5 gm 48s	00168-0154-08	8.57	
30 gm	00168-0154-31	3.00	
LOT,TP, 1%, 118 ml	00168-0287-04	7.90	
OIN,TP, 0.5%, 30 gm	00168-0016-31	2.20	
1%, 30 gm	00168-0181-31	3.00	
(Global Source)			
CRE,TP, 1%, 30 gm	59618-0390-52	2.85	
(Hart Health)			
CRE,TP (25X0.9GM,MAX STRENGTH)			
1%, 0.9 gm 25s UD	50332-0042-02	2.76	
(144X0.9GM,MAX STRENGTH)			
1%, 0.9 gm 144s UD	50332-0042-04	10.39	
(Major)			
CRE,TP, 1%, 30 gm	00904-7623-31	2.95	
(Mericon)			
CRE,TP (EXTRA THICK)			
1%, 120 gm	00394-0855-04	5.38	
LOT,TP (THICK)			
1%, 120 ml	00394-0859-32	5.84	
(Perrigo)			
CRE,TP (MAXIMUM STRENGTH,1X20GM)			
1%, ea	45802-0438-02	3.29	
(MAXIMUM STRNGTH,1X454GM)			
1%, ea	45802-0438-05	31.50	
(1X144UD)			
1%, 0.9 gm 144s UD	45802-0438-70	16.99	
30 gm	45802-0438-03	3.99	
(Prime Marketing)			
CRE,TP, 1%, 30 gm	62107-0010-03	2.65	
(Qualitest)			
CRE,TP (4 PANEL BOX)			
1%, 30 gm	00603-0535-50	2.31	
(6 PANEL BOX)			
1%, 30 gm	00603-0534-50	2.31	
LOT,TP, 1%, 120 ml	00603-7784-54	10.24	
(Rugby)			
CRE,TP, 1%, 30 gm	00536-5108-95	2.85	
LOT,TP, 1%, 120 ml	00536-5105-97	8.09	
(Taro)			
CRE,TP, 0.5%, 15 gm	51672-2010-01	2.50	
30 gm	51672-2010-02	2.75	
(MAX. STR.)			
1%, 15 gm	51672-2013-01	2.25	
(MAX STR W/MOISTURIZERS)			
1%, 28.4 gm	51672-2063-02	3.58	
(MAXIMUM STRENGTH)			
1%, 28.4 gm	51672-2069-02	2.75	
(MAX. STR.)			
1%, 30 gm	51672-2013-02	2.75	
OIN,TP, 0.5%, 30 gm	51672-2015-02	2.93	
(PRESCRIPTION STRENGTH)			
1%, 28.4 gm	51672-2018-02	3.25	
(A-S Medication)			
REPACK			
CRE,TP, 0.5%, 15 gm	54569-3510-00	2.50	
28.35 gm	54569-2632-00	2.87	
1%, 30 gm	54569-1096-00	6.10	
(Dispensing Solutions)			
REPACK			
CRE,TP, 1%, 30 gm	55045-1116-08	7.99	
(Pharma Pac)			
REPACK			
CRE,TP, 0.5%, 30 gm	52959-0581-03	5.39	
1%, 15 gm	52959-0039-15	7.75	
20 gm	52959-0039-01	9.15	
(Phys Total Care)			
REPACK			
CRE,TP, 0.5%, 30 gm	54868-0580-03	5.10	
LOT,TP, 1%, 120 ml	54868-1913-00	23.31	
(Quality Care Prod)			
REPACK			
CRE,TP, 0.5%, 28.35 gm	49999-0413-01	6.08	
1%, 30 gm	49999-0139-01	10.10	
HYDROCORTISONE ACETATE (Cardinal Health)			
CRE,TP (PRIVATE LABEL)			
1%, 30 gm	37205-0162-10	3.20	
(Perrigo)			
OIN,TP, 1%, 30 gm	45802-0276-03	3.99	
454 gm	45802-0276-05	29.99	
(Altura)			
REPACK			
CRE,TP, 0.5%, 15 gm	63874-0044-15	6.29	
30 gm	63874-0044-30	6.29	
1%, 30 gm	63874-0049-30	10.16	
(Phys Total Care)			
REPACK			
CRE,TP, 1%, 1 gm 48s	54868-0228-00	7.20	
(PACKET)			
1%, 1 gm 144s	54868-0228-01	59.25	
30 gm	54868-0228-02	6.48	
454 gm	54868-0228-05	59.24	
OIN,TP (MAX. STR.)			
1%, 454 gm	54868-0327-00	64.96	
HYDROCORTISONE ACETATE W/ALOE (Actavis Mid Atlantic)			
CRE,TP (5 PANEL)			
0.5%, 30 gm	00472-0338-56	2.05	
1%, 30 gm	00472-0339-56	3.48	
(Perrigo)			
CRE,TP, 0.5%, 30 gm	45802-0190-03	2.99	

PROD/MFR	HRI, UPC,NDC	AWP	SRP
HYDROCORTISONE MAXIMUM STRENGTH (Asafi Pharmaceutical)			
OIN,TP, 1%, 30 gm	65557-0206-30	2.25	
(Cardinal Health)			
CRE,TP (W/ALOE VERA) 1%, 30 gm	37205-0272-10	3.35	
OIN,TP (PRIVATE LABEL) 1%, 30 gm	37205-0161-10	1.76	
HYDROCORTISONE PLUS (AmerisourceBergen)			
CRE,TP (W/ALOE,PRIVATE LABEL) 1%, 28.4 gm	24385-0021-03	3.41	3.79
HYDROCORTISONE PLUS 12 (Actavis Mid Atlantic)			
CRE,TP (USP,1X28GM) 1%, 28 gm	00472-0341-56	3.48	
HYDROCORTISONE W/ALOE (G&W)			
CRE,TP, 1%, 30 gm	00713-0626-31	2.93	
OIN,TP, 1%, 30 gm	00713-0290-31	4.18	
HYDROGEN PEROXIDE (Albertson's)			
SOL,TP, 3%, 480 ml	04000-0003-10	0.75	
(AmerisourceBergen)			
SOL,TP (PRIVATE LABEL) 3%, 240 ml	24385-0113-98	0.80	0.89
480 ml	24385-0113-16	12.90	14.30
(Cardinal Health)			
SOL,TP (PRIVATE LABEL) 3%, 240 ml	37205-0871-34	0.56	
480 ml	37205-0871-43	0.67	
960 ml	37205-0871-45	1.11	
(Consolidated Midland)			
SOL,TP, 3%, 120 ml 12s	00223-6520-04	9.75	
240 ml	00223-6520-01	0.95	
480 ml	00223-6520-02	1.50	
3840 ml	00223-6520-03	11.50	
(Denison)			
SOL,TP, 3%, 120 ml	00295-1179-04	0.40	
480 ml	00295-1179-16	0.42	
(Hart Health)			
SOL,TP (1X120ML) 3%, 120 ml	50332-0021-91	1.60	
(Southwood) REPACK			
SOL,TP, 3%, 480 ml	58016-9048-01	3.92	
HYDROLATUM (Denison)			
OIN,TP, 57 gm	00295-1347-96	2.92	
HYDROPEL (Genesis)			
OIN,TP, 30%, 60 gm	00398-0020-02	7.44	
454 gm	00398-0020-16	29.76	
HYDROPHILIC GRX OINTMENT (Geritrex)			
OIN,TP (24X410GM,FRAGRANCE-FREE) 410 gm 24s	54162-0670-14	266.40	
HYDROPHILIC OINTMENT (Consolidated Midland)			
OIN,TP, 454 gm	00223-4134-01	7.50	
2270 gm	00223-4134-02	24.50	
(Gallipot)			
OIN,TP, 454 gm	51552-0675-06	17.85	
(Geritrex)			
OIN,TP, 120 gm	54162-0670-04	3.71	
HYDROPHOR (Geritrex)			
OIN,TP, 100 gm	54162-0500-02	4.85	
42%, 454 gm	54162-0500-01	10.59	11.14
HYLAND'S ARNISPORT (Hyland's)			
TAB,PO, 50s ea	54973-0232-01	4.55	7.59
HYLAND'S ARTHRITIS PAIN FORMULA (Std Homeo)			
TAB,SL, 50s ea	54973-2955-01	3.95	6.59
100s ea	54973-2955-02	5.39	8.99
HYLAND'S BACKACHE WITH ARNICA (Hyland's)			
TAB,PO (CAPLET) 3 x-3 x-6 x-6 x-3 x, 40s ea	54973-2965-02	4.07	6.79
TAB,SL, 100s ea	54973-2965-01	5.51	9.19
HYLAND'S BLADDER IRRITATION (Std Homeo)			
TAB,SL, 100s ea	54973-2953-02	5.39	8.99
HYLAND'S BRONCHIAL COUGH (Std Homeo)			
SL, 100s ea	54973-2954-02	5.39	8.99
HYLAND'S BUG BITE OINTMENT (Hyland's)			
OIN,TP (STICK) 3 x-3 x-3 x-3 x-3 x, 8 gm	54973-7511-01	4.31	7.19
HYLAND'S CALMS (Hyland's)			
TAB,PO, 2 x-1 x-1 x-1 x, 100s ea	54973-1120-01	5.09	8.49
HYLAND'S CALMS FORTE (Hyland's)			
TAB,PO (CAPLET) 32s ea	54973-0112-18	4.07	6.79
50s ea	54973-1121-01	3.71	6.19
100s ea	54973-1121-02	5.09	8.49
HYLAND'S CLEAR AC (Hyland's)			
TAB,PO, 6 x-6 x-6 x-6 x, 50s ea	54973-2202-01	4.55	7.59
HYLAND'S CLEAR-AC (Hyland's)			
LIQ,TP, 120 ml	54973-1123-01	4.55	7.59
HYLAND'S COLD SORES & FEVER BLISTERS (Std Homeo)			
TAB,SL, 100s ea	54973-9127-02	5.39	8.99
HYLAND'S COLD TABLETS W/ZINC (Hyland's)			
TAB,SL, 6 x-6 x-6 x-2 x, 50s ea	54973-0301-01	4.55	7.59
HYLAND'S COLD TABLETS WITH ZINC (Hyland's)			
ODT,SL (QUICK DISSOLVING TABLET) 6 x-6 x-6 x-2 x, 60s ea	54973-3010-02	4.91	8.19
HYLAND'S COMPLETE FLU CARE (Hyland's)			
ODT,SL, 120s ea	54973-0301-52	7.43	12.39
HYLAND'S COUGH (Std Homeo)			
TAB,SL, 100s ea	54973-9104-02	5.39	8.99
HYLAND'S DIARREX (Hyland's)			
TAB,PO, 6 x-6 x-6 x-6 x-6 x, 50s ea	54973-3025-01	4.55	7.59
HYLAND'S EARACHE DROPS (Hyland's)			
SOL,OT (ADULT) 10 ml	54973-0751-62	6.17	10.29
(INFANT) 10 ml	54973-0751-61	6.17	10.29
HYLAND'S ENURAID (Hyland's)			
TAB,PO, 50s ea	54973-3223-01	4.55	7.59
HYLAND'S FLU (Hyland's)			
ODT,SL (QUICK DISSOLVING TABLET) 60s ea	54973-2952-01	4.91	8.19
(Std Homeo)			
TAB,SL, 100s ea	54973-2952-02	5.39	8.99
HYLAND'S GAS (Std Homeo)			
SL, 100s ea	54973-2951-02	5.39	8.99
HYLAND'S HAYFEVER (Std Homeo)			
SL, 100s ea	54973-9138-02	5.39	8.99
HYLAND'S HEADACHE (Std Homeo)			
SL, 100s ea	54973-2950-02	5.39	8.99
HYLAND'S HEMMOREX OINTMENT (Hyland's)			
OIN,RC (HOMEOPATHIC) 1 x-2 x-1 x-1 x, 28 gm	54973-1114-01	5.57	9.29
HYLAND'S HEMORRHOIDS (Std Homeo)			
TAB,SL, 100s ea	54973-9130-02	5.39	8.99
HYLAND'S HIVES (Std Homeo)			
SL, 100s ea	54973-9146-02	5.39	8.99
HYLAND'S INDIGESTION (Std Homeo)			
SL, 100s ea	54973-2958-02	5.39	8.99
HYLAND'S INSOMNIA (Std Homeo)			
SL, 100s ea	54973-9123-02	5.39	8.99
HYLAND'S LEG CRAMPS (Std Homeo)			
SL, 50s ea	54973-2956-01	3.95	6.59
100s ea	54973-2956-02	5.39	8.99
HYLAND'S MENOPAUSE (Std Homeo)			
SL, 100s ea	54973-9113-02	5.39	8.99
HYLAND'S MENSTRUAL CRAMPS (Std Homeo)			
SL, 100s ea	54973-2961-02	5.39	8.99
HYLAND'S MIGRAINE HEADACHE RELIEF (Hyland's)			
TAB,PO 6 x-6 x-6 x-6 x-12 x-6 x, 60s ea	54973-3013-01	4.31	7.19
HYLAND'S MOTION SICKNESS (Std Homeo)			
TAB,SL, 50s ea	54973-9147-01	3.95	6.59
HYLAND'S NERVE TONIC (Hyland's)			
ODT,PO, 3 x-3 x-3 x-3 x-3 x, 100s ea	54973-3014-02	5.09	8.49
500s ea	54973-1129-01	7.73	12.89
TAB,PO (CAPLET) 3 x-3 x-3 x-3 x-3 x, 32s ea	54973-0112-98	4.07	6.79
HYLAND'S PMS (Std Homeo)			
TAB,SL, 50s ea	54973-2957-01	3.95	6.59
100s ea	54973-2957-02	5.39	8.99
HYLAND'S POISON IVY/OAK (Std Homeo)			
SL, 50s ea	54973-1130-01	3.95	6.59
HYLAND'S SINUS (Std Homeo)			
SL, 50s ea	54973-2959-01	3.95	6.59
100s ea	54973-2959-02	5.39	8.99
HYLAND'S SKIN THERAPY (Hyland's)			
OIN,TP (W/CALENDULA) 2 x, 70.9 gm	54973-0751-53	4.55	7.59
HYLAND'S SMILE'S PRID (Hyland's)			
OIN,TP (SALVE) 18 gm	00619-4202-54	2.87	4.79
HYLAND'S SORE THROAT (Std Homeo)			
TAB,SL, 100s ea	54973-9120-02	5.39	8.99
HYLAND'S UPSET STOMACH (Std Homeo)			
SL, 100s ea	54973-9150-02	5.39	8.99
HYLAND'S VAGINITIS (Std Homeo)			
SL, 100s ea	54973-2962-02	5.39	8.99
HYPAFIX (Animas Corp.)			
DEV,NA (4" X 10 YD ROLL) ea	65781-0510-01	32.25	
HYPAFIX POLYESTER (Smith & Nephew)			
DEV,NA (2"X10 YD ROLL) ea	40565-0115-92	11.78	9.42
(2"X2 YD ROLL) ea	40565-0115-95	5.56	4.45
(4"X10 YD ROLL) ea	40565-0115-93	20.24	16.19
(4"X2 YD ROLL) ea	40565-0115-96	9.83	7.86
(6"X10 YD ROLL) ea	40565-0115-94	25.70	20.56
(6"X2 YD ROLL) ea	40565-0115-97	12.50	10.00
HYPERICUM PERF (Luyties)			
TAB,SL (6X) 6 x, 500s ea	00618-4267-03	3.99	
5500s ea	00618-4267-10	30.32	
(30X) 12 x, 500s ea	00622-4267-03	4.19	
5500s ea	00622-4267-10	31.83	
(12X) 30 x, 500s ea	00624-4267-03	4.19	
5500s ea	00624-4267-10	31.83	
HYPOLANCE AST LANCING KIT (Arkray)			
DEV,NA, ea	08317-4100-12	13.50	
HYPOTEARS (Novartis Pharm)			
SOL,OP (1X15ML,DROPS) 1%-1%, 15 ml	00078-0519-24	8.47	
(1X30ML,DROPS) 1%-1%, 30 ml	00078-0519-82	12.32	
(Southwood) REPACK			
SOL,OP, 1%, 15 ml	58016-6107-01	8.50	
HYPROST (A. G. Marin)			
SGL,PO (SOFTGEL) 60s ea	12539-0497-60	29.95	
I-PRIN (Medique)			
TAB,PO (3X2) 200 mg, 6s ea UD	47682-0100-69	0.89	
(12X2) 200 mg, 24s ea UD	47682-0100-64	1.75	
(100X2) 200 mg, 200s ea UD	47682-0100-47	10.34	
(250X2) 200 mg, 500s ea UD	47682-0100-13	24.16	
I-VALEX-1 (Abbott)			
PDR,PO, 400 gm	70074-0511-37	40.46	
I-VALEX-2 (Abbott)			
PDR,PO, 400 gm	70074-0511-39	81.12	
I-VITE LUTEIN (Rugby)			
TAB,PO, 60s ea	00536-5090-08	4.64	
I-VITE PROTECT (Rugby)			
TAB,PO, 120s ea	00536-4178-41	10.31	
I.L.X. B-12 (Kenwood)			
TAB,PO (BLISTER PK,10X10,CAPLET) 100s ea UD	00482-0110-23	56.71	
I.V. START (Medical Action Ind.)			
DEV,NA, 50s ea	73577-0612-23	62.16	
I.V. START W/ACU-DERM (Medical Action Ind.)			
DEV,NA, 50s ea	73577-0612-40	62.28	
50s ea	73577-0612-42	63.60	
50s ea	73577-0612-60	81.60	
I.V. START W/OPSITE (Medical Action Ind.)			
DEV,NA, 50s ea	73577-0612-34	76.08	
(I.V. 3000) 50s ea	73577-0612-65	82.80	

PROD/MFR	HRI, UPC,NDC	AWP	SRP
IBU-2 (Truxton)			
TAB,PO, 200 mg,			
1000s ea	00463-6112-10	36.00	
IBU-DROPS CHILDREN'S (Cardinal Health)			
SUS,PO (PRIVATE LABEL,BERRY)			
50 mg/1.25 ml, 15 ml	37205-0646-05	4.80	
IBUPROFEN (Albertson's)			
TAB,PO, 200 mg, 100s ea	12810-0604-78	4.32	
(AmerisourceBergen)			
TAB,PO (PRIVATE LABEL,CAPLET)			
200 mg, 50s ea	24385-0647-71	4.04	4.49
(PRIVATE LABEL)			
200 mg, 50s ea	24385-0604-71	4.04	4.49
(PRIVATE LABEL,CAPLET)			
200 mg, 100s ea	24385-0647-78	6.29	6.99
(PRIVATE LABEL)			
200 mg, 100s ea	24385-0604-78	6.29	6.99
(Amneal)			
TAB,PO (FILM-COATED)			
200 mg, 100s ea	53746-0140-01	4.95	
500s ea	53746-0140-05	17.25	
1000s ea	53746-0140-10	30.99	
(Asafi Pharmaceutical)			
TAB,PO, 200 mg, 50s ea	65557-0401-50	2.92	
(Basic Vitamins)			
TAB,PO, 200 mg, 50s ea	00761-0373-10	2.00	
100s ea	00761-0373-20	3.20	
(Cardinal Health)			
TAB,PO (PRIVATE LABEL,CAPLET)			
200 mg, 50s ea	37205-0341-71	3.59	
(PRIVATE LABEL)			
200 mg, 50s ea	37205-0345-71	3.65	
50s ea	37205-0350-71	3.59	
(PRIVATE LABEL,CAPLET)			
200 mg, 100s ea	37205-0341-78	5.49	
(PRIVATE LABEL)			
200 mg, 100s ea	37205-0345-78	3.84	
100s ea	37205-0350-78	5.49	
250s ea	37205-0350-85	8.32	
(Chain Drug Marketing)			
TAB,PO (CAPLET)			
200 mg, 24s ea	63868-0341-24	1.14	2.99
50s ea	63868-0341-50	1.66	3.99
100s ea	63868-0341-10	2.39	6.99
(Consolidated Midland)			
TAB,PO, 200 mg, 100s ea	00223-1090-01	5.50	
500s ea	00223-1090-05	22.50	
1000s ea	00223-1090-02	27.50	
(Family Phcy)			
TAB,PO (PRIVATE LABEL)			
200 mg, 120s ea	52735-0751-23	5.75	7.59
120s ea	52735-0758-23	2.85	6.29
(Geri-Care)			
TAB,PO, 200 mg, 100s ea	57896-0941-01	1.60	
(Hart Health)			
TAB,PO (50X2,SF)			
200 mg, 100s ea UD	50332-0118-04	4.25	
(125X2,SF,FILM COATED)			
200 mg, 250s ea UD	50332-0118-07	9.49	
(Magno-Humphries)			
TAB,PO, 200 mg, 50s ea	43292-0556-17	1.62	3.19
100s ea	43292-0556-25	2.33	3.99
250s ea	43292-0556-26	5.20	8.99
(Major)			
SGL,PO (SOFTGEL)			
200 mg, 80s ea	00904-5903-47	6.42	
TAB,PO (12X2)			
200 mg, 24s ea	00904-7914-02	1.43	
(BROWN)			
200 mg, 24s ea	00904-7915-24	2.20	
(CAPLET)			
200 mg, 24s ea	00904-5323-24	2.20	
(BROWN,CAPLET)			
200 mg, 50s ea	00904-7912-51	3.00	
(BROWN)			
200 mg, 50s ea	00904-7915-51	3.00	
(WHITE,COATED)			
200 mg, 50s ea	00904-7914-51	3.00	
(10X10,WHITE,COATED)			
200 mg, 100s ea UD	00904-7914-61	6.77	
(BROWN,CAPLET)			
200 mg, 100s ea	00904-7912-59	5.49	
(BROWN)			
200 mg, 100s ea	00904-7915-59	5.49	
(WHITE,COATED)			
200 mg, 100s ea	00904-7914-59	4.90	
(BROWN)			
200 mg, 250s ea	00904-7915-70	9.45	
500s ea	00904-7915-40	16.45	
(COATED)			
200 mg, 1000s ea	00904-7915-80	29.61	
(Marlex)			
TAB,PO, 200 mg, 100s ea	10135-0143-01	4.17	
100s ea	10135-0183-01	4.16	
(BLISTER PACK)			
200 mg, 100s ea UD	10135-0162-13	2.99	
500s ea	10135-0143-05	18.89	
500s ea	10135-0183-05	18.88	
1000s ea	10135-0183-10	36.55	
(Mason Vit)			
TAB,PO (S.C.,BOTTLED)			
200 mg, 30s ea	11845-0107-28	2.44	
50s ea	11845-0107-29	3.33	
100s ea	11845-0107-21	5.33	
(Ohm)			
TAB,PO, 200 mg, 24s ea	51660-0420-24	2.15	
50s ea	51660-0420-51	2.95	
100s ea	51660-0420-01	1.95	
500s ea	51660-0420-05	7.25	
1000s ea	51660-0420-10	12.00	
(Pfeiffer)			
TAB,PO, 200 mg, 50s ea	00927-0070-53	2.35	4.23
100s ea	00927-0070-01	3.65	6.56
(Rugby)			
TAB,PO (COATED)			
200 mg, 50s ea	00536-3105-06	2.10	
(COATED,COATED)			
200 mg, 100s ea	00536-3105-01	3.36	
250s ea	00536-3105-02	6.72	
(COATED)			
200 mg, 1000s ea	00536-3105-10	21.41	
(SDA)			
TAB,PO (USP,COATED)			
200 mg, 1000s ea	66424-0995-10	34.50	
(UDL)			
TAB,PO (10X10)			
200 mg, 100s ea UD	51079-0731-20	6.86	
(A-S Medication)			
REPACK			
TAB,PO, 200 mg, 15s ea	54569-2005-01	0.76	
20s ea	54569-2005-02	1.02	
(COATED)			
200 mg, 24s ea	54569-2005-03	1.23	
30s ea	54569-2005-05	1.54	
40s ea	54569-2005-04	2.05	
50s ea	54569-2005-00	2.56	
60s ea	54569-2005-07	3.07	
80s ea	54569-4102-00	4.10	
100s ea	54569-2005-08	5.12	
120s ea	54569-4102-01	6.14	
(400 X 2)			
200 mg, 800s ea	54569-3994-00	31.35	
(Altura)			
REPACK			
TAB,PO, 200 mg, 8s ea	63874-0013-08	3.04	
12s ea	63874-0013-12	4.56	
14s ea	63874-0013-14	5.32	
15s ea	63874-0013-15	5.70	
20s ea	63874-0013-20	7.60	
21s ea	63874-0013-21	8.91	
24s ea	63874-0013-24	10.18	
28s ea	63874-0013-28	10.64	
30s ea	63874-0013-30	12.73	
40s ea	63874-0013-40	16.97	
50s ea	63874-0013-50	19.00	
60s ea	63874-0013-60	22.80	
100s ea	63874-0013-01	42.43	
1000s ea	63874-0013-02	424.29	
(Core)			
REPACK			
TAB,PO, 200 mg, 10s ea	33358-0185-10	3.16	
20s ea	33358-0185-20	11.26	
30s ea	33358-0185-30	15.36	
50s ea	33358-0185-50	20.49	
60s ea	33358-0185-60	26.45	
100s ea	33358-0185-00	45.09	
(DHS, Inc.)			
REPACK			
TAB,PO, 200 mg, 30s ea	55887-0961-30	17.95	
50s ea	55887-0961-50	29.95	
100s ea	55887-0961-01	59.90	
(Dispensing Solutions)			
REPACK			
SUS,PO, 100 mg/5 ml,			
120 ml	68258-3005-01	7.85	
TAB,PO, 200 mg, 20s ea	55045-1560-02	7.60	
20s ea	66336-0007-20	6.59	
(COATED)			
200 mg, 24s ea	55045-1560-07	9.12	
30s ea	55045-1560-08	11.40	
30s ea	66336-0007-30	8.82	
(COATED)			
200 mg, 40s ea	55045-1560-03	15.20	
50s ea	55045-1560-04	19.00	
(COATED)			
200 mg, 60s ea	55045-1560-06	22.80	
90s ea	66336-0007-90	18.91	
(COATED)			
200 mg, 90s ea	55045-1560-09	34.20	
100s ea	55045-1560-01	38.00	
120s ea	55045-1560-00	45.60	
(HomeMed)			
REPACK			
TAB,PO, 200 mg, 12s ea	51655-0441-27	3.00	
24s ea	51655-0441-30	3.15	
(Keltman Pharma., Inc.)			
REPACK			
TAB,PO, 200 mg, 30s ea	68387-0205-30	8.90	
50s ea	68387-0205-50	13.11	
(McKesson Packaging)			
REPACK			
TAB,PO, 200 mg,			
100s ea UD	63739-0134-10	6.93	
(BLISTER PACK)			
200 mg, 750s ea UD	63739-0134-01	51.98	
(Nucare Pharm)			
REPACK			
TAB,PO, 200 mg, 20s ea	66267-0115-20	6.28	
24s ea	66267-0115-24	6.28	
30s ea	66267-0115-30	8.45	
40s ea	66267-0115-40	11.27	
50s ea	66267-0115-50	13.86	
90s ea	66267-0115-90	24.95	
(PD-Rx Pharm)			
REPACK			
TAB,PO, 200 mg, 15s ea	55289-0673-15	6.00	
18s ea	55289-0673-18	24.80	
20s ea	55289-0673-20	25.33	
24s ea	55289-0673-24	26.40	
30s ea	55289-0673-30	28.00	
50s ea	55289-0673-50	33.33	
60s ea	55289-0673-60	36.00	
500s ea	55289-0673-94	153.33	
(Pharma Pac)			
REPACK			
TAB,PO, 200 mg, 10s ea	52959-0187-10	4.05	
15s ea	52959-0187-15	5.48	
20s ea	52959-0187-20	6.59	
21s ea	52959-0187-21	6.88	
24s ea	52959-0187-24	7.65	
25s ea	52959-0187-25	7.98	
30s ea	52959-0187-30	8.82	
40s ea	52959-0187-40	9.99	
50s ea	52959-0187-50	11.01	
60s ea	52959-0187-60	13.22	
90s ea	52959-0187-90	18.91	
100s ea	52959-0187-00	23.42	
120s ea	52959-0187-02	28.08	
200s ea	52959-0187-03	43.98	
(Phys Total Care)			
REPACK			
TAB,PO, 200 mg, 50s ea	54868-0984-00	7.05	
100s ea	54868-0984-01	36.65	
100s ea	54868-0984-03	18.75	
500s ea	54868-0984-02	81.69	
1000s ea	54868-0984-04	160.38	
(Physician Partner)			
REPACK			
TAB,PO, 200 mg, 14s ea	21695-0065-14	5.69	
30s ea	21695-0065-30	12.10	
60s ea	21695-0065-60	24.20	
100s ea	21695-0065-00	29.80	
(Quality Care Prod)			
REPACK			
SUS,PO, 100 mg/5 ml,			
120 ml	49999-0928-01	9.14	
TAB,PO, 200 mg, 18s ea	49999-0071-18	6.66	
20s ea	49999-0071-20	7.40	
30s ea	49999-0071-30	11.24	
40s ea	49999-0071-40	14.80	

PROD/MFR	HRI, UPC,NDC	AWP	SRP
50s ea	49999-0071-50	18.50	
60s ea	49999-0071-60	22.20	
90s ea	49999-0071-90	33.30	
100s ea	49999-0071-00	37.00	
(Southwood)			
REPACK			
TAB,PO, 200 mg, 8s ea	58016-0201-08	1.38	
12s ea	58016-0201-12	2.06	
14s ea	58016-0201-14	2.41	
15s ea	58016-0201-15	2.58	
20s ea	58016-0201-20	3.44	
21s ea	58016-0201-21	3.61	
24s ea	58016-0201-24	4.13	
28s ea	58016-0201-28	4.82	
30s ea	58016-0201-30	5.16	
40s ea	58016-0201-40	6.88	
50s ea	58016-0201-50	8.60	
60s ea	58016-0201-60	10.32	
100s ea	58016-0201-00	17.20	
(St. Mary's MPP)			
REPACK			
TAB,PO, 200 mg, 24s ea	60760-0791-24	5.30	
(Stat Rx)			
REPACK			
TAB,PO, 200 mg, 20s ea	16590-0123-20	11.33	
30s ea	16590-0123-30	17.00	
40s ea	16590-0123-40	22.68	
50s ea	16590-0123-50	28.35	
IBUPROFEN 200 (Reese)			
TAB,PO, 200 mg, 24s ea	10956-0678-24	2.46	
50s ea	10956-0678-50	4.00	
100s ea	10956-0678-09	6.15	
IBUPROFEN AND PSEUDOEPHEDRINE COLD AND SINUS (Teva)			
TAB,PO (CAPLET)			
200 mg-30 mg, 20s ea	00182-1195-15	3.99	
40s ea	00182-1195-95	7.05	
IBUPROFEN CHILDREN'S (AmerisourceBergen)			
SUS,PO (AF,PRIVATE LABEL,BERRY)			
100 mg/5 ml, 120 ml	24385-0905-26	4.49	4.99
(Cardinal Health)			
SUS,PO (AF,PRIVATE LABEL,BERRY)			
100 mg/5 ml, 120 ml	37205-0643-26	4.64	
(AF,PRIVATE LABEL,FRUIT)			
100 mg/5 ml, 120 ml	37205-0644-26	4.48	
(Major)			
SUS,PO (AF,BERRY)			
100 mg/5 ml, 120 ml	00904-5309-20	5.39	
(AF,FRUIT)			
100 mg/5 ml, 120 ml	00904-5464-20	4.65	
(AF,GRAPE)			
100 mg/5 ml, 120 ml	00904-5577-20	5.39	
(AF,BERRY)			
100 mg/5 ml, 240 ml	00904-5309-09	7.50	
(BERRY,DROPS)			
50 mg/1.25 ml, 15 ml	00904-5463-35	4.89	
(Altura)			
REPACK			
SUS,PO, 100 mg/5 ml, 120 ml	63874-0053-12	7.49	
(Dispensing Solutions)			
REPACK			
SUS,PO (AF,BERRY) 100 mg/5 ml, 120 ml	55045-2674-08	5.85	
(Pharma Pac)			
REPACK			
SUS,PO (AF,BERRY) 100 mg/5 ml, 120 ml	52959-0298-04	5.25	
IBUPROFEN IB (Family Phcy)			
TAB,PO (PRIVATE LABEL,CAPLET)			
200 mg, 100s ea	52735-0764-01	6.29	6.99
IBUPROFEN PM (Major)			
TAB,PO (COATED CAPLET)			
38 mg-200 mg, 20s ea	00904-5877-95	4.01	
40s ea	00904-5877-39	7.16	
IBUPROHM (Ohm)			
TAB,PO (CAPLET)			
200 mg, 50s ea	51660-0424-51	2.95	
100s ea	51660-0424-01	5.00	
1000s ea	51660-0424-10	42.50	
ICAPS AREDS (Alcon Labs Cons Prod)			
SGL,PO (SOFTGEL)			
60s ea	00658-0046-01	13.84	
TAB,PO (LACTOSE-FREE,COATED)			
120s ea	00658-0040-10	14.29	
ICAPS LUTEIN & ZEAXANTHIN (Alcon Labs Cons Prod)			
TAB,PO (LACTOSE-FREE,COATED)			
60s ea	31928-0040-08	10.44	
120s ea	31928-0040-11	15.13	
ICAPS MV (Alcon Labs Cons Prod)			
TAB,PO (COATED)			
50s ea	00658-0040-82	10.44	
100s ea	00658-0040-83	14.69	
ICAPS ORIGINAL (Alcon Labs Cons Prod)			
SUS,PO (ORIGINAL FORMULA)			
60s ea	31928-0040-06	9.18	
120s ea	31928-0040-10	13.26	
ICAR PEDIATRIC (Hawthorn Pharm)			
CTB,PO (GRAPE)			
15 mg, 60s ea	63717-0103-06	18.12	
SUS,PO, 15 mg/1.25 ml, 118 ml	63717-0102-04	22.29	
(Phys Total Care)			
REPACK			
SUS,PO (1X118ML,GRAPE) 15 mg/1.25 ml, 118 ml	54868-5976-00	27.31	
ICAR-C (Hawthorn Pharm)			
TAB,PO, 250 mg-100 mg, 100s ea	63717-0099-01	36.89	
ICHTHAMMOL (Consolidated Midland)			
OIN,TP, 10%, 30 gm	00223-4135-30	1.80	
454 gm	00223-4135-13	7.50	
20%, 30 gm	00223-4136-30	1.95	
454 gm	00223-4136-13	8.50	
(Perrigo)			
OIN,TP (1X28GM)			
20%, 28 gm	70030-0149-65	5.00	
(Phys Total Care)			
REPACK			
OIN,TP, 20%, 30 gm	54868-2978-02	4.68	
(Quality Care Prod)			
REPACK			
OIN,TP, 20%, 30 gm	49999-0615-01	8.14	
ICY HOT (Chattem)			
CRE,TP, 10%-30%, 37.5 gm	41167-0008-85	2.57	
90 gm	41167-0008-91	4.34	
STI,TP, 7.6%-29%, 105 gm	41167-0008-79	4.34	
(A-S Medication)			
REPACK			
CRE,TP, 10%-30%, 37.5 gm	54569-4483-00	2.92	
(1X37.5GM)			
10%-30%, 37.5 gm	54569-4483-01	2.77	
(Dispensing Solutions)			
REPACK			
CRE,TP (EXTRA STRENGTH)			
10%-30%, 37.5 gm	55045-3408-01	5.25	
(Phys Total Care)			
REPACK			
CRE,TP, 10%-30%, 36 gm	54868-4187-00	4.65	
ICY HOT ARTHRITIS THERAPY (Chattem)			
GEL,TP, 0.025%, 60 gm	41167-0008-61	6.13	
ICY HOT STICK (Chattem)			
STI,TP, 7.6%-29%, 52.5 gm	41167-0008-98	3.41	
(Pharma Pac)			
REPACK			
STI,TP, 7.6%-29%, 52.5 gm	52959-0028-03	12.05	
65.4 gm	52959-0028-04	12.05	
ICY RUB (Teva)			
OIN,TP, 227 gm	00182-5090-44	2.99	
IFEREX 150 (Nnodum)			
CAP,PO (10 X 10)			
150 mg, 100s ea UD	63044-0203-61	13.99	
IGNATIA (Luyties)			
TAB,SL (6X)			
6 x, 500s ea	00618-4415-03	3.99	
5500s ea	00618-4415-10	30.32	
(30X)			
12 x, 500s ea	00622-4415-03	4.19	
5500s ea	00622-4415-10	31.83	
(12X)			
30 x, 500s ea	00624-4415-03	4.19	
5500s ea	00624-4415-10	31.83	
IMMULIFE (Alternativa Natural)			
PDS,PO (NATURAL CHOCOLATE)			
660 gm	91717-0238-33	75.60	105.00
IMMUNE BOOSTER (K-Pax)			
PDS,PO (1X906GM,PROTEIN BLEND)			
906 gm	88856-0005-56	50.54	
IMMUNE SUPPORT PROTEIN BLEND (K-Pax)			
PDR,PO (1X908GM,RASP/LEM)			
908 gm	88856-0004-57	50.54	
IMMUNOCAL (Immunotec)			
PDR,PO (PACKET)			
10 gm 30s	28770-0970-01	78.75	105.00
IMMUNOFIN (Lane Labs)			
CAP,PO (SOFTGEL)			
250 mg, 60s ea	02110-1070-67	9.88	21.95
120s ea	02110-1071-28	16.18	35.95
IMODIUM A-D (McNeil Consumer Healthcare)			
CTB,PO (COOL MINT,EZ CHEWS)			
2 mg, 20s ea	00450-0397-20	7.43	
40s ea	00450-0397-40	12.61	
SOL,PO (AGES 6 & UP,MINT)			
1 mg/7.5 ml, 120 ml	00450-0134-44	5.09	
(MINT)			
1 mg/7.5 ml, 120 ml	00450-0134-04	5.09	
240 ml	00450-0134-08	7.92	
TAB,PO (CAPLET)			
2 mg, 6s ea	00045-0295-06	3.11	
6s ea	00450-0295-06	3.11	
6s ea	50580-0295-06	3.11	
12s ea	00045-0295-12	5.09	
12s ea	00450-0295-12	5.09	
18s ea	00045-0295-18	5.53	
(W/6 FREE TYL FLU,CAPLET)			
2 mg, 18s ea	00045-0295-01	5.53	
(W/FREE GAS AID,CAPLET)			
2 mg, 18s ea	00045-0295-56	5.53	
(CAPLET)			
2 mg, 24s ea	00045-0295-24	7.43	
24s ea	00450-0295-24	7.43	
(W/ 6 FREE,CAPLET)			
2 mg, 24s ea	50580-0295-30	7.43	
(W/6 FREE,CAPLET)			
2 mg, 24s ea	50580-0295-23	6.08	
(W/FREE PEPCID AC,CAPLET)			
2 mg, 24s ea	00045-0295-28	6.47	
(W/TRAVEL CONTAINER)			
2 mg, 24s ea	50580-0295-31	6.79	
(CAPLET)			
2 mg, 30s ea	00045-0295-14	7.43	
48s ea	00045-0295-84	12.61	
48s ea	00450-0295-84	12.61	
(CLUB PACK,CAPLET)			
2 mg, 48s ea	00045-0295-48	10.79	
(36X2,CAPLET)			
2 mg, 72s ea	00450-0295-50	13.07	
(CAPLET)			
2 mg, 72s ea	00045-0295-29	14.39	
72s ea	00450-0295-74	16.06	
(2500X2,CAPLET)			
2 mg, 5000s ea	00045-0295-55	510.60	
IMODIUM ADVANCED (McNeil Consumer Healthcare)			
CTB,PO (2500X2)			
2 mg-125 mg, 5000s ea	00045-0294-25	750.00	
TAB,PO (W/TRAVEL CONTAINER)			
2 mg-125 mg, 18s ea	50580-0922-19	6.84	
(CAPLET)			
2 mg-125 mg, 2500s ea	50580-0922-50	375.00	
IMODIUM MULTI-SYMPTOM RELIEF (McNeil Consumer Healthcare)			
CTB,PO (MINT)			
2 mg-125 mg, 18s ea	00450-0202-18	7.43	
42s ea	00450-0202-42	12.61	
TAB,PO (CAPLET)			
2 mg-125 mg, 12s ea	00450-0212-12	5.76	
18s ea	00450-0212-18	7.43	
30s ea	00450-0212-30	10.33	
42s ea	00450-0212-42	12.61	
IMOGEN (Pharmakon)			
LIQ,PO (AF,SF)			
1 mg/5 ml, 118 ml	55422-0419-04	3.94	9.34

PROD/MFR	HRI, UPC,NDC	AWP	SRP
IMOTIL (Global Source)			
TAB,PO (CAPLET)			
2 mg, 12s ea	59618-0455-02	4.39	
IMPACT (Nestle)			
LIQ,PO (TUBE FEEDING)			
250 ml 24s	00212-3581-51	203.04	
(CLOSED SYSTEM TUBE FDG)			
1000 ml 6s	00212-3581-42	210.17	
SUS,PO (6X1000ML)			
1000 ml 6s	43900-0358-18	210.17	
IMPACT 1.5 (Nestle)			
LIQ,PO (CLOSED SYSTEM TUBE FDG)			
250 ml 24s	00212-3589-51	221.76	
IMPACT ADVANCED RECOVERY (Nestle)			
LIQ,PO (27X237ML,GLUTEN-FREE)			
237 ml 27s	00212-1955-62	97.20	
237 ml 27s	00212-1956-62	97.20	
IMPACT GLUTAMINE (Nestle)			
LIQ,PO (CAN)			
250 ml 24s	00212-1621-51	221.76	
(CLOSED SYSTEM)			
1000 ml 6s	00212-1621-42	228.89	
SUS,PO (6X1000ML)			
1000 ml 6s	43900-0162-88	228.89	
IMPACT W/FIBER (Nestle)			
LIQ,PO (TUBE FEEDING)			
250 ml 24s	00212-3587-51	207.07	
(CLOSED SYSTEM TUBE FDG)			
1000 ml 6s	00212-3587-42	213.98	
IMPACT WITH FIBER (Nestle)			
SUS,PO (6X1000ML)			
1000 ml 6s	43900-0230-51	213.98	
IMPATIENS (Ellon)			
SOL,SL (DROPS)			
10.5 ml	51762-0018-10		9.25
IMPERIM (Prime Marketing)			
TAB,PO (CAPLET)			
2 mg, 12s ea	62107-0012-12	3.75	
IMUPLUS (Swiss Bioceutical)			
PDR,PO, 10 gm 60s	18867-0000-01	92.40	115.00
INCISION/DRAINAGE TRAY (Medical Action Ind.)			
DEV,NA, 20s ea	73577-0612-00	96.66	
(SHARP/BLUNT SCISSORS)			
20s ea	73577-0612-27	106.40	
INFALINIC II (Key Company)			
SOL,PO, 60 ml	11694-0688-01	14.00	
INFANT NEOCATE (Nutricia)			
PDR,PO (4X400GM,HYPOALLERGENIC)			
400 gm 4s	49735-0125-95	148.20	
INFANT NEOCATE FORMULA (Nutricia)			
PDR,PO (USE W/MED SUPV)			
400 gm 4s	49735-0108-04	148.20	
INFANTAIRE (Altaire)			
SOL,PO (DROPS)			
80 mg/0.8 ml,			
15 ml	59390-0001-13	1.25	
30 ml	59390-0001-18	1.50	
INFANTAIRE GAS DROPS (Altaire)			
SUS,PO (DROPS)			
40 mg/0.6 ml,			
30 ml	59390-0042-17	5.95	
INFANTS' ACETAMINOPHEN (Precision Dose)			
SUS,PO (50X0.8ML,AF)			
80 mg/0.8 ml,			
0.8 ml 50s UD	68094-0692-58	60.00	
INFANTS' GAS RELIEF (Major)			
SUS,PO (1X30ML,DYE-FREE,DROP)			
20 mg/0.3 ml, 30 ml	00904-5894-30	3.50	
INFANTS' IBUPROFEN (Actavis)			
SUS,PO (1X15ML,INCLUDES SYRINGE)			
50 mg/1.25 ml, 15 ml	45963-0125-23	4.47	
(1X30ML,INCLUDES SYRINGE)			
50 mg/1.25 ml, 30 ml	45963-0125-24	6.50	
INFANTS' MAPAP DROPS (Major)			
SOL,PO (1X15ML,AF,ASPIRIN-FREE)			
80 mg/0.8 ml, 15 ml	00904-5901-35	3.29	
INFANTS' MYLICON GAS RELIEF (J&J/Merck)			
SOL,PO (NON-STAIN,DYE-FREE)			
20 mg/0.3 ml,			
15 ml	16837-0911-08	6.23	
(ORIGINAL,DROPS)			
20 mg/0.3 ml,			
15 ml	16837-0630-15	6.23	
(NON-STAIN,DYE-FREE)			
20 mg/0.3 ml,			
30 ml	16837-0911-11	10.70	
(ORIGINAL,DROPS)			
20 mg/0.3 ml,			
30 ml	16837-0630-11	10.70	
INFINITY BLOOD GLUCOSE MONITORING SYSTEM (US DIAGNOSTICS, INC)			
DEV,NA (METER KIT)			
ea	08463-5103-01	45.00	
(STARTER KIT)			
ea	08463-5003-01	55.00	
INFINITY BLOOD GLUCOSE TEST STRIPS (US DIAGNOSTICS, INC)			
DEV,NA, 50s ea	08463-5203-50	42.50	
INFINITY HIGH CONTROL SOLUTION (US DIAGNOSTICS, INC)			
DEV,NA (1X3.5ML)			
3.5 ml	08463-5105-01	8.61	
INFINITY LOW CONTROL SOLUTION (US DIAGNOSTICS, INC)			
DEV,NA (1X3.5ML)			
3.5 ml	08463-5205-01	8.61	
INFINITY NORMAL CONTROL SOLUTION (US DIAGNOSTICS, INC)			
DEV,NA, ea	08463-5005-01	10.00	
INFLUDORON (Weleda)			
LIQ,PO, 20 ml	55946-0281-60	5.55	
INJECTION SAFETY GUARD (Apothecary)			
DEV,NA (PROTECTS HANDS)			
ea	25715-0669-56	0.89	1.49
INLINE BURETTE 150 NON-VENTED (Abbott Hosp)			
DEV,NA (18" SOLUSET)			
20s ea	00074-4214-01	327.04	
(W/ADM PORT,19" SOLUSET)			
20s ea	00074-4205-01	343.19	
INLINE BURETTE 150 VENTED (Abbott Hosp)			
DEV,NA (18" SOLUSET)			
20s ea	00074-5831-01	358.86	
INNERMOST NATURE FOR MEN (Reese)			
TAB,PO (PF,SF)			
30s ea	23513-0520-30	8.12	
60s ea	23513-0520-60	12.30	
INNOMED LICE-COMB (Hogil)			
DEV,NA, ea	95814-0900-80	2.40	
INOSITECH (Bio-Tech Pharm)			
CAP,PO, 324 mg, 100s ea	53191-0310-01	4.70	
INOSITOL (Freeda)			
POW,PO (PURE,SF,GLUTEN-FREE)			
900 mg/0.9 gm,			
113 gm	10432-0328-01	11.37	18.95
454 gm	10432-0328-03	32.37	53.95
TAB,PO (PF,SF,DYE-FREE)			
650 mg, 100s ea	10432-0023-01	8.67	14.45
250s ea	10432-0023-02	17.34	28.90
(Nature's Bounty)			
TAB,PO (PF,SF)			
650 mg, 100s ea	74312-0007-10		10.98
(Rugby)			
TAB,PO (PF,SF,DYE-FREE)			
500 mg, 100s ea	00536-3984-01	8.24	
INOSITOL-5 (Key Company)			
TAB,PO, 324 mg, 100s ea	11694-0928-01	5.00	
250s ea	11694-0928-02	10.00	
INSOMNIA (Nuage Labs)			
TAB,SL (TISSUE A)			
125s ea	00634-0901-68	3.05	5.09
INSTA-GLUCOSE (Valeant Pharm Intl)			
GEL,PO, 40%, 31 gm 3s	00187-0746-33	13.99	
(A-S Medication)			
REPACK			
GEL,PO, 40%, 30 gm 3s	54569-5423-00	10.44	
(Phys Total Care)			
REPACK			
GEL,PO, 40%, 31 gm	54868-5125-00	5.14	
INSTACLEAN (Ameriderm Labs)			
SOL,TP (96X118ML)			
118 ml 96s	63921-0240-04	1.71	
(24X473ML)			
473 ml 24s	63921-0240-16	4.43	
(12X800ML)			
800 ml 12s	63921-0240-80	4.68	
(12X1000ML)			
1000 ml 12s	63921-0240-10	5.73	
INSTACORT-10 MAXIMUM STRENGTH (Altaire)			
OIN,TP, 1%, 30 gm	59390-0080-17	2.30	
INSTACORT-5 (Altaire)			
INSTACORT-5			
CRE,TP (W/ALOE VERA)			
0.5%, 30 gm	59390-0022-17	2.10	
INSTANT HAND SANITIZER (Hart Health)			
GEL,TP (1X240ML)			
62%, 240 ml	50332-0261-51	2.97	
(Major)			
GEL,TP (1X237ML)			
62%, 237 ml	00904-5845-09	2.20	
INSTEAD (Instead)			
DEV,NA (CUP W/12 HR. PROTECTION)			
6s ea	07155-0000-60	2.19	3.84
14s ea	07155-0001-60	4.91	8.24
24s ea	07155-0002-40	6.88	11.54
INSTRUMENT TRAY (Medical Action Ind.)			
DEV,NA (STAINLESS STEEL)			
20s ea	73577-0612-07	87.36	
INSTRUMENT TRAY W/KELLY HEMOSTAT (Medical Action Ind.)			
DEV,NA (CURVED)			
20s ea	73577-0612-10	79.44	
(STRAIGHT)			
20s ea	73577-0612-11	79.44	
INSTRUMENT TRAY W/MOSQUITO HEMOSTAT (Medical Action Ind.)			
DEV,NA (CURVED)			
20s ea	73577-0612-08	84.72	
(STRAIGHT)			
20s ea	73577-0612-09	84.72	
INSTY-SPLINT UNIVERSAL (Apothecary)			
DEV,NA (CHILD)			
ea	25715-0975-21	0.86	1.59
(LARGE)			
ea	25715-0975-19	3.68	6.19
(MEDIUM)			
ea	25715-0975-20	3.52	5.89
INSULATED DIABETIC WALLET (Apothecary)			
DEV,NA, ea	25715-0669-70	8.74	14.59
INSULIN HUMULIN 50/50 (Phys Total Care)			
REPACK			
SUS,SC, 50 u/ml-50 u/ml,			
10 ml	54868-5824-00	49.16	
INSURANCE (Health Products Corp)			
TAB,PO (PF,SF)			
60s ea	39686-0012-59	8.07	
INTEGRA (U.S. Pharm)			
CAP,PO (GLUTEN-FREE)			
90s ea	52747-0710-60	35.70	
INTERSORB DRY BURN PAD (Covidien)			
DEV,NA (STER,POLY BACK,24"X36")			
15s ea	08080-6827-00	130.02	
INTERSORB FINE MESH (Covidien)			
DEV,NA (STERILE,4"X25")			
192s ea	08080-6800-00	176.94	
(STERILE,3"X18")			
288s ea	08080-6802-00	141.00	
(STERILE.3"X8")			
864s ea	08080-6801-00	376.54	
INTERSORB WIDE MESH (Covidien)			
DEV,NA (STER,50 PLY,18"X18")			
30s ea	08080-6824-00	301.50	
(STER,10 PLY,18"X18")			
100s ea	08080-6467-00	188.58	
INTESTINEX (A. G. Marin)			
CAP,PO, 600 mg, 30s ea	12539-0108-30	10.80	
INTRADERM (A. G. Marin)			
GEL,TP, 120 gm	12539-0628-04	8.50	
INTRASITE (Smith & Nephew)			
GEL,TP, 8 gm 10s	00223-0438-55	61.53	49.22
(APPLIPAK)			
15 gm 10s	00223-0438-56	87.54	70.03
25 gm 10s	00223-0438-57	104.14	83.31
INTRODUCER GASTROSTOMY (Abbott)			
DEV,NA (18 FR, W/T-FASTENER SET)			
ea	70074-0501-91	207.64	
INVERTA-PEG COMPLETE GASTROSTOMY (Abbott)			
DEV,NA (20FR,COMPLETE KIT,OTG)			
ea	70074-0523-54	164.94	
IODEX (Lee Pharm)			
OIN,TP, 4.7%, 30 gm	23558-0682-10	7.32	
30 gm 36s	23558-0682-11	263.52	
720 gm	23558-0682-21	40.80	

PROD/MFR	HRI, UPC,NDC	AWP	SRP
IODEX W/METHYL SALICYLATE (Lee Pharm)			
OIN,TP, 6%-1.8%, 30 gm	23558-0682-30	7.32	
30 gm 36s	23558-0682-31	263.52	
720 gm	23558-0682-41	40.80	
IODINE (Consolidated Midland)			
TIN,TP, 30 ml	00223-6268-01	2.25	
(MILD)			
480 ml	00223-6268-02	7.95	
(Lex)			
TIN,TP, 2%-2.4%, 30 ml	49523-0008-01	0.70	
(DECOLORIZED)			
2%-2.4%, 30 ml	49523-0009-01	0.73	
(PLASTIC BOTTLE)			
2%-2.4%, 30 ml	49523-0008-11	0.63	
IODINE DECOLORIZED (Denison)			
TIN,TP, 30 ml	00295-1183-31	1.31	
(Lex)			
TIN,TP (PLASTIC BOTTLE)			
2%-2.4%, 30 ml	49523-0009-11	0.66	
IODINE SALICYLIC (Lex)			
LIQ,TP, 2%-0.5%, 30 ml	49523-0014-01	0.75	
IODINE STRONG (AmerisourceBergen)			
TIN,TP (PRIVATE LABEL)			
7%-5%, 30 ml	24385-0934-91	4.85	5.39
IODOCHLORHYDROXYQUIN (Consolidated Midland)			
CRE,TP, 3%, 30 gm	00223-4340-30	3.00	
454 gm	00223-4340-02	18.00	
IONAX ASTRINGENT (Valeant Pharm Intl)			
LIQ,TP, 240 ml	00064-2040-08	12.96	
IONAX SCRUB (Valeant Pharm Intl)			
LIQ,TP, 60 ml	00064-2050-02	12.85	
IONIL (Valeant Pharm Intl)			
LIQ,TP (RINSE)			
360 ml	00064-2100-12	11.49	
2%, 120 ml	00064-2060-04	9.97	
240 ml	00064-2060-08	13.31	
480 ml	00064-2060-16	25.09	
960 ml	00064-2060-32	36.47	
IONIL PLUS (Valeant Pharm Intl)			
LIQ,TP, 2%, 240 ml	00064-2070-08	13.50	
IONIL-T (Valeant Pharm Intl)			
SHA,TP, 240 ml	00064-2080-08	13.31	
480 ml	00064-2080-16	22.40	
960 ml	00064-2080-32	36.47	
(1X473ML)			
5%, 473 ml	00064-2085-16	21.98	
IONIL-T PLUS (Valeant Pharm Intl)			
LIQ,TP, 240 ml	00064-2090-08	15.38	
IPECAC (Luyties)			
TAB,SL (6X)			
6 x, 500s ea	00618-4436-03	3.99	
5500s ea	00618-4436-10	30.32	
(30X)			
12 x, 500s ea	00622-4436-03	4.19	
5500s ea	00622-4436-10	31.83	
(12X)			
30 x, 500s ea	00624-4436-03	4.19	
5500s ea	00624-4436-10	31.83	
(Walker Pharmacal)			
TAB,SL (6X)			
250s ea	00619-4436-02	2.97	
(Dispensing Solutions)			
REPACK			
SYR,PO, 7 gm/100 ml, 30 ml	55045-3692-01	5.00	
IPECAC SYRUP (AmerisourceBergen)			
SYR,PO (PRIVATE LABEL)			
30 ml	24385-0237-91	3.05	3.39
(Denison)			
SYR,PO, 30 ml	00295-1185-01	0.82	
(Humco)			
SYR,PO, 7 gm/100 ml, 30 ml	00395-1237-91	1.71	
(Paddock)			
SYR,PO, 7 mg/5 ml, 30 ml	00574-0012-01	4.70	
(Phys Total Care)			
REPACK			
SYR,PO, 30 ml	54868-0232-00	9.66	
(Southwood)			
REPACK			
SYR,PO, 30 ml	58016-9037-01	5.25	
IRCON (Kenwood)			
TAB,PO (BLISTER PACK,10X10)			
200 mg, 100s ea UD	00482-0628-01	35.90	
IRCON-FA (Kenwood)			
TAB,PO (BLISTER PACK,10X10)			
250 mg-0.8 mg, 100s ea UD	00482-0932-01	43.06	
IRIGATE (Dispensing Solutions)			
REPACK			
SOL,OP, 118 ml	55045-2738-08	5.85	
IROMIN-G (Mission)			
TAB,PO, 100s ea	00178-0081-01	10.03	
IRON (Basic Vitamins)			
TAB,PO, 324 mg, 100s ea	00761-0940-20	2.40	
(Mason Vit)			
TAB,PO (PF)			
90 mg, 100s ea	11845-0127-71	3.89	
(Nature's Bounty)			
TAB,PO (PF,SF)			
325 mg, 100s ea	74312-0012-00	2.67	4.65
IRON ADVANCED (Rexall)			
TAB,PO, 58.5 mg-25 mg, 120s ea	30768-0018-12	2.70	4.08
IRON CHELATED (ADH)			
TAB,PO, 30 mg, 60s ea	60142-0110-06	2.38	4.75
IRON CHEWS (Midlothian Labs)			
CTB,PO (GRAPE)			
15 mg, 60s ea	68308-0910-60	17.12	
IRRIGATION FACEPLATE (Coloplast)			
DEV,NA (1/2"-2")			
ea	11701-0821-15	12.95	13.55
IRRIGATION SET (Abbott Hosp)			
DEV,NA (LATEX,LRG BORE,Y-TYPE)			
20s ea	00074-6599-02	222.96	
(NV,LARGE BORE,Y-TYPE)			
20s ea	00074-6599-01	222.96	
(SECONDARY)			
20s ea	00074-6541-01	72.48	
(Coloplast)			
DEV,NA (DELUXE)			
ea	11701-0820-25	67.07	70.18
(ECONOMY)			
ea	11701-0820-10	52.46	54.90
IRRIGATION SETS DELUXE VERSION (Coloplast)			
DEV,NA, ea	11701-0820-20	74.44	77.90
IRRIGATION SETS ECONOMY VERSION (Coloplast)			
DEV,NA, ea	11701-0820-15	37.48	39.22
IRRIGATION SLEEVES (Coloplast)			
DEV,NA (W/PROD #1291,4560,1120)			
5s ea	11701-0822-25	32.50	34.00
(W/PRODUCT #1201, #4540)			
5s ea	11701-0822-15	32.50	34.00
(W/PRODUCT #1251, #4550)			
5s ea	11701-0822-20	32.50	34.00
(1/2"-2 1/2")			
10s ea	11701-0822-10	28.20	29.50
IRRIGATION Y-CONNECTOR (Abbott Hosp)			
DEV,NA (8")			
20s ea	00074-4694-01	94.80	
ISAGEL (Coloplast)			
GEL,TP (50X6, TOWELETTES)			
60%, 2.5 ml 300s	11701-0032-98	72.00	75.00
(TOWELETTES)			
60%, 2.5 ml 300s	11701-0032-37	78.00	81.00
59 ml 36s	11701-0025-03	56.88	59.76
118 ml 36s	11701-0025-04	68.04	71.28
621 ml 12s	11701-0025-26	98.04	102.60
(REFILL)			
60%, 800 ml 12s	11701-0025-45	123.24	129.00
ISLAND GARD-GRX (Geritrex)			
DEV,NA (4"X4")			
60s ea	92771-0840-44	2.47	
(2"X2")			
100s ea	92771-0840-22	1.41	
ISO-PH (Miller)			
TAB,PO, 250 mg, 100s ea	17204-0415-40	7.56	9.50
ISOLEUCINE (VITAFLO, LLC)			
PDS,PO, 50 mg/4 gm, 30s ea	50600-0543-02	90.00	115.00
ISOLEUCINE 1000 (VITAFLO, LLC)			
POW,NA (30X4GM)			
4 gm 30s	50600-0551-18	120.00	150.00
ISOMIL SOY W/IRON (Abbott)			
LIQ,PO, 390 ml	70074-0421-10	5.09	
ISOPROPYL RUBBING ALCOHOL (Major)			
SOL,TP (1X473ML)			
70%, 473 ml	00904-6045-16	2.05	
ISOPTO TEARS (Alcon Ophthalmic)			
SOL,OP, 0.5%, 15 ml	00998-0408-15	20.88	
ISOSOURCE (Nestle)			
LIQ,PO (TUBE FEEDING)			
250 ml 24s	00212-1825-51	27.94	
(CLOSED SYSTEM TUBE FDG)			
1000 ml 6s	00212-1826-42	35.06	
1500 ml 6s	00212-1826-44	52.63	
(Phys Total Care)			
REPACK			
LIQ,PO (24X250ML,LACTOSE-FREE)			
250 ml 24s	54868-5925-00	40.32	
ISOSOURCE 1.5 CAL (Nestle)			
LIQ,PO (TUBE FEEDING,VANILLA)			
250 ml 24s	00212-1815-51	38.02	
(CLOSED SYSTEM TUBE FDG)			
1000 ml 6s	00212-1816-42	45.07	
1500 ml 6s	00212-1816-44	67.61	
SUS,PO (6X1000ML)			
1000 ml 6s	43900-0181-81	45.07	
(6X1500ML)			
1500 ml 6s	43900-0181-82	67.61	
ISOSOURCE HN (Nestle)			
LIQ,PO (TUBE FEEDING)			
250 ml 24s	00212-1845-51	28.80	
(CLOSED SYSTEM TUBE FDG)			
1000 ml 6s	00212-1846-42	36.00	
1500 ml 6s	00212-1846-44	54.00	
SUS,PO (6X1000ML)			
1000 ml 6s	43900-0184-80	36.00	
(6X1500ML)			
1500 ml 6s	43900-0184-66	54.00	
ISOSOURCE VHN (Nestle)			
LIQ,PO (TUBE FEEDING)			
250 ml 24s	00212-1875-51	36.86	
(CLOSED SYSTEM TUBE FDG)			
1000 ml 6s	00212-1875-42	44.14	
1500 ml 6s	00212-1875-44	66.24	
ITCH-X (Ascher)			
FOA,TP (MAXIMUM STRENGTH)			
1%, 88.7 ml	02250-0498-53	6.48	
GEL,TP, 10%-1%, 35.4 gm	00225-0495-33	3.54	
LOT,TP, 1%, 88.7 ml	02250-0497-53	6.48	
SPR,TP, 10%-1%, 59.1 ml	00225-0516-51	4.74	
IV PREP ANTISEPTIC WIPES (Smith & Nephew)			
PAD,TP, 70%, 50s ea	50484-0210-00	11.84	9.47
IV STAND BASE/HOOK RAMS HORN (Abbott Hosp)			
DEV,NA, ea	00074-2006-04	165.10	
IV STAND UPRIGHT (Abbott Hosp)			
DEV,NA, ea	00074-2006-03	165.10	
IV STAND/BASE ASSEMBLY (Abbott Hosp)			
DEV,NA, ea	00074-2006-02	165.10	
IV STAND/POLE ASSEMBLY (Abbott Hosp)			
DEV,NA, ea	00074-2006-01	165.10	
IV Y-TYPE CONNECTING (Abbott Hosp)			
DEV,NA (10" W OPTION-LOK)			
120s ea	00074-4064-01	388.80	
(6")			
120s ea	00074-4094-01	401.76	
IVEX-2 (Abbott Hosp)			
DEV,NA (0.22MIC W/Y-SITE)			
48s ea	00074-2679-48	498.18	
(H.P./FILTERSET)			
48s ea	00074-4524-58	153.79	
(RAPID FLOW FILTER SET)			
48s ea	00074-1517-48	230.40	
IVY BLOCK (Hyland's)			
LOT,TP, 5%, 120 ml	62333-0111-40	7.62	11.99
(Phys Total Care)			
REPACK			
SUS,TP, 5%, 120 ml	54868-3968-00	10.96	
IVY CLEANSE (Hyland's)			
PAD,TP, 12s ea	62333-0113-12	3.80	5.50
IVY COMPLETE (Hyland's)			
KIT,MR, 5%-1%, ea	62333-0111-49	12.77	22.99
IVY RELIEF (Hyland's)			
TAB,PO, 6 x-6 x-6 x, 50s ea	62333-0114-01	7.62	14.99
IVY SOOTHE (Hyland's)			
CRE,TP (MAXIMUM STRENGTH)			
1%, 28.4 gm	62333-0112-10	3.80	5.50

PROD/MFR	HRI, UPC,NDC	AWP	SRP
IVY-RID (Medique)			
SPR,TP, 0.2%, 82.5 ml	47682-0487-56	4.30	
JELCO INTERMITTENT INJECTION CAP (J&J Medical)			
DEV,NA, ea	56091-0046-00	0.77	
JESSNER'S PLUS (Topix)			
SOL,TP (FOR OFFICE USE ONLY) 14%-14%-14%,			
120 ml	51326-0001-04	22.00	
JEVITY 1 CAL (Abbott)			
LIQ,PO, 240 ml	70074-0401-43	2.38	
1000 ml	70074-0006-82	14.26	
1500 ml	70074-0526-04	21.38	
JEVITY 1.2 CAL (Abbott)			
LIQ,PO, 240 ml	70074-0531-19	2.86	
1000 ml	70074-0531-24	17.11	
1000 ml	70074-0531-25	17.11	
1500 ml	70074-0531-14	25.66	
1500 ml	70074-0531-15	25.66	
JEVITY 1.5 CAL (Abbott)			
LIQ,PO, 237 ml	70074-0573-34	3.01	
(RTH)			
1000 ml	70074-0573-30	18.05	
1500 ml	70074-0573-32	27.07	
JOHNSON & JOHNSON COTTON BALLS (J&J Medical)			
DEV,NA (STERILE,MEDIUM)			
65s ea	56091-0061-01	1.46	
(STERILE,LARGE)			
130s ea	56091-0061-05	2.51	
JOHNSON & JOHNSON EYE STERILE (J&J Medical)			
DEV,NA (2 1/8"X2 5/8")			
12s ea	56091-0087-72	3.12	
(1 5/8"X2 5/8",OVAL)			
50s ea	56091-0087-71	8.90	
(2 1/8"X2 5/8")			
50s ea	56091-0087-73	8.19	
JOHNSON & JOHNSON EYE-AID (J&J Medical)			
SOL,IR, 15 ml	08137-0080-54	1.95	
JOHNSON & JOHNSON FIRST AID (J&J Medical)			
DEV,NA (STANDARD INDUSTRIAL)			
ea	56091-0081-61	20.97	
ea	56091-0081-62	56.01	
ea	56091-0081-63	105.85	
(WEATHERPROOF INDUSTRIAL)			
ea	56091-0081-72	38.54	
JOHNSON & JOHNSON FIRST AID REFILL (J&J Medical)			
DEV,NA, ea	56091-0081-76	13.94	
JOHNSON & JOHNSON GAUZE SPONGE (J&J Medical)			
DEV,NA (STERILE,4X4",12PLY,TRAY)			
10s ea	56091-0023-22	1.06	
(STERILE,4X4",16PLY,TRAY)			
10s ea	56091-0023-29	1.24	
(STERILE,4X4",8-PLY,TRAY)			
10s ea	56091-0023-21	1.06	
(NON-STERILE,2X2",8-PLY)			
200s ea	56091-0076-12	2.41	
(NON-STERILE,4X4",12-PLY)			
200s ea	56091-0076-23	8.80	
(NON-STERILE,4X4",8-PLY)			
200s ea	56091-0076-10	6.07	
JOHNSON & JOHNSON GAUZE STERILE (J&J Medical)			
DEV,NA (4"X4",12-PLY,2X25)			
50s ea	56091-0023-17	3.47	
(2"X2",8-PLY,2X50)			
100s ea	56091-0023-18	3.01	
(4"X4",8-PLY,2X50)			
100s ea	56091-0023-15	5.78	
JOHNSON & JOHNSON INSTANT COLD PACK (J&J Medical)			
DEV,NA (SMALL)			
ea	08137-0080-45	1.32	
JOHNSON & JOHNSON NON-STICK STERILE (J&J Medical)			
DEV,NA (3"X4",LARGE)			
100s ea	56091-0047-31	13.25	
JOHNSON & JOHNSON REACH TOTAL CARE (Johnson & Johnson)			
DEV,NA (30YD,FRESH MINT)			
ea	81371-0093-96	2.51	
(90YD,MINT)			
ea	81371-0092-06	5.20	
JOHNSON & JOHNSON TRIANGULAR (J&J Medical)			
DEV,NA (51")			
ea	08137-0080-68	1.47	
JOHNSON & JOHNSON WATERPROOF (J&J Medical)			
DEV,NA (3"X10YD)			
4s ea	56091-0051-35	25.89	
(2"X10YD)			
6s ea	56091-0051-34	25.89	
(1"X10YD)			
12s ea	56091-0051-32	25.89	
(1/2"X10YD)			
24s ea	56091-0051-31	25.89	
JOHNSON'S BABY BAR (Johnson & Johnson)			
SOA,TP, 85 gm	81370-0032-62	1.60	
JOHNSON'S BABY BUBBLE BATH & WASH (Johnson & Johnson)			
SOA,TP, 444 ml	81371-0021-25	3.42	
828 ml	81371-0021-26	5.81	
JOHNSON'S BABY COLOGNE (Johnson & Johnson)			
SOL,TP (1X200ML)			
200 ml	81370-0031-43	2.29	
JOHNSON'S BABY CREAM (Johnson & Johnson)			
CRE,TP (1X226GM)			
226 gm	81370-0029-93	3.42	
JOHNSON'S BABY LOTION (Johnson & Johnson)			
LOT,TP (1X29ML)			
29 ml	81370-0035-11	0.61	
(1X118ML)			
118 ml	81370-0035-08	1.60	
(1X266ML)			
266 ml	81370-0035-13	2.29	
(1X444ML)			
444 ml	81370-0035-17	3.42	
(1X798ML)			
798 ml	81370-0030-85	5.81	
JOHNSON'S BABY OIL (Johnson & Johnson)			
OIL,TP, 118 ml	81370-0033-07	1.67	
(1X414ML)			
414 ml	81370-0033-14	3.26	
(1X592ML)			
592 ml	81370-0033-20	4.08	
JOHNSON'S BABY OIL ALOE VERA & VITAMIN E (Johnson & Johnson)			
OIL,TP (1X414ML)			
414 ml	81370-0033-32	3.26	
(1X592ML)			
592 ml	81370-0033-39	4.08	
JOHNSON'S BABY OIL GEL (Johnson & Johnson)			
GEL,TP (1X192ML)			
192 ml	81370-0012-58	3.26	
JOHNSON'S BABY OIL GEL ALOE VERA & VITAMIN E (Johnson & Johnson)			
GEL,TP (1X192ML)			
192 ml	81370-0032-96	3.26	
JOHNSON'S BABY OIL GEL SHEA & COCOA BUTTER (Johnson & Johnson)			
GEL,TP (1X192ML)			
192 ml	81371-0020-65	3.26	
JOHNSON'S BABY OIL LAVENDER (Johnson & Johnson)			
OIL,TP (1X414ML)			
414 ml	81370-0033-16	3.26	
JOHNSON'S BABY POWDER (Johnson & Johnson)			
POW,TP (1X42GM)			
42 gm	81370-0030-01	0.61	
(1X113GM)			
113 gm	81370-0030-11	1.32	
(1X255GM)			
255 gm	81370-0030-21	2.17	
(1X425GM)			
425 gm	81370-0030-16	3.26	
(1X624GM)			
624 gm	81370-0030-14	4.08	
JOHNSON'S BABY POWDER COOLING CUCUMBER MELON (Johnson & Johnson)			
POW,TP (1X425GM)			
425 gm	81370-0052-38	3.26	
JOHNSON'S BABY POWDER LAVENDER & CHAMOMILE (Johnson & Johnson)			
POW,TP (1X425GM;CALMING)			
425 gm	81370-0030-17	3.26	
(1X624M;CALMING)			
624 gm	81370-0030-43	4.08	
JOHNSON'S BABY POWDER PURE CORNSTARCH (Johnson & Johnson)			
POW,TP (WITH ALOE & VITAMIN E)			
42 gm	81370-0052-56	0.61	
113 gm	81370-0030-44	1.32	
255 gm	81370-0030-48	2.17	
425 gm	81370-0030-58	3.26	
624 gm	81370-0030-59	4.08	
JOHNSON'S BABY RELIEF (Johnson & Johnson)			
KIT,MR (DROPS)			
ea	81370-0026-42	25.96	
JOHNSON'S BABY SHAMPOO (Johnson & Johnson)			
SHA,TP (1X44ML,NO MORE TEARS)			
44 ml	81370-0037-12	0.61	
(1X103ML,NO MORE TEARS)			
103 ml	81370-0037-15	1.50	
(1X207ML,NO MORE TEARS)			
207 ml	81370-0037-18	2.29	
(1X444ML)			
444 ml	81370-0037-24	3.42	
(WITH NATURAL LAVENDER)			
444 ml	81370-0037-47	8.42	
(1X591ML,NO MORE TEARS)			
591 ml	81370-0037-40	4.30	
(WITH NATURAL LAVENDER)			
591 ml	81370-0037-75	4.30	
(1X751ML,NO MORE TEARS)			
751 ml	81370-0052-44	4.66	
JOHNSON'S BATHTIME (Johnson & Johnson)			
KIT,MR, 10%, ea	81370-0027-38	19.40	
JOHNSON'S BEDTIME BATH (Johnson & Johnson)			
SOA,TP, 266 ml	81370-0032-10	3.42	
444 ml	81370-0032-11	4.30	
828 ml	81370-0032-58	6.74	
JOHNSON'S BEDTIME LOTION (Johnson & Johnson)			
LOT,TP (1X266ML)			
266 ml	81370-0035-03	3.42	
(1X444ML)			
444 ml	81370-0035-26	4.30	
(1X798ML)			
798 ml	81370-0039-68	6.74	
JOHNSON'S BEDTIME MOISTURE WASH (Johnson & Johnson)			
SOA,TP, 444 ml	81370-0027-79	4.30	
JOHNSON'S BEDTIME SWEET SLEEP SET (Johnson & Johnson)			
KIT,MR, ea	81370-0043-55	24.29	
KIT,TP, ea	81371-0022-86	21.01	
JOHNSON'S BODY CARE 24 HOUR (Johnson & Johnson)			
LOT,TP (1X59ML)			
59 ml	81370-0027-40	0.92	
(1X230ML)			
230 ml	81370-0024-70	3.38	
(1X414ML)			
414 ml	81370-0031-11	4.36	
(1X591ML)			
591 ml	81370-0052-41	5.54	
SOA,TP (1X600ML;MOISTURIZING)			
600 ml	81370-0026-77	4.57	
JOHNSON'S BODY CARE BE RADIANT (Johnson & Johnson)			
LOT,TP (1X414ML;COCOA&SHEABUTER)			
414 ml	81370-0031-09	4.36	
SOA,TP (1X532ML;EXFOLIATING)			
532 ml	81370-0059-83	4.57	
JOHNSON'S BODY CARE DEEP HYDRATION (Johnson & Johnson)			
LOT,TP (1X414ML;EXTRA DRY SKIN)			
414 ml	81370-0027-84	4.36	
SOA,TP (1X600ML;INTENSEMOISTURE)			
600 ml	81370-0027-37	4.57	
JOHNSON'S BODY CARE FEELING HEALTHY (Johnson & Johnson)			
LOT,TP (1X414ML;NOURISHING)			
414 ml	81370-0031-69	4.36	
SOA,TP (1X600ML;NOURISHING)			
600 ml	81370-0031-70	4.57	
JOHNSON'S BODY CARE FOREVER FRESH (Johnson & Johnson)			
SOA,TP (1X600ML;REFRESHING)			
600 ml	81371-0021-38	4.57	
JOHNSON'S BODY CARE MELT AWAY STRESS (Johnson & Johnson)			
LOT,TP (1X59ML;RELAXING)			
59 ml	81370-0041-59	0.92	

PROD/MFR | HRI, UPC,NDC | AWP | SRP

(1X325ML;RELAXING)
325 ml 81370-0043-06 4.36
SOA,TP (1X59ML;RELAXING)
59 ml.............. 81370-0041-58 0.92
(1X600ML;RELAXING)
600 ml 81370-0043-34 4.57

JOHNSON'S BUDDIES EASY-COMB (Johnson & Johnson)
SHA,TP (1X248ML,NO MORE TANGLES)
248 ml 81370-0028-20 2.84
SPR,TP (1X236ML)
236 ml 81370-0028-21 2.84

JOHNSON'S BUDDIES EASY-COMB CONDITIONER (Johnson & Johnson)
CRE,TP (1X221ML)
221 ml 81370-0028-19 2.84

JOHNSON'S BUDDIES EASY-GRIP SUDZING BAR (Johnson & Johnson)
SOA,TP (1X70GM)
70 gm.............. 81370-0028-15 0.86

JOHNSON'S BUDDIES MOISTURIZING BODY WASH (Johnson & Johnson)
SOA,TP (1X248ML)
248 ml 81370-0029-89 2.77

JOHNSON'S COTTON SWABS (Johnson & Johnson)
DEV,NA, 30s ea 81370-0026-94 0.77

JOHNSON'S CREAMY BABY OIL (Johnson & Johnson)
OIL,TP (1X444ML)
444 ml 81370-0033-19 3.26

JOHNSON'S CUCUMBER MELON BABY LOTION (Johnson & Johnson)
LOT,TP (1X444ML)
444 ml 81370-0052-33 3.42
(1X798ML)
798 ml 81370-0052-34 5.81

JOHNSON'S CUCUMBER MELON BABY WASH (Johnson & Johnson)
SOA,TP, 444 ml......... 81370-0052-35 3.42
(1X828ML)
828 ml 81370-0052-36 5.81

JOHNSON'S FIRST TOUCH (Johnson & Johnson)
KIT,TP, 10%, ea......... 81370-0027-57 9.08

JOHNSON'S HEAD-TO-TOE BABY LOTION (Johnson & Johnson)
LOT,TP (1X266ML,FRAGRANCE-FREE)
266 ml 81370-0051-49 2.29
(1X444ML,FRAGRANCE-FREE)
444 ml 81370-0051-51 3.42
(1X798ML,FRAGRANCE-FREE)
798 ml 81370-0051-58 5.81

JOHNSON'S HEAD-TO-TOE BABY WASH (Johnson & Johnson)
SOA,TP (1X29ML,DYE-FREE)
29 ml.............. 81370-0032-68 0.61
118 ml 81370-0031-07 1.60
(1X266ML,DYE-FREE)
266 ml 81370-0032-36 2.29
(1X444ML,DYE-FREE)
444 ml 81370-0032-37 3.42
(1X828ML,DYE-FREE)
828 ml 81370-0031-95 5.81

JOHNSON'S HEAD-TO-TOE FOAMING WASH (Johnson & Johnson)
SOA,TP (1X266ML)
266 ml 81371-0021-27 4.30

JOHNSON'S KIDS HEAD-TO-TOE (Johnson & Johnson)
SOA,TP (1X265ML,TROPICAL BLAST)
265 ml 81370-0040-74 2.80

JOHNSON'S KIDS NO MORE TANGLES (Johnson & Johnson)
SPR,TP (STRAWBERRY SENSATION)
300 ml 81370-0040-58 2.80

JOHNSON'S KIDS SUPER SUDZER E-Z GRIP SOAP (Johnson & Johnson)
SOA,TP (3X70GM,BERRY BREEZE,BAR)
70 gm 3s 81370-0040-66 2.80

JOHNSON'S MOISTURE CARE BABY WASH (Johnson & Johnson)
SOA,TP (1X443ML)
443 ml 81370-0029-95 3.42
(1X828ML)
828 ml 81370-0031-57 5.81

PROD/MFR | HRI, UPC,NDC | AWP | SRP

JOHNSON'S NO MORE TANGLES (Johnson & Johnson)
CRE,TP (LEAVE-IN CONDITIONER)
150 ml 81370-0051-76 3.42
SHA,TP (1X384ML,CURLY HAIR)
384 ml 81370-0043-51 3.42
(1X384ML,STRAIGHT HAIR)
384 ml 81370-0043-48 3.42
(1X532ML,CURLY HAIR)
532 ml 81370-0043-52 4.30
(1X532ML,STRAIGHT HAIR)
532 ml 81370-0043-49 4.30
SPR,TP (1X295ML)
295 ml 81370-0040-97 2.98

JOHNSON'S NURSING PADS (Johnson & Johnson)
DEV,NA, 36s ea 81370-0017-74 3.68
60s ea 81370-0017-75 5.36

JOHNSON'S PURE COTTON (Johnson & Johnson)
DEV,NA (COTTON ROUNDS)
80s ea 81370-0082-51 1.66
200s ea 81370-0082-63 1.66
375s ea 81370-0082-28 2.24
525s ea 81370-0082-38 3.01

JOHNSON'S SAFETY SWABS (Johnson & Johnson)
DEV,NA, 55s ea 81370-0082-56 1.26
185s ea 81370-0029-48 3.84

JOHNSON'S SHEA & BUTTER BABY CREAM (Johnson & Johnson)
CRE,TP (1X226GM)
226 gm............. 81370-0052-37 3.42

JOHNSON'S SHEA & COCOA BUTTER BABY LOTION (Johnson & Johnson)
LOT,TP (1X444ML)
444 ml 81370-0024-92 3.42
(1X798ML)
798 ml 81370-0024-89 5.81

JOHNSON'S SHEA & COCOA BUTTER BABY WASH (Johnson & Johnson)
SOA,TP (1X444ML)
444 ml 81370-0024-94 3.42
(1X828ML)
828 ml 81370-0024-93 5.81

JOHNSON'S SOFTLOTION (Johnson & Johnson)
LOT,TP (1X266ML)
266 ml 81370-0031-10 3.42

JOHNSON'S SOOTHING NATURALS HAIR AND BODY WASH (Johnson & Johnson)
SOA,TP (1X236ML)
236 ml 81370-0031-58 4.04

JOHNSON'S SOOTHING NATURALS NOURISHING LOTION (Johnson & Johnson)
LOT,TP (1X236ML)
236 ml 81370-0029-82 4.04

JOHNSON'S SOOTHING NATURALS SOOTHE & PROTECT BALM (Johnson & Johnson)
OIN,TP (1X15GM)
15 gm.............. 81370-0029-84 4.04

JOHNSON'S SOOTHING VAPOR BATH (Johnson & Johnson)
SOA,TP (1X444ML)
444 ml 81370-0032-98 4.30

JOHNSON'S TAKE ALONG PACK (Johnson & Johnson)
KIT,MR, 10%, ea......... 81370-0034-34 2.40

JOHNSON'S TRAVEL KIT (Johnson & Johnson)
KIT,MR, ea 81370-0043-56 5.69

JOHNSON'S VANILLA OATMEAL BABY LOTION (Johnson & Johnson)
LOT,TP (1X444ML)
444 ml 81370-0041-46 3.42
(1X798ML)
798 ml 81370-0041-47 5.81

JOHNSON'S VANILLA OATMEAL BABY WASH (Johnson & Johnson)
SOA,TP (1X444ML)
444 ml 81370-0040-23 3.42
(1X828ML)
828 ml 81370-0040-24 5.81

JOINT BOOST (Freeda)
TAB,PO (PF,SF,DYE-FREE)
100s ea............ 10432-0325-01 6.87 11.45
250s ea............ 10432-0325-02 13.74 22.90

JOINT GUARD (Advanced Nutr)
SGL,PO (SOFTGEL)
60s ea............. 62617-0635-02 15.75 28.00

PROD/MFR | HRI, UPC,NDC | AWP | SRP

JR. TYLENOL (McNeil Consumer Healthcare)
ODT,PO (MELTAWAYS,ASPIRIN-FREE)
160 mg, 24s ea 00450-0513-24 4.85
24s ea 00450-0514-24 4.85

JUICE+FIBRE (Nutra/Balance)
LIQ,PO (27X236ML,APPLE)
236 ml 27s 07249-0501-01 49.28
(27X236ML,GRAPE)
236 ml 27s 07249-0501-03 49.28

JUNIOR MAALOX PLUS (Novartis Consumer)
CTB,PO (WILD BERRY)
400 mg-24 mg,
24s ea............. 00067-6242-24 4.19

JUNIOR NEOCATE (Nutricia)
PDR,PO (4X400GM,TROPICAL FRUIT)
400 gm 4s.......... 49735-0121-24 146.90

JUNIOR STRENGTH MUCINEX MINI-MELTS (Reckitt Benckiser)
PKT,PO (BUBBLEGUM)
100 mg, 12s ea 63824-0254-12 6.83

JUST FOR KIDS (Omnii Intl)
GEL,DE (BUBBLEGUM)
0.4%, 121.9 gm...... 48878-4070-03 7.30
(FRUIT)
0.4%, 121.9 gm...... 48878-4080-03 7.30
(GRAPEY GRAPE)
0.4%, 121.9 gm...... 48878-4020-03 7.30

JUVEN (Abbott)
PDR,PO (23GM PKT,GRAPE)
23 gm.............. 59781-0208-64 2.46
(23GM PKT,ORANGE)
23 gm.............. 59781-0225-50 2.46
(23GMX30,GRAPE)
23 gm 30s.......... 59781-0580-11 85.82
(23GMX30,ORANGE)
23 gm 30s.......... 59781-0580-12 85.82
(GRAPE)
23 gm 30s.......... 59781-0208-65 75.25
(ORANGE)
23 gm 30s.......... 59781-0225-51 75.25

K-99 (Bio-Tech Pharm)
CAP,PO, 99 mg, 100s ea... 53191-0242-01 3.15

K-GLUCON (Wesley)
TAB,PO, 500 mg, 100s ea.. 00917-0269-01 4.95

K-MAG (Bio-Tech Pharm)
CAP,PO, 40 mg-40 mg,
100s ea............ 53191-0074-01 7.35

K-MAG-60 (Bio-Tech Pharm)
CAP,PO, 60 mg-60 mg,
100s ea............ 53191-0136-01 9.95

K-MART VALUE PLUS LANCETS (Can-Am Care)
DEV,NA (21G,PRIVATE LABEL)
100s ea............ 38396-0918-25 5.85
(SUPER THIN,30G)
100s ea............ 38396-0323-25 5.85
(SUPER THIN)
100s ea............ 38396-0311-25 5.85
(THIN,26G,PRIVATE LABEL)
100s ea............ 38396-0312-25 5.85
(21G,PRIVATE LABEL)
200s ea............ 38396-0919-25 9.50
(COLORED,PRIVATE LABEL)
200s ea............ 38396-0900-25 9.50
(THIN,26G,PRIVATE LABEL)
200s ea............ 38396-0322-25 9.50

K-MART VALUE PLUS LANCING (Can-Am Care)
DEV,NA (SUPER THIN,30G)
ea................. 38396-0004-25 6.49

K-MART-VALUE PLUS INSULIN SYRINGES (Can-Am Care)
DEV,NA (29G, ULTRA COMFORT)
100s ea............ 38396-0403-25 17.50
100s ea 38396-0405-25 17.50
(30G, ULTRA COMFORT)
100s ea............ 38396-0406-25 17.50
100s ea 38396-0407-25 17.50
100s ea 38396-0408-25 17.50

K-PAX (K-Pax)
PKT,PO (SINGLE STR,4 CAP PAK)
60s ea............. 88856-0000-01 67.44
(DOUBLE STR,8 CAP PAK)
60s ea............. 88856-0000-02 122.44

K-Y INTENSE (Johnson & Johnson)
GEL,VG (1X10ML, AROUSAL GEL)
10 ml.............. 80040-0086-95 22.04

PROD/MFR	HRI. UPC.NDC	AWP	SRP
K-Y JELLY (Johnson & Johnson)			
GEL,TP, 56 gm	08137-0089-02	1.86	
113 gm	08137-0089-12	3.02	
K-Y LIQUID PERSONAL LUBRICANT (Johnson & Johnson)			
GEL,TP, 142 gm	80040-0089-26	7.92	
K-Y LUBRICATING STERILE (J&J Medical)			
GEL,TP (SINGLE USE FOIL PACK)			
2.7 gm 150s	56091-0089-42	11.37	
(SINGLE USE TUBE)			
5 gm 48s	56091-0089-46	17.34	
(SINGLE USE FOIL PACK)			
5 gm 150s	56091-0089-44	19.19	
(SINGLE USE TUBE)			
60 gm 12s	56091-0089-17	9.62	
(FLIP-TOP TUBE)			
120 gm 12s	56091-0089-19	11.98	
K-Y SENSITIVE (Johnson & Johnson)			
GEL,VG (FRAGRANCE-FREE)			
85 gm	80040-0085-50	5.14	
K.P.N. PRENATAL WITH EXTRA CALCIUM (Freeda)			
TAB,PO (SF,GLUTEN-FREE)			
100s ea	10432-0033-01	5.97	9.95
250s ea	10432-0033-02	11.94	19.90
KAISER PERMANENTE (Natl Vitamin)			
CALCIUM CITRATE			
TAB,PO, 950 mg, 100s ea	79854-0617-25	1.72	
CALCIUM CITRATE W/D			
TAB,PO (PF,SF)			
200 mg-125 iu,			
100s ea	79854-0617-28	1.74	
MACUVITE			
TAB,PO, 60s ea	79854-0619-31	1.48	
MULTIVITAMIN CHILDREN'S			
CTB,PO, 100s ea	79854-0061-90	1.50	
KALA (Freeda)			
TAB,PO (PF,SF,DYE-FREE)			
200 million u, 100s ea	10432-0161-01	5.37	8.95
250s ea	10432-0161-02	10.35	17.25
500s ea	10432-0161-03	17.97	29.95
KALI BICHROMICUM (Luyties)			
TAB,SL (6X)			
6 x, 500s ea	00618-5213-03	3.99	
(12X)			
6 x, 5500s ea	00624-5213-10	31.83	
(30X)			
6 x, 5500s ea	00622-5213-10	31.83	
(6X)			
6 x, 5500s ea	00618-5213-10	30.32	
(30X)			
12 x, 500s ea	00622-5213-03	4.19	
(12X)			
30 x, 500s ea	00624-5213-03	4.19	
KALI CARBONICUM (Luyties)			
TAB,SL (6X)			
6 x, 500s ea	00618-5215-03	3.99	
5500s ea	00618-5215-10	30.32	
30 x, 500s ea	00624-5215-03	4.19	
(30X)			
30 x, 500s ea	00622-5215-03	4.19	
5500s ea	00624-5215-10	31.83	
(30X)			
30 x, 5500s ea	00622-5215-10	31.83	
KALI MUR (Hyland's)			
TAB,PO, 500s ea	54973-1026-01	5.87	9.79
1000s ea	54973-1026-02	10.49	17.49
(Nuage Labs)			
TAB,SL (6X)			
125s ea	00634-5224-68	3.05	5.09
KALI PHOS (Hyland's)			
TAB,PO, 500s ea	54973-1031-01	5.87	9.79
1000s ea	54973-1031-02	10.49	17.49
(Nuage Labs)			
TAB,SL (6X)			
125s ea	00634-5228-68	3.05	5.09
KALI SULPH (Hyland's)			
TAB,PO, 500s ea	54973-1037-01	5.87	9.79
1000s ea	54973-1037-02	10.49	17.49
(Nuage Labs)			
TAB,SL (6X)			
125s ea	00634-5230-68	3.05	5.09
KALTOSTAT (Convatec)			
DEV,NA (3"X4 3/4")			
10s ea	68455-0102-27	80.38	105.64
(4"X8")			
10s ea	68455-0107-39	175.11	230.17
(6"X9 1/2")			
10s ea	68455-0102-31	354.94	466.53
(5X2GM)			
2 gm 5s	68455-0102-24	50.66	66.59
KALTOSTAT FORTEX (Convatec)			
DEV,NA (4"X4")			
10s ea	68455-0102-34	171.19	225.01
KAMELEON (Line One Labs)			
DEV,NA (LUBRICATED,3COLOR,ASTD)			
3s ea	05632-0892-04	2.25	
(TRI-COLOR, LUBRICATED)			
3s ea	05632-0892-00	2.25	
KAMINOS (Key Company)			
TAB,PO, 168s ea	11694-0972-01	9.00	
1000s ea	11694-0972-04	35.00	
KANGAROO (Covidien)			
DEV,NA (FEEDING TUBE 10FR-36")			
10s ea	08080-7115-50	85.32	
(FEEDING TUBE 8FR-36")			
10s ea	08080-7115-68	85.32	
(FEEDING TUBE,12FR-36")			
10s ea	08080-7115-01	78.75	
(FEEDING TUBE,14FR-36")			
10s ea	08080-7115-19	82.04	
(FEED&IRRIG W/SYRG,60CC)			
20s ea	08080-7001-08	27.57	
(GRAVITY,STER,1000ML)			
24s ea	08080-7123-01	141.95	
(1000MLCAP-W/O/ICEPOUCH)			
30s ea	08080-7736-67	177.59	
(1000MLCAPACITY-W/ICEPCH)			
30s ea	08080-7025-05	100.60	
(500ML CAPACITY)			
30s ea	08080-7026-05	90.97	
(50CC IRRIG SRN)			
30s ea	08080-7001-24	21.88	
(AFF PUMP,1000ML,AF)			
30s ea	08080-7736-10	119.63	
(AFF PUMP,500ML,AF)			
30s ea	08080-7020-15	119.63	
(AFF PUMP,DEHP FR,1000ML)			
30s ea	08080-7736-20	132.00	
(AFF PUMP,DEHP FR,500ML)			
30s ea	08080-7020-25	132.00	
(AFF PUMP,DEHP FR,SPIKE)			
30s ea	08080-7046-25	98.44	
(AFF PUMP,GRAVITY,1000ML)			
30s ea	08080-7025-20	98.44	
(AFF PUMP,SPIKE SET,AF)			
30s ea	08080-7046-15	111.38	
(DELUX EZ CAP PUMP,500ML)			
30s ea	08080-7021-05	157.50	
(DELUX EZCAP PUMP,1200ML)			
30s ea	08080-7043-05	207.50	
(DELUX EZCAP PUMP,1600ML)			
30s ea	08080-7048-05	187.04	
(EXTEN SET,4 FT)			
30s ea	08080-7002-07	76.55	
(EZ CAP BAG ONLY,1000ML)			
30s ea	08080-7039-04	87.28	
(EZ CAP PUMP SET,500 ML)			
30s ea	08080-7020-05	170.10	
(FEEDING& IRRIGATION)			
30s ea	08080-7001-16	36.75	
(GRAVITY,EZ CAP,1000ML)			
30s ea	08080-7025-00	91.88	
(PROXIMAL SPIKE PUMP)			
30s ea	08080-7046-05	120.75	
(PUMP,1000 ML)			
30s ea	08080-7736-00	177.59	
(PUMP,NON-STER 1000 ML)			
30s ea	08080-7036-00	177.59	
(RIGID CONT ONLY,1200ML)			
30s ea	08080-7062-12	83.95	
(RIGID CONT ONLY,600 ML)			
30s ea	08080-7062-38	89.25	
(RIGID CONT W/PUMP,600ML)			
30s ea	08080-7062-20	118.33	
(RIGID CONT W/PUMP1200ML)			
30s ea	08080-7062-04	177.59	
(SCREW CAP PUMP /GLS BOT)			
30s ea	08080-7047-05	140.44	
(SCREW CAP PUMP)			
30s ea	08080-7068-00	88.34	
(Y-SITE EXTENSION SET)			
30s ea	08080-7050-08	53.69	
(DELUX EZCAP STER,1200ML)			
36s ea	08080-7143-01	343.98	
(DELUX EZCAP STER,1600ML)			
36s ea	08080-7148-01	306.98	
(EZ CAP STER PUMP,1000ML)			
36s ea	08080-7136-01	206.39	
(STER BURETTE W/PMP100ML)			
36s ea	08080-7161-01	251.88	
(STER DELUX EZ CAP,500ML)			
36s ea	08080-7121-01	286.39	
(STER PROXIMAL SPIKE PMP)			
36s ea	08080-7146-00	184.84	
(STER, EZ CAP PUMP,500ML)			
36s ea	08080-7120-04	232.00	
KANGAROO 224 ENTERAL FEEDING PUMP (Covidien)			
DEV,NA (SIMPLIFIED SET-UP 0.224)			
ea	08080-3224-24	485.63	
KANGAROO 324 ENTERAL FEEDING PUMP (Covidien)			
DEV,NA (PRESET DOSE DELIVERY)			
ea	08080-3324-23	616.87	
KANGAROO EPUMP (Covidien)			
DEV,NA (1000MLPUMPSET&FLUSHBAG)			
30s ea	08080-7736-62	216.57	
(PROXIMALSPIKE,1000MLBAG)			
30s ea	08080-7746-69	196.88	
KANGAROO JOEY ENTERAL FEEDING PUMP (Covidien)			
DEV,NA (WITH POLE CAMP)			
ea	08080-3834-00	1640.62	
KANGAROO PET (Covidien)			
DEV,NA (CARRY CSE W/FRM PET PMP)			
ea	08080-3504-09	265.13	
(CHARGE CORD-PET PUMP)			
ea	08080-3504-90	56.82	
(FRAME ONLY FOR PET PUMP)			
ea	08080-3504-82	198.84	
KAO-TIN (Major)			
SGL,PO (SODIUM-FREE,SOFTGEL)			
240 mg, 100s ea	00904-5779-60	13.50	
(SOFTGEL)			
240 mg, 500s ea	00904-5779-40	39.59	
SUS,PO (MINT)			
262 mg/15 ml, 236 ml	00904-5709-09	3.40	
473 ml	00904-5709-16	5.24	
(Pharma Pac)			
REPACK			
SUS,PO, 750 mg/15 ml,			
240 ml	52959-0297-08	5.25	
KAODENE A-D (Pfeiffer)			
TAB,PO (CAPLET)			
2 mg, 6s ea	00927-0043-16	1.76	3.17
KAODENE NN (Pfeiffer)			
SUS,PO (AF)			
120 ml	00927-0421-12	1.65	2.96
KAOLINPEC (Truxton)			
SUS,PO, 480 ml	00463-9013-16	3.75	
3840 ml	00463-9013-28	22.00	
KAOPECTATE (Pfizer)			
SUS,PO (PEPPERMINT)			
262 mg/15 ml, 236 ml	00009-5214-02	4.40	
(A-S Medication)			
REPACK			
SUS,PO, 262 mg/15 ml,			
240 ml	54569-5519-00	4.34	
KAOPECTATE ADVANCED FORMULA (Pharmacia Consumer)			
SUS,PO (AF)			
750 mg/15 ml,			
90 ml 36s	00009-3785-04	57.50	
240 ml	00009-3785-01	4.12	
(PEPPERMINT)			
750 mg/15 ml,			
240 ml	00009-3786-01	4.12	
(AF)			
750 mg/15 ml,			
360 ml	00009-3785-02	5.59	
(PEPPERMINT)			
750 mg/15 ml,			
360 ml	00009-3786-02	5.59	
(Phys Total Care)			
REPACK			
SUS,PO, 750 mg/15 ml,			
360 ml	54868-2298-00	8.68	
KAOPECTATE CHILDREN'S (Pharmacia Consumer)			
SUS,PO (CHERRY)			
262 mg/15 ml, 180 ml	00009-5271-01	4.27	

PROD/MFR	HRI. UPC.NDC	AWP	SRP
KAOPEK (Phys Total Care)			
REPACK			
SUS,PO, 600 mg/15 ml,			
360 ml	54868-2040-01	9.37	
480 ml	54868-2040-02	11.79	
KAPECTOLIN (Consolidated Midland)			
SUS,PO, 120 ml	00223-6273-01	2.10	
240 ml	00223-6273-02	3.25	
480 ml	00223-6273-03	4.00	
KARAYA GUM (Geritrex)			
POW,TP, 80 gm	92771-0728-00	6.49	
KARBOZYME (Miller)			
TAB,PO, 167 mg-173 mg-346 mg,			
100s ea	17204-0819-40	6.00	10.00
KAVA KAVA (Botanical Labs.)			
CAP,PO, 50s ea	41954-0032-66	6.50	12.99
LIQ,PO, 30 ml	41954-0032-06	8.25	16.49
(Lex)			
CAP,PO, 500 mg, 60s ea	58537-0027-06	4.10	
(Marlex)			
CAP,PO, 250 mg, 100s ea	10135-0291-01	1.93	
500 mg, 100s ea	10135-0292-01	3.24	
(Mason Vit)			
CAP,PO (PF,SF)			
100 mg, 60s ea	11845-0129-85	10.00	
500 mg, 60s ea	11845-0118-25	7.78	
KAVA KAVA ROOT (Cardinal Health)			
CAP,PO (PRIVATE LABEL)			
233 mg, 60s ea	37205-0056-72	9.30	
KEEP ALERT (Magno-Humphries)			
TAB,PO, 200 mg, 60s ea	43292-0558-59	1.95	3.99
KELP (Basic Vitamins)			
TAB,PO, 0.15 mg,			
200s ea	00761-0450-40	1.80	
(Carlson,J.R.)			
TAB,PO (PF,SF,CORN-FREE)			
10 mg-150 mcg,			
300s ea	88395-0085-73	5.75	11.50
1000s ea	88395-0085-76	16.25	32.50
(Marlex)			
TAB,PO, 300s ea	10135-0360-03	1.66	
(Mason Vit)			
TAB,PO, 250s ea	11845-0055-52	3.22	
(Nature's Bounty)			
TAB,PO (PF,SF)			
0.15 mg, 250s ea	74312-0006-23		4.49
KELP-TABS (Key Company)			
TAB,PO, 0.15 mg,			
100s ea	11694-0739-01	4.25	
KELP/LECITHIN/B6 (Mason Vit)			
TAB,PO (EXT. STR.)			
100s ea	11845-0059-81	6.33	
(SF)			
100s ea	11845-0062-31	5.22	
(Rexall)			
TAB,PO (LECITHIN KELP B-6)			
60s ea	30768-0011-08	2.26	3.77
KENGUARD ADD-A-FOLEY (Covidien)			
KENGUARD ADD-A-FOLEY TRAY			
DEV,NA (W/10CC SRN/DRAIN BAG)			
10s ea	08080-3515-00	97.49	
(W/30CC SRN/DRAIN BAG)			
10s ea	08080-3531-00	94.54	
KENGUARD ADD-A-FOLEY CATHETER TRAY (Covidien)			
DEV,NA (LATEX-FREE,POWDER-FREE)			
20s ea	08080-7600-00	68.17	
KENGUARD DRAINAGE BAG WITH ANTI-REFLUX CHAMBER (Covidien)			
DEV,NA (2000ML,LATEX-FREE)			
20s ea	08080-3512-00	52.89	
KENGUARD I.V. POLE POUCH WITH PISTON SYRINGE (Covidien)			
DEV,NA, 30s ea	08080-8406-40	26.40	
KENGUARD SILICONE ELASTOMER FOLEY (Covidien)			
KENGUARD SILICONE ELASTOME FOLEY			
DEV,NA (18FR,16")			
10s ea	08080-4027-18	35.87	
KENGUARD SILICONE-COATED FOLEY (Covidien)			
DEV,NA (14FR,5CC,2 WAY)			
10s ea	08080-3558-00	21.00	
(16FR,30CC,2 WAY)			
10s ea	08080-3601-00	21.00	
KENGUARD URETHRAL CATHETER TRAY (Covidien)			
DEV,NA (LATEX-FREE,POWDER-FREE)			
20s ea	08080-7503-00	77.94	
KERI ADVANCED (B/M Squibb Cons Med)			
LOT,TP (EXTRA DRY SKIN,OIL-FREE)			
241 gm	19810-0300-64	4.58	
425 gm	19810-0300-68	6.77	
567 gm	19810-0300-73	7.79	
(Novartis Consumer)			
LOT,TP (1X450ML)			
450 ml	00067-2107-15	6.77	
KERI AGE DEFY & PROTECT (B/M Squibb Cons Med)			
LOT,TP (ALPHA HYDROXY+SPF15)			
7.5%-2%, 425 gm	19810-0300-70	6.77	
KERI NOURISHING SHEA BUTTER & VITAMIN E (Novartis Consumer)			
LOT,TP (1X450ML)			
450 ml	00067-2100-15	6.77	
KERI ORIGINAL (Novartis Consumer)			
LOT,TP (1X450ML, DRY SKIN)			
450 ml	00067-2105-15	6.77	
KERI ORIGINAL FORMULA (B/M Squibb Cons Med)			
LOT,TP, 241 gm	19810-0300-62	4.58	
425 gm	19810-0300-66	6.77	
567 gm	19810-0300-72	7.79	
(Phys Total Care)			
REPACK			
LOT,TP, 195 ml	54868-4345-00	5.46	
KERI OVERNIGHT (Novartis Consumer)			
LOT,TP (1X450ML)			
450 ml	00067-2112-15	6.77	
KERI RENEWAL MILK BODY (Novartis Consumer)			
LOT,TP (1X241GM)			
241 gm	00672-0605-83	7.94	
KERI RENEWAL SERUM (Novartis Consumer)			
LOT,TP (1X113GM)			
113 gm	00672-0152-04	7.94	
KERI RENEWAL STRETCH MARK MINIMIZER (Novartis Consumer)			
TP (1X255ML)			
255 ml	00067-2708-50	7.94	
KERI SENSITIVE SKIN (B/M Squibb Cons Med)			
LOT,TP (FRAGRANCE-FREE)			
241 gm	19810-0300-65	4.58	
(DYE-FREE,FRAGRANCE-FREE)			
425 gm	19810-0300-69	6.77	
(Novartis Consumer)			
LOT,TP (1X450ML,DYE-FREE)			
450 ml	00067-2109-15	6.77	
KERI SHAVE MINIMIZING (B/M Squibb Cons Med)			
LOT,TP, 425 gm	19810-0301-55	6.77	
KERLIX BOLT NON-STERILE (Covidien)			
DEV,NA (9"X100YDS,3 PLY)			
4s ea	08080-2671-00	218.49	
KERLIX FIVE PACKS - LARGE ROLLS (Covidien)			
KERLIX FIVE PACKS - LARGE ROLLS			
NA (4.5"X4.1YD,STERILE)			
80s ea	08080-6760-00	132.50	
KERLIX LARGE ROLL (Covidien)			
DEV,NA (4.5"X4.1YD,NON-STERILE)			
48s ea	08080-3324-00	97.57	
(4.5"X3.1YDS,8-PLY)			
100s ea	08080-6716-00	172.03	
KERLIX LITE CONFORMING GAUZE BANDAGES (Covidien)			
KERLIX LITE CONFORMING GAUZE BANDAGES			
NA (6"X4.5YD,NON-STERILE)			
48s ea	08080-8056-00	62.83	
(6"X4.5YD,STERILE)			
48s ea	08080-8076-00	62.40	
(3"X4.1YD,STERILE)			
72s ea	08080-8073-00	53.10	
(4"X4.1YD,STERILE)			
72s ea	08080-8074-00	65.07	
(2"X3.5YD,NON-STERILE)			
96s ea	08080-8052-00	40.00	
(2"X3.5YD,STERILE)			
96s ea	08080-8072-00	53.10	
(3"X4.1YD,NON-STERILE)			
96s ea	08080-8053-00	54.17	
(4"X4.1YD,NON-STERILE)			
96s ea	08080-8054-00	77.84	
KERLIX MEDIUM ROLL (Covidien)			
KERLIX MEDIUM ROLL			
NA (3.4"X3.6YD,NON-STERILE)			
96s ea	08080-6735-00	101.72	
(3.4"X3.6YD,STERILE)			
96s ea	08080-6725-00	115.94	
KERLIX ROLL IN RIGID PLASTIC TRAY (Covidien)			
DEV,NA (4.5"X4.1YDS,6 PLY)			
60s ea	08080-6730-00	137.87	
KERLIX ROLL IN SOFT POUCH (Covidien)			
DEV,NA (4.5"X4.1YDS,6 PLY)			
100s ea	08080-6715-00	173.75	
KERLIX ROLL NON-STERILE (Covidien)			
DEV,NA (4.5"X4.1YDS,6 PLY)			
100s ea	08080-1892-00	149.04	
KERLIX ROUND SPONGES (Covidien)			
DEV,NA (RADIOPAQUE-XL)			
640s ea	08080-4935-00	237.40	
1000s ea	08080-2949-00	276.40	
KERLIX SMALL ROLLS (Covidien)			
DEV,NA (2.25"X3YDS,6PLY,STERILE)			
96s ea	08080-6720-00	94.34	
(2.25"X3YDS,NON-STERILE)			
96s ea	08080-1801-00	70.00	
KERLIX SPONGE STERILE (Covidien)			
DEV,NA (4"X4",12 PLY,PLSTC TRAY)			
1280s ea	08080-6120-00	144.04	
(4"X4",16 PLY,PLSTC TRAY)			
1280s ea	08080-4588-00	175.68	
KERLIX SPONGES (Covidien)			
DEV,NA (4"X4",12 PLY,STERILE)			
1200s ea	08080-5072-00	93.55	
(4"X4",12PLY,NON-STERILE)			
2000s ea	08080-4032-00	98.13	
(4"X4",16 PLY)			
2000s ea	08080-5042-00	128.85	
KERLIX SUPER SPONGE STERILE (Covidien)			
DEV,NA (MEDIUM,IN PLASTIC TRAY)			
480s ea	08080-7310-00	218.98	
KERLIX SUPER SPONGES (Covidien)			
DEV,NA (XL,NON-STERILE)			
200s ea	08080-6035-00	104.63	
(LARGE,NON-STERILE)			
400s ea	08080-1272-00	131.77	
(LARGE,STERILE)			
400s ea	08080-4308-00	197.03	
(MED,SOFT POUCH,STERILE)			
480s ea	08080-2585-00	161.69	
(MEDIUM,NON-STERILE)			
600s ea	08080-1167-00	145.69	
(MEDIUM,STERILE)			
600s ea	08080-3085-00	174.78	
KERLIX WET DRESSINGS SALINE (Covidien)			
DEV,NA (6"X6.75", MEDIUM)			
192s ea	08080-3338-00	222.50	
KERODEX 51 (Medtech)			
CRE,TP, 120 gm	75137-0010-10	3.56	
KERODEX 71 (Medtech)			
CRE,TP, 120 gm	75137-0015-10	3.56	
KERR INSTA-CHAR (VistaPharm, Inc.)			
SUS,PO (PEDIATRIC DOSE,CHERRY)			
25 gm/120 ml,			
120 ml UD	66689-0203-04	8.82	
(PEDIATRICDOSE,AQ BASE)			
25 gm/120 ml,			
120 ml UD	66689-0202-04	7.62	
(AQUEOUS BASE,CHERRY)			
25 gm/120 ml,			
240 ml UD	66891-0202-08	8.52	
(AQUEOUS BASE)			
25 gm/120 ml,			
240 ml UD	66689-0201-08	8.40	
(CHERRY)			
25 gm/120 ml,			
240 ml UD	66689-0203-08	9.84	
KERR PRESTIGE SMART SYSTEM (Home Diag)			
DEV,NA (STRIP)			
50s ea	56151-0304-50	28.60	
KERR PRESTIGE SMART SYSTEM STARTER (Home Diag)			
DEV,NA (MTR,STRP,LANCET,DEV,SOL)			
ea	56151-0204-01	22.18	
KETO-DIASTIX (Bayer Diabetes Care)			
DEV,NA, 50s ea	00193-2882-50	12.48	
100s ea	00193-2882-21	21.96	

PROD/MFR	HRI, UPC,NDC	AWP	SRP
KETOCAL 3:1 (Nutricia)			
PDS,PO (6X300GM)			
300 gm 6s	49735-0166-72	184.60	
KETOCAL 4:1 (Nutricia)			
PDR,PO (6X300GM, MEDICAL FOOD)			
300 gm 6s	49735-0166-70	191.10	
KETOCARE (Home Diag)			
DEV,NA, 50s ea	56151-0601-50	7.04	
100s ea	56151-0601-01	13.00	
KETOCONAZOLE (Palmetto)			
REPACK			
CRE,TP, 2%, 15 gm	23490-5785-01	37.84	
30 gm	23490-5785-02	75.68	
60 gm	23490-5785-03	151.36	
SHA,TP, 2%, 120 ml	23490-5786-01	32.05	
TAB,PO, 200 mg, 30s ea	23490-5784-00	110.00	
60s ea	23490-5784-01	220.00	
(Pharma Pac)			
REPACK			
TAB,PO, 200 mg, 60s ea	52959-0699-60	63.21	
KETONEX-1 (Abbott)			
PDR,PO, 400 gm	70074-0511-13	42.18	
KETONEX-2 (Abbott)			
PDR,PO, 400 gm	70074-0511-15	81.12	
KETOSTIX (Bayer Diabetes Care)			
DEV,NA (STRIP)			
20s ea	00193-2640-20	7.80	
50s ea	00193-2880-50	10.32	
100s ea	00193-2880-21	18.00	
KETOTIFEN FUMARATE (Akorn)			
SOL,OP (1X5ML)			
0.025%, 5 ml	17478-0717-10	12.19	
KETOVOLVE (Solace)			
PDS,PO (1X300GM)			
300 gm	57771-0001-23	24.00	40.00
KEY-E (Carlson,J.R.)			
CRE,TP, 120 gm	88395-0005-14	6.45	12.90
CTB,PO, 400 iu, 100s ea	88395-0001-41	11.25	22.50
250s ea	88395-0001-42	49.90	
OIN,TP, 113 gm	88395-0005-24	6.45	12.90
PDS,PO, 700 iu/dose,			
1000 gm	88395-0002-06	157.50	315.00
SUP,RC, 30 iu, 12s ea	88395-0005-55	4.44	8.88
24s ea	88395-0005-54	7.20	14.40
KEY-E-KAPS (Carlson,J.R.)			
SGL,PO, 400 iu, 100s ea	88395-0002-41	13.45	26.90
250s ea	88395-0002-42	29.95	59.90
KEY-PHOS-425 (Key Company)			
SGL,PO (SOFTGEL)			
425 mg-100 mg-75 mg,			
30s ea	11694-0721-30	3.50	
100s ea	11694-0721-01	8.00	
300s ea	11694-0721-03	23.00	
KEYGESIC-10 (Key Company)			
TAB,PO, 650 mg, 25s ea	11694-0908-02	1.50	
100s ea	11694-0908-01	4.25	
1000s ea	11694-0908-05	31.00	
KEYOMEGA (VITAFLO, LLC)			
POW,NA (30X4GM)			
30s ea	50600-0555-07	75.00	93.75
KEYTABS (Key Company)			
TAB,PO (SF)			
180s ea	11694-0787-02	14.00	
KEYTABS W/O IRON (Key Company)			
TAB,PO, 180s ea	11694-0771-02	14.00	
KIDKARE COUGH/COLD (Rugby)			
LIQ,PO (AF,CHERRY)			
120 ml	00536-2310-97	3.15	
KIDNEY (Key Company)			
CAP,PO, 200 mg, 100s ea	11694-0850-01	5.25	
500s ea	11694-0850-03	22.00	
(Miller)			
TAB,PO, 280 mg, 100s ea	17204-0507-40	7.56	12.00
KIMONO MAXX (Mayer)			
DEV,NA, 3s ea	16169-0020-03	2.04	
12s ea	16169-0020-12	8.46	
KIMONO MICROTHIN (Mayer)			
DEV,NA, 3s ea	16169-0050-03	2.04	
(LARGE)			
3s ea	16169-0080-03	2.04	
(W/AQUA LUBE)			
3s ea	16169-0060-03	2.04	
12s ea	16169-0050-12	8.46	
(LARGE)			
12s ea	16169-0080-12	8.46	
(W/AQUA LUBE)			
12s ea	16169-0060-12	8.46	
24s ea	16169-0050-24	12.90	
(W/AQUA LUBE)			
24s ea	16169-0060-24	12.90	
KIMONO THIN (Mayer)			
DEV,NA, 3s ea	16169-0010-03	2.04	
12s ea	16169-0010-12	8.46	
KIMONO TYPE E (Mayer)			
DEV,NA (TEXTURED)			
3s ea	16169-0070-03	2.04	
12s ea	16169-0070-12	8.46	
KINERASE (Valeant Pharm Intl)			
CRE,TP, 0.1%, 80 gm	00187-0401-48	126.89	
LOT,TP, 0.1%, 80 ml	00187-0403-55	126.89	
(Phys Total Care)			
REPACK			
CRE,TP, 0.1%, 40 gm	54868-0139-00	88.74	
KINNEY BRAND LANCETS (Owen Mumford)			
DEV,NA (PRIVATE LABEL)			
100s ea	08214-0187-18	4.70	
KINNEY BRAND THIN LANCETS (Owen Mumford)			
DEV,NA (PRIVATE LABEL)			
100s ea	08214-0207-18	4.70	
KINRAY PREFERRED PLUS LANCETS (Can-Am Care)			
DEV,NA (COLORED,PRIVATE LABEL)			
100s ea	38396-0355-06	5.85	
(SUPER THIN)			
100s ea	38396-0311-56	5.85	
(THIN,PRIVATE LABEL)			
100s ea	38396-0315-06	5.85	
(COLORED,PRIVATE LABEL)			
200s ea	38396-0366-06	9.50	
KLB6 (Nature's Bounty)			
CAP,PO (PF,SF,SOFTGEL)			
100s ea	74312-0012-10		6.79
KLB6 GRAPEFRUIT DIET (Nature's Bounty)			
TAB,PO (PF,SF)			
100s ea	74312-0039-70		7.99
KLEENITE (Regent Labs)			
POW,NA (DENTAL CLEANSER)			
170 gm	83272-0008-46	2.98	
255 gm	83272-0008-49	3.95	
KLING CONFORMING GAUZE (J&J Medical)			
DEV,NA (BULK NS,6"X131",2-PLY)			
6s ea	56091-0069-06	6.65	
(BULK NS,2"X131",2-PLY)			
12s ea	56091-0069-02	4.36	
(BULK NS,3"X131",2-PLY)			
12s ea	56091-0069-03	5.90	
(BULK NS,4"X131",2-PLY)			
12s ea	56091-0069-04	8.48	
(STERILE,2"X131",2-PLY)			
12s ea	56091-0069-22	6.99	
(STERILE,3"X131",2-PLY)			
12s ea	56091-0069-23	9.32	
(STERILE,4"X131",2-PLY)			
12s ea	56091-0069-24	11.42	
(STERILE,6"X131",2-PLY)			
12s ea	56091-0069-26	16.43	
(BULK NS,1"X131",2-PLY)			
24s ea	56091-0069-01	6.54	
KLING FLUFF GAUZE ROLLS NONSTERILE (J&J Medical)			
DEV,NA (4.5"X4.1YD,STRETCH,COTT)			
100s ea	56091-0069-37	117.00	
KLING FLUFF GAUZE ROLLS STERILE (J&J Medical)			
DEV,NA (4.5"X4.1YD,STRETCH,TRAY)			
ea	56091-0069-31	2.05	
(3.4"X3.6YD,STRETCHED)			
96s ea	56091-0069-28	108.36	
(4.5"X3.1YD,STRETCHED)			
100s ea	56091-0069-29	148.20	
(4.5"X4.1YD,STRETCH,COTT)			
100s ea	56091-0069-30	148.20	
KLING FLUFF SPONGES (J&J Medical)			
DEV,NA (6"X6.75",10X48X10/TRAY)			
4800s ea	56091-0023-34	19.24	
KLING FLUFF SPONGES STERILE (J&J Medical)			
DEV,NA (6X6.25",STRETCHED,2X20)			
40s ea	56091-0023-35	11.77	
(6X6.25",STRETCHED,5X10)			
50s ea	56091-0023-36	12.44	
KLING ROLLS (Johnson & Johnson)			
DEV,NA (3"X75",2.1YDS)			
5s ea	81370-0055-21	6.07	
(4"X75",2.1YDS)			
5s ea	81370-0055-22	8.04	
KLUTCH (Oakhurst)			
POW,NA, 22.5 gm	23558-0689-80	2.40	3.60
52.5 gm	23558-0689-70	4.72	7.08
KODET SE (Pfeiffer)			
TAB,PO, 30 mg, 24s ea	00927-0118-24	1.17	2.11
KOLA EXTRACT (Lex)			
LIQ,PO, 1.11%, 30 ml	49523-0043-02	1.10	
KOLA-PECTIN (Seyer Pharmatec)			
SUS,PO, 300 mg/15 ml,			
118 ml	11026-2638-04	6.90	
KOLDETS COUGH SUPPRESANT (Pfeiffer)			
LOZ,MM (CHERRY)			
6.1 mg, 30s ea	00927-0183-07	0.82	1.47
(MENTHOL-EUCALYPTUS)			
6.1 mg, 30s ea	00927-0182-07	0.82	1.47
(HONEY LEMON)			
8.4 mg, 30s ea	00927-0184-07	0.82	1.47
KOLEPHRIN (Pfeiffer)			
TAB,PO, 325 mg-2 mg-30 mg,			
24s ea	00927-0224-24	2.59	4.65
36s ea	00927-0224-63	3.41	6.14
KOLEPHRIN GG/DM (Pfeiffer)			
LIQ,PO, 10 mg/5 ml-150 mg/5 ml,			
120 ml	00927-0637-12	2.33	4.19
KOLEPHRIN/DM (Pfeiffer)			
TAB,PO (CAPLET)			
325 mg-2 mg-10 mg-30 mg,			
30s ea	00927-0187-07	2.80	5.04
KONDREMUL (Heritage/Insight)			
LIQ,PO, 480 ml	00235-0121-00	6.57	
(Southwood)			
REPACK			
LIQ,PO, 480 ml	58016-5713-01	11.39	
KONSYL (Konsyl)			
CAP,PO (EZ-CAPS)			
0.52 gm, 100s ea	00224-1847-10	5.50	
PDR,PO (30X5.8GM,SF,ORANGE)			
3.5 gm/dose,			
5.8 gm 30s	02241-0855-30	7.50	
(1X450GM,SF,ORANGE)			
3.5 gm/dose,			
450 gm	00224-1855-07	7.50	
(EASY MIX FORMULA)			
4.3 gm/dose,			
300 gm	00224-1856-06	8.50	
(W/SHAKER CUP,SF)			
6 gm/dose, 7s ea	00224-1801-37	2.00	
(PACKET)			
6 gm/dose,			
6 gm 30s	00224-1801-35	9.00	12.07
300 gm	00224-1801-06	10.00	13.09
450 gm	00224-1801-07	13.00	16.91
KONSYL FIBER (Konsyl)			
TAB,PO, 625 mg, 90s ea	00224-0500-90	7.25	9.53
KONSYL ORANGE ORIGINAL TEXTURE (Konsyl)			
PDR,PO (1X397GM,ORANGE)			
3.4 gm/dose,			
397 gm	00224-1841-03	3.75	
KONSYL-D (Konsyl)			
PDR,PO (W/DEXTROSE)			
3.4 gm/dose,			
325 gm	00224-1822-06	7.25	10.17
500 gm	00224-1822-07	9.25	13.09
KONSYL-ORANGE (Konsyl)			
PDR,PO (W/SUCROSE,PACKET)			
3.4 gm/dose,			
12 gm 30s	00224-1852-13	6.75	7.54
(W/SUCROSE)			
3.4 gm/dose,			
538 gm	00224-1852-06	7.50	8.73
KROGER ANTISEPTIC ALCOHOL (Triad)			
SWA,TP (PRIVATE LABEL)			
70%, 100s ea	11110-0794-49		1.99

PROD/MFR	HRI, UPC,NDC	AWP	SRP
KROGER BLOOD GLUCOSE TEST STRIPS (Abbott)			
DEV,NA (PRIVATE LABEL)			
50s ea	66004-0850-04	31.20	
100s ea	66004-0851-05	62.40	
KROGER GLUCOSE GEL (Can-Am Care)			
GEL,PO (PRIVATE LABEL)			
15 gm, 114 gm 3s	38396-0550-18	8.11	
KROGER LANCETS (Can-Am Care)			
DEV,NA (SUPER THIN)			
100s ea	38396-0303-18	5.85	
(THIN,PRIVATE LABEL)			
100s ea	38396-0301-18	5.85	
(PRIVATE LABEL)			
200s ea	38396-0304-18	9.50	
(THIN,PRIVATE LABEL)			
200s ea	38396-0302-18	9.50	
KROGER NICOTINE TRANSDERMAL SYSTEM (Novartis Consumer)			
TDM,TD (STEP 1,PRIVATE LABEL)			
21 mg/24 hr,			
14s ea	00067-5020-14	29.87	
KROGER PEN NEEDLE (Can-Am Care)			
DEV,NA (31G,6MM,(1/4"))			
100s ea	38396-0706-18	19.98	
KROGER ULTRA COMFORT INSULIN SYRINGES (Can-Am Care)			
DEV,NA (29G,1/2",1/2ML)			
100s ea	38396-0403-18	17.50	
(29G,1/2",1ML)			
100s ea	38396-0405-18	17.50	
(29G,1/2",3/10ML)			
100s ea	38396-0402-18	17.50	
(30G,5/16",1/2ML)			
100s ea	38396-0407-18	17.50	
(30G,5/16",1ML)			
100s ea	38396-0406-18	17.50	
(30G,5/16",3/10ML)			
100s ea	38396-0408-18	17.50	
(31G,5/16",1/2ML)			
100s ea	38396-0410-18	17.50	
(31G,5/16",1ML)			
100s ea	38396-0411-18	17.50	
(31G,5/16",3/10ML)			
100s ea	38396-0409-18	17.50	
KRUSCHEN SALTS (Consolidated Midland)			
PDR,PO, 120 gm	00223-9250-00	7.50	
KUTKIT STYPTIC (Majestic Drug)			
SWA,TP, 21.3%, 12s ea	10705-0300-50	2.25	4.99
KYOLIC AGED GARLIC EXTRACT (Pharmaton)			
TAB,PO (CAPLET)			
600 mg, 30s ea	93190-0170-01	5.85	6.92
L-ALANINE (Carlson,J.R.)			
PDR,PO (PF,SF,CORN-FREE)			
2000 mg, 100 gm	88395-0067-25	14.95	29.90
L-ARGININE (Carlson,J.R.)			
PDR,PO (PF,SF,CORN-FREE)			
3000 mg, 1000 gm	88395-0067-36	70.00	140.00
(Rexall)			
CAP,PO, 500 mg, 90s ea	30768-0036-59	4.28	6.49
L-ASPARAGINE (Carlson,J.R.)			
PDR,PO (PF,SF,DAIRY-FREE)			
2 gm/tsp, 100 gm	88395-0067-45	12.45	24.90
L-CARNITINE (Rexall)			
TAB,PO, 500 mg, 30s ea	30768-0040-43	13.09	19.79
(Rugby)			
CAP,PO, 250 mg, 60s ea	00536-7410-08	37.99	
L-EMENTAL (Hormel Healthlabs)			
PDR,PO (ENTERAL FORMULA)			
80.4 gm	61678-0160-01	5.60	
L-EMENTAL HEPATIC (Hormel Healthlabs)			
PDR,PO (ENTERAL FORMULA)			
86.2 gm	61678-0124-16	20.21	
L-O-M MUS (Panatoz)			
CAP,PO (SOFTGEL)			
30s ea	25349-0117-52	36.00	60.00
L-TRYPTOPHAN (Freeda)			
TAB,PO (SF,GLUTEN-FREE)			
500 mg, 50s ea	10432-0220-00	19.17	31.95
LABEAUTE (Scandinavian)			
TAB,PO, 60s ea	51137-0060-60	23.97	39.95

PROD/MFR	HRI, UPC,NDC	AWP	SRP
180s ea	51137-0060-65	59.97	99.95
LABSTIX (Siemens)			
DEV,NA, 100s ea	08620-2181-21	79.60	79.60
LAC-DOSE (Rugby)			
TAB,PO (CAPTAB)			
3000 u, 50s ea	00536-7811-06	5.70	
LAC-HYDRIN FIVE (Ranbaxy Labs)			
LOT,TP (1X113GM)			
113 gm	10631-0286-04	6.80	
(1X226GM)			
226 gm	10631-0286-05	11.84	
(Dispensing Solutions)			
REPACK			
LOT,TP, 5%, 240 ml	55045-3690-01	15.00	
LACHESIS (Luyties)			
TAB,SL (6X)			
6 x, 500s ea	00618-5423-03	3.99	
5500s ea	00618-5423-10	30.32	
(30X)			
12 x, 500s ea	00622-5423-03	4.19	
5500s ea	00622-5423-10	31.83	
(12X)			
30 x, 500s ea	00624-5423-03	4.19	
5500s ea	00624-5423-10	31.83	
LACRI LUBE (Physician Partner)			
REPACK			
OIN,OP (1X3.5GM)			
3.5 gm	21695-0681-35	28.90	
LACRI-LUBE S.O.P. (Allergan Inc)			
OIN,OP, 3.5 gm	00023-0312-04	9.61	
7 gm	00023-0312-07	16.62	
(Phys Total Care)			
REPACK			
OIN,OP, 4 gm	54868-1663-00	12.09	
(Physician Partner)			
REPACK			
OIN,OP, 7 gm	21695-0681-07	31.36	
LACROSSE ALL BODY CLEANSER (Aplicare)			
LIQ,TP (SPRAY & FOAM)			
473 ml	52380-1805-06	9.58	
LACROSSE ISOPROPYL ALCOHOL (Aplicare)			
GEL,TP, 70%, 237 ml	52380-1771-08	4.74	
LACTAID (McNeil Consumer Healthcare)			
TAB,PO, 3300 u, 120s ea	00045-0080-02	11.83	17.34
(Phys Total Care)			
REPACK			
TAB,PO (CAPLET)			
3000 u, 100s ea	54868-2430-00	14.78	
LACTAID FAST ACT (McNeil)			
CTB,PO (VANILLA TWIST)			
9000 u, 32s ea	00450-0930-32	6.95	
60s ea	00450-0930-60	11.78	
TAB,PO (CAPLET)			
9000 u, 12s ea	00450-0910-12	3.17	
32s ea	00450-0910-32	6.95	
60s ea	00450-0910-60	11.83	
LACTAID ORIGINAL (McNeil)			
TAB,PO (CAPLET)			
9000 u, 120s ea	00450-0080-02	11.83	
LACTALINS (Health Products Corp)			
CAP,PO (SOFTGEL)			
125 mg, 30s ea	39686-0015-05	3.41	6.95
30s ea	39686-0015-07	5.77	
100s ea	39686-0015-06	7.00	
LACTASE (Major)			
TAB,PO (CAPLET)			
30 mg, 60s ea	00904-5224-52	7.75	
(FAST ACTING,CAPLET)			
9000 iu, 32s ea	09045-0908-87	6.83	
LACTIC ACID (Core)			
REPACK			
LOT,TP, 10%, 360 ml	33358-0201-12	51.35	
LACTICARE (Stiefel Consumer HealthCare)			
LOT,TP, 5%, 222 ml	00145-0626-05	7.62	11.49
340 ml	00145-0626-07	9.90	14.99
LACTINOL HX (Pedinol)			
CRE,TP (1X113.4GM)			
113.4 gm	40185-0750-80		15.00

PROD/MFR	HRI, UPC,NDC	AWP	SRP
LACTO-BICEL (Innovative Health)			
CAP,PO, 50s ea	24038-0100-12	4.19	6.99
TAB,PO, 50s ea	56871-0011-01	4.40	
LACTO-KEY-100 (Key Company)			
CAP,PO, 1 billion u,			
60s ea	11694-0777-01	4.50	
120s ea	11694-0777-02	7.25	
500s ea	11694-0777-05	25.00	
LACTO-KEY-600 (Key Company)			
PO, 6 billion u,			
60s ea	11694-0776-01	9.00	
120s ea	11694-0776-02	17.00	
LACTO-PECTIN (Bio-Tech Pharm)			
CAP,PO, 100s ea	53191-0094-01	8.90	
LACTO-TRI BLEND (Key Company)			
POW,PO, 60 gm	11694-0756-02	16.00	
LACTO-TRI BLEND-100 (Key Company)			
CAP,PO, 60s ea	11694-0758-01	6.50	
120s ea	11694-0758-02	11.75	
LACTO-TRI BLEND-600 (Key Company)			
PO, 60s ea	11694-0757-01	11.50	
120s ea	11694-0757-02	23.00	
LACTOSE INTOLERANCE (Mason Vit)			
CAP,PO (PF,SF,SOFTGEL)			
250 mg, 50s ea	11845-0118-79	6.89	
LACTRASE (UCB)			
CAP,PO, 250 mg, 100s ea	00091-3505-01	51.71	
LACTROL (Advanced Nutr)			
CAP,PO (SOFTGEL)			
125 mg, 100s ea	62617-0620-06	11.25	15.00
LADY ESTHER (Lee Pharm)			
CRE,TP, 120 gm	23558-0681-90	8.40	
120 gm 12s	23558-0681-91	100.80	
225 gm	23558-0682-00	13.44	
225 gm 12s	23558-0682-01	161.28	
LADY-LITE LANCETS (Medicore)			
DEV,NA, 100s ea	32671-0201-22	7.00	
200s ea	32671-0202-22	12.00	12.95
LAMISIL AT (Novartis Consumer)			
CRE,TP (1X30GM)			
1%, 30 gm	00067-3998-30	12.23	
GEL,TP (1X12GM)			
1%, 12 gm	00067-6239-42	8.72	
SPR,TP (ATHLETE'S FOOT)			
1%, 125 ml	00067-6292-83	8.15	
(JOCK ITCH)			
1%, 125 ml	00067-6293-83	8.15	
(A-S Medication)			
REPACK			
CRE,TP, 1%, 12 gm	54569-4755-00	8.49	
LAMISIL AT ATHLETE'S FOOT (Novartis Consumer)			
CRE,TP, 1%, 12 gm	00067-3998-42	8.15	
24 gm	00067-3998-85	12.23	
(Altura)			
REPACK			
CRE,TP, 1%, 15 gm	63874-0964-15	32.61	
(Dispensing Solutions)			
REPACK			
CRE,TP, 1%, 12 gm	55045-2723-07	12.99	
(Pharma Pac)			
REPACK			
CRE,TP, 1%, 12 gm	52959-0632-12	10.75	
(Quality Care Prod)			
REPACK			
CRE,TP, 1%, 12 gm	49999-0506-12	28.16	
LAMISIL AT JOCK ITCH (Novartis Consumer)			
CRE,TP, 1%, 12 gm	00067-3999-42	8.15	
LAN-O-SOOTHE (Geritrex)			
OIN,TP (1X28GM)			
28 gm	92771-0590-01	4.08	
(1X56GM)			
56 gm	92771-0590-02	5.76	5.75

PROD/MFR	HRI. UPC.NDC	AWP	SRP
LANACANE ANTI-ITCH CREAM (Combe)			
CRE,TP (1X28GM,ORIG STRENGTH)			
0.2%-6%, 28 gm	11509-0050-05	3.42	
(1X74GM,ORIG STRENGTH)			
0.2%-6%, 74 gm	11509-0050-06	5.65	
(1X28GM,MAX STRENGTH)			
0.2%-20%, 28 gm	11509-0050-07	4.28	
LANACANE FIRST AID (Combe)			
SPR,TP (WITH, VIT E,&ALOE)			
0.2%-20%, 113 gm	11509-0000-00	6.44	
LANACANE FIRST AID SPRAY (Combe)			
SPR,TP (1X99GM,MAX STRENGTH)			
0.2%-20%, 99 gm	11509-0003-81	4.94	
LANAFLEX (Nutricia)			
PDS,PO (PRIVATE LABEL,ORANGE)			
15.8 gm 40s	49735-0126-43	135.20	
LANAPHILIC (Medco Lab)			
OIN,TP, 454 gm	11940-1203-06	7.25	
LANAPHILIC W/UREA (Medco Lab)			
OIN,TP, 10%, 454 gm	11940-2118-06	8.25	
20%, 454 gm	11940-2112-06	8.75	
LANCETS (AmerisourceBergen)			
DEV,NA (THIN,PRIVATE LABEL)			
100s ea	24385-0394-78	4.49	4.99
(Cardinal Health)			
DEV,NA (THIN,PRIVATE LABEL)			
100s ea	37205-0142-78	5.83	
(PRIVATE LABEL)			
200s ea	37205-0142-82	9.79	
(Medical Plastic)			
DEV,NA (THIN SINGLE USE)			
100s ea	08271-0351-00	2.10	
(ULTRA THIN SINGLE USE)			
100s ea	08271-0361-00	2.20	
(THIN SINGLE USE)			
200s ea	08271-0331-00	4.20	
(ULTRA THIN SINGLE USE)			
200s ea	08271-0362-00	4.40	
LANEX (Carma Labs)			
OIN,TP, 30 gm	83078-0211-11	1.30	2.50
LANOLIN (Consolidated Midland)			
CRE,TP, 30 gm	00223-4138-01	1.50	
454 gm	00223-4137-02	8.50	
454 gm	00223-4138-02	7.50	
LANOLIN HYDROUS (Geritrex)			
OIN,TP, 480 gm	54162-0596-16	10.05	
LANOLIN-GRX (Geritrex)			
TP (48X28GM,USP)			
28 gm 48s	54162-0595-01	1.54	
LANOLOR (Numark)			
CRE,TP, 60 gm	38485-0517-41	4.62	
240 gm	38485-0517-61	13.20	
LANSINOH FOR BREAST FEEDING MOTHERS (Lansinoh)			
OIN,TP, 56 gm	44677-0102-01		9.99
LANTISEPTIC ALL BODY WASH (Summit Industries)			
LIQ,TP, 3840 ml	12090-0017-02	10.79	20.75
SPR,TP, 240 ml	12090-0017-01	2.17	4.29
LANTISEPTIC SKIN PROTECTANT (Summit Industries)			
OIN,TP, 5 gm	12090-0019-06	0.25	0.47
15 gm	12090-0019-01	0.49	0.91
70 gm	12090-0009-02	2.63	4.89
113 gm	12090-0019-03	3.74	7.09
130 gm	12090-0019-04	3.33	6.24
400 gm	12090-0019-05	7.80	14.79
LANTISEPTIC THERAPEUTIC (Summit Industries)			
CRE,TP, 5 gm	12090-0016-02	0.49	0.91
120 gm	12090-0016-01	3.74	7.09
236 ml	12090-0016-03	5.19	9.68
LAP G LAPAROSCOPIC GASTROSTOMY (Abbott)			
DEV,NA (18 FR, W/T-FASTENER SET)			
ea	70074-0511-75	237.60	
LARCH (Ellon)			
SOL,SL (DROPS)			
10.5 ml	51762-0020-10		9.25
LAXA-BASIC 100 (Basic Vitamins)			
SGL,PO (SOFTGEL)			
100 mg, 100s ea	00761-0414-20	2.60	
LAXA-BASIC PLUS (Basic Vitamins)			
SGL,PO, 30 mg-100 mg,			
100s ea	00761-0416-20	2.60	
LAXAGEL (Advanced Nutr)			
SGL,PO (SOFTGEL)			
100s ea	62617-0610-06	15.00	22.50
LAXATIVE (Cardinal Health)			
ECT,PO (PRIVATE LABEL)			
5 mg, 25s ea	37205-0128-63	4.10	
SUP,RC, 10 mg, 25s ea	37205-0102-53	6.43	
(Rugby)			
ECT,PO, 5 mg, 100s ea	00536-3381-01	7.41	
1000s ea	00536-3381-10	27.55	
SUP,RC, 10 mg, 12s ea	00536-1355-12	4.17	
100s ea	00536-1355-01	15.75	
LAXATIVE & STOOL SOFTENER (AmerisourceBergen)			
SGL,PO (PRIVATE LABEL)			
30 mg-100 mg, 100s ea	24385-0495-78	6.29	6.99
LAXATIVE FEMININE (Cardinal Health)			
ECT,PO (PRIVATE LABEL)			
5 mg, 30s ea	37205-0298-65	3.17	
LAXATIVE FOR WOMEN (AmerisourceBergen)			
ECT,PO (PRIVATE LABEL)			
5 mg, 30s ea	24385-0193-65	3.14	3.49
LAXATIVE MAXIMUM STRENGTH (Cardinal Health)			
TAB,PO (PRIVATE LABEL)			
25 mg, 24s ea	37205-0294-62	2.88	
LAXMAR (Marlop)			
PDR,PO (SF)			
3.4 gm/dose, 397 gm	12939-0214-14	7.45	
420 gm	12939-0215-14	6.50	
(ORANGE)			
3.4 gm/dose,			
420 gm	12939-0216-14	6.95	
LAZERCREME (Pedinol)			
CRE,TP, 60 gm	00884-3886-02		13.00
LC-65 (Allergan Inc)			
SOL,NA, 15 ml	11980-0013-15	5.19	
LE-GUME (3 B's Limited)			
CAP,PO, 850 mg, 100s ea	30371-0000-31	9.75	15.95
LEADER 8 HOUR PAIN RELIEVER (Cardinal Health)			
TER,PO (PRIVATE LABEL,CAPLET)			
650 mg, 100s ea	37205-0477-78	8.00	
LEADER ACID CONTROL (Cardinal Health)			
TAB,PO (MAXIMUM STRENGTH,SF)			
150 mg, 24s ea	32705-0844-62	4.96	
LEADER ACID REDUCER (Cardinal Health)			
TAB,PO (MAXIMUM STRENGTH)			
20 mg, 25s ea	37205-0861-63	6.40	
LEADER ADVANCED LANCING (Cardinal Health)			
DEV,NA, ea	08214-0707-34	11.05	
LEADER ALCOHOL (Cardinal Health)			
SWA,TP (PRIVATE LABEL)			
6%-70%, 80s ea	37205-0989-57	2.40	
LEADER ALL DAY ALLERGY D-12 (Cardinal Health)			
TER,PO (ORIGPRESCRPTIONSTRENGTH)			
5 mg-120 mg, 24s ea	32705-0827-62	18.72	
LEADER ALL DAY CALCIUM (Cardinal Health)			
TER,PO (PRIVATE LABEL,CAPLET)			
600 mg-500 iu,			
60s ea	37205-0982-72	3.84	
LEADER ALL DAY GLUCOSAMINE & CHONDROITIN (Cardinal Health)			
TER,PO (PRIVATE LABEL,CAPLET)			
400 mg-500 mg-45 mg,			
90s ea	37205-0714-75	16.00	
LEADER ALLERGY MULTI-SYMPTOM (Cardinal Health)			
TAB,PO (COOL ICE,PRIVATE LABEL)			
325 mg-2 mg-5 mg,			
24s ea	37205-0940-62	1.84	
LEADER ALLERGY RELIEF (Cardinal Health)			
ODT,PO (NON-DROWSY)			
10 mg, 10s ea	37205-0387-52	7.44	
12s ea	37205-0381-53	7.60	
SYR,PO (CHILDRENS,PRIVATE LABEL)			
5 mg/5 ml, 118 ml	96295-0112-26	9.84	
(W/DOSAGE CUP)			
5 mg/5 ml, 120 ml	37205-0378-26	10.00	
LEADER ALLERGY RELIEF D-12 (Cardinal Health)			
T12,PO (PRIVATE LABEL)			
5 mg-120 mg, 10s ea	96295-0112-24	6.96	
20s ea	96295-0112-25	11.84	
LEADER ALLERGY RELIEF D-24 (Cardinal Health)			
T24,PO (NON-DROWSY)			
10 mg-240 mg, 10s ea	37205-0348-52	4.10	9.19
15s ea	37205-0348-88	14.08	
LEADER ANKLE ELASTIC SUPPORT COMPRESSION (Cardinal Health)			
DEV,NA (LARGE-X-LARGE)			
ea	96295-0113-09	5.12	
(SMALL-MEDIUM)			
ea	96295-0113-10	5.12	
LEADER ANKLE NEOPRENE SUPPORT ADJUSTABLE (Cardinal Health)			
DEV,NA (ONE SIZE FITS ALL)			
ea	96295-0109-55	7.12	
LEADER ANTACID (Cardinal Health)			
SUS,PO (PRIVATE LABEL,CHERRY)			
355 ml	37205-0536-40	3.52	
LEADER ANTI-DIARRHEAL (Cardinal Health)			
TAB,PO (PRIVATE LABEL)			
2 mg, 48s ea	96295-0112-80	6.00	
LEADER ANTI-DIARRHEAL PLUS ANTI-GAS (Cardinal Health)			
TAB,PO (PRIVATE LABEL,CAPLET)			
2 mg-125 mg, 12s ea	37205-0964-53	4.48	
LEADER ANTIFUNGAL (Cardinal Health)			
SPR,TP (SPRAY POWDER)			
1%, 130 gm	37205-0344-66	3.60	
LEADER ARTHRITIS PAIN RELIEVER (Cardinal Health)			
TER,PO (CAPLET)			
650 mg, 100s ea	37205-0034-78	8.00	
(Dispensing Solutions)			
REPACK			
TER,PO (CAPLET)			
650 mg, 60s ea	55045-3374-06	16.80	
LEADER ASPIRIN (Cardinal Health)			
CTB,PO (ADULT LOW STRENGTH)			
81 mg, 36s ea	37205-0369-68	1.20	
LEADER ATHLETE'S FOOT AF (Cardinal Health)			
CRE,TP (1X12GM,PRIVATE LABEL)			
1%, 12 gm	37205-0941-14	7.60	
(1X15GM,PRIVATE LABEL)			
1%, 15 gm	37205-0941-99	7.60	
LEADER CALCIUM 600+D (Cardinal Health)			
TAB,PO (PRIVATE LABEL)			
600 mg-400 iu, 60s ea	37205-0829-72	4.14	
LEADER CENTURY (Cardinal Health)			
TAB,PO (100+30EA,PRIVATE LABEL)			
130s ea	37205-0847-81	6.80	
(PRIVATE LABEL)			
300s ea	37205-0847-87	12.96	
LEADER CENTURY SENIOR (Cardinal Health)			
TAB,PO (PRIVATE LABEL)			
100s ea	32705-0846-78	6.08	
300s ea	37205-0846-87	15.20	
LEADER CHEST CONGESTION RELIEF PLUS DM (Cardinal Health)			
TAB,PO (PRIVATE LABEL)			
20 mg-400 mg, 50s ea	37205-0538-71	6.56	
LEADER CHILDREN'S IBUPROFEN (Cardinal Health)			
SUS,PO (1X120ML, W/ DOSAGE CUP)			
100 mg/5 ml, 120 ml	37205-0848-26	5.44	
LEADER CHILDREN'S IBUPROFEN COLD (Cardinal Health)			
SUS,PO (FOR AGES 2-11,AF)			
100 mg/5 ml-15 mg/5 ml,			
120 ml	37205-0399-26	4.56	
LEADER CHILDREN'S MUCUS RELIEF (Cardinal Health)			
SOL,PO (1X118ML,W/DOSAGE CUP,AF)			
100 mg/5 ml, 118 ml	37205-0992-26	2.32	
LEADER CHILDREN'S MUCUS RELIEF COUGH (Cardinal Health)			
SOL,PO (1X118ML,W/DOSAGE CUP,AF)			
5 mg/5 ml-100 mg/5 ml,			
118 ml	37205-0993-26	2.40	
LEADER CHILDREN'S PAIN RELIEVER (Cardinal Health)			
CTB,PO (BUBBLE GUM)			
80 mg, 30s ea	96251-0133-59	1.76	

PROD/MFR	HRI, UPC,NDC	AWP	SRP
LEADER CHILDREN'S TRIACTING DAYTIME COLD & COUGH (Cardinal Health)			
SOL,PO (1X118ML,PRIVATE LABEL)			
5 mg/5 ml-2.5 mg/5 ml,			
118 ml	37205-0994-26	2.80	
LEADER CHILDREN'S TRIACTING NIGHTTIME COLD & COUGH (Cardinal Health)			
SOL,PO (1X118ML,W/DOSAGE CUP,AF)			
6.25 mg/5 ml-2.5 mg/5 ml,			
118 ml	37205-0850-26	2.88	
LEADER CITRUS ISOPROPYL RUBBING ALCOHOL (Cardinal Health)			
SOL,TP (1X473ML,PRIVATE LABEL)			
70%, 473 ml	37205-0974-43	1.98	
LEADER CLEARLAX (Cardinal Health)			
PDS,PO (1X119GM,ORIG PRESCN STR)			
17 gm/dose, 119 gm	37205-0612-71	4.67	
(1X238GM,ORIG PRESCN STR)			
17 gm/dose, 238 gm	37205-0612-72	8.24	
(1X510GM,ORIG PRESCN STR)			
17 gm/dose, 510 gm	37205-0612-73	14.40	
LEADER COLD MULTI-SYMPTOM (Cardinal Health)			
CAP,PO (DAYTIME,NON-DROWSY)			
325 mg-10 mg-5 mg,			
24s ea	37205-0618-62	2.24	
LEADER COLD SORE TREATMENT (Cardinal Health)			
SOL,TP (2X0.6ML,PRIVATE LABEL)			
0.13%, 0.6 ml 2s	37205-0973-19	13.76	
LEADER COLOR LANCETS (Can-Am Care)			
DEV,NA (PRIVATE LABEL)			
200s ea	38396-0306-08	9.50	
LEADER CORN AND CALLUS REMOVER (Cardinal Health)			
SOL,TP (LIQUID,3 CUSHIONS)			
12.6%, 15 ml	96295-0112-86	2.96	
LEADER COUGH DROPS (Cardinal Health)			
LOZ,MM (20% MORE FREE,SF)			
5 mg, 30s ea	96295-0106-59	1.52	
5.8 mg, 30s ea	96295-0106-60	1.52	
LEADER CRANBERRY (Cardinal Health)			
TAB,PO (PRIVATE LABEL)			
50s ea	37205-0606-71	4.72	
LEADER DAY-TIME MULTI-SYMPTOM COLD/FLU (Cardinal Health)			
SGL,PO (NON-DROWSY,AF)			
325 mg-15 mg-30 mg,			
12s ea	37205-0428-53	2.84	
LEADER DAY-TIME PE (Cardinal Health)			
SGL,PO (NON-DROWSY,AF)			
325 mg-10 mg-5 mg,			
12s ea	37205-0705-53	2.84	
LEADER DIABETIC SOCKS (Cardinal Health)			
DEV,NA (BLACK,LARGE)			
2s ea	96295-0116-59	40.95	
(BLACK,MEDIUM)			
2s ea	96295-0116-58	40.95	
(WHITE,LARGE)			
2s ea	96295-0116-56	40.95	
(WHITE,MEDIUM)			
2s ea	96295-0116-55	40.95	
(WHITE,X-LARGE)			
2s ea	96295-0116-57	40.95	
LEADER ELBOW ELASTIC SUPPORT COMPRESSION (Cardinal Health)			
DEV,NA (MEDIUM-LARGE)			
ea	96295-0113-11	5.52	
LEADER ELBOW NEOPRENE SUPPORT ADJUSTABLE (Cardinal Health)			
DEV,NA (ONE SIZE FITS ALL)			
ea	96295-0109-56	7.12	
LEADER ESSENTIAL ONE DAILY (Cardinal Health)			
TAB,PO (PRIVATE LABEL)			
365s ea	37205-0080-82	11.49	
LEADER ESTROPLUS (Cardinal Health)			
PO (EX. STRENGTH)			
56s ea	37205-0506-31	11.60	
LEADER EYE ITCH RELIEF DROPS (Cardinal Health)			
SOL,OP (1X5ML,PRIVATE LABEL)			
0.025%, 5 ml	37205-0849-17	8.96	
LEADER FIBER (Cardinal Health)			
POW,NA (CLEAR SOLUBLE,1X350GM)			
350 gm	37205-0480-04	11.04	
LEADER FIBER LAXATIVE (Cardinal Health)			
CAP,PO (100% NATURAL)			
0.52 gm, 100s ea	37205-0372-78	6.00	
LEADER FOOT (Cardinal Health)			
POW,TP (1X120GM,PRIVATE LABEL)			
1%, 120 gm	37205-0997-26	2.72	
LEADER GARLIC (Cardinal Health)			
TAB,PO (PRIVATE LABEL)			
400 mg, 30s ea	37205-0881-65	2.56	
LEADER GLUCOSAMINE CHONDROITIN (Cardinal Health)			
TAB,PO, 90s ea	37205-0972-75	12.16	
100 mg-750 mg-1.65 mg,			
80s ea	37205-0971-57	12.32	
LEADER GLUCOSAMINE CHONDROITIN COMPLEX (Cardinal Health)			
TAB,PO (DOUBLE STRENGTH)			
50s ea	37205-0985-71	8.64	
(TRIPLE STRENGTH)			
80s ea	37205-0986-57	18.08	
LEADER GLUCOSE (Can-Am Care)			
CTB,PO (CAFFEINE-FREE)			
4 gm, 10s ea	38396-0501-08	1.56	
10s ea	38396-0502-08	1.56	
10s ea	38396-0503-08	1.56	
(QUICK DISSOLVE)			
4 gm, 40s ea	38396-0560-08	4.33	
(CAFFEINE-FREE)			
4 gm, 50s ea	38396-0541-08	6.08	
50s ea	38396-0542-08	6.08	
50s ea	38396-0543-08	6.08	
LEADER HAIR, SKIN & NAILS (Cardinal Health)			
TAB,PO (PRIVATE LABEL,CAPLET)			
60s ea	37205-0716-72	5.52	
LEADER IBU-DROPS INFANTS' (Cardinal Health)			
SUS,PO (W/SYRINGE DOSING DEVICE)			
50 mg/1.25 ml, 30 ml	37205-0436-10	7.36	
LEADER IBUPROFEN PM (Cardinal Health)			
TAB,PO (PRIVATE LABEL)			
38 mg-200 mg, 20s ea	37205-0360-60	3.89	
LEADER INTENSE COUGH RELIEVER (Cardinal Health)			
SOL,PO (EXTRA STRENGTH,NONDRWSY)			
20 mg/5 ml-300 mg/5 ml,			
120 ml	37205-0610-26	4.83	
LEADER IRON (Cardinal Health)			
TER,PO (SLOW RELEASE)			
160 mg, 30s ea	37205-0368-65	6.00	
LEADER IRON TABLETS (Cardinal Health)			
TAB,PO (PRIVATE LABEL,COATED)			
65 mg, 125s ea	37205-0419-96	4.40	
LEADER KNEE ELASTIC SUPPORT COMPRESSION (Cardinal Health)			
DEV,NA (LARGE-X-LARGE)			
ea	96295-0113-12	5.92	
(SMALL-MEDIUM)			
ea	96295-0113-13	5.92	
LEADER KNEE OPEN PATELLA NEOPRENE ADJUSTABLE (Cardinal Health)			
DEV,NA (ONE SIZE FITS ALL)			
ea	96295-0109-58	9.28	
LEADER KNEE STABILIZER NEOPRENE ADJUSTABLE (Cardinal Health)			
DEV,NA (ONE SIZE FITS ALL)			
ea	96295-0109-57	15.12	
LEADER LANCETS (Can-Am Care)			
DEV,NA (THIN,PRIVATE LABEL)			
100s ea	38396-0301-08	5.85	
200s ea	38396-0302-08	9.50	
LEADER LORATADINE (Cardinal Health)			
TAB,PO (NON-DROWSY,USP)			
10 mg, 10s ea	37205-0346-52	3.30	
20s ea	37205-0346-60	5.40	
30s ea	37205-0346-65	7.40	
60s ea	37205-0346-72	12.60	
90s ea	37205-0346-75	14.40	
150s ea	37205-0346-47	20.40	
LEADER MAGNESIUM DR (Cardinal Health)			
TCP,PO (SF,STARCH-FREE)			
112 mg-187 mg-64 mg,			
60s ea	37205-0981-72	6.40	
LEADER MICONAZOLE NITRATE (Cardinal Health)			
SPR,TP (1X131GM,PRIVATE LABEL)			
2%, 131 gm	37205-0998-66	3.68	
LEADER MIGRAINE FORMULA (Cardinal Health)			
TAB,PO (PRIVATE LABEL)			
250 mg-250 mg-65 mg,			
24s ea	37205-0280-62	2.80	
100s ea	37205-0280-78	6.40	
LEADER MILK OF MAGNESIA (Cardinal Health)			
SOL,PO (OVERNIGHT RELIEF)			
400 mg/5 ml, 355 ml	37250-0459-40	3.42	
LEADER MULTI-PURPOSE MOISTURE BARRIER OINTMENT (Cardinal Health)			
OIN,TP (1X113GM,PRIVATE LABEL)			
0.45%-20%, 113 gm	37205-0611-26	5.52	
LEADER NASAL DECONGESTANT PE (Cardinal Health)			
TAB,PO, 10 mg, 18s ea	37205-0473-89	3.79	
LEADER NASAL STRIPS (Cardinal Health)			
DEV,NA (MEDIUM/LARGE)			
12s ea	96295-0109-31	3.92	
(SMALL/MEDIUM)			
12s ea	96295-0109-33	3.92	
(MEDIUM/LARGE)			
30s ea	96295-0109-32	10.40	
LEADER NATURAL B COMPLEX WITH VITAMIN C (Cardinal Health)			
TAB,PO (USP,PRIVATE LABEL)			
100s ea	37205-0489-78	3.68	
LEADER NATURAL FISH OIL (Cardinal Health)			
SGL,PO (PRIVATE LABEL,SOFTGEL)			
300 mg, 120s ea	37205-0354-76	6.16	
LEADER NATURAL HERB (Cardinal Health)			
LOZ,MM (PRIVATE LABEL,NATURAL)			
4.8 mg, 24s ea	96295-0106-96	1.04	
LEADER NATURAL OYSTER SHELL CALCIUM (Cardinal Health)			
TAB,PO (PRIVATE LABEL)			
500 mg-400 iu,			
300s ea	37205-0083-87	6.88	
LEADER NATURAL SUPER OMEGA-3 (Cardinal Health)			
SGL,PO (PRIVATE LABEL,SOFTGEL)			
60s ea	37205-0472-65	7.12	
LEADER NATURAL VITAMIN B12 (Cardinal Health)			
TAB,PO (PRIVATE LABEL)			
500 mcg, 100s ea	37205-0491-78	3.60	
TER,PO, 1000 mcg,			
60s ea	37205-0495-72	4.56	
LEADER NICOTINE POLACRILEX (Cardinal Health)			
LOZ,PO (PRIVATE LABEL,MINT)			
2 mg, 72s ea	37205-0987-69	39.04	
4 mg, 72s ea	37205-0988-69	93.04	
LEADER NICOTINE POLACRILEX GUM (Cardinal Health)			
GUM,PO (PRIVATE LABEL)			
2 mg, 50s ea	37205-0203-71	27.84	
110s ea	37205-0203-77	44.08	
4 mg, 50s ea	37205-0204-71	31.68	
110s ea	37205-0204-77	53.68	
LEADER NICOTINE TRANSDERMAL SYSTEM (Cardinal Health)			
TDM,TD (STEP 3,PRIVATE LABEL)			
7 mg/24 hr, 14s ea	37205-0363-74	41.20	39.99
(STEP 2,PRIVATE LABEL)			
14 mg/24 hr, 14s ea	37205-0361-74	41.20	39.99
(PRIVATE LABEL)			
21 mg/24 hr, 14s ea	37205-0358-74	41.20	39.99
LEADER NITE TIME (Cardinal Health)			
SOL,PO (1X177ML,PRIVATE LABEL)			
177 ml	37205-0781-37	2.73	
LEADER NITE-TIME (Cardinal Health)			
SGL,PO (PRIVATE LABEL,SOFTGELS)			
325 mg-15 mg-6.25 mg,			
12s ea	37205-0707-53	3.11	
LEADER OMEPRAZOLE (Cardinal Health)			
TCP,PO (PRIVATE LABEL)			
20 mg, 14s ea	37205-0837-74	12.24	
28s ea	37205-0837-06	21.60	
42s ea	37205-0837-15	29.28	
LEADER ONE-STEP PREGNANCY TEST (Cardinal Health)			
DEV,NA (ONE TEST,PRIVATE LABEL)			
ea	96295-0103-13	4.80	
(TWO TESTS,PRIVATE LABEL)			
2s ea	96295-0104-70	7.52	

PROD/MFR	HRI, UPC,NDC	AWP	SRP
LEADER ORAL PAIN RELIEF (Cardinal Health)			
GEL,MM (MAXIMUM STRENGTH)			
20%, 14.2 gm	37205-0607-05	3.12	
LEADER ORAL SALINE LAXATIVE (Cardinal Health)			
SOL,PO (1X45ML, SINGLE DOSE,SF)			
45 ml	37205-0306-13	2.08	
LEADER PAIN RELIEF ALLERGY SINUS PE (Cardinal Pharm)			
TAB,PO (PRIVATE LABEL,CAPLET)			
500 mg-2 mg-5 mg, 24s ea	96295-0113-72	1.84	
LEADER PAIN RELIEF COLD PE (Cardinal Health)			
TAB,PO (CAPLET)			
325 mg-2 mg-15 mg-5 mg, 24s ea	37205-0561-62	2.64	
(COOL ICE,PRIVATE LABEL)			
325 mg-15 mg-5 mg, 24s ea	96295-0113-73	2.24	
LEADER PAIN RELIEF SINUS PE (Cardinal Health)			
TAB,PO (DAYTIME,PRIVATE LABEL)			
500 mg-5 mg, 24s ea	37205-0571-62	1.76	
LEADER PAIN RELIEVER (Cardinal Health)			
SGL,PO (EXTRA STRENGTH)			
500 mg, 100s ea	37205-0980-78	5.52	
TAB,PO (EXTRA STRENGTH,EASYTABS)			
500 mg, 50s ea	37205-0711-71	2.16	
100s ea	37205-0711-78	3.36	
(EXTRA STRENGTH)			
500 mg, 100s ea	37205-0488-78	3.20	
LEADER PAIN RELIEVING (Cardinal Health)			
GEL,TP (1X120ML,EXTRA STRENGTH)			
3.5%, 120 ml	37205-0824-26	5.12	
LEADER PEDIATRIC ELECTROLYTE (Cardinal Health)			
SOL,PO (4X237ML,AF)			
237 ml 4s	37205-0220-34	4.16	
LEADER PEDIATRIC ELECTROLYTE FREEZER POPS (Cardinal Health)			
PO (16X62.5ML,VARIETY PACK)			
62.5 ml 16s	37205-0963-16	4.16	
LEADER PEN NEEDLES (Cardinal Health)			
DEV,NA (31G,1/4",6MM,SHORT)			
100s ea	37205-0702-78	18.40	
LEADER POISON IVY WASH (Cardinal Health)			
CRE,TP (1X29GM,FAST ACTING)			
29 gm	37205-0608-10	7.60	
LEADER PRENATAL (Cardinal Health)			
TAB,PO (USP,PRIVATE LABEL)			
365s ea	37205-0395-82	13.60	
LEADER PREPARATION CLEANSING KIT (Cardinal Health)			
SOL,PO (SF,PRIVATE LABEL)			
ea	37205-0996-03	10.08	
LEADER PRESTIGE SMART SYSTEM (Home Diag)			
DEV,NA (STRIP)			
50s ea	56151-0302-50	28.60	
100s ea	56151-0302-01	45.99	
LEADER PROTECTIVE UNDERWEAR (Cardinal Health)			
DEV,NA (DISPOSABLE, SM/MED)			
18s ea	96295-0111-61	15.44	
LEADER PSS STARTER (Home Diag)			
DEV,NA (MTR,STRP,LANCET,DEV,SOL)			
ea	56151-0202-01	17.50	
LEADER RANITIDINE HCL (Cardinal Health)			
TAB,PO (PRIVATE LABEL)			
75 mg, 60s ea	37205-0531-72	8.40	
LEADER SELF-ADHERING ELASTIC BANDAGE (Cardinal Health)			
DEV,NA (3"X1.5YDS,PRIVATE LABEL)			
ea	96295-0109-34	2.28	
(4"X1.5YDS,PRIVATE LABEL)			
ea	96295-0109-35	2.80	
LEADER SEVERE CONGESTION PAIN RELIEF COLD (Cardinal Health)			
TAB,PO (DAY NON-DROWSY)			
325 mg-10 mg-200 mg-5 mg, 24s ea	37205-0828-62	2.87	
LEADER SUPER MOLESKIN (Cardinal Health)			
DEV,NA (4 5/8"X3 3/8")			
3s ea	96295-0112-85	1.60	
LEADER SUPER THIN LANCETS (Can-Am Care)			
DEV,NA (SUPER THIN)			
100s ea	38396-0305-08	5.85	
LEADER THIN LANCETS (Can-Am Care)			
DEV,NA (PRIVATE LABEL)			
100s ea	36652-0301-08	5.36	
200s ea	36652-0302-08	8.96	
LEADER WART REMOVER (Cardinal Health)			
SOL,TP (MAXIMUM STRENGTH)			
17%, 15 ml	96295-0112-87	3.52	
LEADER WILD CHERRY (Cardinal Health)			
LOZ,MM (PRIVATE LABEL)			
6 mg, 30s ea	96295-0116-44	1.06	
LEADER WRIST ELASTIC SUPPORT ADJUSTABLE (Cardinal Health)			
DEV,NA (ONE SIZE FITS ALL)			
ea	96295-0113-17	4.00	
LEADER WRIST SPLINT SUPPORT ELASTIC REVERSIBLE (Cardinal Health)			
DEV,NA (LARGE-XLARGE)			
ea	96295-0113-14	12.48	
(SMALL-MEDIUM)			
ea	96295-0113-15	12.48	
LEADER WRIST SPLINT SUPPORT NEOPRENE ADJUSTABLE (Cardinal Health)			
DEV,NA (LEFT WRIST,ONE SIZE)			
ea	96295-0109-59	12.96	
(RIGHT WRIST,ONE SIZE)			
ea	96295-0109-60	12.96	
LEADER WRIST SPLINT SUPPORT NEOPRENE REVERSIBLE (Cardinal Health)			
DEV,NA (CARPAL TUNNEL,ONE SIZE)			
ea	96295-0113-16	13.04	
LEADER ZOO CHEWS GUMMIES (Cardinal Health)			
CTB,PO (PRIVATE LABEL)			
60s ea	37205-0718-72	5.12	
LEAN ON ME (Pharm Innov)			
DEV,NA (CANE/CRUTCH TIP-1")			
ea	00036-8800-10	14.19	20.28
(CANE/CRUTCH TIP-3/4")			
ea	00036-8800-34	14.19	20.28
(CANE/CRUTCH TIP-7/8")			
ea	00036-8800-78	14.19	20.28
LECI-KEY (Carlson,J.R.)			
POW,PO (VEGETARIAN,SF)			
360 gm	88395-0086-01	7.10	14.20
1200 gm	88395-0086-05	19.95	39.90
LECITHIN (ADH)			
SGL,PO (SOFTGEL)			
1200 mg, 100s ea	60142-0100-10	5.98	11.95
(Advanced Nutr)			
SGL,PO (PF,SF,SOFTGEL)			
1200 mg, 60s ea	62617-0075-02	6.30	8.40
(Basic Vitamins)			
SGL,PO (SOFTGEL)			
1200 mg, 100s ea	00761-0445-20	3.00	
(Carlson,J.R.)			
SGL,PO (SOFTGEL)			
1200 mg, 100s ea	88395-0086-21	4.95	9.90
300s ea	88395-0086-23	12.10	24.20
(Consolidated Midland)			
SGL,PO (SOFTGEL)			
1200 mg, 100s ea	00223-0890-01	4.95	
500s ea	00223-0890-05	17.50	
(Health Products Corp)			
SGL,PO (PF,SF,SOFTGEL)			
1200 mg, 100s ea	39686-0014-15	3.00	
(Key Company)			
GRA,PO, 240 gm	11694-0871-08	3.50	
454 gm	11694-0871-01	6.00	
(Major)			
SGL,PO, 1200 mg, 100s ea	00904-3163-60	3.75	
(Mason Vit)			
GRA,PO, 420 gm	11845-0627-00	12.22	
SGL,PO (SOFTGEL)			
520 mg, 100s ea	11845-0053-01	5.00	
1200 mg, 100s ea	11845-0052-91	6.00	
250s ea	11845-0052-92	13.89	
(Rexall)			
SGL,PO (PF,SF,SOFTGEL)			
1200 mg, 60s ea	30768-0000-47	1.80	2.73
LECITHIN EXTRA STRENGTH (Mason Vit)			
SGL,PO (PF,SF,SOFTGEL)			
3500 mg, 60s ea	11845-0075-35	9.78	
LECITHIN-19 (Key Company)			
SGL,PO (SOFTGEL)			
1200 mg, 100s ea	11694-0927-01	4.50	
200s ea	11694-0927-02	8.00	
650s ea	11694-0927-07	24.00	
LECITHIN/KELP-B6 W/CIDER VINEGAR (Natl Vitamin)			
TAB,PO (PF,SF)			
100s ea	54629-0666-07	2.99	4.99
LECTRON II (Pharm Innov)			
GEL,TP, 60 ml	00036-3000-60	1.31	1.87
90 ml	00036-3000-90	1.57	2.25
150 ml	00036-3000-15	2.06	2.94
250 ml	00036-3000-25	2.43	3.48
3840 ml	00036-3000-28	29.92	42.75
LEDUM PAL (Luyties)			
TAB,SL (6X)			
6 x, 500s ea	00618-5448-03	3.99	
5500s ea	00618-5448-10	30.32	
(30X)			
12 x, 500s ea	00622-5448-03	4.19	
5500s ea	00622-5448-10	31.83	
(12X)			
30 x, 500s ea	00624-5448-03	4.19	
5500s ea	00624-5448-10	31.83	
LEG-GESIC (MAGNA Pharm)			
SOL,PO (1X473ML,VANILLA)			
473 ml	58407-0915-16	19.93	23.95
LENS PLUS DAILY CLEANER (Allergan Inc)			
SOL,NA, 15 ml	11980-0426-15	4.76	
LENS PLUS REWETTING DROPS (Allergan Inc)			
SOL,OP, 0.3 ml 30s UD	00023-0745-01	5.81	
LENS PLUS SALINE (Allergan Inc)			
SOL,NA, 90 ml	00023-0825-03	2.29	
360 ml	00023-0825-12	4.99	
LENSEPT (Ciba Vision)			
SOL,NA, 240 ml	47113-0607-08	4.30	
240 ml	47113-0688-08	4.30	
360 ml	47113-0609-00	5.45	
LEUCINE (VITAFLO, LLC)			
PDS,PO, 0.1 gm/4 gm, 30s ea	50600-0549-20	120.00	150.00
LEV-TOV (Freeda)			
TAB,PO (SF,GLUTEN-FREE)			
250 mcg-800 mcg-25 mg, 100s ea	10432-0358-01	7.77	12.95
LEVOCARNITINE (Key Company)			
CARNITINE-300			
CAP,PO (PF,SF)			
300 mg, 60s ea	11694-0769-01	15.00	
180s ea	11694-0769-02	42.00	
(Freeda)			
L-CARNITINE			
TAB,PO (PF,SF,DYE-FREE)			
500 mg, 50s ea	10432-0303-00	17.97	29.95
100s ea	10432-0303-01	29.31	48.85
(Nature's Bounty)			
CAP,PO (PF,SF)			
250 mg, 30s ea	74312-0041-40		10.89
LEXAGRAN-M (Lex)			
TAB,PO, 30s ea	49523-0041-03	1.05	
130s ea	49523-0041-13	2.57	
LEXATUSSIN DM (Lex)			
SYR,PO, 120 ml	49523-0022-04	1.10	
LEXICHOL (Lex)			
CAP,PO, 100s ea	49523-0090-10	2.70	
LEXVISOL POLIVITAMINES (Lex)			
LIQ,PO, 120 ml	49523-0023-04	0.94	
LICE CONTROL (Cardinal Health)			
SPR,NA (BEDDING/FURNITURE)			
0.5%, 141.8 gm	37205-0166-28	4.24	
LICE KILLING (Cardinal Health)			
LIQ,TP (W/COMB,PRIVATE LABEL)			
4%-0.33%, 120 ml	37205-0165-26	6.87	
LICE KILLING SHAMPOO (Major)			
SHA,TP (W/NIT COMB)			
4%-0.33%, 118 ml	00904-2528-20	6.09	
LICE TREATMENT (AmerisourceBergen)			
LIQ,TP (PRIVATE LABEL)			
60 ml	24385-0116-06	5.39	5.99
120 ml	24385-0116-03	8.36	9.29

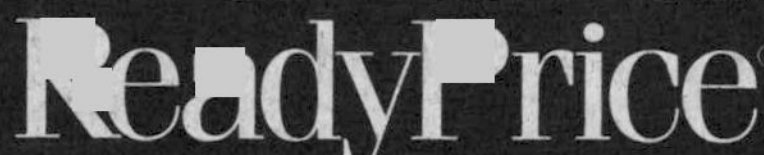

PROD/MFR	HRI, UPC,NDC	AWP	SRP
LICE TREATMENT MAXIMUM STRENGTH (Cardinal Health)			
LIQ,TP (CREME RINSE W/COMB)			
4%-0.33%, 60 ml	37205-0285-16	8.16	
120 ml	37205-0285-26	13.12	
(Teva)			
KIT,NA, ea	00182-6167-99	13.65	
(A-S Medication)			
REPACK			
LIQ,TP (W/COMB)			
4%-0.33%, 120 ml	54569-4599-00	8.13	
(Phys Total Care)			
REPACK			
LIQ,TP, 4%-0.33%, 59 ml	54868-4886-00	17.07	
LICEFREEE SPRAY! (Tec)			
SPR,TP (1X177.4ML)			
2 x, 177.4 ml	51879-0180-06	6.00	12.99
LICEFREEE! (Tec)			
GEL,TP (1X118.3ML,1APPLICATION)			
1 x, 118.3 ml	51879-0120-04	6.00	11.99
(2X118.3ML,2APPLICATIONS)			
1 x, 118.3 ml 2s	51879-0120-08	10.00	19.99
LICEGUARD EGG REMOVER (M D C Associates)			
SHA,TP, 100 ml	63580-0000-80	6.00	9.99
LICEGUARD ROBICOMB (M D C Associates)			
DEV,NA, ea	63580-0000-01	18.00	29.95
LICEMD (Combe)			
GEL,TP (INCLUDES LICE COMB)			
118 ml	11509-0003-48	9.35	
LICIDE (Reese)			
SHA,TP, 3%-0.3%, 120 ml	10956-0711-04	5.66	
SPR,NA, 1%-0.2%, 150 ml	10956-0613-05	4.43	
LICORICE (Botanical Labs.)			
LIQ,PO, 30 ml	41954-0020-31	4.00	7.99
60 ml	41954-0020-14	6.50	12.99
LIDOCREAM (MCR American)			
CRE,TP (5X5GM,W/5 TAGADERM)			
4%, 5 gm 5s	66870-0402-07	32.81	
(1X15GM)			
4%, 15 gm	66870-0402-15	16.56	
LIFE MEDICAL PSS STARTER (Home Diag)			
DEV,NA (MTR,STRP,LANCET,DEV,SOL)			
ea	56151-0214-01	22.18	
LIFE START (Natren)			
POW,PO, 1 billion org/0.5 gm,			
37.5 gm	53983-0500-65	9.00	15.00
75 gm	53983-0500-70	13.20	22.00
LIFE-LINE (Natl Vitamin)			
DINO-LIFE			
CTB,PO (PF,SF)			
100s ea	54629-2059-01	2.96	4.99
DINO-LIFE W/EXTRA C			
PO (PF,SF)			
100s ea	79854-0759-21	3.31	5.59
DINO-LIFE W/IRON/ZINC			
CTB,PO (SF)			
100s ea	79854-0759-11	3.07	5.19
KIDZTUFF HONEY BEARS MULTIVITAMIN			
PO (W/IRON& ZINC,PF,SF)			
100s ea	79854-0733-11	3.07	5.19
(PF,SF)			
100s ea	54629-2033-01	2.96	4.99
100s ea	79854-0733-21	2.96	4.99
MEN'S LIFE-PACK			
KIT,PO (5 X 30 PACKETS,PF,SF)			
150s ea	72499-0525-00	6.23	10.39
MUSCLE BUILD-UP			
PDR,PO (E,CHOCOLATE)			
528 gm	54629-0711-34	5.97	9.99
(VANILLA)			
528 gm	54629-0711-26	5.97	9.99
WOMEN'S LIFE-PACK			
KIT,PO (5 X 30 PACKETS,PF,SF)			
150s ea	72499-0527-00	6.23	10.39
ZINC W/VITAMIN A & VITAMIN C			
LOZ,MM (CHERRY, PF, SF,PF,SF)			
100s ea	79854-0738-51	3.28	5.49
LIFE-LINE DOCUSATE SODIUM (Natl Vitamin)			
SGL,PO (USP,PRIVATE LABEL)			
250 mg, 100s ea	54629-0601-01	4.11	6.89
LIFE-PACK MEN'S (Natl Vitamin)			
TAB,PO (GLUTEN-FREE)			
30s ea	54629-0616-30	5.19	8.99
LIFE-PACK WOMEN'S (Natl Vitamin)			
PO (PF,SF,GLUTEN-FREE)			
30s ea	54629-0617-30	5.19	8.99
LIFEAID BABY DIGITAL THERMOMETER (Faichney)			
DEV,NA (FLEXIBLE W/ BEEPER)			
ea	40814-0065-14	2.24	5.99
LIFEAID BASAL DIGITAL THERMOMETER (Faichney)			
DEV,NA (FLEXIBLE)			
ea	40814-0065-21	2.23	6.49
LIFEAID DIGITAL CLINICAL THERMOMETER (Faichney)			
DEV,NA (W/5 PROBE COVERS)			
ea	40814-0065-12	2.19	4.99
LIFEAID DIGITAL DUAL SCALE THERMOMETER (Faichney)			
DEV,NA, ea	40814-0055-22	2.19	4.99
LIFEAID DIGITAL PROBE COVERS (Faichney)			
DEV,NA, 30s ea	40814-0060-25	0.83	1.69
LIFEAID FLEXIBLE DIGITAL (Faichney)			
DEV,NA (15 SECOND)			
ea	40814-0057-43	2.43	6.49
LIFECARE ADDS RACK (Abbott Hosp)			
DEV,NA, ea	00074-4329-01	130.86	
LIFECARE SHELF STORAGE TRAY (Abbott Hosp)			
DEV,NA, 50s ea	00074-4328-01	55.80	
LIFESTYLES (Ansell)			
DEV,NA (ASSORTED COLORS)			
3s ea	70907-0028-03	1.12	
(LARGE,LUBRICATED)			
3s ea	70907-0011-03	1.12	
(LARGE/SPERMICIDE)			
3s ea	70907-0022-03	1.12	
(LUBRICATED)			
3s ea	70907-0015-03	1.12	
(LUSCIOUS FLAVORS)			
3s ea	70907-0027-03	1.12	
(RIBBED/SPERMICIDE)			
3s ea	70907-0042-03	1.12	
(SPERMICIDALLY LUBR)			
3s ea	70907-0018-03	1.12	
(STUDDED)			
3s ea	70907-0024-03	1.12	
(ULTRA RIBBED)			
3s ea	70907-0041-03	1.12	
(ULTRA SENSITIVE)			
3s ea	70907-0017-03	1.12	
(ULTRA STRENGTH)			
3s ea	70907-0043-03	1.12	
(ASSORTED COLORS)			
12s ea	70907-0028-12	3.98	
(CLASSIC COLLECTION)			
12s ea	70907-0029-12	3.98	
(LARGE,LUBRICATED)			
12s ea	70907-0011-12	3.98	
(LARGE/SPERMICIDE)			
12s ea	70907-0022-12	3.98	
(LUBRICATED)			
12s ea	70907-0015-12	3.98	
(LUSCIOUS FLAVORS)			
12s ea	70907-0027-12	3.98	
(RIBBED/SPERMICIDE)			
12s ea	70907-0042-12	3.98	
(SENSITIVE/SPERMICIDE)			
12s ea	70907-0020-12	3.98	
(SPERMICIDALY LUBRICATED)			
12s ea	70907-0018-12	3.98	
(STUDDED)			
12s ea	70907-0024-12	3.98	
(ULTRA RIBBED)			
12s ea	70907-0041-12	3.98	
(ULTRA SENSITIVE)			
12s ea	70907-0017-12	3.98	
(ULTRA STRENGTH)			
12s ea	70907-0043-12	3.98	
(SPERMICIDALLY LUBRICATE)			
24s ea	70907-0018-24	6.96	
(ULTRA SEN./SPERMICIDE)			
24s ea	70907-0020-24	6.96	
(LUBRICATED)			
36s ea	70907-0015-46	9.36	
(SPERMICIDALY LUBRICATED)			
36s ea	70907-0018-46	9.36	
(ULTRA SENS./SPERMICIDE)			
36s ea	70907-0020-46	9.36	
(ULTRA SENSITIVE)			
36s ea	70907-0017-46	9.36	
LIFESTYLES CONDOM DISCS (Ansell)			
DEV,NA (ASST.COLORS,LUBRICATED)			
3s ea	70907-0012-43	1.32	
(ASST.FLAVORS/LUBRICATED)			
3s ea	70907-0012-23	1.32	
(EX.SENSITIVE/LUBRICATED)			
3s ea	70907-0012-03	1.32	
(EX.SENSITIVE/SPERMICIDE)			
3s ea	70907-0012-13	1.32	
(ASST.COLORS/LUBRICATED)			
6s ea	70907-0012-46	2.51	
(ASST.FLAVORS/LUBRICATED)			
6s ea	70907-0012-26	2.51	
(EX.SENSITIVE/SPERMICIDE)			
6s ea	70907-0012-16	2.51	
(EX.SENSITIVE/LUBRICATED)			
72s ea	70907-0012-06	2.51	
LIFESTYLES SNUGGER FIT (Ansell)			
DEV,NA (LUBRICATED)			
3s ea	70907-0031-03	1.12	
12s ea	70907-0031-12	3.98	
LIFESTYLES TUXEDO (Ansell)			
DEV,NA (BLACK,LUBRICATED)			
3s ea	70907-0026-03	1.12	
12s ea	70907-0026-12	3.98	
LIFESTYLES XTRA PLEASURE (Ansell)			
DEV,NA (LUBRICATED)			
3s ea	70907-0013-03	1.12	
(SPERMICIDE)			
3s ea	70907-0023-03	1.12	
(LUBRICATED)			
12s ea	70907-0013-12	3.98	
(SPERMICIDE)			
12s ea	70907-0023-12	3.98	
LIFESTYLES XTREME PLEASURE (Ansell)			
DEV,NA (DISCS,LUBRICATED)			
3s ea	70907-0012-33	1.32	
6s ea	70907-0012-36	2.51	
LINIMIST (Mead-Raymond)			
SPR,TP, 1.64%-6.25%-12.5%,			
170 gm	11883-0001-01		10.75
LINUM-20 (Key Company)			
SGL,PO (PF,SOFTGEL)			
1130 mg, 100s ea	11694-0782-01	6.50	
650s ea	11694-0782-05	37.00	
LIP IVO (LIPIVO)			
STI,TP (BLISTER PACK,CHERRY)			
4.25 gm	72577-0200-05	0.64	
(BULK,CHERRY)			
4.25 gm	72577-0100-05	0.37	
LIP IVO ALOE VERA (LIPIVO)			
STI,TP (1X4.25GM)			
7.5%-3%, 4.25 gm	72577-0200-02	0.65	
(SPF15, BULK PACKAGE)			
7.5%-3%, 4.25 gm	72577-0100-02	0.38	
LIP IVO ORIGINAL (LIPIVO)			
STI,TP (BLISTER PACK)			
4.25 gm	72577-0200-01	0.61	
(BULK PACKAGE)			
4.25 gm	72577-0100-01	0.35	
LIP TREATMENT (Pfeiffer)			
OIN,TP, 10 gm	00927-0068-35	0.66	1.19
(SPF 15)			
10 gm	00927-0683-50	0.66	1.19
LIPASE-100 (Key Company)			
TAB,PO (UNCOATED)			
100 mg, 60s ea	11694-0774-01	4.50	
LIPISTART (VITAFLO, LLC)			
PDR,PO (400GM)			
ea	50600-0502-05	28.75	39.75
LIPO-B-C (Legere)			
TAB,PO, 100s ea	25332-1129-02	13.50	
LIPO-KEY (Key Company)			
TAB,PO (SF)			
100s ea	11694-0883-01	5.00	
1000s ea	11694-0883-05	40.00	
LIPODASE (Freeda)			
GRA,PO (PF,SF,DYE-FREE)			
7000 mg/15 ml,			
480 gm	10432-0119-03	10.17	16.95
LIPOFLAVONOID (DSE Healthcare)			
GEL,TP, 100s ea	38485-0501-17	21.06	
500s ea	38485-0501-19	90.42	
LIPOGEN (Rugby)			
SGL,PO (SOFTGEL)			
60s ea	00536-3908-08	6.45	
LIPOMUL (Lee Pharm)			
LIQ,PO, 480 ml	23558-0560-40	29.40	
480 ml 12s	23558-0560-41	352.80	

PROD/MFR	HRI, UPC,NDC	AWP	SRP
LIPOTRIAD (Numark)			
TAB,PO (CAPLET)			
60s ea	38485-0500-60	7.50	
LIQ-10 (Tishcon)			
SYR,PO (ORANGE-PINEAPPLE)			
50 mg/5 ml-15 iu/5 ml,			
500 ml	54023-8121-07	59.95	
LIQUA-GEL PUMP (Paddock)			
DEV,NA (PINT)			
ea	00574-1922-16	2.35	
LIQUACEL (Global)			
LIQ,PO (SF,CITRUS ORANGE)			
30s ea	82028-0030-91	53.00	
(SF,CONCORD GRAPE)			
30s ea	82028-0030-95	44.00	
(6X976ML,SF,GRAPE)			
976 ml 6s	82028-0006-94	158.99	
(6X976ML,SF,ORANGE)			
976 ml 6s	82028-0006-92	158.99	
LIQUAFIBER (Global)			
LIQ,PO (100X15ML)			
15 ml 100s	82028-0100-13	57.00	
(6X488ML)			
488 ml 6s	82028-0006-12	64.00	
LIQUI-CAL (Advanced Nutr)			
CAP,PO, 600 mg, 60s ea	62617-0304-02	7.35	14.00
LIQUIBID (Capellon)			
TAB,PO, 400 mg, 100s ea	64543-0130-01	36.52	
LIQUIBID D-R (Capellon)			
TAB,PO (MAXIMUM ADULT STRENGTH)			
400 mg-10 mg,			
90s ea	64543-0350-90	73.75	
LIQUIBID PD-R (Capellon)			
TAB,PO, 200 mg-5 mg,			
90s ea	64543-0340-90	56.25	
LIQUID CAL-600 (Carlson,J.R.)			
SGL,PO (PF,SF,CORN-FREE)			
600 mg, 100s ea	88395-0051-51	5.45	10.90
250s ea	88395-0051-52	12.45	24.90
LIQUID CAL-MAG (Carlson,J.R.)			
SGL,PO (PF,SF,SALT-FREE)			
200 mg-100 mg-500 iu,			
100s ea	88395-0051-71	4.95	9.90
250s ea	88395-0051-72	10.95	21.90
LIQUID CALCIUM (Carlson,J.R.)			
SGL,PO (PF,SF,SALT-FREE)			
100s ea	88395-0051-61	6.45	12.90
250s ea	88395-0051-62	12.25	24.50
LIQUID MAGNESIUM (Carlson,J.R.)			
SGL,PO (PF,SF,CORN-FREE)			
400 mg, 100s ea	88395-0052-01	4.95	9.90
250s ea	88395-0052-02	11.75	23.50
LIQUID MULTIPLE MINERALS (Carlson,J.R.)			
SGL,PO (SOFTGEL)			
90s ea	88395-0050-51	6.45	12.90
180s ea	88395-0050-52	12.25	24.50
360s ea	88395-0050-53	22.00	44.00
LIQUILUBE TEARS (Global Source)			
SOL,OP, 1.4%, 15 ml	59618-0515-28	2.65	
LIQUIMAT MEDIUM (Summers)			
LOT,TP, 5%, 45 ml	11086-0028-01	12.67	
LIQUITEARS (Major)			
SOL,OP, 1.4%, 15 ml	00904-5017-35	3.79	
LISCO NON-STERILE (Covidien)			
DEV,NA (4"X4")			
2000s ea	08080-3208-00	123.24	
(2"X2")			
8000s ea	08080-3041-00	122.95	
LISSAMINE GREEN (HUB Pharma)			
TES,OP, 1.5 mg, 100s ea	64334-1122-01	25.00	
LISTER'S SUTURE REMOVAL STERILE (J&J Medical)			
DEV,NA (LITTAUER SCISSORS)			
ea	56091-0014-41	2.01	
(SHARP/SHARP SCISSORS)			
ea	56091-0014-40	2.01	
(12X4 DISP,LITTAUER SCIS)			
48s ea	56091-0014-42	8.92	
LISTERINE (Johnson & Johnson)			
SOL,MM (1X95ML,ORIGINAL)			
95 ml	12547-0708-95	1.13	
(1X250ML,ORIGINAL)			
250 ml	12547-0701-28	2.83	
(VANILLA MINT)			
250 ml	12547-0521-20	2.83	

PROD/MFR	HRI, UPC,NDC	AWP	SRP
(1X500ML,FRESHBURST)			
500 ml	12547-0428-25	3.91	
(1X500ML,ORIGINAL)			
500 ml	12547-0701-31	3.91	
(VANILLA MINT)			
500 ml	12547-0521-25	3.91	
(1X1000ML,FRESHBURST)			
1000 ml	12547-0428-35	5.40	
(1X1000ML,ORIGINAL)			
1000 ml	12547-0701-52	5.40	
(VANILLA MINT)			
1000 ml	12547-0521-35	5.40	
(1X1500ML,FRESHBURST)			
1500 ml	12547-0428-55	7.60	
(1X1500ML,ORIGINAL)			
1500 ml	12547-0701-53	7.60	
(VANILLA MINT)			
1500 ml	12547-0521-55	7.60	
LISTERINE ADVANCED ANTISEPTIC (Johnson & Johnson)			
SOL,MM (WITH TARTAR PROTECTION)			
95 ml	12547-0429-95	1.13	
(W/TARTER PROTECTION)			
250 ml	12547-0429-20	3.25	
500 ml	12547-0429-25	4.50	
1000 ml	12547-0429-35	5.95	
1500 ml	12547-0429-55	8.35	
LISTERINE AGENT COOL BLUE (Johnson & Johnson)			
SOL,MM (1X500ML,BUBBLE BLAST)			
500 ml	12547-0445-27	4.50	
(1X500ML,GLACIER MINT)			
500 ml	12547-0445-67	4.50	
(GLACIER MINT)			
500 ml	12547-0445-65	4.25	
LISTERINE ANTISEPTIC (Johnson & Johnson)			
SOL,MM (FRESHBURST)			
250 ml	12547-0428-20	2.69	
LISTERINE ESSENTIAL CARE (Johnson & Johnson)			
GEL,DE (MINT)			
119 gm	12547-0434-55	4.21	
(TARTER CONTROL,MINT)			
119 gm	12547-0434-75	4.21	
PAS,DE (MINT)			
119 gm	12547-0434-05	4.21	
LISTERINE POCKETMIST (Johnson & Johnson)			
SPR,PO (1X7.7ML,140 MISTS,SF)			
7.7 ml	12547-0339-09	2.51	
(SF,COOL MINT)			
7.7 ml	12547-0339-01	2.51	
(SF,FRESH CITRUS)			
7.7 ml	12547-0339-51	2.51	
(7.7MLX2,SF,COOL MINT)			
7.7 ml 2s	12547-0339-02	4.40	
(7.7MLX2,SF,FRESH CITRUS)			
7.7 ml 2s	12547-0339-52	4.40	
LISTERINE POCKETPAKS (Johnson & Johnson)			
FIL,MM (SF,CINNAMON,STRIPS)			
24s ea	12547-0437-11	1.32	
(SF,COOL MINT,STRIPS)			
24s ea	12547-0433-10	1.32	
24s ea	12547-0433-65	1.32	
(SF,FRESH CITRUS,STRIPS)			
24s ea	12547-0444-11	1.32	
(SF,FRESHBURST,STRIPS)			
24s ea	12547-0436-10	1.32	
24s ea	12547-0436-11	1.32	
(3X24,SF,CINNAMON,STRIPS)			
72s ea	12547-0437-20	3.53	
(3X24,SF,COOL MINT)			
72s ea	12547-0433-20	3.53	
(3X24,SF,FRESH CITRUS)			
72s ea	12547-0444-20	3.53	
(3X24,SF,FRESHBURST)			
72s ea	12547-0436-20	3.53	
LISTERINE RESTORING (Johnson & Johnson)			
SOL,MM (MINT SHIELD)			
0.0221%, 250 ml	12547-0306-73	3.25	
1000 ml	12547-0306-75	5.95	
LISTERINE SMART RINSE (Johnson & Johnson)			
SOL,MM (1X250ML,BERRY SHIELD)			
0.0221%, 250 ml	12547-0115-20	3.25	
(1X250ML,MINT SHIELD)			
0.0221%, 250 ml	12547-0113-20	3.25	
(1X500ML,BERRY SHIELD)			
0.0221%, 500 ml	12547-0115-25	4.50	
(1X500ML,MINT SHIELD)			
0.0221%, 500 ml	12547-0113-25	4.50	

PROD/MFR	HRI, UPC,NDC	AWP	SRP
LISTERINE TOTAL CARE (Johnson & Johnson)			
SOL,MM (1X95ML,FRESH MINT)			
0.0221%, 95 ml	12547-0306-95	1.13	
(1X250ML,CINNAMINT)			
0.0221%, 250 ml	12547-0306-53	3.25	
(1X250ML,ICY MINT)			
0.0221%, 250 ml	12547-0306-13	3.25	
(FRESH MINT)			
0.0221%, 250 ml	12547-0306-20	3.25	
(1X500ML,CINNAMINT)			
0.0221%, 500 ml	12547-0306-54	4.50	
(1X500ML,ICY MINT)			
0.0221%, 500 ml	12547-0306-14	4.50	
(FRESH MINT)			
0.0221%, 500 ml	12547-0306-25	4.50	
(1X1000ML,CINNAMINT)			
0.0221%, 1000 ml	12547-0306-55	5.95	
(1X1000ML,ICY MINT)			
0.0221%, 1000 ml	12547-0306-15	5.95	
(FRESH MINT)			
0.0221%, 1000 ml	12547-0306-35	5.95	
LISTERINE WHITENING (Johnson & Johnson)			
FIL,DE (CLEAN MINT)			
56s ea	12547-0425-60	16.24	
SOL,MM (PRE-BRUSH RINSE)			
236 ml	12547-0425-20	3.91	
473 ml	12547-0425-25	5.40	
946 ml	12547-0425-35	7.60	
LISTERINE WHITENING PEN (Johnson & Johnson)			
GEL,DE (1X2.2ML)			
2.2 ml	12547-0425-80	9.65	
LISTERINE WHITENING PLUS RESTORING (Johnson & Johnson)			
SOL,MM (CLEAN MINT)			
0.0221%, 473 ml	12547-0425-91	5.94	
946 ml	12547-0425-92	8.35	
LISTERINE WHITENING VIBRANT WHITE (Johnson & Johnson)			
SOL,MM (PRE-BRUSH RINSE)			
473 ml	12547-0425-16	5.94	
946 ml	12547-0425-32	8.35	
LISTERMINT (Johnson & Johnson)			
SOL,MM (AF,FRESH MINT)			
960 ml	12547-0700-56	3.92	
LITE TOUCH INSULIN PEN (Medicore)			
DEV,NA (31G,3/16")			
100s ea	32671-0005-32	2.30	2.39
LITE TOUCH LANCING DEVICE (Medicore)			
DEV,NA (AURORA HEALTH CARE)			
ea	32671-0200-44	12.00	
(PEN TYPE)			
ea	32671-0000-20	12.00	
LITE'N UP 50 (Lee Pharm)			
DEV,NA (NICOTINE FILTERS)			
ea	23558-0693-30	1.80	
6s ea	23558-0693-31	10.80	
LITE'N UP 90 (Lee Pharm)			
DEV,NA (NICOTINE FIITFRS)			
ea	23558-0693-50	1.80	
6s ea	23558-0693-51	10.80	
LITH-ORO (Bio-Tech Pharm)			
CAP,PO, 5 mg, 100s ea	53191-0450-01	7.50	
LITTLE ANIMALS (Mason Vit)			
CTB,PO, 60s ea	11845-0091-85	4.67	
LITTLE ANIMALS PLUS IRON (Mason Vit)			
CTB,PO, 60s ea	11845-0091-95	4.89	
LITTLE NURSE COLD SEASON BATH KIDS (Mentholatum)			
LIQ,TP, 225 ml	10742-0006-31	3.60	
LITTLE ONES (Convatec)			
DEV,NA (0-9/10",TWO-PIECE)			
5s ea	68455-0105-86	19.32	25.14
(1/5"-1 1/4",TWO-PIECE)			
5s ea	68455-0105-92	18.90	24.60
5s ea	68455-0105-93	18.90	24.60
(CLOSED END POUCH)			
10s ea	68455-0105-90	13.71	17.85
10s ea	68455-0105-91	13.71	17.85
(DRAINABLE POUCH)			
10s ea	68455-0105-85	19.25	25.14
10s ea	68455-0105-87	27.63	35.96
10s ea	68455-0105-88	27.48	35.76
10s ea	68455-0105-89	27.48	35.76
LITTLE ONES ACTIVELIFE (Convatec)			
DEV,NA (DRAINABLE POUCH 6")			
10s ea	68455-0104-16	30.08	39.54

PROD/MFR	HRI. UPC.NDC	AWP	SRP
LITTLE ONES ONE-PIECE (Convatec)			
DEV,NA (5/16"-1",TRANS,UROSTOMY)			
15s ea	68455-0108-69	55.28	71.95
(TRANSP,5/16"-2")			
15s ea	68455-0101-39	46.51	60.54
LIVER (Miller)			
TAB,PO, 455 mg, 100s ea	17204-0506-40	5.70	9.00
LMD (Mead Johnson & Co)			
PDR,PO (LEUCINE FREE)			
454 gm	00087-0078-41	52.80	
LMX 4 (Ferndale)			
CRE,TP, 4%, 5 gm	00496-0882-05	9.90	
5 gm 5s	00496-0882-07	48.07	
15 gm	00496-0882-15	25.03	
30 gm	00496-0882-30	46.30	
30 gm	00496-0882-71	49.46	
(Dispensing Solutions)			
REPACK			
CRE,TP, 4%, 15 gm	55045-3705-01	26.00	
LMX 5 (Ferndale)			
CRE,TP, 5%, 15 gm	00496-0883-15	30.53	
30 gm	00496-0883-30	54.53	
LO-DOSE ASPIRIN (Chain Drug Marketing)			
ECT,PO, 81 mg, 120s ea	63868-0360-20	1.56	4.99
LOBANA HAND SOAP (Lobana)			
LIQ,TP, 0.5%, 120 ml	00127-3220-02	1.07	1.77
800 ml	00127-3220-16	5.45	9.08
LOBANA PERI-GARDE (Lobana)			
OIN,TP, 120 gm	00127-1366-06	3.56	5.70
LOBOB HARD LENS CLEANING (Lobob)			
SOL,NA (NON-ABRASIVE,PF)			
60 ml	34672-0101-53	5.10	8.50
120 ml	34672-0101-55	7.90	13.00
LOBOB HARD LENS SOAKING (Lobob)			
SOL,NA, 120 ml	34672-0101-66	5.10	8.50
LOBOB HARD LENS WETTING (Lobob)			
SOL,OP, 60 ml	34672-0101-88	5.10	8.50
LOBOB INSERTION/REMOVAL (Lobob)			
KIT,NA (SOFT CONTACT LENS)			
ea	34672-0400-14	4.20	6.30
LOBOB SOFT LENS CLEANER (Lobob)			
SOL,NA, 60 ml	34672-0103-54	4.65	7.75
LOMA ASTHMA (Loma Lux)			
TAB,PO, 3 x-1 x-3 x-6 x-3 x,			
100s ea	61480-0215-05	17.00	
LOMA LUX ACNEPILL (Loma Lux)			
PO, 9 x-1 x-2 x-6 x-6 x,			
100s ea	61480-0135-05	17.00	
LOMA LUX ECZEMA (Loma Lux)			
PO, 1 x-4 x-4 x-2 x-6 x,			
100s ea	61480-0115-05	17.00	
LOMA LUX PSORIASIS (Loma Lux)			
LIQ,PO, 1 x-4 x-2 x-3 x-4 x,			
237 ml	61480-0125-03	17.00	
LOMA LUX SINUS & ALLERGY (Loma Lux)			
TAB,PO, 1 x-6 x-6 x-1 x-3 x-6 x,			
100s ea	61480-0235-05	17.00	
LONG PRESTIGE SMART SYSTEM (Home Diag)			
DEV,NA (STRIP)			
50s ea	56151-0312-50	28.60	
LONG PRESTIGE SMART SYSTEM STARTER (Home Diag)			
DEV,NA (MTR,STRP,LANCET,DEV,SOL)			
ea	56151-0212-01	22.18	
LONG-ACTING COUGH SUPPRESSANT (Major)			
SYR,PO (1X118ML,AF,ORANGE)			
15 mg/5 ml, 118 ml	00904-5875-20	8.25	
LONGS GLUCOSE (Can-Am Care)			
TAB,PO (CAFFEINE-FREE)			
4 gm, 50s ea	38396-0552-70	6.49	
(DEX4 FAST ACTING)			
4 gm, 50s ea	38396-0554-70	6.49	
LONGS STANDARD LANCETS (Can-Am Care)			
DEV,NA (21G)			
200s ea	38396-0328-70	7.99	
LONGS THIN LANCETS (Can-Am Care)			
DEV,NA (26G)			
200s ea	38396-0329-70	7.99	
LONGS ULTRA COMFORT INSULIN SYRINGE (Can-Am Care)			
DEV,NA (31G,5/16",1/2ML)			
100s ea	38396-0410-70	17.50	
(31G,5/16",3/10ML)			
100s ea	38396-0409-70	17.50	
LONGS ULTRA THIN LANCETS (Can-Am Care)			
DEV,NA (30G)			
100s ea	38396-0330-70	11.59	
LOPERAMIDE HCL (Hi-Tech)			
LIQ,PO, 1 mg/5 ml,			
120 ml	50383-0618-04	5.60	
(Marlex)			
TAB,PO (CAPLET)			
2 mg, 12s ea	10135-0158-12	1.20	
12s ea UD	10135-0158-51	3.00	
(BLISTER PACK)			
2 mg, 100s ea UD	10135-0159-13	15.18	
(Ohm)			
TAB,PO (CAPLET)			
2 mg, 6s ea	51660-0122-06	3.05	
12s ea	51660-0122-12	5.10	
(Roxane)			
SOL,PO, 1 mg/5 ml,			
5 ml 40s UD	00054-8534-16	39.75	
10 ml 40s UD	00054-8535-16	54.75	
(A-S Medication)			
REPACK			
LIQ,PO, 1 mg/5 ml,			
118 ml	54569-3708-00	5.61	
(Nucare Pharm)			
REPACK			
LIQ,PO, 1 mg/5 ml,			
120 ml	68071-1327-04	6.58	
LOPERAMIDE HYDROCHLORIDE (Precision Dose)			
SOL,PO (1X5ML,CHERRY MINT)			
1 mg/5 ml, 5 ml UD	68094-0106-59	1.00	
(30X5ML,CHERRY MINT)			
1 mg/5 ml,			
5 ml 30s UD	68094-0106-62	29.94	
(1X10ML,CHERRY MINT)			
1 mg/5 ml, 10 ml UD	68094-0217-59	1.38	
(30X10ML,CHERRY MINT)			
1 mg/5 ml,			
10 ml 30s UD	68094-0217-62	41.26	
(Advanced Pharm Serv, Inc.)			
REPACK			
CAP,PO, 2 mg, 10s ea	13411-0171-01	6.82	
20s ea	13411-0171-02	13.64	
30s ea	13411-0171-03	20.46	
60s ea	13411-0171-06	40.92	
100s ea	13411-0171-10	68.20	
(AQ)			
REPACK			
CAP,PO, 2 mg, 15s ea	66105-0609-15	13.25	
30s ea	66105-0609-03	24.50	
60s ea	66105-0609-06	47.01	
100s ea	66105-0609-10	77.02	
500s ea	66105-0609-50	329.91	
LOPHLEX (Nutricia)			
PDR,PO (PHENYLANINE-FREE,BERRY)			
30s ea	49735-0121-69	127.40	
POW,PO (PHENYLANINE-FREE,ORANGE)			
14.3 gm 30s	49735-0121-67	127.40	
LOPHLEX LQ 20 (Nutricia)			
SOL,PO (PKU, READY TO DRINK)			
125 ml 30s	49735-0195-35	200.40	
LORADAMED (Medique)			
TAB,PO, 10 mg,			
50s ea UD	47682-0203-50	18.45	
LORATADINE (Apotex Corp.)			
TAB,PO, 10 mg, 100s ea	60505-0147-01	82.50	
1000s ea	60505-0147-08	825.00	
(Major)			
SYR,PO (FRUIT)			
5 mg/5 ml, 120 ml	00904-5727-20	15.98	
TAB,PO (10X10)			
10 mg, 100s ea UD	00904-5793-61	79.95	
(McKesson)			
TAB,PO (NON-DROWSY, 24HR)			
10 mg, 10s ea	49348-0542-01	4.99	
30s ea	49348-0542-44	11.99	
60s ea	49348-0542-12	19.99	
(Novartis Consumer)			
TAB,PO, 10 mg, 10s ea	00067-6070-10	0.77	
30s ea	00670-0674-30	1.44	
(NON-DROWSY)			
10 mg, 30s ea	00067-6070-30	1.44	
(Ohm)			
TAB,PO, 10 mg, 100s ea	51660-0526-01	6.90	
(Perrigo)			
TAB,PO, 10 mg, 30s ea	45802-0650-65	9.02	
(NON-DROWSY)			
10 mg, 100s ea	45802-0650-78	30.07	
300s ea	45802-0650-87	90.20	
(Sandoz)			
TAB,PO (24 HOUR ALLERGY)			
10 mg, 100s ea	00781-5077-01	82.50	
(Silarx)			
SYR,PO (FRUITY)			
5 mg/5 ml, 120 ml	54838-0538-40	8.50	
(TriMarc Labs)			
TAB,PO (USP)			
10 mg, 90s ea	68752-0008-90	12.99	
(UDL)			
TAB,PO (10X10)			
10 mg, 100s ea UD	51079-0538-20	85.50	
(Vision)			
TAB,PO, 10 mg, 100s ea	68013-0017-01	82.50	
(A-S Medication)			
REPACK			
TAB,PO (24 HOUR ALLERGY)			
10 mg, 5s ea	54569-5497-02	4.13	
10s ea	54569-5497-00	8.25	
15s ea	54569-5497-03	12.38	
(24 HOUR ALLERGY)			
10 mg, 20s ea	54569-5497-01	16.50	
30s ea	54569-5497-04	24.75	
30s ea	54569-5497-05	74.25	
(Altura)			
REPACK			
TAB,PO, 10 mg, 10s ea	63874-0545-10	24.62	
12s ea	63874-0545-12	28.08	
14s ea	63874-0545-14	32.58	
15s ea	63874-0545-15	34.31	
20s ea	63874-0545-20	44.00	
24s ea	63874-0545-24	50.00	
30s ea	63874-0545-30	61.27	
(American Health)			
REPACK			
TAB,PO (10X10)			
10 mg, 100s ea	68084-0248-01	70.23	
(DHS, Inc.)			
REPACK			
TAB,PO (24 HOUR ALLERGY)			
10 mg, 10s ea	55887-0607-10	12.99	
15s ea	55887-0607-15	18.20	
30s ea	55887-0607-30	36.69	
(Dispensing Solutions)			
REPACK			
TAB,PO, 10 mg, 10s ea	55045-3340-01	4.00	
20s ea	66336-0422-20	16.58	
30s ea	66336-0422-30	24.75	
(24 HOUR ALLERGY)			
10 mg, 30s ea	55045-3340-08	12.00	
100s ea	55045-3340-00	40.00	
(Nucare Pharm)			
REPACK			
TAB,PO, 10 mg, 14s ea	66267-0653-14	18.68	
30s ea	66267-0653-30	37.89	
(PD-Rx Pharm)			
REPACK			
TAB,PO (24 HOUR ALLERGY)			
10 mg, 10s ea	55289-0728-10	10.86	
15s ea	55289-0728-15	13.80	
30s ea	55289-0728-30	20.45	
30s ea	58864-0799-30	20.45	
90s ea	55289-0728-90	51.35	
(Pharma Pac)			
REPACK			
TAB,PO, 10 mg, 10s ea	52959-0740-10	10.70	
14s ea	52959-0740-14	16.50	
30s ea	52959-0740-30	22.05	
(Phys Total Care)			
REPACK			
TAB,PO, 10 mg, 30s ea	54868-5268-00	15.00	
(Physician Partner)			
REPACK			
SYR,PO (1X120ML,FRUITY)			
5 mg/5 ml, 120 ml	21695-0498-04	17.00	
TAB,PO, 10 mg, 15s ea	21695-0499-15	29.12	
20s ea	21695-0499-20	38.82	
30s ea	21695-0499-30	49.50	

PROD/MFR	HRI, UPC,NDC	AWP	SRP
(Quality Care Prod)			
REPACK			
TAB,PO (24 HOUR ALLERGY)			
10 mg, 10s ea	49999-0229-10	32.90	
20s ea	49999-0229-20	65.80	
30s ea	49999-0229-30	98.70	
90s ea	49999-0229-90	296.10	
(Southwood)			
REPACK			
TAB,PO, 10 mg, 30s ea	58016-4718-01	5.32	
(24 HOUR ALLERGY)			
10 mg, 30s ea	58016-0800-30	24.75	
60s ea	58016-0800-60	49.50	
90s ea	58016-0800-90	74.25	
100s ea	58016-0800-00	82.50	
(Stat Rx)			
REPACK			
TAB,PO, 10 mg, 10s ea	16590-0142-10	13.25	
20s ea	16590-0142-20	26.50	
30s ea	16590-0142-30	36.10	
(Vibranta)			
REPACK			
TAB,PO, 10 mg, 30s ea	57866-3501-02	67.48	
LORATADINE D (Phys Total Care)			
REPACK			
T24,PO, 10 mg-240 mg,			
10s ea	54868-5656-01	31.44	
30s ea	54868-5656-00	69.72	
LORATADINE-D (Major)			
T24,PO (ORIGPRESCRPTIONSTRENGTH)			
10 mg-240 mg, 10s ea	00904-5833-15	11.13	
15s ea	00904-5833-48	16.35	
(Pharma Pac)			
REPACK			
T24,PO, 10 mg-240 mg,			
10s ea	52959-0981-10	8.05	
LORATADINE/PSE (Southwood)			
REPACK			
T24,PO, 10 mg-240 mg,			
10s ea	00490-0071-10	7.39	
LOSO PREP (E-Z-EM)			
KIT,MR (CITRUS)			
ea	10361-0376-40	5.99	
LOTRIMIN AF (Schering Plough)			
CRE,TP, 1%, 12 gm	00085-0963-15	6.80	
(JOCK ITCH)			
1%, 12 gm	11017-0963-30	6.80	
24 gm	00085-0963-17	9.77	
POW,TP, 2%, 90 gm	11523-0919-01	5.77	
LOW DOSE ASPIRIN (Qualitest)			
ECT,PO, 81 mg, 120s ea	00603-0026-22	5.75	
1000s ea	00603-0026-32	54.65	
(Dispensing Solutions)			
REPACK			
ECT,PO, 81 mg, 120s ea	66336-0323-94	6.95	
(Physician Partner)			
REPACK			
ECT,PO, 81 mg, 100s ea	21695-0684-00	25.00	
120s ea	21695-0684-72	30.00	
LUBREX (Allerderm Labs.)			
CRE,TP (FRAGRANCE-FREE)			
114 gm	34674-0033-04	6.54	8.39
LOT,TP, 240 ml	34674-0031-08	5.53	4.39
480 ml	34674-0031-16	9.88	7.85
LUBREX CLEANSER (Allerderm Labs.)			
LOT,TP (FRAGRANCE-FREE)			
356 ml	34674-0035-12	6.24	8.00
LUBRI SILK (Dermarite)			
LOT,TP, 480 ml	61924-0166-16	7.36	
LUBRI SKIN (Geritrex)			
LOT,TP, 240 ml	54162-0810-08	1.56	1.56
LUBRICATING JELLY (AmerisourceBergen)			
GEL,TP (PRIVATE LABEL)			
120 gm	24385-0071-44	2.87	3.19
(G&W)			
GEL,TP, 120 gm	00713-0264-04	2.87	
(Taro)			
GEL,VG (AF,GREASELESS)			
113 gm	51672-0200-64	3.25	
LUBRICATING SKIN LOTION (Medicine Shoppe)			
LOT,TP, 480 ml	49614-0422-43	2.27	3.99
LUBRIDERM ADVANCED THERAPY			
(Johnson & Johnson)			
LOT,TP (1X100ML)			
100 ml	52800-0482-42	2.35	
(1X177ML)			
177 ml	52800-0482-31	3.14	
(TRIPLE SMOOTHING BODY)			
400 ml	52800-0482-33	7.33	
(1X473ML)			
473 ml	52800-0482-34	7.33	
LUBRIDERM ADVANCED THERAPY HAND CREAM			
(Johnson & Johnson)			
CRE,TP (1X100GM)			
100 gm	52800-0482-65	5.05	
LUBRIDERM ADVANCED THERAPY MOISTURIZING CREAM (Johnson & Johnson)			
CRE,TP (1X453GM)			
453 gm	52800-0482-24	10.84	
LUBRIDERM DAILY MOISTURE			
(Johnson & Johnson)			
LOT,TP (NORMAL-DRY SKIN)			
30 ml	52800-0488-81	0.44	
(FRAGRANCE-FREE)			
100 ml	52800-0488-63	2.35	
(1X177ML,FRAGRANCE-FREE)			
177 ml	52800-0488-26	3.14	
(1X177ML)			
177 ml	52800-0488-16	3.14	
(1X473ML,FRAGRANCE-FREE)			
473 ml	52800-0488-56	7.33	
(1X473ML)			
473 ml	52800-0488-46	7.33	
(SPF15)			
7.5%-4%-3%, 100 ml	52800-0486-16	2.35	
473 ml	52800-0486-12	7.33	
LUBRIDERM INTENSE SKIN REPAIR			
(Johnson & Johnson)			
CRE,TP (1X140GM)			
140 gm	52800-0482-70	7.33	
LOT,TP (1X473ML)			
473 ml	52800-0482-68	7.33	
(W/ ITCH RELIEF)			
473 ml	52800-0482-71	7.33	
OIN,TP (1X50GM)			
40%, 50 gm	52800-0482-01	4.25	
LUBRIDERM SENSITIVE SKIN THERAPY			
(Johnson & Johnson)			
LOT,TP (DYE-FREE,FRAGRANCE-FREE)			
473 ml	52800-0483-16	7.33	
LUBRIDERM SKIN NOURISHING			
(Johnson & Johnson)			
LOT,TP (W/ PREMIUM OAT EXTRACT)			
473 ml	52800-0480-56	7.33	
(W/SEA KELP EXTRACT)			
473 ml	52800-0497-56	7.33	
(W/SHEA & COCOA BUTTERS)			
473 ml	52800-0498-56	7.33	
LUBRIFRESH P.M. (Major)			
OIN,OP (PF)			
3.5 gm	00904-5168-38	6.49	
LUBRIN (Kenwood)			
SUP,VG, 5s ea	00482-0118-19	13.84	
12s ea	00482-0118-12	28.62	
LUBRISKIN (Geritrex)			
LOT,TP (FRAGRANCE-FREE)			
480 ml	54162-0810-16	3.06	
(PUMP,PF)			
480 ml	54162-0810-18	3.83	
LUBRISOFT (Major)			
LOT,TP (UNSCENTED)			
473 ml	00904-5300-16	5.49	
LUDEN'S (Johnson & Johnson)			
LOZ,MM (WILD CHERRY,SF)			
1.5 mg, 14s ea	42300-0066-07	0.59	
25s ea	42300-0066-13	1.49	
(CITRUS ASSORTMENT)			
1.7 mg, 30s ea	42300-0065-11	1.27	
(HONEY LICORICE)			
2.5 mg, 14s ea	42300-0058-07	0.47	
(McNeil Consumer Healthcare)			
LOZ,MM (BERRY ASSORTMENT,DROPS)			
30s ea	42300-0064-11	1.39	
(HONEY LEMON,DROPS)			
1.6 mg, 14s ea	42300-0059-07	0.47	
30s ea	42300-0059-11	1.39	
(HONEY LICORICE,DROP)			
1.6 mg, 30s ea	42300-0058-11	1.39	
(WILD CHERRY,DROP)			
1.7 mg, 14s ea	42300-0052-07	0.47	
30s ea	42300-0052-11	1.39	
(ORIGINAL MENTHOL,DROP)			
2.5 mg, 14s ea	42300-0057-07	0.47	
LUMINEB I NEBULIZER (Lumiscope)			
DEV,NA, ea	38673-0055-00	49.99	99.99
LUMINEB I NEBULIZER MASK PEDIATRIC (Lumiscope)			
DEV,NA, ea	38673-0055-03	4.99	9.99
LUMINEB I NEBULIZER REPLACEMENT (Lumiscope)			
DEV,NA (DISPOSABLE)			
ea	38673-0055-01	4.99	8.99
LUMINEB I REPLACEMENT FILTERS (Lumiscope)			
DEV,NA (FOR NEBULIZER)			
10s ea	38673-0055-02	3.49	6.99
LUMITENE (Tishcon)			
CAP,PO, 30 mg, 100s ea	01465-4658-08	44.95	
LUNG (Miller)			
TAB,PO, 180 mg, 100s ea	17204-0538-40	6.00	9.50
LUPICARE (Alwyn)			
CRE,TP (MOISTURIZING SKIN)			
56 gm	62420-0009-02	9.07	16.50
227 gm	62420-0009-08	17.88	32.50
LUPICARE DANDRUFF (Alwyn)			
CRE,TP, 2.5%, 113 gm	62420-0018-04	13.72	24.95
227 gm	62420-0018-08	19.80	36.00
LUPICARE II PSORIASIS SKIN (Alwyn)			
CRE,TP, 2.5%, 56 gm	62420-0015-02	9.97	18.50
227 gm	62420-0015-08	19.80	36.00
LUPICARE PSORIASIS (Alwyn)			
LIQ,TP, 2%, 118 ml	62420-0016-04	5.48	9.95
237 ml	62420-0016-08	8.22	14.95
LUPICARE PSORIASIS SCALP (Alwyn)			
CRE,TP, 2.5%, 113 gm	62420-0017-04	13.72	24.95
227 gm	62420-0017-08	19.80	36.00
LUTEIN (Apothecary)			
SGL,PO (LUTEINPURE,PF,SF)			
20 mg, 30s ea	18833-0900-10	10.65	
60s ea	18833-0900-20	19.35	
(Carlson,J.R.)			
SGL,PO (SOFTGEL)			
6 mg-1 iu-0.264 mg,			
60s ea	88395-0086-50	6.45	12.90
180s ea	88395-0086-52	14.95	29.90
(Freeda)			
TAB,PO (SF)			
20 mg, 50s ea	10432-0352-00	17.07	28.45
100s ea	10432-0352-01	28.77	47.95
(Major)			
SGL,PO (SOFTGEL)			
6 mg, 50s ea	00904-5599-51	5.36	
(Mason Pharm)			
SGL,PO (SOFTGEL)			
6 mg, 60s ea	11845-0136-65	7.00	
LUTEIN + KALE (Carlson,J.R.)			
CAP,PO (PF)			
15 mg-900 mcg,			
60s ea	88395-0086-66	10.95	21.90
180s ea	88395-0086-62	32.20	64.40
LYC-2000 (Key Company)			
PDR,PO (SF)			
150 gm	11694-0717-01	10.50	
LYC-CAPSULES (Key Company)			
CAP,PO (SF)			
100s ea	11694-0717-02	9.00	
LYCOPENE (Carlson,J.R.)			
SGL,PO (TOMATO FREE,PF,SF)			
15 mg, 60s ea	88395-0087-16	9.95	19.90
(PF,SF,CORN-FREE)			
15 mg, 180s ea	88395-0087-12	24.95	49.90
(Freeda)			
TAB,PO (PF,SF)			
10 mg, 100s ea	10432-0344-01	22.77	37.95
LYCOPODIUM (Luyties)			
TAB,SL (6X)			
6 x, 500s ea	00618-5491-03	3.99	
5500s ea	00618-5491-10	30.32	
(30X)			
12 x, 500s ea	00622-5491-03	4.19	
5500s ea	00622-5491-10	31.83	
(12X)			
30 x, 500s ea	00624-5491-03	4.19	
5500s ea	00624-5491-10	31.83	

PROD/MFR	HRI. UPC.NDC	AWP	SRP
LYDIA PINKHAM (Numark)			
LIQ,PO, 240 ml	38485-0502-08	6.30	
480 ml	38485-0502-16	10.08	
TAB,PO, 60 mg-500 mg-6 mg-30 iu,			
72s ea	38485-0504-07	7.14	
150s ea	38485-0504-15	13.20	
LYMPH (Miller)			
TAB,PO, 100s ea	17204-0518-40	9.48	15.00
LYNAE CALCIUM/VITAMIN C (Boscogen)			
CTB,PO (SF,DYE-FREE)			
250 mg-250 mg,			
100s ea	85714-0011-22	3.99	
LYNAE CHONDROITIN/GLUCOSAMINE (Boscogen)			
CAP,PO (SF)			
400 mg-500 mg,			
60s ea	85714-0041-09	10.80	
LYNAE CO Q-10 (Boscogen)			
SGL,PO, 30 mg, 60s ea	85714-0044-00	9.00	
LYNAE GINSE-COOL (Boscogen)			
CTB,PO (PF,SF)			
200 mg, 100s ea	85714-0010-23	3.33	
LYNAE GRAPE SEED EXTRACT (Boscogen)			
CAP,PO, 80 mg-300 mg-60 mg,			
90s ea	85714-0040-00	6.98	
LYNAE SILYMARIN (Boscogen)			
CAP,PO, 120s ea	85714-0017-19	7.75	
LYSINE (ADH)			
L-LYSINE			
CAP,PO, 500 mg, 100s ea	60142-0119-10	3.98	7.95
250s ea	60142-0119-11	8.25	16.58
(Cardinal Health)			
TAB,PO (PF,PRIVATE LABEL)			
500 mg, 100s ea	37205-0189-78	5.24	
(Carlson,J.R.)			
CAP,PO, 500 mg, 100s ea	88395-0068-81	4.38	8.75
300s ea	88395-0068-83	11.45	22.90
POW,PO, 100 gm	88395-0068-85	3.45	6.90
(Freeda)			
TAB,PO (PF,SF,DYE-FREE)			
500 mg, 100s ea	10432-0242-01	5.25	8.75
250s ea	10432-0242-02	10.50	17.50
(Health Products Corp)			
TAB,PO (PF,SF)			
500 mg, 100s ea	39686-0014-69	3.73	
(Mason Vit)			
TAB,PO, 500 mg, 100s ea	11845-0072-11	6.67	
(PF,SF)			
1000 mg, 60s ea	11845-0121-15	8.78	
(Miller)			
CAP,PO, 500 mg, 100s ea	17204-0915-40	6.30	10.50
(Nature's Bounty)			
TAB,PO (PF,SF)			
500 mg, 100s ea	74312-0030-60		6.75
1000 mg, 60s ea	74312-0060-11		6.89
(Neurovites)			
TAB,PO, 500 mg, 100s ea	93595-2028-01	8.50	
(Rexall)			
TAB,PO (PF,SF)			
500 mg, 60s ea	30768-0000-66	2.16	3.27
1000 mg, 60s ea	30768-0001-70	3.49	5.28
(Rugby)			
TAB,PO (PF,SF,DYE-FREE)			
500 mg, 100s ea	00536-6731-01	3.52	
LYSINE (Bio-Tech Pharm)			
CAP,PO, 500 mg, 100s ea	53191-0232-01	5.25	
(Major)			
TAB,PO, 500 mg, 100s ea	00904-2687-60	3.77	
(Marlex)			
TAB,PO, 500 mg, 100s ea	10135-0185-01	1.58	
1000s ea	10135-0185-10	11.98	
LYSINE 500 (Basic Vitamins)			
TAB,PO, 500 mg, 100s ea	00761-0006-10	2.40	
LYSINE-500 (Key Company)			
TAB,PO (SF)			
500 mg, 60s ea	11694-0922-01	4.00	
500s ea	11694-0922-04	23.00	
LYSIPLEX PLUS (Kramer-Novis)			
SOL,PO (1X178ML,SF)			
178 ml	52083-0843-06	11.00	
(SF)			
474 ml	52083-0843-16	20.00	
M S M (Freeda)			
TAB,PO (PURE,SF,GLUTEN-FREE)			
250 mg, 250s ea	10432-0346-02	9.54	15.90
M-SPRAY 2000 (Pharm Innov)			
SPR,NA (FOR MAMMOGRAPHY)			
60 ml	00036-2100-60	1.75	2.50
250 ml	00036-2100-25	5.63	8.05
M-ZOLE 3 COMBINATION PACK (Cardinal Health)			
KIT,NA (3 SUPPS/CREAM W/APPLIC)			
ea	37205-0589-03	9.68	
M.F.A. (Natren)			
PDR,PO, 70 gm	53983-0400-60	13.20	22.00
126 gm	53983-0400-65	19.20	32.00
M2 B125 (Miller)			
TAB,PO, 60s ea	17204-0809-20	11.34	14.60
M2 CALCIUM (Miller)			
TAB,PO, 280 mg, 100s ea	17204-0808-40	5.04	8.40
M2 CHROMIUM (Miller)			
CAP,PO, 500 mcg,			
100s ea	17204-0862-40	5.04	8.40
M2 MAGNESIUM (Miller)			
CAP,PO, 100 mg, 100s ea	17204-0821-40	5.04	8.40
250s ea	17204-0820-65	11.34	18.90
M2 POTASSIUM (Miller)			
CAP,PO, 60 mg, 100s ea	17204-0833-40	5.04	8.40
M2 ZINC 50 (Miller)			
CAP,PO, 50 mg, 100s ea	17204-0829-40	6.30	10.50
MAALOX (Novartis Consumer)			
CTB,PO (REGULAR STRENGTH)			
600 mg, 150s ea	00067-6211-59	4.56	
SUS,PO, 225 mg/5 ml-200 mg/5 ml,			
150 ml	00067-0330-62	2.33	
360 ml	00067-0330-71	4.19	
360 ml	00067-0331-71	4.19	
780 ml	00067-0330-44	7.42	
MAALOX ADVANCED (Novartis Consumer)			
CTB,PO (MAXIMUM STRENGTH)			
1000 mg-60 mg,			
65s ea	00067-6291-65	3.66	
SUS,PO (MINT)			
148 ml	00067-6281-62	2.33	
(1X355ML,MAXIMUMSTRENGTH)			
355 ml	00067-6290-12	4.79	
MAALOX EXTRA STRENGTH (Novartis Consumer)			
SUS,PO, 360 ml	00067-0333-71	5.52	
360 ml	00067-0336-71	4.79	
360 ml	00067-0338-71	4.79	
780 ml	00067-0333-44	9.61	
(CHERRY)			
780 ml	00067-0336-44	9.61	
MACA (Mason Vit)			
CAP,PO (PF,SF)			
500 mg, 60s ea	11845-0125-45	11.00	
MACK'S AQUABLOCK EARPLUGS (McKeon)			
DEV,NA (ULTRASOFT,CLEAR,1PAIR)			
2s ea	33732-0011-31	1.26	3.99
(ULTRASOFT,PURPLE,1PAIR)			
2s ea	33732-0011-12	1.26	3.99
(CLEAR)			
4s ea	33732-0000-13	1.80	5.99
(PURPLE,FLANGED)			
4s ea	33732-0000-12	1.80	5.99
MACK'S DREAMGIRL (McKeon)			
DEV,NA (CONTOUR,EARPLUG,FUCHSIA)			
ea	33732-0020-21	3.36	7.99
MACK'S DREAMGIRL EARPLUGS (McKeon)			
DEV,NA (SOFT FOAM,3 PAIRS,PINK)			
6s ea	33732-0009-33	0.99	2.59
(SOFT FOAM,5 PAIRS,PINK)			
10s ea	33732-0009-35	1.40	3.69
MACK'S DREAMGIRL SOFT FOAM EARPLUGS (McKeon)			
DEV,NA (PINK,CONTOURED)			
20s ea	33732-0000-93	2.28	5.49
MACK'S DREAMWEAVER (McKeon)			
DEV,NA (CONTOUR,W/EARPLUG,BLACK)			
ea	33732-0020-34	3.36	7.99
MACK'S DRY-N-CLEAR EAR DRYING AID (McKeon)			
SOL,OT (EAR DROPS)			
5%-95%, 30 ml	33732-0000-86	2.34	5.99
MACK'S EAR SAVER (McKeon)			
DEV,NA (ORANGE)			
ea	33732-0006-53	5.40	11.99
(WHITE)			
ea	33732-0006-52	5.40	11.99
MACK'S EAR SEALS EARPLUGS (McKeon)			
DEV,NA (W/REMOVABLE CORD)			
2s ea	33732-0000-11	1.86	4.69
MACK'S EARDRYER (McKeon)			
DEV,NA (CORDLESS/RECHARGEABLE)			
ea	33732-0007-47	43.00	69.99
MACK'S EARPHONE ANCHORS (McKeon)			
DEV,NA (2X1 PAIR)			
2s ea	33732-0006-01	1.02	2.49
MACK'S HEAR PLUGS EARPLUGS (McKeon)			
DEV,NA (LARGE,HI-FIDELITY)			
2s ea	33732-0000-15	5.50	13.79
(SMALL,HI-FIDELITY)			
2s ea	33732-0000-14	3.30	7.99
MACK'S LENS WIPES (McKeon)			
DEV,NA (PRE-MOISTENED)			
6s ea	33732-0000-76	0.60	1.49
30s ea	33732-0000-72	1.80	4.49
MACK'S ORIGINAL SAFESOUND FOAM EARPLUGS (McKeon)			
DEV,NA (SOFT FOAM)			
200s ea	33732-0011-09	24.00	84.00
MACK'S PILLOW SOFT EARPLUGS (McKeon)			
DEV,NA (BEIGE,MOLDABLE SILICONE)			
4s ea	33732-0000-08	1.34	3.49
(WHITE,MOLDABLE SILICONE)			
4s ea	33732-0000-05	1.34	3.49
12s ea	33732-0000-07	3.09	6.99
(ORANGE,MOLDABLESILICONE)			
400s ea	33732-0002-06	79.00	150.00
(WHITE,MOLDABLE SILICONE)			
400s ea	33732-0002-00	79.00	150.00
MACK'S PILLOW SOFT KIDS EARPLUGS (McKeon)			
DEV,NA (ORANGE,MOLDABLESILICONE)			
12s ea	33732-0000-10	1.86	4.69
(BRIGHT,MOLDABLESILICONE)			
400s ea	33732-0002-10	64.00	128.00
MACK'S ROCKIN' ROLL-UPS WALLET EARPLUGS (McKeon)			
DEV,NA (4PAIRS,SILKY SMOOTH)			
8s ea	33732-0098-76	1.98	4.99
MACK'S SAFE SOUND FOAM EARPLUGS (McKeon)			
DEV,NA (SOFT FOAM)			
20s ea	33732-0000-09	2.16	5.49
60s ea	33732-0000-39	4.50	11.29
MACK'S SAFE SOUND SLIM FIT EARPLUGS (McKeon)			
DEV,NA (2X3 PAIR,SOFT FOAM)			
6s ea	33732-0009-13	0.96	2.49
(2X5 PAIR,SOFT FOAM)			
10s ea	33732-0009-15	1.34	3.49
MACK'S SAFESOUND SLIM FIT SOFT FOAM EARPLUGS (McKeon)			
DEV,NA (SMALL)			
20s ea	33732-0000-91	2.16	5.49
(SMALL SIZE EARS)			
200s ea	33732-0001-91	24.00	45.00
MACK'S SAFESOUND ULTRA SOFT FOAM EARPLUGS (McKeon)			
DEV,NA (HIGH PERFORMANCE)			
20s ea	33732-0000-92	2.28	5.69
60s ea	33732-0000-32	4.74	11.99
200s ea	33732-0001-92	25.50	48.00
MACK'S SHUT-EYE SHADE SLEEP AID KIT (McKeon)			
DEV,NA, ea	33732-0000-79	3.90	9.75
MACK'S SHUT-EYE SHADE SLEEP MASK (McKeon)			
DEV,NA (PADDED,ADJUSTABLE,BLACK)			
ea	33732-0000-70	3.60	8.99
MACK'S SNORE BLOCKERS (McKeon)			
DEV,NA (SOFT FOAM,12 PAIRS)			
24s ea	33732-0028-10	2.94	6.99
MACK'S SOUNDASLEEP (McKeon)			
DEV,NA (SOFT FOAM,12 PAIRS,BLUE)			
24s ea	33732-0021-40	2.94	6.99
MACK'S ULTRA SAFE SOUND EARPLUGS (McKeon)			
NA (SOFT FOAM,2X3 PAIR)			
6s ea	33732-0009-23	0.99	2.59
(SOFT FOAM,2X5 PAIR)			
10s ea	33732-0009-25	1.40	3.69
MACK'S WAX AWAY EARWAX REMOVAL AID			

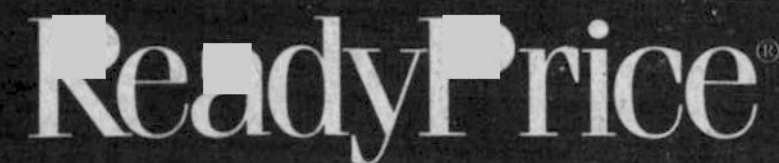

PROD/MFR	HRI, UPC,NDC	AWP	SRP
(McKeon)			
SOL,OT (EAR DROPS)			
6.5%, 15 ml	33732-0000-81	3.18	7.99
MACK'S WAX AWAY EARWAX REMOVAL SYSTEM (McKeon)			
SOL,OT (W/EAR WASHER)			
6.5%, 15 ml	33732-0000-80	4.02	9.89
MAG 200 (Optimox)			
TAB,PO, 150 mg-200 mg,			
120s ea	50520-0006-02	7.50	5.50
MAG DELAY (Major)			
ECT,PO, 110 mg-186.8 mg-64 mg,			
60s ea	00904-7911-52	7.19	
MAG PHOS (Nuage Labs)			
TAB,SL, 125s ea	00634-6020-68	3.05	5.09
MAG-AL (Pharm Assoc Inc)			
SUS,PO (20X10X4;ULTIMATE STRGHT)			
500 mg/5 ml-500 mg/5 ml,			
20 ml 40s UD	00121-4800-20	27.60	
MAG-G (Cypress Pharm)			
TAB,PO, 500 mg, 100s ea	60258-0172-01	9.99	
MAG-ORO (Bio-Tech Pharm)			
CAP,PO, 39.5 mg,			
100s ea	53191-0386-01	12.00	
MAG-OX 400 (Blaine)			
TAB,PO, 400 mg, 60s ea	00165-0022-60	8.70	
100s ea UD	00165-0022-41	22.50	
(SF)			
400 mg, 120s ea	00165-0022-12	13.50	
1000s ea	00165-0022-10	107.70	
(Phys Total Care)			
REPACK			
TAB,PO, 400 mg, 60s ea	54868-3168-00	13.09	
MAG-SR (Cypress Pharm)			
TER,PO (SF)			
535 mg, 60s ea	60258-0173-06	7.99	
MAG-SR PLUS CALCIUM (Cypress Pharm)			
TER,PO (SF)			
380 mg-535 mg,			
60s ea	60258-0174-06	7.99	
MAG-TAB SR (Niche)			
TER,PO, 84 mg, 60s ea	59016-0420-16	15.00	
100s ea	59016-0420-17	22.50	
100s ea UD	59016-0420-19	23.15	
1000s ea	59016-0420-18	181.25	
MAG64 (Rising)			
ECT,PO, 110 mg-186.8 mg-64 mg,			
60s ea	68585-0005-75	6.95	
MAGELLAN SAFETY BLOOD COLLECTOR (Covidien)			
DEV,NA (22GX1")			
300s ea	08080-2251-22	150.25	
MAGGEL (Azur Pharma, Inc.)			
SGL,PO (SOFT GEL)			
600 mg, 60s ea	66663-0211-01	21.46	
MAGIMIN (Key Company)			
TAB,PO (SF)			
80 mg, 100s ea	11694-0138-12	5.00	
1000s ea	11694-0138-15	42.00	
MAGIMIN-FORTE (Key Company)			
TAB,PO, 250 mg, 100s ea	11694-0764-01	5.50	
250s ea	11694-0764-25	12.00	
1000s ea	11694-0764-05	46.00	
MAGINEX (Logan Pharma)			
TAB,PO, 615 mg,			
100s ea UD	09198-0133-03	22.02	
(SUGAR FREE)			
615 mg, 100s ea UD	09198-0133-01	22.23	
MAGINEX DS (Logan Pharma)			
PKT,PO (GRANULES)			
1230 mg/packet,			
30s ea	09198-0134-03	18.90	
MAGLEX (Lex)			
TAB,PO, 500 mg, 100s ea	49523-0004-01	4.95	
1000s ea	49523-0004-10	39.00	
MAGNA-PORT GASTROSTOMY TUBE (Abbott)			
DEV,NA (14 FR)			
ea	70074-0513-59	46.10	
(16 FR)			
ea	70074-0513-61	46.10	
(18 FR)			
ea	70074-0513-63	46.10	
(20 FR)			
ea	70074-0513-65	46.10	
(22 FR)			
ea	70074-0513-67	46.10	
(24 FR)			
ea	70074-0547-39	46.10	
(26FR,W/ LUBRICANT)			
ea	70074-0594-72	46.10	
MAGNA-PORT Y-PORT CONNECTOR (Abbott)			
DEV,NA (14 FR-16 FR)			
ea	70074-0524-41	6.29	
(18 FR-20 FR)			
ea	70074-0524-43	6.29	
MAGNACAPS (Key Company)			
CAP,PO (SF)			
100 mg, 100s ea	11694-0835-01	6.00	
250s ea	11694-0835-25	13.25	
1000s ea	11694-0835-06	49.00	
MAGNEBIND 300 (Nephro-Tech)			
TAB,PO, 250 mg-300 mg,			
150s ea	59528-0508-05	22.00	
MAGNESIA PHOS (Hyland's)			
TAB,PO, 500s ea	54973-1043-01	5.87	9.79
1000s ea	54973-1043-02	10.49	17.49
MAGNESIUM (Carlson,J.R.)			
CAP,PO (PF,SF,CORN-FREE)			
350 mg, 90s ea	88395-0052-21	3.45	6.90
180s ea	88395-0052-22	6.45	12.90
(Mason Vit)			
TAB,PO, 200 mg, 100s ea	11845-0096-11	4.33	
550 mg, 100s ea	11845-0061-71	5.22	
(Medicine Shoppe)			
TAB,PO, 250 mg, 100s ea	49614-0644-78	2.99	2.99
(Nature's Bounty)			
TAB,PO (PF,SF)			
250 mg, 100s ea	74312-0058-30		3.79
(HIGH POTENCY,PF,SF)			
500 mg, 100s ea	74312-0055-35		4.99
(Pharmavite)			
TAB,PO, 250 mg, 100s ea	31604-0012-69	2.11	
MAGNESIUM & B6 (Key Company)			
TAB,PO, 250 mg-125 mg,			
60s ea	11694-0700-01	3.50	
250s ea	11694-0700-02	12.00	
MAGNESIUM ASPARTATE (Miller)			
TAB,PO, 500 mg, 100s ea	17204-0357-40	7.56	12.60
MAGNESIUM CARBONATE (Bio-Tech Pharm)			
CAP,PO, 125 mg, 100s ea	53191-0288-01	7.00	
(Freeda)			
POW,PO, 250 mg/gm,			
448 gm	10432-0224-03	11.97	19.95
MAGNESIUM CHELATED (Freeda)			
TAB,PO (PF,SF,DYE-FREE)			
100 mg, 100s ea	10432-0210-01	5.37	8.95
250s ea	10432-0210-02	10.74	17.90
500s ea	10432-0210-03	18.27	30.45
(Nature's Bounty)			
TAB,PO (PF,SF)			
30 mg, 100s ea	74312-0011-00		6.19
(Rexall)			
TAB,PO (PF,SF)			
100 mg, 100s ea	30768-0000-56	1.46	2.22
(Rugby)			
TAB,PO (PF,SF,DYE-FREE)			
27 mg, 100s ea	00536-6680-01	3.37	
MAGNESIUM CITRATE (Cardinal Health)			
SOL,PO (PRIVATE LABEL,LEMON)			
1.75 gm/30 ml, 296 ml	37205-0362-38	1.24	
(Freeda)			
POW,PO (PURE,SF,GLUTEN-FREE)			
420 mg/2.7 gm,			
454 gm	10432-0360-03	10.05	16.75
TAB,PO (SF,GLUTEN-FREE)			
100 mg, 100s ea	10432-0306-01	5.76	9.60
250s ea	10432-0306-02	11.52	19.20
(Major)			
SOL,PO (1X296ML,LOW SODIUM)			
1.75 gm/30 ml, 296 ml	00904-6042-77	1.92	
(1X296ML,SUCROSE-FREE)			
1.75 gm/30 ml, 296 ml	00904-6043-77	1.92	
(Medicine Shoppe)			
SOL,PO (PASTEURIZED,CHERRY)			
1.75 gm/30 ml, 296 ml	49614-0135-42	1.49	1.49
(Phys Total Care)			
REPACK			
SOL,PO (SF,CHERRY)			
1.75 gm/30 ml,			
300 ml	54868-0010-00	8.01	
MAGNESIUM EC DR (Phys Total Care)			
ECT,PO, 106 mg-186.5 mg-64 mg,			
60s ea	54868-3697-01	21.48	
MAGNESIUM GLUCONATE (Freeda)			
TAB,PO (SF,GLUTEN-FREE)			
27.5 mg, 100s ea	10432-0175-01	4.56	7.60
500s ea	10432-0175-03	15.90	26.50
(RLC)			
TAB,PO, 500 mg, 100s ea	64727-8801-01	13.14	
1000s ea	64727-8801-02	47.94	
MAGNESIUM OXIDE (Basic Vitamins)			
TAB,PO, 250 mg, 100s ea	00761-0283-20	2.00	
(Breckenridge Pharm)			
TAB,PO (SF,GLUTEN-FREE)			
400 mg, 120s ea	51991-0081-36	9.99	
(Cypress Pharm)			
TAB,PO, 400 mg, 120s ea	60258-0171-01	9.99	
(Freeda)			
POW,PO (SF,GLUTEN-FREE)			
390 mg/0.65 gm,			
448 gm	10432-0130-01	11.97	19.95
(Major)			
TAB,PO, 400 mg, 120s ea	00904-5311-18	11.59	
500 mg, 100s ea	00904-4239-60	4.44	
(Qualitest)			
TAB,PO (SF,GLUTEN-FREE)			
400 mg, 120s ea	00603-0209-22	10.84	
420 mg, 100s ea	00603-0213-21	10.84	
(Rising)			
TAB,PO (10X10)			
400 mg, 100s ea UD	68585-0006-41	14.75	
120s ea	68585-0006-12	10.99	
(Rugby)			
TAB,PO (PF,SF,GLUTEN-FREE)			
400 mg, 120s ea	00536-3521-41	7.15	
(McKesson Packaging)			
REPACK			
TAB,PO, 400 mg,			
100s ea UD	63739-0354-10	18.44	
750s ea UD	63739-0354-01	138.28	
(Phys Total Care)			
REPACK			
TAB,PO, 400 mg, 120s ea	54868-5110-00	23.76	
(Southwood)			
REPACK			
TAB,PO, 400 mg, 30s ea	58016-0448-30	3.42	
60s ea	58016-0448-60	6.83	
90s ea	58016-0448-90	10.25	
100s ea	58016-0448-00	11.38	
120s ea	58016-0448-02	13.66	
MAGONATE (Fleming)			
TAB,PO, 87.5 mg-27 mg-66 mg,			
100s ea	00256-0172-01		20.65
MAGONATE MAGNESIUM SUPPLEMENT (Fleming)			
SOL,PO, 54 mg/5 ml,			
355 ml	00256-0184-07		14.99
MAGTRATE (Mission)			
TAB,PO, 500 mg, 100s ea	00178-0299-01	6.56	
MAJOR COMFORT LANCETS (Major)			
DEV,NA, 200s ea	00904-4375-25	12.95	
MAJOR-GESIC (Major)			
TAB,PO, 325 mg-30 mg,			
1000s ea	00904-0392-80	40.43	
MALIC B6 (Bio-Tech Pharm)			
CAP,PO, 103 mg-41 mg,			
100s ea	53191-0222-01	8.00	
MALPOTANE (Health Products Corp)			
TAB,PO, 60s ea	39686-0012-65	9.97	24.50
MALT EXTRACT W/HEMOGLOBIN (Lex)			
SYR,PO (CHERRY)			
45 ml	58537-0070-12	2.50	
MAMMARY (Miller)			
TAB,PO, 150 mg, 100s ea	17204-0510-40	8.52	13.50
MANDELAY MAXIMUM STRENGTH (Majestic Drug)			
GEL,TP, 7.5%, 28.35 gm	10705-0800-77	2.25	5.99
MANGANESE ASPARTATE (Miller)			
TAB,PO, 25 mg, 100s ea	17204-0358-40	10.08	16.80

PROD/MFR	HRI, UPC,NDC	AWP	SRP
MANGANESE CHELATED (Freeda)			
TAB,PO (PF,SF,DYE-FREE)			
50 mg, 100s ea	10432-0236-01	5.37	8.95
MANGANESE GLUCONATE (Freeda)			
PO, 5.7 mg, 100s ea	10432-0010-01	4.17	6.95
(Mason Vit)			
TAB,PO, 600 mg, 100s ea	11845-0061-61	4.22	
MANGIMIN (Key Company)			
TAB,PO (SF)			
10 mg, 100s ea	11694-0137-12	5.00	
1000s ea	11694-0137-15	42.00	
MANIFOLD III-SECURE LOCK (Abbott Hosp)			
DEV,NA (15")			
50s ea	00074-6462-01	208.80	
MANLY MACHOVITES (Neurovites)			
TAB,PO, 126s ea	93595-2030-01	10.50	
MANN EMOLLIENT (Mann)			
OIN,TP, 100 gm	99709-0100-07	10.35	15.50
MANTECA DE UBRE "LA LECHERITA" (Flar Medicine)			
OIN,TP, 70 gm	53154-0175-07	2.00	
MAOX (Manne)			
TAB,PO, 420 mg, 100s ea	10706-0837-00	3.55	
250s ea	10706-0837-01	9.08	
1000s ea	10706-0837-02	35.39	
MAPAP (Major)			
CTB,PO (RAPID TABS,BUBBLE GUM)			
80 mg, 30s ea	00904-5751-46	2.95	
(BUBBLE GUM,RAPID TABS)			
160 mg, 24s ea	00904-5754-24	4.05	
ELI,PO (BOXED,CHERRY)			
160 mg/5 ml, 120 ml	00904-1985-20	4.79	
(CHERRY)			
160 mg/5 ml, 120 ml	00904-1985-00	4.79	
SGL,PO (ASPIRIN-FREE,GELCAP)			
500 mg, 50s ea	00904-5816-51	3.29	
100s ea	00904-5816-60	5.69	
SYR,PO (AF,ASPIRIN-FREE,CHERRY)			
160 mg/5 ml, 480 ml	00904-1985-16	5.49	
TAB,PO (12X2)			
325 mg, 24s ea	00904-1982-02	1.13	
(ASPIRIN-FREE)			
325 mg, 50s ea	00904-1982-51	3.22	
100s ea	00904-1982-60	6.44	
(10X10)			
325 mg, 100s ea UD	00904-1982-61	6.54	
(BOXED)			
325 mg, 100s ea	00904-1982-59	6.44	
1000s ea	00904-1982-80	18.50	
500 mg, 100s ea	00904-1988-60	8.03	
(CAPLET)			
500 mg, 100s ea	00904-1983-60	5.95	
1000s ea	00904-1983-80	26.95	
MAPAP ARTHRITIS PAIN (Major)			
TER,PO (CAPLET)			
650 mg, 100s ea	00904-5769-60	7.01	
MAPAP CHILDREN'S (Major)			
CTB,PO (FRUIT)			
80 mg, 30s ea	00904-5256-46	2.25	
SUS,PO (AF,CHERRY)			
160 mg/5 ml, 120 ml	00904-5116-20	2.89	
MAPAP EXTRA STRENGTH (Major)			
CAP,PO (#100/BOXED)			
500 mg, 100s ea	00904-1987-59	6.99	
(#100/UNBOXED)			
500 mg, 100s ea	00904-1987-60	6.99	
TAB,PO (CAPLET)			
500 mg, 24s ea	00904-1983-24	1.50	
50s ea	00904-1983-51	2.90	
(10X10)			
500 mg, 100s ea UD	00904-1988-61	7.96	
(CAPLET)			
500 mg, 100s ea	00904-1983-59	4.50	
100s ea	00904-1988-59	8.03	
175s ea	00904-1983-94	7.10	
500s ea	00904-1983-40	13.99	
1000s ea	00904-1988-80	25.95	
MAPAP EXTRA STRENGTH ACETAMINOPHEN (Major)			
SOL,PO (RAPID BURST,CHERRY)			
500 mg/15 ml, 237 ml	00904-5847-09	4.19	
MAPAP INFANTS' (Major)			
SUS,PO (AF,CHERRY,DROPS)			
80 mg/0.8 ml, 15 ml	00904-5255-35	3.91	
30 ml	00904-5255-30	3.75	
MAPAP MULTI-SYMPTOM COLD FORMULA (Major)			
TAB,PO (DAYTIME,NON-DROWSY)			
325 mg-10 mg-5 mg,			
24s ea	00904-5786-24	2.65	
MAPAP SINUS CONGESTION AND PAIN (Major)			
TAB,PO (MAX STRENGTH,DAYTIME)			
325 mg-5 mg,			
24s ea	00904-5783-24	3.96	
MAPAP-PM (Major)			
TAB,PO, 500 mg-25 mg,			
50s ea	00904-7651-51	3.55	
MAPLE MELTS (Green Turtle)			
CTB,PO, 90s ea	59074-0800-01	14.40	23.99
MAPO (Merz)			
OIL,TP, 480 ml	02596-0005-16	14.95	
MAR-COF BP (Marnel)			
SOL,PO (1X473ML,AF,SF)			
473 ml	00682-0480-16		54.80
MAR-COF CG EXPECTORANT (Marnel)			
SOL,PO (1X473ML,AF,SUCROSE-FREE)			
7.5 mg/5 ml-225 mg/5 ml,			
473 ml	00682-0475-16	51.03	
MAREPA (A. G. Marin)			
SGL,PO (SOFTGEL)			
1200 mg, 60s ea	12539-0400-01	26.10	
MARJORAM COMPOUND (Weleda)			
LIQ,PO, 50 ml	55946-0310-15	7.20	
MASON NATURAL ADVANCED TART CHERRY (Mason Vit)			
CAP,PO (PRIVATE LABEL)			
90s ea	11845-0150-09	14.44	
MASON NATURAL B-12 (Mason Vit)			
TAB,SL (WHEAT-FREE)			
5000 mcg, 30s ea	11845-0148-18	7.22	
MASON NATURAL BIOTIN PLUS (Mason Vit)			
TAB,PO (PF,CORN-FREE,DAIRY-FREE)			
60s ea	11845-0148-55	7.78	
MASON NATURAL BODYSHAPERS DIETER'S DETOX (Mason Vit)			
CAP,PO (PF,SF,CORN-FREE)			
60s ea	11845-0149-65	16.67	
MASON NATURAL BODYSHAPERS SOUTH AFRICAN HOODIA (Mason Vit)			
CAP,PO (CURBAPPTITE,STOPCRVINGS)			
250 mg, 60s ea	11845-0145-45	22.11	
MASON NATURAL CINNAMON (Mason Vit)			
CAP,PO (PF,CORN-FREE,DAIRY-FREE)			
500 mg, 100s ea	11845-0146-51	7.77	
MASON NATURAL CO Q-10 (Mason Vit)			
SGL,PO (PRIVATE LABEL,SOFTGEL)			
50 mg, 30s ea	11845-0146-08	17.66	
75 mg, 30s ea	11845-0146-18	22.11	
(FOR A HEALTHY HEART,PF)			
100 mg, 60s ea	11845-0131-95	57.15	
MASON NATURAL COLLAGEN (Mason Pharm)			
CAP,PO (PF,CORN-FREE,DAIRY-FREE)			
125 mg-740 mg, 120s ea	11845-0145-62	19.88	
MASON NATURAL COLLAGEN BEAUTY (Mason Vit)			
CRE,TP (PRIVATE LABEL)			
57 gm	11845-0147-57	8.77	
MASON NATURAL CORTISURE (Mason Pharm)			
CAP,PO (ANTI-STRESS WEIGHT LOSS)			
100 mg-150 mg-50 mcg,			
60s ea	11845-0144-95	22.20	
MASON NATURAL D2000 (Mason Vit)			
SGL,PO (ULTRA STRENGTH D3)			
2000 iu, 60s ea	11845-0150-15	11.66	
MASON NATURAL DAILY MULTIPLE VITAMINS WITH IRON (Mason Vit)			
TAB,PO (SF)			
100s ea	11845-0000-01	13.31	
MASON NATURAL DONG QUAI (Mason Vit)			
CAP,PO (WHEAT-FREE)			
500 mg, 60s ea	11845-0113-55	7.22	
MASON NATURAL DRINKIN' BUDDY (Mason Pharm)			
TAB,PO (PF,SF,FRAGRANCE-FREE)			
350 mg-650 mg,			
40s ea	11845-0144-44	4.44	
MASON NATURAL EAR HEALTH FORMULA (Mason Vit)			
TAB,PO (CAPLET)			
100s ea	11845-0149-41	18.89	14.99
MASON NATURAL FERROUS SULFATE (Mason Vit)			
TAB,PO (SF,PRIVATE LABEL)			
325 mg, 100s ea	11845-0149-71	4.99	
MASON NATURAL FRUIT & VEGETABLE DAILY (Mason Vit)			
SGL,PO (PF,SF,CORN-FREE)			
30s ea	11845-0148-68	13.22	
MASON NATURAL GLUCOSAMINE CHONDROITIN (Mason Vit)			
CAP,PO (FAST ACTING,PF,SF)			
300 mg-375 mg-2 mg-50 mg,			
90s ea	11845-0145-39	33.22	
MASON NATURAL GLUCOSAMINE CHONDROITIN 1500 COMPLEX (Mason Vit)			
CAP,PO (80 FREE,MAX STRENGTH,PF)			
280s ea	11845-0130-38	64.33	
MASON NATURAL GREEN TEA SLIM (Mason Vit)			
TAB,PO (SF,CORN-FREE,DAIRY-FREE)			
30s ea	11845-0143-58	4.44	
MASON NATURAL HOODIA PLUS (Mason Vit)			
CAP,PO (750 PLUSEGCG,WHEAT-FREE)			
60s ea	11845-0149-05	33.22	
MASON NATURAL INNER BEAUTY FORMULA (Mason Vit)			
CAP,PO (BODY,HAIR,SKIN&NAILS,PF)			
90s ea	11845-0144-09	19.88	
MASON NATURAL L-TRYPTOPHAN SLEEP FORMULA (Mason Vit)			
CAP,PO (PF,SF,CORN-FREE)			
500 mg, 60s ea	11845-0149-35	19.88	
MASON NATURAL LIQUITHIN (Mason Vit)			
SGL,PO (PROMOTES FAT BREAKDOWN)			
50s ea	11845-0143-49	4.44	
MASON NATURAL LUTEIN (Mason Vit)			
SGL,PO (EXTRASTRGTH,ANTIOXIDANT)			
20 mg, 30s ea	11845-0140-28	17.75	
MASON NATURAL MEN'S DAILY FORMULA (Mason Vit)			
CAP,PO (WHEAT-FREE)			
100s ea	11845-0147-81	10.99	7.59
MASON NATURAL NIACIN (Mason Vit)			
CAP,PO (PRIVATE LABEL)			
141 mg-500 mg,			
60s ea	11845-0149-95	9.67	
MASON NATURAL OMEGA-3 FISH OIL (Mason Vit)			
SGL,PO (SF,CHOLESTEROL-FREE)			
1000 mg-1 iu, 200s ea	11845-0122-30	17.66	
(PF,SF,LACTOSE-FREE)			
1200 mg, 120s ea	11845-0149-22	16.79	
MASON NATURAL OMEGA-3 SALMON OIL (Mason Vit)			
SGL,PO (PF,SF,LACTOSE-FREE)			
1000 mg, 120s ea	11845-0148-82	13.88	
MASON NATURAL OMEGA-3-6-9 (Mason Vit)			
SGL,PO (PRIVATE LABEL,SOFTGEL)			
60s ea	11845-0150-35	13.22	
MASON NATURAL OMEGA-3-6-9 FISH OIL (Mason Vit)			
SGL,PO (NO BURP,SF,LACTOSE-FREE)			
1000 mg-1 iu, 100s ea	11845-0149-51	14.33	
MASON NATURAL PROSTATE THERAPY COMPLEX (Mason Vit)			
SGL,PO (PF,SF,CORN-FREE)			
60s ea	11845-0144-35	24.33	
MASON NATURAL RED WINE EXTRACT PLUS (Mason Vit)			
CAP,PO (PF,SF,CORN-FREE)			
60 mg-200 mg,			
60s ea	11845-0148-95	11.00	
MASON NATURAL RED YEAST RICE 1200 (Mason Vit)			
CAP,PO (PRIVATE LABEL)			
600 mg, 120s ea	11845-0146-62	18.64	
MASON NATURAL RELAX & SLEEP (Mason Vit)			
TAB,PO (PRIVATE LABEL)			
90s ea	11845-0149-89	7.77	
MASON NATURAL SMOKE NO MORE (Mason Pharm)			
TAB,PO (PF,SF,CORN-FREE)			
100s ea	11845-0144-61	4.44	
MASON NATURAL SUPER MULTIPLE (Mason Vit)			
CAP,PO (PF,SF,CORN-FREE)			
60s ea	11845-0146-45	9.88	

PROD/MFR HRI, UPC,NDC AWP SRP

MASON NATURAL SUPER OMEGA-3 (Mason Vit)
SGL,PO (PF,SF,CHOLESTEROL-FREE)
1000 mg, 30s ea **11845-0146-38** 7.22

MASON NATURAL ULTRA COLLAGEN (Mason Vit)
CAP,PO (PF,SF,CORN-FREE)
100s ea............ **11845-0149-11** 26.55

MASON NATURAL VITAMIN D (Mason Vit)
SGL,PO (WHEAT-FREE)
1000 iu, 60s ea....... **11845-0147-75** 7.77 5.39

MASON NATURAL VITATRUM (Mason Vit)
CTB,PO (WHEAT-FREE)
50s ea............... **11845-0148-39** 5.53

MASON REMEDIES DOCUSATE SODIUM WITH SENNOSIDES (Mason Vit)
TAB,PO (PRIVATE LABEL)
50 mg-8.6 mg, 100s ea **11845-0148-71** 4.33

MASONATAL (Mason Vit)
TAB,PO (PF,SF)
100s ea............ **11845-0127-91** 10.00

MASOPHEN (Mason Vit)
TAB,PO, 325 mg, 100s ea.. **11845-0596-01** 2.78

MASSENGILL DOUCHE (Glaxo)
SOL,VG (BABY PWD, TWIN, 2X177ML)
177 ml 2s........... **53100-0515-90** 1.54
(FLOWER, TWIN, 2X177ML)
177 ml 2s........... **53100-0515-50** 1.54
(EXTRA MILD)
180 ml **53100-0520-00** 1.04
(EXTRA CLEANSING,TWIN)
180 ml 2s........... **53100-0520-62** 1.54
(EXTRA MILD,TWIN)
180 ml 2s........... **53100-0520-50** 1.54
(BABY POWDER,4-PACK)
180 ml 4s........... **53100-0516-72** 2.41
(EXTRA CLEANSING,4-PACK)
180 ml 4s........... **53100-0520-25** 2.41
(EXTRA MILD,4-PACK)
180 ml 4s........... **53100-0520-65** 2.41
(FLOWER,4-PACK)
180 ml 4s........... **53100-0516-01** 2.41
(WASH)
240 ml **53100-0001-10** 2.25

MASSENGILL TOWELETTES (Glaxo)
PAD,TP (BABY POWDER,SOAP-FREE)
16s ea.............. **53100-0540-00** 1.58

MASTISOL (Ferndale)
LIQ,TP (VIAL)
0.666 ml 48s......... **00496-0523-48** 127.56
15 ml UD........... **00496-0523-15** 12.55
60 ml **00496-0523-06** 32.46
SPR,TP, 15 ml **00496-0523-16** 13.42

MAXAM (Med-Derm)
LOT,TP (PF)
480 ml **45565-0800-17** 7.81

MAXEPA (Basic Vitamins)
SGL,PO (SOFTGEL)
1000 mg, 100s ea **00761-0237-20** 5.40

(Mason Vit)
CAP,PO, 5 mg-120 mg-180 mg,
100s ea........... **11845-0079-21** 12.78
SGL,PO (SF,SOFTGEL)
1000 mg, 50s ea **11845-0125-10** 6.89
90s ea............ **11845-0125-19** 11.44

MAXI FAT BURNING SYSTEM (Action Labs)
TAB,PO (SF)
60s ea.............. **24675-0427-61** 7.49 14.99
120s ea **24675-0427-21** 13.99 27.99

MAXI VISION (MedOp)
CAP,PO (WHOLE BODY FORMULA)
120s ea............. **53012-0015-32** 26.95

MAXICARE DISPOSABLE BELTLESS UNDERGARMENTS (Covidien)
DEV,NA (SINGLE USE)
120s ea............ **08080-1810-30** 47.08

MAXICARE DISPOSABLE UNDERPADS (Covidien)
DEV,NA (36"X36",4X12)
48s ea............. **08080-0968-00** 36.07
(30"X36")
50s ea............. **08080-9580-10** 26.59
100s ea **08080-9480-00** 50.33

MAXICHLOR DM (MCR American)
TAB,PO, 4 mg-20 mg,
100s ea........... **58605-0448-01** 103.21

MAXICHLOR PEH (MCR American)
TAB,PO, 4 mg-10 mg,
100s ea......... **58605-0444-01** 105.21

MAXICHLOR PEH DM (MCR American)
TAB,PO, 4 mg-20 mg-10 mg,
100s ea........... **58605-0445-01** 108.60

MAXICHLOR PSE (MCR American)
TAB,PO, 4 mg-60 mg,
100s ea........... **58605-0442-01** 109.66

MAXICHLOR PSE DM (MCR American)
TAB,PO, 4 mg-20 mg-60 mg,
100s ea........... **58605-0443-01** 111.71

MAXIFED (MCR American)
TAB,PO, 400 mg-60 mg,
100s ea........... **58605-0406-01** 115.63

MAXIFED DM (MCR American)
TAB,PO, 20 mg-400 mg-40 mg,
100s ea........... **58605-0409-01** 117.39

MAXIFED DMX (MCR American)
PO, 20 mg-400 mg-60 mg,
100s ea........... **58605-0407-01** 118.86

(Phys Total Care)
REPACK
TAB,PO, 20 mg-400 mg-60 mg,
30s ea............ **54868-6084-00** 45.52

MAXIFED-G (MCR American)
TAB,PO, 400 mg-40 mg,
100s ea........... **58605-0408-01** 114.97

(Phys Total Care)
REPACK
TAB,PO, 400 mg-40 mg,
20s ea............ **54868-6068-00** 31.18

(Stat Rx)
REPACK
TAB,PO, 400 mg-40 mg,
20s ea............ **16590-0639-20** 32.50

MAXIFLO DISPOSABLE UNDERPADS (Covidien)
DEV,NA (30"X36",10X6)
60s ea............. **08080-0984-00** 58.38
(23"X36",6X12)
72s ea.............. **08080-0988-00** 59.68

MAXIFLU DM (MCR American)
TAB,PO, 100s ea.......... **58605-0432-01** 110.84

MAXILUBE (Mission)
GEL,VG, 90 gm **00178-0301-03** 2.25
150 gm **01780-0301-05** 3.00

MAXIMA BLOOD GLUCOSE MONITORING SYSTEM (US DIAGNOSTICS, INC)
DEV,NA, ea.............. **08463-4103-01** 45.00

MAXIMA BLOOD GLUCOSE TEST STRIPS (US DIAGNOSTICS, INC)
DEV,NA, 50s ea **08463-4203-50** 42.50

MAXIMA DISPOSABLE UNDERPADS (Covidien)
DEV,NA (23"X36",10X10)
100s ea........... **08080-9820-10** 39.57

MAXIMA NORMAL CONTROL SOLUTION (US DIAGNOSTICS, INC)
DEV,NA, ea.............. **08463-4005-01** 8.61

MAXIMUM D3 (Propharma)
CAP,PO, 10000 iu, 5s ea... **66594-0999-05** 3.88

MAXIMUM ENERGY (Mason Vit)
TAB,PO (PF,SF)
60s ea.............. **11845-0121-85** 13.22

MAXIPHEN (MCR American)
TAB,PO, 400 mg-10 mg,
100s ea........... **58605-0422-01** 103.93

MAXIPHEN DM (MCR American)
TAB,PO, 20 mg-400 mg-10 mg,
100s ea........... **58605-0423-01** 108.65

MAXORB EXTRA ALGINATE (Medline)
DEV,NA (2"X2")
ea.................. **53329-0561-39** 2.48
(4"X4")
ea.................. **53329-0562-40** 4.14
(4"X8")
ea.................. **53329-0563-37** 9.51
(ROPE 12")
ea.................. **53329-0560-49** 7.38

MAXXUS LATEX SURGICAL GLOVES (J&J Medical)
DEV,NA (STERILE,25 PR,SZ 5.5)
50s ea.............. **56091-0505-51** 56.16
(STERILE,25 PR,SZ 6.5)
50s ea.............. **56091-0050-65** 56.16
(STERILE,25 PR,SZ 6)
50s ea.............. **56091-0050-60** 56.16
(STERILE,25 PR,SZ 8.5)
50s ea.............. **56091-0050-85** 56.16
(STERILE,25 PR,SZ 8)
50s ea.............. **56091-0050-80** 56.16
(STERILE,25 PR,SZ 9)
50s ea.............. **56091-0050-90** 56.16
(STERILE,50 PR,SZ 7.5)
50s ea.............. **56091-0050-75** 56.16
(STERILE,50 PR,SZ 7)
50s ea.............. **56091-0050-70** 56.16

MAXXUS PF LATEX SURGICAL GLOVES (J&J Medical)
DEV,NA (STERILE,25 PR,SZ 5.5)
50s ea.............. **56091-0039-55** 107.02
(STERILE,25 PR,SZ 6.5)
50s ea.............. **56091-0039-65** 107.02
(STERILE,25 PR,SZ 6)
50s ea.............. **56091-0039-60** 107.02
(STERILE,25 PR,SZ 7.5)
50s ea.............. **56091-0039-75** 107.02
(STERILE,25 PR,SZ 7)
50s ea.............. **56091-0039-70** 107.02
(STERILE,25 PR,SZ 8.5)
50s ea.............. **56091-0039-85** 107.02
(STERILE,25 PR,SZ 8)
50s ea.............. **56091-0039-80** 107.02
(STERILE,25 PR,SZ 9)
50s ea.............. **56091-0039-90** 107.02

MCT PRO-CAL (VITAFLO, LLC)
POW,PO (16GM)
25s ea.............. **50600-0502-36** 62.50 75.00

MECHOLYL (Gordon)
OIN,TP, 0.25%, 120 gm.... **10481-1049-02** 33.75

MECLIZINE (Nucare Pharm)
REPACK
CTB,PO, 25 mg, 30s ea.... **68071-0763-30** 22.84
60s ea **68071-0763-60** 45.68

MECLIZINE HCL (Rugby)
TAB,PO (USP,CAPLET)
12.5 mg, 100s ea..... **00536-3985-01** 3.59

(GSMS)
REPACK
TAB,PO (UNIT OF USE)
25 mg, 90s ea........ **60429-0608-90** 14.70
120s ea **60429-0608-12** 18.60

(Pharma Pac)
REPACK
TAB,PO (CAPLET)
12.5 mg, 30s ea...... **52959-0995-30** 12.20

MECLIZINE HYDROCHLORIDE (Rugby)
TAB,PO (CAPLET)
12.5 mg, 1000s ea.... **00536-3985-10** 26.90

MEDEBRAL (Med Prods Panamer)
CAP,PO, 60s ea **00576-0254-60** 9.60

MEDENT-PEI (SJ)
TAB,PO, 400 mg-10 mg,
100s ea........... **24839-0340-01** 79.81

MEDERMA (Merz)
CRE,TP (1X20GM)
3%-10%-6%, 20 gm.. **02593-0192-82** 16.64
(1X50GM)
3%-10%-6%, 50 gm.. **02593-0447-25** 29.56
GEL,TP (1X20GM)
20 gm.............. **02590-0303-20** 15.83
50 gm............ **02590-0303-50** 24.60

(A-S Medication)
REPACK
GEL,TP, 50 gm........... **54569-4636-00** 24.60

MEDERMA FOR KIDS (Merz)
GEL,TP (SCENTED)
20 gm **02590-0309-21** 15.23

MEDFIX DRESSING RETENTION SHEET (Medline)
DEV,NA (2"X11YDS)
ea.................. **53329-0552-51** 4.18
(4"X11YDS)
ea.................. **53329-0552-52** 15.45
(6"X11YDS)
ea.................. **53329-0552-53** 10.00

MEDFIX EZ DRESSING RETENTION ROLL (Medline)
DEV,NA (2"X11YRDS)
ea.................. **08327-0506-09** 10.47
(2"X2YDS)
12s ea.............. **08327-0517-09** 22.27
(4"X11YDS)
12s ea.............. **08327-0514-09** 149.38
(4"X2YDS)
12s ea.............. **08327-0518-09** 34.11
(6"X11YDS)
12s ea.............. **08327-0515-09** 225.58
(6"X2YDS)
12s ea.............. **08327-0519-09** 65.82

PROD/MFR	HRI, UPC,NDC	AWP	SRP
MEDI-COOLER (Technological Investments)			
DEV,NA, ea	08605-0102-02	15.63	
MEDI-CORTISONE MAXIMUM STRENGTH (Medicine Shoppe)			
CRE,TP, 1%, 30 gm	49614-0404-10	2.99	2.99
MEDI-FIRST ANTACID (Medique)			
CTB,PO (50X2,PRIVATE LABEL) 420 mg, 100s ea UD	47682-0802-33	3.64	
(125X2,PRIVATE LABEL) 420 mg, 250s ea UD	47682-0802-48	7.81	
(250X2,PRIVATE LABEL) 420 mg, 500s ea UD	47682-0802-13	14.29	
MEDI-FIRST ASPIRIN (Medique)			
TAB,PO (50X2,PRIVATE LABEL) 325 mg, 100s ea UD	47682-0805-33	3.09	
(125X2,PRIVATE LABEL) 325 mg, 250s ea UD	47682-0805-48	6.76	
(250X2,PRIVATE LABEL) 325 mg, 500s ea UD	47682-0805-13	11.81	
MEDI-FIRST CHERRY COUGH DROPS (Medique)			
LOZ,MM (PRIVATE LABEL,CHERRY) 7.6 mg, 50s ea	47682-0815-50	3.16	
125s ea	47682-0815-25	6.98	
MEDI-FIRST CRAMP (Medique)			
TAB,PO (MICRO-COATED,50X2) 325 mg-25 mg, 100s ea UD	47682-0810-33	5.00	
(125X2,PRIVATE LABEL) 325 mg-25 mg, 250s ea UD	47682-0810-48	10.10	
(250X2,PRIVATE LABEL) 325 mg-25 mg, 500s ea UD	47682-0810-13	19.96	
MEDI-FIRST HYDROCORTISONE (Medique)			
CRE,TP (PRIVATE LABEL) 1%, 6s ea UD	47682-0243-69	1.79	
25s ea UD	47682-0211-73	3.78	
144s ea UD	47682-0211-35	14.61	
MEDI-FIRST IBUPROFEN (Medique)			
TAB,PO (4X2,PRIVATE LABEL) 200 mg, 8s ea UD	47682-0808-30	0.84	
(50X2 USP,PRIVATE LABEL) 200 mg, 100s ea UD	47682-0808-33	5.54	
(125X2,PRIVATE LABEL) 200 mg, 250s ea UD	47682-0808-48	13.26	
(250X2,PRIVATE LABEL) 200 mg, 500s ea UD	47682-0808-13	22.81	
MEDI-FIRST NON-ASPIRIN (Medique)			
TAB,PO (50X2,PRIVATE LABEL) 325 mg, 100s ea UD	47682-0803-33	3.70	
(125X2,PRIVATE LABEL) 325 mg, 250s ea UD	47682-0803-48	7.91	
(250X2,PRIVATE LABEL) 325 mg, 500s ea UD	47682-0803-13	13.29	
(EXTRA-STRENGTH,50X2) 500 mg, 100s ea UD	47682-0804-33	4.20	
(EXTRA-STRENGTH,125X2) 500 mg, 250s ea UD	47682-0804-48	9.41	
(EXTRA-STRENGTH,250X2) 500 mg, 500s ea UD	47682-0804-13	18.36	
MEDI-FIRST NON-PSEUDO COLD RELIEF (Medique)			
TAB,PO (50X2,PRIVATE LABEL) 325 mg-15 mg-200 mg-5 mg, 100s ea UD	47682-0822-33	5.96	
(125X2,PRIVATE LABEL) 325 mg-15 mg-200 mg-5 mg, 250s ea UD	47682-0822-48	14.01	
(250X2,PRIVATE LABEL) 325 mg-15 mg-200 mg-5 mg, 500s ea UD	47682-0822-13	27.14	
MEDI-FIRST NON-PSEUDO SINUS DECONGESTANT (Medique)			
TAB,PO (COATED) 10 mg, 24s ea UD	47682-0809-64	1.86	
(2X50,COATED) 10 mg, 100s ea UD	47682-0809-33	6.09	
(2X125,COATED) 10 mg, 250s ea UD	47682-0809-48	12.90	
(2X250,COATED) 10 mg, 500s ea UD	47682-0809-13	24.04	
MEDI-FIRST NON-PSEUDO SINUS PAIN & PRESSURE (Medique)			
TAB,PO (50X2,PRIVATE LABEL) 500 mg-5 mg, 100s ea UD	47682-0819-33	6.09	
(125X2,PRIVATE LABEL) 500 mg-5 mg, 250s ea UD	47682-0819-48	11.69	
(250X2,PRIVATE LABEL) 500 mg-5 mg, 500s ea UD	47682-0819-13	21.21	
MEDI-FIRST PAIN RELIEF (Medique)			
TAB,PO (EXTRA-STRENGTH,50X2) 100s ea UD	47682-0811-33	3.80	
(EXTRA-STRENGTH,125X2) 250s ea UD	47682-0811-48	8.16	
(EXTRA-STRENGTH,250X2) 500s ea UD	47682-0811-13	16.09	
MEDI-FIRST SORE THROAT RELIEF (Medique)			
LOZ,MM (50X2,PRIVATE LABEL) 10 mg-0.5 mg, 100s ea UD	47682-0812-33	4.91	
(125X2,PRIVATE LABEL) 10 mg-0.5 mg, 250s ea UD	47682-0812-48	10.49	
(250X2,PRIVATE LABEL) 10 mg-0.5 mg, 500s ea UD	47682-0812-13	18.99	
MEDI-FIRST TRI-BUFFERED ASPIRIN (Medique)			
TAB,PO (50X2,PRIVATE LABEL) 325 mg, 100s ea UD	47682-0806-33	3.50	
(125X2,PRIVATE LABEL) 325 mg, 250s ea UD	47682-0806-48	8.04	
(250X2,PRIVATE LABEL) 325 mg, 500s ea UD	47682-0806-13	14.91	
MEDI-FRIDGE IIX (Technological Investments)			
DEV,NA (MF-MRIIX, PORTABLE) ea	08605-0100-01	62.50	
MEDI-JECTOR VISION (Antares Pharma)			
DEV,NA (NEEDLE-FREE INJECTOR) ea	55948-0123-10	335.00	335.00
MEDI-LANCE LANCETS (Medicore)			
DEV,NA, 100s ea	32671-0201-00	12.00	8.95
200s ea	32671-0202-00	12.00	12.95
MEDI-LYTE (Medique)			
TAB,PO (2X50,MICRO-COATED) 18 mg-9 mg-40 mg, 100s ea UD	47682-0030-33	5.19	
(2X250,MICRO-COATED) 18 mg-9 mg-40 mg, 500s ea UD	47682-0030-13	21.11	
MEDI-MECLIZINE (Medique)			
TAB,PO (50X2) 25 mg, 100s ea UD	47682-0479-33	9.91	
(PACKET,500X2) 25 mg, 1000s ea	47682-0479-15	53.30	
MEDI-PADS (Major)			
PAD,TP, 100s ea	00904-5059-60	5.31	
MEDI-PHENYL (Medique)			
TAB,PO (50X2,MICRO-COATED) 5 mg, 100s ea UD	47682-0205-33	7.05	
(250X2,MICRO-COATED) 5 mg, 500s ea UD	47682-0205-13	23.84	
MEDI-PROFEN (Medicine Shoppe)			
TAB,PO, 200 mg, 100s ea	49614-0116-78	6.29	6.29
(CAPLET) 200 mg, 100s ea	49614-0647-78	6.29	6.29
250s ea	49614-0488-85	10.49	10.49
MEDI-SELTZER (Medique)			
TAB,PO (18X2) 324 mg, 36s ea UD	47682-0135-20	5.41	
(36X2) 324 mg, 72s ea UD	47682-0135-24	9.94	
MEDICAINE (Alexander, James)			
SWA,TP, 20%-0.95%, 10s ea	46414-2040-03	2.11	3.69
MEDICATED BODY POWDER (Major)			
POW,TP, 300 gm	00904-5098-77	5.55	
MEDICHOICE SAFETY LANCET (Owens & Minor, Inc.)			
DEV,NA (DUAL USE,PRE-SET) 200s ea	08214-5047-12	40.00	
(EXTRA,PRIVATE LABEL) 200s ea	08214-5017-12	38.50	
(LOW FLOW,PRE-SET) 200s ea	08214-5027-12	40.00	
(MEDIUM FLOW,PRE-SET) 200s ea	08214-5037-12	40.00	
(MODERATE FLOW,PRE-SET) 200s ea	08214-5067-12	42.00	
(NORMAL,PRIVATE LABEL) 200s ea	08214-5007-12	38.50	
MEDICIDIN-D (Medique)			
TAB,PO (12X2,MICRO-COATED) 325 mg-2 mg-5 mg, 24s ea UD	47682-0120-64	1.69	
(50X2,MICRO-COATED) 325 mg-2 mg-5 mg, 100s ea UD	47682-0120-33	8.29	
(100X2,MICRO-COATED) 325 mg-2 mg-5 mg, 200s ea UD	47682-0120-47	14.95	
(250X2,MICRO-COATED) 325 mg-2 mg-5 mg, 500s ea UD	47682-0120-13	31.01	
MEDICINE SHOPPE 12 HR DECONGESTANT (Medicine Shoppe)			
TER,PO (MAX STRENGTH,NON-DROWSY) 120 mg, 10s ea	49614-0433-62	3.79	3.69
MEDICINE SHOPPE EAR WAX REMOVAL SYSTEM (Medicine Shoppe)			
SOL,OT, 6.5%, 15 ml	49614-0148-05	4.69	
MEDICINE SHOPPE GLUCOSE (Can-Am Care)			
CTB,PO (QUICK DISSOLVE) 4 gm, 40s ea	38396-0560-12	4.33	
MEDICINE SHOPPE GLUCOSE TABLETS (Can-Am Care)			
PO (CAFFEINE-FREE) 4 gm, 10s ea	38396-0501-12	1.59	
10s ea	38396-0502-12	1.59	
50s ea	38396-0541-12	5.99	
50s ea	38396-0542-12	5.99	
MEDICINE SHOPPE INSULIN SYRINGES (Can-Am Care)			
DEV,NA (29G,1/2CC,1/2") 100s ea	38396-0404-12	23.90	
(29G,1CC,1/2",LATEX-FREE) 100s ea	38396-0405-12	17.50	
(29G,3/10CC,1/2") 100s ea	38396-0402-12	17.50	
(30G,1/2CC,5/16") 100s ea	38396-0407-12	17.50	
(30G,1CC,5/16") 100s ea	38396-0408-12	17.50	
(30G,3/10CC,5/16") 100s ea	38396-0406-12	17.50	
(31G,1/2CC,5/16") 100s ea	38396-0430-12	17.50	
(31G,1CC,5/16") 100s ea	38396-0431-12	17.50	
(31G,3/10CC,5/16") 100s ea	38396-0429-12	17.50	
MEDICINE SHOPPE LANCETS (Can-Am Care)			
DEV,NA (STANDARD 21G) 100s ea	38396-0303-12	5.85	5.99
(SUPER THIN 30G) 100s ea	38396-0305-12	5.85	
(THIN 26G,UNIVERSAL 1) 100s ea	38396-0301-12	5.85	5.99
(STANDARD 21G) 200s ea	38396-0304-12	9.50	9.99
MEDICINE SHOPPE MAGNESIUM CITRATE (Medicine Shoppe)			
SOL,PO (PASTEURIZED) 1.75 gm/30 ml, 296 ml	49614-0134-42	1.49	
MEDICINE SHOPPE NITE TIME SLEEP (Medicine Shoppe)			
TAB,PO (PRIVATE LABEL) 25 mg, 24s ea	49614-0146-62	2.79	
MEDICONE (Dickinson Brands)			
SUP,RC, 0.25%, 18s ea	02590-0396-18	4.70	
24s ea	02590-0396-24	9.00	
MEDICONE MAXIMUM STRENGTH (Dickinson Brands)			
OIN,TP, 20%, 30 gm	02590-0397-01	4.70	
MEDIKOFF DROPS (Medique)			
LOZ,MM, 75s ea	47682-0050-22	4.71	
600s ea	47682-0050-60	37.61	
(BULK,CHERRY) 600s ea	47682-0506-01	28.05	
(SUGAR-FREE,SF) 6.1 mg, 300s ea UD	47682-0109-03	30.26	
(MENTHOL/EUCALYPTUS) 7.6 mg, 6s ea	47682-0050-69	0.95	
24s ea	47682-0050-64	1.81	
MEDIPHEDRYL (Chain Drug Marketing)			
CAP,PO, 25 mg, 24s ea	63868-0087-24	1.20	3.39
100s ea	63868-0087-01	2.52	8.99
MEDIPLAST (Beiersdorf)			
PAD,TP, 40%, 25s ea	72140-0014-96	24.06	

PROD/MFR	HRI, UPC,NDC	AWP	SRP
MEDIPORE + PAD SOFT CLOTH ADHESIVE (3M Health Care)			
DEV,NA (3 1/2"X10")			
25s ea	08333-3571-01	37.20	
(3 1/2"X13 3/4") 25s ea	08333-3573-01	54.00	
(3 1/2"X4") 25s ea	08333-3566-01	18.60	
(3 1/2"X6") 25s ea	08333-3569-01	28.70	
(3 1/2"X8") 25s ea	08333-3570-01	32.10	
(6"X6") 25s ea	08333-3568-01	39.90	
(2 3/8"X4") 50s ea	08333-3564-01	26.40	
(2"X2 3/4") 50s ea	08333-3562-01	12.90	
MEDIPORE H SOFT CLOTH SURGICAL (3M Health Care)			
DEV,NA (8"X10 YDS)			
6s ea	08333-2868-01	163.20	
(2"X10 YDS) 12s ea	08333-2862-01	81.60	
(3"X10 YDS) 12s ea	08333-2863-01	122.00	
(4"X10 YDS) 12s ea	08333-2864-01	163.20	
(6"X10 YDS) 12s ea	08333-2866-01	243.95	
(6"X2 YDS) 16s ea	08333-2866-03	90.10	
(1"X10 YDS) 24s ea	08333-2861-01	81.60	
(4"X2 YDS) 24s ea	08333-2864-03	90.10	
(2"X2 YDS) 48s ea	08333-2862-03	90.10	
MEDIPORE SOFT CLOTH DRESSING COVERS (3M Health Care)			
DEV,NA (3 7/8"X4 5/8")			
25s ea	08333-2954-01	23.00	
(3 7/8"X7 7/8") 25s ea	08333-2955-01	37.83	
(5 7/8"X11") 25s ea	08333-2957-01	70.55	
(5 7/8"X5 7/8") 25s ea	08333-2956-01	37.83	
(7 7/8"X11") 25s ea	08333-2958-01	88.63	
MEDIPORE SOFT CLOTH SURGICAL TAPE (3M Health Care)			
DEV,NA (8"X10 YDS)			
6s ea	08333-2968-01	163.20	
(2"X10 YDS) 12s ea	08333-2962-01	81.60	
(3"X10 YDS) 12s ea	08333-2963-01	122.00	
(4"X10 YDS) 12s ea	08333-2964-01	163.20	
(6"X10 YDS) 12s ea	08333-2966-01	243.95	
(6"X2 YDS) 16s ea	08333-2966-03	90.10	
(1"X10 YDS) 24s ea	08333-2961-01	81.60	
(4"X2 YDS) 24s ea	08333-2964-03	90.10	
(2"X2 YDS) 48s ea	08333-2962-03	90.10	
MEDIPROXEN (Medique)			
TAB,PO (50X1) 220 mg, 50s ea UD	47682-0237-50	12.06	
(100X1) 220 mg, 100s ea UD	47682-0237-33	17.26	
MEDISENSE CONTROL SOLUTION (Abbott)			
DEV,NA (3ML MID) ea	57599-0552-01	7.38	
(3MLXLO,HI) ea	57599-0550-01	8.28	
(3MLXLO,MID,HI) ea	57599-0551-01	10.50	
MEDISENSE THIN LANCETS (Abbott)			
DEV,NA (28-GAUGE) 100s ea	57599-0043-05	5.88	
100s ea	57599-8681-05	5.88	
200s ea	57599-8682-06	10.72	
MEDIWASH EYE IRRIGANT (Medique)			
SOL,OP (BUFFERED-ISOTONIC) 30 ml	47682-0198-28	2.30	
120 ml	47682-0198-18	2.11	
MEDLANCE PLUS SAFETY AND COMFORT FIRST (Medical Plastic)			
DEV,NA (EXTRA,21G,2.4MM) 200s ea	28465-0013-83	25.99	
(LITE,25G,1.5MM) 200s ea	28465-0013-81	25.99	
(UNIVERSAL,21G,1.8MM) 200s ea	28465-0013-82	25.99	
MEDOTAR (Medco Lab)			
OIN,TP, 1%, 454 gm	11940-1318-06	9.50	
MEDROX (Pharmaceutica North)			
OIN,TP (1X60GM) 0.0375%-5%-20%, 60 gm	45861-0001-60	122.80	
(1X120GM) 0.0375%-5%-20%, 120 gm	45861-0001-01	295.00	
(Nucare Pharm) REPACK			
OIN,TP (1X60GM) 0.0375%-5%-20%, 60 gm	68071-1341-00	148.16	
(1X120GM) 0.0375%-5%-20%, 120 gm	68071-1342-00	299.12	
(Pharma Pac) REPACK			
OIN,TP (1X120GM) 0.0375%-5%-20%, 120 gm	52959-0095-02	300.00	
MEDSEPTIC SKIN PROTECTANT (Medline)			
CRE,TP (MOISTURIZING BARRIER) 15 gm 144s	53329-0042-77	84.56	
113.4 gm 24s	53329-0042-44	93.40	
MEGA ENERGY (Rexall)			
TAB,PO (PF,SF) 45s ea	30768-0000-70	4.99	7.57
MEGA VM-80 (Nature's Bounty)			
TAB,PO (PF,SF) 60s ea	74312-0027-81		13.35
MEGA-B (Arco)			
TAB,PO, 100s ea	00275-0150-06	13.50	20.25
MEGA-C (Merit)			
TER,PO, 1000 mg, 100s ea	30727-0447-07	17.95	
MEGA-HEALTH 75 (Health Products Corp)			
TAB,PO, 60s ea	39686-0013-25	8.27	
MEGA-MULTI (Innovative Health)			
CAP,PO, 60s ea	24038-0000-11	13.77	22.95
MEIJER LANCETS (Can-Am Care)			
DEV,NA (PRIVATE LABEL) 100s ea	38396-0303-20	5.85	
(SUPER THIN 30G) 100s ea	38396-0305-20	5.85	
(THIN,PRIVATE LABEL) 100s ea	38396-0301-20	5.85	
(PRIVATE LABEL) 200s ea	38396-0304-20	9.50	
(THIN,PRIVATE LABEL) 200s ea	38396-0302-20	9.50	
MEIJER PRESTIGE SMART SYSTEM (Home Diag)			
DEV,NA (STRIP) 50s ea	56151-0319-50	28.60	
MEIJER PSS STARTER (Home Diag)			
DEV,NA (MTR,STRP,LANCET,DEV,SOL) ea	56151-0219-01	22.18	
MEIJERS PEN NEEDLES (Owen Mumford)			
DEV,NA (12MM,1/2",29G) 100s ea	08214-0567-17	19.24	
(6MM,1/4",31G) 100s ea	08214-0587-17	19.24	
(8MM,5/16",31G) 100s ea	08214-0577-17	19.24	
MELATIN (Mason Vit)			
TAB,PO (PF,SF) 3 mg-1 mg, 60s ea	11845-0112-85	5.00	
MELATONIN (Advanced Nutr)			
TAB,PO (PF,SF) 3 mg, 60s ea	62617-0428-02	9.60	12.80
(Bio-Tech Pharm)			
CAP,PO, 1 mg, 100s ea	53191-0226-01	5.50	
3 mg, 100s ea	53191-0227-01	11.00	
5 mg, 100s ea	53191-0214-01	15.00	
20 mg, 100s ea	53191-0424-01	35.00	
(Breckenridge Pharm)			
TAB,PO, 3 mg, 60s ea	51991-0014-06	5.00	
(Lex)			
TAB,PO, 3 mg, 30s ea	58537-0035-03	2.50	
(Major)			
TAB,PO, 3 mg, 60s ea	00904-5182-52	7.49	
(Mason Vit)			
TAB,PO (PF,SF) 3 mg-1 mg, 60s ea	11845-0111-35	5.00	
SL (PF,ORANGE) 2.5 mg-500 mcg, 60s ea	11845-0111-55	5.56	
(Nature's Bounty)			
TAB,PO (90 TABLETS FREE,PF,SF) 1 mg, 90s ea	74312-0028-32		5.19
(60 TABLETS FREE,PF,SF) 3 mg, 60s ea	74312-0079-01		6.19
(120 TABLETS FREE,PF,SF) 3 mg, 120s ea	74312-0079-03		8.89
(PF,SF) 200 mcg, 60s ea	74312-0079-00		2.59
(Rexall)			
TAB,PO (PF,SF) 0.3 mg, 75s ea	30768-0000-87	1.62	2.70
3 mg, 60s ea	30768-0040-50	2.20	3.29
(Rugby)			
TAB,PO, 3 mg, 60s ea	00536-6412-08	12.95	
(Stat Rx) REPACK			
TAB,PO (PF,SF) 3 mg, 100s ea	16590-0869-71	13.75	
MELATONIN EXTRA STRENGTH (Mason Vit)			
TAB,PO (PF,SF) 5 mg-1 mg, 60s ea	11845-0111-45	7.22	
MELISSENGEIST (Weleda)			
LIQ,PO, 50 ml	55946-0315-15	7.20	
MELLOW-TONE (KRS)			
FIL,MM, 24s ea	03216-0302-24	13.20	20.00
MEMOR-X MEMORY BOOSTING (Health Products Corp)			
TAB,PO, 60s ea	39686-0015-11	9.94	17.50
MEN-PHOR (Geritrex)			
LOT,TP (144X59ML) 0.5%-0.5%, 59 ml 144s	54162-0550-02	203.04	
222 ml	54162-0550-09	4.73	
225 ml	54162-0550-07	4.96	
MEN'S MULTIVITAMIN/MULTIMINERAL (Rexall)			
TAB,PO (WITH HERBS,CAPLET) 60s ea	30768-0040-51	4.67	6.99
MEN'S POTENT FORMULA (Mason Vit)			
TAB,PO (PF,SF) 60s ea	11845-0120-25	15.44	
MEN'S ROGAINE (Johnson & Johnson)			
FOA,TP (3MONTHSUPPLY,3X60GM) 5%, 60 gm 3s	12547-0781-35	48.12	
SOL,TP (UNSCENTED,1MONTHSUPPLY) 5%, 60 ml	12547-0700-20	26.88	
(UNSCENTED,3MONTHSUPPLY) 5%, 60 ml 3s	12547-0700-60	48.12	
MENOPAUSE TRIO (Mason Vit)			
TER,PO (CAPLET) 30s ea	11845-0142-88	17.67	
MENTHODERM (Pharmaceutica North)			
OIN,TP (1X60GM) 10%-15%, 60 gm	45861-0003-60	119.45	
MENTHOL (Family Phcy)			
GEL,TP (PRIVATE LABEL) 2%, 105 gm	52735-0424-48	3.95	4.39
MENTHOL AID (Rose)			
GEL,TP, 2%, 240 gm	42037-0330-08	6.75	
MENTHOLATUM (Mentholatum)			
OIN,TP (JAR) 9%-1.35%, 30 gm	10742-0000-11	1.93	1.39
(TUBE) 9%-1.35%, 30 gm	10742-0000-13	1.93	1.39
(JAR) 9%-1.35%, 90 gm	10742-0000-12	4.43	3.39
MENTHOLATUM CHEST RUB FOR KIDS (Mentholatum)			
OIN,TP, 4.7%-1.2%-2.7%, 30 gm	10742-0005-01	1.93	
MENTHOLATUM DEEP HEATING (Mentholatum)			
LOT,TP, 6%-20%, 60 ml	10742-0000-31	2.92	2.19

PROD/MFR	HRI, UPC,NDC	AWP	SRP
OIN,TP, 37.5 gm	10742-0000-21	2.69	1.99
99.9 gm	10742-0000-22	5.08	3.79
MEPIFORM (Molnlycke Healthcare)			
DRE,TP, ea	83180-2934-09	16.80	
MEPITEL (Molnlycke Healthcare)			
DRE,TP, ea	83180-2907-01	7.24	
MERCURIUS (Walker Pharmacal)			
TAB,SL (6X)			
250s ea	00619-6090-02	2.97	
MERCURIUS VIV (Luyties)			
TAB,SL (6X)			
6 x, 500s ea	00618-6090-03	3.99	
5500s ea	00618-6090-10	30.32	
(30X)			
12 x, 500s ea	00622-6090-03	4.19	
5500s ea	00622-6090-10	31.83	
(12X)			
30 x, 500s ea	00624-6090-03	4.19	
5500s ea	00624-6090-10	31.83	
MERCUROCHROME (Lex)			
SOL,TP, 2%, 30 ml	49523-0007-01	0.75	
(PLASTIC BOTTLE)			
2%, 30 ml	49523-0007-11	0.57	
SPR,TP, 2%, 60 ml	49523-0080-02	1.20	
MERIBIN (Mericon)			
CAP,PO, 5 mg, 120s ea	00394-0130-12	33.49	
MERTHIOLATE (Lex)			
LIQ,TP (PLASTIC BOTTLE)			
1:1000, 30 ml	49523-0006-11	0.60	
SPR,TP, 1:1000, 60 gm	49523-0006-02	1.20	
TIN,TP, 1:1000, 30 ml	49523-0006-01	0.75	
MET-RX FOOD (Met-Rx)			
BAR,PO (CHOCOLATE)			
ea	86560-0050-01	1.96	
(FUDGE BROWNIE)			
ea	86560-0020-01	1.96	
(PEANUT BUTTER)			
ea	86560-0040-01	1.96	
(VANILLA)			
ea	86560-0030-01	1.96	
(CHOCOLATE)			
12s ea	86560-0050-12	23.47	
(FUDGE BROWNIE)			
12s ea	86560-0020-12	23.47	
(PEANUT BUTTER)			
12s ea	86560-0040-12	23.47	
(VANILLA)			
12s ea	86560-0030-12	23.47	
MET-RX TOTAL NUTRITION DRINK MIX (Met-Rx)			
PDR,PO (CHOCOLATE MOCHA)			
72 gm	86560-0000-04	1.96	
(EXTREME CHOCOLATE)			
72 gm	86560-0000-05	1.96	
(PEACH)			
72 gm	86560-0000-09	1.96	
(VANILLA)			
72 gm	86560-0000-01	1.96	
(EXTREME CHOCOLATE)			
72 gm 12s	86560-0000-15	23.47	
(VANILLA)			
72 gm 12s	86560-0000-12	23.47	
(CHOCOLATE MOCHA)			
72 gm 20s	86560-0000-24	39.12	
(EXTREME CHOCOLATE)			
72 gm 20s	86560-0000-25	39.12	
(PEACH)			
72 gm 20s	86560-0000-29	39.12	
(VANILLA)			
72 gm 20s	86560-0000-20	39.12	
METAFIBER (Prime Marketing)			
PDR,PO (ORANGE)			
3.4 gm/dose, 368 gm	62107-0078-04	5.60	
(REGULAR)			
3.4 gm/dose, 368 gm	62107-0079-04	5.60	
METAMUCIL (P & G Company)			
CAP,PO, 0.52 gm,			
100s ea	37000-0458-10	9.83	
160s ea	37000-0458-16	12.94	
PDR,PO, 3.4 gm/dose,			
390 gm	37000-0010-08	8.17	
570 gm	37000-0010-09	10.13	
570 gm	37000-0013-08	8.17	
870 gm	37000-0010-10	13.30	
870 gm	37000-0013-09	10.13	
(ORANGE)			
3.4 gm/dose,			
1254 gm	37000-0013-10	13.30	
WAF,PO (APPLE)			
1.7 gm, 24s ea	37000-0030-01	4.43	
(CINNAMON SPICE)			
1.7 gm, 24s ea	37000-0029-01	4.43	
METAMUCIL SMOOTH TEXTURE (P & G Company)			
PDR,PO (PACKET,ORANGE)			
3.4 gm/dose,			
30s ea	37000-0023-04	8.57	
(PACKET)			
3.4 gm/dose,			
30s ea	37000-0024-04	8.57	
(SF,ORANGE)			
3.4 gm/dose,			
300 gm	37000-0024-01	8.17	
(SF)			
3.4 gm/dose,			
300 gm	37000-0048-01	8.17	
450 gm	37000-0048-02	10.13	
(SF,ORANGE)			
3.4 gm/dose,			
450 gm	37000-0024-02	10.13	
(ORANGE)			
3.4 gm/dose,			
609 gm	37000-0023-05	8.17	
(SF,ORANGE)			
3.4 gm/dose,			
660 gm	37000-0024-06	13.30	
(SF)			
3.4 gm/dose,			
699 gm	37000-0048-05	13.30	
(ORANGE)			
3.4 gm/dose,			
912 gm	37000-0023-06	10.13	
1368 gm	37000-0023-07	13.30	
METED (Sirius Labs)			
SHA,TP, 3%-5%, 120 ml	65880-0610-04	7.80	
METHACHOLINE (Mason Vit)			
SGL,PO, 100s ea	11845-0056-01	8.22	
METHAGUAL (Gordon)			
OIN,TP, 2%-8%, 60 gm	10481-1023-01	13.75	
METHIONAID (Nutricia)			
PDR,PO (USE W/MED SUPV)			
200 gm 10s	49735-0102-42	354.90	
METHIONINE (Carlson,J.R.)			
L-METHIONINE			
CAP,PO, 500 mg, 100s ea	88395-0068-91	8.45	16.90
360s ea	88395-0068-93	21.88	43.75
POW,PO, 100 gm	88395-0068-95	13.45	26.90
(Mason Vit)			
CAP,PO, 500 mg, 60s ea	11845-0082-65	5.89	
METHIONINE (VITAFLO, LLC)			
POW,NA (30X4GM)			
30s ea	50600-0554-40	120.00	150.00
METHIONINE-500 (Key Company)			
TAB,PO (SF)			
500 mg, 60s ea	11694-0917-01	8.25	
120s ea	11694-0917-02	15.00	
500s ea	11694-0917-04	48.00	
METHYLCOBALAMIN (Merit)			
TAB,SL (CHERRY)			
400 mcg-1000 mcg,			
60s ea	30727-0434-06	14.00	
400 mcg-5000 mcg,			
60s ea	30727-0435-06	38.00	
METHYLENE BLUE (Lex)			
SOL,TP, 2%, 30 ml	49523-0050-01	0.63	
MG 217 MEDICATED TAR (Triton Consumer Prod)			
LOT,TP, 1%, 120 ml	79511-0501-04	6.20	
OIN,TP, 2%, 107 gm	79511-0500-04	8.00	
SHA,TP (SF)			
3%, 120 ml	79511-0502-04	3.90	
240 ml	79511-0502-08	6.50	
MG PLUS PROTEIN (Miller)			
TAB,PO, 100s ea	17204-0434-40	5.28	8.40
(Phys Total Care)			
REPACK			
TAB,PO, 100s ea	54868-4933-00	25.02	
MG-225 (Bio-Tech Pharm)			
CAP,PO, 225 mg, 100s ea	53191-0403-01	7.85	
MG/TAURINE FORTE (Miller)			
CAP,PO, 60s ea	17204-0885-20	7.56	
180s ea	17204-0803-50	20.76	
MG217 SAL-ACID (Triton Consumer Prod)			
OIN,TP, 3%, 56 gm	79511-0506-02	4.70	
MGB (Electrolyte)			
TAB,PO, 100s ea	60049-0518-44	10.25	17.10
MI-ACID (Major)			
CTB,PO, 200 mg-200 mg-25 mg,			
100s ea	00904-5068-60	4.45	
SUS,PO, 360 ml	00904-0004-14	2.80	
MI-ACID DOUBLE STRENGTH (Major)			
CTB,PO (COOL MINT)			
700 mg-300 mg,			
70s ea	00904-5115-71	4.19	
MI-ACID II (Major)			
SUS,PO, 360 ml	00904-0005-14	3.80	
MICADERM (Altaire)			
CRE,TP, 2%, 30 gm	59390-0067-17	5.50	
MICONAZOLE 3 COMBINATION PACK (Cardinal Health)			
KIT,NA (3 SUPPS/CRM W/DISP APPL)			
ea	37205-0583-03	10.24	
(Major)			
KIT,NA (3 SUPPS/CRM W/DISP APPL)			
400 mg, ea	00904-5415-01	11.85	
(Phys Total Care)			
REPACK			
KIT,NA (3 SUPPS/CRM W/APPL)			
ea	54868-4333-00	29.13	
MICONAZOLE 7 (Cardinal Health)			
CRE,VG (W/APPLICATOR)			
2%, 45 gm	37205-0590-29	8.44	
(Chain Drug Marketing)			
CRE,VG (W/7 APPLICATORS)			
2%, 45 gm	63868-0200-46	4.50	7.99
(Rugby)			
CRE,VG, 2%, 45 gm	00536-1423-26	12.82	
(Taro)			
CRE,VG (W/APPLICATOR)			
2%, 45 gm	51672-2035-06	11.45	
(Altura)			
REPACK			
CRE,VG, 2%, 45 gm	63874-0045-45	23.94	
(DHS, Inc.)			
REPACK			
CRE,VG, 2%, 45 gm	55887-0852-45	45.01	
(Pharma Pac)			
REPACK			
CRE,VG, 2%, 45 gm	52959-0825-01	11.95	
(Phys Total Care)			
REPACK			
CRE,VG (W/APPLICATOR)			
2%, 60 gm	54868-2999-01	18.45	
SUP,VG, 100 mg, 7s ea	54868-3621-00	28.29	
MICONAZOLE NITRATE (Actavis Mid Atlantic)			
CRE,TP, 2%, 15 gm	00472-0735-14	2.36	
(5 PANEL)			
2%, 30 gm	00472-0735-56	3.30	
45 gm	00472-0735-42	4.79	
VG (W/1 PLASTIC APPLICATOR)			
2%, 45 gm	00472-0730-63	10.98	
(W/7 APPLICATORS)			
2%, 45 gm	00472-0730-41	11.48	
(G&W)			
CRE,VG, 2%, 45 gm	00713-0252-37	7.73	
SUP,VG, 100 mg, 7s ea	00713-0197-57	5.87	
(Major)			
CRE,VG, 2%, 47.7 gm	00904-7734-45	11.79	
(W/APPLICATOR)			
2%, 47.7 gm	00904-7734-57	11.00	
(Qualitest)			
CRE,TP, 2%, 28.4 gm	00603-7805-50	6.95	
(Taro)			
CRE,TP, 2%, 15 gm	51672-2001-01	3.50	
30 gm	51672-2001-02	4.80	
(A-S Medication)			
REPACK			
CRE,VG, 2%, 45 gm	54569-3725-00	11.45	
(Dispensing Solutions)			
REPACK			
CRE,TP (1X30ML)			
2%, 30 gm	68258-3004-01	6.50	
CRE,VG, 2%, 45 gm	55045-2726-05	14.25	
(Palmetto)			
REPACK			
CRE,TP, 2%, 15 gm	23490-5930-02	6.95	
30 gm	23490-5930-03	9.95	
CRE,VG, 2%, 45 gm	23490-6699-01	20.46	

PROD/MFR	HRI, UPC,NDC	AWP	SRP
(Phys Total Care)			
REPACK			
CRE,TP, 2%, 30 gm	54868-2471-01	18.45	
(Physician Partner)			
REPACK			
CRE,VG (1X45GM)			
2%, 45 gm	21695-0854-45	15.46	
(Quality Care Prod)			
REPACK			
CRE,TP, 2%, 45 gm	49999-0165-45	64.80	
(Stat Rx)			
REPACK			
CRE,VG, 2%, 30 gm	16590-0425-30	8.46	
MICONAZOLE-7 (Actavis Mid Atlantic)			
SUP,VG, 100 mg, 7s ea	00472-1736-07	11.57	
MICRO PUMP IV W/HP FILTER (Abbott Hosp)			
DEV,NA (115", VENTED)			
24s ea	00074-9244-68	313.63	
MICRO PUMP LIFECARE (Abbott Hosp)			
DEV,NA (W/RS485)			
ea	00074-1917-04	4703.71	
MICRO PUMP MICRODRIP-SL (Abbott Hosp)			
DEV,NA (W/INLINE CASSETTE)			
24s ea	00074-9289-68	379.87	
MICRO-BUMINTEST (Bayer Diabetes Care)			
DEV,NA (100 TEST KIT)			
ea	00193-2230-21	126.84	
(20 TEST KIT)			
ea	00193-2229-20	30.42	
MICRO-GUARD (Coloplast)			
CRE,TP, 2%, 57 gm 12s	11701-0037-23	93.24	97.68
POW,TP, 2%, 85 gm 12s	11701-0038-16	106.56	111.48
MICRO-GUARD ANTI (Quality Care Prod)			
REPACK			
POW,TP, 2%, 90 gm	35356-0057-03	10.66	
MICRO-TOUCH LATEX MEDICAL GLOVES (J&J Medical)			
DEV,NA (NON-STERILE,LARGE)			
100s ea	56091-0057-61	11.88	
(NON-STERILE,MEDIUM)			
100s ea	56091-0057-41	11.88	
(NON-STERILE,SMALL)			
100s ea	56091-0057-21	8.47	
MICRO-TOUCH NITRILE SYNTHETIC GLOVES (J&J Medical)			
DEV,NA (NON-STER,LARGE)			
100s ea	56091-0040-06	9.75	
(NON-STER,MED)			
100s ea	56091-0040-04	9.75	
(NON-STER,SMALL)			
100s ea	56091-0040-02	9.75	
(NON-STER,X-LG)			
100s ea	56091-0040-08	9.75	
(NON-STER,X-SM)			
100s ea	56091-0040-00	9.75	
MICRO-TOUCH PLUS LATEX GLOVES (J&J Medical)			
DEV,NA (NON-STER,LARGE)			
100s ea	56091-0050-06	8.79	
(NON-STER,MED)			
100s ea	56091-0050-04	8.79	
(NON-STER,SMALL)			
100s ea	56091-0050-02	8.79	
(NON-STER,X-LG)			
100s ea	56091-0050-08	8.79	
(NON-STER,X-SM)			
100s ea	56091-0050-00	8.79	
MICRO-TOUCH ULTRA LATEX EXAM GLOVES (J&J Medical)			
DEV,NA (NON-STER, X-SM)			
100s ea	56091-0053-20	8.79	
(NON-STER,LARGE)			
100s ea	56091-0053-26	8.79	
(NON-STER,MED)			
100s ea	56091-0053-24	8.79	
(NON-STER,SMALL)			
100s ea	56091-0053-22	8.79	
(NON-STER,X-LG)			
100s ea	56091-0053-28	8.79	
MICROBORE EXTENSION (Abbott Hosp)			
DEV,NA (12" W/OPTION-LOK)			
50s ea	00074-6457-01	105.60	
(20" W/OPTION LOK)			
50s ea	00074-6458-01	416.22	
(36" W/OPTION-LOK)			
50s ea	00074-6460-01	133.80	
(72" W/OPTION-LOK)			
50s ea	00074-6461-01	142.20	
(5" W/LOCKING LUER "T")			
120s ea	00074-4616-02	1130.03	
(5" W/T-CONNECTOR)			
120s ea	00074-4612-04	1038.83	
MICROCORT (Alto)			
LOT,TP, 0.5%, 120 ml	00731-0501-04	4.80	
MICRODRIP MICRO PUMP IV (Abbott Hosp)			
DEV,NA (102", VENTED)			
48s ea	00074-9243-48	482.69	
MICROFOAM SURGICAL TAPE (3M Health Care)			
DEV,NA (4"X5 1/2 YDS)			
3s ea	08333-1528-04	29.35	
(3"X5 1/2 YDS)			
4s ea	08333-1528-03	29.35	
(2"X5 1/2 YDS)			
6s ea	08333-1528-02	29.35	
(1"X5 1/2 YDS)			
12s ea	08333-1528-01	29.35	
(4"X7",PATCH)			
25s ea	08333-1562-01	54.25	
MICROKLENZ (Carrington)			
SPR,TP, 0.1%, 236 ml	53303-0007-08	11.22	
MICROLET (Bayer Diabetes Care)			
DEV,NA, ea	00193-6540-01	16.60	
(COLORED)			
100s ea	00193-6586-21	9.96	
MICROLET LANCETS (Bayer Diabetes Care)			
DEV,NA, 100s ea	00193-6546-21	9.96	
MICROPORE SURGICAL (3M Health Care)			
DEV,NA (3"X10 YDS,DISPENSER PAK)			
4s ea	08333-1535-03	10.90	
(3"X10 YDS)			
4s ea	08333-1530-03	9.30	
(2"X10 YDS,DISPENSER PAK)			
6s ea	08333-1535-02	10.90	
(2"X10 YDS,TAN)			
6s ea	08333-1533-02	19.35	
(2"X10 YDS)			
6s ea	08333-1530-02	9.30	
(1"X10 YDS,DISPENSER PAK)			
12s ea	08333-1535-01	10.90	
(1"X10 YDS,TAN)			
12s ea	08333-1533-01	19.35	
(1"X10 YDS)			
12s ea	08333-1530-01	9.30	
(1/2"X10 YDS,DISP PACK)			
24s ea	08333-1535-00	10.90	
(1/2"X10 YDS,TAN)			
24s ea	08333-1533-00	19.35	
(1/2"X10 YDS)			
24s ea	08333-1530-00	9.30	
(2"X1 1/2 YDS)			
50s ea	08333-1530-12	33.90	
(1"X1 1/2 YDS)			
100s ea	08333-1530-11	33.90	
MICROTOUCH PF LATEX SURGICAL GLOVES (J&J Medical)			
DEV,NA (STERILE,50 PR,SZ 5.5)			
100s ea	56091-0058-55	33.80	
100s ea	56091-0065-55	97.50	
(STERILE,50 PR,SZ 6.5)			
100s ea	56091-0058-65	33.80	
100s ea	56091-0065-65	97.50	
(STERILE,50 PR,SZ 6)			
100s ea	56091-0058-60	33.80	
100s ea	56091-0065-60	97.50	
(STERILE,50 PR,SZ 7 1/2)			
100s ea	56091-0058-75	33.80	
(STERILE,50 PR,SZ 7.5)			
100s ea	56091-0065-75	97.50	
(STERILE,50 PR,SZ 7)			
100s ea	56091-0058-70	33.80	
100s ea	56091-0065-70	97.50	
(STERILE,50 PR,SZ 8.5)			
100s ea	56091-0058-85	33.80	
100s ea	56091-0065-85	97.50	
(STERILE,50 PR,SZ 8)			
100s ea	56091-0058-80	33.80	
100s ea	56091-0065-80	97.50	
(STERILE,50 PR,SZ 9)			
100s ea	56091-0058-90	33.80	
100s ea	56091-0065-90	97.50	
MIDOL CRAMP FORMULA (Bayer HealthCare)			
TAB,PO (MAX. STR.,AF)			
200 mg, 24s ea	12843-0143-52	3.88	
MIDOL MAXIMUM STRENGTH (Bayer HealthCare)			
TAB,PO (CAPLET)			
500 mg-60 mg-15 mg,			
8s ea	12843-0158-58	1.58	
16s ea	12843-0024-71	2.75	
24s ea	12843-0158-59	3.88	
(GELCAPLET)			
500 mg-60 mg-15 mg,			
24s ea	12843-0172-53	3.88	
(CAPLET)			
500 mg-60 mg-15 mg,			
40s ea	12843-0501-32	4.92	
MIDOL PMS MAXIMUM STRENGTH (Bayer HealthCare)			
TAB,PO (CAPLET)			
500 mg-25 mg-15 mg,			
24s ea	12843-0163-48	3.88	
MIDOL TEEN FORMULA (Bayer HealthCare)			
TAB,PO (CAPLET)			
400 mg-25 mg,			
24s ea	12843-0166-73	3.88	
MIGRAINE ICE (Mentholatum)			
DEV,NA (BACK OF NECK,1 3/4"X8")			
4s ea	10742-0007-52	5.94	
(TEMPLE,1 1/4"X2 3/4")			
4s ea	10742-0007-53	5.94	
(FOREHEAD,1 3/4"X4 1/2")			
5s ea	10742-0007-51	5.94	
MIL ADREGEN (Miller)			
TAB,PO, 60s ea	17204-0541-20	9.48	15.00
120s ea	17204-0515-55	17.04	27.00
180s ea	17204-0549-50	25.50	40.50
500s ea	17204-0513-90	68.04	108.00
MIL ADRENE (Miller)			
TAB,PO, 80 mg, 100s ea	17204-0502-40	6.00	9.50
MIL ADRENE FORTE (Miller)			
TAB,PO, 160 mg, 100s ea	17204-0503-40	7.56	12.00
MILANTEX (Prime Marketing)			
SUS,PO (ORIGINAL)			
355 ml	62107-0022-11	2.90	
MILANTEX MAXIMUM STRENGTH (Prime Marketing)			
PO (ORIGINAL)			
355 ml	62107-0023-11	3.75	
MILCO-ZYME (Miller)			
TAB,PO, 100s ea	17204-0444-40	8.52	
MILD-C (Carlson,J.R.)			
CAP,PO, 500 mg-56 mg,			
100s ea	88395-0030-61	6.45	12.90
250s ea	88395-0030-62	12.75	
CTB,PO (ORANGE)			
250 mg-25 mg,			
60s ea	88395-0030-50	3.95	7.90
120s ea	88395-0030-51	7.25	14.50
240s ea	88395-0030-52	13.85	27.70
PDR,PO (CRYSTALS,PF,SF)			
3600 mg-400 mg,			
170 gm	88395-0030-86	8.45	16.90
1000 gm	88395-0030-84	27.50	55.00
TER,PO, 1000 mg-111 mg,			
100s ea	88395-0030-71	10.75	21.50
300s ea	88395-0030-73	27.50	55.00
MILK DIGESTANT (Major)			
TAB,PO (PF,SF,GLUTEN-FREE)			
40 mg-2 mg-25 mg,			
200s ea	00904-4324-25	8.35	
MILK OF MAGNESIA (Albertson's)			
SUS,PO, 400 mg/5 ml,			
360 ml	12810-0396-40	2.64	
(AmerisourceBergen)			
SUS,PO (PRIVATE LABEL,MINT)			
400 mg/5 ml, 360 ml	24385-0332-40	3.14	3.49
(PRIVATE LABEL)			
400 mg/5 ml, 360 ml	24385-0396-40	3.23	3.59
(Cardinal Health)			
SUS,PO (PRIVATE LABEL,MINT)			
400 mg/5 ml, 360 ml	37205-0834-40	3.42	
(PRIVATE LABEL)			
400 mg/5 ml, 360 ml	37205-0833-40	3.42	
(Consolidated Midland)			
SUS,PO, 400 mg/5 ml,			
360 ml	00223-6279-12	2.50	
480 ml	00223-6279-01	2.95	
(Cypress Pharm)			
SUS,PO, 400 mg/5 ml,			
473 ml	60258-0960-16	4.99	
(Humco)			
SUS,PO, 400 mg/5 ml,			
480 ml	00395-1670-16	2.01	
(MINT)			
400 mg/5 ml, 480 ml	00395-1671-16	2.28	
3840 ml	00395-1670-28	16.16	

PROD/MFR	HRI, UPC,NDC	AWP	SRP
(Major)			
SOL,PO, 400 mg/5 ml,			
480 ml	00904-0788-16	2.65	
SUS,PO, 400 mg/5 ml,			
360 ml	00904-0788-14	4.03	
(MINT)			
400 mg/5 ml, 360 ml	00904-0789-14	2.40	
(Paddock)			
SUS,PO, 400 mg/5 ml,			
480 ml	00574-0018-16	2.90	
960 ml	00574-0018-32	8.00	
(Pharm Assoc Inc)			
SUS,PO (SF,SPEARMINT)			
400 mg/5 ml,			
30 ml 100s UD	00121-0431-30	43.00	
(Prime Marketing)			
SUS,PO (MINT)			
400 mg/5 ml, 355 ml	62107-0024-11	2.70	
(R.I.J.)			
SUS,PO, 400 mg/5 ml,			
360 ml	53807-0125-01	1.84	
480 ml	53807-0125-02	1.98	
3840 ml	53807-0125-03	14.30	
(Roxane)			
SUS,PO, 400 mg/5 ml,			
100 ml	00054-3567-49	4.85	
(CONCENTRATED)			
400 mg/5 ml, 400 ml	00054-3567-61	9.06	
(Rugby)			
SUS,PO (MINT)			
400 mg/5 ml, 360 ml	00536-2470-83	2.92	
480 ml	00536-2470-85	3.60	
(Phys Total Care)			
REPACK			
SUS,PO, 400 mg/5 ml,			
360 ml	54868-2345-02	7.50	
480 ml	54868-2345-00	12.36	
3840 ml	54868-2345-01	38.28	
(Quality Care Prod)			
REPACK			
SUS,PO (MINT)			
400 mg/5 ml,			
480 ml	49999-0769-16	7.44	
(Southwood)			
REPACK			
SUS,PO, 400 mg/5 ml,			
360 ml	58016-1129-01	9.65	
MILK OF MAGNESIA CONCENTRATE			
(Pharm Assoc Inc)			
SUS,PO (AF,DYE-FREE,LEMON)			
1200 mg/5 ml,			
10 ml 100s UD	00121-0527-10	46.60	
MILK THISTLE (Botanical Labs.)			
CAP,PO, 50s ea	41954-0032-67	7.50	14.99
LIQ,PO, 30 ml	41954-0020-33	5.00	9.99
60 ml	41954-0020-26	8.00	15.99
(Cardinal Health)			
CAP,PO (PRIVATE LABEL)			
180 mg, 40s ea	37205-0052-58	7.02	
(Key Company)			
TAB,PO, 200 mg, 60s ea	11694-0677-01	10.50	
(Major)			
CAP,PO, 175 mg, 60s ea	00904-5665-52	8.93	
(Mason Vit)			
CAP,PO (PF,SF)			
150 mg, 60s ea	11845-0129-95	13.22	
500 mg, 60s ea	11845-0115-05	7.89	
(Nature's Bounty)			
CAP,PO, 100s ea	74312-0034-91		14.79
MILK THISTLE COMPLEX (Rexall)			
CAP,PO (PF,SF)			
50s ea	30768-0000-80	3.62	5.48
MILK THISTLE EXTRA STRENGTH (Yerba)			
CAP,PO, 80 mg, 50s ea	46352-0004-57	10.17	16.95
MILPAN (Miller)			
TAB,PO, 325 mg, 100s ea	17204-0525-40	10.08	16.00
MILTUSS (Seyer Pharmatec)			
SYR,PO (HONEY)			
15 mg/5 ml, 118 ml	11026-2810-04	7.80	
MIMULUS (Ellon)			
SOL,SL (DROPS)			
10.5 ml	51762-0023-10		9.25
MIN-O-EAR (Geritrex)			
SOL,OT (1X22ML,DROPS)			
22 ml	92771-0188-22	2.11	2.08
MINCOL-K (Key Company)			
CAP,PO (CORN-FREE,RYE-FREE)			
105 mg, 100s ea	11694-0847-01	8.00	
250s ea	11694-0847-02	16.00	
MINERAL COMPLEET (Carlson,J.R.)			
TAB,PO (PF,SF,CORN-FREE)			
90s ea	88395-0054-24	9.75	19.50
360s ea	88395-0054-23	34.95	69.90
MINERAL COMPLEET CHELATED (Carlson,J.R.)			
TAB,PO, 120s ea	88395-0054-21	12.45	24.90
MINERAL ICE (Novartis Consumer)			
GEL,TP (1X226.8GM,GREASELESS)			
2%, 226.8 gm	00067-2067-08	7.40	
(1X453.6M,GREASELESS)			
2%, 453.6 gm	00067-2067-16	11.50	
MINERAL OIL (Cardinal Health)			
OIL,PO (PRIVATE LABEL)			
480 ml	37205-0831-43	2.86	
(Geritrex)			
OIL,PO (LUBRI LAXATIVE)			
99.9%, 473 ml 24s	54162-0190-16	106.08	
(Pharm Assoc Inc)			
OIL,PO (AF,SF,DYE-FREE)			
30 ml 100s UD	00121-0462-30	62.95	
MINERAL OIL LIGHT (Geritrex)			
OIL,TP (USP,STERILE)			
25 ml	54162-0185-25	2.48	
480 ml	54162-0185-16	3.19	
MINERALS FOR MEN (Freeda)			
TAB,PO (PF,SF,DYE-FREE)			
100s ea	10432-0337-01	5.67	9.45
MINI CAL-CITRATE (Freeda)			
TAB,PO (PURE,SF,GLUTEN-FREE)			
125 mg, 100s ea	10432-0359-01	3.90	6.50
250s ea	10432-0359-02	7.77	12.95
500s ea	10432-0359-03	13.50	22.50
MINI PRENATAL (Freeda)			
TAB,PO (TINY TABLET,SF)			
120s ea	10432-0350-01	4.17	6.95
250s ea	10432-0350-02	8.34	13.90
500s ea	10432-0350-03	14.37	23.95
MINI-MULTI (Carlson,J.R.)			
TAB,PO (PF,SF,CORN-FREE)			
90s ea	88395-0041-31	7.20	14.40
180s ea	88395-0041-32	12.45	24.90
MINIDROPS EYE THERAPY (Optics)			
SOL,OP (30X0.5ML,PF,DROPS)			
14 mg/ml-6 mg/ml,			
0.5 ml 30s	64108-0212-12	7.95	9.95
MINILET LANCETS (Medtronic Minimed)			
DEV,NA (THIN)			
100s ea	63706-0011-10	18.00	
MINIMED INFUSION PUMP (Medtronic Minimed)			
DEV,NA (W/1 YR WARR,CHARCOL/BLK)			
ea	76300-0407-13	8125.00	
MINIMED INSULIN INFUSION PUMP (Medtronic Minimed)			
DEV,NA (W/VIBRATOR,CHARC/BLACK)			
ea	76300-0508-13	6868.75	
(W/VIBRATOR,TEAL)			
ea	76300-0508-18	6868.75	
(W/VIBRATOR,TRANSL BLUE)			
ea	76300-0508-12	6868.75	
(W/VIBRATOR,WHITE)			
ea	76300-0508-21	6868.75	
MINIPRIN (Time-Cap)			
ECT,PO, 81 mg, 120s ea	49483-0054-12	3.36	
1000s ea	49483-0054-10	14.44	
MINOR DRESSING TRAY (Medical Action Ind.)			
DEV,NA, 20s ea	73577-0612-05	58.80	
MINOR PROCEDURE TRAY (Medical Action Ind.)			
DEV,NA (KELLY HEMOSTAT CURVED)			
20s ea	73577-0612-04	138.96	
(MOSQUITO HEMOST.,CURVED)			
20s ea	73577-0612-14	144.54	
(SERRATED NEEDLE HOLDER)			
20s ea	73577-0612-03	97.26	
(STAINLESS STEEL INSTRUM)			
20s ea	73577-0612-18	162.54	
(WEBSTER NEEDLE HOLDER)			
20s ea	73577-0612-13	98.04	
MINOXIDIL (Actavis Mid Atlantic)			
SOL,TP (FOR MEN)			
2%, 60 ml	00472-0066-73	9.70	
(FOR MEN, TWINPAK)			
2%, 60 ml 2s	00472-0066-75	15.50	
(FOR MEN)			
5%, 60 ml	00472-0094-73	25.20	
(FOR MEN,TWIN PACK)			
5%, 60 ml 2s	00472-0094-75	42.72	
(Phys Total Care)			
REPACK			
SOL,TP, 2%, 120 ml	54868-3781-00	59.47	
MINTOX (Major)			
SUS,PO, 355 ml	00904-5721-14	2.50	
(MAXIMUM STRENGTH)			
355 ml	00904-5725-14	3.60	
TAB,PO (12X2)			
300 mg-150 mg,			
24s ea	00904-6006-02	1.50	
MINTOX PLUS (Major)			
CTB,PO, 200 mg-200 mg-25 mg,			
100s ea	00904-0478-60	4.65	
MIRAFLOW (Ciba Vision)			
SOL,NA, 12 ml	47113-0125-12	3.25	
20 ml	47113-0125-15	4.25	
MIRALAX (Schering Plough)			
PDS,PO, 17 gm/dose,			
12s ea	11523-7234-05	19.68	
17 gm 10s	11523-7268-03	10.08	
(ORIGPRSCRPTNSTRNGTH,CUP)			
17 gm/dose, 119 gm	11523-7234-02	5.70	
238 gm	11523-7234-03	10.08	
510 gm	11523-7234-04	19.68	
(2X510GM,TWIN PACK)			
17 gm/dose,			
510 gm 2s	11523-7234-09	29.64	
(Dispensing Solutions)			
REPACK			
PDS,PO, 17 gm/dose,			
238 gm	55045-3947-01	14.00	
(1X238GM)			
17 gm/dose, 238 gm	68258-3019-04	14.00	
(1X510GM)			
17 gm/dose, 510 gm	68258-3019-08	28.00	
(Stat Rx)			
REPACK			
PDS,PO (1X510GM)			
17 gm/dose, 510 gm	16590-0542-51	35.09	
MIRASORB GAUZE SPONGES (Johnson & Johnson)			
DEV,NA (4"X4")			
50s ea	81370-0055-31	5.32	
MIRASORB NONSTERILE (J&J Medical)			
DEV,NA (2"X2",3-PLY)			
200s ea	56091-0676-12	1.99	
(2"X2",4-PLY)			
200s ea	56091-0676-13	2.29	
(3"X3",4-PLY)			
200s ea	56091-0676-22	5.20	
(4"X4",3-PLY)			
200s ea	56091-0676-10	4.95	
(4"X4",4-PLY)			
200s ea	56091-0676-23	8.58	
MIRASORB STERILE (J&J Medical)			
DEV,NA (4"X4",4-PLY,TRAY)			
10s ea	56091-0623-26	0.94	
(4"X4",4PLY,2X25)			
50s ea	56091-0623-17	2.99	
(3"X3",4-PLY,2X40)			
80s ea	56091-0623-19	3.44	
(2"X2",4-PLY,2X50)			
100s ea	56091-0623-18	3.01	
MISSION PRENATAL (Mission)			
TAB,PO, 100s ea	00178-0132-01	12.73	
MISSION PRENATAL F.A. (Mission)			
TAB,PO, 100s ea	00178-0153-01	13.20	
MISSION PRENATAL H.P. (Mission)			
TAB,PO, 100s ea	00178-0161-01	13.34	
MITRAZOL (Healthpoint)			
POW,TP, 2%, 30 gm	00064-0650-01	9.76	
MK-7 (Bio-Tech Pharm)			
CAP,PO, 150 mcg,			
100s ea	53191-0469-01	45.95	
MLK-1000 (Key Company)			
SGL,PO (SOFTGEL)			
120 mg-180 mg,			
100s ea	11694-0797-01	7.00	
650s ea	11694-0797-05	35.00	

PROD/MFR	HRI, UPC,NDC	AWP	SRP
MM-ZYME (Miller)			
TAB,PO, 100s ea	17204-0539-40	8.22	13.00
MMA/PA EXPRESS (VITAFLO, LLC)			
PDR,PO (30X25GM,UNFLAVORED)			
25 gm 30s	50600-0543-71	265.50	349.75
MN-50 (Bio-Tech Pharm)			
CAP,PO, 50 mg, 100s ea	53191-0263-01	4.20	
MNP-8 (Rx Vitamins)			
CAP,PO, 90s ea	08429-0800-90	10.98	21.95
MOBISYL (Ascher)			
CRE,TP, 10%, 100 gm	00225-0360-11	5.94	
226.8 gm	00225-0360-35	12.00	
MODULEN IBD (Nestle)			
PDR,PO, 400 gm	00065-9084-91	24.00	
MOI-STIR (Kingswood)			
SPR,MM, 120 ml	55299-0601-04	7.40	7.80
MOIST AGAIN (Lake Pharm)			
GEL,VG (W/APPLICATOR)			
75 gm	12277-0518-47	4.19	6.99
MOISTUR-EYES (Carlson,J.R.)			
SGL,PO (PF,SF,CORN-FREE)			
360s ea	88395-0048-23	34.95	69.90
MOISTURE THERAPY CONDITIONER (Dartmouth)			
SOL,TP (1X360ML)			
360 ml	58869-0230-12	12.00	14.99
MOISTURE THERAPY PRE-WASH (Dartmouth)			
TP (1X180ML)			
180 ml	58869-0210-06	12.00	14.99
MOISTURE THERAPY REPLENISHING MASQUE (Dartmouth)			
TP (1X360ML)			
360 ml	58869-0240-08	12.00	14.99
MOISTURE THERAPY SHAMPOO (Dartmouth)			
SHA,TP (1X360ML)			
360 ml	58869-0220-12	12.00	14.99
MOISTUREL (Warner Chilcott)			
CRE,TP (FRAGRANCE-FREE)			
1%, 113 gm	00430-3500-08	6.93	
453 gm	00430-3500-11	15.49	
LOT,TP, 397 gm	00430-3100-11	9.73	
3%, 240 ml	00430-3100-10	7.76	
MOISTUREL SKIN CLEANSER (Warner Chilcott)			
LOT,TP (FRAGRANCE-FREE)			
262.5 ml	00430-3420-10	7.79	
MOISTURIZING CREME (AmerisourceBergen)			
CRE,TP (FRAGRANCE-FREE)			
454 gm	24385-0353-43	6.29	6.99
MOISTURIZING LOTION (AmerisourceBergen)			
LOT,TP (W/PUMP,PRIVATE LABEL)			
473 ml	24385-0354-43	6.29	6.99
MOISTURIZING SUNBLOCK (AmerisourceBergen)			
LOT,TP (SPF 30,AF,SF)			
118 ml	24385-0081-26	3.42	4.99
MOLLIFENE (Pfeiffer)			
SOL,OT, 6.5%, 15 ml	00927-0676-23	2.39	4.29
MOLY-B (Carlson,J.R.)			
TAB,PO (PF,SF,CORN-FREE)			
500 mcg, 300s ea	88395-0056-43	10.80	21.60
MOMENTUM (Medtech)			
TAB,PO (CAPLET)			
467 mg, 24s ea	75137-0212-10	4.84	
48s ea	75137-0212-20	8.43	
MONISTAT 1 COMBO PACK (Johnson & Johnson)			
KIT,MR, ea	80045-0541-10	15.58	
(COOL WIPES)			
ea	80045-0494-00	18.02	
(PREFILLED APPLICATOR)			
ea	80045-0410-20	16.82	
MONISTAT 1 COMINBATION PACK (Johnson & Johnson)			
KIT,MR, ea	62341-5418-00	18.02	
ea	80045-0418-00	18.65	
(INSERT W/APP+EXTRNL CRM)			
ea	62341-5411-00	16.81	
MONISTAT 1-DAY (Johnson & Johnson)			
OIN,VG (PREFILLED APPLICATOR)			
6.5%, 4.6 gm	80045-0410-01	14.41	
MONISTAT 3 (Johnson & Johnson)			
CRE,VG (PREFILLED APPLICATORS)			
4%, 5 gm 3s	00625-0402-01	13.24	
(WITH 3 APPLICATORS)			
4%, 25 gm	00625-0401-01	13.24	
MONISTAT 3 COMBINATION PACK (Johnson & Johnson)			
KIT,NA, ea	80045-0403-10	14.41	
(3 PREFILLED APPLICATORS)			
ea	80045-0403-00	15.61	
KIT,VG, ea	00625-0430-01	14.41	
ea	00625-0430-05	14.41	
ea	80045-0486-00	16.82	
ea	80045-0498-00	18.02	
MONISTAT 7 (Johnson & Johnson)			
CRE,VG (1X45GM)			
2%, 45 gm	00625-0426-35	9.60	
(W/REUSEABLE APPLICATOR)			
2%, 45 gm	00625-0426-05	9.60	
(Phys Total Care) REPACK			
SUP,VG (W/APPLICATOR)			
100 mg, 7s ea	54868-0434-01	12.35	
(Southwood) REPACK			
CRE,VG, 2%, 45 gm	58016-3049-01	12.08	
SUP,VG, 100 mg, 7s ea	58016-3052-01	12.08	
MONISTAT 7 COMBINATION PACK (Johnson & Johnson)			
CRE,VG, ea	80045-0470-04	12.01	
(TRIPLE ACTION SYSTEM)			
ea	80045-0496-00	12.01	
KIT,VG (WITH 7 SUPPOSITORIES)			
ea	00625-0422-02	10.80	
MONISTAT SOOTHING CARE CHAFING RELIEF POWDER (Johnson & Johnson)			
GEL,TP (FRAGRANCE-FREE)			
1.2%, 42 gm	80045-0472-00	5.83	
MONISTAT SOOTHING CARE ITCH RELIEF (Johnson & Johnson)			
CRE,TP (1X28GM,FRAGRANCE-FREE)			
1%, 28 gm	80045-0407-00	3.97	
MONISTAT SOOTHING CARE MEDICATED POWDER (Johnson & Johnson)			
POW,TP (MICRO-FINE)			
10%, 255 gm	80045-0419-00	4.46	
MONO-FLO BEDSIDE DRAIN BAG (Covidien)			
DEV,NA (W/ANTI-REFLUX DEVICE)			
20s ea	08080-6300-00	106.15	
MONO-FLO DRAINAGE BAG (Covidien)			
DEV,NA (W/ ANTI-REFLUX,2000ML)			
20s ea	08080-6209-00	102.04	
MONOCAL (Mericon)			
TAB,PO, 250 mg-3 mg,			
100s ea	00394-0105-02	12.05	
MONOCAPS (Freeda)			
TAB,PO (PF,SF,DYE-FREE)			
100s ea	10432-0037-01	7.77	12.95
250s ea	10432-0037-02	15.54	25.90
500s ea	10432-0037-03	25.77	42.95
MONOFILAMENTS (Owen Mumford)			
DEV,NA (FOR USE W/NEUROPEN,10GM)			
5s ea	08470-0104-01	18.75	23.00
(FOR USE W/NEUROPEN,15GM)			
5s ea	08470-0105-01	18.75	23.00
MONOGEN (Nutricia)			
PDR,PO (6X400GM,MEDICALFOOD)			
400 gm 6s	49735-0170-97	241.80	
MONOJECT (Covidien)			
DEV,NA (GLOVE BOX)			
2s ea	08881-6766-32	78.75	
(WALL CABINET/SHARPS CNT)			
2s ea	08881-6766-24	45.00	
(BN MRW BIOP TRAY 11GX4")			
10s ea	08881-8470-19	455.30	
10s ea	08881-8471-18	309.83	
(BN MRW BIOP TRAY 8GX4")			
10s ea	08881-8470-35	455.30	
10s ea	08881-8470-84	343.75	
(BN MRW BIOP TRY W/O NDL)			
10s ea	08881-8479-93	184.64	
(BNE MRW BIOP TRAY 16G)			
10s ea	08881-8471-67	251.79	
(BNE MRW BIOP TRY 16GX2")			
10s ea	08881-8461-69	246.19	
(BRACKET FOR SHARPS CONT)			
10s ea	08881-6760-12	93.75	
(BONE MARR ASP 16GX3/4")			
20s ea	08881-2400-17	244.55	
(BONE MRW ASPIR 16G X2")			
20s ea	08881-2400-09	221.72	
(PISTON CATH TIP 140CC)			
20s ea	08881-1140-55	66.94	
(PISTON LOCK LUER 140CC)			
20s ea	08881-1140-30	66.94	
(PISTON REG LUER 140CC)			
20s ea	08881-1140-14	66.94	
(60CC CATH TIP)			
100s ea	08881-5601-41	103.94	
(60CC ECCENTRIC LUER)			
100s ea	08881-5601-82	103.94	
(60CC LUER LOCK)			
100s ea	08881-5601-25	103.94	
(60CC REG LUER)			
100s ea	08881-5602-24	103.94	
(60CC TOOMEY TIP)			
100s ea	08881-5602-65	126.50	
(BLUNT CANNULA,15GX1.5")			
100s ea	08881-2023-14	88.20	
(BLUNT CANNULA,16GX1.5")			
100s ea	08881-2023-22	88.20	
(BLUNT CANNULA,17GX1.5")			
100s ea	08881-2023-30	88.20	
(BLUNT CANNULA,18GX1")			
100s ea	08881-2023-48	88.20	
(BLUNT CANNULA,19GX1.5")			
100s ea	08881-2023-55	88.20	
(BLUNT CANNULA,20GX1.5")			
100s ea	08881-2023-63	88.20	
(BLUNT CANNULA,21GX1.5")			
100s ea	08881-2023-71	88.18	
(BLUNT CANNULA,22GX1.5")			
100s ea	08881-2023-89	88.18	
(BLUNT CANNULA,23GX1")			
100s ea	08881-2023-97	88.18	
(CONTROL LUER LOCK 20CC)			
100s ea	08881-5201-78	289.80	
(FILTER ASP 5UM 18G X3")			
100s ea	08881-3051-09	33.62	
(HYPODERMIC,20GX3")			
100s ea	08881-2002-35	93.50	
(NON-STER CATH TIP 60CC)			
100s ea	08881-1601-57	39.85	
(NON-STER ECCEN LUER35CC)			
100s ea	08881-1350-68	67.53	
(NON-STER LUER 35CC)			
100s ea	08881-1350-84	67.53	
(60CC CATHETER TIP)			
120s ea	08080-0004-44	62.60	
(60CC LUER LOCK)			
120s ea	08080-0007-77	62.60	
(60CC REG LUER)			
120s ea	08080-0005-55	62.60	
(PHCY TRAY 355CC LUERLCK)			
120s ea	08881-5351-01	87.57	
(PHCY TRAY 60CC LUERLOCK)			
120s ea	08881-5602-32	130.38	
(20CC ONLY-LUER LOCK)			
160s ea	08080-2000-77	64.38	
(20CC ONLY-REG LUER)			
160s ea	08080-2000-55	64.38	
(35CC CATHETER TIP)			
160s ea	08080-5008-88	76.25	
(35CC LUER LOCK)			
160s ea	08080-5007-77	76.25	
(35CC REG LUER)			
160s ea	08080-5005-55	76.25	
(35CC ECCENTRIC LUERLOCK)			
180s ea	08881-5357-88	119.48	
(35CC LUER LOCK)			
180s ea	08881-5357-62	119.48	
(35CC ONLY CATH TIP)			
180s ea	08881-5357-70	119.48	
(35CC REG LUER)			
180s ea	08881-5357-96	119.48	
(CONTROL LUER 12CC)			
200s ea	08881-5129-77	235.83	
(PHCY TRAY 12CC)			
200s ea	08881-5122-58	44.63	
(PHCY TRAY 20CC)			
200s ea	08881-5202-51	123.38	
(PHCY TRAY 3CC SRN)			
200s ea	08881-5132-07	33.72	
(PHCY TRAY 6CC SRN)			
200s ea	08881-5162-00	40.75	
(EXTEND CAP FOR 1 OR 3CC)			
250s ea	08881-9121-02	45.77	
(NON-STER ECCEN LUER20CC)			
250s ea	08881-1200-29	140.99	
(NON-STER REG LUER 20CC)			
250s ea	08881-1200-37	140.99	
(20CC ECCENTRIC LUERLOCK)			
300s ea	08881-5206-65	170.07	

PROD/MFR	HRI, UPC,NDC	AWP	SRP
(20CC LUER LOCK)			
300s ea	**08881-5206-57**	170.07	
(20CC REG LUER)			
300s ea	**08881-5206-73**	170.07	
(30GX5/16", 3/10CC)			
300s ea	**08881-6008-00**	51.75	
(30GX5/16",1/2CC)			
300s ea	**08881-6007-00**	51.75	
(30GX5/16",1CC)			
300s ea	**08881-6016-00**	51.75	
(6CC SAFETY 20GX1.5")			
300s ea	**08881-5660-15**	142.50	
(6CC SAFETY 21GX1.5")			
300s ea	**08881-5660-23**	142.50	
(6CC SAFETY ONLY LUERLCK)			
300s ea	**08881-5660-07**	112.50	
(FILTER NDL 5UM 18G X1")			
300s ea	**08881-3052-08**	255.94	
(SAFETY 12CC 20GX1.5")			
300s ea	**08881-5220-18**	180.45	
(SAFETY 12CC 21GX.5")			
300s ea	**08881-5220-26**	180.45	
(SAFETY ONLY 12CC LUERLK)			
300s ea	**08881-5220-00**	153.75	
(U100,1/2CC,28GX1/2")			
300s ea	**08881-6000-04**	46.95	
(U100,1/2CC,29GX1/2")			
300s ea	**08881-6003-50**	49.30	
(U100,1CC,28GX1/2")			
300s ea	**08881-6011-01**	46.95	
(U100,1CC,29GX1/2")			
300s ea	**08881-6013-58**	49.30	
(U100,3/10CC,29GX1/2")			
300s ea	**08881-6001-45**	49.30	
(U100,BULKPACK,1/2CC)			
300s ea	**08881-7004-08**	27.65	
(U100,HARDPACK,1CC)			
300s ea	**08881-7014-06**	27.14	
(ULTRACOMFORT,30GX5/16")			
300s ea	**08080-3003-00**	51.75	
(VARISTOP 20CC LUER LOCK)			
300s ea	**08881-5201-86**	354.38	
(6CC 20GX1.5")			
400s ea	**08080-6201-12**	83.68	
(6CC 21GX1.5")			
400s ea	**08080-6211-12**	83.68	
(6CC 21GX1")			
400s ea	**08080-6211-00**	83.68	
(6CC 22GX1.5")			
400s ea	**08080-6221-12**	83.68	
(6CC ONLY-LUER LOCK)			
400s ea	**08080-6007-77**	54.58	
(6CC ONLY-REG LUER)			
400s ea	**08080-6005-55**	54.58	
(12CC 18GX1")			
480s ea	**08080-2181-00**	105.48	
480s ea	**08881-5125-97**	144.97	
(12CC 20GX1.5")			
480s ea	**08080-2201-12**	105.48	
(12CC 21GX1.5")			
480s ea	**08080-2211-12**	105.48	
480s ea	**08881-5127-46**	144.97	
(12CC 21GX1")			
480s ea	**08080-2211-00**	105.48	
480s ea	**08881-5127-38**	144.97	
(12CC 22GX1.5")			
480s ea	**08080-2221-12**	105.48	
(12CC 22GX1.5)			
480s ea	**08881-5128-11**	144.97	
(12CC ONLY ECC LUER)			
480s ea	**08881-5128-60**	97.50	
(12CC ONLY LUER LOCK)			
480s ea	**08881-5128-78**	97.50	
(12CC ONLY REG LUER)			
480s ea	**08881-5128-52**	97.50	
(12CC ONLY-LUER LOCK)			
480s ea	**08080-2007-77**	71.00	
(12CC ONLY-REG LUER)			
480s ea	**08080-2005-55**	71.00	
(12CC VARI-STOP LUER TIP)			
480s ea	**08881-5126-47**	504.00	
(BLUNT CANNULA W/SRN)			
480s ea	**08881-2021-32**	301.74	
(28GX1/2",U100)			
500s ea	**08881-5012-10**	98.25	
(6CC 20GX1.5")			
500s ea	**08881-5160-51**	143.75	
(6CC 21GX1.5")			
500s ea	**08881-5161-50**	143.75	
(6CC 21GX1")			
500s ea	**08881-5161-35**	143.75	
(6CC LUER LOCK)			
500s ea	**08881-5169-37**	94.75	
(6CC ONLY-REG LUER)			
500s ea	**08881-5169-11**	94.75	
(6CC22GX1.5")			
500s ea	**08881-5162-59**	143.75	
(BLUNT CANNULA W/SRN)			
500s ea	**08881-2020-25**	237.32	
500s ea	**08881-2021-16**	265.32	
(ECC LUER 12CC)			
500s ea	**08881-1120-75**	90.28	
(FINGER GRIP EXTEND 20CC)			
500s ea	**08881-8200-08**	93.02	
(FINGER GRIP EXTEND 35CC)			
500s ea	**08881-8350-06**	93.02	
(FINGER GRIP EXTEND 60CC)			
500s ea	**08881-8600-04**	93.02	
(INSULIN, 29GX5", 1/2CC)			
500s ea	**08881-5111-36**	231.44	
(INSULIN, 29GX5", 3/10CC)			
500s ea	**08881-5111-44**	231.44	
(INSULIN,25GX5/8",1CC)			
500s ea	**08080-8125-05**	59.53	
(INSULIN,27GX1/2",1CC)			
500s ea	**08080-8127-01**	59.53	
(INSULIN,28GX1/2",1/2CC)			
500s ea	**08080-8528-01**	59.53	
(INSULIN,28GX1/2",1CC)			
500s ea	**08080-8128-01**	59.53	
(INSULIN,REG,LUER,1CC)			
500s ea	**08080-8100-55**	57.52	
(ORAL MEDICATION 1ML,AMB)			
500s ea	**08881-9010-06**	75.00	
(ORAL MEDICATION 1ML,CLR)			
500s ea	**08881-9010-14**	51.88	
(ORAL MEDICATION 3ML,AMB)			
500s ea	**08881-9030-10**	63.79	
(ORAL MEDICATION 3ML,CLR)			
500s ea	**08881-9030-02**	42.53	
(ORAL MEDICATION 6ML,AMB)			
500s ea	**08881-9060-05**	78.75	
(ORAL MEDICATION 6ML,CLR)			
500s ea	**08881-9061-04**	58.12	
(ORAL MEDICATN 10ML,AMB)			
500s ea	**08881-9070-03**	99.43	
(ORAL MEDICATN 10ML,CLR)			
500s ea	**08881-9071-02**	69.57	
(REG LUER 6CC)			
500s ea	**08881-1060-28**	82.69	
(SAFETY 3CC 20GX1.5")			
500s ea	**08881-5330-56**	184.38	
(SAFETY 3CC 21GX1.5")			
500s ea	**08881-5331-55**	184.38	
(SAFETY 3CC 21GX1")			
500s ea	**08881-5331-30**	184.38	
(SAFETY 3CC 22GX1.5")			
500s ea	**08881-5332-54**	184.38	
(SAFETY 3CC 22GX1")			
500s ea	**08881-5332-39**	184.38	
(SAFETY 3CC 23GX1")			
500s ea	**08881-5333-38**	184.38	
(SAFETY 3CC 25GX5/8")			
500s ea	**08881-5335-10**	184.38	
(SAFETY ONLY 3CC LUERLCK)			
500s ea	**08881-5339-08**	125.32	
(SYRINGE REG LUER 12 CC)			
500s ea	**08881-1120-59**	90.28	
(TUBER 1CC27GX1/2",U100)			
500s ea	**08881-5013-68**	98.19	
(TUBERC 27GX1/2")			
500s ea	**08881-5016-08**	98.19	
(TUBERC,1CC 25GX5/8",DET)			
500s ea	**08080-1250-58**	72.17	
(TUBERCUL,1/2CC 28GX1/2")			
500s ea	**08080-5280-12**	72.17	
(TUBERCUL,1CC 25GX5/8")			
500s ea	**08080-1251-58**	72.17	
(TUBERCUL,1CC 26GX3/8")			
500s ea	**08080-1260-38**	72.17	
(TUBERCUL,1CC 27GX1/2")			
500s ea	**08080-1270-12**	72.17	
(TUBERCUL,1CC 28GX1/2")			
500s ea	**08080-1280-12**	72.17	
(TUBERCUL,1CC REG LUER)			
500s ea	**08080-1005-55**	70.23	
(TUBERCULIN SE,25GX5/8)			
500s ea	**08881-5112-35**	216.82	
(U100 1CC 25GX1.5")			
500s ea	**08881-5018-22**	117.25	
(U100 27GX1/2")			
500s ea	**08881-5019-70**	117.25	
(U100 SE 29GX1/2")			
500s ea	**08881-5111-10**	218.94	
(U100 TUBERC 26GX3/8")			
500s ea	**08881-5011-78**	98.19	
(U100 TUBERC 28GX1/2")			
500s ea	**08881-5001-05**	98.19	
(U100 TUBERC,LUER TIP)			
500s ea	**08881-5014-00**	65.00	
(U100,1CC)			
500s ea	**08881-5013-84**	91.38	
(U100,28G X1/2")			
500s ea	**08881-5000-14**	98.25	
(U100SE TUBERC28GX5/8")			
500s ea	**08881-5112-01**	216.82	
(U100TUBERC 1CC25GX5/8")			
500s ea	**08881-5011-60**	98.19	
(3CC 20GX1.5")			
800s ea	**08080-3201-12**	85.39	
(3CC 20GX1")			
800s ea	**08080-0320-10**	85.39	
(3CC 20GX3/4")			
800s ea	**08080-3200-34**	85.39	
(3CC 21GX1.5")			
800s ea	**08080-3211-12**	85.39	
(3CC 21GX1")			
800s ea	**08080-3211-00**	85.39	
(3CC 22GX1 1/4")			
800s ea	**08080-3221-14**	85.39	
(3CC 22GX1.5")			
800s ea	**08080-3221-12**	85.39	
(3CC 22GX1")			
800s ea	**08080-3221-00**	85.39	
(3CC 23GX1.5")			
800s ea	**08080-3231-12**	85.39	
(3CC 23GX1")			
800s ea	**08080-3231-00**	85.39	
(3CC 25GX1 1/4")			
800s ea	**08080-3251-14**	85.39	
(3CC 25GX1")			
800s ea	**08080-3251-00**	85.39	
(3CC 25GX5/8")			
800s ea	**08080-3250-58**	85.39	
(3CC 27GX1 1/4")			
800s ea	**08080-3271-14**	85.39	
(3CC ONLY-LUER LOCK)			
800s ea	**08080-3007-77**	58.00	
(3CC ONLY-REG LUER)			
800s ea	**08080-3005-55**	58.00	
(3CC 20GX1.5")			
1000s ea	**08881-5130-58**	146.50	
(3CC 20GX1")			
1000s ea	**08881-5130-33**	146.50	
(3CC 20GX3/4")			
1000s ea	**08881-5130-25**	146.50	
(3CC 21GX1.5")			
1000s ea	**08881-5131-57**	146.50	
(3CC 21GX1")			
1000s ea	**08881-5131-32**	146.50	
(3CC 22GX1.5")			
1000s ea	**08881-5132-56**	146.50	
(3CC 23GX1")			
1000s ea	**08881-5133-30**	146.50	
(3CC 25GX1.25")			
1000s ea	**08881-5135-46**	146.50	
(3CC 25GX1")			
1000s ea	**08881-5135-38**	146.50	
(3CC 25GX5/8")			
1000s ea	**08881-5135-12**	146.50	
(3CC 27GX1.25")			
1000s ea	**08881-5137-44**	146.50	
(3CC ONLY-LUER LOCK)			
1000s ea	**08881-5139-34**	99.50	
(3CC ONLY-REG LUER)			
1000s ea	**08881-5139-18**	99.50	
(3CC,22GX1.25")			
1000s ea	**08881-5132-49**	146.50	
(3CC,22GX1")			
1000s ea	**08881-5132-31**	146.50	
(ALLER TRAY 1CC 26GX3/8")			
1000s ea	**08881-5015-58**	121.95	
(ALLER TRAY 1CC 27GX1/2")			
1000s ea	**08881-5019-62**	149.10	
(ALLER TRAY W/1CC SRN)			
1000s ea	**08881-5012-36**	121.90	
(ALLER TRY W/1/2CC SRN)			
1000s ea	**08881-5004-93**	128.22	
1000s ea	**08881-5005-01**	128.17	
(BLUNT CANNULA 18GX1")			
1000s ea	**08881-2020-17**	360.00	
(BLUNT CANNULA W/SRN)			
1000s ea	**08881-2020-33**	452.34	
(BLUNT CANNULA,18GX1&1/2)			
1000s ea	**08881-5401-99**	437.50	
(FILTER NDL 5UM 20GX1.5")			
1000s ea	**08881-3050-18**	257.25	
(FILTER NDL 5UM18GX1-1/2)			
1000s ea	**08881-3051-17**	257.25	

PROD/MFR	HRI, UPC,NDC	AWP	SRP
(HYPODER NDL 18GX1 1/2"A)			
1000s ea	08080-8181-12	65.68	
(HYPODER NDL 18GX1 1/2"B)			
1000s ea	08080-8181-13	65.68	
(HYPODERM NDL 18GX1",A)			
1000s ea	08080-8181-00	65.68	
1000s ea	08080-8191-00	65.68	
(HYPODERM NDL 18GX1",B)			
1000s ea	08080-8181-01	65.68	
(HYPODERM,19TWX1 1/2" B)			
1000s ea	08080-8191-13	65.68	
(HYPODERM,19TWX1 1/2", A)			
1000s ea	08080-8191-12	65.68	
(HYPODERMIC, 14GX1 1/2")			
1000s ea	08881-2000-11	208.44	
(HYPODERMIC, 15GX1.5")			
1000s ea	08881-2000-29	208.44	
(HYPODERMIC, 16GX1.5")			
1000s ea	08881-2000-37	225.12	
1000s ea	08881-2000-45	208.44	
(HYPODERMIC, 16GX1")			
1000s ea	08881-2000-52	225.12	
(HYPODERMIC, 16GX3/4")			
1000s ea	08881-2000-60	208.44	
(HYPODERMIC, 18GX1.5")			
1000s ea	08881-2000-86	119.32	
(HYPODERMIC, 18GX1.5")			
1000s ea	08881-2000-78	120.50	
(HYPODERMIC, 18GX1")			
1000s ea	08881-2001-10	119.32	
(HYPODERMIC,14GX1")			
1000s ea	08881-2008-05	208.44	
(HYPODERMIC,14GX2")			
1000s ea	08881-2005-73	208.44	
(HYPODERMIC,16GX5/8")			
1000s ea	08881-2007-55	208.44	
(HYPODERMIC,18GX1.5")			
1000s ea	08881-2500-16	89.94	12.55
1000s ea	08881-2500-24	89.94	
(HYPODERMIC,18GX1")			
1000s ea	08881-2007-14	120.50	
1000s ea	08881-2500-40	89.94	
1000s ea	08881-2500-57	89.94	
(HYPODERMIC,19TW X1.25")			
1000s ea	08881-2001-51	208.44	
(HYPODERMIC,19TW X1.5")			
1000s ea	08881-2001-36	120.50	
1000s ea	08881-2001-44	119.32	
1000s ea	08881-2500-65	89.94	
1000s ea	08881-2500-73	89.94	
(HYPODERMIC,19TW X1")			
1000s ea	08881-2001-69	120.50	
1000s ea	08881-2500-81	89.94	
1000s ea	08881-2500-99	89.94	
(HYPODERMIC,19TW X1",B)			
1000s ea	08080-8191-01	65.68	
(HYPODERMIC,20GX1 1/2",A)			
1000s ea	08080-8201-12	65.68	
(HYPODERMIC,20GX1 1/2",B)			
1000s ea	08080-8201-13	65.68	
(HYPODERMIC,20GX1.5")			
1000s ea	08881-2001-85	120.50	
1000s ea	08881-2001-93	119.32	
1000s ea	08881-2002-27	119.32	
1000s ea	08881-2501-07	89.94	
1000s ea	08881-2501-15	89.94	
(HYPODERMIC,20GX1")			
1000s ea	08881-2002-19	120.50	
1000s ea	08881-2501-23	89.94	
1000s ea	08881-2501-31	89.94	
(HYPODERMIC,20GX1",A)			
1000s ea	08080-8201-00	65.68	
(HYPODERMIC,20GX1",B)			
1000s ea	08080-8201-01	65.68	
(HYPODERMIC,20GX3/4")			
1000s ea	08881-2511-88	85.63	
(HYPODERMIC,21GX1 1/2 A)			
1000s ea	08080-8211-12	65.68	
(HYPODERMIC,21GX1.5")			
1000s ea	08881-2002-68	120.50	
1000s ea	08881-2501-49	89.94	
1000s ea	08881-2501-98	89.94	
(HYPODERMIC,21GX1.5",B)			
1000s ea	08080-8211-13	65.68	
(HYPODERMIC,21GX1")			
1000s ea	08881-2002-92	120.50	
1000s ea	08881-2501-72	89.94	
1000s ea	08881-2501-80	89.94	
(HYPODERMIC,21GX1", A)			
1000s ea	08080-8211-00	65.68	
(HYPODERMIC,21GX1", B)			
1000s ea	08080-8211-01	65.68	
(HYPODERMIC,21GX2")			
1000s ea	08881-2003-18	225.12	
(HYPODERMIC,22GX1.5")			
1000s ea	08881-2003-26	120.50	
1000s ea	08881-2502-06	89.94	
(HYPODERMIC,22GX1.5",A)			
1000s ea	08080-8221-12	65.68	
(HYPODERMIC,22GX1.5",B)			
1000s ea	08080-8221-13	65.68	
(HYPODERMIC,22GX1.5")			
1000s ea	08881-2502-14	89.94	
(HYPODERMIC,22GX1")			
1000s ea	08881-2003-42	120.50	
1000s ea	08881-2502-22	89.94	
1000s ea	08881-2502-30	89.94	
(HYPODERMIC,22GX1",A)			
1000s ea	08080-8221-00	65.68	
(HYPODERMIC,22GX1",B)			
1000s ea	08080-8221-01	65.68	
(HYPODERMIC,23G1",A)			
1000s ea	08080-8231-00	65.68	
(HYPODERMIC,23GX1")			
1000s ea	08881-2003-83	120.50	
1000s ea	08881-2502-55	89.94	
(HYPODERMIC,23GX1/2")			
1000s ea	08080-8230-12	65.68	
(HYPODERMIC,23GX3/4")			
1000s ea	08881-2502-89	89.94	
(HYPODERMIC,23GX3/4",A)			
1000s ea	08080-8230-34	65.68	
(HYPODERMIC,25GX1.25")			
1000s ea	08881-2004-33	120.50	
(HYPODERMIC,25GX1.5")			
1000s ea	08881-2505-45	89.94	
(HYPODERMIC,25GX1.5",A)			
1000s ea	08080-8251-12	65.68	
(HYPODERMIC,25GX1")			
1000s ea	08881-2503-05	89.94	
(HYPODERMIC,25GX1",A)			
1000s ea	08080-8251-00	65.68	
(HYPODERMIC,25GX2")			
1000s ea	08881-2004-41	208.44	
(HYPODERMIC,25GX5/8")			
1000s ea	08881-2004-66	120.50	
1000s ea	08881-2503-13	89.94	
(HYPODERMIC,25GX5/8",A)			
1000s ea	08080-8250-58	65.68	
(HYPODERMIC,26GX1.5",A)			
1000s ea	08080-8261-12	65.68	
(HYPODERMIC,26GX1/2")			
1000s ea	08881-2503-21	89.94	
(HYPODERMIC,26GX1/2")			
1000s ea	08080-8260-12	65.68	
(HYPODERMIC,27GX.5")			
1000s ea	08881-2005-16	118.13	
(HYPODERMIC,27GX1.25")			
1000s ea	08881-2005-08	130.14	
(HYPODERMIC,27GX1/2")			
1000s ea	08881-2503-62	89.94	
(HYPODERMIC,27GX1/2",A)			
1000s ea	08080-8270-12	65.68	
(HYPODERMIC,30GX3/4")			
1000s ea	08881-2500-32	107.24	
(HYPODERMIC,30GX3/4",A)			
1000s ea	08080-8303-40	87.32	
(MEDICATION TRANSF 20G)			
1000s ea	08881-2040-05	212.63	
(REG LUER 3CC)			
1000s ea	08881-1030-25	89.58	
(TIP CAPS-FLEX LUER TIP)			
1000s ea	08881-6820-85	55.89	
1000s ea	08881-6821-01	59.07	
1000s ea	08881-6821-19	61.82	

MONOJECT ASPIRATION NEEDLE (Covidien)

PROD/MFR	HRI, UPC,NDC	AWP	SRP
DEV,NA (BN MRW BIOP,11GX4")			
10s ea	08881-2471-11	218.22	
(BN MRW BIOP,13GX2.5")			
10s ea	08881-2471-29	218.22	
(BN MRW BIOP,13GX3.5")			
10s ea	08881-2471-37	232.03	
(BN MRW BIOP,8GX4")			
10s ea	08881-2470-87	218.22	
(IL. STERNAL-ILLIAC,16G)			
10s ea	08881-2451-64	136.87	

MONOJECT BLOOD COLLECTION HOLDER (Covidien)

PROD/MFR	HRI, UPC,NDC	AWP	SRP
DEV,NA, 100s ea	08080-6101-02	11.08	
100s ea	08080-6101-10	11.08	

MONOJECT BLOOD COLLECTION NEEDLE AND TUBE (Covidien)

PROD/MFR	HRI, UPC,NDC	AWP	SRP
DEV,NA, 1200s ea	08080-6101-28	96.10	

MONOJECT BLOOD COLLECTION NEEDLES (Covidien)

PROD/MFR	HRI, UPC,NDC	AWP	SRP
DEV,NA (20G,1",SINGLE)			
1000s ea	08080-1211-18	170.53	
(20G,1")			
1000s ea	08080-2160-17	171.97	
(20G,1&1/2",MULTIPLE)			
1000s ea	08080-2160-25	171.97	
(20G,1&1/2",SINGLE)			
1000s ea	08080-2110-26	170.53	
(21G,1",MULTIPLE)			
1000s ea	08080-2160-33	151.45	
(21G,1",SINGLE)			
1000s ea	08080-2111-17	217.95	
(21G,1&1/2",MULTIPLE)			
1000s ea	08080-2160-41	134.64	
(21G,1&1/2",SINGLE)			
1000s ea	08080-2111-25	248.73	
(22G,1",MULTIPLE)			
1000s ea	08080-2160-66	151.45	
(22G,1",SINGLE)			
1000s ea	08080-2112-16	229.97	
(22G,1&1/2",MULTIPLE)			
1000s ea	08080-2160-58	151.90	

MONOJECT BLOOD COLLECTION TUBE (Covidien)

PROD/MFR	HRI, UPC,NDC	AWP	SRP
DEV,NA (RED/YELLOW STOPPER)			
500s ea	08080-3800-03	220.99	
1000s ea	08080-3619-95	301.83	
(13X100MM)			
1000s ea	08080-3405-85	177.09	
(13X75MM)			
1000s ea	08080-3406-76	120.68	
(BLACK STOPPER)			
1000s ea	08080-3425-65	205.52	
1000s ea	08080-3425-73	292.08	
(GRAY STOPPER)			
1000s ea	08080-3545-86	218.63	
(GREY STOPPER)			
1000s ea	08080-3522-83	177.34	
1000s ea	08080-3524-81	134.54	
1000s ea	08080-3525-80	165.70	
1000s ea	08080-3527-88	401.02	
1000s ea	08080-3535-88	233.75	
(YELLOW STOPPER)			
1000s ea	08080-3619-87	335.23	

MONOJECT BLOOD COLLECTION TUBES (Covidien)

PROD/MFR	HRI, UPC,NDC	AWP	SRP
DEV,NA (10.25X50,RED)			
1000s ea	08080-3011-16	142.84	
(10.25X64,3ML,RED)			
1000s ea	08080-3012-15	147.13	
(10.25X82,4ML,RED)			
1000s ea	08080-3012-14	156.54	
(13X100,RED)			
1000s ea	08080-3015-12	136.13	
1000s ea	08080-3025-10	154.64	
(13X75,RED)			
1000s ea	08080-3014-13	144.29	
1000s ea	08080-3024-11	154.64	
(16X100,RED)			
1000s ea	08080-3017-10	158.59	
(16X125,RED)			
1000s ea	08080-3018-19	197.92	
(16X75,RED)			
1000s ea	08080-3016-11	170.39	

MONOJECT BLUNTIP (Covidien)

PROD/MFR	HRI, UPC,NDC	AWP	SRP
DEV,NA (W/12ML LUER LOCK SYRNGE)			
480s ea	08080-5411-25	168.75	
(W/6ML LUER LOCK SYRINGE)			
500s ea	08080-5410-67	162.50	
1000s ea	08080-5401-01	231.25	
(W/3ML LUER LOCK SYRINGE)			
1000s ea	08080-5410-34	275.00	

MONOJECT BLUNTITE IV SECURITY (Covidien)

PROD/MFR	HRI, UPC,NDC	AWP	SRP
DEV,NA, 800s ea	08080-5409-03	415.80	

MONOJECT CRAWFORD POINT EPIDURAL NEEDLE METAL HUB (Covidien)

PROD/MFR	HRI, UPC,NDC	AWP	SRP
DEV,NA (18G TWX2-1/2",4X25)			
100s ea	08080-2210-25	267.10	
(18G TWX3-1/2",4X25)			
100s ea	08080-2210-41	267.10	
(20G TWX3-1/2",4X25)			
100s ea	08080-2210-74	267.10	

MONOJECT DIAMOND POINT SPINAL NEEDLE W/METAL HUB (Covidien)

PROD/MFR	HRI, UPC,NDC	AWP	SRP
DEV,NA (4X25,18GX3-1/2")			
100s ea	08080-2200-19	218.39	
(4X25,19GX3-1/2")			
100s ea	08080-2200-27	218.39	
(4X25,20GX2-1/2")			
100s ea	08080-2200-35	218.39	

PROD/MFR	HRI, UPC,NDC	AWP	SRP
(4X25,22GX1-1/2")			
100s ea	08080-2200-76	218.39	
(4X25,22GX2-1/2")			
100s ea	08080-2200-84	218.39	
(4X25,22GX3-1/2")			
100s ea	08080-2201-01	218.39	
(4X25,25GX3-1/2")			
100s ea	08080-2201-18	218.39	
MONOJECT INTERMITTENT INFUSION PLUG (Covidien)			
DEV,NA (W/18GX1"NEEDLE,STERILE)			
300s ea	08080-1052-02	204.75	
MONOJECT INTRODUCER (Covidien)			
DEV,NA (18GX1-1/4",10X100)			
1000s ea	08080-2050-10	707.83	
MONOJECT LIFESHIELD (Kendall)			
DEV,NA (W/12ML LUERLCKSYR18GX1")			
480s ea	88812-0021-32	301.74	
MONOJECT LUER LOCK SYRINGE (Covidien)			
DEV,NA (W/NEEDLE,20X1 1/2",12ML)			
480s ea	08080-5126-62	144.97	
(W/NEEDLE,23GX1 1/2",3ML)			
1000s ea	08080-5132-64	146.50	
MONOJECT LUER LOCK WITH TIP CAP (Covidien)			
DEV,NA (1ML,LATEX-FREE)			
240s ea	08080-1007-77	151.25	
MONOJECT MAGELLAN (Covidien)			
DEV,NA (W/NEEDLE,18GX1",6ML)			
200s ea	08881-8668-10	104.20	
MONOJECT MAGELLAN SAFETY BLOOD COLLECTOR (Covidien)			
DEV,NA (21GX1.25",6X50)			
300s ea	08881-2261-21	137.50	
(21GX1")			
300s ea	08080-2251-21	150.25	
(22GX1.25",6X50)			
300s ea	08881-2261-22	137.50	
MONOJECT MONOLETTOR SAFETY LANCET (Covidien)			
DEV,NA, 400s ea	08080-6020-91	153.04	
MONOJECT MULTIPLE SAMPLE-LUER ADAPTERS (Covidien)			
DEV,NA (LATEX-FREE)			
1000s ea	08080-2252-57	162.78	
MONOJECT PEDIATRIC TUBE ADAPTER (Covidien)			
DEV,NA, 100s ea	08080-6120-09	14.62	
MONOJECT PHARMACY (Covidien)			
DEV,NA (25 SYRINGES PER TRAY)			
1000s ea	08080-5014-59	178.44	
MONOJECT SAFETY SYRINGE (Covidien)			
DEV,NA (30G,5/16",1/2ML)			
500s ea	08881-5113-36	231.44	
(30G,5/16",1ML)			
500s ea	08881-5113-10	218.94	
(30G,5/16",3/10ML)			
500s ea	08881-5113-44	231.44	
MONOJECT SAFETY SYRINGE TIP (Covidien)			
DEV,NA (STERILE)			
250s ea	08881-6820-10	93.39	
MONOJECT SHARPS (Covidien)			
DEV,NA (REDCHMNYTOPW/WNDW 14QRT)			
10s ea	08080-6764-34	73.75	
(RED HORZNTAL ENTRY 8QRT)			
20s ea	08080-6768-22	95.03	
(RED HORZNTAL ENTRY 4QRT)			
30s ea	08080-6768-14	90.00	
(1.1 QUART)			
40s ea	08080-6764-67	90.00	
(REDCHMNY TOPW/WNDW 4QRT)			
40s ea	08080-6762-36	112.50	
MONOJECT SHARPS CONTAINER (Covidien)			
DEV,NA (8 QUART)			
20s ea	08881-6762-85	93.75	
MONOJECT SMARTIP (Covidien)			
DEV,NA (6ML,W/NEEDLELESSCANNULA)			
400s ea	08881-5401-66	125.00	
(12MLW/NEEDLELESSCANNULA)			
480s ea	08881-5401-22	162.50	
(3ML,W/NEEDLELESSCANNULA)			
800s ea	08881-5401-33	225.00	
(STERILE,100X10)			
1000s ea	08080-5401-11	321.25	
MONOJECT STOPPER (Covidien)			
DEV,NA (CORVACRED/GREYMOTTLED)			
500s ea	08080-3030-50	226.25	
(BLUE,LIQUID ADDITIVE)			
1000s ea	08080-3402-70	136.34	
1000s ea	08080-3402-88	147.94	
1000s ea	08080-3403-12	153.04	
1000s ea	08080-3404-78	120.39	
1000s ea	08080-3404-86	109.98	
1000s ea	08080-3405-77	177.09	
(BROWN,DRY ADDITIVE)			
1000s ea	08080-3067-35	357.50	
(GREEN,LIQUID ADDITIVE)			
1000s ea	08080-3201-57	204.05	
1000s ea	08080-3202-56	196.77	
1000s ea	08080-3204-54	287.42	
1000s ea	08080-3205-53	287.42	
1000s ea	08080-3207-51	298.79	
1000s ea	08080-3212-54	210.18	
1000s ea	08080-3214-52	209.30	
1000s ea	08080-3215-51	287.42	
1000s ea	08080-3217-59	254.94	
(LAVENDER,LIQUID ADDTVE)			
1000s ea	08080-3111-49	147.94	
(LAVENDER,LIQUIDADDITIVE)			
1000s ea	08080-3112-48	157.63	
1000s ea	08080-3113-47	156.28	
1000s ea	08080-3114-46	164.70	
1000s ea	08080-3114-79	103.00	
1000s ea	08080-3114-87	208.64	
1000s ea	08080-3115-45	155.38	
1000s ea	08080-3116-44	208.87	
1000s ea	08080-3117-43	215.72	
1000s ea	08080-3144-40	143.10	
(LAVENDER,PWDERADDITIVE)			
1000s ea	08080-3102-40	180.07	
1000s ea	08080-3104-48	164.70	
1000s ea	08080-3105-47	178.34	
1000s ea	08080-3106-46	335.78	
1000s ea	08080-3107-45	342.93	
(PINK,NONSILICNE,NOADDTV)			
1000s ea	08080-3047-22	218.39	
(RED,NONSILICNE,NOADDTVE)			
1000s ea	08080-3027-18	175.64	
(ROYALBLUE,TRACEELEMENT)			
1000s ea	08080-3070-06	522.99	
1000s ea	08080-3070-14	666.37	
1000s ea	08080-3070-22	541.65	
MONOJECT SYRINGE (Covidien)			
DEV,NA (W/REGLUERTIP,60ML,SMPLE)			
100s ea	08080-1604-05	101.47	
MONOJECT THE NEEDLE BANK (Covidien)			
DEV,NA, 24s ea	08080-5999-90	133.57	
MONOJECT TUBERCULIN (Covidien)			
DEV,NA (W/NEEDLE,25GX5/8",1ML)			
500s ea	08080-5016-40	98.19	
MONOJECT ULTRA COMFORT (Can-Am Care)			
DEV,NA (31G,1ML)			
100s ea	08881-6091-31	23.90	
(31GX1/2",0.5ML)			
100s ea	08881-6092-31	23.90	
(31GX3/10",0.5ML)			
100s ea	08881-6093-31	23.90	
(Covidien)			
DEV,NA (28GX1/2",1/2CC)			
300s ea	08881-6090-04	71.70	
(28GX1/2",1CC)			
300s ea	08881-6091-01	71.70	
(29GX1/2",1/2CC)			
300s ea	08881-6093-50	71.70	
(29GX1/2",1CC)			
300s ea	08881-6093-58	71.70	
(29GX1/2",3/10CC)			
300s ea	08881-6091-45	71.70	
MONOJECTOR ENDCAPS FOR LANCET DEVICE (Covidien)			
DEV,NA (OPD,SINGLE-USE)			
1000s ea	08080-6022-40	261.82	
(SINGLE-USE)			
1000s ea	08080-6022-24	62.50	
MONOJECTOR LANCET (Covidien)			
DEV,NA, 60s ea	08881-6021-17	8.68	7.95
MONOLAURIN & OLIVE LEAF (Key Company)			
CAP,PO, 300 mg-250 mg,			
90s ea	11694-0645-01	12.00	
MONOLET LANCETS (Covidien)			
DEV,NA (21G)			
2400s ea	08881-6021-25	174.15	
(THIN)			
2400s ea	08881-6022-08	149.72	
(O.P.D.)			
5000s ea	08881-6024-22	258.68	
(STERILE)			
5000s ea	08881-6020-18	298.45	
(THIN)			
5000s ea	08881-6022-16	263.34	
MOSCO CORN & CALLUS REMOVER (Medtech)			
LIQ,TP, 17.6%, 10 ml	75137-0183-05	2.42	
MOTHERS FRIEND (S.S.S.)			
CRE,TP, 60 gm	12258-0114-02	3.99	
LOT,TP, 90 ml	12258-0113-03	3.99	
MOTION SICKNESS (Cardinal Health)			
TAB,PO (PRIVATE LABEL)			
50 mg, 12s ea	37205-0111-53	1.36	
(Family Phcy)			
TAB,PO (PRIVATE LABEL)			
50 mg, 12s ea	52735-0707-02	2.69	2.99
(Teva)			
TAB,PO, 50 mg, 12s ea	00182-1437-11	1.39	
MOTION SICKNESS RELIEF (AmerisourceBergen)			
TAB,PO (PRIVATE LABEL)			
50 mg, 12s ea	24385-0004-12	2.69	2.99
MOTRIN CHILDREN'S (McNeil Consumer Healthcare)			
SUS,PO (36X4, HOSPITAL PRODUCT)			
100 mg/5 ml,			
120 ml 36s	50580-0601-50	287.81	
(Dispensing Solutions)			
REPACK			
SUS,PO (AF,BERRY)			
100 mg/5 ml,			
120 ml	55045-2072-02	9.99	
(Phys Total Care)			
REPACK			
CTB,PO (ORANGE)			
50 mg, 24s ea	54868-4362-00	5.11	
MOTRIN IB (McNeil Consumer Healthcare)			
TAB,PO, 200 mg, 24s ea	00450-0463-02	3.30	
(CAPLET)			
200 mg, 24s ea	00450-0481-03	3.30	
24s ea	50580-0110-38	2.96	
30s ea	50580-0110-64	3.30	
50s ea	00450-0463-03	5.69	
(CAPLET)			
200 mg, 50s ea	00450-0481-02	5.69	
60s ea	50580-0110-60	5.18	
(W/24 FREE,GELCAPLET)			
200 mg, 74s ea	00045-0770-74	5.09	
100s ea	00450-0463-04	9.16	
(50X2)			
200 mg, 100s ea	00450-0481-52	8.54	
(CAPLET)			
200 mg, 100s ea	00450-0481-01	9.16	
(100+24 FREE)			
200 mg, 124s ea	50580-0109-09	8.06	
(W/24 FREE,GELCAPLET)			
200 mg, 124s ea	50580-0770-09	8.06	
(100+25 FREE,CAPLET)			
200 mg, 125s ea	50580-0110-95	9.16	
(100+25 FREE)			
200 mg, 125s ea	50580-0109-29	9.16	
(CAPLET)			
200 mg, 165s ea	00450-0481-09	10.68	
(EASY OPEN CAP,CAPLET)			
200 mg, 225s ea	00450-0481-62	13.96	
(CAPLET)			
200 mg, 300s ea	50580-0110-37	14.77	
(2X2500,CAPLET)			
200 mg, 5000s ea	50580-0110-19	403.20	
MOTRIN INFANTS' (McNeil Consumer Healthcare)			
SUS,PO (W/IRC,BERRY,DROPS)			
50 mg/1.25 ml,			
15 ml	50580-0100-20	4.97	
MOTRIN JUNIOR (Dispensing Solutions)			
REPACK			
CTB,PO (GRAPE)			
100 mg, 24s ea	55045-3477-02	7.00	
MOTRIN JUNIOR STRENGTH (McNeil Consumer Healthcare)			
CTB,PO (AGES 6-11)			
100 mg, 24s ea	00450-0494-24	4.85	
(GRAPE)			
100 mg, 24s ea	00450-0909-24	4.85	
TAB,PO (CAPLET)			
100 mg, 24s ea	00450-0498-24	4.85	

PROD/MFR	HRI, UPC,NDC	AWP	SRP
MOTRIN MIGRAINE PAIN (McNeil Consumer Healthcare)			
TAB,PO (50+24 FREE,CAPLET)			
200 mg, 74s ea	50580-0915-74	5.09	
(50+50 FREE,CAPLET)			
200 mg, 100s ea	50580-0915-52	5.09	
(2X100,CAPLET)			
200 mg, 200s ea	50580-0915-20	12.53	
MOUTHKOTE (Parnell)			
SOL,PO (50 X 5ML)			
5 ml 50s UD	50930-0098-05	10.85	16.00
60 ml	50930-0098-02	5.10	7.99
237 ml	50930-0098-08	10.95	15.00
MOVEEN BEDSIDE NIGHT (Coloplast)			
DEV,NA (STERILE)			
10s ea	11701-0878-56	58.70	61.40
(NON-STERILE)			
30s ea	11701-0878-46	128.10	133.80
MOVEEN NIGHT BAG (Coloplast)			
DEV,NA (2000ML)			
10s ea	11701-0878-70	71.20	74.50
MOVEEN SYPHON BAG (Coloplast)			
DEV,NA (STERILE)			
10s ea	11701-0877-92	88.60	92.70
(NON-STERILE, 17 OZ.)			
30s ea	11701-0877-62	190.50	199.20
(NON-STERILE, 26 OZ.)			
30s ea	11701-0877-82	217.80	228.00
MPS (Bio-Tech Pharm)			
CAP,PO, 86 mg-400000 u,			
100s ea	53191-0065-01	9.45	
MSM (Freeda)			
TAB,PO (SF)			
250 mg, 100s ea	10432-0346-01	4.77	7.95
(Key Company)			
CAP,PO, 1000 mg,			
100s ea	11694-0682-01	8.00	
250s ea	11694-0682-02	18.00	
500s ea	11694-0682-05	35.00	
(Rexall)			
TAB,PO, 18 mg-500 mg,			
60s ea	30768-0036-58	2.72	4.12
MSM SULFUR (Carlson,J.R.)			
CAP,PO (PF,SF,CORN-FREE)			
900 mg, 90s ea	88395-0087-21	6.25	12.50
180s ea	88395-0087-22	11.45	22.90
MSM W/ARNICA (Key Company)			
LOT,TP, 90 ml	16946-0676-03	5.75	
240 ml	16946-0676-08	8.75	
960 ml	16946-0676-32	25.00	
MSM-PLUS (Miller)			
CAP,PO (SF)			
1000 mg-0.075 mg,			
120s ea	17204-0847-55	15.12	
MSUD 1 (Milupa North America)			
PDR,PO (2X500GM)			
500 gm 2s	81361-9350-01	150.00	
MSUD 2 (Nutricia)			
PDR,PO (2X500GM)			
500 gm 2s	81361-9351-01	280.80	
MSUD AID (Nutricia)			
PDR,PO (USE W/MED SUPV)			
200 gm 10s	49735-0101-43	354.90	
MSUD ANALOG (Nutricia)			
PDR,PO (1X400GM)			
400 gm	49735-0018-86	60.00	
(USE W/MED SUPV)			
400 gm 4s	49735-0118-86	252.20	
(6X400GM)			
400 gm 6s	49735-0183-02	360.00	
MSUD COOLER (VITAFLO, LLC)			
SOL,PO (15GM PROTEIN EQUIVALENT)			
130 ml 30s	50600-0546-54	265.50	349.75
MSUD EXPRESS (VITAFLO, LLC)			
PDR,PO (ENTERAL,UNFLAVORED)			
25 gm 30s	50600-0535-34	265.50	349.75
MSUD GEL (VITAFLO, LLC)			
PO (UNFLAVORED)			
20 gm 30s	50600-0534-04	148.68	239.00
MSUD MAXAMAID (Nutricia)			
PDR,PO (1X454GM,ORANGE)			
454 gm	49735-0023-60	74.10	
(MED. SUPERVISION,ORANGE)			
454 gm 4s	49735-0123-60	312.00	
(6X454GM,ORANGE)			
454 gm 6s	49735-0177-81	444.60	
MSUD MAXAMUM (Nutricia)			
PDR,PO (1X454GM,ORANGE)			
454 gm	49735-0023-40	117.30	
(6X454GM,ORANGE)			
454 gm 6s	49735-0177-89	703.80	
MT-UD PACKETS (Safecor)			
DEV,NA (AMBER/FOIL)			
1000s ea	48433-0104-00	38.40	
(FILM/FOIL)			
1000s ea	48433-0100-00	32.40	
MUCINEX (Reckitt Benckiser)			
TER,PO (BI-LAYER TAB)			
600 mg, 20s ea	63824-0008-32	9.31	
40s ea	63824-0008-34	17.59	
(12 HOUR)			
600 mg, 60s ea	63824-0008-61	26.36	
100s ea	63824-0008-10	43.86	
500s ea	63824-0008-50	219.66	
(MAXIMUM STRENGTH)			
1200 mg, 14s ea	63824-0023-14	10.20	
28s ea	63824-0023-28	19.37	
(A-S Medication)			
REPACK			
TER,PO, 600 mg, 40s ea	54569-5463-00	17.59	
60s ea	54569-5463-01	25.26	
(Dispensing Solutions)			
REPACK			
TER,PO, 600 mg, 30s ea	55045-3133-08	18.00	
(PD-Rx Pharm)			
REPACK			
TER,PO, 600 mg, 20s ea	55289-0087-20	18.60	
(REDI-SCRIPT)			
600 mg, 30s ea	58864-0196-30	21.00	
(Phys Total Care)			
REPACK			
TER,PO, 600 mg, 20s ea	54868-4750-01	11.36	
40s ea	54868-4750-00	19.77	
(Quality Care Prod)			
REPACK			
TER,PO, 600 mg, 20s ea	35356-0195-20	23.40	
(Southwood)			
REPACK			
TER,PO, 600 mg, 40s ea	58016-4794-01	17.59	
(Stat Rx)			
REPACK			
TER,PO, 600 mg, 20s ea	16590-0651-20	17.20	
30s ea	16590-0651-30	26.00	
40s ea	16590-0651-40	34.67	
60s ea	16590-0651-60	52.00	
MUCINEX D (Reckitt Benckiser)			
TER,PO (BI-LAYER)			
600 mg-60 mg,			
18s ea	63824-0057-18	10.20	
36s ea	63824-0057-36	19.37	
(MAXIMUM STRENGTH)			
1200 mg-120 mg,			
24s ea	63824-0041-24	21.29	
(A-S Medication)			
REPACK			
TER,PO (BI-LAYER)			
600 mg-60 mg,			
18s ea	54569-5984-00	10.20	
36s ea	54569-5985-00	19.37	
(DHS, Inc.)			
REPACK			
TER,PO, 600 mg-60 mg,			
18s ea	55887-0047-18	14.95	
36s ea	55887-0047-36	29.90	
(Phys Total Care)			
REPACK			
TER,PO, 600 mg-60 mg,			
18s ea	54868-5849-00	16.63	
(Quality Care Prod)			
REPACK			
TER,PO (BI-LAYER)			
600 mg-60 mg,			
18s ea	35356-0201-18	48.72	
(Southwood)			
REPACK			
TER,PO, 600 mg-60 mg,			
18s ea	00490-0060-18	14.76	
(Stat Rx)			
REPACK			
TER,PO (BI-LAYER)			
600 mg-60 mg,			
20s ea	16590-0791-20	13.78	
MUCINEX DM (Reckitt Benckiser)			
TER,PO (BI-LAYER)			
30 mg-600 mg, 20s ea	63824-0056-32	10.20	
40s ea	63824-0056-34	19.37	
(BI-LAYER TABLET)			
60 mg-1200 mg,			
14s ea	63824-0072-35	11.22	
28s ea	63824-0072-36	21.19	
(A-S Medication)			
REPACK			
TER,PO (BI-LAYER)			
30 mg-600 mg,			
20s ea	54569-5986-00	10.20	
40s ea	54569-5987-00	19.37	
(Phys Total Care)			
REPACK			
TER,PO, 30 mg-600 mg,			
20s ea	54868-5853-00	13.01	
(Physician Partner)			
REPACK			
TER,PO (BI-LAYER)			
30 mg-600 mg,			
20s ea	21695-0396-20	20.40	
(Southwood)			
REPACK			
TER,PO, 30 mg-600 mg,			
20s ea	58016-4799-01	7.99	
MUCINEX FULL FORCE (Reckitt Benckiser)			
SPR,NS, 0.05%, 22 ml	63824-0123-75	9.31	
MUCINEX MOISTURE SMART (Reckitt Benckiser)			
SPR,NS, 0.05%, 22 ml	63824-0122-75	9.31	
MUCUS RELIEF (Major)			
TAB,PO, 400 mg, 30s ea	00904-5758-46	11.52	
60s ea	00904-5758-52	23.04	
500s ea	00904-5758-40	172.80	
MUCUS RELIEF DM (Major)			
TAB,PO, 20 mg-400 mg,			
30s ea	00904-6013-46	12.68	
60s ea	00904-6013-52	25.36	
500s ea	00904-6013-40	209.33	
MUCUS RELIEF SINUS (Major)			
MUCUS RELIEF SINUS			
TAB,PO, 400 mg-10 mg,			
30s ea	00904-5792-46	12.10	
60s ea	00904-5792-52	24.20	
MULTI FORMULA 50 (Rexall)			
TAB,PO (PF,SF)			
50s ea	30768-0011-11	4.41	6.68
MULTI PURPOSE (AmerisourceBergen)			
SOL,NA (PRIVATE LABEL)			
360 ml	24385-0294-40	5.39	5.99
MULTI VITAMINS (Quality Care Prod)			
REPACK			
TAB,PO, 30s ea	49999-0399-30	4.06	
MULTI VITAMINS W/IRON CHILDREN'S (Cardinal Health)			
CTB,PO (PRIVATE LABEL)			
100s ea	37205-0390-78	4.98	
MULTI-BETIC (Health Care Products)			
TAB,PO (PF,SF,DYE-FREE)			
60s ea	60569-0816-04	10.50	15.99
MULTI-BETIC DIABETES (Health Care Products)			
TAB,PO (SF,CORN-FREE)			
50s ea	60569-0081-50	7.72	11.99
MULTI-DAY (Nature's Bounty)			
TAB,PO, 100s ea	74312-0015-70		3.89
365s ea	74312-0015-74		10.99
(Physician Partner)			
REPACK			
TAB,PO, 30s ea	21695-0390-30	5.85	
100s ea	21695-0390-00	13.10	
MULTI-DAY PLUS IRON (Nature's Bounty)			
TAB,PO (PF,SF)			
100s ea	74312-0015-80		4.09
365s ea	74312-0015-84		11.49
MULTI-DAY PLUS MINERALS (Nature's Bounty)			
PO (PF)			
100s ea	74312-0041-30		7.85

PROD/MFR	HRI, UPC,NDC	AWP	SRP
MULTI-DAY VITAMINS (Dispensing Solutions)			
REPACK			
TAB,PO, 30s ea	66336-0365-30	3.52	
90s ea	66336-0365-90	8.79	
MULTI-DAY W/CALCIUM/EXTRA IRON (Nature's Bounty)			
TAB,PO (PF)			
100s ea	74312-0042-40		7.59
MULTI-DAY WEIGHT TRIM (Rexall)			
TAB,PO, 50s ea	30768-0138-51	3.95	5.99
MULTI-DELYN (Silarx)			
LIQ,PO (AF,SF)			
237 ml	54838-0008-70	6.10	
473 ml	54838-0008-80	9.15	
MULTI-DELYN W/IRON (Silarx)			
LIQ,PO (AF,SF)			
237 ml	54838-0009-70	6.50	
473 ml	54838-0009-80	9.99	
MULTI-FLAVOR CHILDREN'S VITAMINS (Marlex)			
CTB,PO, 60s ea	10135-0170-60	2.84	
100s ea	10135-0170-01	2.13	
250s ea	10135-0170-69	3.65	
1000s ea	10135-0170-10	12.37	
MULTI-LANCET DEVICE (Arkray)			
DEV,NA, ea	08317-6600-15	10.85	
MULTI-SYMPTOM COLD/COUGH (Contract Pharmacal)			
TAB,PO, 500 mg-2 mg-15 mg-30 mg,			
60s ea	10267-2635-07	4.50	
MULTI-VITAMINS (Rugby)			
TAB,PO (PF,SF)			
1000s ea	00536-4046-10	19.12	
MULTI-VITS/FLOUR/IRON (Phys Total Care)			
REPACK			
CTB,PO, 100s ea	54868-3021-00	30.18	
MULTILEX (Rugby)			
TAB,PO, 100s ea	00536-4044-01	5.70	
MULTILEX T/M (Rugby)			
TAB,PO, 100s ea	00536-4060-01	6.83	
MULTIMINERALS (Freeda)			
TAB,PO (PF,SF,DYE-FREE)			
100s ea	10432-0035-01	4.77	7.95
250s ea	10432-0035-02	9.54	15.90
MULTIPLE VITAMIN (Southwood)			
REPACK			
TAB,PO, 30s ea	58016-0918-30	3.38	
60s ea	58016-0918-60	6.75	
90s ea	58016-0918-90	10.13	
100s ea	58016-0918-00	11.25	
MULTIPLE VITAMINS (Albertson's)			
TAB,PO, 100s ea	04000-0002-60	3.16	
(Consolidated Midland)			
SOL,PO (DROPS)			
50 ml	00223-6228-50	3.95	
(Lex)			
TAB,PO, 100s ea	49523-0011-10	1.10	
365s ea UD	49523-0011-05	2.60	
(Medicine Shoppe)			
TAB,PO, 130s ea	49614-0632-81	5.99	5.99
365s ea	49614-0632-88	8.49	8.49
(Phys Total Care)			
REPACK			
TAB,PO, 100s ea	54868-3872-00	14.64	
MULTIPLE VITAMINS & MINERALS (Albertson's)			
TAB,PO, 100s ea	04000-0002-14	6.87	
130s ea	04000-0001-37	8.16	
MULTIPLE VITAMINS CHILDREN'S (ADH)			
CTB,PO, 100s ea	60142-0094-10	3.95	7.90
(Health Products Corp)			
CTB,PO (FRUIT)			
100s ea	39686-0012-47	3.50	
MULTIPLE VITAMINS W/IRON (Consolidated Midland)			
LIQ,PO (DROPS)			
50 ml	00223-6558-01	4.00	
(Lex)			
TAB,PO, 100s ea	49523-0018-10	1.15	
365s ea UD	49523-0018-05	2.68	
(A-S Medication)			
REPACK			
TAB,PO, 100s ea	54569-2342-00	3.59	
(PD-Rx Pharm)			
REPACK			
TAB,PO, 30s ea	55289-0868-30	6.42	
100s ea	55289-0868-01	9.64	
MULTIPLE VITAMINS W/IRON CHILDREN'S (Health Products Corp)			
CTB,PO, 100s ea	39686-0012-50	3.05	
MULTIPLE VITAMINS WITH FLUORIDE (Southwood)			
REPACK			
CTB,PO, 30s ea	58016-0438-30	3.90	
60s ea	58016-0438-60	7.80	
90s ea	58016-0438-90	11.70	
100s ea	58016-0438-00	13.00	
MULTIPLE VITAMINS WOMEN'S (Medicine Shoppe)			
TAB,PO, 100s ea	49614-0246-78	5.99	5.99
MULTIPLE VITAMNS W/IRON (Albertson's)			
TAB,PO, 100s ea	04000-0002-54	3.18	
MULTISTIX (Siemens)			
DEV,NA, 100s ea	08620-2179-21	94.60	94.60
MULTISTIX 10 SG (Siemens)			
DEV,NA, 100s ea	08620-2161-21	86.10	86.10
(Southwood)			
REPACK			
DEV,NA, 100s ea	58016-9061-01	68.44	
MULTISTIX 5 (Siemens)			
DEV,NA, 100s ea	08620-2309-21	39.00	39.00
MULTISTIX 7 (Siemens)			
DEV,NA, 100s ea	08620-2165-21	79.40	79.40
MULTISTIX 8 SG (Siemens)			
DEV,NA, 100s ea	08620-2164-21	88.80	88.80
MULTISTIX 9 (Siemens)			
DEV,NA, 100s ea	08620-2162-21	93.00	93.00
MULTISTIX 9 SG (Siemens)			
DEV,NA, 100s ea	08620-2163-21	93.00	93.00
MULTIVITAMIN (Basic Vitamins)			
TAB,PO, 100s ea	00761-0361-20	2.00	
250s ea	00761-0361-50	3.60	
(Numark)			
SGL,PO (SOFTGEL)			
100s ea UD	38485-0120-41	7.62	
100s ea	38485-0120-42	5.52	
(PD-Rx Pharm)			
REPACK			
TAB,PO, 100s ea	55289-0530-01	12.59	
MULTIVITAMIN W/IRON (Basic Vitamins)			
TAB,PO, 100s ea	00761-0362-20	2.00	
250s ea	00761-0362-50	3.60	
MULTIVITAMINS (Geri-Care)			
TAB,PO, 30s ea	57896-0505-30	0.57	
100s ea	57896-0505-01	0.75	
1000s ea	57896-0505-10	4.95	
MULTIVITAMINS CHILDREN'S (Cardinal Health)			
CTB,PO (ANIMAL SHAPES)			
100s ea	37205-0388-78	4.38	
MULTIVITAMINS W/EXTRA C CHILDREN'S (Basic Vitamins)			
CTB,PO, 120s ea	00761-0121-24	3.00	
MURO-128 (Bausch & Lomb Inc.)			
OIN,OP, 5%, 3.5 gm	24208-0385-55	18.16	
3.5 gm 2s	24208-0385-56	27.98	
SOL,OP, 2%, 15 ml	24208-0276-15	17.25	
5%, 15 ml	24208-0277-15	18.16	
30 ml	24208-0277-30	23.40	
(Phys Total Care)			
REPACK			
SOL,OP, 5%, 15 ml	54868-1172-00	18.61	
MUROCEL (Bausch & Lomb Inc.)			
SOL,OP, 1%, 15 ml	24208-0280-15	7.97	
MUSCLE & WEIGHT GAINER (Nature's Bounty)			
PDR,PO (CHOCOLATE)			
680.4 gm	74312-0054-63		14.39
MUSCLE POWER (Mason Vit)			
POW,PO, 5 gm/tsp,			
150 gm	11845-0130-15	18.87	
MUSCLE RELIEF CREAM (Actavis Mid Atlantic)			
CRE,TP (1X56GM)			
0.075%, 56 gm	00472-0103-57	7.47	
MUSCLE RUB (Family Phcy)			
OIN,TP (PRIVATE LABEL)			
10%-15%, 90 gm	52735-0728-27	2.87	3.19
(Perrigo)			
CRE,TP, 10%-15%, 90 ml	45802-0174-53	2.26	
(Teva)			
CRE,TP, 4%-10%-30%,			
120 gm	00182-5091-57	5.69	
(Nucare Pharm)			
REPACK			
CRE,TP (1X90GM)			
10%-15%, 90 gm	68071-1329-03	3.38	
(St. Mary's MPP)			
REPACK			
CRE,TP (1X90GM)			
10%-15%, 85 gm	60760-0017-03	5.39	
MUSCLE RUB ULTRA STRENGTH (AmerisourceBergen)			
CRE,TP (PRIVATE LABEL)			
10%-30%, 113 gm	24385-0141-26	5.39	5.99
(Cardinal Health)			
CRE,TP (PRIVATE LABEL)			
120 gm	37205-0460-26	2.99	
MUSCLE RUB X/S (Core)			
REPACK			
CRE,TP, 10%-15%, 90 gm	33358-0250-03	6.12	
MUSTARD (Ellon)			
SOL,SL (DROPS)			
10.5 ml	51762-0033-10		9.25
MY-B-TABS (Legere)			
TAB,PO, 50 mg-0.05 mg-0.01 mg,			
90s ea	25332-1043-05	16.00	
MYBEC (Mason Vit)			
TAB,PO, 60s ea	11845-0076-75	7.44	
MYCELEX-7 (Phys Total Care)			
REPACK			
TAB,VG (W/APPLICATOR)			
100 mg, 7s ea	54868-1086-00	9.28	
MYCIN SCALP (Pfeiffer)			
LIQ,TP, 1%, 60 ml	00927-0643-30	2.55	4.59
MYCINAIRE (Pfeiffer)			
SPR,NS, 0.69%, 30 ml	00927-0350-31	2.47	4.44
MYCINETTE (Pfeiffer)			
LOZ,MM, 15 mg, 12s ea	00927-0548-08	1.86	3.34
12s ea	00927-0648-08	1.86	3.34
SPR,MM, 0.3%-1.4%,			
174 ml	00927-0148-06	1.95	3.50
174 ml	00927-0149-06	1.95	3.50
(CHERRY)			
0.3%-1.4%, 174 ml	00927-0150-06	1.95	3.50
(COOL BLUE)			
0.5%-1.4%, 174 ml	00927-0249-06	1.95	3.50
MYCO NAIL A (Kramer-Novis)			
SOL,TP, 25%, 30 ml	52083-0242-30	11.00	
MYCO-NAIL (Kramer-Novis)			
LIQ,TP, 25%, 30 ml	52083-0241-30	11.00	
MYCOCIDE NS (Woodward Labs)			
SOL,TP, 30 ml	60193-0010-30	11.30	
MYGREX (Medique)			
TAB,PO (2X150,SF,LACTOSE-FREE)			
500 mg-32.5 mg-5 mg,			
300s ea	47682-0155-09	31.29	
MYKIDZ IRON (NextWave)			
SUS,PO (W/DISPENSER,AF,SF)			
118 ml	24478-0101-04	15.00	18.00
MYKIDZ IRON 10 (NextWave)			
SUS,PO (W/DROPPER,AF,DYE-FREE)			
15 mg/1.5 ml, 118 ml	24478-0103-04	20.00	24.00
MYLANTA (J&J/Merck)			
SUS,PO (CLASSIC)			
150 ml	16837-0610-55	2.99	
355 ml	16837-0610-12	4.97	
(MINT)			
355 ml	16837-0629-12	4.97	
360 ml	16837-0621-12	4.90	
720 ml	16837-0610-24	8.89	
720 ml	16837-0621-24	8.89	
TAB,PO (SOD.FREE,SF,DYE-FREE)			
550 mg-125 mg,			
24s ea	16837-0850-24	2.77	
50s ea	16837-0850-50	4.43	
(A-S Medication)			
REPACK			
SUS,PO, 360 ml	54569-0036-00	5.04	
MYLANTA DOUBLE STRENGTH (J&J/Merck)			
CTB,PO (CHERRY)			
700 mg-300 mg,			
70s ea	16837-0869-70	4.43	

PROD/MFR	HRI, UPC,NDC	AWP	SRP
(MINT)			
700 mg-300 mg,			
70s ea	16837-0849-70	4.43	
(WAREHOUSE PKG,MINT)			
700 mg-300 mg,			
70s ea	16837-0849-71	4.78	
MYLANTA GAS MAXIMUM STRENGTH (J&J/Merck)			
CTB,PO (CHERRY)			
125 mg, 24s ea	16837-0861-24	3.78	
(MINT)			
125 mg, 24s ea	16837-0455-24	3.78	
60s ea	16837-0455-48	6.72	
SGL,PO (SOFTGEL)			
125 mg, 24s ea	16837-0611-24	3.78	
(Phys Total Care)			
REPACK			
CTB,PO (MINT)			
125 mg, 24s ea	54868-3322-00	5.98	
MYLANTA MAXIMUM STRENGTH (J&J/Merck)			
SUS,PO (CHERRY)			
355 ml	16837-0622-12	5.96	
(MINT)			
355 ml	16837-0624-12	5.96	
(ORIGINAL)			
355 ml	16837-0652-12	5.96	
(W/COOLTEK,ORANGE CREME)			
355 ml	16837-0623-12	5.96	
(CLASSIC)			
710 ml	16837-0652-24	9.77	
(WAREHOUSE PKG)			
720 ml	16837-0652-25	9.25	
MYLANTA SUPREME (J&J/Merck)			
SUS,PO (W/CALCIUM,CHERRY)			
400 mg/5 ml-135 mg/5 ml,			
355 ml	16837-0825-12	5.96	
(CHERRY)			
400 mg/5 ml-135 mg/5 ml,			
360 ml 3s	16837-0825-36	12.64	
(W/CALCIUM,CHERRY)			
400 mg/5 ml-135 mg/5 ml,			
710 ml	16837-0825-24	9.77	
MYLANTA ULTIMATE STRENGTH (J&J/Merck)			
CTB,PO (CHERRY,CHERRY)			
700 mg-300 mg,			
35s ea	16837-0615-35	3.11	
(COOL MINT,COOL MINT)			
700 mg-300 mg,			
35s ea	16837-0613-35	3.11	
(CHERRY,CHERRY)			
700 mg-300 mg,			
70s ea	16837-0615-70	4.61	
(COOL MINT,COOL MINT)			
700 mg-300 mg,			
70s ea	16837-0613-70	4.61	
SUS,PO (CHERRY)			
500 mg/5 ml-500 mg/5 ml,			
355 ml	16837-0644-12	6.52	
(MINT)			
500 mg/5 ml-500 mg/5 ml,			
355 ml	16837-0643-12	6.52	
MYLICON INFANTS (Dispensing Solutions)			
REPACK			
SUS,PO (DROPS)			
40 mg/0.6 ml,			
30 ml	55045-3478-01	12.00	
MYLICON INFANTS' (J&J/Merck)			
SUS,PO (AF,DROPS)			
40 mg/0.6 ml,			
15 ml	16837-0630-05	6.22	
(NON-STAIN,CARD,AF,DROPS)			
40 mg/0.6 ml,			
15 ml	16837-0911-05	6.22	
(AF,DROPS)			
40 mg/0.6 ml,			
30 ml	16837-0630-01	10.68	
30 ml	16837-0630-03	10.68	
(NON-STAINING,AF,DROPS)			
40 mg/0.6 ml,			
30 ml	16837-0911-03	10.68	
(NON-STAINING FORMULA,AF)			
40 mg/0.6 ml,			
30 ml 2s	16837-0911-13	18.13	
MYOFLEX (Novartis Consumer)			
CRE,TP, 10%, 60 gm	00235-1170-02	4.18	
120 gm	00235-1170-04	7.34	
(A-S Medication)			
REPACK			
CRE,TP, 10%, 60 gm	54569-0778-00	4.58	
(Altura)			
REPACK			
CRE,TP, 10%, 60 gm	63874-1036-06	9.93	
(Dispensing Solutions)			
REPACK			
CRE,TP, 10%, 60 gm	55045-3176-02	8.85	
120 gm	55045-3176-04	14.00	
(Pharma Pac)			
REPACK			
CRE,TP, 10%, 60 gm	52959-0025-02	9.93	
120 gm	52959-0025-03	18.78	
120 gm	52959-0025-04	18.78	
(Quality Care Prod)			
REPACK			
CRE,TP, 10%, 60 gm	49999-0424-02	10.06	
(Southwood)			
REPACK			
CRE,TP, 10%, 60 gm	58016-3061-01	3.94	
60 gm	58016-9116-01	5.69	
MYTAB GAS (Qualitest)			
CTB,PO, 80 mg, 100s ea	00603-0210-21	2.88	
MYVITALIFE (ME Pharm)			
CAP,PO (SOFTGEL)			
30s ea	58607-0520-57	6.05	
60s ea	58607-0520-60	8.89	
N.A.C. (Carlson,J.R.)			
CAP,PO (PF,SF,CORN-FREE)			
500 mg, 60s ea	88395-0067-70	7.75	15.50
N'ICE (Heritage/Insight)			
LOZ,MM (ASSORTED,SF)			
5 mg, 24s ea	63736-0859-18	1.53	
(SF,CHERRY)			
5 mg, 24s ea	63736-0860-04	1.53	
(SF,CITRUS)			
5 mg, 24s ea	63736-0859-46	1.53	
(SF,HONEY,LEMON)			
5 mg, 24s ea	63736-0856-22	1.53	
(SF,PEPPERMINT)			
5 mg, 24s ea	63736-0859-48	1.53	
(VITAMIN C,SF,ORANGE)			
5 mg, 24s ea	63736-0859-58	1.53	
NA-ZONE (Snuva)			
SPR,NS (STERILE)			
0.75%, 60 ml	58291-0011-01	2.65	3.85
NAC (Carlson,J.R.)			
POW,PO (PF,SF,CORN-FREE)			
1700 mg, 100 gm	88395-0067-75	19.40	38.80
NAIL SCRUB (Pedinol)			
LIQ,TP (BLISTER PAK, W/BRUSH)			
60 ml	00884-4891-02		14.00
NAIL-EX (Rising)			
TAB,PO, 2.5 mg, 30s ea	64980-0126-03	18.10	
84s ea	64980-0126-84	19.42	
NAILS NAILS NAILS (Health Products Corp)			
CTB,PO (PF)			
60s ea	39686-0015-12	3.05	
NALDECON SENIOR DX EXPECTORANT (Southwood)			
REPACK			
LIQ,PO, 10 mg/5 ml-200 mg/5 ml,			
118 ml	58016-4058-01	6.88	
NANOVM (Solace)			
POW,PO (2X100GM,1-3 YEARS)			
100 gm 2s	57771-0001-13	35.94	59.90
(2X100GM,4-8 YEARS)			
100 gm 2s	57771-0001-48	35.94	59.90
NANOVM T/F (Solace)			
SOL,NA (1X480ML,9-18 YEARS)			
480 ml	57771-0001-90	42.00	70.00
NAPHCON (Alcon Ophthalmic)			
SOL,OP, 0.012%, 15 ml	00998-0078-15	26.76	
NAPHCON-A (Alcon Labs Cons Prod)			
SOL,OP (2X5ML)			
0.025%-0.3%,			
5 ml 2s	00650-0085-42	6.06	
15 ml	00650-0085-15	8.04	
(A-S Medication)			
REPACK			
SOL,OP, 0.025%-0.3%,			
15 ml	54569-0862-00	8.13	
(Pharma Pac)			
REPACK			
SOL,OP, 0.025%-0.3%,			
15 ml	52959-0107-03	19.01	
30 ml	52959-0107-01	19.01	
(Phys Total Care)			
REPACK			
SOL,OP, 0.025%-0.3%,			
15 ml	54868-0637-00	6.76	
(Southwood)			
REPACK			
SOL,OP, 0.025%-0.3%,			
15 ml	58016-6304-01	8.13	
NAPROXEN SODIUM (AmerisourceBergen)			
TAB,PO (PRIVATE LABEL,CAPLET)			
220 mg, 50s ea	24385-0368-71	4.49	4.99
(PRIVATE LABEL)			
220 mg, 50s ea	24385-0490-71	4.49	4.99
(PRIVATE LABEL,CAPLET)			
220 mg, 100s ea	24385-0368-78	8.06	8.99
(PRIVATE LABEL)			
220 mg, 100s ea	24385-0490-78	8.09	8.99
(Cardinal Health)			
TAB,PO (PRIVATE LABEL,CAPLET)			
220 mg, 50s ea	37205-0261-71	4.56	
100s ea	37205-0261-78	8.00	
(Chain Drug Marketing)			
TAB,PO, 220 mg, 50s ea	63868-0465-50	3.47	4.59
100s ea	63868-0465-01	5.92	7.49
(Family Phcy)			
TAB,PO (PRIVATE LABEL,CAPLET)			
220 mg, 100s ea	52735-0791-01	6.65	7.39
(PRIVATE LABEL)			
220 mg, 100s ea	52735-0790-01	6.65	7.39
(Major)			
TAB,PO, 220 mg, 50s ea	00904-5229-51	4.88	
(CAPLET)			
220 mg, 50s ea	00904-5230-51	4.88	
100s ea	00904-5229-59	8.25	
(CAPLET)			
220 mg, 100s ea	00904-5230-59	8.25	
(Teva)			
TAB,PO (CAPLET)			
220 mg, 50s ea	00182-1106-19	6.85	
(A-S Medication)			
REPACK			
TAB,PO, 220 mg, 10s ea	54569-5119-01	0.83	
30s ea	54569-5119-00	2.48	
(Altura)			
REPACK			
TAB,PO (CAPLET)			
220 mg, 10s ea	63874-0030-10	2.92	
20s ea	63874-0030-20	5.83	
24s ea	63874-0030-24	7.00	
30s ea	63874-0030-30	8.75	
(CAPLET)			
220 mg, 40s ea	63874-0030-40	11.66	
50s ea	63874-0030-50	14.58	
60s ea	63874-0030-60	17.49	
90s ea	63874-0030-90	26.24	
100s ea	63874-0030-01	29.17	
300s ea	63874-0030-77	87.60	
(Bryant Ranch)			
REPACK			
TAB,PO, 220 mg, 20s ea	63629-1793-02	2.07	
30s ea	63629-1793-03	3.06	
(DHS, Inc.)			
REPACK			
TAB,PO, 220 mg, 30s ea	55887-0505-30	14.00	
(Dispensing Solutions)			
REPACK			
TAB,PO, 220 mg, 24s ea	55045-2737-02	6.00	
30s ea	55045-2737-08	7.50	
30s ea	66336-0002-30	11.03	
50s ea	55045-2737-05	12.50	
60s ea	55045-2737-06	15.00	
(Keltman Pharma., Inc.)			
REPACK			
TAB,PO (CAPLET)			
220 mg, 40s ea	68387-0570-40	12.85	
(Nucare Pharm)			
REPACK			
TAB,PO, 220 mg, 20s ea	66267-0343-20	15.99	
28s ea	66267-0343-28	17.99	
30s ea	66267-0343-30	18.99	
(PD-Rx Pharm)			
REPACK			
TAB,PO, 220 mg, 20s ea	55289-0579-20	16.00	
30s ea	55289-0579-30	18.77	

PROD/MFR	HRI, UPC,NDC	AWP	SRP
(Pharma Pac)			
REPACK			
TAB,PO, 220 mg, 15s ea	52959-0469-15	5.88	
(CAPLET)			
220 mg, 20s ea	52959-0469-20	7.83	
24s ea	52959-0469-24	9.39	
(CAPLET)			
220 mg, 28s ea	52959-0469-28	10.59	
30s ea	52959-0469-30	10.98	
40s ea	52959-0469-40	14.64	
60s ea	52959-0469-60	16.13	
(Phys Total Care)			
REPACK			
TAB,PO (CAPLET)			
220 mg, 100s ea	54868-5308-00	27.48	
(Physician Partner)			
REPACK			
TAB,PO, 220 mg, 14s ea	21695-0088-14	9.07	
30s ea	21695-0088-30	19.43	
100s ea	21695-0637-00	24.78	
(Quality Care Prod)			
REPACK			
TAB,PO, 220 mg, 30s ea	49999-0068-30	28.60	
(Southwood)			
REPACK			
TAB,PO (CAPLET)			
220 mg, 10s ea	58016-0450-10	1.78	
15s ea	58016-0450-15	2.66	
20s ea	58016-0450-20	3.55	
30s ea	58016-0450-30	5.33	
40s ea	58016-0450-40	7.11	
50s ea	58016-0450-50	8.88	
60s ea	58016-0450-60	10.66	
80s ea	58016-0450-80	14.21	
90s ea	58016-0450-90	15.99	
100s ea	58016-0450-00	17.76	
120s ea	58016-0450-02	21.32	
150s ea	58016-0450-03	26.64	
200s ea	58016-0450-89	35.53	
300s ea	58016-0450-73	53.29	
NASACON (Consolidated Midland)			
SPR,NS, 0.05%, 15 ml	00223-6365-15	2.75	
15 ml 12s	00223-6560-01	30.00	
NASAFLO NETI POT (NeilMed)			
PKT,NS (WITH NETIPOT DEVICE,PF)			
50s ea	05928-0008-16		14.99
NASAL (Albertson's)			
SPR,NS, 0.05%, 30 ml	12810-0667-34	2.46	
(AmerisourceBergen)			
SPR,NS (PRIVATE LABEL)			
0.05%, 30 ml	24385-0304-10	5.39	5.99
(Bayer HealthCare)			
SOL,NS, 0.65%, 15 ml 6s	00024-1315-01	1.71	
SPR,NS, 0.65%, 30 ml	00024-1316-30	2.75	
(Medicine Shoppe)			
SPR,NS (12-HR NASAL DECONGEST)			
0.05%, 30 ml	49614-0314-10	3.99	3.99
NASAL 12 HOUR (Cardinal Health)			
SPR,NS (PRIVATE LABEL)			
0.05%, 15 ml	37205-0304-05	1.52	
29.57 ml	37205-0304-10	3.49	
NASAL ASPIRATOR & EAR SYRINGE (Apothecary)			
DEV,NA, ea	25715-0671-93	3.52	5.89
NASAL DECONGESTANT (Major)			
SPR,NS (12-HOUR)			
0.05%, 15 ml	00904-5711-35	2.05	
30 ml	00904-5711-30	2.95	
(Rugby)			
TAB,PO, 30 mg, 24s ea	00536-4391-35	1.87	
NASAL DECONGESTANT CHILDREN'S (A-S Medication)			
REPACK			
SYR,PO, 30 mg/5 ml,			
120 ml	54569-1064-00	2.33	
NASAL EASE ALLERGY BLOCKER (Health Care Products)			
POW,NS (200 DOSES)			
500 ml	60569-0482-50	9.43	15.99
NASAL EXTRA MOISTURISING 12 HOUR (Cardinal Health)			
SPR,NS (PRIVATE LABEL)			
0.05%, 30 ml	37205-0067-10	4.82	
NASAL EXTRA MOISTURIZING (AmerisourceBergen)			
SPR,NS (PRIVATE LABEL)			
0.05%, 30 ml	24385-0067-10	4.49	4.99
NASAL MOIST (Blairex)			
GEL,TP (AF,DYE-FREE)			
0.65%, 28.5 gm	50486-0027-35	2.51	
NASAL MOISTURIZING (Phys Total Care)			
REPACK			
SPR,NS, 0.65%, 45 ml	54868-3132-01	6.81	
NASAL RELIEF (Chain Drug Marketing)			
SPR,NS, 0.05%, 30 ml	63868-0056-30	1.31	4.99
(NO DRIP,PRIVATE LABEL)			
0.05%, 30 ml	63868-0058-30	1.62	4.99
NASAL RELIEF 12 HOUR (Altaire)			
SPR,NS, 0.05%, 15 ml	59390-0036-13	3.25	
30 ml	59390-0036-18	4.25	
NASAL STRIPS (AmerisourceBergen)			
DEV,NA (MEDIUM/LARGE)			
12s ea	24385-0246-52	3.68	4.09
30s ea	24385-0246-65	8.81	9.79
NASALCROM (McNeil Consumer Healthcare)			
SPR,NS, 5.2 mg/actuation,			
13 ml	00450-0300-13	8.40	
26 ml	00450-0300-26	13.93	
(Dispensing Solutions)			
REPACK			
SPR,NS, 5.2 mg/actuation,			
13 ml	55045-2854-01	12.25	
NASIN (Global Source)			
SPR,NS, 0.05%, 15 ml	59618-0620-28	2.25	
NAT MUR (Nuage Labs)			
TAB,SL (6X)			
125s ea	00634-6433-68	3.05	5.09
NAT PHOS (Nuage Labs)			
SL (6X)			
125s ea	00634-6436-68	3.05	5.09
NAT SULPH (Nuage Labs)			
SL (6X)			
125s ea	00634-6440-68	3.05	5.09
NATALEX (Lex)			
TAB,PO, 30s ea	49523-0102-03	1.02	
100s ea	49523-0102-10	3.29	
NATRUM MUR (Hyland's)			
TAB,PO, 500s ea	54973-1049-01	5.87	9.79
1000s ea	54973-1049-02	10.49	17.49
NATRUM PHOS (Hyland's)			
TAB,PO, 500s ea	54973-1055-01	5.87	9.79
1000s ea	54973-1055-02	10.49	17.49
NATRUM SULPH (Hyland's)			
TAB,PO, 500s ea	54973-1061-01	5.87	9.79
1000s ea	54973-1061-02	10.49	17.49
NATURAL BALANCE TEARS (Major)			
SOL,OP, 0.4%, 15 ml	00904-5018-35	3.30	
NATURAL FIBER LAXATIVE (Phys Total Care)			
REPACK			
PDR,PO (SMOOTH TEXTURE)			
3.4 gm/dose,			
370 gm	54868-3026-02	16.18	
420 gm	54868-3026-00	13.68	
570 gm	54868-3026-01	15.58	
NATURAL FIBER THERAPY (Major)			
PDR,PO (ORANGE)			
3.4 gm/dose, 369 gm	00904-5200-65	4.75	
(REGULAR)			
3.4 gm/dose, 369 gm	00904-5199-65	4.75	
(ORANGE)			
3.4 gm/dose, 539 gm	00904-5200-66	6.85	
(REGULAR)			
3.4 gm/dose, 539 gm	00904-5199-66	6.85	
NATURAL HERBAL DIURETIC (Mason Vit)			
TAB,PO (EXT. STR.,PF,SF)			
90s ea	11845-0068-49	6.11	
TER,PO (PF)			
60s ea	11845-0121-45	6.11	
NATURAL ICE LIP PROTECTANT (Mentholatum)			
STI,TP (SPF 15, BLISTER PACK,SF)			
4.8 gm	10742-0004-82	0.89	0.95
NATURAL ICE MEDICATED LIPBALM (Mentholatum)			
STI,TP (SPF 15, BLISTER PACK,SF)			
4.8 gm	10742-0000-41	0.89	0.95
NATURAL ICE SPORT (Mentholatum)			
STI,TP (SPF 30, BLISTER PACK,AF)			
3%-1%-7.5%-5%,			
4.5 gm	10742-0007-31	1.66	
(SPF 30,LOOSE,AF,SF)			
3%-1%-7.5%-5%,			
4.5 gm	10742-0007-32	1.66	
NATURAL VEGETABLE FIBER (Qualitest)			
PDR,PO (1X283GM,SF,REGULAR)			
3.4 gm/dose, 283 gm	00603-0992-63	6.10	
(1X283GM,SF)			
3.4 gm/dose, 283 gm	00603-0994-63	6.25	
(1X368GM,ORANGE)			
3.4 gm/dose, 368 gm	00603-0993-89	6.31	
(1X368GM,REGULAR)			
3.4 gm/dose, 368 gm	00603-0991-89	6.31	
NATURALYTE (Unico)			
SOL,PO (BUBBLEGUM)			
1000 ml 8s	37513-0000-25	13.30	
(FRUIT)			
1000 ml 8s	37513-0000-01	13.30	
(GRAPE)			
1000 ml 8s	37513-0000-29	13.30	
(UNFLAVORED)			
1000 ml 8s	37513-0000-23	13.30	
NATURE DE FRANCE ALGOLI (Grandpa Soap)			
SOA,TP (3.5 OZ.,DRY/NORMAL SKIN)			
24s ea	10486-0007-40	58.80	
NATURE DE FRANCE ARGILE BLANCHE (Grandpa Soap)			
SOA,TP (3.5 OZ.,DRY SKIN)			
24s ea	10486-0007-42	58.80	
NATURE DE FRANCE ARGIMIEL (Grandpa Soap)			
SOA,TP (3.5 OZ.,COMBINATION)			
24s ea	10486-0007-38	58.80	
NATURE'S BLEND (Natl Vitamin)			
ACIDOPHILUS			
CTB,PO, 200 mg-1 billion u,			
100s ea	54629-0011-56	3.53	5.89
ALPHA-LIPOIC ACID			
CAP,PO, 100 mg, 60s ea	54629-0110-76	3.95	6.59
AMINO ACTION			
TAB,PO (PF,SF)			
100s ea	54629-0240-01	5.87	9.79
B COMPLEX #1			
TAB,PO (PF,SF)			
100s ea	79854-0201-85	3.75	6.29
B-50 FORMULA			
TAB,PO (PF,SF)			
250s ea	54629-0036-10	11.75	19.59
BALANCE B-100			
TAB,PO (PF,SF)			
50s ea	79854-0200-95	5.39	8.99
BALANCE B-50			
PO (PF,SF)			
100s ea	79854-0200-90	5.23	8.79
BEE POLLEN			
CAP,PO (PF,SF)			
500 mg, ea	54629-0340-01	4.19	6.99
BETA CAROTENE			
SGL,PO (PF,SF)			
25000 iu, 100s ea	54629-0103-02	3.69	6.19
BILBERRY EXTRACT			
CAP,PO (PF)			
40 mg-25 mg-10 mg-10 mg,			
60s ea	54629-0691-00	5.66	9.49
BORAGE OIL			
SGL,PO (PF,SF)			
1000 mg, 60s ea	54629-0804-66	6.59	10.99
C COMPLEX			
TAB,PO (PF,SF)			
500 mg, 100s ea	54629-0097-01	3.95	6.59
CALCIUM CARBONATE			
TAB,PO (PF)			
600 mg, 100s ea	54629-0684-01	3.60	6.09
200s ea	54629-0720-00	6.11	10.19
CALCIUM CARBONATE/VITAMIN D			
TAB,PO (PF)			
600 mg-125 iu,			
100s ea	54629-0016-81	3.71	6.19
200s ea	54629-0732-00	6.29	10.49
500s ea	54629-0017-32	13.97	23.29
CALCIUM HIGH POTENCY			
TAB,PO (PF)			
600s ea	54629-0036-11	9.92	16.59
CALCIUM/VITAMIN D			
SGL,PO, 600 mg-200 iu,			
200s ea	54629-0735-00	8.65	14.49
CARDIOVASCULAR SUPPORT			
CAP,PO (PF,SF)			
60s ea	54629-0695-00	3.83	6.39

PROD/MFR	HRI, UPC,NDC	AWP	SRP
CAT'S CLAW			
CAP,PO (PF,SF)			
400 mg, 90s ea	**54629-0014-30**	4.50	7.59
CAYENNE			
CAP,PO (PF)			
450 mg, 90s ea	**54629-0011-00**	2.07	3.49
CHITOSAN SUPERIOR			
CAP,PO (PF,SF)			
90s ea	**54629-0121-69**	4.79	7.99
CHOLESTEROL FIGHTER			
CAP,PO (PF,SF)			
60s ea	**54629-0696-00**	3.95	6.59
CHONDROITIN SULFATE COMPLEX			
CAP,PO (PF,SF)			
60 mg-400 mg-2.5 mg,			
60s ea	**54629-0784-00**	6.28	10.49
CHONDROITIN/GLUCOSAMINE COMPLEX			
CAP,PO (PF,SF)			
60s ea	**54629-0011-18**	5.87	9.79
CHONDROITIN/GLUCOSAMINE/MSM			
TAB,PO (PF,SF,CORN-FREE)			
333.33 mg-200 mg-400 mg,			
120s ea	**54629-0287-12**	6.94	11.59
CHROMIUM PICOLINATE			
CAP,PO (PF)			
200 mcg, 60s ea	**54629-0758-06**	3.93	6.59
COD LIVER OIL			
SGL,PO (PF,SF)			
1250 iu-135 iu,			
100s ea	**54629-0124-01**	2.97	4.99
COENZYME Q10			
CAP,PO (PF,SF)			
50 mg, 30s ea	**54629-0848-00**	6.59	10.99
90s ea	**54629-0673-90**	15.95	
COLD & FLU FIGHTER IMMUNE SYSTEM			
CAP,PO (PF)			
60s ea	**54629-0693-00**	4.54	7.59
CORTISOL			
CAP,PO (SLENDER)			
100 mg-150 mg-0.05 mg,			
60s ea	**54629-0393-36**	6.59	10.99
CRANBERRY CONCENTRATE			
SGL,PO (PF,SF,SOFTGEL)			
500 mg, 60s ea	**54629-0000-20**	3.11	5.19
DAILY MULTI-VITAMIN & MINERALS			
TAB,PO (PF)			
350s ea	**54629-0019-38**	12.76	21.29
DAILY VITE			
TAB,PO (PF)			
250s ea	**54629-0067-02**	3.90	6.59
DAILY VITE PLUS IRON			
PO (PF,SF)			
250s ea	**54629-0068-02**	4.10	6.89
DHEA			
TAB,PO (PF,SF)			
25 mg, 60s ea	**54629-0250-00**	4.19	6.99
DOCUSATE SODIUM			
SGL,PO (SOFTGEL)			
100 mg, 1000s ea	**54629-0600-99**	23.40	32.79
250 mg, 1000s ea	**54629-0601-99**	35.55	
ECHINACEA			
CAP,PO (PF,SF)			
400 mg, 90s ea	**54629-0141-50**	4.50	7.59
180s ea	**54629-0620-00**	8.37	
ECHINACEA/GOLDEN SEAL ROOT			
CAP,PO (PF,SF)			
350 mg-100 mg,			
60s ea	**54629-0141-70**	5.08	8.49
ESTER-C			
TAB,PO (PF,SF)			
500 mg-50 mg,			
90s ea	**54629-0110-80**	4.79	7.99
FLAXSEED OIL			
SGL,PO (PF,SF,SOFTGEL)			
1000 mg, 90s ea	**54629-0080-38**	4.91	8.19
FOLIC ACID			
TAB,PO (PF,SF)			
0.4 mg, 250s ea	**54629-0650-02**	3.00	5.09
FRUITY C			
CTB,PO (PF)			
250 mg, 150s ea	**54629-0870-01**	3.40	5.69
FULL SPECTRUM B			
TAB,PO (W/VITAMIN C)			
100s ea	**54629-0126-91**	3.56	6.49
GARLIC			
TAB,PO (PF,SF)			
500 mg, 250s ea	**54629-0642-00**	9.16	15.29
1250 mg, 100s ea	**54629-0154-00**	4.07	6.79
GARLIC OIL			
SGL,PO (PF,SF)			
500 mg, 100s ea	**54629-0152-01**	2.56	4.29
GARLIC/PARSLEY			
TAB,PO (PF,SF)			
100 mg-50 mg,			
100s ea	**54629-0153-01**	2.75	4.59
GELATIN			
CAP,PO (PF,SF)			
650 mg, 100s ea	**54629-0078-01**	3.75	6.29
GINGER ROOT EXTRACT			
CAP,PO (SF)			
250 mg, 60s ea	**54629-0110-10**	3.83	6.39
GINKGO BILOBA EXTRACT			
CAP,PO, 40 mg, 60s ea	**54629-0142-50**	6.42	10.79
(PF)			
40 mg, 180s ea	**54629-0060-70**	14.49	24.19
GINSENG			
CAP,PO (PF)			
250 mg, 50s ea	**54629-0140-05**	3.40	5.69
200s ea	**79854-0008-88**	11.56	19.29
GLUCOSAMINE SULFATE			
CAP,PO (PF,SF)			
500 mg, 60s ea	**54629-0078-70**	5.39	8.99
GLUCOSAMINE/MSM COMPLEX			
CAP,PO (PF,SF)			
120s ea	**54629-0011-53**	6.11	10.19
GOLDEN SEAL			
CAP,PO (PF,SF)			
500 mg, 60s ea	**79854-0610-62**	6.50	10.89
GOTU KOLA			
CAP,PO (PF,SF)			
500 mg, 60s ea	**79854-0014-35**	3.29	5.49
GRAPE SEED EXTRACT			
TAB,PO (PF,SF)			
50 mg, 60s ea	**54629-0687-00**	5.86	9.79
GREEN TEA EXTRACT			
CAP,PO (PF,SF)			
250 mg, 60s ea	**54629-0110-40**	2.86	4.79
HAWTHORNE BERRY			
CAP,PO (PF,SF)			
450 mg, 60s ea	**54629-0690-00**	2.85	4.79
HI-POTENCY SOFT MULTIPLE VITAMIN			
SGL,PO (PF,SF,SOFTGEL)			
60s ea	**54629-0810-76**	6.53	10.89
IRON			
TAB,PO (PF,SF)			
65 mg, 100s ea	**54629-0110-90**	2.56	4.29
1000s ea	**54629-0775-00**	9.89	
KOREAN GINSENG			
CAP,PO (PF,SF)			
350 mg, 60s ea	**54629-0121-76**	4.48	7.49
L-CARNITINE			
CAP,PO (PF,SF)			
200 mg, 60s ea	**54629-0011-67**	7.79	12.99
L-GLUTAMINE			
CAP,PO (PF,SF)			
500 mg, 100s ea	**54629-0011-68**	4.65	7.79
LECITHIN			
SGL,PO (PF,SF,SOFTGEL)			
1200 mg, 200s ea	**54629-0275-00**	5.65	9.49
LUTEIN			
SGL,PO (PF,SF)			
15 mg-0.7 mg,			
60s ea	**54629-0080-36**	7.64	12.79
LYCOPENE			
SGL,PO (PF,SF,SOFTGEL)			
6 mg, 60s ea	**54629-0080-37**	7.78	12.99
LYSINE			
TAB,PO (PF,SF)			
500 mg, 100s ea	**54629-0765-01**	3.40	5.69
1000 mg, 50s ea	**54629-0770-05**	3.60	6.09
MEGA MULTIVITAMIN W/MINERALS			
TAB,PO, 60s ea	**54629-0760-06**	5.75	9.59
MELATONIN			
TAB,PO (PF,SF)			
3 mg, 60s ea	**54629-0609-00**	3.89	6.49
SL, 5 mg, 60s ea	**54629-0615-00**	5.39	8.99
METABO-STYLE			
TAB,PO (SF,CAPLET)			
0.075 mg-75 mg-6 iu-5 mg,			
90s ea	**54629-0361-20**	6.59	10.99
MILK THISTLE EXTRACT			
CAP,PO (PF)			
140 mg, 60s ea	**54629-0145-10**	4.79	7.99
MSM			
CAP,PO (PF,SF)			
1000 mg, 100s ea	**54629-3592-00**	5.39	8.99
MULTI-VITAMIN W/MINERALS			
SGL,PO (PF,SF,SOFTGEL)			
100s ea	**54629-0780-01**	5.25	8.79
TAB,PO (PF, SF, YEAST-FREE,PF)			
250s ea	**54629-0750-02**	7.11	11.89
MULTIPLE VITAMIN W/MINERALS NO IRON			
PO (PF,SF)			
100s ea	**54629-0111-30**	2.90	4.89
MULTIVITAMIN CHILDREN'S			
CTB,PO (PF)			
100s ea	**54629-0050-01**	2.62	4.39
300s ea	**54629-0501-02**	6.93	11.59
NIACIN			
TAB,PO (PF,SF)			
500 mg, 100s ea	**54629-0712-01**	3.10	5.19
TER,PO, 500 mg, 100s ea	**54629-0711-01**	3.25	5.49
300s ea	**54629-0714-03**	8.30	13.89
NIACIN NO FLUSH			
CAP,PO (PF,SF)			
100 mg-400 mg,			
60s ea	**54629-0705-00**	5.27	8.79
OMEGA-3			
CAP,PO (PF,SF,SOFTGEL)			
1000 mg-5 iu,			
90s ea	**54629-0893-09**	5.00	8.39
SGL,PO, 1000 mg-5 iu,			
300s ea	**54629-0018-93**	12.86	21.49
OYSTER SHELL CALCIUM			
TAB,PO (PF)			
500 mg, 200s ea	**54629-0715-00**	5.15	8.59
OYSTER SHELL CALCIUM/VITAMIN D			
TAB,PO (PF)			
500 mg-125 iu,			
200s ea	**54629-0316-30**	5.33	8.89
1000s ea	**54629-0681-10**	15.10	21.19
PAPAYA ENZYME			
TAB,PO (PF)			
ea	**54629-0122-01**	2.67	4.49
PMS WOMEN'S FORMULA			
TAB,PO (PF)			
60s ea	**54629-0113-10**	5.95	9.99
POTASSIUM GLUCONATE			
TAB,PO (PF,SF)			
500 mg, 100s ea	**54629-0850-01**	2.92	4.89
PRENATAL			
TAB,PO (PF)			
100s ea	**54629-0052-01**	4.49	7.49
REST & RELAXATION			
CAP,PO (PF,SF)			
60s ea	**54629-0692-00**	4.43	7.39
ROYAL JELLY			
CAP,PO (SOFTGEL CAPSULE,SOFTGEL)			
250 mg, 90s ea	**54629-0000-14**	4.06	6.79
SAW PALMETTO			
SGL,PO (PF,SF,SOFTGEL)			
100 mg-160 mg,			
120s ea	**54629-0672-00**	12.45	20.79
SELENIUM			
TAB,PO (PF,SF)			
50 mcg, 100s ea	**54629-0164-01**	2.85	4.79
SOY ISOFLAVONES			
TAB,PO (PF,SF)			
40 mg, 90s ea	**54629-0011-43**	9.44	15.79
ST. JOHN'S WORT EXTRACT			
CAP,PO (PF,SF)			
300 mg, 180s ea	**54629-0682-00**	10.49	17.49
STRESS W/IRON			
TAB,PO (PF,SF)			
60s ea	**54629-0596-06**	3.48	5.89
STRESS W/ZINC			
TAB,PO (PF,SF)			
60s ea	**54629-0597-06**	3.60	6.09
SUPER B COMPLEX/VITAMIN C			
CAP,PO (PF,SF)			
100s ea	**54629-0080-01**	4.11	6.89
TEMP TAB			
TAB,PO, 287 mg-15 mg-180 mg,			
100s ea	**54629-0126-81**	3.16	5.29
THERATRUM COMPLETE			
TAB,PO, 130s ea	**54629-0011-70**	4.19	6.99
(PF)			
250s ea	**54629-0015-99**	9.25	15.49
THERATRUM COMPLETE 50 PLUS			
TAB,PO (PF)			
100s ea	**54629-0011-71**	3.92	6.59
180s ea	**54629-0009-38**	6.92	11.59
ULTRA ENERGY FORMULA			
TAB,PO (PF,SF)			
60s ea	**54629-0350-00**	3.16	5.29
VALERIAN ROOT			
CAP,PO, 500 mg, 90s ea	**54629-0610-90**	3.75	6.29
VITAMIN A			
SGL,PO (PF,SF)			
8000 iu, 100s ea	**54629-0110-01**	1.73	2.89
VITAMIN B1			
TAB,PO (PF,SF)			
100 mg, 100s ea	**54629-0057-01**	2.40	4.09
VITAMIN B12			
TAB,PO (PF,SF)			
100 mcg, 100s ea	**54629-0058-01**	1.90	3.19
1000s ea	**54629-0580-10**	19.10	

PROD/MFR	HRI, UPC,NDC	AWP	SRP
250 mcg, 100s ea	54629-0580-01	2.52	4.29
500 mcg, 100s ea	54629-0585-01	2.99	4.99
1000s ea	54629-0585-10	19.10	
(PF)			
1000 mcg, 50s ea	54629-0586-05	2.86	4.79
VITAMIN B6			
TAB,PO (PF,SF)			
50 mg, 100s ea	54629-0063-01	2.36	3.99
1000s ea	54629-0063-10	15.10	21.19
100 mg, 100s ea	54629-0630-01	2.97	4.99
VITAMIN C			
CTB,PO (PF)			
250 mg, 100s ea	54629-0070-01	2.51	4.19
250s ea	54629-0087-02	5.63	9.39
(PF,SF)			
500 mg, 60s ea	54629-0308-20	2.87	4.79
(PF,BERRY)			
500 mg, 100s ea	54629-0873-01	3.95	6.59
(PF)			
500 mg, 100s ea	54629-0700-01	3.45	5.79
TAB,PO (PF,SF)			
250 mg, 250s ea	54629-0085-02	3.71	6.19
500 mg, 100s ea	54629-0076-01	1.99	3.39
250s ea	54629-0086-02	4.45	7.49
1000s ea	54629-0092-10	14.95	20.99
1000 mg, 100s ea	54629-0093-01	3.60	6.09
TER,PO, 1500 mg, 50s ea	54629-0932-05	3.78	6.39
VITAMIN E			
SGL,PO (PF,SF,SOFTGEL)			
200 iu, 100s ea	54629-0200-01	2.75	4.59
400 iu, 250s ea	54629-0410-02	8.12	13.59
500s ea	54629-0015-35	14.69	24.49
(S,F,PF,SF,SOFTGEL)			
1000 iu, 50s ea	54629-0105-05	4.76	7.99
(PF,SF,SOFTGEL)			
1000 iu, 100s ea	54629-0001-01	8.81	14.69
200s ea	54629-0015-40	15.95	26.59
VITAMIN E MIXED TOCOPHEROL			
PO (PF,SF,SOFTGEL)			
400 iu, 100s ea	54629-0411-01	4.54	7.59
VITAMIN E WATER SOLUBLE			
PO (PF,SF,SOFTGEL)			
400 iu, 100s ea	54629-0405-01	5.74	9.59
VITAMINS FOR HAIR			
CAP,PO (PF,SF)			
50s ea	54629-0156-05	3.75	6.29
WOMEN'S CONTROL & RELIEF			
CAP,PO (PF)			
75 mg-50 mg,			
50s ea	54629-0694-00	4.97	8.29
ZINC GLUCONATE			
TAB,PO, 50 mg, 100s ea	54629-0176-01	2.39	3.99
(PF,SF)			
100 mg, 100s ea	54629-0180-01	3.46	5.79
NATURE'S BLEND ALOE VERA (Natl Vitamin)			
SGL,PO (PF,SF,CORN-FREE)			
25 mg, 100s ea	54629-0000-18	4.81	8.09
NATURE'S BLEND CALCIUM OYSTER SHELL (Natl Vitamin)			
TAB,PO (PF,GLUTEN-FREE)			
500 mg, 100s ea	54629-0683-01	2.98	4.99
NATURE'S BLEND CHEWABLE CALCIUM (Natl Vitamin)			
CTB,PO (PF,PRIVATE LABEL)			
500 mg, 100s ea	54629-0687-01	4.45	7.49
NATURE'S BLEND FOLIC ACID (Natl Vitamin)			
TAB,PO (PF)			
1 mg, 100s ea	54629-0128-10	1.65	2.79
1000s ea	54629-0128-00	6.92	11.59
NATURE'S BLEND GLUCOSAMINE CHONDROITIN (Natl Vitamin)			
CAP,PO (MAX. STR.,PF)			
60s ea	54629-0080-44	10.19	16.99
(MAXIMUM STRENGTH,PF)			
120s ea	54629-0804-12	16.78	27.99
NATURE'S BLEND LACTOBACILLIN ACIDOPHILUS (Natl Vitamin)			
CAP,PO (PF,GLUTEN-FREE)			
25 million u, 100s ea	54629-0111-01	3.50	5.89
NATURE'S BLEND MACUVITE (Natl Vitamin)			
TAB,PO (GLUTEN-FREE)			
60s ea	54629-0755-06	4.37	7.29
NATURE'S BLEND MACUVITE EYE CARE (Natl Vitamin)			
TAB,PO (GLUTEN-FREE)			
120s ea	79854-0012-45	6.32	10.59
NATURE'S BLEND MULTIPLE VITAMIN WITH FOLIC ACID (Natl Vitamin)			
TAB,PO, 100s ea	54629-0333-01	2.39	3.89
NATURE'S BLEND NAC 600 (Natl Vitamin)			
CAP,PO (PF,GLUTEN-FREE)			
600 mg, 60s ea	54629-4097-06	5.86	9.79
NATURE'S BLEND OYSTER SHELL CALCIUM + D (Natl Vitamin)			
TAB,PO (GLUTEN-FREE)			
500 mg-400 iu, 100s ea	54629-0681-01	3.15	5.29
NATURE'S BLEND OYSTER SHELL CALCIUM D (Natl Vitamin)			
TAB,PO (PF,GLUTEN-FREE)			
250 mg-125 iu, 100s ea	54629-0168-01	2.63	4.39
NATURE'S BLEND OYSTER SHELL CALCIUM WITH VITAMIN D (Natl Vitamin)			
PO (USP,CORN-FREE)			
250 mg-250 iu,			
100s ea	54629-3688-01	2.63	4.29
NATURE'S BLEND RED YEAST RICE EXTRACT (Natl Vitamin)			
CAP,PO (PF,GLUTEN-FREE)			
600 mg, 60s ea	54629-1215-06	6.56	10.99
NATURE'S BLEND SUPER ANTIOXIDENT (Natl Vitamin)			
CAP,PO, 90s ea	54629-0011-57	5.98	9.79
NATURE'S BLEND SUPER THERAVITE-M (Natl Vitamin)			
TAB,PO (GLUTEN-FREE)			
130s ea	54629-0082-01	5.86	9.79
NATURE'S BLEND VITAMIN D (Natl Vitamin)			
TAB,PO (GLUTEN-FREE)			
400 iu, 100s ea	54629-0011-62	1.93	3.29
NATURE'S BLEND VITAMIN D3 (Natl Vitamin)			
TAB,PO (PF,SF,CORN-FREE)			
1000 iu, 100s ea	79854-0050-24	2.98	4.99
NATURE'S BLEND VITAMIN E (Natl Vitamin)			
SGL,PO (PF,GLUTEN-FREE)			
400 iu, 100s ea	54629-0400-01	4.07	6.79
NATURE'S BOUNTY ABC PLUS (Nature's Bounty)			
TAB,PO (100+30 FREE TABS)			
130s ea	74312-0417-72		8.99
NATURE'S BOUNTY FISH OIL PLUS CO Q-10 (Nature's Bounty)			
SGL,PO (SODIUM-FREE)			
30 mg-1000 mg,			
50s ea	74312-0148-76		13.99
NATURE'S BOUNTY VITAMIN D (Nature's Bounty)			
TAB,PO (PRIVATE LABEL)			
120 mg-1000 iu,			
100s ea	74312-0156-05		6.59
NATURE'S NATURALS (Natl Vitamin)			
ACIDOPHILUS			
CAP,PO (FREEZE DRIED,PF)			
100s ea	54629-0664-77	3.15	5.29
ALFALFA			
TAB,PO, 250 mg, 90s ea	54629-0112-02	3.41	5.69
ALOE VERA			
CRE,TP, 113.4 gm	54629-4401-04	1.79	2.99
GEL,TP, 240 gm	54629-4440-08	1.97	3.29
240 gm	54629-4450-08	2.09	3.49
B COMPLEX #1			
TAB,PO (PF,SF)			
100s ea	54629-0563-01	3.75	6.29
BALANCE B-100			
PO (PF,SF)			
50s ea	54629-0131-05	5.39	8.99
BALANCE B-50			
PO (PF,SF)			
100s ea	54629-0130-01	5.23	8.79
BEE POLLEN			
CAP,PO (PF,SF)			
500 mg, 100s ea	54629-0664-87	3.45	5.79
BETA CAROTENE			
SGL,PO (PF,SF,SOFTGEL)			
25000 iu, 100s ea	54629-0664-88	3.38	5.69
BILBERRY EXTRACT			
CAP,PO (PF)			
40 mg-25 mg-10 mg-10 mg,			
60s ea	54629-0666-91	5.09	8.49
BREWER'S YEAST			
TAB,PO (PF,SF)			
250s ea	54629-0666-60	2.86	4.79
C COMPLEX			
TER,PO (PF,SF)			
500 mg, 100s ea	54629-0663-50	3.49	5.89
60s ea	54629-0663-60	3.65	6.09
CALCIUM 500			
CTB,PO (PF,BAVARIAN CREAM)			
500 mg, 100s ea	54629-0662-48	3.39	5.69
CALCIUM 600/VITAMIN D			
CAP,PO (SOFTGEL)			
100s ea	54629-0165-01	4.79	7.99
CALCIUM CARBONATE			
TAB,PO (PF)			
600 mg, 100s ea	54629-0662-15	3.49	5.89
CALCIUM CITRATE			
TAB,PO, 950 mg, 100s ea	54629-1686-01	3.71	6.19
CALCIUM/MAGNESIUM			
TAB,PO, 100s ea	54629-0685-01	2.33	3.89
(PF,SF)			
250 mg-155 mg,			
100s ea	54629-0662-35	2.34	3.99
CALCIUM/MAGNESIUM/ZINC			
TAB,PO (PF,SF)			
250 mg-125 mg-5 mg,			
100s ea	54629-0016-89	2.42	4.09
CALCIUM/VITAMIN D			
SGL,PO (PF,SF,SOFTGEL)			
600 mg-200 iu,			
100s ea	54629-0662-49	4.55	7.59
CAT'S CLAW			
CAP,PO (PF,SF)			
400 mg, 90s ea	54629-0666-67	4.28	7.19
CHOLESTEROL FIGHTER			
CAP,PO (PF,SF)			
60s ea	54629-0666-96	3.52	5.89
CHROMIUM PICOLINATE			
CAP,PO (PF,SF)			
200 mcg, 60s ea	54629-0667-58	3.53	5.89
COCOA BUTTER			
CRE,TP, 120 gm	54629-4951-04	1.67	2.79
COD LIVER OIL			
SGL,PO (PF,SF,SOFTGEL)			
100s ea	54629-0665-00	2.51	4.19
COENZYME Q10			
CAP,PO (PF,SF)			
50 mg, 30s ea	54629-0668-48	8.49	14.19
COMPLEX B100			
TER,PO, 50s ea	54629-0132-05	5.57	9.29
COMPLEX C			
TER,PO, 1000 mg, 60s ea	54629-0931-06	4.07	6.79
DAILY VITE			
TAB,PO (PF)			
250s ea	54629-0664-30	3.77	6.29
DAILY VITE PLUS IRON			
PO (PF)			
250s ea	54629-0664-40	3.87	6.49
DHEA			
TAB,PO (PF,SF)			
25 mg, 60s ea	54629-0660-25	4.19	6.99
DOCUSATE SODIUM			
SGL,PO (SOFTGEL)			
100 mg, 100s ea	54629-0600-01	2.75	4.59
ECHINACEA			
CAP,PO (PF,SF)			
400 mg, 90s ea	54629-0667-15	4.28	7.19
ECHINACEA/GOLDEN SEAL ROOT			
CAP,PO (PF,SF)			
350 mg-100 mg,			
60s ea	54629-0667-20	5.08	8.49
FAT BURNER ULTIMATE			
TAB,PO (PF,SF)			
60s ea	54629-0666-79	4.97	8.29
FERROUS GLUCONATE			
TAB,PO, 324 mg, 100s ea	54629-0645-01	2.99	4.99
FOLIC ACID			
TAB,PO (PF,SF)			
0.4 mg, 250s ea	54629-0663-75	3.19	5.39
GARLIC			
SGL,PO (PF,SF,SOFTGEL)			
500 mg, 100s ea	54629-0665-90	2.25	3.79
TAB,PO (PF,SF)			
1250 mg, 100s ea	54629-0661-54	4.10	6.89
GARLIC/PARSLEY			
TAB,PO (PF,SF)			
100 mg-50 mg,			
100s ea	54629-0665-95	2.20	3.69
GELATIN			
CAP,PO (PF,SF)			
650 mg, 100s ea	54629-0663-80	3.13	5.29
GERIATRIC HIGH POTENCY			
TAB,PO, 100s ea	54629-0106-01	3.71	6.19
GINKGO BILOBA			
CAP,PO (PF)			
40 mg, 60s ea	54629-0667-00	6.21	10.39
GINSENG			
SGL,PO (PF,SF)			
250 mg, 50s ea	54629-0666-00	3.14	5.29
GLUCOSAMINE SULFATE			
CAP,PO (PF,SF)			
500 mg, 60s ea	54629-0667-87	7.91	13.19

PROD/MFR	HRI, UPC,NDC	AWP	SRP
GOLDEN SEAL			
CAP,PO (S.F,PF,SF)			
500 mg, 60s ea	54629-0666-69	6.19	10.39
GUARANA			
TAB,PO, 1000 mg,			
100s ea	54629-0145-01	4.66	7.79
HAWTHORNE BERRY			
CAP,PO (PF,SF)			
450 mg, 60s ea	54629-0666-90	2.85	4.79
KELP			
TAB,PO, 200s ea	54629-0149-02	2.64	4.49
(PF,SF)			
0.15 mg, 200s ea	54629-0666-05	2.13	3.59
KELP/LECITHIN/B6			
SGL,PO (SOFTGEL)			
100s ea	54629-0251-01	3.71	6.19
LECITHIN			
SGL,PO (PF,SF,SOFTGEL)			
1200 mg, 100s ea	54629-0666-10	2.99	4.99
LYSINE			
TAB,PO (PF,SF)			
500 mg, 100s ea	54629-0666-20	2.81	4.69
1000 mg, 50s ea	54629-0666-25	2.97	4.99
MAGNESIUM ELEMENTAL			
CAP,PO, 300 mg, 100s ea	54629-0854-01	3.95	6.59
TAB,PO, 30 mg, 100s ea	54629-0853-01	2.91	4.89
MEGA MULTIVITAMIN W/MINERALS			
TAB,PO, 60s ea	54629-0664-10	5.75	9.59
MELATONIN			
TAB,PO (PF,SF)			
3 mg, 60s ea	54629-0666-11	3.89	6.49
MULTI-VITAMIN W/MINERALS			
SGL,PO (PF,SF,SOFTGEL)			
100s ea	54629-0664-60	4.65	7.79
TAB,PO (PF)			
100s ea	54629-0664-50	2.75	4.59
MULTIVITAMIN CHILDREN'S			
CTB,PO, 100s ea	54629-0664-20	2.37	3.99
300s ea	54629-0664-21	6.28	10.49
NIACIN			
TAB,PO, 50 mg, 100s ea	54629-0051-01	1.50	2.59
(PF,SF)			
100 mg, 100s ea	54629-0663-90	1.97	3.29
250 mg, 100s ea	54629-0710-01	2.75	4.59
500 mg, 300s ea	54629-0713-03	7.90	13.19
TER,PO, 250 mg, 100s ea	54629-0709-01	2.92	4.89
(PF,SF)			
500 mg, 100s ea	54629-0663-11	2.99	4.99
300s ea	54629-0663-12	5.93	9.89
NIACIN NO FLUSH			
CAP,PO (PF,SF)			
100 mg-400 mg,			
60s ea	54629-0667-05	4.96	8.29
OAT BRAN			
CTB,PO, 500 mg, 120s ea	54629-0203-01	3.53	5.89
OMEGA-3			
SGL,PO (PF,SF,SOFTGEL)			
1000 mg-5 iu,			
90s ea	54629-0668-93	5.00	8.39
OYSTER SHELL CALCIUM			
TAB,PO (PF)			
500 mg, 100s ea	54629-0662-47	2.80	4.69
OYSTER SHELL CALCIUM/VITAMIN D			
TAB,PO (PF,SF)			
250 mg-125 iu,			
100s ea	54629-0662-40	2.00	3.39
250s ea	54629-0682-02	5.08	8.49
(PF,SF)			
500 mg-125 iu,			
100s ea	54629-0662-46	2.86	4.79
PANTOTHENIC ACID			
TAB,PO, 100 mg, 200s ea	54629-0159-02	3.71	6.19
PAPAYA ENZYME			
TAB,PO (PF,SF)			
100s ea	54629-0666-31	1.95	3.29
POTASSIUM GLUCONATE			
TAB,PO (PF,SF)			
500 mg, 100s ea	54629-0666-40	2.66	4.49
PRENATAL			
TAB,PO (PF,SF)			
100s ea	54629-0663-42	4.04	6.79
PROTEIN			
PDR,PO, 448 gm	54629-0500-16	5.90	9.89
TAB,PO, 200s ea	54629-0550-02	3.75	6.29
(PF,HONEY)			
200s ea	54629-0666-44	3.23	5.39
ROYAL JELLY			
CAP,PO (PF)			
250 mg, 90s ea	54629-0660-14	4.05	6.79
SAW PALMETTO			
SGL,PO (PF,SF,SOFTGEL)			
160 mg, 30s ea	54629-0700-00	3.89	6.49
SELENIUM			
TAB,PO (PF,SF)			
50 mcg, 100s ea	54629-0666-50	2.51	4.19
200 mcg, 100s ea	54629-0163-00	3.17	5.29
SHARK CARTILAGE			
CAP,PO (PF,SF)			
700 mg, 60s ea	54629-0007-95	7.10	11.89
ST. JOHN'S WORT EXTRACT			
CAP,PO (PF,SF)			
250 mg, 60s ea	54629-0014-45	4.07	6.79
300 mg, 60s ea	54629-0664-45	4.07	6.79
STRESS FORMULA			
TAB,PO, 60s ea	54629-0595-06	3.40	5.69
STRESS W/IRON			
TAB,PO (PF,SF)			
60s ea	54629-0662-10	3.50	5.89
STRESS W/ZINC			
TAB,PO (PF,SF)			
60s ea	54629-0662-20	3.59	5.99
SUPER ANTIOXIDANT			
TAB,PO (SOFTGEL,PF,SF)			
60s ea	54629-0936-06	3.95	6.59
SUPER B/VITAMIN C			
CAP,PO (PF,SF)			
100s ea	54629-0661-70	3.71	6.19
SUPER THERAVITE-M			
TAB,PO (PF,SF)			
130s ea	54629-0664-00	4.40	7.39
ULTRA ENERGY FORMULA			
TAB,PO (PF,SF)			
60s ea	54629-0660-35	3.12	5.29
VALERIAN ROOT			
CAP,PO (PF,SF)			
500 mg, 90s ea	54629-0666-16	3.75	6.19
VITAMIN A			
SGL,PO (PF,SF,SOFTGEL)			
8000 iu, 100s ea	54629-0661-00	1.64	2.79
VITAMIN B COMPLEX			
CAP,PO, 100s ea	54629-0560-01	2.99	4.99
250s ea	54629-0561-02	6.36	10.69
VITAMIN B1			
TAB,PO (PF)			
100 mg, 100s ea	54629-0661-20	2.26	3.79
250 mg, 100s ea	54629-0570-01	4.12	6.89
VITAMIN B12			
TAB,PO (PF,SF)			
100 mcg, 100s ea	54629-0661-50	1.97	3.29
250 mcg, 100s ea	54629-0661-55	2.26	3.79
(PF)			
500 mcg, 100s ea	54629-0661-60	2.98	4.99
1000 mcg, 50s ea	54629-0661-65	2.75	4.59
50s ea	79854-0611-45	1.56	
100s ea	79854-0611-46	2.48	
VITAMIN B2			
TAB,PO, 25 mg, 100s ea	54629-0055-01	2.54	4.29
VITAMIN B6			
TAB,PO (PF,SF)			
50 mg, 100s ea	54629-0661-37	2.12	3.59
(P.F,PF,SF)			
100 mg, 100s ea	54629-0661-40	2.89	4.89
(PF,SF)			
250 mg, 100s ea	54629-0632-01	5.34	8.99
VITAMIN C			
CER,PO (PF)			
500 mg, 100s ea	54629-0920-01	4.34	7.29
CTB,PO, 100 mg, 100s ea	54629-0054-01	1.60	2.69
(TANGERINE)			
100 mg, 250s ea	54629-0056-02	3.59	5.99
(PF,FRUIT)			
250 mg, 150s ea	54629-0663-65	3.26	5.43
(PF)			
250 mg, 250s ea	54629-0663-05	4.78	7.99
(PF,BERRY)			
500 mg, 100s ea	54629-0663-63	3.45	5.79
(PF)			
500 mg, 100s ea	54629-0663-10	3.35	5.59
PDR,PO, 250 gm	54629-0926-02	9.85	16.49
TAB,PO, 100 mg, 100s ea	54629-0066-01	1.12	1.89
250 mg, 100s ea	54629-0069-01	1.75	2.99
(PF)			
250 mg, 250s ea	54629-0662-50	3.28	5.49
(PF,SF)			
500 mg, 100s ea	54629-0662-60	1.85	3.09
(PF)			
500 mg, 250s ea	54629-0662-70	4.25	7.09
500s ea	54629-0096-05	8.25	13.79
(PF)			
1000 mg, 100s ea	54629-0662-80	3.68	6.19
250s ea	54629-0930-02	8.27	13.79
TER,PO, 1500 mg,			
100s ea	54629-0320-01	6.95	11.59
VITAMIN C W/ROSE HIPS			
TAB,PO (PF,SF)			
250 mg, 100s ea	54629-0663-15	1.79	2.99
(P.F,PF,SF)			
500 mg, 250s ea	54629-0663-35	5.99	10.09
(PF,SF)			
1000 mg, 100s ea	54629-0663-40	4.40	7.39
VITAMIN C/BIOFLAVONOID/ROSE HIPS			
CAP,PO (PF,SF)			
1000 mg-25 mg-50 mg,			
90s ea	54629-0513-09	5.40	9.09
VITAMIN E			
OIL,TP (24,000 I.U.)			
ea	54629-0331-00	2.68	4.49
(49,000 I.U.)			
52 ml	54629-0331-10	4.80	8.09
SGL,PO (SOFTGEL; PF; SF,PF,SF)			
100 iu, 100s ea	54629-0100-01	2.02	3.39
(PF,SF,SOFTGEL)			
200 iu, 100s ea	54629-0665-20	2.81	4.69
(SOFTGEL)			
200 iu, 250s ea	54629-0210-02	6.40	10.69
(PF,SF,SOFTGEL)			
400 iu, 100s ea	54629-0665-40	3.29	5.49
250s ea	54629-0665-50	8.09	13.49
1000 iu, 50s ea	54629-0665-60	4.65	7.79
100s ea	54629-0665-70	8.56	14.29
VITAMIN E MTC			
PO (PF,SF,SOFTGEL)			
400 iu, 100s ea	54629-0665-86	4.15	6.99
(SOFTGEL)			
1000 iu, 100s ea	54629-0010-01	9.17	15.29
VITAMIN E WATER SOLUBLE			
PO (SF,SOFTGEL)			
400 iu, 100s ea	54629-0665-80	5.45	9.09
VITAMIN E400 D ALPHA			
PO (PF,SF,SOFTGEL)			
400 iu, 100s ea	54629-0665-82	7.55	12.59
VITAMINS FOR HAIR			
TAB,PO (PF,SF)			
50s ea	54629-0666-14	4.15	6.99
YEAST			
TAB,PO, 250s ea	54629-0172-02	3.29	5.49
YUCCA EXTRACT			
CAP,PO (PF,SF)			
500 mg, 100s ea	54629-0666-89	4.54	7.59
ZINC			
LOZ,MM (LEMON - P.F.,PF,LEMON)			
60 mg-5 mg-27 mg,			
120s ea	54629-0171-01	3.47	5.79
ZINC GLUCONATE			
TAB,PO, 20 mg, 100s ea	54629-0174-01	1.67	2.79
(PF,SF)			
50 mg, 100s ea	54629-0666-70	2.06	3.49
100 mg, 100s ea	54629-0666-80	3.07	5.19
NATURE'S TEARS (Rugby)			
SOL,OP, 0.4%, 15 ml	00536-6237-72	4.35	
NATURE'S WASH PLUS (Geritrex)			
LIQ,TP (BODY WASH/SHAMPOO)			
3840 ml	92771-0145-01	23.54	
NATURES REWARD GINKOGIN (Blairex)			
TAB,PO (CAPLET)			
300 mg-60 mg-100 mg,			
30s ea	50486-0370-30	7.91	
NAVARRO PRESTIGE SMART SYSTEM (Home Diag)			
DEV,NA (STRIP)			
50s ea	56151-0308-50	26.12	
NAVARRO PSS STARTER (Home Diag)			
DEV,NA (MTR,STRP,LANCET,DEV,SOL)			
ea	56151-0208-01	22.18	
NECKLACE (American)			
DEV,NA (10KT.,CLASSIC)			
ea	08590-0049-00		229.95
(10KT.,DOG TAG,BLUE)			
ea	08590-0072-00		399.95
(10KT.,DOGTAG,EMBOSSED)			
ea	08590-0070-00		399.95
(10KT.,DOGTAG,RED)			
ea	08590-0071-00		399.95
(10KT.,PREMIER A)			
ea	08590-0106-00		279.95
(10KT.,PREMIER B)			
ea	08590-0108-00		279.95
(10KT.,PREMIER C)			
ea	08590-0107-00		279.95
(14KT.,CLASSIC)			
ea	08590-0052-00		229.95
(14KT.,DOGTAG,BLUE)			
ea	08590-0075-00		499.95
(14KT.,DOGTAG,EMBOSSED)			
ea	08590-0073-00		499.95

PROD/MFR HRI, UPC,NDC AWP SRP

(14KT.,DOGTAG,RED)
ea 08590-0074-00 499.95
(14KT.,PREMIER A)
ea 08590-0113-00 349.95
(14KT.,PREMIER B)
ea 08590-0115-00 349.95
(14KT.,PREMIER C)
ea 08590-0114-00 349.95
(GOLD FILLED,DOGTAG,BLUE)
ea 08590-0077-00 69.95
(GOLD FILLED,DOGTAG,RED)
ea 08590-0078-00 69.95
(GOLD FILLED,PREMIER A)
ea 08590-0121-00 69.95
(GOLD FILLED,PREMIER B)
ea 08590-0120-00 69.95
(GOLD FILLED,PREMIER C)
ea 08590-0122-00 69.95
(GOLD-FILLED,CLASSIC)
ea 08590-0055-00 59.95
(GOLDFIL,DOGTAG,EMBOSSED)
ea 08590-0076-00 69.95
(SILVER CLASSIC)
ea 08590-0059-00 49.95
(SILVER,DOGTAG,BLUE)
ea 08590-0080-00 59.95
(SILVER,DOGTAG,EMBOSSED)
ea 08590-0081-00 59.95
(SILVER,DOGTAG,RED)
ea 08590-0079-00 59.95
(SILVER,PREMIER A)
ea 08590-0129-00 59.95
(SILVER,PREMIER B)
ea 08590-0127-00 59.95
(SILVER,PREMIER C)
ea 08590-0128-00 59.95
(STAINLES,CLASIC,SML,HEX)
ea 08590-0066-00 24.95
(STAINLES,CLASSIC,LRG,LH)
ea 08590-0064-00 29.95
(STAINLESS,BLUE,DOG TAG)
ea 08590-0082-00 39.95
(STAINLESS,DOGTAG,EMBOSS)
ea 08590-0084-00 39.95
(STAINLESS,DOGTAG,RED)
ea 08590-0083-00 39.95

NEEDLE-FREE SYRINGES (Antares Pharma)
DEV,NA (MEDI-JECTOR VISION,A)
6s ea 55948-0295-10 31.95 31.95
(MEDI-JECTOR VISION,B)
6s ea 55948-0300-10 31.95 31.95
(MEDI-JECTOR VISION,C)
6s ea 55948-0305-10 31.95 31.95

NEO-SYNEPHRINE (Bayer HealthCare)
SOL,NS (REG. STR.)
0.5%, 15 ml 00024-1351-05 3.05
(EXT. STR.)
1%, 15 ml 00024-1355-05 3.42
SPR,NS (MILD FORMULA,DYE-FREE)
0.25%, 15 ml 00024-1348-03 3.05
(REG. STR.)
0.5%, 15 ml 00024-1353-01 3.05
(EXT. STR.)
1%, 15 ml 00024-1352-02 3.42

(Phys Total Care)
REPACK
SOL,NS (MILD FORMULA,DYE-FREE)
0.25%, 15 ml 54868-1899-00 5.41
SPR,NS, 0.25%, 15 ml 54868-3717-00 4.81

(Southwood)
REPACK
SOL,NS, 0.25%, 15 ml 58016-6225-01 4.99

NEO-SYNEPHRINE 12 HOUR (Bayer HealthCare)
SPR,NS (EXTRA MOISTURIZING)
0.05%, 15 ml 00024-1754-01 3.42
(MAX. STR.)
0.05%, 15 ml 00024-1390-03 3.42

NEOCATE JUNIOR (Nutricia)
PDR,PO (4X400GM,CHOCOLATE)
400 gm 4s 49735-0126-90 146.90
(USE W/MED SUPV)
400 gm 4s 49735-0117-90 146.90

NEOCATE NUTRA (Nutricia)
POW,PO (3X400GM)
400 gm 3s 49735-0029-10 108.00
400 gm 3s 49735-0129-10 99.00

NEOCATE ONE + (Nutricia)
PDR,PO (60GMX15)
60 gm 15s 49735-0110-48 91.00

NEOMYCIN SULFATE (Consolidated Midland)
OIN,TP, 5 mg/gm, 30 gm .. 00223-4139-30 1.95

NEOPHE LNAA (Solace)
POW,PO (1X376.7GM,LEMON)
376.7 gm 57771-0001-44 360.00 600.00
TAB,PO, 550s ea 57771-0001-43 360.00 600.00

NEOPORACIN (Prime Marketing)
OIN,TP, 15 gm 62107-0007-15 4.25
30 gm 62107-0007-03 5.40

NEOSPORIN (Johnson & Johnson)
OIN,TP (ORIGINAL)
14.2 gm 00810-0730-88 3.97
14.2 gm 12547-0237-40 3.97
(W/APPLICATOR)
15 gm 00081-0730-88 3.97
(ORIGINAL)
28.3 gm 00810-0730-87 6.49
30 gm 00081-0730-87 6.49

(Southwood)
REPACK
OIN,TP, 15 gm 58016-3381-01 8.90

NEOSPORIN + PAIN RELIEF (Johnson & Johnson)
CRE,TP (FOR KIDS 2 & UP)
14.2 gm 12547-0407-40 4.42
(MAXIMUM STRENGTH)
14.2 gm 00810-0737-94 4.42
28.3 gm 12547-0237-79 7.14
OIN,TP, 14.2 gm 00810-0746-88 4.42
28.3 gm 00810-0746-87 7.14

NEOSPORIN AF (Johnson & Johnson)
CRE,TP (JOCK ITCH)
2%, 14 gm 12547-0237-73 4.94

NEOSPORIN LIP HEALTH (Johnson & Johnson)
STI,TP (SPF 20)
7.5%-3%, 10 gm 12547-0238-73 3.90

NEOSPORIN LIP HEALTH OVERNIGHT RENEWAL THERAPY (Johnson & Johnson)
OIN,TP, 77.4%, 7.7 gm 12547-0238-71 3.90

NEOSPORIN LIP TREATMENT (Johnson & Johnson)
OIN,TP, 1.5%-1%, 7 gm ... 00810-0731-01 3.42
(1X7GM)
1.5%-1%, 7 gm 12547-0237-53 3.42

NEOSPORIN NEO TO GO (Johnson & Johnson)
OIN,TP (10X0.9GM)
0.9 gm 10s 12547-0237-21 4.42
SPR,TP (140 SPRAYS)
0.13%-1%, 7.7 ml 12547-0237-22 4.42
(1X7:7ML)
0.13%-1%, 7.7 ml 12547-0237-56 4.42
(FOR KIDS 2 & UP)
0.13%-1%, 7.7 ml 12547-0407-43 4.42

NEOSPORIN PLUS MAXIMUM STRENGTH (Johnson & Johnson)
OIN,TP, 30 gm 00081-0746-87 7.14

(A-S Medication)
REPACK
OIN,TP, 30 gm 54569-4773-00 7.14

NEOTUSS (A. G. Marin)
LOZ,MM (GRAPE-MENTHOL)
6 mg, 16s ea 12539-0666-16 2.00

NEOTUSS S/F (A. G. Marin)
LIQ,PO (AF,SF,DYE-FREE)
30 mg/5 ml-200 mg/5 ml,
480 ml 12539-0555-16 39.60

NEPHRO-VITE (Phys Total Care)
REPACK
TAB,PO, 100s ea 54868-3466-00 18.53

NEPHRO-VITE VITAMIN B AND C COMPLEX (Rugby)
TAB,PO, 100s ea 00536-7300-01 16.54

NEPHRONEX (Llorens Pharma Int)
SOL,PO (AF,SF,DYE-FREE)
236 ml 54859-0516-08 16.00

NEPRO (Abbott)
LIQ,PO (SPECIALIZED COMPLETE)
237 ml 24s 70074-0506-32 96.29
(CHERRY)
240 ml 70074-0541-07 4.03
(PECAN)
240 ml 70074-0541-05 4.03
(VANILLA)
240 ml 70074-0506-33 4.03
(RTH,VANILLA)
1000 ml 70074-0570-50 18.14

NEPRO WITH CARB STEADY (Abbott)
LIQ,PO (GLUTEN-FREE)
237 ml 70074-0596-63 4.03
237 ml 70074-0596-67 4.03
273 ml 70074-0596-61 4.03
1000 ml 70074-0596-78 18.14

NESTLE FLAVOR PACKET (Nestle)
PDR,PO (CHOCOLATE DELUXE)
4 gm 24s 00065-9051-95 14.40
(ORANGE CREAM)
4 gm 24s 00065-9052-95 14.40
(VARIETY PACK)
4 gm 24s 00065-9050-95 1.74

NESTLE FLAVOR PACKET EXTRA STRENGTH (Nestle)
PDR,PO (VARIETY PACK)
4 gm 24s 00065-9070-95 14.40

NESTLE FLAVOR PACKET FOR KIDS (Nestle)
PDR,PO (VARIETY PACK)
4 gm 24s 00065-9060-95 1.74

NESTLE GOOD START 2 ESSENTIALS SOY W/IRON (Nestle)
PDR,PO, 396 gm 00065-9293-70 10.26

NESTLE GOOD START 2 ESSENTIALS W/IRON (Nestle)
LIQ,PO (CONCENTRATE)
384 ml 00065-9292-90 2.97
(RTF)
946 ml 00065-9292-80 4.96
PDR,PO, 340 gm 00065-9292-70 7.84

NESTLE GOOD START 2 SUPREME SOY W/IRON (Nestle)
PDR,PO (LACTOSE-FREE)
366 gm 00066-9201-70 11.25

NESTLE GOOD START 2 SUPREME W/IRON (Nestle)
LIQ,PO (CONCENTRATE)
384 ml 00065-9298-90 4.72
(READY-TO-FEED)
946 ml 00065-9298-80 7.22
PDR,PO, 340 gm 00065-9298-70 14.66

NESTLE GOOD START ESSENTIALS W/IRON (Nestle)
PDR,PO, 340 gm 00065-9295-70 7.84

NESTLE GOOD START SUPREME (Nestle)
SOL,PO (48X90ML)
90 ml 48s 50000-0855-30 86.40
5%, 90 ml 48s 50000-0859-10 86.40

NESTLE GOOD START SUPREME DHA & ARA W/IRON (Nestle)
LIQ,PO (CONCENTRATE)
384 ml 00065-9294-90 4.72
(RTF)
946 ml 00065-9294-80 7.22
PDR,PO, 340 gm 00065-9294-70 14.66

NESTLE GOOD START SUPREME FEEDER (Nestle)
DEV,NA (DUAL PURPOSE,LATEX-FREE)
100s ea 50000-0592-85 120.00

NESTLE GOOD START SUPREME NATURAL B CULTURES (Nestle)
PDR,PO, 340 gm 50000-0625-50 15.06
680 gm 50000-0625-70 28.82

NESTLE GOOD START SUPREME NIPPLE (Nestle)
DEV,NA (PREMATURE,LATEX-FREE)
48s ea 50000-0685-81 52.80

NESTLE GOOD START SUPREME SOY DHA & ARA W/IRON (Nestle)
LIQ,PO (CONCENTRATE)
384 ml 00065-9297-90 4.77
(RTF)
946 ml 00065-9297-80 7.30
PDR,PO, 366 gm 00065-9297-70 15.73

NESTLE GOOD START SUPREME W/IRON (Nestle)
LIQ,PO (CONCENTRATE)
384 ml 00065-9290-90 3.88
(RTF)
946 ml 00065-9290-80 5.81
PDR,PO, 340 gm 00065-9290-70 11.08

NESTLE NAN W/IRON (Nestle)
PDR,PO, 340 gm 00065-9299-70 14.66

NETTLE (Botanical Labs.)
CAP,PO, 100s ea 41954-0030-11 4.25 8.50
LIQ,PO, 30 ml 41954-0020-35 4.00 7.99

NEURODEP (Med Prods Panamer)
CAP,PO, 50s ea 00576-0272-50 12.60

PROD/MFR	HRI, UPC,NDC	AWP	SRP
NEUROFOLIC (Med Prods Panamer)			
TAB,SL, 1 mg-0.8 mg-125 mg,			
60s ea	00576-0625-60	11.87	
NEUROPEN (Owen Mumford)			
DEV,NA (NEUROLOGICAL TESTER)			
ea	08470-0100-01	21.56	28.00
NEUROTIPS NEUROLOGICAL TESTERS (Owen Mumford)			
DEV,NA (STERILE,SINGLE USE)			
100s ea	08470-5405-01	6.88	8.00
NEUTRACARE (Oral B Lab)			
GEL,DE (GRAPE)			
0.15%, 60 gm	00041-0240-22	4.30	
60 gm	00041-0241-22	4.30	
NEUTRALON 50 LATEX SURGICAL GLOVES (J&J Medical)			
DEV,NA (BROWN,STER,50 PR,SZ 5.5)			
100s ea	56091-0066-55	143.91	
(BROWN,STER,50 PR,SZ 6.5)			
100s ea	56091-0066-65	143.91	
(BROWN,STER,50 PR,SZ 6)			
100s ea	56091-0066-60	143.91	
(BROWN,STER,50 PR,SZ 7.5)			
100s ea	56091-0066-75	143.91	
(BROWN,STER,50 PR,SZ 7)			
100s ea	56091-0066-70	143.91	
(BROWN,STER,50 PR,SZ 8.5)			
100s ea	56091-0066-85	143.91	
(BROWN,STER,50 PR,SZ 8)			
100s ea	56091-0066-80	143.91	
(BROWN,STER,50 PR,SZ 9)			
100s ea	56091-0066-90	143.91	
NEUTRALON BROWN LATEX SURG GLOVES (J&J Medical)			
DEV,NA (STERILE,50 PR,SZ 5.5)			
100s ea	56091-0053-55	143.91	
(STERILE,50 PR,SZ 6.5)			
100s ea	56091-0053-65	143.91	
(STERILE,50 PR,SZ 6)			
100s ea	56091-0053-60	143.91	
(STERILE,50 PR,SZ 7.5)			
100s ea	56091-0053-75	143.91	
(STERILE,50 PR,SZ 7)			
100s ea	56091-0053-70	143.91	
(STERILE,50 PR,SZ 8.5)			
100s ea	56091-0053-85	143.91	
(STERILE,50 PR,SZ 8)			
100s ea	56091-0053-80	143.91	
(STERILE,50 PR,SZ 9)			
100s ea	56091-0053-90	143.91	
NEUTRALON PF LATEX SURGICAL GLOVES (J&J Medical)			
DEV,NA (BROWN,STER,50 PR,SZ 5.5)			
100s ea	56091-0059-55	287.82	
(BROWN,STER,50 PR,SZ 6.5)			
100s ea	56091-0059-65	287.82	
(BROWN,STER,50 PR,SZ 6)			
100s ea	56091-0059-60	287.82	
(BROWN,STER,50 PR,SZ 7.5)			
100s ea	56091-0059-75	287.82	
(BROWN,STER,50 PR,SZ 7)			
100s ea	56091-0059-70	287.82	
(BROWN,STER,50 PR,SZ 8.5)			
100s ea	56091-0059-85	287.82	
(BROWN,STER,50 PR,SZ 8)			
100s ea	56091-0059-80	287.82	
(BROWN,STER,50 PR,SZ 9)			
100s ea	56091-0059-90	287.82	
NEUTROGENA (Neutrogena)			
LIQ,TP (TUBE)			
120 ml	70501-0013-80	3.90	4.37
240 ml	70501-0011-70	7.39	8.27
(FRAGRANCE-FREE)			
240 ml	70501-0011-80	7.39	8.27
NEUTROGENA ACNE MASK (Neutrogena)			
CRE,TP (TUBE)			
5%, 60 gm	70501-0097-00	5.63	6.92
NEUTROGENA ACNE WASH (Neutrogena)			
LIQ,TP (AF)			
2%, 180 ml	70501-0017-10	5.25	5.88
NEUTROGENA ANTISEPTIC (Neutrogena)			
SOL,TP (AF,FRAGRANCE-FREE)			
240 ml	70501-0511-90	3.88	4.34
NEUTROGENA BABY SKIN FORMULA (Neutrogena)			
SOA,TP (3.5 OZ.)			
ea	70501-0014-10	2.18	2.68
NEUTROGENA BODY (Neutrogena)			
LOT,TP, 255 ml	70501-0617-20	4.49	5.03
960 ml	70501-0017-60	15.00	16.80
OIL,TP, 255 ml	70501-0618-20	8.06	9.03
(FRAGRANCE-FREE)			
255 ml	70501-0618-30	8.06	9.03
480 ml	70501-0018-45	13.13	14.70
NEUTROGENA CLEANSING (Neutrogena)			
LOT,TP (NON-DRYING,SOAP-FREE)			
165 ml	70501-0026-00	6.00	7.38
NEUTROGENA CLEANSING WASH (Neutrogena)			
LIQ,TP, 180 ml	70501-0013-20	6.90	8.49
NEUTROGENA CLEAR PORE (Neutrogena)			
GEL,TP (TUBE,AF)			
2%, 60 gm	70501-0097-30	5.25	5.88
NEUTROGENA DRY SKIN FORMULA (Neutrogena)			
SOA,TP (3.5 OZ.,FRAGRANCE-FREE)			
ea	70501-0014-70	2.31	2.59
(3.5 OZ.)			
ea	70501-0014-50	2.31	2.59
(5.5 OZ.)			
ea	70501-0014-60	3.00	3.36
NEUTROGENA EMULSION NORWEGIAN FORM (Neutrogena)			
CRE,TP (FRAGRANCE-FREE)			
45 gm	70501-0019-80	7.69	8.61
157.5 gm	70501-0012-60	4.69	5.25
(FRAGRANCE-FREE)			
157.5 gm	70501-0012-30	4.69	5.25
315 gm	70501-0012-80	7.69	8.61
NEUTROGENA FOR ACNE PRONE SKIN (Neutrogena)			
SOA,TP, ea	70501-0013-30	2.44	2.73
NEUTROGENA FRESH FOAMING CLEANSER (Neutrogena)			
LIQ,TP (SOAP-FREE)			
201 ml	70501-0028-10	5.36	6.01
NEUTROGENA GLOW SUNLESS TANNING (Neutrogena)			
LOT,TP (SPF 8,FACE&BODY,DEEP)			
6%, 120 ml	86800-0000-27	7.83	8.76
(SPF 8,FACE&BODY,LIGHT)			
6%, 120 ml	86800-0000-13	7.83	8.76
(SPF8,FACE/BOD,MED/DEEP)			
6%, 120 ml	86800-0000-35	7.83	8.76
SPR,TP (BODY,DEEP)			
105 ml	86800-0000-28	7.83	8.76
(BODY,LIGHT)			
105 ml	86800-0000-14	7.83	8.76
(BODY,MEDIUM/DEEP)			
105 ml	86800-0000-36	7.83	8.76
NEUTROGENA HEALTHY SCALP (Neutrogena)			
SHA,TP, 1.8%, 90 ml	70501-0091-20	3.50	4.31
180 ml	70501-0091-10	5.19	5.81
NEUTROGENA HEALTHY SKIN (Neutrogena)			
LOT,TP (FOR FACE,PUMP,SPF 15,SF)			
75 ml	70501-0062-30	10.00	11.20
(FOR FACE,PUMP)			
75 ml	70501-0052-70	10.00	11.20
NEUTROGENA INTENSIFIED DAY MOISTURE (Neutrogena)			
CRE,TP (SPF 15,SF)			
67.5 gm	70501-0055-40	10.39	11.63
NEUTROGENA INTENSIFIED EYE MOISTURE (Neutrogena)			
CRE,TP (TUBE,FRAGRANCE-FREE)			
15 gm	70501-0022-00	7.50	8.40
NEUTROGENA LIGHT NIGHT (Neutrogena)			
CRE,TP (FRAGRANCE-FREE)			
67.5 gm	70501-0055-50	10.39	11.63
NEUTROGENA LIP MOISTURIZER (Neutrogena)			
STI,TP (SPF 15,SF)			
4.5 gm	70501-0042-00	2.48	2.73
NEUTROGENA MOISTURE UNTINTED (Neutrogena)			
LOT,TP (SPF 15,SF)			
120 ml	70501-0056-50	9.38	10.50
NEUTROGENA MOISTURE W/SHEER TINT (Neutrogena)			
LOT,TP (SPF 15,SF)			
120 ml	70501-0056-00	9.38	10.50
NEUTROGENA MOISTURE/SENSITIVE SKIN (Neutrogena)			
LOT,TP (FRAGRANCE-FREE)			
60 ml	70501-0053-00	5.63	6.30
120 ml	70501-0054-00	9.38	10.50
NEUTROGENA NO-STICK SUNSCREEN (Neutrogena)			
LOT,TP (SPF 30,OIL,OIL-FREE)			
120 ml	86800-0000-31	7.50	8.40
NEUTROGENA NORWEGIAN FORMULA HAND (Neutrogena)			
CRE,TP, 60 gm	70501-0012-90	3.71	4.16
(FRAGRANCE-FREE)			
60 gm	70501-0013-00	3.71	4.16
NEUTROGENA OILY SKIN FORMULA (Neutrogena)			
SOA,TP (3.5 OZ.)			
ea	70501-0011-20	2.31	2.59
NEUTROGENA ON-THE-SPOT ACNE (Neutrogena)			
CRE,TP (TINTED)			
2.5%, 22.5 gm	70501-0022-70	5.25	5.88
(VANISHING)			
2.5%, 22.5 gm	70501-0017-90	5.25	5.88
NEUTROGENA ORIGINAL FORMULA (Neutrogena)			
SOA,TP (3.5 OZ.,FRAGRANCE-FREE)			
ea	70501-0013-50	2.31	2.59
(3.5 OZ.)			
ea	70501-0010-10	2.31	2.59
(5.5 OZ.,FRAGRANCE-FREE)			
ea	70501-0012-20	3.00	3.36
(5.5 OZ.)			
ea	70501-0012-10	3.00	3.36
NEUTROGENA RAINBATH (Neutrogena)			
GEL,TP (TUBE,STARTER KIT)			
120 gm	70501-0049-10	3.86	4.75
255 gm	70501-0610-30	6.71	7.52
(FRAGRANCE-FREE)			
255 gm	70501-0611-50	6.71	7.52
480 gm	70501-0611-60	9.38	10.50
960 gm	70501-0011-30	22.50	25.20
NEUTROGENA RAINBATH DRY OIL (Neutrogena)			
SPR,TP, 105 ml	70501-0045-00	6.38	7.14
NEUTROGENA RAINBATH MOISTURIZING (Neutrogena)			
SPR,TP (SF)			
240 ml	70501-0020-30	5.81	6.51
NEUTROGENA SENSITIVE SKIN SUNBLOCK (Neutrogena)			
LOT,TP (SPF 17,FRAGRANCE-FREE)			
120 ml	86800-0000-11	7.50	8.40
NEUTROGENA SUNBLOCK STICK (Neutrogena)			
STI,TP (SPF 25,SF)			
12.6 gm	70501-0097-70	5.48	6.74
NEUTROGENA T/DERM (Neutrogena)			
LIQ,TP (AF)			
1.2%, 120 ml	10812-0950-04	8.44	
NEUTROGENA T/GEL (Neutrogena)			
LIQ,TP (CONDITIONER)			
1.2%, 132 ml	70501-0092-70	4.69	5.25
SHA,TP, 2%, 132 ml	70501-0092-00	4.69	5.25
255 ml	70501-0092-20	7.44	8.33
480 ml	10812-0920-11	12.19	13.65
(Phys Total Care) REPACK			
SHA,TP, 2%, 150 ml	54868-3631-00	5.75	
NEUTROGENA T/GEL EXTRA STRENGTH (Neutrogena)			
SHA,TP, 1%, 180 ml	70501-0094-50	7.44	8.33
360 ml	70501-0094-80	12.19	13.65
NEUTROGENA T/SAL MAXIMUM STRENGTH (Neutrogena)			
LIQ,TP, 3%, 135 ml	70501-0096-50	5.63	6.30
NEUTROGENA T/SCALP (Neutrogena)			
LIQ,TP, 1%, 60 ml	70501-0964-00	6.30	7.75
NEUTROGENA TONER (Neutrogena)			
SOL,TP (AF)			
240 ml	70501-0027-00	6.00	6.72
NEW IMAGE FLEXTEND SKIN BARRIER (Hollister)			
DEV,NA (FLNGE&TPE,1-3/4",1-1/4")			
5s ea	08380-0147-06	31.18	35.52
(FLNGE&TPE,1-3/4",1-1/8")			
5s ea	08380-0147-05	31.18	35.52
(FLNGE&TPE,2-1/4",1-1/2")			
5s ea	08380-0147-08	31.18	35.52
(FLNGE&TPE,2-1/4",1-3/8")			
5s ea	08380-0147-07	31.18	35.52
(W/FLANGE,1-3/4",1-1/4")			
5s ea	08380-0161-06	31.18	35.52
(W/FLANGE,1-3/4",1-1/8")			
5s ea	08380-0161-05	31.18	35.52
(W/FLANGE,1-3/4",3/4")			
5s ea	08380-0161-02	31.18	35.52
(W/FLANGE,1-3/4",5/8")			
5s ea	08380-0161-01	31.18	35.52
(W/FLANGE,1-3/4",7/8")			
5s ea	08380-0161-03	31.18	35.52

PROD/MFR	HRI, UPC,NDC	AWP	SRP
(W/FLANGE,2-1/4",1-1/2")			
5s ea	08380-0161-08	31.18	35.52
(W/FLANGE,2-1/4",1-3/8")			
5s ea	08380-0161-07	31.18	35.52
(W/FLANGE&TAPE,1-3/4",1")			
5s ea	08380-0147-04	31.18	35.52
(W/FLNGE&TPE,1-3/4",3/4")			
5s ea	08380-0147-02	31.18	35.52
(W/FLNGE&TPE,1-3/4",5/8")			
5s ea	08380-0147-01	31.18	35.52
(W/FLNGE&TPE,1-3/4",7/8")			
5s ea	08380-0147-03	31.18	35.52
(W/FLTNG FLNGE,1-3/4",1")			
5s ea	08380-0161-04	31.18	35.52
NEW IMAGE FLEXWEAR SKIN BARRIER (Hollister)			
DEV,NA (FLNGE&TPE,1-3/4",1-1/4")			
5s ea	08380-0143-06	25.79	29.38
(FLNGE&TPE,1-3/4",1-1/8")			
5s ea	08380-0143-05	25.79	29.38
(FLNGE&TPE,2-1/4",1-1/2")			
5s ea	08380-0143-08	25.79	29.38
(FLNGE&TPE,2-1/4",1-3/8")			
5s ea	08380-0143-07	25.79	29.38
(W/ FLTNG FLNG 1-3/4",1")			
5s ea	08380-0164-04	25.79	29.38
(W/FLANGE 1-3/4",1-1/4")			
5s ea	08380-0164-06	25.79	29.38
(W/FLANGE 1-3/4",1-1/8")			
5s ea	08380-0164-05	25.79	29.38
(W/FLANGE 1-3/4",3/4")			
5s ea	08380-0164-02	25.79	29.38
(W/FLANGE 1-3/4",5/8")			
5s ea	08380-0164-01	25.79	29.38
(W/FLANGE 1-3/4",7/8")			
5s ea	08380-0164-03	25.79	29.38
(W/FLANGE 2-1/4",1-1/2")			
5s ea	08380-0164-08	25.79	29.38
(W/FLANGE 2-1/4",1-3/8")			
5s ea	08380-0164-07	25.79	29.38
(W/FLANGE&TAPE,1-3/4",1")			
5s ea	08380-0143-04	25.79	29.38
(W/FLNGE&TPE,1-3/4",3/4")			
5s ea	08380-0143-02	25.79	29.38
(W/FLNGE&TPE,1-3/4",5/8")			
5s ea	08380-0143-01	25.79	29.38
(W/FLNGE&TPE,1-3/4",7/8")			
5s ea	08380-0143-03	25.79	29.38
NEW LIFE HAIR (Rexall)			
TAB,PO (PF,SF)			
50s ea	30768-0000-65	3.59	5.43
NEW-SKIN (Medtech)			
LIQ,TP, 3.6 ml	75137-0070-40	2.65	2.98
9 ml	75137-0703-35	2.29	2.98
30 ml	75137-0703-31	3.29	3.98
SPR,TP, 30 ml	75137-0704-01	3.29	4.29
NEXCARE ABSOLUTE WATERPROOF (3M Consumer)			
DEV,NA (1"X5 YDS)			
ea	51131-0667-75	2.98	
NEXCARE ACTIVE FLEXIBLE FOAM BRIGHT (3M Health Care)			
DEV,NA (3/4"X3" STRIPS)			
30s ea	08333-0554-30	2.52	
(ASSORTED STRIPS)			
30s ea	08333-0556-30	2.52	
(3/4"X3" STRIPS)			
100s ea	08333-1703-00	6.20	
NEXCARE ACTIVE FLEXIBLE FOAM STRIPS (3M Health Care)			
DEV,NA (1 7/8"X4")			
10s ea	08333-0510-10	2.52	
(1"X3")			
30s ea	08333-0512-30	2.52	
(3/4"X3")			
38s ea	08333-0514-38	2.52	
(ASSORTED)			
45s ea	08333-0516-45	2.52	
(7/8" SPOTS)			
60s ea	08333-0518-60	2.52	
(1"X3")			
100s ea	08333-1702-10	6.44	
(3/4"X3")			
100s ea	08333-1702-00	5.64	
(7/8" SPOTS)			
100s ea	08333-1702-20	6.22	
NEXCARE ACTIVE STRIPS (3M Consumer)			
DEV,NA (KNEE/ELBOW)			
10s ea	51131-0620-34	2.47	
(1"X3")			
30s ea	51131-0620-36	2.47	
(3/4"X3")			
35s ea	55131-0835-33	2.59	
(ASSORTED)			
45s ea	51131-0620-30	2.47	
(SPOTS)			
60s ea	51131-0640-68	2.47	
NEXCARE ACTIVE STRIPS BRIGHTS (3M Consumer)			
DEV,NA (3/4"X3")			
30s ea	51131-0641-06	2.47	
(ASSORTED)			
30s ea	51131-0641-07	2.47	
NEXCARE ADVANCED HOLDING POWER (3M Consumer)			
DEV,NA (1"X6 YDS)			
ea	51131-0667-77	2.98	
NEXCARE ALL PURPOSE MASK (3M Consumer)			
DEV,NA, 5s ea	51131-0015-94	4.14	
NEXCARE ANTIBACTERIAL COMFORT STRIP (3M Consumer)			
DEV,NA (ASSORTED)			
30s ea	51131-0668-01	2.47	
NEXCARE ATHLETIC (3M Consumer)			
DEV,NA (1-1/2"X12.5 YDS)			
ea	51131-0620-98	2.77	
NEXCARE ATHLETIC CLOTH (3M Health Care)			
DEV,NA (1 1/2"X12 1/2 YDS)			
12s ea	08333-0870-00	34.18	
NEXCARE ATHLETIC WRAP (3M Consumer)			
DEV,NA (3"X5 YDS, BLACK)			
ea	51131-0598-50	4.03	
(3"X5 YDS, BLUE)			
ea	51131-0566-51	4.03	
(3"X5 YDS, RED)			
ea	51131-0566-52	4.03	
(3"X5 YDS, WHITE)			
ea	51131-0567-86	4.03	
(3"X5 YDS,TAN)			
ea	51131-0666-86	3.78	
(3M Health Care)			
DEV,NA (3"X5 YDS,BLACK)			
ea	08333-3183-70	4.01	
(3"X5 YDS,BLUE)			
ea	08333-3183-20	4.01	
(3"X5 YDS,RED)			
ea	08333-3183-30	4.01	
(3"X5 YDS,WHITE)			
ea	08333-3183-60	4.01	
NEXCARE BLENDERM WATERPROOF (3M Health Care)			
DEV,NA (1"X7 1/2 YDS+DISPENSER)			
ea	08333-0007-01	2.92	
(1/2"X7 1/2 YD+DISPENSER)			
ea	08333-0007-00	1.71	
NEXCARE CARDED DURABLE CLOTH (3M Consumer)			
DEV,NA (1"X10 YDS)			
2s ea	51131-0913-89	2.28	
NEXCARE CARDED FLEXIBLE CLEAR (3M Consumer)			
DEV,NA (1"X10 YDS)			
2s ea	51131-0913-82	2.28	
NEXCARE CARDED GENTLE PAPER (3M Consumer)			
DEV,NA (1"X10 YDS)			
2s ea	51131-0913-86	2.28	
NEXCARE COBAN SELF-ADHERENT WRAP (3M Consumer)			
DEV,NA (2"X5 YDS, TAN)			
ea	51131-0641-35	2.46	
(3"X5 YDS, TAN)			
ea	51131-0641-19	3.11	
(1"X5 YDS, TAN)			
5s ea	51131-0641-20	5.80	
(3M Health Care)			
DEV,NA (2"X5 YDS,TAN)			
ea	08333-1582-09	2.32	
(3"X5 YDS,TAN)			
ea	08333-1583-09	2.93	
(1"X5 YDS,TAN)			
5s ea	08333-1581-09	5.48	
NEXCARE COLD PACK (3M Consumer)			
DEV,NA (INSTANT AND REUSABLE)			
ea	51131-0083-11	5.32	
(INSTANT)			
ea	51131-0082-95	1.62	
(REUSABLE)			
ea	51131-0184-13	4.51	
NEXCARE COLD/HOT PACK (3M Consumer)			
DEV,NA (REUSABLE)			
ea	51131-0666-88	5.32	
NEXCARE COMFORT STRIPS (3M Consumer)			
DEV,NA (KNEE/ELBOW)			
10s ea	51131-0652-88	2.47	
(1"X3")			
30s ea	51131-0652-86	2.47	
(3/4"X3")			
35s ea	51131-0835-37	2.59	
(ASSORTED)			
50s ea	51131-0652-89	2.47	
(3M Health Care)			
DEV,NA (1"X3")			
100s ea	08333-1704-10	6.44	
(3/4"X3")			
100s ea	08333-1704-00	5.64	
NEXCARE DURAPORE CLOTH (3M Health Care)			
DEV,NA (1"X7 1/2 YDS+DISPENSER)			
12s ea	08333-2611-01	34.99	
(1/2"X7 1/2 YD+DISPENSER)			
12s ea	08333-2610-00	20.57	
NEXCARE DURAPORE DURABLE CLOTH (3M Health Care)			
DEV,NA (1"X10 YDS,CARDED)			
12s ea	08333-0791-01	26.73	
NEXCARE DURAPORE WRAPPED CLOTH (3M Health Care)			
DEV,NA (1"X10 YDS,PHARMACY PACK)			
ea	08333-0538-01	2.24	
(2"X10 YDS,PHARMACY PACK)			
ea	08333-0538-02	4.16	
NEXCARE HOLDFAST ROLL (3M Consumer)			
DEV,NA (2"X4.1 YDS)			
ea	51131-0667-70	2.11	
(3"X4.1 YDS)			
ea	51131-0667-71	2.84	
NEXCARE MICROPORE GENTLE PAPER (3M Health Care)			
DEV,NA (1"X10 YDS,CARDED)			
12s ea	08333-0781-01	26.73	
(1/2"X10 YDS,CARDED)			
12s ea	08333-0785-00	16.36	
(2"X10 YDS,CARDED)			
12s ea	08333-0782-02	43.58	
NEXCARE MICROPORE PAPER (3M Health Care)			
DEV,NA (1"X7 1/2 YDS+DISPENSER)			
ea	08333-0008-01	2.92	
(1/2"X7 1/2 YD+DISPENSER)			
ea	08333-0008-00	1.71	
NEXCARE MICROPORE WRAPPED PAPER (3M Health Care)			
DEV,NA (1"X10 YDS,PHARMACY PACK)			
ea	08333-0530-01	2.24	
(1/2"X10 YDS,PHARM PACK)			
ea	08333-0530-00	1.33	
(2"X10 YDS,PHARMACY PACK)			
ea	08333-0530-02	4.16	
NEXCARE NON-STICK (3M Consumer)			
DEV,NA (2"X3")			
12s ea	51131-0605-92	1.73	
(3"X4")			
12s ea	51131-0641-34	2.68	
(3M Health Care)			
DEV,NA (2"X3")			
12s ea	08333-0412-01	1.81	
(3"X4")			
12s ea	08333-0413-01	2.79	
NEXCARE OPTICLUDE ORTHOPTIC PATCH (3M Consumer)			
DEV,NA (JUNIOR)			
20s ea	51131-0000-22	4.67	
(REGULAR)			
20s ea	51131-0000-23	4.67	
NEXCARE STERI-STRIP SKIN CLOSURE (3M Consumer)			
DEV,NA (1/2"X4")			
18s ea	51131-0641-24	6.32	
(1/4"X4")			
30s ea	51131-0641-25	6.32	
(3M Health Care)			
DEV,NA (1/2"X4")			
18s ea	08333-1547-09	5.86	
(1/4"X4")			
30s ea	08333-1546-09	5.86	
NEXCARE STOMASEAL COLOSTOMY (3M Consumer)			
DEV,NA (4"X4")			
30s ea	51119-0000-25	7.67	

PROD/MFR	HRI, UPC,NDC	AWP	SRP
(3M Health Care)			
DEV,NA (4"X4")			
30s ea	08333-1507-01	7.70	
NEXCARE TATTOO WATERPROOF (3M Consumer)			
DEV,NA (ASSORTED,COOL)			
20s ea	51131-0669-90	2.59	
NEXCARE TATTOO WATERPROOF STRIPS (3M Health Care)			
DEV,NA (1 3/4"X2 3/4" COOL)			
50s ea	08333-1706-20	19.00	
(1 1/16"X2 1/4" WILDLIFE)			
100s ea	08333-1706-10	19.25	
NEXCARE TEGADERM TRANSPARENT (3M Consumer)			
DEV,NA (4"X4-3/4")			
4s ea	51131-0641-13	8.93	
(2-3/8"X2-3/4")			
8s ea	51131-0641-14	5.51	
NEXCARE TEGADERM TRANSPARENT FRAME (3M Health Care)			
DEV,NA (4"X4-3/4")			
4s ea	08333-1626-09	8.28	
(2-3/8"X2-3/4")			
8s ea	08333-1624-09	5.10	
NEXCARE TRANSPORE CLEAR (3M Health Care)			
DEV,NA (1"X10 YDS,PHARMACY PAK)			
ea	08333-0527-01	2.24	
(1"X7 1/2 YDS+DISPENSER)			
ea	08333-0006-01	2.92	
(1/2"X7 1/2 YD+DISPENSER)			
ea	08333-0006-00	1.71	
(2"X10 YDS,PHARMACY PAK)			
ea	08333-0527-02	4.16	
NEXCARE TRANSPORE FLEXIBLE CLEAR (3M Health Care)			
DEV,NA (1"X10 YDS,CARDED)			
12s ea	08333-0771-01	26.73	
NEXCARE TRIPLE LAYER PADS (3M Consumer)			
DEV,NA (2"X2")			
10s ea	51131-0667-72	1.66	
(3"X3")			
10s ea	51131-0667-73	2.24	
(4"X4")			
10s ea	51131-0667-74	3.43	
NEXCARE WATERPROOF (3M Consumer)			
DEV,NA (KNEE/ELBOW)			
10s ea	51131-0664-24	3.40	
(1"X2 1/4")			
20s ea	51131-0664-26	2.47	
(ASSORTED)			
30s ea	51131-0664-27	2.47	
NEXCARE WATERPROOF ADHESIVE (3M Health Care)			
DEV,NA (1"X12 1/2 YDS)			
12s ea	08333-0861-00	41.63	
(1"X7 1/2 YDS)			
12s ea	08333-0851-00	26.57	
(1/2"X12 1/2 YDS)			
12s ea	08333-0860-00	26.57	
(1/2"X7 1/2 YDS)			
12s ea	08333-0850-00	16.04	
NEXCARE WRAPPED DURAPORE CLOTH (3M Consumer)			
DEV,NA (1"X10 YDS)			
ea	51131-0000-20	2.23	
(2"X10 YDS)			
ea	51131-0000-21	4.14	
NEXCARE WRAPPED MICROPORE PAPER (3M Consumer)			
DEV,NA (1"X10 YDS)			
ea	51131-0000-15	2.23	
(1/2"X10 YDS)			
ea	51131-0000-14	1.33	
(2"X10 YDS)			
ea	51131-0000-16	4.14	
NEXCARE WRAPPED TRANSPORE CLEAR (3M Consumer)			
DEV,NA (1"X10 YDS)			
ea	51131-0566-60	2.23	
(2"X10 YDS)			
ea	51131-0566-61	4.14	
NIA-CHROM (Miller)			
TAB,PO, 200 mcg,			
100s ea	17204-0886-40	3.78	
NIACIN (ADH)			
TAB,PO (PF,SF)			
100 mg, 100s ea	60142-0194-01	2.25	4.50
100s ea	60142-0195-01	2.48	4.95
(Albertson's)			
TAB,PO, 50 mg, 100s ea	04000-0001-17	1.71	
100 mg, 100s ea	04000-0001-18	1.92	
100s ea	04000-0002-18	3.75	
(Basic Vitamins)			
CER,PO, 250 mg, 100s ea	00761-0677-20	3.00	
500 mg, 90s ea	00761-0049-20	3.60	
TAB,PO, 100 mg, 100s ea	00761-0239-20	1.60	
(Cardinal Health)			
TAB,PO (PRIVATE LABEL)			
100 mg, 100s ea	37205-0078-78	2.83	
(Carlson,J.R.)			
TAB,PO, 50 mg, 100s ea	88395-0027-60	1.95	3.90
(VEGETARIAN,PF,SF)			
50 mg, 300s ea	88395-0027-63	4.70	9.40
100 mg, 100s ea	88395-0027-71	2.60	5.20
(VEGETARIAN,PF,SF)			
100 mg, 300s ea	88395-0027-73	5.60	11.20
(PF,SF,CORN-FREE)			
500 mg, 100s ea	88395-0027-81	4.45	8.90
250s ea	88395-0027-82	9.10	18.20
(Contract Pharmacal)			
TAB,PO, 500 mg, 100s ea	10267-0053-01	9.80	
(Freeda)			
TAB,PO (PF,SF,DYE-FREE)			
50 mg, 100s ea	10432-0133-01	3.27	5.45
100 mg, 100s ea	10432-0038-01	3.90	6.50
500 mg, 100s ea	10432-0302-01	6.27	10.45
TER,PO, 250 mg, 100s ea	10432-0286-01	5.67	9.45
250s ea	10432-0286-02	11.34	18.90
(Health Products Corp)			
TAB,PO (PF,SF)			
500 mg, 100s ea	39686-0014-23	4.00	
(Major)			
CER,PO, 250 mg, 100s ea	00904-0629-60	6.21	
500 mg, 100s ea	00904-0631-60	7.80	
TAB,PO (PF,SF,LACTOSE-FREE)			
37 mg-500 mg-29 mg,			
100s ea	00904-2272-60	4.30	
50 mg, 100s ea	00904-2270-60	2.78	
64 mg-500 mg,			
1000s ea	00904-2272-80	27.35	
100 mg, 100s ea	00904-2271-60	2.40	
(Marlex)			
TAB,PO, 50 mg, 100s ea	10135-0192-01	0.86	
1000s ea	10135-0192-10	4.95	
100 mg, 100s ea	10135-0186-01	0.96	
1000s ea	10135-0186-10	7.54	
500 mg, 60s ea	10135-0191-60	1.76	
90s ea	10135-0191-90	2.00	
100s ea	10135-0191-01	2.01	
270s ea	10135-0191-68	5.00	
1000s ea	10135-0191-10	13.70	
(Mason Vit)			
CER,PO (PF)			
250 mg, 60s ea	11845-0088-25	5.44	
TAB,PO, 100 mg, 100s ea	11845-0057-81	4.11	
500 mg, 60s ea	11845-0107-55	7.44	
100s ea	11845-0074-21	6.78	
TER,PO (PF,SF)			
500 mg, 60s ea	11845-0094-15	7.00	
(Nature's Bounty)			
CAP,PO (FLUSH FREE,PF,SF)			
500 mg, 50s ea	74312-0016-60		10.99
CER,PO (PF)			
250 mg, 90s ea	74312-0058-00		7.35
TAB,PO (PF,SF)			
100 mg, 100s ea	74312-0014-80		3.45
250s ea	74312-0014-83		6.89
250 mg, 100s ea	74312-0007-20		4.69
(Pharmavite)			
TAB,PO, 100 mg, 100s ea	31604-0013-22	1.93	
(Qualitest)			
CER,PO, 250 mg, 100s ea	00603-4736-21	9.84	
1000s ea	00603-4736-32	67.11	
(Rexall)			
TER,PO (TIMED RELEASE,PF,SF)			
500 mg, 50s ea	30768-0000-61	2.95	4.47
(Rugby)			
CER,PO, 250 mg, 100s ea	00536-4074-01	8.42	
(PF)			
500 mg, 100s ea	00536-4077-01	11.21	
TAB,PO (PF,DYE-FREE)			
50 mg, 100s ea	00536-4070-01	2.10	
(PF,SF,DYE-FREE)			
100 mg, 100s ea	00536-4076-01	2.55	
1000s ea	00536-4076-10	7.51	
(PF,DYE-FREE)			
500 mg, 1000s ea	00536-4078-10	18.02	
TER,PO, 500 mg, 100s ea	00536-7030-01	6.30	
750 mg, 100s ea	00536-7033-01	7.42	
(PF,DYE-FREE,CAPTAB)			
1000 mg, 100s ea	00536-7038-01	8.25	
(Teva)			
CER,PO, 250 mg, 100s ea	00182-0811-01	6.39	
500 mg, 100s ea	00182-4418-01	8.49	
1000s ea	00182-4418-10	62.99	
TER,PO (CAPLET)			
500 mg, 100s ea	00182-4417-01	5.59	
(Time-Cap)			
CER,PO, 250 mg, 100s ea	49483-0014-01	9.20	
1000s ea	49483-0014-10	68.95	
500 mg, 100s ea	49483-0018-01	12.16	
(PD-Rx Pharm)			
REPACK			
TAB,PO, 500 mg, 100s ea	55289-0620-01	18.68	
(Phys Total Care)			
REPACK			
CER,PO, 125 mg, 100s ea	54868-5184-00	13.89	
250 mg, 100s ea	54868-1881-01	18.24	
500 mg, 100s ea	54868-1880-01	12.60	
TAB,PO, 100 mg, 100s ea	54868-2164-00	5.93	
1000s ea	54868-2164-01	30.58	
(Quality Care Prod)			
REPACK			
TER,PO (PF,DYE-FREE,CAPTAB)			
1000 mg, 30s ea	49999-0741-30	8.06	
NIACIN TIME RELEASE (Major)			
TER,PO (CAPLET)			
500 mg, 100s ea	00904-4342-60	5.90	
250s ea	00904-4342-70	14.39	
NIACIN-TIME (Carlson,J.R.)			
TER,PO, 500 mg, 100s ea	88395-0027-91	6.20	12.40
250s ea	88395-0027-92	11.95	23.90
500s ea	88395-0027-95	22.60	45.20
NIACINAMIDE (ADH)			
TAB,PO (PF,SF)			
500 mg, 1000s ea	60142-0203-01	2.98	5.95
(Bio-Tech Pharm)			
CAP,PO, 500 mg, 100s ea	53191-0478-01	4.90	
(Carlson,J.R.)			
TAB,PO (PF,SF,CORN-FREE)			
500 mg, 100s ea	88395-0027-51	3.45	6.90
250s ea	88395-0027-52	7.48	14.95
(Consolidated Midland)			
TAB,PO, 50 mg, 100s ea	00223-1341-01	1.75	
1000s ea	00223-1341-02	8.50	
100 mg, 100s ea	00223-1342-01	2.10	
1000s ea	00223-1342-02	9.50	
(Freeda)			
TAB,PO (PF,SF,DYE-FREE)			
100 mg, 100s ea	10432-0039-01	3.24	5.40
(PF,SF)			
250 mg, 100s ea	10432-0322-01	4.47	7.45
250s ea	10432-0322-02	8.94	14.90
500s ea	10432-0322-03	15.30	25.50
(PF,SF,DYE-FREE)			
500 mg, 100s ea	10432-0134-01	5.37	8.95
250s ea	10432-0134-02	10.74	17.90
(Major)			
TAB,PO, 500 mg, 100s ea	00904-4202-60	4.37	
(Marlex)			
TAB,PO, 500 mg, 100s ea	10135-0193-01	2.01	
1000s ea	10135-0193-10	19.58	
(Mason Vit)			
TAB,PO, 500 mg, 100s ea	11845-0058-01	5.89	
(Nature's Bounty)			
TAB,PO (PF,SF)			
500 mg, 100s ea	74312-0007-30		5.09
(Rugby)			
TAB,PO, 100 mg, 100s ea	00536-4068-01	2.40	
500 mg, 100s ea	00536-4069-01	3.24	
(Rx Vitamins)			
TAB,PO (PF,SF)			
500 mg, 90s ea	08429-0031-01	3.98	10.95
NICODERM CQ (Glaxo)			
TDM,TD (STEP2)			
14 mg/24 hr,			
28s ea	07661-0430-54	62.78	
21 mg/24 hr, 7s ea	00135-0145-01	28.57	
7s ea	00766-1450-10	27.22	
14s ea	00766-1450-20	46.90	

PROD/MFR	HRI, UPC,NDC	AWP	SRP
21s ea	07661-0470-20	59.80	
(STEP1)			
21 mg/24 hr,			
28s ea	07661-0470-24	62.78	
(A-S Medication)			
REPACK			
TDM,TD, 7 mg/24 hr,			
14s ea	54569-5658-00	46.90	
14 mg/24 hr,			
14s ea	54569-4835-01	47.41	
21 mg/24 hr,			
14s ea	54569-4389-01	46.90	
(Phys Total Care)			
REPACK			
TDM,TD, 7 mg/24 hr,			
14s ea	54868-4978-00	56.75	
NICODERM CQ CLEAR (Glaxo)			
TDM,TD, 7 mg/24 hr,			
14s ea	00135-0196-02	49.24	
14 mg/24 hr,			
14s ea	00135-0195-02	49.24	
21 mg/24 hr, 7s ea	07661-0420-50	27.22	
14s ea	00766-1420-20	46.90	
NICOMIDE-T (Sirius Labs)			
CRE,TP, 4%, 30 gm	65880-0406-30	34.33	
NICORELIEF (Major)			
GUM,PO (MINT)			
2 mg, 50s ea	00904-5736-51	29.49	
(ORIGINAL)			
2 mg, 50s ea	00904-5734-51	29.49	
(MINT,MINT)			
2 mg, 110s ea	00904-5736-11	56.99	
(ORIGINAL)			
2 mg, 110s ea	00904-5734-11	56.99	
(MINT,MINT)			
4 mg, 50s ea	00904-5737-51	29.49	
(ORIGINAL,ORIGINAL)			
4 mg, 50s ea	00904-5735-51	29.49	
(MINT,MINT)			
4 mg, 110s ea	00904-5737-11	56.99	
(ORIGINAL,ORIGINAL)			
4 mg, 110s ea	00904-5735-11	56.99	
NICORETTE (Glaxo)			
GUM,PO (FRESH MINT)			
2 mg, 40s ea	07667-0847-20	29.24	
(FRUIT CHILL,COATED)			
2 mg, 40s ea	07667-0857-30	29.24	
(REFILL KIT,MINT)			
2 mg, 50s ea	07667-0843-30	27.22	
(REFILL KIT,ORANGE)			
2 mg, 50s ea	07667-0845-48	27.22	
(CINNAMON SURGE,COATED)			
2 mg, 100s ea	07667-0858-40	49.43	
(FRESH MINT)			
2 mg, 100s ea	07667-0847-30	49.43	
(FRUIT CHILL,COATED)			
2 mg, 100s ea	07667-0857-50	49.43	
(MINT)			
2 mg, 110s ea	07667-0843-20	46.90	
(STARTER KIT,ORANGE)			
2 mg, 110s ea	07667-0843-50	46.90	
(STARTER KIT,ORIGINAL)			
2 mg, 110s ea	07667-0845-08	46.90	
(MINT)			
2 mg, 170s ea	07667-0843-40	61.99	
(ORIGINAL)			
2 mg, 170s ea	07667-0845-60	61.99	
(FRESH MINT,COATED)			
2 mg, 210s ea	07667-0849-57	70.20	
(FRUIT CHILL,COATED)			
2 mg, 210s ea	07667-0867-55	70.20	
(ORIGINAL)			
2 mg, 220s ea	07662-0862-14	63.77	
(FRESH MINT)			
4 mg, 40s ea	07667-0847-40	29.24	
(FRUIT CHILL,COATED)			
4 mg, 40s ea	07667-0857-40	29.24	
(REFILL KIT,MINT)			
4 mg, 50s ea	07667-0844-30	30.62	
(REFILL PACK,ORIGINAL)			
4 mg, 50s ea	07667-0847-48	30.62	
(CINNAMON SURGE,COATED)			
4 mg, 100s ea	07667-0858-70	49.43	
(FRESH MINT)			
4 mg, 100s ea	07667-0847-50	49.43	
(FRUIT CHILL,COATED)			
4 mg, 100s ea	07667-0857-60	49.43	
(STARTER KIT,MINT)			
4 mg, 110s ea	07667-0844-20	52.76	
(STARTER KIT,ORANGE)			
4 mg, 110s ea	07667-0844-50	52.76	
(STARTER KIT,ORIGINAL)			
4 mg, 110s ea	07667-0847-08	52.76	
(MINT)			
4 mg, 170s ea	07667-0844-40	69.76	
(ORIGINAL)			
4 mg, 170s ea	07667-0847-60	69.76	
(FRESH MINT,COATED)			
4 mg, 210s ea	07667-0849-61	70.20	
(FRUIT CHILL,COATED)			
4 mg, 210s ea	07667-0867-65	70.20	
(ORIGINAL)			
4 mg, 220s ea	07662-0862-24	71.74	
(A-S Medication)			
REPACK			
GUM,PO (MINT,ORANGE)			
2 mg, 110s ea	54569-5700-00	46.90	
(MINT)			
4 mg, 110s ea	54569-6150-00	49.43	
NICOTINE (Phys Total Care)			
REPACK			
TDM,TD, 7 mg/24 hr,			
7s ea	54868-5819-00	67.38	
14 mg/24 hr, 7s ea	54868-5820-00	67.38	
21 mg/24 hr, 7s ea	54868-5821-00	67.38	
NICOTINE POLACRILEX (Rugby)			
GUM,PO (ORIGINAL,USP,SF)			
2 mg, 20s ea	00536-3029-34	10.79	
(USP, MINT,SF,MINT)			
2 mg, 20s ea	00536-1362-34	11.99	
(USP,SF,CINNAMON,COATED)			
2 mg, 40s ea	00536-3404-37	21.06	
(USP,SF,COATED)			
2 mg, 40s ea	00536-3112-37	21.06	
(USP,SF,FRUIT,COATED)			
2 mg, 40s ea	00536-3386-37	21.06	
(ORIGINAL,USP,SF)			
2 mg, 50s ea	00536-3029-06	19.22	
(REFILL, U.S.P., MINT)			
2 mg, 50s ea	00536-1362-06	21.36	
(USP,SF,CINNAMON,COATED)			
2 mg, 100s ea	00536-3404-01	35.56	
(USP,SF,COATED)			
2 mg, 100s ea	00536-3112-01	35.56	
(USP,SF,FRUIT,COATED)			
2 mg, 100s ea	00536-3386-01	35.56	
110s ea	00536-3106-23	30.98	
(STARTER KIT, USP, MINT)			
2 mg, 110s ea	00536-1362-23	30.98	
(USP, MINT,SF,MINT)			
4 mg, 20s ea	00536-1372-34	13.32	
(USP,SF,CINNAMON,COATED)			
4 mg, 40s ea	00536-3405-37	22.16	
(USP,SF,COATED)			
4 mg, 40s ea	00536-3113-37	22.16	
(USP,SF,FRUIT,COATED)			
4 mg, 40s ea	00536-3387-37	22.16	
(ORIGINAL,SF)			
4 mg, 50s ea	00536-3030-06	23.23	
(REFILL, U.S.P., MINT)			
4 mg, 50s ea	00536-1372-06	25.81	
(USP,SF,CINNAMON,COATED)			
4 mg, 100s ea	00536-3405-01	37.43	
(USP,SF,COATED)			
4 mg, 100s ea	00536-3113-01	37.43	
(USP,SF,FRUIT,COATED)			
4 mg, 100s ea	00536-3387-01	37.43	
110s ea	00536-3107-23	41.96	
(STARTER KIT, USP, MINT)			
4 mg, 110s ea	00536-1372-23	41.96	
(A-S Medication)			
REPACK			
GUM,PO (MINT)			
2 mg, 110s ea	54569-6151-00	34.99	
4 mg, 110s ea	54569-6161-00	40.59	
LOZ,PO, 2 mg, 72s ea	54569-6162-00	33.59	
4 mg, 72s ea	54569-6163-00	33.59	
NICOTINE TRANSDERMAL SYSTEM (Novartis Consumer)			
NICOTINE TRANSDERMAL SYSTEM			
TDM,TD, 56s ea	00067-6045-56	102.35	
7 mg/24 hr, 7s ea	00067-5124-07	17.63	
14s ea	00067-5124-14	29.87	
14 mg/24 hr, 7s ea	00067-5125-07	17.63	
14s ea	00067-5125-14	29.87	
21 mg/24 hr, 7s ea	00067-5126-07	17.63	
14s ea	00067-5126-14	29.87	
(Rugby)			
TDM,TD (STEP THREE)			
7 mg/24 hr, 14s ea	00536-5894-88	28.79	
(STEP TWO)			
14 mg/24 hr, 14s ea	00536-5895-88	28.79	
(STEP ONE)			
21 mg/24 hr, 14s ea	00536-5896-88	28.79	
(A-S Medication)			
REPACK			
TDM,TD, 7 mg/24 hr,			
14s ea	54569-6154-00	31.35	
14 mg/24 hr,			
14s ea	54569-6155-00	32.22	
21 mg/24 hr,			
14s ea	54569-6156-00	31.70	
NICOTINIC ACID (Consolidated Midland)			
TAB,PO, 50 mg, 100s ea	00223-1351-01	1.75	
1000s ea	00223-1351-02	8.75	
100 mg, 100s ea	00223-1352-01	2.25	
1000s ea	00223-1352-02	10.75	
TER,PO, 500 mg, 100s ea	00223-1353-01	5.75	
1000s ea	00223-1353-02	37.95	
NICOTROL (Pharmacia Consumer)			
TDM,TD (CHECKPOINT REFILL)			
15 mg/16 hr, 7s ea	00045-0602-08	24.71	
(CHECKPOINT)			
15 mg/16 hr, 7s ea	00045-0602-02	25.76	
(NON-EAS REFILL)			
15 mg/16 hr, 7s ea	00045-0602-07	24.71	
(NON-EAS)			
15 mg/16 hr, 7s ea	00045-0602-01	25.76	
(SENSORMATIC REFILL)			
15 mg/16 hr, 7s ea	00045-0602-09	24.71	
(STARTER KIT, SECUR TAG)			
15 mg/16 hr, 7s ea	00009-5197-02	25.76	
(STARTER KIT)			
15 mg/16 hr, 7s ea	00009-5197-01	24.71	
NIFEREX (Ther-RX)			
CAP,PO (10X10)			
40 mg-20 mg,			
100s ea UD	64011-0134-11	70.56	
ELI,PO (SF,DYE-FREE)			
100 mg/5 ml,			
236 ml	64011-0160-05	62.52	
NIFEREX-150 (Phys Total Care)			
REPACK			
CAP,PO, 50 mg-80 mg-70 mg,			
100s ea	54868-3687-00	105.61	
NIGHT TIME MULTI-SYMPTOM COLD/FLU (AmerisourceBergen)			
SGL,PO (PRIVATE LABEL,SOFTGEL)			
12s ea	24385-0530-53	3.14	3.49
20s ea	24385-0530-60	3.95	2.27
NIGHT TIME SLEEP AID (Chain Drug Marketing)			
TAB,PO, 25 mg, 32s ea	63868-0611-32	1.50	3.99
NIGHT-TIME PAIN RELIEVER/SLEEP AID (Basic Vitamins)			
TAB,PO (CAPLET)			
500 mg-25 mg,			
50s ea	00761-0399-10	2.00	
NIGHT-TIME SLEEP AID (Teva)			
SGL,PO (MAX. STR.,SOFTGEL)			
50 mg, 32s ea	00182-1131-93	6.99	
NIGHTTIME COLD (Teva)			
SGL,PO (SOFTGEL)			
12s ea	00182-1361-11	3.49	
NIGHTTIME SLEEP AID (AmerisourceBergen)			
TAB,PO (PRIVATE LABEL,CAPLET)			
25 mg, 24s ea	24385-0431-26	2.87	3.19
NITE TIME (Albertson's)			
SOL,PO, 180 ml	12810-0305-30	2.73	
NITE TIME COLD MEDICINE (Family Phcy)			
SOL,PO (PRIVATE LABEL)			
180 ml	52735-0415-43	2.60	2.89
NITE TIME COLD/FLU MEDICINE (AmerisourceBergen)			
SOL,PO (ORIGINAL,PRIVATE LABEL)			
180 ml	24385-0305-30	2.60	2.89
(PRIVATE LABEL,CHERRY)			
180 ml	24385-0322-30	2.60	2.89
(ORIGINAL,PRIVATE LABEL)			
300 ml	24385-0305-38	4.40	4.89
(PRIVATE LABEL,CHERRY)			
300 ml	24385-0322-38	4.49	4.99
NITRATEST PAPER (Bristol-Myers Squibb Mature Brands)			
DEV,NA (15 FT W/DISPENSER)			
ea	00003-0526-20	37.52	
(FILLED DISPENSER,4X15FT)			
ea	00003-0526-50	127.44	

PROD/MFR	HRI, UPC,NDC	AWP	SRP
NIVEA (Beiersdorf)			
CRE,TP, 60 gm	72140-0406-14	4.84	
60 gm	72140-0407-76	2.06	
120 gm	72140-0001-40	3.45	
180 gm	72140-0002-40	4.70	
LOT,TP, 120 ml	72140-0004-02	3.80	
120 ml	72140-0004-03	4.49	
120 ml	72140-0004-04	5.73	
(SUN-SPF 25)			
120 ml	72140-0431-01	5.13	
120 ml 12s	72140-0003-55	29.52	
120 ml 12s	72140-0400-45	68.76	
120 ml 12s	72140-0401-51	29.52	
240 ml	72140-0003-50	3.45	
240 ml	72140-0401-49	3.45	
360 ml	72140-0003-76	4.70	
360 ml	72140-0402-87	4.70	
OIL,TP, 120 ml 12s	72140-0406-17	29.52	
240 ml	72140-0406-18	3.45	
360 ml	72140-0406-19	4.70	
NIX CREME RINSE (A-S Medication)			
REPACK			
LIQ,TP, 1%, 60 ml	54569-1085-01	9.08	
NIZORAL A-D (McNeil Consumer Healthcare)			
SHA,TP, 1%, 125 ml	00450-0895-04	9.02	
200 ml	00450-0895-07	13.74	
NO FUNGUS (Mericon)			
OIN,TP, 15%, 85.5 gm	03940-0865-03	9.88	
NO PAIN (A. F. Hauser)			
TAB,PO, 10s ea UD	52637-0123-10	0.69	0.98
36s ea	52637-0123-11	4.98	
800s ea	52637-0123-15	69.98	
NODOZ (Novartis Consumer)			
TAB,PO (MAXIMUM STRENGTH)			
200 mg, 36s ea	00067-2070-36	4.46	
60s ea	00672-0070-60	6.38	
NON-ASPIRIN (Albertson's)			
ELI,PO, 160 mg/5 ml,			
120 ml	41280-0220-65	2.22	
NON-ASPIRIN CHILDREN'S (Chain Drug Marketing)			
LIQ,PO (AF,CHERRY)			
160 mg/5 ml, 118 ml	63868-0839-54	1.80	3.99
SUS,PO, 160 mg/5 ml,			
118 ml	63868-0175-26	1.98	4.99
(R.I.J.)			
SOL,PO (DROPS)			
80 mg/0.8 ml, 15 ml	53807-0143-01	1.86	
(Dispensing Solutions)			
REPACK			
SOL,PO (AF)			
80 mg/2.5 ml,			
118 ml	55045-1245-02	5.45	
NON-ASPIRIN EXTRA STRENGTH (Chain Drug Marketing)			
TAB,PO, 500 mg, 60s ea	63868-0315-60	1.19	3.99
100s ea	63868-0315-10	1.79	4.99
NON-ASPIRIN INFANTS (Chain Drug Marketing)			
SOL,PO (AF,DROPS)			
80 mg/0.8 ml, 15 ml	63868-0838-73	1.26	2.99
NON-ASPIRIN PAIN RELIEVER (AmerisourceBergen)			
TAB,PO (EXT. STR.,PRIVATE LABEL)			
500 mg, 50s ea	24385-0187-71	3.86	4.29
50s ea	24385-0484-71	3.95	4.39
60s ea	24385-0405-72	3.86	4.29
100s ea	24385-0405-78	5.84	6.49
100s ea	24385-0433-78	6.98	7.79
100s ea	24385-0484-78	5.84	6.49
500s ea	24385-0484-90	9.89	11.00
NON-ASPIRIN PAIN RELIEVER CHILDRENS (AmerisourceBergen)			
CTB,PO (PRIVATE LABEL,GRAPE)			
80 mg, 30s ea	24385-0481-65	2.33	2.59
NON-ASPIRIN PAIN RELIEVER INFANT'S (AmerisourceBergen)			
SOL,PO (AF,PRIVATE LABEL,FRUIT)			
80 mg/0.8 ml, 15 ml	24385-0313-05	3.41	3.79
(AF,PRIVATE LABEL,GRAPE)			
80 mg/0.8 ml, 15 ml	24385-0289-05	3.41	3.79
NON-ASPIRIN PM EXTRA STRENGTH (Chain Drug Marketing)			
TAB,PO (GELTAB)			
500 mg-25 mg, 50s ea	63868-0090-50	2.40	5.39
NON-ASPIRIN REGULAR STRENGTH (Chain Drug Marketing)			
TAB,PO, 325 mg, 100s ea	63868-0314-10	1.31	3.99
NON-ASPIRIN SINUS MAXIMUM STRENGTH (AmerisourceBergen)			
TAB,PO (NON-DROWSY)			
500 mg-30 mg, 24s ea	24385-0438-62	3.32	3.69
NORFORMS (Fleet,C.B.)			
SUP,VG (FRESH FLOWERS)			
12s ea	41608-0005-32	2.83	
(ISLAND ESCAPE)			
12s ea	41608-0005-22	2.83	
NORMALEX (Lex)			
TAB,PO (PF,SF)			
325 mg, 50s ea	49523-0042-05	0.85	
100s ea	49523-0042-01	1.24	
NORMLSHIELD (MPM Medical Inc.)			
CRE,TP, 4.5%, 113 gm	66977-0022-04	4.21	4.68
NORTEMP INFANTS' (Ballay Pharm., Inc)			
SOL,PO (CONCENTRATED,1X30ML,AF)			
80 mg/0.8 ml, 30 ml	63162-0518-30	6.70	
NORWEGIAN SALMON OIL AND GLA (Carlson,J.R.)			
SGL,PO (PF,SOFT GELS)			
40 mg-260 mg-10 iu,			
60s ea	88395-0015-10	5.95	11.90
120s ea	88395-0015-11	10.95	21.90
240s ea	88395-0015-12	19.95	39.90
NORWICH ASPIRIN (Chattem)			
TAB,PO, 325 mg, 100s ea	41167-0093-01	1.46	
250s ea	41167-0932-05	3.12	
500s ea	41167-0931-01	5.51	
500 mg, 150s ea	01490-0108-15	3.70	
NOSE DROPS EXTRA STRENGTH (AmerisourceBergen)			
SOL,NS (PRIVATE LABEL)			
1%, 30 ml	24385-0390-10	3.23	3.59
NOSTRILLA (Heritage/Insight)			
SPR,NS, 0.05%, 15 ml	00083-7300-52	3.75	4.44
NOURIVA REPAIR (Ferndale)			
CRE,TP (MOISTURIZING)			
30 gm	00496-0865-30	14.56	
NOVA MAX BLOOD GLUCOSE MONITORING SYSTEM (Nova)			
DEV,NA, ea	85480-0434-35	61.00	
(MAIL ORDER)			
ea	85480-0434-36	61.00	
NOVA MAX GLUCOSE TEST STRIPS (Nova)			
DEV,NA, 50s ea	85480-0434-37	47.50	
(MAIL ORDER)			
50s ea	85480-0435-23	45.31	
100s ea	85480-0434-16	87.50	
NOVA MAX NORMAL GLUCOSE CONTROL SOLUTION (Nova)			
DEV,NA, 4 ml	85480-0434-46	8.75	
NOVA SUREFLEX (Nova)			
DEV,NA, ea	08548-0434-33	8.45	
ea	08548-0434-47	11.20	
NOVAFLOR (Med Prods Panamer)			
CAP,PO, 200 mg, 30s ea	00576-0278-30	8.25	
NOVASOURCE PULMONARY (Nestle)			
LIQ,PO (LACTOSE-FREE,VANILLA)			
250 ml 24s	00212-1885-51	69.70	
(CLOSED SYSTEM)			
1000 ml 6s	00212-1885-42	80.57	
1500 ml 6s	00212-1885-44	120.89	
NOVASOURCE RENAL (Nestle)			
LIQ,PO (VANILLA)			
240 ml 27s	00212-3511-62	104.65	
(CLOSED SYSTEM)			
1000 ml 6s	00212-3511-42	111.96	
SUS,PO (6X1000ML)			
1000 ml 6s	43900-0351-80	111.96	
NOVOFINE AUTOCOVER 30G (Novo Nordisk)			
DEV,NA (30G,1/3",DISPOSABLE)			
100s ea	00169-1852-75	57.66	
NOVOFINE TIP (Novo Nordisk)			
DEV,NA (32G,6MM)			
100s ea	01691-0851-89	40.61	
NOVOLIN 70/30 (Novo Nordisk)			
SUS,SC (VIAL)			
70 u/ml-30 u/ml,			
10 ml	00169-1837-11	59.12	
(A-S Medication)			
REPACK			
SUS,SC (VIAL)			
70 u/ml-30 u/ml,			
10 ml	54569-2918-00	51.33	
(10X10ML)			
70 u/ml-30 u/ml,			
10 ml 10s	54569-2918-02	412.50	
(Dispensing Solutions)			
REPACK			
SUS,SC, 70 u/ml-30 u/ml,			
10 ml	55045-3508-01	41.00	
(Phys Total Care)			
REPACK			
SUS,SC (VIAL)			
70 u/ml-30 u/ml,			
10 ml	54868-3474-00	63.72	
NOVOLIN N (Novo Nordisk)			
SUS,SC (VIAL)			
100 u/ml, 10 ml	00169-1834-11	59.12	
(A-S Medication)			
REPACK			
SUS,SC (VIAL)			
100 u/ml, 10 ml	54569-3835-00	51.33	
(Phys Total Care)			
REPACK			
SUS,SC, 100 u/ml, 10 ml	54868-2380-01	48.52	
NOVOLIN R (Novo Nordisk)			
SOL,IJ (VIAL)			
100 u/ml, 10 ml	00169-1833-11	59.12	
(A-S Medication)			
REPACK			
SOL,IJ (VIAL)			
100 u/ml, 10 ml	54569-3833-00	51.33	
(Phys Total Care)			
REPACK			
SOL,IJ, 100 u/ml, 10 ml	54868-3598-00	38.74	
NOVOPEN 3 (Novo Nordisk)			
DEV,NA (INSULIN DELIVERY SYSTEM)			
ea	00169-1852-90	31.89	
NOVOPEN 3 PENMATE (Novo Nordisk)			
DEV,NA, ea	00169-1852-42	12.50	
NOVOPEN JR (Novo Nordisk)			
DEV,NA (GREEN)			
ea	00169-1852-58	37.49	
(YELLOW)			
ea	00169-1852-59	37.49	
NOZOVENT (Scandinavian)			
DEV,NA (MEDIUM, ANTI-SNORING)			
ea	51137-0000-40	5.97	9.95
2s ea	51137-0000-46	8.97	14.95
NRS-NASAL RELIEF (Rugby)			
SPR,NS, 0.05%, 15 ml	00536-5005-72	3.38	
30 ml	00536-5005-75	4.42	
NU-GAUZE GENERAL-USE NONSTERILE (J&J Medical)			
DEV,NA (2"X2",3-PLY)			
200s ea	56091-0076-35	1.97	
(2"X2",4-PLY)			
200s ea	56091-0076-32	2.44	
(3"X3",4-PLY)			
200s ea	56091-0076-33	4.80	
(4"X4",3-PLY)			
200s ea	56091-0076-36	5.56	
(4"X4",4-PLY)			
200s ea	56091-0076-34	8.13	
(8"X4",4-PLY)			
200s ea	56091-0076-37	20.62	
NU-GAUZE GENERAL-USE STERILE (J&J Medical)			
DEV,NA (2"X2",4-PLY,2X25)			
50s ea	56091-0023-38	1.46	
(3"X3",4-PLY,2X25)			
50s ea	56091-0023-39	2.02	
(4"X4",4-PLY,2X25)			
50s ea	56091-0023-37	2.90	
(4"X4",4-PLY,TRAY)			
576s ea	56091-0023-44	73.23	
NU-GAUZE PACKING STRIP SELVAGE EDGE (J&J Medical)			
DEV,NA (STER,IODOFORM,1"X5YD)			
ea	56091-0087-57	4.72	
(STER,IODOFORM,1/2"X5YD)			
ea	56091-0087-56	4.15	
(STER,IODOFORM,1/4"X5YD)			
ea	56091-0087-55	3.90	

PROD/MFR	HRI, UPC, NDC	AWP	SRP
(STER,IODOFORM,2"X5YD)			
ea	56091-0087-58	6.58	
(STER,PLAIN,1"X5YD)			
ea	56091-0087-52	4.15	
(STER,PLAIN,1/2"X5YD)			
ea	56091-0087-51	3.66	
(STER,PLAIN,1/4"X5YD)			
ea	56091-0087-50	3.67	
(STER,PLAIN,2"X5YD)			
ea	56091-0087-53	5.57	
NU-GAUZE UTERINE PACKING STRIPS (J&J Medical)			
DEV,NA (STER,IODOFORM,8"X10YD)			
ea	56091-0017-60	29.24	
NU-GEL (J&J Medical)			
GEL,TP (3 3/4"X3 3/4")			
5s ea	56091-0024-97	16.90	
(6"X8")			
5s ea	56091-0024-98	32.50	
(COLLAGEN)			
30 gm 5s	56091-0024-89	25.68	
90 gm	56091-0024-99	11.39	
NU-IRON 150 (Merz)			
CAP,PO, 150 mg, 100s ea	02590-0291-01	51.36	
NU-TEARS (Southwood)			
REPACK			
OIN,OP, 3.5 gm	58016-6437-01	3.49	
NUBASICS (Nestle)			
LIQ,PO (STRAWBERRY BURST)			
250 ml	00065-9202-70	1.90	
(VANILLA)			
250 ml	00065-9200-70	1.90	
NUBASICS JUICE DRINK (Nestle)			
LIQ,PO (ORANGE)			
163 ml	00065-9241-74	1.49	
(SWEET BERRY)			
163 ml	00065-9240-74	1.49	
NUBASICS PLUS (Nestle)			
LIQ,PO (CHOCOLATE SPLASH)			
250 ml	00065-9251-70	2.12	
(STRAWBERRY BURST)			
250 ml	00065-9252-70	2.12	
(VANILLA)			
250 ml	00065-9250-70	2.12	
NULLO (Monticello)			
TAB,PO, 33.3 mg, 60s ea	11868-0009-60	4.71	
135s ea	11868-0009-01	9.33	
NUMOL (S.S.S.)			
LIQ,TP, 9.6%-3.1%-9.7%,			
60 ml	12258-0125-02	2.39	3.59
120 ml	12258-0125-04	4.66	6.99
NUMOTIZINE CATAPLASM (Hobart)			
OIN,TP (POULTICE)			
0.3%-0.3%-1.3%,			
99 gm	10546-0100-35	5.24	7.88
228 gm	10546-0100-08	9.66	14.49
680 gm	10546-0100-24	17.20	25.81
NUPERCAINAL (Novartis Consumer)			
OIN,TP, 1%, 30 gm	00083-5812-96	5.15	
60 gm	00083-5812-86	8.75	
NUTR-E-SOL (Advanced Nutr)			
LIQ,PO, 400 iu/15 ml,			
480 ml	62617-0515-20	32.00	42.00
NUTRA-SUPPORT BONE (Carlson,J.R.)			
SGL,PO (PF,SF,CORN-FREE)			
90s ea	88395-0046-11	5.95	11.90
180s ea	88395-0046-12	9.95	19.90
360s ea	88395-0046-13	18.85	37.70
NUTRA-SUPPORT JOINT (Carlson,J.R.)			
TAB,PO (PF)			
90s ea	88395-0046-71	13.85	27.70
180s ea	88395-0046-72	24.95	49.90
360s ea	88395-0046-73	47.50	95.00
NUTRA-SUPPORT PROSTATE (Carlson,J.R.)			
SGL,PO (SOFT GELS)			
60s ea	88395-0046-40	12.38	24.75
120s ea	88395-0046-41	22.22	44.44
NUTRA/PRO (Nutra/Balance)			
POW,NA (24X26GM,CHOCOLATE)			
24s ea	07249-0911-06		82.43
(24X26GM,STRAWBERRY)			
24s ea	07249-0911-05		82.43
(24X26GM,VANILLA)			
24s ea	07249-0911-04		82.43
NUTRADERM (Valeant Pharm Intl)			
CRE,TP, 85 gm	00064-2800-03	9.32	
453 gm	00064-2800-16	21.03	
LOT,TP, 236 ml	00064-2700-08	7.80	
473 ml	00064-2700-16	10.73	
NUTRADERM ADVANCED FORMULA (Valeant Pharm Intl)			
LOT,TP, 240 ml	00064-2600-08	7.80	
480 ml	00064-2600-16	10.73	
NUTRALOX (Hart Health)			
CTB,PO (2X50,MINT)			
420 mg, 100s ea UD	50332-0106-04	2.72	
(2X125,MINT)			
420 mg, 250s ea UD	50332-0106-02	6.07	
(2X500,MINT)			
420 mg, 1000s ea UD	50332-0106-01	23.37	
NUTRAMENT (Nestle)			
LIQ,PO (12X360ML,BANANA)			
360 ml 12s	41679-0635-01	20.52	
(12X360ML,CARAMEL)			
360 ml 12s	41679-0603-01	20.52	
(12X360ML,CHOCOLATE)			
360 ml 12s	41679-0632-01	20.52	
(12X360ML,COCONUT)			
360 ml 12s	41679-0636-01	20.52	
(12X360ML,EGG NOG)			
360 ml 12s	41679-0637-01	20.52	
(12X360ML,STRAWBERRY)			
360 ml 12s	41679-0634-01	20.52	
(12X360ML,VANILLA)			
360 ml 12s	41679-0633-01	20.52	
NUTRAMIGEN AA LIPIL (Mead Johnson & Co)			
PDR,PO (IRON FORTIFIED,1X400GM)			
400 gm	00087-1290-49	43.33	
NUTRAMIGEN LIPIL (Mead Johnson & Co)			
LIQ,PO (6X59ML,NURSETTE,20CAL)			
59 ml 6s	00087-1437-41	10.15	
(NURSETTE, 20 CAL)			
177 ml	00087-0263-24	2.33	
(CONCENTRATE)			
384 ml	00087-0498-01	8.62	
(R.T.U.)			
946 ml	00087-0499-01	11.14	
NUTRAPLUS (Valeant Pharm Intl)			
CRE,TP, 10%, 90 gm	00064-2110-03	9.69	
454 gm	00064-2110-16	26.67	
LOT,TP, 10%, 240 ml	00064-2120-08	10.33	
480 ml	00064-2120-16	17.06	
NUTREN 1.0 (Nestle)			
LIQ,PO (UNFLAVORED,GLUTEN-FREE)			
250 ml	00065-9030-70	2.17	
(250MLX24EA,GLUTEN-FREE)			
250 ml 24s	00065-9024-70	27.36	
NUTREN 1.0 ULTRAPAK (Nestle)			
LIQ,PO (1000MLX6,BAG)			
1000 ml 6s	00065-9150-72	34.49	
(1500MLX4,BAG)			
1500 ml 4s	00065-9150-73	34.46	
NUTREN 1.0 WITH FIBER (Nestle)			
LIQ,PO (UNFLAVORED,GLUTEN-FREE)			
250 ml	00065-9031-70	2.24	
(VANILLA, 250MLX24EA)			
250 ml 24s	00065-9025-70	28.80	
NUTREN 1.0 WITH FIBER ULTRAPAK (Nestle)			
LIQ,PO (1000MLX6,BAG)			
1000 ml 6s	00065-9152-72	36.00	
(1500MLX4,BAG)			
1500 ml 4s	00065-9152-73	35.95	
NUTREN 1.5 (Nestle)			
LIQ,PO (UNFLAVORED,GLUTEN-FREE)			
250 ml	00065-9038-70	2.22	
(250MLX24,GLUTEN-FREE)			
250 ml 24s	00065-9032-70	33.41	
(6X1000ML,ULTRAPAK)			
1000 ml 6s	98716-0263-54	40.54	
NUTREN 1.5 FIBER (Nestle)			
LIQ,PO (250MLX24,W/PREBIO1)			
250 ml 24s	00065-9035-70	38.02	
(1000MLX6,WITH PREBIO1)			
1000 ml 6s	00065-9035-72	45.07	
(1500MLX4,WITH PREBIO1)			
1500 ml 4s	00065-9035-73	45.02	
NUTREN 1.5 ULTRAPAK (Nestle)			
LIQ,PO (1000MLX6)			
1000 ml 6s	00065-9154-72	40.54	
(1500MLX4)			
1500 ml 4s	00065-9154-73	40.51	
NUTREN 2.0 (Nestle)			
LIQ,PO (GLUTEN-FREE)			
250 ml	00065-9040-70	2.36	
(ULTRAPAK BAG)			
1000 ml	00065-9040-72	12.25	
NUTREN GLYTROL (Nestle)			
LIQ,PO (250MLX24,VANILLA)			
250 ml 24s	00065-9085-70	56.45	
NUTREN JUNIOR (Nestle)			
LIQ,PO (250MLX24,GLUTEN-FREE)			
250 ml 24s	00065-9043-70	42.62	
(1000MLX6,ULTRAPAK)			
1000 ml 6s	00065-9043-90	49.90	
NUTREN JUNIOR FIBER (Nestle)			
LIQ,PO (1000MLX6,ULTRAPAK)			
1000 ml 6s	00065-9045-90	52.63	
NUTREN JUNIOR ULTRAPAK SPIKERIGHT (Nestle)			
SOL,PO (UNFLAVORED)			
1000 ml 6s	98716-0773-80	49.90	
NUTREN JUNIOR W/FIBER (Nestle)			
LIQ,PO (250MLX24EA,VANILLA)			
250 ml 24s	00065-9045-70	45.50	
NUTREN PROBALANCE (Nestle)			
LIQ,PO (250MLX24,GLUTEN-FREE)			
250 ml 24s	00065-9162-70	30.24	
NUTREN PULMONARY (Nestle)			
LIQ,PO (250MLX24,GLUTEN-FREE)			
250 ml 24s	00065-9141-70	69.70	
(1000MLX6,ULTRAPAK)			
1000 ml 6s	00065-9141-72	80.57	
NUTREN PULMONARY ULTRAPAK SPIKERIGHT (Nestle)			
SOL,PO, 1000 ml 6s	98716-0223-92	80.57	
NUTREN RENAL (Nestle)			
LIQ,PO (250MLX24,GLUTEN-FREE)			
250 ml 24s	00065-9142-70	89.86	
(ULTRAPAK BAG)			
1000 ml	00065-9142-72	18.43	
NUTREN REPLETE (Nestle)			
LIQ,PO (250MLX24,GLUTEN-FREE)			
250 ml 24s	00065-9022-70	36.29	
(6X1000ML,ULTRAPAK)			
1000 ml 6s	98716-0163-56	43.56	
NUTREN REPLETE FIBER ULTRAPAK (Nestle)			
LIQ,PO (1000MLX6)			
1000 ml 6s	00065-9158-72	44.14	
(1500MLX4)			
1500 ml 4s	00065-9158-73	44.16	
NUTREN REPLETE FIBER ULTRAPAK SPIKERIGHT (Nestle)			
SOL,PO, 1000 ml 6s	98716-0263-58	44.14	
NUTREN REPLETE WITH FIBER (Nestle)			
LIQ,PO (250MLX24,GLUTEN-FREE)			
250 ml 24s	00065-9023-70	36.86	
NUTRI-CLAMP LOCKING DEVICE (Abbott Hosp)			
DEV,NA (GREEN)			
400s ea	00074-7915-01	218.50	
(RED)			
400s ea	00074-7914-01	327.75	
NUTRI-DRINK (Unico)			
LIQ,PO (BERRY)			
237 ml	37513-0000-18	0.79	
(CHOCOLATE)			
237 ml	37513-0000-17	0.79	
(VANILLA)			
237 ml	37513-0000-16	0.79	
NUTRI-DRINK PLUS (Unico)			
PO (BERRY)			
237 ml	37513-0000-21	0.83	
(CHOCOLATE)			
237 ml	37513-0000-20	0.83	
(VANILLA)			
237 ml	37513-0000-19	0.83	
NUTRIFOCUS (Abbott)			
LIQ,PO (CHOCOLATE)			
237 ml	70074-0558-61	2.42	
(VANILLA)			
237 ml	70074-0558-59	2.42	
NUTRIHEP (Nestle)			
LIQ,PO (250MLX24, UNFLAVORED)			
250 ml 24s	00065-9078-70	380.74	
NUTRIMIX (Abbott Hosp)			
DEV,NA (MACRO EMPTY CONT 1000ML)			
50s ea	00074-4419-02	894.78	

PROD/MFR	HRI, UPC,NDC	AWP	SRP
(MACRO EMPTY CONT 2000ML)			
50s ea	**00074-4425-01**	947.63	
(MACRO EMPTY CONT 250 ML)			
50s ea	**00074-4417-01**	841.94	
(MACRO EMPTY CONT 3000ML)			
50s ea	**00074-4430-01**	975.53	
(MACRO EMPTY CONT 4000ML)			
50s ea	**00074-4432-01**	1017.09	
(MACRO EMPTY CONT 500 ML)			
50s ea	**00074-4418-01**	868.06	
NUTRIPORT BALLOON GASTROSTOMY TUBE (Covidien)			
DEV,NA (12FR X 0.80CM)			
ea	**08080-7120-80**	144.38	
(12FR X 1.2CM,SKIN LEVEL)			
ea	**08080-7121-20**	144.38	
(12FR X 1.5CM,SKIN LEVEL)			
ea	**08080-7121-50**	144.38	
(12FR X 1.7CM,SKIN LEVEL)			
ea	**08080-7121-70**	144.38	
(12FR X 1CM,SKIN LEVEL)			
ea	**08080-7121-00**	144.38	
(12FR X 2.0CM,SKIN LEVEL)			
ea	**08080-7122-00**	144.38	
(12FR X 2.3CM,SKIN LEVEL)			
ea	**08080-7122-30**	144.38	
(12FR X 2.5CM,SKIN LEVEL)			
ea	**08080-7122-50**	144.38	
(12FR X 2.7CM,SKIN LEVEL)			
ea	**08080-7122-70**	144.38	
(12FR X 3.5CM,SKIN LEVEL)			
ea	**08080-7123-50**	144.38	
(12FR X 4.0CM,SKIN LEVEL)			
ea	**08080-7124-00**	144.38	
(12FR X 4.5CM,SKIN LEVEL)			
ea	**08080-7124-50**	144.38	
(12FR X 5.0CM,SKIN LEVEL)			
ea	**08080-7125-00**	144.38	
(14FR X 0.80CM)			
ea	**08080-7140-80**	144.38	
(14FR X 1.0CM,SKIN LEVEL)			
ea	**08080-7141-00**	144.38	
(14FR X 1.2CM,SKIN LEVEL)			
ea	**08080-7141-20**	144.38	
(14FR X 1.5CM,SKIN LEVEL)			
ea	**08080-7141-50**	144.38	
(14FR X 1.7CM,SKIN LEVEL)			
ea	**08080-7141-70**	144.38	
(14FR X 2.0CM,SKIN LEVEL)			
ea	**08080-7142-00**	144.38	
(14FR X 2.3CM,SKIN LEVEL)			
ea	**08080-7142-30**	144.38	
(14FR X 2.5CM,SKIN LEVEL)			
ea	**08080-7142-50**	144.38	
(14FR X 2.7CM,SKIN LEVEL)			
ea	**08080-7142-70**	144.38	
(14FR X 3.0CM,SKIN LEVEL)			
ea	**08080-7143-00**	144.38	
(14FR X 3.5CM,SKIN LEVEL)			
ea	**08080-7143-50**	144.38	
(14FR X 4.0CM,SKIN LEVEL)			
ea	**08080-7144-00**	144.38	
(14FR X 4.5CM,SKIN LEVEL)			
ea	**08080-7144-50**	144.38	
(14FR X 5.0CM,SKIN LEVEL)			
ea	**08080-7145-00**	144.38	
(16FR X 0.80CM)			
ea	**08080-7160-80**	144.38	
(16FR X 1.0CM,SKIN LEVEL)			
ea	**08080-7161-00**	144.38	
(16FR X 1.2CM,SKIN LEVEL)			
ea	**08080-7161-20**	144.38	
(16FR X 1.5CM,SKIN LEVEL)			
ea	**08080-7161-50**	144.38	
(16FR X 1.7CM,SKIN LEVEL)			
ea	**08080-7161-70**	144.38	
(16FR X 2.0CM,SKIN LEVEL)			
ea	**08080-7162-00**	144.38	
(16FR X 2.3CM,SKIN LEVEL)			
ea	**08080-7162-30**	144.38	
(16FR X 2.5CM,SKIN LEVEL)			
ea	**08080-7162-50**	144.38	
(16FR X 2.7CM,SKIN LEVEL)			
ea	**08080-7162-70**	144.38	
(16FR X 3.0CM,SKIN LEVEL)			
ea	**08080-7163-00**	144.38	
(16FR X 3.5CM,SKIN LEVEL)			
ea	**08080-7163-50**	144.38	
(16FR X 4.0CM,SKIN LEVEL)			
ea	**08080-7164-00**	144.38	
(16FR X 4.5CM,SKIN LEVEL)			
ea	**08080-7164-50**	144.38	
(16FR X 5.0CM,SKIN LEVEL)			
ea	**08080-7165-00**	144.38	
(18FR X 0.80CM)			
ea	**08080-7180-80**	144.38	
(18FR X 1.0CM,SKIN LEVEL)			
ea	**08080-7181-00**	144.38	
(18FR X 1.2CM,SKIN LEVEL)			
ea	**08080-7181-20**	144.38	
(18FR X 1.5CM,SKIN LEVEL)			
ea	**08080-7181-50**	144.38	
(18FR X 1.7CM,SKIN LEVEL)			
ea	**08080-7181-70**	144.38	
(18FR X 2.0CM,SKIN LEVEL)			
ea	**08080-7182-00**	144.38	
(18FR X 2.3CM,SKIN LEVEL)			
ea	**08080-7182-30**	144.38	
(18FR X 2.5CM,SKIN LEVEL)			
ea	**08080-7182-50**	144.38	
(18FR X 2.7CM,SKIN LEVEL)			
ea	**08080-7182-70**	144.38	
(18FR X 3.0CM,SKIN LEVEL)			
ea	**08080-7183-00**	144.38	
(18FR X 3.5CM,SKIN LEVEL)			
ea	**08080-7183-50**	144.38	
(18FR X 4.0CM,SKIN LEVEL)			
ea	**08080-7184-00**	144.38	
(18FR X 4.5CM,SKIN LEVEL)			
ea	**08080-7184-50**	144.38	
(18FR X 5.0CM,SKIN LEVEL)			
ea	**08080-7185-00**	144.38	
(20FR X 0.80CM)			
ea	**08080-7200-80**	144.38	
(20FR X 1.0CM,SKIN LEVEL)			
ea	**08080-7201-00**	144.38	
(20FR X 1.2CM,SKIN LEVEL)			
ea	**08080-7201-20**	144.38	
(20FR X 1.5CM,SKIN LEVEL)			
ea	**08080-7201-50**	144.38	
(20FR X 1.7CM,SKIN LEVEL)			
ea	**08080-7201-70**	144.38	
(20FR X 2.0CM,SKIN LEVEL)			
ea	**08080-7202-00**	144.38	
(20FR X 2.3CM,SKIN LEVEL)			
ea	**08080-7202-30**	144.38	
(20FR X 2.5CM,SKIN LEVEL)			
ea	**08080-7202-50**	144.38	
(20FR X 2.7CM,SKIN LEVEL)			
ea	**08080-7202-70**	144.38	
(20FR X 3.0CM,SKIN LEVEL)			
ea	**08080-0720-30**	144.38	
(20FR X 3.5CM,SKIN LEVEL)			
ea	**08080-7203-50**	144.38	
(20FR X 4.0CM,SKIN LEVEL)			
ea	**08080-7204-00**	144.38	
(20FR X 4.5CM,SKIN LEVEL)			
ea	**08080-7204-50**	144.38	
(20FR X 5.0CM,SKIN LEVEL)			
ea	**08080-7205-00**	144.38	
(24FR X 0.80CM)			
ea	**08080-7240-80**	144.38	
(24FR X 1.0CM,SKIN LEVEL)			
ea	**08080-7241-00**	144.38	
(24FR X 1.2CM,SKIN LEVEL)			
ea	**08080-7241-20**	144.38	
(24FR X 1.5CM,SKIN LEVEL)			
ea	**08080-7241-50**	144.38	
(24FR X 1.7CM,SKIN LEVEL)			
ea	**08080-7241-70**	144.38	
(24FR X 2.0CM,SKIN LEVEL)			
ea	**08080-7242-00**	144.38	
(24FR X 2.3CM,SKIN LEVEL)			
ea	**08080-7242-30**	144.38	
(24FR X 2.5CM,SKIN LEVEL)			
ea	**08080-7242-50**	144.38	
(24FR X 2.7CM,SKIN LEVEL)			
ea	**08080-7242-70**	144.38	
(24FR X 3.0CM,SKIN LEVEL)			
ea	**08080-7243-00**	144.38	
(24FR X 3.5CM,SKIN LEVEL)			
ea	**08080-7243-50**	144.38	
(24FR X 4.0CM,SKIN LEVEL)			
ea	**08080-7244-00**	144.38	
(24FR X 4.5CM,SKIN LEVEL)			
ea	**08080-7244-50**	144.38	
(24FR X 5.0CM,SKIN LEVEL)			
ea	**08080-7245-00**	144.38	
NUTRISION (Westlake Labs.)			
CAP,PO, 60s ea	**10539-0702-63**	42.00	60.00
NUTRISURE OTC (Westlake Labs.)			
TAB,PO (PF,SF)			
180s ea	**10539-0834-59**	26.60	38.00
NUTRITIONAL SUPPLEMENT (AmerisourceBergen)			
LIQ,PO (PRIVATE LABEL,BERRY)			
240 ml	**24385-0222-34**	32.40	36.00
(PRIVATE LABEL,CHOCOLATE)			
240 ml	**24385-0153-34**	32.40	36.00
(PRIVATE LABEL,VANILLA)			
240 ml	**24385-0152-34**	32.40	36.00
NUTRITIONAL SUPPLEMENT PLUS (AmerisourceBergen)			
PO (PRIVATE LABEL,BERRY)			
240 ml	**24385-0223-34**	28.76	31.96
(PRIVATE LABEL,CHOCOLATE)			
240 ml	**24385-0151-34**	36.00	40.00
(PRIVATE LABEL,VANILLA)			
240 ml	**24385-0150-34**	36.00	40.00
NUTRIVIR (Bionexus)			
PDR,PO (VANILLA)			
560 gm	**53110-0980-03**	31.95	39.95
NUTRIVIR NSA (Bionexus)			
PDR,PO (VANILLA)			
401 gm	**53110-0030-11**	31.95	39.95
NUVORAWHITE (Nuvora)			
LOZ,MM, 12s ea	**91124-0002-04**	20.00	
NUX VOMICA (Luyties)			
TAB,SL (6X)			
6 x, 500s ea	**00618-6465-03**	3.99	
5500s ea	**00618-6465-10**	30.32	
(30X)			
12 x, 500s ea	**00622-6465-03**	4.19	
5500s ea	**00622-6465-10**	31.83	
(12X)			
30 x, 500s ea	**00624-6465-03**	4.19	
5500s ea	**00624-6465-10**	31.83	
(Walker Pharmacal)			
TAB,SL (6X)			
250s ea	**00619-6465-02**	2.97	
NYTOL QUICKCAPS (Glaxo)			
TAB,PO, 25 mg, 16s ea	**10158-0043-02**	3.32	
32s ea	**10158-0043-04**	5.59	
72s ea	**10158-0043-06**	8.08	
NYTOL QUICKGELS MAXIMUM STRENGTH (Glaxo)			
SGL,PO (SOFTGEL)			
50 mg, 8s ea	**10158-0042-01**	3.32	
O-CAL-ETTE NURSING CUPS (Pharmics)			
DEV,NA, 2s ea	**00813-0099-00**	6.03	11.95
O.A.D. (Coloplast)			
DEV,NA, 59 ml 24s	**11701-0029-19**	104.88	109.68
118 ml 12s	**11701-0029-04**	136.20	142.56
237 ml 12s	**11701-0029-05**	242.76	254.04
O.B. PRO COMFORT (Johnson & Johnson)			
DEV,NA (REGULAR, SILK TOUCH)			
40s ea	**80045-0509-00**	6.26	
(SUPER, SILKTOUCH)			
40s ea	**80045-0510-00**	6.26	
OA 1 (Mead Johnson & Co)			
PDR,PO, 454 gm	**00087-0085-41**	39.60	
OA 2 (Mead Johnson & Co)			
PDR,PO (GALACTOSE-FREE)			
454 gm	**00087-0191-41**	66.00	
OAK (Ellon)			
SOL,SL (DROPS)			
10.5 ml	**51762-0029-10**		9.25
OASIS BURN MATRIX (Healthpoint)			
DEV,NA (7X20CM,MESHED)			
5s ea	**08213-3000-20**	444.78	
OASIS MOISTURIZING (Glaxo)			
SPR,MM (FOR DRY MOUTH,TRI HYDRA)			
35%, 30 ml	**10158-0117-20**	4.87	
OASIS MOISTURIZING MOUTHWASH (Glaxo)			
SOL,MM (FOR DRY MOUTH,TRI HYDRA)			
473 ml	**10158-0117-00**	5.23	
OASIS WOUND MATRIX (Healthpoint)			
DEV,NA (7X10CM,FENESTRATED)			
5s ea	**08213-1000-10**	243.18	
(7X10CM,MESHED)			
5s ea	**08213-1000-15**	243.18	
(7X20CM,FENESTRATED)			
5s ea	**08213-1000-20**	367.92	
(7X20CM,MESHED)			
5s ea	**08213-1000-25**	367.92	
(3X3.5CM,FENESTRATED)			
10s ea	**08213-1000-33**	94.50	
(3X7CM,FENESTRATED)			
10s ea	**08213-1000-37**	157.50	

PROD/MFR	HRI, UPC,NDC	AWP	SRP
OAT BRAN (Mason Vit)			
TAB,PO (SF)			
500 mg, 100s ea	11845-0094-31	3.89	
(Nature's Bounty)			
TAB,PO (PF,SF)			
850 mg, 100s ea	74312-0060-90		4.49
OATMEAL BATH (AmerisourceBergen)			
PDR,TP (PRIVATE LABEL)			
1.5 gm 8s	24385-0133-95	4.94	5.49
(Family Phcy)			
PDR,TP (PRIVATE LABEL)			
45 gm 8s	52735-0244-16	4.49	4.99
OATMEAL BATH TREATMENT (Cardinal Health)			
PDR,TP (PRIVATE LABEL)			
0.5 gm 8s	37205-0178-51	4.16	
OATSTRAW (Botanical Labs.)			
CAP,PO, 100s ea	41954-0030-12	3.75	7.50
LIQ,PO, 30 ml	41954-0020-69	3.50	6.99
OCEAN (Phys Total Care)			
REPACK			
SOL,NS, 0.65%, 45 ml	54868-1843-01	3.44	
OCEAN COMPLETE (Fleming)			
SPR,NS (PF)			
177 ml	02560-0215-01		13.99
OCEAN FOR KIDS PREMIUM SALINE (Fleming)			
SPR,NS (AF)			
0.65%, 37.5 ml	02560-0211-01		4.79
OCEAN PREMIUM SALINE (Fleming)			
SPR,NS, 0.65%, 45 ml	00256-0152-01		3.57
(1X45ML)			
0.65%, 45 ml	02560-0152-18		3.57
473 ml	00256-0152-02		15.75
(Stat Rx)			
REPACK			
SPR,NS, 0.65%, 45 ml	16590-0792-45	4.38	
OCEAN ULTRA (Fleming)			
SPR,NS (PF)			
90 ml	02560-0212-01		7.99
OCEAN ULTRA MOISTURIZING (Fleming)			
GEL,TP, 14 gm	00256-0213-01		4.99
OCTACO-SANOL (Bio-Tech Pharm)			
CAP,PO, 4000 mcg,			
100s ea	53191-0213-01	8.90	
OCTOGEN (Octogen)			
OIN,TP, 6%-3%-15%-15%,			
37.5 gm	53152-0100-01	2.80	4.19
97.5 gm	53152-0100-03	6.67	9.95
450 gm	53152-0100-15	22.08	32.95
OCTOGEN-2 (Octogen)			
CRE,TP, 3.1%-6%-15%-6%,			
37.5 gm	53152-0200-01	2.80	4.19
97.5 gm	53152-0200-03	6.67	9.95
450 gm	53152-0200-15	22.08	32.95
OCTYCINE-100 (Truxton)			
SGL,PO, 100 mg, 100s ea	00463-2030-01	6.00	
1000s ea	00463-2030-10	24.00	
OCTYCINE-250 (Truxton)			
SGL,PO, 250 mg, 100s ea	00463-2037-01	7.20	
1000s ea	00463-2037-10	39.00	
OCU-WASH (Geritrex)			
SOL,OP (24X113ML)			
113 ml 24s	54162-0150-04	153.36	
OCUBASIC (Basic Vitamins)			
TAB,PO, 100s ea	00761-0188-20	3.60	
OCUFRESH EYE SHOWER (Optics)			
SOL,OP (60X20ML,PF)			
9 mg/ml, 20 ml 60s	64108-0311-12	37.95	
OCUFRESH EYE WASH (Optics)			
SOL,OP (6X20ML,W/CUP,PF)			
9 mg/ml, 20 ml 6s	64108-0311-11	4.95	5.95
(PF)			
9 mg/ml, 473 ml	64108-0321-21	16.50	
OCULAR FORMULA (Rx Vitamins)			
CAP,PO, 60s ea	08429-0140-60	14.98	29.95
OCUSOFT FACIAL/SKIN CLEANSER (Ocusoft)			
SOL,TP, 30 ml	54799-0207-10	5.63	
240 ml	54799-0207-80	13.69	
OCUSOFT HAND SOAP (Ocusoft)			
LIQ,TP, 0.5%, 30 ml	54799-0208-10	5.63	
240 ml	54799-0208-80	9.94	
(REFILL)			
0.5%, 960 ml	54799-0208-95	27.44	
OCUSOFT IRRIGATING SOLUTION I (Ocusoft)			
SOL,OP, 30 ml	54799-0565-01	6.19	
120 ml	54799-0565-59	7.44	
OCUSOFT VMS (Ocusoft)			
TAB,PO, 60s ea	54799-0481-03	10.63	
OCUVITE (Bausch & Lomb Inc.)			
TAB,PO, 60s ea	24208-0387-60	8.29	
120s ea	24208-0387-62	11.32	
(Phys Total Care)			
REPACK			
TAB,PO, 60s ea	54868-1673-00	11.18	
OCUVITE ADULT 50+ (Bausch & Lomb Inc.)			
SGL,PO (SOFTGEL)			
50s ea	24208-0465-30	10.79	
OCUVITE EXTRA (Bausch & Lomb Inc.)			
TAB,PO, 50s ea	24208-0388-19	9.54	
OCUVITE LUTEIN (Bausch & Lomb Inc.)			
CAP,PO, 36s ea	24208-0403-19	10.79	
(Phys Total Care)			
REPACK			
CAP,PO, 36s ea	54868-4299-00	12.71	
OCUVITE PRESERVISION (Bausch & Lomb Inc.)			
TAB,PO, 120s ea	24208-0432-62	15.28	
240s ea	24208-0432-72	24.79	
(Phys Total Care)			
REPACK			
TAB,PO, 120s ea	54868-4709-00	17.35	
ODOR CLEANSE (Yerba)			
CAP,PO, 75 mg, 50s ea	46352-0004-52	5.37	8.95
ODOR-EATERS FOOT POWDER WITH ZORBITEX (Combe)			
POW,NA, 170 gm	11509-0004-46	4.00	
ODOR-EATERS ULTRA-COMFORT (Combe)			
DEV,NA (TRIM FIT, W/O CROWDING)			
2s ea	11509-0004-04	2.62	
6s ea	11509-0067-10	6.48	
ODOR-EATERS ULTRA-DURABLE (Combe)			
DEV,NA (HEAVY DUTY, TRIM TO FIT)			
2s ea	11509-0067-09	3.84	
OHM ALLERGY RELIEF (Ohm)			
TAB,PO, 10 mg, 500s ea	51660-0526-05	96.00	
OHMNI-CEN (Ohm)			
TAB,PO, 400 mg-32 mg,			
100s ea	51660-0015-01	1.75	
1000s ea	51660-0015-10	9.25	
OHMNI-GESIC (Ohm)			
TAB,PO, 325 mg-30 mg,			
24s ea	51660-0078-24	1.35	
90s ea	51660-0078-90	2.70	
1000s ea	51660-0078-01	2.95	
OIL OF EVENING PRIMROSE (Health Products Corp)			
CAP,PO (PF,SF,SOFTGEL)			
50s ea	39686-0016-09	5.25	
OILATUM-AD (Stiefel Consumer HealthCare)			
LOT,TP, 237 ml	00145-1157-08	7.98	11.99
OINTMENT BASE (Medco Lab)			
OIN,TP, 454 gm	11940-1520-06	8.00	
OLBAS (Penn Herb)			
OIL,TP, 9.6 ml	15486-0500-10	3.90	6.50
24.6 ml	15486-0500-20	7.50	12.50
49.5 ml	15486-0500-30	13.17	21.95
OLBAS ANALGESIC SALVE (Penn Herb)			
OIN,TP, 30 gm	15486-0502-10	4.17	6.95
OLBAS COUGH (Penn Herb)			
SYR,PO, 118 ml	15486-0504-20	3.57	5.95
OLBAS HERBAL BATH (Penn Herb)			
OIL,TP, 120 ml	15486-0503-10	3.90	6.50
240 ml	15486-0503-20	6.57	10.95
OLBAS INHALER (Penn Herb)			
DEV,NA, ea	15486-0505-10	2.37	3.95
OLBAS PASTILLES MAXIMUM STRENGTH (Penn Herb)			
LOZ,MM, 10 mg, 27s ea	15486-0506-10	2.37	3.95
OLBAS SPORT (Penn Herb)			
OIL,TP, 60 ml	15486-0501-10	3.90	6.50
120 ml	15486-0501-20	6.57	10.95
240 ml	15486-0501-30	11.97	19.95
OLEEVA (Allerderm Labs.)			
DEV,NA (SCAR MANAGEMENT)			
ea	34674-0025-00	55.95	69.95
OLEEVA CLEAR (Allerderm Labs.)			
DEV,NA (5"X5")			
ea	34674-0025-25	39.59	61.95
OLIVE (Ellon)			
SOL,SL (DROPS)			
10.5 ml	51762-0024-10		9.25
OLIVE LEAF (Key Company)			
CAP,PO, 500 mg, 60s ea	11694-0657-01	10.00	
120s ea	11694-0657-02	19.00	
OLIVE LEAF EXTRACT (Bio-Tech Pharm)			
CAP,PO, 500 mg, 100s ea	53191-0334-01	14.00	
OMEGA 3 (ADH)			
SGL,PO (PF,SF,SOFTGEL)			
1000 mg, 100s ea	60142-0700-01	6.98	13.95
OMEGA-3 1450 (Ocean Blue)			
SGL,PO (NATURAL ORANGE,SOFTGEL)			
725 mg, 60s ea	27912-0085-36	9.49	
120s ea	27912-0085-37	13.49	
OMEGA-3 2100 (Ocean Blue)			
PO (NATURAL ORANGE,SOFTGEL)			
1050 mg, 60s ea	27912-0086-17	13.00	
120s ea	27912-0086-16	22.05	
OMEGA-3 2100+ B VITAMINS (Ocean Blue)			
SGL,PO (NATURAL ORANGE,SOFTGEL)			
6 mcg-1050 mg-8 mg,			
60s ea	27912-0086-15	14.99	
120s ea	27912-0086-14	24.26	
OMEGALINIC (Key Company)			
SGL,PO (SOY-FREE,YEAST-FREE)			
100s ea	11694-0743-01	10.75	
OMEPRAZOLE (Major)			
TCP,PO, 20 mg, 14s ea	00904-5834-41	123.03	
28s ea	00904-5834-71	160.53	
42s ea	00904-5834-42	208.69	
(Perrigo)			
TCP,PO, 20 mg, 28s ea	45802-0888-30	19.21	
42s ea	45802-0888-55	26.06	
(Phys Total Care)			
REPACK			
TCP,PO, 20 mg, 42s ea	54868-5911-00	95.50	
OMNII GEL (Omnii Intl)			
GEL,DE (CINNAMON)			
0.4%, 129 gm	48878-4041-03	7.30	
(GRAPE)			
0.4%, 129 gm	48878-4021-03	7.30	
(MINT)			
0.4%, 129 gm	48878-4061-03	7.30	
(NATURAL)			
0.4%, 129 gm	48878-4051-03	7.30	
(RASPBERRY)			
0.4%, 129 gm	48878-4031-03	7.30	
OMNITROPE PEN 10 (Sandoz)			
DEV,NA, ea	00500-0138-20	180.00	
ea	94922-0201-33	180.00	
OMNITROPE PEN 5 (Sandoz)			
DEV,NA, ea	00781-9602-49	180.00	
ea	94922-0201-34	180.00	
ONCE DAILY (Prime Marketing)			
TAB,PO, 1000s ea	62107-0039-10	24.25	
100s ea	62107-0040-01	3.50	
1000s ea	62107-0040-10	19.95	
100s ea	62107-0039-01	3.60	
ONCE DAILY MULTI-VITAMIN (Altura)			
REPACK			
TAB,PO, 10s ea	63874-0021-10	1.26	
14s ea	63874-0021-14	1.58	
15s ea	63874-0021-15	1.68	
20s ea	63874-0021-20	2.25	
30s ea	63874-0021-30	3.38	
100s ea	63874-0021-01	11.25	
ONCOVITE (Mission)			
TAB,PO, 100s ea	00178-0550-01	20.00	
ONE DAILY (Cardinal Health)			
TAB,PO (PRIVATE LABEL)			
100s ea	37205-0080-78	2.54	
ONE DAILY + IRON (21st Century)			
TAB,PO, 365s ea	40985-0227-33		7.99
(Palmetto)			
REPACK			
TAB,PO, 365s ea	23490-5008-01	9.00	
ONE DAILY ESSENTIAL (21st Century)			
TAB,PO, 100s ea	40985-0226-60		4.99

PROD/MFR	HRI, UPC,NDC	AWP	SRP
(AmerisourceBergen)			
TAB,PO (PRIVATE LABEL)			
100s ea	24385-0139-78	4.49	4.99
250s ea	24385-0139-85	6.29	6.99
(Palmetto)			
REPACK			
TAB,PO, 30s ea	23490-7853-00	4.12	
ONE DAILY MAXIMUM (AmerisourceBergen)			
TAB,PO (PRIVATE LABEL)			
100s ea	24385-0679-78	6.29	6.99
ONE DAILY MULTIPLE VITAMIN WITH IRON (Amneal)			
TAB,PO (SF,STARCH-FREE)			
100s ea	65162-0400-10	3.55	
1000s ea	65162-0400-11	21.35	
ONE DAILY PLUS IRON (AmerisourceBergen)			
TAB,PO (PRIVATE LABEL)			
100s ea	24385-0148-78	6.29	6.99
250s ea	24385-0148-85	6.29	6.99
ONE DAILY PLUS MINERALS (Basic Vitamins)			
TAB,PO, 60s ea	00761-0124-12	2.40	
ONE DAILY W/CALCIUM/IRON/ZINC (Cardinal Health)			
TAB,PO (PRIVATE LABEL)			
100s ea	37205-0081-78	4.29	
ONE DAILY WOMEN'S (AmerisourceBergen)			
TAB,PO (PRIVATE LABEL)			
100s ea	24385-0680-78	6.29	6.99
ONE STEP AT A TIME (Lee Pharm)			
DEV,NA (NICOTINE FILTERS)			
4s ea	23558-0693-10	12.00	
(NICOTINE FILTERS,6X4)			
24s ea	23558-0693-11	72.00	
ONE STEP PREGNANCY TEST KIT (Reese)			
DEV,NA, ea	23513-0774-01	5.54	7.99
(VALUE PAK)			
2s ea	23513-0774-02		11.99
ONE TOUCH (Lifescan)			
DEV,NA (STRIP)			
25s ea	53885-0197-25	29.10	
(STRIP,2X25)			
50s ea	53885-0198-50	58.50	
(STRIP,4X25)			
100s ea	53885-0374-10	117.00	
(A-S Medication)			
REPACK			
DEV,NA (STRIP)			
50s ea	54569-4208-00	69.55	
ONE TOUCH BASIC SYSTEM (Lifescan)			
DEV,NA, ea	53885-0325-01	50.00	
ONE TOUCH FINE POINT LANCETS (Lifescan)			
DEV,NA, 100s ea	53885-0046-10	10.08	
ONE TOUCH GLUCOSE CONTROL (Lifescan)			
DEV,NA (NORMAL)			
2s ea	53885-0272-02	7.38	
ONE TOUCH PROFILE SYSTEM (Lifescan)			
DEV,NA, ea	53885-0372-01	118.75	
ONE TOUCH ULTRA (Lifescan)			
DEV,NA (STRIP)			
25s ea	53885-0994-25	29.10	
(STRIP,2X25)			
50s ea	53885-0244-50	58.86	
(STRIP,4X25)			
100s ea	53885-0245-10	117.72	
(A-S Medication)			
REPACK			
DEV,NA, 50s ea	54569-6080-00	58.44	
(Phys Total Care)			
REPACK			
DEV,NA, 100s ea	54868-5265-00	138.18	
ONE TOUCH ULTRA GLUCOSE CONTROL (Lifescan)			
DEV,NA, ea	53885-0416-01	4.68	
2s ea	53885-0458-02	8.70	
ONE TOUCH ULTRA SYSTEM (Lifescan)			
DEV,NA (METER,SOL,LANCETS)			
ea	53885-0247-01	68.75	
ONE TOUCH ULTRASMART (Arkray)			
DEV,NA (PRIVATE LABEL)			
ea	08317-7100-01	12.00	
(Lifescan)			
DEV,NA, ea	53885-0524-01	75.00	
ONE TOUCH ULTRASOFT LANCET (Lifescan)			
DEV,NA, 100s ea	53885-0393-10	10.32	
(Phys Total Care)			
REPACK			
DEV,NA, 100s ea	54868-5798-00	11.54	
ONE-A-DAY 50 PLUS (Bayer HealthCare)			
TAB,PO, 50s ea	16500-0081-05	4.66	
80s ea	16500-0081-08	6.39	
ONE-A-DAY ACTIVE (Bayer HealthCare)			
TAB,PO, 50s ea	16500-0503-79	6.39	
ONE-A-DAY ESSENTIAL (Bayer HealthCare)			
TAB,PO, 75s ea	16500-0073-17	4.66	
130s ea	16500-0073-03	6.39	
ONE-A-DAY KIDS SCOOBY-DOO COMPLETE (Bayer HealthCare)			
CTB,PO, 50s ea	16500-0506-03	4.31	
ONE-A-DAY MAXIMUM (Bayer HealthCare)			
TAB,PO, 60s ea	16500-0075-13	4.66	
100s ea	16500-0075-11	6.39	
ONE-A-DAY MEN'S (Bayer HealthCare)			
TAB,PO (NO IRON)			
60s ea	16500-0080-04	4.66	
100s ea	16500-0080-12	6.39	
200s ea	16500-0080-14	11.53	
ONE-A-DAY SCOOBY-DOO W/CALCIUM (Bayer HealthCare)			
CTB,PO, 50s ea	16500-0506-04	4.31	
ONE-A-DAY WOMEN'S (Bayer HealthCare)			
TAB,PO, 60s ea	16500-0074-06	4.66	
100s ea	16500-0074-10	6.39	
200s ea	16500-0074-12	11.53	
ONE-GRAM C (Carlson,J.R.)			
TAB,PO, 1000 mg,			
100s ea	88395-0033-01	7.20	14.40
250s ea	88395-0033-02	15.60	31.20
500s ea	88395-0033-05	32.20	64.40
ONE-TIME CENTRAL LINE DRESSING TRAY (Medical Action Ind.)			
DEV,NA (10CMX14CM,W/OPSITE)			
20s ea	73577-0612-29	105.12	
(10CMX28CM,W/OPSITE)			
20s ea	73577-0612-28	119.88	
(I.V DRESS,NON-OCCLUSIVE)			
20s ea	73577-0612-24	158.76	
(I.V. DRESS,OCCLUSIVE)			
20s ea	73577-0612-26	116.28	
(W/ACCESSORIES)			
20s ea	73577-0612-45	90.00	
20s ea	73577-0612-47	106.80	
20s ea	73577-0612-48	82.08	
(W/AIRSTRIP)			
20s ea	73577-0612-30	103.80	
(W/BIOCLUSIVE)			
20s ea	73577-0612-56	100.56	
(W/TEGADERM)			
20s ea	73577-0612-49	99.12	
ONE-TIME FINE POINT TISSUE SCISSORS (Medical Action Ind.)			
DEV,NA (4 1/4")			
20s ea	73577-0562-54	37.01	
ONE-TIME KELLY HEMOSTAT (Medical Action Ind.)			
DEV,NA (CURVED,5 1/2")			
20s ea	73577-0562-25	50.16	
(STRAIGHT,5 1/2")			
20s ea	73577-0562-21	50.16	
ONE-TIME LITTAUER SCISSORS (Medical Action Ind.)			
DEV,NA (4 1/2")			
20s ea	73577-0562-47	20.22	
ONE-TIME MEDICAL SUTURE REMOVAL (Medical Action Ind.)			
DEV,NA (FAIR-LINE,PLSTIC HANDLE)			
50s ea	73577-0614-01	39.72	
(FAIR-LINE)			
50s ea	73577-0613-00	49.20	
ONE-TIME MOSQUITO HEMOSTAT (Medical Action Ind.)			
DEV,NA (CURVED,4 3/4")			
20s ea	73577-0562-24	50.16	
(STRAIGHT,4 3/4")			
20s ea	73577-0562-20	50.16	
ONE-TIME MOUSE TOOTH FORCEPS (Medical Action Ind.)			
DEV,NA (5")			
20s ea	73577-0562-41	15.60	
ONE-TIME NEEDLE HOLDER (Medical Action Ind.)			
DEV,NA (SERRATED,5")			
20s ea	73577-0562-28	52.92	
ONE-TIME SCALPEL ASSEMBLY (Medical Action Ind.)			
DEV,NA (METAL HANDLE,10" BLADE)			
20s ea	73577-0562-14	27.60	
(METAL HANDLE,11" BLADE)			
20s ea	73577-0562-73	27.60	
(METAL HANDLE,15" BLADE)			
20s ea	73577-0562-16	27.60	
ONE-TIME SHARP/BLUNT SCISSORS (Medical Action Ind.)			
DEV,NA (5 1/4")			
20s ea	73577-0562-49	30.84	
ONE-TIME STAPLE REMOVER (Medical Action Ind.)			
DEV,NA (STAINLESS STEEL,4")			
10s ea	73577-0562-66	18.60	
ONE-TIME SUTURE REMOVAL TRAY (Medical Action Ind.)			
DEV,NA, 50s ea	73577-0611-00	60.54	
50s ea	73577-0611-02	50.04	
50s ea	73577-0611-04	93.12	
50s ea	73577-0611-05	79.50	
50s ea	73577-0611-06	103.20	
50s ea	73577-0611-07	84.00	
50s ea	73577-0611-08	45.90	
50s ea	73577-0611-09	80.22	
50s ea	73577-0611-11	63.54	
50s ea	73577-0611-12	111.60	
ONE-TIME THUMB FORCEPS (Medical Action Ind.)			
DEV,NA (METAL,ETCHED TIP,5")			
20s ea	73577-0562-44	16.92	
(PLASTIC,5")			
20s ea	73577-0562-36	10.80	
(W/INSERT,5")			
20s ea	73577-0562-38	18.00	
ONE-TIME WEBSTER NEEDLE HOLDER (Medical Action Ind.)			
DEV,NA (5")			
20s ea	73577-0562-30	55.80	
ONETOUCH SURESOFT (Lifescan)			
DEV,NA (DUAL SITE)			
100s ea	53885-0141-10		17.00
(GENTLE)			
200s ea	53885-0140-20		34.00
(REGULAR)			
200s ea	53885-0139-20		34.00
ONETOUCH ULTRA 2 BLOOD GLUCOSE MONITORING SYSTEM (Lifescan)			
DEV,NA, ea	53885-0448-01	68.75	
ONETOUCH ULTRAMINI BLOOD GLUCOSE MONITORING SYSTEM (Lifescan)			
DEV,NA, ea	53885-0208-01	18.75	
(BLACK)			
ea	53885-0001-30	18.75	
(GREEN)			
ea	53885-0001-29	18.75	
(PINK)			
ea	53885-0001-28	18.75	
ONSET FORTE (Medique)			
TAB,PO (50X2)			
162.5 mg-2 mg-5 mg,			
100s ea UD	47682-0102-33	7.71	
(250X2)			
162.5 mg-2 mg-5 mg,			
500s ea UD	47682-0102-13	31.71	
OPCON-A ALLERGY (Bausch & Lomb Inc.)			
SOL,OP (1X15ML,DROPS)			
0.027%-0.315%,			
15 ml	10119-0020-90	5.23	
OPERAND POVIDONE-IODINE DOUCHE (Aplicare)			
SOL,VG, 10%, 237 ml	52380-1730-08	5.51	
OPERAND POVIDONE-IODINE PERIWASH (Aplicare)			
SOL,TP (W/EMPTY APPLICATOR BOT)			
10%, 237 ml	52380-1880-07	8.35	
OPERAND POVIDONE-IODINE SCRUB (Aplicare)			
SOL,TP (W/HAND PUMP)			
7.5%, 473 ml	52380-1855-03	7.01	
OPERAND POVIDONE-IODINE WHIRLPOOL (Aplicare)			
SOL,TP (LATEX-FREE)			
1%, 3800 ml	18407-0002-28	34.66	

PROD/MFR	HRI, UPC,NDC	AWP	SRP
OPSITE FLEXIGRID TRANSPARENT (Smith & Nephew)			
DEV,NA (4"X4 3/4")			
10s ea	**00223-0438-51**	21.04	16.83
(6"X8")			
10s ea	**00223-0438-54**	46.48	37.18
(4 3/4"X10")			
20s ea	**00230-0438-53**	97.06	77.65
(4"X4 3/4")			
50s ea	**00223-0438-52**	86.13	68.90
(2 3/8"X2 3/4")			
100s ea	**00223-0438-50**	53.60	42.88
OPSITE IV3000 HIGH MVP TRANSPARENT (Animas Corp.)			
DEV,NA (2 3/8" X 2 3/4")			
100s ea	**65781-0420-00**	83.85	
(Smith & Nephew)			
DEV,NA (4"X4 3/4")			
50s ea	**40565-0115-63**	109.30	87.44
(2 3/8"X2 3/4")			
100s ea	**40565-0115-62**	53.73	42.98
(2"X1 1/2")			
100s ea	**40565-0115-71**	55.93	44.74
OPSITE IV3000 TAPE HANDLES (Smith & Nephew)			
DEV,NA (4"X5")			
10s ea	**40565-0115-76**	24.80	19.84
50s ea	**40565-0115-77**	109.30	87.44
(4"X8")			
50s ea	**40565-0115-70**	175.26	140.21
OPSITE POST-OP COMPOSITE (Smith & Nephew)			
DEV,NA (3 3/4"X3 3/8")			
20s ea	**00223-0410-92**	29.15	23.32
(6 1/8"X3 3/8")			
20s ea	**00223-0410-93**	44.21	35.37
(2 1/2"X2")			
100s ea	**00223-0410-91**	73.71	58.97
OPSITE TRANSPARENT ADHESIVE (Smith & Nephew)			
DEV,NA (11"X11 3/4")			
10s ea	**00223-0049-87**	83.70	66.96
(11"X17 3/4")			
10s ea	**00223-0049-88**	112.70	90.16
(11"X4")			
10s ea	**00223-0403-79**	38.61	30.89
(11"X6")			
10s ea	**00223-0049-86**	56.69	45.35
(17 3/4"X21 5/8")			
10s ea	**00223-0049-89**	125.84	100.67
(5 1/2"X4")			
10s ea	**00223-0049-63**	19.85	15.88
(5 1/2"X10")			
20s ea	**00223-0049-67**	85.68	68.54
(5 1/2"X4")			
50s ea	**00223-0049-75**	83.61	66.89
OPTI-C (Key Company)			
TAB,PO (FILM-COATED)			
30s ea	**11694-0737-30**	3.00	
90s ea	**11694-0737-90**	6.00	
OPTI-CLEAN II (Alcon Labs Cons Prod)			
SOL,NA, 20 ml	**00650-0104-20**	8.58	
OPTI-CLEAR (Major)			
SOL,OP, 0.05%, 15 ml	**00904-2992-35**	2.15	
OPTI-FREE DAILY CLEANER (Alcon Labs Cons Prod)			
SOL,NA, 20 ml	**00650-0106-20**	8.58	
OPTI-FREE EXPRESS (Alcon Labs Cons Prod)			
SOL,NA (NO RUB FORMULA)			
120 ml	**00650-0132-04**	4.09	
OPTI-FREE EXPRESS REWETTING DROPS (Alcon Labs Cons Prod)			
SOL,OP (THIMEROSAL-FREE)			
10 ml	**00650-0193-10**	5.24	
20 ml	**00650-0193-20**	7.62	
OPTI-FREE LENS CASE (Alcon Labs Cons Prod)			
DEV,NA, ea	**00650-0180-02**	5.04	
OPTI-FREE REPLENISH (Alcon Labs Cons Prod)			
SOL,OP, 118 ml	**00650-0356-04**	4.09	
300 ml	**00650-0356-10**	8.42	
(TWIN PAC,2X300ML)			
300 ml 2s	**00650-0356-05**	15.41	
OPTI-FREE REPLENISH REWETTING DROPS (Alcon Labs Cons Prod)			
SOL,OP (THIMEROSAL-FREE)			
10 ml	**00650-0192-29**	5.24	
OPTI-FREE SUPRACLENS (Alcon Labs Cons Prod)			
SOL,NA, 3 ml	**00650-0285-03**	6.42	

PROD/MFR	HRI, UPC,NDC	AWP	SRP
OPTI-PLUS (Key Company)			
CAP,PO (CORN-FREE,GLUTEN-FREE)			
60s ea	**11694-0665-01**	7.50	
180s ea	**11694-0665-18**	19.50	
OPTI-VITAMINS (AmerisourceBergen)			
TAB,PO (PRIVATE LABEL)			
60s ea	**24385-0809-72**	6.29	6.99
OPTICLUDE ORTHOPTIC EYE PATCH (3M Health Care)			
DEV,NA (JUNIOR)			
20s ea	**08333-1537-01**	4.56	
(REGULAR)			
20s ea	**08333-1539-01**	4.56	
OPTIFOAM ADHESIVE FOAM (Medline)			
DEV,NA (4"X4")			
10s ea	**53329-0450-40**	45.56	
(6"X6")			
10s ea	**53329-0450-42**	78.82	
OPTIFOAM NON-ADHESIVE FOAM (Medline)			
DEV,NA (4"X4")			
10s ea	**08327-0451-40**	44.82	
(6"X6")			
10s ea	**08327-0451-42**	77.27	
OPTIGENE 3 (Pfeiffer)			
SOL,OP, 0.05%, 15 ml	**00927-0167-23**	1.74	3.13
OPTIGENE EYE WASH (Pfeiffer)			
SOL,OP, 1.11%, 120 ml	**00927-0281-12**	2.47	4.44
OPTIMENTAL (Abbott)			
LIQ,PO (RTF,VANILLA)			
240 ml	**70074-0546-39**	7.84	
(RTH,VANILLA)			
1000 ml	**70074-0570-46**	33.85	
OPTIMUM ACIDOPHILUS (Magno-Humphries)			
CAP,PO (PRIVATE LABEL)			
500 million org,			
100s ea	**43292-0500-22**	2.50	4.99
OPTIMUM CARE SYSTEM (Lobob)			
KIT,NA (W/LID SCRUB & LENS CASE)			
ea	**34672-0102-40**	12.90	18.95
OPTIMUM CLEANING/DISINFECT/STORAGE (Lobob)			
SOL,NA (FOR RIGID GAS PERM LENS)			
118 ml	**34672-0102-68**	5.00	9.50
OPTIMUM EXTRA STRENGTH CLEANER (Lobob)			
LIQ,NA (FOR RIGID GAS PERM LENS)			
60 ml	**34672-0102-50**	5.00	9.50
OPTIMUM WETTING/REWETTING (Lobob)			
LIQ,NA (FOR RIGID GAS PERM LENS)			
30 ml	**34672-0102-70**	5.00	9.50
OPTIPORE (Convatec)			
DEV,NA (WOUND CLEANSING)			
25s ea	**68455-0108-10**	37.39	49.14
OPTIQUE 1 (Boiron)			
SOL,OP (AMP)			
0.4 ml 10s UD	**06962-0193-71**	4.04	6.79
0.4 ml 20s	**06969-0277-71**	6.07	10.19
OPTISOURCE (Nestle)			
CTB,PO (120X12)			
1440s ea	**43900-0175-00**	308.88	
OPTIUM (Abbott)			
DEV,NA, ea	**57599-0899-01**	71.94	
(STRIP)			
50s ea	**57599-9134-04**	46.92	
100s ea	**57599-9135-05**	85.79	
OPTIUM MONITORING SYSTEM (Abbott)			
DEV,NA, ea	**57599-9132-01**	71.94	
OPTIVE (Allergan Inc)			
SOL,OP (2X5ML,DROPS)			
0.5%-0.9%, 5 ml 2s	**00023-3240-10**	7.84	
5 ml 2s	**00233-0240-10**	7.46	
(1X15ML,DROPS)			
0.5%-0.9%, 15 ml	**00023-3240-15**	9.14	
(1X30ML,DROPS)			
0.5%-0.9%, 30 ml	**00023-3240-30**	13.43	
30 ml	**00233-0240-30**	12.67	
OPTIVE SENSITIVE (Allergan Inc)			
SOL,OP (30X0.4ML,SINGLE-USE,PF)			
0.5%-0.9%,			
0.4 ml 30s	**00023-3416-30**	9.54	
OPTIVITE P.M.T. (Optimox)			
TAB,PO, 180s ea	**50520-0001-03**	13.00	18.00
(Phys Total Care)			
REPACK			
TAB,PO, 180s ea	**54868-1567-00**	19.28	

PROD/MFR	HRI, UPC,NDC	AWP	SRP
OPTULLE (Consolidated Midland)			
DRE,TP (5 MTR/19 CM)			
ea	**00223-3503-00**	17.50	
(7 MTR/10 CM)			
ea	**00223-3502-00**	12.50	
36s ea	**00223-3500-03**	5.50	
ORA FILM (Apothecus)			
FIL,MM (FREE 12 EXTRA STRIPS)			
6%, 24s ea	**48723-0042-57**	3.32	
ORABASE SOOTHE-N-SEAL (Colgate Oral)			
LIQ,MM (W/10 APPLICATORS)			
1 ml	**38341-0104-06**	8.11	
ORABASE-B (Colgate Oral)			
GEL,MM, 20%, 7 gm	**38341-0066-57**	3.63	
ORABASE-B MAXIMUM STRENGTH (Colgate Oral)			
PAS,MM, 20%, 6 gm	**38341-0065-45**	3.75	3.06
ORAFIX SPECIAL (Hogil)			
CRE,NA (MAXIMUM HOLD)			
42 gm	**95814-0699-08**	2.28	
72 gm	**95814-0699-09**	3.55	
ORAFIX ULTRA (Hogil)			
CRE,NA (SUPER HOLD)			
96 gm	**95814-0700-01**	4.20	
ORAGESIC (Parnell)			
SOL,MM (SF)			
1%, 237 ml	**50930-0099-08**	5.30	7.99
ORAJEL (Del)			
GEL,MM (REGULAR STRENGTH)			
10%, 5.3 gm	**10310-0320-49**	3.56	5.35
7 gm	**10310-0222-40**	3.56	5.35
9.4 gm	**10310-0222-13**	4.64	6.97
ORAJEL ADVANCED TOOTH DESENSITIZER (Del)			
GEL,DE (W/APPLICATORS)			
1 ml	**10310-0324-39**	3.60	5.40
ORAJEL ANTI-BACTERIAL BLEEDING GUM RINSE (Del)			
SOL,MM (MINT)			
0.1%, 473.6 ml	**10310-0324-98**	5.39	8.09
ORAJEL ANTISEPTIC MOUTH SORE RINSE (Del)			
SOL,PO, 1.5%, 473.6 ml	**10310-0324-99**	5.39	8.09
ORAJEL BABY DAY&NIGHT (Del)			
GEL,MM (AF)			
ea	**10310-0319-55**	4.79	7.18
ORAJEL BABY LIQUID TEETHING MEDICINE (Del)			
GEL,MM (W/CHAMOMILE)			
7.5%, 13.3 ml	**10310-0318-56**	4.19	6.28
ORAJEL BABY NIGHTTIME TEETHING PAIN MEDICINE (Del)			
GEL,MM (AF)			
10%, 5.3 gm	**10310-0339-40**	4.19	6.28
ORAJEL BABY TEETHING MEDICINE (Del)			
GEL,MM, 7.5%, 9.4 gm	**10310-0033-13**	4.19	6.28
(CHERRY FLAVOR)			
7.5%, 11.9 gm	**10310-0321-94**	4.19	6.28
ORAJEL BABY TEETHING SWABS (Del)			
SWA,MM, 7.5%, 12s ea	**10310-0340-38**	4.07	6.10
ORAJEL BABY TOOTH & GUM CLEANSER (Del)			
GEL,MM (FLUORIDE-FREE)			
28.3 gm	**10310-0322-50**	3.29	4.93
ORAJEL BABY TOOTH/GUM CLEANSER (Del)			
GEL,MM (MIXED FRUIT)			
19.8 gm	**10310-0322-70**	2.93	4.39
ORAJEL DENTURE PLUS (Del)			
GEL,MM, 15%-2%, 9 gm	**10310-0377-53**	2.23	3.35
ORAJEL DRY MOUTH MOISTURIZING (Del)			
SPR,PO (SF,MINT)			
18%, 48.8 ml	**10310-0323-54**	4.56	6.84
ORAJEL DRY MOUTH MOISTURIZING GEL (Del)			
GEL,MM (SF)			
18%, 42 gm	**10310-0322-80**	4.56	6.84
ORAJEL KIDS SORE THROAT RELIEF STRIPS (Del)			
FIL,MM (SF,CHERRY)			
28 mg, 20s ea	**10310-0324-58**	3.48	5.22
ORAJEL KIDS SORE THROAT RELIEF STRIPS W/ VITAMIN C (Del)			
FIL,MM (SF,ORANGE)			
28 mg, 20s ea	**10310-0325-24**	3.48	5.22
ORAJEL MAXIMUM STRENGTH (Del)			
GEL,MM, 20%, 5.3 gm	**10310-0320-50**	4.79	7.18
7 gm	**10310-0283-40**	4.79	7.18
9.4 gm	**10310-0320-68**	5.39	8.08
11.9 gm	**10310-0283-13**	5.39	8.08
SOL,MM, 20%, 13.5 ml	**10310-0329-45**	5.39	8.08

PROD/MFR	HRI, UPC,NDC	AWP	SRP
ORAJEL MEDICATED COLD SORE BRUSH (Del)			
SOL,TP, 0.5%-20%-2%-65%,			
1.48 ml	10310-0325-23	5.39	8.08
ORAJEL MEDICATED MOUTH SORE SWAB (Del)			
SWA,MM (MAXIMUM STRENGTH)			
20%, 8s ea	10310-0340-06	4.79	7.18
ORAJEL MEDICATED TOOTHACHE SWAB (Del)			
SWA,MM (MAXIMUM STRENGTH)			
20%, 8s ea	10310-0374-41	4.79	7.18
ORAJEL MOUTH SORE MEDICINE (Del)			
GEL,MM, 0.02%-20%-0.1%,			
5.3 gm	10310-0318-40	3.85	5.78
9.4 gm	10310-0320-52	4.99	7.49
11.9 gm	10310-0318-05	4.99	7.49
(Phys Total Care)			
REPACK			
GEL,MM (1X5.3GM)			
0.02%-20%-0.1%,			
5.3 gm	54868-2603-00	7.14	
ORAJEL MULTI-ACTION COLD SORE (Del)			
GEL,MM, 0.5%-20%-3%-2%-65%,			
9.4 gm	10310-0071-62	5.08	7.61
ORAJEL PM MAXIMUM STRENGTH (Del)			
CRE,MM, 20%, 5.3 gm	10310-0320-51	5.39	8.08
ORAJEL PROTECTIVE MOUTH SORE DISCS (Del)			
LOZ,MM (MAXIMUM STRENGTH)			
15 mg, 8s ea UD	10310-0324-49	5.39	8.08
ORAJEL SENSITIVE TOOTHPASTE FOR ADULTS (Del)			
GEL,DE (FRESH MINT)			
113 gm	10310-0319-54	2.40	3.60
ORAJEL SEVERE PAIN FORMULA (Del)			
GEL,MM, 20%, 9.4 gm	10310-0325-01	6.58	9.88
ORAJEL TODDLER TRAINING TOOTHPASTE (Del)			
PAS,DE (FLUORIDE-FREE)			
2%-0.12%, 42.5 gm	10310-0339-72	2.81	4.21
42.5 gm	10310-0339-73	2.81	4.21
ORAJEL TOOTHACHE POWDER (Del)			
POW,PO (MAXIMUM STRENGTH,CITRUS)			
1000 mg, 8s ea UD	10310-0324-50	5.39	8.08
ORAJEL ULTRA MOUTH SORE (Del)			
GEL,MM, 15%-2%, 9.4 gm	10310-0322-24	5.39	8.08
ORAL PAIN RELIEF (Major)			
SOL,MM (1X15ML,MAX STRENGTH)			
20%, 15 ml	00904-5899-35	4.23	
ORAL PEROXIDE (Major)			
SOL,MM, 10%, 60 ml	00904-4062-03	5.50	
ORALYTE (Rugby)			
SOL,PO (BUBBLE GUM)			
1000 ml	00536-0936-86	6.58	
(FRUIT)			
1000 ml	00536-0935-86	6.58	
(GRAPE)			
1000 ml	00536-1385-86	6.58	
(UNFLAVORED)			
1000 ml	00536-0004-86	6.58	
ORALYTE FREEZE POPS (Rugby)			
PO (CHERRY,GRAPE,ORANGE)			
62.5 ml 16s	00536-1395-17	6.58	
ORAMAGIC PLUS (MPM Medical Inc.)			
PDR,MM (AF,LEMON LIME)			
10%, 60 ml	66977-0223-02	7.96	8.85
210 ml	66977-0223-08	19.88	22.09
ORANYL PE PLUS (Medique)			
TAB,PO (150X2,SF,LACTOSE-FREE)			
500 mg-5 mg, 300s ea	10244-0548-63	30.86	
ORASEPT (Pharmakon)			
LIQ,MM, 1.53%-1.53%,			
15 ml	55422-0201-15	2.52	5.25
ORASEPT MOUTHWASH/GARGLE (Pharmakon)			
LIQ,PO (AF,SF)			
0.1%, 120 ml	55422-0202-04	0.90	1.52
240 ml	55422-0202-08	1.09	2.25
ORASEPT THROAT (Pharmakon)			
SPR,MM, 0.99%-53.82%-1.03%,			
45 ml	55422-0501-45	2.31	4.78
ORAZINC 110 (Mericon)			
TAB,PO, 110 mg, 100s ea	00394-0124-02	4.41	
ORAZINC 220 (Mericon)			
CAP,PO, 220 mg, 100s ea	00394-0499-02	7.85	
OREXIN (Lee Pharm)			
CTB,PO, 100s ea	23558-0560-60	66.00	

PROD/MFR	HRI, UPC,NDC	AWP	SRP
ORNEX (Ascher)			
TAB,PO (CAPLET)			
325 mg-30 mg,			
24s ea	00225-0590-08	6.18	
48s ea	00225-0590-04	11.22	
ORNEX MAXIMUM-STRENGTH (Ascher)			
TAB,PO, 500 mg-30 mg,			
24s ea	00225-0600-08	7.44	
ORNITHINE (Key Company)			
L-ORNITHINE-500			
CAP,PO (SF)			
500 mg, 60s ea	11694-0812-01	8.00	
500s ea	11694-0812-05	48.00	
ORTHO ALL-FLEX DIAPHRAGM (Ortho-McNeil Pharm)			
DEV,NA (65MM,LATEX-FREE)			
ea	00062-3310-00	41.60	
(70MM,LATEX-FREE)			
ea	00062-3311-00	41.60	
(75MM,LATEX-FREE)			
ea	00062-3312-00	41.60	
(80MM,LATEX-FREE)			
ea	00062-3313-00	41.60	
ORTHO ALL-FLEX DIAPHRAGM FITTING SET (Ortho-McNeil Pharm)			
DEV,NA, ea	00062-3644-03	47.94	
ORTHO-NESIC (Blaine)			
GEL,TP (1X89GM)			
0.2%-3.5%, 89 gm	65373-0400-02	17.00	31.00
ORTHOGEL (Southwood)			
REPACK			
GEL,TP, 0.2%-3.5%,			
105 ml	00490-0063-01	4.66	
(COLD THERAPY)			
0.2%-3.5%,			
113.4 gm	58016-4836-01	15.00	
ORUDIS KT (Wyeth Consumer)			
TAB,PO, 12.5 mg, 24s ea	00573-0130-20	2.96	
50s ea	00573-0130-30	5.10	
100s ea	00573-0130-40	8.57	
(Pharma Pac)			
REPACK			
TAB,PO, 12.5 mg, 30s ea	52959-0529-30	15.00	
100s ea	52959-0529-00	29.66	
OS 1 (Milupa North America)			
PDR,PO (2X500GM)			
500 gm 2s	81361-9348-01	150.00	
OS 2 (Nutricia)			
PDR,PO (2X500GM)			
500 gm 2s	81361-9349-01	291.20	
OS-CAL 500 (Glaxo)			
CTB,PO, 500 mg, 60s ea	00088-1657-41	6.11	
TAB,PO, 500 mg, 75s ea	00088-1651-75	6.79	
160s ea	00766-1651-60	12.24	
OS-CAL 500 + D (Glaxo)			
TAB,PO, 500 mg-200 iu,			
75s ea	00088-1654-75	6.79	
160s ea	00766-1654-60	12.24	
OS-CAL 500+D (Glaxo)			
CTB,PO (SF,GLUTEN-FREE)			
500 mg-400 iu,			
60s ea	00881-0663-01	7.13	
120s ea	07661-0663-10	12.24	
TAB,PO (GLUTEN-FREE)			
500 mg-200 iu,			
75s ea	00881-0654-75	7.13	
160s ea	07661-0654-60	12.85	
210s ea	07661-0656-75	15.10	
500 mg-400 iu,			
60s ea	00881-0651-25	6.79	
120s ea	00881-0651-49	12.24	
OSCAL ULTRA 600 (Glaxo)			
TAB,PO, 60s ea	07661-0658-10	6.79	
120s ea	07661-0658-20	12.85	
OSCILLOCOCCINUM (Boiron)			
PEL,PO, 200 c, 3s ea	06969-0999-01	4.79	7.99
6s ea	06969-0998-51	8.76	14.59
OSCO ALCOHOL PREP (Albertson's)			
DEV,NA, 100s ea	41280-0230-60	2.61	
OSCO ASPERCIN (Albertson's)			
TAB,PO, 325 mg, 100s ea	41280-0220-74	2.94	
OSCO CONFORM (Albertson's)			
DEV,NA, ea	04000-0002-85	2.13	
OSCO SORE THROAT (Albertson's)			
SPR,MM, 1.4%, 180 ml	41280-0211-41	2.72	

PROD/MFR	HRI, UPC,NDC	AWP	SRP
OSHA (Botanical Labs.)			
LIQ,PO, 30 ml	41954-0020-71	5.00	9.99
OSMOLITE (Abbott)			
LIQ,PO, 240 ml	70074-0407-09	2.12	
OSMOLITE 1 CAL (Abbott)			
LIQ,PO, 240 ml	70074-0407-35	2.21	
1000 ml	70074-0806-68	13.27	
1500 ml	70074-0526-01	19.91	
OSMOLITE 1.2 CAL (Abbott)			
LIQ,PO, 240 ml	70074-0531-21	2.50	
1000 ml	70074-0531-23	15.02	
1500 ml	70074-0531-17	22.54	
OSMOLITE 1.5 CAL (Abbott)			
LIQ,PO, 240 ml	70074-0574-70	2.35	
OSMOLITE ROSS READY-TO-HANG (Abbott)			
LIQ,PO, 1000 ml	70074-0503-50	12.66	
OSTEO-PORETICAL (TriMarc Labs)			
TAB,PO, 600 mg-1000 iu,			
60s ea	68752-0011-60	9.65	
OSTEO-TECH (Bio-Tech Pharm)			
CAP,PO, 100s ea	53191-0406-01	15.00	
OSTIDERM ROLL-ON (Pedinol)			
LOT,TP, 90 ml	00884-2052-03		13.50
OSTOMY BELT (Coloplast)			
DEV,NA (ADJUSTABLE)			
ea	11701-0825-10	9.37	9.81
OSTOMY PASTE (Coloplast)			
DEV,NA (12X57GM)			
57 gm 12s	11701-0801-51	133.08	139.32
60 gm 12s	11701-0801-23	79.08	82.68
OSTOMY STRIP (Coloplast)			
DEV,NA (10X8,AF)			
57 gm 80s	11701-0910-03	94.96	99.36
OTHER SONIC (Pharm Innov)			
GEL,TP, 60 ml	00036-1111-60	1.23	1.61
250 ml	00036-1111-25	1.61	2.09
5000 ml	00036-1111-05	11.58	16.00
OTIX EAR WAX REMOVAL AID (Monticello)			
SOL,OT, 6.5%, 15 ml	11868-0040-11	2.90	
(W/IRRIGATOR& EAR PLUGS)			
6.5%, 15 ml	11868-0040-21	3.99	
OUTGRO (Medtech)			
LIQ,TP, 20%, 9.3 ml	75137-0531-10	4.63	
OVARY (Key Company)			
CAP,PO, 180 mg, 100s ea	11694-0901-01	6.00	
500s ea	11694-0901-03	22.00	
(Miller)			
TAB,PO, 125 mg, 100s ea	17204-0512-40	7.26	12.00
OVER-THE-GUIDEWIRE GASTROSTOMY (Ross Nutr)			
DEV,NA (16 FR, W/WEBBED BUMPER)			
ea	70074-0507-25	150.54	
OVER-THE-GUIDEWIRE JEJUNAL (Abbott)			
DEV,NA (10FR)			
ea	70074-0507-73	76.19	
(12FR)			
ea	70074-0551-65	76.19	
(8 FR)			
ea	70074-0514-81	76.19	
OVER-THE-GUIDEWIRE NASOJEJUNAL (Abbott)			
DEV,NA (FEEDING TUBE,10 FR)			
ea	70074-0513-35	78.00	
OX-BILE (Key Company)			
POW,RC, 85 gm	11694-0652-01	8.25	
OXALIS (Weleda)			
OIN,TP, 36 gm	55946-0322-50	5.70	
OXEPA (Abbott)			
LIQ,PO, 237 ml 24s	70074-0543-87	273.60	
(RTH)			
1000 ml	70074-0570-44	47.88	
OXI-FREEDA (Freeda)			
TAB,PO (PF,SF,DYE-FREE)			
100s ea	10432-0279-01	15.57	25.95
250s ea	10432-0279-02	29.97	49.95
OXIPLEN (Med Prods Panamer)			
CAP,PO, 50s ea	00576-0593-50	12.60	
OXIPOR VHC (Medtech)			
LOT,TP, 120 ml	75137-0541-20	19.40	
25%, 57 ml	75137-0541-10	11.72	
OXY-OTIC (Consolidated Midland)			
SOL,OT, 6.5%, 15 ml	00223-6573-15	2.25	
OXYMETAZOLINE HCL (Consolidated Midland)			
SOL,NS, 0.05%, 15 ml	00223-6366-15	2.50	

PROD/MFR	HRI, UPC,NDC	AWP	SRP
(Perrigo)			
SPR,NS, 0.05%, 30 ml	45802-0410-59	3.99	
(Taro)			
SPR,NS, 0.05%, 15 ml	51672-2030-05	2.85	
30 ml	51672-2030-03	4.05	
(Dispensing Solutions)			
REPACK			
SPR,NS, 0.05%, 15 ml	55045-1328-05	2.85	
(Phys Total Care)			
REPACK			
SPR,NS, 0.05%, 15 ml	54868-2053-00	6.03	
(Physician Partner)			
REPACK			
SPR,NS, 0.05%, 30 ml	21695-0875-30	8.10	
OXYZAL (Gordon)			
LIQ,TP, 1:2000, 120 ml	10481-1025-02	5.65	
OYSCO 500 (Rugby)			
TAB,PO, 500 mg, 60s ea	00536-4106-08	4.35	
250s ea	00536-4106-02	13.42	
OYSCO 500 + D (Rugby)			
TAB,PO, 500 mg-200 iu,			
60s ea	00536-7817-08	4.35	
1000s ea	00536-7817-10	14.38	
OYSCO D (Rugby)			
TAB,PO, 250 mg-125 iu,			
100s ea	00536-4103-01	3.52	
250s ea	00536-4103-02	7.95	
1000s ea	00536-4103-10	22.43	
OYST-CAL 500 (Teva)			
TAB,PO, 500 mg, 60s ea	00182-1576-26	3.25	
120s ea	00182-1576-07	4.25	
1000s ea	00182-1576-10	28.79	
OYST-CAL-D (Teva)			
TAB,PO, 250 mg-125 iu,			
100s ea	00182-0418-01	2.69	
1000s ea	00182-0418-10	16.36	
OYST-CAL-D 500 (Teva)			
PO (PF,SF)			
500 mg-125 iu, 60s ea	00182-4439-26	3.25	
120s ea	00182-4439-07	5.99	
1000s ea	00182-4439-10	23.06	
OYSTER CALCIUM (Nature's Bounty)			
TAB,PO (PF,SF)			
100s ea	74312-0030-30		4.29
OYSTER SHELL CALCIUM (Albertson's)			
TAB,PO, 250 mg, 100s ea	04000-0002-12	2.88	
500 mg, 120s ea	04000-0001-38	4.23	
(Health Products Corp)			
TAB,PO (PF,SF)			
500 mg, 60s ea	39686-0012-92	2.50	
(Lex)			
TAB,PO, 250 mg, 100s ea	49523-0030-01	0.70	
(Major)			
TAB,PO, 500 mg, 60s ea	00904-1883-52	3.40	
(10X10)			
500 mg, 100s ea UD	00904-1883-61	10.84	
150s ea	00904-1883-92	4.45	
300s ea	00904-1883-72	7.45	
1000s ea	00904-1883-80	23.99	
(Marlex)			
TAB,PO, 500 mg, 60s ea	10135-0211-60	1.00	
100s ea	10135-0211-01	2.00	
100s ea UD	10135-0211-13	3.02	
150s ea	10135-0211-64	2.01	
300s ea	10135-0211-03	3.52	
1000s ea	10135-0211-10	8.25	
(Mason Vit)			
TAB,PO (PF,SF,DYE-FREE)			
500 mg, 100s ea	11845-0091-51	6.67	
500 mg-125 iu,			
250s ea	11845-0075-52	11.44	
(Nature's Bounty)			
TAB,PO (PF,SF)			
500 mg, 100s ea	74312-0068-50		5.99
(Prime Marketing)			
TAB,PO, 500 mg, 100s ea	62107-0049-01	5.40	
500s ea	62107-0049-05	19.90	
(Rexall)			
TAB,PO (SUPPORTS HEALTHY BONES)			
500 mg, 60s ea	30768-0000-33	1.70	2.59
(Truxton)			
TAB,PO, 250 mg, 100s ea	00463-6303-01	3.00	
500 mg, 100s ea	00463-6304-01	3.00	
(Core)			
REPACK			
TAB,PO, 500 mg, 60s ea	33358-0282-60	8.30	
(GSMS)			
REPACK			
TAB,PO, 500 mg, 180s ea	60429-0610-18	13.95	
OYSTER SHELL CALCIUM 1000/VITAMIN D (Mason Vit)			
TAB,PO (PF,SF)			
380 mg-250 iu, 90s ea	11845-0123-99	5.33	
180s ea	11845-0123-97	8.78	
OYSTER SHELL CALCIUM NATURAL (Cardinal Health)			
TAB,PO (PRIVATE LABEL)			
500 mg, 100s ea	37205-0082-78	2.67	
OYSTER SHELL CALCIUM NATURAL/VIT D (Cardinal Health)			
TAB,PO (PRIVATE LABEL)			
500 mg-200 iu,			
100s ea	37205-0083-78	2.02	
OYSTER SHELL CALCIUM W/VITAMIN D (GSMS)			
REPACK			
TAB,PO, 500 mg-200 iu,			
180s ea	60429-0612-18	14.25	
OYSTER SHELL CALCIUM WITH VITAMIN D (Major)			
TAB,PO, 500 mg-200 iu,			
60s ea	00904-5460-52	3.70	
(10X10)			
500 mg-200 iu,			
100s ea UD	00904-5460-61	10.38	
150s ea	00904-5460-92	6.69	
300s ea	00904-5460-72	11.25	
1000s ea	00904-5460-80	29.85	
OYSTER SHELL CALCIUM/VITAMIN D (ADH)			
TAB,PO, 500 mg-400 iu,			
100s ea	60142-0109-10	2.70	5.40
(Basic Vitamins)			
TAB,PO, 250 mg-125 iu,			
100s ea	00761-0894-20	1.80	
240s ea	00761-0894-48	3.40	
(Major)			
TAB,PO (10X10)			
250 mg-125 iu,			
100s ea UD	00904-1882-61	7.69	
250s ea	00904-1882-60	2.70	
300s ea	00904-1882-72	5.45	
1000s ea	00904-1882-80	14.81	
(Mason Vit)			
TAB,PO (SF)			
250 mg-125 iu,			
100s ea	11845-0061-11	3.22	
500 mg-125 iu,			
250s ea	11845-0061-12	6.44	
(Prime Marketing)			
TAB,PO, 250 mg-125 iu,			
100s ea	62107-0073-01	3.25	
(Reese)			
TAB,PO (CAPLET)			
500 mg-200 iu, 60s ea	10956-0682-60	4.31	
100s ea	10956-0682-09	5.84	
(Rexall)			
TAB,PO (PF,SF)			
250 mg-125 iu,			
100s ea	30768-0001-71	1.54	2.33
(McKesson Packaging)			
REPACK			
TAB,PO (BLISTER PACK, 25X30)			
500 mg-200 iu,			
750s ea UD	63739-0291-01	73.26	
(Phys Total Care)			
REPACK			
TAB,PO, 500 mg-125 iu,			
60s ea	54868-4081-00	6.27	
150s ea	54868-4081-01	13.41	
OYSTERCAL 500 (Nature's Bounty)			
TAB,PO (PF,SF)			
500 mg, 60s ea	74312-0039-10		4.79
OYSTERCAL-D 250 (Nature's Bounty)			
TAB,PO (PF,SF)			
250 mg-125 iu,			
100s ea	74312-0039-00		4.45
OYSTERCAL-D 500 (Nature's Bounty)			
PO, 500 mg-125 iu,			
60s ea	74312-0070-90	2.80	4.79
P & S (Teva)			
LIQ,TP, 2%, 120 ml	00575-4007-04	10.99	
240 ml	00575-4007-08	17.69	
TAB,PO (PF,SF)			
500 mg-125 iu,			
120 ml	00575-4001-04	14.29	
240 ml	00575-4001-08	23.99	
P-1000 (Bio-Tech Pharm)			
CAP,PO, 500 mg, 100s ea	53191-0006-01	4.75	
P-A-C ANALGESIC (Lee Pharm)			
TAB,PO, 400 mg-32 mg,			
100s ea	23558-0540-20	9.96	
1000s ea	23558-0540-22	81.60	
(100X48)			
400 mg-32 mg,			
4800s ea	23558-0540-21	478.08	
(1000X12)			
400 mg-32 mg,			
12000s ea	23558-0540-23	979.20	
P.M. MULTIVIT/MULTIMINERAL (ADH)			
TAB,PO, 60s ea	60142-0096-06	7.48	14.95
PABA (Freeda)			
TAB,PO (PF,SF,DYE-FREE)			
100 mg, 100s ea	10432-0223-01	3.45	5.75
PABA 500 (Bio-Tech Pharm)			
CAP,PO, 500 mg, 100s ea	53191-0381-01	6.10	
PACIFIC KELP (Freeda)			
TAB,PO (SF,GLUTEN-FREE)			
0.15 mg, 100s ea	10432-0136-01	3.57	5.95
250s ea	10432-0136-02	7.14	11.90
PACQUIN PLUS (Johnson & Johnson)			
CRE,TP (WITH ALOE)			
42.5 gm	74300-0000-76	0.79	
PAIN & FEVER (Rugby)			
SOL,PO (W/DROPPER,AF)			
80 mg/0.8 ml, 15 ml	00536-1936-72	2.51	
PAIN & FEVER RELIEF (Rugby)			
TAB,PO, 325 mg, 100s ea	00536-3222-01	4.20	
1000s ea	00536-3222-10	22.42	
PAIN & FEVER RELIEF CHILDREN'S (Rugby)			
SOL,PO (CHERRY)			
160 mg/5 ml, 120 ml	00536-0122-97	3.78	
(AF,CHERRY)			
160 mg/5 ml, 480 ml	00536-0122-85	8.25	
PAIN & FEVER RELIEF EXTRA STRENGTH (Rugby)			
TAB,PO, 500 mg, 100s ea	00536-3231-01	4.72	
(CAPTAB)			
500 mg, 100s ea	00536-3218-01	5.10	
1000s ea	00536-3231-10	29.85	
(CAPTAB)			
500 mg, 1000s ea	00536-3218-10	29.93	
PAIN BUST-R II EXTRA STRENGTH (Continental Quest)			
CRE,TP, 12%-17%, 90 gm	14788-0331-30	3.87	
PAIN ENZ (Med Gen Inc)			
LOT,TP, 0.075%, 88.7 ml	32246-0303-03	5.40	9.95
PAIN PATCH (Mentholatum)			
PAD,TP (4"X5 1/2")			
4.26%, 5s ea	10742-0004-92	4.80	
PAIN RELIEF (Basic Vitamins)			
TAB,PO (EXT. STR.,CAPLET)			
500 mg, 100s ea	00761-0904-20	1.80	
(Family Phcy)			
GEL,TP (PRIVATE LABEL)			
10%-15%, 120 gm	52735-0718-41	3.86	4.29
LIQ,TP, 45 ml	52735-0809-28	4.13	4.59
(Major)			
GEL,MM (1X14.2GM)			
20%, 14.2 gm	00904-6021-36	3.75	
TEF,PO, 325 mg-1000 mg-1916 mg,			
36s ea	00904-7948-73	3.95	
(Rose)			
CRE,TP, 10%, 240 gm	42037-0430-08	4.55	
(A-S Medication)			
REPACK			
CRE,TP, 10%, 85 gm	54569-5277-00	3.04	
(Physician Partner)			
REPACK			
GEL,TP, 16%, 85 gm	21695-0642-03	15.09	
PAIN RELIEF MAXIMUM STRENGTH (Cardinal Health)			
GEL,TP (PRIVATE LABEL)			
16%, 60 gm	37205-0704-21	4.63	

PROD/MFR	HRI, UPC,NDC	AWP	SRP
PAIN RELIEVER (Cardinal Health)			
TAB,PO (PRIVATE LABEL)			
325 mg, 100s ea	37205-0031-78	5.72	
(Magno-Humphries)			
TAB,PO, 325 mg, 100s ea	43292-0555-91	1.62	3.29
250s ea	43292-0555-87	3.00	5.89
PAIN RELIEVER & SLEEP AID (AmerisourceBergen)			
TAB,PO (EXT. STR.,PRIVATE LABEL)			
500 mg-25 mg, 50s ea	24385-0437-71	4.67	5.19
PAIN RELIEVER ADDED STRENGTH (AmerisourceBergen)			
TAB,PO (PRIVATE LABEL)			
250 mg-250 mg-65 mg, 100s ea	24385-0430-78	6.74	7.49
(Major)			
TAB,PO, 250 mg-250 mg-65 mg, 100s ea	00904-5135-59	3.90	
PAIN RELIEVER CHILD'S (Family Phcy)			
SUS,PO (PRIVATE LABEL,CHERRY)			
160 mg/5 ml, 120 ml	52735-0759-41	3.95	4.39
PAIN RELIEVER CHILDREN'S (Cardinal Health)			
LIQ,PO (AF,PRIVATE LABEL,CHERRY)			
160 mg/5 ml, 120 ml	37205-0508-26	4.02	
(AF,PRIVATE LABEL,GRAPE)			
160 mg/5 ml, 120 ml	37205-0518-26	3.72	
(AF,PRIVATE LABEL)			
160 mg/5 ml, 120 ml	37205-0717-26	4.02	
(McKesson)			
SUS,PO (SUNMARK,AF,ASPIRIN-FREE)			
160 mg/5 ml, 118 ml	49348-0266-34	4.29	
PAIN RELIEVER COLD/COUGH CHILDREN'S (Cardinal Health)			
CTB,PO (PRIVATE LABEL,CHERRY)			
24s ea	37205-0207-62	3.54	
PAIN RELIEVER EXTRA STRENGTH (Cardinal Health)			
TAB,PO (PRIVATE LABEL,CAPLET)			
500 mg, 50s ea	37205-0020-71	4.42	
(PRIVATE LABEL,GELTAB)			
500 mg, 50s ea	37205-0187-71	2.96	
(PRIVATE LABEL)			
500 mg, 60s ea	37205-0035-72	5.10	
(PRIVATE LABEL,CAPLET)			
500 mg, 100s ea	37205-0020-78	6.52	
(PRIVATE LABEL,GELTAB)			
500 mg, 100s ea	37205-0187-78	4.80	
(PRIVATE LABEL)			
500 mg, 100s ea	37205-0035-78	6.72	
(PRIVATE LABEL,CAPLET)			
500 mg, 500s ea	37205-0020-90	10.92	
(Magno-Humphries)			
TAB,PO, 500 mg, 100s ea	43292-0555-92	1.80	3.89
(CAPLET)			
500 mg, 100s ea	43292-0555-89	1.80	3.89
250s ea	43292-0556-18	3.31	5.99
(CAPLET)			
500 mg, 250s ea	43292-0556-15	3.40	5.99
PAIN RELIEVER INFANTS' (AmerisourceBergen)			
SUS,PO (PRIVATE LABEL,DROPS)			
80 mg/0.8 ml, 30 ml	24385-0289-10	5.39	5.99
(Cardinal Health)			
SUS,PO (AF,PRIVATE LABEL,CHERRY)			
80 mg/0.8 ml, 15 ml	37205-0008-05	3.70	
PAIN RELIEVER PM EXTRA STRENGTH (Cardinal Health)			
TAB,PO (PRIVATE LABEL,CAPLET)			
500 mg-25 mg, 50s ea	37205-0060-71	5.09	
(Chain Drug Marketing)			
TAB,PO (CAPLET)			
500 mg-25 mg, 50s ea	63868-0325-50	1.50	5.39
(Magno-Humphries)			
TAB,PO, 500 mg-25 mg, 100s ea	43292-0558-31	2.26	4.99
PAIN RELIEVER W/O ASPIRIN (AmerisourceBergen)			
TAB,PO (PRIVATE LABEL)			
325 mg, 100s ea	24385-0403-78	5.66	6.29
PAIN RELIEVER W/O ASPIRIN CHILDREN (AmerisourceBergen)			
SUS,PO (AF,PRIVATE LABEL,GRAPE)			
160 mg/5 ml, 118 ml	24385-0130-26	4.04	4.49
(AF,PRIVATE LABEL)			
160 mg/5 ml, 118 ml	24385-0105-26	4.04	4.49
PAIN RELIEVING GEL (AmerisourceBergen)			
GEL,TP (PRIVATE LABEL)			
2%, 90 gm	24385-0209-53	3.86	4.29
(Medicine Shoppe)			
GEL,TP, 10%-15%, 120 gm	49614-0412-26	4.79	4.79
PAIN RELIEVING RUB (G&W)			
CRE,TP (STAINLESS)			
10%-15%, 120 gm	00713-0283-04	4.18	
(Major)			
CRE,TP (1X57GM)			
4%-10%-30%, 57 gm	00904-5848-02	4.39	
PAIN RELIEVING RUB ULTRA STRENGTH (G&W)			
CRE,TP, 4%-10%-30%, 120 gm	00713-0625-04	4.33	
PAIN-EZE +/RHEU-THRITIS (Reese)			
TAB,PO (CAPLET)			
650 mg, 25s ea	10956-0762-25	3.26	
50s ea	10956-0762-50	4.31	
PAIN-GESIC (Mason Vit)			
TAB,PO, 325 mg-30 mg, 100s ea	11845-0867-01	5.00	
PAIN-OFF (Medique)			
TAB,PO (50X2,SF)			
250 mg-250 mg-65 mg, 100s ea UD	47682-0228-33	6.29	
(100X2,SF)			
250 mg-250 mg-65 mg, 200s ea UD	47682-0228-47	11.30	
(250X2,SF)			
250 mg-250 mg-65 mg, 500s ea UD	47682-0228-13	28.51	
PAINALAY (Lee Pharm)			
LIQ,PO, 1.4%, 236 ml	23558-0680-70	5.52	
240 ml 24s	23558-0680-71	132.48	
532 ml	23558-0680-80	9.12	
532 ml 6s	23558-0680-81	54.72	
SPR,MM, 1.4%, 177 ml	23558-0680-60	5.52	
180 ml 24s	23558-0680-61	132.48	
PALADIN (Pal Midwest)			
OIN,TP, 15 gm	49015-0300-00	1.06	1.89
60 gm	49015-0100-00	2.19	3.75
PALMER'S COCOA BUTTER BODY WASH (E.T. Browne)			
LIQ,TP (SOAP-FREE)			
255 ml	10181-0044-44	2.93	
PALMER'S COCOA BUTTER FORMULA (E.T. Browne)			
CRE,TP, 33 gm	10181-0043-60	0.54	
105 gm	10181-0040-00	2.66	
112.5 gm	10181-0043-50	2.40	
(FACIAL)			
113 gm	10181-0041-00	3.73	
217.5 gm	10181-0040-08	4.58	
LOT,TP, 51 ml	10181-0041-82	1.61	
255 ml	10181-0041-80	2.66	
(W/AHA)			
255 ml	10181-0041-95	3.05	
(W/VIT E,FRAGRANCE-FREE)			
255 ml	10181-0041-87	2.66	
405 ml	10181-0041-65	3.56	
OIL,TP, 51 ml	10181-0041-75	2.11	
255 ml	10181-0041-70	3.14	
STI,TP, 4.5 gm	10181-0042-20	0.75	
15 gm	10181-0042-00	1.59	
PALMER'S COCOA BUTTER HAND FORMULA (E.T. Browne)			
CRE,TP, 60 gm	10181-0044-35	2.94	
PALMER'S COCOA BUTTER MASSAGE (E.T. Browne)			
CRE,TP, 132 gm	10181-0040-35	3.11	
PALMER'S COCOA BUTTER NURSING (E.T. Browne)			
CRE,TP, 33 gm	10181-0040-37	2.33	
PALMER'S COCOA BUTTER SOAP FORMULA (E.T. Browne)			
LIQ,TP, 255 ml	10181-0045-08	2.16	
SOA,TP (3.5 OZ)			
ea	10181-0045-55	1.49	
PALMER'S SKIN SUCCESS ACNE (E.T. Browne)			
LOT,TP (INVISIBLE,MAX. STR.)			
10%, 30 ml	10181-0080-10	3.22	
PALMER'S SKIN SUCCESS ACNE CLEANSER (E.T. Browne)			
LIQ,TP, 0.5%, 240 ml	10181-0080-11	3.22	
PALMER'S SKIN SUCCESS FADE CREAM (E.T. Browne)			
CRE,TP (DRY)			
2%, 81 gm	10181-0075-09	3.08	
81 gm	10181-0075-10	3.08	
(OILY)			
2%, 81 gm	10181-0075-05	3.08	
81 gm	10181-0075-06	3.08	
(REGULAR)			
2%, 81 gm	10181-0075-00	3.08	
81 gm	10181-0075-01	3.08	
(DRY)			
2%, 132 gm	10181-0076-09	4.79	
(OILY)			
2%, 132 gm	10181-0076-05	4.79	
(REGULAR)			
2%, 132 gm	10181-0076-00	4.79	
PALMER'S SKIN SUCCESS FADE SERUM (E.T. Browne)			
LOT,TP (SPF 30,SF)			
30 ml	10181-0077-00	6.60	
PALMER'S SKIN SUCCESS MOISTURIZING (E.T. Browne)			
CRE,TP (SPF 30,SF)			
54 gm	10181-0077-02	3.85	
PALOMAR E (Pal Midwest)			
OIN,TP, 60 gm	49015-0500-00	2.19	3.75
PAMPRIN MAXIMUM PAIN RELIEF (Chattem)			
TAB,PO (CAPLET)			
250 mg-250 mg-25 mg, 16s ea	41167-0300-21	2.93	2.25
32s ea	41167-0300-23	4.64	3.40
PAMPRIN MULTI-SYMPTOM (Chattem)			
TAB,PO (CAPLET)			
500 mg-25 mg-15 mg, 10s ea	41167-0300-17	1.74	1.60
(MAX. STR.,GELCAP)			
500 mg-25 mg-15 mg, 16s ea	41167-0300-61	2.99	
(CAPLET)			
500 mg-25 mg-15 mg, 20s ea	41167-0300-12	3.12	2.50
20s ea	41167-0301-12	3.12	
40s ea	41167-0300-14	4.70	3.75
40s ea	41167-0301-14	4.70	
PAN C500 (Freeda)			
TAB,PO (PF,SF,DYE-FREE)			
500 mg-100 mg-100 mg, 100s ea	10432-0202-01	7.47	12.45
250s ea	10432-0202-02	14.94	24.90
500s ea	10432-0202-03	23.37	38.95
PAN-2400 (Bio-Tech Pharm)			
CAP,PO, 2400 mg, 100s ea	53191-0038-01	10.50	
PANADOL ES (Glaxo)			
TAB,PO (CAPLET)			
500 mg, 10s ea	09711-0500-05	1.14	
24s ea	09711-0500-06	1.94	
50s ea	09711-0500-07	3.76	
PANCREATIN (Key Company)			
TAB,PO (SF)			
325 mg, 100s ea	11694-0872-01	4.25	
1000s ea	11694-0872-05	32.00	
PANCREATIN-1200 (Key Company)			
PO (SF)			
1200 mg, 100s ea	11694-0803-01	7.75	
160s ea	11694-0803-16	11.25	
1000s ea	11694-0803-10	59.00	
PANOXYL AQUA GEL (Stiefel Consumer HealthCare)			
GEL,TP, 10%, 42.5 gm	00145-2657-02	4.50	6.79
PANOXYL BAR 10 (Stiefel Consumer HealthCare)			
SOA,TP, 10%, 113 gm	00145-0983-05	5.10	7.69
(Phys Total Care) REPACK			
SOA,TP, 10%, ea	54868-2656-00	7.94	
PANOXYL BAR 5 (Stiefel Consumer HealthCare)			
SOA,TP, 5%, 113 gm	00145-0982-05	4.92	7.39
(Phys Total Care) REPACK			
SOA,TP, 5%, ea	54868-2655-00	7.71	
PANTETHINE 500 (Westlake Labs.)			
CAP,PO (P.F, S.F,PF)			
500 mg, 100s ea	10539-0827-95	44.80	64.00
PANTETHINE TIME (Carlson,J.R.)			
TER,PO, 300 mg, 60s ea	88395-0029-20	19.95	39.90
PANTOTHENIC ACID (ADH)			
TAB,PO (PF,SF)			
500 mg, 100s ea	60142-0222-01	6.38	12.75

PROD/MFR	HRI, UPC,NDC	AWP	SRP
(Carlson,J.R.)			
TER,PO, 500 mg, 100s ea	88395-0029-01	7.45	14.90
250s ea	88395-0029-02	16.50	33.00
(Major)			
TAB,PO, 200 mg, 100s ea	00904-3153-60	3.85	
(Mason Vit)			
TAB,PO, 100 mg, 100s ea	11845-0054-01	5.00	
250 mg, 100s ea	11845-0058-91	7.56	
(PF,SF)			
500 mg, 60s ea	11845-0072-65	6.56	
(Nature's Bounty)			
TAB,PO (PF,SF)			
200 mg, 100s ea	74312-0006-80		5.99
(Pharmavite)			
TAB,PO, 100 mg, 100s ea	31604-0012-65	2.44	
(Rugby)			
TAB,PO (PF,SF,DYE-FREE)			
500 mg, 100s ea	00536-6717-01	5.62	
PANTOTHENIC-250 (Key Company)			
TAB,PO (CORN-FREE,DAIRY-FREE)			
250 mg, 100s ea	11694-0114-21	6.50	
1000s ea	11694-0114-24	45.00	
PAPAYA (Freeda)			
TAB,PO (PF,SF,DYE-FREE)			
100 mg, 100s ea	10432-0211-01	4.77	7.95
250s ea	10432-0211-02	9.54	15.90
(Health Products Corp)			
CTB,PO (PF,SF)			
250s ea	39686-0014-39	2.75	
(Major)			
TAB,PO, 130s ea	00904-1354-13	3.05	
(Marlex)			
CTB,PO, 100s ea	10135-0198-01	3.10	
130s ea	10135-0198-63	1.39	
1000s ea	10135-0198-10	8.25	
(Rugby)			
TAB,PO, 0.05 mg-10 mg-5 mg-1 mg,			
100s ea	00536-6506-01	2.90	
PAPAYA ENZYME (ADH)			
CTB,PO (PF,SF)			
100s ea	60142-0581-01	2.48	4.95
(Nature's Bounty)			
CTB,PO (PF)			
60 mg-60 mg, 100s ea	74312-0011-30		4.49
PAPAYA ENZYME DOUBLE STRENGTH (Rexall)			
TAB,PO (PF,SF)			
60s ea	30768-0011-95	1.99	3.32
PAPAYA ENZYME W/PAPAIN (Mason Vit)			
TAB,PO, 100s ea	11845-0054-71	4.11	
PARADIGM LINK GLUCOSE MONITOR			
(Medtronic Minimed)			
DEV,NA, ea	08290-3332-00	124.55	
PARVA-CAL 250 (Freeda)			
TAB,PO (PF,SF,DYE-FREE)			
250 mg-100 iu,			
100s ea	10432-0042-01	3.87	6.45
250s ea	10432-0042-02	7.74	12.90
PARVA-CAL 500 (Freeda)			
PO (PF,SF,DYE-FREE)			
500 mg-200 iu, 100s ea	10432-0275-01	5.37	8.95
250s ea	10432-0275-02	10.74	17.90
PARVENZYME (Freeda)			
TAB,PO (PF,SF,DYE-FREE)			
100s ea	10432-0044-01	5.67	9.45
250s ea	10432-0044-02	11.34	18.90
PARVLEX (Freeda)			
TAB,PO, 100s ea	10432-0047-01	5.97	9.95
PASSIFLORA INCARNATA (Luyties)			
TAB,SL (6X)			
6 x, 500s ea	00618-7024-03	3.99	
5500s ea	00618-7024-10	30.32	
(30X)			
12 x, 500s ea	00622-7024-03	4.19	
5500s ea	00622-7024-10	31.83	
(12X)			
30 x, 500s ea	00624-7024-03	4.19	
5500s ea	00624-7024-10	31.83	
PASTILLAS MCCOY (McCoy's)			
TAB,PO, 24s ea	31088-0770-24	1.51	2.27
40s ea	31088-0770-40	2.09	3.13
60s ea	31088-0770-60	2.57	3.85
100s ea	31088-0771-00	3.87	5.80

PROD/MFR	HRI, UPC,NDC	AWP	SRP
PATROL ENTERAL NUTRITION PUMP (Abbott)			
DEV,NA, ea	70074-0520-34	1227.60	
(W/PIERCING PIN)			
ea	70074-0520-41	7.99	
PAU D'ARCO (ADH)			
CAP,PO (BRAZILIAN,PF,SF)			
500 mg, 100s ea	60142-0936-71	6.48	12.95
(Botanical Labs.)			
LIQ,PO, 30 ml	41954-0020-37	4.00	7.99
60 ml	41954-0020-16	6.50	12.99
PC TAR (Geritrex)			
LIQ,TP, 1%, 180 ml	54162-0200-06	6.44	
PCN-200 (Bio-Tech Pharm)			
CAP,PO, 200 mg, 100s ea	53191-0217-01	15.75	
PEAK AIR (Omron)			
DEV,NA (ADULT AND PEDIATRIC)			
ea	73796-0699-40	10.08	14.95
PEARSON SAKRIN (Oakhurst)			
LIQ,PO (DROPS)			
34.5 ml	11169-0567-89	2.69	4.03
(DROPS,DROPS)			
85.2 ml	11169-0033-23	4.62	6.93
PECTIN (Freeda)			
APPLE PECTIN			
TAB,PO (PF,SF,DYE-FREE)			
300 mg, 100s ea	10432-0258-01	5.55	9.25
250s ea	10432-0258-02	11.10	18.50
PED ELECTROLYTE (Cardinal Health)			
SOL,PO (PRIVATE LABEL,FRUIT)			
1000 ml	37205-0220-08	4.83	
(PRIVATE LABEL,GRAPE)			
1000 ml	37205-0221-08	4.83	
(UNFLAVORED)			
1000 ml	37205-0222-08	4.83	
PEDI-BORO (Phys Total Care)			
REPACK			
PDR,TP (SOAK PAKS)			
49%-51%, 12s ea	54868-4996-00	15.73	
PEDI-BORO SOAK PAKS (Pedinol)			
PKT,TP (12X2.1GM)			
2.1 gm 12s	00884-1706-27		15.00
(100X2.1GM)			
2.1 gm 100s	00884-1706-10		65.00
PEDIA RELIEF (Cardinal Health)			
LIQ,PO (AF,PRIVATE LABEL,DROPS)			
7.5 mg/0.8 ml, 15 ml	37205-0001-05	3.62	
PEDIA RELIEF COUGH-COLD (AmerisourceBergen)			
LIQ,PO (AF,PRIVATE LABEL,CHERRY)			
120 ml	24385-0007-26	3.59	3.99
PEDIA-POP (Lcm)			
SOL,PO (16X62.5ML,FREEZER POPS)			
62.5 ml 16s	12471-0000-16	4.91	
PEDIA-RELIEF (Major)			
LIQ,PO (AF,CHERRY)			
120 ml	00904-5050-20	3.65	
PEDIACARE CHILDREN'S ALLERGY			
(McNeil Consumer Healthcare)			
SYR,PO (AF,CHERRY)			
12.5 mg/5 ml,			
118 ml	12547-0466-04	5.50	
PEDIACARE CHILDREN'S ALLERGY & COLD			
(McNeil Consumer Healthcare)			
SOL,PO (AF,GRAPE)			
12.5 mg/5 ml-5 mg/5 ml,			
118 ml	00450-0552-04	5.50	
PEDIACARE CHILDREN'S DECONGESTANT			
(Johnson & Johnson)			
SOL,PO (RASPBERRY)			
2.5 mg/5 ml,			
118 ml	00501-2430-04	4.87	
(McNeil Consumer Healthcare)			
SOL,PO (NON-DROWSY,RASPBERRY)			
2.5 mg/5 ml,			
118 ml	00450-0554-04	5.50	
PEDIACARE CHILDREN'S LONG-ACTING COUGH			
(McNeil Consumer Healthcare)			
SOL,PO (NON-DROWSY,AF,GRAPE)			
7.5 mg/5 ml,			
118 ml	00450-0465-04	5.50	
PEDIACARE CHILDREN'S MULTI-SYMPTOM COLD			
(Johnson & Johnson)			
SOL,PO (W/DOSAGE CUP,GRAPE)			
5 mg/5 ml-2.5 mg/5 ml,			
118 ml	00501-2427-04	4.87	

PROD/MFR	HRI, UPC,NDC	AWP	SRP
(McNeil Consumer Healthcare)			
SOL,PO (NON-DROWSY,AF,GRAPE)			
5 mg/5 ml-2.5 mg/5 ml,			
118 ml	00450-0556-05	5.50	
(Dispensing Solutions)			
REPACK			
LIQ,PO, 120 ml	55045-3474-04	7.00	
PEDIACARE COUGH + COLD CHILDREN'S			
(Johnson & Johnson)			
LIQ,PO (NON-DROWSY,AF,GRAPE)			
7.5 mg/5 ml-15 mg/5 ml,			
120 ml	00009-5209-02	4.87	
PEDIACARE DECONGESTANT & COUGH			
(Johnson & Johnson)			
LIQ,PO (W/DROPPER,AF,DYE-FREE)			
15 ml	00501-2410-05	4.87	
PEDIACARE DECONGESTANT DROPS			
(A-S Medication)			
REPACK			
SOL,PO, 1.25 mg/0.8 ml,			
15 ml	54569-5890-00	4.87	
PEDIACARE GENTLE VAPORS			
(McNeil Consumer Healthcare)			
PAD,IH (REFILLS ONLY)			
5s ea	12547-0600-14	4.21	
(W/VAPOR PLUG UNIT)			
5s ea	12547-0600-13	7.24	
PEDIACARE INFANT DECONGESTANT & COUGH			
(Johnson & Johnson)			
SOL,PO (GRAPE,DROPS)			
15 ml	00501-2428-05	4.87	
PEDIACARE INFANT DROPPER DECONGESTANT			
(Johnson & Johnson)			
SOL,PO (RASPBERRY,DROPS)			
1.25 mg/0.8 ml,			
15 ml	00501-2429-05	4.87	
PEDIACARE LONG-ACTING COUGH			
(Johnson & Johnson)			
SOL,PO (NON-DROWSY,AF,DYE-FREE)			
3.75 mg/0.8 ml,			
15 ml	00501-2421-05	4.87	
PEDIACARE MULTI-SYMPTOM COLD			
(Johnson & Johnson)			
LIQ,PO (AF,CHERRY)			
120 ml	00097-0716-01	4.87	
(Pharmacia Consumer)			
LIQ,PO (AF,CHERRY)			
120 ml	00009-7716-02	4.49	
PEDIACARE NIGHTREST (Johnson & Johnson)			
LIQ,PO (AF,CHERRY)			
120 ml	00501-2412-04	4.87	
PEDIALYTE (Abbott)			
SOL,PO, 237 ml 6s	70074-0401-60	16.06	
1000 ml	70074-0803-36	7.07	
(FRUIT)			
1000 ml	70074-0803-65	7.07	
(GRAPE)			
1000 ml	70074-0802-40	7.07	
(Southwood)			
REPACK			
SOL,PO, 240 ml 6s	58016-7037-01	18.74	
PEDIALYTE FREEZER POPS (Abbott)			
SOL,PO (ASSORTED FLAVORS)			
63 ml 16s	70074-0002-46	7.07	
PEDIALYTE SINGLES (Abbott)			
SOL,PO (CHERRY)			
237 ml	70074-0549-82	7.07	
(APPLE FLAVOR,APPLE)			
237 ml 32s	70074-0574-26	47.12	
PEDIASURE (Abbott)			
LIQ,PO (6X237ML,CHOCOLATE)			
237 ml 6s	70074-0580-59	14.83	
(6X237ML,LACTOSE-FREE)			
237 ml 6s	70074-0570-15	14.83	
237 ml 6s	70074-0580-65	14.83	
(6X237ML,VANILLA)			
237 ml 6s	70074-0580-50	14.83	
(6X237ML,W/FIBER,VANILLA)			
237 ml 6s	70074-0580-62	15.34	
(NEWRCLOSBLEBOTTLE)			
237 ml 6s	70074-0580-53	14.83	
PEDIASURE ENTERAL (Abbott)			
LIQ,PO (TUBE FEEDING,VANILLA)			
240 ml	70074-0518-05	2.36	
(VANILLA)			
500 ml	70074-0597-84	7.78	

PROD/MFR	HRI, UPC,NDC	AWP	SRP
PEDIASURE NUTRIPALS (Abbott)			
BAR,PO (PEANUT BUTTER AND JELLY)			
6s ea	70074-0595-67	6.96	
(S'MORES)			
6s ea	70074-0595-61	6.96	
(STRAWBERRY YOGURT)			
6s ea	70074-0595-64	6.96	
6s ea	70074-0595-70	6.96	
LIQ,PO (4X237ML,CHOCOLATE)			
237 ml 4s	70074-0595-58	6.96	
(4X237ML,STRAWBERRY)			
237 ml 4s	70074-0595-55	6.96	
(4X237ML,VANILLA)			
237 ml 4s	70074-0595-49	6.96	
PEDIASURE W/FIBER (Abbott)			
LIQ,PO (1X237ML,VANILLA)			
237 ml	70074-0582-21	2.47	
(VANILLA)			
240 ml 6s	70074-0506-53	15.34	
PEDIASURE W/FIBER ENTERAL (Abbott)			
LIQ,PO (TUBE FEEDING,VANILLA)			
240 ml	70074-0518-07	2.47	
PEDIASURE WITH FIBER AND FOS (Abbott)			
LIQ,PO (ENTERAL FORMULA,VANILLA)			
500 ml	70074-0597-86	8.04	
PEDIATRIC ELECTROLYTE (Chain Drug Marketing)			
SOL,PO (AF,FRUIT)			
1000 ml	63868-0606-33	2.58	3.99
(AF)			
1000 ml	63868-0261-33	2.58	3.99
(Major)			
SOL,PO (1X1000ML,AF,GRAPE)			
1000 ml	00904-5276-69	39.20	
(8X1000ML,AF,BUBBLE GUM)			
1000 ml 8s	00904-5768-69	39.20	
PEDIATRIC FORMULA CHILDRENS COUGH AND CONGESTION AID (Reese)			
SOL,PO (1X240ML,AF,SF,DYE-FREE)			
10 mg/5 ml-100 mg/5 ml,			
240 ml	10956-0776-08	5.17	7.29
PEG 3350 (Major)			
PDS,PO (100X17GM)			
17 gm/dose,			
17 gm 100s	00904-6025-61	152.68	
(1X238GM)			
17 gm/dose, 238 gm	00904-6025-77	10.99	
(1X510GM)			
17 gm/dose, 510 gm	00904-6025-76	19.89	
(1X850GM)			
17 gm/dose, 850 gm	00904-6025-84	29.12	
PELEVERUS (Eli Rutledge, Inc.)			
OIN,TP, 100 gm	61598-0100-10	33.50	
SPR,TP, 0.25%, 240 ml	61598-0500-25	21.35	
PELEVERUS GOLD (Eli Rutledge, Inc.)			
OIN,TP, 100 gm	61598-0200-10	33.50	
PEN NEEDLE (Aurora)			
DEV,NA (28GX12MM,ORIGINAL)			
100s ea	08214-0297-24	19.25	
(31GX6MM,ULTRA SHORT)			
100s ea	08214-0907-24	19.25	
(31GX8MM)			
100s ea	08214-0307-24	19.25	
PEN NEEDLES (Atlanta & Pacific)			
DEV,NA (29GX12MM)			
100s ea	08214-0297-26	21.25	
(31GX6MM)			
100s ea	08214-0907-26	21.25	
(31GX8MM)			
100s ea	08214-0307-26	21.25	
PEN-KERA (Ascher)			
CRE,TP (DYE-FREE)			
120 gm	00225-0440-34	5.29	
240 gm	00225-0440-35	9.54	
PENETRAN (Transdermal Tech)			
LOT,TP (ASPIRIN-FREE,GREASELESS)			
2.5%, 120 ml	62511-0000-01	7.50	12.50
PENLET PLUS BLOOD SAMPLER (Lifescan)			
DEV,NA (W/25 LANCETS)			
ea	53885-0356-01	18.75	
PEPCID AC (J&J/Merck)			
CTB,PO, 10 mg, 60s ea	16837-0873-61	16.18	
(WAREHOUSE PKG)			
10 mg, 60s ea	16837-0873-60	16.18	
(EZ CHEWS/MAX STRENGTH)			
20 mg, 8s ea	16837-0854-08	4.63	
25s ea	16837-0854-25	9.92	
25s ea	16837-0867-25	9.92	
50s ea	16837-0854-50	17.81	
TAB,PO, 10 mg, 6s ea	16837-0872-06	2.88	
(GELCAPLET)			
10 mg, 6s ea	16837-0856-06	2.88	
18s ea	16837-0872-18	6.71	
30s ea	16837-0872-30	9.44	
(GELCAPLET)			
10 mg, 30s ea	16837-0856-30	8.99	
(30+10 FREE)			
10 mg, 40s ea	16837-0872-31	8.99	
(W/10 FREE,GELCAPLET)			
10 mg, 40s ea	16837-0856-31	8.99	
(25X2,ROLLPACK)			
10 mg, 50s ea	16837-0872-09	14.58	
60s ea	16837-0872-60	16.98	
(GELCAPLET)			
10 mg, 60s ea	16837-0856-61	16.18	
90s ea	16837-0872-90	21.66	
(60+30 FREE)			
10 mg, 90s ea	16837-0872-63	16.18	
(GELCAPLET)			
10 mg, 90s ea	16837-0856-90	21.60	
20 mg, 5s ea	16837-0855-05	2.88	
(MAX STRENGTH,W/FREE 5)			
20 mg, 5s ea	16837-0855-06	5.76	
(MAX STRENGTH)			
20 mg, 8s ea	16837-0855-08	4.63	
(25+10 FREE,MAX STRENGTH)			
20 mg, 25s ea	16837-0855-28	8.99	
(25+15,BERRY,MAXSTRNGTH)			
20 mg, 25s ea	16837-0855-41	8.99	
(25+5 BERRY,MAXSTRNGTH)			
20 mg, 25s ea	16837-0855-38	8.99	
(MAX STRENGTH)			
20 mg, 25s ea	16837-0855-25	9.92	
(MAX STRNGT; 25+6)			
20 mg, 25s ea	16837-0855-31	9.90	
(25+5 FREE,MAX STRENGTH)			
20 mg, 30s ea	16837-0855-29	9.90	
(25+5 FREE)			
20 mg, 30s ea	16837-0855-26	9.90	
(MAX STRGTH,25 W/FREE15)			
20 mg, 40s ea	16837-0855-40	9.90	
(MAX STRENGTH)			
20 mg, 50s ea	16837-0855-50	17.81	
(MAX STRENGTH,50 +10)			
20 mg, 60s ea	16837-0855-51	17.76	
(MAXIMUM STRENGTH)			
20 mg, 65s ea	16837-0855-65	20.70	
(MAX STRENGTH,W/FREE10)			
20 mg, 75s ea	16837-0855-85	21.60	
(Palmetto)			
REPACK			
TAB,PO, 10 mg, 30s ea	23490-7900-03	9.90	
(Phys Total Care)			
REPACK			
TAB,PO, 10 mg, 6s ea	54868-4881-00	4.86	
PEPCID COMPLETE (J&J/Merck)			
CTB,PO (BERRY FLAVOR)			
800 mg-10 mg-165 mg,			
5s ea	16837-0291-05	2.88	
(DUAL ACTION)			
800 mg-10 mg-165 mg,			
5s ea	16837-0246-05	2.95	
8s ea	16837-0246-08	4.63	
15s ea	16837-0291-15	7.38	
(MINT)			
800 mg-10 mg-165 mg,			
15s ea	16837-0888-15	7.38	
(25 W/5 FREE,BERRY)			
800 mg-10 mg-165 mg,			
25s ea	16837-0291-26	9.90	
(25+25 FREE BERRY FLAVOR)			
800 mg-10 mg-165 mg,			
25s ea	16837-0291-28	10.80	
(25+25 FREE MINT FLAVOR)			
800 mg-10 mg-165 mg,			
25s ea	16837-0888-28	10.80	
(25X1,MINT)			
800 mg-10 mg-165 mg,			
25s ea	16837-0888-54	11.99	
(BERRY FLAVOR)			
800 mg-10 mg-165 mg,			
25s ea	16837-0291-25	9.92	
(BERRY,25X1)			
800 mg-10 mg-165 mg,			
25s ea	16837-0291-53	11.99	
(COOL MINT,MINT)			
800 mg-10 mg-165 mg,			
25s ea	16837-0888-25	9.92	
(DUAL ACTION)			
800 mg-10 mg-165 mg,			
25s ea	16837-0246-25	9.92	
(25+5FREE,MINT)			
800 mg-10 mg-165 mg,			
30s ea	16837-0888-26	9.90	
(25 W/FREE 10)			
800 mg-10 mg-165 mg,			
35s ea	16837-0291-24	9.90	
(MINT,25 W/FREE 15,MINT)			
800 mg-10 mg-165 mg,			
40s ea	16837-0888-40	9.90	
(BERRY FLAVOR)			
800 mg-10 mg-165 mg,			
50s ea	16837-0291-50	17.81	
(COOL MINT,MINT)			
800 mg-10 mg-165 mg,			
50s ea	16837-0888-50	17.81	
(DUAL ACTION)			
800 mg-10 mg-165 mg,			
50s ea	16837-0246-50	17.81	
(BERRY FLAVOR 10 FREE)			
800 mg-10 mg-165 mg,			
60s ea	16837-0291-51	16.17	
(W/10 FREE,MINT)			
800 mg-10 mg-165 mg,			
60s ea	16837-0888-51	17.76	
(W/FREE 10)			
800 mg-10 mg-165 mg,			
85s ea	16837-0291-85	21.60	
(BERRY FLAVOR,2500X1)			
800 mg-10 mg-165 mg,			
2500s ea	16837-0291-21	585.00	
PEPDITE JUNIOR (Nutricia)			
PDR,PO (DAIRY-FREE,LACTOSE-FREE)			
51 gm 15s	49735-0117-66	81.90	68.00
51 gm 15s	49735-0117-80	81.90	
PEPTAMEN (Nestle)			
LIQ,PO (250MLX24,GLUTEN-FREE)			
250 ml 24s	00065-9014-70	143.42	
250 ml 24s	00065-9067-70	143.42	
PEPTAMEN 1.5 (Nestle)			
LIQ,PO (250MLX24,GLUTEN-FREE)			
250 ml 24s	00065-9087-70	214.56	
(250X24,UNFLAVORED)			
250 ml 24s	00065-9088-70	214.56	
PEPTAMEN 1.5 ULTRAPAK (Nestle)			
LIQ,PO (1000MLX6EA)			
1000 ml 6s	00065-9089-72	221.69	
PEPTAMEN 1.5 ULTRAPAK SPIKERIGHT (Nestle)			
SOL,PO, 1000 ml 6s	98716-0281-94	221.69	
PEPTAMEN AF LIQ (Nestle)			
LIQ,PO (FPO,PREBIO1,ENTERAL USE)			
250 ml 24s	00065-9092-71	181.15	
1000 ml 6s	00065-9092-72	188.42	
PEPTAMEN AF ULTRAPAK SPIKERIGHT (Nestle)			
SOL,PO, 1000 ml 6s	98716-0763-90	188.42	
PEPTAMEN JUNIOR (Nestle)			
LIQ,PO (250MLX24,GLUTEN-FREE)			
250 ml 24s	00065-9070-70	162.14	
250 ml 24s	00065-9070-71	162.14	
250 ml 24s	00065-9070-72	162.14	
(250MLX24,UNFLAVORED)			
250 ml 24s	00065-9069-70	162.14	
PDS,PO (400GMX12,GLUTEN-FREE)			
400 gm 12s	00065-9169-70	532.80	
PEPTAMEN JUNIOR 1.5 WITH PREBIO1 (Nestle)			
LIQ,PO (1X250ML,GLUTEN-FREE)			
250 ml	98716-0073-63	9.43	
(24X250ML,GLUTEN-FREE)			
250 ml 24s	00212-8473-15	226.42	
(1X1000ML,ULTAPAK)			
1000 ml	98716-0085-43	38.96	
(6X1000ML,ULTAPAK)			
1000 ml 6s	00212-8415-15	233.77	
PEPTAMEN JUNIOR FIBER W/ PREBIO1 (Nestle)			
LIQ,PO (250MLX24,GLUTEN-FREE)			
250 ml 24s	00065-9068-71	166.18	
PEPTAMEN JUNIOR ULTRAPAK (Nestle)			
LIQ,PO (1000MLX6)			
1000 ml 6s	00065-9070-90	169.34	
PEPTAMEN JUNIOR ULTRAPAK SPIKERIGHT (Nestle)			
SOL,PO (UNFLAVORED)			
1000 ml 6s	98716-0773-60	169.34	
PEPTAMEN JUNIOR W/PREBIO1 (Nestle)			
LIQ,PO (250MLX24,GLUTEN-FREE)			
250 ml 24s	00065-9068-70	166.18	

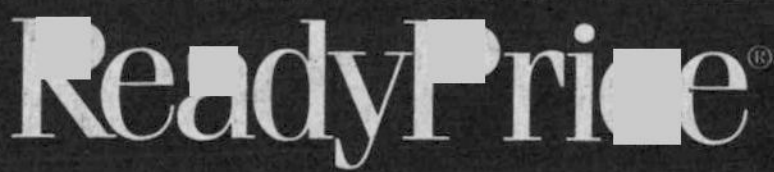

PROD/MFR	HRI, UPC,NDC	AWP	SRP
PEPTAMEN OS (Nestle)			
LIQ,PO (1X237ML,CREAMY VANILLA)			
237 ml	43900-0337-94	5.95	
(1X237ML,RICH CHOCOLATE)			
237 ml	43900-0371-29	5.95	
(24X237ML,CREAMY VANILLA)			
237 ml 24s	43900-0337-99	142.88	
(24X237ML,RICH CHOCOLATE)			
237 ml 24s	43900-0372-19	142.88	
PEPTAMEN OS 1.5 (Nestle)			
LIQ,PO (1X237ML,VANILLA)			
237 ml	43900-0371-22	8.48	
(24X237ML,VANILLA)			
237 ml 24s	43900-0372-29	203.47	
PEPTAMEN ULTRAPAK (Nestle)			
LIQ,PO (BAG)			
1000 ml	00065-9066-72	39.44	
1500 ml	00065-9066-73	59.16	
PEPTAMEN VHP (Nestle)			
LIQ,PO (UNFLAVORED)			
250 ml	00065-9073-70	9.85	
(VANILLA)			
250 ml	00065-9071-70	9.85	
PEPTAMEN VHP ULTRAPAK (Nestle)			
LIQ,PO (BAG)			
1000 ml	00065-9068-72	43.82	
1500 ml	00065-9068-73	65.73	
PEPTAMEN W PREBIO1 (Nestle)			
LIQ,PO (250MLX24,GLUTEN-FREE)			
250 ml 24s	00065-9076-70	148.61	
(1000MLX6,ULTRAPAK)			
1000 ml 6s	00065-9076-72	155.74	
(1500MLX4,ULTRAPAK)			
1500 ml 4s	00065-9076-73	155.71	
PEPTAMEN WITH PREBIO1 ULTRAPAK SPIKERIGHT (Nestle)			
SOL,PO, 1000 ml 6s	98716-0228-04	155.74	
1500 ml 4s	98716-0228-05	155.71	
PEPTIC RELIEF (Rugby)			
CTB,PO (CHERRY)			
262 mg, 30s ea	00536-4301-07	2.93	
SUS,PO (SF,MINT)			
262.5 mg/15 ml,			
240 ml	00536-1810-59	3.12	
(Phys Total Care)			
REPACK			
CTB,PO, 262 mg, 30s ea	54868-4104-00	7.02	
(Physician Partner)			
REPACK			
CTB,PO, 262 mg, 30s ea	21695-0639-30	11.89	
PEPTINEX DT (Nestle)			
LIQ,PO (RTU,TUBE FEEDING)			
250 ml 24s	00212-3701-51	150.62	
(RTU, TUBE FEEDING)			
1000 ml 6s	00212-3701-42	157.82	
1500 ml 6s	00212-3701-44	236.74	
PEPTINEX DT PEDIATRIC (Nestle)			
LIQ,PO (WITH FIBER,LACTOSE-FREE)			
250 ml 24s	00212-3752-51	166.18	
(WITHOUT FIBER)			
250 ml 24s	00212-3751-51	162.14	
PEPTO BISMOL (P & G Company)			
CTB,PO (CAPLET)			
262 mg, 24s ea	37000-0452-02	3.26	
30s ea	37000-0021-04	3.26	
30s ea	37000-0033-09	3.26	
(CAPLET)			
262 mg, 40s ea	37000-0452-03	5.15	
48s ea	37000-0021-06	5.15	
48s ea	37000-0033-10	5.15	
SUS,PO, 262 mg/15 ml,			
120 ml	37000-0032-01	2.26	
240 ml	37000-0032-02	3.32	
360 ml	37000-0032-03	4.44	
480 ml	37000-0032-04	5.21	
(Altura)			
REPACK			
SUS,PO, 262 mg/15 ml,			
240 ml	63874-0090-24	5.70	
PEPTO BISMOL MAXIMUM STRENGTH (P & G Company)			
SUS,PO, 525 mg/15 ml,			
120 ml	37000-0019-01	3.32	
240 ml	37000-0019-02	4.44	
360 ml	37000-0019-03	5.21	
PEPTO RELIEF (Advance)			
CTB,PO, 262 mg, 30s ea	17714-0045-30	3.15	
PEPTO-BISMOL (P & G Company)			
TAB,PO (SF,CAPLET)			
262 mg, 24s ea	37000-0476-02	3.26	
(A-S Medication)			
REPACK			
CTB,PO (CHERRY)			
262 mg, 30s ea	54569-4236-00	3.26	
SUS,PO, 262 mg/15 ml,			
120 ml	54569-3285-00	2.26	
(Southwood)			
REPACK			
SUS,PO, 262 mg/15 ml,			
240 ml	58016-7016-01	5.43	
PERATIVE (Abbott)			
LIQ,PO, 240 ml	70074-0506-29	3.90	
PERATIVE ROSS READY-TO-HANG (Abbott)			
LIQ,PO, 1000 ml	70074-0519-49	18.30	
1500 ml	70074-0576-36	27.46	
PERCOGESIC (Medtech)			
TAB,PO, 325 mg-30 mg,			
24s ea	75137-0904-92	2.33	
50s ea	75137-0004-93	3.86	
90s ea	75137-0004-95	5.79	
PERCOGESIC EXTRA STRENGTH (Medtech)			
TAB,PO (CAPLET)			
500 mg-12.5 mg,			
40s ea	75137-0004-97	3.86	
PERCY MEDICINE (Merrick)			
SUS,PO, 525 mg/5 ml,			
90 ml	00322-2222-03	3.39	4.56
PERDIEM (Novartis Consumer)			
PDR,PO (PACKET)			
6s ea	00067-0690-16	4.36	
TAB,PO (OVERNIGHT RELIEF)			
15 mg, 60s ea	00067-6025-60	8.78	
PERI-COLACE (Purdue Products L.P.)			
TAB,PO, 50 mg-8.6 mg,			
10s ea	67618-0106-10	3.94	
30s ea	67618-0106-30	11.31	
60s ea	67618-0106-60	19.60	
PERI-WASH (Coloplast)			
LIQ,TP, 118 ml 36s	11701-0014-04	89.64	93.96
237 ml 12s	11701-0014-05	40.08	41.88
PERICLEAN (Ameriderm Labs)			
SPR,TP (W/ALOE)			
240 ml	63921-0510-08	1.18	
3840 ml	63921-0510-01	14.04	
PERIDIN-C (Beutlich)			
TAB,PO, 200 mg-200 mg,			
100s ea	00283-0597-01	17.39	26.77
PERIES (Xttrium Labs)			
PAD,TP, 40s ea	00116-0810-01	1.56	2.60
100s ea	00116-0810-02	2.53	5.50
PERIFLEX ADVANCE (Nutricia)			
PDR,PO (4X454GM,CHOCOLATE)			
454 gm 4s	49735-0126-51	288.60	
(4X454GM,ORANGE)			
454 gm 4s	49735-0126-52	288.60	
(UNFLAVORED,4X454GM)			
454 gm 4s	49735-0126-50	288.60	
PERIFLEX JUNIOR (Nutricia)			
PDR,PO (4X454GM,CHOCOLATE)			
454 gm 4s	49735-0125-31	206.70	
(FOR PKU, ORANGE,ORANGE)			
454 gm 4s	49735-0114-01	206.70	
(FOR PKU,UNFLAVORED)			
454 gm 4s	49735-0114-02	206.70	
PERIFRESH (Dermarite)			
LIQ,TP, 237 ml	61924-0199-08	2.32	
3840 ml	61924-0199-01	13.45	
PERIGIENE (Dermarite)			
SOL,TP (DYE-FREE,FRAGRANCE-FREE)			
237 ml	61924-0198-08	1.60	
3840 ml	61924-0198-01	21.00	
PERIGUARD (Dermarite)			
OIN,TP, 120 gm	61924-0204-04	3.69	
454 gm	61924-0204-16	16.38	
PERISCENT (Ameriderm Labs)			
SOL,TP (48X237ML,AF,DYE-FREE)			
237 ml 48s	63921-0520-08	1.19	
PERISHIELD (Ameriderm Labs)			
OIN,TP (W/ALOE)			
113 gm	63921-0500-04	2.75	
(24X452GM)			
452 gm 24s	63921-0505-16	6.25	
PERMA GRIP (Lee Pharm)			
POW,NA, 120 gm	23558-0686-50	9.60	
120 gm 12s	23558-0686-51	115.20	
PERMETHRIN (Actavis Mid Atlantic)			
LOT,TP, 1%, 60 ml	00472-5242-67	8.19	
60 ml 2s	00472-5242-69	12.75	
PERNOX (Ranbaxy Labs)			
SOA,TP (1X113GM,FOR OILY SKIN)			
113 gm	10631-0107-04	21.83	
113 ml	10631-0288-04	21.83	
PERNOX LATHERING ABRADANT SCRUB CLEANSER (Ranbaxy Labs)			
SOA,TP (1X141GM FRESHLY SCENTED)			
141 gm	10631-0289-05	22.47	
PERNOX SCRUB CLEANSER (Ranbaxy Labs)			
CRE,TP (1X56GM)			
1.5%-2%, 56 gm	10631-0288-02	13.26	
PEROXYL (Colgate Oral)			
GEL,MM, 1.5%, 15 gm	38341-0081-88	4.44	
LIQ,PO (ORIGINAL MINT)			
1.5%, 236 ml	38341-0080-08	4.44	
(REFRESHING,COOL MINT)			
1.5%, 236 ml	38341-0103-80	4.44	
(ORIGINAL MINT)			
1.5%, 473 ml	38341-0080-16	7.50	
(REFRESHING,COOL MINT)			
1.5%, 473 ml	38341-0103-79	7.50	
PERRY PRENATAL (Perry Med)			
TAB,PO (CAPSULE)			
200s ea	11763-0522-01	6.60	
PETERSON'S OINTMENT (Lee Pharm)			
OIN,TP (W/APPLICATOR)			
27 gm	23558-0689-00	6.00	
27 gm 12s	23558-0689-01	72.00	
37.5 gm	23558-0689-10	6.00	
37.5 gm 12s	23558-0689-11	72.00	
90 gm	23558-0689-20	9.96	
90 gm 12s	23558-0689-21	119.52	
PETROLATUM (Amend)			
OIN,TP (YELLOW 2A)			
454 gm	17317-1055-01	4.90	
(Consolidated Midland)			
DRE,TP (5/19CM)			
ea	00223-3502-05	14.00	
(7/10CM)			
ea	00223-3503-07	12.50	
OIN,OP, 3.75 gm	00223-4390-03	2.75	
TP (FOILPACK)			
4 gm 144s	00223-0053-46	13.00	
5 gm 144s	00223-0053-45	22.50	
30 gm	00223-4140-15	1.60	
120 gm	00223-4140-11	2.00	
454 gm	00223-4140-04	3.25	
(Denison)			
OIN,TP, 30 gm	00295-1232-95	0.57	
(Fougera)			
OIN,TP (UNIT OF USE)			
5 gm 144s	00168-0053-45	20.11	
30 gm	00168-0053-21	1.21	
454 gm	00168-0053-16	8.63	
PETROLATUM HYDRATED (Denison)			
OIN,TP (HYDROLATUM)			
454 gm	00295-1347-97	5.69	
PETROLATUM OINTMENT BASE (Carolina)			
OIN,TP, 454 gm	46287-0508-16	10.55	
PETROLEUM JELLY (Cardinal Health)			
OIN,TP (PRIVATE LABEL)			
390 gm	37205-0069-27	2.96	
PEVIDERM (Stratus)			
SPR,TP, 177 ml	58980-0731-61	39.75	
PFD 1 (Mead Johnson & Co)			
PDR,PO (PROTEIN/AMINO ACID FREE)			
454 gm	00087-0994-41	19.80	
PFD 2 (Mead Johnson & Co)			
PDR,PO, 454 gm	00087-0079-41	9.31	
PH INDICATOR TEST PAPERS (Apothecary)			
DEV,NA (UNIVERSAL)			
ea	25715-0669-90	5.21	8.69
PH PAPER (Beutlich)			
DEV,NA (1/4" X15)			
180s ea	00283-0074-97	22.19	34.13
PH STRIPS UNIVERSAL (Apothecary)			
DEV,NA, ea	25715-0669-89	25.20	41.99

PROD/MFR	HRI, UPC,NDC	AWP	SRP
PHANASIN (Pharmakon)			
SYR,PO (AF,SF)			
100 mg/5 ml,			
120 ml	55422-0408-04	1.78	4.25
240 ml	55422-0408-08	2.60	5.42
PHANASIN DIABETIC CHOICE (Pharmakon)			
SYR,PO (SOD.FREE,AF,SF,DYE-FREE)			
100 mg/5 ml,			
118 ml	55422-0778-04	2.39	5.98
PHANATUSS (Pharmakon)			
SYR,PO (AF,SF)			
10 mg/5 ml-100 mg/5 ml,			
120 ml	55422-0401-04	1.98	4.70
240 ml	55422-0401-08	2.69	5.62
PHANATUSS DM DIABETIC CHOICE (Pharmakon)			
SYR,PO (SORBITAL/SOD.FREE,AF,SF)			
10 mg/5 ml-100 mg/5 ml,			
118 ml	55422-0777-04	2.59	6.48
PHARMACIST'S CREME (Reese)			
CRE,TP, 0.025%-10%-15%,			
60 gm	10956-0680-02	5.84	
PHARMACY COUNTER LANCETS (Can-Am Care)			
DEV,NA (PRIVATE LABEL)			
100s ea	38396-0305-05	5.85	
PHARMASSURE B-50 COMPLEX (Rite Aid)			
TER,PO (PRIVATE LABEL)			
60s ea	48107-0049-89	7.99	9.99
PHARMASSURE CHELATED ZINC (Rite Aid)			
TAB,PO (SODIUM-FREE,YEAST-FREE)			
30 mg, 100s ea	48107-0049-86	4.99	3.99
PHARMASSURE COENZYME Q-10 (Rite Aid)			
SGL,PO (PRIVATE LABEL,SOFTGEL)			
50 mg, 30s ea	48107-0023-91	13.59	16.99
100 mg, 30s ea	48107-0023-92	21.59	26.99
(PF,SF,CORN-FREE)			
200 mg, 30s ea	48107-0064-35	27.19	33.99
PHARMASSURE FISH OIL (Rite Aid)			
SGL,PO (PRIVATE LABEL,SOFTGEL)			
120 mg-180 mg, 100s ea	48107-0050-13	8.39	10.49
PHARMASSURE FLAX SEED OIL (Rite Aid)			
SGL,PO (PRIVATE LABEL,SOFTGEL)			
1030 mg, 100s ea	48107-0070-87	9.27	11.59
PHARMASSURE FOLIC ACID (Rite Aid)			
TAB,PO (VEGETARIAN,PF,CORN-FREE)			
0.4 mg, 100s ea	48107-0049-50	3.19	3.99
250s ea	48107-0049-51	4.79	5.99
(VEGETARIAN)			
0.8 mg, 100s ea	48107-0010-16	3.99	4.99
PHARMASSURE GARLIC (Rite Aid)			
TAB,PO (PF,SF,DAIRY-FREE)			
500 mg, 100s ea	48107-0049-71	7.19	8.99
PHARMASSURE GINKGO BILOBA (Rite Aid)			
CAP,PO (STANDARDIZED)			
50 mg, 100s ea	48107-0051-27	10.79	13.49
PHARMASSURE GLUCOSAMINE SULFATE (Rite Aid)			
TAB,PO (PF,SF,CORN-FREE)			
500 mg, 60s ea	48107-0049-56	7.59	9.49
(PRIVATE LABEL)			
1000 mg-100 mg, 60s ea	48107-0010-43	12.79	15.99
PHARMASSURE GLUCOSAMINE/CHONDROITIN (Rite Aid)			
CAP,PO (PRIVATE LABEL)			
200 mg-250 mg,			
60s ea	48107-0050-21	10.39	12.99
TAB,PO, 400 mg-500 mg,			
60s ea	48107-0050-22	17.59	21.99
100s ea	48107-0049-55	27.99	34.99
600 mg-750 mg,			
60s ea	48107-0010-24	31.19	38.99
PHARMASSURE GOLDENSEAL (Rite Aid)			
CAP,PO (PRIVATE LABEL)			
500 mg, 60s ea	48107-0049-57	12.39	15.49
PHARMASSURE GRAPE SEED (Rite Aid)			
CAP,PO (STANDARDIZED,SF)			
25 mg-50 mg, 60s ea	48107-0049-59	7.19	8.99
PHARMASSURE GREEN TEA (Rite Aid)			
CAP,PO (STANDARDIZED)			
315 mg, 60s ea	48107-0049-60	5.19	6.49
PHARMASSURE L-LYSINE (Rite Aid)			
TAB,PO (VEGETARIAN,PF,SF)			
500 mg, 100s ea	48107-0049-64	5.19	6.49
PHARMASSURE LECITHIN (Rite Aid)			
SGL,PO (PRIVATE LABEL,SOFTGEL)			
1200 mg, 100s ea	48107-0051-30	6.79	8.49

PROD/MFR	HRI, UPC,NDC	AWP	SRP
PHARMASSURE LUTEIN (Rite Aid)			
SGL,PO (PF,SF,DAIRY-FREE)			
6 mg, 60s ea	48107-0070-88	7.99	9.99
PHARMASSURE MAGNESIUM (Rite Aid)			
CAP,PO (SF,CORN-FREE,DAIRY-FREE)			
500 mg, 100s ea	48107-0010-19	7.19	8.99
PHARMASSURE MELATONIN (Rite Aid)			
TAB,PO (VEGETARIAN,PF,SF)			
3 mg-2 mg, 60s ea	48107-0049-67	4.39	5.49
(VEGETARIAN)			
3 mg-2 mg, 100s ea	48107-0049-68	5.19	6.49
PHARMASSURE MILK THISTLE (Rite Aid)			
SGL,PO (STANDARDIZED)			
200 mg, 60s ea	48107-0049-69	9.19	11.49
PHARMASSURE MSM 1000 (Rite Aid)			
CAP,PO (PRIVATE LABEL)			
1000 mg, 60s ea	48107-0010-44	11.19	13.99
PHARMASSURE NIACIN (Rite Aid)			
TAB,PO (VEGETARIAN,PF,SF)			
100 mg, 100s ea	48107-0049-70	4.39	5.49
PHARMASSURE PAPAYA ENZYME (Rite Aid)			
CTB,PO (PF,DAIRY-FREE)			
250s ea	48107-0049-72	4.79	5.99
PHARMASSURE POTASSIUM (Rite Aid)			
TAB,PO (VEGETARIAN,PF,CORN-FREE)			
99 mg, 100s ea	48107-0049-73	4.79	5.99
PHARMASSURE PREMIUM WOMEN'S BIOMULTIPLE (Rite Aid)			
TAB,PO (PRIVATE LABEL)			
60s ea	48107-0000-08	11.19	13.99
PHARMASSURE SAW PALMETTO (Rite Aid)			
SGL,PO (STANDARDIZED)			
160 mg, 60s ea	48107-0051-34	9.99	12.49
100s ea	48107-0051-35	13.59	16.99
PHARMASSURE SELENIUM (Rite Aid)			
TAB,PO (VEGETARIAN)			
100 mcg, 100s ea	48107-0049-77	4.39	5.49
200 mcg, 100s ea	48107-0049-76	6.79	8.49
PHARMASSURE SIBERIAN ROOT (Rite Aid)			
SGL,PO (CONCENTRATED,PF,SF)			
1000 mg, 100s ea	48107-0050-24	7.99	9.99
PHARMASSURE VALERIAN (Rite Aid)			
SGL,PO (STANDARDIZED,PF,SF)			
250 mg, 60s ea	48107-0049-83	8.79	10.99
PHARMASSURE VITAMIN A (Rite Aid)			
SGL,PO (PF,SF,CORN-FREE)			
10000 iu, 100s ea	48107-0048-93	3.99	4.99
PHARMASSURE VITAMIN B-12 (Rite Aid)			
TAB,PO (VEGETARIAN)			
500 mcg, 100s ea	48107-0048-99	5.19	6.49
TER,PO (VEGETARIAN,PF,SF)			
1000 mcg, 60s ea	48107-0049-05	6.87	8.59
PHARMASSURE VITAMIN B-6 (Rite Aid)			
TAB,PO (PRIVATE LABEL)			
100 mg, 100s ea	48107-0049-00	5.19	6.49
200 mg, 60s ea	48107-0049-01	5.59	6.99
PHARMASSURE VITAMIN C (Rite Aid)			
TAB,PO (PF,SF,CORN-FREE)			
500 mg, 100s ea	48107-0049-14	3.83	4.79
250s ea	48107-0049-15	6.39	7.99
(VEGETARIAN,PF,SF)			
1000 mg, 100s ea	48107-0049-92	7.99	9.99
100s ea	48107-0051-21	6.95	8.69
PHARMASSURE VITAMIN E (Rite Aid)			
SGL,PO (PRIVATE LABEL,SOFTGEL)			
200 iu, 100s ea	48107-0049-40	5.19	6.49
400 iu, 100s ea	48107-0049-38	9.19	11.49
(PF,SF,CORN-FREE)			
1000 iu, 60s ea	48107-0049-37	8.79	10.99
PHARMASSURE ZINC (Rite Aid)			
TAB,PO (PRIVATE LABEL)			
50 mg, 100s ea	48107-0049-85	5.99	4.79
PHARMASSURE ZINC LOZENGES (Rite Aid)			
LOZ,MM (YEAST-FREE)			
60 mg-10 mg, 30s ea	48107-0049-87	3.59	4.49
PHEN-LAX (Global Source)			
TAB,PO, 90 mg, 30s ea	59618-0703-07	2.39	
PHENAGESIC (Global Source)			
TAB,PO, 325 mg-30 mg,			
90s ea	59618-0700-13	4.60	
(Major)			
TAB,PO, 325 mg-30 mg,			
100s ea	00904-5141-59	3.90	

PROD/MFR	HRI, UPC,NDC	AWP	SRP
PHENASEPTIC (Rugby)			
LIQ,PO (CHERRY)			
1.4%, 180 ml	00536-2425-58	2.72	
PHENAZO (Contract Pharmacal)			
TAB,PO, 95 mg, 30s ea	10267-0064-30	4.50	
PHENEX (Abbott)			
CTB,PO (CHOCOLATE MINT)			
350s ea	70074-0582-11	67.20	
(LEMON-LIME)			
350s ea	70074-0582-09	67.20	
PHENEX-1 (Abbott)			
PDR,PO, 400 gm	70074-0511-21	23.14	
PHENEX-2 (Abbott)			
PDR,PO, 400 gm	70074-0511-23	45.43	
(VANILLA)			
400 gm	70074-0557-56	45.43	
PHENFLU DM (MCR American)			
TAB,PO, 100s ea	58605-0435-01	114.26	
PHENYL-FREE 1 (Mead Johnson & Co)			
PDR,PO, 454 gm	00087-0074-47	29.03	
PHENYL-FREE 2 (Mead Johnson & Co)			
PDR,PO, 454 gm	00087-0080-41	33.52	
PHENYL-FREE 2HP (Mead Johnson & Co)			
PDR,PO, 454 gm	00087-0081-41	60.26	
PHENYLADE 40 DRINK MIX (Applied Nutr. Corp.)			
POW,PO (PHENYLALANINE FREE)			
25 gm 20s	00847-0954-04	82.63	
25 gm 20s	00847-0954-14	82.63	
PHENYLADE 60 DRINK MIX (Applied Nutr. Corp.)			
POW,PO (30X16.7GM,UNFLAVORED)			
16.7 gm 30s	00847-0956-04	107.88	
(30X16.7GM,VANILLA)			
16.7 gm 30s	00847-0956-24	107.88	
(4X454GM, VANILLA)			
454 gm 4s	00847-0956-22	337.50	
(4X454GM,UNFLAVORED)			
454 gm 4s	00847-0956-02	337.50	
PHENYLADE AMINO ACID (Applied Nutr. Corp.)			
BAR,PO (MED SUPV,CHOCOLATE)			
47 gm 12s	00847-0959-06	105.88	
(MED SUPV)			
47 gm 12s	00847-0957-06	105.88	
50 gm 12s	00847-0958-06	105.88	
PHENYLADE AMINO ACID BLEND (Applied Nutr. Corp.)			
POW,PO (30X12.4GM,UNFLAVORED)			
30s ea	00847-0950-04	153.75	
(USE W/MED SUPV)			
454 gm 4s	00847-0950-00	579.38	
PHENYLADE DRINK MIX (Applied Nutr. Corp.)			
POW,PO (MED. SUPERV,STRAWBERRY)			
454 gm 4s	00847-0954-42	185.38	
(MED. SUPERV.,VANILLA)			
454 gm 4s	00847-0952-22	185.38	
(MED. SUPV,ORANGE CREME)			
454 gm 4s	00847-0953-32	185.38	
(PHENYLALANINE FREE)			
454 gm 4s	00847-0951-12	185.38	
PHENYLADE ESSENTIAL DRINK MIX (Applied Nutr. Corp.)			
POW,PO (W/FLAX&FIBER,CHOCOLATE)			
40 gm 16s	00847-0950-14	71.13	
(W/FLAX&FIBER,STRAWBERRY)			
40 gm 16s	00847-0950-44	71.13	
(W/FLAX&FIBER,VANILLA)			
40 gm 16s	00847-0950-24	71.13	
(W/FLAX&FIBER)			
40 gm 16s	00847-0950-34	71.13	
(W/ FLAX&FIBER)			
454 gm 4s	00847-0950-42	187.50	
(W/FLAX&FIBER,CHOCOLATE)			
454 gm 4s	00847-0950-12	187.50	
(W/FLAX&FIBER,VANILLA)			
454 gm 4s	00847-0950-22	187.50	
(W/FLAX&FIBER)			
454 gm 4s	00847-0950-32	187.50	
PHENYLADE MTE AMINO ACID BLEND (Applied Nutr. Corp.)			
POW,PO (30X12.8GM,UNFLAVORED)			
30s ea	00847-0959-64	153.75	
(USE W/MED SUPV)			
454 gm 4s	00847-0959-60	579.38	

PROD/MFR	HRI, UPC,NDC	AWP	SRP
PHENYLADE PHEBLOC (Applied Nutr. Corp.)			
TAB,PO (PHENYLALANINE FREE)			
550s ea	00847-0955-01	303.00	
PHENYLALANINE (Freeda)			
L-PHENYLALANINE			
TAB,PO (PF,SF,DYE-FREE)			
500 mg, 100s ea	10432-0197-01	15.57	25.95
(Miller)			
CAP,PO, 500 mg, 100s ea	17204-0902-40	15.78	26.30
PHENYLALANINE (Carlson,J.R.)			
CAP,PO (SF,CORN-FREE,SALT-FREE)			
500 mg, 60s ea	88395-0079-16	7.22	14.44
180s ea	88395-0079-12	19.44	38.88
(VITAFLO, LLC)			
PDS,PO, 50 mg/4 gm,			
30s ea	50600-0549-44	120.00	150.00
PHENYLEPHRINE HYDROCHLORIDE (Consolidated Midland)			
SOL,NS, 0.12%, 15 ml	00223-6694-15	2.50	
(Truxton)			
SOL,NS, 1%, 480 ml	00463-9019-16	9.60	
(A-S Medication)			
REPACK			
TAB,PO, 10 mg, 36s ea	54569-5820-00	1.81	
PHENYLGESIC (Teva)			
TAB,PO, 325 mg-30 mg,			
100s ea	00182-1027-01	4.39	
PHICON (T-Lite)			
KIT,TP (COLD SORE)			
0.5%-7500 iu-2000 iu,			
ea	51189-0092-25	59.95	
(PAPER CUT)			
0.5%-7500 iu-2000 iu,			
ea	51189-0094-25	59.95	
(POISON IVY)			
0.5%-7500 iu-2000 iu,			
ea	51189-0095-25	59.95	
(SUNBURN)			
0.5%-7500 iu-2000 iu,			
ea	51189-0093-25	59.95	
PHICON E (T-Lite)			
LIQ,TP, 15 ml	51189-0078-15	4.95	
PHILLIPS MILK OF MAGNESIA (Bayer HealthCare)			
SUS,PO, 400 mg/5 ml,			
120 ml	12843-0353-01	1.97	
(FRESH MINT)			
400 mg/5 ml,			
120 ml	12843-0363-04	1.97	
(WILD CHERRY)			
400 mg/5 ml,			
120 ml	12843-0393-22	1.97	
(STRAWBERRY)			
400 mg/5 ml,			
240 ml	12843-0347-10	3.95	
360 ml	12843-0353-02	3.67	
(FRESH MINT)			
400 mg/5 ml,			
360 ml	12843-0363-05	3.67	
(WILD CHERRY)			
400 mg/5 ml,			
360 ml	12843-0393-24	3.67	
780 ml	12843-0353-03	6.01	
(FRESH MINT)			
400 mg/5 ml,			
780 ml	12843-0363-06	6.01	
(WILD CHERRY)			
400 mg/5 ml,			
780 ml	12843-0393-25	6.01	
PHILLIPS' (Bayer HealthCare)			
CTB,PO (MINT)			
311 mg, 100s ea	12843-0373-12	3.95	
PHILLIPS' HALEY'S M-O (Bayer HealthCare)			
LIQ,PO (FLAVORED)			
300 mg/5 ml-1.25 ml/5 ml,			
360 ml	12843-0360-68	4.75	
780 ml	12843-0360-69	7.22	
PHILLIPS' STOOL SOFTENER LAXATIVE (Bayer HealthCare)			
SGL,PO (LIQUIGEL)			
100 mg, 10s ea	12843-0035-10	1.62	
30s ea	12843-0035-20	3.24	
PHISO-PUFF (Chattem)			
DEV,NA (CLEANING SPONGE)			
ea	41167-0528-01	3.01	
PHISODERM (Chattem)			
LIQ,TP (OILY SKIN,SOAP-FREE)			
120 ml	41167-0523-02	3.42	
(UNSCENTED,SOAP-FREE)			
120 ml	41167-0521-02	3.42	
(OILY SKIN,SOAP-FREE)			
240 ml	41167-0523-04	5.15	
(UNSCENTED,SOAP-FREE)			
240 ml	41167-0521-04	5.14	
(OILY SKIN,SOAP-FREE)			
420 ml	41167-0523-06	7.54	
(UNSCENTED,SOAP-FREE)			
420 ml	41167-0521-06	7.54	
LOT,TP (BABY)			
120 ml	41167-0525-03	3.13	
SOA,TP (SCENTED)			
ea	41167-0531-03	1.93	
(UNSCENTED)			
ea	41167-0532-03	1.93	
PHISODERM ANTIBACTERIAL CLEANSER (Chattem)			
LIQ,TP, 0.5%, 180 ml	41167-0537-03	1.61	
(REFILL)			
0.5%, 360 ml	41167-0537-05	2.52	
PHISODERM CLEANSER & CONDITIONER (Chattem)			
LIQ,TP (SENS.SKIN,DYE-FREE)			
180 ml	41167-0526-02	3.42	
240 ml	41167-0526-04	5.17	
420 ml	41167-0526-06	7.54	
PHLEXY-10 (Nutricia)			
BAR,PO (USE W/MED SUPV)			
20s ea	49735-0100-77	117.00	
CAP,PO, 200s ea	49735-0118-09	53.30	
TAB,PO, 75s ea	49735-0119-51	40.30	
PHLEXY-10 ADD-INS (Nutricia)			
POW,NA, 17 gm 40s	49735-0118-10	254.80	
PHLEXY-10 DRINK MIX (Nutricia)			
PDR,PO (APPLE,BLACK CURRANT)			
20 gm 30s	49735-0114-67	119.60	
(TROPICAL SURPRISE)			
20 gm 30s	49735-0119-10	119.60	
PHLEXY-VITS (Nutricia)			
PDR,PO (PACKET)			
7 gm 30s	49735-0106-85	40.30	
PHOS-FLUR (Colgate Oral)			
SOL,PO (BUBBLEGUM)			
1 mg/5 ml, 500 ml	00126-0139-46	9.28	
(COOL MINT)			
1 mg/5 ml, 500 ml	00126-0135-46	9.28	
(WINTERGREEN)			
1 mg/5 ml, 500 ml	00126-0138-46	9.28	
500 ml	00126-0144-46	9.28	
PHOS-NAK (Cypress Pharm)			
PDR,PO (SF,FRUIT,PACKETS)			
1.5 gm 100s UD	60258-0006-01	38.80	
PHOSPHATE LAXATIVE (Major)			
SOL,PO (SINGLE DOSE,SF)			
45 ml	00904-5666-75	2.99	
PHOSPHATIDYL CHOLINE (Carlson,J.R.)			
SGL,PO (PF,SF,DAIRY-FREE)			
400 mg, 100s ea	88395-0087-61	7.45	14.90
(PF,SF,CORN-FREE)			
1200 mg, 250s ea	88395-0087-62	16.95	33.90
PHOSPHATIDYL SERINE (Carlson,J.R.)			
SGL,PO (PF,SF,CORN-FREE)			
100 mg, 30s ea	88395-0087-70	11.45	22.90
90s ea	88395-0087-71	32.75	65.50
PHOSPHATIDYL-CHOLINE (Miller)			
CAP,PO, 420 mg, 100s ea	17204-0924-40	12.60	16.80
PHOSPHATIDYL-SERINE (Westlake Labs.)			
CAP,PO (PF,SF)			
60s ea	10539-0830-04	54.60	78.00
PHOSPHO-SODA (Fleet,C.B.)			
LIQ,PO (GINGER-LEMON)			
900 mg/5 ml-2400 mg/5 ml,			
45 ml	00132-0109-15	2.60	
(UNFLAVORED)			
900 mg/5 ml-2400 mg/5 ml,			
45 ml	00132-0108-15	2.60	
(Phys Total Care)			
REPACK			
LIQ,PO, 45 ml	54868-4235-00	4.38	
90 ml	54868-4235-01	3.60	
(UNFLAVORED)			
900 mg/5 ml-2400 mg/5 ml,			
90 ml	54868-5393-00	10.38	
PHOSPHORUS (Luyties)			
TAB,SL (6X)			
6 x, 500s ea	00618-7051-03	3.99	
5500s ea	00618-7051-10	30.32	
(30X)			
12 x, 500s ea	00622-7051-03	4.19	
5500s ea	00622-7051-10	31.83	
(12X)			
30 x, 500s ea	00624-7051-03	4.19	
5500s ea	00624-7051-10	31.83	
(Walker Pharmacal)			
TAB,SL (6X)			
250s ea	00619-7051-02	2.97	
PHYLLO QUINONE (Bio-Tech Pharm)			
CAP,PO, 100 mcg,			
100s ea	53191-0354-01	4.50	
PHYTOLACCA DECANDRA (Luyties)			
TAB,SL (6X)			
6 x, 500s ea	00618-7058-03	3.99	
5500s ea	00618-7058-10	30.32	
(30X)			
12 x, 500s ea	00622-7058-03	4.19	
5500s ea	00622-7058-10	31.83	
(12X)			
30 x, 500s ea	00624-7058-03	4.19	
5500s ea	00624-7058-10	31.83	
PIC INDOLOR INSUPEN (Medical Plastic)			
DEV,NA (SENSITIVE 32G 6MM)			
100s ea	08271-4504-00	21.99	
(SENSITIVE 32G 8MM)			
100s ea	08271-4505-00	21.99	
(ULTRAFIN 29G 12MM)			
100s ea	08271-4500-00	15.99	
(ULTRAFIN 30G 8MM)			
100s ea	08271-4501-00	15.99	
(ULTRAFIN 31G 6MM)			
100s ea	08271-4502-00	15.99	
(ULTRAFIN 31G 8MM)			
100s ea	08271-4503-00	15.99	
PIC INDULOR INSUMED (Medical Plastic)			
DEV,NA (1/2CC,31G,5/16")			
100s ea	08271-3522-00	34.45	
(1CC,30G,1/2")			
100s ea	08271-3520-00	34.45	
(1CC,30G,5/16")			
100s ea	08271-3521-00	34.45	
(3/10CC,31G,5/16")			
100s ea	08271-3523-00	34.45	
PIN-X (Penn Labs)			
CTB,PO (PINWORM TREATMENT)			
720.5 mg, 12s ea	13893-0689-08	13.44	17.99
SUS,PO (EQUIV 50 MG/ML PYRANTEL)			
144 mg/ml, 30 ml	13893-0691-45	8.61	
60 ml	13893-0691-49	12.94	
PINE (Ellon)			
SOL,SL (DROPS)			
10.5 ml	51762-0026-10		9.25
PINEAPPA (Key Company)			
TAB,PO (YEAST-FREE)			
15 mg-300 mg,			
100s ea	11694-0860-01	5.00	
250s ea	11694-0860-25	10.00	
PINK BISMUTH (Chain Drug Marketing)			
CTB,PO (SF)			
262 mg, 30s ea	63868-0989-30	1.92	2.99
SUS,PO, 262 mg/15 ml,			
237 ml	63868-0302-34	2.21	4.79
(Pharm Assoc Inc)			
SUS,PO (10 CUPS/TRAY,SF)			
262 mg/15 ml,			
30 ml 10s UD	00121-4803-30	17.19	
PINK EYE RELIEF (Similasan Corp.)			
SOL,OP (DROPS)			
6 x-6 x-12 x,			
10 ml	59262-0348-11	6.21	10.99
PINWORM (Reese)			
SUS,PO, 144 mg/ml,			
30 ml	10956-0618-01	7.32	
PIOXIL (A. G. Marin)			
SHA,TP, 240 ml	12539-0819-08	15.30	
PITUITARY (Key Company)			
CAP,PO, 40 mg, 100s ea	11694-0920-01	7.50	
PITUITARY WHOLE (Miller)			
TAB,PO, 35 mg, 100s ea	17204-0526-40	8.82	14.00
PIVOT 1.5 CAL (Abbott)			
LIQ,PO, 237 ml	70074-0580-14	9.01	
(RTH)			
1000 ml	70074-0580-16	38.93	

PROD/MFR	HRI, UPC,NDC	AWP	SRP
PKU 1 (Milupa North America)			
PDR,PO (2X500GM)			
500 gm 2s	81361-9345-01	156.25	
PKU 2 (Nutricia)			
PDR,PO (2X500GM)			
500 gm 2s	81361-9346-01	235.30	
PKU 3 (Nutricia)			
PO (2X500GM)			
500 gm 2s	81361-9347-01	239.20	
PKU COOLER 10 (VITAFLO, LLC)			
LIQ,PO (10GM PROTEIN EQUIVALENT)			
87 ml 30s	50600-0548-52	112.50	159.33
87 ml 30s	50600-0548-76	112.50	159.33
87 ml 30s	50600-0549-99	112.50	159.33
SOL,PO (30X87ML)			
87 ml 30s	50600-0513-18	112.50	159.33
PKU COOLER 15 (VITAFLO, LLC)			
LIQ,PO (15GM PROTEIN EQUIVALENT)			
130 ml 30s	50600-0545-00	168.75	239.00
130 ml 30s	50600-0545-62	168.75	239.00
130 ml 30s	50600-0549-75	168.75	239.00
SOL,PO (30X130ML)			
130 ml 30s	50600-0519-98	168.75	239.00
PKU COOLER 20 (VITAFLO, LLC)			
LIQ,PO (20GM PROTEIN EQUIVALENT)			
174 ml 30s	50600-0548-14	225.00	318.67
174 ml 30s	50600-0548-38	225.00	318.67
174 ml 30s	50600-0550-19	225.00	318.67
SOL,PO (30X174ML)			
174 ml 30s	50600-0520-01	225.00	318.67
PKU EXPRESS (VITAFLO, LLC)			
PDR,PO (ENTERAL, UNFLAVORED)			
25 gm 30s	50600-0532-06	168.75	239.00
(ENTERAL,LEMON,SACHET)			
25 gm 30s	50600-0533-05	168.75	239.00
(ENTERAL,ORANGE,SACHET)			
25 gm 30s	50600-0532-20	168.75	239.00
(TROPICAL)			
25 gm 30s	50600-0533-36	168.75	239.00
PKU GEL (VITAFLO, LLC)			
PO (ENTERAL, UNFLAVORED)			
20 gm 30s UD	50600-0512-02	94.50	149.00
(ENTERAL,ORANGE,SACHET)			
20 gm 30s	50600-0512-64	94.50	149.00
(ENTERAL,RASPBERRY)			
20 gm 30s UD	50600-0512-33	94.50	149.00
PLACEBO (Consolidated Midland)			
CAP,PO, 1000s ea	00223-1459-02	100.00	
1000s ea	00223-1465-02	100.00	
TAB,PO, 1000s ea	00223-1453-02	85.00	
1000s ea	00223-1454-02	100.00	
1000s ea	00223-1461-02	85.00	
1000s ea	00223-1464-02	85.00	
1000s ea	00223-1469-02	85.00	
(Truxton)			
CAP,PO, 1000s ea	00463-2039-10	30.00	
PLASTABASE 50W (Neurovites)			
GEL,TP, 454 gm	93595-2152-01	45.20	
PLASTIC STRIPS (AmerisourceBergen)			
DEV,NA (3/4",PRIVATE LABEL)			
60s ea	24385-0164-72	1.50	1.89
PLATELET CONCENTRATE INFUSION (Abbott Hosp)			
DEV,NA (14")			
48s ea	00074-4510-58	211.97	
PLAX ADVANCED FORMULA (Johnson & Johnson)			
SOL,MM (SOFTMINT)			
120 ml	86414-0001-40	1.00	
(MINT SENSATION,MINT)			
480 ml	86414-0001-73	3.40	
(ORIGINAL,ORIGINAL)			
480 ml	86414-0000-16	3.56	
(SOFTMINT)			
480 ml	86414-0001-16	3.56	
(MINT SENSATION,MINT)			
720 ml	86414-0001-74	4.68	
(ORIGINAL,ORIGINAL)			
720 ml	86414-0001-95	4.92	
(SOFT MINT,SOFTMINT)			
720 ml	86414-0001-96	4.92	
PLENAMINS PLUS (Rexall)			
TAB,PO (SUPER PLENAMINS PLUS,PF)			
130s ea	01220-0975-39	7.47	4.32
PLUMBUM MET (Luyties)			
TAB,SL (6X)			
6 x, 500s ea	00618-7088-03	3.99	
5500s ea	00618-7088-10	30.32	
12 x, 500s ea	00622-7088-03	4.19	
5500s ea	00622-7088-10	31.83	
30 x, 500s ea	00624-7088-03	4.19	
5500s ea	00624-7088-10	31.83	
PMS FORMULA (ADH)			
TAB,PO, 60s ea	60142-0099-06	6.98	13.95
(Neurovites)			
TAB,PO, 126s ea	93595-2032-01	10.50	
PMS FORMULA W/BETA CAROTENE (Neurovites)			
PO, 126s ea	93595-2033-01	10.50	
POCION JACCOUD (Lex)			
LIQ,PO (SWEET VERMOUTH)			
10%-5%, 120 ml	58537-0246-04	1.55	
POCKETCHEM EZ (Arkray)			
DEV,NA, ea	08317-6311-01	52.50	
50s ea	08317-6300-50	38.50	
(LEVEL 1)			
3 ml	08317-6300-05	7.20	
PODACTIN (Reese)			
POW,TP, 1%, 45 gm	10956-0642-45	3.94	
PODACTIN ANTI-FUNGAL (Reese)			
CRE,TP (MAX. STR.)			
2%, 30 gm	10956-0708-01	4.31	
PODICLENS (Woodward Labs)			
SPR,TP (AF)			
0.13%, 16 ml	60193-0440-16	7.20	
PODOPHYLLUM (Luyties)			
TAB,SL (6X)			
6 x, 500s ea	00618-7090-03	3.99	
5500s ea	00618-7090-10	30.32	
(30X)			
12 x, 500s ea	00622-7090-03	4.19	
5500s ea	00622-7090-10	31.83	
(12X)			
30 x, 500s ea	00624-7090-03	4.19	
5500s ea	00624-7090-10	31.83	
POISON IVY WASH (Major)			
SOA,TP (1X29GM)			
29 gm	00904-5989-31	24.75	
POLAR FROST (Mettler)			
GEL,TP (1X75ML)			
4%, 75 ml	67138-0533-75	6.75	
(1X150ML)			
4%, 150 ml	67138-0533-15	6.75	
POLI-GRIP (Glaxo)			
CRE,NA (ULTRA FRESH,AF)			
42 gm	10158-0058-01	2.87	
72 gm	10158-0058-03	4.26	
POLI-GRIP FREE (Glaxo)			
CRE,NA (SUPER POLI-GRIP FREE)			
42 gm	10158-0062-02	2.87	
72 gm	10158-0062-04	4.26	
POLI-GRIP SUPER (Glaxo)			
CRE,NA (ULTIMATE HOLD, ORIGINAL)			
42 gm	10158-0054-02	2.87	
72 gm	10158-0054-04	4.26	
POW,NA (ULTIMATE HOLD)			
48 gm	10158-0078-01	2.87	
POLICOSANOL (Miller)			
CAP,PO (PF,SF,SALT-FREE)			
10 mg, 60s ea	17204-0586-20	9.45	
POLIDENT (Glaxo)			
TEF,NA (MINT)			
40s ea	10158-0053-06	3.04	
60s ea	10158-0053-10	4.25	
78s ea	10158-0320-78	5.66	
108s ea	10158-0053-15	6.54	
POLIDENT 3 MINUTE (Glaxo)			
TEF,NA, 84s ea	10158-0053-08	5.66	
POLIDENT DENTU-CREME (Glaxo)			
PAS,NA (MINT)			
117 gm	10158-0092-06	2.88	
153 gm	10158-0092-13	4.04	
POLIDENT DENTU-GEL (Glaxo)			
PAS,NA (FRESH MINT)			
102 gm	10158-0095-06	2.88	
153 gm	10158-0095-08	4.04	
POLIDENT FOR PARTIALS (Glaxo)			
CRY,NA (MINT)			
36s ea	10158-0033-03	3.04	
POLIDENT FRESH CLEANSE (Glaxo)			
FOA,TP, 125 ml	10158-0096-10	4.26	
POLIDENT OVERNIGHT (Glaxo)			
TEF,NA (MINT)			
36s ea	10158-0034-03	3.04	
78s ea	10158-0034-07	5.66	
102s ea	10158-0034-09	6.54	
POLIDENT SMOKERS' (Glaxo)			
TEF,NA (MINT)			
36s ea	10158-0032-03	3.04	
POLY VITAMIN (Rugby)			
CTB,PO, 100s ea	00536-4304-01	4.43	
LIQ,PO (FRUIT,DROPS)			
50 ml	00536-8450-80	5.24	
(Pharma Pac) REPACK			
LIQ,PO (1X50ML,FRUIT,DROPS)			
50 ml	52959-0634-50	6.55	
(Phys Total Care) REPACK			
LIQ,PO (1X50ML,FRUIT,DROPS)			
50 ml	54868-6001-00	15.62	
POLY VITAMIN W/IRON (Rugby)			
CTB,PO (CHERRY-BERRY)			
100s ea	00536-7816-01	4.65	
LIQ,PO (FRUIT,DROPS)			
50 ml	00536-8530-80	5.24	
POLY-IRON 150 (Cypress Pharm)			
CAP,PO, 150 mg, 100s ea	60258-0185-01	27.95	
POLY-VENT DM (Poly)			
TAB,PO, 15 mg-400 mg-45 mg,			
60s ea	50991-0309-60	40.41	
POLY-VENT IR (Poly)			
TAB,PO, 400 mg-45 mg,			
60s ea	50991-0561-60	40.41	
POLY-VENT PLUS (Poly)			
TAB,PO, 500 mg-200 mg-45 mg,			
100s ea	50991-0500-01	70.15	
POLY-VI-SOL (Mead Johnson & Co)			
LIQ,PO (AF,DROPS)			
50 ml	00087-0402-03	7.73	
POLY-VI-SOL W/IRON (Mead Johnson & Co)			
LIQ,PO (AF,DROPS)			
50 ml	00087-0405-01	7.73	
POLY-VITAMIN CHILDREN'S (Silarx)			
LIQ,PO (DROPS)			
50 ml	54838-0003-50	4.70	
POLY-VITAMIN DROPS W/IRON LIQ (Hi-Tech)			
LIQ,PO (CHERRY,DROPS)			
50 ml	50383-0632-50	10.80	
POLY-VITAMIN W/IRON CHILDREN'S (Silarx)			
LIQ,PO (DROPS)			
50 ml	54838-0004-50	4.70	
POLYCAL (Nutricia)			
PDS,PO (WITH SPOON)			
400 gm	49735-0111-52	81.90	
POLYCOSE (Abbott)			
LIQ,PO, 126 ml	70074-0804-31	18.61	
PDR,PO, 350 gm	70074-0607-46	8.11	
POLYETHYLENE GLYCOL (3350) (UDL)			
PDS,PO (30X17GM)			
17 gm/dose, 17 gm 30s	51079-0306-30	52.61	
POLYETHYLENE GLYCOL 3350 (Perrigo)			
PDS,PO (1X119GM)			
17 gm/dose, 119 gm	45802-0868-01	5.13	
(1X238GM)			
17 gm/dose, 238 gm	45802-0868-02	9.07	
(1X510GM)			
17 gm/dose, 510 gm	45802-0868-03	17.71	
POLYETHYLENE GLYCOL 3350-GRX (Geritrex)			
POW,NA (12X250GM)			
250 gm 12s	54162-0335-02	16.38	
(12X500GM)			
500 gm 12s	54162-0335-05	23.04	
POLYMEM (Ferris)			
DEV,NA (1.5"X2" MEMB 4X2" CLOTH)			
ea	08195-7042-01	1.69	
(1.5"X2"MEMB/4"X2" CLEAR)			
ea	08195-3042-30	1.69	
(1"X1" MEMB/2X2 CLOTHDOT)			
ea	08195-7203-01	0.84	
(1"X1"MEMB ON 3"X1"CLEAR)			
ea	08195-3031-50	0.90	
(1"X1"MEMB/2X2 CLEAR DOT)			
ea	08195-0203-12	0.84	
(1X1" MEMB ON 3X1" CLOTH)			
ea	08195-7031-01	0.90	

PROD/MFR	HRI, UPC,NDC	AWP	SRP
(2"X3"MEMB ON 4"X5"FILM)			
ea	08195-0405-01	4.66	
(2X3" MEMB ON 4X5" CLOTH)			
ea	08195-7405-01	4.66	
(3.5X3.5" TUBE PAD)			
ea	08195-5335-01	3.41	
(3.5X3.5"MEMB ON6X6"FILM)			
ea	08195-0606-01	7.72	
(3.5X3.5"MEMB,6X6" CLOTH)			
ea	08195-7606-01	7.87	
(3"X3" PAD)			
ea	08195-5033-01	3.00	
(4"X12.5" PAD)			
ea	08195-5124-01	16.00	
(4"X24" ROLL)			
ea	08195-5244-01	31.44	
(4"X4" PAD)			
ea	08195-5044-01	4.04	
(5"X5" PAD)			
ea	08195-5055-01	6.13	
(6.5"X7.5" PAD)			
ea	08195-5077-01	12.38	
POLYMEM ALGINATE (Ferris)			
DEV,NA (3"X3" PAD)			
ea	08195-5833-01	3.19	
(5"X5" PAD)			
ea	08195-5855-01	6.33	
POLYMEM POLYWIC WOUND FILLER (Ferris)			
DEV,NA (3"X3")			
ea	08195-5733-01	5.20	
POLYSACC IRON 150 COMPLEX (Phys Total Care)			
REPACK			
CAP,PO, 150 mg, 100s ea	54868-5012-00	42.99	
POLYSACCHARIDE IRON (Contract Pharmacal)			
CAP,PO, 150 mg, 100s ea	10267-1465-01	32.18	
POLYSACCHARIDE IRON COMPLEX (United Research)			
CAP,PO, 150 mg, 100s ea	00677-1597-01	23.55	
POLYSKIN (Medtronic Minimed)			
DEV,NA (TRANSPARENT)			
50s ea	76300-0134-50	40.80	
POLYSONIC (Parker)			
LOT,TP (12X250ML)			
250 ml 12s	00341-0021-08	20.92	34.00
(W/ALOE VERA, 12X250ML)			
250 ml 12s	00341-0020-08	20.92	34.00
(W/ALOE VERA & DISPENSER)			
3840 ml	00341-0020-28	15.29	25.45
(W/DISPENSER)			
3840 ml	00341-0021-28	13.77	22.60
(POLYPAC W/ALOE VERA)			
3840 ml 4s	00341-0020-50	57.33	95.55
(POLYPAC, 4X3840ML)			
3840 ml 4s	00341-0021-50	51.91	86.35
POLYSPORIN (Johnson & Johnson)			
OIN,TP, 500 u/gm-10000 u/gm,			
0.9 gm 144s	00081-0798-58	34.22	
(1X14.2GM)			
500 u/gm-10000 u/gm,			
14.2 gm	00810-0798-88	4.42	
15 gm	00081-0798-88	4.22	
30 gm	00081-0798-87	6.67	
POW,TP, 500 u/gm-10000 u/gm,			
10 gm	00501-3793-10	11.20	
(A-S Medication)			
REPACK			
OIN,TP, 500 u/gm-10000 u/gm,			
15 gm	54569-4023-00	4.61	
129.6 gm 144s	54569-2003-00	34.22	
(Pharma Pac)			
REPACK			
POW,TP, 500 u/gm-10000 u/gm,			
10 gm	52959-0564-03	14.36	
(Phys Total Care)			
REPACK			
OIN,TP, 500 u/gm-10000 u/gm,			
15 gm	54868-0986-00	4.85	
(Quality Care Prod)			
REPACK			
OIN,OP, 500 u/gm-10000 u/gm,			
3.5 gm	49999-0209-35	77.94	
OIN,TP, 500 u/gm-10000 u/gm,			
0.9 gm	49999-0592-44	47.18	
15 gm	49999-0270-12	16.13	
(Southwood)			
REPACK			
POW,TP, 500 u/gm-10000 u/gm,			
10 gm	58016-3165-01	8.96	
POLYTAR (Stiefel Consumer HealthCare)			
SHA,TP, 177 ml	00145-0411-06	9.12	13.79
SOA,TP, 0.5%, 100 gm	00145-1092-03	3.84	5.79
POLYTRACIN (Consolidated Midland)			
OIN,TP, 500 u/gm-10000 u/gm,			
15 gm	00223-4395-15	2.25	
30 gm	00223-4395-30	3.25	
POLYVINYL ALCOHOL (Altaire)			
SOL,OP (STERILE)			
1.4%, 15 ml	59390-0196-13	8.23	
POLYVITAMIN (Hi-Tech)			
SOL,PO (DROPS)			
50 ml	50383-0625-50	10.80	
POMEGRANATE WITH EGCG & GRAPE SEED (Mason Vit)			
CAP,PO (WHEAT-FREE)			
5 mg-5 mg-60 mg-100 mg,			
60s ea	11845-0148-25	10.00	
PONARIS (Jamol)			
SOL,NS, 30 ml	10592-0001-01	10.09	14.42
PORTAGEN (Mead Johnson & Co)			
PDR,PO, 454 gm	00087-0387-01	21.90	
POST PEEL BALM (Topix)			
CRE,TP, 1%, 30 gm	51326-0107-30	5.40	
POST-OP DRAINAGE POUCH TWO PIECE (Coloplast)			
DEV,NA (1/2"- 4")			
10s ea	11701-0805-15	31.00	32.40
(1/2"-2 3/4")			
10s ea	11701-0805-10	29.60	31.00
POST-OP SET (Coloplast)			
DEV,NA (1/2"- 4")			
5s ea	11701-0804-15	80.95	84.70
(1/2"-2 3/4")			
5s ea	11701-0804-10	67.40	70.55
POST-OP SKIN BARRIER FLANGE (Coloplast)			
DEV,NA (1/2"- 2 3/4")			
5s ea	11701-0806-10	30.80	32.20
(1/2"- 4")			
5s ea	11701-0806-15	30.80	32.20
POST-OP/WOUND MANAGEMENT POUCH (Coloplast)			
DEV,NA (CURAGARD, 1/2"-4")			
10s ea	11701-0803-10	67.90	71.10
(SECURELIFE, 1/2"-4")			
10s ea	11701-0803-15	67.90	71.10
POSTURE (Inverness)			
TAB,PO, 600 mg, 90s ea	36652-0730-20	8.45	
POTASSIMIN (Key Company)			
TAB,PO, 75 mg, 100s ea	11694-0143-01	5.00	
POTASSIUM (Carlson,J.R.)			
TAB,PO (PF,SF,CORN-FREE)			
99 mg, 100s ea	88395-0052-31	2.75	5.50
250s ea	88395-0052-32	5.95	11.90
(Key Company)			
PDS,PO (3-MIX)			
100 gm	11694-0821-01	7.00	
(Major)			
TER,PO, 95 mg, 60s ea	00904-5353-52	2.85	
POTASSIUM ASPARTATE (Miller)			
TAB,PO, 500 mg, 100s ea	17204-0359-40	6.96	11.60
POTASSIUM BENZOATE (Bio-Tech Pharm)			
CAP,PO, 99 mg, 100s ea	53191-0303-01	8.90	
POTASSIUM CHELATED (ADH)			
TAB,PO (PF,SF)			
99 mg, 60s ea	60142-0377-56	2.48	4.95
(Freeda)			
TAB,PO (PF,SF,DYE-FREE)			
95 mg, 100s ea	10432-0077-01	5.07	8.45
(Health Products Corp)			
TAB,PO (PF,SF)			
99 mg, 100s ea	39686-0014-36	2.33	
POTASSIUM CHLORIDE (Legere)			
TAB,PO, 180 mg,			
1000s ea	25332-1119-01	24.95	
POTASSIUM CHLORIDE ER (Pharma Pac)			
REPACK			
TER,PO, 10 meq, 30s ea	52959-0842-30	10.20	
POTASSIUM FORTIFIED (Rexall)			
TAB,PO (PF,SF)			
99 mg, 60s ea	30768-0000-82	1.94	2.93
POTASSIUM GLUCONATE (Basic Vitamins)			
TAB,PO, 595 mg, 100s ea	00761-0847-20	2.00	
(Freeda)			
TAB,PO (PF,SF,DYE-FREE)			
80 mg, 100s ea	10432-0176-01	4.17	6.95
250s ea	10432-0176-02	8.34	13.90
(Mason Vit)			
TAB,PO, 595 mg, 100s ea	11845-0061-81	5.00	
TER,PO, 595 mg, 100s ea	11845-0080-41	5.89	
(Medicine Shoppe)			
TAB,PO, 595 mg, 100s ea	49614-0239-78	2.89	2.89
(Nature's Bounty)			
TAB,PO (PF,SF)			
610 mg, 100s ea	74312-0011-10		3.99
250s ea	74312-0011-13		7.99
(Pharmavite)			
TAB,PO, 550 mg, 500s ea	31604-0017-97	8.99	
(Rexall)			
TAB,PO (PF,SF)			
595 mg, 60s ea	30768-0000-57	1.33	2.02
(Southwood)			
REPACK			
TAB,PO, 500 mg, 30s ea	58016-0982-30	4.88	
POTASSIUM GLUCONATE NATURAL (Cardinal Health)			
TAB,PO (PF,PRIVATE LABEL)			
550 mg, 100s ea	37205-0174-78	3.11	
POTASSIUM-99 (Key Company)			
TAB,PO (SF)			
99 mg, 100s ea	11694-0894-01	2.75	
1000s ea	11694-0894-03	15.00	
POUCHKINS DRAINABLE POUCH (Hollister)			
DEV,NA (TRANSPARENT,44MM)			
10s ea	08380-0037-71	19.77	
POUCHKINS OSTOMY BELT PEDIATRIC (Hollister)			
DEV,NA, ea	08380-0037-74	7.34	
POUCHKINS SOFTFLEX BARRIER (Hollister)			
DEV,NA (1 3/4"FLANGE)			
5s ea	08380-0037-70	22.24	
POUCHKINS UROSTOMY POUCH (Hollister)			
DEV,NA, 10s ea	08380-0037-72	30.34	
POVIDONE (Consolidated Midland)			
OIN,TP, 10%, 1 gm 144s	00223-0090-09	17.50	
SOL,TP, 1%, 3840 ml	00223-6299-08	34.00	
10%, 480 ml	00223-6841-01	5.75	
3840 ml	00223-6841-02	34.00	
SOL,VG (DOUCHE)			
10%, 240 ml	00223-6298-08	5.25	
POVIDONE DOUCHE (R.I.J.)			
SOL,VG, 10%, 240 ml	53807-0159-01	4.30	
POVIDONE IODINE SCRUB (Dispensing Solutions)			
REPACK			
SOL,TP, 7.5%, 473 ml	55045-3295-01	5.99	
POVIDONE-IODINE (Albertson's)			
OIN,TP, 10%, 30 gm	41280-0210-91	2.34	
(Alexander, James)			
SWA,TP, 10%, 10s ea	46414-7777-03	2.00	3.51
100s ea	46414-7777-02	14.50	33.58
(Asafi Pharmaceutical)			
SOL,TP, 10%, 473 ml	65557-0779-16	5.83	
(Cardinal Health)			
SOL,TP (PRIVATE LABEL)			
10%, 240 ml	37205-0186-34	2.96	
(Consolidated Midland)			
OIN,TP (FOILPACK)			
10%, 1 gm 144s	00223-0090-01	16.00	
1.5 gm 144s	00223-4400-01	22.50	
30 gm	00223-4400-30	2.00	
454 gm	00223-4400-13	12.00	
(Major)			
OIN,TP, 10%, 30 gm	00904-1102-31	3.12	
SOL,TP, 1%, 240 ml	00904-1103-09	4.19	
(Perrigo)			
SOL,TP, 10%, 480 ml	45802-0052-07	6.99	
(Qualitest)			
OIN,TP, 10%, 30 gm	00603-0599-50	6.40	
SOL,TP, 10%, 240 ml	00603-1550-56	3.10	
480 ml	00603-1550-58	4.98	

PROD/MFR	HRI, UPC,NDC	AWP	SRP
(R.I.J.)			
SOL,TP, 10%, 240 ml	53807-0136-01	2.28	
480 ml	53807-0136-02	3.70	
3840 ml	53807-0136-03	24.98	
(Altura)			
REPACK			
OIN,TP, 10%, 100 gm	63874-0857-10	14.88	
(Phys Total Care)			
REPACK			
SOL,TP, 10%, 480 ml	54868-2914-01	13.13	
(Southwood)			
REPACK			
OIN,TP, 10%, 30 gm	58016-3013-01	6.60	
SOL,TP, 10%, 3840 ml	58016-3117-01	12.58	
POVIDONE-IODONE (AmerisourceBergen)			
SOL,TP (PRIVATE LABEL)			
10%, 240 ml	24385-0053-55	6.29	6.99
POWER KIT DISPOSABLE (Medtronic Minimed)			
DEV,NA (1.5 VOLT BATTERIES)			
9s ea	76300-0104-01	33.00	
POWERMATE (Green Turtle)			
TAB,PO (PF,SF,DYE-FREE)			
50s ea	59074-0200-01	14.40	23.99
POWERSLEEP (Green Turtle)			
TAB,PO (PF,SF,DYE-FREE)			
60s ea	59074-0600-01	22.80	37.99
POWERVITES (Green Turtle)			
TAB,PO (NO IRON,PF,SF,DYE-FREE)			
100s ea	59074-0100-01	12.00	19.99
200s ea	59074-0100-03	20.40	33.99
PRAMEGEL (Doak)			
GEL,TP, 0.5%-1%, 120 gm	10337-0808-41	22.87	
PRAMOXINE HYDROCHLORIDE (United Research)			
FOA,RC, 1%, 15 gm	00677-1965-79	33.50	
(Phys Total Care)			
REPACK			
FOA,RC (1X15GM)			
1%, 15 gm	54868-5865-00	91.59	
PRAX (Ferndale)			
LOT,TP, 1%, 15 ml	00496-0748-15	7.70	
120 ml	00496-0748-04	19.07	
240 ml	00496-0748-03	30.68	
PRE SUN ULTRA W/PARSOL (Cutix)			
CRE,TP (SPF 15,FRAGRANCE-FREE)			
3%-5%-5%-6%,			
120 gm	00072-9440-04	7.24	
GEL,TP, 3%-5%-5%-6%,			
120 gm	00072-8840-04	7.24	
SPR,TP (SPF 27,FRAGRANCE-FREE)			
3%-7.5%-5%-6%,			
180 ml	00072-9301-19	7.24	
PRE TAC (Pharm Innov)			
LIQ,TP, 5 ml	00036-9400-05	1.69	2.41
15 ml	00036-9400-15	4.87	6.96
PRE-NATAL (Rexall)			
TAB,PO, 60s ea	30768-0018-18	2.93	4.43
PRE-PROTEIN (Kramer-Novis)			
LIQ,PO, 240 ml	52083-0533-08	13.60	
480 ml	52083-0533-16	25.00	
(SF,PEACH)			
240 ml	52083-0933-08	13.60	
480 ml	52083-0933-16	25.00	
TAB,PO (PF,SF)			
90s ea	52083-0540-90	25.00	
PREAN (Dermasave)			
CRE,TP, 70 gm	61705-0650-36	7.50	
PRECISION 200 PEDIATRIC URINE METER (Covidien)			
DEV,NA (LATEX-FREE)			
10s ea	08080-1000-08	168.54	
PRECISION 200 URINE METER ADD-A-FOLEY CATHETER TRAY (Covidien)			
DEV,NA (LATEX-FREE)			
10s ea	08080-2000-04	190.58	
PRECISION CATHETER (Kendall)			
DEV,NA, 100s ea	94393-0006-45	225.63	
PRECISION DISPOSABLE TISSUE GRINDER (Covidien)			
DEV,NA, 10s ea	08080-3500-01	104.13	
(SMALL,STERILE)			
10s ea	08080-3505-01	94.67	
PRECISION FOLEY CATHETER TRAY (Covidien)			
DEV,NA (14FR, 5CC)			
10s ea	08080-2431-03	257.13	
(14FR,5CC)			
10s ea	08080-2401-02	192.19	
10s ea	08080-2401-03	198.76	
10s ea	08080-2401-04	192.19	
10s ea	08080-2401-13	198.76	
10s ea	08080-2411-03	204.87	
10s ea	08080-2412-02	166.74	
10s ea	08080-2412-03	172.34	
10s ea	08080-2412-04	166.74	
10s ea	08080-2412-13	172.43	
10s ea	08080-2431-05	257.13	
(16FR, 5CC)			
10s ea	08080-2631-03	257.13	
(16FR,5CC)			
10s ea	08080-2601-02	192.19	
10s ea	08080-2601-03	198.76	
10s ea	08080-2601-12	192.19	
10s ea	08080-2601-13	198.76	
10s ea	08080-2611-03	204.87	
10s ea	08080-2612-02	166.74	
10s ea	08080-2612-03	172.43	
10s ea	08080-2612-04	166.74	
10s ea	08080-2612-13	172.43	
10s ea	08080-2614-03	198.14	
10s ea	08080-2631-05	257.13	
(18FR, 5CC)			
10s ea	08080-2831-03	257.13	
(18FR,5CC)			
10s ea	08080-2801-02	192.19	
10s ea	08080-2801-03	198.76	
10s ea	08080-2801-09	198.76	
10s ea	08080-2801-12	192.19	
10s ea	08080-2811-03	204.87	
10s ea	08080-2812-02	166.74	
10s ea	08080-2812-03	172.43	
10s ea	08080-2812-04	166.74	
10s ea	08080-2812-09	172.43	
10s ea	08080-2831-05	257.13	
PRECISION MID-STREAM PRESERVATIVE KIT (Kendall)			
DEV,NA, 200s ea	94393-0006-44	465.79	
PRECISION MID-STREAM URINE COLLECTOR (Kendall)			
DEV,NA, 100s ea	94390-0008-41	347.21	
PRECISION OPERATING ROOM SPECIMEN CONTAINER (Kendall)			
DEV,NA, 100s ea	94393-0006-48	135.51	
PRECISION PCX (Abbott)			
DEV,NA (STRIP,PAC)			
100s ea	57599-9565-05	84.60	
PRECISION PCX PLUS TEST STRIPS (Abbott)			
DEV,NA (PAC)			
100s ea	93815-0803-39	84.60	
PRECISION Q-I-D (Abbott)			
DEV,NA (STRIP)			
50s ea	57599-7400-04	59.03	
50s ea	59599-8732-04	50.38	
100s ea	57599-7401-05	108.66	
100s ea	57599-8733-05	92.72	
PRECISION SPECIMEN CONTAINER (Kendall)			
DEV,NA, 200s ea	94393-0008-04	106.99	
200s ea	94393-0008-05	104.14	
(STERILE,WIDEMOUTH)			
200s ea	94393-0007-15	114.31	
300s ea	94393-0008-07	107.66	
400s ea	94393-0008-06	172.90	
PRECISION SPUTUM COLLECTOR (Kendall)			
DEV,NA, 50s ea	94393-0006-42	129.18	
PRECISION STOOL SPECIMEN COLLECTOR (Kendall)			
DEV,NA, 100s ea	94393-0007-14	116.86	
PRECISION URINE COLLECTION KIT FOR CULTURE (Kendall)			
DEV,NA, 200s ea	94393-0006-43	252.65	
PRECISION XTRA (Abbott)			
DEV,NA (STRIP)			
50s ea	57599-9695-04	55.45	
50s ea	57599-9728-04	60.44	
100s ea	57599-9877-05	113.09	
100s ea	57599-9878-05	113.09	
PRECISION XTRA BLOOD B-KETONE (Abbott)			
DEV,NA (TEST STRIP W/CALIBRATOR)			
10s ea	57599-0745-01	44.26	
PRECISION XTRA MONITOR (Abbott)			
DEV,NA, ea	57599-8814-01	18.00	
ea	57599-9837-01	30.00	
PRECISION400 URNMTR CATHETRIZTIONTRAY W/ TEMPSNSOR (Covidien)			
DEV,NA (14FR, 5CC)			
10s ea	08080-2431-10	574.75	
(16FR, 5CC)			
10s ea	08080-2635-06	574.75	
(18FR, 5CC)			
10s ea	08080-2835-06	574.75	
PREFERRED PLUS INSULIN SYRINGES (Can-Am Care)			
DEV,NA (28G, ULTRA COMFORT)			
100s ea	38396-0408-04	15.50	
(28G,1/2CC,MONOJECT)			
100s ea	38396-0408-01	15.50	
(29G,1/2CC,MONOJECT)			
100s ea	38396-0408-03	17.50	
(29G,1CC,MONOJECT)			
100s ea	38396-0408-05	17.50	
(29G,3/10CC,MONOJECT)			
100s ea	38396-0408-02	17.50	
(30G,1/2CC,MONOJECT)			
100s ea	38396-0408-07	17.50	
(30G,1CC,MONOJECT)			
100s ea	38396-0408-06	17.50	
(30G,3/10CC,MONOJECT)			
100s ea	38396-0408-08	17.50	
PREFERRED PLUS PHARMACY TEST STRIPS (Home Diag)			
DEV,NA (PRESTIGE SMART SYSTEM)			
50s ea	56151-0327-50	28.60	
PREFERRED PLUS ULTRA COMFORT INSULIN SYRINGES (Can-Am Care)			
DEV,NA (31G,5/16",1/2ML)			
100s ea	38396-0006-06	17.50	
(31G,5/16",1ML)			
100s ea	38396-0007-06	17.50	
(31G,5/16",3/10ML)			
100s ea	38396-0005-06	17.50	
PREFERRED PLUS UNIFINE PENTIPS (Kinray)			
DEV,NA (12MM)			
100s ea	61059-0527-19	22.00	
(6MM)			
100s ea	61059-0597-19	22.00	
(8MM)			
100s ea	61059-0537-19	22.00	
PREFRIN LIQUIFILM (Allergan Inc)			
SOL,OP, 0.12%, 21 ml	11980-0036-07	9.89	
PREGESTIMIL IRON FORTIFIED (Mead Johnson & Co)			
PDR,PO (LIPIL)			
454 gm	00087-0367-01	33.10	
PREGESTIMIL LIPIL (Mead Johnson & Co)			
LIQ,PO (6X59ML,NURSETTE,20CAL)			
59 ml 6s	00087-1433-41	10.15	
(6X59ML,NURSETTE,24CAL)			
59 ml 6s	00087-1434-41	10.15	
PREKUNIL LNAA (Solace)			
TAB,PO, 550s ea	57771-0001-42	360.00	600.00
PRELIEF (Akpharma)			
TAB,PO, 333 mg, 60s ea	41383-0220-01	3.65	6.85
120s ea	41383-0260-01	6.50	11.99
PREMIERE VALUE PEN NEEDLES (Chain Drug)			
DEV,NA (29GX12MM,PRIVATE LABEL)			
100s ea	68016-0297-28	21.25	
(31GX6MM,PRIVATE LABEL)			
100s ea	68016-0907-28	21.25	
(31GX8MM,PRIVATE LABEL)			
100s ea	68016-0307-28	21.25	
PREMJACT (Pound Intl)			
SPR,TP, 9.6%,			
13.13 ml 12s	48132-0800-24	71.40	
PREMSYN PMS (Chattem)			
TAB,PO, 500 mg-25 mg-15 mg,			
20s ea	41167-0310-21	3.06	
40s ea	41167-0310-23	4.82	
PREMSYN PMS MAXIMUM STRENGTH (Chattem)			
TAB,PO (GELCAPLET)			
500 mg-25 mg-15 mg,			
16s ea	41167-0310-61	2.99	
PRENATAL (21st Century)			
TAB,PO (GLUTEN-FREE)			
60s ea	40985-0223-75	3.00	4.99
(Major)			
TAB,PO, 100s ea	00904-5313-60	7.52	
30s ea	00904-5313-46	2.79	

PROD/MFR	HRI, UPC, NDC	AWP	SRP
(Phys Total Care)			
REPACK			
TAB,PO, 100s ea	54868-4188-00	14.49	
(Physician Partner)			
REPACK			
TAB,PO (GLUTEN-FREE)			
60s ea	21695-0480-60	19.98	
(Quality Care Prod)			
REPACK			
TAB,PO, 30s ea	35356-0366-30	7.98	
90s ea	35356-0366-90	12.60	
PRENATAL FORMULA (ADH)			
TAB,PO, 100s ea	60142-0029-10	4.14	
(Consolidated Midland)			
TAB,PO, 100s ea	00223-1455-01	4.75	
1000s ea	00223-1455-02	32.50	
(Family Phcy)			
TAB,PO (PRIVATE LABEL)			
100s ea	52735-0035-01	7.19	9.39
PRENATAL LOW IRON (Prime Marketing)			
TAB,PO, 100s ea	62107-0063-01	16.50	
PRENATAL ONE DAILY (Freeda)			
TAB,PO (SF,GLUTEN-FREE)			
100s ea	10432-0313-01	8.37	13.95
250s ea	10432-0313-02	16.74	27.90
PRENATAL VITAMIN (Altura)			
REPACK			
TAB,PO, 30s ea	63874-0016-30	8.03	
100s ea	63874-0016-01	26.78	
300s ea	63874-0016-03	80.34	
PRENATAL VITAMINS (AmerisourceBergen)			
TAB,PO (PRIVATE LABEL)			
100s ea	24385-0078-78	7.19	7.99
(Basic Vitamins)			
TAB,PO, 90s ea	00761-0513-18	4.20	
(Medicine Shoppe)			
TAB,PO, 100s ea	49614-0613-78	6.99	6.99
(Nature's Bounty)			
TAB,PO, 100s ea	74312-0037-00		9.99
PRENATAL-S (Teva)			
TAB,PO, 100s ea	00182-4039-01	5.95	
(Dispensing Solutions)			
REPACK			
TAB,PO, 100s ea	55045-2264-00	9.99	
PRENAVITE (Rugby)			
TAB,PO (PF,SF)			
100s ea	00536-4063-01	6.21	
100s ea	00536-4085-01	6.21	
PREP N' STAY (Pharm Innov)			
LIQ,TP, 15 ml	00036-3440-15	4.87	6.96
50 ml	00036-3440-50	14.23	20.33
PREP TRODE (Pharm Innov)			
LIQ,TP, 250 ml	00036-3400-25	5.21	7.44
4000 ml	00036-3400-04	51.64	73.78
PREP-HEM (Perrigo)			
OIN,TP (1X57GM)			
14.0%-71.9%-0.25%-3.0%,			
57 gm	45802-0354-10	4.99	
PREPARATION H (Wyeth Consumer)			
CRE,RC (MAXIMUM STRENGTH)			
14.4%-15%-0.25%-1%,			
26 gm	05732-0868-10		5.99
OIN,TP, 0.25%-3%, 30 gm	00573-2871-10		5.49
60 gm	00573-2871-20		9.49
SUP,RC, 85.5%-0.25%-3%,			
12s ea	00573-2883-10		6.93
24s ea	00573-2883-20		10.29
48s ea	00573-2883-30		18.99
PREPARATION H HYDROCORTISONE (Wyeth Consumer)			
CRE,TP, 1%, 27 gm	00573-2830-10		5.49
PREPPIES ADHESIVE REMOVER PREP (Covidien)			
PAD,NA (LARGE,2 PLY)			
1000s ea	08080-2148-00	136.58	
PREPTIC PREP RAZORS (J&J Medical)			
DEV,NA (DOUBLE EDGE)			
24s ea	56091-0098-88	16.99	
PREPTIC SHAVE PREP PAK (J&J Medical)			
DEV,NA, ea	56091-0014-25	1.53	
PRESERVE PAK (HVS Labs)			
LIQ,PO (24 WEEKS PROGRAM)			
240 ml	52386-9629-04	40.00	

PROD/MFR	HRI, UPC, NDC	AWP	SRP
PRESERVISION (Bausch & Lomb Inc.)			
SGL,PO (SOFTGEL)			
60s ea	24208-0532-10	15.28	
PRESERVISION AREDS (Bausch & Lomb Inc.)			
SGL,PO (SOFTGEL)			
60s ea	24208-0532-20	15.28	
PRESERVISION LUTEIN (Bausch & Lomb Inc.)			
SGL,PO (SOFTGEL)			
50s ea	24208-0632-10	15.28	
PRESTIGE LX METER (Home Diag)			
DEV,NA (W/CASE)			
ea	56151-0527-01	70.68	
PRESTIGE LX STARTER (Home Diag)			
DEV,NA (W/LANCETS,SOL,STRIPS)			
ea	56151-0504-01	110.00	
PRESTIGE METER (Home Diag)			
DEV,NA (W/CASE)			
ea	56151-0525-01	70.68	
PRESTIGE SMART SYST GLUCOSE CONTROL (Home Diag)			
DEV,NA (HIGH CONTROL)			
ea	56151-0566-01	6.00	
(LOW CONTROL)			
ea	56151-0561-01	4.75	
ea	56151-0563-01	6.00	
PRESTIGE SMART SYSTEM (Home Diag)			
DEV,NA, 50s ea	56151-0950-50	28.60	
(NOT FOR FORMULARY USE)			
50s ea	56151-0555-50	25.99	
(STRIP)			
50s ea	56151-0310-50	28.60	
50s ea	56151-0550-50	25.99	
100s ea	56151-0310-01	45.99	
100s ea	56151-0550-01	45.99	
PRESTIGE SMART SYSTEM CO-BRANDED (Home Diag)			
DEV,NA (STRIP)			
100s ea	56151-0910-01	50.00	
PRESTIGE SMART SYSTEM IQ (Home Diag)			
DEV,NA (STARTER KIT)			
ea	56151-0999-90	17.50	
PRESTIGE SMART SYSTEM VALUE PACK (Home Diag)			
DEV,NA (MTR,STRP,LANCET,DEV,SOL)			
ea	56151-0578-01	71.10	
PRESTIGE STARTER (Home Diag)			
DEV,NA, ea	56151-0505-01	110.00	
PRESUN SENSITIVE SUNBLOCK (Cutix)			
CRE,TP (SPF 28,FRAGRANCE-FREE)			
16%, 100 gm	95193-0001-03		9.99
PRESUN ULTRA SUNSCREEN (Cutix)			
CRE,TP (SPF 30,FRAGRANCE-FREE)			
3%-7.5%-5%-3%,			
113.4 gm	95193-0001-02		9.99
GEL,TP, 3%-7.5%-5%-6%,			
118.3 ml	95193-0001-01		9.99
PRETTY FEET & HANDS (Ascher)			
CRE,TP (ROUGH SKIN REMOVER)			
90 gm	00225-0520-53	5.35	
PRETZ (Parnell)			
SPR,NS, 3%-0.75%, 50 ml	50930-0280-50	3.95	5.50
(REFILL)			
3%-0.75%, 1000 ml	50930-0280-32	23.50	32.00
PRETZ CONCENTRATE (Parnell)			
POW,NS (1X360GM)			
360 gm	50930-0280-12	14.00	19.99
PRETZ IRRIGATION (Parnell)			
SOL,NS, 0.75%, 240 ml	50930-0280-08	11.65	16.50
PREVACARE ANTIMICROBIAL HAND (J&J Medical)			
GEL,TP, 60%, 118 ml	56091-0370-04	3.24	
236 ml	56091-0370-08	6.10	
946 ml	56091-0374-32	23.92	
1500 ml	56091-0374-51	30.58	
PREVACARE ANTIMICROBIAL HANDWASH (J&J Medical)			
LIQ,TP, 0.25%, 60 ml	56091-0310-02	1.63	
240 ml	56091-0311-08	3.28	
480 ml	56091-0311-16	6.14	
1500 ml	56091-0314-51	13.49	
3840 ml	56091-0312-50	24.55	
PREVACARE BOTTLE HOLDER (J&J Medical)			
DEV,NA (USE W/16 OZ. BOTTLE)			
ea	56091-0630-00	2.93	

PROD/MFR	HRI, UPC, NDC	AWP	SRP
PREVACARE EXTRA PROTECTIVE (J&J Medical)			
OIN,TP (NON-GREASY)			
65 gm	56091-0530-02	4.93	
PREVACARE GENTLE SKIN CLEANSER (J&J Medical)			
LIQ,TP (SOAP-FREE)			
60 ml	56091-0330-02	1.49	
240 ml	56091-0331-08	2.97	
480 ml	56091-0331-16	4.67	
1500 ml	56091-0334-51	10.60	
3840 ml	56091-0332-50	15.64	
PREVACARE MOISTURIZING (J&J Medical)			
CRE,TP (SENSITIVE SKIN)			
60 gm	56091-0540-02	2.34	
120 gm	56091-0540-04	4.16	
LOT,TP, 60 ml	56091-0420-02	1.90	
480 ml	56091-0421-16	10.62	
1500 ml	56091-0424-51	20.04	
PREVACARE NO-RINSE CLEANSER (J&J Medical)			
LIQ,TP (DYE-FREE,FRAGRANCE-FREE)			
240 ml	56091-0513-08	4.48	
PREVACARE PERSONAL PROTECTIVE (J&J Medical)			
CRE,TP (FRAGRANCE-FREE)			
56 gm	56091-0520-02	2.73	
112 gm	56091-0520-04	4.83	
PREVACARE PERSONNEL HANDWASH (J&J Medical)			
LIQ,TP, 1%, 60 ml	56091-0320-02	1.82	
240 ml	56091-0321-08	4.08	
480 ml	56091-0321-16	7.55	
1500 ml	56091-0320-51	20.30	
3840 ml	56091-0320-50	39.59	
PREVACARE SKIN CONDITIONER CLEANSER (J&J Medical)			
LOT,TP (FRAGRANCE-FREE)			
60 ml	56091-0340-02	1.71	
240 ml	56091-0341-08	3.69	
480 ml	56091-0341-16	6.76	
1500 ml	56091-0344-51	16.22	
3840 ml	56091-0342-50	31.10	
PREVACARE TOTAL SOLUTION SKIN CARE (J&J Medical)			
SPR,TP, 236 ml	56091-0550-08	9.75	
PREVACARE WALL MOUNTED DISPENSER (J&J Medical)			
DEV,NA (USE W/50 OZ. CANISTER)			
ea	56091-0610-00	19.24	
PREVACID (Novartis Consumer)			
ECC,PO (24HOUR,SODIUM-FREE)			
15 mg, 14s ea	00067-6286-14	12.05	
28s ea	00067-6286-28	21.34	
(24 HR,3X14,SODIUM-FREE)			
15 mg, 42s ea	00676-0286-43	28.96	
(24HOUR,SODIUM-FREE)			
15 mg, 42s ea	00676-0286-42	28.96	
PREVENT (A. G. Marin)			
SGL,PO (SOFTGEL)			
60s ea	12539-0533-01	27.90	
PREVENZYME (Legere)			
TAB,PO, 100s ea	25332-1064-02	15.00	
PRICE CHOPPER ULTRA THIN LANCETS (Price Chopper)			
DEV,NA (28 GAUGE,PRIVATE LABEL)			
100s ea	08214-5357-16	4.70	
PRICE CHOPPER UNIFINE PENTIPS (Price Chopper)			
DEV,NA (G29,12MM,PRIVATE LABEL)			
100s ea	08214-0567-16	19.25	
(G31,6MM,ULTRA SHORT)			
100s ea	08214-0587-16	19.25	
(G31,8MM,PRIVATE LABEL)			
100s ea	08214-0577-16	19.25	
PRILOSEC (A-S Medication)			
REPACK			
TCP,PO, 20 mg, 14s ea	54569-5582-00	12.06	
PRILOSEC OTC (P & G Company)			
TCP,PO, 20 mg, 14s ea	37000-0455-02	12.06	
28s ea	37000-0455-03	21.34	
42s ea	37000-0455-04	28.96	
(Dispensing Solutions)			
REPACK			
TCP,PO, 20 mg, 14s ea	55045-3109-01	13.99	
28s ea	55045-3109-02	20.99	
42s ea	55045-3109-04	27.99	
(Nucare Pharm)			
REPACK			
TCP,PO, 20 mg, 28s ea	68071-1331-08	42.68	

PROD/MFR | HRI, UPC,NDC | AWP | SRP

(Quality Care Prod)
REPACK
TCP,PO, 20 mg, 14s ea....49999-0742-14 15.59

PRIMAPORE IV ADHESIVE (Smith & Nephew)
DEV,NA (2"X3")
100s ea..............00223-0713-30 38.08 30.46

PRIMAPORE SPECIALTY ABSORBENT (Smith & Nephew)
DEV,NA (11 3/4"X4")
20s ea..............00223-0420-36 42.38 33.90
(4"X3 1/8")
20s ea..............00223-0420-24 21.25 17.00
(6"X3 1/8")
20s ea..............00223-0420-27 22.75 18.20
(8"X4")
20s ea..............00223-0420-30 34.84 27.87

PRIMARY PAK (HVS Labs)
LIQ,PO (48 DAYS PROGRAM)
240 ml..............52386-9628-04 40.00

PRIMATENE (Wyeth Consumer)
TAB,PO, 12.5 mg-200 mg,
24s ea..............00573-2952-10 4.91
60s ea..............00573-2952-20 8.56

PRIMATENE MIST (Armstrong Pharm.)
AER,IH (INHALER REFILL)
0.22 mg/actuation,
15 ml..............17270-0504-00 14.88
(W/MOUTHPIECE)
0.22 mg/actuation,
15 ml..............17270-0503-00 15.78

(Wyeth Consumer)
AER,IH, 0.22 mg/actuation,
15 ml..............00573-2910-20 14.38

(Phys Total Care)
REPACK
AER,IH, 0.22 mg/actuation,
15 ml..............54868-2400-02 13.91

PRIMER MODIFIED UNNA BOOT (Western Medical)
DEV,NA (3"X10 YD W/CALAMINE)
12s ea..............16926-0300-10 115.56
(3"X10 YDS)
12s ea..............16926-0300-01 100.43
(4"X10 YD W/CALAMINE)
12s ea..............16926-0400-10 127.14
(4"X10 YD)
12s ea..............16926-0100-01 110.65

PRIMROSE OILE (Green Turtle)
SGL,PO (PF,SF,DYE-FREE)
500 mg, 180s ea.....59074-0500-01 16.20 26.99

PRIVINE (Heritage/Insight)
SOL,NS, 0.05%, 25 ml....63736-0662-07 3.54
SPR,NS, 0.05%, 20 ml....63736-0662-55 4.04

PRO-CAL (VITAFLO, LLC)
PDS,PO (30X15GM,GLUTEN-FREE)
15 gm 30s..............50600-0500-76 35.70 44.69

PRO-CEPTION (Cooper Surgical)
DEV,NA (FERTILITY PAK, SM/LRG)
12s ea..............00396-3910-00 32.00

PRO-OX #7 ANTIOXIDANT FORMULA (Health Products Corp)
TAB,PO (PF,SF)
50s ea..............39686-0014-83 6.00

PRO-PEPTIDE (Hormel Healthlabs)
LIQ,PO, 250 ml..............61678-0224-02 7.75
(VANILLA)
250 ml..............61678-0224-15 7.75

PRO-PEPTIDE FOR KIDS (Hormel Healthlabs)
LIQ,PO (VANILLA)
250 ml..............61678-0224-21 8.16

PRO-PEPTIDE VHN (Hormel Healthlabs)
LIQ,PO, 250 ml..............61678-0224-12 8.16

PRO-PHREE (Abbott)
PDR,PO, 400 gm..............70074-0511-49 9.96

PRO-RITE (Carlson,J.R.)
TAB,PO, 500 mg-500 mg,
60s ea..............88395-0042-30 7.95 15.90
180s ea..............88395-0042-32 21.95 43.90

PRO-STAT 101 (Medical Nutrition USA)
LIQ,PO (30MLX96)
30 ml 96s..............26974-0410-18 115.00 115.00
SOL,NA (6X887ML,GLUTEN-FREE)
887 ml 6s..............26974-0410-08 130.00
887 ml 6s..............26974-0410-10 130.00
887 ml 6s..............26974-0410-41 130.00
(GLUTEN-FREE)
887 ml 6s..............26974-0410-08 130.00 130.00

PRO-STAT 64 (Medical Nutrition USA)
LIQ,PO (30MLX96,SF,GLUTEN-FREE)
30 ml 96s..............26974-0410-17 115.00 115.00
(30MLX96,SF)
30 ml 96s..............26974-0410-42 115.00
(PROTEIN SUPPLEMENT,SF)
887 ml..............26974-0410-40 21.66
(SF,LACTOSE-FREE)
887 ml..............26974-0410-09 21.66
SOL,NA (SF,GLUTEN-FREE)
887 ml 6s..............26974-0410-07 130.00 130.00

PRO-STAT AWC (Medical Nutrition USA)
LIQ,PO (ADVANCED WOUND CARE)
887 ml 4s..............26974-0410-30 181.67

PRO-STAT AWC WITH CITRULLINE (Medical Nutrition USA)
LIQ,PO (30MLX96,GLUTEN-FREE)
30 ml 96s..............26974-0410-31 190.97 190.87

PRO-STAT PROFILE (Medical Nutrition USA)
LIQ,PO (30MLX96,GLUTEN-FREE)
30 ml 96s..............26974-0410-21 119.92 119.92
(887MLX4,GLUTEN-FREE)
887 ml 4s..............26974-0410-12 106.80 106.80

PRO-STAT RC (Medical Nutrition USA)
LIQ,PO (96X30ML,SF,GLUTEN-FREE)
30 ml 96s..............26974-0410-61 119.95 171.88
(6X887ML,SF,GLUTEN-FREE)
887 ml 6s..............26974-0410-60 171.88 171.88

PROBALANCE ULTRAPAK (Nestle)
LIQ,PO (1000MLX6)
1000 ml 6s..............00065-9166-72 37.51
(1500MLX4)
1500 ml 4s..............00065-9166-73 37.49

PROBIATA (Pharmaton)
TAB,PO (PF)
1 billion u,
30s ea..............93190-0180-01 6.50 8.41

PROBIOTIC FORMULA (Rugby)
CAP,PO, 30s ea..............00536-3116-07 9.54

PROBIOTICA (Ortho-McNeil Pharm)
CTB,PO (LEMON)
100 million org,
60s ea..............00045-0128-60 11.99

PROCEL (Global)
POW,PO (100X6.6GM)
6.6 gm 100s..............82028-0100-82 82.00
285 gm..............82028-0000-80 13.00
(6X285GM)
285 gm 6s..............82028-0006-80 77.00

PROCYCLE (Cyclin)
TAB,PO, 120s ea..............53409-0292-56 17.95

PROCYCLE GOLD (Cyclin)
TAB,PO, 120s ea..............53409-0292-55 17.95 7.95

PRODERM (UDL)
SPR,TP, 113.4 gm..............51079-0622-82 16.40

PRODIGY AUTOCODE (Diagnostic)
DEV,NA (ENGLISH&SPANISH TALKING)
ea..............08484-0518-90 123.00
ea..............08484-0701-20 21.46

PRODIGY AUTOCODE BLOOD GLUCOSE MONITORING SYSTEM (Diagnostic)
DEV,NA (ENGLISH&SPANISH TALKING)
ea..............08484-0518-85 117.90
(NON-TALKING)
ea..............08484-0518-10 118.20
ea..............08484-0518-20 123.00
(TALKING)
ea..............08484-0518-50 118.20

PRODIGY AUTOCODE BLOOD GLUCOSE MONITORING SYSTEM KIT (Diagnostic)
DEV,NA (TALKING)
ea..............08484-0518-80 123.00

PRODIGY AUTOCODE POCKET BLOOD GLUCOSE TEST STRIPS (Diagnostic)
DEV,NA, 50s ea..............08484-0725-00 21.54

PRODIGY AUTOCODE VOICE (Diagnostic)
DEV,NA, 32s ea..............08484-0528-35 33.18
50s ea..............08484-0528-00 51.84

PRODIGY BLOOD GLUCOSE MONITORING SYSTEM (Diagnostic)
DEV,NA (NON TALKING)
ea..............08484-0516-00 85.92
ea..............08484-0516-50 91.85
(TALKING)
ea..............08484-0517-20 117.90
ea..............08484-0517-50 123.00

PRODIGY BLOOD GLUCOSE TEST STRIPS (Diagnostic)
DEV,NA, 32s ea..............08484-0523-00 33.18
50s ea..............08484-0524-00 51.84

PRODIGY CONTROL SOLUTION (Diagnostic)
DEV,NA (HIGH)
ea..............08484-0533-50 8.40
(LOW)
ea..............08484-0533-10 8.40

PRODIGY CONTROL SOLUTION LOW (Diagnostic)
DEV,NA, ea..............08484-9903-10 8.40

PRODIGY INSULIN SYRINGES (Diagnostic)
DEV,NA (28G,SINGLE USE)
100s ea..............08484-9904-30 26.21
(31G,SHORT NEEDLE)
100s ea..............08484-9904-38 26.21
(31G,SINGLE USE)
100s ea..............08484-9904-35 26.21

PRODIGY LANCING DEVICE (Diagnostic)
DEV,NA, ea..............08484-9903-55 16.37

(Prodigy)
DEV,NA, ea..............08484-0832-25 16.37

PRODIGY NO CODING BLOOD GLUCOSE TEST STRIPS (Diagnostic)
DEV,NA, 50s ea..............08484-0528-70 21.46
50s ea..............08484-9902-50 37.20

PRODIGY POCKET (Diagnostic)
DEV,NA (BLACK, NO CODING)
ea..............08484-0503-60 41.94
(BLACK)
ea..............08484-0708-00 14.34
(BLUE, NO CODING)
ea..............08484-0503-62 41.94
(BLUE)
ea..............08484-0708-02 14.34
(CAMOUFLAGE, NO CODING)
ea..............08484-0503-64 41.94
(CAMOUFLAGE)
ea..............08484-0708-04 13.14
(GREEN, NO CODING)
ea..............08484-0503-63 41.94
(GREEN)
ea..............08484-0708-03 13.14
(PINK, NO CODING)
ea..............08484-0503-61 41.94
(PINK)
ea..............08484-0708-01 14.34

PRODIGY POCKET BLOOD GLUCOSE MONITORING SYSTEM (Diagnostic)
DEV,NA (BLACK, NO CODING)
ea..............08484-0503-00 35.94
(BLUE)
ea..............08484-0503-02 35.94
(CAMOUFLAGE)
ea..............08484-0503-04 35.94
(GREEN)
ea..............08484-0503-03 35.94
(PINK)
ea..............08484-0503-01 35.94

PRODIGY PREFERRED BLOOD GLUCOSE MONITORING SYSTEM (Prodigy)
DEV,NA, ea..............08484-0561-00 35.94
ea..............08484-0561-50 41.94

PRODIGY PRESSURE ACTIVATED SAFETY LANCETS (Prodigy)
DEV,NA (21G,SINGLE USE)
100s ea..............08484-0823-21 19.19
100s ea..............08484-0823-41 19.19
(26G,SINGLE USE)
100s ea..............08484-0823-16 19.19
(28G,SINGLE USE)
100s ea..............08484-9903-38 18.53

PRODIGY SAFETY LANCETS (Prodigy)
DEV,NA (26G,SINGLE USE)
100s ea..............08484-0820-26 19.19

PRODIGY SAFTEY SYRINGES WITH FINE NEEDLES (Prodigy)
DEV,NA (29G,SINGLE USE)
100s ea..............08484-9904-80 28.13

PRODIGY TWIST TOP LANCETS (Diagnostic)
DEV,NA (28G)
100s ea..............08484-9903-28 10.30

(Prodigy)
DEV,NA (28G)
100s ea..............08484-0810-28 10.30

PROD/MFR	HRI, UPC,NDC	AWP	SRP
PRODIGY VOICE BLOOD GLUCOSE TEST STRIPS (Diagnostic)			
DEV,NA, 50s ea	08484-0729-00	28.26	
PRODIGY VOICE TOTALLY AUDIBLE (Diagnostic)			
DEV,NA, ea	08484-0519-00	183.00	
ea	08484-0719-50	66.00	
PROFE (Propharma)			
CAP,PO, 180 mg, 100s ea	66594-0777-01	20.00	
PROFERRIN ES (Colorado Biolabs)			
TAB,PO, 12 mg, 30s ea	67181-0201-30	19.20	
90s ea	67181-0201-90	47.57	
PROFORE (Smith & Nephew)			
DEV,NA (FOUR LAYER)			
ea	00223-0411-24	24.60	19.68
PROFREE/GP ENZYMATIC CLEANER (Allergan Inc)			
TEF,NA (WEEKLY)			
16s ea	11980-0797-16	7.65	
PROGAINE (Pharmacia Consumer)			
SHA,TP (PERM/COLOR TREATED)			
300 ml	00009-7355-01	3.60	
(W/CONDITIONER)			
300 ml	00009-7353-01	3.60	
300 ml	00009-7356-01	3.60	
PROGAINE 2 IN 1 SHAMPOO (Johnson & Johnson)			
SHA,TP, 360 ml	00097-0353-02	5.15	
PROGAINE DEEP CLEANSING SHAMPOO (Johnson & Johnson)			
SHA,TP, 300 ml	00094-0719-60	5.15	
PROGAINE VOLUMIZING FOAM (Johnson & Johnson)			
FOA,TP, 200 ml	00094-0725-25	5.15	
PROGAINE VOLUMIZING SHAMPOO (Johnson & Johnson)			
SHA,TP, 360 ml	00097-0354-06	5.15	
PROGAINE WEIGHTLESS CONDITIONER (Johnson & Johnson)			
LIQ,TP, 360 ml	00097-0356-02	5.15	
PROGARD ANTIOXIDANT (ADH)			
TAB,PO, 60s ea	60142-0107-06	5.48	10.95
PROHERBS BLOOD SUGAR BALANCE (Mason Vit)			
TAB,PO (PF,SF)			
30s ea	11845-0133-38	19.98	
PROLINE (Carlson,J.R.)			
L-PROLINE			
PDR,PO, 100 gm	88395-0069-25	18.30	36.60
PROLINE (Carlson,J.R.)			
CAP,PO (PF,SF,CORN-FREE)			
500 mg, 100s ea	88395-0069-21	9.95	19.90
PROLINIC (Key Company)			
SGL,PO (SOFTGEL)			
1000 mg, 100s ea	11694-0747-01	10.00	
240s ea	11694-0747-24	22.00	
PROMENSIL (Novogen)			
TAB,PO (PF,SF)			
40 mg, 30s ea	49197-0000-01	14.95	19.95
60s ea	49197-0000-02	23.95	29.95
(6X30,PF,SF)			
40 mg, 180s ea	49197-0000-06	89.70	119.70
PROMOD (Abbott)			
LIQ,PO (GLUTEN-FREE)			
946 ml	70074-0597-22	27.76	
PDR,PO, 275 gm	70074-0607-75	15.22	
PROMOTE (Abbott)			
LIQ,PO (VANILLA)			
240 ml	70074-0507-75	2.32	
(RTH,VANILLA)			
1500 ml	70074-0576-32	21.71	
PROMOTE ROSS READY-TO-HANG (Abbott)			
LIQ,PO, 1000 ml	70074-0516-16	14.47	
PROMOTE W/FIBER (Abbott)			
LIQ,PO (VANILLA)			
240 ml	70074-0518-73	2.32	
(RTH,VANILLA)			
1500 ml	70074-0576-34	21.71	
PROMOTE W/FIBER ROSS READY-TO-HANG (Abbott)			
LIQ,PO, 1000 ml	70074-0518-74	14.47	
PROMPT RELIEF HEMORRHOIDAL (Phys Total Care)			
REPACK			
OIN,TP, 0.25%-3%, 30 gm	54868-2311-01	12.06	
PRONTO (Del)			
SPR,NA, 0.4%, 142 gm	10310-0328-50	4.55	6.82
PRONTO MAXIMUM STRENGTH LICE KILLING (Del)			
LIQ,TP, 4%-0.33%, 60 ml	10310-0230-02	6.16	9.23
PRONTO PLUS LICE EGG REMOVER (Del)			
SOL,TP (KIT)			
0.1%, 59 ml	10310-0321-93	6.85	10.28
PRONTO PLUS LICE KILLING MOUSSE (Del)			
SHA,TP (MAXIMUM STRENGTH)			
4%-0.33%, 118 ml	10310-0340-14	8.40	12.60
PRONTO PLUS PINWORM TREATMENT (Del)			
SUS,PO (SF,CHERRY)			
144 mg/ml, 30 ml	10310-0324-05	6.00	9.00
PRONTO PLUS WARM OIL TREATMENT & CONDITIONER (Del)			
SHA,TP (MAXIMUM STRENGTH)			
4%-0.33%, 36 ml 2s	10310-0323-59	6.85	10.28
PRONUTRA (Immunotec)			
PDR,PO (W/BIOACTIVE CYSTINE)			
37 gm	28770-0004-00	3.00	
PROPASS (Hormel Healthlabs)			
POW,PO (GLUTEN-FREE)			
8 gm 100s	99459-0153-09	56.35	
225 gm 4s	99429-0131-26	36.80	
PROPIMEX-1 (Abbott)			
PDR,PO, 400 gm	70074-0511-33	40.46	
PROPIMEX-2 (Abbott)			
PDR,PO, 400 gm	70074-0511-35	81.12	
PROPRINAL (Hart Health)			
TAB,PO (2X8)			
200 mg, 16s ea UD	50332-0109-05	1.49	
(2X50)			
200 mg, 100s ea UD	50332-0109-04	5.49	
(2X125)			
200 mg, 250s ea UD	50332-0109-07	12.18	
(2X400)			
200 mg, 800s ea UD	50332-0109-01	37.75	
PROS-TECH PLUS (Bio-Tech Pharm)			
CAP,PO, 10 mg-25 mg,			
100s ea	53191-0145-01	11.55	
PROSHIELD CLEANSER (Healthpoint)			
SPR,TP, 120 ml	00064-0700-04	3.06	
PROSHIELD FOAM CLEANSER (Healthpoint)			
SPR,TP, 240 ml	00064-0150-08	7.44	
PROSHIELD GLOVE SKIN PROTECTANT (Healthpoint)			
LOT,TP, 180 gm	00064-0850-06	10.56	
PROSHIELD PLUS SKIN PROTECTANT (Healthpoint)			
GEL,TP (FRAGRANCE-FREE)			
1.11%, 120 gm	00064-0300-04	9.04	
PROSHIELD SKIN CARE KIT (Healthpoint)			
KIT,TP, ea	00064-0300-25	16.45	
PROSIGHT (Major)			
TAB,PO, 60s ea	00904-7735-52	4.79	
120s ea	00904-7735-18	9.49	
PROSIGHT LUTEIN (Major)			
CAP,PO, 36s ea	00904-5494-73	6.89	
PROSOBEE LIPIL (Mead Johnson & Co)			
LIQ,PO (RTU,4X237ML)			
237 ml 4s	00087-0309-51	11.64	
(CONCENTRATE)			
384 ml	00087-1195-41	5.56	
(READY TO USE)			
946 ml	00087-0309-74	8.45	
PDR,PO (LACTOSE-FREE)			
366 gm	00087-1214-41	16.69	
729 gm	00087-1214-42	31.58	
PROSOBEE LIPIL IRON FORTIFIED (Mead Johnson & Co)			
LIQ,PO (NURSETTE, 20 CAL)			
177 ml	00087-0261-24	2.11	
PROSOURCE NOCARB (National Nutrition)			
SOL,PO (4X946ML,GLUTEN-FREE)			
946 ml 4s	94688-0115-25	120.00	
946 ml 4s	94688-0115-35	120.00	
946 ml 4s	94688-0115-45	120.00	
PROSOURCE PLUS (National Nutrition)			
SOL,PO (4X946ML,GLUTEN-FREE)			
946 ml 4s	94688-0116-51	120.00	
946 ml 4s	94688-0116-61	120.00	
946 ml 4s	94688-0116-71	120.00	
PROSTAPLEX HERBAL COMPLEX (ADH)			
CAP,PO (PF,SF)			
10 mg-40 mg-225 mg-5 mg,			
50s ea	60142-0979-01	8.98	17.95
PROSTATE (Key Company)			
CAP,PO, 140 mg, 100s ea	11694-0903-01	5.00	
(Miller)			
TAB,PO, 130 mg, 100s ea	17204-0528-40	7.26	11.50
PROSTATE FORMULA ADVANCED (Rx Vitamins)			
SGL,PO (PF,SF,SOFTGEL)			
90s ea	08429-0100-90	18.48	36.95
PROSTATONIN (Pharmaton)			
CAP,PO (SF)			
25 mg-300 mg,			
56s ea	93190-0070-98	12.97	14.72
PROSTEX (Metabolic Prods)			
CAP,PO, 100s ea	48433-0002-01	11.97	19.95
250s ea	48433-0002-02	23.97	39.95
PROSURE (Abbott)			
LIQ,PO (BANANA)			
237 ml	70074-0557-81	2.11	
(VANILLA)			
237 ml	70074-0557-76	2.11	
(4X237ML,CHOCOLATE)			
237 ml 4s	70074-0557-78	12.67	
PROTEC (Mason Vit)			
TAB,PO, 50s ea	11845-0099-29	10.33	
PROTECT U-2000 (Dihoma Inc.)			
SPR,NA, 3%-0.3%, 142 gm	62294-1003-04	8.85	12.99
PROTECTION PLUS SOAP (Medline)			
LOT,TP, 800 ml 12s	53329-0012-20	54.20	
3840 ml 4s	53329-0012-25	40.50	
PROTECTIVE OINTMENT WITH VITAMINS A & D (Ameriderm Labs)			
OIN,TP (24X113GM)			
113 gm 24s	63921-0160-04	1.20	
PROTECTIVE W/VITAMIN A & D (Ameriderm Labs)			
OIN,TP, 425 gm	63921-0160-15	3.39	
PROTEGRA ANTIOXIDANT (Inverness)			
SGL,PO, 75s ea	36652-0377-18	7.94	
PROTEIN (Mason Vit)			
TAB,PO (PF,SF)			
60s ea	11845-0119-75	6.56	
(Nature's Bounty)			
TAB,PO (PF)			
250 mg, 100s ea	74312-0002-40		4.25
PROTEIN AMINOS (Health Products Corp)			
CTB,PO (PF,SF)			
100s ea	39686-0014-42	6.00	
PROTEIN POWDER (Major)			
PDR,PO (VANILLA)			
480 gm	00904-4246-16	8.20	
PROTEINEX (Llorens Pharma Int)			
LIQ,PO (PREDIGESTED,SF)			
236 ml	54859-0515-08	12.50	12.26
472 ml	54859-0515-16	22.60	22.00
TAB,PO (SF,PHOSPHORUS-FREE)			
120s ea	54859-0715-12	25.00	
(Victus, Inc.)			
PDS,PO, 275 gm 12s	12197-0500-00	180.60	
PKT,PO, 40s ea	12197-0500-10	30.00	
PROTEOLYTIC ENZYMES (Miller)			
TAB,PO, 100s ea	17204-0951-40	8.22	13.00
PROTEXIN (Seyer Pharmatec)			
SYR,PO (ORANGE)			
500 mg/15 ml,			
118.3 ml	11026-2870-04	7.80	
PROTIFAR (Nutricia)			
PDS,PO (WITH SPOON)			
225 gm	49735-0111-34	156.00	
PROTOCOL PAK (HVS Labs)			
KIT,PO (48 DAY)			
ea	52386-9624-04	40.00	
PROVIEW EYE PRESSURE MONITOR (Bausch & Lomb Inc.)			
DEV,NA, ea	24208-0428-01	71.86	
PROVIL (Prime Marketing)			
TAB,PO, 200 mg, 100s ea	62107-0002-01	5.50	
PROVIMIN (Abbott)			
PDR,PO, 150 gm	70074-0502-61	15.80	
PROXACOL (Johnson & Johnson)			
SOL,TP, 3%, 240 ml	00071-3066-20	1.45	
480 ml	00071-3066-23	2.23	
PRUNE SENNA CONCENTRATE (Mason Vit)			
SGL,PO, 100s ea	11845-0111-61	8.11	

PROD/MFR	HRI, UPC,NDC	AWP	SRP
PRUNUS SPINOSA (Weleda)			
LIQ,PO, 50 ml	55946-0370-15	7.20	
PSEUDOCOT (Truxton)			
TAB,PO, 60 mg, 1000s ea	00463-6271-10	22.80	
PSEUDOEPH/TRIPROLIDINE			
(Dispensing Solutions)			
REPACK			
TAB,PO, 60 mg-2.5 mg,			
30s ea	55045-1311-08	7.50	
PSEUDOEPHEDRINE (Dispensing Solutions)			
TAB,PO, 60 mg, 28s ea	55045-1773-08	11.20	
PSEUDOEPHEDRINE HCL (Cardinal Health)			
TAB,PO (NON-DROWSY)			
30 mg, 24s ea	37205-0445-62	3.25	
96s ea	37205-0445-80	8.10	
(Consolidated Midland)			
SYR,PO, 30 mg/5 ml,			
480 ml	00223-6348-01	4.50	
480 ml	00223-6348-04	4.50	
3840 ml	00223-6348-02	27.00	
TAB,PO, 30 mg, 100s ea	00223-1476-01	3.00	
1000s ea	00223-1476-02	19.95	
60 mg, 100s ea	00223-1475-01	2.75	
1000s ea	00223-1475-02	25.00	
(Ohm)			
TAB,PO, 30 mg, 24s ea	51660-0403-24	0.95	
100s ea	51660-0403-01	1.75	
1000s ea	51660-0403-10	8.25	
60 mg, 100s ea	51660-0076-01	1.90	
1000s ea	51660-0076-10	9.55	
(Pharm Assoc Inc)			
SYR,PO (CHERRY)			
30 mg/5 ml, 118 ml	00121-0421-04	2.29	
(Roxane)			
TAB,PO, 30 mg, 100s ea	00054-4743-25	4.54	
60 mg, 100s ea	00054-4744-25	5.70	
(Rugby)			
SYR,PO (RASPBERRY)			
30 mg/5 ml, 120 ml	00536-1850-97	3.15	
480 ml	00536-1850-85	7.42	
(Sandoz)			
TAB,PO, 30 mg, 100s ea	00781-1533-01	6.75	
60 mg, 100s ea	00781-1535-01	10.13	
(A-S Medication)			
REPACK			
TAB,PO, 30 mg, 15s ea	54569-0650-05	1.01	
24s ea	54569-0650-01	1.62	
48s ea	54569-0650-00	3.24	
60 mg, 12s ea	54569-0626-03	1.22	
15s ea	54569-0626-05	1.52	
20s ea	54569-0626-04	2.03	
30s ea	54569-0626-01	3.04	
(Altura)			
REPACK			
TAB,PO, 30 mg, 15s ea	63874-0025-15	6.24	
30s ea	63874-0025-30	12.48	
60 mg, 15s ea	63874-0009-15	6.48	
30s ea	63874-0009-30	12.96	
(Dispensing Solutions)			
REPACK			
LIQ,PO, 30 mg/5 ml,			
118 ml	55045-2307-08	4.25	
SYR,PO (1X120ML,RASPBERRY)			
30 mg/5 ml, 120 ml	68258-8000-04	4.41	
TAB,PO, 30 mg, 24s ea	55045-2678-07	8.65	
60 mg, 20s ea	66336-0096-20	6.84	
30s ea	66336-0096-30	13.79	
(HomeMed)			
REPACK			
TAB,PO, 30 mg, 30s ea	51655-0478-24	3.77	
60 mg, 30s ea	51655-0317-24	3.94	
(Nucare Pharm)			
REPACK			
TAB,PO, 30 mg, 30s ea	66267-0186-30	10.89	
60 mg, 20s ea	66267-0187-20	9.56	
30s ea	66267-0187-30	10.99	
(PD-Rx Pharm)			
REPACK			
TAB,PO, 30 mg, 12s ea	55289-0558-12	6.17	
15s ea	55289-0558-15	6.45	
30s ea	55289-0558-30	7.48	
60 mg, 15s ea	55289-0864-15	6.38	
24s ea	55289-0864-24	7.32	
30s ea	55289-0864-30	7.42	
40s ea	55289-0864-40	8.22	
56s ea	58864-0647-56	9.15	

PROD/MFR	HRI, UPC,NDC	AWP	SRP
(Pharma Pac)			
REPACK			
TAB,PO, 30 mg, 15s ea	52959-0515-15	6.17	
20s ea	52959-0515-20	7.88	
30s ea	52959-0515-30	11.29	
60 mg, 20s ea	52959-0260-20	9.19	
24s ea	52959-0260-24	9.63	
25s ea	52959-0260-25	11.47	
30s ea	52959-0260-30	13.79	
40s ea	52959-0260-40	17.46	
100s ea	52959-0260-00	43.60	
(Phys Total Care)			
REPACK			
TAB,PO, 30 mg, 100s ea	54868-1876-00	14.58	
1000s ea	54868-1876-03	107.65	
60 mg, 30s ea	54868-1973-04	8.64	
100s ea	54868-1973-03	18.27	
1000s ea	54868-1973-00	141.45	
(Southwood)			
REPACK			
SYR,PO, 30 mg/5 ml,			
120 ml	58016-4033-04	3.58	
TAB,PO, 30 mg, 10s ea	58016-0434-10	1.12	
12s ea	58016-0434-12	1.34	
14s ea	58016-0434-14	1.56	
15s ea	58016-0434-15	1.67	
20s ea	58016-0434-20	2.23	
21s ea	58016-0434-21	2.34	
24s ea	58016-0434-24	2.68	
24s ea	58016-4816-01	0.95	
28s ea	58016-0434-28	3.12	
30s ea	58016-0434-30	3.35	
40s ea	58016-0434-40	4.46	
60s ea	58016-0434-60	6.70	
100s ea	58016-0434-00	11.16	
60 mg, 10s ea	58016-0435-10	2.04	
12s ea	58016-0435-12	2.45	
14s ea	58016-0435-14	2.85	
15s ea	58016-0435-15	3.06	
20s ea	58016-0435-20	4.08	
21s ea	58016-0435-21	4.28	
28s ea	58016-0435-28	4.89	
30s ea	58016-0435-30	6.12	
40s ea	58016-0435-40	8.15	
50s ea	58016-0435-50	10.19	
60s ea	58016-0435-60	12.23	
100s ea	58016-0435-00	20.38	
PSEUDOEPHEDRINE HCL 12 HOUR			
(Cardinal Health)			
TER,PO (COATED,NON-DROWSY)			
120 mg, 10s ea	37205-0446-52	3.84	
PSEUDOEPHEDRINE HCL CHILDREN'S (Pharma Pac)			
REPACK			
LIQ,PO, 30 mg/5 ml,			
120 ml	52959-0261-04	4.75	
PSEUDOEPHEDRINE HYDROCHLORIDE (Perrigo)			
TAB,PO, 30 mg, 24s ea	45802-0432-62	2.45	
(Palmetto)			
REPACK			
TAB,PO, 60 mg, 20s ea	23490-6214-01	9.19	
30s ea	23490-6214-02	13.79	
PSEUDOEPHEDRINE/TRIPROLIDINE			
(A-S Medication)			
REPACK			
SYR,PO, 30 mg/5 ml-1.25 mg/5 ml,			
120 ml	54569-4209-00	3.59	
(Phys Total Care)			
REPACK			
TAB,PO, 60 mg-2.5 mg,			
100s ea	54868-2423-00	10.62	
(Southwood)			
REPACK			
SYR,PO, 30 mg/5 ml-1.25 mg/5 ml,			
120 ml	58016-4001-01	4.18	
TAB,PO, 60 mg-2.5 mg,			
8s ea	58016-0401-08	3.30	
12s ea	58016-0401-12	3.69	
25s ea	58016-0401-25	4.25	
30s ea	58016-0401-30	4.70	
40s ea	58016-0401-40	5.05	
100s ea	58016-0401-00	7.62	
PSEUDOEPHEDRINE/ TRIPROLIDINE HYDROCHLORIDE (Altura)			
REPACK			
TAB,PO, 60 mg-2.5 mg,			
8s ea	63874-0010-08	3.47	
12s ea	63874-0010-12	3.87	
15s ea	63874-0010-15	4.83	
20s ea	63874-0010-20	6.45	

PROD/MFR	HRI, UPC,NDC	AWP	SRP
24s ea	63874-0010-24	7.74	
25s ea	63874-0010-25	8.06	
30s ea	63874-0010-30	9.68	
40s ea	63874-0010-40	12.90	
60s ea	63874-0010-60	19.35	
100s ea	63874-0010-01	32.25	
1000s ea	63874-0010-02	322.50	
PSEUDOTABS (Concord Labs)			
TAB,PO, 30 mg, 24s ea	20254-0210-24	1.89	
100s ea	20254-0210-01	2.97	
1000s ea	20254-0210-04	17.40	
PSYLDEX (Contract Pharmacal)			
PDR,PO, 3.4 gm/dose,			
398 gm	10267-0407-14	8.00	
(ORANGE)			
3.4 gm/dose, 398 gm	10267-0858-14	8.00	
595 gm	10267-0407-21	10.21	
(ORANGE)			
3.4 gm/dose, 595 gm	10267-0858-21	10.21	
PSYLLIUM (Carlson,J.R.)			
CAP,PO, 500 mg, 100s ea	88395-0085-34	4.45	8.90
PSYLLIUM HUSK (Yerba)			
CAP,PO, 180s ea	46352-0001-06	6.57	10.95
PDR,PO, 340 gm	46352-0001-04	5.37	8.95
PSYLLIUM HYDROPHILIC MUCILLOID			
(Asafi Pharmaceutical)			
PDR,PO, 3.4 gm/dose,			
371 gm	65557-0778-13	4.25	
PSYLLIUM SEED INDIAN HUSKS (Freeda)			
PDS,PO, 4100 mg/4.1 gm,			
453.6 gm	10432-0122-03	8.97	14.95
PUBLIX ADVANCED LANCING (Owen Mumford)			
DEV,NA (PRIVATE LABEL)			
ea	08214-0707-29	11.05	
PUBLIX EXTRA SHORT PEN NEEDLES			
(Can-Am Care)			
DEV,NA (6MM,PRIVATE LABEL)			
100s ea	38396-0706-01	19.98	
PUBLIX GLUCOSE (Can-Am Care)			
CTB,PO (CAFFEINE-FREE)			
4 gm, 50s ea	38396-0551-01	6.49	
50s ea	38396-0552-01	6.49	
50s ea	38396-0556-01	6.49	
50s ea	38396-0557-01	6.49	
PUBLIX PENNEEDLES (Can-Am Care)			
DEV,NA (SHORT LENGTH,31GX8MM)			
100s ea	38396-0621-03	19.98	
(STANDARD LENGTH)			
100s ea	38396-0621-02	19.98	
PUBLIX PRESTIGE SMART SYSTEM (Home Diag)			
DEV,NA (STRIP)			
50s ea	56151-0320-50	26.12	
PUBLIX PSS STARTER (Home Diag)			
DEV,NA (MTR,STRP,LANCET,DEV,SOL)			
ea	56151-0220-01	22.18	
PUBLIX STERILE TIP LANCETS (Owen Mumford)			
DEV,NA (28G,ULTRA THIN)			
100s ea	08214-0357-29	4.05	
PULMOCARE (Abbott)			
LIQ,PO (BERRY)			
240 ml	70074-0406-99	2.64	
240 ml	70074-0501-81	2.64	
PULMOCARE ROSS READY-TO-HANG (Abbott)			
LIQ,PO, 1000 ml	70074-0512-04	14.82	
PULSATILLA (Luyties)			
TAB,SL (6X)			
6 x, 500s ea	00618-7121-03	3.99	
5500s ea	00618-7121-10	30.32	
(30X)			
12 x, 500s ea	00622-7121-03	4.19	
5500s ea	00622-7121-10	31.83	
(12X)			
30 x, 500s ea	00624-7121-03	4.19	
5500s ea	00624-7121-10	31.83	
(Walker Pharmacal)			
TAB,SL (6X)			
250s ea	00619-7121-02	2.97	
PUMP BATTERY (Animas Corp.)			
DEV,NA (#357, 12 PACK)			
12s ea	65781-0320-12	30.96	
PUMP W/PIERCING PIN (Abbott)			
DEV,NA, ea	70074-0506-19	7.21	
PURALIN DECONGESTANT (Apothecus)			
TAB,SL (HOMEOPATHIC)			
48s ea	52925-0836-38	3.99	

PROD/MFR	HRI, UPC, NDC	AWP	SRP
PURALIN ONE-STEP PREGNANCY (Apothecus)			
DEV,NA, 2s ea	48723-0334-97	3.39	
PURALUBE TEARS (Quality Care Prod)			
REPACK			
SOL,OP, 1.4%, 15 ml	49999-0336-15	8.36	
PURE & GENTLE LUBRICANT EYE DROPS (Altaire)			
PURE & GENTLE			
SOL,OP (STERILE)			
0.3%, 15 ml	59390-0197-13	7.06	
30 ml	59390-0197-18	11.00	
PURE NIACINAMIDE (Freeda)			
TAB,PO, 500 mg, 500s ea	10432-0134-03	17.97	29.95
PURE VITAMIN D3 (Freeda)			
TAB,PO, 3000 iu,			
100s ea	10432-0369-01	6.57	10.95
250s ea	10432-0369-02	13.14	21.90
PURELL DEEP CLEANING (Johnson & Johnson)			
SHE,TP (ON-THE-GO WIPE)			
65%, 18s ea	52800-0658-89	2.69	
PURELL INSTANT HAND SANITIZER (Johnson & Johnson)			
GEL,TP (ORIGINAL FORMULA)			
62%, 30 ml	00501-4050-01	0.68	
(W/2-GO CARRIER)			
62%, 30 ml	52800-0658-10	0.92	
(WITH ALOE)			
62%, 30 ml	52800-0658-84	0.70	
(ORIGINAL)			
62%, 59 ml	73852-0096-50	1.18	
(WITH ALOE)			
62%, 59 ml	00501-4051-02	1.18	
(W/MOISTURIZER&VITAMIN E)			
62%, 60 ml	00501-4050-02	1.18	
118 ml	00501-4051-04	1.64	
(1X118ML)			
62%, 118 ml	73852-0030-40	1.68	
(AMERICAN RED CROSS)			
62%, 118 ml	00501-4050-04	1.64	
(MOISTURE THERAPY)			
62%, 236 ml	52800-0658-09	2.69	
(ORIGINAL,W/PUMP)			
62%, 236 ml	52800-0658-80	2.69	
(W/ALOE & VIT E)			
62%, 236 ml	52800-0658-81	2.69	
(W/MOISTURIZER & VIT E)			
62%, 236 ml	52800-0005-20	2.69	
(W/ALOE & VIT E)			
62%, 473 ml	52800-0658-16	4.30	
(1X30ML)			
65%, 30 ml	52800-0658-71	0.70	
(1X59ML)			
65%, 59 ml	52800-0658-62	2.03	
59 ml	52800-0658-63	2.03	
(W/ALOE & VIT E)			
65%, 59 ml	52800-0658-67	1.20	
(W/MOISTURIZERS & VIT E)			
65%, 59 ml	52800-0658-66	1.20	
KIT,TP, ea	52800-0659-53	1.84	
SPR,TP (1X24ML)			
65%, 24 ml	52800-0658-65	2.69	
PURELL OCEAN MIST INSTANT HAND SANITIZER (Johnson & Johnson)			
GEL,TP (OCEAN MIST)			
62%, 60 ml	00501-4055-02	1.18	
240 ml	00501-4055-08	2.63	
PURELL SPRING BLOOM HAND SANITIZER (Johnson & Johnson)			
GEL,TP (SPRING BLOOM)			
62%, 60 ml	00501-4056-02	1.18	
240 ml	00501-4056-08	2.63	
PURPOSE DUAL TREATMENT (Johnson & Johnson)			
LOT,TP (MOISTURE LOT W/SPF15)			
120 ml	81370-0034-51	7.42	
PURPOSE GENTLE CLEANSING BAR (Johnson & Johnson)			
SOA,TP (1X170GM,OIL-FREE)			
170 gm	81370-0034-55	2.96	
(OIL-FREE)			
170 gm	81370-0034-54	1.94	
PURPOSE GENTLE CLEANSING WASH (Johnson & Johnson)			
SOL,TP (1X180ML,OIL-FREE)			
180 ml	81370-0034-75	4.66	
PYCNOGENOL (ADH)			
CAP,PO (PF,SF)			
30 mg, 30s ea	60142-0497-53	11.48	22.95
(Mason Vit)			
CAP,PO (PF,SF)			
154 mg-25 mg, 30s ea	11845-0123-08	15.44	
(Nature's Bounty)			
CAP,PO (PF,SF)			
30 mg, 30s ea	74312-0071-30		16.99
PYCNOGENOL & GRAPE W/ESTER C (Linus)			
CAP,PO, 50 mg-5 mg-26 mg-15 mg,			
50s ea	10363-0253-22	6.57	11.35
PYCNOGENOL PLUS (Rexall)			
TAB,PO (PF,SF)			
45s ea	30768-0001-78	8.31	12.58
PYRI-500 (Miller)			
TAB,PO, 500 mg, 100s ea	17204-0935-40	12.31	19.50
PYRIDOXINE (DHS, Inc.)			
REPACK			
TAB,PO, 100 mg, 90s ea	55887-0824-90	11.25	
(Quality Care Prod)			
REPACK			
TAB,PO, 50 mg, 30s ea	49999-0894-30	4.23	
PYRIDOXINE HCL (HomeMed)			
REPACK			
TAB,PO, 50 mg, 30s ea	51655-0498-24	3.32	
PYRIDOXINE HCL/MINERALS (Miller)			
CAP,PO, 100s ea	17204-0939-40	10.08	14.70
PYRINEX (Consolidated Midland)			
LIQ,TP, 2%-0.2%, 60 ml	00223-4409-60	2.25	
120 ml	00223-4409-11	3.00	
PYRINYL (Consolidated Midland)			
LIQ,TP, 2%-0.2%, 60 ml	00223-6605-00	3.50	
120 ml	00223-6605-04	6.50	
PYRROXATE EXTRA STRENGTH (Lee Pharm)			
TAB,PO (CAFFEINE FREE,AF,CAPLET)			
650 mg-50 mg-60 mg,			
24s ea	23558-0551-20	6.96	
500s ea	23558-0551-22	106.80	
(CAFF. FREE,24X72,AF)			
650 mg-50 mg-60 mg,			
1728s ea	23558-0551-21	501.12	
(CAFF.FREE,500X12,AF)			
650 mg-50 mg-60 mg,			
6000s ea	23558-0551-23	1281.60	
Q-DRYL (Qualitest)			
CAP,PO, 25 mg, 24s ea	00603-0241-18	2.84	
SOL,PO (AF,CHERRY)			
12.5 mg/5 ml, 120 ml	00603-0823-54	1.92	
(UNBOXED,AF,CHERRY)			
12.5 mg/5 ml, 120 ml	00603-0823-94	1.92	
240 ml	00603-0823-81	3.75	
473 ml	00603-0823-58	4.66	
(Nucare Pharm)			
REPACK			
SOL,PO (AF,CHERRY)			
12.5 mg/5 ml,			
120 ml	68071-1325-04	10.49	
(Physician Partner)			
REPACK			
SOL,PO, 12.5 mg/5 ml,			
480 ml	21695-0689-16	24.84	
Q-NAFTATE (Qualitest)			
CRE,TP, 1%, 15 gm	00603-0618-73	2.94	
Q-PAP (Qualitest)			
SOL,PO (DROPS)			
80 mg/0.8 ml,			
15 ml	00603-0838-73	2.14	
TAB,PO, 325 mg, 100s ea	00603-0263-21	3.41	
(REGULAR STRENGTH)			
325 mg, 100s ea	00603-0263-29	3.41	
1000s ea	00603-0263-32	16.40	
(EXTRA STRENGTH)			
500 mg, 100s ea	00603-0268-29	4.28	
Q-PAP CHILDREN'S (Qualitest)			
SUS,PO (BUBBLEGUM)			
160 mg/5 ml, 120 ml	00603-0841-54	2.50	
(CHERRY)			
160 mg/5 ml, 120 ml	00603-0842-54	2.50	
(GRAPE)			
160 mg/5 ml, 120 ml	00603-0843-54	2.50	
Q-PAP ES (Qualitest)			
TAB,PO (CAPLET)			
500 mg, 100s ea	00603-0265-21	5.85	
1000s ea	00603-0268-32	21.68	
(CAPLET)			
500 mg, 1000s ea	00603-0265-32	26.91	
Q-PAP EXTRA STRENGTH (Qualitest)			
TAB,PO, 500 mg, 100s ea	00603-0268-21	4.28	
Q-TAPP (Qualitest)			
ELI,PO (AF,GRAPE)			
1 mg/5 ml-15 mg/5 ml,			
118 ml	00603-0851-54	4.55	
237 ml	00603-0851-56	7.72	
(UNBOXED,AF,GRAPE)			
1 mg/5 ml-15 mg/5 ml,			
237 ml	00603-0851-81	7.72	
SOL,PO (1X118ML,AF,GRAPE)			
1 mg/5 ml-15 mg/5 ml,			
118 ml	00603-0851-94	4.55	
Q-TAPP DM (Qualitest)			
LIQ,PO (AF,GRAPE)			
118 ml	00603-0852-54	4.55	
SOL,PO (UNBOXED,1X118ML,AF)			
118 ml	00603-0852-94	3.11	
Q-TIPS (Covidien)			
DEV,NA (SINGLETIP-STER,2/PK,6")			
2000s ea	08080-5413-00	40.65	
(SINGLETIP,2/PK DISP,6")			
2000s ea	08080-5414-00	46.89	
(SINGLETIP APPL,BULK,3")			
10000s ea	08080-5404-00	62.97	
(SINGLETIP APPL,BULK,6")			
10000s ea	08080-5405-00	67.33	
Q-TUSSIN (Qualitest)			
LIQ,PO (AF,CHERRY)			
100 mg/5 ml, 120 ml	00603-0857-54	1.88	
(UNBOXED,AF,CHERRY)			
100 mg/5 ml, 120 ml	00603-0857-94	1.88	
(AF,CHERRY)			
100 mg/5 ml, 240 ml	00603-0857-56	3.70	
(UNBOXED,AF,CHERRY)			
100 mg/5 ml, 240 ml	00603-0857-81	3.70	
(AF,CHERRY)			
100 mg/5 ml, 480 ml	00603-0857-58	6.65	
Q-TUSSIN DM (Qualitest)			
LIQ,PO (CHERRY)			
10 mg/5 ml-100 mg/5 ml,			
120 ml	00603-0855-54	2.38	
(UNBOXED,CHERRY)			
10 mg/5 ml-100 mg/5 ml,			
120 ml	00603-0855-94	2.38	
(CHERRY)			
10 mg/5 ml-100 mg/5 ml,			
240 ml	00603-0855-56	4.60	
(UNBOXED,CHERRY)			
10 mg/5 ml-100 mg/5 ml,			
240 ml	00603-0855-81	4.60	
(CHERRY)			
10 mg/5 ml-100 mg/5 ml,			
480 ml	00603-0855-58	7.88	
QC ANTACID ANTI-GAS (Chain Drug Marketing)			
SUS,PO, 355 ml	63868-0712-57	1.68	3.99
QC ANTACID CALCIUM SUPP (Chain Drug Marketing)			
CTB,PO (ASSORTED FRUIT)			
500 mg, 150s ea	63868-0054-15	2.04	3.49
(ASSORTED BERRY)			
750 mg, 96s ea	63868-0153-96	2.04	3.49
(ASSORTED FRUIT)			
750 mg, 96s ea	63868-0127-22	2.04	3.49
QC ANTI GAS (Chain Drug Marketing)			
QC ANTI-GAS			
SGL,PO (ULTRA STRENGTH)			
180 mg, 60s ea	63868-0180-23	3.90	5.99
QC ANTI-DIARRHEAL (Chain Drug Marketing)			
TAB,PO, 2 mg, 12s ea	63868-0338-12	1.56	3.99
24s ea	63868-0338-24	2.22	5.99
QC ENEMA (Chain Drug Marketing)			
NMA,RC (COMPLETE, READY TO USE)			
133 ml	63868-0380-45	0.66	0.99
QC IBUPROFEN (Chain Drug Marketing)			
TAB,PO, 200 mg, 500s ea	63868-0983-03	8.10	12.99
QC NATURAL VEGETABLE (Chain Drug Marketing)			
PDR,PO (ORIGINAL)			
3.4 gm/dose, 368 gm	63868-0347-17	2.99	5.99
(SMOOTH TEXTURE,ORANGE)			
3.4 gm/dose, 368 gm	63868-0347-18	2.99	5.99
QC NON-ASPIRIN EXTRA STRENGTH (Chain Drug Marketing)			
TAB,PO, 500 mg, 24s ea	63868-0088-24	0.95	2.99
50s ea	63868-0088-50	1.26	3.49
100s ea	63868-0088-01	1.79	4.99
500s ea	63868-0088-03	5.10	11.99

PROD/MFR	HRI, UPC,NDC	AWP	SRP
QC PAIN RELIEVER (Chain Drug Marketing)			
TAB,PO (EXTRA STRENGTH)			
250 mg-250 mg-65 mg,			
100s ea	63868-0485-01	1.91	5.99
QC PINK BISMUTH (Chain Drug Marketing)			
TAB,PO, 262 mg, 40s ea	63868-0172-28	2.57	3.99
QC SORE THROAT LOZENGES (Chain Drug Marketing)			
LOZ,MM (CHERRY)			
6 mg-10 mg, 18s ea UD	63868-0983-18	1.62	2.99
QC SUGAR FREE NATURAL VEGETABLE (Chain Drug Marketing)			
PDR,PO (SMOOTH TEXTURE,ORANGE)			
3.4 gm/dose, 283 gm	63868-0347-19	3.59	5.99
QUAD STAND ADAPTER (Abbott Hosp)			
DEV,NA (DUAL-DESIGN CLAMP)			
ea	00074-2003-01	99.03	
QUALITY CHOICE A & D (Chain Drug Marketing)			
OIN,TP (PRIVATE LABEL)			
15.5%-53.4%, 113 gm	63868-0204-04	1.80	3.99
QUALITY CHOICE ACID CONTROLLER (Chain Drug Marketing)			
TAB,PO (ORIGINAL STRENGTH)			
10 mg, 30s ea	63868-0714-30	2.59	6.99
QUALITY CHOICE ADVANCED LANCING (Chain Drug Marketing)			
DEV,NA (PRIVATE LABEL)			
ea	35515-0959-34	11.05	
QUALITY CHOICE ALLERGY & SINUS HEADACHE (Chain Drug Marketing)			
TAB,PO (PRIVATE LABEL,CAPLET)			
325 mg-12.5 mg-5 mg,			
24s ea	63868-0985-24	2.10	4.99
QUALITY CHOICE ALLERGY RELIEF (Chain Drug Marketing)			
ODT,PO (PRIVATE LABEL)			
10 mg, 10s ea	63868-0157-10	3.00	6.99
QUALITY CHOICE ALLERGY RELIEF MULTI-SYMPTOM (Chain Drug Marketing)			
TAB,PO (DAYTIME,PRIVATE LABEL)			
325 mg-2 mg-5 mg,			
24s ea	63868-0981-24	2.04	4.99
QUALITY CHOICE ANTACID (Chain Drug Marketing)			
SUS,PO (MINT CREME)			
360 ml	63868-0694-57	1.68	3.99
QUALITY CHOICE ANTI-DIARRHEAL (Chain Drug Marketing)			
SGL,PO (PRIVATE LABEL,SOFTGEL)			
2 mg, 12s ea	63868-0756-12	1.62	4.99
QUALITY CHOICE ARTHRITIS PAIN RELIEF (Chain Drug Marketing)			
TER,PO (PRIVATE LABEL,CAPLET)			
650 mg, 50s ea	63868-0089-50	3.72	7.99
100s ea	63868-0089-01	6.30	10.99
QUALITY CHOICE AZO (Chain Drug Marketing)			
TAB,PO (PRIVATE LABEL)			
95 mg, 32s ea	63868-0100-32	2.76	5.99
QUALITY CHOICE BACITRACIN (Chain Drug Marketing)			
OIN,TP (USP,PRIVATE LABEL)			
500 u/gm, 28.4 gm	63868-0916-28	2.39	3.99
QUALITY CHOICE BACKACHE RELIEF (Chain Drug Marketing)			
TAB,PO (MAXIMUM STRENGTH)			
580 mg, 24s ea	63868-0508-24	2.94	4.99
QUALITY CHOICE BORIC ACID (Chain Drug Marketing)			
POW,NA (NF,PRIVATE LABEL)			
170 gm	63868-0205-06	2.38	4.99
QUALITY CHOICE CALCIUM (Chain Drug Marketing)			
TAB,PO (PRIVATE LABEL)			
600 mg, 60s ea	63868-0626-60	2.39	3.59
QUALITY CHOICE CALCIUM WITH VITAMIN D (Chain Drug Marketing)			
TAB,PO (USP,PRIVATE LABEL)			
600 mg-400 iu, 60s ea	63868-0615-60	2.39	4.99
300s ea	63868-0615-30	5.87	9.99
QUALITY CHOICE CALCIUM WITH VITAMIN D AND MINERALS (Chain Drug Marketing)			
TAB,PO (PRIVATE LABEL)			
60s ea	63868-0630-60	3.30	5.49
QUALITY CHOICE CHILDREN'S CHEWABLE VITAMINS COMPLETE (Chain Drug Marketing)			
QUALITY CHOICE CHILDREN'S CHEW VITAMINS COMPLETE			
CTB,PO, 60s ea	63868-0629-60	3.35	4.99
QUALITY CHOICE CHILDREN'S CHEWABLE VITAMINS W/EXTRA VITAMIN C (Chain Drug Marketing)			
QUALITY CHOICE CHILDREN'S CHEW VIT W/EXTRA VIT C			
CTB,PO (PRIVATE LABEL)			
60s ea	63868-0616-60	3.30	4.99
QUALITY CHOICE CHILDREN'S CHEWABLE VITAMINS W/IRON (Chain Drug Marketing)			
CTB,PO (PRIVATE LABEL)			
60s ea	63868-0628-60	3.59	5.99
QUALITY CHOICE CHILDREN'S IBUPROFEN (Chain Drug Marketing)			
SUS,PO (1X118ML,AF)			
100 mg/5 ml, 118 ml	63868-0756-18	2.88	4.99
QUALITY CHOICE COLD RELIEF (Chain Drug Marketing)			
TAB,PO (PRIVATE LABEL,CAPLET)			
500 mg-12.5 mg, 24s ea	63868-0506-24	1.92	3.99
QUALITY CHOICE COLD RELIEF PLUS (Chain Drug Marketing)			
SYR,PO (1X118ML,PRIVATE LABEL)			
118 ml	63868-0063-04	2.16	4.99
TEF,PO (PRIVATE LABEL)			
250 mg-2 mg-5 mg,			
20s ea	35515-0957-04	2.70	3.99
QUALITY CHOICE COMPLETE ALLERGY MEDICINE (Chain Drug Marketing)			
TAB,PO (PRIVATE LABEL,CAPLET)			
25 mg, 100s ea	63868-0500-01	2.34	8.99
QUALITY CHOICE COUGH & SORE THROAT (Chain Drug Marketing)			
SYR,PO (NIGHTTIME,W/DOSE CUP,AF)			
237 ml	63868-0065-08	2.70	3.99
QUALITY CHOICE COUGH RELIEF (Chain Drug Marketing)			
SYR,PO (1X118ML,8 HOUR RELIEF)			
15 mg/5 ml, 118 ml	63868-0069-04	3.12	6.99
118 ml	63868-0070-04	3.12	6.99
QUALITY CHOICE DAILY MULTIVITAMINS WITH IRON (Chain Drug Marketing)			
TAB,PO (USP,PRIVATE LABEL)			
100s ea	63868-0624-01	2.87	3.99
QUALITY CHOICE DAYTIME (Chain Drug Marketing)			
SGL,PO (AF,PRIVATE LABEL)			
325 mg-10 mg-5 mg,			
12s ea	63868-0386-12	1.91	3.49
20s ea	63868-0386-20	2.39	4.49
QUALITY CHOICE DYE-FREE ALLERGY MEDICINE (Chain Drug Marketing)			
SGL,PO (DYE-FREE,SOFTGEL)			
25 mg, 24s ea	63868-0995-24	1.40	3.39
QUALITY CHOICE EFFERVESCENT PAIN RELIEF (Chain Drug Marketing)			
TEF,PO (PRIVATE LABEL)			
325 mg-1000 mg-1916 mg,			
36s ea	63868-0229-36	2.46	3.99
QUALITY CHOICE EPSOM SALT (Chain Drug Marketing)			
CRY,NA (1X454GM,PRIVATE LABEL)			
454 gm	63868-0937-16	1.08	1.49
(1X1810GM,PRIVATE LABEL)			
1810 gm	63868-0937-04	2.34	3.29
QUALITY CHOICE ESSENTIALS (Chain Drug Marketing)			
TAB,PO (PRIVATE LABEL)			
100s ea	63868-0623-01	2.87	3.99
QUALITY CHOICE FERROUS SULFATE (Chain Drug Marketing)			
TAB,PO (PRIVATE LABEL)			
325 mg, 100s ea	63868-0617-01	3.36	5.99
QUALITY CHOICE FIBER (Chain Drug Marketing)			
CAP,PO (PRIVATE LABEL)			
0.52 gm, 160s ea	63868-0348-01	4.20	6.99
QUALITY CHOICE GAS RELIEF (Chain Drug Marketing)			
CTB,PO (PRIVATE LABEL,MINT)			
80 mg, 100s ea	63868-0103-16	2.22	6.99
(EXTRA STRENGTH)			
125 mg, 18s ea	63868-0853-18	1.74	3.99
QUALITY CHOICE HEARTBURN 150 (Chain Drug Marketing)			
TAB,PO (MAXIMUM STRENGTH)			
150 mg, 24s ea	63868-0487-24	4.75	7.99
QUALITY CHOICE HEMORRHOIDAL COOLING (Chain Drug Marketing)			
GEL,TP (GREASELESS)			
0.25%-50%, 51 gm	63868-0206-18	2.64	7.99
QUALITY CHOICE HYDROCORTISONE (Chain Drug Marketing)			
CRE,TP (MAX.STRENGTH,W/ALOE)			
1%, 28.4 gm	63868-0200-01	1.38	3.99
QUALITY CHOICE HYDROGEN PEROXIDE (Chain Drug Marketing)			
SOL,TP (1X237ML,USP)			
3%, 237 ml	63868-0926-08	0.47	0.99
(1X473ML,USP)			
3%, 473 ml	63868-0926-16	0.59	0.99
(1X946ML,USP)			
3%, 946 ml	63868-0926-32	0.98	1.79
QUALITY CHOICE IBUPROFEN (Chain Drug Marketing)			
TAB,PO (USP,COATED)			
200 mg, 24s ea	63868-0983-24	1.14	2.99
50s ea	63868-0983-50	1.59	3.99
100s ea	63868-0983-09	2.39	6.99
QUALITY CHOICE INFANTS' DROPS (Chain Drug Marketing)			
SUS,PO (W/DROPPER,AF)			
80 mg/0.8 ml, 30 ml	63868-0838-01	2.16	6.99
QUALITY CHOICE INFANTS' NON-ASPIRIN DROPS (Chain Drug Marketing)			
SOL,PO (1X30ML,AF,DYE-FREE)			
80 mg/0.8 ml, 30 ml	63868-0837-01	2.16	6.99
QUALITY CHOICE INSTANT ANTISEPTIC PAIN RELIEF (Chain Drug Marketing)			
LIQ,TP (PRIVATE LABEL)			
10.8%-4.7%, 45 ml	63868-0060-45	2.34	4.99
QUALITY CHOICE INSULIN SYRINGES (Can-Am Care)			
DEV,NA (ULTRA COMFORT,29G,1/2CC)			
100s ea	38396-0402-05	17.50	
(ULTRA COMFORT,29G,1CC)			
100s ea	38396-0401-05	17.50	
(ULTRA COMFORT,29G)			
100s ea	38396-0403-05	17.50	
(ULTRA COMFORT,31G,1/2CC)			
100s ea	38396-0406-05	17.50	
(ULTRA COMFORT,31G,1CC)			
100s ea	38396-0404-05	17.50	
QUALITY CHOICE IODIDES TINCTURE (Chain Drug Marketing)			
TIN,TP (1X60ML,PRIVATE LABEL)			
60 ml	63868-0331-02	2.16	4.99
QUALITY CHOICE ISOPROPYL RUBBING ALCOHOL (Chain Drug Marketing)			
SOL,TP (1X473ML,PRIVATE LABEL)			
50%, 473 ml	63868-0939-16	0.82	1.29
70%, 473 ml	63868-0936-16	1.19	2.19
(1X473ML,USP)			
70%, 473 ml	63868-0925-16	1.10	1.79
(1X946ML,USP)			
70%, 946 ml	63868-0925-32	2.34	2.19
(1X473ML,USP)			
91%, 473 ml	63868-0933-16	1.80	1.99
QUALITY CHOICE LANCETS (Can-Am Care)			
DEV,NA (PRIVATE LABEL)			
100s ea	38396-0303-22	5.85	
(THIN,PRIVATE LABEL)			
100s ea	38396-0301-22	5.85	
(COLORED,PRIVATE LABEL)			
200s ea	38396-0306-22	9.50	
(THIN,PRIVATE LABEL)			
200s ea	38396-0302-22	9.50	
QUALITY CHOICE LAXATIVE MAXIMUM STRENGTH (Chain Drug Marketing)			
TAB,PO, 25 mg, 24s ea	63868-0549-24	1.71	4.99
QUALITY CHOICE LO-DOSE ASPIRIN (Chain Drug Marketing)			
ECT,PO (PRIVATE LABEL)			
81 mg, 120s ea	63868-0361-20	1.56	4.99
QUALITY CHOICE LORATADINE (Chain Drug Marketing)			
TAB,PO, 10 mg, 10s ea	63868-0151-10	1.18	6.99
(PRIVATE LABEL)			
10 mg, 30s ea	63868-0151-30	2.20	13.99
(NON-DROWSY)			
10 mg, 100s ea	63868-0151-01	7.62	27.99

PROD/MFR	HRI, UPC,NDC	AWP	SRP
QUALITY CHOICE LORATADINE-D (Chain Drug Marketing)			
T24,PO (NON-DROWSY)			
10 mg-240 mg, 10s ea	63868-0154-10	5.22	9.99
QUALITY CHOICE MAGNESIUM CITRATE (Chain Drug Marketing)			
SOL,PO (1X296ML,PRIVATE LABEL)			
1.75 gm/30 ml, 296 ml	63868-0934-10	1.19	1.99
296 ml	63868-0935-10	1.19	1.99
QUALITY CHOICE MAXIMUM DAILY MULTIVITAMIN (Chain Drug Marketing)			
TAB,PO (USP,PRIVATE LABEL)			
100s ea	63868-0613-01	3.95	5.99
QUALITY CHOICE MEDIFIN (Chain Drug Marketing)			
TAB,PO (PRIVATE LABEL)			
200 mg, 60s ea	63868-0754-60	2.91	6.99
QUALITY CHOICE MEDIFIN CP (Chain Drug Marketing)			
TAB,PO (DYE-FREE,PRIVATE LABEL)			
650 mg-400 mg, 50s ea	63868-0762-50	4.44	9.99
QUALITY CHOICE MEDIFIN DM (Chain Drug Marketing)			
TAB,PO (DYE-FREE,PRIVATE LABEL)			
20 mg-400 mg, 50s ea.	63868-0753-50	4.44	9.99
QUALITY CHOICE MEDIFIN PE (Chain Drug Marketing)			
TAB,PO (DYE-FREE,PRIVATE LABEL)			
400 mg-10 mg, 50s ea.	63868-0752-50	4.44	9.99
QUALITY CHOICE MEN'S DAILY MULTIVITAMIN (Chain Drug Marketing)			
TAB,PO (USP,PRIVATE LABEL)			
60s ea	63868-0621-60	4.20	5.99
QUALITY CHOICE MICONAZOLE 7 (Chain Drug Marketing)			
SUP,VG (PRIVATE LABEL)			
100 mg, 7s ea	63868-0199-07	3.48	7.99
QUALITY CHOICE MILK OF MAGNESIA (Chain Drug Marketing)			
SUS,PO (STIMULANT-FREE)			
400 mg/5 ml, 355 ml	63868-0310-12	1.73	3.99
QUALITY CHOICE MINERAL OIL (Chain Drug Marketing)			
OIL,PO (USP,1X473ML)			
473 ml	63868-0938-16	2.28	4.99
QUALITY CHOICE MULTI VITE W/ LYCOPENE AND LUTEIN (Chain Drug Marketing)			
TAB,PO (USP,PRIVATE LABEL)			
130s ea	63868-0619-13	6.60	7.99
QUALITY CHOICE MULTI-VITE 50 & OVER (Chain Drug Marketing)			
TAB,PO (IRON-FREE,PRIVATE LABEL)			
60s ea	63868-0620-60	4.08	5.99
100s ea	63868-0620-01	5.70	8.99
QUALITY CHOICE MULTIVITAMIN FOR CHOLESTEROL (Chain Drug Marketing)			
PO (USP,PRIVATE LABEL)			
50s ea	63868-0622-50	4.50	6.99
QUALITY CHOICE NAPROXEN SODIUM (Chain Drug Marketing)			
TAB,PO, 220 mg, 24s ea	63868-0465-24	2.20	2.99
QUALITY CHOICE NIGHTTIME (Chain Drug Marketing)			
SGL,PO (PRIVATE LABEL,SOFTGEL)			
325 mg-15 mg-6.25 mg, 12s ea	63868-0384-12	1.91	3.49
20s ea	63868-0384-20	2.39	4.49
QUALITY CHOICE NIGHTTIME COLD MEDICINE (Chain Drug Marketing)			
SOL,PO (PRIVATE LABEL,CHERRY)			
177 ml	63868-0803-06	1.86	3.49
(PRIVATE LABEL,ORIGINAL)			
177 ml	63868-0804-06	1.86	3.49
(PRIVATE LABEL,CHERRY)			
295 ml	63868-0803-10	2.34	5.49
(PRIVATE LABEL,ORIGINAL)			
295 ml	63868-0804-10	2.34	5.49
QUALITY CHOICE NIGHTTIME COUGH (Chain Drug Marketing)			
SYR,PO (1X177ML,PRIVATE LABEL)			
177 ml	63868-0807-55	1.86	3.49
(1X296ML,PRIVATE LABEL)			
296 ml	63868-0807-63	2.34	5.49
QUALITY CHOICE NIGHTTIME SINUS (Chain Drug Marketing)			
SGL,PO (AF,PRIVATE LABEL)			
325 mg-6.25 mg-5 mg, 12s ea	63868-0388-12	1.91	3.49
20s ea	63868-0388-20	2.39	4.49
QUALITY CHOICE NON-ASPIRIN (Chain Drug Marketing)			
TAB,PO (EXTRA STRENGTH)			
500 mg, 50s ea	63868-0503-50	2.04	4.99
QUALITY CHOICE NON-ASPIRIN 8 HOUR (Chain Drug Marketing)			
TER,PO (PRIVATE LABEL,CAPLET)			
650 mg, 100s ea	63868-0089-10	6.30	10.99
QUALITY CHOICE NON-ASPIRIN PAIN RELIEF (Chain Drug Marketing)			
TAB,PO (EXTRA STRENGTH,EASYTABS)			
500 mg, 100s ea	63868-0507-01	3.00	6.49
QUALITY CHOICE PEDIATRIC ELECTROLYTE (Chain Drug Marketing)			
SOL,PO (GRAPE)			
1000 ml	63868-0007-33	2.58	3.99
QUALITY CHOICE PEN NEEDLES (Chain Drug Marketing)			
DEV,NA (29G,1/2",ORIGINAL)			
100s ea	35515-0959-37	21.25	
(31G,1/4",MINI)			
100s ea	35515-0959-39	21.25	
(31G,5/16",SHORT)			
100s ea	35515-0959-38	21.25	
QUALITY CHOICE PINK BISMUTH (Chain Drug Marketing)			
SUS,PO (REGULAR STRENGTH)			
262 mg/15 ml, 237 ml	63868-0302-23	1.74	3.49
QUALITY CHOICE PRE-MOISTENED MEDICATED WIPES (Chain Drug Marketing)			
PAD,TP, 50%, 48s ea	63868-0950-49	2.79	4.99
QUALITY CHOICE PRENATAL (Chain Drug Marketing)			
TAB,PO (PRIVATE LABEL)			
100s ea	63868-0001-01	4.55	8.79
QUALITY CHOICE REST SIMPLY (Chain Drug Marketing)			
TAB,PO (CAPLET)			
25 mg, 24s ea	63868-0789-24	1.19	3.99
QUALITY CHOICE SEVERE ALLERGY (Chain Drug Marketing)			
TAB,PO (PRIVATE LABEL,CAPLET)			
500 mg-12.5 mg, 24s ea	63868-0502-24	1.74	3.99
QUALITY CHOICE SINUS PAIN RELIEF (Chain Drug Marketing)			
TAB,PO (NON-DROWSY,DAYTIME)			
325 mg-5 mg, 24s ea	63868-0984-24	2.04	4.99
QUALITY CHOICE SLEEP AID (Chain Drug Marketing)			
SGL,PO (PRIVATE LABEL,SOFTGEL)			
50 mg, 32s ea	63868-0612-32	1.80	5.99
QUALITY CHOICE STOOL SOFTENER (Chain Drug Marketing)			
SGL,PO (LIQUICAP)			
100 mg, 100s ea	63868-0110-01	2.39	8.99
QUALITY CHOICE STOOL SOFTENER PLUS LAXATIVE (Chain Drug Marketing)			
SGL,PO (LIQUICAP)			
30 mg-100 mg, 100s ea	63868-0131-01	2.40	9.99
(LIQUID CAPS)			
30 mg-100 mg, 250s ea	63868-0131-25	5.40	15.99
QUALITY CHOICE SUPER THIN (Chain Drug Marketing)			
QUALITY CHOICE SUPER THIN LANCET			
DEV,NA (30G,PRIVATE LABEL)			
100s ea	35515-0959-35	4.75	
QUALITY CHOICE SUPHEDRINE (Chain Drug Marketing)			
TAB,PO (NON-DROWSY)			
30 mg, 48s ea	63868-0146-48	1.79	5.99
QUALITY CHOICE SUPHEDRINE PE (Chain Drug Marketing)			
TAB,PO (NON-DROWSY)			
10 mg, 36s ea	63868-0144-36	1.08	5.99
QUALITY CHOICE SWEET OIL (Chain Drug Marketing)			
OIL,NA (1X118ML,PRIVATE LABEL)			
118 ml	63868-0346-04	3.00	4.99
QUALITY CHOICE THERIN-M (Chain Drug Marketing)			
TAB,PO (PRIVATE LABEL)			
130s ea	63868-0625-13	6.12	7.99
QUALITY CHOICE TOLNAFTATE (Chain Drug Marketing)			
CRE,TP (GREASELESS,ODOR-FREE)			
1%, 30 gm	63868-0104-46	1.80	4.99
QUALITY CHOICE TUSSIN CF (Chain Drug Marketing)			
SYR,PO (PSEUDOEPHEDRINE-FREE,AF)			
237 ml	63868-0244-08	2.40	5.99
QUALITY CHOICE ULTRA THIN LANCET (Chain Drug Marketing)			
DEV,NA (28G,PRIVATE LABEL)			
100s ea	35515-0959-36	4.65	
QUALITY CHOICE WITCH HAZEL (Chain Drug Marketing)			
SOL,TP (1X473ML,PRIVATE LABEL)			
86%, 473 ml	63868-0927-16	1.98	3.99
QUALITY CHOICE WOMEN'S DAILY MULTIVITAMIN (Chain Drug Marketing)			
TAB,PO (USP,PRIVATE LABEL)			
60s ea	63868-0614-60	3.35	5.99
QUENALIN (Qualitest)			
SOL,PO, 12.5 mg/5 ml, 120 ml	00603-0860-54	2.90	
QUENCH (Bio-Tech Pharm)			
CAP,PO, 120s ea	53191-0366-12	25.00	
QUERCETIN (Bio-Tech Pharm)			
CAP,PO, 500 mg, 100s ea	53191-0418-01	22.00	
(Freeda)			
TAB,PO (PF,SF,DYE-FREE)			
50 mg, 100s ea	10432-0270-01	5.04	8.40
250s ea	10432-0270-02	10.08	16.80
250 mg, 100s ea	10432-0287-01	14.25	23.75
250s ea	10432-0287-02	28.50	47.50
QUICK MELTS (AmerisourceBergen)			
ODT,PO (CHILDREN'S NON-ASPIRIN)			
80 mg, 30s ea	87701-0399-99	2.24	2.49
QUICK RECOVERY (Pharm Innov)			
GEL,TP, 20 ml	00036-7002-20	1.05	1.50
90 ml	00036-7002-90	2.62	3.75
QUICK-SERTER (Medtronic Minimed)			
DEV,NA (INFUSION SET)			
ea	76300-0395-01	31.19	
QUICKLANCE (Arkray)			
DEV,NA (ALL-IN-ONE W/LANCET)			
50s ea	08317-9150-50	10.05	
QUICKTEK (Arkray)			
DEV,NA (CONTROL SOLUTION)			
ea	08317-3305-01	7.20	
(METER,10 STRIPS/LANCETS)			
ea	08317-3311-00	18.00	
(METER)			
ea	08317-3300-01	18.00	
(TEST STRIPS)			
50s ea	08317-3350-50	23.25	
100s ea	08317-3300-00	46.50	
QUIETUDE (Boiron)			
TAB,PO, 3 x-4 c-3 x-6 x, 60s ea	06962-6106-00	5.73	9.59
QUIK LOK (Abbott Hosp)			
DEV,NA (STERILE)			
120s ea	00074-5833-01	67.68	
QUIN B STRONG WITH C & ZINC (Freeda)			
TAB,PO, 100s ea	10432-0027-01	9.57	15.95
250s ea	10432-0027-02	19.14	31.90
QUINTABS (Freeda)			
TAB,PO (PF,SF,DYE-FREE)			
100s ea	10432-0139-01	8.64	14.40
250s ea	10432-0139-02	17.28	28.80
QUINTABS-M (Freeda)			
TAB,PO (HIGH POTENCY, IRON FREE)			
100s ea	10432-0336-01	9.15	15.25
250s ea	10432-0336-02	18.30	30.50
(PF,SF,DYE-FREE)			
100s ea	10432-0050-01	9.27	15.45
250s ea	10432-0050-02	18.54	30.90
500s ea	10432-0050-03	29.85	49.75
R A LOTION (Medco Lab)			
LOT,TP, 120 ml	11940-1801-01	2.85	
240 ml	11940-1801-02	5.00	
480 ml	11940-1801-03	9.00	
R.N.A.-180 (Key Company)			
TAB,PO (SF)			
180 mg, 100s ea	11694-0889-01	4.25	

PROD/MFR	HRI, UPC,NDC	AWP	SRP
RADIABLOCK (Carrington)			
STI,TP (SPF 15,LIP BALM,SF)			
3%-7%, 4 gm	53303-0142-15	2.63	
RADIACREAM (Carrington)			
CRE,TP, 56 gm	53303-0030-41	6.41	
RADIADRES HYDROGEL (Carrington)			
DRE,TP (4"X4")			
ea	53303-0141-41	6.51	
RADIAKLENZ (Carrington)			
SPR,TP, 236 ml	53303-0082-80	11.55	
RAGUS (Miller)			
TAB,PO, 100s ea	17204-0438-40	7.56	12.60
RANITIDINE (Major)			
TAB,PO (MAXIMUM STRENGTH,SF)			
150 mg, 24s ea	00904-5832-24	7.19	
50s ea	00904-5832-51	13.62	
(Pharma Pac)			
REPACK			
TAB,PO, 75 mg, 20s ea	52959-0599-20	6.99	
30s ea	52959-0599-30	10.48	
RANITIDINE 75 (Major)			
TAB,PO (SF,SODIUM-FREE)			
75 mg, 30s ea UD	00904-5399-46	7.19	
30s ea	00904-5818-46	7.19	
60s ea UD	00904-5399-52	13.49	
60s ea	00904-5818-52	13.49	
RANITIDINE HCL (AmerisourceBergen)			
TAB,PO (PRIVATE LABEL)			
75 mg, 30s ea	24385-0296-65	5.75	6.39
60s ea	24385-0296-72	9.89	11.00
(Cardinal Health)			
TAB,PO (PRIVATE LABEL)			
75 mg, 10s ea	37205-0529-52	2.40	
RASH-CARE (Weleda)			
OIN,TP, 30 gm	55946-0160-50	3.90	
RAY-TEC X-RAY DETECTABLE (J&J Medical)			
DEV,NA (4"X4",16-PLY,TRAY)			
10s ea	56091-0025-15	1.43	
(8"X4",16-PLY,TRAY)			
10s ea	56091-0025-27	2.90	
(8"X4",12-PLY,TRAY)			
480s ea	56091-0025-20	114.62	
RAY-TEC X-RAY DETECTABLE NONSTERILE (J&J Medical)			
DEV,NA (4"X4",12-PLY,BANDED)			
100s ea	56091-0074-37	1.99	
(4"X4",16-PLY,BANDED)			
100s ea	56091-0074-38	2.46	
(4"X4",16-PLY)			
100s ea	56091-0074-03	10.65	
(8"X4",12-PLY,BANDED)			
100s ea	56091-0074-39	3.46	
(8"X4",16-PLY,BANDED)			
100s ea	56091-0074-07	19.22	
(8"X4",24-PLY,BANDED)			
100s ea	56091-0074-06	28.09	
RCF (Abbott)			
LIQ,PO, 390 ml	70074-0401-08	5.09	
RCRA HAZARDOUS WASTE (Covidien)			
DEV,NA (SINGLE USE,2 GALLON)			
20s ea	08080-8602-00	161.67	
RE-AZO (Reese)			
TAB,PO, 95 mg, 32s ea	10956-0551-32	4.24	
RE/GEN (Nutra/Balance)			
LIQ,PO (25X118ML,FROZEN)			
118 ml 25s	07249-0600-21		64.07
(27X177ML,LACTOSE-FREE)			
177 ml 27s	72493-0040-11		94.54
177 ml 27s	72493-0040-12		94.54
(27X177ML,REDUCEDSUGAR)			
177 ml 27s	72493-0040-10		95.14
RE/GEN FREE (Nutra/Balance)			
LIQ,PO (25X118ML,LACTOSE-FREE)			
118 ml 25s	07249-0600-22		79.31
REA-LO (Med-Derm)			
CRE,TP (MOISTURIZING)			
30%, 60 gm	45565-0730-11	9.83	
240 gm	45565-0730-23	23.31	
REACH CLEANPASTE (Johnson & Johnson)			
DEV,NA (ORIGINAL,50YDS,ICY MINT)			
ea	81370-0097-23	2.51	
REACH CRYSTAL CLEAN (Johnson & Johnson)			
DEV,NA (SOFT)			
4s ea	81371-0031-19	2.50	
REACH TOTAL CARE (Johnson & Johnson)			
DEV,NA (30YDS,MICRO-GROOVES)			
ea	81370-0095-60	2.51	
(MEDIUM)			
ea	81371-0991-95	2.83	
(SOFT)			
ea	81371-0991-94	2.83	
2s ea	81371-0991-93	4.87	
REAL MCCOY (McCoy's)			
TAB,PO, 60s ea	31088-0780-60	2.60	3.90
REALITY FEMALE CONDOM (Female Health Co)			
DEV,NA (W/LUBRICANT)			
3s ea	11423-0070-00	6.36	10.59
6s ea	11423-0070-70	12.00	20.00
RECAPIT (Majestic Drug)			
CRE,DE (MAXIMUM STRENGTH)			
1 gm	10705-0400-70	2.15	4.85
RECOFEN D (Reese)			
SOL,PO, 5 mg/5 ml-100 mg/5 ml,			
120 ml	10956-0634-04	3.81	
240 ml	10956-0634-08	6.03	
RECORT PLUS (Reese)			
CRE,TP, 1%, 30 gm	10956-0673-01	4.31	
RECOVER (Key Company)			
TAB,PO (SF)			
120s ea	11694-0751-02	5.00	
RECTACAINE (Reese)			
SUP,RC, 0.25%, 12s ea	10956-0692-12	4.00	
RECTAGENE (Pfeiffer)			
OIN,TP, 60 gm	00927-0571-17	2.41	4.34
RECTAGENE II (Pfeiffer)			
SUP,RC, 12s ea	00927-0677-08	2.45	4.40
RECTASOL (Bio-Pharm)			
SUP,RC, 0.25%, 12s ea	59741-0302-12	5.50	
24s ea	59741-0302-24	9.95	
RED CHESTNUT (Ellon)			
SOL,SL (DROPS)			
10.5 ml	51762-0002-10		9.25
RED CLOVER (Botanical Labs.)			
LIQ,PO, 30 ml	41954-0020-39	3.75	7.49
60 ml	41954-0020-18	6.00	11.99
RED CROSS CANKER SORE (Mentholatum)			
OIN,MM (MAX. STR.)			
20%, 7.5 gm	10742-0005-41	3.35	
RED CROSS COTTON STERILE (J&J Medical)			
DEV,NA (PROFESSIONAL)			
ea	56091-0060-26	11.33	
RED CROSS TOOTHACHE KIT (Mentholatum)			
LIQ,MM, 3.75 ml	10742-0000-91	3.35	1.59
RED RASPBERRY (Botanical Labs.)			
LIQ,PO, 30 ml	41954-0020-41	3.75	7.49
RED WINE WITH POMEGRANATE (Major)			
CAP,PO, 60s ea	09046-0038-52	6.79	
RED YEAST RICE (Major)			
CAP,PO (PF,SF,LACTOSE-FREE)			
600 mg, 60s ea	00904-5826-60	9.41	
REDUTEMP (Intl Ethical)			
SOL,PO, 500 mg/15 ml,			
120 ml	11584-0430-05	12.44	
TAB,PO, 500 mg, 60s ea	11584-1022-06	5.73	
REESE'S ONETAB INTENSE STRENGTH ALLERGY & SINUS (Reese)			
TAB,PO (DYE-FREE,CAPLET)			
650 mg-25 mg-10 mg,			
30s ea	10956-0812-30	4.92	7.49
REESE'S ONETAB INTENSE STRENGTH COLD & FLU (Reese)			
TAB,PO (DYE-FREE,CAPLET)			
650 mg-25 mg-10 mg,			
30s ea	10956-0813-30	4.92	7.49
REESE'S ONETAB INTENSE STRENGTH CONGESTION & COUGH (Reese)			
TAB,PO (DYE-FREE,CAPLET)			
400 mg-10 mg,			
30s ea	10956-0814-30	4.92	7.49
REESE'S PINWORM MEDICINE (Reese)			
SUS,PO (2X30ML, FAMILY PACK)			
144 mg/ml, 30 ml 2s	10956-0618-21	12.55	19.99
REFENESEN (Reese)			
TAB,PO, 200 mg, 30s ea	10956-0752-30	2.77	
60s ea	10956-0752-60	4.06	
REFENESEN 400 (Reese)			
TAB,PO (DYE-FREE,CAPLET)			
400 mg, 50s ea	10956-0788-50	5.23	
100s ea	10956-0788-09	8.24	
REFENESEN DM (Reese)			
TAB,PO (DYE-FREE,CAPLET)			
20 mg-400 mg,			
50s ea	10956-0761-50	5.84	8.98
100s ea	10956-0761-09	8.92	13.98
REFENESEN PE (Reese)			
TAB,PO (DYE-FREE,CAPLET)			
400 mg-10 mg,			
50s ea	10956-0791-50	5.84	8.98
REFENESEN PLUS (Reese)			
TAB,PO (DYE-FREE,CAPLET)			
400 mg-60 mg, 20s ea	10956-0757-20	4.53	
REFILIT (Majestic Drug)			
CRE,DE (MAXIMUM STRENGTH,CHERRY)			
2 gm	10705-0400-88	2.15	4.85
REFRESH (Allergan Inc)			
SOL,OP, 1 ml 30s UD	00023-0506-01	9.61	
1 ml 50s UD	00023-0506-50	14.68	
REFRESH CELLUVISC (Allergan Inc)			
SOL,OP, 30s ea UD	00023-4554-30	10.97	
REFRESH CONTACTS (Allergan Inc)			
SOL,OP, 12 ml	00023-1822-12	5.30	
REFRESH DRY EYE THERAPY (Allergan Inc)			
SOL,OP (1X15ML,DROPS)			
1%-1%, 15 ml	00023-9291-15	7.57	
REFRESH EYE ITCH RELIEF (Allergan Inc)			
SOL,OP (1X5ML,DROPS)			
0.035%, 5 ml	00023-3468-05	11.02	
REFRESH LIQUIGEL (Allergan Inc)			
GEL,OP, 1%, 15 ml	00023-9205-15	7.96	
(1X30ML)			
1%, 30 ml	00023-9205-30	11.68	
REFRESH PLUS (Allergan Inc)			
SOL,OP, 30s ea UD	00023-5487-30	8.10	
50s ea UD	00023-5487-50	12.60	
(70X0.4ML,SINGLE-USE,PF)			
0.5%, 0.4 ml 70s	00023-0403-70	17.17	
(Phys Total Care)			
REPACK			
SOL,OP, 50s ea	54868-2816-01	10.26	
REFRESH PM (Allergan Inc)			
OIN,OP (1X3.5GM,PF)			
42.5%-57.3%,			
3.5 gm	00023-0240-04	8.48	
REFRESH REDNESS RELIEF (Allergan Inc)			
SOL,OP (1X15ML,DROPS)			
0.12%-1.4%, 15 ml	00023-3414-15	7.96	
REFRESH TEARS (Allergan Inc)			
SOL,OP, 0.5%, 15 ml	00023-0798-15	7.96	
(1X30ML)			
0.5%, 30 ml	00023-0798-30	11.68	
(2X30ML)			
0.5%, 30 ml 2s	00023-0798-60	20.47	
(Phys Total Care)			
REPACK			
SOL,OP, 0.5%, 15 ml	54868-1686-00	9.95	
REFUAH PLUS BLOOD GLUCOSE MONITORING SYSTEM (SMC)			
DEV,NA, ea	37654-0497-26	47.36	
REFUAH PLUS BLOOD GLUCOSE TEST STRIPS (SMC)			
DEV,NA, 50s ea	37654-0497-27	45.20	
REFUAH PLUS GLUCOSE CONTROL SOLUTION (SMC)			
DEV,NA, ea	37654-0497-28	6.89	
REGENECARE (MPM Medical Inc.)			
GEL,TP (1X4ML)			
2%, 4 ml	66977-0100-25	1.50	1.67
REGENECARE HA (MPM Medical Inc.)			
TP (1X4ML)			
2%, 4 ml	66977-0107-25	1.50	1.67
85 gm	66977-0107-03	18.25	20.28
SPR,TP (1X120GM)			
2%, 120 gm	66977-0107-04	18.25	20.28
REGENECARE HA SATURATED (MPM Medical Inc.)			
PAD,TP (4"X4")			
2%, ea	66977-0107-44	4.21	4.68
REGULOID (Rugby)			
CAP,PO, 0.52 gm,			
160s ea	00536-1500-60	9.70	

PROD/MFR	HRI, UPC,NDC	AWP	SRP
PDR,PO (SF,ORANGE)			
3.4 gm/dose,			
300 gm	00536-1875-79	6.42	
(SF,REGULAR)			
3.4 gm/dose,			
300 gm	00536-1881-79	6.42	
390 gm	00536-4444-54	5.68	
(ORANGE)			
3.4 gm/dose,			
390 gm	00536-4445-54	5.68	
(SF,ORANGE)			
3.4 gm/dose,			
450 gm	00536-1875-16	9.22	
(SF,REGULAR)			
3.4 gm/dose,			
450 gm	00536-1881-16	9.22	
570 gm	00536-4444-89	8.02	
(ORANGE)			
3.4 gm/dose,			
570 gm	00536-4445-89	8.02	
(A-S Medication)			
REPACK			
PDR,PO, 3.4 gm/dose,			
371 gm	54569-3684-00	5.55	
REHYDRALYTE (Abbott)			
SOL,PO, 240 ml 6s	70074-0401-62	17.57	
REJUVENESS (Richmark)			
DEV,NA (10 CM X 20 CM)			
ea	08179-0102-04	115.50	137.50
(10 CM X 30 CM)			
ea	08179-0103-03	135.66	161.50
(11 PC PACK)			
ea	08179-0098-88	720.72	861.50
(15 CM X 20 CM)			
ea	08179-0152-09	137.34	163.50
(2 PC PACK)			
ea	08179-0098-81	73.08	87.00
(4 CM X 18 CM)			
ea	08179-0418-02	72.66	86.50
(4 CM X 8 CM)			
ea	08179-0480-09	36.54	43.50
(40 CM X 25 CM)			
ea	08179-0425-02	86.10	102.50
(4CM X 12CM)			
ea	08179-0412-08	54.18	64.50
(6 PC PACK)			
ea	08179-0098-64	198.07	235.80
(7.5 CM X 12 CM)			
ea	08179-0712-05	86.10	102.50
(7.5 CM X 25 CM)			
ea	08179-0725-09	108.78	129.50
(8 PC PACK)			
ea	08179-0098-26	455.95	531.60
(BREAST SCAR, 1 PIECE)			
ea	08179-0028-10	134.56	149.50
(BREAST SCAR, 2 PIECES)			
ea	08179-0028-27	242.20	269.10
(LG BREAST SCAR, 1 PIECE)			
ea	08179-0028-34	152.56	169.50
(LG BREAST SCAR)			
ea	08179-0028-41	269.56	299.50
REJUVENESS ADHESIVE TAPE (Richmark)			
DEV,NA, ea	08179-0500-02	8.32	9.90
RELEASE NON-ADHERING STERILE (J&J Medical)			
DEV,NA (2"X3")			
50s ea	56091-0020-52	4.45	
(4"X3")			
50s ea	56091-0020-54	7.51	
(8"X3")			
75s ea	56091-0020-58	14.75	
RELI ON INSULIN SYRINGES (Wal-Mart)			
DEV,NA (1/2ML,29G,1/2")			
10s ea	08113-1311-65	2.39	
(1/2ML,30G,5/16")			
10s ea	08113-1311-71	2.39	
(1/2ML,31G,5/16")			
10s ea	08113-1311-77	2.39	
(1ML,29G,1/2",LATEX-FREE)			
10s ea	08113-1311-63	2.39	
(1ML,30G,5/16")			
10s ea	08113-1311-69	2.39	
(1ML,31G,5/16")			
10s ea	08113-1311-75	2.39	
(3/10ML,29G,1/2")			
10s ea	08113-1311-67	2.39	
(3/10ML,30G,5/16")			
10s ea	08113-1311-73	2.39	
(3/10ML,31G,5/16")			
10s ea	08113-1311-79	2.39	
(1/2ML,29G,1/2")			
100s ea	08113-1311-64	18.02	
(1/2ML,30G,5/16")			
100s ea	08113-1311-70	18.02	
(1/2ML,31G,5/16")			
100s ea	08113-1311-76	18.02	
(1ML,29G,1/2",LATEX-FREE)			
100s ea	08113-1311-62	18.02	
(1ML,30G,5/16")			
100s ea	08113-1311-68	18.02	
(1ML,31G,5/16")			
100s ea	08113-1311-74	18.02	
(3/10ML,29G,1/2")			
100s ea	08113-1311-66	18.02	
(3/10ML,30G,5/16")			
100s ea	08113-1311-72	18.02	
(3/10ML,31G,5/16")			
100s ea	08113-1311-78	18.02	
RELI ON LANCET DEVICE (Can-Am Care)			
DEV,NA (W/10 ULTRATHIN LANCETS)			
ea	38396-0505-01	8.00	
RELI ON LANCETS (Can-Am Care)			
DEV,NA (ULTRA THIN,30G)			
100s ea	38396-0451-02	5.85	
(STANDARD,21G)			
200s ea	38396-0450-02	9.50	
(ULTRA THIN,30G)			
200s ea	38396-0452-02	9.50	
RELI ON NEWTEK (Arkray)			
DEV,NA (DISP W/100 STRIPS)			
ea	08480-4501-00	55.90	
RELI ON PEN NEEDLES UNIVERSAL 1 (Can-Am Care)			
DEV,NA (29GX1/2",PRIVATE LABEL)			
50s ea	38396-0470-01	12.00	
(31GX5/16",PRIVATE LABEL)			
50s ea	38396-0470-02	12.00	
RELIABLE GENTLE LAXATIVE (Teva)			
ECT,PO, 5 mg, 100s ea	00182-1992-01	3.00	
RELIADOSE (Blaine)			
DEV,NA, ea	01650-0500-00	8.70	
RELIEF-SF (Hart Health)			
TAB,PO (50X2,FILM COATED)			
500 mg-2 mg-30 mg,			
100s ea UD	50332-0122-04	5.62	
(125X2,FILM COATED)			
500 mg-2 mg-30 mg,			
250s ea UD	50332-0122-07	12.71	
RELIEVE ENEMA (Unico)			
NMA,RC, 133 ml	59640-0016-04	0.62	
RELION CONFIRM BLOOD GLUCOSE MONITORING SYSTEM (Arkray)			
DEV,NA (PRIVATE LABEL)			
ea	08317-7120-02	12.00	
ea	08317-7120-03	12.00	
RELION CONFIRM/MICRO TEST STRIPS (Arkray)			
DEV,NA (PRIVATE LABEL)			
50s ea	08317-7100-50	21.94	
RELION INSULIN SYRINGES (Can-Am Care)			
DEV,NA (1/2ML,29G,1/2")			
100s ea	38396-0412-02	17.50	
(1ML,29G,1/2")			
100s ea	38396-0413-02	17.50	
(3/10ML,29G,1/2")			
100s ea	38396-0411-02	17.50	
RELION MINI PEN NEEDLES (Can-Am Care)			
DEV,NA (31GX6MM)			
50s ea	38396-0472-02	12.00	
RELION ULTRA-THIN PLUS (Can-Am Care)			
DEV,NA (32G)			
100s ea	38396-0314-02	5.85	
RELION ULTRATHIN (Can-Am Care)			
DEV,NA (COLORED,PRIVATE LABEL)			
100s ea	38396-0453-02	5.75	
REMBRANDT (Johnson & Johnson)			
FIL,DE (MINT)			
14s ea	49336-0006-51	18.70	
GEL,DE (WHITENING KIT)			
ea	49336-0653-00	18.70	
REMBRANDT WHITENING (Johnson & Johnson)			
PAS,DE (1X85GM)			
0.243%, 85 gm	49336-0617-00	6.01	
(1X74GM,FRESH MINT)			
0.884%, 74 gm	49336-0436-00	6.01	
(1X74GM,WINTERGREEN)			
0.884%, 74 gm	49336-0437-00	6.01	
SOL,MM (1X474ML,FRESH MINT)			
0.02%, 474 ml	49336-0059-58	6.01	
REME-T (Valeant Pharm Intl)			
SHA,TP, 5%, 236 ml	00064-2500-08	14.89	
REMOVE (Smith & Nephew)			
LIQ,TP (WIPES)			
50s ea	40565-0115-66	10.94	8.75
240 ml	40565-0112-43	13.88	11.10
REMOVER LOTION (3M Health Care)			
LOT,TP, 15 ml 20s	08333-8610-01	17.58	
120 ml	08333-8611-01	4.87	
RENA-VITE (Cypress Pharm)			
TAB,PO, 100s ea	60258-0160-01	13.99	
RENALCAL (Nestle)			
LIQ,PO (250MLX24,UNFLAVORED)			
250 ml 24s	00065-9013-70	180.86	
RENEW ADVANCED LANCING SYSTEM CARTRIDGE REFILLS (Can-Am Care)			
DEV,NA (PRIVATE LABEL)			
5s ea	38396-0444-55	15.00	
RENEW ADVANCED LANCING SYSTEM LANCING (Can-Am Care)			
DEV,NA (PRIVATE LABEL)			
ea	38396-0511-55	14.00	
RENU 1 STEP DAILY PROTEIN REMOVER (Bausch & Lomb Inc.)			
LIQ,NA, 5 ml	10119-0040-49	4.78	
RENU LEAK PROOF LENS CASE (Bausch & Lomb Inc.)			
DEV,NA, ea	10119-0403-07	3.36	
RENU MULTI-PURPOSE (Bausch & Lomb Inc.)			
SOL,NA, 118 ml	10119-0030-48	3.73	
355 ml	10119-0030-18	8.72	
RENU MULTIPLUS (Bausch & Lomb Inc.)			
SOL,NA (LUBE/REWETTING)			
8 ml	10119-0052-20	3.83	
118 ml	10119-0031-18	3.73	
355 ml	10119-0031-22	8.72	
RENU REWETTING DROPS (Bausch & Lomb Inc.)			
SOL,OP, 15 ml	10119-0052-08	5.04	
REPLACE (Key Company)			
SGL,PO (SF)			
100s ea	11694-0842-01	11.50	
500s ea	11694-0842-05	41.00	
REPLACE W/O IRON (Key Company)			
SGL,PO (SF)			
100s ea	11694-0703-01	11.50	
500s ea	11694-0703-05	41.00	
REPLENS (Lil Drug Store)			
CRE,VG (8 APPLICATORS)			
6.3 gm 8s	66715-0830-08		12.99
(14 APPLICATORS)			
36.9 gm	66715-0830-35		10.29
REPLETE ULTRAPAK (Nestle)			
LIQ,PO (1000MLX6)			
1000 ml 6s	00065-9156-72	43.56	
(1500MLX4)			
1500 ml 4s	00065-9156-73	43.54	
REPLICARE HYDROCOLLOID (Smith & Nephew)			
DEV,NA (4"X4")			
5s ea	40565-0115-72	32.40	25.92
(6"X6")			
5s ea	40565-0115-73	68.86	55.09
(6"X8")			
5s ea	40565-0115-87	49.61	39.69
(8"X8")			
5s ea	40565-0115-74	114.66	91.73
(2"X2 3/4")			
10s ea	40565-0115-85	33.70	26.96
(3 1/2"X5 1/2")			
10s ea	40565-0115-86	59.65	47.72
(1 1/2"X2 1/2")			
30s ea	40565-0115-31	91.58	73.26
REQUA ACTIVATED CHARCOAL (Young, W.F.)			
TAB,PO, 250 mg, 125s ea	10961-0001-02	8.40	13.49
RES-OFF (Pharm Innov)			
LOT,TP, 10 ml	00036-3990-10	1.69	2.41
60 ml	00036-3990-60	4.08	5.83
RESCON-DM (Capellon)			
LIQ,PO (AF,SF,DYE-FREE)			
120 ml	64543-0105-04	10.56	
480 ml	64543-0105-16	35.86	
RESCON-GG (Capellon)			
LIQ,PO, 100 mg/5 ml-5 mg/5 ml,			
120 ml	64543-0044-04	10.06	
(AF,DYE-FREE,CHERRY)			
100 mg/5 ml-5 mg/5 ml,			
480 ml	64543-0044-16	34.24	

PROD/MFR	HRI, UPC,NDC	AWP	SRP
RESOLVE/GP (Allergan Inc)			
SOL,NA (DAILY CLEANER,PF)			
30 ml	00023-0515-30	7.65	
RESOURCE 2.0 (Nestle)			
LIQ,PO (237MLX27,LACTOSE-FREE)			
237 ml 27s	00212-1801-62	47.63	
237 ml 27s	43900-0180-40	47.63	
(946MLX12,LACTOSE-FREE)			
946 ml 12s	00212-2760-65	64.08	
946 ml 12s	43900-0277-00	64.08	
RESOURCE ARGINAID EXTRA (Nestle)			
LIQ,PO (ORANGE BURST)			
4.5 gm/237 ml,			
237 ml 27s	00212-1966-62	62.86	
(WILD BERRY)			
4.5 gm/237 ml,			
237 ml 27s	00212-1967-62	62.86	
RESOURCE BENECALORIE (Nestle)			
POW,PO (24 X 1.5OZ,NEUTRAL)			
42 gm 24s	00212-2825-80	39.17	
RESOURCE BENEFIBER (Nestle)			
PDR,PO (MEDICAL SUPV.,PACKET,SF)			
4 gm 75s	00212-2823-74	35.70	
(MEDICAL SUPERVISION,SF)			
205 gm 4s	00212-2821-07	45.89	
RESOURCE BENEPROTEIN (Nestle)			
PKT,PO (PRIVATE LABEL)			
75s ea	00212-2843-71	48.90	
RESOURCE BREEZE (Nestle)			
LIQ,PO (27X237ML,VARIETY)			
237 ml 27s	00212-1860-62	42.77	
(27X237ML)			
237 ml 27s	00212-1862-62	38.88	
237 ml 27s	00212-1864-62	38.88	
(CHOLESTEROL-FREE)			
237 ml 27s	00212-1866-62	38.88	
RESOURCE DIABETISHIELD (Nestle)			
LIQ,PO (CHOLESTEROL-FREE)			
237 ml 27s	00212-3491-62	51.84	
237 ml 27s	00212-3493-61	51.84	
RESOURCE JUST FOR KIDS (Nestle)			
LIQ,PO (27X237ML, 1.5 CAL)			
237 ml 27s	00212-3319-62	63.83	
(LACTOSE-FREE,CHOCOLATE)			
237 ml 27s	00212-3312-62	47.63	
(LACTOSE-FREE,VANILLA)			
237 ml 27s	00212-3311-62	47.63	
(LACTOSE-FREE)			
237 ml 27s	00212-3313-62	47.63	
RESOURCE JUST FOR KIDS W/FIBER (Nestle)			
LIQ,PO (27X237ML, 1.5 CAL)			
237 ml 27s	00212-3320-62	66.42	
(LACTOSE-FREE,VANILLA)			
237 ml 27s	00212-3314-62	50.54	
RESOURCE OPTISOURCE HIGH PROTEIN DRINK (Nestle)			
LIQ,PO (1X237ML, TETRA PAK)			
237 ml	43900-0174-71	2.58	
237 ml	43900-0174-81	2.58	
(237MLX27,LACTOSE-FREE)			
237 ml 27s	43900-0174-71	69.66	
RESOURCE OPTISOURCE MINI NUTRITION BAR (Nestle)			
BAR,PO (30X12,LACTOSE-FREE)			
360s ea	43900-0175-30	472.08	
(237X27,LACTOSE-FREE)			
237 ml 27s	43900-0174-81	69.66	
RESOURCE ORIGINAL DAIRY THICK (Nestle)			
LIQ,PO (HONEY CONSISTENCY,HONEY)			
236 ml	00212-2330-62	27.86	
(NECTAR CONSISTENCY)			
236 ml	00212-2320-62	27.86	
RESOURCE PROTEIN (Nestle)			
PDR,PO ((TUBE FEEDING),6X227GM)			
227 gm 6s	00212-2841-07	73.94	
RESOURCE SUPPORT (Nestle)			
LIQ,PO (237MLX27,CHOCOLATE MINT)			
237 ml 27s	43900-0176-20	91.18	
(237MLX27,VERY VANILLA)			
237 ml 27s	43900-0175-80	91.18	
(237MLX27)			
237 ml 27s	43900-0175-20	91.18	
RESOURCE THICKENED APPLE JUICE (Nestle)			
LIQ,PO (HONEY CONSISTENCY,HONEY)			
236 ml	00212-2280-62	25.60	
(NECTAR CONSISTENCY)			
236 ml	00212-2290-62	25.60	
RESOURCE THICKENED COFFEE (Nestle)			
PDR,PO (PKTS,NECTAR CONSISTENCY)			
10.8 gm 75s	00212-2242-75	34.80	
(PKTS,HONEY CONSISTENCY)			
12.5 gm 75s	00212-2243-75	34.80	
RESOURCE THICKENED CRANBERRY JUICE (Nestle)			
LIQ,PO (HONEY CONSISTENCY,HONEY)			
236 ml	00212-2310-62	27.22	
(NECTAR CONSISTENCY)			
236 ml	00212-2300-62	27.22	
RESOURCE THICKENED LEMON WATER (Nestle)			
LIQ,PO (HONEY CONSISTENCY,HONEY)			
236 ml	00212-2250-62	20.09	
(NECTAR CONSISTENCY)			
236 ml	00212-2240-62	20.09	
RESOURCE THICKENED ORANGE JUICE (Nestle)			
LIQ,PO (HONEY CONSISTENCY,HONEY)			
236 ml	00212-2260-62	28.84	
(NECTAR CONSISTENCY)			
236 ml	00212-2270-62	28.84	
RESOURCE THICKENUP (Nestle)			
PDR,PO, 6.5 gm	00212-2254-71	22.20	
227 gm	00212-2251-07	47.23	
RESOURCE VANILLA DAIRY THICK (Nestle)			
LIQ,PO (HONEY CONSISTENCY,HONEY)			
236 ml	00212-2331-62	23.98	
(NECTAR CONSISTENCY)			
236 ml	00212-2321-62	23.98	
RESTON SELF-ADHERING FOAM PAD (3M Health Care)			
DEV,NA (6 1/4"X7 7/8",HIGH)			
2s ea	08333-2851-01	7.59	
(7 7/8"X11 13/4",HIGH)			
5s ea	08333-1561-01	20.35	
(7 7/8"X11 3/4",MEDIUM)			
10s ea	08333-1560-01	29.60	
RESTON SELF-ADHERING FOAM ROLL (3M Health Care)			
DEV,NA (4"X196",LIGHT SUPPORT)			
ea	08333-1563-01	14.30	
RESTORE WOUND CLEANSER (Hollister)			
SPR,TP, 236 ml	08380-0099-75	7.40	9.44
354 ml	08380-0099-76	10.65	13.65
RESURFIX (Topix)			
CRE,TP, 71 gm	58211-0358-02	15.50	
OIN,TP (PACKET)			
1.75 gm 100s	58211-0353-01	34.50	
100 gm	58211-0353-03	22.25	
RESURGEX (Millennium)			
PDS,PO, 25 gm 15s	18757-0002-11	48.00	
RETINYL PALMITATE (Health Products Corp)			
CRE,TP, 120 gm	39686-0014-78	5.50	
REVITALIZE (Rx Vitamins)			
CAP,PO, 90s ea	08429-0410-90	16.00	29.95
REZAMID (Summers)			
LOT,TP, 2%-5%, 60 ml	11086-0022-01	15.28	
RHINALL (Scherer Labs)			
SOL,NS, 0.25%, 30 ml	00274-7525-31	1.94	
SPR,NS, 0.25%, 40 ml	00274-7540-31	2.02	
RHINARIS (Pharmascience Labs)			
GEL,NS, 15%-20%,			
28.35 gm	51817-0072-02	4.20	5.99
SPR,NS, 15%-5%, 30 ml	51817-0071-02	5.75	7.99
RHUS TOX (Luyties)			
TAB,SL (6X)			
6 x, 500s ea	00618-7637-03	3.99	
5500s ea	00618-7637-10	30.32	
(30X)			
12 x, 500s ea	00622-7637-03	4.19	
5500s ea	00622-7637-10	31.83	
(12X)			
30 x, 500s ea	00624-7637-03	4.19	
5500s ea	00624-7637-10	31.83	
(Walker Pharmacal)			
TAB,SL (6X)			
250s ea	00619-7637-02	2.97	
RHYTHM RIGHT (Carlson,J.R.)			
SGL,PO (PF,SF,SALT-FREE)			
60s ea	88395-0043-26	9.95	19.90
120s ea	88395-0043-21	17.75	35.50
RI-GEL (R.I.J.)			
SUS,PO, 150 ml	53807-0126-05	1.76	
360 ml	53807-0126-01	2.20	
3840 ml	53807-0126-03	22.38	
RI-GEL II (R.I.J.)			
PO, 360 ml	53807-0158-01	2.90	
3840 ml	53807-0158-03	28.68	
RI-MAG (R.I.J.)			
SUS,PO, 540 mg/5 ml,			
360 ml	53807-0134-01	2.76	
RI-MAG PLUS (AmerisourceBergen)			
SUS,PO (PRIVATE LABEL)			
540 mg/5 ml-40 mg/5 ml,			
355 ml	24385-0409-40	3.41	3.79
(R.I.J.)			
SUS,PO, 540 mg/5 ml-20 mg/5 ml,			
360 ml	53807-0135-01	3.00	
RI-MOX (R.I.J.)			
SUS,PO, 225 mg/5 ml-200 mg/5 ml,			
150 ml	53807-0128-05	1.66	
360 ml	53807-0128-01	2.12	
3840 ml	53807-0128-03	21.40	
RI-MOX PLUS (R.I.J.)			
SUS,PO, 360 ml	53807-0151-01	2.34	
RI-TUSSIN (R.I.J.)			
SYR,PO, 100 mg/5 ml,			
120 ml	53807-0153-01	1.34	
240 ml	53807-0153-02	2.40	
480 ml	53807-0153-04	3.18	
3840 ml	53807-0153-03	18.28	
RI-TUSSIN DM (R.I.J.)			
SYR,PO, 10 mg/5 ml-100 mg/5 ml,			
120 ml	53807-0139-01	1.84	
240 ml	53807-0139-02	3.36	
480 ml	53807-0139-04	4.98	
3840 ml	53807-0139-03	33.18	
RIBO-100 (Key Company)			
TAB,PO, 100 mg, 100s ea	11694-0929-01	5.00	
RID (Bayer HealthCare)			
KIT,NA (COMBO)			
4%-0.33%, ea	16500-0504-92	13.55	
SHA,TP, 4%-0.33%, 60 ml	74300-0004-12	5.66	
120 ml	74300-0004-14	8.41	
240 ml	74300-0003-20	11.79	
SPR,NA, 0.5%, 150 ml	74300-0004-21	4.11	
(Phys Total Care)			
REPACK			
LIQ,TP, 4%-0.33%,			
240 ml	54868-3573-00	17.00	
RID LICE EGG LOOSENER (Bayer HealthCare)			
GEL,TP (W/COMB)			
57 gm	74300-0004-46	5.44	
RID MOUSSE (Bayer HealthCare)			
FOA,TP (W/COMB)			
4%-0.33%, 156 gm	74300-0012-60	9.66	
RID-A-PAIN (Pfeiffer)			
CRE,TP, 0.025%, 60 gm	00927-0356-45	4.93	8.89
RID-A-PAIN COMPOUND (Pfeiffer)			
TAB,PO (CAPLET)			
226.8 mg-32.4 mg-97.2 mg,			
24s ea	00927-0378-24	2.27	4.08
RID-A-PAIN DENTAL (Pfeiffer)			
LIQ,TP (DROPS)			
6.3%-0.5%, 30 ml	00927-0403-30	3.27	5.89
RID-A-PAIN RUB (Pfeiffer)			
OIN,TP, 15%, 60 gm	00927-0256-39	2.83	5.08
RID-A-PAIN-HP (Pfeiffer)			
CRE,TP, 0.075%, 45 gm	00927-0357-45	6.94	12.49
RIGHT FOR THE MACULA (Carlson,J.R.)			
SGL,PO (PF,SF,SOFTGEL)			
60s ea	88395-0086-86	14.40	28.80
120s ea	88395-0086-81	27.75	55.50
RIGHTSTEP PRENATAL VITAMINS (TriMarc Labs)			
TAB,PO, 100s ea	68752-0827-01	16.59	
RIGINIC (R.I.J.)			
SUS,PO, 360 ml	53807-0137-01	3.92	
RINOFLOW (Respironics)			
DEV,NA, ea	08373-6320-00	110.00	
RISABAL-PH CREAM (Rising)			
CRE,TP (1X455GM)			
455 gm	64980-0321-45	44.31	
RISACAL-D (Rising)			
TAB,PO (PF,SF,LACTOSE-FREE)			
105 mg-81 mg-120 iu,			
100s ea	64980-0150-01	19.98	

PROD/MFR	HRI, UPC,NDC	AWP	SRP
RISAMINE (Rising)			
OIN,TP (1X113GM)			
0.44%-20.625%,			
113 gm	64980-0322-12	4.45	
RISANOID PLUS (Rising)			
TAB,PO, 100s ea	64980-0148-01	19.06	
RISAQUAD (Rising)			
CAP,PO (PF,GLUTEN-FREE)			
30s ea	64980-0147-03	26.45	
RITE AID 600 CALCIUM PLUS VITAMIN D (Rite Aid)			
TAB,PO (PRIVATE LABEL)			
600 mg-400 iu, 60s ea	11822-0770-39	5.59	6.99
300s ea	11822-0778-45	9.59	11.99
RITE AID ACETAMINOPHEN (Rite Aid)			
TAB,PO (EXTRA STRENGTH,EASY TAB)			
500 mg, 50s ea	11822-0303-00	3.59	4.49
(EXTRA STRENGTH)			
500 mg, 50s ea	11822-0040-31	3.59	4.49
50s ea	11822-0041-24	4.39	5.49
100s ea	11822-0412-50	5.99	7.49
(FREE20%MORE)			
500 mg, 120s ea	11822-0740-05	5.19	6.49
TER,PO (PRIVATE LABEL,CAPLET)			
650 mg, 100s ea	11822-0301-92	5.99	7.49
RITE AID ACETAMINOPHEN PM (Rite Aid)			
TAB,PO (EXTRA STRENGTH)			
500 mg-25 mg,			
100s ea	11822-3171-01	7.59	9.49
300s ea	11822-3169-00	11.19	13.99
RITE AID ACID REDUCER (Rite Aid)			
TAB,PO (USP,SF,SODIUM-FREE)			
75 mg, 160s ea	11822-0399-05	15.99	19.99
(MAXIMUM STRENGTH)			
150 mg, 24s ea	11822-0505-18	5.59	6.99
(FREE 33%,MAX STRENGTH)			
150 mg, 32s ea	11822-0976-80	5.59	6.99
(MAXIMUM STRENGTH)			
150 mg, 50s ea	11822-0505-21	9.59	11.99
65s ea	11822-0505-22	12.79	15.99
RITE AID ACNE CLEANSER (Rite Aid)			
SOL,TP (OIL-FREE)			
2%, 236 ml	11822-0650-30	3.99	4.99
RITE AID ACNEPADS (Rite Aid)			
PAD,TP (MAXIMUM,PRIVATE LABEL)			
2%, 90s ea	11822-0296-73	3.59	4.49
RITE AID ACTA-TABS PE (Rite Aid)			
TAB,PO (PRIVATE LABEL)			
4 mg-10 mg, 24s ea	11822-0415-04	3.59	4.49
48s ea	11822-0416-02	5.19	6.49
72s ea	11822-8744-07	5.19	6.49
RITE AID ADVANCED HEALING (Rite Aid)			
LOT,TP (PRIVATE LABEL)			
1%, 725 ml	11822-3726-01	3.99	4.99
RITE AID ALCOHOL SWABS ANTISEPTIC (Rite Aid)			
SWA,TP (PRIVATE LABEL)			
70%, 120s ea	11822-0253-72	1.99	2.49
RITE AID ALLERGY (Rite Aid)			
SOL,PO (AF,SF,DYE-FREE)			
12.5 mg/5 ml, 118 ml	11822-0527-10	3.59	4.49
RITE AID ALLERGY MULTI-SYMPTOM (Rite Aid)			
TAB,PO (PRIVATE LABEL,COOL)			
325 mg-2 mg-5 mg,			
36s ea	11822-0083-34	3.59	4.49
RITE AID ALLERGY MULTI-SYMPTOM NIGHTTIME (Rite Aid)			
TAB,PO (PRIVATE LABEL,CAPLET)			
325 mg-25 mg-5 mg,			
24s ea	11822-0071-40	3.43	4.29
RITE AID AM/PM LOCKING PILL REMINDER (Rite Aid)			
DEV,NA (7-DAY,PRIVATE LABEL)			
ea	11822-0575-54	3.99	4.99
RITE AID ANGLE EDGE+ (Rite Aid)			
DEV,NA (MEDIUM,PRIVATE LABEL)			
ea	11822-3985-09	1.99	2.49
(SOFT,PRIVATE LABEL)			
ea	11822-3986-00	1.99	2.49
RITE AID ANTACID & ANTI-GAS (Rite Aid)			
SUS,PO (1X710ML,PRIVATE LABEL)			
710 ml	11822-0329-76	5.59	
RITE AID ANTI-FUNGAL (Rite Aid)			
SOL,TP (1X30ML,PRIVATE LABEL)			
12.5%, 30 ml	11822-0342-87	7.19	8.99
RITE AID ANTI-ITCH (Rite Aid)			
GEL,TP (1X118ML,EXTRA STRENGTH)			
2%, 118 ml	11822-0039-24	3.99	4.99
SPR,TP (1X59ML,EXTRA STRENGTH)			
2%-0.1%, 59 ml	11822-0392-03	3.99	4.99
RITE AID ANTI-SNORE (Rite Aid)			
SPR,MM (DYE-FREE,PRIVATE LABEL)			
59 ml	11822-3174-04	7.99	9.99
RITE AID ANTIBIOTIC CREAM PLUS (Rite Aid)			
CRE,TP (PRIVATE LABEL)			
28 gm	11822-0988-99	4.39	5.49
RITE AID ANTICAVITY FLUORIDE RINSE (Rite Aid)			
SOL,PO (AF,PRIVATE LABEL,MINT)			
0.05%, 474 ml	11822-4448-09	2.79	3.49
(AF,PRIVATE LABEL)			
0.05%, 530 ml	11822-2225-07	2.79	3.49
RITE AID ANTIFUNGAL CREAM (Rite Aid)			
CRE,TP (1X28GM,PRIVATE LABEL)			
2%, 28 gm	11822-0125-56	6.15	7.69
RITE AID ANTISEPTIC (Rite Aid)			
SOL,TP (1X354ML,PRIVATE LABEL)			
10%, 354 ml	11822-0895-28	6.39	7.99
RITE AID ANTISEPTIC MOUTH CLEANSER (Rite Aid)			
SOL,MM, 10%, 15 ml	11822-0316-97	3.99	4.99
RITE AID ANTISEPTIC MOUTH RINSE (Rite Aid)			
SOL,MM (1X1000ML,PRIVATE LABEL)			
1000 ml	11822-0310-82	2.79	
1000 ml	11822-0311-98	2.79	
RITE AID ARTHRITIS PAIN RELIEF (Rite Aid)			
CRE,TP (1X56GM,PRIVATE LABEL)			
0.075%, 56 gm	11822-0506-03	10.39	12.99
RITE AID ASPIRIN (Rite Aid)			
ECT,PO (ADULT,LOW STRENGTH)			
81 mg, 180s ea	11822-3169-02	5.99	7.49
(PRIVATE LABEL)			
81 mg, 500s ea	11822-3169-01	11.19	13.99
RITE AID ATHLETE'S FOOT (Rite Aid)			
CRE,TP (GREASELESS)			
1%, 15 gm	11822-4712-05	5.59	6.99
(PRIVATE LABEL)			
1%, 28 gm	11822-0470-95	6.79	8.49
(GREASELESS)			
1%, 30 gm	11822-3078-02	7.19	8.99
RITE AID B-12 (Rite Aid)			
LOZ,PO (PF,PRIVATE LABEL,CHERRY)			
1000 mcg-400 mcg,			
30s ea	11822-0576-05	3.99	4.99
RITE AID B-COMPLEX (Rite Aid)			
TAB,PO (PF,PRIVATE LABEL)			
125s ea	11822-0884-04	3.51	4.39
RITE AID BABY SUNSCREEN SPF 45 (Rite Aid)			
LOT,TP (PRIVATE LABEL)			
7.5%-5%-9%-6%, 89 ml	11822-0707-40	3.99	4.99
(PRIVATE LABEL,SPRAY)			
8%-7.5%-5%-2%-6%,			
237 ml	11822-0356-58	6.39	7.99
RITE AID BABY WASH & SHAMPOO (Rite Aid)			
SHA,TP (NATURAL OAT, TEAR FREE)			
236 ml	11822-0237-08	2.63	3.29
RITE AID BABY WIPES (Rite Aid)			
DEV,NA (PRIVATE LABEL)			
80s ea	11822-0340-68	2.39	2.99
(TWIN PACK,PRIVATE LABEL)			
80s ea	11822-0576-20	3.99	4.99
RITE AID BACK & NECK COLD REUSABLE PAD (Rite Aid)			
DEV,NA (12"X12",PRIVATE LABEL)			
ea	11822-0370-60	23.99	29.99
RITE AID BALANCED B 100 (Rite Aid)			
TAB,PO, 60s ea	11822-0043-07	7.59	9.49
RITE AID BANDAGES (Rite Aid)			
DEV,NA (PRIVATE LABEL)			
30s ea	11822-0370-20	2.39	2.99
36s ea	11822-0952-60	2.39	2.99
RITE AID BEE POLLEN (Rite Aid)			
CTB,PO (PF,PRIVATE LABEL)			
500 mg, 100s ea	11822-0002-38	7.43	9.29
RITE AID BRANDS (Rite Aid)			
OIL,PO (EX-HVY MINERAL)			
480 ml	11822-3306-07	3.99	4.99
960 ml	11822-3319-01	1.95	
SOL,NS (NOSE)			
1%, 30 ml	11822-3202-04	3.99	4.99
SUS,PO (PINK BISMUTH)			
240 ml	11822-3330-08	2.95	3.69
SYR,PO (TUSSIN COUGH)			
100 mg/5 ml, 120 ml	11822-3253-05	5.19	6.49
RITE AID BUTTERFLY (Rite Aid)			
DEV,NA (MEDIUM,LATEX-FREE)			
10s ea	11822-0985-71	1.59	1.99
RITE AID CALCIUM (Rite Aid)			
CTB,PO (PRIVATE LABEL,CARAMEL)			
60s ea	11822-0345-96	6.39	7.99
(PRIVATE LABEL)			
60s ea	11822-0345-95	6.39	7.99
RITE AID CALCIUM AND MINERALS WITH VITAMIN D (Rite Aid)			
TAB,PO (PF,PRIVATE LABEL)			
60s ea	11822-0004-07	5.19	6.49
RITE AID CENTRAL-VITE CARDIO (Rite Aid)			
TAB,PO (WITH ANTIOXIDANTS)			
60s ea	11822-0371-23	6.39	7.99
RITE AID CENTRAL-VITE PERFORMANCE (Rite Aid)			
TAB,PO (PRIVATE LABEL)			
75s ea	11822-0022-71	7.99	9.99
RITE AID CENTRAL-VITE WITH ANTIOXIDANTS (Rite Aid)			
TAB,PO (W/ LYCOPENE)			
130s ea	11822-6031-00	6.39	7.99
(PF,PRIVATE LABEL)			
300s ea	11822-6031-01	11.19	13.99
RITE AID CENTRAL-VITE WITH LYCOPENE (Rite Aid)			
TAB,PO (PRIVATE LABEL)			
300s ea	11822-0663-11	11.19	13.99
RITE AID CETIRI-D (Rite Aid)			
TER,PO (PRIVATE LABEL)			
5 mg-120 mg, 12s ea	11822-0505-40	8.79	10.99
(ORIGPRESCRIPTIONSTRNGTH)			
5 mg-120 mg, 24s ea	11822-0505-41	13.59	16.99
RITE AID CETIRIZINE HYDROCHLORIDE (Rite Aid)			
RITE AID CETIRIZINE HYDROCHLORIDE			
TAB,PO (PRIVATE LABEL)			
10 mg, 14s ea	11822-0505-37	7.99	9.99
30s ea	11822-0505-38	14.39	17.99
60s ea	11822-0505-39	18.39	22.99
RITE AID CHEST RUB (Rite Aid)			
OIN,TP (MEDICATED,PRIVATE LABEL)			
4.8%-1.2%-2.6%,			
100 gm	11822-0319-72	4.39	5.49
RITE AID CHILDREN'S CETIRIZINE (Rite Aid)			
SOL,PO (1X120ML,ALLERGY)			
1 mg/ml, 120 ml	11822-0505-36	7.99	9.99
RITE AID CHILDREN'S CHEWABLE VITAMINS WITH IRON (Rite Aid)			
CTB,PO (PRIVATE LABEL)			
60s ea	11822-0323-42	4.79	5.99
RITE AID CHILDREN'S IBUPROFEN (Rite Aid)			
SUS,PO (1X240ML,W/DOSAGE CUP,AF)			
100 mg/5 ml, 240 ml	11822-0512-88	7.19	8.99
(W/MEASURING CUP,AF)			
100 mg/5 ml, 240 ml	11822-3169-04	7.19	8.99
RITE AID CHILDREN'S NON-ASPIRIN (Rite Aid)			
SUS,PO (1X118ML,PRIVATE LABEL)			
160 mg/5 ml, 118 ml	11822-0309-68	4.39	5.49
118 ml	11822-0989-54	4.39	5.49
RITE AID CHILDREN'S PLUS (Rite Aid)			
SUS,PO (W/ DOSAGE CUP)			
118 ml	11822-0540-73	3.99	4.99
RITE AID CHILDREN'S PLUS MULTI-SYMPTOM (Rite Aid)			
SUS,PO (W/ DOSAGE CUP)			
118 ml	11822-0504-72	3.99	4.99
RITE AID CHROMIUM PICOLINATE (Rite Aid)			
TAB,PO (PRIVATE LABEL)			
400 mcg, 100s ea	11822-0375-41	6.39	7.99
RITE AID CLEAR (Rite Aid)			
DEV,NA (ASSORTED SIZES)			
45s ea	11822-0985-61	2.39	2.99
RITE AID CLEAR BANDAGES (Rite Aid)			
DEV,NA (ALL ONE SIZE)			
30s ea	11822-0037-03	2.39	2.99
(FREE 20% MORE,ONE SIZE)			
36s ea	11822-0095-27	2.39	2.99

PROD/MFR	HRI, UPC,NDC	AWP	SRP
RITE AID CLOTH FIRST AID TAPE (Rite Aid)			
DEV,NA (2X1"X360",LATEX-FREE)			
2s ea	**11822-0370-70**	3.59	4.49
RITE AID COD LIVER OIL (Rite Aid)			
SOL,PO (PF,SF,PRIVATE LABEL)			
4000 iu/5 ml-400 iu/5 ml, 350 ml	**11822-3045-07**	8.79	10.99
RITE AID COENZYME Q-10 (Rite Aid)			
SGL,PO (NATURAL,FREE 33% MORE)			
100 mg, 30s ea	**11822-0119-58**	15.19	18.99
(NATURAL,PRIVATE LABEL)			
100 mg, 30s ea	**11822-0449-58**	15.19	18.99
RITE AID COL-RITE (Rite Aid)			
SGL,PO, 100 mg, 400s ea	**11822-0316-50**	11.99	14.99
RITE AID COLD & ALLERGY (Rite Aid)			
SOL,PO (AF,PRIVATE LABEL,GRAPE)			
1 mg/5 ml-2.5 mg/5 ml, 237 ml	**11822-0525-94**	6.39	7.99
RITE AID COLD & COUGH DM (Rite Aid)			
SOL,PO (AF,PRIVATE LABEL)			
118 ml	**11822-0525-93**	3.99	4.99
237 ml	**11822-0527-06**	5.99	7.49
RITE AID COLD REMEDY MULTI-SYMPTOM (Rite Aid)			
ODT,PO (PRIVATE LABEL,CITRUS)			
1 x-1 x-1 x, 25s ea	**11822-0434-19**	7.19	8.99
RITE AID COMFORT CARE PLUS HOT & COLD COMPRESS (Rite Aid)			
DEV,NA (5.75"X11",REUSABLE)			
ea	**11822-0370-40**	6.39	7.99
RITE AID COMFORT-FOAM EAR PLUGS (Rite Aid)			
DEV,NA (PRIVATE LABEL)			
20s ea	**11822-0513-16**	3.19	3.99
RITE AID COOL HEAT (Rite Aid)			
CRE,TP (EXTRA STRENGTH)			
10%-30%, 85 gm	**11822-0386-79**	4.39	5.49
RITE AID CORAL CALCIUM (Rite Aid)			
CAP,PO (PRIVATE LABEL)			
200 mg-100 mg-100 iu, 60s ea	**11822-1100-07**	5.59	6.99
RITE AID COTTON GLOVES (Rite Aid)			
DEV,NA (MEDIUM,PRIVATE LABEL)			
ea	**11822-0370-52**	3.19	3.99
RITE AID COTTON SWABS (Rite Aid)			
DEV,NA (PRIVATE LABEL)			
375s ea	**11822-0002-12**	1.99	2.49
600s ea	**11822-0741-04**	2.55	3.19
RITE AID DAILY (Rite Aid)			
TAB,PO (PF,PRIVATE LABEL)			
365s ea	**11822-8810-03**	7.99	9.99
RITE AID DAILY FACE WASH (Rite Aid)			
SOA,TP (1X184GM,OIL-FREE)			
184 gm	**11822-0648-30**	3.19	3.99
RITE AID DAIRY RELIEF (Rite Aid)			
CTB,PO (PRIVATE LABEL,VANILLA)			
9000 u, 32s ea	**11822-0002-03**	5.99	7.49
RITE AID DANDRUFF (Rite Aid)			
RITE AID DANDRUFF			
SHA,TP (PRIVATE LABEL)			
1%, 325 ml	**11822-0353-36**	5.59	6.99
RITE AID DARK TANNING (Rite Aid)			
OIL,TP (SPF 2,PRIVATE LABEL)			
1.6%, 237 ml	**11822-9049-03**	4.79	5.99
RITE AID DAY TIME COLD/FLU FORMULA (Rite Aid)			
SOL,PO (NON-DROWSY,MULTISYMPTOM)			
177 ml	**11822-0057-02**	2.79	3.49
296 ml	**11822-0564-03**	4.79	5.99
RITE AID DAYTIME COLD/FLU FORMULA (Rite Aid)			
SGL,PO (MULTISYMPTOM,ND,AF)			
325 mg-10 mg-5 mg, 20s ea	**11822-0063-56**	4.39	5.49
40s ea	**11822-0059-19**	7.19	8.99
RITE AID DECONGESTANT INHALER (Rite Aid)			
STI,NS (1X198MG,PRIVATE LABEL)			
50 mg, 198 ml	**11822-0302-94**	3.19	
RITE AID DISPOSABLE PROBE COVERS (Rite Aid)			
DEV,NA (PRIVATE LABEL)			
50s ea	**11822-0395-28**	3.19	3.99
RITE AID DISPOSABLE PROTECTIVE UNDERWEAR (Rite Aid)			
DEV,NA (SM/MED,SUPER ABSORBENCY)			
18s ea	**11822-3616-03**	10.39	12.99
RITE AID E-ZJECT LANCETS (Rite Aid)			
DEV,NA (ALTERNATE SITE,26G)			
100s ea	**11822-0236-60**	4.79	5.99
(THIN,28G,PRIVATE LABEL)			
100s ea	**11822-0399-28**	4.79	5.99
200s ea	**11822-9894-00**	7.99	9.99
RITE AID EAR DROPS (Rite Aid)			
SOL,OT (PRIVATE LABEL,DROPS)			
10 x-15 x-12 x, 10 ml	**11822-0370-27**	5.59	6.99
RITE AID EAR WAX CLEANSING (Rite Aid)			
KIT,OT (PARABEN-FREE)			
6.5%, ea	**11822-0372-28**	10.39	12.99
RITE AID EARWAX REMOVAL KIT (Rite Aid)			
SOL,OT (1X15ML)			
6.5%, 15 ml	**11822-0371-10**	4.79	5.99
RITE AID EPSOM SALT (Rite Aid)			
CRY,NA (PRIVATE LABEL)			
624 gm	**11822-0037-10**	2.39	2.99
PDR,NA (1X120ML,PRIVATE LABEL)			
120 ml	**11822-0334-30**	2.39	
(1X34560GM,USP)			
34560 gm	**11822-0370-90**	3.19	3.99
RITE AID EXFOLIATING MOISTURIZER (Rite Aid)			
OIN,TP (1X15GM,PRIVATE LABEL)			
5%-10%, 15 gm	**11822-0329-60**	3.59	4.49
RITE AID EYE ALLERGY RELIEF (Rite Aid)			
SOL,OP (PRIVATE LABEL,DROPS)			
0.027%-0.315%, 15 ml	**11822-0386-56**	4.39	5.49
RITE AID EYE PATCH (Rite Aid)			
DEV,NA (PRIVATE LABEL)			
ea	**11822-0351-41**	2.39	2.99
RITE AID EZJECT LANCETS (Can-Am Care)			
DEV,NA (ALTERNATE SITE,26G)			
100s ea	**38396-0301-14**	5.85	
(THIN,28G,PRIVATE LABEL)			
100s ea	**38396-0311-14**	5.85	
(ULTRA THIN,30G)			
100s ea	**38396-0305-14**	5.85	
(THIN,28G,PRIVATE LABEL)			
200s ea	**38396-0312-14**	9.50	
RITE AID FAMOTIDINE ACID REDUCER (Rite Aid)			
TAB,PO (MAXIMUM STRENGTH)			
20 mg, 25s ea	**11822-5279-03**	5.59	6.99
50s ea	**11822-5279-04**	9.59	11.99
170s ea	**11822-5279-05**	15.19	18.99
RITE AID FIBER (Rite Aid)			
CAP,PO (PRIVATE LABEL)			
0.52 gm, 320s ea	**11822-3165-01**	12.79	15.99
PDR,PO (SF,PRIVATE LABEL,ORANGE)			
3.4 gm/dose, 660 gm	**11822-0330-98**	8.79	10.99
(PRIVATE LABEL,ORANGE)			
3.4 gm/dose, 1366 gm	**11822-0330-97**	8.79	10.99
RITE AID FINGER SPLINTS (Rite Aid)			
DEV,NA (TWO-SIDED,M,L,XL)			
3s ea	**11822-0039-47**	3.99	4.99
RITE AID FIRST AID TAPE SELF GRIP (Rite Aid)			
DEV,NA (1"X66",PRIVATE LABEL)			
ea	**11822-0370-48**	2.39	2.99
RITE AID FISH OIL (Rite Aid)			
SGL,PO (PF,SF,PRIVATE LABEL)			
1000 mg, 500s ea	**11822-3652-03**	18.39	22.99
RITE AID FLAX SEED OIL 1000 (Rite Aid)			
SGL,PO (SF,SODIUM-FREE)			
1000 mg, 100s ea	**11822-0372-13**	6.39	7.99
RITE AID FLEXIBLE FABRIC (Rite Aid)			
DEV,NA (2"X3",XTRALRGE)			
12s ea	**11822-0086-11**	2.39	2.99
(3/4"X3",PRIVATE LABEL)			
36s ea	**11822-0086-12**	2.39	2.99
(ASSORTEDSIZES)			
36s ea	**11822-0086-13**	2.39	2.99
RITE AID FLU (Rite Aid)			
TAB,PO (MAXIMUM STRENGTH)			
500 mg-2 mg-15 mg, 20s ea	**11822-0422-00**	3.99	4.99
RITE AID FLU FORMULA (Rite Aid)			
TAB,PO (DAYTIME/NIGHTTIME)			
24s ea	**11822-0341-57**	3.99	4.99
RITE AID FOAMING HAND SOAP (Rite Aid)			
LIQ,TP (HOSPITAL STRENGTH)			
0.6%, 946 ml	**11822-0372-65**	3.59	4.49
RITE AID FOLIC ACID (Rite Aid)			
TAB,PO (PF,PRIVATE LABEL)			
0.4 mg, 350s ea	**11822-0576-06**	5.99	7.49
RITE AID FOOT POWDER (Rite Aid)			
POW,TP (1X198.4GM,PRIVATE LABEL)			
198.4 gm	**11822-0324-54**	3.35	4.19
RITE AID GARLIC OIL (Rite Aid)			
SGL,PO (NATURAL,PF)			
3 mg, 100s ea	**11822-8808-03**	4.79	5.99
RITE AID GAS RELIEF (Rite Aid)			
CTB,PO (EXTRA STRENGTH)			
125 mg, 48s ea	**11822-0505-54**	5.59	6.99
SGL,PO, 125 mg, 30s ea	**11822-3300-08**	4.79	5.99
72s ea	**11822-0505-56**	7.99	9.99
RITE AID GAS RELIEF INFANTS' (Rite Aid)			
SOL,PO (W/DROPPER,AF)			
20 mg/0.3 ml, 30 ml	**11822-0512-68**	7.19	8.99
RITE AID GAUZE BANDAGE (Rite Aid)			
DEV,NA (3INCHESX2.4YARD,FREE20%)			
ea	**11822-0893-99**	2.15	2.69
RITE AID GENTLE INFANT FORMULA W/ IRON (Rite Aid)			
PDR,PO (1X681GM,PRIVATE LABEL)			
681 gm	**11822-0962-37**	15.19	18.99
RITE AID GERM DEFENSE (Rite Aid)			
GEL,TP (PRIVATE LABEL)			
62%, 15 ml	**11822-0575-62**	1.59	1.99
TEF,PO (PRIVATE LABEL,ORANGE)			
10s ea	**11822-0405-20**	4.39	5.49
20s ea	**11822-0525-77**	7.19	8.99
(PRIVATE LABEL)			
10s ea	**11822-0525-75**	4.39	5.49
RITE AID GINKGO BILOBA (Rite Aid)			
TAB,PO (PF,PRIVATE LABEL)			
40 mg, 50s ea	**11822-3196-00**	5.43	6.79
RITE AID GLUCOSAMINE/CHONDROITIN/MSM (Rite Aid)			
TAB,PO (NATURAL,PRIVATE LABEL)			
240s ea	**11822-0165-24**	39.99	49.99
RITE AID GLUCOSE (Rite Aid)			
GEL,PO (3X15GM,CAFFEINE-FREE)			
15 gm 3s	**11822-0575-81**	8.79	10.99
TAB,PO (GLUTEN-FREE)			
4 gm, 10s ea	**11822-0236-80**	1.59	1.99
50s ea	**11822-0253-71**	5.59	6.99
RITE AID HAIR REGROWTH TREATMENT FOR MEN (Rite Aid)			
SOL,TP (4X60ML,PRIVATE LABEL)			
5%, 60 ml 4s	**11822-0741-05**	31.99	39.99
RITE AID HAIR REGROWTH TREATMENT FOR WOMEN (Rite Aid)			
TP (4X60ML,PRIVATE LABEL)			
2%, 60 ml 4s	**11822-0741-03**	23.99	29.99
RITE AID HAIR, SKIN & NAILS (Rite Aid)			
TAB,PO (YEAST-FREE)			
120s ea	**11822-0229-56**	8.79	10.99
RITE AID HAND SANITIZER WITH ALOE (Rite Aid)			
GEL,TP (PRIVATE LABEL)			
62%, 59 ml	**11822-3733-09**	1.51	1.89
RITE AID HEATWRAPS (Rite Aid)			
DEV,NA (NECK,SHOULDER,WRIST)			
4s ea	**11822-0800-93**	3.99	4.99
RITE AID HEMORRHOIDAL COOLING GEL (Rite Aid)			
GEL,TP (PRIVATE LABEL)			
0.25%-50%, 51 gm	**11822-0849-05**	5.59	6.99
RITE AID HEMORRHOIDAL CREAM (Rite Aid)			
CRE,RC (1X51GM,MAX STRENGTH)			
14.4%-15%-0.25%-1%, 51 gm	**11822-0505-23**	5.59	6.99
RITE AID HEMORRHOIDAL MEDICATED PAD (Rite Aid)			
PAD,TP (PRIVATE LABEL)			
50%, 100s ea	**11822-3323-03**	4.79	5.99
RITE AID HI-CAL PLUS VITAMIN D (Rite Aid)			
TAB,PO (PF,PRIVATE LABEL)			
500 mg-200 iu, 60s ea	**11822-3036-05**	5.19	6.49
(PRIVATE LABEL)			
500 mg-200 iu, 60s ea	**11822-0304-79**	5.19	6.49
RITE AID HYDRATING HEALING OINTMENT (Rite Aid)			
OIN,TP (PRIVATE LABEL)			
41%, 396 gm	**11822-0022-47**	11.19	13.99

PROD/MFR	HRI, UPC,NDC	AWP	SRP
RITE AID HYDROCORTISONE (Rite Aid)			
CRE,TP (W/ NAT OATMEAL)			
1%, 28.4 gm	11822-0512-23	3.43	4.29
RITE AID HYDROCORTISONE PLUS 12 (Rite Aid)			
TP (MAXIMUM STRENGTH)			
1%, 56.8 gm	11822-0642-03	5.59	6.99
RITE AID HYDROGEN PEROXIDE WIPES (Rite Aid)			
PAD,TP (PRIVATE LABEL)			
3%, 40s ea	11822-0370-58	2.39	2.99
RITE AID IBUPROFEN (Rite Aid)			
CTB,PO (JUNIOR STRENGTH)			
100 mg, 24s ea	11822-3025-01	3.99	4.99
TAB,PO (PRIVATE LABEL,COATED)			
200 mg, 50s ea	11822-0001-82	3.59	4.49
(FILM-COATED)			
200 mg, 100s ea	11822-0008-13	5.19	6.49
500s ea	11822-0003-22	11.19	13.99
RITE AID IMMUNE SUPPORT INFANT FORMULA W/ IRON (Rite Aid)			
PDR,PO (1X658GM,PRIVATE LABEL)			
658 gm	11822-0862-37	15.19	18.99
RITE AID INFANT'S ACETAMINOPHEN PAIN RELIEF (Rite Aid)			
SUS,PO (WITH DROPPER,AF)			
80 mg/0.8 ml, 30 ml	11822-0241-73	5.59	6.99
RITE AID INFANT'S IBUPROFEN (Rite Aid)			
SUS,PO (W/ SYRINGE,AF)			
50 mg/1.25 ml, 15 ml	11822-0320-65	4.39	5.49
RITE AID INSTANT EAR THERMOMETER (Rite Aid)			
DEV,NA (INFRARED,PRIVATE LABEL)			
ea	11822-3223-06	31.99	39.99
RITE AID INSTANT HAND SANITIZER (Rite Aid)			
GEL,TP (PRIVATE LABEL)			
62%, 59 ml	11822-0319-25	1.43	1.79
(1X236ML,PRIVATE LABEL)			
62%, 236 ml	11822-0390-48	2.39	2.99
RITE AID INSTY-SPLINT FINGER SPLINT (Rite Aid)			
DEV,NA (MEDIUM & LARGE)			
2s ea	11822-4535-04	3.19	3.99
RITE AID INSULIN SYRINGE (Rite Aid)			
DEV,NA (0.5CC,29G,1/2")			
100s ea	11822-3215-07	18.29	16.99
(0.5CC,30G,5/16")			
100s ea	11822-0576-43	18.29	16.99
(1CC,29G,1/2")			
100s ea	11822-3215-08	18.29	16.99
(1CC,30G,5/16")			
100s ea	11822-0576-44	18.29	16.99
RITE AID IRON (Rite Aid)			
TAB,PO (HIGH POTENCY,PF)			
27 mg, 100s ea	11822-0070-50	4.79	5.99
250s ea	11822-0357-09	6.39	7.99
(PRIVATE LABEL)			
65 mg, 100s ea	11822-0110-99	5.92	7.49
RITE AID ISOPROPYL ALCOHOL WIPES (Rite Aid)			
PAD,TP, 70%, 40s ea	11822-0370-59	2.39	2.99
RITE AID JOCK ITCH (Rite Aid)			
CRE,TP (PRIVATE LABEL)			
1%, 14 gm	11822-0392-60	5.19	6.49
RITE AID KID PANTS (Rite Aid)			
DEV,NA (BOYS,X-LARGE,JUMBO)			
21s ea	11822-3033-02	7.19	
(GIRLS,X-LARGE,JUMBO)			
21s ea	11822-3096-07	7.19	
(GIRL,MDIUM,JUMBO)			
29s ea	11822-3013-09	7.19	
RITE AID KIDS SUNSCREEN (Rite Aid)			
SPR,TP (PRIVATE LABEL)			
3%-15%-5%-6%, 177 ml	11822-0376-43	6.39	7.99
RITE AID LIQUID BANDAGE (Rite Aid)			
LIQ,TP (1X10ML,PRIVATE LABEL)			
0.2%-0.75%, 10 ml	11822-0370-00	3.19	3.99
RITE AID LORATADINE (Rite Aid)			
ODT,PO (NON-DROWSY,MELTEEZ)			
10 mg, 30s ea	11822-0527-12	11.99	
SYR,PO (PRIVATE LABEL)			
5 mg/5 ml, 118 ml	11822-0098-03	6.39	7.99
TAB,PO, 10 mg, 30s ea	11822-3201-05	11.19	14.99
120s ea	11822-3164-05	23.99	29.99
RITE AID LUBRICANT EYE (Rite Aid)			
SOL,OP (PRIVATE LABEL,DROPS)			
0.3%-1%, 30 ml	11822-0985-49	8.79	10.99
RITE AID LYCOPENE (Rite Aid)			
SGL,PO (PRIVATE LABEL,SOFTGEL)			
15 mg, 60s ea	11822-0576-08	15.99	19.99
RITE AID MAGNESIUM (Rite Aid)			
CAP,PO (PRIVATE LABEL)			
500 mg, 100s ea	11822-0576-03	6.39	7.99
RITE AID MENSTRUAL RELIEF (Rite Aid)			
TAB,PO (MAXIMUM STRENGTH)			
500 mg-60 mg-15 mg,			
24s ea	11822-3211-02	3.59	4.49
40s ea	11822-3211-00	4.63	5.79
RITE AID MILK OF MAGNESIA (Rite Aid)			
SUS,PO (1X355ML,STIMULANT-FREE)			
400 mg/5 ml, 355 ml	11822-0039-94	3.59	4.49
(1X769ML,STIMULANT-FREE)			
400 mg/5 ml, 769 ml	11822-0505-53	5.59	6.99
RITE AID MILK THISTLE (Rite Aid)			
CAP,PO (DAIRY-FREE,GLUTEN-FREE)			
200 mg, 50s ea	11822-0089-50	5.59	6.99
RITE AID MILK-BASED INFANT FORMULA W/ IRON (Rite Aid)			
PDR,PO (1X730GM)			
730 gm	11822-0023-74	14.39	17.99
RITE AID MOISTURIZING NASAL SPRAY (Rite Aid)			
SPR,NS (1X37ML,PRIVATE LABEL)			
0.05%, 37 ml	11822-0894-75	4.39	5.49
RITE AID MOTION SICKNESS RELIEF (Rite Aid)			
CTB,PO (PRIVATE LABEL,RASPBERRY)			
25 mg, 8s ea	11822-3169-08	2.39	2.99
TAB,PO (PRIVATE LABEL)			
50 mg, 36s ea	11822-0512-66	5.59	6.99
RITE AID MSM (Rite Aid)			
CAP,PO (PRIVATE LABEL)			
1000 mg, 120s ea	11822-0576-09	12.79	15.99
RITE AID MUCUS RELIEF (Rite Aid)			
TAB,PO (PRIVATE LABEL)			
400 mg, 30s ea	11822-0654-06	7.19	8.99
60s ea	11822-0654-07	10.39	12.99
RITE AID MULTI-PURPOSE (Rite Aid)			
SOL,NA (PRIVATE LABEL)			
355 ml	11822-0145-15	5.19	6.49
355 ml 2s	11822-0334-53	7.99	9.99
RITE AID MULTI-SYMPTOM COLD DAYTIME (Rite Aid)			
TAB,PO (NON-DROWSY)			
325 mg-10 mg-5 mg,			
24s ea	11822-0041-73	3.59	4.49
(PRIVATE LABEL,COOL)			
325 mg-10 mg-5 mg,			
36s ea	11822-0083-36	3.59	4.49
(NON-DROWSY)			
325 mg-10 mg-200 mg-5 mg,			
24s ea	11822-0504-69	3.59	4.49
RITE AID MULTI-SYMPTOM COLD NIGHTTIME (Rite Aid)			
TAB,PO (PRIVATE LABEL,COOL)			
325 mg-2 mg-10 mg-5 mg,			
24s ea	11822-0561-40	3.99	4.99
RITE AID MULTI-SYMPTOM NITE TIME COLD/FLU FORMULA (Rite Aid)			
SYR,PO (FREE 20%,PRIVATE LABEL)			
355 ml	11822-0083-30	4.39	5.49
RITE AID MULTI-USE COLD REUSABLE PAD (Rite Aid)			
DEV,NA (5.25"X10.5")			
ea	11822-0370-50	11.99	14.99
RITE AID NAPROXEN SODIUM (Rite Aid)			
TAB,PO (100+20FREE)			
220 mg, 120s ea	11822-0074-06	6.39	7.99
(FREE 20% MORE)			
220 mg, 120s ea	11822-0740-04	5.99	7.49
(PRIVATE LABEL)			
220 mg, 200s ea	11822-3169-03	9.59	11.99
RITE AID NASAL DECONGESTANT PE (Rite Aid)			
TAB,PO (WITHOUT DROWSINESS)			
10 mg, 36s ea	11822-0417-05	4.79	5.99
72s ea	11822-0417-06	7.19	8.99
RITE AID NASAL SPRAY (Rite Aid)			
SPR,NS (ULTRA FINE MIST)			
0.05%, 30 ml	11822-3174-05	3.59	4.49
RITE AID NASAL STRIPS (Rite Aid)			
DEV,NA (MEDIUM CLEAR)			
30s ea	11822-0330-50	7.99	9.99
(MEDIUM LARGE)			
30s ea	11822-0330-49	7.99	9.99
RITE AID NIACIN (Rite Aid)			
TAB,PO (PF,PRIVATE LABEL)			
100 mg, 100s ea	11822-8810-06	3.43	4.29
RITE AID NICOTINE POLACRILEX (Rite Aid)			
GUM,PO (PRIVATE LABEL,COOL MINT)			
2 mg, 40s ea	11822-3534-06	21.59	26.99
(PRIVATE LABEL)			
2 mg, 50s ea	11822-0321-13	19.99	24.99
(PRIVATE LABEL,CINNAMON)			
2 mg, 100s ea	11822-0558-93	31.99	39.99
(PRIVATE LABEL,COOL MINT)			
2 mg, 100s ea	11822-2534-07	31.99	39.99
(PRIVATE LABEL,FRUIT)			
2 mg, 100s ea	11822-0635-69	31.99	39.99
(USP,PRIVATE LABEL)			
2 mg, 100s ea	11822-0575-70	31.99	39.99
(PRIVATE LABEL)			
2 mg, 170s ea	11822-0320-92	43.99	54.99
(PRIVATE LABEL,COOL MINT)			
4 mg, 40s ea	11822-3534-05	19.99	24.99
(PRIVATE LABEL)			
4 mg, 50s ea	11822-0321-14	19.99	24.99
(PRIVATE LABEL,CINNAMON)			
4 mg, 100s ea	11822-0558-96	31.99	39.99
(PRIVATE LABEL,COOL MINT)			
4 mg, 100s ea	11822-2534-08	31.99	39.99
(PRIVATE LABEL,FRUIT)			
4 mg, 100s ea	11822-0655-69	31.99	39.99
(USP,PRIVATE LABEL)			
4 mg, 100s ea	11822-0575-69	31.99	39.99
(REFILL,168+2)			
4 mg, 170s ea	11822-3209-03	43.99	54.99
LOZ,PO (PRIVATE LABEL,MINT)			
2 mg, 72s ea	11822-3239-01	27.99	34.99
4 mg, 72s ea	11822-3239-00	27.99	34.99
RITE AID NITE TIME COLD/FLU FORMULA (Rite Aid)			
SGL,PO (PRIVATE LABEL,SOFTGEL)			
325 mg-15 mg-6.25 mg,			
20s ea	11822-0635-05	4.39	5.49
40s ea	11822-0592-00	6.39	7.99
SOL,PO (PRIVATE LABEL,ORIGINAL)			
355 ml	11822-0832-80	4.39	5.49
RITE AID NUTRITIONAL PLUS DRINK (Rite Aid)			
LIQ,PO (PRIVATE LABEL,CHOCOLATE)			
237 ml	11822-3919-05	0.93	1.17
(PRIVATE LABEL,VANILLA)			
237 ml	11822-3919-02	0.93	1.17
(PRIVATE LABEL)			
237 ml	11822-3005-03	0.93	1.17
RITE AID OATMEAL MOISTURIZING (Rite Aid)			
LOT,TP (1X237ML,PRIVATE LABEL)			
1.6%, 237 ml	11822-0700-14	3.99	4.99
RITE AID OMEGA 3-6-9 (Rite Aid)			
SGL,PO (PRIVATE LABEL,LEMON)			
60s ea	11822-0095-50	8.79	10.99
RITE AID OMEPRAZOLE (Rite Aid)			
TCP,PO (PRIVATE LABEL)			
20 mg, 14s ea	11822-0505-25	8.79	10.99
28s ea	11822-0505-26	15.19	18.99
42s ea	11822-0505-27	19.19	23.99
RITE AID ONE DAILY (Rite Aid)			
TAB,PO (MAXIMUM,PRIVATE LABEL)			
100s ea	11822-3228-06	5.99	7.49
RITE AID ONE DAILY ENERGY FORMULA (Rite Aid)			
TAB,PO (PRIVATE LABEL)			
50s ea	11822-0371-31	6.39	7.99
RITE AID ONE DAILY MEN'S MULTI (Rite Aid)			
TAB,PO (PRIVATE LABEL)			
100s ea	11822-0110-09	5.59	6.99
RITE AID ONE DAILY MULTI-VITAMIN PLUS IRON (Rite Aid)			
TAB,PO (PRIVATE LABEL)			
100s ea	11822-8810-04	4.79	5.99
365s ea	11822-8810-05	8.39	10.49
RITE AID ONE STEP PREGNANCY TEST (Rite Aid)			
DEV,NA (TWIN PACK,PRIVATE LABEL)			
2s ea	11822-3066-04	10.39	12.99
RITE AID ORAL RINSE (Rite Aid)			
SOL,MM (AF,PRIVATE LABEL,MINT)			
0.07%, 500 ml	11822-0576-11	1.79	2.99
1000 ml	11822-0576-12	3.19	3.99
RITE AID ORAL SALINE LAXATIVE (Rite Aid)			
SOL,PO (SF,PRIVATE LABEL)			
45 ml	11822-0652-01	3.03	3.79

PROD/MFR	HRI, UPC,NDC	AWP	SRP
RITE AID OVER NITES (Rite Aid)			
DEV,NA (YOUTH,LARGE/XL-X)			
14s ea	11822-3216-04	7.19	8.99
(JUMBO,YOUTH,MEDIUM)			
17s ea	11822-3216-05	7.19	8.99
RITE AID OYSTER SHELL CALCIUM (Rite Aid)			
TAB,PO (NATURAL,PF,SF)			
250 mg-125 iu, 100s ea	11822-0041-00	3.59	4.49
RITE AID PAIN RELIEF (Rite Aid)			
GEL,MM (MAXIMUM STRENGTH)			
20%, 14 gm	11822-3109-02	4.79	5.99
RITE AID PEDIATRIC BALANCED NUTRITION DRINK (Rite Aid)			
LIQ,PO (PRIVATE LABEL,VANILLA)			
237 ml	11822-0030-05	1.33	1.66
RITE AID PEDIATRIC ELECTROLYTE (Rite Aid)			
SOL,PO (4X237ML,PRIVATE LABEL)			
237 ml 4s	11822-3144-09	0.89	4.49
237 ml 4s	11822-3235-04	3.19	3.99
(1X1000ML,AF)			
1000 ml	11822-0396-84	3.99	4.99
(AF,PRIVATE LABEL,CHERRY)			
1000 ml	11822-3968-03	3.99	4.99
(AF,PRIVATE LABEL)			
1000 ml	11822-3638-05	3.99	4.99
1000 ml	11822-3639-00	3.99	4.99
RITE AID PEDIATRIC ELECTROLYTE FREEZE POPS (Rite Aid)			
PO (16X62.5ML,PRIVATE LABEL)			
62.5 ml 16s	11822-0323-97	3.99	4.99
RITE AID PEN NEEDLES (Rite Aid)			
DEV,NA (31G,5MM,3/16")			
100s ea	11822-0576-46	22.50	20.99
(31G,8MM,5/16")			
100s ea	11822-0576-45	22.50	20.99
RITE AID PERSONAL LUBRICANT (Rite Aid)			
GEL,TP (PRIVATE LABEL)			
113 gm	11822-0323-53	3.19	3.99
RITE AID PHOSPHA-LAX (Rite Aid)			
SOL,PO (MULTI-DOSE CONTAINER,SF)			
0.9 gm/5 ml-2.4 gm/5 ml, 90 ml	11822-3338-02	3.03	3.79
RITE AID POTASSIUM GLUCONATE (Rite Aid)			
TAB,PO (NATURAL,PRIVATE LABEL)			
99 mg, 100s ea	11822-0881-07	4.23	5.29
RITE AID PREGNANCY TEST (Rite Aid)			
DEV,NA (BONUS PACK)			
2s ea	11822-3829-06	7.99	9.99
RITE AID PROTECTIVE UNDERWEAR (Rite Aid)			
DEV,NA (LRGEOVRNGHT,MALE&FMALE)			
14s ea	11822-3216-09	8.79	10.99
(PRIVATE LABEL)			
20s ea	11822-0339-88	8.79	10.99
(LARGE,MALE&FEMLE)			
32s ea	11822-0311-44	15.99	19.99
(SMALL/MEDIUM)			
40s ea	11822-0312-93	15.99	19.99
RITE AID PUSH 'N POP PILL REMINDER (Rite Aid)			
DEV,NA (PRIVATE LABEL)			
ea	11822-0575-52	3.19	3.99
RITE AID REGULAR NASAL SPRAY (Rite Aid)			
SPR,NS (1X37ML,12 HOUR)			
0.05%, 37 ml	11822-0894-74	4.39	5.49
RITE AID REST ASSURED NITE PROTECTOR (Rite Aid)			
DEV,NA (PRIVATE LABEL)			
ea	11822-0577-55	14.39	17.99
RITE AID SALINE SOLUTION (Rite Aid)			
SOL,NA (1X355ML,THIMEROSAL-FREE)			
355 ml	11822-0505-19	1.99	2.49
RITE AID SAM-E 200 (Rite Aid)			
ECT,PO (PRIVATE LABEL)			
200 mg, 30s ea	11822-0576-00	13.59	16.99
RITE AID SAM-E 400 (Rite Aid)			
PO (PRIVATE LABEL)			
400 mg, 10s ea	11822-0576-04	13.59	16.99
RITE AID SCAR (Rite Aid)			
GEL,TP (1X50GM,PRIVATE LABEL)			
50 gm	11822-0370-80	13.59	16.99
RITE AID SELENIUM (Rite Aid)			
TAB,PO (NATURAL,PF)			
50 mcg, 100s ea	11822-8811-02	3.99	4.99
RITE AID SELF GRIP (Rite Aid)			
DEV,NA (2"X66",FREE20%MORE)			
ea	11822-0895-00	3.19	3.99
(2"X66",MAXIMUM SUPPORT)			
ea	11822-3159-05	3.19	3.99
(3"X66",FREE20%MORE)			
ea	11822-0894-99	3.99	4.99
(3"X66",MAXIMUM SUPPORT)			
ea	11822-3159-04	3.99	4.99
(4"X66",MAXIMUM SUPPORT)			
ea	11822-3159-03	5.19	6.49
RITE AID SENNA (Rite Aid)			
SGL,PO, 8.6 mg, 80s ea	11822-0359-22	8.79	10.99
TAB,PO (20 FREE,PRIVATE LABEL)			
8.6 mg, 120s ea	11822-0846-14	9.59	11.99
200s ea	11822-0165-23	11.99	14.99
(20 FREE,PRIVATE LABEL)			
8.6 mg, 220s ea	11822-0074-08	11.99	14.99
RITE AID SINUS CONGESTION & PAIN (Rite Aid)			
TAB,PO (PRIVATE LABEL)			
24s ea	11822-0904-50	3.99	4.99
RITE AID SINUS CONGESTION & PAIN DAYTIME (Rite Aid)			
TAB,PO (NON-DROWSY)			
325 mg-5 mg, 24s ea	11822-0041-63	3.59	4.49
RITE AID SINUS FORMULA DAYTIME (Rite Aid)			
PO (ASPIRIN-FREE)			
325 mg-5 mg, 36s ea	11822-8745-00	3.59	4.49
RITE AID SINUS NASAL SPRAY (Rite Aid)			
SPR,NS (1X37ML,PRIVATE LABEL)			
0.05%, 37 ml	11822-0894-73	3.99	4.99
RITE AID SOFT-TIP THERMOMETER FEVER ALARM (Rite Aid)			
DEV,NA (PRIVATE LABEL)			
ea	11822-0576-13	7.99	9.99
RITE AID SOLUBLE FIBER (Rite Aid)			
TAB,PO (PRIVATE LABEL,CAPLET)			
500 mg, 100s ea	11822-3183-00	7.99	9.99
RITE AID SOY-BASED INFANT FORMULA W/ IRON (Rite Aid)			
PDR,PO (1X730GM,LACTOSE-FREE)			
730 gm	11822-0023-75	14.39	17.99
RITE AID SPORT SUNSCREEN SPF 30 (Rite Aid)			
LOT,TP (PRIVATE LABEL)			
9%-7.5%-5%-4%, 177 ml	11822-0395-50	4.79	5.99
RITE AID SPORT SUNSCREEN SPF 48 (Rite Aid)			
LOT,TP (PRIVATE LABEL)			
9%-7.5%-5%-3%-6%, 177 ml	11822-0379-12	4.79	5.99
RITE AID ST. JOHN'S WORT (Rite Aid)			
TAB,PO (PRIVATE LABEL)			
300 mg, 50s ea	11822-0011-60	4.63	5.79
120s ea	11822-0011-50	8.39	10.49
RITE AID STERILE EYE WASH (Rite Aid)			
SOL,OP (W/EYE CUP,PRIVATE LABEL)			
99.05%, 118 ml	11822-0986-08	4.79	5.99
RITE AID STERILE PADS (Rite Aid)			
DEV,NA (2"X2",FREE 20% MORE)			
30s ea	11822-0893-96	2.79	3.49
(3"X3",FREE 20% MORE)			
30s ea	11822-0893-98	3.19	3.99
(4"X4",FREE 20% MORE)			
30s ea	11822-0893-97	5.19	6.49
RITE AID STOMACH RELIEF (Rite Aid)			
SUS,PO (PRIVATE LABEL,CHERRY)			
262 mg/15 ml, 355 ml	11822-0083-27	2.79	3.49
(1X473MLREGULARSTRENGTH)			
262 mg/15 ml, 473 ml	11822-0291-07	3.19	3.99
(1X355ML,MAXIMUMSTRENGTH)			
525 mg/15 ml, 355 ml	11822-0239-63	3.59	4.49
RITE AID STOOL SOFTENER (Rite Aid)			
SGL,PO (PRIVATE LABEL,SOFTGEL)			
100 mg, 50s ea	11822-0512-67	5.59	6.99
180s ea	11822-0505-55	15.99	19.99
RITE AID SUNSCREEN SHEER (Rite Aid)			
LOT,TP (SPF 45)			
2%-15%-7.5%-5%-1%-6%, 118 ml	11822-0211-46	6.39	7.99
RITE AID SUNSCREEN SPF 30 (Rite Aid)			
TP (PRIVATE LABEL)			
2%-10%-5%-2%-2%, 237 ml	11822-0924-15	5.59	6.99
RITE AID SUNSCREEN SPF 45 OIL FREE ESSENTIAL DEFENSE (Rite Aid)			
TP (SPF 45 OIL FREE)			
2%-12%-7.5%-5%-6%, 118 ml	11822-0322-43	4.79	5.99
RITE AID SUPER MOLESKIN (Rite Aid)			
DEV,NA (4 5/8"X 3 3/8")			
3s ea	11822-0318-80	3.19	3.99
RITE AID SUPER STRIP (Rite Aid)			
DEV,NA (ALL ONE SIZE,LATEX-FREE)			
20s ea	11822-0350-39	2.39	2.99
RITE AID SUPER STRIP BANDAGES (Rite Aid)			
DEV,NA (1"X3",LATEX-FREE)			
24s ea	11822-0050-39	2.39	2.99
RITE AID SUPHEDRINE (Rite Aid)			
TER,PO (MAXIMUM STRENGTH)			
120 mg, 20s ea	11822-3495-02	4.79	5.99
RITE AID SUPHEDRINE PE (Rite Aid)			
TAB,PO (MAXIMUM STRENGTH)			
4 mg-10 mg, 24s ea	11822-0417-02	3.59	4.49
48s ea	11822-0415-05	4.79	5.99
(MAX STRENGTH,FREE 50%)			
4 mg-10 mg, 72s ea	11822-8744-08	4.79	5.99
(PRIVATE LABEL,CAPLET)			
325 mg-5 mg, 24s ea	11822-0416-08	3.99	4.99
(FREE 50%,PRIVATE LABEL)			
325 mg-5 mg, 36s ea	11822-0083-35	3.99	4.99
RITE AID SURECHOICE BLADDER CONTROL PAD (Rite Aid)			
DEV,NA (MAXIMUM,PRIVATE LABEL)			
16s ea	11822-3021-08	3.59	4.49
(HEAVY,PRIVATE LABEL)			
20s ea	11822-3021-09	3.59	4.49
(MEDIUM,PRIVATE LABEL)			
22s ea	11822-3672-01	3.59	4.49
(PRIVATE LABEL)			
36s ea	11822-0370-84	8.79	10.99
(MAXIMUM LONG)			
42s ea	11822-3022-01	10.39	12.99
(MAXIMUM,PRIVATE LABEL)			
60s ea	11822-3022-00	10.39	12.99
(HEAVY,PRIVATE LABEL)			
72s ea	11822-3021-05	10.39	12.99
RITE AID SURECHOICE PANTILINER (Rite Aid)			
DEV,NA (PRIVATE LABEL)			
26s ea	11822-0018-09	2.63	3.29
56s ea	11822-0031-09	3.99	4.99
RITE AID THERAPEUTIC M PLUS BETA-CAROTENE (Rite Aid)			
TAB,PO (PF,PRIVATE LABEL)			
130s ea	11822-8812-00	6.39	7.99
RITE AID TOOTHSHIELD ANTICAVITY FLUORIDE RINSE (Rite Aid)			
SOL,MM (1X946ML,PRIVATE LABEL)			
0.0221%, 946 ml	11822-0370-54	3.19	3.99
RITE AID TRUETEST BLOOD GLUCOSE TEST STRIPS (Rite Aid)			
DEV,NA (PRIVATE LABEL)			
50s ea	11822-0371-43	31.99	39.99
100s ea	11822-0037-14	55.99	69.99
RITE AID TUSSIN (Rite Aid)			
SOL,PO (1X355ML,AF)			
100 mg/5 ml, 355 ml	11822-0873-78	5.19	6.49
RITE AID TUSSIN CF (Rite Aid)			
SOL,PO (W/DOSAGE CUP,AF)			
118 ml	11822-0525-96	3.59	4.49
237 ml	11822-0525-97	5.19	6.49
355 ml	11822-0525-98	7.19	8.99
(W/DOSAGE CUP,FREE 50%)			
355 ml	11822-0083-33	5.19	6.49
RITE AID TUSSIN COUGH (Rite Aid)			
SGL,PO (NON-DROWSY)			
15 mg, 20s ea	11822-3172-00	3.99	4.99
RITE AID TUSSIN SUGAR-FREE COUGH (Rite Aid)			
SOL,PO (FORDIABETICS,AF,SF)			
10 mg/5 ml-100 mg/5 ml, 118 ml	11822-0317-37	3.59	4.49
RITE AID ULTRA FINE CUT N' CRUSH (Rite Aid)			
DEV,NA (PRIVATE LABEL)			
ea	11822-0377-34	4.79	5.99
RITE AID ULTRAFITS DIAPERS (Rite Aid)			
DEV,NA (JUMBO PACK,STAGE 6)			
26s ea	11822-0059-08	7.19	8.99
(JUMBO PACK,STAGE 5)			
30s ea	11822-1692-07	7.59	9.49

PROD/MFR	HRI, UPC,NDC	AWP	SRP
(MEGA PACK,STAGE 6)			
40s ea	11822-0237-06	10.79	13.49
(MEGA PACK,STAGE 5)			
46s ea	11822-3059-00	10.79	13.49
(JUMBO PACK,STAGE 2)			
48s ea	11822-3457-04	7.59	9.49
(MEGA PACK,STAGE 4)			
52s ea	11822-3090-06	10.79	13.49
(JUMBO PACK,STAGE 1)			
56s ea	11822-3457-05	7.59	9.49
(5,PRIVATE LABEL)			
60s ea	11822-0023-51	12.79	15.99
(MEGA PACK,STAGE 3)			
60s ea	11822-0059-05	10.79	13.49
(4,PRIVATE LABEL)			
68s ea	11822-0023-50	12.79	15.99
(3,PRIVATE LABEL)			
80s ea	11822-0023-49	12.79	15.99
RITE AID URINARY PAIN RELIEF (Rite Aid)			
TAB,PO (PRIVATE LABEL)			
95 mg, 12s ea	11822-0370-86	3.99	4.99
RITE AID VANISHING ACNE TREATMENT (Rite Aid)			
CRE,TP, 10%, 28 gm	11822-0396-06	5.59	6.99
RITE AID VINYL GLOVES (Rite Aid)			
DEV,NA (ONE SIZE FITS ALL)			
50s ea	11822-3236-00	7.99	9.99
RITE AID VINYL MEDICAL GLOVES (Rite Aid)			
DEV,NA (LATEX-FREE)			
50s ea	11822-0359-15	6.39	7.99
RITE AID VISION VITE (Rite Aid)			
TAB,PO (PRIVATE LABEL)			
60s ea	11822-0881-21	6.39	7.99
RITE AID VITAMIN A & D (Rite Aid)			
SGL,PO (PRIVATE LABEL,SOFTGEL)			
5000 iu-400 iu,			
100s ea	11822-0576-07	3.99	4.99
RITE AID VITAMIN B-1 (Rite Aid)			
TAB,PO (PF,PRIVATE LABEL)			
100 mg, 100s ea	11822-0336-07	3.99	4.99
RITE AID VITAMIN B12 (Rite Aid)			
TER,PO (NATURAL,PRIVATE LABEL)			
2000 mcg, 60s ea	11822-0003-34	6.39	7.99
RITE AID VITAMIN E (Rite Aid)			
SGL,PO (NATURAL,PRIVATE LABEL)			
400 iu, 60s ea	11822-0110-10	5.19	6.49
RITE AID VITAMINS A AND D (Rite Aid)			
OIN,TP (PRIVATE LABEL)			
15.5%-53.4%, 113 gm	11822-0472-99	3.99	4.99
RITE AID VITAMINS A&D (Rite Aid)			
OIN,TP (PRIVATE LABEL)			
454 gm	11822-0237-07	7.99	9.99
RITE AID WHOLE SOURCE FOR MEN (Rite Aid)			
TAB,PO (PF,PRIVATE LABEL)			
250s ea	11822-0884-03	13.99	17.49
RITE AID WIPES (Rite Aid)			
PAD,TP (NATALOE,FLUSHBLE,MOIST)			
50s ea	11822-0095-10	1.59	1.99
(FRAGRANCE-FREE)			
72s ea	11822-0576-22	2.39	2.99
(AF,PRIVATE LABEL)			
100s ea	11822-0030-60	2.79	3.49
(FRAGRANCE-FREE)			
216s ea	11822-0576-21	5.19	6.49
RITE AID ZINC (Rite Aid)			
TAB,PO (NATURAL,PF)			
50 mg, 100s ea	11822-8812-03	3.43	4.29
(PF,PRIVATE LABEL)			
50 mg, 200s ea	11822-0576-02	5.99	7.49
RITIFED (R.I.J.)			
SYR,PO, 30 mg/5 ml-1.25 mg/5 ml,			
120 ml	53807-0155-01	1.62	
240 ml	53807-0155-02	2.82	
ROBAFEN (Major)			
SYR,PO, 100 mg/5 ml,			
120 ml	00904-0061-00	2.64	
120 ml	00904-0061-20	2.05	
240 ml	00904-0061-09	3.15	
480 ml	00904-0061-16	4.10	
ROBAFEN CF (Major)			
SOL,PO, 118 ml	00904-5770-20	2.55	
(NON DROWSY)			
237 ml	00904-5770-09	4.19	
ROBAFEN COUGH (Major)			
SGL,PO (NON DROWSY,LIQUIDGELS)			
15 mg, 20s ea	00904-5752-95	5.69	
ROBAFEN DM (Major)			
SYR,PO, 10 mg/5 ml-100 mg/5 ml,			
120 ml	00904-0053-20	2.25	
(BOXED)			
10 mg/5 ml-100 mg/5 ml,			
120 ml	00904-0053-00	3.53	
240 ml	00904-0053-09	2.05	
480 ml	00904-0053-16	8.25	
ROBAFEN DM CLEAR (Major)			
SOL,PO (W/DOSAGE CUP,AF,SF)			
10 mg/5 ml-100 mg/5 ml,			
237 ml	00904-5180-09	3.35	
SYR,PO (AF,SF,DYE-FREE)			
10 mg/5 ml-100 mg/5 ml,			
118 ml	00904-5180-20	2.25	
ROBATHOL (Pharm Spec)			
OIL,TP, 480 ml	45334-0100-16	10.60	15.95
3840 ml	45334-0100-99	38.52	55.84
ROBITUSSIN (Wyeth Consumer)			
LOZ,MM (SUNNY ORANGE)			
60 mg-10 mg,			
25s ea	00031-8647-08		1.59
(SUNNY RASPBERRY)			
60 mg-10 mg,			
25s ea	00031-8648-01		1.59
SYR,PO, 100 mg/5 ml,			
240 ml	00031-8624-18		7.99
ROBITUSSIN CHEST CONGESTION (Wyeth Consumer)			
SYR,PO (USP,NON-DROWSY,AF)			
100 mg/5 ml,			
120 ml	00031-8624-12		5.49
ROBITUSSIN COLD & CONGESTION (Wyeth Consumer)			
TAB,PO (MULTI-SYMPTOM)			
325 mg-2 mg-5 mg,			
20s ea	00031-8696-20		4.99
40s ea	00031-8696-40		7.59
ROBITUSSIN COLD & COUGH (Wyeth Consumer)			
SGL,PO (LIQUIGEL)			
10 mg-200 mg-30 mg,			
12s ea	00031-8600-46		4.81
ROBITUSSIN COLD COUGH & FLU (Wyeth Consumer)			
SGL,PO (NON-DROWSY,LIQUIGEL)			
12s ea	00031-8602-46		4.81
ROBITUSSIN COUGH & ALLERGY (Wyeth Consumer)			
SOL,PO (1X118ML,W/DOSAGE CUP,AF)			
118 ml	00031-8607-12		5.49
ROBITUSSIN COUGH & COLD (Wyeth Consumer)			
SYR,PO (MAX. STR.)			
15 mg/5 ml-30 mg/5 ml,			
120 ml	00031-8671-12		5.49
ROBITUSSIN COUGH & COLD CF (Wyeth Consumer)			
SYR,PO (1X118ML,W/DOSAGE CUP,AF)			
118 ml	00031-8616-12		5.49
(1X237ML,W/DOSAGE CUP,AF)			
237 ml	00031-8616-18		7.99
(1X355ML,W/DOSAGE CUP,AF)			
355 ml	00031-8616-24		9.99
ROBITUSSIN COUGH & COLD LONG ACTING (Wyeth Consumer)			
SOL,PO (1X118ML,W/DOSAGE CUP)			
2 mg/5 ml-15 mg/5 ml,			
118 ml	00031-8667-12		5.49
ROBITUSSIN COUGH & CONGESTION (Wyeth Consumer)			
LIQ,PO (NON-DROWSY,AF)			
10 mg/5 ml-200 mg/5 ml,			
120 ml	00031-8662-12		5.49
(1X240ML,W/DOSAGE CUP,AF)			
10 mg/5 ml-200 mg/5 ml,			
240 ml	00031-8662-18		7.99
ROBITUSSIN COUGH DM (Wyeth Consumer)			
SOL,PO (1X118ML, NON-DROWSY,AF)			
10 mg/5 ml-100 mg/5 ml,			
118 ml	00031-8685-12		5.49
(1X118ML,W/DOSAGE CUP,AF)			
10 mg/5 ml-100 mg/5 ml,			
118 ml	00031-8686-12		5.49
(1X237ML, NON-DROWSY,AF)			
10 mg/5 ml-100 mg/5 ml,			
237 ml	00031-8685-18		7.99
(1X355ML, NON-DROWSY,AF)			
10 mg/5 ml-100 mg/5 ml,			
355 ml	00031-8685-22		9.99
ROBITUSSIN COUGH DROPS (Wyeth Consumer)			
LOZ,MM (SF,CITRUS)			
2.5 mg, 18s ea	00031-8615-01		1.69
(CHERRY)			
5 mg, 25s ea	00031-8623-08		1.59
(HONEY LEMON)			
5 mg, 25s ea	00031-8621-08		1.59
(MENTHOL)			
10 mg, 25s ea	00031-8622-01		1.59
ROBITUSSIN COUGH GELS LONG ACTING (Wyeth Consumer)			
SGL,PO (NON-DROWSY,SOFTGEL)			
15 mg, 20s ea	00031-8687-20		5.49
ROBITUSSIN COUGH LONG ACTING (Wyeth Consumer)			
SYR,PO (NON-DROWSY)			
15 mg/5 ml, 118 ml	00031-8670-12		5.49
ROBITUSSIN COUGH, COLD & FLU NIGHTTIME (Wyeth Consumer)			
SOL,PO (1X118ML,W/DOSAGE CUP,AF)			
118 ml	00031-8642-12		5.49
(1X237ML,W/DOSAGE CUP,AF)			
237 ml	00031-8642-18		7.99
ROBITUSSIN HEAD & CHEST CONGESTION PE (Wyeth Consumer)			
SOL,PO (1X118ML,W/DOSAGE CUP,AF)			
100 mg/5 ml-5 mg/5 ml,			
118 ml	00031-8665-12		5.49
ROBITUSSIN HONEY COUGH (Wyeth Consumer)			
LOZ,MM (HONEY CENTER)			
5 mg, 20s ea	00031-8631-01		1.59
(HONEY LEMON TEA)			
5 mg, 25s ea	00031-8632-01		1.59
ROBITUSSIN INFANT COUGH DM (Wyeth Consumer)			
SOL,PO (1X30ML,W/ORAL SYRINGE)			
30 ml	00031-8681-01		4.99
ROBITUSSIN MAXIMUM STRENGTH (Wyeth Consumer)			
SYR,PO, 15 mg/5 ml,			
240 ml	00031-8670-18		8.59
ROBITUSSIN NIGHT RELIEF (Wyeth Consumer)			
LIQ,PO, 180 ml	00031-8639-15		6.29
ROBITUSSIN PE (Wyeth Consumer)			
SYR,PO (AF)			
100 mg/5 ml-30 mg/5 ml,			
120 ml	00031-8695-12		4.99
240 ml	00031-8695-18		7.59
ROBITUSSIN PEDIATRIC COUGH & COLD (Wyeth Consumer)			
LIQ,PO, 7.5 mg/5 ml-15 mg/5 ml,			
120 ml	00031-8609-12		4.99
(Phys Total Care)			
REPACK			
LIQ,PO, 7.5 mg/5 ml-15 mg/5 ml,			
120 ml	54868-1495-00	6.80	
ROBITUSSIN PEDIATRIC COUGH & COLD CF (Wyeth Consumer)			
SOL,PO (1X30ML,AF,FRUIT PUNCH)			
30 ml	00031-8664-10		5.49
ROBITUSSIN PEDIATRIC COUGH & COLD LONG ACTING (Wyeth Consumer)			
SOL,PO (1X118ML,W/DOSAGE CUP,AF)			
1 mg/5 ml-7.5/5 ml,			
118 ml	00031-8660-12	5.49	
ROBITUSSIN PEDIATRIC COUGH LONG ACTING (Wyeth Consumer)			
SOL,PO (1X118ML, NON-DROWSY)			
7.5 mg/5 ml,			
118 ml	00031-8610-12		5.49
ROBITUSSIN PEDIATRIC NIGHT RELIEF (Wyeth Consumer)			
LIQ,PO (AF,CHERRY)			
120 ml	00031-8608-12		4.99
ROBITUSSIN SEVERE CONGESTION (Wyeth Consumer)			
CAP,PO (LIQUIGEL)			
200 mg-30 mg,			
12s ea	00031-8601-46	3.83	
ROC AGE DIMINISHING DAILY MOISTURIZER (Johnson & Johnson)			
LOT,TP (SPF 15)			
3%-7.5%-2%, 90 ml	81370-0084-01	11.72	

PROD/MFR	HRI, UPC,NDC	AWP	SRP
ROC AGE DIMINISHING FACIAL CLEANSER			
(Johnson & Johnson)			
SOL,TP (1X150ML,OIL-FREE)			
150 ml	**81370-0084-17**	6.31	
ROC AGE DIMINISHING NIGHT CREAM			
(Johnson & Johnson)			
CRE,TP (1X48GM)			
48 gm	**81370-0084-14**	11.72	
ROC COMPLETE LIFT DAILY MOISTURIZER			
(Johnson & Johnson)			
LOT,TP (SPF 30)			
3%-12%-5%-1.7%-3%,			
40 ml	**81370-0084-87**	16.58	
ROC COMPLETE LIFT EYE PEN			
(Johnson & Johnson)			
STI,TP (1X15GM)			
15 gm	**81371-0083-21**	14.42	
ROC COMPLETELIFT SERUM (Johnson & Johnson)			
LOT,TP (1X40ML)			
40 ml	**81370-0059-78**	16.58	
ROC DAILY RESURFACING DISKS			
(Johnson & Johnson)			
PAD,TP, 28s ea	**81371-0083-18**	7.81	
ROC MULTI CORREXION SKIN RENEWING SERUM			
(Johnson & Johnson)			
LOT,TP (1X30ML)			
30 ml	**81371-0083-91**	18.64	
ROC MULTI-CORREXION EXFOLIATING CLEANSER			
(Johnson & Johnson)			
SOL,TP (1X147ML,OIL-FREE)			
147 ml	**81370-0088-21**	7.81	
ROC MULTI-CORREXION EYE TREATMENT			
(Johnson & Johnson)			
LOT,TP (1X15ML)			
15 ml	**81370-0088-61**	18.62	
ROC MULTI-CORREXION NIGHT TREATMENT			
(Johnson & Johnson)			
TP (1X30ML)			
30 ml	**81370-0088-53**	18.62	
ROC RETINOL CORREXION DEEP WRINKLE			
(Johnson & Johnson)			
LOT,TP (1X30ML,SPF 30)			
3%-10%-3%-5%,			
30 ml	**81370-0084-88**	16.58	
ROC RETINOL CORREXION DEEP WRINKLE FILLER			
(Johnson & Johnson)			
CRE,TP (1X30ML)			
30 ml	**81371-0083-22**	16.58	
ROC RETINOL CORREXION DEEP WRINKLE NIGHT CREAM (Johnson & Johnson)			
CRE,TP (1X30ML)			
30 ml	**81370-0083-21**	16.58	
ROC RETINOL CORREXION DEEP WRINKLE SERUM			
(Johnson & Johnson)			
LOT,TP (1X30ML)			
30 ml	**81370-0084-44**	16.58	
ROC RETINOL CORREXION EYE CREAM			
(Johnson & Johnson)			
CRE,TP (1X15ML)			
15 ml	**81370-0084-16**	16.58	
ROCK ROSE (Ellon)			
SOL,SL (DROPS)			
10.5 ml	**51762-0015-10**		9.25
ROCK WATER (Ellon)			
SL (DROPS)			
10.5 ml	**51762-0038-10**		9.25
RODEX (Legere)			
CAP,PO, 150 mg, 100s ea	**25332-1037-02**	12.00	
1000s ea	**25332-1037-01**	89.95	
RODEX FORTE (Legere)			
CER,PO, 100 mg-200 mg,			
30s ea	**25332-1144-03**	7.00	
90s ea	**25332-1144-09**	14.00	
ROGAINE (Johnson & Johnson)			
FOA,TP (MEN'S,EXTRA STRENGTH)			
5%, 60 gm	**12547-0781-29**	23.02	
(MEN'S,EXTRASTRENGTH)			
5%, 60 gm	**12547-0781-30**	23.02	
60 gm	**12547-0781-31**	23.02	
SOL,TP (MEN'S)			
2%, 60 ml	**00093-0779-01**	23.02	
(MEN'S/CHECKPOINT)			
2%, 60 ml	**00093-0779-07**	23.02	
(MEN'S/SENSORMATIC)			
2%, 60 ml	**00093-0779-08**	23.02	
(MEN'S/TRIPLE/UNTAGGED)			
2%, 60 ml 3s	**00093-0779-06**	48.96	
(MEN/TRIPLE/CHECKPOINT)			
2%, 60 ml 3s	**00093-0779-11**	48.96	
(MEN/TRIPLE/SENSORMATIC)			
2%, 60 ml 3s	**00093-0779-12**	48.96	
ROGAINE FOR MEN EXTRA STRENGTH			
(Johnson & Johnson)			
SOL,TP, 5%, 60 ml	**00097-0700-01**	23.02	
(CHECKPOINT)			
5%, 60 ml	**00097-0700-09**	23.02	
(SENSORMATIC)			
5%, 60 ml	**00097-0700-13**	23.02	
(Pharmacia Consumer)			
SOL,TP (STARTER KIT)			
5%, 60 ml	**00009-5016-01**	28.32	
(STARTER KIT/CHECKPOINT)			
5%, 60 ml	**00009-5016-02**	28.32	
(STARTER KIT/SENSORMATIC)			
5%, 60 ml	**00009-7700-33**	28.32	
ROGAINE WOMEN'S (Johnson & Johnson)			
SOL,TP (CHECKPOINT)			
2%, 60 ml	**00093-0780-07**	19.56	
(SENSORMATIC)			
2%, 60 ml	**00093-0780-08**	19.56	
(UNTAGGED)			
2%, 60 ml	**00093-0780-01**	19.56	
ROLAIDS (Johnson & Johnson)			
CTB,PO (SODIUM-FREE,CHERRY)			
550 mg-110 mg,			
36s ea	**12547-0652-38**	1.44	
(McNeil Consumer Healthcare)			
CTB,PO (3X12,PEPPERMINT)			
220 mg, 36s ea	**12547-0651-55**	1.44	
(PEPPERMINT)			
220 mg, 36s ea	**12546-0651-31**	0.54	
(SODIUM-FREE,CHERRY)			
550 mg-110 mg,			
12s ea	**12547-0652-36**	0.54	
(SODIUM-FREE,PEPPERMINT)			
550 mg-110 mg,			
12s ea	**12547-0651-21**	0.54	
(SODIUM-FREE,CHERRY)			
550 mg-110 mg,			
150s ea	**12547-0652-42**	3.61	
(SODIUM-FREE,PEPPERMINT)			
550 mg-110 mg,			
150s ea	**12547-0651-15**	3.61	
ROLAIDS EXTRA STRENGTH (Johnson & Johnson)			
CTB,PO (TROPICAL PUNCH)			
675 mg-135 mg,			
10s ea	**12547-0654-21**	0.55	
(FRESHMINT 2X10 W/CASE)			
675 mg-135 mg,			
20s ea	**00501-5421-20**	1.43	
(TROPICAL PUNCH)			
675 mg-135 mg,			
30s ea	**12547-0654-29**	1.44	
(McNeil Consumer Healthcare)			
CTB,PO (FRESHMINT)			
675 mg-135 mg,			
10s ea	**12547-0650-30**	0.54	
(FRUIT)			
675 mg-135 mg,			
10s ea	**12547-0650-34**	0.54	
(3X10,FRESHMINT)			
675 mg-135 mg,			
30s ea	**12547-0650-26**	1.44	
(3X10,FRUIT)			
675 mg-135 mg,			
30s ea	**12547-0650-29**	1.44	
(FRESHMINT)			
675 mg-135 mg,			
100s ea	**12547-0650-21**	3.61	
(FRUIT)			
675 mg-135 mg,			
100s ea	**12547-0650-24**	3.61	
(TROPICAL PUNCH)			
675 mg-135 mg,			
100s ea	**12546-0654-23**	3.62	
ROLAIDS MULTI-SYMPTOM (Johnson & Johnson)			
CTB,PO (BERRY,BERRY)			
675 mg-135 mg-60 mg,			
10s ea	**00501-5441-10**	0.68	
(COOL MINT, 3X12)			
675 mg-135 mg-60 mg,			
36s ea	**00501-5440-30**	1.90	
(COOL MINT,COOL MINT)			
675 mg-135 mg-60 mg,			
100s ea	**00501-5440-99**	4.98	
(McNeil Consumer Healthcare)			
CTB,PO (BERRY)			
675 mg-135 mg-60 mg,			
10s ea	**12547-0654-61**	0.67	
(3X10,BERRY)			
675 mg-135 mg-60 mg,			
30s ea	**12547-0654-65**	1.90	
(BERRY)			
675 mg-135 mg-60 mg,			
100s ea	**12547-0654-57**	4.98	
ROLAIDS PLUS GAS RELIEF			
(McNeil Consumer Healthcare)			
CTB,PO (TROPICAL FRUIT)			
1177 mg-80 mg,			
6s ea	**12547-0065-73**	1.02	
(2X6,TROPICAL FRUIT)			
1177 mg-80 mg,			
12s ea	**12547-0065-75**	2.39	
(EXTRA STRENGTH)			
1177 mg-80 mg,			
36s ea	**12547-0065-77**	4.98	
ROLAIDS SOFTCHEWS (Johnson & Johnson)			
CTB,PO (WILD CHERRY)			
1177 mg, 6s ea	**12547-0655-17**	0.68	
(3X6,VANILLA CREME)			
1177 mg, 18s ea	**12547-0655-22**	2.40	
(7X6,WILD CHERRY)			
1177 mg, 42s ea	**12547-0655-28**	4.98	
(McNeil Consumer Healthcare)			
CTB,PO (ES,WILD CHERRY)			
1177 mg, 6s ea	**12547-0655-20**	0.67	
(3X6, EXSTRENGTH)			
1177 mg, 18s ea	**12547-0655-25**	2.39	
(7X6,EXSTRENGTH)			
1177 mg, 42s ea	**12547-0655-31**	4.98	
RON-ACID (Major)			
SUS,PO, 540 mg/5 ml,			
360 ml	**00904-3235-14**	4.49	
RON-ACID PLUS (Major)			
SUS,PO (COOL MINT)			
540 mg/5 ml-40 mg/5 ml,			
360 ml	**00904-7726-14**	5.49	
ROSE MILK (Lee Pharm)			
LOT,TP, 240 ml	**23558-0681-70**	5.88	
240 ml 24s	**23558-0681-71**	141.12	
ROSS STOMATE DECOMPRESSION TUBE (Abbott)			
DEV,NA, ea	**70074-0503-73**	12.96	
ROSS STOMATE GASTROSTOMY (Abbott)			
DEV,NA (18 FR,EX SHORT,LOW PROF)			
ea	**70074-0500-73**	117.48	
(18 FR,LONG,LOW PROFILE)			
ea	**70074-0501-03**	117.48	
(18 FR,MED,LOW PROFILE)			
ea	**70074-0500-93**	117.48	
(18 FR,SHORT,LOW PROFILE)			
ea	**70074-0500-83**	117.48	
(22 FR,LONG,LOW PROFILE)			
ea	**70074-0501-01**	117.48	
(22 FR,MED,LOW PROFILE)			
ea	**70074-0500-91**	117.48	
(22 FR,SHORT,LOW PROFILE)			
ea	**70074-0500-81**	117.48	
(Ross Nutr)			
DEV,NA (26 FR, MED.,LOW PROFILE)			
ea	**70074-0507-33**	117.48	
(26 FR,EX SHORT,LOW PROF)			
ea	**70074-0507-31**	117.48	
(26 FR,LONG,LOW PROFILE)			
ea	**70074-0507-35**	117.48	
ROXALIA (Boiron)			
TAB,PO, 60s ea	**06962-0611-60**	5.73	9.59
ROYAL BRITTANY EVENING PRIMROSE OIL			
(Nature's Bounty)			
SGL,PO (PF,SF,SOFTGEL)			
365 mg-45 mg,			
50s ea	**74312-0036-31**		12.95
100s ea	**74312-0036-32**		19.95
ROYAL JELLY (Mason Vit)			
CAP,PO, 70 mg-100 mg-500 mg,			
60s ea	**11845-0079-85**	6.11	
TAB,PO (PF,SF)			
70 mg-100 mg-500 mg,			
60s ea	**11845-0124-25**	8.78	
(Nature's Bounty)			
SGL,PO (PF,SF,SOFTGEL)			
100 mg, 50s ea	**74312-0043-70**		7.59

PROD/MFR	HRI, UPC,NDC	AWP	SRP
RULOX (Rugby)			
SUS,PO (USP,1X355ML,MINT)			
355 ml	**00536-1945-83**	2.16	
RUTA GRAV (Luyties)			
TAB,SL (6X)			
6 x, 500s ea	**00618-7649-03**	3.99	
5500s ea	**00618-7649-10**	30.32	
(30X)			
12 x, 500s ea	**00622-7649-03**	4.19	
5500s ea	**00622-7649-10**	31.83	
(12X)			
30 x, 500s ea	**00624-7649-03**	4.19	
5500s ea	**00624-7649-10**	31.83	
RUTIN (Carlson,J.R.)			
TAB,PO (CONTAINS QUERCETIN)			
500 mg, 50s ea	**88395-0088-40**	3.45	6.90
150s ea	**88395-0088-41**	9.75	19.50
250s ea	**88395-0088-42**	13.95	27.90
(Freeda)			
TAB,PO (PF,SF,DYE-FREE)			
50 mg, 100s ea	**10432-0054-01**	3.87	6.45
(Mason Vit)			
TAB,PO, 500 mg, 100s ea	**11845-0073-01**	7.22	
RUTIN-50 (Key Company)			
TAB,PO, 50 mg, 100s ea	**11694-0877-01**	4.25	
RUTIPLEN-C (Med Prods Panamer)			
CAP,PO, 30s ea	**00576-0305-30**	7.50	
RX CHOICE FERROUS SULFATE IRON SUPPLEMENT (Hi-Tech)			
SOL,PO (1X50ML,GLUTEN-FREE)			
15 mg/ml, 50 ml	**50383-0627-50**	8.95	
RYNATAN PEDIATRIC (Meda)			
SUS,PO (1X473ML)			
4.5 mg/5 ml-5 mg/5 ml, 473 ml	**00037-0714-16**	344.71	
S-2 INHALANT (Nephron)			
SOL,IH (UNIT OF USE,ROBOT READY)			
2.25%, 30s ea	**00487-5901-02**	46.80	
(UNIT OF USE)			
2.25%, 30s ea	**00487-5901-99**	37.50	
S.S.S. ANTIOXIDANT COMPLETE (S.S.S.)			
TAB,PO (PF,SF)			
120s ea	**12258-0139-12**	8.66	12.99
S.S.S. ANTIOXIDANT FORMULA (S.S.S.)			
SGL,PO (SOFTGEL)			
60s ea	**12258-0138-60**	8.63	
S.S.S. TONIC (S.S.S.)			
LIQ,PO, 300 ml	**12258-0111-10**	3.99	5.99
600 ml	**12258-0111-20**	6.59	9.89
S.S.S. VITAMIN (S.S.S.)			
TAB,PO, 20s ea	**12258-0112-20**	3.73	
40s ea	**12258-0112-40**	5.57	
80s ea	**12258-0112-80**	8.38	
SABADIL (Boiron)			
TAB,PO, 5 c-5 c-9 c-5 c-5 c-5 c, 60s ea	**06962-0612-60**	5.73	9.59
SACCHARIN (Consolidated Midland)			
TAB,PO, 15 mg, 100s ea	**00223-1650-01**	3.25	
1000s ea	**00223-1650-02**	11.95	
30 mg, 100s ea	**00223-1651-01**	3.50	
1000s ea	**00223-1651-02**	12.50	
60 mg, 100s ea	**00223-1652-01**	4.00	
1000s ea	**00223-1652-02**	12.95	
SAF-GEL (Convatec)			
GEL,TP (12X85GM, HYDRATING)			
85 gm 12s	**68455-0107-89**	197.83	260.02
SAFE TRAVELS FIRST AID KIT (Johnson & Johnson)			
DEV,NA, ea	**81370-0082-74**	4.57	
SAFESNAP ALLERGY SYRINGES (US Medical Instruments)			
DEV,NA (1CC,27GX1/2")			
100s ea	**08595-0527-00**	64.00	
SAFESNAP INSULIN SYRINGES (US Medical Instruments)			
DEV,NA (1/2CC,29GX1/2",10X10)			
100s ea	**08595-0229-10**	73.45	
(1/2CC,29GX1/2")			
100s ea	**08595-0229-01**	67.19	
(1/2CC,30GX5/16",10X10)			
100s ea	**08595-0230-10**	73.54	
(1/2CC,30GX5/16")			
100s ea	**08595-0230-01**	67.19	
(1/3CC,30GX5/16",10X10)			
100s ea	**08595-0130-10**	73.54	
(1/3CC,30GX5/16")			
100s ea	**08595-0130-01**	67.19	
(1CC,28GX1/2",10X10)			
100s ea	**08595-0328-10**	73.45	
(1CC,28GX1/2")			
100s ea	**08595-0328-01**	67.19	
(1CC,29GX1/2",10X10)			
100s ea	**08595-0329-10**	73.54	
(1CC,29GX1/2")			
100s ea	**08595-0329-01**	67.19	
SAFESNAP SYRINGES (US Medical Instruments)			
DEV,NA (10CC,20GX1.5")			
50s ea	**08595-0806-50**	32.60	
(10CC,20GX1")			
50s ea	**08595-0805-50**	32.60	
(10CC,21GX1.5")			
50s ea	**08595-0804-50**	32.60	
(10CC,21GX1")			
50s ea	**08595-0803-50**	32.60	
(10CC,22GX1.5")			
50s ea	**08595-0802-50**	32.60	
(10CC,22GX1")			
50s ea	**08595-0801-50**	32.60	
(10CC,NO NEEDLE)			
50s ea	**08595-0800-50**	31.99	
(5CC,20GX1.5")			
50s ea	**08595-0705-50**	36.20	
(5CC,20GX1")			
50s ea	**08595-0703-50**	36.20	
(5CC,21GX1.5")			
50s ea	**08595-0704-50**	36.20	
(5CC,21GX1")			
50s ea	**08595-0702-50**	36.20	
(5CC,22GX1.5")			
50s ea	**08595-0701-50**	36.20	
(5CC,22GX1")			
50s ea	**08595-0700-50**	36.20	
(5CC)			
50s ea	**08595-0000-50**	29.33	
(3CC,20GX1.5")			
100s ea	**08595-0609-00**	58.63	
(3CC,20GX1")			
100s ea	**08595-0608-00**	58.63	
(3CC,21GX1.5")			
100s ea	**08595-0607-00**	58.63	
(3CC,21GX1")			
100s ea	**08595-0606-00**	58.63	
(3CC,22GX1.5")			
100s ea	**08595-0605-00**	58.63	
(3CC,22GX1")			
100s ea	**08595-0604-00**	58.63	
(3CC,23GX1.5")			
100s ea	**08595-0603-00**	58.63	
(3CC,23GX1")			
100s ea	**08595-0602-00**	58.63	
(3CC,25GX1")			
100s ea	**08595-0601-00**	58.63	
(3CC,25GX5/8")			
100s ea	**08595-0600-00**	58.63	
(3CC,NO NEEDLE)			
100s ea	**08595-0000-00**	53.38	
SAFESNAP TUBERCULIN SYRINGES (US Medical Instruments)			
DEV,NA (1CC,25GX5/8")			
100s ea	**08595-0425-00**	64.00	
(1CC,27GX1/2")			
100s ea	**08595-0427-00**	64.00	
SAFETUSSIN CD (Kramer Labs)			
SOL,PO (AF,SF,ORANGE)			
15 mg/5 ml-2.5 mg/5 ml, 120 ml	**53076-0141-33**	5.98	6.97
SAFETUSSIN DM (Kramer Labs)			
SOL,PO (AF,SF,ORANGE)			
15 mg/5 ml-100 mg/5 ml, 120 ml	**53076-0137-20**	5.58	6.51
(DOSING CUP INCLUDED,AF)			
15 mg/5 ml-100 mg/5 ml, 120 ml	**53076-0111-12**	5.58	6.52
SAL-PLANT GEL (Pedinol)			
GEL,TP, 17%, 14 gm	**00884-5192-15**		19.50
SALACTIC FILM (Pedinol)			
LIQ,TP, 17%, 15 ml	**00884-2592-15**		17.25
SALESE (Nuvora)			
LOZ,MM (AF,SF,PEPPERMINT)			
12s ea	**91124-0002-31**	15.00	
120s ea	**91124-0002-34**	150.00	
SALICYLIC ACID (Quality Care Prod)			
REPACK			
SOL,TP, 17%, 14 ml	**49999-0733-14**	32.57	
SALICYLIC ACID CLEANSING (Stiefel Consumer HealthCare)			
SOA,TP, 2%, 100 gm	**00145-1021-03**	3.84	5.79
SALINE (Cardinal Health)			
SPR,NS (PRIVATE LABEL)			
0.65%, 45 ml	**37205-0930-13**	2.12	
90 ml	**37205-0930-21**	2.80	
(Southwood)			
REPACK			
SPR,NS, 1%-0.35%, 45 ml	**58016-4896-01**	1.99	
SALINE MIST (Perrigo)			
SPR,NS, 0.65%, 45 ml	**45802-0357-58**	3.99	
(Rugby)			
SPR,NS, 0.65%, 45 ml	**00536-2506-76**	2.32	
(A-S Medication)			
REPACK			
SPR,NS, 0.65%, 45 ml	**54569-5200-00**	2.29	
(Phys Total Care)			
REPACK			
SPR,NS, 0.65%, 45 ml	**54868-1947-00**	8.42	
(Physician Partner)			
REPACK			
SPR,NS, 0.65%, 45 ml	**21695-0353-45**	17.98	
SALINE SOLUTION (Automatic Liq Pkg)			
SOL,IH (AL7453)			
0.45%, 3 ml 1000s UD	**48879-0002-01**	80.00	100.00
(AL7455)			
0.45%, 5 ml 1000s UD	**48879-0002-02**	80.00	100.00
(AL7093)			
0.9%, 3 ml 1000s UD	**48879-0003-01**	80.00	100.00
(AL7095)			
0.9%, 5 ml 1000s UD	**48879-0003-02**	80.00	100.00
(AL4015)			
0.9%, 15 ml 144s UD	**48879-0003-07**	34.56	46.08
SALIVA SUBSTITUTE (Roxane)			
SOL,PO, 120 ml	**00054-3769-50**	4.82	
SALIVASURE (Scandinavian)			
LOZ,MM, 90s ea	**51137-0060-28**	5.40	8.99
SALMON OIL 1000 (Key Company)			
SGL,PO (PF,SF,SOFTGEL)			
1000 mg, 100s ea	**11694-0851-01**	5.50	
650s ea	**11694-0851-05**	28.00	
SALTAIRE (Pincgold, Inc.)			
SOL,NS (HYPERTONIC)			
2.16%, 375 ml	**00274-0100-12**	6.50	12.50
960 ml	**00274-0100-30**	7.50	15.00
SAM-E (Pharmavite)			
ECT,PO (BLISTER PACK)			
200 mg, 20s ea	**31604-0016-18**	17.98	
SAM-EPA (Bio-Tech Pharm)			
SGL,PO, 100s ea	**53191-0073-01**	15.75	
SAMBUCUS COMPOUND (Weleda)			
LIQ,PO, 50 ml	**55946-0394-15**	7.20	
SAMOLINIC (Key Company)			
SGL,PO (PF,SF,SOFTGEL)			
100s ea	**11694-0843-01**	10.50	
240s ea	**11694-0843-24**	23.00	
650s ea	**11694-0843-05**	57.00	
SANABALM (Denison)			
POW,TP (MEDICATED)			
120 gm	**00295-7523-04**	3.37	
SANAFITIL (Tarmac)			
CRE,TP, 1.0%-27.5%, 15 gm	**11096-0191-01**	3.84	
GEL,TP (NAIL CONTROL)			
30 gm	**11096-0327-01**	6.12	
LIQ,TP (SOAP)			
105 ml	**11096-0210-01**	2.10	
2%-10%, 30 ml	**11096-0163-01**	3.90	
60 ml	**11096-0163-02**	6.30	
OIN,TP, 2%-10%, 30 gm	**11096-0190-01**	5.10	
60 gm	**11096-0190-02**	7.32	
POW,TP (FOOT DEODORANT)			
60 gm	**11096-0242-01**	2.58	
20%-2%, 60 gm	**11096-0222-01**	3.90	
120 gm	**11096-0222-02**	6.00	
SPR,TP, 10%, 30 ml	**11096-0163-11**	4.14	
SANI-PADS (G&W)			
PAD,TP (W/ALOE)			
100s ea	**00713-0308-98**	4.63	

PROD/MFR	HRI, UPC,NDC	AWP	SRP
SANI-SUPP (G&W)			
SUP,RC, 10s ea	**00713-0101-09**	2.20	
10s ea	**00713-0102-09**	2.14	
25s ea	**00713-0101-25**	3.05	
25s ea	**00713-0102-25**	3.30	
50s ea	**00713-0101-50**	5.01	
SARATOGA (Numark)			
OIN,TP, 30 gm	**38485-0500-10**	7.50	
60 gm	**38485-0500-20**	11.76	
SARNA (Stiefel Consumer HealthCare)			
LOT,TP, 0.5%-0.5%, 222 ml	**00145-0628-05**	7.80	11.79
(Phys Total Care) REPACK			
LOT,TP (1X222ML) 0.5%-0.5%, 222 ml	**54868-1587-00**	11.49	
(Quality Care Prod) REPACK			
LOT,TP, 0.5%-0.5%, 225 ml	**49999-0510-75**	12.86	
SARNA SENSITIVE (Stiefel Consumer HealthCare)			
LOT,TP (FRAGRANCE-FREE) 1%, 222 ml	**00145-0630-05**	9.36	13.99
SARNA ULTRA ANTI-ITCH (Stiefel Labs)			
CRE,TP, 0.5%-30%-1%, 56.6 gm	**00145-0629-02**	7.80	11.79
SARNOL-HC MAXIMUM STRENGTH (Stiefel Consumer HealthCare)			
LOT,TP, 1%, 59 ml	**00145-0622-02**	8.82	13.29
SARSAPARILLA (ADH)			
CAP,PO (PF,SF) 425 mg, 100s ea	**60142-0946-01**	4.98	9.95
SASTID (Stiefel Consumer HealthCare)			
SOA,TP, 3%-5%, 100 gm	**00145-1087-03**	3.84	5.79
SAW PALMETTO (ADH)			
CAP,PO, 450 mg, 100s ea	**60142-0106-10**	5.38	10.75
(AmerisourceBergen)			
SGL,PO (PF,PRIVATE LABEL) 160 mg, 50s ea	**24385-0971-71**	6.29	6.99
(Botanical Labs.)			
CAP,PO (SOFTGEL) 30s ea	**41954-0032-69**	7.50	14.99
60s ea	**41954-0032-70**	12.50	24.99
LIQ,PO, 30 ml	**41954-0020-43**	3.75	7.49
60 ml	**41954-0020-46**	6.00	11.99
(Cardinal Health)			
SGL,PO (PRIVATE LABEL,SOFTGEL) 160 mg, 30s ea	**37205-0096-65**	4.88	
(Key Company)			
SGL,PO (PF,SF,SOFTGEL) 160 mg, 60s ea	**11694-0684-01**	6.50	
250s ea	**11694-0684-02**	23.00	
(Lex)			
CAP,PO, 500 mg, 60s ea	**58537-0036-06**	3.60	
(Luyties)			
TAB,SL (6X) 6 x, 500s ea	**00618-8012-03**	3.99	
5500s ea	**00618-8012-10**	30.32	
(30X) 12 x, 500s ea	**00622-8012-03**	4.19	
5500s ea	**00622-8012-10**	31.83	
(12X) 30 x, 500s ea	**00624-8012-03**	4.19	
5500s ea	**00624-8012-10**	31.83	
(Mason Vit)			
CAP,PO (PF,SF) 500 mg, 60s ea	**11845-0115-15**	8.33	
90s ea	**11845-0115-19**	10.89	
SGL,PO (PF,SOFTGEL) 160 mg, 60s ea	**11845-0129-05**	14.56	
(Nature's Bounty)			
CAP,PO, 100s ea	**74312-0035-31**		6.99
(Rexall)			
CAP,PO (PF,SF) 450 mg, 75s ea	**30768-0000-28**	4.17	6.32
(Sundown)			
CAP,PO, 450 mg, 100s ea	**30768-0004-74**		4.99
(PD-Rx Pharm) REPACK			
CAP,PO, 500 mg, 30s ea	**55289-0408-30**	10.24	
(Phys Total Care) REPACK			
SGL,PO, 160 mg, 30s ea	**54868-5516-00**	14.34	
SAW PALMETTO COMPLEX (Rexall)			
CAP,PO (PF,SF) 50s ea	**30768-0001-09**	4.39	6.65
SAW PALMETTO EXTRACT (Freeda)			
TAB,PO (SF) 160 mg, 100s ea	**10432-0343-01**	13.17	21.95
SAW PALMETTO STANDARDIZED (Rexall)			
CAP,PO (PF,SF) 450 mg, 45s ea	**30768-0001-27**	5.28	9.00
SAYMAN CLEANSING W/LANOLIN (Dickinson Brands)			
SOA,TP (DRY SKIN) ea	**02590-0398-01**	1.45	
SAYMAN CLEANSING W/WITCH HAZEL (Dickinson Brands)			
SOA,TP (OILY SKIN) ea	**02590-0399-01**	1.45	
SAYMAN SALVE (Dickinson Brands)			
OIN,TP, 60 gm	**02590-0394-02**	1.93	
120 gm	**02590-0394-04**	2.82	
SCALP RELIEF (AmerisourceBergen)			
LIQ,TP (NON-GREASY) 3%, 74 ml	**24385-0678-27**	6.02	6.69
SCALPANA (Mericon)			
SOL,TP (1X85.5GM) 1%, 85.5 gm	**00394-0870-03**	6.56	
SCALPCORT (Family Phcy)			
LOT,TP (PRIVATE LABEL) 1%, 120 ml	**52735-0753-38**	5.93	6.59
SCALPICIN (Combe)			
SOL,TP (1X44ML,MAX STRENGTH) 1%, 44 ml	**11509-0054-00**	6.12	
3%, 44 ml	**11509-0003-25**	5.11	
(1X74ML) 3%, 74 ml	**11509-0003-27**	7.58	
SCAN (Parker)			
GEL,TP, 240 ml 12s	**00341-0011-08**	21.06	35.05
(W/DISPENSER, 4X3840ML) 3840 ml 4s	**00341-0011-28**	13.47	21.85
SCANDICAL (Axcan)			
PDR,PO, 227 gm	**58914-0830-08**	6.63	
SCANDISHAKE (Axcan)			
PDR,PO (BERRY) 85 gm 4s	**58914-0802-44**	7.67	
(CHOCOLATE) 85 gm 4s	**58914-0801-44**	7.67	
(VANILLA) 85 gm 4s	**58914-0800-44**	7.67	
(W/ASPARTAME,CHOCOLATE) 510 gm	**58914-0821-18**	11.51	
(W/ASPARTAME,VANILLA) 510 gm	**58914-0820-18**	11.51	
SCANDISHAKE LACTOSE-FREE (Axcan)			
PDR,PO (CHOCOLATE) 85 gm 4s	**58914-0811-44**	7.67	
(VANILLA) 85 gm 4s	**58914-0810-44**	7.67	
SCD B COMPLEX WITH C & ZINC (Freeda)			
TAB,PO (SF,GLUTEN-FREE) 100s ea	**10432-0353-01**	9.39	15.65
250s ea	**10432-0353-02**	18.78	31.30
SCD CALCIUM COMPLETE (Freeda)			
TAB,PO (EASY TO DIGEST,SF) 100s ea	**10432-0364-01**	6.30	10.50
250s ea	**10432-0364-02**	12.57	20.95
SCD EXPRESS FOOT CUFFS (Covidien)			
DEV,NA (LARGE,LATEX-FREE) 10s ea	**08080-5898-01**	437.50	
(REGULAR,LATEX-FREE) 10s ea	**08080-5897-01**	437.50	
SCD MULTIVITAMIN (Freeda)			
TAB,PO (HIGH POTENCY,SF) 90s ea	**10432-0354-01**	13.11	21.85
180s ea	**10432-0354-02**	21.57	35.95
SCHIRMER TEAR TEST (Alcon Ophthalmic)			
DEV,NA, 250s ea UD	**00065-0898-04**	356.88	
SCHNUCKS INSULIN SYRINGES (UltiMed)			
DEV,NA (1/2CC,G29X1/2",ULTIFINE) 100s ea	**08474-9259-00**	18.95	
(1/2CC,G30X5/16"ULTIFINE) 100s ea	**08474-9359-00**	20.95	
SCHUESSLER'S ACIDITY (Luyties)			
TAB,SL (TISSUE C) 3 x-3 x-3 x, 500s ea	**00618-0903-03**	4.19	
5500s ea	**00618-0903-10**	33.50	
SCHUESSLER'S ACNE REMEDY (Luyties)			
TAB,SL (TISSUE D) 3 x-6 x-3 x-12 x, 500s ea	**00618-0904-03**	4.19	
5500s ea	**00618-0904-10**	33.50	
SCHUESSLER'S BILIOUSNESS REMEDY (Luyties)			
TAB,SL (TISSUE H) 3 x-3 x-2 x, 500s ea	**00618-0908-03**	4.19	
5500s ea	**00618-0908-10**	33.50	
SCHUESSLER'S CALCAREA FLUOR (Luyties)			
TAB,SL (TISSUE SALT, 6X) 5500s ea	**00618-2033-10**	30.32	
6 x, 500s ea	**00618-2033-03**	3.99	
(TISSUE SALT) 12 x, 500s ea	**00622-2033-03**	4.19	
5500s ea	**00622-2033-10**	31.83	
30 x, 500s ea	**00624-2033-03**	4.19	
(TISSUE SALT, 12X) 30 x, 5500s ea	**00624-2033-10**	31.83	
SCHUESSLER'S CALCAREA PHOS (Luyties)			
TAB,SL (TISSUE SALT, 6X) 6 x, 500s ea	**00618-2043-03**	3.99	
5500s ea	**00618-2043-10**	30.32	
(TISSUE SALT, 30X) 12 x, 500s ea	**00622-2043-03**	4.19	
5500s ea	**00622-2043-10**	31.83	
(TISSUE SALT) 30 x, 500s ea	**00624-2043-03**	4.19	
5500s ea	**00624-2043-10**	31.83	
SCHUESSLER'S CALCAREA SULPH (Luyties)			
TAB,SL (TISSUE SALT, 6X) 6 x, 500s ea	**00618-2049-03**	3.99	
5500s ea	**00618-2049-10**	30.32	
(TISSUE SALT) 12 x, 500s ea	**00622-2049-03**	4.19	
5500s ea	**00622-2049-10**	31.83	
30 x, 500s ea	**00624-2049-03**	4.19	
5500s ea	**00624-2049-10**	31.83	
SCHUESSLER'S COLDS REMEDY (Luyties)			
TAB,SL (TISSUE J) 3 x-3 x-3 x, 500s ea	**00618-0910-03**	4.19	
5500s ea	**00618-0910-10**	33.50	
SCHUESSLER'S DEBILITY REMEDY (Luyties)			
TAB,SL (TISSUE B) 3 x-3 x-3 x, 500s ea	**00618-0902-03**	4.19	
5500s ea	**00618-0902-10**	33.50	
SCHUESSLER'S ELASTIC TISSUE REMEDY (Luyties)			
TAB,SL (TISSUE G) 3 x-3 x-3 x-6 x, 500s ea	**00618-0907-03**	4.19	
5500s ea	**00618-0907-10**	33.50	
SCHUESSLER'S FERRUM PHOS (Luyties)			
TAB,SL (TISSUE SALT, 6X) 6 x, 500s ea	**00618-3431-03**	3.99	
5500s ea	**00618-3431-10**	30.32	
(TISSUE SALT, 30X) 12 x, 500s ea	**00622-3431-03**	4.19	
5500s ea	**00622-3431-10**	31.83	
(TISSSUE SALT, 12X) 30 x, 500s ea	**00624-3431-03**	4.19	
(TISSUE SALT, 12X) 30 x, 5500s ea	**00624-3431-10**	31.83	
SCHUESSLER'S FEVER REMEDY (Luyties)			
TAB,SL (TISSUE M) 3 x-3 x-1 x, 500s ea	**00618-0912-03**	4.19	
5500s ea	**00618-0912-10**	33.50	
SCHUESSLER'S INSOMNIA REMEDY (Luyties)			
TAB,SL (TISSUE A) 3 x-3 x-3 x, 500s ea	**00618-0901-03**	4.19	
5500s ea	**00618-0901-10**	33.50	
SCHUESSLER'S KALI MUR (Luyties)			
TAB,SL (TISSUE SALT, 6X) 6 x, 500s ea	**00618-5224-03**	3.99	
5500s ea	**00618-5224-10**	30.32	
(TISSUE SALT) 12 x, 500s ea	**00622-5224-03**	4.19	
5500s ea	**00622-5224-10**	31.83	
30 x, 500s ea	**00624-5224-03**	4.19	
5500s ea	**00624-5224-10**	31.83	
SCHUESSLER'S KALI PHOS (Luyties)			
TAB,SL (TISSUE SALT, 6X) 6 x, 500s ea	**00618-5228-03**	3.99	
5500s ea	**00618-5228-10**	30.32	
(TISSUE SALT, 30X) 12 x, 500s ea	**00622-5228-03**	4.19	
5500s ea	**00622-5228-10**	31.83	

PROD/MFR	HRI, UPC,NDC	AWP	SRP
(TISSUE SALT, 12X)			
30 x, 500s ea	00624-5228-03	4.19	
5500s ea	00624-5228-10	31.83	
SCHUESSLER'S KALI SULPH (Luyties)			
TAB,SL (TISSUE SALT, 6X)			
6 x, 500s ea	00618-5230-03	3.99	
5500s ea	00618-5230-10	30.32	
(TISSUE SALT, 30X)			
12 x, 500s ea	00622-5230-03	4.19	
5500s ea	00622-5230-10	31.83	
(TISSUE SALT, 12X)			
30 x, 500s ea	00624-5230-03	4.19	
5500s ea	00624-5230-10	31.83	
SCHUESSLER'S MAGNESIA PHOS (Luyties)			
TAB,SL (TISSUE SALT, 12X)			
500s ea	00624-6020-03	4.19	
5500s ea	00624-6020-10	31.83	
(TISSUE SALT, 6X)			
6 x, 500s ea	00618-6020-03	3.99	
5500s ea	00618-6020-10	30.32	
(TISSUE SALT, 30X)			
12 x, 500s ea	00622-6020-03	4.19	
5500s ea	00622-6020-10	31.83	
SCHUESSLER'S MUSCULAR REMEDY (Luyties)			
TAB,SL (TISSUE I)			
3 x-3 x-3 x, 500s ea	00618-0909-03	4.19	
5500s ea	00618-0909-10	33.50	
SCHUESSLER'S NATRUM MUR (Luyties)			
TAB,SL (TISSUE SALT, 6X)			
6 x, 500s ea	00618-6433-03	3.99	
5500s ea	00618-6433-10	30.32	
(TISSUE SALT)			
12 x, 500s ea	00622-6433-03	4.19	
(TISSUE SALT, 30X)			
12 x, 5500s ea	00622-6433-10	31.83	
(TISSUE SALT, 12X)			
30 x, 500s ea	00624-6433-03	4.19	
5500s ea	00624-6433-10	31.83	
SCHUESSLER'S NATRUM PHOS (Luyties)			
TAB,SL (TISSUE SALT, 6X)			
6 x, 500s ea	00618-6436-03	3.99	
5500s ea	00618-6436-10	30.32	
(TISSUE SALT)			
12 x, 500s ea	00622-6436-03	4.19	
5500s ea	00622-6436-10	31.83	
30 x, 500s ea	00624-6436-03	4.19	
5500s ea	00624-6436-10	31.83	
SCHUESSLER'S NATRUM SULPH (Luyties)			
TAB,SL (TISSUE SALT, 6X)			
6 x, 500s ea	00618-6440-03	3.99	
5500s ea	00618-6440-10	30.32	
(TISSUE SALT, 30X)			
12 x, 500s ea	00622-6440-03	4.19	
(TISSUE SALT)			
12 x, 5500s ea	00622-6440-10	31.83	
30 x, 500s ea	00624-6440-03	4.19	
5500s ea	00624-6440-10	31.83	
SCHUESSLER'S NERVOUS REMEDY (Luyties)			
TAB,SL (TISSUE P)			
3 x-3 x-3 x-3 x,			
500s ea	00618-0915-03	4.19	
5500s ea	00618-0915-10	33.50	
SCHUESSLER'S NEURALGIC REMEDY (Luyties)			
TAB,SL (TISSUE O)			
3 x-2 x-2 x, 500s ea	00618-0914-03	4.19	
5500s ea	00618-0914-10	33.50	
SCHUESSLER'S SILICA (Luyties)			
TAB,SL (TISSUE SALT, 6X)			
6 x, 500s ea	00618-8081-03	3.99	
5500s ea	00618-8081-10	30.32	
(TISSUE SALT)			
12 x, 500s ea	00622-8081-03	4.19	
5500s ea	00622-8081-10	31.83	
30 x, 500s ea	00624-8081-03	4.19	
5500s ea	00624-8081-10	31.83	
SCHUESSLER'S THROAT REMEDY (Luyties)			
TAB,SL (TISSUE K)			
3 x-3 x-3 x, 500s ea	00618-0911-03	4.19	
5500s ea	00618-0911-10	33.50	
SCHUESSLER'S TONIC (Luyties)			
TAB,SL (TISSUE E)			
3 x-2 x-2 x-2 x-2 x,			
500s ea	00618-0905-03	4.19	
5500s ea	00618-0905-10	33.50	
SCHUESSLER'S VAGINAL REMEDY (Luyties)			
TAB,SL (TISSUE N)			
3 x-3 x-3 x-3 x,			
500s ea	00618-0913-03	4.19	
5500s ea	00618-0913-10	33.50	
SCLERANTHUS (Ellon)			
SOL,SL (DROPS)			
10.5 ml	51762-0032-10		9.25
SCLEREX (Miller)			
TAB,PO, 60s ea	17204-0439-20	10.02	16.70
SCOPE SINGLE HEAD (Lumiscope)			
DEV,NA (LIGHTWEIGHT)			
ea	38673-0040-01	3.99	9.99
SCOPODEX (Consolidated Midland)			
CAP,PO, 0.5 mg,			
24s ea UD	00223-1630-01	12.50	
SCOT-TUSSIN DIABETES CF (Scot-Tussin)			
LIQ,PO (AF,SF,DYE-FREE)			
10 mg/5 ml,			
118.3 ml	00372-0043-04	3.98	5.99
SCOT-TUSSIN DM (Scot-Tussin)			
SOL,PO (AF,SF,DYE-FREE)			
2 mg/5 ml-15 mg/5 ml,			
118.3 ml	00372-0036-04	3.98	5.99
SCOT-TUSSIN EXPECTORANT (Scot-Tussin)			
SOL,PO (AF,SF,DYE-FREE)			
100 mg/5 ml,			
118.3 ml	00372-0006-04	3.98	5.99
SCOT-TUSSIN ORIGINAL (Scot-Tussin)			
SOL,PO (COLD/ALLERGY FORMULA,AF)			
118 ml	00372-0002-04	3.98	5.99
SCOT-TUSSIN SENIOR (Scot-Tussin)			
SOL,PO (AF,SF,DYE-FREE)			
15 mg/5 ml-200 mg/5 ml,			
118.3 ml	00372-0050-04	3.98	5.99
SCYTERA (Promius)			
FOA,TP (CALIFORNIA ONLY)			
2%, 100 gm	67857-0801-26	30.00	35.00
(NON-CALIFORNIA)			
2%, 100 gm	67857-0801-52	30.00	35.00
SE ASPARTATE (Miller)			
TAB,PO, 50 mcg, 100s ea	17204-0361-40	7.50	12.50
SE PLUS PROTEIN (Miller)			
TAB,PO, 100s ea	17204-0462-40	6.60	11.00
SE-100 (Bio-Tech Pharm)			
CAP,PO, 100 mcg,			
100s ea	53191-0184-01	4.75	
SE-CURE (Everett)			
TAB,PO (CAPLET)			
60s ea	00642-0103-60	14.95	
SEA BREEZE ASTRINGENT (Clairol, Inc.)			
SOL,TP (ORIGINAL)			
180 ml	19810-0004-23	1.84	
(SENSITIVE)			
180 ml	19810-0004-27	1.84	
(OILY)			
300 ml	19810-0004-26	3.59	
(ORIGINAL)			
300 ml	19810-0004-24	3.59	
(SENSITIVE)			
300 ml	19810-0004-28	3.59	
(ORIGINAL)			
480 ml	19810-0004-25	4.73	
SEA BREEZE BREEZERS (Clairol, Inc.)			
PAD,TP (PACKET,ORIGINAL)			
24s ea	19810-0075-31	3.59	
SEA BREEZE EXFOLIATING FACIAL SCRUB (Clairol, Inc.)			
CRE,TP, 105 gm	19810-0053-21	3.59	
SEA BREEZE FACIAL CLEANSING (Clairol, Inc.)			
SOA,TP (NORMAL/OILY)			
ea	19810-0057-11	1.98	
(SENSITIVE)			
ea	19810-0057-21	1.98	
SEA BREEZE TONER (Clairol, Inc.)			
SOL,TP, 300 ml	19810-0004-29	3.59	
SEA MIST (Altura)			
REPACK			
SPR,NS, 0.65%, 45 ml	63874-0085-45	1.79	
SEA OMEGA 30 (Rugby)			
SGL,PO (PF,SF,DYE-FREE,SOFTGEL)			
1200 mg-2 iu,			
100s ea	00536-7186-01	6.75	
SEA OMEGA 50 (Rugby)			
SGL,PO (PF,SF,DYE-FREE,SOFTGEL)			
1000 mg-1 iu,			
50s ea	00536-7187-06	7.07	
SEA SOFT MIST (Qualitest)			
SPR,NS, 0.65%, 45 ml	00603-0380-46	1.79	
SEA-BAND (Sea-Band)			
DEV,NA (WRISTBAND,1PAIR)			
2s ea	08471-0510-01	5.25	
SEA-BAND FOR CHILDREN (Sea-Band)			
DEV,NA (WRISTBAND,PAIR)			
ea	87279-0005-19	5.25	
SEA-BOND DENTURE ADHESIVE WAFERS (Combe)			
DEV,NA (LOWERS,FRESH MINT)			
15s ea	11509-0065-03	2.90	
(LOWERS,ORIGINAL)			
15s ea	11509-0001-63	2.90	
(UPPERS,FRESH MINT)			
15s ea	11509-0065-02	2.90	
(UPPERS,ORIGINAL)			
15s ea	11509-0001-62	2.90	
(LOWERS, ORIGINAL)			
30s ea	11509-0002-06	5.23	
(LOWERS,FRESH MINT)			
30s ea	11509-0065-08	5.23	
(UPPERS, ORIGINAL)			
30s ea	11509-0002-05	5.23	
(UPPERS,FRESH MINT)			
30s ea	11509-0065-07	5.23	
SEA-BOND DENTURE BRUSH (Combe)			
DEV,NA (DEEP-CLEAN PICK)			
ea	11509-0149-00	1.91	
SEA-BOND DENTURITE CUSTOM-FIT DENTURE RELINER (Combe)			
DEV,NA (UPPER OR LOWER)			
2s ea	11509-0198-00	3.92	
SEA-CLENS (Coloplast)			
SOL,TP, 178 ml 12s	11701-0159-36	104.04	108.84
355 ml 12s	11701-0159-35	161.04	168.48
SEACURE HYDROLYZED WHITE FISH (Proper)			
CAP,PO, 180s ea	60599-0006-37		39.95
SEAMLESS ROBINSON PLASTIC URETHRAL CATHETER (Covidien)			
DEV,NA (VINYL 16FR,LATEX-FREE)			
100s ea	08080-4006-16	88.10	
SEASORB ALGINATE (Coloplast)			
DEV,NA (STERILE,2"X2")			
30s ea	11701-0836-11	109.50	114.60
SEASORB ALGINATE FILLER (Coloplast)			
DEV,NA (STERILE,17-1/2" ROPE)			
6s ea	11701-0836-70	46.14	48.30
SEBA-NIL (Valeant Pharm Intl)			
SOL,TP, 240 ml	00064-2150-08	10.70	
SEBASORB (Summers)			
LOT,TP, 10%-2%, 45 ml	11086-0009-01	11.88	
SEBEX (Rugby)			
LIQ,TP, 2%-2%, 120 ml	00536-1962-97	4.43	
SEBULEX (Ranbaxy Labs)			
LIQ,TP (W/CONDITIONERS)			
2%-2%, 210 ml	00072-2600-07	13.51	
SHA,TP, 2%-2%, 200 gm	10631-0108-07	12.87	
(Phys Total Care)			
REPACK			
LIQ,TP, 2%-2%, 120 ml	54868-2791-01	7.34	
SECURA ANTIFUNGAL EXTRA THICK (Smith & Nephew)			
CRE,TP, 2%, 92 gm	50484-0329-00	8.30	6.64
SECURA ANTIFUNGAL GREASELESS (Smith & Nephew)			
CRE,TP, 2%, 57 gm	50484-0328-00	6.48	5.18
SECURA DIMETHICONE PROTECTANT (Smith & Nephew)			
CRE,TP (FRAGRANCE-FREE)			
5%, 114 gm	50484-0322-00	10.20	8.16
SECURA EPC SKIN CARE STARTER KIT (Smith & Nephew)			
KIT,TP, 0.13%-30.6%, ea	50484-0341-00	13.26	10.61
SECURA EXTRA PROTECTIVE CREAM (Smith & Nephew)			
CRE,TP, 30.6%, 92 gm	50484-0324-00	9.89	7.91
220 gm	50484-0325-00	16.25	13.00
SECURA MOISTURIZING CLEANSER (Smith & Nephew)			
SPR,TP, 0.13%, 118 ml	50484-0308-00	3.84	3.07
236 ml	50484-0309-00	5.80	4.64
SECURA MOISTURIZING CREAM (Smith & Nephew)			
CRE,TP (GREASELESS)			
85 gm	40565-0121-79	3.81	3.05
184 gm	40565-0121-80	6.01	4.81

PROD/MFR	HRI, UPC,NDC	AWP	SRP
SECURA MOISTURIZING LOTION (Smith & Nephew)			
LOT,TP (FRAGRANCE-FREE)			
236 ml	**40565-0121-99**	3.06	2.45
SECURA PERSONAL CLEANSER (Smith & Nephew)			
SPR,TP, 0.13%, 236 ml	**50484-0304-00**	2.95	2.36
3780 ml	**50484-0305-00**	29.00	23.20
SECURA PERSONAL SKIN CARE KIT (Smith & Nephew)			
KIT,TP, 0.13%-98.79%, ea	**50484-0343-00**	8.23	6.58
SECURA PROTECTIVE CREAM (Smith & Nephew)			
CRE,TP, 10%, 50 gm	**50484-0311-00**	5.13	4.10
78 gm	**50484-0312-00**	7.86	6.29
SECURA PROTECTIVE OINTMENT (Smith & Nephew)			
OIN,TP, 98.79%, 70 gm	**50484-0315-00**	3.24	2.59
159 gm	**50484-0316-00**	6.55	5.24
SECURA STARTER KIT (Smith & Nephew)			
KIT,TP (GREASELESS)			
0.13%-98.79%, ea	**50484-0342-00**	14.24	11.39
SECURA TOTAL BODY FOAM CLEANSER (Smith & Nephew)			
FOA,TP, 0.13%, 133 ml	**50484-0302-00**	7.14	5.71
250 ml	**50484-0303-00**	8.46	6.77
SECURA TWO-STEP KIT (Smith & Nephew)			
KIT,TP, 0.13%-10%, ea	**50486-0344-00**	12.73	10.18
SEDALIA (Boiron)			
TAB,PO, 6 c-6 c-6 c-6 c-6 c-6 c, 60s ea	**06962-0614-60**	5.73	9.59
SEDATIVE PILULES (Weleda)			
GRA,PO, 18 gm	**55946-0137-60**	5.55	
SELECT LITE (Arkray)			
DEV,NA, ea	**08317-6600-01**	11.18	
(LANCING DEV/10 LANCETS) ea	**08317-6612-01**	12.00	
SELENICAPS-200 (Key Company)			
CAP,PO (SF)			
200 mcg, 100s ea	**11694-0791-01**	8.00	
SELENIMIN (Key Company)			
TAB,PO (SF)			
125 mcg, 100s ea	**11694-0941-01**	6.75	
SELENIMIN-200 (Key Company)			
PO (SF)			
200 mcg, 100s ea	**11694-0890-01**	7.25	
SELENIMIN-50 (Key Company)			
PO, 50 mcg, 100s ea	**11694-0891-01**	4.25	
SELENIUM (ADH)			
TAB,PO (PF,SF)			
200 mcg, 100s ea	**60142-0395-01**	3.25	6.50
(Basic Vitamins)			
TAB,PO, 50 mcg, 100s ea	**00761-0021-20**	2.40	
(Cardinal Health)			
TAB,PO (PRIVATE LABEL)			
200 mcg, 100s ea	**37205-0087-78**	7.32	
(Carlson,J.R.)			
CAP,PO, 200 mcg, 60s ea	**88395-0052-80**	3.95	7.90
180s ea	**88395-0052-82**	10.75	21.50
TAB,PO, 200 mcg, 90s ea	**88395-0052-91**	4.45	8.90
180s ea	**88395-0052-92**	7.95	15.90
360s ea	**88395-0052-93**	14.45	28.90
(Major)			
TAB,PO, 50 mcg, 100s ea	**00904-3162-60**	4.70	
TER,PO, 200 mcg, 60s ea	**00904-4203-52**	4.86	
(Marlex)			
TAB,PO, 50 mcg, 100s ea	**10135-0200-01**	1.32	
1000s ea	**10135-0200-10**	7.22	
100 mcg, 100s ea	**10135-0201-01**	2.48	
1000s ea	**10135-0201-10**	9.28	
TER,PO, 200 mcg, 60s ea	**10135-0350-60**	1.10	
(Mason Vit)			
TAB,PO, 50 mcg, 100s ea	**11845-0070-81**	4.33	
(SF) 100 mcg, 100s ea	**11845-0079-61**	5.89	
(Nature's Bounty)			
TAB,PO (PF,SF)			
50 mcg, 100s ea	**74312-0021-20**		4.49
200 mcg, 50s ea	**74312-0032-00**		4.49
(Rexall)			
TAB,PO (PF,SF)			
100 mcg, 60s ea	**30768-0001-48**	1.88	2.85
SELENIUM OCEANIC (Freeda)			
TAB,PO (PF,SF,DYE-FREE)			
50 mcg, 100s ea	**10432-0243-01**	4.77	7.95
250s ea	**10432-0243-02**	9.54	15.90
100 mcg, 100s ea	**10432-0291-01**	6.87	11.45
250s ea	**10432-0291-02**	13.74	22.90
200 mcg, 100s ea	**10432-0265-01**	8.82	14.70
250s ea	**10432-0265-02**	17.64	29.40
SELENIUM SULFIDE (Consolidated Midland)			
LOT,TP, 1%, 240 ml	**00223-6607-01**	3.25	
(Rugby)			
SHA,TP, 1%, 210 ml	**00536-1995-53**	4.57	
SELENOMAX (Mason Vit)			
TAB,PO (PF,SF)			
200 mcg, 60s ea	**11845-0124-95**	5.00	
SELSUN BLUE MEDICATED TREATMENT (Phys Total Care)			
REPACK			
SHA,TP, 1%, 210 ml	**54868-2202-01**	7.41	
SEN-O-TABS (Mason Vit)			
TAB,PO, 8.6 mg, 100s ea	**11845-0879-01**	4.67	
SENEXON (Rugby)			
TAB,PO, 8.6 mg, 100s ea	**00536-5904-01**	4.77	
1000s ea	**00536-5904-10**	27.75	
SENEXON LIQUID (Rugby)			
SYR,PO, 8.8 mg/5 ml, 237 ml	**00536-1275-59**	17.52	
SENEXON-S (Rugby)			
TAB,PO, 50 mg-8.6 mg, 100s ea	**00536-4086-01**	4.74	
1000s ea	**00536-4086-10**	18.30	
SENIOR TOPIX SANIX (Topix)			
GEL,TP, 118 ml	**58211-0362-04**	2.25	
SENIORTOPIX AQUIX MOISTURIZING (Topix)			
OIN,TP (TUBE)			
120 gm	**58211-0355-04**	5.46	
(JAR) 450 gm	**58211-0355-15**	11.79	
SENIORTOPIX EMOLLIX MOISTURIZING (Topix)			
LOT,TP, 480 ml	**58211-0351-16**	6.97	
SENIORTOPIX EURIX MOISTURIZING (Topix)			
CRE,TP, 120 gm	**58211-0354-04**	4.55	
480 gm	**58211-0354-16**	6.62	
SENIORTOPIX GUARDIX SKIN PROTECTANT (Topix)			
OIN,TP (TUBE)			
120 gm	**58211-0357-40**	11.93	
SENIORTOPIX HEALIX DIAPER RASH (Topix)			
OIN,TP, 120 gm	**58211-0356-04**	3.71	
480 gm	**58211-0356-16**	9.36	
SENIORTOPIX VESTIX SKIN PROTECTANT (Topix)			
OIN,TP, 120 gm	**58211-0352-04**	5.09	
SENNA (Altaire)			
SYR,PO (NATURAL VEG. LAXATIVE)			
8.8 mg/5 ml, 237 ml	**59390-0125-41**	7.92	
(AmerisourceBergen)			
TAB,PO (PRIVATE LABEL)			
8.6 mg, 100s ea	**24385-0404-78**	6.29	6.99
(Cardinal Health)			
TAB,PO (PRIVATE LABEL)			
8.6 mg, 100s ea	**37205-0241-78**	5.50	
(Chain Drug Marketing)			
TAB,PO, 8.6 mg, 100s ea	**63868-0263-01**	2.39	9.99
(Concord Labs)			
TAB,PO, 5.6 mg, 100s ea	**20254-0209-01**	3.38	
1000s ea	**20254-0209-04**	23.65	
8.6 mg, 100s ea	**20254-0215-01**	4.73	
1000s ea	**20254-0215-04**	28.35	
(Cypress Pharm)			
TAB,PO, 8.6 mg, 100s ea	**60258-0950-01**	3.28	
(Family Phcy)			
TAB,PO (PRIVATE LABEL)			
8.6 mg, 100s ea	**52735-0522-01**	6.29	6.99
(Major)			
SYR,PO, 8.8 mg/5 ml, 240 ml	**00904-5452-09**	17.99	
TAB,PO, 8.6 mg, 100s ea	**00904-5165-59**	4.90	
100s ea UD	**00904-5165-61**	7.70	
1000s ea	**00904-5165-80**	21.59	
(Ohm)			
TAB,PO, 8.6 mg, 100s ea	**51660-0117-01**	1.95	
1000s ea	**51660-0117-10**	9.95	
(Pharm Assoc Inc)			
SYR,PO (40X15ML,AF,DYE-FREE)			
176 mg/5 ml, 15 ml 40s UD	**00121-4722-15**	76.00	
(AF,DYE-FREE)			
176 mg/5 ml, 237 ml	**00121-0722-08**	17.05	
(Dispensing Solutions)			
REPACK			
TAB,PO, 8.6 mg, 30s ea	**55045-3429-08**	3.00	
60s ea	**55045-3429-06**	6.00	
(Nucare Pharm)			
REPACK			
TAB,PO, 8.6 mg, 30s ea	**66267-0730-30**	8.80	
60s ea	**66267-0730-60**	12.65	
120s ea	**66267-0730-91**	25.25	
(PD-Rx Pharm)			
REPACK			
TAB,PO, 8.6 mg, 10s ea	**55289-0840-10**	4.74	
(Phys Total Care)			
REPACK			
TAB,PO, 8.6 mg, 100s ea	**54868-4929-00**	4.19	
(Quality Care Prod)			
REPACK			
TAB,PO, 8.6 mg, 30s ea	**35356-0382-30**	19.56	
(Stat Rx)			
REPACK			
TAB,PO, 8.6 mg, 20s ea	**16590-0205-20**	4.75	
30s ea	**16590-0205-30**	7.14	
60s ea	**16590-0205-60**	14.25	
90s ea	**16590-0205-90**	21.37	
112s ea	**16590-0205-73**	21.65	
120s ea	**16590-0205-72**	28.50	
SENNA CONCENTRATE (Amneal)			
TAB,PO, 8.6 mg, 100s ea	**65162-0440-10**	4.80	
(Physician Partner)			
REPACK			
TAB,PO, 8.6 mg, 60s ea	**21695-0722-60**	23.60	
(Southwood)			
REPACK			
TAB,PO, 8.6 mg, 30s ea	**58016-0492-30**	1.56	
60s ea	**58016-0492-60**	3.12	
90s ea	**58016-0492-90**	4.68	
100s ea	**58016-0492-00**	5.20	
120s ea	**58016-0492-02**	6.24	
SENNA LAXATIVE (Basic Vitamins)			
TAB,PO, 8.6 mg, 100s ea	**00761-0220-20**	3.00	
(PD-Rx Pharm)			
REPACK			
TAB,PO, 8.6 mg, 30s ea	**55289-0840-30**	6.00	
60s ea	**55289-0840-60**	9.00	
SENNA PLUS (Major)			
TAB,PO, 50 mg-8.6 mg, 100s ea	**00904-5512-61**	12.89	
1000s ea	**00904-5512-80**	121.91	
(American Health)			
REPACK			
TAB,PO (10X10)			
50 mg-8.6 mg, 100s ea UD	**68084-0050-01**	11.13	
(IPI)			
REPACK			
TAB,PO, 50 mg-8.6 mg, 60s ea	**18837-0264-60**	11.50	
120s ea	**18837-0264-98**	22.95	
SENNA SOFT (Novartis Consumer)			
TAB,PO (PILL)			
15 mg, 24s ea	**00067-6285-24**	5.17	
SENNA-GEN (Teva)			
TAB,PO, 8.6 mg, 100s ea	**00182-1093-01**	3.59	
1000s ea	**00182-1093-10**	25.19	
SENNA-LAX (Qualitest)			
TAB,PO, 8.6 mg, 100s ea	**00603-0282-21**	4.11	
(CAPLET) 8.6 mg, 1000s ea	**00603-0282-32**	39.86	
SENNA-PLUS (Cardinal Health)			
TAB,PO (PRIVATE LABEL)			
50 mg-8.6 mg, 60s ea	**37205-0251-72**	5.50	
(Major)			
TAB,PO, 50 mg-8.6 mg, 60s ea	**00904-5512-52**	6.99	
(Dispensing Solutions)			
REPACK			
TAB,PO, 50 mg-8.6 mg, 120s ea	**55045-3192-01**	14.99	

PROD/MFR | HRI, UPC,NDC | AWP | SRP

(Physician Partner)
REPACK
TAB,PO, 50 mg-8.6 mg,
60s ea............21695-0790-60 22.90
240s ea..........21695-0790-64 111.08
SENNA-S (Cypress Pharm)
TAB,PO, 50 mg-8.6 mg,
60s ea............60258-0951-06 22.12
(Teva)
TAB,PO, 50 mg-8.6 mg,
100s ea...........00182-1113-01 10.99
(10X10)
50 mg-8.6 mg,
100s ea UD........00182-8642-89 10.99
1000s ea..........00182-1113-10 99.99
(Stat Rx)
REPACK
TAB,PO, 50 mg-8.6 mg,
20s ea............16590-0518-20 4.75
30s ea...........16590-0518-30 7.14
60s ea...........16590-0518-60 14.25
90s ea...........16590-0518-90 21.37
120s ea..........16590-0518-72 28.50
SENNA-TIME (McKesson Packaging)
REPACK
TAB,PO (MICRO-COATED)
8.6 mg, 100s ea UD...63739-0431-10 12.34
SENNA-TIME S (McKesson Packaging)
TAB,PO (FILM-COATED)
50 mg-8.6 mg,
100s ea UD........63739-0432-10 18.13
750s ea UD.......63739-0432-01 92.46
750s ea..........63739-0432-03 92.46
SENNALAX-S (Qualitest)
TAB,PO, 50 mg-8.6 mg,
100s ea...........00603-0283-21 29.94
1000s ea..........00603-0283-32 284.43
SENNAPROMPT (Konsyl)
CAP,PO (EZ-CAPS)
500 mg-9 mg,
90s ea............00224-1860-90 7.75 10.69
SENNATURAL (G&W)
TAB,PO, 8.6 mg, 100s ea...00713-0419-99 5.25
SENNO (Prime Marketing)
TAB,PO, 8.6 mg, 100s ea...62107-0031-01 3.90
SENNOSIDES (Altura)
REPACK
TAB,PO, 8.6 mg, 10s ea...63874-0682-10 5.64
30s ea...........63874-0682-30 16.92
60s ea...........63874-0682-60 33.84
(Quality Care Prod)
REPACK
TAB,PO, 8.6 mg, 30s ea...49999-0711-30 20.30
100s ea..........49999-0711-00 67.67
SENOKOT (Purdue Products L.P.)
TAB,PO, 8.6 mg, 20s ea...67618-0300-20 5.56
50s ea...........67618-0300-50 11.27
100s ea..........67618-0300-10 21.04
(STRIP PACK)
8.6 mg, 100s ea UD...67618-0300-11 24.62
SENOKOT S (Purdue Products L.P.)
TAB,PO, 50 mg-8.6 mg,
10s ea............67618-0310-01 5.56
30s ea...........67618-0310-30 14.73
60s ea...........67618-0310-60 25.98
(STRIP PACK)
50 mg-8.6 mg,
100s ea UD........67618-0310-11 39.39
(Phys Total Care)
REPACK
TAB,PO, 50 mg-8.6 mg,
60s ea............54868-4069-00 30.10
SENOKOTXTRA (Purdue Products L.P.)
TAB,PO (DOUBLE STRENGTH)
17.2 mg, 12s ea......67618-0315-12 5.56
36s ea............67618-0315-36 15.02
SENSITIVE EYES (Bausch & Lomb Inc.)
SOL,OP, 15 ml..........10119-0073-60 3.70
30 ml..............10119-0011-40 5.34
SENSITIVE EYES CONCENTRATED CLEANER (Bausch & Lomb Inc.)
SOL,NA (RGP)
30 ml..............10119-0054-03 5.40

PROD/MFR | HRI, UPC,NDC | AWP | SRP

SENSITIVE EYES SALINE (Bausch & Lomb Inc.)
SOL,NA (THIMEROSAL-FREE)
355 ml............10119-0001-07 3.30
SENSITIVE EYES WETTING AND SOAKING (Bausch & Lomb Inc.)
SOL,NA (RGP)
120 ml............10119-0056-03 5.40
SENSODYNE (Glaxo)
PAS,DE (TRIAL SIZE,FRESH IMPACT)
5%-0.15%, 23 gm....10158-0083-51 0.97
(FRESH IMPACT)
5%-0.15%, 113 gm...10158-0083-50 4.48
SENSODYNE FULL PROTECTION (Glaxo)
PAS,DE, 5%-0.145%,
113 gm............10158-0083-75 4.48
SENSODYNE PRONAMEL (Glaxo)
PAS,DE (SF,MINT ESSENCE)
5%-0.15%, 113 gm...10158-0830-50 4.70
SENSODYNE W/FLUORIDE (Glaxo)
GEL,DE (SF,MINT)
120 gm............10158-0082-04 4.48
PAS,DE, 120 gm.........10158-0077-04 4.48
(EXTRA WHITENING)
120 gm............10158-0084-04 4.48
(SF,FRESH MINT)
120 gm............10158-0081-11 4.70
(EXTRA WHITENING)
180 gm............10158-0084-06 6.01
SENSODYNE W/FLUORIDE TARTAR CONTROL (Glaxo)
PAS,DE (SF)
120 gm............10158-0085-04 4.48
SENSODYNE W/FLUORIDE/BAKING SODA (Glaxo)
PAS,DE, 120 gm.........10158-0074-04 4.48
SENTRY PRESTIGE SMART SYSTEM (Home Diag)
DEV,NA (STRIP)
50s ea............56151-0322-50 26.12
SENTRY PRESTIGE SMART SYTEM STARTER (Home Diag)
DEV,NA (MTR,STRP,LANCET,DEV,SOL)
ea................56151-0222-01 22.18
SEPASOOTHE (Medique)
LOZ,MM (12X2)
10 mg-0.5 mg,
24s ea UD........47682-0180-64 1.54
(50X2)
10 mg-0.5 mg,
100s ea UD........47682-0180-33 5.79
(125X2)
10 mg-0.5 mg,
250s ea UD........47682-0180-48 13.00
(250X2)
10 mg-0.5 mg,
500s ea UD........47682-0180-13 25.75
SEPIA (Luyties)
TAB,SL (6X)
6 x, 500s ea.........00618-8073-03 3.99
5500s ea..........00618-8073-10 30.32
(30X)
12 x, 500s ea........00622-8073-03 4.19
5500s ea..........00622-8073-10 31.83
(12X)
30 x, 500s ea........00624-8073-03 4.19
5500s ea..........00624-8073-10 31.83
SERABRINA LA FRANCE (Larkspur)
LIQ,PO, 50 mg/15 ml,
480 ml............18864-0211-03 5.64
SERINE (Carlson,J.R.)
L-SERINE
POW,PO, 100 gm.........88395-0069-35 27.75 55.50
SHARK CARTILAGE (ADH)
CAP,PO, 740 mg, 60s ea...60142-0092-06 9.98 19.95
(Nature's Bounty)
CAP,PO (30 TABLETS FREE,SF)
740 mg, 30s ea......74312-0065-81 11.69
(Progressive Labs.)
CAP,PO, 750 mg, 100s ea..51821-0482-01 12.50 25.00
300s ea...........51821-0483-01 35.00 70.00
SHARK EDGE (Health Products Corp)
CAP,PO (PF,SF)
750 mg, 30s ea......39686-0016-06 7.00
SHARK FIN CARTILAGE (Mason Vit)
CAP,PO, 500 mg, 30s ea...11845-0099-18 7.22
50s ea............11845-0099-19 12.22
(PF,SF)
740 mg, 30s ea......11845-0119-08 7.78

PROD/MFR | HRI, UPC,NDC | AWP | SRP

SHARK LIVER OIL (Scandinavian)
CAP,PO (GELCAP)
250 mg, 60s ea......51137-0060-20 9.57 15.95
120s ea...........51137-0060-22 17.97 29.95
(PF,DYE-FREE,GELCAP)
500 mg, 120s ea.....51137-0000-24 23.97 39.95
SHARPS DISPOSAL BY MAIL SYSTEM (Sharps)
DEV,NA (1 GALLON)
ea................08568-0011-00 44.00
(1 QUART)
ea................08568-0001-12 10.00
ea................08568-0010-10 29.00
(2 GALLON)
ea................08568-0012-00 54.00
(3 GALLON)
ea................08568-0010-03 77.00
(2X2 GALLON)
2s ea.............08568-0012-02 106.38
(3X1 GALLON)
3s ea.............08568-0012-27 99.00
SHEER STRIPS (AmerisourceBergen)
DEV,NA (EXTRA LARGE)
10s ea............24385-0180-10 1.79 1.99
(ASSORTED,PRIVATE LABEL)
60s ea............24385-0166-72 1.69 1.79
SHEPARD'S (Dermik)
LOT,TP, 240 ml.........00066-0105-66 19.54
480 ml............00066-0105-74 37.33
SHERI-B-12 (Poly)
LIQ,PO (CHERRY)
480 ml............50991-0022-16 19.50
SHIELD SKIN (Mentor)
PAD,TP, 50s ea.........81317-0440-05 7.71
SHOP RITE TEST STRIPS (Home Diag)
DEV,NA (PRESTIGE SMART SYSTEM)
50s ea............56151-0324-50 28.60
100s ea...........56151-0324-01 45.99
SHOWER TO SHOWER BREEZE FRESH (Johnson & Johnson)
POW,TP (1X368GM)
368 gm............81370-0009-17 3.60
SHOWER TO SHOWER ISLAND FRESH (Johnson & Johnson)
POW,TP (1X226GM)
226 gm............81370-0007-68 2.51
(1X368GM)
368 gm............81370-0007-11 3.60
SHOWER TO SHOWER MORNING FRESH (Johnson & Johnson)
POW,TP (1X28GM)
28 gm.............81370-0009-30 0.58
(1X368GM)
226 gm............81370-0007-38 2.51
368 gm............81370-0007-43 3.60
SHOWER TO SHOWER ORIGINAL FRESH (Johnson & Johnson)
POW,TP (1X226GM)
226 gm............81370-0007-08 2.51
(1X368GM)
368 gm............81370-0007-13 3.60
SHOWER TO SHOWER SHIMMER EFFECTS (Johnson & Johnson)
POW,TP (1X368GM)
368 gm............81370-0009-73 3.60
SHOWER TO SHOWER SPORT (Johnson & Johnson)
POW,TP (1X226GM)
226 gm............81370-0009-64 2.51
(1X368GM)
368 gm............81370-0009-63 3.60
SHOWER-PAK PLASTIC POUCHES (Medtronic Minimed)
DEV,NA (SINGLE USE)
30s ea............76300-0117-30 27.60
SIDEKICK BLOOD GLUCOSE METER (Home Diag)
DEV,NA, ea.............56151-0880-50 35.38
SIGHT SAVERS LENS CLEANER (Bausch & Lomb Inc.)
SPR,NA, 15 ml..........10119-0430-02 0.96
SIGHT SAVERS LENS CLEANER/CLOTH (Bausch & Lomb Inc.)
KIT,NA (W/SPRAY)
ea................10119-0815-01 2.27
SIGHT SAVERS LENS CLEANING CLOTHS (Bausch & Lomb Inc.)
PAD,NA (DISPOSABLE,2 BKLT/24EA)
48s ea............10119-0430-20 0.66

PROD/MFR | HRI, UPC,NDC | AWP | SRP

SIGHT SAVERS LENS CLEANING TISSUES
(Bausch & Lomb Inc.)
PAD,NA (PRE-MOISTENED)
14s ea.............. **10119-0415-02** 1.01

SIGNA PAD (Parker)
DEV,NA (400 ELECTRODE PAD DISP.)
20s ea.............. **00341-0016-40** 195.00 310.00

SIGNACREME (Parker)
CRE,TP (12X142GM)
142 gm 12s.......... **00341-0017-05** 22.03 36.70
(W/DISPENSER&PUMP)
1900 ml............ **00341-0017-20** 15.30 25.50

SIGNAGEL (Parker)
GEL,TP (12X60GM)
60 gm 12s.......... **00341-0015-60** 12.96 21.60
(12X250GM)
250 gm 12s.......... **00341-0015-25** 23.53 39.20

SIGNAL 369 (Green Turtle)
SGL,PO (PF,SF,DYE-FREE,SOFTGEL)
90s ea.............. **59074-0700-01** 21.00 35.00

SIGNASPRAY (Parker)
LIQ,TP (W/DISPENSER)
3840 ml............ **00341-0018-28** 23.40 39.00
(2 SPR/DISP PUMP)
3840 ml 4s.......... **00341-0018-04** 84.00 140.00
SPR,TP, 250 ml 12s...... **00341-0018-25** 36.00 60.00

SIGTAB (Lee Pharm)
TAB,PO, 90s ea.......... **23558-0560-80** 42.00
500s ea.......... **23558-0560-82** 198.00

(Phys Total Care)
REPACK
TAB,PO, 90s ea.......... **54868-0771-00** 74.41

SILACE (Silarx)
LIQ,PO, 150 mg/15 ml,
473 ml.......... **54838-0116-80** 15.99
SYR,PO, 60 mg/15 ml,
473 ml.......... **54838-0107-80** 6.70

SILADRYL ALLERGY (Silarx)
SOL,PO (LIQUID MEDICATION,AF,SF)
12.5 mg/5 ml,
118 ml.......... **54838-0135-40** 2.45
237 ml.......... **54838-0135-70** 3.52
(AF,SF)
12.5 mg/5 ml, 473 ml. **54838-0135-80** 6.65

SILAFED (Silarx)
SYR,PO, 30 mg/5 ml-1.25 mg/5 ml,
118 ml.......... **54838-0101-40** 3.15
237 ml.......... **54838-0101-70** 5.59

SILAPAP CHILDREN'S (Silarx)
ELI,PO, 160 mg/5 ml,
118 ml.......... **54838-0144-40** 2.50
237 ml.......... **54838-0144-70** 3.75
473 ml.......... **54838-0144-80** 7.95

(Physician Partner)
REPACK
ELI,PO (1X120ML)
160 mg/5 ml,
120 ml.......... **21695-0244-04** 5.25

SILAPAP INFANT'S (Silarx)
SOL,PO (DROPS)
80 mg/0.8 ml,
15 ml.......... **54838-0145-15** 2.50
(AF,DROPS)
80 mg/0.8 ml,
30 ml.......... **54838-0145-30** 4.85

SILFEDRINE CHILDREN'S (Silarx)
LIQ,PO (GRAPE)
15 mg/5 ml, 118 ml .. **54838-0104-40** 2.30
237 ml.......... **54838-0104-70** 4.10

SILICA (Freeda)
TAB,PO (PF,SF,DYE-FREE)
25 mg, 100s ea...... **10432-0264-01** 7.47 12.45
250s ea.......... **10432-0264-02** 14.94 24.90

SILICEA (Hyland's)
TAB,PO, 1000s ea.......... **54973-1065-02** 10.49 17.49

SILICIA (Nuage Labs)
TAB,SL (6X)
125s ea.......... **00634-8081-68** 3.05 5.09

SILPHEN (Silarx)
SYR,PO, 12.5 mg/5 ml,
118 ml.......... **54838-0154-40** 2.50
237 ml.......... **54838-0154-70** 3.60
473 ml.......... **54838-0154-80** 6.70

PROD/MFR | HRI, UPC,NDC | AWP | SRP

SILPHEN DM (Silarx)
SYR,PO, 10 mg/5 ml,
118 ml.......... **54838-0105-40** 2.59

SILTUSSIN DAS (Silarx)
LIQ,PO (AF,SF,DYE-FREE)
100 mg/5 ml,
118 ml.......... **54838-0130-40** 2.49

SILTUSSIN DM (Silarx)
SYR,PO, 10 mg/5 ml-100 mg/5 ml,
118 ml.......... **54838-0209-40** 2.60
237 ml.......... **54838-0209-70** 4.75
473 ml.......... **54838-0209-80** 7.90

SILTUSSIN DM DAS COUGH FORMULA (Silarx)
SYR,PO (AF,SF,DYE-FREE)
10 mg/5 ml-100 mg/5 ml,
118 ml.......... **54838-0133-40** 3.10

SILTUSSIN SA (Silarx)
SYR,PO (AF,SF)
100 mg/5 ml,
118 ml.......... **54838-0117-40** 1.90
237 ml.......... **54838-0117-70** 3.70
473 ml.......... **54838-0117-80** 6.30

SILVASORB (Medline)
DRE,TP (SR,4.25"X4.25")
25s ea.......... **53329-0310-94** 392.27
(SR,4"X10",LATEX-FREE)
25s ea.......... **08327-0310-98** 892.28
(SR,SUPERABSORBENT,2"X2")
25s ea.......... **53329-0310-89** 212.73
(SR,SUPERABSORBENT,4"X8")
25s ea.......... **53329-0310-37** 713.82
(SRPERFORATED4.25"X4.25")
25s ea.......... **53329-0311-94** 362.00

SILVASORB ANTIMICROBIAL WOUND GEL (Medline)
GEL,TP (SUSTAINED-RELEASE)
6s ea.......... **08327-0309-08** 475.00
8s ea.......... **08327-0309-06** 1021.25
(LATEX-FREE)
45 ml 12s.......... **08327-0309-09** 269.10

SILVASORB CAVITY (Medline)
DRE,TP (LATEX-FREE)
40s ea.......... **08327-0312-76** 598.91

SILVER WING DELUXE (PHR)
DEV,NA (NOSE-EAR HAIR TRIMMER)
ea.......... **44582-0200-00** 4.98 9.95

SILVERMED ANTIMICROBIAL HYDROGEL
(MPM Medical Inc.)
GEL,TP, 44 ml.......... **66977-0140-15** 25.59 28.44
89 ml.......... **66977-0140-03** 51.22 56.91

SILVERMED ANTIMICROBIAL WOUND CLEANSER
(MPM Medical Inc.)
SPR,TP, 240 ml.......... **66977-0141-08** 17.69 19.66

SILYMARIN (Neurovites)
CRE,TP, 10%, 30 gm...... **93595-2042-01** 18.60 31.00

SIMEPED (Kramer-Novis)
SUS,PO (DROPS)
40 mg/0.6 ml,
30 ml.......... **52083-0517-01** 9.20

SIMETHICONE (Advance)
CTB,PO, 80 mg, 100s ea... **17714-0019-01** 2.99

(Carolina)
SUS,PO (DROPS)
40 mg/0.6 ml,
30 ml 12s.......... **46287-0506-30** 85.20

(Marlex)
CTB,PO, 80 mg, 24s ea.... **10135-0203-24** 1.20
90s ea.......... **10135-0203-90** 2.10
100s ea.......... **10135-0203-01** 2.00
(BLISTER PACK)
80 mg, 100s ea UD... **10135-0203-13** 7.11
150s ea.......... **10135-0203-64** 3.00

(Qualitest)
SUS,PO (DROPS)
40 mg/0.6 ml, 30 ml.. **00603-0894-50** 5.94

(R.I.J.)
SUS,PO (DROPS)
40 mg/0.6 ml, 30 ml.. **53807-0162-01** 6.30

(Rugby)
CTB,PO (PEPPERMINT)
80 mg, 100s ea...... **00536-4533-01** 6.30
125 mg, 60s ea...... **00536-4534-08** 5.02
SUS,PO (STRAWBERRY,DROPS)
40 mg/0.6 ml, 30 ml.. **00536-2220-75** 7.05

PROD/MFR | HRI, UPC,NDC | AWP | SRP

(Teva)
CTB,PO (10X10)
80 mg, 100s ea UD... **00182-8643-89** 17.99

(A-S Medication)
REPACK
CTB,PO, 80 mg, 15s ea.... **54569-2163-02** 0.69
30s ea.......... **54569-2163-03** 1.39

(McKesson Packaging)
REPACK
CTB,PO, 80 mg,
100s ea UD.......... **63739-0225-10** 8.93

(Physician Partner)
REPACK
CTB,PO (PEPPERMINT)
125 mg, 50s ea...... **21695-0482-50** 18.37
100s ea.......... **21695-0482-00** 26.74

(Southwood)
REPACK
SUS,PO (DROPS)
20 mg/0.3 ml,
30 ml.......... **58016-4820-01** 2.33

SIMETHICONE INFANTS' (Cardinal Health)
SUS,PO (PRIVATE LABEL,DROPS)
40 mg/0.6 ml, 30 ml.. **37205-0119-10** 4.48

SIMETHICONE MAXIMUM STRENGTH (Advance)
CTB,PO, 125 mg, 60s ea... **17714-0040-60** 3.99

SIMILAC 2 ADVANCE (Abbott)
PDR,PO (MILK-BASED W/IRON)
365 gm.......... **70074-0577-10** 15.49
728 gm.......... **70074-0577-08** 30.88

SIMILAC 2 W/IRON (Ross Nutr)
PDR,PO, 850 gm.......... **70074-0555-07** 28.82

SIMILAC ADVANCE EARLYSHIELD (Abbott)
PDR,PO, 658 gm.......... **70074-0533-60** 30.80

SIMILAC ADVANCE W/IRON (Abbott)
LIQ,PO (RTF)
59 ml 8s.......... **70074-0576-01** 8.80
(RTF,6X118ML)
118 ml 6s.......... **70074-0577-16** 12.32
(RTF,6X237ML)
237 ml 6s.......... **70074-0575-19** 12.90
(CL)
384 ml.......... **70074-0569-74** 5.35
(RTF)
946 ml.......... **70074-0559-62** 8.12
PDR,PO (POWDER PACKET SINGLES)
17 gm 16s.......... **70074-0579-39** 11.06
365 gm.......... **70074-0559-58** 15.49
728 gm.......... **70074-0559-60** 30.88

SIMILAC ALIMENTUM ADVANCE W/IRON (Abbott)
LIQ,PO (RTF)
237 ml.......... **70074-0575-09** 2.84
946 ml.......... **70074-0575-13** 11.22

SIMILAC ALIMENTUM WITH IRON (Abbott)
PDR,PO (HYPOALLERGENIC FORMULA)
454 gm.......... **70074-0576-64** 33.13

SIMILAC HUMAN MILK FORTIFIER (Abbott)
PKT,PO, 50s ea.......... **70074-0545-99** 62.40

SIMILAC ISOMIL 2 ADVANCE (Abbott)
PDR,PO (SOY W/IRON,DAIRY-FREE)
365 gm.......... **70074-0577-14** 16.48
728 gm.......... **70074-0577-12** 31.94

SIMILAC ISOMIL ADVANCE SOY W/IRON (Abbott)
LIQ,PO (RTF,LACTOSE-FREE)
59 ml.......... **70074-0569-80** 2.47
237 ml 6s.......... **70074-0575-32** 8.60
(READY TO EAT)
946 ml.......... **70074-0559-68** 8.32
PDR,PO (POWDER PACKET SINGLES)
17.4 gm 16s.......... **70074-0569-83** 11.06
(LACTOSE-FREE)
365 gm.......... **70074-0559-64** 16.48
727 gm.......... **70074-0559-66** 31.94

SIMILAC ISOMIL SOY W/IRON (Abbott)
PDR,PO (PACKET,8X30.1GM)
30.1 gm 8s.......... **70074-0547-47** 10.75
365 gm.......... **70074-0577-63** 15.35

PROD/MFR	HRI, UPC,NDC	AWP	SRP
SIMILAC LOW-IRON (Abbott)			
LIQ,PO (RTF,PLASTIC BOTTLE)			
960 ml	70074-0514-77	8.15	
PDR,PO, 365 gm	70074-0578-38	14.84	
SIMILAC NEOSURE ADVANCE W/IRON (Abbott)			
LIQ,PO (RTF)			
118 ml 6s	70074-0579-49	16.62	
118 ml 12s	70074-0518-49	26.90	
(READY TO FEED)			
946 ml	70074-0574-56	9.25	
PDR,PO, 363 gm	70074-0574-31	18.62	
SIMILAC NEOSURE WITH IRON 22 (Abbott)			
LIQ,PO (8X59ML)			
59 ml 8s	70074-0596-46	13.69	
SIMILAC PM 60/40 (Abbott)			
PDR,PO, 480 gm	70074-0608-50	19.20	
SIMILAC SENSITIVE (Abbott)			
LIQ,PO (CONCENTRATED LIQUID)			
390 ml	70074-0575-36	6.28	
(RTF,LACTOSE-FREE)			
946 ml	70074-0575-34	8.62	
PDR,PO (LACTOSE-FREE)			
365 gm	70074-0575-41	18.08	
728 gm	70074-0575-44	34.54	
SIMILAC SENSITIVE RS (Abbott)			
LIQ,PO (LACTOSE-FREE)			
946 ml	70074-0567-31	8.36	
SIMILAC SPECIAL CARE W/IRON 24 (Abbott)			
LIQ,PO (PREMATURE INFANT)			
120 ml 6s	70074-0802-14	15.19	
SIMILAC SPECIAL CARE WITH IRON 24 (Abbott)			
LIQ,PO (8X59ML)			
59 ml 8s	70074-0595-83	13.81	
SIMILAC W/IRON (Abbott)			
LIQ,PO, 390 ml	70074-0404-14	5.30	
(RTF)			
960 ml	70074-0514-79	7.69	
PDR,PO, 365 gm	70074-0577-61	14.72	
728 gm	70074-0578-31	27.68	
SIMPLICITY ADULT BRIEFS (Covidien)			
DEV,NA (EXTRA LARGE,3D)			
60s ea	08080-6301-05	43.63	
(LARGE,3D,LATEX-FREE)			
72s ea	08080-6301-04	44.88	
(MEDIUM,3D,LATEX-FREE)			
96s ea	08080-6301-03	43.40	
SIMPLICITY COTTON/POLY SNAP PANTS (Covidien)			
DEV,NA (LARGE,BLUE,36"-40")			
12s ea	08080-6940-01	101.33	
(MEDIUM,WHITE,30"-34")			
12s ea	08080-6910-01	101.33	
(SMALL,RED,24"-28")			
12s ea	08080-6890-01	101.33	
(X-LARGE,GREEN,42"-48")			
12s ea	08080-6980-01	101.33	
(XX-LARGE,BLACK,50"-54")			
12s ea	08080-6990-01	101.33	
SIMPLICITY DISPOSABLE UNDERPADS (Covidien)			
DEV,NA (30"X36")			
100s ea	08080-7157-01	30.68	
(23"X36",5X30)			
150s ea	08080-1505-02	46.89	
(30"X30",5X30)			
150s ea	08080-3030-05	48.94	
SIMPLICITY PLUS (Covidien)			
DEV,NA (EXTRA LARGE)			
60s ea	08080-6302-50	33.20	
SIMPLICITY PLUS ADULT BRIEF (Covidien)			
DEV,NA (3D,LARGE)			
72s ea	08080-6302-40	35.70	
(3D,MEDIUM)			
96s ea	08080-6302-30	35.70	
SIMPLY SALINE (Blairex)			
SPR,NS (PF)			
0.9%, 44 ml	50486-0291-57	4.22	
SIMPLY SLEEP (McNeil Consumer Healthcare)			
TAB,PO (CAPLET)			
25 mg, 24s ea	00450-0843-24	3.88	
24s ea	50580-0843-24	3.88	
48s ea	00450-0843-48	6.62	
48s ea	50580-0843-48	6.62	
72s ea	50580-0843-72	9.01	
100s ea	00450-0843-10	10.99	
100s ea	50580-0843-10	10.99	
SINADRIN PE (Reese)			
TAB,PO (CAPLET)			
650 mg-2 mg-10 mg, 30s ea	10956-0793-30	4.92	7.49
SINE-OFF (Hogil)			
TAB,PO (CAPLET)			
500 mg-2 mg-30 mg, 24s ea	95814-0270-24	3.59	3.85
SINE-OFF MAXIMUM STRENGTH (Hogil)			
TAB,PO (NON-DROWSY,CAPLET)			
500 mg-30 mg, 24s ea	95814-0269-20	3.59	
SINGLE-LET DISPOSABLE LANCETS (Bayer Diabetes Care)			
DEV,NA, 200s ea	01936-0568-31	39.29	
SINUS RELIEF (Similasan Corp.)			
SPR,NS, 6 x-6 x-6 x, 15 ml	59262-0248-21	6.21	10.99
SINUS TABLETS NO DROWSINESS (Basic Vitamins)			
TAB,PO, 325 mg-30 mg, 50s ea	00761-0674-10	1.80	
SINUS/ALLERGY FORMULA (Weleda)			
GRA,PO, 4 gm	55946-0154-61	2.97	
SINUSALIA (Boiron)			
PEL,PO, 3 x-3 x-3 x, 80s ea	06962-0013-03	3.87	6.49
TAB,PO, 3 x-3 x-3 x, 60s ea	06962-0613-60	5.73	9.59
SINUTAB SINUS (McNeil Consumer Healthcare)			
TAB,PO (NON-DROWSY)			
325 mg-5 mg, 24s ea	12547-0364-75	4.49	
SKEETER STIK (Triton Consumer Prod)			
LIQ,TP, 5%-1%, 14 ml	79511-0100-03	1.44	
SKIN ANSWER (Lane Labs)			
CRE,TP, 15 gm	02110-2071-64	22.05	49.00
SKIN BARRIER (Coloplast)			
DEV,NA (6"X6")			
3s ea	11701-0800-90	31.62	33.09
(8"X8")			
3s ea	11701-0800-91	52.05	54.48
(4"X4")			
5s ea	11701-0800-80	21.65	22.70
SKIN BARRIER FLANGE W/SECURELIFE + (Coloplast)			
DEV,NA (W/TAPE, UP TO 1-1/4")			
5s ea	11701-0810-10	28.70	30.05
(W/TAPE, UP TO 1-3/4")			
5s ea	11701-0810-15	28.70	30.05
(W/TAPE, UP TO 2")			
5s ea	11701-0810-20	28.70	30.05
SKIN BARRIER RINGS (Coloplast)			
DEV,NA (1-1/8")			
30s ea	11701-0802-30	71.10	74.40
(1-5/8")			
30s ea	11701-0802-40	71.10	74.40
(1")			
30s ea	11701-0802-25	71.10	74.40
(2")			
30s ea	11701-0802-50	71.10	74.40
(3/4")			
30s ea	11701-0802-20	71.10	74.40
(3/8")			
30s ea	11701-0802-10	71.10	74.40
(5/8")			
30s ea	11701-0802-15	71.10	74.40
SKIN CARE (Mentor)			
KIT,TP, ea	81317-0020-02	28.01	
SKIN SHIELD (Del)			
LIQ,TP, 0.2%-0.75%, 13.5 ml	10310-0293-45	2.52	3.78
SKIN-PREP (Smith & Nephew)			
SPR,TP, 118 ml	40565-0111-84	11.91	9.53
SWA,TP, 50s ea	40565-0115-67	26.15	20.92
SKIN-PREP WIPES (Smith & Nephew)			
PAD,TP, 50s ea	40565-0114-52	9.73	7.78
SKINTEGRITY (Medline)			
SPR,TP, 237 ml 6s	53329-0003-08	42.55	
473 ml 6s	53329-0003-06	41.25	
SKINTEGRITY HYDROGEL (Medline)			
DEV,NA (STERILE, 4"X4")			
ea	08327-0487-33	26.25	
(STERILE,"2X2")			
ea	08327-0487-88	47.45	
(4OZ)			
12s ea	53329-0001-04	81.23	
(1OZ)			
30s ea	53329-0001-03	44.60	
(4"X4", 12-PLY)			
30s ea	53329-0600-40	96.85	
(2X2)			
50s ea	08327-0487-89	38.39	
SKULLCAP (Botanical Labs.)			
LIQ,PO, 30 ml	41954-0020-45	3.75	7.49
SLEEP AID (AmerisourceBergen)			
TAB,PO (PRIVATE LABEL)			
25 mg, 32s ea	24385-0441-64	6.20	6.89
(Cardinal Health)			
TAB,PO (PRIVATE LABEL)			
25 mg, 32s ea	37205-0121-64	5.82	
SLEEP AND GET TRIM (Health Products Corp)			
TAB,PO, 60s ea	39686-0015-13	4.50	
SLEEP FORMULA (Albertson's)			
TAB,PO, 25 mg, 72s ea	41280-0220-59	2.72	
SLEEP TABLETS (AmerisourceBergen)			
TAB,PO (PRIVATE LABEL)			
25 mg, 16s ea	24385-0406-73	1.88	2.79
SLEEP TABS (Major)			
TAB,PO, 25 mg, 50s ea	00904-4274-51	3.99	
SLEEP TONITE (Basic Vitamins)			
TAB,PO (CAPLET)			
60s ea	00761-0441-10	3.00	
SLEEP-ETTES D (Reese)			
TAB,PO, 50 mg, 24s ea	10956-0750-24	3.69	
(NIGHTTIME SLEEP AID)			
50 mg, 24s ea	10956-0750-26	3.94	
48s ea	10956-0750-48	5.23	
SLEEP-TABS (Magno-Humphries)			
TAB,PO, 25 mg, 36s ea	43292-0557-19	1.32	2.59
100s ea	43292-0557-78	2.06	3.99
SLEEPINAL (Blairex)			
CAP,PO, 50 mg, 16s ea	50486-0616-16	2.78	
32s ea	50486-0616-32	5.70	
SLEEPLESSNESS RELIEF (Similasan Corp.)			
PEL,PO (1X15GM)			
12 x-12 x-15 x-12 x, 15 gm	59262-0601-30	6.21	10.99
SLENDER-MIST (Mayor Pharma Labs)			
SPR,PO (ARCTICMINT)			
13.5 ml	45601-0004-30	10.80	15.96
(BERRY SUPREME)			
13.5 ml	45601-0004-50	10.80	15.96
(CHOCOLATE FUDGE)			
13.5 ml	45601-0004-20	10.80	15.96
(TROPICAL DELITE)			
13.5 ml	45601-0004-40	10.80	15.96
SLIM W/FIBER (Nature's Bounty)			
TAB,PO, 120s ea	74312-0041-22		5.65
SLO-NIACIN (Upsher-Smith)			
TER,PO (CAPLET)			
250 mg, 100s ea	00245-0062-11	9.11	
TANNICUM ACIDUM			
PO, 250s ea	54973-9015-01	4.37	7.29
TARENTULA CUBENSIS			
PO, 250s ea	54973-9018-01	4.37	7.29
TARENTULA HISPANA			
PO, 250s ea	54973-9019-01	4.37	7.29
TAXUS BACCATA			
PO, 250s ea	54973-9022-01	4.37	7.29
TELLURIUM METALLICUM			
PO, 250s ea	54973-9025-01	4.37	7.29
TEREBINTHINA			
PO, 250s ea	54973-0902-01	4.37	7.29
THALLIUM METALLICUM			
PO, 250s ea	54973-9034-01	4.37	7.29
THIOSINAMINUM			
PO, 250s ea	54973-9041-01	4.37	7.29
THUJA OGR			
PO, 250s ea	54973-9045-01	4.37	7.29
THYMOLUM			
PO, 250s ea	54973-9046-01	4.37	7.29
THYMUS SERP			
PO, 250s ea	54973-9047-01	4.37	7.29
TITANIUM METALLICUM			
PO, 250s ea	54973-9051-01	4.37	7.29
TOXICOPHIS PUGNAX			
PO, 250s ea	54973-9054-01	4.37	7.29
TRIFOLIUM PRAT			
PO, 250s ea	54973-9062-01	4.37	7.29
TRILLIUM REND			
PO, 250s ea	54973-9067-01	4.37	7.29
TRIOSTEUM PERF			
PO, 250s ea	54973-9071-01	4.37	7.29
TUBERCULINUM			
PO, 250s ea	54973-9076-01	4.37	7.29

PROD/MFR	HRI, UPC,NDC	AWP	SRP
USTILAGO MAIDIS			
PO, 250s ea	54973-9227-01	4.37	7.29
VANADIUM METALLICUM			
PO, 250s ea	54973-9414-01	4.37	7.29
VERATRUM ALBUM			
PO, 250s ea	54973-9420-01	4.37	7.29
VERATRUM VIRIDE			
PO, 250s ea	54973-9422-01	4.37	7.29
VESPA CRAB			
PO, 250s ea	54973-9427-01	4.37	7.29
VIBURNUM OP			
PO, 250s ea	54973-9429-01	4.37	7.29
VINCA MINOR			
PO, 250s ea	54973-9433-01	4.37	7.29
VISCUM ALBUM			
PO, 250s ea	54973-9444-01	4.37	7.29
X-RAY			
PO, 250s ea	54973-9714-01	4.37	7.29
YOHIMBINUM			
PO, 250s ea	54973-9716-01	4.37	7.29
ZINCUM CARBONICUM			
PO, 250s ea	54973-9828-01	4.37	7.29
ZINCUM IODATUM			
PO, 250s ea	54973-9818-01	4.37	7.29
ZINCUM METALLICUM			
PO, 250s ea	54973-9819-01	4.37	7.29
ZINCUM MURIATICUM			
PO, 250s ea	54973-9820-01	4.37	7.29
ZINCUM PHOSPHORATUM			
PO, 250s ea	54973-9822-01	4.37	7.29
ZINCUM PICRICUM			
PO, 250s ea	54973-9823-01	4.37	7.29
ZINCUM SULFURICUM			
PO, 250s ea	54973-9824-01	4.37	7.29
ZINCUM VALERIANICUM			
PO, 250s ea	54973-9825-01	4.37	7.29
SLO-NIACIN (Upsher-Smith)			
TER,PO (CAPLET)			
500 mg, 100s ea	00245-0063-11	13.93	
750 mg, 100s ea	00245-0064-11	18.54	
SLOAN'S LINIMENT (Lee Pharm)			
LIQ,TP, 0.025%-47%,			
120 ml	23558-0682-90	3.72	
120 ml 12s	23558-0682-91	44.64	
SLOW FE (Novartis Consumer)			
TAB,PO (SLOW RELEASE)			
45 mg, 30s ea	00674-0347-30	8.24	
60s ea	00674-0347-60	13.97	
90s ea	00674-0347-90	20.86	
TER,PO (BLISTER PACK)			
160 mg, 30s ea	00083-0125-47	8.24	
60s ea	00083-0125-74	13.97	
90s ea	00083-0125-75	20.86	
(Phys Total Care)			
REPACK			
TER,PO, 160 mg, 30s ea	54868-4513-00	10.78	
SLOW RELEASE IRON (Teva)			
TER,PO (BLISTER PACK)			
160 mg, 90s ea	00182-4476-29	12.99	
SLOW-MAG (Purdue Products L.P.)			
ECT,PO, 106 mg-186.5 mg-64 mg,			
60s ea	67618-0107-60	9.95	
(Phys Total Care)			
REPACK			
ECT,PO, 106 mg-186.5 mg-64 mg,			
60s ea	54868-2259-00	13.03	
SM CALCIUM CITRATE + D (McKesson)			
TAB,PO (PRIVATE LABEL,CAPLET)			
315 mg-200 iu, 60s ea	49348-0324-12	5.59	
SMALL DRAINABLE POUCH ONE PIECE (Coloplast)			
DEV,NA (OPAQUE, 1-1/8")			
10s ea	11701-0808-21	42.70	44.60
(OPAQUE, 1-3/8")			
10s ea	11701-0808-22	42.70	44.60
(OPAQUE, 1-5/8")			
10s ea	11701-0808-23	42.70	44.60
(OPAQUE, 1")			
10s ea	11701-0808-20	42.70	44.60
(OPAQUE, 1/2"-1-1/4")			
10s ea	11701-0808-17	42.70	44.60
10s ea	11701-0808-18	42.70	44.60
(OPAQUE, 3/4")			
10s ea	11701-0808-19	42.70	44.60
(TRANSPARENT, 1-1/8")			
10s ea	11701-0808-14	42.70	44.60
(TRANSPARENT, 1-3/8")			
10s ea	11701-0808-15	42.70	
(TRANSPARENT, 1-5/8")			
10s ea	11701-0808-16	42.70	44.60
(TRANSPARENT, 1")			
10s ea	11701-0808-13	42.70	44.60
(TRANSPARENT, 3/4")			
10s ea	11701-0808-12	42.70	44.60
(TRANSPARENT,1/2"-1-1/4")			
10s ea	11701-0808-10	42.70	44.60
10s ea	11701-0808-11	42.70	44.60
SMALL DRAINABLE POUCH TWO PIECE (Coloplast)			
DEV,NA (OPAQUE, UP TO 1-1/2")			
10s ea	11701-0813-10	28.70	30.10
(OPAQUE, UP TO 1-3/4")			
10s ea	11701-0813-15	28.70	30.10
(OPAQUE, UP TO 2")			
10s ea	11701-0813-20	28.70	30.10
SMARTEST CONTROL SOLUTION (Progressive)			
DEV,NA (MEDIUM)			
3 ml	08524-0002-01	15.00	
SMARTEST LANCET (Progressive)			
DEV,NA, 50s ea	08524-0004-03	11.00	
SMARTEST TEST STRIPS (Progressive)			
DEV,NA, 50s ea	08521-0001-03	37.00	
SMARTEST-EJECT METER (Progressive)			
DEV,NA, ea	08524-0012-01	30.00	
SMARTEST-EJECT STARTER KIT (Progressive)			
DEV,NA; ea	08524-0022-01	45.00	
SMARTEST-PROTEGE METER (Progressive)			
DEV,NA, ea	08524-0013-01	30.00	
SMARTEST-PROTEGE STARTER KIT (Progressive)			
DEV,NA, ea	08524-0023-01	45.00	
SMILAX (Botanical Labs.)			
LIQ,PO, 30 ml	41954-0020-49	3.75	7.49
60 ml	41954-0020-20	6.00	11.99
SMOKER (Health Products Corp)			
TAB,PO (PF,SF)			
250 mg-200 iu, 60s ea	39686-0014-87	4.78	
SMOKERS BREATH-AIDE (Parnell)			
SPR,MM, 60 ml	50930-0095-02	15.00	19.95
SNAP LOCK (Abbott Hosp)			
DEV,NA, 800s ea	00074-8076-01	336.00	
SNORENZ (Med Gen Inc)			
LIQ,PO (REFILL,PF,MINT)			
120 ml	32246-0202-04	8.40	14.95
SPR,MM (PF,MINT)			
60 ml	32246-0202-02	5.20	9.95
SNUG (Mentholatum)			
DEV,NA (2 DENTURE CUSHIONS)			
ea	10742-0000-61	3.11	2.29
SOCHLOR (Ocusoft)			
OIN,OP, 5%, 3.5 gm	54799-0926-35	12.81	
SOL,OP (HYPERTONIC)			
5%, 15 ml	54799-0925-15	14.38	
SOD (Bio-Tech Pharm)			
CAP,PO, 1000 iu-2000 iu,			
100s ea	53191-0373-01	5.25	
SOD-K (Key Company)			
TAB,PO, 0.125 mg,			
100s ea	11694-0852-01	5.50	
SODIUM BICARBONATE (Consolidated Midland)			
TAB,PO, 325 mg, 100s ea	00223-1720-01	5.00	
1000s ea	00223-1720-02	45.00	
650 mg, 100s ea	00223-1721-01	5.50	
1000s ea	00223-1721-02	50.00	
(Rugby)			
TAB,PO, 325 mg,			
1000s ea	00536-4540-10	11.55	
650 mg, 1000s ea	00536-4544-10	13.65	
(United Research)			
TAB,PO, 650 mg,			
1000s ea	00677-0131-10	13.36	
(Phys Total Care)			
REPACK			
TAB,PO, 325 mg, 100s ea	54868-5923-00	25.15	
648 mg, 100s ea	54868-3193-00	25.32	
(Southwood)			
REPACK			
TAB,PO, 325 mg, 30s ea	58016-0055-30	11.55	
60s ea	58016-0055-60	23.10	
90s ea	58016-0055-90	34.65	
100s ea	58016-0055-00	38.50	
SODIUM BICARBONATE POTASSIUM BICARBONATE COMBINATION (Bio-Tech Pharm)			
CAP,PO, 125 mg-88 mg,			
100s ea	53191-0273-01	7.25	
SODIUM CHLORIDE (Akorn)			
OIN,OP (PF)			
5%, 3.5 gm	17478-0622-35	12.11	
SOL,OP, 5%, 15 ml	17478-0623-12	12.11	
(Consolidated Midland)			
TAB,PO, 1 gm, 100s ea	00223-1760-01	5.50	
1000s ea	00223-1760-02	50.00	
(Dey, L.P.)			
SOL,IH, 0.9%,			
3 ml 100s UD	49502-0830-03	14.50	
5 ml 100s UD	49502-0830-05	14.50	
(S.D.V.,PF)			
0.9%, 15 ml 50s UD	49502-0830-50	14.50	
(Nephron)			
SOL,IH, 0.9%,			
3 ml 30s UD	00487-9301-33	4.80	
(ROBOT READY,30X3ML)			
0.9%, 3 ml 30s	00487-9301-02	8.44	
(VIAL)			
0.9%, 3 ml 100s UD	00487-9301-03	12.50	
(A-S Medication)			
REPACK			
SOL,IH, 0.9%,			
5 ml 100s UD	54569-3078-00	20.09	
(Phys Total Care)			
REPACK			
OIN,OP, 5%, 3.5 gm	54868-4698-00	44.04	
SOL,OP, 5%, 15 ml	54868-3293-00	40.78	
TAB,PO, 1 gm, 100s ea	54868-6058-00	45.12	
(Southwood)			
REPACK			
SOL,IH, 0.9%, 3 ml	58016-0603-01	5.27	
SODIUM CHLORIDE HYPERTONICITY (HUB Pharma)			
OIN,OP, 5%, 3.5 gm	17238-0620-35	11.25	
SOL,OP, 5%, 15 ml	17238-0625-15	10.94	
(Major)			
OIN,OP, 5%, 3.5 gm	00904-5315-38	14.75	
SOL,OP, 5%, 15 ml	00904-5314-35	14.75	
SODIUM CHLORIDE TABLETS (Lannett)			
TAB,PO, 1 gm, 1000s ea	00527-1116-10	107.94	
SODIUM FLUORIDE (Southwood)			
REPACK			
CRE,DE, 1.1%, 53.2 gm	58016-4821-01	7.99	
SODIUM SALICYLATE (Consolidated Midland)			
ECT,PO, 325 mg, 100s ea	00223-1821-01	5.75	
1000s ea	00223-1821-02	37.50	
650 mg, 100s ea	00223-1825-01	7.50	
1000s ea	00223-1825-02	44.50	
SOF-BAND BULKY NONSTERILE (J&J Medical)			
DEV,NA (4"X84",6-PLY)			
24s ea	56091-0069-74	15.54	
SOF-BAND BULKY STERILE (J&J Medical)			
DEV,NA (4"X84",6-PLY,TRAY)			
ea	56091-0069-54	1.92	
(4"X84",6-PLY,FLEX POUCH)			
24s ea	56091-0069-64	15.68	
SOF-FOAM HYDROPHILLIC POLYURETHANE (J&J Medical)			
DEV,NA (STERILE,3 1/8"X3 5/8")			
10s ea	56091-0025-93	18.20	
(STERILE,3"X3")			
10s ea	56091-0025-90	15.60	
(STERILE,4"X5")			
10s ea	56091-0025-91	20.80	
(STERILE,4"X8")			
10s ea	56091-0025-92	28.60	
SOF-KLING CONFORMING (J&J Medical)			
DEV,NA (BULK NS,6"X85",2-PLY)			
6s ea	56091-0069-86	5.16	
(BULK NS,2"X65",2-PLY)			
12s ea	56091-0069-82	3.38	
(BULK NS,3"X75",2-PLY)			
12s ea	56091-0069-83	4.59	
(BULK NS,4"X75",2-PLY)			
12s ea	56091-0069-84	6.60	
(STERILE,2"X65",2-PLY)			
12s ea	56091-0069-92	6.35	
(STERILE,3"X75",2-PLY)			
12s ea	56091-0069-93	8.47	
(STERILE,4"X75",2-PLY)			
12s ea	56091-0069-94	10.16	
(STERILE,6"X85",2-PLY)			
12s ea	56091-0069-96	15.05	
(STERILE,1"X60",2-PLY)			
18s ea	56091-0069-91	9.98	
(BULK NS,1"X60",2-PLY)			
24s ea	56091-0069-81	5.18	

PROD/MFR	HRI, UPC,NDC	AWP	SRP
SOF-LOOP FACE MASK (J&J Medical)			
DEV,NA (DESIGNER ANTI-FOG)			
ea	56091-0042-61	0.30	
(EXTRA PROTECTION PLUS)			
25s ea	56091-0042-67	26.00	
(EXTRA PROTECTION)			
50s ea	56091-0042-24	13.65	
SOF-TACT (Abbott)			
DEV,NA (STRIP)			
50s ea	57599-9586-04	49.68	
SOF-WICK DRAIN STERILE (J&J Medical)			
DEV,NA (4"X4",6-PLY,2X25)			
50s ea	56091-0023-91	10.77	
SOF-WICK DRESSING STERILE (J&J Medical)			
DEV,NA (4"X3",6-PLY,2X25)			
50s ea	56091-0023-70	6.50	
(4"X4",6-PLY,2X25)			
50s ea	56091-0023-75	7.74	
(2"X2",6-PLY,2X35)			
70s ea	56091-0023-74	6.10	
SOF-WICK IV STERILE (J&J Medical)			
DEV,NA (2"X2",6-PLY,2X35)			
70s ea	56091-0023-92	8.84	
SOFENOL 5 (Genesis)			
LOT,TP, 240 ml	00398-0090-08	6.66	
SOFLOOP FACE MASK (J&J Medical)			
DEV,NA (REGULAR)			
50s ea	56091-0042-28	8.58	
SOFNET CLEANERS (J&J Medical)			
DEV,NA (MEDIUM)			
30s ea	56091-0041-21	2.21	
(MEDIUM,BULK)			
200s ea	56091-0041-23	10.31	
SOFT TOUCH SAFE-T-STIX LANCETS (Roche Diag)			
DEV,NA, 200s ea	50924-0951-20	52.50	
SOFTDEN (Denison)			
LOT,TP, 180 ml	00295-1250-06	1.02	
SOFTLIPS FRENCH VANILLA (Mentholatum)			
STI,TP (SPF 20, BLISTER CARD,SF)			
2%-7.5%-3%-3%,			
2 gm	10742-0005-11	1.74	
SOFTLIPS ICED CAPPUCCINO (Mentholatum)			
STI,TP (SPF 20, BLISTER CARD,SF)			
2%-7.5%-3%-3%,			
2 gm	10742-0007-71	1.74	
SOFTLIPS LEMON SORBET (Mentholatum)			
STI,TP (SPF 20, BLISTER CARD,SF)			
2%-7.5%-3%-3%,			
2 gm	10742-0005-21	1.74	
SOFTLIPS LIP CONDITIONER (Mentholatum)			
STI,TP (SPF 20, SHEER COLOR,SF)			
2.1 gm	10742-0006-01	1.74	
SOFTLIPS LIP PROTECTANT (Mentholatum)			
STI,TP (SPF 20,SF,CHERRY)			
2%, 2.1 gm	10742-0004-51	1.74	
(SPF 20,SF,MINT)			
2%-5%, 2.1 gm	10742-0004-71	1.74	
SOFTLIPS NIGHTLY CARE EXFOLIATOR (Mentholatum)			
CRE,TP (BLISTERCARD)			
9 gm	10742-0007-01	2.10	
SOFTLIPS UNDERCOVER LIPSTICK PRIMER (Mentholatum)			
CRE,TP (BLISTERCARD)			
9 gm	10742-0006-11	2.10	
SOFTWEAR SALINE (Ciba Vision)			
SOL,NA, 120 ml	47113-0608-04	1.29	
240 ml	47113-0608-08	2.10	
360 ml	47113-0608-12	2.85	
SOLARCAINE COOL ALOE (Schering Plough)			
GEL,TP, 0.5%, 113 gm	41100-0090-55	4.20	
(ALOE EXTRA)			
0.5%, 226 gm	41100-0081-38	5.52	
SPR,TP, 0.5%, 127 ml	41100-0086-47	5.52	
SOLARCAINE FIRST AID (Schering Plough)			
SPR,TP, 20%-0.13%,			
85 gm	41100-0088-82	5.04	
SOLARTEK GLUCOSE CONTROL SOLUTIONS (Abbott)			
DEV,NA (1-LOW,1-HIGH)			
2s ea	66004-9874-01	8.28	
SOLBAR PF SPF30 (Person & Covey)			
LIQ,TP, 114 ml	00096-0685-04	6.54	
SOLBAR PF SPF50 (Person & Covey)			
CRE,TP, 120 gm	00096-0686-04	6.58	
SOLBAR SHIELD SUNSCREEN (Person & Covey)			
CRE,TP (UNSCENTED,SPF 40)			
5%-7.5%, 126 gm	00096-0682-04	6.99	
SOLBAR ZINC SPF38 (Person & Covey)			
CRE,TP, 10%-7.5%-7.5%,			
113 gm	00096-0688-04	6.63	
SOLBAR-AVO (Person & Covey)			
LOT,TP (SPF 32,PABA-FREE)			
3%-8%-7.5%-6%,			
120 ml	00096-0687-04	6.61	
SOLO SITE WOUND (Smith & Nephew)			
GEL,TP, 90 gm	40565-0115-27	14.18	11.34
210 gm	40565-0115-28	32.16	25.73
SOLTICE QUICK-RUB (Oakhurst)			
CRE,TP, 5.1%-5.1%,			
37 gm	11169-0100-11	2.32	3.49
(STAINLESS,GREASELESS)			
5.1%-5.1%, 84 gm	11169-0100-12	4.10	6.15
SOLUBLE FIBER THERAPY (Major)			
PDR,PO (ORANGE)			
2 gm/dose, 454 gm	00904-5675-16	6.50	
SOLUSET (Abbott Hosp)			
DEV,NA (100X15 W/CAIR, VENTED)			
20s ea	00074-1726-02	98.88	
(100X60 W/CAIR, VENTED)			
20s ea	00074-4965-68	563.83	
(150X60 W/CAIR CLAMP)			
20s ea	00074-1882-68	581.16	
20s ea	00074-4966-68	619.16	
(150X60/IVEX-2 FILT&CAIR)			
20s ea	00074-1991-68	687.09	
(250X15 W/CAIR CLAMP)			
20s ea	00074-1717-02	138.24	
(NV,150X60 FILTER W/CAIR)			
20s ea	00074-1864-68	578.79	
(NV,150X60 W/CAIR CLAMP)			
20s ea	00074-1876-68	526.78	
(150X15 PUMP SET, VENTED)			
24s ea	00074-1753-02	307.58	
(150X60 I.V. PUMP SET)			
24s ea	00074-9247-68	323.14	
(50X60 MICRO PUMP/Y/IVEX)			
24s ea	00074-9246-68	453.31	
SOLUTION ADDITIVE INLINE FILTER (Abbott Hosp)			
DEV,NA (18", 1 MICRON FILTER)			
48s ea	00074-4525-48	115.20	
SOLUTION-PLUS (Covidien)			
DEV,NA (3-WAY W/MALE LUER LOCK)			
50s ea	08080-1700-31	95.13	
(4-WAY W/EXTENSION KIT)			
50s ea	08080-1700-42	136.92	
(STERILE,3-WAY)			
50s ea	08080-1700-30	60.49	
SOLVIL (VITAFLO, LLC)			
PDS,PO (30X5GM)			
30s ea	50600-0552-79	87.95	109.94
SOMBRA (Quality Care Prod)			
REPACK			
GEL,TP, 3%-3%, 120 gm	49999-0806-04	25.80	
SOMBRA COOL THERAPY (Sombra)			
GEL,TP (1X14.2GM)			
6%, 14.2 gm	61577-3221-05	1.00	2.00
(1X56.8GM)			
6%, 56.8 gm	61577-3221-02	2.65	5.30
(1X85.05GM)			
6%, 85.05 gm	61577-3221-03	5.20	10.40
(1X113.6GM)			
6%, 113.6 gm	61577-3221-04	4.70	9.40
(1X227.2GM)			
6%, 227.2 gm	61577-3221-08	8.50	17.00
(1X908.8GM)			
6%, 908.8 gm	63669-0140-32	25.00	50.00
(1X3630GM)			
6%, 3630 gm	63669-0141-28	88.40	176.80
(Physician Partner)			
REPACK			
GEL,TP (1X113.6GM)			
6%, 113.6 gm	21695-0713-04	19.95	
SOMBRA NATURAL PAIN RELIEVING (Sombra)			
GEL,TP (1X14.2GM,WARM THERAPY)			
3%-3%, 14.2 gm	61577-3216-05	1.00	2.00
(1X56.7GM)			
3%-3%, 56.7 gm	61577-3216-02	2.65	5.30
(1X85.05GM)			
3%-3%, 85.05 gm	61577-3216-03	5.20	10.40
(1X113.4GM)			
3%-3%, 113.4 gm	61577-3216-04	4.70	9.40
(1X226.8GM)			
3%-3%, 226.8 gm	61577-3216-08	8.50	17.00
(1X908.8GM,WARM THERAPY)			
3%-3%, 908.8 gm	63669-0000-93	25.00	50.00
(1X3785GM)			
3%-3%, 3785 gm	63669-0001-10	88.40	176.80
SOMINEX (Glaxo)			
TAB,PO, 25 mg, 16s ea	53100-0128-22	2.30	
32s ea	53100-0128-32	3.89	
72s ea	53100-0128-51	5.62	
50 mg, 16s ea	53100-0128-75	3.89	
SOOTHADERM (Pharmakon)			
LOT,TP, 0.21%-0.21%-4.16%,			
118 ml	55422-0301-04	2.36	4.91
SOOTHE & COOL COMPLETE TBC (Medline)			
SPR,TP (NO-RINSE)			
473 ml 12s	53329-0017-06	78.75	
SOOTHE & COOL INZO (Medline)			
CRE,TP (ES, INVISIBLE)			
7.5 gm 144s UD	53329-0013-17	60.95	
120 gm 12s	53329-0013-04	74.08	
SOOTHE & COOL INZO ANTIFUNGAL (Medline)			
CRE,TP, 2%, 56.7 gm 24s	53329-0013-13	153.00	
141.75 gm 12s	53329-0013-77	126.00	
SOOTHE & COOL MOISTURE BARRIER (Medline)			
OIN,TP, 5 gm	53329-0022-16	17.51	
60 gm 12s	53329-0011-14	27.25	
210 gm 12s	53329-0011-15	47.15	
SOOTHE & COOL MOISTURIZING (Medline)			
CRE,TP (ALOE,EXTRA THICK)			
113.4 gm 24s	08327-0491-04	120.43	
SOOTHE & COOL PERI FRESH 3 IN 1 (Medline)			
TP (NO-RINSE)			
ea	53329-0018-18	83.05	
SOOTHE & COOL PERINEAL WASH (Medline)			
FOA,TP (ALOE,SCRUBBING BUBBLES)			
227 gm 24s	08327-0545-08	117.58	
SOOTHE & COOL PERINEAL WASH W/ALOE (Medline)			
SOL,TP, 240 ml 12s	53329-0027-08	22.80	
3840 ml 4s	53329-0027-25	39.80	
SOOTHE & COOL SHAMPOO/BODY WASH (Medline)			
SOL,TP (W/ALOE)			
120 ml 48s	53329-0023-44	73.98	
(NO-RINSE)			
240 ml 12s	53329-0960-08	25.10	
(W/ALOE)			
480 ml 12s	53329-0023-08	26.80	
(NO-RINSE)			
3840 ml 4s	53329-0960-25	51.85	
(W/ALOE)			
3840 ml 4s	53329-0023-25	51.80	
SOOTHE & COOL SKIN PASTE (Medline)			
PAS,TP (W/ALLANTOIN)			
70.8 gm 12s	53329-0004-10	60.90	
SOOTHING NON-STICK DRESSING (Johnson & Johnson)			
DEV,NA (3"X3",NON-ADHERING)			
12s ea	81371-0040-29	6.76	
SORBIDON HYDRATE (Gordon)			
CRE,TP, 120 gm	10481-2007-04	12.50	
(1X454GM)			
454 gm	50217-0001-57	48.75	
SORBITOL (Geritrex)			
SOL,PO (24X474ML)			
70%, 474 ml 24s	54162-0700-17	4.67	
SORBSAN (UDL)			
DEV,NA (1/4"X1/4"X12")			
5s ea	62794-0093-47	29.47	
(WOUND-4"X8")			
5s ea	62794-0092-32	46.24	
(WOUND-2"X2")			
10s ea	62794-0092-04	26.50	
(WOUND-3"X3")			
10s ea	62794-0092-09	37.32	
(WOUND-4"X4")			
10s ea	62794-0092-18	45.97	
SORE NO MORE (Sore No More)			
GEL,TP (1X120GM,AF)			
3%-3%, 120 gm	80207-0000-50	23.00	
(1X240GM,AF)			
3%-3%, 240 gm	80207-0000-51	29.00	
SORE THROAT (Albertson's)			
LOZ,MM, 2.4 mg, 24s ea	04000-0002-50	3.90	

PROD/MFR	HRI, UPC,NDC	AWP	SRP
(AmerisourceBergen)			
LOZ,MM (PRIVATE LABEL,CHERRY)			
6 mg-10 mg, 18s ea	**24385-0045-62**	2.15	2.39
SPR,MM, 1.4%, 180 ml	**24385-0328-30**	3.23	3.59
(PRIVATE LABEL,MENTHOL)			
1.4%, 180 ml	**24385-0532-30**	3.23	3.59
(Cardinal Health)			
SPR,MM (AF,SF,PRIVATE LABEL)			
1.4%, 177 ml	**37205-0326-30**	3.26	
177 ml	**37205-0327-30**	3.26	
(Chain Drug Marketing)			
SPR,MM (CHERRY)			
1.4%, 177 ml	**63868-0811-55**	1.92	5.49
(MENTHOL)			
1.4%, 177 ml	**63868-0812-55**	1.92	5.49
(Major)			
LOZ,MM (CHERRY)			
6 mg-10 mg, 18s ea	**00904-5021-98**	2.93	
SPR,MM, 1.4%, 180 ml	**00904-1771-21**	2.50	
(MENTHOL)			
1.4%, 180 ml	**00904-1770-21**	2.50	
(Medicine Shoppe)			
SPR,MM (CHERRY)			
180 ml	**49614-0328-30**	3.99	3.99
(Pharm Assoc Inc)			
SPR,MM (AF,SF,CHERRY)			
1.4%, 177 ml	**00121-0628-06**	2.48	
(Phys Total Care)			
REPACK			
LOZ,MM, 6 mg-10 mg,			
18s ea	**54868-5811-00**	9.18	
SORE THROAT MAXIMUM STRENGTH (AmerisourceBergen)			
LOZ,MM (PRIVATE LABEL,MINT)			
2.4 mg, 18s ea	**24385-0010-89**	2.15	2.39
SORE THROAT SPRAY (Perrigo)			
SPR,MM (1X177ML,AF,SF)			
1.4%, 177 ml	**45802-0282-82**	3.10	
SOURCE ABDEK (SoucreCF, Inc.)			
SGL,PO (SOFTGEL)			
60s ea	**68212-0500-60**	20.55	
720s ea	**58676-0000-02**	246.60	
SOURCE COOKIE BAR (SoucreCF, Inc.)			
BAR,PO (HIGH CAL W/WHEY PROTEIN)			
128 gm	**58676-0000-10**	3.02	
128 gm	**58676-0000-12**	3.02	
128 gm 12s	**58676-0000-11**	36.19	
128 gm 12s	**58676-0000-13**	36.19	
SOURCECF (SoucreCF, Inc.)			
LIQ,PO (PEDIATRIC,MULTIVITAMINS)			
60 ml	**68212-0300-60**	21.55	19.95
SOURCECF CHEWABLES (SoucreCF, Inc.)			
CTB,PO (BUBBLE GUM)			
90s ea	**68212-0600-90**	32.35	29.95
1080s ea	**58676-0000-22**	388.20	359.40
6480s ea	**58676-0000-23**	2329.20	2156.40
SOUTH AFRICAN HOODIA (Natl Vitamin)			
CAP,PO (PF,GLUTEN-FREE)			
250 mg, 60s ea	**54629-4091-06**	8.96	14.99
SOY (Mason Vit)			
TAB,PO (PF,SF,DYE-FREE)			
40 mg, 30s ea	**11845-0126-18**	8.84	
SOY CARE FOR MENOPAUSE (Inverness)			
CAP,PO (PF,SF)			
25 mg-185 mg,			
60s ea	**36652-0201-00**	9.35	
SOY ISOFLAVONES (Rexall)			
TAB,PO, 68 mg-40 mg,			
30s ea	**30768-0035-95**	4.87	6.99
SOYA LECITHIN (Nature's Bounty)			
SGL,PO (PF,SF,SOFTGEL)			
1200 mg, 100s ea	**74312-0003-00**		6.45
SPAN C (Freeda)			
TAB,PO (PF,SF,DYE-FREE)			
200 mg-300 mg,			
100s ea	**10432-0056-01**	7.17	11.95
250s ea	**10432-0056-02**	14.34	23.90
SPECTRA 360 (Parker)			
GEL,TP, 60 gm 12s	**00341-0012-02**	12.96	21.60
250 gm 12s	**00341-0012-08**	23.47	39.10
SPEEDICATH CATHETER (Coloplast)			
DEV,NA (COUDE MALE,10FR,14")			
30s ea	**11701-0903-47**	104.70	109.50
(COUDE MALE,12FR,14")			
30s ea	**11701-0903-48**	104.70	109.50
(COUDE MALE,14FR,14")			
30s ea	**11701-0903-49**	104.70	109.50
(FEMALE,10FR,6",NON-LATX)			
30s ea	**11701-0903-52**	95.40	99.90
(FEMALE,10FR,6")			
30s ea	**11701-0903-72**	94.50	99.90
(FEMALE,12FR,6")			
30s ea	**11701-0903-53**	95.40	99.90
(FEMALE,14FR,6")			
30s ea	**11701-0903-54**	95.40	99.90
(FEMALE,16FR,6"NON-LATEX)			
30s ea	**11701-0903-55**	95.40	99.90
(FEMALE,6FR,6",NON-LATEX)			
30s ea	**11701-0903-50**	95.40	99.90
(FEMALE,8FR,6",NON-LATEX)			
30s ea	**11701-0903-51**	95.40	99.90
(MALE,10FR,14")			
30s ea	**11701-0903-41**	95.40	99.90
(MALE,12FR,14")			
30s ea	**11701-0903-42**	95.40	99.90
(MALE,14FR,14")			
30s ea	**11701-0903-43**	95.40	99.90
(MALE,16FR,14",NON-LATEX)			
30s ea	**11701-0903-44**	95.40	99.90
(MALE,18FR,14",NON-LATEX)			
30s ea	**11701-0903-45**	95.40	99.90
(MALE,8FR,6",NON-LATEX)			
30s ea	**11701-0903-40**	95.40	99.90
(PEDIATRIC,6FR,6")			
30s ea	**11701-0903-70**	94.50	99.90
(PEDIATRIC,8FR,6")			
30s ea	**11701-0903-71**	94.50	99.90
SPEEDICATH CATHETER WITH ACCESSORIES (Coloplast)			
DEV,NA (FEMALE,FR10,6")			
100s ea	**11701-0913-01**	645.00	675.00
(FEMALE,FR12,6")			
100s ea	**11701-0913-02**	645.00	675.00
(FEMALE,FR14,6")			
100s ea	**11701-0913-03**	645.00	675.00
(FEMALE,FR16,6")			
100s ea	**11701-0913-04**	645.00	675.00
(FEMALE,FR6,6")			
100s ea	**11701-0913-99**	645.00	675.00
(FEMALE,FR8,6")			
100s ea	**11701-0913-00**	645.00	675.00
(MALE,FR 8,14")			
100s ea	**11701-0913-81**	645.00	675.00
(MALE,FR10,14")			
100s ea	**11701-0913-82**	645.00	675.00
(MALE,FR12,14")			
100s ea	**11701-0913-83**	645.00	675.00
(MALE,FR14,14")			
100s ea	**11701-0913-84**	645.00	675.00
(MALE,FR16,14")			
100s ea	**11701-0913-85**	645.00	675.00
(MALE,FR18,14")			
100s ea	**11701-0913-86**	645.00	675.00
SPIGELIA (Luyties)			
TAB,SL (6X)			
6 x, 500s ea	**00618-8108-03**	3.99	
5500s ea	**00618-8108-10**	30.32	
(30X)			
12 x, 500s ea	**00622-8108-03**	4.19	
5500s ea	**00622-8108-10**	31.83	
(12X)			
30 x, 500s ea	**00624-8108-03**	4.19	
5500s ea	**00624-8108-10**	31.83	
SPIRULINA (ADH)			
TAB,PO (PF,SF)			
500 mg, 100s ea	**60142-0947-51**	5.98	11.95
(Mason Vit)			
TAB,PO, 500 mg, 100s ea	**11845-0076-61**	8.56	
SPLEEN (Key Company)			
CAP,PO, 200 mg, 100s ea	**11694-0849-01**	5.25	
500s ea	**11694-0849-03**	21.50	
(Miller)			
TAB,PO, 250 mg, 100s ea	**17204-0530-40**	6.00	9.50
SPONGIA TOSTA (Luyties)			
TAB,SL (6X)			
6 x, 500s ea	**00618-8114-03**	3.99	
5500s ea	**00618-8114-10**	30.32	
(30X)			
12 x, 500s ea	**00622-8114-03**	4.19	
5500s ea	**00622-8114-10**	31.83	
(12X)			
30 x, 500s ea	**00624-8114-03**	4.19	
5500s ea	**00624-8114-10**	31.83	
SPONIX ARTHRITIS & MUSCLE RELIEF (BioRx)			
CRE,TP (1X113GM)			
0.025%-10%, 113 gm	**63132-0016-04**	11.98	
LOT,TP (1X85GM,GREASELESS)			
0.045%-10%, 85 gm	**63132-0015-03**	11.98	
SPONIX FOOT THERAPY (BioRx)			
POW,TP (1X58ML)			
58 ml	**01434-0123-69**	12.98	
SPONIX NAIL (BioRx)			
GEL,TP (1X58.8GM)			
58.8 gm	**01434-0123-68**	11.98	
SPONIX SUNSCREEN (BioRx)			
CRE,TP (1X113GM,FRAGRANCE-FREE)			
8%-3.5%, 113 gm	**63132-0017-04**	8.97	
SPOONS (Paddock)			
DEV,NA, ea	**00574-9240-01**	0.55	
SPORTBALM (Gordon)			
LOT,TP, 120 ml	**10481-2003-01**	6.25	
SPORTENINE (Boiron)			
CTB,PO (2X11)			
9 c-6 x-6 x,			
22s ea	**06969-0710-61**	6.74	11.29
SPORTGUARD PROTECTIVE CASE (Medtronic Minimed)			
DEV,NA (WATERPROOF)			
ea	**76300-0145-01**	72.00	
SPORTS PAIN RELIEF RUB (AmerisourceBergen)			
CRE,TP (FRESH SCENT)			
10%, 85 gm	**24385-0248-53**	3.32	3.69
SPORTZ BLOC (Med-Derm)			
CRE,TP (SPF 20,DARK,AF,SF)			
15 gm	**15978-0981-03**	5.18	
(SPF 20,LIGHT,AF,SF)			
15 gm	**15978-0981-01**	5.18	
(SPF 20,MEDIUM,AF,SF)			
15 gm	**15978-0981-02**	5.18	
SPRAIN-CARE (Weleda)			
OIN,TP, 10%, 30 gm	**55946-0005-59**	3.90	
SPRAY APPLICATOR KIT (ZymoGenetics)			
DEV,NA (LATEX-FREE)			
ea	**28400-0700-17**	36.00	
SPRAY BANDAGE (Hart Health)			
SPR,TP, 0.2%-3.2%,			
90 ml	**50332-0218-01**	3.05	
SPRAY EXTENSION TUBE (Beutlich)			
DEV,NA (FOR HURRICAINE)			
200s ea	**00283-1185-20**	15.08	23.20
SPRAYTRODE (Pharm Innov)			
SPR,TP, 60 ml	**00036-3300-60**	1.87	2.63
250 ml	**00036-3300-25**	4.46	6.37
4000 ml	**00036-3300-04**	44.90	64.15
SPRAYZOIN (Geritrex)			
TIN,TP, 118 ml	**54162-0105-04**	9.28	
SPROAM (Coloplast)			
SPR,TP (ALL BODY CLEANSER)			
0.1%, 178 ml 12s	**11701-0156-36**	82.92	86.88
355 ml 12s	**11701-0156-35**	130.80	136.92
3800 ml 4s	**11701-0156-09**	254.16	265.96
ST-37 (Numark)			
LIQ,TP, 0.1%, 240 ml	**38485-0860-00**	6.96	
480 ml	**38485-0860-01**	9.78	
ST. JOHN'S WORT (AmerisourceBergen)			
TAB,PO (PF,PRIVATE LABEL,CAPLET)			
300 mg, 50s ea	**24385-0972-71**	5.57	6.19
(Cardinal Health)			
CAP,PO (PRIVATE LABEL)			
375 mg, 50s ea	**37205-0097-71**	5.76	
(Contract Pharmacal)			
TAB,PO, 300 mg, 50s ea	**10267-0504-06**	9.00	
(Key Company)			
CAP,PO (SF)			
400 mg, 60s ea	**11694-0698-01**	7.90	
(Marlex)			
CAP,PO, 300 mg, 60s ea	**10135-0317-60**	3.06	
(Mason Vit)			
CAP,PO (PF,SF)			
300 mg, 60s ea	**11845-0125-25**	11.00	
60s ea	**11845-0130-05**	11.00	
180s ea	**11845-0130-07**	29.44	
(Rexall)			
CAP,PO (PF,SF)			
150 mg, 50s ea	**30768-0001-18**	3.94	5.97

PROD/MFR	HRI, UPC,NDC	AWP	SRP
(Zayco, Inc.)			
TDM,TD, 900 mg/24 hr,			
30s ea	77987-0990-00	7.80	
ST. JOSEPH (McNeil Consumer Healthcare)			
CTB,PO (ADULT,ORANGE)			
81 mg, 36s ea	00450-0173-36	2.10	
(ADULT,3X36,ORANGE)			
81 mg, 108s ea	00450-0173-08	5.59	
ECT,PO (ADULT)			
81 mg, 36s ea	00450-0126-36	2.10	
100s ea	00450-0126-10	5.33	
(ADULT)			
81 mg, 180s ea	00450-0126-18	8.65	
300s ea	00450-0126-03	13.12	
ST. JOSEPH PAIN RELIEVER (McNeil Consumer Healthcare)			
CTB,PO (ADULT,3X36,ORANGE)			
81 mg, 108s ea	50580-0173-08	5.59	
(ORANGE)			
81 mg, 2500s ea	50580-0173-25	240.00	
ECT,PO, 81 mg, 100s ea	50580-0126-10	5.33	
360s ea	50580-0126-20	10.98	
STA-PUT DISPOSABLE UNDERPADS (Covidien)			
DEV,NA (36"X70",8X6)			
48s ea	08080-9950-00	48.20	
(30"X36",12X6)			
72s ea	08080-0995-00	40.62	
STAIN-AWAY FOR PARTIALS (Regent Labs)			
POW,NA, 238 gm	83272-0981-01	3.95	
STAIN-AWAY PLUS (Regent Labs)			
NA, 113 gm	83272-0982-04	2.74	
230 gm	83272-0981-02	3.95	
STANBACK ANALGESIC (Glaxo)			
PDR,PO, 2s ea	11530-0002-02	0.34	
6s ea	11530-0002-06	0.97	
24s ea	11530-0002-24	2.44	
50s ea	11530-0002-50	3.82	
STANDARD DRAINABLE POUCH ONE PIECE (Coloplast)			
DEV,NA (OPAQUE, 1-1/8")			
10s ea	11701-0807-24	42.70	44.60
(OPAQUE, 1-3/8")			
10s ea	11701-0807-25	42.70	44.60
(OPAQUE, 1-5/8")			
10s ea	11701-0807-26	42.70	44.60
(OPAQUE, 1-7/8")			
10s ea	11701-0807-27	42.70	44.60
(OPAQUE, 1")			
10s ea	11701-0807-23	42.70	44.60
(OPAQUE, 1/2"-2-1/4")			
10s ea	11701-0807-20	42.70	44.60
10s ea	11701-0807-21	42.70	44.60
(OPAQUE, 2-3/8")			
10s ea	11701-0807-29	42.70	44.60
(OPAQUE, 2")			
10s ea	11701-0807-28	42.70	44.60
(OPAQUE, 3/4")			
10s ea	11701-0807-22	42.70	44.60
(TRANSPARENT, 1-1/8")			
10s ea	11701-0807-14	42.70	44.60
(TRANSPARENT, 1-3/8")			
10s ea	11701-0807-15	42.70	44.60
(TRANSPARENT, 1-5/8")			
10s ea	11701-0807-16	44.70	44.60
(TRANSPARENT, 1-7/8")			
10s ea	11701-0807-17	42.70	44.60
(TRANSPARENT, 1")			
10s ea	11701-0807-13	42.70	44.60
(TRANSPARENT, 2-3/8")			
10s ea	11701-0807-19	42.70	44.60
(TRANSPARENT, 2")			
10s ea	11701-0807-18	42.70	44.60
(TRANSPARENT, 3/4")			
10s ea	11701-0807-12	42.70	44.60
(TRANSPARENT,1/2"-2-1/4")			
10s ea	11701-0807-10	42.70	44.60
10s ea	11701-0807-11	42.70	44.60
STANDARD DRAINABLE POUCH TWO PIECE (Coloplast)			
DEV,NA (OPAQUE, UP TO 1-1/2")			
10s ea	11701-0812-25	28.70	30.10
(OPAQUE, UP TO 1-3/4")			
10s ea	11701-0812-30	28.70	30.10
(OPAQUE, UP TO 2")			
10s ea	11701-0812-35	28.70	30.10
(TRANSPAR., UP TO 1-1/2")			
10s ea	11701-0812-10	28.70	30.10
(TRANSPAR., UP TO 1-3/4")			
10s ea	11701-0812-15	28.70	30.10

PROD/MFR	HRI, UPC,NDC	AWP	SRP
(TRANSPARENT, UP TO 2")			
10s ea	11701-0812-20	28.70	30.10
STANDARD HOMEOPATHIC (Std Homeo)			
ABSINTHIUM			
TAB,PO, 250s ea	54973-0015-01	4.37	7.29
ACETICUM ACIDUM			
PO, 250s ea	54973-0024-01	4.37	7.29
ACONITUM NAPELLUS			
PO, 250s ea	54973-0032-01	4.37	7.29
ADONIS VERNALIS			
PO, 250s ea	54973-0042-01	4.37	7.29
ADRENALIUM			
PO, 250s ea	54973-0044-01	4.37	7.29
AESCULUS HIPP			
PO, 250s ea	54973-0047-01	4.37	7.29
AETHIOPS MERCURIAL MIN			
PO, 250s ea	54973-0049-01	4.37	7.29
AETHUSA CYNAPIUM			
PO, 250s ea	54973-0050-01	4.37	7.29
AGARICUS MUSCARUS			
PO, 250s ea	54973-0057-01	4.37	7.29
ALUMEN			
PO, 250s ea	54973-0088-01	4.37	7.29
AMMONIUM IODATUM			
PO, 250s ea	54973-0102-01	4.37	7.29
AMYLNITROSUM			
PO, 250s ea	54973-0129-01	4.37	7.29
ANACARDIUM OCCIDENTALE			
PO, 250s ea	54973-0131-01	4.37	7.29
ANACARDIUM ORIENTALE			
PO, 250s ea	54973-0132-01	4.37	7.29
ANGUSTURA VERA			
PO, 250s ea	54973-0153-01	4.37	7.29
ANILINUM			
PO, 250s ea	54973-0156-01	4.37	7.29
ANTIMON SULFURAT AUREUM			
PO, 250s ea	54973-0176-01	4.37	7.29
ANTIMONIUM ARSENICICUM			
PO, 250s ea	54973-0170-01	4.37	7.29
ANTIMONIUM CRUDUM			
PO, 250s ea	54973-0172-01	4.37	7.29
ANTIMONIUM MURIATICUM			
PO, 250s ea	54973-0174-01	4.37	7.29
ANTIMONIUM OXYDATUM			
PO, 250s ea	54973-0175-01	4.37	7.29
ANTIMONIUM TARTARICUM			
PO, 250s ea	54973-0177-01	4.37	7.29
APIS VENENUM PURUM			
PO, 250s ea	54973-0186-01	4.37	7.29
APOCYNUM ANDROSAEMIFOL			
PO, 250s ea	54973-0187-01	4.37	7.29
APOCYNUM CANNABINUM			
PO, 250s ea	54973-0188-01	4.37	7.29
ARANEA DIADEMA TINC			
PO, 250s ea	54973-0203-01	4.37	7.29
ARGENTUM METALLICUM			
PO, 250s ea	54973-0221-01	4.37	7.29
ARGENTUM MURIATICUM			
PO, 250s ea	54973-0222-01	4.37	7.29
ARGENTUM NITRICUM			
PO, 250s ea	54973-0223-01	4.37	7.29
ARGENTUM PHOSPHORICUM			
PO, 250s ea	54973-0224-01	4.37	7.29
ARNICA MONTANA			
PO, 250s ea	54973-0229-01	4.37	7.29
ARNICATED OIL			
OIL,TP, 10%, 30 ml	05497-3115-61	4.43	7.39
120 ml	05497-3115-62	10.19	16.99
ARSENIC SULFURAT RUBRUM			
TAB,PO, 250s ea	54973-0241-01	4.37	7.29
ARSENICUM ALBUM			
PO, 250s ea	54973-0230-01	4.37	7.29
ARSENICUM BROMATUM			
PO, 250s ea	54973-0231-01	4.37	7.29
ARSENICUM IODATUM			
PO, 250s ea	54973-0237-01	4.37	7.29
ARSENICUM SULFURATUM FL			
PO, 250s ea	54973-0240-01	4.37	7.29
ARTEMESIA ABRO			
PO, 250s ea	54973-0114-01	4.37	7.29
ARTEMESIA VULG			
PO, 250s ea	54973-0249-01	4.37	7.29
ARUM MAC			
PO, 250s ea	54973-0252-01	4.37	7.29
ARUM TRI			
PO, 250s ea	54973-0254-01	4.37	7.29
ASCLEPIAS CURASSAVICA			
PO, 250s ea	54973-0261-01	4.37	7.29
ASCLEPIAS TUBEROSA			
PO, 250s ea	54973-0263-01	4.37	7.29
ASCLEPIAS VINCETOXICUM			
PO, 250s ea	54973-0264-01	4.37	7.29

PROD/MFR	HRI, UPC,NDC	AWP	SRP
ASTERIAS RUBENS			
PO, 250s ea	54973-0270-01	4.37	7.29
ATROPINUM			
PO, 250s ea	54973-0275-01	4.37	7.29
ATROPINUM SULFURICUM			
PO, 250s ea	54973-0274-01	4.37	7.29
AURUM IODATUM			
PO, 250s ea	54973-0281-01	4.37	7.29
AURUM SULFURATUM			
PO, 250s ea	54973-0286-01	4.37	7.29
BACILLINUM			
PO, 250s ea	54973-1011-01	4.37	7.29
BADIAGA			
PO, 250s ea	54973-1016-01	4.37	7.29
BARYTA ACETICA			
PO, 250s ea	54973-1028-01	4.37	7.29
BARYTA CARBONICA			
PO, 250s ea	54973-1029-01	4.37	7.29
BARYTA IODATA			
PO, 250s ea	54973-1030-01	4.37	7.29
BARYTA MURIATICA			
PO, 250s ea	54973-1031-04	4.37	7.29
BENZINUM			
PO, 250s ea	54973-1035-01	4.37	7.29
BENZOIN ODORIFERUM			
PO, 250s ea	54973-1039-01	4.37	7.29
BISMUTH METALLICUM			
PO, 250s ea	54973-1051-01	4.37	7.29
BISMUTH SUBNITRICUM			
PO, 250s ea	54973-1092-01	4.37	7.29
BLATTA AMERICANA			
PO, 250s ea	54973-1054-01	4.37	7.29
BLATTA ORIENTALIS			
PO, 250s ea	54973-1467-04	4.37	7.29
BORAX			
PO, 250s ea	54973-1065-01	4.37	7.29
BOVISTA			
PO, 250s ea	54973-1070-01	4.37	7.29
BROMIUM			
PO, 250s ea	54973-1090-01	4.37	7.29
BROMIUM IOD			
PO, 250s ea	54973-1076-01	4.37	7.29
BRYONIA			
PO, 250s ea	54973-1080-01	4.37	7.29
CACTUS GRAND			
PO, 250s ea	54973-2013-01	4.37	7.29
CADMIUM METALLICUM			
PO, 250s ea	54973-2016-01	4.37	7.29
CADMIUM MURIATICUM			
PO, 250s ea	54973-2017-01	4.37	7.29
CADMIUM SULFURATUM			
PO, 250s ea	54973-2019-01	4.37	7.29
CADMIUM SULFURICUM			
PO, 250s ea	54973-2275-01	4.37	7.29
CALADIUM SEGUINUM			
PO, 250s ea	54973-2025-01	4.37	7.29
CALCAREA ARSENICICA			
PO, 250s ea	54973-2027-01	4.37	7.29
CALCAREA CARBONICA			
PO, 250s ea	54973-2030-01	4.37	7.29
CALCAREA CAUSTICA			
PO, 250s ea	54973-2031-01	4.37	7.29
CALCAREA FLUORICA			
TAB,PO, 6 x, 250s ea	54973-2033-01	4.37	7.29
CALCAREA IODATA			
TAB,PO, 250s ea	54973-2036-01	4.37	7.29
CALCAREA MURIATICA			
PO, 250s ea	54973-2039-01	4.37	7.29
CALCAREA OXALICA			
PO, 250s ea	54973-2042-01	4.37	7.29
CALCAREA PHOS			
TAB,PO, 6 x, 250s ea	54973-2043-01	4.37	7.29
CALCAREA SULF			
TAB,PO, 6 x, 500s ea	54973-2049-01	5.69	9.49
CALCEARA PIC			
TAB,PO, 250s ea	54973-2045-01	4.37	7.29
CALENDULA			
SPR,TP, 22%, 30 ml	05497-3115-31	3.77	6.29
120 ml	05497-3115-32	5.99	9.99
TAB,PO, 250s ea	54973-2052-01	4.37	7.29
CALENDULATED OIL			
OIL,TP, 10%, 30 ml	05497-3115-41	4.37	7.29
120 ml	05497-3115-42	8.69	14.49
CAMPHORA			
TAB,PO, 250s ea	54973-2060-01	4.37	7.29
CANTHARIS			
PO, 250s ea	54973-2068-01	4.37	7.29
CAPSICUM ANNUUM			
PO, 250s ea	54973-2072-01	4.37	7.29
CARBO VEGETABILIS			
PO, 250s ea	54973-2075-01	4.37	7.29
CARBOLICUM ACIDUM			
PO, 250s ea	54973-2676-01	4.37	7.29

PROD/MFR	HRI, UPC,NDC	AWP	SRP
CARBONEUM			
PO, 250s ea	**54973-2077-01**	4.37	7.29
CARBONEUM SULFURATUM			
PO, 250s ea	**54973-2082-01**	4.37	7.29
CASTOR EQUI			
PO, 250s ea	**54973-2100-01**	4.37	7.29
CASTOREUM			
PO, 250s ea	**54973-2101-01**	4.37	7.29
CAULOPHYLLUM THALIC			
PO, 250s ea	**54973-2105-01**	4.37	7.29
CAUSTICUM			
PO, 250s ea	**54973-2107-01**	4.37	7.29
CENCHRIS CONTORTRIX			
PO, 250s ea	**54973-2113-01**	4.37	7.29
CHAMOMILLA			
PO, 250s ea	**54973-2127-01**	4.37	7.29
CHELIDONIUM MAJ			
PO, 250s ea	**54973-2133-01**	4.37	7.29
CHENOPODIUM ANTH			
PO, 250s ea	**54973-2135-01**	4.37	7.29
CHININUM ARSENICOSUM			
PO, 250s ea	**54973-2147-01**	4.37	7.29
CHININUM SALICYLICUM			
PO, 250s ea	**54973-2150-01**	4.37	7.29
CHIONANTHUS VIRG			
PO, 250s ea	**54973-2175-01**	4.37	7.29
CHLORALUM			
PO, 250s ea	**54973-2154-01**	4.37	7.29
CHLORINUM			
PO, 250s ea	**54973-2156-01**	4.37	7.29
CHLOROFORMUM			
PO, 250s ea	**54973-2157-01**	4.37	7.29
CHROMIUM OXYDATUM			
PO, 250s ea	**54973-2163-01**	4.37	7.29
CHROMIUM SULFURICUM			
PO, 250s ea	**54973-2164-01**	4.37	7.29
CHRYSAROBINUM			
PO, 250s ea	**54973-2168-01**	4.37	7.29
CINA			
PO, 250s ea	**54973-2176-01**	4.37	7.29
CINCHONA OFFICINALIS			
PO, 250s ea	**54973-2144-01**	4.37	7.29
CLEMATIS ERECTA			
PO, 250s ea	**54973-2188-01**	4.37	7.29
COBALTUM METALLICUM			
PO, 250s ea	**54973-2192-00**	4.37	7.29
COBALTUM NITRICUM			
PO, 250s ea	**54973-2193-01**	4.37	7.29
COCCULUS INDICUS			
PO, 250s ea	**54973-2196-01**	4.37	7.29
COCCUS CACTI			
PO, 250s ea	**54973-2198-01**	4.37	7.29
COCHLEARIA AMOR			
PO, 250s ea	**54973-2199-01**	4.37	7.29
COFFEA CRUDA			
PO, 250s ea	**54973-2203-01**	4.37	7.29
COFFEA TOSTA			
PO, 250s ea	**54973-2204-01**	4.37	7.29
COLCHICINUM			
PO, 250s ea	**54973-2206-01**	4.37	7.29
COLCHICUM AUTUMNALE			
PO, 250s ea	**54973-2207-01**	4.37	7.29
COLLINSONIA CAN			
PO, 250s ea	**54973-2211-01**	4.37	7.29
COLOCYNTHIS			
PO, 250s ea	**54973-2212-01**	4.37	7.29
CONINUM			
PO, 250s ea	**54973-2219-01**	4.37	7.29
CONVALLARIA MAJALIS			
PO, 250s ea	**54973-2220-01**	4.37	7.29
COPAIVA OFF			
PO, 250s ea	**54973-2223-01**	4.37	7.29
CORALLIUM RUB			
PO, 250s ea	**54973-2225-01**	4.37	7.29
CORTISONE ACETICUM			
PO, 250s ea	**54973-2234-01**	4.37	7.29
COTYLEDON UMBILICUS			
PO, 250s ea	**54973-2236-04**	4.37	7.29
CRATAEGUS OXYCANTHA			
PO, 250s ea	**54973-2240-01**	4.37	7.29
CROCUS SATIVUS			
PO, 250s ea	**54973-2241-01**	4.37	7.29
CROTALLUS HORRIDUS			
PO, 250s ea	**54973-2243-01**	4.37	7.29
CROTALUS CASCAVELLA			
PO, 250s ea	**54973-2242-01**	4.37	7.29
CROTON CHLORALUM			
PO, 250s ea	**54973-2244-01**	4.37	7.29
CUCURBITA PEP			
PO, 250s ea	**54973-2248-01**	4.37	7.29
CUPRUM ACETICUM			
PO, 250s ea	**54973-2255-01**	4.37	7.29
CUPRUM ARSENICOSUM			
PO, 250s ea	**54973-2257-01**	4.37	7.29
CUPRUM METALLICUM			
PO, 250s ea	**54973-2260-01**	4.37	7.29
CUPRUM NITRICUM			
PO, 250s ea	**54973-2262-01**	4.37	7.29
CUPRUM OXYDATUM NIGRUM			
PO, 250s ea	**54973-2263-01**	4.37	7.29
CUPRUM SULFURICUM			
PO, 250s ea	**54973-2264-01**	4.37	7.29
CYCLAMEN EVROPAEUM			
PO, 250s ea	**54973-2269-01**	4.37	7.29
DAMIANA			
PO, 250s ea	**54973-3011-01**	4.37	7.29
DAPHNE INDICA			
PO, 250s ea	**54973-3012-01**	4.37	7.29
DELPHININUM			
PO, 250s ea	**54973-3021-01**	4.37	7.29
DIGITALINUM			
PO, 250s ea	**54973-3029-01**	4.37	7.29
DIGITALIS PURPUREA			
PO, 250s ea	**54973-3030-01**	4.37	7.29
DIOSCOREA			
PO, 250s ea	**54973-3033-01**	4.37	7.29
DIPHTHERINUM			
PO, 250s ea	**54973-3037-01**	4.37	7.29
DISTEMPERINUM			
PO, 250s ea	**54973-3041-01**	4.37	7.29
DOLICHOS			
PO, 250s ea	**54973-3043-01**	4.37	7.29
DROSERA ROTUND			
PO, 250s ea	**54973-3048-01**	4.37	7.29
DUBOISIA MYOPOROIDES			
PO, 250s ea	**54973-3049-01**	4.37	7.29
DULCAMARA			
PO, 250s ea	**54973-3053-01**	4.37	7.29
ECHINACEA ANG			
PO, 250s ea	**54973-3212-01**	4.37	7.29
ELAPS CORALLINUS			
PO, 250s ea	**54973-3219-01**	4.37	7.29
EMETINUM			
PO, 250s ea	**54973-3227-01**	4.37	7.29
EPHEDRA VULG			
PO, 250s ea	**54973-3231-01**	4.37	7.29
EPIPHEGUS			
PO, 250s ea	**54973-3235-01**	4.37	7.29
EQUISETUM HYEMALE			
PO, 250s ea	**54973-3237-01**	4.37	7.29
ERIODICTION			
PO, 250s ea	**54973-3243-01**	4.37	7.29
ESCHOLTZIN CALIF			
PO, 250s ea	**54973-3265-01**	4.37	7.29
EUCALYPTUS GLOB			
PO, 250s ea	**54973-3261-01**	4.37	7.29
EUPATORIUM PERF			
PO, 250s ea	**54973-3270-01**	4.37	7.29
EUPATORIUM PURP			
PO, 250s ea	**54973-3271-01**	4.37	7.29
EUPHORBIA HYPERICIFOLIA			
PO, 250s ea	**54973-3276-01**	4.37	7.29
EUPHORBIUM OFFICINARUM			
PO, 250s ea	**54973-3280-01**	4.37	7.29
FERRUM ACETICUM			
PO, 250s ea	**54973-6419-01**	4.37	7.29
FERRUM IODATUM			
PO, 250s ea	**54973-3425-01**	4.37	7.29
FERRUM METALLICUM			
PO, 250s ea	**54973-3427-01**	4.37	7.29
FERRUM MURIATICUM			
PO, 250s ea	**54973-3428-01**	4.37	7.29
FERRUM PHOSPHORICUM			
TAB,PO, 6 x, 250s ea	**54973-3431-01**	4.37	7.29
FERRUM PICRICUM			
TAB,PO, 250s ea	**54973-3432-01**	4.37	7.29
FILIX MAS			
PO, 250s ea	**54973-3444-01**	4.37	7.29
FORMICA RUFA			
PO, 250s ea	**54973-3452-01**	4.37	7.29
FUCUS VES			
PO, 250s ea	**54973-3460-01**	4.37	7.29
GELSEMIUM SEMPERVIRENS			
PO, 250s ea	**54973-4024-01**	4.37	7.29
GENTIANA			
PO, 250s ea	**54973-4028-01**	4.37	7.29
GERANIUM MAC			
PO, 250s ea	**54973-4032-01**	4.37	7.29
GLONOINUM			
PO, 250s ea	**54973-4038-01**	4.37	7.29
GNAPHALIUM POLY			
PO, 250s ea	**54973-4040-01**	4.37	7.29
GRATIOLA			
PO, 250s ea	**54973-4045-01**	4.37	7.29
GUIACUM			
PO, 250s ea	**54973-4050-01**	4.37	7.29
HAMAMELIS			
PO, 250s ea	**54973-4214-01**	4.37	7.29
HEDERA HELIX			
PO, 250s ea	**54973-4219-01**	4.37	7.29
HELLEBORUS FOETIDUS			
PO, 250s ea	**54973-4225-01**	4.37	7.29
HELLEBORUS NIGER			
PO, 250s ea	**54973-4227-01**	4.37	7.29
HELODERMA			
PO, 250s ea	**54973-0423-01**	4.37	7.29
HEPAR SULFURIS			
PO, 250s ea	**54973-4233-01**	4.37	7.29
HISTAMINUM			
PO, 250s ea	**54973-4269-01**	4.37	7.29
HUMULUS LUP			
PO, 250s ea	**54973-0424-01**	4.37	7.29
HYDRANGEA			
PO, 250s ea	**54973-4250-01**	4.37	7.29
HYDRASTININUM MURIATICU			
PO, 250s ea	**54973-4252-01**	4.37	7.29
HYOSCYAMUS NIGER			
PO, 250s ea	**54973-4265-01**	4.37	7.29
HYPERICUM PERFORATUM			
PO, 250s ea	**54973-4267-01**	4.37	7.29
ICHTHYOLUM			
PO, 250s ea	**54973-4412-01**	4.37	8.99
IGNATIA AMARA			
PO, 250s ea	**54973-4415-01**	4.37	7.29
INDIUM METALLICUM			
PO, 250s ea	**54973-4426-01**	4.37	7.29
INFLUENZINUM			
PO, 250s ea	**54973-4428-01**	4.37	7.29
IODIUM			
PO, 250s ea	**54973-4433-01**	4.37	7.29
IPECACUANHA			
PO, 250s ea	**05497-4436-01**	4.37	7.29
IRIDIUM METALLICUM			
PO, 250s ea	**54973-4440-01**	4.37	7.29
IRIS VERS			
PO, 250s ea	**54973-4447-01**	4.37	7.29
JABORANDI			
PO, 250s ea	**54973-5011-01**	4.37	7.29
JUGLANS CIN			
PO, 250s ea	**54973-5029-01**	4.37	7.29
JUGLANS REG			
PO, 250s ea	**54973-5030-01**	4.37	7.29
JUNIPERUS COMM			
PO, 250s ea	**54973-5033-01**	4.37	7.29
KALI ARSENICOSUM			
PO, 250s ea	**54973-5212-01**	4.37	7.29
KALI BICHROMICUM			
PO, 250s ea	**54973-5213-01**	4.37	7.29
KALI CAUSTICUM			
PO, 250s ea	**54973-5257-01**	4.37	7.29
KALI CHLORICUM			
PO, 250s ea	**54973-5216-01**	4.37	7.29
KALI CHROMICUM			
PO, 250s ea	**54973-5218-01**	4.37	7.29
KALI CYANATUM			
PO, 250s ea	**54973-5220-01**	4.37	7.29
KALI IOD			
PO, 250s ea	**54973-5222-01**	4.37	7.29
KALI MUR			
TAB,PO, 6 x, 250s ea	**54973-5224-01**	4.37	7.29
KALI NITRICUM			
TAB,PO, 250s ea	**54973-5225-01**	4.37	7.29
KALI PHOSPHORICUM			
TAB,PO, 6 x, 250s ea	**54973-5228-01**	4.37	7.29
KALI SILICATUM			
TAB,PO, 250s ea	**54973-5232-01**	4.37	7.29
KALMIA LATIFOLIA			
PO, 250s ea	**54973-5236-01**	4.37	7.29
KOUSSO			
PO, 250s ea	**54973-5252-01**	4.37	7.29
KREOSOTUM			
PO, 250s ea	**54973-5254-01**	4.37	7.29
LAC CANINUM			
PO, 250s ea	**54973-5413-01**	4.37	7.29
LAC DEFLORATUM			
PO, 250s ea	**54973-5420-01**	4.37	7.29
LAC VACCINUM			
PO, 250s ea	**54973-5417-01**	4.37	7.29
LACHESIS MUTUS			
PO, 250s ea	**54973-5423-01**	4.37	7.29
LACTICUM ACIDUM			
PO, 250s ea	**54973-5425-01**	4.37	7.29
LACTUCA VIROSA			
PO, 250s ea	**54973-5427-01**	4.37	7.29
LAPIS ALBUS			
PO, 250s ea	**54973-5435-01**	4.37	7.29

PROD/MFR	HRI, UPC,NDC	AWP	SRP
LATRODECTUS MACTANS			
PO, 250s ea	54973-5443-01	4.37	7.29
LAUROCERASUS			
PO, 250s ea	54973-5444-01	4.37	7.29
LILIUM TIG			
PO, 250s ea	54973-5460-01	4.37	7.29
LITHIUM CARBONICUM			
PO, 250s ea	54973-5469-01	4.37	7.29
LITHIUM MURIATICUM			
PO, 250s ea	54973-5471-01	4.37	7.29
LOBELIA INFLATA			
PO, 250s ea	54973-5477-01	4.37	7.29
LOLIUM TEMULENTUM			
PO, 250s ea	54973-5482-01	4.37	7.29
LUPULUS			
PO, 250s ea	54973-5490-01	4.37	7.29
LYCOPODIUM CLAV			
PO, 250s ea	54973-5491-01	4.37	7.29
LYCOPUS VIRG			
PO, 250s ea	54973-5492-01	4.37	7.29
MAGNESIA CARBONIC			
PO, 250s ea	54973-6018-01	4.37	7.29
MAGNESIA PHOS			
TAB,PO, 6 x, 250s ea	54973-6020-01	4.37	7.29
MAGNESIUM METALLICUM			
TAB,PO, 250s ea	54973-6019-01	4.37	7.29
MANCINELLA			
PO, 250s ea	54973-6035-01	4.37	7.29
MANGANUM ACETICUM			
PO, 250s ea	54973-6037-01	4.37	7.29
MANGANUM MURIATICUM			
PO, 250s ea	54973-6039-01	4.37	7.29
MANGANUM SULFURICUM			
PO, 250s ea	54973-6040-01	4.37	7.29
MEDORRHINUM			
PO, 250s ea	54973-6055-01	4.37	7.29
MELILOTUS ALBA			
PO, 250s ea	05497-6056-01	4.37	7.29
MELILOTUS OFFICINALIS			
PO, 250s ea	54973-6057-01	4.37	7.29
MEPHITIS MEPHITICA			
PO, 250s ea	54973-6066-01	4.19	6.99
MERCURIUS CYANATUS			
PO, 250s ea	54973-6075-01	4.37	7.29
MERCURIUS DULCIS			
PO, 250s ea	54973-6076-01	4.37	7.29
MERCURIUS IODATUS FLAVUS			
PO, 250s ea	54973-6078-04	4.37	7.29
MERCURIUS IODATUS RUBER			
PO, 250s ea	54973-6079-01	4.37	7.29
MERCURIUS METHYLENUS			
PO, 250s ea	54973-6080-01	4.37	7.29
MERCURIUS NITRICUS			
PO, 250s ea	54973-6081-01	4.37	7.29
MERCURIUS PRAECIPITATUS			
PO, 250s ea	54973-6084-00	4.37	7.29
MERCURIUS SOLUBILIS			
PO, 250s ea	54973-6086-01	4.37	7.29
MERCURIUS SULFOCYANATUS			
PO, 250s ea	54973-6089-01	4.37	7.29
MERCURIUS SULFURICUS			
PO, 250s ea	54973-6087-01	4.37	7.29
MERCURIUS VIVUS			
PO, 250s ea	54973-6090-01	4.37	7.29
MILLEFOLIUM			
PO, 250s ea	54973-6102-01	4.37	7.29
MITCHELLA REP			
PO, 250s ea	54973-6104-01	4.37	7.29
MORBILLINUM			
PO, 250s ea	54973-6107-01	4.37	7.29
MOSCHUS			
PO, 250s ea	54973-6114-01	4.37	7.29
MUREX PURPUREA			
PO, 250s ea	54973-6116-01	4.37	7.29
MURIATICUM ACIDUM			
PO, 250s ea	54973-6117-01	4.37	7.29
NAJA TRIPUDIANS			
PO, 250s ea	54973-6411-01	4.37	7.29
NAPTHALIUNUM			
PO, 250s ea	54973-0641-01	4.37	7.29
NATRUM ARSENICICUM			
PO, 250s ea	54973-6423-01	4.37	7.29
NATRUM CARBONICUM			
PO, 250s ea	54973-6427-01	4.37	7.29
NATRUM CAUST			
PO, 250s ea	05497-6468-01	4.37	7.29
NATRUM FLUORATUM			
PO, 250s ea	54973-6429-01	4.37	7.29
NATRUM IODATUM			
PO, 250s ea	54973-6431-01	4.37	7.29
NATRUM MUR			
TAB,PO, 6 x, 250s ea	54973-6433-01	4.37	7.29
NATRUM PHOS			
TAB,PO, 6 x, 250s ea	54973-6436-01	4.37	7.29
NATRUM SULF			
TAB,PO, 6 x, 250s ea	54973-6440-01	4.37	7.29
NICCOLUM CARBONICUM			
TAB,PO, 250s ea	54973-6471-01	4.37	7.29
NICCOLUM METALLICUM			
PO, 250s ea	54973-0644-01	4.37	7.29
NICCOLUM SULFURICUM			
PO, 250s ea	54973-6448-01	4.37	7.29
NICOTINUM			
PO, 250s ea	54973-6450-01	4.37	7.29
NITRICUM ACIDUM			
PO, 250s ea	54973-6451-01	4.37	7.29
NITROMURIATICUM ACIDUM			
PO, 250s ea	54973-6457-01	4.37	7.29
NUX VOMICA			
PO, 250s ea	54973-6465-01	4.37	7.29
NYMPHEA OCORATA			
PO, 250s ea	54973-6467-01	4.37	7.29
OENANTHE CROCATA			
PO, 250s ea	54973-6613-01	4.37	7.29
OLEANDER			
PO, 250s ea	54973-6616-01	4.37	7.29
OLEUM ANIMALE			
PO, 250s ea	54973-6617-01	4.37	7.29
OOPHORINUM			
PO, 250s ea	54973-6624-01	4.37	7.29
ORCHITINUM			
PO, 250s ea	54973-6631-01	4.37	7.29
OSMIUM METALLICUM			
PO, 250s ea	54973-6636-01	4.37	7.29
OXALICUM ACIDUM			
PO, 250s ea	54973-6640-01	4.37	7.29
OXYDENDRON ARB			
PO, 250s ea	54973-6642-01	4.37	7.29
OXYTROPIS LAMBERTII			
PO, 250s ea	54973-6645-01	4.37	7.29
PALLADIUM METALLICUM			
PO, 250s ea	54973-7012-01	4.37	7.29
PANCREATINUM			
PO, 250s ea	54973-7014-01	4.37	7.29
PARIS QUADRIFOLIA			
PO, 250s ea	54973-7020-01	4.37	7.29
PASSIFLORA INC			
PO, 250s ea	54973-7024-01	4.37	7.29
PERTUSSINUM			
PO, 250s ea	54973-7040-01	4.37	7.29
PETROSELINUM			
PO, 250s ea	54973-7044-01	4.37	7.29
PHOSPHORICUM ACIDUM			
PO, 250s ea	54973-7140-01	4.37	7.29
PHOSPHORUS			
PO, 250s ea	54973-7051-01	4.37	7.29
PHYSOSTIGMA VENENOSUM			
PO, 250s ea	54973-7057-01	4.37	7.29
PHYTOLACCA DECANDRA			
PO, 250s ea	54973-7058-01	4.37	7.29
PICRICUM ACIDUM			
PO, 250s ea	54973-7060-01	4.37	7.29
PILOCARPINUM MURIATICUM			
PO, 250s ea	54973-7063-01	4.37	7.29
PILOCARPINUM NITRICUM			
PO, 250s ea	54973-7131-01	4.37	7.29
PINUS SYLV			
PO, 250s ea	54973-7068-01	4.37	7.29
PIPER NIG			
PO, 250s ea	54973-7072-01	4.37	7.29
PITUTARUM POSTERIUM			
PO, 250s ea	54973-7075-01	4.37	7.29
PLANTAGO MAJ			
PO, 250s ea	54973-7077-01	4.37	7.29
PLATINUM METALLICUM			
PO, 250s ea	54973-7081-01	4.37	7.29
PLATINUM MURIATICUM			
PO, 250s ea	54973-7082-01	4.37	7.29
PLUMBUM ACETICUM			
PO, 250s ea	54973-7084-01	4.37	7.29
PLUMBUM CHROMICUM			
PO, 250s ea	54973-7085-01	4.37	7.29
PLUMBUM IODATUM			
PO, 250s ea	54973-7086-01	4.37	7.29
PLUMBUM METALLICUM			
PO, 250s ea	54973-7088-01	4.37	7.29
PODOPHYLLINUM			
PO, 250s ea	54973-7135-01	4.37	7.29
PODOPHYLLUM PELTATUM			
PO, 250s ea	54973-7090-01	4.37	7.29
PRUNUS SPIN			
PO, 250s ea	54973-7112-01	4.37	7.29
PRUNUS VIRG			
PO, 250s ea	54973-7113-01	4.37	7.29
PSORINUM			
PO, 250s ea	54973-7116-01	4.37	7.29
PYROGENIUM			
PO, 250s ea	54973-7126-01	4.37	7.29
QUILLAJA SAPONARIA			
PO, 250s ea	54973-7414-01	4.37	7.29
RADIUM BROMATUM			
PO, 250s ea	54973-7611-01	4.37	7.29
RANUNCULUS BULBOSUS			
PO, 250s ea	54973-7614-01	4.37	7.29
RANUNCULUS SCELERATUS			
PO, 250s ea	54973-7619-01	4.37	7.29
RATANHIA			
PO, 250s ea	54973-7621-01	4.37	7.29
RHAMNUS FRANGULA			
PO, 250s ea	54973-7626-01	4.37	7.29
RHODODENDRON CHRYSANTHU			
PO, 250s ea	54973-7632-01	4.37	7.29
RHUS AROMATICA			
PO, 250s ea	54973-7633-01	4.37	7.29
RHUS GLABRA			
PO, 250s ea	54973-7635-01	4.37	7.29
RHUS TOXICODENDRON			
PO, 250s ea	54973-7637-01	4.37	7.29
RHUS VENENATA			
PO, 250s ea	54973-7638-01	4.37	7.29
RUMEX CRISP			
PO, 250s ea	54973-7646-01	4.37	7.29
RUTA GRAVEOLENS			
PO, 250s ea	54973-7649-01	4.37	7.29
SABADILLA			
PO, 250s ea	54973-8011-01	4.37	7.29
SABAL SER			
PO, 250s ea	54973-8012-01	4.37	7.29
SABINA			
PO, 250s ea	54973-8013-01	4.37	7.29
SALICYLICUM ACIDUM			
PO, 250s ea	54973-8021-01	4.37	7.29
SALIX NIGER			
PO, 250s ea	54973-8023-01	4.37	7.29
SALVIA OFF			
PO, 250s ea	54973-8027-01	4.37	7.29
SAMBUCUS CAN			
PO, 250s ea	05497-8029-00	4.37	7.29
SAMBUCUS NIG			
PO, 250s ea	54973-8030-01	4.37	7.29
SANGUINARIA CANADENSIS			
PO, 250s ea	54973-8033-01	4.37	7.29
SANGUINARIA NITRICA			
PO, 250s ea	54973-8034-01	4.37	7.29
SANTONINUM			
PO, 250s ea	54973-8039-01	4.37	7.29
SAPONARIA OFF			
PO, 250s ea	54973-8042-01	4.37	7.29
SARSASPARILLA			
PO, 250s ea	54973-8048-01	4.37	7.29
SCILLA MARITIMA			
PO, 250s ea	54973-8116-01	4.37	7.29
SECALE CORNUTUM			
PO, 250s ea	54973-8062-01	4.37	7.29
SELENIUM METALLICUM			
PO, 250s ea	54973-8065-01	4.37	7.29
SENECIO CINERARIA			
PO, 250s ea	54973-2179-01	4.37	7.29
SEPIA			
PO, 250s ea	54973-8073-01	4.37	7.29
SILICEA			
TAB,PO, 6 x, 250s ea	54973-8081-01	4.37	7.29
SOLANINUM			
TAB,PO, 250s ea	54973-8092-01	4.37	7.29
SOLANUM NIGRUM			
PO, 250s ea	54973-8099-01	4.37	7.29
SPARTEINUM SULFURICUM			
PO, 250s ea	54973-8165-00	4.37	7.29
SPIGELIA ANTHELMIA			
PO, 250s ea	54973-8108-01	4.37	7.29
SPIREA ULM			
PO, 250s ea	54973-8112-01	4.37	7.29
SPONGIA			
PO, 250s ea	54973-8114-01	4.37	7.29
STANNUM METALLICUM			
PO, 250s ea	54973-8121-01	4.37	7.29
STAPHYSAGRIA			
PO, 250s ea	54973-8124-01	4.37	7.29
STICTA PULM			
PO, 250s ea	54973-8127-01	4.37	7.29
STIGMATA MAY			
PO, 250s ea	54973-8128-01	4.37	7.29
STRAMONIUM			
PO, 250s ea	54973-8132-01	4.37	7.29
STRONTIUM CARBONICUM			
PO, 250s ea	54973-8136-01	4.37	7.29

PROD/MFR	HRI, UPC,NDC	AWP	SRP
STROPHANTHUS HISPIDUS			
PO, 250s ea	54973-8139-01	4.37	7.29
STRYCHNINUM			
PO, 250s ea	54973-8146-01	4.37	7.29
STRYCHNINUM PHOSPHORICUM			
PO, 250s ea	54973-8143-01	4.37	7.29
STRYCHNINUM SULFURICUM			
PO, 250s ea	54973-8144-01	4.37	7.29
SULFANILAMIDUM			
PO, 250s ea	54973-8148-01	4.37	7.29
SULFUR HYDROGENISATUM			
PO, 250s ea	54973-8152-01	4.37	7.29
SULFUR ICUM ACIDUM			
PO, 250s ea	54973-8157-01	4.37	7.29
SULFUR IODATUM			
PO, 250s ea	54973-8156-01	4.37	7.29
SULFUROSUM ACIDUM			
PO, 250s ea	54973-8158-01	4.37	7.29
SYMPHYTUM OFF			
PO, 250s ea	54973-8161-01	4.37	7.29
SYPHILINUM			
PO, 250s ea	54973-8160-01	4.37	7.29
SYZYGIUM JAMBOLANUM			
PO, 250s ea	54973-8163-01	4.37	7.29
TABACUM			
PO, 250s ea	54973-9011-01	4.37	7.29
TAMUS COMMUNIS			
PO, 250s ea	54973-9012-01	4.37	7.29
TANACETUM VULGARE			
PO, 250s ea	54973-9013-01	4.37	7.29
STAPHA+SEPTIC (Tec)			
GEL,TP (1X56.7GM)			
0.2%-2.5%, 56.7 gm	51879-0170-02	8.00	14.99
STAPHYSAGRIA (Luyties)			
TAB,SL (6X)			
6 x, 500s ea	00618-8124-03	3.99	
5500s ea	00618-8124-10	30.32	
(30X)			
12 x, 500s ea	00622-8124-03	4.19	
5500s ea	00622-8124-10	31.83	
(12X)			
30 x, 500s ea	00624-8124-03	4.19	
5500s ea	00624-8124-10	31.83	
STAR OF BETHLEHEM (Ellon)			
SOL,SL (DROPS)			
10.5 ml	51762-0025-10		9.25
STAY AWAKE (AmerisourceBergen)			
TAB,PO (PRIVATE LABEL)			
200 mg, 16s ea	24385-0601-73	2.06	2.29
(Basic Vitamins)			
TAB,PO, 200 mg, 50s ea	00761-0500-10	2.00	
STAY AWAKE MAXIMUM STRENGTH (Chain Drug Marketing)			
TAB,PO, 200 mg, 16s ea	63868-0102-16	1.07	2.99
(Major)			
TAB,PO, 200 mg, 16s ea	00904-7955-44	2.25	
STEP 1 CLEANSER & DEODORIZER (Mentor)			
SPR,TP, 240 ml	81317-0026-80	9.88	
STEP 2 MOISTURE (Mentor)			
CRE,TP, 120 gm	81317-0022-40	12.80	
STEP 3 MOISTURE BARRIER (Mentor)			
OIN,TP, 120 gm	81317-0024-40	13.64	
STERI-OPTICS EYE WASH (Hi-Tech)			
SOL,OP, 118 ml	50383-0018-04	3.75	
(Nucare Pharm) REPACK			
SOL,OP, 120 ml	66267-0974-04	9.24	
STERI-PAD GAUZE STERILE (J&J Medical)			
DEV,NA (2"X2",12-PLY)			
100s ea	56091-0085-13	8.44	
(3"X3",12-PLY)			
100s ea	56091-0085-16	10.70	
(4"X4",12-PLY)			
100s ea	56091-0085-19	17.89	
STERI-STRIP REINFORCED SKIN CLOSURE (3M Health Care)			
DEV,NA (1"X5",4X25)			
100s ea	08333-1548-01	88.80	
(1/4"X3",3X50)			
150s ea	08333-1541-01	56.30	
(1/8"X3",5X50)			
250s ea	08333-1540-01	56.30	
(1/2"X2",6X50)			
300s ea	08333-1549-01	79.90	
(1/2"X4",6X50)			
300s ea	08333-1547-01	87.90	

PROD/MFR	HRI, UPC,NDC	AWP	SRP
(1/4"X1 1/2",6X50)			
300s ea	08333-1542-01	56.30	
(1/4"X4",10X50)			
500s ea	08333-1546-01	87.90	
STERI-STRIP WOUND CLOSURE (3M Health Care)			
DEV,NA (1 CLOSURE/ENVELOPE)			
25s ea	08333-8512-01	57.00	
(3 CLOSURES/ENVELOPE)			
25s ea	08333-8514-01	98.10	
(5 CLOSURES/ENVELOPE)			
25s ea	08333-8516-01	156.75	
STERI-TAMP (APP)			
DEV,NA (13MM,FORBOTTLE&VIAL,RED)			
1000s ea	63323-0210-03	83.65	
(20MM,BOTTLE&VIAL,SILVER)			
1000s ea	63323-0909-01	83.65	
(28MM,FORBOTLE&VIAL,BLUE)			
1000s ea	63323-0111-02	83.65	
(FOR SYRINGES,RED)			
1000s ea	63323-0410-03	83.65	
(FORLARGEBAGPORTS,BLUE)			
1000s ea	63323-0511-02	83.65	
(FORLARGEBAGPORTS,RED)			
1000s ea	63323-0511-03	83.65	
STERILE CATHETER INSERTION (Coloplast)			
DEV,NA, 80s ea	11701-0883-10	89.60	93.60
STERILE LANCETS (Home Diag)			
DEV,NA, 100s ea	56151-0142-60	6.50	
STERILE PADS (AmerisourceBergen)			
DEV,NA (3"X3",PRIVATE LABEL)			
10s ea	24385-0218-52	1.34	1.49
STETHOSCOPE (Lumiscope)			
DEV,NA (MED SPRAGUE RAPPAPORT)			
ea	38673-0040-25	9.99	19.99
STIK-IT (Gordon)			
LIQ,TP (AMP)			
0.5 ml 100s	10481-6107-05	85.00	
STIMULEN (Southwest)			
POW,TP (10X10)			
1 gm 100s	45713-0995-01	875.00	
20 gm 12s	45713-0695-20	2100.00	
40 gm 4s	45713-0395-40	1400.00	
STIMULIN (Marlyn)			
TAB,PO, 100 mg-1875 mg-100 mg,			
60s ea	32115-0609-05	17.50	34.99
120s ea	32115-0609-06	30.00	59.99
STING KILL (Dispensing Solutions) REPACK			
SWA,TP, 20%-1%, 5s ea	55045-3522-01	5.25	
STING-KILL (Randob)			
PAD,TP (WIPES)			
20%-1%, 8s ea	30103-0052-00	2.16	3.25
SWA,TP, 20%-1%, 5s ea	30103-0050-00	2.16	3.25
STOMA CAP ONE PIECE (Coloplast)			
DEV,NA (1-1/2"-2-1/4")			
30s ea	11701-0816-15	64.50	68.70
(UP TO 1-1/4")			
30s ea	11701-0816-10	65.40	68.70
STOMA CAP TWO PIECE (Coloplast)			
DEV,NA (OPAQUE, UP TO 1-1/2")			
30s ea	11701-0817-10	72.30	75.60
(OPAQUE, UP TO 1-3/4")			
30s ea	11701-0817-15	72.30	75.60
(OPAQUE, UP TO 2")			
30s ea	11701-0817-20	72.30	75.60
STOMA CONE W/TUBING (Coloplast)			
DEV,NA, ea	11701-0821-10	13.45	14.08
STOMAHESIVE (Convatec)			
DEV,NA (1X56.7GM,SKIN BARRIER)			
56.7 gm	68455-0106-90	9.46	12.32
STOMAHESIVE PROTECTIVE (Convatec)			
DEV,NA, 30 gm	68455-0108-26	7.46	9.71
STOMAHESIVE SKIN BARRIER (Convatec)			
DEV,NA (8"X8",NONSTERILE,WAFERS)			
3s ea	68455-0106-96	43.01	55.99
(4"X4",NONSTERILE,WAFERS)			
5s ea	68455-0106-94	18.11	23.58
(4"X4",STERILE,WAFERS)			
5s ea	68455-0106-95	21.33	27.76
STOMAHESIVE STRIPS (Convatec)			
DEV,NA (MOLDABLE ADHESIVE)			
15s ea	68455-0107-02	18.76	24.42
STOMATE EXTENSION TUBE (Abbott)			
DEV,NA (STRAIGHT)			
ea	70074-0513-37	10.56	

PROD/MFR	HRI, UPC,NDC	AWP	SRP
STOOL SOFTENER (Albertson's)			
SGL,PO (SOFTGEL)			
100 mg, 100s ea	41280-0201-71	4.62	
(AmerisourceBergen)			
SGL,PO (PRIVATE LABEL)			
100 mg, 100s ea	24385-0486-78	4.49	5.99
SYR,PO, 60 mg/15 ml, 473 ml	24385-0469-43	5.39	5.99
(Cardinal Health)			
SGL,PO (PRIVATE LABEL,SOFTGEL)			
240 mg, 100s ea	37205-0148-78	14.37	
(Major)			
SGL,PO (SOFTGEL)			
100 mg, 100s ea	00904-6039-60	3.98	
1000s ea	00904-6039-80	20.46	
(Mason Vit)			
SGL,PO (SOFTGEL)			
100 mg, 1000s ea	11845-0553-04	28.78	
STOOL SOFTENER EXTRA STRENGTH (AmerisourceBergen)			
SGL,PO (PRIVATE LABEL)			
250 mg, 100s ea	24385-0497-78	5.84	7.69
STOOL SOFTENER LAXATIVE (Cardinal Health)			
SGL,PO (PRIVATE LABEL,SOFTGEL)			
100 mg, 100s ea	37205-0265-01	5.72	
STOOL SOFTENER PLUS LAXATIVE (Albertson's)			
SGL,PO (SOFTGEL)			
30 mg-100 mg, 100s ea	41280-0201-72	5.37	
STOOL SOFTENER PLUS STIMULANT LAXATIVE (Cardinal Health)			
SGL,PO (PRIVATE LABEL,SOFTGEL)			
30 mg-100 mg, 100s ea	37205-0487-78	4.74	
STRATASORB COMPOSITE (Medline)			
DEV,NA (4"X10",STERILE)			
100s ea	08327-0507-09	322.23	
(4"X14",STERILE)			
100s ea	08327-0508-09	327.30	
(4"X4", STERILE)			
100s ea	53329-0006-40	120.00	
(6"X6", STERILE)			
100s ea	53329-0006-42	140.00	
(6"X7.5",STERILE)			
100s ea	53329-0006-46	372.12	
STRESS & TENSION RELIEF (Similasan Corp.)			
PEL,PO (1X15GM)			
4 x-3 x-4 x-4 x, 15 gm	59262-0600-30	6.21	10.99
STRESS 28 (Legere)			
TAB,PO, 100s ea	25332-1077-02	10.00	
1000s ea	25332-1077-01	59.95	
STRESS 600 (Upsher-Smith)			
TAB,PO, ea	00245-0132-89	0.10	
STRESS 600 W/ZINC (Consolidated Midland)			
TAB,PO, 100s ea	00223-1847-01	6.50	
1000s ea	00223-1847-02	57.50	
(Upsher-Smith)			
TAB,PO, ea	00245-0133-89	0.11	
STRESS FORMULA (Mason Vit)			
TAB,PO (PF,SF)			
60s ea	11845-0062-85	6.11	
(Nature's Bounty)			
TAB,PO (SF)			
60s ea	74312-0018-00		7.49
(Rexall)			
TAB,PO (PF,SF)			
60s ea	30768-0001-90	3.31	5.02
STRESS FORMULA + IRON (Cardinal Health)			
TAB,PO (PRIVATE LABEL)			
60s ea	37205-0181-72	5.60	
STRESS FORMULA 500 PLUS IRON (Marlex)			
TAB,PO (CAPLET,CAPLET)			
60s ea	10135-0319-60	1.69	
STRESS FORMULA 500 W/IRON (Basic Vitamins)			
TAB,PO (SF)			
60s ea	00761-0127-12	3.00	
STRESS FORMULA 500 W/ZINC/BIOTIN (Basic Vitamins)			
PO (SF)			
60s ea	00761-0189-12	3.00	

PROD/MFR	HRI, UPC,NDC	AWP	SRP
STRESS FORMULA VITAMINS (Albertson's)			
TAB,PO, 60s ea	04000-0001-93	5.04	
(Family Phcy)			
TAB,PO (PRIVATE LABEL)			
60s ea	52735-0037-13	4.76	6.39
60s ea	52735-0039-13	6.02	6.69
STRESS FORMULA W/IRON (Mason Vit)			
TAB,PO, 60s ea	11845-0070-45	6.11	
STRESS FORMULA W/ZINC (Mason Vit)			
TAB,PO, 60s ea	11845-0074-55	6.11	
(Nature's Bounty)			
TAB,PO (SF)			
60s ea	74312-0003-50		7.49
STRESS TABS (Teva)			
TAB,PO, 60s ea	00182-4487-26	5.99	
STRESS TABS W/VITAMIN B/IRON (Southwood)			
REPACK			
TAB,PO, 130s ea	58016-0634-99	25.31	
STRESS W/ IRON (Teva)			
TAB,PO, 60s ea	00182-4481-26	6.19	
STRESS W/ ZINC (Teva)			
TAB,PO, 60s ea	00182-4491-26	6.39	
STRESSFREE (Health Products Corp)			
TAB,PO (PF,SF)			
60s ea	39686-0013-34	4.85	
STRESSTABS (Inverness)			
TAB,PO, 60s ea	36652-0124-19	7.74	7.30
STRESSTABS W/IRON (Inverness)			
TAB,PO, 60s ea	36652-0126-19	7.74	7.30
STRIP-EASE ADHESIVE REMOVER (Oakhurst)			
LIQ,TP, 473 ml	11169-0048-16	5.82	8.72
STRIX-BILBERRY EXTRACT (Scandinavian)			
TAB,PO, 180 mg-80 mg-5 mg,			
60s ea	51137-0000-00	11.97	19.95
STRONTIUM (Bio-Tech Pharm)			
CAP,PO, 340 mg, 100s ea	53191-0477-01	15.95	
STUART PRENATAL (Xanodyne Pharma)			
TAB,PO, 100s ea	64731-0795-01	24.61	
STUD 100 (Pound Intl)			
SPR,TP, 9.6%,			
13.13 ml 12s	48132-0100-24	71.40	
STYE (Del)			
OIN,OP, 3.75 gm	10310-0143-08	5.98	8.96
STYE EYE RELIEF (Similasan Corp.)			
SOL,OP (DROPS)			
6 x-12 x-12 x,			
10 ml	59262-0350-11	6.21	10.99
STYGIENE (Del)			
LIQ,TP (W/PADS)			
120 ml	10310-0325-30	5.16	7.74
SUCRETS CHILDREN'S FORMULA			
(Heritage/Insight)			
LOZ,MM (CHERRY)			
1.2 mg, 18s ea	53100-0009-02	2.53	
SUCRETS MAXIMUM STRENGTH (Heritage/Insight)			
LOZ,MM (CHERRY)			
3 mg, 18s ea	53100-0009-16	2.91	
(WINTERGREEN)			
3 mg, 18s ea	53100-0009-15	2.91	
SUCRETS ORIGINAL REGULAR STRENGTH			
(Heritage/Insight)			
LOZ,MM (MINT)			
2.4 mg, 18s ea	53100-0008-51	2.53	
SUCRETS REGULAR STRENGTH (Heritage/Insight)			
LOZ,MM (ASSORTED)			
2 mg, 18s ea	53100-0009-17	2.53	
(CHERRY)			
2 mg, 18s ea	53100-0008-85	2.53	
SUDACARE ADVANCED VAPOR-PLUG			
(McNeil Consumer Healthcare)			
PAD,IH (REFILL ONLY)			
ea	12547-0230-02	5.04	
(VAPOR-PLUG UNIT)			
ea	12547-0230-01	7.18	
SUDACARE NIGHTTIME VAPOR PLUG			
(Johnson & Johnson)			
PAD,IH (REFILLS ONLY)			
5s ea	12547-0228-91	4.19	
(W/VAPOR PLUG UNIT)			
5s ea	12547-0228-90	7.19	

PROD/MFR	HRI, UPC,NDC	AWP	SRP
SUDACARE NIGHTTIME VAPOR PLUG CHILDREN'S			
(Johnson & Johnson)			
PAD,IH (REFILLS ONLY)			
5s ea	12547-0228-93	4.19	
(W/VAPOR PLUG UNIT)			
5s ea	12547-0228-92	7.19	
SUDACARE SHOWER SOOTHERS			
(McNeil Consumer Healthcare)			
TEF,IH (NON-MEDICATED)			
3s ea	12547-0230-04	4.16	
(VAPOR SHOWER TABS)			
3s ea	12547-0230-03	4.16	
7s ea	12547-0230-07	8.36	
SUDAFED (McNeil Consumer Healthcare)			
TAB,PO (MAX STRENGTH/NON-DROWSY)			
30 mg, 24s ea	00810-0865-24	4.46	
48s ea	00810-0865-48	7.45	
96s ea	00819-0600-24	12.47	
SUDAFED 12 HOUR			
(McNeil Consumer Healthcare)			
TER,PO (NON-DROWSY,CAPLET)			
120 mg, 10s ea	00810-0670-13	4.46	
20s ea	00810-0670-20	7.45	
(A-S Medication)			
REPACK			
TER,PO (CAPLET)			
120 mg, 10s ea	54569-6088-00	4.49	
SUDAFED 12HR (Phys Total Care)			
REPACK			
TER,PO, 120 mg, 10s ea	54868-1805-00	6.51	
SUDAFED 24 HOUR (Johnson & Johnson)			
TER,PO (NON-DROWSY)			
240 mg, 5s ea	00081-9600-26	4.22	
(McNeil Consumer Healthcare)			
TER,PO (NON-DROWSY)			
240 mg, 10s ea	00819-0600-27	7.45	
SUDAFED CHILDREN'S (Johnson & Johnson)			
SOL,PO (NON-DROWSY,AF,SF,GRAPE)			
15 mg/5 ml, 118 ml	00501-2880-04	4.87	
SUDAFED CHILDREN'S COLD & COUGH			
(Johnson & Johnson)			
SOL,PO (AF,SF,BERRY-CHERRY)			
5 mg/5 ml-15 mg/5 ml,			
118 ml	00081-0875-82	4.87	
SUDAFED OM SINUS COLD			
(McNeil Consumer Healthcare)			
SPR,NS (12HR)			
0.05%, 15 ml	00450-0520-05	5.94	
SUDAFED OM SINUS CONGESTION			
(McNeil Consumer Healthcare)			
SPR,NS (12HR)			
0.05%, 15 ml	00450-0528-05	5.94	
SUDAFED PE (Johnson & Johnson)			
FIL,MM (QUICK-DISSOLVE)			
10 mg, 10s ea	12547-0229-00	4.22	
TAB,PO (MAX STRENGTH,NON-DROWSY)			
10 mg, 18s ea	00501-2902-18	4.22	
36s ea	00501-2902-31	6.79	
72s ea	00501-2902-79	11.76	
(McNeil Consumer Healthcare)			
TAB,PO (MAX STRENGTH,NON-DROWSY)			
10 mg, 18s ea	00819-0600-65	4.46	
36s ea	00819-0600-66	7.15	
72s ea	00819-0600-67	11.95	
(Quality Care Prod)			
REPACK			
TAB,PO, 10 mg, 36s ea	49999-0827-36	6.24	
SUDAFED PE COLD & COUGH (Johnson & Johnson)			
TAB,PO (NON-DROWSY)			
325 mg-10 mg-100 mg-5 mg,			
10s ea	00501-2909-10	3.40	
20s ea	00501-2909-20	5.95	
(McNeil Consumer Healthcare)			
TAB,PO (NON-DROWSY)			
325 mg-10 mg-100 mg-5 mg,			
10s ea	12547-0227-30	3.38	
20s ea	12547-0227-31	5.94	
SUDAFED PE DAY & NIGHT			
(McNeil Consumer Healthcare)			
TAB,PO (18+12,ULTRATAB)			
30s ea	00450-0113-30	7.15	
SUDAFED PE DAY & NIGHT COLD			
(McNeil Consumer Healthcare)			
TAB,PO (CAPLET,COATED CAPLET)			
20s ea	00450-0115-20	5.94	

PROD/MFR	HRI, UPC,NDC	AWP	SRP
SUDAFED PE NIGHTTIME COLD			
(Johnson & Johnson)			
TAB,PO (MAX STRENGTH,CAPLET)			
325 mg-25 mg-5 mg,			
20s ea	00501-2907-20	4.22	
(McNeil Consumer Healthcare)			
TAB,PO (MAX STRENGTH)			
325 mg-25 mg-5 mg,			
20s ea	12547-0227-36	4.46	
SUDAFED PE NON-DRYING SINUS			
(McNeil Consumer Healthcare)			
TAB,PO (MAX STRENGTH/NON-DROWSY)			
200 mg-5 mg,			
24s ea	12547-0227-32	4.76	
SUDAFED PE SEVERE COLD			
(McNeil Consumer Healthcare)			
TAB,PO (MULTI-SYMPTOM)			
325 mg-12.5 mg-5 mg,			
12s ea	12547-0227-33	3.38	
24s ea	12547-0227-34	5.94	
SUDAFED PE SINUS & ALLERGY			
(Johnson & Johnson)			
TAB,PO (MAX STRENGTH)			
4 mg-10 mg, 24s ea	00501-2912-24	4.69	
(McNeil Consumer Healthcare)			
TAB,PO (MAX STRENGTH)			
4 mg-10 mg, 24s ea	00819-0600-70	4.76	
SUDAFED PE SINUS HEADACHE			
(McNeil Consumer Healthcare)			
TAB,PO (MAX STRENGTH/NON-DROWSY)			
325 mg-5 mg,			
24s ea	12547-0227-38	4.76	
48s ea	12547-0227-39	7.45	
SUDAFED PE TRIPLE ACTION			
(McNeil Consumer Healthcare)			
TAB,PO (NON-DROWSY,12DOSES)			
325 mg-200 mg-5 mg,			
24s ea	00450-0526-24	5.94	
SUDAFED SINUS & PAIN			
(McNeil Consumer Healthcare)			
T12,PO (NON-DROWSY,CAPLET)			
220 mg-120 mg,			
16s ea	00450-0358-16	7.45	
SUDAFED TRIPLE ACTION			
(McNeil Consumer Healthcare)			
TAB,PO (NON-DROWSY,18DOSES)			
325 mg-200 mg-30 mg,			
36s ea	00450-0546-36	7.45	
SUDATEX G (Larken Labs, Inc.)			
TAB,PO, 400 mg-40 mg,			
100s ea	68047-0243-01	70.79	
SUDATUSS DM (Pharmakon)			
SYR,PO (AF,CHERRY)			
118 ml	55422-0404-04	2.38	4.95
SUDO GEST CHILDREN'S (Major)			
SOL,PO (AF,SF,GRAPE)			
15 mg/5 ml, 118 ml	00904-5367-20	2.50	
SUDO-TAB (Hart Health)			
TAB,PO (2X8)			
30 mg, 16s ea UD	50332-0104-05	0.97	
(2X50)			
30 mg, 100s ea UD	50332-0104-04	3.39	
(2X125)			
30 mg, 250s ea UD	50332-0104-02	7.59	
SUDO-TAB PE (Hart Health)			
TAB,PO (50 PACKETSX2)			
5 mg, 100s ea UD	50332-0126-04	3.49	
(125 PACKETSX2)			
5 mg, 250s ea UD	50332-0126-07	7.91	
SUDODRINE (Global Source)			
TAB,PO, 30 mg, 24s ea	59618-0800-06	1.70	
SUDOGEST (Major)			
TAB,PO, 30 mg, 24s ea	00904-5053-24	1.65	
(UNBOXED)			
30 mg, 100s ea	00904-5053-59	3.15	
60 mg, 30s ea	00904-5125-46	3.69	
100s ea	00904-5125-59	4.90	
SUDOGEST 12 HOUR (Major)			
TER,PO (MAX STRENGTH)			
120 mg, 10s ea	00904-5803-15	4.17	
SUDOGEST CHILDREN'S (Major)			
SYR,PO (WITHOUT DROWSINESS,AF)			
30 mg/5 ml, 118 ml	00904-5987-20	2.50	

PROD/MFR	HRI, UPC,NDC	AWP	SRP
SUDOGEST COLD & ALLERGY (Major)			
TAB,PO (MAXIMUM STRENGTH)			
4 mg-60 mg, 24s ea	00904-5351-24	2.10	
SUDOGEST PE (Major)			
TAB,PO (12X1)			
10 mg, 12s ea	00904-5733-05	1.35	
18s ea	00904-5733-49	3.79	
36s ea	00904-5733-73	2.95	
72s ea	00904-5733-62	10.58	
SUGAR-DOWN (3 B's Limited)			
CAP,PO, 0.68 gm-0.02 gm,			
200s ea	30371-0000-33	18.10	27.85
SULFO-LO (Med-Derm)			
SOA,TP, ea	45565-0710-20	4.96	
SULFOAM (Doak)			
SHA,TP, 2%, 240 ml	10337-0022-51	29.27	
SULFOIL (Genesis)			
LIQ,TP (SOAP-FREE)			
480 ml	00398-0041-16	9.24	
3840 ml	00398-0041-28	58.14	
SULFUR (Consolidated Midland)			
OIN,TP, 30 gm	00223-4148-30	1.60	
454 gm	00223-4148-13	6.50	
SULFUR SOAP (Stiefel Consumer HealthCare)			
SOA,TP (3.5OZ)			
10%, 100 gm	00145-1024-03	3.84	5.79
(Phys Total Care)			
REPACK			
SOA,TP, 10%, ea	54868-1588-00	6.91	
SULMASQUE (Genesis)			
CRE,TP, 6.4%, 150 gm	00398-0222-50	15.96	
SULPHO-LAC SOAP (Doak)			
LIQ,TP, 5%, 90 ml	10337-0023-61	15.18	
SULPHUR (Luyties)			
TAB,SL (6X)			
6 x, 500s ea	00618-8155-03	3.99	
5500s ea	00618-8155-10	30.32	
(30X)			
12 x, 500s ea	00622-8155-03	4.19	
5500s ea	00622-8155-10	31.83	
30 x, 500s ea	00624-8155-03	4.19	
5500s ea	00624-8155-10	31.83	
(Walker Pharmacal)			
TAB,SL (6X)			
250s ea	00619-8155-02	2.97	
SUMA (Botanical Labs.)			
LIQ,PO, 30 ml	41954-0020-51	5.00	9.99
60 ml	41954-0020-24	8.00	15.99
SUMMER'S EVE ANTI-ITCH (Fleet,C.B.)			
GEL,TP (MAXIMUM STRENGTH)			
39%-1%, 28 gm	41608-0087-82	3.29	
SUMMER'S EVE ANTI-ITCH CLOTHS (Fleet,C.B.)			
PAD,TP (MAXIMUM STRENGTH)			
1%, 12s ea	41608-0087-83	3.29	
SUMMER'S EVE BATH & SHOWER (Fleet,C.B.)			
GEL,TP (GREEN TEA & CUCUMBER)			
354 ml	41608-0001-05	2.30	
(SENSITIVE SKIN)			
354 ml	41608-0001-06	2.30	
SUMMER'S EVE DOUCHE (Fleet,C.B.)			
SOL,VG (ISLAND SPLASH,4 UNITS)			
133 ml	41608-0875-46	2.27	
(ISLAND SPLASH,TWO UNTS)			
133 ml	41608-0087-54	1.48	
(SWEET ROMANCE,FOUR UNTS)			
133 ml	41608-0875-86	2.27	
(SWEET ROMANCE,TWO UNTS)			
133 ml	41608-0087-58	1.48	
(TROPICAL RAIN,TWO UNTS)			
133 ml	41608-0087-55	1.48	
(TROPICL RAIN,FOUR UNTS)			
133 ml	41608-0875-56	2.27	
(FRESH SCENT)			
135 ml	41608-0087-20	0.85	
(VINEGAR& WATER)			
135 ml	41608-0087-22	0.85	
(FRESH SCENT,TWIN)			
135 ml 2s	41608-0087-40	1.48	
(VINEGAR& WATER,TWIN)			
135 ml 2s	41608-0087-42	1.48	
(FRESH SCENT,4-PACK)			
135 ml 4s	41608-0874-04	2.27	
(VINEGAR & WATER,4-PACK)			
135 ml 4s	41608-0874-24	2.27	
(MEDICATED,TWIN)			
0.3%, 135 ml 2s	41608-0087-43	2.29	
SUMMER'S EVE DOUCHE EXTRA CLEANSING (Fleet,C.B.)			
SOL,VG (VINEGAR & WATER)			
135 ml	41608-0087-27	0.85	
(VINEGAR & WATER,TWIN)			
135 ml 2s	41608-0087-47	1.48	
(VINEGAR & WATER,4-PACK)			
135 ml 4s	41608-0874-74	2.27	
SUMMER'S EVE DOUCHE ULTRA (Fleet,C.B.)			
SOL,VG (TWIN)			
135 ml 2s	41608-0087-48	1.48	
(4-PACK)			
135 ml 4s	41608-0874-86	2.27	
SUMMER'S EVE FEMININE (Fleet,C.B.)			
POW,TP (COTTON BREEZE)			
255 gm	41608-0870-99	2.30	
(REGULAR)			
255 gm	41608-0870-85	2.30	
SUMMER'S EVE FEMININE CLEANSING CLOTHS (Fleet,C.B.)			
PAD,TP (SENSITIVE SKIN,AF)			
32s ea	41608-0087-35	2.75	
SUMMER'S EVE FEMININE DEODORANT (Fleet,C.B.)			
SPR,TP (BABY POWDER)			
42.5 gm	41608-0087-65	2.28	
(ISLAND SPLASH)			
42.5 gm	41608-0087-72	2.28	
(TROPICAL RAIN)			
42.5 gm	41608-0087-73	2.28	
(ULTRA EXT. STR.,NO TALC)			
42.5 gm	41608-0087-66	2.28	
SUMMER'S EVE FEMININE WASH (Fleet,C.B.)			
LIQ,TP (NORMAL SKIN,SOAP-FREE)			
450 ml	41608-0087-01	3.00	
SOL,TP (DELICATE BLOSSOM)			
266 ml	41608-0870-39	2.30	
(NORMAL SKIN,SOAP-FREE)			
266 ml	41608-0870-09	2.30	
(SENSITIVE SKIN)			
266 ml	41608-0870-49	2.30	
444 ml	41608-0140-78	3.00	
SUMMER'S EVE FEMININE WASH CLOTHS (Fleet,C.B.)			
PAD,TP (NORMAL SKIN,SOAP-FREE)			
16s ea	41608-0087-10	1.33	
(SENSITIVE SKIN)			
16s ea	41608-0087-11	1.33	
SUMMER'S EVE FOAMING BATH (Fleet,C.B.)			
SOL,TP (SENSITIVE SKIN, BERRY)			
354 ml	41608-0870-52	2.30	
(SOOTHING BOTANICALS)			
354 ml	41608-0870-51	2.30	
SUNBLOCK (AmerisourceBergen)			
LOT,TP (SPF 15,SF,PRIVATE LABEL)			
120 ml	24385-0234-26	4.49	
SUNBLOCK CHILDREN'S (AmerisourceBergen)			
LOT,TP (SPF 45,AF,SF)			
120 ml	24385-0093-26	3.28	5.79
SUNDANCE ALOE VERA (Lee Pharm)			
GEL,TP (FRAGRANCE-FREE)			
120 gm	23558-0684-10	1.79	
120 gm 12s	23558-0684-11	21.46	
240 gm	23558-0684-20	2.51	
240 gm 12s	23558-0684-21	30.10	
SUNMARK ALLERGY RELIEF (McKesson)			
ODT,PO (24 HOUR, NON-DROWSY)			
10 mg, 12s ea	49348-0637-02	8.99	
20s ea	49348-0635-01	16.99	
24s ea	49348-0638-04	15.49	
SUNMARK CLICKFINE UNIVERSAL PEN NEEDLES (Can-Am Care)			
DEV,NA (31G,6MM (1/4"))			
100s ea	08396-9004-00	19.98	
(31G,8MM (5/16"))			
100s ea	08396-9005-00	19.98	
SUNMARK COUGH DROPS (McKesson)			
LOZ,MM (PRIVATE LABEL)			
5 mg, 25s ea	49348-0643-05		1.89
SUNMARK HEADACHE RELIEF (McKesson)			
TAB,PO (COATED)			
250 mg-250 mg-65 mg,			
100s ea	49348-0722-10	6.19	3.99
SUNMARK INSULIN SYRINGE (Can-Am Care)			
DEV,NA (ULTRACMFORT,31G,5/16")			
100s ea	38396-0453-39	17.50	
(ULTRACMFRT,28G,1/2")			
100s ea	38396-0763-39	15.50	
(ULTRACMFRT,29G,1/2")			
100s ea	38396-0793-39	17.50	
(ULTRACOMFORT,28G,1/2")			
100s ea	38396-0773-39	15.50	
(ULTRACOMFORT,29G,1/2")			
100s ea	38396-0803-39	17.50	
(ULTRACOMFRT,30G,5/16")			
100s ea	38396-0833-39	17.50	
(ULTRCMFRT,29G,1/2")			
100s ea	38396-0783-39	17.50	
(ULTRCMFRT,30G,5/16")			
100s ea	38396-0823-39	17.50	
(ULTRCMFRT,31G,5/16")			
100s ea	38396-0463-39	17.50	
(UTRCMFRT,30G,5/16")			
100s ea	38396-0813-39	17.50	
(UTRCMFRT,31G,5/16"1ML)			
100s ea	38396-0473-39	17.50	
SUNMARK LANCETS (Can-Am Care)			
DEV,NA (STANDARD,21G)			
100s ea	38396-0703-39	5.85	
(SUPER THIN,30G)			
100s ea	38396-0723-39	5.85	
(THIN,26G)			
100s ea	38396-0713-39	5.85	
(COLOR,21G)			
200s ea	38396-0743-39	9.50	
(STANDARD,21G)			
200s ea	38396-0733-39	9.50	
(THIN,26G)			
200s ea	38396-0753-39	9.50	
SUNMARK MICONAZOLE 7 (McKesson)			
CRE,VG (1X45GM, W/APPLICATOR)			
2%, 45 gm	49348-0872-77	7.99	
SUNMARK NASAL DECONGESTANT PE (McKesson)			
TAB,PO (ND,MAX STRENGTH)			
10 mg, 18s ea	49348-0700-48		3.79
SUNMARK NICOTINE (McKesson)			
GUM,PO (USP,PRIVATE LABEL,MINT)			
2 mg, 110s ea	49348-0691-36		43.99
4 mg, 110s ea	49348-0692-36		43.99
SUNMARK NICOTINE LOZENGE (McKesson)			
LOZ,PO (PRIVATE LABEL,MINT)			
2 mg, 72s ea	49348-0852-16		33.59
4 mg, 72s ea	49348-0853-16		33.59
SUNMARK SINUS 12 HOUR (McKesson)			
TER,PO (NON-DROWSY)			
120 mg, 10s ea	49348-0361-01		3.89
SUNMARK STOOL SOFTENER (McKesson)			
TAB,PO (PLUS STIMULANT LAXATIVE)			
50 mg-8.6 mg, 100s ea	49348-0544-10	5.79	
250s ea	49348-0544-19	9.69	
SUNMARK ULTRA-COMFORT INSULIN SYRINGES (Can-Am Care)			
DEV,NA (28G,1/2"(12.7MM),1/2CC)			
100s ea	08396-8001-00	17.50	
(28G,1/2"(12.7MM),1CC)			
100s ea	08396-8002-00	17.50	
(29G,1/2"(12.7MM),1/2CC)			
100s ea	08396-8004-00	17.50	
(29G,1/2"(12.7MM),1CC)			
100s ea	08396-8005-00	17.50	
(29G,1/2"(12.7MM),3/10CC)			
100s ea	08396-8003-00	17.50	
(30G, 5/16"(8MM), 1/2CC)			
100s ea	08396-8007-00	17.50	
(30G, 5/16"(8MM), 1CC)			
100s ea	08396-8008-00	17.50	
(30G, 5/16"(8MM), 3/10CC)			
100s ea	08396-8006-00	17.50	
(31G, 5/16"(8MM), 3/10CC)			
100s ea	08396-8009-00	17.50	
(31G, 5/16"(8MM),1/2CC)			
100s ea	08396-8010-00	17.50	
(31G, 5/16"(8MM),1CC)			
100s ea	08396-8011-00	17.50	
SUNNIE (Green Turtle)			
TAB,PO (PF,SF,DYE-FREE)			
120s ea	59074-0400-01	23.40	38.99
SUNSHIELD (Hart Health)			
LOT,TP (1X44ML,SPF 30,OIL-FREE)			
5%-7.5%-5%-3%,			
44 ml	50332-0253-11	1.53	
SUNVITE (Rexall)			
TAB,PO (PF,SF)			
90s ea	30768-0000-64	3.36	5.08

PROD/MFR	HRI, UPC,NDC	AWP	SRP
SUNVITE PLATINUM (Rexall)			
TAB,PO (PF,SF)			
60s ea	30768-0000-67	3.00	4.55
SUPER 2 DAILY (Carlson,J.R.)			
SGL,PO (PF,SF,CORN-FREE)			
60s ea	88395-0040-50	9.45	18.90
120s ea	88395-0040-51	17.95	35.90
SUPER ANTIOXIDANT FORMULA (Linus)			
CAP,PO, 50s ea	10363-0253-19	5.37	9.79
SUPER B100 (Teva)			
TER,PO, 60s ea	00182-4505-26	9.39	
SUPER BETA-CAROTENE (Carlson,J.R.)			
SGL,PO (PF,SF,DAIRY-FREE)			
25000 iu-1 iu, 100s ea	88395-0011-81	7.88	15.75
250s ea	88395-0011-82	17.75	35.50
SUPER C1000 COMPLEX (Mason Vit)			
TER,PO (PF,SF)			
90s ea	11845-0117-89	14.89	
SUPER C500 COMPLEX (Mason Vit)			
PO (PF,SF)			
90s ea	11845-0117-79	9.56	
SUPER CALCIUM (Linus)			
TAB,PO (CAPLET)			
90s ea	10363-0253-18	4.17	7.79
(Mason Vit)			
TAB,PO, 600 mg, 100s ea	11845-0085-31	6.89	
SUPER CALCIUM 600 W/IRON/VITAMIN D (Mason Vit)			
TAB,PO (PF,SF)			
600 mg-18 mg-125 iu, 60s ea	11845-0095-35	5.22	
SUPER CALCIUM EXTRA STRENGTH (Mason Vit)			
TAB,PO (PF,SF)			
600 mg, 60s ea	11845-0085-35	4.22	
SUPER CALCIUM W/D (Dispensing Solutions)			
REPACK			
TAB,PO, 600 mg-200 iu, 100s ea	55045-3507-01	8.00	
SUPER COD LIVER OIL (Carlson,J.R.)			
SGL,PO (SOFTGEL)			
1000 mg, 100s ea	88395-0013-01	6.20	12.40
250s ea	88395-0013-02	11.20	22.40
SUPER COLD (Reese)			
TAB,PO, 325 mg-2 mg-5 mg, 36s ea	10956-0771-36	4.00	
SUPER ENERGY HERBAL COMPLEX (Mason Vit)			
TAB,PO (PF,SF)			
60s ea	11845-0119-65	12.22	
SUPER EPA 1200 (Advanced Nutr)			
SGL,PO, 1200 mg, 90s ea	62617-0045-03	20.30	
SUPER EPA 2000 (Advanced Nutr)			
SGL,PO, 2000 mg, 90s ea	62617-0050-03	27.00	36.00
SUPER FAT BURNERS (Action Labs)			
TAB,PO, 60s ea	24675-0227-61	6.99	13.99
120s ea	24675-0227-21	12.49	24.99
200s ea	24675-0227-81	16.99	33.99
SUPER FIT BURNERS (Action Labs)			
TAB,PO (SF)			
60s ea	24675-0317-61	7.49	14.99
120s ea	24675-0317-21	13.99	27.99
SUPER GINKGO BILOBA PLUS GOTA KOLA (Action Labs)			
TAB,PO (SF)			
50s ea	24675-0170-51	6.49	12.99
100s ea	24675-0171-01	11.99	23.99
SUPER GINSENG MULTIVITAMIN (Mason Vit)			
CAP,PO (PF,SF)			
60s ea	11845-1137-05	13.22	
SUPER GLUCOSAMINE COMPLEX (Action Labs)			
TAB,PO (PF,SF)			
100 mg-500 mg-5 mg, 60s ea	24675-0505-61	10.49	20.99
200 mg-1000 mg-5 mg, 60s ea	24675-0501-60	19.49	38.99
SUPER MALIC PLUS (Optimox)			
TAB,PO, 180s ea	50520-0015-01	13.00	
SUPER MELATONIN PLUS (Action Labs)			
TAB,PO (SF)			
60s ea	24675-0131-61	3.99	7.99
SUPER MILK THISTLE PLUS (Action Labs)			
TAB,PO, 50s ea	24675-0190-51	6.49	12.99
SUPER MSM PLUS (Action Labs)			
TAB,PO (SF)			
60s ea	24675-0544-10	10.00	19.99
SUPER MULTI MINERAL FORMULA (Freeda)			
TAB,PO (IRON FREE,IRON-FREE)			
200s ea	10432-0357-01	12.87	21.45
SUPER MULTI MINERAL FORMULA WITH IRON (Freeda)			
PO (SF,GLUTEN-FREE)			
200s ea	10432-0356-01	13.17	21.95
SUPER MULTI-VITAMIN & MINERALS (Linus)			
TAB,PO (CAPLET)			
120s ea	10363-0253-15	5.98	10.95
SUPER MULTIPLE (Mason Vit)			
TAB,PO, 50s ea	11845-0099-89	11.56	
60s ea	11845-0056-25	9.89	
100s ea	11845-0056-21	13.89	
100s ea	11845-0099-81	14.22	
SUPER MULTIPLE 33 W/MINERALS (Rexall)			
TAB,PO, 60s ea	30768-0011-10	5.06	7.67
SUPER OMEGA-3 (Carlson,J.R.)			
SGL,PO (PF,SOFTGEL)			
1000 mg-10 iu, 50s ea	88395-0015-20	6.45	12.90
100s ea	88395-0015-21	12.75	25.50
250s ea	88395-0015-22	28.95	57.90
SUPER PAPAYA ENZYME (ADH)			
CTB,PO, 100s ea	60142-0098-10	2.48	4.95
SUPER SAW PALMETTO PLUS (Action Labs)			
TAB,PO (SF)			
50s ea	24675-0160-51	5.99	11.99
100s ea	24675-0161-01	10.99	21.99
SUPER SINADRIN (Reese)			
TAB,PO, 325 mg-2 mg-5 mg, 36s ea	10956-0770-36	4.00	
SUPER THIN LANCET (Atlanta & Pacific)			
DEV,NA (30G)			
100s ea	08214-0657-26	4.75	
(Aurora)			
DEV,NA (30G)			
100s ea	08214-0657-24	4.65	
SUPER VIKAPS (Reese)			
TAB,PO (PF,SF,CAPLET)			
50s ea	10956-0617-50	4.61	
100s ea	10956-0617-09	6.77	
SUPER-1-DAILY (Carlson,J.R.)			
TAB,PO (VEGETARIAN,PF,SF)			
30s ea	88395-0040-00	6.45	12.90
60s ea	88395-0040-09	10.75	21.50
120s ea	88395-0040-11	19.95	39.90
180s ea	88395-0040-02	29.95	59.90
SUPER-C-COMPLEX (Carlson,J.R.)			
TAB,PO, 500 mg-500 mg, 100s ea	88395-0032-51	6.45	12.90
250s ea	88395-0032-52	14.95	29.90
500s ea	88395-0032-55	27.95	55.90
SUPERDOPHILUS (Natren)			
CAP,PO (PF)			
60s ea	53983-0600-15	13.20	22.00
PDR,PO, 1.2 billion org/gm, 70 gm	53983-0100-15	12.60	21.00
(PF) 1.2 billion org/gm, 84 gm	53983-0600-35	18.00	30.00
126 gm	53983-0100-25	18.00	30.00
(PF) 2 billion org/gm, 49 gm	53983-0600-25	12.00	20.00
SUPERFATTED SOAP W/LANOLIN (Mann)			
SOA,TP, 12s ea	99743-0012-04	11.20	16.75
SUPERIOR 35 (Mason Vit)			
TER,PO (PF,SF)			
60s ea	11845-0125-05	11.33	
SUPERIOR TRACHEOSTOMY CARE (Covidien)			
DEV,NA, 50s ea	08080-4789-20	51.74	
SUPERMINS (Key Company)			
TAB,PO (CORN-FREE,GLUTEN-FREE)			
100s ea	11694-0714-01	10.00	
250s ea	11694-0714-02	22.50	
SUPERPLEX-T (Major)			
TAB,PO, 100s ea	00904-2253-60	8.65	
SUPERSOFT (Ameriderm Labs)			
LOT,TP (24X473ML,FRAGRANCE-FREE)			
473 ml 24s	63921-0120-16	3.39	
SUPHEDRIN (AmerisourceBergen)			
SYR,PO (PRIVATE LABEL)			
30 mg/5 ml, 118 ml	24385-0410-26	3.41	3.79
TAB,PO, 30 mg, 48s ea	24385-0432-67	4.49	5.99
96s ea	24385-0432-80	8.81	9.79
SUPHEDRIN 12 HOUR (AmerisourceBergen)			
TER,PO (NON-DROWSY)			
120 mg, 10s ea	24385-0054-52	3.59	3.99
SUPHEDRIN COLD & COUGH (AmerisourceBergen)			
SGL,PO (LIQUICAP,NON-DROWSY)			
10s ea	24385-0915-52	2.60	2.89
SUPHEDRIN PLUS (AmerisourceBergen)			
TAB,PO (PRIVATE LABEL)			
4 mg-60 mg, 24s ea	24385-0450-62	4.49	4.99
SUPHEDRIN SINUS MAXIMUM STRENGTH (AmerisourceBergen)			
TAB,PO (NON-DROWSY)			
500 mg-30 mg, 24s ea	24385-0643-62	3.50	3.89
SUPHEDRINE (Chain Drug Marketing)			
TAB,PO (NON-DROWSY)			
30 mg, 24s ea	63868-0146-24	0.83	3.99
SUPLENA (Abbott)			
LIQ,PO (VANILLA)			
240 ml	70074-0501-65	3.20	
SUPLENA WITH CARB STEADY (Abbott)			
LIQ,PO (GLUTEN-FREE)			
237 ml	70074-0596-65	3.20	
SUPLEVIT (Gil Pharmaceutical)			
LIQ,PO (AF,SF,BUTTERSCOTCH)			
237 ml	58552-0101-08	15.30	
SUPPOSITORY MOLD DISPOSABLE (Paddock)			
DEV,NA (ADULT)			
100s ea	00574-9100-01	12.15	
(PEDIATRIC) 100s ea	00574-9050-01	12.15	
(ADULT) 1000s ea	00574-9100-10	85.00	
SUPREME (Arkray)			
DEV,NA (STRIP)			
50s ea	08317-8850-50	35.40	
SUPREME II (Arkray)			
DEV,NA (HIGH/LOW CONTROL)			
ea	08317-8825-01	12.00	
SUPRESS DX PEDIATRIC (Kramer-Novis)			
LIQ,PO (SF,DROPS)			
30 ml	52083-0055-01	8.00	
SUR-FIT NATURA LOW-PRESSURE ADAPTOR (Convatec)			
DEV,NA (1 3/4")			
10s ea	68455-0108-61	54.83	71.36
(2 1/4") 10s ea	68455-0108-60	54.83	71.36
(2 3/4") 10s ea	68455-0108-59	54.83	71.36
(4") 10s ea	68455-0108-58	54.83	71.36
SUR-FIT NATURA STOMAHESIVE FLEXIBLE COLLAR (Convatec)			
DEV,NA (4"X4", TAN, 5/8", STOMA)			
10s ea	68455-0101-81	49.86	64.91
(4"X4",TAN,1 1/2" WAFER) 10s ea	68455-0101-76	48.85	63.59
(4"X4",TAN,1 1/4" WAFER) 10s ea	68455-0101-75	48.85	63.59
(4"X4",TAN,1 1/4") 10s ea	68455-0101-86	49.86	64.91
(4"X4",TAN,1 1/8") 10s ea	68455-0101-85	49.86	64.91
(4"X4",TAN,1 3/4" WAFER) 10s ea	68455-0101-77	48.85	63.59
(4"X4",TAN,1 3/8",WAFER) 10s ea	68455-0101-87	49.86	64.91
(4"X4",TAN,1",WAFER) 10s ea	68455-0101-84	49.86	64.91
(4"X4",TAN,3/4",WAFER) 10s ea	68455-0101-82	49.86	64.91
(4"X4",TAN,WAFER,7/8") 10s ea	68455-0101-83	49.86	64.91
(4"X4",WAFER,TAN,1/2") 10s ea	68455-0101-80	50.60	65.87
(4"X4",WHT,1 1/2" WAFER) 10s ea	68455-0101-71	48.85	63.59
(4"X4",WHT,1 1/4" WAFER) 10s ea	68455-0101-70	48.85	63.59
(4"X4",WHT,1 3/4" WAFER) 10s ea	68455-0101-72	48.85	63.59

PROD/MFR	HRI, UPC,NDC	AWP	SRP
(5"X5",TAN,1 1/2",WAFER)			
10s ea	68455-0101-88	49.80	64.82
(5"X5",TAN,1 3/4",WAFER)			
10s ea	68455-0101-90	49.80	64.82
(5"X5",TAN,1 5/8",WAFER)			
10s ea	68455-0101-89	49.80	64.82
(5"X5",TAN,2 1/4" WAFER)			
10s ea	68455-0101-78	48.85	63.59
(5"X5",TAN,2 3/4" WAFER)			
10s ea	68455-0101-79	48.85	63.59
(5"X5",WHT,2 1/4" WAFER)			
10s ea	68455-0101-73	48.85	63.59
(5"X5",WHT,2 3/4" WAFER)			
10s ea	68455-0101-74	48.85	63.59
SURE CARE DISPOSABLE UNDERPADS (Covidien)			
DEV,NA (30"X36")			
30s ea	08080-1552-01	19.52	
54s ea	08080-1550-00	19.90	
SURECARE GUARDS (Covidien)			
DEV,NA (FOR MEN,6&1/2"X13")			
84s ea	08080-2324-60	37.24	
SURECARE PRESENCE (Covidien)			
DEV,NA (4"X12&1/2",EXTRA PLUS)			
96s ea	08080-1140-16	24.50	
(EXTRA ABSORBENCY)			
120s ea	08080-1110-20	25.00	
(REGULAR)			
132s ea	08080-1100-22	25.00	
SURECARE PROTECTIVE UNDERWEAR (Covidien)			
DEV,NA (XLARGEREGULARABSORBENCY)			
56s ea	08080-1625-00	47.85	
(LARGE,FOR MEN & WOMEN)			
64s ea	08080-1215-00	60.00	
(LARGE,REGULARABSORBENCY)			
72s ea	08080-1615-00	54.94	
(SMALL/MEDIUMFORMENWOMEN)			
72s ea	08080-1205-00	60.00	
(MED,REGULAR ABSORBENCY)			
80s ea	08080-1605-00	54.94	
SURECARE UNDERGARMENTS (Covidien)			
DEV,NA, 60s ea	08080-1527-01	23.85	
(SUPER ABSORBENCY)			
60s ea	08080-1528-01	22.90	
SURECATH INTERMITTENT CATHETER (Coloplast)			
DEV,NA (STERILE,10FR,14")			
20s ea	11701-0899-06	116.00	121.40
(STERILE,12FR,14")			
20s ea	11701-0899-07	116.00	121.40
20s ea	11701-0899-27	564.00	590.00
(STERILE,12FR,6")			
20s ea	11701-0899-03	116.00	121.40
(STERILE,14FR,14")			
20s ea	11701-0899-08	116.00	121.40
20s ea	11701-0899-28	564.00	590.00
(STERILE,14FR,6")			
20s ea	11701-0899-04	116.00	121.40
(STERILE,16FR,14")			
20s ea	11701-0899-09	116.00	121.40
(STERILE,6FR,6")			
20s ea	11701-0899-11	116.00	121.40
(STERILE,8FR,14")			
20s ea	11701-0899-05	116.00	121.40
(STERILE,10FR,14")			
100s ea	11701-0899-26	564.00	590.00
(STERILE,16FR,14")			
100s ea	11701-0899-29	564.00	590.00
(STERILE,8FR,14")			
100s ea	11701-0899-25	564.00	590.00
SURECATH SET W/ACCESSORIES (Coloplast)			
DEV,NA (STERILE,10FR,14")			
100s ea	11701-0899-23	592.00	619.00
(STERILE,12FR,14")			
100s ea	11701-0899-24	592.00	619.00
(STERILE,14FR,14")			
100s ea	11701-0899-32	592.00	619.00
100s ea	11701-0899-36	592.00	619.00
(STERILE,14FR,6")			
100s ea	11701-0899-34	592.00	619.00
(STERILE,16FR,14")			
100s ea	11701-0899-33	592.00	619.00
100s ea	11701-0899-37	592.00	619.00
(STERILE,8FR,14")			
100s ea	11701-0899-22	592.00	619.00
SURESITE (Medline)			
DEV,NA (TRANSPARENT,4"X5")			
ea	53329-0026-45	1.35	
SURESITE IV (Medline)			
DEV,NA (TRANSPARENT,2"X3")			
ea	53329-0026-39	0.36	
SURESITE MATRIX TRANSPARENT FILM DRESSING (Medline)			
DEV,NA (4"X4.5")			
50s ea	53329-0026-50	1.40	
(6"X8")			
100s ea	08327-0026-46	256.24	
SURESITE WINDOW (Medline)			
DEV,NA (TRANSPARENT,4"X4 1/2")			
50s ea	53329-0026-35	32.19	
(TRANSPRNT,2 3/8"X2 3/4")			
50s ea	53329-0026-38	64.82	
SURESTEP (Lifescan)			
DEV,NA (STRIP,2X25)			
50s ea	53885-0359-50	61.38	
(STRIP,4X25)			
100s ea	53885-0052-10	122.76	
SURESTEP GLUCOSE CONTROL (Lifescan)			
DEV,NA, 2s ea	53885-0637-02	7.44	
SURESTEP PRO GLUCOSE CONTROL (Lifescan)			
DEV,NA (DUO PACK,HIGH/LOW)			
2s ea	53885-0850-02	7.50	
(DUO PACK,NORMAL)			
2s ea	53885-0851-02	7.50	
(HIGH)			
25s ea	53885-0793-25	65.00	
(LOW)			
25s ea	53885-0795-25	65.00	
(NORMAL)			
25s ea	53885-0794-25	65.00	
SURESTEP PRO LINEARITY (Lifescan)			
DEV,NA, 5s ea	53885-0798-05	80.00	
SURESTEP SYSTEM (Lifescan)			
DEV,NA, ea	53885-0341-01	62.50	
SURGEL (Ulmer)			
GEL,TP, 120 ml	00127-1786-06	2.05	3.42
240 gm	00127-1786-12	3.03	5.05
3840 ml	00127-1786-16	27.83	44.30
SURGIGRIP TUBULAR ELASTIC SUPPORT (Western Medical)			
DEV,NA (2 1/2"X10 METER,NATURAL)			
ea	16926-0000-02	45.30	
(2 3/4"X10 METER,NATURAL)			
ea	16926-0000-03	49.53	
(3 1/2"X10 METER,NATURAL)			
ea	16926-0000-05	64.05	
(3"X10 METER,NATURAL)			
ea	16926-0000-04	56.53	
(4 1/2"X10 METER,NATURAL)			
ea	16926-0000-07	83.72	
(4"X10 METER,NATURAL)			
ea	16926-0000-06	70.02	
SURGIKOS TIP CLEANER (J&J Medical)			
DEV,NA (ELECTRO-SURG,STERILE)			
36s ea	56091-0043-15	27.32	
SURGILAST TUBULAR ELASTIC RETAINER (Western Medical)			
DEV,NA (10 YARD, SIZE A)			
ea	16926-0072-00	6.65	
(10 YARD, SIZE B)			
ea	16926-0072-20	8.57	
(10 YARD, SIZE C)			
ea	16926-0072-40	14.35	
(10 YARD, SIZE D)			
ea	16926-0072-60	23.96	
(25 YARD, SIZE 1)			
ea	16926-0070-10	13.77	
(25 YARD, SIZE 10)			
ea	16926-0071-10	62.03	
(25 YARD, SIZE 2)			
ea	16926-0070-20	14.82	
(25 YARD, SIZE 3)			
ea	16926-0070-30	17.09	
(25 YARD, SIZE 4)			
ea	16926-0070-40	20.07	
(25 YARD, SIZE 5.5)			
ea	16926-0070-60	28.12	
(25 YARD, SIZE 5)			
ea	16926-0070-50	22.39	
(25 YARD, SIZE 6)			
ea	16926-0070-70	37.26	
(25 YARD, SIZE 7)			
ea	16926-0070-80	43.74	
(25 YARD, SIZE 8)			
ea	16926-0070-90	47.28	
(25 YARD, SIZE 9)			
ea	16926-0071-00	55.84	
SURGILUBE (Savage)			
GEL,TP (1X3GM,FOILPAC)			
3 gm	00281-0205-43	11.12	
(144X5GM,FOILPAC)			
5 gm 144s	00281-0205-45	17.08	
(144X5GM)			
5 gm 144s	00281-0205-55	109.28	
(1X56.7GM,FLIPCAP)			
56.7 gm	00281-0205-12	15.08	
(1X56.7GM)			
56.7 gm	00281-0205-02	13.85	
(12X120.49GM,FLIP CAP)			
120.49 gm 12s	00281-0205-37	21.29	
(12X120.49GM)			
120.49 gm 12s	00281-0205-36	21.11	
SURGINE FACE MASK (J&J Medical)			
DEV,NA, 50s ea	56091-0042-39	9.10	
(ANTI-FOG)			
50s ea	56091-0042-38	11.88	
(FASHION)			
50s ea	56091-0042-37	12.18	
SURGINE II FACE MASK (J&J Medical)			
DEV,NA, 50s ea	56091-0042-30	9.75	
(ANTI-FOG)			
50s ea	56091-0042-31	14.11	
(CONE)			
50s ea	56091-0042-35	11.11	
(DESIGNER ANTI-FOG)			
50s ea	56091-0042-60	12.18	
(SOFT ARCH)			
50s ea	56091-0042-33	11.22	
SURGIPAD COMBINE STERILE (J&J Medical)			
DEV,NA (8"X10")			
20s ea	56091-0021-48	6.71	
(8"X7 1/2")			
20s ea	56091-0021-44	4.78	
(5"X9")			
25s ea	56091-0021-45	5.37	
SURGIPAD SURGICAL DRESSINGS (Johnson & Johnson)			
DEV,NA (5"X9")			
12s ea	81370-0055-11	4.00	
SURGITUBE TUBULAR GAUZE (Western Medical)			
DEV,NA (1 1/2"X10 YD,WHITE)			
ea	16926-0003-10	6.94	
(1 1/2"X5 YD,FLESH)			
ea	16926-0013-05	3.82	
(1 1/2"X5 YD,WHITE)			
ea	16926-0003-05	3.65	
(1 1/2"X50 YD,WHITE)			
ea	16926-0003-50	23.78	
(1 1/2"X50YD,USE APPL,FL)			
ea	16926-0135-05	26.39	
(1 1/2"X50YD,USE APPL,WH)			
ea	16926-0350-50	23.78	
(1 1/2"X5YD,WHT,TIGHT WV)			
ea	16926-0004-05	3.82	
(1 1/8"X50 YD,WHITE)			
ea	16926-0225-00	21.29	
(1-1/2"X50YD,WHT,TIGHTWV)			
ea	16926-0004-50	26.97	
(1"X50 YD,USE APPL,FLSH)			
ea	16926-0125-05	22.16	
(1"X50 YD,USE APPL,WHITE)			
ea	16926-0250-50	20.66	
(2 5/8"X50YD,USE APPL,FL)			
ea	16926-0145-05	32.05	
(2 5/8"X50YD,USE APPL,WH)			
ea	16926-0022-20	31.08	30.17
(2"X50 YD,FLESH)			
ea	16926-0005-50	35.01	
(2"X50 YD,WHITE)			
ea	16926-0055-50	29.86	
(3 5/8"X50YD,USE APPL,WH)			
ea	16926-0550-50	33.42	
(5"X50YD,USE APPL,WHITE)			
ea	16926-0224-00	41.36	
(5/8"X10 YD,WHITE)			
ea	16926-0001-10	5.15	
(5/8"X50 YD,FLESH)			
ea	16926-0015-50	18.52	
(5/8"X50 YD,USE APPL,FL)			
ea	16926-0115-05	18.52	
(5/8"X50 YD,USE APPL,WH)			
ea	16926-0150-50	16.25	
(5/8"X50 YD,WHITE)			
ea	16926-0001-50	16.25	15.78
(7"X50YD,USE APPL,WHITE)			
ea	00516-2250-05	47.64	
(7/8"X10 YD,FLESH)			
ea	16926-0210-10	6.25	
(7/8"X10 YD,WHITE)			
ea	16926-0002-10	5.49	

PROD/MFR	HRI, UPC,NDC	AWP	SRP
(7/8"X50 YD,FLESH)			
ea	**16926-0025-50**	20.66	
(7/8"X50 YD,WHITE)			
ea UD	**16926-0002-50**	17.76	17.24
(5/8"X5 YD,FLESH)			
12s ea	**16926-0210-50**	36.99	
(5/8"X5 YD,WHITE)			
12s ea	**16926-0255-80**	34.53	
(7/8"X5 YD,FLESH)			
12s ea	**16926-0220-50**	38.42	
(7/8"X5 YD,WHITE)			
12s ea	**16926-0260-50**	36.99	
SWAMP ROOT (Oakhurst)			
LIQ,TP, 120 ml	**11169-0702-04**	4.29	6.44
240 ml	**11169-0702-08**	5.88	8.81
SWAN CITROMA (Vi-Jon)			
SOL,PO (LEMON)			
1.75 gm/30 ml,			
296 ml	**00869-0686-38**	1.08	
(LEMONY)			
1.75 gm/30 ml,			
296 ml	**00869-0667-38**	1.08	
(VERY LOW SODIUM,CHERRY)			
1.75 gm/30 ml,			
296 ml	**00869-0693-38**	1.08	
SWAN EPSOM SALT (Vi-Jon)			
PDR,NA (PRIVATE LABEL)			
1814.37 gm	**08693-0108-10**	2.87	3.29
SWAN GENTIAN VIOLET (Vi-Jon)			
SOL,TP (1X30ML,USP)			
1%, 30 ml	**08693-0400-10**	1.28	3.29
SWAN HYDROGEN PEROXIDE (Vi-Jon)			
SOL,TP (PRIVATE LABEL)			
3%, 237 ml	**08694-0704-10**	0.54	0.99
(1X473ML,USP)			
3%, 473 ml	**00869-0871-43**	0.58	0.99
SWAN RUBBING ALCOHOL (Cumberland-Swan)			
LIQ,TP (PRIVATE LABEL)			
70%, 473 ml	**00869-0810-43**	1.10	
SWEEN 24 (Coloplast)			
CRE,TP (4GM X 300)			
6%, 4 gm 300s	**11701-0063-22**	150.00	156.00
(57GM X 12)			
6%, 57 gm 12s	**11701-0063-23**	31.80	33.24
(142GM X 12)			
6%, 142 gm 12s	**11701-0063-14**	68.88	72.12
(270GM X 12)			
6%, 270 gm 12s	**11701-0063-13**	114.72	120.12
SWEEN BATH (Coloplast)			
OIL,TP, 59 ml 36s	**11701-0001-03**	36.36	38.16
237 ml 36s	**11701-0001-05**	184.68	192.96
473 ml 12s	**11701-0001-06**	112.32	117.48
621 ml 12s	**11701-0001-26**	130.08	136.08
3840 ml 4s	**11701-0001-09**	242.80	254.08
SWEEN BODY (Coloplast)			
POW,TP, 85 gm 36s	**11701-0005-16**	55.08	57.60
227 gm 36s	**11701-0005-05**	101.52	106.20
SWEEN CREAM (Coloplast)			
CRE,TP (PACKET,FRESH SCENT)			
2 gm 300s	**11701-0043-21**	87.00	93.00
(PACKET)			
2 gm 300s	**11701-0002-21**	87.00	93.00
14 gm 36s	**11701-0002-01**	72.36	75.96
(FRESH SCENT)			
57 gm 12s	**11701-0043-23**	59.64	62.40
(JAR,FRAGRANCE-FREE)			
57 gm 12s	**11701-0019-03**	76.80	80.40
(JAR)			
85 gm	**11701-0002-15**	6.88	7.20
(TUBE)			
85 gm	**11701-0002-16**	5.12	5.36
(FRESH SCENT)			
142 gm 12s	**11701-0043-14**	107.28	112.32
(TUBE)			
184 gm	**11701-0002-38**	9.20	9.63
(JAR)			
339 gm	**11701-0002-35**	11.59	12.13
SWEET CHESTNUT (Ellon)			
SOL,SL (DROPS)			
10.5 ml	**51762-0008-10**		9.25
SWEET EASE NATURAL THE SUCROSE SOLUTION (Philips Children's)			
SYR,PO (PF)			
24%, 15 ml 50s	**00906-9904-41**		34.50
SWEETA (Numark)			
SOL,PO, 22.7%, 120 ml	**38485-0806-30**	12.60	
SWIM-EAR (Fougera)			
SOL,OT, 5%-95%, 30 ml	**00168-0126-91**	4.35	
(Phys Total Care) REPACK			
SOL,OT (1X29.57ML)			
5%-95%, 29.57 ml	**54868-0128-00**	5.50	
(Southwood) REPACK			
SOL,OT, 5%-95%, 1 ml	**58016-4841-01**	4.38	
SWIRL (Pfeiffer)			
SOL,MM (COOL MINT)			
180 ml	**00927-0152-06**	1.11	1.99
SWISS KRISS (Modern Prod)			
FLA,PO, 45 gm	**75820-0160-15**	3.60	5.99
97.5 gm	**75820-0158-35**	6.00	9.99
TAB,PO, 24s ea	**75820-0162-01**	2.70	4.49
120s ea	**75820-0162-12**	5.10	8.49
250s ea	**75820-0186-30**	9.60	15.99
SWORD FLOSS (Majestic Drug)			
DEV,NA (MINT)			
40s ea	**10705-0000-25**	1.10	2.39
(REGULAR)			
40s ea	**10705-0000-24**	1.10	2.39
SWORD FLOSS PROXI-PLUS (Majestic Drug)			
DEV,NA, 20s ea	**10705-0000-28**	3.50	4.99
SYMPHYTUM (Luyties)			
TAB,SL (6X)			
6 x, 500s ea	**00618-8161-03**	3.99	
5500s ea	**00618-8161-10**	30.32	
(30X)			
12 x, 500s ea	**00622-8161-03**	4.19	
5500s ea	**00622-8161-10**	31.83	
(12X)			
30 x, 500s ea	**00624-8161-03**	4.19	
5500s ea	**00624-8161-10**	31.83	
SYMPT-X (Baxter)			
PDS,PO (USE W/MED SUPV)			
10 gm/packet,			
60s ea	**00338-9177-91**	97.20	
SYMPT-X G.I. (Baxter)			
PDS,PO (PACKET,USE W/MED SUPV)			
10 gm/packet,			
60s ea	**00338-9178-91**	97.20	
SYRINGE CARRYING CASE (Apothecary)			
DEV,NA (PRE-LOADED)			
ea	**25715-0669-20**	8.74	14.59
SYRINGE MAGNIFIER (Apothecary)			
DEV,NA (CLIPS TO SYRINGE BARREL)			
ea	**25715-0669-55**	3.33	5.59
SYST-AMUNE (Baxter)			
PDR,PO (PACKET)			
15 gm 60s	**00338-9180-91**	138.00	
SYSTANE (Alcon Labs Cons Prod)			
OIN,OP (1X3.5GM,PF)			
3%-94%, 3.5 gm	**00650-0509-35**	8.76	
SOL,OP (PRESERVATIVE FREE)			
0.4%-0.3%, 28s ea	**00650-0431-32**	9.54	
(2X5ML)			
0.4%-0.3%, 5 ml 2s	**00650-0429-21**	7.56	
15 ml	**00650-0429-15**	8.76	
(2X20ML)			
0.4%-0.3%,			
20 ml 2s	**00650-0429-67**	20.39	
30 ml	**00650-0429-30**	13.44	
SYSTANE LUBRICANT EYE DROPS (Southwood) REPACK			
SOL,OP, 0.4%-0.3%, 5 ml	**58016-4683-01**	8.69	
SYSTANE ULTRA (Alcon Labs Cons Prod)			
SOL,OP (1X10ML,1X5ML)			
0.4%-0.3%, ea	**00651-0431-06**	13.50	
(1X10ML)			
0.4%-0.3%, 10 ml	**00651-0431-05**	8.70	
T-LITE (T-Lite)			
SGL,PO, 60s ea	**94007-0134-68**	8.40	
T-PAINOL (Global Source)			
TAB,PO, 325 mg, 100s ea	**59618-0848-15**	3.00	
T-SPRAY (Pharm Innov)			
SPR,NA, 250 ml	**00036-3200-25**	5.63	8.05
(W/SPRAY BOTTLE)			
3840 ml	**00036-3200-28**	73.78	105.39
T-SPRAY II (Pharm Innov)			
SPR,NA (FOR ULTRASOUND & MAMMO)			
60 ml	**00036-2102-60**	1.75	2.50
250 ml	**00036-2102-25**	5.63	8.05
T-VITES (Freeda)			
TAB,PO (PF,SF,DYE-FREE)			
100s ea	**10432-0148-01**	7.17	11.95
(IMPROVED, WITHOUT A & E)			
250s ea	**10432-0148-02**	14.34	23.90
T.E.D. ANTI-EMBOLISM (Covidien)			
DEV,NA (THIGH LENGTH,MEDIUM,REG)			
36s ea	**08080-3416-10**	70.05	
(KNEELNGTHW/INSPCTIONTOE)			
72s ea	**08080-7203-00**	77.85	
TAB A VITE MAXIMUM (Major)			
TAB,PO, 60s ea	**00904-5647-52**	4.23	
TAB A VITE WEIGHT SLIM (Major)			
TAB,PO (WITH EGCG)			
50s ea	**00904-5689-51**	4.10	
TAB A VITE WOMEN'S FORMULA (Major)			
TAB,PO (WITH CALCIUM & IRON)			
60s ea	**00904-5713-52**	4.96	
TAB-A-VITE (Major)			
TAB,PO, 30s ea	**00904-0530-46**	1.95	
100s ea	**00904-0530-60**	3.10	
(10X10)			
100s ea UD	**00904-0530-61**	6.01	
1000s ea	**00904-0530-80**	20.65	
TAB-A-VITE W/IRON (Major)			
TAB,PO, 100s ea	**00904-0531-60**	3.30	
1000s ea	**00904-0531-80**	20.85	
TAC GEL (Pharm Innov)			
GEL,TP, 10 gm	**00036-9000-10**	1.69	2.41
50 gm	**00036-9000-50**	4.08	5.83
TACTINAL (Prime Marketing)			
TAB,PO, 325 mg, 100s ea	**62107-0052-01**	2.75	
1000s ea	**62107-0052-10**	14.96	
(CAPLET)			
500 mg, 100s ea	**62107-0051-01**	3.90	
1000s ea	**62107-0051-10**	21.75	
TACTINAL CHILDREN'S (Prime Marketing)			
CTB,PO (FRUIT)			
80 mg, 30s ea	**62107-0053-30**	2.90	
TACTINAL EXTRA STRENGTH (Prime Marketing)			
TAB,PO, 500 mg, 100s ea	**62107-0050-01**	3.60	
1000s ea	**62107-0050-10**	19.95	
TAGAMET HB (Glaxo)			
TAB,PO, 200 mg, 6s ea	**00766-5016-06**	2.98	
30s ea	**00766-5016-30**	9.25	
50s ea	**00766-5016-50**	13.91	
70s ea	**00766-5016-70**	17.30	
TANAC (Del)			
LIQ,MM (AF)			
0.5%-1%, 15 ml	**10310-0011-01**	5.08	7.61
TANDEM (U.S. Pharm)			
CAP,PO, 162 mg-115.2 mg,			
90s ea	**52747-0900-90**	35.04	
(Phys Total Care) REPACK			
CAP,PO (DUAL ACTION)			
162 mg-115.2 mg,			
90s ea	**54868-5919-00**	43.88	
TAPE/ELASTIC BANDAGE (Dome)			
DEV,NA (SELFGRIP/JHOOKS, RED 1")			
ea	**78509-0033-51**	2.02	3.37
(SELFGRIP/JHOOKS, RED 2")			
ea	**78509-0033-52**	2.90	4.83
(SELFGRIP/JHOOKS, RED 3")			
ea	**78509-0033-53**	3.66	5.97
(SELFGRIP/JHOOKS, RED 4")			
ea	**78509-0033-54**	4.61	6.95
(SELFGRIP/JHOOKS,BEIGE1")			
ea	**78509-0013-51**	2.02	3.37
(SELFGRIP/JHOOKS,BEIGE2")			
ea	**78509-0013-52**	2.90	4.83
(SELFGRIP/JHOOKS,BEIGE3")			
ea	**78509-0013-53**	3.66	5.97
(SELFGRIP/JHOOKS,BEIGE4")			
ea	**78509-0013-54**	4.61	6.95
(SELFGRIP/JHOOKS,BLUE 1")			
ea	**78509-0023-51**	2.02	3.37
(SELFGRIP/JHOOKS,BLUE 2")			
ea	**78509-0023-52**	2.90	4.83
(SELFGRIP/JHOOKS,BLUE 3")			
ea	**78509-0023-53**	3.66	5.97
(SELFGRIP/JHOOKS,BLUE 4")			
ea	**78509-0023-54**	4.61	6.95
(SELFGRIP/JHOOKS,WHITE1")			
ea	**78509-0043-51**	2.02	3.37
(SELFGRIP/JHOOKS,WHITE2")			
ea	**78509-0043-52**	2.90	4.83

PROD/MFR	HRI, UPC,NDC	AWP	SRP
(SELFGRIP/JHOOKS,WHITE3")			
ea	**78509-0043-53**	3.66	5.97
(SELFGRIP/JHOOKS,WHITE4")			
ea	**78509-0043-54**	4.61	6.95
TAR GARD CARTRIDGE FILTER SYSTEM (Venturi)			
DEV,NA, ea	**11120-0010-01**	4.35	
ea	**11120-0010-31**	1.95	
TAR GARD DISPOSABLE FILTER SYSTEM (Venturi)			
DEV,NA, ea	**11120-0049-11**	1.50	2.95
TAR GARD INVISIBLE FILTER SYSTEM (Venturi)			
DEV,NA, ea	**11120-0020-11**	0.90	1.95
TAR GARD PERMANENT FILTER SYSTEM (Venturi)			
DEV,NA, ea	**11120-0012-00**	2.10	4.35
TARAPHILIC (Medco Lab)			
OIN,TP, 1%, 16 gm	**11940-8183-06**	8.25	
TARGET ADVANCED LANCING (Target)			
DEV,NA (PRIVATE LABEL)			
ea	**61059-0270-20**	10.99	
TARGET ALTERNATE SITE LANCETS (Target)			
DEV,NA (26G,PRIVATE LABEL)			
100s ea	**61059-0435-20**	4.75	
TARGET LANCING DEVICE (Target)			
DEV,NA (PRIVATE LABEL)			
ea	**16730-0707-20**	10.99	
TARGET SUPER THIN LANCETS (Target)			
DEV,NA (30G,PRIVATE LABEL)			
100s ea	**61059-0465-20**	4.75	
(33G, SINGLE USE)			
100s ea	**16730-0657-20**	4.75	
TARGET THIN LANCET (Target)			
DEV,NA (28G,PRIVATE LABEL)			
100s ea	**16730-0157-20**	4.60	
TARGET ULTRA THIN LANCET (Target)			
DEV,NA (28G,PRIVATE LABEL)			
100s ea	**16730-0357-20**	4.69	
(28G)			
100s ea	**61059-0257-20**	4.75	
(28G,PRIVATE LABEL)			
200s ea	**16730-0307-20**	8.30	
TARGON SMOKERS' MOUTHWASH (Glaxo)			
SOL,MM (MINTY FRESH)			
480 ml	**10158-0037-01**	3.46	
720 ml	**10158-0037-02**	4.61	
TARSUM GEL (Summers)			
SHA,TP, 10%-5%, 120 ml	**11086-0011-01**	9.86	
240 ml	**11086-0011-02**	16.46	
TAURINE (Bio-Tech Pharm)			
CAP,PO, 500 mg, 100s ea	**53191-0143-01**	6.30	
(Carlson,J.R.)			
POW,PO (PF,SALT-FREE)			
100 gm	**88395-0069-45**	4.95	9.90
(Miller)			
CAP,PO, 500 mg, 60s ea	**17204-0883-20**	5.04	
TAURINE-500 (Key Company)			
TAB,PO (PF,SF)			
500 mg, 60s ea	**11694-0733-01**	4.00	
TAVIST-1 (Novartis Consumer)			
TAB,PO, 1.34 mg, 8s ea	**00043-0119-08**	4.24	
16s ea	**00043-0119-16**	7.49	
TEAR FLO (HUB Pharma)			
DEV,NA, 100s ea	**64334-0090-06**	15.56	
TEARS AGAIN (Ocusoft)			
OIN,OP (PF)			
3.5 gm	**54799-0906-35**	14.38	
SOL,OP, 0.7%, 15 ml	**54799-0909-15**	12.81	
1.4%, 15 ml	**54799-0904-15**	7.44	
TEARS AGAIN LIPOSOME (Ocusoft)			
SPR,TP, 10 ml	**54799-0901-10**	17.44	
TEARS AGAIN MC (Ocusoft)			
SOL,OP, 0.4%, 15 ml	**54799-0905-15**	14.94	
TEARS AGAIN NIGHT & DAY (Ocusoft)			
GEL,OP, 1.5%, 3.5 gm	**54799-0903-35**	12.81	
TEARS NATURALE (Southwood)			
REPACK			
SOL,OP, 15 ml	**58016-2098-01**	7.13	
TEARS NATURALE FORTE (Alcon Labs Cons Prod)			
SOL,OP (DROPS)			
0.1%-0.2%-0.3%,			
15 ml	**00650-0426-22**	8.64	
30 ml	**00650-0426-23**	12.78	
TEARS NATURALE FREE (Alcon Labs Cons Prod)			
SOL,OP (RECLOSABLE VIAL,PF)			
0.1%-0.3%, 36s ea	**00650-0416-25**	9.06	
(PF,DROPS)			
0.1%-0.3%, 60s ea	**00650-0416-36**	12.90	
TEARS NATURALE II (Alcon Labs Cons Prod)			
SOL,OP (POLYQUAD)			
0.1%-0.3%, 15 ml	**00650-0418-15**	8.64	
30 ml	**00650-0418-30**	12.78	
(A-S Medication)			
REPACK			
SOL,OP, 0.1%-0.3%,			
15 ml	**54569-4379-00**	9.00	
TEARS NATURALE PM (Alcon Labs Cons Prod)			
OIN,OP (PF)			
3%-94%, 3.5 gm	**00650-0420-05**	8.39	
TEARS PLUS (Allergan Inc)			
SOL,OP, 15 ml	**11980-0165-15**	8.19	
30 ml	**11980-0165-30**	11.19	
TEARS PURE LUBRICANT (Cardinal Health)			
SOL,OP (PRIVATE LABEL)			
0.4%, 15 ml	**37205-0603-05**	3.44	
TEARS RENEWED (Akorn)			
OIN,OP (PF)			
3.5 gm	**17478-0063-35**	5.39	
SOL,OP, 0.1%-0.3%,			
15 ml	**17478-0061-12**	4.94	
TEARS RENEWED LUBRICANT EYE DROPS (Dispensing Solutions)			
REPACK			
SOL,OP (DROPS)			
0.1%-0.3%, 15 ml	**55045-1349-00**	6.99	
TECHLITE AST LANCETS (Arkray)			
DEV,NA, 100s ea	**08317-8803-00**	2.03	
TECHLITE LANCETS (Arkray)			
DEV,NA (25G, TRI-BEVEL POINT)			
100s ea	**08317-8801-25**	2.03	
(28G)			
100s ea	**08317-8801-28**	2.03	
(25G, TRI-BEVEL POINT)			
200s ea	**08317-8802-25**	4.05	
(28G)			
200s ea	**08317-8802-28**	4.05	
TECNU (Tec)			
LIQ,TP, 120 ml	**83926-0141-00**	3.40	5.99
360 ml	**83926-0112-00**	6.12	9.99
(Phys Total Care)			
REPACK			
LIQ,TP, 120 ml	**54868-4966-00**	6.23	
TECNU EXTREME MEDICATED POISON IVY SCRUB (Tec)			
SOA,TP (1X113.4GM)			
3 x, 113.4 gm	**51879-0140-04**	8.00	14.99
TECNU RASH RELIEF MEDICATED ANTI-ITCH (Tec)			
SPR,TP (1X177ML)			
3 x-4 x, 177 ml	**51879-0160-06**	8.00	14.99
TEGA FOAM NON-ADHESIVE (3M Health Care)			
DEV,NA (8"X8")			
5s ea	**08333-9060-30**	86.41	
(4"X24" ROLL)			
6s ea	**08333-9060-50**	174.60	
(2"X2")			
10s ea	**08333-9060-00**	35.00	
(3.5"X3.5",FENESTRATED)			
10s ea	**08333-9060-40**	46.68	
(4"X4")			
10s ea	**08333-9060-10**	46.69	
(4"X8")			
10s ea	**08333-9060-20**	97.73	
TEGADERM + PAD TRANSPARENT (3M Health Care)			
DEV,NA (3 1/2"X10")			
25s ea	**08333-3591-01**	71.90	
(3 1/2"X4 1/8")			
25s ea	**08333-3587-01**	29.40	
(3 1/2"X4")			
25s ea	**08333-3586-01**	29.40	
(3 1/2"X6")			
25s ea	**08333-3589-01**	43.90	
(3 1/2"X8")			
25s ea	**08333-3590-01**	58.40	
(3-1/2"X13-3/4", W/PAD)			
25s ea	**08333-3593-01**	94.50	
(6"X6")			
25s ea	**08333-3588-01**	70.20	
(2 3/8"X4")			
50s ea	**08333-3584-01**	40.50	
(2"X2 3/4")			
50s ea	**08333-3582-01**	23.00	
TEGADERM HP TRANSPARENT (3M Health Care)			
DEV,NA (2 3/8"X2 3/8" W/STRIPS)			
100s ea	**08333-9519-01**	49.13	
(Animas Corp.)			
DEV,NA (4" X 4 3/4")			
50s ea	**65781-0413-50**	148.35	
(2 3/8" X 2 3/4")			
100s ea	**65781-0412-50**	126.42	
TEGADERM HP TRANSPARENT FRAME STYLE (3M Health Care)			
DEV,NA (5-1/2"X6 1/2")			
10s ea	**08333-9548-01**	36.46	
(4 1/2"X4 3/4")			
12s ea	**08333-9543-01**	19.33	
(2 1/8"X2 1/2")			
50s ea	**08333-9545-01**	23.33	
(4"X4 1/2")			
50s ea	**08333-9546-01**	80.48	
(4"X4 3/4")			
50s ea	**08333-9536-01**	80.48	
(2 3/8"X2 3/4")			
100s ea	**08333-9534-01**	48.16	
TEGADERM IV TRANSPARENT (3M Health Care)			
DEV,NA (3 1/2"X4 1/4")			
50s ea	**08333-1635-01**	81.50	
(2 3/4"X3 1/4")			
100s ea	**08333-1633-01**	52.40	
TEGADERM PLUS TRANSPARENT (3M Health Care)			
DEV,NA (W/IODOPHOR,4"X5 7/8")			
25s ea	**08333-9526-01**	44.10	
(W/IODOPHOR,2 3/8X2 3/4")			
50s ea	**08333-9524-01**	26.40	
TEGADERM TRANSPARENT (Animas Corp.)			
DEV,NA (4" X 4 3/4")			
50s ea	**65781-0411-50**	141.90	
(2 3/8" X 2 3/4")			
100s ea	**65781-0410-00**	96.75	
TEGADERM TRANSPARENT FIRST AID (3M Health Care)			
DEV,NA (4"X5 1/2",IV DRESSING)			
50s ea	**08333-1621-01**	78.20	
(2 3/8"X2 3/4",IV DRESS)			
100s ea	**08333-1620-01**	46.80	
TEGADERM TRANSPARENT FRAME STYLE (3M Health Care)			
DEV,NA (4"X4 3/4", EASY APPL.)			
10s ea	**08333-9506-05**	15.60	
(6"X8")			
10s ea	**08333-1628-01**	34.75	
(8"X12")			
10s ea	**08333-1629-01**	45.50	
(2 3/8"X2 3/4",EASY APPL)			
20s ea	**08333-9505-05**	9.36	
(4"X10")			
20s ea	**08333-1627-01**	63.40	
(4"X4 1/2",EASY APPL)			
50s ea	**08333-1630-05**	76.65	
(4"X4 3/4",EASY APPL)			
50s ea	**08333-1626-05**	76.65	
(4"X4 3/4")			
50s ea	**08333-1626-01**	76.65	
(1 3/4"X1 3/4",EASY APPL)			
100s ea	**08333-1622-05**	44.50	
(2 3/8"X2 3/4",EASY APPL)			
100s ea	**08333-1624-05**	45.90	
(2 3/8"X2 3/4")			
100s ea	**08333-1634-01**	45.90	
(Quality Care Prod)			
REPACK			
DEV,NA (4"X4&3/4")			
10s ea	**35356-0185-10**	76.80	
(2.37"X2.75")			
20s ea	**35356-0184-20**	49.00	
(4"X4&3/4")			
50s ea	**35356-0185-50**	233.46	
(2.37"X2.75")			
100s ea	**35356-0184-00**	159.81	
(Stat Rx)			
REPACK			
DEV,NA (4X4)			
10s ea	**16590-0725-10**	22.75	
TEGAGEL HYDROGEL WOUND FILLER (3M Health Care)			
DRE,TP (85 GM TUBE)			
ea	**08333-9041-20**	15.62	
(25GM HYDROGEL 4"X4" PAD)			
15s ea	**08333-9041-40**	100.06	

PROD/MFR HRI, UPC,NDC AWP SRP

TEGAGEN HG ALGINATE (3M Health Care)
DEV,NA (12" ROPE)
5s ea ... 08333-9022-00 27.13
(4"X8")
5s ea ... 08333-9021-40 41.39
(2"X2")
10s ea ... 08333-9021-00 24.43
(4"X4")
10s ea ... 08333-9021-20 42.18

TEGAGEN HI ALGINATE (3M Health Care)
DEV,NA (12" ROPE)
5s ea ... 08333-9012-00 27.13
(4"X8")
5s ea ... 08333-9011-40 41.39
(2'X2")
10s ea ... 08333-9011-00 24.43
(4"X4")
10s ea ... 08333-9011-20 42.18

TEGAPORE WOUND CONTACT MATERIAL
(3M Health Care)
DEV,NA (8"X10")
10s ea ... 08333-5640-01 134.55
(3"X4")
25s ea ... 08333-5634-01 83.25
(3"X8")
25s ea ... 08333-5638-01 125.65

TEGASORB HYDROCOLLOID (3M Health Care)
DEV,NA (5 1/2"X6 3/4",OVAL)
3s ea ... 08333-9000-40 46.95
(6"X6",SQUARE)
3s ea ... 08333-9000-50 34.45
(2 3/4"X3 1/2",OVAL)
5s ea ... 08333-9000-10 20.50
(4"X4",SQUARE)
5s ea ... 08333-9000-20 20.50
(4"X43/4",OVAL)
5s ea ... 08333-9000-30 28.65
(4.9"X5.5",SACRAL)
6s ea ... 08333-9000-70 64.40

TEGASORB THIN HYDROCOLLOID (3M Health Care)
DEV,NA (6"X6",SQUARE)
3s ea ... 08333-9002-50 31.27
(4"X4",SQUARE)
5s ea ... 08333-9002-20 18.00
(5 1/2"X6 3/4",OVAL)
6s ea ... 08333-9002-40 49.49
(2 3/4"X3 1/2",OVAL)
10s ea ... 08333-9002-10 36.00
(4"X4 3/4",OVAL)
10s ea ... 08333-9002-30 53.25

TELDRIN HBP (Hogil)
TAB,PO, 4 mg, 24s ea ... 95814-0826-24 3.40

TELFA CLEAR NON-ADHERENT WOUND DRESSINGS
(Covidien)
TELFA CLEAR NON-ADHEREN WOUND DRESSINGS
DEV,NA (39"X25YD,NON-STERILE)
4s ea ... 08080-1115-00 328.32
(12"X12",STERILE)
50s ea ... 08080-1113-00 154.50
(12"X24",STERILE)
50s ea ... 08080-1114-00 221.45
(3"X3",STERILE)
50s ea ... 08080-1109-00 64.38
(4"X5",STERILE)
50s ea ... 08080-1111-00 70.82

TELFA ISLAND DRESSINGS (Covidien)
DEV,NA (4"X14",STERILE)
50s ea ... 08080-7544-00 111.62
(4"X10",STERILE)
100s ea ... 08080-7542-00 186.02
(4"X8",STERILE)
100s ea ... 08080-7541-00 161.79
(6"X6",STERILE)
100s ea ... 08080-7551-00 175.73
(4"X4",STERILE)
200s ea ... 08080-7550-00 172.13
(4"X5",STERILE)
200s ea ... 08080-7540-00 200.93

TELFA MINI ISLAND DRESSINGS (Covidien)
DEV,NA (2"X3.75",LATEX-FREE)
400s ea ... 08080-7539-01 67.02

TELFA NON-ADHERENT DRESSINGS (Covidien)
DEV,NA (8"X10",NON-STERILE)
500s ea ... 08080-3279-00 257.94
(3"X8",STERILE)
600s ea ... 08080-1238-00 140.44
(3"X6",STERILE)
750s ea ... 08080-1169-00 148.79
(3"X4",STERILE)
900s ea ... 08080-1050-00 160.89
(3"X8",NON-STERILE)
1000s ea ... 08080-2891-00 147.90
4000s ea ... 08080-1238-80 578.19

TELFA OUCHLESS ADHESIVE PADS (Covidien)
DEV,NA (3"X4YDS,STERILE)
50s ea ... 08080-2394-00 70.59
(2"X3",100X24)
2400s ea ... 08080-6017-00 299.99
(3"X4",STERILE)
2400s ea ... 08080-7643-00 250.43

TELFA OUCHLESS NON-ADHERENT (Covidien)
DEV,NA (2"X3",STERILE)
2400s ea ... 08080-1961-00 258.82
(3"X4",STERILE)
2400s ea ... 08080-2132-00 417.28

TELFA PLUS BARRIER ISLAND DRESSING
(Covidien)
DEV,NA (8"X8",STERILE)
60s ea ... 08080-2565-00 216.30
(4"X6",STERILE)
100s ea ... 08080-2562-00 251.07
(6"X10",STERILE)
100s ea ... 08080-2564-00 354.07
(6"X7",STERILE)
100s ea ... 08080-2563-00 296.13

TENA ADJUSTABLE BRIEFS (Johnson & Johnson)
DEV,NA (LARGE, ULTIMATE)
16s ea ... 80040-0619-00 14.80
(MED,ULTIMATE)
18s ea ... 80040-0618-00 14.80

TENA MEN PROTECTIVE GUARDS
(Johnson & Johnson)
DEV,NA, 48s ea ... 80040-0527-00 16.38

TENA MEN PROTECTIVE UNDERWEAR
(Johnson & Johnson)
DEV,NA (XL, SUPER PLUS)
12s ea ... 80040-0819-00 13.64
(M/L, SUPER PLUS)
14s ea ... 80040-0817-00 13.64

TENA MODERATE ABSORBENCY PADS
(Johnson & Johnson)
DEV,NA (LONG)
16s ea ... 80040-0416-00 5.21

TENA SERENITY DRIACTIVE PLUS PADS
(Johnson & Johnson)
DEV,NA (ULTRA THIN, LONG)
24s ea ... 80040-0482-00 5.21

TENA SERENITY DRIACTIVE SLENDER PADS
(Johnson & Johnson)
DEV,NA (ULTRA THIN, REGULAR)
30s ea ... 80040-0465-00 5.21

TENA SERENITY MALE GUARDS
(Johnson & Johnson)
DEV,NA (ODASORB PLUS)
20s ea ... 80040-0507-00 7.06

TENA SERENITY PADS (Johnson & Johnson)
DEV,NA (HEAVY, LONG)
12s ea ... 80040-0473-00 5.21
(HEAVY,REGULAR)
14s ea ... 80040-0428-00 5.21
(MODERATE, REGULAR)
20s ea ... 80040-0413-00 5.21
(ULTIMATE, OVERNIGHT)
30s ea ... 80040-0574-00 16.38
(ULTIMATE, REGULAR)
36s ea ... 80040-0498-00 16.38
(HEAVY, LONG)
42s ea ... 80040-0476-00 16.38
(ULTRA)
56s ea ... 80040-0494-00 16.38
(MODERATE,LONG)
60s ea ... 80040-0469-00 16.38
60s ea ... 80040-0806-00 16.38
(EXTRA)
72s ea ... 80040-0489-00 16.38

TENA SERENITY PANTILINERS
(Johnson & Johnson)
DEV,NA (LONG)
24s ea ... 80040-0564-00 3.17
(REGULAR)
26s ea ... 80040-0563-00 3.17
(LONG)
44s ea ... 80040-0649-00 5.45
(REGULAR)
48s ea ... 80040-0648-00 5.45

TENA SERENITY UNDERWEAR (Johnson & Johnson)
DEV,NA (SUPER PLUS LARGE)
7s ea ... 80040-0579-00 6.83
(SUPER PLUS, MED)
8s ea ... 80040-0539-00 6.83
(SUPER PLUS, XL)
12s ea ... 80040-0538-00 13.64
(ULTRA PLUS, LARGE)
16s ea ... 80040-0509-00 13.64
(SUPER PLUS, LARGE)
28s ea ... 80040-0626-00 25.00
(SUPER PLUS SMALL/MED)
32s ea ... 80040-0625-00 25.00

TENA WIPES (Johnson & Johnson)
PAD,TP (PRE-MOISTENED)
48s ea ... 80040-0710-00 4.67

TENA WOMEN PROTECTIVE UNDERWEAR
(Johnson & Johnson)
DEV,NA (LARGE, SUPER PLUS)
14s ea ... 80040-0534-00 13.64
(L,ULTIMATE COVERAGE)
16s ea ... 80040-0617-00 13.64
(S/M, SUPER PLUS)
16s ea ... 80040-0533-00 13.64
(M,ULTIMATE FULLCOVERAGE)
18s ea ... 80040-0616-00 13.64

TENDERFIX HYPOALLERGENIC CLOTH (Tyco)
DEV,NA (20.3CM X 9.1M)
6s ea ... 08080-9418-00 75.08
(10CM X 9.1M)
12s ea ... 08080-9414-10 75.08
(15CM X 9.1M)
12s ea ... 08080-9416-10 75.08
(5CM X 9.1M)
12s ea ... 08080-9412-10 66.94
(7.5CM X 9.1M)
12s ea ... 08080-9413-10 75.08
(15CM X 1.8M)
16s ea ... 08080-9416-11 73.90
(10CM X 1.8M)
24s ea ... 08080-9414-11 73.90
(2.5CM X 9.1M)
24s ea ... 08080-9411-10 66.94
(5CM X 1.8M)
48s ea ... 08080-9412-11 73.90

TENDERSKIN HYPOALLERGENIC PAPER (Covidien)
DEV,NA (3"X10YDS)
40s ea ... 08080-3394-10 84.68
(2"X10YDS, TAN)
60s ea ... 08080-2419-12 129.94
(2"X10YDS)
60s ea ... 08080-2419-10 83.91
(1"X10YDS, TAN)
120s ea ... 08080-1914-12 103.95
(1"X10YDS)
120s ea ... 08080-1914-10 76.13
(1/2"X10YDS, TAN)
240s ea ... 08080-1596-11 76.13
(1/2"X10YDS)
240s ea ... 08080-1596-10 76.13
(1"X2 1/2YDS)
250s ea ... 08080-2419-11 99.63
(1/2"X10YDS)
288s ea ... 08080-1596-00 96.34
(1"X1 1/2YDS)
500s ea ... 08080-1914-11 76.13

TENDERSORB DISPOSABLE UNDERPADS (Covidien)
DEV,NA (23"X36",15X10)
150s ea ... 08080-7176-00 35.25
(23"X36",3X50)
150s ea ... 08080-7174-00 33.09
(30"X30",15X10)
150s ea ... 08080-8490-10 40.42
(23"X24",20X10)
200s ea ... 08080-7136-00 33.72
(23"X24",4X50)
200s ea ... 08080-7134-00 30.90
(17"X24",30X10)
300s ea ... 08080-7107-01 39.79
(17"X24")
300s ea ... 08080-7105-00 35.17

TENDERSORB WET PRUF ABDOMINAL (Covidien)
DEV,NA (8"X10",NON-STERILE)
432s ea ... 08080-8194-10 100.50
(7 1/2"X8",NON-STERILE)
648s ea ... 08080-8192-10 112.58
(5"X9",NON-STERILE)
880s ea ... 08080-8190-10 159.33

PROD/MFR	HRI, UPC,NDC	AWP	SRP
(Kendall)			
DEV,NA (7.5"X8")			
216s ea	08080-9192-10	61.04	
(8"X10")			
216s ea	08080-9194-10	101.61	
(5"X9")			
432s ea	08080-9190-10	126.14	
TENDERWET ACTIVE (Medline)			
REPACK			
DEV,NA (3"X8")			
42s ea	08327-0030-95	533.55	
(4"X5")			
42s ea	08327-0030-82	320.00	
42s ea	08327-0031-82	279.82	
TENDERWET SYSTEM (Medline)			
DEV,NA (W/1.6" PAD)			
ea	53329-0992-54	139.38	
(W/2.2" PAD)			
ea	53329-0991-24	175.88	
(W/3"X3"PAD)			
ea	53329-0992-50	155.40	
(W/4"X4" PAD)			
ea	53329-0992-40	364.25	
TENDERWRAP UNNA BOOT BANDAGE (Covidien)			
DEV,NA (3INX10YDS)			
12s ea	08080-8033-00	75.37	
(4INX10YD)			
12s ea	08080-8034-00	82.37	
TENSIVE (Parker)			
GEL,TP, 50 gm 12s	00341-0022-60	36.00	60.00
TENSOR ELASTIC ROLL BANDAGES (Covidien)			
DEV,NA (6"X4.5YD,W/REMVBLE CLPS)			
72s ea	08080-4206-00	164.10	
(6"X4.5YDS,NON-STERILE)			
72s ea	08080-3930-00	275.72	
(2"X4.1YDS,NON-STERILE)			
144s ea	08080-3302-00	226.57	
(2"X4.1YDW/REMVBLE CLIPS)			
144s ea	08080-4202-00	134.17	
(3"X4.1YD,W/REMVBLE CLPS)			
144s ea	08080-4203-00	173.17	
(3"X4.1YDS,NON-STERILE)			
144s ea	08080-3550-00	320.67	
(4"X4.5YD,W/REMVBLE CLPS)			
144s ea	08080-4204-00	215.73	
(4"X4.5YDS,NON-STERILE)			
144s ea	08080-3616-00	393.57	
TERA GEL (Geritrex)			
SHA,TP, 0.5%, 120 ml	54162-0250-04	3.67	
235 ml	54162-0250-80	124.32	
TERBINAFINE HCL (Taro)			
CRE,TP (1X15GM)			
1%, 15 gm	51672-2080-01	5.71	
(1X30GM)			
1%, 30 gm	51672-2080-02	8.56	
(Phys Total Care)			
REPACK			
CRE,TP, 1%, 30 gm	54868-5992-00	29.93	
TERIX (Topix)			
LOT,TP, 227 gm	58211-0361-08	6.43	
TERSASEPTIC (Doak)			
LIQ,TP (SOAP-FREE)			
480 ml	10337-0600-42	23.81	
SOA,TP (3 OZ.)			
ea	10337-0666-73	10.20	
TETRA-FORMULA/TETRA-ETTES (Reese)			
LOZ,MM, 15 mg-7.5 mg,			
10s ea	10956-0714-10	3.57	
TETRAHYDROZOLINE (Stat Rx)			
REPACK			
SOL,OP, 0.05%, 15 ml	16590-0218-15	6.25	
TETRAHYDROZOLINE HCL (Rugby)			
SOL,OP, 0.05%, 15 ml	00536-0940-94	2.10	
(Altura)			
REPACK			
SOL,OP, 0.05%, 15 ml	63874-0955-15	5.31	
(Pharma Pac)			
REPACK			
SOL,OP, 0.05%, 15 ml	52959-0597-01	6.30	
(Southwood)			
REPACK			
SOL,OP, 0.05%, 15 ml	58016-4734-01	1.31	
15 ml	58016-4777-01	1.25	
15 ml	58016-4831-01	1.90	
15 ml	58016-6079-01	5.28	
TETTERINE (S.S.S.)			
OIN,TP (GREEN)			
2%, 30 gm	12258-0141-01	2.77	
(WHITE)			
2%, 30 gm	12258-0142-01	2.77	
TETTERINE SOAP (S.S.S.)			
SOA,TP (3 OZ.)			
ea	12258-0143-03	1.50	
THE DOCTOR'S BRUSHPICKS (Medtech)			
DEV,NA, 120s ea	42037-0411-12	1.56	
THE DOCTOR'S NIGHTGUARD (Medtech)			
DEV,NA, ea	42037-0789-12	17.99	
THE DOCTOR'S ORAPIK INTERDENTAL PICK & MIRROR (Medtech)			
DEV,NA, ea	42037-0500-25	3.90	
THE DOCTOR'S ORAPIK TRAVELER (Medtech)			
DEV,NA, ea	42037-0100-01	1.80	
THE DOCTOR'S SULCUSBRUSH (Medtech)			
DEV,NA, ea	42037-0500-00	3.30	
THE MEDICINE SHOPPE 100% NATURAL FIBER (Medicine Shoppe)			
CAP,PO (PRIVATE LABEL)			
0.52 gm, 100s ea	49614-0408-78	7.49	
THE MEDICINE SHOPPE ACID CONTROL (Cardinal Health)			
TAB,PO (MAXIMUM STRENGTH)			
20 mg, 25s ea	49614-0237-63	7.99	
THE MEDICINE SHOPPE ACID REDUCER (Cardinal Health)			
TAB,PO (MAXIMUM STRENGTH,SF)			
150 mg, 24s ea	49614-0255-51	6.99	
(Medicine Shoppe)			
TAB,PO (PRIVATE LABEL)			
75 mg, 30s ea	49614-0220-65	6.59	
THE MEDICINE SHOPPE ALCOHOL SWABS (Cardinal Health)			
SWA,TP (PRIVATE LABEL)			
6%-70%, 80s ea	49614-0221-44	2.49	
THE MEDICINE SHOPPE ALL DAY ALLERGY D-12 (Cardinal Health)			
TER,PO (PRIVATE LABEL)			
5 mg-120 mg, 24s ea	49614-0235-62	18.99	
THE MEDICINE SHOPPE ALL DAY COLD & SINUS (Medicine Shoppe)			
TER,PO (NON-DROWSY)			
220 mg-120 mg, 10s ea	49614-0381-52	3.79	
THE MEDICINE SHOPPE ALLERGY RELIEF (Cardinal Health)			
TAB,PO (ORIG PRSCRPTN STRNGTH)			
10 mg, 90s ea	49614-0170-75	24.99	
THE MEDICINE SHOPPE ALLERGY RELIEF 24 HOUR (Medicine Shoppe)			
ODT,PO (PRIVATE LABEL,CHERRY)			
10 mg, 10s ea	49614-0176-52	7.99	7.99
THE MEDICINE SHOPPE ANTACID (Cardinal Health)			
SUS,PO (REGULARSTRNGTH,1X355ML)			
355 ml	49614-0361-40	3.59	
(Medicine Shoppe)			
SUS,PO (FAST ACTING)			
355 ml	49614-0358-40	3.09	
THE MEDICINE SHOPPE ANTI-NAUSEA (Cardinal Health)			
SOL,PO (1X118ML,PRIVATE LABEL)			
118 ml	49614-0228-26	5.99	
THE MEDICINE SHOPPE ARTHRITIS PAIN RELIEVER (Cardinal Health)			
TER,PO (PRIVATE LABEL,CAPLET)			
650 mg, 50s ea	49614-0473-71	4.99	
100s ea	49614-0473-78	7.49	
THE MEDICINE SHOPPE AZO-TABS (Medicine Shoppe)			
TAB,PO (PROMPT RELIEF)			
95 mg, 32s ea	49614-0173-66	4.99	
THE MEDICINE SHOPPE BANDAGE ROLL (Cardinal Health)			
DEV,NA (4.5"X4YD,STRETCHED)			
ea	49614-0616-80	3.29	
THE MEDICINE SHOPPE CALCIUM CITRATE + (Medicine Shoppe)			
TAB,PO (PRIVATE LABEL,CAPLET)			
315 mg-200 iu, 120s ea	91899-0515-76	8.99	
THE MEDICINE SHOPPE CENTURY (Cardinal Health)			
TAB,PO (ADVANCED FORMULA)			
300s ea	49614-0257-87	12.99	
THE MEDICINE SHOPPE CENTURY MATURE (Cardinal Health)			
TAB,PO (ADVANCED FORMULA)			
100s ea	49614-0258-78	7.59	
300s ea	49614-0258-87	14.99	
THE MEDICINE SHOPPE CHEST CONGESTION AND SINUS RELIEF (Cardinal Health)			
TAB,PO (DYE-FREE)			
400 mg-10 mg, 50s ea	49614-0471-71	8.99	
THE MEDICINE SHOPPE CHEST CONGESTION RELIEF (Medicine Shoppe)			
TAB,PO (DYE-FREE,PRIVATE LABEL)			
400 mg, 50s ea	49614-0448-71	7.99	
THE MEDICINE SHOPPE CHEST CONGESTION&COUGH RELIEF (Cardinal Health)			
TAB,PO (DYE-FREE,PRIVATE LABEL)			
20 mg-400 mg, 50s ea	49614-0472-71	8.99	
THE MEDICINE SHOPPE CHILDREN'S COLD & ALLERGY (Cardinal Health)			
SOL,PO (1X118ML,AF)			
1 mg/5 ml-2.5 mg/5 ml,			
118 ml	49614-0376-26	3.79	
THE MEDICINE SHOPPE CHILDREN'S MEDI-PROFEN (Medicine Shoppe)			
SUS,PO (W/DOSAGE CUP,AF)			
100 mg/5 ml, 118 ml	49614-0897-26	4.69	
THE MEDICINE SHOPPE CO Q-10 (Cardinal Health)			
SGL,PO (PRIVATE LABEL,SOFTGEL)			
200 mg, 30s ea	49614-0252-65	21.99	
THE MEDICINE SHOPPE COUGH & SORE THROAT LOZENGES (Medicine Shoppe)			
LOZ,MM (PRIVATE LABEL)			
15 mg-10 mg, 10s ea	49614-0997-52	3.69	
THE MEDICINE SHOPPE COUGHTAB (Cardinal Health)			
TAB,PO (PRIVATE LABEL)			
200 mg, 60s ea	49614-0745-72	5.99	
THE MEDICINE SHOPPE DECONGESTANT INHALER (Medicine Shoppe)			
STI,NS (PRIVATE LABEL)			
50 mg, ea	49614-0436-12	2.79	
THE MEDICINE SHOPPE ENEMA (Medicine Shoppe)			
NMA,RC (SINGLE,READY-TO-USE)			
7 gm/118 ml-19 gm/118 ml,			
133 ml	49614-0331-27	0.99	
(TWINPACK,RDYTOUSE)			
7 gm/118 ml-19 gm/118 ml,			
133 ml,2s	49614-0331-28	1.79	
THE MEDICINE SHOPPE FIBER (Medicine Shoppe)			
TAB,PO (BULK FORMING LAXATIVE)			
625 mg, 90s ea	49614-0350-75	8.19	
THE MEDICINE SHOPPE FIBER POWDER (Cardinal Health)			
POW,NA (CLEAR SOLUBLE,1X350GM)			
350 gm	49614-0227-17	12.99	
THE MEDICINE SHOPPE HEADACHE RELIEF (Medicine Shoppe)			
TAB,PO (ADDED STRENGTH)			
250 mg-250 mg-65 mg,			
100s ea	49614-0114-78	4.69	
THE MEDICINE SHOPPE HYDROGEN PEROXIDE (Medicine Shoppe)			
SOL,TP (PRIVATE LABEL)			
3%, 473 ml	49614-0335-43	0.79	0.79
THE MEDICINE SHOPPE IBUPROFEN PM (Cardinal Health)			
TAB,PO (PRIVATE LABEL)			
38 mg-200 mg, 20s ea	49614-0155-60	3.89	
THE MEDICINE SHOPPE INFANTS' CONCENTRATED MEDI-PROFEN (Medicine Shoppe)			
SUS,PO (CONCENT./NON-STAINING)			
50 mg/1.25 ml, 30 ml	49614-0898-10	6.99	
THE MEDICINE SHOPPE INTENSE COUGH RELIEVER (Cardinal Health)			
SOL,PO (1X120ML,DOUBLESTRENGTH)			
20 mg/5 ml-300 mg/5 ml,			
120 ml	49614-0317-26	5.99	

PROD/MFR HRI, UPC,NDC AWP SRP

(Medicine Shoppe)
SOL,PO (AF,SF,PRIVATE LABEL)
30 mg/5 ml-200 mg/5 ml,
120 ml 49614-0307-26 5.99

THE MEDICINE SHOPPE IPECAC
(Medicine Shoppe)
SYR,PO (PRIVATE LABEL)
30 ml................ 49614-0200-10 1.99

THE MEDICINE SHOPPE LATEX (Cardinal Health)
DEV,NA (GENERAL PURPOSE)
50s ea............... 49614-0997-71 2.99

THE MEDICINE SHOPPE LORATADINE
(Medicine Shoppe)
TAB,PO (NON-DROWSY,ORIG STRGTH)
10 mg, 10s ea........ 49614-0170-52 6.99

THE MEDICINE SHOPPE MEDI-LICE COMBING
(Medicine Shoppe)
GEL,TP (W/SPECIAL NIT COMB)
59.1 ml.............. 49614-0532-16 5.99

THE MEDICINE SHOPPE MEDI-NATURAL
(Medicine Shoppe)
TAB,PO (PRIVATE LABEL)
8.6 mg, 100s ea...... 49614-0132-78 6.99

THE MEDICINE SHOPPE MEDI-NATURAL PLUS
(Medicine Shoppe)
TAB,PO (PRIVATE LABEL)
50 mg-8.6 mg, 60s ea 49614-0145-72 10.99

THE MEDICINE SHOPPE MEDI-PHEDRYL
(Medicine Shoppe)
SOL,PO (MAY CAUSE DROWSINESS,AF)
12.5 mg/5 ml, 118 ml. 49614-0379-26 3.29

THE MEDICINE SHOPPE MEDI-PROFEN
(Medicine Shoppe)
CTB,PO (JUNIOR STRENGTH)
100 mg, 24s ea 49614-0466-62 4.19

THE MEDICINE SHOPPE MEDI-SLEEP
(Medicine Shoppe)
TAB,PO (PRIVATE LABEL)
25 mg, 32s ea........ 49614-0143-66 6.99

THE MEDICINE SHOPPE MEDI-TABS
(Cardinal Health)
TAB,PO (EXTRA STRENGTH,CAPLET)
500 mg, 125s ea 49614-0123-00 5.29

THE MEDICINE SHOPPE MEDI-TABS PM
(Medicine Shoppe)
TAB,PO (EXTRA STRENGTH)
500 mg-25 mg, 50s ea. 49614-0439-71 4.59

THE MEDICINE SHOPPE MEDICOOL'S DIASOX
(Cardinal Health)
DEV,NA (LARGE,BLACK)
2s ea................ 49614-0999-10 7.99
(LARGE,WHITE)
2s ea................ 49614-0999-08 7.99
(MEDIUM,WHITE)
2s ea................ 49614-0999-06 7.99

THE MEDICINE SHOPPE MILK OF MAGNESIA
(Cardinal Health)
SUS,PO (1X355ML,SF)
400 mg/5 ml, 355 ml . 49614-0339-40 3.99
(1X355ML,STIMULANT-FREE)
400 mg/5 ml, 355 ml . 49614-0338-40 3.99

THE MEDICINE SHOPPE MULTI-SYMPTOM DAY-TIME
(Cardinal Health)
SOL,PO (1X177ML,AF)
177 ml 49614-0329-30 3.29

THE MEDICINE SHOPPE NASAL (Cardinal Health)
DEV,NA (LARGE,PRIVATE LABEL)
12s ea............... 49614-0998-18 3.99

THE MEDICINE SHOPPE NASAL DECONGESTANT
(Cardinal Health)
TAB,PO (MAXIMUM STRENGTH,PILL)
10 mg, 18s ea........ 49614-0440-89 3.09

THE MEDICINE SHOPPE NATURAL FIBER LAXATIVE
(Cardinal Health)
PDR,PO (SMOOTH TEXTURE, 48DOSES)
3.4 gm/dose, 283 gm . 49614-0366-38 5.99
(ORIGINAL TEXTURE)
3.4 gm/dose, 368 gm . 49614-0345-27 5.99
(SMOOTH TEXTURE, 30DOSES)
3.4 gm/dose, 368 gm . 49614-0347-27 5.99

THE MEDICINE SHOPPE NATURAL FISH OIL
(Cardinal Health)
SGL,PO (PRIVATE LABEL,SOFTGEL)
300 mg, 120s ea 49614-0423-76 8.79

THE MEDICINE SHOPPE NATURAL SUPER OMEGA-3
(Cardinal Health)
SGL,PO (PRIVATE LABEL,SOFTGEL)
60s ea............... 49614-0852-72 8.69

THE MEDICINE SHOPPE NATURAL VITAMIN B12
(Cardinal Health)
TER,PO (PRIVATE LABEL)
1000 mcg, 60s ea 49614-0655-72 5.99

THE MEDICINE SHOPPE NATURAL VITAMIN D
(Cardinal Health)
SGL,PO (PRIVATE LABEL,SOFTGEL)
400 iu, 100s ea...... 49614-0578-78 2.49

THE MEDICINE SHOPPE NICOTINE TRANSDERMAL SYSTEM (Medicine Shoppe)
TDM,TD (STOP SMOKING AID)
7 mg/24 hr, 14s ea ... 91899-0440-74 39.99
14 mg/24 hr,
14s ea............ 91899-0684-74 39.99
21 mg/24 hr,
14s ea............ 91899-0684-10 39.99

THE MEDICINE SHOPPE NITE-TIME COLD/FLU RELIEF (Cardinal Health)
SYR,PO (1X295ML,AF)
295 ml 49614-0326-38 3.99

THE MEDICINE SHOPPE NON-STICK PADS
(Cardinal Health)
DEV,NA (3"X4",PRIVATE LABEL)
10s ea............... 49614-0616-76 3.19

THE MEDICINE SHOPPE OMEPRAZOLE
(Cardinal Health)
TCP,PO (PRIVATE LABEL)
20 mg, 14s ea........ 49614-0238-66 9.59
28s ea............ 49614-0238-30 16.99

THE MEDICINE SHOPPE PAIN RELIEVER
(Cardinal Health)
SGL,PO (EXTRA STRENGTH,GELCAP)
500 mg, 50s ea 49614-0169-71 4.19

THE MEDICINE SHOPPE PAPER FIRST AID
(Cardinal Health)
DEV,NA (2.5CMX4.5CM,LATEX-FREE)
ea................... 49614-0805-05 2.89

THE MEDICINE SHOPPE PEDIATRIC ELECTROLYTE
(Medicine Shoppe)
SOL,PO (AF,PF,PRIVATE LABEL)
1000 ml 49614-0222-08 4.49
1000 ml 49614-0223-08 4.49

THE MEDICINE SHOPPE PEN NEEDLE
(Medicine Shoppe)
DEV,NA (29G, 12MM,PRIVATE LABEL)
100s ea.............. 08214-9989-01 18.99 18.99
(31G, 8MM,PRIVATE LABEL)
100s ea.............. 08214-9989-21 18.99 18.99

THE MEDICINE SHOPPE PEN NEEDLES
(Cardinal Health)
DEV,NA (31G,1/4",6MM,SHORT)
100s ea.............. 08214-9989-11 18.40

THE MEDICINE SHOPPE SORE THROAT LOZENGES
(Cardinal Health)
LOZ,MM (FAST-ACTING)
6 mg-10 mg, 18s ea .. 91899-0019-18 3.19

THE MEDICINE SHOPPE STERILE ADHESIVE PADS
(Cardinal Health)
DEV,NA (3"X4",LATEX-FREE)
10s ea............... 49614-0613-52 3.29

THE MEDICINE SHOPPE STERILE GAUZE
(Cardinal Health)
DEV,NA (76MMX2.28M,UNSTRETCHED)
ea................... 49614-0617-00 2.89

THE MEDICINE SHOPPE STERILE PADS
(Cardinal Health)
DEV,NA (4"X4",PRIVATE LABEL)
10s ea............... 49614-0616-86 3.19

THE MEDICINE SHOPPE TUSSIN CF
(Cardinal Health)
SYR,PO (1X237ML,W/DOSAGE CUP,AF)
237 ml 49614-0321-34 5.19

THE MEDICINE SHOPPE TUSSIN DM
(Cardinal Health)
SYR,PO (1X118ML,W/DOSAGE CUP,AF)
10 mg/5 ml-100 mg/5 ml,
118 ml 49614-0311-26 3.29

THE MEDICINE SHOPPE VINYL GLOVES
(Cardinal Health)
DEV,NA (DISPOSABLE,POWDER-FREE)
50s ea............... 49614-0998-71 2.99

THE MEDICINE SHOPPE VITAMIN B12
(Cardinal Health)
TER,PO (PRIVATE LABEL)
2000 mcg, 60s ea 49614-0657-72 6.99

THE MEDICINE SHOPPE VITAMIN C
(Cardinal Health)
CTB,PO (PRIVATE LABEL)
500 mg-35 mg, 100s ea 91899-0618-85 5.09

THE VERY FINEST FISH OIL OMEGA-3
(Carlson,J.R.)
OIL,PO (LEMON)
1600 mg/5 ml, 200 ml 88395-0015-40 12.45 24.90
500 ml 88395-0015-45 24.25 48.50

THERA (Major)
TAB,PO (10X10)
100s ea UD 00904-0539-61 10.56
130s ea 00904-0539-13 6.21
1000s ea 00904-0539-80 37.46

THERA DERM (Major)
OIL,TP (1X473ML)
473 ml 00904-4303-16 9.01

THERA MULTIVITAMIN (Major)
SOL,PO, 120 ml 00904-0538-00 4.29

THERA PLUS (Cardinal Health)
TAB,PO (PRIVATE LABEL)
130s ea.............. 37205-0185-81 7.36

THERA TABS (Prime Marketing)
TAB,PO (CAPLET)
100s ea.............. 62107-0066-01 4.40
500s ea.............. 62107-0066-05 17.20

THERA-DERM (Major)
LOT,TP, 240 ml 00904-4299-09 3.00
OIL,TP, 240 ml........... 00904-4303-09 4.50

THERA-GESIC (Mission)
CRE,TP (MAXIMUM STRENGTH)
1%-15%, 85 gm...... 00178-0320-03 3.61
142 gm 00178-0320-05 4.91

(DHS, Inc.)
REPACK
CRE,TP, 1%-15%, 60 gm .. 55887-0706-02 13.25
90 gm............ 55887-0706-03 17.26
120 gm 55887-0706-04 23.01

(Southwood)
REPACK
CRE,TP, 1%-15%, 90 gm .. 58016-3169-01 6.95

THERA-GESIC EXTRA STRENGTH
(Dispensing Solutions)
REPACK
CRE,TP, 1%-15%, 90 gm .. 55045-2579-03 14.20

(Nucare Pharm)
REPACK
CRE,TP, 1%-15%, 90 gm .. 66267-0938-03 10.47

(Pharma Pac)
REPACK
CRE,TP, 1%-15%, 90 gm .. 52959-0147-03 14.85

THERA-GESIC PLUS (Mission)
CRE,TP (ALOE VERA ENRICHED,FAST)
4%-25%, 85 gm...... 00178-0350-03 5.04

THERA-M (Phys Total Care)
REPACK
TAB,PO (SF)
100s ea.............. 54868-3458-00 12.65

THERA-M ENHANCED (Major)
TAB,PO (W/BETA CAROTENE)
100s ea UD 00904-5492-61 10.66
130s ea 00904-5492-13 8.00
1000s ea 00904-5492-80 44.27

THERA-M MULTIPLE (ADH)
TAB,PO, 100s ea.......... 60142-0076-10 2.95

THERA-M MULTIVITAMINS (A-S Medication)
REPACK
TAB,PO, 100s ea.......... 54569-2181-00 6.80

THERA-M W/MINERALS (Prime Marketing)
TAB,PO (CAPLET)
130s ea.............. 62107-0038-13 8.24
500s ea.............. 62107-0038-05 28.42

THERA-P (Perrigo)
LOT,TP, 240 ml 45802-0593-55 5.99

THERA-PLUS (Hi-Tech)
SOL,PO, 120 ml 50383-0683-04 4.30

THERA-SAL (Major)
SHA,TP (ORIG FORMULA,1X177ML)
3%, 177 ml 00904-5846-21 4.88

PROD/MFR	HRI, UPC,NDC	AWP	SRP
THERABASIC M (Basic Vitamins)			
TAB,PO (PF,SF)			
100s ea	00761-0425-20	3.00	
THERACAPS INTENSE COUGH & COLD RELIEVER (Reese)			
TAB,PO, 500 mg-2 mg-15 mg-30 mg,			
30s ea	10956-0772-30	4.92	
THERACOF PLUS (Reese)			
SOL,PO (INTENSE STRENGTH,AF,SF)			
118 ml	10956-0790-04	4.37	
240 ml	10956-0790-08	6.77	
THERADEX (Mason Vit)			
TAB,PO, 100s ea	11845-0063-31	7.78	
THERADEX M (Mason Vit)			
TAB,PO, 30s ea	11845-0058-38	3.11	
(PF)			
130s ea	11845-0058-33	8.78	
THERAFLU (Novartis Consumer)			
PDS,PO (MAX. STR., NON-DROWSY)			
6s ea	00043-0472-06	4.39	
THERAFLU COLD & COUGH (Novartis Consumer)			
PKT,PO (NATURAL LEMON)			
20 mg-20 mg-10 mg,			
6s ea	00067-6616-06	4.61	
THERAFLU DAYTIME SEVERE COLD & COUGH (Novartis Consumer)			
PKT,PO (BERRY/MENTHOL&GREEN TEA)			
650 mg-20 mg-10 mg,			
6s ea	00043-6257-06	4.61	
TAB,PO (COATED CAPLET)			
325 mg-10 mg-5 mg,			
24s ea	00043-6294-24	4.61	
THERAFLU FLU & CHEST CONGESTION (Novartis Consumer)			
PKT,PO (NATURAL CITRUS)			
1000 mg-400 mg,			
6s ea	00043-0483-06	4.61	
THERAFLU FLU & COLD (Novartis Consumer)			
PDS,PO (MAX. STR.,APPLE)			
6s ea	00043-0479-06	4.39	
(PACKET)			
6s ea	00043-0467-06	3.95	
THERAFLU FLU COLD & COUGH (Novartis Consumer)			
PDS,PO (PACKET)			
6s ea	00043-0466-06	3.95	
TAB,PO (MAX STR,NON-DR,CAPLET)			
500 mg-15 mg-30 mg,			
12s ea	00043-0476-12	2.93	
24s ea	00043-0476-24	4.90	
THERAFLU NIGHTTIME MAXIMUM STRENGTH (Novartis Consumer)			
PDS,PO, 6s ea	00043-0471-06	4.39	
TAB,PO (CAPLET)			
500 mg-2 mg-15 mg-30 mg,			
12s ea	00043-0136-12	2.93	
24s ea	00043-0136-24	4.90	
THERAFLU NIGHTTIME SEVERE COLD (Novartis Consumer)			
TAB,PO (COATED CAPLET)			
325 mg-2 mg-10 mg-5 mg,			
24s ea	00043-6258-24	4.61	
THERAFLU NIGHTTIME SEVERE COLD & COUGH (Novartis Consumer)			
PKT,PO (HONEYLEMON/CHAMOMILE)			
650 mg-25 mg-10 mg,			
6s ea	00043-6256-06	4.61	
THERAFLU SUGAR-FREE NIGHTTIME SEVERE COLD & COUGH (Novartis Consumer)			
PKT,PO (SF,SORBITOL-FREE)			
650 mg-25 mg-10 mg,			
6s ea	00067-6318-06	4.61	
THERAFLU WARMING RELIEF COLD & CHEST CONGESTION (Novartis Consumer)			
SOL,PO (ORANGE)			
245.5 ml	00043-6296-08	4.61	
THERAFLU WARMING RELIEF FLU & SORE THROAT (Novartis Consumer)			
SOL,PO (CHERRY)			
245.5 ml	00043-6265-08	4.61	
THERAFLU WARMING RELIEF SEVERE NIGHTTIME COLD&COUGH (Novartis Consumer)			
SOL,PO (1X245.5ML,CHERRY)			
245.5 ml	00043-0460-08	4.61	
THERAGEN (Altura)			
REPACK			
CRE,TP, 0.025%, 60 gm	63874-1052-06	18.60	
(Pharma Pac)			
REPACK			
CRE,TP, 0.025%, 60 gm	52959-0815-02	11.75	
(Southwood)			
REPACK			
CRE,TP, 0.025%, 60 gm	58016-3547-01	18.60	
THERAHEALTH (Health Products Corp)			
TAB,PO, 130s ea	39686-0013-40	5.32	
THERAHEALTH M (Health Products Corp)			
TAB,PO, 130s ea	39686-0013-37	5.50	
THERAMILL FORTE (Miller)			
SGL,PO, 90s ea	17204-0546-85	12.00	15.80
180s ea	17204-0547-50	20.16	29.30
THERAMILL PLUS (Miller)			
SGL,PO, 180s ea	17204-0548-50	21.78	
THERAMINERALS (Truxton)			
TAB,PO, 100s ea	00463-6174-01	4.20	
1000s ea	00463-6174-10	42.00	
THERAPATCH COOL (Lec Tec)			
PAD,TP (2"X3")			
3.5%-2%-11%, 5s ea	40100-0100-01	3.75	7.50
20s ea	40100-0010-01	13.00	26.00
(2"X3",BULK PACKAGE)			
3.5%-2%-11%,			
1000s ea	40100-0030-01	550.00	1000.00
THERAPATCH WARM (Lec Tec)			
PAD,TP (4"X5")			
0.09%, 20s ea	40100-0020-01	19.40	38.80
(4"X5",BULK PACKAGE)			
0.09%, 500s ea	40100-0040-01	435.00	975.00
THERAPAUSE HOT FLASH COOL DOWN STRIPS (Del)			
GEL,TP, 5s ea	10310-0324-12	6.90	10.35
THERAPAUSE PERSONAL LUBRICANT COMFORT FOAM (Del)			
GEL,VG, 103.5 ml	10310-0324-13	4.80	7.20
THERAPEUTIC (Teva)			
TAB,PO, 130s ea	00182-4518-06	7.99	
1000s ea	00182-4518-10	39.59	
THERAPEUTIC BATH (Teva)			
OIL,TP, 480 ml	00182-6019-40	4.39	
THERAPEUTIC BLUE (Family Phcy)			
GEL,TP (PRIVATE LABEL)			
2%, 240 gm	52735-0716-44	4.94	5.49
(Pharma Pac)			
REPACK			
GEL,TP, 2%, 240 gm	52959-0203-03	5.99	
THERAPEUTIC FORMULA (Albertson's)			
TAB,PO, 130s ea	04000-0001-35	8.64	
THERAPEUTIC ICE (Pfeiffer)			
GEL,TP, 2%, 240 gm	00927-0081-09	2.41	4.34
THERAPEUTIC SHAMPOO (Major)			
SHA,TP (1X251ML)			
0.5%, 251 ml	00904-5259-44	5.79	
THERAPEUTIC-M (Teva)			
TAB,PO, 130s ea	00182-4519-06	7.39	
1000s ea	00182-4519-10	47.99	
THERAPY ICE (Major)			
GEL,TP (1X227GM,GREASELESS)			
2%, 227 gm	00904-5732-26	3.75	
THERASEAL (Valeant Pharm Intl)			
LOT,TP, 1%, 180 ml	00064-3700-06	12.70	
THERASOFT ANTI-ACNE (SFC)			
CRE,TP (AF,FRAGRANCE-FREE)			
0.5%, 45 gm	66822-0101-15	4.77	7.95
THERASOFT ANTI-ITCH & DERMATITIS (SFC)			
OIN,TP, 1%, 30 gm	66822-0104-01	4.17	6.95
THERASOFT ANTIFUNGAL (SFC)			
OIN,TP, 2%, 22.5 gm	66822-0103-75	5.10	8.50
THERASOFT FIRST AID (SFC)			
OIN,TP, 500 u/gm,			
22.5 gm	66822-0102-75	3.30	5.50
THERASOFT SKIN PROTECTANT (SFC)			
CRE,TP (AF,DYE-FREE)			
0.5%, 120 gm	66822-0100-04	6.57	10.95
THERASOFT THERAPEUTIC TOTAL SKIN (SFC)			
CRE,TP, 195 gm	51743-0437-14	12.00	20.00
THERASTAT (Hart Health)			
LOZ,MM, 6 mg, 50s ea	50332-0113-04	2.58	
(CHERRY)			
6 mg, 50s ea	50332-0123-04	2.58	
125s ea	50332-0113-02	5.60	
(CHERRY)			
6 mg, 125s ea	50332-0123-02	5.60	
THERATEARS (Advanced Vision)			
SOL,OP (PF)			
0.6 ml 32s UD	58790-0000-32		12.49
0.25%, 15 ml	58790-0001-15	7.32	9.99
THERATEARS STERILID (Advanced Vision)			
FOA,TP (1X48ML,PRIVATE LABEL)			
48 ml	58790-0005-50		18.99
THERAVIM-M (Nature's Bounty)			
TAB,PO, 130s ea	74312-0016-32		9.29
THEREMS (Rugby)			
TAB,PO, 130s ea	00536-4660-38	7.35	
1000s ea	00536-4660-10	36.83	
THEREMS H (Rugby)			
TAB,PO, 90s ea	00536-4667-11	8.50	
THEREMS M (Rugby)			
TAB,PO, 130s ea	00536-4661-38	7.60	
1000s ea	00536-4661-10	39.02	
THEREMS-M (DHS, Inc.)			
REPACK			
TAB,PO, 130s ea	55887-0082-13	7.60	
THERMA-KOOL HOT/COLD COMPRESS (Nortech)			
DEV,NA (4"X18", FREEDOM WRAP)			
ea	10824-0044-18	6.95	
(4"X6", FREEDOM WRAP)			
ea	10824-0004-46	3.59	
(4"X9", FREEDOM WRAP)			
ea	10824-0004-49	4.59	
(6"X9", FREEDOM WRAP)			
ea	10824-0006-69	5.15	
(8.5"X10.5",FREEDOM WRAP)			
ea	10824-0088-10	6.15	
(4"X18")			
6s ea	10824-0004-18	24.00	
(4"X9")			
12s ea	10824-0000-49	21.60	
(6"X9")			
12s ea	10824-0000-69	26.70	
(8.5"X10.5")			
12s ea	10824-0008-10	37.50	
(4"X6")			
25s ea	10824-0000-46	21.60	
THERMACARE (P & G Company)			
DEV,NA (L/XL,ADHESIVE WRAP)			
2s ea	37000-0345-63	6.40	
(S/M,ADHESIVE WRAP)			
2s ea	37000-0345-62	6.40	
(MENSTRUAL PATCH)			
3s ea	37000-0345-64	6.34	
(NECK TO ARM WRAP)			
3s ea	37000-0345-65	6.34	
THERMACARE HEATWRAPS (Wyeth Consumer)			
DEV,NA (NECK, WRIST & SHOULDER)			
3s ea	05733-0015-02		6.99
THERMASONIC (Parker)			
DEV,NA (GEL WARMER/GEL)			
ea	00341-0082-04	145.00	198.00
THERMOMETER DIGITAL (Lumiscope)			
DEV,NA (W/PEAK TEMP BEEPER)			
ea	38673-0000-08	4.49	9.99
THERMOMETER MEDICAL (Lumiscope)			
DEV,NA (TWO-PART STYLE,W/BEEPER)			
ea	38673-0000-48	8.99	19.99
THERMOMETER PROBE COVER (Lumiscope)			
DEV,NA, 50s ea	38673-0011-10	1.49	2.99
THERMOTABS (Numark)			
TAB,PO (BUFFERED)			
287 mg-15 mg-180 mg,			
100s ea	38485-0863-35	5.10	
THEVIMINE-T (Mason Vit)			
TAB,PO, 100s ea	11845-0058-41	8.11	
THEX FORTE (Lee Pharm)			
TAB,PO (CAPLET)			
75s ea	23558-0681-00	16.20	
(75X24,CAPLET)			
1800s ea	23558-0681-02	388.80	
THICK-IT (Precision Milani)			
POW,PO (ORIGINAL)			
240 gm	72058-0040-75	4.58	
900 gm	72058-0040-76	12.89	

PROD/MFR	HRI, UPC,NDC	AWP	SRP
THICK-IT 2 (Precision Milani)			
POW,PO (CONCENTRATED)			
240 gm	72058-0040-80	7.04	
900 gm	72058-0040-81	19.76	
THIK & CLEAR (Nutra/Balance)			
POW,NA (12X227GM,STARCH-FREE)			
227 gm 12s	07249-0222-27		112.38
THIK & CLEAR HONEY (Nutra/Balance)			
NA (200X5GM,STARCH-FREE)			
5 gm 200s	07249-0222-24		93.63
THIK & CLEAR NECTAR (Nutra/Balance)			
NA (200X5GM,STARCH-FREE)			
5 gm 200s	07249-0222-25		93.63
THIMEROSAL (Consolidated Midland)			
SWA,TP, 2%, 10s ea	00223-4004-01	4.50	
(Truxton)			
TIN,TP, 1:1000, 480 ml	00463-9028-16	16.80	
3840 ml	00463-9028-28	30.00	
THIN LANCET (Aurora)			
DEV,NA (23G)			
100s ea	08214-0157-24	4.60	
THINNING HAIR SYSTEM (Dartmouth)			
KIT,MR (LACTOSE-FREE)			
5000 mcg-50 mg-100 mg, ea	58869-0270-00	39.90	49.99
THINNING HAIR SYSTEM WITH MULTI (Dartmouth)			
KIT,MR (LACTOSE-FREE)			
ea	58869-0270-11	43.80	54.99
THISILIBIN (Bio-Tech Pharm)			
CAP,PO, 300 mg, 100s ea	53191-0228-01	17.75	
THORACOL (Hart Health)			
LOZ,MM, 7 mg, 50s ea	50332-0112-04	2.51	
125s ea	50332-0112-02	5.49	
THREE FLOWERS BRILLIANTINE (Johnson & Johnson)			
OIL,TP, 120 ml	52800-0116-04	2.89	
OIN,TP, 97.5 gm	52800-0116-05	2.89	
THREE-WAY STOPCOCK (Abbott Hosp)			
DEV,NA (STERILE PACK)			
50s ea	00074-3232-01	72.00	
THREE-WAY STOPCOCK EXTENSION (Abbott Hosp)			
DEV,NA (20" W/OPTION-LOK)			
50s ea	00074-3230-01	117.60	
(36" W/OPTION-LOK)			
50s ea	00074-3231-01	121.80	
THREE-WAY STOPCOCK EXTENSION 20-SL (Abbott Hosp)			
DEV,NA (W/NON-REMOVABLE RESEAL)			
50s ea	00074-3234-01	117.60	
THREE-WAY STOPCOCK EXTENSION 36-SL (Abbott Hosp)			
DEV,NA (W/NON-REMOVABLE RESEAL)			
50s ea	00074-3235-01	121.80	
THREE-WAY STOPCOCK W/MALE LUER LOCK (Abbott Hosp)			
DEV,NA, 50s ea	00074-3233-01	87.00	
THREONINE (Carlson,J.R.)			
L-THREONINE			
POW,PO, 100 gm	88395-0069-55	14.95	29.90
(Freeda)			
TAB,PO (PF,SF,DYE-FREE)			
500 mg, 100s ea	10432-0288-01	15.57	25.95
THRIVE (Novartis Consumer)			
GUM,PO (MINT,COATED)			
2 mg, 100s ea	00067-5605-95	42.00	
4 mg, 100s ea	00067-5606-95	42.00	
THROAT (Nuage Labs)			
TAB,SL ((TISSUE K, 6X)			
125s ea	00634-0911-68	3.05	5.09
THROAT LOZENGES (Major)			
THROAT LOZENGES			
LOZ,MM (12X1)			
10 mg-0.5 mg, 12s ea	00904-6005-05	1.52	
THROAT SPRAY RED (Perrigo)			
SPR,MM (AF)			
1.4%, 180 ml	45802-0327-82	3.10	
THROMBI-PAD (King Pharm)			
DEV,NA, 10s ea	60793-0916-03	648.24	
THROTO-CEPTIC (S.S.S.)			
SPR,MM (AF,SF,CHERRY)			
0.5%-1.4%, 117 ml	12258-0150-06	2.33	3.50
(AF,SF,COOL MENTHOL)			
0.5%-1.4%, 117 ml	12258-0151-06	2.33	3.50
(AF,SF,MINT)			
0.5%-1.4%, 117 ml	12258-0149-06	2.33	3.50
(REGULAR,AF,SF)			
0.5%-1.4%, 117 ml	12258-0148-06	2.33	3.50
THUJA (Boiron)			
OIN,TP, 1 x, 30 gm	00220-5001-51	3.71	6.19
THUJA OCC (Luyties)			
TAB,SL (6X)			
6 x, 500s ea	00618-9045-03	3.99	
5500s ea	00618-9045-10	30.32	
12 x, 500s ea	00622-9045-03	4.19	
5500s ea	00622-9045-10	31.83	
30 x, 500s ea	00624-9045-03	4.19	
5500s ea	00624-9045-10	31.83	
THUM (Oakhurst)			
LIQ,TP, 6 ml	11169-0100-01	2.17	3.26
THUROCLENS (Woodward Labs)			
SOL,TP, 355 ml	60193-0160-12	7.45	
800 ml	60193-0160-08	8.65	
THYLOX ACNE TREATMENT SOAP (Grandpa Soap)			
SOA,TP, 3%, 92 gm 24s	10486-0012-12	71.28	
THYMUS (Bio-Tech Pharm)			
CAP,PO, 300 mg, 100s ea	53191-0341-01	7.00	
(Miller)			
TAB,PO, 140 mg, 100s ea	17204-0514-40	7.56	12.00
THYROSHIELD (Fleming)			
SOL,PO (BLACK RASPBERRY)			
65 mg/ml, 30 ml	02560-0210-01		16.56
TI-CREME (Bethany Pharmacal)			
CRE,TP (HEELS, SOLES, BODY)			
120 gm	51687-0140-04	7.50	12.98
TI-SCREEN SPORTS W/PARSOL (Pedinol)			
GEL,TP (SPF 20,AF)			
2%-7.5%-5%-6%, 118.28 ml	00884-2099-04		9.75
TI-SEB (Allerderm Labs.)			
LIQ,TP, 2%, 240 ml	34674-0365-08	7.63	
TIELLE HYDROPOLYMER (J&J Medical)			
DEV,NA (5 7/8"X 7 3/4")			
5s ea	56091-0024-41	69.68	
(7"X7",SACRUM)			
5s ea	56091-0024-43	88.40	
(7"X7")			
5s ea	56091-0024-42	91.65	
(4 1/4"X4 1/4")			
10s ea	56091-0024-40	59.54	
(STERILE,2 3/4X3 1/2")			
10s ea	56091-0024-39	39.00	
TIELLE PLUS HYDROPOLYMER (J&J Medical)			
DEV,NA (5 7/8"X7 3/4")			
5s ea	56091-0054-41	69.68	
(4 1/4"X4 1/4")			
10s ea	56091-0054-40	59.54	
(5 7/8"X5 7/8")			
10s ea	56091-0054-44	112.58	
TIGER BALM (Prince Of Peace)			
OIN,TP (EXTRA STRENGTH)			
18 gm	66403-0308-35		5.95
TIGER BALM ARTHRITIS RUB (Prince Of Peace)			
LOT,TP (AF,GREASELESS)			
11%-11%, 113 ml	62003-0422-04		11.99
TIGER BALM PATCH (Prince Of Peace)			
TDM,TP (4"X2.75")			
5s ea	62003-0322-05		5.25
TIGER BALM ULTRA (Prince Of Peace)			
OIN,TP, 18 gm	49906-0315-10		6.95
(Pharma Pac)			
REPACK			
OIN,TP, 18 gm	52959-0624-01	7.51	
TIME-C (Carlson,J.R.)			
CER,PO (TIME RELEASED,PF)			
500 mg, 100s ea	88395-0034-51	5.95	11.90
250s ea	88395-0034-52	13.45	26.90
TIME-C-BIO (Carlson,J.R.)			
TER,PO, 1000 mg-100 mg,			
100s ea	88395-0034-11	7.75	15.50
250s ea	88395-0034-12	17.75	35.50
TINACTIN (Schering Plough)			
CRE,TP, 1%, 15 gm	00085-0715-05	5.82	
30 gm	00085-0715-07	8.68	
POW,TP, 1%, 90 gm	00085-0444-06	5.41	
133 gm	11523-4161-02	5.52	
SOL,TP, 1%, 156.47 ml	11523-0165-03	5.52	
(Phys Total Care)			
REPACK			
CRE,TP, 1%, 96 gm	54868-3620-00	20.79	
(Southwood)			
REPACK			
CRE,TP, 1%, 15 gm	58016-3264-01	8.44	
TINACTIN JOCK ITCH (Schering Plough)			
CRE,TP, 1%, 15 gm	00085-0934-05	5.82	
TINEACIDE (Blaine)			
CRE,TP (PHYSICIAN FORMULA)			
13%, 35 gm	65373-0100-01	9.44	21.50
(Quality Care Prod)			
REPACK			
CRE,TP, 15 gm	49999-0320-35	30.40	
TING (Heritage/Insight)			
CRE,TP, 1%, 15 gm	63736-0051-45	2.00	
SPR,TP, 1%, 90 ml	63736-0532-61	2.00	
90 ml	63736-0819-61	2.00	
TISIT (Pfeiffer)			
KIT,TP, 2%-0.3%, ea	00927-0235-53	7.20	12.95
LIQ,TP, 2%-0.3%, 60 ml	00927-0147-39	2.65	4.76
120 ml	00927-0147-12	4.33	7.79
SHA,TP, 3%-0.3%, 60 ml	00927-0053-39	2.45	4.40
120 ml	00927-0053-12	4.04	7.26
SPR,NA, 2%-0.3%, 150 ml	00927-0235-25	3.22	5.79
TISIT BLUE GEL (Pfeiffer)			
GEL,TP, 3%-0.3%, 30 gm	00927-0045-30	2.16	3.89
TITRALAC (3M Consumer)			
CTB,PO, 420 mg, 100s ea	21200-0765-91	4.36	
TITRALAC EXTRA STRENGTH (3M Consumer)			
CTB,PO, 750 mg, 100s ea	51131-0572-32	5.70	
TITRALAC PLUS (3M Consumer)			
CTB,PO (MINT)			
420 mg-21 mg, 100s ea	51131-0539-37	4.74	
TOCOTRIENOLS (Carlson,J.R.)			
SGL,PO (PF,SOFT GELS)			
100 iu, 30s ea	88395-0008-80	9.95	19.90
90s ea	88395-0008-81	24.95	49.90
180s ea	88395-0008-82	46.00	92.00
TODAY SPONGE (Mayer)			
SPG,VG, 1000 mg, 3s ea	44376-0100-01	10.80	
12s ea	44376-0100-02	43.20	
TODDLER'S DIMETAPP DECONGESTANT (Wyeth Consumer)			
SOL,PO (AF,GRAPE,DROPS)			
1.25 mg/0.8 ml, 15 ml	00031-2236-12		5.49
TODDLER'S DIMETAPP DECONGESTANT PLUS COUGH (Wyeth Consumer)			
SOL,PO (AF,GRAPE,DROPS)			
15 ml	00031-2243-12		5.49
TOLEREX (Nestle)			
PDR,PO (PACKET)			
80 gm 60s	00212-4580-72	493.92	
TOLNAFTATE (Actavis Mid Atlantic)			
CRE,TP, 1%, 15 gm	00472-1900-15	1.88	
(AmerisourceBergen)			
CRE,TP (PRIVATE LABEL)			
1%, 15 gm	24385-0032-01	3.59	3.99
(Asafi Pharmaceutical)			
CRE,TP, 1%, 15 gm	65557-0209-30	1.80	
POW,TP, 1%, 45 gm	65557-0775-45	2.62	
(Cardinal Health)			
CRE,TP (PRIVATE LABEL)			
1%, 30 gm	37205-0197-10	4.49	
(Consolidated Midland)			
CRE,TP, 1%, 15 gm	00223-4432-15	2.75	
POW,TP, 1%, 45 gm	00223-2086-45	3.00	
SOL,TP, 1%, 10 ml	00223-6315-10	2.75	
(G&W)			
CRE,TP, 1%, 30 gm	00713-0292-31	2.24	
(Major)			
CRE,TP, 1%, 15 gm	00904-0722-36	2.75	
POW,TP, 1%, 45 gm	00904-0726-45	3.69	
(Mericon)			
CRE,TP, 1%, 114 gm	00394-0857-04	3.52	
(Perrigo)			
CRE,TP, 1%, 15 gm	45802-0032-01	2.99	
30 gm	45802-0032-03	4.99	
POW,TP, 1%, 45 gm	45802-0034-86	5.99	
SOL,TP, 1%, 10 ml	45802-0033-85	4.60	

PROD/MFR	HRI, UPC,NDC	AWP	SRP
(R.I.J.)			
POW,TP, 1%, 45 gm	53807-0123-01	2.30	
(Rugby)			
POW,TP, 1%, 45 gm	00536-5150-26	3.37	
(Taro)			
CRE,TP, 1%, 15 gm	51672-2020-01	2.55	
30 gm	51672-2020-02	4.35	
(A-S Medication)			
REPACK			
CRE,TP, 1%, 15 gm	54569-0756-00	3.34	
(Altura)			
REPACK			
CRE,TP, 1%, 15 gm	63874-0041-15	8.86	
(Palmetto)			
REPACK			
CRE,TP, 1%, 15 gm	23490-6775-01	8.44	
(Phys Total Care)			
REPACK			
CRE,TP, 1%, 15 gm	54868-2422-01	8.16	
30 gm	54868-2422-03	6.33	
POW,TP, 1%, 45 gm	54868-3331-00	8.98	
SOL,TP, 1%, 10 ml	54868-2078-00	6.67	
(Quality Care Prod)			
REPACK			
CRE,TP, 1%, 30 gm	49999-0273-30	9.70	
TOLNAFTIN (Prime Marketing)			
CRE,TP, 1%, 15 gm	62107-0008-15	2.90	
TONOSEX (Tarmac)			
TAB,PO, 50s ea	11096-0125-01	8.04	
TONSILINE (Oakhurst)			
LIQ,PO (GARGLE)			
120 ml	11169-0040-36	4.75	7.15
TOP CARE CLICKFINE UNIVERSAL PEN NEEDLES (Can-Am Care)			
DEV,NA (31G,6MM,1/4")			
100s ea	38396-0706-37	19.98	
(31G,8MM,5/16")			
100s ea	38396-0702-37	19.98	
TOP CARE ULTRA COMFORT INSULIN SYRINGES (Can-Am Care)			
DEV,NA (29G,1/2CC,1/2")			
100s ea	38396-0412-37	17.50	
(29G,1CC,1/2")			
100s ea	38396-0413-37	17.50	
(29G,3/10CC,1/2")			
100s ea	38396-0411-37	17.50	
(30G,1/2CC,5/16")			
100s ea	38396-0415-37	17.50	
(30G,1CC,5/16")			
100s ea	38396-0416-37	17.50	
(30G,3/10CC,5/16")			
100s ea	38396-0414-37	17.50	
(31G,1/2CC,5/16")			
100s ea	38396-0420-37	17.50	
(31G,1CC,5/16")			
100s ea	38396-0421-37	17.50	
(31G,3/10CC,5/16")			
100s ea	38396-0419-37	17.50	
TOP CARE UNIVERSAL 1 LANCETS (Can-Am Care)			
DEV,NA (26G,SINGLE USE,THIN)			
100s ea	38396-0301-37	5.85	
(30G,SINGLEUSE,ULTRATHIN)			
100s ea	38396-0305-37	5.85	
TOP-FILL BAG (Abbott)			
DEV,NA, ea	70074-0090-01	6.26	
(W/GRAVITY FEEDING)			
ea	70074-0000-89	10.76	
TOP-FILL BAG W/COMPANION PUMP (Abbott)			
DEV,NA (1000 ML)			
ea	70074-0000-71	14.95	
(500 ML)			
ea	70074-0504-31	14.95	
TOP-FILL BAG W/PATROL PUMP (Abbott)			
DEV,NA (1000 ML)			
ea	70074-0520-43	14.56	
TOP-FILL BAG/FLEXIFLO QUANTUM PUMP (Abbott)			
DEV,NA, ea	70074-0506-09	14.69	
(W/FLUSH BAG)			
ea	70074-0506-07	19.58	
TOPICAINE (ESBA Labs)			
GEL,TP, 4%, 10 gm	63135-0312-13	8.50	15.99
30 gm	63135-0312-30	24.00	39.99
113 gm	63135-0312-04	48.00	79.99
TOPICAINE 5 (ESBA Labs)			
TP, 5%, 10 gm	63135-0581-10	10.00	18.99
30 gm	63135-0581-30	29.00	47.50
TOPICLEAR (Med-Derm)			
LOT,TP, 60 ml	45565-0800-11	5.58	
TOPPER DRESSING NONSTERILE (J&J Medical)			
DEV,NA (3X3",GAUZE COVER FACING)			
100s ea	56091-0064-13	3.29	
(3X3",NONWOVEN FACING)			
100s ea	56091-0064-17	3.03	
(4X3",NONWOVEN FACING)			
100s ea	56091-0064-18	3.91	
(4X4",GAUZE COVER FACING)			
100s ea	56091-0064-11	6.06	
(4X4",NONWOVEN FACING)			
100s ea	56091-0064-15	5.39	
(8X4",NONWOVEN FACING)			
100s ea	56091-0064-16	6.13	
TOPPER DRESSING STERILE (J&J Medical)			
DEV,NA (4"X3",2X25)			
50s ea	56091-0024-35	3.12	
(4"X4",2X25)			
50s ea	56091-0024-36	3.89	
TOPTAINER ENTERAL CONTAINER (Abbott)			
DEV,NA, ea	70074-0004-90	6.20	
(W/GRAVITY FEEDING)			
ea	70074-0004-89	10.51	
TOPTAINER W/COMPANION PUMP (Abbott)			
DEV,NA, ea	70074-0004-94	14.50	
TOPTAINER W/FLEXIFLO QUANTUM PUMP (Abbott)			
DEV,NA, ea	70074-0506-11	14.27	
(W/FLUSH BAG)			
ea	70074-0506-15	19.16	
TOPTAINER W/PATROL PUMP (Abbott)			
DEV,NA (1000 ML)			
ea	70074-0520-47	14.03	
TOTAL B W/C (Major)			
TAB,PO (CAPLET)			
130s ea	00904-0260-13	5.55	
1000s ea	00904-0260-80	35.10	
TOTAL GERIATRIC FORMULA (Health Products Corp)			
TAB,PO (PF,SF)			
50s ea	39686-0012-74	7.50	
TOTAL NUTRITION (Health Products Corp)			
PO (PF,SF)			
50s ea	39686-0012-77	7.50	
TOUCH-TROL SUCTION CATHETER (Covidien)			
DEV,NA (10FR GLOVES)			
100s ea	08080-1409-80	93.75	
(10FR)			
100s ea	08080-1419-00	65.00	
(14FR GLOVES)			
100s ea	08080-1409-82	93.75	
(14FR)			
100s ea	08080-1419-02	65.00	
(18FR)			
100s ea	08080-1419-04	78.75	
(6FR GLOVES)			
100s ea	08080-1409-86	110.00	
(6FR)			
100s ea	08080-1419-06	85.32	
(8FR GLOVES)			
100s ea	08080-1409-88	104.50	
(8FR)			
100s ea	08080-1419-08	80.00	
TOUGH PADS (Johnson & Johnson)			
DEV,NA (3"X2.25")			
4s ea	81370-0085-26	3.91	
TRANQUIL-EZE (Reese)			
TAB,PO (CAPLET)			
20s ea	23513-0640-20	4.00	5.49
TRANS-VER-SAL (Doak)			
TDM,TD (20 MM)			
15%, 10s ea	10337-0203-02	29.62	
(12 MM)			
15%, 12s ea	10337-0202-03	22.79	
(6 MM)			
15%, 15s ea	10337-0201-15	19.40	
(20 MM)			
15%, 25s ea	10337-0203-05	68.22	
(12 MM)			
15%, 40s ea	10337-0202-06	69.83	
(6 MM)			
15%, 40s ea	10337-0201-06	47.72	
(Southwood)			
REPACK			
TDM,TD (12 MM)			
15%, 40s ea	58016-3233-01	29.50	
(6 MM)			
15%, 40s ea	58016-3234-01	20.94	
TRANSEPTIC (Parker)			
SPR,NA (12250ML)			
250 ml 12s	00341-0009-25	50.04	83.40
TRANSFER DEVICE 2-WAY (Abbott Hosp)			
DEV,NA, 400s ea	00074-3002-04	456.00	
TRANSFER SET (Abbott Hosp)			
DEV,NA (3 LEG, VENTED)			
10s ea	00074-4403-01	526.54	
(4 LEG, NON-VENTED)			
10s ea	00074-4402-01	631.99	
(4 LEG, VENTED)			
10s ea	00074-4401-01	631.99	
(14")			
48s ea	00074-1718-48	374.40	
(36")			
48s ea	00074-6402-48	238.46	
TRANSPORE SURGICAL (3M Health Care)			
DEV,NA (3"X10 YDS)			
4s ea	08333-1527-03	18.30	
(2"X10 YDS)			
6s ea	08333-1527-02	18.30	
(1"X10 YDS)			
12s ea	08333-1527-01	18.30	
(1/2"X10 YDS)			
24s ea	08333-1527-00	18.30	
(2"X1 1/2 YDS)			
50s ea	08333-1527-12	38.50	
(1"X1 1/2 YDS)			
100s ea	08333-1527-11	38.50	
TRAUMEEL (Heel/BHI)			
LIQ,PO (DROPS)			
48 ml	50114-1160-04	6.65	11.85
TAB,PO, 100s ea	50114-6150-02	6.95	11.95
TRAVEL SICKNESS (Chain Drug Marketing)			
TAB,PO, 50 mg, 12s ea	63868-0160-12	0.96	1.99
(Rugby)			
CTB,PO (RASPBERRY)			
25 mg, 100s ea	00536-3990-01	4.80	
1000s ea	00536-3990-10	32.83	
TRAVEL-EZE (Mason Vit)			
TAB,PO, 50 mg, 12s ea	11845-0131-20	2.22	
TRENEV TRIO (Natren)			
CAP,PO, 30s ea	53983-0600-30	30.00	50.00
TRI ACTING (Medicine Shoppe)			
LIQ,PO (COLD & COUGH)			
118 ml	49614-0144-26	3.69	3.69
TRI-B (Carlson,J.R.)			
TAB,PO, 0.4 mg-0.8 mg-25 mg,			
120s ea	88395-0020-01	3.88	7.75
360s ea	88395-0020-03	9.95	19.90
TRI-BIOZENE (Reese)			
OIN,TP, 15 gm	10956-0709-15	5.47	
TRI-PSEUDAFED (Concord Labs)			
TAB,PO, 60 mg-2.5 mg,			
24s ea	20254-0204-24	2.30	
100s ea	20254-0204-01	4.32	
1000s ea	20254-0204-04	29.57	
TRI-SALTS (Bio-Tech Pharm)			
CAP,PO, 50 mg-97 mg-102 mg,			
100s ea	53191-0417-01	4.50	
POW,PO (1X120GM)			
120 gm	53191-0267-12	3.90	
TRI-SUPER FLAVONS (Freeda)			
TAB,PO (PF,SF,DYE-FREE)			
1000 mg, 100s ea	10432-0234-01	8.97	14.95
250s ea	10432-0234-02	17.94	29.90
TRI-VI-SOL (Mead Johnson & Co)			
LIQ,PO (DROPS)			
50 ml	00087-0403-03	7.00	
TRI-VI-SOL W/IRON (Mead Johnson & Co)			
LIQ,PO (AF,DROPS)			
50 ml	00087-0453-03	7.00	
TRI-VITAMIN (Hi-Tech)			
LIQ,PO (DROPS)			
50 ml	50383-0635-50	10.80	
(Pharma Pac)			
REPACK			
LIQ,PO (1X50ML,DROPS)			
50 ml	52959-0967-50	7.95	

PROD/MFR	HRI, UPC,NDC	AWP	SRP
TRI-VITAMINS (Rugby)			
LIQ,PO (CHERRY,DROPS)			
50 ml	**00536-8501-80**	8.07	
(Phys Total Care)			
REPACK			
LIQ,PO (1X50ML,CHERRY,DROPS)			
50 ml	**54868-6000-00**	21.55	
TRIACTING CHEST CONGESTION (AmerisourceBergen)			
LIQ,PO (AF,PRIVATE LABEL,CITRUS)			
50 mg/5 ml-15 mg/5 ml,			
118 ml	**24385-0523-26**	3.50	3.89
TRIACTING NITE TIME (AmerisourceBergen)			
LIQ,PO (AF,PRIVATE LABEL,GRAPE)			
120 ml	**24385-0048-26**	3.50	3.89
TRIAD WOUND CARE (Coloplast)			
GEL,TP (WOUND DRESSING)			
71 gm 12s	**11701-0031-33**	196.92	206.04
170 gm 12s	**11701-0031-32**	298.20	312.12
TRIAMIN (Key Company)			
TAB,PO (SF)			
100s ea	**11694-0796-01**	5.50	
250s ea	**11694-0796-25**	11.75	
1000s ea	**11694-0796-05**	40.00	
TRIAMINIC ALLERCHEWS (Novartis Consumer)			
ODT,PO (24 HOUR NON-DROWSY)			
10 mg, 8s ea	**00067-6099-08**	5.10	
TRIAMINIC AM-COUGH/DECONGESTANT (Novartis Consumer)			
LIQ,PO, 7.5 mg/5 ml-15 mg/5 ml,			
120 ml	**00043-0558-04**	4.85	
TRIAMINIC CHEST & NASAL CONGESTION (Novartis Consumer)			
SYR,PO (ASPIRIN-FREE,TROPICAL)			
50 mg/5 ml-15 mg/5 ml,			
118 ml	**00067-6081-04**	4.85	
TRIAMINIC COLD & ALLERGY (Novartis Consumer)			
SYR,PO (ASPIRIN-FREE,ORANGE)			
1 mg/5 ml-15 mg/5 ml,			
118 ml	**00067-0216-04**	4.85	
TRIAMINIC COLD & COUGH (Novartis Consumer)			
SYR,PO (ASPIRIN-FREE,CHERRY)			
236 ml	**00067-0211-08**	8.00	
TRIAMINIC COUGH (Novartis Consumer)			
SYR,PO (ASPIRIN-FREE,BERRY)			
5 mg/5 ml-15 mg/5 ml,			
118 ml	**00067-0217-04**	4.85	
TRIAMINIC COUGH & NASAL CONGESTION (Novartis Consumer)			
SYR,PO (ASPIRIN-FREE)			
7.5 mg/5 ml-15 mg/5 ml,			
118 ml	**00067-6080-04**	4.85	
TRIAMINIC COUGH & SORE THROAT (Novartis Consumer)			
SYR,PO (ASPIRIN-FREE,GRAPE)			
118 ml	**00067-0230-04**	4.85	
TRIAMINIC FLU (Novartis Consumer)			
SOL,PO (COUGH & FEVER)			
118 ml	**00067-0750-04**	4.85	
TRIAMINIC NIGHT TIME (Novartis Consumer)			
LIQ,PO, 120 ml	**00043-0548-04**	4.85	
240 ml	**00043-0548-08**	8.00	
TRIAMINIC NIGHT TIME COUGH & COLD (Novartis Consumer)			
SYR,PO (ASPIRIN-FREE,GRAPE)			
118 ml	**00067-6102-04**	4.85	
TRIAMINIC SOFTCHEW ALLERGY RUNNY NOSE & CONGESTION (Novartis Consumer)			
CTB,PO (ASPIRIN-FREE,ORANGE)			
1 mg-15 mg, 18s ea	**00067-0296-18**	4.85	
TRIAMINIC SOFTCHEWS COLD & COUGH (Novartis Consumer)			
CTB,PO (ASPIRIN-FREE,CHERRY)			
1 mg-5 mg-15 mg,			
18s ea	**00067-6015-18**	4.85	
TRIAMINIC SOFTCHEWS COUGH & SORE THROAT (Novartis Consumer)			
CTB,PO (ASPIRIN-FREE,GRAPE)			
160 mg-5 mg-15 mg,			
18s ea	**00067-6014-18**	4.85	
TRIAMINIC SORE THROAT (Novartis Consumer)			
SPR,MM (AF,SF,ASPIRIN-FREE)			
0.5%, 118 ml	**00067-6085-04**	4.85	
TRIAMINIC SORE THROAT FORMULA (Novartis Consumer)			
LIQ,PO, 120 ml	**00043-0555-04**	4.40	
TRIAMINO (Freeda)			
TAB,PO (SF)			
200 mg-200 mg-200 mg,			
100s ea	**10432-0177-01**	7.77	12.95
(PF,SF,DYE-FREE)			
200 mg-200 mg-200 mg,			
250s ea	**10432-0177-02**	15.54	25.90
TRICARDIO B (Miller)			
CAP,PO (SF)			
0.25 mg-0.4 mg-25 mg,			
60s ea	**17204-0581-20**	5.04	
TRICHLOR FRESH PAC (Topix)			
SOL,TP (OFFICE USE ONLY)			
ea	**51326-0011-30**	8.50	
ea	**51326-0012-30**	9.50	
ea	**51326-0013-30**	10.00	
ea	**51326-0016-30**	12.25	
ea	**51326-0030-30**	8.00	
ea	**51326-0031-30**	8.25	
TRICODENE (Pfeiffer)			
SYR,PO, 2 mg/5 ml-10 mg/5 ml,			
120 ml	**00927-0406-12**	3.10	5.57
(SF)			
2 mg/5 ml-10 mg/5 ml,			
120 ml	**00927-0698-12**	2.86	5.14
TRIMO-SAN (Cooper Surgical)			
GEL,VG, 0.025%,			
113.4 gm	**59365-5030-00**	15.60	
TRINOVIN (Novogen)			
TAB,PO, 40 mg, 30s ea	**49197-0010-01**	14.95	19.95
(6X30)			
40 mg, 180s ea	**49197-0010-06**	89.70	119.70
TRIPHED (Global Source)			
TAB,PO, 60 mg-2.5 mg,			
24s ea	**59618-0861-06**	2.80	
TRIPLE A/B (Stat Rx)			
REPACK			
OIN,TP, 15 gm	**16590-0241-15**	9.00	
TRIPLE ANTIBIOTIC (Actavis Mid Atlantic)			
OIN,TP, 0.9 gm 144s UD	**00472-0179-09**	45.72	
(5 PANEL)			
15 gm	**00472-0179-34**	5.38	
30 gm	**00472-0179-56**	7.62	
(Albertson's)			
OIN,TP, 30 gm	**41280-0200-77**	2.42	
(Altaire)			
OIN,TP, 30 gm	**59390-0027-17**	5.05	
(AmerisourceBergen)			
OIN,TP (PRIVATE LABEL)			
14 gm	**24385-0061-01**	3.05	3.39
28 gm	**24385-0061-03**	4.49	4.99
(Asafi Pharmaceutical)			
OIN,TP, 30 gm	**65557-0207-30**	2.20	
(Cardinal Health)			
OIN,TP (PRIVATE LABEL)			
30 gm	**37205-0273-10**	3.92	
(G&W)			
OIN,TP, 30 gm	**00713-0268-31**	3.18	
(Global Source)			
OIN,TP, 30 gm	**59618-0870-52**	2.40	
(Hart Health)			
OIN,TP, 144s ea UD	**50332-0032-05**	10.91	
(25X0.9GM)			
0.9 gm 25s UD	**50332-0032-02**	3.63	
(Major)			
OIN,TP, 15 gm	**00904-0734-36**	2.25	
30 gm	**00904-0734-31**	3.25	
(Medicine Shoppe)			
OIN,TP, 30 gm	**49614-0409-10**	4.99	4.99
(Perrigo)			
OIN,TP, 0.9 gm 144s	**45802-0061-70**	39.99	
15 gm	**45802-0061-01**	4.25	
30 gm	**45802-0061-03**	6.15	
(Pfeiffer)			
OIN,TP, 30 gm	**00927-0025-30**	1.62	2.92
(Qualitest)			
OIN,TP, 30 gm	**00603-0644-50**	6.95	
(Rugby)			
OIN,TP, 30 gm	**00536-1100-95**	4.95	
(Taro)			
OIN,TP, 15 gm	**51672-2016-01**	3.71	
28.4 gm	**51672-2016-02**	5.45	
(Truxton)			
OIN,TP, 15 gm	**00463-8009-15**	1.50	
30 gm	**00463-8009-30**	2.22	
(A-S Medication)			
REPACK			
OIN,TP			
0.9375 gm 144s UD	**54569-3398-00**	39.99	
14.2 gm	**54569-2295-00**	3.51	
30 gm	**54569-1111-00**	5.45	
(Aidarex)			
REPACK			
OIN,TP (1X15GM)			
15 gm	**33261-0607-01**	5.25	
(1X30GM)			
30 gm	**33261-0360-01**	7.50	
(Altura)			
REPACK			
OIN,TP, 15 gm	**63874-0083-15**	7.99	
30 gm	**63874-0083-30**	9.37	
(DHS, Inc.)			
REPACK			
OIN,TP, 15 gm	**55887-0844-15**	8.00	
(Dispensing Solutions)			
REPACK			
OIN,TP, 15 gm	**55045-1436-05**	8.25	
(Nucare Pharm)			
REPACK			
OIN,TP, 15 gm	**66267-0931-15**	6.27	
30 gm	**66267-0930-30**	7.95	
(Palmetto)			
REPACK			
OIN,TP, 15 gm	**23490-7859-01**	8.95	
30 gm	**23490-7859-00**	10.27	
(Phys Total Care)			
REPACK			
OIN,TP, 0.9 gm 144s	**54868-0582-01**	115.96	
15 gm	**54868-0582-03**	10.32	
30 gm	**54868-0582-02**	11.46	
454 gm	**54868-0582-00**	49.56	
(Physician Partner)			
REPACK			
OIN,TP, 15 gm	**21695-0194-15**	12.48	
28.35 gm	**21695-0194-28**	24.96	
(Quality Care Prod)			
REPACK			
OIN,OP, 3.5 gm	**49999-0184-35**	12.96	
OIN,TP, 15 gm	**49999-0154-15**	9.59	
30 gm	**49999-0154-30**	25.70	
(Southwood)			
REPACK			
OIN,TP, 15 gm	**58016-3062-01**	4.47	
30 gm	**58016-3063-01**	4.86	
TRIPLE ANTIBIOTIC EXTRA (Altaire)			
OIN,TP, 30 gm	**59390-0096-17**	5.74	
(Cardinal Health)			
OIN,TP (MAX. STR.,PRIVATE LABEL)			
30 gm	**37205-0266-10**	6.08	
TRIPLE ANTIBIOTIC OINTMENT (Hart Health)			
OIN,TP (FIRST AID ANTIBIOTIC)			
0.5 gm 25s UD	**50332-0032-03**	2.59	
TRIPLE ANTIBIOTIC PLUS (AmerisourceBergen)			
OIN,TP (MAX. STR.,PRIVATE LABEL)			
30 gm	**24385-0143-03**	5.39	5.99
(G&W)			
OIN,TP, 30 gm	**00713-0622-31**	3.88	
(Taro)			
OIN,TP, 14.2 gm	**51672-2027-02**	6.72	
(Pharma Pac)			
REPACK			
OIN,TP, 30 gm	**52959-0682-30**	3.75	
TRIPLE CREAM (Summers)			
CRE,TP (1X99GM,PREMIUM)			
99 gm	**11086-0042-35**	7.56	
(1X114GM,PREMIUM)			
114 gm	**11086-0042-04**	8.46	
(1X227GM,PREMIUM)			
227 gm	**11086-0042-08**	14.40	
TRIPLE PAPAYA COMPLEX (Mason Vit)			
TAB,PO (PF)			
120s ea	**11845-0118-92**	8.11	

PROD/MFR	HRI, UPC,NDC	AWP	SRP
TRIPLE PASTE (Summers)			
PAS,TP (FRAGRANCE-FREE)			
12.8%, 56.7 gm	11086-0021-01	6.23	
(1X227GM,FRAGRANCE-FREE)			
12.8%, 227 gm	11086-0021-03	13.32	
(FRAGRANCE-FREE)			
12.8%, 454 gm	11086-0021-02	22.68	
(Phys Total Care)			
REPACK			
PAS,TP, 60 gm	54868-4927-00	85.92	
454 gm	54868-4927-01	85.92	
TRIPLE PASTE AF (Summers)			
OIN,TP (1X56.7GM)			
2%, 56.7 gm	11086-0040-02	21.60	
TRIPTONE (Del)			
TAB,PO, 50 mg, 15s ea	10310-0333-15	2.40	3.60
TRIXAICIN (Qualitest)			
CRE,TP, 0.025%, 60 gm	00603-0648-88	16.50	
TRIXAICIN HP (Qualitest)			
CRE,TP, 0.075%, 60 gm	00603-0649-88	26.95	
(Nucare Pharm)			
REPACK			
CRE,TP (1X60GM)			
0.075%, 60 gm	68071-1336-02	28.95	
TRONOLANE (Phys Total Care)			
REPACK			
CRE,TP, 1%, 28 gm	54868-0772-00	5.20	
TRUE CARE PRESTIGE SMART SYSTEM (Home Diag)			
DEV,NA (STRIP)			
50s ea	56151-0317-50	28.60	
TRUE CARE PSS STARTER (Home Diag)			
DEV,NA (MTR,STRP,LANCET,DEV,SOL)			
ea	56151-0217-01	22.18	
TRUE WHITE WHITENING TOOTHPASTE (Health Products Corp)			
PAS,DE, 135 gm	39686-0015-17	5.25	
TRUE2GO BLOOD GLUCOSE MONITORING SYSTEM (Home Diag)			
DEV,NA (W/10 TEST STRIPS)			
ea	56151-1340-01	15.00	
TRUECONTROL GLUCOSE CONTROL (Home Diag)			
DEV,NA (LEVEL 0)			
3 ml	56151-0864-01	6.90	
(LEVEL 1)			
3 ml	56151-0865-01	6.90	
TRUERESULT BLOOD GLUCOSE MONITORING SYSTEM (Home Diag)			
DEV,NA (GOLDSENSOR,10TESTSTRIP)			
ea	56151-1240-01	37.50	
TRUETEST (Home Diag)			
DEV,NA (GOLDSENSOR)			
50s ea	21292-0002-70	36.00	
50s ea	56151-1813-05	36.00	
100s ea	56151-1030-01	67.50	
TRUETEST GLUCOSE CONTROL LEVEL 1 (Home Diag)			
DEV,NA, ea	56151-0871-01	6.90	
TRUETEST GLUCOSE CONTROL LEVEL 2 (Home Diag)			
DEV,NA, ea	56151-0872-01	6.90	
TRUETEST GLUCOSE CONTROL LEVEL 3 (Home Diag)			
DEV,NA, ea	56151-0873-01	6.90	
TRUETRACK (Home Diag)			
DEV,NA, 50s ea	56151-0813-05	33.23	
TRUETRACK SMART SYSTEM (Home Diag)			
DEV,NA, ea	56151-0888-01	17.60	
(HIGH)			
ea	56151-0863-01	6.90	
(LEVEL 0)			
ea	56151-0860-01	6.90	
(LOW)			
ea	56151-0861-01	6.90	
(MONITOR)			
ea	56151-0888-80	20.60	
(STRIP)			
50s ea	56151-0850-50	33.23	
100s ea	56151-0810-01	57.97	
(A-S Medication)			
REPACK			
DEV,NA, 50s ea	54569-5703-00	33.23	
TRUSTEX (Line One Labs)			
DEV,NA (LUBRICATED W/SPERMICIDE)			
3s ea	05632-0830-10	2.00	
3s ea	05632-0830-30	2.00	
(LUBRICATED,BERRY)			
3s ea	05632-0840-15	2.25	
(LUBRICATED,CHOCOLATE)			
3s ea	05632-0840-20	2.25	
3s ea	05632-0840-25	2.25	
(LUBRICATED,COLA)			
3s ea	05632-0840-35	2.25	
(LUBRICATED,GRAPE)			
3s ea	05632-0840-30	2.25	
(LUBRICATED,MINT)			
3s ea	05632-0840-05	2.25	
(LUBRICATED,RIB&STUD)			
3s ea	05632-0830-60	1.85	
(LUBRICATED,VANILLA)			
3s ea	05632-0840-10	2.25	
(LUBRICATED)			
3s ea	05632-0830-20	2.00	
3s ea	05632-0830-40	2.00	
(NONLUBRICATED)			
3s ea	05632-0830-50	1.85	
(ASSTCLOR,LBRCTED,NON9)			
12s ea	05632-0980-82	7.50	
(ASTDDUALCLOR,LBRCTED)			
12s ea	05632-0880-80	7.50	
12s ea	05632-0880-82	7.50	
(LUBRICATED W/SPERMICIDE)			
12s ea	05632-0830-15	5.50	
12s ea	05632-0830-35	6.00	
(LUBRICATED,ASST FLAVORS)			
12s ea	05632-0840-40	7.50	
(LUBRICATED,RIB&STUD)			
12s ea	05632-0830-65	6.25	
(LUBRICATED)			
12s ea	05632-0830-25	5.50	
12s ea	05632-0830-45	6.00	
(NON-LUB,ASSTD FLAVORS)			
12s ea	05632-0841-40	7.00	
(NONLUBRICATED)			
12s ea	05632-0830-55	5.25	
TRUSTEX ES (Line One Labs)			
DEV,NA (ASORTD FLAVRS,LUBRICATD)			
12s ea	05632-0842-40	7.75	
(ASST CLR,EXTRA STRENGTH)			
12s ea	05632-0830-87	6.50	
(ASST COLORS W/NON-9,ES)			
12s ea	05632-0830-67	6.50	
(LUBRICATED W/NON-9,ES)			
12s ea	05632-0830-27	6.00	
(LUBRICATED,XTRA STRNGTH)			
12s ea	05632-0830-47	6.00	
TRUSTEX FLAVORED NON-LUBRICATED (Line One Labs)			
DEV,NA (RESERVOIR TIP,BANANA)			
12s ea	05632-0841-56	6.75	
(RESERVOIR TIP,CHOCOLATE)			
12s ea	05632-0841-54	6.75	
(RESERVOIR TIP,MINT)			
12s ea	05632-0841-58	6.75	
(RESERVOIR TIP,VANILLA)			
12s ea	05632-0841-50	6.75	
(RESERVOIR TIP)			
12s ea	05632-0841-52	6.75	
TRUSTEX XL (Line One Labs)			
DEV,NA (ASST CLR,EXTRA LARGE)			
12s ea	05632-0831-97	6.25	
(ASST COLORS W/NON-9,XL)			
12s ea	05632-0831-77	6.25	
(LUBRICATED W/NON-9,XL)			
12s ea	05632-0831-37	6.00	
(LUBRICATED,EXTRA LARGE)			
12s ea	05632-0831-57	6.00	
TRYPTOPHAN (Bio-Tech Pharm)			
CAP,PO, 500 mg, 100s ea	53191-0451-01	27.50	
1000s ea	53191-0451-10	225.00	
TUB O' RUB (Monticello)			
OIN,TP, 5.5%-2%-2.8%-5%-4%,			
9 gm	11868-0003-19	0.55	
TUCKS (Johnson & Johnson)			
OIN,TP (1X19.8GM)			
1%, 19.8 gm	42002-0301-07	4.63	
(FORMERLY ANUSOL)			
1%, 19.8 gm	00501-4105-07	4.62	
(1X28.3GM)			
46.6%-1%-12.5%,			
28.3 gm	42002-0300-01	3.97	
(FORMERLY ANUSOL)			
46.6%-1%-12.5%,			
28.3 gm	00501-4104-01	3.96	
PAD,TP, 50%, 12s ea	00071-1704-01	2.41	
(TAKE ALONG TOWELETTES)			
50%, 12s ea	12547-0150-42	2.41	
40s ea	00501-4100-40	3.68	
40s ea	12547-0150-40	3.68	
40s ea	42002-0302-68	3.54	
100s ea	00071-1703-24	5.48	
100s ea	12547-0150-20	5.51	
SUP,RC, 51%, 12s ea	42002-0303-12	5.10	
(FORMERLY ANUSOL)			
51%, 12s ea	00501-4106-12	5.09	
24s ea	12547-0150-24	9.47	
(FORMERLY ANUSOL)			
51%, 24s ea	00501-4106-24	9.43	
TUMS (Glaxo)			
CTB,PO (ASSORTED)			
500 mg, 12s ea	00766-0741-20	0.52	
(PEPPERMINT)			
500 mg, 12s ea	00766-0740-20	0.52	
(3X8,ASSORTED)			
500 mg, 24s ea	00766-0741-62	1.44	
(3X12,PEPPERMINT)			
500 mg, 36s ea	00766-0740-62	1.44	
(ASSORTED)			
500 mg, 75s ea	00766-0741-51	2.45	
(PEPPERMINT)			
500 mg, 75s ea	00766-0740-51	2.45	
(ASSORTED)			
500 mg, 150s ea	00766-0741-52	3.96	
(PEPPERMINT)			
500 mg, 150s ea	00766-0740-52	3.96	
TUMS CALCIUM FOR LIFE BONE HEALTH (Glaxo)			
CTB,PO (ASSORTED FRUIT)			
500 mg, 90s ea	00766-0747-30	5.78	
TUMS E-X (Glaxo)			
CTB,PO (ASSORTED BERRY)			
750 mg, 8s ea	00766-7388-08	0.52	
(ASSORTED)			
750 mg, 8s ea	00766-0739-19	0.52	
(TROPICAL)			
750 mg, 8s ea	00766-7393-05	0.52	
(3X8,ASSORTED BERRY)			
750 mg, 24s ea	00766-7388-24	1.44	
(3X8,ASSORTED)			
750 mg, 24s ea	00766-0739-21	1.44	
(3X8,TROPICAL)			
750 mg, 24s ea	00766-7393-24	1.44	
(ARTIC MINT)			
750 mg, 24s ea	00766-0739-80	1.91	
(ASSORTED BERRY)			
750 mg, 48s ea	00766-7388-48	2.45	
(ASSORTED)			
750 mg, 48s ea	00766-0739-23	2.45	
(TROPICAL)			
750 mg, 48s ea	00766-7391-48	2.45	
(WITH FRIVA CRYSTALS)			
750 mg, 72s ea	00766-7373-50	3.96	
(ASSORTED BERRY)			
750 mg, 96s ea	00766-7388-96	3.96	
(ASSORTED)			
750 mg, 96s ea	00766-0739-66	3.96	
(TROPICAL)			
750 mg, 96s ea	00766-7391-96	3.96	
(WINTERGREEN)			
750 mg, 96s ea	00766-7394-66	4.00	
TUMS EX (Glaxo)			
CTB,PO (ASSORTED BERRIES)			
750 mg, 200s ea	07667-0392-70	7.25	
(TROPICAL)			
750 mg, 200s ea	07667-0392-30	7.25	
TUMS KIDS (Glaxo)			
CTB,PO (CHERRY BLAST)			
750 mg, 36s ea	07667-0980-00	3.78	
TUMS SMOOTH DISSOLVE (Glaxo)			
CTB,PO (TROPICAL SMOOTHIES)			
750 mg, 45s ea	07667-0429-80	3.96	
TUMS SMOOTHIES (Glaxo)			
CTB,PO (ASSORTED FRUIT)			
750 mg, 12s ea	07660-0740-60	1.26	
(ASSORTED TROPICAL FRUIT)			
750 mg, 12s ea	07667-0412-55	1.26	
(COCOA CREME)			
750 mg, 12s ea	07667-0520-15	1.26	
(EXTRA STRENGTH)			
750 mg, 12s ea	07660-0740-65	1.26	
12s ea	07667-0520-23	1.26	
(PEPPERMINT)			
750 mg, 12s ea	07667-0392-99	1.26	
(BERRY FUSION)			
750 mg, 60s ea	07667-0250-00	3.96	

PROD/MFR	HRI, UPC,NDC	AWP	SRP
(COCOA CREME)			
750 mg, 60s ea	07667-0520-20	3.96	
(2BOTTLE,2FREETRAVELPCK)			
750 mg, 72s ea	07667-0492-10	16.66	
(2BTL,2 FREETRAVELPACK)			
750 mg, 72s ea	07667-0492-05	8.33	
TUMS ULTRA (Glaxo)			
CTB,PO (ASSORTED BERRIES)			
1000 mg, 12s ea	07660-0746-70	0.80	
(PEPPERMINT)			
1000 mg, 12s ea	07660-0746-80	0.80	
(ASSORTED FRUIT)			
1000 mg, 36s ea	00766-0745-75	2.45	
(MAXIMUMSTRNGTH,3ROLLX12)			
1000 mg, 36s ea	07660-0746-43	2.40	
36s ea	07660-0746-81	2.40	
(ASSORTED BERRIES)			
1000 mg, 72s ea	07660-0746-50	3.96	
(ASSORTED FRUIT)			
1000 mg, 72s ea	00766-0745-65	3.96	
(PEPPERMINT)			
1000 mg, 72s ea	00766-0745-85	3.96	
(TROPICAL FRUIT)			
1000 mg, 72s ea	07660-0746-30	3.96	
(ASSORTED BERRY)			
1000 mg, 160s ea	00766-0746-55	7.25	
(ASSORTED FRUIT)			
1000 mg, 160s ea	00766-0746-10	7.25	
(FRUIT,TROPICAL)			
1000 mg, 160s ea	00766-0746-25	7.25	
(SPEARMINT)			
1000 mg, 160s ea	00766-0746-40	7.25	
TUR IRRIGATION (Abbott Hosp)			
DEV,NA (98", Y-TYPE)			
20s ea	00074-6543-01	195.12	
(LATEX,NONVENTED)			
20s ea	00074-6543-02	195.12	
TUR SYSTEM W/FLOW POUCH RESERVOIR (Abbott Hosp)			
DEV,NA (38")			
20s ea	00074-6542-02	159.36	
TUR-BI-CAL (Humco)			
SOL,NS, 0.17%, 30 ml	00395-3921-91	5.64	
TUSSI PRES-B (Kramer-Novis)			
SOL,PO (1X120ML,AF,SF,DYE-FREE)			
120 ml	52083-0237-04	5.00	
(1X480ML,AF,SF,DYE-FREE)			
480 ml	52083-0237-16	18.30	
TUSSIN (Albertson's)			
SYR,PO, 100 mg/5 ml,			
240 ml	41280-0200-61	3.03	
(Cardinal Health)			
SYR,PO (PRIVATE LABEL)			
100 mg/5 ml, 120 ml	37205-0960-26	3.65	
240 ml	37205-0960-34	5.60	
TUSSIN CF (AmerisourceBergen)			
LIQ,PO (AF,PRIVATE LABEL)			
118 ml	24385-0572-26	2.69	2.99
TUSSIN COLD & COUGH (AmerisourceBergen)			
SGL,PO (NON-DROWSY)			
10 mg-200 mg-30 mg,			
12s ea	24385-0226-53	2.87	3.19
TUSSIN COUGH (Cardinal Health)			
SYR,PO (NON-DROWSY)			
10 mg/5 ml, 118 ml	37205-0962-26	3.65	
TUSSIN DAC (Bryant Ranch)			
REPACK			
LIQ,PO, 120 ml	63629-2960-01	9.60	
240 ml	63629-2960-02	19.20	
TUSSIN DM (Albertson's)			
SYR,PO, 10 mg/5 ml-100 mg/5 ml,			
240 ml	41280-0200-60	3.93	
(AmerisourceBergen)			
SYR,PO (PRIVATE LABEL)			
10 mg/5 ml-100 mg/5 ml,			
240 ml	24385-0359-34	4.49	4.99
(Cardinal Health)			
SYR,PO (PRIVATE LABEL)			
10 mg/5 ml-100 mg/5 ml,			
120 ml	37205-0970-26	4.60	
240 ml	37205-0970-34	6.45	
(Chain Drug Marketing)			
SYR,PO, 10 mg/5 ml-100 mg/5 ml,			
118 ml	63868-0855-54	1.50	3.99
236 ml	63868-0855-56	3.06	5.99
TUSSIN DM CLEAR (Cardinal Health)			
LIQ,PO (AF,SF,DYE-FREE)			
10 mg/5 ml-100 mg/5 ml,			
120 ml	37205-0712-26	5.25	
TUSSIN EXPECTORANT (Chain Drug Marketing)			
SYR,PO, 100 mg/5 ml,			
118 ml	63868-0857-54	1.50	3.99
236 ml	63868-0857-56	3.06	5.49
TUSSIN PEDIATRIC COUGH/COLD (AmerisourceBergen)			
LIQ,PO (PRIVATE LABEL)			
7.5 mg/5 ml-15 mg/5 ml,			
120 ml	24385-0575-26	2.96	3.29
TWELVE RESIN-K (Key Company)			
TAB,PO, 1000 mcg,			
60s ea	11694-0829-01	6.25	
250s ea	11694-0829-02	17.50	
1000s ea	11694-0829-06	62.00	
TWILITE (Pfeiffer)			
TAB,PO, 50 mg, 20s ea	00927-0616-34	2.41	4.34
TWIN-SITE EXTENSION (Abbott Hosp)			
DEV,NA (32", SLIDE CLAMPS)			
48s ea	00074-4522-58	327.75	
TWOCAL HN (Abbott)			
LIQ,PO (PECAN)			
237 ml	70074-0540-65	2.45	
(VANILLA)			
240 ml	70074-0407-29	2.45	
(RTH,PECAN)			
1000 ml	70074-0570-48	11.75	
TYCOLENE (Pfeiffer)			
TAB,PO (CAPLET)			
325 mg, 50s ea	00927-0186-53	1.53	2.75
100s ea	00927-0186-01	2.22	3.99
500 mg, 50s ea	00927-0174-53	2.17	3.91
100s ea	00927-0174-01	3.47	6.24
TYLENOL (McNeil Consumer Healthcare)			
TAB,PO, 325 mg, 100s ea	00450-0496-60	7.54	
TYLENOL 8 HOUR (McNeil Consumer Healthcare)			
TER,PO (CAPLET)			
650 mg, 24s ea	00450-0297-24	3.89	
50s ea	00450-0297-50	6.71	
(W/FREE CLIP)			
650 mg, 50s ea	50580-0297-55	6.29	
50s ea	50580-0505-45	5.88	
(CAPLET)			
650 mg, 100s ea	00450-0297-10	10.94	
150s ea	00450-0297-15	13.86	
200s ea	50580-0297-20	13.84	
TYLENOL ALLERGY MULTI-SYMPTOM (McNeil Consumer Healthcare)			
CAP,PO (RAPID RELEASE)			
325 mg-2 mg-5 mg,			
24s ea	00450-0238-24	5.44	
48s ea	00450-0238-48	8.54	
TAB,PO (12+12,COOL BURST,CAPLET)			
24s ea	00450-0284-24	5.44	
(COOL BURST,CAPLET)			
325 mg-2 mg-5 mg,			
24s ea	00450-0273-24	4.79	
72s ea	50580-0273-72	9.37	
(50X2,COOL BURST,CAPLET)			
325 mg-2 mg-5 mg,			
100s ea	00450-0273-50	16.21	
TYLENOL ALLERGY MULTI-SYMPTOM NIGHTTIME (McNeil Consumer Healthcare)			
TAB,PO (COOL BURST,CAPLET)			
325 mg-25 mg-5 mg,			
24s ea	00450-0283-24	4.79	
TYLENOL ARTHRITIS (McNeil Consumer Healthcare)			
TER,PO (GELTAB)			
650 mg, 20s ea	00450-0292-20	3.89	
(CAPLET)			
650 mg, 24s ea	00450-0838-24	3.89	
(GELTAB)			
650 mg, 40s ea	00450-0292-40	6.71	
(CAPLET)			
650 mg, 50s ea	00450-0838-50	6.71	
(GELTAB)			
650 mg, 80s ea	00450-0292-80	10.94	
(EZ-OPEN CAP,CAPLET)			
650 mg, 100s ea	00450-0838-21	10.94	
(W/FREE TYL PM,CAPLET)			
650 mg, 100s ea	00045-0838-11	9.58	
(CAPLET)			
650 mg, 150s ea	00450-0838-15	13.87	
170s ea	50580-0112-26	12.88	
(150+40 FREE,CAPLET)			
650 mg, 190s ea	50580-0112-59	13.87	
(W/FREE TYLENOL PM 50'S)			
650 mg, 200s ea	50580-0112-05	12.88	
(CAPLET)			
650 mg, 225s ea	00450-0838-37	16.50	
290s ea	50580-0112-29	17.17	
5000s ea	50580-0112-22	478.80	
TYLENOL CHILDREN'S (McNeil Consumer Healthcare)			
CTB,PO (ASPIRIN-FREE)			
80 mg, 30s ea	50580-0518-30	3.61	
30s ea	50580-0519-30	3.61	
(BUBBLEGUM)			
80 mg, 30s ea	00045-0430-30	2.92	
SUS,PO (ACCOUNT SPECIFIC,AF)			
160 mg/5 ml,			
120 ml	50580-0407-07	5.95	
(AF,CHERRY)			
160 mg/5 ml,			
240 ml	50580-0123-08	9.86	
TYLENOL COLD CHILDREN'S (McNeil Consumer Healthcare)			
KIT,PO (AF,ASPIRIN-FREE)			
120 ml	50580-0372-45	9.91	
SUS,PO (BOGO 2X120ML,AF)			
120 ml 2s	50580-0372-42	9.24	
TYLENOL COLD HEAD CONGESTION (McNeil Consumer Healthcare)			
TAB,PO (DAY/NIGHT,COOL BURST)			
20s ea	00450-0282-20	5.45	
(NIGHTTIME,COOL BURST)			
325 mg-2 mg-10 mg-5 mg,			
24s ea	00450-0278-24	4.80	
(DAYTIME, COOL BURST)			
325 mg-10 mg-5 mg,			
24s ea	00450-0277-24	4.80	
TYLENOL COLD HEAD CONGESTION SEVERE (McNeil Consumer Healthcare)			
TAB,PO (DAYTIME,COOL BURST)			
325 mg-10 mg-200 mg-5 mg,			
24s ea	00450-0261-24	5.45	
100s ea	00450-0261-50	16.21	
TYLENOL COLD MULTI-SYMPTOM (McNeil Consumer Healthcare)			
CAP,PO (GELCAP)			
20s ea	00450-0396-20	5.45	
(NIGHTTIME,GELCAP)			
325 mg-2 mg-10 mg-5 mg,			
24s ea	00450-0395-24	5.45	
(DAYTIME)			
325 mg-10 mg-5 mg,			
24s ea	00450-0251-24	5.45	
SOL,PO (DAYTIME,CITRUS BURST)			
240 ml	00450-0257-08	5.45	
(NIGHTTIME,COOL BURST)			
240 ml	00450-0269-08	5.45	
TAB,PO (DAYTIME, CAPLET,CAPLET)			
325 mg-10 mg-5 mg,			
24s ea	00450-0271-24	4.80	
TYLENOL COLD MULTI-SYMPTOM SEVERE (McNeil Consumer Healthcare)			
SOL,PO (DAYTIME,COOL BURST)			
240 ml	00450-0521-08	5.45	
TAB,PO			
325 mg-10 mg-200 mg-5 mg,			
24s ea	00450-0270-24	5.45	
TYLENOL COLD PLUS COUGH CHILDREN'S (McNeil Consumer Healthcare)			
SUS,PO (W/IRC)			
120 ml	50580-0203-10	9.94	
(BOGO,AF,CHERRY)			
120 ml 2s	00045-0372-42	4.62	
TYLENOL COLD PLUS COUGH INFANTS' (McNeil Consumer Healthcare)			
SUS,PO (AF,ASPIRIN-FREE)			
15 ml	50580-0829-02	4.97	
30 ml	50580-0829-30	9.94	
TYLENOL COLD SEVERE CONGESTION (McNeil Consumer Healthcare)			
TAB,PO (COOLBURST/DAYTIME)			
24s ea	00450-0214-24	5.02	
TYLENOL DAY & NIGHT (McNeil Consumer Healthcare)			
TAB,PO (VALUE PACK,CAPLET)			
74s ea	00450-0527-10	9.02	

PROD/MFR	HRI, UPC,NDC	AWP	SRP
TYLENOL ES (Altura)			
REPACK			
TAB,PO (RAPID RELEASE)			
500 mg, 24s ea	63874-1160-04	7.25	
TYLENOL EXTRA STRENGTH			
(McNeil Consumer Healthcare)			
CAP,PO (RAPID RELEASE,GELCAP)			
500 mg, 24s ea	00450-0488-24	3.89	
50s ea	00450-0488-50	6.72	
100s ea	00450-0488-10	10.96	
150s ea	00450-0488-15	13.88	
225s ea	00450-0488-25	16.50	
(RAPID RELEASE,2500X2)			
500 mg, 5000s ea	00450-0488-02	478.80	
SOL,PO (RAPID BLAST,CHERRY)			
500 mg/15 ml,			
240 ml	00450-0500-08	5.23	
TAB,PO (3X2,CAPLET)			
500 mg, 6s ea	50580-0449-13	0.90	
(BLISTER VIAL)			
500 mg, 10s ea	00450-0449-15	1.64	
(VIAL RACK)			
500 mg, 10s ea	50580-0449-12	1.64	
(ASPIRIN-FREE,CAPLET)			
500 mg, 24s ea	00450-0449-05	3.54	
(COOL CAPLET)			
500 mg, 24s ea	00450-0444-24	3.54	
(EZ TABS,COATED)			
500 mg, 24s ea	00450-0422-24	3.54	
(ASPIRIN-FREE,CAPLET)			
500 mg, 50s ea	00450-0449-07	6.11	
(COOL CAPLET)			
500 mg, 50s ea	00450-0444-50	6.11	
(EZ TABS,COATED)			
500 mg, 50s ea	00450-0422-50	6.11	
(W/ FREE 25,COOL CAPLET)			
500 mg, 50s ea	50580-0710-75	6.11	
(CRUSHABLE,DYE-FREE)			
500 mg, 60s ea	00450-0499-68	5.09	
(50X2,ASPIRIN-FREE)			
500 mg, 100s ea	00450-0449-10	9.92	
(ASPIRIN-FREE,CAPLET)			
500 mg, 100s ea	00450-0449-09	9.96	
(COOL CAPLET)			
500 mg, 100s ea	00045-0444-10	9.46	
100s ea	00450-0444-10	9.96	
(EZ TABS,COATED)			
500 mg, 100s ea	00450-0422-10	9.96	
(W/ FREE 25,COOL CAPLET)			
500 mg, 100s ea	50580-0710-12	9.46	
(100+8 FREE,COOL CAPLET)			
500 mg, 108s ea	50580-0710-09	8.92	
(ASPIRIN-FREE,CAPLET)			
500 mg, 150s ea	00450-0449-23	12.61	
(COOL CAPLET)			
500 mg, 150s ea	00450-0444-55	12.61	
(EZ TABS,SWEET COATING)			
500 mg, 150s ea	00450-0422-16	12.61	
(150+50 FREE,CAPLET)			
500 mg, 200s ea	50580-0449-46	12.61	
(ASPIRIN-FREE,CAPLET)			
500 mg, 225s ea	00450-0444-27	15.01	
(EZ TABS,COATED)			
500 mg, 225s ea	00450-0422-37	15.01	
(CAPLET)			
500 mg, 320s ea	50580-0449-81	16.28	
325s ea	50580-0449-83	16.19	
(A-S Medication)			
REPACK			
TAB,PO (CAPLET)			
500 mg, 24s ea	54569-0023-00	3.51	
TYLENOL FLU CHILDREN'S			
(McNeil Consumer Healthcare)			
SUS,PO (BOGO,AF,BUBBLEGUM)			
120 ml 2s	00045-0803-42	4.62	
TYLENOL FLU NIGHT TIME MAX STRENGTH			
(McNeil Consumer Healthcare)			
LIQ,PO (AF,CHERRY)			
240 ml	50580-0145-08	5.27	
TYLENOL INFANTS'			
(McNeil Consumer Healthcare)			
SUS,PO (AF,GRAPE,DROPS)			
80 mg/0.8 ml,			
30 ml	50580-0144-01	8.00	
TYLENOL JUNIOR (McNeil Consumer Healthcare)			
CTB,PO (ASPIRIN-FREE)			
160 mg, 48s ea	50580-0514-48	7.72	
TYLENOL PM (McNeil Consumer Healthcare)			
CAP,PO (RAPID RELEASE,GELCAP)			
500 mg-25 mg,			
20s ea	00450-0244-20	4.00	
40s ea	00450-0244-40	7.03	
80s ea	00450-0244-80	11.27	
TYLENOL PM EXTRA STRENGTH			
(McNeil Consumer Healthcare)			
SYR,PO (GOLDEN VANILLA)			
500 mg/15 ml-25 mg/15 ml,			
240 ml	00450-0427-08	5.96	
TAB,PO (CAPLET)			
500 mg-25 mg,			
10s ea	00045-0482-20	1.64	
24s ea	00045-0482-24	4.00	
24s ea	00450-0482-24	4.00	
(GELTAB,GELTAB)			
500 mg-25 mg,			
24s ea	00450-0176-24	4.00	
(GELTAB)			
500 mg-25 mg,			
24s ea	00045-0176-24	3.86	
(CAPLET)			
500 mg-25 mg,			
50s ea	00450-0482-50	7.03	
(GELTAB)			
500 mg-25 mg,			
50s ea	00045-0176-50	7.03	
50s ea	00450-0176-50	7.03	
(W/FREE 20'S,CAPLET)			
500 mg-25 mg,			
70s ea	50580-0482-70	7.03	
(W/FREE 20'S,GELTAB)			
500 mg-25 mg,			
70s ea	00045-0176-70	7.03	
(CAPLET)			
500 mg-25 mg,			
100s ea	00045-0482-10	11.27	
100s ea	00450-0482-10	11.27	
(GELTAB,GELTAB)			
500 mg-25 mg,			
100s ea	00450-0176-10	11.27	
(GELTAB)			
500 mg-25 mg,			
100s ea	00045-0176-10	11.27	
(W/24 FREE,GELTAB)			
500 mg-25 mg,			
124s ea	50580-0176-08	9.58	
(CAPLET)			
500 mg-25 mg,			
150s ea	00045-0482-15	14.21	
150s ea	00450-0482-15	14.21	
(GELTAB,GELTAB)			
500 mg-25 mg,			
150s ea	00450-0176-15	14.21	
(W/ FREE VANILLA 24)			
500 mg-25 mg,			
150s ea	50580-0482-26	12.80	
(WHOLESALE PACK,CAPLET)			
500 mg-25 mg,			
150s ea	00045-0482-16	11.86	
(CAPLET)			
500 mg-25 mg,			
225s ea	50580-0482-35	16.70	
(TRAY,CAPLET)			
500 mg-25 mg,			
225s ea	00045-0482-35	16.70	
TYLENOL SEVERE ALLERGY			
(McNeil Consumer Healthcare)			
TAB,PO (CAPLET)			
500 mg-12.5 mg,			
24s ea	00450-0211-24	5.44	
48s ea	00450-0211-48	8.54	
TYLENOL SINUS CHILDREN'S			
(McNeil Consumer Healthcare)			
SUS,PO (AF,ASPIRIN-FREE)			
160 mg/5 ml-15 mg/5 ml,			
120 ml	50580-0107-14	4.97	
120 ml	50580-0107-15	4.97	
TYLENOL SINUS CONGESTION & PAIN			
(McNeil Consumer Healthcare)			
CAP,PO (RAPID RELEASE,GELCAP)			
325 mg-5 mg,			
24s ea	00450-0229-24	5.44	
48s ea	00450-0229-48	8.54	
TAB,PO (DAY/NIGHT,COOL BURST)			
20s ea	00450-0266-20	5.44	
(COOLBURST,NIGHTTIME)			
325 mg-2 mg-5 mg,			
24s ea	00450-0264-24	4.79	
(DAYTIME,COOL BURST)			
325 mg-5 mg,			
24s ea	00450-0275-24	4.79	
TYLENOL SINUS CONGESTION & PAIN SEVERE			
(McNeil Consumer Healthcare)			
TAB,PO (DAYTIME,COOL BURST)			
325 mg-200 mg-5 mg,			
24s ea	00450-0262-24	5.44	
48s ea	00450-0262-48	8.54	
(DAYTIME, 50X2)			
325 mg-200 mg-5 mg,			
100s ea	00450-0262-50	16.21	
TYLENOL SINUS MAXIMUM STRENGTH			
(McNeil Consumer Healthcare)			
TAB,PO (W/NT SAMPLE,CAPLET)			
500 mg-30 mg,			
48s ea	50580-0432-49	7.25	
(50X2,GELTAB)			
500 mg-30 mg,			
100s ea	00045-0290-55	14.17	
TYLENOL SINUS SEVERE CONGESTION			
(McNeil Consumer Healthcare)			
TAB,PO (COOLBURST,DAYTIME)			
325 mg-200 mg-30 mg,			
24s ea	00450-0442-24	5.00	
TYLENOL SORE THROAT			
(McNeil Consumer Healthcare)			
SYR,PO (DAYTIME,COOLBURST)			
500 mg/15 ml,			
240 ml	00450-0813-08	5.48	
TYLENOL WARMING COLD MULTI-SYMPTOM			
(McNeil Consumer Healthcare)			
SOL,PO (NIGHTTIME,AF)			
240 ml	00450-0523-08	5.48	
TYLENOL WARMING COUGH & SEVERE CONGESTION (McNeil Consumer Healthcare)			
SOL,PO (DAYTIME,HONEY LEMON)			
240 ml	00450-0525-08	5.48	
TYLENOL XSTR (Phys Total Care)			
REPACK			
TAB,PO, 500 mg, 100s ea.	54868-3337-00	11.88	
TYLEX (Lex)			
TAB,PO, 325 mg, 100s ea.	49523-0034-10	1.32	
1000s ea	49523-0034-00	9.89	
TYLEX EXTRA-STRENGTH (Lex)			
PO, 500 mg, 100s ea	49523-0033-10	1.63	
1000s ea	49523-0033-00	13.36	
TYLOPHEN (Mason Vit)			
TAB,PO, 325 mg,			
1000s ea	11845-0596-04	14.44	
TYLTABS (Medicine Shoppe)			
TAB,PO, 325 mg, 100s ea.	49614-0118-78	3.99	3.99
TYLTABS CHILDREN'S (Medicine Shoppe)			
CTB,PO (GRAPE)			
80 mg, 30s ea	49614-0125-65	2.49	2.49
ELI,PO, 160 mg/5 ml,			
120 ml	49614-0393-26	4.39	4.39
SUS,PO, 160 mg/5 ml,			
120 ml	49614-0175-26	4.39	4.39
TYLTABS EXTRA STRENGTH (Medicine Shoppe)			
TAB,PO (CAPLET)			
500 mg, 50s ea	49614-0123-71	3.59	3.59
(GELTAB)			
500 mg, 100s ea	49614-0188-78	6.99	6.99
TYR 1 (Milupa North America)			
PDR,PO (2X500GM)			
500 gm 2s	81361-9352-01	181.25	
TYR 2 (Nutricia)			
PDR,PO (2X500GM)			
500 gm 2s	81361-9353-01	327.60	
TYR COOLER (VITAFLO, LLC)			
SOL,PO (15GM PROTEIN EQUIVALENT)			
130 ml 30s	50600-0539-92	265.50	349.75
TYR EXPRESS (VITAFLO, LLC)			
PDR,PO (ENTERAL,UNFLAVORED)			
25 gm 25s	50600-0538-48	265.50	349.75
TYR GEL (VITAFLO, LLC)			
PO (ENTERAL,UNFLAVORED)			
20 gm 30s	50600-0538-00	148.68	239.00
TYREX-1 (Abbott)			
PDR,PO, 400 gm	70074-0511-29	40.46	
TYREX-2 (Abbott)			
PDR,PO, 400 gm	70074-0511-27	81.12	

PROD/MFR	HRI, UPC,NDC	AWP	SRP
TYROMINE-K (Key Company)			
CAP,PO, 475 mg-225 mg,			
100s ea	**11694-0720-01**	13.25	
250s ea	**11694-0720-25**	27.00	
TYROS 1 (Mead Johnson & Co)			
PDR,PO, 454 gm	**00087-0194-41**	39.60	
TYROS 2 (Mead Johnson & Co)			
PDR,PO, 454 gm	**00087-0082-41**	68.99	
TYROSINE (Freeda)			
L-TYROSINE			
TAB,PO (PF,SF,DYE-FREE)			
500 mg, 100s ea	**10432-0152-01**	11.97	19.95
250s ea	**10432-0152-02**	23.94	39.90
1000 mg, 100s ea	**10432-0154-01**	22.17	36.95
(Miller)			
CAP,PO, 500 mg, 100s ea	**17204-0903-40**	11.34	18.90
(Neurovites)			
CAP,PO, 500 mg, 100s ea	**93595-2029-01**	25.00	
(Rugby)			
TAB,PO (PF,SF,DYE-FREE,CAPTAB)			
500 mg, 50s ea	**00536-7049-06**	6.30	
TYROSINE (Bio-Tech Pharm)			
CAP,PO, 500 mg, 100s ea	**53191-0059-01**	9.45	
(Carlson,J.R.)			
CAP,PO (PF,SF,CORN-FREE)			
500 mg, 100s ea	**88395-0069-71**	7.45	14.90
200s ea	**88395-0069-72**	12.45	24.90
(VITAFLO, LLC)			
PDS,PO, 1 gm/4 gm,			
30s ea	**50600-0547-91**	120.00	150.00
TYROSINE-500 (Key Company)			
TAB,PO (SF)			
500 mg, 60s ea	**11694-0783-01**	6.00	
250s ea	**11694-0783-25**	20.00	
U-LACTIN (Allerderm Labs.)			
LOT,TP, 240 ml	**34674-0253-08**	7.13	5.82
480 ml	**34674-0253-16**	10.58	9.71
UCD 1 (Milupa North America)			
PDR,PO (2X500GM)			
500 gm 2s	**81361-9360-01**	225.00	
UCD 2 (Nutricia)			
PDR,PO (2X500GM)			
500 gm 2s	**81361-9361-01**	348.40	
UICE+FIBRE (Nutra/Balance)			
JUICE+FIBRE			
LIQ,PO (27X236ML,ORANGE)			
236 ml 27s	**07249-0501-04**		49.28
ULCEREASE (Med-Derm)			
SOL,TP, 30 ml	**45565-0100-09**	1.32	
180 ml	**45565-0100-21**	6.59	
(Phys Total Care)			
REPACK			
SOL,TP, 178 ml	**54868-5571-00**	8.77	
ULTEC HYDROCOLLOID (Covidien)			
DEV,NA (STERILE,6"X6")			
30s ea	**08080-4756-02**	193.75	
(STERILE,6"X8")			
30s ea	**08080-4758-00**	280.50	
(STERILE,8"X8")			
30s ea	**08090-4758-26**	331.50	
(STERILE,4"X4")			
50s ea	**08080-4754-00**	172.13	
ULTICARE (UltiMed)			
DEV,NA (1/2CC,G31X5/16")			
100s ea	**08222-0945-99**	21.95	
(1/2ML,30GX1/2")			
100s ea	**08222-0735-56**	25.70	
100s ea	**08222-0935-54**	20.95	
(1CC,G31X5/16")			
100s ea	**08222-0941-93**	21.95	
(1ML,30GX1/2",LATEX-FREE)			
100s ea	**08222-0731-50**	25.70	
100s ea	**08222-0931-58**	20.95	
(3/10CC,G31X5/16")			
100s ea	**08222-0943-91**	21.95	
(3/10ML,30GX1/2")			
100s ea	**08222-0733-58**	25.70	
100s ea	**08222-0933-56**	20.95	
ULTICARE LANCETS (UltiMed)			
DEV,NA (28G)			
100s ea	**08222-0072-08**	8.99	
200s ea	**08222-0072-01**	14.99	
ULTICARE PEN NEEDLES (UltiMed)			
DEV,NA (G29X1/2",ORIGINAL)			
100s ea	**08222-0951-21**	25.17	
(G31X1/4"MINI,ULTIFINEIV)			
100s ea	**08222-0956-33**	28.75	
(G31X5/16",SHORT)			
100s ea	**08222-0958-31**	27.01	
ULTICARE THIN LANCETS (UltiMed)			
DEV,NA (G30,ULTI-THIN)			
100s ea	**08222-0730-15**	8.99	
ULTIGUARD INSULIN SYRINGE DISPENSER & SHARPS (UltiMed)			
DEV,NA (0.3CC,G31X5/16")			
100s ea	**08222-0743-93**	26.35	
(0.5CC,G31X5/16")			
100s ea	**08222-0745-91**	26.35	
(1CC,G31X5/16")			
100s ea	**08222-0741-95**	26.35	
ULTILET INSULIN SYRINGE (Boca Pharmacal)			
DEV,NA (30G X 5/16"; 1/2ML)			
100s ea	**08326-3002-50**	26.50	
ULTRA B-100 COMPLEX (Mason Vit)			
TER,PO (PF,SF)			
60s ea	**11845-0807-50**	12.56	
ULTRA CAROTENOIDS (Westlake Labs.)			
SGL,PO (PF,SF)			
15000 iu, 60s ea	**10539-0745-86**	11.90	17.00
ULTRA COMFORT (Covidien)			
DEV,NA (1/2CC, 30GX5/16")			
300s ea	**08881-6097-00**	71.70	
(1CC, 30GX5/16")			
300s ea	**08881-6096-00**	71.70	
(3/10CC, 30GX5/16")			
300s ea	**08881-6098-00**	71.70	
ULTRA DIABLESS (Advanced Nutr)			
TAB,PO, 60s ea	**62617-0630-02**	26.00	39.00
ULTRA ENERGY (Rexall)			
TAB,PO (PF,SF)			
45s ea	**30768-0001-32**	4.22	6.40
ULTRA FRESH (Altaire)			
SOL,OP, 0.5%, 15 ml	**59390-0185-13**	6.95	
30 ml	**59390-0185-18**	10.00	
ULTRA G.I. (Westlake Labs.)			
CAP,PO (PF,SF)			
90s ea	**10539-0827-52**	26.60	38.00
ULTRA MIDE 25 (Teva)			
OIN,TP, 120 ml	**00575-4020-04**	11.99	
240 ml	**00575-4020-08**	18.99	
ULTRA THIN LANCET (Atlanta & Pacific)			
DEV,NA (28G)			
100s ea	**08214-0357-26**	4.65	
ULTRA VITA-TIME (Nature's Bounty)			
TAB,PO, 50s ea	**74312-0005-60**		7.39
100s ea	**74312-0005-62**		13.35
(SF)			
100s ea	**74312-0005-00**		12.69
ULTRA ZN PROSTATE FORMULA (Advanced Nutr)			
TAB,PO, 60s ea	**62617-0460-02**	27.00	49.00
ULTRA-FREEDA IRON FREE (Freeda)			
TAB,PO (PF,SF,DYE-FREE)			
90s ea	**10432-0281-01**	13.17	21.95
180s ea	**10432-0281-02**	21.54	35.90
270s ea	**10432-0281-03**	29.82	49.70
ULTRA-FREEDA W/IRON (Freeda)			
TAB,PO (PF,SF,DYE-FREE)			
90s ea	**10432-0257-01**	13.32	22.20
180s ea	**10432-0257-02**	21.57	35.95
270s ea	**10432-0257-03**	29.97	49.95
ULTRA-LIPOIC FORTE (Westlake Labs.)			
CAP,PO (PF,SF)			
333 mg, 60s ea	**10539-0630-05**	55.30	79.00
ULTRA/PHONIC (Pharm Innov)			
GEL,TP, 20 ml	**00036-1000-20**	0.90	1.28
60 ml	**00036-1000-60**	1.31	1.87
90 ml	**00036-1000-90**	1.57	2.25
90 ml	**00036-1001-90**	1.57	2.25
250 ml	**00036-1000-25**	2.06	2.94
250 ml	**00036-1001-25**	2.06	2.94
4000 ml	**00036-1000-04**	15.17	21.67
4000 ml	**00036-1001-04**	15.17	21.67
5000 ml	**00036-1000-05**	17.04	24.34
5000 ml	**00036-1001-05**	17.04	24.34
10000 ml	**00036-1000-10**	32.77	46.81
10000 ml	**00036-1001-10**	32.77	46.81
ULTRA/PHONIC BP BREAST PHANTOM (Pharm Innov)			
DEV,NA (BIOPSY TRAINING DEVICE)			
ea	**00036-1400-01**	131.08	187.25
ULTRA/PHONIC FOCUS (Pharm Innov)			
PAD,TP (1.5 CMX9 CM)			
5s ea	**00036-1300-15**	48.87	69.82
(2.5 CMX9 CM)			
5s ea	**00036-1300-25**	31.83	45.48
ULTRA/PHONIC FREE (Pharm Innov)			
GEL,TP, 60 ml	**00036-1200-60**	1.31	1.87
250 ml	**00036-1200-25**	2.06	2.94
5000 ml	**00036-1200-05**	17.04	24.34
ULTRA/PHONIC WHITE (Pharm Innov)			
LOT,TP, 90 ml	**00036-6101-90**	1.57	2.25
250 ml	**00036-6101-25**	2.06	2.94
4000 ml	**00036-6101-04**	15.17	21.67
ULTRA/WARMER (Pharm Innov)			
DEV,NA (WHITE,NAVY,RED,YELLOW)			
ea	**00036-1100-01**	69.26	98.95
ULTRACARE DISINFECTING/NEUTRALIZER (Allergan Inc)			
SOL,NA, 360 ml	**00023-2152-02**	8.35	
ULTRAHEAL (Johnson & Johnson)			
DEV,NA (2 3/4"X3 1/2",MULTI-DAY)			
ea	**81371-0040-03**	3.64	
(4 1/3"X4 1/3",MULTI-DAY)			
ea	**81371-0055-20**	4.84	
3s ea	**81371-0055-24**	14.22	
(2 3/4"X3 1/2",MULTI-DAY)			
4s ea	**81371-0055-23**	14.22	
ULTRAKLENZ (Carrington)			
SPR,TP (SKIN/WOUND CLEANSER)			
236 ml	**53303-0080-80**	10.71	
354 ml	**53303-0080-12**	14.18	
ULTRALINIC (Key Company)			
SGL,PO (SOFTGEL)			
1000 mg, 60s ea	**11694-0726-01**	12.50	
ULTRALON PF LATEX SURGICAL GLOVES (J&J Medical)			
DEV,NA (STER,50 PR,SZ 5.5)			
100s ea	**56091-0032-55**	141.70	
(STER,50 PR,SZ 6.5)			
100s ea	**56091-0032-65**	141.70	
(STER,50 PR,SZ 6)			
100s ea	**56091-0032-60**	141.70	
(STER,50 PR,SZ 7.5)			
100s ea	**56091-0032-75**	141.70	
(STER,50 PR,SZ 7)			
100s ea	**56091-0032-70**	141.70	
(STER,50 PR,SZ 8.5)			
100s ea	**56091-0032-85**	141.70	
(STER,50 PR,SZ 8)			
100s ea	**56091-0032-80**	141.70	
(STER,50 PR,SZ 9)			
100s ea	**56091-0032-90**	141.70	
ULTRAMINO (Freeda)			
PDR,PO (PF,SF,DYE-FREE)			
453.6 gm	**10432-0194-03**	10.65	17.75
ULTRAPRIN (Medique)			
TAB,PO (250X2,SF)			
200 mg, 500s ea	**47682-0255-02**	19.41	18.50
ULTRASONE (Gordon)			
CRE,TP, 240 gm	**10481-3017-08**	10.00	
3840 gm	**10481-3017-01**	46.25	
ULTRASONIC NEBULIZER (Lumiscope)			
DEV,NA, ea	**38673-0065-00**	79.99	159.90
ULTRASONIC PORTABLE NEBULIZER (Bestmed)			
DEV,NA (COMPACT,W/CARRYING CASE)			
ea	**08466-0921-00**	100.00	
ULTRATRAK PRO (Vertex)			
DEV,NA, ea	**08593-2111-02**	19.90	
50s ea	**08593-2110-02**	55.50	
ULTRATRAK PRO CONTROL (Vertex)			
SOL,NA (1X4ML, HIGH AND LOW)			
0.03%-0.3%, 4 ml	**08593-2113-02**	9.50	
ULTRAZYME (ENZYMATIC CLEANER) (Allergan Inc)			
TEF,NA, 5s ea	**00023-0212-05**	6.05	
10s ea	**00023-0212-10**	9.15	
20s ea	**00023-0212-20**	14.30	
ULTREX (Carrington)			
DEV,NA (HYDROGELPRESERVATV FREE)			
8 gm	**53303-0170-08**	7.13	
15 gm	**53303-0170-15**	9.68	
UNDELENIC (Gordon)			
OIN,TP, 5%-20%, 60 gm	**10481-1037-02**	6.60	
TIN,TP, 0.5%-10%, 30 ml	**10481-1038-01**	7.60	

PROD/MFR	HRI, UPC, NDC	AWP	SRP
UNI DERM (Smith & Nephew)			
CRE,TP (MOISTURIZER)			
90 gm	50484-0435-00	6.36	5.09
UNI-SOLVE (Animas Corp.)			
PAD,TP (WIPES)			
50s ea	65781-0620-50	19.35	
(Smith & Nephew)			
DEV,NA (WIPES)			
50s ea	40565-0115-65	10.75	8.60
SOL,TP (ADHESIVE REMOVER,BTL)			
240 ml	40565-0117-16	11.16	8.93
UNICARE (Smith & Nephew)			
LOT,TP, 60 ml	50484-0454-00	2.00	1.60
240 ml	50484-0450-00	7.19	5.75
UNICOMPLEX-M (Rugby)			
TAB,PO, 90s ea	00536-4750-11	4.50	
UNICON MULTIVITAMINS (Consolidated Midland)			
CAP,PO, 100s ea	00223-1955-01	4.50	
1000s ea	00223-1955-02	37.50	
UNIFIBER (Alaven)			
POW,PO (GLUTEN-FREE)			
3 gm/4 gm, 240 gm	68220-0044-08	10.25	
UNIFINE PENTIPS (Owen Mumford)			
DEV,NA (12MM,29G,ORIGINAL)			
90s ea	08470-2029-01	20.50	
(6MM,31G,MINI)			
90s ea	08470-2090-01	20.50	
(8MM,31G,SHORT)			
90s ea	08470-2030-01	20.50	
UNIGARD DISPOSABLE ADULT INCONTINENT PADS (Covidien)			
DEV,NA (10"X24")			
100s ea	08080-5874-00	33.32	
UNIGARD DISPOSABLE BOOSTER PADS (Covidien)			
DEV,NA (8"X17")			
100s ea	08080-6426-01	23.60	
UNIGARD PLUS ADULT INCONTINENT BRIEFS (Covidien)			
DEV,NA, 100s ea	08080-6229-01	56.79	
UNILET COMFORTOUCH LANCETS (Owen Mumford)			
DEV,NA (26G,PURPLE,ULTRA THIN)			
100s ea	08470-0465-01	5.63	6.95
(ALTERNATE SITE)			
100s ea	08470-0435-01	5.63	
(26G,PURPLE,ULTRA THIN)			
200s ea	08470-0460-01	9.31	11.95
(ALTERNATE SITE)			
200s ea	08470-0430-01	9.31	
UNILET EXCELITE II (Owen Mumford)			
DEV,NA (28G,CLEAR)			
100s ea	08470-0535-01	4.18	
(ULTRA THIN)			
100s ea	08214-0535-01	3.63	5.99
(28G,CLEAR)			
200s ea	08470-0530-01	8.26	
(ULTRA THIN)			
200s ea	08214-0530-01	7.25	9.99
UNILET EXELITE (Owen Mumford)			
DEV,NA (23 GAUGE,ORANGE)			
100s ea	08470-0515-01	4.18	
200s ea	08470-0510-01	8.26	
UNILET G.P. LANCETS (Owen Mumford)			
DEV,NA (21G,BLUE)			
100s ea	08470-0414-01	5.06	7.00
200s ea	08470-0418-01	8.25	10.00
UNILET G.P. SUPERLITE LANCETS (Owen Mumford)			
DEV,NA (THIN CANNULA,23G,0.66MM)			
100s ea	08470-0455-01	5.38	7.00
200s ea	08470-0450-01	9.63	10.50
UNILET GP ULTRALITE (Owen Mumford)			
DEV,NA (28G,NATURAL)			
100s ea	08470-0925-01	5.63	5.99
200s ea	08470-0920-01	9.31	8.99
UNILET LANCETS (Owen Mumford)			
DEV,NA (21G, 0.81MM,YELLOW)			
200s ea	08470-0400-01	9.31	12.00
UNILET SUPERLITE LANCETS (Owen Mumford)			
DEV,NA (THIN CANNULA,23G,0.66MM)			
100s ea	08470-0445-01	5.38	6.75
200s ea	08470-0440-01	9.94	12.25
UNISOL 4 SALINE (Alcon Labs Cons Prod)			
SOL,NA (3X120ML,PF)			
120 ml 3s	00580-0527-30	6.24	

PROD/MFR	HRI, UPC, NDC	AWP	SRP
UNISOM (Phys Total Care)			
REPACK			
TAB,PO, 25 mg, 8s ea	54868-4882-00	5.34	
UNISTIK 2 LANCETS (Owen Mumford)			
DEV,NA (21G,YELLOW,NORMAL,2.4MM)			
50s ea	08470-0700-01	13.83	12.25
(18G,NEONATAL,1.8MM)			
100s ea	08470-0762-01	23.13	25.00
(21G,BURGUNDY,SUPER,30MM)			
100s ea	08470-0752-01	26.25	19.95
(21G,YELLOW,NORMAL,2.4MM)			
100s ea	08470-0702-01	26.25	18.75
(26G, LAVENDER, 1.8MM)			
100s ea	08470-0742-01	26.25	18.75
(21G,YELLOW,NORMAL,2.4MM)			
200s ea	08470-0704-01	46.69	
UNISTIK 3 COMFORT LANCET (Owen Mumford)			
DEV,NA, 50s ea	08470-1047-01	13.84	
UNISTIK 3 EXTRA (Owen Mumford)			
DEV,NA, 100s ea	08470-1012-01	26.25	
200s ea	08470-1014-01	46.49	
UNISTIK 3 LANCETS (Owen Mumford)			
DEV,NA (18G,BURGUNDY,NEONATAL)			
100s ea	08470-1062-01	26.25	
(21G,YELLOW,NORMAL,1.8MM)			
100s ea	08470-1002-01	26.25	
(26G,LAVENDER,COMFORT)			
100s ea	08470-1042-01	26.25	
(18G,BURGUNDY,NEONATAL)			
200s ea	08470-1064-01	46.69	
(21G,YELLOW,NORMAL,1.8MM)			
200s ea	08470-1004-01	46.69	
(26G,LAVENDER,COMFORT)			
200s ea	08470-1044-01	46.69	
UNISTIK 3 NORMAL LANCET (Owen Mumford)			
DEV,NA, 50s ea	08470-1007-01	13.84	
UNISTIK CZT COMFORT LANCET (Owen Mumford)			
DEV,NA, 25s ea	08470-1048-01	7.00	
UNISTIK CZT NORMAL LANCET (Owen Mumford)			
DEV,NA, 25s ea	08470-1008-01	7.00	
UNISTIK I LANCETS (Owen Mumford)			
DEV,NA (ORANGE,3.0MM)			
50s ea	08470-0610-01	10.63	13.75
(YELLOW,2.4MM)			
50s ea	08470-0600-01	10.63	13.75
UNIVERSAL CVP MANOMETER (Abbott Hosp)			
DEV,NA (49", GRADUATIONS IN CM)			
24s ea	00074-4607-02	376.70	
UNJURY (ProSynthesis Labs)			
PDR,PO (UNFLAVORED)			
330 gm	68905-0330-33	13.00	
(CHOCOLATE)			
422 gm	68905-0110-11	15.00	
(VANILLA)			
422 gm	68905-0220-22	15.00	
PKT,PO (22GM SINGLE-DOSE PACK)			
ea	68905-0110-44	1.50	
ea	68905-0220-55	1.50	
ea	68905-0330-66	1.50	
UNNA-PAK TWO LAYER UNNA BOOT SYSTEM (Western Medical)			
DEV,NA (3" PRIMER + 3" COPRESS)			
12s ea	16926-0141-51	143.77	
(4" PRIMER + 4" COPRESS)			
12s ea	16926-0141-52	157.12	
UPCAL D (Global)			
POW,PO (120X4;GOPACK)			
480s ea	82028-0004-88	44.88	
(6X568GM)			
568 gm 6s	82028-0006-87	59.91	
UPVITE-AM (Freeda)			
TAB,PO (SF,GLUTEN-FREE)			
100s ea	10432-0347-01	9.57	15.95
UPVITE-PM (Freeda)			
PO (SF,GLUTEN-FREE)			
100s ea	10432-0348-01	7.77	12.95
UREA (Bio-Tech Pharm)			
POW,PO (USP)			
2.3 gm/tsp,			
453.59 gm	53191-0161-10	10.50	
2267.96 gm	53191-0161-05	39.40	
UREACIN-10 (Pedinol)			
LOT,TP, 10%, 236.56 ml	00884-3249-08		16.00
UREACIN-20 (Pedinol)			
CRE,TP, 20%, 120 gm	00884-0449-04		21.00

PROD/MFR	HRI, UPC, NDC	AWP	SRP
UREZE-M (Key Company)			
TAB,PO, 60s ea	11694-0706-01	5.25	
180s ea	11694-0706-18	12.50	
URIN-TEK (Siemens)			
DEV,NA (CASE CAPS ONLY-500X6)			
ea	00193-4205-23	119.50	119.50
(SYSTEM,100X5)			
500s ea	00193-4202-21	95.05	95.05
(TUBES)			
500s ea	00193-4204-23	55.55	55.55
URISTIX (Siemens)			
DEV,NA, 100s ea	08620-2184-21	36.40	36.40
URISTIX 4 (Siemens)			
DEV,NA, 100s ea	08620-2166-21	45.70	45.70
URO-2 (Bio-Tech Pharm)			
CAP,PO, 2 mg, 100s ea	53191-0361-01	4.50	
URO-MAG (Blaine)			
CAP,PO, 140 mg, 100s ea	00165-0054-01	12.06	
(SF)			
140 mg, 100s ea UD	00165-0054-41	22.50	
1000s ea	00165-0054-10	107.70	
URO-PRO (Westlake Labs.)			
CAP,PO (PF,SF)			
60s ea	10539-0682-04	25.20	36.00
UROSTOMY POUCH (Coloplast)			
DEV,NA (TRANSPAR., SM., 1-1/2")			
10s ea	11701-0815-25	42.10	44.10
(TRANSPAR., SM., 1-3/4")			
10s ea	11701-0815-15	42.10	44.10
(TRANSPAR., STD., 1-1/2")			
10s ea	11701-0815-10	42.10	44.10
(TRANSPAR., STD., 1-3/4")			
10s ea	11701-0815-30	42.10	44.10
(TRANSPAR., STD., 2")			
10s ea	11701-0815-20	42.10	44.10
URTICA URENS (Luyties)			
TAB,SL (12X)			
500s ea	00624-9225-03	4.19	
5500s ea	00624-9225-10	31.83	
12 x, 500s ea	00622-9225-03	4.19	
5500s ea	00622-9225-10	31.83	
30 x, 500s ea	00618-9225-03	3.99	
5500s ea	00618-9225-10	30.32	
US DIAGNOSTICS LANCET (US DIAGNOSTICS, INC)			
DEV,NA (28G)			
100s ea	08463-7012-28	6.00	
(30G)			
100s ea	08463-7029-30	6.00	
(SINGLE USE,PRE-COCKED)			
100s ea	82783-0303-18	12.50	
USNEA (Botanical Labs.)			
LIQ,PO, 30 ml	41954-0020-75	4.00	7.99
UTI CRANBERRY (Consumer Choice)			
CAP,PO (SF)			
480 mg, 50s ea	18149-0508-50	4.55	6.59
UTI HOMESCREENING TEST STICK (Consumer Choice)			
DEV,NA, 2s ea	60369-0506-20	6.20	10.95
UTI-STAT (Medical Nutrition USA)			
SOL,PO (96X30ML,GLUTEN-FREE)			
30 ml 96s	26974-0410-67	116.10	
(4X887ML,GLUTEN-FREE)			
887 ml 4s	26974-0410-66	30.50	
UVA URSI LEAF (ADH)			
CAP,PO (PF,SF)			
455 mg, 100s ea	60142-0977-01	4.98	9.95
VAGI-GARD (Lake Pharm)			
GEL,VG, 120 gm	12277-0544-04	2.09	3.49
SPR,TP (MAXIMUM STRENGTH)			
59.25 ml	12277-0525-02	3.00	5.00
(SENSITIVE FORMULA)			
59.25 ml	12277-0524-02	3.00	5.00
VAGI-GARD DOUCHE (Lake Pharm)			
SOL,VG, 10%, 237 ml	12277-0517-08	4.79	7.99
VAGI-GARD DOUCHE MAXIMUM STRENGTH (Lake Pharm)			
SOL,VG (TILT BOTTLE/DISP NOZZLE)			
10%, 177.75 ml 2s	12277-0517-05	2.39	3.99
VAGI-GARD DOUCHE NON-STAINING (Lake Pharm)			
LIQ,VG (DISP BOTTLE/DISP NOZZLE)			
177.75 ml 2s	12277-0521-08	2.99	4.99
VAGI-GARD MAXIMUM STRENGTH FORMULA (Lake Pharm)			
CRE,TP, 0.13%-20%,			
45 gm	12277-0521-01	3.99	6.69

PROD/MFR	HRI, UPC,NDC	AWP	SRP
VAGI-GARD SENSITIVE FORMULA (Lake Pharm)			
CRE,TP, 0.13%-5%, 45 gm	12277-0516-01	2.99	4.99
VAGI-GARD TOWELETTES (Lake Pharm)			
PAD,TP, 24s ea	12277-0526-24	1.80	2.99
VAGISIL DEODORANT POWDER (Combe)			
POW,TP (EASY HOLD BOTTLE)			
227 gm	11509-0003-92	2.51	
VAGISIL FEMININE MOISTURIZER (Combe)			
LOT,TP (VITAMIN E PLUS ALOE)			
59 ml	11509-0060-00	3.76	
VAGISIL SCREENING KIT (Combe)			
DEV,NA, 2s ea	11509-0003-20	12.31	
VAGISTAT-1 (Novartis Consumer)			
OIN,VG (1X4.6,1-DOSE TREATMENT)			
6.5%, 4.6 gm	00067-2090-46	14.39	
VALERIAN (Botanical Labs.)			
LIQ,PO, 30 ml	41954-0020-53	4.00	7.99
30 ml	41954-0032-02	5.25	10.49
60 ml	41954-0020-42	6.50	12.99
60 ml	41954-0032-32	8.25	16.49
(Mason Vit)			
CAP,PO (PF,SF)			
500 mg, 60s ea	11845-0115-25	5.33	
VALERIAN ROOT (ADH)			
CAP,PO (PF,SF)			
450 mg, 100s ea	60142-0978-51	4.98	9.95
(Cardinal Health)			
CAP,PO (PRIVATE LABEL)			
445 mg, 100s ea	37205-0049-78	5.14	
(Mason Vit)			
CAP,PO (PF,SF)			
100 mg, 60s ea	11845-0129-15	6.67	
(Nature's Bounty)			
CAP,PO, 450 mg, 100s ea	74312-0033-90		4.99
(Rexall)			
CAP,PO (PF,SF)			
530 mg, 75s ea	30768-0000-79	2.26	3.43
VALERIAN ROOT COMPLEX (Rexall)			
CAP,PO (PF,SF)			
50s ea	30768-0001-15	2.34	3.55
VALERIAN ROOT STANDARDIZED (Rexall)			
CAP,PO (PF,SF)			
530 mg, 45s ea	30768-0001-28	3.09	4.68
VALIHIST (Medique)			
TAB,PO (150X2,SF)			
325 mg-45 mg-2 mg-5 mg,			
300s ea	10244-0543-63	41.79	
VALINE (VITAFLO, LLC)			
PDS,PO, 50 mg/4 gm,			
30s ea	50600-0543-33	90.00	115.00
VALINE 1000 (VITAFLO, LLC)			
POW,NA (30X4GM)			
30s ea	50600-0551-32	120.00	150.00
VALU-RITE (McKesson)			
12-HOUR NASAL			
SPR,NS, 0.05%, 30 ml	49348-0028-27	4.09	2.99
ACID REDUCER			
TAB,PO, 10 mg, 30s ea	49348-0442-44	6.49	
60s ea	49348-0442-12	8.99	
ADHESIVE TAPE			
DEV,NA (1"X5 YD)			
ea	49348-0587-83	1.99	
(1/2"X10 YD)			
ea	49348-0586-86	1.99	
ALCOHOL ETHYL			
LIQ,TP (RUBBING)			
70%, 480 ml	49348-0003-38	1.59	
ALCOHOL ISOPROPYL			
LIQ,TP, 70%, 480 ml	49348-0007-38	1.33	
480 ml	49348-0030-38	0.73	1.19
(RUBBING)			
70%, 3840 ml	49348-0030-40	10.49	
91%, 480 ml	49348-0004-38	1.69	
99%, 480 ml	49348-0005-38	2.57	
ALCOHOL PREP			
DEV,NA, 120s ea	49348-0077-53	1.69	2.19
ALLERGY			
TAB,PO, 4 mg, 24s ea	49348-0025-04	4.19	1.99
100s ea	49348-0025-10	7.49	
ANIMAL SHAPES			
CTB,PO, 100s ea	49348-0105-10	5.59	3.99
ANTACID			
SUS,PO (MINT)			
225 mg/5 ml-200 mg/5 ml,			
360 ml	49348-0019-39	2.99	2.09
780 ml	49348-0019-97	5.49	
TAB,PO (ASSORTED)			
500 mg, 150s ea	49348-0170-21	3.29	2.99
(PEPPERMINT)			
500 mg, 150s ea	49348-0169-21	3.29	2.99
ANTACID EXTRA STRENGTH			
PO (ASSORTED)			
750 mg, 96s ea	49348-0865-13	3.29	
ANTACID W/SIMETHICONE			
SUS,PO, 360 ml	49348-0020-39	2.99	2.39
360 ml	49348-0035-39	4.39	2.99
780 ml	49348-0020-97	5.49	
ANTI-DIARRHEAL			
LIQ,PO, 1 mg/5 ml,			
120 ml	49348-0277-34	5.19	
TAB,PO (CAPLET)			
2 mg, 12s ea	49348-0529-02	4.29	
(EZ OPEN,CAPLET)			
2 mg, 24s ea	49348-0083-04	5.19	
ANTIFUNGAL			
CRE,TP, 1%, 15 gm	49348-0155-29	4.69	2.99
ANTISEPTIC CLEANSER FOR MOUTH			
SOL,MM, 10%, 60 ml	49348-0619-30	6.69	
ARTHRICREAM			
CRE,TP, 10%, 90 gm	49348-0156-84	3.79	2.79
ARTIFICIAL TEARS			
SOL,OP, 1.4%, 15 ml	49348-0699-29	6.19	
ASPIRIN			
ECT,PO, 325 mg, 100s ea	49348-0034-10	5.19	2.99
250s ea	49348-0034-19	7.79	5.99
500s ea	49348-0283-14	10.79	
TAB,PO, 325 mg, 100s ea	49348-0001-10	1.89	1.69
300s ea	49348-0001-23	3.59	
500s ea	49348-0001-14	5.99	
ASPIRIN CHILDREN'S			
CTB,PO (CHERRY)			
81 mg, 36s ea	49348-0191-07	1.89	
(ORANGE)			
81 mg, 36s ea	49348-0757-07	1.89	
ASPIRIN LOW STRENGTH			
ECT,PO, 81 mg, 120s ea	49348-0756-53	4.99	
180s ea	49348-0756-15	6.69	
300s ea	49348-0284-23	8.69	
ASPIRIN MAXIMUM STRENGTH			
PO, 500 mg, 60s ea	49348-0784-12	5.19	
ASTRINGENT			
PDR,TP (PACKET)			
12s ea	49348-0358-02	8.99	
BACITRACIN			
OIN,TP, 500 u/gm, 30 gm	49348-0154-72	2.99	2.99
BANDAGES CLEAR			
DEV,NA (ASSORTED)			
40s ea	49348-0581-59	1.99	
BANDAGES FLEXIBLE			
NA (ASSORTED)			
20s ea	49348-0075-47	2.17	
30s ea	49348-0582-44	1.99	
BANDAGES PLASTIC			
NA (EXTRA LARGE)			
10s ea	49348-0585-01	1.99	
(3/4")			
60s ea	49348-0583-12	1.89	
BANDAGES SHEER			
NA (1")			
40s ea	49348-0684-59	1.99	
(ASSORTED)			
60s ea	49348-0685-12	1.99	
BENZOIN			
TIN,TP, 60 ml	49348-0801-30	2.89	
BENZOYL PEROXIDE			
LOT,TP, 10%, 30 ml	49348-0186-27	3.89	2.99
BETA CAROTENE			
SGL,PO (SOFTGEL)			
25000 iu, 100s ea	49348-0438-10	6.59	5.19
BRONCHIAL MIST			
AER,IH (REFILL)			
0.22 mg/actuation,			
15 ml	49348-0025-29	9.53	
BRONCHIAL MIST W/PUMP			
IH, 0.22 mg/actuation,			
15 ml	49348-0751-29	9.79	
CALAMINE			
LOT,TP, 120 ml	49348-0011-34	1.69	
CALAMINE PHENOLATED			
LOT,TP, 8%-1%, 120 ml	49348-0802-34	1.99	
CALCIUM 500 + D			
TAB,PO, 500 mg-125 iu,			
60s ea	49348-0264-12	5.69	4.49
CALCIUM 600			
CAP,PO, 600 mg, 60s ea	49348-0233-12	5.09	4.29
CALCIUM 600/VITAMIN D			
CAP,PO (PF,SF)			
600 mg-125 iu,			
60s ea	49348-0110-12	5.23	4.19
CALCIUM PLUS			
TAB,PO (PF,SF)			
60s ea	49348-0139-12	5.19	
CALCIUM/MAGNESIUM/ZINC			
TAB,PO, 333 mg-333 mg-8.3 mg,			
100s ea	49348-0238-10	4.49	3.89
CALDYPHEN			
LOT,TP, 8%-0.1%-1%,			
180 ml	49348-0337-36	3.99	2.99
CALDYPHEN CLEAR			
LOT,TP, 180 ml	49348-0610-36	3.99	
CASTOR OIL			
OIL,PO, 120 ml	49348-0016-34	3.23	
CENTRAL-VITE			
TAB,PO, 130s ea	49348-0103-45	7.19	7.29
CHROMIUM PICOLINATE			
TAB,PO, 200 mcg,			
100s ea	49348-0826-10	6.19	
CLOTRIMAZOLE			
CRE,VG, 1%, 15 gm	49348-0827-69	5.69	
30 gm	49348-0279-72	7.49	
45 gm	49348-0793-76	6.29	
CO Q-10			
SGL,PO (SOFTGEL)			
10 mg, 30s ea	49348-0326-44	12.39	
COLD & HOT THERAPY PAIN RELIEF			
STI,TP, 7.6%-29%,			
105 gm	49348-0420-96	3.99	
COLD INFANTS'			
LIQ,PO (AF,BUBBLEGUM,DROPS)			
15 ml	49348-0207-29	3.99	
COMPLETE MAXIMUM STRENGTH			
TAB,PO, 500 mg-2 mg-15 mg-30 mg,			
24s ea	49348-0167-04	4.19	
COMPLETE SENIOR			
TAB,PO, 100s ea	49348-0335-10	7.79	
CONTACT LENS CLEANER			
SOL,NA, 30 ml	49348-0082-27	5.39	
CONTACT LENS CONDITIONING			
NA, 120 ml	49348-0081-34	5.39	
COOL GEL			
GEL,TP, 2%, 240 gm	49348-0147-91	5.29	4.99
COSMETIC PUFFS TRIPLE SIZE			
DEV,NA, 100s ea	49348-0160-22	1.23	
COSMETIC SQUARES			
NA (RESEALABLE)			
200s ea	49348-0159-22	3.49	
COTTON BALLS STERILE			
NA (BOX)			
130s ea	49348-0590-45	2.99	
COTTON BALLS TRIPLE SIZE			
NA (RESEALABLE)			
100s ea	49348-0157-22	1.69	
DAILYHIST-1			
TAB,PO, 1.34 mg, 16s ea	49348-0686-03	5.79	
DAIRY DIGESTIVE SUPPLEMENT ULTRA			
TAB,PO (CAPLET)			
60 mg, 32s ea	49348-0291-06	6.29	
60s ea	49348-0291-12	11.49	
DAY TIME			
CAP,PO (AF,SOFTGEL)			
250 mg-10 mg-10 mg-30 mg,			
12s ea	49348-0772-02	2.89	
LIQ,PO (AF)			
180 ml	49348-0837-36	3.19	
DECONGESTANT COUGH FORMULA D			
LIQ,PO, 10 mg/5 ml-20 mg/5 ml,			
240 ml	49348-0039-37	4.99	4.09
DOCUSATE CALCIUM			
SGL,PO, 240 mg, 100s ea	49348-0280-10	10.69	
EAR DROPS			
SOL,OT, 6.5%, 15 ml	49348-0143-29	4.79	
ELECTROLYTE PEDIATRIC			
SOL,PO, 960 ml	49348-0571-41	4.17	
(FRUIT)			
960 ml	49348-0570-41	4.29	
(BUBBLEGUM)			
1014 ml	49348-0880-62	4.29	
(GRAPE)			
1014 ml	49348-0161-62	4.29	
ENEMA RTU			
NMA,RC, 135 ml	49348-0527-20	0.99	
EVENING PRIMROSE OIL			
SGL,PO (SOFTGEL)			
500 mg, 75s ea	49348-0325-43	6.19	
EXPECTORANT			
SYR,PO, 100 mg/5 ml,			
120 ml	49348-0278-34	2.59	
240 ml	49348-0278-37	4.39	3.99
EXPECTORANT DM			
LIQ,PO, 10 mg/5 ml-100 mg/5 ml,			
120 ml	49348-0017-34	3.39	
120 ml	49348-0861-34	4.19	

PROD/MFR	HRI, UPC,NDC	AWP	SRP
240 ml	49348-0017-37	5.19	3.99
SYR,PO (W/DOSAGE CUP,AF,SF)			
10 mg/5 ml-100 mg/5 ml,			
355 ml	49348-0295-98	6.19	
EYE,DROPS			
SOL,OP, 0.05%, 15 ml	49348-0037-29	2.29	2.19
EYE DROPS ALLERGY RELIEF			
SOL,OP, 0.05%-0.25%,			
15 ml	49348-0697-29	2.29	
EYE WASH			
SOL,OP, 120 ml	49348-0783-34	3.29	
FIBER LAXATIVE			
TAB,PO, 625 mg, 90s ea	49348-0759-13	9.49	
FISH OIL CONCENTRATE			
SGL,PO (SOFTGEL)			
60s ea	49348-0132-12	6.69	
FLU/COLD/COUGH MEDICINE PAKS			
PDR,PO, 6s ea	49348-0400-95	3.49	
FLU/COLD/COUGH NIGHTTIME MEDICINE			
PDS,PO (MAX. STR.,PACKET,LEMON)			
6s ea	49348-0209-95	3.89	
FOLIC ACID			
TAB,PO, 0.4 mg, 250s ea	49348-0825-19	4.29	
GARLIC			
TAB,PO (PF,SF,DYE-FREE)			
400 mg, 30s ea	49348-0303-44	7.09	
GARLIC OIL			
SGL,PO (SOFTGEL)			
1 mg, 100s ea	49348-0078-10	4.09	2.99
GAS RELIEF EXTRA STRENGTH			
SGL,PO (SOFTGEL)			
125 mg, 30s ea	49348-0263-44	4.59	
GAS RELIEF INFANTS'			
SUS,PO (DROPS)			
40 mg/0.6 ml,			
30 ml	49348-0577-34	9.19	
GAS RELIEF MAXIMUM STRENGTH			
SGL,PO (SOFTGEL)			
166 mg, 60s ea	49348-0380-12	9.29	
GENTLE LAXATIVE			
ECT,PO, 5 mg, 25s ea	49348-0599-05	4.19	
SUP,RC, 10 mg, 8s ea	49348-0598-67	5.39	
GINSENG			
SGL,PO (SOFTGEL)			
100 mg, 30s ea	49348-0824-44	7.79	
GLUCOSAMINE COMPLEX			
TAB,PO (CAPLET)			
200 mg-300 mg,			
60s ea	49348-0218-12	13.89	
GLUCOSE			
CTB,PO (ORANGE)			
4 gm, 10s ea	49348-0913-01	1.67	
(RASPBERRY)			
4 gm, 10s ea	49348-0915-01	1.67	
(ORANGE)			
4 gm, 50s ea	49348-0914-09	6.03	
(RASPBERRY)			
4 gm, 50s ea	49348-0916-09	6.03	
GLYCERIN SUPPOSITORIES			
SUP,RC, 25s ea	49348-0159-05	1.87	1.99
(INFANT)			
25s ea	49348-0158-05	1.87	1.99
50s ea	49348-0159-09	3.29	3.09
HEADACHE FORMULA ADDED STRENGTH			
TAB,PO, 250 mg-250 mg-65 mg,			
50s ea	49348-0293-09	4.39	
HEARTBURN RELIEF 200			
TAB,PO, 200 mg, 30s ea	49348-0246-44	7.19	
50s ea	49348-0247-09	10.19	
HEMORRHOIDAL			
CRE,RC, 0.25%-3%, 54 gm	49348-0428-32	5.69	
OIN,TP, 60 gm	49348-0720-27	5.69	3.99
SUP,RC, 24s ea	49348-0345-04	6.69	4.59
HOME PREGNANCY			
DEV,NA, ea	49348-0870-00	7.99	
HOSPITAL ANTISEPTIC SOLUTION			
SOL,TP, 10%, 240 ml	49348-0622-37	5.39	
480 ml	49348-0622-38	7.79	
HYDROCORT ACETATE W/ALOE			
CRE,TP, 0.5%, 30 gm	49348-0021-72	3.03	2.69
OIN,TP, 0.5%, 30 gm	49348-0271-72	3.03	2.69
HYDROCORTISONE MAXIMUM STRENGTH			
CRE,TP, 1%, 30 gm	49348-0521-72	3.19	
OIN,TP, 1%, 30 gm	49348-0522-72	3.19	
HYDROGEN PEROXIDE			
SOL,TP, 3%, 120 ml	49348-0031-34	0.49	
240 ml	49348-0031-37	0.57	
480 ml	49348-0031-38	0.73	0.89
HYGIENIC CLEANSING PADS			
PAD,TP, 100s ea	49348-0459-10	5.29	
IBUPROFEN			
TAB,PO, 200 mg, 50s ea	49348-0196-09	4.19	3.09
50s ea	49348-0706-09	3.99	3.09
(WHITE,CAPLET)			
200 mg, 50s ea	49348-0087-09	3.89	
(WHITE)			
200 mg, 50s ea	49348-0086-09	3.89	
100s ea	49348-0196-10	5.69	4.99
100s ea	49348-0706-10	5.69	4.99
100s ea	49348-0808-10	5.69	
(CAPLET)			
200 mg, 100s ea	49348-0809-10	5.69	
250s ea	49348-0706-19	10.99	
(CAPLET)			
200 mg, 250s ea	49348-0196-19	10.99	
500s ea	49348-0706-14	14.29	
(CAPLET)			
200 mg, 500s ea	49348-0196-35	14.29	
IBUPROFEN CHILDREN'S			
SUS,PO (AF,BERRY)			
100 mg/5 ml,			
120 ml	49348-0229-34	4.19	
(AF,FRUIT)			
100 mg/5 ml,			
120 ml	49348-0228-34	4.29	
IODINE			
TIN,TP, 2%, 30 ml	49348-0133-27	1.87	
IRON			
TAB,PO, 65 mg, 100s ea	49348-0180-10	6.69	
L-LYSINE			
TAB,PO, 500 mg, 100s ea	49348-0053-10	5.99	
LANCETS			
DEV,NA, 100s ea	49348-0240-10	5.99	
(THIN)			
100s ea	49348-0241-10	5.99	
200s ea	49348-0563-22	9.59	
(COLORED)			
200s ea	49348-0912-22	9.59	
(THIN)			
200s ea	49348-0911-22	9.59	
LAXATIVE PILLS			
TAB,PO, 15 mg, 30s ea	49348-0225-49	4.49	
LAXATIVE PILLS MAXIMUM STRENGTH			
PO, 25 mg, 24s ea	49348-0224-04	4.29	
LECITHIN			
SGL,PO (SOFTGEL)			
1200 mg, 100s ea	49348-0050-10	5.29	5.09
LICE TREATMENT			
LIQ,TP, 60 ml	49348-0443-30	5.49	
120 ml	49348-0443-34	8.49	
240 ml	49348-0434-37	14.99	
LICE TREATMENT MAXIMUM STRENGTH			
KIT,NA (SHAMPOO,SPRAY,COMB)			
ea	49348-0235-87	10.99	
LUBRICATING JELLY			
GEL,VG, 120 gm	49348-0184-85	2.89	
MAGNESIUM CITRATE			
SOL,PO (LEMON)			
1.75 gm/30 ml,			
300 ml	49348-0696-49	1.19	
MEDICATED BODY POWDER			
POW,TP, 300 gm	49348-0834-92	5.49	
MEDICATED CHEST RUB			
OIN,TP, 4.73%-1.2%-2.6%,			
105 gm	49348-0398-96	3.79	
MICONAZOLE 7			
CRE,TP, 2%, 47.7 gm	49348-0530-77	7.99	
SUP,VG, 100 mg, 7s ea	49348-0833-61	7.99	
MICONAZOLE NITRATE			
CRE,TP, 2%, 30 gm	49348-0689-72	6.49	
MILK OF MAGNESIA			
SUS,PO, 400 mg/5 ml,			
360 ml	49348-0687-39	3.99	
(MINT)			
400 mg/5 ml,			
360 ml	49348-0688-39	3.99	
780 ml	49348-0687-44	6.69	
(MINT)			
400 mg/5 ml,			
780 ml	49348-0688-44	6.69	
MOTION SICKNESS LESS DROWSY			
TAB,PO (BLISTER CARD)			
25 mg, 8s ea	49348-0363-67	3.39	
MULTI-VIT CHILDREN'S			
SOL,PO (DROPS)			
50 ml	49348-0864-32	6.39	
MULTI-VIT W/C			
CTB,PO, 100s ea	49348-0108-10	5.69	5.19
MULTI-VIT W/IRON CHILDREN'S			
LIQ,PO (DROPS)			
50 ml	49348-0863-32	6.39	
MULTI-VIT W/IRON PEDIATRIC			
CTB,PO (PEDIATRIC)			
100s ea	49348-0106-10	5.59	3.99
MULTIPLE VITAMINS			
TAB,PO, 100s ea	49348-0101-10	4.99	3.19
250s ea	49348-0101-19	7.89	6.09
MUSCLE RUB ULTRA STRENGTH			
CRE,TP, 120 gm	49348-0214-85	5.69	
NAPROXEN SODIUM			
TAB,PO, 220 mg, 50s ea	49348-0150-09	4.09	
(CAPLET)			
220 mg, 50s ea	49348-0149-09	4.09	
100s ea	49348-0151-10	6.99	
NASAL			
SPR,NS, 0.05%, 30 ml	49348-0276-27	5.19	2.99
NASAL DECONGESTANT/ANTIHISTAMINE			
TAB,PO, 60 mg-2.5 mg,			
24s ea	49348-0032-04	3.09	2.99
48s ea	49348-0165-08	4.99	
NASAL EXTRA MOISTURIZING 12 HOUR			
SPR,NS, 0.05%, 30 ml	49348-0230-27	4.39	
NATURAL B-COMPLEX W/VITAMIN C			
TAB,PO, 100s ea	49348-0391-10	5.73	
NATURAL SENNA LAXATIVE			
TAB,PO, 8.6 mg, 100s ea	49348-0262-10	10.99	
NAUSEA CONTROL			
SOL,PO (CHERRY)			
120 ml	49348-0576-27	5.49	
NIGHTTIME			
SGL,PO (LIQUICAP)			
12s ea	49348-0533-02	2.99	
SOL,PO, 180 ml	49348-0014-36	2.99	2.99
180 ml	49348-0153-36	2.99	2.99
300 ml	49348-0014-92	3.99	3.99
(CHERRY)			
300 ml	49348-0153-49	3.99	
NON-ASPIRIN			
TAB,PO, 325 mg, 100s ea	49348-0009-10	5.49	2.99
NON-ASPIRIN ALLERGY/SINUS			
CAP,PO (MAX. STR.,GELCAP)			
500 mg-2 mg-30 mg,			
24s ea	49348-0300-04	3.39	
TAB,PO (CAPLET)			
325 mg-2 mg-30 mg,			
24s ea	49348-0838-04	3.69	
(MAX. STR.,GELTAB)			
500 mg-2 mg-30 mg,			
24s ea	49348-0299-04	3.39	
NON-ASPIRIN CHILDREN'S			
CTB,PO, 80 mg, 30s ea	49348-0199-44	2.29	1.99
(FRUIT)			
80 mg, 30s ea	49348-0022-44	2.29	1.99
ELI,PO (CHERRY)			
160 mg/5 ml,			
120 ml	49348-0036-34	4.29	2.99
SUP,RC, 120 mg, 12s ea	49348-0796-02	5.49	
SUS,PO (BUBBLEGUM)			
160 mg/5 ml,			
120 ml	49348-0888-34	4.29	
(CHERRY)			
160 mg/5 ml,			
120 ml	49348-0797-34	4.29	
NON-ASPIRIN EXTRA STRENGTH			
TAB,PO, 500 mg, 50s ea	49348-0042-09	4.19	2.99
(GELCAPLET)			
500 mg, 50s ea	49348-0286-09	4.19	3.19
(GELTAB)			
500 mg, 50s ea	49348-0085-09	4.09	
60s ea	49348-0023-12	4.89	2.99
100s ea	49348-0023-10	5.49	3.99
100s ea	49348-0042-10	5.59	3.99
(GELCAPLET)			
500 mg, 100s ea	49348-0286-10	6.19	
(GELTAB)			
500 mg, 100s ea	49348-0871-10	6.19	
(CAPLET)			
500 mg, 250s ea	49348-0042-19	10.79	
500s ea	49348-0042-14	13.89	
NON-ASPIRIN INFANT'S			
SOL,PO (DROPS)			
80 mg/0.8 ml,			
15 ml	49348-0268-29	3.79	
NON-ASPIRIN JR.			
CTB,PO (FRUIT)			
160 mg, 24s ea	49348-0346-04	3.69	
(GRAPE)			
160 mg, 24s ea	49348-0792-04	3.69	
NON-ASPIRIN PM EXTRA STRENGTH			
TAB,PO (CAPLET)			
500 mg-25 mg,			
50s ea	49348-0349-09	5.19	
(GELTAB)			
500 mg-25 mg,			
50s ea	49348-0292-09	5.39	
NON-ASPIRIN SINUS			
TAB,PO (CAPLET)			
500 mg-30 mg,			
24s ea	49348-0860-04	3.69	

PROD/MFR	HRI, UPC,NDC	AWP	SRP
NON-ASPIRIN SINUS MAXIMUM STRENGTH			
PO (GELTAB)			
500 mg-30 mg,			
24s ea	**49348-0297-04**	3.39	
NON-DROWSY SINUS			
PO (MAX. STR.)			
325 mg-30 mg,			
24s ea	**49348-0514-04**	3.99	
NOSE DROPS EXTRA STRENGTH			
SOL,NS, 1%, 30 ml	**49348-0197-27**	4.19	
NUTRITIONAL SUPPLEMENT DRINK			
LIQ,PO (CHOCOLATE)			
240 ml	**10939-0027-22**	7.39	
(VANILLA)			
240 ml	**10939-0026-22**	7.39	
NUTRITIONAL SUPPLEMENT DRINK PLUS			
PO (CHOCOLATE)			
240 ml	**10939-0030-22**	8.19	
(VANILLA)			
240 ml	**10939-0029-22**	8.19	
ONE DAILY MULTI-VIT W/CALCIUM/IRON			
TAB,PO, 100s ea	**49348-0236-10**	6.19	5.59
ONE DAILY MULTI-VIT W/IRON			
TAB,PO, 100s ea	**49348-0102-10**	4.99	3.19
250s ea	**49348-0102-19**	7.99	6.09
ONE DAY PILL BOX			
DEV,NA, ea	**49348-0730-01**	1.39	
ORAL MEDICINE DROPPER			
DEV,NA (1/2 TSP)			
ea	**49348-0735-01**	1.49	
ORAL MEDICINE SPOON			
DEV,NA (2 TSP)			
ea	**49348-0736-01**	1.39	
ORAL MEDICINE SYRINGE			
DEV,NA (2 TSP)			
ea	**49348-0734-01**	1.99	
OYSTER SHELL CALCIUM/VITAMIN D			
TAB,PO, 250 mg-125 iu,			
100s ea	**49348-0061-10**	4.09	3.09
PAIN RELIEF MAXIMUM STRENGTH			
GEL,TP, 16%, 90 gm	**49348-0429-84**	4.89	
PAIN RELIEVING GEL			
TP, 10%-15%, 120 gm	**49348-0446-85**	4.59	
PEDIA RELIEF COUGH-COLD			
LIQ,PO (AF,CHERRY)			
118 ml	**49348-0201-34**	3.69	
PEDIA RELIEF INFANTS'			
LIQ,PO (AF,DROPS)			
7.5 mg/0.8 ml,			
15 ml	**49348-0200-29**	3.69	
PEDIA RELIEF PLUS COUGH INFANTS'			
LIQ,PO (AF,DROPS)			
15 ml	**49348-0290-69**	3.59	
PILL DIVIDER W/PILL BOX			
DEV,NA, ea	**49348-0733-01**	5.19	
PRENATAL VITAMIN FORMULA			
TAB,PO, 100s ea	**49348-0556-10**	10.19	
SALINE			
SPR,NS, 45 ml	**49348-0356-25**	2.09	2.29
SELENIUM			
TAB,PO, 200 mcg,			
100s ea	**49348-0178-10**	7.19	
SLEEP AID			
TAB,PO, 25 mg, 32s ea	**49348-0574-06**	7.29	
SORE THROAT			
LOZ,MM, 2.4 mg, 24s ea	**49348-0040-04**	1.99	1.99
SPR,MM (CHERRY)			
1.4%, 180 ml	**49348-0397-36**	3.79	
(MENTHOL)			
1.4%, 180 ml	**49348-0038-36**	3.79	2.99
SORE THROAT W/BENZOCAINE			
LOZ,MM (CHERRY)			
18s ea	**49348-0160-48**	2.29	1.99
STAY AWAKE			
TAB,PO, 200 mg, 16s ea	**49348-0771-03**	2.19	
STERILE GAUZE			
DEV,NA (4X4)			
10s ea	**49348-0593-01**	2.99	
(2X2)			
25s ea	**49348-0591-05**	2.99	
(3X3)			
25s ea	**49348-0592-05**	3.49	
STERILE STRETCH GAUZE			
NA (2X4 YD)			
ea	**49348-0588-83**	1.99	
(3X4 YD)			
ea	**49348-0589-83**	2.39	
STOMACH RELIEF			
CTB,PO, 262 mg, 30s ea	**49348-0177-44**	2.89	2.39
SUS,PO, 262 mg/15 ml,			
240 ml	**49348-0192-37**	2.59	2.29
STOMACH RELIEF EXTRA STRENGTH			
PO, 525 mg/15 ml,			
240 ml	**49348-0338-37**	3.69	2.99
STOOL SOFTENER			
SGL,PO, 100 mg, 100s ea	**49348-0616-10**	5.79	
STOOL SOFTENER W/LAXATIVE			
SGL,PO, 30 mg-100 mg,			
100s ea	**49348-0617-10**	5.79	
STRESS B & BIOTIN			
TAB,PO, 60s ea	**49348-0226-12**	6.19	5.39
STRESS B W/ZINC & BIOTIN			
TAB,PO, 60s ea	**49348-0095-12**	6.19	5.69
STRESS FORMULA + IRON			
TAB,PO, 60s ea	**49348-0094-12**	6.19	5.49
SUPHEDRINE			
TAB,PO, 30 mg, 24s ea	**49348-0024-04**	3.09	2.39
SUPHEDRINE COUGH/COLD/FLU			
SGL,PO (LIQUICAP)			
10s ea	**49348-0859-01**	3.19	
SUPHEDRINE MAXIMUM STRENGTH			
TAB,PO (NON-DROWSY)			
30 mg, 48s ea	**49348-0296-08**	4.69	
SUPHEDRINE PLUS			
TAB,PO, 4 mg-60 mg,			
24s ea	**49348-0795-04**	3.59	
SUPHEDRINE SEVERE COLD			
TAB,PO (CAPLET)			
10s ea	**49348-0866-01**	3.39	
SUPHEDRINE SINUS			
TAB,PO, 500 mg-30 mg,			
24s ea	**49348-0858-04**	3.79	
THERAPEUTIC M			
TAB,PO, 130s ea	**49348-0260-45**	7.09	6.29
THERMOMETER DIGITAL W/PROBECOVERS			
DEV,NA, ea	**49348-0739-01**	7.99	
THERMOMETER PROBE COVERS			
DEV,NA, 25s ea	**49348-0740-05**	1.39	
TRAVEL SICKNESS			
TAB,PO, 50 mg, 12s ea	**49348-0070-02**	3.39	1.99
TRI-BUFFERED ASPIRIN			
TAB,PO, 325 mg, 100s ea	**49348-0006-10**	4.99	2.49
TRIPLE ANTIBIOTIC			
OIN,TP, 30 gm	**49348-0029-72**	3.79	2.49
TRIPLE ANTIBIOTIC W/LIDOCAINE			
OIN,TP, 30 gm	**49348-0600-72**	4.19	
TUSSIN COUGH/COLD MAXIMUM STRENGTH			
SYR,PO, 15 mg/5 ml-30 mg/5 ml,			
118 ml	**49348-0261-34**	3.99	
TUSSIN COUGH/COLD PEDIATRIC			
LIQ,PO, 7.5 mg/5 ml-15 mg/5 ml,			
118 ml	**49348-0203-34**	3.39	
URINARY PAIN RELIEF			
TAB,PO, 95 mg, 30s ea	**49348-0364-44**	5.89	
VALU-DRYL ALLERGY			
CAP,PO, 25 mg, 24s ea	**49348-0044-04**	3.09	2.69
48s ea	**49348-0282-08**	4.79	
100s ea	**49348-0044-10**	7.59	
TAB,PO, 25 mg, 24s ea	**49348-0564-04**	3.19	
VALU-DRYL ALLERGY CHILDREN'S			
SOL,PO, 12.5 mg/5 ml,			
120 ml	**49348-0045-34**	3.79	2.99
(AF,CHERRY)			
12.5 mg/5 ml,			
236 ml	**49348-0205-37**	5.99	
VALU-DRYL ALLERGY/SINUS HEADACHE			
TAB,PO (CAPLET)			
500 mg-12.5 mg-30 mg,			
24s ea	**49348-0206-04**	3.99	
VALU-DRYL ANTI-ITCH			
CRE,TP, 2%, 30 gm	**49348-0502-72**	3.49	
VEGETABLE POWDER			
PDR,PO (SF,ORANGE)			
3.4 gm/dose,			
280 gm	**49348-0090-92**	5.89	
390 gm	**49348-0047-93**	5.39	4.99
(REGULAR)			
3.4 gm/dose,			
390 gm	**49348-0166-93**	4.79	4.99
538 gm	**49348-0047-65**	5.29	
(SMOOTH,ORANGE)			
3.4 gm/dose,			
568.4 gm	**49348-0091-68**	5.49	
(REGULAR)			
3.4 gm/dose,			
570 gm	**49348-0166-65**	6.89	
VISION			
TAB,PO, 60s ea	**49348-0549-12**	6.19	
VITAMIN A			
SGL,PO (SOFTGEL)			
8000 iu, 100s ea	**49348-0163-10**	3.09	
VITAMIN B-100 NATURAL			
TAB,PO, 50s ea	**49348-0321-09**	8.19	
VITAMIN B-50 NATURAL			
PO, 50s ea	**49348-0322-09**	5.59	
VITAMIN B1			
TAB,PO, 100 mg, 100s ea	**49348-0088-10**	3.99	3.69
VITAMIN B12			
TAB,PO, 500 mcg,			
100s ea	**49348-0821-10**	5.79	
TER,PO, 1000 mcg,			
60s ea	**49348-0407-12**	6.39	
VITAMIN C			
TAB,PO, 250 mg, 100s ea	**49348-0080-10**	2.99	2.79
500 mg, 100s ea	**49348-0083-10**	3.29	2.89
250s ea	**49348-0083-19**	7.19	6.09
500s ea	**49348-0083-14**	12.19	
TER,PO, 1000 mg, 60s ea	**49348-0319-12**	6.19	
VITAMIN E			
SGL,PO (SOFTGEL)			
200 iu, 100s ea	**49348-0098-10**	4.49	4.69
400 iu, 100s ea	**49348-0099-10**	5.69	4.49
100s ea	**49348-0410-10**	10.19	10.99
(NATURAL BLEND,SOFTGEL)			
400 iu, 100s ea	**49348-0318-10**	8.19	
(WATER DISPERS)			
400 iu, 100s ea	**49348-0258-10**	7.69	6.59
(SOFTGEL)			
400 iu, 300s ea	**49348-0328-23**	14.09	
(NATURAL BLEND,SOFTGEL)			
1000 iu, 50s ea	**49348-0317-09**	8.19	
(SOFTGEL)			
1000 iu, 50s ea	**49348-0329-09**	9.99	
100s ea	**49348-0100-10**	14.09	14.39
VITAMIN E NATURAL			
PO (SOFTGEL)			
1000 iu, 50s ea	**49348-0136-09**	14.69	
WEEKLY PILL BOX			
DEV,NA (7 DAYS)			
ea	**49348-0731-01**	1.69	
WEEKLY PILL PLANNER			
NA (7 DAYS)			
ea	**49348-0732-01**	7.99	
WITCH HAZEL			
LIQ,TP, 480 ml	**49348-0805-38**	2.57	
ZINC NATURAL			
TAB,PO, 50 mg, 1000s ea	**49348-0141-10**	5.09	
VALUE DRUG LANCETS (Can-Am Care)			
DEV,NA (PRIVATE LABEL)			
200s ea	**38396-0323-00**	9.50	
VALUE PLUS ASSORTED FRUIT GLUCOSE (Can-Am Care)			
TAB,PO (CAFFEINE-FREE)			
4 gm, 50s ea	**38396-0557-25**	6.49	
VALUE PLUS GLUCOSE (Can-Am Care)			
GEL,PO (TROPICAL FRUIT)			
15 gm, 38 gm 3s	**38396-0550-25**	8.11	
VALUE PLUS GRAPE GLUCOSE (Can-Am Care)			
TAB,PO (CAFFEINE-FREE)			
4 gm, 50s ea	**38396-0543-25**	6.49	
VALUMARK PEN NEEDLES (Owen Mumford)			
DEV,NA (29GX12MM)			
100s ea	**08214-0297-35**	22.00	
(31GX6MM)			
100s ea	**08214-0907-35**	22.00	
(31GX8MM)			
100s ea	**08214-0307-35**	22.00	
VALUMARK SUPER THIN LANCETS (Owen Mumford)			
DEV,NA (30G,SINGLE-USE)			
100s ea	**08214-0657-35**	4.75	
VALUMARK ULTRA THIN LANCETS (Owen Mumford)			
DEV,NA (28G,SINGLE-USE)			
100s ea	**08214-0257-35**	4.75	
VANACHOL (GM Pharm)			
SGL,PO (SOFTGEL)			
240s ea	**58809-0747-90**	43.69	
VANADYL SULFATE (Mason Vit)			
TAB,PO (PF)			
10 mg, 90s ea	**11845-0120-09**	6.89	
(Nature's Bounty)			
CAP,PO (SF)			
60s ea	**74312-0769-00**	6.94	8.68
VANATAB DX (GM Pharm)			
TAB,PO, 12.5 mg-200 mg-30 mg,			
100s ea	**58809-0407-01**	81.55	
VANICREAM (Pharm Spec)			
CRE,TP (DYE-FREE,FRAGRANCE-FREE)			
120 gm	**45334-0300-04**	4.59	6.90
(1X170GM,SENSITIVE SKIN)			
170 gm	**45334-0340-06**	5.92	8.95
454 gm	**45334-0300-01**	10.43	15.70

PROD/MFR	HRI, UPC,NDC	AWP	SRP
(W/PUMP)			
454 gm	45334-0300-16	10.87	16.35
(PAIL,DYE-FREE)			
18160 gm	45334-0300-40	311.80	
SOA,TP (3.9 OZ,DYE-FREE)			
ea	45334-0320-39	2.09	3.15
VANICREAM LIP PROTECTANT (Pharm Spec)			
CRE,TP (SPF 30)			
2%-6%, 10 gm	45334-0330-35	3.29	4.95
VANICREAM LITE (Pharm Spec)			
LOT,TP (DYE-FREE,FRAGRANCE-FREE)			
240 ml	45334-0310-08	5.69	8.60
VANICREAM SPF 30 (Pharm Spec)			
CRE,TP (PF,DYE-FREE)			
5%-5%, 113 gm	45334-0333-04	9.93	14.95
VANICREAM SPF 60 (Pharm Spec)			
CRE,TP (PF,DYE-FREE)			
7.5%-7.5%, 113 gm	45334-0336-04	11.92	17.95
VANICREAM SUNSCREEN (Pharm Spec)			
CRE,TP (SPF 35)			
7.5%-8%, 120 gm	45334-0335-04	9.93	14.95
VANQUISH (Bayer HealthCare)			
TAB,PO (CAPLET)			
194 mg-227 mg-33 mg,			
100s ea	12843-0171-48	6.66	
VAPORX BALM (Geritrex)			
OIN,TP (1X50GM)			
4.8%-1.2%-2.6%, 50 gm	54162-0450-50	3.14	
VARIDIN (Med Prods Panamer)			
CAP,PO, 60s ea	00576-0501-60	6.60	
VARIDIN FORTE (Med Prods Panamer)			
CAP,PO (W/DIOSMIN)			
60s ea	00576-0503-60	11.58	
VARISAN VITALITY (Kramer-Novis)			
TAB,PO, 50s ea	52083-0529-50	7.10	
VASELINE PETROLATUM (Covidien)			
DRE,TP (STRIP,STERILE,.5"X72")			
72s ea	08080-4116-00	125.50	
72s ea	08080-4216-00	142.14	
(STRIP,STERILE,1"X36")			
72s ea	08080-4126-00	75.63	
72s ea	08080-4226-00	90.43	
(STRIP,STERILE,3"X18")			
72s ea	08080-4146-00	66.34	
72s ea	08080-4246-00	82.88	
(STRIP,STERILE,3"X36")			
72s ea	08080-4156-00	94.12	
72s ea	08080-4256-00	125.62	
(STRIP,STERILE,3"X9")			
72s ea	08080-4236-00	94.34	
(STRIP,STERILE,6"X36")			
72s ea	08080-4166-00	136.39	
72s ea	08080-4266-00	181.38	
(1X8")			
200s ea	08080-4176-01	164.47	
200s ea	08080-4276-01	198.93	
(3X9")			
200s ea	08080-4136-05	225.13	
VASELINE PETROLEUM JELLY (Covidien)			
OIN,TP (STERILE,PACKET,576X5GM)			
5 gm 576s	08080-4332-00	177.17	
(BULK PACKAGE,144X18GM)			
18 gm 144s	08080-4301-01	106.84	
(BULK PACKAGE,144X30GM)			
30 gm 144s	08080-4302-01	119.25	
(BULK PACKAGE,72X105GM)			
105 gm 72s	08080-4303-01	87.18	
VASOCON-A (Novartis Pharm)			
SOL,OP, 0.5%-0.05%,			
15 ml	58768-0881-15	5.63	
(Pharma Pac)			
REPACK			
SOL,OP, 0.5%-0.05%,			
15 ml	52959-0248-03	15.60	
15 ml	52959-0591-00	15.32	
VASOFLEX (Kramer-Novis)			
TAB,PO, 60s ea	52083-0335-60	15.00	12.00
VASOFLEX FORTE (Kramer-Novis)			
CAP,PO, 150 mg-150 mg-150 mg,			
90s ea	52083-0336-90	22.00	
VCF (Apothecus)			
FIL,VG (DISSOLVING)			
12s ea	48723-0400-10	4.04	
12s ea	48723-0400-20	4.04	
VCF CONTRACEPTIVE (Apothecus)			
FIL,VG, 28%, 3s ea	52925-0112-03	2.83	
6s ea	52925-0112-02	4.30	
12s ea	52925-0112-01	7.07	
FOA,VG (W/APPLICATOR)			
12.5%, 40 gm	52925-0312-14	9.22	
VCF PERSONAL LUBRICANT (Apothecus)			
GEL,TP, 71 gm	48723-0445-98	3.99	
VEG E-GEMS (Carlson,J.R.)			
SGL,PO (VEGETARIAN,PF,SF)			
400 iu, 90s ea	88395-0003-54	9.95	19.90
200s ea	88395-0003-52	14.95	29.90
VEGETABLE LAXATIVE (Family Phcy)			
PDR,PO (PRIVATE LABEL)			
3.4 gm/dose, 390 gm	52735-0509-54	5.39	5.99
VEGETABLE POWDER SMOOTH TEXTURE (AmerisourceBergen)			
PDR,PO (SF,PRIVATE LABEL,ORANGE)			
3.4 gm/5 ml, 283 gm	24385-0366-38	6.29	6.99
(Medicine Shoppe)			
PDR,PO (CITRUS)			
3.4 gm/dose, 609 gm	49614-0370-37	5.99	5.99
VEHICLE/N (Neutrogena)			
LIQ,TP, 51 ml	10812-0910-01	5.00	
(MILD)			
51 ml	10812-0940-01	5.00	
VEIN ERECT (Mason Vit)			
CAP,PO, 625 mg-12.5 mg-125 mg,			
80s ea	11845-0134-98	23.89	
VELVACHOL (Valeant Pharm Intl)			
CRE,TP, 420 gm	00064-2180-14	20.89	
VENASTAT (Pharmaton)			
CAP,PO, 300 mg, 30s ea	93190-0090-01	7.20	9.50
60s ea	93190-0090-02	11.80	14.40
VENCEDOR (Larkspur)			
OIN,TP, 45 gm	18864-0221-03	3.32	
VENI-PREP I (Abbott Hosp)			
DEV,NA, 60s ea	00074-2681-01	113.04	
VENI-PREP II (Abbott Hosp)			
DEV,NA, 60s ea	00074-2657-01	115.92	
VENI-PREP III (Abbott Hosp)			
DEV,NA (W/SITE-CARE DRESSNG)			
60s ea	00074-2665-01	143.28	
VENILOOP CONNECTOR (Abbott Hosp)			
DEV,NA (5" W/EXTENDED TUBING)			
120s ea	00074-8078-01	230.40	
(5", W/RESEAL)			
120s ea	00074-8079-01	1171.35	
VENTED Y-TYPE BLOOD PUMP (Abbott Hosp)			
DEV,NA (121",SECURE LOCK)			
24s ea	00074-1781-73	286.27	
VENTS (A. F. Hauser)			
LOZ,MM (CHERRY FLAVOR)			
400s ea	52637-0666-14	59.98	
VERACOLATE (Numark)			
ECT,PO, 5 mg, 100s ea	38485-0402-10	4.62	
VERATRUM ALBUM (Luyties)			
TAB,SL (6X)			
6 x, 500s ea	00618-9420-03	3.99	
5500s ea	00618-9420-10	30.32	
12 x, 500s ea	00622-9420-03	4.19	
5500s ea	00622-9420-10	31.83	
30 x, 500s ea	00624-9420-03	4.19	
5500s ea	00624-9420-10	31.83	
VERSALON ALL-PURPOSE SPONGES (Covidien)			
DEV,NA (4"X4",4 PLY,STERILE)			
800s ea	08080-8045-00	87.52	
(3"X4",4 PLY,STERILE)			
1200s ea	08080-8046-00	60.82	
(4"X4",4 PLY,STERILE)			
1200s ea	08080-8044-00	82.28	
1600s ea	08080-8047-00	216.00	
(3"X4",4 PLY,NON-STERILE)			
2000s ea	08080-9026-00	83.82	
(4"X4",4 PLY,NON-STERILE)			
2000s ea	08080-9024-00	98.20	
(3"X3",4 PLY,STERILE)			
2400s ea	08080-8043-00	110.88	
(2"X2",4 PLY,STERILE)			
3000s ea	08080-8042-00	100.14	
(3"X3",4 PLY,NON-STERILE)			
4000s ea	08080-9023-00	113.45	
(3"X4",3 PLY)			
4000s ea	08080-9136-00	118.08	
(4"X4",3 PLY,NON-STERILE)			
4000s ea	08080-9134-00	109.05	
(2"X2",3 PLY)			
5000s ea	08080-9132-00	48.84	
(2"X2",4 PLY,NON-STERILE)			
8000s ea	08080-9022-00	111.65	
VERSALON PERI-PADS (Covidien)			
DEV,NA (ADHESVEWINGDTABS,20X12)			
240s ea	08080-1580-00	32.99	
(REGULAR,3"X11",24X12)			
288s ea	08080-1380-00	38.00	
VERSALON WASHCLOTHS (Covidien)			
DEV,NA, 500s ea	08080-6360-00	31.73	
(10X50)			
500s ea	08080-6361-00	34.83	
VERVAIN (Ellon)			
SOL,SL (DROPS)			
10.5 ml	51762-0036-10		9.25
VEVSIVA XC (Convatec)			
DEV,NA (10"X8",ADHESIVE,SACRAL)			
5s ea	68455-0107-58	93.71	123.18
(6"X6",NON-ADHESIVE)			
5s ea	68455-0107-53	65.36	85.91
(7.5"X7.5",ADHESIVE)			
5s ea	68455-0107-59	72.58	95.39
(8"X7",ADHESIVE,HEEL)			
5s ea	68455-0107-57	82.69	108.68
(8"X8",NON-ADHESIVE)			
5s ea	68455-0107-54	118.13	155.26
(3"X3",NON-ADHESIVE)			
10s ea	68455-0107-51	51.19	67.28
(4.3"X4.3",NON-ADHESIVE)			
10s ea	68455-0107-52	62.30	81.89
(4"X4",ADHESIVE)			
10s ea	68455-0107-55	49.76	65.41
(5.5"X5.5",ADHESIVE)			
10s ea	68455-0107-56	70.80	93.06
VHC 2.25 (Nestle)			
LIQ,PO (VANILLA)			
250 ml	00065-9042-70	2.36	
VI-DAN D.C. (Vita-Rx)			
CAP,PO, 240 mg,			
1000s ea	49727-0153-05	19.95	
VI-STRESS (Rugby)			
TAB,PO, 60s ea	00536-4753-08	5.47	
VIACTIV (Phys Total Care)			
REPACK			
CTB,PO (CARAMEL,CARAMEL)			
500 mg-0.04 mg-100 iu,			
60s ea	54868-4846-00	9.17	
VIACTIV CALCIUM (McNeil)			
CTB,PO (SOFT CHEWS,RASPBERRY)			
500 mg-0.04 mg-100 iu,			
60s ea	00450-0219-60	6.91	
((CARAMEL),SOFT CHEWS)			
60s ea	00045-0103-03	6.91	
((MILK CHOCOLATE),SFTCHW)			
60s ea	00045-0102-03	6.91	
(CHOCOLATE MINT)			
60s ea	00045-0043-76	6.91	
(CARAMEL,SOFT CHEWS)			
90s ea	00045-0103-90	9.78	
(SOFT CHEWS)			
90s ea	00045-0102-90	9.78	
VIACTIV MULTI-VITAMIN (McNeil)			
CTB,PO (SOFT CHEWS)			
60s ea	00450-0162-60	7.38	
60s ea	00450-0164-60	7.38	
VIAL ADAPTERS, METAL SPIKE (Antares Pharma)			
DEV,NA (INT'L,MEDI-JECTORVISION)			
6s ea	55948-0315-10	39.95	39.95
VIAL ADAPTERS, PLASTIC SPIKE (Antares Pharma)			
DEV,NA (DMSTC,MEDI-JECTORVISION)			
6s ea	55948-0310-10	31.95	31.95
VIAL SYRINGE GUIDE (Apothecary)			
DEV,NA (KEEPS NEEDLES SHARP)			
ea	25715-0669-74	4.08	6.79
VIASORB (Covidien)			
DEV,NA, 100s ea	08080-4720-05	429.48	
(2X3")			
100s ea	08080-4726-41	179.90	
(4X6")			
100s ea	08080-4724-01	252.59	
(STERILE,7"X7")			
100s ea	08080-4725-00	374.85	
(Kendall)			
DEV,NA (STERILE,6"X10")			
100s ea	08884-4720-05	401.38	

PROD/MFR	HRI, UPC,NDC	AWP	SRP

VIBRANT HEALTH SAW PALMETTO (Major)
CAP,PO (PF,DAIRY-FREE)
450 mg, 100s ea 00904-5720-60 7.50

VICKS 44 COUGH RELIEF (P & G Company)
LIQ,PO (W/ACCUTIP)
10 mg/5 ml, 120 ml .. 37000-0513-04 4.00

VICKS 44D COUGH & HEAD CONGESTION (P & G Company)
LIQ,PO, 10 mg/5 ml-20 mg/5 ml,
120 ml 37000-0514-04 4.00
240 ml 37000-0514-08 6.38

VICKS 44E COUGH & CHEST CONGESTION (P & G Company)
LIQ,PO (NON-DROWSY)
20 mg/15 ml-200 mg/15 ml,
120 ml 37000-0515-04 4.00
235 ml 37000-0515-08 6.38

VICKS 44E PEDIATRIC (P & G Company)
LIQ,PO (AF,CHERRY)
10 mg/15 ml-100 mg/15 ml,
120 ml 37000-0520-04 4.00

VICKS 44M COUGH COLD & FLU (P & G Company)
SYR,PO, 240 ml 37000-0516-08 6.38
120 ml 37000-0516-04 4.00

VICKS 44M PEDIATRIC (P & G Company)
LIQ,PO (AF)
120 ml 37000-0521-04 4.00

VICKS COUGH DROPS (P & G Company)
LOZ,MM (BOX,CHERRY)
20s ea.............. 37000-0548-04 0.48
(CHERRY)
20s ea.............. 37000-0547-04 0.48

(Phys Total Care)
REPACK
LOZ,MM (MENTHOL)
30s ea.............. 54868-2427-00 1.14

VICKS DAYQUIL MULTI-SYMPTOM (P & G Company)
LIQ,PO (NON-DROWSY,AF)
180 ml 37000-0511-06 4.39
SGL,PO (NON-DROWSY,AF,SOFTGEL)
250 mg-10 mg-30 mg,
12s ea............ 37000-0537-05 4.33
20s ea 37000-0537-07 5.76
36s ea 37000-0018-80 9.25

VICKS NYQUIL CHILDREN'S (P & G Company)
LIQ,PO (AF,CHERRY)
118 ml 37000-0508-04 5.05

(Southwood)
REPACK
LIQ,PO (AF,CHERRY)
118 ml 58016-4149-01 6.10

VICKS NYQUIL MULTI-SYMPTOM (P & G Company)
SGL,PO (LIQUICAP)
12s ea.............. 37000-0539-02 4.33
20s ea 37000-0539-04 5.76
36s ea 37000-0018-90 9.25
SOL,PO, 180 ml 37000-0517-06 4.39
180 ml 37000-0518-06 4.39
300 ml 2s 37000-0517-07 5.82
300 ml 2s 37000-0518-07 5.82

VICKS SINEX (P & G Company)
SPR,NS, 0.5%, 15 ml 37000-0540-05 4.66
(ULTRA FINE MIST PUMP,AF)
0.5%, 15 ml 37000-0541-05 5.24

VICKS SINEX 12 HOUR (P & G Company)
SPR,NS (AF)
0.05%, 15 ml 37000-0542-05 4.68
(ULTRA FINE MIST PUMP,AF)
0.05%, 15 ml 37000-0543-05 5.54

VICKS VAPOR INHALER (P & G Company)
STI,NS, 50 mg, ea 37000-0536-07 3.37

VICKS VAPORUB (P & G Company)
CRE,TP (TUBE)
4.7%-1.2%-2.6%,
60 gm............ 37000-0529-02 4.33
OIN,TP, 4.2%-1.2%-2.6%,
180 gm........... 37000-0544-06 8.42
(1X50GM)
4.8%-1.2%-2.6%,
50 gm............ 23900-0003-61 3.43

VICKS VAPOSTEAM (P & G Company)
LIQ,IH, 120 ml........... 37000-0522-04 4.33
240 ml 37000-0522-08 6.71

VICKS VITAMIN C (P & G Company)
LOZ,MM (ORANGE)
25 mg, 20s ea....... 23900-0001-29 0.48

VIGOMAR FORTE (Marlop)
TAB,PO, 100s ea.......... 12939-0304-10 6.75

VIGOREX (A. G. Marin)
CAP,PO (SF)
60s ea.............. 12539-0050-60 16.65

VIGORTOL (Rugby)
LIQ,PO (SHERRY)
480 ml 00536-2380-85 8.69

VIMAR (Marlop)
SYR,PO, 240 ml 12939-0135-08 6.75

VIMAR W/IRON (Marlop)
SYR,PO, 240 ml 12939-0504-08 7.50

VINCE (Lee Pharm)
PDR,MM, 45 gm.......... 23558-0686-10 5.16
45 gm 24s.......... 23558-0686-11 123.84
120 gm 23558-0686-00 7.68
120 gm 12s 23558-0686-01 92.16

VINE (Ellon)
SOL,SL (DROPS)
10.5 ml............. 51762-0037-10 9.25

VINYL GLOVES HEAVY-DUTY (Allerderm Labs.)
DEV,NA (1PAIR,LARGE)
ea.................. 34674-0413-30 1.18
(1PAIR,MEDIUM)
ea.................. 34674-0413-20 1.18
(1PAIR,SMALL)
ea.................. 34674-0413-10 1.18

VIRA FEMALE (Natl Vitamin)
CAP,PO (PF,SF)
60s ea.............. 54629-0011-69 4.91 8.19

VISCOPASTE PB7 (Smith & Nephew)
PAS,TP (3"X10 YDS)
10%, ea 00223-0415-04 143.79 115.03

VISI-FLOW IRRIGATION SLEEVE TAIL CLOSURE (Convatec)
DEV,NA, 10s ea 68455-0107-07 21.53 28.02

VISI-FLOW STOMA CONE (Convatec)
DEV,NA, ea............... 68455-0107-08 10.96 14.27

VISINE (Johnson & Johnson)
SOL,OP (ORIGINAL)
0.05%, 15 ml 74300-0008-03 4.02
30 ml 74300-0003-08 5.71

(Southwood)
REPACK
SOL,OP, 0.05%, 15 ml..... 58016-9232-01 4.86

VISINE A.C. (Johnson & Johnson)
SOL,OP, 0.05%-0.25%,
15 ml............. 74300-0004-01 4.02
30 ml 74300-0004-02 5.71

VISINE ADVANCED RELIEF (Johnson & Johnson)
SOL,OP (1X8ML)
0.1%-1%-1%-0.05%,
8 ml.............. 74300-0081-48 1.45
15 ml 74300-0008-48 4.02
30 ml 74300-0008-49 5.71

VISINE ALL DAY EYE ITCH RELIEF (Johnson & Johnson)
SOL,OP (1X5ML)
0.025%, 5 ml 12547-0493-17 9.91

VISINE FOR CONTACTS (Johnson & Johnson)
SOL,OP (REWETTING)
15 ml............. 74300-0012-53 4.02
30 ml 74300-0034-71 5.71

VISINE L.R. (Johnson & Johnson)
SOL,OP (LONG LASTING)
0.025%, 15 ml 74300-0004-03 4.02
30 ml 74300-0004-04 5.71

VISINE PURE TEARS (Johnson & Johnson)
SOL,OP (32X0.3ML,DRY EYE RELIEF)
0.2%-0.2%-1%,
0.3 ml 32s......... 12547-0493-32 6.96
(DRY EYE RELIEF)
0.2%-0.2%-1%,
9.5 ml............ 74300-0081-78 6.96

VISINE TEARS (Johnson & Johnson)
SOL,OP (SINGLE USE CONTAINER)
0.2%-0.2%-1%,
0.4 ml 28s........ 74300-0010-70 5.82
(1X15ML)
0.2%-0.2%-1%,
15 ml............ 74300-0010-67 4.96
(1X30ML)
0.2%-0.2%-1%,
30 ml............ 74300-0010-69 6.96
(1X15ML)
0.2%-0.36%-1%,
15 ml............ 42002-0207-05 6.96

VISINE TOTAL EYE SOOTHING WIPES (Johnson & Johnson)
PAD,TP, 30s ea 74300-0493-41 5.71

VISINE TOTALITY (Johnson & Johnson)
SOL,OP (MULTI-SYMPTOM)
15 ml............... 42002-0209-05 5.71

VISINE-A (Johnson & Johnson)
SOL,OP, 0.025%-0.3%,
15 ml.............. 05016-0505-05 4.96
15 ml 74300-0001-58 4.90
(2X15ML,TWIN PACK)
0.025%-0.3%,
15 ml 2s........... 12547-0493-36 7.72

VISION EYE (Global Source)
SOL,OP, 0.05%, 15 ml..... 59618-0930-28 1.95

VISION FORMULA (Cardinal Health)
TAB,PO (PRIVATE LABEL)
60s ea.............. 37205-0079-72 5.18

VISION NEEDLE-FREE KIT A (Antares Pharma)
DEV,NA (4 SRN,SM ORIFICE,ADAPT)
ea................ 55948-0122-10 31.95 31.95
(4SRN,2ADAPT-METAL SPIKE)
ea.................. 55948-0222-10 34.95 34.95

VISION NEEDLE-FREE KIT B (Antares Pharma)
DEV,NA (4 SRN,M ORIFICE,2 ADAPT)
ea................ 55948-0124-10 31.95 31.95
(4SRN,2ADAPT-METAL SPIKE)
ea.................. 55948-0224-10 34.95 34.95

VISION NEEDLE-FREE KIT C (Antares Pharma)
DEV,NA (4 SRN,LG ORIFICE,2ADAPT)
ea................ 55948-0126-10 31.95 31.95
(4SRN,2ADAPT-METAL SPIKE)
ea.................. 55948-0226-10 34.95 34.95

VISION SELECT MULTI-PURPOSE (Allergan Inc)
SOL,NA, 355 ml 00023-7635-12 3.86

VIT A/VIT D (Key Company)
A & D JR.
SGL,PO, 10000 iu-400 iu,
100s ea........... 11694-0693-01 3.75
250s ea........... 11694-0693-02 7.50

(Freeda)
VITAMIN A & D
TAB,PO (PF,SF,DYE-FREE)
10000 iu-400 iu,
100s ea........... 10432-0064-01 4.77 7.95

(Key Company)
SGL,PO (SOFTGEL)
25000 u-1000 u,
100s ea........... 11694-0865-01 4.00
1000s ea 11694-0865-05 31.00

(Mason Vit)
CAP,PO, 10000 iu-400 iu,
100s ea........... 11845-0071-01 5.11
SGL,PO, 100s ea.......... 11845-0053-11 3.67

VIT B COMP/VIT C (Nature's Bounty)
B COMPLEX + C
TER,PO (PF,SF)
100s ea............ 74312-0005-30 8.39

(Basic Vitamins)
B-COMPLEX W/VITAMIN C
CAP,PO, 100s ea.......... 00761-0102-30 3.20
240s ea............ 00761-0102-48 6.00

(Medicine Shoppe)
TAB,PO, 100s ea.......... 49614-0620-78 4.49 4.49
HIGH POTENCY B-COMPLEX W/C
PO (CAPLET)
130s ea............. 49614-0577-81 6.69 6.69

(Mason Vit)
VITAMIN B COMPLEX W/C
CAP,PO, 100s ea.......... 11845-0053-51 7.11

(Consolidated Midland)
VITAMIN B COMPLEX W/VITAMIN C
CAP,PO, 100s ea.......... 00223-0046-01 5.00
1000s ea 00223-0046-02 32.50

(Pharmavite)
VITAMIN B COMPLEX/VITAMIN C
TAB,PO (CAPLET)
100s ea............. 31604-0013-38 4.18

VIT B-6 (Dispensing Solutions)
REPACK
TAB,PO, 100 mg, 9s ea 66336-0312-09 2.50

PROD/MFR	HRI, UPC,NDC	AWP	SRP
VIT C/VIT E (Nature's Bounty)			
C & E			
CAP,PO (PF,SF,SOFTGEL)			
500 mg-400 iu,			
50s ea	74312-0012-60		9.65
250s ea	74312-0012-63		32.99
VITA DROPS INFANTS (Major)			
LIQ,PO, 50 ml	00904-5099-50	14.75	
VITA DROPS W/IRON INFANTS (Major)			
PO, 50 ml	00904-5100-50	14.75	
VITA HEALTH POLYETHYLENE GLYCOL 3350 (Nexgen)			
PDS,PO (1X119GM)			
17 gm/dose, 119 gm	00722-7116-01	5.07	
(1X238GM)			
17 gm/dose, 238 gm	00722-7116-02	8.97	
(1X510GM)			
17 gm/dose, 510 gm	00722-7116-03	17.52	
VITA ZINC (Major)			
TAB,PO, 60s ea	00904-2754-52	7.20	
VITA-BEE W/C (Rugby)			
TAB,PO (CAPTAB)			
100s ea	00536-4763-01	4.46	
VITA-C CRYSTALS (Freeda)			
PDR,PO (PF,SF)			
4 gm/packet, 100 gm	10432-0150-01	7.32	12.20
VITA-COLD (Health Products Corp)			
TAB,PO (PF,SF)			
30s ea	39686-0014-97	3.00	
VITA-MIN (Bio-Tech Pharm)			
CAP,PO, 100s ea	53191-0240-01	19.95	
180s ea	53191-0240-18	29.95	
VITA-RAY (Gordon)			
CRE,TP, 15 gm	10481-3014-01	5.20	
75 gm	10481-3014-02	12.85	
VITABASIC COMPLETE (Basic Vitamins)			
TAB,PO, 100s ea	00761-0873-20	3.60	
VITABASIC SENIOR (Basic Vitamins)			
TAB,PO, 100s ea	00761-0750-20	4.20	
VITABESE (Legere)			
CAP,PO, 1000s ea	25332-1044-01	55.00	
VITACARE (S.S.S.)			
TAB,PO, 30s ea	12258-0136-30	2.90	4.35
VITACARE ANTIOXIDANT (Pfeiffer)			
SGL,PO (P.F,PF,SF,SOFTGEL)			
60s ea	00927-0013-60	7.19	12.84
VITACARE ANTIOXIDANT COMPLETE (Pfeiffer)			
TAB,PO, 120s ea	00927-0012-12	7.22	12.99
VITACARE MULTIPLE VITAMINS/MINERALS (Pfeiffer)			
TAB,PO (PF,SF)			
120s ea	00927-0011-12	7.22	12.99
VITACARE PRENATAL (Pfeiffer)			
TAB,PO, 120s ea	00927-0010-12	7.22	12.99
VITAJOULE (VITAFLO, LLC)			
PDS,PO (1X500GM)			
500 gm	50600-0504-41	12.95	16.19
VITAL HIGH NITROGEN (Abbott)			
PDR,PO (PACKET,VANILLA)			
79 gm 6s	70074-0407-66	50.39	
VITAL JR (Abbott)			
LIQ,PO (GLUTEN-FREE)			
240 ml	70074-0597-61	8.76	
240 ml	70074-0597-63	8.76	
VITALCARE ADJUSTABLE DEPTH SAFETY LANCETS (Diagnostic)			
DEV,NA (26G,PRIVATE LABEL)			
100s ea	08321-0001-70	31.08	
VITALCARE LANCETS (Diagnostic)			
DEV,NA (28G,PULL TOP)			
30s ea	08321-2402-28	3.30	
(28G,TWIST TOP)			
30s ea	08321-2401-28	3.30	
(30G,PULL TOP)			
100s ea	08321-2401-10	10.30	
(30G,TWIST TOP)			
100s ea	08321-0810-30	10.30	
(W/ LANCET ADAPTER)			
100s ea	08321-0001-23	10.30	
(28G,PRIVATE LABEL)			
200s ea	08321-0810-38	14.68	
(Vitalcare)			
DEV,NA (28G,PULL TOP)			
100s ea	08321-0811-28	10.30	
(28G,TWIST TOP)			
100s ea	08321-0810-28	10.30	
VITALCARE LANCING DEVICE (Vitalcare)			
DEV,NA (ADJUSTABLE DEPTH)			
ea	08321-0832-25	16.37	
VITALCARE SAFETY LANCETS (Diagnostic)			
DEV,NA (21G,PRIVATE LABEL)			
100s ea	08321-2401-30	19.19	
(26G,PRIVATE LABEL)			
100s ea	08321-2401-60	19.19	
VITAMIN A (ADH)			
SGL,PO (PF,SF)			
10000 iu, 100s ea	60142-0746-01	2.25	4.50
(Basic Vitamins)			
SGL,PO, 10000 iu,			
100s ea	00761-0433-10	1.60	
(Carlson,J.R.)			
SGL,PO (SF,SALT-FREE,WHEAT-FREE)			
15000 iu, 120s ea	88395-0011-01	4.45	8.90
240s ea	88395-0011-02	7.75	15.50
(WITH PECTIN,PF,SF)			
25000 iu, 100s ea	88395-0011-61	5.45	10.90
(PF,SF,CORN-FREE)			
25000 iu, 250s ea	88395-0011-32	11.25	22.50
(WITH PECTIN,PF,SF)			
25000 iu, 300s ea	88395-0011-63	13.85	27.70
(Consolidated Midland)			
SGL,PO, 10000 iu,			
100s ea	00223-1739-01	3.25	
1000s ea	00223-1739-02	17.50	
(Health Products Corp)			
SGL,PO (PF,SF,SOFTGEL)			
10000 iu, 100s ea	39686-0011-00	2.65	
(Major)			
SGL,PO, 10000 iu,			
100s ea	00904-2085-60	3.05	
(Marlex)			
SGL,PO (SOFTGEL)			
10000 iu, 100s ea	10135-0214-01	1.79	
25000 iu, 100s ea	10135-0128-01	2.57	
(Mason Vit)			
SGL,PO, 10000 iu,			
100s ea	11845-0059-21	3.44	
100s ea	11845-0059-31	4.11	
(PF,SF,SOFTGEL)			
25000 u, 100s ea	11845-0069-01	5.11	
(Nature's Bounty)			
SGL,PO (PF,SF,SOFTGEL)			
10000 iu, 100s ea	74312-0064-80		4.19
(PF,SF)			
10000 iu, 100s ea	74312-0010-20		3.95
(Pharmavite)			
SGL,PO (SOFTGEL)			
8000 iu, 100s ea	31604-0013-06	2.24	
(WATER SOLUBLE,SOFTGEL)			
10000 iu, 100s ea	31604-0013-12	2.40	
(Phys Total Care)			
REPACK			
SGL,PO, 10000 iu,			
100s ea	54868-3740-00	11.94	
(SOLUABLE)			
25000 u, 100s ea	54868-3456-01	9.75	
VITAMIN A & BETA CAROTENE (Freeda)			
TAB,PO, 25000 iu,			
100s ea	10432-0235-01	8.37	13.95
VITAMIN A & D (Basic Vitamins)			
CAP,PO, 10000 iu-400 iu,			
100s ea	00761-0432-10	1.60	
(Consolidated Midland)			
OIN,TP, 4 gm 144s	00223-0035-04	21.00	
60 gm	00223-4100-60	1.80	
120 gm	00223-4100-11	2.25	
454 gm	00223-4100-02	4.50	
SGL,PO, 100s ea	00223-1810-01	2.95	
1000s ea	00223-1810-02	19.50	
(Fougera)			
OIN,TP (UNIT OF USE)			
5 gm 144s	00168-0035-45	25.30	
60 gm	00168-0035-01	2.16	
120 gm	00168-0035-04	3.96	
454 gm	00168-0035-16	11.40	
(Major)			
OIN,TP (1X454GM)			
15.5%-53.4%, 454 gm	00904-5843-27	7.38	
(Qualitest)			
OIN,TP, 120 gm	00603-0410-54	2.40	
(Teva)			
OIN,TP, 60 gm	00182-0763-43	1.80	
454 gm	00182-0763-45	11.00	
(A-S Medication)			
REPACK			
OIN,TP, 57 gm	54569-5639-00	2.84	
(Dispensing Solutions)			
REPACK			
OIN,TP, 57 gm	55045-1738-07	3.59	
(Phys Total Care)			
REPACK			
OIN,TP (1X56.7GM)			
56.7 gm	54868-2877-02	7.82	
VITAMIN A & D NATURAL (Cardinal Health)			
SGL,PO (PRIVATE LABEL,SOFTGEL)			
1250 iu-135 iu,			
100s ea	37205-0070-78	3.51	
VITAMIN A NATURAL (Carlson,J.R.)			
SGL,PO (SOFTGEL)			
10000 iu, 100s ea	88395-0011-11	2.75	5.50
250s ea	88395-0011-12	5.45	10.90
25000 u, 100s ea	88395-0011-31	5.45	10.90
VITAMIN A PALMITATE (Freeda)			
A-PALMITATE-10			
TAB,PO (PF,SF,DYE-FREE)			
10000 iu, 100s ea	10432-0061-01	3.69	6.15
VITAMIN A PALMITATE (Freeda)			
PO (PF,SF,DYE-FREE)			
10000 iu, 250s ea	10432-0061-02	7.38	12.30
15000 iu, 100s ea	10432-0301-01	4.77	7.95
250s ea	10432-0301-02	9.54	15.90
VITAMIN A SOLUBILIZED (Carlson,J.R.)			
SGL,PO (SOFTGEL)			
10000 iu, 100s ea	88395-0011-21	5.95	11.90
250s ea	88395-0011-22	12.45	24.90
VITAMIN A-NATURAL (Key Company)			
SGL,PO (SOFTGEL)			
10000 iu, 100s ea	11694-0127-02	3.25	
VITAMIN A-NATURAL-25 (Key Company)			
PO (SOFTGEL)			
25000 u, 100s ea	11694-0127-01	4.00	
1000s ea	11694-0127-03	30.00	
VITAMIN A/VITAMIN D (Nature's Bounty)			
A & D			
TAB,PO (PF,SF)			
100s ea	74312-0010-40		3.99
VITAMIN A/VITAMIN D (Carlson,J.R.)			
CAP,PO (SOFTGEL)			
10000 iu-400 iu,			
100s ea	88395-0012-11	3.45	6.90
300s ea	88395-0012-13	8.70	17.40
25000 iu-1000 iu,			
100s ea	88395-0012-41	5.95	11.90
250s ea	88395-0012-42	11.75	23.50
(Mason Vit)			
CAP,PO (PF,SF,SOFTGEL)			
25000 iu-400 iu,			
100s ea	11845-0113-11	5.33	
(Pharmavite)			
CAP,PO (SOFTGEL)			
5000 iu-400 iu,			
100s ea	31604-0013-13	2.32	
(Nature's Bounty)			
VITAMINS A & D			
CAP,PO (SOFTGEL)			
5000 iu-400 iu,			
100s ea	74312-0043-01		3.59
VITAMIN A&D (ADH)			
SGL,PO (PF,SF)			
100s ea	60142-0748-01	2.48	4.95
(Geritrex)			
OIN,TP (1X60GM)			
55%, 60 gm	54162-0000-02	1.39	
VITAMIN ABC PLUS (Nature's Bounty)			
TAB,PO, 100s ea	74312-0000-70		7.35
250s ea	74312-0000-73		14.89
VITAMIN ABC PLUS SENIOR (Nature's Bounty)			
PO, 60s ea	74312-0071-90		4.99

PROD/MFR	HRI, UPC, NDC	AWP	SRP
VITAMIN B COMPLEX (Health Products Corp)			
ALL 100 SUPER B COMPLEX			
TAB,PO (PF,SF)			
100s ea	**39686-0012-34**	10.50	
TER,PO, 50s ea	**39686-0012-38**	6.05	
ALL 50 SUPER B COMPLEX			
TAB,PO (PF,SF)			
50s ea	**39686-0012-26**	3.90	
100s ea	**39686-0012-29**	6.00	
(Nature's Bounty)			
B COMPLEX			
TAB,PO (PF,SF)			
100s ea	**74312-0057-60**		5.89
(PF)			
100s ea	**74312-0064-70**		5.59
(Rexall)			
TAB,PO, 75s ea	**30768-0000-55**	1.66	2.52
(Nature's Bounty)			
B COMPLEX & B12			
TAB,PO (PF,SF)			
90s ea	**74312-0001-90**		3.89
(ADH)			
B COMPLEX 50			
TAB,PO, 100s ea	**60142-0116-10**	6.25	12.50
(Rexall)			
B-100 COMPLEX			
TAB,PO (PF,SF)			
50s ea	**30768-0010-92**	4.70	7.12
60s ea	**30768-0012-15**	2.22	3.37
B-50 COMPLEX			
PO (PF,SF)			
60s ea	**30768-0012-14**	3.38	5.12
(Freeda)			
B-COMPLEX			
TAB,PO (PF,SF,DYE-FREE)			
100s ea	**10432-0294-01**	6.27	10.45
250s ea	**10432-0294-02**	12.54	20.90
(Nature's Bounty)			
B100			
TER,PO (PF,SF)			
100s ea	**74312-0028-12**		19.29
(Mason Vit)			
B100 COMPLEX ULTRA			
TAB,PO (PF,SF)			
60s ea	**11845-0064-45**	10.78	
100s ea	**11845-0064-41**	15.89	
(Nature's Bounty)			
B50			
TAB,PO (PF,SF)			
50s ea	**74312-0005-80**		6.39
100s ea	**74312-0005-83**		10.75
TER,PO, 60s ea	**74312-0049-70**		7.85
(Major)			
BALANCED B100			
TAB,PO, 50s ea	**00904-3192-51**	6.60	
BALANCED B50			
PO (CAPLET)			
100s ea	**00904-3177-60**	7.50	
TER,PO, 60s ea	**00904-4184-52**	6.34	
(Freeda)			
KOBEE			
TAB,PO (PF,SF,DYE-FREE)			
100s ea	**10432-0032-01**	5.25	8.75
QUIN B STRONG			
PO (PF,SF,DYE-FREE)			
100s ea	**10432-0052-01**	5.97	9.95
250s ea	**10432-0052-02**	11.94	19.90
500s ea	**10432-0052-03**	20.97	34.95
(Health Products Corp)			
SUPER B COMPLEX W/B-12			
TAB,PO (PF,SF)			
100s ea	**39686-0012-71**	3.50	
(Basic Vitamins)			
SUPER B50 COMPLEX			
CAP,PO, 100s ea	**00761-0839-20**	4.80	
VITAMIN B COMPLEX (Marlex)			
TAB,PO, 100s ea	**10135-0120-01**	1.21	
1000s ea	**10135-0120-10**	5.92	
(Mason Vit)			
CAP,PO, 100s ea	**11845-0060-11**	5.00	
(Rugby)			
SGL,PO (PF,SF,SOFTGEL)			
100s ea	**00536-4787-01**	4.58	
(Consolidated Midland)			
VITAMIN B COMPLEX 100			
ELI,PO, 480 ml	**00223-6217-01**	6.50	

PROD/MFR	HRI, UPC, NDC	AWP	SRP
TAB,PO, 100s ea	**00223-2330-01**	2.50	
1000s ea	**00223-2330-02**	17.50	
(Major)			
VITAMIN B COMPLEX W/B12			
TAB,PO, 100s ea	**00904-4181-60**	3.85	
(Albertson's)			
VITAMIN B COMPLEX WITH E/C/ZINC			
TAB,PO, 60s ea	**04000-0002-20**	6.60	
(Nature's Bounty)			
VITAMIN B100			
TAB,PO (PF,SF)			
50s ea	**74312-0007-70**		9.75
100s ea	**74312-0007-72**		17.99
TER,PO, 50s ea	**74312-0028-10**		10.29
(Mason Vit)			
VITAMIN B50 SUPER COMPLEX			
TAB,PO, 100s ea	**11845-0069-41**	11.67	
VITAMIN B COMPLEX + C (Marlex)			
CAP,PO, 60s ea	**10135-0157-60**	1.90	
100s ea	**10135-0157-01**	2.81	
130s ea	**10135-0157-63**	2.35	
1000s ea	**10135-0157-10**	18.63	
VITAMIN B COMPLEX WITH VITAMIN C			
(Dispensing Solutions)			
REPACK			
CAP,PO, 100s ea	**55045-3476-01**	8.00	
VITAMIN B PLUS+ OMEGA-3 ETHYL ESTER			
(Ocean Blue)			
SGL,PO (NATURAL ORANGE,SOFTGEL)			
6 mcg-725 mg-8 mg,			
60s ea	**27912-0085-40**	9.99	
120s ea	**27912-0085-41**	14.99	
VITAMIN B-1 (Amneal)			
TAB,PO, 100 mg, 100s ea	**65162-0456-10**	3.65	
1000s ea	**65162-0456-11**	32.60	
VITAMIN B-6 (Core)			
REPACK			
TAB,PO, 50 mg, 30s ea	**33358-0357-30**	6.48	
60s ea	**33358-0357-60**	8.86	
80s ea	**33358-0357-80**	11.13	
90s ea	**33358-0357-90**	13.29	
100s ea	**33358-0357-00**	15.45	
120s ea	**33358-0357-01**	20.80	
100 mg, 30s ea	**33358-0358-30**	7.98	
60s ea	**33358-0358-60**	10.51	
100s ea	**33358-0358-00**	17.50	
(Physician Partner)			
REPACK			
TAB,PO, 100 mg, 30s ea	**21695-0190-30**	9.99	
(Vibranta)			
REPACK			
TAB,PO, 50 mg, 30s ea	**57866-3621-01**	8.50	
VITAMIN B1 (Consolidated Midland)			
THIAMINE HCL			
TAB,PO, 50 mg, 100s ea	**00223-2243-01**	1.95	
1000s ea	**00223-2243-02**	10.95	
100 mg, 100s ea	**00223-2244-01**	2.50	
1000s ea	**00223-2244-02**	17.50	
250 mg, 100s ea	**00223-2245-01**	3.75	
1000s ea	**00223-2245-02**	32.50	
500 mg, 100s ea	**00223-2246-01**	7.00	
1000s ea	**00223-2246-02**	57.50	
(Marlex)			
TAB,PO, 50 mg, 100s ea	**10135-0131-01**	1.06	
1000s ea	**10135-0131-10**	6.00	
100 mg, 30s ea	**10135-0132-30**	1.17	
90s ea	**10135-0132-90**	2.65	
100s ea	**10135-0132-01**	1.50	
(BLISTER PACK)			
100 mg, 100s ea UD	**10135-0168-13**	2.20	
1000s ea	**10135-0132-10**	10.08	
250 mg, 100s ea	**10135-0322-01**	2.23	
(Key Company)			
THIAMINE-100			
TAB,PO, 100 mg, 100s ea	**11694-0730-01**	3.00	
1000s ea	**11694-0730-10**	18.00	
VITAMIN B1 (Basic Vitamins)			
TAB,PO, 100 mg, 100s ea	**00761-0555-20**	1.90	
(Cardinal Health)			
TAB,PO (PRIVATE LABEL)			
100 mg, 100s ea	**37205-0084-78**	3.53	
(Carlson,J.R.)			
TAB,PO, 100 mg, 100s ea	**88395-0021-11**	3.25	6.50
250s ea	**88395-0021-12**	6.95	13.90

PROD/MFR	HRI, UPC, NDC	AWP	SRP
(Family Phcy)			
TAB,PO (PRIVATE LABEL)			
100 mg, 100s ea	**52735-0045-01**	1.55	2.99
(Freeda)			
TAB,PO (PF,SF,DYE-FREE)			
100 mg, 100s ea	**10432-0081-01**	4.17	6.95
250 mg, 100s ea	**10432-0082-01**	5.97	9.95
(PURE)			
500 mg, 100s ea	**10432-0083-01**	7.95	13.25
(Health Products Corp)			
TAB,PO (PF,SF)			
250 mg, 100s ea	**39686-0011-12**	4.20	
(Major)			
TAB,PO, 100 mg, 100s ea	**00904-0544-60**	3.41	
1000s ea	**00904-0544-80**	24.25	
250 mg, 100s ea	**00904-4177-60**	5.65	
(Mason Vit)			
TAB,PO, 50 mg, 100s ea	**11845-0056-41**	4.11	
100 mg, 100s ea	**11845-0056-51**	5.89	
250 mg, 100s ea	**11845-0056-61**	8.33	
(PF)			
500 mg, 60s ea	**11845-0073-15**	10.00	
(Nature's Bounty)			
TAB,PO (PF,SF)			
100 mg, 100s ea	**74312-0016-70**		4.65
(Pharmavite)			
TAB,PO, 100 mg, 100s ea	**31604-0012-81**	2.77	
(Prime Marketing)			
TAB,PO, 50 mg, 100s ea	**62107-0060-01**	2.85	
100 mg, 100s ea	**62107-0059-01**	2.95	
(Rugby)			
TAB,PO, 50 mg, 100s ea	**00536-4678-01**	2.17	
(PF,SF,DYE-FREE)			
100 mg, 100s ea	**00536-4680-01**	4.50	
1000s ea	**00536-4680-10**	20.25	
(A-S Medication)			
REPACK			
TAB,PO (PF,SF,DYE-FREE)			
100 mg, 30s ea	**54569-2880-01**	1.35	
100s ea	**54569-2880-00**	4.50	
VITAMIN B12 (Rexall)			
B-12			
TAB,PO (PF,SF)			
500 mcg, 75s ea	**30768-0001-69**	2.52	3.82
(PF)			
1000 mcg, 60s ea	**30768-0001-75**	3.36	5.08
TER,PO (PF,SF)			
1500 mcg, 60s ea	**30768-0013-10**	3.81	5.77
VITAMIN B12 (ADH)			
TAB,SL, 1000 mcg,			
100s ea	**60142-0117-10**	5.25	10.50
(AmerisourceBergen)			
TAB,PO (PRIVATE LABEL)			
500 mcg, 100s ea	**24385-0117-78**	3.77	4.19
(Basic Vitamins)			
TAB,PO, 100 mcg,			
100s ea	**00761-0372-20**	1.80	
500 mcg, 100s ea	**00761-0440-20**	3.00	
TER,PO, 1000 mcg,			
60s ea	**00761-0221-20**	2.30	
(Carlson,J.R.)			
TAB,SL, 1000 mcg,			
90s ea	**88395-0024-34**	5.95	11.90
(Consolidated Midland)			
TAB,PO, 50 mcg, 100s ea	**00223-2283-01**	2.25	
1000s ea	**00223-2283-02**	19.50	
100 mcg, 100s ea	**00223-2285-01**	4.50	
1000s ea	**00223-2285-02**	19.75	
500 mcg, 100s ea	**00223-2286-01**	3.95	
1000s ea	**00223-2286-02**	29.50	
1000 mcg, 100s ea	**00223-2287-01**	4.75	
1000s ea	**00223-2287-02**	42.50	
(Freeda)			
LOZ,MM (PF,SF,DYE-FREE)			
100 mcg, 100s ea	**10432-0070-01**	4.50	7.50
250 mcg, 100s ea	**10432-0158-01**	5.37	8.95
250s ea	**10432-0158-02**	10.74	
500 mcg, 100s ea	**10432-0241-01**	6.27	10.45
250s ea	**10432-0241-02**	12.54	20.90
TAB,PO, 50 mcg, 100s ea	**10432-0091-01**	3.54	5.90
(Health Products Corp)			
TAB,PO (PF,SF)			
1000 mcg, 50s ea	**39686-0011-35**	3.25	

PROD/MFR	HRI, UPC,NDC	AWP	SRP
(Major)			
TAB,PO, 100 mcg,			
130s ea	**00904-1132-13**	2.75	
250 mcg, 130s ea	**00904-4218-13**	4.30	
500 mcg, 130s ea	**00904-3207-13**	6.05	
1000 mcg, 130s ea	**00904-4217-13**	7.75	
(Marlex)			
TAB,PO, 100 mcg,			
130s ea	**10135-0330-63**	1.12	
250 mcg, 130s ea	**10135-0331-63**	1.71	
500 mcg, 130s ea	**10135-0332-63**	2.21	
1000 mcg, 130s ea	**10135-0329-63**	2.88	
(Mason Vit)			
TAB,PO, 50 mcg, 100s ea	**11845-0057-31**	3.00	
(PF)			
68 mg-2 mg, 60s ea	**11845-0076-25**	7.89	
100 mcg, 100s ea	**11845-0057-41**	4.11	
(PF,SF)			
154 mg-1 mg, 60s ea	**11845-0069-35**	6.67	
250 mcg, 100s ea	**11845-0057-51**	5.22	
500 mcg, 100s ea	**11845-0057-61**	6.89	
SL, 1000 mcg,			
100s ea	**11845-0096-61**	8.33	
TER,PO (PF,SF)			
75 mg-1.5 mg, 60s ea	**11845-0116-65**	7.67	
(Medicine Shoppe)			
TAB,PO, 500 mcg,			
100s ea	**49614-0654-78**	5.49	5.49
(Nature's Bounty)			
TAB,PO (PF,SF)			
100 mcg, 100s ea	**74312-0011-70**		3.89
250 mcg, 100s ea	**74312-0006-60**		4.59
500 mcg, 100s ea	**74312-0013-70**		6.79
1000 mcg, 100s ea	**74312-0013-80**		9.39
SL, 2500 mcg,			
50s ea	**74312-0038-60**		7.95
5000 mcg, 30s ea	**74312-0014-71**		8.19
TER,PO, 1500 mcg,			
100s ea	**74312-0020-50**		10.65
(Pharmavite)			
TAB,PO, 100 mcg,			
100s ea	**31604-0012-88**	2.34	
250 mcg, 100s ea	**31604-0012-89**	2.71	
500 mcg, 100s ea	**31604-0012-90**	4.07	
TER,PO, 1000 mcg,			
60s ea	**31604-0016-30**	4.34	
(Rugby)			
TAB,PO (PF,SF,DYE-FREE)			
100 mcg, 100s ea	**00536-3542-01**	2.25	
500 mcg, 100s ea	**00536-3551-01**	3.60	
1000 mcg, 100s ea	**00536-3556-01**	5.02	
(Teva)			
TAB,PO, 1000 mcg,			
100s ea	**00182-1017-01**	5.80	
(A-S Medication)			
REPACK			
TAB,PO (PF,SF,DYE-FREE)			
1000 mcg, 100s ea	**54569-2881-00**	5.09	
(Phys Total Care)			
REPACK			
TAB,PO (PF,SF,DYE-FREE)			
1000 mcg, 100s ea	**54868-3716-00**	20.64	
VITAMIN B2 (Consolidated Midland)			
RIBOFLAVIN			
TAB,PO, 10 mg, 100s ea	**00223-2258-01**	1.40	
25 mg, 100s ea	**00223-2259-01**	3.75	
1000s ea	**00223-2259-02**	27.50	
VITAMIN B2 (Carlson,J.R.)			
TAB,PO, 100 mg, 100s ea	**88395-0022-11**	5.45	10.90
250s ea	**88395-0022-12**	10.75	21.50
(Freeda)			
TAB,PO (PF,SF,DYE-FREE)			
50 mg, 100s ea	**10432-0065-01**	4.77	7.95
100 mg, 100s ea	**10432-0060-01**	6.51	10.85
(Mason Vit)			
TAB,PO, 50 mg, 100s ea	**11845-0071-31**	5.67	
100 mg, 100s ea	**11845-0071-41**	6.33	
(Nature's Bounty)			
TAB,PO (PF,SF)			
100 mg, 100s ea	**74312-0006-40**		6.89
(Pharmavite)			
TAB,PO, 25 mg, 100s ea	**31604-0012-83**	2.43	
VITAMIN B6 (Consolidated Midland)			
PYRIDOXINE HCL			
TAB,PO, 10 mg, 100s ea	**00223-2266-01**	1.95	
1000s ea	**00223-2266-02**	12.50	
25 mg, 100s ea	**00223-2267-01**	2.25	
1000s ea	**00223-2267-02**	16.50	
50 mg, 100s ea	**00223-2268-01**	2.50	
1000s ea	**00223-2268-02**	17.50	
100 mg, 100s ea	**00223-2269-01**	2.95	
1000s ea	**00223-2269-02**	19.50	
250 mg, 100s ea	**00223-2270-01**	4.00	
1000s ea	**00223-2270-02**	42.50	
(Marlex)			
TAB,PO, 25 mg, 100s ea	**10135-0119-01**	0.88	
1000s ea	**10135-0119-10**	5.10	
50 mg, 30s ea	**10135-0139-30**	0.66	
100s ea	**10135-0139-01**	1.26	
(BLISTER PACK)			
50 mg, 100s ea UD	**10135-0167-13**	3.25	
1000s ea	**10135-0139-10**	8.24	
100 mg, 100s ea	**10135-0145-01**	2.21	
1000s ea	**10135-0145-10**	8.61	
(VersaPharm)			
TAB,PO, 25 mg, 30s ea	**61748-0092-30**	3.15	
100s ea	**61748-0092-01**	4.55	
1000s ea	**61748-0092-10**	18.50	
50 mg, 30s ea	**61748-0095-30**	3.15	
100s ea	**61748-0095-01**	4.55	
1000s ea	**61748-0095-10**	18.50	
VITAMIN B6 (ADH)			
TAB,PO, 100 mg, 100s ea	**60142-0118-10**	1.90	4.50
(AmerisourceBergen)			
TAB,PO (PRIVATE LABEL)			
100 mg, 100s ea	**24385-0115-78**	3.50	3.89
(Basic Vitamins)			
TAB,PO, 50 mg, 100s ea	**00761-0436-20**	1.90	
100 mg, 100s ea	**00761-0437-20**	2.75	
TER,PO, 200 mg, 60s ea	**00761-0223-12**	2.60	
(Bio-Tech Pharm)			
TAB,PO, 250 mg, 100s ea	**53191-0070-01**	6.30	
(Carlson,J.R.)			
TAB,PO, 50 mg, 100s ea	**88395-0023-61**	2.25	4.50
250s ea	**88395-0023-62**	5.25	10.50
(Family Phcy)			
TAB,PO (PRIVATE LABEL)			
100 mg, 100s ea	**52735-0049-01**	3.50	3.89
(Freeda)			
TAB,PO (PF,SF,DYE-FREE)			
50 mg, 100s ea	**10432-0087-01**	3.87	6.45
250s ea	**10432-0087-02**	7.74	12.90
100 mg, 100s ea	**10432-0088-01**	5.22	8.70
250s ea	**10432-0088-02**	10.44	17.40
250 mg, 100s ea	**10432-0165-01**	8.55	14.25
(Health Products Corp)			
TAB,PO (PF,SF)			
50 mg, 100s ea	**39686-0011-18**	2.49	
100 mg, 100s ea	**39686-0011-21**	3.70	
(Major)			
TAB,PO, 50 mg, 100s ea	**00904-0520-60**	2.85	
1000s ea	**00904-0520-80**	18.70	
100 mg, 100s ea	**00904-0518-60**	3.75	
(Mason Vit)			
TAB,PO, 50 mg, 100s ea	**11845-0057-01**	4.44	
100 mg, 100s ea	**11845-0057-11**	7.11	
(PF)			
250 mg, 60s ea	**11845-0072-95**	6.78	
500 mg, 60s ea	**11845-0072-85**	10.00	
(Medicine Shoppe)			
TAB,PO, 100 mg, 100s ea	**49614-0593-78**	4.39	4.39
(Nature's Bounty)			
TAB,PO (PF,SF)			
50 mg, 100s ea	**74312-0011-60**		4.49
100 mg, 100s ea	**74312-0006-50**		6.49
200 mg, 100s ea	**74312-0043-50**		9.75
(Pharmavite)			
TAB,PO, 50 mg, 100s ea	**31604-0012-84**	2.71	
100 mg, 100s ea	**31604-0012-85**	3.89	
TER,PO, 200 mg, 60s ea	**31604-0016-28**	4.48	
(Prime Marketing)			
TAB,PO, 100 mg, 100s ea	**62107-0061-01**	3.20	
(Rexall)			
TAB,PO (PF,SF)			
100 mg, 75s ea	**30768-0000-52**	2.65	4.02
(Rugby)			
TAB,PO (PF,SF,DYE-FREE)			
25 mg, 100s ea	**00536-4406-01**	3.44	
50 mg, 100s ea	**00536-4408-01**	3.89	
1000s ea	**00536-4408-10**	15.67	
100 mg, 100s ea	**00536-4409-01**	3.30	
(A-S Medication)			
REPACK			
TAB,PO (PF,SF,DYE-FREE)			
25 mg, 100s ea	**54569-3753-01**	3.44	
100 mg, 30s ea	**54569-2598-02**	1.28	
100s ea	**54569-2598-00**	4.26	
(Dispensing Solutions)			
REPACK			
TAB,PO (PF,SF,DYE-FREE)			
50 mg, 30s ea	**66336-0965-30**	4.25	
100s ea	**55045-2160-00**	6.00	
(Nucare Pharm)			
REPACK			
TAB,PO, 50 mg, 30s ea	**66267-0214-30**	8.48	
100s ea	**68071-1338-00**	12.49	
(Pharma Pac)			
REPACK			
TAB,PO, 50 mg, 30s ea	**52959-0218-30**	3.25	
50s ea	**52959-0218-50**	5.15	
200s ea	**52959-0218-02**	13.50	
100 mg, 20s ea	**52959-0215-20**	3.08	
30s ea	**52959-0215-30**	3.44	
100s ea	**52959-0215-00**	9.87	
(Phys Total Care)			
REPACK			
TAB,PO, 50 mg, 100s ea	**54868-3548-01**	7.87	
100 mg, 100s ea	**54868-3626-01**	10.22	
100s ea	**54868-4843-00**	10.14	
(Quality Care Prod)			
REPACK			
TAB,PO, 100 mg, 30s ea	**49999-0803-30**	16.50	
(Stat Rx)			
REPACK			
TAB,PO, 100 mg, 100s ea	**16590-0864-71**	3.75	
VITAMIN B6 LIQUID (Carlson,J.R.)			
SOL,PO (VEGETARIAN,SF,CORN-FREE)			
200 mg/5 ml, 120 ml	**88395-0023-81**	7.45	14.90
VITAMIN C (Key Company)			
ASCO-TABS-1000			
TAB,PO (SF)			
1000 mg, 100s ea	**11694-0719-01**	6.50	
(Consolidated Midland)			
ASCORBIC ACID			
TAB,PO, 100 mg, 100s ea	**00223-2332-01**	1.75	
1000s ea	**00223-2332-02**	11.50	
250 mg, 100s ea	**00223-2333-01**	2.25	
1000s ea	**00223-2333-02**	16.50	
500 mg, 100s ea	**00223-2334-01**	3.25	
1000s ea	**00223-2334-02**	27.50	
(Marlex)			
CTB,PO, 500 mg, 10s ea	**10135-0237-61**	0.66	
100s ea	**10135-0237-01**	1.88	
300s ea	**10135-0237-03**	4.85	
TAB,PO, 250 mg, 100s ea	**10135-0141-01**	1.67	
1000s ea	**10135-0141-10**	7.44	
500 mg, 30s ea	**10135-0142-30**	0.80	
60s ea	**10135-0142-60**	1.23	
100s ea	**10135-0142-01**	2.21	
(BLISTER PACK)			
500 mg, 100s ea UD	**10135-0165-13**	3.05	
250s ea	**10135-0142-69**	5.16	
300s ea	**10135-0142-03**	4.90	
500s ea	**10135-0142-05**	8.78	
1000s ea	**10135-0142-10**	11.21	
(Freeda)			
C-GRAM			
TAB,PO (PF,SF,DYE-FREE)			
1000 mg, 100s ea	**10432-0076-01**	7.50	12.50
250s ea	**10432-0076-02**	14.97	24.95
(Mason Vit)			
C1000			
TER,PO (PF,SF)			
1000 mg, 90s ea	**11845-0096-39**	9.78	
180s ea	**11845-0117-37**	19.67	
(Nature's Bounty)			
TAB,PO (W/ROSE HIPS,PF,SF)			
1000 mg, 100s ea	**74312-0006-90**		9.89
TER,PO, 1000 mg, 60s ea	**74312-0040-70**		8.19
(Rexall)			
TAB,PO (PF,SF)			
1000 mg, 50s ea	**30768-0000-39**	2.19	3.32
C1000 PLUS ROSE HIPS			
PO, 1000 mg, 50s ea	**30768-0000-45**	2.99	4.53

PROD/MFR	HRI, UPC,NDC	AWP	SRP
(Mason Vit)			
C1000 PLUS ROSE HIPS/BIOFLAVONOIDS			
TAB,PO (PF,SF)			
1000 mg, 60s ea	**11845-0117-35**	7.22	
90s ea	**11845-0117-39**	10.11	
TER,PO, 1000 mg, 60s ea	**11845-0117-45**	9.44	
90s ea	**11845-0117-49**	13.67	
(Rexall)			
C1000 W/ROSE HIPS			
TER,PO (TIMED RELEASE,PF,SF)			
1000 mg, 50s ea	**30768-0000-41**	3.88	5.88
(Mason Vit)			
C1500 PLUS ROSE HIPS/BIOFLAVONOIDS			
TER,PO (PF,SF)			
1500 mg, 60s ea	**11845-0117-55**	11.67	
(Nature's Bounty)			
C250			
CTB,PO (PF)			
250 mg, 100s ea	**74312-0017-30**		4.89
C250 W/ROSE HIPS			
TAB,PO (PF,SF)			
250 mg, 100s ea	**74312-0018-20**		4.09
(Mason Vit)			
C500			
CER,PO (PF)			
500 mg, 180s ea	**11845-0052-67**	17.67	
(Nature's Bounty)			
CER,PO (PF)			
500 mg, 100s ea	**74312-0047-50**		8.99
(Rexall)			
TAB,PO (PF,SF)			
500 mg, 100s ea	**30768-0000-43**	2.37	3.58
(Mason Vit)			
C500 PLUS ROSE HIPS/BIOFLAVONOIDS			
TAB,PO (PF,SF)			
500 mg, 60s ea	**11845-0117-25**	4.89	
90s ea	**11845-0117-29**	5.89	
(Nature's Bounty)			
C500 W/ROSE HIPS			
TAB,PO (PF,SF)			
500 mg, 100s ea	**74312-0004-30**		5.59
250s ea	**74312-0004-33**		12.39
TER,PO, 500 mg, 100s ea	**74312-0024-30**		7.59
(Rexall)			
CTB,PO (ORANGE CHEWABLES,PF)			
500 mg, 60s ea	**30768-0001-46**	2.56	3.88
TAB,PO (PF,SF)			
500 mg, 75s ea	**30768-0000-44**	2.52	3.82
(Key Company)			
CHEW-C			
CTB,PO (ORANGE)			
500 mg, 100s ea	**11694-0976-01**	5.00	
250s ea	**11694-0976-02**	11.50	
500s ea	**11694-0976-03**	21.25	
(Freeda)			
FRUIT C100			
CTB,PO (PF,SF,DYE-FREE)			
100 mg, 100s ea	**10432-0013-01**	4.17	6.95
250s ea	**10432-0013-02**	8.34	13.90
FRUIT C200			
PO (PF,SF,DYE-FREE)			
200 mg, 100s ea	**10432-0012-01**	5.97	9.95
250s ea	**10432-0012-02**	11.94	19.90
FRUIT C500			
PO (PF,SF,DYE-FREE)			
500 mg, 100s ea	**10432-0157-01**	8.37	13.95
250s ea	**10432-0157-02**	16.74	27.90
(Nature's Bounty)			
PURE VITAMIN C-CRYSTALS			
PDR,PO (5000 MG/TSP,PF,SF)			
1000 mg/ml, 168 gm	**74312-0031-60**		11.99
VITAMIN C (ADH)			
CTB,PO (PF)			
100 mg, 100s ea	**60142-0133-01**	1.98	3.95
250 mg, 100s ea	**60142-0134-01**	2.98	5.95
500 mg, 50s ea	**60142-0135-05**	2.88	5.75
100s ea	**60142-0135-01**	3.98	7.95
(Albertson's)			
TAB,PO, 500 mg, 100s ea	**04000-0001-28**	3.75	
1000 mg, 100s ea	**04000-0001-31**	6.51	
(AmerisourceBergen)			
CTB,PO (MULTI-FLAVORED)			
500 mg, 100s ea	**24385-0257-58**	5.39	5.99
(PRIVATE LABEL)			
500 mg, 100s ea	**24385-0293-78**	4.49	4.99
TAB,PO, 250 mg, 100s ea	**24385-0292-78**	3.14	3.49
500 mg, 100s ea	**24385-0295-78**	4.49	4.99
250s ea	**24385-0295-85**	8.09	8.99
500s ea	**24385-0295-90**	14.40	16.00
1000 mg, 100s ea	**24385-0298-78**	6.29	6.99
TER,PO, 500 mg, 100s ea	**24385-0297-78**	5.39	5.99
(Basic Vitamins)			
CER,PO, 500 mg, 100s ea	**00761-0099-20**	3.60	
CTB,PO, 250 mg, 100s ea	**00761-0843-20**	2.10	
500 mg, 100s ea	**00761-0844-20**	3.30	
TAB,PO, 250 mg, 100s ea	**00761-0093-20**	1.55	
500 mg, 100s ea	**00761-0094-20**	2.00	
250s ea	**00761-0094-50**	4.20	
500s ea	**00761-0094-55**	7.80	
1000 mg, 100s ea	**00761-0379-20**	3.60	
TER,PO, 1000 mg,			
100s ea	**00761-0501-20**	4.00	
(Cardinal Health)			
TAB,PO (PRIVATE LABEL)			
250 mg, 100s ea	**37205-0143-78**	3.25	
500 mg, 100s ea	**37205-0089-78**	3.03	
250s ea	**37205-0089-85**	6.24	
1000 mg, 100s ea	**37205-0129-78**	5.87	
(Cypress Pharm)			
CTB,PO (ORANGE)			
250 mg, 100s ea	**60258-0142-01**	2.78	
TAB,PO, 500 mg, 100s ea	**60258-0141-01**	3.89	
(Family Phcy)			
TAB,PO (PRIVATE LABEL)			
500 mg, 250s ea	**52735-0055-07**	5.39	5.99
(Freeda)			
POW,PO, 1060 mg/1.06 gm,			
120 gm	**10432-0186-01**	7.17	11.95
480 gm	**10432-0186-03**	23.25	38.75
TAB,PO (PF,SF,DYE-FREE)			
100 mg, 250s ea	**10432-0067-02**	4.68	7.80
250 mg, 100s ea	**10432-0075-01**	4.05	6.75
500s ea	**10432-0075-03**	12.87	21.45
500 mg, 100s ea	**10432-0250-01**	4.77	7.95
250s ea	**10432-0250-02**	9.54	15.90
500s ea	**10432-0250-03**	16.68	27.80
1000 mg, 500s ea	**10432-0076-03**	25.77	42.95
TER,PO, 500 mg, 100s ea	**10432-0084-01**	6.48	10.80
250s ea	**10432-0084-02**	12.96	21.60
500s ea	**10432-0084-03**	21.57	35.95
1000 mg, 100s ea	**10432-0174-01**	9.30	15.50
250s ea	**10432-0174-02**	18.57	30.95
500s ea	**10432-0174-03**	29.97	49.95
(Health Products Corp)			
CTB,PO (PF,FRUIT)			
250 mg, 100s ea	**39686-0011-87**	2.60	
500 mg, 100s ea	**39686-0011-90**	3.80	
TAB,PO (PF,SF)			
250 mg, 250s ea	**39686-0011-48**	4.00	
500 mg, 50s ea	**39686-0011-49**	1.80	
100s ea	**39686-0030-25**	2.45	
250s ea	**39686-0011-51**	5.25	
TER,PO, 1000 mg, 50s ea	**39686-0011-75**	3.90	
(Hi-Tech)			
LIQ,PO, 500 mg/5 ml,			
480 ml	**50383-0167-16**	14.00	
(Lex)			
TAB,PO, 500 mg, 100s ea	**49523-0084-01**	1.50	
(Major)			
CTB,PO, 250 mg, 100s ea	**00904-0525-60**	4.12	
500 mg, 100s ea	**00904-0526-60**	6.49	
TAB,PO, 250 mg, 100s ea	**00904-0522-60**	2.70	
500 mg, 100s ea	**00904-0523-60**	6.15	
(10X10)			
500 mg, 100s ea UD	**00904-0523-61**	6.74	
300s ea	**00904-0523-72**	12.21	
1000s ea	**00904-0523-80**	37.13	
1000 mg, 100s ea	**00904-5013-60**	10.30	
TER,PO, 500 mg, 100s ea	**00904-0528-60**	8.37	
1000 mg, 100s ea	**00904-2749-60**	11.57	
(Mason Vit)			
CTB,PO, 250 mg, 100s ea	**11845-0051-81**	6.11	
(ORANGE)			
500 mg, 100s ea	**11845-0062-91**	7.44	
TAB,PO, 250 mg, 100s ea	**11845-0051-61**	2.67	
500 mg, 30s ea	**11845-0051-78**	2.11	
100s ea	**11845-0051-71**	4.44	
250s ea	**11845-0051-72**	10.22	
1000 mg, 100s ea	**11845-0071-61**	8.56	
250s ea	**11845-0071-62**	20.56	
TER,PO, 500 mg, 100s ea	**11845-0096-21**	8.78	
(Medicine Shoppe)			
CTB,PO, 500 mg, 100s ea	**49614-0520-78**	4.29	4.29
TAB,PO, 500 mg, 100s ea	**49614-0506-78**	3.19	3.19
(Neurovites)			
CRE,TP, 10%, 60 gm	**93595-2037-01**	22.50	32.50
(Pharmavite)			
TAB,PO, 250 mg, 100s ea	**31604-0014-80**	1.81	
TER,PO, 500 mg, 100s ea	**31604-0014-84**	3.96	
(Prime Marketing)			
TAB,PO, 500 mg, 100s ea	**62107-0046-01**	2.95	
1000s ea	**62107-0046-10**	26.95	
(Rugby)			
CTB,PO (ORANGE)			
500 mg, 100s ea	**00536-3291-01**	5.08	
SYR,PO, 500 mg/5 ml,			
120 ml	**00536-0160-97**	5.26	
480 ml	**00536-0160-85**	14.65	
TAB,PO (PF,SF,DYE-FREE)			
500 mg, 100s ea	**00536-3292-01**	3.61	
1000s ea	**00536-3292-10**	30.91	
(A-S Medication)			
REPACK			
TAB,PO (PF,SF,DYE-FREE)			
500 mg, 100s ea	**54569-2677-00**	3.73	
(Core)			
REPACK			
TAB,PO, 1000 mg,			
100s ea	**33358-0359-00**	15.68	
(Phys Total Care)			
REPACK			
CTB,PO, 500 mg, 100s ea	**54868-2409-01**	11.96	
TAB,PO, 500 mg, 100s ea	**54868-3601-00**	9.09	
1000 mg, 1000s ea	**54868-4433-00**	202.68	
TER,PO, 1000 mg,			
100s ea	**54868-4433-01**	27.81	
(Quality Care Prod)			
REPACK			
TAB,PO, 500 mg, 100s ea	**49999-0352-00**	11.51	
(Mason Vit)			
VITAMIN C PLUS ROSE HIPS			
TAB,PO (PF,SF)			
250 mg, 90s ea	**11845-0117-09**	4.89	
(Freeda)			
VITAMIN C W/ROSE HIPS			
TAB,PO (PF,SF,DYE-FREE)			
500 mg, 100s ea	**10432-0096-01**	5.37	8.95
250s ea	**10432-0096-02**	10.74	17.90
500s ea	**10432-0096-03**	18.57	30.95
1000 mg, 100s ea	**10432-0208-01**	7.77	12.95
250s ea	**10432-0208-02**	15.54	25.90
500s ea	**10432-0208-03**	26.97	44.95
(Health Products Corp)			
TAB,PO (PF,SF)			
250 mg, 100s ea	**39686-0011-60**	2.42	
500 mg, 100s ea	**39686-0011-70**	3.65	
250s ea	**39686-0011-63**	8.06	
1000 mg, 30s ea	**39686-0011-66**	3.15	
100s ea	**39686-0011-69**	6.45	
TER,PO, 1000 mg, 50s ea	**39686-0011-78**	4.55	
(Nature's Bounty)			
SOL,PO (LIME)			
300 mg/5 ml,			
120 ml	**74312-0027-40**		5.89
(Pharmavite)			
TAB,PO, 250 mg, 100s ea	**31604-0012-55**	2.45	
500 mg, 130s ea	**31604-0112-59**	3.74	
250s ea	**31604-0012-60**	7.31	
1000 mg, 60s ea	**31604-0012-64**	3.98	
TER,PO, 500 mg, 60s ea	**31604-0016-45**	3.05	
1000 mg, 60s ea	**31604-0016-50**	4.72	
1500 mg, 60s ea	**31604-0013-48**	6.03	
(Basic Vitamins)			
VITAMIN C W/ROSE HIPS NATURAL			
TAB,PO (SF)			
500 mg, 100s ea	**00761-0381-20**	2.60	
1000 mg, 80s ea	**00761-0382-16**	3.20	
(Nature's Bounty)			
VITAMIN C1000			
TAB,PO (PF,SF)			
1000 mg, 100s ea	**74312-0017-10**		8.15
VITAMIN C250			
PO (PF,SF)			
250 mg, 100s ea	**74312-0015-30**		3.15
VITAMIN C500			
CTB,PO (W/ACEROLA,PF)			
500 mg, 60s ea	**74312-0050-00**		6.99
(W/ROSE HIPS,PF,ORANGE)			
500 mg, 90s ea	**74312-0038-80**		8.35
TAB,PO (PF,SF)			
500 mg, 100s ea	**74312-0015-10**		3.75

PROD/MFR	HRI, UPC,NDC	AWP	SRP
250s ea	74312-0015-13		8.79
500s ea	74312-0015-15		15.49
VITAMIN C BUFFERED (Nature's Bounty)			
TAB,PO (PF,SF)			
500 mg, 100s ea	74312-0028-20		8.69
VITAMIN C CRYSTALS (Carlson,J.R.)			
PDS,PO (VEGETARIAN,PF,SF)			
4000 mg/4 gm, 170 gm	88395-0033-46	8.45	16.90
1000 gm	88395-0033-44	27.50	55.00
VITAMIN C W/BIOFLAVONOID COMPLEX (Linus)			
TER,PO (CAPLET)			
1000 mg, 90s ea	10363-0253-17	5.97	10.95
VITAMIN C W/ROSE HIPS (Marlex)			
TAB,PO, 500 mg, 100s ea	10135-0239-01	1.62	
250s ea	10135-0239-69	4.10	
(Natl Vitamin)			
TAB,PO (PF,SF)			
250 mg, 100s ea	54629-0250-01	1.97	3.29
500 mg, 100s ea	54629-0500-01	2.63	4.39
250s ea	54629-0510-02	5.99	9.99
1000 mg, 100s ea	54629-0511-01	4.50	7.59
250s ea	54629-0477-00	10.67	17.79
500s ea	54629-0014-77	15.28	25.49
VITAMIN C W/ROSE HIPS NATURAL			
(AmerisourceBergen)			
TAB,PO (PRIVATE LABEL)			
500 mg, 100s ea	24385-0311-78	5.21	5.79
TER,PO, 1000 mg, 60s ea	24385-0312-72	5.39	5.99
(Cardinal Health)			
TAB,PO (PF,PRIVATE LABEL)			
500 mg, 100s ea	37205-0147-78	2.96	
1000 mg, 100s ea	37205-0141-78	6.32	
TER,PO, 1000 mg, 60s ea	37205-0133-72	5.25	
VITAMIN C-1000MG WITH ROSE HIPS			
(Nature's Bounty)			
C1000			
TAB,PO (W/ROSE HIPS,PF,SF)			
1000 mg, 30s ea	74312-0028-00		5.19
100s ea	74312-0028-02		15.95
(WITH ROSE HIPS,PF,SF)			
1000 mg, 250s ea	74312-0006-93		21.89
VITAMIN C-500MG WITH ECHINACEA (Major)			
TAB,PO, 500 mg-76 mg-100 mg,			
100s ea	00904-5614-60	15.07	
VITAMIN C/ROSE HIPS (ADH)			
TAB,PO, 500 mg, 100s ea	60142-0115-10	2.78	5.55
TER,PO (AF,PF,SF)			
1000 mg, 100s ea	60142-0116-01	5.75	11.50
1500 mg, 60s ea	60142-0118-06	4.88	9.75
(AF,PF,SF)			
1500 mg, 100s ea	60142-0118-01	7.75	15.50
VITAMIN C500 PLUS (Mason Vit)			
TAB,PO (PF,SF)			
500 mg, 180s ea	11845-0117-27	11.00	
VITAMIN D (Cardinal Health)			
TAB,PO (PRIVATE LABEL)			
400 iu, 60s ea	37205-0091-72	1.89	
(Carlson,J.R.)			
SGL,PO (PF,SF,CORN-FREE)			
1000 iu-400 iu,			
100s ea	88395-0014-41	3.25	6.50
250s ea	88395-0014-42	6.20	12.40
1600 iu-1000 iu,			
100s ea	88395-0014-51	3.95	7.90
250s ea	88395-0014-52	7.45	14.90
(Magno-Humphries)			
TAB,PO, 400 iu, 100s ea	43292-0558-81	1.79	5.69
(Major)			
CAP,PO (PF,SF,STARCH-FREE)			
5000 iu, 100s ea	09045-0986-60	5.99	
TAB,PO, 400 iu, 100s ea	00904-5823-60	2.49	
1000 iu, 100s ea	00904-5824-60	2.89	
(Mason Vit)			
SGL,PO (PF,SF,SOFTGEL)			
400 iu, 100s ea	11845-0118-31	2.89	
(Nature's Bounty)			
TAB,PO (PF)			
400 iu, 100s ea	74312-0011-40		3.35
(Phys Total Care)			
REPACK			
TAB,PO (PF,SF,STARCH-FREE)			
400 iu, 100s ea	54868-5910-00	8.68	
1000 iu, 100s ea	54868-5895-00	9.60	
VITAMIN D NATURAL (Basic Vitamins)			
TAB,PO, 400 iu, 100s ea	07610-0058-20	1.80	
VITAMIN D2 (Freeda)			
TAB,PO (PF,SF,DYE-FREE)			
400 iu, 250s ea	10432-0312-02	6.75	11.25
VITAMIN D3 (Freeda)			
TAB,PO (PF,SF,DYE-FREE)			
1000 iu, 100s ea	10432-0237-01	4.17	6.95
500s ea	10432-0237-03	13.50	22.50
(Rugby)			
SGL,PO (PF,SF,GLUTEN-FREE)			
2000 iu, 100s ea	00536-3790-01	6.12	
(Quality Care Prod)			
REPACK			
TAB,PO (PF,SF,DYE-FREE)			
1000 iu, 100s ea	35356-0563-00	18.80	
VITAMIN E (Key Company)			
ALPH-E			
SGL,PO (SOFTGEL)			
200 iu, 100s ea	11694-0126-71	6.25	
400 iu, 100s ea	11694-0994-01	8.25	
250s ea	11694-0994-02	16.50	
1000s ea	11694-0994-03	62.00	
ALPH-E-MIXED-1000			
PO (SOFTGEL)			
1000 iu, 100s ea	11694-0886-01	16.00	
500s ea	11694-0886-04	71.00	
ALPH-E-MIXED-200			
PO (SOFTGEL)			
200 iu, 100s ea	11694-0924-01	6.00	
ALPH-E-MIXED-400			
PO (SOFTGEL)			
400 iu, 100s ea	11694-0923-01	8.75	
250s ea	11694-0923-02	17.50	
1000s ea	11694-0923-04	63.00	
(Nature's Bounty)			
E100			
SGL,PO (PF,SF,SOFTGEL)			
100 iu, 100s ea	74312-0002-60		5.99
100s ea	74312-0017-50		3.85
E1000			
PO (PF,SF,SOFTGEL)			
1000 iu, 50s ea	74312-0005-51		10.99
50s ea	74312-0017-80		9.59
50s ea	74312-0029-01		14.85
100s ea	74312-0005-50		20.45
100s ea	74312-0017-81		17.95
(Mason Vit)			
E1000 D-ALPHA			
SGL,PO (PF,SF,SOFTGEL)			
1000 iu, 90s ea	11845-0060-69	33.22	
(Rexall)			
E1000 MIXED			
SGL,PO (PF,SF,SOFTGEL)			
1000 iu, 50s ea	30768-0000-35	8.39	12.72
(Nature's Bounty)			
E200			
SGL,PO (PF,SF,SOFTGEL)			
200 iu, 100s ea	74312-0002-70		8.99
100s ea	74312-0017-60		4.99
(Rexall)			
E200 MIXED			
SGL,PO (PF,SF,SOFTGEL)			
200 iu, 50s ea	30768-0000-38	2.27	3.43
(Nature's Bounty)			
E400			
SGL,PO (WATER SOLUBLE BASE,SF)			
400 iu, 50s ea	74312-0023-41		5.99
(PF,SF,SOFTGEL)			
400 iu, 100s ea	74312-0004-60		8.99
100s ea	74312-0005-40		12.45
100s ea	74312-0017-70		5.99
(WATER SOLUBLE BASE,SF)			
400 iu, 100s ea	74312-0023-40		9.69
(PF,SF,SOFTGEL)			
400 iu, 250s ea	74312-0005-43		28.89
250s ea	74312-0017-73		13.75
(Rexall)			
E400 MIXED			
SGL,PO (PF,SF,SOFTGEL)			
400 iu, 50s ea	30768-0000-36	2.81	4.25
E400 NATURAL			
PO (PF,SF,SOFTGEL)			
400 iu, 50s ea	30768-0000-40	3.84	5.82
E400 PLUS FOLIC ACID			
SGL,PO (PF,SF,SOFTGEL)			
50s ea	30768-0000-94	4.13	6.25
(Westlake Labs.)			
TOTAL E-400			
SGL,PO (PF,SF,SOFTGEL)			
400 iu, 60s ea	10539-0705-69	11.90	17.00
(DRY,PF,SF)			
400 iu, 100s ea	10539-0705-91	19.60	28.00
VITAMIN E (Albertson's)			
SGL,PO (SOFTGEL)			
400 iu, 100s ea	04000-0001-24	7.20	
1000 iu, 100s ea	04000-0001-27	15.60	
(AmerisourceBergen)			
SGL,PO (PRIVATE LABEL,SOFTGEL)			
200 iu, 100s ea	24385-0314-78	5.66	6.29
400 iu, 300s ea	24385-0318-87	12.59	13.99
1000 iu, 50s ea	24385-0319-71	9.89	11.00
100s ea	24385-0681-78	12.59	13.99
(Basic Vitamins)			
SGL,PO, 100 iu, 100s ea	00761-0300-20	2.00	
200 iu, 100s ea	00761-0301-20	2.60	
400 iu, 100s ea	00761-0302-20	3.85	
250s ea	00761-0302-50	7.80	
600 iu, 50s ea	00761-0303-10	3.60	
1000 iu, 50s ea	00761-0305-10	4.40	
100s ea	00761-0305-20	8.40	
(Cardinal Health)			
SGL,PO (PRIVATE LABEL,SOFTGEL)			
400 iu, 100s ea	37205-0074-78	5.92	
(WATER DISPERS.)			
400 iu, 100s ea	37205-0076-78	8.80	
(PRIVATE LABEL,SOFTGEL)			
400 iu, 250s ea	37205-0090-85	11.32	
800 iu, 50s ea	37205-0167-71	6.18	
1000 iu, 50s ea	37205-0156-71	7.76	
(Consolidated Midland)			
SGL,PO, 100 iu, 100s ea	00223-1990-01	3.00	
1000s ea	00223-1990-02	25.00	
200 iu, 100s ea	00223-2031-01	4.50	
1000s ea	00223-2031-02	37.50	
400 iu, 100s ea	00223-2032-01	7.75	
1000s ea	00223-2032-02	70.00	
600 iu, 100s ea	00223-2033-01	11.00	
1000s ea	00223-2033-02	105.00	
1000 iu, 100s ea	00223-2040-01	18.50	
1000s ea	00223-2040-02	160.00	
(Family Phcy)			
SGL,PO (PRIVATE LABEL)			
400 iu, 100s ea	52735-0064-01	4.49	5.99
300s ea	52735-0064-09	11.69	12.99
1000 iu, 50s ea	52735-0060-12	6.29	6.99
(Freeda)			
LIQ,PO (PF,SF,DYE-FREE)			
4600 iu/5 ml, 30 ml	10432-0183-01	5.97	9.95
60 ml	10432-0183-02	9.90	16.50
(PF,SF)			
4600 iu/5 ml, 120 ml	10432-0183-03	15.57	25.95
TAB,PO (PF,SF,DYE-FREE)			
100 iu, 100s ea	10432-0109-01	5.37	8.95
250s ea	10432-0109-02	10.74	17.90
200 iu, 100s ea	10432-0066-01	7.47	12.45
250s ea	10432-0066-02	14.94	24.90
500s ea	10432-0066-03	25.68	42.80
400 iu, 100s ea	10432-0110-01	11.67	19.45
250s ea	10432-0110-02	23.37	38.95
500s ea	10432-0110-03	40.77	67.95
500 iu, 100s ea	10432-0111-01	15.57	25.95
250s ea	10432-0111-02	31.14	51.90
(Health Products Corp)			
CRE,TP, 60 gm	39686-0014-73	2.37	
120 gm	39686-0014-74	4.47	
SGL,PO (PF,SF,SOFTGEL)			
400 iu, 30s ea	39686-0011-97	2.75	
100s ea	39686-0012-14	6.75	
250s ea	39686-0012-17	17.05	
1000 iu, 30s ea	39686-0012-20	5.58	
50s ea	39686-0012-02	6.60	
100s ea	39686-0012-23	12.45	
(Lex)			
SGL,PO (SF,SOFTGEL)			
400 iu, 50s ea	49523-0021-05	1.45	
500s ea	49523-0021-10	2.30	
(Major)			
CRE,TP (1X112GM)			
1000 iu, 112 gm	00904-5324-22	2.75	
SGL,PO, 100 iu, 100s ea	00904-0270-60	3.07	
200 iu, 100s ea	00904-0272-60	4.65	
400 iu, 100s ea	00904-0274-60	12.45	
100s ea	00904-2752-60	9.44	
100s ea	00904-3346-60	7.60	
300s ea	00904-0274-72	34.75	

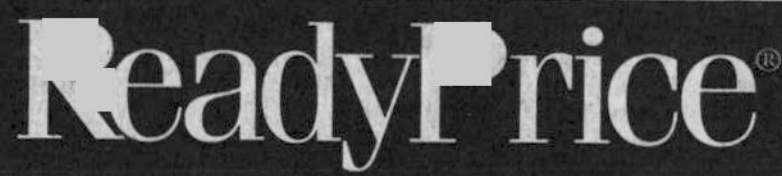

PROD/MFR	HRI, UPC,NDC	AWP	SRP
600 iu, 100s ea	00904-4193-60	9.53	
1000 iu, 30s ea	00904-0277-46	8.64	
100s ea	00904-0277-60	25.36	
(Marlex)			
SGL,PO (SOFTGEL)			
100 iu, 100s ea	10135-0218-01	1.48	
200 iu, 100s ea	10135-0219-01	2.13	
400 iu, 30s ea	10135-0220-30	1.74	
50s ea	10135-0220-50	5.90	
60s ea	10135-0220-60	2.65	
100s ea	10135-0220-01	3.24	
300s ea	10135-0220-03	8.70	
1000s ea	10135-0220-10	18.99	
1000 iu, 30s ea	10135-0217-30	2.79	
100s ea	10135-0217-01	7.81	
(Mason Vit)			
CRE,TP, 50 mg/gm, 60 gm	11845-0811-07	6.11	
OIL,TP, 30 ml	11845-0059-01	9.44	
SGL,PO, 200 iu, 100s ea	11845-0050-81	10.11	
(Medicine Shoppe)			
SGL,PO (SOFTGEL)			
400 iu, 100s ea	49614-0569-78	5.69	5.69
(Nature's Bounty)			
CRE,TP (6,000IU)			
100 iu/gm, 57 gm	74312-0006-10		3.95
OIL,TP (30,000IU)			
60 ml	74312-0008-10		7.39
(Prime Marketing)			
SGL,PO, 400 iu, 100s ea	62107-0064-01	6.95	
(Reese)			
CRE,TP, 500 iu/gm,			
57 gm	23513-0738-02	7.01	
(Rugby)			
OIL,TP, 60 ml	00536-8533-96	6.96	
SGL,PO, 100 iu, 100s ea	00536-4793-01	3.94	
(PF,SF,DYE-FREE,SOFTGEL)			
400 iu, 100s ea	00536-4799-01	7.72	
(Torrance)			
OIN,TP, 30 iu, 60 gm	00389-1465-00	5.99	
(Truxton)			
SGL,PO, 400 iu, 100s ea	00463-2032-01	6.00	
1000s ea	00463-2032-10	45.60	
1000 iu, 100s ea	00463-2033-01	12.00	
1000s ea	00463-2033-10	108.00	
(A-S Medication)			
REPACK			
SGL,PO (SOFTGEL)			
400 iu, 60s ea	54569-4856-00	11.50	
(PD-Rx Pharm)			
REPACK			
SGL,PO (SOFTGEL)			
400 iu, 90s ea	55289-0063-90	8.48	
(Phys Total Care)			
REPACK			
SGL,PO, 1000 iu,			
100s ea	54868-3288-00	38.22	
(Stat Rx)			
REPACK			
CRE,TP, 120 gm	16590-0245-04	11.25	
(Freeda)			
VITAMIN E MIXED			
TAB,PO (PF,SF,DYE-FREE)			
100 iu, 250s ea	10432-0155-02	11.34	18.90
(Health Products Corp)			
VITAMIN E100 DL ALPHA			
SGL,PO (PF,SF,SOFTGEL)			
100 iu, 100s ea	39686-0011-93	2.20	
(Mason Vit)			
VITAMIN E1000 D-ALPHA			
SGL,PO (PF,SF,SOFTGEL)			
1000 iu, 60s ea	11845-0060-65	22.78	
(Health Products Corp)			
VITAMIN E1000 DL ALPHA			
SGL,PO (PF,SF,SOFTGEL)			
1000 iu, 100s ea	39686-0012-05	10.93	
(Mason Vit)			
VITAMIN E1000 DL-ALPHA			
SGL,PO (COLD PRESSED,SF)			
1000 iu, 50s ea	11845-0050-49	12.44	
100s ea	11845-0050-41	22.11	
(Health Products Corp)			
VITAMIN E200 D ALPHA			
SGL,PO (PF,SF,SOFTGEL)			
200 iu, 100s ea	39686-0012-11	5.25	
(Freeda)			
VITAMIN E200 MIXED			
TAB,PO (PF,SF,DYE-FREE)			
200 iu, 100s ea	10432-0156-01	7.77	12.95
250s ea	10432-0156-02	15.54	25.90
(Health Products Corp)			
VITAMIN E400 DL ALPHA			
SGL,PO (PF,SF,SOFTGEL)			
400 iu, 100s ea	39686-0012-35	5.30	
250s ea	39686-0011-99	9.25	
(Freeda)			
VITAMIN E400 MIXED			
TAB,PO (PF,SF,DYE-FREE)			
400 iu, 100s ea	10432-0245-01	12.57	20.95
250s ea	10432-0245-02	25.14	41.90
500s ea	10432-0245-03	43.35	72.25
VITAMIN E ACETATE (Key Company)			
SGL,PO (SOFTGEL)			
400 iu, 100s ea	11694-0951-01	7.00	
1000s ea	11694-0951-03	42.00	
VITAMIN E AQUEOUS (Silarx)			
SOL,PO (DROPS)			
15 iu/0.3 ml, 30 ml	54838-0005-30	40.49	
VITAMIN E NATURAL (AmerisourceBergen)			
SGL,PO (PRIVATE LABEL,SOFTGEL)			
400 iu, 100s ea	24385-0321-78	9.89	10.99
1000 iu, 50s ea	24385-0323-71	14.39	15.99
(Basic Vitamins)			
SGL,PO, 200 iu, 100s ea	00761-0401-20	3.60	
400 iu, 100s ea	00761-0402-20	5.40	
1000 iu, 60s ea	00761-0403-12	7.20	
(Cardinal Health)			
SGL,PO (PRIVATE LABEL,SOFTGEL)			
400 iu, 100s ea	37205-0075-78	6.56	
(Geritrex)			
SOL,PO, 15 iu/0.3 ml,			
12 ml	92771-0725-12	10.36	
(Rugby)			
SGL,PO (PF,SF,DYE-FREE,SOFTGEL)			
400 iu, 100s ea	00536-5440-01	9.65	
(Phys Total Care)			
REPACK			
SGL,PO (SOFTGEL)			
400 iu, 100s ea	54868-2215-01	16.92	
300s ea	54868-2215-00	48.00	
VITAMIN E NATURAL BLEND (AmerisourceBergen)			
SGL,PO (PRIVATE LABEL,SOFTGEL)			
400 iu, 100s ea	24385-0666-78	7.19	7.99
VITAMIN E SKIN CREAM (Southwood)			
REPACK			
CRE,TP, 120 gm	58016-9233-01	13.24	
VITAMIN E SUCCINATE (Key Company)			
ALPH-E-400			
CAP,PO (SF)			
400 iu, 100s ea	11694-0126-31	15.00	
VITAMIN E WATER DISPERSIBLE (AmerisourceBergen)			
SGL,PO (WATER DISPERS)			
400 iu, 100s ea	24385-0996-78	8.09	8.99
VITAMIN E WITH MIXED TOCOPHEROLS (Freeda)			
TAB,PO, 5 mg-100 iu,			
100s ea	10432-0155-01	5.67	9.45
VITAMIN E-SYNTHETIC (Major)			
SGL,PO (10X10,SOFTGEL)			
400 iu, 100s ea UD	00904-0274-61	26.93	
VITAMIN E1000 MIXED (Mason Vit)			
SGL,PO (COLD PRESSED,SF)			
1000 iu, 50s ea	11845-0050-09	13.89	
100s ea	11845-0050-01	24.33	
VITAMIN E200 DL-ALPHA (Mason Vit)			
PO (SF)			
200 iu, 100s ea	11845-0050-61	7.22	
VITAMIN E200 MIXED (Mason Vit)			
PO (PF,SF,SOFTGEL)			
200 iu, 100s ea	11845-0050-21	7.56	
VITAMIN E400 D-ALPHA (Mason Vit)			
PO (PF,SF,SOFTGEL)			
400 iu, 60s ea	11845-0050-95	9.44	
90s ea	11845-0050-99	15.00	
180s ea	11845-0050-97	26.56	
VITAMIN E400 DL-ALPHA (Mason Vit)			
PO (PF,SF,SOFTGEL)			
400 iu, 30s ea	11845-0050-58	4.44	
(COLD PRESSED,SF)			
400 iu, 100s ea	11845-0050-51	8.33	
250s ea	11845-0050-52	19.56	
VITAMIN E400 MIXED (Mason Vit)			
PO (COLD PRESSED,SF)			
400 iu, 100s ea	11845-0050-11	9.78	
250s ea	11845-0050-12	23.22	
VITAMIN E600 DL-ALPHA (Mason Vit)			
PO (COLD PRESSED,SF)			
600 iu, 100s ea	11845-0076-51	13.22	
VITAMIN E800 D-ALPHA (Pharmavite)			
SGL,PO (PF,SOFTGEL)			
800 iu, 60s ea	31604-0014-74	8.95	
VITAMIN HUT OCULAR VITAMINS (Global Source)			
TAB,PO, 60s ea	59618-0650-12	1.74	
VITAMIN K (Mason Vit)			
TAB,PO (SF)			
0.1 mg, 100s ea	11845-0077-91	3.11	
VITAMINS & MINERALS (Consolidated Midland)			
TAB,PO, 100s ea	00223-2365-01	6.50	
1000s ea	00223-2365-02	52.50	
(Major)			
VITAMINS & MINERALS HIGH POTENCY			
TAB,PO, 100s ea	00904-5042-60	5.99	
VITAMINS + IRON CHILDREN'S (Prime Marketing)			
CTB,PO (FRUIT)			
100s ea	62107-0048-01	3.90	
1000s ea	62107-0048-10	23.50	
VITAMINS A & D (AmerisourceBergen)			
OIN,TP (PRIVATE LABEL)			
60 gm	24385-0070-10	2.15	2.39
VITAMINS A AND D (Perrigo)			
OIN,TP (1X57GM)			
15.5%-53.4%, 57 gm	45802-0395-10	2.99	
(1X113GM)			
15.5%-53.4%, 113 gm	45802-0395-04	3.99	
VITAMINS CHILDREN'S (Albertson's)			
CTB,PO, 100s ea	04000-0001-96	3.66	
(Prime Marketing)			
CTB,PO (FRUIT)			
100s ea	62107-0047-01	3.80	
1000s ea	62107-0047-10	22.95	
VITAMINS FOR HAIR (Basic Vitamins)			
TAB,PO, 50s ea	00761-0117-10	3.00	
VITAMINS FOR THE HAIR (Nature's Bounty)			
TAB,PO (PF,SF)			
65s ea	74312-0021-00		8.69
VITAMINS W/EXTRA C CHILDREN'S (Albertson's)			
CTB,PO, 100s ea	04000-0001-98	4.83	
VITAMINS W/IRON CHILDREN'S (Albertson's)			
CTB,PO, 100s ea	04000-0001-97	3.75	
(Marlex)			
CTB,PO, 100s ea	10135-0153-01	1.60	
250s ea	10135-0153-69	3.00	
1000s ea	10135-0153-10	14.00	
VITAMIST ARTHRIFLEX (Mayor Pharma Labs)			
SPR,PO, 13.5 ml	45601-0001-10	10.80	15.96
VITAMIST COLD WEATHER FORMULA (Mayor Pharma Labs)			
SPR,PO, 13.5 ml	45601-0000-80	10.00	15.96
VITAMIST MEN'S FORMULA (Mayor Pharma Labs)			
SPR,PO, 13.5 ml	45601-0000-30	10.80	15.96
VITAMIST PRE-NATAL (Mayor Pharma Labs)			
SPR,PO, 13.5 ml	45601-0001-20	10.80	15.96
VITAMIST RE VITALIZER (Mayor Pharma Labs)			
SPR,PO, 13.5 ml	45601-0000-90	10.80	15.96
VITAMIST WOMEN'S HEALTH (Mayor Pharma Labs)			
SPR,PO, 13.5 ml	45601-0000-20	10.80	15.96
VITAPRO (VITAFLO, LLC)			
POW,PO (1X250GM)			
250 gm	50600-0506-01	19.95	24.94
VITAQUICK (VITAFLO, LLC)			
PDS,PO (1X300GM)			
300 gm	50600-0503-35	18.95	23.69
VITATRUM COMPLETE (Mason Vit)			
TAB,PO (IMPROVED FORMULA)			
30s ea	11845-0141-28	3.67	
130s ea	11845-0141-23	9.67	
VITEC (Pharm Spec)			
LOT,TP, 120 ml	45334-0400-04	9.65	14.55
VITOXAPAP (Vita-Rx)			
TAB,PO, 325 mg-30 mg,			
100s ea	49727-0336-02	3.10	
1000s ea	49727-0336-05	20.45	
VITRON-C (Heritage/Insight)			
TAB,PO, 125 mg-66 mg,			
60s ea	00235-0123-01	76.80	

PROD/MFR	HRI, UPC,NDC	AWP	SRP
(PLUS VIT C,COATED)			
125 mg-200 mg,			
60s ea	63736-0123-01		8.18
VITRUM JR (Mason Vit)			
CTB,PO (SF)			
60s ea	11845-0094-65	5.00	
VITRUM SENIOR (Mason Vit)			
TAB,PO (IMPROVED FORMULA)			
60s ea	11845-0141-35	7.53	
VIVA-DROPS (Vision)			
SOL,OP, 10 ml	54891-0001-02	4.58	5.73
15 ml	54891-0001-01	5.50	6.88
VIVARIN (Glaxo)			
TAB,PO (CLIP STRIP)			
200 mg, 16s ea	53100-0186-24	2.48	
(CAPLET)			
200 mg, 24s ea	53100-0186-60	3.62	
40s ea	53100-0186-31	5.99	
80s ea	53100-0186-51	7.84	
VIVONEX PEDIATRIC (Nestle)			
PDR,PO (TUBE FEEDING, PACKETS)			
48.5 gm 36s	00212-7131-76	212.11	
VIVONEX PEPTINEX 1.0 (Nestle)			
LIQ,PO (TETRA BRIK)			
237 ml	43900-0371-21	355.32	
237 ml	43900-0371-41	355.32	
VIVONEX PEPTINEX 1.5 (Nestle)			
LIQ,PO (TETRA BRIK,VANILLA)			
237 ml	43900-0371-31	426.34	
VIVONEX PEPTINEX DT (Nestle)			
LIQ,PO (24X250ML,W/PREBIOTICS)			
250 ml 24s	00212-3757-51	155.81	
VIVONEX PLUS (Nestle)			
PDR,PO (TUBE FEEDING, PACKETS)			
79.5 gm 36s	00212-7298-18	331.34	
VIVONEX RTF (Nestle)			
LIQ,PO (250MLX24,UNFLAVORED)			
250 ml 24s	43900-0362-50	214.50	
(TUBE FEEDING)			
250 ml 24s	00212-3625-51	166.75	
1000 ml 6s	00212-3625-42	173.88	
1500 ml 6s	00212-3625-44	260.78	
SUS,PO (6X1000ML)			
1000 ml 6s	43900-0362-80	173.88	
(6X1500ML)			
1500 ml 6s	43900-0362-82	260.78	
VIVONEX T.E.N. (Nestle)			
PDR,PO (10X6)			
85.2 gm 60s	43900-0712-74	511.56	
VSL#3 (Sigma-Tau)			
CAP,PO (GLUTEN-FREE)			
112.5 billion org,			
60s ea	00544-8209-31	38.80	48.50
PKT,PO (GLUTEN-FREE,LEMON)			
450 billion org/packet,			
10s ea	00544-8209-11	22.26	29.68
(GLUTEN-FREE)			
450 billion org/packet,			
10s ea	54482-0922-02	22.26	
(GLUTEN-FREE,LEMON)			
450 billion org/packet,			
30s ea	00544-8209-12	63.60	79.50
(GLUTEN-FREE)			
450 billion org/packet,			
30s ea	00544-8209-21	63.60	79.50
VSL#3-DS (Sigma-Tau)			
PKT,PO (GLUTEN-FREE)			
900 billion org/packet,			
20s ea	00544-8209-41	99.75	123.50
W-D PRESTIGE SMART SYSTEM (Home Diag)			
DEV,NA (STRIP)			
50s ea	56151-0313-50	28.60	
W-D PRESTIGE SMART SYSTEM STARTER (Home Diag)			
DEV,NA (MTR,STRP,LANCET,DEV,SOL)			
ea	56151-0213-01	22.18	
WABANA (Key Company)			
TAB,PO, 50 mg-20 mg-500 mg,			
60s ea	11694-0870-01	5.00	
500s ea	11694-0870-05	26.00	
WALGREENS COMFORT ASSURED INSULIN SYRINGES (Walgreens)			
DEV,NA (31GX5/16,0.3CC,THIN II)			
100s ea	11917-0048-15	19.00	
(31GX5/16,0.5CC,THIN II)			
100s ea	11917-0048-14	19.00	
(31GX5/16,1CC,THIN II)			
100s ea	11917-0048-13	19.00	
WALGREENS COMFORT ASSURED LANCETS (Can-Am Care)			
DEV,NA (21G,UNIVERSAL 1)			
100s ea	38396-0501-32	5.85	
(26G,THIN,UNIVERSAL 1)			
100s ea	38396-0502-32	5.85	
(30G,ULTRA THIN)			
100s ea	38396-0504-32	5.85	
(26G,THIN,UNIVERSAL 1)			
200s ea	38396-0503-32	9.50	
WALGREENS PRESTIGE SMART SYSTEM (Home Diag)			
DEV,NA (STRIP)			
50s ea	56151-0301-50	28.60	
WALGREENS PSS STARTER (Home Diag)			
DEV,NA (METR,LANC,DEV,SOL,STRIP)			
ea	56151-0201-01	22.18	
WALNUT (Ellon)			
SOL,SL (DROPS)			
10.5 ml	51762-0019-10		9.25
WART-OFF MAXIMUM STRENGTH (Johnson & Johnson)			
LIQ,TP, 17%, 13.5 ml	74300-0004-31	4.87	
WASSER (S.S.S.)			
TAB,PO, 30s ea	12258-0131-80	3.33	4.99
WATE-ON (Lee Pharm)			
LIQ,PO (BERRY)			
480 ml	23558-0822-00	14.40	
480 ml 12s	23558-0822-01	172.80	
WATE-ON SUPER (Lee Pharm)			
LIQ,PO (BERRY)			
480 ml	23558-0820-10	15.00	
480 ml 12s	23558-0820-11	180.00	
WATER FOR INHALATION (Automatic Liq Pkg)			
SOL,IH (AL7023)			
3 ml 1000s UD	48879-0001-01	80.00	100.00
(AL7025)			
5 ml 1000s UD	48879-0001-02	80.00	100.00
WATER PILL EXTRA STRENGTH (Nature's Bounty)			
TAB,PO, 50s ea	74312-0018-31		7.95
WATER PILL W/POTASSIUM (Nature's Bounty)			
TAB,PO (PF,SF)			
50s ea	74312-0022-10		5.29
WATER VIOLET (Ellon)			
SOL,SL (DROPS)			
10.5 ml	51762-0016-10		9.25
WAVESENSE KEYNOTE BLOOD GLUCOSE MONITORING SYSTEM (AgaMatrix)			
DEV,NA, ea	08554-1317-01	35.00	
WAVESENSE KEYNOTE NORMAL CONTROL SOLUTION (AgaMatrix)			
DEV,NA, 6 ml	08554-1333-01	28.00	
WAVESENSE KEYNOTE TEST STRIP (AgaMatrix)			
DEV,NA, 50s ea	08554-1328-01	28.00	
(2X50)			
100s ea	08554-2265-02	28.00	
WEBCOL ALCOHOL PREP (Covidien)			
PAD,TP (LARGE,1 PLY,STERILE)			
70%, 4000s ea	08080-5033-00	64.25	
(LARGE,2 PLY,STERILE)			
70%, 4000s ea	08080-5110-00	70.50	
(MEDIUM,2 PLY,STERILE)			
70%, 4000s ea	08080-6818-00	42.75	
WEBRIL II UNDERCAST PADDING (Covidien)			
DEV,NA (6"X4YDS,NON-STERILE)			
36s ea	08080-4519-00	77.39	
(2"X4YDS,STERILE)			
50s ea	08080-2666-00	52.23	
(3"X4YDS,STERILE)			
50s ea	08080-2754-00	73.74	
(4"X4YDS,STERILE)			
50s ea	08080-2847-00	93.50	
(2"X4YDS,NON-STERILE)			
72s ea	08080-4095-00	58.88	
(3"X4YDS,NON-STERILE)			
72s ea	08080-4152-00	81.85	
(4"X4YDS,NON-STERILE)			
72s ea	08080-4221-00	102.25	
WEBRIL UNDERCAST PADDING (Covidien)			
DEV,NA (6"X4YDS,NON-STERILE)			
36s ea	08080-3489-00	71.68	
(2"X4YDS,STERILE)			
50s ea	08080-2283-00	51.38	
(4"X4YDS,STERILE)			
50s ea	08080-2502-00	90.40	
(2"X4YDS,NON-STERILE)			
72s ea	08080-1418-00	57.22	
(3"X4YDS,NON-STERILE)			
72s ea	08080-2059-00	77.63	
(4"X4YDS,NON-STERILE)			
72s ea	08080-3175-00	101.18	
WERNET'S SUPER EXTRA STRENGTH (Glaxo)			
POW,NA, 108 gm	10158-0097-08	8.63	
WET-N-SOAK PLUS (Allergan Inc)			
SOL,NA, 120 ml	00023-0080-04	7.65	
WET-PRUF WATERPROOF (Covidien)			
DEV,NA (3"X10YDS)			
48s ea	08080-3354-00	276.89	
(2"X10YDS)			
72s ea	08080-3267-00	281.95	
(1"X10YDS)			
144s ea	08080-3142-00	301.69	
(1/2"X10YDS)			
288s ea	08080-3063-00	306.25	
WHEY PROTEIN (Innovative Health)			
PDR,PO (BERRY)			
6s ea	24038-0000-14	12.57	20.95
(CHOCOLATE)			
6s ea	24038-0000-12	12.57	20.95
(VANILLA)			
6s ea	24038-0000-13	12.57	20.95
WHITE CHESTNUT (Ellon)			
SOL,SL (DROPS)			
10.5 ml	51762-0003-10		9.25
WHITE PETROLEUM (Major)			
GEL,TP, 100%, 390 gm	00904-5731-82	3.15	
WHITE WILLOW BARK (ADH)			
CAP,PO (PF,SF)			
400 mg, 100s ea	60142-0975-51	5.98	11.95
WILD OAT (Ellon)			
SOL,SL (DROPS)			
10.5 ml	51762-0005-10		9.25
WILD OATS (Action Labs)			
LIQ,PO (SF,DROPS)			
1000 mg/ml, 60 ml	24675-0543-20	8.75	17.49
TAB,PO (SF)			
50s ea	24675-0543-50	7.49	14.99
100s ea	24675-0543-00	13.99	27.99
WILD ROSE (Ellon)			
SOL,SL (DROPS)			
10.5 ml	51762-0030-10		9.25
WILD YAM (Neurovites)			
CRE,TP, 3%, 60 gm	93595-2043-01	19.17	31.95
WILLIAMS LECTRIC SHAVE ORIGINAL (Combe)			
SOL,TP (WITH GREEN TEA COMPLEX)			
88 ml	11509-0221-32	2.21	
207 ml	11509-0221-51	4.70	
WILLIAMS MUG SHAVING SOAP (Combe)			
BAR,TP, ea	11509-0230-33	0.77	
WILLOW (Ellon)			
SOL,SL (DROPS)			
10.5 ml	51762-0031-10		9.25
WINGS BARIATRIC ADULT BRIEFS (Tyco)			
DEV,NA, 32s ea	08080-6709-50	87.50	
WINGS CHOICE ADULT INCONTINENT BRIEFS (Covidien)			
DEV,NA (LARGE,LATEX-FREE)			
72s ea	08080-6004-40	57.98	
(MEDIUM,LATEX-FREE)			
96s ea	08080-6004-30	55.19	
WINGS CHOICE PLUS ADULT INCONTINENT BRIEFS (Covidien)			
DEV,NA (XL,W/WETNESSINDICATOR)			
60s ea	08080-6003-50	40.10	
(LARGE)			
72s ea	08080-6003-40	59.23	
(MEDIUM)			
96s ea	08080-6003-30	57.00	
(SMALL)			
96s ea	08080-6003-20	49.69	
WINGS CHOICE PLUS YOUTH INCONTINENT BRIEFS (Covidien)			
DEV,NA (LATEX-FREE)			
96s ea	08080-6003-10	46.64	
WINGS CLASSIC ADULT INCONTINENT BRIEFS (Covidien)			
DEV,NA (LARGE)			
72s ea	08080-6000-40	56.10	
(XL,W/WETNESSINDICATOR)			
72s ea	08080-6001-00	54.67	
(MED,W/WETNESSINDICATOR)			
96s ea	08080-6000-30	54.70	
(SMALL)			
96s ea	08080-6000-20	44.99	
WINGS CLASSIC YOUTH BRIEFS (Covidien)			
DEV,NA (W/WETNESSINDICATOR)			
96s ea	08080-6000-10	42.08	

PROD/MFR	HRI, UPC,NDC	AWP	SRP
WINGS DAY PLUS INSERT PADS (Covidien)			
DEV,NA (LATEX-FREE)			
80s ea	08080-6597-01	37.03	
WINGS DAY REGULAR INSERT PADS (Covidien)			
DEV,NA (LATEX-FREE)			
88s ea	08080-6596-22	38.68	
WINGS HL ADULT BRIEFS (Covidien)			
DEV,NA (L,3D,DUAL AIR SYSTEM)			
72s ea	08080-6306-40	60.48	
(M,3D,DUAL AIR SYSTEM)			
96s ea	08080-6306-03	57.69	
WINGS HL EXTRA LARGE ADULT BRIEFS (Covidien)			
DEV,NA (3D,DUAL AIR SYSTEM)			
60s ea	08080-6306-50	55.13	
WINGS HL ULTRA ADULT BRIEFS (Covidien)			
DEV,NA (XL,3D,DUAL AIR SYSTEM)			
60s ea	08080-6307-05	57.89	
(3D,LARGE,DUAL-AIR SYS)			
72s ea	08080-6307-40	63.50	
(3D,MEDIUM,LATEX-FREE)			
96s ea	08080-6307-30	60.58	
WINGS MAXIMA DISPOSABLE UNDERPADS (Covidien)			
DEV,NA (23"X36",LATEX-FREE)			
72s ea	08080-6418-00	46.60	
(30"X30",LATEX-FREE)			
72s ea	08080-6569-01	31.79	
(23"X36",15X5,LATEX-FREE)			
75s ea	08080-6422-00	44.65	
(30"X30",LATEX-FREE)			
80s ea	08080-9173-00	35.28	
WINGS NIGHT SUPER INSERT PADS (Covidien)			
DEV,NA (2X24,LATEX-FREE)			
48s ea	08080-6598-01	28.42	
WINGS PERSONAL CLEANSING WASHCLOTHS (Covidien)			
PAD,TP, 384s ea	08080-6399-01	33.75	
512s ea	08080-6599-10	39.42	
576s ea	08080-6499-01	42.19	
768s ea	08080-6699-01	51.93	
(Kendall)			
PAD,TP (11.8"X8.7")			
192s ea	08080-6899-00	26.60	
576s ea	08080-6399-10	41.01	
WINGS PLUS LAYERED DISPOSABLE UNDERPADS (Covidien)			
DEV,NA (30"X36",12X5)			
60s ea	08080-7059-01	30.34	
(30"X36")			
60s ea	08080-7159-01	28.55	
(30"X30",15X5)			
75s ea	08080-7058-01	29.50	
(30"X30")			
75s ea	08080-7158-01	27.54	
WINGS QUILTED BREATHABLE UNDERPADS (Covidien)			
DEV,NA (30"X36")			
40s ea	08080-3036-01	73.30	
(30"X30")			
60s ea	08080-3030-01	94.80	
(23"X36")			
72s ea	08080-2336-00	99.68	
72s ea	08080-2336-01	108.40	
WINGS QUILTED UNDERPADS (Covidien)			
DEV,NA (30"X36")			
40s ea	08080-3036-00	67.10	
(30"X30")			
60s ea	08080-3030-02	87.08	
WINGS SEAMLESS KNIT PANTS (Covidien)			
DEV,NA (LARGE/X-LARGE)			
50s ea	08080-7060-00	76.74	
(SMALL/MEDIUM)			
50s ea	08080-7050-00	60.53	
(XXL/XXXL)			
50s ea	08080-7070-00	86.78	
(XXXL)			
50s ea	08080-7080-00	104.13	
(XXXXL)			
50s ea	08080-7080-01	104.13	
(L/XL)			
100s ea	08080-7060-01	76.43	
100s ea	08080-7060-11	97.50	
(XXL/XXXL)			
100s ea	08080-7070-01	89.28	
100s ea	08080-7070-11	114.28	
WINGS STRETCH MESH PANTS (Covidien)			
DEV,NA (LARGE,10X5)			
50s ea	08080-7020-00	76.74	
(MEDIUM,10X5)			
50s ea	08080-7010-00	68.53	
(SMALL,10X5)			
50s ea	08080-7000-00	60.53	
(X-LARGE,10X5)			
50s ea	08080-7030-00	84.65	
WINGS SUPREME ADULT INCONTINENT BRIEFS (Covidien)			
DEV,NA (LARGE,12X6,LATEX-FREE)			
72s ea	08080-9502-00	61.72	
(MEDIUM,12X8,LATEX-FREE)			
96s ea	08080-9501-00	60.18	
WINN DIXIE MEDIC ORIGINAL LANCETS (Can-Am Care)			
DEV,NA (PRIVATE LABEL)			
100s ea	36652-0303-31	4.98	
WINN DIXIE MEDIC THIN LANCETS (Can-Am Care)			
DEV,NA (PRIVATE LABEL)			
100s ea	36652-0301-31	4.99	
200s ea	36652-0302-31	7.99	
WINTERGREEN OIL (AmerisourceBergen)			
OIL,TP (PRIVATE LABEL)			
60 ml	24385-0667-92	2.96	4.19
WITCH HAZEL (AmerisourceBergen)			
LIQ,TP (PRIVATE LABEL)			
473 ml	24385-0214-16	32.30	35.90
(Cardinal Health)			
LIQ,TP (PRIVATE LABEL)			
480 ml	37205-0822-43	27.84	
(Denison)			
LIQ,TP, 480 ml	00295-1221-16	0.96	
WND 1 (Mead Johnson & Co)			
PDR,PO, 454 gm	00087-0092-41	19.80	
WND 2 (Mead Johnson & Co)			
PDR,PO, 454 gm	00087-0093-41	28.15	
WOBENZYM N (Marlyn)			
ECT,PO, 40s ea	32115-0480-47	13.25	26.50
200s ea	32115-0457-29	24.50	49.00
800s ea	32115-0411-78	81.00	162.00
WOMAN'S LAXATIVE (Chain Drug Marketing)			
ECT,PO, 5 mg, 30s ea	63868-0499-30	1.35	2.99
(Family Phcy)			
ECT,PO (PRIVATE LABEL)			
5 mg, 30s ea	52735-0399-08	3.14	3.49
WOMAN'S WELLBEING HYDRA-SMOOTH (Consumer Choice)			
CRE,VG (FRAGRANCE-FREE)			
67.5 ml	60369-0800-25	3.10	6.49
WOMAN'S WELLBEING PERSONAL CREAM LUBRICANT (Consumer Choice)			
CRE,VG (FRAGRANCE-FREE)			
4 ml 8s	60369-0800-02	9.60	14.95
WOMAN'S WELLBEING UTI RELIEF (Consumer Choice)			
TAB,PO (MAX STRENGTH)			
97.2 mg, 24s ea	60369-0505-24	4.15	8.29
WOMEN'S DAILY FORMULA (Mason Vit)			
TAB,PO (PF,SF)			
90s ea	11845-0120-49	7.22	
WOMEN'S MULTIVITAMIN/MULTIMINERAL (Rexall)			
TAB,PO (WITH HERBS,CAPLET)			
60s ea	30768-0040-52	4.67	6.99
WOMEN'S ROGAINE (Johnson & Johnson)			
SOL,TP (UNSCENTED)			
2%, 60 ml	12547-0780-20	19.22	
60 ml 3s	00093-0780-06	41.62	
60 ml 3s	00093-0780-11	41.62	
60 ml 3s	00093-0780-12	41.62	
(UNSCENTED)			
2%, 60 ml 3s	12547-0780-60	40.90	
(Physician Partner)			
REPACK			
SOL,TP, 2%, 60 ml	21695-0429-60	47.96	
WONDERGEL W/ALOE VERA (Lake Pharm)			
GEL,VG, 70.5 gm	12277-0511-23	3.00	4.99
WOUN'DRES (Coloplast)			
GEL,TP (WOUND DRESSING)			
28 gm 36s	11701-0161-95	225.36	235.80
84 gm 12s	11701-0161-16	184.92	193.56
WOUND CLEANSER (Ameriderm Labs)			
SPR,TP, 473 ml	63921-0430-16	6.25	
WOUND GEL DRESSING (Ameriderm Labs)			
SPR,TP (HYDROGEL)			
237 gm	63921-0450-08	15.00	
WOUND GEL WVITAMIN E & ALOE VERA (Ameriderm Labs)			
GEL,TP (HYDROGEL)			
90 gm	63921-0420-03	6.25	
WOUND WASH SALINE (Blairex)			
SPR,IR, 0.9%, 90 ml	50486-0855-39	3.80	
210 ml	50486-0855-28	5.00	
WOUND-CARE (Weleda)			
OIN,TP, 34 gm	55946-0006-60	3.90	
WRIGHT & FILIPPIS ULTRA THIN LANCETS (Can-Am Care)			
DEV,NA (30G)			
100s ea	38396-0501-78	4.24	
X-PREP (Southwood)			
REPACK			
LIQ,PO, 7%, 74 ml	58016-7038-01	10.99	
X-SEB T PEARL (Teva)			
LIQ,TP, 120 ml	00575-1004-04	11.49	
240 ml	00575-1004-08	15.99	
X-SEB T PLUS (Teva)			
SHA,TP, 10%-3%, 120 ml	00575-1015-04	13.89	
240 ml	00575-1015-08	19.29	
XEROFLO DRESSING (Covidien)			
DEV,NA, 36s ea	08080-4373-05	256.59	
XEROFLO GAUZE (Covidien)			
DRE,TP (STERILE,5"X9")			
3%, 72s ea	08080-4371-00	195.09	
(STERILE,1"X8")			
3%, 200s ea	08080-4372-01	415.57	
(STERILE,2"X2")			
3%, 300s ea	08080-4364-00	274.84	
XEROFORM GAUZE (Covidien)			
DRE,TP (PETROLATUM,4"X3YD)			
3%, 36s ea	08080-4320-00	223.15	
(PETROLATUM,2"X2")			
3%, 150s ea	08080-4334-01	143.72	
(PETROLATUM,4"X4"))			
3%, 150s ea	08080-4335-01	205.42	
(PETROLATUM,1"X8")			
3%, 200s ea	08080-4313-02	170.22	
200s ea	08080-4333-01	147.15	
(PETROLATUM,5"X9")			
3%, 200s ea	08080-4316-05	328.94	
200s ea	08080-4336-05	218.57	
XLEU ANALOG (Nutricia)			
PDR,PO (1X400GM)			
400 gm	49735-0018-88	60.00	
(USE W/MED SUPV)			
400 gm 4s	49735-0118-88	252.20	
(6X400GM)			
400 gm 6s	49735-0183-61	360.00	
XLEU MAXAMAID (Nutricia)			
PDR,PO (1X454GM,ORANGE)			
454 gm	49735-0023-64	74.10	
(MED. SUPERVISION,ORANGE)			
454 gm 4s	49735-0123-64	312.00	
(6X454GM,ORANGE)			
454 gm 6s	49735-0177-91	444.60	
XLEU MAXAMUM (Nutricia)			
PDR,PO (1X454GM,ORANGE)			
454 gm	49735-0023-43	115.50	
(6X454GM,ORANGE)			
454 gm 6s	49735-0177-90	693.00	
XLYS XTRP ANALOG (Nutricia)			
PDR,PO (USE W/MED SUPV)			
400 gm 4s	49735-0118-82	252.20	
XLYS XTRP MAXAMAID (Nutricia)			
PDR,PO (MED. SUPERVISION,ORANGE)			
454 gm 4s	49735-0123-59	312.00	
XLYS, XTRP ANALOG (Nutricia)			
PDR,PO (1X400GM)			
400 gm	49735-0018-82	60.00	
(6X400GM)			
400 gm 6s	49735-0183-28	360.00	
XLYS, XTRP MAXAMAID (Nutricia)			
PDR,PO (1X454GM,ORANGE)			
454 gm	49735-0023-59	74.10	
(6X454GM,ORANGE)			
454 gm 6s	49735-0177-80	444.60	
XLYS, XTRP MAXAMUM (Nutricia)			
PDR,PO (1X454GM,ORANGE)			
454 gm	49735-0023-44	115.50	
(6X454GM,ORANGE)			
454 gm 6s	49735-0177-88	693.00	
XMET ANALOG (Nutricia)			
PDR,PO (1X400GM)			
400 gm	49735-0018-81	60.00	
(USE W/MED SUPV)			
400 gm 4s	49735-0118-81	252.20	
(6X400GM)			
400 gm 6s	49735-0183-27	360.00	

PROD/MFR	HRI, UPC,NDC	AWP	SRP
XMET MAXAMAID (Nutricia)			
PDR,PO (1X454GM,ORANGE)			
454 gm	49735-0023-63	74.10	
(MED. SUPERVISION,ORANGE)			
454 gm 4s	49735-0123-63	312.00	
(6X454GM,ORANGE)			
454 gm 6s	49735-0177-87	444.60	
XMET MAXAMUM (Nutricia)			
PDR,PO (1X454GM,ORANGE)			
454 gm	49735-0023-41	115.50	
(6X454GM,ORANGE)			
454 gm 6s	49735-0177-95	693.00	
XMTVI ANALOG (Nutricia)			
PDR,PO (1X400GM)			
400 gm	49735-0018-87	60.00	
(USE W/MED SUPV)			
400 gm 4s	49735-0118-87	252.20	
(6X400GM)			
400 gm 6s	49735-0183-03	360.00	
XMTVI MAXAMAID (Nutricia)			
PDR,PO (1X454GM,ORANGE)			
454 gm	49735-0023-61	74.10	
(MED. SUPERVISION,ORANGE)			
454 gm 4s	49735-0123-61	312.00	
(6X454GM,ORANGE)			
454 gm 6s	49735-0177-85	444.60	
XMTVI MAXAMUM (Nutricia)			
PDR,PO (1X454GM,ORANGE)			
454 gm	49735-0023-42	115.50	
(6X454GM,ORANGE)			
454 gm 6s	49735-0177-79	693.00	
XPECT (Hawthorn Pharm)			
TAB,PO (IMMEDIATE-RELEASE)			
400 mg, 60s ea	63717-0251-06	14.99	
XPHE ANALOG (Nutricia)			
PDR,PO (USE W/MED SUPV)			
400 gm 4s	49735-0118-80	100.10	
XPHE MAXAMAID (Nutricia)			
PDR,PO (1X454GM,ORANGE)			
454 gm	49735-0023-57	43.20	
(1X454GM,STRAWBERRY)			
454 gm	49735-0023-71	43.20	
(1X454GM,UNFLAVORED)			
454 gm	49735-0023-58	43.20	
(454GMX4,MED SUPERVISION)			
454 gm 4s	49735-0123-71	182.00	
(MED. SUPERVISION,ORANGE)			
454 gm 4s	49735-0123-57	182.00	
(USE W/MED SUPV.)			
454 gm 4s	49735-0123-58	182.00	
(6X454GM,ORANGE)			
454 gm 6s	49735-0177-92	259.20	
(6X454GM,STRAWBERRY)			
454 gm 6s	49735-0177-94	259.20	
(6X454GM,UNFLAVORED)			
454 gm 6s	49735-0177-93	259.20	
XPHE MAXAMUM (Nutricia)			
PDR,PO (REQ DR SUPERVISION)			
50 gm 30s	49735-0123-11	226.20	
50 gm 30s	49735-0123-12	226.20	
(1X454GM,ORANGE)			
454 gm	49735-0023-02	68.70	
(1X454GM,UNFLAVORED)			
454 gm	49735-0023-01	68.70	
(6X454GM,ORANGE,ORANGE)			
454 gm 6s	49735-0183-24	412.20	
(6X454GM,UNFLAVORED)			
454 gm 6s	49735-0183-23	412.20	
XPHE MAXAMUM DRINK (Nutricia)			
LIQ,PO (250MLX18,FOREST BERRIES)			
250 ml 18s	49735-0025-24	192.40	
(250MLX18,ORANGE)			
250 ml 18s	49735-0025-51	192.40	
XPHE XTYR ANALOG (Nutricia)			
PDR,PO (USE W/MED SUPV)			
400 gm 4s	49735-0118-85	252.20	
XPHE XTYR MAXAMAID (Nutricia)			
PDR,PO (MED. SUPERVISION,ORANGE)			
454 gm 4s	49735-0123-62	312.00	
XPHE, XTYR ANALOG (Nutricia)			
PDR,PO (1X400GM)			
400 gm	49735-0018-85	60.00	
(6X400GM)			
400 gm 6s	49735-0183-01	360.00	
XPHE, XTYR MAXAMAID (Nutricia)			
PDR,PO (1X454GM,ORANGE)			
454 gm	49735-0023-62	74.10	
(6X454GM,ORANGE)			
454 gm 6s	49735-0177-86	444.60	
XPTM ANALOG (Nutricia)			
PDR,PO (1X400GM)			
400 gm	49735-0018-84	60.00	
(USE W/MED SUPV)			
400 gm 4s	49735-0118-84	252.20	
(6X400GM)			
400 gm 6s	49735-0188-43	360.00	
XTRA-CARE (Coloplast)			
LOT,TP (PACKET)			
2 ml 300s	11701-0004-21	45.00	48.00
59 ml 36s	11701-0004-03	34.20	35.64
118 ml 36s	11701-0004-04	58.32	60.84
237 ml 36s	11701-0004-05	102.24	106.92
621 ml 12s	11701-0004-26	87.72	91.80
(REFILL)			
1000 ml 12s	11701-0004-46	113.28	118.56
3840 ml 4s	11701-0004-09	101.12	105.34
XTRAMINS (Key Company)			
TAB,PO (SF)			
100s ea	11694-0790-01	8.50	
250s ea	11694-0790-25	17.00	
1000s ea	11694-0790-03	65.00	
Y-PORT CONNECTOR (Abbott)			
DEV,NA (W/RIGHT ANGLE ADAPTER)			
5s ea	70074-0503-71	5.50	
(14 FR-16 FR)			
10s ea	70074-0008-35	62.83	
(18 FR-20 FR)			
10s ea	70074-0008-36	62.83	
YAGER'S LINIMENT (Oakhurst)			
LIQ,TP, 120 ml	11169-0000-04	4.00	6.00
240 ml	11169-0000-08	5.40	8.11
YEAST-GARD (Lake Pharm)			
SUP,VG (W/APPLICATOR)			
28 x-28 x-28 x,			
15s ea	55663-0501-15	4.79	7.99
YEASTAWAY (Boiron)			
SUP,VG, 30 x-1 x-1 x-14 x,			
7s ea	06969-7159-80	8.09	13.49
YELETS (Freeda)			
TAB,PO (PF,SF,DYE-FREE)			
100s ea	10432-0063-01	6.27	10.45
YODORA (Numark)			
CRE,TP (NON-IRRITATING)			
60 gm	38485-0672-50	6.06	
YOHIMBE (Mason Vit)			
CAP,PO (PF,SF)			
500 mg, 60s ea	11845-0115-35	10.56	
YOHIMBE POWER MAX 1500 (Action Labs)			
TAB,PO, 30s ea	24675-0880-30	9.49	18.99
60s ea	24675-0880-60	16.99	33.99
YOHIMBE POWER MAX 1500 FOR WOMEN (Action Labs)			
TAB,PO (SF)			
30s ea	24675-0820-30	9.49	18.99
YOHIMBE POWER MAX 2000 (Action Labs)			
CAP,PO, 50s ea	24675-0115-50	10.99	21.99
100s ea	24675-0115-00	19.99	39.99
LIQ,PO, 60 ml	24675-0115-20	13.99	27.99
YOHIMBE SUPER POTENT (Mason Vit)			
TAB,PO (PF,SF)			
800 mg, 30s ea	11845-0120-18	8.78	
YOHIMBIZED 1000 (Action Labs)			
CAP,PO (SF)			
25 mg-25 mg-500 mg,			
50s ea	24675-0240-50	7.99	15.99
YUCCA (ADH)			
CAP,PO (PF,SF)			
450 mg, 100s ea	60142-0978-01	5.48	10.95
Z-BEC (Inverness)			
TAB,PO, 60s ea	36652-0689-62	8.75	
Z-CLINZ CLEANSER (TriMarc Labs)			
SOA,TP (1X60ML)			
60 ml	68752-0770-60	4.50	
Z-GEN (Teva)			
TAB,PO, 60s ea	00182-1407-26	6.29	
Z-SLIM CARB CUTTER (MAGNA Pharm)			
TAB,PO, 400 mg-400 mg,			
90s ea	58407-0176-90	19.93	23.95
Z-XTRA (MAGNA Pharm)			
GEL,TP, 118 ml	58407-0303-04	8.68	9.95
ZADITOR (Novartis Pharm)			
SOL,OP, 0.025%, 5 ml	00078-0476-61	11.70	
(2X5ML)			
0.025%, 5 ml 2s	00078-0476-41	19.50	
6 ml	00078-0476-25	11.70	
(6X6ML)			
0.025%, 6 ml 6s	00078-0476-60	70.20	
(8X6ML)			
0.025%, 6 ml 8s	00078-0476-38	93.60	
6 ml 8s	00078-0476-44	93.60	
ZANFEL (Zanfel)			
SOA,TP (1X30GM)			
30 gm	89901-0537-87		39.99
ZANTAC 150 (Boehr Ingelheim Cons)			
TAB,PO, 150 mg, 8s ea	12547-0686-08		4.99
24s ea	12547-0686-24		9.99
50s ea	12547-0686-50		17.99
65s ea	12547-0686-65		22.99
ZANTAC 75 (Boehr Ingelheim Cons)			
TAB,PO, 75 mg, 4s ea	12547-0684-04		2.99
10s ea UD	12547-0684-10		4.99
20s ea	12547-0684-20		7.99
30s ea	12547-0684-30		9.99
60s ea	12547-0684-62		17.99
80s ea	12547-0684-40		22.99
(Phys Total Care)			
REPACK			
TAB,PO, 75 mg, 30s ea	54868-3877-00	12.49	
60s ea	54868-3877-01	20.12	
ZAPZYT ACNE (Waltman)			
GEL,TP, 10%, 30 gm	10768-0001-10	4.20	
ZAPZYT FACE & BODY WASH (Waltman)			
GEL,TP, 2%, 188.5 gm	10768-0000-70	4.20	
ZAPZYT PORE TREATMENT (Waltman)			
GEL,TP, 2%, 22.5 gm	10768-0000-40	4.20	
ZAPZYT TREATMENT (Waltman)			
SOA,TP (SOAP-FREE)			
10%, ea	10768-0000-60	4.45	
ZE-PLUS (Everett)			
SGL,PO (SF,SOFTGEL)			
60s ea	00642-0102-60	13.50	
ZEASORB (Stiefel Consumer HealthCare)			
POW,TP, 70.9 gm	00145-1504-05	3.00	4.49
312 gm	00145-1504-07	8.70	12.99
ZEASORB AF (Stiefel Labs)			
GEL,TP, 2%, 24 gm	00145-1505-08	7.80	11.79
(Phys Total Care)			
REPACK			
GEL,TP (1X0.85GM)			
2%, 0.85 gm	54868-5877-00	11.49	
ZEASORB-AF (Stiefel Consumer HealthCare)			
LOT,TP, 2%, 56 gm	00145-1606-03	9.60	14.49
POW,TP, 2%, 70 gm	00145-1506-05	5.46	8.29
(Phys Total Care)			
REPACK			
POW,TP (1X70GM)			
2%, 70 gm	54868-5876-00	8.41	
ZEEL (Heel/BHI)			
TAB,SL, 100s ea	50114-6165-02	7.45	12.80
ZEPHIRAN CHLORIDE (Sanofi-Aventis)			
SOL,TP, 1:750, 240 ml	00024-2521-04	23.82	
3840 ml 2s	00024-2521-08	202.42	
(Nucare Pharm)			
REPACK			
SOL,TP (1X240ML)			
1:750, 240 ml	68071-1340-08	47.65	
ZETTS (A. F. Hauser)			
LOZ,MM, 10 mg, 5s ea	52637-0777-05	0.69	0.98
400s ea	52637-0777-14	59.98	
ZIKS ARTHRITIS PAIN RELIEF (Nnodum)			
CRE,TP, 0.025%-1%-12%,			
60 gm	63044-0030-60	15.99	
ZILACTIN (Zila)			
GEL,MM, 10%, 7.5 gm	51284-0468-02	4.60	6.49
ZILACTIN BABY EXTRA STRENGTH (Zila)			
GEL,MM (AF,DYE-FREE,GRAPE)			
10%, 9.9 gm	51284-0570-72	2.84	
ZILACTIN TOOTHACHE MAXIMUM STRENGTH (Zila)			
SWA,MM, 20%, 8s ea	51284-0850-52	3.95	
ZILACTIN-B (Zila)			
GEL,MM, 10%, 7.5 gm	51284-0550-32	4.60	
ZILACTIN-L (Zila)			
LIQ,MM, 2.5%, 7.5 ml	51284-0470-12	4.60	
ZILACTIN-LIP (Zila)			
STI,TP (MENTHOL)			
4.5 gm	51284-0468-80	1.36	
ZIM'S CRACK CREME (Perfecta Prod)			
LOT,TP, 60 ml	81485-0032-04	4.17	5.95
ZINC (ADH)			
TAB,PO (PF,SF)			
22 mg, 60s ea	60142-0368-06	1.88	3.75
100 mg, 60s ea	60142-0372-06	2.98	5.95

PROD/MFR	HRI, UPC,NDC	AWP	SRP
(Basic Vitamins)			
TAB,PO, 50 mg, 150s ea	00761-0078-30	2.40	
(Carlson,J.R.)			
TAB,PO (VEGETARIAN,PF,SALT-FREE)			
15 mg, 100s ea	88395-0053-11	1.95	3.90
250s ea	88395-0053-12	4.50	9.00
(PF,SF,CORN-FREE)			
50 mg, 100s ea	88395-0053-21	3.25	6.50
300s ea	88395-0053-23	8.85	17.70
(Family Phcy)			
TAB,PO (PRIVATE LABEL)			
50 mg, 100s ea	52735-0067-01	2.33	2.59
(Freeda)			
TAB,PO (PF,SF,DYE-FREE)			
30 mg, 100s ea	10432-0207-01	4.77	7.95
250s ea	10432-0207-02	9.54	15.90
(Health Products Corp)			
LOZ,MM (PF,LEMON)			
23 mg, 60s ea	39686-0014-66	4.00	
TAB,PO (PF,SF)			
10 mg, 100s ea	39686-0014-57	1.56	
(Mason Vit)			
LOZ,MM (PF,LEMON)			
23 mg, 60s ea	11845-0121-95	5.67	
(Mericon)			
LOZ,MM (MINT)			
10 mg, 25s ea	00394-0494-25	2.34	
(CHOCOLATE)			
10 mg, 50s ea	00394-0495-50	2.80	
(Rexall)			
LOZ,MM, 60 mg-20 mg-23 mg,			
50s ea	30768-0013-09	3.29	4.98
(Phys Total Care)			
REPACK			
TAB,PO, 50 mg, 100s ea	54868-4877-00	12.51	
ZINC & C (Rugby)			
LOZ,MM, 30 mg-15 mg,			
100s ea	00536-7183-01	3.90	
ZINC & ECHINACEA (Mason Vit)			
LOZ,MM (PF,CHERRY)			
100 mg-100 mg-23 mg,			
60s ea	11845-0127-85	5.56	
ZINC + VITAMIN C (Major)			
LOZ,MM, 300 mg-7 mg,			
100s ea	00904-5683-60	5.60	
ZINC ASPARTATE (Miller)			
TAB,PO, 40 mg, 100s ea	17204-0360-40	10.08	16.80
ZINC CHELATED (Freeda)			
TAB,PO (PF,SF,DYE-FREE)			
22.5 mg, 100s ea	10432-0214-01	4.65	7.75
250s ea	10432-0214-02	9.30	15.50
50 mg, 100s ea	10432-0252-01	5.85	9.75
250s ea	10432-0252-02	11.70	19.50
(Nature's Bounty)			
LOZ,MM (PF,ORANGE)			
23 mg, 60s ea	74312-0041-60		7.39
TAB,PO (PF,SF)			
25 mg, 100s ea	74312-0020-00		3.45
50 mg, 100s ea	74312-0020-60		4.89
(Rexall)			
TAB,PO (P.F,PF,SF)			
50 mg, 60s ea	30768-0000-58	1.53	2.32
(Rugby)			
TAB,PO, 50 mg, 100s ea	00536-6671-01	2.85	
ZINC FOR KIDS (Mason Vit)			
LOZ,MM, 60 mg-32 mg-15 mg,			
50s ea	11845-0131-79	3.44	
ZINC GLUCONATE (ADH)			
TAB,PO, 22 mg, 60s ea	60142-0108-06	0.95	1.60
(Freeda)			
TAB,PO (PF,SF,DYE-FREE)			
15 mg, 100s ea	10432-0168-01	3.87	6.45
500s ea	10432-0168-03	11.97	19.95
(Lex)			
TAB,PO, 50 mg, 100s ea	49523-0028-01	1.20	
(Major)			
TAB,PO, 50 mg, 100s ea	00904-3191-60	3.33	
(Marlex)			
TAB,PO, 50 mg, 100s ea	10135-0210-01	1.35	
1000s ea	10135-0210-10	9.28	
(Mason Vit)			
TAB,PO, 30 mg, 100s ea	11845-0072-01	4.11	
50 mg, 100s ea	11845-0069-11	5.22	
100 mg, 100s ea	11845-0077-51	6.89	
(Nature's Bounty)			
TAB,PO (PF,SF)			
100 mg, 100s ea	74312-0003-70		6.89
(Truxton)			
TAB,PO, 10 mg, 1000s ea	00463-6298-10	12.00	
ZINC GLUCONATE NATURAL (AmerisourceBergen)			
TAB,PO (PRIVATE LABEL)			
50 mg, 100s ea	24385-0346-78	2.51	2.79
ZINC LOZENGES (Freeda)			
LOZ,MM, 10 mg, 100s ea	10432-0274-01	6.57	10.95
250s ea	10432-0274-02	13.14	21.90
ZINC NATURAL (Cardinal Health)			
TAB,PO (PF,PRIVATE LABEL)			
50 mg, 100s ea	37205-0176-78	2.67	
ZINC OXIDE (Actavis Mid Atlantic)			
OIN,TP, 60 gm	00472-1800-57	2.50	
20%, 30 gm	00472-1800-56	1.80	
480 gm	00472-1800-16	13.00	
(Consolidated Midland)			
OIN,TP, 30 gm	00223-4152-30	1.25	
30 gm	00223-4155-30	1.60	
60 gm	00223-4152-60	1.75	
454 gm	00223-4152-13	5.50	
454 gm	00223-4155-13	6.95	
(Family Phcy)			
OIN,TP (PRIVATE LABEL)			
60 gm	52735-0241-36	2.69	2.99
(Fougera)			
OIN,TP, 30 gm	00168-0062-31	1.55	
60 gm	00168-0062-02	2.40	
454 gm	00168-0062-16	11.27	
(G&W)			
OIN,TP, 60 gm	00713-0293-32	2.98	
(Rugby)			
OIN,TP, 20%, 454 gm	00536-5700-98	6.75	
(Teva)			
OIN,TP, 20%, 60 gm	00182-0952-43	2.50	
(Phys Total Care)			
REPACK			
OIN,TP (1X30GM)			
20%, 30 gm	54868-2968-00	8.40	
480 gm	54868-2968-01	17.93	
ZINC PICOLINATE (Mason Vit)			
TAB,PO (PF,SF)			
122 mg-10 mg,			
100s ea	11845-0124-51	5.44	
ZINC SULFATE (Cypress Pharm)			
CAP,PO, 220 mg, 100s ea	60258-0131-01	7.99	
(Major)			
CAP,PO, 220 mg, 100s ea	00904-5332-60	4.34	
(Marlex)			
CAP,PO, 220 mg, 100s ea	10135-0356-01	1.67	
(Rising)			
CAP,PO, 220 mg, 100s ea	68585-0008-01	4.95	
(Rugby)			
TAB,PO (PF,SF,CORN-FREE)			
111 mg-50 mg,			
100s ea	00536-2450-01	4.79	
ZINC SULFATE 15 (Mericon)			
TAB,PO, 66 mg, 100s ea	00394-0122-02	2.18	
ZINC W/VITAMIN C (Rx Vitamins)			
LOZ,MM (PF,CHERRY)			
30 mg-46 mg, 90s ea	08429-0030-01	5.48	10.95
ZINC-220 (Alto)			
CAP,PO, 220 mg, 100s ea	00731-0401-01	7.92	
100s ea UD	00731-0401-06	12.00	
ZINC-50 (Key Company)			
TAB,PO, 50 mg, 100s ea	11694-0141-50	4.75	
250s ea	11694-0141-52	10.00	
ZINC-EASE (Carlson,J.R.)			
LOZ,MM (PF,SF,CORN-FREE)			
10 mg, 42s ea	88395-0053-40	1.72	3.44
84s ea	88395-0053-41	2.94	5.88
ZINCON (Medtech)			
SHA,TP, 1%, 120 ml	75137-0455-58	2.97	
240 ml	75137-0455-61	4.90	
ZINIMIN (Key Company)			
TAB,PO, 15 mg, 100s ea	11694-0141-12	4.50	
ZINX (Auriga)			
LOZ,MM, 2 x, 50s ea	14629-0401-50		6.77
ZMO OIL (ZMO)			
OIL,TP, 120 ml	04691-5139-00	5.17	
240 ml	04691-5161-00	8.67	
ZN PLUS PROTEIN (Miller)			
TAB,PO, 15 mg, 100s ea	17204-0440-40	5.04	8.40
ZN-50 (Bio-Tech Pharm)			
CAP,PO, 50 mg, 100s ea	53191-0249-01	3.70	
ZNP (Stiefel Consumer HealthCare)			
SOA,TP, 2%, 119 gm	00145-0986-05	6.36	9.59
(Phys Total Care)			
REPACK			
SOA,TP, 2%, ea	54868-1594-00	10.69	
ZOEY ASTHMAMENTOR PEAK FLOW METER (Respironics)			
DEV,NA (UNIVERSAL RANGE)			
ea	83730-0742-30	26.50	
ZOEY PERSONAL BEST PEAK FLOW METER (Respironics)			
DEV,NA (FULL RANGE)			
ea	83730-0755-30	26.50	
(LOW RANGE)			
ea	83730-0756-30	26.50	
ZONAS POROUS (J&J Medical)			
DEV,NA (3"X10YD/ROLL)			
4s ea	56091-0051-07	11.87	
(2"X10YD/ROLL)			
6s ea	56091-0051-06	11.87	
(1 1/2"X10YD/ROLL)			
8s ea	56091-0051-05	11.87	
(1"X10YD/ROLL)			
12s ea	56091-0051-04	11.87	
(1/2"X10YD/ROLL)			
24s ea	56091-0051-03	11.87	
ZONITE (Lee Pharm)			
SOL,VG, 240 ml	23558-0680-30	8.40	
240 ml 12s	23558-0680-31	100.80	
360 ml	23558-0680-40	11.04	
360 ml 12s	23558-0680-41	132.48	
ZOSTRIX (Health Care Products)			
CRE,TP (ORIGINAL STRENGTH)			
0.025%, 56.6 gm	61787-0442-02	11.55	16.99
(Rodlen Labs)			
CRE,TP, 0.025%, 60 gm	29936-0602-27	12.44	
STI,TP, 0.025%, 21 gm	99207-0605-04	9.96	
(Pharma Pac)			
REPACK			
CRE,TP, 0.025%, 60 gm	52959-0595-03	14.25	
(Southwood)			
REPACK			
CRE,TP (1X56.6GM,ODOR-FREE)			
0.025%, 56.6 gm	58016-3509-01	10.45	
ZOSTRIX HIGH POTENCY (Rodlen Labs)			
CRE,TP, 0.075%, 60 gm	29936-0601-02	16.88	
STI,TP, 0.075%, 21 gm	99207-0607-04	11.55	
ZOSTRIX NEUROPATHY (Health Care Products)			
CRE,TP (1X60GM)			
0.25%, 60 gm	61787-0711-02	15.74	24.99
ZOSTRIX SPORTS (Rodlen Labs)			
CRE,TP, 0.075%, 30 gm	06601-0567-30	8.31	
ZOSTRIX-HP (Health Care Products)			
CRE,TP (TRIPLE STRENGTH FORMULA)			
0.075%, 56.6 gm	61787-0443-02	14.18	19.99
ZUN SPOT (Kramer Labs)			
CRE,TP (1X60GM)			
1%, 60 gm	53076-0164-29	9.06	10.57
ZURION (Health Products Corp)			
TAB,PO (SF)			
100s ea	39686-0012-98	8.25	15.95
ZYRTEC (McNeil Consumer Healthcare)			
TAB,PO (ALLERGY)			
10 mg, 3s ea	00450-0204-43	3.11	
5s ea	12547-0204-30	6.14	
14s ea	12547-0204-32	13.12	
30s ea	12547-0204-36	18.78	
45s ea	50580-0726-38	24.67	
(75X15 CLUB TRAY)			
10 mg, 1125s ea	12547-0204-64	35.26	
ZYRTEC ITCHY EYE DROPS (McNeil Consumer Healthcare)			
SOL,OP, 0.035%, 5 ml	00450-0208-05	13.12	
ZYRTEC-D (McNeil Consumer Healthcare)			
TER,PO, 5 mg-120 mg,			
12s ea	12547-0204-50	13.12	
(ALLERGY&CONGESTION)			
5 mg-120 mg,			
24s ea	12547-0204-52	18.78	
(24X24 CLUB TRAY)			
5 mg-120 mg,			
576s ea	12547-0204-68	18.52	
(Phys Total Care)			
REPACK			
TER,PO, 5 mg-120 mg,			
24s ea	54868-5879-00	24.19	